AHFS
Drug
Information® 2025

www.ahfsdruginformation.com

Some monographs have been omitted from the print version of AHFS® DI™ because of space limitations. Copies of these monographs are available on the "Print Subscribers" page of the AHFS Drug Information® website, www.ahfsdruginformation.com, in the "Electronic-Only Monographs" section.

A username and password are required to access the subscriber-only portions of the website. For the 2025 edition, the username and password for accessing electronic-only content are as follows:

- **username: ahfs2025**
- **password: ASHP46360**

Associated index entries for monographs that appear on the website are followed by the symbol "§" rather than by a page number. This symbol refers the user to a footnote in the index that also provides the above username and password for the 2025 edition.

AHFS
DRUG
INFORMATION® 2025

Published under the Editorial Authority of ASHP®
American Society of Health-System Pharmacists®

AHFS®

**American Hospital
Formulary Service®**

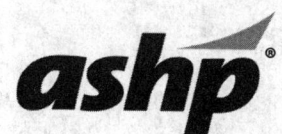

Production Services: Progressive Publishing Services
Printing: Marquis Imprimeur, Inc.
Cover Design: DeVall Advertising
Page Design: David Wade

Library of Congress Catalog Card Number: 59-7620
ISBN: 978-1-58528-761-1
ISSN: 8756-6028

Printed in Canada

10 9 8 7 6 5 4 3 2 1

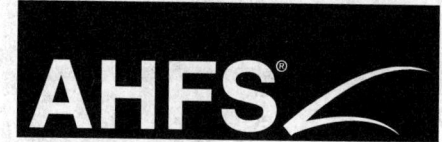

Editorial Staff

Senior Vice President, Professional Development and Publishing: Daniel J. Cobaugh, Pharm.D., DABAT, FAACT

AHFS Editor-in-Chief and Senior Editorial Director: Michael Gabay, Pharm.D., JD, BCPS, FCCP

Deputy Editor-in-Chief: Shingyee Cindy Huang, Pharm.D.

Principal Editorial Contributors: The University of Illinois at Chicago Drug Information Group

Editorial Contributors: Nicole Acquisto, Pharm.D., FASHP, FCCM, FCCP, BCCCP; Linda Bedford Arcuri, Pharm.D.; Heather Draper, Pharm.D., BCPS, BCEMP; Justyna Fydrych, Pharm.D.; Micheline Goldwire Pharm.D., M.S., M.A.; Donna Lisi, Pharm.D.; Natalie A. Mendham, Pharm.D.; Cambrey Bao-Phuong Nguyen, Pharm.D.; Kelly Pillinger, Pharm.D., BCPS, BCIDP; Tonya Scardina, Pharm.D., BCIDP; Margaret Segovia, Pharm.D.; Elaine K. Snow, B.S.Pharm.; Stephanie Weightman, Pharm.D., BCPS, BCPPS, BCEMP; Karen M. Whalen, B.S. Pharm., BCPS, FASHP; and Barbara F. Young, Pharm.D., M.H.A.

Contributors: Auburn University Drug Information Service; Belmont University Drug Information Service; Creighton University Drug Information Service; Medical University of South Carolina Drug Information Service; the University of Arizona Drug Information Service; the University of Missouri, Kansas City Drug Information Service; and the University of Rhode Island Drug Information Service

Assistant Editor for Injectable Drug Information: Natalie C. Rosanelli, Pharm.D.

Clinical Informatics Analyst: Kevin Son, Pharm.D., M.H.I.

Editorial Coordinator: Alexandra Rallo, B.A.

Content Management and Publishing Specialist: Shawna Rafalko, B.A.

Director of Production and Platform Services:: Johnna Hershey, B.A.

Consultant: Elizabeth Shannon, B.A.

FORMER EDITORS

Charles B. Cleveland

Donald E. Francke

William M. Heller

Judith A. Kepler

George P. Provost

Mary Jo Reilly

Gerald K. McEvoy

Elaine K. Snow

AHFS ONCOLOGY EXPERT COMMITTEE

Chase Ayres, Pharm.D., BCOP

Jason Bergsbaken, Pharm.D., MBS, BCOP

Rachel Bubik, Pharm.D., BCOP, BCPS

Caroline Clark, MSN, APRN, OCN, AG-CNS

Sandra Cuellar, Pharm.D., BCOP, FHOPA, FASHP

Christine Gegeckas, RPh, BCOP

Chelsea Gustafson*, Pharm.D., BCOP

Kirollos Hanna, Pharm.D., BCPS, BCOP

Isabel Houlzet*, Pharm.D., BCPS, BCOP

Andrew (Weiyi) Li, Pharm.D.

Donald Moore, Pharm.D., BCPS, BCOP, DPLA, FCCP

Eve Segal, Pharm.D., BCOP

Kate Taucher, Pharm.D., MHS, BCOP, FASHP, FAPO

John Villano, M.D., Ph.D.

Kathleen Wiley, MSN, RN, AOCNS

* Appointed in cooperation with the Hematology/Oncology Pharmacy Association (HOPA)

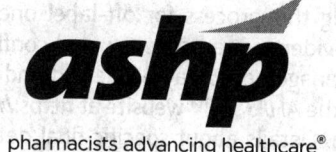

pharmacists advancing healthcare®

PREFACE

An Evidence-based Foundation for Safe and Effective Drug Therapy

With the 2025 edition, *AHFS Drug Information*® (*AHFS*® *DI*™) marks 66 years of continuous publication. The mission of *AHFS*® *DI*™ is to provide an evidence-based foundation for safe and effective drug therapy. Widely trusted for its established record and rigorous editorial process, *AHFS*® *DI*™ has remained true to its mission since the first edition in 1959. This notable achievement has gained *AHFS*® *DI*™ the unique distinction of being the longest published federally designated drug compendium issued by a scientific and professional society.

AHFS® *DI*™ is a collection of drug monographs kept current by ongoing electronic updates and by a revised master print volume issued annually. The *AHFS*® *DI*™ database is maintained continuously throughout the year and updates are issued frequently in electronic formats. (See AHFS® Clinical Drug Information™ [AHFS® CDI™].)

AHFS® was initially published as an adaptation from the *Hospital Formulary of Selected Drugs* by Don E. Francke, and the compendium has its roots in the hospital formulary system. The evidence-based assessments of medically accepted uses of drugs by *AHFS*® predated the US Food and Drug Administration's (FDA's) own authority to evaluate drug effectiveness claims, and established *AHFS*® as one of the first authoritative sources of critical evaluations of drug therapy. Today, it is the sole independent, non-commercial source of such evaluations in the US.

● *AHFS*® *Patient Medication Information*™ (*PMI*™)

ASHP has a long history of providing patients with meaningful information about medications. *AHFS*® *Patient Medication Information*™ (*PMI*™) originated in 1976 as a collaboration among ASHP, the American Hospital Association (AHA), the US Department of Health, and Human Services (DHHS), and the US Centers for Disease Control and Prevention (CDC). It is the only compendium-based PMI database published by a professional and scientific society in the US.

The trust placed in *AHFS*®*PMI*™ has resulted in a strategic alliance with the National Library of Medicine, an institute within the National Institutes of Health (NIH). *AHFS*®*PMI*™, hosted by the National Library of Medicine on MedlinePlus® and MedlinePlus® Connect, is one of few sites of trusted, accurate PMI, provided in both English and Spanish, with an outreach to over 100 million consumers annually. *AHFS*®*PMI*™ also has been adopted as the trusted source of PMI by Sonifi®, a leading provider of bedside patient engagement and education resources in hospitals. This service focuses on improving patient satisfaction, outcomes, and quality as measured by the Hospital Consumer Assessment of Healthcare Providers and Systems (HCAHPS) survey, care measures, and other indicators. Lastly, *AHFS*®*PMI*™ is accessible through ASHP's own website—https://www.safemedication.com.

AHFS®*PMI*™ also includes links within the context of each of its drug monographs in support of CDC's PROTECT initiative on safe medication use. Through PROTECT, CDC, the Consumer Healthcare Products Association Educational Foundation, and other organizations support the Up and Away and Out of Sight campaign aimed at educating families and other caregivers about the importance of storing medications in a safe place to prevent inadvertent overdoses by children.

● *Off-Label Drug Reviews for Oncology*

In 2008, *AHFS*® *DI*™ introduced a process for publishing structured, codified, evidence-based determinations for off-label cancer uses. The decision to create a separate method resulted from the unique characteristics of evidence-based decisions that are applied to serious and life-threatening conditions such as cancer. This process supplements the long-standing evidence-based process used by *AHFS*® to evaluate off-label uses of drugs and biologics. The cancer-specific codified method developed by *AHFS*® is consistent with distinctions applied to evidence-based assessments of cancer treatments by other authoritative sources such as the National Cancer Institute (NCI) and FDA.

The principles of the *AHFS*® *DI*™ evidence-based editorial development process have not changed with this oncology process. However, the codified determinations supplement and enhance the traditional *AHFS*® *DI*™ evaluation of off-label uses with structured determinations that summarize ongoing assessments of new and changing evidence. ASHP appointed an Oncology Expert Committee, comprised of oncologists, oncology pharmacists, and oncology nurses, to assist with the independent review and final recommendations for off-label cancer determinations. Final decisions are made solely by the Oncology Expert Committee for determinations emanating from this supplementary process for oncology uses and by *AHFS*® staff for other information. All processes related to the review and publication of determinations are transparent and designed to mitigate any potential conflict of interest in order to preserve the integrity of *AHFS*® *DI*™ and to minimize bias.

Federal regulations for transparency and conflict of interest disclosure and management became effective January 1, 2010 for off-label oncology determinations. *AHFS*® employs a process for evaluating therapies that is publicly transparent as defined by CFR Section 414.930(a) and that includes criteria used to evaluate the use, a listing of evidentiary materials reviewed by the compendium, and a listing of all individuals who participated substantively in the development, review, or disposition of the request. In the case of balloted determinations made by the *AHFS*® Oncology Expert Committee, conflict of interest disclosure policies follow the definition of a publicly transparent process for identifying potential conflicts of interest as established in this section of the CFR.

Documents describing this process for off-label oncology uses, including levels of evidence, transparency, and conflict of interest disclosure and management, may be viewed under the Off-label Uses section of the *AHFS*® *DI*™ website at https://www.ahfsdruginformation.com. Details about specific final determinations of medical acceptance for off-label oncology uses may also be accessed at this website location.

PREFACE

● Editorial Independence

Information included in *AHFS® DI™* shapes treatment decisions made by clinicians and influences public and private health-care policies and decisions. As a result, it is important that the information be authoritative, objective, and free of undue influence from pharmaceutical companies and other third parties who may seek to use the compendium to promote their own vested interests.

AHFS® DI™ is the only remaining official drug compendium published by a non-commercial, nonprofit, professional and scientific society. ASHP is the national professional organization that represents pharmacists who serve as patient care providers on healthcare teams in acute and ambulatory settings spanning the full spectrum of medication use. ASHP has an over 80 year history of fostering evidence-based medication use and patient medication safety. *AHFS® DI™* and *PMI™* are published in part to support the mission of pharmacists in helping people achieve optimal health outcomes.

AHFS® DI™ is published by ASHP under the authority of its elected Board of Directors. As such, the Board exercises oversight through its ongoing Society considerations. This oversight by the Board also involves review and approval of relevant recommendations originating from its appointed Council on Therapeutics and the advisory and best practices developments of its other Councils, House of Delegates, and other policy-recommending bodies.

ASHP considers it essential that interactions between AHFS® staff and pharmaceutical companies be limited to the legitimate exchange of the scientific and medical information needed to fulfill the mission of *AHFS® DI™*. To maintain independence from the undue influence of the promotional interests of pharmaceutical companies, communications are directed to the scientific and medical information areas within the companies; contact with marketing areas is avoided.

ASHP holds in high regard the responsibilities attendant to the public and private trust placed in the evidence-based editorial deliberations of *AHFS® DI™*. As such, ASHP also considers it essential to protect the integrity and independence of the editorial decisions of AHFS® staff by separating the Society's business activities with pharmaceutical companies (e.g., exhibits at educational meetings, journal advertising) from the editorial activities of its drug compendium. An editorial independence statement, approved by ASHP's Board of Directors and available at https://www.ahfsdruginformation.com, outlines the principles that AHFS® staff apply in ensuring such independence.

● Comparative, Unbiased, Evaluative Drug Information

AHFS® DI™ is a tested and proven source of comparative, unbiased, and evidence-based drug information containing a monograph on virtually every molecular drug entity available in the US. Drug monographs are prepared by a professional editorial and analytical staff, who critically evaluate published evidence on the drug.

AHFS® DI™ monographs incorporate information from pertinent references in the literature and expert therapeutic guidelines. The monographs also address the labeling approved by FDA, in some cases challenging outdated and clinically irrelevant information that may persist in the approved labeling. *AHFS® DI™* monographs continue to include information on uses, dosages, and routes and/or methods of administration that may not be included in the FDA-approved labeling for the drug ("off-label/unlabeled uses"). Monographs may incorporate information from numerous published references.

● Widely Used in Print and Electronic Formats

AHFS® DI™ and its point-of-care derivative database *AHFS® DI™ Essentials™* are used widely as sources of authoritative drug information by physicians, pharmacists, dentists, nurses, and other health care professionals, by schools of pharmacy, nursing, and medicine, and are available in a variety of formats. Electronic formats include UpToDate® Lexidrug™; First DataBank's AHFS Drug Information® monographs available from multiple vendors; *AHFS Drug Information®* from STAT!Ref®, Pepid's Pharmacist Pro with *AHFS® DI™*, and MedicinesComplete®; *Drug Information Fulltext®* (*DIF®*); and *AHFS® DI™* Powered by Skyscape Medpresso. *AHFS® DI™ Essentials™* is available electronically in online and mobile applications.

In hospitals, clinics, extended-care facilities, nursing homes, health maintenance organizations, and other organized health-care settings, *AHFS® DI™* is accessible in patient-care areas for ready use by physicians, nurses, pharmacists, and other health-care professionals. *AHFS® DI™* also is used in community pharmacies, chain drugstores, and other ambulatory care and professional practice settings and is available in most medical libraries.

● AHFS® Clinical Drug Information™ (AHFS® CDI™)

In 2016, ASHP released a comprehensive, electronic suite of its leading drug information databases, including *AHFS® DI™*. AHFS® Clinical Drug Information™ (AHFS® CDI™), expands the availability of these trusted ASHP resources, providing clinicians with real-time drug and safety updates and direct links to a vast number of supporting evidence sources, as well as easy access to the detailed drug information and in-depth coverage of off-label uses found in *AHFS® DI™*. In addition to the monographs of *AHFS® DI™*, subscribers to AHFS® CDI™ have access to *AHFS® DI™ Essentials™*, which offers quick, point-of-care answers. Additional ASHP drug information resources are included in the product, including ASHP's drug shortages resources (which are prepared in conjunction with the University of Utah Drug Information Service) and the AHFS Pharmacologic-Therapeutic Classification system. AHFS® CDI™ features links to additional specialty databases of drug-specific information, including prescribing information, FDA's latest boxed warnings, safety labeling changes, REMS, pharmacogenomic data, a specialty breast-feeding database, and other clinical resources.

PREFACE

AHFS® Clinical Drug Information™ is available for individual and institutional subscribers via web browser and is mobile-optimized for use on iOS and Android devices. AHFS® CDI™ also is available as an iOS app. In addition, the user interface will integrate into clinical workflow solutions in hospitals and ambulatory care settings. An application programming interface (API) is available.

● Highly Recognized Authority

AHFS® DI™ is supported solely through subscriptions. AHFS® DI™ has been officially adopted by the US Public Health Service and the Department of Veterans Affairs; recommended by the National Association of Boards of Pharmacy as part of the standard reference library; recommended by the American College of Physicians as part of a library for internists; included in the Standards for Medicare; approved by the American Pharmacists Association, American Health Care Association, American Hospital Association, and Catholic Health Care Association of the United States; recognized by the US Congress, CMS, AHIP, National Blue Cross and Blue Shield Association, National Association of Insurance Commissioners, and various third-party healthcare insurance providers for coverage decisions on off-label (unlabeled) uses; and included as a required or recommended standard reference for pharmacies in many states.

The authority of AHFS® DI™ also includes Federal recognition through legislation and regulation as an "official" compendium for information on medically accepted uses of drugs. The Federal compendial recognition for AHFS® DI™ originated in the Medicare Catastrophic Coverage Act. CMS determined that AHFS® DI™ met the compendial selection criteria established by Congress and adopted the compendium for carrying out certain aspects of the Act and in meeting the need of the US Secretary of HHS to establish standards based on accepted medical practice for the prescribing, dispensing, and utilization of covered drugs. This established the Federal precedent for use of AHFS® DI™ as a compendial standard in subsequent legislative and regulatory initiatives, including for drug coverage under Medicaid and Medicare Parts B and D.

● Continuously Updated and Revised

The AHFS® DI™ database and annual print edition are updated extensively, incorporating revised information on uses, therapeutic perspectives, cautions, drug interactions, new products, and other new developments. In addition, the database is expanded by dozens of new drug monographs over the course of the year.

The AHFS® DI™ database is also revised and updated extensively throughout the year to address evolving information on medication safety. Manufacturer labeling, FDA safety communications such as MedWatch notices and Risk Evaluation and Mitigation Strategy (REMS) information, published studies and reports, and other safety information are evaluated and addressed. Through semi-automated processes, much of this information is updated on an ongoing basis in electronic versions of the database to reflect more contemporaneous changes made by FDA.

● Recognition and Granularity of the AHFS® Pharmacologic-Therapeutic Classification©

The AHFS® Pharmacologic-Therapeutic Classification© is the most widely used formulary-structure drug classification in the US and Canada. The AHFS® classification is maintained continuously by ASHP and allows the grouping of drugs with similar pharmacologic, therapeutic, and/or chemical characteristics in a 4-tier hierarchy.

For details on class changes and drug monograph assignments and reassignments throughout the year, see the link to the AHFS® Classification Drug Assignments and Reassignments on the homepage at https://www.ahfsdruginformation .com.

In the printed version of the classification in AHFS® DI™, a drug monograph generally is only printed under one classification; however, multiple classifications may apply based on a drug's pharmacology or therapeutic uses. Multiple classifications for a drug in print are represented by cross-references in the table of contents for each chapter/class. If cross-referenced, the drug name is given followed by the classification number that it is printed under. Electronically, all applicable classes for a drug are listed.

CMS' "Guidelines for Reviewing Prescription Drug Plan Formularies and Procedures" and "Medicare Prescription Drug Benefit Manual: Part D Drugs and Formulary Requirements" describe use of the AHFS® Pharmacologic-Therapeutic Classification© as the only named alternative to USP's Model Guidelines for use by prescription drug plans (PDPs) in implementing the formulary portion of the outpatient prescription drug benefit in the Medicare Modernization Act (MMA) of 2003. These Guidelines are part of the MMA Final Guidelines for Formularies that address the "CMS Strategy for Affordable Access to Comprehensive Drug Coverage."

The AHFS® Classification is a registered external code system in the HL7 Vocabulary Repository. (OID: 2.16.840.1. 113883.6.234.)

The AHFS® Classification also is an approved value code of the External Code List for use in the Formulary & Benefit, Telecommunication, Post-Adjudication, & SCRIPT e-Prescribing standards of the National Council for Prescription Drug Programs (NCPDP).

● Selected Content in the Print Edition of AHFS® DI™

As the number of FDA-approved drugs has increased and information about existing drugs has expanded, it has been necessary to omit an increasing number of monographs from the print version of AHFS® DI™ each year. Considerations used to select monographs for print include the following:

- Frequently prescribed drugs (based on prescription drug utilization data estimates for patients in the US)
- Drugs used as first-line therapy or as the mainstay of important treatment regimens (based on therapeutic guidelines and/or labeled indications)

- Drugs with a wider range of established uses or with unique roles as compared with other drugs in the same therapeutic class

- Monograph contains unique information not found in other monographs in the drug class, such as more extensive discussion of guideline recommendations

The Editorial staff wishes to express appreciation to the many consultants and reviewers for their excellent guidance and cooperation and to our subscribers for their support and comments.

● www.ahfsdruginformation.com

Some monographs have been omitted from the print version of *AHFS® DI™* because of space limitations. Copies of these monographs are available on the "Print Subscribers" page of the AHFS Drug Information® website, https://www.ahfsdruginformation.com, in the "Electronic Only Monographs" section. A username and password are required to access the subscriber-only portions of the website. For the 2025 edition, the username and password for accessing electronic-only content are as follows:

- **username: ahfs2025**
- **password: ASHP46360**

Associated index entries for monographs that appear on the website are followed by the symbol "§" rather than by a page number. This symbol refers the user to a footnote in the index that also provides the above username and password for the 2025 edition.

USERS GUIDE

AHFS Drug Information®
Users Guide

ORGANIZATION OF CONTENT

AHFS Drug Information® (*AHFS® DI™*) is a collection of drug monographs on virtually every single-drug entity available in the United States; information on various trademarked preparations and brands of a drug are contained in a single monograph. Drug *combinations* are generally described in the monographs on the principal ingredients; however, they may appear as separate monographs when the combinations are considered important because of therapeutic rationale and/or frequency of use. There are also general statements on groups of drugs whose activities and uses permit their discussion as a class.

Organization of the Book

In the annual print edition of *AHFS® DI™*, drug monographs are arranged by the widely recognized and used *AHFS®* Pharmacologic-Therapeutic Classification©. This arrangement permits easy review of information on a group of drugs with similar activities and uses and allows the reader to determine quickly the similarities and differences among drugs within a group.

A *table of contents* precedes each major class of drugs (e.g., 8:00 Anti-infective Agents) in the book. The table of contents lists each drug monograph included in that major class according to the specific subclass (e.g., Cephalosporins 8:12.06). Within each subclass, monographs are arranged alphabetically by nonproprietary (generic) name and are preceded by the general statement, when present, for that subclass. The names of the drugs are the United States Adopted Names (USAN) and other names for drugs as described in the *USP Dictionary of USAN and International Drug Names*.

In the print edition of *AHFS® DI™*, a monograph must be printed within a single class section. However, multiple classifications may apply to a drug (based on its pharmacology or therapeutic uses); these are represented by cross-references provided in the table of contents for each class to the location of the monograph in the book. Although the print version of *AHFS® DI™* does not include reference notations, all statements appearing in the publication are documented. (See the discussion on References.)

Information on a particular drug can be located via the Index by looking up the drug by its proprietary (trade) or nonproprietary (generic) name. The Index also includes entries for the major *AHFS®* Pharmacologic-Therapeutic Classification© terms. Once the table of contents for a specific major class of drugs has been located, the page number for the beginning of each drug monograph is listed alongside the monograph title in the table; thus, the list of drug monographs in a given subclass can be quickly scanned to locate a specific drug or drugs of interest.

Some monographs are omitted from the print version of *AHFS® DI™* because of space limitations. Associated index entries and listings in the table of contents for each major class of drugs

in the printed book refer users to the website https://www.ahfsdruginformation.com to see these monographs. A username and password are required to access these electronic-only monographs, as follows:

- **username: ahfs2025**
- **password: ASHP46360**

Each year after publication of the print edition of *AHFS® DI™*, new monographs are created, and revisions to existing monographs continue. At the end of the subscription year, any new or revised monographs that were published electronically usually will become incorporated into the upcoming annual edition of *AHFS® DI™* within the appropriate AHFS® Pharmacologic-Therapeutic Classification©. Revised monographs carry the statement "Selected Revisions January 2023" or some other appropriate revision date in the Copyright notice at the end of the monograph. Because information about a drug frequently changes, the manufacturer's labeling should be reviewed periodically.

Organization of Full-length Monographs

Information within each full-length drug monograph is divided into the sections and subsections described below; the types of information that may be included in each major section and subsection within a monograph also are described. Not all sections or subsections are included in each monograph; such subdivisions are used when applicable and necessary. Some information may appear in one or more sections, depending on the type of discussion (e.g., pharmacogenomics information may appear under Dosage, Cautions, and/or Pharmacokinetics depending on the specific information presented). Individual monographs may not contain all of the information described below, or other subsections may be used as needed to organize the text; the absence of specific information within an individual monograph does not imply that such information is unavailable.

The presence or absence of a particular drug or use should *not* be interpreted as indicating any judgment by *AHFS® DI™* on its merits.

● *Monograph Title and Synonyms*

Lists the USAN name or other name for the drug(s) described; salts generally are included even when omitted from the USAN name. If multiple forms (e.g., salts, esters) of the same drug are available, all forms are described within the monograph; the title may include all forms (if only a few) or just the base (active moiety). Occasionally, when several drug entities are described in a single monograph, an alternative title descriptive of the group (e.g., Antacids 56:04) is used. Common synonyms for the drug are listed alongside the USAN or other names.

When recommended by the US Food and Drug Administration (FDA) or the Institute for Safe Medication Practices (ISMP), "tall person" (mixed case) lettering is used for drug names in titles or synonyms (e.g., "diazePAM").

When a graphic formula of the drug or prototype (if multiple drugs) is present, it is in the style adopted by the USAN Council and United States Pharmacopeial Convention.

USERS GUIDE

Occasionally, certain synonyms (e.g., pharmacy equivalent names [PENs]) that apply to specific preparations or combinations rather than to the drug itself are noted parenthetically alongside various preparation headings. (See the discussion on Preparations.)

● *Introductory Description*

Provides a brief chemical, structural, and/or pharmacologic/therapeutic description for the purpose of orientation and introduction.

● *REMS*

Provides a brief description of a Risk Evaluation and Mitigation Strategy (REMS) approved by FDA. Because REMS frequently are modified or rescinded, a cross reference to FDA's list of "Approved Risk Evaluation and Mitigation Strategies (REMS)" is provided to refer users to the most current information. REMS for drug *combinations* are described in the monographs on the principal ingredient that requires the REMS.

● *Uses*

Provides information on uses that are included in the labeling approved by FDA and those that are not (i.e., "off-label" [unlabeled] uses). Off-label uses are identified with daggers† within the text of the monograph; a footnote that describes the use as unlabeled appears at the end of the monograph. The authority of *AHFS® DI*™ to establish medically accepted uses of drugs is recognized through designation as an official federal compendium. (See the Preface for additional information.) Comparisons with other forms of therapy and limitations on use are included when appropriate. This section usually is subdivided by major indication.

Under the Federal Food, Drug, and Cosmetic (FD&C) Act, the labeling approved by FDA for a drug is limited to those uses for which the sponsor has submitted information regarding the safety and efficacy of that product and which has been reviewed by FDA; other uses for which the sponsor has chosen not to submit data to FDA may be demonstrated in the clinical literature before and after the product is approved by FDA. The FD&C Act does not, however, limit the manner in which a clinician may use an approved drug. Once a drug has been approved for marketing, the clinician may prescribe it for uses or in treatment regimens or patient populations (e.g., children) that are not included in approved labeling. Such off-label uses may be appropriate and rational, and may reflect approaches to drug therapy that have been reported extensively in the medical literature.

Valid new uses for drugs often are first discovered via serendipitous observations and therapeutic innovations, and then subsequently may be confirmed by well-designed and controlled studies. Inclusion of such new uses in the FDA-approved labeling for a drug may take considerable time and, without the initiative of the sponsor whose product is involved, may never occur. Therefore, accepted medical practice (state-of-the-art) often includes drug use that is not included in FDA-approved labeling.

Accordingly, *AHFS® DI*™ monographs attempt to describe most uses for a drug, whether or not they are included in FDA-approved labeling; however, the presence or absence of a particular use should *not* be interpreted as indicating any judgment by *AHFS® DI*™ on its merits. Coverage of off-label uses in *AHFS Drug Information*®, an official Federal drug compendium, has been recognized by the US Congress (e.g., in OBRA 90 and OBRA 93), the Centers for Medicare & Medicaid Services (CMS; Section 1861 and 1927 of the Social Security Act), third-party health-care providers, and others. (See Off-label Uses at https://www.ahfs druginformation.com for additional information.)

AHFS Grades of Recommendation

During 2008, *AHFS® DI*™ introduced a new process for publishing structured, codified, evidence-based determinations for off-label cancer uses. In some monographs that subsequently were revised based on Final Off-label Determinations for cancer uses, text describing such uses based on *AHFS® Grades of Recommendation may be noted. Following are the categories of *AHFS® Grades of Recommendation and the definitions of each:

A: Recommended (Accepted) (e.g., should be used, is recommended/indicated, is useful/effective/beneficial in most cases)

B: Reasonable Choice (Accepted, with Possible Conditions) (e.g., treatment option) (e.g., is reasonable to use under certain conditions [e.g., in certain patient groups], can be useful/effective/beneficial, is probably recommended/indicated)

C: Not Fully Established (Unclear risk/benefit, equivocal evidence, inadequate data and/or experience) (e.g., usefulness/effectiveness unknown/unclear/uncertain or not well established relative to standard of care)

D: Not Recommended (Unaccepted) (e.g., considered inappropriate, obsolete, or unproven; is not recommended/indicated/useful/effective/beneficial; or may be harmful)

● *Dosage and Administration*

Includes information on reconstitution and administration of specific dosage forms and on dosage. In addition, pretreatment screening, patient monitoring, premedication and prophylaxis, dispensing and administration precautions, and certain Risk Evaluation and Mitigation Strategies (REMS) program requirements are described in discrete sections to allow quick retrieval of pertinent dosage and administration information.

The Administration subsection describes the routes of administration and, when necessary for clarity, the appropriate dosage form for each route. Instructions for administering the drug (e.g., after meals, with food) and specialized methods of administration are given. Occasionally, instructions for extemporaneous preparation of a dosage form that is not commercially available (e.g., preparation of a pediatric oral suspension from the contents of capsules) are included. For injectable drugs or other dosage forms requiring reconstitution, the Administration subsection is replaced by the Reconstitution and Administration subsection. In addition to information described for the Administration subsection, instructions for reconstitution and, when applicable, further dilution of the dosage form are presented. The rate of injection or infusion of the drug is described, as well as any precautions associated with administration.

USERS GUIDE

The Dosage subsection describes recommended and alternative dosage schedules for each dosage form and route of administration and condition being treated. Information in this subsection often is divided by use. When applicable, dosage equivalencies are described. The initial, maintenance, and maximum dosages are given. When available and applicable, specific dosages for children, geriatric or debilitated patients, or patients with renal and/or hepatic impairment are described. Occasionally, when use of a fixed-dosage combination preparation or concomitant use of the drug with another drug is considered rational, specific regimens may be described. Because information about a drug frequently changes, the manufacturer's labeling should be reviewed periodically.

● Cautions

Includes information about adverse effects, precautions and contraindications, pediatric and geriatric precautions, and pregnancy, fertility, and lactation precautions.

Adverse reactions of a drug are undesirable effects, reasonably associated with use of the drug, that may occur as part of its pharmacologic action or may be unpredictable in occurrence. The general Adverse Effects subsection usually is replaced by multiple subsections that are specifically divided by body system affected (e.g., GI, CNS, Hematologic) or by type of effect (e.g., Sensitivity Reactions).

The Precautions and Contraindications subsection includes any special care to be taken by practitioners and/or patients for safe and effective use of the drug and describes serious adverse effects and potential safety hazards, limitations on use imposed by them, and actions that should be taken if they occur. Those situations or conditions for which the drug should not be used because the risk clearly outweighs any possible benefit also are described. Additional precautions and contraindications are included in other appropriate sections of the drug monograph (e.g., Pediatric; Drug Interactions). Because precautionary information about a drug frequently changes, the manufacturer's labeling should be reviewed periodically.

The Pediatric subsection describes those pediatric age groups for which safety and/or efficacy of the drug have not been established from adequate and well-controlled studies. Risks associated with use of the drug in pediatric age groups also are described.

The Geriatric subsection includes precautions, warnings, and contraindications associated with use of the drug in geriatric individuals and provides some perspective regarding study and experience in this population, including factors that may affect response and tolerance.

Pediatric and geriatric information also may be described within the appropriate major sections of the monograph. For example, information on age-dependent pharmacokinetics of the drug would be described within the Pharmacokinetics section and on age-specific dosage recommendations would be described in the Dosage and Administration section of the monograph. When relevant information on use of the drug in pediatric or geriatric patients is readily available in the medical literature and/or the drug is labeled specifically for use in this age group, details about efficacy generally are described in the Uses section.

The Pregnancy, Fertility, and Lactation subsection describes the safety of the drug in pregnant and/or lactating women and any potential effects on male and female reproduction capacity. Precautionary information regarding use of the drug during pregnancy is included when available. In 2014, FDA amended the requirements for pregnancy and lactation labeling, eliminating the long-recognized lettered categories (A, B, C, D, and X) and replacing the letters with a narrative structure for pregnancy labeling. Therefore, AHFS® DI™ monographs may have varying styles depending on available information. Additional pertinent information regarding use of the drug during pregnancy or effects on labor and delivery also is presented.

A description of whether the drug is distributed into milk is included when available, and any associated precautions regarding use of the drug in nursing women are described. Effects of the drug on lactation and/or the nursing infant also are described.

Evidence from animal studies regarding effects of the drug on fertility is given, and relevant advice regarding the importance of these animal findings is included when available. Pertinent evidence from humans regarding effects of the drug on fertility also is described.

● Acute Toxicity

Describes toxic effects of the drug associated with intentional or accidental ingestion or administration of a large dose. Information on the amount of drug in a single dose that usually is associated with symptoms of overdosage and the amount of drug in a single dose that is likely to be life-threatening is included when available. Manifestations, laboratory findings, and potential complications of acute overdosage are described. Plasma concentrations associated with toxicity are included when well described.

Recommendations for management of acute toxicity, including those for supportive and symptomatic treatment, are described.

● Chronic Toxicity

Includes well-described toxic effects of the drug associated with prolonged use. When information on chronic toxicity is limited, it often is described in the appropriate subsection under Cautions. The pathogenesis, manifestations, and treatment of chronic toxic effects are discussed. Also included is a description of tolerance to and/or physical or psychologic dependence on the drug. Adverse effects associated with abrupt withdrawal of the drug are described, and appropriate measures for management are included.

● Drug Interactions

Describes clinically important drug interactions, including adverse and therapeutically useful interactions. The mechanism of the interaction, associated clinical importance, precautions to be observed, and management of the interaction are described. Generally, potential interactions supported only by animal or in vitro data are not described. Occasionally, theoretical interactions are presented because of the likelihood of their occurrence (e.g., based on evidence from similar drugs) or the potential severity of the effect should it occur.

USERS GUIDE

● Laboratory Test Interferences

Includes information on common, well-established drug/laboratory test interferences. The mechanism of the interaction, effects on test results, and effects on interpretation of these results are included. Alternative laboratory tests are described when appropriate. Alterations in laboratory test results that reflect a pathologic effect of the drug (e.g., aminoglycoside-induced increase in serum creatinine concentration) are described in the appropriate subsections under Cautions. Because of the nature of information on laboratory tests, appropriate specialized references on laboratory methods should be consulted when detailed information is required.

● Pharmacology

Includes a brief statement of pharmacologic activity and/or mechanism of action, often compared with other similar drugs, for the purpose of orientation and introduction. Expanded descriptions of pharmacologic activities and effects are included. When relevant to human pharmacology and therapeutics, animal or in vitro data are presented. Data from human studies are not specified as such unless needed for clarification. Quantitative and qualitative comparative (with other drugs) information is provided when appropriate. Pharmacology usually is subdivided by pharmacologic effect (e.g., Anti-inflammatory, Analgesic) and/or body system affected (e.g., CNS, GI, Hematologic).

For anti-infectives, pharmacology is described under Mechanism of Action, Spectrum, and Resistance.

● Mechanism of Action

Describes the mechanism of anti-infective activity for anti-infective agents.

● Spectrum

Describes the in vitro spectra of activity of anti-infectives. MIC values for clinically important organisms are included in the spectra subsections as appropriate. Spectra often are divided according to class of organism (e.g., Gram-negative Bacteria, Anaerobic Bacteria).

● Resistance

Describes the mechanism of resistance of microorganisms to anti-infective agents. Microbiologic tolerance to these agents also is described. Information on cross-resistance with other anti-infective agents is included.

Resistance of cells to antineoplastic agents generally is described in the Pharmacology section. Resistance or tolerance to the pharmacologic and/or therapeutic effects (e.g., tachyphylaxis) of other drugs generally is described in Pharmacology and/or Uses.

● Pharmacokinetics

Describes absorption, distribution, and elimination (biotransformation and excretion) characteristics of a drug.

The Absorption subsection includes information on extent (bioavailability) and rate of absorption by usual routes of administration and factors (e.g., product formulation) that might influence them. Applicable comparative information on doses, dosage forms, and routes of administration is included. Information on serum concentrations achieved and on the period of time for onset, peak, and duration of pharmacologic and/or therapeutic effect also is included, even when an absorption phase per se does not occur (e.g., following IV administration). Ranges for therapeutic and/or toxic concentrations (e.g., plasma, serum) of the drug are described when established.

The Distribution subsection describes the usual distribution of the drug into body tissue and fluids. Information describing the drug's propensity to cross the blood-brain barrier and placenta and to distribute into milk is included. Protein binding characteristics are presented.

The Elimination subsection describes the biotransformation and excretory characteristics of the drug. Information on elimination half-life and factors influencing it, clearance, site and extent of biotransformation, metabolic products and their activities, and routes of elimination from the body (e.g., urine, feces via bile) and factors affecting them is included. The effect of peritoneal dialysis and hemodialysis on elimination of the drug also is discussed.

● Chemistry and Stability

Includes a brief chemical, structural, and/or pharmacologic description, often compared with other similar drugs, for the purpose of orientation and introduction. Structure-activity relationships are described when applicable. A physical description of drug entities includes physical appearance, taste, odor, and solubility.

If the drug is ionizable, the pK_a is given. Other chemical and/or physical constants such as pH and osmolarity/osmolality of commercially available preparations are included. Dosage equivalencies (e.g., units per mg of drug, mg of base per mg of salt) are given when the dosage of a drug differs from the commercially available form (e.g., salt, ester). Amounts of important ions (e.g., mg/mEq of potassium, sodium) in commercial preparations also are included.

Applicable stability information such as the effect of pH, autoclaving, heat, light, moisture, air, freezing, and microwave thawing is described. Storage requirements (i.e., recommended environmental storage conditions) also are described. Stability information about reconstituted and/or diluted preparations is provided.

● Preparations

Lists commercially available preparations of the drug. Preparations are described under the appropriate heading by USAN or other nonproprietary (generic) name. Combination preparations are described under a separate heading (e.g., Aspirin Combinations) following the appropriate single-entity subsection (e.g., Aspirin); official USP combination names (e.g., Metoprolol Tartrate and Hydrochlorothiazide) are used whenever possible.

Although USP has changed its naming conventions to eliminate salt forms in many official monograph titles (active moiety nomenclature concept), the American Society of Health-System Pharmacists continues to oppose this nomenclature change

USERS GUIDE

because of resulting confusion and loss of important chemical identity cues, and therefore *AHFS® DI*™ will continue to include salts in the Preparations headings for clarity. When recommended by FDA or the Institute for Safe Medication Practices (ISMP), "tall person" (mixed case) lettering is used for generic or brand (trade) names (e.g., "diazePAM").

Preparations are listed hierarchically by route of administration (alphabetically), dosage form (alphabetically), and strength (in order of increasing strength). When potency is described in terms other than those listed in the drug heading (e.g., potency of cefotaxime sodium is expressed in terms of cefotaxime), the labeled moiety is described parenthetically after the strength [e.g., 1 g (of cefotaxime)].

Route of administration and dosage form listings may be modified (e.g., Injection, for IM use only; Tablets, chewable; Capsules, extended-release). Following each preparation description, the proprietary (trade) names are listed alphabetically and include the corresponding manufacturers. Generally, preparations that are available by nonproprietary (generic) name do not include the names of the manufacturers/labelers; these preparations are listed under the generic name and described as being "available by nonproprietary name."

Generally, dosage forms used in the Preparations sections are the pharmaceutical dosage forms described in USP. (See the current edition of the *United States Pharmacopeia–National Formulary*.) Several dosage forms (i.e., elixir, extract, fluid extract, spirit, tincture) are used only when the preparation is official (USP or NF). Solution generally is used to describe all liquid preparations of dissolved drug, regardless of solvent; although syrups occasionally are official (USP or NF), these are listed as solutions and syrup is included only as part of the proprietary name.

Applicable legal descriptions (e.g., drugs subject to control under the Federal Controlled Substances Act of 1970, drugs subject to restricted distribution programs) are included.

● *References*

Includes the bibliography for cited references. Information included in *AHFS® DI*™ is thoroughly referenced. Access to referenced statements and the References section of individual drug monographs for *AHFS® DI*™ and its point-of-care derivative database *AHFS® DI™Essentials*™ can be gained through electronic versions (e.g., AHFS® Clinical Drug Information™ [AHFS® CDI™], eBroselow's SafeDose®, UpToDate® Lexidrug™; First DataBank's AHFS Drug Information® monographs available from multiple vendors; *AHFS Drug Information*® from STAT!Ref®, Pepid's Pharmacist Pro with AHFS DI®, and MedicinesComplete®; *Drug Information Fulltext*® [DIF®]; *AHFS® DI*™ Powered by Skyscape Medpresso).

Reference citations currently are electronically accessible for all monographs published after March 1984. For monographs originally published prior to that time, bibliographic citations are accessible only for selected revisions occurring since 1984. To determine whether a monograph was published or revised after March 1984, see the copyright notice at the end of the monograph in question. In electronic versions of *AHFS® DI*™, approximately 90% of the monographs currently are completely or partially referenced.

For additional information on searching the electronic versions of *AHFS® DI*™, contact the ASHP Customer Service by phone at 1-866-279-0681 or by email at *custserv@ashp.org*.

AHFS®*FIRST*RELEASES™

Certain monographs in *AHFS® DI*™ are designated as AHFS®-*first*Releases™. This designation appears in a boldface footnote preceding the Preparations section of the monograph. The AHFS®*first*Releases™ disseminate timely information on new molecular entities (NMEs) in an expedited format as soon as possible after FDA approval; the principal limitation is availability of final labeling from the manufacturer.

● *Scope*

AHFS®*first*Releases™ are descriptions about new molecular entities that include information drawn from the manufacturer's labeling (package insert); however, the descriptions are not intended to be comprehensive. When additional information on such drugs is needed before publication of a more detailed monograph, the manufacturer's labeling should be consulted. AHFS®*first*Releases™ are intended to provide information that can answer typical basic questions about newly approved drugs. As such, the descriptions are limited to highlights of boxed warnings in labeling; a brief description of a REMS (if one is approved by FDA for the drug); the brand name; an introductory sentence providing a brief pharmacologic/therapeutic description; highlights of labeled dosage and administration information; highlights of labeled contraindications; labeled warnings and precautions, including those for specific populations; highlights of common adverse effects; highlights of interactions; highlights of the actions of the drug; manufacturer-recommended advice to patients; and a product description. As a result, the AHFS®-*first*Releases™ do not provide full disclosure about the respective drugs, and therefore it is essential that the manufacturer's labeling be consulted for more detailed information on usual uses, dosage and administration, cautions, precautions, contraindications, potential drug interactions, and laboratory test interferences. Sections for Preparations and References are similar to those previously described for full-length monographs. Of note, certain medications have an expanded *first* Release™ format (e.g., gene therapies) with a limited summary of clinical trial data and other medications may be permanent *first* Releases™.

OVERVIEWS

Certain monographs in *AHFS® DI*™ are designated as Overviews. This designation appears in a boldface footnote preceding the Preparations section of the monograph.

● *Scope*

The Overview drug monographs are summary descriptions that include information drawn principally from the manufacturer's labeling (package insert) and the principal clinical studies that supported approval of the drug. Pertinent information from other sources such as authoritative therapeutic guidelines, secondary references (e.g., review articles), and a limited number of primary references also are included; however, the overviews are not intended to be comprehensive.

The Overviews are intended to provide subscribers to *AHFS® DI*™ with summaries on new molecular entities (NMEs) that can answer the most common questions about these drugs. As such, the Overviews are limited to basic information on the drugs, including brief descriptions (chemical and pharmacologic) of the type of drug, its labeled uses and associated dosages, administration instructions, product availability, cautionary information (e.g., contraindications; warnings and precautions; sensitivity reactions; cautions applicable to specific populations, common adverse effects), drug interactions, and important advice for patients. Some Overviews have been expanded to include important "unlabeled/off-label" uses. While selected information appears in these monographs, the scope of the Overview format limits the extent of discussion. As a result, the Overviews do not provide full disclosure about the respective drugs, and therefore it is essential that the manufacturer's labeling be consulted for more detailed information on pharmacodynamics, pharmacokinetics, adverse reactions, laboratory test interferences, and acute and chronic toxicity. Sections for Preparations and References are similar to those previously described for full-length monographs.

● *Pregnancy Precautions*

The pregnancy precautions in the Overviews historically have followed FDA's lettered categories (A, B, C, D, or X), as stated in the manufacturer's labeling. Because of the summary format of the Overviews, only the letter designation previously appeared. However, as noted previously FDA amended the requirements for pregnancy and lactation labeling in 2014, eliminating these lettered categories and replacing the letters with a narrative structure for pregnancy labeling. Therefore, some *AHFS® DI*™ Overviews now contain text descriptions of information about use of a drug during pregnancy when the lettered category has not been provided in the labeling.

Following are definitions of the categories FDA previously had designated:

Category A

Adequate and well-controlled studies in pregnant women have failed to demonstrate a risk to the fetus in the first trimester and there is no evidence of risk in later trimesters. If the drug were used during pregnancy, the possibility of fetal harm appears remote.

Category B

Either animal reproduction studies have failed to demonstrate a risk to the fetus and there are no adequate and well-controlled studies in pregnant women or animal reproduction studies have shown an adverse effect (other than on fertility) but adequate and well-controlled studies in pregnant women have failed to demonstrate a risk to the fetus in the first trimester and there is no evidence of risk in later trimesters. In either case, the drug should be used during pregnancy only when clearly needed.

Category C

Either animal reproduction studies have revealed evidence of an adverse fetal effect and there are no adequate and well-controlled studies in pregnant women or animal reproduction studies have not been performed and it is not known whether the drug can cause fetal harm when administered to pregnant women. In the first case, the drug should be used during pregnancy only when the potential benefits justify the possible risks to the fetus. In the latter case, the drug should be used during pregnancy only when clearly needed.

Category D

There is positive evidence of human fetal risk based on adverse reaction data from investigational or postmarketing experience or studies in humans, but the potential benefits from use of the drug in pregnant women may be acceptable in certain conditions despite the possible risks to the fetus. The drug should be used during pregnancy only in life-threatening situations or severe disease for which safer drugs cannot be used or are ineffective. When the drug is administered during pregnancy or if the patient becomes pregnant while receiving the drug, the patient should be informed of the potential hazard to the fetus.

Category X

The drug may (can) cause fetal toxicity when administered to pregnant women based on animal or human studies demonstrating fetal abnormalities or positive evidence of human fetal risk from adverse reaction data from investigational or postmarketing experience, or both, and the risk of use of the drug during pregnancy clearly outweighs any benefit (e.g., safer drugs or alternative therapies are available). Since the risks clearly outweigh any possible benefits in women who are or may become pregnant, the drug is contraindicated in such women. If the drug is inadvertently administered during pregnancy or if the patient becomes pregnant while receiving the drug, the patient should be informed of the potential hazard to the fetus.

SUMMONS®

Certain monographs in *AHFS® DI*™ are designated as SumMons® (summary monographs). This designation appears in a boldface footnote preceding the Preparations section of the monograph. SumMons® are summary descriptions about a drug, which include information that is drawn principally from the manufacturer's labeling (package insert) and/or other pertinent information (such as secondary references [e.g., review articles] and a limited number of primary references [e.g., the principal clinical studies]); however, no attempt is made to be complete, and the information may *not* be evaluative. When additional information on such drugs is needed pending development and publication of a more detailed *AHFS® DI*™ monograph, the manufacturer's labeling should be consulted.

The summaries are intended to provide only basic information on the drugs, and therefore are limited to brief descriptions (chemical and pharmacologic) of the type of drug, its labeled uses and associated dosages, and product availability. While selected precautionary information occasionally may appear in these summaries, no attempt is made to be complete, and therefore it is *essential* that the labeling be consulted for detailed information on the usual cautions, precautions, and contraindications.

USERS GUIDE

Some SumMons® have been expanded to include a detailed Cautions section, but it remains *essential* that the labeling be consulted for information on potential drug interactions, laboratory test interferences, and acute toxicity for such expanded descriptions. Some SumMons® also have been expanded to include important "unlabeled/off-label" uses. Sections for Preparations and References are similar to those previously described for full-length monographs.

Essentials

AHFS DI®Essentials™ is designed to offer clinicians easy access to knowledge that is critical at the point of care. Essentials™ monographs draw on the meticulously evidence-based guidance from the full *AHFS DI®* database, distilling for the clinician the essential information on prescription and key over-the-counter (OTC) drugs in an easy-to-use, highly structured outline format.

Clinically important information that is needed to help clinicians provide safe and effective drug therapy is included. *AHFS DI®Essentials™* is not intended to provide the "full disclosure" safety information provided by US Food and Drug Administration (FDA)-approved professional labeling. Instead, it provides a summary of critical information intended to provide quick, point-of-care answers to common prescribing and monitoring questions. More detailed information generally can be found in full-length *AHFS DI®* monographs and the manufacturers' professional labeling. Users should refer to these resources for more complete information. Information on multiple products containing the same drug (either singly or in combination) often is

included in the same *Essentials™* monograph, incorporating key elements from a variety of professional labeling and other references (e.g., authoritative therapeutic guidelines).

NOTICES

● *Copyright*

AHFS® monographs are copyrighted by the American Society of Health-System Pharmacists (ASHP), Inc., 4500 East-West Highway, Suite 900, Bethesda, MD 20814. All rights reserved.

Subscribers to *AHFS Drug Information®* are authorized to reproduce or retransmit AHFS monographs that are published only electronically on the https://www.ahfsdruginformation.com website, not to exceed the total number of paid subscriptions by the subscriber. For example, if a subscriber pays for 3 subscriptions ("copies"), then the subscriber is authorized to reproduce and distribute and/or retransmit a total of 3 copies of a given document. All material distributed as part of *AHFS Drug Information®*, including AHFS full-length monographs, AHFS®*first* Releases™, Overviews, and Essentials is copyrighted. Reproduction, storage in a retrieval system, or transmission of any such material or any part thereof in any form or by any means except as authorized (see above) or with the express written permission of ASHP is prohibited. Published in the United States of America.

● *Other Notices*

For other notices of warning, see Notices.

AHFS® Pharmacologic-Therapeutic Classification©

AHFS CLASSIFICATION

4:00 - Antihistamine Drugs
4:04 - First Generation Antihistamines
4:08 - Second Generation Antihistamines
4:92 - Other Antihistamines*

8:00 - Anti-infective Agents
8:08 - Anthelmintics
8:12 - Antibacterials
  8:12.02 - Aminoglycosides
  8:12.06 - Cephalosporins
    8:12.06.04 - First Generation Cephalosporins
    8:12.06.08 - Second Generation Cephalosporins
    8:12.06.12 - Third Generation Cephalosporins
    8:12.06.16 - Fourth Generation Cephalosporins
    8:12.06.20 - Fifth Generation Cephalosporins
    8:12.06.28 - Siderophore Cephalosporins
  8:12.07 - Miscellaneous β-Lactams
    8:12.07.04 - Carbacephems*
    8:12.07.08 - Carbapenems
    8:12.07.12 - Cephamycins
    8:12.07.16 - Monobactams
  8:12.08 - Chloramphenicol
  8:12.12 - Macrolides
    8:12.12.04 - Erythromycins
    8:12.12.08 - Other Macrolides
    8:12.12.12 - Ketolides*
  8:12.16 - Penicillins
    8:12.16.04 - Natural Penicillins
    8:12.16.08 - Aminopenicillins
    8:12.16.12 - Penicillinase-resistant Penicillins
    8:12.16.16 - Extended-spectrum Penicillins
  8:12.18 - Quinolones
  8:12.20 - Sulfonamides
  8:12.24 - Tetracyclines
    8:12.24.04 - Aminomethylcyclines
    8:12.24.08 - Fluorocyclines
    8:12.24.12 - Glycylcyclines
  8:12.28 - Antibacterials, Miscellaneous
    8:12.28.04 - Aminocyclitols*
    8:12.28.08 - Bacitracins*
    8:12.28.12 - Cyclic Lipopeptides
    8:12.28.16 - Glycopeptides
    8:12.28.20 - Lincomycins
    8:12.28.24 - Oxazolidinones
    8:12.28.26 - Pleuromutilins
    8:12.28.28 - Polymyxins
    8:12.28.30 - Rifamycins
    8:12.28.32 - Streptogramins
    8:12.28.92 - Other Miscellaneous Antibacterials
8:14 Antifungals
  8:14.04 - Allylamines
  8:14.08 - Azoles
  8:14.16 - Echinocandins
  8:14.20 - Triterpenoids
  8:14.28 - Polyenes
  8:14.32 - Pyrimidines
  8:14.92 - Antifungals, Miscellaneous
8:16 - Antimycobacterials
  8:16.04 - Antituberculosis Agents
  8:16.08 - Antileprosy Agents
  8:16.92 - Antimycobacterials, Miscellaneous*
8:18 - Antivirals
  8:18.04 - Adamantanes
  8:18.08 - Antiretrovirals
    8:18.08.04 - HIV Entry and Fusion Inhibitors
    8:18.08.08 - HIV Protease Inhibitors
    8:18.08.12 - HIV Integrase Inhibitors
    8:18.08.16 - HIV Nonnucleoside Reverse Transcriptase Inhibitors
    8:18.08.20 - HIV Nucleoside and Nucleotide Reverse Transcriptase Inhibitors
    8:18.08.24 - HIV Capsid Inhibitors
    8:18.08.92 - Antiretrovirals, Miscellaneous
  8:18.20 - Interferons
  8:18.24 - Monoclonal Antibodies
  8:18.28 - Neuraminidase Inhibitors
  8:18.30 - Endonuclease Inhibitors
  8:18.32 - Nucleosides and Nucleotides
  8:18.40 - HCV Antivirals
    8:18.40.04 - HCV Cyclophilin Inhibitors*
    8:18.40.08 - HCV Entry Inhibitors*
    8:18.40.16 - HCV Polymerase Inhibitors
    8:18.40.20 - HCV Protease Inhibitors
    8:18.40.24 - HCV Replication Complex Inhibitors
    8:18.40.92 - HCV Antivirals, Miscellaneous*
  8:18.44 - CMV Antivirals
  8:18.48 - Coronavirus (COVID-19)
  8:18.92 - Antivirals, Miscellaneous
8:30 - Antiprotozoals
  8:30.04 - Amebicides
  8:30.08 - Antimalarials
  8:30.12 - Antiprotozoals, Pneumocystis jirovecii Pneumonia
  8:30.16 - Antiprotozoals, Nitroimidazole-derivative
    8:30.16.04 - Nitroimidazole Derivatives, Trypanocidal
    8:30.16.08 - Nitroimidazole Derivatives, Anti-leishmanial
    8:30.16.92 - Nitroimidazole Derivatives, Miscellaneous
  8:30.20 - Antiprotozoals, Cryptosporidiosis
  8:30.92 - Antiprotozoals, Miscellaneous
8:36 - Urinary Anti-infectives
8:92 - Anti-infectives, Miscellaneous*

10:00 - Antineoplastic Agents

12:00 - Autonomic Drugs
12:02 - Smoking Cessation Agents
12:04 - Parasympathomimetic (Cholinergic) Agents
12:08 - Anticholinergic Agents
  12:08.04 - Antiparkinsonian Agents*
  12:08.08 - Antimuscarinics/Antispasmodics
12:12 - Sympathomimetic (Adrenergic) Agents
  12:12.04 - α-Adrenergic Agonists
  12:12.08 - β-Adrenergic Agonists
    12:12.08.04 - Nonselective β-Adrenergic Agonists
    12:12.08.08 - Selective β_1-Adrenergic Agonists
    12:12.08.12 - Selective β_2-Adrenergic Agonists
  12:12.12 - α- and β-Adrenergic Agonists
12:16 - Sympatholytic (Adrenergic Blocking) Agents
  12:16.04 - α-Adrenergic Blocking Agents
    12:16.04.04 - Nonselective α-Adrenergic Blocking Agents
    12:16.04.08 - Nonselective α_1-Adrenergic Blocking Agents*
    12:16.04.12 - Selective α_1-Adrenergic Blocking Agents
  12:16.08 - β-Adrenergic Blocking Agents*
    12:16.08.04 - Nonselective β-Adrenergic Blocking Agents*
    12:16.08.08 - Selective β-Adrenergic Blocking Agents*
12:20 - Skeletal Muscle Relaxants
  12:20.04 - Centrally Acting Skeletal Muscle Relaxants
  12:20.08 - Direct-acting Skeletal Muscle Relaxants
  12:20.10 - Indirect-acting Skeletal Muscle Relaxants
  12:20.12 - GABA-derivative Skeletal Muscle Relaxants
  12:20.20 - Neuromuscular Blocking Agents
    12:20.20.24 - Botulinum Toxins
  12:20.92 - Skeletal Muscle Relaxants, Miscellaneous*
12:92 - Autonomic Drugs, Miscellaneous*

16:00 - Blood Derivatives

* Category is currently not in use in the *AHFS® Pharmacologic-Therapeutic Classification©* system.

© Copyright 1959–2025, American Society of Health-System Pharmacists, Inc.

Table of Contents

4:00 ANTIHISTAMINE DRUGS

Antihistamines General Statement

4:00 • ANTIHISTAMINE DRUGS

■ Antihistamines, which inhibit the effects of histamine at H_1 receptors, have been classified as first generation (i.e., relatively sedating) or second generation (i.e., relatively nonsedating).

USES

Antihistamines are most often used to provide symptomatic relief of allergic symptoms caused by histamine release. The drugs are not curative and merely provide palliative therapy. Antihistamines are used only as adjunctive therapy to epinephrine and other standard measures in the treatment of anaphylactic reactions and laryngeal edema after the acute manifestations have been controlled. Individual patients vary in their response to antihistamines. A specific antihistamine that provides dramatic relief without adverse effects to one patient may produce intolerable adverse effects in another patient. Trial of various antihistamines may be necessary to determine which drug will provide relief while causing minimal adverse effects.

● Nasal Allergies and the Common Cold

Antihistamines are most beneficial in the management of nasal allergies. Seasonal allergic rhinitis (e.g., hay fever) and perennial (nonseasonal) allergic rhinitis are benefited more than perennial nonallergic (vasomotor) rhinitis. Orally administered antihistamines generally provide symptomatic relief of rhinorrhea, sneezing, oronasopharyngeal irritation or itching, lacrimation, and red, irritated, or itching eyes associated with the early response to histamine. The drugs generally are not effective in relieving symptoms of nasal obstruction, which are characteristic of the late allergic reaction, although limited data indicate that cetirizine and levocetirizine may relieve some symptoms of late allergic reactions. Antihistamines (e.g., azelastine) also may be administered intranasally for the symptomatic relief of seasonal allergic rhinitis. (See Uses in Azelastine 52:02.) In comparative studies, intranasal azelastine was more effective than placebo and at least as effective as oral antihistamines (e.g., cetirizine, terfenadine [no longer commercially available in the US]) or intranasal corticosteroids in relieving allergic rhinitis. However, unlike intranasal corticosteroids, azelastine does not appear to exhibit local histologic anti-inflammatory activity; therefore, beneficial effects on nasal obstruction appear to result principally from antihistaminic and/or other activity.

Chronic nasal congestion and headache caused by edema of the paranasal sinus mucosa are often refractory to antihistamine therapy. In the treatment of hay fever, antihistamines are more likely to be beneficial when therapy is initiated at the beginning of the hay fever season when pollen counts are low (e.g., before pollination begins) and if used regularly during the pollen season. Antihistamines are less likely to be effective when pollen counts are high, when pollen exposure is prolonged, and when nasal congestion is prominent.

Although antihistamines frequently are used for symptomatic relief in the common cold, evidence of effectiveness remains to be clearly established. Antihistamines cannot prevent, cure, or shorten the course of the common cold, but may provide some symptomatic relief. Conventional (prototypical, first generation) antihistamines (e.g., those with anticholinergic activity) are considered effective in relieving rhinorrhea and sneezing associated with the common cold, but evidence of efficacy in relieving oronasopharyngeal itching, lacrimation, or itching eyes associated with this condition currently is lacking. Nonsedating (second generation) antihistamines do not appear to be effective in relieving rhinorrhea, suggesting that histamine is not a principal mediator of this manifestation. The extent to which histamine contributes to other manifestations of the common cold currently is unclear, but pathogenesis of the full constellation of symptoms that constitute the common cold appears to be complex, involving a number of mediators and neurologic mechanisms.

Routine, prolonged administration of fixed combinations containing antihistamines, nasal decongestants, anticholinergics, analgesic-antipyretics, caffeine, antitussives, and/or expectorants has been questioned. Single-ingredient products generally are safer than combination products, while also facilitating dosage adjustment. There is no evidence that combinations containing 2 or more antihistamines are more effective than one antihistamine or that combinations of subtherapeutic doses of 2 or more antihistamines are more effective than therapeutic doses of one antihistamine. Oral antihistamine combinations containing an analgesic-antipyretic and/or nasal decongestant; an antitussive and nasal decongestant; an analgesic-antipyretic, antitussive, and nasal decongestant; or an antitussive may be rational if each ingredient has demonstrated clinical effectiveness and is present in therapeutic dosage. Selective use of such combinations can provide a convenient and rational approach for relief of concurrent symptoms (e.g., rhinorrhea, nasal congestion, cough), which often are present in allergic rhinitis and other conditions (e.g., common cold), by allowing the patient to use a single combination rather than multiple single-entity preparations. Combination preparations generally should be used only when symptoms amenable to each ingredient are present concurrently. Combinations containing an antihistamine and an expectorant, anticholinergic agent, or bronchodilator are *not* considered rational.

Although cough and cold preparations that contain antihistamines, nasal decongestants, cough suppressants, and/or expectorants commonly were used in pediatric patients younger than 2 years of age, systematic reviews of controlled trials have concluded that nonprescription (over-the-counter, OTC) cough and cold preparations are *no* more effective than placebo in reducing acute cough and other symptoms of upper respiratory tract infection in these patients. Furthermore, adverse events, including deaths, have been (and continue to be) reported in pediatric patients younger than 2 years of age receiving these preparations. (See Cautions: Pediatric Precautions.)

● Other Allergic Conditions

Antihistamines are often effective in the treatment of allergic dermatoses and other dermatoses associated with histamine release, but effectiveness varies with the causative agent and symptoms may return when the drug is stopped. Antihistamines have been used in the symptomatic treatment of chronic idiopathic urticaria; occasionally, patients who do not experience adequate relief with an antihistamine (H_1-receptor antagonist) alone may benefit from the addition of an H_2-receptor antagonist. However, in one study, the addition of an H_2-receptor antagonist did not provide a substantial increase in response (as determined by reduction in whealing). Some antihistamines also may symptomatically relieve pruritus accompanying atopic dermatitis, contact dermatitis, pruritus ani or vulvae, and insect bites. Some evidence suggests that first generation antihistamines such as hydroxyzine and diphenhydramine may be more effective than second generation antihistamines (e.g., terfenadine [no longer commercially available in the US], loratadine) for the relief of pruritus associated with certain allergic dermatoses (e.g., atopic dermatitis), but additional study is needed to elucidate further the relative efficacy of these drugs as antipruritics. Antihistamines also may be used in the treatment of dermatographism. Patients with dermatographism or other urticarial conditions who do not experience adequate relief with an antihistamine (H_1-receptor antagonist) alone may benefit from the addition of an H_2-receptor antagonist to enhance relief of pruritus and wheal formation.

Antihistamines are useful in the management of allergic conjunctivitis caused by foods or inhaled allergens. Allergic or hypersensitivity reactions to penicillin, streptomycin, sulfonamides, and other drugs may be amenable to antihistamine therapy. Pruritus and urticaria accompanying these conditions usually are temporarily relieved; edema is more resistant and serum sickness is not benefited.

Symptoms of mild transfusion reactions not caused by ABO incompatibility or pyrogens may be alleviated by antihistamines. The drugs should *not* be added to blood being transfused. Antihistamines may be administered prophylactically to patients with a history of transfusion reactions, but the drugs should not be given routinely to patients receiving blood. Antihistamines also may be useful to prevent sequelae following desensitization procedures and allergic reactions to radiographic contrast media. It must be kept in mind that prophylactic use of antihistamines may mask incipient signs of allergic reactions, and the patient's hypersensitivity may not be recognized until a serious reaction occurs.

Although epinephrine is the initial drug of choice for patients with anaphylactic or anaphylactoid reactions, antihistamines are useful in the ancillary treatment of pruritus, urticaria, angioedema, and bronchospasm associated with these reactions. Concurrent use of H_1- and H_2-receptor antagonists appears to reduce the adverse effects of histamine on the peripheral vasculature and myocardium during anaphylaxis.

● Asthma

Antihistamines may provide some benefit in certain asthmatic patients, but the drugs usually are not effective in treating bronchial asthma per se and should *not* be used in the treatment of severe acute asthma attacks. In addition, antihistamines are not included in the usual recommended regimens for the management of asthma, including long-term control of the disease. Antihistamine and decongestant combinations may provide symptomatic relief (e.g., of rhinitis) in patients with chronic rhinitis and persistent asthma, but the drugs have not been shown to have a protective effect on lower airways; other agents (e.g., inhaled corticosteroids) are for protective effects on lower airways. In general, patients with predictable seasonal asthma should receive long-term anti-inflammatory therapy (e.g., inhaled corticosteroids, mast-cell stabilizers), initiated prior to the anticipated onset of exposure to allergens and continued throughout the season. The drugs may be used with caution to treat hay fever or other airway disorder with a histamine-mediated component in patients with such disorders and asthma. Although some clinicians believe that the anticholinergic effects (e.g., reduction of nasal secretions) of some of these drugs may cause thickening of bronchial secretions resulting in further airway obstruction in asthmatics, especially those with status asthmaticus, most experts consider complete avoidance of currently available antihistamines in asthmatics unjustified. (See Cautions: Precautions and Contraindications.)

● Motion Sickness and Vertigo

Some antihistamines (e.g., dimenhydrinate, diphenhydramine, meclizine, promethazine) are useful for the prevention and treatment of nausea, vomiting, and/or vertigo associated with motion sickness and they are considered the drugs of choice for the management of this condition. For additional information on the use of antihistamines for the management of motion sickness, see Dimenhydrinate and see Meclizine Hydrochloride in 56:22.08. Dimenhydrinate and meclizine have also been used in the symptomatic treatment of vertigo associated with diseases affecting the vestibular system (e.g., labyrinthitis, Ménière's disease). Nonphenothiazine antihistamines are less effective than the phenothiazines in controlling nausea and vomiting not related to vestibular stimulation.

● Nausea and Vomiting of Pregnancy

Doxylamine succinate is used in fixed combination with pyridoxine hydrochloride for the management of nausea and vomiting of pregnancy in women who have not responded to conservative management. (See Uses in Doxylamine 4:04.)

● Chemotherapy-induced Nausea and Vomiting

Some antihistamines (e.g., diphenhydramine) may be useful as adjunctive antiemetic agents to prevent chemotherapy-induced nausea and vomiting†; however, the American Society of Clinical Oncology currently does not recommend that antihistamines be used alone as antiemetic agents in patients receiving chemotherapy.

● Insomnia

Some antihistamines, especially the ethanolamines such as diphenhydramine and doxylamine, are used for their sedative effects as nighttime sleep aids. The US Food and Drug Administration (FDA) states that diphenhydramine currently is the only antihistamine commercially available in the US that has been shown to be both safe and effective for *self-medication* as a nighttime sleep aid. In individuals who experience occasional sleeplessness or those who have difficulty falling asleep, diphenhydramine (administered as either the citrate or hydrochloride salt) is more effective than placebo in reducing sleep onset (i.e., time to fall asleep) and increasing the depth and quality of sleep. Although the safety and efficacy of doxylamine as a nighttime sleep aid have not been fully established, the FDA states that, pending further accumulation of data, doxylamine-containing nighttime sleep aids that have been approved for this use may continue to be marketed in the US. Some proprietary sleep aids also may continue to contain pyrilamine despite a lack of substantial evidence of safety and efficacy for use of this antihistamine as a nighttime sleep aid; however, many such preparations have been or are likely to be reformulated with other antihistamines (e.g., diphenhydramine).

● Other Systemic Uses

Some antihistamines such as diphenhydramine have been used effectively as antitussives. Diphenhydramine also may be useful in the management of tremor early in the course of parkinsonian syndrome and in the management of drug-induced extrapyramidal reactions.

● Topical and Other Local Uses

Diphenhydramine and tripelennamine (no longer commercially available in the US; extemporaneous formulation would be necessary) are used topically for temporary relief of pruritus and pain associated with various skin conditions including minor burns, sunburn, minor cuts or scrapes, insect bites, or minor skin irritations. The drugs may provide effective localized antipruritic activity when applied topically if pruritus and discomfort are histamine mediated; the weak local anesthetic action of the drugs also may contribute to the overall effect. However, many clinicians suggest that topical diphenhydramine not be used on large areas of the body or more often than directed, since increased percutaneous absorption of the drug may occur that can result in systemic adverse effects and toxicity. (See Acute Toxicity: Manifestations.) Topical diphenhydramine also should not be used for *self-medication* in the management of varicella (chickenpox) or measles without first consulting a clinician.

Some antihistamines also have been used for their topical or local anesthetic effects in ophthalmic, urologic, proctologic, gastroscopic, otolaryngologic, and dental procedures. However, topical use of antihistamines generally is discouraged because sensitivity reactions (e.g., sensitization, hypersensitivity) may result. (See Cautions: Sensitivity Reactions.) In addition, use of certain antihistamines (e.g., diphenhydramine) for local anesthesia via local infiltration also is discouraged because of the risk of local tissue necrosis. If the drugs are used topically as antipruritics, therapy generally should be short-term (i.e., for no longer than 7 days) because of the increasing risk of sensitivity reactions from prolonged or repeated use. Antihistamines are more effective, especially if pruritus is generalized, and are less likely to cause sensitivity reactions when the drugs are administered systemically rather than applied topically.

DOSAGE AND ADMINISTRATION

● Administration

Antihistamines usually are administered orally. Although some of these drugs may be given IV, IM, or subcutaneously, most antihistamines are not administered parenterally because they frequently cause local irritation. Some antihistamines also may be administered topically or intranasally. Topical use of antihistamines generally is discouraged since sensitivity reactions (e.g., sensitization, hypersensitivity) may result. In addition, topical preparations containing diphenhydramine should not be used more often than directed for any condition, applied on large areas of the body, or used concomitantly with other preparations containing diphenhydramine, including those used orally, since increased serum concentrations of diphenhydramine may occur that can result in CNS toxicity. (See Acute Toxicity: Manifestations.) Topical diphenhydramine also should not be used for *self-medication* in the management of varicella (chickenpox) or measles without first consulting a clinician.

● Dosage

Dosage of antihistamines should be individualized according to the patient's response and tolerance.

CAUTIONS

Adverse effects, which vary in incidence and severity with the individual drug, are caused by all antihistamines, although serious toxicity rarely occurs. Individual patients vary in their susceptibility to the adverse effects of these drugs, and such effects may disappear despite continued therapy. Geriatric patients may be particularly susceptible to dizziness, sedation, and hypotension. Most mild reactions may be relieved by a reduction in dosage or changing to another antihistamine.

Severe cardiovascular effects, including prolongation of the QT interval, arrhythmias, cardiac effects, hypotension, palpitations, syncope, dizziness and/or death have been reported in patients receiving astemizole (no longer commercially available in the US) or terfenadine (no longer commercially available in the US). These cardiotoxic effects usually were associated with higher than recommended dosages and/or increased plasma concentrations of the drugs and their active metabolites.

● CNS Effects

CNS depression is common with usual dosage of antihistamines, especially with the ethanolamine derivatives. Sedation, ranging from mild drowsiness to deep sleep, occurs most frequently; however, in the treatment of allergies, this effect may be therapeutically useful. Dizziness, lassitude, disturbed coordination, and muscular weakness may also occur. In some patients, the sedative effects disappear spontaneously after the antihistamine has been administered for 2–3 days. Individuals who perform potentially hazardous tasks requiring mental alertness or physical coordination (e.g., operating machinery, driving a motor vehicle) should be warned about possible drowsiness, dizziness, or weakness. Patients also should be warned to avoid consuming alcoholic beverages while taking antihistamines, since alcohol may potentiate these CNS effects. In addition, patients already receiving other CNS depressants (e.g., sedatives, tranquilizers) should be warned not to undertake *self-medication* with an antihistamine without first consulting their clinician. Patients using diphenhydramine or doxylamine for *self-medication* should be warned that the drugs may cause *marked* drowsiness. Acrivastine, desloratadine, fexofenadine, loratadine, and, possibly, cetirizine and levocetirizine appear to cause fewer adverse CNS effects, including effects on psychomotor performance and reactivity, than other currently available (first generation) antihistamines and therefore commonly have been referred to as relatively "nonsedating" or second generation antihistamines. However, while most second generation antihistamines do not appear to potentiate the effects of CNS depressants, including alcohol, acrivastine, cetirizine, and levocetirizine may potentiate such effects, although less prominently than first generation antihistamines.

Some patients, especially children, receiving antihistamines may experience paradoxical excitement characterized by restlessness, insomnia, tremors, euphoria, nervousness, delirium, palpitation, and even seizures. There have been several reports of toxic psychosis in children who received concomitant oral and topical diphenhydramine for relief of pruritus associated with varicella (chickenpox), poison ivy, or sunburn. (See Acute Toxicity: Manifestations.) In addition, central anticholinergic syndrome characterized by hallucinations, agitation, and confusion occurred in several children receiving usual or excessive dosages of cyproheptadine. Patients should be warned that phenindamine may be particularly likely to occasionally cause insomnia and nervousness in some individuals. Antihistamines also may precipitate epileptiform seizures in patients with focal lesions of the cerebral cortex, and the drugs should be administered with caution in patients with seizure disorders.

An acute dystonic reaction, which consisted of trismus, difficulty in swallowing, dysarthria, rigidity, and motor incoordination, and was accompanied by mental confusion and tremors, was reported in at least 1 patient receiving IV diphenhydramine.

● GI and Hepatic Effects

Adverse GI effects of antihistamines include epigastric distress, anorexia, nausea, vomiting, diarrhea, or constipation. GI symptoms may be decreased by administering the drug with meals or with milk. Cholestasis, hepatitis, hepatic failure, hepatic function abnormality, and jaundice have been reported rarely in patients receiving antihistamines (e.g., cyproheptadine, terfenadine).

● Sensitivity Reactions

Antihistamines can cause sensitivity reactions (e.g., sensitization, hypersensitivity) following topical application or systemic administration, but such reactions are more likely following topical use of the drugs, especially ethylenediamine derivatives. Antihistamines can act as haptens and cause IgE-mediated (type I) hypersensitivity reactions or T cell-mediated (type IV) sensitization reactions. Type I reactions appear to occur rarely, but type IV reactions occur more frequently, particularly following topical application of the drugs. Sensitization following topical use of antihistamines results in allergic contact dermatitis, which may be manifested as eczema, pruritus, and inflammation, at the site of application. Once local sensitization to an antihistamine occurs, the dermatitis can recur following subsequent topical or systemic exposure to the drug or a chemically related drug (including local anesthetics). Photosensitivity (principally photoallergic dermatitis) reactions, which may be manifested as eczema, pruritus, papular rash, and erythema on exposed skin, also have occurred following topical or systemic administration of antihistamines, and cross-sensitivity with chemically related drugs can occur.

● Cardiovascular Effects

Although antihistamines exhibit anticholinergic and local anesthetic effects, including quinidine-like effects on cardiac conduction, and certain drugs have been investigated for potential antiarrhythmic activity, adverse cardiovascular effects are uncommon and usually limited to overdosage situations. When adverse cardiac effects have occurred, they generally were characteristic anticholinergic and/or local anesthetic (quinidine-like) effects such as tachycardia, palpitation, ECG changes (e.g., widened QRS), and arrhythmias (e.g., extrasystole, heart block). Other cardiovascular effects reported with antihistamines include hypotension and hypertension; in some cases, hypotension may result in part from α-adrenergic blocking activity of the antihistamine.

Serious cardiac effects, including prolongation of the QT interval corrected for rate (QT_c), ST-U abnormalities, arrhythmias (e.g., ventricular tachycardia, atypical ventricular tachycardia [torsades de pointes], ventricular fibrillation, heart block), arrest, hypotension, palpitations, syncope, dizziness, and/or death (secondary to ventricular tachyarrhythmia), have been reported rarely in patients receiving terfenadine or astemizole. Astemizole and terfenadine are no longer commercially available in the US. These cardiotoxic effects usually were associated with higher than recommended dosages and/or increased plasma concentrations of the drugs and their active metabolites, although serious cardiac effects also have been reported occasionally at usual astemizole or terfenadine dosages. While patients with impaired liver function and, possibly, geriatric patients may have been at particular risk of accumulation of these antihistamines and associated cardiotoxic effects, these effects have been reported rarely in apparently healthy individuals with no associated risk factors.

Patients who were receiving concomitant therapy with an azole (including imidazole derivative [e.g., ketoconazole] and triazole derivative [e.g., itraconazole]) antifungal, a macrolide (e.g., clarithromycin, erythromycin, troleandomycin) anti-infective, mibefradil (no longer commercially available in the US), quinine, or grapefruit juice also appeared to be at substantial risk of such toxicity, probably secondary to interference with metabolism of the antihistamine. In addition, concomitant use of terfenadine or astemizole with most human immunodeficiency virus (HIV) protease inhibitors, quinupristin and dalfopristin, zileuton, or serotonin-reuptake inhibitors has not been recommended since HIV protease inhibitors, quinupristin and dalfopristin, zileuton, and serotonin-reuptake inhibitors have been associated with increased plasma concentrations of these antihistamines and potentially serious and/or life-threatening adverse effects could have occurred as a result of these drugs' effects on the metabolism of astemizole or terfenadine.

The potential for similar drug interactions and cardiac effects with loratadine remains to be elucidated more fully. However, acrivastine and loratadine have not been shown to prolong the QT interval when administered alone. Prolongation of the QT_c interval has been reported in a limited number of healthy adults receiving desloratadine dosages of 45 mg daily (9 times the recommended daily dosage) for 10 days; however, the manufacturer states that no clinically relevant adverse events were reported.

The manufacturer of cetirizine states that no clinically important prolongation of the QT_c interval has been reported in healthy adult men receiving cetirizine during controlled clinical studies. The manufacturer of levocetirizine (the *R* enantiomer of cetirizine) states that no clinically important prolongation of the QT_c interval has been reported following administration of a single dose of levocetirizine. The effects of multiple-dose administration are not known, but levocetirizine is not expected to have clinically important effects on the QT_c interval based on results of QT_c studies with cetirizine and the lack of reports of QT_c interval prolongation during postmarketing surveillance of that drug. The manufacturer of cetirizine also states that concomitant administration of the antihistamine with drugs known to inhibit cytochrome P-450 microsomal enzymes (e.g., azithromycin, erythromycin, ketoconazole) has not been associated with clinically important changes in ECG parameters (e.g., QT_c intervals) and that no clinically important interactions have been reported in patients receiving cetirizine concomitantly with azithromycin, erythromycin, or ketoconazole.

The manufacturer of fexofenadine states that no statistically significant mean increases in the QT_c interval have been reported in healthy adults or patients with seasonal allergic rhinitis receiving fexofenadine hydrochloride dosages up to 400 mg twice daily (for 6 days) or 60–240 mg twice daily (for 2 weeks), respectively, during controlled clinical studies.

The mechanism of the cardiotoxic effects of astemizole and terfenadine has not been fully understood, and it appeared to be contrary to what would have been expected from studies on cardiac histamine H₁-receptors; the possibility that H₃-receptors (mediating a regulatory feedback mechanism) may have been involved had been suggested. Limited evidence from animal models using terfenadine has suggested that the cardiotoxic effects of the drug may have resulted at least in part from blockade of the potassium channel involved in repolarization of cardiac cells (i.e., blockade of the delayed rectifier potassium current I_K). Unlike other antihistamines, anticholinergic and/or local anesthetic effects appeared to be unlikely causes of the cardiac effects of these 2 second generation (relatively "nonsedating") antihistamines.

It has been recommended that usual dosages of terfenadine (i.e., 60 mg twice daily) and astemizole (i.e., 10 mg daily) *not* be exceeded because of the risk of potentially life-threatening cardiotoxic effects. Because of this risk, patients were advised *not* to temporarily increase (e.g., double) the prescribed dosage in an attempt to accelerate or improve symptomatic relief provided by these drugs.

Patients with hepatic impairment, geriatric patients, those receiving drugs or who had underlying conditions that might have prolonged the QT interval, and those who were receiving drugs that could have produced electrolyte abnormalities such as hypokalemia or hypomagnesemia may have been at increased risk of cardiac arrhythmias during terfenadine or astemizole therapy. Therefore, administration of these antihistamines was *not* recommended in such patients. Terfenadine or astemizole also should *not* have been used in patients receiving a macrolide (e.g., clarithromycin, erythromycin, troleandomycin) anti-infective, an azole antifungal (including imidazole [e.g., itraconazole] and triazole [e.g., itraconazole] derivatives), or mibefradil; in addition, use of these antihistamines in patients receiving any other drug (e.g., quinine, most HIV protease inhibitors, serotonin-reuptake inhibitors, zileuton) that potentially could inhibit their metabolism was *not* recommended. It also has been recommended that astemizole or terfenadine not be taken with grapefruit juice. Concomitant administration of astemizole with therapeutic doses of quinine was contraindicated.

● *Other Adverse Effects*

Adverse anticholinergic effects of antihistamines include dryness of mouth, nose, and throat; dysuria; urinary retention; impotence; vertigo; visual disturbances; blurred vision; diplopia; tinnitus; acute labyrinthitis; insomnia; tremors; nervousness; irritability; and facial dyskinesia. Tightness of the chest, thickening of bronchial secretions, wheezing, nasal stuffiness, sweating, chills, early menses, toxic psychosis, headache, faintness, and paresthesia have occurred.

Rarely, agranulocytosis, hemolytic anemia, leukopenia, thrombocytopenia, and pancytopenia have been reported in patients receiving some antihistamines. Increased appetite and/or weight gain also occurred in patients receiving antihistamines (cyproheptadine).

● *Precautions and Contraindications*

Antihistamines having substantial anticholinergic activity (usually conventional [prototypical, first generation] including ethanolamines) should be administered with caution, if at all, in patients with angle-closure glaucoma, prostatic hypertrophy (which may result in difficulty in urination), stenosing peptic ulcer, pyloroduodenal obstruction, or bladder neck obstruction. Because it was suggested that the anticholinergic effect of antihistamines might reduce the volume and cause thickening of bronchial secretions and thus result in obstruction of respiratory passages, it had been recommended that the drugs be used with caution and only under the direction of a clinician in patients with asthma or chronic obstructive pulmonary disease if clearance of bronchial secretions was a problem. While some clinicians and manufacturers continue to warn against use of the drugs in patients with asthma because of potential effects of anticholinergic activity on the volume and fluidity of bronchial secretions, most experts and clinicians believe that there currently is little, if any, direct evidence of antihistamine-induced exacerbation of asthma secondary to bronchial drying nor substantiation for avoiding use of currently available antihistamines in asthmatic patients. Antihistamines usually should not be used, unless under the direction of a clinician, in patients who have a breathing problem (e.g., emphysema, chronic bronchitis), and these drugs generally should not be used in asthmatics who previously experienced a serious antihistamine-induced adverse bronchopulmonary effect. In addition, antihistamines should be used with caution in patients with increased intraocular pressure, hyperthyroidism, cardiovascular disease, or hypertension. The drugs are contraindicated in patients with asthmatic attacks. For *self-medication*, cough preparations containing an antihistamine (e.g., diphenhydramine) should not be used for persistent or chronic cough or breathing problems such as those occurring with smoking, asthma, chronic bronchitis, or emphysema, or for cough accompanied by excessive phlegm, unless directed by a clinician. A persistent cough may be indicative of a serious condition. If cough persists for more than one week, is recurrent, or is accompanied by fever, rash, or persistent headache, a clinician should be consulted.

Patients should be advised that CNS depression (e.g., drowsiness) is common with first generation antihistamines, even at usual dosages and particularly with ethanolamine derivatives. (See Cautions: CNS Effects.) In addition, patients should be warned that additive CNS depression may occur when first generation antihistamines or possibly, cetirizine or levocetirizine is administered concomitantly with other CNS depressants, including alcohol. (See Drug Interactions:

CNS Depressants.) Patients receiving acrivastine, a second generation antihistamine, also should be warned of the possibility of such effects.

Diphenhydramine toxicity (e.g., dilated pupils, facial flushing, hallucinations, ataxic gait, urinary retention) has been reported in pediatric patients following topical application of diphenhydramine to large areas of the body (often areas with broken skin) or following concomitant use of topical and oral preparations containing diphenhydramine. (See Acute Toxicity: Manifestations.) Therefore, the US Food and Drug Administration (FDA) and many clinicians warn that oral diphenhydramine should *not* be used concomitantly with any other preparations containing the drug, including those used topically. (See Cautions, in Diphenhydramine 4:04.) In addition, topical preparations containing diphenhydramine should not be used more often than directed for any condition, applied on large areas of the body, or used concomitantly with other preparations containing diphenhydramine, including those used orally, since increased serum concentrations of diphenhydramine may occur that can result in CNS toxicity. (See Acute Toxicity: Manifestations.) Patients should be advised to consult a clinician prior to use of topical diphenhydramine for the management of varicella (chickenpox) or measles.

Although diphenhydramine appears to have low abuse potential, several children, adolescents, and at least one adult with chronic hematologic and antineoplastic diseases have exhibited drug-seeking behavior and anticholinergic effects after chronic intermittent rapid IV administration of the drug.

While astemizole and terfenadine were commercially available in the US, individuals receiving these second generation antihistamines were warned that patients with hepatic impairment (e.g., cirrhosis, hepatitis); geriatric patients; those who were concomitantly receiving an azole-derivative anti-infective (e.g., fluconazole, itraconazole, ketoconazole, metronidazole, miconazole), a macrolide antibiotic (e.g., clarithromycin, erythromycin, troleandomycin), mibefradil (no longer commercially available in the US), or other potent inhibitors of the cytochrome P-450 isoenzyme (CYP3A) (including most HIV protease inhibitors, quinupristin and dalfopristin, zileuton, or serotonin-reuptake inhibitors) responsible for the metabolism of astemizole or terfenadine (see Drug Interactions); those who were having underlying conditions that might prolong the QT interval corrected for rate (QT$_c$) (e.g., hypokalemia, hypomagnesemia, bradycardia, congenital QT syndrome); those who were receiving drugs that might prolong the QT$_c$ interval (e.g., certain antiarrhythmic agents, bepridil hydrochloride, certain psychotropic agents, probucol [no longer commercially available in the US], cisapride, sparfloxacin, pentamidine); or those who were receiving drugs (e.g., diuretics) that could produce electrolyte abnormalities, such as hypokalemia or hypomagnesemia, may have experienced prolongation of the QT$_c$ interval and may have been at increased risk of cardiac arrhythmias (e.g., ventricular tachycardia, atypical ventricular tachycardia [torsades de pointes], ventricular fibrillation) when they were receiving recommended dosages of astemizole or terfenadine. Therefore, administration of astemizole or terfenadine was not recommended in such patients.

In addition, astemizole or terfenadine was contraindicated in patients with disease states (e.g., severe hepatic impairment) or receiving concomitant therapy (e.g., itraconazole, ketoconazole, clarithromycin, erythromycin, troleandomycin, mibefradil) known to impair metabolism of the antihistamine. Astemizole also was contraindicated in patients receiving concomitant therapy with quinine.

For additional cautions, contraindications, and drug interactions with the phenothiazine derivatives, see the Phenothiazines General Statement 28:16.08.24.

● *Pediatric Precautions*

Antihistamines should not be administered to premature or full-term neonates. Young children may be more susceptible than adults to the toxic effects of antihistamines. (See Acute Toxicity.) Adults responsible for the supervision of a child receiving an antihistamine should be warned that children may be at increased risk for experiencing CNS stimulant effects with antihistamines. (See Cautions: CNS Effects.) Although the relationship and possible mechanism(s) have not been elucidated, respiratory depression, sleep apnea, and sudden infant death syndrome (SIDS) have occurred in a number of infants and young children who were receiving usual dosages of phenothiazine-derivative antihistamines (i.e., promethazine, trimeprazine [no longer commercially available in the US]). (See Cautions: Pediatric Precautions, in Promethazine 4:04.) In addition, death has been reported in children younger than 2 years of age receiving carbinoxamine-containing preparations or cough and cold preparations containing an antihistamine with or without other agents (e.g., cough suppressants, expectorants, nasal decongestants). (See Uses: Regulations Governing Carbinoxamine-containing

Preparations, in Carbinoxamine Maleate 4:04 and also see Cautions: Pediatric Precautions, in Pseudoephedrine Hydrochloride 12:12.12.)

In a report published by the US Centers for Disease Control and Prevention (CDC), cough and cold preparations containing carbinoxamine, pseudoephedrine, acetaminophen, and/or dextromethorphan were determined by medical examiners or coroners to be the underlying cause of death in 3 infants 6 months of age or younger during 2005. The actual cause of death might have been overdosage of one drug, interaction of different drugs, an underlying medical condition, or a combination of drugs and underlying medical conditions. In addition, an estimated 1519 children younger than 2 years of age were treated in emergency departments in the US during 2004–2005 for adverse events, including overdoses, associated with cold and cough preparations.

The dosages at which cold and cough preparations can cause illness or death in pediatric patients younger than 2 years of age are not known, and there are no specific dosage recommendations (i.e., approved by the US Food and Drug Administration [FDA]) for the symptomatic treatment of cold and cough for patients in this age group. Because of the absence of dosage recommendations, limited published evidence of effectiveness, and risks for toxicity (including fatal overdosage). FDA stated that nonprescription cough and cold preparations should not be used in children younger than 2 years of age; the agency continues to assess safety and efficacy of these preparations in older children. Meanwhile, because children 2–3 years of age also are at increased risk of overdosage and toxicity, some manufacturers of oral nonprescription cough and cold preparations agreed to voluntarily revise the product labeling to state that such preparations should not be used in children younger than 4 years of age. FDA recommends that parents and caregivers adhere to the dosage instructions and warnings on the product labeling that accompanies the preparation if administering to children and consult with their clinician about any concerns. Clinicians should ask caregivers about use of nonprescription cough and cold preparations to avoid overdosage.

Because antihistamines may cause drowsiness that can be potentiated by other CNS depressants (e.g., sedatives, tranquilizers), an antihistamine should be used in children receiving one of these drugs only under the direction of a clinician. Antihistamines should not be used in children who have a breathing problem (e.g., chronic bronchitis) or glaucoma unless otherwise directed by a clinician. It also has been recommended that antihistamines not be used in children with asthma, liver disease, or seizure disorder unless under the direction of a clinician. Overdosage of doxylamine has been reported in children. Manifestations of doxylamine overdosage in children have included coma, generalized tonic-clonic (grand mal) seizures, cardiorespiratory arrest, and death. Children appear to be at high risk for cardiorespiratory arrest secondary to doxylamine overdosage. For additional information, see the individual monographs in 4:00.

Acute toxicity has been reported in pediatric patients following topical application of diphenhydramine to large areas of the body (often areas with broken skin) or following concomitant use of topical and oral preparations containing diphenhydramine. (See Cautions: Precautions and Contraindications, and also see Acute Toxicity.)

While it is desirable to avoid the use of alcohol-containing antihistamine preparations in children because of potential toxicity, inclusion of alcohol in some preparations may be a pharmaceutical necessity (e.g., as a solvent) and therefore complete avoidance of such preparations may not be possible. According to a final rule issued in 1995 by FDA, over-the-counter (OTC) oral preparations intended for use in children younger than 6 years of age, children 6–11 years of age, or children 12 years of age and older may contain up to 0.5, 5, or 10% alcohol, respectively.

● Pregnancy, Fertility, and Lactation

Pregnancy

Antihistamines should not be used in women who are or may become pregnant unless the potential benefits justify the possible risks to the fetus. Some manufacturers caution that antihistamines should not be used during the third trimester because of the risk of severe reactions (e.g., seizures) to the drugs in neonates and premature infants. For additional information, see the individual monographs in 4:00.

Doxylamine succinate in fixed combination with pyridoxine hydrochloride is intended for use in the management of nausea and vomiting of pregnancy. Historically, there was considerable controversy regarding the teratogenic potential, if any, of doxylamine succinate; however, after evaluating extensive data and information concerning the possible teratogenicity of the drug, FDA concluded that it is unlikely that doxylamine succinate is teratogenic. In addition, FDA states that the removal of products containing doxylamine succinate that previously were

commercially available for the management of nausea and vomiting of pregnancy was not for reasons of safety or effectiveness. Numerous epidemiologic studies (including cohort studies, case-control studies, and meta-analyses) have been performed to investigate possible teratogenic effects of doxylamine succinate in fixed combination with pyridoxine hydrochloride in pregnant women and have found no evidence of an increased risk of fetal malformations.

Lactation

Most manufacturers state that antihistamines should not be administered to nursing women, since the drugs may inhibit lactation and small amounts appear to be distributed into milk. Adverse effects (e.g., excitement, irritability, and sedation) have been reported in infants presumably exposed to antihistamines (e.g., doxylamine) through human milk. Infants with apnea or other respiratory syndromes may be particularly vulnerable to the sedative effects of antihistamines (e.g., doxylamine).

Because of the potential for serious adverse reactions (e.g., CNS effects) to antihistamines in nursing infants, a decision should be made whether to discontinue nursing or antihistamines, taking into account the importance of the drugs to the woman. The manufacturer of doxylamine in fixed combination with pyridoxine states that this preparation should *not* be used in nursing women.

DRUG INTERACTIONS

● CNS Depressants

Additive CNS depression may occur when antihistamines are administered concomitantly with other CNS depressants including barbiturates, tranquilizers, and alcohol. If antihistamines are used concomitantly with other depressant drugs, caution should be used to avoid overdosage. Patients should be advised to avoid alcoholic beverages during antihistamine therapy. Patients already receiving another CNS depressant (e.g., sedatives, tranquilizers) should not undertake *self-medication* with an antihistamine without first consulting a physician. Unlike first generation antihistamines, most second generation antihistamines (e.g., astemizole [no longer commercially available in the US], loratadine, terfenadine [no longer commercially available in the US]) do not appear to potentiate the sedative effects of CNS depressants; however, acrivastine, cetirizine, and levocetirizine, which also have been classified as second generation antihistamines, may potentiate such effects, although less prominently than first generation antihistamines.

It also should be considered that monoamine oxidase (MAO) inhibitors may prolong and intensify some anticholinergic effects (e.g., dryness) of antihistamines. The manufacturer of doxylamine in fixed combination with pyridoxine hydrochloride states that the drug is contraindicated in patients receiving MAO inhibitors.

● Epinephrine

Phenothiazine-type antihistamines (e.g., methdilazine [no longer commercially available in the US], promethazine, trimeprazine [no longer commercially available in the US]) may block and reverse the vasopressor effect of epinephrine. If patients receiving phenothiazines require a vasopressor agent, norepinephrine or phenylephrine should be used; *epinephrine should not be used.*

● Drugs and Foods Affecting Hepatic Microsomal Enzymes

Concomitant administration of astemizole or terfenadine with drugs that can inhibit the metabolism of these antihistamines has resulted in accumulation of potentially cardiotoxic concentrations of astemizole or terfenadine and/or their active metabolites. (See Cautions: Cardiovascular Effects.) Both human and animal data have indicated that associated cardiotoxic effects resulted principally from accumulation of unchanged astemizole (and its main metabolite desmethylastemizole) or unchanged terfenadine.

Serious, potentially life-threatening cardiac effects have occurred when astemizole or terfenadine was used concomitantly with certain azole antifungal (including imidazole derivative [e.g., ketoconazole] and triazole derivative [e.g., itraconazole]) or macrolide (e.g., clarithromycin, erythromycin, troleandomycin) anti-infectives, mibefradil (no longer commercially available in the US), or quinine sulfate (a single dose of 430 mg), probably secondary to inhibition of metabolism of the antihistamine by these drugs. Therefore, while astemizole or terfenadine was commercially available in the US, concomitant therapy with these or other known inhibitors of astemizole or terfenadine metabolism was contraindicated. No clinically adverse effects or changes in the QT_c intervals were reported after concomitant administration of erythromycin or ketoconazole with fexofenadine, the active metabolite of terfenadine. The increased safety profile of fexofenadine compared with the parent drug, terfenadine, may result from the lack of fexofenadine-induced cardiotoxicity in addition to only minimal metabolism of fexofenadine in the liver by the cytochrome P-450 microsomal enzyme system.

Concomitant use of terfenadine or astemizole with other chemically related azole-derivative anti-infective (e.g., fluconazole, miconazole, metronidazole), most human immunodeficiency virus (HIV) protease inhibitors, quinupristin and dalfopristin, zileuton, or serotonin-reuptake inhibitors has not been recommended since these drugs may have increased plasma concentrations of terfenadine and/or astemizole and potentially serious and/or life-threatening adverse effects could have occurred.

Grapefruit juice also may have inhibited metabolism of terfenadine. Increased oral bioavailability of unchanged terfenadine observed with concomitant administration of the drug and grapefruit juice has been associated with prolongation of the QT interval averaging 3.3% (range: −1.6 to 9.5%); mean QT interval corrected for rate (QT_c) increased by 4–14 msec compared with administration of terfenadine with water. Therefore, it has been recommended that astemizole or terfenadine not be taken concomitantly with grapefruit juice.

Ketoconazole and Other Azole Antifungal Agents

Prolongation of the QT interval and QT interval corrected for rate (QT_c) and, rarely, serious cardiovascular effects, including arrhythmias (e.g., ventricular tachycardia, atypical ventricular tachycardia [torsades de pointes, ventricular fibrillation]), cardiac arrest, palpitations, hypotension, dizziness, syncope, and death, have been reported in patients receiving recommended dosages of astemizole or terfenadine concomitantly with ketoconazole. Ketoconazole has markedly inhibited the metabolism of astemizole or terfenadine, probably via inhibition of the cytochrome P-450 microsomal enzyme system, which resulted in increased plasma concentrations of unchanged astemizole (and its principal metabolite desmethylastemizole) or unchanged terfenadine; clearance of the active carboxylic acid metabolite of terfenadine also may have been reduced. Increased plasma concentrations of unchanged astemizole (and its principal metabolite desmethylastemizole) or unchanged terfenadine has been associated with prolongation of the QT and QT_c intervals. Similar alterations in astemizole or terfenadine pharmacokinetics and adverse cardiac effects (prolongation of the QT_c interval, cardiac arrest, and ventricular arrhythmias [e.g., torsades de pointes]) have been reported in patients receiving the antihistamine concomitantly with itraconazole. Therefore, while commercially available in the US, astemizole and terfenadine were contraindicated in patients receiving ketoconazole or itraconazole. In addition, it has been recommended that astemizole and terfenadine also not be used in patients receiving drugs that are structurally related to these antifungals (e.g., triazoles such as fluconazole, imidazoles such as miconazole, nitroimidazoles such as metronidazole).

Increased plasma concentrations of loratadine and its active metabolite desloratadine (descarboethoxyloratadine) also have been reported in controlled clinical studies in healthy men receiving 10 mg of loratadine once daily concomitantly with ketoconazole dosages of 200 mg every 12 hours. In these studies, area under the plasma concentration-time curve (AUC) of loratadine increased by 307% following concomitant administration with ketoconazole while AUC of desloratadine increased by 73% following concomitant administration with ketoconazole. However, no clinically important changes, as measured by ECG and laboratory evaluations, vital signs, and adverse effects, were reported after concomitant administration of ketoconazole with loratadine. In addition, no changes in QT_c intervals, sedation, or syncope were reported in these individuals. Plasma concentrations of ketoconazole appeared to be unchanged in individuals receiving loratadine concomitantly. In addition, increased plasma concentrations of loratadine (AUC increased by 180%) and desloratadine (AUC increased by 56%) have been reported in a limited number of individuals receiving a single 20-mg dose of loratadine concomitantly with a ketoconazole dosage of 200 mg twice daily. However, no changes in QT_c intervals were reported 2, 6, and 24 hours after concomitant administration of the drugs. Adverse effects were similar in individuals receiving loratadine alone compared with those receiving loratadine concomitantly with ketoconazole.

Increased plasma concentrations of desloratadine and 3-hydroxydesloratadine have been reported in a controlled clinical study in healthy individuals receiving 7.5 mg of desloratadine once daily concomitantly with ketoconazole dosages of 200 mg every 12 hours for 10 days. In this study, AUC of desloratadine or 3-hydroxydesloratadine increased by 39 or 72%, respectively, while peak plasma concentrations increased by 45 or 43%, respectively, following concomitant administration with ketoconazole. However, no clinically important changes, as measured by ECG and laboratory evaluations, vital signs, and adverse effects, were reported after concomitant administration of ketoconazole with desloratadine.

The manufacturer of cetirizine states that no clinically important drug interactions have been reported in patients receiving cetirizine concomitantly with ketoconazole.

Increased plasma concentrations of fexofenadine have been reported in 2 studies in healthy individuals receiving 120 mg of fexofenadine twice daily concomitantly with ketoconazole 400 mg once daily. In these studies, AUC of fexofenadine increased by 164% following concomitant administration with ketoconazole while peak plasma concentrations of fexofenadine increased by 135%. However, no clinically important adverse effects or changes in the QT_c intervals were reported after concomitant administration of ketoconazole with fexofenadine.

Macrolides

Erythromycin and clarithromycin have altered the metabolism of astemizole or terfenadine. In some individuals, concomitant administration of erythromycin with astemizole or terfenadine has resulted in increased plasma concentrations of unchanged astemizole (and its principal metabolite desmethylastemizole) or unchanged terfenadine (and its active carboxylic metabolite fexofenadine). Prolongation of the QT_c, ST-U abnormalities, and ventricular tachycardia, including torsades de pointes, have been reported in some patients receiving astemizole or terfenadine concomitantly with erythromycin or the structurally related macrolides clarithromycin, troleandomycin, or josamycin. Cardiac arrest and death have occurred in patients receiving erythromycin concomitantly with astemizole or terfenadine. Therefore, while commercially available in the US, astemizole or terfenadine was contraindicated in patients receiving clarithromycin, erythromycin, or troleandomycin.

Limited data have suggested that azithromycin and dirithromycin did not appear to alter the metabolism of terfenadine.

Increased plasma concentrations of loratadine and its active metabolite desloratadine have been reported in controlled clinical studies in healthy men receiving 10 mg of loratadine once daily concomitantly with erythromycin dosages of 500 mg every 8 hours for 10 days. In these studies, AUC of loratadine increased by 40% following concomitant administration with erythromycin, while AUC of desloratadine increased by 46%. However, no clinically important changes, as measured by ECG and laboratory evaluations, vital signs, and adverse effects, were reported after concomitant administration of erythromycin with loratadine. In addition, no changes in QT_c intervals, sedation, or syncope were reported in these individuals. Although the clinical importance has not been established, decreased plasma concentrations of erythromycin (AUC decreased by 15–18%) have been reported in these patients receiving loratadine concomitantly.

Increased plasma concentrations of loratadine and desloratadine also have been reported in a controlled drug interaction study in healthy men receiving 10 mg of loratadine every 24 hours concomitantly with clarithromycin dosages of 500 mg every 12 hours for 10 days. In this study, peak steady-state plasma concentrations and AUC of loratadine increased by 36 and 76%, respectively, following concomitant administration with clarithromycin for 10 days while peak steady-state plasma concentrations and AUC of desloratadine increased by 69 and 49%, respectively, compared with administration of loratadine alone. Although mean maximum QT_c interval was modestly increased (by less than 3% and not exceeding 439 msec) when loratadine was administered concomitantly with clarithromycin, such increase was similar to that observed when loratadine was administered alone and probably was not clinically important. The pharmacokinetics of clarithromycin were not affected by concomitant loratadine.

Increased plasma concentrations of desloratadine and 3-hydroxydesloratadine have been reported in a controlled clinical study in healthy individuals receiving 7.5 mg of desloratadine once daily concomitantly with erythromycin dosages of 500 mg every 8 hours for 10 days. In this study, AUC of desloratadine or 3-hydroxydesloratadine increased by 14 or 40%, respectively, while peak plasma concentrations increased by 24 or 43%, respectively, following concomitant administration with erythromycin. In another study in healthy individuals receiving 5 mg of desloratadine once daily concomitantly with azithromycin (500 mg followed by 250 mg once daily for 4 days), AUC of desloratadine or 3-hydroxydesloratadine increased by 5 or 4%, respectively, while peak plasma concentrations increased by 15%. However, no clinically important changes, as measured by ECG and laboratory evaluations, vital signs, and adverse effects, were reported after concomitant administration of erythromycin or azithromycin with desloratadine.

The manufacturer of cetirizine states that no clinically important drug interactions have been reported in patients receiving cetirizine concomitantly with azithromycin or erythromycin.

Increased plasma concentrations of fexofenadine have been reported in 2 studies in healthy individuals receiving 120 mg of fexofenadine twice daily concomitantly with erythromycin dosages of 500 mg every 8 hours. In these studies, AUC of fexofenadine increased by 109% following concomitant administration with erythromycin, while peak plasma concentrations of fexofenadine increased by 82%. However, no clinically important adverse effects or changes in the QT$_c$ intervals were reported after concomitant administration of erythromycin with fexofenadine.

HIV Protease Inhibitors

In vitro, ritonavir has been shown to inhibit the metabolism of terfenadine, but the clinical importance of this in vitro finding is not known. Several manufacturers of HIV protease inhibitors and some clinicians state that specific in vivo pharmacokinetic drug interaction studies between these antihistamines and HIV protease inhibitors currently are not available. Concomitant use of astemizole or terfenadine with HIV protease inhibitors (e.g., indinavir, nelfinavir, ritonavir, saquinavir) has not been recommended, because of the theoretical risk that the HIV protease inhibitor could produce substantially increased plasma concentrations of unchanged astemizole or terfenadine resulting in potentially serious and/or life-threatening adverse effects. The manufacturers of indinavir and ritonavir state that concomitant use of either drug with astemizole or terfenadine is contraindicated because such use may precipitate potentially life-threatening adverse effects.

Serotonin-reuptake Inhibitors

In vitro, fluvoxamine, nefazodone, or sertraline and/or their metabolites have been shown to inhibit metabolism of terfenadine probably secondary to inhibition of the cytochrome P-450 (CYP34A) enzyme system, but the clinical importance of these in vitro findings is not known. Concomitant administration of astemizole or terfenadine and any of the serotonin-reuptake inhibitors (i.e., fluoxetine, fluvoxamine, nefazodone, paroxetine, sertraline) has not been recommended since substantially increased plasma concentrations of unchanged astemizole or terfenadine could occur resulting in an increased risk of serious adverse cardiac effects. The manufacturer of fluvoxamine and some clinicians state that concomitant use of the antidepressant with terfenadine or astemizole is contraindicated. However, at least one manufacturer (i.e., of sertraline) states that in vivo drug interaction studies with sertraline and terfenadine have failed to confirm any important alteration in plasma terfenadine concentrations by the antidepressant and that a clinically important interaction is unlikely.

Increased plasma concentrations of desloratadine and 3-hydroxydesloratadine have been reported in a controlled clinical study in healthy individuals who were pretreated with fluoxetine for 23 days prior to receiving 5 mg of desloratadine once daily concomitantly with fluoxetine 20 mg once daily for 7 days. In this study, peak plasma concentrations of desloratadine or 3-hydroxydesloratadine increased by 15 or 17%, respectively, while AUC of 3-hydroxydesloratadine increased by 13%, following concomitant administration with fluoxetine. However, no clinically important changes, as measured by ECG and laboratory evaluations, vital signs, and adverse effects, were reported after concomitant administration of fluoxetine with desloratadine.

Zileuton

Increased plasma concentrations of terfenadine have been reported in one study in healthy individuals receiving 60 mg of terfenadine every 12 hours concomitantly with zileuton dosages of 600 mg every 6 hours for 7 days. In this study, AUC and peak plasma concentrations of terfenadine increased by about 35%, resulting from a 22% decrease in the clearance of unchanged terfenadine. Although no adverse cardiac effects (e.g., substantial changes in QT$_c$ intervals) were reported in these individuals, concomitant administration of astemizole or terfenadine with zileuton is not recommended since pharmacokinetics of the antihistamines may be impaired resulting in an increased risk of serious adverse cardiac effects.

Quinine and Chemically Related Drugs

There has been some evidence indicating that quinine may alter the pharmacokinetics of astemizole. Quinine is extensively metabolized in the liver; however, only limited information exists about the specific cytochrome P-450 microsomal isoenzymes responsible for the drug's metabolism. Increased plasma concentrations of astemizole and desmethylastemizole were reported in a study in healthy men receiving 10 mg of astemizole orally once daily for 24 days and 20 mg of

quinine sulfate every 4 hours for 4 consecutive doses on the 22nd day and then a single 430-mg dose on the 24th day of the study. In this study, slight increases in the maximum plasma concentration and AUC of astemizole were associated with concomitant administration of the 20-mg doses of quinine sulfate; however, no clinically or statistically significant changes in QT interval were observed. Maximum plasma concentrations and AUCs of astemizole and desmethylastemizole increased threefold following concomitant administration of the antihistamine and the 430-mg dose of quinine sulfate; these increases were associated with increases in the QT interval. Therefore, the manufacturer of astemizole has stated that concomitant administration of astemizole and therapeutic doses (i.e., more than 80 mg daily) of quinine sulfate were contraindicated.

Although increases in plasma concentrations of astemizole and its desmethyl metabolite also may occur in patients receiving the antihistamine concomitantly with food products containing quinine (e.g., tonic water), such increases are small and not associated with clinically or statistically significant prolongation of the QT interval when consumption is limited to approximately 1 L (32 oz) of tonic water a day (about 80 mg of quinine sulfate). Since consumption of larger daily amounts of quinine in tonic water may be associated with risk in patients receiving astemizole, patients who consume large amounts of tonic water daily may wish to consult their clinician.

Histamine H$_2$-Receptor Antagonists and Xanthine Derivatives

The manufacturer of terfenadine has stated that detectable plasma concentrations of unchanged terfenadine were not present and mean pharmacokinetic parameters (e.g., AUC, elimination half-life, peak plasma concentration) for the carboxylic acid metabolite fexofenadine did not appear to be affected in a study in which a single dose of terfenadine was given to individuals receiving multiple doses of cimetidine. Other data also suggest that an interaction between the drugs seems unlikely. While the potential for such a drug interaction has not been established, cardiotoxic effects also occurred following a terfenadine overdosage in at least one patient who was receiving cimetidine. In addition, torsades de pointes and prolongation of QT interval were reported in a patient receiving terfenadine 60 mg twice daily concomitantly with cimetidine 400 mg twice daily, and some clinicians state that concomitant use of terfenadine and cimetidine is not recommended.

Increased plasma concentrations of loratadine and its active metabolite desloratadine have been reported in controlled clinical studies in healthy men receiving 10 mg of loratadine once daily concomitantly with cimetidine dosages of 300 mg 4 times daily (every 6 hours) for 10 days. In these studies, AUC of loratadine increased by 103% following concomitant administration with cimetidine, while AUC of descarboethoxyloratadine increased by 6% following concomitant administration with cimetidine. However, no clinically important changes, as measured by ECG and laboratory evaluations, vital signs, and adverse effects, were reported after concomitant administration of cimetidine with loratadine. In addition, no changes in QT$_c$ intervals, sedation, or syncope were reported in these individuals. Plasma concentrations of cimetidine appeared to be unchanged in individuals receiving loratadine concomitantly.

Increased plasma concentrations of desloratadine have been reported in a controlled clinical study in healthy individuals receiving 5 mg of the drug once daily concomitantly with cimetidine (600 mg every 12 hours for 14 days under steady-state conditions). In this study, peak plasma concentrations and AUC of desloratadine increased by 12 and 19%, respectively, following concomitant administration with cimetidine. However, no clinically important changes, as measured by ECG and laboratory evaluations, vital signs, and adverse effects, were reported after concomitant administration of cimetidine with desloratadine.

Other Drugs

To date, the number of patients receiving loratadine concomitantly with ranitidine or theophylline has been too small to rule out a possible drug interaction between loratadine and such drugs and therefore, the manufacturers have recommended that loratadine be used with caution in patients receiving them.

Grapefruit Juice

Concomitant oral administration of grapefruit juice with terfenadine has been reported to increase bioavailability of terfenadine. This increased bioavailability of terfenadine was associated with prolongation of the QT interval averaging 3.3% (range: -1.6 to 9.5%); mean QT$_c$ intervals increased by 4-14 msec compared with administration of terfenadine with water. The interaction between grapefruit juice and terfenadine bioavailability appears to result from inhibition, probably prehepatic, of the cytochrome P-450 enzyme system by some constituent(s) in the juice.

Patients have been discouraged to ingest grapefruit juice concomitantly with terfenadine; in addition, concomitant administration of astemizole with grapefruit juice has not been recommended since substantially increased plasma concentrations of unchanged astemizole also could occur resulting in an increased risk of serious adverse cardiac effects.

Concomitant oral administration of grapefruit juice with desloratadine does not appear to alter bioavailability of the drug.

LABORATORY TEST INTERFERENCES

Antihistamines may suppress inhalation-challenge testing with histamine or antigen as well as the wheal and flare reactions to antigen skin testing. Considerable interindividual variation in the extent and duration of suppression has been reported, depending on the antigen and test technique, antihistamine and dosage regimen, time since the last dose, and individual response to testing. In one study, usual oral dosages of chlorpheniramine or diphenhydramine suppressed the wheal response for about 2 days after the last dose, promethazine or tripelennamine suppressed whealing for about 3 days, and hydroxyzine suppressed whealing for about 4 days. Combined use of an H₁- and H₂-antagonist appears to have a synergistic suppressive effect on immediate and late cutaneous reactions to skin test antigens. Whenever possible, antihistamines should be discontinued about 4 days prior to skin testing procedures since they may prevent otherwise positive reactions to dermal reactivity indicators. Some evidence suggests that loratadine or terfenadine should be discontinued at least 7 days prior to such testing and that the results of such tests should be interpreted with caution even if testing were performed 4–6 weeks after astemizole discontinuance.

In one study, topical application of an antihistamine (i.e., 2% pyrilamine maleate cream) to the skin test site 10 minutes after antigen testing decreased pruritus but did not suppress wheal or flare 10 minutes after application.

ACUTE TOXICITY

● Manifestations

Although antihistamines have relatively high therapeutic indexes, overdosage may result in death, especially in infants and children. There have been several reports of toxicity, often occurring within 24–48 hours of repeated topical application of diphenhydramine, in children with pruritus associated with varicella (chickenpox), poison ivy, or sunburn. Such toxicity included toxic psychosis (sometimes mimicking varicella encephalitis) and occurred in children who received oral and topical diphenhydramine concomitantly. The toxicity usually was associated with increased (60–1900 ng/mL) serum concentration of diphenhydramine. Topical diphenhydramine usually was applied to large areas of the body and usually was contained in Caladryl®, a commercially available lotion containing 1% diphenhydramine and 8% calamine; such combination is no longer commercially available in the US since Caladryl® has been reformulated by the manufacturer to contain pramoxine hydrochloride with calamine or zinc acetate. In general, overdosage of diphenhydramine may cause CNS stimulation and/or depression; in young children, CNS stimulation is dominant. Symptoms of antihistamine toxicity in children may resemble atropine overdosage and include fixed dilated pupils, abnormal eye movements, flushed face, dry mouth, urinary retention, fever, excitation, hallucinations, disorientation, delusions, agitation, bizarre behavior, confusion, jitteriness, restlessness, irritability, hyperactivity, delirium, twitching, tiredness, abnormal tongue movement, unsteady gait, trembling extremities, slurred speech, ataxia, incoordination, athetosis, tonic-clonic seizures, and postictal depression. Children recovered gradually from these adverse CNS effects, usually within 24–48 hours following removal of the topical preparation and discontinuance of all diphenhydramine-containing preparations.

Overdosage in adults usually causes CNS depression with drowsiness or coma which may be followed by excitement, seizures, and finally postictal depression. In children and adults, cerebral edema and upper nephron nephrosis, a deepening coma, tachycardia, QRS widening, heart block, cardiorespiratory collapse/arrest, cardiogenic shock, and death may occur. The risk of cardiotoxicity has been particularly likely with astemizole and terfenadine; however, these 2 antihistamines are no longer commercially available in the US. (See Cautions: Cardiovascular Effects.) Symptoms of overdosage occur within 30 minutes to 2 hours after ingestion; death may occur within 18 hours. Toxic effects may persist for prolonged (e.g., several days) periods after acute overdosage of antihistamines (e.g., astemizole) with long elimination half-lives. Rhabdomyolysis (evidenced by myoglobinuria) has been associated with overdosage of doxylamine. Acute toxicity has been reported following topical overdosage of diphenhydramine or tripelennamine (no longer commercially available in the US) in children.

● Treatment

Treatment of acute antihistamine overdosage consists of symptomatic and supportive therapy including artificial respiration, if necessary. If the patient is conscious, has not lost the gag reflex, and is not having seizures, emesis should be induced; however, the manufacturer of trimeprazine (no longer commercially available in the US) stated that emesis should not be induced because dystonic reaction of the head and neck may cause aspiration of gastric contents. The manufacturer of carbinoxamine maleate also states that emesis should not be induced; activated charcoal should be administered and gastric lavage should be considered following ingestion of a potentially life-threatening amount of carbinoxamine maleate.

While phenothiazine-type antihistamines may exhibit an antiemetic effect, ipecac syrup still may be effective in oral poisonings with these agents if given early (usually within 1 hour) before toxic or antiemetic effects appear. If emesis cannot be induced, gastric lavage and administration of activated charcoal are indicated; an endotracheal tube with cuff inflated should be in place to prevent aspiration of gastric contents. Saline cathartics (e.g., magnesium sulfate) may be administered.

Vasopressor agents, such as norepinephrine or phenylephrine, may be administered if necessary. Epinephrine should *not* be used, especially with phenothiazine overdosage, because epinephrine may lower the blood pressure further. Analeptic agents should *not* be used since they may cause seizures. Physostigmine may be useful to counteract the CNS anticholinergic effects of antihistamine intoxication. Diazepam can be given IV in the management of seizures that do not respond to physostigmine. Hyperthermia may be treated with cold packs or sponging with tepid water; sponging with alcohol should not be used.

If hypotension and/or cardiac arrhythmias occur (reported mainly with overdosage of astemizole or terfenadine), appropriate therapy should be instituted. Antiarrhythmic agents that can prolong the QT interval (e.g., class 1A agents) should be *avoided* in treating overdosage-associated arrhythmias in which prolongation of the QT꜀ interval is a manifestation. While arrhythmias may resolve spontaneously following discontinuance of the antihistamine, when necessary, therapy for ventricular tachyarrhythmias with associated QT prolongation (e.g., torsades de pointes) can include temporary atrial or ventricular pacing, IV magnesium sulfate, IV isoproterenol, and/or DC cardioversion (for initial management of sustained, symptomatic runs).

PHARMACOLOGY

Histamine is a physiologically active, endogenous substance (autacoid) that binds to and activates histamine H₁- and H₂-receptors at various sites in the body. H₃-receptors, which may be involved in feedback control of histamine synthesis and release, also have been described. The principal pharmacologic effects of histamine involve the cardiovascular system, extravascular smooth muscle (e.g., bronchial tree), and exocrine glands (e.g., stimulation of salivary, gastric, lacrimal, and bronchial secretions). Histamine also can stimulate some nerve endings and thus causes pruritus. Characteristic cardiovascular effects of histamine include direct and indirect microvascular dilation, hypotension, tachycardia, and flushing (involving H₁- and H₂-receptors) and increased vascular permeability (thought to principally involve H₁-receptors). Intracutaneous injection of histamine produces a "triple response" of local reddening, a bright halo or flare, and wheal formation. In allergic conditions, histamine and other substances (e.g., leukotrienes, prostaglandins, kinins, serotonin, platelet-activating factor) are secreted from mast cells, basophils, and other cells in response to antigenic stimulation. Histamine binds to and activates specific receptors in the nose, eyes, respiratory tract, and skin, causing characteristic allergic signs and symptoms.

The term antihistamine has historically been used to describe drugs that act as H₁-receptor antagonists. Although drugs that antagonize H₂-receptors also are commercially available (e.g., cimetidine, famotidine, nizatidine, ranitidine), these drugs generally are not referred to as antihistamines but rather as H₂-receptor antagonists. Antihistamines competitively antagonize most of the smooth muscle stimulating actions of histamine on the H₁-receptors of the GI tract, uterus, large blood vessels, and bronchial muscle. Contraction of the sphincter of Oddi and bile duct may be mediated in part by H₁-receptors, and opiate-induced contraction of biliary smooth muscle has been antagonized by antihistamines. The drugs only are feebly antagonistic to bronchospasm induced by antigen-antibody reactions.

Antihistamines also effectively antagonize the action of histamine that results in increased capillary permeability and the formation of edema. H_1-receptor antagonists also suppress flare and pruritus that accompany the endogenous release of histamine. Antihistamines appear to act by blocking H_1-receptor sites, thereby preventing the action of histamine on the cell; they do not chemically inactivate or physiologically antagonize histamine nor do they prevent the release of histamine. Antihistamines do not block the stimulating effect of histamine on gastric acid secretion, which is mediated by H_2-receptors of the parietal cells. **For information on the effects of H_2-receptor antagonists, see Cimetidine 56:28.12, Famotidine 56:28.12, and Nizatidine 56:28.12.**

The basic ethylamine group common to antihistamines also is common to anticholinergics, ganglionic and adrenergic blocking agents, local anesthetics, and antispasmodics; antihistamines therefore may be expected to exhibit some of the activities of these other classes of drugs. Some antihistamines also demonstrate a quinidine-like effect on myocardial conduction, and they may enhance the pressor action of norepinephrine. The antiemetic and antimotion-sickness actions of some antihistamines appear to result, at least in part, from their central anticholinergic and CNS depressant properties. The effects of diphenhydramine on parkinsonian syndrome and drug-induced extrapyramidal reactions are also apparently related to its central anticholinergic effects.

Although the antipruritic effect of systemically administered or locally applied antihistamines in conditions associated with histamine-induced pruritus appears to result from a peripheral antihistaminic effect and possibly a local anesthetic effect, the sedative effect of systemically administered antihistamines also appears to contribute to their antipruritic activity. The drugs are more effective antipruritics when administered systemically than when applied topically, especially when pruritus is generalized. Because pruritus can involve mediators other than histamine, the antipruritic efficacy of antihistamines is not routine.

PHARMACOKINETICS

Limited information is available on the pharmacokinetics of most antihistamines.

● Absorption

Antihistamines generally are well absorbed following oral or parenteral administration, but various salts may differ in activity and toxicity because of differences in solubility or absorption. The least soluble antihistamines are often the least toxic and may have a slow onset but prolonged duration of action. Following oral administration of antihistamines, symptomatic relief of allergic reactions usually begins within 15–30 minutes and usually is maximal within 1 hour. The duration of action is variable but symptoms usually are relieved for 3–6 hours after oral administration of most antihistamines. There may be some decrease in effectiveness with prolonged use of these drugs, although a substantial degree of tolerance to the antihistaminic effects generally does not occur. However, tolerance to the sedative effects may occur.

Some antihistamines (e.g., astemizole [no longer commercially available in the US], cetirizine, desloratadine, loratadine) exhibit a slower onset of action and/or prolonged duration of effect. Following single- and multiple-dose administration, the long-acting antihistamine loratadine exhibits antihistaminic effects beginning within 1–3 hours, reaching a maximum at 8–10 hours, and lasting in excess of 24 hours. Following single- and multiple-dose administration of a 5-mg dose of desloratadine, the antihistaminic effect of the drug is apparent within 1 hour and lasts for 24 hours. Following oral administration of a single 10-mg dose of cetirizine hydrochloride in healthy individuals, the antihistaminic effect of the drug is apparent within 20–60 minutes and lasts for at least 24 hours. Following oral administration of a 5-mg dose of levocetirizine dihydrochloride in patients with allergic rhinitis, the antihistaminic effect of the drug is apparent within 1 hour and lasts for at least 24 hours.

Topically applied antihistamines generally do not readily penetrate intact skin, especially when salts of the drugs are used. However, percutaneous absorption can occur, especially when the stratum corneum is disrupted, and rarely may result in systemic effects and toxicity.

● Distribution

The distribution of most antihistamines has not been fully characterized. Those compounds that have been studied show highest concentrations in the lungs and lower concentrations in spleen, kidneys, brain, muscle, and skin. Protein binding of these agents ranges from 50–99%.

Unlike other currently available antihistamines, second generation (also referred to as relatively "nonsedating") antihistamines such as acrivastine, astemizole, cetirizine, desloratadine, fexofenadine, levocetirizine, loratadine, and terfenadine (no longer commercially available in the US) appear to distribute poorly or not appreciably into the CNS at usual dosages. It is thought that this lack of CNS distribution results principally from the inability of these agents to cross the tightly fused outer membranes of endothelial cells lining the brain capillaries. Cetirizine, because of its substantial polarity, also does not readily cross the blood-brain barrier; however, some data indicate that the drug may cause more somnolence than other second generation antihistamines. Levocetirizine also is considered mildly sedating.

Small amounts of the drugs appear to be distributed into milk.

● Elimination

The metabolic fate of most antihistamines is not clearly established. The drugs usually appear to be extensively metabolized, mainly in the liver. Some second generation antihistamines (e.g., astemizole, loratadine, terfenadine) are metabolized principally by the cytochrome P-450 microsomal enzyme system, mainly by the isoenzyme 3A4 (CYP3A4), although other isoenzymes, including CYP1A2 and CYP2D6, also may be involved. Desloratadine also is extensively metabolized; however, the enzyme(s) responsible for metabolism of the drug has not been identified. Other second generation antihistamines (e.g., cetirizine, fexofenadine, levocetirizine) appear to be only minimally metabolized in the liver.

Metabolism of some antihistamines that are extensively metabolized in the liver (e.g., astemizole, terfenadine) may be substantially reduced in patients with hepatic impairment and possibly in geriatric patients. In addition, metabolism also may be substantially reduced in patients concomitantly receiving foods (e.g., grapefruit juice) or drugs (e.g., certain azole-derivative anti-infective agents, including fluconazole, itraconazole, ketoconazole, metronidazole, and miconazole; certain macrolide antibiotics, including clarithromycin, erythromycin, and troleandomycin; mibefradil [no longer commercially available in the US]; possibly certain human immunodeficiency virus [HIV] protease inhibitors, including indinavir, nelfinavir, ritonavir, and saquinavir; possibly some serotonin-reuptake inhibitors, including fluoxetine, fluvoxamine, nefazodone, paroxetine, and sertraline; zileuton; quinine) that affect the hepatic microsomal enzyme system. Decreased metabolism may result in accumulation of potentially toxic concentrations of the unchanged antihistamines that may be associated with serious adverse cardiac effects. (See Cautions: Cardiovascular Effects and see Drug Interactions.)

Many antihistamines are excreted in urine as inactive metabolites within 24 hours; however, some antihistamines (e.g., terfenadine, desloratadine, loratadine, astemizole, acrivastine) have active H_1-antagonist metabolites. Negligible amounts of most antihistamines are excreted unchanged in urine; however, cetirizine and levocetirizine are excreted in urine mainly as unchanged drug.

● Chemistry

Antihistamines (histamine H_1-receptor antagonists) competitively inhibit most of the pharmacologic actions of histamine.

Antihistamines have been classified chemically and also have been classified according to their propensity to cause sedation, with relatively sedating antihistamines (i.e., conventional, prototypical antihistamines) being classified as first generation and relatively "nonsedating" antihistamines (e.g., acrivastine, astemizole [no longer commercially available in the US], desloratadine, fexofenadine, loratadine, terfenadine [no longer commercially available in the US]) being classified as second generation. Cetirizine also is considered a second generation antihistamine; however, some data indicate that it causes more sedation than other second generation antihistamines. Levocetirizine, the active R enantiomer of cetirizine, is considered a mildly sedating antihistamine and has been found to be slightly more sedating than desloratadine.

First Generation Antihistamines

azatadine*	diphenhydramine
brompheniramine	doxylamine
carbinoxamine	hydroxyzine
chlorpheniramine	meclizine
clemastine	promethazine
cyproheptadine	triprolidine
dimenhydrinate	

Second Generation Antihistamines

acrivastine	fexofenadine
astemizole[a]	levocetirizine
cetirizine	loratadine
desloratadine	terfenadine[a]

[a]*no longer commercially available in the US*

Most antihistamines are substituted ethylamines. In general, these molecules consist of 3 portions: R^1 = nucleus, X = a linkage such as nitrogen, oxygen, or carbon, and the ethylamine group. Antihistamines can be depicted by a general formula:

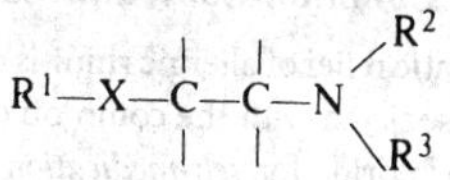

$$R^1-X-\underset{|}{\overset{|}{C}}-\underset{|}{\overset{|}{C}}-N\diagup\overset{R^2}{}\diagdown\underset{R^3}{}$$

R^1 is composed of aromatic and/or heterocyclic groups, which may be separated from X by a methylene group. Hydrogenation of the rings in the R^1 portion of the molecule decreases antihistamine activity. Usually, activity of an antihistamine is increased by substitution of a halogen atom in the *para* position of the phenyl or benzyl group of R^1. For maximum activity, the terminal nitrogen of the ethylamine group should be a tertiary amine with methyl groups or a small cyclic moiety in R^2 and R^3. In optically active compounds, the *dextro* isomer (e.g., dexchlorpheniramine, dexbrompheniramine) usually is more active than the *levo* isomer.

Antihistamines can be classified on the basis of X substitution as follows:

Ethylenediamine Derivatives

antazoline	pyrilamine
methapyrilene	tripelennamine

This group of antihistamines has nitrogen in the X position. Ethylenediamine derivatives have relatively weak CNS effects; however, drowsiness may occur in some patients. Adverse GI effects are common with this group of antihistamines.

Ethanolamine Derivatives (Aminoalkyl Ethers)

bromodiphenhydramine*	diphenhydramine
carbinoxamine	diphenylpyraline
clemastine	doxylamine
dimenhydrinate	phenyltoloxamine

This group of antihistamines, which has oxygen in the X position, has substantial atropine-like activity. Drugs in this group commonly cause CNS depression; with usual doses, drowsiness occurs in about 50% of patients who receive ethanolamine derivative antihistamines. The incidence of adverse GI effects with

these antihistamines is relatively low. Dimenhydrinate (see 56:22.08) and diphenhydramine also are used as antiemetics.

Alkylamines (Propylamine Derivatives)

acrivastine	dimethindene
brompheniramine	pheniramine
chlorpheniramine	pyrrobutamine
dexbrompheniramine	triprolidine
dexchlorpheniramine	

These antihistamines contain a carbon atom in the X position. Alkylamines cause less drowsiness and more CNS stimulation than the other antihistamines and thus are suitable for daytime use.

Phenothiazine Derivatives

promethazine

In this group of antihistamines, nitrogen, as part of a phenothiazine nucleus, is in the X position. Most phenothiazines are used principally as antipsychotics (see 28:16.08); however, some are useful as antihistamines, antipruritics, and antiemetics.

Piperazine Derivatives

cetirizine	levocetirizine
hydroxyzine	meclizine

In this group, nitrogen, as part of a piperazine nucleus, is in the X position. Meclizine is used in the treatment of motion sickness. (See 56:22.08.) Hydroxyzine is used as a tranquilizer, sedative, antipruritic, and antiemetic. (See 28:24.92.)

Others

astemizole[a]	fexofenadine
azatadine[a]	loratadine
cyproheptadine	phenindamine
desloratadine	terfenadine[a]

[a]*no longer commercially available in the US*

For further information on chemistry and stability, pharmacokinetics, uses, and dosage and administration of antihistamines available as single entities, see the individual monographs in 4:00.

diphenhydrAMINE Hydrochloride

4:04 • FIRST GENERATION ANTIHISTAMINES

■ Diphenhydramine is an ethanolamine-derivative, first generation antihistamine.

USES

Diphenhydramine shares the actions and uses of other antihistamines.

Diphenhydramine also is used as an antitussive for temporary relief of cough caused by minor throat and bronchial irritation such as may occur with common colds or inhaled irritants.

Diphenhydramine is effective for the prevention and treatment of nausea, vomiting, and/or vertigo associated with motion sickness.

Diphenhydramine may be useful as an adjunctive antiemetic agent to prevent chemotherapy-induced nausea and vomiting†; however, the American Society of Clinical Oncology (ASCO) currently does not recommend that antihistamines be used alone as antiemetic agents in patients receiving chemotherapy.

Diphenhydramine also is used as a nighttime sleep aid for the short-term management of insomnia. In individuals who experience occasional sleeplessness or those who have difficulty falling asleep, the drug is more effective than placebo in reducing sleep onset (i.e., time to fall asleep) and increasing the depth and quality of sleep.

Diphenhydramine, alone or in conjunction with other antiparkinsonian agents, may be useful as alternative therapy in the management of tremor early in the course of parkinsonian syndrome. The drug also may be useful in the management of drug-induced extrapyramidal reactions.

Diphenhydramine may be used topically for temporary relief of pruritus and pain associated with various skin conditions including minor burns, sunburn, minor cuts or scrapes, insect bites, minor skin irritations, or rashes associated with poison oak, poison ivy, or poison sumac. However, because systemic diphenhydramine toxicity (e.g., psychosis) has been reported in pediatric patients following topical application of the drug to large areas of the body (often areas with broken skin), many clinicians suggest that topical diphenhydramine be used only on limited areas of skin and not used more often than directed to avoid excessive percutaneous absorption of the drug. (See Acute Toxicity: Manifestations, in the Antihistamines General Statement 4:00.) Topical diphenhydramine also should not be used for *self-medication* in the management of varicella (chickenpox) or measles without first consulting a clinician.

DOSAGE AND ADMINISTRATION

● Administration

Diphenhydramine hydrochloride usually is administered orally.

Diphenhydramine citrate usually is administered orally.

When oral therapy is not feasible, diphenhydramine hydrochloride may be given by deep IM or, preferably, IV injection. The drug should not be given subcutaneously, intradermally, or perivascularly because of its irritating effects; local necrosis has been reported following subcutaneous or intradermal administration of parenteral diphenhydramine. IV use of the drug in a home-care setting should be employed under careful supervision. Use of diphenhydramine for local anesthesia via local infiltration is discouraged because of the risk of local tissue necrosis. Diphenhydramine hydrochloride should not be given to premature or full-term neonates. (See Cautions: Pediatric Precautions.)

For the temporary relief of pruritus associated with various skin conditions and disorders, diphenhydramine hydrochloride-containing preparations are applied topically in the form of a cream, lotion, or topical solution. The possibility of clinically important percutaneous absorption of the drug following topical application should be considered. (See Cautions.)

● Dosage

Dosage should be individualized according to the patient's response and tolerance.

Adult Dosage
Usual Dosage

The usual adult oral dosage of diphenhydramine hydrochloride is 25–50 mg 3 or 4 times daily at 4- to 6-hour intervals, not to exceed 300 mg in 24 hours.

The usual adult IM or IV dose of diphenhydramine hydrochloride is 10–50 mg; in a few patients, up to 100 mg may be required. Some experts recommend a dose of 25–50 mg. The rate of IV administration should not exceed 25 mg/minute.

The maximum adult IM or IV dosage of diphenhydramine hydrochloride is 400 mg daily.

Allergic Rhinitis, the Common Cold, and Cough

For temporary symptomatic relief of allergic rhinitis or for temporary relief of rhinorrhea and sneezing associated with the common cold, the usual oral dosage of diphenhydramine hydrochloride for *self-medication* in adults is 25–50 mg every 4–6 hours, not to exceed 300 mg in 24 hours.

For the temporary relief of cough caused by minor throat and bronchial irritation, the usual oral dosage of diphenhydramine hydrochloride for *self-medication* in adults is 25 mg (equivalent to 38 mg of diphenhydramine citrate) every 4 hours, not to exceed 150 mg (equivalent to 228 mg of diphenhydramine citrate) in 24 hours.

When used both for temporary symptomatic relief of allergic rhinitis or rhinorrhea and sneezing associated with the common cold and also for relief of cough caused by minor throat and bronchial irritation, the usual oral dosage of diphenhydramine hydrochloride for *self-medication* in adults is 25 mg (equivalent to 38 mg of diphenhydramine citrate) every 4–6 hours, not to exceed 150 mg (equivalent to 228 mg of diphenhydramine citrate) in 24 hours.

Motion Sickness

For the prevention and treatment of nausea, vomiting, and/or vertigo associated with motion sickness, the usual oral dosage of diphenhydramine hydrochloride for *self-medication* in adults is 25–50 mg every 4–6 hours, not to exceed 300 mg in 24 hours. For the prevention of motion sickness, a dose should be given 30 minutes before exposure to motion; subsequent doses may be given before meals and at bedtime for the duration of the exposure.

Insomnia

As a nighttime sleep aid, the usual oral dosage of diphenhydramine hydrochloride for *self-medication* in adults is 50 mg (equivalent to 76 mg of diphenhydramine citrate) at bedtime as needed, or as directed by a clinician. Higher dosages also occasionally have been used for sedative effects as directed by a clinician, but some evidence suggests that the efficacy of a 100-mg dose is not substantially greater than that of a 50-mg dose, although adverse (e.g., anticholinergic) effects may be increased.

Because insomnia may be indicative of a serious underlying physical, emotional, or psychological condition requiring professional medical attention, patients should be advised to avoid using diphenhydramine for *self-medication* for longer than 7–10 nights and to consult a clinician if insomnia persists continuously for longer than 2 weeks.

Parkinsonian Syndrome

For the symptomatic treatment of parkinsonian syndrome, some clinicians have suggested an initial oral dosage of 25 mg of diphenhydramine hydrochloride 3 times daily; if necessary, dosage is then gradually increased to 50 mg 4 times daily.

Pediatric Dosage
Usual Dosage

When diphenhydramine was available only by prescription, the prescribing information for the drug indicated a usual oral diphenhydramine hydrochloride dosage for children weighing more than 9.1 kg of 12.5–25 mg 3 or 4 times daily at 4- to 6-hour intervals and for children weighing 9.1 kg or less an oral diphenhydramine hydrochloride dosage of 6.25–12.5 mg 3 or 4 times daily at 4- to 6-hour intervals. However, these dosage recommendations are *not* included in the current labeling of *nonprescription* oral diphenhydramine preparations, and clinicians should use caution when considering use of nonprescription oral diphenhydramine in children younger than 4 years of age. (See Cautions: Pediatric Precautions.)

Alternatively, for oral, deep IM, or IV therapy, children (other than premature or full-term neonates) may be given 5 mg/kg daily or 150 mg/m² daily divided in 4 doses; some experts recommend a dosage of 1–2 mg/kg daily. The rate of IV administration should not exceed 25 mg/minute.

The maximum oral, IM, or IV dosage of diphenhydramine hydrochloride in children older than 1 month of age is 300 mg daily.

Allergic Rhinitis, the Common Cold, and Cough

For *self-medication* to provide temporary symptomatic relief of allergic rhinitis or temporary relief of rhinorrhea or sneezing associated with the common cold, children 12 years of age and older may receive the dosage used in adults; children 6 to younger than 12 years of age may receive 12.5–25 mg orally every 4–6 hours, not to exceed 150 mg in 24 hours. Diphenhydramine hydrochloride should not be used for *self-medication* of these conditions in children younger than 6 years of age; when directed by a clinician, the usual oral dosage in children 2 to younger than 6 years of age is 6.25 mg every 4–6 hours, not to exceed 37.5 mg in 24 hours.

For *self-medication* of cough caused by minor throat and bronchial irritation, children 12 years of age and older may receive the dosage used in adults; children 6 to younger than 12 years of age may receive 12.5 mg (equivalent to 19 mg of diphenhydramine citrate) orally every 4 hours, not to exceed 75 mg (equivalent to 114 mg of diphenhydramine citrate) in 24 hours. Diphenhydramine hydrochloride should not be used for *self-medication* of cough in children younger than 6 years of age; when directed by a clinician, the usual oral dosage in children 2 to younger than 6 years of age is 6.25 mg (equivalent to 9.5 mg of diphenhydramine citrate) every 4 hours, not to exceed 37.5 mg (equivalent to 57 mg of diphenhydramine citrate) in 24 hours.

Motion Sickness

For *self-medication* to prevent and treat nausea, vomiting, and/or vertigo associated with motion sickness, children 12 years of age and older may receive the dosage used in adults; children 6 to younger than 12 years of age may receive 12.5–25 mg of diphenhydramine hydrochloride 30–60 minutes before travel and every 4–6 hours, not to exceed 150 mg in 24 hours. Children 2–5 years of age† may receive a dosage of 6.25 mg of diphenhydramine hydrochloride 30–60 minutes before travel and every 4–6 hours during travel, not to exceed 37.5 mg in 24 hours. (See Cautions: Pediatric Precautions.)

Insomnia

For *self-medication* as a nighttime sleep aid, children 12 years of age and older may receive the dosage used in adults. In children 2 to younger than 12 years of age with sleep disorders†, oral diphenhydramine hydrochloride doses of 1 mg/kg (up to a maximum dose of 50 mg) have been given 30 minutes before retiring. (See Cautions: Pediatric Precautions.) Diphenhydramine should not be used for *self-medication* for longer than 7–10 nights.

Topical Dosage

For temporary relief of pruritus and pain associated with various skin conditions in adults and children 2 years of age or older, creams, lotions, or solutions containing 1–2% diphenhydramine hydrochloride are applied to the affected areas 3 or 4 times daily or as directed by a clinician; topical diphenhydramine should not be used more often than directed.

If the condition worsens, or if symptoms persist for longer than 7 days or resolve and then recur within a few days, topical therapy with diphenhydramine hydrochloride should be discontinued and a clinician consulted; the possibility of sensitization by, or hypersensitivity to, the drug should be considered.

Topical preparations containing diphenhydramine hydrochloride should not be used on large areas of the body or concomitantly with other preparations containing the antihistamine, including those used orally, since increased serum concentrations of diphenhydramine may occur that can result in systemic toxicity. (See Acute Toxicity: Manifestations, in the Antihistamines General Statement 4:00.) The drug also should not be used for topical *self-medication* in the management of varicella (chickenpox) or measles without first consulting a clinician.

CAUTIONS

Diphenhydramine shares the toxic potentials of other antihistamines, and the usual precautions of antihistamine therapy should be observed. (See Cautions in the Antihistamines General Statement 4:00.)

When diphenhydramine is used in fixed combination with other agents (e.g., analgesic-antipyretics, nasal decongestants), the usual cautions, precautions, and contraindications associated with these agents must be considered in addition to those associated with diphenhydramine.

Local necrosis has occurred with subcutaneous or intradermal administration of parenteral diphenhydramine.

Diphenhydramine toxicity (e.g., dilated pupils, flushed face, hallucinations, ataxic gait, urinary retention) has been reported in pediatric patients following topical application of diphenhydramine to large areas of the body (often areas with broken skin) or following concomitant use of topical and oral preparations containing the drug. (See Acute Toxicity: Manifestations, in the Antihistamines General Statement 4:00.) Therefore, the US Food and Drug Administration (FDA) and many clinicians warn that oral diphenhydramine should *not* be used concomitantly with any other preparations containing the drug, including those used topically. In December 2002, the FDA issued a final rule requiring that a warning statement regarding such concomitant use be added to all OTC oral antiemetic, antihistamine, antitussive, and nighttime sleep aid preparations containing diphenhydramine.

Diphenhydramine hydrochloride topical solution contains a flammable vehicle, and the solution should not be exposed to an open flame or ignited materials (e.g., a lighted cigarette). Because of the potential for increased systemic exposure and subsequent toxicity, many clinicians state that topical preparations containing diphenhydramine should not be used more often than directed for any condition, applied on large areas of the body, or used concomitantly with other preparations containing the drug, including those used orally, since increased serum concentrations of diphenhydramine may occur that can result in systemic toxicity. (See Acute Toxicity: Manifestations, in the Antihistamines General Statement 4:00.) Patients should be advised to consult a clinician prior to use of topical diphenhydramine for the management of varicella (chickenpox) or measles.

Commercially available formulations of diphenhydramine may contain sodium bisulfite, a sulfite that may cause allergic-type reactions, including anaphylaxis and life-threatening or less severe asthmatic episodes, in certain susceptible individuals. The overall prevalence of sulfite sensitivity in the general population is unknown but probably low; such sensitivity appears to occur more frequently in asthmatic than in nonasthmatic individuals.

Although diphenhydramine appears to have low abuse potential and a favorable adverse effect profile, several children, adolescents, and young adults with chronic hematologic and neoplastic diseases have exhibited drug-seeking behavior or anticholinergic effects after repeated parenteral (e.g., bolus IV injection) administration of diphenhydramine over a prolonged period of time. It has been suggested that such route of administration may be associated with the development of adverse effects and the abuse potential of the drug and therefore, some clinicians recommend oral administration of diphenhydramine whenever possible. Alternatively, if the IV route is indicated, the drug should be infused over 20 minutes or longer and the lowest effective dosage of diphenhydramine should be employed. In addition, some clinicians suggest that IV diphenhydramine should not be used empirically for premedication, but should be reserved for patients with a history of reactions requiring treatment with an antihistamine. It is recommended that IV diphenhydramine be administered under careful supervision in a home-care setting.

● Pediatric Precautions

Diphenhydramine toxicity (e.g., dilated pupils, facial flushing, hallucinations, ataxic gait, urinary retention) has been reported in pediatric patients (19 months to 9 years of age) following topical application of diphenhydramine to large areas of the body (often areas with broken skin) or following concomitant use of topical and oral preparations containing the drug for *self-medication* in the symptomatic management of pain and pruritus associated with varicella (chickenpox), poison ivy, or sunburn. Manifestations typically resolved within 48 hours following discontinuance of the drug, and no deaths have been reported following topical use of diphenhydramine alone. For a complete discussion of acute diphenhydramine toxicity, see Acute Toxicity: Manifestations, in the Antihistamines General Statement 4:00.

Like other antihistamines, diphenhydramine should be used with caution in infants and young children and should not be used in premature or full-term neonates. (See Cautions: CNS Effects and see Pediatric Precautions, in the Antihistamines General Statement 4:00.) Children younger than 6 years of age should receive diphenhydramine only under the direction of a physician. Safety and efficacy of diphenhydramine as a nighttime sleep aid in children younger than 12 years of age have not been established. In addition, children may be more prone than adults to paradoxically experience CNS stimulation rather than sedation when antihistamines are used as nighttime sleep aids. Because diphenhydramine may cause marked drowsiness that may be potentiated by other CNS depressants (e.g., sedatives, tranquilizers), the antihistamine should be used in children receiving one of these drugs only under the direction of a physician.

Depending on the manufacturer and the particular formulation of the drug, topical preparations containing diphenhydramine should be used in children younger than 2, 6, or 12 years of age only under the direction of a clinician.

The possibility of drug-seeking behavior and anticholinergic effects in pediatric patients receiving repeated parenteral diphenhydramine over prolonged periods should be considered.

Overdosage and toxicity (including death) have been reported in children younger than 2 years of age receiving nonprescription (over-the-counter, OTC) preparations containing antihistamines, cough suppressants, expectorants, and nasal decongestants alone or in combination for relief of symptoms of upper respiratory tract infection. There is limited evidence of efficacy for these preparations in this age group, and appropriate dosages (i.e., approved by the US Food and Drug Administration [FDA]) for the symptomatic treatment of cold and cough have not been established. Therefore, FDA stated that nonprescription cough and cold preparations should not be used in children younger than 2 years of age; the agency continues to assess safety and efficacy of these preparations in older children. Meanwhile, because children 2–3 years of age also are at increased risk of overdosage and toxicity, some manufacturers of oral nonprescription cough and cold preparations agreed to voluntarily revise the product labeling to state that such preparations should not be used in children younger than 4 years of age. FDA recommends that parents and caregivers adhere to the dosage instructions and warnings on the product labeling that accompanies the preparation if administering to children and consult with their clinician about any concerns. Clinicians should ask caregivers about use of nonprescription cough and cold preparations to avoid overdosage. For additional information on precautions associated with the use of cough and cold preparations in pediatric patients, see Cautions: Pediatric Precautions in the Antihistamines General Statement 4:00.

● Mutagenicity and Carcinogenicity

Long-term animal studies to determine the carcinogenic and mutagenic potential of diphenhydramine have not been performed to date.

● Pregnancy, Fertility, and Lactation

Pregnancy

Reproduction studies in rats and rabbits receiving diphenhydramine hydrochloride dosages up to 5 times the recommended human dosage have not revealed evidence of harm to the fetus. However, diphenhydramine has been shown to cross the placenta. In one epidemiologic study, use of bromodiphenhydramine (no longer commercially available) but not diphenhydramine was associated with an increased risk of teratogenic effects. In another epidemiologic study, there also was no evidence of increased risk of teratogenicity associated with diphenhydramine use during the first trimester, although a modest association could not be ruled out. Use of diphenhydramine during the first trimester of pregnancy has been associated with an increased risk of cleft palate alone or combined with other fetal abnormalities, and the drug has been reported to potentiate the teratogenic effect of morphine in mice. The manufacturers state that there are no adequate and controlled studies to date using diphenhydramine in pregnant women, and the drugs should be used during pregnancy only when clearly needed.

Fertility

Reproduction studies in rats and rabbits receiving diphenhydramine hydrochloride dosages up to 5 times the recommended human dosage have not revealed evidence of impaired fertility.

Lactation

Diphenhydramine has been detected in milk. Because of the potential for serious adverse reactions to antihistamines in nursing infants, a decision should be made whether to discontinue nursing or diphenhydramine, taking into account the importance of the drug to the woman.

PHARMACOKINETICS

● Absorption

Diphenhydramine hydrochloride is well absorbed following oral administration, but apparently undergoes first-pass metabolism in the liver and only about 40–60% of an oral dose reaches systemic circulation as unchanged diphenhydramine. Diphenhydramine can be absorbed percutaneously following topical administration and rarely may result in systemic effects and toxicity, especially following concomitant oral and topical administration of the drug or when extensive disruption of the epidermal barrier (e.g., blistered or oozing skin) is present. (See Acute Toxicity: Manifestations, in the Antihistamines General Statement 4:00.)

Following oral administration of a single dose of diphenhydramine, the drug appears in plasma within 15 minutes and peak plasma concentrations are attained within 1–4 hours. Following single oral doses of 50 and 100 mg in healthy adults, peak plasma drug concentrations of 37–83 and 81–159 ng/mL, respectively, have been reported. Following oral administration of diphenhydramine hydrochloride dosages of 25 mg every 4 hours or 50 mg every 6 hours, peak steady-state plasma concentrations of the drug were 55 or 85 ng/mL, respectively, and minimum steady-state plasma concentrations were 27.5 or 30 ng/mL, respectively. Following IV injection of a single 50-mg dose over a 1-minute period in healthy adults in one study, plasma diphenhydramine concentration 1 hour after the injection ranged from 99–196 ng/mL. The antihistamine effect, as determined by suppression of the wheal response induced by intradermal injection of histamine, appears to be maximal within 1–3 hours and may persist for up to 7 hours after administration of a single dose of the drug, and appears to be positively correlated with plasma concentration of the drug. The sedative effect also appears to be maximal within 1–3 hours after administration of a single dose of diphenhydramine and appears to be positively correlated with plasma drug concentration, with marked drowsiness and/or sleep occurring at plasma concentrations of 70 ng/mL or greater.

● Distribution

Distribution of diphenhydramine into human body tissues and fluids has not been fully characterized. Following IV administration in rats, highest concentrations of the drug are attained in the lungs, spleen, and brain, with lower concentrations in the heart, muscle, and liver. Following IV administration in healthy adults, diphenhydramine reportedly has an apparent volume of distribution of 188–336 L. Volume of distribution of the drug reportedly is larger in Asian (about 480 L) than white adults. The drug crosses the placenta and has been detected in milk, although the extent of distribution into milk has not been quantitated.

Diphenhydramine is approximately 80–85% bound to plasma proteins in vitro. Less extensive protein binding of the drug has been reported in healthy Asian adults and in adults with liver cirrhosis.

● Elimination

Plasma concentrations of diphenhydramine appear to decline in a monophasic manner, although some pharmacokinetic data suggest a polyphasic elimination. The terminal elimination half-life of diphenhydramine has not been fully elucidated, but appears to range from 2.4–9.3 hours in healthy adults. The terminal elimination half-life reportedly is prolonged in adults with liver cirrhosis.

Diphenhydramine is rapidly and apparently almost completely metabolized. Following oral administration, the drug apparently undergoes substantial first-pass metabolism in the liver. Diphenhydramine appears to be metabolized principally to diphenylmethoxyacetic acid, which may further undergo conjugation. The drug also undergoes dealkylation to form the *N*-demethyl and *N*, *N*-didemethyl derivatives. Diphenhydramine and its metabolites are excreted principally in urine. Following oral administration of a single 100-mg dose in healthy adults, about 50–75% of the dose is excreted in urine within 4 days, almost completely as metabolites and with most urinary excretion occurring within the first 24–48 hours; only about 1% of a single oral dose is excreted unchanged in urine.

CHEMISTRY AND STABILITY

● Chemistry

Diphenhydramine and bromodiphenhydramine (no longer commercially available) are ethanolamine-derivative antihistamines. Bromodiphenhydramine differs structurally from diphenhydramine in the *para*-substitution of a bromine atom for a hydrogen atom on one phenyl group. Diphenhydramine is commercially available as the hydrochloride or citrate salt; the citrate salt is only available in fixed-combination preparations. Diphenhydramine hydrochloride occurs as a white, odorless, crystalline powder which slowly darkens on exposure to light. Diphenhydramine hydrochloride has solubilities of approximately 1 g/mL in water and 0.5 g/mL in alcohol at 25°C. The pK$_a$ of diphenhydramine is approximately 9. Commercially available diphenhydramine hydrochloride injection has a pH of 5–6, which may have been adjusted with either sodium hydroxide or hydrochloric acid.

• Stability

Diphenhydramine hydrochloride preparations generally should be stored at 15–30°C and protected from moisture; freezing of the elixir, injection, oral solution, or topical lotion should be avoided. The injection and elixir should be stored in light-resistant containers. Diphenhydramine hydrochloride capsules and elixir should be stored in tight containers and the elixir, oral solution, and tablets in well-closed containers.

Diphenhydramine hydrochloride injection is reportedly compatible with most IV infusion solutions. The injection has been reported to be physically incompatible with some drugs, but the compatibility depends on several factors (e.g., concentration of the drugs, specific diluents used, resulting pH, temperature). Specialized references should be consulted for specific compatibility information.

For further information on chemistry, pharmacology, pharmacokinetics, uses, cautions, acute toxicity, drug interactions, laboratory test interferences, and dosage and administration of diphenhydramine, see the Antihistamines General Statement 4:00.

PREPARATIONS

Excipients in commercially available drug preparations may have clinically important effects in some individuals; consult specific product labeling for details.

diphenhydrAMINE Hydrochloride

Oral

Capsules	25 mg*	**Diphenhist®**, Rugby
		Diphenhydramine Hydrochloride Capsules
	50 mg*	**Diphenhydramine Hydrochloride Capsules**
		Sleepinal® Night-time Sleep Aid Capsules, Blairex
Capsules, liquid-filled	25 mg	**Benadryl® Allergy Dye-Free Liqui-Gels®**, McNeil Consumer
	50 mg	**Unisom® SleepGels®**, Chattem
Elixir	12.5 mg/5 mL*	**Diphenhydramine Hydrochloride Elixir**
		Hydramine® Elixir, Goldline
Solution	12.5 mg/5 mL*	**AllerMax®**, Pfeiffer
		Diphenhist®, Rugby
		Diphenhydramine Solution
Tablets	25 mg*	**Diphenhist® Captabs®**, Rugby
		diphenhydrAMINE Hydrochloride Tablets
		Nytol® QuickCaps® Caplets®, GlaxoSmithKline
		Sominex® Nighttime Sleep Aid, GlaxoSmithKline
	50 mg	**Compoz® Nighttime Sleep Aid**, Medtech
		Nighttime Sleep Aid®, Rugby
		Sominex® Nighttime Sleep Aid, GlaxoSmithKline
		Twilite® Caplets®, Pfeiffer

Tablets, film-coated	25 mg	**Benadryl® Allergy Ultratab®**, McNeil Consumer
	50 mg	**AllerMax® Caplets®**, Pfeiffer
		Sominex® Caplets® Maximum Strength, GlaxoSmithKline

Parenteral

| Injection | 50 mg/mL* | **Benadryl®**, Pfizer |
| | | **diphenhydrAMINE Hydrochloride Injection** |

* available from one or more manufacturer, distributor, and/or repackager by generic (nonproprietary) name

diphenhydrAMINE Citrate and Acetaminophen

Oral

For solution	38 mg/packet with 500 mg/packet Acetaminophen	**Goody's® PM Powder**, GlaxoSmithKline
Tablets, film-coated	38 mg with Acetaminophen 500 mg	**Excedrin P.M.® Caplets®**, Novartis
		Excedrin P.M.® Gelcaps®, Novartis

Other diphenhydrAMINE Citrate Combinations

Oral

| Tablets, film-coated | 38 mg with Aspirin 500 mg | **Bayer® PM Extra Strength Caplets®**, Bayer |

diphenhydrAMINE Hydrochloride Combinations

Oral

Solution	12.5 mg/5 mL with Acetaminophen 160 mg/5 mL, and Phenylephrine Hydrochloride 2.5 mg/5 mL	**Children's Tylenol® Plus Cold and Allergy**, McNeil
Tablets	25 mg with Acetaminophen 500 mg	**Tylenol® PM Caplets®**, McNeil
		Tylenol® PM Geltabs®, McNeil
		Tylenol® PM Rapid Release Gels®, McNeil
Tablets, film-coated	12.5 mg with Acetaminophen 325 mg and Phenylephrine Hydrochloride 5 mg	**Sudafed® PE Severe Cold Caplets®**, Pfizer
	12.5 mg with Acetaminophen 500 mg	**Percogesic® Aspirin-Free Caplets® Extra Strength**, Medtech
		Tylenol® Severe Allergy Caplets®, McNeil
	25 mg with Acetaminophen 325 mg and Phenylephrine Hydrochloride 5 mg	**Tylenol® Allergy Multi-Symptom Nighttime Cool Burst® Caplets®**, McNeil
	25 mg with Acetaminophen 500 mg	**Tylenol® PM Caplets®**, McNeil

† Use is not currently included in the labeling approved by the US Food and Drug Administration.

Selected Revisions October 13, 2015, © Copyright, January 1, 1979, American Society of Health-System Pharmacists, Inc.

Promethazine Hydrochloride

4:04 • FIRST GENERATION ANTIHISTAMINES

■ Promethazine is a phenothiazine derivative with potent first generation antihistaminic properties.

USES

Promethazine shares the uses of the antihistaminic drugs. (See Uses in the Antihistamines General Statement 4:00.) Promethazine's pronounced sedative effect limits the usefulness of the drug as an antihistamine in many ambulatory patients. In contrast to most other phenothiazines, promethazine is effective in the management of motion sickness.

For the use of promethazine as a sedative and antiemetic, see Promethazine Hydrochloride 28:24.92 and also see the Phenothiazines General Statement 28:16.08.24.

DOSAGE AND ADMINISTRATION

● *Administration*

Promethazine hydrochloride may be administered orally, rectally, or by deep IM injection. Promethazine hydrochloride also is administered by IV injection. However, because IV administration of the drug has been associated with severe tissue injury, including gangrene requiring amputation, the US Food and Drug Administration (FDA) states that deep IM injection is the preferred method for administration of promethazine hydrochloride injections. (See Cautions: Precautions and Contraindications.) If IV administration of promethazine hydrochloride is required, FDA states that the drug should be administered through the tubing of an IV infusion set that is known to be correctly functioning; FDA also states that the *maximum* rate of IV administration is 25 mg/minute, and the *maximum* concentration of the injection is 25 mg/mL. If the patient complains of pain at the injection site during presumed IV injection of the drug, the injection should immediately be stopped, and the possibility of intra-arterial placement of the needle or perivascular extravasation should be evaluated. Promethazine hydrochloride injection is commercially available in 2 strengths: 25 mg/mL and 50 mg/mL. FDA states that the preparation containing 50 mg/mL is for IM injection *only*; the preparation containing 25 mg/mL may be administered by IM or IV injection.

Because of the risk of severe tissue injury and amputations if promethazine hydrochloride is inadvertently administered intra-arterially or if extravasation were to occur, some medication safety experts (e.g., the Institute for Safe Medication Practices [ISMP]) recommend that parenteral administration of the drug be avoided and replaced by safer alternative therapies.

Subcutaneous or intra-arterial injection of promethazine hydrochloride is contraindicated.

Promethazine hydrochloride injection should be inspected visually for particulate matter and discoloration prior to administration whenever solution and container permit. The injection should be discarded if the solution is discolored or contains a precipitate.

● *Dosage*

Dosages of promethazine hydrochloride by the various routes of administration are identical.

Because of the risk of potentially fatal respiratory depression, promethazine hydrochloride should *not* be used in children younger than 2 years of age. The drug should be used cautiously and at the lowest effective dosage in older children (See Cautions: Pediatric Precautions.)

Allergic Conditions

As an antihistamine, promethazine hydrochloride usually is given at bedtime because of its pronounced sedative effects. The usual adult oral dose of promethazine hydrochloride is 25 mg before retiring; if necessary, however, 12.5 mg may be administered before meals and on retiring. Children 2 years of age and older may receive a single bedtime dose of up to 25 mg or up to 12.5 mg 3 times daily depending on the age and weight of the child. Alternatively, children 2 years of age and older may be given 0.5 mg/kg at bedtime or 0.125 mg/kg as needed. Dosage should be adjusted to the smallest amount adequate to relieve symptoms.

When the oral route is not feasible, 25 mg of promethazine hydrochloride may be given rectally or IM; if required, the drug may be administered by IV injection (see Dosage and Administration: Administration and see Cautions: Precautions and Contraindications). This dose may be repeated within 2 hours if necessary, but oral therapy should be instituted as soon as possible if further medication is necessary.

To prevent or control minor allergic transfusion reactions in adults, 25 mg of promethazine hydrochloride may be administered prior to or during a blood transfusion.

Motion Sickness

For the management of motion sickness, adults may be given 25 mg of promethazine hydrochloride and children may receive 12.5–25 mg or 0.5 mg/kg. The first dose should be given at least 30–60 minutes prior to departure. A second dose may be given 8–12 hours later if necessary. Additional doses may be given on arising in the morning and before the evening meal for the duration of the journey.

Common Cold

For the temporary relief of rhinorrhea or sneezing associated with the common cold in adults and children 12 years of age and older, an oral promethazine hydrochloride dosage of 6.25 mg every 4–6 hours, not to exceed 37.5 mg in 24 hours, has been suggested. In children 6 to younger than 12 years of age, an oral dosage of 3.125 mg every 4–6 hours, not to exceed 18.75 mg in 24 hours, has been suggested. When directed by a clinician, an oral dosage of 1.56 mg every 4–6 hours, not to exceed 9.36 mg in 24 hours, has been suggested for children 2 to younger than 6 years of age. (See Cautions: Pediatric Precautions.) Because the toxic potential of long-term therapy with promethazine for the symptomatic relief of the common cold has not been fully elucidated, the drug currently is recommended only for short-term use.

CAUTIONS

● *Adverse Effects*

Promethazine has adverse effects similar to those of other antihistamines and shares the toxic potentials of the phenothiazines; the usual precautions of antihistamine and phenothiazine therapy should be observed. (See Cautions in the Antihistamines General Statement 4:00 and in the Phenothiazines General Statement 28:16.08.24.) Although the risk of adverse reactions (e.g., blood dyscrasias, hepatotoxicity, reactivation of psychotic processes, tachycardia, cardiac arrest, endocrine disturbances, dermatologic disorders, ocular changes, hypersensitivity reactions) that have occurred during long-term administration of antipsychotic phenothiazines appears to be minimal, the possibility that they could occur with prolonged administration of promethazine should be considered.

The most common adverse reactions of promethazine are pronounced sedative effects and confusion or disorientation. Adverse anticholinergic effects of the drug include dryness of mouth, blurring of vision, and, rarely, dizziness. Extrapyramidal reactions may occur with high doses and usually subside with dosage reduction. Lassitude, fatigue, incoordination, tinnitus, diplopia, oculogyric crises, insomnia, excitation, nervousness, euphoria, hysteria, tremors, abnormal movements, nightmares, delirium, agitation, seizures, hallucinations, torticollis, tongue protrusion, oversedation, dystonic reactions, and catatonic-like states have been reported. Restlessness, akathisia, and, occasionally, marked irregular respiration have occurred. Neuroleptic malignant syndrome (NMS) also may occur. Patients with pain who have received inadequate or no analgesia have developed athetoid-like movements of the upper extremities following parenteral administration of promethazine. These symptoms usually disappeared when the pain was controlled.

Leukopenia, thrombocytopenia, thrombocytopenic purpura, and agranulocytosis have been reported in patients receiving promethazine.

Tachycardia, bradycardia, increased or decreased blood pressure, and faintness have occurred in patients receiving promethazine. Although rapid IV administration of promethazine may produce a transient fall in blood pressure, blood pressure usually is maintained or slightly elevated when the drug is given slowly. Venous thrombosis at the injection site also has been reported.

Promethazine has been associated with obstructive jaundice, which was usually reversible following discontinuance of the drug. Cholestatic jaundice, nausea, and vomiting have been reported in patients receiving promethazine. Photosensitivity has been reported and may be a contraindication to further promethazine therapy. Urticaria, dermatitis, angioedema, dermatologic reactions, and asthma also have been reported. Nasal stuffiness, respiratory depression (may be fatal), cardiac arrest, and apnea (may be fatal) also may occur.

Local Reactions Associated with Promethazine Hydrochloride Injection

Severe chemical irritation and damage to tissues (e.g., burning, pain, erythema, swelling, severe spasm of distal vessels, thrombophlebitis, venous thrombosis, phlebitis, abscesses, tissue necrosis, gangrene) may occur with administration of promethazine injection, regardless of the route of administration. Such irritation and damage also may result from perivascular extravasation, unintentional intra-arterial injection, and intraneuronal or perineuronal infiltration. Parenteral administration of promethazine may produce nerve damage (ranging from temporary sensory loss to palsies and paralysis) while injection near or into a nerve may result in permanent tissue damage. In some cases, surgical intervention (e.g., fasciotomy, skin graft, amputation) may be needed. (See Dosage and Administration: Administration and see also Cautions: Precautions and Contraindications.)

● *Precautions and Contraindications*

Promethazine has adverse effects similar to those of other antihistamines and shares the toxic potentials of the phenothiazines; the usual precautions of antihistamine and phenothiazine therapy should be observed. (See Cautions: Precautions and Contraindications in the Antihistamines General Statement 4:00 and in the Phenothiazines General Statement 28:16.08.24.)

Some commercially available formulations of promethazine hydrochloride contain sulfites that may cause allergic-type reactions, including anaphylaxis and life-threatening or less severe asthmatic episodes, in certain susceptible individuals. The overall prevalence of sulfite sensitivity in the general population is unknown but probably low; such sensitivity appears to occur more frequently in asthmatic than in nonasthmatic individuals.

Ambulatory patients should be warned that promethazine may impair their ability to perform hazardous tasks requiring mental alertness or physical coordination such as operating machinery or driving a motor vehicle. It should be kept in mind that the antiemetic effect of promethazine may obscure signs of overdosage of other drugs or of symptoms of conditions such as intestinal obstruction or brain tumor, and thereby interfere with diagnosis.

Promethazine should be used with caution in patients with cardiovascular disease or impaired liver function or who are having an asthmatic attack. Some manufacturers state that the drug should be used cautiously in individuals with peptic ulcer. Some manufacturers also state that the drug should be used with caution in patients with acute or chronic respiratory impairment, particularly children, because the cough reflex may be suppressed. Promethazine should be used with caution, if at all, in patients with a history of sleep apnea. (See Cautions: Pediatric Precautions.)

Because IV administration of the drug has been associated with severe tissue injury, including gangrene requiring amputation, the US Food and Drug Administration (FDA) states that deep IM injection is the preferred method for administration of promethazine hydrochloride injections. If IV administration of promethazine hydrochloride is required, extreme care should be exercised to avoid extravasation or inadvertent intra-arterial injection. (See Dosage and Administration: Administration and see Local Reactions Associated with Promethazine Hydrochloride Injection under Cautions: Adverse Effects.) If the patient complains of pain at the injection site during presumed IV injection of the drug, the injection should immediately be stopped, and the possibility of intra-arterial placement of the needle or perivascular extravasation should be evaluated. Clinicians should be alert for signs and symptoms of potential tissue injury, including burning or pain at the site of injection, phlebitis, swelling, and blistering, and patients should be informed that adverse effects may occur immediately (i.e., while receiving the injection) or may develop hours to days after an injection of promethazine. Although there are no proven successful treatment regimens for the management of extravasation or inadvertent intra-arterial injection of promethazine, sympathetic block and administration of heparin are commonly employed during the acute management.

Because of the risk of severe tissue injury and amputations if promethazine hydrochloride is inadvertently administered intra-arterially or if extravasation were to occur, some medication safety experts (e.g., the Institute for Safe Medication Practices [ISMP]) recommend that parenteral administration of the drug be avoided and replaced by safer alternative therapies.

FDA states that subcutaneous or intra-arterial administration of promethazine hydrochloride is contraindicated. Promethazine hydrochloride should *not* be administered intra-arterially, because chemical irritation may be severe and cause severe arteriospasm, possibly resulting in impairment of circulation and gangrene requiring amputation. Since promethazine discolors blood on contact, aspiration of dark blood at the site of injection does *not* rule out the possibility of intra-arterial placement of the needle.

Promethazine is contraindicated in patients who have exhibited hypersensitivity or idiosyncrasy to promethazine or other phenothiazines. Promethazine also is contraindicated in pediatric patients younger than 2 years of age, because of the risk of developing potentially fatal respiratory depression. (See Cautions: Pediatric Precautions.) In addition, the drug is contraindicated in patients who have received large doses of other CNS depressants and/or who are comatose. The manufacturers state that the drug is contraindicated for use in the treatment of lower respiratory tract symptoms (e.g., asthma). There is some evidence that epileptic patients may experience increased severity of seizures if treated with promethazine, and the drug may be contraindicated in these patients. Since increases in blood pressure may occur, promethazine should be administered with extreme caution, if at all, to patients in hypertensive crisis. Some manufacturers state that promethazine also is contraindicated in patients with bone marrow depression, angle-closure glaucoma, prostatic hypertrophy, stenosing peptic ulcer, pyloroduodenal obstruction, or bladder neck obstruction, while others state that the drug may be used with caution in such patients. Some experts do *not* recommend administering promethazine to pediatric patients who are vomiting, unless the vomiting is prolonged and there is a known cause.

● *Pediatric Precautions*

Promethazine (like other antihistamines) should not be used in premature or full-term neonates. (See Cautions: CNS Effects and see Pediatric Precautions, in the Antihistamines General Statement 4:00.)

Because respiratory depression (sometimes fatal) has been reported in pediatric patients younger than 2 years of age receiving a wide range of weight-adjusted doses of promethazine hydrochloride during postmarketing surveillance, the drug is *contraindicated* in this pediatric age group.

Promethazine should be administered with caution in children 2 years of age and older, because of possible respiratory depression and/or apnea that may be fatal. The lowest effective dose of the drug should be used. Concomitant use of promethazine with other respiratory depressants should be avoided.

Children receiving promethazine should be closely supervised while performing hazardous activities such as bike riding. Adults responsible for the supervision of a child receiving promethazine should be warned that children may be at increased risk for experiencing CNS-stimulant effects with antihistamines. The drug should not be used in acutely ill or dehydrated children or in those with acute infections, since these patients have an increased susceptibility to dystonias. Use of promethazine also should be avoided in children with signs and symptoms that suggest Reye's syndrome, since the potential extrapyramidal effects produced by the drug may obscure the diagnosis of or be confused with the CNS signs and symptoms of this condition, and in children with signs and symptoms of other hepatic disease. Because promethazine may cause marked drowsiness that may be potentiated by other CNS depressants (e.g., sedatives, tranquilizers), the antihistamine should be used in children receiving one of these drugs only under the direction of a clinician. Promethazine should not be used in children with asthma, liver disease, a seizure disorder, or glaucoma unless otherwise directed by a clinician.

Excessively high dosages of promethazine hydrochloride have caused sudden death in pediatric patients, although sleep apnea, and sudden infant death syndrome (SIDS) have been reported in a number of infants and young children who were receiving usual dosages of promethazine hydrochloride or trimeprazine (no longer commercially available in the US). The relationship to the drugs and possible mechanism(s) of such effects have not been elucidated. In one study, the number but not the duration of central apneas during sleep was increased and obstructive apnea during sleep (accompanied by decreased heart rate and arterial oxygen pressure) developed in 4 healthy infants who were receiving 1 mg/kg of promethazine hydrochloride daily for 3 days. Promethazine should be used with caution in children with a history of sleep apnea, those with a family history of SIDS, and those who are less prone than usual to spontaneous arousal from sleep.

Overdosage and toxicity (including death) have been reported in children younger than 2 years of age receiving nonprescription (over-the-counter, OTC) preparations containing antihistamines, cough suppressants, expectorants, and nasal decongestants alone or in combination for relief of symptoms of upper respiratory tract infection. Clinicians should ask caregivers about use of nonprescription cough and cold preparations to avoid overdosage. For additional information on precautions associated with the use of cough and cold preparations in pediatric patients, see Cautions: Pediatric Precautions, in the Antihistamines General Statement 4:00.

● Geriatric Precautions

Clinical studies of promethazine did not include sufficient numbers of patients 65 years of age and older to determine whether geriatric patients respond differently than younger patients. While clinical experience generally has not revealed age-related differences in response to the drug, care should be taken in dosage selection of promethazine. Because of increased risk of sedative effects and confusion (associated with promethazine) and the greater frequency of decreased hepatic, renal, and/or cardiac function and of concomitant disease and drug therapy in geriatric patients, the manufacturers suggest that patients in this age group receive initial dosages of the drug in the lower end of the usual range.

● Mutagenicity and Carcinogenicity

Long-term animal studies to determine the carcinogenic potential of promethazine have not been performed to date. There was no evidence of promethazine-induced mutagenesis in the Ames microbial mutagen test. There are no human or other animal data concerning the carcinogenic or mutagenic potentials of the drug. For information on the carcinogenic potential of phenothiazines, see Cautions: Carcinogenicity, in the Phenothiazines General Statement 28:16.08.24.

● Pregnancy, Fertility, and Lactation

Pregnancy

Safe use of promethazine during pregnancy (except during labor) with respect to possible adverse effects on fetal development has not been established. Although there are no adequate and controlled studies to date in humans, promethazine has not been shown to be teratogenic in rats receiving oral dosages of 6.25–12.5 mg/kg daily (about 2.1–4.2 times the maximum recommended human dosage, depending on the use of the drug). The drug has been shown to produce fetal mortality in rats receiving intraperitoneal dosages of 25 mg/kg daily. Antihistamines, including promethazine, have been fetocidal in rodents, but the pharmacologic effects of histamine in rodents differ from those in humans. Promethazine has been reported to possibly ameliorate the effects of hemolytic disease of the newborn† (erythroblastosis fetalis) when administered during pregnancy in Rh-sensitized women, but the safety and efficacy of the drug for this use have not been clearly established; other methods of management are preferred. Promethazine should be used during pregnancy only when the potential benefits justify the possible risks to the fetus.

Fertility

There are no animal or human data concerning the effect of promethazine on fertility.

Lactation

It is not known whether promethazine is distributed into milk. Because many drugs are distributed in human milk and because of the potential for serious adverse reactions to promethazine in nursing infants if it were distributed, a decision should be made whether to discontinue nursing or the drug, taking into account the importance of the drug to the woman.

DRUG INTERACTIONS

● CNS Depressants

Promethazine hydrochloride is additive with or may potentiate the sedative and respiratory depressant actions of opiates or other analgesics and other CNS depressants such as barbiturates or other sedatives, antihistamines, tranquilizers, or alcohol. When promethazine is used concomitantly with other depressant drugs, caution should be used to avoid overdosage. When promethazine is used concomitantly with barbiturates or opiates, dosage of these drugs should be reduced by at least 50 or 25–50%, respectively.

● Epinephrine

Although reversal of the vasopressor effect of epinephrine has not been reported with promethazine, such possibility should be considered. If patients receiving promethazine require a vasopressor agent, norepinephrine or phenylephrine

should be used; *epinephrine should not be used* since it may further decrease blood pressure in patients with partial adrenergic blockade.

● Anticholinergic Agents

Caution should be used during concomitant use of promethazine with drugs having anticholinergic properties.

● Monoamine Oxidase (MAO) Inhibitors

An increased incidence of extrapyramidal effects has been reported in patients receiving phenothiazines concomitantly with MAO inhibitors.

LABORATORY TEST INTERFERENCES

Promethazine may interfere with several immunologic urinary pregnancy tests. The drug may elicit a false-positive Gravindex® test and false-negative Prepurex® and Dap® test. Promethazine may interfere with blood grouping in the ABO system. The drug significantly alters the flare response in intradermal allergen tests.

ACUTE TOXICITY

● Manifestations

In adults, overdosage of promethazine may range from mild depression of the CNS and cardiovascular system to profound hypotension, respiratory depression, seizures, deep sleep, unconsciousness, and sudden death. Hyperreflexia, hypertonia, ataxia, athetosis, and extensor-plantar reflexes (Babinski reflex) also may occur. In children, a paradoxical reaction characterized by hyperexcitability, abnormal movements, nightmares, and respiratory depression may occur. A 12-year-old patient who had taken 200 mg of the drug exhibited numbness and pain in the left leg, tactile hallucinations, extreme hyperesthesia and hyperalgesia, and sinus tachycardia.

● Treatment

Treatment of promethazine overdosage is similar to that of other phenothiazines. Treatment of phenothiazine overdosage generally involves symptomatic and supportive care. General physiologic measures such as maintenance of adequate ventilation should be instituted if necessary. There is no specific antidote for phenothiazine intoxication; however, anticholinergic antiparkinsonian drugs may be useful in controlling extrapyramidal reactions associated with phenothiazine overdosage.

Following acute ingestion of the drugs, the stomach should be emptied by gastric lavage and consideration also should be given to repeated doses of activated charcoal. If the patient is comatose, having seizures or a dystonic reaction, or lacks the gag reflex, gastric lavage may be performed if an endotracheal tube with cuff inflated is in place to prevent aspiration of gastric contents. Gastric lavage may be useful even several hours after the drug has been ingested, since GI motility may be greatly reduced following overdosage of phenothiazines. Induction of emesis generally should not be attempted, since a phenothiazine-induced dystonic reaction of the head or neck may result in aspiration of vomitus during emesis; centrally acting emetics are of little value in the management of promethazine overdosage. Administration of a saline cathartic may be beneficial in enhancing evacuation of the drug from the GI tract.

Cardiovascular monitoring should begin immediately and should include continuous ECG monitoring to detect possible arrhythmias. Treatment may include correction of electrolyte abnormalities and acid-base balance, lidocaine, phenytoin, isoproterenol, ventricular pacing, and defibrillation. Antiarrhythmic agents that can prolong the QT interval (e.g., class IA [disopyramide, procainamide, quinidine] or III agents) should be avoided in treating overdosage-associated arrhythmias in which prolongation of QTc is a manifestation.

Appropriate therapy (IV fluids and a vasopressor [norepinephrine, phenylephrine]) should be instituted if hypotension occurs; epinephrine, bretylium, or dopamine should not be used. See Cautions: Cardiovascular Effects in the Phenothiazines General Statement 28:16.08.24. For the management of refractory hypotension, vasopressors such as phenylephrine, levarterenol, or metaraminol may be used. Acidosis and electrolyte imbalances should be corrected.

Appropriate therapy should be instituted if excessive sedation occurs; CNS stimulants that may cause seizures should be avoided. If seizures occur, treatment should not include barbiturates because these drugs may potentiate phenothiazine-induced respiratory depression. However, pentobarbital and secobarbital have been used in acute overdosage of promethazine. Hypothermia is common and sometimes difficult to control. Naloxone does not appear to reverse the depressant effects of promethazine overdosage.

In some patients with acute toxicity, exchange transfusions may be useful, but hemodialysis, forced diuresis, hemoperfusion, or manipulation of urine pH is of little value in enhancing elimination of phenothiazines.

PHARMACOLOGY

Promethazine is a phenothiazine derivative with potent antihistaminic properties and shares the actions of the antihistamines.

Although the drug can produce either CNS stimulation or CNS depression, CNS depression manifested by sedation is more common with therapeutic doses of promethazine. The precise mechanism of the CNS effects of the drug is not known. Promethazine also has antiemetic, anticholinergic, and local anesthetic effects. In contrast to most other phenothiazines, promethazine also has an antimotion sickness action, possibly as a result of a central anticholinergic effect on the vestibular apparatus and the integrative vomiting center and medullary chemoreceptive trigger zone of the midbrain. Although it has been reported that the drug has slight antitussive activity, this may result from its anticholinergic and CNS-depressant effects. In therapeutic doses, promethazine appears to have no significant effect on the cardiovascular system. Although rapid IV administration of promethazine may produce a transient fall in blood pressure, blood pressure usually is maintained or slightly elevated when the drug is given slowly.

Promethazine has been reported to inhibit collagen-induced neonatal platelet aggregation in vitro and collagen-induced platelet aggregation in neonates whose mothers had received the drug during labor; however, the clinical importance of this effect is not known. Promethazine also has been reported to possibly ameliorate the effects of hemolytic disease of the newborn (erythroblastosis fetalis) when administered during pregnancy in Rh-sensitized women. The exact mechanism(s) has not been elucidated, but several mechanisms may be involved. In vitro studies indicate that promethazine inhibits the ability of fetal macrophages to bind Rh-positive erythrocytes; inhibits phagocytosis and hexose monophosphate shunt activity in polymorphonuclear leukocytes; inhibits lysis of fetal Rh-positive erythrocytes mediated by lymphocytes and polymorphonuclear leukocytes; and stabilizes the erythrocyte membrane against hemolysis. Promethazine also has been shown to have immunosuppressive activity in animals. Although some data suggested that the drug may reduce the number and function of fetal T-cells when administered chronically during pregnancy, other data indicate that the drug does not affect the number of fetal T- or B-cells; further studies on the potential effects of promethazine on fetal immunocompetence are needed.

PHARMACOKINETICS

● *Absorption*

Promethazine is well absorbed from the GI tract and from parenteral sites. Plasma concentrations of promethazine required for antihistaminic effects are unknown. The onset of antihistaminic effects occurs within 20 minutes following oral, rectal, or IM administration, and within 3–5 minutes following IV administration. The duration of antihistaminic effects usually is about 4–6 hours (depending on the dose and route of administration), but such effects may persist for 12 hours or more.

● *Distribution*

Promethazine is widely distributed in body tissues. Compared with other organs, lower concentrations of the drug are found in the brain, but this concentration is higher than the plasma concentration. Promethazine has been reported to be 93% protein bound when determined by gas chromatography and 76–80% bound when determined by high-performance liquid chromatography.

Promethazine readily crosses the placenta. It is not known whether the drug is distributed into milk.

● *Elimination*

Promethazine is metabolized in the liver. The drug is excreted slowly in the urine (mainly) and feces principally as inactive promethazine sulfoxide and glucuronides.

CHEMISTRY AND STABILITY

● *Chemistry*

Promethazine hydrochloride is an ethylamino derivative of phenothiazine and occurs as a racemic mixture. The drug occurs as a white to faint yellow, practically odorless, crystalline powder that slowly oxidizes and turns blue on prolonged exposure to air. The drug is very soluble in water and in hot dehydrated alcohol. Promethazine hydrochloride injection has a pH of 4–5.5. The pKa of the drug is 9.1.

● *Stability*

Promethazine hydrochloride preparations should be protected from light. Promethazine hydrochloride oral solution and tablets should be stored in tight, light-resistant containers at 15–30 and 20–25°C, respectively, while the rectal suppositories should be stored in well-closed containers at 2–8°C. Freezing of the oral solution should be avoided. Following the date of manufacture, commercially available promethazine preparations have expiration dates of 2–5 years depending on the dosage form and manufacturer.

Promethazine hydrochloride injection should be stored in tight, light-resistant containers at 20–25°C with excursions of 15–30°C permitted. The injection should be discarded if the solution is discolored or contains a precipitate. Promethazine hydrochloride injection has been reported to be chemically incompatible with several drugs, especially those with an alkaline pH. However, the compatibility depends on several factors (e.g., concentration of the drugs, specific diluents used, resulting pH, temperature). Specialized references should be consulted for specific compatibility information.

PREPARATIONS

Excipients in commercially available drug preparations may have clinically important effects in some individuals; consult specific product labeling for details.

Promethazine Hydrochloride

Oral

Solution	6.25 mg/5 mL*	Promethazine Hydrochloride Syrup
Tablets	12.5 mg*	Phenergan® (scored), Wyeth
		Promethazine Hydrochloride Tablets
	25 mg*	Phenergan® (scored), Wyeth
		Promethazine Hydrochloride Tablets
	50 mg*	Phenergan®, Wyeth
		Promethazine Hydrochloride Tablets

Parenteral

Injection	25 mg/mL*	Promethazine Hydrochloride Injection
Injection, for IM use only	50 mg/mL*	Promethazine Hydrochloride Injection

Rectal

Suppositories	12.5 mg*	Phenadoz®, Paddock
		Phenergan®, Wyeth
		Promethazine Hydrochloride Suppositories
	25 mg*	Phenadoz®, Paddock
		Phenergan®, Wyeth
		Promethazine Hydrochloride Suppositories
	50 mg*	Phenergan®, Wyeth
		Promethazine Hydrochloride Suppositories
		Promethegan®, G&W

* available from one or more manufacturer, distributor, and/or repackager by generic (nonproprietary) name

Promethazine Hydrochloride Combinations

Oral

Solution	6.25 mg/5 mL with Phenylephrine Hydrochloride 5 mg/5 mL*	Prometh® VC Syrup, Actavis

* available from one or more manufacturer, distributor, and/or repackager by generic (nonproprietary) name

† Use is not currently included in the labeling approved by the US Food and Drug Administration.

Selected Revisions September 24, 2018, © Copyright, May 1, 1976, American Society of Health-System Pharmacists, Inc.

Table of Contents

8:00 ANTI-INFECTIVE AGENTS

§ Omitted from the print version of *AHFS Drug
Information* because of space limitations. This
monograph is available on the *AHFS Drug Information*
web site, http://www.ahfsdruginformation.com.
See the Preface for details on accessing this site.

Cefadroxil

8:12.06.04 • FIRST GENERATION CEPHALOSPORINS

■ Cefadroxil is a semisynthetic, first generation cephalosporin antibiotic.

USES

● Pharyngitis and Tonsillitis

Oral cefadroxil is used for the treatment of pharyngitis and tonsillitis caused by *Streptococcus pyogenes* (group A β-hemolytic streptococci). Although cefadroxil generally is effective in eradicating *S. pyogenes* from the nasopharynx, efficacy of the drug in prevention of subsequent rheumatic fever has not been established to date.

Selection of an anti-infective for the treatment of *S. pyogenes* pharyngitis and tonsillitis should be based on the drug's spectrum of activity, bacteriologic and clinical efficacy, potential adverse effects, ease of administration, patient compliance, and cost. No regimen has been found to date that effectively eradicates group A β-hemolytic streptococci in 100% of patients.

Because the drugs have a narrow spectrum of activity, are inexpensive, and generally are effective with a low frequency of adverse effects, the American Academy of Pediatrics (AAP), Infectious Diseases Society of America (IDSA), American Heart Association (AHA), and others recommend a penicillin regimen (i.e., 10 days of oral penicillin V or oral amoxicillin or single dose of IM penicillin G benzathine) as the treatment of choice for *S. pyogenes* pharyngitis and tonsillitis and prevention of initial attacks (primary prevention) of rheumatic fever. Other anti-infectives (e.g., oral cephalosporins, oral macrolides, oral clindamycin) are recommended as alternatives in penicillin-allergic individuals.

If an oral cephalosporin is used for the treatment of *S. pyogenes* pharyngitis and tonsillitis, a 10-day regimen of a first generation cephalosporin (cefadroxil, cephalexin) is preferred instead of other cephalosporins with broader spectrums of activity (e.g., cefaclor, cefdinir, cefixime, cefpodoxime, cefuroxime).

● Skin and Skin Structure Infections

Oral cefadroxil is used for the treatment of mild to moderate skin and skin structure infections caused by susceptible staphylococci or streptococci.

● Urinary Tract Infections

Oral cefadroxil is used for the treatment of mild to moderate urinary tract infections, including acute prostatitis, caused by susceptible *Escherichia coli*, *Klebsiella*, or *Proteus mirabilis*.

● Prevention of Bacterial Endocarditis

Oral cefadroxil is used as an alternative for prevention of α-hemolytic (viridans group) streptococcal endocarditis† in penicillin-allergic individuals undergoing certain dental or upper respiratory tract procedures who have underlying cardiac conditions that put them at highest risk of adverse outcomes from endocarditis. Cefadroxil should not be used for such prophylaxis in those with a history of immediate-type hypersensitivity to penicillins (e.g., urticaria, angioedema, anaphylaxis).

For information on which cardiac conditions are associated with highest risk of endocarditis and which procedures require prophylaxis, see Prevention under Uses: Endocarditis, in the Cephalosporins General Statement 8:12.06. When selecting anti-infectives for prophylaxis of bacterial endocarditis, the current recommendations published by the AHA should be consulted.

DOSAGE AND ADMINISTRATION

● Reconstitution and Administration

Cefadroxil is administered orally.

Cefadroxil may be administered without regard to meals. Administration with food may minimize adverse GI effects.

Reconstitution

Cefadroxil powder for oral suspension should be reconstituted at the time of dispensing by adding the amount of water specified on the container to provide a suspension containing 125, 250, or 500 mg of cefadroxil per 5 mL. The water should be added in 2 equal portions and the bottle shaken after each addition.

The oral suspension should be shaken well prior to administration of each dose.

● Dosage

Adult Dosage

Pharyngitis and Tonsillitis

For the treatment of pharyngitis and tonsillitis caused by *Streptococcus pyogenes* (group A β-hemolytic streptococci), the usual adult dosage of cefadroxil is 1 g daily given as a single dose or in 2 equally divided doses for 10 days.

Skin and Skin Structure Infections

For the treatment of skin and skin structure infections, the usual adult dosage of cefadroxil is 1 g daily given as a single dose or in 2 equally divided doses.

Urinary Tract Infections

For the treatment of uncomplicated urinary tract infections (i.e., cystitis), the usual adult dosage of cefadroxil is 1 or 2 g daily given as a single dose or in 2 equally divided doses. The usual adult dosage for the treatment of other urinary tract infections is 2 g daily given in 2 equally divided doses.

Pediatric Dosage

General Pediatric Dosage

The American Academy of Pediatrics (AAP) recommends that pediatric patients beyond the neonatal period receive cefadroxil in a dosage of 30 mg/kg daily in 2 equally divided doses for the treatment of mild or moderate infections. The AAP states that the drug is inappropriate for the treatment of severe infections.

Pharyngitis and Tonsillitis

For the treatment of group A β-hemolytic streptococcal pharyngitis and tonsillitis, the usual pediatric dosage of cefadroxil is 30 mg/kg daily given as a single dose or in 2 equally divided doses for 10 days.

Skin and Skin Structure Infections

For the treatment of impetigo, pediatric patients should receive cefadroxil in a dosage of 30 mg/kg daily given as a single dose or in 2 equally divided doses. For the treatment of other skin and skin structure infections, children should receive 30 mg/kg daily given in divided doses every 12 hours.

Urinary Tract Infections

For the treatment of urinary tract infections, the usual pediatric dosage of cefadroxil is 30 mg/kg daily given in divided doses every 12 hours.

● Dosage in Renal Impairment

In patients with creatinine clearances of 50 mL/minute per 1.73 m² or lower, doses and/or frequency of administration of cefadroxil must be modified in response to the degree of renal impairment. The manufacturers recommend that adults receive an initial dose of 1 g followed by 500-mg maintenance doses at the following dosage intervals based on the patient's creatinine clearance: (See Table 1.)

TABLE 1. Adult Dosage of Cefadroxil in Renal Impairment

Cl$_{cr}$ (mL/min per 1.73 m²)	Initial Dose	Maintenance Dosage
25–50	1 g	500 mg every 12 hours
10–25	1 g	500 mg every 24 hours
0–10	1 g	500 mg every 36 hours

CAUTIONS

Cefadroxil shares the toxic potentials of other cephalosporins, and the usual cautions, precautions, and contraindications associated with cephalosporin therapy should be observed. (See Cautions in the Cephalosporins General Statement 8:12.06.)

SPECTRUM

Based on its spectrum of activity, cefadroxil is classified as a first generation cephalosporin. For information on the classification of cephalosporins and closely related β-lactam antibiotics based on spectra of activity, see Spectrum in the Cephalosporins General Statement 8:12.06. Like other first generation cephalosporins (e.g., cefazolin, cephalexin), cefadroxil is active in vitro against many gram-positive aerobic cocci but has limited activity against gram-negative bacteria.

● In Vitro Susceptibility Testing

Strains of staphylococci resistant to penicillinase-resistant penicillins (methicillin-resistant [oxacillin-resistant] staphylococci) should be considered resistant to cephalexin, although results of in vitro susceptibility tests may indicate that the organisms are susceptible to the drug.

For information on interpreting results of in vitro susceptibility testing (disk susceptibility tests, dilution susceptibility tests) when cefadroxil susceptibility testing is performed according to the standards of the Clinical and Laboratory Standards Institute (CLSI; formerly National Committee for Clinical Laboratory Standards [NCCLS]), see Spectrum: In Vitro Susceptibility Testing, in the Cephalosporins General Statement 8:12.06.

PHARMACOKINETICS

● Absorption

Cefadroxil is acid-stable and is rapidly and almost completely absorbed from the GI tract. The rate of absorption and peak serum concentrations of cefadroxil are not affected when the drug is administered with food.

Following oral administration in healthy adults with normal renal function, peak serum cefadroxil concentrations are attained within 1–2 hours and average about 10–18 mcg/mL following a single 500-mg dose and 24–35 mcg/mL following a single 1-g dose.

In a group of children 13 months to 12 years of age with normal renal function, peak serum concentrations of cefadroxil averaged 13.7 mcg/mL and were attained within 1 hour after a single oral dose of 15 mg/kg; serum concentrations of the drug were 0.6–1.8 mcg/mL at 6 hours.

● Elimination

The serum half-life of cefadroxil is 1.1–2 hours in adults with normal renal function.

Cefadroxil is excreted unchanged in urine. In adults with normal renal function, from 70 to more than 90% of a single 500-mg or 1-g oral dose of the drug is excreted unchanged in urine within 24 hours, principally within the first 6–9 hours after administration. In adults with normal renal function, peak urine concentrations of cefadroxil of 1.8 mg/mL may be attained following a single 500-mg oral dose.

The serum half-life of cefadroxil is prolonged in patients with impaired renal function. The half-life of cefadroxil is 2.5–8.5 hours in patients with creatinine clearances of 20–50 mL/minute per 1.73 m^2 and 13.3–25.5 hours in patients with creatinine clearances less than 20 mL/minute per 1.73 m^2. Renal elimination of cefadroxil is substantially reduced in patients with creatinine clearances less than 20 mL/minute per 1.73 m^2, with about 10–30% of a single oral dose excreted unchanged in urine within 24 hours.

Cefadroxil is removed by hemodialysis.

CHEMISTRY AND STABILITY

● Chemistry

Cefadroxil is a semisynthetic cephalosporin antibiotic. Cefadroxil is commercially available as the monohydrate which occurs as a white to yellowish-white, crystalline powder and is soluble in water and slightly soluble in alcohol.

● Stability

Cefadroxil capsules and tablets should be stored in tight containers at 20–25°C.

Cefadroxil powder for oral suspension should be stored at 20–25°C. After reconstitution, cefadroxil oral suspension should be refrigerated in a tight container; any unused suspension should be discarded if not used within 14 days.

For further information on chemistry, mechanism of action, spectrum, resistance, pharmacokinetics, uses, cautions, drug interactions, laboratory test interferences, and dosage and administration of cefadroxil, see the Cephalosporins General Statement 8:12.06.

PREPARATIONS

Excipients in commercially available drug preparations may have clinically important effects in some individuals; consult specific product labeling for details.

Cefadroxil

Oral		
Capsules	500 mg*	**Cefadroxil Capsules**
For suspension	125 mg/5 mL*	**Cefadroxil for Suspension**
	250 mg/5 mL*	**Cefadroxil for Suspension**
	500 mg/5 mL*	**Cefadroxil for Suspension**
Tablets	1 g*	**Cefadroxil Tablets**

* available from one or more manufacturer, distributor, and/or repackager by generic (nonproprietary) name

† Use is not currently included in the labeling approved by the US Food and Drug Administration.

ceFAZolin Sodium

8:12.06.04 • FIRST GENERATION CEPHALOSPORINS

■ Cefazolin sodium is a semisynthetic, first generation cephalosporin antibiotic.

USES

● Biliary Tract Infections

Cefazolin is used for the treatment of biliary tract infections caused by susceptible *Escherichia coli*, *Klebsiella*, *Proteus mirabilis*, *Staphylococcus aureus*, or various streptococci.

● Bone and Joint Infections

Cefazolin is used for the treatment of bone and joint infections caused by susceptible *S. aureus*.

● Endocarditis

Treatment

Staphylococcal Endocarditis

Cefazolin is used as an alternative to nafcillin or oxacillin for the treatment of staphylococcal endocarditis, including infections caused by coagulase-positive strains (*S. aureus*) or coagulase-negative strains (e.g., *S. epidermidis*, *S. lugdunensis*) in penicillin-allergic patients (nonanaphylactoid type only). Cefazolin should *not* be used in patients with a history of immediate-type penicillin hypersensitivity (urticaria, angioedema, anaphylaxis).

For the treatment of native valve endocarditis caused by oxacillin-susceptible (methicillin-susceptible) staphylococci, the American Heart Association (AHA) and Infectious Diseases Society of America (IDSA) recommend a regimen of IV nafcillin or oxacillin with or without IV or IM gentamicin. For penicillin-allergic patients (nonanaphylactoid type only), a regimen of IV cefazolin with or without IV or IM gentamicin is recommended. In patients with complicated right-sided staphylococcal endocarditis or with left-sided staphylococcal endocarditis, a 6-week regimen of the β-lactam should be used and gentamicin given concomitantly during the first 3–5 days of treatment. In those with uncomplicated right-sided staphylococcal endocarditis (i.e., patients with no evidence of renal failure, extrapulmonary metastatic infections, aortic or mitral valve involvement, meningitis, or oxacillin-resistant strains), a 2-week regimen that includes both the β-lactam and gentamicin can be considered.

Staphylococcal endocarditis in patients with prosthetic valves or other prosthetic material usually is caused by oxacillin-resistant staphylococci, especially when endocarditis develops within 1 year after surgery, and is associated with high morbidity and mortality rates. Unless susceptibility to oxacillin has been demonstrated using in vitro susceptibility testing, it should be assumed that patients with staphylococcal prosthetic valve endocarditis have oxacillin-resistant strains. If prosthetic valve endocarditis is known to be caused by oxacillin-susceptible staphylococci, the AHA and IDSA recommend at least 6 weeks of IV nafcillin or oxacillin in conjunction with IV or oral rifampin and concomitant use of IV or IM gentamicin during the initial 2 weeks of treatment. If the strain is known to be penicillin susceptible (i.e., penicillin MIC 0.1 mcg/mL or less) and does not produce β-lactamase, IV penicillin G sodium can be substituted for nafcillin or oxacillin in this regimen; for penicillin-allergic patients (nonanaphylactoid type only), IV cefazolin can be substituted for nafcillin or oxacillin.

Cefazolin and other cephalosporins should *not* be used for the treatment of endocarditis caused by oxacillin-resistant staphylococci, despite the fact that in vitro testing may indicate the strains are susceptible. If the strain is known or presumed to be oxacillin-resistant, the AHA and IDSA recommend at least 6 weeks of IV vancomycin in conjunction with IV or oral rifampin and concomitant use of IV or IM gentamicin during the initial 2 weeks of treatment.

Streptococcal Endocarditis

Cefazolin is used as an alternative to penicillin G sodium for the treatment of endocarditis caused by susceptible *Streptococcus pyogenes* (group A β-hemolytic streptococci), or *S. pneumoniae*†.

For the treatment of endocarditis caused by highly penicillin-susceptible *S. pneumoniae*†, the AHA and IDSA recommend a 4-week regimen of penicillin G sodium, cefazolin, or ceftriaxone. Vancomycin should only be used in patients who cannot receive a β-lactam. It has been suggested that high-dose treatment with penicillin G sodium or a third-generation cephalosporin can be used in patients with endocarditis caused by penicillin-resistant *S. pneumoniae* provided meningitis is not present. However, penicillin-resistant *S. pneumoniae* often are cross-resistant to cephalosporins, and consultation with an infectious disease specialist is recommended whenever decisions are being made regarding treatment of pneumococcal endocarditis.

For the treatment of endocarditis caused by *S. pyogenes*, the AHA and IDSA recommend a 4-week regimen of IV penicillin G sodium. In penicillin-allergic patients (nonanaphylactoid type only), cefazolin or ceftriaxone are acceptable alternatives. Vancomycin should only be used in patients who cannot receive a β-lactam.

For the treatment of endocarditis caused by groups B, C, or G streptococci, the AHA and IDSA recommend 4–6 weeks of IV penicillin G sodium or, alternatively, a cephalosporin; some clinicians recommend that gentamicin be added to the regimen for at least the first 2 weeks. Consultation with an infections disease specialist is recommended.

Prevention

Cefazolin is used for the prevention of α-hemolytic (viridans group) streptococcal endocarditis† in penicillin-allergic individuals undergoing certain dental or upper respiratory tract procedures who have cardiac conditions that put them at highest risk. Oral amoxicillin is the usual drug of choice for such prophylaxis. Cefazolin is an alternative in penicillin-allergic individuals or when an oral anti-infective cannot be used. Cefazolin should not be used in those with immediate-type penicillin hypersensitivity (e.g., urticaria, angioedema, anaphylaxis).

For information on which cardiac conditions are associated with the highest risk of endocarditis and which procedures require prophylaxis, see Prevention under Uses: Endocarditis, in the Cephalosporins General Statement 8:12.06. When selecting anti-infectives for prophylaxis of bacterial endocarditis, the current recommendations published by the AHA should be consulted.

● Respiratory Tract Infections

Cefazolin is used for the treatment of respiratory tract infections caused by susceptible *S. pneumoniae*, *S. pyogenes* (group A β-hemolytic streptococci), *S. aureus* (including penicillin-resistant strains), *Klebsiella*, or *Haemophilus influenzae*.

● Septicemia

Cefazolin is used for the treatment of septicemia caused by susceptible *S. pneumoniae*, *S. aureus* (including penicillinase-producing strains), *E. coli*, *Klebsiella*, or *P. mirabilis*.

● Skin and Skin Structure Infections

Cefazolin is used for the treatment of skin or skin structure infections caused by susceptible *S. aureus* (including penicillinase-producing strains), *S. pyogenes*, or other streptococci.

● Urinary Tract and Urogenital Infections

Cefazolin is used for the treatment of urinary tract infections caused by susceptible *E. coli*, *P. mirabilis*, *Klebsiella*, some strains of *Enterobacter*, or some strains of enterococci.

Cefazolin is used for the treatment of prostatitis or epididymitis caused by susceptible *E. coli*, *Klebsiella*, *P. mirabilis*, or some strains of enterococci.

● Prevention of Perinatal Group B Streptococcal Disease

In certain penicillin-allergic women, cefazolin is used as an alternative to penicillin G or ampicillin for prevention of perinatal group B streptococcal (GBS) disease†.

Pregnant women who are colonized with GBS in the genital or rectal areas can transmit GBS infection to their infants during labor and delivery resulting in invasive neonatal infection that can be associated with substantial morbidity and mortality. Intrapartum anti-infective prophylaxis for prevention of early-onset neonatal GBS disease is administered *selectively* to women at high risk for transmitting GBS infection to their neonates. The US Centers for Disease Control and Prevention (CDC), American Academy of Pediatrics (AAP), and other experts recommend *routine* universal prenatal culture-based screening for GBS colonization† (vaginal and rectal cultures) in *all* pregnant women at 35–37 weeks of gestation, unless GBS bacteriuria is known to be present during the current pregnancy or the woman had a previous infant with invasive GBS disease. These experts state that anti-infective prophylaxis to prevent perinatal GBS disease is indicated in pregnant women identified as GBS carriers during the routine pre-natal GBS screening performed at 35–37 weeks during the current pregnancy, in women with GBS bacteriuria identified at any time during the current pregnancy, and in women who had a previous infant diagnosed with invasive GBS disease. Anti-infective prophylaxis to prevent perinatal GBS disease also is indicated in women with unknown GBS status at the time of onset of labor (i.e., culture not done, incomplete, or results unknown) if delivery is at less than 37 weeks of gesta-tion, the duration of amniotic membrane rupture is 18 hours or longer, intrapar-tum temperature is 38°C or higher, or an intrapartum nucleic acid amplification test (NAAT) was positive for GBS.

When intrapartum prophylaxis is indicated in the mother to prevent GBS disease in the neonate, it should be given at onset of labor or rupture of mem-branes. The CDC, AAP, and other experts recommend penicillin G as the drug of choice and ampicillin as the preferred alternative for such prophy-laxis. If intrapartum prophylaxis is indicated in a penicillin-allergic woman who is *not* at high risk for anaphylaxis (i.e., does not have a history of ana-phylaxis, angioedema, respiratory distress, or urticaria after receiving a penicil-lin or cephalosporin), IV cefazolin is recommended. If intrapartum prophylaxis is indicated in a penicillin-allergic woman who is at high risk for anaphylaxis (e.g., history of anaphylaxis, angioedema, respiratory distress, or urticaria after receiving a penicillin or cephalosporin), IV clindamycin is recommended if the GBS isolate is susceptible to the drug; alternatively, IV vancomycin can be used if the isolate is resistant to clindamycin.

For additional information regarding prevention of perinatal group B strepto-coccal disease, the current CDC guidelines available at http://www.cdc.gov should be consulted.

• Perioperative Prophylaxis

Cefazolin is used perioperatively to reduce the incidence of infection in patients undergoing certain cardiac surgery (e.g., coronary artery bypass, placement of cardiac devices), noncardiac thoracic surgery (e.g., lobectomy), vascular surgery (arterial surgery involving the abdominal aorta, a prosthesis, or a groin incision or lower extremity amputation for ischemia), head and neck surgery involving incisions through oral or pharyngeal mucosa, neurosurgery (e.g., craniotomy, spi-nal surgery), orthopedic surgery (e.g., total joint replacement, surgical repair of closed fractures, internal fixation of compound or open fractures), GI surgery (gastroduodenal, esophageal, biliary tract, colorectal, appendectomy, bariatric), genitourinary surgery (e.g., open or laparoscopic surgery including percutane-ous renal surgery, procedures with entry into the urinary tract or implantation of a prosthesis), and gynecologic and obstetric surgery (cesarean section or vaginal, abdominal, or laparoscopic hysterectomy). Published guidelines and protocols for perioperative prophylaxis should be consulted for recommendations regarding specific procedures.

Because cefazolin has a narrow spectrum of activity that covers the most likely surgical site pathogens, has a moderately long serum half-life, and has been shown to be effective, it is considered by many clinicians to be the drug of choice for perioperative prophylaxis for a wide variety of contaminated or potentially con-taminated procedures. Cefazolin also is recommended as a drug of choice for perioperative prophylaxis in patients undergoing heart, lung, heart-lung, pan-creas, and pancreas-kidney transplantation.

If cefazolin is used for perioperative prophylaxis in patients undergoing cer-tain GI procedures (e.g., colorectal surgery, appendectomy) that might involve exposure to *Bacteroides fragilis* or other anaerobic bowel bacteria or in patients undergoing head and neck surgery involving incisions through oral or pharyngeal mucosa, it should be used in conjunction with metronidazole to provide anaer-obic coverage. (See Uses: Perioperative Prophylaxis, in the Cephalosporins Gen-eral Statement 8:12.06.)

DOSAGE AND ADMINISTRATION

• Reconstitution and Administration

Cefazolin sodium is administered by IV injection or infusion or by deep IM injec-tion. The drug also has been administered intraperitoneally in dialysis solutions†.

Prior to administration, cefazolin solutions should be inspected visually for particulate matter; if particulate matter is evident, the solution should be discarded.

Intermittent IV Injection

For direct IV injection, vials labeled as containing 500 mg or 1 g of cefazolin should be reconstituted with 2 or 2.5 mL, respectively, of sterile water for injection to provide solutions containing approximately 225 or 330 mg/mL, respectively. These solutions should be further diluted in approximately 5 mL of sterile water for injection, or according to the manufacturers' directions.

The appropriate dose should then be injected over a period of 3–5 minutes directly into a vein or the tubing of a freely flowing compatible IV solution.

Intermittent or Continuous IV Infusion

For intermittent IV infusion, vials labeled as containing 500 mg or 1 g of cefazolin should be reconstituted with 2 or 2.5 mL, respectively, of sterile water for injec-tion to provide solutions containing approximately 225 or 330 mg/mL, respec-tively. The reconstituted solutions should be further diluted in 50–100 mL of a compatible IV solution.

Alternatively, the commercially available Duplex® drug delivery system con-taining 1 or 2 g of cefazolin and 50 mL of dextrose 4 or 3% injection, respectively, in separate chambers should be reconstituted (activated) according to the manu-facturer's directions and administered by IV infusion.

Cefazolin pharmacy bulk vials should be reconstituted according to the man-ufacturer's directions and then further diluted in a compatible IV solution prior to IV infusion. The reconstituted solutions should be used promptly; the pharmacy bulk vial should be discarded within 4 hours after initial entry.

Thawed solutions of the commercially available frozen premixed cefazolin sodium injection in dextrose should be given only by intermittent or continuous IV infusion. The frozen injection should be thawed at room temperature (25°C) or under refrigeration (5°C); the injection should not be thawed by warming in a water bath or by exposure to microwave radiation. Precipitates that may have formed in the frozen injection usually will dissolve with little or no agitation when the injection reaches room temperature; potency is not affected. After thawing to room temperature, the injection should be agitated and the container checked for minute leaks by firmly squeezing the bag. The injection should be discarded if container seals or outlet ports are not intact or leaks are found or if the solution is cloudy or contains an insoluble precipitate. Additives should not be introduced into the injection container. The injection should not be used in series connec-tions with other plastic containers, since such use could result in air embolism from residual air being drawn from the primary container before administration of fluid from the secondary container is complete.

IM Injection

IM injections of cefazolin sodium are prepared by reconstituting vials labeled as con-taining 500 mg or 1 g of cefazolin with 2 or 2.5 mL, respectively, of sterile water for injec-tion to provide solutions containing approximately 225 or 330 mg/mL, respectively.

IM injections of cefazolin should be made deeply into a large muscle mass.

• Dosage

Dosage of cefazolin sodium is expressed in terms of cefazolin and is identical for IM or IV administration.

To avoid unintentional overdosage, the commercially available Duplex® drug delivery system containing cefazolin and dextrose injection and the commercially available frozen premixed cefazolin injection in dextrose should *not* be used in patients who require less than the entire 1- or 2-g dose in the container.

Adult Dosage

General Adult Dosage

The usual adult dosage of cefazolin for the treatment of mild infections caused by susceptible gram-positive cocci is 250–500 mg every 8 hours.

The usual adult dosage of cefazolin for the treatment of moderate to severe infections is 0.5–1 g every 6–8 hours.

The usual adult dosage of cefazolin for the treatment of severe, life-threat-ening infections (e.g., endocarditis, septicemia) is 1–1.5 g every 6 hours. In rare instances, up to 12 g daily has been used.

Endocarditis Treatment

For the treatment of endocarditis caused by staphylococci or *Streptococcus pneu-moniae*, the manufacturers recommend that adults receive 1–1.5 g of cefazolin every 6 hours. Dosage up to 12 g daily has been used.

If IV cefazolin is used for the treatment of native valve staphylococcal endocarditis in penicillin-allergic patients (nonanaphylactoid type only) with oxacillin-susceptible (methicillin-susceptible) strains, the American Heart Association (AHA) and Infectious Diseases Society of America (IDSA) recommend that adults receive 6 g daily given in 3 equally divided doses; cefazolin should be given for 6 weeks and may be used with or without IM or IV gentamicin (3 mg/kg daily in 3 equally divided doses given during the first 3–5 days of the cefazolin regimen).

If IV cefazolin is used for the treatment of prosthetic valve staphylococcal endocarditis in penicillin-allergic patients (nonanaphylactoid type only) with oxacillin-susceptible strains, the AHA and IDSA recommend that adults receive 6 g daily given in 3 equally divided doses; cefazolin should be given for 6 weeks or longer and used in conjunction with IV or IM gentamicin (3 mg/kg daily given in 2 or 3 equally divided doses during the first 2 weeks of treatment) and IV or oral rifampin (900 mg daily given in 3 equally divided doses for 6 weeks or longer).

If cefazolin is used for the treatment of endocarditis caused by susceptible *S. pyogenes* or *S. pneumoniae*†, the AHA recommends a treatment duration of 4 weeks.

If cefazolin is used for the treatment of endocarditis caused by groups B, C, or G streptococci†, a treatment duration of 4–6 weeks is recommended and some clinicians also include gentamicin during at least the first 2 weeks. Consultation with an infectious disease specialist is recommended.

Endocarditis Prevention

If cefazolin is used as an alternative for *prevention* of α-hemolytic (viridans group) streptococcal endocarditis† in individuals considered to be at highest risk for bacterial endocarditis following certain dental or upper respiratory tract procedures, adults should receive a single 1-g IM or IV dose administered 0.5–1 hour prior to the procedure. Cefazolin should *not* be used for such prophylaxis in individuals with a history of immediate-type hypersensitivity reactions to penicillin.

Respiratory Tract Infections

The usual adult dosage of cefazolin for the treatment of pneumonia caused by *S. pneumoniae* is 500 mg every 12 hours.

Septicemia

The usual adult dosage of cefazolin for the treatment of septicemia is 1–1.5 g every 6 hours. Dosage up to 12 g daily has been used.

Urinary Tract Infections

The usual adult dosage of cefazolin for the treatment of acute, uncomplicated urinary tract infections is 1 g every 12 hours.

Prevention of Perinatal Group B Streptococcal Disease

If cefazolin is used for intrapartum anti-infective prophylaxis for prevention of perinatal group B streptococcal (GBS) disease in women with penicillin hypersensitivity who are not at risk for anaphylaxis, the US Centers for Disease Control and Prevention (CDC) recommends that an initial 2-g IV dose of cefazolin be given at the time of onset of labor or rupture of membranes followed by 1 g IV every 8 hours until delivery. (See Uses: Prevention of Perinatal Group B Streptococcal Disease.)

Perioperative Prophylaxis

For perioperative prophylaxis in contaminated or potentially contaminated surgery, the manufacturers recommend that adults receive 1 or 2 g of cefazolin IM or IV 30–60 minutes prior to surgery and state that additional doses of 0.5–1 g may be given IM or IV during the procedure. Although the manufacturers state that 0.5–1 g may be given IM or IV every 6–8 hours for 24 hours postoperatively and, when the occurrence of infection may be particularly devastating (e.g., open-heart surgery, prosthetic arthroplasty), prophylaxis may be continued for 3–5 days postoperatively, most clinicians state that the duration of prophylaxis should be less than 24 hours for most procedures.

For perioperative prophylaxis in adults undergoing certain cardiac surgery, noncardiac thoracic surgery, vascular surgery, head and neck surgery, neurosurgery, orthopedic surgery, GI surgery, genitourinary surgery, or gynecologic and obstetric surgery (see Uses: Perioperative Prophylaxis), cefazolin should be given within 60 minutes before surgical incision to ensure adequate serum and tissue concentrations. Some experts recommend a cefazolin dose of 1 g in adults weighing less than 80 kg and 2 g in those weighing 80 kg or more and suggest that morbidly obese patients may need higher dosage. Other experts recommend a cefazolin dose of 2 g for most adults and 3 g in those weighing 120 kg or more.

During prolonged procedures (longer than 4 hours) or if major blood loss occurs, additional intraoperative doses of cefazolin should be given every 4 hours. The duration of prophylaxis should be less than 24 hours for most procedures; there is no evidence to support continuing prophylaxis after wound closure or until all indwelling drains and intravascular catheters are removed.

If cefazolin is used for perioperative prophylaxis in patients undergoing certain GI procedures (e.g., colorectal surgery, appendectomy) that might involve exposure to *Bacteroides fragilis* or other anaerobic bowel bacteria or in patients undergoing head and neck surgery involving incisions through oral or pharyngeal mucosa, the usual cefazolin dose should be given in conjunction with IV metronidazole (0.5 g) within 60 minutes before surgical incision.

Pediatric Dosage
General Dosage for Neonates

The manufacturers state that safety and efficacy of cefazolin have not been established in premature infants or neonates 1 month of age or younger.

The American Academy of Pediatrics (AAP) recommends that neonates 7 days of age or younger† receive IV or IM cefazolin in a dosage of 25 mg/kg every 12 hours, regardless of weight. For neonates 8–28 days of age†, the AAP recommends a dosage of 25 mg/kg every 12 hours for those weighing 2 kg or less and 25 mg/kg every 8 hours for those weighing more than 2 kg.

General Dosage for Infants and Children

The usual dosage of cefazolin recommended by the manufacturers for the treatment of mild to moderately severe infections in pediatric patients older than 1 month of age is 25–50 mg/kg daily given in 3 or 4 equally divided doses. The manufacturers state that dosage may be increased to 100 mg/kg daily in divided doses for the treatment of severe infections.

The AAP recommends that pediatric patients beyond the neonatal period receive IV or IM cefazolin in a dosage of 25–50 mg/kg daily given in 3 equally divided doses for the treatment of mild to moderate infections or 100–150 mg/kg daily given in 3 equally divided doses for the treatment of severe infections.

Endocarditis Treatment

If IV cefazolin is used for the treatment of native valve staphylococcal endocarditis in penicillin-allergic patients (nonanaphylactoid type only) with oxacillin-susceptible strains, the AHA and IDSA recommend that pediatric patients receive 100 mg/kg daily (up to 6 g daily) given in 3 or 4 equally divided doses; cefazolin should be given for 6 weeks and may be used with or without IM or IV gentamicin (3 mg/kg daily in 3 equally divided doses given during the first 3–5 days of the cefazolin regimen).

If IV cefazolin is used for the treatment of prosthetic valve staphylococcal endocarditis in penicillin-allergic patients (nonanaphylactoid type only) with oxacillin-susceptible strains, the AHA and IDSA recommend that pediatric patients receive 100 mg/kg daily (up to 6 g daily) given in 3 or 4 equally divided doses; cefazolin should be given for 6 weeks or longer and used in conjunction with IV or IM gentamicin (3 mg/kg daily given in 2 or 3 equally divided doses during the first 2 weeks of treatment) and IV or oral rifampin (20 mg/kg daily in 3 equally divided doses given for 6 weeks or longer).

If cefazolin is used for the treatment of endocarditis caused by susceptible *S. pyogenes* or *S. pneumoniae*†, the AHA recommends a treatment duration of 4 weeks.

Endocarditis Prevention

If cefazolin is used as an alternative for *prevention* of α-hemolytic (viridans group) streptococcal endocarditis† in individuals considered to be at highest risk for bacterial endocarditis following certain dental or upper respiratory tract procedures, pediatric patients should receive a single dose of 50 mg/kg given IM or IV 0.5–1 hour prior to the procedure. Cefazolin should *not* be used for such prophylaxis in individuals with a history of immediate-type hypersensitivity reactions to penicillin.

Perioperative Prophylaxis

For perioperative prophylaxis in pediatric patients undergoing certain cardiac surgery, noncardiac thoracic surgery, vascular surgery, head and neck surgery, neurosurgery, orthopedic surgery, GI surgery, or genitourinary surgery (see Uses: Perioperative Prophylaxis), some experts recommend that cefazolin should be given in a dose of 30 mg/kg within 60 minutes before surgical incision to ensure adequate serum and tissue concentrations.

During prolonged procedures (longer than 4 hours) or if major blood loss occurs, additional intraoperative doses of cefazolin should be given every 4 hours. The duration of prophylaxis should be less than 24 hours for most procedures; there is no evidence to support continuing prophylaxis after wound closure or until all indwelling drains and intravascular catheters are removed.

If cefazolin is used for perioperative prophylaxis in patients undergoing certain GI procedures (e.g., colorectal surgery, appendectomy) that might involve exposure to *B. fragilis* or other anaerobic bowel bacteria or in patients undergoing head and neck surgery involving incisions through oral or pharyngeal mucosa, pediatric patients should receive the usual cefazolin dose in conjunction with IV metronidazole (15 mg/kg) within 60 minutes before surgical incision.

● Dosage in Renal Impairment

In patients with impaired renal function, doses and/or frequency of administration of cefazolin must be modified in response to the degree of impairment, severity of the infection, susceptibility of the causative organism, and serum concentrations of the drug.

The manufacturers recommend an initial loading dose appropriate for the severity of the infection followed by dosage based on the degree of renal impairment. (See Table 1 and Table 2.)

TABLE 1. Dosage for Adults with Renal Impairment

Creatinine Clearance (mL/minute)	Dosage After Initial Loading Dose
35–54	Full doses at intervals ≥8 hours
11–34	50% of usual dose every 12 hours
≤10	50% of usual dose every 18–24 hours

TABLE 2. Dosage for Children Older than 1 Month of Age with Renal Impairment

Creatinine Clearance (mL/minute)	Dosage After Initial Loading Dose
40–70	60% of usual daily dosage in divided doses every 12 hours
20–40	25% of usual daily dosage in divided doses every 12 hours
5–20	10% of usual daily dosage once every 24 hours

CAUTIONS

Cefazolin shares the toxic potentials of other cephalosporins, and the usual cautions, precautions, and contraindications associated with cephalosporin therapy should be observed. (See Cautions in the Cephalosporins General Statement 8:12.06.)

SPECTRUM

Based on its spectrum of activity, cefazolin is classified as a first generation cephalosporin. For information on the classification of cephalosporins and closely related β-lactam antibiotics based on spectra of activity, see Spectrum in the Cephalosporins General Statement 8:12.06. Like other first generation cephalosporins (e.g., cefadroxil, cephalexin), cefazolin is active in vitro against many gram-positive aerobic cocci but has limited activity against gram-negative bacteria.

● In Vitro Susceptibility Testing

Strains of staphylococci resistant to penicillinase-resistant penicillins (oxacillin-resistant [methicillin-resistant] staphylococci) should be considered resistant to cefazolin, although results of in vitro susceptibility tests may indicate that the organisms are susceptible to the drug.

For information on interpreting results of in vitro susceptibility testing (disk susceptibility tests, dilution susceptibility tests) when cefazolin susceptibility testing is performed according to the standards of the Clinical and Laboratory Standards Institute (CLSI; formerly National Committee for Clinical Laboratory Standards [NCCLS]), see Spectrum: In Vitro Susceptibility Testing, in the Cephalosporins General Statement 8:12.06.

PHARMACOKINETICS

● Absorption

Cefazolin sodium is not appreciably absorbed from the GI tract and must be administered parenterally. Following IM administration of cefazolin sodium in healthy adults with normal renal function, peak serum cefazolin concentrations are attained within 1–2 hours and average 17 mcg/mL following a single 250-mg dose, 30–44 mcg/mL following a single 500-mg dose, and 64–76 mcg/mL following a single 1-g dose. Following a single 1-g IV dose in adults with normal renal function, serum concentrations of cefazolin average 188 mcg/mL at 5 minutes, 74 mcg/mL at 1 hour, and 46 mcg/mL at 2 hours. In one study in adults with normal renal function, steady-state serum concentrations of cefazolin were reached 3 hours after IV infusion of 3.5 mg/kg over 1 hour followed by 1.5 mg/kg over 2 hours.

In one study in children, peak serum concentrations of cefazolin occurred at 30 minutes and averaged 28 mcg/mL after a single cefazolin IM dose of 5–6.25 mg/kg and 42 mcg/mL after a single IM dose of 10–12.5 mg/kg.

● Elimination

The serum half-life of cefazolin is 1.2–2.2 hours in adults with normal renal function. In one study, half-life was 6.8 hours in 1 adult with a creatinine clearance of 26 mL/minute, 12 hours in 3 adults with creatinine clearances of 12–17 mL/minute, and 57 hours in 3 adults with creatinine clearances less than 5 mL/minute.

Cefazolin is excreted unchanged in urine. Approximately 60% of a single IM or IV dose of cefazolin is excreted within 6 hours and 80–100% of the dose is excreted within 24 hours in adults with normal renal function. In adults with normal renal function, peak urinary cefazolin concentrations of about 2 or 4 mg/mL may be attained following a single 500-mg or 1-g IM dose, respectively, of the drug.

CHEMISTRY AND STABILITY

● Chemistry

Cefazolin sodium is a semisynthetic cephalosporin antibiotic. Cefazolin sodium occurs as a white to off-white, crystalline powder which may have a faint odor or as a white to off-white lyophilized solid. The drug is freely soluble in water and very slightly soluble in alcohol. Each gram of cefazolin as the sodium salt contains 48 mg of sodium.

When the commercially available cefazolin sodium powder for injection is reconstituted as directed, solutions containing 225 or 330 mg/mL are light yellow to yellow and have a pH of 4.5–6.

When the commercially available Duplex® delivery system containing 1 or 2 g of cefazolin and 50 mL of dextrose 4 or 3% injection, respectively, in separate chambers is reconstituted (activated) according to the manufacturer's directions, the resultant solution is iso-osmotic and has an osmolality of approximately 290 mOsm/kg.

Commercially available frozen premixed cefazolin sodium injection in dextrose containing 1 g of cefazolin is a sterile, nonpyrogenic, iso-osmotic solution of the drug provided in a plastic container fabricated from specially formulated multilayered plastic (PL 2040). The 1-g frozen injection of cefazolin contains approximately 2 g of dextrose to adjust osmolality and contains sodium bicarbonate to adjust pH.

● Stability

Cefazolin sodium powder for injection should be stored at 20–25°C and protected from light. Following reconstitution of the commercially available powder for injection with sterile water for injection, solutions containing approximately 225 or 330 mg of cefazolin per mL are pale yellow to yellow in color and are stable for 24 hours at room temperature or 10 days at 5°C. Reconstituted solutions have a pH of approximately 4.5–6; rapid hydrolysis of the drug occurs when pH exceeds 8.5, and precipitation of the insoluble free acid may occur when pH is below 4.5.

Reconstituted solutions containing approximately 225 or 330 mg of cefazolin per mL may be frozen in their original containers immediately after reconstitution with sterile water for injection and are stable for 12 weeks when stored at –20°C. If the solutions are warmed to facilitate thawing, care should be taken to avoid heating after thawing has been completed. Once thawed, solutions should not be refrozen.

The commercially available Duplex® delivery system containing 1 or 2 g of cefazolin and 50 mL of dextrose injection in separate chambers should be stored at 20–25°C, but may be exposed to temperatures ranging from 15–30°C. Following reconstitution (activation), these IV solutions must be used within 24 hours if stored at room temperature or within 7 days if stored in a refrigerator and should not be frozen.

The commercially available frozen premixed cefazolin sodium injection in dextrose should be stored at –20°C or lower. The frozen injection should be thawed at room temperature (25°C) or under refrigeration (5°C) and, once thawed, should not be refrozen. Thawed solutions of the commercially available frozen injection are stable for 48 hours at room temperature (25°C) or 30 days under refrigeration (5°C). The commercially available frozen injection of the drug is provided in plastic containers fabricated from specially formulated multilayered plastic PL 2040 (Galaxy® containers). Solutions in contact with PL 2040 can leach out some of its chemical components in very small amounts within the expiration period of the injection; however, safety of the plastic has been confirmed in tests in animals according to USP biological tests for plastic containers as well as by tissue culture toxicity studies.

Cefazolin sodium powder and solutions of the drug tend to darken, depending on storage conditions; however, such discoloration does not indicate loss of potency.

For further information on chemistry, mechanism of action, spectrum, resistance, pharmacokinetics, uses, cautions, drug interactions, laboratory test interferences, and dosage and administration of cefazolin, see the Cephalosporins General Statement 8:12.06.

PREPARATIONS

Excipients in commercially available drug preparations may have clinically important effects in some individuals; consult specific product labeling for details.

ceFAZolin Sodium

Parenteral

For injection	500 mg (of cefazolin)*	Cefazolin Sodium for Injection
	1 g (of cefazolin)*	Cefazolin Sodium for Injection
	10 g (of cefazolin) pharmacy bulk package*	Cefazolin Sodium for Injection
	20 g (of cefazolin) pharmacy bulk package*	Cefazolin Sodium for Injection
For injection, for IV infusion	1 g (of cefazolin)*	Cefazolin for Injection (available in dual-chambered Duplex® drug delivery system with 4% dextrose injection), B Braun
	2 g (of cefazolin)	Cefazolin for Injection (available in dual-chambered Duplex® drug delivery system with 3% dextrose injection), B Braun

* available from one or more manufacturer, distributor, and/or repackager by generic (nonproprietary) name

ceFAZolin Sodium in Dextrose

Parenteral

Injection (frozen), for IV infusion	20 mg (of cefazolin) per mL (1 g) in 4% Dextrose*	Cefazolin Sodium Iso-osmotic in Dextrose Injection (Galaxy® [Baxter])

* available from one or more manufacturer, distributor, and/or repackager by generic (nonproprietary) name

† Use is not currently included in the labeling approved by the US Food and Drug Administration.

Cephalexin

8:12.06.04 • FIRST GENERATION CEPHALOSPORINS

■ Cephalexin is a semisynthetic, first generation cephalosporin antibiotic.

USES

● Acute Otitis Media

Oral cephalexin is used for the treatment of acute otitis media (AOM) caused by susceptible *Streptococcus pneumoniae*, *Haemophilus influenzae*, *Moraxella catarrhalis*, staphylococci, or streptococci.

When anti-infective therapy is indicated for the treatment of AOM, the American Academy of Pediatrics (AAP) recommends high-dose amoxicillin or amoxicillin and clavulanate potassium as the drugs of first choice for initial treatment. These experts recommend certain cephalosporins (cefdinir, cefpodoxime, cefuroxime, ceftriaxone) as alternatives for initial treatment in penicillin-allergic patients who do not have a history of severe and/or recent penicillin-allergic reactions.

For additional information regarding treatment of AOM, including information on diagnosis and management strategies, anti-infectives for initial treatment, duration of initial treatment, and anti-infectives after initial treatment failure, see Acute Otitis Media under Uses: Otitis Media, in the Cephalosporins General Statement 8:12.06.

● Pharyngitis and Tonsillitis

Oral cephalexin is used for the treatment of pharyngitis and tonsillitis caused by *S. pyogenes* (group A β-hemolytic streptococci). Although cephalexin generally is effective in eradicating *S. pyogenes* from the nasopharynx, efficacy of the drug in prevention of subsequent rheumatic fever has not been established to date.

Selection of an anti-infective for the treatment of *S. pyogenes* pharyngitis and tonsillitis should be based on the drug's spectrum of activity, bacteriologic and clinical efficacy, potential adverse effects, ease of administration, patient compliance, and cost. No regimen has been found to date that effectively eradicates group A β-hemolytic streptococci in 100% of patients.

Because the drugs have a narrow spectrum of activity, are inexpensive, and generally are effective with a low frequency of adverse effects, the AAP, Infectious Diseases Society of America (IDSA), American Heart Association (AHA), and others recommend a penicillin regimen (i.e., 10 days of oral penicillin V or oral amoxicillin or single dose of IM penicillin G benzathine) as the treatment of choice for *S. pyogenes* pharyngitis and tonsillitis and prevention of initial attacks (primary prevention) of rheumatic fever. Other anti-infectives (e.g., oral cephalosporins, oral macrolides, oral clindamycin) are recommended as alternatives in penicillin-allergic individuals.

If an oral cephalosporin is used for the treatment of *S. pyogenes* pharyngitis and tonsillitis, a 10-day regimen of a first generation cephalosporin (cefadroxil, cephalexin) is preferred instead of other cephalosporins with broader spectrums of activity (e.g., cefaclor, cefdinir, cefixime, cefpodoxime, cefuroxime).

● Bone and Joint Infections

Oral cephalexin is used for the treatment of bone and joint infections caused by susceptible staphylococci or *Proteus mirabilis*.

● Respiratory Tract Infections

Oral cephalexin is used for the treatment of mild to moderate respiratory tract infections caused by susceptible *S. pneumoniae*.

● Skin and Skin Structure Infections

Oral cephalexin is used for the treatment of mild to moderate skin and skin structure infections caused by susceptible staphylococci or streptococci.

● Urinary Tract Infections

Oral cephalexin is used for the treatment of mild to moderate urinary tract infections, including acute prostatitis, caused by susceptible *Escherichia coli*, *Klebsiella pneumoniae*, or *P. mirabilis*.

● Prevention of Bacterial Endocarditis

Oral cephalexin is used as an alternative for prevention of α-hemolytic (viridans group) streptococcal endocarditis† in penicillin-allergic individuals undergoing certain dental or upper respiratory tract procedures who have underlying cardiac conditions that put them at highest risk of adverse outcomes from endocarditis. Cephalexin should not be used for such prophylaxis in those with a history of immediate-type hypersensitivity to penicillins (e.g., urticaria, angioedema, anaphylaxis).

For information on which cardiac conditions are associated with highest risk of endocarditis and which procedures require prophylaxis, see Prevention under Uses: Endocarditis, in the Cephalosporins General Statement 8:12.06. When selecting anti-infectives for prophylaxis of bacterial endocarditis, the current recommendations published by AHA should be consulted.

DOSAGE AND ADMINISTRATION

● Reconstitution and Administration

Cephalexin is administered orally.

Although food may decrease the rate of absorption of cephalexin (see Pharmacokinetics: Absorption), the manufacturers state that the drug may be administered without regard to meals.

Reconstitution

Cephalexin powder for oral suspension should be reconstituted at the time of dispensing by adding the amount of water specified on the container to provide a suspension containing 125 or 250 mg of cephalexin per 5 mL. The water should be added in 2 equal portions and the bottle shaken after each addition.

The oral suspension should be shaken well prior to administration of each dose.

● Dosage

Cephalexin is commercially available as the monohydrate; dosage is expressed in terms of cephalexin.

Adult Dosage

General Adult Dosage

The usual adult dosage of cephalexin ranges from 1–4 g daily given in divided doses. Dosage usually is 250 mg every 6 hours or 500 mg every 12 hours. For severe infections or those caused by less susceptible organisms, higher dosage may be needed (up to 4 g daily in adults).

If dosage greater than 4 g daily is required, initial therapy with a parenteral cephalosporin should be considered.

Pharyngitis and Tonsillitis

For the treatment of group A β-hemolytic streptococcal pharyngitis and tonsillitis in patients older than 15 years of age, the usual dosage is 500 mg of cephalexin every 12 hours given for at least 10 days.

Bone and Joint Infections

For the treatment of bone and joint infections in patients older than 15 years of age, the manufacturer recommends 250 mg every 6 hours. Higher dosages may be needed for severe infections or those caused by less susceptible bacteria.

Respiratory Tract Infections

For the treatment of respiratory tract infections in patients older than 15 years of age, the manufacturer recommends 250 mg every 6 hours for mild to moderate infections. Higher dosages may be needed for more severe infections or those caused by less susceptible bacteria.

Skin and Skin Structure Infections

For the treatment of skin and skin structure infections in patients older than 15 years of age, the usual dosage is 500 mg of cephalexin every 12 hours.

Urinary Tract Infections

For the treatment of uncomplicated cystitis in patients older than 15 years of age, the usual dosage is 500 mg of cephalexin every 12 hours given for 7–14 days.

Prevention of Bacterial Endocarditis

If cephalexin is used as an alternative to amoxicillin or ampicillin for prevention of α-hemolytic (viridans group) streptococcal endocarditis† in penicillin-allergic individuals considered to be at highest risk for bacterial endocarditis following certain dental or upper respiratory tract procedures, adults should receive a single 2-g dose administered 0.5–1 hour prior to the procedure.

Pediatric Dosage

General Pediatric Dosage

The manufacturers state that the usual dosage of cephalexin for children is 25–50 mg/kg daily in divided doses; however, these dosages may be doubled for severe infections.

The American Academy of Pediatrics (AAP) recommends that pediatric patients beyond the neonatal period receive cephalexin in a dosage of 25–50 mg/kg daily in 2 or 4 equally divided doses for the treatment of mild or moderate infections and 75–100 mg/kg daily in 3 or 4 equally divided doses for the treatment of severe infections.

Acute Otitis Media

For the treatment of otitis media, the manufacturers recommend a pediatric dosage of 75–100 mg/kg daily in 4 equally divided doses.

Pharyngitis and Tonsillitis

The usual dosage of cephalexin for the treatment of group A β-hemolytic streptococcal pharyngitis in children older than 1 year of age is 25–50 mg/kg daily in equally divided doses every 12 hours given for at least 10 days.

Skin and Skin Structure Infections

For the treatment of skin and skin structure infections in pediatric patients, the usual dosage of cephalexin is 25–50 mg/kg daily in equally divided doses every 12 hours.

Prevention of Bacterial Endocarditis

If cephalexin is used as an alternative to amoxicillin or ampicillin for prevention of α-hemolytic (viridans group) streptococcal endocarditis† in penicillin-allergic individuals considered to be at highest risk for bacterial endocarditis following certain dental or upper respiratory tract procedures, pediatric patients should receive a single 50-mg/kg dose (no more than 2 g) administered 0.5–1 hour prior to the procedure.

• Dosage in Renal Impairment

The manufacturers state that cephalexin should be used with caution in patients with markedly impaired renal function, and close clinical observation and laboratory studies are recommended in such patients because safe dosage may be lower than usual dosages.

Some clinicians state that modification of the usual dosage does not appear to be necessary in patients with creatinine clearances greater than 40 mL/minute. These clinicians suggest that the usual adult dosage be used for the initial dose. Then, for subsequent doses, adults with creatinine clearances of 11–40 mL/minute should receive 500 mg every 8–12 hours, those with creatinine clearances of 5–10 mL/minute should receive 250 mg every 12 hours, and those with creatinine clearances less than 5 mL/minute should receive 250 mg every 12–24 hours.

CAUTIONS

Cephalexin shares the toxic potentials of other cephalosporins, and the usual cautions, precautions, and contraindications associated with cephalosporin therapy should be observed. (See Cautions in the Cephalosporins General Statement 8:12.06.)

• Pediatric Precautions

Cephalexin is labeled for use in pediatric patients; safety and efficacy were established based on clinical trials using recommended dosages of the drug administered as capsules or oral suspension.

Cephalexin capsules should only be used in children and adolescents who are able to ingest capsules.

SPECTRUM

Based on its spectrum of activity, cephalexin is classified as a first generation cephalosporin. For information on the classification of cephalosporins and closely related β-lactam antibiotics based on spectra of activity, see Spectrum in the Cephalosporins General Statement 8:12.06. Like other first generation cephalosporins (e.g., cefadroxil, cefazolin), cephalexin is active in vitro against many gram-positive aerobic cocci but has limited activity against gram-negative bacteria.

• In Vitro Susceptibility Testing

Strains of staphylococci resistant to penicillinase-resistant penicillins (methicillin-resistant [oxacillin-resistant] staphylococci) should be considered resistant to cephalexin, although results of in vitro susceptibility tests may indicate that the organisms are susceptible to the drug.

For information on interpreting results of in vitro susceptibility testing (disk susceptibility tests, dilution susceptibility tests) when cephalexin susceptibility testing is performed according to the standards of the Clinical and Laboratory Standards Institute (CLSI; formerly National Committee for Clinical Laboratory Standards [NCCLS]), see Spectrum: In Vitro Susceptibility Testing, in the Cephalosporins General Statement 8:12.06.

PHARMACOKINETICS

• Absorption

Cephalexin (as the monohydrate) is acid-stable and is rapidly and completely absorbed from the GI tract. Following oral administration in healthy, fasting adults with normal renal function of a single 250-mg, 500-mg, or 1-g dose of cephalexin, peak serum cephalexin concentrations are attained within 1 hour and average 9, 18, or 32 mcg/mL, respectively. Serum concentrations of cephalexin were still detectable 6 hours after the dose.

Peak serum concentrations are slightly lower and are attained later when cephalexin is administered with food, although the total amount of drug absorbed is unchanged. Following oral administration of cephalexin in healthy, fasting adults, serum concentrations 15 and 30 minutes after a single 500-mg dose averaged about 0.2 and 12 mcg/mL, respectively.

Absorption of cephalexin is delayed in young children and may be decreased up to 50% in neonates. Peak serum concentrations of the drug have been reported to occur within 3 hours in infants younger than 6 months of age, within 2 hours in children 9–12 months of age, and within 1 hour in older children.

• Elimination

The serum half-life of cephalexin is 0.5–1.2 hours in adults with normal renal function. The serum half-life of the drug is reported to be about 5 hours in neonates and 2.5 hours in children 3–12 months of age. In one study, the serum half-life was 7.7 hours in adults with creatinine clearances of 13.5 mL/minute, 10.8 hours in adults with creatinine clearances of 9.2 mL/minute, and 13.9 hours in adults with creatinine clearances of 4 mL/minute.

Cephalexin is excreted in urine as unchanged drug via both glomerular filtration and tubular secretion. Approximately 70–90% of a single 250- or 500-mg oral dose is excreted within 8–12 hours in adults with normal renal function. Cephalexin concentrations of 0.2 (range: 0.054–0.67) or 0.11–4 mg/mL have been reported in urine collected over a 6-hour period following a single 250- or 500-mg dose, respectively, in adults with normal renal function. Peak urine concentrations of the drug averaging about 2 mg/mL occur 2 hours after a single 500-mg oral dose of cephalexin.

CHEMISTRY AND STABILITY

• Chemistry

Cephalexin is a semisynthetic cephalosporin antibiotic. Cephalexin is commercially available as the monohydrate. Cephalexin (as the monohydrate) occurs as a white to off-white, crystalline powder and is slightly soluble in water and practically insoluble in alcohol.

• Stability

Cephalexin capsules should be stored in tight, light-resistant containers at 20–25°C, but may be exposed to temperatures ranging from 15–30°C.

Cephalexin powder for oral suspension should be stored at 20–25°C. After reconstitution, cephalexin oral suspension should be refrigerated in a tight container; any unused suspension should be discarded if not used within 14 days.

For further information on chemistry, mechanism of action, spectrum, resistance, pharmacokinetics, uses, cautions, drug interactions, laboratory test interferences, and dosage and administration of cephalexin, see the Cephalosporins General Statement 8:12.06.

PREPARATIONS

Excipients in commercially available drug preparations may have clinically important effects in some individuals; consult specific product labeling for details.

Cephalexin

Oral

Capsules	250 mg*	Cephalexin Capsules
		Keflex®, Shionogi
	333 mg*	Cephalexin Capsules
	500 mg*	Cephalexin Capsules
		Keflex®, Shionogi
	750 mg*	Cephalexin Capsules
		Keflex®, Shionogi
For suspension	125 mg/5 mL*	Cephalexin for Suspension
	250 mg/5 mL*	Cephalexin for Suspension
Tablets, film-coated	250 mg*	Cephalexin Film-coated Tablets
	500 mg*	Cephalexin Film-coated Tablets

* available from one or more manufacturer, distributor, and/or repackager by generic (nonproprietary) name

† Use is not currently included in the labeling approved by the US Food and Drug Administration.

Cefuroxime Axetil
Cefuroxime Sodium

8:12.06.08 • SECOND GENERATION CEPHALOSPORINS

■ Cefuroxime is a semisynthetic, second generation cephalosporin antibiotic.

USES

Cefuroxime axetil is used orally for the treatment of mild to moderate respiratory tract infections (i.e., acute maxillary sinusitis, acute exacerbations of chronic bronchitis, secondary infections of acute bronchitis, community-acquired pneumonia†) caused by susceptible bacteria; acute bacterial otitis media; pharyngitis and tonsillitis caused by *Streptococcus pyogenes* (group A β-hemolytic streptococci); mild to moderate uncomplicated skin and skin structure infections caused by *Staphylococcus aureus* (including β-lactamase-producing strains) or *S. pyogenes*; and uncomplicated urinary tract infections caused by *Escherichia coli* or *Klebsiella pneumoniae*. Cefuroxime axetil also is used orally for the treatment of Lyme disease and has been used for the treatment of uncomplicated gonorrhea. The manufacturers of cefuroxime axetil oral suspension state that safety and efficacy of the suspension have been established only for the treatment of pharyngitis and tonsillitis, acute otitis media, and impetigo caused by susceptible bacteria. and for the treatment of Lyme disease.

Cefuroxime sodium is used parenterally in the treatment of lower respiratory tract infections (including pneumonia), serious skin and skin structure infections, genitourinary tract infections, bone and joint infections, septicemia, and meningitis caused by susceptible organisms. Cefuroxime sodium also has been used parenterally for perioperative prophylaxis.

Because cefuroxime, like other second generation cephalosporins, generally is less active against susceptible gram-positive cocci than are first generation cephalosporins, most clinicians state that cefuroxime probably should not be used in the treatment of infections caused by gram-positive bacteria when a penicillin or a first generation cephalosporin could be used. In addition, because cefuroxime generally is less active in vitro against Enterobacteriaceae than third generation cephalosporins, some clinicians state that a third generation drug such as cefotaxime or ceftriaxone generally is preferred if a parenteral cephalosporin is indicated in the treatment of infections known or suspected to be caused by these gram-negative bacteria.

Prior to initiation of cefuroxime therapy, appropriate specimens should be obtained for identification of the causative organism and in vitro susceptibility tests. If cefuroxime is started pending results of susceptibility tests, it should be discontinued if the causative organism is found to be resistant to the drug. In the treatment of known or suspected sepsis or the treatment of other serious infections when the causative organism is unknown, concomitant therapy with an aminoglycoside may be indicated pending results of in vitro susceptibility tests.

● Acute Otitis Media

Cefuroxime axetil is used orally for the treatment of acute otitis media (AOM) caused by *S. pneumoniae*, *H. influenzae* (including β-lactamase-producing strains), *M. catarrhalis* (including β-lactamase-producing strains), or *S. pyogenes*.

When anti-infective therapy is indicated for the treatment of AOM, the American Academy of Pediatrics (AAP) recommends high-dose amoxicillin and amoxicillin and clavulanate potassium as the drugs of first choice for initial treatment. These experts recommend certain cephalosporins (cefdinir, cefpodoxime, cefuroxime, ceftriaxone) as alternatives for initial treatment in penicillin-allergic patients who do not have a history of severe and/or recent penicillin-allergic reactions.

Results of controlled clinical studies in children 3 months to 12 years of age with AOM indicate that a 10-day regimen of oral cefuroxime axetil is as effective or more effective than a 10-day regimen of oral cefaclor, oral amoxicillin, or oral amoxicillin and clavulanate potassium. In published studies, the overall clinical response rate to a 10-day regimen of oral cefuroxime axetil in pediatric patients with AOM has ranged from 62–94%.

Cefuroxime axetil also has been effective for the treatment of AOM in pediatric patients when administered in a 5-day regimen†. In a randomized study in children 3 months to 12 years of age with AOM, a satisfactory bacteriologic

response (cure or presumed cure) was obtained in 92% of those who received a 5-day regimen of cefuroxime axetil (30 mg/kg daily given in 2 divided doses), 84% of those who received a 10-day regimen or cefuroxime axetil (30 mg/kg daily given in 2 divided doses), or 95% of those who received a 10-day regimen of amoxicillin and clavulanate potassium (40 mg/kg daily given in 3 divided doses). There is evidence from a randomized study in children 6–36 months of age with AOM that a 5-day regimen of oral cefuroxime axetil is as effective as and may be better tolerated than an 8- or 10-day regimen of oral amoxicillin and clavulanate potassium. The AAP states that oral anti-infective regimens of less than 10 days' duration are not recommended for the treatment of AOM in children younger than 2 years of age or in patients with severe symptoms.

For additional information regarding treatment of AOM, including information on diagnosis and management strategies, anti-infectives for initial treatment, duration of initial treatment, and anti-infectives after initial treatment failure, see Acute Otitis Media under Uses: Otitis Media, in the Cephalosporins General Statement 8:12.06.

● Pharyngitis and Tonsillitis

Cefuroxime axetil is used orally for the treatment of pharyngitis and tonsillitis caused by *S. pyogenes* (group A β-hemolytic streptococci). Although cefuroxime usually is effective in eradicating *S. pyogenes* from the nasopharynx, efficacy of the drug in the subsequent prevention of rheumatic fever remains to be established.

Selection of an anti-infective for the treatment of *S. pyogenes* pharyngitis and tonsillitis should be based on the drug's spectrum of activity, bacteriologic and clinical efficacy, potential adverse effects, ease of administration, patient compliance, and cost. No regimen has been found to date that effectively eradicates group A β-hemolytic streptococci in 100% of patients.

Because the drugs have a narrow spectrum of activity, are inexpensive, and generally are effective with a low frequency of adverse effects, the AAP, Infectious Diseases Society of America (IDSA), American Heart Association (AHA), and others recommend a penicillin regimen (i.e., 10 days of oral penicillin V or oral amoxicillin or a single dose of IM penicillin G benzathine) as the treatment of choice for *S. pyogenes* pharyngitis and tonsillitis and prevention of initial attacks (primary prevention) of rheumatic fever. Other anti-infectives (e.g., oral cephalosporins, oral macrolides, oral clindamycin) are recommended as alternatives in penicillin-allergic individuals.

If an oral cephalosporin is used for the treatment of *S. pyogenes* pharyngitis and tonsillitis, a 10-day regimen of a first generation cephalosporin (cefadroxil, cephalexin) is preferred instead of other cephalosporins with broader spectrums of activity (e.g., cefaclor, cefdinir, cefixime, cefpodoxime, cefuroxime).

Although there is some evidence that a shorter duration of therapy with certain oral cephalosporins (e.g., a 5-day regimen of cefadroxil, cefdinir, cefixime, or cefpodoxime proxetil or a 4- or 5-day regimen of cefuroxime axetil) achieves bacteriologic and clinical cure rates equal to or greater than those achieved with the traditional 10-day oral penicillin V regimen, the IDSA and AHA state that use of cephalosporin regimens administered for 5 days or less for the treatment of *S. pyogenes* pharyngitis and tonsillitis cannot be recommended at this time.

A 10-day regimen of oral cefuroxime axetil is at least as effective as a 10-day regimen of oral penicillin V for the treatment of *S. pyogenes* pharyngitis and tonsillitis. In addition, results of a prospective, randomized study in children 2–15 years of age indicate that a 4-day regimen of oral cefuroxime axetil (20 mg/kg of cefuroxime in 2 divided doses daily) is as effective as a 10-day regimen of oral penicillin V (45 mg/kg daily in 3 divided doses). The clinical response rate was 94.8% in those who received the 4-day cefuroxime regimen and 96.1% in those who received the 10-day penicillin regimen; 30 days after treatment, the bacteriologic relapse rate was 2.8 and 2.3%, respectively.

● Respiratory Tract Infections

Cefuroxime axetil is used orally for the treatment of mild to moderate respiratory tract infections, including acute maxillary sinusitis caused by susceptible *Streptococcus pneumoniae* or *Haemophilus influenzae* (non-β-lactamase-producing strains only) and acute exacerbations of chronic bronchitis and secondary infections of acute bronchitis caused by susceptible *S. pneumoniae*, *H. influenzae* (non-β-lactamase-producing strains only), or *H. parainfluenzae* (non-β-lactamase-producing strains only).

Cefuroxime sodium is used parenterally for the treatment of lower respiratory tract infections, including pneumonia, caused by susceptible *S. pneumoniae*, *Staphylococcus aureus* (penicillinase- and nonpenicillinase-producing strains),

S. pyogenes (group A β-hemolytic streptococci), *H. influenzae* (including ampicillin-resistant strains), *Escherichia coli*, and *Klebsiella*.

Acute Sinusitis

Cefuroxime axetil is used orally for the treatment of acute maxillary sinusitis caused by susceptible *S. pneumoniae* or *H. influenzae* (non-β-lactamase-producing strains only). The manufacturers state that insufficient data exist to establish efficacy of cefuroxime axetil in the treatment of acute bacterial maxillary sinusitis that is known or suspected to be caused by β-lactamase-producing strains of *H. influenzae* or *M. catarrhalis*.

When anti-infective therapy is indicated for the treatment of acute bacterial sinusitis, the IDSA recommends amoxicillin and clavulanate potassium and the AAP recommends either amoxicillin or amoxicillin and clavulanate potassium as the drug of choice for initial empiric treatment. Because of variable activity against *S. pneumoniae* and *H. influenzae*, the IDSA no longer recommends second or third generation oral cephalosporins for empiric monotherapy of sinusitis in adults or children. If an oral cephalosporin is used as an alternative for empiric treatment of acute bacterial sinusitis in children (e.g., in penicillin-allergic individuals), the IDSA and AAP recommend a combination regimen that includes a third generation cephalosporin (cefixime or cefpodoxime) and clindamycin (or linezolid).

Community-Acquired Pneumonia

Oral cefuroxime axetil is used for the treatment of mild to moderate community-acquired pneumonia† (CAP). The American Thoracic Society (ATS) and Infectious Diseases Society of America (IDSA) recommended cefuroxime as an alternative for treatment of CAP caused by penicillin-susceptible *S. pneumoniae* and as an alternative in certain combination regimens used for empiric treatment of CAP.

Initial treatment of CAP generally involves use of an empiric anti-infective regimen based on the most likely pathogens and local susceptibility patterns; therapy may then be changed (if possible) to provide a more specific regimen (pathogen-directed therapy) based on results of in vitro culture and susceptibility testing. The most appropriate empiric regimen varies depending on the severity of illness at the time of presentation and whether outpatient treatment or hospitalization in or out of an intensive care unit (ICU) is indicated and the presence or absence of cardiopulmonary disease and other modifying factors that increase the risk of certain pathogens (e.g., penicillin- or multidrug-resistant *Streptococcus pneumoniae*, enteric gram-negative bacilli, *Pseudomonas aeruginosa*). Most experts recommend that an empiric regimen for the treatment of CAP include an anti-infective active against *S. pneumoniae* since this organism is the most commonly identified cause of bacterial pneumonia and causes more severe disease than many other common CAP pathogens.

For empiric *outpatient* treatment of CAP when risk factors for drug-resistant *S. pneumoniae* are present (e.g., comorbidities such as chronic heart, lung, liver, or renal disease, diabetes, alcoholism, malignancies, asplenia, immunosuppression; use of anti-infectives within the last 3 months), ATS and IDSA recommend monotherapy with a fluoroquinolone active against *S. pneumoniae* (moxifloxacin, gemifloxacin, levofloxacin) or, alternatively, a combination regimen that includes a β-lactam active against *S. pneumoniae* (high-dose amoxicillin or fixed combination of amoxicillin and clavulanic acid or, alternatively, ceftriaxone, cefpodoxime, or cefuroxime) given in conjunction with a macrolide (azithromycin, clarithromycin, erythromycin) or doxycycline. Cefuroxime and cefpodoxime may be less active against *S. pneumoniae* than amoxicillin or ceftriaxone.

A sequential regimen of parenteral cefuroxime sodium (given for 48–72 hours) followed by oral cefuroxime axetil (given for 7 days) has been used effectively for the treatment of CAP in adults. If a parenteral cephalosporin is used as an alternative to penicillin G or amoxicillin for treatment of CAP caused by penicillin-susceptible *S. pneumoniae*, ATS and IDSA recommend ceftriaxone, cefotaxime or cefuroxime; if an oral cephalosporin is used for treatment of these infections, ATS and IDSA recommend cefpodoxime, cefprozil, cefuroxime, cefdinir, or cefditoren.

For additional information on treatment of CAP, see Community-Acquired Pneumonia under Uses: Respiratory Tract Infections, in the Cephalosporins General Statement 8:12.06.

Gonorrhea and Associated Infections

IM cefuroxime sodium has been used in conjunction with oral probenecid for the treatment of uncomplicated gonorrhea and disseminated gonococcal infections caused by *Neisseria gonorrhoeae*, including penicillinase-producing strains (PPNG). Cefuroxime axetil has been used orally for the treatment of

uncomplicated urethral and endocervical gonorrhea caused by *N. gonorrhoeae* and for the treatment of uncomplicated rectal gonorrhea in females caused by nonpenicillinase-producing strains of the organism. However, parenteral cefuroxime sodium and oral cefuroxime axetil are not included in current US Centers for Disease Control and Prevention (CDC) recommendations for the treatment of gonococcal infections.

Because of concerns related to recent reports of *N. gonorrhoeae* with reduced susceptibility to cephalosporins, the CDC states that oral cephalosporins are no longer recommended as first-line treatment for uncomplicated gonorrhea. For the treatment of uncomplicated urogenital, anorectal, or pharyngeal gonorrhea, the CDC recommends a combination regimen that includes a single dose of IM ceftriaxone *and* either a single dose of oral azithromycin or a 7-day regimen of oral doxycycline.

The CDC states that cefuroxime axetil at the dosage recommended by the manufacturers (single 1-g oral dose of cefuroxime) meets the minimum efficacy criteria for treatment of urogenital and rectal gonococcal infections, but the pharmacodynamics of this oral drug are less favorable than those of IM ceftriaxone, oral cefixime, or oral cefpodoxime. In addition, cefuroxime axetil has unsatisfactory efficacy in pharyngeal infections.

For additional information on current recommendations for the treatment of gonorrhea and associated infections, see Uses: Gonorrhea and Associated Infections in Ceftriaxone 8:12.06.12.

Lyme Disease

Oral cefuroxime axetil is used in adults and children for the treatment of early Lyme disease manifested as erythema migrans. When an oral regimen is indicated, oral cefuroxime axetil also is used in the treatment of early neurologic Lyme disease† in patients with cranial nerve palsy alone without evidence of meningitis, Lyme carditis†, borrelial lymphocytoma†, and uncomplicated Lyme arthritis† without clinical evidence of neurologic disease.

Lyme disease is a tick-borne spirochetal disease. In the US, Lyme disease is caused by the spirochete *Borrelia burgdorferi*, which is transmitted by the bite of *Ixodes scapularis* or *I. pacificus* ticks. For additional information on Lyme disease, see Lyme Disease in Uses: Spirochetal Infections, in the Tetracyclines General Statement 8:12.24.

Early Lyme Disease
Erythema Migrans

Oral cefuroxime axetil is used for the treatment of early Lyme disease manifested as erythema migrans.

The IDSA, AAP, and other clinicians recommend oral doxycycline, oral amoxicillin, or oral cefuroxime axetil as first-line therapy for the treatment of early localized or early disseminated Lyme disease associated with erythema migrans, in the absence of specific neurologic involvement or advanced atrioventricular (AV) heart block. The IDSA states that a 14-day regimen (range 14–21 days) of any of these oral anti-infectives (doxycycline, amoxicillin, cefuroxime axetil) may be used for initial treatment of early Lyme disease since all 3 drugs have been shown to be effective for the treatment of erythema migrans and associated symptoms in prospective clinical studies. Doxycycline offers the advantage of also being effective for the treatment of human granulocytic anaplasmosis (HGA, formerly known as human granulocytic ehrlichiosis), which may occur simultaneously with early Lyme disease.

Efficacy of cefuroxime axetil for the treatment of early Lyme disease has been evaluated in studies that included adults and pediatric patients 12 years of age or older with physician-documented erythema migrans (with or without systemic manifestations of infection), and results of these studies indicate that the drug is as effective as oral doxycycline in producing resolution of erythema migrans and preventing the development of manifestations of late Lyme disease. The clinical diagnosis of early Lyme disease in study patients was validated objectively by a blinded expert who examined available photographs of skin lesions taken before therapy and/or by serologic evidence of antibodies specific to *B. burgdorferi* identified using enzyme-linked immunosorbent assay (ELISA) and Western immunoblot. Patients were randomized to receive oral cefuroxime axetil (500 mg of cefuroxime twice daily) or oral doxycycline (100 mg 3 times daily) for 20 days and evaluated during treatment (days 8–12) and posttreatment (days 1–5, 1 month, and then at 3-month intervals for up to 1 year). In patients who were evaluated at 1 month posttreatment, a satisfactory clinical response consisting of either clinical success (defined as resolution of erythema migrans and other manifestations of infection within 5 days posttreatment and maintained through follow-up at 1 month posttreatment) or clinical improvement (defined as resolution of erythema migrans within 5 days posttreatment with incomplete resolution of other manifestations of infection at that time but further improvement or complete resolution of manifestations by follow-up at 1 month posttreatment) was attained in 91 or 93% of patients who received cefuroxime axetil or doxycycline, respectively. Clinical success was attained in 72 or 73% of patients receiving cefuroxime axetil or doxycycline, respectively; clinical improvement was attained in 19% of patients receiving either drug. In patients evaluated at 1 year, a satisfactory clinical outcome consisting of success (defined as the absence of signs or symptoms of late Lyme disease throughout the 1-year follow-up) or clinical improvement (defined as the presence of some signs or symptoms consistent with late Lyme disease but no objective evidence of active disease throughout the 1-year follow-up) was attained in 84 or 87% of patients who received cefuroxime axetil or doxycycline, respectively. Success at 1 year was attained in 73% of patients receiving either drug; clinical improvement was attained in 10% of patients receiving cefuroxime axetil and 13% of patients receiving doxycycline.

Early Neurologic Lyme Disease

Oral cefuroxime axetil is used in the treatment of early neurologic Lyme disease† in patients with cranial nerve palsy alone without evidence of meningitis. Parenteral anti-infectives (IV ceftriaxone, IV penicillin G sodium, IV cefotaxime) are recommended for the treatment of early Lyme disease when there are acute neurologic manifestations such as meningitis or radiculopathy. However, some clinicians suggest that a 14-day regimen (range: 14–21 days) of oral anti-infectives (amoxicillin, doxycycline, cefuroxime axetil) may be used in patients with cranial nerve palsy without clinical evidence of meningitis (i.e., those with normal CSF examinations or those for whom CSF examination is deemed unnecessary because there are no clinical signs of meningitis). Although there is some experience using oral anti-infectives in patients with seventh cranial nerve palsy, it is unclear whether an oral regimen would be as effective for patients with other cranial neuropathies. Although anti-infectives may not hasten resolution of seventh cranial nerve palsy associated with *B. burgdorferi* infection, anti-infectives should be given to prevent further sequelae.

Lyme Carditis

Oral cefuroxime axetil is used in the treatment of Lyme carditis†. The IDSA states that patients with AV heart block and/or myopericarditis associated with early Lyme disease may be treated with a 14-day regimen (range: 14–21 days) of oral or parenteral anti-infectives. Although there is no evidence to date to suggest that a parenteral regimen is more effective than an oral regimen for the treatment of Lyme carditis, a parenteral regimen usually is recommended for initial treatment of hospitalized patients; an oral regimen can be used to complete therapy and for the treatment of outpatients. When a parenteral regimen is used, IV ceftriaxone or, alternatively, IV cefotaxime or IV penicillin G sodium is recommended. When an oral regimen is used, oral doxycycline, oral amoxicillin, or oral cefuroxime axetil is recommended.

Borrelial Lymphocytoma

Although experience is limited, the IDSA states that available data indicate that borrelial lymphocytoma† may be treated with a 14-day regimen (range 14–21 days) of oral doxycycline, oral amoxicillin, or oral cefuroxime axetil in the dosages used for the treatment of erythema migrans.

Late Lyme Disease
Lyme Arthritis

Patients with uncomplicated Lyme arthritis† without clinical evidence of neurologic disease generally can be treated with a 28-day regimen of oral doxycycline, oral amoxicillin, or oral cefuroxime axetil. Patients with Lyme arthritis and concomitant neurologic disease should receive a parenteral regimen of IV ceftriaxone or, alternatively, IV cefotaxime or IV penicillin G sodium. While oral regimens are easier to administer, associated with fewer serious adverse effects, and less expensive than IV regimens, some patients with Lyme arthritis treated with oral anti-infectives have subsequently developed overt neuroborreliosis, which may require IV therapy for successful resolution. Therefore, additional study is needed to fully evaluate the comparative safety and efficacy of oral versus IV anti-infectives for the treatment of Lyme arthritis.

In patients who have persistent or recurrent joint swelling after a recommended oral regimen, the IDSA and other clinicians recommend retreatment with the oral regimen or a switch to a parenteral regimen. Some clinicians

prefer retreatment with an oral regimen for patients whose arthritis substantively improved but did not completely resolve; these clinicians reserve parenteral regimens for those patients whose arthritis failed to improve or worsened. It has been suggested that clinicians should consider allowing several months for joint inflammation to resolve after initial treatment before an additional course of anti-infectives is given.

● Meningitis

Parenteral cefuroxime has been used in neonates†, children, and adults for the treatment of meningitis caused by susceptible *S. pneumoniae, H. influenzae* (including ampicillin-resistant strains), *N. meningitidis*, or *S. aureus* (penicillinase- and nonpenicillinase-producing strains); however, cefuroxime is not considered a drug of choice for these infections. Treatment failures have been reported when cefuroxime was used in the treatment of meningitis, especially in meningitis caused by *H. influenzae*. In addition, while results of some studies in pediatric patients with meningitis indicate that the clinical cure rate with IV cefuroxime is similar to that reported for IV ceftriaxone, the bacteriologic response to cefuroxime appears to be slower, which may increase the risk for hearing loss and neurologic sequelae. In a study in children 44 days to 16 years of age with acute bacterial meningitis who were randomized to receive empiric therapy with IV ceftriaxone (100 mg/kg once daily) or IV cefuroxime (240 mg/kg daily in 4 doses), all patients in both groups were considered clinically cured; however, the rate of sterilization of CSF after the first 18–36 hours of therapy was higher in those who received ceftriaxone (98%) than in those who received cefuroxime (88%). When a cephalosporin is indicated for the treatment of bacterial meningitis, a parenteral third generation cephalosporin (usually ceftriaxone or cefotaxime) generally is recommended.

● Perioperative Prophylaxis

IV cefuroxime sodium is used for perioperative prophylaxis in patients undergoing cardiac surgery and is considered a drug of choice for cardiac procedures (e.g., coronary artery bypass, pacemaker or other cardiac device insertion, ventricular assist devices). IV cefuroxime also is considered a drug of choice when used alone for perioperative prophylaxis in patients undergoing clean head and neck surgery involving placement of prosthesis (excluding tympanostomy) and when used in conjunction with metronidazole for perioperative prophylaxis in patients undergoing clean-contaminated cancer surgery of the head and neck or other clean-contaminated head and neck procedures (excluding tonsillectomy and functional endoscopic sinus procedures).

IV cefuroxime also has been used for perioperative prophylaxis in patients undergoing noncardiac thoracic surgery, GI or biliary tract surgery, gynecologic or obstetric surgery (e.g., vaginal hysterectomy), orthopedic procedures, or heart transplantation. However, other anti-infectives (e.g., cefazolin) usually are recommended for perioperative prophylaxis in patients undergoing these procedures. (See Uses: Perioperative Prophylaxis, in the Cephalosporins General Statement 8:12.06.)

DOSAGE AND ADMINISTRATION

● Reconstitution and Administration

Cefuroxime axetil is administered orally. Cefuroxime sodium is administered by IV injection or infusion or by deep IM injection. The drug should be given IV rather than IM in patients with septicemia or other severe or life-threatening infections or in patients with lowered resistance, particularly if shock is present.

Oral Administration

Cefuroxime axetil oral suspension must be administered with food. Although cefuroxime axetil film-coated tablets may be given orally without regard to meals, administration with food maximizes bioavailability of the drug. (See Pharmacokinetics: Absorption.)

In children aged 3 months to 12 years who are unable to swallow tablets, cefuroxime may be administered as the commercially available oral suspension. Although commercially available cefuroxime axetil tablets have been crushed and mixed with food (e.g., applesauce, ice cream), the crushed tablets have a strong, persistent taste and the manufacturers state that the drug should not be administered in this manner. (See Cautions: Pediatric Precautions.) Cefuroxime axetil tablets also have been allowed to disintegrate in a small amount (60–90 mL) of beverage (e.g., apple juice or milk) and the beverage stirred and ingested immediately followed by additional amounts of beverage; disintegration of the tablets is optimal when the beverage is at room temperature.

Limited data from a study conducted by the manufacturer suggest that cefuroxime axetil is stable for 2 hours at room temperature when added as single 125- or 250-mg tablets to 40 mL of Tropicana® orange juice, Welch's® grape juice, or Nestle's® chocolate milk. However, extemporaneous preparation of an oral suspension of the drug intended for *multiple* dosing currently is not recommended since stability information for more prolonged periods currently is not available and because the drug is commercially available as an oral suspension.

The child's tolerance of the taste of cefuroxime axetil should be ascertained by the clinician and parent, preferably when prescription of the drug is being considered (e.g., while the child is still in the physician's office).

Reconstitution

Cefuroxime axetil powder for oral suspension should be reconstituted at the time of dispensing by adding the amount of water specified on the bottle to provide a suspension containing 125 or 250 mg of cefuroxime (as cefuroxime axetil) per 5 mL of suspension. After tapping the bottle to thoroughly loosen the powder for oral suspension, the water should be added in one portion and the suspension agitated well.

The suspension should be agitated well just prior to each use and the cap replaced securely after each opening.

Intermittent IV Injection

For direct intermittent IV injection, vials labeled as containing 750 mg or 1.5 g of cefuroxime should be reconstituted with 8 or 16 mL, respectively, of sterile water for injection to provide solutions containing approximately 90 mg/mL; the entire contents of the vial should be withdrawn for each dose.

The appropriate dose should then be injected directly into a vein over a 3- to 5-minute period or injected slowly into the tubing of a freely flowing compatible IV solution.

Intermittent or Continuous IV Infusion

ADD-Vantage® (TwistVial®) vials labeled as containing 750 mg or 1.5 g of cefuroxime should be reconstituted with 50 or 100 mL of 5% dextrose injection, 0.9% sodium chloride injection, or 0.45% sodium chloride injection in a compatible flexible container according to the manufacturer's directions.

Alternatively, the commercially available Duplex® drug delivery system containing 750 mg or 1.5 g of cefuroxime and 50 mL of dextrose 4.1 or 2.9% injection, respectively, in separate chambers should be reconstituted (activated) according to the manufacturer's directions and administered by IV infusion.

The 7.5-g pharmacy bulk vial should be reconstituted according to the manufacturer's directions. The pharmacy bulk vial is *not* intended for direct IV infusion.

Thawed solutions of the commercially available frozen premixed cefuroxime sodium injection should be administered only by intermittent or continuous IV infusion. The frozen injection should be thawed at room temperature (25°C) or under refrigeration (5°C); the injection should not be thawed by warming in a water bath or by exposure to microwave radiation. Precipitates that may have formed in the frozen injection usually will dissolve with little or no agitation when the injection reaches room temperature; potency is not affected. After thawing to room temperature, the injection should be agitated and the container checked for minute leaks by firmly squeezing the bag; the container may be fragile and should be handled with care. The injection should be discarded if container seals or outlet ports are not intact or leaks are found or if the solution is cloudy or contains an insoluble precipitate. Additives should not be introduced into the injection container. The injection should not be used in series connections with other plastic containers, since such use could result in air embolism from residual air being drawn from the primary container before administration of fluid from the secondary container is complete.

Other IV solutions flowing through a common administration tubing or site should be discontinued while cefuroxime is being infused unless the solutions are known to be compatible and the flow rate is adequately controlled. If an aminoglycoside is administered concomitantly with cefuroxime, the drugs should be administered at separate sites.

Rate of Administration

Intermittent IV infusions of cefuroxime generally are infused over 15–60 minutes.

IM Injection

IM injections of Zinacef® are prepared by adding 3 mL of sterile water for injection to a vial labeled as containing 750 mg of cefuroxime to provide a suspension containing approximately 220 mg/mL. The suspension should be shaken gently prior to administration, and the entire contents of the vial should be withdrawn for each dose.

IM injections should be made deeply into a large muscle mass such as the gluteus or lateral aspect of the thigh. The plunger of the syringe should be drawn back before IM injection to ensure that the needle is not in a blood vessel.

● Dosage

Dosage of cefuroxime axetil is expressed in terms of cefuroxime. Cefuroxime axetil tablets and oral suspension are *not* bioequivalent and are *not* substitutable on a mg/mg basis. (See Pharmacokinetics: Absorption.)

Dosage of cefuroxime sodium also is expressed in terms of cefuroxime and is identical for IM or IV administration.

Adult Dosage
General Oral Adult Dosage

For the treatment of uncomplicated skin and skin-structure infections in adults and adolescents 13 years of age or older, the usual oral dosage of cefuroxime given as cefuroxime axetil tablets is 250 or 500 mg twice daily for 10 days. For the treatment of uncomplicated urinary tract infections (UTIs), the usual oral dosage of cefuroxime given as cefuroxime axetil tablets is 125 or 250 mg twice daily for 7–10 days.

The usual parenteral adult dosage of cefuroxime given as cefuroxime sodium is 750 mg to 1.5 g every 8 hours. Uncomplicated UTIs, skin and skin structure infections, and uncomplicated pneumonia in adults generally respond to a parenteral dosage of 750 mg every 8 hours. Severe or complicated infections or bone and joint infections in adults generally require 1.5 g every 8 hours and life-threatening infections or infections caused by less susceptible organisms may require 1.5 g every 6 hours. Dosage of parenteral cefuroxime for the treatment of bacterial meningitis in adults should not exceed 3 g every 8 hours.

Pharyngitis and Tonsillitis

For the treatment of pharyngitis and tonsillitis caused by *Streptococcus pyogenes* (group A β-hemolytic streptococci) in adults and adolescents 13 years of age or older, the usual oral dosage of cefuroxime given as cefuroxime axetil tablets is 250 mg twice daily for 10 days.

Respiratory Tract Infections

For the treatment of acute bacterial maxillary sinusitis in adults and adolescents 13 years of age or older, the usual oral dosage of cefuroxime given as cefuroxime axetil tablets is 250 mg twice daily for 10 days. For the treatment of acute bacterial exacerbations of chronic bronchitis and secondary bacterial infections of acute bronchitis in adults and adolescents 13 years of age or older, the usual oral dosage of cefuroxime given as cefuroxime axetil tablets is 250 or 500 mg twice daily. The manufacturers recommend that therapy be continued for 10 days for the treatment of acute bacterial exacerbations of chronic bronchitis or for 5–10 days for the treatment of secondary bacterial infections of acute bronchitis. While there is evidence that a 5-day regimen of cefuroxime axetil is as effective as a 10-day regimen of the drug for the treatment of secondary bacterial infections of acute bronchitis, efficacy of the shorter regimen for the treatment of acute exacerbations of chronic bronchitis has not been established.

If cefuroxime axetil is used for the outpatient treatment of community-acquired pneumonia† (CAP) in adults, the American Thoracic Society (ATS) and Infectious Diseases Society of America (IDSA) recommend an oral dosage of 500 mg of cefuroxime twice daily. For empiric treatment of CAP, cefuroxime must be used in conjunction with other anti-infectives. (See Community-acquired Pneumonia under Uses: Respiratory Tract Infections.)

For the treatment of uncomplicated pneumonia in adults, the manufacturers recommend a parenteral cefuroxime dosage of 750 mg every 8 hours. In severe or complicated infections, a dosage of 1.5 g every 8 hours is recommended.

Gonorrhea and Associated Infections

For the parenteral treatment of uncomplicated gonorrhea caused by *Neisseria gonorrhoeae*, including penicillinase-producing strains (PPNG), the manufacturer of Zinacef® recommends that adults receive a single 1.5-g IM dose of cefuroxime and 1 g of oral probenecid; the cefuroxime dose should be divided and given at 2 different sites. For the parenteral treatment of disseminated gono-coccal infections, the manufacturers recommend that adults receive 750 mg of cefuroxime IM or IV every 8 hours.

For the oral treatment of uncomplicated urethral or endocervical gonorrhea caused by *N. gonorrhoeae* or for the oral treatment of uncomplicated rectal gon-orrhea in females caused by nonpenicillinase-producing strains of the organism, adults and adolescents 13 years of age or older have received a single 1-g dose of cefuroxime.

The US Centers for Disease Control and Prevention (CDC) does not recom-mend oral or parenteral cefuroxime for the treatment of gonococcal infections. (See Uses: Gonorrhea and Associated Infections.)

Lyme Disease

For the treatment of early Lyme disease manifested as erythema migrans, the manufacturers recommend that adults and adolescents 13 years of age or older receive 500 mg of oral cefuroxime twice daily for 20 days.

IDSA and other clinicians recommend that adults receive 500 mg of oral cefu-roxime twice daily for 14 days (range: 14–21 days) for the treatment of early local-ized or early disseminated Lyme disease manifested as erythema migrans, in the absence of specific neurologic involvement or advanced atrioventricular (AV) heart block.

If an oral regimen is used for the treatment of early neurologic Lyme disease† in patients with cranial nerve palsy alone without clinical evidence of meningitis (see Early Neurologic Lyme Disease under Uses: Lyme Disease), Lyme carditis†, or borrelial lymphocytoma†, the IDSA recommends that adults receive 500 mg of oral cefuroxime twice daily for 14 days (range: 14–21 days).

If an oral regimen is used for the treatment of uncomplicated Lyme arthritis† in patients without clinical evidence of neurologic disease (see Late Lyme Disease under Uses: Lyme Disease), the IDSA recommends that adults receive 500 mg of oral cefuroxime twice daily for 28 days.

Perioperative Prophylaxis

For perioperative prophylaxis in adults undergoing open-heart surgery, the manu-facturers recommend that a single 1.5-g dose of cefuroxime be given IV at the time of induction of anesthesia and every 12 hours thereafter for a total dosage of 6 g (i.e., up to 48 hours). Some experts recommend that 1.5 g of cefuroxime be given within 1 hour prior to surgical incision and that additional 1.5-g doses be given every 4 hours during prolonged procedures (longer than 4 hours) or if major blood loss occurs. Various data support a duration of perioperative prophylaxis ranging from a single preoperative dose to continuation of prophylaxis for 24 hours postop-eratively; there is no evidence of benefit beyond 48 hours and no evidence to sup-port continuing prophylaxis until all drains and indwelling catheters are removed.

If cefuroxime is used for perioperative prophylaxis in other clean-contami-nated or potentially contaminated surgery (e.g., vaginal hysterectomy), the man-ufacturers recommend that adults receive 1.5 g of cefuroxime IV just prior to surgery (approximately 30–60 minutes before the initial incision) and, in lengthy operations, 750 mg of the drug IV or IM every 8 hours. For most procedures, postoperative doses are usually unnecessary and may increase the risk of bacterial resistance. If the procedure is prolonged (longer than 4 hours) or if major blood loss occurs, 1.5-g doses of cefuroxime may be given IV every 4 hours.

Pediatric Dosage

Cefuroxime axetil film-coated tablets and oral suspension are not bioequivalent and are not substitutable on a mg/mg basis. (See Pharmacokinetics: Absorption.)

General Pediatric Dosage

For the treatment of most susceptible infections (except bone and joint infections or meningitis) in children 3 months of age or older, the manufacturers recommend a cefuroxime dosage of 50–100 mg/kg daily given IM or IV in equally divided doses every 6–8 hours; the manufacturer states that 100 mg/kg should be given IM or IV for more severe infections. The IM or IV dosage of cefuroxime recommended by the manufacturers for the treatment of bone and joint infections in children 3 months of age or older is 150 mg/kg daily in 3 divided doses every 8 hours.

The American Academy of Pediatrics (AAP) recommends that neonates 7 days of age or younger receive IM or IV cefuroxime in a dosage of 50 mg/kg every 12 hours, regardless of weight. Neonates 8–28 days of age should receive a dosage of 50 mg/kg every 8–12 hours if they weigh 2 kg or less or 50 mg/kg every 8 hours if they weigh more than 2 kg.

For pediatric patients beyond the neonatal period, the AAP recommends an IM or IV cefuroxime dosage of 75–100 mg/kg daily given in 3 equally divided doses for the treatment of mild to moderate infections or 100–200 mg/kg daily in 3 or 4 equally divided doses for the treatment of severe infections. These clinicians recommend that children beyond the neonatal period receive oral cefuroxime in a dosage of 20–30 mg/kg daily in 2 equally divided doses for the treatment of mild to moderate infections. The AAP states that oral cefuroxime is inappropriate for the treatment of severe infections.

Acute Otitis Media

For the treatment of acute otitis media in children 3 months to 12 years of age who can swallow tablets whole, the usual oral dosage of cefuroxime as cefuroxime axetil film-coated tablets is 250 mg twice daily for 10 days. Alternatively, children 3 months to 12 years of age with acute otitis media can receive cefuroxime as cefu-roxime axetil oral suspension in a dosage of 30 mg/kg daily (maximum 1 g daily) given in 2 divided doses for 10 days.

Cefuroxime axetil has been administered in a 5-day regimen† for the treat-ment of acute otitis media in children 3 months to 12 years of age. The AAP states that oral anti-infective regimens of less than 10 days' duration are not recom-mended for the treatment of AOM in children younger than 2 years of age or in patients with severe symptoms.

Pharyngitis and Tonsillitis

For the treatment of pharyngitis and tonsillitis caused by *S. pyogenes* (group A β-hemolytic streptococci) in children 3 months to 12 years of age who can swallow tablets whole, the usual oral dosage of cefuroxime as cefuroxime axetil film-coated tablets is 125 mg every 12 hours for 10 days. Alternatively, children 3 months to 12 years of age may receive cefuroxime as cefuroxime axetil oral suspension in a dosage of 20 mg/kg daily (maximum 500 mg daily) in 2 divided doses for 10 days.

Acute Sinusitis

For the treatment of acute bacterial maxillary sinusitis in children 3 months to 12 years of age who can swallow tablets whole, the usual oral dosage of cefuroxime as cefuroxime axetil film-coated tablets is 250 mg twice daily for 10 days. Alterna-tively, children 3 months to 12 years of age may receive cefuroxime as cefuroxime axetil oral suspension in a dosage of 30 mg/kg daily (maximum 1 g daily) given in 2 divided doses for 10 days.

Lyme Disease

For the treatment of early localized or early disseminated Lyme disease mani-fested as erythema migrans, in the absence of specific neurologic involvement or advanced AV heart block, the manufacturer, IDSA, AAP, and other clini-cians recommend that children receive oral cefuroxime in a dosage of 30 mg/kg daily (up to 1 g daily) administered in 2 divided doses for 14 days (range 14–21 days).

If an oral regimen is used for the treatment of early neurologic Lyme disease† in patients with cranial nerve palsy alone without clinical evidence of meningi-tis (see Early Neurologic Lyme Disease under Uses: Lyme Disease), Lyme cardi-tis†, or borrelial lymphocytoma†, the IDSA recommends that children receive oral cefuroxime in a dosage of 30 mg/kg daily in 2 equally divided doses (up to 500 mg per dose) for 14 days (range 14–21 days).

If an oral regimen is used for the treatment of uncomplicated Lyme arthritis† in patients without clinical evidence of neurologic disease (see Late Lyme Disease under Uses: Lyme Disease), the IDSA and AAP recommend that children receive oral cefuroxime in a dosage of 30 mg/kg daily in 2 equally divided doses (up to 500 mg per dose) for 28 days.

Meningitis

For the treatment of bacterial meningitis in children 3 months of age or older, the usual dosage of IV cefuroxime is 200–240 mg/kg daily given in divided doses every 6–8 hours.

Skin and Skin Structure Infections

For the treatment of impetigo in children 3 months to 12 years of age, the usual oral dosage of cefuroxime as cefuroxime axetil oral suspension is 30 mg/kg daily (maximum 1 g daily) in 2 divided doses for 10 days.

Perioperative Prophylaxis

If cefuroxime is used for perioperative prophylaxis in children, some clinicians recommend that 50 mg/kg of cefuroxime be given within 1 hour prior to surgical incision. If the procedure is prolonged (longer than 4 hours) or if major blood loss occurs, additional 50-mg/kg doses may be given IV. Various data support a duration of perioperative prophylaxis ranging from a single preoperative dose to continuation of prophylaxis for 24 hours postoperatively; there is no evidence of benefit beyond 48 hours and no evidence to support continuing prophylaxis until all drains and indwelling catheters are removed.

Duration of Therapy

The duration of cefuroxime therapy depends on the type of infection but should generally be continued for at least 48–72 hours after the patient becomes afebrile or evidence of eradication of the infection is obtained.

For the treatment of uncomplicated UTIs, the manufacturers recommend that therapy with cefuroxime axetil tablets be continued for 7–10 days. For the treatment of uncomplicated skin and skin-structure infections, or acute otitis media caused by susceptible organisms, the manufacturers recommend that therapy with cefuroxime axetil tablets be continued for 10 days.

Chronic urinary tract infections may require several weeks of cefuroxime therapy, and bacteriologic and clinical assessments should be made frequently during therapy and for several months after the drug is discontinued. When cefuroxime is used in the treatment of staphylococcal and other infections involving a collection of pus, surgical drainage should be performed when indicated.

● Dosage in Renal Impairment

Modification of usual dosage of parenteral cefuroxime is unnecessary in patients with creatinine clearances greater than 20 mL/minute. However, in patients with creatinine clearances of 20 mL/minute or less, doses and/or frequency of administration of parenteral cefuroxime must be modified in response to the degree of renal impairment, severity of the infection, and susceptibility of the causative organism. The manufacturers and some clinicians recommend that adults with creatinine clearances of 10–20 mL/minute receive 750 mg IM or IV every 12 hours and that adults with creatinine clearances less than 10 mL/minute receive 750 mg IM or IV every 24 hours. In children with impaired renal function, the manufacturers recommend that the frequency of administration of parenteral cefuroxime be modified based on the recommendations for adults with impaired renal function.

In patients undergoing hemodialysis, a supplemental dose of parenteral cefuroxime should be given after each dialysis period.

Safety and efficacy of oral cefuroxime axetil in patients with renal impairment have not been established.

CAUTIONS

Adverse effects reported with cefuroxime axetil and cefuroxime sodium are similar to those reported with other cephalosporins.

● Dermatologic and Sensitivity Reactions

Hypersensitivity reactions have been reported in less than 1% of patients receiving cefuroxime axetil or cefuroxime sodium. These reactions include rash (e.g., morbilliform), fever, pruritus, erythema, urticaria, Stevens-Johnson syndrome, erythema multiforme, toxic epidermal necrolysis, serum sickness-like reactions, angioedema, and anaphylaxis. At least one case of severe bronchospasm has been reported in a patient who received cefuroxime axetil. Positive direct antiglobulin (Coombs') test results have also been reported in a few patients receiving oral or parenteral cefuroxime; however, it is not clear whether the mechanism of this reaction is immunologic in nature. If a severe hypersensitivity reaction occurs during cefuroxime therapy, the drug should be discontinued and the patient given appropriate therapy (e.g., epinephrine, corticosteroids, maintenance of an adequate airway, oxygen) as indicated.

There is clinical and laboratory evidence of partial cross-allergenicity among cephalosporins and other β-lactam antibiotics including penicillins and cephamycins; however, the true incidence of cross-allergenicity among these anti-infectives has not been established. When cefuroxime axetil was used in patients with a history of delayed hypersensitivity reactions to penicillins and no history of hypersensitivity to cephalosporins, a delayed hypersensitivity reaction occurred in about 3% of these patients. The manufacturer states that when cefuroxime sodium was used in patients with a history of hypersensitivity to penicillin, rash reportedly occurred in 4.4–6.7% of these patients.

● Local Effects

The most frequent adverse reactions to IM or IV cefuroxime sodium are local reactions at the injection site. Mild to moderate pain, which persists for less than 5 minutes, has been reported in up to 95% of patients following IM administration of cefuroxime. Severe pain has been reported occasionally. IM injections of cefuroxime reportedly are less painful when the drug is administered as a suspension rather than a solution and are also less painful when the injection is given into the buttock rather than the thigh.

Thrombophlebitis reportedly occurs in approximately 2% of patients receiving cefuroxime IV.

● GI Effects

Nausea and vomiting have been reported in 2.6–6.7% and diarrhea or loose stools have been reported in 3.7–10.6% of patients receiving oral cefuroxime axetil. A strong, persistent, bitter taste has been reported when cefuroxime axetil was administered as crushed tablets (see Pediatric Precautions). In addition, up to 5% of children receiving the commercially available oral suspension of cefuroxime axetil disliked the taste of the suspension; during clinical trials, discontinuance of therapy because of the taste of the suspension or other problems with administration occurred in 1.4% of patients.

Gagging, epigastric burning, GI bleeding, abdominal pain, flatulence, GI infection, ptyalism, indigestion, mouth ulcers, swollen tongue, anorexia, thirst, dyspepsia, and stomach cramps also have been reported in patients receiving the drug orally.

The frequency of adverse GI effects (particularly diarrhea) may be greater with oral cefuroxime axetil than with oral cefaclor, and nausea appears to be more common when oral cefuroxime axetil is used concomitantly with oral probenecid than when the antibiotic is used alone. In addition, adverse GI effects were reported more frequently with previously available oral formulations of cefuroxime axetil, and, in part, prompted several reformulations of the product. Adverse GI effects including nausea and diarrhea have been reported in less than 1% of patients receiving IM or IV cefuroxime sodium.

Clostridium difficile-associated Diarrhea and Colitis

Treatment with anti-infectives alters normal colon flora and may permit overgrowth of *Clostridium difficile*.

C. difficile infection (CDI) and *C. difficile*-associated diarrhea and colitis (CDAD; also known as antibiotic-associated diarrhea and colitis or pseudomembranous colitis) have been reported with nearly all anti-infectives, including cefuroxime, and may range in severity from mild diarrhea to fatal colitis. *C. difficile* produces toxins A and B which contribute to the development of CDAD; hypertoxin-producing strains of *C. difficile* are associated with increased morbidity and mortality since they may be refractory to anti-infectives and colectomy may be required.

CDAD should be considered in the differential diagnosis in patients who develop diarrhea during or after anti-infective therapy and managed accordingly. Careful medical history is necessary since CDAD has been reported to occur as late as 2 months or longer after anti-infective therapy is discontinued.

If CDAD is suspected or confirmed, anti-infectives not directed against *C. difficile* should be discontinued whenever possible. Patients should be managed with appropriate supportive therapy (e.g., fluid and electrolyte management, protein supplementation), anti-infective therapy directed against *C. difficile* (e.g., metronidazole, vancomycin), and surgical evaluation as clinically indicated.

● Hematologic Effects

Decreased hemoglobin concentration and decreased hematocrit have been reported in about 10% of patients receiving cefuroxime. Transient eosinophilia occurs less frequently, and transient neutropenia, pancytopenia, thrombocytopenia, and leukopenia occur rarely. Thrombocytosis, lymphocytosis, hemolytic anemia, and increased prothrombin time also have been reported.

● CNS Effects

Headache, dizziness, somnolence or sleepiness, hyperactivity, irritable behavior, seizures, myoclonic jerks, and generalized hyperexcitability have been reported rarely in patients receiving cefuroxime.

A psychotic reaction, consisting of disorientation, fluctuating consciousness, and episodes of restlessness, agitation, and anxiety, occurred in a geriatric patient who received IV cefuroxime sodium; symptoms resolved within 24 hours after the drug was discontinued. Some patients who experienced adverse CNS effects while receiving cefuroxime had preexisting renal impairment.

● Hepatic Effects

Transient increases in serum AST (SGOT), ALT (SGPT), alkaline phosphatase, LDH, and bilirubin concentrations have been reported in less than 5% of patients receiving oral or parenteral cefuroxime. Jaundice has been reported rarely.

● Renal and Genitourinary Effects

Acute renal failure and interstitial nephritis have been reported rarely in patients receiving cefuroxime. Although a causal relationship has not been established, transient increases in BUN and/or serum creatinine concentrations and decreased creatinine clearance have been reported in a few patients receiving cefuroxime. Bilateral renal cortical necrosis that appeared to be a hypersensitivity reaction has been reported in at least one patient who received cefuroxime axetil.

Urinary tract infection, kidney pain, urethral pain or bleeding, dysuria, vaginitis, vaginal candidiasis, vulvovaginal pruritus, and vaginal discharge or irritation have been reported in less than 1% of patients receiving oral cefuroxime axetil therapy.

● Other Adverse Effects

Jarisch-Herxheimer reaction has occurred in 5.6% of patients receiving cefuroxime axetil for the treatment of Lyme disease. In a clinical study in patients with early Lyme disease, the Jarisch-Herxheimer reaction occurred in 11.8% of patients receiving cefuroxime axetil and 11.5% of patients receiving doxycycline. These transient reactions generally last only 1–2 days.

Overgrowth with nonsusceptible organisms (e.g., perianal, oral, or vaginal candidiasis; pseudomembranous colitis; superinfection) has occurred in patients receiving cefuroxime sodium or cefuroxime axetil. (See Cautions: GI Effects and also see Precautions and Contraindications.)

Mild to severe hearing loss has been reported in a few pediatric patients receiving cefuroxime sodium for the treatment of meningitis. Persistence of positive CSF cultures at 18–36 hours has been observed with cefuroxime sodium injection; however, the clinical relevance of this finding is unknown.

Muscle spasm of the neck, muscle cramps or stiffness, chest pain or tightness, shortness of breath, tachycardia, chills, lockjaw-type reaction, viral illness, upper respiratory infection, sinusitis, fever, cough, joint swelling, and arthralgia have been reported in less than 1% of patients receiving oral cefuroxime axetil therapy. Diaper rash has been reported in 3.4% of pediatric patients receiving cefuroxime axetil as the commercially available oral suspension.

● Precautions and Contraindications

Prior to initiation of cefuroxime therapy, careful inquiry should be made concerning previous hypersensitivity reactions to cephalosporins, penicillins, or other drugs. Cefuroxime axetil and cefuroxime sodium are contraindicated in patients who are hypersensitive to cefuroxime or other cephalosporins and should be used with caution in patients with a history of hypersensitivity to penicillins. Use of cephalosporins should be avoided in patients who have had an immediate-type (anaphylactic) hypersensitivity reaction to penicillins. Although it has not been definitely proven that allergic reactions to antibiotics are more frequent in atopic individuals, the manufacturer states that parenteral cefuroxime should be used with caution in patients with a history of allergy, particularly to drugs.

To reduce development of drug-resistant bacteria and maintain effectiveness of cefuroxime and other antibacterials, the drug should be used only for the treatment or prevention of infections proven or strongly suspected to be caused by susceptible bacteria. When selecting or modifying anti-infective therapy, results of culture and in vitro susceptibility testing should be used. In the absence of such data, local epidemiology and susceptibility patterns should be considered when selecting anti-infectives for empiric therapy.

Patients should be advised that antibacterials (including cefuroxime) should only be used to treat bacterial infections and not used to treat viral infections (e.g., the common cold). Patients also should be advised about the importance of completing the full course of therapy, even if feeling better after a few days, and that skipping doses or not completing therapy may decrease effectiveness and increase the likelihood that bacteria will develop resistance and will not be treatable with cefuroxime or other antibacterials in the future.

As with other anti-infectives, prolonged use of cefuroxime axetil or cefuroxime sodium may result in overgrowth of nonsusceptible organisms. Careful observation of the patient during cefuroxime therapy is essential. If suprainfection or superinfection occurs, appropriate therapy should be instituted.

Individuals with phenylketonuria (i.e., homozygous genetic deficiency of phenylalanine hydroxylase) and other individuals who must restrict their intake of phenylalanine should be warned that Ceftin® oral suspensions containing 125 or 250 mg of cefuroxime per 5 mL contains aspartame (NutraSweet®), which is metabolized in the GI tract to provide 11.8 or 25.2 mg of phenylalanine/5 mL, respectively.

Like other dextrose-containing solutions, the commercially available Duplex® drug delivery system containing 750 mg or 1.5 g of cefuroxime and 50 mL of dextrose injection should be used with caution in patients with overt or known subclinical diabetes mellitus or in patients with carbohydrate intolerance for any reason.

Because CDAD has been reported with the use of cefuroxime and other cephalosporins, it should be considered in the differential diagnosis of patients who develop diarrhea during or after cefuroxime therapy. (See Clostridium difficile-associated Diarrhea and Colitis under Cautions: GI Effects.) Patients should be advised that diarrhea is a common problem caused by anti-infectives and usually resolves when the drug is discontinued; however, they should contact a clinician if watery and bloody stools (with or without stomach cramps and fever) occur during or as late as 2 months or longer after the last dose. Cefuroxime should be used with caution in patients with a history of GI disease, particularly colitis. The safety and efficacy of cefuroxime axetil therapy in patients with GI malabsorption have not been established.

Although cefuroxime sodium only rarely causes adverse renal effects, the manufacturers state that renal function should be monitored during therapy with the drug, especially when maximum dosage is used in seriously ill patients.

Safety and efficacy of oral cefuroxime axetil in patients with renal impairment have not been established. Because serum concentrations of cefuroxime are higher and more prolonged in patients with renal impairment than in patients with normal renal function, dose and/or frequency of administration of parenteral cefuroxime sodium should be decreased in patients with transient or persistent renal impairment. (See Dosage in Renal Impairment in Dosage and Administration: Dosage.)

Several cephalosporins (including cefuroxime) have been associated with the development of seizures, particularly in patients with renal impairment, in whom dosage of the drug was not reduced. If seizures associated with cefuroxime develop, the drug should be discontinued and anticonvulsant therapy initiated as clinically indicated.

Because some cephalosporins have been associated with a decrease in prothrombin activity, the manufacturers state that prothrombin time (PT) should be monitored when cefuroxime is used in patients with renal or hepatic impairment, in patients with poor nutritional status, in patients receiving a protracted course of anti-infective therapy, or in those previously stabilized on anticoagulant therapy. Vitamin K should be administered if indicated.

● Pediatric Precautions

Safety and efficacy of oral cefuroxime axetil or parenteral cefuroxime sodium in children younger than 3 months of age have not been established.

In vitro studies indicate that cefuroxime does not appear to displace bilirubin appreciably from albumin binding sites in neonates†.

Cefuroxime Axetil

The manufacturers state that safety and efficacy of cefuroxime axetil for the treatment of acute bacterial maxillary sinusitis in pediatric patients 3 months to 12 years of age have been established based on safety and efficacy of the drug in adults. In addition, use of cefuroxime axetil in pediatric patients is supported by pharmacokinetic and safety data in adult and pediatric patients, clinical and microbiologic data from adequate and well-controlled studies of the treatment of acute bacterial maxillary sinusitis in adults and acute otitis media with effusion in pediatric patients, and postmarketing surveillance of adverse effects.

Cefuroxime axetil tablets and oral suspension generally are well tolerated in children aged 3 months to 12 years. Cefuroxime axetil has a strong, persistent, bitter taste and complaints caused by the taste were reported in up to 66% of children who received the drug as crushed tablets and vomiting was induced aversively in some of these children. This bitter taste and/or problems with administering the drug required discontinuance of such cefuroxime axetil therapy in 2–28% of children in clinical trials. Although discontinuance of therapy with the suspension because of its taste or other problems with administration occurred in 1.4% of children receiving the oral suspension, the commercially available oral suspension should be used in children who cannot swallow the tablets whole.

Cefuroxime Sodium

To avoid overdosage, the commercially available Duplex® drug delivery system containing 750 mg or 1.5 g of cefuroxime should not be used in pediatric patients only if the entire 750-mg or 1.5-g dose in the container is required.

● Geriatric Precautions

In clinical studies of cefuroxime axetil, 375 patients were 65 years of age or older and 151 were 75 years of age or older. There were no apparent differences in safety or effectiveness between these individuals and younger adults. Although the group of patients aged 65 years or older experienced a lower incidence of some adverse effects (e.g., vaginal candidiasis, GI effects) compared with patients 12–64 years of age, no clinically important differences were observed between geriatric and younger patients and there have been no reports of differences in response in either group.

In clinical studies of cefuroxime sodium involving over 1900 patients, approximately 47% of the patients were 65 years of age or older and 22% were 75 years of age or older. Although no overall differences in efficacy or safety were observed between geriatric and younger patients, and other clinical experience revealed no evidence of age-related differences, the possibility that some geriatric patients may exhibit increased sensitivity to the drug cannot be ruled out.

Cefuroxime is substantially excreted by the kidney, and renal elimination of the drug may be decreased and the risk of severe adverse reactions may be increased in patients with impaired renal function. Limited data indicate that mean serum elimination half-life of cefuroxime is prolonged in geriatric patients (mean age: 83.9 years) who have a mean creatinine clearance of approximately 35 mL/minute. Despite this prolonged elimination, the manufacturers state that age-based dosage adjustment does not appear to be necessary. However, because geriatric patients are more likely to have decreased renal function, dosage should be selected with caution in these patients and monitoring of renal function may be useful.

● Mutagenicity and Carcinogenicity

No evidence of mutagenicity was observed with cefuroxime in various in vitro and in vivo test systems, including the mouse lymphoma assay, micronucleus test, and bacterial mutation tests. Cefuroxime produced positive results in the in vitro chromosome aberration assay. Studies have not been performed to date to evaluate the carcinogenic potential of cefuroxime.

● Pregnancy, Fertility, and Lactation

Pregnancy

Reproduction studies in mice and rabbits using cefuroxime sodium in dosages up to 6 and 2 times the usual human dosage based on mg/m², respectively, and reproduction studies in mice and rats using cefuroxime axetil in dosages up to 14 and 9 times, respectively, the usual human dosage based on mg/m² have not revealed evidence of impaired fertility or harm to the fetus. There are no adequate and controlled studies to date using cefuroxime in pregnant women, and cefuroxime axetil and cefuroxime sodium should be used during pregnancy only when clearly needed. Cefuroxime axetil has not been studied for use during labor and delivery.

Lactation

Because cefuroxime is distributed into milk, cefuroxime axetil and cefuroxime sodium should be used with caution in nursing women.

DRUG INTERACTIONS

● Aminoglycosides

In vitro studies indicate that the antibacterial activity of cefuroxime and aminoglycosides may be additive or synergistic against some organisms including *Enterobacter*, *Escherichia coli*, *Klebsiella*, *Proteus mirabilis*, and *Serratia marcescens*.

Concurrent use of aminoglycosides and certain cephalosporins reportedly may increase the risk of nephrotoxicity during therapy. Although this effect has not been reported to date with cefuroxime, the possibility that nephrotoxicity may be potentiated should be considered if the drug is used concomitantly with an aminoglycoside.

● Diuretics

The manufacturers state that cefuroxime should be used with caution in patients receiving diuretics because concurrent use of these drugs may increase the risk of adverse renal effects.

● Estrogens or Progestins

Cefuroxime axetil may affect gut flora, leading to decreased estrogen reabsorption and reduced efficacy of oral contraceptives containing estrogen and progestin.

● Probenecid

Oral probenecid administered shortly before or concomitantly with cefuroxime usually slows the rate of tubular secretion of cefuroxime and produces higher and more prolonged serum concentrations of cefuroxime. This effect has been used to therapeutic advantage in the treatment of gonorrhea. Peak serum concentrations of cefuroxime and the half-life of the drug are reportedly increased by up to 30% when probenecid is administered concomitantly; the area under the concentration-time curve (AUC) of cefuroxime is increased by about 50%. Concomitant administration of probenecid also reportedly decreases the apparent volume of distribution of cefuroxime by about 20%.

LABORATORY TEST INTERFERENCES

● Immunohematology Tests

Positive direct antiglobulin (Coombs') test results have been reported in a few patients receiving cefuroxime axetil or cefuroxime sodium. This reaction may interfere with hematologic studies or transfusion cross-matching procedures.

● Tests for Glucose

Like most other cephalosporins, cefuroxime reportedly causes false-positive results in urine glucose determinations using cupric sulfate solution (Benedict's reagent, Clinitest®); however, glucose oxidase tests (Clinistix®) are unaffected by the drug.

Cefuroxime may cause false-negative results when ferricyanide methods are used to determine blood glucose concentrations.

● Tests for Creatinine

Although some cephalosporins reportedly cause falsely elevated serum or urine creatinine values when the Jaffé reaction is used, cefuroxime does not appear to interfere with this laboratory test.

ACUTE TOXICITY

Limited information is available on the acute toxicity of cefuroxime in humans. Overdosage of cephalosporins can cause CNS irritation leading to seizures. If acute overdosage of cefuroxime occurs, hemodialysis and/or peritoneal dialysis can be used to enhance elimination of the drug from the body.

MECHANISM OF ACTION

Cefuroxime is usually bactericidal in action. Like other cephalosporins, the antibacterial activity of the drug results from inhibition of mucopeptide synthesis in the bacterial cell wall. For information on the mechanism of action of cephalosporins, see Mechanism of Action in the Cephalosporins General Statement 8:12.06.

SPECTRUM

Based on its spectrum of activity, cefuroxime is classified as a second generation cephalosporin. For information on the classification of cephalosporins and closely related β-lactam antibiotics based on spectra of activity, see Spectrum in the Cephalosporins General Statement 8:12.06.

Like other currently available second generation cephalosporins (e.g., cefaclor, cefamandole, cefprozil), cefuroxime generally is more active in vitro against gram-negative bacteria than first generation cephalosporins but has a narrower spectrum of activity against gram-negative bacteria than third generation cephalosporins. The spectrum of activity of cefuroxime resembles that of cefamandole and, to a lesser extent, that of cefoxitin. Cefuroxime is more resistant to hydrolysis by β-lactamases than cefamandole and is active against some strains of gram-negative bacteria (e.g., *Escherichia coli, Enterobacter, Klebsiella, Neisseria*) that are resistant to cefamandole. Cefoxitin is active against several organisms that generally are resistant to cefuroxime (e.g., *Serratia marcescens, Proteus vulgaris, Bacteroides fragilis*).

● *In Vitro Susceptibility Testing*

Results of in vitro cefuroxime susceptibility tests are not generally affected by inoculum size, culture media, presence of serum, or pH. However, results of susceptibility tests for some gram-negative bacilli (e.g., *Morganella morganii, Bacteroides fragilis, Serratia*) may be affected by the size of the inoculum.

Different interpretive criteria are used for defining in vitro susceptibility of certain organisms to cefuroxime axetil and cefuroxime sodium, and the appropriate zone diameter or MIC categories should be used when determining whether or not an isolate is susceptible to the parenteral or oral preparation of the drug.

Strains of staphylococci resistant to penicillinase-resistant penicillins (oxacillin-resistant [methicillin-resistant] staphylococci) should be considered resistant to cefuroxime and cefuroxime axetil, although results of in vitro susceptibility tests may indicate that the organisms are susceptible to the drug. In addition, β-lactamase-negative, ampicillin-resistant (BLNAR) strains of *H. influenzae* should be considered resistant to cefuroxime and cefuroxime axetil despite the fact that results of in vitro susceptibility tests may indicate that the organisms are susceptible to the drug.

For information on interpreting results of in vitro susceptibility testing (disk susceptibility tests, dilution susceptibility tests) when cefuroxime and cefuroxime axetil susceptibility testing is performed according to the standards of the Clinical and Laboratory Standards Institute (CLSI; formerly National Committee for Clinical Laboratory Standards [NCCLS]), see Spectrum: In Vitro Susceptibility Testing, in the Cephalosporins General Statement 8:12.06.

● *Gram-Positive Aerobic Bacteria*

In vitro, cefuroxime concentrations of 0.5–1 mcg/mL inhibit most strains of *Staphylococcus aureus* (including penicillinase-producing and nonpenicillinase-producing strains) and concentrations of 1–2 mcg/mL inhibit most strains of *S. epidermidis*. Most strains of staphylococci resistant to penicillinase-resistant penicillins also are resistant to cefuroxime.

In vitro, α-hemolytic and β-hemolytic streptococci are usually inhibited by cefuroxime concentrations of 0.05–0.5 mcg/mL and *Streptococcus pneumoniae* is usually inhibited by concentrations of 0.01–0.13 mcg/mL. Most strains of enterococci, including *E. faecalis* (formerly *S. faecalis*), are generally resistant to cefuroxime.

Listeria monocytogenes generally is resistant to cefuroxime.

● *Gram-Negative Aerobic Bacteria*

Cefuroxime is active in vitro against most gram-negative aerobic cocci and many gram-negative aerobic bacilli including Enterobacteriaceae. *Pseudomonas aeruginosa* is resistant to cefuroxime. *Acinetobacter calcoaceticus* is also usually resistant to the drug.

Generally, cefuroxime is active in vitro against the following Enterobacteriaceae: *Citrobacter diversus, C. freundii, Enterobacter aerogenes, Escherichia coli, Klebsiella pneumoniae, Proteus mirabilis, Providencia stuartii, Salmonella*, and *Shigella*. Although cefuroxime is active in vitro against some strains of *Morganella morganii* (formerly *Proteus morganii*), *Providencia rettgeri* (formerly *Proteus rettgeri*), and *Proteus vulgaris*, most strains of these organisms are resistant to the drug. In addition, *Enterobacter cloacae, Legionella, Pseudomonas, Campylobacter* spp., *Providencia*, and most strains of *Serratia* are usually resistant to cefuroxime. Most susceptible Enterobacteriaceae are inhibited in vitro by cefuroxime concentrations of 1–12.5 mcg/mL. In vitro on a weight basis, the activity of cefuroxime against susceptible Enterobacteriaceae is approximately equal to that of cefoxitin but less than that of cefotaxime. Cefuroxime may be active in vitro against some strains of *E. aerogenes* that are resistant to cefoxitin; however, cefotaxime and, to a lesser extent, cefoxitin may be active in vitro against some strains of *P. vulgaris* and *Serratia* resistant to cefuroxime.

Cefuroxime is active in vitro against *Haemophilus influenzae* (including ampicillin-resistant strains) and *H. parainfluenzae*. Most susceptible strains of *H. influenzae* are inhibited in vitro by cefuroxime concentrations of 0.1–2 mcg/mL.

Cefuroxime is active in vitro against *Neisseria gonorrhoeae* (including both penicillinase-producing and nonpenicillinase-producing strains) and *N. meningitidis*. The MIC$_{90}$ (minimum inhibitory concentration of the drug at which 90% of strains tested are inhibited) of cefuroxime reported for *N. gonorrhoeae* (including both penicillinase-producing and nonpenicillinase-producing strains) is 0.1–0.5 mcg/mL.

● *Anaerobic Bacteria*

Cefuroxime is active in vitro against some anaerobic bacteria including *Actinomyces, Eubacterium, Fusobacterium, Lactobacillus, Peptococcus, Peptostreptococcus, Propionibacterium*, and *Veillonella*. Cefuroxime is active in vitro against some strains of *Clostridium*; however, *C. difficile* is usually resistant to the drug.

Most susceptible anaerobes are inhibited in vitro by cefuroxime concentrations of 0.5–16 mcg/mL. Although cefuroxime concentrations of 16 mcg/mL inhibit some strains of *Bacteroides fragilis* in vitro, most strains of the organism are resistant to the drug.

● *Spirochetes*

Cefuroxime is active in vitro and in vivo against *Borrelia burgdorferi*, the causative organism of Lyme disease. In vitro, the MIC of cefuroxime for *B. burgdorferi* reportedly is 0.13 mcg/mL and the minimum bactericidal concentration (MBC) is 1 mcg/mL.

RESISTANCE

For information on possible mechanisms of bacterial resistance to cephalosporins, see Resistance in the Cephalosporins General Statement 8:12.06.

Because cefuroxime contains a methoxyimino group that protects the β-lactam ring from hydrolysis by many penicillinases and cephalosporinases, the drug is more resistant to hydrolysis by β-lactamases than are first generation cephalosporins or cefamandole. Cefuroxime is generally resistant to hydrolysis by β-lactamases classified as Richmond-Sykes types I, II, III, IV, and V and most β-lactamases produced by *Neisseria gonorrhoeae, Haemophilus influenzae*, and staphylococci. However, cefuroxime is hydrolyzed by β-lactamases produced by *B. fragilis* and some type I β-lactamases produced by *Serratia, P. vulgaris*, and *P. rettgeri*. Results of one in vitro study indicate that cefuroxime is hydrolyzed more rapidly than cefotaxime by β-lactamases produced by *P. vulgaris* and *B. fragilis*. Although cefuroxime is resistant to hydrolysis by β-lactamases produced by *Ps. aeruginosa*, these organisms are resistant to cefuroxime because the drug cannot penetrate their cell wall.

PHARMACOKINETICS

In all studies described in the Pharmacokinetics section, cefuroxime was administered orally as the 1-(acetyloxy)ethyl ester (i.e., cefuroxime axetil) and parenterally as the sodium salt; dosages and concentrations of the drug are expressed in terms of cefuroxime. Because cefuroxime axetil is hydrolyzed rapidly (t$_{1/2}$: 3.5 minutes) in vitro in blood or serum, some clinicians recommend that acetonitrile be added immediately to blood or serum samples intended for pharmacokinetic determinations of the drug in order to prevent further hydrolysis and resultant falsely high concentrations of active drug.

● *Absorption*

Cefuroxime Axetil

Following oral administration of cefuroxime axetil, the drug is absorbed as the 1-(acetyloxy)ethyl ester from the GI tract and rapidly hydrolyzed to cefuroxime by nonspecific esterases in the intestinal mucosa and blood. Cefuroxime remaining within the intestinal lumen following hydrolysis of the ester is not absorbed appreciably. The drug has little, if any, microbiologic activity until hydrolyzed in vivo to cefuroxime.

Bioavailability following oral administration of cefuroxime axetil is variable and depends on the formulation used and presence of food in the GI tract. Many published studies on the pharmacokinetics of the drug used various formulations that provided poorer bioavailability than the currently available tablets and cannot be used to provide information on the currently available preparation.

When tested in healthy adults, the bioavailability of cefuroxime axetil oral suspension was found *not* to be equivalent to that of cefuroxime axetil tablets. Mean area under the concentration-time curve (AUC) for the oral suspension was 91% of the AUC for the tablets, and the mean peak plasma concentration of cefuroxime following administration of the cefuroxime axetil oral suspension was 71%

of that achieved following administration of cefuroxime axetil tablets. Therefore, cefuroxime axetil oral suspension and tablet formulations are not substitutable on a mg/mg basis. (See Dosage: Pediatric Dosage in Dosage and Administration.)

In adults, bioavailability of cefuroxime following oral administration of commercially available cefuroxime axetil tablets averages about 37% when given in the fasting state and 52% when given with or shortly after food. Absorption of the drug is increased when given with milk or infant formula. In one study, the extent but not the rate of absorption was substantially greater when the drug was administered concomitantly with milk compared with applesauce or fasting.

Following oral administration in adults of a single 125-mg, 250-mg, 500-mg, or 1-g dose of commercially available cefuroxime axetil tablets immediately following a meal, peak serum cefuroxime concentrations are attained approximately 2–3 hours after the dose and average 2.1, 4.1, 7, or 13.6 mcg/mL, respectively; serum concentrations 6 hours after the dose average 0.3, 0.7, 2.2, or 3.4 mcg/mL, respectively. AUC of the drug in these individuals averaged 6.7, 12.9, 27.4, or 50 mcg-h/mL, respectively.

Results of a study in healthy adults indicate that cefuroxime axetil oral suspensions containing 125 mg/5 mL or 250 mg/5 mL are bioequivalent. In healthy adults who received a 250-mg dose of cefuroxime axetil given as a suspension containing 125 mg/5 mL or 250 mg/5 mL with food, peak plasma concentrations of cefuroxime were 2.4 or 2.2 mcg/mL, respectively, and were attained 3 hours after the dose.

In pharmacokinetic studies of cefuroxime axetil oral suspension in children, the drug was administered postprandially or with food; no data are available regarding absorption of the suspension in fasting children. Following oral administration to children 3 months to 12 years of age (mean age: 23 months) of a single 10-, 15-, or 20-mg/kg dose of commercially available cefuroxime axetil oral suspension concomitantly with milk or milk products, peak serum cefuroxime concentrations are attained approximately 3.6, 2.7, or 3.1 hours after the dose, respectively, and average 3.3, 5.1, or 7 mcg/mL, respectively.

Cefuroxime Sodium

Cefuroxime sodium is not appreciably absorbed from the GI tract and must be given parenterally. Following IM administration of a single 500-mg, 750-mg, or 1-g dose of cefuroxime in healthy adults with normal renal function, peak serum concentrations of the drug are attained within 15–60 minutes and range from 20.8–25.7, 26–34.9, and 32–40 mcg/mL, respectively. In one study following IM administration of a single 750-mg dose of cefuroxime in healthy adults, serum concentrations of the drug averaged 32.8 mcg/mL 40 minutes after the dose, 19.1 mcg/mL 2 hours after the dose, 6.1 mcg/mL 4 hours after the dose, 1.5 mcg/mL 6 hours after the dose, and 0.7 mcg/mL 8 hours after the dose. IM injection of a single 1.5-g dose of the drug reportedly results in peak serum concentrations averaging 46 mcg/mL. Mean peak serum concentrations of cefuroxime and the areas under the concentration-time curve (AUC) are not substantially different after IM injection of cefuroxime as a suspension or as a solution. The AUC of cefuroxime is proportional to the dose administered and is similar following IM or IV administration of the drug. In one preliminary study in women, serum concentrations of cefuroxime were lower when IM injections of the drug were given into the gluteus maximus than when the same dose was given into the thigh.

In one study in healthy adults with normal renal function, a single 500-mg or 1-g dose of cefuroxime given by IV injection over 3 minutes resulted in serum concentrations of cefuroxime that averaged 66.3 and 99.2 mcg/mL, respectively, immediately after the injection; serum concentrations of the drug averaged 2.1 and 3.6 mcg/mL, respectively, 4 hours after the injection. In another study in healthy adults with normal renal function, IV injection over 2–3 minutes of a single 750-mg dose of cefuroxime resulted in serum concentrations of cefuroxime that averaged 52.6 mcg/mL 15 minutes after the injection, 24 mcg/mL 1 hour after the injection, 9.7 mcg/mL 2 hours after the injection, 3.5 mcg/mL 4 hours after the injection, and 0.5 mcg/mL 8 hours after the injection.

IV infusion over 30 minutes of a single 500- or 750-mg dose of cefuroxime reportedly results in peak serum concentrations of the drug averaging 37.8 and 51.1 mcg/mL, respectively. IV infusion over 1 hour of a single 750-mg or 1-g dose of cefuroxime reportedly results in peak serum concentrations of the drug averaging 38 and 64.4 mcg/mL, respectively.

In one study in neonates, IM administration of a single cefuroxime dose of 25 mg/kg resulted in serum concentrations of the drug that averaged 45 mcg/mL 30 minutes after the injection, 35 mcg/mL 3 hours after the

injection, and 10.5 mcg/mL 12 hours after the injection. IM administration of a single cefuroxime dose of 10 mg/kg in neonates younger than 3 weeks of age reportedly resulted in serum concentrations of the drug that ranged from 15–25 mcg/mL 30–60 minutes after injection.

● Distribution

The apparent volume of distribution of cefuroxime in healthy adults ranges from 9.3–15.8 L/1.73 m².

Following IM or IV administration of usual dosages of cefuroxime, the drug is widely distributed into body tissues and fluids including the kidneys, heart, gallbladder, liver, prostatic adenoma tissue, uterine and ovarian tissue, aqueous humor, saliva, sputum, bronchial secretions, bone, bile, adipose tissue, wound exudates, peritoneal fluid, ascitic fluid, synovial fluid, pericardial fluid, and pleural fluid.

Following oral administration of cefuroxime axetil in pediatric patients with acute otitis media with effusion or with chronic or recurrent otitis media with effusion, cefuroxime is distributed into middle ear effusions. In a study in pediatric patients 1–4 years of age with acute otitis media with effusion who received a single 15 mg/kg dose of cefuroxime as cefuroxime axetil oral suspension, cefuroxime concentrations in middle ear effusions 2–5 hours after a dose ranged from 0.2–3.6 mcg/mL; concurrent serum concentrations were 2.8–7.3 mcg/mL.

Cefuroxime is 33–50% bound to serum proteins.

Cefuroxime concentrations in CSF are low following IV administration of usual dosages of the drug in patients with uninflamed meninges; however, therapeutic concentrations of cefuroxime may be attained following IV administration of the drug in patients with inflamed meninges. In one study in adults receiving 1–2 g of cefuroxime IV every 8 hours, the maximum CSF concentration of cefuroxime in patients with uninflamed or inflamed meninges was 0.1 or 8.28 mcg/mL, respectively. In adults with meningitis receiving 1.5 g of cefuroxime every 6 or 8 hours, mean CSF concentrations of the drug attained within 8 hours after dosing are 6 mcg/mL (range: 1.5–13.5) or 5.2 mcg/mL (range: 2.7–8.9), respectively. In one study in children 1–4 years of age with meningitis receiving rapid IV injection of cefuroxime 50 mg/kg every 6 hours, CSF concentrations of the drug after at least 2 days of therapy ranged from 1.1–9.8 mcg/mL in CSF specimens obtained 2 hours after a dose. In pediatric patients 4 weeks to 6.5 years of age with meningitis receiving 50 mg/kg every 6 hours, mean CSF concentrations of cefuroxime were 6.6 mcg/mL (range: 0.9–17.3). In another study in pediatric patients 7 months to 9 years of age with meningitis receiving 67–77 mg/kg every 8 hours, mean CSF concentrations of cefuroxime were 8.3 mcg/mL (range: less than 2 up to 22.5).

Cefuroxime readily crosses the placenta. Amniotic fluid concentrations of cefuroxime reportedly average 17–18.6 mcg/mL 3–5.5 hours after a single 750-mg IM dose of the drug. Cefuroxime is distributed into milk.

● Elimination

In adults, the serum or plasma half-life of cefuroxime following oral administration of commercially available cefuroxime axetil tablets or oral suspension ranges from 1.2–1.6 hours. In adults with normal renal function, the serum half-life of cefuroxime following IM or IV administration reportedly ranges from 1–2 hours. In adults, approximately 50% of an administered dose of cefuroxime axetil is recovered in the urine within 12 hours.

In patients with renal impairment, the serum half-life of the drug is prolonged and generally ranges from 1.9–16.1 hours depending on the degree of impairment. In one study, the serum half-life of cefuroxime was 1 hour in patients with creatinine clearances of 50–79 mL/minute, 2.55 hours in patients with creatinine clearances of 25–46 mL/minute, 5.1 hours in patients with creatinine clearances of 10–24 mL/minute, and 14.8 hours in patients with creatinine clearances less than 10 mL/minute. A serum half-life of 15–22 hours has been reported in anuric patients.

In neonates and children, the serum half-life of cefuroxime is inversely proportional to age. Following oral administration of cefuroxime axetil oral suspension in children 3 months to 12 years of age, the serum half-life of cefuroxime averages 1.4–1.9 hours. The serum half-life of cefuroxime following IM or IV administration is reportedly 5.1–5.8 hours in neonates 3 days of age or younger, 2–4.2 hours in neonates 6–14 days of age, and 1–1.5 hours in neonates 3–4 weeks of age. The manufacturers of cefuroxime axetil state that the urinary pharmacokinetics of cefuroxime axetil have not been determined in children and that the renal pharmacokinetics of oral cefuroxime axetil as established in the adult population should not be extrapolated to children.

Following oral administration, cefuroxime axetil is rapidly hydrolyzed to cefuroxime by nonspecific esterases in the intestinal mucosa and blood; the axetil moiety is metabolized to acetaldehyde and acetic acid. Cefuroxime is not metabolized and is excreted unchanged principally in urine by both glomerular filtration and tubular secretion. In adults with normal renal function, 90–100% of a single IM or IV dose of cefuroxime is excreted unchanged in urine within 24 hours; most of the dose is excreted within the first 6 hours following administration. Following IM administration of a single 750-mg dose of cefuroxime, urinary concentrations of the drug average 1.3 mg/mL in urine collected during the first 8 hours after administration. Urinary concentrations of cefuroxime average 1.15 or 2.5 mg/mL in urine collected over the first 8 hours following IV administration of a single 750-mg or 1.5-g dose of the drug, respectively.

Concomitant administration of probenecid competitively inhibits renal tubular secretion of cefuroxime and produces higher and more prolonged serum concentrations of the drug. (See Drug Interactions: Probenecid.)

Cefuroxime is removed by hemodialysis and by peritoneal dialysis.

CHEMISTRY AND STABILITY

● Chemistry

Cefuroxime is a semisynthetic cephalosporin antibiotic. cefuroxime contains a methoxyimino group at position 7 on the β-lactam ring and also contains a carbamate group at position 3 on the ring. The methoxyimino group results in stability against hydrolysis by many β-lactamases and the carbamate group results in metabolic stability.

Cefuroxime is commercially available for parenteral administration as the sodium salt. The drug is commercially available for oral administration as film-coated tablets or as a powder for suspension of cefuroxime axetil, the 1-(acetyloxy)ethyl ester of the drug. Potency of cefuroxime sodium and cefuroxime axetil is expressed in terms of cefuroxime.

Cefuroxime Axetil

Cefuroxime axetil is a prodrug of cefuroxime and has little, if any, antibacterial activity until hydrolyzed in vivo to cefuroxime. Esterification of the carboxyl C-4 group of cefuroxime results in a more lipophilic and readily absorbable (from the GI tract) form of the drug. Cefuroxime axetil occurs as a white to cream-colored, amorphous powder.

Cefuroxime Sodium

Cefuroxime sodium occurs as a white to off-white powder. The drug has solubilities of about 200 mg/mL in water and 1 mg/mL in alcohol. The drug has a pK_a of 2.45. The sodium salt of cefuroxime contains 2.4 mEq of sodium per gram of cefuroxime.

Following reconstitution, cefuroxime sodium solutions are light yellow to amber in color and have a pH of 6–8.5, depending on the concentration of the drug and the diluent used. Reconstitution of cefuroxime sodium sterile powder for injection to provide a final concentration of 208 mg/mL results in the formation of a suspension; dilution to at least 100 mg/mL effects complete dissolution of the drug.

When the commercially available Duplex® delivery system containing 750 mg or 1.5 g of cefuroxime and 50 mL of dextrose injection in separate chambers is reconstituted (activated) according to the manufacturer's directions, the resultant solution is iso-osmotic and has an osmolality of approximately 290 mOsm/kg.

The commercially available frozen premixed injection of cefuroxime sodium containing 1.5 g of cefuroxime is a sterile, nonpyrogenic, iso-osmotic solution of the drug provided in a plastic container fabricated from specially formulated multilayered plastic PL 2040. The 1.5-g frozen injection contains 600 mg of sodium citrate hydrous as a buffer and 222 mg (9.7 mEq) of sodium, and has an osmolality of approximately 300 mOsm/kg. After thawing, the injection has a pH to 5–7.5.

● Stability

Cefuroxime Axetil

Cefuroxime axetil tablets should be stored in tight containers at 20–25°C or 15–30°C, depending on the manufacturer. When cefuroxime axetil tablets are allowed to disintegrate in apple juice, the drug is stable for 24 hours at room temperature.

Commercially available cefuroxime axetil powder for oral suspension should be stored at 2–30°C. Following reconstitution, oral suspensions of cefuroxime axetil containing 125 mg/5 mL or 250 mg/5 mL should be stored immediately at 2–8°C in a refrigerator. Any unused oral suspension should be discarded after 10 days.

Cefuroxime Sodium

Commercially available cefuroxime sodium sterile powder for injection should be stored at 15–30°C and protected from light.

Following reconstitution of vials containing 750 mg or 1.5 g of cefuroxime or the pharmacy bulk vial containing 7.5 g of the drug with sterile water for injection according to the manufacturer's directions, solutions for IV administration are stable for 24 hours at room temperature or 48 hours (750-mg and 1.5-g vials) or 7 days (7.5-g pharmacy bulk vial) when refrigerated (5°C). More dilute solutions, such as 750 mg or 1.5 g in 100 mL of sterile water for injection, 5% dextrose injection, or 0.9% sodium chloride injection also are stable for 24 hours at room temperature or 7 days when refrigerated.

Following reconstitution of 750-mg or 1.5-g ADD-Vantage® (TwistVial®) vials of cefuroxime with 5% dextrose injection, 0.9% sodium chloride injection, or 0.45% sodium chloride injection according to the manufacturer's directions, solutions are stable for 24 hours at room temperature or 7 days under refrigeration; joined vials that have not been activated (diluted) may be used within a 14-day period.

IM injections containing 225 mg/mL of cefuroxime prepared using the 750-mg vial and sterile water for injection according to the manufacturer's directions are stable for 24 hours at room temperature or 48 hours when refrigerated (5°C).

Cefuroxime sodium is chemically and physically compatible with the following IV solutions: 0.9% sodium chloride; Ringer's; lactated Ringer's; 5% dextrose; 5% dextrose and 0.2%, 0.45%, or 0.9% sodium chloride; 10% dextrose; 10% invert sugar; or (1/6) M sodium lactate. Reconstituted solutions of cefuroxime that have been further diluted to a concentration of 1–30 mg/mL with one of the above IV solutions are stable for 24 hours at room temperature or at least 7 days when refrigerated.

The manufacturer of Zinacef® states that cefuroxime sodium solutions prepared using the 750-mg or 1.5-g vials or the 7.5-g pharmacy bulk vial may be frozen immediately after reconstitution and dilution; the entire contents from the reconstituted 750-mg or 1.5-g vial or 8 or 16 mL from the 7.5-g vial should be immediately withdrawn and added to a Viaflex® minibag containing 50 or 100 mL of 0.9% sodium chloride injection or 5% dextrose injection and frozen. These extemporaneously prepared solutions are stable for 6 months when frozen at –20°C. After thawing at room temperature, these solutions are stable for 24 hours at room temperature or 7 days when refrigerated; these solutions should not be refrozen.

The commercially available Duplex® drug delivery system containing 750 mg or 1.5 g of cefuroxime and 50 mL of dextrose injection should be stored at 20–25°C, but may be exposed to 15–30°C. Following reconstitution (activation), these IV solutions must be used within 24 hours if stored at room temperature or within 7 days if stored in a refrigerator and should not be frozen.

The commercially available frozen premixed cefuroxime sodium injection should be stored at –20°C or lower. The frozen injection should be thawed at room temperature (25°C) or under refrigeration (5°C) and, once thawed, should not be refrozen. Thawed solutions of the commercially available frozen injection are stable for 24 hours at room temperature (25°C) or 28 days under refrigeration (5°C). The commercially available frozen injection of the drug is provided in a plastic container fabricated from specially formulated multilayered plastic PL 2040 (Galaxy® containers). Solutions in contact with PL 2040 can leach out some of its chemical components in very small amounts within the expiration period of the injection; however, safety of the plastic has been confirmed in tests in animals according to USP biological tests for plastic containers as well as by tissue culture toxicity studies.

Cefuroxime sodium sterile powder and solutions of the drug tend to darken, depending on storage conditions; however, this discoloration does not necessarily indicate a change in potency.

Cefuroxime sodium is potentially physically and/or chemically incompatible with some drugs, including aminoglycosides, but the compatibility depends on several factors (e.g., concentrations of the drugs, specific diluents used, resulting pH, temperature). Specialized references should be consulted for specific compatibility information. Admixtures in 0.9% sodium chloride injection containing cefuroxime sodium and heparin (10 or 50 units/mL) or potassium chloride (10 or 40 mEq/L) are stable for 24 hours at room temperature. The manufacturer of Zinacef® states that cefuroxime sodium not be diluted with sodium bicarbonate injection. Because of the potential for incompatibility, the manufacturers state that cefuroxime sodium and aminoglycosides should not be admixed.

For further information on chemistry, mechanism of action, spectrum, resistance, pharmacokinetics, uses, cautions, drug interactions, laboratory test interferences, and dosage and administration of cefuroxime, see the Cephalosporins General Statement 8:12.06.

PREPARATIONS

Excipients in commercially available drug preparations may have clinically important effects in some individuals; consult specific product labeling for details.

Cefuroxime Axetil

Oral		
For Suspension	125 mg (of cefuroxime) per 5 mL*	**Ceftin®**, GlaxoSmithKline
		Cefuroxime Axetil for Suspension
	250 mg (of cefuroxime) per 5 mL*	**Ceftin®**, GlaxoSmithKline
		Cefuroxime Axetil for Suspension
Tablets, film-coated	125 mg (of cefuroxime)*	**Cefuroxime Axetil Tablets**
	250 mg (of cefuroxime)*	**Ceftin®**, GlaxoSmithKline
		Cefuroxime Axetil Tablets
	500 mg (of cefuroxime)*	**Ceftin®**, GlaxoSmithKline
		Cefuroxime Axetil Tablets

* available from one or more manufacturer, distributor, and/or repackager by generic (nonproprietary) name

Cefuroxime Sodium

Parenteral		
For injection	750 mg (of cefuroxime)*	**Cefuroxime Sodium for Injection**
		Zinacef®, Covis
	1.5 g (of cefuroxime)*	**Cefuroxime Sodium for Injection**
		Zinacef®, Covis
	7.5 g (of cefuroxime) pharmacy bulk package*	**Cefuroxime Sodium for Injection**
		Zinacef®, Covis
For injection, for IV infusion	750 mg (of cefuroxime)*	**Cefuroxime Sodium for Injection** (available in dual-chambered Duplex® drug delivery system with 4.1% dextrose injection), B Braun
		Zinacef® TwistVial®, Covis
	1.5 g (of cefuroxime)*	**Cefuroxime Sodium for Injection** (available in dual-chambered Duplex® drug delivery system with 2.9% dextrose injection), B Braun
		Zinacef® TwistVial®, Covis

* available from one or more manufacturer, distributor, and/or repackager by generic (nonproprietary) name

Cefuroxime Sodium in Water

Parenteral		
Injection (frozen), for IV infusion	30 mg (of cefuroxime) per mL (1.5 g)	**Zinacef® Iso-osmotic in Sterile Water Injection** (Galaxy® [Baxter]), Covis

† Use is not currently included in the labeling approved by the US Food and Drug Administration.

Selected Revisions October 11, 2013, © Copyright, April 1, 1984, American Society of Health-System Pharmacists, Inc.

Cefotaxime Sodium

8:12.06.12 • THIRD GENERATION CEPHALOSPORINS

■ Cefotaxime is a semisynthetic, third generation cephalosporin antibiotic.

USES

Cefotaxime is used for the treatment of serious bone and joint infections, serious intra-abdominal and gynecologic infections (including peritonitis, endometritis, pelvic inflammatory disease, pelvic cellulitis), meningitis and other CNS infections, serious lower respiratory tract infections (including pneumonia), bacteremia/septicemia, serious skin and skin structure infections, and serious urinary tract infections caused by susceptible bacteria. The drug also is used in the treatment of gonorrhea, typhoid fever and other infections caused by Salmonella†, infections caused by Vibrio parahaemolyticus† or V. vulnificus†, and Lyme disease†. Cefotaxime also has been used for perioperative prophylaxis.

Prior to initiation of cefotaxime therapy, appropriate specimens should be obtained for identification of the causative organism and in vitro susceptibility tests. If cefotaxime therapy is started pending results of susceptibility tests, it should be discontinued if the causative organism is found to be resistant to the drug. Because resistant strains of some organisms, especially Enterobacter, Ps. aeruginosa, and Serratia, have developed during cefotaxime therapy, it is important that appropriate specimens be obtained periodically until the infection is eradicated and cefotaxime is discontinued. In certain cases of confirmed or suspected gram-positive or gram-negative sepsis or in the empiric treatment of other serious infections when the causative organism has not been identified, cefotaxime may be used concomitantly with an aminoglycoside pending results of in vitro susceptibility tests. In infections which fail to respond to cefotaxime although in vitro tests indicate that the causative organism is susceptible to the drug, the presence of undrained abscesses or vascular infections should be suspected. The possibility that the organism may be tolerant to cefotaxime should also be considered. (See Resistance.) Use of cefotaxime does not replace surgical procedures such as incision and drainage when indicated.

● Gram-positive Aerobic Bacterial Infections

Cefotaxime is used in the treatment of lower respiratory tract infections caused by susceptible Streptococcus pneumoniae, S. pyogenes (group A β-hemolytic streptococci), other streptococci (except enterococci), or Staphylococcus aureus (penicillinase-producing and nonpenicillinase-producing strains); genitourinary tract infections caused by susceptible S. aureus, S. epidermidis, or enterococci; gynecologic infections caused by susceptible S. epidermidis or streptococci (including enterococci); skin and skin structure infections caused by susceptible S. aureus, S. epidermidis, group A β-hemolytic streptococci, or other streptococci (including enterococci); intra-abdominal infections caused by susceptible streptococci; or bone and joint infections caused by susceptible S. aureus, group A β-hemolytic streptococci, or other streptococci. Cefotaxime generally should not be used in the treatment of infections caused by gram-positive bacteria when a penicillin or a first generation cephalosporin could be used. Although cefotaxime has been effective in the treatment of cellulitis, wound infections, septicemia, and lower respiratory tract infections caused by susceptible staphylococci or streptococci, treatment failures have been reported when the drug was used in the treatment of osteomyelitis caused by S. aureus.

● Gram-negative Aerobic Bacterial Infections

Cefotaxime is used in the treatment of lower respiratory tract infections caused by susceptible Escherichia coli, Klebsiella, Haemophilus influenzae (including ampicillin-resistant strains), H. parainfluenzae, Proteus mirabilis, indole-positive Proteus, Serratia marcescens, or Enterobacter; genitourinary tract infections caused by susceptible Citrobacter, Enterobacter, E. coli, Klebsiella, P. mirabilis, Providencia stuartii (formerly group B Proteus inconstans), Pseudomonas, Morganella morganii, Providencia rettgeri, P. vulgaris, S. marcescens, or Neisseria gonorrhoeae; intra-abdominal and gynecologic infections caused by susceptible E. coli, Enterobacter, Klebsiella, or P. mirabilis; bacteremia or septicemia caused by susceptible E. coli, Klebsiella, or S. marcescens; skin and skin structure infections caused by susceptible E. coli, Enterobacter, Klebsiella, P. mirabilis, M. morganii, P. rettgeri, P. vulgaris, Pseudomonas, or S. marcescens; or bone and joint infections caused by susceptible P. mirabilis.

It has been suggested that certain parenteral cephalosporins (i.e., cefepime, cefotaxime, ceftriaxone, ceftazidime) may be drugs of choice for the treatment of many infections caused by susceptible Enterobacteriaceae, including susceptible E. coli, K. pneumoniae, P. rettgeri, M. morganii, P. vulgaris, P. stuartii, or Serratia; an aminoglycoside (amikacin, gentamicin, tobramycin) usually is used concomitantly in severe infections.

Although cefotaxime has been effective when used in the treatment of infections caused by susceptible Ps. aeruginosa, other anti-infectives generally are preferred for the treatment of pseudomonal infections. Because most strains of Ps. aeruginosa require high concentrations of the drug for in vitro inhibition and resistant strains have developed during cefotaxime therapy, an aminoglycoside should be used concomitantly if cefotaxime is used in any infection where Ps. aeruginosa may be present.

● Anaerobic and Mixed Aerobic-Anaerobic Bacterial Infections

Cefotaxime has been used in the treatment of skin and skin structure infections, intra-abdominal infections, or gynecologic infections caused by susceptible Bacteroides (including B. fragilis), Clostridium, Fusobacterium (including F. nucleatum), or anaerobic gram-positive cocci (including Peptococcus and Peptostreptococcus); however, cefotaxime is not considered a drug of choice for these infections. Cefotaxime has been effective when used in the treatment of mixed aerobic-anaerobic infections, including intra-abdominal and gynecologic infections (see Uses: Pelvic Inflammatory Disease). Because many strains of B. fragilis are resistant to cefotaxime, some clinicians recommend that cefotaxime not be used alone for the treatment of serious intra-abdominal infections when B. fragilis may be present.

● Meningitis and Other CNS Infections

Cefotaxime is used in neonates, children, or adults for the treatment of meningitis and ventriculitis caused by susceptible H. influenzae, N. meningitidis, or S. pneumoniae. The drug also has been used for the treatment of meningitis and other CNS infections caused by susceptible Enterobacteriaceae† (e.g., Escherichia coli, Klebsiella pneumoniae). Cefotaxime is ineffective in and should not be used alone for empiric treatment of meningitis when Listeria monocytogenes, enterococci, staphylococci, or Pseudomonas aeruginosa may be involved.

Empiric Treatment of Meningitis

Pending results of CSF culture and in vitro susceptibility testing, the most appropriate anti-infective regimen for empiric treatment of suspected bacterial meningitis should be selected based on results of CSF Gram stain and antigen tests, age of the patient, the most likely pathogen(s) and source of infection, and current patterns of bacterial resistance within the hospital and local community. When results of culture and susceptibility tests become available and the pathogen is identified, the empiric anti-infective regimen should be modified (if necessary) to ensure that the most effective regimen is being administered. There is some evidence that short-term adjunctive therapy with IV dexamethasone may decrease the incidence of audiologic and/or neurologic sequelae in infants and children with H. influenzae meningitis and possibly may provide some benefit in patients with S. pneumoniae meningitis. The American Academy of Pediatrics (AAP) and other clinicians suggest that use of adjunctive dexamethasone therapy may be considered during the initial 2–4 days of anti-infective therapy in infants and children 6–8 weeks of age or older with known or suspected bacterial meningitis, especially in those with suspected or proven H. influenzae infection. If used, dexamethasone should be initiated before or concurrently with the first dose of anti-infective. (See Uses: Bacterial Meningitis in the Corticosteroids General Statement 68:04 and see Dexamethasone 68:04.)

Bacterial meningitis in neonates usually is caused by S. agalactiae (group B streptococci), L. monocytogenes, or aerobic gram-negative bacilli (e.g., E. coli, K. pneumoniae). The AAP and other clinicians recommend that neonates 4 weeks of age or younger with suspected bacterial meningitis receive an empiric regimen of IV ampicillin and an aminoglycoside pending results of CSF culture and susceptibility testing. Alternatively, neonates can receive an empiric regimen of IV ampicillin and IV cefotaxime or IV ceftazidime (with or without gentamicin). Because frequent use of cephalosporins in neonatal units may result in rapid emergence of resistant strains of some gram-negative bacilli (e.g., Enterobacter cloacae, Klebsiella, Serratia), the AAP cautions that cephalosporins should be used for empiric treatment of meningitis in neonates only if gram-negative bacterial meningitis is strongly suspected. Consideration should be given to including IV vancomycin in the initial empiric regimen if *S. pneumoniae*, enterococci, or staphylococci is suspected. Because ceftriaxone should be used with caution in neonates who are hyperbilirubinemic (especially those born prematurely), cefotaxime may be the preferred cephalosporin in neonates. Alternatively, because premature, low-birthweight neonates are at increased risk for nosocomial infection caused by staphylococci or gram-negative bacilli, some clinicians suggest that these neonates receive an empiric regimen of IV ceftazidime and IV vancomycin.

In infants beyond the neonatal stage who are younger than 3 months of age, bacterial meningitis may be caused by *S. agalactiae*, *L. monocytogenes*, *Haemophilus influenzae*, *S. pneumoniae*, *N. meningitidis*, or aerobic gram-negative bacilli (e.g., *E. coli*, *K. pneumoniae*). An empiric regimen recommended for infants in this age group is IV ampicillin and either IV cefotaxime or IV ceftriaxone. Because of the increased prevalence of *S. pneumoniae* resistant to penicillin, cefotaxime, and ceftriaxone, the initial empiric regimen in children 1 month of age or older should include vancomycin and either cefotaxime or ceftriaxone if meningitis is known or suspected to be caused by *S. pneumoniae*.

In children 3 months through 17 years of age, bacterial meningitis usually is caused by *N. meningitidis*, *S. pneumoniae*, or *H. influenzae*, and the most common cause of bacterial meningitis in adults 18–50 years of age is *N. meningitidis* or *S. pneumoniae*. Most clinicians recommend that children 3 months through 17 years of age and adults 18–50 years of age receive IV cefotaxime or IV ceftriaxone for empiric therapy of suspected bacterial meningitis; an alternative regimen in children 3 months through 17 years of age is IV ampicillin and IV chloramphenicol. In addition, because of the increasing incidence of penicillin-resistant *S. pneumoniae* with reduced susceptibility to cephalosporins, the AAP and others suggest that the initial empiric regimen include IV vancomycin (with or without rifampin) pending results of in vitro susceptibility tests; vancomycin and rifampin should be discontinued if the causative organism is found to be susceptible to cephalosporins.. The US Centers for Disease Control and Prevention (CDC) and some clinicians have recommended that vancomycin be added to the empiric regimen in areas where there have been reports of highly penicillin-resistant strains of *S. pneumoniae*, but other clinicians suggest that use of cefotaxime or ceftriaxone in conjunction with vancomycin provides the optimal initial empiric regimen. While *L. monocytogenes* meningitis is relatively rare in this age group, the empiric regimen should include ampicillin if *L. monocytogenes* is suspected.

In adults older than 50 years of age, bacterial meningitis usually is caused by *S. pneumoniae*, *L. monocytogenes*, *N. meningitidis*, or aerobic gram-negative bacilli, and the empiric regimen recommended for this age group is IV ampicillin given in conjunction with IV cefotaxime or IV ceftriaxone. If *S. pneumoniae* is suspected, the empiric regimen also should include IV vancomycin (with or without rifampin); vancomycin and rifampin should be discontinued if the causative organism is found to be susceptible to the cephalosporin.

Meningitis Caused by Streptococcus pneumoniae

IV cefotaxime and IV ceftriaxone are considered drugs of choice for the treatment of meningitis caused by *S. pneumoniae*. While cefotaxime and ceftriaxone generally have been considered the drugs of choice for the treatment of meningitis caused by penicillin-resistant *S. pneumoniae*, treatment failures have been reported when the drugs were used alone for the treatment of meningitis caused by strains of *S. pneumoniae* with intermediate or high-level penicillin resistance (i.e., penicillin MIC 0.1 mcg/mL or greater). In addition, strains of *S. pneumoniae* with reduced susceptibility to cephalosporins have been reported with increasing frequency, and use of cefotaxime or ceftriaxone alone may be ineffective for the treatment of meningitis caused by these strains. The prevalence of *S. pneumoniae* with reduced susceptibility to penicillin and/or cephalosporins varies geographically, and clinicians should be aware of the prevalence and pattern of *S. pneumoniae* drug resistance in the local community to optimize empiric regimens and initial therapy for serious pneumococcal infections. Because susceptibility can no longer be assumed, *S. pneumoniae* isolates should be routinely tested for in vitro susceptibility.

If anti-infective therapy in a patient with meningitis is initiated with an empiric regimen of IV cefotaxime and IV vancomycin (with or without rifampin) and results of culture and in vitro susceptibility testing indicate that the pathogen involved is a strain of *S. pneumoniae* susceptible to cefotaxime and susceptible or resistant to penicillin, vancomycin can be discontinued and therapy completed using cefotaxime alone. If the isolate is found to have reduced susceptibility to cefotaxime *and* penicillin, both IV cefotaxime and IV vancomycin (with or without rifampin) usually are continued. If the patient's condition does not improve or worsens or results of a second repeat lumber puncture (performed 24–36 hours

after initiation of anti-infective therapy) indicate that the anti-infective regimen has not eradicated or reduced the number of pneumococci in CSF, rifampin probably should be added to the regimen or vancomycin discontinued and replaced with rifampin. If meningitis is caused by *S. pneumoniae* highly resistant to cefotaxime (i.e., MIC 2–4 mcg/mL or greater), consultation with an infectious disease expert is recommended.

Meningitis Caused by Haemophilus influenzae

IV cefotaxime and IV ceftriaxone are considered drugs of choice for the treatment of meningitis caused by susceptible *H. influenzae* (including penicillinase-producing strains). The AAP suggests that children with meningitis possibly caused by *H. influenzae* receive an initial treatment regimen of cefotaxime, ceftriaxone, or a regimen of ampicillin given in conjunction with chloramphenicol; some clinicians prefer cefotaxime or ceftriaxone for the initial treatment of meningitis caused by *H. influenzae* since the drugs are active against both β-lactamase-producing and non-β-lactamase-producing strains. The incidence of *H. influenzae* meningitis in the US has decreased considerably since *H. influenzae* type b conjugate vaccines became available for immunization of infants.

Meningitis Caused by Neisseria meningitidis

Although IV penicillin G or ampicillin generally are considered the drugs of choice for the treatment of meningitis caused by *N. meningitidis*, IV cefotaxime and IV ceftriaxone are acceptable alternatives.

Meningitis Caused by Enterobacteriaceae

Some clinicians recommend that meningitis caused by Enterobacteriaceae (e.g., *E. coli*, *K. pneumoniae*) be treated with a third generation cephalosporins (i.e., cefotaxime, ceftazidime, ceftriaxone) with or without an aminoglycoside. Because ceftazidime or cefepime (but not cefotaxime or ceftriaxone) is effective for the treatment of meningitis caused by *Ps. aeruginosa*, some clinicians suggest that a regimen of ceftazidime or cefepime (with or without an aminoglycoside) may be preferred for the treatment of meningitis caused by gram-negative bacilli pending results of culture and susceptibility testing.

Brain Abscess and Other CNS Infections

IV cefotaxime has been effective when used in conjunction with metronidazole for empiric treatment of brain abscess in patients 6 months of age or older. Bacterial brain abscesses and other CNS infections (e.g., subdural empyema, intracranial epidural abscesses) often are polymicrobial and can be caused by gram-positive aerobic cocci, Enterobacteriaceae (e.g., *E. coli*, *Haemophilus*, *Klebsiella*), and/or anaerobic bacteria (e.g., *Bacteroides*, *Fusobacterium*).

The choice of anti-infectives for empiric therapy of these infections should be based on the predisposing condition and site of primary infection. Some clinicians suggest that the empiric anti-infective regimen in patients who develop the CNS infections after respiratory tract infection (e.g., otitis media, mastoiditis, paranasal sinusitis, pyogenic lung disease) should consist of an appropriate IV third generation cephalosporin (e.g., cefotaxime) given in conjunction with metronidazole, employing the cephalosporin rather than a penicillin to extend coverage to *Haemophilus* and facultative anaerobic gram-negative bacteria; if presence of staphylococci is suspected, a penicillinase-resistant penicillin (e.g., nafcillin, oxacillin) or vancomycin should be added to the empiric regimen. In patients who develop brain abscess, subdural empyema, or intracranial epidural abscess after trauma or neurosurgery, the empiric regimen should consist of an appropriate IV third generation cephalosporin (e.g., cefotaxime) given in conjunction with a penicillinase-resistant penicillin or vancomycin. Prolonged anti-infective therapy (e.g., 3–6 weeks or longer) usually is required for these CNS infections.

● *Gonorrhea and Associated Infections*
Gonococcal Infections in Adults and Adolescents
Uncomplicated Gonorrhea

Cefotaxime has been used for the treatment of uncomplicated cervical, urethral, or rectal gonorrhea caused by susceptible *Neisseria gonorrhoeae*, including penicillinase-producing *N. gonorrhoeae* (PPNG) in adults and adolescents.

For the treatment of uncomplicated urogenital, anorectal, or pharyngeal gonorrhea, the CDC states that a combination regimen that includes a single 250-mg IM dose of ceftriaxone *and* either oral azithromycin (single 1-g dose) or oral doxycycline (100 mg twice daily for 7 days) is the regimen of choice. Although a single 500-mg dose of IM cefotaxime may be effective for the treatment of uncomplicated urogenital and anorectal gonorrhea, the CDC states that the drug does not offer any advantages over IM ceftriaxone for urogenital infections and its efficacy for pharyngeal infections is less certain.

Disseminated Gonococcal Infections

IV cefotaxime has been used for *initial* treatment of disseminated gonococcal infections† in adults and adolescents.

The CDC recommends that treatment of disseminated gonococcal infections in adults and adolescents be initiated with a multiple-dose regimen of IM or IV ceftriaxone; a multiple-dose regimen of IV cefotaxime is considered an alternative. The initial parenteral regimen should be continued for 24–48 hours after improvement begins; therapy can then be switched to oral cefixime and continued to complete at least 1 week of treatment.

The CDC recommends that the patient be hospitalized for initial treatment, especially when compliance may be a problem, when the diagnosis is uncertain, or when the patient has purulent synovial effusions or other complications. Patients should be examined for clinical evidence of endocarditis and meningitis; the recommended regimen for these infections is IV ceftriaxone.

Gonococcal Infections in Neonates and Infants

Cefotaxime is used for the treatment of *N. gonorrhoeae* infections in neonates, including disseminated gonococcal infections and gonococcal scalp abscesses†. The CDC states that IV or IM ceftriaxone or IV or IM cefotaxime are the drugs of choice for these infections in neonates; the AAP states that cefotaxime is preferred in neonates with hyperbilirubinemia. IV or IM ceftriaxone is the drug of choice for the treatment of nondisseminated gonococcal infections in neonates, including gonococcal ophthalmia (ophthalmia neonatorum), and also is the drug of choice for disseminated gonococcal infections (e.g., sepsis, arthritis, meningitis) in children.

Gonococcal infections in neonates usually occur as the result of exposure to the mother's infected cervical exudate and are apparent 2–5 days after birth. The most serious manifestations of *N. gonorrhoeae* infection in neonates are ophthalmia neonatorum and sepsis, arthritis, and meningitis; less serious manifestations include rhinitis, vaginitis, urethritis, and inflammation at sites of fetal monitoring (e.g., scalp). Because a neonate with gonococcal infection usually has acquired the organism from its mother, both the mother and her sexual partner(s) should be evaluated and treated for gonorrhea.

While universal *topical prophylaxis* using 0.5% erythromycin ophthalmic ointment, silver nitrate 1% topical solution (no longer commercially available in the US), or 1% tetracycline ophthalmic ointment (no longer commercially available in the US) is recommended for *all* neonates as soon as possible after birth to prevent gonococcal ophthalmia neonatorum, these topical anti-infectives are inadequate for prophylaxis of gonococcal infections at other sites, and may be ineffective in preventing chlamydial ocular infections. Because neonates born to mothers with untreated gonorrhea are at high risk of infection with *N. gonorrhoeae*, the CDC and AAP recommend that, in addition to *topical prophylaxis*, these neonates should receive *parenteral prophylaxis* against the disease. The CDC and AAP currently recommend that neonates born to mothers with documented peripartum gonococcal infection receive *parenteral prophylaxis* with a single IM or IV dose of ceftriaxone (25–50 mg/kg not to exceed 125 mg).

For additional information on current recommendations for the treatment of gonorrhea and associated infections, see Uses: Gonorrhea and Associated Infections, in Ceftriaxone 8:12.06.12.

● GI Infections

Cefotaxime is used for empiric treatment of infectious diarrhea†. For empiric treatment of severe diarrhea in HIV-infected individuals, the CDC, National Institutes of Health (NIH), and Infectious Diseases Society of America (IDSA) state that ciprofloxacin is the drug of choice and ceftriaxone and cefotaxime are reasonable alternatives. (For information on *Salmonella* gastroenteritis, see Salmonella Gastroenteritis under Uses: Typhoid Fever and Other Salmonella Infections.)

Yersinia Infections

Although GI infections caused by *Yersinia enterocolitica* or *Y. pseudotuberculosis* usually are self-limited and anti-infective therapy unnecessary, the

AAP, IDSA, and others recommend use of anti-infectives in immunocompromised individuals or for the treatment of severe infections or when septicemia or other invasive disease occurs. GI infections caused by *Y. enterocolitica* or *Y. pseudotuberculosis* can occur as the result of ingesting undercooked pork, unpasteurized milk, or contaminated water; infection has occurred in infants whose caregivers handled contaminated chitterlings (raw pork intestines) or tofu. Use of co-trimoxazole, an aminoglycoside (e.g., amikacin, gentamicin, tobramycin), a fluoroquinolone (e.g., ciprofloxacin), doxycycline, or cefotaxime has been recommended when treatment is considered necessary; combination therapy may be necessary. Some clinicians suggest that, while cefotaxime may be effective in the treatment of *Y. enterocolitica* bacteremia, the role of anti-infectives, including oral anti-infectives, in the management of enterocolitis, pseudoappendicitis syndrome, or mesenteric adenitis caused by *Yersinia* needs further evaluation.

● Lyme Disease

Cefotaxime is used in the treatment of Lyme disease†. The IDSA and other clinicians recommend IV cefotaxime as a preferred alternative to IV ceftriaxone for the treatment of early neurologic Lyme disease† with acute neurologic manifestations such as meningitis or radiculopathy, Lyme carditis†, Lyme arthritis†, and late neurologic Lyme disease†.

Lyme disease is a tick-borne spirochetal disease. In the US, Lyme disease is caused by the spirochete *Borrelia burgdorferi*, which is transmitted by the bite of *Ixodes scapularis* or *I. pacificus* ticks. For additional information on Lyme disease, see Lyme Disease in Uses: Spirochetal Infections, in the Tetracyclines General Statement 8:12.24.

Early Lyme Disease
Early Neurologic Lyme Disease

Although oral anti-infectives (doxycycline, amoxicillin, cefuroxime axetil) generally are effective for the treatment of the early localized or early disseminated Lyme disease associated with erythema migrans, in the absence of specific neurologic manifestations or advanced atrioventricular (AV) heart block, parenteral anti-infectives are recommended for the treatment of early Lyme disease when there are acute neurologic manifestations such as meningitis or radiculoneuritis.

The IDSA and other clinicians recommend a 14-day regimen (range: 10–28 days) of IV ceftriaxone as the preferred parenteral regimen for the treatment of acute neurologic Lyme disease manifested by meningitis or radiculopathy; IV cefotaxime and IV penicillin G sodium are the preferred alternatives. In patients with acute neurologic manifestations who are intolerant of cephalosporins and penicillin, there is some evidence that oral doxycycline may be an adequate alternative that can be considered for use in adults and children 8 years of age or older.

Although IV cefotaxime appears to be as effective as IV ceftriaxone for the treatment of acute neurologic Lyme disease and does not cause the biliary complications reported with ceftriaxone, ceftriaxone has the advantage of once-daily dosing. Limited data suggest that IV cefotaxime (6 g daily in divided doses for 10 days) is at least as effective as IV penicillin G (20 million units daily for 10 days) in patients with late complications of Lyme disease (e.g., severe radiculitis and/or meningitis, peripheral neuropathy, arthritis).

Lyme Carditis

Cefotaxime is used as an alternative to ceftriaxone when a parenteral regimen is indicated for the treatment of Lyme carditis†. The IDSA states that patients with AV heart block and/or myopericarditis associated with early Lyme disease may be treated with a 14-day regimen (range: 14–21 days) of oral or parenteral anti-infectives. Although there is no evidence to date to suggest that a parenteral regimen is more effective than an oral regimen for the treatment of Lyme carditis, a parenteral regimen usually is recommended for initial treatment of hospitalized patients; an oral regimen can be used to complete therapy and for the treatment of outpatients. When a parenteral regimen is used, IV ceftriaxone or, alternatively, IV cefotaxime or IV penicillin G sodium is recommended. When an oral regimen is used, oral doxycycline, oral amoxicillin, or oral cefuroxime axetil is recommended.

Because of the potential for life-threatening complications, hospitalization and continuous monitoring is advisable for patients who are symptomatic (syncope, dyspnea, chest pain) and also is recommended for those with second- or third-degree AV block or first-degree heart block when the PR interval is prolonged to 0.3 seconds or longer. Patients with advanced heart block may require a temporary pacemaker and consultation with a cardiologist is recommended.

Late Lyme Disease
Lyme Arthritis

Cefotaxime is used as an alternative to ceftriaxone when a parenteral regimen is indicated for the treatment of Lyme arthritis†. While patients with uncomplicated Lyme arthritis without clinical evidence of neurologic disease generally can be treated with a 28-day regimen of oral anti-infectives (doxycycline, amoxicillin, cefuroxime axetil), the IDSA and other clinicians state that patients with Lyme arthritis and concomitant neurologic disease should receive a 14-day parenteral regimen (range: 14–28 days) of IV ceftriaxone or, alternatively, IV cefotaxime or IV penicillin G. While oral regimens are easier to administer, associated with fewer serious adverse effects, and less expensive than IV regimens, some patients with Lyme arthritis treated with oral anti-infectives have subsequently developed overt neuroborreliosis, which may require IV therapy for successful resolution. Therefore, additional study is needed to fully evaluate the comparative safety and efficacy of oral versus IV anti-infectives for the treatment of Lyme arthritis.

In patients who have persistent or recurrent joint swelling after a recommended oral regimen, the IDSA and other clinicians recommend retreatment with the oral regimen or a switch to a parenteral regimen. Some clinicians prefer retreatment with an oral regimen for patients whose arthritis substantively improved but did not completely resolve; these clinicians reserve parenteral regimens for those patients whose arthritis failed to improve or worsened. It has been suggested that clinicians should consider allowing several months for joint inflammation to resolve after initial treatment before an additional course of anti-infectives is given.

Late Neurologic Lyme Disease

Cefotaxime is used as an alternative to ceftriaxone for the treatment of late neurologic Lyme disease†. The IDSA and other clinicians state that patients with late neurologic Lyme disease affecting the CNS or peripheral nervous system (e.g., encephalopathy, neuropathy) should receive a 14-day regimen (range: 14–28 days) of IV ceftriaxone or, alternatively, IV cefotaxime or IV penicillin G sodium. Response to anti-infective treatment usually is slow and may be incomplete in patients with late neurologic Lyme disease. The IDSA states that retreatment is not recommended unless relapse is shown by reliable objective measures.

● Pelvic Inflammatory Disease

Cefotaxime has been used for the treatment of pelvic inflammatory disease (PID). Because cefotaxime (like other cephalosporins) has no activity against *Chlamydia trachomatis*, it should be given in conjunction with an anti-infective active against this organism (e.g., doxycycline) whenever it is used in the treatment of PID.

PID is an acute or chronic inflammatory disorder in the upper female genital tract and can include any combination of endometritis, salpingitis, tubo-ovarian abscess, and pelvic peritonitis. PID generally is a polymicrobial infection most frequently caused by *N. gonorrhoeae* and/or *Chlamydia trachomatis*; however, organisms that are part of the normal vaginal flora (e.g., anaerobic bacteria, *Gardnerella vaginalis, H. influenzae*, enteric gram-negative bacilli, *S. agalactiae*) or mycoplasma (e.g., *Mycoplasma hominis, Ureaplasma urealyticum*) also may be involved. PID is treated with an empiric regimen that provides broad-spectrum coverage. The regimen should be effective against *N. gonorrhoeae* and *C. trachomatis* and also probably should be effective against anaerobes, gram-negative facultative bacteria, and streptococci. The optimum empiric regimen for the treatment of PID has not been identified. A wide variety of parenteral and oral regimens have been shown to achieve clinical and microbiologic cure in randomized studies with short-term follow-up; however, only limited data are available to date regarding elimination of infection in the endometrium and fallopian tubes or intermediate or long-term outcomes, including the impact of these regimens on the incidence of long-term sequelae of PID (e.g., tubal infertility, ectopic pregnancy, pain).

When a parenteral regimen is indicated for the treatment of PID, the CDC recommends a 2-drug regimen of cefoxitin (2 g IV every 6 hours) or cefotetan (2 g IV every 12 hours) given in conjunction with doxycycline (100 mg IV or orally every 12 hours) or a 2-drug regimen of clindamycin (900 mg IV every 8 hours) and gentamicin (usually a 2-mg/kg IV or IM loading dose followed by 1.5 mg/kg every 8 hours). While there is some evidence that other parenteral cephalosporins (e.g., cefotaxime, ceftriaxone) may be effective for the treatment of PID, the CDC states that these drugs are less active than cefoxitin or cefotetan against anaerobic bacteria.

When an oral regimen is used for the outpatient treatment of mild to moderately severe acute PID, the CDC recommends a regimen that consists of a single IM dose of ceftriaxone, cefoxitin (with oral probenecid), or cefotaxime given with oral

doxycycline (with or without oral metronidazole). The optimal cephalosporin for the regimen is unclear, although cefoxitin has better anaerobic coverage and ceftriaxone has better coverage against *N. gonorrhoeae*.

For additional information on treatment of PID, including information on follow-up and management of sexual partners, see Uses: Pelvic Inflammatory Disease, in the Cephalosporins General Statement 8:12.06.

● Respiratory Tract Infections
Community-acquired Pneumonia

Cefotaxime is used for the treatment of community-acquired pneumonia (CAP). The American Thoracic Society (ATS) and IDSA recommend cefotaxime as an alternative to penicillin G or amoxicillin for treatment of community-acquired pneumonia (CAP) caused by penicillin-susceptible *S. pneumoniae* and as a preferred drug for treatment of CAP caused by penicillin-resistant *S. pneumoniae*, provided in vitro susceptibility has been demonstrated. IDSA and ATS also recommend use of cefotaxime in certain combination regimens used for empiric treatment of CAP.

Initial treatment of CAP generally involves use of an empiric anti-infective regimen based on the most likely pathogens and local susceptibility patterns; therapy may then be changed (if possible) to provide a more specific regimen (pathogen-directed therapy) based on results of in vitro culture and susceptibility testing. The most appropriate empiric regimen varies depending on the severity of illness at the time of presentation and whether outpatient treatment or hospitalization in or out of an intensive care unit (ICU) is indicated and the presence or absence of cardiopulmonary disease and other modifying factors that increase the risk of certain pathogens (e.g., penicillin- or multidrug-resistant *S. pneumoniae*, enteric gram-negative bacilli, *Ps. aeruginosa*).

Most experts recommend that an empiric regimen for treatment of CAP include an anti-infective active against *S. pneumoniae* since this organism is the most commonly identified cause of bacterial pneumonia and causes more severe disease than many other common CAP pathogens. Pathogens most frequently involved in *outpatient* CAP include *S. pneumoniae, M. pneumoniae, Chlamydophila pneumoniae* (formerly *Chlamydia pneumoniae*), respiratory viruses, and *H. influenzae*. Pathogens most frequently involved in *inpatient* CAP in non-ICU patients are *S. pneumoniae, M. pneumoniae, C. pneumoniae, H. influenzae, Legionella*, and respiratory viruses. Patients with severe CAP admitted into the ICU usually have infections caused by *S. pneumoniae, S. aureus, Legionella*, gram-negative bacilli, or *H. influenzae*. Coverage against anaerobic bacteria usually is indicated only in classic aspiration pleuropulmonary syndrome in patients who had loss of consciousness as a result of alcohol or drug overdosage after seizures in patients with concomitant gingival disease or esophageal motility disorders.

Inpatient treatment of CAP is initiated with a parenteral regimen, although therapy may be changed to an oral regimen if the patient is improving clinically, is hemodynamically stable, able to ingest drugs, and has a normally functioning GI tract. CAP patients usually have a clinical response within 3–7 days after initiation of therapy and a switch to oral therapy generally can be made during this period.

For empiric *inpatient* treatment of CAP in non-ICU patients, IDSA and ATS recommend monotherapy with a fluoroquinolone (moxifloxacin, gemifloxacin, levofloxacin) or, alternatively, a combination regimen that includes a β-lactam (usually cefotaxime, ceftriaxone, or ampicillin) given in conjunction with a macrolide (azithromycin, clarithromycin, erythromycin). For empiric *inpatient* treatment of CAP in ICU patients when *Pseudomonas* and oxacillin-resistant (methicillin-resistant) *S. aureus* are *not* suspected, IDSA and ATS recommend a combination regimen that includes a β-lactam (cefotaxime, ceftriaxone, fixed combination of ampicillin and sulbactam) given in conjunction with either azithromycin or fluoroquinolone (gemifloxacin, levofloxacin, moxifloxacin).

For additional information on treatment of CAP, see Community-acquired Pneumonia under Uses: Respiratory Tract Infections, in the Cephalosporins General Statement 8:12.06.

● Septicemia

Cefotaxime is used for the treatment of bacteremia/septicemia caused by *E. coli, Klebsiella, S. marcescens, S. aureus*, and streptococci (including *S. pneumoniae*).

The choice of anti-infective agent for the treatment of sepsis syndrome should be based on the probable source of infection, causative organism, immune status of the patient, and local patterns of bacterial resistance. For initial treatment of life-threatening sepsis in adults, some clinicians recommend that a third or fourth generation cephalosporin (cefepime, cefotaxime, ceftriaxone, ceftazidime), the fixed combination of piperacillin and tazobactam, or a carbapenem (doripenem, imipenem, meropenem) be used in conjunction with vancomycin; some experts also suggest including an aminoglycoside or fluoroquinolone during the initial few days of treatment.

● Typhoid Fever and Other Salmonella Infections

Typhoid Fever

Cefotaxime has been used in adults or children for the treatment of typhoid fever† (enteric fever) or septicemia caused by *Salmonella typhi*† or *S. paratyphi*†, including multidrug-resistant strains. Multidrug-resistant strains of *S. typhi* (i.e., strains resistant to ampicillin, chloramphenicol, and/or co-trimoxazole) have been reported with increasing frequency, and third generation cephalosporins (e.g., cefotaxime, ceftriaxone) and fluoroquinolones (e.g., ciprofloxacin, ofloxacin) are considered the agents of first choice for the treatment of typhoid fever or other severe infections known or suspected to be caused by these strains.

Cefotaxime also has been used in the treatment of infections caused by non-typhi *Salmonella*, including bacteremia, osteomyelitis, and meningitis caused by *S. typhimurium*.

Salmonella Gastroenteritis

Anti-infective therapy generally is not indicated in otherwise healthy individuals with uncomplicated (noninvasive) gastroenteritis caused by non-typhi *Salmonella* (e.g., *S. enteritidis*, *S. typhimurium*) since such therapy may prolong the duration of fecal excretion of the organism and there is no evidence that it shortens the duration of the disease; however, the CDC, AAP, IDSA, and others recommend anti-infective therapy in individuals with severe *Salmonella* gastroenteritis and in those who are at increased risk of invasive disease. These individuals at increased risk include infants younger than 3–6 months of age; individuals older than 50 years of age; individuals with hemoglobinopathies, severe atherosclerosis or valvular heart disease, prostheses, uremia, chronic GI disease, or severe colitis; and individuals who are immunocompromised because of malignancy, immunosuppressive therapy, HIV infection, or other immunosuppressive illness.

When an anti-infective agent is considered necessary in an individual with *Salmonella* gastroenteritis, the CDC, AAP, IDSA, and others recommend use of ceftriaxone, cefotaxime, a fluoroquinolone (should be used in children only if the benefits outweigh the risks and no alternative exists), ampicillin, amoxicillin, co-trimoxazole, or chloramphenicol, depending on the susceptibility of the causative organism.

HIV-Infected Individuals

Because HIV-infected individuals with *Salmonella* gastroenteritis† are at high risk for bacteremia, the CDC, NIH, and IDSA recommend that such patients receive anti-infective treatment. These experts state that the initial drug of choice for the treatment of *Salmonella* gastroenteritis (with or without bacteremia) in HIV-infected adults is ciprofloxacin; other fluoroquinolones (levofloxacin, moxifloxacin) also are likely to be effective, but clinical data are limited. Depending on results of in vitro susceptibility testing of the causative organism, alternatives for treatment of *Salmonella* gastroenteritis in HIV-infected adults are co-trimoxazole or third generation cephalosporins (ceftriaxone, cefotaxime).

HIV-infected individuals who have been treated for *Salmonella* bacteremia should be monitored for recurrence. The CDC, NIH, and IDSA state that long-term maintenance anti-infective therapy (secondary prophylaxis) to prevent recurrence should be considered for those with recurrent *Salmonella* bacteremia and also may be considered for those with recurrent gastroenteritis (with or without bacteremia) or those who have CD4+ T-cell counts less than 200 cells/mm³ and severe diarrhea. However, the value of such prophylaxis has not been established and the possible benefits must be weighed against the risks of long-term anti-infective exposure.

● Capnocytophaga Infections

Based on results of in vitro susceptibility tests that indicate that *Capnocytophaga* generally are inhibited by cefotaxime, some clinicians suggest that cefotaxime can be used in the treatment of infections caused by *Capnocytophaga*†. *Capnocytophaga* is a gram-negative bacilli that can cause life-threatening septicemia, meningitis, and/or endocarditis and often is associated with disseminated intravascular coagulation; splenectomized and immunocompromised individuals are at particularly high risk for serious infections caused by the organism. *C. canimorsus* infection usually occurs as the result of a dog bite. The optimum regimen for the treatment of infections caused by *Capnocytophaga* has not been identified but

some clinicians recommend use of penicillin G or, alternatively, a third generation cephalosporin (cefotaxime, ceftriaxone), a carbapenem (imipenem, meropenem), vancomycin, a fluoroquinolone, or clindamycin.

● Vibrio Infections

Vibrio parahaemolyticus Infections

Cefotaxime is one of several alternatives recommended for the treatment of severe cases of *Vibrio parahaemolyticus*† infection when anti-infective therapy is indicated in addition to supportive care. *V. parahaemolyticus* infection is a relatively rare foodborne illness that can occur as the result of ingestion of undercooked or raw fish or shellfish; the incubation period usually is 2–48 hours. The signs and symptoms of *V. parahaemolyticus* infection are watery diarrhea, abdominal cramps, and nausea and vomiting lasting 2–5 days. Although supportive care usually is sufficient, some clinicians recommend use of tetracycline, doxycycline, gentamicin, or cefotaxime in severe cases.

Vibrio vulnificus Infections

Some clinicians suggest that cefotaxime is a drug of choice for the treatment of infections caused by *V. vulnificus*†. *V. vulnificus* can cause potentially fatal septicemia, wound infections, or gastroenteritis and generally is transmitted through ingestion of contaminated raw or undercooked seafood (especially raw oysters) or through contamination of a wound with seawater or seafood drippings. *V. vulnificus* is naturally present in marine environments, thrives in warm ocean water, and frequently is isolated from oysters and other shellfish harvested from the Gulf of Mexico and from US coastal waters along the Pacific and Atlantic ocean. Individuals with preexisting liver disease are at high risk for developing fatal septicemia following ingestion of seafood contaminated with *V. vulnificus* and debilitated or immunocompromised individuals (e.g., those with chronic renal impairment, cancer, diabetes mellitus, steroid-dependent asthma, chronic GI disease) or individuals with iron overload states (e.g., thalassemia, hemochromatosis) also are at increased risk for fatal infections. The incubation period for *V. vulnificus* infection reportedly is 1–7 days and the duration of illness usually is 2–8 days. In immunocompromised individuals, fever, nausea, myalgia, and abdominal cramps may occur as soon as 24–48 hours after ingestion of seafood contaminated with *V. vulnificus* and sepsis and cutaneous bullae may be present within 36 hours of the onset of symptoms.

Because the case fatality rate for *V. vulnificus* septicemia exceeds 50% in immunocompromised individuals and those with preexisting liver disease, these individuals should be informed about the health hazards of ingesting raw or undercooked seafood (especially oysters), the need to avoid contact with seawater during the warm months, and the importance of using protective clothing (e.g., gloves) when handling shellfish. *V. vulnificus* infection should be considered in the differential diagnosis of fever of unknown etiology, and individuals who present with fever (especially when bullae, cellulitis, or wound infection is present) and who have preexisting liver disease or are immunocompromised should be questioned regarding a history of raw oyster ingestion or seawater contact. While optimum anti-infective therapy for the treatment of *V. vulnificus* infections has not been identified, use of a tetracycline or third generation cephalosporin (e.g., cefotaxime, ceftazidime) is recommended. Because of the high fatality rate associated with *V. vulnificus* infections, anti-infective therapy should be initiated promptly if indicated.

● Perioperative Prophylaxis

Cefotaxime has been used for perioperative prophylaxis in patients undergoing liver transplantation†, and some experts recommend cefotaxime in conjunction with ampicillin as a regimen of choice for such prophylaxis in patients undergoing this procedure.

Cefotaxime has been used perioperatively to reduce the incidence of infection in patients undergoing contaminated or potentially contaminated surgery, including biliary tract, colorectal, and other intra-abdominal or GI procedures (e.g., appendectomy), genitourinary surgery, or abdominal or vaginal hysterectomy, and in patients undergoing cesarean section. However, other anti-infectives (e.g., cefazolin) usually are recommended for perioperative prophylaxis in patients undergoing these procedures.

A first or second generation cephalosporin (cefazolin, cefoxitin, cefotetan, cefuroxime) generally is preferred when a cephalosporin is used for perioperative prophylaxis. Third generation cephalosporins (cefotaxime, ceftriaxone, ceftazidime) and fourth generation cephalosporins (cefepime) are not usually recommended for perioperative prophylaxis because they are expensive, some are less active than first or second generation cephalosporins against staphylococci, they have spectrums of activity wider than necessary for organisms encountered in elective surgery, and their use for prophylaxis may promote emergence of resistant organisms. (See Uses: Perioperative Prophylaxis in the Cephalosporins General Statement 8:12.06.)

DOSAGE AND ADMINISTRATION

● Reconstitution and Administration

Cefotaxime sodium is administered IV or by deep IM injection. The drug should be given IV rather than IM in patients with septicemia, bacteremia, peritonitis, meningitis, or other severe or life-threatening infections or in patients with lowered resistance resulting from debilitating conditions (e.g., malnutrition, trauma, surgery, diabetes, heart failure, malignancy), particularly if shock is present.

Intermittent IV Injection

For direct intermittent IV administration, 10 mL of sterile water for injection should be added to a vial labeled as containing 500 mg, 1 g, or 2 g of cefotaxime to provide a solution containing approximately 50, 95, or 180 mg of cefotaxime per mL, respectively. A solution of 1 g of cefotaxime per 14 mL of sterile water for injection is isotonic.

The appropriate dose may then be injected directly into a vein over a 3- to 5-minute period or slowly into the tubing of a freely flowing compatible IV solution. Cefotaxime should *not* be injected IV over less than 3 minutes since rapid (over less than 1 minute) injection was consistently associated with potentially life-threatening arrhythmias during postmarketing surveillance.

Intermittent or Continuous IV Infusion

For intermittent or continuous IV infusion, 50 or 100 mL of 0.9% sodium chloride injection or 5% dextrose injection should be added to an infusion bottle labeled as containing 1 or 2 g of cefotaxime or, alternatively, reconstituted solutions of cefotaxime may be further diluted with 50 mL to 1 L of a compatible IV solution. ADD-Vantage® vials or infusion bottles labeled as containing 1 or 2 g of cefotaxime or the 10-g pharmacy bulk package of cefotaxime should be reconstituted according to the manufacturer's directions. The cefotaxime bulk package is *not* intended for direct IV infusion; doses of the drug from the reconstituted bulk package must be further diluted in a compatible IV infusion solution prior to administration.

Thawed solutions of the commercially available frozen premixed cefotaxime sodium injection should be administered only by intermittent or continuous IV infusion. The frozen injections should be thawed at room temperature or under refrigeration (5°C or lower); the injection should not be thawed by warming in a water bath or by exposure to microwave radiation. Precipitates that may have formed in the frozen injection usually will dissolve with little or no agitation when the injection reaches room temperature; potency is not affected. After thawing to room temperature, the injection should be agitated and the container checked for minute leaks by firmly squeezing the bag. The injection should be discarded if container seals or outlet ports are not intact or leaks are found or if the solution is cloudy or contains an insoluble precipitate. Additives should not be introduced into the injection container. The injection should not be used in series connections with other plastic containers, since such use could result in air embolism from residual air being drawn from the primary container before administration of fluid from the secondary container is complete.

Other IV solutions flowing through a common administration tubing or site should be discontinued while cefotaxime is being infused unless the solutions are known to be compatible and the flow-rate is adequately controlled.

Rate of Administration

Intermittent IV infusions of cefotaxime are generally infused over 20–30 minutes; solutions should preferably be infused via butterfly or scalp vein-type needles.

IM Injection

IM injections of cefotaxime are prepared by adding 2, 3, or 5 mL of sterile or bacteriostatic water for injection to a vial labeled as containing 500 mg, 1 g, or 2 g of the drug. Resultant solutions contain approximately 230, 300, or 330 mg of cefotaxime per mL, respectively.

IM injections should be made deeply into a large muscle mass such as the upper outer quadrant of the gluteus maximus; aspiration should be performed to avoid inadvertent injection into a blood vessel. The manufacturers state that if an IM dose of 2 g of cefotaxime is indicated, the dose should be divided and administered at 2 different injection sites. However, because large IM doses of cefotaxime may be painful, some clinicians recommend that large doses of the drug be given IV.

● Dosage

Dosage of cefotaxime sodium is expressed in terms of cefotaxime and is identical for IM or IV administration.

Adult Dosage

The usual adult dosage of cefotaxime for the treatment of uncomplicated infections is 1 g IM or IV every 12 hours. Moderate to severe infections usually respond to 1–2 g IM or IV every 8 hours, but some infections (e.g., septicemia) should be treated with 2 g IV every 6–8 hours. Severe or life-threatening infections may require 2 g IV every 4 hours.

The maximum adult dosage recommended by the manufacturers is 12 g daily.

Meningitis and Other CNS Infections

For the treatment of meningitis or other CNS infections caused by susceptible bacteria, the usual adult dosage of cefotaxime is 2 g IV every 6 hours for 7–21 days. Some clinicians recommend that adults receive 8–12 g daily in divided doses every 4–6 hours for the treatment of meningitis. Other clinicians recommend that patients with meningitis known or suspected to be caused by *S. pneumoniae* receive an initial cefotaxime dosage of 350 mg/kg daily given in 4 divided doses; if results of in vitro susceptibility testing indicate that the organism is susceptible to penicillin, dosage can be reduced to 225 mg/kg daily given in 3 divided doses.

While 7 days of cefotaxime therapy may be adequate for the treatment of uncomplicated meningitis caused by susceptible *Haemophilus influenzae* or *Neisseria meningitidis*, at least 10–14 days of therapy is recommended for complicated cases or meningitis caused by *Streptococcus pneumoniae* and at least 21 days of therapy is recommended for meningitis caused by susceptible Enterobacteriaceae (e.g., *Escherichia coli*, *Klebsiella*).

Gonorrhea and Associated Infections

For the treatment of uncomplicated urethral, cervical, or rectal gonorrhea caused by susceptible *N. gonorrhoeae*, adults and adolescents should receive a single 500-mg IM dose of cefotaxime. The manufacturers recommend a single 1-g IM dose for the treatment of rectal gonorrhea in males.

For the treatment of disseminated gonorrhea†, adults and adolescents should receive 1 g of cefotaxime IV every 8 hours. Parenteral cefotaxime should be continued for 24–48 hours after improvement begins; therapy can then be switched to oral cefixime to complete at least 1 week of therapy.

GI Infections

If cefotaxime is used as an alternative for empiric treatment of infectious diarrhea† in HIV-infected adults, the US Centers for Disease Control and Prevention (CDC), National Institutes of Health (NIH), and Infectious Diseases Society of America (IDSA) recommend a dosage of 1 g IV every 8 hours. If there is no clinical response after 5–7 days, stool culture and in vitro susceptibility testing should be considered.

If cefotaxime is used as an alternative for the treatment of *Salmonella* gastroenteritis† (with or without bacteremia) in HIV-infected adults, the CDC, NIH, and IDSA recommend a dosage of 1 g IV every 8 hours. The recommended duration of treatment is 7–14 days in those with CD4+ T-cell counts of 200 cells/mm³ or greater (14 days or longer if the patient is bacteremic or the infection is complicated) or 2–6 weeks in those with CD4+ T-cell counts less than 200 cells/mm³.

Lyme Disease

If cefotaxime is used for the treatment of early Lyme disease† in adults with acute neurologic disease manifested by meningitis or radiculopathy, the Infectious Diseases Society of America (IDSA) and other clinicians recommend a dosage of 2 g IV every 8 hours for 14 days (range: 10–28 days).

If cefotaxime is used when a parenteral regimen is indicated for the treatment of Lyme carditis† in patients with atrioventricular (AV) heart block and/or myopericarditis associated with early Lyme disease, the IDSA and other clinicians recommend a dosage of 2 g IV every 8 hours for 14 days (range: 14–21 days). Although a parenteral regimen is recommended for initial treatment of hospitalized patients, the parenteral regimen can be switched to an oral regimen (doxycycline, amoxicillin, cefuroxime axetil) to complete therapy and for outpatients.

If cefotaxime is used when a parenteral regimen is indicated for the treatment of Lyme arthritis† in patients with evidence of neurologic disease or when arthritis has not responded to an oral regimen, the IDSA recommends that adults receive 2 g IV every 8 hours for 14 days (range: 14–28 days).

If cefotaxime is used for the treatment of late neurologic Lyme disease† affecting the CNS or peripheral nervous system, the IDSA recommends that adults receive 2 g IV every 8 hours for 14 days (range: 14–28 days).

Respiratory Tract Infections

For the treatment of community-acquired pneumonia (CAP) in adults who are hospitalized for inpatient treatment, cefotaxime usually is given in a dosage of 1 g every 6–8 hours.

If used for empiric treatment of CAP, cefotaxime is used in conjunction with other anti-infectives. (See Community-acquired Pneumonia under Uses: Respiratory Tract Infections.)

Perioperative Prophylaxis

If cefotaxime is used for perioperative prophylaxis in contaminated or potentially contaminated surgery, the manufacturers recommend that adults receive 1 g IM or IV given 30–90 minutes prior to surgery. If cefotaxime is used prophylactically in patients undergoing cesarean section, the manufacturers recommend 1 g given IV as soon as the umbilical cord is clamped, followed by 1 g IM or IV 6 and 12 hours after the first dose.

Although not usually considered a drug of choice for perioperative prophylaxis (see Uses: Perioperative Prophylaxis), if cefotaxime is used for perioperative prophylaxis some experts recommend that adults receive 1 g of cefotaxime (2 g in obese patients) within 60 minutes prior to surgical incision. If the procedure is prolonged (longer than 3–4 hours) or if major blood loss occurs, additional intraoperative doses of cefotaxime may be given every 3 hours. The duration of prophylaxis should be less than 24 hours for most procedures; there is no evidence to support continuing prophylaxis after wound closure or until all indwelling drains and intravascular catheters are removed.

Pediatric Dosage

General Dosage for Neonates

The usual dosage of cefotaxime recommended by the manufacturers for premature or full-term neonates less than 1 week of age is 50 mg/kg every 12 hours and the usual dosage for neonates 1–4 weeks of age is 50 mg/kg every 8 hours.

The American Academy of Pediatrics (AAP) recommends that neonates 7 days of age or younger receive IV or IM cefotaxime in a dosage of 50 mg/kg every 12 hours, regardless of weight. For neonates 8–28 days of age, the AAP recommends a dosage of 50 mg/kg every 8–12 hours for those weighing 2 kg or less and 50 mg/kg every 8 hours for those weighing more than 2 kg.

General Dosage for Infants and Children

Children weighing 50 kg or more should receive the usual daily adult dosage, but dosage should not exceed 12 g daily.

The manufacturers recommend that children 1 month to 12 years of age weighing less than 50 kg receive 50–180 mg/kg daily given in 4–6 equally divided doses; the higher dosages should be used for more severe or serious infections, including meningitis.

The AAP recommends that pediatric patients beyond the neonatal period receive cefotaxime in a dosage of 50–180 mg/kg daily given in 3 or 4 equally divided doses for the treatment of mild to moderate infections or 200–225 mg/kg daily given in 4 or 6 equally divided doses for the treatment of severe infections.

Meningitis and Other CNS Infections

For the treatment of meningitis caused by susceptible bacteria, the manufacturers recommend that children 1 month to 12 years of age who weigh less than 50 kg receive a cefotaxime dosage at the high end of the range of 50–180 mg/kg daily.

Some clinicians recommend that infants and children younger than 18 years of age with meningitis receive cefotaxime in a dosage of 50 mg/kg IV every 6 hours. Other clinicians recommend a cefotaxime dosage of 100–150 mg/kg daily

given in divided doses every 8–12 hours in neonates 7 days of age or younger, 150–200 mg/kg daily given in divided doses every 6–8 hours in neonates 8–28 days of age, and 225–300 mg/kg daily given in divided doses every 6–8 hours in older infants and children.

The AAP states that a cefotaxime dosage up to 300 mg/kg daily given in 4 or 6 divided doses can be used for the treatment of meningitis in pediatric patients beyond the neonatal period.

While 7 days of therapy may be adequate for the treatment of uncomplicated meningitis caused by susceptible *H. influenzae* or *N. meningitidis*, at least 10–14 days of therapy is recommended for complicated cases or for meningitis caused by *S. pneumoniae* and at least 21 days is recommended for meningitis caused by susceptible Enterobacteriaceae (e.g., *E. coli*, *Klebsiella*).

Gonorrhea and Associated Infections

The usual dosage of cefotaxime for the treatment of disseminated gonococcal infection† (e.g., sepsis, arthritis, meningitis) or gonococcal scalp abscesses† in neonates is 25 mg/kg IV or IM every 12 hours for 7 days; if meningitis is documented, the drug should be continued for 10–14 days.

Lyme Disease

If cefotaxime is used for the treatment of early Lyme disease† in children with acute neurologic disease manifested by meningitis or radiculopathy, the IDSA and other clinicians recommend a dosage of 150–200 mg/kg daily (up to 6 g daily) given IV in divided doses every 6–8 hours for 14 days (range: 10–28 days).

If cefotaxime is used when a parenteral regimen is indicated for the treatment of Lyme carditis† in patients with atrioventricular (AV) heart block and/or myopericarditis associated with early Lyme disease, the IDSA and other clinicians recommend that children receive a dosage of 150–200 mg/kg daily (up to 6 g daily) given IV in divided doses every 6–8 hours for 14 days (range: 14–21 days). Although a parenteral regimen is recommended for initial treatment of hospitalized patients, the parenteral regimen can be switched to an oral regimen (doxycycline, amoxicillin, cefuroxime axetil) to complete therapy and for outpatients.

If cefotaxime is used when a parenteral regimen is indicated for the treatment of Lyme arthritis† in patients with evidence of neurologic disease or when arthritis has not responded to an oral regimen, the IDSA recommends that children receive a dosage of 150–200 mg/kg daily (up to 6 g daily) given IV in divided doses every 6–8 hours for 14 days (range: 14–28 days).

If cefotaxime is used for the treatment of late neurologic Lyme disease† affecting the CNS or peripheral nervous system, the IDSA recommends that children receive a dosage of 150–200 mg/kg daily (up to 6 g daily) given IV in divided doses every 6–8 hours for 14 days (range: 14–28 days).

Duration of Therapy

The duration of cefotaxime therapy depends on the type of infection but should generally be continued for at least 48–72 hours after the patient becomes afebrile or evidence of eradication of the infection is obtained. Although other drugs generally are preferred, if cefotaxime is used in infections caused by group A β-hemolytic streptococci, therapy should be continued for at least 10 days to decrease the risk of rheumatic fever or glomerulonephritis. Chronic urinary tract infections may require several weeks of therapy, and bacteriologic and clinical assessments should be made frequently during therapy and for several months after therapy is discontinued.

● Dosage in Renal and Hepatic Impairment

Modification of the usual dosage of cefotaxime is unnecessary in patients with creatinine clearances of 20 mL/minute or greater per 1.73 m^2. However, in patients with creatinine clearances less than 20 mL/minute per 1.73 m^2, doses and/or frequency of administration should be modified in response to the degree of renal impairment. The manufacturers recommend that these patients receive half the usual dose of cefotaxime at the usual time interval.

In patients undergoing hemodialysis, some clinicians recommend that 0.5–2 g be given as single daily doses and that a supplemental dose of cefotaxime be given after each dialysis period.

Although serum half-life and clearance of cefotaxime and its major metabolite may be prolonged in patients with impaired hepatic function, dosage adjustments are not necessary in such patients unless renal function also is impaired.

CAUTIONS

● Dermatologic and Sensitivity Reactions

Hypersensitivity reactions have been reported to occur in approximately 2% of patients receiving cefotaxime. These reactions include rash (maculopapular or erythematous), pruritus, fever, and eosinophilia. Urticaria, anaphylaxis, erythema multiforme, Stevens-Johnson syndrome, and toxic epidermal necrolysis have occurred rarely. If a severe hypersensitivity reaction occurs during cefotaxime therapy, the drug should be discontinued and the patient given appropriate therapy (e.g., epinephrine, corticosteroids, maintenance of an adequate airway, oxygen) as indicated.

Positive direct antiglobulin (Coombs') test results have also been reported occasionally in patients receiving cefotaxime; however, it is not clear whether the mechanism of this reaction is immunologic in nature.

● Local Effects

The most frequent adverse reactions to cefotaxime are local reactions at the injection site which occur in approximately 4% of patients. IV administration has caused inflammation, phlebitis, and thrombophlebitis and IM administration has caused pain, induration, and tenderness at the injection site. Extensive perivascular extravasation of cefotaxime may result in tissue damage requiring surgical intervention; however, in most cases, perivascular extravasation responds to changing the infusion site. To minimize the potential for tissue inflammation, the manufacturers recommend that IV infusion sites be monitored regularly and changed appropriately.

● GI Effects

Adverse GI effects including anorexia, diarrhea, nausea, vomiting, abdominal pain, and colitis have occurred in approximately 1% of patients receiving cefotaxime.

Treatment with anti-infectives alters the normal colon flora and may permit overgrowth of *Clostridium difficile*. *C. difficile* infection (CDI) and *C. difficile*-associated diarrhea and colitis (CDAD; also known as antibiotic-associated diarrhea and colitis or pseudomembranous colitis) have been reported with nearly all anti-infectives, including cefotaxime, and may range in severity from mild diarrhea to fatal colitis. *C. difficile* produces toxins A and B which contribute to the development of CDAD; hypertoxin-producing strains of *C. difficile* are associated with increased morbidity and mortality since they may be refractory to anti-infectives and colectomy may be required.

CDAD should be considered in the differential diagnosis in patients who develop diarrhea during or after anti-infective therapy and managed accordingly. Careful medical history is necessary since CDAD has been reported to occur as late as 2 months or longer after anti-infective therapy is discontinued.

If CDAD is suspected or confirmed, anti-infectives not directed against *C. difficile* should be discontinued whenever possible. Patients should be managed with appropriate supportive therapy (e.g., fluid and electrolyte management, protein supplementation), anti-infective therapy directed against *C. difficile* (e.g., metronidazole, vancomycin), and surgical evaluation as clinically indicated.

● Hematologic Effects

Transient neutropenia, granulocytopenia, leukopenia, eosinophilia, or thrombocytopenia have occurred in less than 1% of patients receiving cefotaxime. Agranulocytosis reportedly may occur rarely with cefotaxime treatment, particularly during prolonged therapy; therefore, blood cell counts should be performed in patients receiving treatment courses lasting for more than 10 days. Hemolytic anemia has also been reported rarely. Prolongation of the prothrombin time and hypoprothrombinemia have been reported only rarely in patients receiving cefotaxime.

● Renal Effects

Transient increases in BUN and/or serum creatinine concentrations and interstitial nephritis have been reported in a few patients receiving cefotaxime. A transient increase in urinary concentration of alanine aminopeptidase, which may be an indication of transient tubular damage, has been reported in a few patients receiving the drug. Most studies indicate that cefotaxime is not nephrotoxic and that urine concentrations of alanine aminopeptidase are usually unchanged during therapy with the drug.

● Other Adverse Effects

Transient increases in serum AST (SGOT), ALT (SGPT), LDH, bilirubin, and alkaline phosphatase concentrations have been reported in less than 1% of patients receiving cefotaxime.

Headache, agitation, confusion, fatigue, and nocturnal perspiration have also been reported in less than 1% of patients receiving the drug. Seizures have been reported with some cephalosporins,

During postmarketing surveillance, potentially life-threatening arrhythmias were reported in several patients who received cefotaxime by rapid (less than 1 minute) bolus injection through a central venous catheter.

● Precautions and Contraindications

Prior to initiation of cefotaxime therapy, careful inquiry should be made concerning previous hypersensitivity reactions to cefotaxime, cephalosporins, penicillins, or other drugs. There is clinical and laboratory evidence of partial cross-allergenicity among cephalosporins and other β-lactam antibiotics including penicillins and cephamycins; however, the true incidence of cross-allergenicity among these anti-infectives has not been established. Cefotaxime is contraindicated in patients with a history of allergic reactions to the drug or other cephalosporins and should be used with caution in patients with a history of hypersensitivity to penicillins. Use of cephalosporins should be avoided in patients who have had an immediate-type (anaphylactic) hypersensitivity reaction to penicillins. Although it has not been definitely proven that allergic reactions to antibiotics are more frequent in atopic individuals, the manufacturers state that cefotaxime should be used with caution in patients with a history of allergy, particularly to drugs.

To reduce development of drug-resistant bacteria and maintain effectiveness of cefotaxime and other antibacterials, the drug should be used only for the treatment or prevention of infections proven or strongly suspected to be caused by susceptible bacteria. When selecting or modifying anti-infective therapy, results of culture and in vitro susceptibility testing should be used. In the absence of such data, local epidemiology and susceptibility patterns should be considered when selecting anti-infectives for empiric therapy.

Patients should be advised that antibacterials (including cefotaxime) should only be used to treat bacterial infections and not used to treat viral infections (e.g., the common cold). Patients also should be advised about the importance of completing the full course of therapy, even if feeling better after a few days, and that skipping doses or not completing therapy may decrease effectiveness and increase the likelihood that bacteria will develop resistance and will not be treatable with cefotaxime or other antibacterials in the future.

Like other anti-infectives, prolonged use of cefotaxime may result in overgrowth of nonsusceptible organisms, especially *Candida* and *Pseudomonas*. Vaginitis and moniliasis have occurred in less than 1% of patients receiving cefotaxime. Resistant strains of some organisms, especially *Enterobacter*, *Ps. aeruginosa*, and *Serratia*, have developed during therapy with cefotaxime. Careful observation of the patient during cefotaxime therapy is essential. If suprainfection or superinfection occurs, appropriate therapy should be instituted.

Because CDAD has been reported with the use of cefotaxime or other cephalosporins, it should be considered in the differential diagnosis of patients who develop diarrhea during or after cefotaxime therapy. (See Cautions: GI Effects.) Patients should be advised that diarrhea is a common problem caused by anti-infectives and usually resolves when the drug is discontinued; however, they should contact a clinician if watery and bloody stools (with or without stomach cramps and fever) occur during or as late as 2 months or longer after the last dose. Cefotaxime should be used with caution in patients with a history of GI disease, particularly colitis.

Seizures have been reported with several cephalosporins, particularly in patients with renal impairment in whom dosage of the drug was not reduced. If seizures occur during cephalosporin therapy, the drug should be discontinued and anticonvulsant therapy initiated as clinically indicated.

● Pediatric Precautions

Cefotaxime is well tolerated in pediatric patients, and adverse effects reported in children receiving the drug are similar to those reported in adults. A retrospective review of children 3 months to 18 years of age who received cefotaxime indicates that adverse effects occurred in up to 2.5% of these children and included adverse local reactions, rash, and adverse GI effects such as diarrhea and vomiting.

Safety of the chemical components that may leach out of the plastic containing commercially available frozen cefotaxime sodium injections has not been established in children.

● Geriatric Precautions

In clinical studies of cefotaxime sodium, there were no overall differences in safety or efficacy between geriatric adults 65 years of age or older and younger adults. Other clinical experience revealed no evidence of age-related differences;

however, the possibility that some geriatric patients may exhibit increased sensitivity to the drug cannot be ruled out.

Cefotaxime is substantially excreted by the kidney, and the risk of severe adverse reactions may be increased in patients with impaired renal function. Because geriatric patients are more likely to have decreased renal function, dosage should be selected with caution in these patients and renal function monitoring may be useful.

● Mutagenicity and Carcinogenicity

Cefotaxime was not mutagenic in the mouse micronucleus test or the Ames test. Studies have not been performed to date to evaluate the carcinogenic potential of cefotaxime.

● Pregnancy, Fertility, and Lactation

Pregnancy

Reproduction studies in mice or rats using IV cefotaxime dosages up to 1.2 g/kg daily (0.4 or 0.8 times, respectively, the usual human dosage based on mg/m³) have not revealed evidence of embryotoxicity or teratogenicity. However, the offspring of rats that received 1.2 g/kg of cefotaxime weighed less at birth and also remained smaller during 21 days of nursing than offspring of rats that did not receive the drug. There are no adequate and controlled studies to date using cefotaxime in pregnant women, and the drug should be used during pregnancy only when clearly needed.

Fertility

There was no evidence of impaired fertility in rats given cefotaxime subcutaneously at dosages up to 250 mg/kg daily or in mice given the drug IV at dosages up to 2 g/kg daily (0.2 or 0.7 times, respectively, the recommended human dosage based on mg/m³).

Lactation

Because cefotaxime is distributed into milk, the drug should be used with caution in nursing women.

DRUG INTERACTIONS

● Aminoglycosides

In vitro studies indicate that the antibacterial activity of cefotaxime and aminoglycosides may be additive or synergistic against some organisms including some strains of Ps. aeruginosa and S. marcescens. However, synergism is unpredictable and antagonism has also occurred in vitro when cefotaxime was used in combination with an aminoglycoside.

Concurrent use of aminoglycosides and cephalosporins may increase the risk of nephrotoxicity during therapy. Although this effect has not been reported to date with cefotaxime, the manufacturers state that the possibility that nephrotoxicity may be potentiated if the drug is used concomitantly with an aminoglycoside should be considered.

● Other Anti-infective Agents

In one in vitro study which used the checkerboard technique to assess synergism, a combination of cefotaxime and ampicillin appeared to be partially additive or synergistic against a few strains of group B streptococci. However, when the killing-curve technique was used to assess synergism, the combination was no more effective than cefotaxime alone against these organisms. In one in vitro study, a combination of cefotaxime and clindamycin was neither synergistic nor antagonistic against Enterobacteriaceae.

LABORATORY TEST INTERFERENCES

● Immunohematology Tests

Positive direct antiglobulin (Coombs') test results have been reported in some patients receiving cefotaxime. This reaction may interfere with hematologic studies or transfusion cross-matching procedures.

● Tests for Glucose and Creatinine

Although other currently available cephalosporins reportedly cause false-positive results in urine glucose determinations using cupric sulfate solution (Benedict's reagent, Clinitest®) and may cause falsely elevated serum or urine creatinine

values when the Jaffé reaction is used, cefotaxime does not appear to interfere with these laboratory tests.

ACUTE TOXICITY

In neonatal and adult mice and rats, acute overdosage of cefotaxime resulted in significant mortality at parenteral dosages exceeding 6 g/kg daily. Common toxic signs in those that died included a decrease in spontaneous activity, tonic and clonic convulsions, dyspnea, hypothermia, and cyanosis.

Acute overdosage of cefotaxime in patients has most frequently resulted in increased serum concentrations of BUN and creatinine, but most cases were not associated with overt toxicity. If acute overdosage occurs, the patient should be closely observed and given supportive treatment.

MECHANISM OF ACTION

Cefotaxime has a mechanism of action similar to that of other cephalosporins. For information on the mechanism of action of cephalosporins, see Mechanism of Action in the Cephalosporins General Statement 8:12.06.

The target enzymes of β-lactam antibiotics have been classified as penicillin-binding proteins (PBPs) and appear to vary substantially among bacterial species. Studies evaluating the binding of cefotaxime to PBPs indicate that the drug has a high affinity for PBPs 1a, 1b, and 3 of Escherichia coli and PBPs 1a, 1b, 3, and 4 of Pseudomonas aeruginosa. The affinities of various β-lactam antibiotics for different PBPs appear to explain the differences in morphology which occur in susceptible organisms following exposure to different β-lactam antibiotics and may also explain differences in the spectrum of activity of β-lactam antibiotics which are not due to the presence or absence of β-lactamases.

SPECTRUM

Based on its spectrum of activity, cefotaxime is classified as a third generation cephalosporin. For information on the classification of cephalosporins and closely related β-lactam antibiotics based on spectra of activity, see Spectrum in the Cephalosporins General Statement 8:12.06.

Like other currently available parenteral third generation cephalosporins (e.g., ceftazidime, ceftriaxone), cefotaxime generally is less active in vitro against susceptible staphylococci than first generation cephalosporins but has an expanded spectrum of activity against gram-negative bacteria compared with first and second generation cephalosporins. The spectrum of activity of cefotaxime closely resembles that of ceftriaxone. In vitro on a weight basis, the activity of cefotaxime against most susceptible Enterobacteriaceae is approximately equal to that of ceftriaxone. Cefotaxime is inactive against Chlamydia, fungi, and viruses.

The major metabolite of cefotaxime, desacetylcefotaxime, is also microbiologically active. In vitro, desacetylcefotaxime has only about 10% of the antibacterial activity of cefotaxime. However, desacetylcefotaxime is more active in vitro against susceptible gram-positive aerobic bacteria than is cefazolin or cefoxitin. It has been suggested that the antibacterial activity of desacetylcefotaxime may be clinically important in infections in patients with impaired renal function or in infections in organs or tissues where desacetylcefotaxime accumulates. Preliminary data indicate that the antibacterial activities of cefotaxime and desacetylcefotaxime are additive or synergistic against cefotaxime-susceptible S. aureus and Enterobacteriaceae.

● In Vitro Susceptibility Testing

For most organisms, inoculum size, pH, test media, and presence of serum do not appear to influence results of in vitro cefotaxime susceptibility tests. However, results of susceptibility tests for some gram-negative bacilli (especially Proteus, Providencia, Pseudomonas aeruginosa, Klebsiella, and Serratia marcescens) may be greatly affected by the size of the inoculum.

Strains of staphylococci resistant to penicillinase-resistant penicillins (oxacillin-resistant [methicillin-resistant] staphylococci) should be considered resistant to cefotaxime, although results of in vitro susceptibility tests may indicate that the organisms are susceptible to the drug.

For information on interpreting results of in vitro susceptibility testing (disk susceptibility tests, dilution susceptibility tests) when cefotaxime susceptibility testing is performed according to the standards of the Clinical and Laboratory Standards Institute (CLSI; formerly National Committee for Clinical Laboratory

Standards [NCCLS]), see Spectrum: In Vitro Susceptibility Testing, in the Cephalosporins General Statement 8:12.06.

● Gram-positive Aerobic Bacteria

In vitro, cefotaxime concentrations of 0.5 mcg/mL or less inhibit most strains of *Streptococcus pneumoniae*, *S. pyogenes* (group A β-hemolytic streptococci), and *S. agalactiae* (group B streptococci). Some strains of viridans streptococci are inhibited in vitro by cefotaxime concentrations of 4 mcg/mL or less. In one study, the MIC_{50} and MIC_{90} of cefotaxime for the *S. milleri* group of viridans streptococci (*S. anginosus*, *S. constellatus*, *S. intermedius*) were 0.25 and 0.5 mcg/mL, respectively. Cefotaxime concentrations of 4 mcg/mL or less inhibit most strains of *Staphylococcus aureus* in vitro. Cefotaxime is active in vitro against most strains of penicillinase-producing *S. aureus*; however, almost all strains of staphylococci resistant to penicillinase-resistant penicillins are also resistant to cefotaxime. The MIC_{90} (minimum inhibitory concentration of the drug at which 90% of strains are inhibited) of cefotaxime for *S. epidermidis* generally is 4.8–16 mcg/mL, although lower MIC_{90}s have been reported occasionally; in a few studies, however, the MIC_{90} was 64 mcg/mL or greater. *Listeria monocytogenes* and enterococci, including *E. faecalis* (formerly *S. faecalis*), generally are resistant to the drug. Strains of *S. pneumoniae* with MICs of 2 mcg/mL or greater generally are considered resistant to cefotaxime.

The MIC_{90} of desacetylcefotaxime reported for susceptible *S. pneumoniae* and *S. pyogenes* is 4 mcg/mL or less. *S. aureus* is generally resistant to desacetylcefotaxime.

● Gram-negative Aerobic Bacteria

Cefotaxime is active in vitro against a wide variety of gram-negative bacteria including most Enterobacteriaceae and some strains of *Pseudomonas aeruginosa*. Cefotaxime is active against some gram-negative bacteria that are resistant to first and second generation cephalosporins and currently available penicillins and aminoglycosides, especially *Escherichia coli*, *Klebsiella pneumoniae*, and *Serratia marcescens*.

Enterobacteriaceae

Generally, cefotaxime is active in vitro against the following Enterobacteriaceae: *Citrobacter freundii*, *C. diversus*, *Enterobacter aerogenes*, *E. cloacae*, *Escherichia coli*, *Klebsiella pneumoniae*, *K. oxytoca*, *Morganella morganii* (formerly *Proteus morganii*), *Proteus mirabilis*, *P. vulgaris*, *Providencia stuartii* (formerly group B *Proteus inconstans*), *P. rettgeri* (formerly *Proteus rettgeri*), *Salmonella*, *Serratia marcescens*, *Shigella*, and *Yersinia enterocolitica*. The MIC_{90} of cefotaxime for many of these gram-negative bacilli is 4 mcg/mL or less. However, the MIC_{90} of cefotaxime for *C. freundii*, *E. aerogenes*, *E. cloacae*, *M. morganii*, and *Serratia* generally ranges from 0.1–32 mcg/mL, although higher MIC_{90}s have been reported. The MIC_{90} of desacetylcefotaxime reported for susceptible *E. coli*, *K. pneumoniae*, *P. mirabilis*, and *Providencia stuartii* is 4 mcg/mL or less; *E. aerogenes*, *E. cloacae*, *M. morganii*, *P. vulgaris*, and *S. marcescens* are generally resistant to desacetylcefotaxime.

Pseudomonas

The in vitro activity of cefotaxime against *Pseudomonas* is variable. Although some strains of *Ps. aeruginosa* and *Ps. maltophilia* (*Stenotrophomonas maltophilia*) are inhibited in vitro by cefotaxime concentrations of 32 mcg/mL or less, most strains of these organisms require cefotaxime concentrations of 64 mcg/mL or greater for in vitro inhibition and are therefore considered resistant to the drug. Cefotaxime is less active in vitro against susceptible *Ps. aeruginosa* than is ceftazidime or some extended-spectrum penicillins. *Ps. aeruginosa* generally is resistant to desacetylcefotaxime.

Other Gram-negative Aerobic Bacteria

Cefotaxime is active in vitro against *Haemophilus influenzae* (including ampicillin-resistant strains) and *H. parainfluenzae*. The MIC_{90}s of cefotaxime reported for *H. influenzae* and *H. parainfluenzae* are 0.01–0.8 and 0.024–4 mcg/mL, respectively, and the MIC_{90} of desacetylcefotaxime reported for *H. influenzae* is 4 mcg/mL or less.

Cefotaxime is active in vitro against *Neisseria meningitidis* and *Neisseria gonorrhoeae*. The MIC_{90} of cefotaxime reported for *N. gonorrhoeae* (including both penicillinase-producing and nonpenicillinase-producing strains) is 0.1–0.4 mcg/mL.

Both β-lactamase- and non-β-lactamase-producing strains of *Moraxella catarrhalis* are inhibited in vitro by cefotaxime concentrations of 0.03–0.5 mcg/mL.

Cefotaxime is active in vitro against *Eikenella corrodens*, and the MIC_{90} of the drug for this organism generally is 0.06–0.5 mcg/mL. *Campylobacter fetus* subsp. *jejuni*, an organism that can be microaerophilic or anaerobic, generally is inhibited in vitro by cefotaxime concentrations of 2–6.25 mcg/mL.

Although cefotaxime has some activity in vitro against *Acinetobacter*, the MIC_{90} of the drug generally ranges from 8–32 mcg/mL for *A. calcoaceticus* var. *lwoffi* and from 16–32 mcg/mL for *A. calcoaceticus* var. *anitratus*; higher MIC_{90}s also have been reported.

In vitro, some strains of *Bartonella bacilliformis* are inhibited by cefotaxime concentrations of 0.03–0.12 mcg/mL.

While some strains of *Burkholderia cepacia* (formerly *Pseudomonas cepacia*) are inhibited in vitro by cefotaxime concentrations of 16 mcg/mL, the MIC_{90} of the drug for this organism is 64 mcg/mL and most strains are resistant to the drug.

Cefotaxime is active in vitro against *Capnocytophaga*. In an in vitro study, the MIC_{90} of cefotaxime for *Capnocytophaga* was 0.25 mcg/mL. Cefotaxime-resistant strains of *C. sputigena* (formerly CDC group DF-1) have been reported.

Vibrio vulnificus may be inhibited in vitro by cefotaxime concentrations of 0.03 mcg/mL. While the clinical importance is unclear, results of an in vitro study and a study in mice indicate that the combination of cefotaxime and minocycline is more active against *V. vulnificus* than either anti-infective alone.

● Anaerobic Bacteria

Cefotaxime is active in vitro against *Bacteroides*, *Eubacterium*, *Fusobacterium*, *Peptococcus*, *Peptostreptococcus*, *Propionibacterium*, and *Veillonella*. Cefotaxime is also active against some strains of *Clostridium* including *C. perfringens*; however, *C. difficile* is usually resistant to the drug.

Although the MIC_{90} of cefotaxime reported for most susceptible anaerobes is 16 mcg/mL or less, cefotaxime concentrations of 16–64 mcg/mL are generally required in vitro to inhibit *Bacteroides* (including *B. fragilis*). In vitro, cefotaxime is less active than cefoxitin against susceptible *B. fragilis*.

● Spirochetes

Borrelia burgdorferi, the causative organism of Lyme disease, reportedly may be inhibited in vitro by a cefotaxime concentration of 0.12 mcg/mL.

RESISTANCE

For information on possible mechanisms of bacterial resistance to cephalosporins, see Resistance in the Cephalosporins General Statement 8:12.06.

Because cefotaxime contains an α-*syn*-methoximino group which protects the β-lactam ring from hydrolysis by many penicillinases and cephalosporinases, cefotaxime is more resistant to hydrolysis by most β-lactamases than first and second generation cephalosporins. Cefotaxime is generally resistant to hydrolysis by β-lactamases classified as Richmond-Sykes types I, II, III, IV, and V, and most penicillinases produced by *S. aureus*. However, β-lactamases produced by *B. fragilis* and *P. vulgaris* can slowly hydrolyze cefotaxime.

Resistant strains of some organisms, especially *Enterobacter*, *Ps. aeruginosa*, or *Serratia*, have developed during therapy with cefotaxime. Strains of *Ps. aeruginosa* which are only moderately susceptible to cefotaxime in vitro at the beginning of therapy appear to be especially likely to become resistant during therapy.

Like most cephalosporins and penicillins, cefotaxime is inactivated by inducible, chromosomally mediated β-lactamases produced by some strains of *Citrobacter*, *Enterobacter*, *Pseudomonas*, and *Serratia*. Therefore, organisms that possess inducible β-lactamases are usually resistant to cefotaxime following derepression of the enzymes. Inducible β-lactamases may be derepressed by mutation to a stable derepressed state or may be reversibly derepressed by an enzyme inducer. Cefoxitin and imipenem are potent inducers of these enzymes, and in vitro exposure of organisms possessing these enzymes to these drugs results in resistance to cefotaxime as well as to many other β-lactam antibiotics. Inducible β-lactamases inactivate cephalosporins and penicillins either by hydrolyzing the drugs or by binding to them to prevent access to penicillin-binding proteins (PBPs). The clinical importance of these inducible β-lactamases is unclear, but emergence of cefotaxime resistance in some organisms during therapy with the drug may be related to these enzymes.

Strains of *S. pneumoniae* considered resistant to cefotaxime have been reported with increasing frequency. These strains generally have intermediate- or high-level resistance to penicillin G as well as decreased susceptibility to third generation cephalosporins. Resistance to cefotaxime in *S. pneumoniae* appears to be related to alterations in the PBPs of the organism.

Tolerance to cefotaxime has been reported to occur in some bacteria including some strains of *Enterobacter*, *Proteus*, and *Ps. aeruginosa*. In vitro, tolerant bacteria have a minimum bactericidal concentration (MBC) of cefotaxime which is much greater than the MIC of the drug. Bacteria which are tolerant to cefotaxime appear to be inhibited but not necessarily killed by the drug. Preliminary studies suggest that tolerant organisms may have decreased concentrations of autolysins or an increased concentration of an unidentified inhibitor of autolysis. Tolerance may be important clinically since infections caused by these organisms may persist during cefotaxime therapy despite in vitro susceptibility tests which indicate that the organisms are susceptible to the drug.

PHARMACOKINETICS

In all studies described in the Pharmacokinetics section, cefotaxime was administered as the sodium salt; dosages of the drug are expressed in terms of cefotaxime.

The antibacterial activity of both cefotaxime and its major metabolite, desacetylcefotaxime, must be considered when attempting to correlate the pharmacokinetics with the therapeutic effect of the drug. In early published studies on the pharmacokinetics of cefotaxime, microbiologic assays were used to determine body fluid and tissue concentrations of the drug. Microbiologic assays which used test organisms susceptible to cefotaxime but resistant to desacetylcefotaxime accurately reflect concentrations of the parent drug; however, microbiologic assays used in some published pharmacokinetic studies of cefotaxime actually measured total microbiologic activity since both cefotaxime and desacetylcefotaxime were active against the test organism. Information on body fluid and tissue concentrations of cefotaxime obtained from studies that used nonspecific microbiologic assays or from studies that did not identify the test organism used is reported as *microbiologic activity* in the following sections on the pharmacokinetics of the drug. More recent pharmacokinetic studies generally use high-performance liquid chromatography (HPLC) that differentiates between cefotaxime and desacetylcefotaxime and can specifically measure concentrations of cefotaxime and/or its metabolite.

● **Absorption**

Cefotaxime is not appreciably absorbed from the GI tract and must be given parenterally.

Following IM administration of a single 500-mg or 1-g dose of cefotaxime in healthy adults with normal renal function, peak serum concentrations of the drug are attained within 30 minutes and average 11.7–11.9 mcg/mL and 20.5–25.3 mcg/mL, respectively. Plasma concentrations of cefotaxime are undetectable 8 hours after a single 500-mg IM dose of the drug but average 1 mcg/mL 8 hours after a single 1-g IM dose of the drug. In one multiple-dose study in adults with normal renal function receiving 500-mg doses of cefotaxime by IM injection every 8 hours, steady-state peak serum concentrations of cefotaxime ranged from 9.2–11.9 mcg/mL and steady-state trough serum concentrations of the drug ranged from 0.1–0.6 mcg/mL.

In one study in healthy adults with normal renal function, a single 500-mg, 1-g, or 2-g dose of cefotaxime given by IV injection over 5 minutes resulted in serum concentrations of cefotaxime which averaged 37.9 mcg/mL, 102.4 mcg/mL, and 214.1 mcg/mL, respectively, immediately after the injection; serum concentrations of the drug averaged 1 mcg/mL, 1.9 mcg/mL, and 3.3 mcg/mL, respectively, 4 hours after the injection. In a multiple-dose study in healthy adults with normal renal function receiving 1-g doses of cefotaxime every 6 hours by IV infusion over 30 minutes, steady-state peak serum concentrations of cefotaxime ranged from 40.6–46 mcg/mL and steady-state trough serum concentrations of the drug ranged from 1.1–1.6 mcg/mL.

Following a single cefotaxime dose of 50 mg/kg given by IV infusion over 10 minutes in average birthweight neonates 1–7 days of age, *microbiologic activity* in serum averaged 133 mcg/mL immediately after completion of the infusion, 85 mcg/mL 1 hour later, 52 mcg/mL 4 hours later, and 38 mcg/mL 6 hours later.

In one study in children 1 month to 12 years of age, serum concentrations of cefotaxime averaged 25.3 mcg/mL 30 minutes after a single cefotaxime dose of 25 mg/kg given by IM injection and averaged 53.3 mcg/mL 5 minutes after a single dose of 25 mg/kg of the drug given by IV injection.

● **Distribution**

Following IM or IV administration of usual dosages of cefotaxime, *microbiologic activity* is widely distributed into body tissues and fluids including the aqueous humor, bronchial secretions, sputum, middle ear effusions, bone, bile, and ascitic, pleural, and prostatic fluids. The apparent volume of distribution of cefotaxime in adults is reported to be 0.22–0.29 L/kg.

Cefotaxime is 13–38% bound to serum proteins in vitro.

Cefotaxime and its major metabolite are distributed into CSF following parenteral administration. Following IV administration of a single 2-g IV dose of cefotaxime in patients with *uninflamed* meninges, low concentrations of cefotaxime (0.14–1.81 mcg/mL) and desacetylcefotaxime (0.06–0.38 mcg/mL) are attained in CSF; however, higher concentrations are attained in patients with *inflamed* meninges. In one study in neonates and children 2 weeks to 2 years of age with inflamed meninges, IV injection or infusion over 30 minutes of cefotaxime doses of 50 mg/kg every 4–6 hours resulted in *microbiologic activity* in CSF which ranged from 1–13.2 mcg/mL 1–4 hours after administration. In another study in children 2 months to 12 years of age with meningitis who received cefotaxime in a dosage of 50 mg/kg IV every 6 hours, CSF concentrations of cefotaxime or its major metabolite averaged 6.2 or 5.6 mcg/mL, respectively, 1 hour after a dose; concurrent serum concentrations were 61.44 and 19.3 mcg/mL, respectively. In a study in adults with bacterial meningitis receiving 2 g of cefotaxime IV every 4 hours, trough CSF cefotaxime and desacetylcefotaxime concentrations ranged from 5.6–44.3 mcg/mL and 3.7–44 mcg/mL, respectively, after 1–3 days of therapy.

Following IM or IV administration of usual dosages of cefotaxime, *microbiologic activity* in hepatic bile is reported to be 15–75% of concurrent *microbiologic activity* in serum and *microbiologic activity* in gallbladder bile is reported to be up to 3 times greater than concurrent *microbiologic activity* in serum. *Microbiologic activity* in ascitic fluid is reported to be 40% of concurrent *microbiologic activity* in serum.

In patients receiving 2-g doses of cefotaxime IV every 6 hours, concentrations of cefotaxime and desacetylcefotaxime in bronchial secretions averaged 1.7 and 5.8 mcg/mL, respectively, and plasma concentrations averaged 23.1 and 9.3 mcg/mL, respectively, in samples obtained 1–2 hours after the fourth dose.

Cefotaxime readily crosses the placenta, and *microbiologic activity* in amniotic fluid is reported to be equal to or greater than concurrent *microbiologic activity* in maternal serum following multiple doses of the drug.

Cefotaxime is distributed into milk. In one study, *microbiologic activity* in milk ranged from 0.25–0.52 mcg/mL 2–3 hours after a single 1-g IV dose of cefotaxime.

● **Elimination**

Cefotaxime is partially metabolized in the liver to desacetylcefotaxime which has antibacterial activity. (See Spectrum.) Desacetylation of cefotaxime occurs rapidly in vivo and rapidly in vitro in hemolyzed blood. Following IV injection over 5 minutes of a single 500-mg or 2-g dose of cefotaxime in adults with normal renal function, peak plasma concentrations of desacetylcefotaxime are generally attained within 45 minutes and average 2.7 mcg/mL and 9.8 mcg/mL, respectively. Desacetylcefotaxime is partially converted in the liver to desacetylcefotaxime lactone which is inactive and is further degraded to 2 unidentified inactive metabolites currently designated as UP_1 and its optical isomer UP_2.

Serum concentrations of cefotaxime appear to decline in a biphasic manner. In adults with normal renal function, the serum half-life of cefotaxime in the initial phase ($t_{\frac{1}{2}\alpha}$) averages 0.2–0.4 hours and the serum half-life of the drug in the terminal phase ($t_{\frac{1}{2}\beta}$) averages 0.9–1.7 hours. The $t_{\frac{1}{2}\beta}$ of desacetylcefotaxime is longer than that of the parent drug and is reported to be 1.4–1.9 hours in adults with normal renal function. In adults with renal impairment, the $t_{\frac{1}{2}\alpha}$ of cefotaxime is not affected, and the $t_{\frac{1}{2}\beta}$ is only slightly prolonged in patients with creatinine clearances of 20 mL/min or greater per 1.73 m². In adults with creatinine clearances of 10 mL/min or less per 1.73 m², the $t_{\frac{1}{2}\beta}$ of cefotaxime is reported to range from 1.4–11.5 hours and the $t_{\frac{1}{2}\beta}$ of desacetylcefotaxime is reported to range from 8.2–56.8 hours. The $t_{\frac{1}{2}\beta}$ of both cefotaxime and desacetylcefotaxime may be prolonged in patients with impaired hepatic function. In a study in patients with chronic parenchymal liver disease with or without jaundice, edema, or ascites, the $t_{\frac{1}{2}\beta}$ of the parent drug ranged from 1.49–2.42 hours and the apparent $t_{\frac{1}{2}}$ of the metabolite ranged from 7.1–13.4 hours.

In one study in children 5 months to 1 year of age, the $t_{\frac{1}{2}\alpha}$ of cefotaxime averaged 0.2 hours and the $t_{\frac{1}{2}\beta}$ averaged 1.2 hours. In children 2–12 years of age, the $t_{\frac{1}{2}\alpha}$ averaged 0.3 hours and the $t_{\frac{1}{2}\beta}$ averaged 1.5 hours. In neonates, the half-life of cefotaxime depends principally on gestational and chronologic age. The $t_{\frac{1}{2}\alpha}$ is reported to range from 0.1–0.4 hours in premature or full-term neonates. The $t_{\frac{1}{2}\beta}$ of cefotaxime averages 5–6 hours in premature neonates less than 1 week of age, 3.4–3.5 hours in premature neonates 1–4 weeks of age, 2–3.4 hours in full-term neonates less than 1 week of age, and 2 hours in full-term neonates 1–4 weeks of age.

Cefotaxime and its metabolites are excreted principally in urine; tubular secretion of the drug occurs. In adults with normal renal function, approximately 40–60% of a single IM or IV dose of cefotaxime is excreted in urine as unchanged drug and approximately 24% is excreted as desacetylcefotaxime within 24 hours. The majority of the IM or IV dose is excreted within the first 2 hours following administration.

In one study, urine concentrations of cefotaxime ranged from 90–3261 mcg/mL in urine collected over 2 hours following a single 500-mg IM dose of cefotaxime.

The serum clearance of cefotaxime in adults with normal renal function is reported to be 207–342 mL/minute per 1.73 m². In one study, the serum clearance of the drug averaged 23 mL/minute per 1.73 m² in low birthweight neonates 1–7 days of age and 44 mL/minute per 1.73 m² in average birthweight neonates 1–7 days of age.

Oral probenecid administered shortly before or concomitantly with cefotaxime usually slows the rate of excretion of the antibiotic and its metabolites and produces higher and more prolonged serum concentrations of cefotaxime and its metabolites. The volume of distribution of cefotaxime does not appear to be affected by concomitant administration of oral probenecid.

Cefotaxime and its metabolites are removed by hemodialysis. The amount of cefotaxime removed during hemodialysis depends on several factors (e.g., type of coil used, dialysis flow-rate); however, a 4- to 6-hour period of hemodialysis in one study removed into the dialysate 60% of a single 15 mg/kg dose of cefotaxime when the dose was given by IV injection immediately prior to dialysis. Only minimal amounts of cefotaxime are removed by peritoneal dialysis.

CHEMISTRY AND STABILITY

● Chemistry

Cefotaxime is a semisynthetic cephalosporin antibiotic. Like cefepime, ceftazidime, and ceftriaxone, cefotaxime is a parenteral aminothiazolyl cephalosporin. Cefotaxime contains an aminothiazolyl-acetyl side chain, with an α-*syn*-methoximino group, at position 7 of the cephalosporin nucleus. The aminothiazolyl side chain enhances antibacterial activity, particularly against Enterobacteriaceae, and generally results in enhanced stability against β-lactamases; the methoximino group contributes to stability against hydrolysis by many β-lactamases.

Cefotaxime is commercially available as the sodium salt. Potency of cefotaxime sodium is expressed in terms of cefotaxime. Cefotaxime sodium occurs as an off-white to pale yellow, crystalline powder. Cefotaxime sodium is sparingly soluble in water, slightly soluble in alcohol, and has a pK_a of 3.4. The sodium salt of cefotaxime contains approximately 50.5 mg (2.2 mEq) of sodium per gram of cefotaxime.

Commercially available frozen premixed cefotaxime sodium injections containing 1 or 2 g of cefotaxime are sterile, nonpyrogenic, iso-osmotic solutions of the drug provided in a plastic container fabricated from specially formulated multilayered plastic (PL 2040). The 1- and 2-g frozen injections of cefotaxime contain approximately 1.7 g and 700 mg of dextrose hydrous, respectively, to adjust osmolality. The injections are buffered with sodium citrate hydrous and may contain hydrochloric acid and/or sodium hydroxide to adjust pH. After thawing, the injections are pale yellow to light amber solutions.

● Stability

Cefotaxime sodium powder for injection and solutions of the drug tend to darken, depending on storage conditions, and should be protected from excess heat and light. Discoloration of cefotaxime sodium sterile powder for injection or solutions of the drug may indicate a loss of potency.

Commercially available cefotaxime sodium sterile powder for injection should be stored at 15–30°C.

Following reconstitution as directed by the manufacturer, cefotaxime sodium solutions containing 50–330 mg of cefotaxime per mL have a pH of 4.5–6.5 and are light yellow to amber in color. Following reconstitution with sterile or bacteriostatic water for injection, IM solutions containing 230–330 mg/mL are stable in their original containers for 12 hours at room temperature (22°C or lower) or 7 days when refrigerated (5°C or lower). Following reconstitution with sterile water for injection, IV solutions containing 50 or 95 mg/mL are stable for 24 hours at room temperature (22°C or lower) or 7 days when refrigerated (5°C or lower). When reconstituted as directed in 0.9% sodium chloride injection or 5% dextrose injection, solutions prepared from ADD-Vantage® vials of the drug are stable for 24 hours at a room temperature of 22°C or less; these solutions should not be frozen.

Cefotaxime sodium is physically and chemically compatible with the following IV solutions: 0.9% sodium chloride; 5% or 10% dextrose; 5% dextrose and 0.2%, 0.45%, or 0.9% sodium chloride; lactated Ringer's; ¼ M sodium lactate; 10% invert sugar; or Travasol® 8.5%. Reconstituted solutions of cefotaxime sodium which have been further diluted with 50 mL to 1 liter of one of the above IV solutions are physically and chemically stable for 24 hours at room temperature or

at least 5 days when refrigerated at 5°C or less. Cefotaxime sodium solutions are most stable at a pH of 5–7 and the drug should not be diluted with IV solutions (e.g., sodium bicarbonate) which have a pH greater than 7.5.

Reconstituted solutions of cefotaxime sodium which have been further diluted with 50 mL to 1 liter of 0.9% sodium chloride injection or 5% dextrose injection may be frozen in Viaflex® containers immediately after preparation and are stable for 13 weeks. Frozen solutions of cefotaxime sodium should be thawed at room temperature. Once thawed, solutions are stable for 24 hours at room temperature or 5 days at less than 5°C and should not be refrozen.

The commercially available frozen premixed cefotaxime sodium injection should be stored at –20°C or lower. Thawed solutions of the commercially available frozen injection are stable for 24 hours at room temperature (22°C or lower) or 10 days when refrigerated at 5°C or lower. The commercially available frozen injection of the drug is provided in a plastic container fabricated from specially formulated multilayered plastic PL 2040 (Galaxy® container). Solutions in contact with PL 2040 can leach out some of its chemical components in very small amounts within the expiration period of the injection; however, safety of the plastic has been confirmed in tests in animals according to USP biological tests for plastic containers as well as by tissue culture toxicity studies.

Cefotaxime sodium is potentially physically and/or chemically incompatible with some drugs, including aminoglycosides, but the compatibility depends on several factors (e.g., concentrations of the drugs, specific diluents used, resulting pH, temperature). Specialized references should be consulted for specific compatibility information. Because of the potential for incompatibility, cefotaxime sodium and aminoglycosides should not be admixed.

PREPARATIONS

Excipients in commercially available drug preparations may have clinically important effects in some individuals; consult specific product labeling for details.

Cefotaxime Sodium

Parenteral

For injection	500 mg (of cefotaxime)*	Cefotaxime Sodium for Injection
		Claforan®, Sanofi-Aventis
	1 g (of cefotaxime)*	Cefotaxime Sodium for Injection
		Claforan®, Sanofi-Aventis
	2 g (of cefotaxime)*	Cefotaxime Sodium for Injection
		Claforan®, Sanofi-Aventis
	10 g (of cefotaxime) pharmacy bulk package*	Cefotaxime Sodium for Injection
		Claforan®, Sanofi-Aventis
For injection, for IV infusion	1 g (of cefotaxime)	Claforan®, Sanofi-Aventis
		Claforan® ADD-Vantage®, Sanofi-Aventis
	2 g (of cefotaxime)	Claforan®, Sanofi-Aventis
		Claforan® ADD-Vantage®, Sanofi-Aventis

* available from one or more manufacturer, distributor, and/or repackager by generic (nonproprietary) name

Cefotaxime Sodium in Dextrose

Parenteral

| Injection (frozen), for IV infusion | 20 mg (of cefotaxime) per mL (1 g) in 3.4% Dextrose* | Cefotaxime Sodium Iso-osmotic in Dextrose Injection (Galaxy® [Baxter]) |
| | 40 mg (of cefotaxime) per mL (2 g) in 1.4% Dextrose* | Cefotaxime Sodium Iso-osmotic in Dextrose Injection (Galaxy® [Baxter]) |

* available from one or more manufacturer, distributor, and/or repackager by generic (nonproprietary) name

† Use is not currently included in the labeling approved by the US Food and Drug Administration.

cefTAZidime

8:12.06.12 • THIRD GENERATION CEPHALOSPORINS

■ Ceftazidime is a semisynthetic, third generation cephalosporin antibiotic.

USES

Ceftazidime is used for the treatment of bone and joint infections, intra-abdominal and gynecologic infections, meningitis and other CNS infections, lower respiratory tract infections, skin and skin structure infections, septicemia, and complicated or uncomplicated urinary tract infections caused by susceptible bacteria. The drug also is used for empiric anti-infective agent therapy in febrile neutropenic patients† and has been used for perioperative prophylaxis†.

Ceftazidime therapy may be started pending results of susceptibility tests, but should be discontinued if the organism is found to be resistant to the drug. When the causative organism is unknown, concomitant therapy with another anti-infective agent may be indicated pending results of in vitro susceptibility tests. In severe or life-threatening infections or in immunocompromised patients, ceftazidime may be used concomitantly with other anti-infectives such as aminoglycosides, vancomycin, or clindamycin.

● Gram-positive Aerobic Bacterial Infections

Like other parenteral third generation cephalosporins (cefotaxime, ceftriaxone), ceftazidime is less active than first and second generation cephalosporins against some gram-positive bacteria (e.g., staphylococci) and generally should not be used in the treatment of infections caused by these organisms when a penicillin or first or second generation cephalosporin could be used. Although ceftazidime has been effective when used alone in adults or children for the treatment of septicemia, cellulitis, urinary tract infections, osteomyelitis, or respiratory tract infections (including pneumonia) caused by susceptible gram-positive cocci (e.g., *Staphylococcus aureus*, *S. epidermidis*, groups A and B streptococci, *Streptococcus pneumoniae*), treatment failures also have been reported in some of these infections, especially in immunocompromised patients or patients with cystic fibrosis. Therefore, ceftazidime is not used alone for empiric therapy in infections where gram-positive bacteria may be involved (e.g., community-acquired pneumonia).

● Gram-negative Aerobic Bacterial Infections

Ceftazidime generally has been effective when used alone in adults or children for the treatment of respiratory tract infections (including pneumonia), skin and skin structure infections, osteomyelitis, septicemia, intra-abdominal infections, or urinary tract infections caused by susceptible Enterobacteriaceae (e.g., *Enterobacter, Escherichia coli, Klebsiella, Morganella, Proteus, Serratia*). A principal use of ceftazidime is for the treatment of infections known or suspected to be caused by multidrug-resistant Enterobacteriaceae (e.g., nosocomial urinary tract infections or pneumonia, suspected septicemia in non-neutropenic patients) and serious gram-negative infections when other anti-infectives are contraindicated or ineffective. It has been suggested that certain parenteral cephalosporins (i.e., cefepime, cefotaxime, ceftriaxone, ceftazidime) may be drugs of choice for the treatment of infections caused by susceptible *E. coli, K. pneumoniae, P. rettgeri, M. morganii, P. vulgaris, P. stuartii*, or *Serratia*; an aminoglycoside (amikacin, gentamicin, tobramycin) should be used concomitantly in severe infections. There is some evidence that for the treatment of some infections (e.g., pneumonia, bacteremia) caused by susceptible Enterobacteriaceae, ceftazidime used alone can be as effective as a 2-drug regimen of a third generation cephalosporin or an extended-spectrum penicillin used in conjunction with an aminoglycoside.

● Mixed Aerobic-Anaerobic Bacterial Infections

Ceftazidime has been used with some success in the treatment of mixed aerobic-anaerobic bacterial infections. The manufacturers indicate that ceftazidime may be used in the treatment of polymicrobial intra-abdominal infections caused by aerobic and anaerobic bacteria, including *Bacteroides*; however, the drug should not be used alone for the treatment of any infection when *B. fragilis* may be present, since it generally is inactive against this organism.

● Intra-abdominal and Gynecologic Infections

Ceftazidime is used for the treatment of gynecologic infections (including endometritis, pelvic cellulitis, other infections of the female genital tract) caused by susceptible *E. coli*.

Ceftazidime also is used for the treatment of intra-abdominal infections (including peritonitis) caused by susceptible *S. aureus* (oxacillin-susceptible strains only), *E. coli*, or *Klebsiella*. and polymicrobial infections caused by aerobic and anaerobic bacteria.

For initial empiric treatment of high-risk or severe community-acquired extrabiliary intra-abdominal infections in adults (e.g., those with advanced age, immunocompromise, severe physiologic disturbance), the Infectious Diseases Society of America (IDSA) recommends either monotherapy with a carbapenem (doripenem, imipenem, meropenem) or the fixed combination of piperacillin and tazobactam, or a combination regimen that includes either a cephalosporin (cefepime, ceftazidime) or fluoroquinolone (ciprofloxacin, levofloxacin) in conjunction with metronidazole. IDSA also recommends ceftazidime in conjunction with metronidazole as one of several regimens that can be used for initial empiric treatment of health-care-associated complicated intra-abdominal infections in adults and community-acquired complicated intra-abdominal infections in pediatric patients.

For additional information regarding management of intra-abdominal infections, the current IDSA clinical practice guidelines available at http://www.idsociety.org should be consulted.

● Meningitis and Other CNS Infections

Ceftazidime used in conjunction with an aminoglycoside is considered a regimen of choice for the treatment of meningitis caused by susceptible *Pseudomonas aeruginosa* or susceptible Enterobacteriaceae† (e.g., *E. coli, P. mirabilis, Enterobacter, S. marcescens*). While ceftazidime also has been effective when used alone for the treatment of meningitis caused by susceptible *Haemophilus influenzae, Neisseria meningitidis*, or *S. pneumoniae*, cefotaxime or ceftriaxone generally is preferred when a cephalosporin is indicated for the treatment of meningitis caused by these organisms. (See Uses: Meningitis and Other CNS Infections in the Cephalosporins General Statement 8:12.06.)

Because preterm, low-birthweight neonates are at increased risk for nosocomial infection caused by staphylococci or gram-negative bacilli, some clinicians suggest that these neonates receive an empiric regimen of IV ceftazidime and IV vancomycin for suspected bacterial meningitis. Immunocompromised individuals, geriatric individuals, and individuals with recent head trauma, neurosurgery, or CSF shunts also are at increased risk for meningitis caused by gram-negative bacilli and some clinicians recommend that IV ceftazidime be use for empiric therapy in these patients. If ceftazidime is used for empiric therapy in individuals with meningitis, concomitant use of IV ampicillin should be considered to provide coverage against *Listeria monocytogenes*, especially in patients who are immunocompromised, infants younger than 3 months of age, or adults older than 50 years of age. In addition, for empiric therapy of meningitis in individuals with recent head trauma, neurosurgery, or CSF shunts, concomitant use of vancomycin should be considered to provide coverage against gram-positive bacteria. When results of culture and in vitro susceptibility tests become available and the pathogen is identified, the empiric anti-infective regimen should be modified (if necessary) to ensure that the most effective regimen is being administered.

In patients with meningitis caused by *Ps. aeruginosa*, many clinicians recommend that therapy be initiated with a regimen of ceftazidime and a parenteral aminoglycoside (amikacin, gentamicin, tobramycin). If the patient fails to respond to this regimen, concomitant use of intrathecal or intraventricular aminoglycoside therapy or use of an alternative parenteral anti-infective (e.g., aztreonam, meropenem, a fluoroquinolone) should be considered based on results of in vitro susceptibility tests.

● Septicemia

Ceftazidime is used in adult and pediatric patients for the treatment of septicemia caused by *S. aureus, S. pneumoniae, E. coli, H. influenzae, K. pneumoniae*, or *Ps. aeruginosa*. Some clinicians recommend that an aminoglycoside (amikacin, gentamicin, tobramycin) be used concomitantly for the treatment of gram-negative bacteremia in seriously ill patients.

The choice of anti-infective agent for the treatment of sepsis syndrome should be based on the probable source of infection, causative organism, immune status of the patient, and local patterns of bacterial resistance. For initial treatment of life-threatening sepsis in adults, some clinicians recommend that a third or fourth generation cephalosporin (cefepime, cefotaxime, ceftriaxone, ceftazidime), the fixed combination of piperacillin and tazobactam, or a carbapenem (doripenem, imipenem, meropenem) be used in conjunction with vancomycin; some experts also suggest including an aminoglycoside or fluoroquinolone during the initial few days of treatment.

● Urinary Tract Infections

Ceftazidime is used in adult and pediatric patients for the treatment of complicated and uncomplicated urinary tract infections caused by *Enterobacter, E. coli, Klebsiella, M. morganii, P. mirabilis, P. vulgaris,* or *Ps. aeruginosa.* The most appropriate agent for the treatment of urinary tract infections should be selected based on the severity of the infection and results of culture and in vitro susceptibility testing. It has been suggested that certain parenteral cephalosporins (i.e., cefepime, cefotaxime, ceftriaxone, ceftazidime) may be drugs of choice for the treatment of infections caused by susceptible Enterobacteriaceae, including susceptible *E. coli, K. pneumoniae, P. rettgeri, M. morganii, P. vulgaris, P. stuartii,* or *Serratia*; an aminoglycoside should be used concomitantly in severe infections. However, ceftazidime, like other third generation cephalosporins, generally should not be used in the treatment of uncomplicated urinary tract infections when other anti-infectives with a narrower spectrum of activity could be used.

● Pseudomonas aeruginosa Infections

Ceftazidime is used in adult and pediatric patients for the treatment of septicemia, osteomyelitis, respiratory tract, skin and skin structure, or urinary tract infections caused by susceptible *Ps. aeruginosa.* The drug also is used for the treatment of meningitis caused by *Ps. aeruginosa* (see Uses: Meningitis and Other CNS Infections) and has been used for the treatment of malignant otitis externa† caused by *Ps. aeruginosa* (see Otitis Externa under Uses: Otitis, in the Cephalosporins General Statement 8:12.06).

Ceftazidime generally has been considered a drug of choice for the treatment of infections caused by *Ps. aeruginosa* since it is more active in vitro on a weight basis against the organism than most other currently available cephalosporins and is active against some strains resistant to many other cephalosporins, aminoglycosides, and extended-spectrum penicillins. However, ceftazidime-resistant strains of *Ps. aeruginosa* can emerge during therapy with the drug, and superinfection with resistant strains has occurred. In severe infections, especially in immuno-compromised patients, concomitant use of ceftazidime and an aminoglycoside (e.g., amikacin, gentamicin, tobramycin) is recommended.

For the treatment of community-acquired pneumonia (CAP) caused by *Ps. aeruginosa,* the American Thoracic Society (ATS) and IDSA recommend a combination regimen that includes an antipseudomonal β-lactam (cefepime, ceftazidime, aztreonam, imipenem, meropenem, piperacillin, ticarcillin) given in conjunction with ciprofloxacin, levofloxacin, or an aminoglycoside. For additional information on treatment of CAP, see Community-Acquired Pneumonia under Uses: Respiratory Tract Infections, in the Cephalosporins General Statement 8:12.06.

Ceftazidime is used alone or in conjunction with an aminoglycoside for the treatment of acute exacerbations of bronchopulmonary *Ps. aeruginosa* infections in children and adults with cystic fibrosis and generally is considered a drug of choice for these infections. In cystic fibrosis patients with acute exacerbations of *Ps. aeruginosa* infection, there is some evidence that an empiric regimen of ceftazidime and an aminoglycoside may be more effective than ceftazidime monotherapy; however, ceftazidime monotherapy appears to be as effective or more effective than monotherapy with aztreonam, ciprofloxacin, or meropenem or combination therapy with ticarcillin and tobramycin. Although anti-infective therapy in patients with cystic fibrosis may result in clinical improvement and *Ps. aeruginosa* may be temporarily cleared from the sputum, a bacteriologic cure is rarely obtained and should not be expected. Continuous IV infusion of ceftazidime has been used effectively for the treatment of *Ps. aeruginosa* infections in some adult and pediatric cystic fibrosis patients, including patients who failed to respond to ceftazidime administered by intermittent IV injection or infusion. Because a ceftazidime dosing regimen that consists of an IV loading dose followed by continuous IV infusion may provide more consistent concentrations of the drug than an intermittent dosing regimen, it has been suggested that such a regimen theoretically would be more effective in suppressing *Ps. aeruginosa* and possibly may decrease emergence of drug-resistant strains of the organism. Ceftazidime has been administered on an outpatient basis for the treatment of acute exacerbations of *Ps. aeruginosa* infections in cystic fibrosis patients; such community-based parenteral therapy generally is used to complete a course of ceftazidime therapy initiated during hospitalization.

● Burkholderia Infections

Burkholderia cepacia Infections

Ceftazidime has been used alone or in conjunction with an aminoglycoside for the treatment of septicemia or pulmonary infections caused by *Burkholderia*

cepacia (formerly *Ps. cepacia*)†. Patients with cystic fibrosis often are colonized with *B. cepacia* (with or without *Ps. aeruginosa* colonization). In addition, *B. cepacia* has recently been recognized as a cause of nosocomial pneumonia or nosocomial bacteremia in immunocompromised patients (e.g., patients with malignancy) *B. cepacia* is an aerobic, nonfermenting gram-negative bacilli resistant to many anti-infective agents, and no anti-infective regimen has been identified that effectively eradicates the organism in colonized cystic fibrosis patients. The optimum regimen for the treatment of infections caused by *B. cepacia* has not been identified. Some clinicians consider co-trimoxazole the drug of choice and ceftazidime, chloramphenicol, and imipenem alternative agents for the treatment of *B. cepacia* infections. Ceftazidime monotherapy has been used effectively to treat nosocomial *B. cepacia* bacteremia in a limited number of patients with severe underlying disease (e.g., malignancy); many of these patients had indwelling central venous catheters or recent surgery that may have precipitated the infection.

Melioidosis

Ceftazidime is considered by many clinicians to be a drug of choice for the treatment of severe melioidosis†, a potentially life-threatening disease caused by *B. pseudomallei* (formerly *Ps. pseudomallei*).

B. pseudomallei is an aerobic, nonfermenting gram-negative bacilli resistant to many anti-infective agents (e.g., penicillins, first and second generation cephalosporins, aminoglycosides). *B. pseudomallei* may cause subclinical illness and localized infections or fulminant septicemia; disseminated infections may include hepatic and splenic abscesses. The incubation period usually is 1–21 days (median 9 days), but can be prolonged (years). In some asymptomatic individuals, the disease has remained dormant and active melioidosis was not evident for more than 20 years, usually at a time when the patient was immunosuppressed. If left untreated, severe septicemic infections can be fatal within 24–48 hours after onset. *B. pseudomallei* is widely distributed in water and soil in many tropical and subtropical countries and melioidosis is endemic in Southeast Asia (e.g., Thailand, Malaysia, Singapore) and northern Australia, and also is found in the Indian subcontinent and South and Central America. The disease occurs only rarely in the US. Person-to-person spread occurs only rarely. *B. pseudomallei* usually is transmitted to humans from contaminated materials (e.g., soil) via contact with nasal, oral, or conjunctival mucous membranes, contact with abraded or lacerated skin, or, rarely, by inhalation. Laboratory workers have become infected via aerosols from *B. pseudomallei* cultures.

Melioidosis, regardless of severity, should be treated with an initial parenteral regimen of ceftazidime, imipenem, or meropenem (some clinicians recommend that co-trimoxazole also be included, especially if the patient is septicemic) followed by a prolonged maintenance regimen of oral anti-infectives (e.g., co-trimoxazole with or without doxycycline). In patients with melioidosis septic shock, adjunctive use of filgrastim (granulocyte colony-stimulating factor; G-CSF) during initial treatment has been suggested. *B. pseudomallei* is difficult to eradicate, and relapse of melioidosis commonly occurs. Therefore, after the maintenance regimen is completed, life-long follow-up is recommended since relapse of melioidosis can occur despite effective anti-infective therapy. The fact that resistant strains of *B. pseudomallei* have developed during ceftazidime therapy should be considered.

B. pseudomallei has been studied for and is considered a potential pathogen for aerosol distribution in the context of biologic warfare or bioterrorism. Acute respiratory or systemic infection probably would occur following high-dose aerosol exposure to *B. pseudomallei*. Some experts (e.g., US Army Medical Research Institute of Infectious Diseases [USAMRIID], European Commission's Task Force on Biological and Chemical Agent Threats [BICHAT]) state that the same treatment regimens recommended for naturally occurring melioidosis should be used if the disease occurs in the context of biologic warfare or bioterrorism.

Ceftazidime monotherapy (40 mg/kg or 2 g IV 3 times daily) has been effective for the treatment of severe septicemic or pulmonary melioidosis, and has been associated with a lower mortality rate than a 3-drug regimen of IV chloramphenicol, oral doxycycline, and oral co-trimoxazole. In an open, prospective study in adults with acute severe melioidosis randomized to receive an initial parenteral regimen of IV ceftazidime or IV imipenem followed by an oral maintenance regimen, the survival rate at 48 hours was similar with both drugs (20.8% of those receiving ceftazidime and 25% of those receiving imipenem died within the first 48 hours), and the choice of initial drug did not appear to influence the final outcome; however, a higher percentage of patients receiving ceftazidime were considered to be treatment failures after 48 hours and had to be switched to an alternative drug because of primary treatment failure.

Vibrio vulnificus Infections

Ceftazidime is considered by some clinicians to be a drug of choice for the treatment of infections caused by *Vibrio vulnificus*†. *V. vulnificus*, a gram-negative aerobic bacteria that can cause potentially fatal septicemia, wound infections, or gastroenteritis, generally is transmitted through ingestion of contaminated raw or undercooked seafood (especially raw oysters) or through contamination of a wound with seawater or seafood drippings. *V. vulnificus* is naturally present in marine environments, thrives in warm ocean water, and frequently is isolated from oysters and other shellfish harvested from the Gulf of Mexico and from US coastal waters along the Pacific and Atlantic ocean. Individuals with preexisting liver disease are at high risk for developing fatal septicemia following ingestion of seafood contaminated with *V. vulnificus* and debilitated or immunocompromised individuals (e.g., those with chronic renal impairment, cancer, diabetes mellitus, steroid-dependent asthma, chronic GI disease) or individuals with iron overload states (e.g., thalassemia and hemochromatosis) also are at increased risk for fatal infections. The incubation period for *V. vulnificus* infection reportedly is 1–7 days and the duration of illness usually is 2–8 days. In immunocompromised individuals, fever, nausea, myalgia, and abdominal cramps may occur as soon as 24–48 hours after ingestion of seafood contaminated with *V. vulnificus* and sepsis and cutaneous bullae may be present within 36 hours of the onset of symptoms.

Because the case fatality rate for *V. vulnificus* septicemia exceeds 50% in immunocompromised individuals or those with preexisting liver disease, these individuals should be informed about the health hazards of ingesting raw or undercooked seafood (especially oysters), the need to avoid contact with seawater during the warm months, and the importance of using protective clothing (e.g., gloves) when handling shellfish. *V. vulnificus* infection should be considered in the differential diagnosis of fever of unknown etiology, and individuals who present with fever (especially when bullae, cellulitis, or wound infection is present) and who have preexisting liver disease or are immunocompromised should be questioned regarding a history of raw oyster ingestion or seawater contact. While optimum anti-infective therapy for the treatment of *V. vulnificus* infections has not been identified, use of a tetracycline or third generation cephalosporin (e.g., cefotaxime, ceftazidime) is recommended. Because the high fatality rate associated with *V. vulnificus* infections, anti-infective therapy should be initiated promptly if indicated.

Empiric Therapy in Febrile Neutropenic Patients

Ceftazidime has been effective when used alone or in conjunction with other anti-infectives for empiric anti-infective therapy of presumed bacterial infections in febrile granulocytopenic adults or children†.

Results of several studies in febrile granulocytopenic patients indicate that ceftazidime used alone may be as effective as combination regimens that include ceftazidime and an aminoglycoside (e.g., amikacin, gentamicin, tobramycin) or combination regimens that include some other β-lactam antibiotic (e.g., cefepime, ceftriaxone, piperacillin) and an aminoglycoside for empiric therapy in these patients. Results of a randomized study in adults indicate that ceftazidime monotherapy (2 g IV every 8 hours) is as effective as meropenem monotherapy (1 g IV every 8 hours) for empiric anti-infective therapy in febrile neutropenic patients; at the end of therapy, a satisfactory response was obtained in 49 or 46% of those receiving ceftazidime or meropenem, respectively. Because gram-positive bacteria are being reported with increasing frequency in febrile granulocytopenic patients and because ceftazidime is less active against these organisms than many other cephalosporins and β-lactam antibiotics, some clinicians suggest that an anti-infective agent active against staphylococci (e.g., vancomycin) probably should be used concomitantly if ceftazidime is used for empiric therapy in these patients. However, unlike ceftazidime, other anti-infectives used for empiric therapy (e.g., cefepime, imipenem, meropenem) have good activity against viridans streptococci and *S. pneumoniae*.

Successful treatment of infections in granulocytopenic patients requires prompt initiation of empiric anti-infective therapy (even when fever is the only sign or symptom of infection) and appropriate modification of the initial regimen if the duration of fever and neutropenia is protracted, if a specific site of infection is identified, or if organisms resistant to the initial regimen are present. The initial empiric regimen should be chosen based on the underlying disease and other host factors that may affect the degree of risk; local epidemiologic data regarding the type, frequency of occurrence, and in vitro susceptibility of bacterial isolates recovered from other patients in the same health-care facility; and the individual patient's pattern of colonization and resistance. No empiric regimen has been identified that would be appropriate for initial treatment of all febrile neutropenic patients. Regardless of the initial regimen selected, patients should be reassessed daily and the anti-infective regimen altered (if indicated) based on the presence or absence of fever, identification of the causative organism, and the clinical condition of the patient.

The fact that gram-positive bacteria have become a predominant pathogen in febrile neutropenic patients should be considered when selecting an empiric anti-infective regimen. The IDSA states that ceftazidime is no longer a reliable agent for empiric monotherapy in febrile neutropenic patients because of decreasing potency against gram-negative bacteria and poor activity against many gram-positive bacteria (e.g., streptococci).

Published protocols for the treatment of infections in febrile neutropenic patients should be consulted for specific recommendations regarding selection of the initial empiric anti-infective regimen, when to change the initial regimen, possible subsequent regimens, and duration of therapy in these patients. In addition, consultation with an infectious disease expert knowledgeable about infections in immunocompromised patients is advised.

Perioperative Prophylaxis

Ceftazidime has been used for perioperative prophylaxis† in patients undergoing vaginal hysterectomy, biliary or intra-abdominal surgery, or transurethral resection of the prostate; however, many clinicians state that ceftazidime should not be used prophylactically.

A first or second generation cephalosporin (cefazolin, cefoxitin, cefotetan, cefuroxime) generally is preferred when a cephalosporin is used for perioperative prophylaxis. Third generation cephalosporins (cefotaxime, ceftriaxone, ceftazidime) and fourth generation cephalosporins (cefepime) are not usually recommended for perioperative prophylaxis because they are expensive, some are less active than first or second generation cephalosporins against staphylococci, they have spectrums of activity wider than necessary for organisms encountered in elective surgery, and their use for prophylaxis may promote emergence of resistant organisms. (See Uses: Perioperative Prophylaxis, in the Cephalosporins General Statement 8:12.06.)

DOSAGE AND ADMINISTRATION

Reconstitution and Administration

Ceftazidime sodium (as commercially available formulations of ceftazidime with sodium carbonate) is administered by intermittent IV injection or infusion or by deep IM injection. Ceftazidime sodium premixed with dextrose injection is administered by continuous or intermittent IV infusion. Ceftazidime sodium also has been administered by continuous IV infusion† and has been administered intraperitoneally in dialysis solutions. *Intra-arterial injection should be avoided since distal necrosis can occur.*

The IV route usually is preferred in patients with septicemia, meningitis, peritonitis, or other severe or life-threatening infections and in patients with lowered resistance resulting from malnutrition, trauma, surgery, diabetes, heart failure, or malignancy, particularly if shock is present or impending.

If an aminoglycoside or vancomycin is administered concomitantly with ceftazidime or ceftazidime sodium, the drugs should be administered at separate sites. Reconstituted and diluted solutions of ceftazidime or ceftazidime sodium should be inspected visually for particulate matter prior to administration whenever solution and container permit.

Intermittent IV Infusion

Vials labeled as containing 500 mg, 1 g, or 2 g of ceftazidime with sodium carbonate should be reconstituted with 5.3, 10, or 10 mL, respectively, of sterile water for injection or a compatible IV solution to provide solutions containing approximately 100, 100, or 170 mg/mL, respectively. After adding the diluent to the vial, the vial should be shaken to dissolve the drug. With sodium carbonate formulations of ceftazidime, carbon dioxide is released as the drug dissolves and the solution will become clear within 1–2 minutes. The appropriate dose of the drug should then be added to a compatible IV solution. When withdrawing a dose from reconstituted vials, ensure that the syringe needle opening remains within the solution. The withdrawn solution may contain some carbon dioxide bubbles, which should be expelled from the syringe before injection.

Alternatively, TwistVial® (Fortaz®) or ADD-Vantage® (Tazicef®) vials labeled as containing 1 or 2 g of ceftazidime with sodium carbonate should be reconstituted according to the manufacturer's directions. Carbon dioxide that forms inside the package in sodium carbonate formulations of ceftazidime should be relieved by inserting a vent needle; to preserve sterility, it is important that the vent needle be inserted through the vial closure only after the drug has dissolved. The vent needle should be removed prior to use of the solution.

Alternatively, the commercially available Duplex® drug delivery system containing 1 or 2 g of ceftazidime and 50 mL of 5% dextrose injection in separate chambers should be reconstituted (activated) according to the manufacturer's directions and administered by IV infusion. If stored in the refrigerator after reconstitution (see Chemistry and Stability: Stability), the solution should be allowed to reach room temperature prior to administration.

The 6-g pharmacy bulk vial of ceftazidime as a sodium carbonate formulation should be reconstituted with sterile water for injection according to the manufacturer's directions. The pharmacy bulk vial is *not* intended for direct IV infusion.

Thawed solutions of the commercially available frozen premixed ceftazidime sodium injection in dextrose may be administered by continuous or intermittent IV infusion. The frozen injections should be thawed at room temperature (25°C) or under refrigeration (5°C); the injections should *not* be thawed by warming in a water bath or by exposure to microwave radiation. Precipitates that may have formed in the frozen injections usually will dissolve with little or no agitation when the injections reach room temperature; potency is not affected. After thawing to room temperature, the injection should be agitated and the container checked for minute leaks by firmly squeezing the bag. The injection should be discarded if container seals or outlet ports are not intact or leaks are found or if the solution is cloudy or contains an insoluble precipitate. Additives should not be introduced into the injection container. The injections should not be used in series connections with other plastic containers, since such use could result in air embolism from residual air being drawn from the primary container before administration of fluid from the secondary container is complete.

If a Y-type administration set is used, the other solution flowing through the tubing should be discontinued while ceftazidime or ceftazidime sodium is being infused.

Rate of Administration

Intermittent IV infusions of ceftazidime sodium have generally been infused over 15–30 minutes in adults, neonates, and children.

Intermittent IV Injection

For direct intermittent IV injection, vials labeled as containing 500 mg, 1 g, or 2 g of ceftazidime with sodium carbonate should be reconstituted with sterile water for injection as for initial reconstitution for IV infusion to provide solutions containing 100, 100, or 170 mg/mL, respectively. (See Reconstitution and Administration: Intermittent IV Infusion, in Dosage and Administration.) When withdrawing a dose from reconstituted vials of ceftazidime sodium, ensure that the syringe needle opening remains within the solution. Any carbon dioxide bubbles that may be present in the withdrawn solution of ceftazidime sodium should be expelled from the syringe prior to injection.

The appropriate dose of reconstituted ceftazidime sodium should be injected over a period of 3–5 minutes directly into a vein or the tubing of a compatible IV solution.

IM Injection

For IM injection, vials labeled as containing 500 mg or 1 g of ceftazidime with sodium carbonate (Fortaz®) are prepared by adding 1.5 or 3 mL of sterile or bacteriostatic water for injection or 0.5 or 1% lidocaine hydrochloride injection, respectively, to provide solutions containing approximately 280 mg/mL. When withdrawing a dose from reconstituted vials of ceftazidime sodium, ensure that the syringe needle opening remains within the solution. Any carbon dioxide bubbles that may be present in the withdrawn solution of ceftazidime sodium should be expelled from the syringe prior to injection.

IM injections should be made deeply into a large muscle mass, such as the upper outer quadrant of the gluteus maximus or lateral part of the thigh, using usual techniques and precautions.

Intraperitoneal Instillation

For intraperitoneal instillation, a sodium carbonate formulation of ceftazidime powder for injection can be reconstituted with sterile water for injection as for initial reconstitution for IV infusion. (See Reconstitution and Administration: Intermittent IV Infusion, in Dosage and Administration.) The manufacturers of the sodium carbonate formulations of ceftazidime recommend that the drug then be further diluted in a compatible peritoneal dialysis solution to provide a solution containing 250 mg of ceftazidime in each 2 L of dialysis solution.

● Dosage

Following reconstitution of the commercially available powders for injection containing a mixture of ceftazidime (as the pentahydrate) and sodium carbonate, solutions contain ceftazidime sodium; dosage of the drug is expressed in terms of anhydrous ceftazidime.

To avoid unintentional overdosage, the commercially available Duplex® drug delivery system containing ceftazidime and dextrose injection should *not* be used in patients who require less than the entire 1- or 2-g dose in the container.

Adult Dosage

General Adult Dosage

The usual adult dosage of ceftazidime for the treatment of less severe infections caused by susceptible organisms is 1 g given IV or IM every 8 or 12 hours; however, the dosage and route of administration should be determined by the susceptibility of the causative organism, the severity of the infection, and the condition and renal function of the patient. For severe or life-threatening infections, especially in immunocompromised patients, a dosage of 2 g every 8 hours is recommended.

The maximum adult dosage of ceftazidime recommended by the manufacturers is 6 g daily.

Bone and Joint Infections

For the treatment of bone and joint infections, the usual adult dosage is 2 g IV every 12 hours.

Intra-abdominal and Gynecologic Infections

For the treatment of serious gynecologic and intra-abdominal infections, the usual adult dosage of ceftazidime is 2 g IV every 8 hours.

Meningitis

For the treatment of meningitis, the usual dosage of ceftazidime is 2 g IV every 8 hours. Because of a high rate of relapse, anti-infective therapy in patients with meningitis caused by gram-negative bacilli generally should be continued for at least 3 weeks.

Respiratory Tract Infections

The usual adult dosage of the drug for the treatment of uncomplicated pneumonia is 0.5–1 g IV or IM every 8 hours.

Skin and Skin Structure Infections

The usual adult dosage of the drug for the treatment of mild skin and skin structure infections is 0.5–1 g IV or IM every 8 hours.

Urinary Tract Infections

The manufacturers recommend that adults with uncomplicated urinary tract infections receive 250 mg of ceftazidime IV or IM every 12 hours and that adults with complicated urinary tract infections receive 500 mg IV or IM every 8 or 12 hours.

Pseudomonas aeruginosa Infections

For the treatment of pulmonary infections caused by *Pseudomonas aeruginosa* in patients with cystic fibrosis and normal renal function, the usual dosage of ceftazidime is 30–50 mg/kg given IV every 8 hours up to a maximum dosage of 6 g daily. Clinical improvement may occur, but bacteriologic cures should not be expected in patients with chronic respiratory disease and cystic fibrosis.

Burkholderia Infections

For the treatment of melioidosis† caused by *Burkholderia pseudomallei*, the US Army Medical Research Institute of Infectious Diseases (USAMRIID) recommends a ceftazidime dosage of 40 mg/kg every 8 hours. Other clinicians recommend a ceftazidime dosage of 2 g IV every 8 hours (up to 6 g daily) or 50 mg/kg (up to 2 g) IV every 6 hours. Concomitant co-trimoxazole (6–8 mg/kg of trimethoprim daily in 4 divided doses) or doxycycline (100 mg IV twice daily) may be indicated in septicemic or other severe cases. The initial parenteral regimen should be continued for at least 10–14 days and until there is clinical improvement. Although the median time to fever resolution is 9 days, some patients may remain febrile for prolonged periods despite appropriate antimicrobial therapy. When appropriate, treatment may be changed to an oral maintenance regimen (e.g., oral co-trimoxazole with or without oral doxycycline) and continued for at least 3–6 months to prevent recrudence or relapse. More prolonged oral maintenance therapy (up to 12 months) may be necessary, depending on the response to therapy and severity of initial illness.

Although only limited experience is available regarding the treatment of human cases of glanders†, some clinicians suggest that the regimens recommended for the treatment of severe melioidosis also can be used for the treatment of glanders.

Empiric Therapy in Febrile Neutropenic Patients

If ceftazidime is used for empiric anti-infective therapy in febrile neutropenic patients† (see Uses: Empiric Therapy in Febrile Neutropenic Patients), the usual dosage of the drug is 100 mg/kg daily given IV in 3 divided doses or 2 g IV every 8 hours either alone or in conjunction with an aminoglycoside (amikacin, gentamicin, tobramycin).

Pediatric Dosage

Children 12 years of age and older may receive the usual adult dosage of ceftazidime.

General Dosage for Neonates

The usual dosage of ceftazidime recommended by the manufacturers for neonates up to 4 weeks of age is 30 mg/kg IV every 12 hours.

The American Academy of Pediatrics (AAP) recommends that neonates 7 days of age or younger receive 50 mg/kg of ceftazidime every 12 hours, regardless of weight. For neonates 8–28 days of age, the AAP recommends a dosage of 50 mg every 8–12 hours for those weighing 2 kg or less and 50 mg/kg every 8 hours for those weighing more than 2 kg.

General Dosage for Infants and Children

The usual dosage of ceftazidime for children 1 month to 12 years of age is 25–50 mg/kg IV every 8 hours, depending on the type and severity of infection. The manufacturers state that the maximum ceftazidime dosage for children 1 month to 12 years of age is 6 g daily, and that the higher dosage (i.e., 50 mg/kg every 8 hours) should be used in immunocompromised children or children with cystic fibrosis or meningitis.

The AAP recommends that children beyond the neonatal period receive ceftazidime in a dosage of 90–150 mg/kg daily in 3 equally divided doses for the treatment of mild to moderate infections or 200–300 mg/kg daily in 3 equally divided doses for the treatment of severe infections.

Meningitis

For the treatment of meningitis, some clinicians recommend a ceftazidime dosage of 100–150 mg/kg daily in 2 or 3 equally divided doses for neonates 7 days of age or younger and 150 mg/kg daily in 3 divided doses in older neonates and children. Because of a high rate of relapse, anti-infective therapy in patients with meningitis caused by gram-negative bacilli generally should be continued for at least 3 weeks. For treatment of meningitis in neonates, some clinicians recommend that anti-infective treatment be continued for 2 weeks beyond the first sterile CSF culture or at least 3 weeks, whichever is longer.

Burkholderia Infections

For the treatment of melioidosis† caused by B. pseudomallei, some clinicians recommend a ceftazidime dosage of 60 mg/kg daily given IV in 2 equally divided doses in children younger than 2 months of age or 100 mg/kg daily given IV in 3 equally divided doses in children 2 months of age or older. Concomitant co-trimoxazole (6–8 mg/kg of trimethoprim daily) or doxycycline may be indicated in septicemic or other severe cases. The initial parenteral regimen should be continued for at least 10–14 days and until there is clinical improvement. When appropriate, treatment may be changed to an oral maintenance regimen (e.g., oral co-trimoxazole with or without oral doxycycline) and continued for at least 3–6 months to prevent recrudence or relapse. More prolonged oral maintenance therapy (up to 12 months) may be necessary, depending on the response to therapy and severity of initial illness.

Empiric Therapy in Febrile Neutropenic Patients

For empiric anti-infective therapy in febrile neutropenic patients†, pediatric patients 2 years of age or older have received ceftazidime in a dosage of 50 mg/kg (maximum 2 g) every 8 hours. (See Uses: Empiric Therapy in Febrile Neutropenic Patients.)

Duration of Therapy

The duration of ceftazidime therapy depends on the type and severity of infection and should be determined by the clinical and bacteriologic response of the patient. For most infections, therapy generally should be continued for at least 48 hours after the patient becomes asymptomatic or evidence of eradication of the infection has been obtained. Complicated infections may require more prolonged therapy.

● Dosage in Renal and Hepatic Impairment

In patients with renal impairment, doses and/or frequency of administration of ceftazidime should be modified in response to the degree of renal impairment, severity of the infection, and susceptibility of the causative organism. Excessive dosage and elevated plasma concentrations of the drug in patients with renal impairment can precipitate serious neurotoxicity (e.g., seizures, encephalopathy, coma, asterixis, neuromuscular excitability, myoclonia).

The manufacturers recommend that adults with creatinine clearances of 50 mL/minute or less receive an initial loading dose of 1 g of ceftazidime and a maintenance dosage based on the patient's creatinine clearance. (See Table 1.)

TABLE 1. Maintenance Dosage for Adults with Renal Impairment

Creatinine Clearance (mL/minute)	Dosage
31–50	1 g every 12 h
16–30	1 g every 24 h
6–15	500 mg every 24 h
<5	500 mg every 48 h

In patients with renal impairment and severe infections who would generally receive a ceftazidime dosage of 6 g daily if their renal function were normal, the manufacturers state that doses in the above table may be increased by 50% or the dosing frequency may be increased appropriately.

Alternatively, some clinicians recommend that adults with creatinine clearances of 30–80 mL/minute receive the usual doses of ceftazidime every 12–24 hours, adults with creatinine clearances of 10–29 mL/minute receive the usual doses every 24–36 hours, and adults with creatinine clearances less than 10 mL/minute receive the usual doses every 36–48 hours.

Because ceftazidime is removed by hemodialysis, a supplemental dose of the drug is generally indicated after each dialysis period. The manufacturers recommend that adults undergoing hemodialysis receive an initial 1-g loading dose of ceftazidime followed by a 1-g dose after each dialysis period.

In adults undergoing intraperitoneal dialysis or continuous ambulatory peritoneal dialysis, the manufacturers recommend that an initial 1-g loading dose of ceftazidime be given followed by a 500-mg dose every 24 hours. Some clinicians recommend that patients undergoing peritoneal dialysis receive 500 mg of ceftazidime every 24 hours and a supplemental 500-mg dose of the drug at the end of each dialysis period. If ceftazidime (as a sodium carbonate formulation) is administered intraperitoneally in the dialysis solution, the manufacturers recommend that 250 mg of the drug be added to each 2 L of dialysis solution.

In children with impaired renal function, the frequency of dosing should be decreased based on the degree of impairment.

Modification of the usual dosage of ceftazidime is generally unnecessary in patients with impaired hepatic function, unless renal function is also impaired.

CAUTIONS

Adverse effects reported with ceftazidime are similar to those reported with other cephalosporins. For information on adverse effects reported with cephalosporins, see Cautions in the Cephalosporins General Statement and other monographs in 8:12.06. Ceftazidime is generally well tolerated; adverse effects have been reported in about 9% of patients receiving the drug and have required discontinuance in about 2% of patients.

● Hematologic Effects

Eosinophilia has generally been reported in less than 7% of patients receiving ceftazidime. Thrombocytosis has occurred in about 2% of patients receiving the drug. Transient leukopenia, neutropenia, thrombocytopenia, agranulocytosis, and lymphocytosis have been reported rarely.

Positive direct antiglobulin (Coombs') test results have occurred in about 5% of patients receiving ceftazidime. In most reported cases, there was no clinical or laboratory evidence of hemolysis. However, hemolytic anemia has been reported rarely. In one patient with a positive direct antiglobulin test, mild hemolytic anemia occurred; the serum of this patient reacted with ceftazidime-treated erythrocytes, but did not react with untreated erythrocytes.

Cephalosporins have been reported to cause hypothrombinemia. Patients with renal or hepatic impairment, poor nutritional status, or those receiving a protracted course of anti-infective therapy are at particular risk of cephalosporin-induced hypothrombinemia. Prothrombin time should be monitored and vitamin K administered as indicated in patients who are at risk of developing hypothrombinemia.

● GI Effects

Adverse GI effects, including diarrhea, nausea, vomiting, abdominal pain, and a metallic taste, have been reported in less than 2% of patients receiving ceftazidime.

Clostridium difficile-associated Diarrhea and Colitis

Treatment with anti-infectives alters the normal flora of the colon and may permit overgrowth of *Clostridium difficile*.

C. difficile infection (CDI) and *C. difficile*-associated diarrhea and colitis (CDAD; also known as antibiotic-associated diarrhea and colitis or pseudomembranous colitis) have been reported with nearly all anti-infectives, including ceftazidime, and may range in severity from mild diarrhea to fatal colitis. *C. difficile* produces toxins A and B which contribute to the development of CDAD; hypertoxin-producing strains cause increased morbidity and mortality since these infections may be refractory to anti-infective therapy and may require colectomy.

CDAD should be considered in the differential diagnosis in patients who develop diarrhea during or after anti-infective therapy and managed accordingly. Careful medical history is necessary since CDAD has been reported to occur as late as 2 months or longer after anti-infective therapy is discontinued.

If CDAD is suspected or confirmed, anti-infectives not directed against *C. difficile* should be discontinued whenever possible. Patients should be managed with appropriate supportive therapy (e.g., fluid and electrolyte management, protein supplementation), anti-infective therapy directed against *C. difficile* (e.g., metronidazole, vancomycin), and surgical evaluation as clinically indicated.

● Dermatologic and Sensitivity Reactions

Hypersensitivity reactions have been reported in 1–3% of patients receiving ceftazidime and include pruritus, rash (maculopapular or erythematous), urticaria, photosensitivity, angioedema, and fever.

Immediate hypersensitivity reactions, including anaphylaxis (manifested as bronchospasm and/or hypotension), have occurred rarely with ceftazidime. Toxic epidermal necrolysis, Stevens-Johnson syndrome, and erythema multiforme have been reported with cephalosporins, including ceftazidime.

The manufacturer of the commercially available Duplex® drug delivery system containing ceftazidime and 5% dextrose injection cautions that hypersensitivity reactions, including anaphylaxis, have been reported with administration of dextrose-containing solutions. These reactions have been reported in patients receiving high concentrations of dextrose (i.e., 50% dextrose) and also have been reported when corn-derived dextrose solutions were administered to patients with or without a history of hypersensitivity to corn products.

If a hypersensitivity reaction occurs during ceftazidime therapy, the drug should be discontinued. Severe acute hypersensitivity reactions should be treated with appropriate therapy (e.g., epinephrine, oxygen, antihistamines, corticosteroids, IV fluids, vasopressors, airway management) as indicated.

● Hepatic Effects

Transient increases in serum concentrations of AST (SGOT), ALT (SGPT), alkaline phosphatase, LDH, and/or γ-glutamyltransferase (γ-glutamyl transpeptidase, GGT, GGTP) have been reported in 3–9% of patients receiving ceftazidime. Increased serum concentrations of bilirubin have occurred in less than 1% of patients receiving the drug. Jaundice has been reported with ceftazidime.

● Renal Effects

Transient increases in BUN and/or serum creatinine concentrations have been reported in less than 2% of patients receiving ceftazidime.

A transient, mild to moderate decrease in glomerular filtration rate has occurred in a few patients receiving ceftazidime. Although excretion of thermophilic aminopeptidase (alanine aminopeptidase), an enzyme originating from renal proximal tubular cells, was increased slightly in some of these patients, serum creatinine and urinary β_2-microglobulin concentrations were generally unaffected, suggesting that ceftazidime did not adversely affect proximal tubular cells. In healthy adults who received 6 g of ceftazidime daily for 3 days, urinary excretion of thermophilic aminopeptidase was unaffected by the drug. It has been suggested that ceftazidime's potential to slightly decrease glomerular filtration rate may be clinically important in patients with preexisting renal impairment if adequate dosage adjustments are not made in these patients. (See Dosage and Administration: Dosage in Renal and Hepatic Impairment.)

Renal failure has been reported in a few patients receiving ceftazidime; however, a causal relationship to the drug has not been established. Like cephaloridine (a cephalosporin known to be nephrotoxic; no longer commercially available in the US), ceftazidime contains a methylpyridinium at position 3 of the cephalosporin nucleus; however, there is no evidence to date that this group is associated with nephrotoxicity, and the manufacturers state that ceftazidime has not been shown to be nephrotoxic. Nephrotoxicity of cephaloridine apparently results from accumulation of the drug in renal proximal tubular cells; there is no evidence to date that ceftazidime accumulates in renal tubular cells.

● Nervous System Effects

Coma, encephalopathy, asterixis, hallucinations, neuromuscular excitability, and myoclonia have been reported in patients with renal impairment who received usual dosages of ceftazidime.

● Local Effects

Adverse local reactions, including phlebitis and pain or inflammation at the injection site, have been reported in less than 3% of patients receiving ceftazidime. Following IM injection of the drug, pain at the injection site is reportedly mild to moderate for about 2–5 minutes and subsides within 10–20 minutes.

Distal necrosis can occur after inadvertent intra-arterial administration of ceftazidime.

● Other Adverse Effects

Other adverse effects that have been reported in less than 1% of patients receiving ceftazidime include candidiasis (e.g., oral thrush) and vaginitis.

● Precautions and Contraindications

Ceftazidime shares the toxic potentials of the cephalosporins, and the usual precautions of cephalosporin therapy should be observed. Prior to initiation of therapy with ceftazidime, careful inquiry should be made concerning previous hypersensitivity reactions to cephalosporins, penicillins, or other drugs. There is clinical and laboratory evidence of partial cross-allergenicity among cephalosporins and other β-lactam antibiotics including penicillins and cephamycins. Ceftazidime is contraindicated in patients who are hypersensitive to any cephalosporin and should be used with caution in patients with a history of hypersensitivity reactions to penicillins. Use of cephalosporins should be avoided in patients who have had an immediate-type (anaphylactic) hypersensitivity reaction to penicillins.

To reduce development of drug-resistant bacteria and maintain effectiveness of ceftazidime and other antibacterials, the drug should be used only for the treatment or prevention of infections proven or strongly suspected to be caused by susceptible bacteria. When selecting or modifying anti-infective therapy, results of culture and in vitro susceptibility testing should be used. In the absence of such data, local epidemiology and susceptibility patterns should be considered when selecting anti-infectives for empiric therapy should be considered.

Patients should be advised that antibacterials (including ceftazidime) should only be used to treat bacterial infections and not used to treat viral infections (e.g., the common cold). Patients also should be advised about the importance of completing the full course of therapy, even if feeling better after a few days, and that skipping doses or not completing therapy may decrease effectiveness and increase the likelihood that bacteria will develop resistance and will not be treatable with ceftazidime or other antibacterials in the future.

Like other dextrose-containing solutions, the commercially available Duplex® drug delivery system containing ceftazidime and 5% dextrose injection should be used with caution in patients with overt or known subclinical diabetes mellitus or in patients with carbohydrate intolerance for any reason.

Use of ceftazidime may result in overgrowth of nonsusceptible organisms, especially *Candida*, *Staphylococcus aureus*, enterococci, *Enterobacter*, or *Pseudomonas*. Resistant strains of *Ps. aeruginosa* and *Enterobacter* have developed during therapy with ceftazidime. (See Resistance.) Careful observation of the patient during ceftazidime therapy is essential. If superinfection or suprainfection occurs, appropriate therapy should be instituted.

Because CDAD has been reported with the use of ceftazidime and other cephalosporins, it should be considered in the differential diagnosis of patients who develop diarrhea during or after ceftazidime therapy. (See Cautions: GI Effects.) Patients should be advised that diarrhea is a common problem caused by anti-infectives and usually ends when the drug is discontinued; however, they should contact a clinician if watery and bloody stools (with or without stomach cramps and fever) occur during or as late as 2 months or longer after the last dose. Ceftazidime should be used with caution in patients with a history of GI disease, especially colitis.

As with other extended-spectrum β-lactams, resistance to ceftazidime in some gram-negative bacteria (e.g., *Enterobacter*, *Pseudomonas*) can develop during therapy, leading to clinical failure in some cases. When ceftazidime is used to treat infections caused by these gram-negative bacteria, periodic susceptibility testing should be performed when clinically appropriate. If patients fail to respond to ceftazidime monotherapy, adding an aminoglycoside or similar agent to the regimen should be considered.

High and prolonged serum ceftazidime concentrations may occur if usual dosages of the drug are used in patients with transient or persistent reduction in urinary output because of renal insufficiency. Doses and/or frequency of administration of ceftazidime should be decreased in patients with transient or persistent renal impairment. (See Dosage and Administration: Dosage in Renal and Hepatic Impairment.) Increased serum ceftazidime concentrations can result in serious adverse nervous system effects (e.g., seizures, encephalopathy, coma, asterixis, neuromuscular excitability, myoclonia). (See Cautions: Nervous System Effects.) Continued dosage should be determined by degree of renal impairment, severity of infection, and susceptibility of the causative organisms.

• Geriatric Precautions

Clinical studies of ceftazidime did not include sufficient numbers of patients 65 years of age or older to determine whether geriatric patients respond differently than younger patients. Of the 2221 adults who received ceftazidime in clinical studies, 37% were 65 years of age or older, while 18% were 75 years of age or older. Although no overall differences in efficacy or safety were observed between geriatric and younger patients and other clinical experience revealed no age-related differences, the possibility that some older patients may exhibit increased sensitivity to the drug cannot be ruled out.

Ceftazidime is known to be substantially excreted by the kidney, and the risk of ceftazidime-induced toxicity may be greater in patients with renal impairment. Because geriatric patients may have decreased renal function, initial dosage should be selected carefully and it may be useful to monitor renal function. (See Dosage and Administration: Dosage in Renal and Hepatic Impairment.)

• Mutagenicity and Carcinogenicity

In vitro studies using microbial (i.e., Ames test) or mammalian cell (i.e., mouse micronucleus) systems have not shown ceftazidime to be mutagenic. Studies have not been performed to date to evaluate the carcinogenic potential of ceftazidime.

• Pregnancy, Fertility, and Lactation
Pregnancy

Safe use of ceftazidime during pregnancy has not been definitely established. Reproduction studies in mice and rats using ceftazidime dosages up to 40 times the usual human dosage have not revealed evidence of harm to the fetus. There are no adequate or controlled studies using ceftazidime in pregnant women, and the drug should be used during pregnancy only when clearly needed.

Fertility

Reproduction studies in mice and rats using ceftazidime dosages up to 40 times the usual human dosage have not revealed evidence of impaired fertility.

Lactation

Because ceftazidime is distributed into milk, sodium carbonate formulations of the drug should be used with caution in nursing women.

DRUG INTERACTIONS

• Probenecid

Concomitant administration of 2 g of oral probenecid does not affect the pharmacokinetics of ceftazidime, presumably because ceftazidime is excreted principally by glomerular filtration.

• Anti-infective Agents
Aminoglycosides

In vitro studies indicate that the antibacterial activity of ceftazidime and an aminoglycoside may be additive or synergistic against some strains of Enterobacteriaceae and *Pseudomonas aeruginosa*. Organisms with high-level resistance to both ceftazidime and the aminoglycoside alone are unlikely to be synergistically inhibited by concomitant use of the drugs.

Concomitant use of aminoglycosides and certain cephalosporins reportedly may increase the risk of nephrotoxicity during therapy. Although this effect has not been reported to date with ceftazidime, the manufacturers suggest that renal function be carefully monitored when an aminoglycoside is used concomitantly with ceftazidime, especially if high aminoglycoside dosage is used or if therapy is prolonged.

β-Lactam Antibiotics

Although a synergistic or partially synergistic effect has occurred in vitro against a few strains of *Ps. aeruginosa* when ceftazidime and carbenicillin, cefsulodin, mezlocillin, or piperacillin were used concomitantly, use of ceftazidime and another cephalosporin or an extended-spectrum penicillin has generally resulted in an effect that was only slightly additive or indifferent against *Ps. aeruginosa*. In addition, the combination of ceftazidime and cefoxitin has been antagonistic in vitro against *Ps. aeruginosa*.

The clinical importance is unclear, but concomitant use of ceftazidime and ampicillin in vitro has resulted in antagonism against group B streptococci and *Listeria monocytogenes*.

Quinolones

Although the clinical importance is unclear, in vitro studies indicate that the combination of ceftazidime and ciprofloxacin exerts a synergistic effect against *Burkholderia cepacia*. In an in vitro study using *B. cepacia* isolates from patients with cystic fibrosis, the combination of ceftazidime and ciprofloxacin resulted in increased killing activity against most isolates (except ciprofloxacin-resistant strains). While a 3-drug combination (ceftazidime, ciprofloxacin, and tobramycin or rifampin) resulted in increased killing activity against *B. cepacia* isolates compared with ceftazidime alone, this effect was not substantially greater than that attained with the 2-drug combination of ceftazidime and ciprofloxacin.

Other Anti-infectives

In vitro, the combination of ceftazidime and clindamycin has been reported to be neither synergistic nor antagonistic against *Bacteroides fragilis*.

In vitro results indicate that the combination of ceftazidime and metronidazole may be at least partially synergistic against *Clostridium*, but results against *B. fragilis* are conflicting.

Chloramphenicol has been reported to antagonize the bactericidal activity of β-lactam antibiotics including ceftazidime, in vitro, and the possibility of in vivo antagonism should be considered. Therefore, the manufacturers recommend that combined therapy with chloramphenicol and ceftazidime be avoided, particularly when bactericidal activity is considered important.

● **Clavulanic Acid**

In vitro studies indicate that the combination of ceftazidime and clavulanic acid, a β-lactamase inhibitor, is synergistic against some strains of *B. fragilis* resistant to ceftazidime alone. The combination was not effective against other *Bacteroides*, such as *B. distasonis*, that are not β-lactamase producers. In vitro studies indicate that the combination of ceftazidime and chloramphenicol may be antagonistic against some organisms.

● **Diuretics**

Although concomitant use of cephalosporins and potent diuretics (e.g., furosemide) reportedly may adversely affect renal function, this effect apparently did not occur when furosemide was used concomitantly with ceftazidime in a few patients.

LABORATORY TEST INTERFERENCES

● **Immunohematology Tests**

Positive direct antiglobulin (Coombs') test results have been reported in patients receiving ceftazidime. This reaction may interfere with hematologic studies or transfusion cross-matching procedures.

● **Tests for Glucose**

Like most cephalosporins, ceftazidime interferes with urinary glucose determinations using cupric sulfate (e.g., Benedict's solution, Fehling's solution, Clinitest®). Urinary glucose determinations using glucose oxidase methods (e.g., Clinistix®) are unaffected by the drug. In addition, ceftazidime does not interfere with glucose oxidase or hexokinase methods used to determine serum glucose concentrations.

● **Tests for Creatinine**

Ceftazidime does not appear to interfere with manual or automated methods used to determine serum or urinary creatinine concentrations, including those using the Jaffé reaction.

ACUTE TOXICITY

Limited information is available on the acute toxicity of ceftazidime. Inappropriately large doses of parenteral cephalosporins may cause seizures, especially in patients with renal impairment. Overdosage of ceftazidime in patients with renal failure has produced seizures, encephalopathy, coma, asterixis, neuromuscular excitability, and myoclonia. The drug should be discontinued promptly if seizures occur; anticonvulsant therapy may be administered if indicated. If acute overdosage of ceftazidime occurs, hemodialysis or peritoneal dialysis may be used to enhance elimination of the drug.

MECHANISM OF ACTION

Ceftazidime usually is bactericidal in action. Like other cephalosporins, the antibacterial activity of the drug results from inhibition of mucopeptide synthesis in the bacterial cell wall. For information on the mechanism of action of cephalosporins, see Mechanism of Action in the Cephalosporins General Statement 8:12.06.

Studies evaluating the binding of ceftazidime to penicillin-binding proteins (PBPs), the target enzymes of β-lactam antibiotics, indicate that ceftazidime binds principally to PBP 3 of *Escherichia coli* and *Pseudomonas aeruginosa*. The drug also has some affinity for PBP 1a of these organisms, but has little affinity for PBPs 2, 4, 5, and 6. Ceftazidime binds less well than cefuroxime to PBPs 1, 2, and 3 of *Staphylococcus aureus*.

SPECTRUM

Based on its spectrum of activity, ceftazidime is classified as a third generation cephalosporin. For information on the classification of cephalosporins and closely related β-lactam antibiotics based on spectra of activity, see Spectrum in the Cephalosporins General Statement 8:12.06.

Like other currently available parenteral third generation cephalosporins (e.g., cefotaxime, ceftriaxone), ceftazidime generally is less active in vitro against susceptible staphylococci than first generation cephalosporins but has an expanded spectrum of activity against gram-negative bacteria compared with first and second generation cephalosporins. The spectrum of activity of ceftazidime resembles that of cefotaxime and ceftriaxone; however, ceftazidime is more active in vitro on a weight basis against *Pseudomonas* than most other currently available parenteral third generation cephalosporins, but less active in vitro on a weight basis against anaerobes and gram-positive aerobic cocci than these drugs.

● **In Vitro Susceptibility Testing**

Results of in vitro susceptibility tests with ceftazidime for some Enterobacteriaceae, *Pseudomonas aeruginosa*, and *Bacteroides* may be affected by the size of the inoculum. For most organisms there is generally little difference in MICs of ceftazidime when the size of the inoculum is increased from 10^3 to 10^5 colony-forming units (CFU) per mL, but MICs of some organisms (e.g., *Citrobacter freundii*, *Enterobacter*, *Morganella morganii*, *Proteus*, *Ps. aeruginosa*) may be 8–128 times greater when the size of the inoculum is increased from 10^5 to 10^7 CFU/mL. Results of ceftazidime susceptibility tests are generally unaffected by culture media, pH, or presence of serum.

Strains of staphylococci resistant to penicillinase-resistant penicillins (oxacillin-resistant [methicillin-resistant] staphylococci) should be considered resistant to ceftazidime, although results of in vitro susceptibility tests may indicate that the organisms are susceptible to the drug.

For information on interpreting results of in vitro susceptibility testing (disk susceptibility tests, dilution susceptibility tests) when ceftazidime susceptibility testing is performed according to the standards of the Clinical and Laboratory Standards Institute (CLSI; formerly National Committee for Clinical Laboratory Standards [NCCLS]), see Spectrum: In Vitro Susceptibility Testing, in the Cephalosporins General Statement 8:12.06.

● **Gram-positive Aerobic Bacteria**

Ceftazidime generally is active in vitro against the following gram-positive aerobic cocci: penicillinase-producing and nonpenicillinase-producing strains of *Staphylococcus aureus* and *S. epidermidis*, *Streptococcus pneumoniae*, *S. pyogenes* (group A β-hemolytic streptococci), *S. agalactiae* (group B streptococci), and viridans streptococci. However, in vitro on a weight basis, ceftazidime is slightly less active than most other currently available third generation cephalosporins against these gram-positive bacteria.

Staphylococci resistant to penicillinase-resistant penicillins are resistant to ceftazidime. *Listeria monocytogenes* and enterococci, including *E. faecalis* (formerly *S. faecalis*), also are generally resistant to the drug.

The MIC_{90} (minimum inhibitory concentration of the drug at which 90% of strains tested are inhibited) of ceftazidime for penicillinase-producing and nonpenicillinase-producing *S. aureus* is 8–25 mcg/mL. Although the MIC_{50} of ceftazidime reported for *S. epidermidis* is 8–16 mcg/mL, the MIC_{90} of the drug for *S. epidermidis* or *S. saprophyticus* usually is 8–50 mcg/mL. The MIC_{90} of ceftazidime for group A β-hemolytic streptococci or group B streptococci is 0.06–2 mcg/mL. The MIC_{90} of the drug reported for *Streptococcus pneumoniae* is 0.13–4 mcg/mL, and the MIC_{90} reported for viridans streptococci is 3.1–8 mcg/mL. In one study, the MIC_{50} and MIC_{90} of ceftazidime for the *S. milleri* group of viridans streptococci (*S. anginosus*, *S. constellatus*, *S. intermedius*) were 4 and 8 mcg/mL, respectively.

● **Gram-negative Aerobic Bacteria**

Neisseria

Ceftazidime is active in vitro against *Neisseria meningitidis* and most strains of penicillinase-producing and nonpenicillinase-producing *Neisseria gonorrhoeae*. Ceftazidime concentrations of 0.001–0.06 mcg/mL generally inhibit *N. meningitidis*. The MIC_{90} of ceftazidime is 0.02–0.25 mcg/mL for nonpenicillinase-producing *N. gonorrhoeae* and 0.001–0.03 mcg/mL for penicillinase-producing strains of the organism.

Haemophilus

Ceftazidime is active in vitro against most β-lactamase-producing and non-β-lactamase-producing strains of *Haemophilus influenzae*, *H. parainfluenzae*, and *H. ducreyi*. The MIC_{90} of the drug reported for *H. influenzae* is 0.1–1 mcg/mL. In one study, the MIC_{90} of ceftazidime for *H. ducreyi* was 0.13 mcg/mL.

Enterobacteriaceae

Generally, ceftazidime is active in vitro against the following Enterobacteriaceae: *Citrobacter diversus, C. freundii, Enterobacter agglomerans, E. cloacae, E. aerogenes, Escherichia coli, Klebsiella oxytoca, K. pneumoniae, Morganella morganii* (formerly *Proteus morganii*), *Proteus mirabilis, P. vulgaris, Providencia rettgeri* (formerly *Proteus rettgeri*), *P. stuartii, Serratia marcescens, Salmonella, Shigella,* and *Yersinia enterocolitica.*

The MIC_{90} of ceftazidime for *E. coli, Klebsiella* (including *K. pneumoniae*), *M. morganii, Providencia,* and *S. marcescens* is 0.2–6.3 mcg/mL. The MIC_{90} of the drug for *P. mirabilis, P. vulgaris,* and *Y. enterocolitica* is 0.05–0.8 mcg/mL.

The MIC_{90} of ceftazidime reported for *C. diversus* is 0.2–1 mcg/mL. The in vitro activity of ceftazidime against *C. freundii,* however, varies considerably. In some studies the MIC_{90} of ceftazidime for *C. freundii* was 0.2–8 mcg/mL, and in other studies it was 32 mcg/mL or greater. The in vitro activity of ceftazidime against *Enterobacter* also varies considerably. The MIC_{90} of ceftazidime reported for *E. agglomerans* is 0.5–6.3 mcg/mL, and the MIC_{90} of the drug reported for *E. aerogenes* is 0.2–32 mcg/mL. In some studies the MIC_{90} of ceftazidime reported for *E. cloacae* was 0.5–12.5 mcg/mL, but in other studies it was 32–64 mcg/mL or greater.

The MIC_{90} of ceftazidime reported for *Salmonella enteritidis, S. newport,* and *S. typhi* is 0.1–6.5 mcg/mL. In one study, strains of *S. typhi* resistant to ampicillin and chloramphenicol were susceptible in vitro to ceftazidime concentrations of 0.1–0.2 mcg/mL. The MIC_{90} of ceftazidime reported for *Shigella,* including *Sh. flexneri* and *Sh. sonnei,* is 0.12–6.3 mcg/mL.

Pseudomonas

Ceftazidime is active in vitro against *Pseudomonas aeruginosa.* In vitro on a weight basis, ceftazidime is more active against *Ps. aeruginosa* than most other cephalosporins. In addition, ceftazidime is active in vitro against some strains of *Ps. aeruginosa* resistant to other third generation cephalosporins, aminoglycosides, and extended-spectrum penicillins. The MIC_{90} of ceftazidime reported for *Ps. aeruginosa* is 0.5–32 mcg/mL.

Ceftazidime is also active against *Pseudomonas* other than *Ps. aeruginosa.* The MIC_{90} of ceftazidime reported for *Ps. acidovorans, Ps. fluorescens, Ps. putida,* and *Ps. stutzeri* is 0.5–16 mcg/mL.

Burkholderia

Ceftazidime is active in vitro against some strains of *Burkholderia cepacia* (formerly *Ps. cepacia*). The MIC_{50} and MIC_{90} of ceftazidime reported for some strains of *B. cepacia* are 2–8 and 4–32 mcg/mL, respectively; however, strains of *B. cepacia* isolated from patients with cystic fibrosis generally require higher ceftazidime concentrations for in vitro inhibition than strains isolated from patients who do not have cystic fibrosis and many of these strains have MIC_{90}s of 64 mcg/mL or greater and are resistant to the drug. Although the clinical importance is unclear, in vitro studies indicate that the combination of ceftazidime and amikacin or ciprofloxacin exerts a synergistic effect against *B. cepacia.* (See Quinolones under Drug Interactions: Anti-infective Agents.)

Ceftazidime also has in vitro activity against some strains of *B. pseudomallei* (formerly *Ps. pseudomallei*). Susceptible strains of *B. pseudomallei* are inhibited in vitro by ceftazidime concentrations of 1–8 mcg/mL; other strains are resistant to the drug.

Other Gram-negative Aerobic Bacteria

Ceftazidime has some activity in vitro against *Acinetobacter.* The MIC_{90} of ceftazidime reported for *A. calcoaceticus, A. lwoffi,* and *A. baumannii* is 8–32 mcg/mL.

Moraxella catarrhalis generally is inhibited in vitro by ceftazidime concentrations of 0.06–0.13 mcg/mL. Some strains of *M. osloensis* and *M. nonliquefaciens* are inhibited in vitro by ceftazidime concentrations of 8 mcg/mL.

Ceftazidime also is active in vitro against *Eikenella corrodens* and *Pasteurella multocida.* The MIC_{90} of the drug is 16 mcg/mL for *E. corrodens* and 0.13–1.6 mcg/mL for *P. multocida.*

Campylobacter fetus subsp. *jejuni,* an organism that can be microaerophilic or anaerobic, may be inhibited in vitro by ceftazidime concentrations of 3.1–6.25 mcg/mL.

While some strains of *Alcaligenes denitrificans, A. faecalis,* and *A. xylosoxidans* may be inhibited in vitro by ceftazidime concentrations of 1–16 mcg/mL, the MIC_{90} of the drug reported for *Alcaligenes* ranges from 2 to more than 64 mcg/mL.

In vitro, some strains of *Bartonella bacilliformis* are inhibited by ceftazidime concentrations of 0.12–0.25 mcg/mL.

The MIC_{90} of ceftazidime reported for some strains of *Chryseobacterium gleum* (formerly *Flavobacterium gleum,* CDC group IIb) and *C. indologenes* (formerly *F. indologenes,* CDC group IIb) is 8 mcg/mL and the MIC_{90} reported for *Sphingobacterium multivorum* (formerly *F. multivorum*) is 32 mcg/mL. *C. meningosepticum* (formerly *F. meningosepticum*) generally are resistant to ceftazidime.

Rare strains of *Stenotrophomonas maltophilia* (formerly *Ps. maltophilia* or *Xanthomonas maltophilia*) are inhibited in vitro by ceftazidime concentrations of 4–16 mcg/mL; however, most strains require ceftazidime concentrations of 32 mcg/mL or greater for in vitro inhibition and are considered resistant to the drug. Although the clinical importance is unclear, in vitro studies indicate that the combination of ceftazidime and a quinolone (e.g., ciprofloxacin, levofloxacin, trovafloxacin) exerts a synergistic bactericidal activity against some strains of *S. maltophilia.*

● Anaerobic Bacteria

Ceftazidime is active in vitro against some gram-positive anaerobic bacteria including some strains of *Bifidobacterium, Clostridium, Eubacterium, Lactobacillus, Peptococcus, Peptostreptococcus,* and *Propionibacterium.* The MIC_{90} of ceftazidime reported for most of these gram-positive anaerobic bacteria is 4–32 mcg/mL. *C. perfringens* generally is inhibited in vitro by ceftazidime concentrations of 2–16 mcg/mL; however, *C. difficile* is resistant to the drug. The MIC_{50} of ceftazidime for *Actinomyces* is reportedly 6–8 mcg/mL, but the MIC_{90} is 48–64 mcg/mL.

Ceftazidime has little in vitro activity against gram-negative anaerobic bacteria. Although the MIC_{90} of ceftazidime reported for *Bacteroides melaninogenicus* is 4–16 mcg/mL, other *Bacteroides* (including *B. fragilis*) are generally resistant to the drug. The MIC_{50} of ceftazidime reported for *B. fragilis, B. distasonis, B. ovatus,* and *B. thetaiotaomicron* is 8–32 mcg/mL, and the MIC_{90} of the drug reported for these organisms is usually 64 mcg/mL or greater. Although the MIC_{50} of ceftazidime reported for *Fusobacterium* and *Veillonella* is 4–16 mcg/mL, the MIC_{90} of the drug for these organisms is 32 mcg/mL or greater and many strains are considered resistant to the drug.

RESISTANCE

For information on possible mechanisms of bacterial resistance to cephalosporins, see Resistance in the Cephalosporins General Statement 8:12.06.

Ceftazidime generally is stable against hydrolysis by β-lactamases classified as Richmond-Sykes types I, II, III (TEM type), IV, and V and most PSE types. The drug is hydrolyzed to some extent by chromosomally mediated β-lactamases isolated from *Bacteroides* and *Providencia.* Ceftazidime is more stable than cefotaxime against hydrolysis by β-lactamases, but as stable as or slightly less stable than cefoxitin.

Resistant strains of *Enterobacter* and *Pseudomonas* have developed during therapy with ceftazidime. Resistance to ceftazidime in some Enterobacteriaceae (e.g., *Enterobacter cloacae, Citrobacter freundii*) reportedly results from increased production of chromosomally mediated β-lactamases, nonspecific binding of PBPs, and permeability factors. In vitro studies indicate that resistance to ceftazidime in *Ps. aeruginosa, Acinetobacter,* and some strains of *Serratia* is generally related to permeability factors; however, in a few strains of *Ps. aeruginosa* that developed resistance to ceftazidime during therapy with the drug, resistance appeared to result partly from increased production of chromosomally mediated β-lactamases. *Bacteroides* are generally resistant to ceftazidime because of permeability factors and because the drug has little affinity for the PBPs of this organism.

Ceftazidime-resistant strains of *Klebsiella pneumoniae* have been reported, and these strains have been involved in nosocomial outbreaks in hospitals and chronic care facilities. Resistance in these strains results from acquisition of plasmid-mediated extended-spectrum β-lactamases (TEM- or SHV-derived extended-spectrum β-lactamases).

In vitro studies indicate that ceftazidime can induce β-lactamase production in some strains of *Enterobacter* and *Ps. aeruginosa* that possess these inducible, chromosomally mediated enzymes; however, the drug is not an efficient inducer when compared with cefoxitin.

PHARMACOKINETICS

In all studies described in the Pharmacokinetics section, ceftazidime was administered as ceftazidime sodium; dosages and concentrations of the drug are expressed in terms of ceftazidime.

● *Absorption*

Ceftazidime is not absorbed from the GI tract and must be given parenterally.

Following IM administration of a single 0.5- or 1-g dose of ceftazidime in healthy adults, peak serum concentrations of the drug are attained approximately 1 hour after the dose and average 17 or 29–39 mcg/mL, respectively. Following IM injection into the gluteus maximus or vastus lateralis, ceftazidime may be absorbed more slowly in women than in men. In women, peak serum concentrations of the drug may be lower following IM injection into the gluteus maximus than into the vastus lateralis.

Following IV infusion over 20–30 minutes of a single 0.5- or 1-g dose of ceftazidime in healthy men, peak serum concentrations of the drug at completion of the infusion average 42 or 69 mcg/mL, respectively. IV infusion over 20–30 minutes of a single 2-g dose in healthy adults results in peak serum ceftazidime concentrations at completion of the infusion that average 159–185.5 mcg/mL and serum concentrations at 0.5, 1, 2, 4, and 6 hours after completion of the infusion that average 87.9, 65.2–70.6, 38.7, 16.7–16.9, and 7.7 mcg/mL, respectively.

Following IV injection over 3–5 minutes of a single 0.5- or 1-g dose of ceftazidime in healthy men, serum concentrations of the drug at 0.25, 0.5, 1, 2, 4, 6, and 8 hours after the dose average 34.1, 24.5, 17.1, 11.2, 5.6, 2.1–2.4, and 0.9–1.3 mcg/mL, respectively, after the 0.5-g dose and 59.9–83.3, 45.3–60.9, 32.1–40.9, 22.9–23.2, 9.7, 4.4–5.3, and 1.9–3.2 mcg/mL, respectively, after the 1-g dose.

In adults with suspected gram-negative infections who received a 2-g IV loading dose of ceftazidime followed by 3 g given by continuous IV infusion over 24 hours, steady-state serum concentrations averaged 29.7 mcg/mL. Serum concentrations averaged 21.3–56.4 mcg/mL in cystic fibrosis patients 9–25 years of age who received a 7.5- or 10-mg/kg IV loading dose of ceftazidime followed by 3.4 or 4.5 mg/kg hourly given by continuous IV infusion over 24 hours.

In neonates 1–15 days of age with infections who received a single 50-mg/kg dose of ceftazidime by IM injection, serum concentrations of the drug averaged 67.2, 68.2, 42.1, 23.7, and 8.9 mcg/mL at 0.5, 1, 3, 6, and 12 hours, respectively, after the dose. In neonates and children with infections who received a single 30-mg/kg dose by IV injection, serum concentrations of ceftazidime averaged 54.1, 31.2, and 18.6 mcg/mL at 3, 6, and 9 hours, respectively, after the dose in those less than 2 months of age and 26.5, 12.3, 6.4, and 3.3 mcg/mL at 3, 5, 7, and 9 hours, respectively, after the dose in those 2–12 months of age. In neonates who received 25-mg/kg doses every 12 hours by IV injection, serum ceftazidime concentrations on the third or fourth day of therapy averaged 81.7, 70, 68, 50, 39.5, and 16.1 mcg/mL at 0.25, 0.5, 1, 3, 5, and 12 hours, respectively, after a dose.

In children 5–14 years of age with cystic fibrosis who received 35-mg/kg doses of ceftazidime every 8 hours by IV injection, serum concentrations averaged 110, 86, 50, 25.5, 8.1, 4.3, and 2.3 mcg/mL at 0.25, 0.5, 1, 2, 4, 6, and 8 hours, respectively, after the eighth dose.

In patients with end-stage chronic renal failure who received a single 1-g dose of ceftazidime via an intraperitoneal catheter, peak serum concentrations were attained 2.75 hours after the dose and averaged 44.7 mcg/mL; serum ceftazidime concentrations at 0.25, 2, and 8 hours after the dose averaged 14.2, 40, and 32 mcg/mL, respectively. Following intraperitoneal administration of a 200-mg dose of ceftazidime in 2 L of dialysis fluid in patients with end-stage chronic renal failure undergoing a 12-hour period of peritoneal dialysis (12 cycles of dialysis, each exchanging 2 L of dialysate for 15–20 minutes), serum ceftazidime concentrations averaged 1.3, 25.3, and 18.7 mcg/mL at 1, 12, and 24 hours, respectively, after the start of dialysis. Concentrations of the drug in the dialysis effluent averaged 42.2 mcg/mL.

● *Distribution*

Following IM or IV administration, ceftazidime is widely distributed into body tissues and fluids including the gallbladder, bone, bile, skeletal muscle, prostatic tissue, endometrium, myometrium, heart, skin, adipose tissue, aqueous humor, and sputum, and pleural, peritoneal, synovial, ascitic, lymphatic, and blister fluids.

The volume of distribution of ceftazidime at steady state (V_{ss}) averages 0.18–0.31 L/kg in healthy adults. In neonates 2–9 days of age, the V_{ss} of ceftazidime averaged 0.42–0.55 L/kg. In patients with cystic fibrosis, the volume of distribution of ceftazidime reportedly averages 0.15–0.19 L/kg in the central compartment and 0.17–0.27 L/kg in the peripheral compartment.

Ceftazidime generally diffuses into CSF following IV administration; however, CSF concentrations of the drug are higher in patients with inflamed meninges than in those with uninflamed meninges. CSF concentrations of ceftazidime do not appear to correlate with CSF leukocyte cell counts or CSF protein concentrations. In adults with meningitis who received 2 g of ceftazidime every 8 hours by IV infusion over 30 minutes, CSF concentrations of the drug on days 2–4 of therapy averaged 9.8 mcg/mL in samples obtained 2 hours after a dose and 9.4 mcg/mL in samples obtained 3 hours after a dose. On days 11–20 of therapy, when the meninges were presumably healed, CSF concentrations of ceftazidime averaged 4.1 and 7.2 mcg/mL in samples obtained 2 and 3 hours, respectively, after a dose. In neonates with meningitis who received IV ceftazidime in a dosage of 90–150 mg/kg daily, CSF concentrations 2–4 hours after a dose were 22–30 mcg/mL.

Ceftazidime generally is distributed into bile, but biliary concentrations of the drug following IM or IV administration may be lower than concurrent serum concentrations. In women 36–70 years of age undergoing cholecystectomy who received a single 2-g dose of ceftazidime by IV infusion over 15 minutes, ceftazidime concentrations in gallbladder bile 25–160 minutes after the dose ranged from 6.6–58 mcg/mL and concurrent serum concentrations of the drug ranged from 51.6–108 mcg/mL. In another study in patients 34–72 years of age also undergoing cholecystectomy who received a single 1-g IV dose of the drug, ceftazidime concentrations in gallbladder and bile duct bile 60 minutes following the dose averaged 3.9 mcg/mL (range: 0.1–15.2 mcg/mL) and 31.8 mcg/mL (range: 12.5–55.4 mcg/mL), respectively, and concurrent serum concentrations of the drug averaged 36.1 mcg/mL (range: 23.6–46.8 mcg/mL).

In cystic fibrosis patients aged 5–32 years who received 35- or 50-mg/kg doses of ceftazidime every 8 hours by IV injection, concentrations of ceftazidime in sputum ranged from 0.7–9.8 mcg/mL; peak sputum concentrations were usually attained 1 hour after a dose.

In patients undergoing cataract surgery who received a single 2-g dose of ceftazidime by IV injection over 3–5 minutes, aqueous humor concentrations of the drug averaged 2.8, 4, 3.2, 3.4, and 1.9 mcg/mL at 0.5, 1, 2, 4, and 6 hours, respectively, after the dose.

Ceftazidime is 5–24% bound to serum proteins. The degree of protein binding is independent of the concentration of the drug.

Ceftazidime crosses the placenta and is distributed into amniotic fluid. Ceftazidime is also distributed into milk. In lactating women with endometritis who received 2 g of ceftazidime IV every 8 hours, concentrations of the drug in milk obtained during days 2–4 of therapy averaged 3.8 mcg/mL immediately prior to a dose and 5.2 and 4.5 mcg/mL at 1 and 3 hours, respectively, after a dose.

● *Elimination*

Plasma concentrations of ceftazidime decline in a biphasic manner. In adults with normal renal and hepatic function, the distribution half-life ($t_{\frac{1}{2}\alpha}$) of ceftazidime is 0.1–0.6 hours and the elimination half-life ($t_{\frac{1}{2}\beta}$) is 1.4–2 hours.

Ceftazidime is not metabolized and is excreted unchanged principally in urine by glomerular filtration. Following IM or IV administration of a single 0.5- or 1-g dose of ceftazidime in adults with normal renal function, 80–90% of the dose is excreted in urine unchanged within 24 hours; approximately 50% of the dose is excreted within 2 hours after the dose.

Serum clearance of ceftazidime averages 98–122 mL/minute in healthy adults. In geriatric patients 63–83 years of age with urinary tract infections, serum clearance of ceftazidime averaged 79 mL/minute and the serum half-life of the drug averaged 2.9 hours. In patients with cystic fibrosis, the serum clearance of ceftazidime ranges from 142–316 mL/minute per 1.73 m^2; the serum half-life of the drug in these patients, however, ranges from 1–2.2 hours and is generally within the same range as that for healthy individuals.

The serum half-life of ceftazidime is longer in neonates than in older children and adults, but does not appear to be related to gestational age or birthweight. The $t_{\frac{1}{2}\beta}$ of ceftazidime in neonates 1–23 days of age reportedly ranges from 2.2–4.7 hours. In a group of children 2–12 months of age, the $t_{\frac{1}{2}\beta}$ of ceftazidime averaged 2 hours.

Serum concentrations of ceftazidime are higher and the serum half-life of the drug is prolonged in patients with impaired renal function. The $t_{\frac{1}{2}\beta}$ of ceftazidime ranged from 3–4.6 hours in patients with creatinine clearances of 39–73 mL/minute and 9.4–10.3 hours in patients with creatinine clearances of 13–27 mL/minute. The $t_{\frac{1}{2}\beta}$ of ceftazidime in patients with creatinine clearances less than 10 mL/minute ranges from 11.9–35 hours.

The serum half-life of ceftazidime is only slightly prolonged in patients with impaired hepatic function and accumulation of the drug does not generally occur in these patients unless renal function is also impaired. In a group of patients who had normal renal function but impaired hepatic function (e.g., alcoholic cirrhosis, chronic active hepatitis B, biliary cirrhosis), the serum half-life of ceftazidime averaged 2.9 hours. In another group of patients with ascites who had normal renal function, the $t_{\frac{1}{2}\alpha}$ of ceftazidime averaged 0.4 hours and the $t_{\frac{1}{2}\beta}$ averaged 5.9 hours.

Ceftazidime is readily removed by hemodialysis. The drug is also removed by peritoneal dialysis.

CHEMISTRY AND STABILITY

● Chemistry

Ceftazidime is a semisynthetic cephalosporin antibiotic. Like cefepime, cefotaxime, and ceftriaxone, ceftazidime is a parenteral aminothiazolyl cephalosporin. Ceftazidime contains an aminothiazolyl side chain at position 7 of the cephalosporin nucleus. The aminothiazolyl side chain enhances antibacterial activity, particularly against Enterobacteriaceae, and generally results in enhanced stability against β-lactamases. However, ceftazidime contains a carboxypropyl oxyimino group in the side chain rather than the methoxyimino group contained in many aminothiazolyl cephalosporins. This difference results in increased stability against hydrolysis by β-lactamases, increased activity against *Pseudomonas*, and decreased activity against gram-positive bacteria. Ceftazidime also contains a pyridine at position 3 of the cephalosporin nucleus.

Ceftazidime is commercially available as sterile powders for injection containing a mixture of ceftazidime (as the pentahydrate) and sodium carbonate. In these formulations, sodium carbonate has been admixed with ceftazidime to facilitate its dissolution; ceftazidime sodium is formed *in situ* following reconstitution of the powdered mixture as directed. These preparations contain 118 mg of sodium carbonate per gram of ceftazidime or 54 mg (2.3 mEq) of sodium per gram of ceftazidime. Potency of ceftazidime sodium is expressed in terms of ceftazidime, calculated on the anhydrous basis.

Ceftazidime occurs as a white to off-white powder. The drug has solubilities of 5 mg/mL in water and less than 1 mg/mL in alcohol. Ceftazidime has pK$_a$s of 1.9, 2.7, and 4.1. When reconstituted as directed, ceftazidime sodium solutions have a pH of 5–8, and are light yellow to amber in color depending on the diluent used, concentration of the drug, and length of storage.

When the commercially available Duplex® drug delivery system containing 1 or 2 g of ceftazidime and 50 mL of 5% dextrose injection in separate chambers is reconstituted (activated) according to the manufacturer's directions, the resultant solution has an osmolality of approximately 340 and 400 mOsm/kg, respectively. The solutions are light yellow to amber in color and have a pH of 5–7.5.

Commercially available frozen premixed injections of ceftazidime sodium in dextrose are sterile, nonpyrogenic, iso-osmotic solutions of the drug provided in a plastic container (Galaxy® container) fabricated from specially formulated multilayered plastic (PL 2040). The 1- and 2-g frozen injections of ceftazidime contain approximately 2.2 or 1.6 g of dextrose, respectively, and have osmolalities of approximately 300 mOsm/kg; The frozen injections also contain hydrochloric acid and/or sodium hydroxide to adjust pH to 5–7.5; sodium hydroxide neutralizes ceftazidime pentahydrate free acid to the sodium salt.

● Stability

Ceftazidime powder and solutions of ceftazidime sodium tend to darken depending on storage conditions; however, color changes do not necessarily indicate loss of potency.

The commercially available vials of Fortaz® sterile powder for injection containing ceftazidime (as the pentahydrate) with sodium carbonate should be stored at 15–30°C and protected from light. Following reconstitution with sterile water for injection according to the manufacturer's directions, Fortaz® solutions for IV administration containing 100, 170, or 200 mg of ceftazidime per mL are stable for 12 hours at room temperature or 3 days when refrigerated. IV solutions prepared according to the manufacturer's directions using Fortaz® TwistVial® vials containing 1 or 2 g of ceftazidime and 0.9 or 0.45% sodium chloride injection or 5% dextrose injection are stable for 12 hours at room temperature or 3 days under refrigeration.

Following reconstitution with sterile water for injection, bacteriostatic water for injection, or 0.5 or 1% lidocaine hydrochloride injection, Fortaz® solutions for IM injection containing 280 mg/mL are stable for 12 hours at room temperature or 3 days when refrigerated.

The manufacturer of Fortaz® states that ceftazidime at concentrations of 1–40 mg/mL is chemically and physically stable for 12 hours at room temperature or for 3 days when refrigerated in the following IV solutions: 0.9% sodium chloride; $\frac{1}{6}$ M sodium lactate; 5 or 10% dextrose; 5% dextrose and 0.225, 0.45, or 0.9% sodium chloride; Ringer's; lactated Ringer's; 10% invert sugar; or Normosol®-M and 5% dextrose. Fortaz® solutions in 5% dextrose or 0.9% sodium chloride are stable for at least 6 hours at room temperature in plastic tubing, drip chambers, and volume control devices of common IV infusion sets.

The commercially available vials of Tazicef® sterile powder for injection containing ceftazidime (as the pentahydrate) with sodium carbonate should be stored at 20–25°C and protected from light. Following reconstitution with sterile water for injection according to the manufacturer's directions, Tazicef® solutions for IV or IM administration containing 95, 180, or 280 mg of ceftazidime per mL are stable for 24 hours at room temperature or 7 days when refrigerated. IV solutions prepared according to the manufacturer's directions using Tazicef® ADD-Vantage® vials containing 1 or 2 g of ceftazidime and 0.45 or 0.9% sodium chloride injection or 5% dextrose injection are stable for 24 hours at room temperature.

The commercially available Duplex® drug delivery system containing 1 or 2 g of ceftazidime and 50 mL of 5% dextrose injection in separate chambers should be stored at 20–25°C, but may be exposed to temperatures ranging from 15–30°C. Following reconstitution (activation), these IV solutions must be used within 12 hours if stored at room temperature or within 3 days if stored in a refrigerator and should not be frozen.

The commercially available frozen premixed injections of ceftazidime sodium in dextrose (Fortaz®) should be stored at −20°C or lower. The frozen injections should be thawed at room temperature (25°C) or under refrigeration (5°C) and, once thawed, should not be refrozen. Thawed solutions of the commercially available frozen injections are stable for 8 hours at room temperature or 7 days when refrigerated. The commercially available frozen injections of the drug are provided in plastic containers fabricated from specially formulated multilayered plastic PL 2040 (Galaxy® containers). Solutions in contact with PL 2040 can leach out some of its chemical components in very small amounts within the expiration period of the injections; however, safety of the plastic has been confirmed in tests in animals according to USP biological tests for plastic containers as well as by tissue culture toxicity studies.

Ceftazidime and ceftazidime sodium are potentially physically and/or chemically incompatible with some drugs, including aminoglycosides and vancomycin, but the compatibility depends on several factors (e.g., concentrations of the drugs, specific diluents used, resulting pH, temperature). Specialized references should be consulted for specific compatibility information. Sodium bicarbonate injection should not be used as a diluent for ceftazidime or ceftazidime sodium since the drug is less stable in sodium bicarbonate than in other IV solutions. Because of the potential for incompatibility, the manufacturers state that ceftazidime or ceftazidime sodium should not be admixed with aminoglycosides or vancomycin.

For further information on chemistry, mechanism of action, spectrum, resistance, pharmacokinetics, uses, cautions, drug interactions, laboratory test interferences, and dosage and administration of ceftazidime, see the Cephalosporins General Statement 8:12.06.

PREPARATIONS

Excipients in commercially available drug preparations may have clinically important effects in some individuals; consult specific product labeling for details.

cefTAZidime

Parenteral

For injection	equivalent to anhydrous ceftazidime 500 mg (with sodium carbonate)*	cefTAZidime for Injection Fortaz®, Covis
	equivalent to anhydrous ceftazidime 1 g (with sodium carbonate)*	cefTAZidime for Injection Fortaz®, Covis Tazicef®, Hospira
	equivalent to anhydrous ceftazidime 2 g (with sodium carbonate)*	cefTAZidime for Injection Fortaz®, Covis Tazicef®, Hospira
	equivalent to anhydrous ceftazidime 6 g pharmacy bulk package (with sodium carbonate)*	cefTAZidime for Injection Fortaz®, Covis Tazicef®, Hospira
For injection, for IV infusion	equivalent to anhydrous ceftazidime 1 g (with sodium carbonate)	cefTAZidime for Injection (available in dual-chambered Duplex® drug delivery system with 5% dextrose injection), B Braun Fortaz® TwistVial®, Covis Tazicef® ADD-Vantage®, Hospira
	equivalent to anhydrous ceftazidime 2 g (with sodium carbonate)	cefTAZidime for Injection (available in dual-chambered Duplex® drug delivery system with 5% dextrose injection), B Braun Fortaz® TwistVial®, Covis Tazicef® ADD-Vantage®, Hospira

* available from one or more manufacturer, distributor, and/or repackager by generic (nonproprietary) name

cefTAZidime Sodium in Dextrose

Parenteral

Injection (frozen), for IV infusion	equivalent to 20 mg (of anhydrous ceftazidime) per mL (1 g) in 4.4% Dextrose	Fortaz® Iso-osmotic in Dextrose Injection (Galaxy® [Baxter]), Covis
	equivalent to 40 mg (of anhydrous ceftazidime) per mL (2 g) in 3.2% Dextrose	Fortaz® Iso-osmotic in Dextrose Injection (Galaxy® [Baxter]), Covis

† Use is not currently included in the labeling approved by the US Food and Drug Administration.

Selected Revisions October 10, 2013, © Copyright, June 1, 1986, American Society of Health-System Pharmacists, Inc.

cefTAZidime and Avibactam Sodium

8:12.06.12 • THIRD GENERATION CEPHALOSPORINS

■ Ceftazidime and avibactam sodium is a fixed combination of ceftazidime (a third generation cephalosporin) and avibactam (a non-β-lactam β-lactamase inhibitor); avibactam inactivates certain bacterial β-lactamases and expands ceftazidime's spectrum of activity against some bacteria that produce these β-lactamases.

USES

● Intra-abdominal Infections

Ceftazidime and avibactam is used in conjunction with metronidazole for the treatment of complicated intra-abdominal infections caused by susceptible *Enterobacter cloacae, Escherichia coli, Klebsiella oxytoca, K. pneumoniae, Proteus mirabilis, Providencia stuartii,* or *Pseudomonas aeruginosa.*

Use of ceftazidime and avibactam for the treatment of complicated intra-abdominal infections should be reserved for patients with limited or no alternative treatment options since only limited data are available regarding safety and efficacy of the drug.

Clinical Experience

Efficacy and safety of ceftazidime and avibactam for the treatment of complicated intra-abdominal infections is based on results from a phase 2, randomized, double-blind, active-controlled study in 204 adults with evidence of intra-abdominal infection requiring surgical intervention and anti-infective treatment. Patients were randomized in a 1:1 ratio to receive 5–14 days of treatment with the fixed combination of ceftazidime and avibactam (2.5 g [ceftazidime 2 g and avibactam 0.5 g] given by IV infusion every 8 hours) in conjunction with metronidazole (500 mg given by IV infusion every 8 hours) or treatment with meropenem (1 g given by IV infusion every 8 hours) in conjunction with placebo. Baseline characteristics were generally similar between groups (mean age 43 years, 69–79% male, 55–64% white, 83–87% with peritonitis, 39–44% with visceral perforation, 26–28% with abscess). Clinical response (defined as complete resolution or substantial improvement of signs and symptoms of infection with no requirement for additional antibiotics or surgery at the test-of-cure visit [2 weeks after the last treatment dose]) in the microbiologically evaluable population was achieved by 91.2% of patients treated with ceftazidime and avibactam in conjunction with metronidazole and 93.4% of those treated with meropenem.

● Urinary Tract Infections

Ceftazidime and avibactam is used for the treatment of complicated urinary tract infections, including pyelonephritis, caused by susceptible *E. coli, Citrobacter freundii, C. koseri, E. aerogenes, E. cloacae, K. pneumoniae, Proteus,* or *Ps. aeruginosa.*

Use of ceftazidime and avibactam for the treatment of complicated urinary tract infections should be reserved for patients with limited or no alternative treatment options since only limited data are available regarding safety and efficacy of the drug.

Clinical Experience

Efficacy and safety of ceftazidime and avibactam for the treatment of complicated urinary tract infections is based on results from a phase 2, randomized, double-blind study in 137 adults with complicated urinary tract infection, including pyelonephritis, caused by gram-negative bacteria and requiring parenteral anti-infective treatment. Patients were randomized in a 1:1 ratio to receive treatment with the fixed combination of ceftazidime and avibactam (625 mg [ceftazidime 500 mg and avibactam 125 mg] given by IV infusion every 8 hours) or the fixed combination of imipenem and cilastatin (500 mg of imipenem given by IV infusion every 6 hours). Dosage of ceftazidime and avibactam used in this study is lower than the usually recommended dosage of the drug. After at least 4 days of IV treatment, patients with clinical improvement (afebrile for at least 24 hours, with resolution of nausea and vomiting and improved signs and symptoms) who had pathogens susceptible to both study anti-infectives were permitted to switch

to oral ciprofloxacin (500 mg twice daily). The total duration of IV and/or oral anti-infective treatment was 7–14 days. Baseline characteristics were generally similar between groups (mean age 46–48 years, 25–27% male, 59–61% white, 61–65% diagnosed with acute pyelonephritis). Favorable microbiologic response (defined as eradication of all uropathogens at the test-of-cure visit 5–9 days after the last treatment dose) in the microbiologically evaluable population was achieved by 70.4% of patients treated with ceftazidime and avibactam and 71.4% of those treated with imipenem and cilastatin.

DOSAGE AND ADMINISTRATION

● Administration

Ceftazidime and avibactam is administered by IV infusion.

IV Infusion

Reconstitution and Dilution

Ceftazidime and avibactam powder must be reconstituted and further diluted prior to IV infusion.

Single-dose vials of ceftazidime and avibactam labeled as containing 2.5 g (ceftazidime 2 g and avibactam 0.5 g) should be reconstituted by adding 10 mL of a compatible IV solution (sterile water for injection, 0.9% sodium chloride injection, 5% dextrose injection, 2.5% dextrose and 0.45% sodium chloride injection, lactated Ringer's injection) to the vial and gently mixing. The volume of the reconstituted solution is approximately 12 mL and the approximate concentration is ceftazidime 167 mg/mL and avibactam 42 mg/mL. Reconstituted ceftazidime and avibactam solution may be stored for up to 30 minutes prior to transfer and dilution.

Prior to IV infusion, reconstituted ceftazidime and avibactam solution *must* be further diluted. To prepare the indicated dose, the appropriate volume of reconstituted solution should be withdrawn from the vial and added to a compatible IV solution to achieve a total final volume of 50–250 mL in an IV infusion bag. (See Table 1.) With the exception of sterile water for injection, the same IV solution used for reconstitution should be used for dilution; any other compatible IV solution should be used for dilution if sterile water for injection was used for reconstitution. The diluted solution should be mixed gently to ensure that the drug is completely dissolved.

TABLE 1. Dilution of Reconstituted Ceftazidime and Avibactam

Recommended Dose of Ceftazidime and Avibactam	Volume to Withdraw from Reconstituted Vial for Further Dilution
2.5 g (ceftazidime 2 g and avibactam 0.5 g)	12 mL (entire contents)
1.25 g (ceftazidime 1 g and avibactam 0.25 g)	6 mL
940 mg (ceftazidime 750 mg and avibactam 190 mg)	4.5 mL

The reconstituted and diluted solution of ceftazidime and avibactam should be inspected visually for particulate matter and discoloration prior to administration; the solution should appear clear and colorless to light yellow.

Following reconstitution and dilution, ceftazidime and avibactam solutions may be stored in the IV infusion bag at room temperature for up to 12 hours. Alternatively, these solutions may be stored at 2–8°C for up to 24 hours and then used within 12 hours after removal from refrigeration to room temperature.

Rate of Administration

IV infusions of ceftazidime and avibactam should be given over 2 hours.

Dispensing and Dosage and Administration Precautions

FDA alerted healthcare professionals about the risk of medication errors with ceftazidime and avibactam. There have been reports of errors occurring during preparation of IV solutions of the drug that resulted in administration of incorrect dosage (higher than intended); the errors were due to confusion about how dosage of ceftazidime and avibactam is expressed (total of the dosage of each of the 2 active components) and how drug strength was displayed on vial labels and carton packaging. To prevent such errors, vial labels and carton packaging have been revised to indicate the strength of the fixed combination as the total of the 2 active components.

Healthcare professionals should be aware that dosage of ceftazidime and avibactam is expressed as the total (sum) of the dosage of each of the 2 active components (i.e., dosage of ceftazidime plus dosage of avibactam). This dosage convention should be considered when prescribing, preparing, and dispensing ceftazidime and avibactam. FDA urges healthcare professionals and patients to report any medication errors and adverse effects involving the drug to the FDA MedWatch program.

● Dosage

Ceftazidime and avibactam is a fixed combination containing a 4:1 ratio of ceftazidime to avibactam.

The ceftazidime component is provided as a mixture of ceftazidime pentahydrate and sodium carbonate (dosage of this component is expressed in terms of anhydrous ceftazidime); the avibactam component is provided as avibactam sodium (dosage of this component is expressed in terms of avibactam).

Dosage of the fixed combination of ceftazidime and avibactam is expressed in terms of the total of the ceftazidime and avibactam content.

Each single-dose vial of ceftazidime and avibactam contains a total of 2.5 g (i.e., 2 g of ceftazidime and 0.5 g of avibactam).

Adult Dosage

Intra-abdominal Infections

The recommended dosage of ceftazidime and avibactam for the treatment of complicated intra-abdominal infections in adults is 2.5 g (ceftazidime 2 g and avibactam 0.5 g) every 8 hours given in conjunction with metronidazole. The duration of treatment is 5–14 days.

Urinary Tract Infections

The recommended dosage of ceftazidime and avibactam for the treatment of complicated urinary tract infections, including pyelonephritis, in adults is 2.5 g (ceftazidime 2 g and avibactam 0.5 g) every 8 hours. The duration of treatment is 7–14 days.

● Dosage in Renal Impairment

Dosage of ceftazidime and avibactam must be adjusted in adults with creatinine clearances of 50 mL/minute or less, including those undergoing hemodialysis. (See Table 2.)

Creatinine clearance should be monitored at least once daily in patients with changing renal function and dosage of ceftazidime and avibactam adjusted accordingly.

TABLE 2. Ceftazidime and Avibactam Dosage for Adults with Renal Impairment

Estimated Creatinine Clearance (mL/minute)	Recommended Dosage
31–50	1.25 g (ceftazidime 1 g and avibactam 0.25 g) every 8 hours
16–30	940 mg (ceftazidime 750 mg and avibactam 190 mg) every 12 hours
6–15 [a]	940 mg (ceftazidime 750 mg and avibactam 190 mg) every 24 hours
≤5 [a]	940 mg (ceftazidime 750 mg and avibactam 190 mg) every 48 hours

[a] On hemodialysis days, the dose should be administered after dialysis.

● Dosage in Hepatic Impairment

Dosage adjustments are not needed when ceftazidime and avibactam is used in adults with hepatic impairment.

● Dosage in Geriatric Patients

Dosage adjustments based solely on age are not needed when ceftazidime and avibactam is used in geriatric patients. However, because geriatric patients are more likely to have decreased renal function and because dosage of ceftazidime and avibactam needs to be adjusted based on renal impairment, dosage should be selected with caution and it may be useful to monitor renal function.

CAUTIONS

● Adverse Effects

Adverse effects reported in 5% or more of patients receiving ceftazidime and avibactam in phase 2 clinical trials include GI effects (nausea, vomiting, diarrhea, abdominal pain, constipation), pyrexia, increased AST, increased ALT, increased blood alkaline phosphatase, increased leukocyte count, headache, dizziness, chest pain, hypertension, cough, anxiety, insomnia, and infusion site reactions.

● Precautions and Contraindications

Sensitivity Reactions

Ceftazidime and avibactam is contraindicated in patients with known serious hypersensitivity to ceftazidime and/or avibactam, avibactam-containing preparations, or other cephalosporins.

Serious and occasionally fatal hypersensitivity (anaphylactic) reactions and serious skin reactions have been reported in patients receiving β-lactam antibacterials. Before initiating therapy with ceftazidime and avibactam, the clinician should carefully inquire about the patient's previous hypersensitivity reactions to other cephalosporins, penicillins, or carbapenems. Ceftazidime and avibactam should be used with caution in patients allergic to penicillins or other β-lactams since cross-sensitivity among β-lactams antibacterials has been established.

Patients should be advised that allergic reactions, including serious allergic reactions, could occur and that serious reactions require immediate treatment.

If an allergic reaction occurs, ceftazidime and avibactam should be discontinued.

Reduced Efficacy in Patients with Moderate Renal Impairment

Results of a subgroup analysis of a phase 3 clinical trial in patients with complicated intra-abdominal infections indicated that the clinical cure rate in patients with moderate renal impairment was lower than the clinical cure rate in those with normal renal function or only mild renal impairment, and this difference was more marked in those treated with a regimen of ceftazidime and avibactam in conjunction with metronidazole than in those treated with the comparator drug (meropenem). The clinical cure rate in patients treated with ceftazidime and avibactam in conjunction with metronidazole was 45% in those with baseline creatinine clearances of 30–50 mL/minute compared with 85% in those with baseline creatinine clearances greater than 50 mL/minute. Although the reason for this reduced efficacy is unclear, the dosage of ceftazidime and avibactam used in this study in patients with creatinine clearances of 30–50 mL/minute was 33% lower than the currently recommended dosage of the drug for such patients and it is possible that those with rapidly changing renal function did not receive appropriate dosage.

Creatinine clearance should be monitored at least once daily in patients with changing renal function and dosage of ceftazidime and avibactam adjusted accordingly. (See Other Precautions and Contraindications under Cautions: Precautions and Contraindications.)

Nervous System Effects

Seizures, nonconvulsive status epilepticus, encephalopathy, coma, asterixis, neuromuscular excitability, and myoclonia have been reported in patients receiving ceftazidime, particularly in patients with renal impairment. Dosage of ceftazidime and avibactam should be adjusted based on creatinine clearance. (See Dosage and Administration: Dosage in Renal Impairment.)

Patients should be advised that adverse neurologic reactions can occur while receiving ceftazidime and avibactam and that they should immediately inform a clinician if any neurologic signs and symptoms, including encephalopathy (disturbance of consciousness such as confusion, hallucinations, stupor, coma), myoclonus, or seizures, occur since immediate treatment, dosage adjustment, or discontinuance of ceftazidime and avibactam may be necessary.

Hematologic Effects

In clinical trials, seroconversion from a negative to a positive direct Coombs' test result occurred in 7.3% of patients receiving ceftazidime and avibactam in conjunction with metronidazole and in 1.9% of patients receiving ceftazidime and avibactam alone. Adverse reactions representing hemolytic anemia were not reported in any treatment group.

Eosinophilia and thrombocytopenia have been reported in less than 5% of patients receiving ceftazidime and avibactam.

Superinfection/Clostridium difficile-associated Diarrhea and Colitis (CDAD)

Use of ceftazidime and avibactam may result in emergence and overgrowth of nonsusceptible bacteria or fungi. The patient should be carefully monitored and appropriate therapy instituted if superinfection occurs.

Treatment with anti-infectives alters normal colon flora and may permit overgrowth of *Clostridium difficile*. *C. difficile* infection (CDI) and *C. difficile*-associated diarrhea and colitis (CDAD; also known as antibiotic-associated diarrhea and colitis or pseudomembranous colitis) have been reported in patients receiving nearly all anti-infectives, including ceftazidime and avibactam, and may range in severity from mild diarrhea to fatal colitis. *C. difficile* produces toxins A and B which contribute to development of CDAD; hypertoxin-producing strains of *C. difficile* are associated with increased morbidity and mortality since they may be refractory to anti-infectives and colectomy may be required.

CDAD should be considered in the differential diagnosis of patients who develop diarrhea during or after anti-infective therapy. Careful medical history is necessary since CDAD has been reported to occur as late as 2 months or longer after anti-infective therapy is discontinued.

If CDAD is suspected or confirmed, anti-infective therapy not directed against *C. difficile* should be discontinued whenever possible. Patients should be managed with appropriate supportive therapy (e.g., fluid and electrolyte management, protein supplementation), anti-infective therapy directed against *C. difficile* (e.g., metronidazole, vancomycin), and surgical evaluation as clinically indicated.

Patients should be advised that diarrhea is a common problem caused by anti-infectives and usually resolves when the drug is discontinued; however, they should contact a clinician if watery and bloody stools (with or without stomach cramps and fever) occur during or as late as 2 months or longer after the last dose.

Selection and Use of Anti-infectives

To reduce development of drug-resistant bacteria and maintain effectiveness of ceftazidime and avibactam and other antibacterials, the drug should be used only for treatment of infections proven or strongly suspected to be caused by susceptible bacteria.

When selecting or modifying anti-infective therapy, results of culture and in vitro susceptibility testing should be used. In the absence of such data, local epidemiology and susceptibility patterns should be considered when selecting anti-infectives for empiric therapy.

Patients should be advised that antibacterials (including ceftazidime and avibactam) should only be used to treat bacterial infections and not used to treat viral infections (e.g., the common cold). Patients also should be advised about the importance of completing the full course of therapy, even if feeling better after a few days, and that skipping doses or not completing therapy may decrease effectiveness and increase the likelihood that bacteria will develop resistance and will not be treatable with ceftazidime and avibactam or other antibacterials in the future.

Precautions Related to Use of Fixed Combinations

When ceftazidime and avibactam is used, the cautions, precautions, contraindications, and drug interactions associated with both drugs in the fixed combination must be considered. Cautionary information applicable to specific populations (e.g., pregnant or nursing women, individuals with hepatic or renal impairment, geriatric patients) should be considered for each drug. (For additional cautionary information on ceftazidime, see Cautions in Ceftazidime 8:12.06.12.)

When prescribing, preparing, and dispensing ceftazidime and avibactam, healthcare professionals should consider that dosage of the fixed combination is expressed as the total (sum) of the dosage of each of the 2 active components (i.e., dosage of ceftazidime plus dosage of avibactam). (See Dispensing and Dosage and Administration Precautions under Administration: IV Infusion, in Dosage and Administration.)

Other Precautions and Contraindications

Ceftazidime and avibactam are principally eliminated by the kidneys, and the risk of adverse effects may be greater in patients with renal impairment. In addition,

a lower cure rate has been reported in some patients with moderate renal impairment (see Reduced Efficacy in Patients with Moderate Renal Impairment under Cautions: Precautions and Contraindications). Dosage of ceftazidime and avibactam should be adjusted in patients with moderate or severe renal impairment (creatinine clearances of 50 mL/minute or less), including those undergoing hemodialysis. In patients with changing renal function, creatinine clearance should be monitored at least once daily and dosage adjusted accordingly. (See Dosage and Administration: Dosage in Renal Impairment.)

● *Pediatric Precautions*

Safety and efficacy of ceftazidime and avibactam have not been established in patients younger than 18 years of age.

● *Geriatric Precautions*

In phase 2 clinical trials evaluating ceftazidime and avibactam for the treatment of complicated intra-abdominal infections or complicated urinary tract infections, 10.7% of patients were 65 years of age or older. Since only limited data are available, age-related differences in outcomes or specific risks with ceftazidime and avibactam cannot be ruled out.

Ceftazidime and avibactam are eliminated principally by the kidneys, and the risk of adverse effects may be greater in those with impaired renal function. Because geriatric patients are more likely to have reduced renal function, dosage should be selected with caution and renal function monitoring should be considered. Dosage adjustments in geriatric patients should be based on renal function.

● *Mutagenicity and Carcinogenicity*

Ceftazidime was not mutagenic in a microbial (i.e., Ames test) or mammalian cell (i.e., mouse micronucleus) test. Avibactam was not genotoxic in the Ames assay, unscheduled DNA synthesis test, chromosomal aberration assay, or a rat micronucleus study.

● *Pregnancy, Fertility, and Lactation*
Pregnancy

Reproduction studies in mice and rats using ceftazidime dosages up to 40 times the usual human dose have not revealed evidence of harm to the fetus. Avibactam was not teratogenic in rats or rabbits. In rats, there was no evidence of embryofetal toxicity at an avibactam dosage of 1 g/kg daily (approximately 9 times the human dosage based on area under the concentration-time curve [AUC]) and no effects on pup growth and viability at a dosage of 825 mg/kg daily. In rabbits, there was no evidence of embryofetal toxicity at an avibactam dosage of 100 mg/kg, but increased implantation loss, lower mean fetal weights, delayed ossification of bones, and other anomalies were observed at higher dosages.

There are no adequate and controlled studies using ceftazidime and avibactam in pregnant women, and the drug should be used during pregnancy only if clearly needed.

Fertility

Avibactam had no adverse effects on fertility in male and female rats using dosages up to 1 g/kg daily (approximately 20 times higher than the recommended human dosage based on body surface area). In female rats, IV avibactam dosages of 0.5 g/kg or higher resulted in dose-related increases in the percentage of pre- and post-implantation loss compared with controls.

Lactation

Ceftazidime is distributed into human milk in low concentrations. It is not known whether avibactam is distributed into human milk. (See Pharmacokinetics: Distribution.)

Ceftazidime and avibactam should be used with caution in nursing women.

DRUG INTERACTIONS

The following drug interactions are based on studies using the fixed combination containing ceftazidime and avibactam, ceftazidime alone, or avibactam alone. When ceftazidime and avibactam is used, interactions associated with both drugs in the fixed combination should be considered.

● **Drugs Affecting or Metabolized by Hepatic Microsomal Enzymes**

Ceftazidime does not induce cytochrome P-450 (CYP) 1A1, 1A2, 2B6, or 3A4/5 when tested in vitro in human hepatocytes.

In vitro, avibactam does not inhibit CYP1A2, 2A6, 2B6, 2C8, 2C9, 2C19, 2D6, 2E1, or 3A4/5 and does not induce CYP1A2, 2B6, 2C9, or 3A4. At concentrations exceeding clinically relevant exposures, avibactam shows some potential to induce CYP2E1.

● **Drugs Affecting or Affected by Organic Anion Transporters**

In vitro, avibactam is a substrate of organic anion transporter (OAT) 1 and OAT3 kidney transporters. In vitro, probenecid (a potent OAT1/OAT3 inhibitor) inhibits uptake of avibactam by 56–70% and has the potential to decrease elimination of avibactam. (See Drug Interactions: Probenecid.)

Ceftazidime and avibactam do not inhibit OAT1 or OAT3 and ceftazidime does not inhibit avibactam transport mediated by OAT1 and OAT3.

● **Drugs Affecting or Affected by Other Membrane Transporters**

In vitro, ceftazidime and avibactam do not inhibit multidrug-resistance transporter (MDR) 1, breast cancer resistance protein (BCRP), organic anion transporting polypeptide (OATP) 1B1, OATP1B3, bile salt export pump (BSEP), multidrug resistance-associated protein (MRP) 4, organic cation transporter (OCT) 1, or OCT2 at clinically relevant concentrations. Avibactam is not a substrate of MDR1, BCRP, MRP4, or OCT2.

● **Anti-infectives**

Metronidazole

In healthy males, administration of ceftazidime and avibactam (2.5 g [ceftazidime 2 g and avibactam 0.5 g] given by IV infusion over 2 hours) following metronidazole (500 mg given by IV infusion over 1 hour every 8 hours for 3 days) had no effect on peak plasma concentrations or area under the plasma concentration-time curve (AUC) of ceftazidime or avibactam compared with use of ceftazidime and avibactam alone. Similarly, administration of metronidazole (500 mg given by IV infusion over 1 hour) followed by ceftazidime and avibactam (2.5 g [ceftazidime 2 g and avibactam 0.5 g] given by IV infusion over 2 hours every 8 hours for 3 days) in healthy males had no effect on peak plasma concentrations and AUC of metronidazole compared with use of metronidazole alone.

There is no in vitro evidence of antagonistic antibacterial effects between ceftazidime and avibactam and metronidazole.

Other Anti-infectives

There is no in vitro evidence of antagonistic antibacterial effects between ceftazidime and avibactam and colistin (commercially available in US as colistimethate sodium), levofloxacin, linezolid, tigecycline, tobramycin, or vancomycin.

● **Probenecid**

In vitro studies indicate probenecid (a potent OAT1/OAT3 inhibitor) has the potential to decrease elimination of avibactam by inhibiting renal uptake of the drug. Therefore, concomitant use of probenecid with ceftazidime and avibactam is not recommended.

LABORATORY TEST INTERFERENCES

● **Tests for Urinary Glucose**

Administration of ceftazidime may result in a false-positive reaction for urine glucose when certain testing methods are used. Urine glucose tests based on enzymatic glucose oxidase reactions should be used in patients receiving ceftazidime and avibactam.

MECHANISM OF ACTION

Ceftazidime and avibactam is bactericidal in action.

Like other cephalosporins, the antibacterial activity of ceftazidime results from inhibition of mucopeptide synthesis in the bacterial cell wall and is mediated through binding to penicillin-binding proteins (PBPs). (For information on the mechanism of action of cephalosporins, see Mechanism of Action in the Cephalosporins General Statement 8:12.06.)

Avibactam is a non-β-lactam β-lactamase inhibitor that inactivates certain β-lactamases, including some extended-spectrum β-lactamases (ESBLs). Avibactam inactivates many β-lactamases in Ambler class A (e.g., ESBLs, carbapenemases such as *Klebsiella pneumoniae* carbapenemases [KPCs]), class C (e.g., cephalosporinases such as AmpC), and class D (e.g., some oxacillinases [OXAs]). Avibactam binds to the β-lactamase active site serine residue by covalent acylation, which is partially reversible; subsequently, deacylation can occur resulting in release of intact avibactam allowing additional β-lactamase inhibition. This mechanism of action differs from that of some other β-lactamase inhibitors (e.g., clavulanic acid, sulbactam, tazobactam) that can form covalent, irreversible, acyl-enzyme intermediates that may undergo hydrolysis, resulting in decomposition of the β-lactamase inhibitor. Avibactam cannot inactivate Ambler class B metallo-β-lactamases (MBLs) or certain OXA-type carbapenemases.

Because avibactam inactivates certain β-lactamases, concomitant use with ceftazidime can protect ceftazidime from degradation by these β-lactamases and expand the spectrum of activity of the cephalosporin to include many β-lactamase-producing bacteria that are resistant to ceftazidime alone. Avibactam does not decrease the antibacterial activity of ceftazidime against ceftazidime-susceptible bacteria.

SPECTRUM

Based on its spectrum of activity, ceftazidime and avibactam is classified as a third generation cephalosporin. (For information on the classification of cephalosporins and closely related β-lactam antibiotics based on spectra of activity, see Spectrum in the Cephalosporins General Statement 8:12.06.)

Like other currently available parenteral third generation cephalosporins (e.g., cefotaxime, ceftriaxone), ceftazidime generally is less active against staphylococci but has an expanded spectrum of activity against gram-negative bacteria compared with first and second generation cephalosporins. Ceftazidime is distinguished from many other cephalosporins by its activity against *Pseudomonas aeruginosa*. (For information on the spectrum of activity of ceftazidime used alone, see Spectrum in Ceftazidime 8:12.06.12.)

Ceftazidime and avibactam has a wider spectrum of activity than ceftazidime alone. Ceftazidime and avibactam is active against many β-lactamase-producing gram-negative bacteria that are resistant to ceftazidime alone, including many strains that produce extended-spectrum β-lactamases (ESBLs). The fixed combination is active in vitro against Enterobacteriaceae that produce TEM, SHV, CTX-M, *Klebsiella pneumoniae* carbapenemase (KPC), AmpC, and certain oxacillinase (OXA) β-lactamases and also is active in vitro against *Ps. aeruginosa* that produce certain AmpC β-lactamases.

Ceftazidime and avibactam is active in vitro against some Enterobacteriaceae and *Ps. aeruginosa* that are resistant to carbapenems, other cephalosporins (including ceftazidime alone), or fluoroquinolones.

● **In Vitro Susceptibility Testing**

When in vitro susceptibility testing is performed according to the standards of the Clinical and Laboratory Standards Institute (CLSI; formerly National Committee for Clinical Laboratory Standards [NCCLS]), clinical isolates identified as *susceptible* to ceftazidime and avibactam are inhibited by drug concentrations usually achievable when dosage recommended for the site of infection is used. If results of in vitro susceptibility testing indicate that a clinical isolate is *resistant* to ceftazidime and avibactam, the strain is not likely to be inhibited by drug concentrations generally achievable with usual dosage schedules and other anti-infective therapy should be selected.

Disk Susceptibility Tests

When the disk-diffusion procedure is used to test susceptibility to ceftazidime and avibactam, a disk containing 30 mcg of ceftazidime and 20 mcg of avibactam is used.

When disk-diffusion susceptibility testing is performed according to CLSI standardized procedures, Enterobacteriaceae with growth inhibition zones of 21 mm or greater are susceptible to ceftazidime and avibactam and those with zones of 20 mm or less are resistant to the drug. *Ps. aeruginosa* with growth inhibition zones of 18 mm or greater are susceptible to ceftazidime and avibactam and those with zones of 17 mm or less are resistant to the drug.

Dilution Susceptibility Tests

When dilution susceptibility testing (agar or broth dilution) is used to test susceptibility to ceftazidime and avibactam, tests should be performed using serial dilutions of ceftazidime combined with a fixed avibactam concentration of 4 mcg/mL. If a broth dilution test is used, results should be read within 18 hours because degradation of ceftazidime activity occurs by 24 hours.

When dilution susceptibility testing is performed according to CLSI standardized procedures, Enterobacteriaceae and *Ps. aeruginosa* with MICs of 8 mcg/mL or less of ceftazidime and 4 mcg/mL or less of avibactam are susceptible to ceftazidime and avibactam and those with MICs of 16 mcg/mL or greater of ceftazidime and 4 mcg/mL or greater of avibactam are resistant to the drug.

• Gram-negative Aerobic Bacteria

Ceftazidime and avibactam is active in vitro against many Enterobacteriaceae, including *Citrobacter freundii, C. koseri, Enterobacter aerogenes, E. cloacae, Escherichia coli, K. pneumoniae, K. oxytoca, Morganella morganii, Proteus* (including *P. mirabilis* and *P. vulgaris*), *Providencia rettgeri, P. stuartii,* and *Serratia marcescens.*

Ceftazidime and avibactam is active in vitro against many strains of *Ps. aeruginosa,* including some multidrug-resistant (MDR) and extensively drug-resistant (XDR) *Ps. aeruginosa.*

• Anaerobic Bacteria

Although ceftazidime and avibactam has been active in vitro against a few strains of *Bacteroides fragilis, Prevotella,* and *Porphyromonas,* the fixed combination shows only limited in vitro activity against most anaerobic bacteria.

RESISTANCE

Resistance or reduced susceptibility to ceftazidime and avibactam can occur. The mechanism of resistance to the fixed combination may be multifactorial.

Bacteria that produce Ambler class B metallo-β-lactamases (MBLs) are resistant to ceftazidime and avibactam because avibactam does not inhibit this type of β-lactamase. In addition, bacterial strains producing certain oxacillinase (OXA) β-lactamases (e.g., *Acinetobacter, Pseudomonas aeruginosa*) also are resistant to ceftazidime and avibactam. There is some in vitro evidence that point mutations in existing β-lactamases can result in selection of resistant mutants that have β-lactamases with reduced affinity for avibactam or changes that prevent the β-lactamase inhibitor from binding to and inhibiting the enzyme.

Bacteria resistant to ceftazidime because of altered penicillin-binding proteins (PBPs) may also be resistant to ceftazidime and avibactam. Some strains of gram-negative bacteria (e.g., *Ps. aeruginosa, Serratia marcescens*) that over-express efflux pumps or have porin mutations that result in resistance to ceftazidime may also have reduced susceptibility or resistance to ceftazidime and avibactam.

Cross-resistance between ceftazidime and avibactam and other classes of anti-infectives has not been reported.

PHARMACOKINETICS

Following IV administration of the fixed combination of ceftazidime and avibactam sodium, pharmacokinetic parameters for ceftazidime and avibactam are similar to those reported when each drug is administered alone. In addition, pharmacokinetic parameters are similar following single or multiple IV doses of the fixed combination.

• Absorption

In healthy adult males with normal renal function receiving multiple doses of ceftazidime and avibactam (2.5 g [ceftazidime 2 g and avibactam 0.5 g]) given by IV infusion over 2 hours every 8 hours for 11 days, peak plasma concentrations of ceftazidime were 90.4 mcg/mL and peak plasma concentrations of avibactam were 14.6 mcg/mL.

Peak plasma concentrations and area under the plasma concentration-time curve (AUC) of ceftazidime increase in proportion to the dose; avibactam

demonstrated approximately linear pharmacokinetics when single IV doses ranging from 50 mg to 2 g were given alone.

There is no appreciable accumulation of ceftazidime or avibactam in healthy adults with normal renal function following multiple doses of ceftazidime and avibactam (2.5 g [ceftazidime 2 g and avibactam 0.5 g]) given by IV infusion every 8 hours for up to 11 days.

In healthy adults 65 years of age or older who received a single 0.5-g IV dose of avibactam, the AUC of the drug was 17% higher than the AUC reported in healthy adults 18–45 years of age; peak plasma concentrations of avibactam in these adults were not substantially affected by age.

In a study in healthy adults who received a single 0.5-g IV dose of avibactam, peak plasma concentrations of the drug in males were 18% lower than in females; gender did not affect the AUC of avibactam.

• Distribution

The steady-state volumes of distribution of ceftazidime and avibactam are 17 and 22.2 L, respectively, in healthy adults following multiple doses of ceftazidime and avibactam (2.5 g [ceftazidime 2 g and avibactam 0.5 g]) given by IV infusion every 8 hours for 11 days.

Ceftazidime is less than 10% protein bound; avibactam is approximately 5.7–8.2% bound to plasma proteins.

Ceftazidime is distributed into human milk in low concentrations. In rats, avibactam is distributed into milk in a dose-dependent manner; it is not known whether avibactam is distributed into human milk.

• Elimination

Ceftazidime and avibactam do not undergo clinically important metabolism, and both drugs are principally eliminated unchanged in urine.

There was no evidence of metabolism of avibactam in vitro in human liver preparations (microsomes and hepatocytes), and unchanged avibactam was the major component in human plasma and urine after a single IV dose of 0.5 g of avibactam.

Following an IV dose of ceftazidime, approximately 80–90% of the dose is excreted unchanged by the kidneys over 24 hours. Following an IV dose of avibactam, an average of 97% of the dose is eliminated in urine and 0.2% is eliminated in feces.

The plasma elimination half-lives of ceftazidime and avibactam are 2.8 and 2.7 hours, respectively, in healthy adult males with normal renal function receiving multiple doses of ceftazidime and avibactam (2.5 g [ceftazidime 2 g and avibactam 0.5 g]) given by IV infusion over 2 hours every 8 hours.

The serum half-life of ceftazidime is prolonged in patients with renal impairment. Following a single 100-mg IV dose of avibactam in adults with mild, moderate, or severe renal impairment not requiring hemodialysis, the AUC of avibactam was 2.6-, 3.8-, or 7-fold higher, respectively, compared with the AUC reported in healthy adults with normal renal function. In adults with end-stage renal disease (ESRD) who received a single 100-mg IV dose of avibactam 1 hour after hemodialysis, the AUC of avibactam was 19.5-fold higher than the AUC reported in healthy adults with normal renal function.

Both ceftazidime and avibactam are removed by hemodialysis. In patients with ESRD who received 1 g of ceftazidime or 100 mg of avibactam prior to a 4-hour hemodialysis session, 55% of the ceftazidime dose or 55% of the avibactam dose was recovered in the dialysate.

There was no effect on ceftazidime pharmacokinetics when ceftazidime was given in a dosage of 2 g IV every 8 hours for 5 days in adults with hepatic impairment. Pharmacokinetics of avibactam have not been established in patients with hepatic impairment; however, avibactam does not appear to undergo clinically important hepatic metabolism and systemic clearance of the drug is not expected to be affected by hepatic impairment.

CHEMISTRY AND STABILITY

• Chemistry

Ceftazidime and avibactam sodium is a fixed combination of ceftazidime (a third generation cephalosporin antibiotic) and avibactam (a non-β-lactam β-lactamase inhibitor); avibactam inactivates certain bacterial β-lactamases and expands ceftazidime's spectrum of activity against some bacteria that produce these β-lactamases.

Ceftazidime contains an aminothiadiazole ring that enhances antibacterial activity against gram-negative bacteria, a carboxypropyl-oxyimino group that contributes to stability in the presence of β-lactamases, and a methylpyridinium group responsible for the drug's antipseudomonal activity. (For additional information on ceftazidime, see Ceftazidime 8:12.06.12.)

Avibactam is a diazabicyclooctanone derivative non-β-lactam β-lactamase inhibitor that differs structurally and pharmacologically from β-lactam β-lactamase inhibitors (e.g., sulbactam, clavulanic acid, tazobactam). Avibactam does not contain a β-lactam core, but does resemble β-lactams in key areas (i.e., carbonyl at position 7, sulfate at position 6, carboxamide at position 2), which allows binding to and inactivation of certain β-lactamases produced by bacteria.

Ceftazidime and avibactam is commercially available as a white to yellow sterile powder for IV infusion containing a 4:1 ratio of ceftazidime to avibactam. The ceftazidime component is provided as a mixture of ceftazidime (as the pentahydrate) and sodium carbonate (facilitates dissolution of ceftazidime); the avibactam component is provided as avibactam sodium. Drug strength and dosage are expressed as the total of the 2 active components. (See Dispensing and Dosage and Administration Precautions under Administration: IV Infusion, in Dosage and Administration.)

Each single-dose vial of ceftazidime and avibactam contains 2.5 g (2 g of ceftazidime [equivalent to 2.635 g of the ceftazidime pentahydrate and sodium carbonate mixture] and 0.5 g of avibactam [equivalent to 0.551 g of avibactam sodium]). The total sodium content is approximately 146 mg (6.4 mEq) per single-dose vial.

● Stability

Ceftazidime and avibactam powder for IV infusion should be stored at 25°C, but may be exposed to temperatures ranging from 15–30°C. Vials should be protected from light.

Following reconstitution and dilution, ceftazidime and avibactam solutions should be used within 12 hours when stored at room temperature. Alternatively, reconstituted and diluted solutions of the drug may be stored for up to 24 hours at 2–8°C and then used within 12 hours after removal from refrigeration to room temperature.

For further information on chemistry, mechanism of action, spectrum, resistance, uses, cautions, acute toxicity, drug interactions, or laboratory test interferences of cephalosporins, see the Cephalosporins General Statement 8:12.06.

PREPARATIONS

Excipients in commercially available drug preparations may have clinically important effects in some individuals; consult specific product labeling for details.

cefTAZidime and Avibactam Sodium

Parenteral

For injection, for IV infusion	2.5 g (2 g of ceftazidime and 0.5 g of avibactam)	Avycaz®, Forest

Selected Revisions October 16, 2015, © Copyright, October 16, 2015, American Society of Health-System Pharmacists, Inc.

cefTRIAXone Sodium

8:12.06.12 • THIRD GENERATION CEPHALOSPORINS

■ Ceftriaxone is a semisynthetic, third generation cephalosporin antibiotic.

USES

Ceftriaxone is used for the treatment of bone and joint infections, endocarditis†, intra-abdominal infections, meningitis and other CNS infections, otitis media, respiratory tract infections, septicemia, skin and skin structure infections, and urinary tract infections caused by susceptible bacteria. The drug also is used for the treatment of chancroid†, gonorrhea and associated infections, pelvic inflammatory disease, infections caused by *Neisseria meningitidis*†, infections caused by *Shigella*†, and typhoid fever† and other infections caused by *Salmonella*†. In addition, ceftriaxone is used for the treatment of Lyme disease† and has been used for empiric anti-infective therapy in febrile neutropenic patients† and for perioperative prophylaxis.

Ceftriaxone has a wide spectrum of activity and is effective for the treatment of infections caused by a variety of gram-positive and gram-negative bacteria. Like other parenteral third generation cephalosporins (cefotaxime, ceftazidime), ceftriaxone is less active than first and second generation cephalosporins against some gram-positive aerobic bacteria (e.g., staphylococci) and generally should not be used in the treatment of infections caused by these organisms when a penicillin or first or second generation cephalosporin could be used. However, ceftriaxone may be a drug of choice for serious infections caused by certain other gram-positive bacteria, including *Streptococcus pneumoniae*. Ceftriaxone is considered a drug of choice for many infections caused by gram-negative bacteria, and a principal use of the drug is for the treatment of serious gram-negative bacterial infections, especially nosocomial infections, when other anti-infectives are ineffective or contraindicated.

Because ceftriaxone has a long serum half-life and can be administered once daily, the drug has been used for community-based parenteral anti-infective therapy for the treatment of infections that require prolonged therapy (e.g., community-acquired pneumonia, osteomyelitis, endocarditis†). Ceftriaxone has been administered parenterally to adults and children in outpatient settings, including clinicians' office, outpatient clinics, infusion centers, skilled nursing facilities, rehabilitation centers, and the patient's home. Outpatient parenteral anti-infective therapy generally is used to complete a course of ceftriaxone therapy initiated during hospitalization, but ceftriaxone therapy also has been initiated on an outpatient basis in patients who were clinically stable. When considering use of community-based ceftriaxone therapy, the benefits and risks of such therapy should be considered.

Prior to initiation of ceftriaxone therapy, appropriate specimens should be obtained for identification of the causative organism and in vitro susceptibility tests. Ceftriaxone therapy may be started pending results of susceptibility tests, but should be discontinued if the organism is found to be resistant to the drug.

● Bone and Joint Infections

Ceftriaxone is used in adults and pediatric patients for the treatment of bone and joint infections (e.g., osteomyelitis, septic arthritis) caused by susceptible *Staphylococcus aureus*, *Streptococcus pneumoniae*, *Escherichia coli*, *Proteus mirabilis*, *Klebsiella pneumoniae*, or *Enterobacter*.

For the treatment of native vertebral osteomyelitis or prosthetic joint infections caused by oxacillin-susceptible staphylococci, the Infectious Diseases Society of America (IDSA) recommends IV nafcillin (or oxacillin), IV cefazolin, or IV ceftriaxone as the drugs of choice. If native vertebral osteomyelitis or prosthetic joint infections are caused by β-hemolytic streptococci†, IDSA recommends IV penicillin G or IV ceftriaxone. For the treatment of native vertebral osteomyelitis or prosthetic joint infections caused by *Cutibacterium acnes*† (formerly *Propionibacterium acnes*), IDSA recommends IV penicillin G or IV ceftriaxone. These experts also recommend IV ceftriaxone as an alternative to ciprofloxacin for the treatment of native vertebral osteomyelitis caused by susceptible *Salmonella*†.

For additional information on management of bone and joint infections, current clinical practice guidelines from IDSA available at http://www.idsociety.org should be consulted.

● Endocarditis

Ceftriaxone is used for the treatment of endocarditis† caused by various streptococci, including viridans group streptococci (e.g., *S. milleri* group, *S. mutans*, *S. salivarius*, *S. sanguis*), nonenterococcal group D streptococci (e.g., *S. gallolyticus* [formerly *S. bovis*]), *S. pneumoniae*, *S. pyogenes* (group A β-hemolytic streptococci; GAS), *S. agalactiae* (group B streptococci; GBS), or streptococci groups C, F, or G. The drug also is used for the treatment of endocarditis† caused by enterococci (e.g., *Enterococcus faecalis*, *E. faecium*) or fastidious gram-negative bacilli of the HACEK group (i.e., *Haemophilus*, *Aggregatibacter*, *Cardiobacterium hominis*, *Eikenella corrodens*, *Kingella*). Ceftriaxone has been administered on an outpatient basis for the treatment of endocarditis† caused by susceptible bacteria.

Ceftriaxone also is used for prevention of α-hemolytic (viridans group) streptococcal endocarditis† in individuals undergoing certain dental or upper respiratory tract procedures who have cardiac conditions that put them at highest risk of adverse outcomes from endocarditis. (See Uses: Prevention of Bacterial Endocarditis.)

The American Heart Association (AHA) recommends that treatment of endocarditis be managed in consultation with an infectious disease expert, especially when endocarditis is caused by *S. pneumoniae*, β-hemolytic streptococci, staphylococci, or enterococci.

For additional information on management of endocarditis, current guidelines from AHA should be consulted.

Endocarditis Caused by Viridans Group Streptococci or S. gallolyticus

For the treatment of native valve endocarditis† caused by viridans group streptococci or *S. gallolyticus* (formerly *S. bovis*) highly susceptible to penicillin (penicillin MIC 0.12 mcg/mL or less), AHA states that a 4-week regimen of IV penicillin G or IV or IM ceftriaxone is reasonable in adults and pediatric patients. If necessary in those unable to tolerate penicillin G or ceftriaxone, a 4-week regimen of IV vancomycin can be used. In *selected* adults, AHA states that a 2-week regimen that consists of IV penicillin G or IV or IM ceftriaxone in conjunction with IV or IM gentamicin is reasonable. The 2-week regimen should be considered only in adults with uncomplicated native valve endocarditis caused by highly penicillin-susceptible viridans group streptococci or *S. gallolyticus* who are at low risk for gentamicin adverse effects; the 2-week regimen is *not* recommended in those with known cardiac or extracardiac abscess, creatinine clearance less than 20 mL/minute, impaired eighth cranial nerve function, or infections caused by *Abiotrophia*, *Granulicatella*, or *Gemella*. In addition, AHA states that the 2-week regimen is *not* recommended in pediatric patients because of lack of clinical data.

For the treatment of native valve endocarditis† caused by viridans group streptococci or *S. gallolyticus* relatively resistant to penicillin (penicillin MIC greater than 0.12 mcg/mL but less than 0.5 mcg/mL), AHA states that a 4-week regimen of either IV penicillin G (or IV ampicillin) or IV or IM ceftriaxone in conjunction with IV or IM gentamicin given during the initial 2 weeks of treatment is reasonable in adults and pediatric patients. If the isolate is susceptible to ceftriaxone, AHA states that a 4-week regimen of ceftriaxone alone may be considered in adults. A 4-week regimen of vancomycin alone is a reasonable alternative only in adults unable to tolerate β-lactam anti-infectives.

If native valve endocarditis is caused by viridans group streptococci, *Abiotrophia defectiva*, or *Granulicatella* that are resistant to penicillin (penicillin MIC 0.5 mcg/mL or greater), AHA states that a regimen of IV penicillin G (or ampicillin) in conjunction with gentamicin is reasonable in adults. These experts state that a regimen of ceftriaxone in conjunction with gentamicin may be a reasonable alternative in adults for the treatment of native valve endocarditis† caused by viridans group streptococci that are resistant to penicillin but susceptible to ceftriaxone.

For the treatment of endocarditis† involving prosthetic valves or other prosthetic material caused by viridans group streptococci or *S. gallolyticus* highly susceptible to penicillin (penicillin MIC 0.12 mcg/mL or less), AHA states that a 6-week regimen of IV penicillin G or IV or IM ceftriaxone given with or without IV or IM gentamicin during the initial 2 weeks of treatment is reasonable in adults. When highly penicillin-susceptible strains are involved, there is no evidence that use of the combination regimen that includes gentamicin during the first 2 weeks is more effective than use of the β-lactam alone. If endocarditis† involving prosthetic valves or other prosthetic material is caused by viridans group streptococci or *S. gallolyticus* relatively or highly resistant to penicillin (penicillin MIC greater than 0.12 mcg/mL), AHA states that it is reasonable for adults to receive a 6-week regimen of IV penicillin G or IV or IM ceftriaxone given with a 6-week regimen of IV or IM gentamicin. In adults unable to tolerate penicillin G, ceftriaxone, or gentamicin, a 6-week regimen of IV vancomycin can be used.

Endocarditis Caused by S. pneumoniae, S. pyogenes, S. agalactiae, or Groups C, F, and G Streptococci

For the treatment of endocarditis† involving native valves or prosthetic valves or other prosthetic material caused by *S. pneumoniae* highly susceptible to penicillin (penicillin MIC 0.1 mcg/mL or less), AHA states that penicillin G, ceftriaxone, or cefazolin are reasonable choices in adults. If endocarditis is caused by *S. pneumoniae* with penicillin resistance (penicillin MIC greater than 0.1 mcg/mL), AHA states that treatment with high-dose penicillin G or a third generation cephalosporin (cefotaxime, ceftriaxone) is reasonable in adults if meningitis is not present; cefotaxime or ceftriaxone is reasonable if meningitis is present. AHA states that use of cefotaxime or ceftriaxone in conjunction with vancomycin and rifampin may be considered in adults if endocarditis is caused by *S. pneumoniae* resistant to cefotaxime (cefotaxime MIC greater than 2 mcg/mL).

For the treatment of endocarditis† caused by *S. pyogenes*, AHA states that penicillin G is a reasonable regimen in adults and ceftriaxone is a reasonable alternative. Vancomycin is a reasonable alternative only for those unable to tolerate β-lactam anti-infectives.

AHA states that penicillin G or ceftriaxone is a reasonable regimen for the treatment of endocarditis† caused by *S. agalactiae* or groups C and G streptococci in adults, but concomitant use of gentamicin during the initial weeks of treatment should be considered.

Enterococcal Endocarditis

For the treatment of enterococcal endocarditis†, AHA states that a double-β-lactam regimen of ampicillin and ceftriaxone is a reasonable option in certain adults.

Enterococcus (e.g., *E. faecalis*, *E. faecium*) are relatively resistant to penicillins and vancomycin and a synergistic combination regimen of penicillin, ampicillin, or vancomycin in conjunction with an aminoglycoside (gentamicin or streptomycin) has usually been used for the treatment of enterococcal endocarditis. However, enterococci resistant to aminoglycosides have been reported with increasing frequency and AHA states that all enterococcal isolates should be routinely tested for in vitro susceptibility to penicillin and vancomycin and for high-level resistance to gentamicin to predict synergistic interactions and aid in selection of the most appropriate treatment regimen.

Although there are few therapeutic alternatives to aminoglycoside-containing regimens for the treatment of enterococcal endocarditis, there are some data from in vitro and in vivo studies and limited clinical experience indicating that a double β-lactam regimen of ampicillin and ceftriaxone can be effective for the treatment of endocarditis caused by *E. faecalis*, including gentamicin-resistant strains. The major advantages of the ampicillin and ceftriaxone regimen are the lower risk of nephrotoxicity and the lack of any need to measure aminoglycoside serum concentrations; a potential disadvantage of this regimen is the possibility of hypersensitivity reactions to 2 separate β-lactam anti-infectives.

For the treatment of enterococcal endocarditis† involving native valves, prosthetic valves, or other prosthetic material caused by strains susceptible to penicillin and gentamicin in adults who can tolerate β-lactam anti-infectives, AHA states that either a regimen of IV ampicillin or IV penicillin G given in conjunction with gentamicin for 4–6 weeks or a double β-lactam regimen of IV ampicillin and IV ceftriaxone given for 6 weeks is reasonable. The most appropriate regimen should be selected based on characteristics of the individual patient. The double β-lactam regimen is recommended in adults who should not receive an aminoglycoside (i.e., creatinine clearance less than 50 mL/minute [pretreatment or developed during treatment with a gentamicin-containing regimen], impaired eighth cranial nerve function).

For the treatment of enterococcal endocarditis† involving native valves, prosthetic valves, or other prosthetic material caused by strains susceptible to penicillin but resistant to gentamicin in adults who can tolerate β-lactam anti-infectives, AHA states that a double β-lactam regimen of IV ampicillin and IV ceftriaxone given for 6 weeks is reasonable. If enterococcal endocarditis is caused by penicillin-susceptible strains that are gentamicin-resistant but streptomycin-susceptible, a double β-lactam regimen of IV ampicillin and IV ceftriaxone given for 6 weeks is reasonable in adults; alternatively, a regimen of IV ampicillin or IV penicillin G given in conjunction with IV or IM streptomycin for 4–6 weeks can be considered if the patient has a creatinine clearance of 50 mL/minute or greater and rapid tests for streptomycin serum concentrations

are available. A 6-week regimen of vancomycin in conjunction with gentamicin should be considered only when enterococcal endocarditis is caused by strains intrinsically resistant to penicillin or the patient cannot tolerate β-lactam anti-infectives.

Endocarditis Caused by the HACEK Group

AHA states that ceftriaxone is a reasonable option for the treatment of endocarditis† caused by the HACEK group in adults and pediatric patients.

The slow-growing fastidious gram-negative bacilli known as the HACEK group (i.e., *Haemophilus*, *Aggregatibacter*, *C. hominis*, *E. corrodens*, *Kingella*) account for approximately 5–10% of cases of community-acquired native valve endocarditis in patients who are not IV drug abusers and also rarely cause prosthetic valve endocarditis. Because β-lactamase-producing strains have been reported with increasing frequency, AHA states that the HACEK group should be considered ampicillin-resistant and penicillin and ampicillin should not be used for the treatment of HACEK endocarditis unless results of in vitro susceptibility testing are available.

AHA states that a 4-week regimen of IV or IM ceftriaxone alone is a reasonable choice for the treatment of native valve endocarditis† caused by the HACEK group and a 6-week regimen of the drug is a reasonable choice for the treatment of endocarditis involving prosthetic valves or other prosthetic material† caused by the HACEK group since most strains are susceptible to ceftriaxone or other third or fourth generation cephalosporins. Although ceftriaxone is preferred in such patients, cefotaxime or another third or fourth generation cephalosporin could be substituted and IV ampicillin is an option if in vitro susceptibility testing is performed and the isolate is susceptible. For the treatment of HACEK endocarditis in adults unable to tolerate ceftriaxone or other appropriate cephalosporin, AHA states that a fluoroquinolone (ciprofloxacin, levofloxacin, moxifloxacin) may be considered as an alternative since the HACEK group usually is susceptible to fluoroquinolones in vitro; however, such patients should be treated in consultation with an infectious disease specialist.

In pediatric patients with endocarditis caused by the HACEK group, AHA recommends a 4-week regimen of ceftriaxone or another third-generation cephalosporin (e.g., cefotaxime) used alone or a regimen of ampicillin in conjunction with gentamicin (or amikacin or tobramycin).

● GI Infections

Ceftriaxone has been used for the treatment of gastroenteritis† caused by *Salmonella* or *Shigella*. Ceftriaxone also is recommended as an alternative for empiric treatment of infectious diarrhea† in individuals with human immunodeficiency virus (HIV) infection or for long-term suppressive antibacterial therapy† (secondary prophylaxis) in such individuals.

Salmonella Gastroenteritis

Anti-infective therapy generally is not indicated in otherwise healthy individuals with uncomplicated (noninvasive) gastroenteritis caused by nontyphoidal *Salmonella* (e.g., *Salmonella* serovars Enteritidis or Typhimurium) since such therapy may prolong the duration of fecal excretion of the organism and there is no evidence that it shortens the duration of the disease; however, the US Centers for Disease Control and Prevention (CDC), National Institutes of Health (NIH), IDSA, and others recommend anti-infective therapy in individuals with severe *Salmonella* gastroenteritis and in those who are at increased risk for invasive disease. These individuals include infants younger than 3–6 months of age; individuals older than 50 years of age; individuals with hemoglobinopathies, severe atherosclerosis or valvular heart disease, prostheses, uremia, chronic GI disease, or severe colitis; and individuals who are immunocompromised because of malignancy, immunosuppressive therapy, HIV infection, or other immunosuppressive illness.

When an anti-infective agent is considered necessary in an individual with *Salmonella* gastroenteritis, CDC, AAP, IDSA, and others recommend ceftriaxone, cefotaxime, a fluoroquinolone (should be used in children only if benefits outweigh risks and no other alternative exists), ampicillin, amoxicillin, co-trimoxazole, or chloramphenicol, depending on susceptibility of the causative organism. Some experts recommend that patients with presumed or proven nontyphoidal *Salmonella* gastroenteritis receive an initial dose of ceftriaxone followed by oral azithromycin pending results of diagnostic evaluation. The fact that multidrug-resistant *Salmonella* have been reported with increasing frequency in the US should be considered.

Because HIV-infected individuals with *Salmonella* infections are at increased risk for bacteremia and mortality compared with patients without HIV infection,

CDC, NIH, and IDSA recommend that *all* HIV-infected patients with salmonellosis receive antibacterial treatment. In addition, some clinicians suggest that long-term suppressive antibacterial therapy (secondary prophylaxis) can be considered in HIV-infected adults and adolescents with recurrent *Salmonella* gastroenteritis (with or without bacteremia) and in those with CD4+ T-cell counts less than 200 cells/mm³ and severe diarrhea. However, the value of secondary prophylaxis has not been established and possible benefits must be weighed against the risks of long-term antibacterial exposure. CDC, NIH, and IDSA state that ciprofloxacin is the drug of choice for the treatment of *Salmonella* gastroenteritis (with or without bacteremia) and for long-term suppressive therapy in HIV-infected adults and adolescents; other fluoroquinolones (e.g., levofloxacin, moxifloxacin) are likely to be effective, but clinical data are limited. Depending on in vitro susceptibility of the causative organism, these experts recommend co-trimoxazole, ceftriaxone, or cefotaxime as alternatives for such treatment or secondary prophylaxis in HIV-infected adults and adolescents.

For information on the treatment of typhoid and paratyphoid fever (enteric fever) or bacteremia caused by *Salmonella*, see Uses: Typhoid Fever and Other Invasive Salmonella Infections.

Shigella Infections

Ceftriaxone has been effective when used for the treatment of shigellosis† caused by susceptible *Shigella sonnei* or *S. flexneri* and has been recommended as an alternative when anti-infectives are indicated for the treatment of shigella infections.

Infections caused by *S. sonnei* usually are self-limited (48–72 hours), and mild cases may not require treatment with anti-infectives. However, since anti-infectives may shorten the duration of diarrhea and period of fecal excretion of *Shigella*, anti-infective treatment generally is recommended in addition to fluid and electrolyte replacement in patients with severe shigellosis, dysentery, or underlying immunosuppression.

Although an empiric regimen can be used initially when anti-infectives are indicated in the treatment of *Shigella* infections, in vitro susceptibility testing of clinical isolates is indicated since resistance to ampicillin and co-trimoxazole is common and strains resistant to ciprofloxacin, ceftriaxone, or azithromycin have been reported with increasing frequency. For infections caused by *Shigella* resistant to ampicillin and co-trimoxazole or when in vitro susceptibility of the isolate is unknown, ceftriaxone, a fluoroquinolone (e.g., ciprofloxacin), or azithromycin is recommended.

For the treatment of *Shigella* infections in HIV-infected adults and adolescents, CDC, NIH, and IDSA state that the drug of choice is ciprofloxacin and alternatives are levofloxacin, moxifloxacin, co-trimoxazole, or azithromycin.

Empiric Treatment of Infectious Diarrhea

CDC, NIH, and IDSA recommend that adults and adolescents with advanced HIV disease (CD4+ T-cell counts less than 200 cells/mm³ or concomitant AIDS-defining illness) who have clinically severe diarrhea (i.e., 6 or more liquid stools per day, bloody stools, or any number of liquid stools per day accompanied by fever or chills) should undergo diagnostic evaluation to determine the etiology of the diarrheal illness and receive appropriate anti-infective treatment. These experts state that ciprofloxacin is preferred and ceftriaxone and cefotaxime are reasonable alternatives when empiric treatment of severe bacterial diarrhea is indicated in HIV-infected adults and adolescents. Treatment should be adjusted if needed when results of diagnostic testing are available. If diarrhea persists for longer than 14 days without other clinical signs of severity (e.g., bloody stool, dehydration), additional evaluation is indicated and pathogen-directed therapy should be initiated after a diagnosis is confirmed.

The possibility of resistant infections should be considered when selecting an empiric anti-infective regimen for treatment of diarrhea in HIV-infected travelers during travel or after return to the US.

● Intra-abdominal Infections

Ceftriaxone is used for the treatment of intra-abdominal infections caused by susceptible *E. coli*, *K. pneumoniae*, *Clostridium*, or *Peptostreptococcus*. The drug also has been used for the treatment of various gynecologic infections, including pelvic inflammatory disease. (See Uses: Pelvic Inflammatory Disease.) Although the manufacturers state that ceftriaxone can be used for the treatment of intra-abdominal infections caused by *Bacteroides fragilis*, the drug has been ineffective in the treatment of intra-abdominal infections when *B. fragilis* was present and superinfection with this organism has been reported occasionally.

Although monotherapy with ceftriaxone is an option for initial empiric treatment of mild to moderate community-acquired biliary tract infections (acute cholecystitis or cholangitis), ceftriaxone should be used in conjunction with metronidazole for initial empiric treatment of mild to moderate extrabiliary community-acquired intra-abdominal infections.

For additional information on management of intra-abdominal infections, current clinical practice guidelines from IDSA available at http://www.idsociety.org should be consulted.

● Meningitis and Other CNS Infections

Ceftriaxone is used in neonates, children, and adults for the treatment of meningitis caused by susceptible *H. influenzae*, *N. meningitidis*, or *S. pneumoniae*. The drug also has been used for the treatment of meningitis and other CNS infections caused by susceptible Enterobacteriaceae† (e.g., *E. coli*, *Klebsiella*†) or *S. epidermidis*.

IV cefotaxime with or without other anti-infectives (e.g., ampicillin, gentamicin, vancomycin) has been recommended for empiric treatment of meningitis†. Pending results of CSF culture and in vitro susceptibility testing, the most appropriate anti-infective regimen for empiric treatment of suspected bacterial meningitis should be selected based on results of CSF gram stain and antigen tests, age of the patient, the most likely pathogen(s) and source of infection, and current patterns of bacterial resistance within the hospital and local community. When results of culture and susceptibility tests become available and the pathogen is identified, the empiric anti-infective regimen should be modified (if necessary) to ensure that the most effective regimen is being administered. Ceftriaxone should *not* be used alone for empiric treatment of meningitis when *Listeria monocytogenes*, enterococci, staphylococci, or *Pseudomonas aeruginosa* may be involved.

Meningitis Caused by Streptococcus pneumoniae

IV ceftriaxone and IV cefotaxime are considered drugs of choice for the treatment of meningitis caused by susceptible *S. pneumoniae*. While cefotaxime and ceftriaxone generally have been considered the drugs of choice when meningitis is caused by penicillin-resistant *S. pneumoniae*, treatment failures have been reported when these cephalosporins were used alone for the treatment of meningitis caused by *S. pneumoniae* with intermediate or high-level penicillin resistance (i.e., penicillin MIC 0.1 mcg/mL or greater). In addition, strains of *S. pneumoniae* with reduced susceptibility to cephalosporins have been reported with increasing frequency and use of cefotaxime or ceftriaxone alone may be ineffective for the treatment of meningitis caused by these strains. The prevalence of *S. pneumoniae* with reduced susceptibility to penicillin and/or cephalosporins varies geographically, and clinicians should be aware of the prevalence and pattern of *S. pneumoniae* drug resistance in the local community to optimize empiric and initial treatment regimens for serious pneumococcal infections. Because susceptibility can no longer be assumed, *S. pneumoniae* isolates should be routinely tested for in vitro susceptibility.

If anti-infective therapy in a patient with meningitis is initiated with an empiric regimen of IV ceftriaxone and IV vancomycin (with or without rifampin) and results of culture and in vitro susceptibility testing indicate that the pathogen involved is a strain of *S. pneumoniae* susceptible to ceftriaxone and susceptible or resistant to penicillin, vancomycin and rifampin can be discontinued and therapy completed using ceftriaxone alone. If the isolate is found to have reduced susceptibility to ceftriaxone *and* penicillin, both IV ceftriaxone and IV vancomycin usually are continued and consideration given to adding rifampin to the regimen. If meningitis is caused by *S. pneumoniae* highly resistant to ceftriaxone (i.e., MIC 4 mcg/mL or greater), consultation with an infectious disease expert is recommended.

Meningitis Caused by Haemophilus influenzae

IV ceftriaxone and IV cefotaxime are considered drugs of choice for initial treatment of meningitis caused by susceptible *H. influenzae* (including penicillinase-producing strains). In children, AAP suggests that ampicillin may be substituted if the isolate is susceptible; however, because of the prevalence of ampicillin-resistant *H. influenzae*, ampicillin should not be used alone for empiric treatment of meningitis when *H. influenzae* may be involved. The incidence of *H. influenzae* meningitis in the US has decreased considerably since *H. influenzae* type b (Hib) conjugate vaccines became available for immunization of infants.

Meningitis Caused by Neisseria meningitidis

IV ceftriaxone and IV cefotaxime are considered drugs of choice for empiric treatment of meningitis when *N. meningitidis* may be involved. If a diagnosis of *N. meningitidis* meningitis is confirmed, AAP and other clinicians suggest treatment with penicillin G or, alternatively, ampicillin, ceftriaxone, or cefotaxime. Chloramphenicol, if available, is recommended by AAP for the treatment of *N. meningitidis* meningitis in patients with a history of anaphylactoid-type hypersensitivity reactions to penicillin.

Meningitis Caused by Enterobacteriaceae

Some clinicians recommend that meningitis caused by Enterobacteriaceae† (e.g., *E. coli*, *K. pneumoniae*†) be treated with a third generation cephalosporins (i.e., cefotaxime, ceftazidime, ceftriaxone) with or without an aminoglycoside. Because ceftazidime (but not cefotaxime or ceftriaxone) is effective for the treatment of meningitis caused by *Ps. aeruginosa*, some clinicians suggest that a regimen of ceftazidime and an aminoglycoside may be preferred for the treatment of meningitis caused by gram-negative bacilli pending results of culture and in vitro susceptibility testing.

Meningitis Caused by Streptococcus agalactiae

Third generation cephalosporins (i.e., ceftriaxone, cefotaxime) have been suggested as an alternative for the treatment of meningitis caused by *S. agalactiae*†.

For initial treatment of meningitis or other severe infection caused by *S. agalactiae*, a regimen of IV ampicillin or IV penicillin G given in conjunction with an aminoglycoside is recommended. Some clinicians suggest that IV ampicillin is the drug of choice for the treatment of *S. agalactiae* meningitis and that an aminoglycoside (IV gentamicin) should be used concomitantly during the first 72 hours until in vitro susceptibility testing is completed and a clinical response is observed; thereafter, ampicillin can be given alone if the strain is susceptible to the drug.

Meningitis Caused by Listeria monocytogenes

The optimal regimen for the treatment of meningitis caused by *L. monocytogenes* has not been established. Ceftriaxone is ineffective in and should not be used alone for the treatment of meningitis caused by *L. monocytogenes*. AAP and other clinicians generally recommend that meningitis or other severe infection caused by *L. monocytogenes* be treated with a regimen of IV ampicillin with or without an aminoglycoside (usually gentamicin); alternatively, a regimen of penicillin G in conjunction with gentamicin can be used. In patients hypersensitive to penicillin, the preferred alternative regimen for treatment of meningitis caused by *L. monocytogenes* is co-trimoxazole.

Other CNS Infections

Ceftriaxone is a drug of choice for the treatment of healthcare-associated ventriculitis and meningitis caused by susceptible β-lactamase-producing *H. influenzae* or susceptible Enterobacteriaceae†. Ceftriaxone also is a drug of choice for the treatment of healthcare-associated ventriculitis and meningitis caused by susceptible *S. pneumoniae* when penicillin G is not the preferred anti-infective (i.e., penicillin MIC 0.12 mcg/mL or greater). Some experts state that ceftriaxone can be used alone if the infection is caused by *S. pneumoniae* with penicillin MIC less than 1 mcg/mL, but should be used in conjunction with vancomycin if the strain has a penicillin MIC 1 mcg/mL or greater and that consideration should be given to also including rifampin in the regimen if the strain has a ceftriaxone MIC greater than 2 mcg/mL.

Although penicillin G usually is the drug of choice, ceftriaxone is recommended as an alternative for the treatment of healthcare-associated ventriculitis and meningitis caused by susceptible *C. acnes*† (formerly *P. acnes*).

● Acute Otitis Media

IM ceftriaxone is used for the treatment of acute otitis media (AOM) caused by *S. pneumoniae*, *H. influenzae* (including β- lactamase-producing strains), or *Moraxella catarrhalis* (including β-lactamase-producing strains).

When anti-infective therapy is indicated for the treatment of AOM, AAP recommends high-dose amoxicillin or amoxicillin and clavulanate potassium as the drug of first choice for initial treatment. These experts recommend certain cephalosporins (cefdinir, cefpodoxime, cefuroxime, ceftriaxone) as alternatives for initial treatment in penicillin-allergic patients who do not have a history of severe and/or recent penicillin-allergic reactions.

Ceftriaxone has been shown to be effective for initial or repeat treatment of AOM, and is a good choice when the patient has persistent vomiting or cannot otherwise tolerate an oral regimen. The manufacturers recommend a single-dose regimen of IM ceftriaxone for the treatment of AOM, but caution that

the potential advantages of this single-dose parenteral regimen should be balanced against its potentially lower clinical cure rate compared with a 10-day oral anti-infective regimen. AAP states that either a 1- or 3-day regimen† of IM or IV ceftriaxone can be used for initial treatment of AOM, but cautions that there is some evidence that more than a single dose of the drug may be required to prevent recurrence of middle ear infections within 5–7 days after the initial dose. A 3-day regimen† of ceftriaxone is recommended for retreatment in patients who fail to respond to initial treatment with other anti-infectives.

Results of several controlled clinical studies in pediatric patients with AOM indicate that the short-term clinical response rate to a single-dose IM ceftriaxone regimen is similar to that of a 10-day regimen of oral cefaclor (40 mg/kg daily), a 7- or 10-day regimen of oral amoxicillin (40 mg/kg daily), a 10-day regimen of oral co-trimoxazole (8 mg/kg trimethoprim and 40 mg/kg of sulfamethoxazole daily), or a 10-day regimen of oral amoxicillin and clavulanate potassium; however, in one study, the single-dose IM ceftriaxone regimen had a lower clinical cure rate than a 10-day regimen of oral amoxicillin and clavulanate potassium.

A 3-day regimen of IM ceftriaxone has been shown to be more effective than a 1-day regimen for retreatment in patients who fail to respond to initial treatment with another anti-infective. The 3-day ceftriaxone regimen has been effective for the treatment of persistent or relapsing otitis media caused by *H. influenzae*, *M. catarrhalis*, *S. pyogenes*, or penicillin-susceptible *S. pneumoniae*; however, treatment failures have been reported when the causative agent was *S. pneumoniae* with reduced susceptibility to penicillin.

For additional information on diagnosis and management of AOM, current AAP clinical practice guidelines for AOM should be consulted.

● Respiratory Tract Infections

Ceftriaxone is used in adults and pediatric patients for the treatment of lower respiratory tract infections (including pneumonia) caused by susceptible gram-positive cocci (e.g., *S. pneumoniae*, *S. aureus*) or gram-negative bacteria (e.g., *H. influenzae*, *H. parainfluenzae*, *K. pneumoniae*, *E. coli*, *Enterobacter aerogenes*, *P. mirabilis*, *Serratia marcescens*). Ceftriaxone generally has been effective in the treatment of pneumonia caused by *S. pneumoniae* with intermediate resistance to penicillin (i.e., penicillin MIC less than 0.1–2 mcg/mL), but treatment failures have been reported when the drug was used alone in the treatment of severe infections (e.g., meningitis) caused by strains with intermediate or high-level penicillin resistance (i.e., penicillin MIC 0.12 mcg/mL or greater). (See Uses: Meningitis and Other CNS Infections.)

Acute Sinusitis

Ceftriaxone is used as an alternative for the treatment of acute bacterial sinusitis†.

When anti-infective therapy is indicated for the treatment of acute bacterial sinusitis, IDSA recommends amoxicillin and clavulanate potassium and AAP recommends either amoxicillin or amoxicillin and clavulanate potassium as the drug of choice for initial empiric treatment. Because of variable activity against *S. pneumoniae* and *H. influenzae*, IDSA no longer recommends second or third generation oral cephalosporins for empiric monotherapy of sinusitis in adults or children. If an oral cephalosporin is used as an alternative for empiric treatment of acute bacterial sinusitis in children (e.g., in penicillin-allergic individuals), IDSA and AAP recommend a combination regimen that includes a third generation cephalosporin (cefixime or cefpodoxime) and clindamycin (or linezolid). In children who are vomiting, unable to tolerate oral therapy, or unlikely to adhere to the initial doses, treatment of acute sinusitis can be initiated with a single dose of IV or IM ceftriaxone and then switched to an oral regimen if clinical improvement is observed at 24 hours. IV ceftriaxone also is an alternative for severe sinusitis requiring hospitalization.

Community-acquired Pneumonia

IDSA and the American Thoracic Society (ATS) recommend ceftriaxone as an alternative to penicillin G, ampicillin, or amoxicillin for the treatment of community-acquired pneumonia (CAP) caused by penicillin-susceptible *S. pneumoniae* and as a preferred drug for the treatment of CAP caused by penicillin-resistant *S. pneumoniae*, provided in vitro susceptibility has been demonstrated. These experts state that ceftriaxone is a preferred anti-infective for the treatment of CAP caused by β-lactamase-producing *H. influenzae*. IDSA and ATS also recommend use of ceftriaxone in certain combination regimens used for empiric treatment of CAP. The drug has been administered on an outpatient basis for empiric anti-infective therapy in adults with CAP who did not require hospitalization.

Initial treatment of CAP generally involves use of an empiric anti-infective regimen based on the most likely pathogens and local susceptibility patterns; therapy may then be changed (if possible) to provide a more specific regimen (pathogen-directed therapy) based on results of in vitro culture and susceptibility testing. The most appropriate empiric regimen varies depending on the severity of illness at the time of presentation and whether outpatient treatment or hospitalization in or out of an intensive care unit (ICU) is indicated and the presence or absence of cardiopulmonary disease and other modifying factors that increase the risk of certain pathogens (e.g., penicillin- or multidrug-resistant *S. pneumoniae*, enteric gram-negative bacilli, *Ps. aeruginosa*).

Most experts recommend that an empiric regimen for treatment of CAP include an anti-infective active against *S. pneumoniae* since this organism is the most commonly identified cause of bacterial pneumonia and causes more severe disease than many other common CAP pathogens. Pathogens most frequently involved in *outpatient* CAP include *S. pneumoniae*, *M. pneumoniae*, *Chlamydophila pneumoniae* (formerly *Chlamydia pneumoniae*), respiratory viruses, and *H. influenzae*. Pathogens most frequently involved in *inpatient* CAP in non-ICU patients are *S. pneumoniae*, *M. pneumoniae*, *C. pneumoniae*, *H. influenzae*, *Legionella*, and respiratory viruses. Patients with severe CAP admitted into the ICU usually have infections caused by *S. pneumoniae*, *S. aureus*, *Legionella*, gram-negative bacilli, or *H. influenzae*. Coverage against anaerobic bacteria usually is indicated only in classic aspiration pleuropulmonary syndrome in patients who had loss of consciousness as a result of alcohol or drug overdosage or after seizures in patients with concomitant gingival disease or esophageal motility disorders.

Inpatient treatment of CAP is initiated with a parenteral regimen, although therapy may be changed to an oral regimen if the patient is improving clinically, is hemodynamically stable, able to ingest drugs, and has a normally functioning GI tract. CAP patients usually have a clinical response within 3–7 days after initiation of therapy and a switch to oral therapy generally can be made during this period.

For empiric *outpatient* treatment of CAP in adults when risk factors for drug-resistant *S. pneumoniae* are present (e.g., comorbidities such as chronic heart, lung, liver, or renal disease, diabetes, alcoholism, malignancies, asplenia, immunosuppression, use of anti-infectives within the last 3 months), ATS and IDSA recommend monotherapy with a fluoroquinolone active against *S. pneumoniae* (moxifloxacin, gemifloxacin, levofloxacin) or, alternatively, a combination regimen that includes a β-lactam active against *S. pneumoniae* (high-dose amoxicillin or fixed combination of amoxicillin and clavulanic acid or, alternatively, ceftriaxone, cefpodoxime, or cefuroxime) given in conjunction with a macrolide (azithromycin, clarithromycin, erythromycin) or doxycycline.

For empiric *inpatient* treatment of CAP in adult non-ICU patients, IDSA and ATS recommend monotherapy with a fluoroquinolone (moxifloxacin, gemifloxacin, levofloxacin) or, alternatively, a combination regimen that includes a β-lactam (usually cefotaxime, ceftriaxone, or ampicillin) given in conjunction with a macrolide (azithromycin, clarithromycin, erythromycin). For empiric *inpatient* treatment of CAP in adult ICU patients when *Pseudomonas* and methicillin-resistant *S. aureus* (MRSA; also known as oxacillin-resistant *S. aureus* or ORSA) are *not* suspected, IDSA and ATS recommend a combination regimen that includes a β-lactam (cefotaxime, ceftriaxone, fixed combination of ampicillin and sulbactam) given in conjunction with either azithromycin or a fluoroquinolone (gemifloxacin, levofloxacin, moxifloxacin).

For additional information on management of respiratory tract infections, including CAP, current clinical practice guidelines from IDSA available at http://www.idsociety.org should be consulted.

● Septicemia

Ceftriaxone is used in adults and pediatric patients for the treatment of septicemia caused by *S. aureus*, *S. pneumoniae*, *H. influenzae*, *E. coli*, or *K. pneumoniae*.

● Skin and Skin Structure Infections

Ceftriaxone is used for the treatment of skin and skin structure infections caused by susceptible *S. aureus*, *S. epidermidis*, *S. pyogenes*, viridans group streptococci, *E. cloacae*, *E. coli*, *K. oxytoca*, *K. pneumoniae*, *P. mirabilis*, *Morganella morganii*, *S. marcescens*, *Acinetobacter calcoaceticus*, *B. fragilis*, or *Peptostreptococcus*.

Ceftriaxone has been recommended for use in multiple-drug anti-infective regimens for empiric treatment of necrotizing infections of the skin, fascia, and muscle†. Because necrotizing fasciitis (including Fornier gangrene) may be polymicrobial (e.g., mixed aerobic-anaerobic infections) or monomicrobial (e.g., *S. pyogenes*, *S. aureus*, *Vibrio vulnificus*, *Aeromonas hydrophila*, *Peptostreptococcus*),

IDSA recommends that empiric anti-infective regimens be selected to provide broad-spectrum coverage.

Ceftriaxone in conjunction with metronidazole has been recommended as an option for the treatment of surgical site infections that occur following GI or genitourinary surgery. For the treatment of surgical site infections that occur following procedures involving the axilla or perineum, ceftriaxone is recommended as an option; concomitant vancomycin may also be needed for coverage against methicillin-resistant *S. aureus*.

Ceftriaxone also is one of several options recommended for empiric treatment of infected animal bite wounds or for empiric treatment of moderate or severe diabetic foot infections.

Although the manufacturers state that ceftriaxone can be used for the treatment of skin and skin structure infections caused by *Ps. aeruginosa*, treatment failures have been reported when ceftriaxone was used alone in the treatment of urinary tract infections or respiratory tract infections caused by *Ps. aeruginosa*. Some of these failures occurred because superinfection with resistant strains of *Ps. aeruginosa* occurred during treatment with the drug. Because many strains of *Ps. aeruginosa* are only susceptible to high concentrations of ceftriaxone in vitro and because resistant strains of the organism have developed during treatment with the drug, many clinicians state that ceftriaxone should not be used alone in any infection where *Ps. aeruginosa* may be present.

For additional information on management of skin and skin structure infections, current clinical practice guidelines from IDSA available at http://www.idsociety.org should be consulted.

● Urinary Tract Infections

Ceftriaxone is used in adult and pediatric patients for the treatment of complicated and uncomplicated urinary tract infections caused by *E. coli*, *K. pneumoniae*, *M. morganii*, *P. mirabilis*, or *P. vulgaris*.

The most appropriate anti-infective for the treatment of urinary tract infections should be selected based on the severity of the infection and results of culture and in vitro susceptibility testing. It has been suggested that certain parenteral cephalosporins (i.e., cefepime, cefotaxime, ceftriaxone, ceftazidime) may be drugs of choice for the treatment of complicated urinary tract infections caused by susceptible Enterobacteriaceae, including susceptible strains of *E. coli*, *K. pneumoniae*, *P. rettgeri*, *M. morganii*, *P. vulgaris*, or *P. stuartii*; an aminoglycoside usually is used concomitantly in severe infections. Ceftriaxone may be particularly useful as initial therapy for the treatment of nosocomial urinary tract infections known or suspected to be caused by multidrug-resistant Enterobacteriaceae. However, ceftriaxone, like other third generation cephalosporins, generally should *not* be used in the treatment of uncomplicated urinary tract infections when other anti-infectives with a narrower spectrum of activity could be used.

● Chancroid

A single IM dose of ceftriaxone is used for the treatment of chancroid† (genital ulcers caused by *H. ducreyi*).

CDC and other clinicians state that a single IM dose of ceftriaxone, a single oral dose of azithromycin, a 3-day oral ciprofloxacin regimen (contraindicated in pregnant or lactating women), or a 7-day oral erythromycin regimen are recommended for the treatment of chancroid.

HIV-infected individuals and patients who are uncircumcised may not respond to treatment of chancroid as well as those who are HIV-negative or circumcised. Clinicians should consider that, although treatment failures can occur with any of the recommended regimens, only limited data are available regarding efficacy of the single-dose ceftriaxone and single-dose azithromycin regimens for the treatment of chancroid in HIV-infected individuals. Because treatment failures and slow healing of ulcers are more likely in HIV-infected individuals, such patients should be monitored closely and more prolonged treatment or retreatment may be necessary.

Data are limited regarding the prevalence of *H. ducreyi* resistant to the anti-infectives recommended for treatment. Some treatment failures that have occurred in HIV-infected individuals who received the single-dose ceftriaxone regimen for the treatment of chancroid did not appear to be related to ceftriaxone resistance since isolates of *H. ducreyi* obtained from these individuals were susceptible to ceftriaxone in vitro.

For additional information on management of chancroid, current CDC sexually transmitted diseases treatment guidelines available at http://www.cdc.gov/std should be consulted.

● *Gonorrhea and Associated Infections*

Ceftriaxone is used in adults, adolescents, and pediatric patients for the treatment of uncomplicated gonorrhea, disseminated gonorrhea (including meningitis and endocarditis), and various other gonococcal infections caused by *Neisseria gonorrhoeae*, including infections caused by penicillin-, fluoroquinolone-, and tetracycline-resistant strains. Ceftriaxone in conjunction with azithromycin is the regimen of choice for the treatment of gonococcal infections in most patients. Unlike the majority of other drugs that have been used for the treatment of gonococcal infections, ceftriaxone usually is effective for the treatment of gonorrhea at all sites, including cervical, urethral, rectal, and pharyngeal gonococcal infections.

Recommendations for the treatment of gonorrhea have changed multiple times over the last several decades because of the ability of *N. gonorrhoeae* to develop resistance to anti-infectives. Ceftriaxone has been considered a drug of choice for the treatment of uncomplicated and disseminated gonococcal infections since 1989 when CDC first altered their guidelines to no longer recommend use of penicillins or tetracyclines for these infections because of the widespread prevalence of antibiotic-resistant *N. gonorrhoeae*, including penicillinase-producing *N. gonorrhoeae* resistant to penicillins (PPNG), strains with plasmid-mediated resistance to tetracyclines (TRNG), and strains with chromosomally mediated resistance to multiple anti-infectives (CMRNG).

In 2007, CDC altered their guidelines to no longer recommend use of fluoroquinolones for the treatment of gonococcal infections because quinolone-resistant *N. gonorrhoeae* (QRNG) had become widespread in the US and elsewhere. As a result, cephalosporins became the only remaining class of anti-infectives that could be considered for the treatment of gonococcal infections. However, *N. gonorrhoeae* with reduced susceptibility to ceftriaxone and/or cefixime or other cephalosporins have also been reported with increasing frequency in the US and elsewhere (e.g., Asia, Europe, Canada) and there have been rare reports of *N. gonorrhoeae* with high-level ceftriaxone resistance in some countries (Japan, France, Spain).

In 2012, based on evidence of declining cefixime susceptibility among urethral *N. gonorrhoeae* isolates collected during 2006–2011 in the US and elsewhere and reports of treatment failures with cefixime and other oral cephalosporins in some countries, CDC again altered their guidelines to state that IM ceftriaxone is the cephalosporin of choice for the treatment of uncomplicated urogenital, anorectal, and pharyngeal gonorrhea and that cefixime and other oral cephalosporins should not be used for first-line treatment.

Currently, CDC and other clinicians state that dual combination treatment with ceftriaxone *and* azithromycin is the regimen of choice for gonococcal infections in the US. The theoretical basis of dual combination treatment is that the use of 2 anti-infectives with different mechanisms of action against *N. gonorrhoeae* may improve treatment efficacy and potentially delay emergence and spread of cephalosporin resistance. In addition, because individuals with *N. gonorrhoeae* infection frequently are coinfected with *Chlamydia trachomatis*, a dual regimen that includes azithromycin provides coverage against such infections. Although CDC previously stated that either a single dose of oral azithromycin or a 7-day regimen of oral doxycycline could be used as the second anti-infective in dual treatment regimens, single-dose azithromycin is now preferred because of convenience and compliance advantages and because the prevalence of *N. gonorrhoeae* resistant to tetracyclines is substantially higher than that reported for azithromycin. In patients allergic to azithromycin, multiple-dose doxycycline can be substituted for single-dose azithromycin in recommended or alternative dual treatment regimens. Dual treatment regimens should be used in all adults and adolescents with gonorrhea, regardless of the presence or absence of chlamydial coinfection.

HIV-infected individuals should receive the same treatment regimens recommended for other individuals with gonococcal infections.

CDC recommends that health-care providers treating gonorrhea remain vigilant for treatment failures (evidenced by persistent symptoms or a positive follow-up test despite treatment). If there is evidence of treatment failure and reinfection is unlikely, relevant clinical specimens should be obtained for culture (preferable with simultaneous nucleic acid amplification test [NAAT]) and in vitro susceptibility testing should be performed if *N. gonorrhoeae* is isolated. Whenever treatment failure is suspected, an infectious disease specialist, an STD/HIV Prevention Training Center (http://www.nnptc.org), local or state health department STD program, or CDC (404-639-8659) should be consulted for advice on obtaining cultures, in vitro susceptibility testing, and treatment. Suspected treatment failures should be reported to CDC through local or state health departments within 24 hours of diagnosis and clinical isolates should be sent to CDC and stored at local laboratories for possible further testing.

For additional information on management of gonococcal infections, current CDC sexually transmitted diseases treatment guidelines available at http://www.cdc.gov/std should be consulted.

Gonococcal Infections in Adults and Adolescents
Uncomplicated Cervical, Urethral, and Rectal Gonorrhea

For the treatment of uncomplicated cervical, urethral, or rectal gonorrhea in adults and adolescents, CDC states that a dual combination regimen that includes a single 250-mg IM dose of ceftriaxone *and* a dose of azithromycin (single 1-g oral dose) is the regimen of choice. In clinical trials, a single 250-mg IM dose of ceftriaxone was associated with a 99.2% cure rate in patients with uncomplicated urogenital and anorectal gonorrhea. There are no clinical data to support a ceftriaxone dose greater than 250 mg for the treatment of uncomplicated gonorrhea. Although other parenteral cephalosporins (e.g., a single 500-mg IM dose of cefotaxime or single 2-g IM dose of cefoxitin) are safe and generally effective for the treatment of uncomplicated urogenital and anorectal gonorrhea, these drugs offer no advantage over ceftriaxone for urogenital infections.

If necessary because ceftriaxone is not available or cannot be used, CDC states that adults and adolescents can receive an alternative dual combination regimen that includes a single 400-mg dose of oral cefixime *and* a dose of azithromycin (single 1-g oral dose) for the treatment of uncomplicated urogenital or anorectal gonorrhea. The oral cefixime regimen does not provide the high, sustained bactericidal blood concentrations provided by IM ceftriaxone and has been associated with a cure rate of 97.5% in patients with uncomplicated urogenital and anorectal gonorrhea.

In adults and adolescents with cephalosporin allergy, CDC states that a dual treatment regimen that includes a single dose of oral gemifloxacin (320 mg) and a single dose of oral azithromycin (2 g) or a dual treatment regimen that includes a single dose of IM gentamicin (240 mg) and a single dose of oral azithromycin (2 g) could be considered for the treatment of uncomplicated urogenital gonorrhea; however, GI effects may limit use of these regimens. If available, spectinomycin (no longer commercially available in the US) is an effective alternative for the treatment of urogenital and anorectal gonorrhea. Although monotherapy with a single 2-g dose of oral azithromycin was previously recommended for the treatment of uncomplicated urogenital gonorrhea in patients with cephalosporin allergy, CDC states that monotherapy is no longer recommended because of concerns related to development of resistance and because there have been documented treatment failures with azithromycin monotherapy.

A test-of-cure follow-up (culture or NAAT) is not usually needed in patients with uncomplicated urogenital or rectal gonorrhea who receive a recommended or alternative dual treatment regimen.

Uncomplicated Pharyngeal Gonorrhea

For the treatment of uncomplicated gonorrhea of the pharynx† in adults and adolescents, CDC states that a dual combination regimen that includes a single 250-mg IM dose of ceftriaxone *and* a dose of azithromycin (single 1-g oral dose) is the regimen of choice.

Pharyngeal gonococcal infections are more difficult to eradicate than cervical, urethral, or rectal infections. Ceftriaxone generally has been effective in the treatment of pharyngeal gonococcal infections; most other anti-infectives, including oral cephalosporins, do not reliably cure such infections. In clinical trials, a single 250-mg IM dose of ceftriaxone was associated with a cure rate of 98.9% in patients with pharyngeal infections.

A test-of-cure follow-up is not usually needed in patients with uncomplicated pharyngeal gonorrhea who receive the recommended ceftriaxone dual treatment regimen; however, if an alternative regimen is used in patients with pharyngeal gonorrhea, a test-of-cure follow-up (culture or NAAT) is recommended 14 days after treatment.

Gonococcal Conjunctivitis

The regimen of choice for the treatment of gonococcal conjunctivitis† in adults and adolescents is a dual combination regimen that includes a single IM dose of ceftriaxone *and* a single dose of oral azithromycin. As an adjunct to anti-infective therapy, the infected eye can be irrigated once with sterile sodium chloride solution. Because only limited data are available regarding treatment of gonococcal conjunctivitis, consultation with an infectious disease specialist should be considered.

Disseminated Gonococcal Infections

For initial treatment of disseminated gonococcal infections that include arthritis and arthritis-dermatitis syndrome†, CDC recommends that adults and adolescents receive a dual combination regimen that includes a multiple-dose regimen of IM or IV ceftriaxone *and* a single dose of oral azithromycin. The alternative for initial treatment is a multiple-dose regimen of IV cefotaxime *and* a single dose of oral azithromycin. The initial parenteral regimen should be continued for 24–48 hours after substantial improvement occurs; treatment can then be switched to an oral regimen that is selected based on in vitro susceptibility testing and continued to complete at least 1 week of treatment.

For the treatment of gonococcal meningitis† or gonococcal endocarditis†, CDC recommends that adults and adolescents receive a dual combination regimen that includes a multiple-dose regimen of IV ceftriaxone *and* a single dose of oral azithromycin. The parenteral regimen should be continued for 10–14 days in patients with meningitis and for at least 4 weeks in patients with endocarditis.

Initial treatment of disseminated gonococcal infections should be undertaken in consultation with an infectious disease specialist, especially if the diagnosis is uncertain, purulent synovial effusions or other complications are present, or adherence to the regimen is uncertain. Evaluation for clinical evidence of endocarditis and meningitis is recommended in all patients with disseminated gonorrhea.

Gonococcal Epididymitis

Ceftriaxone is a drug of choice for the treatment of acute epididymitis†. Although acute epididymitis in sexually active men younger than 35 years of age is most frequently caused by *C. trachomatis* or *N. gonorrhoeae*, epididymitis can also be caused by other organisms (e.g., sexually transmitted enteric bacteria, *Mycoplasma*, *Ureaplasma*). Presumptive treatment is usually initiated prior to availability of all diagnostic laboratory test results and is selected based on the patient's risk for chlamydia, gonorrhea, and/or enteric bacteria (e.g., *E. coli*).

For empiric treatment of acute epididymitis most likely caused by sexually transmitted chlamydia and gonorrhea†, CDC recommends that adults receive a single dose of IM ceftriaxone given in conjunction with a 10-day regimen of oral doxycycline.

For empiric treatment of acute epididymitis most likely caused by sexually transmitted chlamydia, gonorrhea, and enteric bacteria†, CDC recommends that adults receive a single dose of IM ceftriaxone given in conjunction with a 10-day regimen of oral levofloxacin or oral ofloxacin. CDC states that levofloxacin or ofloxacin monotherapy can be considered for empiric treatment of acute epididymitis most likely caused by enteric bacteria if gonorrhea has been ruled out using gram, methylene blue, or gentian violet microscopy stain.

Gonococcal Proctitis

For presumptive treatment of acute proctitis† prior to availability of diagnostic laboratory test results, CDC recommends that adults receive a single dose of IM ceftriaxone given in conjunction with a 7-day regimen of oral doxycycline.

Gonococcal Infections in Neonates

Gonococcal infections in neonates usually occur as the result of exposure to the mother's infected cervical exudate and are apparent 2–5 days after birth. The most serious manifestations of *N. gonorrhoeae* infection in neonates are ophthalmia neonatorum and sepsis, arthritis, and meningitis; less serious manifestations include rhinitis, vaginitis, urethritis, and reinfection at sites of fetal monitoring (e.g., scalp). Because a neonate with gonococcal infection usually has acquired the organism from their mother, both the mother and her sexual partner(s) should be evaluated and treated for gonorrhea.

Prophylaxis and Presumptive Treatment of Gonococcal Infections in Neonates

CDC and AAP recommend routine topical prophylaxis using 0.5% erythromycin ophthalmic ointment in *all* neonates as soon as possible after birth to prevent gonococcal ophthalmia neonatorum; however, topical anti-infectives are inadequate for prophylaxis of gonococcal infections at other sites and may be ineffective in preventing chlamydial neonatal conjunctivitis.

Because neonates born to women with untreated gonorrhea are at high risk of infection with *N. gonorrhoeae*, CDC and AAP recommend that such neonates receive a single dose of IM or IV ceftriaxone for *parenteral prophylaxis*† and presumptive treatment of gonorrhea†. The single-dose ceftriaxone regimen also is recommended in other neonates if topical ophthalmic erythromycin is unavailable, especially for neonates born to women who are at risk for gonococcal infection or received no prenatal care. Topical erythromycin prophylaxis is unnecessary in neonates who receive parenteral prophylaxis with ceftriaxone.

CDC states that data are not available regarding the use of dual combination treatment regimens in neonates born to women with gonorrhea.

Gonococcal Ophthalmia Neonatorum

For the *treatment* of ophthalmia neonatorum† caused by *N. gonorrhoeae*, CDC and AAP recommend that neonates receive a single dose of IM or IV ceftriaxone.

As an adjunct to parenteral treatment of gonococcal ophthalmia neonatorum, the neonate's eyes should be irrigated with sterile sodium chloride solution immediately and at frequent intervals until the discharge is eliminated. Topical anti-infectives are inadequate for the treatment of gonococcal ophthalmia neonatorum and are unnecessary when appropriate systemic anti-infective therapy is given.

Infants born to mothers with untreated gonorrhea are at increased risk for gonococcal ophthalmia neonatorum if they do not receive appropriate parenteral prophylaxis at birth. Other neonates at increased risk for gonococcal ophthalmia neonatorum include those with mothers who received no prenatal care or have a history of sexually transmitted diseases or substance abuse. In all cases of neonatal conjunctivitis, conjunctival exudate should be cultured for *N. gonorrhoeae* and tested for anti-infective susceptibility and both mother and infant should be tested for chlamydial infection. Although the single-dose ceftriaxone regimen is adequate for treatment of gonococcal conjunctivitis, infants with ophthalmia neonatorum be hospitalized and evaluated for signs of disseminated infection (e.g., sepsis, arthritis, meningitis). CDC recommends that infants with gonococcal ophthalmia be managed in consultation with an infectious disease specialist.

Disseminated Gonococcal Infections and Gonococcal Scalp Abscesses in Neonates

Neonates with documented gonococcal infection at any site (including the eyes or scalp) should be evaluated for the possibility of disseminated infection (e.g., sepsis, arthritis, meningitis). If disseminated gonococcal infection is present, CDC and AAP recommend a multiple-dose regimen of IV or IM ceftriaxone or IV or IM cefotaxime. While either ceftriaxone or cefotaxime can be used for the treatment of disseminated gonococcal infections in neonates, ceftriaxone is contraindicated in certain neonates (see Cautions: Pediatric Precautions). AAP states that cefotaxime is preferred in infants with hyperbilirubinemia.

CDC states that data are not available regarding the use of dual combination regimens for the treatment of disseminated gonococcal infections or gonococcal scalp abscesses in neonates.

Gonococcal Infections in Infants and Children
Uncomplicated Gonorrhea

For the treatment of uncomplicated gonococcal vulvovaginitis, cervicitis, epididymitis, urethritis, pharyngitis, or proctitis in infants and children, CDC and AAP recommend a single dose of IM ceftriaxone. AAP states that a dual combination treatment regimen that includes a single dose of IM ceftriaxone *and* a single dose of oral azithromycin can be used for the treatment of uncomplicated gonorrhea in children weighing at least 45 kg. CDC states that data are not available regarding the use of dual combination regimens for the treatment of uncomplicated gonorrhea in children weighing 45 kg or less.

CDC and AAP state that adolescents with uncomplicated gonorrhea should receive a dual combination treatment regimen recommended for adults. (See Gonococcal Infections in Adults and Adolescents under Uses: Gonorrhea.)

Disseminated Gonococcal Infections

For the treatment of disseminated gonococcal infections† (e.g., bacteremia, arthritis) in infants and children, CDC and AAP recommend a multiple-dose regimen of IM or IV ceftriaxone. AAP states that a dual combination treatment regimen that includes IM or IV ceftriaxone *and* oral erythromycin can be used for the treatment of complicated gonococcal infections in children weighing less than 45 kg and a dual combination treatment regimen that includes IM or IV ceftriaxone *and* oral azithromycin can be used in children weighing at least 45 kg. CDC states that data are not available regarding the use of dual combination regimens for the treatment of complicated gonorrhea in children weighing 45 kg or less.

CDC and AAP state that adolescents with disseminated gonococcal infections should receive a dual combination treatment regimen recommended for adults. (See Gonococcal Infections in Adults and Adolescents under Uses: Gonorrhea.)

Prophylaxis in Sexual Assault Victims

A single dose of IM ceftriaxone is used in conjunction with a single dose of oral azithromycin and a single dose of either oral metronidazole or oral tinidazole for empiric anti-infective prophylaxis in adult or adolescent victims of sexual assault†. Gonorrhea, genital chlamydial infection, trichomoniasis, and bacteria vaginosis are the sexually transmitted diseases most commonly diagnosed in women following sexual assault; however, the prevalence of these infections is substantial among sexually active women and their presence after assault does not necessarily indicate that the infections were acquired during the assault. Gonococcal and chlamydial infections among females are of special concern because of the possibility of ascending infection.

CDC recommends routine empiric prophylaxis after a sexual assault, and use of such prophylaxis probably benefits most patients since follow-up of assault victims can be difficult and such prophylaxis allays the patient's concerns about possible infections. The 3-drug empiric anti-infective prophylaxis regimen recommended for adults and adolescents (ceftriaxone, azithromycin, and either metronidazole or tinidazole) provides coverage against gonorrhea, chlamydia, trichomoniasis, and bacterial vaginosis, but efficacy in preventing these infections after sexual assault has not been evaluated. Patients should be counseled regarding the potential benefits and toxicities associated with the regimen (e.g., GI effects).

Routine postexposure vaccination with hepatitis B virus (HBV) vaccine also is recommended for adult and adolescent sexual assault victims who have not previously received the vaccine or whose immunity against HBV is uncertain; hepatitis B immune globulin also should be given to previously unvaccinated individuals if the assailant is known to be hepatitis B surface antigen (HBsAg)-positive. In addition, vaccination with human papillomavirus (HPV) vaccine is recommended for previously unvaccinated or incompletely vaccinated female assault victims 9–26 years of age and male assault victims 9–21 years of age. CDC states that a decision to offer antiretroviral postexposure prophylaxis against HIV should be individualized taking into account the probability of HIV transmission (e.g., likelihood of the assailant having HIV, exposure characteristics that might increase the risk for HIV transmission, time elapsed after the event) and potential benefits and risks of such prophylaxis. (See Guidelines for Use of Antiretroviral Agents: Antiretrovirals for Postexposure Prophylaxis following Sexual, Injection Drug Use, or other Nonoccupational Exposures to HIV [nPEP], in the Antiretroviral Agents General Statement 8:18.08.)

● Pelvic Inflammatory Disease

Ceftriaxone is used for the treatment of pelvic inflammatory disease (PID) caused by *N. gonorrhoeae*. Ceftriaxone, like other cephalosporins, generally is inactive against *C. trachomatis* and should not be used alone in the treatment of PID.

PID is an acute or chronic inflammatory disorder in the upper female genital tract and can include any combination of endometritis, salpingitis, tubo-ovarian abscess, and pelvic peritonitis. PID generally is a polymicrobial infection most frequently caused by *N. gonorrhoeae* and/or *Chlamydia trachomatis*; however, organisms that can be part of the normal vaginal flora (e.g., anaerobic bacteria, *Gardnerella vaginalis*, *H. influenzae*, enteric gram-negative bacilli, *S. agalactiae*) or mycoplasma (e.g., *Mycoplasma hominis*, *Ureaplasma urealyticum*) also may be involved. PID is treated with an empiric regimen that provides broad-spectrum coverage. The regimen should be effective against *N. gonorrhoeae* and *C. trachomatis* and also probably should be effective against anaerobes. The optimum empiric regimen for the treatment of PID has not been identified. A variety of parenteral and oral regimens have been shown to achieve clinical and microbiologic cure in randomized studies with short-term follow-up.

IV Regimens for PID

When a parenteral regimen is indicated for the treatment of PID, CDC and other clinicians generally recommend a 2-drug regimen of cefoxitin (2 g IV every 6 hours) or cefotetan (2 g IV every 12 hours) given in conjunction with doxycycline (100 mg IV or orally every 12 hours) or a 2-drug regimen of clindamycin (900 mg IV every 8 hours) and gentamicin (usually a 2-mg/kg IV or IM loading dose followed by 1.5 mg/kg every 8 hours; regimen of 3–5 mg/kg once daily can be substituted). While certain parenteral cephalosporins (e.g., cefotaxime, ceftriaxone) also have been used and may be effective for the treatment of PID, CDC states that there is less experience with use of these cephalosporins in patients with PID and these drugs may be less active than cefotetan or cefoxitin against anaerobic bacteria.

The parenteral regimen should be continued until 24–48 hours after the patient improves clinically and then, based on clinical experience, a transition to an oral regimen can be considered to complete 14 days of treatment. If tubo-ovarian abscess is present, at least 24 hours of inpatient observation is recommended.

IM and Oral Regimens for PID

In women with mild to moderately severe acute PID, CDC states that an IM and oral regimen can be considered since clinical outcomes with these regimens are similar to IV regimens in such patients. However, if there is no response to the IM and oral regimen within 72 hours, the patient should be reevaluated to confirm the diagnosis and an IV regimen initiated.

If an IM and oral regimen is used, CDC recommends a single dose of an IM cephalosporin (e.g., ceftriaxone, cefoxitin with oral probenecid, cefotaxime) given in conjunction with a 14-day regimen of oral doxycycline (with or without oral metronidazole). The optimal cephalosporin is unclear; although cefoxitin usually has better anaerobic coverage, ceftriaxone has better coverage against *N. gonorrhoeae*.

For additional information on management of PID, current CDC sexually transmitted diseases treatment guidelines available at http://www.cdc.gov/std should be consulted.

● Actinomycosis

Ceftriaxone has been used in a limited number of patients to treat infections caused by *Actinomyces*†. IV ceftriaxone has been effective when given on an outpatient basis for the treatment of thoracic actinomycosis. However, IV penicillin G generally is the drug of choice for initial treatment of all forms of actinomycosis, including thoracic, abdominal, genitourinary, CNS, and cervicofacial infections. Alternative anti-infectives that can be used for the treatment of actinomycosis include amoxicillin, tetracyclines, erythromycins, chloramphenicol, clindamycin, third generation cephalosporins, and meropenem.

● Bartonella Infections

IM or IV ceftriaxone has been used in conjunction with oral erythromycin or oral azithromycin for the treatment of bacteremia caused by *Bartonella quintana*† (formerly *Rochalimaea quintana*). *B. quintana*, a gram-negative bacilli, can cause cutaneous bacillary angiomatosis, trench fever, bacteremia, endocarditis, and chronic lymphadenopathy. *B. quintana* infections have been reported most frequently in immunocompromised patients (e.g., HIV-infected individuals), homeless individuals in urban areas, and chronic alcohol abusers. Optimum anti-infective regimens for the treatment of infections caused by *B. quintana* have not been identified, and various drugs have been used or are recommended to treat these infections, including doxycycline, erythromycin, azithromycin, clarithromycin, chloramphenicol, or cephalosporins. There is evidence that these *B. quintana* infections tend to persist or recur and prolonged therapy (several months or longer) usually is necessary.

The possible role of ceftriaxone in the treatment of infections caused by *Bartonella henselae*† (formerly *Rochalimaea henselae*) (e.g., cat scratch disease, bacillary angiomatosis, peliosis hepatitis) has not been determined. Cat scratch disease generally is a self-limited illness in immunocompetent individuals and may resolve spontaneously in 2–4 months; however, some clinicians suggest that anti-infective therapy be considered for acutely or severely ill patients with systemic symptoms, particularly those with hepatosplenomegaly or painful lymphadenopathy, and such therapy probably is indicated in immunocompromised patients. Anti-infectives also are indicated in patients with *B. henselae* infections who develop bacillary angiomatosis, neuroretinitis, or Parinaud's oculoglandular syndrome. While the optimum anti-infective regimen for the treatment of cat scratch disease or other *B. henselae* infections has not been identified, some clinicians recommend azithromycin, clarithromycin, erythromycin, doxycycline, ciprofloxacin, rifampin, co-trimoxazole, gentamicin, or third generation cephalosporins.

In HIV-infected patients, *Bartonella* infections occur most frequently in those with median CD4+ T-cell counts less than 50 cells/mm³. CDC, NIH, and IDSA recommend that all HIV-infected adults and adolescents diagnosed with a *Bartonella* infection receive at least 3 months of antibacterial treatment; if relapse occurs, long-term suppressive antibacterial treatment (secondary prophylaxis) may be needed. For initial treatment or long-term suppressive therapy of *Bartonella* infections in HIV-infected adults or adolescents, doxycycline or a macrolide (erythromycin, azithromycin, clarithromycin) is recommended. Although pregnant HIV-infected women should usually receive a macrolide (erythromycin) for treatment of these infections, CDC, NIH, and IDSA state that ceftriaxone may be a possible alternative when macrolides cannot be used.

● Capnocytophaga Infections

Based on results of in vitro susceptibility tests that indicate that *Capnocytophaga* generally is inhibited by ceftriaxone, some clinicians suggest that ceftriaxone can be used in the treatment of infections caused by *C. canimorsus*† (formerly CDC group DF-2). *Capnocytophaga* is a gram-negative bacilli that can cause life-threatening septicemia, meningitis, and/or endocarditis and often is associated with disseminated intravascular coagulation; splenectomized and immunocompromised individuals are at particularly high risk for serious *Capnocytophaga* infections. *C. canimorsus* infection usually occurs as the result of a dog bite or other close contact with a dog. The optimum regimen for the treatment of infections caused by *Capnocytophaga* has not been identified, but some clinicians recommend penicillin G or, alternatively, a third generation cephalosporin (cefotaxime, ceftriaxone), a carbapenem (imipenem or meropenem), vancomycin, a fluoroquinolone, or clindamycin.

● Leptospirosis

Ceftriaxone is used in the treatment of severe leptospirosis† caused by *Leptospira*. Leptospirosis is a spirochete infection that may range in severity from an asymptomatic or subclinical illness that is self-limited to a severe, life-threatening illness that includes jaundice, renal failure, hemorrhage, cardiac arrhythmias, pneumonitis, and hemodynamic collapse (Weil syndrome).

Penicillin G generally has been considered the drug of choice for the treatment of moderate to severe leptospirosis, and doxycycline has been used in less severe infections. Other anti-infectives recommended for the treatment of severe leptospirosis include cephalosporins (ceftriaxone, cefotaxime), aminopenicillins (ampicillin, amoxicillin), tetracyclines (doxycycline, tetracycline), or macrolides (azithromycin).

In one randomized study in adults, IV ceftriaxone was as effective as IV penicillin G for the treatment of severe leptospirosis. The duration of fever was decreased to 3 days in both treatment groups, and there were comparable improvements in complications associated with the infection (renal failure, respiratory failure, liver impairment, thrombocytopenia).

● Lyme Disease

Ceftriaxone is used in the treatment of Lyme disease†. IDSA, AAP, and other clinicians recommend IV ceftriaxone as a drug of choice for the treatment of early neurologic Lyme disease† with acute neurologic manifestations such as meningitis or radiculopathy, Lyme carditis†, Lyme arthritis†, and late neurologic Lyme disease†.

Lyme disease is a tick-borne spirochetal disease. In the US, Lyme disease is caused by the spirochete *Borrelia burgdorferi*, which is transmitted by the bite of *Ixodes scapularis* or *I. pacificus* ticks. For additional information on Lyme disease, see Lyme Disease in Uses: Spirochetal Infections, in the Tetracyclines General Statement 8:12.24.

Early Lyme Disease
Erythema Migrans

Oral anti-infectives (doxycycline, amoxicillin, cefuroxime axetil) generally are effective for the treatment of early localized or early disseminated Lyme disease associated with erythema migrans, in the absence of specific neurologic manifestations or advanced atrioventricular (AV) heart block. Although IV ceftriaxone is effective for early Lyme disease manifested as erythema migrans, it is not superior to the recommended oral drugs and is more likely to cause serious adverse effects; therefore, ceftriaxone is not usually recommended for the treatment of early Lyme disease in the absence of neurologic involvement or advanced AV heart block.

Early Neurologic Lyme Disease

Ceftriaxone is a drug of choice for the treatment of early neurologic Lyme disease†. Parenteral anti-infectives are recommended for the treatment of early Lyme disease when there are acute neurologic manifestations such as meningitis or radiculoneuritis.

IDSA and other clinicians recommend a 14-day regimen (range: 10–28 days) of IV ceftriaxone as the preferred parenteral regimen for the treatment of acute neurologic Lyme disease manifested by meningitis or radiculopathy; IV cefotaxime and IV penicillin G sodium are the preferred alternatives. In patients with acute neurologic manifestations who are intolerant of cephalosporins and penicillin, there is some evidence that oral doxycycline may be an adequate alternative that can be considered for use in adults and children 8 years of age or older.

Lyme Carditis

Ceftriaxone is the drug of choice when a parenteral regimen is indicated for the treatment of Lyme carditis†. IDSA states that patients with AV heart block and/or myopericarditis associated with early Lyme disease may be treated with a 14-day regimen (range: 14–21 days) of oral or parenteral anti-infectives. Although there is no evidence to date to suggest that a parenteral regimen is more effective than an oral regimen for the treatment of Lyme carditis, a parenteral regimen usually is recommended for initial treatment of hospitalized patients; an oral regimen can be used to complete therapy and for the treatment of outpatients. When a parenteral regimen is used, IV ceftriaxone or, alternatively, IV cefotaxime or IV penicillin G sodium is recommended. When an oral regimen is used, doxycycline, amoxicillin, or cefuroxime axetil is recommended.

Because of the potential for life-threatening complications, hospitalization and continuous monitoring is advisable for patients who are symptomatic (syncope, dyspnea, chest pain) and also is recommended for those with second- or third-degree AV block or first-degree heart block when the PR interval is prolonged to 0.3 seconds or longer. Patients with advanced heart block may require a temporary pacemaker and consultation with a cardiologist is recommended.

Late Lyme Disease
Lyme Arthritis

Ceftriaxone is the drug of choice when a parenteral regimen is indicated for the treatment of Lyme arthritis†. While patients with uncomplicated Lyme arthritis without clinical evidence of neurologic disease generally can be treated with a 28-day oral regimen (doxycycline, amoxicillin, or cefuroxime axetil), IDSA and other clinicians state that patients with Lyme arthritis and concomitant neurologic disease should receive a 14-day parenteral regimen (range: 14–28 days) of IV ceftriaxone or, alternatively, IV cefotaxime or IV penicillin G. While oral regimens are easier to administer, associated with fewer serious adverse effects, and less expensive than IV regimens, some patients with Lyme arthritis treated with oral anti-infectives have subsequently developed overt neuroborreliosis, which may require IV therapy for successful resolution. Therefore, additional study is needed to fully evaluate the comparative safety and efficacy of oral versus IV anti-infectives for the treatment of Lyme arthritis.

In patients who have persistent or recurrent joint swelling after a recommended oral regimen, IDSA and other clinicians recommend retreatment with the oral regimen or a switch to a parenteral regimen. Some clinicians prefer retreatment with an oral regimen for patients whose arthritis substantively improved but did not completely resolve; these clinicians reserve parenteral regimens for those patients whose arthritis failed to improve or worsened. It has been suggested that clinicians should consider allowing several months for joint inflammation to resolve after initial treatment before an additional course of anti-infectives is given.

Late Neurologic Lyme Disease

Ceftriaxone is the drug of choice for the treatment of late neurologic Lyme disease†. IDSA and other clinicians state that patients with late neurologic Lyme disease affecting the CNS or peripheral nervous system (e.g., encephalopathy, neuropathy) should receive 2–4 weeks of IV ceftriaxone or, alternatively, IV cefotaxime or IV penicillin G sodium. Response to anti-infective treatment usually is slow and may be incomplete in patients with late neurologic Lyme disease. IDSA states that retreatment is not recommended unless relapse is documented with reliable objective measures.

In a limited number of adults with late complications of Lyme disease (i.e., CNS dysfunction, peripheral neuropathy, and/or arthritis), most of whom failed to respond adequately to other anti-infectives (e.g., penicillin, tetracycline), ceftriaxone therapy (1 or 2 g IM or IV twice daily for 14 days) resulted in clinical improvement, including resolution of arthritis and chronic fatigue. A regimen of IV ceftriaxone (2 g once daily for 30 days) has been used with some success for the treatment of Lyme encephalopathy. Although IV penicillin G therapy can be effective in treating neurologic abnormalities of Lyme disease, central or peripheral neurologic deficits associated with disease progression have been noted in a few patients after such therapy, and some clinicians suggest that therapy with IV ceftriaxone may be preferred for serious manifestations (i.e., involving major organs) of disseminated or late Lyme disease because of its greater in vitro and in vivo activity against *B. burgdorferi* compared with IV penicillin G and the prolonged serum concentrations and excellent CSF penetration achievable with once-daily administration of ceftriaxone.

● Neisseria meningitidis Infections

Ceftriaxone is used in the treatment of invasive infections caused by *N. meningitidis* and also is used to eliminate nasopharyngeal carriage of *N. meningitidis*† and for chemoprophylaxis to prevent meningococcal disease in close contacts of patients with invasive disease†.

For suspected meningococcal disease, including presumptive *N. meningitidis* meningitis, AAP and IDSA recommend a third generation cephalosporin (ceftriaxone or cefotaxime) for initial empiric treatment. If the infection is found to be caused by penicillin-susceptible *N. meningitidis*, IV penicillin G or ampicillin can be substituted or the third generation cephalosporin can be continued. Although IV penicillin G generally has been considered the drug of choice for the treatment of meningitis known to be caused by susceptible *N. meningitidis*, some experts recommend ampicillin, ceftriaxone, or cefotaxime.

Patients with invasive meningococcal disease who have been treated with penicillin G or any anti-infective agent other than ceftriaxone or another third generation cephalosporin may still be carriers of *N. meningitidis* and should receive an anti-infective regimen to eradicate nasopharyngeal carriage of the organism prior to hospital discharge. The treatments of choice to eradicate nasopharyngeal carriage of *N. meningitidis* are ceftriaxone (single IM dose), rifampin (2-day regimen), and ciprofloxacin (single oral dose). These regimens are all 90–95% effective and any of these is an acceptable regimen in appropriate patients.

Chemoprophylaxis in Household and Other Close Contacts of Individuals with Invasive Meningococcal Disease

Chemoprophylaxis in close contacts of a patients with invasive meningococcal disease is an important means of preventing secondary cases in household and other close contacts. Recommended regimens for chemoprophylaxis against meningococcal disease include a single dose of IM ceftriaxone, 2-day regimen of oral rifampin (not recommended in pregnant women), or a single dose of oral ciprofloxacin (not recommended in individuals younger than 18 years of age unless no other regimen can be used and not recommended for pregnant or lactating women). These regimens are all 90–95% effective and any of these is an acceptable regimen for chemoprophylaxis. AAP suggests that rifampin may be the drug of choice for chemoprophylaxis in most children.

The attack rate for household contacts who do not receive chemoprophylaxis has been estimated to be 4 cases per 1000 individuals exposed, which is 500–800 times greater than that for the general population. A decision to administer chemoprophylaxis to close contacts of an individual with invasive meningococcal disease is based on the degree of risk. Throat and nasopharyngeal cultures are *not* useful in determining the need for chemoprophylaxis and may unnecessarily delay administration of the regimen.

The USPHS Advisory Committee on Immunization Practices (ACIP), AAP, and others recommend that chemoprophylaxis be administered to contacts of patients with invasive meningococcal disease who are considered at high risk of infection. These high risk individuals include household contacts (especially children younger than 2 years of age) and any individual who has slept or eaten frequently in the same dwelling with the index case; child care and nursery school contacts who were exposed during the 7 days before the onset of disease in the index case; individuals exposed directly to oropharyngeal secretions of the index case (e.g., through kissing or sharing toothbrushes, eating utensils, or drinking containers) during the 7 days before the onset of disease in the index case; and medical personnel and others who had intimate exposure (e.g., through mouth to mouth resuscitation or unprotected contact during endotracheal intubation or suctioning) to the index case during the 7 days before the onset of disease. For travelers, chemoprophylaxis should be considered for any passenger who had direct contact with respiratory secretions from an index case or for anyone seated directly next to an index case on a prolonged flight (i.e., lasting 8 hours or longer).

Chemoprophylaxis is *not* routinely recommended for contacts of patients with invasive meningococcal disease who are considered at low risk of infection. Individuals considered in most circumstances as being at low risk include casual contacts with no history of direct exposure to the index case's oral secretions (e.g., school or work contacts); individuals who had only indirect contact with the index case (only contact was with a high-risk contact of the index case); and medical personnel who had no direct exposure to the index case's oral secretions. Because reports of secondary cases after close contact with patients with noninvasive pneumonia or conjunctivitis caused by *N. meningitidis* are rare, chemoprophylaxis is not recommended for close contacts of patients who only have evidence of *N. meningitidis* in nonsterile sites (e.g., oropharyngeal, conjunctival, endotracheal secretions).

When chemoprophylaxis is indicated in high-risk contacts, it must be administered promptly (ideally within 24 hours after identification of the index case) since the attack rate of secondary disease is greatest in the few days following disease onset in the index case. All high-risk contacts should be informed that even if chemoprophylaxis is taken or started, the development of any suspicious clinical manifestation warrants early, rapid medical attention. Chemoprophylaxis probably is of limited or no value if administered more than 14 days after contact with the index case. If high-risk exposure to a new index case occurs more than 2 weeks after initial chemoprophylaxis, additional chemoprophylaxis is indicated.

Outbreak Control

When an outbreak of meningococcal disease occurs in the US and the outbreak is caused by a vaccine-preventable meningococcal strain (e.g., serogroups A, C, Y, or W-135), large-scale vaccination programs with meningococcal polysaccharide vaccine in the appropriate target group may be indicated. (See Uses: Outbreak Control in Meningococcal Polysaccharide Vaccine 80:12.) Mass chemoprophylaxis programs (i.e., administration of ceftriaxone, rifampin, or ciprofloxacin to large population groups) are not recommended to control large outbreaks since the disadvantages of such programs (e.g., costs, difficulty in ensuring simultaneous administration of the anti-infectives to large populations, adverse effects of the drugs, emergence of resistant organisms) probably outweigh any possible benefit in disease prevention. However, when outbreaks involve limited populations (e.g., a single school), administration of chemoprophylaxis to all individuals in the population may be considered, especially if the outbreak involves a meningococcal serogroup not represented in currently available meningococcal vaccines. Other measures, such as restricting travel to areas with a suspected meningococcal outbreak, closing schools or universities, or canceling sporting or social events, are not usually recommended to control meningococcal outbreaks in the US.

While the vast majority of cases of meningococcal disease in the US are sporadic, localized outbreaks of meningococcal disease do occur. When a suspected outbreak of meningococcal disease occurs in the US, public health authorities will then determine whether mass vaccinations (with or without mass chemoprophylaxis) is indicated and delineate the target population based on risk assessment.

● Nocardia Infections

Ceftriaxone has been used for the treatment of nocardiosis† caused by *Nocardia*.

Co-trimoxazole (fixed combination of sulfamethoxazole and trimethoprim) usually is considered the drug of choice for the treatment of nocardiosis. Other drugs that have been used alone or in combination regimens for the treatment of nocardiosis include a sulfonamide alone (sulfamethoxazole [not commercially available in the US], sulfadiazine), amikacin, tetracyclines, cephalosporins (ceftriaxone, cefotaxime, cefuroxime), cefoxitin, carbapenems (imipenem, meropenem), fixed combination of amoxicillin and clavulanate, clarithromycin, cycloserine, or linezolid. A regimen of amikacin and ceftriaxone has been effective for the treatment of disseminated *N. asteroides* infection complicated by cerebral abscess.

Ceftriaxone has been recommended as one of several alternatives to co-trimoxazole for the treatment of skin and skin structure infections caused by *Nocardia*† (e.g., *N. farcinica*, *N. brasiliensis*). Prolonged anti-infective treatment (6–24 months) and/or a multiple-drug anti-infective regimen may be necessary for severe or disseminated infections or in patients with immunosuppression.

In vitro susceptibility testing, if available, is recommended to guide selection of anti-infectives for the treatment of severe nocardiosis or for treatment in patients who cannot tolerate or failed to respond to sulfonamide treatment.

Relapsing Fever

Ceftriaxone may be effective for the treatment of relapsing fever† caused by *Borrelia recurrentis*; however, other drugs (e.g., tetracycline, penicillin G) are considered the drugs of choice for the treatment of the disease.

Syphilis

Ceftriaxone has some activity against *Treponema pallidum* and there is some limited evidence that the drug may be effective for the treatment of syphilis†.

IM penicillin G benzathine is the drug of choice for the treatment of primary syphilis (i.e., ulcer or chancre at infection site), secondary syphilis (i.e., manifestations that include, but are not limited to, rash, mucocutaneous lesions, and lymphadenopathy), and tertiary syphilis (i.e., cardiac, gummatous lesions, tabes dorsalis, and general paresis) in adults, adolescents, and children. IM penicillin G benzathine also is the drug of choice for the treatment of latent syphilis (i.e., detected by serologic testing but lacking clinical manifestations), including both early latent syphilis (latent syphilis acquired within the preceding year) and late latent syphilis (i.e., all other cases of latent syphilis or syphilis of unknown duration) in all age groups. For the treatment of neurosyphilis and otic or ocular syphilis, IV penicillin G potassium or sodium is the drug of choice and IM penicillin G procaine (with oral probenecid) is an alternative if compliance can be ensured.

CDC states that limited clinical studies as well as biologic and pharmacologic evidence suggest that a multiple-dose ceftriaxone regimen may be effective for the treatment of primary and secondary syphilis† and, on the basis of biologic plausibility and pharmacologic properties, may also be effective for the treatment of latent syphilis† in penicillin-allergic patients. However, optimal dosage and duration of ceftriaxone for the treatment of syphilis have not been defined and there is more extensive clinical experience using tetracyclines (doxycycline, tetracycline) as alternatives for the treatment of primary, secondary, or latent syphilis in penicillin-allergic patients.

CDC states that limited data suggest that a multiple-dose ceftriaxone regimen can be used as an alternative for the treatment of neurosyphilis† in penicillin-allergic patients.

Decisions regarding the treatment of syphilis in penicillin-allergic patients should be made in consultation with a specialist. Because of limited experience with penicillin alternatives, close follow-up is essential if ceftriaxone is used for the treatment of syphilis in penicillin-allergic patients and the possibility of cross-sensitivity between penicillin and ceftriaxone should be considered. If compliance with an alternative regimen or follow-up cannot be ensured, CDC recommends desensitization and treatment with the appropriate penicillin G preparation.

Data are insufficient to recommend use of ceftriaxone or other alternatives for the treatment of any stage of syphilis in penicillin-allergic pregnant women or for the treatment of congenital syphilis in neonates, infants, or children with known or suspected penicillin allergy; CDC recommends that such patients be desensitized and treated with the appropriate penicillin G preparation.

In certain circumstance when there is a penicillin shortage and penicillin G is not available, CDC states that a multiple-dose ceftriaxone regimen can be considered for the treatment of congenital syphilis. In such situations, CDC recommends that ceftriaxone be used with close clinical, serologic, and CSF follow-up and in consultation with a specialist in the treatment of infants with congenital syphilis.

For additional information on management of syphilis, current CDC sexually transmitted diseases treatment guidelines available at http://www.cdc.gov/std should be consulted.

Typhoid Fever and Other Invasive Salmonella Infections

Ceftriaxone has been effective when used in adults or children for the treatment of typhoid fever† or paratyphoid fever† (enteric fever) or septicemia caused by *Salmonella* serovars Typhi or Paratyphi, respectively, including multidrug-resistant strains. Ceftriaxone also has been used and is recommended for the treatment of invasive infections (e.g., bacteremia, osteomyelitis) caused by nontyphoidal *Salmonella*, including *Salmonella* serovar Typhimurium.

Multidrug-resistant strains of *Salmonella* serovar Typhi (i.e., strains resistant to ampicillin, chloramphenicol, and/or co-trimoxazole) have been reported with increasing frequency, and third generation cephalosporins (e.g., ceftriaxone, cefotaxime) and fluoroquinolones (e.g., ciprofloxacin, ofloxacin) are considered the drugs of first choice for the treatment of typhoid fever or other severe infections known or suspected to be caused by these strains. AAP states that ceftriaxone is a drug of choice for empiric treatment of enteric fever pending results of in vitro

susceptibility tests. Strains of *S. typhi* resistant to ceftriaxone have been reported rarely in the US,

IV ceftriaxone (3 or 4 g once daily in adults or 75 mg/kg once daily in children) given for 5–7 days has been as effective as a 14-day course of oral or IV chloramphenicol in the treatment of typhoid fever caused by susceptible *S. typhi*. Although bacteremia resolved sooner with ceftriaxone in some patients, the time to defervescence was faster with chloramphenicol.

Whipple's Disease

Ceftriaxone has been effective when used in the treatment of Whipple's disease†, a progressive systemic infection caused by *Tropheryma whipplei* (formerly *Tropheryma whippelii*). Optimal regimens for the treatment of Whipple's disease have not been identified, in part because of difficulties in identifying and cultivating the causative agent and because relapses commonly occur, even after adequate and long-term anti-infective treatment. Some clinicians recommend an initial parenteral regimen (e.g., ceftriaxone or penicillin G used with or without streptomycin) followed by a long-term regimen of oral co-trimoxazole given for 1–2 years.

Ceftriaxone has been effective for the treatment of Whipple's disease when the CNS was involved. For the treatment of encephalitis caused by *T. whipplei*, IDSA recommends initial treatment with ceftriaxone given for 2–4 weeks followed by co-trimoxazole or cefixime for 1–2 years. Some clinicians suggest that ceftriaxone may be a drug of choice for patients who experience cerebral relapse during or after treatment with penicillin G or co-trimoxazole.

Empiric Therapy in Febrile Neutropenic Patients

Ceftriaxone has been used in conjunction with an aminoglycoside for empiric anti-infective therapy of presumed bacterial infections in febrile neutropenic adults or pediatric patients†. While ceftriaxone has been used alone for empiric therapy in some febrile neutropenic patients considered to be at low risk, use of ceftriaxone monotherapy may not provide adequate coverage against some potential pathogens (e.g., *Ps. aeruginosa*) and generally is *not* recommended for empiric anti-infective therapy in febrile neutropenic patients.

In studies in febrile neutropenic cancer patients 1 year of age or older, the overall response rate to a once-daily regimen of IV ceftriaxone (30 mg/kg once daily in adults or 80 mg/kg once daily in children) given in conjunction with IV amikacin (20 mg/kg daily) was similar to that of a regimen of IV ceftazidime (100–150 mg/kg daily given in 3 divided doses) given in conjunction with amikacin (20 mg/kg given once daily or in 3 divided doses).

Published protocols for the treatment of infections in febrile neutropenic patients should be consulted for specific recommendations regarding selection of the initial empiric anti-infective regimen, when to change the initial regimen, possible subsequent regimens, and duration of therapy in these patients. In addition, consultation with an infectious disease expert knowledgeable about infections in immunocompromised patients is advised.

Prevention of Bacterial Endocarditis

Ceftriaxone is used as an alternative for *prevention* of α-hemolytic (viridans group) streptococcal endocarditis† in adults and children undergoing certain dental or upper respiratory tract procedures who have certain cardiac conditions that put them at the highest risk of adverse outcome from endocarditis.

The cardiac conditions identified by AHA as those associated with highest risk of adverse outcomes from endocarditis and for which anti-infective prophylaxis is reasonable are prosthetic cardiac valves or prosthetic material used for cardiac valve repair, previous infective endocarditis, cardiac valvulopathy after cardiac transplantation, and certain forms of congenital heart disease (i.e., unrepaired cyanotic congenital heart disease including palliative shunts and conduits; a completely repaired congenital heart defect where prosthetic material or device was placed by surgery or catheter intervention within the last 6 months; repaired congenital heart disease with residual defects at the site or adjacent to the site of a prosthetic patch or prosthetic device that inhibits endothelialization).

AHA states that anti-infective prophylaxis for prevention of α-hemolytic (viridans group) streptococcal bacterial endocarditis is reasonable for patients with the above cardiac risk factors if they are undergoing any dental procedures that involve manipulation of gingival tissue or the periapical region of teeth or perforation of the oral mucosa (e.g., biopsies, suture removal, placement of orthodontic bands). AHA states that anti-infective prophylaxis is *not* needed for routine anesthetic injections through noninfected tissue, dental radiographs, placement of removable prosthodontic or orthodontic appliances, adjustment of orthodontic appliances, placement of orthodontic brackets, shedding of deciduous teeth, or bleeding from trauma to the lips or oral mucosa.

AHA states that anti-infective prophylaxis for prevention of bacterial endocarditis also is reasonable for patients with the above cardiac risk factors if they are undergoing invasive procedures of the respiratory tract that involve incision or biopsy of respiratory mucosa (e.g., tonsillectomy, adenoidectomy) and may be reasonable for such patients if they are undergoing surgical procedures that involve infected skin, skin structure, or musculoskeletal tissue. However, anti-infective prophylaxis solely to prevent infective endocarditis is no longer recommended by AHA for GI or genitourinary tract procedures.

Oral amoxicillin is the drug of choice when prevention of bacterial endocarditis is indicated in patients undergoing certain dental or upper respiratory tract procedures who have certain cardiac conditions that put them at highest risk of adverse outcomes from endocarditis. If an oral regimen cannot be used in such patients, AHA recommends IM or IV ampicillin or IM or IV cefazolin or ceftriaxone. Alternatives for penicillin-allergic patients include oral cephalexin, oral azithromycin or clarithromycin, oral or parenteral clindamycin, or parenteral cefazolin or ceftriaxone; cephalosporins should not be used for such prophylaxis in individuals with a history of anaphylaxis, angioedema, or urticaria after receiving a penicillin.

For additional information on which cardiac conditions are associated with the highest risk of adverse outcomes from endocarditis and additional information regarding use of prophylaxis to prevent bacterial endocarditis, current recommendations published by AHA should be consulted.

● *Perioperative Prophylaxis*

Ceftriaxone has been used perioperatively to reduce the incidence of infection in patients undergoing certain contaminated or potentially contaminated surgical procedures, including biliary tract procedures (e.g., cholecystectomy), colorectal procedures, intra-abdominal surgery, or vaginal or abdominal hysterectomy, and in those undergoing certain clean surgical procedures in which the development of infection at the surgical site would represent a serious risk, including coronary artery bypass, open heart surgery, thoracic surgery, or orthopedic surgery. The drug also has been used perioperatively in patients undergoing transurethral resection of the prostate† or renal transplantation†.

Ceftriaxone in conjunction with metronidazole is one of several options recommended for perioperative prophylaxis in patients undergoing colorectal surgery. Ceftriaxone also is one of several options recommended for perioperative prophylaxis in patients undergoing biliary tract procedures, but should not be used in those undergoing cholecystectomy for noninfected biliary conditions, including biliary colic or dyskinesia without infection.

A first or second generation cephalosporin (e.g., cefazolin, cefuroxime) generally is preferred when a cephalosporin is used for perioperative prophylaxis. Third generation cephalosporins (e.g., cefotaxime, ceftriaxone, ceftazidime) and fourth generation cephalosporins (e.g., cefepime) are not usually recommended for routine perioperative prophylaxis because they are expensive, some are less active than first or second generation cephalosporins against staphylococci, they have spectrums of activity wider than necessary for organisms encountered in elective surgery, and their use for prophylaxis may promote emergence of resistant organisms. (See Uses: Perioperative Prophylaxis, in the Cephalosporins General Statement 8:12.06.)

DOSAGE AND ADMINISTRATION

● *Reconstitution and Administration*

Ceftriaxone sodium is administered by IV infusion or deep IM injection.

Ceftriaxone should *not* be administered intrathecally.

Ceftriaxone has been administered IM or IV to adults or children in outpatient settings, including clinicians' offices, outpatient clinics, infusion centers, skilled nursing facilities, rehabilitation centers, or the patient's home, for the treatment of certain infections suitable for community-based parenteral anti-infective agent therapy (e.g., community-acquired pneumonia, osteomyelitis, endocarditis†). Outpatient parenteral anti-infective therapy often is used to complete a course of ceftriaxone therapy initiated during hospitalization, but ceftriaxone therapy also has been initiated on an outpatient basis. Ceftriaxone usually is administered in the outpatient setting by a healthcare provider; however, the drug has been self-administered in the patients' home by the patient, family member, or other responsible person.

Ceftriaxone should *not* be reconstituted with or further diluted with diluents containing calcium (e.g., Ringer's/lactated Ringer's solution, Hartmann's solution)

because a precipitate can form. (See Interaction with Calcium-containing Products under Cautions: Precautions and Contraindications.)

Because precipitation of ceftriaxone-calcium can occur, ceftriaxone must *not* be admixed with calcium-containing solutions and must *not* be administered *simultaneously* with calcium-containing IV solutions, including continuous infusions of calcium-containing solutions such as parenteral nutrition, even via different infusion lines at different sites in any patient (irrespective of age). In adult and pediatric patients older than 28 days of age, ceftriaxone and calcium-containing solutions may be administered *sequentially* if the infusion lines are thoroughly flushed between infusions with a compatible fluid (e.g., 0.9% sodium chloride injection, 5% dextrose injection).

Ceftriaxone is contraindicated in neonates (28 days of age or younger) if they are receiving (or expected to require) treatment with calcium-containing IV solutions, including continuous calcium-containing infusions such as parenteral nutrition.

Patients receiving ceftriaxone should be adequately hydrated.

Intermittent IV Infusion

For intermittent IV infusion, vials labeled as containing 250 mg, 500 mg, 1 g, or 2 g of ceftriaxone should be reconstituted with 2.4, 4.8, 9.6, or 19.2 mL, respectively, of a compatible IV solution to provide solutions containing approximately 100 mg/mL. The reconstituted solution should then be further diluted to the desired concentration by withdrawing the entire contents of the vial and adding it to an appropriate IV diluent. Ceftriaxone solutions for IV infusion containing 10–40 mg/mL are recommended; however, lower concentrations may be used.

Alternatively, ADD-Vantage® vials containing 1 or 2 g of ceftriaxone should be reconstituted with 0.9% sodium chloride or 5% dextrose injection in ADD-Vantage® flexible containers according to the manufacturer's directions and administered by IV infusion.

Alternatively, the commercially available Duplex® drug delivery system containing 1 or 2 g of lyophilized ceftriaxone and 50 mL of dextrose 3.74 or 2.22% injection, respectively, in separate chambers should be reconstituted (activated) according to the manufacturer's directions and administered by IV infusion. If stored in the refrigerator after reconstitution (see Chemistry and Stability: Stability), the solution should be allowed to reach room temperature prior to administration.

The 10-g pharmacy bulk package of ceftriaxone is reconstituted by adding 95 mL of a compatible IV solution to provide a solution containing approximately 100 mg/mL. Reconstituted solutions in the ceftriaxone pharmacy bulk package should *not* be used for direct IV infusion; these reconstituted solutions must be further diluted in a compatible IV infusion solution, generally to a concentration of 10–40 mg/mL, although lower concentrations may be used if desired.

Thawed solutions of the commercially available frozen premixed ceftriaxone sodium injection in dextrose should be administered only by intermittent IV infusion. The commercially available frozen injection should be thawed at room temperature (25°C) or under refrigeration (5°C); the injection should not be thawed by warming in a water bath or by exposure to microwave radiation. The container may be fragile in the frozen state and should be handled with care. Precipitates that may have formed in the frozen injection usually will dissolve with little or no agitation when the injection reaches room temperature; potency is not affected. After thawing at room temperature, the injection should be agitated and the container checked for minute leaks by firmly squeezing the bag. The injection should be discarded if container seals or outlet ports are not intact or leaks are found or if the solution is cloudy or contains an insoluble precipitate. Additives should not be introduced into the injection container. The injection should not be used in series connections with other plastic containers, since such use could result in air embolism from residual air being drawn from the primary container before administration of fluid from the secondary container is complete.

Rate of Administration

The manufacturers recommend that intermittent IV infusions of ceftriaxone sodium be infused over 30 minutes (except in neonates).

In neonates, the manufacturers recommend that intermittent IV infusions of ceftriaxone be given over 60 minutes. (See Cautions: Pediatric Precautions.)

IM Injection

IM injections of ceftriaxone sodium should be prepared by adding 0.9, 1.8, 3.6, or 7.2 mL of compatible diluent (e.g., sterile water for injection, 0.9% sodium chloride injection, 5% dextrose injection, bacteriostatic water for injection containing 0.9% benzyl alcohol, 1% lidocaine hydrochloride without epinephrine) to vials labeled as containing 250 mg, 500 mg, 1 g, or 2 g of ceftriaxone, respectively, to provide solutions containing approximately 250 mg/mL or by adding 1, 2.1, or 4.2 mL of one of these diluents to vials labeled as containing 500 mg, 1 g, or 2 g of ceftriaxone, respectively, to provide solutions containing approximately 350 mg/mL. More dilute solutions of the drug may be used for IM injection if required.

Solutions of the drug for IM injection that have been reconstituted with bacteriostatic water containing benzyl alcohol should not be used in neonates. (See Cautions: Pediatric Precautions.)

IM injections of ceftriaxone should be made deeply into a large muscle mass, using usual techniques and precautions.

● Dosage

Dosage of ceftriaxone sodium is expressed in terms of ceftriaxone and is identical for IM or IV administration.

To avoid unintentional overdosage, the commercially available Duplex delivery system containing ceftriaxone and dextrose injection should *not* be used in patients who require less than the entire 1- or 2-g dose in the container.

Pediatric Dosage
General Pediatric Dosage

The American Academy of Pediatrics (AAP) recommends that neonates 28 days of age or younger receive ceftriaxone in a dosage of 50 mg/kg once daily, regardless of weight.

For pediatric patients beyond the neonatal period, AAP recommends a ceftriaxone dosage of 50–75 mg/kg once daily for the treatment of mild to moderate infections or a dosage of 100 mg/kg daily given in 1 or 2 doses for the treatment of severe infections.

The manufacturers state that the usual dosage of ceftriaxone for the treatment of serious infections (other than meningitis) in pediatric patients is 50–75 mg/kg daily given in divided doses every 12 hours. The maximum dosage recommended by the manufacturers for pediatric patients is 2 g daily.

Endocarditis

For the treatment of native valve endocarditis† caused by streptococci highly susceptible to penicillin (penicillin MIC 0.1 mcg/mL or less), including *Streptococcus pyogenes* (group A β-hemolytic streptococci; GAS), *S. agalactiae* (group B streptococci; GBS), streptococci groups C or G, most viridans group streptococci, or nonenterococcal group D streptococci (e.g., *S. gallolyticus* [formerly *S. bovis*], *S. equinas*), the American Heart Association (AHA) states that pediatric patients may receive IV ceftriaxone in a dosage of 100 mg/kg daily in divided doses every 12 hours for 4 weeks. Alternatively, AHA states that IV ceftriaxone can be given in a dosage of 80 mg/kg once daily (up to 4 g daily), but doses greater than 2 g should be given in divided doses every 12 hours.

For the treatment of native valve endocarditis† caused by streptococci relatively resistant to penicillin (penicillin MIC greater than 0.1 but less than 0.5 mcg/mL), AHA states that pediatric patients may receive IV ceftriaxone in a dosage of 100 mg/kg daily in divided doses every 12 hours for 4 weeks in conjunction with gentamicin (3–6 mg/kg daily IV in divided doses every 8 hours given concomitantly during the first 2 weeks of ceftriaxone treatment). Alternatively, AHA states that IV ceftriaxone can be given in a dosage of 80 mg/kg once daily (up to 4 g daily) in this regimen.

For the treatment of endocarditis† involving prosthetic valves or other prosthetic material caused by penicillin-susceptible streptococci (penicillin MIC 0.1 mcg/mL or less), AHA states that pediatric patients may receive IV ceftriaxone in a dosage of 100 mg/kg daily in divided doses every 12 hours for 6 weeks in conjunction with gentamicin (3–6 mg/kg daily IV in divided doses every 8 hours given concomitantly during the first 2 weeks of ceftriaxone treatment). Alternatively, AHA states that IV ceftriaxone can be given in a dosage of 80 mg/kg once daily (up to 4 g daily) in this regimen. If endocarditis involving prosthetic valves or other prosthetic material is caused by streptococci with penicillin MIC greater than 0.1 mcg/mL or caused by *Abiotrophia* or *Granulicatella*, AHA recommends that ceftriaxone be given for 6 weeks in conjunction with gentamicin (given concomitantly for the entire 6 weeks of ceftriaxone treatment).

For the treatment of endocarditis† caused by the HACEK group (i.e., *Haemophilus, Aggregatibacter, Cardiobacterium hominis, Eikenella corrodens, Kingella*), AHA states that pediatric patients may receive IV ceftriaxone in a dosage of 100 mg/kg daily in divided doses every 12 hours for 4 weeks. Alternatively, AHA

states that IV ceftriaxone can be given in a dosage of 80 mg/kg once daily (up to 4 g daily) for 4 weeks.

GI Infections

If ceftriaxone is used as an alternative for the treatment of *Salmonella* gastroenteritis† (with or without bacteremia) in adolescents with human immunodeficiency virus (HIV) infection, the US Centers for Disease Control and Prevention (CDC), National Institutes of Health (NIH), and Infectious Diseases Society of America (IDSA) recommend a dosage of 1 g IV every 24 hours. The recommended duration of treatment is 7–14 days in those with CD4+ T-cell counts of 200 cells/mm³ or greater (14 days or longer if bacteremia is present or the infection is complicated) or 2–6 weeks in those with CD4+ T-cell counts less than 200 cells/mm³.

For the treatment of shigellosis† caused by *Shigella sonnei* or *S. flexneri*, pediatric patients have received ceftriaxone in a dosage of 50 mg/kg once daily for 2–5 days.

If ceftriaxone is used as an alternative for empiric treatment of infectious diarrhea† in HIV-infected adolescents, CDC, NIH, and IDSA recommend a dosage of 1 g IV every 24 hours. If there is no clinical response after 5–7 days, stool culture and in vitro susceptibility testing should be considered.

Intra-abdominal Infections

If ceftriaxone is used for empiric treatment of complicated intra-abdominal infections in pediatric patients, a dosage of 50–75 mg/kg once or twice daily is recommended. Although ceftriaxone may be used alone for initial empiric treatment of community-acquired biliary tract infections (cholecystitis or cholangitis), the drug should be used in conjunction with metronidazole for initial empiric treatment of extrabiliary community-acquired intra-abdominal infections.

Meningitis and Other CNS Infections

For the treatment of meningitis caused by susceptible bacteria, the manufacturers and some clinicians recommend that pediatric patients receive an initial ceftriaxone dosage of 100 mg/kg (up to 4 g) followed by 100 mg/kg daily (up to 4 g daily) given once daily or in equally divided doses every 12 hours for 7–21 days. Other clinicians recommend a dosage of 80–100 mg/kg daily (up to 4 g daily) given once daily or in divided doses every 12 hours. A twice-daily dosing regimen may be preferred for the treatment of meningitis caused by *S. pneumoniae*.

While 7 days of anti-infective therapy may be adequate for the treatment of uncomplicated meningitis caused by susceptible *H. influenzae* or *N. meningitidis*, at least 10–14 days of therapy is suggested for complicated cases or meningitis caused by *S. pneumoniae* and at least 21 days is suggested for meningitis caused by susceptible Enterobacteriaceae† (e.g., *Escherichia coli, Klebsiella*†). In neonates, some experts state that treatment of meningitis should be continued for 2 weeks beyond the first sterile CSF culture or for at least 3 weeks, whichever is longer.

If IV ceftriaxone is used for the treatment of healthcare-associated ventriculitis and meningitis caused by susceptible bacteria (see Uses: Meningitis and Other CNS Infections), IDSA recommends that infants and children receive a dosage of 100 mg/kg daily as a single dose or in divided doses every 12 hours. The duration of treatment depends on the causative organism and patient characteristics. The recommended treatment duration is 10–14 days for infections caused by gram-negative bacilli (with or without significant CSF pleocytosis, CSF hypoglycorrhachia, or clinical symptoms or systemic features); some experts recommend a duration of 21 days.

Respiratory Tract Infections

If ceftriaxone is used in children for the treatment of severe acute bacterial rhinosinusitis† requiring hospitalization, IDSA recommends a dosage of 50 mg/kg daily given IV in divided doses every 12 hours.

For the treatment of community-acquired pneumonia (CAP) caused by *S. pneumoniae* in pediatric patients 3 months of age or older, IDSA recommends that ceftriaxone be given in a dosage of 50–100 mg/kg daily as a single dose or in divided doses every 12 hours if the infection is caused by penicillin-susceptible strains or a dosage of 100 mg/kg daily as a single dose or in divided doses every 12 hours if the infection is caused by penicillin-resistant strains. Treatment usually is continued for 10 days.

For the treatment of CAP caused by susceptible *S. pyogenes* (group A β-hemolytic streptococci; GAS) or *H. influenzae* in pediatric patients 3 months of age or older, IDSA recommends that ceftriaxone be given in a dosage of 50–100 mg/kg daily as a single daily dose or in divided doses every 12 hours. Treatment usually is continued for 10 days.

Skin and Skin Structure Infections

The usual dosage of ceftriaxone for the treatment of skin and skin structure infections caused by susceptible organisms in pediatric patients is 50–75 mg/kg daily given as a single daily dose or in equally divided doses every 12 hours.

Acute Otitis Media

For the treatment of acute otitis media (AOM), the manufacturers recommend that pediatric patients receive a single 50-mg/kg IM dose of ceftriaxone (maximum dose 1 g).

For initial treatment of AOM, AAP recommends a ceftriaxone dosage of 50 mg/kg daily given IM or IV for 1 to 3 days†. AAP cautions that more than a single dose may be required to prevent recurrence.

For retreatment in patients with AOM who failed to respond to an initial anti-infective regimen, AAP recommends a ceftriaxone dosage of 50 mg/kg daily given for 3 days†.

Chancroid

When ceftriaxone is used for the treatment of chancroid† (genital ulcers caused by *H. ducreyi*), AAP recommends that infants and children weighing less than 45 kg receive a single 50-mg/kg IM dose (up to 250 mg) and that pediatric patients weighing 45 kg or more receive a single 250-mg IM dose.

Gonococcal Infections in Neonates

When ceftriaxone is used for parenteral *prophylaxis*† or presumptive treatment of gonorrhea† in neonates born to mothers with gonorrhea, CDC and AAP recommend that a single dose of 25–50 mg/kg (maximum 125 mg) of the drug be given IM or IV at birth.

For the *treatment* of gonococcal ophthalmia neonatorum†, CDC and AAP recommend that neonates receive a single IM or IV dose of 25–50 mg/kg (maximum 125 mg) of ceftriaxone.

For the treatment of disseminated gonococcal infections (e.g., sepsis, arthritis, meningitis) or gonococcal scalp abscess in neonates†, the usual dosage of ceftriaxone is 25–50 mg/kg IM or IV once daily for 7 days. If meningitis is documented, ceftriaxone should be continued for 10–14 days.

Gonococcal Infections in Infants and Children

For the treatment of uncomplicated gonorrhea in children beyond the neonatal age (prepubertal), AAP recommends that those weighing less than 45 kg receive a single 125-mg IM dose of ceftriaxone and that those weighing 45 kg or more receive a single 250-mg IM dose of ceftriaxone *and* a dose of azithromycin (single 1-g oral dose). CDC recommends that infants and children with uncomplicated gonococcal infections (vulvovaginitis, cervicitis, urethritis, pharyngitis, proctitis) weighing 45 kg or less receive a single IV or IM ceftriaxone dose of 25–50 mg/kg (up to 125 mg IM) and that those weighing more than 45 kg receive a single 250-mg IM dose of ceftriaxone *and* a dose of azithromycin (single 1-g oral dose).

For the treatment of disseminated or complicated gonococcal infections† (e.g., arthritis-dermatitis syndrome) in children beyond the neonatal period (prepubertal), AAP recommends that those weighing less than 45 kg receive IV or IM ceftriaxone in a dosage of 50 mg/kg once daily (up to 1 g daily) for 7 days in conjunction with erythromycin (30 mg/kg daily given orally in 4 divided doses [up to 2 g daily] for 14 days) and that those weighing 45 kg or more receive IV or IM ceftriaxone in a dosage of 1 g once daily for 7 days in conjunction with a dose of azithromycin (single 1-g oral dose). If meningitis or endocarditis is present, AAP recommends that dosage and duration of ceftriaxone in these regimens be increased to 50 mg/kg IV or IM every 12–24 hours for 10–14 days in those weighing less than 45 kg or 1–2 g IV every 12–24 hours for 10–14 days in those weighing 45 kg or more.

For the treatment of gonococcal bacteremia or arthritis in children, CDC recommends that those weighing 45 kg or less receiving IM or IV ceftriaxone in a dosage of 50 mg/kg daily (maximum 1 g daily) for 7 days and that those weighing more than 45 kg receive an IM or IV ceftriaxone dosage of 1 g once daily for 7 days.

Gonorrhea and Associated Infections in Adolescents

For the treatment of uncomplicated cervical, urethral, rectal, or pharyngeal gonorrhea, CDC recommends that adolescents receive a single 250-mg IM dose of ceftriaxone *and* a dose of azithromycin (single 1-g oral dose).

For the treatment of gonococcal conjunctivitis†, adolescents should receive a single 1-g IM dose of ceftriaxone *and* a dose of azithromycin (single 1-g oral dose).

For the treatment of gonococcal arthritis and arthritis-dermatitis syndrome†, CDC recommends that adolescents receive 1 g of ceftriaxone IV or IM once daily *and* a dose of azithromycin (single 1-g oral dose). Ceftriaxone should be continued until 24–48 hours after substantial clinical improvement; treatment can then be switched to an oral antibacterial selected based on in vitro susceptibility testing and given to complete a total treatment duration of at least 7 days.

For the treatment of gonococcal meningitis† or gonococcal endocarditis†, CDC recommends that adolescents receive 1–2 g of ceftriaxone IV every 12–24 hours *and* a dose of azithromycin (single 1-g oral dose). Ceftriaxone should be continued for 10–14 days in those with meningitis and for at least 4 weeks in those with endocarditis.

Prophylaxis in Sexual Assault Victims

For empiric anti-infective prophylaxis for gonorrhea, chlamydia, and trichomoniasis in adolescent sexual assault victims†, CDC recommends that a single 250-mg IM dose of ceftriaxone be given in conjunction with azithromycin (single 1-g oral dose) and either metronidazole (single 2-g oral dose) or tinidazole (single 2-g oral dose).

Lyme Disease

If IV ceftriaxone is used for the treatment of early Lyme disease† in children with acute neurologic disease manifested by meningitis or radiculopathy, IDSA and AAP recommend a dosage of 50–75 mg/kg (up to 2 g) once daily for 14 days (range: 10–28 days).

When a parenteral regimen is indicated for the treatment of Lyme carditis† in patients with atrioventricular (AV) heart block and/or myopericarditis associated with early Lyme disease, IDSA recommends that children receive IV ceftriaxone in a dosage of 50–75 mg/kg (up to 2 g) once daily for 14 days (range: 14–21 days). Although a parenteral regimen is recommended for initial treatment of hospitalized patients, the parenteral regimen can be switched to an oral regimen (doxycycline, amoxicillin, cefuroxime axetil) to complete therapy and for outpatients.

When a parenteral regimen is indicated for the treatment of Lyme arthritis† in patients with evidence of neurologic disease or when arthritis has not responded to an oral regimen, IDSA and AAP recommend that children receive IV ceftriaxone in a dosage of 50–75 mg/kg (up to 2 g) once daily for 14 days (range: 14–28 days).

For the treatment of late neurologic Lyme disease† affecting the central or peripheral nervous system, IDSA and AAP recommend that children receive IV ceftriaxone in a dosage of 50–75 mg/kg (up to 2 g) once daily for 2–4 weeks.

Neisseria meningitidis Infections

When ceftriaxone is used to eliminate nasopharyngeal carriage of *N. meningitidis*† or for chemoprophylaxis in close contacts of individuals with invasive meningococcal disease†, a single 125-mg IM dose should be used in children and adolescents younger than 15 years of age and a single 250-mg IM dose should be used in adolescents 15 years of age or older.

For dosage recommendations for the treatment of meningitis caused by *N. meningitidis*, see Meningitis and Other CNS Infections under Dosage: Pediatric Dosage, in Dosage and Administration.)

Pelvic Inflammatory Disease

For the treatment of mild to moderately severe acute pelvic inflammatory disease (PID) when an IM and oral regimen is indicated, adolescents may receive a single 250-mg IM dose of ceftriaxone followed by a 14-day regimen of doxycycline (100 mg orally twice daily) with or without metronidazole (500 mg orally twice daily). If there is no clinical response within 72 hours, the patient should be reevaluated to confirm the diagnosis and an IV regimen should be administered if indicated.

Syphilis

If ceftriaxone is used as an alternative in infants or children with clinical evidence of congenital syphilis† when penicillin G is not available, dosage should be based on age and weight. CDC states that infants 30 days of age or older may receive a dosage of 75 mg/kg IV or IM once daily for 10–14 days (dosage adjustments may be needed based on weight) and children may receive 100 mg/kg IV or IM once daily for 10–14 days. Clinicians should consider that ceftriaxone is contraindicated in certain neonates (see Cautions: Pediatric Precautions). Ceftriaxone should be used for the treatment of congenital syphilis *only* when necessary (i.e., during a penicillin shortage) and should be used in consultation with a specialist in the treatment of infants with congenital syphilis and with close clinical, serologic, and CSF follow-up.

If ceftriaxone is used as an alternative to IM penicillin G benzathine for the treatment of primary or secondary syphilis† in penicillin-allergic nonpregnant adolescents, CDC and other clinicians recommend a ceftriaxone dosage of 1–2 g IM or IV once daily for 10–14 days. Some clinicians suggest that this ceftriaxone dosage also can be used as an alternative in penicillin-allergic nonpregnant adolescents with early latent syphilis.

If ceftriaxone is used as an alternative to IV penicillin G for the treatment of neurosyphilis† in penicillin-allergic nonpregnant adolescents, CDC and others suggest a dosage of 2 g IM or IV daily for 10–14 days based on limited data.

CDC cautions that the optimal dosage and duration of ceftriaxone for the treatment of syphilis have not been defined and close follow-up is essential. (See Uses: Syphilis.)

Typhoid Fever and Other Invasive Salmonella Infections

For the treatment of typhoid fever† (enteric fever) or septicemia caused by Salmonella serovar Typhi†, including multidrug-resistant strains, pediatric patients have received ceftriaxone in a dosage of 50–75 mg/kg given IM or IV once daily. While ceftriaxone has been effective for the treatment of typhoid fever when administered for 3–7 days, anti-infective therapy for the treatment of typhoid fever usually is continued for at least 14 days to prevent relapse and a duration of at least 4–6 weeks may be necessary for the treatment of immunocompromised individuals (including HIV-infected individuals) or for the treatment of Salmonella meningitis.

Empiric Therapy in Febrile Neutropenic Patients

When used for empiric anti-infective therapy in febrile neutropenic patients†, children have received ceftriaxone in a dosage of 80 mg/kg (up to 2 g) once daily in conjunction with amikacin (20 mg/kg IV daily).

Prevention of Bacterial Endocarditis

If ceftriaxone is used as an alternative for prevention of α-hemolytic (viridans group) streptococcal endocarditis† in individuals with certain cardiac conditions who are undergoing certain dental or upper respiratory tract procedures (see Uses: Prevention of Bacterial Endocarditis), AHA recommends that children receive a single dose of 50 mg/kg given IV or IM 30–60 minutes prior to the procedure.

Adult Dosage
General Adult Dosage

The usual adult dosage of ceftriaxone for the treatment of most infections caused by susceptible organisms is 1–2 g given once daily or in equally divided doses twice daily, depending on the type and severity of the infection.

One manufacturer recommends that adults receive ceftriaxone in a dosage of 50–75 mg/kg every 12 hours (maximum 2 g daily) for the treatment of serious infections other than meningitis.

The maximum adult dosage of ceftriaxone recommended by the manufacturers is 4 g daily.

Bone and Joint Infections

For the treatment of native vertebral osteomyelitis caused by susceptible staphylococci, β-hemolytic streptococci†, or Cutibacterium acnes† (formerly Propionibacterium acnes), IDSA recommends that adults receive ceftriaxone in a dosage of 2 g IV once daily for 6 weeks.

If ceftriaxone is used as an alternative for the treatment of native vertebral osteomyelitis caused by susceptible Salmonella† (nalidixic acid-resistant strains), IDSA recommends that adults receive a dosage of 2 g IV once daily for 6–8 weeks.

For the treatment of prosthetic joint infections caused by susceptible staphylococci, IDSA recommends that adults receive ceftriaxone in a dosage of 1–2 g IV once daily for 2–4 weeks in conjunction with rifampin (300–450 mg orally twice daily) and that this regimen be followed by an oral anti-infective regimen (e.g., rifampin and ciprofloxacin or levofloxacin) to complete a total treatment duration of 3 months for infections related to total hip arthroplasty or 6 months for infections related to total knee arthroplasty.

For the treatment of prosthetic joint infections caused by susceptible β-hemolytic streptococci or C. acnes†, IDSA recommends that adults receive 2 g IV once daily for 4–6 weeks.

Endocarditis

For the treatment of native valve endocarditis† caused by viridans group streptococci or S. gallolyticus highly susceptible to penicillin (penicillin MIC 0.12 mcg/mL or less), AHA recommends that adults receive IV or IM ceftriaxone in a dosage of 2 g once daily for 4 weeks. Alternatively, adults with uncomplicated endocarditis† caused by highly penicillin-susceptible viridans group streptococci or S. gallolyticus who are at low risk for adverse effects related to aminoglycoside therapy may receive a 2-week regimen consisting of IV or IM ceftriaxone in a dosage of 2 g once daily in conjunction with gentamicin (3 mg/kg daily IV or IM given as a single daily dose or as 1 mg/kg every 8 hours). The 2-week regimen is not recommended for patients with known cardiac or extracardiac abscesses, creatinine clearance less than 20 mL/minute, impaired eighth cranial nerve function, or infection with Abiotrophia, Granulicatella, or Gemella.

For the treatment of endocarditis† involving prosthetic valves or other prosthetic material caused by viridans group streptococci or S. gallolyticus highly susceptible to penicillin (penicillin MIC 0.12 mcg/mL or less), AHA states that adults can receive IV or IM ceftriaxone in a dosage of 2 g once daily for 6 weeks with or without gentamicin (3 mg/kg daily IV or IM as a single daily dose or as 1 mg/kg every 8 hours given concomitantly during the first 2 weeks of ceftriaxone treatment). When endocarditis involving prosthetic valves or other prosthetic material is caused by viridans group streptococci or S. gallolyticus relatively or highly resistant to penicillin (penicillin MIC greater than 0.12 mcg/mL), AHA states that it is reasonable to extend the duration of concomitant gentamicin to the entire 6 weeks of ceftriaxone treatment.

When a double β-lactam regimen is used for the treatment of enterococcal endocarditis† involving native valves or prosthetic valves or other prosthetic material (see Enterococcal Endocarditis under Uses: Endocarditis), AHA recommends that adults receive ceftriaxone in a dosage of 2 g IV every 12 hours in conjunction with ampicillin (2 g IV every 4 hours). Both drugs should be continued for 6 weeks.

For the treatment of endocarditis† caused by the HACEK group (i.e., Haemophilus, Aggregatibacter, C. hominis, E. corrodens, Kingella), AHA recommends that adults receive IV or IM ceftriaxone in a dosage of 2 g once daily. A duration of 4 weeks is reasonable for the treatment of native valve endocarditis and 6 weeks is reasonable for the treatment of endocarditis involving prosthetic valves or other prosthetic material.

GI Infections

If ceftriaxone is used as an alternative for the treatment of Salmonella gastroenteritis† (with or without bacteremia) in HIV-infected adults, CDC, NIH, and IDSA recommend a dosage of 1 g IV every 24 hours. The recommended duration of treatment is 7–14 days in those with CD4+ T-cell counts of 200 cells/mm³ or greater (14 days or longer if the patient is bacteremic or the infection is complicated) or 2–6 weeks in those with CD4+ T-cell counts less than 200 cells/mm³.

If ceftriaxone is used as an alternative for empiric treatment of infectious diarrhea† in HIV-infected adults, CDC, NIH, and IDSA recommend a dosage of 1 g IV every 24 hours. If there is no clinical response after 5–7 days, stool culture and in vitro susceptibility testing should be considered.

Intra-abdominal Infections

If ceftriaxone is used for empiric treatment of complicated intra-abdominal infections, a dosage of 1–2 g once or twice daily is recommended. Although ceftriaxone may be used alone for initial empiric treatment of community-acquired biliary tract infections (cholecystitis or cholangitis), the drug should be used in conjunction with metronidazole for initial empiric treatment of extrabiliary community-acquired intra-abdominal infections.

Meningitis and Other CNS Infections

For the treatment of meningitis caused by susceptible bacteria, the usual adult dosage of ceftriaxone is 2 g IV every 12 hours. Some manufacturers and clinicians suggest a ceftriaxone dosage of 50–100 mg/kg (up to 4 g) once daily or in 2 equally divided doses every 12 hours; some clinicians suggest a dosage of 4 g daily given in 1 or 2 equally divided doses.

While 7 days of anti-infective therapy may be adequate for the treatment of uncomplicated meningitis caused by susceptible H. influenzae or N. meningitidis, at least 10–14 days of therapy is suggested for complicated cases or meningitis caused by S. pneumoniae and at least 21 days of therapy is suggested for meningitis caused by susceptible Enterobacteriaceae† (e.g., E. coli, Klebsiella†).

If ceftriaxone is used for the treatment of healthcare-associated ventriculitis and meningitis caused by susceptible bacteria (see Uses: Meningitis and Other CNS Infections), IDSA recommends that adults receive a dosage of 4 g daily given in divided doses every 12 hours. The duration of treatment depends on the causative organism and patient characteristics. The recommended treatment duration is 10–14 days for infections caused by gram-negative bacilli (with or without significant CSF pleocytosis, CSF hypoglycorrhachia, or clinical symptoms or systemic features); some experts recommend a duration of 21 days.

Respiratory Tract Infections

If ceftriaxone is used for the treatment of severe acute bacterial rhinosinusitis† requiring hospitalization, IDSA recommends that adults receive a dosage of 1–2 g IV every 12–24 hours.

Skin and Skin Structure Infections

For the treatment of skin and skin structure infections, adults should receive ceftriaxone in a dosage of 50–75 mg/kg once daily or in 2 equally divided doses every 12 hours (maximum 2 g daily).

If ceftriaxone is used for the treatment of necrotizing fasciitis involving *Aeromonas hydrophila*†, IDSA recommends that adults receive a dosage of 1–2 g IV once daily in conjunction with doxycycline (100 mg IV every 12 hours). If necrotizing fasciitis involves *Vibrio vulnificus*†, IDSA recommends that adults receive ceftriaxone in a dosage of 1 g IV once daily in conjunction with doxycycline (100 mg IV every 12 hours).

If ceftriaxone is used for the treatment of surgical site infections following intestinal or genitourinary tract surgery, IDSA recommends a dosage of 1 g once daily in conjunction with metronidazole (500 mg IV every 8 hours). For the treatment of surgical site infections following procedures involving the axilla or perineum, IDSA recommends that ceftriaxone be given in a dosage of 1 g once daily; concomitant vancomycin (15 mg/kg every 12 hours) may also be needed.

If ceftriaxone is used for the treatment of an infected animal bite wound, IDSA recommends a dosage of 1 g IV every 12 hours.

Urinary Tract Infections

For the treatment of acute pyelonephritis (e.g., pending results of in vitro susceptibility testing), a single 1-g IV dose of ceftriaxone has been recommended followed by an appropriate oral anti-infective regimen given for 7–14 days.

Chancroid

If ceftriaxone is used for the treatment of chancroid† (genital ulcers caused by *H. ducreyi*), CDC and other clinicians recommend that adults receive a single 250-mg IM dose of the drug.

Gonorrhea and Associated Infections

For the treatment of uncomplicated cervical, urethral, rectal, or pharyngeal gonorrhea, adults should receive a single 250-mg IM dose of ceftriaxone *and* a dose of azithromycin (single 1-g oral dose). (See Gonococcal Infections in Adults and Adolescents in Uses: Gonorrhea and Associated Infections.)

For the treatment of gonococcal conjunctivitis†, adults should receive a single 1-g IM dose of ceftriaxone *and* a dose of azithromycin (single 1-g oral dose).

For the treatment of gonococcal arthritis and arthritis-dermatitis syndrome†, CDC recommends that adults receive 1 g of ceftriaxone IV or IM once daily *and* a dose of azithromycin (single 1-g oral dose). Ceftriaxone should be continued until 24–48 hours after substantial clinical improvement; treatment can then be switched to an oral antibacterial (selected based on in vitro susceptibility testing) to complete a total treatment duration of at least 7 days.

For the treatment of gonococcal meningitis† or gonococcal endocarditis†, CDC recommends that adults receive 1–2 g of ceftriaxone IV every 12–24 hours in conjunction with a dose of azithromycin (single 1-g oral dose). Ceftriaxone should be continued for 10–14 days in those with meningitis and for at least 4 weeks in those with endocarditis.

For presumptive treatment of acute epididymitis most likely caused by sexually transmitted chlamydia and gonorrhea†, adults should receive a single 250-mg IM dose of ceftriaxone given in conjunction with doxycycline (100 mg orally twice daily for 10 days).

For presumptive treatment of acute epididymitis most likely caused by sexually transmitted chlamydia, gonorrhea, and enteric bacteria† (e.g., *E. coli*), adults should receive a single 250-mg IM dose of ceftriaxone given in conjunction with levofloxacin (500 mg orally once daily for 10 days) or ofloxacin (300 mg orally twice daily for 10 days).

For presumptive treatment of acute proctitis†, adults should receive a single 250-mg IM dose of ceftriaxone given in conjunction with doxycycline (100 mg orally twice daily for 7 days).

Prophylaxis in Sexual Assault Victims

For empiric anti-infective prophylaxis for gonorrhea, chlamydia, and trichomoniasis in adult sexual assault victims†, CDC recommends that a single 250-mg IM dose of ceftriaxone be given in conjunction with azithromycin (single 1-g oral dose) and either metronidazole (single 2-g oral dose) or tinidazole (single 2-g oral dose).

Leptospirosis

For the treatment of severe leptospirosis†, adults have received ceftriaxone in a dosage of 1 g IV once daily for 7 days.

Lyme Disease

If ceftriaxone is used for the treatment of early Lyme disease† in adults with acute neurologic disease manifested by meningitis or radiculopathy, IDSA and other clinicians recommend a dosage of 2 g IV once daily for 14 days (range: 10–28 days).

When a parenteral regimen is indicated for the treatment of Lyme carditis† in adults with AV heart block and/or myopericarditis associated with early Lyme disease, IDSA and other clinicians recommend a ceftriaxone dosage of 2 g IV once daily for 14 days (range: 14–21 days). Although a parenteral regimen is recommended for initial treatment of hospitalized patients, the parenteral regimen can be switched to an oral regimen (doxycycline, amoxicillin, cefuroxime axetil) to complete therapy and for outpatients.

When a parenteral regimen is indicated for the treatment of Lyme arthritis† in patients with evidence of neurologic disease or when arthritis has not responded to an oral regimen, IDSA and other clinicians recommend that adults receive a ceftriaxone dosage of 2 g IV once daily for 14 days (range: 14–28 days).

For the treatment of late neurologic Lyme disease† affecting the central or peripheral nervous system, IDSA and other clinicians recommend that adults receive ceftriaxone in a dosage of 2 g IV once daily for 2–4 weeks.

Neisseria meningitidis Infections

When ceftriaxone is used to eliminate nasopharyngeal carriage of *N. meningitidis*† or for chemoprophylaxis in close contacts of individuals with invasive meningococcal disease†, adults should receive a single 250-mg IM dose.

For dosage recommendations for the treatment of meningitis caused by *N. meningitidis*, see Meningitis and Other CNS Infections under Dosage: Adult Dosage, in Dosage and Administration.)

Pelvic Inflammatory Disease

For the treatment of mild to moderately severe acute pelvic inflammatory disease (PID) when an IM and oral regimen is indicated, adults may receive a single 250-mg IM dose of ceftriaxone followed by a 14-day regimen of doxycycline (100 mg orally twice daily) with or without oral metronidazole (500 mg twice daily). If there is no clinical response within 72 hours, the patient should be reevaluated to confirm the diagnosis and an IV regimen should be administered if indicated.

Syphilis

If ceftriaxone is used as an alternative to IM penicillin G benzathine for the treatment of primary or secondary syphilis† in penicillin-allergic nonpregnant adults, CDC and other clinicians recommend a ceftriaxone dosage of 1–2 g IM or IV once daily for 10–14 days. Some clinicians suggest that this ceftriaxone dosage also can be used as an alternative in penicillin-allergic nonpregnant adults with early latent syphilis.

If ceftriaxone is used as an alternative to IV penicillin G for the treatment of neurosyphilis† in penicillin-allergic nonpregnant adults, a dosage of 2 g IM or IV daily for 10–14 days has been suggested by CDC and others based on limited data.

CDC cautions that the optimal dosage and duration of ceftriaxone for the treatment of syphilis have not been defined and close follow-up is essential. (See Uses: Syphilis.)

Typhoid Fever and Other Invasive Salmonella Infections

For the treatment of typhoid fever† or septicemia caused by *Salmonella* serovars Typhi† or Paratyphi†, including infections caused by multidrug-resistant strains, adults have received ceftriaxone in a dosage of 2–4 g IM or IV once daily for 3–7 days. Alternatively, adults have received a dosage of 1 g once daily for 15 days.

While ceftriaxone has been effective for the treatment of typhoid fever when administered for 3–7 days, anti-infective therapy for the treatment of typhoid fever usually is continued for at least 14 days to prevent relapse and a duration of at least 4–6 weeks may be necessary for the treatment of immunocompromised individuals (including those with HIV infection) or for the treatment of *Salmonella* meningitis.

Whipple's Disease

For the treatment of Whipple's disease† caused by *Tropheryma whipplei* (formerly *Tropheryma whippelii*), some clinicians recommend that ceftriaxone be given in a dosage of 2 g IV once daily for 2–4 weeks followed by oral co-trimoxazole given for 1–2 years. For the treatment of encephalitis caused by *T. whipplei*, IDSA recommends initial treatment with ceftriaxone given for 2–4 weeks followed by co-trimoxazole or cefixime for 1–2 years.

Empiric Therapy in Febrile Neutropenic Patients

When used for empiric anti-infective therapy in febrile neutropenic patients†, adults have received ceftriaxone in a dosage of 30 mg/kg (up to 2 g) given IV once daily in conjunction with amikacin (20 mg/kg IV once daily).

Perioperative Prophylaxis

If ceftriaxone is used for perioperative prophylaxis in adults, the manufacturers and some clinicians recommend that a single 1-g dose be given IV 0.5–2 hours prior to surgery.

For perioperative prophylaxis in patients undergoing cholecystectomy, adults have received a single 1-g dose of ceftriaxone given IV 0.5–2 hours prior to surgery; however, higher doses (e.g., 2 g) also have been used.

For perioperative prophylaxis in adults undergoing colorectal procedures, some experts recommend that a single 2-g dose of ceftriaxone be given IV in conjunction with metronidazole (single 500-mg IV dose) within 1 hour prior to surgery.

Prevention of Bacterial Endocarditis

If ceftriaxone is used as an alternative for prevention of α-hemolytic (viridans group) streptococcal endocarditis† in individuals with certain cardiac conditions who are undergoing certain dental or upper respiratory tract procedures (see Uses: Prevention of Bacterial Endocarditis), AHA recommends that adults receive a single dose of 1 g given IM or IV 30–60 minutes prior to the procedure.

● Dosage in Renal and Hepatic Impairment

Modification of the usual dosage of ceftriaxone is not usually necessary in adults with impaired renal or hepatic function alone who are receiving the drug in dosages up to 2 g daily. However, if the drug is used in patients with hepatic impairment *and* clinically important renal impairment, caution is advised and dosage should not exceed 2 g daily.

Some clinicians state that serum concentrations of the drug should be monitored when ceftriaxone is used in patients with severe renal impairment (e.g., dialysis patients) or in patients with both hepatic and substantial renal impairment.

Because ceftriaxone is not removed by hemodialysis or peritoneal dialysis, supplemental doses of the drug are unnecessary during or after dialysis.

CAUTIONS

Adverse effects reported with ceftriaxone are similar to those reported with other cephalosporins. For information on adverse effects reported with cephalosporins, see Cautions in the Cephalosporins General Statement 8:12.06. Ceftriaxone generally is well tolerated; adverse effects have been reported in about 10% of patients receiving ceftriaxone and have required discontinuance of the drug in less than 2% of these patients.

● Hematologic Effects

Hematologic effects are among the most frequent adverse effects reported with ceftriaxone. Eosinophilia has been reported in about 6%, thrombocytosis in about 5%,

and leukopenia in about 2% of patients receiving ceftriaxone. Anemia, neutropenia, lymphopenia, and thrombocytopenia have been reported in less than 1% and leukocytosis, lymphocytosis, monocytosis, agranulocytosis, basophilia, and coagulopathy have been reported in less than 0.1% of patients receiving ceftriaxone.

Hypoprothrombinemia or prolongation of prothrombin time (PT), with or without bleeding, has been reported in patients receiving ceftriaxone. (See Other Precautions and Contraindications under Cautions: Precautions and Contraindications.) Although very high concentrations of ceftriaxone (3–4 g/L) inhibited platelet aggregation in an in vitro study, in vivo studies indicate that the drug does not interfere with platelet function.

Immune-mediated hemolytic anemia has been reported in patients receiving ceftriaxone. Severe cases of hemolytic anemia, including fatalities, have occurred in both adults and children. Some cases occurred shortly after administration of a ceftriaxone dose, and some reactions have consisted of severe intravascular hemolysis and anemia, decreased hemoglobin concentrations, reticulocytosis, hemoglobinuria, and cardiac arrest. In at least one case, the direct antiglobulin (Coombs') test was strongly positive and the patient's serum agglutinated washed erythrocytes in the presence of complement and ceftriaxone. (See Other Precautions and Contraindications under Cautions: Precautions and Contraindications.)

● GI Effects

Diarrhea or loose stools has generally been reported in 2–4% of patients receiving ceftriaxone. However, transient diarrhea was reported in 42–44% of children receiving ceftriaxone in 2 studies and in 28% (10/36) of adults receiving the drug in another study. Nausea, vomiting, and dysgeusia have been reported in less than 1% and abdominal pain, flatulence, dyspepsia, colitis, gallbladder sludge, and biliary lithiasis have been reported in less than 0.1% of patients receiving the drug. Stomatitis and glossitis also have been reported.

Pancreatitis, possibly secondary to biliary obstruction, has been reported in patients treated with ceftriaxone. Most patients presented with risk factors for biliary stasis and biliary sludge (preceding major therapy, severe illness, total parenteral nutrition). A cofactor role of ceftriaxone-related biliary precipitation cannot be ruled out.

Clostridium difficile-associated Diarrhea and Colitis

Treatment with anti-infectives alters the normal colon flora and may permit overgrowth of *Clostridium difficile*.

C. difficile infection (CDI) and *C. difficile*-associated diarrhea and colitis (CDAD; also known as antibiotic-associated diarrhea and colitis or pseudomembranous colitis) have been reported with nearly all anti-infectives, including ceftriaxone, and may range in severity from mild diarrhea to fatal colitis. *C. difficile* produces toxins A and B, which contribute to the development of CDAD; hypertoxin-producing strains of *C. difficile* are associated with increased morbidity and mortality since these infections may be refractory to anti-infective therapy and may require colectomy.

CDAD should be considered in the differential diagnosis in patients who develop diarrhea during or after anti-infective therapy. Careful medical history is necessary since CDAD has been reported to occur as late as 2 months or longer after anti-infective therapy is discontinued.

If CDAD is suspected or confirmed, anti-infectives not directed against *C. difficile* should be discontinued as soon as possible. Patients should be managed with appropriate anti-infective therapy directed against *C. difficile* (e.g., vancomycin, fidaxomicin, metronidazole), supportive therapy (e.g., fluid and electrolyte management, protein supplementation), and surgical evaluation as clinically indicated. (See Superinfection/Clostridium difficile-associated Diarrhea and Colitis under Cautions: Precautions and Contraindications.)

Gallbladder Pseudolithiasis

Ceftriaxone-calcium precipitates in the gallbladder have been observed in patients receiving ceftriaxone. These precipitates appear on sonography as an echo without acoustical shadowing suggesting sludge or as an echo with acoustical shadowing which may be misinterpreted as gallstones. Although patients may be asymptomatic, symptoms of gallbladder disease (e.g., colic, nausea, vomiting, anorexia) can occur and may be severe enough to require discontinuance of ceftriaxone therapy.

The condition appears to be reversible and generally resolves following discontinuance of the drug and conservative management; surgery may not be necessary. The time to resolution, however, is variable and may range from a few days to several months. Upper abdominal ultrasonography should be considered for patients who develop biliary colic while receiving ceftriaxone therapy; biliary precipitates of ceftriaxone may be detected by ultrasonography after only 4 days of ceftriaxone therapy. The risk of precipitation may depend on the dose and rate of IV administration of ceftriaxone, occurring more frequently with relatively high dosages and rapid (e.g., over several minutes) rates of administration. In some patients with renal impairment or those receiving higher than usual dosages of the drug, precipitates containing traces of ceftriaxone, possibly combined with calcium, have been recovered in surgical specimens.

The probability of gallbladder precipitates associated with ceftriaxone therapy appears to be greatest in pediatric patients. In one study in children with various infections who received IV ceftriaxone in a dosage of 60–100 mg/kg daily, gallbladder precipitates developed in 43% of patients. The typical abnormality observed sonographically in these children was a strikingly hyperechogenic material with postacoustic shadowing; the precipitates differed from typical biliary sludge or cholelithiasis, usually were mobile, and tended to clump in the most dependent part of the gallbladder.

In a retrospective study of more than 1300 patients admitted to the hospital during a 2-year period with a diagnosis of Lyme disease, biliary symptoms (e.g., cholecystitis, cholelithiasis) or cholecystectomy occurred in approximately 2% of patients (84% were female with a median age of 12 years [range: 3–40 years]); 56% of these patients underwent laparoscopic cholecystectomy, mainly for cholelithiasis. Among cases and controls who received anti-infective therapy for treatment of suspected Lyme disease, each patient had received a median of 3 courses of oral and/or IV anti-infectives. All patients with biliary symptoms had received IV ceftriaxone therapy within 90 days prior to the occurrence of biliary disease; daily ceftriaxone dosage at the time of onset of biliary symptoms in these patients averaged 57 mg/kg (range: 27–96 mg/kg), and the median duration of therapy was 28 days (range: 4–170 days). These data suggest an association between biliary complications and the repeated and often prolonged courses of IV ceftriaxone therapy used in these patients, most of whom lacked documented objective clinical or laboratory evidence of Lyme disease. (See Lyme Disease in Uses: Spirochetal Infections.)

In studies in dogs and baboons receiving high dosages of ceftriaxone sodium, concretions consisting of the precipitated calcium salt of ceftriaxone have been found in gallbladder bile. These appeared as gritty sediment in dogs who received ceftriaxone in a dosage of 100 mg/kg daily for 4 weeks but were evident in the baboon only after a daily dosage of 335 mg/kg or more for 6 months. The likelihood of this occurrence in humans has been considered to be low since ceftriaxone has a longer plasma half-life in humans, the calcium salt of ceftriaxone is more soluble in human gallbladder bile, and the calcium content of human gallbladder bile is relatively low.

● Dermatologic and Sensitivity Reactions

Rash (e.g., erythematous, urticarial) has been reported in about 2% of patients receiving ceftriaxone and pruritus, fever, and chills have been reported in less than 1% of patients receiving the drug.

Serious, occasionally fatal, hypersensitivity reactions (anaphylaxis or anaphylactoid) have been reported in patients receiving ceftriaxone. Bronchospasm and serum sickness have been reported in less than 0.1% of patients receiving the drug.

Exanthema, allergic dermatitis, urticaria, and edema have been reported in patients receiving ceftriaxone. There also have been postmarketing reports of generalized exanthematous pustulosis and isolated reports of severe cutaneous adverse reactions (e.g., erythema multiforme, Stevens-Johnson syndrome, Lyell's syndrome/toxic epidermal necrolysis).

● Hepatic Effects

Increased serum concentrations of AST (SGOT) and ALT (SGPT) have been reported in about 3% of patients and increased serum concentrations of alkaline phosphatase and bilirubin have been reported in less than 1% of patients receiving ceftriaxone. Jaundice has been reported in less than 0.1% of patients receiving the drug and there have been postmarketing reports of hepatitis.

● Renal Effects

Increased concentrations of BUN have been reported in about 1% of patients receiving ceftriaxone and increased concentrations of serum creatinine and the presence of casts in urine have been reported in less than 1% of patients receiving the drug. Glycosuria, hematuria, renal precipitates, and nephrolithiasis have

been reported in less than 0.1% of patients receiving the drug. Oliguria, ureteric obstruction, and post-renal acute renal failure also have been reported.

Ceftriaxone-calcium precipitates in the urine have been observed in patients receiving ceftriaxone and may be detected as sonographic abnormalities. The probability of such precipitates appears to be greatest in pediatric patients. Patients may be asymptomatic or may develop symptoms of urolithiasis, ureteral obstruction, and post-renal acute renal failure. The condition appears to be reversible following discontinuance of the drug and conservative management.

● Pulmonary and Renal Precipitates

Fatalities have been reported in some neonates who received ceftriaxone and calcium-containing IV solutions. A crystalline material was observed in the lungs and kidneys of these neonates at autopsy. In some cases, the same IV infusion line had been used for both ceftriaxone and the calcium-containing fluid and, in some, a precipitate was observed in the IV infusion line. At least 1 fatality occurred in a neonate who received ceftriaxone and calcium-containing fluids administered at different times and through different infusion lines; no crystalline material was observed at autopsy in this neonate. (See Interactions with Calcium-containing Products under Cautions: Precautions and Contraindications.) There have been no similar reports in patients other than neonates treated with ceftriaxone and calcium-containing IV solutions.

To date, there have been no reports of an interaction between ceftriaxone and oral calcium-containing preparations or between IM ceftriaxone and calcium-containing preparations (IV or oral).

● Local Effects

Local reactions, including pain, induration, ecchymosis, and tenderness at the injection site have been reported in patients receiving IM ceftriaxone. The overall incidence of pain, induration, and tenderness following IM injection of the drug is 1–2%. The incidence of warmth, tightness, or induration reported following IM injection of ceftriaxone doses of 250 or 350 mg/mL was 5 or 17%, respectively. Local reactions occur less frequently and are less intense when IM injections of ceftriaxone are reconstituted with 1% lidocaine hydrochloride (without epinephrine) rather than sterile water for injection. (See Other Precautions and Contraindications under Cautions: Precautions and Contraindications.)

Results of a cross-over study involving IM injection into the buttock of 1-g doses of ceftriaxone diluted in 2 mL of sterile water for injection, 1% lidocaine, or 1% lidocaine buffered with sodium carbonate indicate that the pharmacokinetics of ceftriaxone are not affected by the diluent; however, use of a lidocaine diluent was associated with a 50–78% reduction in injection pain scores compared with use of sterile water for injection. Buffered lidocaine did not appear to offer any advantages over unbuffered lidocaine.

Phlebitis has been reported in less than 1% of patients receiving IV ceftriaxone.

● Other Adverse Effects

Other adverse effects that have been reported in less than 1% of patients receiving ceftriaxone include diaphoresis and flushing, headache, dizziness, oral candidiasis, and candidal vaginitis. Palpitation and epistaxis have been reported in less than 0.1% of patients receiving the drug.

In at least one patient, inadvertent IV injection over 5 minutes of a 2-g dose of ceftriaxone resulted in a reaction that consisted of restlessness, shivering, diaphoresis with dilated pupils, and palpitations; this reaction did not occur when the drug was administered by IV infusion over 30 minutes as recommended by the manufacturer.

● Precautions and Contraindications

Ceftriaxone is contraindicated in patients with known hypersensitivity to ceftriaxone, any other cephalosporin, or any ingredient in the formulation. Patients with previous hypersensitivity reactions to penicillin and other β-lactam anti-infectives may be at greater risk of hypersensitivity to ceftriaxone. Some manufacturers state that ceftriaxone is contraindicated in patients with a history of anaphylaxis to ceftriaxone, other cephalosporins, penicillins, or other β-lactam anti-infectives. (See Sensitivity Reactions under Cautions: Precautions and Contraindications.)

Ceftriaxone is contraindicated in certain neonates (e.g., premature or hyperbilirubinemic neonates, those requiring calcium-containing IV solutions). (See Cautions: Pediatric Precautions.)

Ceftriaxone shares the toxic potentials of the cephalosporins, and the usual precautions of cephalosporin therapy should be observed.

Sensitivity Reactions

Prior to initiation of therapy with ceftriaxone, careful inquiry should be made concerning previous hypersensitivity reactions to ceftriaxone, cephalosporins, penicillins, other β-lactam anti-infectives, or other drugs. There is clinical and laboratory evidence of partial cross-allergenicity among cephalosporins and other β-lactam antibiotics including penicillins and cephamycins.

As with all β-lactam anti-infectives, serious and occasionally fatal hypersensitivity reactions, including anaphylaxis, have been reported with ceftriaxone.

Although it has not been proven that allergic reactions to antibiotics are more frequent in atopic individuals, some manufacturers state that ceftriaxone should be used with caution in patients with a history of allergy, particularly to drugs.

The manufacturer of the commercially available frozen premixed ceftriaxone injection in dextrose states that dextrose-containing solutions may be contraindicated in patients with known allergy to corn or corn products. Hypersensitivity reactions, including anaphylaxis, have been reported with administration of dextrose products. These reactions have been reported in patients receiving high concentrations of dextrose (i.e., 50% dextrose) and also have been reported when corn-derived dextrose solutions were administered to patients with or without a history of hypersensitivity to corn products.

Patients should be advised that allergic reactions, including serious allergic reactions, could occur and that serious reactions require immediate treatment.

If a severe hypersensitivity reaction occurs during ceftriaxone therapy, the drug should be discontinued immediately and the patient treated with appropriate therapy (e.g., epinephrine, corticosteroids, maintenance of an adequate airway, oxygen) as indicated.

Interaction with Calcium-containing Products

Because of the risk of precipitation of ceftriaxone-calcium and because fatalities associated with ceftriaxone-calcium precipitates in lungs and kidneys have been reported in neonates (see Cautions: Pulmonary and Renal Precipitates), ceftriaxone is contraindicated in neonates (28 days of age or younger) who are receiving (or are expected to require) treatment with calcium-containing IV solutions, including continuous calcium-containing infusions such as parenteral nutrition.

Intravascular or pulmonary ceftriaxone-calcium precipitates have not been reported to date in patients other than neonates treated with ceftriaxone and calcium-containing IV solutions. There is some evidence that neonates have an increased risk for precipitation of ceftriaxone-calcium. In vitro studies evaluating the combination of ceftriaxone and calcium in adult plasma and neonatal plasma from umbilical cord blood indicate that recovery of ceftriaxone from plasma was reduced in adult plasma when calcium concentrations were 24 mg/dL or greater and was reduced in neonatal plasma when calcium concentrations were 16 mg/dL or greater. This may reflect ceftriaxone-calcium precipitation.

Ceftriaxone must *not* be admixed with calcium-containing IV solutions and must *not* be administered *simultaneously* with calcium-containing IV solutions, including continuous infusions of calcium-containing solutions such as parenteral nutrition, even via different infusion lines or sites in any patient (irrespective of age). In adults or pediatric patients older than 28 days of age, ceftriaxone and calcium-containing solutions may be administered *sequentially* if the IV infusion lines are thoroughly flushed between infusions with a compatible fluid. (See Dosage and Administration: Reconstitution and Administration.)

Selection and Use of Anti-infectives

To reduce development of drug-resistant bacteria and maintain effectiveness of ceftriaxone and other antibacterials, the drug should be used only for the treatment or prevention of infections proven or strongly suspected to be caused by susceptible bacteria. When selecting or modifying anti-infective therapy, results of culture and in vitro susceptibility testing should be used. In the absence of such data, local epidemiology and susceptibility patterns should be considered when selecting anti-infectives for empiric therapy.

Patients should be advised that antibacterials (including ceftriaxone) should only be used to treat bacterial infections and not used to treat viral infections (e.g., the common cold). Patients also should be advised about the importance of completing the full course of therapy, even if feeling better after a few days, and that skipping doses or not completing therapy may decrease effectiveness and increase the likelihood that bacteria will develop resistance and will not be treatable with ceftriaxone or other antibacterials in the future.

Superinfection/Clostridium difficile-associated Diarrhea and Colitis

Use of ceftriaxone may result in overgrowth of nonsusceptible organisms, especially *Candida*, enterococci, *Bacteroides fragilis*, or *Pseudomonas aeruginosa*. Resistant strains of *Ps. aeruginosa* and *Enterobacter* have developed during therapy with ceftriaxone. (See Resistance.) Careful observation of the patient during ceftriaxone therapy is essential. If superinfection or suprainfection occurs, appropriate therapy should be instituted.

Because CDAD has been reported with the use of ceftriaxone or other cephalosporins, it should be considered in the differential diagnosis of patients who develop diarrhea during or after ceftriaxone therapy. (See Clostridium difficile-associated Diarrhea and Colitis under Cautions: GI Effects.) Patients should be advised that diarrhea is a common problem caused by anti-infectives and usually ends when the drug is discontinued; however, they should contact a clinician if watery and bloody stools (with or without stomach cramps and fever) occur during or as late as 2 months or longer after the last dose.

Some manufacturers state that ceftriaxone should be used with caution in patients with a history of GI disease, particularly colitis.

Other Precautions and Contraindications

Because potentially fatal immune-mediated hemolytic anemia has been reported with cephalosporins, including ceftriaxone, the diagnosis of cephalosporin-associated anemia should be considered if anemia occurs in a patient receiving ceftriaxone. The drug should be discontinued until the etiology of the anemia is determined.

Ceftriaxone can precipitate in the gallbladder. (See Cautions: GI Effects.) Some clinicians recommend that ceftriaxone be used with caution in patients with preexisting disease of the gallbladder, biliary tract, liver, or pancreas, and, if the drug is used in such patients, serial abdominal ultrasonography should be performed during therapy. Ceftriaxone should be discontinued and conservative management considered in any patient who develops signs and symptoms suggestive of gallbladder disease, including sonographic abnormalities.

Ceftriaxone can precipitate in the urinary tract. (See Cautions: Renal Effects.) Patients receiving the drug should be adequately hydrated. Ceftriaxone should be discontinued if there are signs and symptoms suggestive of urolithiasis, oliguria, or renal failure and/or if sonographic abnormalities are detected.

Because prolonged PT has been reported in patients receiving ceftriaxone, the manufacturers state that PT should be monitored when the drug is used in patients with impaired vitamin K synthesis or low vitamin K stores (e.g., patients with chronic hepatic disease, malnutrition). The manufacturers state that administration of vitamin K (10 mg weekly) may be necessary if the PT is prolonged before or during ceftriaxone therapy. Concomitant use of ceftriaxone and vitamin K antagonists may increase the risk of bleeding. (See Drug Interactions: Anticoagulants.)

Seizures have been reported with some cephalosporins, including ceftriaxone. Ceftriaxone should be discontinued if seizures occur and anticonvulsant therapy should be administered if clinically indicated. Patients should be advised that adverse neurologic events can occur and to immediately contact a clinician if any neurologic signs and symptoms, including encephalopathy (disturbance of consciousness including confusion, hallucinations, stupor, coma), myoclonus, or seizures, occur since immediate treatment, dosage adjustment, or discontinuance of ceftriaxone therapy is required.

Like other dextrose-containing solutions, the commercially available Duplex® drug delivery system containing 1 or 2 g of lyophilized ceftriaxone and 50 mL of dextrose 3.74 or 2.22% injection should be used with caution in patients with overt or known subclinical diabetes mellitus or in patients with carbohydrate intolerance for any reason.

Although IM injections of ceftriaxone may be prepared using diluents containing 1% lidocaine hydrochloride (see IM Injection under Dosage and Administration: Reconstitution and Administration), all contraindications to lidocaine should be considered before administering such injections. IV administration of ceftriaxone solutions containing lidocaine is contraindicated.

Dosage adjustments are not usually necessary when ceftriaxone is used in patients with renal impairment or hepatic impairment alone. Some clinicians recommend that serum concentrations of the drug be monitored when ceftriaxone is used in patients with severe renal impairment (e.g., dialysis patients) or in patients with hepatic impairment and clinically important renal impairment. (See Dosage and Administration: Dosage in Renal and Hepatic Impairment.)

● Pediatric Precautions

Ceftriaxone is contraindicated in premature neonates up to postmenstrual age 41 weeks (i.e., time elapsed since first day of the mother's last menstrual period to birth plus time elapsed after birth).

Ceftriaxone is contraindicated in hyperbilirubinemic neonates, particularly those who are premature. Ceftriaxone, at therapeutic concentrations, has been shown to displace bilirubin from albumin binding sites in vitro. Because ceftriaxone can displace bilirubin from serum albumin, there is a risk that bilirubin encephalopathy could develop if the drug is used in hyperbilirubinemic neonates. Addition of ceftriaxone to blood samples obtained from hyperbilirubinemic neonates resulted in increased free and erythrocyte-bound bilirubin concentrations and decreased unconjugated (albumin-bound) bilirubin concentrations.

Ceftriaxone is contraindicated in neonates (28 days of age or younger) if they are receiving (or expected to require) treatment with calcium-containing IV solutions, including continuous infusions of calcium-containing solutions such as parenteral nutrition, because of the risk of precipitation of a ceftriaxone-calcium salt. Fatalities associated with ceftriaxone-calcium precipitates in lungs and kidneys have been reported in neonates who received ceftriaxone and calcium-containing IV solutions. (See Cautions: Pulmonary and Renal Precipitates and see Interaction with Calcium-containing Products under Cautions: Precautions and Contraindications.)

To reduce the risk of bilirubin encephalopathy, IV infusions of ceftriaxone should be given over 60 minutes in neonates. (See Dosage and Administration: Reconstitution and Administration.)

Ceftriaxone that has been reconstituted for IM use with bacteriostatic water for injection containing benzyl alcohol should *not* be used in neonates. Although a causal relationship has not been established, administration of injections preserved with benzyl alcohol has been associated with toxicity in neonates. Toxicity appears to have resulted from administration of large amounts (i.e., about 100–400 mg/kg daily) of benzyl alcohol in these neonates.

To avoid unintentional overdosage, the commercially available Duplex® drug delivery system containing 1 or 2 g of ceftriaxone and 50 mL of dextrose injection in separate chambers should *not* be used in pediatric patients who require less than the entire 1- or 2-g dose in the container.

● Geriatric Precautions

In clinical studies, safety and efficacy of ceftriaxone in geriatric adults 60 years of age or older have been similar to those observed in younger adults. Although other clinical experience has revealed no evidence of age-related differences, the possibility that some older patients may exhibit increased sensitivity to the drug cannot be ruled out.

The pharmacokinetics of ceftriaxone are only minimally altered in geriatric patients compared with healthy younger adults. Dosage adjustments based solely on age are not necessary in geriatric patients receiving ceftriaxone dosages up to 2 g daily, provided they do not have severe renal and hepatic impairment.

Ceftriaxone is substantially eliminated by the kidneys, and the risk of adverse effects may be greater in those with impaired renal function. Because geriatric patients are more likely to have reduced renal function, dosage should be selected with caution and monitoring of renal function should be considered.

● Mutagenicity and Carcinogenicity

In vitro studies using microbial (i.e., Ames test) or mammalian cell (i.e., human lymphoblasts) systems have not shown ceftriaxone to be mutagenic. Specific studies to determine the carcinogenic potential of ceftriaxone have not been performed to date, and animal toxicity studies have been performed to a maximum duration of only 6 months.

● Pregnancy, Fertility, and Lactation

Pregnancy

Reproduction studies in mice, rats, and primates have not revealed evidence of embryotoxicity, fetotoxicity, or teratogenicity. There are no adequate or controlled studies using ceftriaxone in pregnant women, and the drug should be used during pregnancy only when clearly needed.

Fertility

Studies in rats using IV ceftriaxone have not revealed evidence of impaired fertility.

Lactation

Because ceftriaxone is distributed into milk, the drug should be used with caution in nursing women.

DRUG INTERACTIONS

● Alcohol

A disulfiram-like reaction reportedly occurred in one patient who ingested alcohol while receiving ceftriaxone. However, this effect generally has been reported only with β-lactam antibiotics that contain an N-methylthiotetrazole (NMTT) side chain (e.g., cefamandole, cefoperazone, cefotetan).

● Aminoglycosides

In vitro studies indicate that the antibacterial activity of ceftriaxone and aminoglycosides (amikacin, gentamicin, tobramycin) may be additive or synergistic against some strains of Enterobacteriaceae and some strains of *Pseudomonas aeruginosa*. Although the clinical importance has not been determined to date, antagonism has also occurred rarely in vitro when ceftriaxone was used in combination with an aminoglycoside. Organisms with high-level resistance to both the aminoglycoside and the β-lactam antibiotic alone are unlikely to be synergistically inhibited by concomitant use of the drugs.

● Anticoagulants

Concomitant use of ceftriaxone and vitamin K antagonists may increase the risk of bleeding. Increased international normalized ratio (INR) has been reported in patients receiving warfarin and ceftriaxone concomitantly. In one patient who had been receiving long-term warfarin therapy with stable INR, administration of a single 1-g IM dose of ceftriaxone for the treatment of a urinary tract infection resulted in a substantially increased INR that was managed by withholding a warfarin dose and administering vitamin K. If ceftriaxone is used in patients receiving a vitamin K antagonist (e.g., warfarin), coagulation parameters should be monitored frequently and dosage of the anticoagulant adjusted as needed, both during and after ceftriaxone treatment.

● Chloramphenicol

Antagonism has been reported in vitro when ceftriaxone was used in combination with chloramphenicol.

● Probenecid

Concomitant administration of oral probenecid (500 mg daily) does not appear to affect the pharmacokinetics of ceftriaxone, presumably because ceftriaxone is excreted principally by glomerular filtration and nonrenal mechanisms. However, higher dosages of oral probenecid (1 or 2 g daily) administered concomitantly reportedly may partially block biliary secretion of ceftriaxone as well as displace the drug from plasma proteins. As a result, serum clearance of ceftriaxone may be increased by about 30% and elimination half-life of ceftriaxone may be decreased by about 20%.

● Quinolones

Although the clinical importance is unclear, results of an in vitro study indicate that the combination of ceftriaxone and trovafloxacin (not commercially available in the US) is synergistic against both penicillin-susceptible and penicillin-resistant *Streptococcus pneumoniae*, including some strains that also were resistant to ceftriaxone alone. There was no evidence of antagonism with the combination of ceftriaxone and trovafloxacin.

LABORATORY TEST INTERFERENCES

● Tests for Glucose

False-positive results for urinary glucose may occur in patients receiving ceftriaxone if nonenzymatic glucose test methods are used. Like most cephalosporins, ceftriaxone interferes with urinary glucose determinations using cupric sulfate (e.g., Benedict's solution, Clinitest®); however, glucose oxidase methods (e.g., Clinistix®, Tes-Tape®) are unaffected by the drug. Enzymatic methods should be used to test for urinary glucose in patients receiving ceftriaxone.

The presence of ceftriaxone may result in falsely low estimated blood glucose concentrations measured using some blood glucose monitoring systems. The manufacturer's instructions for the glucose monitoring system should be consulted and alternative testing methods should be used if necessary.

● Tests for Creatinine

In one in vitro study, high concentrations of ceftriaxone (50 mcg/mL or greater) caused falsely elevated serum creatinine values when a manual method was used; however, other studies indicate that the drug does not interfere with automated methods for determining serum or urinary creatinine concentrations.

ACUTE TOXICITY

Limited information is available on the acute toxicity of ceftriaxone; there is no specific antidote. If acute overdosage of ceftriaxone occurs, supportive and symptomatic treatment should be initiated. Ceftriaxone is not removed by hemodialysis or peritoneal dialysis, and these procedures would be ineffective in reducing ceftriaxone concentrations following overdosage.

MECHANISM OF ACTION

Ceftriaxone usually is bactericidal in action. Like other cephalosporins, the antibacterial activity of the drug results from inhibition of mucopeptide synthesis in the bacterial cell wall. For information on the mechanism of action of cephalosporins, see Mechanism of Action in the Cephalosporins General Statement 8:12.06.

SPECTRUM

Based on its spectrum of activity, ceftriaxone is classified as a third generation cephalosporin. For information on the classification of cephalosporins and closely related β-lactam antibiotics based on spectra of activity, see Spectrum in the Cephalosporins General Statement 8:12.06.

Like other currently available parenteral third generation cephalosporins (e.g., cefotaxime, ceftazidime), ceftriaxone generally is less active in vitro against susceptible staphylococci than first generation cephalosporins but has an expanded spectrum of activity against gram-negative bacteria compared with first and second generation cephalosporins. The spectrum of activity of ceftriaxone closely resembles that of cefotaxime and ceftazidime. In vitro on a weight basis, the activity of ceftriaxone against most susceptible organisms, including most Enterobacteriaceae, is approximately equal to that of cefotaxime.

● In Vitro Susceptibility Testing

Results of in vitro susceptibility tests with ceftriaxone for some bacteria (e.g., *Enterobacter cloacae, Klebsiella pneumoniae, Proteus, Pseudomonas, Serratia,* staphylococci) may be affected by the size of the inoculum. Although results of ceftriaxone susceptibility tests do not appear to be affected by culture media, results may be affected by pH or the presence of serum. MICs of ceftriaxone for *Staphylococcus aureus, Pseudomonas aeruginosa,* or Enterobacteriaceae may be 4–8 times higher when tested in the presence of serum.

Strains of staphylococci resistant to penicillinase-resistant penicillins (methicillin-resistant [oxacillin-resistant] staphylococci) should be considered resistant to ceftriaxone, although results of in vitro susceptibility tests may indicate that the organisms are susceptible to the drug.

For information on interpreting results of in vitro susceptibility testing (disk susceptibility tests, dilution susceptibility tests) when ceftriaxone susceptibility testing is performed according to the standards of the Clinical and Laboratory Standards Institute (CLSI; formerly National Committee for Clinical Laboratory Standards [NCCLS]), see Spectrum: In Vitro Susceptibility Testing, in the Cephalosporins General Statement 8:12.06.

● Gram-positive Aerobic Bacteria

Ceftriaxone is active in vitro against most gram-positive aerobic cocci including penicillinase-producing and nonpenicillinase-producing strains of *Staphylococcus aureus* and *S. epidermidis; Streptococcus pneumoniae; S. pyogenes* (group A

β-hemolytic streptococci; GAS); *S. agalactiae* (group B streptococci; GBS); and viridans streptococci (including the *S. milleri* group [*S. anginosus, S. constellatus, S. intermedius*]). Staphylococci resistant to penicillinase-resistant penicillins also generally are resistant to ceftriaxone. Group D streptococci and enterococci, including *E. faecalis* (formerly *S. faecalis*), generally are resistant to ceftriaxone.

The MIC$_{90}$ (minimum inhibitory concentration of the drug at which 90% of strains tested are inhibited) of ceftriaxone for penicillinase-producing and nonpenicillinase-producing *S. aureus* is 3–8 mcg/mL. The MIC$_{90}$ of the drug reported for *S. epidermidis* is 16–50 mcg/mL and the MIC$_{50}$ of the drug reported for this organism is 3.1–7.3 mcg/mL.

The MIC$_{90}$ of ceftriaxone for *S. pyogenes* is 0.15–0.25 mcg/mL, and the MIC$_{90}$ of the drug reported for *S. agalactiae* is 0.06–0.78 mcg/mL. The MIC$_{90}$ reported for viridans streptococci is 0.5–4 mcg/mL. In one study, the MIC$_{50}$ and MIC$_{90}$ of ceftriaxone for the *S. milleri* group of viridans streptococci were 0.25 and 0.5 mcg/mL, respectively.

Although the MIC$_{90}$ reported for *S. pneumoniae* generally is 0.15–0.25 mcg/mL, some strains have reduced susceptibility and require ceftriaxone concentrations of 0.5–2 mcg/mL or greater for in vitro inhibition. Strains of *S. pneumoniae* with MICs of 2 mcg/mL or greater generally are considered resistant to ceftriaxone; however, strains with MICs of 0.5–1 mcg/mL that are isolated from patients with meningitis generally also are considered resistant to the drug.

Other Gram-positive Bacteria

Although a few strains of *Listeria monocytogenes* may be inhibited in vitro by ceftriaxone concentrations of 0.8–32 mcg/mL, most strains of the organism are resistant to the drug.

Ceftriaxone is active in vitro against some strains of *Nocardia,* including some strains of *N. asteroides* and *N. brasiliensis.* However, resistance to ceftriaxone also has been reported in environmental isolates of *N. asteroides* and clinical isolates of *N. farcinica.*

● Gram-negative Aerobic Bacteria

Neisseria

Ceftriaxone is active in vitro against *Neisseria meningitidis,* and most strains of this organism are inhibited by ceftriaxone concentrations of 0.001–0.025 mcg/mL.

Ceftriaxone is active in vitro against penicillinase-producing (PPNG) and nonpenicillinase-producing *Neisseria gonorrhoeae* and those with chromosomally mediated resistance (e.g., to penicillin) (CMRNG) or plasmid-mediated tetracycline resistance (TRNG). The MIC$_{90}$ of ceftriaxone reported for *N. gonorrhoeae* usually is 0.001–0.05 mcg/mL. However, *N. gonorrhoeae* with reduced susceptibility to ceftriaxone (MICs 0.125 mcg/mL or greater), including some ceftriaxone-resistant strains, have been reported with increasing frequency during the last decade; some treatment failures have been reported. (See Resistance.)

Haemophilus

Ceftriaxone is active in vitro against most β-lactamase-producing and non-β-lactamase-producing strains of *Haemophilus influenzae, H. parainfluenzae,* and *H. ducreyi.* The MIC$_{90}$ of the drug reported for *H. influenzae* is 0.003–0.03 mcg/mL. *H. ducreyi* generally is inhibited in vitro by ceftriaxone concentrations of 0.002–0.06 mcg/mL.

Enterobacteriaceae

Generally, ceftriaxone is active in vitro against the following Enterobacteriaceae: *Citrobacter diversus, C. freundii, Enterobacter cloacae, E. aerogenes, Escherichia coli, Klebsiella pneumoniae, Morganella morganii* (formerly *Proteus morganii*), *Proteus mirabilis, P. vulgaris, Providencia rettgeri* (formerly *Proteus rettgeri*), *P. stuartii, Serratia marcescens, Salmonella, Shigella,* and *Yersinia enterocolitica.*

The MIC$_{90}$ of ceftriaxone for most of these Enterobacteriaceae, including *Citrobacter, E. coli, Klebsiella, M. morganii, P. vulgaris, Providencia,* and *Yersinia enterocolitica,* is 0.05–4 mcg/mL. The MIC$_{90}$ of the drug for *P. mirabilis* is 0.006–0.1 mcg/mL. Although the MIC$_{90}$ of ceftriaxone reported for *E. aerogenes* generally is 0.12–8 mcg/mL, the MIC$_{90}$ of the drug reported for *E. cloacae* is 0.5–25 mcg/mL. The MIC$_{90}$ of ceftriaxone for *S. marcescens* is 0.25–32 mcg/mL.

The MIC$_{90}$ of ceftriaxone reported for *Salmonella enteritidis, S. paratyphi, S. sendai, S. typhi,* and *S. typhimurium* is 0.04–0.1 mcg/mL. Strains of *Salmonella* resistant to ceftriaxone have been reported rarely. Multidrug-resistant *Salmonella* serotype Newport has been reported with increasing frequency in the US. These strains usually are resistant to ampicillin, amoxicillin clavulanate, cefoxitin, cephalothin, chloramphenicol, streptomycin, sulfamethoxazole, or tetracycline and have either decreased susceptibility or resistance to ceftriaxone.

The MIC_{90} of ceftriaxone reported for *Shigella*, including *Sh. sonnei*, is 0.02–0.5 mcg/mL.

Pseudomonas

Although ceftriaxone is active in vitro against some strains of *Ps. aeruginosa*, many strains of the organism require ceftriaxone concentrations of 64 mcg/mL or greater for in vitro inhibition and are therefore considered resistant to the drug. Ceftriaxone generally is less active in vitro against susceptible *Ps. aeruginosa* than ceftazidime or extended-spectrum penicillins (e.g., piperacillin). In some in vitro studies, the MIC_{50} of ceftriaxone for *Ps. aeruginosa* was 4–16 mcg/mL and the MIC_{90} of the drug was 16–32 mcg/mL. However, in other studies, the MIC_{50} was 16–64 mcg/mL and the MIC_{90} was 64 mcg/mL or greater.

Ceftriaxone has some activity against *Pseudomonas* other than *Ps. aeruginosa*. The MIC_{90} of ceftriaxone reported for *Ps. acidovorans* and *Ps. stutzeri* is 2–16 mcg/mL, but *Ps. fluorescens* and *Ps. putida* generally are resistant to the drug.

Other Gram-Negative Aerobic Bacteria

Ceftriaxone is active in vitro against *Moraxella* and *Eikenella corrodens*, and the MIC_{90} of the drug reported for these organisms is 1–2 mcg/mL.

While ceftriaxone has some activity in vitro against *Acinetobacter* and the MIC_{90} of ceftriaxone reported for *A. calcoaceticus* and *A. lwoffi* is 8–32 mcg/mL, the MIC_{90} reported for *A. baumannii* is 64 mcg/mL and this organism is considered resistant to the drug.

Alcaligenes faecalis may be inhibited in vitro by ceftriaxone concentrations of 0.5 mcg/mL or less; however, *A. denitrificans* and *A. xylosoxidans* generally are resistant to the drug.

Bartonella henselae and *B. quintana* may be inhibited in vitro by ceftriaxone concentrations of 0.06–0.25 mcg/mL. Some strains of *B. bacilliformis* are inhibited in vitro by ceftriaxone concentrations of 0.003–0.006 mcg/mL.

In one study, all strains of *Burkholderia cepacia* (formerly *Pseudomonas cepacia*) tested were resistant to ceftriaxone.

Ceftriaxone is active in vitro against *Capnocytophaga*, including *C. canimorsus* (formerly CDC group DF-2). The MIC_{90} of ceftriaxone reported for *Capnocytophaga* is 4 mcg/mL.

Stenotrophomonas maltophilia (formerly *Ps. maltophilia* or *Xanthomonas maltophilia*) generally is resistant to ceftriaxone.

Some strains of *Weeksella virosa* are inhibited in vitro by ceftriaxone concentrations of 0.5 mcg/mL or lower.

● Anaerobic Bacteria

Ceftriaxone is active in vitro against some anaerobic bacteria including *Actinomyces*, *Fusobacterium*, *Lactobacillus*, *Peptococcus*, *Peptostreptococcus*, *Propionibacterium*, and *Veillonella*. The MIC_{90} of ceftriaxone reported for most of these anaerobic bacteria is 0.5–16 mcg/mL.

Some strains of *Clostridium*, including *C. perfringens*, are inhibited in vitro by ceftriaxone concentrations of 0.5–16 mcg/mL; however, *C. difficile* generally is resistant to the drug.

Most strains of *Bacteroides fragilis* are resistant to ceftriaxone. Although the MIC_{50} of ceftriaxone reported for *B. fragilis*, *B. distasonis*, *B. ovatus*, *B. thetaiotaomicron*, and *B. vulgatus* is 2–64 mcg/mL, the MIC_{90} is 32 mcg/mL or greater.

The MIC_{90} of ceftriaxone reported for *Prevotella melaninogenica* (formerly *Bacteroides melaninogenicus*) is 4–16 mcg/mL.

● Spirochetes

Studies in rabbits with experimentally induced syphilis indicate that ceftriaxone has some activity against *Treponema pallidum*.

Borrelia burgdorferi, the causative organism of Lyme disease, reportedly may be inhibited in vitro by ceftriaxone concentrations of 0.1–1 mcg/mL; minimum bactericidal concentrations (MBCs) of ceftriaxone for *B. burgdorferi* generally have ranged from 0.02–0.16 mcg/mL.

Ceftriaxone is active in vitro against *Leptospira*. In one study, all strains of *L. interrogans* and *L. weilii* tested were inhibited in vitro by ceftriaxone concentrations of 0.06 mcg/mL or less.

● Chlamydia

Studies using a limited number of isolates indicate that some strains of *Chlamydia trachomatis* are inhibited in vitro by ceftriaxone concentrations of 8–32 mcg/mL; however, the clinical importance of this in vitro activity is unclear. Ceftriaxone generally is considered to be inactive against *C. trachomatis*.

RESISTANCE

For information on possible mechanisms of bacterial resistance to cephalosporins, see Resistance in the Cephalosporins General Statement 8:12.06.

Ceftriaxone generally is stable against hydrolysis by β-lactamases classified as Richmond-Sykes types II, III (TEM types), and V; some PSE types; and most β-lactamases produced by *Neisseria gonorrhoeae*, *Haemophilus influenzae*, and staphylococci. Ceftriaxone may be inactivated by Richmond type IV β-lactamases, and in vitro studies indicate that some β-lactamases produced by *Bacteroides*, *Citrobacter*, *Enterobacter*, *Morganella*, *Proteus*, and *Pseudomonas* can inactivate the drug. Ceftriaxone generally is as stable as cefotaxime against inactivation by β-lactamases but less stable than cefoxitin.

Resistant strains of some organisms, including *Enterobacter* and *Ps. aeruginosa*, have developed during therapy with ceftriaxone. Although further study is needed, it has been suggested that resistance may develop in many of these organisms because they possess inducible β-lactamases. These inducible enzymes generally are chromosomally mediated cephalosporinases classified as Richmond-Sykes type I. In vitro studies indicate that following exposure to certain β-lactam antibiotics (e.g., cefoxitin), inducible β-lactamases are derepressed. Inducible β-lactamases appear to inactivate β-lactam antibiotics by binding to the drugs, which prevents them from binding to penicillin-binding proteins of the organism. Most β-lactam antibiotics, including second and third generation cephalosporins and extended-spectrum penicillins, are inactivated by inducible β-lactamases.

Strains of *S. pneumoniae* considered resistant to ceftriaxone have been reported with increasing frequency. These strains generally have intermediate- or high-level resistance to penicillin G as well as decreased susceptibility to third generation cephalosporins. Resistance to ceftriaxone in *S. pneumoniae* appears to be related to alterations in the target enzymes, penicillin-binding proteins (PBPs), of the organism.

N. gonorrhoeae with reduced susceptibility to ceftriaxone and/or cefixime or other cephalosporins have been reported with increasing frequency in the US and elsewhere (e.g., Asia, Europe, Canada). Strains with reduced susceptibility to ceftriaxone generally have ceftriaxone MICs of 0.125 mcg/mL or greater. There also have been rare reports of *N. gonorrhoeae* with high-level ceftriaxone resistance (MICs 1–4 mcg/mL) in some countries (Japan, France, Spain), including at least one patient with pharyngeal gonorrhea. Susceptibility of *N. gonorrhoeae* in the US is being monitored by CDC Gonococcal Isolate Surveillance Project (GISP). GISP data from 2000–2010 indicate that the percentage of US *N. gonorrhoeae* isolates with elevated ceftriaxone MICs (MICs 0.125 mcg/mL or greater) increased from 0.1% to 0.3% and the percentage with elevated cefixime MICs (MICs 0.25 mcg/mL or greater) increased from 0.2% to 1.4%. GISP data regarding *N. gonorrhoeae* isolates from men who have sex with men indicate that the percentage of isolates with elevated ceftriaxone MICs increased from 0% in 2006 to 1% in 2011 and the percentage of isolates with elevated cefixime MICs increased from 0.2% in 2006 to 3.8% in 2011.

PHARMACOKINETICS

In all studies described in the Pharmacokinetics section, ceftriaxone was administered as ceftriaxone sodium; dosages and concentrations of the drug are expressed in terms of ceftriaxone.

Ceftriaxone exhibits nonlinear dose-dependent pharmacokinetics. Serum concentrations, the area under the serum concentration-time curve (AUC), and most pharmacokinetic parameters (except elimination half-life and the fraction excreted unchanged in urine) of total ceftriaxone (both protein-bound and unbound drug) are dose dependent and increase nonlinearly with increases in dosage. However, pharmacokinetic parameters of free (unbound) ceftriaxone are not dose dependent and increase linearly with dosage. Dose-dependent changes in the pharmacokinetic parameters of ceftriaxone apparently occur because the drug exhibits concentration-dependent protein binding. (See Pharmacokinetics: Distribution.) Some clinicians suggest that because of this concentration-dependent protein binding, distribution and clearance parameters calculated with data obtained using concentrations of total ceftriaxone may be invalid and misleading. Other clinicians suggest that concentration-dependent protein binding and dose-related changes in the pharmacokinetic parameters of ceftriaxone over the usual dosage range of the drug are small and not clinically important.

● Absorption

Ceftriaxone is not appreciably absorbed from the GI tract and must be given parenterally.

Following IM administration of a single ceftriaxone dose of 0.5–1 g in healthy adults, the drug appears to be completely absorbed, and peak serum concentrations are attained 1.5–4 hours after the dose. In one study in healthy adults who received a single 1-g IM dose of ceftriaxone, serum concentrations of the drug averaged 28.9, 43.7, 62.3, 83.2, 40.6, 35.5, and 7.8 mcg/mL at 0.25, 0.5, 1, 2, 6, 12, and 24 hours, respectively, after the dose.

Following IV infusion over 30 minutes of a single 1-g dose of ceftriaxone in healthy adults, peak serum concentrations of the drug at completion of the infusion average 123.2–150.7 mcg/mL and serum concentrations at 1, 2, 6, 12, and 24 hours after start of the infusion average 109.5–111, 60.8–88.2, 33–52.5, 20.2–28.1, and 4.6–9.3 mcg/mL, respectively. IV infusion over 30 minutes of a single 2-g dose of ceftriaxone in healthy adults results in peak serum concentrations of the drug at completion of the infusion that range from 223–276 mcg/mL and serum concentrations at 1, 2, 6, 12, and 24 hours after start of the infusion that range from 166–209, 135–173, 75–104, 32–58, and 7–22 mcg/mL, respectively.

In one study in healthy adults, a ceftriaxone dosage of 2 g daily was given either as 1 g every 12 hours or 2 g every 24 hours; each dose was administered by IV infusion over 30 minutes. At steady state, peak serum concentrations of the drug ranged from 132–213 mcg/mL in those who received 1 g every 12 hours and from 216–281 mcg/mL in those who received 2 g every 24 hours; trough serum concentrations ranged from 23–58 and 7–27 mcg/mL, respectively. Average steady-state serum concentrations of ceftriaxone were similar for both regimens and were 72 mcg/mL when 1 g was given every 12 hours and 63 mcg/mL when 2 g was given every 24 hours.

In multiple-dose studies in healthy adults who received a ceftriaxone dosage of 0.5–2 g given every 12 or 24 hours by IM injection or IV infusion over 30 minutes, serum concentrations of the drug at steady state on the fourth day of therapy were 15–36% higher than serum concentrations attained with single doses of the drug.

In one study in adults with neoplastic disease, IM administration of a single 500-mg dose of ceftriaxone resulted in serum concentrations of the drug averaging 28, 31.9, 32.9, 28.3, and 25.5 mcg/mL at 0.5, 1, 2, 4, and 6 hours, respectively, after the dose. IV infusion over 5 minutes of a single ceftriaxone dose of 500 mg or 1 g in these patients resulted in serum concentrations of the drug at 0.5, 1, 2, 4, and 8 hours that averaged 54.4, 44.7, 33.5, 25.4, and 16.8 mcg/mL, respectively, after the 500-mg dose and 79.3, 65.7, 52.2, 28.7, and 22.3 mcg/mL, respectively, after the 1-g dose.

In one study in neonates and children 1–45 days of age with meningitis who received a single ceftriaxone dose of 50 mg/kg by IV infusion over 15 minutes, serum concentrations of the drug immediately following the infusion and 1, 2, 4, and 6 hours later averaged 136–173, 91–116, 80–112, 70–86, and 66–74 mcg/mL, respectively. In another study in neonates 1–4 days of age with meningitis who received a single 50-mg/kg dose of ceftriaxone by IV infusion over 5 minutes, serum concentrations of the drug 1, 12, and 24 hours after the dose ranged from 108–141, 43–76, and 20–52 mcg/mL, respectively. Serum concentrations of ceftriaxone in neonates 9–30 days of age with meningitis who received a single 100-mg/kg dose of the drug by IV infusion over 5 minutes ranged from 100–262, 43–140, and 8–33 mcg/mL at 1, 12, and 24 hours, respectively, after the dose.

In one study in children 7–15 months of age who received a single ceftriaxone dose of 50 mg/kg by IV infusion over 5 minutes, serum concentrations of the drug ranged from 139–197, 66.6–99.2, 31.3–58.9, 2.4–14.8, and 0.85–8.4 mcg/mL at 0.5, 4, 8, 24, and 32 hours, respectively, after the dose. When the same dose was administered by IV infusion over 5 minutes to children 2–6 years of age, serum concentrations of the drug at the same time intervals ranged from 180–209,

74.4–108, 32.5–70.2, 5.1–16.1, and 2.4–7.3 mcg/mL, respectively. In another study in children 2 months to 16 years of age with CNS infections who received a single ceftriaxone dose of 50 or 75 mg/kg by IV infusion over 15 minutes, peak serum concentrations of the drug occurred immediately following the infusion and ranged from 162–370 mcg/mL after the 50-mg/kg dose and 218–348 mcg/mL after the 75-mg/kg dose; serum concentrations of the drug 12 hours after the dose ranged from 8–56.7 and 13.4–51.2 mcg/mL, respectively.

● Distribution

The volume of distribution of ceftriaxone is dose dependent and ranges from 5.8–13.5 L in healthy adults. The volume of distribution of the drug averages 8.5–9.4 L in healthy adults following a single 500-mg dose of the drug and 10–11.4 L following a single 2-g dose. The volume of distribution of ceftriaxone is 0.497–0.608 L/kg in neonates 1–45 days of age and 0.26–0.54 L/kg in children 1.5 months to 16 years of age following a single ceftriaxone dose of 50–100 mg/kg.

Following IM or IV administration, ceftriaxone is widely distributed into body tissues and fluids including the gallbladder, lungs, bone, heart, bile, prostate adenoma tissue, uterine tissue, atrial appendage, sputum, tears, middle ear fluid, and pleural, peritoneal, synovial, ascitic, and blister fluids.

In pediatric patients with otitis media who received a single 50-mg/kg IM dose of ceftriaxone, peak concentrations of ceftriaxone (both protein-bound and unbound drug) in middle ear fluid were attained 24–30 hours after the dose and averaged 35 mcg/mL; middle ear fluid concentrations 48–52 hours after the dose averaged 19 mcg/mL.

In one study in adults with normal hepatobiliary and renal function who received a single 500-mg IV dose of ceftriaxone, peak concentrations of the drug in bile occurred 1–2 hours after the dose and concentrations in bile were generally 2–5 times higher than concurrent serum concentrations. In another study in patients who received a single 1-g IV dose of ceftriaxone, concentrations of the drug in specimens obtained 1–3 hours after the dose averaged 62.1 mcg/mL in plasma, 78.2 mcg/g in the gallbladder wall, and 581, 788, and 898 mcg/mL in gallbladder, common duct, and cystic duct biles, respectively.

In one study in patients undergoing open heart surgery who received a single 1-g IV dose of ceftriaxone approximately 1 hour prior to surgery, concentrations of the drug in the right atrial appendage ranged from 3.6–10.2 mcg/g in samples obtained 1.5–3 hours after the dose. In a study in patients undergoing abdominal or vaginal hysterectomy who received a single 2-g IV dose of ceftriaxone, peak concentrations of the drug in gynecologic tissue occurred during the first 2 hours after the dose and concentrations of the drug were higher in the salpinges than in myometrium or endometrium. Ceftriaxone concentrations in the salpinges averaged 53.1 and 31.3 mcg/mL at 1–2 and 4–5 hours, respectively, after the dose, and concentrations in myometrium or endometrium averaged 29.8–36.6 and 21.4–24.9 mcg/mL at 1–2 and 4–5 hours, respectively, after the dose.

Only low concentrations of ceftriaxone are distributed into aqueous humor following IV or IM administration of the drug. In one study in patients undergoing cataract surgery who received a single 1- or 2-g dose of ceftriaxone by IV infusion over 10 minutes, peak concentrations of the drug in aqueous humor were attained approximately 2 hours after the dose and averaged 0.93 and 2.47 mcg/mL, respectively. Aqueous humor concentrations averaged 0.88 mcg/mL 12 hours after the 1-g dose and were 2.1 and 2.5 mcg/mL in two patients 12 hours after the 2-g dose.

Ceftriaxone generally diffuses into CSF following IM or IV administration of the drug; however, CSF concentrations of the drug are higher in patients with inflamed meninges than in those with uninflamed meninges. Studies in neonates and children with meningitis indicate that peak CSF concentrations of ceftriaxone generally are attained 3–6 hours after an IV dose of the drug, and CSF concentrations of ceftriaxone may be 1–32% of concurrent serum concentrations. CSF concentrations of ceftriaxone do not generally correlate with CSF leukocyte cell counts or CSF protein or glucose concentrations. In one study in neonates and children with meningitis who received a single 50- or 100-mg/kg dose of ceftriaxone, CSF concentrations of the drug were 5–31.6 and 1.4–4.5 mcg/mL at 4 and 24 hours, respectively, after the dose. In another study in children 2–42 months of age with meningitis who received a single ceftriaxone dose of 50 mg/kg given by IV infusion over 10–15 minutes, CSF concentrations of the drug averaged 1.2–3, 1.4–4.3, and 2.8–7.2 mcg/mL at 1, 4, and 6 hours, respectively, after the dose. In one adult with meningitis who received 2 g of the drug once daily, the concentration in CSF was 8.5 mcg/mL in a specimen obtained 5 hours after the third dose of the drug.

The degree of protein binding of ceftriaxone is concentration dependent and decreases nonlinearly with increasing concentrations of the drug. It has been suggested that ceftriaxone may have more than one concentration-dependent protein binding site. The drug is 93–96% bound to plasma proteins at a concentration less than 70 mcg/mL, 84–87% bound at a concentration of 300 mcg/mL, and 58% or less bound at a concentration of 600 mcg/mL. Ceftriaxone binds mainly to albumin. Protein binding of ceftriaxone is lower in neonates and children than in adults because of decreased plasma albumin concentrations in this age group. In one study in children 7 months to 6 years of age with ceftriaxone plasma concentrations of 118–202 mcg/mL, ceftriaxone was 80–87% bound to plasma proteins. Ceftriaxone also is less protein bound in patients with renal or hepatic impairment as the result of decreased plasma albumin concentrations or displacement from protein binding sites by bilirubin and other endogenous compounds that may accumulate.

Ceftriaxone crosses the placenta and is distributed into amniotic fluid. In one study in women who received a single 2-g dose of ceftriaxone given by IV injection over 2–5 minutes during labor, peak concentrations of the drug in cord blood, amniotic fluid, and the placenta occurred 4–8 hours after the dose; ceftriaxone concentrations in the first voided urine of infants born to these women ranged from 6–92 mcg/mL. Ceftriaxone also is distributed into milk in low concentrations. In one study in lactating women who received a single 1-g IM or IV dose of ceftriaxone, peak concentrations of the drug in milk occurred 4–6 hours after the dose and the AUC for milk was 3–4% of the AUC for serum.

● Elimination

Plasma concentrations of ceftriaxone decline in a biphasic manner. In adults with normal renal and hepatic function, the distribution half-life ($t_{\frac{1}{2}\alpha}$) of ceftriaxone is 0.12–0.7 hours and the elimination half-life ($t_{\frac{1}{2}\beta}$) is 5.4–10.9 hours.

Ceftriaxone is excreted both by renal and nonrenal mechanisms. The drug is excreted principally in urine by glomerular filtration and also is excreted in feces via bile. Following IM or IV administration of a single dose of ceftriaxone in adults with normal renal and hepatic function, 33–67% of the dose is excreted in urine as unchanged drug and the remainder of the dose is excreted in feces as unchanged drug and microbiologically inactive metabolites.Ceftriaxone is metabolized to a small extent in the intestines after biliary excretion.

Following IM or IV administration of a single 1-g dose of ceftriaxone in healthy adults, urinary concentrations of the drug average 504–995 mcg/mL in urine collected over the first 2 hours after the dose, 293–418 mcg/mL in urine collected 4–8 hours after the dose, and 132 mcg/mL in urine collected 12–24 hours after the dose.

Serum clearance of ceftriaxone is dose dependent and ranges from 9.7–25 mL/minute in healthy adults. The serum clearance of the drug averages 10.2–16.7 mL/minute in healthy adults following a single 500-mg IV dose and 19.8–21.6 mL/minute following a single 2-g IV dose. In children 2 months to 16 years of age who receive a single ceftriaxone dose of 50–100 mg/kg, the serum clearance of ceftriaxone averages 32–40.8 mL/minute per 1.73 m². Preliminary studies in patients with cystic fibrosis suggest that serum clearance of ceftriaxone is higher in these patients than in healthy individuals.

The serum half-life of ceftriaxone is longer in neonates than in older children and adults. In one study, the serum half-life of ceftriaxone was longer in neonates weighing less than 1.5 kg than in heavier neonates. Results of another study in neonates 1–8 days of age weighing 1.8–3.9 kg suggested that there was no correlation between weight and serum half-life of the drug at this weight range. In one study, the serum half-life of the drug averaged 16.2 hours in neonates 1–4 days of age and 9.2 hours in those 9–30 days of age. The serum half-life of ceftriaxone in children is similar to that reported in adults, and the elimination half-life of the drug averages 4–7.7 hours in children 1.5 months to 16 years of age. In one study in children 2–42 months of age, the $t_{\frac{1}{2}\alpha}$ of ceftriaxone averaged 0.25 hours and the $t_{\frac{1}{2}\beta}$ of the drug averaged 4 hours.

The elimination half-life of ceftriaxone is only slightly prolonged in patients with moderately impaired renal function and has been reported to range from 10–16 hours in adults with creatinine clearances of 5–73 mL/minute. In patients with creatinine clearances less than 5 mL/minute, the elimination half-life of ceftriaxone has generally been reported to average 12.2–18.2 hours. However, the elimination half-life of ceftriaxone was 15–57 hours in several uremic patients with creatinine clearances less than 5 mL/minute who had no apparent liver impairment.

Studies in patients with hepatic impairment (e.g., patients with fatty liver, liver fibrosis, compensated liver cirrhosis) indicate that the pharmacokinetics of ceftriaxone are not generally altered in these patients. Although the elimination half-life of ceftriaxone was not prolonged in patients with ascites, the volume of distribution and plasma clearance of the drug were increased slightly compared with healthy individuals and averaged 22 L and 28 mL/minute, respectively.

Ceftriaxone is not removed by hemodialysis or peritoneal dialysis.

CHEMISTRY AND STABILITY

● Chemistry

Ceftriaxone is a semisynthetic cephalosporin antibiotic. Like cefepime, cefotaxime, and ceftazidime, ceftriaxone is a parenteral aminothiazolyl cephalosporin. Ceftriaxone contains an aminothiazolyl-acetyl side chain, with a methoxyimino group, at position 7 of the cephalosporin nucleus. The aminothiazolyl side chain enhances antibacterial activity, particularly against Enterobacteriaceae, and generally results in enhanced stability against β-lactamases; the methoxyimino group contributes to stability against hydrolysis by many β-lactamases. Ceftriaxone also has an acidic enol in the triazine moiety at position 3 of the cephalosporin nucleus, which presumably is responsible for the long serum half-life of the drug.

Ceftriaxone is commercially available as the disodium salt; however, the drug is referred to as ceftriaxone sodium. Potency of ceftriaxone sodium is expressed in terms of ceftriaxone. Each mg of ceftriaxone sodium contains not less than 776 mcg of ceftriaxone, calculated on the anhydrous free acid basis.

Ceftriaxone sodium is readily soluble in water, having an aqueous solubility of 400 mg/mL at 25°C. The drug has a solubility of 1 mg/mL in alcohol at 25°C. Ceftriaxone sodium has pK$_a$s of 3, 3.2, and 4.1. Ceftriaxone sodium contains approximately 83 mg (3.6 mEq) of sodium per gram of ceftriaxone.

Commercially available sterile ceftriaxone sodium powder for injection occurs as a white to yellowish or yellowish-orange crystalline powder. When reconstituted as directed, solutions of the drug are light yellow to amber in color depending on the diluent used, concentration of the drug, and length of storage. The pH of an aqueous solution containing 10 mg of ceftriaxone per mL is approximately 6.7.

When the commercially available Duplex® drug delivery system that contains 1 or 2 g of ceftriaxone powder and 50 mL of dextrose injection in separate chambers is reconstituted (activated) according to the manufacturer's directions, the resultant solution is iso-osmotic and has an osmolality of approximately 290 mOsm/kg.

Commercially available frozen premixed ceftriaxone sodium injections in dextrose are sterile, nonpyrogenic, iso-osmotic solutions of the drug provided in a plastic container (Galaxy® containers) fabricated from specially formulated multilayered plastic PL 2040 plastic. The 1- and 2-g frozen injections of ceftriaxone contain approximately 1.9 and 1.2 g of dextrose hydrous, respectively, to adjust osmolality and may contain sodium hydroxide and/or hydrochloric acid to adjust pH. After thawing, the injections are light yellow to amber in color and have a pH of 6–8.

● Stability

Commercially available ceftriaxone sodium sterile powder for injection should be stored at 20–25°C and protected from light. It is unnecessary to protect reconstituted solutions of the drug from normal light.

Following reconstitution of ceftriaxone powder for injection with sterile water for injection, 0.9% sodium chloride injection, or 5% dextrose injection, ceftriaxone sodium solutions for IM injection containing approximately 250 or 350 mg of ceftriaxone per mL are stable for 24 hours at room temperature (25°C) or 3 days refrigerated at 4°C and solutions containing approximately 100 mg/mL are stable for 2 days at 25°C or 10 days at 4°C. Following reconstitution with 1% lidocaine hydrochloride injection (without epinephrine) or bacteriostatic water for injection (containing 0.9% benzyl alcohol), solutions of the drug for IM injection containing 250 or 350 mg/mL are stable for 24 hours at 25°C or 3 days at 4°C and solutions containing 100 mg/mL are stable for 24 hours at 25°C or 10 days at 4°C.

Following reconstitution of ceftriaxone powder for injection as directed by the manufacturer and further dilution with sterile water for injection, 0.9% sodium chloride injection, or 5 or 10% dextrose injection, solutions containing 10–40 mg of ceftriaxone per mL are stable in glass or PVC containers for 2 days at room temperature (25°C) or 10 days when refrigerated at 4°C. If 5% dextrose in 0.45 or 0.9% sodium chloride is used for dilution, solutions of the drug containing 10–40 mg/mL are stable for 2 days at room temperature when stored in glass or PVC containers but are unstable at 4°C. Solutions of the drug containing 10–40 mg/mL are stable for 24 hours at room temperature (25°C) in 10% invert sugar, 5% sodium bicarbonate, 5 or 10% mannitol, FreAmine® III, Normosol®-M in 5% dextrose, or Ionosol® B in 5% dextrose when stored in glass containers. The same concentrations of the drug are stable for 24 hours at room temperature in sodium lactate or Normosol®-M in 5% dextrose when stored in PVC containers.

The manufacturers state that following reconstitution with 0.9% sodium chloride injection or 5% dextrose injection, extemporaneously prepared ceftriaxone sodium solutions containing 10–40 mg of ceftriaxone per mL are stable for 26 weeks when frozen at –20°C in PVC or polyolefin containers. Frozen solutions of ceftriaxone sodium should be thawed at room temperature; once thawed, unused portions should be discarded and should not be refrozen.

Commercially available 10-g pharmacy bulk packages of ceftriaxone that have been reconstituted to a concentration of 100 mg/mL with a compatible IV solution should be further diluted in a compatible IV infusion solution without delay; any unused portions of the reconstituted solution should be discarded after 4 hours.

Following reconstitution of ADD-Vantage® vials containing 1 or 2 g of ceftriaxone with 0.9% sodium chloride injection or 5% dextrose injection according to the manufacturer's directions, IV solutions containing 10–40 mg/mL in 0.9% sodium chloride or 5% dextrose in ADD-Vantage® flexible containers are stable for 2 days at room temperature (25°C) or 10 days refrigerated at 4°C.

The commercially available Duplex® drug delivery system that contains 1 or 2 g of lyophilized ceftriaxone and 50 mL of dextrose injection should be stored at 20–25°C, but may be exposed to 15–30°C. Following reconstitution (activation), these IV solutions must be used within 24 hours if stored at room temperature or within 7 days if stored in a refrigerator and should not be frozen.

The commercially available frozen premixed ceftriaxone sodium injection in dextrose should be stored at –20°C or lower. The frozen injection should be thawed at room temperature (25°C) or under refrigeration (5°C) and, once thawed, should not be refrozen. Thawed solutions of the commercially available frozen injection are stable for 48 hours at room temperature (25°C) or 21 days under refrigeration (5°C). The commercially available frozen injection of the drug is provided in a plastic container fabricated from specially formulated multilayered plastic PL 2040 (Galaxy®). Solutions in contact with PL 2040 can leach out some of its chemical components in very small amounts within the expiration period of the injection; however, safety of the plastic has been confirmed in tests in animals according to USP biological tests for plastic containers as well as by tissue culture toxicity studies.

Ceftriaxone is physically incompatible with aminoglycosides, fluconazole, and vancomycin, and the manufacturers state that ceftriaxone should not be admixed with these drugs. If an aminoglycoside, fluconazole, or vancomycin is to be administered in a patient receiving ceftriaxone by intermittent IV infusion, the drugs should be given sequentially and IV infusion lines should be thoroughly flushed with a compatible infusion fluid before administering the other drug. Admixtures containing ceftriaxone 10 mg/mL and metronidazole hydrochloride 5–7.5 mg/mL in 0.9% sodium chloride injection or 5% dextrose injection are stable for 24 hours at room temperature; however, precipitation will occur if these admixtures are refrigerated or if metronidazole concentrations greater than 8 mg/mL are used.

Ceftriaxone is incompatible with calcium-containing diluents or solutions (e.g. Ringer's/lactated Ringer's solution, Hartmann's solution); particulate formation can result if the drug is admixed with calcium-containing diluents or solutions.

Specialized references should be consulted for specific compatibility information.

PREPARATIONS

Excipients in commercially available drug preparations may have clinically important effects in some individuals; consult specific product labeling for details.

cefTRIAXone Sodium

Parenteral

For injection	250 mg (of ceftriaxone)*	cefTRIAXone for Injection
	500 mg (of ceftriaxone)*	cefTRIAXone for Injection
	1 g (of ceftriaxone)*	cefTRIAXone for Injection
	2 g (of ceftriaxone)*	cefTRIAXone for Injection
For injection, for IV infusion	1 g (of ceftriaxone)*	cefTRIAXone ADD-Vantage®, Hospira
		cefTRIAXone for Injection, for IV Infusion (available in dual-chambered Duplex® drug delivery system with 3.74% dextrose injection), B Braun
		cefTRIAXone for Injection, for IV Infusion
	2 g (of ceftriaxone)*	cefTRIAXone ADD-Vantage®, Hospira
		cefTRIAXone for Injection, for IV Infusion (available in dual-chambered Duplex® drug delivery system with 2.22% dextrose injection), B Braun
		cefTRIAXone for Injection, for IV Infusion
	10 g (of ceftriaxone) pharmacy bulk package*	cefTRIAXone for Injection, for IV Infusion
	100 g (of ceftriaxone) pharmacy bulk package*	cefTRIAXone for Injection, for IV Infusion

* available from one or more manufacturer, distributor, and/or repackager by generic (nonproprietary) name

cefTRIAXone Sodium in Dextrose

Parenteral

| Injection (frozen), for IV infusion | 20 mg (of ceftriaxone) per mL (1 g) in 3.8% Dextrose* | cefTRIAXone Iso-osmotic in Dextrose Injection (Galaxy® [Baxter]) |
| | 40 mg (of ceftriaxone) per mL (2 g) in 2.4% Dextrose* | cefTRIAXone Iso-osmotic in Dextrose Injection (Galaxy® [Baxter]) |

* available from one or more manufacturer, distributor, and/or repackager by generic (nonproprietary) name

† Use is not currently included in the labeling approved by the US Food and Drug Administration.

Selected Revisions October 1, 2018, © Copyright, August 1, 1985, American Society of Health-System Pharmacists, Inc.

Cefepime Hydrochloride

8:12.06.16 • FOURTH GENERATION CEPHALOSPORINS

■ Cefepime is a semisynthetic, fourth generation cephalosporin antibiotic.

USES

Cefepime is used for the treatment of uncomplicated and complicated urinary tract infections (including pyelonephritis), uncomplicated skin and skin structure infections, and moderate to severe pneumonia caused by susceptible organisms. For the treatment of complicated intra-abdominal infections, cefepime is used in conjunction with IV metronidazole. In addition, cefepime is used alone or in conjunction with other anti-infectives for empiric anti-infective therapy in febrile neutropenic patients.

● Intra-abdominal Infections

IV cefepime is used in conjunction with IV metronidazole for the treatment of complicated intra-abdominal infections caused by *Escherichia coli*, viridans streptococci, *Pseudomonas aeruginosa*, *Klebsiella pneumoniae*, *Enterobacter*, or *Bacteroides fragilis* in adults. Safety and efficacy of cefepime used in conjunction with metronidazole has been evaluated in a randomized, double-blind, multicenter study in adults with surgically confirmed complicated intra-abdominal infections who were randomized to receive cefepime (2 g IV every 12 hours) and metronidazole (7.5 mg/kg or 500 mg IV every 6 hours) or monotherapy with imipenem and cilastatin sodium (500 mg IV every 6 hours). The overall clinical cure rate was 88% in those who received combination therapy with cefepime and metronidazole and 76% in those who received monotherapy with imipenem and cilastatin sodium.

For initial empiric treatment of high-risk or severe community-acquired extrabiliary intra-abdominal infections in adults (e.g., those with advanced age, immunocompromised state, severe physiologic disturbance), the Infectious Diseases Society of America (IDSA) recommends either monotherapy with a carbapenem (doripenem, imipenem, meropenem) or the fixed combination of piperacillin and tazobactam, or a combination regimen that includes either a cephalosporin (cefepime, ceftazidime) or fluoroquinolone (ciprofloxacin, levofloxacin) in conjunction with metronidazole. IDSA also recommends cefepime in conjunction with metronidazole as one of several regimens that can be used for initial empiric treatment of health-care associated complicated intra-abdominal infections in adults and community-acquired complicated intra-abdominal infections in pediatric patients. For additional information regarding management of intra-abdominal infections, the current IDSA clinical practice guidelines available at http://www.idsociety.org should be consulted.

While cefepime has been effective when used alone for the treatment of acute obstetric and gynecologic infections† (e.g., pelvic inflammatory disease, pelvic surgical wound infection, postpartum endometritis), safety and efficacy of the drug for use as monotherapy in the treatment of such infections have not been established.

● Respiratory Tract Infections

Cefepime is used in adult and pediatric patients 2 months of age or older for the treatment of moderate to severe pneumonia, including that associated with concurrent bacteremia, caused by susceptible *Streptococcus pneumoniae*. The drug also is used in adult and pediatric patients 2 months of age or older for the treatment of moderate to severe pneumonia caused by susceptible *Ps. aeruginosa*, *K. pneumoniae*, or *Enterobacter*.

Community-acquired Pneumonia

Cefepime appears to be at least as effective and as well tolerated as ceftriaxone or ceftazidime for the treatment of community-acquired pneumonia (CAP). In an open-label, randomized study in hospitalized adults who were randomized to receive 5–10 days (14 days maximum) of therapy with either cefepime (2 g IV every 12 hours) or ceftriaxone (1 g IV every 12 hours) for empiric treatment of CAP, a satisfactory clinical response (cure or improvement) was achieved in 95% of those receiving cefepime and 97.8% of those receiving ceftriaxone. When

cefepime (1 g IV or IM every 12 hours) was compared with ceftazidime (1 g IV every 8 hours) for empiric therapy in adults 21–90 years of age with community-acquired lower respiratory tract infections, the clinical cure rate was 87% in those who received cefepime and 86% in those who received ceftazidime. The most common pathogens in these studies were *S. pneumoniae*, *Haemophilus influenzae*, *Moraxella catarrhalis*, and/or *Staphylococcal aureus*.

The American Thoracic Society (ATS) and IDSA recommend use of cefepime in the treatment of CAP only when *Ps. aeruginosa* is known or suspected to be involved. Factors that increase the risk of *Ps. aeruginosa* infection in CAP patients include severe CAP requiring treatment in an intensive care unit (ICU), structural lung disease (bronchiectasis), severe chronic obstructive pulmonary disease (COPD), smoking, alcoholism, chronic corticosteroid therapy, and frequent anti-infective therapy. In CAP patients with risk factors for *Ps. aeruginosa*, the ATS and IDSA recommend use of an empiric combination regimen that includes an antpneumococcal, antipseudomonal β-lactam (cefepime, imipenem, meropenem, fixed combination of piperacillin and tazobactam) given in conjunction with a fluoroquinolone (ciprofloxacin, levofloxacin); a combination regimen that includes one of these antipseudomonal β-lactams, an aminoglycoside, and azithromycin; or a combination regimen that includes one of these antipseudomonal β-lactams, an aminoglycoside, and an antipneumococcal fluoroquinolone. The ATS and IDSA state that if *Ps. aeruginosa* has been identified by appropriate microbiologic testing, the preferred treatment regimen is an antipseudomonal β-lactam (cefepime, ceftazidime, aztreonam, imipenem, meropenem, piperacillin, ticarcillin) given in conjunction with ciprofloxacin, levofloxacin, or an aminoglycoside and the preferred alternative regimen is an aminoglycoside given in conjunction with ciprofloxacin or levofloxacin.

For additional information on use of cephalosporins in the treatment of CAP, see Community-acquired Infections under Uses: Respiratory Tract Infections, in the Cephalosporins General Statement 8:12.06.

Nosocomial Infections

Cefepime is used in the treatment of nosocomial pneumonia. The ATS, IDSA, and other clinicians recommend use of an antipseudomonal cephalosporin (cefepime, ceftazidime), antipseudomonal penicillin (piperacillin and tazobactam, ticarcillin and clavulanate), or an antipseudomonal carbapenem (imipenem or meropenem) for initial therapy of hospital-acquired pneumonia, ventilator-associated pneumonia, or health-care associated pneumonia because these drugs have a broad spectrum of activity against gram-positive, gram-negative, and anaerobic bacteria. In hospitals where methicillin-resistant *S. aureus* (MRSA; also known as oxacillin-resistant *S. aureus* or ORSA) is common or if there are risk factors for these strains, the initial regimen also should include vancomycin or linezolid.

● Skin and Skin Structure Infections

Cefepime is used in adult and pediatric patients 2 months of age or older for the treatment of uncomplicated skin and skin structure infections caused by susceptible *S. aureus* (methicillin-susceptible [oxacillin-susceptible] strains only) or susceptible *Streptococcus pyogenes*.

● Urinary Tract Infections

Cefepime is used in adult and pediatric patients 2 months of age or older for the treatment of severe uncomplicated and complicated urinary tract infections (including those associated with pyelonephritis and/or concurrent bacteremia) caused by susceptible *E. coli* or *K. pneumoniae*. Cefepime also is used in adult and pediatric patients 2 months of age or older for the treatment of mild to moderate uncomplicated and complicated urinary tract infections (including those associated with pyelonephritis and/or with concurrent bacteremia) when the causative organism is *E. coli*, *K. pneumoniae*, or *Proteus mirabilis*.

● Endocarditis

For empiric treatment of culture-negative endocarditis† in prosthetic valve recipients with early onset endocarditis (within 1 year after prosthetic valve placement), the American Heart Association (AHA) recommends a multiple-drug regimen that includes vancomycin, gentamicin, cefepime, and rifampin. Blood cultures are negative in up to 20% of patients with infective endocarditis because of inadequate microbiologic technique, infection with highly fastidious bacteria or nonbacterial pathogens, or administration of anti-infective agents prior to obtaining blood cultures. Selection of the most appropriate anti-infective regimen for the treatment of culture-negative endocarditis is difficult and should be guided by epidemiologic features and clinical course of the infection. Consultation with an infectious diseases specialist is recommended.

● Meningitis and Other CNS Infections

Cefepime has been used in adult and pediatric patients 2 months of age or older for the treatment of meningitis† caused by susceptible gram-negative bacteria (e.g., *H. influenzae, Neisseria meningitidis, E. coli, E. aerogenes, Ps. aeruginosa*) or gram-positive bacteria (e.g., *S. pneumoniae, S. aureus, S. epidermidis*). However, safety and efficacy of cefepime for the treatment of meningitis have not been established, and the manufacturers caution that an alternative anti-infective with demonstrated clinical efficacy in this setting should be used in patients in whom meningeal seeding from a distant infection site or in whom meningitis is suspected or documented.

IDSA states that cefepime is one of several alternatives that can be used for the treatment of meningitis caused by *H. influenzae* or *E. coli* or treatment of meningitis caused by *S. pneumonia* susceptible to penicillins and third generation cephalosporins. For the treatment of meningitis caused by *Ps. aeruginosa*, IDSA and other experts recommend a regimen that consists of an antipseudomonal cephalosporin (cefepime or ceftazidime) or carbapenem (imipenem or meropenem) given with or without an aminoglycoside (amikacin, gentamicin, tobramycin). Treatment of these infections should be guided by results of in vitro susceptibility tests.

IDSA also recommends a regimen of cefepime and vancomycin as one of several regimens that can be used in adult and pediatric patients for empiric treatment of penetrating head trauma or postneurosurgical infections caused by *S. aureus*, coagulase-negative staphylococci (especially *S. epidermidis*), or aerobic gram-negative bacilli (including *Ps. aeruginosa*).

In a prospective, randomized study in infants and children 2 months to 15 years of age, IV cefepime was as effective as IV cefotaxime for the treatment of meningitis caused by susceptible gram-negative or gram-positive bacteria. However, some clinicians suggest that additional study is needed regarding cefepime's efficacy for the treatment of meningitis, particularly for infections caused by penicillin- and/or cefotaxime-resistant *S. pneumoniae*. In addition, it has been suggested that cefepime would not be a good choice for empiric treatment of meningitis if *Acinetobacter* may be involved.

● Septicemia

Cefepime is used for the treatment of septicemia† caused by susceptible gram-negative bacteria.

The choice of anti-infective agent for the treatment of sepsis syndrome should be based on the probable source of infection, causative organism, immune status of the patient, and local patterns of bacterial resistance. For initial treatment of life-threatening sepsis in adults, some clinicians recommend that a third or fourth generation cephalosporin (cefepime, cefotaxime, ceftriaxone, ceftazidime), the fixed combination of piperacillin and tazobactam, or a carbapenem (imipenem or meropenem) be used in conjunction with vancomycin; some experts also suggest including an aminoglycoside or fluoroquinolone during the initial few days of treatment.

● Empiric Therapy in Febrile Neutropenic Patients

Cefepime is used in adult and pediatric patients 2 months of age or older as monotherapy for empiric anti-infective therapy of presumed bacterial infections in febrile neutropenic patients. The manufacturers caution that use of monotherapy for empiric therapy in patients at high risk for *severe* infection (e.g., those with a history of recent bone marrow transplantation, hypotension on presentation, underlying hematologic malignancy, or severe or prolonged neutropenia) may not be appropriate and data regarding efficacy of cefepime monotherapy in these patients is limited to date.

Safety and efficacy of cefepime monotherapy for empiric therapy in febrile neutropenic patients were initially evaluated in a pilot study that involved 84 granulocytopenic cancer patients who received cefepime (2 g IV every 8 hours) for a minimum of 7 days or until infections resolved; the overall response rate in these patients was 71%. Cefepime also has been used in conjunction with amikacin for empiric therapy in febrile neutropenic patients in an open-label, randomized study in adults with chemotherapy-induced neutropenia who were considered at high risk of infection. Patients were randomized to receive empiric therapy with a combination regimen of cefepime (2 g IV every 12 hours) and amikacin (7.5 mg/kg every 12 hours) or ceftazidime (2 g IV every 8 hours) and amikacin (7.5 mg/kg every 12 hours); both regimens were comparable in terms of clinical response, rates of bacteriologic eradication, incidence of new infection, and survival.

There is evidence from open-label, randomized studies in febrile neutropenic patients that empiric therapy with cefepime monotherapy is as effective as empiric monotherapy with ceftazidime, imipenem, or the fixed combination of piperacillin and tazobactam or empiric treatment with combination regimens that consist of piperacillin sodium and gentamicin sulfate or ceftriaxone and amikacin.

Successful treatment of infections in granulocytopenic patients requires prompt initiation of empiric anti-infective therapy (even when fever is the only sign or symptom of infection) and appropriate modification of the initial regimen if the duration of fever and neutropenia is protracted, if a specific site of infection is identified, or if organisms resistant to the initial regimen are present. The initial empiric regimen should be chosen based on the underlying disease and other host factors that may affect the degree of risk and on local epidemiologic data regarding the type, frequency of occurrence, in vitro susceptibility of bacterial isolates recovered from other patients in the same health-care facility, and the individual patient's pattern of colonization and resistance. The fact that gram-positive bacteria have become a predominant pathogen in febrile neutropenic patients should be considered when selecting an empiric anti-infective regimen. However, although gram-positive bacteria reportedly account for about 60% and gram-negative bacteria account for about 35% of microbiologically documented infections, gram-negative infections are associated with greater mortality.

No empiric regimen has been identified that would be appropriate for initial treatment of all febrile neutropenic patients. The IDSA recommends use of a parenteral empiric regimen in most febrile neutropenic patients; use of an oral regimen (e.g., oral ciprofloxacin and oral amoxicillin and clavulanate potassium) should be considered *only* for selected adults at low risk for complications who have adequate and stable renal and hepatic function, an expected duration of neutropenia less than 7 days, and no active medical comorbidities. All other patients are considered high risk and should receive an initial IV empiric regimen consisting of an antipseudomonal β-lactam (e.g., cefepime, imipenem, meropenem, fixed-combination of piperacillin and tazobactam). Other anti-infectives (e.g., aminoglycosides, fluoroquinolones, and/or vancomycin) may be added to the regimen for the management of complications (e.g., pneumonia) or when antimicrobial resistance is suspected or proven. Vancomycin or other anti-infectives active against aerobic gram-positive cocci are not usually included in the initial empiric regimen except in certain clinical scenarios, including suspected catheter-related infections, skin and soft tissue infections, pneumonia, or hemodynamic instability.

Regardless of the initial regimen selected, patients should be reassessed daily and the anti-infective regimen altered (if indicated) based on the presence or absence of fever, identification of the causative organism, and the clinical condition of the patient; anti-infectives active against gram-positive organisms may be discontinued after 2 days if there is no evidence of such infections.

Published protocols for the treatment of infections in febrile neutropenic patients should be consulted for specific recommendations regarding selection of the initial empiric anti-infective regimen, when to change the initial regimen, possible subsequent regimens, and duration of therapy in these patients. In addition, consultation with an infectious disease expert knowledgeable about infections in immunocompromised patients is advised.

For additional information on the role of parenteral cephalosporins in the treatment of these and other infections, see Uses in the Cephalosporins General Statement 8:12.06.

DOSAGE AND ADMINISTRATION

● Reconstitution and Administration

Cefepime preferably is administered by IV infusion but also can be given by deep IM injection when indicated depending on the severity of the infection being treated.

The manufacturer states that IM administration of the drug is indicated *only* for the treatment of mild to moderate uncomplicated or complicated urinary tract infections caused by *Escherichia coli* and *only* when this route is considered more appropriate

If an aminoglycoside, ampicillin (at a concentration exceeding 40 mg/mL), metronidazole, vancomycin, or aminophylline is administered concomitantly with cefepime, the drugs should be administered separately.

Reconstituted and diluted solutions of cefepime should be inspected visually for particulate matter prior to administration whenever solution and container permit.

Intermittent IV Infusion

For intermittent IV infusion, vials labeled as containing 500 mg, 1 g, or 2 g of cefepime should be reconstituted with 5, 10, or 10 mL, respectively, of a compatible IV solution to provide solutions containing approximately 100, 100, or 160 mg/mL of the drug, respectively. The appropriate dose of the drug should then be added to a compatible IV solution.

Alternatively, ADD-Vantage® vials containing 1 or 2 g of cefepime should be reconstituted with 50 or 100 mL, respectively, of 0.9% sodium chloride or 5% dextrose injection according to the manufacturer's directions and administered by IV infusion.

Another alternative is the commercially available Duplex® drug delivery system that contains 1 or 2 g of cefepime and 50 mL of 5% dextrose injection in separate chambers, which should be reconstituted (activated) according to the manufacturer's directions and administered by IV infusion. If stored in the refrigerator after reconstitution (see Chemistry and Stability: Stability), the solution should be allowed to reach room temperature prior to administration.

Thawed solutions of the commercially available frozen premixed cefepime injection in dextrose should be administered only by IV infusion. The frozen injection should be thawed at room temperature (25°C) or under refrigeration (5°C); the injection should not be thawed by warming in a water bath or by exposure to microwave radiation. Precipitates that may have formed in the frozen injection usually will dissolve with little or no agitation when the injection reaches room temperature; potency is not affected. After thawing to room temperature, the injection should be agitated and the container checked for minute leaks by firmly squeezing the bag; the container may be fragile and should be handled with care. The injection should be discarded if container seals or outlet ports are not intact or leaks are found or if the solution is cloudy or contains an insoluble precipitate. Additives should not be introduced into the injection container. The injection should not be used in series connections with other plastic containers, since such use could result in air embolism from residual air being drawn from the primary container before administration of fluid from the secondary container is complete.

If a Y-type administration set is used, the other solution flowing through the tubing should be discontinued while cefepime is being infused.

Rate of Administration

The cefepime dose should be administered by IV infusion over approximately 30 minutes.

IM Injection

IM injections of cefepime are prepared by adding 1.3 or 2.4 mL of an appropriate diluent (i.e., sterile water for injection, 0.9% sodium chloride, 5% dextrose, 0.5 or 1% lidocaine hydrochloride, bacteriostatic water for injection with parabens or benzyl alcohol) to a vial labeled as containing 500 mg or 1 g of cefepime, respectively, to provide a solution containing approximately 280 mg/mL.

● Dosage

Cefepime is commercially available as cefepime hydrochloride, which is monohydrated; dosage is expressed in terms of cefepime, calculated on the anhydrous basis.

Adult Dosage

Intra-abdominal Infections

For the treatment of complicated intra-abdominal infections (in conjunction with IV metronidazole), the usual adult dosage of cefepime is 2 g given IV every 12 hours for 7–10 days.

For the treatment of complicated intra-abdominal infections (in conjunction with IV metronidazole), some experts recommend that adults receive cefepime in a dosage of 2 g every 8–12 hours for 4–7 days. A longer duration of treatment has not been associated with improved outcome and is not recommended unless adequate source control is difficult to achieve.

Respiratory Tract Infections

For the treatment of moderate to severe pneumonia caused by *Streptococcus pneumoniae* (including those with concurrent bacteremia), the usual adult dosage of cefepime is 1–2 g given IV every 12 hours for 10 days.

For initial treatment of hospital-acquired pneumonia, ventilator-associated pneumonia, or health-care associated pneumonia, some clinicians recommend that adults receive a cefepime dosage of 1–2 g every 8–12 hours.

Skin and Skin Structure Infections

For the treatment of moderate to severe uncomplicated skin and skin structure infections caused by *Staphylococcus aureus* or *Streptococcus pyogenes*, the usual adult dosage of cefepime is 2 g IV every 12 hours for 10 days.

Urinary Tract Infections

For the treatment of mild to moderate uncomplicated or complicated urinary tract infections (including those associated with pyelonephritis and/or with concurrent bacteremia), the usual adult dosage of cefepime is 0.5–1 g administered IV or IM every 12 hours for 7–10 days.

For the treatment of severe uncomplicated or complicated urinary tract infections (including those associated with pyelonephritis and/or concurrent bacteremia), adults should received 2 g of cefepime IV every 12 hours for 10 days.

Endocarditis

If cefepime is used in a multiple-drug regimen for empiric treatment of culture-negative endocarditis† in prosthetic valve recipients (see Uses: Endocarditis), the American Heart Association (AHA) recommends that adults receive IV cefepime in a dosage of 6 g daily given in 3 equally divided doses in conjunction with vancomycin (30 mg/kg daily given IV in 2 equally divided doses), gentamicin (3 mg/kg daily given IV or IM in 3 equally divided doses), and rifampin (900 mg daily given orally or IV in 3 equally divided doses). The multiple-drug regimen should be continued for 6 weeks; gentamicin should be discontinued after the first 2 weeks of treatment.

Meningitis and Other CNS Infections

For the treatment of meningitis† in adults, the Infectious Diseases Society of America (IDSA) recommends that IV cefepime be given in a dosage of 2 g every 8 hours.

IDSA states that the duration of therapy should be individualized based on response and recommends a duration of 7 days for infections caused by *Haemophilus influenzae* or *Neisseria meningitidis*, 10–14 days for infections caused by *S. pneumoniae*, or 21 days for infections caused by aerobic gram-negative bacilli.

Empiric Therapy in Febrile Neutropenic Patients

When cefepime is used as monotherapy for empiric anti-infective therapy in febrile neutropenic patients, adults should receive a dosage of 2 g IV every 8 hours for 7 days or until neutropenia resolves. The need for continued anti-infective therapy in patients whose fever resolves but who remain neutropenic for longer than 7 days should be frequently reevaluated.

Pediatric Dosage
General Pediatric Dosage

For the treatment of uncomplicated and complicated urinary tract infections (including pyelonephritis), uncomplicated skin and skin structure infections, or pneumonia, the manufacturers recommend that pediatric patients 2 months to 16 years of age weighing less than 40 kg receive cefepime in a dosage of 50 mg/kg given IV every 12 hours. Pediatric dosage should not exceed the recommended adult dosage.

Although safety and efficacy of cefepime have not been established in neonates or infants younger than 2 months of age, the American Academy of Pediatrics (AAP) states that neonates 28 days of age or younger† may receive IV or IM cefepime in a dosage of 30 mg/kg every 12 hours and that a dosage of 50 mg/kg every 12 hours may be required for *Pseudomonas* infections.

The AAP states that pediatric patients beyond the neonatal period may receive IV or IM cefepime in a dosage of 100 mg/kg daily in 2 equally divided doses for the treatment of mild to moderate infections or a dosage of 100–150 mg/kg daily in 2 or 3 equally divided doses for the treatment of severe infections.

To avoid unintentional overdosage, the manufacturers state that the commercially available Duplex® drug delivery systems containing cefepime and the commercially available frozen premixed cefepime injection should *not* be used in pediatric patients who require less than the entire 1- or 2-g dose in the container.

Intra-abdominal Infections

For the treatment of complicated intra-abdominal infections (in conjunction with IV metronidazole) in pediatric patients, some experts recommend a cefepime dosage of 50 mg/kg every 12 hours for 4–7 days. A longer duration of treatment has not been associated with improved outcome and is not recommended unless adequate source control is difficult to achieve.

Endocarditis

If cefepime is used in a multiple-drug regimen for empiric treatment of culture-negative endocarditis† in prosthetic valve recipients (see Uses: Endocarditis), the AHA recommends that pediatric patients receive IV cefepime in a dosage of 150 mg/kg daily given in 3 equally divided doses in conjunction with vancomycin (40 mg/kg daily given IV in 2 or 3 equally divided doses), gentamicin (3 mg/kg daily given IV or IM in 3 equally divided doses), and rifampin (20 mg/kg daily given orally or IV in 3 equally divided doses). The multiple-drug regimen should be continued for 6 weeks; gentamicin should be discontinued after the first 2 weeks of treatment.

Meningitis and Other CNS Infections

For the treatment of meningitis†, infants and children 2 months to 15 years of age have received IV cefepime in a dosage of 50 mg/kg every 8 hours for 7–10 days.

IDSA states that the duration of therapy should be individualized based on response and recommends a duration of 7 days for infections caused by *H. influenzae* or *N. meningitidis*, 10–14 days for infections caused by *S. pneumoniae*, or 21 days for infections caused by aerobic gram-negative bacilli.

Empiric Therapy in Febrile Neutropenic Patients

When cefepime is used as monotherapy for empiric anti-infective therapy in febrile neutropenic pediatric patients 2 months to 16 years of age who weigh less than 40 kg, the manufacturers recommend a dosage of 50 mg/kg given IV every 8 hours. The need for continued anti-infective therapy in patients whose fever resolves but who remain neutropenic for longer than 7 days should be frequently reevaluated.

• Dosage in Renal and Hepatic Impairment

In patients with renal impairment (i.e., creatinine clearance of 60 mL/minute or less), doses and/or frequency of administration of cefepime should be modified in response to the degree of renal impairment, severity of the infection, and susceptibility of the causative organism.

The manufacturers recommend that adults with creatinine clearance of 60 mL/minute or less (not receiving hemodialysis) receive the same initial dose of cefepime recommended for patients with normal renal function followed by a maintenance dosage of cefepime based on the patient's measured or estimated creatinine clearance. (See Table 1 and Table 2.)

TABLE 1. Maintenance Dosage for Treatment of Infections in Adults with Renal Impairment

Creatinine Clearance (mL/minute)	Initial dose: 500 mg	Initial dose: 1 g	Initial dose: 2 g
30–60	500 mg every 24 h	1 g every 24 h	2 g every 24 h
11–29	500 mg every 24 h	500 mg every 24 h	1 g every 24 h
<11	250 mg every 24 h	250 mg every 24 h	500 mg every 24 h

TABLE 2. Maintenance Dosage for Empiric Therapy in Febrile Neutropenic Adults with Renal Impairment

Creatinine Clearance (mL/minute)	Initial Dose: 2 g
30–60	2 g every 12 h
11–29	2 g every 24 h
<11	1 g every 24 h

The manufacturers recommend that adults undergoing hemodialysis receive an initial 1-g dose of cefepime on day 1, then 500 mg once daily thereafter for the treatment of infections or 1 g once daily for empiric therapy of presumed bacterial infections in febrile neutropenic patients. The manufacturers also recommend

that the daily dose be given at the same time of day whenever possible; on hemodialysis days, the dose should be given after the procedure.

Adults undergoing continuous ambulatory peritoneal dialysis (CAPD) should receive the usual cefepime dose every 48 hours.

Data regarding use of cefepime in pediatric patients with impaired renal function are not available. Because the pharmacokinetics of cefepime are similar in pediatric and adult patients, the manufacturers recommend that dosage modifications proportional to those recommended for adults be used in pediatric patients with impaired renal function.

Since pharmacokinetics of cefepime appear not to be altered in patients with hepatic impairment, the manufacturers state that dosage adjustments are not necessary in such patients.

CAUTIONS

• Adverse Effects

Adverse effects reported with cefepime are similar to those reported with other parenteral cephalosporins. (See Cautions in the Cephalosporins General Statement 8:12.06.) Cefepime generally is well tolerated. Most adverse effects are transient and mild to moderate in severity, but have been severe enough to require discontinuance of the drug in up to 3% of patients. Headache, rash, diarrhea, nausea, and vomiting have been reported in up to 2% and local reactions, including phlebitis, pain and/or inflammation, and rash, have been reported in up to 3% of patients receiving cefepime in a dosage of 0.5–2 g every 12 hours. In patients receiving cefepime in a dosage of 2 g every 8 hours, rash occurred in 4%, diarrhea in 3%, nausea in 2%, and vomiting, headache, pruritus, or fever in 1% of patients. Neutropenia has been reported rarely in patients receiving cefepime.

• Precautions and Contraindications

Cefepime shares the toxic potentials of other cephalosporins, and the usual cautions, precautions, and contraindications associated with cephalosporin therapy should be observed.

Sensitivity Reactions

Prior to initiation of cefepime therapy, careful inquiry should be made concerning previous hypersensitivity reactions to cefepime, cephalosporins, penicillins, or other drugs. There is clinical and laboratory evidence of partial cross-allergenicity among cephalosporins and other β-lactam antibiotics, including penicillins and cephamycins.

Cefepime is contraindicated in patients who are hypersensitive to the drug or other cephalosporins and should be used with caution in patients with a history of hypersensitivity to penicillins. Use of cephalosporins generally should be avoided in patients who have had an immediate-type (anaphylactic) hypersensitivity reaction to penicillins.

The manufacturers of the commercially available Duplex® drug delivery system containing cefepime and dextrose injection and the commercially available frozen premixed cefepime injection in dextrose state that solutions containing dextrose may be contraindicated in patients with known allergy or hypersensitivity to corn or corn products.

Anaphylaxis, including anaphylactic shock, has been reported in a few patients receiving cefepime.

If a hypersensitivity reaction occurs during cefepime therapy, the drug should be discontinued and the patient treated with appropriate therapy (e.g., epinephrine, corticosteroids, and maintenance of an adequate airway and oxygen) as indicated.

Neurotoxicity

Serious adverse events, including life-threatening or fatal encephalopathy (disturbance of consciousness including confusion, hallucinations, stupor, and coma), myoclonus, and seizures, have been reported in patients receiving cefepime during postmarketing experience. Nonconvulsive status epilepticus, characterized by alteration of consciousness without convulsions that is associated with continuous epileptiform EEG activity, also has been reported.

Most cases of cefepime-associated neurotoxicity have occurred in patients with renal impairment who received a cefepime dosage that exceeded the recommended dosage for such patients. However, some cases of neurotoxicity occurred in patients who received a dosage appropriately adjusted for renal impairment or in patients with normal renal function. In most reported cases, symptoms of neurotoxicity were reversible and resolved after discontinuance of cefepime and/or after hemodialysis.

If neurotoxicity associated with cefepime therapy occurs, consideration should be given to discontinuing the drug or making appropriate dosage adjustments based on the patient's renal function. (See Dosage and Administration: Dosage in Renal and Hepatic Impairment.)

Patients should be advised that neurologic adverse events can occur and to immediately contact a clinician if any neurologic signs and symptoms, including encephalopathy (disturbance of consciousness including confusion, hallucinations, stupor, coma), myoclonus, seizures, or nonconvulsive status epilepticus, occur since immediate treatment, dosage adjustment, or discontinuance of cefepime therapy is required.

Increased Mortality

In November 2007, FDA announced that a safety review of cefepime was initiated after a published meta-analysis described a higher risk of all-cause mortality in patients treated with cefepime compared with patients treated with comparator β-lactams. The published meta-analysis looked at all-cause mortality data from 57 randomized controlled trials that compared cefepime with other β-lactams for various indications and found a risk ratio of 1.26 in those who received cefepime. FDA began working with Bristol-Myers Squibb to further evaluate the findings presented in the published meta-analysis and additional safety data.

On June 17, 2009, FDA announced that, although the safety review is ongoing, it has determined that cefepime remains an appropriate therapy for its approved indications based on results of FDA's additional meta-analyses. FDA performed meta-analyses based on both trial- and patient-level data derived from all available cefepime comparative clinical trials. FDA's trial-level meta-analysis included data from 88 clinical trials (total of 9467 cefepime-treated patients and 8288 comparator-treated patients) and found no statistically significant differences in mortality between cefepime and the comparator drugs. Results of the trial-level meta-analysis indicated that all-cause mortality rates 30 days after treatment were 6.21% for cefepime-treated patients and 6% for comparator-treated patients. FDA's patient-level meta-analysis included data from 35 clinical trials and results indicated that all-cause mortality rates 30 days after treatment were 5.63% for cefepime-treated patients and 5.68% for comparator-treated patients. In addition, in a trial-level meta-analysis of 24 febrile neutropenia trials, there was no statistically significant increase in mortality in cefepime-treated patients compared with comparator-treated patients. A review of deaths reported in 7 of these febrile neutropenia trials indicated that most patients appeared to have died from their underlying malignancies and/or comorbid conditions.

Selection and Use of Anti-infectives

To reduce development of drug-resistant bacteria and maintain effectiveness of cefepime and other antibacterials, the drug should be used only for the treatment or prevention of infections proven or strongly suspected to be caused by susceptible bacteria. When selecting or modifying anti-infective therapy, use results of culture and in vitro susceptibility testing. In the absence of such data, consider local epidemiology and susceptibility patterns when selecting anti-infectives for empiric therapy.

Patients should be advised that antibacterials (including cefepime) should only be used to treat bacterial infections and not used to treat viral infections (e.g., the common cold). Patients also should be advised about the importance of completing the full course of therapy, even if feeling better after a few days, and that skipping doses or not completing therapy may decrease effectiveness and increase the likelihood that bacteria will develop resistance and will not be treatable with cefepime or other antibacterials in the future.

Superinfection/Clostridium difficile-associated Diarrhea and Colitis

As with other anti-infectives, prolonged cefepime therapy may result in overgrowth of nonsusceptible organisms. Careful observation of the patient is essential. If superinfection occurs, appropriate therapy should be initiated.

Treatment with anti-infectives alters the normal colon flora and may permit overgrowth of *Clostridium difficile*. *C. difficile* infection (CDI) and *C. difficile*-associated diarrhea and colitis (CDAD; also known as antibiotic-associated diarrhea and colitis or pseudomembranous colitis) have been reported with nearly all anti-infectives, including cefepime, and may range in severity from mild diarrhea to fatal colitis. *C. difficile* produces toxins A and B, which contribute to the development of CDAD; hypertoxin-producing strains of *C. difficile* are associated with increased morbidity and mortality since these infections may be refractory to anti-infective therapy and may require colectomy.

CDAD should be considered in the differential diagnosis of patients who develop diarrhea during or after anti-infective therapy. Careful medical history is necessary since CDAD has been reported to occur as late as 2 months or longer after anti-infective therapy is discontinued.

If CDAD is suspected or confirmed, anti-infective therapy not directed against *C. difficile* should be discontinued whenever possible. Patients should be managed with appropriate supportive therapy (e.g., fluid and electrolyte management, protein supplementation), anti-infective therapy directed against *C. difficile* (e.g., metronidazole, vancomycin), and surgical evaluation as clinically needed.

Patients should be advised that diarrhea is a common problem caused by anti-infectives and usually resolves when the drug is discontinued; however, they should contact a clinician if severe watery or bloody diarrhea develops.

Other Precautions and Contraindications

Cefepime should be used with caution in patients with a history of GI disease, particularly colitis. (See Superinfection/Clostridium difficile-associated Diarrhea and Colitis under Cautions: Precautions and Contraindications.)

Commercially available cefepime preparations contain L-arginine to adjust pH. (See Chemistry and Stability: Chemistry.) At concentrations 33 times higher than the amount provided by the maximum recommended human cefepime dosage, arginine has been shown to alter glucose metabolism and transiently increase serum potassium concentrations. The effect of lower arginine concentrations is not known.

Like other dextrose-containing solutions, the commercially available Duplex® drug delivery system containing cefepime and 5% dextrose injection should be used with caution in patients with overt or known subclinical diabetes mellitus or in patients with carbohydrate intolerance for any reason.

High or prolonged serum cefepime concentrations can occur if usual dosage is used in patients with renal impairment or other conditions that may compromise renal function. Serious adverse events, including life-threatening or fatal encephalopathy, may occur if inappropriate cefepime dosage is used in patients with impaired renal function. (See Neurotoxicity under Cautions: Precautions and Contraindications.) The maintenance dosage of cefepime should be decreased whenever the drug is used in patients with renal impairment (i.e., creatinine clearance 60 mL/minute or less) and continued dosage should be determined by the degree of renal impairment, severity of the infection, and susceptibility of the causative organisms. (See Dosage and Administration: Dosage in Renal and Hepatic Impairment.)

For a more complete discussion of these and other precautions associated with the use of cefepime, see Cautions: Precautions and Contraindications in the Cephalosporins General Statement 8:12.06.

● Pediatric Precautions

Safety and efficacy of cefepime have not been established in neonates or infants younger than 2 months of age.

Safety and efficacy of cefepime have been established for use in pediatric patients 2 months to 16 years of age for the treatment of uncomplicated and complicated urinary tract infections (including pyelonephritis), uncomplicated skin and skin structure infections, and pneumonia and for empiric therapy for febrile neutropenic patients. Use of cefepime in this age group is supported by evidence from adequate and well-controlled studies evaluating the drug in adults and additional pharmacokinetic and safety data from pediatric studies.

Adverse effects reported when cefepime was used in pediatric patients 2 months to 16 years of age have been similar to those reported in adults.

The manufacturers caution that cefepime should not be used in pediatric patients of any age for the treatment of serious infections that are suspected or known to be caused by *Haemophilus influenzae* type b (Hib) and states that pediatric patients in whom meningeal seeding from a distant infection site or in whom meningitis is suspected or documented should receive an alternative anti-infective with demonstrated clinical efficacy in this setting.

Although safety and efficacy for the treatment of meningitis† have not been established, cefepime has been used effectively in a limited number of children 2 months to 15 years of age for the treatment of meningitis caused by susceptible bacteria. (See Uses: Meningitis and Other CNS Infections.) In one study in pediatric patients with meningitis, adverse effects were reported in 18% of patients receiving cefepime and included diarrhea, macular rash, candidal thrush, and eosinophilia.

The manufacturers state that the commercially available Duplex® drug delivery system containing cefepime and the commercially available frozen premixed cefepime injection should be used in pediatric patients *only* if the entire 1- or 2-g dose in the container is required.

● Geriatric Precautions

Studies evaluating safety and efficacy of cefepime indicate that there are no age-related differences when the drug is used in geriatric patients or in younger adults.

Cefepime is substantially eliminated by kidneys, and the risk of toxicity may be greater in those with impaired renal function. Serious adverse effects (e.g., life-threatening or fatal encephalopathy, myoclonus, or seizures) have occurred in geriatric patients with renal impairment who received cefepime dosages that were not adjusted based on the degree of renal impairment.

Whenever cefepime is used in geriatric patients, select dosage with caution and monitor renal function because of age-related decreases in renal function. (See Dosage and Administration: Dosage in Renal and Hepatic Impairment.)

● Mutagenicity and Carcinogenicity

In vivo and in vitro studies evaluating cefepime have not shown evidence of mutagenicity. Long-term animal studies have not been performed to evaluate the carcinogenic potential of the drug.

● Pregnancy, Fertility, and Lactation

Pregnancy

Reproduction studies in rats, rabbits, or mice using cefepime dosages approximately 1.6 times or 0.3 times, or equal to the recommended maximum human dosage (calculated on a mg/m^2 basis), respectively, have not revealed evidence of teratogenicity or embryotoxicity. There are no adequate and controlled studies using cefepime in pregnant women or during labor and delivery, and the drug should be used during pregnancy only when clearly needed.

Fertility

Studies in rats using subcutaneous cefepime dosages 1.6 times the recommended maximum human dosage (calculated on a mg/m^2 basis) have not revealed evidence of impaired fertility.

Lactation

Cefepime is distributed into milk in low concentrations following parenteral administration, and the drug should be used with caution in nursing women.

SPECTRUM

Based on its spectrum of activity and decreased susceptibility to certain β-lactamases, cefepime is classified as a fourth generation cephalosporin. For information on the classification of cephalosporins and closely related β-lactam antibiotics based on spectra of activity, see Spectrum in the Cephalosporins General Statement 8:12.06.

Fourth generation cephalosporins (e.g., cefepime) usually have a spectrum of activity against gram-negative bacteria that includes organisms susceptible to most third generation cephalosporins; however, the drugs also are active against some gram-negative bacteria, including *Pseudomonas aeruginosa* and certain Enterobacteriaceae, that generally are resistant to most third generation cephalosporins. The activity of cefepime against *Ps. aeruginosa* is similar to that of ceftazidime. Cefepime is more active in vitro against some gram-positive bacteria (e.g., staphylococci) than some third generation cephalosporins (e.g., ceftazidime).

● In Vitro Susceptibility Testing

Strains of staphylococci resistant to penicillinase-resistant penicillins (methicillin-resistant [oxacillin-resistant] staphylococci) should be considered resistant to cefepime, although results of in vitro susceptibility tests may indicate that the organisms are susceptible to the drug.

For information on interpreting results of in vitro susceptibility testing (disk susceptibility tests, dilution susceptibility tests) when cefepime susceptibility testing is performed according to the standards of the Clinical and Laboratory Standards Institute (CLSI; formerly National Committee for Clinical Laboratory Standards [NCCLS]), see Spectrum: In Vitro Susceptibility Testing, in the Cephalosporins General Statement 8:12.06.

PHARMACOKINETICS

Studies in adults indicate that cefepime exhibits linear dose-dependent pharmacokinetics over the dosage range of 250 mg to 2 g, and there is no evidence of accumulation following multiple doses in healthy adults with normal renal function receiving usual parenteral dosages of the drug. While there is no evidence of accumulation of cefepime in pediatric patients 2 months to 11 years of age when the drug is given in a dosage of 50 mg/kg every 12 hours, steady-state peak plasma concentration, area under the concentration-time curve (AUC), and plasma half-life are increased about 15% when the drug is given in a dosage of 50 mg/kg every 8 hours.

There is no evidence of gender-related differences in the pharmacokinetics of cefepime, and differences in the pharmacokinetics of the drug in geriatric individuals appear to be related to changes in renal function rather than age.

Studies in adults with impaired renal function indicate that the pharmacokinetics of cefepime are affected by the degree of renal impairment and that total body clearance of the drug decreases in proportion to decreases in creatinine clearance. The pharmacokinetics of cefepime do not appear to be affected by hepatic impairment.

● Absorption

Cefepime is almost completely absorbed following IM administration. In healthy adult males who received single 500-mg, 1-g, or 2-g IM doses of cefepime, peak plasma concentrations of the drug were attained within 1.4–1.6 hours and averaged 13.9, 29.6, or 57.5 mcg/mL, respectively; plasma concentrations averaged 1.9, 4.5, or 8.7 mcg/mL, respectively, 8 hours after the dose. In children 2 months to 16 years of age who received a single 50-mg/kg dose IM, plasma cefepime concentrations averaged 76, 75.2, 64, and 4.8 mcg/mL at 0.5, 0.75, 1, and 8 hours, respectively, after the dose. The absolute bioavailability of cefepime after a single 50-mg/kg IM dose in pediatric patients has been reported to be 82.3%.

Following IV infusion over 30 minutes of a single 500-mg, 1-g, or 2-g dose of cefepime in healthy adult males, peak plasma concentrations of the drug average 31.6–39.1, 65.9–81.7, or 126–163.9 mcg/mL; plasma concentrations were still detectable 8 hours after the dose and averaged 1.4, 2.4, and 3.9 mcg/mL, respectively, in one study.

In pediatric patients 2 months to 15 years of age with bacterial meningitis who received cefepime dosages of 50 mg/kg every 8 hours given by IV infusion over 15–20 minutes, plasma concentrations averaged 67.1, 44.1, 23.9, 11.7, and 4.9 mcg/mL at 0.5, 1, 2, 4, and 8 hours, respectively, after the third dose. The manufacturers state that IV administration of a single 50-mg/kg dose of cefepime in pediatric patients results in cefepime exposure similar to that reported in adults following IV administration of a single 2-g dose of the drug.

● Distribution

The volume of distribution of cefepime at steady state ranges from 13–22 L in healthy adults, and averages 0.3 L/kg in pediatric patients 2 months to 11 years of age.

Following parenteral administration, cefepime is widely distributed into tissues and fluids, including blister fluid, bronchial mucosa, sputum, bile, peritoneal fluid, appendix, gallbladder, and prostate. In adults with acute cholecystitis who received 2 g of cefepime IV every 12 hours, concentrations of the drug in peritoneal fluid, bile, and gallbladder tissue in samples obtained 2–15 hours after a dose averaged 5.66 mcg/mL, 15.51 mcg/mL, and 5.35 mcg/g, respectively; concurrent plasma concentrations averaged 7.6 mcg/mL.

Cefepime is distributed into CSF following IV administration in adult or pediatric patients. In a study in adults who received cefepime in a dosage of 2 g every 12 hours given by IV infusion over 30 minutes, CSF concentrations ranged from 0.34–11.8 mcg/mL and minimum CSF concentrations were 5–58% of minimum serum concentrations. In children 2 months to 15 years of age who received 50-mg/kg doses of cefepime every 8 hours given by IV infusion over 15–20 minutes, CSF concentrations of the drug were 5.7, 4.3, 3.6, 4.2, and 3.3 mcg/mL at 0.5, 1, 2, 4, and 8 hours, respectively, after the third dose. There is evidence from a limited study in neonates with meningitis that cefepime CSF concentrations in premature neonates are higher than those reported in full-term neonates.

Cefepime is distributed into human milk. Following a single 1-g dose of cefepime given by IV infusion over 1 hour, peak concentrations of the drug in milk averaged 1.2 mcg/mL.

Cefepime is approximately 20% bound to serum proteins; binding is independent of drug concentrations.

• Elimination

In healthy adults with normal renal function, the plasma half-life of cefepime averages 2–2.3 hours and total body clearance averages 120 mL/minute. In pediatric patients, the plasma half-life of cefepime averages 1.9 hours in those 2 months up to 6 months of age and 1.5–1.7 hours in those 6 months to 16 years of age. Total body clearance reportedly averages 3.3 mL/minute per kg in pediatric patients 2 months to 11 years of age. Limited data from neonates younger than 2 months of age indicate that the mean plasma half-life of cefepime is 4.9 hours in this age group.

The plasma half-life of cefepime is prolonged in patients with renal impairment and averages 4.9, 10.5, and 13.5 hours in adults with creatinine clearances of 31–60, 11–30, or less than 10 mL/minute, respectively. Results of a single-dose study in a limited number of patients with impaired hepatic function indicate that the pharmacokinetics of cefepime are not affected by hepatic impairment.

Cefepime is partially metabolized in vivo to N-methylpyrrolidine (NMP) which is rapidly converted to the N-oxide (NMP-N-oxide). The drug is eliminated principally unchanged in urine by glomerular filtration. In adults with normal renal function, 80–82% of a single dose of cefepime is excreted unchanged in urine; less than 1% of the dose is eliminated as NMP, 6.8% as NMP-N-oxide, and 2.5% as an epimer of cefepime. In adults with normal renal function who received single 500-mg, 1-g, or 2-g IV doses of cefepime, urine concentrations of the drug in samples obtained within 4 hours after the dose averaged 292, 926, or 3120 mcg/mL, respectively. In pediatric patients 2 months to 11 years of age who received a single 50-mg/kg IV dose of cefepime, 60% of the dose was excreted unchanged in urine and the average renal clearance was 2 mL/minute per kg.

Cefepime is removed by hemodialysis and peritoneal dialysis. The amount of cefepime removed during hemodialysis depends on several factors (e.g., type of coil used, dialysis flow-rate); however, a 3- to 5-hour period of hemodialysis removes into the dialysate approximately 20–68% of a dose of the drug. In a study in patients with end-stage renal failure undergoing continuous ambulatory peritoneal dialysis (CAPD) who received a single 1- or 2-g IV dose of cefepime given over 30 minutes, approximately 25% of the dose was removed into the peritoneal dialysate over 72 hours; the plasma half-life of the drug in these patients ranged from 15.4–22.6 hours.

CHEMISTRY AND STABILITY

• Chemistry

Cefepime is a semisynthetic cephalosporin antibiotic. The drug is a parenteral zwitterionic aminothiazolyl cephalosporin. Cefepime is structurally similar to parenteral third generation cephalosporins that contain an aminothiazolyl side chain at position 7 of the cephalosporin nucleus (e.g., cefotaxime, ceftazidime, ceftriaxone). The aminothiazolyl side chain enhances antibacterial activity, particularly against Enterobacteriaceae, and generally results in enhanced stability against β-lactamases. However, cefepime contains an alkoxyimino group in the side chain rather than the methoxyimino group contained in many aminothiazolyl cephalosporins. The alkoxyimino group results in increased activity against staphylococci. In addition, cefepime contains a quaternary N-methylpyrrolidine (NMP) group at the 3-position, resulting in a zwitterion that enhances stability against certain β-lactamases and penetration through the outer membrane of gram-negative bacteria.

Cefepime is commercially available for parenteral use as cefepime hydrochloride, which is monohydrated; potency of cefepime hydrochloride is expressed in terms of cefepime, calculated on the anhydrous basis. Cefepime hydrochloride occurs as a white to pale yellow powder and contains the equivalent of not less than 825 mcg and not more than 911 mcg of cefepime per mg, calculated on the anhydrous basis. The drug is highly soluble in water and has pK$_a$s of 1.5–1.6 and 3.1–3.2.

Cefepime hydrochloride powder for IM injection or IV infusion that is commercially available in vials contains a mixture of the drug and L-arginine; the powder for injection contains 707 mg of L-arginine per g of cefepime. When vials containing 500 mg, 1 g, or 2 g of cefepime are reconstituted as directed, the resultant cefepime hydrochloride solutions have a pH of 4–6 and range in color from pale yellow to amber.

When the commercially available Duplex® delivery system that contains 1 or 2 g of cefepime powder (with approximately 725 mg of L-arginine per g of cefepime) and 50 mL of 5% dextrose injection in separate chambers is reconstituted (activated) according to the manufacturer's directions, the resultant solution has a pH of 4–6 and an osmolality of approximately 431 or 577 mOsm/kg, respectively. The reconstituted solution may range in color from colorless to amber.

Commercially available frozen premixed injections of cefepime hydrochloride in dextrose are sterile, nonpyrogenic, iso-osmotic solutions of the drug provided in a plastic container fabricated from specially formulated multilayered plastic PL 2040 (Galaxy®). The 1- or 2-g frozen injections of cefepime contain 1.03 or 2.06 g of dextrose, respectively, to adjust osmolality. The 1- or 2-g frozen injections also contain 725 mg or 1.45 g of L-arginine, respectively, and may contain hydrochloric acid to adjust pH to 4–6. These premixed injections may range in color from colorless to amber.

• Stability

Like some other cephalosporins, cefepime hydrochloride powder for injection and solutions of the drug tend to darken, depending on storage conditions; however, such discoloration does not indicate loss of potency.

Vials containing cefepime hydrochloride powder for IM injection or IV infusion should be stored at 20–25°C and protected from light. Following reconstitution and dilution in 0.9% sodium chloride, 5 or 10% dextrose, (1/6) M sodium lactate, 5% dextrose and 0.9% sodium chloride, lactated Ringer's and 5% dextrose, Normosol®-R, or Normosol®-M in 5% dextrose injection, cefepime solutions for IV infusion containing 1–40 mg/mL are stable for 24 hours when stored at a room temperature of 20–25°C or for 7 days when refrigerated at 2–8°C.

Following reconstitution with sterile water for injection, 0.9% sodium chloride, 5% dextrose, 0.5 or 1% lidocaine hydrochloride, sterile bacteriostatic water for injection with parabens or benzyl alcohol, cefepime solutions for IM injection containing 280 mg/mL are stable for 24 hours when stored at a room temperature of 20–25°C or for 7 days when refrigerated at 2–8°C.

Following reconstitution of ADD-Vantage® vials containing 1 or 2 g of cefepime according to the manufacturer's directions, IV solutions containing 10–40 mg/mL in 5% dextrose injection or 0.9% sodium chloride injection are stable for 24 hours at 20–25°C or 7 days at 2–8°C.

The commercially available Duplex® delivery system that contains 1 or 2 g of cefepime and 50 mL of 5% dextrose injection in separate chambers should be stored at 20–25°C, but may be exposed to temperatures ranging from 15–30°C. Following reconstitution (activation), these IV solutions must be used within 12 hours if stored at room temperature or within 5 days if stored in a refrigerator and should not be frozen.

The commercially available frozen premixed cefepime hydrochloride injection in dextrose should be stored at –20°C or lower. The frozen injections should be thawed at room temperature (25°C) or under refrigeration (5°C) and, once thawed, should not be refrozen. Thawed solutions of the commercially available frozen injections are stable for 24 hours at room temperature (25°C) or 7 days under refrigeration (5°C). The commercially available frozen injections of the drug are provided in plastic containers fabricated from specially formulated multilayered plastic PL 2040 (Galaxy®). Solutions in contact with PL 2040 can leach out some of its chemical components in very small amounts within the expiration period of the injection; however, safety of the plastic has been confirmed in tests in animals according to USP biological tests for plastic containers as well as by tissue culture toxicity studies.

For further information on chemistry, mechanism of action, spectrum, resistance, uses, cautions, acute toxicity, drug interactions, or laboratory test interferences of cefepime, see the Cephalosporins General Statement 8:12.06.

PREPARATIONS

Excipients in commercially available drug preparations may have clinically important effects in some individuals; consult specific product labeling for details.

Cefepime Hydrochloride

Parenteral

For injection	500 mg (of anhydrous cefepime)*	Cefepime Hydrochloride for Injection Maxipime®, Hospira
	1 g (of anhydrous cefepime)*	Cefepime Hydrochloride for Injection Maxipime®, Hospira
	2 g (of anhydrous cefepime)*	Cefepime Hydrochloride for Injection Maxipime®, Hospira
For injection, for IV infusion	1 g (of anhydrous cefepime)*	Cefepime Hydrochloride for Injection (available in dual-chambered Duplex® drug delivery system with 5% dextrose injection), B Braun Maxipime® ADD-Vantage®, Hospira
	2 g (of anhydrous cefepime)*	Cefepime Hydrochloride for Injection (available in dual-chambered Duplex® drug delivery system with 5% dextrose injection), B Braun Maxipime® ADD-Vantage®, Hospira

* available from one or more manufacturer, distributor, and/or repackager by generic (nonproprietary) name

Cefepime Hydrochloride in Dextrose

Parenteral

Injection (frozen), for IV infusion	20 mg (of cefepime) per mL (1 g) in 2% Dextrose*	Cefepime Hydrochloride Iso-osmotic in Dextrose Injection (Galaxy® [Baxter])
	20 mg (of cefepime) per mL (2 g) in 2% Dextrose*	Cefepime Hydrochloride Iso-osmotic in Dextrose Injection (Galaxy® [Baxter])

* available from one or more manufacturer, distributor, and/or repackager by generic (nonproprietary) name

† Use is not currently included in the labeling approved by the US Food and Drug Administration.

Selected Revisions August 29, 2013, © Copyright, November 1, 1996, American Society of Health-System Pharmacists, Inc.

Ceftaroline Fosamil

8:12.06.20 • FIFTH GENERATION CEPHALOSPORINS

■ Ceftaroline is a semisynthetic, fifth generation cephalosporin antibiotic.

USES

● Community-acquired Pneumonia

Ceftaroline fosamil is used for the treatment of community-acquired bacterial pneumonia (CABP, CAP) caused by susceptible *Streptococcus pneumoniae* (including cases with concurrent bacteremia), *Staphylococcus aureus* (methicillin-susceptible [oxacillin-susceptible] strains only), *Haemophilus influenzae, Klebsiella pneumoniae, K. oxytoca,* or *Escherichia coli* in adults and pediatric patients 2 months of age and older.

Initial treatment of CAP generally involves use of an empiric anti-infective regimen based on the most likely pathogens and local susceptibility patterns; treatment may then be changed (if possible) to provide a more specific regimen (pathogen-directed therapy) based on results of in vitro culture and susceptibility testing. The most appropriate empiric regimen varies depending on the severity of illness at the time of presentation, whether outpatient treatment or hospitalization in or out of an intensive care unit (ICU) is indicated, and the presence or absence of cardiopulmonary disease and other modifying factors that increase the risk of certain pathogens (e.g., methicillin-resistant *S. aureus* [MRSA; also known as oxacillin-resistant *S. aureus* or ORSA], penicillin-resistant *S. pneumoniae*, multidrug-resistant *S. pneumoniae* [MDRSP], enteric gram-negative bacilli, *Pseudomonas aeruginosa*).

For information regarding the treatment of CAP, including infections caused by MRSA, the current clinical practice guidelines from the Infectious Diseases Society of America (IDSA) available at http://www.idsociety.org should be consulted.

Clinical Experience

Efficacy of ceftaroline fosamil for the treatment of CAP in adults is based on results of 2 randomized, double-blind, active-controlled, phase 3 noninferiority trials in 1231 adults with CAP requiring hospitalization (Pneumonia Outcome Research Team [PORT] risk class III or IV and *not* admitted to an intensive care unit). Patients in each trial (Focus 1 and Focus 2) were randomized to receive either ceftaroline fosamil (600 mg given by IV infusion over 1 hour every 12 hours) or ceftriaxone (1 g given by IV infusion over 30 minutes every 24 hours); patients in the first trial also received oral clarithromycin on the initial day of treatment (500 mg every 12 hours for 2 doses). Treatment duration was 5–7 days (maximum 7 days); a switch to oral therapy was not allowed. Patients with CAP known or suspected to be caused by methicillin-resistant *S. aureus* (MRSA; also known as oxacillin-resistant *S. aureus* or ORSA) or caused by an atypical pathogen (e.g., *Chlamydophila pneumoniae, Mycoplasma pneumoniae, Legionella*) alone were excluded from the trials.

In the first trial (Focus 1), clinical cure rates at the test-of-cure visit (8–15 days after treatment ended) in the clinically evaluable population were similar for ceftaroline- and ceftriaxone-treated patients (87 and 78%, respectively). Similarly, clinical cure rates in the second trial (Focus 2) were 82% with ceftaroline and 77% with ceftriaxone. When results from both adult trials were combined, the overall clinical cure rate in the clinically evaluable population was similar in patients treated with ceftaroline fosamil (84%) compared with those receiving ceftriaxone (78%). In addition, when results from both trials were pooled, the 30-day all-cause mortality rate did not differ between treatment groups.

When results from both adult trials were combined and stratified according to causative organism, the clinical cure rates at the test-of-cure visit in the microbiologically evaluable population that received ceftaroline fosamil were 86% for CAP caused by *S. pneumonia,* 72% for methicillin-susceptible *S. aureus,* 83% for *H. influenzae,* 100% for *K. pneumoniae,* 83% for *K. oxytoca,* and 83% for *E. coli.*

● Skin and Skin Structure Infections

Ceftaroline fosamil is used for the treatment of acute bacterial skin and skin structure infections (ABSSSI) caused by susceptible *S. aureus* (including MRSA), *S. pyogenes* (group A β-hemolytic streptococci, GAS), *S. agalactiae* (group B streptococci, GBS), *E. coli, K. pneumoniae,* or *K. oxytoca* in adults and children 2 months of age and older.

Ceftaroline fosamil is one of several anti-infectives that have been recommended for treatment of skin and skin structure infections caused by MRSA, including empiric treatment of surgical site infections in patients at high risk for MRSA (e.g., nasal colonization, prior MRSA infection, recent hospitalization, recent anti-infective therapy).

For information regarding the treatment of skin and skin structure infections, including infections caused by MRSA, the current IDSA clinical practice guidelines available at http://www.idsociety.org should be consulted.

Clinical Experience

Efficacy of ceftaroline fosamil for the treatment of skin and skin structure infections in adults is based on the results of 2 randomized, double-blind, active-controlled trials in 1396 adults with complicated skin and skin structure infections (e.g., cellulitis, major abscess, infected wound/ulcer/burn). Patients in each trial (Canvas 1 and Canvas 2) were randomized to receive either ceftaroline fosamil with placebo (600 mg of ceftaroline fosamil given by IV infusion over 1 hour followed by placebo given by IV infusion over 1 hour every 12 hours) or a 2-drug regimen of vancomycin and aztreonam (1 g of vancomycin given by IV infusion over 1 hour followed by 1 g of aztreonam given by IV infusion over 1 hour every 12 hours). Treatment duration was 5–14 days (mean approximately 8 days); a switch to oral therapy was not allowed.

In the first trial (Canvas 1), clinical cure rates at the test-of-cure visit in the clinically evaluable population for ceftaroline-treated patients were similar to clinical cure rates for vancomycin- and aztreonam-treated patients (91 and 93%, respectively). Similarly, the clinical cure rate in the second trial (Canvas 2) was 92% in both treatment groups. When results from both adult trials were combined, the overall clinical cure rate in the clinically evaluable population was similar in those treated with ceftaroline fosamil (92%) compared with those treated with vancomycin and aztreonam (93%). Of the 693 patients in the modified intent-to-treat population from both trials, 20 patients had *S. aureus* bacteremia at baseline (11 with methicillin-susceptible strains, 9 with MRSA); 65% of these patients were clinical responders at study day 3 and 90% were considered clinical success at the test-of-cure visit (8–15 days after treatment ended).

When results from both adult trials were combined and stratified according to causative organism, the clinical cure rates in the microbiologically evaluable population that received ceftaroline fosamil were 93% for methicillin-susceptible *S. aureus,* 93% for MRSA, 100% for *S. pyogenes,* 96% for *S. agalactiae,* 95% for *E. coli,* 94% for *K. pneumoniae,* and 83% for *K. oxytoca.*

For additional information on the role of parenteral cephalosporins in the treatment of these and other infections, see Uses in the Cephalosporins General Statement 8:12.06.

DOSAGE AND ADMINISTRATION

● Administration

Ceftaroline fosamil is administered by IV infusion.

Ceftaroline fosamil solutions should not be admixed with or added to solutions containing other drugs.

Reconstitution and Dilution

Ceftaroline fosamil must be reconstituted and further diluted prior to IV infusion. Strict aseptic technique must be observed when preparing IV solutions of the drug.

Single-use vials labeled as containing 400 or 600 mg of ceftaroline fosamil should be reconstituted by adding 20 mL of sterile water for injection, 0.9% sodium chloride injection, 5% dextrose injection, or lactated Ringer's injection, to provide a solution containing approximately 20 or 30 mg/mL, respectively. The vial should be gently mixed; reconstitution should be complete in less than 2 minutes.

Prior to IV administration, the appropriate dose of reconstituted solution must be further diluted in 50–250 mL of an appropriate infusion solution. The same diluent should be used for both reconstitution and further dilution unless the drug was reconstituted with sterile water, in which case the dose should be further diluted using any compatible IV solution (e.g., 0.45 or 0.9% sodium chloride injection, 2.5 or 5% dextrose injection, lactated Ringer's injection).

To prepare a 600-mg dose of ceftaroline fosamil in a 50-mL infusion bag for administration in adults, 20 mL of the diluent should be removed from the infusion bag prior to injecting the entire reconstituted contents of a 600-mg vial of the drug; the concentration of the final infusion solution is approximately 12 mg/mL.

To prepare a 400-mg dose of ceftaroline fosamil in a 50-mL infusion bag for administration in adults or pediatric patients 2 months of age or older weighing more than 33 kg, 20 mL of the diluent should be removed from the infusion bag prior to injecting the entire reconstituted contents of a 400-mg vial of the drug; the concentration of the final infusion solution is approximately 8 mg/mL.

To prepare a dose in a 50-mL infusion bag for administration in pediatric patients 2 months of age or older weighing 33 kg or less, the amount of diluent to be removed from the infusion bag *and* the amount of reconstituted solution of drug to be withdrawn from the vial and added to the diluent vary depending on the age and weight of the child. The concentration of the final infusion solution for these pediatric patients should not exceed 12 mg/mL.

Reconstituted and diluted ceftaroline fosamil solutions should appear clear and light to dark yellow, depending on the concentration and storage conditions. Final ceftaroline fosamil solutions in the IV infusion bag should be used within 6 hours when stored at room temperature or within 24 hours when stored in the refrigerator at 2–8°C. (See Chemistry and Stability: Stability.)

Rate of Administration

IV infusions of ceftaroline fosamil should be given over 5–60 minutes.

● Dosage

Ceftaroline fosamil is commercially available as ceftaroline fosamil monoacetate monohydrate; dosage is expressed in terms of anhydrous ceftaroline fosamil.

Adult Dosage

Community-acquired Pneumonia

The recommended dosage of ceftaroline fosamil for the treatment of community-acquired bacterial pneumonia (CABP, CAP) in adults is 600 mg every 12 hours for 5–7 days.

The duration of therapy should be guided by the severity and site of infection and the patient's clinical and bacteriologic progress.

Skin and Skin Structure Infections

The recommended dosage of ceftaroline fosamil for the treatment of acute bacterial skin and skin structure infections (ABSSSI) in adults is 600 mg every 12 hours for 5–14 days.

The duration of therapy should be guided by the severity and site of infection and the patient's clinical and bacteriologic progress.

Pediatric Dosage

Community-acquired Pneumonia

The recommended dosage of ceftaroline fosamil for the treatment of community-acquired bacterial pneumonia in pediatric patients 2 months to less than 2 years of age is 8 mg/kg every 8 hours. Pediatric patients 2 years to less than 18 years of age weighing 33 kg or less should receive 12 mg/kg every 8 hours and those 2 years to less than 18 years of age weighing more than 33 kg should receive 400 mg every 8 hours or 600 mg every 12 hours.

The manufacturer recommends a treatment duration of 5–14 days in pediatric patients; the duration of therapy should be guided by the severity and site of infection and the patient's clinical and bacteriologic progress.

Skin and Skin Structure Infections

The recommended dosage of ceftaroline fosamil for the treatment of acute bacterial skin and skin structure infections in pediatric patients 2 months to less than 2 years of age is 8 mg/kg every 8 hours. Pediatric patients 2 years to less than 18 years of age weighing 33 kg or less should receive 12 mg/kg every 8 hours and those 2 years to less than 18 years of age weighing more than 33 kg should receive 400 mg every 8 hours or 600 mg every 12 hours.

The manufacturer recommends a treatment duration of 5–14 days in pediatric patients; the duration of therapy should be guided by the severity and site of infection and the patient's clinical and bacteriologic progress.

● Dosage in Renal and Hepatic Impairment

Dosage of ceftaroline fosamil must be modified according to the degree of renal impairment in adults with creatinine clearances of 50 mL/minute or less, including those undergoing hemodialysis. (See Table 1.)

TABLE 1. Ceftaroline Fosamil Dosage for Adults with Renal Impairment

Estimated Creatinine Clearance (mL/minute)	Recommended Dosage
31–50	400 mg every 12 hours
15–30	300 mg every 12 hours
<15 or receiving hemodialysis	200 mg every 12 hours; on hemodialysis days, give dose after hemodialysis

Dosage adjustments are not necessary if ceftaroline fosamil is used in pediatric patients with creatinine clearances greater than 50 mL/minute per 1.73 m². Data are insufficient to make dosage recommendations for pediatric patients with creatinine clearances less than 50 mL/minute per 1.73 m².

Pharmacokinetics of ceftaroline fosamil have not been studied in patients with impaired hepatic function, but hepatic impairment is not expected to have a clinically important effect on systemic clearance of the drug.

● Dosage in Geriatric Patients

Dosage of ceftaroline fosamil should be selected with caution in geriatric patients. Dosage adjustments are not required based on age, but may be required based on age-related changes in renal function. (See Dosage and Administration: Dosage in Renal and Hepatic Impairment.)

CAUTIONS

● Adverse Effects

Adverse effects reported with ceftaroline fosamil are similar to those reported with other cephalosporins. (See Cautions in the Cephalosporins General Statement 8:12.06.) Ceftaroline fosamil generally is well tolerated; serious adverse effects have been reported in up to 7.5% of adults receiving the drug in phase 3 clinical trials and have required discontinuance of the drug in about 3% of patients.

Adverse effects reported in 2% or more of adults receiving ceftaroline fosamil in phase 3 clinical trials include GI effects (diarrhea, nausea, vomiting, constipation), headache, rash, pruritus, hypokalemia, increased transaminases, and phlebitis.

● Precautions and Contraindications

Ceftaroline fosamil shares the toxic potentials of the cephalosporins, and the usual precautions of cephalosporin therapy should be observed.

Sensitivity Reactions

Serious, sometimes fatal hypersensitivity (anaphylactic) reactions and serious skin reactions have been reported in patients receiving β-lactam antibiotics. Anaphylaxis has been reported in some patients receiving ceftaroline fosamil.

Prior to initiation of ceftaroline fosamil therapy, careful inquiry should be made concerning previous hypersensitivity reactions to ceftaroline, other cephalosporins, penicillins, or carbapenems. There is clinical and laboratory evidence of partial cross-sensitivity among β-lactam antibiotics.

Ceftaroline fosamil is contraindicated in patients with known serious hypersensitivity to the drug or other cephalosporins. If ceftaroline fosamil is used in patients allergic to penicillin or other β-lactams, the patient should be closely monitored.

Patients should be advised that allergic reactions, including serious allergic reactions, could occur and that serious reactions require immediate treatment.

If a hypersensitivity reaction occurs, ceftaroline fosamil should be discontinued and appropriate treatment and supportive measures initiated.

Clostridium difficile-associated Diarrhea and Colitis

Treatment with anti-infectives alters normal colon flora and may permit overgrowth of *Clostridium difficile*.

C. difficile infection (CDI) and *C. difficile*-associated diarrhea and colitis (CDAD; also known as antibiotic-associated diarrhea and colitis or pseudomembranous colitis) have been reported with nearly all systemic anti-infectives, including ceftaroline, and may range in severity from mild diarrhea to fatal colitis. *C. difficile* produces toxins A and B which contribute to the development of CDAD; hypertoxin-producing strains of *C. difficile* are associated with increased morbidity and mortality since they may be refractory to anti-infectives and colectomy may be required.

CDAD should be considered in the differential diagnosis in patients who develop diarrhea during or after anti-infective therapy. Careful medical history is necessary since CDAD has been reported to occur as late as 2 months or longer after anti-infective therapy is discontinued.

If CDAD is suspected or confirmed, anti-infective therapy not directed against *C. difficile* should be discontinued whenever possible. Patients should be managed with appropriate supportive therapy (e.g., fluid and electrolyte management, protein supplementation), anti-infective therapy directed against *C. difficile* (e.g., metronidazole, vancomycin), and surgical evaluation as clinically indicated.

Patients should be advised that diarrhea is a common problem caused by anti-infectives and usually resolves when the drug is discontinued; however, they should contact a clinician if severe watery or bloody diarrhea develops.

Hematologic Effects

Neutropenia, leukopenia, and agranulocytosis have been reported in patients receiving ceftaroline fosamil during postmarketing experience.

Seroconversion from negative to positive direct antiglobulin (Coombs') test results was reported in about 10–11% of adults receiving ceftaroline fosamil in phase 3 clinical trials compared with about 4–5% of adults receiving comparator anti-infectives. In pediatric trials, seroconversion from negative to positive direct antiglobulin (Coombs') test results was reported in about 18% of those receiving ceftaroline fosamil compared with about 3% of those receiving comparator anti-infectives. There was no evidence of hemolytic anemia in these adult or pediatric patients.

Drug-induced hemolytic anemia should be considered in patients who develop anemia during or after treatment with ceftaroline fosamil. In such patients, diagnostic studies should be performed and should include a direct antiglobulin test. If drug-induced hemolytic anemia is suspected, discontinuance of ceftaroline fosamil should be considered and supportive treatment (e.g., transfusion) should be administered as clinically indicated.

Selection and Use of Anti-infectives

To reduce development of drug-resistant bacteria and maintain effectiveness of ceftaroline fosamil and other antibacterials, the drug should be used only for the treatment of infections proven or strongly suspected to be caused by susceptible bacteria.

When selecting or modifying anti-infective therapy, results of culture and in vitro susceptibility testing should be used. In the absence of such data, local epidemiology and susceptibility patterns should be considered when selecting anti-infectives for empiric therapy.

Patients should be advised that antibacterials (including ceftaroline fosamil) should only be used to treat bacterial infections and not used to treat viral infections (e.g., the common cold). Patients also should be advised about the importance of completing the full course of therapy, even if feeling better after a few days, and that skipping doses or not completing therapy may decrease effectiveness and increase the likelihood that bacteria will develop resistance and will not be treatable with ceftaroline fosamil or other antibacterials in the future.

Precautions in Patients with Renal Impairment

Because the area under the concentration-time curve (AUC) and plasma half-life of ceftaroline are increased in patients with renal impairment, dosage adjustments are recommended for adults with creatinine clearances less than 50 mL/minute, including those undergoing hemodialysis. Data are insufficient to date to make dosage recommendations for use of ceftaroline fosamil in pediatric patients with creatinine clearances less than 50 mL/minute per 1.73 m². (See Dosage and Administration: Dosage in Renal and Hepatic Impairment.)

● Pediatric Precautions

Safety and efficacy of ceftaroline fosamil have not been established in pediatric patients younger than 2 months of age.

Safety and efficacy of ceftaroline fosamil for the treatment of community-acquired bacterial pneumonia and acute bacterial skin and skin structure infections have been established in pediatric patients 2 months to less than 18 years of age. Use of the drug for these indications in this age group is supported by evidence from adequate and well-controlled studies in adults and additional pharmacokinetic and safety data from pediatric trials.

Data indicate that clinical cure rates reported with ceftaroline fosamil for the treatment of community-acquired bacterial pneumonia or acute bacterial skin and skin structure infections in children 2 months to less than 18 years of age are similar to clinical cure rates reported in adults 18 years of age or older. In addition, adverse effects reported with ceftaroline fosamil in pediatric trials are similar to those reported in adult trials. Adverse effects reported in 3% or more of children 2 months to less than 18 years of age receiving ceftaroline fosamil in clinical trials include GI effects (diarrhea, nausea, vomiting), pyrexia, and rash.

● Geriatric Precautions

In phase 3 trials evaluating ceftaroline fosamil for the treatment community-acquired bacterial pneumonia or acute bacterial skin and skin structure infections in adults, about 31% of patients were 65 years of age or older and no overall differences in efficacy or safety relative to younger adults were observed.

Ceftaroline is substantially eliminated by the kidneys, and the risk of adverse effects may be greater in those with impaired renal function. Because geriatric patients are more likely to have reduced renal function, dosage should be selected with caution and monitoring of renal function should be considered. Dosage adjustments in geriatric patients should be based on renal function. (See Dosage and Administration: Dosage in Renal and Hepatic Impairment.)

● Mutagenicity and Carcinogenicity

In vivo and in vitro studies evaluating ceftaroline fosamil have not shown evidence of mutagenicity. Although ceftaroline fosamil and ceftaroline were clastogenic in the absence of metabolic activation in an in vitro chromosomal aberration assay, this did not occur in the presence of metabolic activation.

Long-term animal studies have not been performed to date to evaluate the carcinogenic potential of ceftaroline fosamil.

● Pregnancy, Fertility, and Lactation

Pregnancy

Adequate data are not available regarding use of ceftaroline fosamil in pregnant women.

Animal studies in rats using ceftaroline fosamil dosages up to 4 times the maximum recommended human dosage (MRHD) or in rabbits using dosages up to approximately equal to the MRHD have not revealed evidence of fetal harm.

Fertility

There was no evidence of impaired fertility in male or female rats receiving ceftaroline fosamil dosages approximately 4 times higher than the MRHD based on body surface area.

Lactation

It is not known whether ceftaroline is distributed into human milk; possible effects of the drug on a breast-fed infant or on milk production are unknown.

Benefits of breast-feeding and the importance of ceftaroline fosamil to the woman should be considered along with the potential adverse effects on the breast-fed infant from the drug or from the underlying maternal condition.

DRUG INTERACTIONS

No formal drug interaction studies have been performed to date using ceftaroline fosamil. Interactions are unlikely between ceftaroline fosamil and drugs that are cytochrome P-450 (CYP) substrates, inhibitors, or inducers or drugs that undergo active renal secretion or alter renal blood flow.

In vitro, ceftaroline does not inhibit CYP isoenzymes 1A1, 1A2, 2A6, 2B6, 2C8, 2C9, 2C19, 2D6, 2E1, or 3A4 and does not induce CYP isoenzymes 1A2, 2B6, 2C8, 2C9, 2C19, or 3A4/5. Therefore, pharmacokinetic interactions with drugs metabolized by these isoenzymes are unlikely.

● Aminoglycosides

In vitro, the antibacterial effects of ceftaroline and amikacin were synergistic against *Escherichia coli* and *Klebsiella pneumoniae* that produce extended-spectrum β-lactamases (ESBL-producing), AmpC-derepressed *Enterobacter cloacae*, and *Pseudomonas aeruginosa*; there was no evidence of antagonism between the drugs.

● Aztreonam

In vitro, the antibacterial effects of ceftaroline and aztreonam were indifferent against ESBL-producing *E. coli* and *K. pneumoniae*, AmpC-derepressed *E. cloacae*, and *Ps. aeruginosa*; there was no evidence of synergism or antagonism between the drugs.

● Carbapenems

In vitro, the antibacterial effects of ceftaroline and meropenem were synergistic against ESBL-producing *E. coli* and indifferent against ESBL-producing *K. pneumoniae*, AmpC-derepressed *E. cloacae*, and *Ps. aeruginosa*; there was no evidence of antagonism between the drugs.

● Other Anti-infectives

To date, there has been no in vitro evidence of antagonism between ceftaroline and azithromycin, daptomycin, levofloxacin, linezolid, tigecycline, or vancomycin.

● Warfarin

Increased prothrombin time (PT) and elevated international normalized ratio (INR) have been reported when ceftaroline fosamil was initiated in a patient receiving a stable warfarin dosage.

MECHANISM OF ACTION

Ceftaroline usually is bactericidal in action. Like other cephalosporins, the antibacterial activity of the drug results from inhibition of mucopeptide synthesis in the bacterial cell wall. For information on the mechanism of action of cephalosporins, see Mechanism of Action in the Cephalosporins General Statement 8:12.06.

Studies evaluating the binding of ceftaroline to penicillin-binding proteins (PBPs), the target enzymes of β-lactam antibiotics, indicate that ceftaroline has high affinity for PBPs 1, 2, 2a, and 3 of *Staphylococcus aureus*. High affinity for PBP2a appears to be associated with bactericidal activity against methicillin-resistant *S. aureus* (MRSA; also known as oxacillin-resistant *S. aureus*, ORSA). Ceftaroline also has high affinity for PBPs 1a, 1b, 2a, 2b, 2x, and 3 of *Streptococcus pneumoniae*. Penicillin resistance in *S. pneumoniae* appears to involve PBP 2b, 2x, and 1a.

For most susceptible bacteria, the minimum bactericidal concentration (MBC) of ceftaroline is only 1–4 times higher than the minimum inhibitory concentration (MIC).

SPECTRUM

Based on its spectrum of activity, ceftaroline is classified as a fifth generation cephalosporin. For information on the classification of cephalosporins and closely related β-lactam antibiotics based on spectra of activity, see Spectrum in the Cephalosporins General Statement 8:12.06.

Like third and fourth generation cephalosporins, fifth generation cephalosporins have an expanded spectrum of activity that includes both gram-positive and gram-negative bacteria. However, unlike first, second, third, and fourth generation cephalosporins, fifth generation cephalosporins have activity against methicillin-resistant *Staphylococcus aureus* (MRSA; also known as oxacillin-resistant *S. aureus*, ORSA).

● In Vitro Susceptibility Testing

For information on interpreting results of in vitro susceptibility testing (disk susceptibility tests, dilution susceptibility tests) when ceftaroline susceptibility testing

is performed according to the standards of the Clinical and Laboratory Standards Institute (CLSI; formerly National Committee for Clinical Laboratory Standards [NCCLS]), see Spectrum: In Vitro Susceptibility Testing, in the Cephalosporins General Statement 8:12.06.

● Gram-positive Aerobic Bacteria

Ceftaroline is active in vitro against *S. aureus*, including MRSA, vancomycin-resistant *S. aureus* [VRSA], and daptomycin-nonsusceptible *S. aureus*. The drug also is active in vitro against coagulase-negative staphylococci (e.g., *S. epidermidis*), including methicillin-resistant (oxacillin-resistant) strains. The MIC_{90} of ceftaroline reported for methicillin-susceptible (oxacillin-susceptible) *S. aureus* is 0.25 mcg/mL, and the MIC_{90} of the drug reported for MRSA is 1–2 mcg/mL.

Ceftaroline is active in vitro against *Streptococcus pneumoniae*, including penicillin-resistant *S. pneumoniae* and multidrug-resistant *S. pneumoniae* (MDRSP). The MIC_{90} of the drug is 0.015–0.12 mcg/mL for penicillin-susceptible *S. pneumoniae* and 0.12–0.25 mcg/mL for penicillin-resistant and multidrug-resistant strains.

Ceftaroline is active in vitro against *S. pyogenes* (group A β-hemolytic streptococci, GAS), *S. agalactiae* (group B streptococci, GBS), viridans streptococci, and *S. dysgalactiae*. The MIC_{90} of the drug reported for *S. pyogenes* and *S. agalactiae* is 0.03 mcg/mL or less.

Ceftaroline has only limited activity against *Enterococcus*. Some strains of *Enterococcus faecalis* are inhibited in vitro by ceftaroline concentrations of 2–4 mcg/mL, but *E. faecium* are resistant to the drug.

● Gram-negative Aerobic Bacteria

Ceftaroline is active in vitro against many Enterobacteriaceae, including some *Citrobacter freundii*, *C. koseri*, *Enterobacter aerogenes*, *E. cloacae*, *Escherichia coli*, *Klebsiella pneumoniae*, *K. oxytoca*, *Morganella morganii*, and *Proteus mirabilis*. The MIC_{90} of ceftaroline for most susceptible Enterobacteriaceae is 0.25–1 mcg/mL. However, the MIC_{90} of the drug has been reported to be 4 mcg/mL or higher for many Enterobacteriaceae, including *P. mirabilis*, *C. freundii* (ceftazidime-nonsusceptible strains), *M. morganii*, and *Serratia*. *Providencia* and *Acinetobacter* usually are resistant. The activity of ceftaroline against gram-negative bacteria is similar to that reported with third generation cephalosporins. Ceftaroline is not active against Enterobacteriaceae that produce extended-spectrum β-lactamases (ESBL-producing), AmpC cephalosporinases, metallo-β-lactamases, or serine carbapenemases.

Ceftaroline is active in vitro against β-lactamase-producing and non-β-lactamase-producing *Haemophilus influenzae*, *H. parainfluenzae*, and *Moraxella catarrhalis*, and the MIC_{90} reported for most of these organisms is 0.015–0.25 mcg/mL. The MIC_{90} of ceftaroline reported for *Neisseria gonorrhoeae* and *N. meningitidis* is 0.004–0.25 mcg/mL.

The MIC_{90} of ceftaroline reported for *Pasteurella multocida* is 0.06 mcg/mL. In vitro studies indicate that *Acinetobacter* is resistant to ceftaroline.

Ceftaroline is not active against *Pseudomonas aeruginosa*.

● Anaerobic Bacteria

Ceftaroline has some in vitro activity against anaerobic bacteria. The MIC_{90} of ceftaroline reported for some gram-positive anaerobic bacteria, including *Actinomyces*, *Eubacterium*, *Lactobacillus*, *Clostridium*, *Peptostreptococcus*, and *Propionibacterium*, has been 0.06–4 mcg/mL. The MIC_{90} of ceftaroline reported for some gram-negative anaerobic bacteria, including *Fusobacterium*, *Porphyromonas*, and *Veillonella*, has been 0.03–0.5 mcg/mL. In vitro studies indicate that *Bacteroides* and *Prevotella* are resistant to ceftaroline.

RESISTANCE

Methicillin-resistant *Staphylococcus aureus* (MRSA; also known as oxacillin-resistant *S. aureus*, ORSA) with reduced susceptibility or resistance to ceftaroline have been produced in vitro and have been reported in clinical isolates. Although resistance to ceftaroline in MRSA generally is associated with modifications in the *mecA*-encoded penicillin-binding protein 2a (PBP2a), other mechanisms of resistance may also be involved.

Gram-negative bacteria that produce extended-spectrum β-lactamases (ESBLs) from the TEM, SHV or CTX-M families, AmpC cephalosporinases, class

B metallo-β-lactamases, or serine carbapenemases (such as KPC) are resistant to ceftaroline.

Although cross-resistance may occur between ceftaroline and other cephalosporins, some bacteria resistant to other cephalosporins may be susceptible to ceftaroline.

PHARMACOKINETICS

● Absorption

Ceftaroline is administered as ceftaroline fosamil, a prodrug that is inactive until converted in vivo to ceftaroline by a plasma phosphatase.

Peak plasma concentrations and area under the concentration-time curve (AUC) of ceftaroline in healthy adults increase approximately in proportion to dose following single IV doses of 50–1000 mg of ceftaroline fosamil.

There is no appreciable accumulation of ceftaroline when 600-mg doses of ceftaroline fosamil are given by IV infusion over 1 hour every 12 hours for up to 14 days in adults with normal renal function.

In healthy adults receiving ceftaroline fosamil in a dosage of 600 mg given by IV infusion over 1 hour every 12 hours for 14 days, peak plasma concentrations of ceftaroline average 21.3 mcg/mL and the median time to peak plasma concentrations is 0.9 hours.

When 600-mg doses of ceftaroline fosamil in 50 mL of compatible infusion solution were given by IV infusion over 5 or 60 minutes every 8 hours for 5 days in healthy adults, mean peak plasma concentrations of ceftaroline were 32.5 mcg/mL after the 5-minute infusions and 17.4 mcg/mL after the 60-minute infusion; the time to peak plasma concentrations (about 5 minutes after the end of the infusion) and AUC were similar for both infusion rates.

In healthy adolescents 12–17 years of age, peak plasma concentrations and AUC after a single 8-mg/kg IV dose (600 mg in those weighing more than 75 kg) are 10 and 23% lower, respectively, compared with healthy adults who received a single 600-mg IV dose.

● Distribution

The steady-state volume of distribution of ceftaroline in healthy adults following a single 600-mg IV dose of ceftaroline fosamil is 20.3 L and is similar to extracellular fluid volume.

Ceftaroline is approximately 20% bound to plasma proteins. Protein binding decreases slightly with increasing ceftaroline concentrations exceeding 1–50 mcg/mL.

Limited data are available regarding tissue distribution of ceftaroline; animal data indicate that the drug is distributed into kidneys, skin, and lungs.

It is not known whether ceftaroline is distributed into milk.

● Elimination

Ceftaroline fosamil is rapidly converted in vivo to ceftaroline by a plasma phosphatase, principally during IV infusion. In addition, the β-lactam ring of ceftaroline is hydrolyzed to an inactive, open-ring metabolite (ceftaroline M-1).

Ceftaroline is not a substrate of cytochrome P-450 (CYP) isoenzymes.

Ceftaroline and its metabolites are principally eliminated in urine by glomerular filtration. Following a single 600-mg IV dose of ceftaroline fosamil, approximately 88% is eliminated in urine (approximately 64% as unchanged drug and 2% as ceftaroline M-1) and 6% is eliminated in feces within 48 hours.

The terminal elimination half-life of ceftaroline is 2.7 hours in healthy adults receiving ceftaroline fosamil in a dosage of 600 mg given by IV infusion over 1 hour every 12 hours for 14 days. When 600-mg doses of ceftaroline fosamil in 50 mL of compatible infusion solution were given by IV infusion over 5 or 60 minutes every 8 hours for 5 days in healthy adults, the terminal elimination half-life of ceftaroline was similar for both infusion rates.

The pharmacokinetics of ceftaroline in pediatric patients 2 months to less than 18 years of age are similar to the pharmacokinetics reported in adults.

The pharmacokinetics of ceftaroline in patients with hepatic impairment have not been established.

In adults with renal impairment, the AUC and plasma half-life of ceftaroline are increased.

Ceftaroline is removed by hemodialysis. In adults with end-stage renal disease who received 400 mg of ceftaroline fosamil, 76.5 mg of the drug (approximately 21.6% of the dose) was recovered in the dialysate following a 4-hour hemodialysis session started 4 hours after the dose.

CHEMISTRY AND STABILITY

● Chemistry

Ceftaroline is a semisynthetic cephalosporin antibiotic. Ceftaroline is structurally similar to parenteral third and fourth generation cephalosporins (e.g., cefepime, cefotaxime, ceftazidime, ceftriaxone). Like many third and fourth generation drugs, ceftaroline contains a 1,2,4-thiadiazole ring that enhances antibacterial activity against gram-negative bacteria and an oxime group that contributes to stability in the presence of β-lactamases. Unlike other commercially available cephalosporins, ceftaroline contains a 1,3-thiazole ring linked to the 3-position of the cephem ring by a sulfur which appears to contribute to activity against methicillin-resistant *Staphylococcus aureus* (MRSA; also known as oxacillin-resistant *S. aureus* or ORSA).

Ceftaroline is commercially available for parenteral use as ceftaroline fosamil monoacetate monohydrate; potency is expressed in terms of anhydrous ceftaroline fosamil. Ceftaroline fosamil is a prodrug that is inactive until converted in vivo to ceftaroline by a plasma phosphatase. Commercially available ceftaroline fosamil powder for IV infusion is a pale yellowish-white to light yellow powder. Each vial of the drug also contains L-arginine as an excipient. When reconstituted as directed, ceftaroline fosamil solutions have a pH of 4.8–6.5. Depending on the concentration and storage conditions, ceftaroline fosamil solutions are clear, light to dark yellow.

● Stability

Ceftaroline fosamil powder for IV infusion should be stored at 25°C, but may be exposed to temperatures ranging from 15–30°C.

Following reconstitution and dilution, ceftaroline fosamil solutions in IV infusion bags should be used within 6 hours when stored at room temperature or within 24 hours when refrigerated at 2–8°C. Stability testing indicates that ceftaroline fosamil solutions containing 4–12 mg/mL diluted in 50- or 100-mL infusion bags containing 0.9% sodium chloride (Baxter Mini-Bag Plus containers) may be stored for up to 6 hours at room temperature or for up to 24 hours at 2–8°C.

For further information on chemistry, mechanism of action, spectrum, resistance, uses, cautions, acute toxicity, drug interactions, or laboratory test interferences of cephalosporins, see the Cephalosporins General Statement 8:12.06.

PREPARATIONS

Excipients in commercially available drug preparations may have clinically important effects in some individuals; consult specific product labeling for details.

Ceftaroline Fosamil

Parenteral		
For injection, for IV infusion	400 mg	Teflaro®, Forest
	600 mg	Teflaro®, Forest

Selected Revisions October 4, 2016, © Copyright, July 15, 2011, American Society of Health-System Pharmacists, Inc.

Ceftolozane Sulfate and Tazobactam Sodium

8:12.06.20 • FIFTH GENERATION CEPHALOSPORINS

■ Ceftolozane sulfate and tazobactam sodium is a fixed combination of ceftolozane (a fifth generation cephalosporin) and tazobactam (a β-lactamase inhibitor); tazobactam inactivates certain bacterial β-lactamases and expands ceftolozane's spectrum of activity against some bacteria that produce these β-lactamases.

USES

● Intra-abdominal Infections

Ceftolozane and tazobactam is used in conjunction with metronidazole for the treatment of complicated intra-abdominal infections caused by susceptible *Enterobacter colacae, Escherichia coli, Klebsiella oxytoca, K. pneumoniae, Proteus mirabilis, Pseudomonas aeruginosa, Bacteroides fragilis, Streptococcus anginosus, S. constellatus,* or *S. salivarius.*

Clinical Experience

Efficacy and safety of ceftolozane and tazobactam for the treatment of complicated intra-abdominal infections are based on results from 2 identical phase 3, randomized, double-blind, placebo-controlled studies in 979 hospitalized adults with complicated intra-abdominal infections, including appendicitis, cholecystitis, diverticulitis, gastric or duodenal perforation, intestinal perforation, or other causes of intra-abdominal abscesses and peritonitis. Patients were randomized in a 1:1 ratio to receive 4–14 days of treatment with the fixed combination of ceftolozane and tazobactam (1.5 g [ceftolozane 1 g and tazobactam 0.5 g] given by IV infusion every 8 hours) in conjunction with metronidazole (500 mg given by IV infusion every 8 hours) or treatment with meropenem (1 g given by IV infusion every 8 hours) in conjunction with placebo. Baseline characteristics were similar between groups (mean age 50–51 years, 56–60% male, 93–94% white, 75% from Eastern Europe, 6.3% from the US, 45–49% with diagnosis of appendiceal perforation or abscess). In a pooled analysis of both studies, the clinical cure rate (defined as complete resolution or marked improvement in signs and symptoms of the index infection at the test-of-cure visit [24–32 days after first treatment dose]) in the microbiological intent-to-treat (MITT) population was 83% in patients treated with ceftolozane and tazobactam in conjunction with metronidazole and 87.3% in those treated with meropenem. Based on clinical cure rate in the MITT population at the test-of-cure visit, ceftolozane and tazobactam in conjunction with metronidazole was noninferior to meropenem. When results were stratified according to causative organism, clinical cure rates at the test-of-cure visit in patients treated with ceftolozane and tazobactam in conjunction with metronidazole were 80.8% for *E. cloacae,* 84.7% for *E. coli,* 87.5% for *K. oxytoca,* 75.6% for *K. pneumoniae,* 91.7% for *P. mirabilis,* 79% for *Ps. aeruginosa,* 89.4% for *B. fragilis,* 84.4% for *B. ovatus,* 84% for *B. thetaiotaomicron,* 80% for *B. vulgatus,* 72.2% for *S. anginosus,* 75% for *S. constellatus,* and 81.8% for *S. salivarius.*

● Urinary Tract Infections

Ceftolozane and tazobactam is used for the treatment of complicated urinary tract infections, including pyelonephritis, caused by susceptible *E. coli, K. pneumoniae, P. mirabilis,* or *Ps. aeruginosa.*

Clinical Experience

Efficacy of ceftolozane and tazobactam for the treatment of complicated urinary tract infections is based on results from a phase 3 randomized, double-blind clinical trial in 1068 hospitalized adults with complicated urinary tract infections, including pyelonephritis. Patients were randomized to receive 7 days of treatment with the fixed combination of ceftolozane and tazobactam (1.5 g [ceftolozane 1 g and tazobactam 0.5 g] given by IV infusion every 8 hours) or levofloxacin (750 mg given by IV infusion once daily). The MITT population had a median age of 51 years, 74% were female, 82% were diagnosed with pyelonephritis, 76% were enrolled in Eastern Europe, and 1.8% were enrolled in the US. The composite end

point of microbiologic and clinical cure rate (defined as complete resolution or marked improvement in signs and symptoms and microbiologic eradication at the test-of-cure visit [approximately 7 days after the last treatment dose]) in the MITT population was 76.9% in patients treated with ceftolozane and tazobactam and 68.4% in those treated with levofloxacin. When results were stratified according to causative organism, the composite end point of microbiologic and clinical cure rates at the test-of-cure visit in patients treated with ceftolozane and tazobactam were 81% for *E. coli,* 66.7% for *K. pneumoniae,* 91.7% for *P. mirabilis,* and 75% for *Ps. aeruginosa.*

DOSAGE AND ADMINISTRATION

● Administration

Ceftolozane and tazobactam is administered by IV infusion.

IV Infusion

IV solutions of ceftolozane and tazobactam should not be admixed with or added to solutions containing other drugs.

Reconstitution and Dilution

Ceftolozane and tazobactam powder must be reconstituted and further diluted prior to IV infusion.

Single-dose vials of ceftolozane and tazobactam labeled as containing 1.5 g (ceftolozane 1 g and tazobactam 0.5 g) should be reconstituted by adding 10 mL of sterile water for injection or 0.9% sodium chloride injection to the vial and shaking gently until the contents are dissolved. Reconstituted ceftolozane and tazobactam solutions may be stored for up to 1 hour prior to transfer and dilution; reconstituted solutions should not be frozen.

Prior to IV infusion, reconstituted ceftolozane and tazobactam solutions *must* be further diluted. To prepare the indicated dose, the appropriate volume of reconstituted solution should be withdrawn from the vial and added to 100 mL of 0.9% sodium chloride or 5% dextrose injection. (See Table 1.)

TABLE 1. Dilution of Reconstituted Ceftolozane and Tazobactam

Recommended Dose of Ceftolozane and Tazobactam	Volume to Withdraw from Reconstituted Vial for Further Dilution
1.5 g (ceftolozane 1 g and tazobactam 0.5 g)	11.4 mL (entire contents)
750 mg (ceftolozane 500 mg and tazobactam 250 mg)	5.7 mL
375 mg (ceftolozane 250 mg and tazobactam 125 mg)	2.9 mL
150 mg (ceftolozane 100 mg and tazobactam 50 mg)	1.2 mL

The reconstituted and diluted solution of ceftolozane and tazobactam should be inspected visually for particulate matter and discoloration prior to administration; the solution should appear clear and colorless to slightly yellow.

Following reconstitution and dilution, ceftolozane and tazobactam solutions may be stored at room temperature for up to 24 hours or at 2–8°C for up to 7 days; diluted solutions should not be frozen.

Rate of Administration

IV infusions of ceftolozane and tazobactam should be given over 1 hour.

Dispensing and Dosage and Administration Precautions

FDA alerted healthcare professionals about the risk of medication errors with ceftolozane and tazobactam. There have been reports of errors occurring during preparation of IV solutions of the drug that resulted in administration of incorrect dosage (50% overdosage in some cases); the errors were due to confusion about how dosage of ceftolozane and tazobactam is expressed (total of the dosage of each of the 2 active components) and how drug strength was displayed on vial labels and carton packaging. To prevent such errors, vial labels and carton packaging have been revised to indicate the strength of the fixed combination as the total of the 2 active components.

Healthcare professionals should be aware that dosage of ceftolozane and tazobactam is expressed as the total (sum) of the dosage of each of the 2 active components (i.e., dosage of ceftolozane plus dosage of tazobactam). This dosage convention should be considered when prescribing, preparing, and dispensing ceftolozane and tazobactam. FDA urges healthcare professionals and patients to report any medication errors and adverse effects involving the drug to the FDA MedWatch program.

● Dosage

Ceftolozane and tazobactam is a fixed combination containing a 2:1 ratio of ceftolozane to tazobactam.

The ceftolozane component is provided as ceftolozane sulfate (dosage of this component is expressed in terms of ceftolozane); the tazobactam component is provided as tazobactam sodium (dosage of this component is expressed in terms of tazobactam).

Dosage of the fixed combination of ceftolozane and tazobactam is expressed in terms of the total of the ceftolozane and tazobactam content.

Each single-dose vial of ceftolozane and tazobactam contains a total of 1.5 g (i.e., 1 g of ceftolozane and 0.5 g of tazobactam).

Adult Dosage

Intra-abdominal Infections

The recommended dosage of ceftolozane and tazobactam for the treatment of complicated intra-abdominal infections in adults is 1.5 g (ceftolozane 1 g and tazobactam 0.5 g) every 8 hours in conjunction with metronidazole (500 mg given by IV infusion every 8 hours).

The recommended duration of treatment is 4–14 days. Duration should be guided by the severity and site of infection and the patient's clinical and bacteriologic progress.

Urinary Tract Infections

The recommended dosage of ceftolozane and tazobactam for the treatment of complicated urinary tract infections in adults is 1.5 g (ceftolozane 1 g and tazobactam 0.5 g) every 8 hours.

The recommended duration of treatment is 7 days. Duration should be guided by the severity and site of infection and the patient's clinical and bacteriologic progress.

● Dosage in Renal Impairment

Dosage of ceftolozane and tazobactam must be adjusted in adults with creatinine clearances of 50 mL/minute or less, including those undergoing hemodialysis. (See Table 2.)

Creatinine clearance should be monitored at least once daily in patients with changing renal function and dosage of ceftolozane and tazobactam adjusted accordingly.

TABLE 2. Ceftolozane and Tazobactam Dosage for Adults with Renal Impairment

Estimated Creatinine Clearance (mL/minute)	Recommended Dosage
30–50	750 mg (ceftolozane 500 mg and tazobactam 250 mg) every 8 hours
15–29	375 mg (ceftolozane 250 mg and tazobactam 125 mg) every 8 hours
End-stage renal disease on hemodialysis	Single loading dose of 750 mg (ceftolozane 500 mg and tazobactam 250 mg) followed by maintenance dosage of 150 mg (ceftolozane 100 mg and tazobactam 50 mg) every 8 hours[a]

[a] On hemodialysis days, the dose should be administered as soon as possible after dialysis.

● Dosage in Hepatic Impairment

Dosage adjustments are not needed when ceftolozane and tazobactam is used in adults with hepatic impairment.

● Dosage in Geriatric Patients

Dosage adjustments based solely on age are not needed when ceftolozane and tazobactam is used in geriatric patients. However, because geriatric patients are more likely to have decreased renal function and because dosage of ceftolozane and tazobactam needs to be adjusted based on renal impairment, dosage should be selected with caution and it may be useful to monitor renal function.

CAUTIONS

● Adverse Effects

Adverse effects reported in 5% or more of patients receiving ceftolozane and tazobactam in phase 3 clinical trials include GI effects (nausea, diarrhea), headache, and pyrexia.

● Precautions and Contraindications

Sensitivity Reactions

Ceftolozane and tazobactam is contraindicated in patients with known serious hypersensitivity to ceftolozane and/or tazobactam, the fixed combination of piperacillin and tazobactam, or other β-lactams.

Serious and occasionally fatal hypersensitivity (anaphylactic) reactions have been reported in patients receiving β-lactam antibacterials. Before initiating therapy with ceftolozane and tazobactam, the clinician should carefully inquire about the patient's previous hypersensitivity reactions to other cephalosporins, penicillins, or other β-lactams. Ceftolozane and tazobactam should be used with caution in patients allergic to cephalosporins, penicillins, or other β-lactams since cross-sensitivity among β-lactam antibacterials has been established.

Patients should be advised that allergic reactions, including serious allergic reactions, could occur and that serious reactions require immediate treatment.

If an anaphylactic reaction occurs, ceftolozane and tazobactam should be discontinued and appropriate therapy initiated.

Reduced Efficacy in Patients with Moderate Renal Impairment

Results of a subgroup analysis of a phase 3 clinical trial in patients with complicated intra-abdominal infections indicated that the clinical cure rate in patients with moderate renal impairment (baseline creatinine clearances of 30–50 mL/minute) was lower than the clinical cure rate in those with normal renal function or only mild renal impairment (creatinine clearances of 50 mL/minute or greater), and this difference was more marked in those treated with ceftolozane and tazobactam in conjunction with metronidazole than in those treated with the comparator drug (meropenem). The clinical cure rate in patients treated with ceftolozane and tazobactam in conjunction with metronidazole was 47.8% in those with baseline creatinine clearances of 30–50 mL/minute compared with 85.2% in those with baseline creatinine clearances of 50 mL/minute or greater. A similar trend also was observed in a clinical trial evaluating ceftolozane and tazobactam for treatment of complicated urinary tract infections.

Creatinine clearance should be monitored at least once daily in patients with changing renal function and dosage of ceftolozane and tazobactam adjusted accordingly. (See Other Precautions and Contraindications under Cautions: Precautions and Contraindications.)

Superinfection/Clostridium difficile-associated Diarrhea and Colitis (CDAD)

Use of ceftolozane and tazobactam may result in emergence and overgrowth of nonsusceptible bacteria or fungi. The patient should be carefully monitored and appropriate therapy instituted if superinfection occurs.

Treatment with anti-infectives alters normal colon flora and may permit overgrowth of Clostridium difficile. C. difficile infection (CDI) and C. difficile-associated diarrhea and colitis (CDAD; also known as antibiotic-associated diarrhea and colitis or pseudomembranous colitis) have been reported in patients receiving nearly all anti-infectives, including ceftolozane and tazobactam, and may range in severity from mild diarrhea to fatal colitis. C. difficile produces toxins A and B which contribute to development of CDAD; hypertoxin-producing strains of *C. difficile* are associated with increased morbidity and mortality since they may be refractory to anti-infectives and colectomy may be required.

CDAD should be considered in the differential diagnosis of patients who develop diarrhea during or after anti-infective therapy. Careful medical history is necessary since CDAD has been reported to occur as late as 2 months or longer after anti-infective therapy is discontinued.

If CDAD is suspected or confirmed, anti-infective therapy not directed against *C. difficile* should be discontinued whenever possible. Patients should be managed with appropriate supportive therapy (e.g., fluid and electrolyte management, protein supplementation), anti-infective therapy directed against *C. difficile* (e.g., metronidazole, vancomycin), and surgical evaluation as clinically indicated.

Patients should be advised that diarrhea is a common problem caused by anti-infectives and usually resolves when the drug is discontinued; however, they should contact a clinician if watery and bloody stools (with or without stomach cramps and fever) occur during or as late as 2 months or longer after the last dose.

Selection and Use of Anti-infectives

To reduce development of drug-resistant bacteria and maintain effectiveness of ceftolozane and tazobactam and other antibacterials, the drug should be used only for treatment of infections proven or strongly suspected to be caused by susceptible bacteria.

When selecting or modifying anti-infective therapy, results of culture and in vitro susceptibility testing should be used. In the absence of such data, local epidemiology and susceptibility patterns should be considered when selecting anti-infectives for empiric therapy.

Patients should be advised that antibacterials (including ceftolozane and tazobactam) should only be used to treat bacterial infections and not used to treat viral infections (e.g., the common cold). Patients also should be advised about the importance of completing the full course of therapy, even if feeling better after a few days, and that skipping doses or not completing therapy may decrease effectiveness and increase the likelihood that bacteria will develop resistance and will not be treatable with ceftolozane and tazobactam or other antibacterials in the future.

Precautions Related to Use of Fixed Combinations

When ceftolozane and tazobactam is used, the cautions, precautions, contraindications, and drug interactions associated with both drugs in the fixed combination must be considered. Cautionary information applicable to specific populations (e.g., pregnant or nursing women, individuals with hepatic or renal impairment, geriatric patients) should be considered for each drug.

When prescribing, preparing, and dispensing ceftolozane and tazobactam, healthcare professionals should consider that dosage of the fixed combination is expressed as the total (sum) of the dosage of each of the 2 active components (i.e., dosage of ceftolozane plus dosage of tazobactam). (See Dispensing and Dosage and Administration Precautions under Administration; IV Infusion, in Dosage and Administration.)

Other Precautions and Contraindications

Ceftolozane and tazobactam are substantially eliminated by the kidneys, and the risk of adverse reactions may be greater in patients with renal impairment. In addition, a lower cure rate has been reported in some patients with moderate renal impairment (see Reduced Efficacy in Patients with Moderate Renal Impairment under Cautions: Precautions and Contraindications). Dosage of ceftolozane and tazobactam should be adjusted in patients with moderate or severe renal impairment (creatinine clearances of 50 mL/minute or less), including those undergoing hemodialysis. In patients with changing renal function, creatinine clearance should be monitored at least once daily and dosage adjusted accordingly. (See Dosage and Administration: Dosage in Renal Impairment.)

● Padiatric Precautions

Safety and efficacy of ceftolozane and tazobactam have not been established in patients younger than 18 years of age.

● Geriatric Precautions

In phase 3 trials evaluating ceftolozane and tazobactam for the treatment of complicated intra-abdominal infections or complicated urinary tract infections, 24.6% of patients were 65 years of age or older, while about 11% were 75 years of

age or older. The incidence of adverse effects reported in geriatric patients treated with ceftolozane and tazobactam was higher than that reported in younger adults treated with the drug. In addition, in adults 65 years of age or older with complicated intra-abdominal infections, the clinical cure rate was 69% in those treated with ceftolozane and tazobactam in conjunction with metronidazole compared with 82.4% in those treated with the comparator drug. A difference in cure rates between the ceftolozane and tazobactam regimen and the comparator regimen was not observed in geriatric patients with complicated urinary tract infections.

Ceftolozane and tazobactam are substantially eliminated by the kidneys, and the risk of adverse effects may be greater in those with impaired renal function. Because geriatric patients are more likely to have reduced renal function, dosage should be selected with caution and renal function monitoring should be considered. Dosage adjustments in geriatric patients should be based on renal function.

● Pregnancy, Fertility, and Lactation

Pregnancy

Embryofetal development studies in mice and rats using ceftolozane dosages associated with exposures approximately 7 and 4 times, respectively, the exposure expected in humans receiving a ceftolozane dosage of 1 g three times daily did not reveal evidence of fetal toxicity. In a study in rats, ceftolozane administered during pregnancy and lactation was associated with decreased auditory startle response in male pups at postnatal day 60.

Embryofetal development studies in rats using tazobactam dosages approximately 19 times the recommended human dosage revealed evidence of maternal toxicity (decreased food consumption and body weight gain), but no evidence of fetal toxicity. In a study in rats, tazobactam administered during pregnancy and lactation in dosages approximately 8 times the recommended human dosage produced decreased maternal food consumption and body weight gain at the end of gestation and an increased incidence of stillbirths. Although pups of dams receiving tazobactam in dosages of 320–1280 mg/kg daily had substantially reduced postnatal body weight at 21 days after delivery, there was no evidence of effects on development, function, learning, or fertility of the pups.

There are no adequate and controlled studies using ceftolozane and tazobactam in pregnant women, and the drug should be used during pregnancy only if potential benefits to the woman justify potential risks to the fetus.

Fertility

Ceftolozane showed no evidence of impaired fertility in male or female rats receiving ceftolozane dosages approximately 3 times higher than the recommended human dosage based on mean plasma exposure.

Tazobactam showed no evidence of impaired fertility in male or female rats receiving tazobactam dosages approximately 4 times higher than the recommended human dosage based on body surface area.

Lactation

Because it is not known whether ceftolozane or tazobactam is distributed into human milk, the fixed combination of ceftolozane and tazobactam should be used with caution in nursing women.

DRUG INTERACTIONS

The following drug interactions are based on studies using the fixed combination containing ceftolozane and tazobactam, ceftolozane alone, or tazobactam alone. When ceftolozane and tazobactam is used, interactions associated with both drugs in the fixed combination should be considered.

● Drugs Affecting or Metabolized by Hepatic Microsomal Enzymes

Drug interactions are not expected between ceftolozane and tazobactam and inhibitors or inducers of cytochrome P-450 (CYP) enzymes.

In vivo data indicate ceftolozane and tazobactam is not a substrate for CYP enzymes. In vitro, ceftolozane, tazobactam, and the M1 metabolite of tazobactam do not inhibit CYP1A2, 2B6, 2C8, 2C9, 2C19, 2D6, or 3A4 and do not induce CYP1A2, 2B6, or 3A4 at therapeutic concentrations.

Results from in vitro induction studies show that ceftolozane, tazobactam, and the M1 metabolite of tazobactam decrease CYP1A2 and 2B6 enzyme activity and mRNA levels in human hepatocytes and decrease CYP3A4 mRNA levels at supratherapeutic plasma concentrations. In addition, the M1 metabolite of tazobactam decreased CYP3A4 activity at supratherapeutic plasma concentrations. A clinical drug interaction study showed that drug interactions involving inhibition of CYP1A2 or 3A4 by ceftolozane and tazobactam are not expected.

● Drugs Affecting or Affected by Organic Anion Transporters

Tazobactam is a substrate of organic anion transporter (OAT) 1 and OAT3. Therefore, concomitant use of OAT1 and/or OAT3 inhibitors (e.g., probenecid) with ceftolozane and tazobactam may increase tazobactam plasma concentrations. (See Drug Interactions: Probenecid.)

In vitro, tazobactam inhibits OAT1 and OAT3; ceftolozane does not inhibit OAT1 or OAT3. Clinically important interactions involving OAT1 or OAT3 inhibition by ceftolozane and tazobactam are not expected.

● Drugs Affecting or Affected by Other Membrane Transporters

In vitro, ceftolozane and tazobactam are not substrates or inhibitors of P-glycoprotein (P-gp) or breast cancer resistance protein (BCRP); tazobactam is not a substrate of organic cation transporter (OCT) 2.

In vitro data indicate that ceftolozane and tazobactam do not inhibit organic anion transporting polypeptide (OATP) 1B1 or 1B3, organic cation transporter (OCT) 1 or 2, or bile salt export pump (BSEP) at therapeutic plasma concentrations. In addition, ceftolozane does not inhibit multidrug resistance-associated protein (MRP) or multidrug and toxin extrusion (MATE) 1 or 2-K.

● Anti-infectives

There is no in vitro evidence of antagonistic antibacterial effects between ceftolozane and tazobactam and amikacin, aztreonam, daptomycin, levofloxacin, linezolid, meropenem, metronidazole, rifampin, tigecycline, or vancomycin.

● Probenecid

Concomitant use of probenecid (an OAT1/OAT3 inhibitor) prolongs the half-life of tazobactam by 71%.

MECHANISM OF ACTION

Ceftolozane and tazobactam is bactericidal in action.

Like other cephalosporins, the antibacterial activity of ceftolozane results from inhibition of mucopeptide synthesis in the bacterial cell wall and is mediated through binding to penicillin-binding proteins (PBPs).

Tazobactam is a β-lactam β-lactamase inhibitor that inactivates certain β-lactamases, including some extended-spectrum β-lactamases (ESBLs). Tazobactam binds to and forms covalent, irreversible, acyl-enzyme intermediates with certain β-lactamases. After this complex is formed, functional inhibition of the β-lactamase depends on the relative rates of deacylation, tautomerization, or hydrolysis of the complex. Tazobactam inactivates many β-lactamases in Ambler class A (e.g., penicillinases, ESBLs) and some in class C (e.g., cephalosporinases such as AmpC). Tazobactam cannot inactivate Ambler class A carbapenemases (e.g., Klebsiella pneumoniae carbapenemases [KPCs]), Ambler class D β-lactamases, or Ambler class B metallo-β-lactamases (MLBs).

Because tazobactam inactivates certain β-lactamases, concomitant use with ceftolozane can protect ceftolozane from degradation by these β-lactamases and expand the spectrum of activity of the cephalosporin to include some β-lactamase-producing bacteria that are resistant to ceftolozane alone.

SPECTRUM

Based on its spectrum of activity, ceftolozane and tazobactam is classified as a fifth generation cephalosporin.

Ceftolozane and tazobactam has a wider spectrum of activity than ceftolozane alone. Ceftolozane and tazobactam is active against many gram-negative aerobic

and anaerobic bacteria and select gram-positive bacteria. Ceftolozane and tazobactam is active in vitro against many β-lactamase-producing gram-negative bacteria that are resistant to ceftolozane alone, including Enterobacteriaceae that produce extended-spectrum β-lactamases (ESBLs).

Some bacteria that are resistant to other cephalosporins and/or other anti-infectives because of β-lactamase production may be susceptible to ceftolozane and tazobactam. The fixed combination also is active in vitro against some bacteria resistant to other β-lactams (e.g., carbapenems) because of loss of outer membrane porin (OprD).

● In Vitro Susceptibility Testing

When in vitro susceptibility testing is performed according to the standards of the Clinical and Laboratory Standards Institute (CLSI; formerly National Committee for Clinical Laboratory Standards [NCCLS]), clinical isolates identified as susceptible to ceftolozane and tazobactam are inhibited by drug concentrations usually achievable when dosage recommended for the site of infection is used. A report of intermediate should be considered equivocal and, if the isolate is not fully susceptible to alternative anti-infectives, the test should be repeated. The intermediate category implies possible clinical applicability in body sites where the drug is physiologically concentrated and provides a buffer zone which should prevent small, uncontrolled technical factors from causing major discrepancies in interpretation. If results of in vitro susceptibility testing indicate that a clinical isolate is resistant to ceftolozane and tazobactam, the strain is not likely to be inhibited by drug concentrations generally achievable with usual dosage schedules and other anti-infective therapy should be selected.

Disk Susceptibility Tests

When the disk-diffusion procedure is used to test susceptibility to ceftolozane and tazobactam, a disk containing 30 mcg of ceftolozane and 10 mcg of tazobactam is used.

When disk-diffusion susceptibility testing is performed according to CLSI standardized procedures, Ps. aeruginosa with growth inhibition zones of 21 mm or greater are susceptible to ceftolozane and tazobactam, those with zones of 17–20 mm have intermediate susceptibility, and those with zones of 16 mm or less are resistant to the drug.

Dilution Susceptibility Tests

When dilution susceptibility testing (agar or broth dilution) is used to test susceptibility to ceftolozane and tazobactam, tests should be performed using serial dilutions of ceftolozane combined with a fixed tazobactam concentration of 4 mcg/mL.

When dilution susceptibility testing is performed according to CLSI standardized procedures, Enterobacteriaceae with ceftolozane MICs of 2 mcg/mL or less in the presence of 4 mcg/mL of tazobactam are susceptible to ceftolozane and tazobactam, isolates with ceftolozane MICs of 4 mcg/mL in the presence of 4 mcg/mL of tazobactam have intermediate resistance, and those with ceftolozane MICs of 8 mcg/mL or greater in the presence of 4 mcg/mL of tazobactam are resistant to the drug.

When susceptibility of Ps. aeruginosa is tested using dilution susceptibility testing, those with ceftolozane MICs of 4 mcg/mL or less in the presence of 4 mcg/mL of tazobactam are susceptible to ceftolozane and tazobactam, isolates with ceftolozane MICs of 8 mcg/mL in the presence of 4 mcg/mL of tazobactam have intermediate susceptibility, and those with ceftolozane MICs of 16 mcg/mL or greater in the presence of 4 mcg/mL of tazobactam are resistant to the drug.

When susceptibility of Bacteroides fragilis, Streptococcus anginosus, S. constellatus, or S. salivarius is tested using dilution susceptibility testing, isolates with ceftolozane MICs of 8 mcg/mL or less in the presence of 4 mcg/mL of tazobactam are susceptible to ceftolozane and tazobactam, those with ceftolozane MICs of 16 mcg/mL in the presence of 4 mcg/mL of tazobactam have intermediate susceptibility, and those with ceftolozane MICs of 32 mcg/mL or greater in the presence of 4 mcg/mL of tazobactam are resistant to the drug.

● Gram-positive Aerobic Bacteria

Ceftolozane and tazobactam is active in vitro against Streptococcus anginosus, S. constellatus, S. salivarius, S. agalactiae (group B streptococci, GBS), S. intermedius, S. pyogenes (group A β-hemolytic streptococci, GAS), and S. pneumoniae.

• Gram-negative Aerobic Bacteria

Ceftolozane and tazobactam is active in vitro against many Enterobacteriaceae, including *Enterobacter aerogenes, E. cloacae, Escherichia coli, Klebsiella oxytoca, K. pneumoniae, Proteus mirabilis, P. vulgaris, Citrobacter freundii, C. koseri, Morganella morganii, Providencia rettgeri, P. stuartii, Serratia liquefacians,* and *S. marcescens.* The fixed combination is active in vitro against some Enterobacteriaceae that produce one or more ESBLs, including certain TEM, SHV, CTX-M, or OXA β-lactamases.

Ceftolozane and tazobactam is active in vitro against *Ps. aeruginosa,* including some multidrug-resistant (MDR) strains. The fixed combination is active in vitro against *Ps. aeruginosa* resistant to some others drugs (e.g., ceftazidime, ciprofloxacin, imipenem, piperacillin and tazobactam, tobramycin) because of chromosomal AmpC β-lactamase, reduction in cell permeability because of loss of OprD, and/or up-regulation of efflux pumps (e.g., MexXY, MexAB).

Ceftolozane and tazobactam is active in vitro against *Acinetobacter baumannii, Burkholderia cepacia, Haemophilus influenzae, Moraxella catarrhalis,* and *Pantoea agglomerans.*

• Anaerobic Bacteria

Ceftolozane and tazobactam is active in vitro against some gram-negative anaerobic bacteria, including some strains of *Bacteroides fragilis, Fusobacterium,* and *Prevotella.*

The fixed combination also is active in vitro against some gram-positive anaerobic bacteria, including *Propionibacterium.*

RESISTANCE

Resistance or reduced susceptibility to ceftolozane and tazobactam can occur.

Bacteria that produce Ambler class B metallo-β-lactamases (MLBs) or serine carbapenemases (such as *Klebsiella pneumoniae* carbapenemase [KPC]) are resistant to ceftolozane and tazobactam because tazobactam does not inhibit these types of β-lactamases. Although some isolates of *Escherichia coli* and *K. pneumoniae* producing β-lactamases in certain enzyme groups (e.g., CTX-M, OXA, TEM, SHV) were susceptible to ceftolozane and tazobactam in vitro, other isolates of *E. coli* and *K. pneumoniae* producing β-lactamases in these enzyme groups were resistant to the drug. *Pseudomonas aeruginosa* with reduced susceptibility or resistance to ceftolozane and tazobactam have been produced in vitro.

Cross-resistance between ceftolozane and tazobactam and other cephalosporins may occur; however, some bacteria resistant to other cephalosporins may be susceptible to ceftolozane and tazobactam.

PHARMACOKINETICS

Following IV administration of the fixed combination of ceftolozane sulfate and tazobactam sodium, pharmacokinetic parameters for ceftolozane and tazobactam are similar to those reported when each drug is administered alone. In addition, pharmacokinetic parameters are similar following single or multiple IV doses of the fixed combination.

• Absorption

Peak plasma concentrations and areas under the plasma concentration-time curve (AUCs) of both ceftolozane and tazobactam increase in proportion to the dose of ceftolozane and tazobactam.

In healthy adults with normal renal function receiving multiple doses of ceftolozane and tazobactam (1.5 g [ceftolozane 1 g and tazobactam 0.5 g]) given by IV infusion over 1 hour every 8 hours for 10 days, peak plasma concentrations of ceftolozane and tazobactam are 74.4 and 18 mcg/mL, respectively, and are attained at approximately 1 hour.

There is no appreciable accumulation of ceftolozane or tazobactam in adults with normal renal function following multiple doses of ceftolozane and tazobactam given by IV infusion every 8 hours for 10 days.

In a population pharmacokinetic analysis, age, gender, and race did not result in clinically important differences in ceftolozane and tazobactam exposures.

• Distribution

The steady-state volumes of distribution of ceftolozane and tazobactam are 13.5 and 18.2 L, respectively, in healthy adult males following a single IV dose of ceftolozane and tazobactam, suggesting that both drugs distribute into extracellular space.

Ceftolozane and tazobactam were both distributed into pulmonary epithelial lining fluid following IV administration of ceftolozane and tazobactam in healthy adults.

Ceftolozane is approximately 16–21% bound to plasma proteins; tazobactam is 30% bound to plasma proteins.

It is not known whether ceftolozane crosses the placenta. Tazobactam crosses the placenta in rats; fetal concentrations in rats are 10% or less of maternal plasma concentrations.

It is not known whether ceftolozane or tazobactam is distributed into human milk.

• Elimination

Ceftolozane does not appear to be metabolized to any appreciable extent. Tazobactam is partially metabolized by hydrolysis of the β-lactam ring to form an inactive metabolite, M1.

Ceftolozane, tazobactam, and the MI metabolite of tazobactam are eliminated by the kidneys. Following a single IV dose of ceftolozane and tazobactam (1.5 g [ceftolozane 1 g and tazobactam 0.5 g]) in healthy adult males, more than 95% of the ceftolozane dose is eliminated in urine unchanged and more than 80% of the tazobactam dose is eliminated in urine unchanged (the remainder is eliminated as the M1 metabolite).

The plasma elimination half-lives of ceftolozane and tazobactam are approximately 3 and 1 hour, respectively, following multiple doses of ceftolozane and tazobactam in healthy adults with normal renal function.

In adults with mild, moderate, or severe renal impairment, the dose-normalized geometric mean AUC of ceftolozane is increased by 1.26-, 2.5-, or 5-fold, respectively, and the dose-normalized geometric mean AUC of tazobactam is increased by 1.3-, 2-, or 4-fold, respectively, compared with AUCs reported in healthy individuals with normal renal function.

Both ceftolozane and tazobactam are removed by hemodialysis. In adults with end-stage renal disease, a 4-hour hemodialysis session decreases the AUC of ceftolozane and tazobactam by approximately 66 and 56%, respectively.

CHEMISTRY AND STABILITY

• Chemistry

Ceftolozane sulfate and tazobactam sodium is a fixed combination of ceftolozane (a fifth generation cephalosporin antibiotic) and tazobactam (a β-lactamase inhibitor); tazobactam inactivates certain bacterial β-lactamases and expands ceftolozane's spectrum of activity against some bacteria that produce these β-lactamases.

Ceftolozane is structurally similar to ceftazidime and contains an aminothiadiazole ring that enhances antibacterial activity against gram-negative bacteria, an oxime group that contributes to stability in the presence of β-lactamases, and a dimethylacetic acid moiety that provides enhanced antipseudomonal activity. Unlike ceftazidime, ceftolozane contains a pyrazole ring at the 3-position of the cephem ring which prevents hydrolysis and improves stability against AmpC β-lactamase-overproducing *Pseudomonas aeruginosa.*

Tazobactam is a penicillanic acid sulfone β-lactamase inhibitor that is structurally similar to sulbactam. Tazobactam contains a β-lactam ring and a triazole group at the C-2 β-methyl position that facilitates binding to β-lactamases.

Ceftolozane and tazobactam is commercially available as a white to yellow powder for IV infusion containing a 2:1 ratio of ceftolozane to tazobactam. The ceftolozane component is provided as ceftolozane sulfate and the tazobactam component is provided as tazobactam sodium. Drug strength and dosage are expressed as the total of the 2 active components. (See Dispensing and Dosage and Administration Precautions under Administration: IV Infusion, in Dosage and Administration.)

Each single-dose vial of ceftolozane and tazobactam contains 1.5 g (1 g of ceftolozane [equivalent to 1.147 g of ceftolozane sulfate] and 0.5 g of tazobactam [equivalent to 0.537 g of tazobactam sulfate]). Each single-dose vial of the drug also contains 487 mg of sodium chloride as a stabilizing agent and 21 mg of citric acid and approximately 600 mg of L-arginine as excipients.

● Stability

Ceftolozane and tazobactam powder for IV infusion should be stored at 2–8°C and protected from light.

Following reconstitution and dilution, ceftolozane and tazobactam solutions may be stored for up to 24 hours at room temperature or for up to 7 days when refrigerated at 2–8°C.

PREPARATIONS

Excipients in commercially available drug preparations may have clinically important effects in some individuals; consult specific product labeling for details.

Ceftolozane Sulfate and Tazobactam Sodium

Parenteral

For injection, for IV infusion	1.5 g (1 g of ceftolozane and 0.5 g of tazobactam)	Zerbaxa®, Cubist

Selected Revisions August 25, 2023, © Copyright, October 19, 2015, American Society of Health-System Pharmacists, Inc.

Cefiderocol Sulfate Tosylate

8:12.06.28 • SIDEROPHORE CEPHALOSPORINS

■ Cefiderocol sulfate tosylate is a siderophore cephalosporin antibiotic.

USES

● Respiratory Tract Infections

Hospital-acquired and Ventilator-associated Bacterial Pneumonia

Cefiderocol sulfate tosylate is used for the treatment of hospital-acquired bacterial pneumonia and ventilator-associated bacterial pneumonia (HABP/VABP) caused by susceptible *Acinetobacter baumannii* complex, *Escherichia coli*, *Enterobacter cloacae* complex, *Klebsiella pneumoniae*, *Pseudomonas aeruginosa*, and *Serratia marcescens*.

Clinical Trials and Experience

Efficacy and safety of cefiderocol for the treatment of HABP/VABP have been evaluated in a multicenter, randomized, double-blind, parallel-group, phase 3 noninferiority trial that included a total of 298 adults hospitalized with acute bacterial pneumonia (hospital-acquired pneumonia, ventilator-associated pneumonia, or healthcare-associated pneumonia) known or suspected to be caused by gram-negative bacteria (NCT03032380; trial 2). Patients were randomized 1:1 to receive cefiderocol (2 g every 8 hours given by IV infusion over 3 hours) or meropenem (2 g every 8 hours given by IV infusion over 3 hours) for 7–14 days; treatment could be extended to 21 days based on clinical assessment of the patient and dosage was adjusted if needed based on renal function. Patients in both treatment arms received open-label treatment with linezolid (600 mg every 12 hours for at least 5 day) for empiric coverage against gram-positive bacteria. The trial protocol permitted prior therapy with other active antibacterials if such therapy lasted no more than 24 hours within 72 hours prior to randomization; however, concomitant antibacterial therapy (systemic or via oral inhalation) was not permitted from the time of randomization until the test-of-cure (TOC) visit 7 days after the end of treatment; the protocol did not permit step-down to oral anti-infectives during the study. The primary efficacy end point was all-cause mortality at day 14 in the modified intention-to-treat (mITT) population, which included all randomized patients who received study drug and had evidence of bacterial pneumonia, except those with only anaerobic or gram-positive aerobic infections; secondary efficacy end points included all-cause mortality at day 28 and clinical cure (defined as resolution or substantial improvement in signs and symptoms associated with pneumonia, with no additional antibacterial treatment required for the current infection through the TOC visit). There were 292 patients in the mITT population (145 in the cefiderocol arm and 147 in the meropenem arm); the median acute physiology and chronic health evaluation II [APACHE II] score was 15 (29% had a baseline APACHE II score of 20 or greater), 68% were in an intensive care unit (60% were mechanically ventilated), and gram-negative bacteremia was present at baseline in 6% of patients. The baseline creatinine clearance was 80 mL/minute or less in 60% of patients (50 mL/minute or less in 34%, and less than 30 mL/minute in 14% of these patients); augmented renal clearance (creatinine clearance greater than 120 mL/minute) was present in 16% of patients. In both treatment groups, most patients (70%) received the study drug for 7–14 days and 18% received the study drug for 15–21 days.

Results indicated that cefiderocol was noninferior to meropenem based on the 14-day all-cause mortality rate in the m-ITT population in patients with HABP/VABP caused by gram-negative bacteria. (See Table 1.)

TABLE 1. All-cause Mortality and Clinical Cure Rates at the TOC Visit in HABP/VABP Patients (m-ITT Population)

Study End Point	Cefiderocol	Meropenem
Day 14 all-cause mortality	12.4%	12.2%
Day 28 all-cause mortality	22.1%	21.1%
Clinical cure at TOC	64.8%	66.7%

Results for cefiderocol and meropenem were stratified according to baseline lower respiratory pathogens that were susceptible to meropenem. (See Table 2 and Table 3.) Data for patients with infections caused by extended-spectrum β-lactamase (ESBL) producers (31% of patients in the cefiderocol arm and 28.6% of patients in the meropenem arm) indicate that all-cause mortality rates at days 14 and 28 were consistent with the overall results. Although there were 51 patients with *A. baumannii* complex at baseline, only 17 of these patients (33.3%) had isolates that were susceptible to meropenem. Results for all 51 patients with *A. baumannii* complex (regardless of susceptibility to meropenem) indicate that all-cause mortality at day 14, all-cause mortality at day 28, and clinical cure rate at the TOC visit were 19, 34.6, and 53.8%, respectively, in the cefiderocol arm compared with 16, 24, and 60%, respectively, in the meropenem arm.

TABLE 2. All-cause Mortality Based on Baseline Pathogen Susceptible to Meropenem[a] in HABP/VABP Patients (mITT Population)

Baseline Pathogen	Day 14 All-cause Mortality: Cefiderocol	Day 14 All-cause Mortality: Meropenem	Day 28 All-cause Mortality: Cefiderocol	Day 28 All-cause Mortality: Meropenem
K. pneumoniae	10.5% (4/28)	11.1% (4/36)	21.1% (8/38)	25% (9/36)
E. coli	16.7% (3/18)	14.3% (3/21)	27.8% (5/18)	19% (4/21)
Other Enterobacterales[b]	12.5% (2/16)	14.3% (2/14)	25% (4/16)	21.4% (3/14)
A. baumannii complex[c]	12.5% (1/8)	0% (0/9)	37.5% (3/8)	0% (0/9)
Ps. aeruginosa	10% (2/20)	23.5% (4/17)	10% (2/20)	29.4% (5/17)

[a] Susceptible defined as meropenem MIC 8 mcg/mL or less.
[b] Includes *E. cloacae* complex (*E. cloacae, E. asburiae, E. kobei*) and *S. marcescens*.
[c] Includes *A. baumannii, A. nosocomialis*, and *A. pittii*.

TABLE 3. Clinical Cure Rate Based on Baseline Pathogen Susceptible to Meropenem[a] in HABP/VABP Patients (mITT Population)

Baseline Pathogen	Cefiderocol	Meropenem
K. pneumoniae	63.2% (24/38)	63.9% (24/36)
E. coli	66.7% (12/18)	61.9% (13/21)
Other Enterobacterales[b]	62.5% (10/16)	57.1% (8/14)
A. baumannii complex[c]	75% (6/8)	77.8% (7/9)
Ps. aeruginosa	65% (13/20)	76.5% (13/17)

[a] Susceptible defined as meropenem MIC 8 mcg/mL or less.
[b] Includes *E. cloacae* complex (*E. cloacae, E. asburiae, E. kobei*) and *S. marcescens*.
[c] Includes *A. baumannii, A. nosocomialis*, and *A. pittii*.

● Urinary Tract Infections

Complicated Urinary Tract Infections

Cefiderocol sulfate tosylate is used for the treatment of complicated urinary tract infections (cUTIs), including pyelonephritis, caused by susceptible *E. cloacae* complex, *E. coli*, *K. pneumoniae*, *Proteus mirabilis*, and *Ps. aeruginosa*. The drug is one of several preferred options for the treatment of cUTIs caused by carbapenem-resistant Enterobacterales (CRE) and cUTIs caused by *Ps. aeruginosa* with difficult-to-treat (DTR) resistance.

Clinical Trials and Experience

Efficacy and safety of cefiderocol for the treatment of cUTIs, including pyelonephritis, were evaluated in a multinational, randomized, double-blind, parallel group phase 2 trial that included a total of 448 hospitalized adults (NCT02321800; trial 1). Patients were randomized 2:1 to receive cefiderocol (2 g every 8 hours given by IV infusion over 1 hour) or the fixed combination of imipenem and cilastatin sodium (1 g of imipenem every 8 hours given as imipenem/cilastatin by IV infusion over 1 hour) for 7–14 days. The trial protocol did not permit a switch from IV to oral antibacterial therapy. Patients were excluded if baseline urine cultures indicated more than 2 uropathogens, fungal UTI, or uropathogens known to be carbapenem resistant. The primary efficacy end point was a composite of microbiologic eradication and clinical cure at the TOC visit in the microbiologic ITT (micro-ITT) population, which included all patients who received at least one dose of study drug and had at least one baseline gram-negative uropathogen. Other efficacy end points included the microbiologic eradication rate and the clinical response rate at TOC in the micro-ITT population. The micro-ITT population included 371 patients (252 in the cefiderocol arm and 119 in the imipenem/cilastatin arm); 25% had cUTI with pyelonephritis, 48% had cUTI without pyelonephritis, and 27% had acute uncomplicated pyelonephritis; complicating conditions included obstructive uropathy, catheterization, and renal stones; the most common baseline pathogens were *E. coli* and *K. pneumoniae*; and concomitant gram-negative bacteremia was identified in 7%. At baseline, creatinine clearance was greater than 50-80 mL/minute in 32%, 30-50 mL/minute in 17%, and less than 30 mL/minute in 3% of the micro-ITT population.

Results indicated that the composite end point of microbiologic eradication (defined as all gram-negative uropathogens found at baseline at concentrations of 10^5 CFU/mL or greater reduced to less than 10^4 CFU/mL) and clinical response (defined as resolution or improvement of cUTI symptoms and no new symptoms assessed by the investigator) at the TOC visit were greater in the cefiderocol arm compared with the imipenem/cilastatin arm. (See Table 4.) Although the microbiologic response at the TOC visit was greater with cefiderocol compared with imipenem/cilastatin, clinical response rates at the TOC visit were similar. Most patients who had microbiologic failure at the TOC visit in either treatment arm did not require further antibacterial treatment.

TABLE 4. Composite, Microbiologic, and Clinical Response Rates at the TOC Visit in cUTI Patients (micro-ITT Population)

Study End Point	Cefiderocol	Imipenem/Cilastatin
Composite response	72.6%	54.6%
Microbiologic response	73%	56.3%
Clinical response	89.7%	87.4%

When results for cefiderocol and imipenem/cilastatin were stratified according to baseline pathogens, results for the composite outcome at the TOC visit were consistent with those in the overall population. (See Table 5.) For bacterial isolates that were ESBL producers (24.2% of isolates in the cefiderocol arm and 26.9% of isolates in the imipenem/cilastatin arm), the composite response rate at the TOC visit also was consistent with the overall results.

TABLE 5. Composite End Point of Microbiologic Eradication and Clinical Response Rates in cUTI Patients Based on Baseline Pathogen[a] (micro-ITT Population)

Baseline Pathogen	Cefiderocol	Imipenem/Cilastatin
E. coli	74.3% (113/152)	57% (45/79)
K. pneumoniae	75% (36/48)	48% (12/25)
P. mirabilis	76.5% (13/17)	0% (0/2)
E. cloacae complex	61.5% (8/13)	60% (3/5)
Ps. aeruginosa	44.4% (8/18)	100% (3/3)

[a] Patients may have had more than one pathogen in the baseline culture.

Additional subgroup analyses examining outcomes by age, gender, and/or outcomes in patients with renal impairment, concomitant bacteremia, or acute uncomplicated pyelonephritis also indicated that results were consistent with those in the overall population.

DOSAGE AND ADMINISTRATION

● Administration

Cefiderocol sulfate tosylate is administered by IV infusion.

Cefiderocol sulfate tosylate is commercially available as a white to off-white, sterile, lyophilized powder that must be reconstituted and diluted prior to IV infusion.

Although the drug is compatible with 0.9% sodium chloride injection and 5% dextrose injection, compatibility with other diluents or other drugs has not been established to date.

IV Infusion
Reconstitution and Dilution

The appropriate number of single-use vials labeled as containing 1 g of cefiderocol should be reconstituted by adding 10 mL of 0.9% sodium chloride injection or 5% dextrose injection to each vial. The vial(s) should be gently shaken to dissolve the powder and then allowed to stand until foaming disappears (typically takes no more than 2 minutes). The final volume in each reconstituted vial is approximately 11.2 mL. Reconstituted cefiderocol preferably should be immediately diluted by transferring to an appropriate IV infusion bag, but may be stored in the vial for up to 1 hour at room temperature.

To prepare the diluted solution, the appropriate volume of reconstituted cefiderocol should be transferred from the vial(s) into a 100-mL IV infusion bag containing 0.9% sodium chloride injection or 5% dextrose injection. (See Table 6.)

TABLE 6. Instructions for Preparing Doses of Cefiderocol Using Reconstituted 1-g Vials of the Drug

Cefiderocol Dose	Required Number of Reconstituted 1-g Vials of Cefiderocol	Total Volume of Reconstituted Cefiderocol to be Transferred from Vial(s) into a 100-mL IV Infusion Bag
2 g	2	22.4 mL (11.2 mL [entire contents] from each vial)
1.5 g	2	16.8 mL (11.2 mL from first vial **and** 5.6 mL from second vial)
1 g	1	11.2 mL (entire contents of vial)
0.75 g	1	8.4 mL

Reconstituted and diluted cefiderocol solutions should be inspected visually for particulate matter and discoloration prior to administration. The solution should appear clear and colorless and should not be used if it is discolored or contains particulates. Any vials containing unused reconstituted cefiderocol solution should be discarded.

The reconstituted and diluted cefiderocol solution is stable in the IV infusion bag for up to 6 hours at room temperature. Although the diluted solution may be stored for up to 24 hours in a refrigerator at 2–8°C protected from light; the IV infusion should be completed within 6 hours after removal from refrigeration.

Rate of Administration

IV infusions of cefiderocol should be given over 3 hours.

● Dosage

Dosage of cefiderocol sulfate tosylate is expressed in terms of cefiderocol.

Adult Dosage
Hospital-acquired and Ventilator-associated Bacterial Pneumonia (HABP/VABP)

For the treatment of HABP/VABP caused by susceptible gram-negative bacteria in adults, the recommended dosage of cefiderocol is 2 g IV every 8 hours in those with creatinine clearance of 60–119 mL/minute. In those with creatinine clearance of 120 mL/minute or greater (e.g., seriously ill patients receiving IV fluid resuscitation), the recommended dosage is 2 g IV every 6 hours.

The recommended duration of cefiderocol treatment is 7–14 days; treatment duration should be guided by the clinical status of the patient.

Complicated Urinary Tract Infections (cUTIs)

For the treatment of cUTIs caused by susceptible gram-negative bacteria in adults, the recommended dosage of cefiderocol is 2 g IV every 8 hours in those with creatinine clearance of 60–119 mL/minute. In those with creatinine clearance of 120 mL/minute or greater (e.g., seriously ill patients receiving IV fluid resuscitation), the recommended dosage is 2 g IV every 6 hours.

The recommended duration of cefiderocol treatment is 7–14 days; treatment duration should be guided by the clinical status of the patient.

● Special Populations

Hepatic Impairment

Adjustment of cefiderocol dosage is not necessary in patients with hepatic impairment. (See Hepatic Impairment under Cautions.)

Renal Impairment

Cefiderocol dosage must be reduced in adults with creatinine clearance less than 60 mL/minute, including those receiving intermitted hemodialysis or continuous renal replacement therapy (CRRT). (See Table 7 and Table 8.)

In those with fluctuating renal function, regularly monitor creatinine clearance during treatment with the drug and adjust dosage as needed. (See Renal Impairment under Cautions.)

TABLE 7. Recommended Cefiderocol Dosage in Adults with Creatinine Clearance less than 60 mL/minute

Estimated Creatinine Clearance[a]	Recommended Dosage
30–59 mL/minute	1.5 g every 8 hours
15–29 mL/minute	1 g every 8 hours
<15 mL/minute (with or without intermittent hemodialysis)[b]	0.75 g every 12 hours

[a] Creatinine clearance estimated by Cockcroft-Gault equation.
[b] Cefiderocol is removed by hemodialysis (60% of a dose removed by 3- to 4-hour hemodialysis session); administer initial dose immediately after a hemodialysis session.

● Dosage in Patients Receiving Continuous Renal Replacement Therapy (CRRT)

Dosage of cefiderocol in patients receiving CRRT, including continuous venovenous hemofiltration (CVVH), continuous venovenous hemodialysis (CVVHD), and continuous venovenous hemodiafiltration (CVVHDF) should be based on the CRRT effluent flow rate. The following dosage recommendations for such patients is intended to provide initial cefiderocol dosage; dosage may need to be adjusted based on residual renal function and the clinical status of the patient. (See Table 8.)

TABLE 8. Recommended Cefiderocol Dosage[a] in Adults with Creatinine Clearance less than 60 mL/minute Receiving CRRT

Effluent Flow Rate[b]	Recommended Dosage
≤2 L/hr	1.5 g every 12 hours
2.1–3 L/hr	2 g every 12 hours
3.1–4 L/hr	1.5 g every 8 hours
≥4.1 L/hr	2 g every 8 hours

[a] Dosage recommendations for CRRT patients are intended to provide initial cefiderocol dosage; may need to adjust dosage based on residual renal function and clinical status of patient.
[b] Ultrafiltrate flow rate for CVVH, dialysis flow rate for CVVHD, ultrafiltrate flow rate plus dialysis flow rate for CVVHDF.

Geriatric Patients

Dosage of cefiderocol should be selected with caution in geriatric patients. Dosage adjustments are not required based on age, but dosage should be adjusted based on renal function. (See Geriatric Use under Cautions.)

CAUTIONS

● Contraindications

Cefiderocol sulfate tosylate is contraindicated in patients with known history of severe hypersensitivity to cefiderocol or other β-lactam antibacterials or other components of the preparation.

● Warnings/Precautions

Increased All-cause Mortality in Patients with Carbapenem-resistant Gram-negative Bacterial Infections

An increase in all-cause mortality was observed in patients treated with cefiderocol compared with best available therapy (BAT) in a multinational, randomized, open-label trial in critically-ill patients with carbapenem-resistant gram-negative bacterial infections (NCT02714595). Patients with nosocomial pneumonia, bloodstream infections†, sepsis†, or complicated UTIs (cUTIs) were included in the trial. BAT regimens varied according to local practices and consisted of 1–3 antibacterials with activity against gram-negative bacteria; most of the BAT regimens contained colistin (commercially available in the US as colistimethate sodium).

The increase in all-cause mortality occurred in patients treated for nosocomial pneumonia, bloodstream infections, or sepsis. The 28-day all-cause mortality was higher in patients treated with cefiderocol (24.8%) than in those treated with BAT (18.4%); all-cause mortality through day 49 remained higher in those treated with cefiderocol. Generally, deaths were in patients with infections caused by gram-negative bacteria, including non-fermenters such as *A. baumannii* complex, *Stenotrophomonas maltophilia*, and *Ps. aeruginosa*, and were the result of worsening or complications of infection or underlying comorbidities. The cause of the increase in mortality has not been established.

Clinical response should be closely monitored in patients receiving cefiderocol for the treatment of hospital-acquired and ventilator-associated bacterial pneumonia (HABP/VABP) or cUTIs.

Hypersensitivity Reactions

Serious and occasionally fatal hypersensitivity (anaphylactic) reactions and serious skin reactions have been reported in patients receiving β-lactam antibacterials. In clinical trials, hypersensitivity reactions were observed in some cefiderocol-treated patients. Such reactions are more likely to occur in individuals with a history of β-lactam hypersensitivity and/or a history of sensitivity to multiple allergens. There have been reports of individuals with a history of penicillin hypersensitivity who experienced severe reactions when treated with cephalosporins.

Prior to initiation of cefiderocol therapy, patients should be queried about previous hypersensitivity reactions to cephalosporins, penicillins, or other β-lactam antibacterials.

Cefiderocol should be discontinued if an allergic reaction occurs.

Superinfection/Clostridioides difficile-associated Diarrhea

Use of cefiderocol may result in emergence and overgrowth of nonsusceptible organisms (e.g., *Candida*).

Treatment with anti-infectives alters normal colon flora and may permit overgrowth of *Clostridioides difficile* (formerly *Clostridium difficile*). *C. difficile* infection (CDI) and *C. difficile*-associated diarrhea and colitis (CDAD; also known as antibiotic-associated diarrhea and colitis or pseudomembranous colitis) have been reported with nearly all anti-infectives, including cefiderocol, and may range in severity from mild diarrhea to fatal colitis. *C. difficile* produces toxins A and B which contribute to development of CDAD; hypertoxin-producing strains of *C. difficile* are associated with increased morbidity and mortality since they may be refractory to anti-infectives and colectomy may be required.

CDAD should be considered in the differential diagnosis of patients who develop diarrhea during or after anti-infective therapy. Careful medical history is necessary since CDAD has been reported to occur as late as 2 months or longer after anti-infective therapy is discontinued.

If CDAD is suspected or confirmed, antibacterial therapy not directed against *C. difficile* should be discontinued whenever possible. Patients should be managed with appropriate anti-infective therapy directed against *C. difficile* (e.g., fidaxomicin, vancomycin, metronidazole), supportive therapy (e.g., fluid and electrolyte management, protein supplementation), and surgical evaluation as clinically indicated.

Seizures and Other CNS Adverse Reactions

Cephalosporins, including cefiderocol, have been implicated in triggering seizures. Nonconvulsive status epilepticus (NCSE), encephalopathy, coma, asterixis, neuromuscular excitability, and myoclonia have been reported with cephalosporins, particularly in patients with a history of epilepsy and/or when recommended dosages of cephalosporins were exceeded in patients with renal impairment.

Cefiderocol dosage should be based on creatinine clearance (see Dosage under Dosage and Administration). In patients with known seizure disorder, anticonvulsant therapy should be continued during cefiderocol therapy.

If CNS adverse reactions (including seizures) occur, patients should undergo a neurological evaluation to determine whether cefiderocol should be discontinued.

Selection and Use of Anti-infectives

To reduce development of drug-resistant bacteria and maintain effectiveness of cefiderocol and other antibacterials, the drug should be used only for the treatment of infections proven or strongly suspected to be caused by susceptible bacteria.

When selecting or modifying anti-infective therapy, results of culture and in vitro susceptibility testing should be used. In the absence of such data, local epidemiology and susceptibility patterns should be considered when selecting anti-infectives for empiric therapy.

Information on test methods and quality control standards for in vitro susceptibility testing of antibacterial agents and specific interpretive criteria for such testing recognized by FDA is available at https://www.fda.gov/STIC. For most antibacterial agents, including cefiderocol, FDA recognizes the standards published by the Clinical and Laboratory Standards Institute (CLSI).

Laboratory Test Interference

Cefiderocol may cause false-positive results in urine dipstick tests (e.g., urine protein, ketones, or occult blood). If positive results are reported for such dipstick tests, alternative clinical laboratory methods of testing should be used to confirm the results.

Specific Populations

Pregnancy

There are no data available on use of cefiderocol in pregnant women to evaluate for a drug-associated risk of major birth defects, miscarriage, or adverse maternal or fetal outcomes.

Although available studies cannot definitively establish an absence of risk, published data from prospective cohort studies, case series, and case reports over several decades regarding use of cephalosporins in pregnant women have not identified an association between cephalosporin use during pregnancy and major birth defects, miscarriage, or other adverse maternal or fetal outcomes. Available studies have methodologic limitations, including small sample size, retrospective data collection, and inconsistent comparator groups.

In developmental toxicity studies in rats and mice, there was no evidence of embryofetal toxicity, including drug-induced fetal malformations or reductions in fetal viability, when cefiderocol was administered during organogenesis at dosages providing mean AUCs 0.9 times (rats) or 1.3 times (mice) higher than the daily mean plasma exposure reported in patients with cUTIs receiving 2 g of cefiderocol by IV infusion every 8 hours. In a pre- and postnatal development study, cefiderocol was administered IV at doses up to 1 g/kg daily to rats from day 6 of pregnancy until weaning. No adverse effects on parturition, maternal function, or pre- and postnatal development and viability of the pups were observed.

Cefiderocol crosses the placenta in pregnant rats (less than 0.5% of a dose detected in fetuses).

Lactation

It is not known whether cefiderocol distributes into human milk, affects breast-fed infants, or affects milk production.

Cefiderocol is distributed into milk in rats (peak concentrations in milk are reported to be approximately 6% of peak plasma concentrations).

The developmental and health benefits of breast-feeding should be considered along with the mother's clinical need for cefiderocol and any potential adverse effects on the breast-fed child from cefiderocol or from the underlying maternal condition.

Pediatric Use

Safety and efficacy of cefiderocol have not been established in patients younger than 18 years of age.

Geriatric Use

Of the 148 patients with HABP/VABP who received cefiderocol in a clinical trial, 83 (56.1%) were 65 years of age and older, and 40 (27%) were 75 years of age and older. The incidence of adverse reactions reported in patients 65 years of age or older was similar to that reported in younger adults, and the incidence did not differ between those 65 years of age and older and those 75 years of age and older.

Of the 300 patients with cUTIs who received cefiderocol in a clinical trial, 158 (52.7%) were 65 years of age and older, and 67 (22.3%) were 75 years of age and older. No overall differences in safety or efficacy were observed between these patients and younger adults.

Cefiderocol is known to be substantially excreted by the kidneys, and the risk of adverse reactions to the drug may be greater in patients with impaired renal function. Because elderly patients are more likely to have decreased renal function, care should be taken when selecting dosage and it may be useful to monitor renal function. Although dosage adjustments are not required based on age, dosage should be based on renal function. (See Renal Impairment under Dosage and Administration.)

Hepatic Impairment

Although the effects of hepatic impairment on the pharmacokinetics of cefiderocol have not been evaluated, hepatic impairment is not expected to alter cefiderocol elimination since hepatic metabolism/excretion represents a minor pathway of elimination for the drug.

Renal Impairment

Dosage adjustment of cefiderocol is required in patients with creatinine clearance less than 60 mL/minute, including those receiving hemodialysis.

Dosage adjustment of cefiderocol is required in patients receiving CRRT, including CVVH, CVVHD, and CVVHDF; dosage in such patients should be based on the effluent flow rate. (See Renal Impairment under Dosage.) Consider that residual renal function may change in patients receiving CRRT and improvements or reductions in residual renal function may warrant a change in cefiderocol dosage. A total of 16 patients receiving CRRT were included in cefiderocol clinical trials to date.

Renal function should be monitored regularly during cefiderocol therapy and dosage should be adjusted as needed.

● Common Adverse Effects

Patients with HABP/VABP: The most frequent adverse effects reported in 4% or more of patients treated with cefiderocol were elevated liver enzymes, hypokalemia, diarrhea, hypomagnesemia, and atrial fibrillation.

Patients with cUTIs: The most frequently reported adverse effects reported in 2% or more of patients treated with cefiderocol include diarrhea, infusion site reactions, constipation, rash, candidiasis (oral or vulvovaginal candidiasis, candiduria), cough, elevated liver enzymes, headache, hypokalemia, nausea, and vomiting.

DRUG INTERACTIONS

In vitro, cefiderocol does not inhibit cytochrome P-450 (CYP) isoenzymes 1A2, 2B6, 2C8, 2C9, 2C19, 2D6, 2E1, or 3A4. The drug is not an inducer of CYP1A2, 2B6, or 3A4 in vitro.

In vitro, cefiderocol is not an inhibitor of P-glycoprotein (P-gp), breast cancer resistance protein (BCRP), bile salt export pump transporters, organic anion transporting polypeptide (OATP) 1B1, or multidrug and toxin extrusion (MATE) 1, and is not a substrate of P-gp, BCRP, organic anion transporter (OAT) 1, OAT3, organic cation transporter (OCT) 2, MATE1, or MATE2-K.

Concomitant use of cefiderocol did not result in clinically important effects on the pharmacokinetics of furosemide (OAT1 and OAT3 substrate), metformin (OCT1, OCT2, and MATE2-K substrate), or rosuvastatin (OATP1B3 substrate).

● *Antibacterials*

There was no in vitro evidence of antagonism between cefiderocol and amikacin, the fixed combination of ceftazidime and avibactam (ceftazidime/avibactam), the fixed combination of ceftolozane sulfate and tazobactam sodium (ceftolozane/tazobactam), ciprofloxacin, clindamycin, colistin, daptomycin, linezolid, meropenem, metronidazole, tigecycline, or vancomycin against Enterobacterales, *Ps. aeruginosa*, or *A. baumannii*.

Synergism between cefiderocol and some antibacterials (e.g., levofloxacin, polymyxin B, co-trimoxazole) against *S. maltophilia* has been demonstrated in vitro.

● *β-Lactamase Inhibitors*

In vitro studies indicate that combined use of cefiderocol and a β-lactamase inhibitor (e.g., avibactam, clavulanic acid, dipicolinic acid [not commercially available in the US]) results in lower MICs than use of the drug alone.

DESCRIPTION

Cefiderocol sulfate tosylate is a siderophore cephalosporin antibacterial. The drug is a conjugate that contains a cephalosporin core with side chains similar to those in some other cephalosporins (cefepime, ceftazidime) and a catechol group that functions as an iron-chelating siderophore. This structure and the unique mechanism of action of cefiderocol results in enhanced stability against hydrolysis by many β-lactamases, including extended-spectrum β-lactamases (ESBLs) (e.g., TEM, SHV, CTX-M) and carbapenemases (e.g., KPC, NDM, VIM, IMP, OXA-23, OXA-48-like, OXA-51-like, OXA-58).

Cefiderocol is actively transported across the outer bacterial cell membrane into the periplasmic space by a siderophore iron uptake mechanism. In addition, passive diffusion of the drug into bacterial cells occurs via porin channels. After entry into the periplasmic space, cefiderocol dissociates from the iron and binds to penicillin-binding proteins (PBPs), primarily PBP3, and inhibits peptidoglycan synthesis. In vitro studies indicate that cefiderocol usually is bactericidal in action.

Following IV infusion of cefiderocol sulfate tosylate, peak plasma concentrations and AUC of cefiderocol increase proportionally with dose. Mean peak plasma concentrations of cefiderocol in patients with hospital-acquired and ventilator-associated bacterial pneumonia (HABP/VABP) or complicated urinary tract infections (cUTIs) receiving 2 g of cefiderocol every 8 hours given by IV infusion over 3 hours (dosage adjusted based on renal function) were 111 or 115 mg/L, respectively. In patients with pneumonia requiring mechanical ventilation who received a 2-g dose by IV infusion over 3 hours (dose adjusted based on renal function) at steady state, cefiderocol concentrations in epithelial lining fluid ranged from 3.1–20.7 mg/L and 7.2–15.9 mg/L at the end of the IV infusion and at 2 hours after completion of the infusion, respectively. Cefiderocol is 40–60% bound to plasma proteins, primarily albumin. Cefiderocol is minimally metabolized (less than 10% of a dose). The drug is primarily excreted by the kidneys. After a single 1-g radiolabeled dose of cefiderocol given by IV infusion over 1 hour, 98.6% of total radioactivity was excreted in urine (90.6% as unchanged drug) and 2.8% was excreted in feces. The terminal elimination half-life of cefiderocol is 2–3 hours. The AUC of cefiderocol increases with decreasing renal function. In vitro data indicate that the effluent flow rate of CRRT is the major determinant of cefiderocol clearance. In patients receiving CRRT, dosage recommendations based on flow rate (see Renal Impairment under Dosage and Administration) are predicted to provide cefiderocol exposures similar to those observed when a dosage of 2 g every 8 hours is used in patients not receiving CRRT. Increased cefiderocol clearance has been observed in patients with creatinine clearances of

120 mL/minute or greater (e.g., seriously ill patients receiving IV fluids); increasing dosage to 2 g every 6 hours in such patients provides cefiderocol exposures comparable to those observed in patients with creatinine clearances of 90–119 mL/minute receiving a dosage of 2 g every 8 hours. Age (18–19 years of age), sex, and race do not have clinically important effects on the pharmacokinetics of the drug. The effect of hepatic impairment on the pharmacokinetics of cefiderocol has not been evaluated.

● *Spectrum*

Cefiderocol has a spectrum of activity that includes various gram-negative aerobic bacteria, including some multidrug-resistant gram-negative aerobic bacteria. Although cefiderocol has variable activity against some gram-positive bacteria and anaerobes in vitro, this activity is not considered clinically relevant.

Cefiderocol is active in vitro and in clinical infections (HABP/VABP, cUTIs) against *E. coli, E. cloacae* complex, *K. pneumoniae*, and *Ps. aeruginosa*. The drug also is active in vitro and in clinical infections (HABP/VABP) against *A. baumannii* complex and *S. marcescens* and is active in vitro and in clinical infections (cUTIs) caused by *P. mirabilis*.

Although cefiderocol is active in vitro against some other gram-negative aerobes, including *Achromobacter, Burkholderia cepacia* complex, *Citrobacter freundii* complex, *C. koseri, K. aerogenes, K. oxytoca, Morganella morganii, P. vulgaris, Providencia rettgeri*, and *Stenotrophomonas maltophilia*, the clinical importance of this in vitro activity is not known and efficacy for the treatment of infections caused by these bacteria has not been established in adequate and well-controlled clinical studies.

Cefiderocol has been active in vitro against some *S. maltophilia* isolates and a subset of isolates of Enterobacterales and *Ps. aeruginosa* resistant to other antibacterials (meropenem, fluoroquinolones, amikacin, cefepime, ceftazidime/avibactam, ceftolozane/tazobactam) and has been active in vitro against a subset of isolates of *A. baumannii* complex resistant to meropenem, ciprofloxacin, and amikacin. Cefiderocol is active against some colistin-resistant *E. coli* isolates containing *mcr*-1.

Cefiderocol demonstrated in vitro activity against a subgroup of Enterobacterales genetically confirmed to contain the following resistance mechanisms: ESBLs (TEM, SHV, CTX-M, oxacillinase [OXA]), AmpC, AmpC-type ESBL (CMY), serine-carbapenemases (such as KPC, OXA-48), and metallo-carbapenemases (such as NDM and VIM). The drug also demonstrated in vitro activity against a subgroup of *Ps. aeruginosa* genetically confirmed to contain VIM, IMP, GES, and AmpC; a subgroup of *A. baumannii* containing OXA-23, OXA-24/40, OXA-51, OXA-58, and AmpC; and a subgroup of *S. maltophilia* containing metallo-carbapenemase (L1) and serine β-lactamases.

In vitro, cefiderocol remained active against *K. pneumoniae* in the presence of porin channel deletions (OmpK35/36) and against *Ps. aeruginosa* in the presence of porin channel deletions (OprD) and efflux pump up-regulation (MexAB-OprM, MexCD-OprJ, MexEF-OprN, and MexXY).

● *Resistance*

In vitro studies indicate that a combination of β-lactamases (including AmpC β-lactamase overproduction), modifications of PBPs, and mutations of transcriptional regulators that impact siderophore or efflux pump expression can result in increased cefiderocol MICs and may result in resistance to the drug in gram-negative bacteria.

A. baumannii with reduced in vitro susceptibility or resistance to cefiderocol has been reported. In one study, there was no clear relationship between cefiderocol resistance in *A. baumannii* and the presence of acquired β-lactamases (TEM-1, SHV-5 or SHV-12, or OXA-23) or with the expression of chromosomal β-lactamases.

Cefiderocol does not induce AmpC β-lactamase in *P. aeruginosa* or *E. cloacae*. Following in vitro exposure of gram-negative bacteria (including carbapenemase producers) to cefiderocol concentrations 10 times the MIC, the frequency of resistance development in these bacteria ranged from 10^{-6} to less than 10^{-8}.

E. cloacae complex with AmpC-mediated resistance to ceftazidime/avibactam that also was resistant to cefepime and had reduced susceptibility to cefiderocol in vitro has been reported. Cross-resistance between cefiderocol and other antibacterial classes has not been reported to date.

ADVICE TO PATIENTS

Advise patients that antibacterials, including cefiderocol, should only be used to treat bacterial infections and not used to treat viral infections (e.g., the common cold).

Importance of completing full course of therapy, even if feeling better after a few days.

Advise patients that skipping doses or not completing the full course of therapy may decrease effectiveness and increase the likelihood that bacteria will develop resistance and will not be treatable with cefiderocol or other antibacterials in the future.

Advise patients and their families that allergic reactions, including serious allergic reactions, could occur with cefiderocol and that serious reactions require immediate treatment. Ask patients about any previous hypersensitivity reactions to cefiderocol, other β-lactams (including cephalosporins), or other allergens.

Advise patients that diarrhea is a common problem caused by antibacterials. Sometimes, frequent watery or bloody diarrhea may occur and may be a sign of a more serious intestinal infection. Importance of contacting a clinician if severe watery or bloody diarrhea develops.

Inform patients that cephalosporins have been implicated in triggering seizures, particularly in patients with renal impairment when dosage was not reduced and in patients with a history of epilepsy.

Importance of informing clinicians of existing or contemplated concomitant therapy, including prescription and OTC drugs and dietary or herbal supplements, as well as any concomitant illnesses.

Importance of women informing clinicians if they are or plan to become pregnant or plan to breast-feed.

Importance of informing patients of other important precautionary information. (See Cautions.)

PREPARATIONS

Excipients in commercially available drug preparations may have clinically important effects in some individuals; consult specific product labeling for details.

Cefiderocol Sulfate Tosylate

Parenteral

For Injection, for IV use	1 g (of cefiderocol)	**Fetroja®** Shionogi

† Use is not currently included in the labeling approved by the US Food and Drug Administration.

Meropenem and Vaborbactam

8:12.07.08 • CARBAPENEMS

■ Meropenem and vaborbactam is a fixed combination of meropenem (a carbapenem β-lactam antibiotic) and vaborbactam (a non-β-lactam β-lactamase inhibitor); vaborbactam inactivates certain bacterial β-lactamases and expands meropenem's spectrum of activity against some bacteria that produce these β-lactamases.

USES

● Urinary Tract Infections

Meropenem and vaborbactam is used for the treatment of complicated urinary tract infections, including pyelonephritis, caused by susceptible *Escherichia coli*, *Klebsiella pneumoniae*, or *Enterobacter cloacae* species complex.

Clinical Experience

Efficacy and safety of meropenem and vaborbactam for the treatment of complicated urinary tract infections is based on results from a phase 3, randomized, double-blind, noninferiority study in 545 adults with complicated urinary tract infections, including pyelonephritis. Patients were randomized in a 1:1 ratio to receive treatment with the fixed combination of meropenem and vaborbactam (4 g [meropenem 2 g and vaborbactam 2 g] given by IV infusion every 8 hours) or the fixed combination of piperacillin and tazobactam (4.5 g [piperacillin 4 g and tazobactam 0.5 g] given by IV infusion every 8 hours). After at least 15 doses of IV treatment, patients with clinical improvement (afebrile for at least 24 hours, urinary tract infection symptoms and leukocytosis improved, urine culture at 24 hours with growth less than 10^4 CFU/mL, negative blood culture in those with bacteremia, able to tolerate oral medications) were permitted to switch to an oral antibacterial (e.g., levofloxacin). The planned total duration of IV and oral anti-infective treatment was 10 days; patients with bacteremia could receive up to 14 days of treatment. The primary efficacy end point was overall success at the end of IV treatment visit (defined as the composite end point of successful clinical outcome [investigator judgment of cure or improvement] *and* microbiologic outcome [baseline pathogen(s) reduced to less than 10^4 CFU/mL on urine culture]). Baseline characteristics were generally similar between treatment groups (mean age 54 years, 93% white, 66% female, 17–19% with diabetes mellitus, 6–8% with bacteremia identified at baseline, 59% with pyelonephritis, 40% with complicated urinary tract infection). The mean duration of IV treatment was 8 days and the mean total treatment duration (IV and oral antibacterial treatment) was 10 days in both groups. Overall success at the end of IV treatment visit was achieved by substantially more patients receiving meropenem and vaborbactam compared with those receiving piperacillin and tazobactam (98.4% versus 94.3%, respectively). At the test-of-cure visit 7 days after completion of treatment in a subset of patients that excluded those with baseline pathogens resistant to piperacillin and tazobactam, the overall success rate in patients receiving meropenem and vaborbactam was noninferior to the success rate in those receiving piperacillin and tazobactam (76.5% versus 73.2%, respectively). In the microbiologically modified intent-to-treat population, the rate of clinical and microbiologic response in patients with bacteremia at baseline who received meropenem and vaborbactam was 83.3%.

DOSAGE AND ADMINISTRATION

● Administration

Meropenem and vaborbactam is administered by IV infusion.

IV Infusion
Reconstitution and Dilution

Meropenem and vaborbactam powder for injection must be reconstituted and further diluted prior to IV infusion.

Single-dose vials of meropenem and vaborbactam labeled as containing 2 g (meropenem 1 g and vaborbactam 1 g) should be reconstituted by withdrawing 20 mL of 0.9% sodium chloride injection from an infusion bag and adding that to the vial and gently mixing. The volume of reconstituted solution in the vial is approximately 21.3 mL and the approximate concentration is meropenem 50 mg/mL and vaborbactam 50 mg/mL.

Immediately after reconstitution and prior to IV infusion, the reconstituted meropenem and vaborbactam solution *must* be further diluted. To prepare the indicated dose, the appropriate volume of reconstituted solution should be withdrawn from the vial(s) and added back into the 0.9% sodium chloride injection infusion bag. (See Table 1.) The final concentration of meropenem and of vaborbactam in the infusion solution is approximately 2–8 mg/mL.

TABLE 1. Dilution of Reconstituted Meropenem and Vaborbactam

Recommended Dose of Meropenem and Vaborbactam	Volume to Withdraw from Reconstituted Vial(s) for Further Dilution	Volume of Infusion Bag
4 g (meropenem 2 g and vaborbactam 2 g)	Entire contents of 2 reconstituted vials (approximately 21 mL from *each* vial)	250–1000 mL
2 g (meropenem 1 g and vaborbactam 1 g)	Entire contents of 1 reconstituted vial (approximately 21 mL)	125–500 mL
1 g (meropenem 0.5 g and vaborbactam 0.5 g)	10.5 mL of reconstituted solution	70–250 mL

The reconstituted and diluted solution of meropenem and vaborbactam should be inspected visually for particulate matter and discoloration prior to administration; the solution should appear colorless to light yellow.

Unused portions of the reconstituted and diluted solution should be discarded.

Following reconstitution and dilution, IV infusion of meropenem and vaborbactam solutions *must* be completed within 4 hours if stored at room temperature. Alternatively, IV infusion of these solutions *must* be completed within 22 hours if stored under refrigeration (2–8°C).

Rate of Administration

IV infusions of meropenem and vaborbactam should be given over 3 hours.

Dispensing and Dosage and Administration Precautions

Healthcare professionals should be aware that dosage of meropenem and vaborbactam is expressed as the total (sum) of the dosage of each of the 2 active components (i.e., dosage of meropenem plus dosage of vaborbactam). This dosage convention should be considered when prescribing, preparing, and dispensing meropenem and vaborbactam.

● Dosage

Meropenem and vaborbactam is a fixed combination containing a 1:1 ratio of meropenem to vaborbactam.

The meropenem component is provided as meropenem trihydrate (dosage of this component is expressed in terms of meropenem).

Dosage of the fixed combination of meropenem and vaborbactam is expressed in terms of the total of the meropenem and vaborbactam content.

Each single-dose vial of meropenem and vaborbactam contains a total of 2 g (i.e., 1 g of meropenem and 1 g of vaborbactam).

Adult Dosage
Urinary Tract Infections

The recommended dosage of meropenem and vaborbactam for the treatment of complicated urinary tract infections, including pyelonephritis, in adults with normal renal function is 4 g (meropenem 2 g and vaborbactam 2 g) every 8 hours for up to 14 days.

● **Special Populations**

Renal Impairment

Dosage adjustments are recommended in adults with an estimated glomerular filtration rate (eGFR) less than 50 mL/minute per 1.73 m². (See Table 2.) The duration of treatment is up to 14 days.

For patients with changing renal function, serum creatinine concentrations and eGFR should be monitored at least daily and dosage of meropenem and vaborbactam should be adjusted accordingly.

TABLE 2. Dosage of Meropenem and Vaborbactam in Adults with Renal Impairment

eGFR (mL/minute per 1.73 m²)	Recommended Dosage of Meropenem and Vaborbactam
30–49	2 g (meropenem 1 g and vaborbactam 1 g) every 8 hours
15–29	2 g (meropenem 1 g and vaborbactam 1 g) every 12 hours
Less than 15	1 g (meropenem 0.5 g and vaborbactam 0.5 g) every 12 hours

For patients receiving hemodialysis, meropenem and vaborbactam should be administered after a hemodialysis session.

Geriatric Patients

Dosage adjustments based solely on age are not needed when meropenem and vaborbactam is used in geriatric patients. However, because geriatric patients are more likely to have decreased renal function and because dosage of meropenem and vaborbactam needs to be adjusted based on renal impairment, dosage should be selected with caution and it may be useful to monitor renal function.

CAUTIONS

● **Contraindications**

Meropenem and vaborbactam is contraindicated in patients with known hypersensitivity to any component of the drug or other drugs in the same class and in patients who have demonstrated anaphylactic reactions to β-lactam antibacterials.

● **Warnings/Precautions**

Sensitivity Reactions

Hypersensitivity reactions were reported in patients receiving meropenem and vaborbactam in clinical trials. Serious and occasionally fatal hypersensitivity (anaphylactic) reactions and serious skin reactions have been reported in patients receiving β-lactam antibacterials. These reactions are more likely to occur in individuals with a history of sensitivity to multiple allergens. There have been reports of individuals with a history of penicillin hypersensitivity who experienced severe hypersensitivity reactions when treated with another β-lactam antibacterial.

Before initiating meropenem and vaborbactam treatment, the clinician should carefully inquire about the patient's previous hypersensitivity reactions to cephalosporins, penicillins, other β-lactams, or other allergens.

If an allergic reaction to meropenem and vaborbactam occurs, the drug should be immediately discontinued.

CNS Effects

Seizures and other adverse CNS effects have been reported during treatment with meropenem, a component of meropenem and vaborbactam. These adverse effects have occurred most commonly in patients with underlying CNS disorders (e.g., brain lesions, history of seizures), bacterial meningitis, and/or compromised renal function.

The recommended dosage of meropenem and vaborbactam should be closely followed, especially in patients with known factors that predispose the patient to seizures. Anticonvulsant therapy should be continued in those with known seizure disorders. (See Risk of Breakthrough Seizures under Cautions: Warnings/Precautions.) If focal tremors, myoclonus, or seizures occur, the patient should be evaluated neurologically, anticonvulsant therapy should be initiated, and meropenem and vaborbactam dosage should be reexamined to determine if it should be decreased or if the drug should be discontinued.

Adverse effects, including seizures, delirium, headaches, and/or paresthesias, can occur in patients receiving meropenem and vaborbactam and may interfere with mental alertness and/or cause motor impairment. Patients receiving meropenem and vaborbactam in an outpatient setting should be informed of the potential for such adverse effects and advised not to operate machinery or motorized vehicles until it is reasonably well established that meropenem and vaborbactam is well tolerated.

Risk of Breakthrough Seizures

Case reports have shown that concomitant use of carbapenems, including meropenem, in patients receiving valproic acid or divalproex sodium results in reduced valproic acid concentrations. As a result of this interaction, valproic acid concentrations may fall below the therapeutic range and increase the risk of breakthrough seizures. Increased dosages of valproic acid or divalproex sodium may not be sufficient to overcome this interaction.

Concomitant use of meropenem and vaborbactam with valproic acid or divalproex sodium is generally not recommended. (See Drug Interactions: Valproic Acid and Divalproex Sodium.)

Hematologic Effects

Thrombocytopenia has been observed in patients with renal impairment receiving meropenem, but clinical bleeding has not been reported.

Superinfection/Clostridium difficile-associated Diarrhea and Colitis (CDAD)

Prolonged use of meropenem and vaborbactam may result in emergence and overgrowth of nonsusceptible bacteria or fungi. The patient should be carefully monitored and appropriate therapy instituted if superinfection occurs.

Treatment with anti-infectives alters normal colon flora and may permit overgrowth of *Clostridium difficile*. *C. difficile* infection (CDI) and *C. difficile*-associated diarrhea and colitis (CDAD; also known as antibiotic-associated diarrhea and colitis or pseudomembranous colitis) have been reported in patients receiving nearly all anti-infectives, including meropenem and vaborbactam, and may range in severity from mild diarrhea to fatal colitis. *C. difficile* produces toxins A and B which contribute to development of CDAD; hypertoxin-producing strains of *C. difficile* are associated with increased morbidity and mortality since they may be refractory to anti-infectives and colectomy may be required.

CDAD should be considered in the differential diagnosis of patients who develop diarrhea during or after anti-infective therapy. Careful medical history is necessary since CDAD has been reported to occur as late as 2 months or longer after anti-infective therapy is discontinued.

If CDAD is suspected or confirmed, anti-infective therapy not directed against *C. difficile* should be discontinued whenever possible. Patients should be managed with appropriate supportive therapy (e.g., fluid and electrolyte management, protein supplementation), anti-infective therapy directed against *C. difficile* (e.g., metronidazole, vancomycin), and surgical evaluation as clinically indicated.

Patients should be advised that diarrhea is a common problem caused by anti-infectives and usually resolves when the drug is discontinued; however, they should contact a clinician if watery and bloody stools (with or without stomach cramps and fever) occur during or as late as 2 months or longer after the last dose.

Selection and Use of Anti-infectives

To reduce development of drug-resistant bacteria and maintain effectiveness of meropenem and vaborbactam and other antibacterials, the drug should be used only for treatment of infections proven or strongly suspected to be caused by susceptible bacteria.

When selecting or modifying anti-infective therapy, results of culture and in vitro susceptibility testing should be used. In the absence of such data, local epidemiology and susceptibility patterns should be considered when selecting anti-infectives for empiric therapy.

Patients should be advised that antibacterials (including meropenem and vaborbactam) should only be used to treat bacterial infections and not used to treat viral infections (e.g., the common cold). Patients also should be advised about the importance of completing the full course of therapy, even if feeling better after a few days, and that skipping doses or not completing therapy may decrease effectiveness and increase the likelihood that bacteria will develop resistance and will not be treatable with meropenem and vaborbactam or other antibacterials in the future.

Precautions Related to Use of Fixed Combinations

When meropenem and vaborbactam is used, the cautions, precautions, contraindications, and drug interactions associated with both drugs in the fixed combination must be considered. Cautionary information applicable to specific populations (e.g., pregnant or nursing women, individuals with hepatic or renal impairment, geriatric patients) should be considered for each drug. (For additional cautionary information on meropenem, see Cautions in Meropenem 8:12.07.08.)

When prescribing, preparing, and dispensing meropenem and vaborbactam, healthcare professionals should consider that dosage of the fixed combination is expressed as the total (sum) of the dosage of each of the 2 active components (i.e., dosage of meropenem plus dosage of vaborbactam). (See Dispensing and Dosage and Administration Precautions under Administration: IV Infusion, in Dosage and Administration.)

Specific Populations

Pregnancy

Fetal malformations (e.g., supernumerary lung lobes, interventricular septal defect) were observed in rabbits receiving IV vaborbactam during organogenesis at doses approximately equivalent to or greater than the maximum recommended human dose. Similar malformations or fetal toxicity were not observed in offspring from pregnant rats receiving IV vaborbactam during organogenesis or from late pregnancy and through lactation at doses equivalent to approximately 1.6 times the maximum recommended human dose. No fetal toxicity or malformations were observed in pregnant rats or cynomolgus monkeys receiving IV meropenem during organogenesis at doses up to 1.6 or 1.2 times the maximum recommended human dose, respectively.

Human data are insufficient to determine whether there is a drug-associated risk of major birth defects or miscarriages if the fixed combination of meropenem and vaborbactam, meropenem alone, or vaborbactam alone is used in pregnant women.

Lactation

Meropenem has been reported to be distributed into human milk. It is not known whether vaborbactam is distributed into human milk.

The benefits of breast-feeding and the importance of meropenem and vaborbactam to the woman should be considered along with potential adverse effects on the breast-fed child from the drug or from the underlying maternal condition.

Pediatric Use

Safety and efficacy of meropenem and vaborbactam have not been established in pediatric patients younger than 18 years of age.

Geriatric Use

No overall differences in safety and efficacy of meropenem and vaborbactam were observed in patients 65 years of age and older compared with younger adults, but greater sensitivity in some older individuals cannot be ruled out.

Meropenem is substantially eliminated by the kidneys, and the risk of adverse reactions to the drug may be greater in patients with renal impairment. Because geriatric patients are more likely to have decreased renal function, dosage should be selected with caution and renal function monitoring should be considered. Dosage adjustments in geriatric patients should be based on renal function.

Population pharmacokinetic analysis indicates that the pharmacokinetics of meropenem and vaborbactam in geriatric patients is similar to that in younger adults.

Hepatic Impairment

Hepatic impairment does not affect the pharmacokinetics of meropenem; vaborbactam does not undergo hepatic metabolism. Hepatic impairment is not expected to affect the clearance of meropenem and vaborbactam.

Renal Impairment

Plasma exposures of both meropenem and vaborbactam are increased in patients with renal impairment, and dosage adjustments are recommended in those with estimated glomerular filtration rate (eGFR) less than 50 mL/minute per 1.73 m².

(See Renal Impairment under Dosage and Administration: Special Populations, in Dosage and Administration.)

Following a single dose of meropenem and vaborbactam in patients with mild, moderate, or severe renal impairment, the area under the plasma concentration-time curve (AUC) of meropenem was 1.3-, 2.1-, or 4.6-fold higher, respectively, and the AUC of vaborbactam was 1.2-, 2.3-, and 7.8-fold higher, respectively, compared with AUCs in individuals with normal renal function.

Hemodialysis removes 38% of the meropenem dose and 53% of the vaborbactam dose.

● *Common Adverse Effects*

Adverse effects reported in 1% or more patients receiving meropenem and vaborbactam include headache, phlebitis or infusion site reactions, diarrhea, hypersensitivity, nausea, increased ALT concentrations, increased AST concentrations, pyrexia, and hypokalemia.

DRUG INTERACTIONS

● *Drugs Affecting or Metabolized by Hepatic Microsomal Enzymes*

Studies evaluating the potential for meropenem to interact with CYP isoenzymes have not been conducted. Carbapenems as a class have not shown potential for inhibition or induction of CYP isoenzymes and clinical experience suggests such effects are unlikely.

Vaborbactam does not inhibit cytochrome P-450 (CYP) isoenzymes 1A2, 2B6, 2C8, 2C9, 2C19, 2D6, or 3A4 in vitro at therapeutic concentrations and does not show potential to induce CYP1A2, 2B6, or 3A4.

● *Drugs Affecting or Affected by Organic Anion Transporters*

Meropenem is a substrate of organic anion transporter (OAT) 1 and OAT3. Therefore, concomitant use of OAT1 and/or OAT3 inhibitors (e.g., probenecid) with meropenem and vaborbactam may increase meropenem plasma concentrations. (See Drug Interactions: Probenecid.)

Vaborbactam is not a substrate or inhibitor of OAT1 or OAT3.

● *Drugs Affecting or Affected by Other Membrane Transporters*

Studies evaluating the potential for meropenem to interact with active transport systems have not been conducted.

In vitro, vaborbactam is not a substrate or inhibitor of P-glycoprotein (P-gp), breast cancer resistance protein (BCRP), or organic cation transporter (OCT) 2. Vaborbactam does not inhibit OCT1, organic anion transporting polypeptide (OATP) 1B1 or 1B3, or bile salt export pump (BSEP).

● *Anti-infectives*

There is no in vitro evidence of antagonistic antibacterial effects between meropenem and vaborbactam and amikacin, azithromycin, daptomycin, levofloxacin, linezolid, polymyxin, tigecycline, or vancomycin.

● *Probenecid*

Probenecid competes with meropenem for active tubular secretion, resulting in a 56% increase in mean systemic exposure and a 38% increase in mean elimination half-life of meropenem.

Concomitant use of probenecid with meropenem and vaborbactam is not recommended.

● *Valproic Acid and Divalproex Sodium*

Concomitant use of carbapenems, including meropenem, and valproic acid or divalproex sodium, has resulted in decreased valproic acid concentrations. Valproic acid concentrations may fall below the therapeutic range and increase the risk of breakthrough seizures. Although the mechanism of this interaction is not known, data from in vitro and animal studies suggest that carbapenems may inhibit the hydrolysis of valproic acid's glucuronide metabolite (VPA-g) back to valproic acid, which decreases serum concentrations of valproic acid.

Concomitant use of meropenem and vaborbactam with valproic acid or divalproex sodium generally is not recommended. In patients whose seizures are well controlled on valproic acid or divalproex sodium, an alternative to carbapenems should be considered. If use of meropenem and vaborbactam is necessary, alternative or supplemental anticonvulsant therapy should be considered.

DESCRIPTION

Meropenem and vaborbactam is a fixed combination of meropenem (a carbapenem) and vaborbactam (a non-β-lactam β-lactamase inhibitor). Vaborbactam inactivates certain bacterial β-lactamases and expands meropenem's spectrum of activity against some bacteria that produce these β-lactamases. Meropenem and vaborbactam is bactericidal in action.

Meropenem is a synthetic carbapenem antibiotic structurally and pharmacologically related to other carbapenems (e.g., doripenem, ertapenem, imipenem). Like other β-lactam antibiotics, the antibacterial activity of meropenem results from inhibition of bacterial cell wall synthesis and is mediated through binding to penicillin-binding proteins (PBPs). Meropenem is stable to hydrolysis by most β-lactamases, including penicillinases and cephalosporinases produced by gram-negative and gram-positive bacteria, but can be hydrolyzed by carbapenemases.

Vaborbactam is a cyclic boronic acid non-β-lactam β-lactamase inhibitor that protects meropenem from degradation by certain β-lactamases, primarily Ambler class A serine carbapenemases (e.g., *Klebsiella pneumoniae* carbapenemase [KPC]) and some class C serine carbapenemases. Vaborbactam's boronate moiety forms a covalent bond with the catalytic serine side chain of the β-lactamase, thereby inhibiting the enzyme from degrading meropenem. This mechanism of action differs from that of β-lactam β-lactamase inhibitors (e.g., clavulanic acid, sulbactam, tazobactam) and some other non-β-lactam β-lactamase inhibitors (e.g., avibactam). In animal models of infection, vaborbactam restored activity of meropenem against some meropenem non-susceptible KPC-producing Enterobacteriaceae. The drug does *not* inhibit class D carbapenemases (e.g., OXA-48) or class B β-lactamases (e.g., metallo β-lactamases [MBLs]). Vaborbactam does not have antibacterial activity and does not decrease the activity of meropenem against meropenem-susceptible organisms.

Each single-dose vial of meropenem and vaborbactam contains 2 g (1 g of meropenem [equivalent to 1.14 g of meropenem trihydrate] and 1 g of vaborbactam) and also contains 575 mg of sodium carbonate. The total sodium content is approximately 250 mg (10.9 mEq) per single-dose vial.

Following IV administration of 4 g of meropenem and vaborbactam (meropenem 2 g and vaborbactam 2 g) given by IV infusion over 3 hours every 8 hours for 7 days in healthy adults with normal renal function, peak plasma concentrations of the drugs were 43.4 and 55.6 mcg/mL, respectively, and there was no accumulation of either drug. Meropenem is partially metabolized by hydrolysis of the β-lactam ring to a microbiologically inactive hydrolysis product; vaborbactam is not metabolized. The plasma protein binding of meropenem is approximately 2% and the plasma protein binding of vaborbactam is approximately 33%. Both drugs are principally eliminated by the kidneys. Approximately 40–60% of a meropenem dose is eliminated unchanged in urine, 22% is eliminated in urine as the microbiologically inactive hydrolysis product, and approximately 2% is eliminated in feces. Approximately 75–95% of a vaborbactam dose is eliminated unchanged in urine. In healthy adults, meropenem has a plasma half-life of 1.2 hours and vaborbactam has a plasma half-life of 1.7 hours.

SPECTRUM

Meropenem and vaborbactam is active in vitro and in clinical studies against *Enterobacter cloacae* species complex, *Escherichia coli*, and *K. pneumoniae*.

Although the clinical importance is not known, meropenem and vaborbactam is active in vitro against other gram-negative bacteria, including *Citrobacter freundii*, *C. koseri*, *E. aerogenes*, *K. oxytoca*, *Morganella morganii*, *Proteus mirabilis*, *Providencia*, *Pseudomonas aeruginosa*, and *Serratia marcescens*. Efficacy of meropenem and vaborbactam for treatment of clinical infections caused by these bacteria has not been established in adequate and well-controlled clinical studies.

In vitro, meropenem and vaborbactam is active against Enterobacteriaceae in the presence of some β-lactamases and extended-spectrum β-lactamases (ESBLs), including KPC, SME, TEM, SHV, CTX-M, CMY, and ACT. Meropenem and vaborbactam is *not* active against bacteria that produce MBLs or oxacillinases with carbapenemase activity.

RESISTANCE

Resistance or reduced susceptibility to meropenem and vaborbactam can occur. Mechanisms of resistance to carbapenems include production of β-lactamases, modification of PBPs by gene acquisition or target alteration, up-regulation of efflux pumps, and loss of outer membrane porin. Meropenem and vaborbactam may not be active against gram-negative bacteria with porin mutations *and* overexpression of efflux pumps. Clinical isolates may produce multiple β-lactamases, express varying levels of β-lactamases, have amino acid sequence variations, or have other resistance mechanisms that have not been identified.

Some isolates resistant to carbapenems (including meropenem) and to cephalosporins may be susceptible to meropenem and vaborbactam. Cross-resistance with other classes of anti-infectives has not been reported.

ADVICE TO PATIENTS

Advise patients that antibacterials (including meropenem and vaborbactam) should only be used to treat bacterial infections and not used to treat viral infections (e.g., the common cold).

Importance of completing full course of therapy, even if feeling better after a few days.

Advise patients that skipping doses or not completing the full course of therapy may decrease effectiveness and increase the likelihood that bacteria will develop resistance and will not be treatable with meropenem and vaborbactam or other antibacterials in the future.

Advise patients that allergic reactions, including serious allergic reactions, can occur and that serious reactions require immediate treatment. Ask patients about previous hypersensitivity reactions to meropenem and vaborbactam, penicillins, cephalosporins, other β-lactams, or other allergens.

Inform patients receiving meropenem and vaborbactam on an outpatient basis that adverse effects, including seizures, delirium, headaches, and/or paresthesias, can occur and interfere with mental alertness and/or cause motor impairment. Advise patients to not operate machinery or motorized vehicles until it is reasonably established that meropenem and vaborbactam is well tolerated.

Advise patients that diarrhea is a common problem caused by anti-infectives and usually ends when the drug is discontinued. Importance of contacting a clinician if watery and bloody stools (with or without stomach cramps and fever) occur during or as late as 2 months or longer after the last dose.

Importance of informing clinician if currently being treated with valproic acid or divalproex sodium. If meropenem and vaborbactam used concomitantly with these drugs, valproic acid concentrations in the blood may drop below therapeutic range and increase the risk of seizures. (See Drug Interactions: Valproic Acid and Divalproex Sodium.)

Importance of informing clinicians of existing or contemplated concomitant therapy, including prescription and OTC drugs and dietary or herbal supplements, as well as any concomitant illnesses.

Importance of women informing their clinician if they are or plan to become pregnant or plan to breast-feed.

Importance of informing patients of other important precautionary information. (See Cautions.)

PREPARATIONS

Excipients in commercially available drug preparations may have clinically important effects in some individuals; consult specific product labeling for details.

Meropenem and Vaborbactam

Parenteral

For injection, for IV infusion	2 g (1 g of meropenem and 1 g of vaborbactam)	Vabomere®, Medicines Company

Selected Revisions September 17, 2018, © Copyright, October 9, 2017, American Society of Health-System Pharmacists, Inc.

Aztreonam

8:12.07.16 • MONOBACTAMS

■ Aztreonam is a synthetic monocyclic β-lactam (i.e., monobactam) antibiotic.

USES

Aztreonam is used for the treatment of infections caused by susceptible gram-negative pathogens including *Pseudomonas aeruginosa*; such infections include intra-abdominal infections (e.g., peritonitis), gynecologic infections (e.g., endometritis, pelvic cellulitis), lower respiratory tract infections (e.g., pneumonia, bronchitis), septicemia, skin and skin structure infections (including those associated with postoperative wounds or ulcers and burns), and complicated and uncomplicated urinary tract infections (e.g., pyelonephritis, cystitis).

Aztreonam is commercially available as a parenteral preparation for IM or IV use; the drug is also available as an inhalation solution for administration via nebulization to improve respiratory symptoms in cystic fibrosis patients with *Pseudomonas aeruginosa* in the lungs.

Aztreonam has no useful activity against gram-positive bacteria or anaerobes, and therefore should *not* be used alone for empiric therapy in seriously ill patients if there is a possibility that the infection may be caused by gram-positive bacteria, or if a mixed aerobic-anaerobic bacterial infection is suspected. If potential pathogens also include gram-positive or anaerobic bacteria, an anti-infective active against such bacteria should be used concomitantly with aztreonam pending results of in vitro culture and susceptibility testing. Aztreonam has been used safely and effectively in conjunction with vancomycin, clindamycin, an aminoglycoside, erythromycin, metronidazole, or a penicillin. However, anti-infectives that have been shown to be potent inducers of β-lactamase production in gram-negative aerobes in vitro (e.g., cefoxitin, imipenem) should *not* be used concomitantly with aztreonam since the drugs may antagonize the antibacterial activity of aztreonam. If an aminoglycoside is used concomitantly with aztreonam, renal function should be monitored, especially if high aminoglycoside dosage is used or if concomitant therapy is prolonged.

● Intra-abdominal Infections

Aztreonam is used parenterally for the treatment of intra-abdominal infections (e.g., peritonitis) caused by susceptible gram-negative aerobic bacteria, including *Citrobacter* (including *C. freundii*), *Enterobacter* (including *E. cloacae*), *E. coli*, *Klebsiella* (including *K. pneumoniae*), *Ps. aeruginosa*, or *Serratia* (including *S. marcescens*).

Because intra-abdominal infections generally are polymicrobial and frequently are mixed aerobic-anaerobic bacterial infections, aztreonam should *not* be used alone for empiric treatment of these infections.

The Surgical Infection Society (SIS) has issued guidelines on the management of intra-abdominal infections. The guidelines state to use antimicrobial regimens that cover the typical gram-negative Enterobacteriaceae, gram-positive cocci, and obligate anaerobes involved in these infections. Aztreonam is generally recommended in treatment regimens for higher-risk patients. Although aztreonam has good in vitro activity against many gram-negative bacteria, the drug has relatively poor activity against extended-spectrum β-lactamase (ESBL)-producing strains of *E. coli* and *K. pneumoniae*. The SIS guidelines state to consider the use of aztreonam plus metronidazole and vancomycin as an option for empiric therapy in adults and children with intra-abdominal infections, but suggests that this regimen be reserved for higher-risk patients with serious β-lactam allergies.

For the treatment of peritonitis in patients undergoing peritoneal dialysis, aztreonam has been administered intraperitoneally†. Some clinicians suggest that intraperitoneal administration is the preferred route for empiric antibiotic therapy unless the patient has systemic sepsis. An intraperitoneal regimen of vancomycin and aztreonam has been used for the treatment of peritoneal dialysis-associated peritonitis.

● Gynecologic Infections

Aztreonam is used parenterally for the treatment of gynecologic infections (e.g., endometritis, pelvic cellulitis) caused by susceptible gram-negative aerobic bacteria, including *Enterobacter* (including *E. cloacae*), *E. coli*, *Klebsiella pneumoniae*, or *P. mirabilis*.

Because gynecologic infections generally are polymicrobial and frequently are mixed aerobic-anaerobic bacterial infections, aztreonam should *not* be used alone for empiric treatment of these infections.

For the treatment of endometritis, an empiric regimen active against all likely mixed aerobic and anaerobic pathogens is generally selected. The combination of clindamycin and gentamicin has been considered the gold standard for this type of infection; however, a regimen consisting of aztreonam plus clindamycin has been used.

Oral or topical antibiotics (e.g., clindamycin, metronidazole) are generally used for the treatment of other common gynecologic infections (e.g., bacterial vaginosis).

● Respiratory Tract Infections

Aztreonam is used for the treatment of lower respiratory tract infections (e.g., pneumonia, bronchitis) caused by susceptible gram-negative aerobic bacteria including *Enterobacter*, *E. coli*, *H. influenzae*, *K. pneumoniae*, *P. mirabilis*, *Ps. aeruginosa*, or *S. marcescens*. The drug also has been effective for the treatment of lower respiratory tract infections caused by susceptible *Citrobacter*†, *Hafnia*†, *K. oxytoca*†, *Morganella*†, *P. vulgaris*†, *Providencia stuartii*†, or *Moraxella catarrhalis*†.

Because lower respiratory tract infections frequently are caused by gram-positive and/or anaerobic bacteria, aztreonam should *not* be used alone for empiric treatment of these infections.

The American Thoracic Society (ATS) and the Infectious Diseases Society of America (IDSA) have published a joint clinical practice guideline on the treatment of adults with community-acquired pneumonia. Aztreonam is included as an empiric treatment option for *Ps. aeruginosa* in adults with community-acquired pneumonia who are being treated in the inpatient setting. The guideline recommends empiric coverage for *Ps. aeruginosa* only if locally validated risk factors for the pathogen are present.

IDSA also has published a clinical practice guideline on the management of adults with hospital-acquired and ventilator-associated pneumonia. Aztreonam is suggested as an empiric treatment option for gram-negative/antipseudomonal coverage; if the patient has a severe penicillin allergy and aztreonam is used instead of a β-lactam-based antibiotic, coverage for methicillin-sensitive *S. aureus* (MSSA) should be included.

Cystic Fibrosis

Aztreonam also has been used alone or in conjunction with an aminoglycoside for the treatment of acute exacerbations of bronchopulmonary *Ps. aeruginosa* infections in some patients with cystic fibrosis. As with other anti-infective agents, a bacteriologic cure is rarely obtained and should not be expected in cystic fibrosis patients.

Oral Inhalation via Nebulization

Aztreonam for inhalation solution (Cayston®) is used via nebulization to improve respiratory symptoms in cystic fibrosis patients 7 years of age or older with *Ps. aeruginosa* in the lungs. Safety and efficacy of aztreonam oral inhalation therapy have *not* been established in pediatric patients younger than 7 years of age, in patients with forced expiratory volume in 1 second (FEV_1) less than 25% or exceeding 75% of predicted values, or in patients colonized with *Burkholderia cepacia*. Aggressive management of chronic airway infections in patients with cystic fibrosis has been shown to prevent lung function decline. Nebulized antibiotics such as aztreonam can be used as suppressive therapy for such individuals with chronic infection or colonization with *Ps. aeruginosa* and/or other gram-negative organisms.

Efficacy of aztreonam oral inhalation therapy in cystic fibrosis patients was evaluated in a randomized, double-blind, placebo-controlled, multicenter trial. The trial enrolled 164 adults and pediatric patients 7 years of age or older with FEV_1 of 25–75% of predicted values (mean age 30 years [77% were 18 years of age or older], 43% female, 96% Caucasian, mean baseline FEV_1 55% of predicted values). Patients were randomized in a 1:1 ratio to receive a 28-day regimen of aztreonam (75 mg 3 times daily) or volume-matched placebo (3 times daily) administered by oral inhalation via nebulization. All patients were required to take a dose of an inhaled bronchodilator (β-agonist) prior to each inhaled dose of aztreonam or placebo. Patients were receiving standard care for cystic fibrosis, including drugs for obstructive airway diseases; those who had received an anti-infective within the last 28 days were excluded. The primary efficacy end point was improvement in respiratory symptoms on the last day of oral inhalation treatment with aztreonam or placebo; respiratory symptoms also were assessed 2 weeks after completion of treatment. Changes in respiratory symptoms (e.g., cough, wheezing, sputum production) were assessed using a patient questionnaire.

On the last day of oral inhalation treatment, improvement in respiratory symptoms was noted in aztreonam-treated patients relative to placebo-treated patients. Statistically significant improvements were seen in both adult and pediatric patients, but were substantially smaller in adults. At 2 weeks after completion of treatment, a difference in respiratory symptoms between treatment groups was still present, but the difference was smaller. Pulmonary function, as measured by FEV_1 (L), increased from baseline in patients treated with aztreonam and decreased in those treated with placebo. On the last day of treatment, there was a 10% difference between aztreonam-treated and placebo-treated patients in percent change in FEV_1 (L); improvements in FEV_1 were comparable between adult and pediatric patients. At 2 weeks after completion of treatment, the difference in FEV_1 between aztreonam-treated and placebo-treated patients had decreased to 6%.

● Septicemia

Aztreonam is used parenterally for the treatment of septicemia caused by susceptible gram-negative aerobic bacteria, including *Enterobacter*, *E. coli*, *K. pneumoniae*, *Ps. aeruginosa*, *P. mirabilis*, and *S. marcescens*. The drug also has been effective when used parenterally in a limited number of adults for the treatment of septicemia caused by susceptible *Citrobacter*† or *H. influenzae*†.

Aztreonam has generally been effective in either community-acquired or nosocomial septicemia known to be caused by susceptible gram-negative aerobes, and has been as effective as gentamicin or ceftazidime in the treatment of these infections.

The Surviving Sepsis Campaign has published guidelines on the management of sepsis and septic shock. The guidelines recommend immediate administration of appropriate antimicrobials in adults with possible sepsis or septic shock. Empiric antimicrobials with adequate coverage for likely pathogens should be selected based on the patient's risk for certain pathogens (e.g., MRSA, multidrug-resistant organisms).

● Skin and Skin Structure Infections

Aztreonam is used parenterally for the treatment of skin and skin structure infections, including those associated with postoperative wounds or ulcers and burns, caused by susceptible gram-negative aerobic bacteria, including *Citrobacter*, *Enterobacter*, *E. coli*, *K. pneumoniae*, *P. mirabilis*, *Ps. aeruginosa*, or *S. marcescens*.

Aztreonam is also used as an adjunct to surgery in the management of abscesses, cutaneous infections, infections complicating hollow viscus perforations, or infections of serous surfaces caused by susceptible gram-negative aerobic bacteria.

The Infectious Diseases Society of America (IDSA) has published guidelines on the management of skin and skin structure infections. Such infections include purulent skin and soft tissue infections (e.g., cutaneous abscesses, furuncles, carbuncles, inflamed epidermoid cysts). Aztreonam is not included as a potential antimicrobial of choice in these guidelines; when broad-spectrum empiric treatment is necessary for suspected polymicrobial infection, other antibiotics are generally recommended.

IDSA also has published a clinical practice guideline for the diagnosis and treatment of diabetic foot infections. When empiric treatment of moderate or severe diabetic foot infections is indicated, IDSA recommends use of a broad-spectrum regimen pending results of in vitro culture and susceptibility testing. When probable pathogens include methicillin-resistant *Staphylococcus aureus* (MRSA), Enterobacteriaceae, *Pseudomonas*, and obligate anaerobes, IDSA recommends an empiric regimen of vancomycin used in conjunction with ceftazidime, cefepime, piperacillin/tazobactam, aztreonam, or a carbapenem. If aztreonam,

ceftazidime, or cefepime is used in conjunction with vancomycin, the empiric regimen should also include an additional anti-infective for anaerobic coverage.

● Urinary Tract Infections

Aztreonam is used parenterally for the treatment of complicated or uncomplicated urinary tract infections (UTIs), including pyelonephritis and initial and recurrent cystitis, caused by susceptible gram-negative aerobes, including *Citrobacter*, *E. cloacae*, *E. coli*, *K. oxytoca*, *K. pneumoniae*, *P. mirabilis*, *Ps. aeruginosa*, and *S. marcescens*. The drug also has been effective when used parenterally in a limited number of adults for the treatment of UTIs caused by susceptible *E. aerogenes*†, *Morganella morganii*†, *P. vulgaris*†, or *Providencia*†. Aztreonam has been effective in the treatment of cystitis or pyelonephritis caused by gram-negative aerobic bacteria resistant to aminopenicillins, first or second generation cephalosporins, and/or aminoglycosides.

In controlled studies in men and women with UTIs, 5–14 days of aztreonam therapy was at least as effective as 5–14 days of therapy with an aminoglycoside (i.e., gentamicin, tobramycin) or a parenteral cephalosporin (i.e., cefotaxime, ceftriaxone). Although aztreonam therapy generally is associated with less toxicity than aminoglycoside therapy, colonization or superinfection with gram-positive bacteria (especially *Enterococcus faecalis* [formerly *Streptococcus faecalis*]) has been reported more frequently with aztreonam than with aminoglycosides.

In a controlled study in women with uncomplicated cystitis caused by *E. coli*, a single 1-g IM dose of aztreonam was as effective as 10 days of therapy with oral amoxicillin (250 mg 3 times daily); however, efficacy of a single dose of aztreonam in the treatment of these infections has not been established.

● Bone and Joint Infections

Aztreonam has been effective when used parenterally in adults for the treatment of bone and joint infections† caused by susceptible aerobic gram-negative bacteria, including osteomyelitis or septic arthritis, caused by susceptible *Enterobacter*, *Escherichia coli*, *Klebsiella*, *Proteus mirabilis*, *Ps. aeruginosa*, or *Serratia marcescens*. The drug also has been effective when used parenterally in a limited number of children for the treatment of osteomyelitis, osteochondritis, or septic arthritis caused by susceptible *Ps. aeruginosa* or *Haemophilus influenzae*†. An antistaphylococcal anti-infective agent (e.g., a penicillinase-resistant penicillin, vancomycin) should be used concomitantly with aztreonam if gram-positive bacteria are known or suspected to also be involved.

The Infectious Diseases Society of America (IDSA) states that aztreonam can be considered an alternative for the treatment of native vertebral osteomyelitis† caused by *Ps. aeruginosa* when a drug of first choice (i.e., cefepime, meropenem, doripenem) cannot be used because the patient has severe penicillin allergy and when ciprofloxacin cannot be used because the infection is caused by a quinolone-resistant strain.

● CNS Infections

Aztreonam is a treatment option for healthcare-associated ventriculitis and meningitis† caused by susceptible aerobic gram-negative bacteria in patients with anaphylaxis or other contraindications to β-lactam therapy (including carbapenems). Case reports and cohort studies support the use of using aztreonam as an alternative to β-lactams in adults and children with meningitis due to *Ps. aeruginosa*, *H. influenzae*, and other Enterobacteriaceae.

Guidelines from IDSA suggest that the choice between aztreonam and other alternatives (such as ciprofloxacin for *Ps. aeruginosa* or trimethoprim-sulfamethoxazole for β-lactamase-producing Enterobacteriacea) should consider local susceptibility patterns and known co-infecting organisms.

● Antimicrobial Prophylaxis in Surgery

Aztreonam has been used parenterally in conjunction with other anti-infectives for antimicrobial prophylaxis during surgery† in patients undergoing certain surgical procedures in which aerobic gram-negative bacteria are common pathogens.

Some clinicians state that a regimen of vancomycin (or clindamycin) in conjunction with aztreonam can be used as an alternative regimen for perioperative prophylaxis in patients undergoing gastroduodenal or biliary tract surgery, hysterectomy (vaginal or abdominal), or certain organ transplant procedures (liver, pancreas, pancreas-kidney). These clinicians state that a regimen of clindamycin and aztreonam can be used as an alternative regimen in patients undergoing appendectomy, colorectal or small intestine surgery, or urologic surgery involving an implanted prosthesis.

Some clinicians recommend that an anti-infective active against enteric gram-negative bacilli (e.g., aztreonam, an aminoglycoside, a fluoroquinolone) be used concomitantly when vancomycin is used for perioperative prophylaxis in patients undergoing neurosurgery or cardiac, orthopedic, or vascular surgery.

● **Empiric Therapy in Febrile Neutropenic Patients**

Aztreonam has been used parenterally in conjunction with vancomycin (with or without amikacin) for empiric anti-infective therapy in febrile granulocytopenic adults†. Because gram-positive bacteria (especially *S. epidermidis*) are being reported with increasing frequency in febrile granulocytopenic patients and because aztreonam is inactive against these organisms, an anti-infective agent active against staphylococci (e.g., vancomycin) should be used in conjunction with aztreonam if the drug is used for empiric therapy in these patients. Some guidelines have suggested a regimen of aztreonam and vancomycin as an alternative empiric regimen in patients with immediate-type penicillin hypersensitivity.

DOSAGE AND ADMINISTRATION

● **Administration**

Administer aztreonam by IV injection or infusion, or by deep IM injection.

Aztreonam also is administered by oral inhalation via nebulization in patients with cystic fibrosis.

Aztreonam has been administered intraperitoneally† in dialysis fluid.

Parenteral

Administer IV or IM depending on the type and severity of infection, susceptibility of the causative organism, and condition of the patient.

The manufacturers recommend that aztreonam be given IV (rather than IM) in patients with septicemia, localized parenchymal abscess (such as intra-abdominal abscess), peritonitis, or other severe systemic or life-threatening infection and when individual doses greater than 1 g are indicated.

Inspect aztreonam solutions visually for particulate matter and discoloration prior to IV or IM administration. Discard any unused solution.

When aztreonam is given IV via a common administration tubing used to administer another drug, especially one that is incompatible with aztreonam, flush the tubing before and after aztreonam administration with an IV infusion solution compatible with both drugs; do not give the drugs simultaneously. When a Y-type IV administration set is used to administer aztreonam, give careful attention to the calculated volume of aztreonam solution to ensure that the entire dose is infused.

Intermittent IV Injection

For direct intermittent IV injection, reconstitute the contents of a single-dose vial labeled as containing 500 mg, 1 g, or 2 g of aztreonam by adding 6–10 mL of sterile water for injection. Shake the vial vigorously immediately after the diluent is added.

Inject the appropriate dose of reconstituted solution slowly over a period of 3–5 minutes either directly into a vein or into the tubing of a compatible IV solution.

Intermittent IV Infusion

For intermittent IV infusion, reconstitute a single-dose vial labeled as containing 500 mg, 1 g, or 2 g of aztreonam by adding at least 1.5, 3, or 6 mL, respectively, of sterile water for injection. Shake the vial vigorously immediately after the diluent is added. Further dilute the reconstituted solution in a compatible IV infusion solution. A volume control IV administration set may be used to add the appropriate dose of reconstituted aztreonam solution to the compatible IV infusion solution during administration; this final dilution should provide a solution with a concentration of 20 mg/mL or less.

Infuse intermittent IV infusions of aztreonam over 20–60 minutes.

IM Injection

For IM administration, reconstitute a single-dose vial labeled as containing 500 mg, 1 g, or 2 g of aztreonam by adding at least 1.5, 3, or 6 mL, respectively, of sterile water for injection, 0.9% sodium chloride injection, bacteriostatic water for injection (with benzyl alcohol or parabens), or bacteriostatic sodium chloride injection (with benzyl alcohol). Shake the vial vigorously immediately after the diluent is added.

Administer the appropriate dose of reconstituted solution by deep IM injection into a large muscle (e.g., upper outer quadrant of the gluteus maximus, lateral part of the thigh). Aztreonam generally is well tolerated when given IM and should not be admixed with local anesthetic agents.

Oral Inhalation by Nebulization

For administration by oral inhalation via nebulization, aztreonam is commercially available in a kit containing single-dose vials of lyophilized aztreonam powder for inhalation solution and single-dose ampuls of 0.17% sodium chloride diluent. Reconstitute the powder for inhalation solution using *only* the diluent provided by the manufacturer and just before it is time to administer a dose.

Following reconstitution, administer aztreonam inhalation solution via nebulization using only an Altera® nebulizer system. The manufacturer states that the reconstituted inhalation solution should not be administered using any other type of nebulizer and should not be administered IV or IM.

Patients receiving aztreonam oral inhalation therapy should use a bronchodilator before aztreonam is administered. Short-acting bronchodilators can be taken between 15 minutes and 4 hours prior to each aztreonam dose. Alternatively, long-acting bronchodilators can be taken 0.5–12 hours prior to administration of aztreonam. For patients taking multiple inhaled therapies, the recommended order of administration is a bronchodilator, mucolytics, and, lastly, aztreonam.

To prepare a dose of aztreonam inhalation solution for oral inhalation via nebulization, add the contents of a single-dose ampul of diluent provided by the manufacturer to a single-dose vial of aztreonam powder for inhalation solution. Swirl the vial gently until the powder has completely dissolved.

Pour the reconstituted aztreonam inhalation solution into the handset of the Altera® nebulizer system and turn on the unit. The reconstituted inhalation solution should not be mixed with any other drug in the Altera® nebulizer handset.

Administer the dose with the patient seated in a relaxed, upright position. Place the mouthpiece of the nebulizer handset into the mouth; with lips closed around the mouthpiece, the patient should breathe normally through the mouthpiece.

A period of about 2–3 minutes usually is required to administer the complete dose of reconstituted inhalation solution via the nebulizer. Consult the manufacturer's labeling for additional information on how to administer aztreonam inhalation solution. Instructions on testing nebulizer functionality and cleaning the handset are provided in the instructions for use included with the nebulizer system.

Compatibility

Admixtures containing aztreonam (10 or 20 mg/mL) and clindamycin phosphate (3, 6, or 9 mg/mL) or cefazolin (5 or 20 mg/mL) in 0.9% sodium chloride injection or 5% dextrose injection are stable for up to 48 hours at room temperature (25°C) or for 7 days when refrigerated at 4–5°C. Admixtures containing aztreonam (10 or 20 mg/mL) and ampicillin (5 or 20 mg/mL) in 0.9% sodium chloride injection are stable for 24 hours at room temperature (25°C) or for 48 hours when refrigerated at 4°C; similar admixtures of these drugs in 5% dextrose injection are stable for only 2 hours at room temperature or for 8 hours when refrigerated at 4°C. Admixtures containing aztreonam (10 or 20 mg/mL) and cefoxitin (10 or 20 mg/mL) in one of these diluents are stable for 12 hours at 25°C or 7 days at 4°C.

Although many bicyclic β-lactam antibiotics (e.g., penicillins) are physically and/or chemically incompatible with aminoglycosides and can inactivate the drugs in vitro, aztreonam appears to be less likely to inactivate aminoglycosides in vitro. Admixtures containing aztreonam (10 or 20 mg/mL) and tobramycin (0.2 or 0.8 mg/mL) in 0.9% sodium chloride injection or 5% dextrose injection are stable for up to 48 hours at room temperature (25°C) or for 7 days at 4°C. The manufacturer states that similar solutions containing gentamicin (0.2 or 0.8 mg/mL) are also stable for up to 48 hours at room temperature or for 7 days when refrigerated. However, there is evidence that loss of gentamicin potency may occur with such admixtures at these storage temperatures and times; therefore, it has been suggested that solutions containing aztreonam (10 or 20 mg/mL) and gentamicin (0.2 or 0.8 mg/mL) be considered stable for only 8 hours at 25°C or for 24 hours at 4°C.

Admixtures containing aztreonam and vancomycin hydrochloride in Dianeal® 137 (Peritoneal Dialysis Solution) with 4.25% dextrose are stable for up to 24 hours at room temperature. At the Y-site, aztreonam (10 and 20 mg/mL) is compatible with ceftazidime-avibactam (8, 25, and 50 mg/mL).

Aztreonam is physically and/or chemically incompatible with some drugs, but the compatibility depends on several factors (e.g., concentrations of the drugs, specific diluents used, resulting pH, temperature). Aztreonam is incompatible with nafcillin sodium, and metronidazole, and these drugs should be administered separately.

● Dosage

Dosage and route of administration of aztreonam should be determined by the type and severity of infection, susceptibility of the causative organism, and patient condition. Do not use dosages lower than those usually recommended.

For most infections, continue parenteral aztreonam treatment for at least 48 hours after the patient becomes asymptomatic or evidence of eradication of the infection has been obtained. Persistent infections may require several weeks of treatment.

Parenteral Adult Dosage

General Adult Dosage

The usual parenteral dosage of aztreonam for the treatment of moderately severe systemic infections in adults is 1 g IV or IM or 2 g IV every 8 or 12 hours. For the treatment of severe systemic or life-threatening infections, including infections caused by *Pseudomonas aeruginosa*, the usual adult dosage of aztreonam is 2 g IV every 6 or 8 hours.

The manufacturers state that the maximum recommended IV or IM dosage of aztreonam in adults is 8 g daily.

Intra-abdominal Infections

The standard dosage of aztreonam in the treatment of intra-abdominal infections is 1–2 g IV every 8 hours. In patients with impaired renal function, an initial dose of 1–2 g IV followed by 0.5–1 g IV every 6–12 hours is usually given.

Urinary Tract Infections

The usual adult IV or IM dosage of aztreonam for the treatment of urinary tract infections is 500 mg or 1 g every 8 or 12 hours.

The usual duration of aztreonam therapy for the treatment of uncomplicated urinary tract infections is 5–10 days; continue therapy for at least 10–18 days for the treatment of complicated urinary tract infections.

Bone and Joint Infections

If aztreonam is used as an alternative for the treatment of osteomyelitis† caused by *Ps. aeruginosa*, the Infectious Diseases Society of America (IDSA) recommends that adults receive 2 g IV every 8 hours for 6 weeks.

Antimicrobial Prophylaxis in Surgery

If aztreonam is used for antimicrobial prophylaxis in surgery†, some clinicians recommend that adults receive 2 g within 1 hour prior to initial incision. During prolonged procedures (longer than 4 hours) or if major blood loss occurs, administer additional intraoperative doses of aztreonam every 4 hours. The duration of prophylaxis should be less than 24 hours for most procedures; there is no evidence to support continuing prophylaxis after wound closure or until all indwelling drains and intravascular catheters are removed.

Parenteral Pediatric Dosage

General Pediatric Dosage

The manufacturers recommend that pediatric patients 9 months of age or older with normal renal function receive aztreonam in a dosage of 30 mg/kg IV every 8 hours for the treatment of mild to moderate infections or 30 mg/kg IV every 6 or 8 hours for the treatment of moderate to severe infections. The manufacturers state that the maximum recommended dosage of aztreonam for pediatric patients is 120 mg/kg daily; however, higher dosages may be warranted in those with cystic fibrosis.

A dosage of 50 mg/kg IV every 6 or 8 hours (i.e., 150–200 mg/kg daily) has been suggested by some clinicians for the treatment of infections in children with cystic fibrosis.

Although safe use of aztreonam in neonates† has not been established, the American Academy of Pediatrics (AAP) states that neonates 7 days of age or younger may receive 30 mg/kg of aztreonam IV every 12 hours if their gestational age is less than 34 weeks or 30 mg/kg IV every 8 hours if their gestational age is 34 weeks or more. Neonates 8–28 days of age may receive 30 mg/kg IV every 8 hours if their gestational age is less than 34 weeks or 30 mg/kg IV every 6 hours if their gestational age is 34 weeks or more.

For pediatric patients beyond the neonatal period, AAP recommends an aztreonam dosage of 90–120 mg/kg daily given IV or IM in 3 or 4 divided doses.

Intra-abdominal Infections

Aztreonam dosage of 30 mg/kg IV every 6–8 hours has been used in pediatric patients >9 months of age. Higher doses may be reasonable in critically ill pediatric patients who may have an increased volume of distribution and/or accelerated clearance of antimicrobial agents.

Oral Inhalation Dosage

Adult and Pediatric Dosage

When the commercially available aztreonam powder for inhalation solution is used in cystic fibrosis patients with *Ps. aeruginosa* in the lungs, the recommended dosage for adults and pediatric patients 7 years of age or older is 75 mg of aztreonam 3 times daily for 28 days via nebulization. Administer oral inhalation doses at least 4 hours apart (e.g., in the morning, after school, at bedtime).

In clinical trials, adults and pediatric patients with cystic fibrosis received up to 9 courses of aztreonam oral inhalation therapy; each course consisted of 28 days of aztreonam oral inhalation therapy (75 mg 3 times daily), followed by 28 days without such therapy.

Intraperitoneal Dosage

If aztreonam is administered intraperitoneally† for the treatment of peritonitis in adults undergoing continuous ambulatory peritoneal dialysis (CAPD), some clinicians recommend that a 1-g loading dose of the drug be given IV followed by maintenance doses of 500 mg intraperitoneally in 2 L of dialysate every 6 hours. For empiric gram-negative coverage in the treatment of peritonitis in patients undergoing CAPD, some clinicians recommend a continuous aztreonam dosage regimen consisting of a loading dose of 1 g per L of dialysate followed by maintenance doses of 250 mg per L of dialysate.

● Special Populations

Renal Impairment

In adults with renal impairment, modify doses and/or frequency of administration of IV or IM aztreonam in response to the degree of renal impairment.

Data are insufficient to date to make dosage recommendations for parenteral aztreonam in pediatric patients with impaired renal function.

When aztreonam is administered by oral inhalation via nebulization, dosage adjustments are not necessary in adults or pediatric patients 7 years of age or older with mild, moderate, or severe renal impairment.

Because serum creatinine concentrations alone may not be sufficiently accurate to assess the degree of renal impairment, especially in geriatric adults, the dosage of IV or IM aztreonam preferably should be based on the patient's measured or estimated creatinine clearance.

Adults with creatinine clearances greater than 30 mL/minute per 1.73 m² may receive the usual adult dosage of IV or IM aztreonam. Adults with creatinine clearances of 10–30 mL/minute per 1.73 m² should receive an initial 1- or 2-g IV or IM loading dose of aztreonam followed by maintenance doses equal to one-half the usual dose (i.e., 250 mg, 500 mg, or 1 g) given at the usual dosage intervals. In adults with severe renal failure (creatinine clearances less than 10 mL/minute per 1.73 m^2) and adults undergoing hemodialysis, follow an initial IV or IM loading dose equal to the usual dose (i.e., 500 mg, 1 g, or 2 g) with maintenance doses equal to one-fourth the usual dose (i.e., 125 mg, 250 mg, or 500 mg) given at the usual dosage intervals.

Because aztreonam is removed by hemodialysis, patients with serious or life-threatening infections undergoing hemodialysis should receive a supplemental IV or IM dose of the drug equal to one-eighth the initial dose (i.e., 62.5 mg, 125 mg, or 250 mg) immediately after each dialysis period in addition to the recommended maintenance doses. In contrast to dosing recommendations from the manufacturer, results of a study found that aztreonam 1 g (for MICs up to 4 mg/L) or 2 g (for MICs up to 8 mg/L) administered once daily after hemodialysis had >90% probability of achieving target concentrations.

In adults undergoing CAPD, some clinicians recommend an initial IV loading dose of aztreonam equal to the usual dose (i.e., 500 mg, 1 g, or 2 g) followed by maintenance doses equal to one-fourth the usual dose (i.e., 125 mg, 250 mg, or 500 mg) given at the usual dosage intervals.

Hepatic Impairment

The serum half-life of aztreonam is only slightly prolonged in patients with hepatic impairment. Modification of usual IV or IM dosage probably is unnecessary in patients with stable primary biliary cirrhosis or other chronic hepatic disease, unless renal function also is impaired. Although some clinicians recommend that parenteral aztreonam dosage be decreased by 20–25% in patients with alcoholic cirrhosis, especially if long-term therapy with the drug is required, others state that this decrease in dosage is unnecessary unless renal function also is impaired.

Geriatric Patients

Select dosage in geriatric patients with caution because of the greater frequency of decreased hepatic, renal, and/or cardiac function and of concomitant disease and drug therapy observed in these patients. Aztreonam is substantially eliminated by the kidneys and the risk of adverse reactions may be greater in patients with impaired renal function. Because geriatric patients are more likely to have renal impairment, monitor renal function and make appropriate dosage modifications if necessary.

CAUTIONS

● *Contraindications*
● Known hypersensitivity to aztreonam or any component of the formulation.

● *Warnings/Precautions*
Hypersensitivity

Treatment with aztreonam can result in hypersensitivity reactions in patients with or without prior exposure to the drug. In addition, hypersensitivity reactions to aztreonam (e.g., localized or urticarial rash) have occurred rarely when the drug was used in patients with a history of hypersensitivity to penicillins and/or cephalosporins. There is clinical and laboratory evidence of partial cross-allergenicity among bicyclic β-lactam antibiotics (e.g., carbapenems, cephalosporins, cephamycins, penicillins). Although cross-allergenicity between aztreonam and bicyclic β-lactam antibiotics has been reported only rarely, aztreonam should be used with caution in patients with a history of hypersensitivity to β-lactam antibiotics. Retrospective data suggest that there is a low potential for cross-reactivity with aztreonam among patients with an allergy to ceftazidime.

In a study that included 212 individuals with documented immediate (IgE-mediated) hypersensitivity to penicillins who had positive skin test reactions to at least 1 penicillin reagent, all individuals had negative skin test reactions to aztreonam; there was no reaction to aztreonam in 211 of these individuals who were willing to receive an IM aztreonam challenge. In another study that included 214 individuals with nonimmediate (T cell-mediated) hypersensitivity to penicillins who had positive patch and/or delayed-reading skin test responses to at least 1 penicillin reagent, all individuals had negative skin test reactions to aztreonam and all tolerated IM aztreonam challenges. Studies in rabbits and humans suggest that antibodies produced in response to penicillin G (including IgE antibodies to major and minor determinants) show negligible cross-reactivity with aztreonam. Likewise, antibodies produced in response to aztreonam have had negligible cross-reactivity with penicillin G,, cephalothin and cefotaxime. In one study in healthy men who had not previously received aztreonam, no IgE antibody response to aztreonam was detectable after therapy with the drug (500-mg or 1-g doses every 8 hours for 7 days). A few of these individuals did have naturally occurring side-chain-specific IgG antibodies to aztreonam, but only one demonstrated an IgG response to the drug.

Prior to initiation of aztreonam, assess whether the patient has had a previous hypersensitivity reaction to β-lactam antibiotics, other drugs, or allergens.

If a hypersensitivity reaction occurs during aztreonam therapy, discontinue the drug and initiate appropriate therapy (e.g., vasopressors, antihistamines, corticosteroids, maintenance of ventilation). Serious hypersensitivity reactions may require the use of epinephrine and other emergency measures.

C. difficile-associated Diarrhea and Colitis

C. difficile infection (CDI) and *C. difficile*-associated diarrhea and colitis (CDAD; also known as antibiotic-associated diarrhea and colitis or pseudomembranous colitis) have been reported with nearly all systemic anti-infectives, including aztreonam, and may range in severity from mild diarrhea to fatal colitis. *C. difficile* produces toxins A and B, which contribute to the development of CDAD; hypertoxin-producing strains of *C. difficile* are associated with increased morbidity and mortality since they may be refractory to anti-infectives and colectomy may be required.

CDAD should be considered in the differential diagnosis of patients who develop diarrhea during or after parenteral aztreonam therapy. Careful medical history is necessary since CDAD has been reported to occur as late as 2 months or longer after anti-infective therapy is discontinued. If CDAD is suspected or confirmed, discontinue anti-infective therapy not directed against *C. difficile* whenever possible. Manage patients with appropriate supportive therapy (e.g., fluid and electrolytes management, protein supplementation), anti-infective therapy directed against C. difficile (e.g., metronidazole, vancomycin), and surgical evaluation as clinically indicated. Other causes of colitis also should be considered.

Advise patients that diarrhea is a common problem caused by systemic anti-infectives and usually ends when the drug is discontinued; however, it is important to contact a clinician if watery and bloody stools (with or without stomach cramps and fever) occur during or as late as 2 months or longer after the last dose.

Toxic Epidermal Necrolysis

Toxic epidermal necrolysis has been reported rarely when parenteral aztreonam was used in patients undergoing bone marrow transplantation; these patients had multiple risk factors, including sepsis, radiation therapy, and concomitant treatment with drugs associated with toxic epidermal necrolysis.

Selection and Use of Anti-infectives

To reduce development of drug-resistant bacteria and maintain effectiveness of parenteral aztreonam and other antibacterials, use aztreonam only for the treatment or prevention of infections proven or strongly suspected to be caused by susceptible bacteria.

When selecting or modifying anti-infective therapy, consider results of culture and in vitro susceptibility testing. In the absence of such data, consider local epidemiology and susceptibility patterns when selecting anti-infectives for empiric therapy. Culture and susceptibility testing performed periodically during therapy provides information on the therapeutic effect of the anti-infective agent and the possible emergence of bacterial resistance.

Patients should be advised to only use antibacterials (including aztreonam) to treat bacterial infections and not to treat viral infections (e.g., the common cold). Patients also should be advised about the importance of completing the full course of therapy, even if feeling better after a few days, and that skipping doses or not completing therapy may decrease effectiveness and increase the likelihood that bacteria will develop resistance and will not be treatable with aztreonam or other antibacterials in the future.

Because aztreonam has little or no activity against gram-positive bacteria and anaerobes, use another anti-infective active against such bacteria concomitantly if aztreonam is used empirically in infections that may involve gram-positive bacteria or anaerobes (e.g., gynecologic, intra-abdominal, or respiratory tract infections).

Overgrowth of Nonsusceptible Organisms

As with other anti-infective agents, use of parenteral aztreonam may result in overgrowth of nonsusceptible organisms, especially gram-positive bacteria (e.g., enterococci, *Staphylococcus aureus*, *Streptococcus pneumoniae*) or fungi. Colonization or superinfection with aztreonam-resistant organisms has occurred in up to 60% of patients receiving the drug, and superinfections have required treatment with another anti-infective agent in about 4–11% of patients. Use of indwelling catheters or the presence of tracheotomy sites or open, draining wounds appears to contribute to the occurrence of superinfections during aztreonam therapy. Resistant strains of some organisms (e.g., *Pseudomonas aeruginosa*, *Klebsiella pneumoniae*) have developed during parenteral aztreonam therapy. If superinfection occurs, institute appropriate therapy.

Precautions Related to Oral Inhalation Therapy

Aztreonam powder for inhalation solution should only be used to treat patients with cystic fibrosis who are known to have *Ps. aeruginosa* in the lungs. Use of aztreonam oral inhalation therapy in the absence of known *Ps. aeruginosa* infection is unlikely to provide benefit and increases the risk of development of drug-resistant bacteria.

Clinicians should consider that bronchospasm is a known complication associated with nebulized therapies, including aztreonam inhalation solution. In clinical trials in patients pretreated with a bronchodilator, a reduction of 15% or more in FEV_1 was reported in 3% of patients immediately following administration of a dose of aztreonam inhalation solution administered by oral inhalation via nebulization.

In clinical trials, patients with increases in FEV_1 during a 28-day course of aztreonam oral inhalation therapy were sometimes treated for pulmonary exacerbations when FEV_1 declined after the treatment period. When evaluating whether a change in FEV_1 after treatment is caused by a pulmonary exacerbation, consider the patient's baseline FEV_1 measured prior to initiation of aztreonam oral inhalation therapy and the presence of other symptoms.

Specific Populations

Pregnancy

There are no adequate and controlled studies to date using parenteral aztreonam or aztreonam administered by oral inhalation via nebulization in pregnant women. Use parenteral or orally inhaled aztreonam during pregnancy only when clearly needed. Aztreonam crosses the placenta in pregnant women and enters fetal circulation.

No evidence of embryotoxicity, fetotoxicity, or teratogenicity was found in reproduction studies in pregnant rats and rabbits using daily parenteral aztreonam dosages up to 1.8 and 1.2 g/kg, respectively; these aztreonam dosages were 2.2- and 2.9-fold greater than the maximum recommended human dosage (MRHD) based on body surface area. There was no evidence of drug-induced changes in any maternal, fetal, or neonatal parameters when parenteral aztreonam was used in a perinatal/postnatal study in rats; the highest dosage used in this study (1.8 g/kg daily) was 2.2 times the MRHD based on body surface area. However, in a 2-generation reproduction study in rats using parenteral aztreonam dosages up to 2.4 g/kg daily (2.9-fold greater than the MRHD), there was a slightly reduced survival rate during the lactation period in offspring of rats that received the highest dosage, but not in offspring of rats that received lower dosages.

Lactation

Because aztreonam is distributed into milk in low (<1%) concentrations following parenteral administration and because safety of aztreonam in neonates has not been fully evaluated to date, consider temporary discontinuance of nursing if parenteral aztreonam is used in lactating women.

Aztreonam 75 mg administered by oral inhalation via nebulization in lactating women produced peak plasma concentrations approximately 1% of peak plasma concentrations reported following a 500-mg IV dose of the drug. Systemic absorption of aztreonam following inhaled administration is likely minimal, but the effects on the infant or on milk production are unknown.

Pediatric Use

The manufacturers state that use of IV aztreonam in children 9 months of age or older is supported by evidence from adequate and well-controlled studies in adults and additional efficacy, safety, and pharmacokinetic data from noncomparative clinical studies in pediatric patients. However, data are insufficient to date to determine safety and efficacy of IV aztreonam in pediatric patients 9 months of age or older for the treatment of septicemia or skin and skin structure infections (when skin infection suspected or known to be caused by *Haemophilus influenzae* type b). In addition, the manufacturers state that data are insufficient to date to evaluate IM administration of aztreonam in pediatric patients or use of the drug in pediatric patients with impaired renal function.

In clinical studies evaluating parenteral aztreonam in pediatric patients, discontinuance of the drug because of adverse effects was required in less than 1% of patients. Rash, diarrhea, and fever have been reported in 1–4.3% of pediatric patients. In pediatric patients receiving IV aztreonam, pain was reported in 12% and erythema, induration, or phlebitis were reported in 0.9–2.9% of patients overall; in US patients, pain occurred in 1.5% and other local reactions occurred in about 0.5%. Eosinophilia, neutropenia, or increased platelet count has been reported in 6.3, 3.2, or 3.6% of pediatric patients, respectively, and increased serum AST, ALT, or serum creatinine has been reported in 3.8–6.5%. In US pediatric studies, neutropenia (absolute neutrophil count less than $1000/mm^3$) occurred in 11.3% of patients younger than 2 years of age receiving aztreonam in a dosage of 30 mg/kg every 6 hours and increased serum AST and ALT (greater than 3 times the upper limit of normal) occurred in 15–20% of patients 2 years of age or older receiving a dosage of 50 mg/kg every 6 hours. It is unclear whether the increased frequency of these adverse effects was related to increased severity of illness in the patients or aztreonam dosage administered.

Aztreonam has been used IM or IV in a limited number of neonates and infants as young as 1 month of age† without unusual adverse effects.

Safety and efficacy of aztreonam administered by oral inhalation via nebulization have not been established in pediatric patients younger than 7 years of age. The drug has been used by oral inhalation via nebulization for the treatment of newly acquired *Ps. aeruginosa* respiratory tract infections in a limited number of cystic fibrosis patients 3 months through 6 years of age† without unusual adverse effects. In clinical trials evaluating aztreonam inhalation therapy in cystic fibrosis patients 7 years of age or older, pyrexia was reported more frequently in pediatric patients than in adults.

Geriatric Use

Clinical studies evaluating IV or IM aztreonam or aztreonam administered by oral inhalation via nebulization did not include sufficient numbers of patients 65 years of age and older to determine whether they respond differently than younger patients. Other reported clinical experience with parenteral aztreonam has not identified differences in responses between geriatric patients and younger adults.

Aztreonam is substantially eliminated by the kidneys, and the risk of adverse effects may be greater in those with impaired renal function. Because geriatric patients are more likely to have reduced renal function, select IV or IM dosage of aztreonam with caution and monitor renal function.

Hepatic Impairment

Monitor appropriate laboratory tests when aztreonam is used in patients with impaired hepatic function. Some clinicians suggest that liver function tests (i.e., serum hepatic enzyme concentrations) be determined once weekly in patients receiving IV or IM aztreonam; however, the manufacturer and other clinicians question the necessity of this precaution.

Renal Impairment

Monitor appropriate laboratory tests when aztreonam is used in patients with impaired renal function. Decrease doses and/or frequency of administration of IV or IM aztreonam in patients with impaired renal function, since serum concentrations of the drug are higher and prolonged in these patients compared with patients with normal renal function.

● Common Adverse Effects

Adverse effects reported with IV or IM aztreonam are similar to those reported with other β-lactam antibiotics, and the drug generally is well tolerated. Adverse effects have been reported in 7% or less of patients receiving parenteral aztreonam and have required discontinuance in about 2% of patients.

DRUG INTERACTIONS

Drug interactions reported are based on parenteral aztreonam. Formal drug interaction studies have not been conducted to date using aztreonam administered by oral inhalation via nebulization.

● Antibacterial Agents

Aminoglycosides

In a study in healthy adults who received a single 1-g IV dose of aztreonam concomitantly with a single 80-mg IV dose of gentamicin, peak serum concentrations of aztreonam were decreased by about 13%, but other pharmacokinetic parameters of the drugs (e.g., half-lives, AUCs) were not affected by concomitant administration. This was not considered clinically important. Further study using multiple doses of the drugs and/or higher doses is probably needed to confirm that there are no clinically important pharmacokinetic interactions between aztreonam and gentamicin.

The antibacterial activity of aztreonam and aminoglycosides is additive or synergistic in vitro against most strains of *Pseudomonas aeruginosa* and some strains of *Ps. cepacia*, *Ps. fluorescens*, and *Ps. maltophilia*. The combination of aztreonam and an aminoglycoside also is synergistic against some Enterobacteriaceae, including some strains of *Enterobacter*, *Escherichia coli*, *Klebsiella*, and *Serratia*.

In vitro, the combination of aztreonam and an aminoglycoside has occasionally been synergistic against *Acinetobacter*, although the combination more frequently is only additive or indifferent against this organism.

The combination of aztreonam and an aminoglycoside generally is indifferent against gram-positive bacteria, including *Staphylococcus aureus*, *S. epidermidis*, and *Enterococcus faecalis* (formerly *Streptococcus faecalis*).

β-Lactam Antibiotics

In a single-dose IV study, there were no clinically important pharmacokinetic interactions between nafcillin sodium and aztreonam.

An additive or synergistic effect has occurred in vitro against some strains of *Ps. aeruginosa* when aztreonam was used concomitantly with piperacillin or cefotaxime. The combination of aztreonam and ampicillin, piperacillin, or cefotaxime generally is indifferent or only slightly additive against Enterobacteriaceae, including *Enterobacter*, *E. coli*, *S. marcescens*, and *Klebsiella*.

In vitro, the combination of aztreonam and cefoxitin has been synergistic against some strains of *Enterobacter*, *E. coli*, *Klebsiella*, *S. marcescens*, *Salmonella*, and *Shigella*. However, antagonism has occurred in vitro when aztreonam was used in combination with cefoxitin against *Enterobacter* or *S. marcescens*. Antagonism also has occurred in vitro when imipenem was used in combination with aztreonam against *Ps. aeruginosa*. Antagonism between aztreonam and these anti-infectives may occur because cefoxitin and imipenem are potent β-lactamase inducers and can derepress inducible, chromosomally mediated β-lactamases in gram-negative bacteria that possess these enzymes (e.g., *Enterobacter*, *Serratia*, *Ps. aeruginosa*). Although aztreonam is relatively stable against hydrolysis by inducible β-lactamases, it has been suggested that the enzymes may inactivate aztreonam by binding to the drug and preventing access to penicillin-binding proteins (PBPs). Because the combinations may be antagonistic, anti-infective agents that are potent inducers of β-lactamase production (e.g., cefoxitin, imipenem) should not be used concomitantly with aztreonam.

Chloramphenicol

Results of an in vitro study using *K. pneumoniae* indicate that chloramphenicol can antagonize the bactericidal activity of aztreonam. It has been suggested that if concomitant use of the drugs is indicated, chloramphenicol should be administered a few hours after aztreonam; however, the necessity of this precaution has not been established.

Clindamycin

In a study in healthy adults who received a single IV dose of aztreonam concomitantly with a single IV dose of clindamycin, total urinary excretion of aztreonam was increased by about 5%. This was not considered clinically important, and other parameters (e.g., half-lives, AUCs) were not affected by concomitant administration of the drugs. Further study using multiple and/or higher doses of the drugs probably are needed to confirm that there are no clinically important pharmacokinetic interactions between aztreonam and clindamycin.

In vitro, the antibacterial activity of aztreonam and clindamycin has been synergistic against some strains of *E. coli*, *Klebsiella*, and *Enterobacter*, although the combination more frequently is indifferent or additive against these organisms. Indifferent or slightly additive effects also have been reported when aztreonam was used in conjunction with clindamycin against anaerobic bacteria.

Metronidazole

In a study in healthy adults who received a single IV dose of aztreonam concomitantly with a single IV dose of metronidazole, peak serum concentrations of aztreonam were decreased by about 10%. This was not considered clinically important, and other parameters (e.g., half-lives, AUCs) were not affected by concomitant administration of the drugs. Further study using multiple and/or higher doses of the drugs probably are needed to confirm that there are no clinically important pharmacokinetic interactions between aztreonam and metronidazole.

In vitro, indifferent or slightly additive effects have been reported when aztreonam was used in conjunction with metronidazole against anaerobic bacteria.

● Clavulanic Acid

In vitro studies indicate that the combination of aztreonam and clavulanic acid, a β-lactamase inhibitor, is synergistic against some strains of β-lactamase-producing *Enterobacter*, *Klebsiella*, and *Bacteroides fragilis* resistant to aztreonam alone. The combination of aztreonam and clavulanic acid may also be antagonistic against some organisms. Clavulanic acid can induce production of chromosomally mediated β-lactamases in some gram-negative bacteria (e.g., *Enterobacter*, *Ps. aeruginosa*) and therefore could interfere with the antibacterial activity of aztreonam by a mechanism similar to that seen with cefoxitin or imipenem. Concomitant use of clavulanic acid and aztreonam does not alter the in vitro susceptibility of *S. aureus* to aztreonam since resistance to the drug in these organisms is intrinsic.

● Furosemide

Concomitant use of furosemide can increase serum concentrations of aztreonam, but this effect is not considered clinically important.

● Probenecid

Concomitant use of probenecid slows the rate of renal tubular secretion of aztreonam and can increase serum concentrations of aztreonam. This effect, however, is not sufficient to be of therapeutic benefit since it produces only a 5% increase in serum aztreonam concentrations and an 11% increase in the serum half-life of the drug. Concomitant probenecid also appears to decrease the binding of aztreonam to plasma proteins by about 13%, presumably by competing with the drug for plasma and tissue protein binding sites, and decreases the steady-state volume of distribution of aztreonam by about 16%.

PHARMACOLOGY

● Description

Aztreonam is a synthetic monobactam antibiotic.

Like bicyclic β-lactam antibiotics, the antibacterial activity of aztreonam results from inhibition of mucopeptide synthesis in the bacterial cell wall. Aztreonam has a high affinity for and preferentially binds to penicillin-binding protein 3 (PBP 3) of susceptible gram-negative bacteria. The drug also has some affinity for PBP 1a of these bacteria, but little or no affinity for PBPs 1b, 2, 4, 5, or 6. Because PBP 3 is involved in septation, aztreonam causes the formation of abnormally elongated or filamentous forms in susceptible gram-negative bacteria. As a consequence, cell division is inhibited and breakage of the cell wall occurs resulting in lysis and death. Studies using *Staphylococcus aureus* indicate that aztreonam does not bind to the essential PBPs of gram-positive bacteria. Aztreonam also has poor affinity for the PBPs of anaerobic bacteria. The drug, therefore, generally is inactive against these organisms.

Aztreonam usually is bactericidal in action. Since aztreonam has poor affinity for PBPs 1a and 1b of susceptible gram-negative bacteria, it is not as rapidly bactericidal as some other β-lactam antibiotics (e.g., imipenem, cefotaxime, cefoxitin, ceftriaxone) against these organisms. For most susceptible Enterobacteriaceae, the minimum bactericidal concentration (MBC) of aztreonam is equal to or only 2–4 times higher than the minimum inhibitory concentration (MIC) of the drug. For *Pseudomonas aeruginosa*, the MBC of aztreonam is usually only 2 times higher than the MIC, but may be up to 125 times higher than the MIC for some strains of the organism.

● Spectrum

Aztreonam has a narrow spectrum of activity. The drug is active in vitro against many gram-negative aerobic bacteria, including most Enterobacteriaceae and Pseudomonas aeruginosa, but has little or no activity against gram-positive aerobic bacteria or against anaerobic bacteria. Aztreonam is inactive against Chlamydia Mycoplasma, fungi, and viruses.

● Resistance

Aztreonam has a high degree of stability against hydrolysis by bacterial β-lactamases, including both plasmid-mediated and chromosomally mediated enzymes, and retains activity in the presence of some penicillinases and cephalosporinases produced by gram-negative and gram-positive bacteria. The drug generally is more stable against inactivation by β-lactamases than cefotaxime. Aztreonam generally is stable against hydrolysis by β-lactamases classified as Richmond-Sykes types I, III (TEM-1, TEM-2, SHV-1), and V (PSE and OXA types). The drug is stable against hydrolysis by most chromosomally mediated Richmond-Sykes type I enzymes produced by Citrobacter, Enterobacter, Morganella, Proteus, Providencia, Serratia, and Proteus. The drug also is stable against hydrolysis by staphylococcal β-lactamases and most β-lactamases produced by Bacteroides.

Aztreonam in combination with other β-lactams or β-lactam/β-lactamase inhibitors (such as ceftazidime-avibactam) has shown synergistic efficacy against metallo-β-lactamase, serine-β-lactamase, and extended-spectrum β-lactamase-producing organisms, including Enterobacteriaceae and other Enterobacterales species, *K. pneumoniae* and *Ps. aeruginosa*

Aztreonam is hydrolyzed by a chromosomally mediated Richmond-Sykes type IV enzyme (K-1) produced by some strains of Klebsiella oxytoca, and strains that produce this enzyme generally are resistant to the drug. Aztreonam also is hydrolyzed to some extent by PSE 2, a Richmond-Sykes type V plasmid-mediated β-lactamase produced by Ps. aeruginosa; the drug generally is stable against hydrolysis by PSE 1, 3, and 4. A chromosomally mediated β-lactamase produced by Bacteroides (B1) can also slowly hydrolyze aztreonam.

In vitro studies indicate that aztreonam is a poor inducer of β-lactamase production and generally does not derepress inducible, chromosomally mediated enzymes in gram-negative bacteria that possess these enzymes (e.g., some strains of Pseudomonas, Citrobacter, Enterobacter, and Serratia). Although aztreonam is relatively stable against hydrolysis by inducible β-lactamases, it has been suggested that the enzymes may inactivate the drug by binding to it and preventing access to penicillin-binding proteins (PBPs). Therefore, gram-negative bacteria that possess these inducible β-lactamases may be resistant to aztreonam following derepression of the enzymes.

Resistance to aztreonam has been produced in vitro in some strains of E. cloacae initially susceptible to the drug, and aztreonam-resistant strains of the organism have emerged during aztreonam therapy. E. cloacae resistant to aztreonam may also be resistant to third generation cephalosporins and extended-spectrum penicillins, but may be susceptible to imipenem. Aztreonam resistance in some strains of E. cloacae appears to be related to alterations in outer-membrane porin proteins and/or other factors that affect permeability of the organism to the drug.

PHARMACOKINETICS

Aztreonam exhibits linear, dose-independent pharmacokinetics. The pharmacokinetics of the drug after IV administration are best described by an open, linear, 2-compartment model and pharmacokinetics after IM administration are best described by an open, one-compartment model with first-order absorption and elimination. The pharmacokinetics of aztreonam in pediatric patients 9 months of age or older are similar to those in adults. Aztreonam is rapidly and completely absorbed following IM administration, and peak serum concentrations of the drug generally are attained within 1 hour after an IM dose. Although peak serum concentrations of aztreonam attained with an IM dose are slightly lower than those attained with an equivalent IV dose, serum aztreonam concentrations 1 hour or longer after dosing are similar.

Multiple-dose studies in adults with normal renal and hepatic function receiving an IM or IV aztreonam dosage of 0.5–1 g every 8 hours for 7 days indicate that neither peak nor trough serum concentrations of the drug increase after repeated dosing and that the drug does not accumulate.

Data from adults and pediatric patients with cystic fibrosis indicate that variable concentrations of aztreonam enter systemic circulation when the drug is administered by oral inhalation via nebulization, but accumulation does not occur following multiple doses.

Aztreonam is widely distributed into body tissues and fluids following IM or IV administration. At serum concentrations of 1–100 mcg/mL, aztreonam is 46–60% bound to serum proteins in healthy adults. In adults with impaired renal function and decreased serum albumin concentrations, aztreonam is 22–49% bound to serum proteins. Aztreonam crosses the placenta and is distributed into amniotic fluid. The drug is distributed into milk in low concentrations. In lactating women who received a single 1-g IM or IV dose of aztreonam, peak milk concentrations were attained 2–6 hours after the dose.

When aztreonam is administered by oral inhalation via nebulization in adult and pediatric patients with cystic fibrosis, sputum concentrations of the drug exhibit considerable interindividual variation, but accumulation does not occur following multiple doses.

Aztreonam is partially metabolized to several microbiologically inactive metabolites; no active metabolites of the drug have been found in serum or urine. The principal metabolite of aztreonam, which is formed by nonspecific hydrolysis of the β-lactam ring, is 2-[[(2-amino-4-thiazolyl)[(1-carboxy-1-methylethoxy)imino]acetyl]amino]-3-(sulfoamino)butanoic acid (SQ 26,992). Other inactive metabolites, which have not been identified, reportedly may be demethylated products of SQ 26,992.

Serum concentrations of aztreonam decline in a biphasic manner after IV administration. In adults with normal renal and hepatic function, the distribution half-life ($t_{1/2\alpha}$) of aztreonam averages 0.2–0.7 hours and the elimination half-life ($t_{1/2\beta}$) averages 1.3–2.2 hours. The $t_{1/2\beta}$ of SQ 26,992 is longer than that of aztreonam and is about 26 hours in adults with normal renal and hepatic function.

In geriatric adults, renal clearance of aztreonam is decreased and the $t_{1/2}$ of the drug is prolonged compared with younger adults. The $t_{1/2\beta}$ of aztreonam ranges from 1.7–4.3 hours in adults 64–82 years of age with renal function normal for their age.

The $t_{1/2\beta}$ of aztreonam averages 1.7 hours in children 2 months to 12 years of age. Half-life of the drug is longer in neonates than in older children and adults and is inversely related to age and birthweight. In neonates younger than 7 days of age, $t_{1/2\beta}$ of aztreonam averages 5.5–9.9 hours in those weighing less than 2.5 kg and 2.6 hours in those weighing more than 2.5 kg. In neonates 1 week to 1 month of age, $t_{1/2\beta}$ of the drug averages 2.4 hours.

In patients with renal impairment, serum concentrations of aztreonam are higher and the serum half-life prolonged.

In patients with hepatic impairment, serum half-life of aztreonam is only slightly prolonged since the liver is a minor pathway of elimination for the drug. In a study in patients with cirrhosis but with normal renal function, the $t_{1/2\beta}$ of aztreonam averaged 2.2 hours in those with primary biliary cirrhosis and 3.2 hours in those with alcoholic cirrhosis.

Aztreonam is excreted principally in urine as unchanged drug via both glomerular filtration and tubular secretion. Following IM or IV administration of a single 0.5-, 1-, or 2-g dose of aztreonam in adults with normal renal function, approximately 58–74% of the dose is excreted in urine unchanged, 1–7% is excreted as SQ 26,992, and 3–4% is excreted as unidentified inactive metabolites. Urinary excretion of unchanged aztreonam is essentially complete 8–12 hours after a single dose of the drug, but SQ 26,992 is excreted for up to 48 hours after the dose.

Aztreonam is partially excreted in feces, presumably via biliary elimination. Approximately 1% of a single 500-mg IV dose of the drug is excreted in feces unchanged, 3% as SQ 26,992, and 7.5–10.8% as unidentified inactive metabolites.

Cystic fibrosis patients may eliminate aztreonam at a faster rate than healthy individuals. Serum half-life of the drug averaged 1–1.3 hours in several patients with cystic fibrosis.

Aztreonam and SQ 26,992 are removed by hemodialysis. The amount of the drug and its metabolites removed during hemodialysis depends on several factors (e.g., type of coil used, dialysis flow rate). In one group of patients with end-stage renal disease undergoing hemodialysis, the serum half-life of aztreonam averaged 2.7 hours during hemodialysis and 7.9 hours between dialysis sessions. A 4-hour period of hemodialysis generally removes into the dialysate about 27–58% of a single 1-g IV dose of aztreonam when the dose is given 1 hour prior to dialysis.

Aztreonam is removed to a lesser extent by peritoneal dialysis. In patients with chronic renal failure undergoing CAPD with a 6-hour dwell time, about 10% of a single 1-g IV dose of aztreonam is removed into the dialysate within 48 hours after the dose.

When the commercially available aztreonam powder for inhalation solution is administered by oral inhalation via nebulization, approximately 10% of the total dose is excreted unchanged in urine; glomerular filtration and tubular secretion are equally involved in elimination of systemically absorbed drug.

In adults with cystic fibrosis receiving aztreonam by oral inhalation via nebulization, the plasma elimination half-life of systemically absorbed drug is approximately 2.1 hours.

ADVICE TO PATIENTS

- Advise patients that antibacterials (including aztreonam) should only be used to treat bacterial infections and not used to treat viral infections (e.g., the common cold).

- Advise patients to complete the full course of therapy, even if feeling better after a few days.

- Advise patients that skipping doses or not completing the full course of therapy may decrease effectiveness and increase the likelihood that bacteria will develop resistance and will not be treatable with aztreonam or other antibacterials in the future.

- Advise patients to discontinue therapy and inform their clinician if an allergic reaction occurs.

- Advise patients that diarrhea is a common problem caused by systemic anti-infectives and usually ends when the drug is discontinued. Advise patients to contact a clinician if watery and bloody stools (with or without stomach cramps and fever) occur during or as late as ≥2 months after the last dose.

- Oral inhalation via nebulization: Advise patients to reconstitute the powder for inhalation solution using *only* the diluent provided by the manufacturer and to administer reconstituted solution *only* with the Altera® nebulizer system.

- Oral inhalation via nebulization: Advise patients to complete the full 28-day oral inhalation regimen, even if feeling better; if a dose is missed, advise patient to take all 3 daily doses as long as the doses are at least 4 hours apart.

- Oral inhalation via nebulization: Advise patients to inform their clinician if they have new or worsening symptoms and to immediately contact a clinician if a possible allergic reaction occurs.

- Advise patient to inform their clinician of existing or contemplated concomitant therapy, including prescription and OTC drugs and dietary or herbal supplements, as well as any concomitant illnesses.

- Advise women to inform their clinician if they are or plan to become pregnant or plan to breast-feed.

- Inform patients of other important precautionary information.

PREPARATIONS

Aztreonam oral inhalation (Cayston®) can only be obtained through designated specialty pharmacies. Contact manufacturer or consult the Cayston® website (https://www.caystonhcp.com/programs/cayston-access-program) for specific availability information.

Excipients in commercially available drug preparations may have clinically important effects in some individuals; consult specific product labeling for details.

Aztreonam

Oral-inhalation		
Kit	Aztreonam 75 mg powder for inhalation solution for nebulization	Cayston®, Gilead
	0.17% sodium chloride diluent	
Parenteral		
For injection	1 g*	Azactam®, Squibb
		Aztreonam for Injection
	2 g*	Azactam®, Squibb
		Aztreonam for Injection

* available from one or more manufacturer, distributor, and/or repackager by generic (nonproprietary) name

† Use is not currently included in the labeling approved by the US Food and Drug Administration.

Selected Revisions July 25, 2023, © Copyright, September 1, 1987, American Society of Health-System Pharmacists, Inc.

Chloramphenicol Sodium Succinate

8:12.08 • CHLORAMPHENICOL

■ Chloramphenicol is a broad-spectrum antibacterial agent.

USES

Chloramphenicol must be used only for the treatment of serious infections caused by susceptible bacteria or Rickettsia when potentially less toxic anti-infectives are contraindicated or ineffective. The drug must not be used for the treatment of trivial infections or when it is not indicated (e.g., treatment of colds, influenza, throat infections) and must not be used as a prophylactic agent to prevent bacterial infections.

Prior to initiation of chloramphenicol therapy, appropriate specimens should be collected for identification of the causative organism and in vitro susceptibility tests. Chloramphenicol may be started pending results of in vitro susceptibility testing, but the drug should be discontinued as soon as possible if results indicate that the causative organism is resistant to chloramphenicol or if the organism is found to be susceptible to potentially less toxic anti-infectives. If results of in vitro susceptibility testing indicate that chloramphenicol and another anti-infective are both likely to be effective, a decision to continue use of chloramphenicol rather than switching to the other anti-infective should be based on the severity of the infection, comparative in vitro susceptibility of the drugs, expected efficacy of the drugs in the specific infection, and comparative safety profiles of the drugs.

● Meningitis

Chloramphenicol is used as an alternative for the treatment of meningitis caused by susceptible bacteria, including susceptible *Haemophilus influenzae, Neisseria meningitidis,* or *Streptococcus pneumoniae.* Chloramphenicol is not considered a drug of first choice for the treatment of meningitis and generally is used only when penicillins and cephalosporins are contraindicated or ineffective. Despite evidence of in vitro activity against *Listeria monocytogenes,* chloramphenicol has been ineffective for the treatment of systemic infections caused by this organism. Chloramphenicol should not be used for the treatment of meningitis caused by gram-negative bacilli.

Pending results of CSF culture and in vitro susceptibility testing, the most appropriate anti-infective regimen for empiric treatment of suspected bacterial meningitis should be selected based on results of CSF gram stain and antigen tests, age of the patient, the most likely pathogen(s) and source of infection, and current patterns of bacterial resistance within the hospital and local community. When results of culture and susceptibility tests become available and the pathogen is identified, the empiric anti-infective regimen should be modified (if necessary) to ensure that the most effective regimen is being administered.

Although chloramphenicol has been recommended as an alternative to penicillins and third generation cephalosporins for the treatment of meningitis caused by susceptible β-lactamase-producing or non-β-lactamase-producing *H. influenzae,* strains of chloramphenicol-resistant *H. influenzae* have been reported in some areas of the world and this limits use of the drug, including for empiric treatment when *H. influenzae* may be involved. There also is some evidence that third generation cephalosporins are as effective or more effective than chloramphenicol for the treatment of meningitis caused by susceptible *H. influenzae.*

IV penicillin G, ampicillin, and third generation cephalosporins usually are considered the drugs of choice for the treatment of meningitis caused by *N. meningitidis,* and chloramphenicol is recommended as one of several alternatives when penicillins and cephalosporins cannot be used. Strains of *N. meningitidis* resistant to chloramphenicol have been reported.

Chloramphenicol has been used as an alternative to penicillins and third generation cephalosporins for the treatment of meningitis caused by penicillin-susceptible *S. pneumoniae.* However, treatment failures have been reported when chloramphenicol was used in the treatment of infections caused by penicillin-resistant *S. pneumoniae,* despite the fact that in vitro susceptibility tests indicated that the clinical isolates were susceptible to chloramphenicol.

● Rickettsial Infections

Chloramphenicol has been used for the treatment of rickettsial infections and has been recommended as a possible alternative to tetracyclines in certain situations. The US Centers for Disease Control and Prevention (CDC) and other experts state that doxycycline is the drug of choice for the treatment of *all* rickettsial infections in *all* age groups (including children younger than 8 years of age). These experts state that empiric treatment with a tetracycline (preferably doxycycline) should be initiated immediately in patients with known or suspected rickettsial disease and should not be delayed while waiting for confirmatory testing since some of these infections can be rapidly progressive and may be fatal or lead to long-term sequelae. If an alternative to doxycycline is being considered for the treatment of a rickettsial infection, CDC recommends consultation with an expert.

Rocky Mountain Spotted Fever and Other Tickborne Spotted Fevers

CDC and the American Academy of Pediatrics (AAP) state that doxycycline is the drug of choice for the treatment of *all* tickborne rickettsial infections, including Rocky Mountain spotted fever (RMSF) caused by *Rickettsia rickettsii,* regardless of patient age. Chloramphenicol has been recommended as a possible alternative to doxycycline for the treatment of RMSF in patients who have had potentially life-threatening allergic reactions to the drug (e.g., anaphylaxis, Stevens-Johnson syndrome) and in pregnant women. However, there is some epidemiologic evidence that the risk of death in patients with RMSF is higher in those treated with chloramphenicol than in those treated with a tetracycline and close monitoring is required if chloramphenicol is used. CDC states that the risks and benefits of chloramphenicol versus doxycycline in patients with a history of allergic reactions to tetracyclines should be considered for the individual patient. For those with a history of non-life-threatening reactions to tetracyclines, CDC states that administering doxycycline in an observed setting is a possible option. Although data are limited, CDC states that rapid doxycycline desensitization in consultation with an allergy and immunology specialist may be an option for individuals with a history of life-threatening hypersensitivity reactions to tetracyclines.

CDC states that, although chloramphenicol is a potential alternative to doxycycline for the treatment of RMSF in pregnant women, chloramphenicol must be used with caution during the third trimester of pregnancy because of the theoretical risk of gray syndrome (see Cautions: Gray Syndrome).

Endemic, Epidemic, and Scrub Typhus

Chloramphenicol has been recommended as a possible alternative to doxycycline for the treatment of endemic typhus (murine typhus; fleaborne typhus) caused by *R. typhi* or *R. felis,* but may be less effective than doxycycline. Doxycycline is the drug of choice for the treatment of endemic typhus, regardless of patient age.

Chloramphenicol has been recommended as a possible alternative to doxycycline for the treatment of epidemic typhus (louseborne typhus; sylvatic typhus) caused by *R. prowazekii* (e.g., in patients with life-threatening allergic reactions to doxycycline). Doxycycline is the drug of choice for the treatment of epidemic typhus, regardless of patient age.

Although chloramphenicol has been used for the treatment of scrub typhus caused by *Orientia tsutsugamushi* and is recommended as a possible alternative to doxycycline for the treatment of such infections, chloramphenicol resistance and persistence or relapse of the infection has been reported.

Anaplasmosis and Ehrlichiosis

Chloramphenicol should *not* be used for the treatment of anaplasmosis caused by *Anaplasma phagocytophilum* (also known as human granulocytic anaplasmosis; HGA) or ehrlichiosis caused by *Ehrlichia chaffeensis* (also known as human monocytic ehrlichiosis; HME). CDC and other experts state that doxycycline is the drug of choice for the treatment of human ehrlichiosis and anaplasmosis, regardless of patient age.

Although chloramphenicol has been used in some patients for the treatment of ehrlichiosis† caused by *E. chaffeensis* or *E. canis* and was recommended in the past as a possible alternative to tetracyclines for these infections, such use is not supported by results of in vitro susceptibility testing for these organisms and the drug is considered ineffective for these infections.

● Typhoid Fever and Other Severe Salmonella Infections

Chloramphenicol has been used for the treatment of typhoid fever (enteric fever) caused by susceptible *Salmonella enterica* serovar Typhi. The drug also has been used for the treatment of paratyphoid fever caused by *S. enterica* serovar Paratyphi.

Various anti-infectives have been used for the treatment of typhoid fever, including ampicillin, amoxicillin, chloramphenicol, co-trimoxazole, cefotaxime, ceftriaxone, fluoroquinolones, and azithromycin. Although chloramphenicol was a drug of choice for the treatment of infections caused by typhoidal *Salmonella* in the past, multidrug-resistant strains of *S. enterica* serovar Typhi (i.e., strains resistant to ampicillin, chloramphenicol, and/or co-trimoxazole) are reported worldwide and are common in many regions of the world. In addition, strains with decreased susceptibility or resistance to other drugs used for the treatment of typhoid fever (e.g., fluoroquinolones, third generation cephalosporins) have been reported. Whenever possible, anti-infectives for the treatment of typhoid fever should be selected based on results of in vitro susceptibility testing. For empiric treatment of typhoid fever known or likely to be caused by multidrug-resistant strains, azithromycin or a parenteral third generation cephalosporin (e.g., ceftriaxone, cefotaxime) has been recommended.

Chloramphenicol should *not* be used for the treatment of typhoid carriers. Depending on susceptibility of the strain, a fluoroquinolone (e.g., ciprofloxacin), ampicillin, amoxicillin, or co-trimoxazole usually is recommended to treat the typhoid carrier state.

Chloramphenicol should *not* be used for the treatment of uncomplicated *Salmonella* gastroenteritis.

● *Anthrax*

Chloramphenicol has been recommended as an alternative for the *treatment* of anthrax†. Although there is evidence that chloramphenicol has in vitro activity against *Bacillus anthracis*, limited clinical data exist regarding use of the drug in the treatment of anthrax.

Penicillins generally have been considered the drugs of choice for the treatment of anthrax (inhalational, GI, meningitis) caused by penicillin-susceptible *B. anthracis* that occurs as the result of natural or endemic exposures, although a fluoroquinolone (e.g., ciprofloxacin) or doxycycline also has been recommended for the treatment of naturally occurring anthrax. A multiple-drug regimen may be indicated in patients with severe infections. Chloramphenicol has been suggested as an alternative for the treatment of naturally occurring anthrax in patients hypersensitive to penicillins or as one of several options for use in multiple-drug regimens for the treatment of anthrax; however, the World Health Organization (WHO) states that chloramphenicol is no longer recommended as an alternative for the treatment of naturally occurring anthrax because evidence of in vivo efficacy in the treatment of severe anthrax is lacking and the drug is associated with serious adverse effects.

For the treatment of inhalational anthrax that occurs as the result of exposure to *B. anthracis* spores in the context of biologic warfare or bioterrorism, CDC, AAP, and the US Working Group on Civilian Biodefense recommend that treatment be initiated with a multiple-drug parenteral regimen that includes a fluoroquinolone (preferably ciprofloxacin) or doxycycline and 1 or 2 additional anti-infective agents predicted to be effective. Based on in vitro data, drugs that have been suggested as possibilities to augment ciprofloxacin or doxycycline in such multiple-drug regimens include clindamycin, rifampin, a carbapenem (doripenem, imipenem, meropenem), chloramphenicol, vancomycin, penicillin, ampicillin, linezolid, gentamicin, and clarithromycin. IV anti-infective therapy is recommended for initial treatment of clinically apparent GI, inhalational, septicemic, or meningeal anthrax and also is indicated for the treatment of cutaneous anthrax when there are signs of systemic involvement, extensive edema, or head and neck lesions.

For the treatment of systemic anthrax with possible or confirmed meningitis, CDC and AAP recommend a regimen of IV ciprofloxacin with an IV bactericidal anti-infective (preferably meropenem) and an IV protein synthesis inhibitor (preferably linezolid). These experts state that IV chloramphenicol is a possible alternative to linezolid in this regimen, but should be used only if clindamycin and rifampin are not available.

● *Burkholderia Infections*

Burkholderia cepacia Infections

Chloramphenicol has been used in patients with cystic fibrosis and has been recommended as an alternative for the treatment of infections caused by *Burkholderia cepacia*† (formerly *Ps. cepacia*). However, *B. cepacia* usually is resistant to chloramphenicol in vitro.

Patients with cystic fibrosis often are chronically infected or colonized with species within the *B. cepacia* complex. In addition, the *B. cepacia* complex has been associated with infections in immunocompromised patients (e.g., those with chronic granulomatous disease, hemoglobinopathies, malignant neoplasms) and in preterm infants. Optimum regimens for the treatment of chronic *B. cepacia* complex infections have not been identified and anti-infectives should be selected based on in vitro susceptibility data and previous clinical responses. Anti-infectives that have been recommended for the treatment of these infections include meropenem, imipenem, co-trimoxazole, ceftazidime, doxycycline, and chloramphenicol; some experts recommend that multiple-drug regimens be used.

Melioidosis

Chloramphenicol has been used in conjunction with doxycycline and co-trimoxazole for the treatment of melioidosis†, a life-threatening disease caused by *B. pseudomallei* (formerly *Ps. pseudomallei*); however, chloramphenicol is not usually recommended. *B. pseudomallei* is an aerobic, nonfermentative gram-negative bacilli resistant to many anti-infectives. The drugs of choice for the treatment of melioidosis depend on the type of infection, results of in vitro susceptibility tests, and the presence of comorbidities (e.g., diabetes mellitus, liver or renal disease, malignancies, hemoglobinopathies, cystic fibrosis). Many clinicians recommend ceftazidime or a carbapenem (either meropenem or imipenem) as the drugs of choice for initial treatment of severe melioidosis, followed by long-term treatment with an oral anti-infective (e.g., co-trimoxazole, amoxicillin and clavulanate potassium, doxycycline) given for at least 3 months to reduce the risk of relapse. There is some evidence that ceftazidime monotherapy has been associated with a lower mortality rate than a 3-drug regimen of IV chloramphenicol, oral doxycycline, and oral co-trimoxazole. In addition, there is evidence that a 2-drug oral regimen of co-trimoxazole and doxycycline is as effective and better tolerated for follow-up treatment than a 3-drug oral regimen of co-trimoxazole, doxycycline, and chloramphenicol (oral preparation no longer available in the US). *B. pseudomallei* may be difficult to eradicate, and relapse of melioidosis may occur, especially if there is poor compliance with the follow-up regimen.

● *Plague*

Chloramphenicol is used as an alternative for the treatment of plague† caused by *Yersinia pestis*.

Streptomycin (or gentamicin) historically has been considered the drug of choice for the treatment of plague. Alternatives recommended when these aminoglycosides are not used include fluoroquinolones (ciprofloxacin, levofloxacin, moxifloxacin), doxycycline (or tetracycline), chloramphenicol, or co-trimoxazole (may be less effective than other alternatives). Chloramphenicol is considered a drug of choice for the treatment of plague meningitis.

Anti-infective regimens recommended for the treatment of naturally occurring or endemic bubonic, septicemic, or pneumonic plague also are recommended for the treatment of plague that occurs following exposure to *Y. pestis* in the context of biologic warfare or bioterrorism. Such exposures would most likely result in primary pneumonic plague, and prompt initiation of anti-infective therapy (within 18–24 hours of onset of symptoms) is essential in the treatment of pneumonic plague. Some experts (e.g., the US Working Group on Civilian Biodefense, US Army Medical Research Institute of Infectious Diseases [USAMRIID]) recommend that treatment of plague in the context of biologic warfare or bioterrorism be initiated with a parenteral anti-infective regimen of streptomycin (or gentamicin) or, alternatively, doxycycline, a fluoroquinolone (ciprofloxacin, levofloxacin, moxifloxacin), or chloramphenicol. An oral regimen of doxycycline (or tetracycline) or a fluoroquinolone (ciprofloxacin, levofloxacin, moxifloxacin, ofloxacin) may be substituted when the patient's condition improves or when parenteral therapy is unavailable (e.g., when there are supply or logistic problems because large numbers of individuals require treatment in a mass casualty setting). Although oral chloramphenicol has been recommended as an alternative in these situations, an oral preparation of chloramphenicol is no longer commercially available in the US.

In the context of biologic warfare or bioterrorism, some experts (e.g., the US Working Group on Civilian Biodefense, USAMRIID) recommend that asymptomatic individuals with exposure to plague aerosol or asymptomatic individuals with household, hospital, or other close contact (within about 2 m) with an individual who has pneumonic plague receive an oral anti-infective for postexposure prophylaxis; however, any exposed individual who develops a temperature of 38.5°C or higher or new cough should promptly receive a parenteral anti-infective for treatment of the disease. If postexposure prophylaxis is indicated, these experts recommend an oral regimen of doxycycline (or tetracycline) or a fluoroquinolone (ciprofloxacin, levofloxacin, moxifloxacin, ofloxacin). Although oral chloramphenicol has been recommended as an alternative for postexposure prophylaxis following exposure to *Y. pestis* in the context of biologic warfare or bioterrorism, an oral preparation of chloramphenicol is no longer commercially available in the US.

• Tularemia

Chloramphenicol is used as an alternative for the treatment of tularemia† caused by *Francisella tularensis*.

Streptomycin generally has been considered the drug of choice for the treatment of tularemia; however, gentamicin is more readily available and is considered an alternative drug of choice when streptomycin is unavailable. Alternatives recommended for the treatment of tularemia when these aminoglycosides are not used include tetracyclines (doxycycline), chloramphenicol, or ciprofloxacin. Some clinicians state that chloramphenicol should be reserved for the treatment of tularemic meningitis (usually used in conjunction with streptomycin), and should not be used for other forms of tularemia.

Anti-infective regimens recommended for the treatment of naturally occurring or endemic tularemia also are recommended for the treatment of tularemia that occurs following exposure to *F. tularensis* in the context of biologic warfare or bioterrorism. However, the fact that a fully virulent streptomycin-resistant strain of *F. tularensis* was developed in the past for use in biologic warfare should be considered. Exposures to *F. tularensis* in the context of biologic warfare or bioterrorism would most likely result in inhalational tularemia with pleuropneumonitis, although the organism also can infect humans through the skin, mucous membranes, and GI tract.

DOSAGE AND ADMINISTRATION

• Reconstitution and Administration

Chloramphenicol sodium succinate is administered IV.

Although chloramphenicol has been administered IM†, plasma concentrations following IM injection are unpredictable. The manufacturer states that chloramphenicol sodium succinate should *not* be given IM since the drug may be ineffective when administered by this route.

Chloramphenicol has been administered orally as the base or as chloramphenicol palmitate; however, oral preparations of the drug are no longer commercially available in the US.

IV Administration

Prior to IV administration, chloramphenicol sodium succinate vials labeled as containing 1 g of chloramphenicol should be reconstituted by adding 10 mL of aqueous diluent (e.g., sterile water for injection, 5% dextrose injection) to provide a solution containing 100 mg of chloramphenicol per mL.

Rate of Administration

The appropriate dose of reconstituted chloramphenicol solution should be injected IV over a period of at least 1 minute.

The drug also has been given by intermittent IV infusion† over 15–60 minutes.

• Dosage

Dosage of chloramphenicol sodium succinate is expressed in terms of chloramphenicol.

Because the difference between therapeutic and toxic plasma concentrations of chloramphenicol is narrow (i.e., a narrow therapeutic index) and because of interindividual differences in chloramphenicol metabolism and elimination, most clinicians recommend that plasma concentrations of chloramphenicol be monitored in all patients receiving the drug and dosage adjusted accordingly. Blood samples to measure peak plasma concentrations of chloramphenicol usually are obtained 0.5–1.5 hours after an IV dose.

Chloramphenicol dosage generally should be adjusted to maintain plasma concentrations of 5–20 mcg/mL (usually 10–20 mcg/mL). When used in pediatric patients beyond the neonatal period, the American Academy of Pediatrics (AAP) suggests that chloramphenicol dosage be adjusted to maintain target plasma concentrations of 15–25 mcg/mL. Some clinicians suggest that dosage in pediatric patients be adjusted to maintain peak plasma concentrations of 15–25 mcg/mL for the treatment of meningitis

or 10–20 mcg/mL for the treatment of other infections. Chloramphenicol plasma concentrations greater than 25 mcg/mL have been associated with toxicity.

Chloramphenicol should be used no longer than is necessary to eradicate the infection with little or no risk of relapse. IV chloramphenicol should be switched to an appropriate oral anti-infective as soon as feasible.

Repeated courses of chloramphenicol should be avoided if possible.

Pediatric Dosage
General Dosage for Neonates

The manufacturer states that an IV chloramphenicol dosage of 25 mg/kg daily given in 4 equally divided doses every 6 hours usually provides and maintains blood and tissue concentrations of the drug that are adequate for most indications. The manufacturer also states that, after the first 2 weeks of life, full-term neonates usually may receive a dosage up to 50 mg/kg daily given in 4 equally divided doses every 6 hours. If a higher dosage is required for the treatment of severe infections in neonates, the manufacturer recommends that such dosage be given only to maintain blood concentrations within a therapeutically effective range.

Some clinicians recommend that neonates receive an IV loading dose of chloramphenicol of 20 mg/kg followed 12 hours later by maintenance dosage based on age and weight. These clinicians recommend a maintenance dosage of 25 mg/kg once every 24 hours in neonates 7 days of age or younger, 25 mg/kg once every 24 hours in neonates older than 7 days of age weighing 2 kg or less, and 25 mg/kg once every 12 hours in those older than 7 days of age weighing more than 2 kg.

Other clinicians recommend that neonates receive an IV loading dose of 20 mg/kg followed 12 hours later by maintenance dosage based on age and weight. These clinicians recommend that premature neonates weighing 1.2 kg or less receive a maintenance dosage of 22 mg/kg once every 24 hours and that premature neonates 1 week of age or younger weighing 2 kg or less receive a maintenance dosage of 25 mg/kg once every 24 hours. These clinicians recommend that full-term neonates younger than 2 weeks of age receive a maintenance dosage of 25 mg/kg daily in divided doses every 12 hours and that full-term neonates 2–4 weeks of age receive a maintenance dosage of 25–50 mg/kg daily in divided doses every 12 hours.

Chloramphenicol should be used with caution in neonates because immature metabolic processes in this age group may result in excessive plasma concentrations of the drug. (See Cautions: Pediatric Precautions.)

General Dosage for Pediatric Patients Beyond the Neonatal Period

The manufacturer states that an IV chloramphenicol dosage of 50 mg/kg daily given in 4 divided doses every 6 hours provides blood concentrations of the drug that are adequate for most indications in pediatric patients. For the treatment of severe infections (e.g., bacteremia, meningitis), especially when adequate CSF concentrations are desired, the manufacturer states that a dosage up to 100 mg/kg daily may be required; however, this dosage should be reduced to 50 mg/kg daily as soon as possible.

If IV chloramphenicol is used for the treatment of severe infections in pediatric patients beyond the neonatal period, AAP recommends a dosage of 50–100 mg/kg daily given in 4 divided doses.

General Dosage for Pediatric Patients with Immature Metabolic Processes

The manufacturer states that IV chloramphenicol given in a dosage of 25 mg/kg daily will usually produce therapeutic blood concentrations of the drug in young infants and other pediatric patients in whom immature metabolic functions are suspected.

Chloramphenicol plasma concentrations should be carefully monitored in patients with immature metabolic processes because high concentrations of the drug may occur and tend to increase with succeeding doses. (See Cautions: Pediatric Precautions.)

Rickettsial Infections

If IV chloramphenicol is used as an alternative for the treatment of rickettsial infections, including Rocky Mountain spotted fever (RMSF) in children, a dosage of 12.5–25 mg/kg every 6 hours for 5–10 days has been recommended.

In patients with known or suspected RMSF, anti-infective treatment should be initiated promptly and should be continued for at least 3 days after fever subsides and until there is evidence of clinical improvement. The minimum duration of treatment is 5–7 days; a longer duration may be required for severe or complicated disease.

When considering use of chloramphenicol for the treatment of rickettsial infections, consultation with an expert is recommended. (See Uses: Rickettsial Infections.)

Typhoid Fever and other Severe Salmonella Infections

For the treatment of typhoid fever, pediatric patients 14 years of age or older have received IV chloramphenicol in a dosage of 50 mg/kg daily in 4 divided doses (up to 3 g daily) for 14 days. In children 2 years of age or older with typhoid fever, the drug has been given in a dosage of 60 mg/kg daily until defervescence, followed by 40 mg/kg daily to complete 14 days of treatment.

To lessen the possibility of relapse, some clinicians recommend that chloramphenicol dosage be adjusted to provide therapeutic plasma concentrations of the drug and be continued for 8–10 days after the patient becomes afebrile.

Anthrax

If IV chloramphenicol is used as an alternative for the treatment of anthrax† (inhalational, GI, meningitis) that occurs as the result of natural or endemic exposures to *Bacillus anthracis* (see Uses: Anthrax), some clinicians recommend that children receive a dosage of 50–75 mg/kg daily given in divided doses every 6 hours. Treatment of naturally occurring or endemic anthrax generally should be continued for at least 14 days after symptoms abate.

If IV chloramphenicol is used as an alternative in a multiple-drug regimen for initial treatment of severe anthrax† (inhalational, GI, meningitis, or cutaneous with systemic involvement, extensive edema, or head or neck lesions) that occurs in the context of biologic warfare or bioterrorism, AAP recommends that full-term or preterm neonates 7 days of age or younger receive IV chloramphenicol in a dosage of 25 mg/kg once daily and that those 1–4 weeks of age receive 50 mg/kg daily in divided doses every 12 hours. AAP recommends that children 1 month of age or older receive IV chloramphenicol in a dosage of 100 mg/kg daily in divided doses every 6 hours. The multiple-drug parenteral regimen should be continued for at least 2–3 weeks until the patient is clinically stable; treatment can then be switched to appropriate oral anti-infectives.

Plague

If IV chloramphenicol is used as an alternative for the treatment of pneumonic plague† that occurs as the result of exposure to *Yersinia pestis* in the context of biologic warfare or bioterrorism, some experts (e.g., the US Working Group on Civilian Biodefense) recommend that children 2 years of age or older receive a dosage of 25 mg/kg 4 times daily and that dosage be adjusted to maintain plasma chloramphenicol concentrations of 5–20 mcg/mL. Other experts (e.g., US Army Medical Research Institute of Infectious Diseases [USAMRIID]) recommend that children 2 years of age or older receive an IV loading dose of 25 mg/kg followed by 15 mg/kg IV every 6 hours and that dosage be adjusted based on plasma concentrations.

Treatment can be switched to an appropriate oral anti-infective when clinically indicated; the total duration of treatment usually is 10–14 days.

Tularemia

If IV chloramphenicol is used as an alternative for the treatment of tularemia† that occurs as the result of exposure to *Francisella tularensis* in the context of biologic warfare or bioterrorism, some experts (e.g., US Working Group on Civilian Biodefense) recommend that children receive a dosage of 15 mg/kg 4 times daily. Treatment can be switched to an appropriate oral anti-infective when clinically indicated; the total duration of treatment usually is 14–21 days.

If IV chloramphenicol is used in conjunction with streptomycin (or gentamicin) for the treatment of tularemic meningitis in children, some clinicians recommend a dosage of 15 mg/kg every 6 hours (maximum 4 g daily) given for 14–21 days.

Adult Dosage
General Dosage for Adults

The manufacturer recommends that adults with normal renal and hepatic function receive an IV chloramphenicol dosage of 50 mg/kg daily given in divided doses every 6 hours.

In infections caused by less susceptible organisms, the manufacturer states that an IV chloramphenicol dosage up to 100 mg/kg daily may be required. However, because toxic plasma concentrations of the drug may occur in many patients receiving dosages of 100 mg/kg daily, some clinicians suggest that a dosage of 75 mg/kg daily be used initially for the treatment of such infections. Dosage should be reduced to 50 mg/kg daily as soon as possible.

Rickettsial Infections

If IV chloramphenicol is used as an alternative for the treatment of rickettsial infections, including endemic typhus or epidemic typhus, in adults, a dosage of 60–75 mg/kg daily in 4 divided doses for 5–10 days has been recommended. For the treatment of scrub typhus caused by *Orientia tsutsugamushi*, a dosage of 50–100 mg/kg daily (up to 3 g daily) in divided doses every 6 hours has been recommended.

In patients with known or suspected RMSF, anti-infective treatment should be initiated promptly and should be continued for at least 3 days after fever subsides and until there is evidence of clinical improvement. The minimum duration of treatment is 5–7 days; a longer duration may be required for severe or complicated disease.

When considering use of chloramphenicol for the treatment of a rickettsial infection, consultation with an expert is recommended. (See Uses: Rickettsial Infections.)

Typhoid Fever and Other Salmonella Infections

For the treatment of typhoid fever in adults, IV chloramphenicol has been given in a dosage of 50 mg/kg daily in 4 divided doses for 14 days. The drug also has been given in a dosage of 60 mg/kg daily in 4 divided doses until defervescence followed by 40 mg/kg daily in 4 divided doses to complete 14 days of treatment.

To lessen the possibility of relapse, some clinicians recommend that chloramphenicol be given in a dosage that provides therapeutic plasma concentrations of the drug and treatment be continued for 8–10 days after the patient becomes afebrile.

Anthrax

If IV chloramphenicol is used as an alternative in a multiple-drug regimen for the treatment of anthrax† (inhalational, GI, meningitis) that occurs as the result of natural or endemic exposures to *B. anthracis* (see Uses: Anthrax), some clinicians recommend that adults receive a dosage of 50–100 mg/kg daily given in divided doses every 6 hours. Treatment of naturally occurring or endemic anthrax generally should be continued for at least 14 days after symptoms abate.

If IV chloramphenicol is used as an alternative in a multiple-drug regimen for initial treatment of severe anthrax† (inhalational, GI, meningitis, or cutaneous with systemic involvement, extensive edema, or head or neck lesions) that occurs in the context of biologic warfare or bioterrorism, the US Centers for Disease Control and Prevention (CDC) recommends that adults receive a dosage of 1 g every 6–8 hours. The multiple-drug parenteral regimen should be continued for at least 2–3 weeks until the patient is clinically stable; treatment can then be switched to appropriate oral anti-infectives.

Plague

If IV chloramphenicol is used as an alternative for the treatment of pneumonic plague† that occurs as the result of exposure to *Y. pestis* in the context of biologic warfare or bioterrorism, some experts (e.g., the US Working Group on Civilian Biodefense) recommend that adults receive a dosage of 25 mg/kg 4 times daily and that dosage be adjusted to maintain plasma chloramphenicol concentrations of 5–20 mcg/mL. Other experts (e.g., USAMRIID) recommend an IV loading dose of 25 mg/kg followed by 15 mg/kg IV every 6 hours and that dosage be adjusted based on plasma concentrations.

Treatment can be switched to an appropriate oral anti-infective when clinically indicated; total duration of treatment usually is 10–14 days.

Tularemia

If IV chloramphenicol is used as an alternative for the treatment of tularemia† that occurs as the result of exposure to *F. tularensis* in the context of biologic warfare or bioterrorism, some experts (e.g., the US Working Group on Civilian Biodefense) recommend that adults receive a dosage of 15 mg/kg 4 times daily. Other experts (e.g., USAMRIID) recommend a dosage of 15–25 mg/kg IV every 6 hours.

Treatment can be switched to an appropriate oral anti-infective when clinically indicated; the total duration of treatment usually is 14–21 days.

If IV chloramphenicol is used in conjunction with streptomycin (or gentamicin) for the treatment of tularemic meningitis, some clinicians recommend that adults receive a dosage of 15–25 mg/kg every 6 hours (maximum 4 g daily) given for 14–21 days.

● Dosage in Renal and Hepatic Impairment

Because patients with renal and/or hepatic impairment may have reduced ability to metabolize and eliminate chloramphenicol, dosage should be based on plasma chloramphenicol concentrations and adjusted accordingly.

Clinicians should consider that pediatric patients with impaired renal or hepatic function may retain excessive amounts of the drug. (See General Dosage for Pediatric Patients with Immature Metabolic Processes under Dosage: Pediatric Dosage, in Dosage and Administration.)

CAUTIONS

● Hematologic Effects

Serious and fatal blood dyscrasias (aplastic anemia, hypoplastic anemia, thrombocytopenia, granulocytopenia) have occurred in patients receiving both short-term and prolonged treatment with chloramphenicol. Aplastic anemia attributed to chloramphenicol, which later terminated in leukemia, has been reported.

Two forms of hematologic toxicity may occur with chloramphenicol. The first type is the most common and is a dose-related bone marrow suppression that appears to be a direct pharmacologic effect of chloramphenicol and usually is reversible upon discontinuance of the drug. This type of bone marrow suppression is characterized by anemia, leukopenia, reticulocytopenia, thrombocytopenia, increased concentrations of serum iron, increased serum iron-binding capacity, and vacuolation of erythroid and myeloid precursors. It is more likely to occur in patients receiving a chloramphenicol dosage of 4 g daily or higher and in those with plasma chloramphenicol concentrations greater than 25 mcg/mL.

The second type of hematologic toxicity that can occur in patients receiving chloramphenicol is a rare, but often fatal, irreversible aplastic anemia that does not appear to be dose related. This type of bone marrow effect leading to aplastic anemia has been reported with oral or parenteral chloramphenicol and has been associated with a mortality rate greater than 50%. Bone marrow aplasia or hypoplasia may occur weeks or months after the drug has been discontinued. Pancytopenia is frequently observed peripherally, but in some cases only 1 or 2 of the major cell types (erythrocytes, leukocytes, platelets) may be depressed.

Paroxysmal nocturnal hemoglobinuria has been reported in patients receiving chloramphenicol. Hemolytic anemia has been reported when chloramphenicol was used in patients with glucose-6-phosphate dehydrogenase deficiency.

● Gray Syndrome

A type of circulatory collapse, referred to as the gray syndrome, has occurred in neonates and premature infants receiving chloramphenicol. In most cases, chloramphenicol therapy had been instituted within the first 48 hours of life; however, the gray syndrome has occurred in older infants and in infants born to mothers who received chloramphenicol during the late stages of pregnancy or during labor. In addition, a similar syndrome has been reported in older children and adults following chloramphenicol overdosage.

Symptoms of the gray syndrome in infants usually develop 2–9 days after chloramphenicol therapy is initiated and include abdominal distention (with or without vomiting), progressive pallid cyanosis, flaccidity, and vasomotor collapse which may frequently be accompanied by irregular respiration. Gray syndrome can be fatal within a few hours after onset of symptoms. However, if chloramphenicol is discontinued when early evidence of symptoms becomes apparent, the process may be reversible and complete recovery may follow.

The gray syndrome may occur because chloramphenicol impairs myocardial contractility by directly interfering with myocardial tissue respiration and oxidative phosphorylation. It has been attributed to high plasma concentrations of chloramphenicol and is believed to occur more frequently in neonates and young infants because of their inability to conjugate chloramphenicol and excrete the unconjugated drug.

● Nervous System Effects

Optic neuritis, rarely resulting in optic atrophy and blindness, has been reported in patients receiving chloramphenicol, usually following long-term therapy with the drug. Although symptoms tend to be reversible, permanent vision loss may occur.

Peripheral neuritis has occurred following long-term chloramphenicol therapy. Headache, ophthalmoplegia, depression, confusion, and delirium have been reported.

● GI and Hepatic Effects

Adverse GI effects, including nausea, vomiting, diarrhea, glossitis, stomatitis, and enterocolitis have been reported rarely with chloramphenicol.

● Sensitivity Reactions

Hypersensitivity reactions, including anaphylaxis, rash (macular and vesicular), angioedema, urticaria, and fever, have occurred in patients receiving chloramphenicol.

Herxheimer-like reactions have occurred in patients receiving chloramphenicol for the treatment of typhoid fever.

● Precautions and Contraindications

Chloramphenicol is contraindicated in patients with a history of hypersensitivity and/or toxic reactions to the drug.

Because serious, sometimes fatal, reactions have been reported in patients who received chloramphenicol, patients should be hospitalized during therapy with the drug so that appropriate laboratory studies and clinical observations can be made. Chloramphenicol *must not* be used for the treatment of trivial infections or when it is not indicated (e.g., treatment of colds, influenza, throat infections) and *must not* be used for prophylaxis. The drug should be administered no longer than is necessary to eradicate the infection with little or no risk of relapse, and repeated courses should be avoided if possible.

Because of the narrow margin between effective therapeutic and toxic dosages of chloramphenicol and because there are interindividual differences in metabolism and elimination of the drug, most clinicians recommend that plasma concentrations of chloramphenicol be monitored in all patients receiving the drug. In general, plasma chloramphenicol concentrations should be maintained at 5–20 mcg/mL to ensure efficacy and avoid toxicity. (See Dosage and Administration: Dosage.)

It is essential that adequate hematologic studies be performed prior to and approximately every 2 days during chloramphenicol therapy. The drug should be discontinued if reticulocytopenia, leukopenia, thrombocytopenia, anemia, or other hematologic abnormalities attributable to chloramphenicol occur. Although peripheral blood studies may detect leukopenia, reticulocytopenia, or granulocytopenia before these become irreversible, such studies cannot be relied on to detect bone marrow depression prior to development of aplastic anemia.

If optic or peripheral neuritis occurs during chloramphenicol therapy (see Cautions: Nervous System Effects), the drug should be discontinued immediately.

Chloramphenicol should be used with caution in patients with impaired renal and/or hepatic function and in neonates and infants or other pediatric patients with immature metabolic processes. Plasma chloramphenicol concentrations should be monitored closely in these patients and dosage should be adjusted accordingly.

When selecting or modifying anti-infective therapy, results of culture and in vitro susceptibility testing should be used. In the absence of such data, local epidemiology and susceptibility patterns should be considered when selecting anti-infectives for empiric therapy.

As with other anti-infectives, use of chloramphenicol may result in overgrowth of nonsusceptible organisms, including fungi. If infection caused by nonsusceptible organisms occurs, appropriate therapy should be instituted.

● Pediatric Precautions

Chloramphenicol should be used with caution in premature and full-term neonates and infants to avoid potential toxicity, including a type of circulatory collapse referred to as the gray syndrome. (See Cautions: Gray Syndrome.)

Excessive plasma concentrations of chloramphenicol may occur in neonates and infants or other pediatric patients with immature metabolic processes, even when recommended chloramphenicol dosage is used. Plasma concentration of the drug should be determined at appropriate intervals during chloramphenicol treatment and dosage should be adjusted accordingly. (See Dosage and Administration: Dosage.)

● *Geriatric Precautions*

Clinical studies of chloramphenicol did not include sufficient numbers of patients 65 years of age or older to determine whether geriatric adults respond differently than younger patients. Other reported clinical experience has not identified differences in responses between geriatric and younger adults.

Chloramphenicol is substantially eliminated by the kidneys, and the risk of adverse effects may be greater in those with impaired renal function. Dosage in geriatric patients should be selected with caution, usually starting at the low end of the dosage range, and it may be useful to monitor renal function during chloramphenicol treatment. The greater frequency of decreased renal, hepatic, and/or cardiac function and of concomitant disease and drug therapy observed in geriatric patients should be considered.

● *Mutagenicity and Carcinogenicity*

Animal and human studies have not been performed to evaluate the mutagenic and carcinogenic potential of chloramphenicol.

● *Pregnancy, Fertility, and Lactation*

Pregnancy

There are no adequate and well-controlled studies evaluating use of chloramphenicol in pregnant women. Animal reproduction studies have not been conducted using the drug.

Studies using oral chloramphenicol (no longer commercially available in the US) indicate that the drug crosses the placenta.

Use of chloramphenicol during late pregnancy and during labor has been associated with the gray syndrome and other adverse effects in the fetus or infant. (See Cautions: Gray Syndrome.)

Because of potential toxic effects on the fetus, the manufacturer states that chloramphenicol should be used during pregnancy only if potential benefits justify potentials risks to the fetus.

Fertility

Animal and human studies have not been performed to evaluate whether chloramphenicol affects fertility.

Lactation

Studies using oral chloramphenicol (no longer commercially available in the US) indicate that the drug is distributed into human milk.

Because chloramphenicol potentially could cause serious adverse effects in breast-fed infants (see Cautions: Gray Syndrome), the manufacturer states that a decision should be made whether to discontinue nursing or chloramphenicol, taking into account the importance of the drug to the woman.

DRUG INTERACTIONS

● *Drugs Affecting or Metabolized by Hepatic Microsomal Enzymes*

Chloramphenicol inhibits cytochrome P-450 (CYP) isoenzymes 2C9 and 3A4.

● *Antianemia Drugs*

When administered concurrently with iron preparations, vitamin B_{12}, or folic acid, chloramphenicol may delay the response to these drugs.

● *Anticoagulants*

Chloramphenicol may prolong the half-life of warfarin.

● *Anticonvulsants*

Concomitant use of fosphenytoin and chloramphenicol may result in altered (increased or decreased) chloramphenicol concentrations.

Concomitant use of phenobarbital and chloramphenicol has resulted in decreased plasma concentrations of chloramphenicol. Concomitant use of the drugs may increase clearance of chloramphenicol resulting in a 30–40% reduction in plasma concentrations of the drug. In addition, phenobarbital plasma concentrations may be increased by up to 50%.

Concomitant use of phenytoin and chloramphenicol may result in altered (increased or decreased) chloramphenicol concentrations and may result in potentially toxic plasma chloramphenicol concentrations. In addition, concomitant use of the drugs may increase plasma concentrations and prolong the half-life of phenytoin resulting in phenytoin toxicity.

● *Antidiabetic Agents*

Chloramphenicol may decrease metabolism of some sulfonylurea antidiabetic agents (e.g., chlorpropamide, tolbutamide) and may increase plasma half-lives of these drugs.

● *Anti-infective Agents*

Chloramphenicol has been reported to antagonize the bactericidal activity of certain penicillins, cephalosporins, fluoroquinolones, and aminoglycosides in vitro. Although the clinical importance of this in vitro data is unclear, some clinicians recommend that chloramphenicol and these anti-infectives be used concomitantly with caution or that concomitant use be avoided.

Results of an in vitro study using *Klebsiella pneumoniae* indicate that chloramphenicol can antagonize the bactericidal activity of aztreonam. It has been suggested that if concomitant use of the drugs is indicated, chloramphenicol should be administered a few hours after aztreonam; however, the necessity of this precaution has not been established.

Concomitant use of chloramphenicol and rifampin may increase clearance of chloramphenicol resulting in decreased plasma concentrations of the drug.

● *Cyclophosphamide*

Concomitant use of cyclophosphamide and chloramphenicol may prolong the half-life of cyclophosphamide and result in decreased concentrations of the active cyclophosphamide metabolite and reduced effectiveness of the drug.

● *Immunosuppressive Agents*

Concomitant use of cyclosporine and chloramphenicol may result in increased cyclosporine concentrations and increased risk of renal dysfunction, cholestasis, and paresthesias.

Concomitant use of tacrolimus and chloramphenicol may result in increased tacrolimus concentrations.

● *Myelosuppressive Agents*

Because of potential additive effects on bone marrow, concomitant use of chloramphenicol and other drugs associated with bone marrow depression should be avoided.

● *Typhoid Vaccine*

Concomitant use of chloramphenicol and typhoid vaccine live oral Ty21a may decrease efficacy of the live, attenuated vaccine.

MECHANISM OF ACTION

Chloramphenicol usually is bacteriostatic in action, but may be bactericidal against some organisms.

Chloramphenicol inhibits protein synthesis in susceptible organisms by reversibly binding to the peptidyl transferase cavity of the 50S ribosomal subunit of the bacterial 70S ribosome. This prevents the aminoacyl-tRNA from binding to the ribosome and terminates polypeptide chain synthesis.

Chloramphenicol also appears to inhibit protein synthesis in rapidly proliferating mammalian cells. It has been suggested that dose-related bone marrow depression due to chloramphenicol is the result of inhibition of protein synthesis in mitochondria of bone marrow cells.

SPECTRUM

Chloramphenicol has a broad spectrum of activity and is active in vitro against many gram-positive and gram-negative aerobic bacteria, some anaerobic bacteria, and some other organisms, including some *Rickettsia*, *Chlamydia*, and *Mycoplasma*. The drug is inactive against *Mycobacterium* and protozoa.

● Gram-positive Bacteria

Chloramphenicol is active in vitro against many gram-positive aerobic cocci, including *Staphylococcus aureus*, *S. epidermidis*, *Streptococcus pneumoniae*, *S. pyogenes* (group A β-hemolytic streptococci; GAS), *S. agalactiae* (group B streptococci; GBS), α-hemolytic streptococci, and *Enterococcus faecalis*. Chloramphenicol may be active in vitro against some methicillin-resistant *S. aureus* (MRSA; also known as oxacillin-resistant *S. aureus* or ORSA) and some *S. aureus* resistant to vancomycin.

Chloramphenicol also is active in vitro against some other gram-positive bacteria, including *Corynebacterium diphtheriae* and *Listeria monocytogenes*. The drug is not active against *Nocardia*.

Chloramphenicol has in vitro activity against *Bacillus anthracis*. Results of in vitro susceptibility testing of 11 *B. anthracis* isolates that were associated with cases of inhalational or cutaneous anthrax that occurred in the US (Florida, New York, District of Columbia) during September and October 2001 in the context of an intentional release of anthrax spores (biologic warfare, bioterrorism) indicate that these strains had chloramphenicol MICs of 4 mcg/mL and were considered susceptible to the drug. Limited clinical data are available to date regarding in vivo activity of chloramphenicol against *B. anthracis* or use of the drug in the treatment of anthrax.

● Gram-negative Bacteria

Chloramphenicol is active in vitro against some gram-negative aerobic bacteria, including *Haemophilus influenzae*, *H. parainfluenzae*, *Moraxella catarrhalis*, *Neisseria gonorrhoeae*, and *N. meningitidis*.

Although chloramphenicol is active against some Enterobacteriaceae, including some *Citrobacter*, *Enterobacter*, *Escherichia coli*, *Hafnia*, *Klebsiella*, *Proteus*, *Providencia*, *Salmonella*, and *Shigella*, susceptibility is variable and many strains are resistant to the drug.

Yersinia pestis and *Y. enterocolitica* usually are susceptible to chloramphenicol, but resistant strains have been reported.

Burkholderia pseudomallei generally is susceptible to chloramphenicol. *B. cepacia* and *Pseudomonas aeruginosa* usually are resistant to the drug.

Chloramphenicol usually is active against *Aeromonas*, *Bordetella pertussis*, *Brucella*, *Campylobacter jejuni*, *Francisella tularensis*, *Helicobacter pylori*, *Legionella pneumophila*, *Pasteurella multocida*, and *Vibrio parahaemolyticus*. Although *V. cholerae* usually are susceptible to chloramphenicol, resistance has been reported.

● Anaerobic Bacteria

Chloramphenicol is active in vitro against many gram-positive anaerobic bacteria, including *Actinomyces*, *Bifidobacterium*, *Clostridium*, *Eubacterium*, *Lactobacillus*, *Peptococcus*, *Peptostreptococcus*, and *Propionibacterium*.

Chloramphenicol also is active in vitro against some gram-negative anaerobic bacteria, including *Bacteroides fragilis*, *Fusobacterium*, *Prevotella*, and *Veillonella*.

● Other Organisms

Treponema pallidum, *Chlamydia*, and *Mycoplasma* are susceptible to chloramphenicol.

Chloramphenicol is active against some *Rickettsia*, including *R. rickettsii* and causative agents of various typhus fevers. The drug also is active against *Coxiella burnetii*.

● In Vitro Susceptibility Testing

When in vitro susceptibility testing is performed according to the standards of the Clinical and Laboratory Standards Institute (CLSI; formerly National Committee for Clinical Laboratory Standards [NCCLS]), clinical isolates identified as *susceptible* to chloramphenicol are inhibited by drug concentrations usually achievable when the recommended dosage is used for the site of infection. Clinical isolates classified as *intermediate* have minimum inhibitory concentrations (MICs) that approach usually attainable blood and tissue concentrations and response rates may be lower than for strains identified as susceptible. Therefore, the intermediate category implies clinical applicability in body sites where the drug is physiologically concentrated or when a higher than usual dosage can be used. This

intermediate category also includes a buffer zone which should prevent small, uncontrolled technical factors from causing major discrepancies in interpretation, especially for drugs with narrow pharmacotoxicity margins. If results of in vitro susceptibility testing indicate that a clinical isolate is *resistant* to chloramphenicol, the strain is not inhibited by drug concentrations generally achievable with usual dosage schedules and/or MICs fall in the range where specific microbial resistance mechanisms are likely and clinical efficacy of the drug against the isolate has not been reliably demonstrated in clinical studies.

Disk Susceptibility Tests

When the disk-diffusion procedure is used to test susceptibility to chloramphenicol, a disk containing 30 mcg/mL of the drug should be used.

When disk-diffusion susceptibility testing is performed according to CLSI standardized procedures using CLSI interpretive criteria, *Staphylococcus* or *Enterococcus* with growth inhibition zones of 18 mm or greater are susceptible to chloramphenicol, those with zones of 13–17 mm have intermediate susceptibility, and those with zones of 12 mm or less are resistant to the drug.

When the disk-diffusion procedure is performed according to CLSI standardized procedures, *Haemophilus* with growth inhibition zones of 29 mm or greater are susceptible to chloramphenicol, those with zones of 26–28 mm have intermediate susceptibility, and those with zones of 25 mm or less are resistant to the drug.

When testing susceptibility of *S. pneumoniae* according to CLSI standardized procedures, *S. pneumoniae* with growth inhibition zones of 21 mm or greater are susceptible to chloramphenicol and those with zones of 20 mm or less are resistant to the drug. When testing streptococci other than *S. pneumoniae*, those with zones of 21 mm or greater are susceptible to chloramphenicol, those with zones of 18–20 mm have intermediate susceptibility, and those with zones of 17 mm or less are resistant to the drug.

When the disk-diffusion procedure is performed according to CLSI standardized procedures, *N. meningitidis* with growth inhibition zones of 26 mm or greater are susceptible to chloramphenicol, those with zones of 20–25 mm have intermediate susceptibility, and those with zones of 19 mm or less are resistant to the drug.

Dilution Susceptibility Tests

When dilution susceptibility testing (agar or broth dilution) is performed according to CLSI standardized procedures, *Staphylococcus*, *Enterococcus*, Enterobacteriaceae, non-Enterobacteriaceae gram-negative bacilli (e.g., *B. cepacia* complex, *Pseudomonas* spp. other than *Ps. aeruginosa*) with MICs of 8 mcg/mL or less are susceptible to chloramphenicol, those with MICs of 16 mcg/mL have intermediate susceptibility, and those with MICs of 32 mcg/mL or greater are resistant to the drug.

When broth dilution susceptibility testing is performed according to CLSI standardized procedures, *Haemophilus* or *N. meningitidis* with MICs of 2 mcg/mL or less are susceptible to chloramphenicol, those with MICs of 4 mcg/mL have intermediate susceptibility, and those with MICs of 8 mcg/mL or greater are resistant to the drug.

When testing susceptibility of *S. pneumoniae* according to CLSI standardized procedures, *S. pneumoniae* with MICs of 4 mcg/mL or less are susceptible to chloramphenicol and those with MICs of 8 mcg/mL or greater are resistant to the drug. Streptococci other than *S. pneumoniae* with MICs of 4 mcg/mL or less are susceptible to chloramphenicol, those with MICs of 8 mcg/mL have intermediate susceptibility, and those with MICs of 16 mcg/mL or greater are resistant to the drug.

When broth dilution susceptibility testing is performed according to CLSI standardized procedures, anaerobes with MICs of 8 mcg/mL or less are susceptible to chloramphenicol, those with MICs of 16 mcg/mL have intermediate susceptibility, and those with MICs of 32 mcg/mL or greater are resistant to the drug.

RESISTANCE

Resistance to chloramphenicol has been induced in vitro and has been shown to be induced in a stepwise manner. The reported incidence of chloramphenicol resistance in clinical isolates varies considerably worldwide and may be reported more frequently in regions of the world where the drug is still commonly used and has not been reserved for the treatment of serious infections.

Several mechanisms of resistance to chloramphenicol have been reported. A common mechanism of resistance to the drug is enzymatic acetylation and inactivation by chloramphenicol acetyltransferases (CATs). CATs have been identified in many different bacteria and may be readily transmitted to other bacteria. Other mechanisms of resistance to chloramphenicol involve transmembrane efflux pumps, decreased membrane permeability, or alterations in the 50S ribosomal subunit.

Staphylococcus aureus, *S. epidermidis*, *S. hemolyticus*, *Streptococcus pneumoniae*, *S. pyogenes*, and *Enterococcus faecium* resistant to chloramphenicol have been reported.

Escherichia coli, *Salmonella*, and *Shigella* resistant to chloramphenicol have been reported with increasing frequency. Chloramphenicol-resistant strains of *Haemophilus influenzae* and *Neisseria meningitidis* have been reported rarely.

Clostridium difficile and *C. perfringens* resistant to chloramphenicol have been reported.

PHARMACOKINETICS

● Absorption

Following IV administration of chloramphenicol sodium succinate, there is considerable interindividual variation in plasma chloramphenicol concentrations attained in adults, children, or neonates. (For information on monitoring plasma chloramphenicol concentrations, see Dosage and Administration: Dosage.) Chloramphenicol sodium succinate is a prodrug and is hydrolyzed in vivo to active chloramphenicol. The rate and extent of hydrolysis of the ester are highly variable. Bioavailability of chloramphenicol following IV administration of chloramphenicol sodium succinate also depends on renal clearance of the unchanged ester, which also is highly variable.

● Distribution

Chloramphenicol is widely distributed into body tissues and fluids including ascitic fluid, pleural fluid, synovial fluid, saliva, and aqueous and vitreous humor. Highest concentrations of the drug are found in the liver and kidneys.

Chloramphenicol is distributed into CSF, even in the absence of meningeal inflammation. CSF concentrations of chloramphenicol have been reported to be at least 50% of concurrent plasma concentrations in patients with uninflamed meninges. In 3 neonates 2–6 weeks of age receiving IV chloramphenicol for the treatment of meningitis or ventriculitis, CSF concentrations of the drug were 45–89% of concurrent plasma concentrations.

Chloramphenicol crosses the placenta.

Chloramphenicol is distributed into milk.

Chloramphenicol is approximately 60% bound to plasma proteins.

● Elimination

Chloramphenicol sodium succinate is hydrolyzed in vivo, presumably by esterases in the liver, kidneys, and lungs, to form active chloramphenicol. Chloramphenicol is then metabolized primarily in the liver to chloramphenicol glucuronide, an inactive metabolite.

Following IV administration of chloramphenicol sodium succinate in adults with normal renal and hepatic function, approximately 30% of the dose is excreted unchanged in urine; however, the fraction of the dose excreted unchanged in urine varies considerably and may range from 6–80%. Small amounts of the dose (2–3%) are eliminated in bile and about 1% is eliminated in feces.

The plasma half-life of chloramphenicol in adults with normal renal and hepatic function is 1.2–4.1 hours.

Because neonates and premature infants have immature mechanisms for glucuronide conjugation and renal excretion, usual doses of chloramphenicol may produce high and prolonged plasma concentrations of the drug in such neonates and infants. The plasma half-life of chloramphenicol is inversely related to age. In one study, plasma half-life was 10–36 hours in neonates 1–8 days of age and 5.5–15.7 hours in infants 11 days to 8 weeks of age.

The elimination half-life of chloramphenicol is prolonged and clearance of the drug is decreased in patients with reduced hepatic function.

In patients with impaired renal function, the elimination half-life of chloramphenicol is not significantly prolonged, although accumulation of the inactive conjugated metabolite may occur. Following IV administration of chloramphenicol sodium succinate in patients with renal impairment, plasma chloramphenicol concentrations may be increased since renal excretion of the succinate ester is reduced in these patients.

Increased chloramphenicol clearance has been reported in patients undergoing hemodialysis. Plasma half-life of chloramphenicol is not affected by peritoneal dialysis. The drug appears to be readily removed by charcoal hemoperfusion.

CHEMISTRY AND STABILITY

● Chemistry

Chloramphenicol is a broad-spectrum antibiotic originally isolated from *Streptomyces venezuelae* and now produced synthetically. Chloramphenicol occurs as fine, white to grayish or yellowish white, needle-like crystals or elongated plates, has a solubility of approximately 2.5 mg/mL in water at 25°C, and is freely soluble in alcohol. The pK_a of the drug is 5.5. Chloramphenicol sodium succinate occurs as a white to light yellow powder and is freely soluble in water and in alcohol.

Chloramphenicol sodium succinate is commercially available as a lyophilized powder that should be reconstituted as directed by the manufacturer to provide an IV solution containing 100 mg of chloramphenicol per mL. Each 1 g of chloramphenicol in the reconstituted solution contains approximately 52 mg (2.25 mEq) of sodium.

● Stability

Chloramphenicol sodium succinate powder for injection should be stored at 20–25°C.

Chloramphenicol has been reported to be physically incompatible with some drugs, but the compatibility depends on several factors (e.g., the concentration of the drugs, specific diluents used, resulting pH, temperature). Specialized references should be consulted for specific compatibility information.

PREPARATIONS

Excipients in commercially available drug preparations may have clinically important effects in some individuals; consult specific product labeling for details.

Chloramphenicol Sodium Succinate

Parenteral		
For injection, for IV use only	1 g (of chloramphenicol)*	Chloramphenicol Sodium Succinate

* available from one or more manufacturer, distributor, and/or repackager by generic (nonproprietary) name

† Use is not currently included in the labeling approved by the US Food and Drug Administration.

Selected Revisions June 24, 2019, © Copyright, August 1, 1980, American Society of Health-System Pharmacists, Inc.

Preface to the Penicillins

8:12.16 • PENICILLINS

CLASSIFICATION OF PENICILLINS BASED ON SPECTRA OF ACTIVITY

Penicillins are natural or semisynthetic antibiotics produced by or derived from certain species of the fungus *Penicillium*. The drugs are β-lactam antibiotics structurally and pharmacologically related to other β-lactam antibiotics, including cephalosporins and cephamycins. Penicillins contain a 6-aminopenicillanic acid (6-APA) nucleus, which is composed of a β-lactam ring fused to a 5-membered thiazolidine ring. Although the 6-APA nucleus has little antibacterial activity itself, it is a major structural requirement for antibacterial activity of penicillins. In currently available penicillins, cleavage at any point in the penicillin nucleus, including the β-lactam ring, results in complete loss of antibacterial activity. A free carboxyl group in the thiazolidine ring and one or more substituted amino side chains at R are also essential for antibacterial activity.

Addition of various side chains at R on the penicillin nucleus results in penicillin derivatives with differences in spectra of activity, stability against hydrolysis by β-lactamases, acid stability, GI absorption, and protein binding.

Currently available penicillins can be divided into 4 groups based principally on their spectra of activity:

- Natural Penicillins
- Penicillinase-Resistant Penicillins
- Aminopenicillins
- Extended-Spectrum Penicillins

Natural Penicillins

penicillin G   penicillin V

Natural penicillins are produced by fermentation of mutant strains of *Penicillium chrysogenum*. Natural penicillins with different side chains at R are produced by altering the composition of the culture media of *Penicillium*. Although various natural penicillins have been produced (e.g., penicillins F, G, N, O, V, X), only penicillin G and penicillin V are used clinically.

Natural penicillins are active in vitro against many gram-positive aerobic cocci including nonpenicillinase-producing *Staphylococcus aureus* and *S. epidermidis*, *Streptococcus pneumoniae*, *S. pyogenes* (group A β-hemolytic streptococci; GAS), *S. agalactiae* (group B streptococci; GBS), other β-hemolytic streptococci (e.g., groups C, G, H, L, R), viridans streptococci, and nonenterococcal group D streptococci. Although some strains of enterococci are susceptible to penicillin G in vitro, many strains are resistant and penicillin tolerance has been reported. Natural penicillins are readily hydrolyzed by staphylococcal penicillinases and are therefore inactive against penicillinase-producing strains of *S. aureus* and *S. epidermidis*. The drugs are active in vitro against some gram-positive aerobic bacilli including *Bacillus anthracis*, *Corynebacterium diphtheriae*, *Erysipelothrix rhusiopathiae*, and *Listeria monocytogenes*.

Natural penicillins also are active in vitro against some gram-negative aerobic cocci including *Neisseria meningitidis*. Although natural penicillins may be active in vitro against strains of nonpenicillinase-producing *N. gonorrhoeae*, penicillinase-producing strains of *N. gonorrhoeae* (PPNG) are resistant. The drugs are active in vitro against some gram-negative aerobic bacilli including some strains of *Haemophilus influenzae*, *Pasteurella multocida*, *Streptobacillus moniliformis*, and *Spirillum minus*. However, *Pseudomonas* and most Enterobacteriaceae are resistant to natural penicillins.

Natural penicillins are active in vitro against many gram-positive anaerobic bacteria, including *Actinomyces israelii*, *Clostridium* (*C. botulinum*, *C. perfringens*, and *C. tetani*), *Cutibacterium acnes* (formerly *Propionibacterium acnes*), *Eubacterium*, *Lactobacillus*, *Peptococcus*, and *Peptostreptococcus*. Gram-negative anaerobic bacteria vary in their susceptibility to the drugs. Although penicillin G is active

in vitro against some strains of *Fusobacterium*, *Veillonella*, and *Bacteroides oralis*, the *B. fragilis* group (e.g., *B. fragilis*, *B. distasonis*, *B. ovatus*, *B. thetaiotaomicron*, *B. vulgatus*) require high penicillin G concentrations for in vitro inhibition and usually are resistant.

The drugs also are active against spirochetes, including *Treponema pallidum* subsp *pallidum*, *T. pallidum* subsp *pertenue*, *T. carateum*, *Leptospira*, *Borrelia burgdorferi* (causative agent of Lyme disease), *B. hermsii*, and *B. recurrentis*.

Penicillinase-Resistant Penicillins

dicloxacillin   oxacillin

nafcillin

Penicillinase-resistant penicillins are semisynthetic derivatives of 6-APA that are stable against hydrolysis by staphylococcal penicillinases. These penicillins have bulky side chains at R on the 6-APA nucleus that result in steric hindrance and help to prevent attachment of penicillinases to the β-lactam ring.

Because penicillinase-resistant penicillins are not hydrolyzed by most staphylococcal penicillinases, these drugs are active in vitro against many penicillinase-producing strains of *S. aureus* and *S. epidermidis* that are resistant to natural penicillins, aminopenicillins, and extended-spectrum penicillins.

Penicillinase-resistant penicillins also have some in vitro activity against other gram-positive bacteria and some gram-negative bacteria and spirochetes; however, the drugs generally are less active on a weight basis against these organisms than natural penicillins, and use of penicillinase-resistant penicillins generally is limited to the treatment of infections caused by susceptible penicillinase-producing staphylococci.

Aminopenicillins

amoxicillin   ampicillin

Aminopenicillins are semisynthetic derivatives of 6-APA which have a free amino group at the α-position at R on the penicillin nucleus. Partly because of this polar group, aminopenicillins have enhanced activity against gram-negative bacteria compared with natural penicillins and penicillinase-resistant penicillins.

In vitro, aminopenicillins are generally active against gram-positive aerobic cocci and gram-positive aerobic bacilli that are susceptible to natural penicillins. However, with the possible exception of enterococcal infections, natural penicillins are generally the penicillins of choice for the treatment of infections caused by gram-positive cocci that are susceptible to both natural penicillins and aminopenicillins. Like natural penicillins and extended-spectrum penicillins, aminopenicillins are readily hydrolyzed by staphylococcal penicillinases and are therefore inactive against penicillinase-producing strains of *S. aureus* and *S. epidermidis*.

Aminopenicillins are generally active in vitro against gram-negative aerobic cocci, gram-negative aerobic bacilli, and anaerobic bacteria that are susceptible to natural penicillins. In addition, aminopenicillins are active in vitro against some Enterobacteriaceae including some strains of *Escherichia coli*, *Proteus mirabilis*, *Salmonella*, and *Shigella*. Aminopenicillins are generally inactive against other Enterobacteriaceae, *B. fragilis*, and *Pseudomonas*.

Because clavulanic acid and sulbactam are β-lactamase inhibitors that can inhibit certain β-lactamases that inactivate aminopenicillins, fixed combinations of amoxicillin and clavulanate potassium (amoxicillin/clavulanate) and fixed combinations of ampicillin sodium and sulbactam sodium (ampicillin/sulbactam) are active in vitro against many β-lactamase-producing organisms that are resistant to the aminopenicillin alone.

Extended-Spectrum Penicillins

piperacillin   ticarcillin (no longer commercially available in the US)

Extended-spectrum penicillins are semisynthetic derivatives of 6-APA that have a wider spectra of activity than natural penicillins, penicillinase-resistant penicillins, and aminopenicillins.

The group of extended-spectrum penicillins is composed of 2 different subgroups: Acylaminopenicillins (piperacillin) and α-carboxypenicillins (ticarcillin; no longer commercially available in the US). Acylaminopenicillins have basic groups on the side chain at R on the penicillin nucleus and α-carboxypenicillins have a carboxylic acid group at the α-position at R on the penicillin nucleus. Partly because of these polar groups, extended-spectrum penicillins are more active against gram-negative aerobic and gram-negative anaerobic bacilli than aminopenicillins, and use of extended-spectrum penicillins is generally limited to the treatment of serious infections caused by susceptible gram-negative bacilli or mixed aerobic-anaerobic bacterial infections.

In vitro, extended-spectrum penicillins are generally active against gram-positive and gram-negative aerobic cocci that are susceptible to natural penicillins and aminopenicillins. Like natural penicillins and aminopenicillins, extended-spectrum penicillins are hydrolyzed by staphylococcal penicillinases and are therefore inactive when used alone against penicillinase-producing strains of S. aureus and S. epidermidis. Extended-spectrum penicillins have some activity against gram-positive aerobic and gram-positive anaerobic bacilli, but the drugs are generally less active in vitro on a weight basis against these organisms than are natural penicillins and aminopenicillins.

Extended-spectrum penicillins are generally active in vitro against gram-negative bacilli that are susceptible to aminopenicillins. The drugs are also active against many Enterobacteriaceae and some Pseudomonas that are resistant to other currently available penicillins. α-Carboxypenicillins are active in vitro against some strains of E. coli, Morganella morganii, P. mirabilis, P. vulgaris, Providencia rettgeri, Salmonella, Shigella, and Ps. aeruginosa. In addition to these organisms, acylaminopenicillins are generally active in vitro against some strains of Citrobacter, Enterobacter, Klebsiella, and Serratia. Extended-spectrum penicillins are more active in vitro against B. fragilis than other currently available penicillins.

The only extended-spectrum penicillin commercially available in the US is piperacillin sodium in fixed combination with tazobactam sodium (piperacillin/tazobactam). Because tazobactam has a high affinity for and irreversibly binds to certain β-lactamases that can inactivate extended-spectrum penicillins, piperacillin/tazobactam is active against many β-lactamase-producing bacteria that are resistant to piperacillin alone.

For more complete information on the spectra of activity of penicillins and additional information on the drugs, see the General Statements on Natural Penicillins, Aminopenicillins, and Penicillinase-Resistant Penicillins and the individual monographs in 8:12.16.04, 8:12.16.08, 8:12.16.12, and 8:12.16.16.

---

† Use is not currently included in the labeling approved by the US Food and Drug Administration.

Penicillin G Benzathine

8:12.16.04 • NATURAL PENICILLINS

■ Penicillin G benzathine, a natural penicillin, is a β-lactam antibiotic. The drug is the benzathine tetrahydrate salt of penicillin G and is a long-acting formulation of penicillin G.

USES

Penicillin G benzathine is used only for the treatment of mild to moderately severe infections caused by organisms that are susceptible to the low, prolonged concentrations of penicillin G provided by IM penicillin G benzathine and for prophylaxis of certain infections caused by these organisms. When high, sustained concentrations of penicillin G are required for the treatment of severe infections, parenteral penicillin G potassium or sodium should be used.

The fixed combinations of penicillin G benzathine and penicillin G procaine are used for the treatment of moderately severe to severe infections caused by susceptible streptococci (e.g., upper respiratory tract infections, scarlet fever, erysipelas, skin and skin structure infections). The fixed combinations should *not* be used for *initial* treatment of severe pneumococcal infections, including pneumonia, empyema, bacteremia, pericarditis, meningitis, peritonitis, or arthritis. In addition, fixed combinations of penicillin G benzathine and penicillin G procaine should *not* be used for the treatment of syphilis, yaws, bejel, pinta, or gonorrhea.

For additional information on the uses of penicillin G benzathine, see Uses in the Natural Penicillins General Statement 8:12.16.04.

● Pharyngitis and Tonsillitis

IM penicillin G benzathine is a drug of choice for the treatment of pharyngitis and tonsillitis caused by *Streptococcus pyogenes* (group A β-hemolytic streptococci; GAS) and prevention of initial attacks (primary prevention) of rheumatic fever.

Selection of an anti-infective for the treatment of *S. pyogenes* pharyngitis and tonsillitis should be based on the drug's spectrum of activity, bacteriologic and clinical efficacy, potential adverse effects, ease of administration, patient compliance, and cost. No regimen has been found to date that effectively eradicates group A β-hemolytic streptococci in 100% of patients.

Because the drugs have a narrow spectrum of activity, are inexpensive, and generally are effective with a low frequency of adverse effects, the American Academy of Pediatrics (AAP), Infectious Diseases Society of America (IDSA), and American Heart Association (AHA) recommend a penicillin regimen (i.e., 10 days of oral penicillin V or oral amoxicillin or a single dose of IM penicillin G benzathine) as the treatment of choice for *S. pyogenes* pharyngitis and tonsillitis. Other anti-infectives (narrow-spectrum oral cephalosporins, oral macrolides, oral clindamycin) are recommended as alternatives in penicillin-allergic patients.

Experts state that the single-dose IM penicillin G benzathine regimen may be the preferred regimen in patients who are unlikely to complete the recommended 10-day regimen of oral penicillin V potassium or amoxicillin and in patients with a personal or family history of rheumatic fever or rheumatic heart disease or with other environmental factors (e.g., crowded living conditions) that place them at increased risk for development of rheumatic fever.

If signs and symptoms of pharyngitis recur shortly after initial treatment and presence of *S. pyogenes* is documented, retreatment with the original or an alternative anti-infective is recommended. Initial treatment failures may occur more frequently with oral penicillins than with IM penicillin G benzathine because of poor adherence to the oral regimen. Alternative regimens recommended for retreatment include a narrow-spectrum oral cephalosporin, oral clindamycin, oral fixed combination of amoxicillin and clavulanate, oral macrolide, or IM penicillin G benzathine.

If there are multiple, recurrent episodes of symptomatic pharyngitis within a period of several months to years, it may be difficult to determine whether these are true episodes of *S. pyogenes* infection or whether the patient is a long-term pharyngeal carrier of *S. pyogenes* who is experiencing repeated episodes of non-streptococcal (e.g., viral) pharyngitis.

Treatment of asymptomatic chronic pharyngeal carriers of *S. pyogenes* is not usually indicated and these individuals should not receive repeated courses of anti-infective therapy. However, eradication of the carrier state may be desirable in certain situations (e.g., during a community outbreak of acute rheumatic fever, acute poststreptococcal glomerulonephritis, or invasive *S. pyogenes* infections; during an outbreak of *S. pyogenes* pharyngitis in a closed or partially closed community; when multiple episodes of documented symptomatic *S. pyogenes* pharyngitis are occurring within a family for many weeks despite appropriate treatment; when there is a personal or family history of acute rheumatic fever). In such situations, recommended regimens include oral clindamycin, oral fixed combination of amoxicillin and clavulanate, or oral rifampin used in conjunction with either IM penicillin G benzathine or oral penicillin V.

● Prevention of Rheumatic Fever Recurrence

IM penicillin G benzathine is used for prevention of recurrent attacks of rheumatic fever (secondary prophylaxis) in individuals who have had a previous attack of rheumatic fever.

IM penicillin G benzathine generally is considered the drug of choice for secondary prophylaxis of rheumatic fever because it ensures compliance; alternatives include oral penicillin V or oral sulfadiazine. Sulfadiazine is recommended when hypersensitivity precludes the use of a penicillin; however, a macrolide (azithromycin, clarithromycin, erythromycin) should be used in patients allergic to penicillins *and* sulfonamides. Even with optimal patient adherence, the risk of recurrence of rheumatic fever is higher in individuals receiving an oral prophylaxis regimen than in those receiving IM penicillin G benzathine.

AHA and AAP recommend long-term (continuous) secondary prophylaxis in patients who have been treated for documented acute rheumatic fever (even if manifested solely by Sydenham chorea) and in those with evidence of rheumatic heart disease (even after prosthetic valve replacement).

Prophylaxis should be initiated as soon as the diagnosis of rheumatic fever or rheumatic heart disease is made, although patients with acute rheumatic fever should first receive the usually recommended anti-infective treatment for *S. pyogenes* pharyngitis and tonsillitis (see Uses: Pharyngitis and Tonsillitis).

● Syphilis

IM penicillin G benzathine is used for the treatment of syphilis.

The US Centers for Disease Control and Prevention (CDC) and other experts state that IM penicillin G benzathine is the drug of choice for the treatment of primary syphilis (i.e., ulcer or chancre at infection site), secondary syphilis (i.e., manifestations that include, but are not limited to, rash, mucocutaneous lesions, and lymphadenopathy), and tertiary syphilis (i.e., cardiac syphilis, gummatous lesions, tabes dorsalis, and general paresis) in adults, adolescents, and children.

IM penicillin G benzathine also is the drug of choice for the treatment of latent syphilis (i.e., detected by serologic testing but lacking clinical manifestations), including both early latent syphilis (latent syphilis acquired within the preceding year) and late latent syphilis (i.e., all other cases of latent syphilis or syphilis of unknown duration) in all age groups.

For the treatment of neurosyphilis and otic or ocular syphilis, CDC and other experts state that IV penicillin G potassium or sodium is the drug of choice and IM penicillin G procaine (with oral probenecid) is an alternative if compliance can be ensured.

For the treatment of congenital syphilis, CDC recommends IV penicillin G potassium or sodium or IM penicillin G procaine in neonates with proven or highly probable congenital syphilis (i.e., abnormal physical examination consistent with congenital syphilis, serum quantitative nontreponemal serologic titer fourfold higher than the mother's titer, or positive darkfield test or polymerase chain reaction [PCR] of lesions or body fluids). CDC recommends IV penicillin G potassium or sodium, IM penicillin G procaine, or IM penicillin G benzathine in neonates with possible congenital syphilis (i.e., normal physical examination and serum quantitative nontreponemal serologic titer no more than fourfold higher than the mother's titer and the mother received a recommended treatment regimen less than 4 weeks before delivery; the mother was not treated or was inadequately treated, including treatment with erythromycin or any regimen not included in CDC recommendations; or there is no documentation that the mother received treatment).

Neonates with human immunodeficiency virus (HIV) infection who have congenital syphilis and HIV-infected children, adolescents, and adults who have neurosyphilis or primary, secondary, early latent, late latent, or tertiary syphilis should receive the same treatment regimens as those without HIV infection. Available data indicate that additional treatment doses of IM penicillin G benzathine do not enhance efficacy, including in HIV-infected patients. Because serologic nonresponse and neurologic complications may be more frequent in HIV-infected individuals, close follow-up is essential in those coinfected with syphilis and HIV. In addition, careful neurologic examinations are indicated in all HIV-infected patients coinfected with syphilis.

Limited data support the use of certain alternatives to IM penicillin G benzathine for treatment of primary or secondary syphilis in patients with penicillin hypersensitivity (e.g., doxycycline, tetracycline); however, if compliance with alternative regimens or follow-up cannot be ensured, CDC recommends desensitization and treatment with IM penicillin G benzathine. Some experts state that efficacy of alternatives to IM penicillin G benzathine for the treatment of early syphilis in HIV-infected individuals has not been well studied and use of alternatives in such patients should be undertaken only with close clinical and serologic monitoring.

There are no proven alternatives to penicillin G for the treatment of congenital syphilis in infants and children with known or suspected penicillin hypersensitivity and no proven alternatives to penicillin G for the treatment of any stage of syphilis in pregnant women with penicillin hypersensitivity; therefore, CDC recommends desensitization and treatment with the appropriate penicillin G preparation.

Fixed combinations of penicillin G benzathine and penicillin G procaine (Bicillin® C-R, Bicillin® C-R 900/300) should not be used for the treatment of any form of syphilis; inadvertent use of one of these fixed-combination preparations may not provide the sustained serum concentrations of penicillin G required for treatment of syphilis and could increase the risk of treatment failure and neurosyphilis, especially in HIV-infected patients.

For additional information regarding treatment of syphilis, the current CDC sexually transmitted diseases treatment guidelines available at https://www.cdc.gov/std/syphilis/treatment.htm should be consulted.

DOSAGE AND ADMINISTRATION

● Administration

Penicillin G benzathine and fixed combinations containing penicillin G benzathine and penicillin G procaine are administered *only* by deep IM injection.

Special precaution should be taken to avoid inadvertent intravascular or intra-arterial administration of penicillin G benzathine or fixed combinations of penicillin G benzathine and penicillin G procaine or injection into or near major peripheral nerves or blood vessels because this may result in severe and/or permanent neurovascular damage. (See Cautions: Adverse Effects.)

Penicillin G benzathine and fixed combinations containing penicillin G benzathine and penicillin G procaine must *not* be given IV or admixed with IV solutions because inadvertent IV administration of penicillin G benzathine has been associated with cardiorespiratory arrest and death.

IM Injection

Penicillin G benzathine and fixed combinations containing penicillin G benzathine and penicillin G procaine are provided in prefilled syringes and the appropriate dose should be administered undiluted according to the manufacturer's directions.

In adults, IM injections of penicillin G benzathine or fixed combinations of penicillin G benzathine and penicillin G procaine generally should be made deeply into the gluteus maximus (upper outer quadrant of the buttock) or into the midlateral thigh. In neonates, infants, and small children, IM injections of these preparations should be given preferably into the midlateral muscles of the thigh.

To minimize the possibility of damage to the sciatic nerve, one manufacturer of penicillin G benzathine recommends that the periphery of the upper outer quadrant of the gluteal regions be used in infants and small children only when necessary (e.g., in burn patients) and recommends that the deltoid area be used only if well developed, such as in certain adults and older children, and only with caution to avoid radial nerve injury. This manufacturer also suggests that the penicillin G benzathine dose can be divided and administered at 2 separate sites if necessary in children younger than 2 years of age.

IM injections may be less painful if penicillin G benzathine is warmed to room temperature before administration.

IM injections of penicillin G benzathine or fixed combinations of penicillin G benzathine and penicillin G procaine should be made at a slow, steady rate to avoid blockage of the needle.

When the fixed combination of penicillin G benzathine and penicillin G procaine (Bicillin® C-R) is used, the manufacturer states that the dose usually is given at a single session using multiple IM sites; alternatively, if compliance regarding the return visit is ensured, the total dose can be divided and half given on day 1 and half on day 3.

When repeated doses are given, IM injection sites should be rotated. Repeated IM injection into the anterolateral thigh, especially in neonates and infants, should be avoided because quadriceps femoris fibrosis and atrophy have been reported.

● Dosage

Dosage of penicillin G benzathine usually is expressed in terms of penicillin G units, but also has been expressed as mg of penicillin G.

Dosage of the fixed combinations containing penicillin G benzathine and penicillin G procaine (Bicillin® C-R, Bicillin® C-R 900/300) usually is expressed in terms of the total (sum) of penicillin G units of penicillin G benzathine and penicillin G units of penicillin G procaine.

Pediatric Dosage
General Pediatric Dosage

The American Academy of Pediatrics (AAP) states that the usual dosage of IM penicillin G benzathine for the treatment of mild to moderate infections in pediatric patients beyond the neonatal period is a single dose of 300,000–600,000 units in those weighing less than 27 kg or a single dose of 900,000 units in those weighing 27 kg or more. AAP states that IM penicillin G benzathine is inappropriate for the treatment of severe infections.

If the fixed combination of penicillin G benzathine and penicillin G procaine (Bicillin® C-R) is used in pediatric patients beyond the neonatal period, AAP recommends a single IM dose of 600,000 penicillin G units in those weighing less than 14 kg and a single IM dose of 900,000 to 1.2 million penicillin G units in those weighing 14–27 kg. If this fixed-combination preparation is used in those weighing 27 kg or more, AAP recommends a single dose of 2.4 million penicillin G units.

Pharyngitis and Tonsillitis

For the treatment of pharyngitis or tonsillitis caused by *Streptococcus pyogenes* (group A β-hemolytic streptococci; GAS) and prevention of initial attacks (primary prevention) of rheumatic fever in children, AAP, Infectious Diseases Society of America (IDSA), and American Heart Association (AHA) recommend that IM penicillin G benzathine be given as a single dose of 600,000 units in those weighing less than 27 kg and a single dose of 1.2 million units in those weighing 27 kg or more.

The manufacturers recommend a single IM penicillin G benzathine dose of 300,000–600,000 units in children weighing less than 27 kg and a single dose of 900,000 units in older children for the treatment of *S. pyogenes* pharyngitis.

Although anti-infective treatment is not recommended for most individuals identified as chronic pharyngeal carriers of *S. pyogenes* (see Uses: Pharyngitis and Tonsillitis), IDSA states that a single IM penicillin G benzathine dose of 600,000 units in those weighing less than 27 kg or 1.2 million units in those weighing 27 kg or more given in conjunction with oral rifampin (20 mg/kg daily given in 2 doses [up to 600 mg daily] for 4 days) is an option when eradication of the carrier state is desirable.

Streptococcal Infections

If IM penicillin G benzathine is used for the treatment of mild to moderate infections of the upper respiratory tract caused by susceptible *S. pyogenes*, one manufacturer recommends a single dose of 300,000–600,000 units in children weighing less than 27 kg and 900,000 units in older pediatric patients.

If the fixed combination of penicillin G benzathine and penicillin G procaine (Bicillin® C-R) is used for the treatment of moderately severe to severe infections caused by susceptible *S. pyogenes* (e.g., upper respiratory tract infections, scarlet fever, erysipelas, skin and skin structure infections), the manufacturer recommends that children weighing less than 13.6 kg receive a single IM dose of 600,000 penicillin G units, those weighing 13.6–27.2 kg receive a single IM dose of 900,000 to 1.2 million penicillin G units, and those weighing more than 27.2 kg receive a single IM dose of 2.4 million penicillin G units. If this fixed-combination preparation is used for the treatment of moderately severe infections caused by susceptible *S. pneumoniae* (pneumonia, otitis media), the manufacturer recommends that pediatric patients receive an IM dose of 600,000 penicillin G units once every 2 or 3 days until the patient has been afebrile for 48 hours. Other penicillins are recommended for severe *S. pneumoniae* infections (e.g., pneumonia, empyema, bacteremia, pericarditis, meningitis, peritonitis, arthritis).

If the fixed combination of penicillin G benzathine and penicillin G procaine (Bicillin® C-R 900/300) is used for the treatment of moderately severe to severe infections caused by susceptible *S. pyogenes* (e.g., upper respiratory tract infections, scarlet fever, erysipelas, skin and skin structure infections), the manufacturer states that a single IM dose of 1.2 million penicillin G units usually is sufficient in pediatric patients. If this fixed-combination preparation is used for the treatment of moderately severe infections caused by susceptible *S. pneumoniae* (pneumonia, otitis media), the manufacturer recommends that pediatric patients receive an IM dose of 1.2 million penicillin G units once every 2 or 3 days until the patient has been afebrile for 48 hours. Other penicillins are recommended for severe *S. pneumoniae* infections (e.g., pneumonia, empyema, bacteremia, pericarditis, meningitis, peritonitis, arthritis).

Diphtheria

If IM penicillin G benzathine is used for prevention of diphtheria† in asymptomatic household or close contacts of patients with respiratory or cutaneous diphtheria caused by *Corynebacterium diphtheriae*, the US Centers for Disease Control and Prevention (CDC) and AAP recommend that children younger than 6 years of age or those weighing less than 30 kg receive a single dose of 600,000 units and that children 6 years of age or older or those weighing 30 kg or more receive a single dose of 1.2 million units. Household or close contacts of patients with diphtheria should receive anti-infective prophylaxis regardless of their immunization status and should be closely monitored for symptoms of diphtheria for 7 days. Contacts who are inadequately immunized against diphtheria or whose immunization status is unknown should receive an immediate dose of an age-appropriate preparation containing diphtheria toxoid adsorbed and the primary series should be completed according to the recommended schedule. Contacts who are fully immunized should receive an immediate booster dose of an age-appropriate preparation containing diphtheria toxoid adsorbed if it has been 5 years or longer since their last booster dose.

When IM penicillin G benzathine is used to eliminate the diphtheria carrier state† in identified carriers of toxigenic *C. diphtheriae*, CDC and AAP recommend that children younger than 6 years of age or those weighing less than 30 kg receive a single dose of 600,000 units and that children 6 years of age or older or those weighing 30 kg or more receive a single dose of 1.2 million units. Follow-up cultures should be obtained at least 2 weeks after treatment of diphtheria carriers; if cultures are positive, a 10-day course of oral erythromycin should be given and additional follow-up cultures obtained.

Syphilis

If IM penicillin G benzathine is used for the treatment of possible congenital syphilis or when congenital syphilis is less likely (see Uses: Syphilis), CDC and the manufacturers recommend a single dose of 50,000 units/kg. Neonates with proven or highly probable congenital syphilis (see Uses: Syphilis) should receive a 10-day regimen of IV penicillin G potassium or sodium or IM penicillin G procaine.

In infants and children 1 month of age or older with reactive serologic tests for syphilis but no clinical manifestation of congenital syphilis and a normal evaluation (including CSF examination), CDC states that treatment with IM penicillin G benzathine given in a dosage of 50,000 units/kg (up to 2.4 million units) once weekly for up to 3 weeks can be considered. If a 10-day regimen of IV penicillin G potassium or sodium is used in such patients, a single dose of IM penicillin G benzathine (50,000 units/kg) may be considered after completion of the IV regimen.

For the treatment of primary, secondary, or early latent syphilis in infants and children 1 month of age or older, CDC and others recommend that IM penicillin G benzathine be given as a single dose of 50,000 units/kg (up to 2.4 million units).

For the treatment of late latent syphilis in infants and children 1 month of age or older, CDC and others recommend that IM penicillin G benzathine be given in a dosage of 50,000 units/kg (up to 2.4 million units) administered once weekly for 3 consecutive weeks (up to a maximum total dosage of 7.2 million units).

CDC recommends that treatment of syphilis diagnosed in infants and children 1 month of age or older should be managed by a pediatric infectious disease specialist and that CSF should be examined in those with latent syphilis.

In adolescents 10–19 years of age, some experts state that those with early syphilis (primary, secondary, or early latent syphilis) should receive a single IM penicillin G benzathine dose of 2.4 million units and that those with late latent syphilis or syphilis of unknown duration should receive IM penicillin G benzathine in a dosage of 2.4 million units once weekly for 3 consecutive weeks. The interval between consecutive doses of IM penicillin G benzathine should not exceed 14 days.

Neonates with human immunodeficiency virus (HIV) infection who have congenital syphilis and HIV-infected children and adolescents with any stage of syphilis should receive the same treatment regimens recommended for those without HIV infection.

Fixed combinations of penicillin G benzathine and penicillin G procaine (Bicillin® C-R, Bicillin® C-R 900/300) should not be used for the treatment of any form of syphilis.

Yaws, Pinta, and Bejel

For the treatment of yaws, pinta, and bejel in children, IM penicillin G benzathine has been given as a single dose of 600,000 units in those younger than 10 years of age or 1.2 million units in those 10 years of age or older. A single IM dose of 50,000 units/kg (up to 2.4 million units) also has been used for the treatment of yaws in children.

Fixed combinations of penicillin G benzathine and penicillin G procaine (Bicillin® C-R, Bicillin® C-R 900/300) should not be used for the treatment of yaws, pinta, or bejel.

Prevention of Rheumatic Fever Recurrence

For prevention of recurrent rheumatic fever (secondary prophylaxis), AAP and AHA state that the usual dosage of IM penicillin G benzathine is 600,000 units once every 4 weeks in children weighing 27 kg or less and 1.2 million units once every 4 weeks in those weighing more than 27 kg. The manufacturers recommend that penicillin G benzathine be given in a dosage of 1.2 million units once monthly or 600,000 units once every 2 weeks for such prophylaxis.

AAP and AHA state that an IM penicillin G benzathine regimen that uses a 4-week dosing interval seems adequate and is recommended for most patients in the US, but a 3-week dosing interval may be warranted and is recommended when there is a particularly high risk of rheumatic fever (e.g., recurrent acute rheumatic fever despite adherence to a 4-week regimen). There is some evidence that serum penicillin concentrations may decline to subtherapeutic concentrations before the fourth week in some patients and there is limited evidence of an increased frequency of prophylactic failure with a 4-week interval compared with a 3-week interval in areas with a high risk of rheumatic fever.

Prevention of recurrent rheumatic fever requires long-term, continuous prophylaxis. (See Table 1.) Some clinicians use IM penicillin G benzathine initially and change to oral prophylaxis (usually oral penicillin V) when the patient reaches late adolescence or young adulthood and has remained free of rheumatic attacks for at least 5 years.

TABLE 1. Recommended Duration of Prophylaxis for Prevention of Rheumatic Fever Recurrence

Patient Category	Duration
Rheumatic fever without carditis	5 years since last episode or until 21 years of age, whichever is longer
Rheumatic fever with carditis but no residual heart disease (no valvular disease)	10 years since last episode or until 21 years of age, whichever is longer
Rheumatic fever with carditis and residual heart disease (persistent valvular disease)	10 years since last episode or until 40 years of age, whichever is longer; sometimes for life

Adult Dosage

Pharyngitis and Tonsillitis

For the treatment of pharyngitis or tonsillitis caused by *S. pyogenes* (group A β-hemolytic streptococci; GAS) and prevention of initial attacks (primary prevention) of rheumatic fever, the usual adult dosage of penicillin G benzathine is a single IM dose of 1.2 million units.

Although anti-infective treatment is not recommended for most individuals identified as chronic pharyngeal carriers of *S. pyogenes* (see Uses: Pharyngitis and Tonsilitis), IDSA states that a single IM penicillin G benzathine dose of 600,000 units in those weighing less than 27 kg or 1.2 million units in those weighing 27 kg or more given in conjunction with oral rifampin (20 mg/kg daily given in 2 doses [up to 600 mg daily] for 4 days) is an option when eradication of the carrier state is desirable.

Streptococcal Infections

If IM penicillin G benzathine is used for the treatment of mild to moderate upper respiratory tract infections caused by susceptible *S. pyogenes* (group A β-hemolytic streptococci; GAS), adults should receive a single dose of 1.2 million units.

If the fixed combination of penicillin G benzathine and penicillin G procaine (Bicillin® C-R) is used for the treatment of moderately severe to severe infections caused by susceptible *S. pyogenes* (e.g., upper respiratory tract infections, scarlet fever, erysipelas, skin and skin structure infections), the manufacturer recommends that adults receive a single IM dose of 2.4 million penicillin G units. If this fixed-combination preparation is used for the treatment of moderately severe infections caused by susceptible *S. pneumoniae* (pneumonia, otitis media) in adults, the manufacturer recommends an IM dose of 1.2 million penicillin G units once every 2 or 3 days until the patient has been afebrile for 48 hours. Other penicillins are recommended for severe *S. pneumoniae* infections (e.g., pneumonia, empyema, bacteremia, pericarditis, meningitis, peritonitis, arthritis).

Diphtheria

If IM penicillin G benzathine is used for prevention of diphtheria† in asymptomatic household or close contacts of patients with respiratory or cutaneous diphtheria, CDC recommends that adults receive a single dose of 1.2 million units. Household or close contacts of patients with diphtheria should receive anti-infective prophylaxis regardless of their immunization status and should be closely monitored for symptoms of diphtheria for 7 days. Contacts who are inadequately immunized against diphtheria or whose immunization status is unknown should receive an immediate dose of an age-appropriate preparation containing diphtheria toxoid adsorbed and the primary series should be completed according to the recommended schedule. Contacts who are fully immunized should receive an immediate booster dose of an age-appropriate preparation containing diphtheria toxoid adsorbed if it has been 5 years or longer since their last booster dose.

When IM penicillin G benzathine is used to eliminate the diphtheria carrier state† in identified carriers of toxigenic *C. diphtheriae*, adults should receive a single dose of 1.2 million units. Follow-up cultures should be obtained at least 2 weeks after treatment of diphtheria carriers; if cultures are positive, a 10-day course of oral erythromycin should be given and additional follow-up cultures obtained.

Syphilis

For the treatment of primary, secondary, or early latent syphilis in adults, CDC, the manufacturers, and others recommend that IM penicillin G benzathine be given as a single dose of 2.4 million units. For pregnant women with primary, secondary, or early latent syphilis, some clinicians recommend that a second IM penicillin G benzathine dose of 2.4 million units be given 1 week after the initial dose. If retreatment of primary, secondary, or early latent syphilis is necessary and there is no evidence that neurosyphilis is present, CDC and others recommend that adults receive IM penicillin G benzathine in a dosage of 2.4 million units once weekly for 3 consecutive weeks.

For the treatment of late latent syphilis, latent syphilis of unknown duration, or tertiary syphilis, CDC and others recommend that adults receive IM penicillin G benzathine in a dosage of 2.4 million units once weekly for 3 consecutive weeks (total dosage 7.2 million units). The interval between consecutive doses of IM penicillin G benzathine should not exceed 14 days.

Although the manufacturers state that adults can receive 2.4 or 3 million units of penicillin G benzathine IM once weekly for 3 successive weeks for the treatment of neurosyphilis, treatment failures have been reported when penicillin G

benzathine was used alone for the treatment of neurosyphilis. CDC and others state that IV penicillin G potassium or sodium is the drug of choice for the treatment of neurosyphilis and IM penicillin G procaine (with oral probenecid) is an alternative if compliance can be ensured. Some clinicians recommend that the IV penicillin G potassium or sodium regimen or IM penicillin G procaine regimen be followed by a regimen of IM penicillin G benzathine (2.4 million units once weekly for up to 3 weeks).

HIV-infected adults with any stage of syphilis should receive the same treatment regimens recommended for those without HIV infection.

Fixed combinations of penicillin G benzathine and penicillin G procaine (Bicillin® C-R, Bicillin® C-R 900/300) should not be used for the treatment of any form of syphilis.

Yaws, Pinta, and Bejel

For the treatment of yaws, pinta, and bejel in adults, IM penicillin G benzathine has been given as a single dose of 1.2 million units. A single IM dose of 2.4 million units also has been used for the treatment of yaws.

Fixed combinations of penicillin G benzathine and penicillin G procaine (Bicillin® C-R, Bicillin® C-R 900/300) should not be used for the treatment of yaws, pinta, or bejel.

Prevention of Rheumatic Fever Recurrence

For prevention of rheumatic fever recurrence (secondary prophylaxis) in adults, AHA states that the usual dosage of IM penicillin G benzathine is 1.2 million units once every 4 weeks. The manufacturers recommend that IM penicillin G benzathine be given in a dosage of 1.2 million units once monthly or 600,000 units once every 2 weeks for such prophylaxis.

AHA and AAP state that an IM penicillin G benzathine regimen that uses a 4-week dosing interval seems adequate and is recommended for most patients in the US, but a 3-week dosing interval may be warranted and is recommended when there is a particularly high risk of rheumatic fever (e.g., recurrent acute rheumatic fever despite adherence to a 4-week regimen). There is some evidence that serum penicillin concentrations may decline to subtherapeutic concentrations before the fourth week in some patients and there is limited evidence of an increased frequency of prophylactic failure with a 4-week interval compared with a 3-week interval in areas with a high risk of rheumatic fever.

Prevention of recurrent rheumatic fever requires long-term, continuous prophylaxis. (See Table 2.)

TABLE 2. Recommended Duration of Prophylaxis for Prevention of Rheumatic Fever Recurrence

Patient Category	Duration
Rheumatic fever without carditis	5 years since last episode or until 21 years of age, whichever is longer
Rheumatic fever with carditis but no residual heart disease (no valvular disease)	10 years since last episode or until 21 years of age, whichever is longer
Rheumatic fever with carditis and residual heart disease (persistent valvular disease)	10 years since last episode or until 40 years of age, whichever is longer; sometimes for life

CAUTIONS

● Adverse Effects

Adverse effects reported with penicillin G benzathine are similar to those reported with other natural penicillins.

Serious and occasionally fatal hypersensitivity reactions, including anaphylaxis, have been reported with penicillins. Rash (maculopapular), exfoliative dermatitis, urticaria, laryngeal edema, fever, eosinophilia, other serum sickness-like reactions (e.g., chills, fever, edema, arthralgia, prostration), and anaphylaxis (including shock and death) have been reported with penicillin G. Fever and eosinophilia may frequently be the only reaction observed.

Inadvertent IV administration of penicillin G benzathine has been associated with cardiorespiratory arrest and death.

Inadvertent intravascular administration (including inadvertent direct intra-arterial injection or injection immediately adjacent to arteries) of penicillin G benzathine or fixed combinations containing penicillin G benzathine and penicillin G procaine has resulted in severe neurovascular damage (e.g., transverse myelitis with permanent paralysis, gangrene requiring amputation of digits and more proximal portions of extremities, necrosis and sloughing at and surrounding the injection site). These severe effects have been reported following injections into the buttock, thigh, and deltoid areas. Other serious complications of suspected intravascular administration include immediate pallor, mottling, or cyanosis of the extremity (both distal and proximal to the injection site), followed by bleb formation or severe edema requiring anterior and/or posterior compartment fasciotomy in the lower extremity. These severe effects and complications have occurred most often in infants and small children.

For additional information on adverse effects reported with natural penicillins, see Cautions in the Natural Penicillins General Statement 8:12.16.04.

● Precautions and Contraindications

Penicillin G benzathine and fixed combinations of penicillin G benzathine and penicillin G procaine are contraindicated in patients hypersensitive to any penicillin. The fixed combinations also are contraindicated in patients hypersensitive to procaine.

Penicillin G benzathine shares the toxic potentials of the penicillins, including the risk of hypersensitivity reactions, and the usual precautions of penicillin therapy should be observed.

Prior to administration of penicillin G benzathine or a fixed combination of penicillin G benzathine and penicillin G procaine, careful inquiry should be made concerning previous hypersensitivity reactions to penicillins, cephalosporins, or other allergens. There is clinical and laboratory evidence of partial cross-allergenicity among penicillins and other β-lactam antibiotics, including cephalosporins and cephamycins.

Hypersensitivity reactions to penicillins are more likely to occur in individuals with a history of penicillin hypersensitivity and/or a history of sensitivity to multiple allergens. Penicillin G benzathine and fixed combinations of penicillin G benzathine and penicillin G procaine should be used with caution in individuals with a history of clinically important allergies and/or asthma.

If a hypersensitivity reaction occurs, the drug should be discontinued immediately and appropriate therapy instituted as indicated (e.g., epinephrine, corticosteroids, maintenance of an adequate airway and oxygen).

If use of a fixed combination containing penicillin G benzathine and penicillin G procaine is being considered in a patient with a history of procaine sensitivity, a test dose of procaine (0.1 mL of a 1–2% solution of procaine) should be administered intradermally prior to IM administration of full doses of the fixed combination. Development of erythema or a wheal, flare, or eruption at the intradermal test site indicates procaine sensitivity and the patient should *not* receive a preparation containing penicillin G procaine. If a hypersensitivity reaction to procaine occurs, it should be treated by usual methods; antihistamines may be beneficial and barbiturates may be indicated if seizures occur.

Special precaution should be taken to avoid IV, intravascular, or intra-arterial administration or injection of penicillin G benzathine or fixed combinations containing the drug into or near major peripheral nerves or blood vessels since inadvertent intravascular or intra-arterial injection may produce severe and/or permanent neurovascular damage and inadvertent IV administration has been associated with cardiorespiratory arrest and death. If evidence of compromise of the blood supply occurs at or proximal or distal to the site of injection, an appropriate specialist should be consulted immediately.

Renal and hematologic systems should be evaluated periodically during prolonged therapy with a fixed combination containing penicillin G benzathine and penicillin G procaine, particularly if high dosage is used.

For additional information on precautions associated with the use of penicillin G benzathine, see Cautions: Precautions and Contraindications, in the Natural Penicillins General Statement 8:12.16.04.

● Pediatric Precautions

Penicillin G benzathine should be used with caution in neonates and organ system function should be evaluated frequently in such patients.

Renal clearance of penicillin G may be delayed in neonates and young infants because of incompletely developed renal function.

● Geriatric Precautions

Clinical studies of penicillin G benzathine or penicillin G procaine did not include sufficient numbers of patients 65 years of age or older to determine whether geriatric patients respond differently than younger patients. Other clinical experience has not identified differences in responses between geriatric and younger patients.

Penicillin G is substantially eliminated by the kidneys and the risk of adverse effects may be greater in those with impaired renal function. Because geriatric patients are more likely to have reduced renal function, dosage should be selected with caution, usually starting at the low end of the dosage range, and renal function monitoring may be useful.

● Pregnancy, Fertility, and Lactation

Pregnancy

Reproduction studies evaluating penicillin G in mice, rats, and rabbits have not revealed evidence of impaired fertility or harm to the fetus. Although experience with use of penicillins during pregnancy has not shown any evidence of adverse effects on the fetus, there are no adequate or controlled studies using penicillin G benzathine in pregnant women.

Some clinicians state that IM penicillin G benzathine is considered low risk and safe for use during pregnancy. The drug is included in the US Centers for Disease Control and Prevention (CDC) recommendations for the treatment of syphilis during pregnancy.

The manufacturers state that penicillin G benzathine and fixed combinations containing penicillin G benzathine and penicillin G procaine should be used during pregnancy only when clearly needed.

Lactation

Penicillin G is distributed into milk. Some clinicians state that IM penicillin G benzathine usually is considered compatible with breast-feeding. The manufacturers and others state that penicillin G benzathine and fixed combinations of penicillin G benzathine and penicillin G procaine should be used with caution in nursing women.

SPECTRUM

Based on its spectrum of activity, penicillin G benzathine is classified as a natural penicillin. For information on the classification of penicillins based on spectra of activity, see the Preface to the General Statements on Penicillins 8:12.16.

For specific information on the spectrum of activity of penicillin G and resistance to the drug, see the sections on Spectrum and on Resistance in the Natural Penicillins General Statement 8:12.16.04.

PHARMACOKINETICS

For additional information on the absorption, distribution, and elimination of penicillin G, see Pharmacokinetics in the Natural Penicillins General Statement 8:12.16.04.

● Absorption

Because penicillin G benzathine is relatively insoluble, IM administration of the drug provides a tissue depot from which the drug is slowly absorbed and hydrolyzed to penicillin G. IM administration of penicillin G benzathine results in serum concentrations of penicillin G that are more prolonged, but lower, than those attained with an equivalent IM dose of penicillin G procaine or penicillin G potassium or sodium.

Following IM administration of a single dose of penicillin G benzathine in adults, children, or neonates, peak serum concentrations of penicillin G are attained in 13–24 hours and usually are detectable for 1–4 weeks (depending on the dose).

In adults, a single IM penicillin G benzathine dose of 1.2 million units results in serum penicillin G concentrations of 0.15, 0.03, and 0.003 units/mL at 1, 14, and 32 days, respectively, after the dose. In one study in adults who received IM penicillin G benzathine in a dosage of 2.4 million units administered once weekly for 3 successive weeks, serum penicillin G concentrations ranged from 0.04–0.48 units/mL at 7 days after the first dose, 0.06–0.48 units/mL at 7 days after the second dose, and 0.17–0.52 units/mL at 7 days after the third dose. In adults receiving IM penicillin G benzathine in a dosage of 1.2 million units once every 4 weeks, mean serum penicillin G concentrations were at least 0.02 mcg/mL for 21 days after a dose; however, at 28 days after a dose, the drug was detectable in serum in only 44% of samples and was at least 0.02 mcg/mL in only 36% of samples.

Following a single IM dose of a fixed combination containing 1.2 million penicillin G units (i.e., 600,000 units as penicillin G benzathine and 600,000 units as penicillin G procaine; Bicillin® C-R) in adults, peak blood penicillin G concentrations were 2.1–2.6 units/mL within 3 hours and blood concentrations averaged 0.75 units/mL at 12 hours, 0.28 units/mL at 24 hours, and 0.04 units/mL at 7 days.

Following a single IM dose of a fixed combination containing 1.2 million penicillin G units (i.e., 900,000 units as penicillin G benzathine and 300,000 units as penicillin G procaine; Bicillin® C-R 900/300) in patients weighing 45–64 kg, average blood penicillin G concentrations were 0.24 units/mL at 24 hours, 0.039 units/mL at 7 days, and 0.024 units/mL at 10 days after the dose.

In a study in children 1.8–10.7 years of age who received a single IM penicillin G benzathine dose of 600,000 units if they weighed less than 27 kg or 1.2 million units if they weighed more than 27 kg, peak serum penicillin G concentrations occurred 24 hours after the dose and ranged from 0.11–0.2 mcg/mL. In these children, serum penicillin G concentrations ranged from 0.04–0.19 mcg/mL at 1, 2, and 4 hours after the dose and from 0.03–0.13, 0.02–0.09, and 0–0.02 mcg/mL at 5, 10, and 18 days, respectively, after the dose. In children weighing 11.9–22.6 kg, IM administration of a single dose of a fixed combination containing 1.2 million penicillin G units (900,000 units as penicillin G benzathine and 300,000 units as penicillin G procaine) resulted in peak serum penicillin G concentrations that occurred 1 hour after the dose and averaged 3.9 mcg/mL. Serum penicillin G concentrations in these children ranged from 2.5–5.5, 2.5–5.5, 0.7–3.7, and 0.17–0.48 mcg/mL at 1, 2, 4, and 24 hours, respectively, after the dose and from 0.08–0.12, 0.01–0.09, and 0–0.1 mcg/mL at 5, 10, and 18 days, respectively, after the dose.

In one study in neonates who received a single IM penicillin G benzathine dose of 50,000 units/kg, peak serum penicillin G concentrations occurred 24 hours after the dose and ranged from 0.38–2.1 mg/mL; serum penicillin G concentrations ranged from 0.07–0.09 mcg/mL 12 days after the dose. In another study in neonates, IM administration of a single penicillin G benzathine dose of 100,000 units resulted in serum penicillin G concentrations that ranged from 1.18–3.9 mcg/mL at 24 hours after the dose and were still detectable 5 days after the dose.

● Distribution

Following IM administration of penicillin G benzathine, penicillin G is widely distributed throughout the body in varying amounts. Highest concentrations generally are attained in the kidneys, with lower amounts in the liver, skin, and intestines.

Minimal concentrations of penicillin G generally are attained in CSF following IM administration of penicillin G benzathine in patients with inflamed or uninflamed meninges. The minimum treponemicidal concentration of penicillin G is generally defined as 0.03 units/mL or 0.02 mcg/mL. In one study in adults who received IM penicillin G benzathine given in a dosage of 3.6 million units once weekly for up to 4 weeks, penicillin G was undetectable in the CSF of 12/13 patients in specimens obtained following administration of the last dose. In another study in adults who received IM penicillin G benzathine in a dosage of 2.4 or 4.8 million units administered once weekly for 3 successive weeks, CSF penicillin G concentrations were less than 0.03 units/mL in specimens obtained 7 days after the last dose of the drug. In a study in neonates who received a single IM dose of penicillin G benzathine of 100,000 units/kg, peak CSF penicillin G concentrations occurred 12–24 hours after the dose and ranged from 0.012–0.2 mcg/mL; however, CSF penicillin G concentrations were less than 0.01 mcg/mL 48 hours after the dose.

In a study in children who received a single IM dose of penicillin G benzathine of 600,000 units to 1.2 million units, penicillin G concentrations in tonsils were 0.042 mcg/mL or less in specimens obtained 24 hours after the dose; concurrent serum concentrations ranged from 0.03–0.17 mcg/mL.

Penicillin G is about 60% bound to serum proteins.

Penicillin G crosses the placenta and is distributed into milk.

● Elimination

Following IM administration of penicillin G benzathine, the drug is slowly absorbed and hydrolyzed to penicillin G and elimination of penicillin G in urine continues over a prolonged period of time. Penicillin G and its metabolites are excreted in urine mainly by tubular secretion.

Penicillin G has been detected in urine for up to 12 weeks after a single IM penicillin G benzathine dose of 1.2 million units. In a study in children 1.8–10.7 years of age who received a single IM dose of penicillin G benzathine of 600,000 units or 1.2 million units, urinary penicillin G concentrations 30 days after the dose ranged from 0.6–12.5 mcg/mL. Following IM administration of a single

penicillin G benzathine dose of 50,000 units/kg in neonates, urinary penicillin G concentrations ranged from 4.3–17.2 mcg/mL during the first 4 days after the dose and were 1.4–6 mcg/mL at 12 days after the dose.

The serum half-life of penicillin G may be prolonged in patients with impaired renal function.

Renal clearance of penicillin G is delayed in neonates and young infants.

Renal clearance of penicillin G may be increased in pregnant women during the second and third trimesters.

CHEMISTRY AND STABILITY

● Chemistry

Penicillin G benzathine is a natural penicillin. The drug is the benzathine tetrahydrate salt of penicillin G. Penicillin G benzathine is hydrolyzed in vivo to penicillin G and is frequently referred to as a long-acting, depot, or repository form of penicillin G.

Penicillin G benzathine occurs as a white, crystalline powder. The drug is very slightly soluble in water and sparingly soluble in alcohol. Potency of penicillin G benzathine generally is expressed in terms of penicillin G units, but also has been expressed as mg of penicillin G.

Commercially available penicillin G benzathine suspension for IM injection is a viscous, opaque suspension of the drug in sterile water for injection. The IM suspension has a pH of 5–7.5 and is buffered with sodium citrate. The suspension contains methylparaben and propylparaben as preservatives and also contains povidone, lecithin, and carboxymethylcellulose.

Penicillin G benzathine also is commercially available in fixed combination with penicillin G procaine as a viscous, opaque, aqueous suspension for IM injection. Each 2 mL of fixed-combination suspension contains the equivalent of 1.2 million units of penicillin G in a formulation containing the equivalent of 600,000 units of penicillin G as the benzathine salt and 600,000 units of penicillin G as the procaine salt (Bicillin® C-R) or a formulation containing the equivalent of 900,000 units of penicillin G as the benzathine salt and 300,000 units of penicillin G as the procaine salt (Bicillin® C-R 900/300).

● Stability

Commercially available penicillin G benzathine suspension for IM injection should be stored at 2–8°C; freezing should be avoided.

The fixed combinations of penicillin G benzathine and penicillin G procaine for IM injection should be stored at 2–8°C; freezing should be avoided.

For further information on chemistry and stability, mechanism of action, spectrum, resistance, pharmacokinetics, uses, cautions, drug interactions, laboratory test interferences, and dosage and administration of penicillin G benzathine, see the Natural Penicillins General Statement 8:12.16.04.

PREPARATIONS

Excipients in commercially available drug preparations may have clinically important effects in some individuals; consult specific product labeling for details.

Penicillin G Benzathine

Parenteral		
Suspension, for IM Injection	600,000 units (of penicillin G) per mL	**Bicillin® L-A**, Pfizer
		Permapen®, Casper

Penicillin G Benzathine and Penicillin G Procaine

Parenteral		
Suspension, for IM Injection	1.2 million units of penicillin G per 2 mL (600,000 units as penicillin G benzathine and 600,000 units as penicillin G procaine)	**Bicillin® C-R**, Pfizer
	1.2 million units of penicillin G per 2 mL (900,000 units as penicillin G benzathine and 300,000 units as penicillin G procaine)	**Bicillin® C-R 900/300**, Pfizer

† Use is not currently included in the labeling approved by the US Food and Drug Administration.

Penicillin G Potassium
Penicillin G Sodium

8:12.16.04 · NATURAL PENICILLINS

■ Penicillin G, a natural penicillin, is a β-lactam antibiotic.

USES

Penicillin G potassium and penicillin G sodium are used parenterally when rapid and high concentrations of penicillin G are required, as in the treatment of endocarditis, meningitis, pericarditis, septicemia, severe pneumonia, or other serious infections caused by organisms susceptible to penicillin G.

For additional information on the uses of penicillin G potassium and penicillin G sodium, see Uses in the Natural Penicillins General Statement 8:12.16.04.

● Endocarditis

IV penicillin G potassium or sodium is used for the treatment of endocarditis caused by susceptible *Streptococcus pyogenes* (group A β-hemolytic streptococci; GAS), other β-hemolytic streptococci (including groups C, H, G, L, and M), or *S. pneumoniae*. The American Heart Association (AHA) states that IV penicillin G is a reasonable regimen for the treatment of endocarditis caused by susceptible *S. pyogenes*, *S. agalactiae*† (group B streptococci; GBS), groups C and G streptococci, and highly penicillin-susceptible *S. pneumoniae* (penicillin MIC 0.1 mcg/mL or less), but concomitant use of gentamicin during the initial weeks of penicillin G treatment should be considered if endocarditis is caused by streptococci groups B, C, or G.

For the treatment of endocarditis caused by viridans group streptococci† or nonenterococcal group D streptococci† (including *S. gallolyticus*† [formerly *S. bovis*]) that are highly susceptible to penicillin (penicillin MIC 0.12 mcg/mL or less), AHA states that IV penicillin G (with or without gentamicin) is a regimen of choice. If endocarditis is caused by viridans group streptococci† or *S. gallolyticus*† relatively resistant to penicillin (penicillin MIC greater than 0.12 mcg/mL but less than 0.5 mcg/mL), AHA states that IV penicillin G should be used in conjunction with gentamicin. These recommendations include endocarditis involving native valves or prosthetic valves or other prosthetic material caused by these gram-positive bacteria.

AHA states that IV penicillin G in conjunction with gentamicin is a reasonable regimen for the treatment of native valve endocarditis caused by viridans group streptococci†, *Abiotrophia defectiva*†, or *Granulicatella*† with penicillin MIC 0.5 mcg/mL or greater.

For the treatment of endocarditis involving native valves or prosthetic valves or other prosthetic material caused by *Enterococcus faecalis*†, *E. faecium*†, or other enterococcal species susceptible to both penicillin G *and* gentamicin, AHA states that IV penicillin G in conjunction with gentamicin is a regimen of choice. AHA states that it is reasonable to substitute streptomycin for gentamicin in this regimen if enterococci are susceptible to penicillin *and* streptomycin, but resistant to gentamicin.

IV penicillin G has been used for the treatment of endocarditis caused by nonpenicillinase-producing staphylococci. AHA states that IV penicillin G may be considered for the treatment of native valve endocarditis caused by penicillin-susceptible *S. aureus* or coagulase-negative staphylococci in pediatric patients; however, penicillin G is not included in current AHA recommendations for the treatment of staphylococcal endocarditis in adults.

AHA recommends that treatment of endocarditis should be managed in consultation with an infectious disease expert, especially when endocarditis is caused by *S. pneumoniae*, β-hemolytic streptococci, staphylococci, or enterococci.

For additional information on management of endocarditis, current guidelines from AHA should be consulted.

● Syphilis

IV penicillin G potassium or sodium is used for the treatment of syphilis caused by *Treponema pallidum*.

For the treatment of neurosyphilis and otic or ocular syphilis, the US Centers for Disease Control and Prevention (CDC) and other clinicians state that IV penicillin G potassium or sodium is the drug of choice and IM penicillin G procaine (with oral probenecid) is an alternative if compliance can be ensured.

For the treatment of congenital syphilis, CDC recommends IV penicillin G potassium or sodium or IM penicillin G procaine in neonates with proven or highly probable congenital syphilis (i.e., abnormal physical examination consistent with congenital syphilis, serum quantitative nontreponemal serologic titer fourfold higher than the mother's titer, or positive darkfield test or polymerase chain reaction [PCR] of lesions or body fluids). CDC recommends IV penicillin G potassium or sodium, IM penicillin G procaine, or IM penicillin G benzathine in neonates with possible congenital syphilis (i.e., normal physical examination and serum quantitative nontreponemal serologic titer no more than fourfold higher than the mother's titer and the mother received a recommended treatment regimen less than 4 weeks before delivery; the mother was not treated or was inadequately treated, including treatment with erythromycin or any regimen not included in CDC recommendations; or there is no documentation that the mother received treatment).

CDC and other clinicians state that IM penicillin G benzathine is the drug of choice for the treatment of primary syphilis (i.e., ulcer or chancre at infection site), secondary syphilis (i.e., manifestations that include, but are not limited to, rash, mucocutaneous lesions, and lymphadenopathy), and tertiary syphilis (i.e., cardiac syphilis, gummatous lesions, tabes dorsalis, and general paresis) in adults, adolescents, and children.

IM penicillin G benzathine also is the drug of choice for the treatment of latent syphilis (i.e., detected by serologic testing but lacking clinical manifestations), including both early latent syphilis (latent syphilis acquired within the preceding year) and late latent syphilis (i.e., all other cases of latent syphilis or syphilis of unknown duration) in all age groups.

Neonates with human immunodeficiency virus (HIV) infection who have congenital syphilis and HIV-infected children, adolescents, or adults who have neurosyphilis or primary, secondary, early latent, late latent, or tertiary syphilis should receive the same treatment regimens as those without HIV infection. Because serologic nonresponse and neurologic complications may be more frequent in HIV-infected individuals, close follow-up is essential in those coinfected with syphilis and HIV. In addition, careful neurologic examinations are indicated in all HIV-infected patients coinfected with syphilis.

There are no proven alternatives to penicillin G for the treatment of congenital syphilis in infants and children with known or suspected penicillin hypersensitivity and no proven alternatives to penicillin G for the treatment of any stage of syphilis in pregnant women with penicillin hypersensitivity; therefore, CDC recommends that such patients be desensitized and treated with the appropriate penicillin G preparation.

For additional information on management of syphilis, current CDC sexually transmitted diseases treatment guidelines available at https://www.cdc.gov/std/syphilis/treatment.htm should be consulted.

● Prevention of Perinatal Group B Streptococcal Disease

IV penicillin G potassium or sodium is used in pregnant women during labor (intrapartum) for prevention of early-onset neonatal group B streptococcal (GBS) disease†.

GBS infection is a leading cause of neonatal morbidity and mortality in the US. Pregnant women who are colonized with GBS in the genital or rectal areas can transmit GBS infection to their infants during labor and delivery, resulting in invasive neonatal infection that can be associated with substantial morbidity and mortality.

CDC, AAP, and other experts recommend *routine* universal prenatal screening for GBS colonization (e.g., vaginal and rectal cultures) in *all* pregnant women at 35–37 weeks of gestation, unless GBS bacteriuria is known to be present during the current pregnancy or the woman had a previous infant with invasive GBS disease. These experts state that intrapartum anti-infective prophylaxis for prevention of perinatal GBS is indicated in pregnant women identified as GBS carriers during the routine prenatal GBS screening performed at 35–37 weeks during the current pregnancy, in women with GBS bacteriuria identified at any time during the current pregnancy, and in women who had a previous infant diagnosed with invasive GBS disease. Intrapartum anti-infective prophylaxis also is indicated in women with unknown GBS status at the time of onset of labor (i.e., culture not done, incomplete, or results unknown) if delivery is at less than 37 weeks of gestation, the duration of amniotic membrane rupture is 18 hours or longer, or intrapartum temperature is 38°C or higher. If an intrapartum nucleic acid amplification test (NAAT) is performed in a woman with unknown GBS status at the time of onset of labor (may not be available in all settings) and results are positive for GBS, intrapartum anti-infective prophylaxis is indicated; if an intrapartum NAAT is negative for GBS, anti-infective prophylaxis is indicated if any of the above risk factors for perinatal GBS infection are present.

When intrapartum anti-infective prophylaxis is indicated in the mother for prevention of GBS in the neonate, it should be initiated at the onset of labor or rupture of membranes. If cesarean delivery is performed *before* onset of labor in a woman with intact amniotic membranes, anti-infective prophylaxis is not usually indicated, regardless of the GBS colonization status of the woman or gestational age.

CDC, AAP, and other experts recommend IV penicillin G as the drug of choice and state that IV ampicillin is the preferred alternative for such prophylaxis. Penicillin G is considered the drug of choice because it has a narrower spectrum of activity than ampicillin and is less likely to select for antibiotic-resistant organisms.

Regardless of whether the mother received intrapartum anti-infective prophylaxis, appropriate diagnostic evaluations and anti-infective therapy should be initiated in the neonate if signs or symptoms of active infection develop.

For additional information regarding prevention of perinatal group B streptococcal disease, current guidelines from CDC and AAP should be consulted.

DOSAGE AND ADMINISTRATION

● Reconstitution and Administration

Penicillin G potassium and penicillin G sodium are administered by IM injection or by intermittent IV injection or infusion or continuous IV infusion. Penicillin G has been administered by intrapleural, intraperitoneal, intra-articular, or other local instillations. Although the drug has been administered intrathecally, this route is *not* recommended because of possible neurotoxicity (e.g., seizures).

Vials containing penicillin G potassium or penicillin G sodium powder for injection should be reconstituted to the desired concentration using the amount of diluent specified by the manufacturer. Depending on the specific product and route of administration, the powders generally are reconstituted with sterile water for injection, 0.9% sodium chloride injection, or dextrose injection. The powder should be loosened in the vial and the vial held horizontally and rotated while slowly directing the stream of diluent against the wall of the vial. After the diluent has been added, the vial should be shaken vigorously. Because penicillin G is unstable in solutions at room temperature, reconstituted penicillin G potassium and penicillin G sodium solutions should be used immediately or refrigerated. (See Chemistry and Stability: Stability.)

IM Injection

To prepare solutions for IM administration, vials labeled as containing 1 or 5 million units of penicillin G (as penicillin G potassium) or vials labeled as containing 5 million units of penicillin G (as penicillin G sodium) should be reconstituted to the desired concentration using the amount of diluent specified by the manufacturer. If not used immediately, vials reconstituted for IM use should be refrigerated (see Chemistry and Stability: Stability).

Vials labeled as containing 20 million units of penicillin G (as penicillin G potassium) are intended *only* for IV infusion and should *not* be used to prepare solutions for IM injection.

For IM administration, penicillin G potassium solutions containing up to 100,000 penicillin G units/mL may be used with a minimum of discomfort; higher concentrations are physically possible and may be used when needed.

If large doses of penicillin G are required, the drug should be administered IV (not IM).

IV Administration

To prepare solutions for IV administration, vials labeled as containing 1, 5, or 20 million units of penicillin G (as penicillin G potassium) or 5 million units of penicillin G (as penicillin G sodium) should be reconstituted according to the manufacturer's directions. If not used immediately, vials reconstituted for IV use should be refrigerated (see Chemistry and Stability: Stability).

For intermittent IV administration, the daily dosage usually is given in equally divided doses every 4–6 hours; however, daily dosage may be given in equally divided doses every 2–3 hours for the treatment of severe infections (e.g., meningitis).

For continuous IV infusion, the volume of IV fluid and rate of administration required by the patient in a 24-hour period should be determined and the

appropriate daily dosage of penicillin G should be added to the fluid. For example, if an adult patient requires 2 L of fluid in 24 hours and a dosage of 10 million penicillin G units daily, 5 million units can be added to 1 L of IV solution and the rate of administration adjusted so that the liter of fluid will be infused over 12 hours.

Thawed solutions of the commercially available frozen premixed penicillin G potassium injection in dextrose should be administered *only* by IV infusion. The commercially available frozen injection should be thawed at room temperature (25°C) or under refrigeration (5°C); the injection should not be thawed by warming in a water bath or by exposure to microwave radiation. Precipitates that may have formed in the frozen injection usually will dissolve with little or no agitation when the injection reaches room temperature; potency is not affected. After thawing at room temperature, the injections should be agitated and the container checked for minute leaks by firmly squeezing the bag. The injection should be discarded if the container seals or outlet ports are not intact or leaks are found or if the solution is cloudy or contains a precipitate. Additives should not be introduced into the injection container. The premixed injection should not be used in series connections with other plastic containers since such use could result in air embolism from residual air being drawn from the primary container before administration of fluid from the secondary container is complete.

Rate of Administration

Large IV doses of penicillin G potassium or sodium (greater than 10 million penicillin G units) should be administered slowly because of the potential for serious electrolyte disturbances from the potassium and/or sodium content of these preparations. (See Cautions: Adverse Effects.)

For intermittent IV administration, penicillin G potassium or sodium has been given by IV infusion over 1–2 hours or by IV infusion over 10–30 minutes. Although doses of the drug also have been injected IV over 3–5 minutes, large doses should be administered slowly.

● Dosage

Dosage of penicillin G potassium and penicillin G sodium usually is expressed in terms of penicillin G units, but also has been expressed as mg of penicillin G.

Pediatric Dosage
General Pediatric Dosage

Dosage of IM or IV penicillin G potassium or sodium for pediatric patients should be individualized and generally is based on weight and the severity of the infection.

The manufacturers state that penicillin G potassium or sodium should *not* be used in pediatric patients requiring less than 1 million penicillin G units per dose.

The American Academy of Pediatrics (AAP) states that the usual dosage of IV or IM penicillin G potassium or sodium in neonates 7 days of age or younger is 25,000–50,000 units/kg every 12 hours. In neonates 8–28 days of age, AAP recommends a dosage of 25,000–50,000 units/kg every 8 hours. Higher dosages may be necessary for the treatment of meningitis in neonates.

In pediatric patients beyond the neonatal period, AAP states that the usual dosage of IV or IM penicillin G potassium or sodium is 100,000–150,000 units/kg daily given in 4 equally divided doses for the treatment of mild to moderate infections or 200,000–300,000 units/kg daily given in 4–6 equally divided doses for the treatment of severe infections. AAP states that the highest dosage recommended for pediatric patients beyond the neonatal period should be used for the treatment of meningitis.

Endocarditis

For the treatment of native valve endocarditis caused by highly penicillin-susceptible streptococci (penicillin MIC 0.1 mcg/mL or less), including *Streptococcus pyogenes* (group A β-hemolytic streptococci; GAS), other β-hemolytic streptococci (e.g., groups C, G), *S. agalactiae*† (group B streptococci; GBS), viridans group streptococci†, or nonenterococcal group D streptococci† (e.g., *S. gallolyticus*† [formerly *S. bovis*], *S. equinus*†), the American Heart Association (AHA) states that pediatric patients may receive IV penicillin G in a dosage of 200,000–300,000 units/kg daily (up to 12–24 million units daily) given in divided doses every 4 hours for 4 weeks.

For the treatment of native valve endocarditis caused by streptococci that are relatively resistant to penicillin† (penicillin MIC greater than 0.1 but less than 0.5 mcg/mL), AHA states that pediatric patients may receive IV penicillin G in a dosage of 200,000–300,000 units/kg daily (up to 12–24 million units daily) given in divided doses every 4 hours for 4 weeks in conjunction with gentamicin (3–6 mg/

kg daily IV in divided doses every 8 hours given concomitantly during the first 2 weeks of penicillin G treatment).

For the treatment of native valve endocarditis caused by viridans group streptococci†, Abiotrophia†, or Granulicatella† with penicillin MIC 0.5 mcg/mL or greater, AHA states that pediatric patients may receive IV penicillin G in a dosage of 200,000–300,000 units/kg daily (up to 12–24 million units daily) given in divided doses every 4 hours for 4–6 weeks in conjunction with gentamicin (3–6 mg/kg IV daily in divided doses every 8 hours given concomitantly during the first 2 weeks of penicillin G treatment).

For the treatment of endocarditis involving prosthetic valves or other prosthetic material caused by penicillin-susceptible viridans group streptococci†, other streptococci, Abiotrophia†, or Granulicatella† with penicillin MIC 0.1 mcg/mL or greater, AHA states that pediatric patients may receive IV penicillin G in a dosage of 200,000–300,000 units/kg daily (up to 12–24 million units daily) given in divided doses every 4 hours for 6 weeks in conjunction with gentamicin (3–6 mg/kg IV daily in divided doses every 8 hours given concomitantly for the entire 6 weeks of penicillin G treatment).

For the treatment of enterococcal endocarditis† (native valve or prosthetic valve or other prosthetic material), AHA states that pediatric patients may receive IV penicillin G in a dosage of 200,000–300,000 units/kg daily (up to 12–24 million units daily) given in divided doses every 4 hours in conjunction with gentamicin (3–6 mg/kg IV daily in divided doses every 8 hours). The recommended duration of treatment with the 2-drug regimen is 4–6 weeks for native valve enterococcal endocarditis; a longer duration of treatment with both drugs is recommended if prosthetic valves or other prosthetic material is involved.

If IV penicillin G is used for the treatment of endocarditis caused by susceptible S. aureus or coagulase-negative staphylococci (penicillin MIC 0.1 mcg/mL or less) in pediatric patients, AHA recommends a dosage of 200,000–300,000 units/kg daily (up to 12–24 million units daily) given in divided doses every 4 hours.

The manufacturers recommend that pediatric patients with endocarditis caused by susceptible streptococci (including S. pyogenes, streptococci groups C, H, G, L, and M, or S. pneumoniae) receive penicillin G potassium or sodium in a dosage of 150,000–300,000 units/kg daily given in divided doses every 4–6 hours.

Meningitis and Other CNS Infections

For the treatment of meningitis caused by susceptible Listeria monocytogenes, the Infectious Diseases Society of America (IDSA) recommends that neonates 7 days of age or younger receive IV penicillin G in a dosage of 150,000 units/kg daily given in divided doses every 8–12 hours and that those 8–28 days of age receive a dosage of 200,000 units/kg daily given in divided doses every 6–8 hours; these experts recommend that treatment in neonates be continued for 2 weeks beyond the first sterile CSF culture or for at least 3 weeks, whichever is longer. In infants and children with L. monocytogenes meningitis, IDSA recommends a dosage of 300,000 units/kg daily given in divided doses every 4–6 hours for a duration of at least 21 days. Concomitant use of an aminoglycoside should be considered.

For the treatment of meningitis caused by susceptible Neisseria meningitidis (penicillin MIC less than 0.1 mcg/mL), IDSA recommends that neonates 7 days of age or younger receive IV penicillin G in a dosage of 150,000 units/kg daily given in divided doses every 8–12 hours and that those 8–28 days of age receive a dosage of 200,000 units/kg daily given in divided doses every 6–8 hours; these experts recommend that treatment in neonates be continued for 2 weeks beyond the first sterile CSF culture or for at least 3 weeks, whichever is longer. In infants and children with N. meningitidis meningitis, a dosage of 300,000 units/kg daily (up to 12 million units daily) given in divided doses every 4–6 hours for a duration of 7 days has been recommended.

For the treatment of meningitis caused by susceptible S. agalactiae† (group B streptococci; GBS), AAP recommends that neonates 7 days of age or younger receive IV penicillin G in a dosage of 250,000–450,000 units/kg daily given in 3 divided doses and that those older than 7 days of age receive a dosage of 450,000–500,000 units/kg daily given in 4 divided doses and states that treatment should be continued for at least 14 days. IDSA recommends that neonates 7 days of age or younger receive IV penicillin G in a dosage of 150,000 units/kg daily given in divided doses every 8–12 hours and that those 8–28 days of age receive a dosage of 200,000 units/kg daily given in divided doses every 6–8 hours; these experts recommend that treatment in neonates be continued for 2 weeks beyond the first sterile CSF culture or for at least 3 weeks, whichever is longer. In infants and children with S. agalactiae meningitis, IDSA recommends a dosage of 300,000 units/

kg daily given in divided doses every 4–6 hours for a duration of 14–21 days. Concomitant use of an aminoglycoside should be considered.

For the treatment of meningitis caused by susceptible S. pneumoniae, IDSA recommends that neonates 7 days of age or younger receive IV penicillin G in a dosage of 150,000 units/kg daily given in divided doses every 8–12 hours and that those 8–28 days of age receive a dosage of 200,000 units/kg daily given in divided doses every 6–8 hours; these experts recommend that treatment in neonates be continued for 2 weeks beyond the first sterile CSF culture or for at least 3 weeks, whichever is longer. AAP recommends that infants and children 1 month of age or older with S. pneumoniae meningitis receive IV penicillin G in a dosage of 250,000–400,000 units/kg daily given in divided doses every 4–6 hours. IDSA recommends that infants and children receive a dosage of 300,000 units/kg daily given in divided doses every 4–6 hours for a duration of 10–14 days.

For the treatment of healthcare-associated ventriculitis and meningitis caused by susceptible Cutibacterium acnes† (formerly Propionibacterium acnes), IDSA recommends that pediatric patients receive IV penicillin G in a dosage of 300,000 units/kg daily given in divided doses every 4–6 hours. The recommended treatment duration is 10 days in those with no or minimal CSF pleocytosis, normal CSF glucose, and few clinical symptoms or systemic features or 10–14 days in those with significant CSF pleocytosis, CSF hypoglycorrhachia, or clinical symptoms or systemic features.

The manufacturers recommend that pediatric patients with meningitis caused by susceptible N. meningitidis or S. pneumoniae receive penicillin G potassium or sodium in a dosage of 250,000 units/kg daily (up to 12–20 million units daily) given in divided doses every 4 hours for 7–14 days.

Respiratory Tract Infections

For the treatment of community-acquired pneumonia (CAP) caused by susceptible S. pyogenes (group A β-hemolytic streptococci; GAS) in pediatric patients 3 months of age or older, IDSA recommends that IV penicillin G be given in a dosage of 100,000–200,000 units daily in divided doses every 4–6 hours. For severe infections, 200,000–250,000 units/kg daily may be used.

For the treatment of CAP caused by susceptible S. pneumoniae (penicillin MIC 2 mcg/mL or lower) in pediatric patients 3 months of age or older, IDSA recommends that IV penicillin G be given in a dosage of 200,000–250,000 units/kg daily in divided doses every 4–6 hours. AAP recommends that infants and children 1 month of age or older with nonmeningeal infections caused by S. pneumoniae receive penicillin G in a dosage of 250,000–400,000 units/kg daily given in divided doses every 4–6 hours. Penicillin G should not be used for empiric treatment of CAP if local epidemiologic data indicate that invasive S. pneumoniae have high-level penicillin resistance.

If penicillin G potassium or sodium is used for the treatment of serious respiratory tract infections (e.g., pneumonia) caused by susceptible S. pyogenes, streptococci groups C, H, G, L, and M, or S. pneumoniae, in pediatric patients, the manufacturers recommend a dosage of 150,000–300,000 units/kg daily in divided doses every 4–6 hours.

Skin and Skin Structure Infections

For the treatment of necrotizing infections of the skin, fascia, and muscle caused by susceptible S. pyogenes, IDSA recommends that pediatric patients receive a regimen of IV penicillin G given in a dosage of 60,000–100,000 units/kg every 6 hours in conjunction with clindamycin (10–13 mg/kg IV every 8 hours).

Anthrax

For the treatment of anthrax (inhalational, GI, meningitis) caused by penicillin-susceptible Bacillus anthracis that occurs as the result of natural or endemic exposures to anthrax, some clinicians recommend that children receive IV penicillin G in a dosage of 100,000–150,000 units/kg daily given in divided doses every 4–6 hours. For the treatment of severe or life-threatening systemic anthrax (inhalational, GI, meningoencephalitis, sepsis) or the treatment of cutaneous anthrax with signs of systemic involvement, lesions on the head or neck, or extensive edema caused by penicillin-susceptible B. anthracis that occurs as the result of natural or endemic anthrax exposure, some experts recommend that children receive IV penicillin G in a dosage of 300,000–400,000 units/kg daily given in divided doses every 4–6 hours. Concomitant use of other anti-infectives (e.g., streptomycin or other aminoglycoside, clindamycin, clarithromycin, rifampin, vancomycin) may also be indicated. Treatment of naturally occurring or endemic anthrax generally should be continued for at least 14 days after symptoms abate.

If IV penicillin G is used in a multiple-drug parenteral regimen for initial treatment of systemic anthrax (inhalational, GI, meningitis, cutaneous anthrax with systemic involvement, lesions on the head or neck, or extensive edema) caused by penicillin-susceptible *B. anthracis* that occurs in the context of biologic warfare or bioterrorism, AAP states that full-term neonates 7 days of age or younger should receive a dosage of 300,000 units/kg daily given in divided doses every 8 hours and those 1–4 weeks of age should receive 400,000 units/kg daily given in divided doses every 6 hours. For the treatment of these systemic anthrax infections in premature neonates, AAP recommends that those with gestational age of 32–34 weeks receive 200,000 units/kg daily given in divided doses every 12 hours from birth until 7 days of age and 300,000 units/kg daily given in divided doses every 8 hours from 1–4 weeks of age; those with gestational age of 34–37 weeks should receive 300,000 units/kg daily given in divided doses every 8 hours from birth until 7 days of age and 400,000 units/kg daily given in divided doses every 6 hours from 1–4 weeks of age. In infants and children 1 month of age or older, AAP recommends that IV penicillin G be given in a dosage of 400,000 units/kg daily in divided doses every 4 hours (up to 4 million units per dose). The multiple-drug parenteral regimen should be continued for at least 2–3 weeks until the patient is clinically stable; treatment can then be switched to an oral regimen. Because of the possible persistence of anthrax spores in lung tissue following an aerosol exposure in the context of biologic warfare or bioterrorism, the US Centers for Disease Control and Prevention (CDC) and other experts state that the total duration of anti-infective treatment should be 60 days.

For additional information on the treatment of anthrax and recommendations for postexposure prophylaxis following exposure to anthrax spores, see Uses: Anthrax, in Ciprofloxacin 8:12.18.

Clostridium Infections

For the treatment of myonecrosis and gas gangrene caused by *Clostridium perfringens* or other clostridium in children, IDSA recommends that IV penicillin G be given in a dosage of 60,000–100,000 units/kg every 6 hours in conjunction with clindamycin (10–13 mg/kg IV every 8 hours). AAP recommends that children with myonecrosis caused by *C. perfringens* receive IV penicillin G in a dosage of 250,000–400,000 units/kg daily and states that concomitant use of clindamycin may be more effective than penicillin G alone. Surgical debridement and/or surgery should be performed as indicated.

If IV penicillin G is used as an adjunct to tetanus immune globulin (TIG) in the management of tetanus caused by *C. tetani*, AAP recommends that children receive a dosage of 100,000 units/kg daily (up to 12 million units daily) given in divided doses every 4–6 hours for 7–10 days. The role of anti-infectives in the adjunctive treatment of tetanus is unclear; metronidazole usually is preferred if an anti-infective is used.

Diphtheria

If penicillin G potassium or sodium is used as an adjunct to diphtheria antitoxin (not commercially available in the US, but may be available from CDC) for the treatment of diphtheria caused by *Corynebacterium diphtheriae* and prevention of the diphtheria carrier state, the manufacturers recommend that pediatric patients receive a dosage of 150,000–250,000 units/kg daily given in divided doses every 6 hours for 7–10 days. CDC recommends a 14-day regimen of IM penicillin G procaine if a penicillin is used for adjunctive treatment of diphtheria. Patients usually are no longer contagious 48 hours after initiation of anti-infective treatment. Eradication of *C. diphtheriae* should be confirmed 24 hours after completion of treatment by 2 consecutive negative cultures taken 24 hours apart.

Lyme Disease

If IV penicillin G is used as an alternative to IV ceftriaxone for the treatment of early Lyme disease† in children with acute neurologic disease manifested as meningitis or radiculopathy, IDSA recommends a dosage of 200,000–400,000 units/kg daily (up to 18–24 million units daily) given in divided doses every 4 hours for 10–28 days.

If IV penicillin G is used as an alternative to IV ceftriaxone or IV cefotaxime for the treatment of late Lyme disease† in children with recurrent Lyme arthritis and objective evidence of neurologic disease, AAP and IDSA recommend a dosage of 200,000–400,000 units/kg daily (up to 18–24 million units daily) given in divided doses every 4 hours for 14–28 days.

For the treatment of late neurologic Lyme disease† affecting the central or peripheral nervous system, IDSA, AAP, and others state that children can receive

IV penicillin G in a dosage of 200,000–400,000 units/kg daily (up to 18–24 million units daily) given in divided doses every 4 hours for 14–28 days as an alternative to IV ceftriaxone. IDSA states that retreatment is not recommended unless relapse of neurologic disease is documented with reliable objective measures.

Neisseria meningitidis Infections

For the treatment of serious infections (e.g. endocarditis, pneumonia) caused by susceptible *N. meningitidis*, the manufacturers recommend that pediatric patients receive penicillin G potassium or sodium in a dosage of 150,000–300,000 units/kg daily given in divided doses every 4–6 hours.

For dosage recommendations for the treatment of meningitis caused by *N. meningitidis* in pediatric patients, see Meningitis and Other CNS Infections under Dosage: Pediatric Dosage, in Dosage and Administration.

Rat-Bite Fever

For the treatment of rat-bite fever caused by *Streptobacillus moniliformis* (erythema arthriticum epidemicum, Haverhill fever) or *Spirillum minus* (sodoku), the manufacturers recommend that pediatric patients receive penicillin G potassium or sodium in a dosage of 150,000–250,000 units/kg daily given in divided doses every 4 hours for 4 weeks.

Some clinicians suggest that pediatric patients with rat-bite fever receive IV penicillin G in a dosage of 20,000–50,000 units/kg daily for 5–7 days followed by oral penicillin V (25–50 mg/kg daily [up to 3 g daily] in 4 divided doses for 7 days). For the treatment endocarditis caused by *S. moniliformis* strains that are less susceptible to penicillin G (MIC greater than 0.1 mcg/mL), some clinicians state that pediatric patients should receive IV penicillin G in a dosage of 160,000–240,000 units/kg daily (up to 20 million units daily) for 6 weeks; concomitant use of an aminoglycoside (streptomycin or gentamicin) may be indicated for initial treatment.

Syphilis

For the treatment of proven or highly probable congenital syphilis in neonates (see Uses: Syphilis), CDC recommends an IV penicillin G dosage of 50,000 units/kg every 12 hours during the first 7 days of life and 50,000 units/kg every 8 hours thereafter for a total duration of 10 days. If more than 1 day of treatment is missed in such neonates, the entire course of treatment should be restarted. If IV penicillin G is used in neonates with possible congenital syphilis (see Uses: Syphilis), CDC recommends 50,000 units/kg every 12 hours during the first 7 days of life and 50,000 units/kg every 8 hours thereafter for a total duration 10 days.

In infants and children 1 month of age or older with reactive serologic tests for syphilis, CDC recommends that IV penicillin G be given in a dosage of 200,000–300,000 units/kg daily (50,000 units/kg every 4–6 hours) for 10 days.

CDC, AAP, and the manufacturers recommend that penicillin G potassium or sodium be given in a dosage of 200,000–300,000 units/kg daily (50,000 units every 4–6 hours) for 10–14 days for the treatment of congenital syphilis diagnosed after the neonatal period or for the treatment of neurosyphilis in infants and children 1 month of age or older. Some clinicians recommend that this regimen be followed by a single dose of IM penicillin G benzathine (50,000 units/kg [up to 2.4 million units]).

For the treatment of neurosyphilis and otic or ocular syphilis in adolescents with human immunodeficiency virus (HIV) infection, some clinicians recommend that IV penicillin G be given a dosage of 18–24 million units daily (by continuous IV infusion or given as 3–4 million units every 4 hours) for 10–14 days. Some clinicians recommend that this regimen be followed by a regimen of IM penicillin G benzathine (2.4 million units once weekly for 1–3 weeks).

HIV-infected neonates with congenital syphilis and HIV-infected children and adolescents with any stage of syphilis should receive the same treatment regimens recommended for those without HIV infection.

Adult Dosage
Bone and Joint Infections

For the treatment of native vertebral osteomyelitis or prosthetic joint infections caused by susceptible β-hemolytic streptococci†, IDSA recommends that adults receive IV penicillin G in a dosage of 20–24 million units daily (by continuous IV infusion or in 6 divided doses). The recommended duration of treatment is 6 weeks in patients with native vertebral osteomyelitis or 4–6 weeks in those with prosthetic joint infections.

For the treatment of native vertebral osteomyelitis or prosthetic joint infections caused by susceptible *Enterococcus*†, IDSA recommends that adults receive IV penicillin G in a dosage of 20–24 million units daily (by continuous IV infusion or in 6 divided doses) for 4–6 weeks. Concomitant treatment with an aminoglycoside given for 4–6 weeks also can be considered and is recommended if infective endocarditis also in present.

For the treatment of native vertebral osteomyelitis or prosthetic joint infections caused by susceptible *C. acnes*† (formerly *P. acnes*), IDSA recommends that adults receive IV penicillin G in a dosage of 20 million units daily (by continuous IV infusion or in 6 divided doses). The recommended duration of treatment is 6 weeks in patients with native vertebral osteomyelitis or 4–6 weeks in those with prosthetic joint infections.

Endocarditis

For the treatment of native valve endocarditis caused by viridans group streptococci† or *S. gallolyticus*† (formerly *S. bovis*) that are highly penicillin-susceptible (penicillin MIC 0.12 mcg/mL or less), AHA recommends that adults receive IV penicillin G in a dosage of 12–18 million units daily (by continuous IV infusion or in 4 or 6 divided doses) given for 4 weeks. Alternatively, adults with uncomplicated endocarditis caused by highly penicillin-susceptible viridans group streptococci† or *S. gallolyticus*† who are at low risk for adverse effects related to aminoglycoside therapy may receive a 2-week regimen consisting of IV penicillin G in a dosage of 12–18 million units daily (by continuous IV infusion or in 6 divided doses) in conjunction with gentamicin (3 mg/kg daily IV or IM given as a single daily dose or as 1 mg/kg every 8 hours). The 2-week regimen is not recommended for patients with known cardiac or extra-cardiac abscesses, creatinine clearance less than 20 mL/minute, impaired eighth cranial nerve function, or infection with *Abiotrophia*, *Granulicatella*, or *Gemella*.

For the treatment of native valve endocarditis caused by viridans streptococci† or *S. gallolyticus*† that are relatively resistant to penicillin G (penicillin MIC greater than 0.12 mcg/mL but less than 0.5 mcg/mL), AHA recommends that adults receive IV penicillin G in a dosage of 24 million units daily (by continuous IV infusion or in 4–6 divided doses) given for 4 weeks in conjunction with gentamicin (3 mg/kg daily IV or IM given as a single daily dose or as 1 mg/kg every 8 hours during the first 2 weeks of penicillin G treatment).

For the treatment of native valve endocarditis caused by viridans streptococci†, *A. defectiva*†, or *Granulicatella*† with penicillin MIC 0.5 mcg/mL or greater, AHA states that IV penicillin G given in a dosage of 18–30 million units daily (by continuous IV infusion or in 6 divided doses) in conjunction with gentamicin (3 mg/kg daily IV or IM in 2 or 3 divided doses) is a reasonable regimen for adults. AHA states that consultation with an infectious disease expert is recommended to determine the duration of treatment for such infections.

For the treatment of endocarditis involving prosthetic valves or other prosthetic material caused by viridans streptococci† or *S. gallolyticus*† that are highly penicillin-susceptible (penicillin MIC 0.12 mcg/mL or less), AHA states that adults can receive IV penicillin G in a dosage of 24 million units daily (by continuous IV infusion or in 4–6 divided doses) given for 6 weeks with or without gentamicin (3 mg/kg daily IV or IM as a single daily dose or as 1 mg/kg every 8 hours given concomitantly during the first 2 weeks of penicillin G treatment). When endocarditis involving prosthetic valves or other prosthetic material is caused by viridans streptococci† or *S. gallolyticus*† relatively or highly resistant to penicillin G (penicillin MIC greater than 0.12 mcg/mL), AHA states that it is reasonable to extend the duration of concomitant gentamicin to 6 weeks.

For the treatment of enterococcal endocarditis† (native valve or prosthetic valve or other prosthetic material) caused by *Enterococcus* susceptible to penicillin *and* gentamicin, AHA states that adults may receive IV penicillin G in a dosage of 18–30 million units daily (by continuous IV infusion or in 6 divided doses) in conjunction with gentamicin (3 mg/kg daily IV or IM in 2 or 3 divided doses; dose adjusted to achieve gentamicin peak serum concentrations of 3–4 mcg/mL and trough concentrations less than 1 mcg/mL). In patients with native valve enterococcal endocarditis, treatment with both drugs should be continued for 4 weeks in those who had symptoms of infection for less than 3 months prior to treatment or for 6 weeks in those who had symptoms for 3 months or longer prior to treatment. In patients with enterococcal endocarditis involving prosthetic heart valves or other prosthetic material, continuation of both drugs for 6 weeks is reasonable. If endocarditis is caused by enterococci resistant to gentamicin but susceptible to penicillin *and* streptomycin, AHA states that streptomycin (15 mg/kg daily IV or IM in 2 divided doses; dose adjusted to achieve streptomycin peak serum concentrations of 20–35 mcg/mL and trough concentrations less than 10 mcg/mL) can

be substituted for gentamicin in recommended regimens. Alternative regimens (e.g., double β-lactam regimens) should be considered in patients with creatinine clearance less than 50 mL/minute.

The manufacturers state that penicillin G potassium or sodium can be given in a dosage of 5–24 million units daily in divided doses every 4–6 hours for the treatment of endocarditis caused by susceptible staphylococci. However, penicillin G is not included in current AHA recommendations for the treatment of staphylococcal endocarditis in adults.

The manufacturers state that penicillin G potassium or sodium can be given in a dosage of 12–24 million units daily in divided doses every 4–6 hours for the treatment of endocarditis caused by susceptible streptococci, including *S. pyogenes*, streptococci groups C, H, G, L, and M, and *S. pneumoniae*.

Meningitis and Other CNS Infections

For the treatment of meningitis caused by susceptible *L. monocytogenes*, IDSA and other clinicians recommend that adults receive IV penicillin G in a dosage of 24 million units daily (4 million units every 4 hours). IDSA recommends a treatment duration of at least 21 days and states that concomitant use of an aminoglycoside should be considered. The manufacturers recommend that adults with meningitis caused by susceptible *L. monocytogenes* receive a penicillin G dosage of 15–20 million units daily given in divided doses every 4–6 hours for 2 weeks.

For the treatment of meningitis caused by susceptible *N. meningitidis*, IDSA recommends that adults receive IV penicillin G in a dosage of 24 million units daily (4 million units every 4 hours) for 7 days. The manufacturers recommend that adults receive a dosage of 24 million units daily (2 million units every 2 hours).

If meningitis is caused by susceptible *S. agalactiae*† (group B streptococci; GBS), IDSA recommends that adults receive IV penicillin G in a dosage of 24 million units daily (4 million units every 4 hours) for 14–21 days. IDSA states that concomitant use of an aminoglycoside should be considered.

For the treatment of meningitis caused by susceptible *S. pneumonia* (penicillin MIC less than 0.1 mcg/mL), IDSA and other clinicians recommend that adults receive IV penicillin G in a dosage of 24 million units daily (4 million units every 4 hours) for 10–14 days. The manufacturers recommend that adults receive a dosage of 12–24 million units daily given in divided doses every 4–6 hours. One manufacturer recommends a dosage of 5–24 million units daily given in divided doses every 4–6 hours.

For the treatment of healthcare-associated ventriculitis and meningitis caused by *C. acnes*† (formerly *P. acnes*), IDSA recommends that adults receive IV penicillin G in a dosage of 24 million units daily given in divided doses every 4 hours. Treatment should be continued for 10 days in those with no or minimal CSF pleocytosis, normal CSF glucose, and few clinical symptoms or systemic features or for 10–14 days in those with significant CSF pleocytosis, CSF hypoglycorrhachia, or clinical symptoms or systemic features.

Respiratory Tract Infections

If penicillin G potassium or sodium is used for the treatment of serious respiratory tract infections (e.g., empyema, pneumonia) caused by susceptible non-penicillinase-producing staphylococci, the manufacturers recommend that adults receive a dosage of 5–24 million units daily in divided doses every 4–6 hours depending on severity.

If penicillin G potassium is used for the treatment of serious respiratory tract infections (e.g., empyema, pneumonia) caused by susceptible *S. pyogenes*, streptococci groups C, H, G, L, and M, or *S. pneumoniae*, the manufacturers recommend that adults receive a dosage of 12–24 million units daily in divided doses every 4–6 hours depending on severity. If penicillin G sodium is used for the treatment of these infections, the manufacturer recommends a dosage of 5–24 million units daily in divided doses every 4–6 hours depending on severity.

Septicemia

If penicillin G potassium or sodium is used for the treatment of septicemia caused by susceptible nonpenicillinase-producing staphylococci, the manufacturers recommend that adults receive a dosage of 5–24 million units daily in divided doses every 4–6 hours depending on severity.

If penicillin G potassium is used for the treatment of septicemia caused by susceptible *S. pyogenes*, streptococci groups C, H, G, L, and M, or *S. pneumoniae*, the manufacturers recommend that adults receive a dosage of 12–24 million units daily in divided doses every 4–6 hours depending on severity. If penicillin

G sodium is used for the treatment of these infections, the manufacturer recommends a dosage of 5–24 million units daily in divided doses every 4–6 hours depending on severity.

Skin and Skin Structure Infections

For the treatment of necrotizing infections of the skin, fascia, and muscle caused by susceptible *S. pyogenes*, IDSA recommends that adults receive a regimen of IV penicillin G given in a dosage of 2–4 million units every 4–6 hours in conjunction with clindamycin (600–900 mg IV every 8 hours).

Actinomycosis

For the treatment of actinomycosis caused by *Actinomyces* in adults, the manufacturers recommend that penicillin G potassium or sodium be given in a dosage of 1–6 million units daily in divided doses every 4–6 hours for cervicofacial disease or 10–20 million units daily in divided doses every 4–6 hours for thoracic or abdominal disease.

Some clinicians state that, although dosage and duration of therapy should be individualized, a reasonable treatment regimen for pulmonary actinomycosis or other severe infections caused by *Actinomyces* is IV penicillin G given in a dosage of 18–24 million units daily (3–4 million units every 4 hours) for at least 2–6 weeks followed by 6–12 additional months of an oral regimen (penicillin V or amoxicillin). A shorter duration of treatment may be sufficient for less extensive disease (e.g., cervicofacial region). Surgical procedures should be performed as indicated.

Anthrax

For the treatment of anthrax (inhalational, GI, meningitis) caused by penicillin-susceptible *B. anthracis* that occurs as the result of naturally occurring or endemic anthrax exposure, some clinicians recommend that adults receive IV penicillin G in a dosage of 8–12 million units daily given in divided doses every 4–6 hours. For the treatment of severe or life-threatening systemic anthrax (inhalational, GI, meningoencephalitis, sepsis) or the treatment of cutaneous anthrax with signs of systemic involvement or extensive edema caused by penicillin-susceptible *B. anthracis* that occurs as the result of natural or endemic anthrax exposure, some clinicians recommend that adults receive IV penicillin G in a dosage of 4 million units every 4–6 hours (16–24 million units daily). Concomitant use of other anti-infectives (e.g., streptomycin or other aminoglycoside, clindamycin, clarithromycin, rifampin, vancomycin) may also be indicated. Treatment of naturally occurring or endemic anthrax generally should be continued for at least 14 days after symptoms abate.

If IV penicillin G is used in a multiple-drug parenteral regimen for initial treatment of systemic anthrax (inhalational, GI, meningitis, cutaneous anthrax with systemic involvement, lesions on the head or neck, or extensive edema) caused by penicillin-susceptible *B. anthracis* that occurs in the context of biologic warfare or bioterrorism, CDC recommends that adults (including pregnant and postpartum women) receive a dosage of 4 million units every 4 hours. The multiple-drug parenteral regimen should be continued for at least 2–3 weeks until the patient is clinically stable; treatment can then be switched to an oral regimen. Because of the possible persistence of anthrax spores in lung tissue following an aerosol exposure in the context of biologic warfare or bioterrorism, CDC and other experts state that the total duration of anti-infective treatment should be 60 days.

The manufacturers state that the minimum dosage of penicillin G potassium or sodium for the treatment of anthrax in adults is 8 million units daily given in divided doses every 6 hours and that higher dosage may be required depending on susceptibility of the organism.

For additional information on the treatment of anthrax and recommendations for postexposure prophylaxis following exposure to anthrax spores, see Uses: Anthrax, in Ciprofloxacin 8:12.18.

Clostridium Infections

For the treatment of myonecrosis and gas gangrene caused by *C. perfringens* or other clostridium, IDSA recommends that adults receive IV penicillin G in a dosage of 2–4 million units every 4–6 hours in conjunction with clindamycin (600–900 mg IV every 8 hours). The manufacturers recommend that adults receive penicillin G potassium or sodium in a dosage of 20 million units daily given in divided doses every 4–6 hours. Surgical debridement and/or surgery should be performed as indicated.

If penicillin G potassium or sodium is used as an adjunct to TIG in the management of tetanus caused by *C. tetani*, the manufacturers recommend that adults receive 20 million units daily given in divided doses every 4–6 hours. The role of anti-infectives in the adjunctive treatment of tetanus is unclear; metronidazole usually is preferred if an anti-infective is used.

If penicillin G potassium or sodium is used as an adjunct in the management of botulism caused by *C. botulinum*, the manufacturers recommend that adults receive 20 million units daily given in divided doses every 4–6 hours. Although the role of anti-infectives is unclear, some clinicians recommend a penicillin G dosage of 10–20 million units daily for adjunctive management of wound botulism. Botulism antitoxin (not commercially available in the US, but may be available from CDC) is the recommended treatment for foodborne and wound botulism and for botulism that occurs in the context of biologic warfare or bioterrorism.

Diphtheria

If penicillin G potassium or sodium is used as an adjunct to diphtheria antitoxin (not commercially available in the US, but may be available from CDC) for the treatment of diphtheria caused by *C. diphtheriae*, the manufacturers recommend that adults receive a dosage of 2–3 million units daily given in divided doses every 4–6 hours for 10–12 days. CDC recommends a 14-day regimen of IM penicillin G procaine if a penicillin is used for adjunctive treatment of diphtheria. Patients usually are no longer contagious 48 hours after initiation of anti-infective treatment. Eradication of *C. diphtheriae* should be confirmed 24 hours after completion of treatment by 2 consecutive negative cultures taken 24 hours apart.

Erysipelothrix Infections

If penicillin G potassium or sodium is used for the treatment of *Erysipelothrix* endocarditis, the manufacturers recommend that adults receive 12–20 million units daily given in divided doses every 4–6 hours for 4–6 weeks.

Fusobacterium Infections

If penicillin G potassium or sodium is used for the treatment of severe *Fusobacterium* infections of the oropharynx (including acute necrotizing ulcerative gingivitis [Vincent's infection], trench mouth, *Fusobacterium* gingivitis or pharyngitis), lower respiratory tract, or genital area, the manufacturers recommend that adults receive 5–10 million units daily in divided doses every 4–6 hours. Penicillin G is not recommended for empiric treatment of such infections because, although the drug may be effective against *Fusobacterium*, other organisms may also be involved (e.g., *Bacteroides fragilis, Prevotella, Porphyromonas*) that usually are resistant to penicillin G.

Leptospirosis

For the treatment of severe leptospirosis†, IV penicillin G has been given in a dosage of 6 million units daily (1.5 million units every 6 hours) for 7 days. Anti-infective treatment should be initiated as soon as possible after symptom onset; however, the benefits of anti-infective therapy are uncertain, especially if initiated in patients with late and/or severe disease.

Listeria Infections

For the treatment of serious infections caused by susceptible *L. monocytogenes* (e.g., endocarditis, meningitis) in adults, the manufacturers recommend that penicillin G potassium or sodium be given in a dosage of 15–20 million units daily in divided doses every 4–6 hours.

For additional dosage recommendations regarding the treatment of meningitis caused by *L. monocytogenes* in adults, see Meningitis and Other CNS Infections under Dosage: Adult Dosage, in Dosage and Administration.

Lyme Disease

If IV penicillin G is used as an alternative to IV ceftriaxone for the treatment of early Lyme disease† in adults with acute neurologic disease manifested as meningitis or radiculopathy, IDSA recommends a dosage of 18–24 million units daily given in divided doses every 4 hours for 10–28 days.

If IV penicillin G is used as an alternative to IV ceftriaxone for the treatment of late Lyme disease† in adults with recurrent Lyme arthritis and objective evidence of neurologic disease, IDSA recommends a dosage of 18–24 million units daily given in divided doses every 4 hours for 14–28 days.

For the treatment of late neurologic Lyme disease† affecting the central or peripheral nervous system, IDSA and others state that adults can receive IV penicillin G in a dosage of 18–24 million units daily given in divided doses every 4 hours for 14–28 days as an alternative to IV ceftriaxone. IDSA states that retreatment is not recommended unless relapse of neurologic disease is documented with reliable objective measures.

Neisseria meningitidis Infections

For the treatment of septicemia and/or meningitis caused by susceptible *N. meningitidis*, the manufacturers recommend that adults receive penicillin G potassium or sodium in a dosage of 24 million units daily (2 million units every 2 hours).

For additional dosage recommendations regarding the treatment of meningitis caused by *N. meningitidis* in adults, see Meningitis and Other CNS Infections under Dosage: Adult Dosage, in Dosage and Administration.

Pasteurella multocida Infections

For the treatment of serious infections caused by *Pasteurella multocida*, including bacteremia and meningitis, the manufacturers recommend that adults receive penicillin G potassium or sodium in a dosage of 4–6 million units daily given in divided doses every 4–6 hours for 2 weeks.

Rat-Bite Fever

For the treatment of rat-bite fever caused by susceptible *S. moniliformis* (erythema arthriticum epidemicum, Haverhill fever) or *S. minus* (sodoku), the manufacturers recommend that adults receive penicillin G potassium or sodium in a dosage of 12–20 million units daily given in divided doses every 4–6 hours for 3–4 weeks.

CDC recommends that adults with rat-bite fever caused by *S. moniliformis* receive IV penicillin G in a dosage of 1.2 million units daily for 5–7 days; if improvement occurs, treatment can be switched to oral penicillin V or oral ampicillin (500 mg 4 times daily for 7 days). Some clinicians suggest that adults with rat-bite fever can receive IV penicillin G in a dosage of 400,000–600,000 units daily for at least 7 days, but that dosage should be increased to 1.2 million units daily if there is no response to the lower dosage within 2 days.

For the treatment of *S. moniliformis* endocarditis caused by a strain that is less susceptible to penicillin G (MIC greater than 0.1 mcg/mL), some clinicians recommend that adults receive IV penicillin G in a dosage of 20 million units daily for 4 weeks; concomitant use of an aminoglycoside (streptomycin or gentamicin) may be indicated for initial treatment.

Syphilis

For the treatment of neurosyphilis and otic or ocular syphilis, CDC and other clinicians recommend that adults receive IV penicillin G in a dosage of 18–24 million units daily (by continuous IV infusion or given as 3–4 million units every 4 hours) for 10–14 days. Some clinicians recommend that this regimen be followed by a regimen of IM penicillin G benzathine (2.4 million units once weekly for up to 3 weeks).

The manufacturers recommend that adults with neurosyphilis receive penicillin G potassium or sodium in a dosage of 12–24 million units daily (2–4 million units every 4 hours) for 10–14 days; this may be followed by a regimen of IM penicillin G benzathine (2.4 million units once weekly for up to 3 weeks).

HIV-infected adults with any stage of syphilis should receive the same treatment regimens recommended for those without HIV infection.

Whipple's Disease

For initial treatment of Whipple's disease† caused by *Tropheryma whipplei*, some clinicians recommend that IV penicillin G be given in a dosage of 10 million units daily. Others recommend a dosage of 12–24 million units daily (2–4 million units every 4 hours). A regimen of IV penicillin G given in a dosage of 1.2 million units daily in conjunction with parenteral streptomycin (1 g daily) also has been recommended. The initial parenteral regimen usually is continued for 2–4 weeks and should be followed by 1–2 years of treatment with an oral regimen (e.g., co-trimoxazole).

Optimal regimens for treatment of Whipple's disease have not been identified and relapses may occur, even after adequate and long-term anti-infective treatment.

Prevention of Perinatal Group B Streptococcal Disease

When intrapartum anti-infective prophylaxis for prevention of perinatal group B streptococcal (GBS) disease† is indicated in the mother to prevent early-onset GBS disease in her neonate (see Uses: Prevention of Perinatal Group B Streptococcal Disease), CDC and AAP recommend that an initial dose of 5 million units of penicillin G be given IV at the onset of labor or rupture of membranes followed by 2.5–3 million units IV every 4 hours until delivery.

Regardless of whether anti-infective prophylaxis was administered to the mother, appropriate diagnostic evaluations and anti-infective therapy should be initiated in the neonate if signs or symptoms of active infection develop.

● Dosage in Renal and Hepatic Impairment

In patients with impaired renal function, doses and/or frequency of administration of penicillin G may need to be modified in response to the degree of impairment.

The manufacturers state that dosage of IM or IV penicillin G potassium or sodium should be adjusted in patients with severe renal impairment. These manufacturers and others recommend that patients with creatinine clearance less than 10 mL/minute per 1.73 m² receive a loading dose of penicillin G using the usually recommended dose followed by 50% of the usually recommended dose given every 8–10 hours. In uremic patients with creatinine clearance greater than 10 mL/minute per 1.73 m², the manufacturers and others recommend a loading dose of penicillin G using the usually recommended dose followed by 50% of the usually recommended dose given every 4–5 hours.

Alternatively, some clinicians suggest that if the usual dosing interval for penicillin G potassium or sodium in patients with normal renal function (creatinine clearance greater than 50 mL/minute) is every 6 or 8 hours, then the usual dose should be given every 8–12 hours in those with creatinine clearance of 10–50 mL/minute or every 12–18 hours in those with creatinine clearance less than 10 mL/minute.

Some clinicians suggest a maximum daily dosage of 4–10 million penicillin G units in adults with severe renal failure.

In patients with impaired hepatic function in addition to impaired renal function, further dosage reductions may be advisable.

CAUTIONS

● Adverse Effects

Adverse effects reported with penicillin G potassium and penicillin G sodium are similar to those reported with other natural penicillins.

Serious and occasionally fatal hypersensitivity reactions, including anaphylaxis, have been reported with penicillins. Hypersensitivity reactions to penicillins may be immediate reactions (usually occurring within 20 minutes after administration) that range in severity from urticaria and pruritus to angioedema, laryngospasm, bronchospasm, hypotension, vascular collapse, and death; accelerated reactions (usually occurring between 20 minutes and 48 hours after administration) that may include urticaria, pruritus, fever, and, occasionally, laryngeal edema; or delayed reactions (usually occurring within 1–2 weeks after initiation of penicillin therapy) that may include serum sickness-like symptoms (i.e., fever, malaise, urticaria, myalgia, arthralgia, abdominal pain) and rash ranging from maculopapular eruptions to exfoliative dermatitis.

Jarisch-Herxheimer reactions may occur in patients receiving penicillin G potassium or sodium for the treatment of syphilis or other spirochetal infections (e.g., leptospirosis†, Lyme disease†, relapsing fever†).

Because of the potassium and sodium content, penicillin G potassium and penicillin G sodium may cause serious and potentially fatal electrolyte disturbances, particularly if high IV dosage is used. Penicillin G potassium powders for injection contain approximately 66 mg (1.7 mEq) of potassium and approximately 7 mg (0.3 mEq) of sodium in each 1 million units of penicillin G. Frozen premixed penicillin G potassium injections in dextrose contain approximately 1.7 mEq of potassium and approximately 1 mEq of sodium in each 1 million units of penicillin G. Penicillin G sodium powder for injection contains approximately 1.7 mEq of sodium in each 1 million units of penicillin G.

For additional information on adverse effects reported with penicillin G, see Cautions in the Natural Penicillins General Statement 8:12.16.04.

● Precautions and Contraindications

Penicillin G potassium and sodium are contraindicated in patients hypersensitive to any penicillin.

The manufacturer of the commercially available frozen premixed penicillin G potassium injections in dextrose states that dextrose-containing solutions may be contraindicated in patients with known allergy to corn or corn products.

Penicillin G potassium and sodium share the toxic potentials of the penicillins, including the risk of hypersensitivity reactions, and the usual precautions of penicillin therapy should be observed.

Prior to initiation of therapy with penicillin G potassium or sodium, careful inquiry should be made concerning previous hypersensitivity reactions to penicillins, cephalosporins, or other drugs. There is clinical and laboratory evidence of partial cross-allergenicity among penicillins and other β-lactam antibiotics including cephalosporins and cephamycins.

Hypersensitivity reactions to penicillins are more likely to occur in individuals with a history of penicillin hypersensitivity and/or a history of sensitivity to multiple allergens. Penicillin G potassium or sodium should be used with caution in individuals with a history of allergies and/or asthma.

If a hypersensitivity reaction occurs, penicillin G should be discontinued immediately and appropriate therapy instituted as indicated (e.g., epinephrine, maintenance of an adequate airway and oxygen, corticosteroids). Desensitization has been used to enable a penicillin to be administered to penicillin-hypersensitive patients who have life-threatening infections for which other effective anti-infective agents are not available (e.g., endocarditis, neurosyphilis or congenital syphilis, syphilis during pregnancy). Such procedures are usually performed in a hospital setting and expert consultation may be indicated. Specialized references should be consulted for specific information on sensitivity testing and desensitization protocols.

During prolonged therapy with high dosage of penicillin G potassium or sodium, the patient's organ system functions should be assessed periodically, including frequent evaluation of hepatic, renal, and hematologic systems, electrolyte balance, and cardiac and vascular status. If any impairment of function is suspected or known to exist, a reduction in total dosage should be considered. (See Dosage and Administration: Dosage in Renal and Hepatic Impairment.)

For a more complete discussion of these and other precautions associated with the use of penicillin G potassium or sodium, see Cautions: Precautions and Contraindications, in the Natural Penicillins General Statement 8:12.16.04.

● Pediatric Precautions

Renal clearance of penicillin G may be delayed in neonates and premature or young infants because of incompletely developed renal function. Appropriate reductions in dosage and frequency of administration should be made in such patients.

Neonates receiving penicillin G potassium or sodium should be monitored closely for clinical and laboratory evidence of toxic or adverse effects.

● Geriatric Precautions

Clinical studies of penicillin G potassium did not include sufficient numbers of patients 65 years of age or older to determine whether geriatric patients respond differently than younger patients. Other clinical experience has not identified differences in responses between geriatric and younger patients.

Penicillin G is substantially eliminated by the kidneys and the risk of adverse effects may be greater in those with impaired renal function. Because geriatric patients are more likely to have reduced renal function, dosage should be selected with caution, usually starting at the low end of the dosage range, and renal function monitoring may be useful.

The potassium and/or sodium content of penicillin G potassium or sodium preparations and the potential for electrolyte imbalance should be considered. Geriatric patients may respond to salt loading with a blunted natriuresis that may be clinically important in those with certain conditions (e.g., congestive heart failure).

● Pregnancy, Fertility, and Lactation
Pregnancy

Reproduction studies evaluating penicillin G in mice, rats, and rabbits have not revealed evidence of impaired fertility or harm to the fetus. Although experience with use of penicillins during pregnancy has not shown any evidence of adverse effects on the fetus, there are no adequate or controlled studies using penicillin G in pregnant women.

Some clinicians state that penicillin G is considered low risk and safe for use during pregnancy. The drug is included in the US Centers for Disease Control and Prevention (CDC) recommendations for the treatment of syphilis during pregnancy.

The manufacturers state that penicillin G potassium or sodium should be used during pregnancy only when clearly needed.

Lactation

Penicillin G is distributed into milk. Some clinicians state that penicillin G is usually considered compatible with breast-feeding. The manufacturers and others state that penicillin G potassium or sodium should be used with caution in nursing women.

SPECTRUM

Based on its spectrum of activity, penicillin G is classified as a natural penicillin. For information on the classification of penicillins based on spectra of activity, see the Preface to the General Statements on Penicillins 8:12.16.

For specific information on the spectrum of activity of penicillin G and resistance to the drug, see the sections on Spectrum and on Resistance in the Natural Penicillins General Statement 8:12.16.04.

PHARMACOKINETICS

For additional information on the absorption, distribution, and elimination of penicillin G, see Pharmacokinetics in the Natural Penicillins General Statement 8:12.16.04.

● Absorption

Penicillin G potassium and penicillin G sodium are rapidly absorbed followed IM administration, and serum concentrations of penicillin G generally are the same following IM administration of equivalent doses of either salt. Following IM administration in adults of a single dose of 600,000 or 1 million units of penicillin G (as either salt), peak serum concentrations of penicillin G generally are attained within 15–30 minutes and average 6–8 or 20 units/mL, respectively. In one study in neonates 6 days of age or younger who received IM penicillin G in a dosage of 25,000 units/kg every 12 hours as the potassium salt, serum penicillin G concentrations ranged from 12.5–36, 7.8–35.1, 4.4–35.1, 0.7–21.9, and 0.3–9.2 mcg/mL at 30 minutes, 1 hour, 2 hours, 4 hours, and 12 hours, respectively, after a dose.

Following IV infusion of penicillin G, peak serum concentrations are attained immediately after completion of the infusion. In a study in 10 patients who received 5 million units of penicillin G given IV over 3–5 minutes, mean serum concentrations were 400, 273, and 3 mcg/mL at 5–6 minutes, 10 minutes, and 4 hours after administration, respectively. In a study in 5 healthy adults who received 1 million units of penicillin G given IV over 4 minutes or 60 minutes, mean serum concentrations 8 minutes after administration were 45 or 14.4 mcg/mL, respectively.

Following intermittent IV infusion of 2 million units of penicillin G every 2 hours or 3 million units of penicillin G every 3 hours (as either salt), serum penicillin G concentrations reportedly average 20 mcg/mL.

Penicillin G potassium or sodium is absorbed from the peritoneal cavity following local instillation and also is absorbed from pleural surfaces, pericardium, and joint cavities.

● Distribution

Penicillin G is widely distributed throughout the body in varying amounts following parenteral administration. Penicillin G is distributed into the lungs, liver, kidneys, muscle, bone, and pleural, pericardial, peritoneal, ascitic, synovial, and interstitial fluids. The volume of distribution of penicillin G is reportedly 0.53–0.67 L/kg in adults with normal renal function.

Minimal concentrations of penicillin G generally are attained in CSF following administration of penicillin G potassium or sodium in patients with uninflamed meninges; however, higher penicillin G concentrations are attained in CSF when the meninges are inflamed. Following IV administration of penicillin G sodium, concentrations of penicillin G in CSF reportedly range from 0–10% of concurrent serum concentrations of the drug in patients with normal meninges. In 2 adults with syphilis who received a daily IV dosage of 5 or 10 million units of penicillin G (as the potassium salt) for at least 10 days, penicillin G concentrations in CSF immediately following completion of therapy were 0.3 or 2.4 mcg/mL, respectively. In one study in children 2 weeks to 11 years of age with meningitis who received penicillin G potassium in a dosage of 250,000 units/kg daily given in 6 divided doses by IV infusion over 15 minutes, penicillin G concentrations in CSF specimens obtained between doses averaged 0.8, 0.7, and 0.3 mcg/mL on the first, fifth, and tenth days of therapy, respectively.

Penicillin G is approximately 45–68% bound to serum proteins.

Penicillin G crosses the placenta, although cord blood concentrations of the drug may be less than maternal serum concentrations.

Penicillin G is distributed into milk.

● **Elimination**

The serum half-life of penicillin G in adults with normal renal function is 0.4–0.9 hours.

Approximately 16–30% of an IM dose of penicillin G sodium is metabolized to penicilloic acid which is microbiologically inactive. Small amounts of 6-aminopenicillanic acid (6-APA) have also been found in the urine of patients receiving penicillin G. In addition, the drug appears to be hydroxylated to a small extent to one or more microbiologically active metabolites which also are excreted in urine.

Penicillin G and its metabolites are excreted in urine mainly by tubular secretion. Small amounts of the drug are also excreted in bile. Following IM or IV administration of a single dose of penicillin G in adults with normal renal function, 58–85% of the dose is excreted in urine as unchanged drug and active metabolites within 6 hours.

Serum concentrations of penicillin G may be higher and the serum half-life prolonged in patients with impaired renal function. The serum half-life of the drug is reportedly 1–2 hours in azotemic patients with serum creatinine concentrations less than 3 mg/dL and ranges from 6–20 hours in anuric patients. In anuric patients with hepatic impairment, the serum half-life of penicillin G may be 2–3 times more prolonged than in anuric patients with normal hepatic function.

Renal clearance of penicillin G is delayed in neonates and premature or young infants. The serum half-life of penicillin G varies inversely with age and appears to be independent of birthweight. The serum half-life of the drug is reportedly 3.2–3.4 hours in neonates 6 days of age or younger, 1.2–2.2 hours in neonates 7–13 days of age, and 0.9–1.9 hours in neonates 14 days of age or older.

Renal clearance of penicillin G may be delayed in geriatric patients because of diminished tubular secretion ability.

Renal clearance of penicillin G may be increased in pregnant women during the second and third trimesters.

Penicillin G is removed by hemodialysis and may be removed to a lesser extent by peritoneal dialysis.

CHEMISTRY AND STABILITY

● **Chemistry**

Penicillin G is a natural penicillin produced by fermentation of *Penicillium chrysogenum* in a medium containing phenylacetic acid. Penicillin G potassium and penicillin G sodium are frequently referred to as aqueous, crystalline forms of penicillin G.

Penicillin G potassium occurs as colorless or white crystals or a white, crystalline powder that is odorless or practically odorless and moderately hygroscopic. Penicillin G potassium is very soluble in water. Penicillin G potassium

is commercially available as a sterile powder for injection in vials containing the equivalent of 1, 5, or 20 million units of penicillin G. Each 1 million units of penicillin G (as penicillin G potassium) contains approximately 66 mg (1.7 mEq) of potassium and approximately 7 mg (0.3 mEq) of sodium. The sterile powders are buffered with sodium citrate and/or citric acid. Following reconstitution according to the manufacturer's directions, penicillin G potassium solutions have a pH of 6–8.5. Penicillin G potassium also is commercially available as a frozen premixed solution in dextrose.

Penicillin G sodium occurs as a white to almost white, crystalline powder that is almost odorless. Penicillin G sodium is commercially available as a sterile powder for injection in vials containing the equivalent of 5 million units of penicillin G. Each 1 million units of penicillin G (as penicillin G sodium) contains approximately 1.7 mEq of sodium. Following reconstitution according to the manufacturer's directions, penicillin G sodium solutions are colorless and have a pH of 5–7.5.

Commercially available frozen premixed penicillin G potassium injections in dextrose are sterile, iso-osmotic, nonpyrogenic solutions of the drug provided in single-dose plastic containers (Galaxy® containers) fabricated from specially formulated multilayered plastic (PL 2040). The frozen injections containing 1, 2, or 3 million units of penicillin G contain approximately 2, 1.2, or 350 mg of dextrose hydrous, respectively, to adjust osmolality and also contain sodium citrate as a buffer. Hydrochloric acid and/or sodium hydroxide may have been added to adjust pH to 5.5–8. The frozen premixed penicillin G potassium injections in dextrose contain approximately 1.7 mEq of potassium and approximately 1 mEq of sodium in each 1 million units of penicillin G.

Potency of penicillin G potassium and penicillin G sodium generally is expressed in terms of penicillin G units, but also has been expressed as mg of penicillin G. Each mg of penicillin G potassium has a potency of 1440–1680 USP penicillin G units; each mg of penicillin G potassium powder for injection buffered with sodium citrate has a potency of 1355–1595 USP penicillin G units. Each mg of penicillin G sodium has a potency of 1500–1750 USP penicillin G units.

● **Stability**

Commercially available penicillin G potassium sterile powder for injection should be stored at less than 30°C. Following reconstitution, penicillin G potassium solutions should be stored at 2–8°C and are stable for 7 days at this temperature.

Commercially available penicillin G sodium powder for injection should be stored at 20–25°C. Following reconstitution, penicillin G sodium solutions should be stored at 2–8°C and are stable for 3 days at this temperature.

The commercially available frozen premixed penicillin G potassium injections in dextrose should be stored at –20°C or lower. The frozen premixed injections should be thawed at room temperature (25°C) or under refrigeration (5°C) and, once thawed, should not be refrozen. Thawed solutions of the commercially available frozen injections are stable for 24 hours at room temperature (25°C) or 14 days when refrigerated at 5°C. The commercially available frozen injections of the drug are provided in a plastic container fabricated from specially formulated multilayered plastic PL 2040 (Galaxy® containers). Solutions in contact with the polyethylene layer can leach out some of its chemical components in very small amounts within the expiration period of the injection; however, safety of the plastic has been confirmed in tests in animals according to USP biological tests for plastic containers as well as by tissue culture toxicity studies.

Penicillin G is unstable in solution at room temperature and is rapidly inactivated in carbohydrate solutions at alkaline pH. Small amounts of polymer conjugation products reportedly form in solutions of penicillin G during in vitro storage, especially when high concentrations of the drug are stored at room temperature. Penicillin degradation products may be more potent antigens than penicillin G and may play a role in hypersensitivity reactions to the drug. Therefore, reconstituted solutions of penicillin G potassium or penicillin G sodium should be refrigerated as directed by the manufacturer or used shortly following reconstitution.

Penicillin G is potentially physically and/or chemically incompatible with some drugs, including aminoglycosides and tetracyclines, but the compatibility depends on several factors (e.g., concentrations of the drugs, specific diluents used, resulting pH, temperature). Specialized references should be consulted for specific compatibility information.

For further information on chemistry and stability, mechanism of action, spectrum, resistance, pharmacokinetics, uses, cautions, drug interactions, laboratory test interferences, and dosage and administration of penicillin G potassium or sodium, see the Natural Penicillins General Statement 8:12.16.04.

PREPARATIONS

Excipients in commercially available drug preparations may have clinically important effects in some individuals; consult specific product labeling for details.

Penicillin G Potassium

Parenteral		
For injection	1 million units (of penicillin G)*	Penicillin G Potassium for Injection
	5 million units (of penicillin G)*	Penicillin G Potassium for Injection Pfizerpen®, Pfizer
	20 million units (of penicillin G)*	Penicillin G Potassium for Injection Pfizerpen®, Pfizer

* available from one or more manufacturer, distributor, and/or repackager by generic (nonproprietary) name

Penicillin G Potassium in Dextrose

Parenteral		
Injection (frozen), for IV infusion	20,000 units (of penicillin G) per mL (1 million units) in 4% Dextrose*	Penicillin G Potassium in Iso-osmotic Dextrose Injection Galaxy®
	40,000 units (of penicillin G) per mL (2 million units) in 2.4% Dextrose*	Penicillin G Potassium in Iso-osmotic Dextrose Injection Galaxy®
	60,000 units (of penicillin G) per mL (3 million units) in 0.7% Dextrose*	Penicillin G Potassium in Iso-osmotic Dextrose Injection Galaxy®

* available from one or more manufacturer, distributor, and/or repackager by generic (nonproprietary) name

Penicillin G Sodium

Parenteral		
For injection	5 million units (of penicillin G)*	Penicillin G Sodium for Injection

* available from one or more manufacturer, distributor, and/or repackager by generic (nonproprietary) name

† Use is not currently included in the labeling approved by the US Food and Drug Administration.

Selected Revisions October 1, 2018, © Copyright, January 1, 1985, American Society of Health-System Pharmacists, Inc.

Penicillin G Procaine

8:12.16.04 • NATURAL PENICILLINS

■ Penicillin G procaine, a natural penicillin, is a β-lactam antibiotic. The drug is the procaine monohydrate salt of penicillin G and is a long-acting formulation of penicillin G.

USES

Penicillin G procaine is used only for the treatment of moderately severe infections caused by organisms that are susceptible to the low, prolonged serum concentrations of penicillin G provided by IM penicillin G procaine. When high, sustained concentrations of penicillin G are required for the treatment of severe infections, parenteral penicillin G potassium or sodium should be used.

The fixed combinations of penicillin G benzathine and penicillin G procaine are used for the treatment of moderately severe to severe infections caused by susceptible streptococci (e.g., upper respiratory tract infections, scarlet fever, erysipelas, skin and skin structure infections). The fixed combinations should *not* be used for *initial* treatment of severe pneumococcal infections, including pneumonia, empyema, bacteremia, pericarditis, meningitis, peritonitis, or arthritis. In addition, fixed combinations of penicillin G benzathine and penicillin G procaine should *not* be used for the treatment of syphilis, yaws, bejel, pinta, or gonorrhea.

For additional information on the uses of penicillin G procaine, see Uses in the Natural Penicillins General Statement 8:12.16.04.

● Anthrax

IM penicillin G procaine is used for inhalational anthrax (postexposure) to reduce the incidence or progression of disease following suspected or confirmed exposure to aerosolized *Bacillus anthracis* spores. Ciprofloxacin or doxycycline are the initial drugs of choice for postexposure prophylaxis following suspected or confirmed exposure to aerosolized anthrax spores, including exposures that occur in the context of biologic warfare or bioterrorism. If penicillin susceptibility is confirmed, consideration can be given to changing prophylaxis to a penicillin in infants and children, pregnant or lactating women, or when the drugs of choice are not tolerated or not available; however, oral amoxicillin or penicillin V usually is recommended.

IM penicillin G procaine is used for the treatment of mild, uncomplicated cutaneous anthrax caused by susceptible *B. anthracis* that occurs as the result of naturally occurring or endemic exposure to anthrax. If cutaneous anthrax occurs in the context of biologic warfare or bioterrorism, the initial drugs of choice are ciprofloxacin and doxycycline. If penicillin susceptibility is confirmed, consideration can be given to changing treatment to a penicillin in infants and children, pregnant or lactating women, or when the drugs of choice are not tolerated or not available; however, oral amoxicillin or penicillin V usually is recommended.

For additional information on the treatment of anthrax and recommendations for postexposure prophylaxis following exposure to anthrax spores, see Uses: Anthrax, in Ciprofloxacin 8:12.18.

● Syphilis

IM penicillin G procaine is used for the treatment of syphilis.

The US Centers for Disease Control and Prevention (CDC) and other clinicians state that IM penicillin G benzathine is the drug of choice for the treatment of primary syphilis (i.e., ulcer or chancre at infection site), secondary syphilis (i.e., manifestations that include, but are not limited to, rash, mucocutaneous lesions, and lymphadenopathy), and tertiary syphilis (i.e., cardiac syphilis, gummatous lesions, tabes dorsalis, and general paresis) in adults, adolescents, and children.

IM penicillin G benzathine also is the drug of choice for the treatment of latent syphilis (i.e., detected by serologic testing but lacking clinical manifestations), including both early latent syphilis (latent syphilis acquired within the preceding year) and late latent syphilis (i.e., all other cases of latent syphilis or syphilis of unknown duration) in all age groups.

For the treatment of neurosyphilis and otic or ocular syphilis, CDC and other clinicians state that IV penicillin G potassium or sodium is the drug of choice and IM penicillin G procaine (with oral probenecid) is an alternative if compliance can be ensured.

For the treatment of congenital syphilis, CDC recommends IV penicillin G potassium or sodium or IM penicillin G procaine in neonates with proven or highly probable congenital syphilis (i.e., abnormal physical examination consistent with congenital syphilis, serum quantitative nontreponemal serologic titer fourfold higher than the mother's titer, or positive darkfield test or polymerase chain reaction [PCR] of lesions or body fluids). CDC recommends IV penicillin G potassium or sodium, IM penicillin G procaine, or IM penicillin G benzathine in neonates with possible congenital syphilis (i.e., normal physical examination and serum quantitative nontreponemal serologic titer no more than fourfold higher than the mother's titer and the mother received a recommended treatment regimen less than 4 weeks before delivery; the mother was not treated or was inadequately treated, including treatment with erythromycin or any regimen not included in CDC recommendations; or there is no documentation that the mother received treatment).

Neonates with human immunodeficiency virus (HIV) infection who have congenital syphilis and HIV-infected children, adolescents, or adults who have neurosyphilis or primary, secondary, early latent, late latent, or tertiary syphilis should receive the same treatment regimens as those without HIV infection. Because serologic nonresponse and neurologic complications may be more frequent in HIV-infected individuals, close follow-up is essential in those coinfected with syphilis and HIV. In addition, careful neurologic examinations are indicated in all HIV-infected patients coinfected with syphilis.

There are no proven alternatives to penicillin G for the treatment of congenital syphilis in infants and children with known or suspected penicillin hypersensitivity and no proven alternatives to penicillin G for the treatment of any stage of syphilis in pregnant women with penicillin hypersensitivity; therefore, CDC recommends desensitization and treatment with the appropriate penicillin G preparation.

Fixed combinations of penicillin G benzathine and penicillin G procaine (Bicillin® C-R, Bicillin® C-R 900/300) should not be used for the treatment of any form of syphilis; inadvertent use of one of these fixed-combination preparations may not provide the sustained serum concentrations of penicillin G required for treatment of syphilis and could increase the risk of treatment failure and neurosyphilis, especially in HIV-infected patients.

For additional information regarding treatment of syphilis, the current CDC sexually transmitted diseases treatment guidelines available at https://www.cdc.gov/std/syphilis/treatment.htm should be consulted.

DOSAGE AND ADMINISTRATION

● Administration

Penicillin G procaine and fixed combinations containing penicillin G benzathine and penicillin G procaine are administered *only* by deep IM injection.

Special precaution should be taken to avoid inadvertent intravascular or intra-arterial administration of penicillin G procaine or fixed combinations of penicillin G benzathine and penicillin G procaine or injection into or near major peripheral nerves or blood vessels because this may result in severe and/or permanent neurovascular damage. (See Cautions: Adverse Effects.)

Fixed combinations containing penicillin G benzathine and penicillin G procaine must *not* be given IV or admixed with IV solutions because inadvertent IV administration of penicillin G benzathine has been associated with cardiorespiratory arrest and death.

IM Injection

Penicillin G procaine and fixed combinations containing penicillin G benzathine and penicillin G procaine are provided in prefilled syringes and the appropriate dose should be administered undiluted according to the manufacturer's directions.

In adults, IM injections of penicillin G procaine or fixed combinations of penicillin G benzathine and penicillin G procaine generally should be made deeply into the gluteus maximus (upper outer quadrant of the buttock) or into the midlateral thigh. In neonates, infants, and small children, IM injections of these preparations should be given preferably into the midlateral muscles of the thigh.

IM injections of penicillin G procaine or fixed combinations of penicillin G benzathine and penicillin G procaine should be made at a slow, steady rate to avoid blockage of the needle.

When the fixed combination of penicillin G benzathine and penicillin G procaine (Bicillin® C-R) is used, the manufacturer states that the dose usually is given at a single session using multiple IM sites; alternatively, if compliance regarding the return visit is ensured, the total dose can be divided and half given on day 1 and half on day 3.

When repeated doses are given, IM injection sites should be varied. Repeated IM injection into the anterolateral thigh, especially in neonates and infants, should be avoided since quadriceps femoris fibrosis and atrophy may occur.

● Dosage

Dosage of penicillin G procaine usually is expressed in terms of penicillin G units, but also has been expressed as mg of penicillin G.

Dosage of the fixed combinations containing penicillin G benzathine and penicillin G procaine (Bicillin® C-R, Bicillin® C-R 900/300) usually is expressed in terms of the total (sum) of penicillin G units of penicillin G benzathine and penicillin G units of penicillin G procaine.

Pediatric Dosage
General Pediatric Dosage

The American Academy of Pediatrics (AAP) states that the usual dosage of IM penicillin G procaine in neonates 28 days of age or younger is 50,000 units/kg once every 24 hours.

For the treatment of mild to moderate infections in pediatric patients beyond the neonatal period, AAP states that the usual dosage of IM penicillin G procaine is 50,000 units/kg daily given in 1 or 2 divided doses. AAP states that IM penicillin G procaine is inappropriate for the treatment of severe infections.

If the fixed combination of penicillin G benzathine and penicillin G procaine (Bicillin® C-R) is used in pediatric patients beyond the neonatal period, AAP recommends a single IM dose of 600,000 penicillin G units in those weighing less than 14 kg and a single IM dose of 900,000 to 1.2 million penicillin G units in those weighing 14–27 kg. If this fixed-combination preparation is used in those weighing 27 kg or more, AAP recommends a single dose of 2.4 million penicillin G units.

Staphylococcal Infections

If IM penicillin G procaine is used for the treatment of moderately severe skin and skin structure infections caused by susceptible staphylococci, the manufacturer recommends a dosage of 300,000 units daily in children weighing less than 27 kg and 600,000 to 1 million units daily in others. Because of the high incidence of resistant strains, in vitro culture and susceptibility testing should be performed when treating suspected staphylococcal infections.

Streptococcal Infections

If IM penicillin G procaine is used for the treatment of infections caused by *Streptococcus pyogenes* (group A β-hemolytic streptococci; GAS), such as moderately severe to severe upper respiratory tract infections, tonsillitis, scarlet fever, erysipelas, and skin and skin structure infections, the manufacturer recommends a dosage of 300,000 units daily for at least 10 days in children weighing less than 27 kg and 600,000 to 1 million units daily for at least 10 days in others.

If IM penicillin G procaine is used for the treatment of moderately severe, uncomplicated respiratory tract infections (pneumonia) caused by susceptible *S. pneumoniae*, the manufacturer recommends a dosage of 300,000 units daily in children weighing less than 27 kg and 600,000 to 1 million units daily in others.

If the fixed combination of penicillin G benzathine and penicillin G procaine (Bicillin® C-R) is used for the treatment of moderately severe to severe infections caused by susceptible *S. pyogenes* (e.g., upper respiratory tract infections, scarlet fever, erysipelas, skin and skin structure infections), the manufacturer recommends that children weighing less than 13.6 kg receive a single IM dose of 600,000 penicillin G units, those weighing 13.6–27.2 kg receive a single IM dose of 900,000 to 1.2 million penicillin G units, and those weighing more than 27.2 kg receive a single IM dose of 2.4 million penicillin G units. If this fixed-combination preparation is used for the treatment of moderately severe infections caused by susceptible *S. pneumoniae* (pneumonia, otitis media), the manufacturer recommends that pediatric patients receive an IM dose of 600,000 penicillin G units once every 2 or 3 days until the patient has been afebrile for 48 hours. Other penicillins are recommended for severe *S. pneumoniae* infections (e.g., pneumonia, empyema, bacteremia, pericarditis, meningitis, peritonitis, arthritis).

If the fixed combination of penicillin G benzathine and penicillin G procaine (Bicillin® C-R 900/300) is used for the treatment of moderately severe to severe infections caused by susceptible *S. pyogenes* (e.g., upper respiratory tract infections, scarlet fever, erysipelas, skin and skin structure infections), the manufacturer states that a single IM dose of 1.2 million penicillin G units usually is sufficient in pediatric patients. If this fixed-combination preparation is used for the treatment of moderately severe infections caused by susceptible *S. pneumoniae* (pneumonia, otitis media), the manufacturer recommends that pediatric patients receive an IM dose of 1.2 million penicillin G units once every 2 or 3 days until the patient has been afebrile for 48 hours. Other penicillins are recommended for severe *S. pneumoniae* infections (e.g., pneumonia, empyema, bacteremia, pericarditis, meningitis, peritonitis, arthritis).

Anthrax

If IM penicillin G procaine is used for inhalational anthrax (postexposure) to reduce the incidence or progression of disease following exposure to aerosolized *Bacillus anthracis* spores, the manufacturer recommends that children receive 25,000 units/kg (up to 1.2 million units) every 12 hours. Because of the possible persistence of anthrax spores in lung tissue following an aerosol exposure, the US Centers for Disease Control and Prevention (CDC) and other experts recommend that the total duration of anti-infective prophylaxis should be at least 60 days. The manufacturer states that safety data for penicillin G procaine administered at the dosage recommended for inhalational anthrax (postexposure) supports a duration of 2 weeks or less, and clinicians must consider the risks versus benefits of administering IM penicillin G procaine for longer than 2 weeks or switching to an appropriate alternative anti-infective.

If IM penicillin G procaine is used for the treatment of mild, uncomplicated cutaneous anthrax caused by susceptible *B. anthracis* that occurs as the result of naturally occurring or endemic anthrax exposure, some experts recommend a dosage of 25,000–50,000 units/kg daily (single or 2 divided doses daily) in children weighing less than 20 kg. Although 3–10 days of anti-infective therapy may be adequate for the treatment of mild, uncomplicated cutaneous anthrax that occurs as the result of naturally occurring or endemic exposures to anthrax, some experts recommend a duration of 7–14 days. CDC and other experts state that anti-infectives should be continued for 60 days if cutaneous anthrax occurred as the result of exposure to aerosolized *B. anthracis* spores in the context of biologic warfare or bioterrorism since the possibility of inhalational anthrax would also exist. Although anti-infective therapy may limit the size of the cutaneous anthrax lesion and it usually becomes sterile within the first 24 hours of treatment, the lesion will still progress through the black eschar stage despite effective treatment.

For additional information on treatment of anthrax and recommendations for postexposure prophylaxis following exposure to anthrax spores, see Uses: Anthrax, in Ciprofloxacin 8:12.18.

Diphtheria

When IM penicillin G procaine is used as an adjunct to diphtheria antitoxin (not commercially available in the US, but may be available from CDC) for the treatment of diphtheria caused by *Corynebacterium diphtheriae*, the manufacturer recommends a dosage of 300,000–600,000 units daily. CDC recommends a 14-day regimen of IM penicillin G procaine given in a dosage of 300,000 units daily in those weighing 10 kg or less and 600,000 units daily in those weighing more than 10 kg for adjunctive treatment of diphtheria. Patients usually are no longer contagious 48 hours after initiation of anti-infective therapy. Eradication of *C. diphtheriae* should be confirmed 24 hours after completion of treatment by 2 consecutive negative cultures taken 24 hours apart.

If IM penicillin G procaine is used to eliminate the diphtheria carrier state in identified carriers of toxigenic *C. diphtheriae*, the manufacturer recommends a dosage of 300,000 units daily for 10 days. CDC and AAP recommend IM penicillin G benzathine if a penicillin G preparation is used for elimination of the diphtheria carrier state. Follow-up cultures should be obtained at least 2 weeks after treatment of diphtheria carriers; if cultures are positive, a 10-day course of oral erythromycin should be given and additional follow-up cultures obtained.

Syphilis

For the treatment of proven or highly probable congenital syphilis in neonates (see Uses: Syphilis), CDC states that IM penicillin G procaine should be given in a dosage of 50,000 units/kg once daily for 10 days. If more than 1 day of treatment is missed in such neonates, the entire course of treatment should be restarted. If IM penicillin G procaine is used in neonates with possible congenital syphilis (see Uses: Syphilis), CDC recommends a dosage of 50,000 units/kg once daily for 10 days.

CDC recommends that treatment of syphilis diagnosed in infants and children 1 month of age or older should be managed by a pediatric infectious disease specialist and that CSF should be examined in those with latent syphilis.

The manufacturer states that children older than 12 years of age with primary, secondary, or latent syphilis with a negative CSF test for syphilis may receive IM penicillin G procaine in a dosage of 600,000 units daily for 8 days (total dosage 4.8 million units) and those with tertiary or latent syphilis with a positive CSF examination or no CSF examination may receive 600,000 units of daily for 10–15 days (total dosage 6–9 million units). CDC and others state that IM penicillin G benzathine is the drug of choice for the treatment of primary, secondary, tertiary, and latent syphilis.

If IM penicillin G procaine is used as an alternative for the treatment of syphilis in adolescents 10–19 years of age, some experts state that those with early syphilis (primary, secondary, or early latent syphilis) can receive a dosage of 1.2 million units once daily for 10–14 days and those with late latent syphilis or syphilis of unknown duration can receive 1.2 million units once daily for 20 days.

Neonates with human immunodeficiency virus (HIV) infection who have congenital syphilis and HIV-infected children and adolescents with any stage of syphilis should receive the same treatment regimens recommended for those without HIV infection.

Fixed combinations of penicillin G benzathine and penicillin G procaine (Bicillin® C-R, Bicillin® C-R 900/300) should not be used for the treatment of any form of syphilis.

Adult Dosage

Staphylococcal Infections

If IM penicillin G procaine is used for the treatment of moderately severe to severe skin and skin structure infections caused by susceptible staphylococci, the manufacturer recommends that adults receive a dosage of 600,000 to 1 million units daily. Because of high incidence of resistant strains, in vitro culture and susceptibility testing should be performed when treating suspected staphylococcal infections.

Streptococcal Infections

If IM penicillin G procaine is used for the treatment of infections caused by susceptible *S. pyogenes* (group A β-hemolytic streptococci; GAS), such as moderately severe to severe upper respiratory tract infections, tonsillitis, pharyngitis, scarlet fever, erysipelas, and skin and skin structure infections, the manufacturer recommends that adults receive a dosage of 600,000 to 1 million units daily for at least 10 days.

The manufacturer states that bacterial endocarditis caused by extremely susceptible *S. pyogenes* may be treated with an IM penicillin G procaine dosage of 600,000 to 1 million units daily. AHA recommends IV penicillin G potassium or sodium if a penicillin G preparation is used for the treatment of endocarditis.

If IM penicillin G procaine is used for the treatment of moderately severe, uncomplicated respiratory tract infections (pneumonia) caused by susceptible *S. pneumoniae*, the manufacturer recommends that adults receive a dosage of 600,000 to 1 million units daily.

If the fixed combination of penicillin G benzathine and penicillin G procaine (Bicillin® C-R) is used for the treatment of moderately severe to severe infections caused by susceptible *S. pyogenes* (e.g., upper respiratory tract infections, scarlet fever, erysipelas, skin and skin structure infections), the manufacturer recommends that adults receive a single IM dose of 2.4 million penicillin G units. If this fixed-combination preparation is used for the treatment of moderately severe infections caused by susceptible *S. pneumoniae* (pneumonia, otitis media) in adults, the manufacturer recommends an IM dosage of 1.2 million penicillin G units given once every 2 or 3 days until the patient has been afebrile for 48 hours. Other penicillins are recommended for severe *S. pneumoniae* infections (e.g., pneumonia, empyema, bacteremia, pericarditis, meningitis, peritonitis, arthritis).

Anthrax

If IM penicillin G procaine is used for inhalational anthrax (postexposure) to reduce the incidence or progression of disease following exposure to aerosolized *B. anthracis* spores, the manufacturer recommends that adults receive 1.2 million units every 12 hours. Because of the possible persistence of anthrax spores in lung

tissue following an aerosol exposure, CDC and other experts recommend that the total duration of anti-infective prophylaxis should be at least 60 days. The manufacturer states that safety data for IM penicillin G procaine administered at the dosage recommended for inhalational anthrax (postexposure) supports a duration of 2 weeks or less, and clinicians must consider the risks versus benefits of administering penicillin G procaine for longer than 2 weeks or switching to an appropriate alternative anti-infective.

If IM penicillin G procaine is used for the treatment of mild, uncomplicated cutaneous anthrax caused by susceptible *B. anthracis* in adults, the manufacturer recommends a dosage of 600,000 to 1 million units daily. Some experts recommend that adults receive a dosage of 600,000 to 1.2 million units every 12–24 hours for the treatment of mild, uncomplicated cutaneous anthrax caused by susceptible *B. anthracis* that occurs as the result of naturally occurring or endemic exposure to anthrax. Although 3–10 days of anti-infective therapy may be adequate for the treatment of mild, uncomplicated cutaneous anthrax that occurs as the result of naturally occurring or endemic exposures to anthrax, some experts recommend a duration of 7–14 days. CDC and other experts state that anti-infectives should be continued for 60 days if cutaneous anthrax occurred as the result of exposure to aerosolized *B. anthracis* spores since the possibility of inhalational anthrax would also exist. Although anti-infective therapy may limit the size of the cutaneous anthrax lesion and it usually becomes sterile within the first 24 hours of treatment, the lesion will still progress through the black eschar stage despite effective treatment.

For additional information on treatment of anthrax and recommendations for postexposure prophylaxis following exposure to anthrax spores, see Uses: Anthrax, in Ciprofloxacin 8:12.18.

Diphtheria

When IM penicillin G procaine is used as an adjunct to diphtheria antitoxin (not commercially available in the US, but may be available from CDC) for the treatment of diphtheria caused by *C. diphtheriae*, the manufacturer recommends a dosage of 300,000–600,000 units daily. CDC recommends a 14-day regimen of IM penicillin G procaine given in a dosage of 600,000 units daily in those weighing more than 10 kg for adjunctive treatment of diphtheria. Patients usually are no longer contagious 48 hours after initiation of anti-infective therapy. Eradication of *C. diphtheriae* should be confirmed 24 hours after completion of treatment by 2 consecutive negative cultures taken 24 hours apart.

If IM penicillin G procaine is used to eliminate the diphtheria carrier state in identified carriers of toxigenic *C. diphtheriae*, the manufacturer recommends a dosage of 300,000 units daily for 10 days. CDC and AAP recommend IM penicillin G benzathine if a penicillin G preparation is used for elimination of the diphtheria carrier state. Follow-up cultures should be obtained at least 2 weeks after treatment of diphtheria carriers; if cultures are positive, a 10-day course of oral erythromycin should be given and additional follow-up cultures obtained.

Erysipeloid

If IM penicillin G procaine is used in the treatment of erysipeloid caused by *Erysipelothrix rhusiopathiae*, the manufacturer recommends a dosage of 600,000 to 1 million units daily.

Necrotizing Ulcerative Gingivitis

If IM penicillin G procaine is used for the treatment of moderately severe infections of the oropharynx caused by *Fusobacterium*, including Vincent's gingivitis and pharyngitis, the manufacturer recommends a dosage of 600,000 to 1 million units daily.

Rat-Bite Fever

For the treatment of rat-bite fever caused by *Streptobacillus moniliformis* (erythema arthriticum epidemicum, Haverhill fever) or *Spirillum minus* (sodoku), the manufacturer recommends that IM penicillin G procaine be given in a dosage of 600,000 to 1 million units daily. Although IM penicillin G procaine has been given in a dosage of 600,000 units every 12 hours for 10–14 days for the treatment of rat-bite fever, CDC and some clinicians state that IV penicillin G potassium or sodium is preferred.

Syphilis

The manufacturer states that adults with primary, secondary, or latent syphilis with a negative CSF test for syphilis may receive IM penicillin G procaine in a dosage of

600,000 units daily for 8 days (total dosage 4.8 million units) and that those with tertiary syphilis or latent syphilis with a positive CSF examination or no CSF examination may receive 600,000 units daily for 10–15 days (total dosage 6–9 million units). CDC and others state that IM penicillin G benzathine is the drug of choice for the treatment of primary, secondary, tertiary, and latent syphilis in adults.

If IM penicillin G procaine is used as an alternative for the treatment of syphilis in adults, some experts state that those with early syphilis (primary, secondary, or early latent syphilis) can receive a dosage of 1.2 million units once daily for 10–14 days and those with late latent syphilis or syphilis of unknown duration can receive 1.2 million units once daily for 20 days.

For the treatment of neurosyphilis in adults when compliance with the regimen can be ensured (see Uses: Syphilis), CDC recommends that IM penicillin G procaine be given in a dosage of 2.4 million units once daily for 10–14 days in conjunction with oral probenecid (500 mg every 6 hours for 10–14 days). Some clinicians recommend that the penicillin G procaine regimen be followed by a regimen of IM penicillin G benzathine (2.4 million units once weekly for up to 3 weeks).

HIV-infected adults with any stage of syphilis should receive the same treatment regimens recommended for those without HIV infection.

Fixed combinations of penicillin G benzathine and penicillin G procaine (Bicillin® C-R, Bicillin® C-R 900/300) should not be used for the treatment of any form of syphilis.

Yaws, Pinta, and Bejel

The manufacturer states that the usual dosage of IM penicillin G procaine for the treatment of yaws, pinta, or bejel is the same as that recommended for the corresponding stage of syphilis.

Fixed combinations of penicillin G benzathine and penicillin G procaine (Bicillin® C-R, Bicillin® C-R 900/300) should not be used for the treatment of yaws, pinta, or bejel.

CAUTIONS

● Adverse Effects

Adverse effects reported with penicillin G procaine are similar to those reported with other natural penicillins.

Serious and occasionally fatal hypersensitivity reactions, including anaphylaxis, have been reported with penicillins. Rash (maculopapular), exfoliative dermatitis, urticaria, laryngeal edema, fever, eosinophilia, other serum sickness-like reactions (e.g., chills, fever, edema, arthralgia, prostration), and anaphylaxis (including shock and death) have been reported with penicillin G. Fever and eosinophilia may frequently be the only reaction observed.

Jarisch-Herxheimer reactions have been reported in patients receiving IM penicillin G procaine for the treatment of syphilis.

Immediate toxic reactions to procaine have been reported rarely with IM penicillin G procaine, especially when a large single dose (4.8 million penicillin G units) was administered. These reactions may be manifested by mental disturbances (anxiety, confusion, agitation, depression, weakness, seizures, hallucinations, combativeness, fear of impending death) and usually are transient (lasting about 15–30 minutes). A small percentage of the population is hypersensitive to procaine, and sensitivity reactions to IM penicillin G procaine have been reported. (See Cautions: Precautions and Contraindications.)

Inadvertent intravascular administration (including inadvertent direct intra-arterial injection or injection immediately adjacent to arteries) of penicillin G procaine or fixed combinations of penicillin G benzathine and penicillin G procaine has resulted in severe neurovascular damage (e.g., transverse myelitis with permanent paralysis, gangrene requiring amputation of digits and more proximal portions of extremities, necrosis and sloughing at and surrounding the injection site). These severe effects have been reported following injections into the buttock, thigh, and deltoid areas. Other serious complications of suspected intravascular administration include immediate pallor, mottling, or cyanosis of the extremity (both distal and proximal to the injection site), followed by bleb formation or severe edema requiring anterior and/or posterior compartment fasciotomy in the lower extremity. These severe effects and complications have occurred most often in infants and small children.

For additional information on adverse effects reported with natural penicillins, see Cautions in the Natural Penicillins General Statement 8:12.16.04.

● Precautions and Contraindications

Penicillin G procaine and fixed combinations of penicillin G benzathine and penicillin G procaine are contraindicated in patients hypersensitive to any penicillin or to procaine.

Penicillin G procaine shares the toxic potentials of the penicillins, including the risk of hypersensitivity reactions, and the usual precautions of penicillin therapy should be observed.

Prior to administration of penicillin G procaine or a fixed combination of penicillin G benzathine and penicillin G procaine, careful inquiry should be made concerning previous hypersensitivity reactions to penicillins, cephalosporins, or other allergens. There is clinical and laboratory evidence of partial cross-allergenicity among penicillins and other β-lactam antibiotics, including cephalosporins and cephamycins.

Hypersensitivity reactions to penicillins are more likely to occur in individuals with a history of penicillin hypersensitivity and/or a history of sensitivity to multiple allergens. Penicillin G procaine and fixed combinations of penicillin G benzathine and penicillin G procaine should be used with caution in individuals with a history of clinically important allergies and/or asthma.

If a hypersensitivity reaction occurs, the drug should be discontinued immediately and appropriate therapy instituted as indicated (e.g., epinephrine, corticosteroids, maintenance of an adequate airway and oxygen).

If use of penicillin G procaine or a fixed combination containing penicillin G procaine is being considered in a patient with a history of procaine sensitivity, a test dose of procaine (0.1 mL of a 1–2% solution of procaine) should be administered intradermally prior to IM administration of full doses of penicillin G procaine or a fixed combination containing penicillin G procaine. Development of erythema or a wheal, flare, or eruption at the intradermal test site indicates procaine sensitivity and the patient should *not* receive a preparation containing penicillin G procaine. If a hypersensitivity reaction to procaine occurs, it should be treated by usual methods; antihistamines may be beneficial and barbiturates may be indicated if seizures occur.

Special precaution should be taken to avoid IV, intravascular, or intra-arterial administration or injection of penicillin G procaine or fixed combinations containing the drug into or near major peripheral nerves or blood vessels since inadvertent intravascular or intra-arterial injection may produce severe and/or permanent neurovascular damage. In addition, inadvertent IV administration of preparations containing penicillin G benzathine has been associated with cardiorespiratory arrest and death. If evidence of compromise of blood supply occurs at or proximal or distal to the site of injection, an appropriate specialist should be consulted immediately.

Renal and hematologic systems should be evaluated periodically during prolonged therapy with penicillin G procaine or a fixed combination containing penicillin G benzathine and penicillin G procaine, particularly if high dosage is used. In such situations, use of penicillin G procaine for longer than 2 weeks may be associated with an increased risk of neutropenia and an increased incidence of serum sickness-like reactions.

For additional information on precautions associated with the use of penicillin G procaine, see Cautions: Precautions and Contraindications, in the Natural Penicillins General Statement 8:12.16.04.

● Pediatric Precautions

Renal clearance of penicillin G may be delayed in neonates and young infants because of incompletely developed renal function.

● Geriatric Precautions

Clinical studies of penicillin G procaine or penicillin G benzathine did not include sufficient numbers of patients 65 years of age or older to determine whether geriatric patients respond differently than younger patients. Other clinical experience has not identified differences in responses between geriatric and younger patients.

Penicillin G is substantially eliminated by the kidneys and the risk of adverse effects may be greater in those with impaired renal function. Because geriatric patients are more likely to have reduced renal function, dosage should be selected with caution, usually starting at the low end of the dosage range, and renal function monitoring may be useful.

● Pregnancy, Fertility, and Lactation

Pregnancy

Reproduction studies evaluating penicillin G in mice, rats, and rabbits have not revealed evidence of impaired fertility or harm to the fetus. Although experience with use of penicillins during pregnancy has not shown any evidence of adverse effects on the fetus, there are no adequate or controlled studies using penicillin G procaine in pregnant women.

Some clinicians state that IM penicillin G procaine is considered low risk and safe for use during pregnancy. The drug is included in the US Centers for Disease Control and Prevention (CDC) recommendations for the treatment of syphilis during pregnancy.

The manufacturers state that penicillin G procaine and fixed combinations containing penicillin G benzathine and penicillin G procaine should be used during pregnancy only when clearly needed.

Lactation

Penicillin G is distributed into milk. Some clinicians state that IM penicillin G procaine usually is considered compatible with breast-feeding. The manufacturers and others state that penicillin G procaine and fixed combinations containing penicillin G benzathine and penicillin G procaine should be used with caution in nursing women.

SPECTRUM

Based on its spectrum of activity, penicillin G procaine is classified as a natural penicillin. For information on the classification of penicillins based on spectra of activity, see the Preface to the General Statements on Penicillins 8:12.16.

For specific information on the spectrum of activity of penicillin G and resistance to the drug, see the sections on Spectrum and on Resistance in the Natural Penicillins General Statement 8:12.16.04.

PHARMACOKINETICS

For additional information on the absorption, distribution, and elimination of penicillin G, see Pharmacokinetics in the Natural Penicillins General Statement 8:12.16.04.

● Absorption

Because penicillin G procaine is relatively insoluble, IM administration of the drug provides a tissue depot from which the drug is slowly absorbed and hydrolyzed to penicillin G. IM administration of penicillin G procaine results in serum concentrations of penicillin G that are generally more prolonged, but lower, than those attained with an equivalent IM dose of penicillin G potassium or sodium.

Following IM administration of a single dose of penicillin G procaine in adults or neonates, peak serum penicillin G concentrations are attained in 1–4 hours and the drug is usually detectable in serum for 1–2 days; however, penicillin G may be detectable in serum for up to 5 days (depending on the dose). In general, increasing the dose of penicillin G procaine to more than 600,000 units tends to prolong the duration of penicillin G serum concentrations rather than increase peak serum concentrations.

Following a single IM dose of a fixed combination containing 1.2 million penicillin G units (i.e., 600,000 units as penicillin G benzathine and 600,000 units as penicillin G procaine; Bicillin® C-R) in adults, peak blood penicillin G concentrations were 2.1–2.6 units/mL within 3 hours and blood concentrations averaged 0.75 units/mL at 12 hours, 0.28 units/mL at 24 hours, and 0.04 units/mL at 7 days.

Following a single IM dose of a fixed combination containing 1.2 million penicillin G units (i.e., 900,000 units as penicillin G benzathine and 300,000 units as penicillin G procaine; Bicillin® C-R 900/300) in patients weighing 45–64 kg, average blood penicillin G concentrations were 0.24 units/mL at 24 hours, 0.039 units/mL at 7 days, and 0.024 units/mL at 10 days after the dose.

In children weighing 11.9–22.6 kg, IM administration of a single dose of a fixed combination containing 1.2 million penicillin G units (900,000 units as penicillin G benzathine and 300,000 units as penicillin G procaine) resulted in peak serum penicillin G concentrations that occurred 1 hour after the dose and averaged 3.9 mcg/mL. Serum penicillin G concentrations in these children ranged from 2.5–5.5, 2.5–5.5, 0.7–3.7, and 0.17–0.48 mcg/mL at 1, 2, 4, and 24 hours, respectively, after the dose and from 0.08–0.12, 0.01–0.09, and 0–0.1 mcg/mL at 5, 10, and 18 days, respectively, after the dose.

In a study in neonates younger than 1 week of age with congenital syphilis who received a penicillin G procaine dosage of 50,000 units/kg IM once daily for 7 days, serum penicillin G concentrations averaged 7.4–8.8 mcg/mL 2–12 hours after a dose and 1.5 mcg/mL 24 hours after a dose in neonates younger than 1 week of age. In neonates older than 1 week of age who received the same dosage of penicillin G procaine, serum penicillin G concentrations averaged 5–6 mcg/mL during the first 4 hours after administration of a dose and 0.4 mcg/mL 24 hours after a dose. In another study in neonates who received a single IM penicillin G procaine dose of 50,000 units/kg, peak serum concentrations of penicillin G occurred 4 hours after the dose and ranged from 7.7–41.9 mcg/mL; serum concentrations of the drug ranged from 0.2–5.8 mcg/mL 24 hours after the dose.

● Distribution

Following IM administration of penicillin G procaine, penicillin G is widely distributed throughout the body in varying amounts. Highest concentrations generally are attained in the kidneys, with lower amounts in the liver, skin, and intestines.

Minimal concentrations of penicillin G are generally attained in CSF following IM administration of penicillin G procaine in patients with uninflamed meninges. Higher penicillin G concentrations are attained in CSF when the meninges are inflamed or when oral probenecid is administered concomitantly. The minimum treponemicidal concentration of penicillin G is generally defined as 0.03 units/mL or 0.02 mcg/mL. In one study, CSF concentrations of penicillin G were undetectable to 0.6% of concurrent serum concentrations in patients receiving IM penicillin G procaine in a dosage of 600,000 units once daily without probenecid; however, CSF concentrations of the drug were 2.1–6.6% of concurrent serum concentrations in patients receiving 600,000 units IM once daily with concomitant oral probenecid (500 mg every 6 hours). In a study in adults following IM administration of penicillin G procaine in a dosage of 2.4 million units once daily with oral probenecid (500 mg every 6 hours), CSF concentrations of penicillin G ranged from 0.12–0.6 mcg/mL in specimens obtained 3–3.5 hours after a dose on the third or fourth day of therapy. In another study in adults with syphilis who received IM penicillin G procaine in a dosage of 2.4 million units once daily with oral probenecid (500 mg every 6 hours), CSF penicillin G concentrations ranged from 0.07–1.5 mcg/mL in specimens obtained 2–10 hours after a dose on the second through ninth day of therapy; concurrent serum penicillin G concentrations ranged from 6.3–7.9 mcg/mL.

In a study in neonates younger than 3 days of age who received a single IM penicillin G procaine dose of 10,000 units/kg, penicillin G concentrations in CSF 4 hours after the dose averaged 0.06 mcg/mL and concurrent serum concentrations averaged 6.1 mcg/mL. IM administration of a single penicillin G procaine dose of 50,000 units/kg in these neonates resulted in CSF concentrations averaging 0.14 mcg/mL 4 hours after the dose and concurrent serum concentrations averaging 13.2 mcg/mL. In another study in neonates who received a single penicillin G procaine dose of 50,000 units/kg, peak CSF concentrations of penicillin G occurred 12 hours after the dose and ranged from 0.09–1.98 mcg/mL; CSF concentrations of the drug 24 hours after the dose ranged from 0.03–0.27 mcg/mL.

Penicillin G is about 60% bound to serum proteins.

Penicillin G crosses the placenta and is distributed into milk.

● Elimination

Following IM administration of penicillin G procaine, the drug is slowly absorbed and hydrolyzed to penicillin G and elimination of penicillin G in urine continues over a prolonged period of time. Penicillin G and its metabolites are excreted in urine mainly by tubular secretion.

Concurrent administration of oral probenecid increases and prolongs serum penicillin G concentrations by decreasing the apparent volume of distribution and slowing the rate of excretion by competitively inhibiting renal tubular secretion of penicillin.

The serum half-life of penicillin G may be prolonged in patients with impaired renal function.

Renal clearance of penicillin G is delayed in neonates and young infants.

Renal clearance of penicillin G may be increased in pregnant women during the second and third trimesters.

CHEMISTRY AND STABILITY

● Chemistry

Penicillin G procaine is a natural penicillin. The drug is the procaine monohydrate salt of penicillin G which is prepared by reacting equimolar amounts of penicillin G sodium or potassium and procaine hydrochloride. Penicillin G procaine is hydrolyzed in vivo to penicillin G and is frequently referred to as a long-acting, depot, or repository form of penicillin G.

Penicillin G procaine occurs as white crystals or a white, microcrystalline powder. The drug is slightly soluble in water. Potency of penicillin G procaine generally is expressed in terms of penicillin G units, but also has been expressed as mg of penicillin G.

Commercially available penicillin G procaine sterile suspension for injection is a viscous, opaque suspension of the drug in sterile water for injection. The IM suspension is buffered with sodium citrate and contains methylparaben and propylparaben as preservatives, povidone, lecithin, and carboxymethylcellulose.

Penicillin G procaine also is commercially available in fixed combination with penicillin G benzathine as a viscous, opaque, aqueous suspension for IM injection. Each 2 mL of fixed-combination suspension contains the equivalent of 1.2 million units of penicillin G in a formulation containing the equivalent of 600,000 units of penicillin G as the benzathine salt and 600,000 units of penicillin G as the procaine salt (Bicillin® C-R) or a formulation containing the equivalent of 900,000 units of penicillin G as the benzathine salt and 300,000 units of penicillin G as the procaine salt (Bicillin® C-R 900/300).

● Stability

Commercially available penicillin G procaine suspension for IM injection should be stored at 2–8°C; freezing should be avoided.

The fixed combinations of penicillin G benzathine and penicillin G procaine for IM injection should be stored at 2–8°C; freezing should be avoided.

For further information on chemistry and stability, mechanism of action, spectrum, resistance, pharmacokinetics, uses, cautions, drug interactions, laboratory test interferences, and dosage and administration of penicillin G procaine, see the Natural Penicillins General Statement 8:12.16.04.

PREPARATIONS

Excipients in commercially available drug preparations may have clinically important effects in some individuals; consult specific product labeling for details.

Penicillin G Procaine

Parenteral Suspension, for IM Injection	600,000 units (of penicillin G) per mL*	Penicillin G Procaine Suspension

* available from one or more manufacturer, distributor, and/or repackager by generic (nonproprietary) name

Penicillin G Benzathine and Penicillin G Procaine

Parenteral Suspension, for IM Injection	1.2 million units of penicillin G per 2 mL (600,000 units as penicillin G benzathine and 600,000 units as penicillin G procaine)	Bicillin® C-R, Pfizer
	1.2 million units of penicillin G per 2 mL (900,000 units as penicillin G benzathine and 300,000 units as penicillin G procaine)	Bicillin® C-R 900/300, Pfizer

Selected Revisions October 1, 2018, © Copyright, January 1, 1985, American Society of Health-System Pharmacists, Inc.

Penicillin V Potassium

8:12.16.04 • NATURAL PENICILLINS

■ Penicillin V, a natural penicillin, is a β-lactam antibiotic.

USES

Penicillin V potassium is used for the treatment of mild to moderately severe upper respiratory tract infections caused by susceptible streptococci or mild skin and skin structure infections caused by susceptible streptococci or staphylococci and for prophylaxis of certain streptococcal infections.

For some infections, oral penicillin V is used after an initial response is obtained with parenteral penicillin G. Penicillin V should *not* be used for *initial* treatment of severe infections, including pneumonia, empyema, bacteremia, pericarditis, meningitis, or arthritis. In addition, the high incidence of staphylococci resistant to the drug should be considered.

For additional information on the uses of penicillin V potassium, see Uses in the Natural Penicillins General Statement 8:12.16.04.

● Pharyngitis and Tonsillitis

Penicillin V is a drug of choice for the treatment of pharyngitis and tonsillitis caused by *Streptococcus pyogenes* (group A β-hemolytic streptococci; GAS) and prevention of initial attacks (primary prevention) of rheumatic fever.

Selection of an anti-infective for the treatment of *S. pyogenes* pharyngitis and tonsillitis should be based on the drug's spectrum of activity, bacteriologic and clinical efficacy, potential adverse effects, ease of administration, patient compliance, and cost. No regimen has been found to date that effectively eradicates group A β-hemolytic streptococci in 100% of patients.

Because the drugs have a narrow spectrum of activity, are inexpensive, and generally are effective with a low frequency of adverse effects, the American Academy of Pediatrics (AAP), Infectious Diseases Society of America (IDSA), and American Heart Association (AHA) recommend a penicillin regimen (i.e., 10 days of oral penicillin V or oral amoxicillin or a single dose of IM penicillin G benzathine) as the treatment of choice for *S. pyogenes* pharyngitis and tonsillitis. Other anti-infectives (narrow-spectrum oral cephalosporins, oral macrolides, oral clindamycin) are recommended as alternatives in penicillin-allergic patients.

If signs and symptoms of pharyngitis recur shortly after initial treatment and presence of *S. pyogenes* is documented, retreatment with the original or an alternative anti-infective is recommended. Initial treatment failures may occur more frequently with oral penicillins than with IM penicillin G benzathine because of poor adherence to the oral regimen. Alternative regimens recommended for retreatment include a narrow-spectrum oral cephalosporin, oral clindamycin, oral fixed combination of amoxicillin and clavulanate, oral macrolide, or IM penicillin G benzathine.

If there are multiple, recurrent episodes of symptomatic pharyngitis within a period of several months to years, it may be difficult to determine whether these are true episodes of *S. pyogenes* infection or whether the patient is a long-term pharyngeal carrier of *S. pyogenes* who is experiencing repeated episodes of non-streptococcal (e.g., viral) pharyngitis.

Treatment of asymptomatic chronic pharyngeal carriers of *S. pyogenes* is not usually indicated and these individuals should not receive repeated courses of anti-infective therapy. However, eradication of the carrier state may be desirable in certain situations (e.g., during a community outbreak of acute rheumatic fever, acute poststreptococcal glomerulonephritis, or invasive *S. pyogenes* infections; during an outbreak of *S. pyogenes* pharyngitis in a closed or partially closed community; when multiple episodes of documented symptomatic *S. pyogenes* pharyngitis are occurring within a family for many weeks despite appropriate treatment; when there is a personal or family history of acute rheumatic fever). In such situations, recommended regimens include oral clindamycin, oral fixed combination of amoxicillin and clavulanate, or oral rifampin used in conjunction with either IM penicillin G benzathine or oral penicillin V.

● Prevention of Rheumatic Fever Recurrence

Penicillin V is used as an alternative for prevention of recurrent attacks of rheumatic fever (secondary prophylaxis) in individuals who have had a previous attack of rheumatic fever.

IM penicillin G benzathine generally is considered the drug of choice for secondary prophylaxis of rheumatic fever because it ensures compliance; alternatives include oral penicillin V or oral sulfadiazine. Sulfadiazine is recommended when hypersensitivity precludes the use of a penicillin; however, a macrolide (azithromycin, clarithromycin, erythromycin) should be used in patients allergic to penicillins *and* sulfonamides. Even with optimal patient adherence, the risk of recurrence of rheumatic fever is higher in individuals receiving an oral prophylaxis regimen than in those receiving IM penicillin G benzathine.

AHA and AAP recommend long-term (continuous) secondary prophylaxis in patients who have been treated for documented acute rheumatic fever (even if manifested solely by Sydenham chorea) and in those with evidence of rheumatic heart disease (even after prosthetic valve replacement).

Prophylaxis should be initiated as soon as the diagnosis of rheumatic fever or rheumatic heart disease is made, although patients with acute rheumatic fever should first receive the usually recommended anti-infective treatment for *S. pyogenes* pharyngitis and tonsillitis (see Uses: Pharyngitis and Tonsillitis).

● Prevention of Invasive Pneumococcal Disease in Asplenic Individuals

Penicillin V is used for prevention of invasive *S. pneumoniae* disease in children with anatomic or functional asplenia† (e.g., congenital asplenia or polysplenia, splenectomy, sickle cell disease, thalassemia). AAP recommends that such prophylaxis be continued until at least 5 years of age in those with sickle cell disease and continued for at least 1 year after splenectomy in all age groups.

Penicillin V also is used for prevention of invasive *S. pneumoniae* disease in certain asplenic adults†. Some clinicians recommend that such prophylaxis be continued for at least 1–2 years after splenectomy in adults.

Asplenic infants, children, adolescents, and adults are at increased risk of fulminant septicemia, most commonly caused by *S. pneumoniae*. Age-appropriate vaccination against pneumococcal disease with pneumococcal 13-valent conjugate vaccine (PCV13) and pneumococcal 23-valent polysaccharide vaccine (PPSV23) is recommended in *all* asplenic individuals. AAP states that anti-infective prophylaxis for prevention of invasive pneumococcal disease is recommended for young children with anatomic or functional asplenia, regardless of vaccination status.

Although penicillin V usually is considered a drug of choice for prevention of pneumococcal infections in asplenic children, some experts recommend amoxicillin.

● Anthrax

Penicillin V has been recommended as an alternative for postexposure prophylaxis of anthrax† following exposure to *Bacillus anthracis* spores (inhalational anthrax). Ciprofloxacin or doxycycline are the initial drugs of choice for prophylaxis following suspected or confirmed exposure to aerosolized anthrax spores, including exposures that occur in the context of biologic warfare or bioterrorism. If penicillin susceptibility is confirmed, consideration can be given to changing prophylaxis to a penicillin (oral amoxicillin or penicillin V) in infants and children, pregnant or lactating women, or when the drugs of choice are not tolerated or not available; oral amoxicillin may be preferred, especially in infants and children.

Penicillin V is used for the treatment of mild, uncomplicated cutaneous anthrax† caused by susceptible *B. anthracis* that occurs as the result of naturally occurring or endemic exposure to anthrax. If cutaneous anthrax occurs in the context of biologic warfare or bioterrorism, the initial drugs of choice are ciprofloxacin or doxycycline. If penicillin susceptibility is confirmed, consideration can be given to changing treatment to a penicillin (oral amoxicillin or penicillin V) in infants and children, pregnant or lactating women, or when the drugs of choice are not tolerated or not available; oral amoxicillin may be preferred, especially in infants and children.

For additional information on recommendations for postexposure prophylaxis following exposure to anthrax spores and treatment of anthrax, see Uses: Anthrax, in Ciprofloxacin 8:12.18.

DOSAGE AND ADMINISTRATION

● Reconstitution and Administration

Penicillin V potassium is administered orally.

Although the manufacturers state that penicillin V potassium may be given with meals, the drug generally should be administered in the fasting state (preferably 1 hour before meals). Maximum oral absorption is achieved when the drug is administered at least 1 hour before or 2 hours after meals.

Oral penicillin V potassium should *not* be used for initial treatment of severe infections and should *not* be relied on in patients with nausea, vomiting, gastric dilatation, cardiospasm, or intestinal hypermotility.

Penicillin V potassium powder for oral solution should be reconstituted at the time of dispensing by adding the amount of water specified on the bottle to provide a solution containing 125 or 250 mg of penicillin V per 5 mL. The water should be added to the powder for oral solution in 2 portions and the solution agitated vigorously immediately after each addition.

● **Dosage**

Dosage of penicillin V potassium is expressed in terms of penicillin V. Although dosage of the drug is usually expressed as mg of penicillin V, it may be expressed in terms of penicillin V units.

Potency of penicillin V potassium preparations containing 125, 250, or 500 mg of penicillin V is approximately equivalent to 200,000, 400,000, or 800,000 penicillin V units, respectively.

Pediatric Dosage
General Pediatric Dosage

The American Academy of Pediatrics (AAP) states that the usual dosage of oral penicillin V for the treatment of mild to moderate infections in pediatric patients beyond the neonatal period is 25–75 mg/kg daily given in 3 or 4 divided doses.

Some clinicians recommend that children younger than 5 years of age receive oral penicillin V in a dosage of 125 mg 4 times daily and that those older than 5 years of age receive a dosage of 250–500 mg every 6 hours.

The manufacturers state that pediatric patients 12 years of age or older may receive the usual adult dosage of penicillin V. Some clinicians state that children older than 5 years of age may receive the usual adult dosage of the drug.

Pharyngitis and Tonsillitis

For the treatment of *Streptococcus pyogenes* (group A β-hemolytic streptococci; GAS) pharyngitis and tonsillitis and prevention of initial attacks (primary prevention) of rheumatic fever in children, AAP, American Heart Association (AHA), and Infectious Diseases Society of America (IDSA) recommend that oral penicillin V be given in a dosage of 250 mg 2 or 3 times daily for 10 days. Some experts recommend a dosage of 500 mg 2 or 3 times daily in children weighing more than 27 kg.

When used for the treatment of *S. pyogenes* pharyngitis and tonsillitis and prevention of initial attacks (primary prevention) of rheumatic fever in adolescents, oral penicillin V should be given in a dosage of 500 mg 2 or 3 times daily for 10 days or 250 mg 4 times daily for 10 days.

Although anti-infective treatment is not recommended for most individuals identified as chronic pharyngeal carriers of *S. pyogenes* (see Uses: Pharyngitis and Tonsillitis), IDSA states that a regimen of oral penicillin V given in a dosage of 50 mg/kg daily (up to 2 g daily) in 4 divided doses for 10 days used in conjunction with oral rifampin (20 mg/kg daily as a single dose [up to 600 mg daily] given during the last 4 days of penicillin V treatment) is an option when eradication of the carrier state is desirable.

Respiratory Tract Infections

If oral penicillin V is used for the treatment of mild community-acquired pneumonia (CAP) caused by susceptible *S. pyogenes* or for step-down treatment of CAP caused by *S. pyogenes* after initial parenteral treatment, IDSA recommends that children 3 months of age or older receive 50–75 mg/kg daily in 3 or 4 divided doses.

For the treatment of mild to moderate upper respiratory tract infections (including scarlet fever) caused by susceptible streptococci in adolescents 12 years of age or older, the manufacturers recommend that oral penicillin V be given in a dosage of 125–250 mg every 6–8 hours for 10 days.

For the treatment of mild to moderately severe respiratory tract infections (including otitis media) caused by susceptible *Streptococcus pneumoniae* in adolescents 12 years of age or older, the manufacturers recommend that oral penicillin V be given in a dosage of 250–500 mg every 6 hours until the patient has been afebrile for at least 2 days.

Skin and Skin Structure Infections

For the treatment of mild to moderate erysipelas caused by susceptible streptococci in adolescents 12 years of age or older, the manufacturers recommend that oral penicillin V be given in a dosage of 125–250 mg every 6–8 hours for 10 days.

If oral penicillin V is used for the treatment of mild skin or skin structure infections caused by susceptible non-penicillinase-producing staphylococci in adolescents 12 years of age or older, the manufacturers recommend a dosage of 250–500 mg every 6–8 hours. Because of the high incidence of resistant strains, in vitro culture and susceptibility testing should be performed when treating suspected staphylococcal infections.

Necrotizing Ulcerative Gingivitis

If oral penicillin V is used for the treatment of mild to moderate infections of the oropharynx caused by *Fusobacterium*, including acute necrotizing ulcerative gingivitis (Vincent's infection, trench mouth, *Fusobacterium* gingivitis or pharyngitis), in adolescents 12 years of age or older, the manufacturers recommend a dosage of 250–500 mg every 6–8 hours.

Prevention of Rheumatic Fever Recurrence

For prevention of recurrent rheumatic fever (secondary prophylaxis), AAP and AHA recommend that children receive oral penicillin V in a dosage of 250 mg twice daily. The manufacturers recommend that adolescents 12 years of age or older receive oral penicillin V in a dosage of 125–250 mg twice daily for such prophylaxis.

Prevention of recurrent rheumatic fever requires long-term, continuous prophylaxis. (See Table 1.) Some clinicians use IM penicillin G benzathine initially and change to oral prophylaxis (usually with oral penicillin V) when the patient reaches late adolescence or young adulthood and has remained free of rheumatic attacks for at least 5 years.

TABLE 1. Recommended Duration of Prophylaxis for Prevention of Rheumatic Fever Recurrence

Patient Category	Duration
Rheumatic fever without carditis	5 years since last episode or until 21 years of age, whichever is longer
Rheumatic fever with carditis but no residual heart disease (no valvular disease)	10 years since last episode or until 21 years of age, whichever is longer
Rheumatic fever with carditis and residual heart disease (persistent valvular disease)	10 years since last episode or until 40 years of age, whichever is longer; sometimes for life

Prevention of Invasive Pneumococcal Disease in Asplenic Individuals

If oral penicillin V is used for prevention of invasive pneumococcal disease† in children with anatomic or functional asplenia, AAP recommends a dosage of 125 mg twice daily in those younger than 3 years of age and 250 mg twice daily in those 3 years of age or older.

In infants with sickle cell anemia, AAP recommends that penicillin V prophylaxis be initiated as soon as the diagnosis is established (preferably by 2 months of age). At 5 years of age, discontinuance of prophylaxis can be considered if the child is receiving regular medical attention, is fully immunized against pneumococcal disease, and has not had a severe pneumococcal infection or surgical splenectomy.

In children with asplenia from causes other than sickle cell anemia, the appropriate duration of prophylaxis is unknown. Some experts recommend that such children receive prophylaxis throughout childhood and into adulthood. AAP recommends that prophylaxis be continued for at least 1 year after splenectomy.

Anthrax

If oral penicillin V is used as an alternative for postexposure prophylaxis of anthrax† following exposure to aerosolized *Bacillus anthracis* spores in the context of biologic warfare or bioterrorism when penicillin-susceptible strains are involved, AAP recommends that infants and children 1 month of age or older receive 50–75 mg/kg daily given in divided doses every 6–8 hours. Because of the possible persistence of anthrax spores in lung tissue following an aerosol exposure, the US Centers for Disease Control and Prevention (CDC), AAP, and other experts recommend that the total duration of anti-infective prophylaxis should be at least 60 days.

If oral penicillin V is used for the treatment of mild, uncomplicated cutaneous anthrax† caused by penicillin-susceptible *B. anthracis* that occurs as the result of naturally occurring or endemic exposure to anthrax and when IV therapy is not considered necessary, the recommended dosage in children is 25–50 mg/kg daily given in 2 or 4 divided doses. For the treatment of cutaneous anthrax without systemic involvement† caused by penicillin-susceptible strains that occurs in the context of biologic warfare or bioterrorism, AAP recommends that infants and children 1 month of age or older receive oral penicillin V in a dosage of 50–75 mg/kg daily given in divided doses every 6–8 hours.

If oral penicillin V is used in full-term neonates as an alternative for postexposure prophylaxis† following exposure to aerosolized *B. anthracis* spores in the context of biologic warfare or bioterrorism when penicillin-susceptible strains are involved or for the treatment of cutaneous anthrax† without systemic involvement caused by penicillin-susceptible strains that occurred in the context of biologic warfare or bioterrorism, AAP recommends a dosage of 75 mg/kg daily given in divided doses every 6–8 hours in those up to 1 week of age and 75 mg/kg daily given in divided doses every 8 hours in those 1–4 weeks of age. In preterm neonates (gestational age 32–37 weeks), AAP recommends a dosage of 50 mg/kg daily given in divided doses every 12 hours in those up to 1 week of age and 75 mg/kg daily given in divided doses every 8 hours in those 1–4 weeks of age.

Although 3–10 days of anti-infective therapy may be adequate for the treatment of mild, uncomplicated cutaneous anthrax that occurs as the result of naturally occurring or endemic exposures to anthrax, some experts recommend a duration of 7–14 days. CDC and other experts recommend that anti-infectives be continued for 60 days if cutaneous anthrax occurred as the result of exposure to aerosolized *B. anthracis* spores since the possibility of inhalational anthrax would also exist. Although anti-infective therapy may limit the size of the cutaneous anthrax lesion and it usually becomes sterile within the first 24 hours of treatment, the lesion will still progress through the black eschar stage despite effective treatment. It is not known whether infants and young children are at increased risk of disseminated, systemic disease and/or meningoencephalitis after focal anthrax infection. CDC has recommended that initial treatment of cutaneous anthrax in young children (i.e., younger than 2 years of age) in the context of biologic warfare or bioterrorism should be IV (not oral) and combination anti-infective therapy should be considered.

Rat-bite Fever

If oral penicillin V is used in children for the treatment of rat-bite fever† caused by *Streptobacillus moniliformis* after an initial response is obtained with IV penicillin G, a dosage of 25–50 mg/kg daily (up to 3 g daily) in 4 divided doses has been recommended.

Adult Dosage
Pharyngitis and Tonsillitis

When used for the treatment of *S. pyogenes* (group A β-hemolytic streptococci; GAS) pharyngitis and tonsillitis and prevention of initial attacks (primary prevention) of rheumatic fever in adults, AHA and IDSA recommend that oral penicillin V be given in a dosage of 500 mg 2 or 3 times daily for 10 days or 250 mg 4 times daily for 10 days.

Although anti-infective treatment is not recommended for most individuals identified as chronic pharyngeal carriers of *S. pyogenes* (see Uses: Pharyngitis and Tonsillitis), IDSA states that a regimen of oral penicillin V given in a dosage of 50 mg/kg daily (up to 2 g daily) in 4 divided doses for 10 days used in conjunction with oral rifampin (20 mg/kg daily as a single dose [up to 600 mg daily] given during the last 4 days of penicillin V treatment) is an option when eradication of the carrier state is desirable.

Respiratory Tract Infections

For the treatment of mild to moderate upper respiratory tract infections (including scarlet fever) caused by susceptible streptococci in adults, the manufacturers recommend that oral penicillin V be given in a dosage of 125–250 mg every 6–8 hours for 10 days.

For the treatment of mild to moderately severe respiratory tract infections (including otitis media) caused by susceptible *S. pneumoniae* in adults, the manufacturers recommend that oral penicillin V be given in a dosage of 250–500 mg every 6 hours until the patient has been afebrile for at least 2 days.

Skin and Skin Structure Infections

For the treatment of mild to moderate erysipelas caused by susceptible streptococci in adults, the manufacturers recommend that oral penicillin V be given in a dosage of 125–250 mg every 6–8 hours for 10 days.

For the treatment of nonpurulent skin and skin structure infections (e.g., cellulitis) caused by susceptible streptococci in adults, IDSA recommends that oral penicillin V be given in a dosage of 250–500 mg every 6 hours.

If oral penicillin V is used for the treatment of mild skin or skin structure infections caused by susceptible non-penicillinase-producing staphylococci in adults, the manufacturers recommend a dosage of 250–500 mg every 6–8 hours. Because of the high incidence of resistant strains, in vitro culture and susceptibility tests should be performed when treating suspected staphylococcal infections.

Necrotizing Ulcerative Gingivitis

If oral penicillin V is used in adults for the treatment of mild to moderate infections of the oropharynx caused by *Fusobacterium*, including acute necrotizing ulcerative gingivitis (Vincent's infection, trench mouth, *Fusobacterium* gingivitis or pharyngitis), the manufacturers recommend a dosage of 250–500 mg every 6–8 hours.

Prevention of Rheumatic Fever Recurrence

For prevention of recurrent rheumatic fever (secondary prophylaxis), AHA recommends that oral penicillin V be given in a dosage of 250 mg twice daily. The manufacturers recommend a dosage of 125–250 mg twice daily for such prophylaxis.

Prevention of recurrent rheumatic fever requires long-term, continuous prophylaxis. (See Table 2.)

TABLE 2. Recommended Duration of Prophylaxis for Prevention of Rheumatic Fever Recurrence

Patient Category	Duration
Rheumatic fever without carditis	5 years since last episode or until 21 years of age, whichever is longer
Rheumatic fever with carditis but no residual heart disease (no valvular disease)	10 years since last episode or until 21 years of age, whichever is longer
Rheumatic fever with carditis and residual heart disease (persistent valvular disease)	10 years since last episode or until 40 years of age, whichever is longer; sometimes for life

Anthrax

If oral penicillin V is used as an alternative for postexposure prophylaxis of anthrax† following exposure to aerosolized *B. anthracis* spores in the context of biologic warfare or bioterrorism when penicillin-susceptible strains are involved, CDC recommends that adults (including pregnant and postpartum women) receive a dosage of 500 mg every 6 hours. Because of the possible persistence of anthrax spores in lung tissue following an aerosol exposure, CDC and other experts recommend that the total duration of anti-infective prophylaxis should be at least 60 days.

If oral penicillin V is used for the treatment of mild, uncomplicated cutaneous anthrax† caused by penicillin-susceptible *B. anthracis* that occurs as the result of naturally occurring or endemic exposure to anthrax and when IV therapy is not considered necessary, the recommended dosage in adults is 500 mg 4 times daily, although some clinicians recommend 200–500 mg 4 times daily. For the treatment of cutaneous anthrax without systemic involvement† that occurs in the context of biologic warfare or bioterrorism, CDC recommends that adults (including pregnant and postpartum women) receive oral penicillin V in a dosage of 500 mg 4 times daily.

Although 3–10 days of anti-infective therapy may be adequate for the treatment of mild, uncomplicated cutaneous anthrax that occurs as the result of naturally occurring or endemic exposures to anthrax, some experts recommend a duration of 7–14 days. CDC and other experts recommend that anti-infectives be continued for 60 days if cutaneous anthrax occurred as the result of exposure to aerosolized *B. anthracis* spores since the possibility of inhalational anthrax would also exist. Although anti-infective therapy may limit the size of the cutaneous anthrax lesion and it usually becomes sterile within the first 24 hours of treatment, the lesion will still progress through the black eschar stage despite effective treatment.

Actinomycosis

If oral penicillin V is used for the treatment of actinomycosis† in adults after at least 2–6 weeks of initial treatment with IV penicillin G, a dosage of 2–4 g daily given in divided doses every 6 hours for 6–12 months is recommended.

If oral penicillin V is used for the treatment of mild cervicofacial actinomycosis†, a 2-month regimen of the drug may be adequate.

Rat-bite Fever

If oral penicillin V is used for the treatment of rat-bite fever† caused by *S. moniliformis* in adults after an initial response is obtained with IV penicillin G, a dosage of 500 mg every 6 hours has been recommended.

● *Dosage in Renal Impairment*

Dosage adjustments are not usually necessary in patients with renal impairment. Some clinicians suggest increasing the dosing interval to every 8 hours in patients with creatinine clearance less than 10 mL/minute.

CAUTIONS

● *Adverse Effects*

Adverse effects reported with oral penicillin V potassium are similar to those reported with penicillin G.

The most common adverse effects reported in patients receiving oral penicillins are GI effects (e.g., nausea, vomiting, epigastric distress, diarrhea, black hairy tongue).

Serious and occasionally fatal hypersensitivity reactions, including anaphylaxis, have been reported with penicillins. Hypersensitivity reactions that have been reported with oral penicillins include rash (maculopapular), exfoliative dermatitis, urticaria and other serum sickness-like reactions, laryngeal edema, and anaphylaxis. Fever and eosinophilia may frequently be the only reaction observed.

For additional information on adverse effects reported with penicillin V potassium, see Cautions in the Natural Penicillins General Statement 8:12.16.04.

● *Precautions and Contraindications*

Penicillin V potassium is contraindicated in individuals with known hypersensitivity to any penicillin.

Oral penicillin V potassium shares the toxic potentials of the penicillins, including the risk of hypersensitivity reactions, and the usual precautions of penicillin therapy should be observed.

Prior to initiation of therapy with penicillin V potassium, careful inquiry should be made concerning previous hypersensitivity reactions to penicillins, cephalosporins, or other allergens. There is clinical and laboratory evidence of partial cross-allergenicity among penicillins and other β-lactam antibiotics including cephalosporins and cephamycins.

Hypersensitivity reactions are more likely to occur in individuals with a history of penicillin hypersensitivity and/or a history of sensitivity to multiple allergens. Penicillins should be used with caution in individuals with a history of clinically important allergies and/or asthma.

If a hypersensitivity reaction occurs, penicillin V potassium should be discontinued immediately and appropriate therapy instituted as indicated (e.g., epinephrine, corticosteroids, maintenance of an adequate airway and oxygen).

Some penicillin V potassium oral solutions contain aspartame, which is metabolized in the GI tract to phenylalanine following oral administration. These penicillin V potassium oral solutions containing 125 or 250 mg of penicillin V per 5 mL contain 4.5 mg of phenylalanine per 5 mL. The aspartame content should be considered in individuals with phenylketonuria (i.e., homozygous genetic deficiency of phenylalanine hydroxylase) and other individuals who must restrict their intake of phenylalanine.

For additional information on precautions associated with the use of penicillin V potassium, see Cautions: Precautions and Contraindications, in the Natural Penicillins General Statement 8:12.16.04.

● *Pregnancy, Fertility, and Lactation*

Pregnancy

Available data regarding use of penicillin V in pregnant women, including first-trimester exposures, have not revealed evidence of an association between the drug and congenital defects.

Some clinicians state that penicillin V is considered low risk and safe for use during pregnancy.

Lactation

Penicillin V is distributed into milk. Some clinicians state that oral penicillin V usually is considered compatible with breast-feeding; others state that the drug should be used with caution in nursing women.

SPECTRUM

Based on its spectrum of activity, penicillin V is classified as a natural penicillin. For information on the classification of penicillins based on spectra of activity, see the Preface to the General Statements on Penicillins 8:12.16.

The spectrum of activity of penicillin V is similar to that of penicillin G, but penicillin V is less potent than penicillin G against susceptible bacteria.

For specific information on the spectrum of activity of penicillin V and resistance to the drug, see the sections on Spectrum and on Resistance in the Natural Penicillins General Statement 8:12.16.04.

PHARMACOKINETICS

For additional information on the absorption, distribution, and elimination of penicillin V, see Pharmacokinetics in the Natural Penicillins General Statement 8:12.16.04.

● *Absorption*

Approximately 60–73% of an oral dose of penicillin V (no longer commercially available in the US) or penicillin V potassium is absorbed from the GI tract in healthy, fasting adults. There is considerable interindividual variation in the extent of oral absorption of penicillin V; some patients may not absorb therapeutic concentrations of oral penicillins.

Following oral administration of a single dose of penicillin V or penicillin V potassium in fasting children or adults, peak serum concentrations of penicillin V are generally attained within 30–60 minutes. Peak serum penicillin V concentrations are attained sooner and are slightly higher following administration of the potassium salt than the free acid.

Following oral administration of a single 125-mg tablet of penicillin V potassium in healthy, fasting adults in one study, serum penicillin V concentrations averaged 1.2, 1.2, 0.5, and 0.1 mcg/mL at 30 minutes, 1 hour, 2 hours, and 4 hours, respectively, after the dose. Oral administration of a single 250-mg tablet of penicillin V potassium in healthy, fasting adults results in serum penicillin V concentrations averaging 2.1–2.8, 2.3–2.7, 0.8–0.9, and 0.1–0.2 mcg/mL at 30 minutes, 1 hour, 2 hours, and 4 hours, respectively, after the dose. Following oral administration of a single 500-mg tablet of penicillin V potassium in healthy, fasting adults, serum penicillin V concentrations average 4.7–5, 4.9–6.3, 2.3–3, and 0.04–0.1 mcg/mL at 30 minutes, 1 hour, 2 hours, and 6 hours, respectively, after the dose.

Variable results have been obtained in studies evaluating the effect of food on GI absorption of penicillin V and penicillin V potassium. In most studies, presence of food in the GI tract resulted in lower and delayed peak serum concentrations of penicillin V. If penicillin V is administered 1 hour before a meal, peak serum concentrations may be threefold higher and the total amount absorbed may be twofold higher compared with administration with food.

● *Distribution*

Penicillin V is widely distributed into body tissues with highest concentrations attained in the kidneys and lower amounts in the liver, skin, and intestine. Penicillin V also is distributed into bile, tonsils, maxillary sinus secretions, saliva, and ascitic, synovial, pleural, and pericardial fluids.

Minimal concentrations of penicillin V generally distribute into CSF.

Penicillin V is approximately 75–89% bound to serum proteins.

Penicillin V readily crosses the placenta and is distributed into milk.

● Elimination

The serum half-life of penicillin V in adults with normal renal function is reportedly 0.5 hours.

Approximately 35–70% of an oral dose of penicillin V or penicillin V potassium is metabolized to penicilloic acid which is microbiologically inactive. Small amounts of 6-aminopenicillanic acid (6-APA) have also been found in urine of patients receiving penicillin V. In addition, the drug appears to be hydroxylated to a small extent to one or more microbiologically active metabolites which are also excreted in urine.

Penicillin V and its metabolites are excreted in urine mainly by tubular secretion. Small amounts of the drug are also excreted in feces and bile.

Following oral administration of a single dose of penicillin V or penicillin V potassium in adults with normal renal function, 20–65% of the dose is excreted in urine as unchanged drug and metabolites within 6–8 hours; approximately 32% of the dose is excreted in feces.

Renal clearance of penicillin V is delayed in neonates and young infants and in individuals with impaired renal function.

Renal clearance of penicillin V may be increased in pregnant women during the second and third trimesters.

CHEMISTRY AND STABILITY

● Chemistry

Penicillin V is a natural penicillin produced by fermentation of *Penicillium chrysogenum* in a medium containing phenoxyacetic acid. Penicillin V is the phenoxymethyl analog of penicillin G and is commercially available as the potassium salt.

Although potency of penicillin V potassium generally is expressed in terms of mg of penicillin V, potency of the drug may be expressed in terms of penicillin V units. Potency of penicillin V potassium preparations containing 125, 250, or 500 mg of penicillin V is equivalent to 200,000, 400,000, or 800,000 penicillin V units, respectively.

Each tablet containing 250 mg of penicillin V as the potassium salt contains approximately 0.7 mEq (approximately 28 mg) of potassium; each tablet

containing 500 mg of penicillin V as the potassium salt contains approximately 1.4 mEq (approximately 56 mg) of potassium. When reconstituted as directed, oral solutions of penicillin V potassium have a pH of 5–7.5.

● Stability

Commercially available penicillin V potassium tablets should be stored in a tight container at 20–25°C and protected from moisture.

Penicillin V powder for oral solution should be stored in a tight container at 20–25°C and protected from moisture. Following reconstitution, penicillin V potassium oral solutions should be refrigerated and any unused solution should be discarded after 14 days.

For further information on chemistry and stability, mechanism of action, spectrum, resistance, pharmacokinetics, uses, cautions, drug interactions, laboratory test interferences, and dosage and administration of penicillin V, see the Natural Penicillins General Statement 8:12.16.04.

PREPARATIONS

Excipients in commercially available drug preparations may have clinically important effects in some individuals; consult specific product labeling for details.

Penicillin V Potassium

Oral		
For solution	125 mg (of penicillin V) per 5 mL*	Penicillin V Potassium for Oral Solution
	250 mg (of penicillin V) per 5 mL*	Penicillin V Potassium for Oral Solution
Tablets	250 mg (of penicillin V)*	Penicillin V Potassium Tablets
	500 mg (of penicillin V)*	Penicillin V Potassium Tablets
Tablets, film-coated	250 mg (of penicillin V)*	Penicillin V Potassium Tablets
	500 mg (of penicillin V)*	Penicillin V Potassium Tablets

* available from one or more manufacturer, distributor, and/or repackager by generic (nonproprietary) name

† Use is not currently included in the labeling approved by the US Food and Drug Administration.

Amoxicillin

8:12.16.08 • AMINOPENICILLINS

■ Amoxicillin is an aminopenicillin antibiotic that is structurally related to ampicillin.

USES

Amoxicillin shares the uses of other aminopenicillins and is used principally for the treatment of infections caused by susceptible gram-negative bacteria (e.g., *Haemophilus influenzae, Escherichia coli, Proteus mirabilis, Salmonella*). Amoxicillin also is used for the treatment of infections caused by susceptible gram-positive bacteria (e.g., *Streptococcus pneumoniae*, enterococci, nonpenicillinase-producing staphylococci, *Listeria*); however, like other aminopenicillins, amoxicillin generally should not be used for the treatment of streptococcal or staphylococcal infections when a natural penicillin would be effective.

● Acute Otitis Media

Amoxicillin is used for the treatment of acute otitis media (AOM) caused by *S. pneumoniae, H. influenzae,* or *M. catarrhalis.* Amoxicillin usually is considered the drug of first choice for initial empiric treatment of AOM, unless the infection is suspected of being caused by β-lactamase-producing bacteria resistant to the drug, in which case the fixed combination of amoxicillin and clavulanate potassium is recommended. The American Academy of Pediatrics (AAP), American Academy of Family Physicians (AAFP), US Centers for Disease Control and Prevention (CDC), and others state that, despite the increasing prevalence of multidrug-resistant *S. pneumoniae* and presence of β-lactamase-producing *H. influenzae* or *M catarrhalis* in many communities, amoxicillin remains the anti-infective of first choice for treatment of uncomplicated AOM since it is highly effective, has a narrow spectrum of activity, is well distributed into middle ear fluid, is well tolerated, has an acceptable taste, and is inexpensive. Amoxicillin (when given in a dosage of 80–90 mg/kg daily) usually is effective in the treatment of AOM caused by *S. pneumoniae*, including infections involving strains with intermediate resistance to penicillins, and also usually is effective in the treatment of AOM caused by most strains of *H. influenzae.*

AAP, AAFP, and others recommend that patients who fail to respond to an initial amoxicillin regimen (given in a dosage of 80–90 mg/kg daily) should be retreated using a regimen of amoxicillin and clavulanate potassium (90 mg/kg of amoxicillin and 6.4 mg/kg of clavulanate daily).

For additional information regarding treatment of AOM, including information on diagnosis and management strategies, anti-infectives for initial treatment, duration of initial treatment, and anti-infectives for retreatment and for information on current recommendations regarding management of otitis media with effusion (OME), see Uses: Otitis Media, in the Aminopenicillins General Statement 8:12.16.08.

● Anthrax

Amoxicillin is used as an alternative for *postexposure prophylaxis of anthrax†* following exposure to *Bacillus anthracis* spores, for treatment of anthrax† when a parenteral regimen is not available (e.g., when there are supply or logistic problems because large numbers of individuals require treatment in a mass casualty setting), and for treatment of cutaneous anthrax†. Strains of *B. anthracis* with naturally occurring penicillin resistance have been reported rarely, and there are published reports of *B. anthracis* strains that have been engineered to have penicillin and tetracycline resistance as well as resistance to other anti-infectives (e.g., macrolides, chloramphenicol, rifampin). Therefore, it has been postulated that exposures to *B. anthracis* that occur in the context of biologic warfare or bioterrorism may involve bioengineered resistant strains and this concern should be considered when selecting initial therapy for the treatment of anthrax that occurs as the result of bioterrorism-related exposures or for postexposure prophylaxis following such exposures. For additional information on treatment of anthrax and recommendations for postexposure prophylaxis following exposure to anthrax spores, see Uses: Anthrax, in Ciprofloxacin 8:12.18.

Postexposure Prophylaxis

Ciprofloxacin or doxycycline generally are considered the initial drugs of choice for postexposure prophylaxis following suspected or confirmed exposure to aerosolized *B. anthracis* spores that occurs in the context of biologic warfare or bioterrorism. If exposure is confirmed and results of in vitro testing indicate that the organism is susceptible to penicillin, then consideration can be given to changing the postexposure prophylaxis regimen to a penicillin (e.g., oral amoxicillin, oral penicillin V). Although monotherapy with a penicillin is not recommended for the treatment of clinically apparent inhalational anthrax when high concentrations of the organism are likely to be present, penicillins may be considered an option for anti-infective prophylaxis when ciprofloxacin and doxycycline are contraindicated, since the likelihood of β-lactamase induction resulting in an increase in penicillin MICs is lower when only a small number of vegetative cells are present.

The possible benefits of postexposure prophylaxis against anthrax should be weighed against the possible risks to the fetus when choosing an anti-infective for postexposure prophylaxis in pregnant women. CDC and other experts state that ciprofloxacin should be considered the drug of choice for initial postexposure prophylaxis in pregnant women exposed to *B. anthracis* spores and that, if in vitro studies indicate that the organism is susceptible to penicillin, then consideration can be given to changing the postexposure regimen to amoxicillin. Women who become pregnant while receiving anti-infective prophylaxis should continue the existing regimen and consult with a healthcare provider or public health official to discuss whether an alternative regimen might be more appropriate.

Cutaneous Anthrax

Although natural penicillins (e.g., oral penicillin V, IM penicillin G benzathine, IM penicillin G procaine) generally have been considered drugs of choice for the *treatment* of mild, uncomplicated cutaneous anthrax caused by susceptible strains of *B. anthracis* that occurs as the result of naturally occurring or endemic exposure to anthrax, the initial drugs of choice for the treatment of cutaneous anthrax that occurs following exposure to *B. anthracis* spores in the context of biologic warfare or bioterrorism are ciprofloxacin or doxycycline. If penicillin susceptibility is confirmed, consideration can be given to changing to a penicillin (oral amoxicillin or oral penicillin V) in infants and children, pregnant or lactating women, or when the drugs of choice are not tolerated or not available; oral amoxicillin may be preferred, especially in infants and children.

For more specific information on the uses of amoxicillin, see Uses in the Aminopenicillins General Statement 8:12.16.08.

For information on the uses of amoxicillin in fixed combination with clavulanic acid, see Amoxicillin and Clavulanate Potassium 8:12.16.08.

DOSAGE AND ADMINISTRATION

● Reconstitution and Administration

Amoxicillin trihydrate is administered orally. Amoxicillin has also been given IV as the sodium salt, but a parenteral dosage form of amoxicillin is currently not available in the US.

Amoxicillin may be administered orally without regard to meals. However, in studies evaluating the film-coated tablet containing 875 mg of amoxicillin, the tablet was administered at the start of a light meal.

The required dose of reconstituted amoxicillin oral suspension should be placed directly on the child's tongue for swallowing. Alternatively, the required dose of oral suspension may be added to formula, milk, fruit juice, water, or ginger ale and then administered immediately.

Amoxicillin powder for oral suspension should be reconstituted at the time of dispensing by adding the amount of water specified on the bottle to provide a suspension containing 125, 200, 250, or 400 mg of amoxicillin per 5 mL or 50 mg of amoxicillin per mL. After tapping the bottle to thoroughly loosen the powder for oral suspension, the water should be added to the powder in 2 portions and the suspension agitated well after each addition. The suspension should be agitated well just prior to administration of each dose.

● Dosage

Dosage of amoxicillin, which is available for oral use as the trihydrate, is expressed in terms of anhydrous amoxicillin.

General Adult Dosage

The usual adult dosage of amoxicillin for the treatment of mild to moderate infections of the ear, nose, or throat; skin and skin structure; or genitourinary tract is 500 mg every 12 hours or 250 mg every 8 hours. A dosage of 875 mg every 12 hours or 500 mg every 8 hours should be used for the treatment of severe infections of the ear, nose, or throat; skin and skin structure; or genitourinary tract in adults. The usual adult dosage of amoxicillin for the treatment of mild, moderate, or severe lower respiratory tract infections is 875 mg every 12 hours or 500 mg every 8 hours.

A single 3-g oral dose of amoxicillin has been used effectively for the initial treatment of acute, uncomplicated urinary tract infections in nonpregnant women†.

General Pediatric Dosage

When oral amoxicillin is used in neonates and infants 12 weeks of age or younger, the manufacturer states that a dosage up to 30 mg/kg daily can be given in divided doses every 12 hours.

The usual dosage of oral amoxicillin for pediatric patients 3 months of age or older for the treatment of mild to moderate infections of the ear, nose, throat, skin and skin structure, or genitourinary tract is 20 mg/kg daily in divided doses every 8 hours or 25 mg/kg daily in divided doses every 12 hours. The usual dosage of oral amoxicillin for pediatric patients 3 months of age or older for the treatment of mild, moderate, or severe lower respiratory tract infections or for the treatment of severe infections of the ear, nose, throat, skin and skin structure, or genitourinary tract is 40 mg/kg daily in divided doses every 8 hours or 45 mg/kg daily in divided doses every 12 hours.

When oral amoxicillin is used for the treatment of mild to moderate infections in children beyond the neonatal period, the American Academy of Pediatrics (AAP) recommends a dosage of 25–50 mg/kg daily given in 3 divided doses.

When oral amoxicillin is used for step-down therapy in the treatment of severe infections in children beyond the neonatal period, AAP recommends a dosage of 80–100 mg/kg daily given in 3 divided doses. For highly susceptible pathogens, AAP states that a dosage of 90 mg/kg daily given in 2 divided doses can be used.

Acute Otitis Media

For the treatment of uncomplicated acute otitis media (AOM), the recommended dosage of oral amoxicillin is 80–90 mg/kg daily given in 2 or 3 divided doses†. The drug usually is given for 10 days, but the optimal duration of therapy is uncertain. AAP recommends that a 10-day regimen be used for the treatment of AOM in children younger than 2 years of age and in those with severe symptoms. For the treatment of mild to moderate AOM in older children, AAP states that 7- and 10-day regimens appear equally effective in those 2–5 years of age and a treatment duration of 5–7 days may be adequate in those 6 years of age or older.

Although amoxicillin has been given in a dosage of 40–45 mg/kg daily for 10 days for the treatment of AOM, AAP, AAFP, US Centers for Disease Control and Prevention (CDC), and others recommend use of the higher amoxicillin dosage. The higher amoxicillin dosage (80–90 mg/kg daily) is especially important in patients with AOM known or suspected of being caused by *Streptococcus pneumoniae* with reduced susceptibility to penicillins and in patients with a history of anti-infective treatment of AOM within the previous few months.

Pharyngitis and Tonsillitis

For the treatment of pharyngitis and tonsillitis caused by *Streptococcus pyogenes* (group A β-hemolytic streptococci; GAS), the American Heart Association (AHA) and AAP recommend that oral amoxicillin be given in a dosage of 50 mg/kg (up to 1 g) once daily for 10 days. The Infectious Diseases Society of America (IDSA) recommends that oral amoxicillin be given in a dosage of 50 mg/kg (up to 1 g) once daily for 10 days or 25 mg/kg (up to 500 mg) twice daily for 10 days.

Gonorrhea and Associated Infections

Some manufacturers state that adults and children weighing 40 kg or more may receive a single 3-g oral dose of amoxicillin for the treatment of acute, uncomplicated gonorrhea caused by susceptible nonpenicillinase-producing *Neisseria gonorrhoeae*. and that children weighing less than 40 kg who are 2 years of age or older may receive a single 50-mg/kg (maximum 3 g) dose of oral amoxicillin given with a single 25-mg/kg (up to 1 g) oral dose of probenecid. However, CDC has not

recommended use of penicillins for the treatment of gonorrhea for over 30 years because of the widespread prevalence of penicillinase-producing strains of *Neisseria gonorrhoeae* (PPNG) resistant to penicillins.

Chlamydial Infections

For the treatment of chlamydial urogenital infections during pregnancy, the recommended dosage of oral amoxicillin is 500 mg 3 times daily for 7 days.

Lyme Disease

Amoxicillin is a drug of choice for the treatment of erythema migrans and certain other manifestations of Lyme disease†. (See Lyme Disease under Uses, in the Aminopenicillins General Statement 8:12.16.08.)

If amoxicillin is used for the treatment of erythema migrans in patients with Lyme disease, IDSA, AAP, American Academy of Neurology (AAN), American College of Rheumatology (ACR), and others recommend that adults receive 500 mg 3 times daily for 14 days and that children receive 50 mg/kg daily given in 3 divided doses (maximum 500 mg per dose) for 14 days.

For the treatment of Lyme carditis† in outpatients when an IV regimen is not required, adults should receive amoxicillin 500 mg 3 times daily for 14–21 days and children should receive amoxicillin 50 mg/kg daily in 3 divided doses (maximum 500 mg per dose) for 14–21 days. This dosage of amoxicillin also can be used for follow-up to complete 14–21 days of treatment in patients who required initial treatment with an IV regimen.

For the treatment of Lyme arthritis†, adults should receive amoxicillin 500 mg 3 times daily for 28 days and children should receive amoxicillin 50 mg/kg daily in 3 divided doses (maximum 500 mg per dose) for 28 days.

Helicobacter pylori Infection

For the treatment of *Helicobacter pylori* infection and duodenal ulcer disease (active or 1-year history of duodenal ulcer) in adults, the recommended dosage of amoxicillin is 1 g twice daily in combination with clarithromycin (500 mg twice daily) and lansoprazole (30 mg twice daily) for 14 days (triple therapy). When used in combination with clarithromycin (500 mg twice daily) and omeprazole (20 mg twice daily) for the treatment of *H. pylori* infection and duodenal ulcer disease (active or 1-year history of duodenal ulcer), the recommended dosage of amoxicillin is 1 g twice daily for 10 days (triple therapy). An additional 18 days of omeprazole monotherapy is recommended for ulcer healing and symptom relief in patients with an active duodenal ulcer at the time therapy is initiated.

For the treatment of *H. pylori* infection and duodenal ulcer disease (active or 1-year history of duodenal ulcer) in adults who are either allergic to or intolerant of clarithromycin or in whom resistance to clarithromycin is known or suspected, the recommended dosage of amoxicillin is 1 g 3 times daily in combination with lansoprazole 30 mg 3 times daily for 14 days (dual therapy).

When amoxicillin has been used in other multiple-drug regimens† for the treatment of *H. pylori* infection and peptic ulcer disease in combination with at least one other agent that has activity against *H. pylori*, oral dosages of 500 mg 3 or 4 times daily (or 1 g 2 or 3 times daily) generally have been used; higher dosages of amoxicillin in such regimens reportedly have not been associated with improved results. Studies in which *H. pylori* was eradicated successfully generally have employed regimens consisting of a bismuth salt (e.g., bismuth subsalicylate), a nitroimidazole anti-infective (e.g., metronidazole), and another anti-infective agent (e.g., amoxicillin, tetracycline) or combined therapy with a proton-pump inhibitor (e.g., lansoprazole, omeprazole) and 1 or 2 anti-infective agents (e.g., clarithromycin, amoxicillin).

In a limited number of children with *H. pylori*-associated peptic ulcer disease† (e.g., gastritis, duodenitis/ duodenal ulcer), oral amoxicillin 25–50 mg/kg daily in divided doses (e.g., 250–500 mg 3 times daily) has been administered as part of multiple-drug regimens that included a nitroimidazole anti-infective (e.g., metronidazole) and/or a bismuth salt (e.g., bismuth subsalicylate). Further study is needed to establish an optimal drug regimen for treatment of *H. pylori* infection in children.

Prevention of Bacterial Endocarditis

If oral amoxicillin is used for prevention of bacterial endocarditis† in patients with certain cardiac conditions who are undergoing certain dental procedures or certain other procedures (see Prevention of Bacterial Endocarditis under Uses:

Prophylaxis, in the Aminopenicillins General Statement 8:12.16.08), AHA recommends that adults receive a single dose of 2 g and that children receive a single dose of 50 mg/kg given 30–60 minutes prior to the procedure.

When selecting anti-infectives for prevention of bacterial endocarditis, the current recommendations published by AHA should be consulted.

Anthrax

AAP recommends that infants and children 1 month of age or older receive oral amoxicillin in a dosage of 75 mg/kg daily (up to 1 g daily) given in divided doses every 8 hours if the drug is used as an alternative for postexposure prophylaxis of anthrax† following exposure to aerosolized *Bacillus anthracis* in the context of biologic warfare or bioterrorism when penicillin-susceptible strains are involved or is used as an alternative for treatment of cutaneous anthrax† without systemic involvement or treatment of inhalational anthrax† when these infections are caused by penicillin-susceptible strains.

CDC recommends that adults (including pregnant and postpartum women) receive oral amoxicillin in a dosage of 1 g every 8 hours if the drug is used as an alternative for postexposure prophylaxis of anthrax† in the context of biologic warfare or bioterrorism when penicillin-susceptible *B. anthracis* are involved or is used as an alternative for treatment of cutaneous anthrax† without systemic involvement when the infection is caused by penicillin-susceptible strains.

If oral amoxicillin is used as an alternative for postexposure prophylaxis of anthrax† or for the treatment of anthrax† when a parenteral regimen is not available (e.g., when there are supply or logistic problems because large numbers of individuals require treatment in a mass casualty setting), some experts (e.g., US Working Group on Civilian Biodefense) recommend that adults receive 500 mg 3 times daily and that children receive 80 mg/kg daily (maximum 1.5 mg daily) given in 3 divided doses at 8-hour intervals. Anti-infective postexposure prophylaxis should be continued until exposure to *B. anthracis* has been excluded. If exposure is confirmed, postexposure vaccination with anthrax vaccine (if available) may be indicated in conjunction with prophylaxis. Because of the possible persistence of anthrax spores in lung tissue following an aerosol exposure, CDC and other experts recommend that postexposure prophylaxis be continued for at least 60 days.

If oral amoxicillin is used as an alternative for the treatment of mild, uncomplicated cutaneous anthrax† caused by susceptible *B. anthracis*, some experts (e.g., US Working Group on Civilian Biodefense) recommend that adults receive 500 mg 3 times daily and that children receive 80 mg/kg daily (maximum 1.5 g daily) given in 3 divided doses at 8-hour intervals. CDC has recommended that cutaneous anthrax in infants and children younger than 2 years of age should be treated initially IV. Although 5–10 days of anti-infective therapy may be adequate for the treatment of mild, uncomplicated cutaneous anthrax that occurs as the result of natural or endemic exposures to anthrax, CDC and other experts recommend that therapy be continued for 60 days if the cutaneous infection occurred as the result of exposure to aerosolized anthrax spores since the possibility of inhalational anthrax would also exist. Anti-infective therapy may limit the size of the cutaneous anthrax lesion and it usually becomes sterile within the first 24 hours of treatment, but the lesion will still progress through the black eschar stage despite effective treatment.

DURATION OF THERAPY

The duration of amoxicillin therapy depends on the type and severity of infection and should be determined by the clinical and bacteriologic response of the patient. For most infections, except gonorrhea, therapy should be continued for at least 48–72 hours after the patient becomes asymptomatic or evidence of eradication of the infection has been obtained. Persistent infections may require several weeks of therapy. Amoxicillin usually is continued for 60 days for postexposure prophylaxis or treatment of inhalational or cutaneous anthrax in the context of biologic warfare or bioterrorism.

If amoxicillin is used in the treatment of infections caused by group A β-hemolytic streptococci, therapy should be continued for at least 10 days to decrease the risk of rheumatic fever and glomerulonephritis.

If amoxicillin is used in the treatment of chronic urinary tract infections, frequent bacteriologic and clinical appraisal is necessary during therapy and may be required for several months after therapy.

Dosage in Renal Impairment

In patients with renal impairment, doses and/or frequency of administration of amoxicillin should be modified in response to the degree of renal impairment, severity of the infection, and susceptibility of the causative organisms. The manufacturer states that adults with severe renal impairment and creatinine clearances less than 30 mL/minute should not receive the commercially available film-coated tablets containing 875 mg of amoxicillin. The recommended dosage of amoxicillin for adults with creatinine clearances of 10–30 mL/minute is 250 or 500 mg every 12 hours, depending on the severity of the infection, and the recommended dosage for adults with creatinine clearances less than 10 mL/minute is 250 or 500 mg every 24 hours, depending on the severity of the infection.

Patients undergoing hemodialysis should receive 250 or 500 mg of amoxicillin every 24 hours, depending on the severity of the infection, and should receive an additional dose of the drug during and after each dialysis period.

The manufacturer states that data are insufficient to recommend dosage for pediatric patients with renal impairment.

CAUTIONS

Adverse Effects

Adverse effects reported with amoxicillin are similar to those reported with other aminopenicillins. For information on adverse effects reported with aminopenicillins, see Cautions in the Aminopenicillins General Statement 8:12.16.08.

Precautions and Contraindications

Amoxicillin shares the toxic potentials of the penicillins, including the risk of hypersensitivity reactions, and the usual precautions of penicillin therapy should be observed. Prior to initiation of therapy with amoxicillin, careful inquiry should be made concerning previous hypersensitivity reactions to penicillins, cephalosporins, or other allergens. There is clinical and laboratory evidence of partial cross-allergenicity among penicillins and other β-lactam antibiotics including cephalosporins and cephamycins. Amoxicillin is contraindicated in patients who are hypersensitive to any penicillin.

Because a high percentage of patients with infectious mononucleosis have developed rash during therapy with aminopenicillins, amoxicillin probably should not be used in patients with the disease.

Individuals with phenylketonuria (i.e., homozygous genetic deficiency of phenylalanine hydroxylase) and other individuals who must restrict their intake of phenylalanine should be warned that the amoxicillin 200- and 400-mg chewable tablets contain aspartame which is metabolized in the GI tract to provide 1.82 or 3.64 mg of phenylalanine, respectively, following oral administration. Amoxicillin powder for oral suspension does not contain aspartame.

Renal, hepatic, and hematologic systems should be evaluated periodically during prolonged therapy with amoxicillin.

For a more complete discussion of these and other precautions associated with the use of amoxicillin, see Cautions: Precautions and Contraindications, in the Aminopenicillins General Statement 8:12.16.08.

Pregnancy, Fertility, and Lactation

Pregnancy

Safe use of amoxicillin during pregnancy has not been definitely established. There are no adequate or controlled studies using aminopenicillins in pregnant women, and amoxicillin should be used during pregnancy only when clearly needed. However, amoxicillin has been administered to pregnant women without evidence of adverse effects to the fetus. In addition, amoxicillin is included in the US Centers For Disease Control and Prevention (CDC) recommendations for the treatment of chlamydial infections† during pregnancy and included in CDC recommendations for the treatment of cutaneous anthrax† or for postexposure prophylaxis† following exposure to *Bacillus anthracis* spores.

Lactation

Because amoxicillin is distributed into milk and may lead to sensitization of infants, the drug should be used with caution in nursing women. Because of its general safety in infants, CDC states that amoxicillin is an option for anti-infective prophylaxis in breast-feeding women when *B. anthracis* is known to be penicillin susceptible and there is no contraindication to maternal amoxicillin use.

SPECTRUM

Based on its spectrum of activity, amoxicillin is classified as an aminopenicillin. For information on the classification of penicillins based on spectra of activity, see the Preface to the Penicillins 8:12.16.

Amoxicillin generally has the same spectrum of activity and the same level of activity against susceptible organisms as ampicillin; however, amoxicillin is more active in vitro on a weight basis than ampicillin against enterococci and *Salmonella* but less active than ampicillin against *Shigella* and *Enterobacter*. For specific information on the spectrum of activity of amoxicillin and resistance to the drug, see the sections on Spectrum and on Resistance in the Aminopenicillins General Statement 8:12.16.08.

PHARMACOKINETICS

For additional information on absorption of amoxicillin and for information on distribution and elimination of the drug, see Pharmacokinetics in the Aminopenicillins General Statement 8:12.16.08.

● Absorption

Amoxicillin is generally stable in the presence of acidic gastric secretions, and 74–92% of a single oral dose of the drug is absorbed from the GI tract. Amoxicillin is more completely absorbed from the GI tract than is ampicillin, and peak serum concentrations of amoxicillin are generally 2–2.5 times higher than those attained with an equivalent oral dose of ampicillin. As oral dosage of amoxicillin is increased, the fraction of the dose absorbed from the GI tract decreases only slightly and peak serum concentrations and areas under the serum concentration-time curves (AUCs) increase linearly with increasing dosage.

Peak serum concentrations are usually reached 1–2 hours after oral administration of amoxicillin capsules, film-coated tablets, chewable tablets, or oral suspension in fasting and nonfasting adults. Following oral administration of a single 250- or 500-mg dose of amoxicillin, peak serum concentrations range from 3.5–5 or 5.5–11 mcg/mL, respectively. In one study in healthy, fasting adults who received a single 500-mg oral dose of amoxicillin, serum concentrations of the drug averaged 3.3, 6.7, 9.3, 5.8, and 0.6 mcg/mL at 30 minutes, 1 hour, 2 hours, 3 hours, and 4 hours, respectively, after the dose. The manufacturer states that serum concentrations attained following administration of 125- or 250-mg chewable tablets are similar to those attained when the same dose is given as the oral suspension containing 125 or 250 mg of the drug per 5 mL. In healthy adults who received a single 400-mg dose of amoxicillin given as a 400-mg chewable tablet or the oral suspension containing 400 mg of the drug per 5 mL (dose given at the start of a light meal), peak serum concentrations were attained approximately 1 hour after the dose and averaged 5.18 or 5.92 mcg/mL, respectively, and AUC averaged 17.9 or 17.1 mcg•hr/mL, respectively.

In one study in children 4–45 months of age receiving amoxicillin oral suspension in a dosage of 15 mg/kg daily, serum amoxicillin concentrations ranged from 2.4–8.5, 1.9–11.3, 1.7–6.4, 0.17–1.9, and 0.14–3.3 mcg/mL at 30 minutes, 1 hour, 2 hours, 4 hours, and 6 hours, respectively, after a dose.

Although presence of food in the GI tract reportedly results in lower and delayed peak serum concentrations of amoxicillin, the total amount of drug absorbed does not appear to be affected.

CHEMISTRY AND STABILITY

● Chemistry

Amoxicillin is an aminopenicillin which differs structurally from ampicillin only in the addition of an hydroxyl group on the phenyl ring.

Amoxicillin is commercially available as the trihydrate. Potency of amoxicillin trihydrate is calculated on the anhydrous basis. Amoxicillin occurs as a white, practically odorless, crystalline powder and is sparingly soluble in water. When reconstituted as directed, amoxicillin oral suspensions have a pH of 5–7.5.

Amoxicillin is commercially available for oral administration as capsules, film-coated tablets, chewable tablets, or powder for oral suspension. Amoxicillin also is commercially available for oral administration in fixed-ratio combinations with clavulanate potassium. (See Amoxicillin and Clavulanate Potassium 8:12.16.08.)

Each 125-, 200-, 250-, or 400-mg amoxicillin chewable tablet contains 0.0019 mEq (0.044 mg), 0.0005 mEq (0.0107 mg), 0.0037 mEq (0.085 mg), or 0.0009 mEq (0.0215 mg) of sodium, respectively. The 200- and 400-mg chewable tablets contain aspartame which is metabolized in the GI tract to provide 1.82 or 3.64 mg of phenylalanine, respectively, following oral administration.

● Stability

Amoxicillin capsules, 125- and 250-mg chewable tablets, and powder for oral suspension should be stored in tight containers at 20°C or lower; amoxicillin 200- and 400-mg chewable tablets and amoxicillin film-coated tablets should be stored in tight containers at 25°C or lower.

Following reconstitution, amoxicillin oral suspensions should preferably be refrigerated at 2–8°C, but refrigeration is not necessary and the suspensions are stable for 14 days at room temperature or 2–8°C.

For further information on chemistry and stability, mechanism of action, spectrum, resistance, pharmacokinetics, uses, cautions, drug interactions, laboratory test interferences, and dosage and administration of amoxicillin, see the Aminopenicillins General Statement 8:12.16.08.

PREPARATIONS

Excipients in commercially available drug preparations may have clinically important effects in some individuals; consult specific product labeling for details.

Amoxicillin (Trihydrate)

Oral		
Capsules	250 mg (of amoxicillin)*	**Amoxicillin Capsules** Amoxil®, GlaxoSmithKline
	500 mg (of amoxicillin)*	**Amoxicillin Capsules** Amoxil®, GlaxoSmithKline
For suspension	125 mg (of amoxicillin) per 5 mL*	Amoxicillin for Suspension Amoxil®, GlaxoSmithKline Larotid®
	200 mg (of amoxicillin) per 5 mL*	Amoxicillin for Suspension
	250 mg (of amoxicillin) per 5 mL*	Amoxicillin for Suspension Amoxil®, GlaxoSmithKline Larotid®
	50 mg (of amoxicillin) per mL*	Amoxicillin for Suspension Amoxil®, GlaxoSmithKline
	400 mg (of amoxicillin) per 5 mL*	Amoxicillin for Suspension Amoxil®, GlaxoSmithKline
Tablets, chewable	125 mg (of amoxicillin)*	**Amoxicillin Chewable Tablets**
	250 mg (of amoxicillin)*	**Amoxicillin Chewable Tablets**
Tablets, film-coated	500 mg (of amoxicillin)*	**Amoxicillin Tablets**
	875 mg (of amoxicillin)*	**Amoxicillin Tablets**

* available from one or more manufacturer, distributor, and/or repackager by generic (nonproprietary) name

Amoxicillin (Trihydrate) Combinations

	Capsules, Amoxicillin (trihydrate) 500 mg (of amoxicillin)	Lansoprazole, Amoxicillin, and Clarithromycin
	Capsules, delayed-release (containing enteric-coated granules) Lansoprazole 30 mg	
	Tablets, film-coated, Clarithromycin 500 mg	

† Use is not currently included in the labeling approved by the US Food and Drug Administration.

Amoxicillin and Clavulanate Potassium

8:12.16.08 • AMINOPENICILLINS

■ Amoxicillin and clavulanate potassium (amoxicillin/clavulanate) is a fixed combination of amoxicillin trihydrate (an aminopenicillin antibiotic) and the potassium salt of clavulanic acid (a β-lactamase inhibitor); clavulanic acid synergistically expands amoxicillin's spectrum of activity against many strains of β-lactamase-producing bacteria.

USES

The fixed combination of amoxicillin and clavulanate potassium (amoxicillin/clavulanate) is used orally for the treatment of lower respiratory tract infections, otitis media, sinusitis, skin and skin structure infections, and urinary tract infections caused by susceptible organisms.

Amoxicillin/clavulanate is used principally for the treatment of infections caused by susceptible β-lactamase-producing strains of *Moraxella catarrhalis*, *Escherichia coli*, *Haemophilus influenzae*, *Klebsiella*, and *Staphylococcus aureus*. Although amoxicillin/clavulanate also may be effective in the treatment of infections caused by non-β-lactamase-producing organisms susceptible to amoxicillin alone, most clinicians state that an aminopenicillin used alone is preferred to the combination drug for the treatment of these infections and that amoxicillin/clavulanate should be reserved for use in the treatment of infections caused by, or suspected of being caused by, β-lactamase-producing organisms when an aminopenicillin alone would be ineffective.

Prior to initiation of therapy with amoxicillin/clavulanate, appropriate specimens should be obtained for identification of the causative organism and in vitro susceptibility tests. Amoxicillin/clavulanate may be started pending results of susceptibility tests if the infection is believed to be caused by β-lactamase-producing bacteria susceptible to the drug, but should be discontinued if the organism is found to be resistant to the drug. If the infection is found to be caused by non-β-lactamase-producing organisms susceptible to aminopenicillins, some clinicians suggest that therapy generally should be changed to an aminopenicillin alone, unless this is impractical.

● Gram-positive Aerobic Bacterial Infections

Amoxicillin/clavulanate has been effective for the treatment of abscesses, cellulitis, and impetigo caused by susceptible penicillinase-producing and nonpenicillinase-producing *Staphylococcus aureus* and *S. epidermidis*, *Streptococcus pyogenes* (group A β-hemolytic streptococci), or *Corynebacterium*. Results of several controlled studies indicate that amoxicillin/clavulanate is as effective as cefaclor in the treatment of these infections. However, natural penicillins are generally the drugs of choice for the treatment of infections caused by nonpenicillinase-producing staphylococci or group A β-hemolytic streptococci and penicillinase-resistant penicillins are generally the drugs of choice for the treatment of infections caused by susceptible penicillinase-producing staphylococci.

Amoxicillin/clavulanate should not be used in the treatment of infections caused by methicillin-resistant staphylococci, even though results of in vitro susceptibility tests may indicate that the organism is susceptible to the drug.

● Gram-negative Aerobic Bacterial Infections

Haemophilus Infections

Amoxicillin/clavulanate generally has been effective for the treatment of otitis media or upper and lower respiratory tract infections such as bronchopneumonia, sinusitis, and acute exacerbations of chronic bronchitis caused by susceptible *H. influenzae*. Amoxicillin/clavulanate usually is the drug of choice for empiric anti-infective therapy of otitis media and sinusitis in communities with a high incidence of ampicillin-resistant *H. influenzae* or *M. catarrhalis* and for infections that fail to respond to other regimens. (See Uses: Acute Otitis Media.)

Moraxella catarrhalis Infections

Infections caused by β-lactamase-producing *M. catarrhalis* have been reported with increasing frequency. This organism recently has been recognized as a common cause of otitis media and maxillary sinusitis in children and of bronchitis and pneumonia in adults, especially those with chronic lung disease. Rarely, septicemia, endocarditis, urethritis, meningitis, neonatal ophthalmia, and conjunctivitis caused by *M. catarrhalis* have been reported. Amoxicillin/clavulanate generally has been effective when used in the treatment of upper and lower respiratory tract infections caused by *M. catarrhalis*, and many clinicians consider it a drug of choice for infections caused by the organism.

Amoxicillin/clavulanate generally has been effective when used for the treatment of acute otitis media or acute maxillary sinusitis caused by *M. catarrhalis*. In several controlled studies, amoxicillin/clavulanate was more effective than cefaclor for the empiric treatment of acute otitis media in children 2 months to 12 years of age. Although adverse GI effects occurred more frequently with amoxicillin/clavulanate than with cefaclor, amoxicillin/clavulanate appears to be more active than cefaclor against β-lactamase-producing *M. catarrhalis*. Some clinicians suggest that amoxicillin/clavulanate is a drug of choice for the empiric treatment of otitis media and sinusitis in communities with a high incidence of β-lactamase-producing *M. catarrhalis*.

Gonorrhea

Amoxicillin/clavulanate has been used with some success for the treatment of uncomplicated gonorrhea† caused by penicillinase-producing strains of *N. gonorrhoeae* (PPNG) or nonpenicillinase-producing strains of the organism. Regimens consisting of a single oral dose of amoxicillin (3 g) and clavulanic acid (125–500 mg) with or without oral probenecid (1 g) have been effective in some cases for the treatment of uncomplicated gonorrhea caused by PPNG or nonpenicillinase-producing *N. gonorrhoeae*. However, CDC has not recommended use of penicillins for the treatment of gonococcal infections for over 30 years because of the widespread prevalence of PPNG resistant to penicillins. Ceftriaxone is the drug of choice for the treatment of gonococcal infections.

Urinary Tract Infections

Amoxicillin/clavulanate has been effective for the treatment of uncomplicated or complicated urinary tract infections (UTIs) caused by susceptible organisms, including *E. coli*, *Klebsiella*, *Enterobacter*, or *P. mirabilis*. Because amoxicillin/clavulanate is active in vitro against many urinary pathogens resistant to amoxicillin or ampicillin alone, some clinicians suggest that the combination drug may be preferred over ampicillin or amoxicillin alone for the initial treatment of UTIs; however, further studies are needed to evaluate the relative efficacy of amoxicillin/clavulanate and other anti-infectives used for the treatment of UTIs.

Other Gram-negative Aerobic Bacterial Infections

Amoxicillin/clavulanate has been used in the treatment of infections caused by *Eikenella corrodens*† or *Pasteurella multocida*†.

● Anaerobic and Mixed Aerobic-Anaerobic Bacterial Infections

Amoxicillin/clavulanate has been used with some success for the treatment of anaerobic and mixed aerobic-anaerobic bacterial infections† including intra-abdominal and gynecologic infections such as endometritis, salpingitis, pelvic cellulitis, and acute pelvic inflammatory disease. Although oral amoxicillin/clavulanate has been effective in the treatment of these infections, including infections caused by *Bacteroides fragilis*, further study is needed to evaluate efficacy of the drug in the treatment of anaerobic and mixed aerobic-anaerobic bacterial infections and to determine if serum and tissue concentrations of amoxicillin and clavulanic acid obtained following oral administration of the drug are adequate for the treatment of these infections.

● Acute Otitis Media

Amoxicillin/clavulanate is used for the treatment of acute otitis media (AOM) caused by *S. pneumoniae*†, *H. influenzae* (including β-lactamase-producing strains), or *M. catarrhalis* (including β-lactamase-producing strains). Amoxicillin usually is considered the drug of first choice for initial treatment of AOM, unless the patient has severe illness (moderate to severe otalgia or fever 39°C or higher) or the infection is suspected of being caused by β-lactamase-producing bacteria resistant to the drug, in which case amoxicillin/clavulanate is recommended for initial treatment. The American Academy of Pediatrics (AAP), American Academy of Family Physicians (AAFP), CDC, and others state that, despite the increasing prevalence of multidrug-resistant *S. pneumoniae* and presence of β-lactamase-producing *H. influenzae* or *M. catarrhalis* in many communities, amoxicillin remains the anti-infective of first choice for treatment of uncomplicated AOM since it is highly effective, has a narrow spectrum of activity, is well distributed into middle ear fluid, is well tolerated, has an acceptable taste, and is inexpensive. Amoxicillin (when given in a dosage of 80–90 mg/kg daily) usually is effective in the treatment of AOM caused by *S. pneumoniae*, including infections involving strains with intermediate resistance to penicillins, and also usually is effective in the treatment of AOM caused by most strains of *H. influenzae*.

Alternatives for initial treatment of AOM in patients with a history of non-type I hypersensitivity reactions to penicillins include oral cephalosporins (cefdinir, cefpodoxime, cefuroxime axetil) or parenteral ceftriaxone. Alternatives for patients with type I penicillin hypersensitivity include oral macrolides (azithromycin, clarithromycin, fixed combination of erythromycin and sulfisoxazole), oral co-trimoxazole, or oral clindamycin (especially in those with infections known or presumed to be caused by penicillin-resistant *S. pneumoniae).*

Amoxicillin/clavulanate (given in a dosage of 80–90 mg/kg of amoxicillin and 6.4 mg/kg of clavulanate daily) is the drug of choice for retreatment in patients who fail to respond to an initial amoxicillin regimen (given in a dosage of 80–90 mg/kg daily). The AAP and AAFP recommend that amoxicillin/clavulanate be substituted if there has been no response to amoxicillin within 48–72 hours. A 3-day regimen of IM or IV ceftriaxone also is recommended for retreatment, especially in those who have severe illness (moderate to severe otalgia or fever 39°C or higher) and in those who are vomiting or cannot otherwise tolerate an oral regimen.

● Pharyngitis and Tonsillitis

Although not considered a drug of choice for the treatment of pharyngitis and tonsillitis caused by *S. pyogenes*† (group A β-hemolytic streptococci), amoxicillin/clavulanate is recommended as one of several possible alternatives for the treatment of symptomatic patients who have multiple, recurrent episodes of pharyngitis known to caused by *S. pyogenes*†. Natural penicillins (i.e., 10 days of oral penicillin V or a single IM dose of penicillin G benzathine) is the treatment of choice for streptococcal pharyngitis and tonsillitis, although oral amoxicillin often is used instead of penicillin V in small children because of a more acceptable taste.

If there is recurrence of signs and symptoms of pharyngitis shortly after the initial recommended regimen is completed (i.e., within a few weeks) and presence of *S. pyogenes* is detected, retreatment with the original regimen or another regimen of choice is indicated; if compliance with a 10-day oral regimen is a concern, IM penicillin G benzathine should be used for retreatment. Some clinicians suggest use of an alternative agent (e.g., Amoxicillin/clavulanate, clindamycin, macrolide) for retreatment. However, if there are multiple, recurrent episodes of symptomatic pharyngitis within a period of months to years, it may be difficult to determine whether these are true episodes of *S. pyogenes* infection or whether the patient is a long-term streptococcal pharyngeal carrier who is experiencing repeated episodes of nonstreptococcal pharyngitis (e.g., viral pharyngitis) in whom treatment is not usually indicated. Continuous anti-infective prophylaxis (secondary prophylaxis) to prevent the recurrence of streptococcal pharyngitis is not recommended in these circumstances, unless the patient has a history of rheumatic fever. Instead, use of an alternative regimen is recommended by some clinicians. Although there are no controlled clinical studies evaluating efficacy, the IDSA suggests that symptomatic individuals with multiple, recurrent episodes of documented *S. pyogenes* pharyngitis receive a regimen of oral amoxicillin clavulanate, oral clindamycin, or IM penicillin G benzathine (with or without oral rifampin).

For additional information on treatment of *S. pyogenes* pharyngitis, see Pharyngitis and Tonsillitis under Uses in the Natural Penicillins General Statement 8:12.16.04.

DOSAGE AND ADMINISTRATION

● Reconstitution and Administration

The fixed combination of amoxicillin and clavulanate potassium (amoxicillin/clavulanate) is administered orally. Chewable tablets should be thoroughly chewed before swallowing. Amoxicillin/clavulanate has also been given IV, but a parenteral dosage form of the drug is not available in the US.

Because GI absorption of amoxicillin and clavulanate potassium is not affected by food following oral administration of conventional preparations of amoxicillin/clavulanate, these preparations may be administered orally without regard to meals. However, administration of oral amoxicillin/clavulanate with meals may minimize adverse GI effects. Extended-release tablets of amoxicillin/clavulanate should be administered at the beginning of a meal to enhance GI absorption of amoxicillin and clavulanate and to minimize adverse GI effects; amoxicillin absorption from extended-release tablets is decreased when administered in a fasting state, and clavulanate absorption is decreased when these tablets are administered with a high-fat meal.

Amoxicillin/clavulanate powder for oral suspension should be reconstituted at the time of dispensing by adding the amount of water specified on the bottle to provide a suspension containing 125 mg of amoxicillin and 31.25 mg of clavulanic acid per 5 mL, 200 mg of amoxicillin and 28.5 mg of clavulanic acid per 5 mL, 250 mg of amoxicillin and 62.5 mg of clavulanic acid per 5 mL, or 600 mg of amoxicillin and 42.9 mg of clavulanic acid per 5 mL. After tapping the bottle to thoroughly loosen the powder for oral suspension, the water should be added to the powder in 2 portions and the suspension agitated well after each addition. The suspension should be agitated well just prior to administration of each dose.

● Dosage

Dosage of amoxicillin/clavulanate generally is expressed in terms of the amoxicillin content of the fixed combination. Although commercially available amoxicillin/clavulanate contains amoxicillin as the trihydrate and/or the sodium salt and clavulanic acid as the potassium salt, potency of amoxicillin is calculated on the anhydrous basis and potency of clavulanate potassium is expressed in terms of clavulanic acid.

Amoxicillin/clavulanate is commercially available for oral administration as a powder for oral suspension containing a 4:1, 7:1, or 14:1 ratio of amoxicillin to clavulanic acid; as chewable tablets containing a 4:1 or 7:1 ratio of the drugs; as film-coated tablets containing a 2:1 or 4:1 ratio of the drugs; as scored tablets containing a 7:1 ratio of the drugs; and as extended-release tablets containing a 16:1 ratio of the drugs.

Commercially available amoxicillin/clavulanate powders for oral suspension should not be considered interchangeable since they contain different amounts of clavulanic acid. The powder for oral suspension containing 600 mg of amoxicillin and 42.9 mg of clavulanic acid per 5 mL (Augmentin ES-600®) is indicated only for the treatment of persistent or recurrent acute otitis media (AOM) in certain pediatric patients 3 months to 12 years of age; safety and efficacy of this preparation in younger children or in adolescents or adults have not been established. Because commercially available amoxicillin/clavulanate film-coated tablets containing 250 mg of amoxicillin contain 125 mg of clavulanic acid and commercially available chewable tablets containing 250 mg of amoxicillin contain 62.5 mg of clavulanic acid, these preparations should not be considered interchangeable. In addition, since the 250- and 500-mg film-coated tablets of the drug both contain the same amount of clavulanic acid, two 250-mg film-coated tablets are not equivalent to one 500-mg film-coated tablet. Because extended-release tablets of amoxicillin/clavulanate contain different ratios of the drugs, the extended-release tablets are not equivalent to conventional or chewable tablets of the drug.

Children weighing less than 40 kg should *not* receive the 250-mg film-coated tablets since this formulation contains a higher dose of clavulanic acid. (See Dosage: Pediatric Dosage, under Dosage and Administration.) Safety and efficacy of the extended-release tablets have not been established in pediatric patients younger than 16 years of age.

Adult Dosage

The usual adult oral dosage of amoxicillin/clavulanate is one 250-mg film-coated tablet (containing 250 mg of amoxicillin and 125 mg of clavulanic acid) every 8 hours or one 500-mg film-coated tablet (containing 500 mg of amoxicillin and 125 mg of clavulanic acid) every 12 hours. For more severe infections and infections of the respiratory tract, the usual adult oral dosage is one 500-mg film-coated tablet (containing 500 mg of amoxicillin and 125 mg of clavulanic acid) every 8 hours or one 875-mg scored tablet (containing 875 mg of amoxicillin and 125 mg of clavulanic acid) every 12 hours. Alternatively, adults who have difficulty swallowing tablets may receive the oral suspension containing 125 or 250 mg of amoxicillin/5 mL instead of the 500-mg film-coated tablet or may receive the oral suspension containing 200 or 400 mg of amoxicillin/5 mL instead of the 875-mg scored tablet.

The usual oral dosage of amoxicillin/clavulanate extended-release tablets for the treatment of acute bacterial sinusitis in patients 16 years of age and older is 2 tablets (containing 1 g of amoxicillin and 62.5 mg of clavulanic acid in each tablet) every 12 hours for 10 days. The usual oral dosage of the extended-release tablets for the treatment of community-acquired pneumonia (CAP) in patients 16 years of age and older is 2 tablets (containing 1 g of amoxicillin and 62.5 mg of clavulanic acid in each tablet) every 12 hours for 7–10 days. Dosage adjustment for extended-release tablets of the combination based solely on age is not necessary in geriatric patients.

Pediatric Dosage

Children weighing 40 kg or more may receive the usual adult oral dosage of amoxicillin/clavulanate.

The usual dosage of amoxicillin/clavulanate in neonates and infants younger than 12 weeks of age is 30 mg/kg of amoxicillin daily given in divided doses every 12 hours. Because experience with the oral suspension containing 200 mg of amoxicillin/5 mL is limited in this age group, the manufacturer recommends that the oral suspension containing 125 mg of amoxicillin/5 mL be used in neonates and infants younger than 12 weeks of age.

For the treatment of sinusitis, lower respiratory tract infections, and more severe infections in pediatric patients 12 weeks of age and older, the usual dosage of amoxicillin/clavulanate is 45 mg/kg of amoxicillin daily in divided doses every 12 hours administered as the oral suspension containing 200 or 400 mg of amoxicillin/5 mL or as chewable tablets containing 200 or 400 mg of amoxicillin. Alternatively, these infections in this age group can be treated with a dosage of 40 mg/kg of amoxicillin daily in divided doses every 8 hours administered as the oral suspension containing 125 or 250 mg of amoxicillin/5 mL or as chewable tablets containing 125 or 250 mg of amoxicillin.

For the treatment of less severe infections in pediatric patients 12 weeks of age or older, the usual dosage of amoxicillin/clavulanate is 25 mg/kg of amoxicillin daily in divided doses every 12 hours administered as the oral suspension containing 200 or 400 mg of amoxicillin/5 mL or as chewable tablets containing 200 or 400 mg of amoxicillin. Alternatively, less severe infections in this age group can be treated with a dosage of 20 mg/kg of amoxicillin daily in divided doses every 8 hours administered as the oral suspension containing 125 or 250 mg of amoxicillin/5 mL or as chewable tablets containing 125 or 250 mg of amoxicillin.

Acute Otitis Media

For the treatment of acute otitis media (AOM) in pediatric patients, the recommended dosage of amoxicillin/clavulanate is 90 mg/kg of amoxicillin and 6.4 mg/kg of clavulanate daily given in 2 divided doses†. The drug usually is given for 10 days, but the optimal duration of therapy is uncertain. The American Academy of Pediatrics (AAP) and American Academy of Family Physicians (AAFP) recommend that a 10-day regimen be used for treatment of AOM in children younger than 6 years of age and in those with severe disease, but that a duration of 5–7 days may be appropriate in those 6 years of age or older with mild to moderate AOM.

Although amoxicillin/clavulanate can be administered in a dosage of 40–45 mg/kg of amoxicillin daily given in 2 or 3 divided doses for 10 days for the treatment of AOM, the AAP, AAFP, US Centers for Disease Control and Prevention (CDC), and others recommend use of the higher dosage. The higher dosage is especially important in patients with AOM known or suspected of being caused by *Streptococcus pneumoniae* with reduced susceptibility to penicillins, patients with primary treatment failure or persistent or recurrent AOM after treatment with amoxicillin, and in patients who have received anti-infective therapy within the previous few months.

When amoxicillin/clavulanate is administered in the higher dosage for the treatment of AOM in pediatric patients, commercially available formulations containing a 7:1 or 14:1 ratio of amoxicillin to clavulanic acid should be used since these formulations provide a lower daily dosage of clavulanate potassium and minimize the risk of adverse GI effects associated with the clavulanate potassium component. When the oral suspension containing 600 mg of amoxicillin and 42.9 mg of clavulanic acid per 5 mL is used for the treatment of persistent or recurrent AOM in pediatric patients weighing less than 40 kg, the usual dosage is 90 mg/kg of amoxicillin daily given in divided doses every 12 hours for 10 days.

Pharyngitis and Tonsillitis

If amoxicillin/clavulanate is used for the treatment of symptomatic patients who have multiple, recurrent episodes of pharyngitis known to be caused by *Streptococcus pyogenes*† (group A β-hemolytic streptococci) (see Uses: Pharyngitis and Tonsillitis), the Infectious Diseases Society of America (IDSA) recommends that children receive 40 mg/kg of amoxicillin daily (maximum 750 mg daily) given in 3 equally divided doses for 10 days. Adults should receive amoxicillin/clavulanate in a dosage of 500 mg of amoxicillin twice daily for 10 days; the IDSA states that this dosage has not been specifically studied in adults and was extrapolated from the pediatric dosage.

● Dosage in Renal and Hepatic Impairment

In patients with renal impairment, doses and/or frequency of administration of amoxicillin/clavulanate should be modified in response to the degree of renal impairment. Some clinicians suggest that modification of usual dosage is unnecessary in adults with creatinine clearances greater than 30 mL/minute. These clinicians recommend that adults with creatinine clearances of 15–30 mL/minute receive the usual dose of conventional preparations of the drug every 12–18 hours, adults with creatinine clearances of 5–15 mL/minute receive the usual dose every 20–36 hours, and adults with creatinine clearances less than 5 mL/minute receive the usual dose every 48 hours. However, other clinicians suggest that use of amoxicillin/clavulanate should be avoided in patients with creatinine clearances less than 30 mL/minute until more data are available on use of the drug in these patients.

Some clinicians suggest that adults undergoing hemodialysis receive a 500-mg tablet containing 500 mg of amoxicillin and 125 mg of clavulanic acid halfway through each dialysis period and an additional 500-mg tablet after each dialysis period.

The pharmacokinetics of extended-release tablets of amoxicillin/clavulanate have not been studied in patients with renal impairment, and the manufacturer states that this preparation is contraindicated in patients with severe impairment (creatinine clearance less than 30 mL/minute and those undergoing hemodialysis). The extended-release tablets should be dosed cautiously in patients with hepatic impairment and liver function should be monitored at frequent intervals.

CAUTIONS

● Adverse Effects

Adverse effects reported with the fixed combination of amoxicillin and clavulanate potassium (amoxicillin/clavulanate) are generally dose related and similar to those reported with amoxicillin alone. For information on adverse effects reported with amoxicillin and other aminopenicillins, see Cautions in the Aminopenicillins General Statement 8:12.16.08.

With the exception of adverse GI effects, which have been reported more frequently with amoxicillin/clavulanate than with amoxicillin alone, the frequency and severity of adverse effects reported with the fixed-combination are generally similar to those reported with amoxicillin alone. The manufacturers state that adverse effects reported with oral amoxicillin/clavulanate are generally mild and transient and have required discontinuance of therapy in less than 3% of patients receiving the drug.

GI effects are the most frequent adverse reactions to oral amoxicillin/clavulanate. Diarrhea or loose stools has been reported in about 9% of patients receiving the drug, and nausea and vomiting have been reported in 1–5% of patients. Abdominal discomfort, anorexia, and flatulence, dyspepsia, gastritis, stomatitis, glossitis, black or hairy tongue, and enterocolitis also have been reported. The frequency of nausea and vomiting appears to be related to the dose of clavulanic acid since these effects have been reported in up to 40% of patients when a 250-mg dose of clavulanic acid rather than a 125-mg dose was used in conjunction with amoxicillin. Administration of oral amoxicillin/clavulanate with meals reportedly decreases the frequency and severity of adverse GI effects, and therefore patients should be advised to take the drug with a meal or snack.

Treatment with anti-infectives alters normal colon flora and may permit overgrowth of *Clostridioides difficile* (formerly known as *Clostridium difficile*). *C. difficile*-associated diarrhea and colitis (also known as antibiotic-associated pseudomembranous colitis; CDAD) may occur during or following discontinuance of amoxicillin/clavulanate. *C. difficile* produces toxins A and B which contribute to development of CDAD. If CDAD is suspected or confirmed, anti-infective therapy not directed against *C. difficile* should be discontinued as soon as possible. Patients should be managed with appropriate anti-infective therapy directed against *C. difficile* (e.g., fidaxomicin, vancomycin, metronidazole), supportive therapy (e.g., fluid and electrolyte management, protein supplementation), and surgical evaluation as clinically indicated.

Rash and urticaria have been reported in approximately 3% of patients receiving amoxicillin/clavulanate. Other adverse effects that have been reported in 1% or less of patients receiving the drug include candidal vaginitis, dizziness, headache, fever, and slight thrombocytosis.

Moderate increases in serum concentrations of AST (SGOT) and/or ALT (SGPT), alkaline phosphatase, and/or bilirubin have been reported in patients receiving amoxicillin/clavulanate. Hepatic dysfunction has been reported most frequently in geriatric patients, males, or in patients receiving prolonged therapy with the drug. Histologic findings on liver biopsies have consisted of predominantly cholestatic, hepatocellular, or mixed cholestatic-hepatocellular changes. The onset of manifestations of hepatic dysfunction may occur during or several weeks following discontinuance of amoxicillin/clavulanate therapy and usually is reversible. However, fatal cholestatic hepatitis has been reported rarely; these generally have been cases associated with serious underlying diseases or concomitant drug therapy.

Although not reported to date with amoxicillin/clavulanate, positive direct antiglobulin (Coombs') test results have been reported in patients who received therapy with ticarcillin and clavulanic acid. In one study in immunocompromised patients, positive direct antiglobulin test results occurred during 44% of the courses of therapy with ticarcillin and clavulanic acid and concomitant tobramycin. Positive reactions occurred within 48 hours after initiation of therapy and reverted to negative within 2–4 months after completion of therapy. These reactions appear to result from nonimmunologic adsorption of proteins onto erythrocytes in the presence of clavulanic acid; this nonimmunologic mechanism is similar to that observed with cephalosporins. Nonimmunologic adsorption of proteins onto erythrocyte membranes and positive direct antiglobulin test results also occurred in vitro when erythrocytes obtained from healthy individuals were exposed to clavulanic acid; however, exposure of erythrocytes to ticarcillin alone under various conditions did not result in a positive reaction.

● Precautions and Contraindications

Amoxicillin/clavulanate shares the toxic potentials of the penicillins, including the risk of hypersensitivity reactions, and the usual precautions of penicillin therapy should be observed. Prior to initiation of therapy with amoxicillin/clavulanate, careful inquiry should be made concerning previous hypersensitivity reactions to penicillins, cephalosporins, or other drugs. There is clinical and laboratory evidence of partial cross-allergenicity among penicillins and other β-lactam antibiotics including cephalosporins and cephamycins.

Renal, hepatic, and hematologic function should be evaluated periodically during prolonged therapy with amoxicillin/clavulanate.

Because *C. difficile*-associated diarrhea and colitis has been reported with the use of nearly all anti-infective agents, including amoxicillin/clavulanate, it should be considered in the differential diagnosis of patients who develop diarrhea during or after amoxicillin/clavulanate therapy. Careful medical history is necessary since CDAD has been reported to occur as late as 2 months or longer after anti-infective therapy is discontinued. Patients should be advised that diarrhea is a common problem caused by anti-infectives and usually ends when the drug is discontinued; however, it is important to contact a clinician if watery and bloody stools (with or without stomach cramps and fever) occur during or as late as 2 months or longer after the last dose.

Because a high percentage of patients with infectious mononucleosis have developed rash during therapy with aminopenicillins, amoxicillin/clavulanate should not be used in patients with the disease. amoxicillin/clavulanate is contraindicated in patients who are hypersensitive to any penicillin.

Commercially available amoxicillin/clavulanate chewable tablets containing 200 or 400 mg of amoxicillin and amoxicillin/clavulanate oral suspension containing 200 400, or 600 mg of amoxicillin per 5 mL contain aspartame,

which is metabolized in the GI tract to phenylalanine following oral administration. Individuals with phenylketonuria (i.e., homozygous genetic deficiency of phenylalanine hydroxylase) and other individuals who must restrict their intake of phenylalanine should be warned that each 200- or 400-mg chewable tablet of amoxicillin/clavulanate provides 2.1 or 4.2 mg of phenylalanine, respectively, and each 5 mL of amoxicillin/clavulanate oral suspension containing 200, 400, or 600 mg of amoxicillin provides 7 mg of phenylalanine. While these preparations should not be used in patients with phenylketonuria, other commercially available preparations of amoxicillin/clavulanate do not contain aspartame.

For information on the potassium and sodium content of various amoxicillin/clavulanate preparations, see Chemistry and Stability: Chemistry.

For a more complete discussion of these and other precautions associated with the use of amoxicillin, see Cautions: Precautions and Contraindications in the Aminopenicillins General Statement 8:12.16.08.

● Pediatric Precautions

Adverse effects reported in pediatric patients receiving amoxicillin/clavulanate are similar to those reported in adults.

In a clinical study in pediatric patients 2 months to 12 years of age with acute otitis media who received amoxicillin/clavulanate oral suspension, the incidence of diarrhea was lower in those who received the drug in a dosage of 45 mg/kg of amoxicillin daily in divided doses every 12 hours than in those who received the drug in a dosage of 40 mg/kg of amoxicillin daily in divided doses every 8 hours. Diarrhea occurred in 14.3% of those receiving the twice-daily regimen and 34.3% of those receiving the 3-times-daily regimen, and 3.1% of those receiving the twice-daily regimen and 7.6% of those receiving the 3-times-daily regimen had severe diarrhea or were withdrawn from the study with diarrhea. It is not known whether a similar difference in the incidence of diarrhea occurs when amoxicillin/clavulanate chewable tablets are administered in a twice-daily or 3-times-daily regimen.

Safety and efficacy of the extended-release tablets of amoxicillin/clavulanate have not been established in pediatric patients younger than 16 years of age.

● Mutagenicity and Carcinogenicity

Studies have not been performed to date to evaluate the mutagenic or carcinogenic potential of amoxicillin/clavulanate.

● Pregnancy, Fertility, and Lactation

Pregnancy

Safe use of amoxicillin/clavulanate during pregnancy has not been definitely established. There are no adequate or controlled studies using amoxicillin/clavulanate in pregnant women, and the drug should be used during pregnancy only when clearly needed.

Aminopenicillins are generally poorly absorbed when given orally during labor. Although the mechanism is unclear and the clinical importance has not been determined to date, studies using oral ampicillin indicate that, when administered during pregnancy, the drug interferes with metabolism and enterohepatic circulation of steroids resulting in decreased urinary concentrations of estrogen metabolites. The manufacturers state that this effect could also occur with amoxicillin/clavulanate. IV administration of ampicillin to guinea pigs has decreased uterine tone and decreased the frequency, height, and duration of uterine contractions; however, it is not known whether use of amoxicillin/clavulanate in humans during labor or delivery could have any immediate or delayed adverse effects on the fetus, prolong the duration of labor, or increase the likelihood of forceps delivery, other obstetrical intervention, or resuscitation of the neonate.

Fertility

Reproduction studies in mice and rats using doses up to 10 times the usual human dose have not revealed evidence of impaired fertility or harm to the fetus.

Lactation

Because amoxicillin and clavulanic acid are distributed into milk, amoxicillin/clavulanate should be used with caution in nursing women.

DRUG INTERACTIONS

● Allopurinol

Because an increased incidence of rash reportedly occurs in patients with hyperuricemia who are receiving allopurinol and concomitant amoxicillin or ampicillin compared with those receiving amoxicillin, ampicillin, or allopurinol alone, some clinicians suggest that concomitant use of the drugs should be avoided if possible. The manufacturers state that there are no data to date on concomitant administration of allopurinol and amoxicillin/clavulanate.

● Probenecid

Oral probenecid administered shortly before or concomitantly with the fixed combination of amoxicillin and clavulanate potassium (amoxicillin/clavulanate) slows the rate of renal tubular secretion of amoxicillin and produces higher and prolonged serum concentrations of amoxicillin. However, concomitant administration of probenecid with amoxicillin/clavulanate does not affect the area under the serum concentration-time curve (AUC), half-life, or peak serum concentration of clavulanic acid.

LABORATORY TEST INTERFERENCES

Ampicillin reportedly interferes with urinary glucose determinations using cupric sulfate (e.g., Benedict's solution, Clinitest®), but does not affect glucose oxidase methods (e.g., Clinistix®, Tes-Tape®). Since this laboratory test interference could also occur with amoxicillin, glucose oxidase methods should be used when urinary glucose determinations are indicated in patients receiving the fixed combination of amoxicillin and clavulanate potassium (amoxicillin/clavulanate).

Although not reported to date with amoxicillin/clavulanate, positive direct antiglobulin (Coombs') test results have been reported in patients who received ticarcillin and clavulanic acid and appear to be caused by clavulanic acid. (See Cautions: Adverse Effects.) This reaction may interfere with hematologic studies or transfusion cross-matching procedures and should be considered in patients receiving amoxicillin/clavulanate.

MECHANISM OF ACTION

The fixed combination of amoxicillin and clavulanate potassium (amoxicillin/clavulanate) usually is bactericidal in action. Concurrent administration of clavulanic acid does not alter the mechanism of action of amoxicillin. However, because clavulanic acid has a high affinity for and binds to certain β-lactamases that generally inactivate amoxicillin by hydrolyzing its β-lactam ring, concurrent administration of the drug with amoxicillin results in a synergistic bactericidal effect which expands the spectrum of activity of amoxicillin against many strains of β-lactamase-producing bacteria that are resistant to amoxicillin alone. For information on the mechanism of action of penicillins, see Mechanism of Action in the Natural Penicillins General Statement 8:12.16.04.

In vitro studies indicate that clavulanic acid generally inhibits staphylococcal penicillinases, β-lactamases produced by Bacteroides fragilis, β-lactamases produced by Moraxella catarrhalis, and β-lactamases classified as Richmond-Sykes types II, III (TEM-type), IV, and V. Clavulanic acid can inhibit some cephalosporinases produced by Proteus vulgaris, Bacteroides fragilis, and Burkholderia cepacia, but generally does not inhibit inducible, chromosomally mediated cephalosporinases classified as Richmond-Sykes type I.

Clavulanic acid generally acts as an irreversible, competitive inhibitor of β-lactamases. The mechanism by which clavulanic acid binds to and inhibits β-lactamases varies depending on the specific β-lactamase involved. Because clavulanic acid is structurally similar to penicillins and cephalosporins, it initially acts as a competitive inhibitor and binds to the active site on the β-lactamase. An inactive acyl intermediate is then formed but it is only transiently inactive since the intermediate can be hydrolyzed, resulting in restoration of β-lactamase activity and release of clavulanic acid degradation products. With many types of β-lactamases, however, subsequent reactions occur that lead to irreversible inactivation of the β-lactamase.

Synergism does not generally occur between amoxicillin and clavulanic acid if resistance to aminopenicillins is intrinsic (i.e., results from the presence of a permeability barrier in the outer membrane of the organism or alterations in the properties of the penicillin-binding proteins). Synergism between the drugs also does not generally occur against organisms that are susceptible to amoxicillin alone; however, a slight additive effect has been reported in vitro with amoxicillin and clavulanic acid against some non-β-lactamase-producing strains of Staphylococcus aureus and Haemophilus influenzae and some strains of Streptococcus pneumoniae and group A β-hemolytic streptococci. This additive effect may result from clavulanic acid's intrinsic antibacterial activity, but this activity generally is inadequate for the drug to be therapeutically useful alone.

Clavulanic acid, like cefoxitin and imipenem, can induce production of chromosomally mediated type I cephalosporinases in certain gram-negative bacteria that possess these enzymes (e.g., some strains of Enterobacter, Pseudomonas aeruginosa, Morganella morganii). Concomitant use of clavulanic acid with a β-lactam antibiotic that is inactivated by inducible β-lactamases theoretically could result in an antagonistic effect against organisms that possess these enzymes. However, high concentrations of clavulanic acid generally are required to induce production of these β-lactamases and the clinical importance of this effect has not been determined.

SPECTRUM

The fixed combination of amoxicillin and clavulanate potassium (amoxicillin/clavulanate) is active in vitro against organisms susceptible to amoxicillin alone. In addition, because clavulanic acid can inhibit certain β-lactamases that generally inactivate amoxicillin, amoxicillin/clavulanate is active in vitro against many β-lactamase-producing organisms that are resistant to amoxicillin alone.

Clavulanic acid alone has some antibacterial activity and is active in vitro against some gram-positive and gram-negative bacteria including Moraxella catarrhalis, Bacteroides fragilis, Haemophilus influenzae, Legionella, Neisseria gonorrhoeae, and Staphylococcus aureus. However, high concentrations of clavulanic acid are necessary to inhibit most susceptible organisms and the drug is not therapeutically useful alone.

● In Vitro Susceptibility Testing

The Clinical and Laboratory Standards Institute) states that, for streptococci (including Streptococcus pneumoniae), results of in vitro susceptibility tests using penicillin can be used to predict susceptibility to amoxicillin/clavulanate and, for non-β-lactamase-producing enterococci, results of in vitro susceptibility tests using penicillin or ampicillin can be used to predict susceptibility to amoxicillin/clavulanate. However, to determine susceptibility of staphylococci, Enterobacteriaceae, and Haemophilus to amoxicillin/clavulanate, CLSI recommends that disk-diffusion and dilution susceptibility tests be performed using appropriate combinations of amoxicillin/clavulanate. For information on interpretive criteria specified for ampicillin, see Spectrum: In Vitro Susceptibility Testing, in the Aminopenicillins General Statement 8:12.16.08.

To test in vitro susceptibility to amoxicillin/clavulanate, a 2:1 ratio of amoxicillin to clavulanic acid generally is used for both disk-diffusion and agar or broth dilution procedures.

Results of in vitro susceptibility tests with amoxicillin/clavulanate may be affected by inoculum size or test media. However, results of the tests are not generally affected by pH changes between 6 and 8 or the presence of serum.

CLSI, the manufacturers, and most clinicians recommend that strains of staphylococci resistant to penicillinase-resistant penicillins also be considered resistant to amoxicillin/clavulanate, although results of in vitro susceptibility tests may indicate that the organism is susceptible to the drug. In addition, CLSI recommends that non-β-lactamase-producing strains of Haemophilus influenzae that are resistant to ampicillin (BLNAR H. influenzae) be considered resistant to amoxicillin/clavulanate despite the fact that results of in vitro susceptibility tests may indicate that the organisms are susceptible to the drug.

Disk Susceptibility Tests

When disk-diffusion procedures are used to test susceptibility to amoxicillin/clavulanate, a disk containing 20 mcg of amoxicillin and 10 mcg of clavulanic acid is used.

When disk-diffusion susceptibility tests are performed according to CLSI standardized procedures using CLSI interpretive criteria, *Staphylococcus* with growth inhibition zones of 20 mm or greater are considered susceptible to amoxicillin/clavulanate and those with zones of 19 mm or less are resistant to the drug.

When disk-diffusion susceptibility tests are performed according to CLSI standardized procedures, Enterobacteriaceae with growth inhibition zones of 18 mm or greater are susceptible to amoxicillin/clavulanate, those with zones of 14–17 mm have intermediate susceptibility, and those with zones of 13 mm or less are resistant to the drug.

When disk-diffusion susceptibility testing for *Haemophilus* is performed according to CLSI standardized procedures, *Haemophilus* with growth inhibition zones of 20 mm or greater are considered susceptible to amoxicillin/clavulanate and those with zones of 19 mm or less are resistant to the drug.

Dilution Susceptibility Tests

For dilution susceptibility testing (agar or broth dilution), CLSI recommends that a 2:1 ratio of amoxicillin to clavulanic acid be used with each dilution and that the MIC of amoxicillin/clavulanate be reported as mcg/mL of amoxicillin and mcg/mL of clavulanic acid. The MIC of amoxicillin/clavulanate has also been reported as mcg of amoxicillin plus mcg of clavulanic acid per mL (i.e., mcg of "Augmentin" per mL) or in terms of the MIC of amoxicillin in the presence of a specified concentration of clavulanic acid.

When dilution tests are performed using CLSI standardized procedures and a 2:1 ratio of amoxicillin to clavulanic acid with each dilution, *Staphylococcus* with MICs of 4 mcg/mL or less of amoxicillin and 2 mcg/mL or less of clavulanic acid are considered susceptible to amoxicillin/clavulanate and those with MICs of 8 mcg/mL or greater of amoxicillin and 4 mcg/mL or greater of clavulanic acid are resistant to the drug.

When broth dilution susceptibility for *S. pneumoniae* (from nonmeningeal sites only) is performed using CLSI standardized procedure and cation-adjusted Mueller-Hinton broth (supplemented with 2–5% lysed horse blood), *S. pneumoniae* with MICs of 2 mcg/mL or less of amoxicillin and 1 mcg/mL or less of clavulanic acid are considered susceptible to amoxicillin/clavulanate, those with MICs of 4 mcg/mL of amoxicillin and 2 mcg/mL of clavulanic acid have intermediate susceptibility, and those with MICs of 8 mcg/mL or greater of amoxicillin and 4 mcg/mL or greater of clavulanic acid are resistant to amoxicillin/clavulanate.

When dilution susceptibility tests are performed according to CLSI standardized procedures using CLSI interpretive criteria, Enterobacteriaceae with MICs of 8 mcg/mL or less of amoxicillin and 4 mcg/mL or less of clavulanic acid are susceptible to amoxicillin/clavulanate, those with MICs of 16 mcg/mL of amoxicillin and 8 mcg/mL of clavulanic acid are considered to have intermediate susceptibility, those with MICs of 16 mcg/mL of amoxicillin and 8 mcg/mL of clavulanic acid have intermediate susceptibility, and those with MICs of 32 mcg/mL or greater of amoxicillin and 16 mcg/mL or greater of clavulanic acid are resistant to the drug.

When susceptibility of *Haemophilus* is tested in a broth dilution procedure according to CLSI standardized procedures using HTM, *Haemophilus* with MICs of 4 mcg/mL or less of amoxicillin and 2 mcg/mL or less of clavulanic acid are susceptible to amoxicillin/clavulanate and those with MICs of 8 mcg/mL or greater of amoxicillin and 4 mcg/mL or greater of clavulanic acid are resistant to the drug.

● Gram-positive Aerobic Bacteria

Amoxicillin/clavulanate is active in vitro against most gram-positive aerobic cocci, including penicillinase-producing and nonpenicillinase-producing strains of *Staphylococcus aureus*, *S. epidermidis*, and *S. saprophyticus*; group A β-hemolytic streptococci; *Streptococcus pneumoniae*; *Enterococcus faecalis*; and viridans streptococci. Amoxicillin/clavulanate is active in vitro against many strains of penicillinase-producing staphylococci that are resistant to amoxicillin alone; however, staphylococci resistant to penicillinase-resistant penicillins are generally also resistant to amoxicillin/clavulanate.

In one in vitro study using dilutions containing a 2:1 ratio of amoxicillin to clavulanic acid, the MIC$_{90}$ (minimum inhibitory concentration of the drug at which 90% of strains tested are inhibited) of amoxicillin/clavulanate for both penicillinase-producing and nonpenicillinase-producing strains of *S. aureus* was 8 mcg/mL of amoxicillin and 4 mcg/mL of clavulanic acid and the MIC$_{90}$ of the drug for group A β-hemolytic streptococci, *S. pneumoniae*, and *E. faecalis* was 0.03–1 mcg/mL of amoxicillin and 0.015–0.5 mcg/mL of clavulanic acid. In a

similar in vitro study, the MIC$_{90}$ for penicillinase-producing *S. aureus* was 1.33 mcg/mL of amoxicillin and 0.67 mcg/mL of clavulanic acid.

● Gram-negative Aerobic Bacteria

Neisseria

Amoxicillin/clavulanate is active in vitro against most strains of *Neisseria meningitidis* and penicillinase-producing and nonpenicillinase-producing *N. gonorrhoeae*. Although penicillinase-producing *N. gonorrhoeae* (PPNG) are usually resistant to amoxicillin alone, these strains usually are susceptible in vitro to amoxicillin/clavulanate.

The MIC$_{90}$ of amoxicillin/clavulanate for *N. meningitidis* is reportedly 0.12 mcg/mL of amoxicillin and 0.06 mcg/mL of clavulanic acid. In one in vitro study using dilutions containing a 2:1 ratio of amoxicillin to clavulanic acid, the MIC of amoxicillin/clavulanate for nonpenicillinase-producing *N. gonorrhoeae* ranged from 0.08–2.7 mcg/mL of amoxicillin and 0.04–1.3 mcg/mL of clavulanic acid and the MIC for PPNG ranged from 0.67–2.7 mcg/mL of amoxicillin and 0.33–1.3 mcg/mL of clavulanic acid.

Haemophilus

Amoxicillin/clavulanate is active in vitro against most β-lactamase-producing and non-β-lactamase-producing strains of *Haemophilus influenzae*, *H. parainfluenzae*, and *H. ducreyi*. However, strains of non-β-lactamase-producing*Haemophilus* that are resistant to aminopenicillins may also be resistant to amoxicillin/clavulanate.

In one in vitro study using dilutions containing a 2:1 ratio of amoxicillin to clavulanate potassium, the MIC of amoxicillin/clavulanate for non-β-lactamase-producing strains of *H. influenzae* was 0.06–0.5 mcg/mL of amoxicillin and 0.03–0.25 mcg/mL of clavulanic acid and the MIC of the drug for β-lactamase-producing strains was 0.5–2 mcg/mL of amoxicillin and 0.25–1 mcg/mL of clavulanic acid. In another in vitro study using β-lactamase-producing *H. influenzae* type b, the MIC of amoxicillin alone ranged from 6.25–12.5 mcg/mL and the MIC of clavulanic acid alone ranged from 12.5–25 mcg/mL, but the MIC of amoxicillin/clavulanate was 0.36 mcg/mL of amoxicillin and 0.36 mcg/mL of clavulanic acid.

Moraxella catarrhalis

Amoxicillin/clavulanate is active in vitro against both β-lactamase-producing and non-β-lactamase-producing strains of *Moraxella catarrhalis*. The MIC$_{90}$ of amoxicillin plus clavulanate acid is 0.005 mcg/mL for non-β-lactamase-producing strains of *M. catarrhalis* and 0.125–0.25 mcg/mL for β-lactamase-producing strains. In an in vitro study of β-lactamase-producing *M. catarrhalis*, the MIC of amoxicillin alone was 25–50 mcg/mL, the MIC of clavulanic acid alone was 2.5–12.5 mcg/mL, and the MIC of amoxicillin plus clavulanate acid was 0.02–0.05 mcg/mL.

Enterobacteriaceae

Amoxicillin/clavulanate is active in vitro against Enterobacteriaceae that are susceptible to amoxicillin alone (e.g., some strains of *Escherichia coli*, *Proteus mirabilis*, *Salmonella*, *Shigella*). In addition, amoxicillin/clavulanate is active in vitro against many β-lactamase-producing strains of *Citrobacter diversus*, *K. pneumoniae*, *P. mirabilis*, and *P. vulgaris* and some strains of β-lactamase-producing *E. coli* and *Enterobacter* that are resistant to amoxicillin alone.

In one in vitro study using dilutions containing a 2:1 ratio of amoxicillin to clavulanic acid, the MIC$_{90}$ of amoxicillin/clavulanate for *E. coli* was 32 mcg/mL of amoxicillin and 16 mcg/mL of clavulanic acid, the MIC$_{90}$ for *Klebsiella* and *P. vulgaris* was 8 mcg/mL of amoxicillin and 4 mcg/mL of clavulanic acid, and the MIC$_{90}$ for *C. diversus* and *P. mirabilis* was 1–2 mcg/mL of amoxicillin and 0.5–1 mcg/mL of clavulanic acid.

Although rare strains of *C. freundii*, *Enterobacter cloacae*, *Morganella morganii*, *Providencia*, and *Serratia* are inhibited in vitro by high concentrations of amoxicillin/clavulanate, most strains of these organisms are considered resistant to the drug.

Other Gram-negative Aerobic Bacteria

Amoxicillin/clavulanate has some in vitro activity against *Legionella*, although the drug may not be effective clinically. In one in vitro study using CYEA media containing 2.5 mcg/mL of clavulanic acid, *L. pneumophila*, *L. micdadei*, and

L. bozemanii were inhibited by 0.003 mcg/mL of amoxicillin plus clavulanate potassium. In another in vitro study using *L. pneumophila* and Mueller-Hinton agar, the MIC of amoxicillin alone was 1.95 mcg/mL, the MIC of clavulanic acid alone was 0.2–0.4 mcg/mL, and the MIC of amoxicillin plus clavulanate potassium was 0.61 mcg/mL.

Amoxicillin and clavulanic acid is generally inactive against *Pseudomonas*; however, the drug may be active in vitro against *Burkholderia pseudomallei*.

● Anaerobic Bacteria

Amoxicillin/clavulanate is active in vitro against gram-positive anaerobic bacteria including *Clostridium*, *Peptococcus*, and *Peptostreptococcus*.

Amoxicillin/clavulanate is active in vitro against *Prevotella melaninogenica* and *P. oralis*. Although the *Bacteroides fragilis* group (e.g., *B. fragilis*, *B. distasonis*, *B. ovatus*, *B. thetaiotamicron*, *B. vulgatus*) usually is resistant to amoxicillin alone, amoxicillin/clavulanate is active in vitro against many strains of these organisms. In one in vitro study, the MIC of amoxicillin in the presence of 0.75 mcg/mL of clavulanic acid was 0.5–1 mcg/mL for *B. fragilis*, *B. ovatus*, *B. thetaiotamicron*, and *B. vulgatus* and 4 mcg/mL for *B. distasonis*.

● Mycobacterium

Although the clinical importance has not been determined to date, amoxicillin/clavulanate is active in vitro against some strains of *Mycobacterium tuberculosis* and *M. fortuitum*. *M. tuberculosis* and *M. fortuitum* are β-lactamase producers and are generally resistant to amoxicillin alone. In one in vitro study using dilutions containing a 2:1 ratio of amoxicillin to clavulanic acid, the MIC of amoxicillin/clavulanate for *M. tuberculosis* was 1–2 mcg/mL of amoxicillin and 0.5–1 mcg/mL of clavulanic acid and the minimum bactericidal concentration (MBC) of the drug was 1–4 mcg/mL of amoxicillin and 0.5–2 mcg/mL of clavulanic acid. In another study using *M. fortuitum*, the MIC of amoxicillin/clavulanate for most strains was 4–16 mcg/mL of amoxicillin and 2–8 mcg/mL of clavulanic acid, although some strains had an MIC of 32 mcg/mL or greater of amoxicillin and 16 mcg/mL or greater of clavulanic acid.

RESISTANCE

Gram-negative aerobic bacilli that produce Richmond-Sykes type I chromosomally mediated β-lactamases (e.g., *Citrobacter freundii*, *Enterobacter cloacae*, *Serratia marcescens*, *Pseudomonas aeruginosa*) are generally resistant to amoxicillin/clavulanate, since clavulanic acid does not inhibit most type I β-lactamases. Strains of *E. coli* with chromosomally mediated β-lactamases are also resistant to amoxicillin/clavulanate.

Strains of *E. cloacae* and *Providencia stuartii* that appear to be resistant to amoxicillin/clavulanate but susceptible to ampicillin in vitro have been reported rarely.

PHARMACOKINETICS

Crossover studies using fixed combinations of amoxicillin and clavulanate potassium, amoxicillin alone, and clavulanate potassium alone indicate that concomitant administration of clavulanate potassium does not affect the pharmacokinetics of amoxicillin; however, concomitant administration of amoxicillin reportedly may increase GI absorption and renal elimination of clavulanate potassium compared with administration of clavulanate potassium alone.

For additional information on absorption, distribution, and elimination of amoxicillin, see Pharmacokinetics in the Aminopenicillins General Statement 8:12.16.08 and in Amoxicillin 8:12.16.08.

● Absorption

Amoxicillin trihydrate and clavulanate potassium are both generally stable in the presence of acidic gastric secretions and are well absorbed following oral administration of the fixed combination of amoxicillin and clavulanate potassium (amoxicillin/clavulanate). Peak serum concentrations of amoxicillin and of clavulanic acid are generally attained within 1–2.5 hours following oral administration of a single dose of conventional preparations of amoxicillin/clavulanate

in fasting adults or a single dose of extended-release tablets in adults fed a standardized meal.

Following oral administration of a single conventional tablet containing 250 mg of amoxicillin and 125 mg of clavulanic acid in healthy, fasting adults, peak serum concentrations of amoxicillin and of clavulanic acid average 3.7–4.8 mcg/mL and 2.2–3.5 mcg/mL, respectively. Following oral administration of a single conventional tablet containing 500 mg of amoxicillin and 125 mg of clavulanic acid in healthy, fasting adults, peak serum concentrations of amoxicillin average 6.5–9.7 mcg/mL and peak serum concentrations of clavulanic acid average 2.1–3.9 mcg/mL. The manufacturer states that serum concentrations of the drugs achieved following oral administration of a single chewable tablet containing 250 mg of amoxicillin and 62.5 mg of clavulanic acid or 2 chewable tablets each containing 125 and 31.25 mg of the drugs, respectively, are similar to those achieved following oral administration of a single equivalent dose of the oral suspension. The manufacturer also states that serum concentrations of amoxicillin achieved following oral administration of conventional preparations or extended-release tablets of amoxicillin/clavulanate are similar to those achieved following oral administration of equivalent doses of amoxicillin alone.

Following oral administration of a single dose of 250 mg of amoxicillin and 62.5 mg of clavulanic acid as an oral suspension, peak serum concentrations of amoxicillin average 6.9 mcg/mL and peak concentrations of clavulanic acid average 1.6 mcg/mL. In one study in children 2–5 years of age with urinary tract infections, oral administration of a single dose of 125 mg of amoxicillin and 31.75 mg of clavulanic acid as an oral suspension resulted in serum concentrations of amoxicillin that averaged 9.4, 9.7, and 6.5 mcg/mL and serum concentrations of clavulanic acid that averaged 2.1, 4.4, and 2.5 mcg/mL at 30, 60, and 90 minutes, respectively, after the dose.

Studies in healthy adults using conventional preparations of amoxicillin/clavulanate indicate that presence of food in the GI tract does not affect oral absorption of either amoxicillin or clavulanic acid following administration of fixed-combination preparations of the drugs. However, amoxicillin and clavulanate are optimally absorbed from extended-release tablets of the combination when administered orally at the beginning of a standardized meal (612 kcal, 89.3 g carbohydrate, 24.9 g fat, and 14 g protein); administration of the extended-release tablets with a high-fat meal is not recommended because clavulanate absorption is decreased, and administration of these tablets in the fasting state is not recommended because amoxicillin absorption is decreased. GI absorption of the drugs from extended-release tablets is not affected by administration simultaneously with or 2 hours before a magnesium and aluminum-containing antacid (Maalox®).

● Distribution

Following administration of amoxicillin/clavulanate, amoxicillin and clavulanic acid are both distributed into the lungs, pleural fluid, and peritoneal fluid. Low concentrations (i.e., less than 1 mcg/mL) of each drug are attained in sputum and saliva.

In one study in fasting children who received a single amoxicillin dose of 35 mg/kg given as amoxicillin/clavulanate oral suspension, concentrations of amoxicillin and of clavulanic acid in middle ear effusions averaged 3 and 0.5 mcg/mL, respectively, 2 hours after the dose.

Only minimal concentrations of amoxicillin or clavulanic acid are attained in CSF following oral administration of amoxicillin/clavulanate in patients with uninflamed meninges; higher concentrations may be attained when meninges are inflamed. In one study in patients with uninflamed meninges who received a single 250-mg oral dose of clavulanic acid as the sodium salt, concentrations of clavulanic acid in CSF obtained 1–6 hours after the dose ranged from 0–0.2 mcg/mL. In 2 patients with continuous CSF drainage after neurosurgical procedures who received a similar oral dose of the drug, peak CSF concentrations of clavulanic acid were 2.4 and 0.4 mcg/mL, respectively, and occurred approximately 4 hours after the dose; concurrent serum concentrations of clavulanic acid were 2.3 and 0.3 mcg/mL, respectively.

Amoxicillin is 17–20% bound to serum proteins. In vitro or in vivo following oral administration, clavulanic acid is reportedly 22–30% bound to serum proteins at a concentration of 1–100 mcg/mL.

Amoxicillin and clavulanic acid readily cross the placenta. Amoxicillin and clavulanic acid are distributed into milk in low concentrations.

• Elimination

Serum concentrations of amoxicillin and clavulanic acid both decline in a biphasic manner and half-lives of the drugs are similar. Following oral administration of conventional preparations or extended-release tablets of amoxicillin/clavulanate in adults with normal renal function, amoxicillin has an elimination half-life of 1–1.3 hours and clavulanic acid has a distribution half-life of 0.28 hours and an elimination half-life of 0.78–1.2 hours. In one study in children 2–15 years of age, the elimination half-lives of amoxicillin and of clavulanic acid averaged 1.2 and 0.8 hours, respectively.

The metabolic fate of clavulanate potassium has not been fully elucidated; however, the drug appears to be extensively metabolized. In rats and dogs, the major metabolite of clavulanic acid is 1-amino-4-hydroxybutan-2-one; this metabolite has also been found in human urine following administration of clavulanic acid. Clavulanic acid is excreted in urine principally by glomerular filtration. Studies in dogs and rats using radiolabeled clavulanic acid indicate that 34–52, 25–27, and 16–33% of a dose of the drug is excreted in urine, feces, and respired air, respectively.

Following oral administration of a single oral dose of amoxicillin/clavulanate in adults with normal renal function, approximately 50–73 and 25–45% of the amoxicillin and clavulanic acid doses, respectively, are excreted unchanged in urine within 6–8 hours. In one study in healthy adults who received a single oral dose of 250 mg of amoxicillin and 125 mg of clavulanic acid, urinary concentrations of amoxicillin and of clavulanic acid averaged 381 and 118 mcg/mL, respectively, in urine collected over the first 2 hours after the dose.

Serum concentrations of amoxicillin and of clavulanic acid are higher and the serum half-lives prolonged in patients with renal impairment. In one study in patients with creatinine clearances of 9 mL/minute, the serum half-lives of amoxicillin and of clavulanic acid were 7.5 and 4.3 hours, respectively.

Oral probenecid administered shortly before or with amoxicillin/clavulanate competitively inhibits renal tubular secretion of amoxicillin and produces higher and prolonged serum concentrations of the drug; however, probenecid does not appreciably affect the pharmacokinetics of clavulanic acid. (See Drug Interactions: Probenecid.)

Amoxicillin and clavulanic acid are both removed by hemodialysis. The manufacturers state that clavulanic acid is also removed by peritoneal dialysis. Only minimal amounts of amoxicillin appear to be removed by peritoneal dialysis.

CHEMISTRY AND STABILITY

• Chemistry

Amoxicillin and clavulanate potassium (amoxicillin/clavulanate) is a fixed combination of amoxicillin trihydrate and the potassium salt of clavulanic acid. Amoxicillin is an aminopenicillin. (See Amoxicillin 8:12.16.08.) The fixed combination also is commercially available as extended-release tablets containing the sodium salt and the trihydrate of amoxicillin and the potassium salt of clavulanic acid. Clavulanic acid is a β-lactamase inhibitor produced by fermentation of *Streptomyces clavuligerus*. Clavulanic acid contains a β-lactam ring and is structurally similar to penicillins and cephalosporins; however, the β-lactam ring in clavulanic acid is fused with an oxazolidine ring rather than with a thiazolidine ring as in penicillins or a dihydrothiazine ring as in cephalosporins. Although clavulanic acid has only weak antibacterial activity when used alone, the combined use of clavulanic acid and certain penicillins or cephalosporins (e.g., amoxicillin, ampicillin, carbenicillin, cefoperazone, cefotaxime, penicillin G, ticarcillin) results in a synergistic effect that expands the spectrum of activity of the penicillin or cephalosporin against many strains of β-lactamase-producing bacteria. Clavulanic acid and its salts currently are commercially available in the US only in fixed combination with other drugs.

Amoxicillin/clavulanate is commercially available for oral administration as film-coated tablets containing a 2:1 or 4:1 ratio of amoxicillin to clavulanic acid; as scored tablets containing a 7:1 ratio of amoxicillin to clavulanic acid; as chewable tablets containing a 4:1 or 7:1 ratio of amoxicillin to clavulanic acid; as extended-release tablets containing a 16:1 ratio of the drugs; or a powder for oral suspension containing a 4:1, 7:1, or 14:1 ratio of the drugs.

Although commercially available amoxicillin/clavulanate contains amoxicillin as the trihydrate and clavulanic acid as the potassium salt, potency of amoxicillin is calculated on the anhydrous basis and potency of clavulanate potassium is expressed in terms of clavulanic acid.

Amoxicillin occurs as a white, practically odorless, crystalline powder and is sparingly soluble in water. Clavulanate potassium occurs as an off-white, crystalline powder and is very soluble in water and slightly soluble in alcohol at room temperature. Clavulanic acid has a pK_a of 2.7.

Each amoxicillin/clavulanate film-coated tablet containing 250 or 500 mg of amoxicillin and 125 mg of clavulanic acid or each scored tablet containing 875 mg of amoxicillin and 125 mg of clavulanic acid contains 0.63 mEq of potassium. Following reconstitution as directed, each 5 mL of amoxicillin/clavulanate oral suspension containing 125, 200, 250, 400, or 600 mg of amoxicillin contains 0.16, 0.14, 0.32, 0.29, or 0.23 mEq of potassium, respectively. Each amoxicillin/clavulanate chewable tablet containing 125, 200, 250, 400 mg, or 600 of amoxicillin contains 0.16, 0.14, 0.32, or 0.29 mEq of potassium, respectively. Each amoxicillin/clavulanate extended-release tablet containing 1 g of amoxicillin contains 0.32 mEq of potassium and 1.27 mEq of sodium. When reconstituted as directed, the oral suspensions have a pH of 4.8–6.8.

Amoxicillin/clavulanate chewable tables containing 200, 400, or 600 mg of amoxicillin and amoxicillin/clavulanate oral suspension containing 200 or 400 mg of amoxicillin per 5 mL contain aspartame; following metabolism of aspartame in the GI tract, each 200- or 400-mg chewable tablet provides 2.1 or 4.2 mg of phenylalanine, respectively, and each 5 mL of amoxicillin/clavulanate oral suspension containing 200, 400, or 600 mg of amoxicillin provides 7 mg of phenylalanine.

• Stability

Commercially available amoxicillin/clavulanate film-coated tablets, scored tablets, chewable tablets, extended-release tablets, and powder for oral suspension should be stored in tight containers at a temperature of 25°C or lower; exposure to excessive humidity should be avoided.

Following reconstitution, oral suspensions of amoxicillin/clavulanate should be stored at 2–8°C, and any unused suspension should be discarded after 10 days.

For further information on chemistry and stability, mechanism of action, spectrum, resistance, pharmacokinetics, uses, cautions, drug interactions, and laboratory test interferences of amoxicillin, see the Aminopenicillins General Statement 8:12.16.08 and see Amoxicillin 8:12.16.08.

PREPARATIONS

Excipients in commercially available drug preparations may have clinically important effects in some individuals; consult specific product labeling for details.

Amoxicillin (Trihydrate) and Clavulanate Potassium

Oral

For suspension	125 mg (of amoxicillin) per 5 mL and 31.25 mg (of clavulanic acid) per 5 mL*	**Amoxicillin and Clavulanate Potassium for Oral Suspension** Augmentin®, GlaxoSmithKline
	200 mg (of amoxicillin) per 5 mL and 28.5 mg (of clavulanic acid) per 5 mL*	**Amoxicillin and Clavulanate Potassium for Oral Suspension**
	250 mg (of amoxicillin) per 5 mL and 62.5 mg (of clavulanic acid) per 5 mL*	**Amoxicillin and Clavulanate Potassium for Oral Suspension** Augmentin®, GlaxoSmithKline
	400 mg (of amoxicillin) per 5 mL and 57 mg (of clavulanic acid) per 5 mL*	**Amoxicillin and Clavulanate Potassium for Oral Suspension**
	600 mg (of amoxicillin) per 5 mL and 42.9 mg (of clavulanic acid) per 5 mL*	**Amoxicillin and Clavulanate Potassium for Oral Suspension** Augmentin ES-600®, GlaxoSmithKline

Tablets, chewable	200 mg (of amoxicillin) and 28.5 mg (of clavulanic acid)*	**Amoxicillin and Clavulanate Potassium Chewable Tablets**
	400 mg (of amoxicillin) and 57 mg (of clavulanic acid)*	**Amoxicillin and Clavulanate Potassium Chewable Tablets**
Tablets, film-coated	250 mg (of amoxicillin) and 125 mg (of clavulanic acid)*	**Amoxicillin and Clavulanate Potassium Tablets**
	500 mg (of amoxicillin) and 125 mg (of clavulanic acid)*	**Amoxicillin and Clavulanate Potassium Tablets**
	875 mg (of amoxicillin) and 125 mg (of clavulanic acid)*	**Amoxicillin and Clavulanate Potassium Tablets**
		Augmentin®, GlaxoSmithKline

Amoxicillin (Trihydrate), Amoxicillin Sodium, and Clavulanate Potassium

Oral

Tablets, extended-release	1 g (of amoxicillin) and 62.5 mg (of clavulanic acid)*	**Amoxicillin and Clavulanate Potassium Extended-release Tablets**

† Use is not currently included in the labeling approved by the US Food and Drug Administration.

* available from one or more manufacturer, distributor, and/or repackager by generic (nonproprietary) name

Selected Revisions February 23, 2022, © Copyright, July 1, 2000, American Society of Health-System Pharmacists, Inc.

Ampicillin Sodium, Ampicillin Trihydrate

8:12.16.08 • AMINOPENICILLINS

■ Ampicillin is an aminopenicillin antibiotic.

USES

Ampicillin shares the uses of other aminopenicillins and is used principally for the treatment of infections caused by susceptible gram-negative bacteria (e.g., *Haemophilus influenzae*, *Escherichia coli*, *Proteus mirabilis*, *Salmonella*). Ampicillin also is used for the treatment of infections caused by susceptible gram-positive bacteria (e.g., *Streptococcus pneumoniae*, enterococci, nonpenicillinase-producing staphylococci, *Listeria*); however, like other aminopenicillins, ampicillin generally should not be used for the treatment of streptococcal or staphylococcal infections when a natural penicillin would be effective. Orally administered ampicillin should not be used for the initial treatment of severe, life-threatening infections, but may be used as follow-up therapy after parenteral ampicillin therapy. For specific information on the uses of ampicillin, see Uses in the Aminopenicillins General Statement 8:12.16.08.

DOSAGE AND ADMINISTRATION

● Reconstitution and Administration

Ampicillin trihydrate is administered orally. Although ampicillin may be given orally with meals, maximum absorption is achieved when the drug is administered 1 hour before or 2 hours after meals.

Ampicillin sodium may be administered by IM or slow IV injection or by IV infusion.

Parenteral forms of ampicillin should be used only in the treatment of moderately severe or severe infections. Direct IV injections should be made slowly over 10–15 minutes to avoid the possibility of seizures. For intermittent IV infusion, the concentration of ampicillin and rate of infusion should be adjusted so that the total dose of the drug is administered before 10% or more of the drug is inactivated in the IV solution. (See Chemistry and Stability: Stability.)

Ampicillin sodium preparations for parenteral use should be reconstituted according to the manufacturers' instructions. Ampicillin sodium solutions should be inspected visually for particulate matter and discoloration prior to administration whenever solution and container permit.

● Dosage

Dosage of ampicillin sodium and ampicillin trihydrate is expressed in terms of ampicillin.

The manufacturers' dosage recommendations for adults usually are the same for both parenteral and oral routes; however, higher serum concentrations usually are attained parenterally, and this route is used for severe infections.

General Adult Dosage

The usual adult dosage of ampicillin for the treatment of respiratory tract or skin and skin structure infections is 250–500 mg every 6 hours. For the treatment of GI or urinary tract infections, the usual adult dosage is 500 mg every 6 hours. For severe infections, larger doses may be required.

The usual adult dosage of ampicillin for the treatment of septicemia or bacterial meningitis is 8–14 g or 150–200 mg/kg daily given parenterally in equally divided doses every 3–4 hours. For the initial treatment of septicemia or meningitis, ampicillin should be given IV for at least 3 days but may then be given IM.

General Pediatric Dosage

For oral therapy, most manufacturers state that children weighing more than 20 kg may receive the usual adult dosage of ampicillin. For parenteral therapy, some manufacturers recommend that the usual adult dosage be used in children weighing more than 20 kg, whereas other manufacturers and many clinicians recommend that the usual adult dosage be used in those weighing more than 40 kg. Pediatric dosage should not exceed dosage recommended for similar infections in adults.

For the treatment of respiratory tract or skin and skin structure infections, the usual dosage of ampicillin for children weighing 40 kg or less is 25–50 mg/kg daily administered in equally divided doses every 6 hours. For the treatment of GI or urinary tract infections, the usual dosage for children weighing 40 kg or less is 50–100 mg/kg daily given in equally divided doses every 6 hours.

For the treatment of septicemia or CNS infections, the usual pediatric dosage recommended by the manufacturers is 100–200 mg/kg daily given in divided doses every 3–4 hours, starting with IV administration for 3 days and continuing with IM administration. For empiric treatment of bacterial meningitis in neonates and children younger than 2 months of age, many clinicians recommend that an IV ampicillin dosage of 100–300 mg/kg daily be given in divided doses in conjunction with IM gentamicin pending results of in vitro susceptibility tests. For the empiric treatment of bacterial meningitis in children 2 months to 12 years of age, many clinicians recommend that an IV ampicillin dosage of 200–400 mg/kg daily be given in divided doses every 4–6 hours in conjunction with IV chloramphenicol. If bacterial susceptibility data are not available and clinical and bacteriologic response is unsatisfactory after 24–48 hours, other appropriate anti-infective therapy should be substituted.

When IM or IV ampicillin is used in neonates younger than 7 days of age, the American Academy of Pediatrics (AAP) recommends a dosage of 50 mg/kg every 12 hours in those weighing 2 kg or less or 50 mg/kg every 8 hours in those weighing more than 2 kg. For neonates 8–28 days of age, AAP recommends an IM or IV dosage of 50 mg/kg every 8 hours in those weighing 2 kg or less or 50 mg/kg every 6 hours in those weighing more than 2 kg. AAP states that higher ampicillin dosage may be necessary for the treatment of meningitis in neonates. For the treatment of meningitis caused by *Streptococcus agalactiae* (group B streptococci; GBS), some experts recommend that neonates 28 days of age or younger receive IV ampicillin in a dosage of 75 mg/kg every 6 hours, regardless of weight; others recommend a dosage of 200–300 mg/kg daily given IV in 3 divided doses in neonates 7 days of age or younger or a dosage of 300 mg/kg daily given IV in 4 divided doses in neonates older than 7 days of age. AAP states that a dosage of 100 mg/kg every 12 hours is acceptable for the treatment of early-onset group B streptococcal septicemia *without* meningitis in neonates 7 days of age or younger.

When IM or IV ampicillin is used in pediatric patients beyond the neonatal period, AAP recommends a dosage of 100–150 mg/kg daily given in 4 divided doses for the treatment of mild to moderate infections or a dosage of 200–400 mg/kg daily given in 4 divided doses for the treatment of severe infections. The highest dosage should be used for the treatment of CNS infections. When oral ampicillin is used in pediatric patients beyond the neonatal period, AAP recommends a dosage of 50–100 mg/kg daily in 4 divided doses. AAP states that oral ampicillin is inappropriate for the treatment of severe infections.

Treatment of Enterococcal Endocarditis

If IV ampicillin is used for the treatment of enterococcal endocarditis, the American Heart Association (AHA) and others recommend that adults receive 2 g every 4 hours in conjunction with gentamicin. Treatment with both drugs generally should be continued for 4–6 weeks, but patients who had symptoms of infection for more than 3 months before treatment was initiated and patients with prosthetic heart valves require a minimum of 6 weeks of therapy with both drugs.

Prevention of Perinatal Group B Streptococcal Disease

If IV ampicillin is used as an alternative to IV penicillin G for intrapartum anti-infective prophylaxis for prevention of early-onset neonatal group B streptococcal (GBS) disease† (see Prevention of Perinatal Group B Streptococcal Disease under Uses in the Aminopenicillins General Statement 8:12.16.08), the American College of Obstetricians and Gynecologists (ACOG), AAP, and other experts recommend an initial IV ampicillin loading dose of 2 g at the onset of labor or rupture of membranes followed by 1 g IV every 4 hours until delivery.

Regardless of whether anti-infective prophylaxis was administered to the mother, appropriate diagnostic evaluations and anti-infective therapy should be initiated in the neonate if signs or symptoms of active infection develop.

Prevention of Bacterial Endocarditis

If IM or IV ampicillin is used for prevention of bacterial endocarditis† in patients with certain cardiac conditions who are undergoing certain dental procedures or certain other procedures who cannot receive an oral regimen (see Prevention of

Bacterial Endocarditis under Uses in the Aminopenicillins General Statement 8:12.16.08), AHA recommends that adults receive a single 2-g dose and that children receive a single 50-mg/kg dose of the drug given 30–60 minutes prior to the procedure.

When selecting anti-infectives for prevention of bacterial endocarditis, the current recommendations published by AHA should be consulted.

Duration of Therapy

The duration of ampicillin therapy depends on the type and severity of infection and should be determined by the clinical and bacteriologic response of the patient. For most infections, except gonorrhea, therapy should be continued for at least 48–72 hours after the patient becomes asymptomatic or evidence of eradication of the infection has been obtained. Persistent infections may require several weeks of therapy.

DOSAGE IN RENAL IMPAIRMENT

In patients with renal impairment, doses and/or frequency of administration of ampicillin should be modified in response to the degree of renal impairment, severity of the infection, and susceptibility of the causative organism. Some clinicians suggest that adults with glomerular filtration rates of 10–50 mL/minute receive the usual dose of ampicillin every 6–12 hours and that adults with glomerular filtration rates less than 10 mL/minute receive the usual dose every 12–16 hours. Alternatively, some clinicians suggest that modification of usual dosage of ampicillin is unnecessary in adults with creatinine clearances of 30 mL/minute or greater, but adults with creatinine clearances of 10 mL/minute or less should receive the usual dose of the drug every 8 hours.

Patients undergoing hemodialysis should receive a supplemental dose of ampicillin after each dialysis period.

CAUTIONS

• Adverse Effects

Adverse effects reported with ampicillin are similar to those reported with other aminopenicillins; however, diarrhea and rash have been reported more frequently with ampicillin than with other currently available aminopenicillins. For information on adverse effects reported with aminopenicillins, see Cautions in the Aminopenicillins General Statement 8:12.16.08.

• Precautions and Contraindications

Ampicillin shares the toxic potentials of the penicillins, including the risk of hypersensitivity reactions, and the usual precautions of penicillin therapy should be observed. Prior to initiation of therapy with ampicillin careful inquiry should be made concerning previous hypersensitivity reactions to penicillins, cephalosporins, or other drugs. There is clinical and laboratory evidence of partial cross-allergenicity among penicillins and other β-lactam antibiotics including cephalosporins, cephamycins, and 1-oxa-β-lactams. Ampicillin is contraindicated in patients who are hypersensitive to any penicillin.

Because a high percentage of patients with infectious mononucleosis have developed rash during therapy with aminopenicillins, ampicillin probably should not be used in patients with this disease.

Renal, hepatic, and hematologic systems should be evaluated periodically during prolonged therapy with ampicillin.

For a more complete discussion of these and other precautions associated with the use of ampicillin, see Cautions: Precautions and Contraindications, in the Aminopenicillins General Statement 8:12.16.08.

• Pregnancy, Fertility, and Lactation

Pregnancy

Safe use of ampicillin during pregnancy has not been established. There are no adequate or controlled studies using ampicillin in pregnant women, and the drug should be used during pregnancy only when clearly needed. However, ampicillin has been administered to pregnant women, especially in the treatment of urinary tract infections, without evidence of adverse effects to the fetus.

Lactation

Because ampicillin is distributed into milk, the drug should be used with caution in nursing women.

SPECTRUM

Based on its spectrum of activity, ampicillin is classified as an aminopenicillin. For information on the classification of penicillins based on spectra of activity, see the Preface to the Penicillins 8:12.16.

Ampicillin generally has the same spectrum of activity and the same level of activity against susceptible organisms as amoxicillin; however, ampicillin is less active in vitro on a weight basis than amoxicillin against enterococci and *Salmonella* but more active than amoxicillin against *Shigella* and *Enterobacter*. For specific information on in vitro susceptibility testing and information on the spectrum of activity of ampicillin and resistance to the drug, see the sections on Spectrum and on Resistance in the Aminopenicillins General Statement 8:12.16.08.

PHARMACOKINETICS

For additional information on absorption and distribution of ampicillin and information on elimination of the drug, see Pharmacokinetics in the Aminopenicillins General Statement 8:12.16.08.

• Absorption

Ampicillin trihydrate generally are stable in the presence of acidic gastric secretions, and 30–55% of an oral dose of the drugs is absorbed from the GI tract in fasting adults. Although peak serum concentrations may occur as soon as 1 hour after administration, the maximum serum concentration usually is attained in approximately 2 hours. Two hours after oral administration of 250 mg of ampicillin in fasting individuals, average peak serum concentrations of 1.8–2.9 mcg/mL are attained. A 500-mg oral dose results in average peak serum concentrations of 3–6 mcg/mL. Concentrations of the antibiotic in serum are less than 1 mcg/mL 6 hours after a 500-mg oral dose. Although higher peak serum ampicillin concentrations and larger areas under the serum concentration-time curves (AUCs) have been reported following oral administration of anhydrous ampicillin than following the trihydrate, the differences are generally not considered clinically important. As oral dosage of ampicillin is increased from 500 mg to 2 g, the fraction of the dose absorbed from the GI tract decreases and, there is a nonlinear relationship between dosage and peak serum concentrations or AUCs of ampicillin.

Presence of food in the GI tract generally decreases the rate and extent of absorption of ampicillin.

Following IM administration of ampicillin sodium, peak serum concentrations generally are attained more quickly and are higher than those resulting from equivalent doses of ampicillin given orally. In premature neonates younger than 7 days of age, IM administration of a single ampicillin dose of 50 mg/kg has been reported to produce mean serum concentrations of 104, 87, 60, and 31 mcg/mL at 1, 4, 8, and 12 hours, respectively, after the dose. The same dose in full-term neonates younger than 7 days of age produced mean serum concentrations of 75, 64, 34, and 20 mcg/mL at the same time intervals.

Following IV administration over 20 minutes of a single 2-g dose of ampicillin in healthy adults, serum concentrations of ampicillin averaged 47.6, 23.3, 10.8, and 3.7 mcg/mL at 30 minutes, 1 hour, 2 hours, and 4 hours, respectively, after the infusion.

Serum ampicillin concentrations are higher and the serum half-life is prolonged in patients with impaired renal function. Serum concentrations of the drug also are higher and more prolonged in premature or full-term neonates younger than 6 days of age than in full-term neonates 6 days of age or older.

• Distribution

In one study in neonates with meningitis, average ampicillin concentrations in CSF ranged from 1–28 mcg/mL (11–65% of simultaneous serum concentrations) during the 7-hour period following IV administration of 40–70 mg/kg. Highest CSF concentrations occurred at 3–7 hours.

Ampicillin is distributed into bile. Biliary concentrations of ampicillin in patients with normal biliary function may be 1–30 times greater than simultaneous serum concentrations following a single oral dose of ampicillin.

CHEMISTRY AND STABILITY

● Chemistry

Ampicillin is an aminopenicillin. Ampicillin differs structurally from penicillin G only in the presence of an amino group at the α-position on the benzene ring at R on the penicillin nucleus.

Ampicillin is commercially available as ampicillin trihydrate for oral administration and as the sodium salt for parenteral administration. Potency of ampicillin trihydrate and ampicillin sodium is expressed in terms of ampicillin and is calculated on the anhydrous basis.

Ampicillin trihydrate occurs as a white, practically odorless, crystalline powder that is slightly soluble in water. Ampicillin trihydrate reportedly has aqueous solubility of about 6 mg/mL at 20°C and about 10 mg/mL at 40°C. Ampicillin sodium occurs as a white to off-white, odorless or practically odorless, crystalline, hygroscopic powder and is very soluble in water, in 0.9% sodium chloride, and in dextrose solutions. Reconstituted solutions of ampicillin sodium containing 10 mg of ampicillin per mL have a pH of 8–10. When reconstituted as directed, ampicillin trihydrate oral suspensions have a pH of 5–7.5.

Commercially available ampicillin sodium powder for injection contains 2.9–3.1 mEq of sodium per g of ampicillin.

● Stability

Ampicillin capsules and powder for oral suspension should be stored in tight containers at 15–30°C. Following reconstitution, oral suspension of ampicillin trihydrate preferably should be refrigerated at 2–8°C but is stable for 7 days at room temperature or 14 days at 2–8°C.

Following reconstitution with sterile or bacteriostatic water for injection, ampicillin sodium solutions for IM or direct IV injection should be used within 1 hour after reconstitution and should not be frozen. The stability of ampicillin sodium in solution is concentration dependent and decreases as the concentration of the drug increases. Ampicillin sodium appears to be especially susceptible to inactivation in solutions containing dextrose, which appears to have a catalytic effect on hydrolysis of the drug.

The manufacturers report that when stored at room temperature (25°C), ampicillin sodium solutions containing 30 mg or less of ampicillin per mL in sterile water for injection, 0.9% sodium chloride injection, (1/6) M sodium lactate injection, or lactated Ringer's injection lose less than 10% of activity within 8 hours and solutions containing 2 mg or less of ampicillin per mL in 5% dextrose, 5% dextrose and 0.45% sodium chloride, or 10% invert sugar lose less than 10% of activity within 4 hours. At concentrations of 10–20 mg/mL in 5% dextrose, ampicillin loses less than 10% of its activity within 2 hours at room temperature.

When refrigerated at 4°C, ampicillin sodium solutions containing 30 mg of ampicillin per mL are stable for 48 hours in sterile water for injection or 0.9% sodium chloride injection and solutions containing 30 mg or less per mL are stable for 24 hours in lactated Ringer's or 8 hours in (1/6) M sodium lactate injection. Solutions of the drug containing 20 mg or less of ampicillin per mL are stable

at 4°C for 72 hours in sterile water for injection or 0.9% sodium chloride injection, 4 hours in 5% dextrose, or 3 hours in 10% invert sugar and solutions containing 10 mg or less per mL are stable for 4 hours at 4°C in 5% dextrose and 0.45% sodium chloride.

Ampicillin sodium is potentially physically and/or chemically incompatible with some drugs, including aminoglycosides, but the compatibility depends on several factors (e.g., concentrations of the drugs, specific diluents used, resulting pH, temperature). For information on the in vitro and in vivo incompatibility of penicillins and aminoglycosides, see Drug Interactions: Aminoglycosides, in the Aminopenicillins General Statement 8:12.16.08. Specialized references should be consulted for specific compatibility information. Because of the potential for incompatibility, ampicillin sodium and aminoglycosides should not be admixed.

For further information on chemistry and stability, mechanism of action, spectrum, resistance, pharmacokinetics, uses, cautions, drug interactions, laboratory test interferences, and dosage and administration of ampicillin, see the Aminopenicillins General Statement 8:12.16.08.

PREPARATIONS

Excipients in commercially available drug preparations may have clinically important effects in some individuals; consult specific product labeling for details.

Ampicillin (Trihydrate)

Oral

Capsules	250 mg (of ampicillin)*	**Ampicillin Capsules**
	500 mg (of ampicillin)*	**Ampicillin Capsules**

Ampicillin Sodium

Parenteral

For injection	125 mg (of ampicillin)*	**Ampicillin Sodium for Injection**
	250 mg (of ampicillin)*	**Ampicillin Sodium for Injection**
	500 mg (of ampicillin)*	**Ampicillin Sodium for Injection**
	1 g (of ampicillin)*	**Ampicillin Sodium for Injection**
	2 g (of ampicillin)*	**Ampicillin Sodium for Injection**
	10 g (of ampicillin) pharmacy bulk package*	**Ampicillin Sodium for Injection**
For injection, for IV infusion	1 g (of ampicillin)*	**Ampicillin Sodium ADD-Vantage®,** Ampicillin Sodium Piggyback
	2 g (of ampicillin)*	**Ampicillin Sodium ADD-Vantage®,** Ampicillin Sodium Piggyback

† Use is not currently included in the labeling approved by the US Food and Drug Administration.

*available from one or more manufacturer, distributor, and/or repackager by generic (nonproprietary) name

Ampicillin Sodium and Sulbactam Sodium

8:12.16.08 • AMINOPENICILLINS

■ Ampicillin sodium and sulbactam sodium (ampicillin/sulbactam) is a fixed combination of the sodium salts of ampicillin (an aminopenicillin antibiotic) and sulbactam (a β-lactam β-lactamase inhibitor); sulbactam synergistically expands ampicillin's spectrum of activity against many strains of β-lactamase-producing bacteria.

USES

The fixed combination of ampicillin sodium and sulbactam sodium (ampicillin/sulbactam) is used parenterally for the treatment of skin and skin structure, intra-abdominal, and gynecologic infections caused by susceptible bacteria. The drug also has been used parenterally for the treatment of some other infections, including respiratory tract infections† caused by susceptible bacteria.

Ampicillin/sulbactam is used principally for the treatment of infections caused by, or suspected of being caused by, susceptible β-lactamase-producing strains of staphylococci, Enterobacteriaceae, and/or *Bacteroides*. Although ampicillin/sulbactam also may be effective in the treatment of infections caused by non-β-lactamase-producing bacteria susceptible to ampicillin alone, most clinicians state that an aminopenicillin used alone is preferred to the fixed combination drug for the treatment of these infections and that ampicillin/sulbactam should be reserved for use in the treatment of infections caused by, or suspected of being caused by, β-lactamase-producing bacteria when an aminopenicillin alone would be ineffective. Ampicillin/sulbactam may be particularly useful for empiric treatment of intra-abdominal or gynecologic infections likely to involve anaerobes (e.g., mixed aerobic-anaerobic infections) or for infections suspected of being caused by both ampicillin-resistant and ampicillin-susceptible bacteria. For most other infections caused by susceptible organisms, including *Staphylococcus aureus* or *S. epidermidis*†, *Bacteroides*, *Klebsiella pneumoniae*, *Escherichia coli*, *Proteus vulgaris*†, *Providencia rettgeri*†, *Morganella morganii*†, *Eikenella corrodens*, or *Pasteurella multocida*†, ampicillin/sulbactam generally is considered an alternative to other anti-infectives. When used for the treatment of infections caused by Enterobacteriaceae in *severely ill* patients, some clinicians recommend combined therapy with ampicillin/sulbactam and an aminoglycoside. Because ampicillin/sulbactam is not active against *Pseudomonas*, the drug should not be used alone in infections known or suspected of being caused by *Ps. aeruginosa*.

Prior to initiation of therapy with ampicillin/sulbactam, appropriate specimens should be obtained for identification of the causative organism(s) and in vitro susceptibility tests. Ampicillin/sulbactam may be started pending results of susceptibility tests if the infection is believed to be caused by β-lactamase-producing bacteria susceptible to the drug, but should be discontinued and other appropriate anti-infective therapy substituted if the organism is found to be resistant to the drug. If the infection is found to be caused by non-β-lactamase-producing organisms susceptible to ampicillin, some clinicians suggest that therapy should be changed to an aminopenicillin alone, unless this is impractical.

● Skin and Skin Structure Infections

Ampicillin/sulbactam is used in adults and children 1 year of age or older for the treatment of a variety of skin and skin structure infections, including wound infections, cellulitis, ulcers, abscesses, and furunculosis, caused by susceptible β-lactamase-producing strains of *Staphylococcus aureus*, *E. coli*, *Klebsiella* (including *K. pneumoniae*), *P. mirabilis*, *Bacteroides* (including *B. fragilis*), or *Acinetobacter*. The drug also has been effective when used for the treatment of skin and skin structure infections caused by other susceptible gram-positive bacteria, including *S. epidermidis*†, *S. warneri*†, or *Enterococcus faecalis*†, or other susceptible gram-negative bacteria, including susceptible strains of *Citrobacter*†, *Enterobacter*†, or *Morganella morganii*†.

In controlled studies in adults with serious skin and skin structure infections, ampicillin/sulbactam was at least as effective as a regimen of clindamycin with or without an aminoglycoside. Ampicillin/sulbactam therapy generally results in clinical and bacteriologic cure rates of 86–100% in adults with skin and skin structure infections caused by susceptible bacteria. In a clinical trial in pediatric patients with skin and skin structure infections, initial treatment with IV ampicillin/sulbactam was as effective as IV cefuroxime (clinical success rate of 85 or 87%, respectively); most patients were switched to an oral regimen after initial IV treatment. Although ampicillin/sulbactam appears to be an effective regimen for the treatment of serious skin and skin structure infections, concomitant use of an anti-infective agent that is active against *Pseudomonas* (e.g., an aminoglycoside) may be necessary in some of these infections. In addition, less severe skin and skin structure infections (e.g., cellulitis, impetigo, erysipelas) usually can be treated with other antibacterials that have a narrower spectrum of activity (e.g., penicillinase-resistant penicillins, erythromycin, cephalosporins).

● Intra-abdominal and Gynecologic Infections

Ampicillin/sulbactam is used in adults for the treatment of a variety of intra-abdominal and gynecologic infections caused by susceptible *E. coli*, *Klebsiella* (including *K. pneumoniae*), *Bacteroides* (including *B. fragilis*), or *Enterobacter*. Most intra-abdominal and gynecologic infections are mixed aerobic-anaerobic infections, and efficacy of ampicillin/sulbactam in these polymicrobial infections is based on the drug's broad spectrum of activity against both gram-positive and gram-negative aerobic and anaerobic bacteria and on its distribution into most tissues and fluids. Depending on suspected organisms and severity of the infection, addition of an aminoglycoside may be considered.

Intra-abdominal Infections

Ampicillin/sulbactam has been effective when used in adults as an adjunct to surgical measures (e.g., drainage) in the treatment of appendicitis, peritonitis, perforated appendix, diverticulitis, postoperative bowel infections, small bowel infarct, intra-abdominal or retroperitoneal abscess, cholecystitis, and secondary liver infections caused by susceptible bacteria.

Use of ampicillin/sulbactam in adults with intra-abdominal infections has been associated with clinical and bacteriologic cure rates of 78–96%. In a few studies in adults, ampicillin/sulbactam appeared to be at least as effective as other regimens used in the adjunctive treatment of intra-abdominal infections (e.g., clindamycin or metronidazole and an aminoglycoside, cefoxitin with or without an aminoglycoside, imipenem and cilastatin sodium) and generally was associated with fewer adverse effects than these other regimens. However, in at least one study, ampicillin/sulbactam was less effective than a regimen of clindamycin and gentamicin in the treatment of patients with perforated or gangrenous appendicitis; most treatment failures in patients receiving ampicillin/sulbactam were the result of overgrowth with *Pseudomonas*. Some clinicians suggest that, although ampicillin/sulbactam alone may be as effective as multiple-drug regimens for the treatment of less severe intra-abdominal infections, an aminoglycoside probably should be used concomitantly with the drug for empiric therapy in more serious intra-abdominal infections, including hospital-acquired infections, pending results of in vitro susceptibility tests.

Gynecologic Infections

Ampicillin/sulbactam is used in adults for the treatment of gynecologic infections including endometritis (after abortion or curettage), postpartum endomyometritis, posthysterectomy pelvic cellulitis, vaginal cuff abscess, salpingitis, tubo-ovarian abscess, pelvic peritonitis or abscess, surgical wound sepsis, uncomplicated acute pelvic inflammatory disease (PID), or complicated PID that may include pelvic peritonitis, tubo-ovarian abscesses, endometritis, or posthysterectomy pelvic cellulitis. The clinical and bacteriologic cure rates of ampicillin/sulbactam in the treatment of these gynecologic infections have been 83–100%.

In several studies in patients with mixed aerobic-anaerobic gynecologic infections, ampicillin/sulbactam was as effective as cefoxitin or cefotetan or multiple-drug regimens such as clindamycin or metronidazole and an aminoglycoside in the treatment of these infections and generally was associated with fewer adverse effects. The fact that ampicillin/sulbactam generally is considered to be inactive against *Mycoplasma* and to have incomplete inhibitory activity against *Chlamydia* should be considered if the drug is used in the treatment of gynecologic infections, and concomitant tetracycline (e.g., doxycycline) or, alternatively, macrolide therapy probably should be included if there is a possibility that these organisms are involved in the gynecologic infection being treated.

The US Centers for Disease Control and Prevention (CDC) states that a regimen of IV ampicillin/sulbactam with oral or IV doxycycline is an alternative parenteral regimen for the treatment of PID and provides good coverage against *Chlamydia trachomatis*, *N. gonorrhoeae*, and anaerobes for women with tuboovarian abscess. CDC states that the preferred parenteral regimens for the treatment of PID are a regimen of IV ceftriaxone with oral or IV doxycycline and oral or IV metronidazole or a regimen of IV cefotetan (or IV cefoxitin) with oral or IV doxycycline. For further information on the treatment of PID, see Uses: Pelvic Inflammatory Disease in the Cephalosporins General Statement 8:12.06.

● Gonorrhea and Associated Infections

Ampicillin/sulbactam has been used for the treatment of uncomplicated gonorrhea, including infections caused by penicillinase-producing strains of *Neisseria gonorrhoeae* (PPNG) and nonpenicillinase-producing strains of the organism. However, CDC has not recommended use of penicillins for the treatment of gonococcal infections for over 30 years because of the widespread prevalence of PPNG resistant to penicillins. Ceftriaxone is the drug of choice for the treatment of gonococcal infections.

● Respiratory Tract Infections

Ampicillin/sulbactam has been used for the treatment of lower respiratory tract infections†, including pneumonia, bronchitis, acute exacerbations of chronic bronchitis, and bronchiectasis caused by susceptible staphylococci, streptococci, *Haemophilus influenzae*, *H. parainfluenzae*, *Moraxella catarrhalis*, *E. coli*, *Klebsiella*, or *Proteus mirabilis*. Ampicillin/sulbactam therapy is reported to have clinical and bacteriologic cure rates of 58–100% when used for the treatment of lower respiratory tract infections.

Some clinicians suggest that ampicillin/sulbactam is an effective alternative for the treatment of lower respiratory tract infections known or suspected of being caused by ampicillin-resistant organisms, including community-acquired or nosocomial pneumonia, chronic obstructive pulmonary disease, and exacerbation of severe chronic bronchitis in hospitalized patients. Overgrowth with *Ps. aeruginosa* has been reported in some patients receiving ampicillin/sulbactam alone for the treatment of respiratory infections.

The American Thoracic Society (ATS) and Infectious Diseases Society of America (IDSA) recommend a regimen of ampicillin/sulbactam with a macrolide (azithromycin or clarithromycin) as one of several options for empiric treatment of nonsevere community-acquired pneumonia (CAP) in hospitalized adults who do not have risk factors for methicillin-resistant *S. aureus* (MRSA; also known as oxacillin-resistant *S. aureus* or ORSA) or *Ps. aeruginosa*.

Ampicillin/sulbactam has been effective for the treatment of respiratory tract infections† (e.g., pneumonia, tracheobronchitis) or bacteremia caused by strains of *Acinetobacter baumannii* that were resistant to imipenem and cilastatin sodium as well as most other anti-infectives tested. However, other anti-infectives (e.g., imipenem and cilastatin sodium or meropenem with or without an aminoglycoside) are preferred in the treatment of infections caused by susceptible *Acinetobacter*.

Ampicillin/sulbactam has been used in a limited number of adults and children for the treatment of various ear, nose, and throat infections† including tonsillitis, sinusitis, rhinitis, pharyngitis, acute epiglottitis, and acute and chronic otitis media caused by susceptible staphylococci, streptococci, *Klebsiella*, *Proteus*, *M. catarrhalis*, or *H. influenzae*. Although the drug generally was effective in the treatment of these infections, other anti-infectives are considered drugs of choice for these infections.

● Bone and Joint Infections

Ampicillin/sulbactam has been used for the treatment of bone and joint infections†, including osteomyelitis and/or septic arthritis, caused by susceptible β-lactamase-producing organisms.

● Endocarditis

Ampicillin/sulbactam has been used for the treatment of endocarditis†. Although other regimens are preferred, the American Heart Association (AHA) states that a regimen of ampicillin/sulbactam and an aminoglycoside can be considered as an alternative for the treatment of endocarditis involving native valves or prosthetic

valves or other prosthetic material caused by β-lactamase-producing *Enterococcus*. AHA also states that ampicillin/sulbactam may be considered an option for the treatment of endocarditis cause by fastidious gram-negative bacilli of the HACEK group (i.e., *Haemophilus*, *Aggregatibacter*, *Cardiobacterium hominis*, *Eikenella corrodens*, *Kingella*).

Current guidelines from AHA should be consulted for information on management of endocarditis.

● Meningitis

Ampicillin/sulbactam has been used for the treatment of meningitis† caused by *H. influenzae*, *N. meningitidis*, or *S. pneumoniae*. In one study in infants and children, ampicillin sodium (400 mg/kg daily) and sulbactam sodium (50 mg/kg daily) was as effective as a regimen of IV chloramphenicol (100 mg/kg daily) and IV ampicillin (400 mg/kg daily) for the treatment of meningitis caused by *H. influenzae*, *N. meningitidis*, or *S. pneumoniae*. Although some clinicians suggest that ampicillin/sulbactam therapy may be an effective alternative to therapy with ampicillin and chloramphenicol in infants and children for the treatment of meningitis caused by *H. influenzae*, *S. pneumoniae*, or *N. meningitidis* and might be especially useful in areas where ampicillin- and chloramphenicol-resistant strains have been reported, other drugs are preferred for the treatment of CNS infections. Treatment failures have been reported when ampicillin/sulbactam was used in patients with meningitis caused by *K. pneumoniae*.

● Urinary Tract Infections

Ampicillin/sulbactam has been used for the treatment of uncomplicated urinary tract infections† caused by susceptible bacteria, including *S. epidermidis*, *E. coli*, *K. pneumoniae*, or *P. mirabilis*. Although the drug may be effective for these infections, treatment failures have been reported. Ampicillin/sulbactam is unlikely to be effective for the treatment of urinary tract infections caused by extended-spectrum β-lactamase-producing (ESBL) strains of *E. coli*, *K. pneumoniae*, and *P. mirabilis*.

● Perioperative Prophylaxis

Ampicillin/sulbactam has been used for perioperative prophylaxis† to reduce the incidence of infections in patients undergoing certain contaminated or potentially contaminated surgery† (e.g., GI or biliary tract surgery, vaginal or abdominal hysterectomy).

Ampicillin/sulbactam is recommended as one of several options for perioperative prophylaxis in patients undergoing biliary tact surgery, colorectal surgery, gynecologic and obstetric procedures (e.g., vaginal, abdominal, or laparoscopic hysterectomy), head and neck surgery (involving incisions through oral or pharyngeal mucosa), non-cardiac thoracic surgery (e.g., lobectomy, pneumonectomy, lung resection, thoracotomy), or urologic procedures involving implanted prosthesis. Local susceptibility patterns of potential pathogens should be considered when selecting ampicillin/sulbactam for perioperative prophylaxis in procedures that involve exposure to bowel flora (e.g., *E. coli*) that may be resistant to the drug.

In adults undergoing biliary tract surgery, a single 3-g dose of ampicillin/sulbactam (2 g of ampicillin and 1 g of sulbactam) was as effective as a single dose of cefazolin (1 g) or cefoxitin (2 g) in preventing postoperative wound infection. A single 1.5-g dose of ampicillin/sulbactam (1 g of ampicillin and 0.5 g of sulbactam) has been used effectively for prophylaxis in various gynecologic procedures, including abdominal or vaginal hysterectomy. In a study in adults, ampicillin/sulbactam was as effective as cefoxitin for prevention of postoperative infections in patients undergoing colorectal or transurethral surgery. In a study in children 5–13 years of age undergoing appendectomy, a single dose of ampicillin/sulbactam (15 mg/kg of ampicillin and 7.5 mg/kg of sulbactam) given IV at the time of anesthesia was as effective as a single dose of metronidazole (7.5 mg/kg) and cefotaxime (25 mg/kg) in the prevention of postoperative sepsis; therapy with the drug was continued for 72 hours after surgery in patients with gangrenous or perforated appendixes at the time of surgery. Ampicillin/sulbactam also has been used with some success for perioperative prophylaxis in patients with head and neck cancer undergoing surgery. Although in one study ampicillin/sulbactam appeared to be as effective as a regimen of clindamycin and amikacin in such patients, patients who received ampicillin/sulbactam had a higher incidence of postoperative infection with anaerobes than patients who received the other regimen.

DOSAGE AND ADMINISTRATION

• Reconstitution and Administration

The fixed combination of ampicillin sodium and sulbactam sodium (ampicillin/sulbactam) is administered by IM or slow IV injection or by IV infusion. A combination of ampicillin and sulbactam also have been administered orally as a preparation containing the drugs covalently linked as a double ester in a single molecule (sultamicillin; CP-49,952), but an oral dosage form is not commercially available in the US.

IM or IV solutions of ampicillin/sulbactam should be allowed to stand after dissolution to allow any foaming to dissipate in order to permit visual inspection for complete solubilization.

IM Injection

For IM injection, vials labeled as containing 1.5 or 3 g of ampicillin/sulbactam should be reconstituted with 3.2 or 6.4 mL, respectively, of sterile water for injection or 0.5 or 2% lidocaine hydrochloride injection to provide a solution containing 375 mg of the fixed combination per mL (250 mg of ampicillin and 125 mg of sulbactam per mL). Reconstituting ampicillin/sulbactam with lidocaine hydrochloride can minimize the local pain associated with IM injection of the drug.

IM injections of ampicillin/sulbactam should be made deeply into a large muscle mass within 1 hour after reconstitution.

IV Injection or Infusion

For IV administration, vials labeled as containing 1.5 or 3 g of ampicillin/sulbactam should be reconstituted with sterile water for injection to yield solutions containing 375 mg of the drug per mL (250 mg of ampicillin and 125 mg of sulbactam per mL). An appropriate volume of reconstituted drug then should be diluted immediately with a compatible IV solution to yield solutions containing 3–45 mg of the drug per mL (2–30 mg of ampicillin and 1–15 mg of sulbactam per mL).

IV injections of ampicillin/sulbactam should be given slowly over at least 10–15 minutes.

IV infusions of ampicillin/sulbactam should be administered over 15–30 minutes.

• Dosage

Ampicillin/sulbactam is commercially available for parenteral administration as a sterile powder containing a 2:1 ratio of ampicillin to sulbactam. The ampicillin component is provided as ampicillin sodium and the sulbactam component is provided as sulbactam sodium; potency of each component is expressed in terms of the base.

Dosage of ampicillin/sulbactam usually is expressed in terms of the total (sum) of the dosage of both components of the fixed combination (i.e., dosage of ampicillin plus dosage of sulbactam); pediatric dosage of ampicillin/sulbactam also has been expressed in terms of the ampicillin content.

The manufacturer's dosage recommendations for adults are the same for IM and IV administration; however, higher serum concentrations usually are attained with IV administration of the drug, and this route generally is preferred, especially for severe infections.

Adult Dosage

Intra-abdominal, Gynecologic, or Skin and Skin Structure Infections

The usual adult IM or IV dosage of ampicillin/sulbactam for the treatment of skin and skin structure, intra-abdominal, or gynecologic infections caused by susceptible organisms ranges from 1.5 g (1 of ampicillin and 0.5 g of sulbactam) to 3 g (2 g of ampicillin and 1 g of sulbactam) every 6 hours.

The maximum adult dosage of sulbactam recommended by the manufacturer is 4 g (i.e., 8 g of ampicillin and 4 g of sulbactam in fixed combination) daily. While comparative efficacy of various dosages in the usual range have not been established, patients in many of early clinical studies received a maximum of 3 g (2 g of ampicillin and 1 g of sulbactam).

Pelvic Inflammatory Disease

For the treatment of pelvic inflammatory disease (PID), CDC recommends that IV ampicillin/sulbactam be given in a dosage of 3 g (2 g of ampicillin and 1 g of

sulbactam) every 6 hours in conjunction with doxycycline (100 mg orally or IV every 12 hours). The parenteral regimen may be discontinued 24–48 hours after there is clinical improvement and treatment switched to an oral regimen of doxycycline (100 mg twice daily) and metronidazole (500 mg twice daily) to complete 14 days of therapy.

Respiratory Tract Infections

For empiric treatment of nonsevere community-acquired pneumonia† (CAP) in hospitalized adults without risk factors for MRSA or *Ps. aeruginosa*, ATS and IDSA recommend that ampicillin/sulbactam be given in a dosage of 1.5 g (1 of ampicillin and 0.5 g of sulbactam) to 3 g (2 g of ampicillin and 1 g of sulbactam) every 6 hours in conjunction with azithromycin (500 mg daily) or clarithromycin (500 mg twice daily).

Endocarditis

If IV ampicillin/sulbactam is used as an alternative for the treatment of endocarditis† cause by β-lactamase-producing *Enterococcus*, AHA recommends a dosage of 3 g (2 g of ampicillin and 1 g of sulbactam) every 6 hours given in conjunction with an aminoglycoside.

Perioperative Prophylaxis

For perioperative prophylaxis†, a dosage of 3 g (2 g of ampicillin and 1 g of sulbactam) given within 60 minutes prior to initial incision is recommended.

Although additional intraoperative doses may be given every 2 hours during prolonged procedures, postoperative doses generally are not recommended.

Pediatric Dosage

The manufacturer states that pediatric patients who weigh 40 kg or more may receive the usual adult dosage of ampicillin/sulbactam.

The American Academy of Pediatrics (AAP) suggests that pediatric patients beyond the neonatal period† may receive a dosage of 100–200 mg/kg of ampicillin daily (as ampicillin/sulbactam) in 4 divided doses for the treatment of severe infections. A dosage of 200–400 mg/kg of ampicillin daily (as ampicillin/sulbactam) in 4 divided doses is recommended for meningitis or severe infections caused by resistant *S. pneumoniae*.

For the treatment of skin and skin structure infections in pediatric patients 1 year of age or older, the manufacturer recommends a dosage of 300 mg/kg daily (200 mg of ampicillin and 100 mg of sulbactam) given by IV infusion in equally divided doses every 6 hours. The manufacturer recommends that the duration of IV ampicillin/sulbactam therapy in pediatric patients not exceed 14 days; in clinical studies, most children received an oral anti-infective after an initial regimen of IV ampicillin/sulbactam.

Pelvic Inflammatory Disease

For the treatment of PID in adolescents, CDC recommends that IV ampicillin/sulbactam be given in a dosage of 3 g (2 g of ampicillin and 1 g of sulbactam) every 6 hours in conjunction with doxycycline (100 mg orally or IV every 12 hours). The parenteral regimen may be discontinued 24–48 hours after there is clinical improvement and treatment switched to an oral regimen of doxycycline (100 mg twice daily) and metronidazole (500 mg twice daily) to complete 14 days of therapy.

Perioperative Prophylaxis

For perioperative prophylaxis†, pediatric patients may receive 50 mg/kg of ampicillin (as ampicillin/sulbactam) within 60 minutes prior to initial incision.

Although additional intraoperative doses may be given every 2 hours during prolonged procedures, postoperative doses generally are not recommended.

• Dosage in Renal Impairment

Because the pharmacokinetics of both ampicillin and sulbactam are affected to the same degree in patients with renal impairment, the recommended 2:1 ratio of the drugs remains the same regardless of the degree of renal impairment.

The manufacturer recommends that patients with renal impairment receive the usually recommended doses of ampicillin/sulbactam, but doses should be given less frequently than usual and the dosing intervals should be based on the patient's creatinine clearance. The manufacturer recommends that patients with creatinine clearances of 30 mL/minute per 1.73 m² or greater receive 1.5 g (1 g of ampicillin and 0.5 g of sulbactam) to 3 g (2 g of ampicillin and 1 g of sulbactam) of the drug every 6–8 hours and that patients with creatinine clearances of 15–29 or 5–14 mL/minute per 1.73 m² receive these doses every 12 or 24 hours, respectively.

Because ampicillin and sulbactam are removed by hemodialysis, some clinicians suggest that patients undergoing hemodialysis receive 1.5 g (1 g of ampicillin and 0.5 g of sulbactam) to 3 g (2 g of ampicillin and 1 g of sulbactam) once every 24 hours and that the dose preferably should be given immediately after dialysis.

CAUTIONS

The fixed combination of ampicillin sodium and sulbactam sodium (ampicillin/sulbactam) generally is well tolerated. The frequency and severity of adverse effects reported with the commercially available fixed-combination preparation for parenteral administration generally are similar to those reported with parenteral ampicillin alone. With the exception of local reactions at the IM injection site, adverse effects generally have been reported in 10% or less of patients receiving parenteral ampicillin/sulbactam, and have been severe enough to require discontinuance of the drug in less than 1% of patients. The most frequent adverse effects of parenteral ampicillin/sulbactam are pain at the IM or IV injection site, diarrhea, and rash.

Parenteral sulbactam sodium alone is associated with few adverse effects, principally pain at the injection site and diarrhea.

For information on adverse effects reported with ampicillin and other aminopenicillins as well as the usual precautions and contraindications associated with these drugs, see Cautions in the Aminopenicillins General Statement 8:12.16.08.

● *Dermatologic and Sensitivity Reactions*

Rash has been reported in less than 2% of patients receiving parenteral ampicillin/sulbactam. Urticaria, pruritus, dry skin, and erythema also have been reported with the drug. Severe skin reactions, including toxic epidermal necrolysis, Stevens-Johnson syndrome, angioedema, acute generalized exanthematous pustulosis (AGEP), erythema multiforme, and exfoliative dermatitis, have been reported in patients receiving ampicillin/sulbactam or ampicillin.

Serious and occasionally fatal hypersensitivity reactions, including anaphylaxis, have been reported in patients receiving penicillin therapy. (See Cautions: Precautions and Contraindications.) Systemic allergic reactions have been reported during parenteral ampicillin/sulbactam therapy and required discontinuance of the drug.

● *Hepatotoxicity*

Ampicillin/sulbactam has been associated with hepatic dysfunction, including hepatitis and cholestatic jaundice. Although hepatotoxicity usually is reversible, deaths have been reported.

Transient increases in serum concentrations of AST (SGOT) and/or ALT (SGPT), alkaline phosphatase, LDH, creatine kinase (CK, creatine phosphokinase, CPK), bilirubin, and γ-glutamyltransferase (γ-glutamyltranspeptidase, GT, GGTP) have been reported in up to 11% of patients receiving parenteral ampicillin/sulbactam.

● *GI Effects*

Diarrhea, nausea, and vomiting have been reported in up to 4% of patients receiving parenteral ampicillin/sulbactam. Flatulence, abdominal discomfort or distension, rectal bleeding, and glossitis have been reported in less than 1% of patients receiving the drug parenterally. Gastritis, stomatitis, and black or hairy tongue have been reported in patients receiving ampicillin/sulbactam or ampicillin.

Treatment with anti-infectives alters normal colon flora and may permit overgrowth of *Clostridioides difficile* (formerly known as *Clostridium difficile*). *C. difficile*-associated diarrhea and colitis (CDAD; also known as antibiotic-associated diarrhea and colitis or pseudomembranous colitis) has been reported with parenteral ampicillin/sulbactam. *C. difficile* produces toxins A and B which contribute to development of CDAD; hypertoxin-producing strains of *C. difficile* are associated with increased morbidity and mortality since they may be refractory to anti-infectives and colectomy may be required. (See Cautions: Precautions and Contraindications.)

● *Local Reactions*

The most frequent adverse effect of parenteral ampicillin/sulbactam is pain at the injection site. Pain at the injection site has been reported in 3–16% of patients receiving the drug IM and in up to 3% of patients receiving the drug IV. Pain following IM administration of ampicillin/sulbactam may be minimized or avoided if 0.5 or 2% lidocaine hydrochloride is used as the diluent when preparing IM injections of the drug. Phlebitis, thrombophlebitis, and inflammation at the injection site also have been reported in up to 3% of patients receiving the drug IV.

● *Other Adverse Effects*

Decreased concentrations of serum albumin and total protein have been reported. Increased BUN and serum creatinine concentrations, presence of red blood cells and hyaline casts in urine, urine retention, dysuria, and hematuria have been reported in less than 1% of patients receiving the drug.

Decreased hemoglobin concentration, hematocrit, and erythrocyte, leukocyte, neutrophil, lymphocyte, and platelet counts and increased lymphocyte, monocyte, basophil, eosinophil, and platelet counts have been reported in patients receiving parenteral ampicillin/sulbactam. Although some of these hematologic changes may represent hypersensitivity reactions, many have not been attributed directly to the drug.

Other adverse effects that have been reported in less than 1% of patients receiving parenteral ampicillin/sulbactam include headache, fatigue, malaise, confusion, dizziness, changes in smell or taste perception, chest pain or tightness, edema, facial swelling, chills, throat tightness, substernal pain, epistaxis, and mucosal bleeding.

Reversible glycogenosis has been reported in animals receiving sulbactam. Diffuse hepatocellular glycogen deposits associated with increases in liver enzymes and hepatomegaly have occurred in rats and dogs that received high doses of sulbactam for prolonged periods of time. These adverse effects in animals were dose and time dependent and are not expected to occur in humans with the usually recommended ampicillin/sulbactam dosages and corresponding plasma concentrations of the drug attained during the relatively short periods of therapy. Similar glycogen deposits have not been reported in humans receiving ampicillin/sulbactam, although patients with preexisting liver dysfunction, diabetes mellitus, hypoglycemia, or glycogen storage disease were excluded from most early clinical studies of the drug. In subsequent studies in patients with type I or II diabetes mellitus, sulbactam given at the usually recommended dosages did not appear to affect glucose mobilization or regulation.

● *Precautions and Contraindications*

Ampicillin/sulbactam is contraindicated in individuals with a history of serious hypersensitivity reactions (e.g., anaphylaxis, Stevens-Johnson syndrome) to ampicillin, sulbactam, or other beta-lactam antibacterials (e.g., penicillins, cephalosporins).

Ampicillin/sulbactam also is contraindicated in individuals with a history of cholestatic jaundice/hepatic dysfunction associated with the drug.

Ampicillin/sulbactam shares the toxic potentials of the penicillins, including the risk of hypersensitivity reactions, and the usual precautions of penicillin therapy should be observed. Prior to initiation of therapy with ampicillin/sulbactam, careful inquiry should be made concerning previous hypersensitivity reactions to penicillins, cephalosporins, or other allergens.(See Cautions: Hypersensitivity Reactions, in the Natural Penicillins General Statement 8:12.16.04.) If an allergic reaction occurs, ampicillin/sulbactam should be discontinued and appropriate therapy instituted.

Because a high percentage of patients with infectious mononucleosis have developed rash during therapy with aminopenicillins (see Cautions: Ampicillin Rash, in the Aminopenicillins General Statement 8:12.16.08), the manufacturer states that ampicillin/sulbactam should not be used in patients mononucleosis.

Because hepatotoxicity has been associated with ampicillin/sulbactam, hepatic function should be monitored at regular intervals if the drug is used in patients with hepatic impairment.

As with use of other anti-infectives, use of ampicillin/sulbactam may result in overgrowth of nonsusceptible organisms, especially *Pseudomonas* or *Candida*. If superinfection occurs, the drug should be discontinued and appropriate therapy initiated.

Because CDAD has been reported with nearly all anti-infectives, including ampicillin/sulbactam, it should be considered in the differential diagnosis of patients who develop diarrhea during or after ampicillin/sulbactam therapy. Careful medical history is necessary since CDAD has been reported to occur as late as 2 months or longer after anti-infective therapy is discontinued. If CDAD is suspected or confirmed, anti-infective therapy not directed against *C. difficile* should be discontinued as soon as possible. Patients should be managed with appropriate anti-infective therapy directed against *C. difficile* (e.g., fidaxomicin, vancomycin, metronidazole), supportive therapy (e.g., fluid and electrolyte management, protein supplementation), and surgical evaluation as clinically indicated. Patients should be advised that diarrhea is a common problem caused by anti-infectives and usually ends when the drug is discontinued; however, it is important to contact a clinician if watery and bloody stools (with or without stomach cramps and fever) occur during or as late as 2 months or longer after the last dose.

To reduce development of drug-resistant bacteria and maintain effectiveness of ampicillin/sulbactam and other antibacterials, ampicillin/sulbactam should be used only for the treatment of infections proven or strongly suspected to be caused by susceptible bacteria. Prescribing ampicillin/sulbactam in the absence of a proven or strongly suspected bacterial infection is unlikely to provide benefit to the patient and increases the risk of development of drug-resistant bacteria.

Patients should be advised that antibacterials (including ampicillin/sulbactam) should only be used to treat bacterial infections and not used to treat viral infections (e.g., the common cold). Patients also should be advised about the importance of completing the full course of therapy, even if feeling better after a few days, and that skipping doses or not completing therapy may decrease effectiveness and increase the likelihood that bacteria will develop resistance and will not be treatable with ampicillin/sulbactam or other antibacterials in the future.

When selecting or modifying anti-infective therapy, results of culture and in vitro susceptibility testing should be used. In the absence of such data, local epidemiology and susceptibility patterns should be considered when selecting anti-infectives for empiric therapy.

Information on test methods and quality control standards for in vitro susceptibility testing of antibacterials and specific interpretive criteria for such testing recognized by FDA is available at https://www.fda.gov/STIC. For most antibacterials, including ampicillin/sulbactam, FDA recognizes the standards published by the Clinical and Laboratory Standards Institute (CLSI). (See In Vitro Susceptibility Testing under Spectrum.)

For a more complete discussion of these and other precautions associated with the use of ampicillin, see Cautions: Precautions and Contraindications, in the Aminopenicillins General Statement 8:12.16.08.

● **Pediatric Precautions**

Safety and efficacy of IV ampicillin/sulbactam have been established for the treatment of skin and skin structure infections in children 1 year of age or older. Use of the drug for this use in pediatric patients is supported by evidence from adequate and well-controlled studies in adults with additional data from pediatric pharmacokinetic studies, a controlled clinical trial conducted in pediatric patients, and post-marketing adverse events surveillance.

Safety and efficacy of IV ampicillin/sulbactam for the treatment of intraabdominal infections or any other indication in pediatric patients have not been established.

Safety and efficacy of IM administration of ampicillin/sulbactam have not been established for any indication in pediatric patients.

Various combinations of ampicillin and sulbactam (e.g., 1.3:1, 2:1, 3:1, 4:1, 7:1, and 8:1 ratios of ampicillin to sulbactam) have been administered IM or IV to neonates and children 1 month to 17 years of age without unusual adverse effects. The most frequent adverse effects of parenteral ampicillin/sulbactam in children are transient increases in serum liver enzyme concentrations, diarrhea, and rash.

● **Geriatric Precautions**

Although serum half-lives of ampicillin and sulbactam are slightly longer in geriatric adults than in younger adults, dosage of ampicillin/sulbactam does not need to be modified in geriatric patients with renal function normal for their age. In geriatric adults with renal impairment, doses and/or frequency of administration of ampicillin/sulbactam should be modified in response to the degree of renal impairment.

● **Mutagenicity and Carcinogenicity**

Studies have not been performed to date to evaluate the mutagenic or carcinogenic potential of ampicillin/sulbactam.

● **Pregnancy, Fertility, and Lactation**

Pregnancy

There are no adequate or controlled studies using ampicillin/sulbactam in pregnant women. Reproduction studies in mice, rats, and rabbits using ampicillin and sulbactam doses up to 10 times the usual human dose have not revealed evidence of impaired fertility or harm to the fetus due to ampicillin/sulbactam. Because animal reproduction studies are not always predictive of human response, ampicillin/sulbactam should be used during pregnancy only when clearly needed.

Although the clinical importance is unclear, administration of ampicillin alone to pregnant women has resulted in a transient decrease in plasma concentrations of total conjugated estriol, estriol glucuronide, conjugated estrone, and estradiol; this effect also may occur following administration of ampicillin/sulbactam. IV administration of ampicillin to guinea pigs has resulted in decreased uterine tone and decreased frequency, height, and duration of uterine contractions. It is not known whether use of ampicillin/sulbactam in humans during labor or delivery could have any immediate or delayed adverse effects on the fetus, prolong the duration of labor, or increase the likelihood of forceps delivery, other obstetrical intervention, or resuscitation of the neonate.

Lactation

Because ampicillin and sulbactam are distributed into milk in low concentrations, ampicillin/sulbactam should be used with caution in nursing women.

DRUG INTERACTIONS

For further information on these and other drug interactions reported with aminopenicillins, see Drug Interactions in the Aminopenicillins General Statement 8:12.16.08. In addition, while not all drug interactions reported with other penicillins have been reported with aminopenicillins, the possibility that they could occur with these drugs should be considered.

● **Aminoglycosides**

The antibacterial activity of aminoglycosides and penicillins may be additive or synergistic in vitro against some organisms. In vitro and animal studies indicate that a synergistic bactericidal effect can occur against some strains of enterococci when ampicillin is used in conjunction with amikacin, gentamicin, streptomycin, or tobramycin.

Ampicillin is potentially physically and/or chemically incompatible with aminoglycosides in vitro. In one in vitro study, sulbactam concentrations of 25 mcg/mL had no appreciable affect on aminoglycosides in serum at 37°C; however, at concentrations of 75 mcg/mL, sulbactam inactivated tobramycin (but not other aminoglycosides tested) and, at concentrations of 200 mcg/mL or greater (with or without ampicillin), sulbactam inactivated amikacin, gentamicin, and tobramycin. Some clinicians suggest that in vivo inactivation of aminoglycosides by sulbactam is unlikely to occur since sulbactam concentrations of 25 mcg/mL usually are not achieved clinically.

● **Allopurinol**

An increased incidence of rash reportedly occurs in patients with hyperuricemia who are receiving allopurinol and concomitant ampicillin compared with those receiving either drug alone. It is unclear whether this increased incidence of rash is caused by concomitant use of the drug or the hyperuricemia present in these patients. The manufacturer states that there are no data to date on concomitant use of allopurinol with ampicillin/sulbactam.

● **Methotrexate**

Concomitant use of methotrexate and penicillins may reduce the renal clearance of methotrexate, resulting in increased serum concentrations of methotrexate and increased hematologic and GI toxicity. Patients should be carefully monitored if methotrexate and penicillins are used concomitantly.

• Probenecid

Oral probenecid administered shortly before or concomitantly with the fixed combination of ampicillin sodium and sulbactam sodium (ampicillin/sulbactam) competitively inhibits renal tubular secretion of both ampicillin and sulbactam and produces higher and prolonged serum concentrations of the drugs. The serum half-life of sulbactam may be increased by 18–45% by concomitant probenecid.

LABORATORY TEST INTERFERENCES

For more complete information on these and other laboratory test interferences reported with penicillins, see Laboratory Test Interferences in the Natural Penicillins General Statement 8:12.16.04. Although not all laboratory test interferences reported with other penicillins have been reported with ampicillin, the possibility that these interferences could occur with any of the aminopenicillins should be considered.

Ampicillin can interfere with urinary glucose determinations using cupric sulfate (e.g., Benedict's solution, Clinitest®), but does not affect glucose oxidase methods (e.g., Clinistix®, Tes-Tape®).

ACUTE TOXICITY

Overdosage of ampicillin/sulbactam would be expected to produce manifestations that principally are extensions of the adverse reactions reported with the drug. The fact that high CSF concentrations of β-lactam antibiotics may cause neurologic effects, including seizures, should be considered. Because ampicillin and sulbactam are both removed from the circulation by hemodialysis, these procedures may enhance elimination of the drug from the body if overdosage occurs in patients with impaired renal function; these procedures probably are unnecessary in patients with normal renal function.

MECHANISM OF ACTION

The fixed combination of ampicillin sodium and sulbactam sodium (ampicillin/ sulbactam) usually is bactericidal in action. Concurrent administration of sulbactam does not alter the mechanism of action of ampicillin. However, because sulbactam has a high affinity for and binds to certain β-lactamases that generally inactivate ampicillin by hydrolyzing the β-lactam ring, concurrent administration of the drug with ampicillin results in a synergistic bactericidal effect which expands the spectrum of activity of ampicillin against many strains of β-lactamase-producing bacteria that are resistant to ampicillin alone. For information on the mechanism of action of ampicillin, see Mechanism of Action in the Natural Penicillins General Statement 8:12.16.04 and in the Aminopenicillins General Statement 8:12.16.08.

Sulbactam is a β-lactam β-lactamase inhibitor that is active against a wide range of bacterial β-lactamases and acts as an irreversible inhibitor. The drug is considered a "suicide inhibitor" because the interaction between sulbactam and target β-lactamases causes both the drug and the enzyme to be incapable of further action. Sulbactam inhibition of β-lactamases is concentration and time dependent. At low sulbactam concentrations, a first-order reaction occurs and at high concentrations a zero-order reaction occurs. Results of in vitro studies indicate that ampicillin to sulbactam ratios of 2:1, 1:1, or 1:2 result in optimal β-lactamase inhibition and antibacterial activity.

Sulbactam inactivates both plasmid- and chromosome-mediated β-lactamases. In vitro studies indicate that sulbactam generally inhibits staphylococcal β-lactamases and β-lactamases classified as Richmond-Sykes types II, III (TEM type, HSV-1), IV, V (PSE and OXA types), and VI. The drug generally does not inhibit inducible, chromosomally mediated cephalosporinases classified as Richmond-Sykes type I, which may be produced by Pseudomonas aeruginosa, Citrobacter, Enterobacter, and Serratia.

In addition to its affinity for bacterial β-lactamases, sulbactam has an affinity for and binds to some bacterial penicillin-binding proteins (PBPs). PBPs are the target enzymes of β-lactam antibiotics and this binding may be the mechanism of sulbactam's intrinsic antibacterial activity against some organisms. It also may contribute to the synergistic bactericidal effect that occurs between sulbactam and

ampicillin or other β-lactam anti-infectives. Sulbactam has a strong affinity for PBP 1a of Proteus mirabilis and Escherichia coli and PBP 2 of Acinetobacter. The drug has a lesser affinity for PBPs of Staphylococcus aureus, PBP 1a of E. coli, and PBP 2 of E. coli oP. mirabilis.

The minimum bactericidal concentration (MBC) of ampicillin/sulbactam for ampicillin-resistant strains of S. aureus, Haemophilus influenzae, and Bacteroides fragilis generally is only 1–2 times higher than the minimum inhibitory concentration (MIC); however, the MBC may be 8 times higher than the MIC for some strains.

Unlike clavulanic acid, sulbactam generally does not induce production of type I chromosomally mediated cephalosporinases in Pseudomonas or Enterobacteriaceae, including Citrobacter, Enterobacter, Morganella, and Serratia marcescens.

SPECTRUM

The fixed combination of ampicillin sodium and sulbactam sodium (ampicillin/ sulbactam) has a wide spectrum of activity and is active in vitro against many gram-positive and -negative aerobic and anaerobic bacteria. Ampicillin/sulbactam is active in vitro against organisms susceptible to ampicillin alone. In addition, because sulbactam can inhibit certain β-lactamases that generally inactivate ampicillin, ampicillin/sulbactam is active in vitro against many β-lactamase-producing organisms that are resistant to ampicillin alone, including ampicillin-resistant strains of staphylococci, Haemophilus, Neisseria, and Bacteroides.

Sulbactam alone has some intrinsic antibacterial activity against certain organisms. In vitro, sulbactam concentrations of 0.1–4 mcg/mL inhibit many strains of Neisseria meningitidis, nonpenicillinase- and penicillinase-producing N. gonorrhoeae, non-β-lactamase-producing Moraxella catarrhalis, and some strains of Acinetobacter. In addition, sulbactam concentrations of 8–16 mcg/mL inhibit some strains of Bacteroides and Legionella in vitro. However, sulbactam concentrations of 25 mcg/mL or greater generally are required for in vitro inhibition of other gram-positive or -negative bacteria, and the drug is not therapeutically useful alone.

• In Vitro Susceptibility Testing

When in vitro susceptibility testing is performed according to the standards of the Clinical and Laboratory Standards Institute (CLSI), clinical isolates identified as susceptible are inhibited by drug concentrations usually achievable when the recommended dosage is used for the site of infection, resulting in likely clinical efficacy. Clinical isolates identified as intermediate have MICs or zone diameters that approach usually attainable blood and tissue concentrations and/or for which response rates may be lower than response rates for isolates identified as susceptible. The intermediate category also includes a buffer zone for inherent variability in test methods that should prevent small, uncontrolled technical factors from causing major discrepancies in interpretation, especially for drugs with narrow pharmacotoxicity margins. If results of in vitro susceptibility testing indicate that a clinical isolate is resistant, the strain is not inhibited by drug concentrations generally achievable with usual dosage schedules and/or MICs or zone diameters fall in the range where specific microbial resistance mechanisms are likely and clinical efficacy of the drug against the isolate has not been reliably demonstrated in clinical studies.

Strains of staphylococci resistant to penicillinase-resistant penicillins also should be considered resistant to ampicillin/sulbactam, although results of in vitro susceptibility tests may indicate that the organisms are susceptible to the drug. In addition, CLSI currently recommends that non-β-lactamase-producing strains of H. influenzae that are resistant to ampicillin (BLNAR H. influenzae) be considered resistant to ampicillin/sulbactam despite the fact that results of in vitro susceptibility tests may indicate that the organisms are susceptible to the drug.

CLSI states that, for streptococci and non-β-lactamase-producing enterococci, results of in vitro susceptibility tests using ampicillin can be used to predict susceptibility to ampicillin/sulbactam. However, to determine susceptibility of staphylococci and gram-negative enteric bacteria to ampicillin/sulbactam, CLSI recommends that disk-diffusion and dilution susceptibility tests be performed using appropriate combinations of ampicillin sodium and sulbactam sodium. For information on interpretive criteria specified for ampicillin, see Spectrum: In Vitro Susceptibility Testing in the Aminopenicillins General Statement 8:12.16.08.

To test in vitro susceptibility to ampicillin/sulbactam, a 1:1 ratio of ampicillin to sulbactam generally is used for disk-diffusion procedures and a 2:1 ratio of the drugs is used for agar or broth dilution procedures.

Disk Susceptibility Tests

When the disk-diffusion procedure is used to test susceptibility to ampicillin/sulbactam, a disk containing 20 mcg of the drug (10 mcg of ampicillin and 10 mcg of sulbactam) is used.

When disk-diffusion susceptibility testing is performed according to CLSI standardized procedures using CLSI interpretive criteria, *Staphylococcus*, Enterobacterales, and *Acinetobacter* with growth inhibition zones of 15 mm or greater are susceptible to ampicillin/sulbactam, those with zones of 12–14 mm have intermediate susceptibility, and those with zones of 11 mm or less are resistant to the drug.

When disk-diffusion susceptibility testing is performed according to CLSI standardized procedures, *Haemophilus* with growth inhibition zones of 20 mm or greater are considered susceptible to ampicillin/sulbactam and those with zones of 19 mm or less are considered resistant to the drug.

Dilution Susceptibility Tests

When dilution susceptibility testing (agar or broth dilution) is performed according to CLSI standardized procedures using CLSI interpretive criteria, *Staphylococcus*, Enterobacterales, and *Acinetobacter* with MICs of 8 mcg/mL or less of ampicillin in the presence of sulbactam at a constant 2:1 ratio are susceptible to ampicillin/sulbactam, those with MICs of 16 mcg/mL of ampicillin have intermediate susceptibility, and those with MICs of 32 mcg/mL or greater of ampicillin are resistant to the drug.

When susceptibility of *Haemophilus* is tested according to CLSI standardized procedures, *Haemophilus* with MICs of 2 mcg/mL or less of ampicillin in the presence of sulbactam at a constant 2:1 ratio are susceptible to ampicillin/sulbactam and those with MICs of 4 mcg/mL or greater of ampicillin in the presence of sulbactam at a constant 2:1 ratio are resistant to the drug.

● Gram-positive Aerobic Bacteria

Gram-positive Aerobic Cocci

Ampicillin/sulbactam is active in vitro against many gram-positive aerobic cocci including *Streptococcus pneumoniae*, *S. pyogenes* (group A β-hemolytic streptococci), *S. agalactiae* (group B streptococci), viridans streptococci, and penicillinase-producing and nonpenicillinase-producing strains of *Staphylococcus aureus*, *S. epidermidis*, *S. saprophyticus*, and *S. warneri*. The drug is active in vitro against some strains of *Enterococcus faecalis*. Ampicillin/sulbactam is active in vitro against most strains of penicillinase-producing staphylococci that are resistant to ampicillin alone. Although ampicillin/sulbactam may be active in vitro against some strains of staphylococci resistant to penicillinase-resistant penicillins including methicillin-resistant *S. aureus* (MRSA; also known as oxacillin-resistant *S. aureus* or ORSA) and methicillin-resistant *S. epidermidis*, in vitro activity against these organisms does not necessarily correlate with in vivo activity and the manufacturer, CLSI, and most clinicians state that strains of staphylococci resistant to penicillinase-resistant penicillins (e.g., nafcillin, oxacillin) should be considered resistant to ampicillin/sulbactam.

In in vitro studies using dilutions containing a 2:1 ratio of ampicillin to sulbactam, the MIC_{90} (minimum inhibitory concentration of the drug at which 90% of strains tested are inhibited) of ampicillin/sulbactam for penicillinase-producing and nonpenicillinase-producing strains of *S. aureus* and *S. epidermidis* is 0.12–8 mcg/mL of ampicillin in the presence of sulbactam at a constant 2:1 ratio of the drugs. The MIC_{90} of ampicillin/sulbactam for group A β- hemolytic streptococci, group B streptococci, *S. pneumoniae*, and *E. faecalis* is 0.03–1 mcg/mL of ampicillin in the presence of sulbactam at a constant 2:1 ratio of the drugs. Although some strains of *E. faecium* are inhibited in vitro by 0.5–8 mcg/mL of ampicillin in the presence of sulbactam at a constant 2:1 ratio of the drugs, many strains of the organism require concentrations of 16 mcg/mL or greater for in vitro inhibition and are considered resistant to the drug. (See Resistance.)

Gram-positive Aerobic Bacilli

Ampicillin/sulbactam is active in vitro against *Listeria monocytogenes*. The drug reportedly is inactive against *Nocardia asteroides*.

● Gram-negative Aerobic Bacteria

Neisseria

Ampicillin/sulbactam is active in vitro against most strains of *Neisseria meningitidis* and penicillinase-producing and nonpenicillinase-producing *N. gonorrhoeae*.

In in vitro studies using dilutions containing a 2:1 ratio of ampicillin to sulbactam, the MIC_{90} of ampicillin/sulbactam for *N. meningitidis* is 0.12–2 mcg/mL or less of ampicillin in the presence of sulbactam at a constant 2:1 ratio of the drugs. The MIC_{90} of the drug for PPNG is 4 mcg/mL of ampicillin in the presence of 2 mcg/mL of sulbactam.

Haemophilus

Ampicillin/sulbactam is active in vitro against most β-lactamase-producing and non-β-lactamase-producing strains of *Haemophilus influenzae* and *H. ducreyi*. Although some strains of non-β-lactamase-producing *H. influenzae* that are resistant to ampicillin (BLNAR *H. influenzae*) may be susceptible to ampicillin/sulbactam in vitro, CLSI currently recommends that these strains be considered resistant to the drug.

The MIC_{90} of ampicillin/sulbactam reported for non-β-lactamase-producing strains of *H. influenzae* is 0.25–0.5 mcg/mL and the MIC_{90} of the drug for β-lactamase producing strains is 0.78–2 mcg/mL of ampicillin in the presence of sulbactam at a constant 2:1 ratio of the drugs.

Moraxella catarrhalis

Ampicillin/sulbactam is active in vitro against both β-lactamase-producing and non-β-lactamase-producing strains of *Moraxella catarrhalis*. The MIC_{90} of the drug reported for these organisms is 0.015–0.8 mcg/mL of ampicillin in the presence of sulbactam at a constant 2:1 ratio of the drugs.

Enterobacteriaceae

Ampicillin/sulbactam is active in vitro against Enterobacteriaceae that are susceptible to ampicillin alone (e.g., some strains of *Escherichia coli*, *Proteus mirabilis*, *Salmonella*, *Shigella*). In addition, ampicillin/sulbactam is active in vitro against many β-lactamase-producing Enterobacteriaceae that are resistant to ampicillin alone, including many strains of β-lactamase-producing *Citrobacter,Klebsiella*, *Morganella morganii*, *Proteus*, *Providencia*, and *Yersinia enterocolitica* and some strains of β-lactamase-producing *E. coli*. Although ampicillin/sulbactam is active in vitro against some strains of *Enterobacter cloacae*, *E. aerogenes*, and *E. agglomerans*, many strains of *Enterobacter* as well as most strains of *Serratia* are resistant to the drug. (See Resistance.)

In in vitro studies using dilutions containing a 2:1 ratio of ampicillin to sulbactam, the MIC_{90} of ampicillin/sulbactam for *E. coli*, including multiple-drug resistant strains, generally is 4–16 mcg/mL of ampicillin in the presence of sulbactam at a constant 2:1 ratio of the drugs. However, the MIC_{90} for *E. coli* occasionally has been reported as 16–32 mcg/mL. The MIC_{90} of the drug for*Klebsiella*, including *K. pneumoniae* and *K. oxytoca*, and for *Citrobacter* and *Proteus* is 1–16 mcg/mL of ampicillin in the presence of sulbactam at a constant 2:1 ratio of the drugs. *Serratia marcescens* usually has an MIC_{90} of 16–32 mcg/mL or greater of ampicillin in the presence of sulbactam at a constant 2:1 ratio and generally is considered resistant to the drug.

Other Gram-negative Aerobic Bacteria

Ampicillin/sulbactam is active in vitro against some strains of *Acinetobacter*. The MIC_{90} of the drug reported for *Acinetobacter baumannii* (*A. calcoaceticus* subsp. *anitratus*), *A. lwoffi* (*A. calcoaceticus* subsp. *lwoffi*), and *A. haemolyticus* is 1–8 mcg/mL of ampicillin in the presence of sulbactam at a constant 2:1 ratio of the drugs.

Ampicillin/sulbactam generally is inactive against *Pseudomonas*, including *Ps. aeruginosa*.

Some strains of *Burkholderia pseudomallei* and *B. cepacia* may be inhibited in vitro by the drug.

In one study, the MIC_{90} of ampicillin/sulbactam reported for *Legionella*, including *L. pneumophila*, was 2 mcg/mL of ampicillin in the presence of 1 mcg/mL of sulbactam.

Ampicillin/sulbactam has some in vitro activity against *Campylobacter fetus* subsp. *jejuni*.

● *Anaerobic Bacteria*

Ampicillin/sulbactam is active in vitro against both gram-positive and -negative anaerobic bacteria and is active against some anaerobes that are resistant to many other anti-infectives, including other β-lactam antibiotics, metronidazole, and clindamycin.

Ampicillin/sulbactam is active in vitro against gram-positive anaerobic bacteria including *Actinomyces, Bifidobacterium, Clostridium, Eubacterium, Lactobacillus, Peptococcus, Peptostreptococcus,* and *Propionibacterium.* The MIC$_{90}$ of ampicillin/sulbactam reported for *Clostridium* (including *C. clostridioforme, C. innocuum, C. perfringens, C. ramosum, C. subterminale,* and *C. tertium*) is 0.5–8 mcg/mL of ampicillin in the presence of sulbactam in a constant 2:1 ratio of the drugs. Most other susceptible gram-positive anaerobes are inhibited in vitro by ampicillin/sulbactam concentrations of 0.25–2 mcg/mL of ampicillin in the presence of sulbactam at a constant 2:1 ratio of the drugs.

Ampicillin/sulbactam is active in vitro against gram-negative anaerobic bacteria including most strains of *Bacteroides, Porphyromonas, Prevotella,* and *Fusobacterium.* The MIC$_{90}$ of the drug reported for most *Bacteroides* in the *B. fragilis* group (e.g., *B. fragilis, B. caccae, B. distasonis, B. ovatus, B. thetaiotamicron, B. uniformis, B. vulgatus*) is 1.6–16 mcg/mL of ampicillin in the presence of sulbactam at a constant 2:1 ratio of the drugs. The MIC$_{90}$ of the drug reported for *B. capillosus* and *B. ureolyticus* is 0.25–4 mcg/mL of ampicillin in the presence of sulbactam at a constant 2:1 ratio of the drugs. Ampicillin/sulbactam concentrations of 32 mcg/mL of ampicillin in the presence of 16 mcg/mL of sulbactam may be required for in vitro inhibition of *B. gracilis,* and this organism generally is considered resistant to the drug.

The MIC$_{90}$ of ampicillin/sulbactam for *Porphyromonas asaccharolyticus* (*B. asaccharolytica*), *Prevotella bivius* (*B. bivia*), *P. disiens* (*B. disiens*), *P. intermedius* (*B. intermedia*), *P. loescheii* (*B. loescheii*), *P. melaninogenicus* (*B. melaninogenica*), and *P. oralis* (*B. oralis*) is 0.25–4 mcg/mL of ampicillin in the presence of sulbactam at a constant 2:1 ratio of the drugs.

Fusobacterium, including *F. nucleatum,* generally is inhibited in vitro by concentrations of 0.1–8 mcg/mL of ampicillin in the presence of sulbactam at a constant 2:1 ratio of the drugs; however, some strains of *F. necrophorum* may be resistant to ampicillin/sulbactam.

● *Chlamydia and Mycoplasma*

Ampicillin/sulbactam generally is considered inactive against *Mycoplasma* and *Chlamydia,* including *C. trachomatis.* Like most other penicillins (e.g., amoxicillin, penicillin G), ampicillin reportedly has an incomplete inhibitory effect against *Chlamydia* and may be bacteriostatic but not bactericidal against these organism.

RESISTANCE

Gram-negative aerobic bacilli that produce Richmond-Sykes type I chromosomally mediated β-lactamases (e.g., *Pseudomonas aeruginosa, Citrobacter, Enterobacter, Serratia*) generally are resistant to the fixed combination of ampicillin sodium and sulbactam sodium (ampicillin/sulbactam) because sulbactam does not inhibit most type I β-lactamases.

Some strains of *Klebsiella, Escherichia coli,* and *Acinetobacter* and rare strains of *Neisseria gonorrhoeae* are resistant to ampicillin/sulbactam. Rarely, strains of *Bacteroides fragilis* resistant to ampicillin/sulbactam have been reported.

Results of in vitro studies using ampicillin-resistant strains of *Staphylococcus aureus, Haemophilus influenzae,* and *B. fragilis* indicate that serial passage of these strains in the presence of ampicillin/sulbactam or continuous culture in the presence of subinhibitory concentrations of the drug does not result in resistance to ampicillin/sulbactam.

Enterococcus faecium generally is resistant to ampicillin/sulbactam. Resistance to aminopenicillins in some enterococci (e.g., *E. faecalis, E. faecium*) can result from β-lactamase production or from decreased binding to and/or increased production of penicillin-binding proteins with a low affinity for the drugs (e.g., PBP 5 or 6). Enterococci that exhibit ampicillin resistance secondary to β-lactamase production may be susceptible in vitro when the aminopenicillin is combined with a β-lactamase inhibitor (e.g., clavulanic acid, sulbactam). Strains that exhibit ampicillin resistance secondary to alterations in PBPs remain resistant when the drug is combined with a -lactamase inhibitor such as sulbactam or clavulanic acid,

and some evidence suggests that such strains occasionally may emerge secondary to high-dose drug exposure. In addition, enterococci resistant to multiple drugs (e.g., vancomycin, teicoplanin, aminoglycosides, ampicillin, penicillin G, imipenem, tetracyclines, synergistic combinations of β-lactam anti-infectives) have been reported with increasing frequency.

PHARMACOKINETICS

Cross-over studies using fixed combinations of ampicillin sodium and sulbactam sodium, ampicillin sodium alone, and sulbactam sodium alone indicate that concomitant administration of sulbactam sodium does not appreciably affect the pharmacokinetics of either drug. Dosage of the fixed combination of ampicillin sodium and sulbactam sodium (ampicillin/sulbactam) generally is expressed in terms of the total of the ampicillin and sulbactam content of the fixed combination.

The pharmacokinetics of ampicillin and sulbactam following parenteral administration are similar and reportedly are best described by an open, 2-compartment model. For additional information on absorption, distribution, and elimination of ampicillin, see Pharmacokinetics in the Aminopenicillins General Statement 8:12.16.08 and in Ampicillin 8:12.16.08.

● *Absorption*

Sulbactam sodium is not absorbed appreciably from the GI tract and must be given parenterally. Although sulbactam is orally bioavailable following administration of an oral formulation containing ampicillin and sulbactam covalently linked as a double ester in a single molecule (sultamicillin; CP-49,952), this oral dosage formulation is not commercially available in the US.

Peak serum concentrations of ampicillin and sulbactam are attained immediately following completion of a 15-minute IV infusion of ampicillin/sulbactam. In adults with normal renal function, peak serum concentrations of ampicillin are 40–71 mcg/mL following administration of a 1.5-g dose of ampicillin/sulbactam (1 g of ampicillin and 0.5 g of sulbactam) or 109–150 mcg/mL following a 3-g dose of the drug (2 g of ampicillin and 1 g of sulbactam); peak serum concentrations of sulbactam following these doses are 21–40 or 48–88 mcg/mL, respectively.

Following IM injection of ampicillin/sulbactam, both drugs are rapidly and almost completely absorbed. Peak serum concentrations of ampicillin and sulbactam generally are attained within 30–40 and 30–52 minutes, respectively. In healthy adults with normal renal function, IM injection of 1.5 g of ampicillin/sulbactam (1 g of ampicillin and 0.5 g of sulbactam) results in peak serum concentrations of ampicillin of 8–37 mcg/mL and of sulbactam of 6–24 mcg/mL.

Peak serum concentrations and areas under the concentration-time curve (AUCs) of ampicillin and sulbactam are slightly higher in geriatric patients than in younger adults; this presumably occurs because of reduced renal clearance in the elderly. In a study in healthy geriatric adults 65–85 years of age, a single 3-g dose of ampicillin/sulbactam (2 g of ampicillin and 1 g of sulbactam) given IV over 30 minutes resulted in peak serum concentrations of ampicillin and sulbactam that averaged 112.4 and 59.1 mcg/mL, respectively; the same dose administered to healthy adults 20–64 years of age resulted in peak serum concentrations of 82.4–99.8 and 42.5–52.2 mcg/mL, respectively.

In a study in neonates who received ampicillin/sulbactam in a 1:1 ratio (50 mg/kg of each drug) given by rapid IV injection every 12 hours, plasma concentrations of ampicillin at 3, 8, and 12 hours after a dose averaged 86.8, 77.3, and 56.8 mcg/mL, respectively, and those of sulbactam at the same intervals averaged 110.2, 72.8, and 38.4 mcg/mL, respectively.

There is no evidence that sulbactam accumulates in serum following IM or IV administration of 0.5-g doses every 6 hours for 3 days in adults with normal renal function.

In a few patients with chronic renal failure undergoing continuous ambulatory peritoneal dialysis, intraperitoneal administration of a single 3-g dose of ampicillin/sulbactam (2 g of ampicillin and 1 g of sulbactam) instilled over 6 hours resulted in peak plasma concentrations of ampicillin and sulbactam of 87.5 and 27.8 mcg/mL, respectively.

● *Distribution*

Following IM or IV administration of ampicillin/sulbactam, both ampicillin and sulbactam are well distributed into fluids and tissues. Ampicillin and sulbactam distribute into peritoneal fluid, blister fluid, tissue fluid, sputum, middle ear effusion, intestinal mucosa, bronchial wall, alveolar lining fluid, sternum, pericardium, myocardium, endocardium, prostate, gallbladder, bile, myometrium, salpinges, ovaries, and appendix. Concentrations of the drugs in most of these tissues and fluids generally are 53–100% of concurrent serum concentrations.

In adults with normal renal function, the apparent volume of distribution at steady state of ampicillin is 0.28–0.33 L/kg and that of sulbactam is 0.24–0.4 L/kg. The apparent volume of distribution of sulbactam at steady state in infants and children is 0.31–0.38 L/kg.

Both ampicillin and sulbactam are distributed into CSF in low concentrations following IV or IM administration in adults and children. CSF concentrations of the drugs generally are higher in patients with inflamed meninges than in those with uninflamed meninges. In a study in adults receiving 0.8- to 2-g doses of ampicillin IV every 4 hours and 1-g doses of sulbactam IV every 6 hours, ampicillin concentrations in CSF ranged from less than 0.3 to 9.6 mcg/mL in those with mild meningeal inflammation and 1.4–23.8 mcg/mL in those with marked inflammation; sulbactam CSF concentrations in these patients ranged from less than 0.5 to 4.7 mcg/mL and from 1–10.7 mcg/mL, respectively.

In patients undergoing cholecystectomy who received a single 1.5-g IV dose of ampicillin/sulbactam (1 g of ampicillin and 0.5 g of sulbactam), concentrations of ampicillin 0.25–1.5 hours after the dose averaged 15.9 mcg/mL in gallbladder bile, 7.7 mcg/g in gallbladder, and 20.2 mcg/mL in serum; concentrations of sulbactam in these samples averaged 4.3 mcg/mL, 6.3 mcg/g, and 19.9 mcg/mL, respectively.

Ampicillin is approximately 15–28% bound to serum proteins and sulbactam is approximately 38% bound to serum proteins.

Ampicillin and sulbactam both readily cross the placenta and concentrations in umbilical cord blood may be similar to serum concentrations. Ampicillin and sulbactam are distributed into milk in low concentrations. In lactating women who received 500-mg or 1-g doses of sulbactam by IV infusion over 20 minutes every 6 hours, concentrations of the drug in milk averaged 0.52 mcg/mL in samples obtained at random intervals between the first and thirteenth doses.

● **Elimination**

Serum concentrations of ampicillin and sulbactam both decline in a biphasic manner and half-lives of the drugs are similar. In healthy adults with normal renal function, both ampicillin and sulbactam have a distribution half-life ($t_{\frac{1}{2}\alpha}$) of about 15 minutes and an elimination half-life ($t_{\frac{1}{2}\beta}$) of about 1 hour. In some studies, the $t_{\frac{1}{2}\beta}$ of ampicillin ranged from 0.8–1.3 hours and that of sulbactam ranged from 0.97–1.4 hours. The $t_{\frac{1}{2}\beta}$ of ampicillin and sulbactam are slightly longer in geriatric adults than in younger adults. In a study in healthy geriatric adults 65–85 years of age with renal function normal for their age, the elimination half-life of ampicillin averaged 1.4 hours and that of sulbactam averaged 1.6 hours.

In infants and children younger than 12 years of age, sulbactam has a $t_{\frac{1}{2}\beta}$ of 0.92–1.9 hours. In neonates, the half-lives of ampicillin and sulbactam vary inversely with age; as renal tubular function matures, the drugs are cleared more rapidly.

The major route of elimination of both sulbactam and ampicillin is glomerular filtration and tubular secretion. Only small amounts of the drugs are eliminated in feces and bile. Following IM or IV administration of ampicillin/sulbactam in adults with normal renal function, approximately 75–92% of the dose of ampicillin and the dose of sulbactam is excreted unchanged in urine within 8 hours.

Serum concentrations of both ampicillin and sulbactam are higher and the half-lives of the drugs prolonged in patients with renal impairment. The elimination kinetics of both drugs appear to be affected to the same degree by impaired renal function. In one study, the half-lives of ampicillin and sulbactam averaged 1.6 and 1.6 hours, respectively, in adults with creatinine clearances of 30–60 mL/minute and 3.4 and 3.7 hours, respectively, in those with clearances of 7–30 mL/minute. In adults with creatinine clearances less than 7 mL/minute, the $t_{\frac{1}{2}\beta}$ of ampicillin and sulbactam averaged 17.4 and 13.4 hours, respectively.

Oral probenecid administered shortly before or with ampicillin/sulbactam competitively inhibits renal tubular secretion of both ampicillin and sulbactam and produces higher and prolonged serum concentrations of the drugs. (See Drug Interactions: Probenecid.)

Cystic fibrosis patients may eliminate sulbactam at faster rates than healthy individuals. In a study in children with cystic fibrosis, plasma clearance and apparent volume of distribution of sulbactam were about 1.5–2 times higher, peak plasma sulbactam concentrations were about 50% lower, and $t_{\frac{1}{2}\beta}$ of the drug slightly shorter in these children than in children without cystic fibrosis.

In healthy adults with normal renal function, renal clearance of ampicillin is 203–319 mL/minute and that of sulbactam is 169–204 mL/minute.

Ampicillin and sulbactam are both removed by hemodialysis. The amount of the drugs removed during hemodialysis depends on several factors (e.g., type of coil used, dialysis flow rate). In a few patients undergoing chronic dialysis, a 4-hour period of hemodialysis removed into the dialysate about 35% of the ampicillin dose and 45% of the sulbactam dose when a single 3-g dose of ampicillin/sulbactam (2 g of ampicillin and 1 g of sulbactam) was given 2 hours prior to dialysis.

CHEMISTRY AND STABILITY

● **Chemistry**

Ampicillin sodium and sulbactam sodium (ampicillin/sulbactam) is a fixed combination of the sodium salts of ampicillin and sulbactam. Ampicillin is an aminopenicillin. (See Ampicillin 8:12.16.08.) Sulbactam, a β-lactam β-lactamase inhibitor, is a synthetic penicillinate sulfone containing a β-lactam ring and derived from 6-aminopenicillanic acid. Although sulbactam has minimal antibacterial activity when used alone, the combined use of sulbactam sodium and certain penicillins or cephalosporins (e.g., amoxicillin, ampicillin, cefazolin, ceftizoxime, ceftriaxone, penicillin G) results in a synergistic effect that expands the spectrum of activity of the penicillin or cephalosporin against many strains of β-lactamase-producing bacteria.

The fixed combination of ampicillin sodium and sulbactam sodium (ampicillin/sulbactam) is commercially available as a sterile powder for parenteral use containing a 2:1 ratio of ampicillin to sulbactam. Potency of the fixed combination is expressed in terms of the total ampicillin content plus the total sulbactam content.

Ampicillin/sulbactam for parenteral use occurs as a white to off-white powder that is freely soluble in aqueous diluents. Each 1.5 g of ampicillin/sulbactam (1 g of ampicillin and 0.5 g of sulbactam) contains approximately 5 mEq (115 mg) of sodium; 3 g of the drug (2 g of ampicillin and 1 g of sulbactam) contains approximately 10 mEq (230 mg) of sodium. Following reconstitution, ampicillin/sulbactam solutions containing 375 mg/mL (250 mg of ampicillin and 125 mg of sulbactam per mL) occur as pale yellow to yellow solutions and have a pH of 8–10. Dilute solutions of the drug containing up to 30 mg of ampicillin and 15 mg of sulbactam are essentially colorless to pale yellow and have a pH of 8–10.

● **Stability**

Commercially available ampicillin/sulbactam sterile powder should be stored at 20–25°C.

The stability of ampicillin sodium in solution is concentration dependent, decreasing as the concentration of the drug increases. Ampicillin sodium appears to be especially susceptible to inactivation in solutions containing dextrose, which appears to have a catalytic effect on hydrolysis of the drug. Sulbactam sodium is much more stable in aqueous solution than ampicillin sodium, but when combined with ampicillin sodium, sulbactam sodium does not substantially improve nor adversely affect the stability of the aminopenicillin. Therefore, the stability of ampicillin/sulbactam solutions is similar to that of ampicillin sodium solutions.

Following reconstitution with sterile water for injection or 0.5 or 2% lidocaine hydrochloride injection, ampicillin/sulbactam solutions for IM injection containing 375 mg/mL (250 mg of ampicillin and 125 mg of sulbactam per mL) are stable for at least 1 hour, and the manufacturer recommends that such solutions be used within 1 hour after reconstitution.

Following reconstitution with sterile water for injection or 0.9% sodium chloride injection, ampicillin/sulbactam solutions for IV administration containing 45 mg/mL (30 mg of ampicillin and 15 mg of sulbactam per mL) are stable for 8 hours at 25°C or 48 hours at 4°C, and solutions containing 30 mg/mL (20 mg of ampicillin and 10 mg of sulbactam per mL) are stable for 72 hours at 4°C. The manufacturer states that solutions for IV administration containing 45 mg/mL (30 mg of ampicillin and 15 mg of sulbactam per mL) in lactated Ringer's injection or (1/6) M sodium lactate injection are stable for 24 or 8 hours, respectively, when refrigerated at 4°C and for 8 hours at 25°C, although some investigators have reported more prolonged stability. Likewise, the manufacturer states that solutions in 5% dextrose injection containing 30 mg/mL (20 mg of ampicillin and 10 mg of sulbactam per mL) are stable for 2 hours at 25°C or 4 hours when refrigerated at 4°C and those containing 3 mg/mL (2 mg of ampicillin and 1 mg of sulbactam per mL) are stable for 4 hours at 25°C, despite some data suggesting more prolonged stability. The manufacturer also states that solutions of the combination in 5% dextrose with 0.45% sodium chloride injection containing 3 mg/mL are stable for 4 hours at 25°C and those containing 15 mg/mL (10 mg of ampicillin and 5 mg of sulbactam per mL) are stable for 4 hours at 4°C, although some investigators also have reported more prolonged stability with such solutions. Similarly, while some data indicate more prolonged stability than that recommended by the manufacturer, the manufacturer states that solutions diluted in 10% invert sugar and containing 3 mg/mL (2 mg of ampicillin and 1 mg of sulbactam per mL) are stable for 4 hours at 25°C and those containing 30 mg/mL (20 mg of ampicillin and 10 mg of sulbactam per mL) are stable for 3 hours when refrigerated.

Ampicillin/sulbactam is potentially physically and/or chemically incompatible with some drugs, but the compatibility depends on several factors (e.g., concentrations of the drugs, specific diluents used, resulting pH, temperature). Specialized references should be consulted for specific compatibility information. Because of the potential for incompatibility, ampicillin/sulbactam and aminoglycosides should not be admixed..

For further information on chemistry and stability, mechanism of action, spectrum, resistance, pharmacokinetics, uses, cautions, drug interactions, and laboratory test interferences of ampicillin, see the Aminopenicillins General Statement 8:12.16.08 and see Ampicillin 8:12.16.08.

PREPARATIONS

Excipients in commercially available drug preparations may have clinically important effects in some individuals; consult specific product labeling for details.

Ampicillin Sodium and Sulbactam Sodium

Parenteral

For injection	1 g (of ampicillin) and 0.5 g (of sulbactam) (labeled as a combined total potency of 1.5 g)*	**Ampicillin and Sulbactam for Injection**
		Unasyn®, Pfizer
	2 g (of ampicillin) and 1 g (of sulbactam) (labeled as a combined total potency of 3 g)*	**Ampicillin and Sulbactam for Injection**
		Unasyn®, Pfizer
	10 g (of ampicillin) and 5 g (of sulbactam) (labeled as a combined total potency of 15 g) pharmacy bulk package*	**Ampicillin and Sulbactam for Injection**
		Unasyn®, Pfizer

† Use is not currently included in the labeling approved by the US Food and Drug Administration.

* available from one or more manufacturer, distributor, and/or repackager by generic (nonproprietary) name

Dicloxacillin Sodium

8:12.16.12 • PENICILLINASE-RESISTANT PENICILLINS

■ Dicloxacillin is a semisynthetic penicillinase-resistant penicillin antibiotic.

USES

Dicloxacillin shares the uses of other penicillinase-resistant penicillins and generally is used only in the treatment of infections caused by, or suspected of being caused by, susceptible penicillinase-resistant staphylococci. Oral dicloxacillin should not be used for the initial treatment of severe, life-threatening infections, including endocarditis, but may be used as follow-up after therapy with a parenteral penicillinase-resistant penicillin (e.g., nafcillin, oxacillin). For specific information on the uses of dicloxacillin, see Uses in the Penicillinase-Resistant Penicillins General Statement 8:12.16.12.

DOSAGE AND ADMINISTRATION

● Reconstitution and Administration

Dicloxacillin sodium is administered orally at least 1 hour before or 2 hours after meals. Although the drug also has been given parenterally by slow IV injection or infusion or by IM injection, a parenteral dosage form is no longer commercially available in the US.

Oral dicloxacillin should not be used for the initial treatment of severe infections and should not be relied on in patients with nausea, vomiting, gastric dilatation, cardiospasm, or intestinal hypermotility.

● Dosage

Dosage of dicloxacillin sodium is expressed in terms of dicloxacillin. Dosage of the drug should be adjusted according to the type and severity of infection.

Adult Dosage

The usual adult oral dosage of dicloxacillin for the treatment of mild to moderate infections caused by susceptible penicillinase-producing staphylococci is 125 mg every 6 hours. For more severe infections, the usual adult oral dosage of dicloxacillin is 250 mg every 6 hours; higher dosage may be necessary depending on the severity of the infection.

Pediatric Dosage

Children weighing 40 kg or more may receive the usual adult dosage of dicloxacillin.

In children who weigh less than 40 kg, the usual oral dosage of dicloxacillin for the treatment of mild to moderate infections caused by susceptible penicillinase-producing staphylococci is 12.5 mg/kg daily given in divided doses every 6 hours. The usual oral dosage for the treatment of more severe infections is 25 mg/kg daily given in divided doses every 6 hours; higher dosage may be necessary depending on the severity of the infection. If dicloxacillin is used in neonates, they should be monitored closely for clinical and laboratory evidence of toxic or adverse effects, and serum concentrations of the drug should be determined frequently and appropriate reductions in dosage and frequency of administration made when indicated. (See Cautions: Pediatric Precautions.)

The American Academy of Pediatrics (AAP) suggests that children older than 1 month of age receive oral dicloxacillin in a dosage of 25–50 mg/kg daily in 4 divided doses for the treatment of mild to moderate infections; the AAP states that the oral drug is inappropriate for severe infections.

Some clinicians suggest that, when dicloxacillin is used as follow-up therapy to parenteral penicillinase-resistant penicillin therapy in the treatment of acute or chronic osteomyelitis caused by susceptible staphylococci, children should receive an oral dosage of 50–100 mg/kg daily given in divided doses every 6 hours. If oral anti-infective therapy is used in the treatment of osteomyelitis, compliance must be assured and some clinicians suggest that serum bactericidal titers (SBTs) be used to monitor adequacy of therapy and to adjust dosage. (See Uses: Staphylococcal Infections, in the Penicillinase-Resistant Penicillins General Statement 8:12.16.12.)

Duration of Therapy

The duration of dicloxacillin therapy depends on the type and severity of infection and should be determined by the clinical and bacteriologic response of the patient. Dicloxacillin therapy usually should be continued for at least 48 hours after cultures are negative and the patient becomes afebrile and asymptomatic. For severe staphylococcal infections, therapy should be continued for at least 14 days; more prolonged therapy is necessary for the treatment of osteomyelitis, endocarditis, or other metastatic infections. When oral dicloxacillin is used as follow-up therapy to parenteral penicillinase-resistant therapy in the treatment of acute osteomyelitis, the drug generally is given for 3–6 weeks or until the total duration of parenteral and oral therapy is at least 6 weeks; when used as follow-up therapy in the treatment of chronic osteomyelitis, the drug generally is given for at least 1–2 months and has been given for as long as 1–2 years.

● Dosage in Renal Impairment

Adjustment of dicloxacillin dosage in patients with renal impairment generally is unnecessary.

CAUTIONS

● Adverse Effects

Adverse effects reported with dicloxacillin are similar to those reported with other penicillinase-resistant penicillins. For information on adverse effects reported with penicillinase-resistant penicillins, see Cautions in the Penicillinase-Resistant Penicillins General Statement 8:12.16.12.

● Precautions and Contraindications

Dicloxacillin is contraindicated in patients who are hypersensitive to any penicillin.

Dicloxacillin shares the toxic potentials of the penicillins, including the risk of hypersensitivity reactions, and the usual precautions of penicillin therapy should be observed. Prior to initiation of therapy with dicloxacillin, careful inquiry should be made concerning previous hypersensitivity reactions to penicillins, cephalosporins, or other drugs. There is clinical and laboratory evidence of partial cross-allergenicity among penicillins and other β-lactam antibiotics including cephalosporins and cephamycins.

Renal, hepatic, and hematologic systems should be evaluated periodically during prolonged therapy with dicloxacillin. Because adverse hematologic effects have occurred during therapy with penicillinase-resistant penicillins, white blood cell (WBC) count and differential should be performed prior to initiation of therapy and 1–3 times weekly during therapy. In addition, urinalysis should be performed and BUN, serum creatinine, AST (SGOT), and ALT (SGPT) concentrations should be determined prior to and periodically during therapy.

Patients should be advised to discontinue dicloxacillin and notify their clinicians if they develop shortness of breath, wheezing, rash, mouth irritation, black tongue, sore throat, nausea, vomiting, diarrhea, fever, swollen joints, or any unusual bleeding or bruising during therapy with the drug.

For a more complete discussion of these and other precautions associated with the use of dicloxacillin, see Cautions: Precautions and Contraindications, in the Penicillinase-Resistant Penicillins General Statement 8:12.16.12.

● Pediatric Precautions

Elimination of penicillins is delayed in neonates because of immature mechanisms for renal excretion, and abnormally high serum concentrations of the drugs may occur in this age group. If dicloxacillin is used in neonates, they should be monitored closely for clinical and laboratory evidence of toxic or adverse effects, and serum concentrations of the drug should be determined frequently and appropriate reductions in dosage and frequency of administration made when indicated.

● Pregnancy, Fertility, and Lactation
Pregnancy

Safe use of penicillinase-resistant penicillins during pregnancy has not been definitely established. Clinical experience with use of penicillins during pregnancy in humans has not revealed evidence of adverse effects on the fetus. However, there are no adequate and controlled studies using penicillinase-resistant penicillins in pregnant women, and dicloxacillin should be used during pregnancy only when clearly needed.

Lactation

Because dicloxacillin is distributed into milk, the drug should be used with caution in nursing women.

SPECTRUM

Based on its spectrum of activity, dicloxacillin is classified as a penicillinase-resistant penicillin. For information on the classification of penicillins based on spectra of activity, see the Preface to the General Statements on Penicillins 8:12.16.

Like other penicillinase-resistant penicillins, dicloxacillin is resistant to inactivation by staphylococcal penicillinases and is active against many penicillinase-producing strains of *Staphylococcus aureus* and *S. epidermidis* that are resistant to other commercially available penicillins. For specific information on the spectrum of activity of dicloxacillin and resistance to the drug, see the sections on Spectrum and on Resistance in the Penicillinase-Resistant Penicillins General Statement 8:12.16.12.

PHARMACOKINETICS

In all studies described in the Pharmacokinetics section, dicloxacillin was administered as the sodium salt; dosages and concentrations of the drug are expressed in terms of dicloxacillin.

● Absorption

Dicloxacillin is resistant to inactivation in the presence of acidic gastric secretions and is rapidly but incompletely absorbed from the GI tract. In healthy, fasting adults, 35–76% of an orally administered dose of dicloxacillin is absorbed from the GI tract and peak serum concentrations of the drug are generally attained within 0.5–2 hours.

Presence of food in the GI tract generally decreases the rate and extent of absorption of dicloxacillin.

Following oral administration of a single 500-mg dose of dicloxacillin in fasting adults, peak serum concentrations of the drug average 10–18 μg/mL; serum concentrations of the drug decline rapidly and are generally low 6 hours after the drug is administered. In fasting adults who receive a single 250-mg oral dose of dicloxacillin as a capsule, serum concentrations of the drug average 2.9–3, 4.6–5.5, 3–5.6, and 1.5–1.7 μg/mL at 30 minutes, 1 hour, 2 hours, and 4 hours, respectively, after the dose.

In one study in children with acute osteomyelitis who received oral dicloxacillin in a dosage of 100 mg/kg daily given in divided doses every 6 hours, serum concentrations of the drug ranged from 12–40 μg/mL 1 hour after dosing and 6.5–20 μg/mL 3 hours after dosing.

● Distribution

Dicloxacillin is distributed into bone, bile, pleural fluid, ascitic fluid, and synovial fluid. In one study in children 2–16 years of age with acute osteomyelitis who received dicloxacillin IM in a dosage of 50 mg/kg daily, dicloxacillin concentrations in bone ranged from 1.8–21.6 μg/g and concurrent serum concentrations of the drug ranged from 7–9 μg/mL in samples taken 1–3 hours after a dose. In children 7 months to 14 years of age with suppurative arthritis who received a single oral dicloxacillin dose of 25 mg/kg, dicloxacillin concentrations in synovial fluid obtained 2 hours after the dose were 70% of concurrent serum concentrations; synovial fluid concentrations averaged 9.5 μg/mL and serum concentrations averaged 13.6 μg/mL. Like other penicillins, only minimal concentrations of dicloxacillin are attained in CSF.

Dicloxacillin is 95–99% bound to serum proteins.

Dicloxacillin reportedly distributes into amniotic fluid in therapeutic concentrations following usual dosages. The drug also crosses the placenta and is distributed into milk. Following oral administration of a single 250-mg dose of dicloxacillin in lactating women, milk concentrations of the drug were 0.1–0.3 μg/mL 2 and 4 hours after the dose and undetectable 6 hours after the dose.

● Elimination

The serum half-life of dicloxacillin in adults with normal renal function is 0.6–0.8 hours. In one study in children 2–16 years of age, the serum half-life of the drug averaged 1.9 hours.

Dicloxacillin is partially metabolized to active and inactive metabolites. In one study following administration of a single 500-mg oral dose of dicloxacillin, 10% of the absorbed drug was hydrolyzed to penicilloic acids which are microbiologically inactive. Dicloxacillin is also hydroxylated to a small extent to a microbiologically active metabolite which appears to be slightly less active than dicloxacillin.

Dicloxacillin and its metabolites are rapidly excreted in urine mainly by tubular secretion and glomerular filtration. The drug is also partly excreted in feces via biliary elimination. Following oral administration of a single 250-mg, 500-mg, or 1-g dose of dicloxacillin in adults with normal renal function, 31–65% of the dose is excreted in urine as unchanged drug and active metabolites within 6–8 hours; approximately 10–20% of this is the active metabolite.

The serum half-life of dicloxacillin is slightly prolonged in patients with impaired renal function and has been reported to range from 1–2.2 hours in patients with severe renal impairment.

Serum concentrations of dicloxacillin are higher and the serum half-life longer in neonates than in older children.

Patients with cystic fibrosis eliminate dicloxacillin approximately 3 times faster than healthy individuals. In one study following oral administration of a single 6.25-mg/kg dose of the drug, peak serum concentrations and areas under the serum concentration-time curves (AUCs) were, on average, 2.5 times lower in patients with cystic fibrosis than in healthy individuals. Patients with cystic fibrosis had renal clearances of the drug averaging 282 mL/minute per 1.73 m² while healthy individuals had renal clearances averaging 95 mL/minute per 1.73 m².

Dicloxacillin is only minimally removed by hemodialysis or peritoneal dialysis.

CHEMISTRY AND STABILITY

● Chemistry

Dicloxacillin is a semisynthetic penicillinase-resistant penicillin. Dicloxacillin, like cloxacillin (no longer commercially available in the US) and oxacillin, is an isoxazolyl penicillin.

Dicloxacillin is commercially available as the monohydrate sodium salt. Potency of dicloxacillin sodium is expressed in terms of dicloxacillin. Each mg of dicloxacillin sodium contains not less than 850 μg of dicloxacillin. Dicloxacillin sodium occurs as a white to off-white, crystalline powder. The drug is freely soluble in water. Dicloxacillin sodium has a pK$_a$ of 2.7–2.8.

Each 250-mg capsule of dicloxacillin contains approximately 0.6 mEq of sodium.

● Stability

Commercially available dicloxacillin sodium capsules should be stored in tight containers at a temperature less than 40°C, preferably between 15–30°C.

For further information on chemistry and stability, mechanism of action, spectrum, resistance, pharmacokinetics, uses, cautions, drug interactions, laboratory test interferences, and dosage and administration of dicloxacillin sodium, see the Penicillinase-Resistant Penicillins General Statement 8:12.16.12.

PREPARATIONS

Excipients in commercially available drug preparations may have clinically important effects in some individuals; consult specific product labeling for details.

Dicloxacillin Sodium

Oral		
Capsules	250 mg (of dicloxacillin)*	**Dicloxacillin Sodium**
	500 mg (of dicloxacillin)*	**Dicloxacillin Sodium**

* available from one or more manufacturer, distributor, and/or repackager by generic (nonproprietary) name

Selected Revisions January 1, 2009, © Copyright, January 1, 1985, American Society of Health-System Pharmacists, Inc.

Nafcillin Sodium

8:12.16.12 • PENICILLINASE-RESISTANT PENICILLINS

■ Nafcillin is a semisynthetic penicillinase-resistant penicillin antibiotic.

USES

Nafcillin shares the uses of other parenteral penicillinase-resistant penicillins (e.g., oxacillin) and generally is used only in the treatment of infections caused by, or suspected of being caused by, susceptible penicillinase-producing staphylococci. For specific information on the uses of nafcillin, see Uses in the Penicillinase-Resistant Penicillins General Statement 8:12.16.12.

DOSAGE AND ADMINISTRATION

● Reconstitution and Administration

Nafcillin sodium is administered by IM injection or by IV injection or infusion. Although nafcillin also has been administered orally, the drug is poorly absorbed from the GI tract and an oral preparation of the drug is no longer commercially available in the US.

Reconstituted, diluted, and thawed solutions of nafcillin sodium should be inspected visually for particulate matter and discoloration prior to administration whenever solution and container permit.

To reduce the risk of thrombophlebitis and other adverse local reactions associated with IV administration of nafcillin sodium, particularly in geriatric patients, the drug should be administered slowly and care should be taken to avoid extravasation. In addition, the IV route should be used for relatively short periods of time (e.g., 24–48 hours). For additional information, see Cautions: Local Reactions, in the Penicillinase-Resistant Penicillins General Statement 8:12.16.12.

IM Injection

For IM injection, nafcillin sodium powder for injection is reconstituted by adding 3.4 or 6.8 mL of sterile water for injection, bacteriostatic water for injection (with benzyl alcohol or parabens), or 0.9% sodium chloride injection to a vial labeled as containing 1 or 2 g of nafcillin, respectively, to provide solutions containing 250 mg/mL.

IM injections of nafcillin sodium should be made deeply into a large muscle (e.g., gluteus maximus) and care should be taken to avoid sciatic nerve injury.

Intermittent IV Injection

For direct intermittent IV injection, nafcillin sodium powder for injection should be reconstituted as for IM administration and, when dissolved, the appropriate dose of the drug should be further diluted with 15–30 mL of sterile water for injection or sodium chloride injection.

The appropriate dose of *diluted* nafcillin sodium should then be injected slowly over 5–10 minutes into the tubing of a free-flowing compatible IV solution.

Intermittent IV Infusion

For intermittent IV infusion, vials labeled as containing 1 or 2 g of nafcillin should be reconstituted as for IM injection and, when dissolved, should be further diluted with a compatible IV solution according to the manufacturer's directions. Alternatively, ADD-Vantage vials containing 1 or 2 of the drug may be reconstituted according to the manufacturer's directions.

Pharmacy bulk packages containing 10 g of nafcillin should be reconstituted with 93 mL of sterile water for injection or 0.9% sodium chloride injection to provide a solution containing 100 mg/mL. Pharmacy bulk packages of the drug are not intended for direct IV infusion; doses of the drug from the reconstituted pharmacy bulk package must be further diluted in a compatible IV infusion solution prior to administration.

Thawed solutions of the commercially available frozen nafcillin sodium injection are administered by intermittent IV infusion. Commercially available frozen nafcillin sodium injections should not be thawed by warming them in a water bath or by exposure to microwave radiation. A precipitate may form while the commercially available frozen injection in dextrose is frozen; however, this usually will dissolve with little or no agitation upon reaching room temperature, and the potency of the injection is not affected. After thawing at room temperature or under refrigeration, the container should be checked for minute leaks by firmly squeezing the bag. The injection should be discarded if the container seal is not intact or leaks are found or if the solution is cloudy or contains a precipitate. Additives should not be introduced into the injection. The injection should not be used in series connections with other plastic containers, since such use could result in air embolism from residual air being drawn from the primary container before administration of fluid from the secondary container is complete.

Intermittent IV infusions of nafcillin sodium generally are infused over at least 30–60 minutes. (See Chemistry and Stability: Stability.)

● Dosage

Dosage of nafcillin sodium is expressed in terms of nafcillin. Dosage of the drug should be adjusted according to the type and severity of infection.

Adult Dosage

The usual adult IM dosage of nafcillin for the treatment of infections caused by susceptible penicillinase-producing staphylococci is 500 mg every 4–6 hours; severe infections may require 1 g IM every 4 hours.

The usual adult IV dosage of nafcillin for the treatment of infections caused by susceptible penicillinase-producing staphylococci is 500 mg every 4 hours; severe infections may require 1 g every 4 hours. When nafcillin is used for the treatment of acute or chronic osteomyelitis caused by susceptible penicillinase-producing staphylococci, many clinicians recommend that adults receive 1–2 g of the drug IV every 4 hours. If nafcillin is used for the treatment of staphylococcal infections related to intravascular catheters, some clinicians recommend that adults receive 2 g every 4 hours. Some clinicians recommend that adults receive IV dosages of at least 100–200 mg/kg daily given in equally divided doses every 4–6 hours for the treatment of meningitis.

Staphylococcal Endocarditis

For the treatment of native valve endocarditis caused by staphylococci susceptible to penicillinase-resistant penicillins, the American Heart Association (AHA) recommends that adults receive nafcillin in a dosage of 2 g IV every 4 hours for 4–6 weeks. Although the benefits of concomitant aminoglycoside therapy have not been clearly established in these infections, the AHA states that gentamicin (1 mg/kg IM or IV every 8 hours) may be given concomitantly during the first 3–5 days of nafcillin therapy.

For the treatment of staphylococcal endocarditis in the presence of prosthetic valves or other prosthetic material in patients with infections caused by isolates susceptible to penicillinase-resistant penicillins, the AHA states that adults should receive nafcillin in a dosage of 2 g IV every 4 hours for 6 weeks or longer in conjunction with rifampin (300 mg orally every 8 hours for 6 weeks or longer) and gentamicin (1 mg/kg IM or IV every 8 hours during the first 2 weeks of nafcillin therapy). However, because coagulase-negative staphylococci causing prosthetic valve endocarditis usually are resistant to penicillinase-resistant penicillins (especially when endocarditis develops within 1 year after surgery), coagulase-negative staphylococci involved in prosthetic valve endocarditis should be assumed to be resistant to penicillinase-resistant penicillins unless results of in vitro testing indicate that the isolates are susceptible to the drugs. (See Uses: Endocarditis in the Penicillinase-resistant Penicillins General Statement 8:12.16.12.)

Pediatric Dosage

Children weighing 40 kg or more may receive the usual adult dosage of nafcillin.

The manufacturer recommends that pediatric patients weighing less than 40 kg receive IM nafcillin in a dosage of 25 mg/kg twice daily and that neonates receive an IM dosage of 10 mg/kg twice daily.

The American Academy of Pediatrics (AAP) recommends that children 1 month of age or older receive IM or IV nafcillin in a dosage of 50–100 mg/kg daily in 4 equally divided doses for the treatment of mild to moderate infections or 100–150 mg/kg daily in 4 equally divided doses for the treatment of severe infections. Other clinicians recommend that children receive nafcillin in a dosage of 100–200 mg/kg daily given in 4–6 equally divided doses for severe infections.

The AAP and other clinicians recommend that neonates younger than 1 week of age receive IM or IV nafcillin in a dosage of 25 mg/kg every 12 hours if they weigh 2 kg or less or 25 mg/kg every 8 hours if they weigh more than 2 kg. Neonates 1–4 weeks should receive 25 mg/kg every 8 hours if they weigh 2 kg or less (25 mg/kg every 12 hours for those less than 1.2 kg) or 25–35 mg/kg every 6 hours if they weigh more than 2 kg. The higher dosages are recommended for meningitis.

Staphylococcal Endocarditis

For the treatment of native valve endocarditis caused by staphylococci susceptible to penicillinase-resistant penicillins, the AHA recommends that pediatric patients receive nafcillin in a dosage of 200 mg/kg daily given IV in divided doses every 4–6 hours for 6 weeks (maximum daily dosage 12 g). In addition, during the first 3–5 days of oxacillin therapy, gentamicin (3 mg/kg daily given IM or IV in divided doses every 8 hours; dosage adjusted to achieve peak serum gentamicin concentrations approximately 3 mcg/mL and trough concentrations less than 1 mcg/mL) may be given concomitantly if the causative organism is susceptible to the drug.

For the treatment of staphylococcal endocarditis in the presence of prosthetic valves or other prosthetic material in patients with infections caused by isolates susceptible to penicillinase-resistant penicillins, the AHA recommends that pediatric patients receive nafcillin in a dosage of 200 mg/kg daily given IV in divided doses every 4–6 hours for 6 weeks or longer (maximum daily dosage 12 g) in conjunction with rifampin (20 mg/kg daily given orally in divided doses every 8 hours for 6 weeks or longer) and gentamicin (3 mg/kg daily given IM or IV in divided doses every 8 hours during the first 2 weeks of oxacillin therapy; dosage adjusted to achieve peak serum gentamicin concentrations approximately 3 mcg/mL and trough concentrations less than 1 mcg/mL).

Duration of Therapy

The duration of nafcillin therapy depends on the type and severity of infection and should be determined by the clinical and bacteriologic response of the patient. In severe staphylococcal infections, therapy should be continued for at least 2 weeks; more prolonged therapy is necessary for the treatment of osteomyelitis, endocarditis, or other metastatic infections.

When nafcillin is used in the treatment of acute or chronic osteomyelitis caused by susceptible penicillinase-producing staphylococci, the drug is generally given for 3–8 weeks; follow-up therapy with an oral penicillinase-resistant penicillin after nafcillin therapy generally is recommended for the treatment of chronic osteomyelitis.

● Dosage in Renal and Hepatic Impairment

Modification of nafcillin dosage generally is unnecessary in patients with either renal impairment or hepatic impairment alone; however, modification of dosage may be necessary in patients with both severe renal impairment and hepatic impairment.

CAUTIONS

● Adverse Effects

Adverse effects reported with nafcillin are similar to those reported with other penicillinase-resistant penicillins. For information on adverse effects reported with penicillinase-resistant penicillins, see Cautions in the Penicillinase-Resistant Penicillins General Statement 8:12.16.12.

● Precautions and Contraindications

Nafcillin is contraindicated in patients who are hypersensitive to any penicillin.

Nafcillin shares the toxic potentials of the penicillins, including the risk of hypersensitivity reactions, and the usual precautions of penicillin therapy should be observed. Prior to initiation of therapy with nafcillin, careful inquiry should be made concerning previous hypersensitivity reactions to penicillins, cephalosporins, or other drugs. There is clinical and laboratory evidence of partial cross-allergenicity among penicillins and other β-lactam antibiotics including cephalosporins and cephamycins.

Renal, hepatic, and hematologic systems should be evaluated periodically during prolonged therapy with nafcillin. Because adverse hematologic effects have occurred during therapy with penicillinase-resistant penicillins, white blood cell (CBC) count and differential should be performed prior to initiation of therapy and 1–3 times weekly during therapy. In addition, urinalysis should be performed and BUN, serum creatinine, AST (SGOT), and ALT (SGPT) concentrations should be determined prior to and periodically during therapy. If eosinophilia, suspected drug fever, rash, arthralgia, hematuria, or unexplained elevations of BUN or serum creatinine occur during penicillinase-resistant penicillin therapy, alternative anti-infective therapy should be considered.

For a more complete discussion of these and other precautions associated with the use of nafcillin, see Cautions: Precautions and Contraindications, in the Penicillinase-Resistant Penicillins General Statement 8:12.16.12.

● Pediatric Precautions

If nafcillin is used in neonates, they should be monitored closely for clinical and laboratory evidence of toxic or adverse effects. In addition, serum concentrations of the drug should be determined frequently and appropriate reductions in dosage and frequency of administration made when indicated.

● Pregnancy, Fertility, and Lactation

Pregnancy

Safe use of nafcillin during pregnancy has not been definitely established. Reproduction studies using nafcillin in rats and rabbits have not revealed evidence of impaired fertility or harm to the fetus. Clinical experience with use of penicillins during pregnancy in humans has not revealed evidence of adverse effects on the fetus. However, there are no adequate and controlled studies using penicillinase-resistant penicillins in pregnant women, and nafcillin should be used during pregnancy only when clearly needed.

Lactation

Because penicillins are distributed into milk, nafcillin should be used with caution in nursing women.

SPECTRUM

Based on its spectrum of activity, nafcillin is classified as a penicillinase-resistant penicillin. For information on the classification of penicillins based on spectra of activity, see the Preface to the Penicillins General Statements 8:12.16.

Like other penicillinase-resistant penicillins, nafcillin is resistant to inactivation by most staphylococcal penicillinases and is active against many penicillinase-producing strains of *Staphylococcus aureus* and *S. epidermidis* that are resistant to other commercially available penicillins. For specific information on the spectrum of activity of nafcillin and resistance to the drug, see the sections on Spectrum and on Resistance in the Penicillinase-Resistant Penicillins General Statement 8:12.16.12.

PHARMACOKINETICS

In all studies described in the Pharmacokinetics section, nafcillin was administered as the sodium salt; dosages and concentrations of the drug are expressed in terms of nafcillin.

● Absorption

Nafcillin is poorly absorbed from the GI tract, and oral preparations of the drug are no longer commercially available in the US.

IM injection of a single 1-g dose of nafcillin results in peak serum concentrations of 7.6 mcg/mL at 30–60 minutes after the dose.

Following IV injection over 5 minutes of a single 500-mg dose of nafcillin in healthy adults, serum concentrations of the drug average approximately 40, 10, 4.5, and 1.7 mcg/mL at 5 minutes, 30 minutes, 1 hour, and 2 hours, respectively, after the injection.

In one study in children 1 month to 14 years of age who received nafcillin in a dosage of 150 mg/kg daily in divided doses every 6 hours, serum concentrations of the drug averaged 48.1, 23.6, 6.4, and 1.8 mcg/mL at 30 minutes, 1 hour, 2 hours, and 4 hours, respectively, after a dose.

● Distribution

Nafcillin is distributed into synovial, pleural, pericardial, and ascitic fluids. The drug also is distributed into liver, bone, and bile. The volume of distribution of nafcillin reportedly ranges from 0.57–1.55 L/kg in adults, 0.85–0.91 L/kg in children 1 month to 14 years of age, and 0.24–0.53 L/kg in neonates. In one study, the volume of distribution of nafcillin at steady state averaged 27.1 L in adults with normal renal and hepatic function, 19.9 L in adults with cirrhosis, and 15.9 L in adults with extrahepatic biliary obstruction.

Concentrations of nafcillin in bile are generally equal to or greater than concurrent serum concentrations unless biliary obstruction is present.

Like other penicillins, only low concentrations of nafcillin are attained in CSF; however, CSF concentrations of the drug are generally higher when meninges are inflamed than when meninges are uninflamed. In one study following IV administration of 1- or 2-g doses of nafcillin every 4 hours in adults with inflamed or uninflamed meninges, CSF concentrations of the drug ranged from 0.1–58 mcg/mL in specimens obtained approximately 1–2 hours after a dose. In one study in adults with uninflamed meninges who received a single 40-mg/kg dose of nafcillin IV over 30 minutes, CSF concentrations of the drug ranged from 0.02–0.09, 0.03–0.17, 0.06–0.12, and 0–0.07 mcg/mL in specimens obtained 1, 2, 3, and 4 hours, respectively, after the dose. In hydrocephalic children 3 weeks to 8.5 years of age with suspected ventriculoperitoneal shunt infections who received 50 mg/kg of nafcillin every 6 hours given by IV infusion over 30–40 minutes, peak concentrations of the drug in ventricular fluid were generally attained 2–2.5 hours after a dose and ranged from 0.2–10.3 mcg/mL.

Only negligible concentrations of nafcillin are distributed into aqueous humor following parenteral administration. In patients with uninflamed eyes undergoing cataract surgery, IV administration of a single 2-g dose over 10 minutes resulted in serum and aqueous humor concentrations of the drug ranging from 70–120 mcg/mL and unmeasurable to 1.9 mcg/mL, respectively, 30–50 minutes after administration.

Nafcillin is 70–90% bound to serum proteins.

Nafcillin crosses the placenta. Nafcillin, like other penicillins, probably is distributed into milk.

● Elimination

The serum half-life of nafcillin in adults with normal renal and hepatic function averages 0.5–1.5 hours. In one study in healthy adults, nafcillin had a distribution half-life ($t_{1/2}\alpha$) of 0.17 hours and an elimination half-life ($t_{1/2}\beta$) of 1.02 hours.

Approximately 60% of a dose of nafcillin is metabolized in the liver to inactive metabolites. Although small amounts of nafcillin are excreted in urine, the drug is eliminated mainly via bile and undergoes enterohepatic circulation. About 27–31% of a single IM or IV dose of nafcillin is excreted in urine as unchanged drug and active metabolites within 12 hours in adults with normal renal and hepatic function.

Serum clearance of nafcillin is reportedly 410–583 mL/minute per 1.73 m² in adults with normal renal and hepatic function.

Serum concentrations of nafcillin may be higher and the serum half-life slightly prolonged in patients with impaired renal function. The serum half-life of the drug is reportedly 1.2–1.9 hours in patients with creatinine clearances of 3–59 mL/minute per 1.73 m² and 1.8–2.8 hours in patients with creatinine clearances less than 3 mL/minute per 1.73 m².

In one study in patients with cirrhosis or extrahepatic biliary obstruction, the $t_{1/2}\alpha$ of nafcillin averaged 0.26 or 0.29 hours, respectively, and the $t_{1/2}\beta$ averaged 1.2 and 1.7 hours, respectively. Serum clearance of the drug in these patients was lower than in patients with normal renal and hepatic function and averaged 291.5 mL/minute in those with cirrhosis and 163.4 mL/minute in those with extrahepatic obstruction.

In children 1 month to 14 years of age, the serum half-life of nafcillin ranges from 0.75–1.9 hours. Serum concentrations of nafcillin are generally higher and the serum half-life is longer in neonates than in older children. In one study, the serum half-life of nafcillin ranged from 2.2–5.5 hours in neonates 3 weeks of age or younger and 1.2–2.3 hours in neonates 4–9 weeks of age.

Nafcillin is only minimally removed by hemodialysis or peritoneal dialysis.

CHEMISTRY AND STABILITY

● Chemistry

Nafcillin is a semisynthetic penicillinase-resistant penicillin.

Nafcillin is commercially available as the monohydrate sodium salt. Potency of nafcillin sodium is expressed in terms of nafcillin. Each mg of nafcillin sodium contains not less than 820 mcg of nafcillin. Nafcillin sodium occurs as a white to yellowish white powder which may have a slight characteristic odor. The drug

is freely soluble in water and soluble in alcohol. Nafcillin sodium has a pK_a of approximately 2.7.

Commercially available frozen nafcillin sodium in dextrose injections are sterile, nonpyrogenic, iso-osmotic solutions of the drug; about 1.8 or 1 g of dextrose has been added to the 1- or 2-g injections of nafcillin sodium, respectively, to adjust osmolality to about 300 mOsm/kg. Nafcillin sodium in dextrose frozen injections also contain sodium citrate as a buffer and hydrochloric acid and/or sodium hydroxide to adjust pH to 6–8.5.

● Stability

Following reconstitution with sterile water for injection, bacteriostatic water for injection, or 0.9% sodium chloride injection, nafcillin sodium solutions containing 250 mg of nafcillin per mL are stable for 3 days at room temperature, 7 days when refrigerated, or 90 days when frozen. The manufacturer states that solutions containing 10–200 mg/mL are stable for 24 hours at room temperature, 7 days when refrigerated, or 90 days when frozen.

The manufacturer states that the stability of the commercially available frozen nafcillin sodium injection may vary. These injections are stable for at least 90 days from the date of shipment when stored at –20°C. The frozen injection should be thawed at room temperature (25°C) or under refrigeration (5°C) and, once thawed, should not be refrozen. Thawed solutions of the commercially available frozen injection are stable for 72 hours at room temperature (25°C) or 21 days when refrigerated at 5°C. The commercially available frozen injection of the drug in dextrose is provided in a plastic container fabricated from specially formulated multilayered plastic PL 2040 (Galaxy®). Solutions in contact with the plastic can leach out some of its chemical components in very small amounts within the expiration period of the injection; however, safety of the plastic has been confirmed in animals according to USP biological tests for plastic containers as well as by tissue culture toxicity studies.

Nafcillin sodium is potentially physically and/or chemically incompatible with some drugs, including aminoglycosides and admixtures resulting in a pH greater than 8 or less than 5, but the compatibility depends on several factors (e.g., concentrations of the drugs, specific diluents used, resulting pH, temperature). For information on the in vitro and in vivo incompatibility of penicillins and aminoglycosides, see Drug Interactions: Aminoglycosides, in the Penicillinase-Resistant Penicillins General Statement 8:12.16.12. Specialized references should be consulted for specific compatibility information. Because of the potential for incompatibility, nafcillin sodium and other drugs should not be admixed.

For further information on chemistry and stability, mechanism of action, spectrum, resistance, pharmacokinetics, uses, cautions, drug interactions, laboratory test interferences, and dosage and administration of nafcillin sodium, see the Penicillinase-Resistant Penicillins General Statement 8:12.16.12.

PREPARATIONS

Excipients in commercially available drug preparations may have clinically important effects in some individuals; consult specific product labeling for details.

Nafcillin Sodium in Dextrose

Parenteral		
For injection	1 g (of nafcillin)*	**Nafcillin Sodium for Injection**
	2 g (of nafcillin)*	**Nafcillin Sodium for Injection**
	10 g (of nafcillin) pharmacy bulk package*	**Nafcillin Sodium for Injection**
For injection, for IV infusion	1 g (of nafcillin)*	**Nafcillin Sodium for Injection ADD-Vantage®, Sandoz**
	2 g (of nafcillin)*	**Nafcillin Sodium for Injection ADD-Vantage®, Sandoz**
Injection (frozen), for IV infusion	20 mg (of nafcillin) per mL (1 g) in 3.6% Dextrose*	**Nafcillin Sodium in Iso-osmotic Dextrose Injection Galaxy®, Baxter**
	20 mg (of nafcillin) per mL (2 g) in 3.6% Dextrose*	**Nafcillin Sodium in Iso-osmotic Dextrose Injection Galaxy®, Baxter**

* available from one or more manufacturer, distributor, and/or repackager by generic (nonproprietary) name

Selected Revisions January 1, 2009, © Copyright, January 1, 1985, American Society of Health-System Pharmacists, Inc.

Oxacillin Sodium

8:12.16.12 • PENICILLINASE-RESISTANT PENICILLINS

■ Oxacillin is a semisynthetic penicillinase-resistant penicillin antibiotic.

USES

Oxacillin shares the uses of other parenteral penicillinase-resistant penicillins (e.g., nafcillin) and generally is used only in the treatment of infections caused by, or suspected of being caused by, susceptible penicillinase-producing staphylococci. For specific information on the uses of oxacillin, see Uses in the Penicillinase-Resistant Penicillins General Statement 8:12.16.12.

DOSAGE AND ADMINISTRATION

● Reconstitution and Administration

Oxacillin sodium is administered by IM injection or slow IV injection or infusion. Although oxacillin has been administered orally, an oral preparation of the drug is no longer commercially available in the US.

IM Injection

For IM injection, oxacillin sodium powder for injection is reconstituted by adding 5.7 or 11.4 mL of sterile water for injection to a vial containing 1 or 2 g of oxacillin, respectively, to provide solutions containing 167 mg of oxacillin per mL (250 mg/1.5 mL). The vials should be shaken well until a clear solution is obtained.

IM injections of oxacillin sodium should be made deeply into a large muscle (e.g., gluteus maximus) and care should be taken to avoid sciatic nerve injury.

Intermittent IV Injection

For direct intermittent IV injection, a solution containing approximately 100 mg/mL may be prepared by adding 10 or 20 mL of sterile water for injection or 0.45 or 0.9% sodium chloride injection to vials containing 1 or 2 g of oxacillin, respectively.

The appropriate dose should then be injected slowly over a period of about 10 minutes. Particular attention to the risk of thrombophlebitis should be given when oxacillin is administered IV to geriatric patients.

Intermittent or Continuous IV Infusion

For intermittent IV infusion, vials containing 1 or 2 g of oxacillin should be reconstituted as for direct IV injection and then further diluted with a compatible IV solution to a concentration of 0.5–40 mg/mL. (See Chemistry and Stability: Stability.) Alternatively, ADD-Vantage® vials containing 1 or 2 g of the drug should be reconstituted according to the manufacturer's directions. Pharmacy bulk packages containing 10 g of oxacillin usually are reconstituted by adding 93 mL of sterile water for injection or 0.9% sodium chloride injection to provide a solution containing 100 mg/mL. Pharmacy bulk packages of the drug are *not* intended for direct IV infusion; doses of the drug from the reconstituted pharmacy bulk package must be further diluted in a compatible IV infusion solution prior to administration.

Thawed solutions of the commercially available frozen oxacillin sodium in dextrose injection should be administered by continuous or intermittent IV infusion. These frozen oxacillin sodium injections should not be thawed by warming them in a water bath or by exposure to microwave radiation. A precipitate may form while the commercially available injection in dextrose is frozen; however, this usually will dissolve with little or no agitation upon reaching room temperature, and the potency of the injection is not affected. After thawing at room temperature or under refrigeration, the containers should be checked for minute leaks by firmly squeezing the bag. The injection should be discarded if the container seal is not intact or leaks are found or if the solution is cloudy, discolored, or contains a precipitate. Additives should not be introduced into the injection. The injections should not be used in series connections with other plastic containers, since such use could result in air embolism from residual air being drawn from the primary container before administration of fluid from the secondary container is complete.

For IV infusion of oxacillin, the rate of infusion should be adjusted so that the total dose of oxacillin is administered before the drug is inactivated in the IV solution. (See Chemistry and Stability: Stability.)

● Dosage

Dosage of oxacillin sodium is expressed in terms of oxacillin. Dosage of the drug should be adjusted according to the type and severity of infection.

Adult Dosage

For the treatment of infections caused by susceptible penicillinase-producing staphylococci, the usual adult IM or IV dosage of oxacillin is 250–500 mg every 4–6 hours for mild to moderate infections or 1 g every 4–6 hours for severe infections. When oxacillin is used for the treatment of acute or chronic osteomyelitis caused by susceptible penicillinase-producing staphylococci, some clinicians recommend that adults receive 1.5–2 g of the drug IV every 4 hours. If oxacillin is used for the treatment of staphylococcal infections related to intravascular catheters, some clinicians recommend that adults receive 2 g every 4 hours.

Staphylococcal Endocarditis

For the treatment of native valve endocarditis caused by staphylococci susceptible to penicillinase-resistant penicillins, the American Heart Association (AHA) recommends that adults receive oxacillin in a dosage of 2 g IV every 4 hours for 4–6 weeks. Although the benefits of concomitant aminoglycoside therapy have not been clearly established in these infections, the AHA states that gentamicin (1 mg/kg IM or IV every 8 hours) may be given concomitantly during the first 3–5 days of oxacillin therapy.

For the treatment of staphylococcal endocarditis in the presence of prosthetic valves or other prosthetic material in patients with infections caused by isolates susceptible to penicillinase-resistant penicillins, the AHA states that adults should receive oxacillin in a dosage of 2 g IV every 4 hours for 6 weeks or longer in conjunction with rifampin (300 mg orally every 8 hours for 6 weeks or longer) and gentamicin (1 mg/kg IM or IV every 8 hours during the first 2 weeks of oxacillin therapy). However, because coagulase-negative staphylococci causing prosthetic valve endocarditis usually are resistant to penicillinase-resistant penicillins (especially when endocarditis develops within 1 year after surgery), coagulase-negative staphylococci involved in prosthetic valve endocarditis should be assumed to be resistant to penicillinase-resistant penicillins unless results of in vitro testing indicate that the isolates are susceptible to the drugs. (See Uses: Endocarditis in the Penicillinase-resistant Penicillins General Statement 8:12.16.12.)

Pediatric Dosage

Children weighing 40 kg or more may receive the usual adult dosage of oxacillin.

The usual IM or IV dosage of oxacillin for the treatment of mild to moderate infections caused by susceptible penicillinase-producing staphylococci in children weighing less than 40 kg is 50 mg/kg daily given in equally divided doses every 6 hours. For severe infections, the usual IM or IV dosage in children weighing less than 40 kg is 100–200 mg/kg daily given in equally divided doses every 4–6 hours. The American Academy of Pediatrics (AAP) recommends that children 1 month of age or older receive IM or IV oxacillin in a dosage of 100–150 mg/kg daily in 4 divided doses for the treatment of mild to moderate infections or 150–200 mg/kg daily in 4 divided doses for the treatment of severe infections.

The manufacturer recommends that neonates receive IM or IV oxacillin in a dosage of 25 mg/kg daily. The AAP and other clinicians recommend that neonates younger than 1 week of age receive IM or IV oxacillin in a dosage of 25–50 mg/kg every 12 hours if they weigh 2 kg or less (25 mg/kg every 12 hours for those less than 1.2 kg) or 25–50 mg/kg every 8 hours if they weigh more than 2 kg. Neonates 1–4 weeks should receive 25–50 mg/kg every 8 hours if they weigh 2 kg or less (25 mg/kg every 12 hours for those less than 1.2 kg) or 25–50 mg/kg every 6 hours if they weigh more than 2 kg. The higher dosages are recommended for meningitis.

Staphylococcal Endocarditis

For the treatment of native valve endocarditis caused by staphylococci susceptible to penicillinase-resistant penicillins, the AHA recommends that pediatric patients receive oxacillin in a dosage of 200 mg/kg daily given IV in divided doses every 4–6 hours for 6 weeks (maximum daily dosage 12 g). In addition, during the first 3–5 days of oxacillin therapy, gentamicin (3 mg/kg daily given IM or IV in divided doses every 8 hours; dosage adjusted to achieve peak serum gentamicin concentrations approximately 3 mcg/mL and trough concentrations less than 1 mcg/mL) may be given concomitantly if the causative organism is susceptible to the drug.

For the treatment of staphylococcal endocarditis in the presence of prosthetic valves or other prosthetic material in patients with infections caused by isolates susceptible to penicillinase-resistant penicillins, the AHA recommends that pediatric patients receive oxacillin in a dosage of 200 mg/kg daily given IV in divided doses every 4–6 hours for 6 weeks or longer (maximum daily dosage 12 g) in conjunction with rifampin (20 mg/kg daily given orally in divided doses every 8 hours for 6 weeks or longer) and gentamicin (3 mg/kg daily given IM or IV in divided doses every 8 hours during the first 2 weeks of oxacillin therapy; dosage adjusted to achieve peak serum gentamicin concentrations approximately 3 mcg/mL and trough concentrations less than 1 mcg/mL).

Duration of Therapy

The duration of oxacillin therapy depends on the type and severity of infection and should be determined by the clinical and bacteriologic response of the patient. In serious staphylococcal infections, therapy should be continued for at least 1–2 weeks; more prolonged therapy is necessary for the treatment of osteomyelitis or endocarditis.

When oxacillin is used parenterally in the treatment of acute or chronic osteomyelitis caused by susceptible penicillinase-producing staphylococci, the drug generally is given for 3–8 weeks; follow-up therapy with an oral penicillinase-resistant penicillin (e.g., dicloxacillin) generally is recommended for the treatment of osteomyelitis. In the treatment of acute osteomyelitis, a shorter course of parenteral penicillinase-resistant therapy (5–28 days) followed by 3–6 weeks of oral penicillinase-resistant penicillin therapy also has been effective.

● Dosage in Renal Impairment

Modification of dosage generally is unnecessary when oxacillin is used in patients with renal impairment; however, some clinicians suggest that the lower range of the usual dosage (1 g IM or IV every 4–6 hours) be used in adults with creatinine clearances less than 10 mL/minute.

CAUTIONS

● Adverse Effects

Adverse effects reported with oxacillin are similar to those reported with other penicillinase-resistant penicillins. However, adverse hepatic effects have been reported more frequently with IV oxacillin than with other commercially available penicillinase-resistant penicillins. For information on adverse effects reported with penicillinase-resistant penicillins, see Cautions in the Penicillinase-Resistant Penicillins General Statement 8:12.16.12.

● Precautions and Contraindications

Oxacillin is contraindicated in patients who are hypersensitive to any penicillin.

Oxacillin shares the toxic potentials of the penicillins, including the risk of hypersensitivity reactions, and the usual precautions of penicillin therapy should be observed. Prior to initiation of therapy with oxacillin, careful inquiry should be made concerning previous hypersensitivity reactions to penicillins, cephalosporins, or other drugs. There is clinical and laboratory evidence of partial cross-allergenicity among penicillins and other β-lactam antibiotics including cephalosporins and cephamycins.

Renal, hepatic, and hematologic systems should be evaluated periodically during prolonged therapy with oxacillin. Because adverse hematologic effects have occurred during therapy with penicillinase-resistant penicillins, CBCs and differential should be performed prior to initiation of therapy and 1–3 times weekly during therapy. In addition, urinalysis should be performed and BUN and serum creatinine, AST (SGOT), and ALT (SGPT) concentrations should be determined prior to and periodically during therapy.

For a more complete discussion of these and other precautions associated with the use of oxacillin, see Cautions: Precautions and Contraindications, in the Penicillinase-Resistant Penicillins General Statement 8:12.16.12.

● Pediatric Precautions

Elimination of penicillins is delayed in neonates because of immature mechanisms for renal excretion, and abnormally high serum concentrations of the drugs may occur in this age group. If oxacillin is used in neonates, they should be monitored closely for clinical and laboratory evidence of toxic or adverse effects including renal impairment; organ systems and serum concentrations of the drug should be monitored frequently and appropriate reductions in dosage and frequency of administration made when indicated.

● Pregnancy, Fertility, and Lactation

Pregnancy

Safe use of penicillinase-resistant penicillins during pregnancy has not been definitely established. Clinical experience with use of penicillins during pregnancy in humans has not revealed evidence of adverse effects on the fetus. However, there are no adequate and controlled studies using penicillinase-resistant penicillins in pregnant women, and oxacillin should be used during pregnancy only when clearly needed.

Lactation

Because oxacillin is distributed into milk, the drug should be used with caution in nursing women.

SPECTRUM

Based on its spectrum of activity, oxacillin is classified as a penicillinase-resistant penicillin. For information on the classification of penicillins based on spectra of activity, see the Preface to the General Statements on Penicillins 8:12.16.

Like other penicillinase-resistant penicillins, oxacillin is resistant to inactivation by most staphylococcal penicillinases and is active against many penicillinase-producing strains of *Staphylococcus aureus* and *S. epidermidis* that are resistant to other commercially available penicillins. For specific information on the spectrum of activity of oxacillin and resistance to the drug, see the sections on Spectrum and on Resistance in the Penicillinase-Resistant Penicillins General Statement 8:12.16.12.

PHARMACOKINETICS

In all studies described in the Pharmacokinetics section, oxacillin was administered as the sodium salt; dosages and concentrations of the drug are expressed in terms of oxacillin.

● Absorption

Oxacillin is resistant to inactivation in the presence of acidic gastric secretions and is rapidly but incompletely absorbed from the GI tract. In healthy, fasting adults, 30–35% of an orally administered dose of oxacillin is absorbed from the GI tract and peak serum concentrations of the drug are generally attained within 0.5–2 hours. Presence of food in the GI tract generally decreases the rate and extent of absorption of oxacillin.

Following oral administration of a single 250- or 500-mg dose of oxacillin as capsules (no longer commercially available in the US) in healthy, fasting adults, peak serum concentrations of the drug average 1.65 or 2.6–3.9 mcg/mL, respectively. Following oral administration of oxacillin as an oral solution (no longer commercially available in the US), peak serum concentrations occur about 30 minutes after the dose and average 1.9 mcg/mL after a single 250-mg dose and 4.8 mcg/mL after a single 500-mg dose.

Oxacillin is rapidly absorbed from IM injection sites. Following IM injection of a single 250- or 500-mg dose of oxacillin in healthy adults with normal renal function, peak serum concentrations of the drug are generally attained within 30 minutes and average 5.3 and 10.9 mcg/mL, respectively. Following IM administration of a single 500-mg dose of oxacillin in healthy adults, serum concentrations of the drug averaged 7.4, 7.4, 4.3, and 0.8 mcg/mL at 30 minutes, 1 hour, 2 hours, and 4 hours, respectively, after the dose.

Following rapid IV injection of a single 500-mg dose of oxacillin in healthy adults, peak serum concentrations of the drug average 52–63 mcg/mL.

In one study in children 1 week to 2 years of age with staphylococcal infections who received an IM oxacillin dosage of 100 mg/kg daily in divided doses every 6 hours, peak serum concentrations of the drug occurred 30 minutes after a dose and ranged from 45–86 mcg/mL; trough serum concentrations ranged from 2.5–7.5 mcg/mL. Following IM injection of a single 20-mg/kg dose of oxacillin in neonates, peak serum concentrations of the drug reportedly average 51.5 mcg/mL in those 8–15 days of age and 47 mcg/mL in those 20–21 days of age.

● Distribution

Oxacillin is distributed into synovial, pleural, pericardial, and ascitic fluids. The drug is also distributed into bone, lungs, sputum, and bile. The volume of distribution of oxacillin is reportedly 0.39–0.43 L/kg in healthy adults.

Following IM or IV administration, oxacillin concentrations in bone may be 5–20% of concurrent serum concentrations. In one study in adults who received a single 2-g IV dose of oxacillin, concentrations of the drug in bone ranged from 1.1–18.5 mcg/g.

Like other penicillins, only low concentrations of oxacillin are attained in CSF. Following IM administration, oxacillin does not appear to distribute into aqueous humor in measurable concentrations; in animals, the drug is not distributed into aqueous humor even in the presence of inflammation. In rabbits, subconjunctival injection of a 100-mg dose of oxacillin produced aqueous humor concentrations of 145 mcg/mL 1 hour after the injection and 70 mcg/mL 2 hours after the injection.

Oxacillin is 89–94% bound to serum proteins.

Oxacillin is distributed into cord serum and amniotic fluid and crosses the placenta Oral administration of a single 500-mg dose of oxacillin to pregnant women in labor has resulted in fetal serum concentrations of the drug of 1.4 mcg/mL and amniotic fluid concentrations of 3.2 mcg/mL. Oxacillin is distributed into milk. Following IM administration of a single 500-mg dose of oxacillin in lactating women, milk concentrations of the drug were 0.2–0.7 mcg/mL 1 and 2 hours after the dose and 0.2–0.4 mcg/mL 4 hours after the dose.

● Elimination

The serum half-life of oxacillin in adults with normal renal function is 0.3–0.8 hours.

Oxacillin is partially metabolized to active and inactive metabolites. In one study following a single 500-mg oral dose of oxacillin (no longer commercially available in the US), 49% of the absorbed dose was hydrolyzed to penicilloic acids which are microbiologically inactive. Oxacillin is also hydroxylated to a small extent to a microbiologically active metabolite which appears to be slightly less active than oxacillin.

Oxacillin and its metabolites are rapidly excreted in urine mainly by tubular secretion and glomerular filtration. Following oral administration of a single 500-mg dose of oxacillin in adults with normal renal function, 17–24% of the dose is excreted in urine as unchanged drug and active metabolites within 6 hours; approximately 21% of the antibacterial activity in urine is represented by the active metabolite. Following IM administration of a single 500-mg or 1-g dose of oxacillin in adults with normal renal function, 40–70% of the dose is excreted in urine as unchanged drug and active metabolites within 6 hours.

In one study, serum clearance of oxacillin averaged 380 mL/minute per 1.73 m^2 in adults with normal renal function.

Serum concentrations of oxacillin may be higher and the serum half-life slightly prolonged in patients with impaired renal function. The serum half-life of the drug is reportedly 0.5–2 hours in patients with creatinine clearances less than 10 mL/minute per 1.73 m^2.

In one study in children 1 week to 2 years of age, the elimination half-life of oxacillin ranged from 0.9–1.8 hours. Serum concentrations of oxacillin are generally higher and the serum half-life is longer in neonates than in older children. The serum half-life of oxacillin reportedly is 1.6 hours in neonates 8–15 days of age and 1.2 hours in neonates 20–21 days of age.

Oxacillin is only minimally removed by hemodialysis or peritoneal dialysis.

CHEMISTRY AND STABILITY

● Chemistry

Oxacillin is a semisynthetic penicillinase-resistant penicillin. Oxacillin, like cloxacillin (no longer commercially available in the US) and dicloxacillin, is an isoxazolyl penicillin.

Oxacillin is commercially available as the monohydrate sodium salt. Potency of oxacillin sodium is expressed in terms of oxacillin. Each mg of oxacillin sodium contains 815–950 mcg of oxacillin. Oxacillin sodium occurs as a fine, white, crystalline powder which is odorless or may have a slight odor. The drug is freely soluble in water. Oxacillin sodium has a pK_a of approximately 2.8.

Each gram of commercially available oxacillin sodium powder for injection contains approximately 2.5 mEq of sodium and is buffered with 20 mg of dibasic sodium phosphate.

Commercially available frozen oxacillin sodium in dextrose injection are sterile, nonpyrogenic, iso-osmotic solutions of the drug; about 1.5 or 0.3 g of dextrose has been added to the 1- or 2-g injection of oxacillin sodium, respectively, to adjust osmolality to about 300 mOsm/kg. Frozen oxacillin sodium in dextrose injection also contains sodium citrate as a buffer and hydrochloric acid and/or sodium hydroxide to adjust pH to 6–8.5.

● Stability

Commercially available oxacillin sodium powder for IM or IV injection should be stored at controlled room temperature; the pharmacy bulk package containing 10 g of the drug should be stored at 15–30°C.

When oxacillin sodium powder for injection is reconstituted with sterile water for injection, solutions for IM injection containing 167 mg of oxacillin per mL (250 mg/1.5 mL) are stable for 3 days at room temperature or 7 days when refrigerated. When reconstituted as directed in 0.9% sodium chloride injection or 5% dextrose injection, solutions prepared from ADD-Vantage® vials of the drug are stable for 4 days or 6 hours, respectively, at room temperature.

At concentrations of 0.5–4 mg/mL, oxacillin loses less than 10% of its activity within 6 hours at room temperature in the following IV solutions: 5% dextrose and 0.9% sodium chloride; 10% fructose or 10% fructose and 0.9% sodium chloride; 10% invert sugar and 0.9% sodium chloride or 0.3% potassium chloride; or 10% invert sugar with electrolytes (Travert® 10% with Electrolytes No. 1, 2, or 3).

The commercially available preparations of frozen oxacillin sodium in dextrose injection should be stored at –20°C or lower and are stable for at least 90 days from the date of shipment when stored at –20°C. The frozen injection should be thawed at room temperature (25°C) or under refrigeration (5°C) and, once thawed, should not be refrozen. Thawed solutions of the commercially available frozen injection are stable for 48 hours at room temperature (25°C) or 21 days when refrigerated at 5°C. The commercially available frozen injections of the drug are provided in a plastic container fabricated from specially formulated multilayered plastic PL 2040 (Galaxy®). Solutions in contact with the plastic can leach out some of its chemical components in very small amounts within the expiration period of the injection; however, safety of the plastic has been confirmed in tests in animals according to USP biological tests for plastic containers as well as by tissue culture toxicity studies.

Oxacillin sodium is potentially physically and/or chemically incompatible with some drugs, including aminoglycosides and tetracyclines, but the compatibility depends on several factors (e.g., concentrations of the drugs, specific diluents used, resulting pH, temperature). For information on the in vitro and in vivo incompatibility of penicillins and aminoglycosides, see Drug Interactions: Aminoglycosides, in the Penicillinase-Resistant Penicillins General Statement 8:12.16.12. Specialized references should be consulted for specific compatibility information.

For further information on chemistry and stability, mechanism of action, spectrum, resistance, pharmacokinetics, uses, cautions, drug interactions, laboratory test interferences, and dosage and administration of oxacillin sodium, see the Penicillinase-Resistant Penicillins General Statement 8:12.16.12.

PREPARATIONS

Excipients in commercially available drug preparations may have clinically important effects in some individuals; consult specific product labeling for details.

Oxacillin Sodium

Parenteral		
For injection	1 g (of oxacillin)*	Oxacillin Sodium for Injection
	2 g (of oxacillin)*	Oxacillin Sodium for Injection
	10 g (of oxacillin) pharmacy bulk package*	Oxacillin Sodium for Injection
For injection, for IV infusion	1 g (of oxacillin)*	Oxacillin Sodium ADD-Vantage®, Sandoz
	2 g (of oxacillin)*	Oxacillin Sodium ADD-Vantage®, Sandoz

* available from one or more manufacturer, distributor, and/or repackager by generic (nonproprietary) name

Oxacillin Sodium in Dextrose

Parenteral		
Injection (frozen), for IV infusion	20 mg (of oxacillin) per mL (1 g) in 3% Dextrose*	Oxacillin Sodium® in Iso-osmotic Dextrose Injection, Baxter
	40 mg (of oxacillin) per mL (2 g) in 0.6% Dextrose*	Oxacillin Sodium® in Iso-osmotic Dextrose Injection, Baxter

* available from one or more manufacturer, distributor, and/or repackager by generic (nonproprietary) name

Selected Revisions January 1, 2009, © Copyright, January 1, 1985, American Society of Health-System Pharmacists, Inc.

Piperacillin Sodium and Tazobactam Sodium

8:12.16.16 • EXTENDED-SPECTRUM PENICILLINS

■ Piperacillin sodium and tazobactam sodium (piperacillin/tazobactam) is a fixed combination of the sodium salts of piperacillin (an extended-spectrum penicillin antibiotic) and tazobactam (a β-lactamase inhibitor); tazobactam inactivates certain bacterial β-lactamases and expands piperacillin's spectrum of activity against some bacteria that produce these β-lactamases.

USES

The fixed combination of piperacillin sodium and tazobactam sodium (piperacillin/tazobactam) is used for the treatment of moderate to severe infections caused by susceptible β-lactamase-producing bacteria and certain other gram-negative or anaerobic bacteria. Piperacillin/tazobactam is used principally for the treatment of infections caused by susceptible gram-negative bacteria and for empiric treatment of polymicrobial infections such as mixed aerobic-anaerobic infections.

When piperacillin/tazobactam is used for the treatment of infections known or suspected of being caused by *Pseudomonas aeruginosa*, the drug usually is used in conjunction with another anti-infective with antipseudomonal activity (e.g., antipseudomonal fluoroquinolone, aminoglycoside).

● Gynecologic and Obstetric Infections

Piperacillin/tazobactam is used for the treatment of postpartum endometritis or pelvic inflammatory disease (PID) caused by susceptible β-lactamase-producing *Escherichia coli*.

Piperacillin/tazobactam is not included in US Centers for Disease Control and Prevention (CDC) recommendations for the treatment of PID. If a penicillin is used for empiric treatment of PID, CDC and other clinicians recommend a parenteral regimen that includes the fixed combination of ampicillin sodium and sulbactam sodium (ampicillin/sulbactam) in conjunction with doxycycline.

● Intra-abdominal Infections

Piperacillin/tazobactam is used for the treatment of appendicitis (complicated by rupture or abscess) and peritonitis caused by susceptible β-lactamase-producing *E. coli*, *Bacteroides fragilis*, *B. ovatus*, *B. thetaiotaomicron*, or *B. vulgatus*.

Piperacillin/tazobactam has been used for the treatment of various intra-abdominal infections, and has been recommended as one of several options for initial empiric treatment of high-risk or severe community-acquired extrabiliary intra-abdominal infections (e.g., in patients with advanced age, immunocompromise, severe physiologic disturbance), community-acquired biliary tract infections (e.g., acute cholecystitis), and complicated healthcare-associated intra-abdominal infections.

● Respiratory Tract Infections

Community-acquired Pneumonia

Piperacillin/tazobactam is used for the treatment of moderately severe community-acquired pneumonia (CAP) caused by susceptible β-lactamase-producing *Haemophilus influenzae*. The drug also is used for the treatment of CAP caused by susceptible Enterobacteriaceae† or anaerobic bacteria†.

Piperacillin/tazobactam has been recommended as one of several options for empiric treatment of CAP in hospitalized patients requiring treatment in an intensive care unit (ICU). If *Ps. aeruginosa* is known or suspected to be involved, the Infectious Diseases Society of America (IDSA) and American Thoracic Society (ATS) state that piperacillin/tazobactam should be used in conjunction with a fluoroquinolone with antipseudomonal activity (ciprofloxacin, levofloxacin) with or without an aminoglycoside or in conjunction with an aminoglycoside and azithromycin. Factors that increase the risk of *Ps. aeruginosa* infection in CAP patients include severe CAP requiring treatment in an ICU, structural lung disease (e.g., bronchiectasis), repeated exacerbations of severe chronic obstructive pulmonary disease (COPD), alcoholism, chronic corticosteroid therapy, and frequent anti-infective therapy.

Nosocomial Pneumonia

Piperacillin/tazobactam is used for the treatment of moderate to severe nosocomial pneumonia caused by susceptible β-lactamase-producing *Staphylococcus aureus* or susceptible *Acinetobacter baumannii*, *H. influenzae*, *Klebsiella pneumoniae*, or *Ps. aeruginosa*. If *Ps. aeruginosa* is involved, piperacillin/tazobactam should be used in conjunction with an aminoglycoside or a fluoroquinolone with antipseudomonal activity (e.g., ciprofloxacin, levofloxacin).

IDSA and ATS state that piperacillin/tazobactam is one of several options for initial empiric treatment of hospital-acquired pneumonia (HAP) not associated with mechanical ventilation and initial empiric treatment of ventilator-associated bacterial pneumonia (VAP).

In adults with HAP (not associated with mechanical ventilation) who are not at high risk of mortality, IDSA and ATS state that use of piperacillin/tazobactam alone (monotherapy) can be considered for initial empiric treatment if no factors are present that increase the likelihood of methicillin-resistant *S. aureus* (MRSA; also known as oxacillin-resistant *S. aureus* or ORSA); however, these experts state that piperacillin/tazobactam should be used in conjunction with an antibacterial active against MRSA (vancomycin, linezolid) if such factors are present or if the patient is at high risk of mortality or has received IV anti-infectives during the prior 90 days.

In adults with clinically suspected VAP, IDSA and ATS state that use of piperacillin/tazobactam alone (monotherapy) can be considered for initial empiric treatment in those not at increased risk for MRSA. However, in patients with factors that increase the risk of MRSA or multidrug-resistant gram-negative bacteria, these experts state that piperacillin/tazobactam should be used in conjunction with an anti-infective active against MRSA (vancomycin, linezolid) plus an antipseudomonal fluoroquinolone (ciprofloxacin, levofloxacin), aminoglycoside (amikacin, gentamicin, tobramycin), or polymyxin B.

● Septicemia

Piperacillin/tazobactam has been used for the treatment of septicemia†. The drug has been recommended as one of several options for initial empiric treatment of sepsis and bacteremia.

● Skin and Skin Structure Infections

Piperacillin/tazobactam is used for the treatment of uncomplicated and complicated skin and skin structure infections (including cellulitis, cutaneous abscesses, ischemic/diabetic foot infections) caused by susceptible β-lactamase-producing *S. aureus*. Piperacillin/tazobactam has been recommended as a possible option for empiric monotherapy of complicated skin and skin structure infections that could be polymicrobial and are unlikely to involve MRSA; the drug should not be used alone in infections that may be caused by MRSA.

Although the fixed combination of amoxicillin and clavulanate potassium (amoxicillin/clavulanate) usually is the drug of choice, piperacillin/tazobactam has been suggested as an alternative for the treatment of infected human or animal (e.g., dog, cat, reptile) bite wounds† when a parenteral anti-infective is used. Purulent bite wounds are likely to be polymicrobial and broad-spectrum anti-infective coverage is recommended. Nonpurulent infected bite wounds usually are caused by staphylococci and streptococci, but can be polymicrobial.

Piperacillin/tazobactam used in conjunction with vancomycin is considered one of several possible regimens for empiric treatment of severe cellulitis or treatment of clostridial myonecrosis† (gas gangrene).

Piperacillin/tazobactam used in conjunction with vancomycin or linezolid also is one of several possible regimens for empiric treatment of necrotizing fasciitis†.

● Urinary Tract Infections

Piperacillin/tazobactam has been used with or without an aminoglycoside for the treatment of urinary tract infections† in hospitalized patients.

● Empiric Therapy in Febrile Neutropenic Patients

Piperacillin/tazobactam has been used alone (monotherapy) or in conjunction with other anti-infectives (e.g., an aminoglycoside) for empiric anti-infective therapy in febrile neutropenic patients†.

Piperacillin/tazobactam has been recommended as one of several options for initial outpatient management of febrile neutropenia in adults receiving treatment for malignancy.

● Perioperative Prophylaxis

Piperacillin/tazobactam has been used for perioperative prophylaxis† to decrease postoperative infections in patients undergoing various urologic procedures (e.g., prostate biopsy), gastroduodenal procedures (e.g., pancreatic duodenectomy), or liver transplantation. However, piperacillin/tazobactam generally is not recommended for perioperative prophylaxis.

DOSAGE AND ADMINISTRATION

● Administration

The fixed combination of piperacillin sodium and tazobactam sodium (piperacillin/tazobactam) is administered by IV infusion.

Piperacillin/tazobactam usually is administered by intermittent IV infusion, but also has been administered by continuous IV infusion†.

The drug should not be given by rapid IV injection.

IV Infusion

Piperacillin/tazobactam should *not* be admixed with other drugs in a syringe or infusion bottle and should *not* be added to blood products or albumin hydrolysates.

If concomitant use of an aminoglycoside is indicated (e.g., treatment of nosocomial pneumonia), the drugs should be reconstituted, diluted, and administered separately. (See Concomitant Use with Aminoglycosides under Administration: IV Infusion, in Dosage and Administration.)

Piperacillin/tazobactam (Zosyn®) and generic preparations of piperacillin/tazobactam commercially available in the US are *not* identical. Piperacillin/tazobactam (Zosyn®) is formulated with edetate disodium dihydrate (EDTA) and sodium citrate; the generic preparations do not contain EDTA or sodium citrate. Because EDTA acts as a metal-chelating agent and sodium citrate acts as a buffer, certain aspects of chemical degradation and particulate formation are inhibited and there is a lower risk of particulate matter formation and accumulation following reconstitution of Zosyn® with commonly used diluents or storage of solutions of the drug. In addition, the presence of EDTA and sodium citrate allows coadministration of Zosyn® and lactated Ringer's injection via Y-site infusion.

Reconstitution and Dilution

Single-dose vials of piperacillin/tazobactam (Zosyn®, generic) labeled as containing 2.25 g (2 g of piperacillin and 0.25 g of tazobactam), 3.375 g (3 g of piperacillin and 0.375 g of tazobactam), or 4.5 g (4 g of piperacillin and 0.5 g of tazobactam) should be reconstituted with 10, 15, or 20 mL, respectively, of compatible diluent and swirled until the contents are dissolved. Diluents that can be used for reconstitution include 0.9% sodium chloride injection, sterile water for injection, 5% dextrose injection, bacteriostatic water for injection (with parabens or benzyl alcohol), or bacteriostatic sodium chloride injection (with parabens or benzyl alcohol). Reconstituted solutions prepared from single-dose vials of piperacillin/tazobactam should be further diluted and any unused reconstituted solution should be discarded after 24 hours if stored at room temperature (20–25°C) or after 48 hours if refrigerated at 2–8°C. Prior to IV infusion, reconstituted piperacillin/tazobactam solutions should be diluted to the desired volume (usually 50–150 mL) with a compatible diluent (0.9% sodium chloride injection, sterile water for injection [maximum recommended volume is 50 mL], 5% dextrose injection, or 6% dextran in sodium chloride injection). Lactated Ringer's injection is compatible *only* with piperacillin/sodium solutions prepared using piperacillin/tazobactam formulated with EDTA (i.e., Zosyn®) for coadministration via Y-site infusion; lactated Ringer's injection is incompatible with and cannot be used with generic piperacillin/tazobactam preparations that do not contain EDTA.

Single-dose ADD-Vantage® vials of piperacillin/tazobactam (generic) should be reconstituted and diluted according to the manufacturer's labeling. When reconstituted as directed in 0.9% sodium chloride injection or 5% dextrose injection, piperacillin/tazobactam solutions prepared from ADD-Vantage® vials are stable for 24 hours at room temperature; these reconstituted solutions should not be refrigerated or frozen.

Pharmacy bulk vials or bottles of piperacillin/tazobactam (Zosyn®, generic) containing 40.5 g (36 g of piperacillin and 4.5 g of tazobactam) should be reconstituted by adding 152 mL of a compatible IV solution to the vial to provide a solution containing 200 mg/mL of piperacillin and 25 mg/mL of tazobactam. Pharmacy bulk vials or bottles of the drug are not intended for direct IV infusion; prior to administration, solutions reconstituted in the pharmacy bulk package must be further diluted with a compatible IV solution.

The commercially available single-dose frozen premixed injections of piperacillin/tazobactam in dextrose (Zosyn® in Galaxy® containers) should be thawed at room temperature (20–25°C) or under refrigeration (2–8°C); frozen injections should not be thawed by immersion in water baths or by microwave irradiation. Precipitates that may have formed in the frozen injection usually will dissolve with little or no agitation when the injection reaches room temperature; potency is not affected. After thawing at room temperature, the injection should be agitated and the container checked for minute leaks by firmly squeezing the bag. The injection should be discarded if container seals or outlet ports are not intact or leaks are found or if the solution is cloudy or contains an insoluble precipitate. The injection should not be used in series connections with other plastic containers, since such use could result in air embolism from residual air being drawn from the primary container before administration of fluid from the secondary container is complete. Once thawed, the solutions are stable for 24 hours at a room temperature of 20–25°C or 14 days when refrigerated at 2–8°C and should not be refrozen.

Rate of Administration

IV infusions of piperacillin/tazobactam usually are given over 30 minutes.

Piperacillin/tazobactam has been administered by IV infusion over 3–4 hours† and by continuous IV infusion†. Some clinicians suggest that 4-hour intermittent IV infusions or continuous IV infusion of piperacillin/tazobactam may be beneficial in certain clinical situations (e.g., critically ill patients, pathogen with high piperacillin/tazobactam minimum inhibitory concentration [MIC]); there is some evidence that lengthening the duration of piperacillin/tazobactam infusions may maximize the pharmacokinetic/pharmacodynamic properties of the drug.

Concomitant Use with Aminoglycosides

Because piperacillin/tazobactam and aminoglycosides are physically and/or chemically incompatible in vitro, the drugs should be reconstituted, diluted, and administered separately if concomitant use is indicated (e.g., treatment of nosocomial pneumonia).

In certain situations when coadministration of piperacillin/tazobactam and an aminoglycoside via Y-site infusion is considered necessary, this can be accomplished using *only* certain dosages of amikacin or gentamicin and *only* certain acceptable diluents. (See Tables 1 and 2.) For Y-site coadministration, tobramycin or any aminoglycoside other than amikacin or gentamicin should *not* be used. Coadministration via Y-site infusion in any manner other than that specified in the tables may result in inactivation of the aminoglycoside.

TABLE 1. Y-site Compatibility of Piperacillin/tazobactam in Single-dose Vials and Bulk Vials or Bottles (Zosyn®, generics) with Aminoglycosides

Aminoglycoside	Piperacillin/tazobactam Dose (g)	Piperacillin/tazobactam Diluent (mL)	Aminoglycoside Concentration Range (mg/mL) [a]	Acceptable Diluents
Amikacin	2.25	50	1.75–7.5	0.9% sodium chloride injection or 5% dextrose injection
	3.375	100		
	4.5	150		
Gentamicin	2.25	50	0.7–3.32	0.9% sodium chloride injection or 5% dextrose injection
	3.375	100		
	4.5	150		

[a] Based on amikacin dosage of 10–15 mg/kg daily given in 2 divided doses or gentamicin dosage of 3–5 mg/kg daily given in 3 divided doses; higher dosage or once-daily dosage has not been evaluated for Y-site compatibility.

TABLE 2. Y-site Compatibility of Piperacillin/tazobactam (Frozen) Premixed Injections in Dextrose (Zosyn® in Galaxy® Containers) with Aminoglycosides

Aminoglyco-side	Zosyn® Dose (g)	Aminoglycoside Concentration Range (mg/mL) [a]	Acceptable Diluents
Amikacin	2.25, 3.375, or 4.5	1.75–7.5	0.9% sodium chloride injection or 5% dextrose injection
Gentamicin	2.25 or 4.5 [b]	0.7–3.32	0.9% sodium chloride injection or 5% dextrose injection

[a] Based on amikacin dosage of 10–15 mg/kg daily given in 2 divided doses or gentamicin dosage of 3–5 mg/kg daily given in 3 divided doses; higher dosage or once-daily dosage has not been evaluated for Y-site compatibility.

[b] Frozen premixed Zosyn® injections in Galaxy® containers that contain 3.375 g/50 mL are *not* compatible with gentamicin and should *not* be used for Y-site coadministration with gentamicin.

● Dosage

Piperacillin/tazobactam is a fixed combination of piperacillin sodium and tazobactam sodium; potency of each component is expressed in terms of the base. The commercially available fixed combination contains an 8:1 ratio of piperacillin to tazobactam.

Dosage of piperacillin/tazobactam usually is expressed as the total (sum) of the dosage of each of the 2 components (i.e., dosage of piperacillin plus dosage of tazobactam). However, dosage of piperacillin/tazobactam for pediatric patients often is expressed in terms of the piperacillin component.

Pediatric Dosage

General Neonatal Dosage

The American Academy of Pediatrics (AAP) recommends that dosage of IV piperacillin/tazobactam in neonates 28 days of age or younger† should be based on postmenstrual age (i.e., gestational age plus chronologic age). AAP recommends that neonates with postmenstrual age of 30 weeks or less receive IV piperacillin/tazobactam in a dosage of 100 mg/kg (of piperacillin) every 8 hours and that those with postmenstrual age greater than 30 weeks receive a dosage of 80 mg/kg (of piperacillin) every 6 hours.

In neonates weighing less than 1 kg†, some clinicians recommend that those 14 days of age or younger receive IV piperacillin/tazobactam in a dosage of 100 mg/kg (of piperacillin) every 12 hours and that those 15–28 days of age receive 100 mg/kg (of piperacillin) every 8 hours. These clinicians recommend that neonates weighing 1 kg or greater† receive a dosage of 100 mg/kg (of piperacillin) every 12 hours if they are 7 days of age or younger or 100 mg/kg (of piperacillin) every 8 hours if they are 8–28 days of age.

For the treatment of severe infections in neonates and infants younger than 2 months of age†, some clinicians suggest that IV piperacillin/tazobactam be given in a dosage of 80 mg/kg (of piperacillin) every 6 hours and others recommend a dosage of 80 mg/kg (of piperacillin) every 4 hours. Some clinicians suggest that shortening the dosing interval to every 6 hours and prolonging the duration of the IV infusion to 4 hours will maximize the pharmacokinetic/pharmacodynamic properties of the drug.

General Pediatric Dosage

AAP states that the usual dosage of IV piperacillin/tazobactam in pediatric patients beyond the neonatal period is 240–300 mg/kg (of piperacillin) daily in 3 or 4 divided doses. These experts state that a dosage of 400–600 mg/kg (of piperacillin) daily in 6 divided doses may be appropriate in some cystic fibrosis patients.

For the treatment of severe infections, some clinicians suggest that pediatric patients 2–9 months of age receive IV piperacillin/tazobactam in a dosage of 80 mg/kg (of piperacillin) every 6–8 hours and that those older than 9 months of age receive a dosage of 100 mg/kg (of piperacillin) every 6–8 hours.

AAP and some other clinicians state that the maximum recommended dosage of IV piperacillin/tazobactam in most pediatric patients is 16 g (of piperacillin) daily; however, AAP states that a maximum dosage of 24 g (of piperacillin) daily may be appropriate in some cystic fibrosis patients.

Intra-abdominal Infections

For the treatment of appendicitis and/or peritonitis in pediatric patients 2–9 months of age, the manufacturer recommends that IV piperacillin/tazobactam be given in a dosage of 80 mg/kg (of piperacillin) and 10 mg/kg (of tazobactam) every 8 hours.

For the treatment of appendicitis and/or peritonitis in pediatric patients 9 months of age or older weighing 40 kg or less with normal renal function, the manufacturer recommends that IV piperacillin/tazobactam be given in a dosage of 100 mg/kg (of piperacillin) and 12.5 mg/kg (of tazobactam) every 8 hours. The manufacturer states that pediatric patients with normal renal function weighing more than 40 kg should receive the usual adult dosage of piperacillin/tazobactam.

For the treatment of complicated intra-abdominal infections in pediatric patients, some clinicians recommend that IV piperacillin/tazobactam be given in a dosage of 200–300 mg/kg (of piperacillin) daily in divided doses every 6–8 hours.

Some clinicians state that the usual duration of treatment for intra-abdominal infections is 4–7 days, unless it is difficult to achieve adequate source control. These clinicians state that longer treatment durations have not been associated with improved outcomes.

Skin and Skin Structure Infections

If IV piperacillin/tazobactam is used for the treatment of necrotizing infections of the skin, fascia, and muscle†, some clinicians recommend that pediatric patients receive a dosage of 60–75 mg/kg (of piperacillin) every 6 hours in conjunction with vancomycin.

Adult Dosage

General Adult Dosage

The manufacturer states that the usual dosage of IV piperacillin/tazobactam for adults is 3.375 g (3 g of piperacillin and 0.375 g of tazobactam) every 6 hours for 7–10 days.

The maximum dosage of IV piperacillin/tazobactam recommended in adults usually is 3.375 g (3 g of piperacillin and 0.375 g of tazobactam) every 4 hours or 4.5 g (4 g of piperacillin and 0.5 g of tazobactam) every 6 hours. The manufacturer recommends a maximum dosage of 18 g (16 g of piperacillin and 2 g of tazobactam) daily.

Gynecologic and Obstetric Infections

For the treatment of postpartum endometritis or pelvic inflammatory disease (PID), the manufacturer states that the usual dosage of IV piperacillin/tazobactam in adults is 3.375 g (3 g of piperacillin and 0.375 g of tazobactam) every 6 hours for 7–10 days.

Intra-abdominal Infections

For the treatment of appendicitis and/or peritonitis, the manufacturer states that the usual dosage of IV piperacillin/tazobactam in adults is 3.375 g (3 g of piperacillin and 0.375 g of tazobactam) every 6 hours for 7–10 days.

For the treatment of complicated intra-abdominal infections in adults, some clinicians recommend that IV piperacillin/tazobactam be given in a dosage of 3.375 g (3 g of piperacillin and 0.375 g of tazobactam) every 6 hours; however, if *Pseudomonas aeruginosa* is identified, these clinicians state that dosage of the drug may be increased to 3.375 g (3 g of piperacillin and 0.375 g of tazobactam) every 4 hours or 4.5 g (4 g of piperacillin and 0.5 g of tazobactam) every 6 hours.

Some clinicians state that the usual duration of treatment for intra-abdominal infections is 4–7 days, unless it is difficult to achieve adequate source control. These clinicians state that longer treatment durations have not been associated with improved outcomes.

Community-acquired Pneumonia

For the treatment of moderately severe community-acquired pneumonia (CAP), the manufacturer states that the usual dosage of IV piperacillin/tazobactam in adults is 3.375 g (3 g of piperacillin and 0.375 g of tazobactam) every 6 hours for 7–10 days.

Nosocomial Pneumonia

For initial empiric treatment of nosocomial pneumonia in adults, the manufacturer recommends that IV piperacillin/tazobactam be given in a dosage of 4.5 g (4 g of piperacillin and 0.5 g of tazobactam) every 6 hours in conjunction with an aminoglycoside. The manufacturer states that the recommended duration of piperacillin/tazobactam therapy for the treatment of nosocomial pneumonia is 7–14 days; if *Ps. aeruginosa* is identified, the aminoglycoside should be continued concomitantly for the full duration of piperacillin/tazobactam treatment.

When IV piperacillin/tazobactam is used with or without other anti-infectives for initial empiric treatment of hospital-acquired pneumonia (HAP) not associated with mechanical ventilation or initial empiric treatment of ventilator-associated pneumonia (VAP), some clinicians recommend that adults receive a dosage of 4.5 g (4 g of piperacillin and 0.5 g of tazobactam) every 6 hours. These experts recommend a treatment duration of 7 days; however, depending on clinical response, a longer or shorter duration may be indicated.

Skin and Skin Structure Infections

For the treatment of skin and skin structure infections in adults, the manufacturer states that the usual dosage of IV piperacillin/tazobactam is 3.375 g (3 g of piperacillin and 0.375 g of tazobactam) every 6 hours for 7–10 days.

For the treatment of incisional surgical site infections†, some clinicians recommended that adults receive IV piperacillin/tazobactam in a dosage of 3.375 g (3 g of piperacillin and 0.375 g of tazobactam) every 6 hours or 4.5 g (4 g of piperacillin and 0.5 g of tazobactam) every 8 hours.

If IV piperacillin/tazobactam is used for the treatment of infected human or animal bite wounds†, a dosage of 3.375 g (3 g of piperacillin and 0.375 g of tazobactam) every 6–8 hours has been recommended.

If IV piperacillin/tazobactam is used for the treatment of necrotizing infections of the skin, fascia, and muscle†, some clinicians recommend that adults receive a dosage of 3.375 g (3 g of piperacillin and 0.375 g of tazobactam) every 6–8 hours in conjunction with vancomycin.

● Dosage in Renal and Hepatic Impairment

Renal Impairment

Because serum concentrations of piperacillin and tazobactam are higher and prolonged in patients with renal impairment than in patients with normal renal function, doses and/or frequency of administration of piperacillin/tazobactam should be decreased in patients with renal impairment.

In adults with creatinine clearances of 40 mL/minute or less, including patients undergoing hemodialysis or continuous ambulatory peritoneal dialysis (CAPD), dosage of piperacillin/tazobactam should be decreased based on the degree of renal impairment. (See Table 3.)

The manufacturer makes no dosage recommendations for pediatric patients with impaired renal function.

TABLE 3. Dosage of Piperacillin/tazobactam for Adults with Renal Impairment

Creatinine Clearance (mL/minute)	Daily Dosage (Except Nosocomial Pneumonia)	Daily Dosage (Nosocomial Pneumonia)
20–40	2.25 g every 6 hours	3.375 g every 6 hours
<20	2.25 g every 8 hours	2.25 g every 6 hours
Hemodialysis Patients [a]	2.25 g every 12 hours; also give 0.75 g after each hemodialysis session	2.25 g every 8 hours; also give 0.75 g after each hemodialysis session
CAPD Patients [b]	2.25 g every 12 hours	2.25 g every 8 hours

[a] Hemodialysis removes approximately 30–40% of a dose of piperacillin/tazobactam (see Pharmacokinetics: Elimination); a supplemental dose of the drug is necessary after each hemodialysis session.

[b] Supplemental doses of piperacillin/tazobactam are not necessary in CAPD patients.

Hepatic Impairment

Although serum half-lives of piperacillin and tazobactam are prolonged in patients with hepatic cirrhosis compared with healthy patients, this effect is not clinically important and does not necessitate a change in dosage of piperacillin/tazobactam when the drug is used in patients with hepatic cirrhosis.

CAUTIONS

Adverse effects reported with the fixed combination of piperacillin sodium and tazobactam sodium (piperacillin/tazobactam) are similar to those reported with piperacillin alone and generally are transient and mild to moderate in severity. Adverse effects have been severe enough to require discontinuance of piperacillin/tazobactam in 3% or less of patients receiving the drug. The most frequent adverse effects (reported in more than 5% of patients receiving piperacillin/tazobactam) include GI effects (diarrhea, nausea, constipation), headache, and insomnia.

● GI Effects

Diarrhea, nausea, and constipation have been reported in up to 11% of patients receiving IV piperacillin/tazobactam. Vomiting, dyspepsia, and abdominal pain have been reported in up to 3%.

C. difficile-associated Diarrhea and Colitis

Treatment with anti-infectives alters normal colon flora and may permit overgrowth of *Clostridioides difficile* (formerly known as *Clostridium difficile*).

C. difficile infection (CDI) and *C. difficile*-associated diarrhea and colitis (CDAD; also known as antibiotic-associated diarrhea and colitis or pseudomembranous colitis) have been reported with nearly all anti-infectives, including piperacillin/tazobactam, and may range in severity from mild diarrhea to fatal colitis. *C. difficile* produces toxins A and B, which contribute to the development of CDAD; hypertoxin-producing strains cause increased morbidity and mortality since these infections may be refractory to anti-infective therapy and may require colectomy. CDAD should be considered if diarrhea develops during or after therapy and managed accordingly. (See Precautions Related to C. difficile-associated Diarrhea and Colitis under Cautions: Precautions and Contraindications.)

● Dermatologic and Sensitivity Reactions

Rash (maculopapular, bullous, urticarial), pruritus, and fever have been reported in up to 4% of patients receiving piperacillin/tazobactam. There also have been postmarketing reports of erythema multiforme, Stevens-Johnson syndrome, toxic epidermal necrolysis, drug reaction with eosinophilia and systemic symptoms (DRESS), acute generalized exanthematous pustulosis, and exfoliative dermatitis in patients receiving the drug. (See Precautions Related to Dermatologic and Sensitivity Reactions under Cautions: Precautions and Contraindications.)

Serious and occasionally fatal hypersensitivity reactions, including anaphylaxis or anaphylactoid reactions, have been reported in patients receiving piperacillin/tazobactam. Such reactions are more likely to occur in individuals with a history of penicillin, cephalosporin, or carbapenem hypersensitivity or a history of sensitivity to multiple allergens. (See Precautions Related to Dermatologic and Sensitivity Reactions under Cautions: Precautions and Contraindications.)

● Hematologic Effects

Decreased hemoglobin and hematocrit, anemia, thrombocytopenia, increased platelet count, transient eosinophilia, transient leukopenia, and neutropenia have been reported in patients receiving piperacillin/tazobactam. In most reported cases, leukopenia and neutropenia occurred after prolonged therapy with the drug (e.g., 21 days or longer) and generally were reversible; systemic symptoms (e.g., fever, rigors, chills) also occurred in some patients. There have been postmarketing reports of hemolytic anemia, agranulocytosis, and pancytopenia in patients receiving the drug.

Positive direct antiglobulin (Coombs') test results, prolonged prothrombin time, and prolonged partial thromboplastin time have been reported in patients receiving piperacillin/tazobactam.

Epistaxis and purpura have been reported in 1% or less of patients receiving the drug. Manifestations of bleeding, occasionally associated with abnormal results in coagulation tests (e.g., clotting time, platelet aggregation, prothrombin time), have occurred in some patients receiving β-lactam anti-infectives, including piperacillin. Bleeding manifestations are more likely to occur in patients with renal failure than in patients with normal renal function. (See Precautions Related to Hematologic Effects under Cautions: Precautions and Contraindications.)

● Nervous System Effects

Headache and insomnia have been reported in up to 8% of patients receiving piperacillin/tazobactam. There have been postmarketing reports of delirium in patients receiving the drug.

As with other penicillins, neuromuscular excitability or seizures could occur if higher than recommended doses of IV piperacillin/tazobactam are given, especially in patients with renal failure.

● Renal and Electrolyte Effects

Increased concentrations of serum creatinine and BUN have been reported in patients receiving piperacillin/tazobactam. Renal failure has been reported rarely and there have been postmarketing reports of interstitial nephritis in patients receiving the drug.

When used in critically ill patients, piperacillin/tazobactam has been found to be an independent risk factor for renal failure and was associated with delayed recovery of renal function compared with other β-lactam anti-infectives in such patients. In addition, concomitant use of vancomycin with piperacillin/tazobactam in critically ill patients has been associated with an increased incidence of acute kidney injury. (See Drug Interactions: Vancomycin.)

Changes in serum electrolytes, including increased and decreased serum sodium, potassium, and calcium concentrations, have occurred in patients receiving piperacillin/tazobactam. (See Precautions Related to Renal and Electrolyte Effects under Cautions: Precautions and Contraindications.)

● Local Reactions

Adverse reactions at the IV infusion site, including phlebitis and thrombophlebitis, have been reported in 1% or less of patients receiving piperacillin/tazobactam.

● Hepatic Effects

Transient increases in AST, ALT, alkaline phosphatase, and bilirubin have been reported in patients receiving piperacillin/tazobactam. There have been postmarketing reports of hepatitis and jaundice.

● Other Adverse Effects

Candidiasis, including oral candidiasis, has been reported in 2–4% of patients receiving piperacillin/tazobactam. Stomatitis has been reported in 1% or less of patients receiving the drug.

Hypotension, rigors, myalgia, arthralgia, hypoglycemia, and flushing have been reported in 1% or less of patients receiving piperacillin/tazobactam. There have been postmarketing reports of eosinophilic pneumonia in patients receiving the drug.

● Precautions and Contraindications

Piperacillin/tazobactam is contraindicated in patients hypersensitive to any penicillin, cephalosporin, or β-lactamase inhibitor.

Precautions Related to Dermatologic and Sensitivity Reactions

Piperacillin/tazobactam shares the toxic potentials of the penicillins, including the risk of hypersensitivity reactions, and the usual precautions of penicillin therapy should be observed. (See Cautions: Hypersensitivity Reactions, in the Natural Penicillins General Statement 8:12.16.04.) Serious hypersensitivity reactions are more likely to occur in individuals with a history of penicillin, cephalosporin, or carbapenem hypersensitivity.

Prior to initiation of piperacillin/tazobactam, careful inquiry should be made concerning previous hypersensitivity reactions to the drug, other β-lactams (including cephalosporins), or other allergens.

Patients should be advised that serious hypersensitivity reactions, including serious allergic cutaneous reactions, could occur that require immediate treatment.

If a severe hypersensitivity reaction occurs during piperacillin/tazobactam therapy, the drug should be discontinued and the patient given appropriate treatment as indicated.

Precautions Related to Hematologic Effects

Because manifestations of bleeding have been reported with some β-lactam anti-infectives, including piperacillin, the possibility of bleeding complications should be considered in patients receiving piperacillin/tazobactam, especially when the drug is used in patients with renal impairment. If bleeding manifestations occur, piperacillin/tazobactam should be discontinued and appropriate therapy instituted.

Hematologic function should be evaluated periodically during piperacillin/tazobactam therapy, especially in patients receiving prolonged therapy with the drug (i.e., 21 days or longer).

Precautions Related to Renal and Electrolyte Effects

Renal systems should be evaluated periodically during prolonged therapy with piperacillin/tazobactam.

Because there is evidence that piperacillin/tazobactam is an independent risk factor for renal failure and has been associated with delayed recovery of renal function compared with other β-lactam anti-infectives when used in critically ill patients, the manufacturer states that alternatives to piperacillin/tazobactam should be considered in such patients. If use of piperacillin/tazobactam is considered necessary in critically ill patients because alternative treatment options are inadequate or unavailable, renal function should be monitored during treatment with the drug.

Serum electrolytes should be determined periodically when piperacillin/tazobactam is used in patients with low potassium reserves, and the possibility of hypokalemia should be considered when the drug is used in those with potentially low potassium reserves who are receiving cytotoxic therapy or diuretics.

The sodium content of piperacillin/tazobactam should be considered when the drug is used in geriatric patients or patients whose sodium intake is restricted. Piperacillin/tazobactam (Zosyn®) contains 2.84 mEq (65 mg) of sodium per gram of piperacillin. Most generic preparations of piperacillin/tazobactam contain 2.35 mEq (54 mg) of sodium per gram of piperacillin; some contain 2.43 mEq (56 mg) of sodium per gram of piperacillin.

Precautions Related to C. difficile-associated Diarrhea and Colitis

Because CDAD has been reported with the use of nearly all anti-infectives, including piperacillin/tazobactam, it should be considered in the differential diagnosis of patients who develop diarrhea during or after anti-infective therapy. Careful medical history is necessary since CDAD has been reported to occur as late as 2 months or longer after anti-infective therapy is discontinued.

If CDAD is suspected or confirmed, anti-infective therapy not directed against *C. difficile* should be discontinued as soon as possible. Patients should be managed with appropriate anti-infective therapy directed against *C. difficile* (e.g., vancomycin, fidaxomicin, metronidazole), supportive therapy (e.g., fluid and electrolyte management, protein supplementation), and surgical evaluation as clinically indicated.

Patients should be advised that diarrhea is a common problem caused by anti-infectives and usually resolves when the drug is discontinued; however, they should contact a clinician if watery and bloody stools (with or without stomach cramps and fever) occur during or as late as 2 months or longer after the last dose.

Selection and Use of Anti-infectives

To reduce development of drug-resistant bacteria and maintain effectiveness of piperacillin/tazobactam and other antibacterials, the drug should be used only for the treatment of infections proven or strongly suspected to be caused by bacteria.

When selecting or modifying anti-infective therapy, results of culture and in vitro susceptibility testing should be used. In the absence of such data, local epidemiology and susceptibility patterns when selecting anti-infectives for empiric therapy patterns should be considered.

Patients should be advised that antibacterials (including piperacillin/tazobactam) should only be used to treat bacterial infections and not used to treat viral infections (e.g., the common cold). Patients also should be advised about the importance of completing the full course of therapy, even if feeling better after a few days, and that skipping doses or not completing therapy may decrease effectiveness and increase the likelihood that bacteria will develop resistance and will not be treatable with piperacillin/tazobactam or other antibacterials in the future.

Information on test methods and quality control standards for in vitro susceptibility testing of antibacterial agents and specific interpretive criteria for such testing recognized by FDA is available at https://www.fda.gov/STIC.

● Pediatric Precautions

Safety and efficacy of piperacillin/tazobactam in children younger than 2 months of age have not been established.

The manufacturer states that use of piperacillin/tazobactam for the treatment of appendicitis and/or peritonitis in pediatric patients 2 months of age or older is supported by evidence from well-controlled studies and pharmacokinetic studies in adults and pediatric patients.

Adverse effects reported when piperacillin/tazobactam was used in pediatric patients 2–12 years of age with severe intra-abdominal infections (including appendicitis and/or peritonitis) have been similar to those reported in adults.

● *Geriatric Precautions*

Geriatric patients older than 65 years of age receiving piperacillin/tazobactam are not at increased risk of developing adverse effects based solely on their age. However, geriatric patients are more likely to have decreased renal function compared with younger adults and the risk of toxic reactions to the drug may be greater in patients with impaired renal function.

Because of the greater frequency of decreased hepatic, renal, or cardiac function and of concomitant disease and drug therapy in geriatric patients, dosage of piperacillin/tazobactam generally should be selected cautiously in these patients, usually initiating therapy at the low end of the dosage range, and it may be useful to monitor renal function. In geriatric patients with renal impairment, dosage should be modified in response to the degree of renal impairment. (See Renal Impairment under Dosage and Administration: Dosage in Renal and Hepatic Impairment.)

When piperacillin/tazobactam is used in geriatric patients, the sodium content of the specific preparation used should be considered. Geriatric patients may respond to salt loading with a blunted natriuresis and this may be clinically important in patients with diseases such as heart failure. Piperacillin/tazobactam (Zosyn®) contains 65 mg (2.84 mEq) of sodium per gram of piperacillin; patients would receive 780–1040 mg (34.1–45.5 mEq) of sodium daily with usually recommended dosages of this preparation. The sodium content of commercially available generic preparations of piperacillin/tazobactam differs depending on the manufacturer. (See Precautions Related to Renal and Electrolyte Effects under Cautions: Precautions and Contraindications.)

● *Mutagenicity and Carcinogenicity*

The mutagenic potential of piperacillin/tazobactam has been evaluated in vitro and in vivo. There was no in vitro evidence of mutagenicity when the fixed combination was used in microbial mutagenicity assays, unscheduled DNA synthesis tests, mammalian point mutation assays in Chinese hamster ovary cell HPRT, or mammalian cell (BALB/c-3T3) transformation assays. In addition, in vivo studies in rats using piperacillin/tazobactam indicated that the drug did not induce chromosomal aberrations.

Long-term studies have not been performed to evaluate the carcinogenic potential of piperacillin, tazobactam, or piperacillin/tazobactam.

● *Pregnancy, Fertility, and Lactation*

Pregnancy

Available human data regarding use of piperacillin/tazobactam during pregnancy are inadequate to inform a drug-associated risk for major birth defects and miscarriage. Piperacillin and tazobactam both cross the human placenta.

Reproduction studies in pregnant mice and rats using IV piperacillin/tazobactam (up to 1–2 times the human dosage of piperacillin and 2–3 times the human dosage of tazobactam based on body surface area) did not reveal evidence of teratogenicity or fetal structural abnormalities; however, intraperitoneal administration in rats at doses less than the maximum recommended human daily dosage based on body surface area given prior to mating and throughout gestation or from gestation day 17 through lactation day 21 resulted in maternal toxicity, reduced litter size, and effects on peri- and postnatal development (e.g., reduced pup weights, increased stillbirths, increased pup mortality, ossification delays, rib variations).

Fertility

There was no evidence of impaired fertility in reproduction studies in rats using IV piperacillin/tazobactam in dosages similar to the maximum recommended human daily dosage based on body surface area.

Lactation

Piperacillin is distributed into human milk; it is not known whether tazobactam is distributed into human milk. Effects of the drugs on breast-fed infants or milk production are not known.

The developmental and health benefits of breast-feeding should be considered along with the woman's clinical need for piperacillin/tazobactam and potential adverse effects on the breast-fed infant from the drug or from the underlying maternal condition.

DRUG INTERACTIONS

● *Aminoglycosides*

The antibacterial activities of piperacillin and aminoglycosides (e.g., amikacin, gentamicin, tobramycin) have been synergistic in vitro against some strains of Enterobacteriaceae and *Pseudomonas aeruginosa*.

The fixed combination of piperacillin sodium and tazobactam sodium (piperacillin/tazobactam) is physically and/or chemically incompatible with aminoglycosides and can inactivate aminoglycosides in vitro if the drugs are admixed or administered using the same IV infusion line. If concomitant therapy with piperacillin/tazobactam and an aminoglycoside is indicated, the drugs should be reconstituted, diluted, and administered separately. Piperacillin/tazobactam can be coadministered with amikacin or gentamicin (but not tobramycin or other aminoglycosides) via Y-site infusion *only* under certain specific conditions. (See Concomitant Use with Aminoglycosides under Administration: IV Infusion, in Dosage and Administration.)

Piperacillin also can inactivate aminoglycosides in vivo. Decreased aminoglycoside serum concentrations and half-lives have been reported in patients receiving concomitant piperacillin therapy, usually when high piperacillin dosage was used or the patient had impaired renal function. Although *sequential* administration of piperacillin/tazobactam and tobramycin in patients with normal renal function or mild to moderate renal impairment has resulted in modestly decreased serum tobramycin concentrations, the manufacturer of piperacillin/tazobactam states that dosage adjustments are not needed.

Because concomitant use of piperacillin and an aminoglycoside in patients with end-stage renal disease (ESRD) requiring hemodialysis may result in substantially decreased serum concentrations of the aminoglycoside (especially tobramycin), aminoglycoside serum concentrations should be monitored closely in patients receiving piperacillin/tazobactam and an aminoglycoside.

● *Anticoagulants*

Coagulation parameters should be monitored more frequently if piperacillin/tazobactam is used concomitantly with oral anticoagulants, high doses of heparin, or other drugs that affect blood coagulation or thrombocyte function.

● *Methotrexate*

Concomitant use of methotrexate and piperacillin may result in decreased renal clearance of methotrexate due to competition for renal secretion; the effect of tazobactam on methotrexate elimination has not been evaluated.

If concurrent therapy with methotrexate and piperacillin/tazobactam is necessary, serum methotrexate concentrations should be evaluated frequently and the patient should be monitored for signs and symptoms of methotrexate toxicity.

● *Neuromuscular Blocking Agents*

Prolonged neuromuscular blockade has been reported when vecuronium was used concomitantly with piperacillin, and this also could occur if vecuronium is used concomitantly with piperacillin/tazobactam. Because other nondepolarizing muscle relaxants have similar mechanisms of action, a similar effect could occur if piperacillin/tazobactam is used concomitantly with any of these drugs.

If piperacillin/tazobactam is used concomitantly with a neuromuscular blocking agent, the patient should be monitored for adverse effects related to neuromuscular blockade.

● *Probenecid*

Probenecid inhibits tubular renal secretion of both piperacillin and tazobactam and prolongs their half-lives by 21 and 71%, respectively.

Concomitant use of probenecid and piperacillin/tazobactam is not recommended unless benefits outweigh risks.

● *Vancomycin*

Concomitant use of vancomycin and piperacillin/tazobactam in critically ill patients has been associated with an increased incidence of acute kidney injury compared with use of vancomycin alone.

If vancomycin and piperacillin/tazobactam are used concomitantly, renal function should be monitored. In addition, because vancomycin and some piperacillin/tazobactam preparations may be physically and/or chemically incompatible, it has been recommended that the drugs should be administered separately.

Pharmacokinetic interactions between vancomycin and piperacillin/tazobactam have not been reported.

LABORATORY TEST INTERFERENCES

● Tests for Aspergillus

False-positive test results for *Aspergillus* were reported when the Bio-Rad Laboratories Platelia *Aspergillus* EIA test was performed in patients receiving the fixed combination of piperacillin sodium and tazobactam sodium (piperacillin/tazobactam). Cross reactions with non-*Aspergillus* polysaccharides and polyfuranoses have been reported with the Bio-Rad Laboratories Platelia *Aspergillus* EIA test. Positive Platelia *Aspergillus* EIA test results in patients receiving piperacillin/tazobactam should be interpreted with caution and confirmed using other diagnostic methods.

● Tests for Urinary Glucose

As with other penicillins, piperacillin/tazobactam may result in false-positive urinary glucose determinations with tests that use copper reduction (e.g., Clinitest®). Glucose tests based on enzymatic glucose oxidase reactions should be used.

ACUTE TOXICITY

There have been postmarketing reports of overdosage of the fixed combination of piperacillin sodium and tazobactam sodium (piperacillin/tazobactam). Adverse effects reported with such overdosages have included adverse effects reported with usual dosages of the drug (e.g., nausea, vomiting, diarrhea). Neuromuscular excitability or convulsions may occur if higher than recommended dosages of IV piperacillin/tazobactam are given, especially in patients with renal failure.

If acute overdosage of piperacillin/tazobactam occurs, supportive and symptomatic treatment should be initiated as indicated. Because piperacillin and tazobactam are removed by hemodialysis (see Pharmacokinetics: Elimination), this procedure may be effective in reducing excessive serum concentrations of the drugs.

MECHANISM OF ACTION

The fixed combination of piperacillin sodium and tazobactam sodium (piperacillin/tazobactam) is bactericidal in action.

Like other penicillins, piperacillin inhibits bacterial septum formation and cell wall synthesis in susceptible bacteria. The mechanism of action of penicillins is mediated through binding to penicillin-binding proteins (PBPs).

Tazobactam alone has only limited intrinsic antibacterial activity because of reduced affinity for PBPs. However, tazobactam is a β-lactamase inhibitor that generally acts as an irreversible inhibitor and can inactivate both plasmid- and chromosome-mediated β-lactamases. In vitro studies indicate that tazobactam can inhibit staphylococcal β-lactamases and β-lactamases classified as Richmond-Sykes types II, III (TEM type, HSV-1), IV, and V (PSE and OXA types). Tazobactam is effective against some type I β-lactamases, including type IC, and may be slightly more active against type I enzymes than some other β-lactamase inhibitors (e.g., clavulanic acid, sulbactam). Unlike clavulanic acid, tazobactam generally does not induce production of type I chromosomally mediated cephalosporins in *Pseudomonas* or Enterobacteriaceae.

Because tazobactam inactivates certain β-lactamases, concomitant use with piperacillin can protect the penicillin from degradation by these β-lactamases and expand its spectrum of activity to include some β-lactamase-producing bacteria that are resistant to piperacillin alone.

SPECTRUM

Based on its spectrum of activity, the fixed combination of piperacillin sodium and tazobactam sodium (piperacillin/tazobactam) is classified as an extended-spectrum penicillin. For information on the classification of penicillins based on spectrum of activity, see the Preface to the Penicillins 8:12.16.

Piperacillin/tazobactam has a wide spectrum of activity and is active in vitro against various gram-positive and -negative aerobic and anaerobic bacteria. The fixed combination is active against bacteria susceptible to piperacillin alone. In addition, because tazobactam has a high affinity for and binds to certain β-lactamases that generally inactivate piperacillin, piperacillin/tazobactam is active against many β-lactamase-producing bacteria that are resistant to piperacillin alone, including piperacillin-resistant strains of staphylococci, *Haemophilus*, Enterobacteriaceae, and *Bacteroides*.

Piperacillin/tazobactam is not active against *Mycoplasma* and *Chlamydia*.

● Gram-positive Aerobic Bacteria

Piperacillin/tazobactam is active in vitro and in clinical infections against *Staphylococcus aureus* (methicillin-susceptible strains only).

Piperacillin/tazobactam also is active in vitro against *S. epidermidis* (methicillin-susceptible strains only), *Streptococcus pyogenes* (group A β-hemolytic streptococci; GAS), *S. agalactiae* (group B streptococci; GBS), *S. pneumoniae* (penicillin-susceptible strains only), viridans group streptococci, and *Enterococcus faecalis* (ampicillin- or penicillin-susceptible strains only).

Although piperacillin/tazobactam is active against β-lactamase-producing *S. aureus* and *S. epidermidis*, the fixed combination is not active against methicillin-resistant *S. aureus* (MRSA; also known as oxacillin-resistant *S. aureus* or ORSA) or methicillin-resistant *S. epidermidis*.

● Gram-negative Aerobic Bacteria

Enterobacteriaceae

Piperacillin/tazobactam is active in vitro and in clinical infections against *Escherichia coli* and *Klebsiella pneumoniae*.

Piperacillin/tazobactam also is active in vitro against *Citrobacter koseri*, *Enterobacter*, *Morganella morganii*, *Proteus mirabilis*, *P. vulgaris*, *Providencia stuartii*, *P. rettgeri*, *Salmonella*, *Shigella*, and *Serratia marcescens*.

Pseudomonas

Piperacillin/tazobactam is active in vitro and in clinical infections against *Pseudomonas aeruginosa*.

Other Gram-negative Aerobic Bacteria

Piperacillin/tazobactam is active in vitro and in clinical infections against *Acinetobacter* (including *A. baumannii*) and *Haemophilus influenzae* (except β-lactamase negative, ampicillin-resistant strains; BLNAR). The drug also is active in vitro against *Moraxella catarrhalis* and *Neisseria*.

Piperacillin/tazobactam has some in vitro activity against *Legionella*; however, the drug is not effective against intracellular *Legionella* and is unlikely to be effective for the treatment of *Legionella* infections.

● Anaerobic Bacteria

Piperacillin/tazobactam is active in vitro and in clinical infections against some gram-negative anaerobic bacteria, including *Bacteroides fragilis*, *B. ovatus*, *B. thetaiotaomicron*, and *B. vulgatus*. The drug also is active in vitro against *B. distasonis*, *Fusobacterium*, and *Prevotella melaninogenica*.

Piperacillin/tazobactam is active in vitro against some gram-positive anaerobic bacteria, including *Bacillus*, *Clostridium perfringens*, *Cutibacterium acnes* (formerly *Propionibacterium acnes*), and *Peptostreptococcus*.

RESISTANCE

Resistance or reduced susceptibility to the fixed combination of piperacillin sodium and tazobactam sodium (piperacillin/tazobactam) can occur.

The major mechanism of resistance to piperacillin/tazobactam in gram-positive bacteria is alteration in penicillin-binding proteins (PBPs). Methicillin-resistant *Staphylococcus aureus* (MRSA; also known as oxacillin-resistant *S. aureus* or ORSA) and *Enterococcus faecium* are intrinsically resistant to piperacillin/tazobactam because of low affinity of PBPs.

Resistance to piperacillin/tazobactam in gram-negative bacteria may be multifactorial and may involve β-lactamases, transferable multidrug-resistance genes, alterations in outer membrane porins, and antibiotic efflux. Piperacillin/tazobactam may be active against some Enterobacteriaceae that produce extended-spectrum β-lactamases (ESBLs), but strains that produce multiple ESBLs or have additional mechanisms of resistance (e.g., AmpC β-lactamases) may have reduced susceptibility or resistance to the drug. *Pseudomonas* resistant to piperacillin generally also are resistant to piperacillin/tazobactam.

β-Lactamase-negative, ampicillin-resistant *Haemophilus influenzae* (BLNAR *H. influenzae*) are resistant to piperacillin/tazobactam.

PHARMACOKINETICS

● Absorption

Following IV infusion of the fixed combination of piperacillin sodium and tazobactam sodium (piperacillin/tazobactam), peak plasma concentrations of piperacillin and tazobactam are attained immediately or 1–2 hours after completion of the infusion. Studies in adults indicate that piperacillin plasma concentrations attained following IV infusion of piperacillin/tazobactam over 30 minutes are similar to those attained with equivalent doses of piperacillin administered alone.

● Distribution

Both piperacillin and tazobactam are widely distributed into tissues and body fluids, including intestinal mucosa, gallbladder, female reproductive tissues (uterus, ovary, fallopian tube), lung, skin, bone, interstitial fluid, synovial fluid, and bile. Mean tissue concentrations generally are 50–100% of plasma concentrations.

Only low concentrations of piperacillin and tazobactam are distributed into CSF in patients with uninflamed meninges.

Both piperacillin and tazobactam cross the placenta.

Piperacillin is distributed into milk; it is not known whether tazobactam is distributed into milk.

The mean volume of distribution of piperacillin is 0.243 L/kg and is independent of age.

Both piperacillin and tazobactam are approximately 30% bound to plasma proteins.

● Elimination

Piperacillin is metabolized to a minor microbiologically active desethyl metabolite and an inactive metabolite.

Tazobactam is metabolized to a single metabolite that lacks pharmacologic and antibacterial activity.

Both piperacillin and tazobactam are eliminated in urine by glomerular filtration and tubular secretion. In addition, piperacillin, desethylpiperacillin, and tazobactam are eliminated in bile.

Following IV administration, 68 and 80% of the piperacillin and tazobactam doses, respectively, are eliminated unchanged in urine.

Plasma half-lives of piperacillin and tazobactam range from 0.7–1.2 hours in healthy adults.

In adults with cirrhosis, the half-lives of piperacillin and tazobactam are increased by approximately 25 and 18%, respectively, compared with adults with normal hepatic function.

In adults with renal impairment, the half-lives of piperacillin and tazobactam increase with decreasing creatinine clearance. In adults with creatinine clearances less than 20 mL/minute, the half-life of piperacillin is twofold higher and the half-life of tazobactam is fourfold higher compared with adults with normal renal function.

In geriatric adults 65–80 years of age, the mean half-lives of piperacillin and tazobactam are increased by 32 and 55%, respectively, compared with adults 18–35 years of age; this increase may be the result of age-related changes in creatinine clearance.

In children 9 months to 12 years of age, clearance of piperacillin and tazobactam is comparable to that reported in adults; piperacillin clearance in children 2–9 months of age is estimated to be 80% of that value. Clearance is slower in patients younger than 2 months of age compared with older children.

Both piperacillin and tazobactam are removed by hemodialysis and, to a lesser extent, by peritoneal dialysis. Hemodialysis removes approximately 31 and 39% of the piperacillin and tazobactam dose, respectively; an additional 5% of the tazobactam dose is removed as the tazobactam metabolite. Peritoneal dialysis removes approximately 6 and 21% of the piperacillin and tazobactam dose, respectively; up to 16% of the tazobactam dose is removed as the tazobactam metabolite.

CHEMISTRY AND STABILITY

● Chemistry

Piperacillin sodium and tazobactam sodium (piperacillin/tazobactam) is a fixed combination of the sodium salts of piperacillin and tazobactam.

Piperacillin, a piperazine derivative of ampicillin, is an extended-spectrum penicillin. Piperacillin is commercially available in the US only in fixed combination with tazobactam.

Tazobactam, a β-lactamase inhibitor, is a synthetic penicillanic acid sulfone that is structurally similar to sulbactam. Although tazobactam has only limited intrinsic antibacterial activity alone, the combined use of tazobactam and certain penicillins or cephalosporins (e.g., amoxicillin, ampicillin, ceftazidime, ceftolozane, piperacillin) results in a synergistic effect that expands the spectrum of activity of the penicillin or cephalosporin against many strains of β-lactamase-producing bacteria.

Piperacillin/tazobactam contains an 8:1 ratio of piperacillin to tazobactam; potency of the fixed combination is expressed in terms of the piperacillin content plus the tazobactam content.

Piperacillin/tazobactam (Zosyn®) and generic preparations of piperacillin/tazobactam commercially available in the US are *not* identical. Piperacillin/tazobactam (Zosyn®) is formulated with edetate disodium dihydrate (EDTA) and sodium citrate; the generic preparations do not contain EDTA or sodium citrate. Because EDTA acts as a metal-chelating agent and sodium citrate acts as a buffer, certain aspects of chemical degradation and particulate formation are inhibited and there is a lower risk of particulate matter formation and accumulation following reconstitution of Zosyn® with commonly used diluents or storage of solutions of the drug. In addition, the presence of EDTA and sodium citrate allows coadministration of Zosyn® and lactated Ringer's injection via Y-site infusion. (See IV Infusion under Dosage and Administration: Administration.)

Each single-dose vial of piperacillin/tazobactam sterile powder (Zosyn®) contains 2.84 mEq (65 mg) of sodium and 0.25 mg of EDTA per gram of piperacillin.

Commercially available piperacillin/tazobactam sterile powder (generic) in single-dose ADD-Vantage® vials contains 2.35 mEq (54 mg) of sodium per gram of piperacillin.

Bulk vials of piperacillin/tazobactam (Zosyn®) containing 40.5 g (36 g of piperacillin and 4.5 g of tazobactam) contain 100.4 mEq (2304 mg) of sodium and 9 mg of EDTA. Bulk bottles of piperacillin/tazobactam (generic) containing 40.5 g (36 g of piperacillin and 4.5 g of tazobactam) contain 84.6 mEq (1945 mg) of sodium and do not contain EDTA.

Commercially available single-dose frozen premixed piperacillin/tazobactam injections in dextrose (Zosyn® in Galaxy® containers) are sterile, nonpyrogenic, iso-osmotic solutions of the drug formulated with EDTA. The single-dose frozen injection contains 2.79 mEq (64 mg) of sodium and 0.25 mg of EDTA per gram of piperacillin. Sodium bicarbonate and/or hydrochloric acid may have been added to adjust the pH of the injections to 5.5–6.8.

● Stability

Piperacillin/tazobactam powder for injection provided in single-dose vials (Zosyn®, generic) should be stored at 20–25°C. Following reconstitution, the solutions should be used immediately; any unused portions should be discarded after 24 hours if stored at 20–25°C or after 48 hours if refrigerated at 2–8°C. These reconstituted solutions should not be frozen.

Single-dose ADD-Vantage® vials of piperacillin/tazobactam (generic) should be stored at 20–25°C. Following reconstitution with 0.9% sodium chloride injection or 5% dextrose injection according to the manufacturer's directions, these IV solutions are stable for 24 hours at room temperature and should not be refrigerated or frozen.

Piperacillin/tazobactam powder for injection provided in bulk vials or bottles (Zosyn®, generic) should be stored at 20–25°C. Following reconstitution, the solutions should be used promptly; any unused portions should be discarded after 24 hours if stored at 20–25°C or after 48 hours if refrigerated at 2–8°C. These reconstituted solutions should not be frozen.

The commercially available single-dose frozen premixed piperacillin/tazobactam injections in dextrose (Zosyn® in Galaxy® containers) should be stored at −20°C or lower. The frozen premixed injections should be thawed at room temperature (20–25°C) or under refrigeration (2–8°C) and, once thawed, should not be refrozen. Thawed solutions of the commercially available frozen injection are stable for 24 hours at room temperature (20–25°C) or 14 days at 2–8°C.

Piperacillin/tazobactam is potentially physically and/or chemically incompatible with some drugs, including aminoglycosides, but the compatibility depends on several factors (e.g., concentration of the drugs, specific diluents used, resulting pH, temperature). Specialized references should be consulted for specific compatibility information.

PREPARATIONS

Excipients in commercially available drug preparations may have clinically important effects in some individuals; consult specific product labeling for details.

Piperacillin Sodium and Tazobactam Sodium

Parenteral		
For injection, for IV infusion	2.25 g (2 g of piperacillin and 0.25 g of tazobactam)*	Piperacillin Sodium and Tazobactam Sodium for Injection
		Piperacillin Sodium and Tazobactam Sodium for Injection ADD-Vantage®, Hospira
		Zosyn®, Wyeth
	3.375 g (3 g of piperacillin and 0.375 g of tazobactam)*	Piperacillin Sodium and Tazobactam Sodium for Injection
		Piperacillin Sodium and Tazobactam Sodium for Injection ADD-Vantage®, Hospira
		Zosyn®, Wyeth
	4.5 g (4 g of piperacillin and 0.5 g of tazobactam)*	Piperacillin Sodium and Tazobactam Sodium for Injection
		Piperacillin Sodium and Tazobactam Sodium for Injection ADD-Vantage®, Hospira
		Zosyn®, Wyeth
	40.5 g (36 g of piperacillin and 4.5 g of tazobactam) pharmacy bulk package*	Piperacillin Sodium and Tazobactam Sodium for Injection
		Zosyn®, Wyeth

* available from one or more manufacturer, distributor, and/or repackager by generic (nonproprietary) name

Piperacillin Sodium and Tazobactam Sodium in Dextrose

Parenteral		
Injection (frozen), for IV infusion	2.25 g (40 mg of piperacillin per mL [2 g] and 5 mg of tazobactam per mL [0.25 g]) in 2% Dextrose	Zosyn® Iso-osmotic in Dextrose Injection (Galaxy®), Wyeth
	3.375 g (60 mg of piperacillin per mL [3 g] and 7.5 mg of tazobactam per mL [0.375 g]) in 0.7% Dextrose	Zosyn® Iso-osmotic in Dextrose Injection (Galaxy®), Wyeth
	4.5 g (40 mg of piperacillin per mL [4 g] and 5 mg of tazobactam per mL [0.5 g]) in 2% Dextrose	Zosyn® Iso-osmotic in Dextrose Injection (Galaxy®), Wyeth

† Use is not currently included in the labeling approved by the US Food and Drug Administration.

Selected Revisions September 2, 2019, © Copyright, May 1, 1994, American Society of Health-System Pharmacists, Inc.

Ciprofloxacin, Ciprofloxacin Hydrochloride

8:12.18 • QUINOLONES

■ Ciprofloxacin is a fluoroquinolone anti-infective agent.

USES

Ciprofloxacin is used orally or IV for the treatment of urinary tract infections (UTIs), chronic bacterial prostatitis, acute sinusitis, lower respiratory tract infections (including nosocomial pneumonia and acute exacerbations of chronic bronchitis), GI infections, skin and skin structure infections, or bone and joint infections caused by susceptible gram-negative and gram-positive aerobic bacteria. Ciprofloxacin is used orally or IV for inhalational anthrax (postexposure) following suspected or confirmed exposure to aerosolized *Bacillus anthracis* spores and also is used for prophylaxis following ingestion of *B. anthracis* spores† and for the treatment of inhalational anthrax†, cutaneous anthrax†, or GI and oropharyngeal anthrax†. Ciprofloxacin is used orally or IV for the treatment or prophylaxis of plague. In addition, ciprofloxacin is used orally or IV in conjunction with metronidazole for the treatment of complicated intra-abdominal infections caused by *Escherichia coli*, *Pseudomonas aeruginosa*, *Proteus mirabilis*, *Klebsiella pneumoniae*, or *Bacteroides fragilis*. Because ciprofloxacin is inactive against most anaerobic bacteria, the drug is ineffective in and should not be used alone if a mixed aerobic-anaerobic bacterial infection is suspected. Ciprofloxacin has been used in conjunction with other anti-infectives for empiric anti-infective therapy in febrile neutropenic patients.

Ciprofloxacin extended-release tablets containing both the hydrochloride and the base are used in adults for the treatment of uncomplicated UTIs (acute cystitis), complicated UTIs, or acute uncomplicated pyelonephritis. Safety and efficacy of ciprofloxacin extended-release tablets have been established *only* for infections involving the urinary tract; the extended-release tablets should *not* be used for the treatment of infections at other sites (e.g., respiratory tract, skin and skin structure, bone and joint, GI tract, intra-abdominal) that are treated with ciprofloxacin conventional tablets or oral suspension or with IV ciprofloxacin.

Prior to initiation of ciprofloxacin therapy, appropriate specimens should be obtained for identification of the causative organism(s) and in vitro susceptibility tests. Ciprofloxacin therapy may be started pending results of susceptibility tests, but should be discontinued and other appropriate anti-infective therapy substituted if the organism is found to be resistant to ciprofloxacin. Because resistant strains of *Pseudomonas aeruginosa* have developed during ciprofloxacin therapy, in vitro susceptibility tests should be performed periodically when the drug is used in the treatment of infections caused by this organism. Because staphylococci may develop resistance to ciprofloxacin during prolonged therapy with the drug, in vitro susceptibility tests should be repeated during therapy, especially when infections are caused by methicillin-resistant strains of *Staphylococcus aureus* (MRSA; also known as oxacillin-resistant *S. aureus* or ORSA).

● *Bone and Joint Infections*

Ciprofloxacin (IV, conventional tablets, oral suspension) is used in adults for the treatment of bone and joint infections, including osteomyelitis, caused by susceptible *E. aerogenes*†, *E. cloacae*, *E. coli*†, *K. pneumoniae*†, *M. morganii*†, *P. mirabilis*†, *Ps. aeruginosa*, or *S. marcescens*.

For the treatment of native vertebral osteomyelitis caused by Enterobacteriaceae or *Ps. aeruginosa*, the Infectious Diseases Society of America (IDSA) recommends ciprofloxacin as an alternative to the drugs of choice (cefepime, carbapenems). For the treatment of native vertebral osteomyelitis caused by *Salmonella*†, these experts recommend ciprofloxacin as the drug of choice and ceftriaxone as an alternative.

For the treatment of prosthetic joint infections caused by *Enterobacter* or *Ps. aeruginosa*, IDSA states that cefepime or a carbapenem is preferred and ciprofloxacin is recommended as an alternative. These experts state that ciprofloxacin may be a preferred drug for the treatment of prosthetic joint infections caused by other Enterobacteriaceae.

For additional information on management of bone and joint infections, current clinical practice guidelines from IDSA available at http://www.idsociety.org should be consulted.

Clinical Experience

Clinical response has been reported in 61–86% and bacteriologic cure has been reported in 75–81% of patients with bone and joint infections (caused principally by gram-negative aerobes) who received oral ciprofloxacin. Treatment failures have been reported most frequently in patients with an underlying metal appliance at the site of infection and in patients with ciprofloxacin-resistant *Ps. aeruginosa* or *S. aureus*. However, there is evidence from a randomized, controlled study in patients with culture-proven staphylococcal infections associated with stable orthopedic implants that a long-term regimen (3–6 weeks) of ciprofloxacin and rifampin given after initial debridement and a 2-week IV regimen of flucloxacillin (not commercially available in the US) or vancomycin with rifampin or placebo can result in cure of the infection without removal of the implant.

● *Endocarditis*

Endocarditis Caused by the HACEK Group

Ciprofloxacin is used as an alternative for the treatment of endocarditis† (native or prosthetic valve or other prosthetic material) caused by fastidious gram-negative bacilli known as the HACEK group (*Haemophilus*, *Aggregatibacter*, *Cardiobacterium hominis*, *Eikenella corrodens*, *Kingella*). The HACEK group accounts for up to 10% of cases of community-acquired native valve endocarditis in patients who are not IV drug abusers. These organisms should be considered ampicillin-resistant, but may be susceptible to third or fourth generation cephalosporins or fluoroquinolones.

The American Heart Association (AHA) and IDSA recommend ceftriaxone (or other third or fourth generation cephalosporin) for the treatment of endocarditis caused by the HACEK group, but state that a fluoroquinolone (ciprofloxacin, levofloxacin, moxifloxacin) may be considered in patients who cannot tolerate cephalosporins. Because only limited data are available regarding use of fluoroquinolones for the treatment of HACEK endocarditis, an infectious disease specialist should be consulted when treating such infections in patients who cannot tolerate cephalosporins.

● *GI Infections*

Infectious Diarrhea

Ciprofloxacin is used in adults for the treatment of infectious diarrhea caused by susceptible enterotoxigenic *E. coli*, *Campylobacter*, *Salmonella*†, *Shigella* (*S. flexneri*, *S. boydii*, *S. sonnei*, *S. dysenteriae*), or *Vibrio*† (see Uses: Vibrio Infections).

Because ciprofloxacin is active in vitro against many pathogens associated with infectious diarrhea, including some strains of *Campylobacter*, *E. coli*, *Shigella*, *Salmonella*, *Aeromonas*, *Vibrio*, and *Yersinia enterocolitica*, some clinicians suggest that it may be a drug of choice for empiric treatment of the disease in adults. However, because of concerns about increasing emergence of fluoroquinolone-resistant strains in some enteric pathogens (e.g., *Campylobacter*, *Salmonella*, *Shigella*) secondary to widespread use of the drugs, a decision to use a fluoroquinolone for empiric treatment of infectious diarrhea should be based on local susceptibility patterns.

Campylobacter Infections

Ciprofloxacin is used for the treatment of campylobacteriosis caused by susceptible *Campylobacter*.

Optimal treatment of campylobacteriosis in patients with human immunodeficiency virus (HIV) infection has not been identified. Some clinicians withhold anti-infective treatment in HIV-infected patients with CD4+ T-cell counts exceeding 200 cells/mm³ if they have only mild campylobacteriosis, but initiate treatment if symptoms persist for more than several days. In HIV-infected patients with mild to moderate campylobacteriosis, treatment with a fluoroquinolone (preferably ciprofloxacin or, alternatively, levofloxacin or moxifloxacin) or azithromycin is reasonable. Anti-infective therapy should be modified based on results of in vitro susceptibility testing. In the US, resistance to fluoroquinolones has been reported in 22% of *C. jejuni* and 35% of *C. coli* isolates tested. To limit emergence of resistance, some clinicians suggest that it may be prudent to use an aminoglycoside concomitantly in patients with bacteremic infections.

Cyclospora Infections

Ciprofloxacin is recommended by some clinicians as an alternative to co-trimoxazole for the treatment of cyclosporiasis† caused by *Cyclospora cayetanensis*.

Cystoisospora Infections

Ciprofloxacin has been used for the treatment of cystoisosporiasis† (formerly isosporiasis) caused by *Cystoisospora belli* (formerly *Isospora belli*).

Although co-trimoxazole is the drug of choice for the treatment of cystoisosporiasis, pyrimethamine, ciprofloxacin, and nitazoxanide are recommended as alternatives. Ciprofloxacin may not be as effective as co-trimoxazole, but may be useful for the treatment of cystoisosporiasis in patients who cannot tolerate co-trimoxazole.

In HIV-infected patients, ciprofloxacin is recommended as an alternative to co-trimoxazole for treatment and chronic maintenance therapy (secondary prophylaxis) of cystoisosporiasis.

Salmonella Gastroenteritis

Ciprofloxacin is used for the treatment of *Salmonella* gastroenteritis† (with or without bacteremia).

Anti-infective therapy is not usually indicated in otherwise healthy individuals with uncomplicated (noninvasive) gastroenteritis caused by *Salmonella* since such therapy may prolong the duration of fecal excretion of the organism and there is no evidence that it shortens the duration of the disease; however, the US Centers for Disease Control and Prevention (CDC), American Academy of Pediatrics (AAP), IDSA, and others recommend anti-infective therapy in individuals with severe *Salmonella* gastroenteritis and in those who are at increased risk of invasive disease. These individuals include infants younger than 3–6 months of age; individuals older than 50 years of age; individuals with hemoglobinopathies, severe atherosclerosis or valvular heart disease, prostheses, uremia, chronic GI disease, or severe colitis; and individuals who are immunocompromised because of malignancy, immunosuppressive therapy, HIV infection, or other immunosuppressive illness. When an anti-infective agent is considered necessary in an individual with *Salmonella* gastroenteritis, CDC, AAP, IDSA, and others recommend ceftriaxone, cefotaxime, ciprofloxacin, ampicillin, amoxicillin, co-trimoxazole, chloramphenicol, or azithromycin depending on the susceptibility of the causative organism. If invasive disease is suspected or confirmed, IDSA recommends ceftriaxone over ciprofloxacin because of the increasing incidence of resistance to fluoroquinolones.

Because HIV-infected individuals with *Salmonella* gastroenteritis are at high risk for bacteremia, CDC, National Institutes of Health (NIH), and the HIV Medicine Association of IDSA recommend that such patients receive anti-infective treatment. These experts state that the initial drug of choice for the treatment of salmonella gastroenteritis (with or without bacteremia) in HIV-infected adults is ciprofloxacin; other fluoroquinolones (levofloxacin, moxifloxacin) also are likely to be effective in these patients, but clinical data are limited. Depending on results of in vitro susceptibility testing of the causative organism, alternatives for treatment of *Salmonella* gastroenteritis in HIV-infected adults are co-trimoxazole or third generation cephalosporins (ceftriaxone, cefotaxime).

The role of long-term treatment (secondary prophylaxis) against *Salmonella* in HIV-infected individuals is not well established, and possible benefits of such prophylaxis should be weighed against the risks of long-term anti-infective exposure. CDC, NIH, and IDSA state that secondary prophylaxis should be considered in those with recurrent bacteremia and may also be considered in those with recurrent gastroenteritis (with or without bacteremia) and in those with CD4+ T-cell counts less than 200 cells/mm³ and severe diarrhea. These experts state that secondary prophylaxis should be discontinued if the *Salmonella* infection resolves and there has been a sustained response to antiretroviral therapy with CD4+ T-cell counts greater than 200 cells/mm³.

Shigella Infections

Ciprofloxacin is used for the treatment of shigellosis caused by susceptible *Shigella*.

Infections caused by *S. sonnei* usually are self-limited (48–72 hours), and mild cases may not require treatment with anti-infectives. However, because there is some evidence that anti-infectives may shorten the duration of diarrhea and the period of fecal excretion of *Shigella*, anti-infective treatment generally is recommended in addition to fluid and electrolyte replacement in patients with severe shigellosis, dysentery, or underlying immunosuppression. An empiric treatment regimen can be used initially, but in vitro susceptibility testing of clinical isolates is indicated since resistance is common. A fluoroquinolone (preferably ciprofloxacin or, alternatively, levofloxacin or moxifloxacin) generally has been recommended for the treatment of shigellosis. However, fluoroquinolone-resistant *Shigella* have been reported in the US, especially in international travelers, the homeless, and men who have sex with men (MSM). Depending on in vitro susceptibility, other drugs recommended for the treatment of shigellosis include co-trimoxazole, ceftriaxone, azithromycin (not recommended in those with bacteremia), or ampicillin.

Yersinia Infections

Although GI infections caused by *Y. enterocolitica* or *Y. pseudotuberculosis* usually are self-limited and anti-infective therapy is unnecessary, some experts recommend use of anti-infectives in immunocompromised individuals or for the treatment of severe infections or when septicemia or other invasive disease occurs. GI infections caused by *Y. enterocolitica* or *Y. pseudotuberculosis* can occur as the result of ingesting undercooked pork, unpasteurized milk, or contaminated water; infection has occurred in infants whose caregivers handled contaminated chitterlings (raw pork intestines) or tofu. When treatment is considered necessary, some clinicians recommend co-trimoxazole as the drug of choice and cefotaxime and ciprofloxacin as alternatives.

Travelers' Diarrhea

Ciprofloxacin is used for the short-term treatment of travelers' diarrhea† and has been used for the prevention of travelers' diarrhea† in adults traveling for relatively short periods of time to high-risk areas.

The most common cause of travelers' diarrhea worldwide is noninvasive enterotoxigenic strains of *E. coli* (ETEC), but travelers' diarrhea also can be caused by various other bacteria including enteroaggregative and other *E. coli* pathotypes, *C. jejuni*, *Shigella*, *Salmonella*, *Aeromonas*, *Plesiomonas*, *Y. enterocolitica*, or *V. parahaemolyticus* or non-O-group 1 *V. cholerae*, and, possibly, *Acrobacter*, *Larobacter*, and enterotoxigenic *Bacteroides fragilis*. In some cases, travelers' diarrhea is caused by parasitic enteric pathogens (e.g., *Giardia*, *Cryptosporidium*, *Entamoeba histolytica*) or viral enteric pathogens (e.g., rotavirus, norovirus, astrovirus).

Countries where travelers are at low risk of travelers' diarrhea include the US, Canada, Australia, New Zealand, Japan, and countries in Northern and Western Europe. Travelers are at intermediate risk for travelers' diarrhea in Eastern Europe, South Africa, and some of the Caribbean islands, but are at high risk in most of Asia, the Middle East, Africa, Mexico, and Central and South America.

Treatment

Travelers' diarrhea caused by bacteria may be self-limited and often resolves within 3–7 days without anti-infective treatment. CDC states that anti-infective treatment is *not* recommended in patients with mild travelers' diarrhea. However, CDC and other clinicians state that empiric short-term anti-infective treatment (single dose or up to 3 days) may be used if diarrhea is moderate or severe, associated with high fever or bloody stools, or extremely disruptive to travel plans. Since bacteria are the most common cause of travelers' diarrhea (80–90% of cases), an anti-infective directed against enteric bacterial pathogens usually is used. Fluoroquinolones (e.g., ciprofloxacin, levofloxacin) generally have been considered the anti-infectives of choice for empiric treatment, including self-treatment, of travelers' diarrhea in adults; alternatives include azithromycin and rifaximin.

If the causative pathogen is susceptible to the anti-infective chosen for empiric treatment, the duration of illness may be reduced by about a day. However, the increasing incidence of enteric bacteria resistant to fluoroquinolones and other anti-infectives may limit the usefulness of empiric treatment in individuals traveling in certain geographic areas, and the possible adverse effects of the anti-infective and adverse consequences of such treatment (e.g., development of resistance, effect on normal gut microflora) should be considered.

Prophylaxis

CDC and most experts do *not* recommend anti-infective prophylaxis to prevent travelers' diarrhea in most individuals traveling to areas of risk. However, anti-infective prophylaxis may be considered for short-term travelers who are high-risk individuals (e.g., HIV-infected or other immunocompromised individuals, travelers with poorly controlled diabetes mellitus or chronic renal failure) and those who are taking critical trips during which even a short period of diarrhea could adversely affect the purpose of the trip.

The risks of use of anti-infective prophylaxis in travelers should be weighed against the use of prompt, early self-treatment with an empiric anti-infective if moderate to severe travelers' diarrhea occurs. If anti-infective prophylaxis is used, fluoroquinolones (e.g., ciprofloxacin, levofloxacin) usually have been recommended; alternatives include azithromycin and rifaximin. The increasing incidence of fluoroquinolone resistance in pathogens that cause travelers' diarrhea (e.g., Campylobacter, Salmonella, Shigella) should be considered and may limit their potential usefulness.

● **Intra-abdominal Infections**

Ciprofloxacin (IV, conventional tablets, oral suspension) is used in conjunction with metronidazole for the treatment of complicated intra-abdominal infections caused by E. coli, Ps. aeruginosa, P. mirabilis, K. pneumoniae, or Bacteroides fragilis.

For additional information on management of intra-abdominal infections, the current clinical practice guidelines from IDSA available at http://www.idsociety.org should be consulted.

● **Meningitis and Other CNS Infections**

IV ciprofloxacin has been used for the treatment of meningitis† caused by gram-negative bacteria.

Ciprofloxacin has been effective when used alone or in conjunction with other drugs (e.g., antipseudomonal aminoglycosides) to treat meningitis and other CNS infections† caused by susceptible Ps. aeruginosa. Some clinicians suggest that a regimen of ciprofloxacin (with or without an aminoglycoside) can be used as an alternative for the treatment of Ps. aeruginosa meningitis when cefepime or ceftazidime cannot be used.

Ciprofloxacin has been recommended as a preferred alternative for the treatment of healthcare-associated ventriculitis and meningitis† caused by Enterobacteriaceae or Ps. aeruginosa when the drugs of choice cannot be used.

Ciprofloxacin also has been used for the treatment of meningitis and other CNS infections† caused by susceptible Salmonella. Some clinicians suggest that ciprofloxacin alone or in conjunction with a third generation cephalosporin (cefotaxime, ceftriaxone) may be a drug of choice for the treatment of Salmonella meningitis in pediatric patients†, especially when the causative organism is resistant to other drugs.

Because only low concentrations of ciprofloxacin are distributed into CSF and because efficacy and safety of the drug for the treatment of CNS infections have not been established, fluoroquinolones (including ciprofloxacin) should be considered for the treatment of meningitis *only* when the infection is caused by multidrug-resistant gram-negative bacilli or when the usually recommended anti-infectives cannot be used or have been ineffective.

For additional information on management of meningitis and other CNS infections, the current clinical practice guidelines from IDSA available at http://www.idsociety.org should be consulted.

● **Ophthalmic and Otic Infections**

Oral or IV ciprofloxacin is used in the treatment of malignant otitis externa† caused by Ps. aeruginosa. Bacterial otitis externa usually is caused by Ps. aeruginosa or S. aureus. Although acute bacterial otitis externa localized in the external auditory canal may be effectively treated using topical anti-infectives (e.g., ciprofloxacin otic suspension, ofloxacin otic solution), malignant otitis externa is an invasive, potentially life-threatening infection, especially in immunocompromised patients such as those with diabetes mellitus or HIV infection, and requires prompt diagnosis and long-term treatment with systemic anti-infectives. The treatment of choice for malignant otitis externa usually is ciprofloxacin or an antipseudomonal β-lactam (e.g., ceftazidime, imipenem). Because ciprofloxacin-resistant Ps. aeruginosa have been reported with increasing frequency in patients with malignant otitis externa and has been associated with treatment failure, clinical isolates should be tested for in vitro susceptibility, especially if there is an inadequate response to treatment.

● **Respiratory Tract Infections**

Ciprofloxacin (IV, conventional tablets, oral suspension) is used in adults for the treatment of respiratory tract infections, including acute sinusitis, acute

exacerbations of chronic bronchitis), bronchiectasis, lung abscess, and pneumonia, caused by susceptible E. aerogenes†, E. cloacae, E. coli, Haemophilus influenzae, H. parainfluenzae, K. oxytoca†, K. pneumoniae, P. mirabilis, Ps. aeruginosa, S. aureus†, or S. pneumoniae (penicillin-susceptible strains). The drug also is used for the treatment of respiratory tract infections caused by susceptible Moraxella catarrhalis.

IV ciprofloxacin is used for the treatment of nosocomial pneumonia caused by susceptible H. influenzae or K. pneumoniae and for the treatment of acute bacterial sinusitis caused by H. influenzae, S. pneumoniae (penicillin-susceptible strains), or M. catarrhalis.

Ciprofloxacin should be used for the treatment of acute bacterial sinusitis or acute bacterial exacerbations of chronic bronchitis only when there are no other treatment options. Because systemic fluoroquinolones, including ciprofloxacin, have been associated with disabling and potentially irreversible serious adverse reactions (e.g., tendinitis and tendon rupture, peripheral neuropathy, CNS effects) that can occur together in the same patient and because acute bacterial sinusitis and acute bacterial exacerbations of chronic bronchitis may be self-limiting in some patients, the risks of serious adverse reactions outweigh the benefits of fluoroquinolones for patients with these infections.

In controlled studies in adults with respiratory tract infections, oral ciprofloxacin therapy was as effective as therapy with oral amoxicillin, oral ampicillin, IV cefamandole, oral doxycycline, or IV imipenem and cilastatin sodium. Oral ciprofloxacin therapy generally resulted in a bacteriologic cure rate of 80–98% in adults with respiratory tract infections. Oral ciprofloxacin has been most effective in the treatment of respiratory tract infections caused by H. influenzae or M. catarrhalis; treatment failures have occurred when the drug was used in the treatment of infections caused by S. pneumoniae or Ps. aeruginosa. Treatment failure of S. pneumoniae respiratory tract infections may be related to the moderate in vitro susceptibility of this organism to ciprofloxacin. Although ciprofloxacin may be effective, it is not a drug of first choice for the treatment of presumed or confirmed pneumonia secondary to S. pneumoniae, and some clinicians suggest that ciprofloxacin generally *not* be used for empiric treatment of community-acquired pneumonia when S. pneumoniae is likely or suspected as the causative organism. A β-lactam antibiotic generally is preferred for empiric treatment of these infections and also is preferred in other respiratory tract infections known or suspected to be caused by pneumococci or streptococci. Ciprofloxacin probably should not be used in the treatment of aspiration pneumonia because these infections generally involve anaerobic bacteria.

Acute Exacerbations of Chronic Bronchitis

Clinical improvement has occurred when oral ciprofloxacin was used alone for the treatment of acute exacerbations of bronchopulmonary Ps. aeruginosa infections in adults with cystic fibrosis. As with other anti-infectives, Ps. aeruginosa may be cleared temporarily from the sputum, but a bacteriologic cure rarely is obtained and should not be expected in these patients.

Resistant strains of Ps. aeruginosa have developed during ciprofloxacin therapy; in one study, up to 45% of cystic fibrosis patients developed resistance after 2 weeks of therapy with the drug. Clinical improvement occurred in some patients despite the emergence of resistant Ps. aeruginosa; in some cases, the resistant organisms reverted to being susceptible after ciprofloxacin therapy was discontinued. Further study is necessary to determine if emergence of resistance will limit use of ciprofloxacin in the treatment of Ps. aeruginosa infections in cystic fibrosis patients. Some clinicians caution against long-term use of ciprofloxacin in these patients and recommend that the drug be used in short courses (e.g., 14 days), alternated with other anti-infectives active against Ps. aeruginosa (e.g., aztreonam, extended-spectrum penicillins, third generation cephalosporins) and/or used in conjunction with one of these agents. If ciprofloxacin is used, it is important that susceptibility of isolates be tested carefully in subsequent exacerbations.

Nosocomial Pneumonia

IV ciprofloxacin is used for the treatment of nosocomial pneumonia, including hospital-acquired pneumonia (HAP) not associated with mechanical ventilation and ventilator-associated pneumonia (VAP).

Local susceptibility data should be used when selecting initial empiric regimens for the treatment of nosocomial pneumonia, including HAP and VAP.

For initial empiric treatment of HAP in adults, IDSA states that ciprofloxacin should be used in conjunction with an anti-infective active against MRSA (vancomycin, linezolid) if factors that increase the likelihood of MRSA are present or if the patient is at high risk of mortality or has received IV anti-infectives during the prior 90 days.

For initial empiric treatment in adults with clinically suspected VAP and factors that increase the risk of MRSA or multidrug-resistant gram-negative bacteria, IDSA states that ciprofloxacin should be used in conjunction with an anti-infective active against MRSA (vancomycin, linezolid) plus an antipseudomonal β-lactam (fixed combination of piperacillin and tazobactam [piperacillin/tazobactam], cefepime, ceftazidime, imipenem, meropenem, aztreonam).

For additional information on management of nosocomial pneumonia, the current clinical practice guidelines from IDSA available at http://www.idsociety.org should be consulted.

● **Skin and Skin Structure Infections**

Ciprofloxacin (IV, conventional tablets, oral suspension) is used in adults for the treatment of skin and skin structure infections caused by susceptible *C. freundii, E. cloacae, E. coli, K. oxytoca†, K. pneumoniae, M. morganii, P. mirabilis, P. vulgaris, P. stuartii, Ps. aeruginosa, Serratia marcescens†, S. aureus* (methicillin-susceptible strains), *S. epidermidis* (methicillin-susceptible strains), or *S. pyogenes* (group A β-hemolytic streptococci). The drug has been effective in the treatment of cellulitis, abscesses, folliculitis, furunculosis, pyoderma, postoperative wound infections, and infected ulcers, burns, or wounds.

Ciprofloxacin may be particularly useful as an oral agent for the treatment of skin and skin structure infections caused by susceptible gram-negative bacteria. Because staphylococci, streptococci, and anaerobes are only moderately susceptible to ciprofloxacin, ciprofloxacin generally should not be used alone and other anti-infectives remain the drugs of choice for skin and skin structure infections caused by these bacteria. Treatment failures have been reported in patients with skin or skin structure infections caused by *S. aureus* and the increasing emergence of strains of staphylococci resistant to quinolones limits the usefulness of the drugs in the treatment of these infections. Some clinicians suggest that ciprofloxacin therapy may be particularly useful for the treatment of hospital-acquired decubitus ulcers when anti-infective therapy is indicated.

In several controlled studies, oral ciprofloxacin was at least as effective as IV cefotaxime in the treatment of skin and skin structure infections caused by susceptible organisms. Oral ciprofloxacin resulted in a bacteriologic cure rate of 80–92% in patients with skin and skin structure infections.

Although ciprofloxacin is active in vitro against most common aerobic pathogens isolated from animal and human bite wounds, including *Flavobacterium†* and *Eikenella corrodens†*, the in vitro activity of the drug against streptococci, which frequently are isolated from such wounds (usually in mixed cultures), and against anaerobes generally is poor. Therefore, use of the drug as monotherapy in these infections is not recommended pending accumulation of additional efficacy data.

For additional information on management of skin and skin structure infections, the current clinical practice guidelines from IDSA available at http://www.idsociety.org should be consulted.

● **Urinary Tract Infections and Prostatitis**

Uncomplicated and Complicated Urinary Tract Infections

Ciprofloxacin extended-release tablets containing both the hydrochloride and the base are used *only* for the treatment of uncomplicated UTIs (acute cystitis) caused by susceptible *E. faecalis, E. coli, P. mirabilis,* or *S. saprophyticus,* complicated UTIs caused by susceptible *E. coli, K. pneumoniae, P. mirabilis, Ps. aeruginosa,* or *E. faecalis,* or acute uncomplicated pyelonephritis caused by *E. coli* in adults.

Ciprofloxacin (IV, conventional tablets, oral suspension) is used in adults for the treatment of complicated or uncomplicated UTIs caused by susceptible *Citrobacter koseri* (formerly *C. diversus*), *C. freundii, Enterobacter cloacae, E. aerogenes†, E. coli, Klebsiella oxytoca†, K. pneumoniae, Morganella morganii, Proteus mirabilis, Providencia*

rettgeri, P. stuartii†, Pseudomonas aeruginosa, or *Serratia marcescens.* The drug also is used in adults for the treatment of UTIs caused by susceptible gram-positive bacteria, including *Staphylococcus aureus†, S. epidermidis* (methicillin-susceptible strains), *S. saprophyticus,* or *E. faecalis.*

Ciprofloxacin (IV, conventional tablets, oral suspension) is used in pediatric patients 1 year of age or older for the treatment of complicated UTIs and pyelonephritis caused by susceptible *E. coli.* Although effective in UTIs, ciprofloxacin

is not a drug of first choice for these infections in pediatric patients because of the risk of adverse effects (e.g., musculoskeletal effects) reported in this patient population.

Ciprofloxacin should be used for the treatment of uncomplicated UTIs only when there are no other treatment options. Because systemic fluoroquinolones, including ciprofloxacin, have been associated with disabling and potentially irreversible serious adverse reactions (e.g., tendinitis and tendon rupture, peripheral neuropathy, CNS effects) that can occur together in the same patient and because uncomplicated UTIs may be self-limiting in some patients, the risk of serious adverse reactions outweigh the benefits of fluoroquinolones for patients with uncomplicated UTIs.

Some clinicians suggest that ciprofloxacin be reserved for the treatment of complicated UTIs, especially those caused by multidrug-resistant bacteria. IDSA and other experts state that fluoroquinolones (ciprofloxacin, levofloxacin, ofloxacin) generally should be considered alternatives for the treatment of uncomplicated UTIs (e.g., acute cystitis) and should be used in these infections only when other urinary anti-infectives are likely to be ineffective or are contraindicated or not tolerated.

Clinical Experience

In controlled studies in men and women, oral ciprofloxacin therapy was as effective as therapy with oral co-trimoxazole in the treatment of uncomplicated UTIs; bacteriologic cure rates and rate of relapse and/or reinfection were similar with both drugs. Oral ciprofloxacin therapy generally results in a bacteriologic cure in 80–100% of patients with UTIs. Oral ciprofloxacin is more effective in the treatment of uncomplicated UTIs than in complicated infections, and most treatment failures occur in patients with underlying structural abnormalities of the urinary tract (e.g., obstructions, neurogenic bladder) or indwelling catheters.

Oral ciprofloxacin has been as effective as oral co-trimoxazole in the treatment of complicated UTIs, and has been effective in the treatment of UTIs caused by organisms resistant to co-trimoxazole. Prolonged, high-dose oral ciprofloxacin therapy (500–750 mg every 12 hours) has been effective in the treatment of complicated UTIs caused by multidrug-resistant *Ps. aeruginosa.*

A 3-day regimen of oral ciprofloxacin (conventional tablets) generally is effective for the treatment of acute, uncomplicated cystitis caused by susceptible *E. coli, E. faecalis, P. mirabilis,* or *S. saprophyticus* (bacteriologic eradication rate 81–100%). Oral ciprofloxacin (conventional tablets) has been effective in women for the treatment of uncomplicated UTIs when given as a single 100- or 250-mg dose†. However, efficacy of a single dose of the drug for the treatment of these infections has not been clearly established; single-dose therapy was less effective in the treatment of UTIs caused by gram-positive bacteria than in those caused by gram-negative bacteria.

Safety and efficacy of ciprofloxacin extended-release tablets for the treatment of uncomplicated UTIs (acute cystitis) have been evaluated in a randomized, double-blind, controlled study in adults. In this study, adults were randomized to receive ciprofloxacin extended-release tablets (500 mg once daily for 3 days) or conventional ciprofloxacin tablets (250 mg twice daily for 3 days). The bacteriologic eradication rate with no new infections or superinfections at the time of test of cure (post-therapy day 4–11) was 94.5% in those who received the extended-release tablets and 93.7% in those who received conventional tablets. Safety and efficacy of ciprofloxacin extended-release tablets for the treatment of complicated UTIs or acute uncomplicated pyelonephritis also have been evaluated in a randomized, double-blind study. In this study, adults were randomized to receive ciprofloxacin extended-release tablets (1 g once daily for 7–14 days) or conventional ciprofloxacin tablets (500 mg twice daily for 7–14 days). In the per-protocol population, the bacteriologic eradication rate with no new infections or superinfections at the time of test of cure (post-therapy day 5–11) in those who received the extended-release tablets was 89.2 or 87.5% in those with complicated UTIs or uncomplicated pyelonephritis, respectively; in those who received the conventional tablets, the rates were 81.4 or 98.1%, respectively.

In clinical studies evaluating IV or oral ciprofloxacin for the treatment of complicated UTIs and pyelonephritis in pediatric patients 1–17 years of age, the bacteriologic eradication rate was about 84% in those receiving ciprofloxacin compared with about 78% in those receiving a cephalosporin.

Prostatitis

Ciprofloxacin (IV, conventional tablets, oral suspension) is used in men for the treatment of recurrent UTIs and chronic prostatitis caused by *E. coli* or *P.*

mirabilis. Ciprofloxacin has been most effective in the treatment of prostatitis caused by *E. coli* or other Enterobacteriaceae, and has been effective in infections that did not respond to co-trimoxazole therapy. Prostatitis caused by *Ps. aeruginosa*, enterococci, or staphylococci may respond poorly to the drug. Because high concentrations of ciprofloxacin are attained in prostatic tissues, the drug may become a drug of choice for the treatment of recurrent UTIs associated with prostatitis; however, further study is needed to compare efficacy of ciprofloxacin with that of other anti-infectives used in the treatment of these infections.

● Anthrax

Ciprofloxacin (conventional tablets, oral suspension) is used for inhalational anthrax (postexposure) to reduce the incidence or progression of disease following suspected or confirmed exposure to aerosolized *Bacillus anthracis* spores in adults and pediatric patients. Ciprofloxacin (IV, conventional tablets, oral suspension) is used for the treatment of clinically apparent inhalational anthrax†, other systemic anthrax infections (GI, meningitis, or cutaneous with systemic involvement, head or neck lesions, or extensive edema), or uncomplicated cutaneous anthrax†, and for prophylaxis following ingestion of *B. anthracis* spores in contaminated meat†.

Naturally occurring or endemic cutaneous anthrax in humans can occur after exposure to *B. anthracis* spores following contact with contaminated soil or infected animals (e.g., goats, sheep, cattle, swine, horses, buffalo, deer) or animal by-products (e.g., hides, hair, wool, carcasses, bone meal); GI or oropharyngeal anthrax can occur after ingestion of anthrax spores (e.g., in contaminated, raw or undercooked meat); and inhalational anthrax can occur after exposure to *B. anthracis* spores aerosolized during industrial processing of contaminated animal by-products or in the laboratory. Inhalational or cutaneous anthrax also may occur as the result of exposure to aerosolized *B. anthracis* spores in the context of biologic warfare or bioterrorism, including exposure to mail or other fomites contaminated with anthrax spores.

Following exposure to aerosolized *B. anthracis* spores, inhalational anthrax may develop if spore-containing particles are deposited into alveolar spaces. Macrophages ingest the spores and some undergo lysis and destruction. Surviving spores are transported via the lymph system to mediastinal lymph nodes where germination and vegetative growth may occur after a period of spore dormancy. Monkey studies have demonstrated that viable spores can persist in a dormant state in alveolar surface epithelium and mediastinal lymph nodes for up to 100 days after inhalation. The process responsible for the delayed transformation of spores to vegetative cells remains to be elucidated. Once germination occurs, disease follows rapidly. Replicating *B. anthracis* release toxins that can result in hemorrhage, edema, and necrosis. Cutaneous anthrax may occur if *B. anthracis* spores are introduced into a cut or abrasion (e.g., on the face, neck, or arms). Septicemia and meningeal anthrax result from hematogenous spread of the organism from the primary cutaneous, GI, or inhalation site. Although discharge from cutaneous lesions might be infectious, the risk for person-to-person transmission of cutaneous anthrax is low. Person-to-person transmission and secondary cases of anthrax (e.g., in medical personnel) have not been documented to date.

For the treatment of clinically apparent inhalational, GI, or meningeal anthrax and anthrax septicemia that occurs as the result of natural or endemic exposures to *B. anthracis*, parenteral penicillin historically has been considered the drug of choice and IV ciprofloxacin or IV doxycycline have been suggested as alternatives. However, it has been postulated that exposures to *B. anthracis* that occur in the context of biologic warfare or bioterrorism may involve bioengineered resistant strains and this concern should be considered when selecting initial anti-infective regimens for the treatment of anthrax that occurs as the result of bioterrorism-related exposures or when selecting anti-infectives for postexposure prophylaxis following such exposures. *B. anthracis* with natural resistance to penicillins have been reported and there are published reports of *B. anthracis* strains that have been engineered to have tetracycline and penicillin resistance as well as resistance to other anti-infectives (e.g., macrolides, chloramphenicol, rifampin). In addition, reduced susceptibility to ofloxacin (4-fold increase in MICs from baseline) has been produced in vitro following sequential subculture of the Sterne strain of *B. anthracis* in subinhibitory concentrations of the fluoroquinolone.

Recommendations for the treatment and prophylaxis of anthrax have evolved based on experience gained in treating US patients who developed inhalational or cutaneous anthrax during September and October 2001 following bioterrorism-related exposures to *B. anthracis* spores as well results of animal studies and concerns related to treating large numbers of individuals in a mass casualty setting.

For additional information on management of anthrax, including postexposure prophylaxis of anthrax, the current guidelines from CDC and AAP should be consulted.

Postexposure Prophylaxis of Anthrax

Ciprofloxacin is used for inhalational anthrax (postexposure) to reduce the incidence or progression of disease following suspected or confirmed exposure to aerosolized *B. anthracis* spores in adults and pediatric patients. CDC, AAP, US Working Group on Civilian Biodefense, and US Army Medical Research Institute of Infectious Diseases (USAMRIID) recommend oral ciprofloxacin and oral doxycycline as the initial drugs of choice for postexposure prophylaxis following exposure to aerosolized anthrax spores, including exposures that occur in the context of biologic warfare or bioterrorism. Other oral fluoroquinolones (levofloxacin, moxifloxacin, ofloxacin) are alternatives for postexposure prophylaxis when ciprofloxacin or doxycycline cannot be used.

Following natural, occupational, or bioterrorism-related exposures to aerosolized *B. anthracis* spores, anti-infective postexposure prophylaxis should be initiated immediately or as soon as possible. Postexposure vaccination with anthrax vaccine (if available) may be indicated in conjunction with anti-infective postexposure prophylaxis in some individuals. Vaccine-induced immunity provides protection if there are issues related to the anti-infective postexposure prophylaxis regimen (e.g., poor adherence, early discontinuance because of adverse effects) or if there are residual spores that germinate after the anti-infective regimen has been completed.

Because of the possible persistence of anthrax spores in lung tissue following an aerosol exposure, prolonged postexposure prophylaxis usually is required. Based on a competing-risks model, some clinicians suggest that the optimum duration of prophylaxis depends on the dose of inhaled spores. These clinicians state that a duration of 60 days may be adequate for a low-dose exposure, but that a duration exceeding 4 months may be necessary to reduce the risk following a high-dose exposure. CDC, AAP, US Working Group on Civilian Biodefense, and USAMRIID recommend that postexposure prophylaxis following a confirmed exposure (including in laboratory workers with confirmed exposures to *B. anthracis* cultures) should be continued for 60 days.

Postexposure anti-infective prophylaxis may be indicated in laboratory workers and other individuals who work in occupations that result in exposure to *B. anthracis* and may also be considered following a naturally occurring GI exposure to *B. anthracis* (e.g., ingestion of meat from an undercooked carcass of an anthrax-infected animal).

Pediatric Patients

Ciprofloxacin (IV, conventional tablets, oral suspension) is labeled by FDA for inhalational anthrax (postexposure) in neonates, infants, and children 17 years of age or younger. Although ciprofloxacin generally is not recommended for use in infants and children, the benefits of ciprofloxacin in reducing the incidence or progression of disease following exposure to aerosolized *B. anthracis* spores outweigh the risks in pediatric patients.

For initial anti-infective prophylaxis following a suspected exposure to *B. anthracis* spores that occurs in the context of biologic warfare or bioterrorism, AAP states that oral ciprofloxacin is the drug of choice in neonates 4 weeks of age or younger and oral ciprofloxacin or oral doxycycline are the drugs of choice in pediatric patients 1 month of age or older (prior to susceptibility testing and when penicillin-resistant strains have been identified). If exposure has been confirmed and in vitro tests indicate that the organism is susceptible to penicillin, the postexposure prophylaxis regimen in pediatric patients may be switched to oral amoxicillin or, alternatively, oral penicillin V.

Pregnant and Breast-feeding Women

If anti-infective postexposure prophylaxis following a suspected exposure to aerosolized *B. anthracis* spores in the context of biologic warfare or bioterrorism is indicated in pregnant women, postpartum women, and women who are breast-feeding, CDC states that oral ciprofloxacin is preferred over oral doxycycline, unless oral ciprofloxacin is unavailable. If in vitro studies indicate that the organism is susceptible to penicillin, consideration can be given to changing the postexposure regimen to oral amoxicillin or oral penicillin V.

Individuals at Contaminated Sites

For the bioterrorism-related exposures to *B. anthracis* spores that occurred in the US during the fall of 2001, CDC recommended that anti-infective prophylaxis be initiated (pending additional information) in individuals exposed to an air space where a suspicious material may have been aerosolized (e.g., near a suspicious powder-containing letter during opening) and in individuals who shared the air spaces likely to be the source of an inhalational anthrax case. While culture of nasal swabs can occasionally document exposure and provide clues to help assess the exposure circumstances, these nasal swabs are investigative tools only and results cannot be used to rule out exposure to *B. anthracis*. Following confirmation of the presence of *B. anthracis* spores, CDC recommended that a full 60-day postexposure regimen be completed in individuals exposed to an air space known to be contaminated with aerosolized *B. anthracis*, in individuals exposed to an air space known to be the source of an inhalational anthrax case, and in individuals along the transit path of an envelope or other vehicle containing *B. anthracis* that may have been aerosolized (e.g., a postal sorting facility in which an envelope containing *B. anthracis* was processed).

Remediation workers with repeated entries into contaminated sites over a prolonged period of time may require anti-infective prophylaxis for considerably longer than the 60 days recommended for individuals with a single exposure. Some remediation workers exposed during the bioterrorism-related events that occurred in the US during the fall of 2001 received anti-infective prophylaxis for more than 6 months. At that time, CDC recommended that anti-infective prophylaxis be continued throughout the period of risk and for 60 days after the risk of exposure ended, unless a 6-dose series of anthrax vaccine had been completed and annual boosters were up to date.

Laboratory Workers and Other Individuals

Laboratory workers and other individuals who work in occupations that might result in repeated exposure to aerosolized *B. anthracis* spores should receive preexposure vaccination with anthrax vaccine adsorbed. ACIP states that anti-infective postexposure prophylaxis is not necessary in fully vaccinated workers who wear appropriate personal protective equipment (PPE) while working in environments contaminated with *B. anthracis* spores, unless PPE is disrupted. If there is any type of disruption of PPE in a worker who is fully or partially vaccinated against anthrax, ACIP recommends that anti-infective postexposure prophylaxis be given for at least 30 days in conjunction with any remaining indicated doses of anthrax vaccine. Following an occupational exposure to *B. anthracis* spores in previously unvaccinated workers, ACIP recommends that anti-infective postexposure prophylaxis be given for 60 days in conjunction with postexposure vaccination and states that the anti-infective prophylaxis regimen should be continued for 14 days after the third vaccine dose (even if this results in more than 60 days of anti-infective prophylaxis).

Following a bioterrorism-related event, use of anti-infective prophylaxis in asymptomatic individuals in the general population is *not* indicated unless appropriate public health or law-enforcement agencies have ascertained that a risk of exposure to *B. anthracis* spores exists. In addition, CDC states that postexposure prophylaxis is *not* indicated for the prevention of cutaneous anthrax, for autopsy personnel examining bodies infected with anthrax when appropriate isolation precautions and procedures are followed, for hospital personnel caring for patients with anthrax, or for individuals who routinely open or handle mail in the absence of a suspicious letter or credible threat.

Clinical Experience

Although controlled studies evaluating ciprofloxacin for aerosolized anthrax exposure in humans have not been conducted for ethical reasons, the indication for use of ciprofloxacin is based on serum concentrations of the drug achieved in humans, a surrogate end point reasonably likely to predict clinical benefit. Efficacy of ciprofloxacin has been evaluated in a rhesus monkey model of inhalational anthrax. In this study, rhesus monkeys were exposed to an inhaled mean dose of 11 LD_{50} (approximately 5.5×10^5) spores (range: 5–30 LD_{50}) of *B. anthracis* and then received a 30-day regimen of placebo or oral ciprofloxacin beginning 24 hours after exposure. Mortality due to anthrax was significantly lower in monkeys that received ciprofloxacin (1/9) compared with those that received placebo (9/10); the one ciprofloxacin-treated monkey that died of anthrax did so following the 30-day drug administration period. In the monkeys studied, mean serum concentrations of ciprofloxacin 1 hour after dosing (at the expected time of peak serum concentrations) following oral dosing to steady state ranged from 0.98–1.69 mcg/mL; mean steady-state trough concentrations at 12 hours after dosing ranged from 0.12–0.19 mcg/mL. The mean serum concentrations of ciprofloxacin associated with a statistically significant improvement in survival in this rhesus

monkey model of inhalational anthrax are reached or exceeded in adult and pediatric patients receiving oral or IV ciprofloxacin.

Some data regarding efficacy of ciprofloxacin for postexposure prophylaxis in humans following exposure to aerosolized *B. anthracis* spores is available since the drug was used for postexposure prophylaxis in individuals in the US who were exposed to *B. anthracis* spores in bioterrorism-related incidences that occurred during September and October 2001. Approximately 300 postal or other facilities were tested for *B. anthracis* spores and anti-infective prophylaxis with ciprofloxacin or other anti-infectives was initiated in approximately 32,000 individuals in Florida, New Jersey, New York, and the District of Columbia who had potential exposures. A full 60-day postexposure prophylaxis regimen was recommended for approximately 8424 of these individuals. To date, no individual who received anti-infective prophylaxis following these bioterrorism-related exposures developed microbiologically confirmed anthrax. Although ciprofloxacin postexposure prophylaxis generally was well tolerated, the incidence of adverse effects was higher than that reported previously in controlled clinical trials evaluating the drug for other indications.

Treatment of Systemic Anthrax

The rapid course of symptomatic inhalational anthrax and high mortality rate make early initiation of anti-infective therapy essential. Because of the difficulty in making a rapid microbiologic diagnosis of anthrax, high-risk individuals who develop fever or other evidence of systemic infection should promptly receive therapy for possible anthrax infection while waiting for results of laboratory studies.

Based on clinical experience from the bioterrorism-related anthrax exposures of 2001 and the possibility that a *B. anthracis* strain resistant to one or more anti-infectives might be used in a future bioterrorism event, CDC, AAP, and other experts (e.g., US Working Group on Civilian Biodefense, USAMRIID) state that treatment of clinically apparent systemic anthrax (inhalational, GI, meningitis, or cutaneous with systemic involvement, head or neck lesions, or extensive edema) in adults and pediatric patients that occurs as the result of exposure to anthrax spores in the context of biologic warfare or bioterrorism should be initiated with a multiple-drug parenteral regimen that includes ciprofloxacin or doxycycline and 1 or 2 additional anti-infectives predicted to be effective. Other drugs to be included in the initial treatment regimen with ciprofloxacin or doxycycline should be selected based on in vitro susceptibility, possibility of efficacy, adverse effects, and cost. Based on in vitro data, other drugs that have been suggested as possibilities to augment ciprofloxacin or doxycycline in such multiple-drug regimens include carbapenems (doripenem, imipenem, meropenem), penicillin G, ampicillin, linezolid, clindamycin, rifampin, chloramphenicol, vancomycin, macrolides (azithromycin, clarithromycin, erythromycin), daptomycin, quinupristin and dalfopristin, and aminoglycosides (gentamicin).

For initial empiric treatment of systemic anthrax (with possible or confirmed meningitis), CDC and AAP recommend use of a multiple-drug parenteral regimen that includes at least 3 anti-infectives with activity against *B. anthracis* and good CNS penetration, including at least one drug that has bactericidal activity against the organism and at least one drug classified as a protein synthesis inhibitor. These experts state that IV ciprofloxacin is recommended as the primary bactericidal component of these regimens. The preferred multiple-drug regimen for the treatment of systemic anthrax (with possible or confirmed meningitis) in adults and pediatric patients (including neonates) is IV ciprofloxacin in conjunction with another IV bactericidal anti-infective (preferably meropenem) and an IV protein synthesis inhibitor (preferably linezolid).

For initial empiric treatment of systemic anthrax when meningitis has been excluded, CDC and AAP recommend use of a multiple-drug parenteral regimen that includes at least 2 anti-infectives with activity against *B. anthracis*, including at least one drug with bactericidal activity against the organism and at least one drug classified as a protein synthesis inhibitor. The preferred multiple-drug regimen for the treatment of systemic anthrax in adults and pediatric patients (including neonates) when meningitis has been excluded is IV ciprofloxacin in conjunction with an IV protein synthesis inhibitor (preferably clindamycin or linezolid in adults or clindamycin in pediatric patients).

If the *B. anthracis* strain is tested and found to be susceptible to penicillin, CDC and AAP state that IV penicillin G and IV ampicillin are acceptable alternatives for the second bactericidal agent (i.e., the carbapenem) used in multiple-drug regimens for the treatment of systemic anthrax (with possible or confirmed meningitis) or the bactericidal agent used in multiple-drug regimens for the treatment of systemic anthrax when meningitis has been excluded.

Some experts suggest that oral ciprofloxacin or other oral fluoroquinolones (levofloxacin, moxifloxacin, ofloxacin) can be considered for the treatment of inhalational anthrax† when a parenteral regimen is not available. Although a multiple-drug parenteral regimen should be used for the treatment of inhalational anthrax that occurs as the result of exposure to *B. anthracis* spores in the context of biologic warfare or bioterrorism, use of these parenteral regimens may not be possible if large numbers of individuals require treatment in a mass casualty setting and it may be necessary to use an oral regimen.

Because of the possible persistence of anthrax spores in lung tissue, anti-infective therapy for the treatment of systemic anthrax that occurs as the result of exposure to aerosolized *B. anthracis* spores in the context of biologic warfare or bioterrorism should be continued for 60 days. The initial multiple-drug parenteral regimen should be continued for at least 2–3 weeks until the patient is clinically stable and can be switched to an appropriate oral anti-infective.

Clinical Experience

A multiple-drug parenteral regimen that was used in 2 patients who survived inhalational anthrax following the bioterrorism-related exposures in 2001 was a 3-drug regimen of ciprofloxacin (400 mg every 8 hours), rifampin (300 mg every 12 hours), and clindamycin (900 mg every 8 hours). Other multiple-drug regimens that were used for the initial treatment of patients who survived inhalational anthrax following these bioterrorism-related anthrax exposures were ciprofloxacin/cefotaxime/azithromycin (1 patient); levofloxacin/rifampin initially then ciprofloxacin rifampin/vancomycin (1 patient); and oral levofloxacin (prior to diagnosis), then ciprofloxacin/azithromycin, then clindamycin/ceftriaxone/azithromycin, then doxycycline (1 patient). Although it is unclear whether the deaths were related to ineffective regimens and/or delays in initiation of therapy, the regimens used in patients who died of inhalational anthrax following these exposures were levofloxacin/clindamycin/penicillin G (1 patient, initiated on the second day of hospitalization after various anti-infectives, died 3 days after admission); levofloxacin monotherapy (1 patient, died day of admission); levofloxacin/rifampin/penicillin G/ceftriaxone (1 patient, died day of admission); levofloxacin monotherapy, then levofloxacin/rifampin/gentamicin/nafcillin, then ciprofloxacin/rifampin/clindamycin/ceftazidime (1 patient, died 3 days after admission); ampicillin-sulbactam/ciprofloxacin/clindamycin (1 patient, initiated on the third day of hospitalization after various other regimens, died 4 days after admission) and ampicillin-sulbactam/ciprofloxacin (1 patient, initiated on the day of hospitalization and clindamycin added on the third day, died 4 days after admission).

Results of in vitro susceptibility testing of strains of *B. anthracis* that were associated with cases of inhalational or cutaneous anthrax that occurred in the US (Florida, New York, District of Columbia) during September and October 2001 in the context of bioterrorism-related exposures to anthrax spores indicated that these strains were susceptible to ciprofloxacin, doxycycline, tetracycline, rifampin, clindamycin, vancomycin, and chloramphenicol. Isolates were susceptible to clarithromycin, azithromycin (borderline susceptibility), and imipenem, but had only intermediate susceptibility to erythromycin. Although these *B. anthracis* strains were susceptible to penicillin and amoxicillin in vitro, additional tests indicated that some of these strains had constitutive and inducible β-lactamases and there is in vitro evidence that exposure of some penicillin-susceptible *B. anthracis* strains to penicillins can induce β-lactamases. Therefore, CDC states that use of a penicillin *alone* is not recommended for the treatment of anthrax that occurs as the result of biologic warfare or bioterrorism when high concentrations of the organism are likely to be present, although penicillin can be included in appropriate combination regimens. *B. anthracis* strains resistant to sulfamethoxazole, trimethoprim, cephalosporins (i.e., cefuroxime, cefotaxime, ceftazidime), or aztreonam have been reported, and these anti-infectives should *not* be used in the treatment of anthrax.

Treatment of Uncomplicated Cutaneous Anthrax

Natural penicillins (e.g., oral penicillin V, IM penicillin G benzathine, IM penicillin G procaine) generally have been considered drugs of choice for the treatment of mild, uncomplicated cutaneous anthrax caused by susceptible *B. anthracis* that occurs as the result of naturally occurring or endemic exposure to anthrax, although some clinicians suggest use of oral fluoroquinolones (ciprofloxacin, levofloxacin, ofloxacin), oral amoxicillin, or oral doxycycline if in vitro tests indicate susceptibility.

For the treatment of uncomplicated cutaneous anthrax† (without systemic involvement) that occurs following exposure to *B. anthracis* spores in the context of biologic warfare or bioterrorism, CDC recommends that adults receive an oral regimen of ciprofloxacin, doxycycline, levofloxacin, or moxifloxacin; alternatives include oral amoxicillin or penicillin V (if penicillin susceptibility is confirmed) or oral clindamycin.

For the treatment of uncomplicated cutaneous anthrax† (without systemic involvement) that occurs following exposure to *B. anthracis* spores in the context of biologic warfare or bioterrorism, AAP recommends that pediatric patients (including neonates) receive an oral regimen of ciprofloxacin; alternatives include oral amoxicillin or penicillin V (if penicillin susceptibility is confirmed) or oral doxycycline, clindamycin, or levofloxacin.

CDC, AAP, and other experts recommend that anti-infective treatment be continued for 60 days if the cutaneous infection occurred as the result of exposure to aerosolized anthrax spores since the possibility of inhalational anthrax would also exist. For the treatment of mild, uncomplicated cutaneous anthrax that occurs as the result of natural or endemic exposures to anthrax (e.g., known exposure to infected livestock or their products), a treatment duration of 3–10 days may be sufficient. Anti-infective therapy may limit the size of the cutaneous anthrax lesion and it usually becomes sterile within the first 24 hours of treatment, but the lesion will still progress through the black eschar stage despite effective treatment.

Treatment of GI and Oropharyngeal Anthrax Following Natural or Endemic Exposures

Although penicillin usually is considered the drug of choice for the treatment of GI anthrax† that occurs as the result of ingesting contaminated, undercooked meat, ciprofloxacin is considered an alternative for the treatment of these infections. Ciprofloxacin has been used for prophylaxis following ingestion of *B. anthracis* spores† in contaminated meat.

● Brucellosis

Ciprofloxacin has been used in the treatment of brucellosis† caused by *Brucella melitensis*, and some clinicians suggest that a regimen of ciprofloxacin and rifampin can be used as an alternative regimen for the treatment of the disease. Most experts recommend a regimen of doxycycline and streptomycin (or gentamicin) or a regimen of doxycycline and rifampin; alternative regimens include co-trimoxazole with or without gentamicin or rifampin; ciprofloxacin (or ofloxacin) and rifampin; or chloramphenicol with or without streptomycin. Monotherapy with any drug usually is associated with a high relapse rate and is not recommended.

In a study in adults with brucellosis, a 30-day regimen of oral ciprofloxacin (500 mg twice daily) and rifampin (600 mg once daily) was as effective as a regimen of oral doxycycline (100 mg twice daily) and rifampin (600 mg once daily). Oral ciprofloxacin has been used in patients with acute brucellosis or acute brucella arthritis-diskitis†. Although oral ciprofloxacin therapy resulted in an initial apparent response in most patients and defervescence within 7 days, at least one patient was considered a treatment failure because blood cultures remained positive and about 25% of patients (generally those with arthritis-diskitis) had relapse or reinfection within 8–32 weeks after the drug was discontinued.

● Chancroid

Ciprofloxacin (conventional tablets, oral suspension) has been effective in men for the treatment of chancroid†, genital ulcers caused by *Haemophilus ducreyi*. Although a single 500-mg oral dose of the drug was effective in some men for the treatment of chancroid, multiple-dose regimens generally have been associated with fewer treatment failures.

CDC states that a single IM dose of ceftriaxone, a single oral dose of azithromycin, a 3-day regimen of oral ciprofloxacin (not recommended in pregnant or lactating women), or a 7-day regimen of oral erythromycin are the regimens of choice for the treatment of chancroid.

HIV-infected patients and patients who are uncircumcised may not respond to treatment as well as those who are HIV-negative or circumcised. Clinicians should consider that, although treatment failures can occur with any of these recommended regimens, only limited data are available regarding efficacy of the single-dose ceftriaxone and single-dose azithromycin regimens in HIV-infected patients. Because treatment failures and slow healing of ulcers are more likely in

HIV-infected individuals, such patients should be monitored closely and more prolonged treatment or retreatment may be necessary.

Data are limited regarding the prevalence of *H. ducreyi* resistant to the anti-infectives recommended for treatment. Isolates of *H. ducreyi* with intermediate resistance to ciprofloxacin have been reported rarely.

For additional information on management of chancroid, current CDC sexually transmitted diseases treatment guidelines available at http://www.cdc.gov/std should be consulted.

Chlamydial and Mycoplasmal Infections

Multiple-dose oral ciprofloxacin therapy has been used for the treatment of non-gonococcal urethritis†, but results have been conflicting. Although 7–10 days of oral ciprofloxacin appeared to be effective for the treatment of nongonococcal urethritis in some men, efficacy of the drug was unpredictable when *Chlamydia* was present, and the rate of relapse was high. If a fluoroquinolone is used as an alternative for the treatment of nongonococcal urethritis when the regimens of choice (azithromycin, doxycycline) are not used, CDC recommends a 7-day regimen of oral ofloxacin or oral levofloxacin.

Oral ciprofloxacin was used with some success in a limited number of women for the treatment of urethral and cervical infections caused by *C. trachomatis* or *Mycoplasma hominis*†. The drug generally has been ineffective in both men and women for the treatment of urogenital infections caused by *Ureaplasma urealyticum*†. If a fluoroquinolone is used as an alternative for the treatment of *C. trachomatis* urogenital infections, CDC recommends a 7-day regimen of oral levofloxacin or oral ofloxacin.

Crohn's Disease

Oral ciprofloxacin (administered with or without metronidazole) has been used for induction of remission of mildly to moderately active Crohn's disease†; the drug also has been used for refractory perianal Crohn's disease. Because intestinal flora appear to have an association with intestinal inflammation, and because ciprofloxacin appears to have immunosuppressive effects, the drug may be useful in the management of Crohn's disease as an adjunct to conventional therapies. However, there currently is no established standard therapy with ciprofloxacin for the management of active Crohn's disease, and further larger studies are needed to confirm study results to date and to establish management criteria and safety considerations for the disease.

Results of several open-label, comparative, retrospective, and at least 1 placebo-controlled study indicate that ciprofloxacin (with or without metronidazole) can result in clinical response (e.g., improvement of clinical condition, clinical remission) in patients with mildly to moderately active Crohn's disease. It appears that the combination of ciprofloxacin and metronidazole is more effective than ciprofloxacin alone. Safety and efficacy of ciprofloxacin in the management of active Crohn's disease were evaluated in a small 6-month preliminary, placebo-controlled, randomized study that included 47 adults with moderately active Crohn's disease who had an inadequate response to conventional therapies (e.g., prednisone, mesalamine, mercaptopurine). To be included in the study, patients had to have had symptomatic disease and a Crohn's Disease Activity Index [CDAI]) greater than 150 at the time of study entry. The CDAI score is based on subjective observations by the patient (e.g., the daily number of liquid or very soft stools, severity of abdominal pain, general well-being) and objective evidence (e.g., number of extraintestinal manifestations, presence of an abdominal mass, use or nonuse of antidiarrheal drugs, the hematocrit, body weight). Patients were randomized to receive ciprofloxacin 500 mg twice daily or placebo while they continued to receive conventional therapy for the disease. Clinical response was described as achievement of a CDAI score of less than 150. Only 37 patients completed the study; 25 of those were receiving ciprofloxacin and 12 were receiving placebo. Mean CDAI score at the end of 6 months was 112 or 205 in those receiving ciprofloxacin or placebo, respectively.

Results of a small, randomized, comparator-drug (ciprofloxacin versus mesalamine) controlled study (patients having a median CDAI score of 217 [range:160–305]) indicate that clinical improvement in patients receiving ciprofloxacin in a dosage of 1 g daily was similar to that in those receiving mesalamine controlled-release capsules in a dosage of 4 g daily. At 6 weeks of therapy, complete remission (defined as a CDAI score of 150 or less, associated with a reduction from baseline CDAI of more than 75 points) was reported in 56 or 55% of patients receiving ciprofloxacin or mesalamine, respectively, while partial remission (defined as a CDAI score of 150 or less, associated with a reduction from baseline CDAI of greater than 50 but less than 70 points) was reported in 17 (3 out of 18 patients) or 4.5% (1 out of 22) patients receiving ciprofloxacin or mesalamine, respectively.

In addition, safety and efficacy of concomitant use of ciprofloxacin and metronidazole have been evaluated in a 12-week comparative (versus methylprednisolone) study in 41 patients with active Crohn's disease (CDAI of more than 200 at the time of study entry). Patients were randomized to receive ciprofloxacin 500 mg twice daily in conjunction with metronidazole 250 mg 4 times daily (22 patients) or methylprednisolone (0.7–1 mg/kg daily initially, followed by variable tapering to 40 mg, and subsequent tapering of 4 mg weekly; 19 patients). At 12 weeks of therapy, clinical remission (defined as a CDAI of 150 points or less) was reported in 63 or 46% of patients receiving the corticosteroid or the combination therapy, respectively. It has been suggested that combination therapy with ciprofloxacin and metronidazole could be an alternative to corticosteroids, although a high incidence of adverse effects (27% discontinued therapy because of such effects) was associated with the anti-infectives.

Limited data indicate that ciprofloxacin may be more effective in patients with ileitis than in those with colitis. It has been suggested that reduced efficacy of ciprofloxacin in colitis may be associated with the low activity of the drug against anaerobic bacteria.

Ciprofloxacin has been used in the management of refractory perianal Crohn's disease†. Anecdotal reports suggest that ciprofloxacin may be useful in the long-term treatment of active perianal Crohn's disease; however, the drug generally is used for short-term administration for this condition. Relapse usually occurs when the anti-infective is discontinued. Limited data indicate that short-term (8 weeks) combination therapy with ciprofloxacin and metronidazole given with, or followed by, azathioprine (up to about 20 weeks) in patients with perianal Crohn's disease may result in rapid reduction of fistula drainage (induced by the anti-infectives) and beneficial maintenance (associated with the azathioprine).

Gonorrhea and Associated Infections

Although oral ciprofloxacin (conventional tablets, oral suspension) was used in the past for the treatment of uncomplicated urethral, endocervical, rectal†, or pharyngeal† gonorrhea caused by susceptible *Neisseria gonorrhoeae*, quinolone-resistant *N. gonorrhoeae* (QRNG) is widely disseminated throughout the world, including in the US. Therefore, CDC states that fluoroquinolones are no longer recommended for the treatment of gonorrhea and should not be used routinely for any associated infections that may involve *N. gonorrhoeae* (e.g., pelvic inflammatory disease [PID], epididymitis).

From 1993–2000, CDC recommended fluoroquinolones as drugs of choice for the treatment of uncomplicated gonorrhea in the US; however, because of reports of QRNG, subsequent CDC recommendations regarding use of the drugs for the treatment of gonorrhea became more restrictive. Beginning in 2000, CDC no longer recommended use of fluoroquinolones for the treatment of gonorrhea in individuals who acquired their infections in Asia or the Pacific Islands (including Hawaii) because of the high incidence QRNG in these areas. In 2002, this restriction was broadened to include individuals who acquired gonorrhea in California. In 2004, CDC recommended that fluoroquinolones not be used to treat gonorrhea in men who have sex with men because of the increased prevalence of QRNG in this population. Beginning in April 2007, CDC stated that fluoroquinolones should *not* be used for the treatment of gonorrhea or any associated infections that may involve *N. gonorrhoeae* (e.g., PID, epididymitis).

Granuloma Inguinale (Donovanosis)

Oral ciprofloxacin is considered an alternative for the treatment of granuloma inguinale (donovanosis)† caused by *Klebsiella granulomatis* (formerly *Calymmatobacterium granulomatis*).

CDC recommends that granuloma inguinale be treated with a regimen of oral azithromycin or, alternatively, a regimen of oral doxycycline, oral ciprofloxacin, oral erythromycin, or oral co-trimoxazole. Anti-infective treatment should be continued until all lesions have healed completely; a minimum duration of 3 weeks usually is necessary. If improvement is not evident within the first few days of treatment, CDC states that consideration can be given to adding a parenteral aminoglycoside (e.g., IV gentamicin) to the regimen. Anti-infective therapy appears to halt progression of lesions, although prolonged duration of therapy often is required to enable granulation and re-epithelization of ulcers. Despite effective anti-infective therapy, granuloma inguinale may relapse 6–18 months later.

Individuals with HIV infection should receive the same treatment regimens recommended for other individuals with granuloma inguinale; however, CDC suggests that addition of a parenteral aminoglycoside to the regimen can be considered if improvement is not evident within the first few days of treatment.

For additional information on management of granuloma inguinale, current CDC sexually transmitted diseases treatment guidelines available at http://www.cdc.gov/std should be consulted.

● Legionnaires' Disease

Ciprofloxacin has been used for the treatment of Legionnaires' Disease† caused by *Legionella pneumophila*, including in immunocompromised patients (e.g., transplant recipients).

● Malaria

Although ciprofloxacin reportedly has some activity in vitro against *Plasmodium falciparum*, oral ciprofloxacin (750 mg every 12 hours) has been ineffective when used alone in the treatment of uncomplicated malaria caused by chloroquine-resistant *P. falciparum*†.

● Mycobacterial Infections

Treatment of Active Tuberculosis

Ciprofloxacin has been used in multiple-drug regimens for the treatment of active tuberculosis† caused by *Mycobacterium tuberculosis*.

Although the potential role of fluoroquinolones and the optimal length of therapy have not been fully defined, the American Thoracic Society (ATS), CDC, IDSA, and others state that use of fluoroquinolones as alternative (second-line) agents can be considered for the treatment of active tuberculosis in patients intolerant of certain first-line agents and in those with relapse, treatment failure, or *M. tuberculosis* resistant to certain first-line agents. If a fluoroquinolone is used in multiple-drug regimens for the treatment of active tuberculosis, ATS, CDC, IDSA, and others recommend levofloxacin or moxifloxacin. Some experts state that ciprofloxacin is no longer recommended for treatment of tuberculosis.

The most recent ATS, CDC, and IDSA recommendations for the treatment of tuberculosis should be consulted for more specific information.

Other Mycobacterial Infections

Ciprofloxacin has been used alone or in conjunction with amikacin for the treatment of cutaneous infections caused by *M. fortuitum*†. Although ciprofloxacin appeared to be effective in a few patients with *M. fortuitum* infections, ciprofloxacin-resistant strains of the organism have developed when the drug was used alone or in conjunction with amikacin in the treatment of these infections. Although optimum regimens have not been identified, ATS and IDSA recommend that *M. fortuitum* pulmonary infections be treated with a regimen consisting of at least 2 anti-infectives selected based on results of in vitro susceptibility testing and tolerability (e.g., amikacin, ciprofloxacin or ofloxacin, a sulfonamide, cefoxitin, imipenem, doxycycline).

Ciprofloxacin has been used in multiple-drug regimens for the treatment of pulmonary and extrapulmonary (localized or disseminated) *M. avium* complex† (MAC) infections. However, ATS and IDSA state that the role of fluoroquinolones in the treatment of MAC infections has not been established. If a fluoroquinolone is included in a treatment regimen (e.g., for macrolide-resistant MAC infections), moxifloxacin may be preferred, although many strains are resistant in vitro.

Based on results of in vitro susceptibility testing, ciprofloxacin may be considered for use in combination antimycobacterial regimens used for the treatment of infections caused by *M. chelonae*†, *M. haemophilum*†, or *M. terrae*†. Optimal treatment regimens for these infections have not been identified. Because of considerations related to resistance, ciprofloxacin is not recommended for treatment of *M. marinum* infections.

The most recent ATS, CDC, and IDSA recommendations for the treatment of other mycobacterial infections should be consulted for more specific information.

● Neisseria meningitidis Infections

Ciprofloxacin (conventional tablets, oral suspension) is used in adults to eliminate nasopharyngeal carriage of *Neisseria meningitidis*† and for chemoprophylaxis to prevent meningococcal disease in household or other close contacts of patients with invasive disease†.

Patients with invasive meningococcal disease who have been treated with penicillin G or any anti-infective other than ceftriaxone or another third generation cephalosporin may still be carriers of *N. meningitidis* and should receive an anti-infective regimen to eradicate nasopharyngeal carriage of the organism prior to hospital discharge. The treatments of choice to eradicate nasopharyngeal carriage of *N. meningitidis* are ceftriaxone (single IM dose), rifampin (2-day regimen), and ciprofloxacin (single oral dose). These regimens are all 90–95% effective and any of these is an acceptable regimen in appropriate patients.

Chemoprophylaxis in close contacts of a patients with invasive meningococcal disease is an important means of preventing secondary cases in household and other close contacts. Recommended regimens for chemoprophylaxis against meningococcal disease include a single dose of IM ceftriaxone, 2-day regimen of oral rifampin (not recommended in pregnant women), or a single dose of oral ciprofloxacin (not recommended in individuals younger than 18 years of age unless no other regimen can be used and not recommended for pregnant or lactating women). These regimens are all 90–95% effective and any of these is an acceptable regimen for chemoprophylaxis. AAP suggests that rifampin may be the drug of choice for chemoprophylaxis in most children.

The attack rate for household contacts who do not receive chemoprophylaxis has been estimated to be 4 cases per 1000 individuals exposed, which is 500–800 times greater than that for the general population. A decision to administer chemoprophylaxis to close contacts of an individual with invasive meningococcal disease is based on the degree of risk. Throat and nasopharyngeal cultures are not useful in determining the need for chemoprophylaxis and may unnecessarily delay administration of the regimen.

When chemoprophylaxis is indicated in high-risk contacts, it must be administered promptly (ideally within 24 hours after identification of the index case) since the attack rate of secondary disease is greatest in the few days following disease onset in the index case. All high-risk contacts should be informed that even if chemoprophylaxis is taken or started, the development of any suspicious clinical manifestation warrants early, rapid medical attention. Chemoprophylaxis probably is of limited or no value if administered more than 14 days after contact with the index case. If high-risk exposure to a new index case occurs more than 2 weeks after initial chemoprophylaxis, additional chemoprophylaxis is indicated.

Fluoroquinolone-resistant *N. meningitidis* has been reported rarely in the US and elsewhere (e.g., India). Ciprofloxacin should not be used for prophylaxis in close contacts of individuals with meningococcal disease in areas where fluoroquinolone-resistant strains have been reported (e.g., selected counties of North Dakota and Minnesota).

● Plague

Ciprofloxacin (IV, conventional tablets, oral suspension) is used for the treatment of plague, including pneumonic and septicemic plague, caused by *Yersinia pestis* and for postexposure prophylaxis of plague in adults and children. Based on results of in vitro and animal testing, fluoroquinolones (ciprofloxacin, levofloxacin, moxifloxacin, ofloxacin) are recommended as alternatives for the treatment of plague and for postexposure prophylaxis following a high-risk exposure to *Y. pestis*, including exposures that occur in the context of biologic warfare or bioterrorism.

Efficacy of ciprofloxacin for treatment or prophylaxis of plague has not be evaluated in clinical trials in humans for ethical and feasibility reasons. The drug is labeled by FDA for this indication based on an efficacy study in animals that demonstrated a survival benefit. In a placebo-controlled study, African green monkeys were exposed to an inhaled dose of *Y. pestis* (mean dose of 110 LD_{50} [range 92–127 LD_{50}]) and then randomized to receive either ciprofloxacin (15 mg/kg IV for 10 days) or placebo initiated when fever started or 76 hours post-challenge, whichever occurred first. In vitro testing indicated that the *Y. pestis* strain used in this study (CO92 strain) had a ciprofloxacin MIC of 0.015 mcg/mL. Pharmacokinetic data indicated that mean peak serum concentrations of ciprofloxacin attained in the monkeys at the end of a single 60-minute IV infusion of the drug were approximately 3.5, 3.9, and 4 mcg/mL on days 2, 6, and 10 of treatment, respectively; trough concentrations on these days were all less than 0.5 mcg/mL. Study results indicated that mortality in the ciprofloxacin treatment group was significantly lower (1 out of 10) compared with the placebo group (2 out of 2). The single ciprofloxacin-treated monkey that died had not received the protocol-directed ciprofloxacin dosage because of a failure of the administration catheter; ciprofloxacin serum concentrations in this monkey were less than 0.5 mcg/mL at all time points tested. Although this monkey became culture negative on day 2 of treatment and terminal blood cultures were negative, the animal had a resurgence of low grade bacteremia on day 6 after initiation of ciprofloxacin.

Treatment of Plague

For the treatment of plague, IM streptomycin (or IM or IV gentamicin) historically has been considered the regimen of choice. Alternatives recommended for the treatment of plague when aminoglycosides are not used include IV doxycycline (or IV tetracycline), IV chloramphenicol (a drug of choice for plague meningitis), an IV fluoroquinolone (ciprofloxacin [a drug of choice for plague meningitis], levofloxacin, moxifloxacin), or co-trimoxazole (may be less effective than other alternatives).

Anti-infective regimens recommended for the treatment of naturally occurring or endemic bubonic, septicemic, or pneumonic plague also are recommended for the treatment of plague that occurs following exposure to *Y. pestis* in the context of biologic warfare or bioterrorism. Such exposures would most likely result in primary pneumonic plague, and prompt initiation of anti-infective therapy (within 18–24 hours of onset of symptoms) is essential in the treatment of pneumonic plague. Some experts (e.g., US Working Group on Civilian Biodefense, USAMRIID) recommend that treatment of plague in the context of biologic warfare or bioterrorism be initiated with a parenteral anti-infective regimen of streptomycin (or gentamicin) or, alternatively, doxycycline, a fluoroquinolone (ciprofloxacin, levofloxacin, moxifloxacin) or chloramphenicol. However, an oral regimen of doxycycline (or tetracycline) or a fluoroquinolone (ciprofloxacin, levofloxacin, moxifloxacin, ofloxacin) may be substituted when the patient's condition improves or when a parenteral regimen is unavailable (e.g., when there are supply or logistic problems because large numbers of individuals require treatment in a mass casualty setting); oral chloramphenicol is considered an alternative in these situations.

Postexposure Prophylaxis of Plague

In the context of biologic warfare or bioterrorism, some experts (e.g., US Working Group on Civilian Biodefense, USAMRIID) recommend that asymptomatic individuals with exposure to plague aerosol or asymptomatic individuals with household, hospital, or other close contact (within about 2 m) with an individual who has pneumonic plague receive an oral anti-infective regimen for postexposure prophylaxis; however, any exposed individual who develops a temperature of 38.5°C or higher or new cough should promptly receive a parenteral anti-infective for treatment of the disease. If postexposure prophylaxis is indicated, these experts recommend a regimen of oral doxycycline (or tetracycline) or an oral fluoroquinolone (ciprofloxacin, levofloxacin, moxifloxacin, ofloxacin).

Although plague vaccine (no longer commercially available in the US) was previously recommended to provide protection against *Y. pestis* infection, the vaccine was effective for preventing or ameliorating bubonic plague but was not effective for prophylaxis against exposure to aerosolized *Y. pestis* and therefore did not provide protection against pneumonic plague.

● Rickettsial Infections

Ciprofloxacin has been used with some success in a limited number of patients for the treatment of various rickettsial infections†, including Mediterranean spotted fever† caused by *Rickettsia conorii*. CDC and other clinicians state that doxycycline is the drug of choice for the treatment of all tickborne rickettsial diseases. Although some fluoroquinolones have in vitro activity against Rickettsiae and some clinicians have suggested that fluoroquinolones (e.g., ciprofloxacin, ofloxacin) may be considered alternatives for the treatment of some rickettsial infections (e.g., Rocky Mountain spotted fever caused by *R. rickettsii*) when doxycycline cannot be used, CDC states that fluoroquinolones are *not* recommended for the treatment of Rocky Mountain spotted fever.

Ciprofloxacin has been used for the long-term treatment of Q fever endocarditis caused by *Coxiella burnetii*†. However, CDC states that doxycycline is the drug of choice when treatment of acute Q fever is indicated and doxycycline in conjunction with hydroxychloroquine is the regimen of choice for the treatment of chronic Q fever, including endocarditis.

● Tularemia

Treatment of Tularemia

Ciprofloxacin (IV, conventional tablets, oral suspension) is recommended as an alternative to aminoglycosides (streptomycin or gentamicin) for the treatment of tularemia† caused by *Francisella tularensis*. Streptomycin generally has been considered the drug of choice for the treatment of tularemia; however, gentamicin is more readily available and is considered an alternative drug of choice when streptomycin is unavailable. Other alternatives for the treatment of tularemia include tetracyclines (doxycycline), chloramphenicol, or ciprofloxacin. Anti-infective regimens recommended for the treatment of naturally occurring or endemic tularemia also are recommended for the treatment of tularemia that occurs following exposure to *F. tularensis* in the context of biologic warfare or bioterrorism. However, the fact that a fully virulent streptomycin-resistant strain of *F. tularensis* was developed in the past for use in biologic warfare should be considered. Exposures to *F. tularensis* in the context of biologic warfare or bioterrorism would most likely result in inhalational tularemia with pleuropneumonitis, although the organism also can infect humans through the skin, mucous membranes, and GI tract.

Postexposure Prophylaxis of Tularemia

Postexposure prophylaxis with anti-infectives usually is not recommended after possible exposure to natural or endemic tularemia (e.g., tick bite, rabbit or other animal exposure) and is unnecessary in close contacts of tularemia patients since human-to-human transmission of the disease is not known to occur. However, postexposure prophylaxis is recommended following a high-risk laboratory exposure to *F. tularensis* (e.g., spill, centrifuge accident, needlestick injury). In the context of biologic warfare or bioterrorism, some experts (e.g., US Working Group on Civilian Biodefense, USAMRIID) recommend that asymptomatic individuals with exposure to *F. tularensis* receive postexposure anti-infective prophylaxis; however, any individual who develops an otherwise unexplained fever or flu-like illness within 14 days of presumed exposure should promptly receive a parenteral anti-infective for treatment of the disease. Oral ciprofloxacin or oral doxycycline (or oral tetracycline) usually is recommended for postexposure prophylaxis of tularemia† following such exposures.

● Typhoid Fever and Other Invasive Salmonella Infections

Ciprofloxacin (conventional tablets, oral suspension) is used in adults for the treatment of typhoid fever (enteric fever) or paratyphoid fever† caused by susceptible *Salmonella enterica* serovars Typhi or Paratyphi, respectively. Although fluoroquinolones have been recommended for empiric treatment of *Salmonella* enteric fever in adults, resistance to fluoroquinolones has been reported in more than 80% of such infections in travelers to South and Southeast Asia and treatment failures will occur.

Oral ciprofloxacin has been effective when used to treat chronic typhoid carriers†; however, the manufacturer of ciprofloxacin cautions that efficacy of the drug in the eradication of the chronic typhoid carrier state has not been demonstrated.

Ciprofloxacin is recommended as a drug of choice for the treatment of native vertebral osteomyelitis caused by *Salmonella*†.

Ciprofloxacin has been used to treat meningitis caused by susceptible *Salmonella*†.

● Vibrio Infections

Cholera

Ciprofloxacin has been used for the treatment of cholera† caused by *Vibrio cholerae* 01 or 0139 in adults or children†. Doxycycline generally is considered the drug of choice when anti-infective therapy is indicated as an adjunct to fluid and electrolyte replacement in patients with cholera; alternatives include azithromycin, co-trimoxazole, ciprofloxacin, or ceftriaxone.

In a controlled study in adults, a 1-g oral dose of oral ciprofloxacin (given as a single dose or in 2 divided doses 12 hours apart) was at least as effective as a 3-day regimen of oral doxycycline (100 mg twice daily for 3 days) for the treatment of cholera. In another study in adults, a single 1-g dose of oral ciprofloxacin was more effective than a single 300-mg oral dose of doxycycline in eradicating *V. cholerae* from stool; although there was no difference between the regimens in terms of duration of diarrhea in those with *V. cholerae* 0139 infections, the duration of diarrhea was shorter in those with *V. cholerae* 01 infections who received ciprofloxacin.

Although further study is needed to evaluate safety and efficacy in children, a single dose of oral ciprofloxacin (20 mg/kg) was as effective as a 3-day regimen of oral erythromycin (12.5 mg/kg every 6 hours) for the treatment of *V. cholerae* 01 or 0139 in children 2–15 years of age. The overall clinical success rate was 60% for ciprofloxacin and 55% for erythromycin; although the bacteriologic eradication rate was lower with ciprofloxacin (42%) than with erythromycin (70%) and erythromycin was associated with a more rapid clearance of *V. cholerae*, there was no difference in duration of diarrhea.

Other Vibrio Infections

Some clinicians suggest that fluoroquinolones (e.g., ciprofloxacin) may be an alternative to tetracyclines for the treatment of other *Vibrio* infections, including gastroenteritis or wound infections caused by *V. parahaemolyticus*† or *V. vulnificus*†.

Although optimum anti-infective therapy for *V. vulnificus* infections has not been identified, a tetracycline or third generation cephalosporin (e.g., cefotaxime, ceftazidime), a fluoroquinolone, or aminoglycoside has been recommended. Because the case fatality rate associated with *V. vulnificus* is high, anti-infective therapy should be initiated promptly if indicated.

● Perioperative Prophylaxis

Ciprofloxacin is used for perioperative prophylaxis† to reduce the risk of postoperative infections in patients undergoing certain genitourinary surgery.

Perioperative prophylaxis is not recommended for patients with sterile urine undergoing cystoscopy without manipulation. However, if the patient has positive (or unavailable) urine cultures or an indwelling urinary catheter or is undergoing cystoscopy with manipulation (dilation, biopsy, fulguration, resection, or ureteral instrumentation), some clinicians recommend pretreatment to sterilize the urine before surgery or perioperative prophylaxis with a single preoperative dose of an anti-infective (e.g., ciprofloxacin) active against the most likely urologic pathogens.

Perioperative prophylaxis using an appropriate anti-infective (e.g., ciprofloxacin) is recommended in patients undergoing transurethral prostatectomy, transrectal prostatic biopsies, ureteroscopy, shock wave lithotripsy, percutaneous renal surgery, open laparoscopic procedures, or procedures that involve placement of a urologic prosthesis (e.g., penile implant, artificial sphincter, synthetic pubovaginal sling, bone anchors for pelvic floor reconstruction). Because of increasing resistance of *E. coli* to fluoroquinolones, local susceptibility patterns should be considered when selecting an anti-infective for prophylaxis in patients undergoing genitourinary surgery.

● Empiric Therapy in Febrile Neutropenic Patients

Ciprofloxacin is used for empiric therapy of presumed bacterial infections in febrile neutropenic patients.

IV ciprofloxacin has been used in conjunction with IV piperacillin sodium (no longer commercially available in the US as a single-entity preparation) for empiric anti-infective therapy in febrile neutropenic patients. Safety and efficacy of combination therapy with ciprofloxacin and piperacillin sodium for empiric therapy in febrile neutropenic patients have been evaluated in a multicenter, randomized study in adults. Patients were randomized to receive a regimen of ciprofloxacin (400 mg IV every 8 hours) and piperacillin sodium (50 mg/kg IV every 4 hours) or a regimen of tobramycin (2 mg/kg IV every 8 hours) and piperacillin sodium (50 mg/kg IV every 4 hours). There was clinical resolution of the initial febrile episode (resolution of fever, microbiologic eradication of infection if such infection was microbiologically documented, resolution of signs and symptoms of infection) without modification of the empiric regimen in 27% of those who received ciprofloxacin and piperacillin and in 21.9% of those who received tobramycin and piperacillin; the overall survival rate was 96.1 or 94.1%, respectively.

Anti-infective prophylaxis with a fluoroquinolone during periods of expected neutropenia is recommended by some experts in patients who are at high risk for febrile neutropenia or profound, protracted neutropenia (e.g., most patients with acute myeloid leukemia/myelodysplastic syndromes [AML/MDS] or hematopoietic stem-cell transplantation [HSCT] treated with myeloablative conditioning regimens). These experts state that prophylaxis with a fluoroquinolone is not routinely recommended in patients with solid tumors because the benefits do not outweigh risks in these patients, but may be considered for some patients with solid tumors or lymphoma who are expected to experience profound neutropenia for at least 7 days and are not receiving granulocyte colony-stimulating factor (G-CSF).

An empiric regimen that includes a fluoroquinolone (ciprofloxacin or levofloxacin) in conjunction with the fixed combination of amoxicillin and clavulanate potassium (or clindamycin in those with penicillin allergy) has been recommended for outpatient management of febrile neutropenic adults receiving

treatment for malignancy. Use of a fluoroquinolone alone is not recommended for initial empiric therapy for outpatient management in febrile neutropenic patients; however, some studies have shown that monotherapy may be effective in low-risk outpatients.

Published protocols on anti-infective prophylaxis in febrile neutropenic patients should be consulted for specific recommendations regarding when anti-infective prophylaxis is appropriate for immunosuppressed patients with cancer and options for such prophylaxis.

DOSAGE AND ADMINISTRATION

● Administration

Ciprofloxacin is administered orally as conventional tablets containing the hydrochloride, as a conventional oral suspension containing the base, and as extended-release tablets containing both the hydrochloride and the base. Ciprofloxacin is given by IV infusion as the base.

Patients receiving initial therapy with IV ciprofloxacin may be switched to oral ciprofloxacin (conventional tablets, oral suspension) when clinically appropriate.

Ciprofloxacin extended-release tablets are used *only* for the treatment of certain urinary tract infections (UTIs) in adults and should *not* be used for any indication in pediatric patients. The extended-release tablets are *not* interchangeable with other oral ciprofloxacin preparations (conventional tablets, oral suspension).

Patients receiving oral or IV ciprofloxacin should be adequately hydrated and should be instructed to drink fluids liberally to prevent highly concentrated urine and formation of crystals in urine.

Oral Administration

Ciprofloxacin conventional tablets, extended-release tablets, or oral suspension may be given without regard to meals.

Ciprofloxacin conventional tablets, extended-release tablets, or oral suspension should *not* be administered concurrently with dairy products (e.g., milk, yogurt) or calcium-fortified products (e.g., juices) alone (without a meal) since absorption of the drug may be substantially reduced. Doses should preferably be taken 2 hours before or after these calcium-fortified products or substantial calcium intake (greater than 800 mg).

Conventional tablets and extended-release tablets should be swallowed whole and should *not* be split, crushed, or chewed.

Following reconstitution, ciprofloxacin oral suspension containing 250 or 500 mg of ciprofloxacin per 5 mL should be administered using the graduated spoon provided by the manufacturer that has markings for 2.5 and 5 mL. The microcapsules contained in the reconstituted oral suspensions should be swallowed whole and should not be chewed. Water may be ingested after the oral suspension is swallowed.

Reconstitution

Ciprofloxacin microcapsules for oral suspension are provided in a kit that contains a bottle of microcapsules, a bottle of oral suspension diluent, and a graduated dosing spoon. At the time of dispensing, the bottle containing the microcapsules (either 5 or 10 g of ciprofloxacin) should be added to the bottle of diluent according to the manufacturer's directions and shaken vigorously for about 15 seconds to provide a suspension containing 250 or 500 mg of ciprofloxacin per 5 mL, respectively. Only the diluent supplied in the kit should be used; water should *not* be added to the oral suspension.

Prior to administration of each dose, the reconstituted oral suspension should be shaken vigorously for about 15 seconds.

IV Infusion

Prior to IV infusion, commercially available ciprofloxacin concentrate for injection containing 10 mg/mL must be diluted with a compatible IV solution (e.g., sterile water for injection, 5% or 10% dextrose injection, 0.9% sodium chloride injection, 5% dextrose and 0.225 or 0.45% sodium chloride injection, or lactated Ringer's injection) to provide a solution containing 1–2 mg/mL.

Alternatively, commercially available premixed ciprofloxacin injection for IV infusion containing 2 mg/mL in 5% dextrose injection may be used without further dilution.

IV infusions should be given into a large vein to minimize discomfort and reduce the risk of venous irritation. If a Y-type administration set is used, the other IV solution flowing through the tubing should be discontinued while ciprofloxacin is being infused. If concomitant use of IV ciprofloxacin and another parenteral drug is necessary, each drug should be given separately.

Rate of Administration

IV infusions of ciprofloxacin should be infused over 1 hour.

Because local reactions (e.g., thrombophlebitis, burning, pain, pruritus, paresthesia, erythema, swelling) at the site of IV infusion are more frequent when the drug is administered rapidly (e.g., over 30 minutes or less) or via a small vein, ciprofloxacin should be infused IV *slowly* over a period of 1 hour as a dilute solution (1–2 mg of ciprofloxacin per mL) via a large vein. If such reactions occur despite these precautions, they generally resolve rapidly following completion of the infusion; the manufacturers state that subsequent IV administration of ciprofloxacin is not contraindicated unless the reaction recurs or worsens.

● Dosage

Dosage of ciprofloxacin hydrochloride and ciprofloxacin is expressed in terms of ciprofloxacin.

Unless otherwise specified, oral ciprofloxacin dosage is for the conventional tablets or oral suspension of the drug.

The extended-release tablets are *not* interchangeable with the conventional tablets or oral suspension.

Dosage of oral and IV ciprofloxacin is *not* identical. Based on pharmacokinetic parameters (i.e., area under the plasma concentration-time curve [AUC]), the following oral and IV ciprofloxacin regimens are considered equivalent: 250 mg orally every 12 hours (conventional tablets) is equivalent to 200 mg IV every 12 hours; 500 mg orally every 12 hours (conventional tablets) is equivalent to 400 mg IV every 12 hours; and 750 mg orally every 12 hours (conventional tablets) is equivalent to 400 mg IV every 8 hours.

The duration of ciprofloxacin therapy depends on the type and severity of infection, and should be determined by the clinical and bacteriologic response of the patient.

Pediatric Dosage
Complicated Urinary Tract Infections and Pyelonephritis

If ciprofloxacin is used for the treatment of complicated UTIs or pyelonephritis in pediatric patients 1–17 years of age, dosage and route of administration should be based on infection severity. The manufacturers recommend a total treatment duration of 10–21 days; the mean total duration of treatment (IV and/or oral) in clinical trials was 11 days (range 10–21 days).

If IV ciprofloxacin is used for the treatment of complicated UTIs or pyelonephritis in pediatric patients 1–17 years of age, the manufacturer recommends a dosage of 6–10 mg/kg (up to 400 mg) every 8 hours.

If oral ciprofloxacin is used for the treatment of complicated UTIs or pyelonephritis in pediatric patients 1–17 years of age, the manufacturer recommends a dosage of 10–20 mg/kg (up to 750 mg) every 12 hours.

If ciprofloxacin oral suspension containing 250 mg/5 mL is used for the treatment of complicated UTIs or pyelonephritis in pediatric patients 1–17 years of age, the manufacturer recommends a dosage of 125 mg every 12 hours in those weighing 9–12 kg, 250 mg every 12 hours in those weighing 13–18 kg, 250–375 mg every 12 hours in those weighing 19–24 kg, 375–500 mg every 12 hours in those weighing 25–31 kg, 375–625 mg every 12 hours in those weighing 32–37 kg, and 500–750 mg every 12 hours in those weighing 38 kg or more.

If ciprofloxacin oral suspension containing 500 mg/5 mL is used for the treatment of complicated UTIs or pyelonephritis in pediatric patients 1–17 years of age, the manufacturer recommends a dosage of 250 mg every 12 hours in those weighing 13–24 kg, 250–500 mg every 12 hours in those weighing 25 kg, 500 mg every 12 hours in those weighing 26–37 kg, and 500–750 mg every 12 hours in those weighing 38 kg or more.

Postexposure Prophylaxis of Anthrax

If oral ciprofloxacin is used for inhalational anthrax (postexposure) to reduce the incidence or progression of disease following exposure to aerosolized *Bacillus*

anthracis spores in the context of biologic warfare or bioterrorism, the manufacturer recommends that neonates, infants, and children 17 years of age or younger receive 15 mg/kg (up to 500 mg) every 12 hours.

If ciprofloxacin oral suspension containing 250 mg/5 mL is used for inhalational anthrax (postexposure) in neonates, infants, and children 17 years of age or younger, the manufacturer recommends a dosage of 125 mg every 12 hours in those weighing 9–12 kg, 250 mg every 12 hours in those weighing 13–18 kg, 250–375 mg every 12 hours in those weighing 19–24 kg, and 500 mg every 12 hours in those weighing 25 kg or more.

If ciprofloxacin oral suspension containing 500 mg/5 mL is used for inhalational anthrax (postexposure) in neonates, infants, and children 17 years of age or younger, the manufacturer recommends a dosage of 250 mg every 12 hours in those weighing 13–24 kg and 500 mg every 12 hours in those weighing 25 kg or more.

If IV ciprofloxacin is used for inhalational anthrax (postexposure) in neonates, infants, and children 17 years of age or younger, the manufacturer recommends a dosage of 10 mg/kg (up to 400 mg) every 12 hours.

For postexposure prophylaxis of anthrax in neonates up to 4 weeks of age following an exposure that occurred in the context of biologic warfare or bioterrorism, the American Academy of Pediatrics (AAP) recommends that oral ciprofloxacin be given in a dosage of 10 mg/kg every 12 hours in preterm neonates (gestational age 32–37 weeks) and 15 mg/kg every 12 hours in full-term neonates. AAP recommends that pediatric patients 1 month of age or older receive oral ciprofloxacin in a dosage of 15 mg/kg (up to 500 mg) every 12 hours for such postexposure prophylaxis.

Postexposure anti-infective prophylaxis should be initiated as soon as possible following suspected or confirmed anthrax exposure.

Because of possible persistence of *B. anthracis* spores in lung tissue following an aerosol exposure, the US Centers for Disease Control and Prevention (CDC), AAP, and others recommend that anti-infective prophylaxis be continued for 60 days following a confirmed exposure.

Treatment of Systemic Anthrax

If IV ciprofloxacin is used in neonates up to 4 weeks of age as part of a multiple-drug parenteral regimen for initial treatment of systemic anthrax† (inhalational, GI, meningitis, or cutaneous with systemic involvement, extensive edema, or head or neck lesions) that occurs in the context of biologic warfare or bioterrorism, AAP recommends a dosage of 10 mg/kg every 12 hours in preterm neonates (gestational age 32–37 weeks) and 15 mg/kg every 12 hours in full-term neonates.

If IV ciprofloxacin is used in pediatric patients 1 month of age or older as part of a multiple-drug parenteral regimen for initial treatment of systemic anthrax† (inhalational, GI, meningitis, or cutaneous with systemic involvement, lesions on the head or neck, or extensive edema) that occurs in the context of biologic warfare or bioterrorism, AAP recommends a dosage of 10 mg/kg (up to 400 mg) every 8 hours.

The multiple-drug parenteral regimen should be continued for at least 2–3 weeks until the patient is clinically stable and treatment can be switched to an appropriate oral anti-infective. If systemic anthrax occurred as the result of exposure to aerosolized *B. anthracis* spores (e.g., in the context of biologic warfare or bioterrorism), the oral follow-up regimen should be continued until 60 days after onset of the illness.

When oral ciprofloxacin is used for follow-up treatment of systemic anthrax after an initial parenteral regimen in neonates up to 4 weeks of age, AAP recommends a dosage of 10 mg/kg every 12 hours in preterm neonates (gestational age 32–37 weeks) and 15 mg/kg every 12 hours in full-term neonates. AAP recommends a dosage of 15 mg/kg (up to 500 mg) every 12 hours when oral ciprofloxacin is used for such follow-up treatment in pediatric patients 1 months of age or older.

Treatment of Uncomplicated Cutaneous Anthrax

If oral ciprofloxacin is used in neonates up to 4 weeks of age for the treatment of uncomplicated cutaneous anthrax† (without systemic involvement) that occurs in the context of biologic warfare or bioterrorism, AAP recommends a dosage of 10 mg/kg every 12 hours in preterm neonates (gestational age 32–37 weeks) and 15 mg/kg every 12 hours in full-term neonates.

If oral ciprofloxacin is used in pediatric patients 1 month of age or older for the treatment of uncomplicated cutaneous anthrax† (without systemic involvement) that occurs in the context of biologic warfare or bioterrorism, AAP recommends a dosage of 15 mg/kg (up to 500 mg) every 12 hours.

If uncomplicated cutaneous anthrax occurred after exposure to aerosolized *B. anthracis* spores in the context of biologic warfare or bioterrorism, anti-infective treatment should be continued for 60 days after onset of the illness. A treatment duration of 7–10 days may be sufficient if uncomplicated cutaneous anthrax occurred as the result of naturally occurring or endemic exposures.

Treatment of Plague

When IV ciprofloxacin is used for the treatment of plague (including pneumonic and septicemic plague) caused by *Yersinia pestis*, the manufacturer recommends that neonates, infants, and children 17 years of age or younger receive a dosage of 10 mg/kg (up to 400 mg) every 8–12 hours.

If oral ciprofloxacin is used for the treatment of plague, the manufacturer recommends that neonates, infants, and children 17 years of age or younger receive a dosage of 15 mg/kg (up to 500 mg) every 8–12 hours.

If ciprofloxacin oral suspension containing 250 mg/5 mL is used for the treatment of plague in neonates, infants, and children 17 years of age or younger, the manufacturer recommends a dosage of 125 mg every 12 hours in those weighing 9–12 kg, 250 mg every 12 hours in those weighing 13–18 kg, 250–375 mg every 12 hours in those weighing 19–24 kg, 375–500 mg every 12 hours in those weighing 25–31 kg, 375–625 mg every 12 hours in those weighing 32–37 kg, and 500–750 mg every 12 hours in those weighing 38 kg or more.

If ciprofloxacin oral suspension containing 500 mg/5 mL is used for the treatment of plague in neonates, infants, and children 17 years of age or younger, the manufacturer recommends a dosage of 250 mg every 12 hours in those weighing 13–24 kg, 250–500 mg every 12 hours in those weighing 25 kg, 500 mg every 12 hours in those weighing 26–37 kg, and 500–750 mg every 12 hours in those weighing 38 kg or more.

Some experts (e.g., US Working Group on Civilian Biodefense, US Army Medical Research Institute of Infectious Diseases [USAMRIID]) recommend that children receive IV ciprofloxacin in a dosage of 15 mg/kg every 12 hours (up to 1 g daily) for the treatment of pneumonic plague that occurs as the result of exposure to *Y. pestis* in the context of biologic warfare or bioterrorism. If oral ciprofloxacin is used for the treatment of plague when the patient's clinical condition improves or when a parenteral regimen is not available (e.g., in mass casualty settings), some experts (e.g., US Working Group on Civilian Biodefense) recommend that children receive 20 mg/kg twice daily (up to 1 g daily).

A parenteral regimen is preferred for initial treatment of plague; an oral regimen can be used after clinical improvement occurs or when a parenteral regimen is not available (e.g., mass casualty setting).

The manufacturer recommends a total treatment duration (IV and oral) of 10–21 days in pediatric patients; some experts state that the total treatment duration should be 10–14 days.

Postexposure Prophylaxis of Plague

When oral ciprofloxacin is used for prophylaxis of plague, the manufacturer recommends that neonates, infants, and children 17 years of age or younger receive a dosage of 15 mg/kg (up to 500 mg) every 8–12 hours for 10–21 days.

If ciprofloxacin oral suspension containing 250 mg/5 mL is used for prophylaxis of plague in neonates, infants, and children 17 years of age or younger, the manufacturer recommends a dosage of 125 mg every 12 hours in those weighing 9–12 kg, 250 mg every 12 hours in those weighing 13–18 kg, 250–375 mg every 12 hours in those weighing 19–24 kg, 375–500 mg every 12 hours in those weighing 25–31 kg, 375–625 mg every 12 hours in those weighing 32–37 kg, and 500–750 mg every 12 hours in those weighing 38 kg or more.

If ciprofloxacin oral suspension containing 500 mg/5 mL is used for the prophylaxis of plague in neonates, infants, and children 17 years of age or younger, the manufacturer recommends a dosage of 250 mg every 12 hours in those weighing 13–24 kg, 250–500 mg every 12 hours in those weighing 25 kg, 500 mg every 12 hours in those weighing 26–37 kg, and 500–750 mg every 12 hours in those weighing 38 kg or more.

If IV ciprofloxacin is used for prophylaxis of plague, the manufacturer recommends that neonates, infants, and children 17 years of age or younger receive a dosage of 10 mg/kg (up to 400 mg) every 8–2 hours for 10–21 days.

Some experts (e.g., US Working Group on Civilian Biodefense, USAMRIID) recommend that children receive oral ciprofloxacin in a dosage of 20 mg/kg twice daily (up to 1 g daily) for postexposure prophylaxis following exposure to *Y. pestis* in the context of biologic warfare or bioterrorism.

Postexposure prophylaxis of plague should be initiated as soon as possible after a suspected or confirmed exposure to *Y. pestis*.

In close contacts of patients with pneumonic plague or individuals exposed to plague aerosol (e.g., in the context of biologic warfare or bioterrorism), prophylaxis should be continued for 7 days or for the duration of the risk of exposure plus 7 days. If fever or cough develops during prophylaxis, the regimen should be switch to that used for treatment of plague.

Treatment of Tularemia

If IV ciprofloxacin is used for the treatment of tularemia† that occurs as the result of exposure to *Francisella tularensis* in the context of biologic warfare or bioterrorism, some experts (e.g., US Working Group on Civilian Biodefense, USAMRIID) recommend that children receive 15 mg/kg every 12 hours (up to 1 g daily) for at least 10–14 days. Oral therapy may be substituted when the patient's condition improves.

If oral ciprofloxacin is used for the treatment of tularemia when the patient's clinical condition improves or if a parenteral regimen is not available, experts recommend that children receive 15 mg/kg twice daily (up to 1 g daily) for a total treatment duration of at least 10–14 days.

Postexposure Prophylaxis of Tularemia

If oral ciprofloxacin is used for postexposure prophylaxis of tularemia† following exposure to *F. tularensis* that occurs in the context of biologic warfare or bioterrorism, some experts (e.g., US Working Group on Civilian Biodefense, USAMRIID) recommend that children receive 15 mg/kg orally twice daily (up to 1 g daily).

Postexposure prophylaxis of tularemia ideally should be initiated within 24 hours of exposure and continued for at least 14 days.

Cystoisospora Infections

If oral ciprofloxacin is used as an alternative for the treatment of infections caused by *Cystoisospora belli*† (formerly *Isospora belli*) in pediatric patients with human immunodeficiency virus (HIV) infection, the recommended dosage is 10–20 mg/kg (up to 500 mg) twice daily for 7 days.

If oral ciprofloxacin is used for chronic maintenance therapy (secondary prophylaxis) of cystoisosporiasis in HIV-infected pediatric patients†, a dosage of 10–20 mg/kg (up to 500 mg) 3 times weekly is recommended. Consideration can be given to discontinuing such prophylaxis in pediatric patients if there is no evidence of active *Cystoisospora* infection and there has been sustained improvement in immunologic status (CDC immunologic category 1 or 2) for more than 6 months in response to antiretroviral therapy.

Meningitis and Other CNS Infections

Although safety and efficacy have not been established, if use of IV ciprofloxacin is considered necessary for the treatment of healthcare-associated ventriculitis and meningitis† caused by susceptible gram-negative bacteria when the drugs of choice cannot be used, the Infectious Diseases Society of America (IDSA) recommends that pediatric patients receive a dosage of 30 mg/kg daily given in divided doses every 8–12 hours.

Neisseria meningitidis Infections

If use of ciprofloxacin is considered necessary in children and infants 1 month of age or older to eliminate nasopharyngeal carriage of *Neisseria meningitidis*† or for chemoprophylaxis in household or other close contacts of individuals with invasive meningococcal disease† when other anti-infectives (e.g., rifampin, ceftriaxone) cannot be used, AAP recommends a single oral dose of 20 mg/kg (up to 500 mg). Ciprofloxacin should be used only if fluoroquinolone-resistant *N. meningitis* have not been identified in the community.

Vibrio Infections

If use of ciprofloxacin is considered necessary in pediatric patients for the treatment of cholera†, AAP recommends a dosage of 15 mg/kg (up to 500 mg) twice daily for 3 days. Children 2–12 years of age have received a single oral ciprofloxacin dose of 20 mg/kg (up to 750 mg) for the treatment of cholera caused by *V. cholerae* 01 or 0139.

Adult Dosage

Bone and Joint Infections

If IV ciprofloxacin is used for the treatment of bone and joint infections in adults, the manufacturer recommends a dosage of 400 mg every 8 to 12 hours for 4–8 weeks.

If oral ciprofloxacin is used for the treatment of bone and joint infections in adults, the manufacturer recommends a dosage of 500–750 mg every 12 hours for 4–8 weeks.

For the treatment of native vertebral osteomyelitis, IDSA recommends that IV ciprofloxacin be given in a dosage of 400 mg every 8 hours for 6 weeks for infections caused by *Ps. aeruginosa* or a dosage of 400 mg every 12 hours for the treatment of infections caused by Enterobacteriaceae. If oral ciprofloxacin is used for the treatment of native vertebral osteomyelitis, IDSA recommends a dosage of 750 mg every 12 hours for 6 weeks for infections caused by *Ps. aeruginosa*, 500 mg every 12 hours for 6–8 weeks for infections caused by *Salmonella*, and 500–750 mg every 12 hours for 6 weeks for infections caused by other Enterobacteriaceae.

For the treatment of prosthetic joint infections, IDSA recommends that IV ciprofloxacin be given in a dosage of 400 mg every 12 hours for 4–6 weeks for infections caused by *Ps. aeruginosa* or *Enterobacter*. If oral ciprofloxacin is used for the treatment of prosthetic joint infections, IDSA recommends a dosage of 750 mg twice daily for 4–6 weeks for infections caused by *Ps. aeruginosa* and for infections caused by *Enterobacter* or other Enterobacteriaceae.

Endocarditis

For the treatment of endocarditis† (native or prosthetic valve or other prosthetic material) caused by fastidious gram-negative bacilli of the HACEK group when ceftriaxone (or other third or fourth generation cephalosporin) cannot be used, the American Heart Association (AHA) and IDSA suggest that adults receive IV ciprofloxacin in a dosage of 800 mg daily given in 2 equally divided doses or oral ciprofloxacin in a dosage of 1 g daily given in 2 equally divided doses.

Treatment should be continued for 4 weeks in those with native valve endocarditis or for 6 weeks in those with endocarditis involving prosthetic cardiac valves or other prosthetic cardiac material. Because only limited data are available regarding use of ciprofloxacin for the treatment of these infections, AHA and IDSA recommend that patients with HACEK endocarditis who cannot receive ceftriaxone be treated in consultation with an infectious disease specialist.

Infectious Diarrhea

The usual oral dosage of ciprofloxacin for the treatment of infectious diarrhea in adults is 500 mg every 12 hours for 5–7 days.

Campylobacter Infections

For the treatment of campylobacteriosis caused by susceptible *Campylobacter* in HIV-infected adults, the recommended dosage of oral ciprofloxacin is 500–750 mg every 12 hours. If IV ciprofloxacin is used, the recommended dosage is 400 mg every 12 hours.

The recommended duration of treatment in HIV-infected adults is 7–10 days for gastroenteritis or at least 14 days for bacteremic infections. A duration of 2–6 weeks is recommended for recurrent infections.

Cyclospora Infections

If oral ciprofloxacin is used for the treatment of infections caused by *Cyclospora cayetanensis*†, some clinicians recommend that adults receive 500 mg twice daily for 7 days.

Cystoisospora Infections

If oral ciprofloxacin is used as an alternative for the treatment of infections caused by *C. belli*† (formerly *I. belli*) in HIV-infected adults, the recommended dosage is 500 mg twice daily for 7 days.

If oral ciprofloxacin is used as an alternative for chronic maintenance therapy (secondary prophylaxis) of cystoisosporiasis† in HIV-infected adults with CD4+ T-cell counts less than 200 cells/mm³, a dosage of 500 mg 3 times weekly is recommended based on limited data. Consideration can be given to discontinuing such

prophylaxis if CD4+ T-cell counts exceed 200 cells/mm³ for more than 6 months in response to antiretroviral therapy.

Salmonella Gastroenteritis

For the treatment of *Salmonella* gastroenteritis† (with or without bacteremia) in HIV-infected adults, the recommended dosage of oral ciprofloxacin is 500–750 mg every 12 hours. Alternatively, 400 mg can be given IV every 12 hours.

The recommended duration of treatment in HIV-infected adults is 7–14 days in those with CD4+ T-cell counts of 200 cells/mm³ or greater (14 days or longer if the patient is bacteremic or the infection is complicated) or 2–6 weeks in those with CD4+ T-cell counts less than 200 cells/mm³.

Shigella Infections

For the treatment of shigellosis caused by susceptible *Shigella* in HIV-infected adults, the recommended dosage of oral ciprofloxacin is 500–750 mg every 12 hours. Alternatively, 400 mg can be given IV every 12 hours.

The recommended duration of treatment in HIV-infected adults is 7–10 days for gastroenteritis or at least 14 days for bacteremic infections. Recurrent infections, especially in patients with CD4+ T-cell counts less than 200 cells/mm³, may require up to 6 weeks of treatment.

Travelers' Diarrhea

If oral ciprofloxacin (conventional tablets or oral suspension) is used for the treatment of travelers' diarrhea† in adults, some clinicians recommend a dosage of 500 once or twice daily for 1–3 days or 750 mg once daily for 1–3 days. Alternatively, if ciprofloxacin extended-release tablets are used, some clinicians recommend a dosage of 500 mg or 1 g once daily for 1–3 days.

If ciprofloxacin is used for empiric treatment of travelers' diarrhea† in HIV-infected adults, an oral dosage of 500–750 mg every 12 hours or IV dosage of 400 mg every 12 hours is recommended. If there is no clinical response after 3–4 days of treatment, stool culture and in vitro susceptibility testing should be considered.

Although the use of anti-infectives for prophylaxis of travelers' diarrhea† generally is discouraged, if oral ciprofloxacin (conventional tablets or oral suspension) is used, the recommended adult dosage is 500 mg once daily during the period of risk (not exceeding 2–3 weeks) beginning the day of travel and continuing for 1 or 2 days after leaving the area of risk.

Intra-abdominal Infections

When IV ciprofloxacin is used for the treatment of complicated intra-abdominal infections, the recommended dosage for adults is 400 mg every 12 hours given in conjunction with metronidazole. If oral ciprofloxacin is used for the treatment of complicated intra-abdominal infections, the recommended dosage for adults is 500 mg every 12 hours in conjunction with metronidazole.

The manufacturers recommend a total treatment duration of 7–14 days. IDSA states that the usual duration of treatment for intra-abdominal infections is 4–7 days. A longer duration of treatment has not been associated with improved outcome and is not recommended unless adequate source control is difficult to achieve.

Meningitis and Other CNS Infections

Although efficacy and safety have not been established, some clinicians suggest that adults can receive IV ciprofloxacin in a dosage of 400 mg every 8 hours for the treatment of meningitis† caused by susceptible gram-negative bacteria. Other clinicians recommend a dosage of 800–1200 mg daily for the treatment of meningitis in adults.

If IV ciprofloxacin is used for the treatment of healthcare-associated ventriculitis and meningitis† caused by susceptible gram-negative bacteria when the drugs of choice cannot be used, IDSA recommends that adults receive a dosage of 800–1200 mg daily given in divided doses every 8–12 hours.

Malignant Otitis Externa

If oral ciprofloxacin is used for the treatment of malignant otitis externa†, some clinicians recommend a dosage of 750 mg twice daily. Although there may be rapid relief of symptoms (pain, otorrhea), treatment should be continued for 6–8 weeks.

Because ciprofloxacin-resistant *Pseudomonas aeruginosa* have been isolated from patients with malignant otitis externa with increasing frequency, in vitro susceptibility testing is indicated, especially if there is an inadequate response to treatment.

Acute Sinusitis

If oral ciprofloxacin is used for the treatment of acute sinusitis, dosage in adults is 500 mg every 12 hours for 10 days.

The usual IV dosage of ciprofloxacin for the treatment of acute sinusitis in adults is 400 mg every 12 hours for 10 days.

Lower Respiratory Tract Infections

The usual dosage of oral ciprofloxacin for the treatment of lower respiratory tract infections in adults is 500–750 mg every 12 hours for 7–14 days.

The usual IV dosage of ciprofloxacin for the treatment of lower respiratory tract infections in adults is 400 mg every 8 to 12 hours; severe or complicated lower respiratory tract infections should be treated with 400 mg IV every 8 hours. The usual duration of treatment is 7–14 days.

Nosocomial Pneumonia

The usual dosage of IV ciprofloxacin for the treatment of nosocomial pneumonia in adults, including hospital-acquired pneumonia (HAP) not associated with mechanical ventilation and ventilator-associated pneumonia (VAP), is 400 mg every 8 hours.

The manufacturer recommends a treatment duration of 10–14 days. IDSA states that a treatment duration of 7 days is recommended in patients with HAP or VAP; however, a longer or shorter duration may be indicated depending on clinical response.

Skin and Skin Structure Infections

For the treatment of skin and skin structure infections, the usual dosage of oral ciprofloxacin for adults is 500–750 mg every 12 hours for 7–14 days.

The usual IV dosage of ciprofloxacin for the treatment of skin and skin structure infections in adults is 400 mg every 8 to 12 hours for 7–14 days.

Acute, Uncomplicated Cystitis

If ciprofloxacin (conventional tablets or oral suspension) is used for the treatment of acute, uncomplicated cystitis, dosage in adults is 250 mg every 12 hours for 3 days.

If ciprofloxacin extended-release tablets are used for the treatment of uncomplicated UTIs (acute cystitis) caused by susceptible E. faecalis, Escherichia coli, Proteus mirabilis, or Staphylococcus saprophyticus, the recommended dosage in adults is 500 mg once every 24 hours for 3 days.

Complicated Urinary Tract Infections and Pyelonephritis

The usual oral dosage of ciprofloxacin (conventional tablets or oral suspension) for the treatment of UTIs in adults is 250–500 mg every 12 hours for 7–14 days.

If ciprofloxacin extended-release tablets are used for the treatment of complicated UTIs or acute, uncomplicated pyelonephritis caused by susceptible bacteria, the usual adult dosage is 1 g once every 24 hours for 7–14 days.

The usual IV dosage of ciprofloxacin for the treatment of UTIs in adults is 200–400 mg every 8 to 12 hours for 7–14 days.

Prostatitis

For the treatment of chronic bacterial prostatitis in men, the usual oral dosage of ciprofloxacin (conventional tablets or oral suspension) is 500 mg every 12 hours for 28 days.

The usual IV dosage of ciprofloxacin for the treatment of chronic bacterial prostatitis is 400 mg every 12 hours for 28 days.

Postexposure Prophylaxis of Anthrax

When oral ciprofloxacin is used for inhalational anthrax (postexposure) to reduce the incidence or progression of disease following exposure to aerosolized B. anthracis spores in the context of biologic warfare or bioterrorism, adults should receive 500 mg every 12 hours. If IV ciprofloxacin is used for inhalational anthrax (postexposure), adults should receive 400 mg IV every 12 hours.

CDC recommends that adults (including pregnant and postpartum women) receive oral ciprofloxacin in a dosage of 500 mg every 12 hours for postexposure prophylaxis of anthrax.

Postexposure anti-infective prophylaxis should be initiated as soon as possible following suspected or confirmed anthrax exposure.

Because of possible persistence of B. anthracis spores in lung tissue following an aerosol exposure, CDC and other experts recommend that anti-infective prophylaxis be continued for 60 days following a confirmed exposure.

For prophylaxis following ingestion of B. anthracis spores† in contaminated meat, a ciprofloxacin dosage of 500 mg orally twice daily has been recommended for adults.

If anti-infective prophylaxis is used following a naturally occurring GI exposure to B. anthracis (e.g., ingestion of meat from an undercooked carcass of an anthrax-infected animal), ACIP states that a duration of 7–14 days can be considered.

Treatment of Systemic Anthrax

When IV ciprofloxacin is used in a multiple-drug parenteral regimen for initial treatment of systemic anthrax† (inhalational, GI, meningitis, or cutaneous anthrax with systemic involvement, lesions on the head or neck, or extensive edema) that occurs in the context of biologic warfare or bioterrorism, CDC recommends that adults (including pregnant and postpartum women) receive a dosage of 400 mg every 8 hours.

The multiple-drug parenteral regimen should be continued for at least 2–3 weeks until the patient is clinically stable and treatment can be switched to an oral anti-infective. If systemic anthrax occurred as the result of exposure to aerosolized B. anthracis spores (e.g., in the context of biologic warfare or bioterrorism), the oral follow-up regimen should be continued until 60 days after onset of the illness.

If oral ciprofloxacin is used for follow-up after an initial parenteral regimen or as an alternative for the treatment of inhalational anthrax† when a parenteral regimen is not available (e.g., when there are supply or logistic problems because large numbers of individuals require treatment in a mass casualty setting), some experts (US Working Group on Civilian Biodefense, USAMRIID) recommend that adults receive an oral dosage of 500 mg every 12 hours.

Treatment of Uncomplicated Cutaneous Anthrax

For the treatment of uncomplicated cutaneous anthrax† (without systemic involvement) that occurs in the context of biologic warfare or bioterrorism, CDC recommends that adults (including pregnant and postpartum women) receive oral ciprofloxacin in a dosage of 500 mg every 12 hours.

If uncomplicated cutaneous anthrax occurred after exposure to aerosolized B. anthracis spores in the context of biologic warfare or bioterrorism, anti-infective treatment should be continued for 60 days after onset of the illness. A treatment duration of 3–10 days may be sufficient if uncomplicated cutaneous anthrax occurred as the result of naturally occurring or endemic exposures.

Treatment of GI or Oropharyngeal Anthrax

For treatment of GI and oropharyngeal anthrax† that occurs in the context of biologic warfare or bioterrorism, CDC and other experts (US Working Group on Civilian Biodefense, USAMRIID) recommend that therapy be initiated with the same parenteral multiple-drug regimen recommended for treatment of inhalational anthrax.

Brucellosis

For the treatment of brucellosis† caused by Brucella melitensis, some clinicians recommend that oral ciprofloxacin be given in a dosage of 500 mg twice daily in conjunction with oral rifampin (600 mg once daily). Oral ciprofloxacin also has been given in a dosage of 500 mg 2 or 3 times daily for 6–12 weeks or 750 mg 3 times daily for 6–8 weeks for the treatment of brucellosis or acute brucella arthritis-diskitis†. Monotherapy or treatment regimens shorter than 4–6 weeks are not recommended.

Chancroid

When oral ciprofloxacin is used in the treatment of chancroid†, CDC recommends that adults receive 500 mg twice daily for 3 days.

Crohn's Disease

Oral ciprofloxacin has been given in a dosage of 500 mg twice daily (with or without metronidazole) for induction of remission of mildly to moderately active Crohn's disease†.

Gonorrhea and Associated Infections

Although ciprofloxacin is no longer recommended for the treatment of gonorrhea, the manufacturer recommends a single 250-mg dose of oral ciprofloxacin for the treatment of uncomplicated urethral or endocervical gonorrhea caused by susceptible *Neisseria gonorrhoeae*.

Granuloma Inguinale (Donovanosis)

For the treatment of granuloma inguinale† (donovanosis) caused by *Klebsiella granulomatis* (formerly *Calymmatobacterium granulomatis*), 750 mg of oral ciprofloxacin should be given twice daily for at least 3 weeks and until all lesions have completely healed. Consideration can be given to adding a parenteral aminoglycoside (e.g., gentamicin 1 mg/kg IV every 8 hours) if improvement is not evident within the first few days of treatment.

Legionnaires' Disease

For the treatment of Legionnaires' disease†, some clinicians recommend that 500 mg of ciprofloxacin be given orally every 12 hours or 400 mg be given IV every 12 hours for 2–3 weeks.

Mycobacterial Infections

When used in multiple-drug regimens for the treatment of *Mycobacterium avium* complex (MAC) infections†, oral ciprofloxacin has been given to adults in a dosage of 750 mg twice daily.

Neisseria meningitidis Infections

When ciprofloxacin is used to eliminate nasopharyngeal carriage of *N. meningitidis*† or for chemoprophylaxis in household or other close contacts of individuals with invasive meningococcal disease†, adults should receive a single 500-mg oral dose.

Treatment of Plague

When IV ciprofloxacin is used for the treatment of plague caused by *Y. pestis*, the manufacturer recommends that adults receive a dosage of 400 mg every 8 to 12 hours for 14 days.

If oral ciprofloxacin is used for the treatment of plague, the manufacturer recommends that adults receive 500–750 mg orally every 12 hours for 14 days.

Some experts (e.g., US Working Group on Civilian Biodefense, USAMRIID) recommend that adults receive a dosage of 400 mg every 12 hours if IV ciprofloxacin is used for as an alternative for the treatment of pneumonic plague that occurs as the result of exposure to *Y. pestis* in the context of biologic warfare or bioterrorism. If oral ciprofloxacin is used for the treatment of plague when the patient's clinical condition improves or when a parenteral regimen is not available (e.g., in mass casualty settings), these experts recommend that adults receive 500–750 mg orally twice daily.

A parenteral regimen is preferred for initial treatment of plague; an oral regimen can be used after clinical improvement occurs or when a parenteral regimen is not available (e.g., mass casualty setting).

The manufacturer recommends a total treatment duration (IV and oral) of 14 days in adults; some experts state that the total treatment duration should be 10–14 days.

Postexposure Prophylaxis of Plague

When oral ciprofloxacin is used for prophylaxis of plague, the manufacturer recommends that adults receive a dosage of 500–750 mg orally every 12 hours for 14 days.

If IV ciprofloxacin is used for prophylaxis of plague, the manufacturer recommends that adults receive a dosage of 400 mg every 8 to 12 hours for 14 days.

Some experts (e.g., US Working Group on Civilian Biodefense, USAMRIID) recommend that oral ciprofloxacin be given in a dosage of 500 mg twice daily if the drug is used for postexposure prophylaxis following exposure to *Y. pestis* in the context of biologic warfare or bioterrorism.

Postexposure prophylaxis of plague should be initiated as soon as possible after a suspected or confirmed exposure to *Y. pestis*.

In close contacts of patients with pneumonic plague or individuals exposed to plague aerosol (e.g., in the context of biologic warfare or bioterrorism), prophylaxis should be continued for 7 days or for the duration of the risk of exposure plus 7 days. If fever or cough develops during prophylaxis, the regimen should be switch to that used for treatment of plague.

Treatment of Tularemia

If IV ciprofloxacin is used for the treatment of tularemia† that occurs as the result of exposure to *F. tularensis* in the context of biologic warfare or bioterrorism, some experts (e.g., US Working Group on Civilian Biodefense, USAMRIID) recommend that adults receive a dosage of 400 mg every 12 hours. Oral therapy may be substituted when the patient's condition improves.

If oral ciprofloxacin is used for the treatment of tularemia when the patient's clinical condition improves or if a parenteral regimen is not available, adults should receive 500 mg orally twice daily.

Postexposure Prophylaxis of Tularemia

If oral ciprofloxacin is used for postexposure prophylaxis of tularemia† following exposure to *F. tularensis* that occurs in the context of biologic warfare or bioterrorism, some experts (e.g., US Working Group on Civilian Biodefense, USAMRIID) recommend that adults receive 500 mg orally every 12 hours.

Postexposure prophylaxis ideally should be initiated within 24 hours of exposure and continued for at least 14 days.

Typhoid Fever and Other Invasive Salmonella Infections

The usual adult oral dosage of ciprofloxacin for the treatment of mild to moderate typhoid fever is 500 mg every 12 hours for 10 days.

Although the optimum dosage and duration of therapy have not been established, oral ciprofloxacin dosages of 750 mg twice daily for 28 days have been used in adults for the treatment of chronic typhoid carriers†.

Vibrio Infections

For the treatment of cholera† caused by *Vibrio cholerae* 01 or 0139, adults have received oral ciprofloxacin in a dosage of 1 g given either as a single dose or in 2 divided doses 12 hours apart.

Perioperative Prophylaxis

If ciprofloxacin is used for perioperative prophylaxis† in high risk patients undergoing genitourinary procedures, some clinicians recommend that a single 500-mg oral dose or a single 400-mg IV dose of ciprofloxacin be given prior to the procedure. If IV ciprofloxacin is used, the dose should be given within 1–2 hours prior to the procedure or initial incision. Postoperative doses generally are unnecessary and should not be used.

Empiric Therapy in Febrile Neutropenic Patients

For empiric anti-infective therapy in febrile neutropenic patients, the manufacturer recommends that adults receive ciprofloxacin in a dosage of 400 mg IV every 8 hours for 7–14 days given in conjunction with piperacillin sodium (50 mg/kg IV every 4 hours, not to exceed 24 g/daily or 300 mg/kg daily; no longer commercially available in the US as a single-entity preparation).

● Dosage in Renal and Hepatic Impairment

Renal Impairment

Dosage adjustments may be necessary when ciprofloxacin is used in adults with renal impairment, especially those with severe impairment.

Dosage recommendations are not available for use of ciprofloxacin in pediatric patients with impaired renal function (creatinine clearances less than 50 mL/minute).

When ciprofloxacin conventional tablets or oral suspension is used in adults, modification of the usual dosage is unnecessary in patients with creatinine clearances exceeding 50 mL/minute. However, dosage should be decreased in adults with creatinine clearances of 50 mL/minute or less. (See Table 1.) The manufacturer states that a dosage of 750 mg administered at the intervals noted in Table 1 may be used with close monitoring in adults with severe infections and severe renal impairment.

TABLE 1. Dosage of Ciprofloxacin Conventional Tablets or Oral Suspension in Adults with Renal Impairment

Creatinine Clearance (mL/minute)	Dosage
>50	No dosage adjustment
30–50	250–500 mg every 12 hours
5–29	250–500 mg every 18 hours
Hemodialysis or peritoneal dialysis patients	250–500 mg once every 24 hours; give dose after dialysis

Dosage adjustments are not needed when ciprofloxacin 500-mg extended-release tablets are used for the treatment of uncomplicated UTIs (acute cystitis) in adults with renal impairment. However, a decreased dosage of 500 mg once daily is recommended when extended-release tablets are used for the treatment of complicated UTIs or acute uncomplicated pyelonephritis in adults with creatinine clearances of 30 mL/minute or less. (See Table 2.) The maximum dosage of ciprofloxacin extended-release tablets in adults undergoing hemodialysis or peritoneal dialysis (including continuous ambulatory peritoneal dialysis) is 500 mg once daily. The manufacturers state that the 1-g extended-release tablets are *not* recommended in adults who have creatinine clearances of 30 mL/minute or less or are undergoing hemodialysis or peritoneal dialysis.

TABLE 2. Dosage of Ciprofloxacin Extended-release Tablets in Adults with Renal Impairment

Creatinine Clearance (mL/minute)	Dosage
≤30 (complicated UTIs or acute uncomplicated pyelonephritis)	500 mg once daily
Hemodialysis or peritoneal dialysis patients	Give dose after dialysis period (maximum 500 mg once daily)
Continuous ambulatory peritoneal dialysis	Maximum 500 mg once daily

Dosage adjustments are not needed when IV ciprofloxacin is used in adults with creatinine clearances exceeding 30 mL/minute. However, dosage should be decreased in those with creatinine clearances less than 30 mL/minute. (See Table 3.)

TABLE 3. Dosage of IV Ciprofloxacin in Adults with Renal Impairment

Creatinine Clearance (mL/minute)	Dosage
>30	No dosage adjustment
5–29	200–400 mg every 18–24 hours

Hepatic Impairment

The manufacturers make no specific dosage recommendations for patients with impaired hepatic function. Patients with both hepatic and renal impairment should be carefully monitored.

In preliminary studies in patients with stable chronic liver cirrhosis, no clinically important changes in ciprofloxacin pharmacokinetics were observed; however, the pharmacokinetics of the drug in patients with acute hepatic insufficiency have not been fully studied.

CAUTIONS

Adverse effects reported with ciprofloxacin are similar to those reported with other fluoroquinolone anti-infectives (e.g., gemifloxacin, levofloxacin, moxifloxacin, ofloxacin). Adverse effects have been reported in 5–14% of patients receiving ciprofloxacin, and have been severe enough to require discontinuance in up to 3.5% of patients. The most frequent adverse effects of the drug include nausea, diarrhea, vomiting, abnormal liver function test results and rash.

Systemic fluoroquinolones, including ciprofloxacin, have been associated with disabling and potentially irreversible serious adverse reactions (e.g., tendinitis and tendon rupture, peripheral neuropathy, CNS effects) that can occur together in the same patient. These serious reactions may occur within hours to weeks after a systemic fluoroquinolone is initiated and have occurred in all age groups and in patients without preexisting risk factors for such adverse reactions.

● *Tendinitis and Tendon Rupture*

Systemic fluoroquinolones, including ciprofloxacin, are associated with an increased risk of tendinitis and tendon rupture in all age groups.

The risk of developing fluoroquinolone-associated tendinitis and tendon rupture is increased in older adults (usually those older than 60 years of age), individuals receiving concomitant corticosteroids, and kidney, heart, or lung transplant recipients. Other factors that may independently increase the risk of tendon rupture include strenuous physical activity, renal failure, and previous tendon disorders such as rheumatoid arthritis. However, tendinitis and tendon rupture have been reported in patients receiving fluoroquinolones who did not have any risk factors for such adverse effects.

Fluoroquinolone-associated tendinitis and tendon rupture most frequently involve the Achilles tendon and have also been reported in the rotator cuff (shoulder), hand, biceps, thumb, and other tendon sites. Tendinitis or tendon rupture can occur within hours or days after ciprofloxacin is initiated or as long as several months after completion of therapy and can occur bilaterally.

Ciprofloxacin should be discontinued immediately if pain, swelling, inflammation, or rupture of a tendon occurs.

● *Peripheral Neuropathy*

Systemic fluoroquinolones, including ciprofloxacin, have been associated with an increased risk of peripheral neuropathy.

Sensory or sensorimotor axonal polyneuropathy affecting small and/or large axons resulting in paresthesias, hypoesthesias, dysesthesias, and weakness has been reported in patients receiving systemic fluoroquinolones, including ciprofloxacin. Symptoms may occur soon after initiation of ciprofloxacin and, in some patients, may be irreversible.

Ciprofloxacin should be discontinued immediately if symptoms of peripheral neuropathy (e.g., pain, burning, tingling, numbness, and/or weakness) occur or if there are other alterations in sensations (e.g., light touch, pain, temperature, position sense, vibratory sensation).

● *CNS Effects*

Systemic fluoroquinolones, including ciprofloxacin, have been associated with an increased risk of adverse psychiatric effects, including toxic psychosis, psychotic reactions progressing to suicidal ideations/thoughts, hallucinations, paranoia, depression, self-injurious behavior such as attempted or completed suicide, anxiety, agitation, delirium, confusion, disorientation, disturbances in attention, nervousness, insomnia, nightmares, and memory impairment. These adverse effects may occur after the first dose.

Systemic fluoroquinolones, including ciprofloxacin, have been associated with an increased risk of seizures (convulsions), increased intracranial pressure (including pseudotumor cerebri), dizziness, and tremors. Ciprofloxacin, like other fluoroquinolones, is known to trigger seizures or lower the seizure threshold. Status epilepticus has been reported.

Headache, dizziness, and restlessness have been reported in 1–3% or more of patients receiving ciprofloxacin. Lightheadedness, insomnia, nightmares, hallucinations, paranoia, manic reaction, toxic psychosis, irritability, tremor, ataxia, seizures, lethargy, drowsiness, vertigo, anxiety, nervousness, agitation, confusion, weakness, malaise, phobia, depersonalization, depression, psychotic reactions, suicidal thoughts or acts, paresthesia, and increased intracranial pressure (including pseudotumor cerebri) have also been reported.

Some adverse nervous system effects of ciprofloxacin may be related to the fact that the drug, like other fluoroquinolones, is a γ-aminobutyric acid (GABA) inhibitor. In addition, it has been suggested that some CNS stimulant effects reported in patients receiving the drug may have resulted from ciprofloxacin-induced alterations in caffeine pharmacokinetics.

If psychiatric or other CNS effects occur during ciprofloxacin therapy, the drug should be discontinued immediately and appropriate measures instituted.

● Exacerbation of Myasthenia Gravis

Fluoroquinolones, including ciprofloxacin, have neuromuscular blocking activity and may exacerbate muscle weakness in individuals with myasthenia gravis. Use of fluoroquinolones in myasthenia gravis patients has resulted in requirements for ventilatory support and in death.

● Dermatologic and Sensitivity Reactions

Mild, transient rash has been reported in 1–4% and eosinophilia, pruritus, urticaria, cutaneous candidiasis, hyperpigmentation, erythema nodosum, angioedema, and edema of the face, neck, lips, conjunctivae, or hands have been reported in less than 1% of patients. Flushing, fever, and chills also have been reported in less than 1% of patients receiving the drug.

Hypersensitivity Reactions

Severe hypersensitivity reactions characterized by rash, fever, eosinophilia, jaundice, and hepatic necrosis and that were fatal have been reported rarely in patients receiving ciprofloxacin and other drugs concomitantly. Toxic epidermal necrolysis (Lyell's syndrome) also has been reported rarely in patients receiving ciprofloxacin. The possibility that these reactions were related to ciprofloxacin therapy could not be excluded. Other serious and occasionally fatal hypersensitivity (anaphylactic and anaphylactoid) reactions have occurred, some with the initial dose, in patients receiving quinolone therapy, including ciprofloxacin.

Some hypersensitivity reactions reported in patients receiving fluoroquinolones, including ciprofloxacin, have been accompanied by cardiovascular collapse, loss of consciousness, paresthesia, pharyngeal or facial edema, dyspnea, urticaria, and/or pruritus.

Other serious and sometimes fatal adverse reactions that have been reported with fluoroquinolones, including ciprofloxacin, and that may or may not be related to hypersensitivity reactions include one of more of the following: fever, rash or severe dermatologic reaction (e.g., toxic epidermal necrolysis, Stevens-Johnson syndrome); vasculitis, arthralgia, myalgia, serum sickness; allergic pneumonitis; interstitial nephritis, acute renal insufficiency or failure; hepatitis, jaundice, acute hepatic necrosis or failure; anemia (including hemolytic and aplastic anemia), thrombocytopenia (including thrombotic thrombocytopenic purpura), leukopenia, agranulocytosis, pancytopenia, and/or other hematologic abnormalities.

Ciprofloxacin should be discontinued immediately at the first appearance of rash, jaundice, or any other sign of hypersensitivity. Appropriate therapy (e.g., epinephrine, corticosteroids, maintenance of an adequate airway, oxygen, maintenance of blood pressure) should be initiated as indicated.

Photosensitivity Reactions

Moderate to severe photosensitivity/phototoxicity reactions have been reported in patients receiving fluoroquinolones, including ciprofloxacin.

Phototoxicity may manifest as exaggerated sunburn reactions (e.g., burning, erythema, exudation, vesicles, blistering, edema) on areas exposed to sun or artificial ultraviolet (UV) light (usually the face, neck, extensor surfaces of forearms, dorsa of hands).

Ciprofloxacin should be discontinued if photosensitivity or phototoxicity (sunburn-like reaction, skin eruption) occurs.

● Hepatotoxicity

Severe hepatotoxicity, including hepatic necrosis, life-threatening hepatic failure, and fatal events, has been reported in patients receiving ciprofloxacin. Most fatalities have occurred in adults older than 55 years of age.

Acute liver injury has a rapid onset (range 1–39 days) and is often associated with hypersensitivity. The pattern of injury can be hepatocellular, cholestatic, or

mixed. Temporary increase in aminotransferase or alkaline phosphatase concentrations or cholestatic jaundice may occur, especially in patients with previous liver damage.

Increased serum concentrations of AST (SGOT) and ALT (SGPT) have been reported in about 2% and increased serum concentrations of alkaline phosphatase, LDH, bilirubin, and γ-glutamyltransferase (GGT, γ-glutamyl transpeptidase, GGTP) have been reported in less than 1% of patients receiving the drug. In addition, fulminant and occasionally fatal hepatic failure has occurred rarely in patients receiving ciprofloxacin.

Ciprofloxacin should be discontinued immediately if any signs or symptoms of hepatitis (e.g., anorexia, jaundice, dark urine, pruritus, tender abdomen) occur.

● Aortic Aneurysm and Dissection

Rupture or dissection of aortic aneurysms has been reported in patients receiving systemic fluoroquinolones. Epidemiologic studies indicate an increased risk of aortic aneurysm and dissection within 2 months following use of systemic fluoroquinolones, particularly in elderly patients. The cause for this increased risk has not been identified.

If a patient reports adverse effects suggestive of aortic aneurysm or dissection, fluoroquinolone treatment should be discontinued immediately.

● Cardiovascular Effects

Prolonged QT interval leading to ventricular arrhythmias, including torsades de pointes, has been reported with some fluoroquinolones, including ciprofloxacin. Patients with known prolongation of the QT interval or with risk factors for QT interval prolongation or torsades de pointes, patients receiving drugs known to prolong the QT interval (e.g., class IA or III antiarrhythmic agents, tricyclic antidepressants, macrolides, antipsychotics), and geriatric patients may be more susceptible to drug-associated effects on the QT interval.

Palpitation, atrial flutter, ventricular ectopy, syncope, hypertension, angina pectoris, chest pain, myocardial infarction, cardiopulmonary arrest, and cerebral thrombosis have been reported in less than 1% of patients receiving ciprofloxacin.

● Hypoglycemia or Hyperglycemia

Systemic fluoroquinolones, including ciprofloxacin, have been associated with alterations in blood glucose concentrations, including symptomatic hypoglycemia and hyperglycemia. Blood glucose disturbances during fluoroquinolone therapy usually have occurred in patients with diabetes mellitus receiving an oral antidiabetic agent (e.g., glyburide) or insulin.

Severe cases of hypoglycemia resulting in coma or death have been reported with some systemic fluoroquinolones. Although most reported cases of hypoglycemic coma have involved patients with risk factors for hypoglycemia, (e.g., older age, diabetes mellitus, renal insufficiency, concomitant use of antidiabetic agents [especially sulfonylureas]), some cases have occurred in patients receiving a fluoroquinolone who were not diabetic and were not reported to be receiving an oral antidiabetic agent or insulin.

If a hypoglycemic reaction occurs, ciprofloxacin should be discontinued and appropriate therapy initiated immediately.

● GI Effects

Nausea, diarrhea, vomiting, and abdominal pain/discomfort have been reported in 1–10% of patients receiving ciprofloxacin. These effects generally are mild and transient and occur most frequently in geriatric patients and/or when high dosage is used. Anorexia, dyspepsia, flatulence, GI erosion and bleeding, dysphagia, bad taste, intestinal perforation, painful oral mucosa, and oral candidiasis have been reported in less than 1% of patients receiving the drug.

Effects on Fecal Flora

Ciprofloxacin exerts a selective effect on normal bowel flora.

Total bacterial counts of normal anaerobic fecal flora generally are unaffected during or following ciprofloxacin therapy. However, total bacterial counts of normal aerobic fecal flora are decreased within 2–5 days following initiation of therapy with the drug and generally return to pretreatment levels within 1–4 weeks after the drug is discontinued. Ciprofloxacin therapy generally markedly reduces or completely eradicates normal fecal Enterobacteriaceae; the drug reduces fecal aerobic gram-positive bacteria to a lesser extent. Ciprofloxacin therapy does not appear to affect total bacterial counts of normal salivary flora, including strepto-cocci, staphylococci, and anaerobic bacteria.

C. difficile-associated Diarrhea and Colitis

Treatment with anti-infectives alters normal colon flora and may permit over-growth of *Clostridioides difficile* (formerly known as *Clostridium difficile*.

C. difficile infection (CDI) and *C. difficile*-associated diarrhea and coli-tis (CDAD; also known as antibiotic-associated diarrhea and colitis or pseudo-membranous colitis) have been reported with nearly all anti-infectives, including ciprofloxacin, and may range in severity from mild diarrhea to fatal colitis. *C. difficile* produces toxins A and B, which contribute to the development of CDAD; hypertoxin-producing strains of *C. difficile* are associated with increased morbid-ity and mortality since they may be refractory to anti-infectives and colectomy may be required.

C. difficile generally is resistant to ciprofloxacin. When fluoroquinolones were first marketed, there appeared to be a relative lack of association between use of the drugs and CDAD and the risk of CDAD appeared to be lower than that reported with some other anti-infectives. However, there now is some evidence that increasing use of the drugs may have resulted in emergence of *C. difficile* that are more resistant and/or more virulent than previous strains. Outbreaks of severe CDAD caused by fluoroquinolone-resistant *C. difficile* have been reported in US health-care facilities with increasing frequency over the last several years. Many of these CDAD cases occurred in patients who had received a fluoroquinolone (cip-rofloxacin, gatifloxacin [no longer commercially available in the US], levofloxacin, moxifloxacin) or cephalosporin within the prior 4–6 weeks.

● Genitourinary Effects

Increased serum creatinine and BUN concentrations have occurred in about 1% of patients receiving ciprofloxacin. Interstitial nephritis, nephritis, renal failure, dysuria, polyuria, urinary retention, albuminuria, urethral bleeding, vaginitis, and acidosis have been reported in less than 1% of patients receiving the drug. In at least one patient, acute renal failure associated with interstitial nephritis occurred within about 2 weeks after initiating ciprofloxacin and appeared to be a hypersen-sitivity reaction to ciprofloxacin; renal biopsy showed marked interstitial edema, with extensive lymphocytic infiltrations and occasional eosinophils.

Crystalluria, cylindruria, and hematuria have been reported rarely in patients receiving ciprofloxacin. Crystalluria generally occurs in patients with alkaline urine who receive high dosage of the drug, and has not been associated with changes in renal function. The risk of crystal formation and crystalluria in patients receiving usual recommended dosages of the drug (250–750 mg) is low if urine pH is within the usual range (i.e., less than 6.8). Patients receiving the drug, par-ticularly at relatively high dosages, should maintain adequate fluid intake; in addi-tion, alkaline urine should be avoided. Crystalluria, sometimes associated with nephropathy, occurs in animals receiving ciprofloxacin. This may be related to the fact that ciprofloxacin has reduced solubility under alkaline conditions and the urine of test animals (e.g., rats, monkeys) is predominantly alkaline. In studies in rhesus monkeys, crystalluria (without evidence of nephropathy) has occurred after a single oral ciprofloxacin dose as low as 5 mg/kg (approximately 0.07 times the highest recommended therapeutic dosage based on body surface area [BSA]). Nephropathy did not occur when these monkeys received 6 months of IV cip-rofloxacin at a dosage of 10 mg/kg daily; however, nephropathy occurred after 6 months of therapy at a dosage of 20 mg/kg daily (approximately 0.2 times the highest recommended therapeutic dosage based on BSA).

● Musculoskeletal Effects

Arthralgia, joint or back pain, joint inflammation, joint stiffness, achiness, vascu-litis, neck or chest pain, and flare-up of gout have been reported in less than 1% of patients receiving ciprofloxacin.

An increased incidence of musculoskeletal disorders related to joints and/or surrounding tissues (e.g., arthralgia, abnormal gait, abnormal joint exam, joint sprains, leg pain, back pain, arthrosis, bone pain, myalgia, arm pain, decreased range of motion in a joint) has been reported in pediatric patients receiving cip-rofloxacin. These events usually were mild to moderate in intensity and those that occurred by week 6 usually resolved (clinical resolution of signs and symptoms) within 30 days after treatment ended.

Fluoroquinolones, including ciprofloxacin, cause arthropathies (arthrosis) in immature animals of various species. In young beagles, ciprofloxacin given in a

dosage of 100 mg/kg daily for 4 weeks caused degenerative articular changes of the knee joint; in a daily dosage of 30 mg/kg, effects on the joint were minimal, although some damage to weight-bearing joints was observed even at the lower dosage. In another study, removal of weight bearing from the joint reduced the lesions, but did not totally prevent them. In a subsequent study in young bea-gle dogs, oral ciprofloxacin in a dosage of 30 mg/kg or 90 mg/kg daily for 2 weeks (approximately 1.3 or 3.5 times the pediatric dosage based on comparative plasma AUCs) caused articular changes that were still evident on histologic evaluation after a treatment-free period of 5 months. However, a dosage of 10 mg/kg (approx-imately 0.6 times the pediatric dosage based on comparative plasma AUCs) had no effects on joints and was not associated with arthrotoxicity after an additional treatment-free period of 5 months.

Morphologic changes observed in animals with quinolone-induced arthrop-athies include erosions in joint cartilage accompanied by noninflammatory, cell-free effusion of the joint space; the cartilage is incapable of regeneration and may serve as a site for the development of arthropathy deformans. In addition, break-down products of the cartilage may irritate the synovia. The relationship of these effects in animals and the rheumatologic symptoms associated with use of cipro-floxacin in humans is unknown.

● Hematologic Effects

Eosinophilia, leukopenia, neutropenia, increased or decreased platelet count, and pancytopenia have been reported in less than 1% of patients receiving ciproflox-acin. Anemia, decreased hemoglobin, increased monocytes, leukocytosis, and bleeding diathesis have been reported in less than 1% of patients receiving the drug. In at least one patient, decreased hemoglobin was associated with GI bleed-ing, although there was no evidence of such bleeding in some other patients with hemoglobin reductions. In addition, transient acquired von Willebrand's disease has been reported rarely in patients receiving ciprofloxacin; factor VIII concen-tration returned to normal values several months (i.e., 5–6 months) following dis-continuance of the drug in these patients.

● Local Effects

Local adverse effects have been reported at the site of infusion following IV admin-istration of ciprofloxacin. These reactions generally resolve rapidly after comple-tion of the infusion and have been reported most frequently when IV infusions of the drug were given over 30 minutes or less. The manufacturers state that adverse local reactions to IV ciprofloxacin do not contraindicate subsequent IV adminis-tration of the drug, unless the reactions recur or worsen.

● Other Adverse Effects

Epistaxis, laryngeal or pulmonary edema, hiccups, hemoptysis, dyspnea, bron-chospasm, and pulmonary embolism have been reported in less than 1% of patients receiving ciprofloxacin.

Blurred vision, disturbed vision (e.g., change in color perception, overbright-ness of lights), decreased visual acuity, diplopia, and eye pain have been reported in less than 1% of patients receiving ciprofloxacin. Although reported with some other quinolones, there has been no evidence of ocular toxicity in animal studies using ciprofloxacin. Tinnitus, increased serum amylase, and increased serum uric acid concentrations have been reported rarely (i.e., in less than 0.1% of patients).

● Adverse Effects Reported when Used for Inhalational Anthrax (Postexposure)

Some information regarding the safety of ciprofloxacin for long-term postex-posure prophylaxis of anthrax are available based on use of the drug in the fall of 2001 following bioterrorism-related exposures to *Bacillus anthracis* spores. Among individuals surveyed by the US Centers for Disease Control and Pre-vention (CDC), adverse GI effects (nausea, vomiting, diarrhea, stomach pain), neurologic effects (problems sleeping, nightmares, headache, dizziness, lighthead-edness), and musculoskeletal effects (muscle or tendon pain and joint swelling or pain) were reported more frequently than in controlled clinical studies eval-uating the drug for other indications. This higher incidence in the absence of a control group could be the result of report bias, concurrent medical conditions, other concomitant drug therapy, emotional stress or other confounding factors, and/or the long duration of ciprofloxacin treatment required for prophylaxis. In response to a questionnaire given to 490 such individuals in Florida on approxi-mately day 7 or 14 of anti-infective prophylaxis, 19% sought medical attention for any anti-infective related adverse effect or reported one or more of the following: pruritus, breathing problems, or swelling of the face, neck, or throat. Although the percentage of patients in this subgroup who received ciprofloxacin versus other anti-infectives was not reported, 86% of all patients (i.e., those who did or did not answer the questionnaire) received ciprofloxacin and 80% continued to receive prophylaxis beyond 14 days.

In an epidemiologic evaluation in 8424 postal workers who were offered 60 days of prophylaxis for anthrax and given a questionnaire in New Jersey, New York City, and the District of Columbia on days 7–10 of anti-infective prophylaxis, 5819 completed or were administered the questionnaire, of whom 3863 had initiated prophylaxis (3428 with ciprofloxacin). Of the ciprofloxacin-treated individuals, 19% reported severe nausea, vomiting, diarrhea, and/or abdominal pain; 14% reported fainting, lightheadedness, and/or dizziness; 7% reported heartburn or acid reflux; 6% reported rash, urticaria, or/or pruritus; and 8% discontinued therapy with the drug (3% for adverse effects, 1% for fear of developing an adverse effect, and 1% because they were confused about the need). Only 2% of those on any anti-infective sought medical attention for possible manifestations of anaphylaxis, none of whom required hospitalization.

● Precautions and Contraindications

Ciprofloxacin is contraindicated in patients with a history of hypersensitivity to the drug, other quinolones, or any ingredient in the formulation.

Systemic fluoroquinolones, including ciprofloxacin, have been associated with disabling and potentially irreversible serious adverse reactions (e.g., tendinitis and tendon rupture, peripheral neuropathy, CNS effects) that can occur together in the same patient. These serious reactions may occur within hours to weeks after a systemic fluoroquinolone is initiated and have occurred in all age groups and in patients without preexisting risk factors for such adverse reactions. Patients receiving ciprofloxacin should be informed about these serious adverse reactions and advised to immediately discontinue ciprofloxacin and contact a clinician if they experience any signs or symptoms of serious adverse effects (e.g., unusual joint or tendon pain, muscle weakness, a "pins and needles" tingling or pricking sensation, numbness of the arms or legs, confusion, hallucinations) while taking the drug. Systemic fluoroquinolones, including ciprofloxacin, should be avoided in patients who have experienced any of the serious adverse reactions associated with fluoroquinolones.

Because fluoroquinolones, including ciprofloxacin, are associated with an increased risk of tendinitis and tendon rupture in all age groups, patients receiving ciprofloxacin should be informed of this potentially irreversible adverse effect and the drug should be discontinued immediately if pain, swelling, inflammation, or rupture of a tendon occurs. The risk of developing fluoroquinolone-associated tendinitis and tendon rupture is increased in adults older than 60 years of age, individuals receiving concomitant corticosteroids, and kidney, heart, or lung transplant recipients. Patients should be advised to rest and refrain from exercise at the first sign of tendinitis or tendon rupture (e.g., pain, swelling, or inflammation of a tendon or weakness or inability to use a joint) and advised to immediately discontinue the drug and contact a clinician. Systemic fluoroquinolones, including ciprofloxacin, should be avoided in patients who have a history of tendon disorders or have experienced tendinitis or tendon rupture.

Because fluoroquinolones, including ciprofloxacin, are associated with an increased risk of peripheral neuropathy, ciprofloxacin should be discontinued immediately if symptoms of peripheral neuropathy (e.g., pain, burning, tingling, numbness, and/or weakness) occur or if there are other alterations in sensations (e.g., light touch, pain, temperature, position sense, vibratory sensation) and/or motor strength since this may minimize development of an irreversible condition. Patients receiving ciprofloxacin should be advised that peripheral neuropathies have been reported in patients receiving systemic fluoroquinolones, including ciprofloxacin, and that symptoms may occur soon after initiation of therapy and, in some patients, may be irreversible. Patients should be advised of the importance of immediately discontinuing the drug and contacting a clinician if such symptoms occur. Systemic fluoroquinolones, including ciprofloxacin, should be avoided in patients who have experienced peripheral neuropathy.

Because fluoroquinolones, including ciprofloxacin, have been associated with an increased risk of adverse CNS effects, ciprofloxacin should be used with caution in epileptic patients, in patients with known or suspected CNS disorders that predispose to seizures or lower the seizure threshold (e.g., severe cerebral arteriosclerosis, history of convulsions, reduced cerebral blood flow, altered brain structure, stroke), and in the presence of other risk factors that predispose to seizures

or lower the seizure threshold (e.g., certain drug therapies, renal dysfunction). Patients should be informed that seizures have been reported in patients receiving ciprofloxacin and advised to inform their clinician of any history of seizures before initiating therapy with the drug. Because increased intracranial pressure has been reported, patients receiving ciprofloxacin should be advised to notify their clinician if persistent headache (with or without blurred vision) occurs. Patients receiving ciprofloxacin also should be advised that ciprofloxacin may cause dizziness or lightheadedness and cautioned not to engage in activities requiring mental alertness and motor coordination (e.g., driving or operating machinery) until they experience how the drug affects them. If seizures or other CNS effects occur, ciprofloxacin should be discontinued immediately and appropriate measures instituted. Systemic fluoroquinolones, including ciprofloxacin, should be avoided in patients who have experienced CNS effects associated with fluoroquinolones.

Ciprofloxacin should be avoided in patients with a known history of myasthenia gravis since fluoroquinolones may exacerbate myasthenia gravis symptoms. Patients should be advised of the importance of informing their clinician of any history of myasthenia gravis. Patients also should be advised to immediately contact a clinician if any symptoms of muscle weakness, including respiratory difficulties, occur.

Because severe hepatotoxicity, including acute hepatitis and fatalities, has been reported in patients receiving ciprofloxacin, the drug should be discontinued immediately if any sign or symptom of hepatitis (e.g., anorexia, jaundice, dark urine, pruritus, tender abdomen) occurs. Patients should be advised to contact their clinician if any sign or symptom of hepatotoxicity (e.g., loss of appetite, nausea, vomiting, fever, weakness, tiredness, right upper quadrant tenderness, itching, yellowing of skin or eyes, light colored bowel movements, dark colored urine) occurs.

Because an increased risk of aortic aneurysm and dissection has been reported with systemic fluoroquinolones, ciprofloxacin should not be used in patients who have an aortic aneurysm or are at increased risk for an aortic aneurysm unless there are no other treatment options. This includes elderly patients and patients with peripheral atherosclerotic vascular disease, hypertension, or certain genetic conditions (e.g., Marfan syndrome, Ehlers-Danlos syndrome). Patients should be informed that systemic fluoroquinolones may increase the risk of aortic aneurysm and dissection and of the importance of informing their clinician of any history of aneurysms, blockages or hardening of the arteries, high blood pressure, or genetic conditions such as Marfan syndrome or Ehlers-Danlos syndrome. Patients receiving ciprofloxacin should be advised to seek immediate medical treatment if they experience sudden, severe, and constant pain in the stomach, chest, or back.

Because prolongation of the QT interval has been reported in patients receiving ciprofloxacin, the drug should be avoided in patients with known prolongation of the QT interval or with risk factors for QT interval prolongation or torsades de pointes (e.g., congenital long QT syndrome, uncorrected electrolyte imbalance such as hypokalemia or hypomagnesemia, cardiac disease such as heart failure, myocardial infarction, or bradycardia). Ciprofloxacin also should be avoided in patients receiving drugs known to prolong the QT interval, including class IA antiarrhythmic agents (quinidine, procainamide), class III antiarrhythmic agents (amiodarone, sotalol), tricyclic antidepressants, macrolides, and antipsychotics. Patients should be advised of the importance of informing their clinician of a personal or family history of QT interval prolongation or proarrhythmic conditions (e.g., hypokalemia, bradycardia, recent myocardial ischemia) or current therapy with any class IA (e.g., quinidine, procainamide) or class III (amiodarone, sotalol) antiarrhythmic agents; patients should be advised to contact their clinician if any symptoms of prolongation of QT interval, including prolonged heart palpitations or loss of consciousness, occur.

Blood glucose concentrations should be carefully monitored when systemic fluoroquinolones, including ciprofloxacin, are used in patients with diabetes mellitus receiving antidiabetic agents. Patients should be informed that hypoglycemia has been reported when systemic fluoroquinolones were used in some patients receiving antidiabetic agents. Patients with diabetes mellitus receiving oral antidiabetic agents or insulin should be advised to discontinue ciprofloxacin and contact a clinician if they experience hypoglycemia or symptoms of hypoglycemia. Appropriate therapy should be initiated immediately.

Ciprofloxacin inhibits cytochrome P-450 (CYP) isoenzyme 1A2, and concomitant use with drugs metabolized by this enzyme (e.g., clozapine, methylxanthines [e.g., caffeine, theophylline], olanzapine, ropinirole, tizanidine) may result in increased plasma concentrations of the concomitant drug and could lead to clinically important adverse effects. Because of an increased risk of adverse effects, ciprofloxacin is contraindicated in patients receiving tizanidine. Concomitant use with theophylline should be avoided since serious and sometimes fatal reactions (e.g., cardiac arrest, seizures, status epilepticus, respiratory failure) have occurred in patients receiving the drugs concomitantly. In addition, concomitant use of ciprofloxacin and other drugs metabolized by CYP1A2 should be avoided or requires particular caution.

Sensitivity Reactions

Ciprofloxacin, like other quinolones, can cause serious, potentially fatal hypersensitivity reactions, occasionally following the initial dose. Patients receiving ciprofloxacin should be advised of this possibility and instructed to immediately discontinue the drug and contact a clinician at the first sign of rash, hives, other skin reaction, jaundice, rapid heartbeat, difficulty swallowing or breathing, any swelling suggesting angioedema (e.g., swelling of lips, tongue, or face; tightness of throat; hoarseness), or any other sign of hypersensitivity. Serious anaphylactic reactions require immediate emergency treatment with epinephrine and other resuscitation measures (e.g., oxygen, IV fluids, IV antihistamines, corticosteroids, pressor amines, airway management such as intubation) as indicated.

Because photosensitivity/phototoxicity reactions have been reported with fluoroquinolones, unnecessary or excessive exposure to sunlight or artificial UV light (sunlamps, tanning beds, UVA/UVB treatment) should be avoided during ciprofloxacin therapy. If the patient needs to be outdoors, they should use sunscreen and wear a hat and clothing that protects skin from sun exposure. Patients should be advised to discontinue ciprofloxacin and contact a clinician if photosensitivity or phototoxicity (sunburn-like reaction, skin eruption) occurs.

Selection and Use of Anti-infectives

Ciprofloxacin should be used for the treatment of acute bacterial sinusitis, acute bacterial exacerbations of chronic bronchitis, or uncomplicated urinary tract infections (UTIs) *only* when no other treatment options are available. Because ciprofloxacin, like other systemic fluoroquinolones, has been associated with disabling and potentially irreversible serious adverse reactions (e.g., tendinitis and tendon rupture, peripheral neuropathy, CNS effects) that can occur together in the same patient, the risks of serious adverse reactions outweigh the benefits of ciprofloxacin for patients with these infections.

To reduce development of drug-resistant bacteria and maintain effectiveness of ciprofloxacin and other antibacterials, the drug should be used only for the treatment or prevention of infections proven or strongly suspected to be caused by susceptible bacteria.

Patients should be advised that antibacterials (including ciprofloxacin) should only be used to treat bacterial infections and not used to treat viral infections (e.g., the common cold). Patients also should be advised about the importance of completing the full course of therapy, even if feeling better after a few days, and that skipping doses or not completing therapy may decrease effectiveness and increase the likelihood that bacteria will develop resistance and will not be treatable with ciprofloxacin or other antibacterials in the future.

When selecting or modifying anti-infective therapy, use results of culture and in vitro susceptibility testing. In the absence of such data, consider local epidemiology and susceptibility patterns when selecting anti-infectives for empiric therapy. Culture and susceptibility testing performed periodically during therapy provides information on the therapeutic effect of the anti-infective agent and the possible emergence of bacterial resistance.

Information on test methods and quality control standards for in vitro susceptibility testing of antibacterial agents and specific interpretive criteria for such testing recognized by FDA is available at https://www.fda.gov/STIC.

Superinfection/C. difficile-associated Diarrhea and Colitis

As with other anti-infectives, use of ciprofloxacin may result in overgrowth of nonsusceptible organisms, especially enterococci or *Candida*. Resistant strains of some organisms (e.g., *Pseudomonas aeruginosa*, staphylococci) have developed during ciprofloxacin therapy. Careful monitoring of the patient and periodic in vitro susceptibility tests are essential.

Because CDAD has been reported with the use of nearly all anti-infectives, including ciprofloxacin, it should be considered in the differential diagnosis in patients who develop diarrhea during or after ciprofloxacin therapy. Careful medical history is necessary since CDAD has been reported to occur as late as 2 months or longer after anti-infective therapy is discontinued.

If CDAD is suspected or confirmed, anti-infective therapy not directed against *C. difficile* should be discontinued as soon as possible. Patients should be managed with appropriate anti-infective therapy directed against *C. difficile* (e.g., vancomycin, fidaxomicin, metronidazole), supportive therapy (e.g., fluid and electrolyte management, protein supplementation), and surgical evaluation as clinically indicated.

Patients should be advised that diarrhea is a common problem caused by anti-infectives and usually ends when the drug is discontinued; however, it is important to contact a clinician if watery and bloody stools (with or without stomach cramps and fever) occur during or as late as 2 months or longer after the last dose.

Other Precautions and Contraindications

Crystalluria has been reported rarely in patients receiving ciprofloxacin. Although crystalluria is not expected to occur under usual conditions with the usual recommended dosages of the drug, patients should be instructed to drink sufficient quantities of fluids to ensure proper hydration and adequate urinary output during ciprofloxacin therapy. Measures also should be taken to avoid alkaline urine.

Ciprofloxacin has *not* been shown to be effective in the treatment of syphilis. Because use of anti-infectives given in high dosage for short periods of time to treat gonorrhea may mask or delay symptoms of incubating syphilis, serologic tests for syphilis should be performed at the time of diagnosis of gonorrhea. If ciprofloxacin is used for the treatment of gonorrhea, follow-up serologic tests for syphilis should be performed 3 months after gonorrhea treatment is completed.

Doses and/or frequency of administration of ciprofloxacin should be decreased in patients with severe renal impairment since serum concentrations of the drug are higher and prolonged in these patients compared with patients with normal renal function.

● Pediatric Precautions

Ciprofloxacin, like other fluoroquinolones, is associated with arthropathy and histopathologic changes in weight-bearing joints of juvenile animals. Oral ciprofloxacin caused lameness in immature dogs; histologic evaluation of the weight-bearing joints of these dogs revealed permanent lesions of the cartilage. When used in pediatric patients younger than 18 years of age, ciprofloxacin has been associated with an increased rate of adverse effects involving joints and/or surrounding tissue (e.g., tendons) compared with comparator anti-infectives.

The manufacturers state that ciprofloxacin (IV, conventional tablets, oral suspension) should be used in pediatric patients younger than 18 years of age *only* for the treatment of complicated UTIs and pyelonephritis caused by susceptible *Escherichia coli*, inhalational anthrax (postexposure), and treatment and prophylaxis of plague. However, the American Academy of Pediatrics (AAP) and other experts (e.g., the American Heart Association [AHA], Infectious Diseases Society of America [IDSA]) state that use of fluoroquinolones in pediatric patients younger than 18 years of age also may be justified in certain other infections (e.g., endocarditis, multidrug-resistant gram-negative infections). Parents should be advised to inform their child's clinician if the child has a history of joint-related problems present before ciprofloxacin is initiated or if such problems occur during or after therapy with the drug.

Ciprofloxacin extended-release tablets should *not* be used in children and adolescents younger than 18 years of age since safety and efficacy of the extended-release preparation have *not* been established for any indication in pediatric patients.

● Urinary Tract Infections

Ciprofloxacin (IV, conventional tablets, oral suspension) is labeled by FDA for the treatment of complicated UTIs and pyelonephritis caused by susceptible *E. coli* in pediatric patients 1–17 years of age. However, ciprofloxacin is not considered a drug of first choice for these infections in pediatric patients because an increased incidence of adverse effects has been reported in such patients. In clinical studies evaluating IV or oral ciprofloxacin for the treatment of complicated UTIs and pyelonephritis in pediatric patients 1–17 years of age, the rate of adverse effects (including events related to joints and/or surrounding tissues) occurring during 6 weeks of follow-up was 9.3% in those receiving ciprofloxacin compared with 6% in those receiving a cephalosporin. The rate of adverse effects occurring at any time up to 1 year was 13.7% or 9.5%, respectively and the rate of all adverse effects (regardless of drug relationship) at 6 weeks was 41 or 31%, respectively.

● Anthrax

Ciprofloxacin (IV, conventional tablets, oral suspension) is labeled by FDA for inhalational anthrax (postexposure) to reduce the incidence or progression of disease following exposure to aerosolized *Bacillus anthracis* spores in pediatric patients from birth to 17 years of age. The manufacturers state that risk-benefit assessment indicates that use of ciprofloxacin is appropriate for this indication in pediatric patients. AAP states that ciprofloxacin is a drug of choice for postexposure prophylaxis of anthrax in pediatric patients. Because of potential adverse effects from prolonged use of ciprofloxacin in pediatric patients and because postexposure prophylaxis should be continued for 60 days following exposures to aerosolized *B. anthracis* spores that occur in the context of biologic warfare or bioterrorism, the postexposure prophylaxis regimen can be changed to oral amoxicillin or oral penicillin V if penicillin susceptibility is confirmed.

AAP states that oral ciprofloxacin is a drug of choice for the treatment of cutaneous anthrax without systemic involvement† in pediatric patients. Because of potential adverse effects from prolonged use of ciprofloxacin in pediatric patients and because a treatment duration of 60 days is recommended when cutaneous anthrax occurs following exposures to aerosolized *B. anthracis* spores that occur in the context of biologic warfare or bioterrorism, the treatment regimen can be changed to oral amoxicillin or oral penicillin V if penicillin susceptibility is confirmed.

IV ciprofloxacin also is considered a drug of choice for use in multiple-drug parenteral regimens for initial treatment of systemic anthrax† (inhalational, GI, meningitis, or cutaneous with systemic involvement, extensive edema, or head or neck lesions) that occurs in the context of biologic warfare or bioterrorism. Because of potential adverse effects from prolonged use of ciprofloxacin in pediatric patients, IV penicillin G or IV ampicillin can replace IV ciprofloxacin in the multiple-drug regimen if penicillin susceptibility is confirmed.

● Plague

Ciprofloxacin (IV, conventional tablets, oral suspension) is labeled by FDA for treatment of plague, including pneumonic and septicemic plague, and for prophylaxis of plague in pediatric patients from birth to 17 years of age. The manufacturers state that risk-benefit assessment indicates that use of ciprofloxacin is appropriate for this indication in pediatric patients.

● Other Infections

Some clinicians suggest that quinolones may be used cautiously in adolescents if skeletal growth is complete, and that the potential benefits of ciprofloxacin therapy may outweigh the possible risks in certain children 9–18 years of age with serious infections when the causative organism is resistant to other available anti-infectives.

AAP states that use of a systemic fluoroquinolone may be justified in children younger than 18 years of age in certain specific circumstances when there are no safe and effective alternatives and the drug is known to be effective. AAP states that use of fluoroquinolones may be justified in pediatric patients when parenteral therapy is not practical and no other safe and effective oral agent is available or when the pediatric patient has an infection caused by a multidrug-resistant organism (e.g., *Pseudomonas*, *Mycobacterium*) for which there is no safe and effective alternative. Therefore, in addition to use after exposure to aerosolized *B. anthracis* (to decrease the incidence or progression of the disease), other possible uses of fluoroquinolones in pediatric patients include the treatment of urinary tract infections caused by *Ps. aeruginosa* or other multidrug-resistant gram-negative bacteria, infections caused by multidrug-resistant *Streptococcus pneumoniae*, chronic suppurative otitis media or malignant otitis externa caused by *Ps. aeruginosa*, chronic or acute osteomyelitis or osteochondritis caused by *Ps. aeruginosa* or other multidrug-resistant gram-negative bacteria known to be susceptible to fluoroquinolones and resistant to other alternatives, mycobacterial infections caused by isolates known to be susceptible to fluoroquinolones, gram-negative bacterial infections in immunocompromised patients when oral therapy is desired or when the causative agent is resistant to other alternatives, GI infections known or suspected to be caused by multidrug-resistant *Shigella*, *Salmonella*, *Vibrio cholerae*, or *Campylobacter*, or serious infections caused by fluoroquinolone-susceptible pathogens in pediatric patients with severe allergy to alternative anti-infectives.

● Geriatric Precautions

Retrospective analysis of 23 multiple-dose controlled clinical studies evaluating ciprofloxacin in over 3500 patients revealed that 25% of patients included in these studies were 65 years of age or older and 10% were 75 years of age or older. In a large, prospective, randomized study evaluating use of ciprofloxacin extended-release tablets for treatment of complicated UTIs, 49% of patients were 65 years of age or older and 30% were 75 years of age or older. Although no overall differences in safety or efficacy were observed between geriatric individuals and younger adults in these studies and other clinical experience revealed no evidence of age-related differences, the possibility that some older patients may exhibit increased sensitivity to the drug cannot be ruled out.

The risk of fluoroquinolone-associated tendon disorders, including tendon rupture, is increased in geriatric adults older than 60 years of age. This risk is further increased in those receiving concomitant corticosteroids. Ciprofloxacin should be used with caution in geriatric adults, especially those receiving concomitant corticosteroids.

The risk of prolonged QT interval leading to ventricular arrhythmias may be increased in geriatric patients. Ciprofloxacin should be used with caution in those receiving concurrent therapy with drugs that can prolong the QT interval (e.g., class IA or III antiarrhythmic agents) or those with risk factors for torsades de pointes (e.g., known QT prolongation, uncorrected hypokalemia).

The risk of fluoroquinolone-associated aortic aneurysm and dissection may be increased in geriatric patients.

Ciprofloxacin is substantially eliminated by the kidney, and the risk of adverse reactions may be greater in patients with impaired renal function. Although dosage of ciprofloxacin does not need to be modified in individuals older than 65 years of age with normal renal function, the greater frequency of decreased renal function observed in the elderly should be considered and dosage carefully selected in geriatric patients; monitoring renal function may be useful in these patients.

● Mutagenicity and Carcinogenicity

Ciprofloxacin was not mutagenic in vivo in the rat hepatocyte DNA repair assay or dominant lethal or micronucleus tests in mice. Although ciprofloxacin was positive for mutagenicity in vitro in the mouse lymphoma cell forward mutation assay and rat hepatocyte DNA repair assay, the drug was not mutagenic in other in vitro studies, including the *Salmonella* microsome test, mouse lymphoma cell forward mutation assay, *Escherichia coli* DNA repair assay, Chinese hamster V-79 cell HGPRT test, Syrian hamster embryo cell transformation assay, *Saccharomyces cerevisiae* point mutation assay, and *S. cerevisiae* mitotic crossover and gene conversion assay.

In 2-year carcinogenicity studies in rats or mice, there was no evidence of carcinogenic or tumorigenic potential with oral ciprofloxacin in a dosage of 250 or 750 mg/kg daily (equivalent to approximately 2 or 3 times, respectively, a human dosage of 1 g daily based on BSA).

● Pregnancy, Fertility, and Lactation

Pregnancy

There are no adequate and controlled studies to date using ciprofloxacin in pregnant women. Because ciprofloxacin, like most other fluoroquinolones, causes arthropathy in immature animals, the drug should *not* be used in pregnant women unless potential benefits justify potential risks to the fetus and mother.

CDC states that oral ciprofloxacin is the preferred drug for initial anti-infective postexposure prophylaxis in pregnant and postpartum women following a suspected or confirmed exposure to aerosolized *B. anthracis* spores in the context of biologic warfare or bioterrorism. CDC also states that oral ciprofloxacin is the preferred drug for treatment of uncomplicated cutaneous anthrax and IV ciprofloxacin is the preferred bactericidal component of a multiple-drug regimen for treatment of systemic anthrax in pregnant and postpartum women when such infections occur in the context of biologic warfare or bioterrorism.

An expert review of published data regarding clinical experience with use of ciprofloxacin during pregnancy concluded that therapeutic doses of the drug during pregnancy are unlikely to pose a substantial teratogenic risk, but that data are insufficient to state that there is no risk. Although some safety data are available from several postmarketing epidemiology studies involving short-term, first-trimester exposures to ciprofloxacin, these studies are insufficient to evaluate the risk for less common defects or to permit reliable and definitive conclusions regarding the safety of ciprofloxacin in pregnant women and their developing fetuses. In one controlled prospective observational study of 200 women exposed to fluoroquinolones during pregnancy (68% were first-trimester exposures,

52.5% of exposures involved ciprofloxacin), in utero exposure to fluoroquino-lones during embryogenesis did not appear to be associated with an increased risk of major congenital malformations (incidence was 2.2% in the fluoroquino-lone group and 2.6% in the control group; background incidence is 1–5%). There also was no evidence of increases in the rates of spontaneous abortion, prema-turity, or low birthweight and no clinically important increase in musculoske-tal dysfunction in the ciprofloxacin-exposed children followed to 1 year of age. In another prospective follow-up study that included 549 pregnancies with fluoro-quinolone exposure (93% were first-trimester exposures, 70 first-trimester expo-sures involved ciprofloxacin), there was no increase in the rates of spontaneous abortion, prematurity, or low birthweight, and the malformation rate was similar to the background incidence rate with no evidence of any specific patterns of con-genital abnormalities.

Reproduction studies in rats and mice using oral ciprofloxacin dosages up to 100 mg/kg (0.6 and 0.3 times, respectively, the maximum daily human dosage of 1 g based on BSA) have not revealed evidence of harm to the fetus. In rabbits, oral ciprofloxacin dosages of 30 and 100 mg/kg (approximately 0.4 and 1.3 times, respectively, the highest recommended therapeutic dosage based on BSA) caused GI toxicity resulting in maternal weight loss and an increased incidence of abor-tion, but there was no evidence of teratogenicity. IV ciprofloxacin given to rabbits at dosages up to 20 mg/kg (approximately 0.3 times the highest recommended therapeutic dosage based on BSA) has not resulted in maternal toxicity, embryo-toxicity, or teratogenicity.

● Fertility

Fertility studies in rats using oral ciprofloxacin dosages up to 100 mg/kg (equiva-lent to the highest recommended daily human dose of 1 g based on BSA) did not reveal evidence of impaired fertility.

Administration of high dosages (100 mg/kg daily) of some quinolones (e.g., norfloxacin [no longer commercially available in the US], pefloxacin [not commer-cially available in the US] and pipemidic acid [not commercially available in the US]) has been associated with impaired spermatogenesis and/or testicular dam-age (atrophy in rats and dogs) in chronic (for 3 months or longer) toxicity studies.

Lactation

Ciprofloxacin is distributed into milk, but the amount of the drug absorbed by a nursing infant is unknown. Because of the potential for serious adverse effects of ciprofloxacin (including articular damage) in nursing infants, a decision should be made whether to discontinue nursing or the drug, taking into account the importance of the drug to the woman.

AAP considers ciprofloxacin to be usually compatible with breast-feeding since the amount of the fluoroquinolone potentially absorbed by nursing infants would be small and no observable change in infants associated with such expo-sure has been reported to date.

CDC states that recommendations for use of ciprofloxacin in breast-feeding women for postexposure prophylaxis following a suspected or confirmed expo-sure to aerosolized *B. anthracis* spores in the context of biologic warfare or bio-terrorism and for treatment of uncomplicated cutaneous anthrax or systemic anthrax in such situations are the same as those for other adults.

DRUG INTERACTIONS

● Drugs Metabolized by Hepatic Microsomal Enzymes

Ciprofloxacin inhibits cytochrome P-450 (CYP) isoenzyme 1A2. Concomitant use with CYP1A2 substrates (e.g., clozapine, methylxanthines [e.g., caffeine, the-ophylline], olanzapine, ropinirole, tizanidine) may result in increased plasma con-centrations and increased pharmacologic or adverse effects of the concomitant drug.

● Drugs that Prolong the QT Interval

Concomitant use of ciprofloxacin and drugs known to prolong the QT interval, including class IA antiarrhythmics (e.g., quinidine, procainamide), class III anti-arrhythmics (e.g., amiodarone, sotalol), tricyclic antidepressants, macrolides, and antipsychotics, may result in additive effects on QT interval prolongation. Con-comitant use with these drugs should be avoided; if concomitant use is necessary, caution is advised.

● Antacids

Antacids containing magnesium, aluminum, or calcium decrease absorption of oral ciprofloxacin, resulting in decreased serum and urine concentrations of the anti-infective agent. Ciprofloxacin bioavailability may be decreased by as much as 90% and serum ciprofloxacin concentrations generally are decreased by 14–50% in patients receiving an antacid concomitantly; anti-infective treatment fail-ure may occur as a result of reduced quinolone absorption in these patients. The mechanism of this interaction has not been fully elucidated to date, but magne-sium, aluminum, and other divalent ions may bind to, and form insoluble com-plexes with, quinolones in the GI tract.

The manufacturers state that ciprofloxacin conventional tablets, extended-release tablets, or oral suspension should be administered at least 2 hours before or 6 hours after antacids containing magnesium or aluminum. Some clinicians suggest that patients be instructed not to ingest antacids containing magnesium, aluminum, or calcium concomitantly with or within 2–4 hours of a ciprofloxa-cin dose; however, other clinicians state that these antacids should *not* be used in patients receiving ciprofloxacin and that ciprofloxacin probably should not be used in patients with renal failure who require aluminum hydroxide or aluminum carbonate for intestinal binding of phosphate.

● Aminoglycosides

The antibacterial activities of ciprofloxacin and aminoglycosides have been addi-tive or synergistic in vitro against some strains of Enterobacteriaceae and *Pseudo-monas aeruginosa*. However, synergism between the drugs is unpredictable, and indifference generally occurs when ciprofloxacin is used in conjunction with ami-kacin, gentamicin, or tobramycin against *Ps. aeruginosa* or Enterobacteriaceae. Indifference also generally occurs when the drug is used in conjunction with tobramycin against *Acinetobacter*.

● Antiarrhythmic Agents

Use ciprofloxacin with caution in those receiving concurrent therapy with drugs that can prolong the QT interval (e.g., class IA or III antiarrhythmic agents).

● Anticoagulants

Initiation of oral ciprofloxacin therapy in patients stabilized on warfarin has resulted in prolongation of the prothrombin time; hematemesis occurred in at least 1 patient. The mechanism of this interaction has not been determined to date, but ciprofloxacin may displace the anticoagulant from serum albumin bind-ing sites. The risk may vary with the underlying infection, age, and general status of the patient so that the contribution of ciprofloxacin to the increase in interna-tional normalized ratio (INR) is difficult to assess.

Ciprofloxacin should be used with caution in patients receiving warfarin, and prothrombin time and international normalized ratio (INR) should be monitored frequently during and shortly after concomitant therapy.

● Antidiabetic Agents

Concomitant use of ciprofloxacin and oral antidiabetic agents (e.g., sulfonylurea agents such as glimepiride or glyburide) has resulted in hypoglycemia, presum-ably by potentiating the glucose-lowering effect of the antidiabetic agent. Severe hypoglycemia and some fatalities have been reported.

Ciprofloxacin should be used with caution in patients receiving oral antidiabetic agents, and blood glucose concentrations should be monitored. Patients receiving an oral antidiabetic agent and ciprofloxacin concomitantly should be advised to contact their clinician if low blood glucose occurs during ciprofloxacin therapy so that the clinician can determine whether the anti-infective should be changed.

● Antimuscarinics

Although the clinical importance has not been determined and further study is needed to evaluate the interactions, concomitant administration of antimusca-rinics (e.g., pirenzepine, scopolamine) delays GI absorption of the anti-infective.

● Bismuth Subsalicylate

Concomitant administration of a single dose of oral bismuth subsalicylate (428 mg) and a single dose of oral ciprofloxacin (750 mg) results in a slight decrease in peak plasma concentrations and area under the concentration-time curve (AUC) of ciprofloxacin, but this is not considered clinically important.

● Clindamycin

The combination of ciprofloxacin and clindamycin has been synergistic in vitro against many strains of *Peptostreptococcus*, *Lactobacillus*, and *B. fragilis* tested.

● Corticosteroids

Concomitant use of corticosteroids increases the risk of severe tendon disorders (e.g., tendinitis, tendon rupture), especially in geriatric patients older than 60 years of age.

● Clozapine

Concomitant use of ciprofloxacin (250 mg) and clozapine (304 mg) for 7 days increased serum concentrations of clozapine and *N*-desmethylclozapine by 29 and 31%, respectively, potentially resulting in adverse effects.

Clozapine and ciprofloxacin should be used concomitantly with caution; patients should be carefully monitored for clozapine adverse effects during and shortly after concomitant therapy and appropriate clozapine dosage adjustments made.

● Cyclosporine

Concomitant use of cyclosporine and ciprofloxacin may result in transient increases in serum creatinine. Acute renal failure occurred within 4 days after initiation of ciprofloxacin in a patient receiving cyclosporine maintenance therapy. The mechanism of this potential interaction has not been elucidated, but could involve synergistic nephrotoxic effects of the drugs and/or interference of cyclosporine metabolism by ciprofloxacin.

Cyclosporine and ciprofloxacin should be used concomitantly with caution and renal function (especially serum creatinine concentrations) should be monitored.

● Didanosine

Concomitant use of oral ciprofloxacin and buffered didanosine preparations (pediatric oral solution admixed with antacid) may decrease absorption of ciprofloxacin resulting in decreased serum and urine concentrations of the quinolone.

The manufacturers state that ciprofloxacin conventional tablets, extended-release tablets, or oral suspension should be administered at least 2 hours before or 6 hours after buffered didanosine preparations.

● Duloxetine

Concomitant use of duloxetine and potent CYP1A2 inhibitors may result in increased mean peak concentrations and AUC of duloxetine. Although clinical data are not available regarding a possible interaction between duloxetine and ciprofloxacin, similar effects on duloxetine exposure can be expected if duloxetine and ciprofloxacin are administered concomitantly.

Concomitant use of duloxetine and ciprofloxacin should be avoided. If concomitant use cannot be avoided, patients should be monitored for duloxetine toxicity.

● Histamine H₂-receptor Antagonists

Histamine H_2-receptor antagonists do not appear to have a clinically important effect on bioavailability of ciprofloxacin. Concomitant cimetidine or ranitidine does not appear to alter GI absorption of ciprofloxacin.

● Iron, Multivitamins, and Mineral Supplements

Oral multivitamin and mineral supplements containing divalent or trivalent cations such as calcium, iron, or zinc may interfere with oral absorption of ciprofloxacin resulting in decreased serum and urine concentrations of the quinolone. Therefore, these multivitamins and/or mineral supplements should not be ingested concomitantly with ciprofloxacin.

The manufacturers state that ciprofloxacin conventional tablets, extended-release tablets, or oral suspension should be administered at least 2 hours before or 6 hours after preparations containing calcium, iron, or zinc.

● β-Lactam Antibiotics

An additive or synergistic effect has occurred occasionally in vitro against some strains of *Ps. aeruginosa* and *Ps. maltophilia* when ciprofloxacin was used concomitantly with an extended-spectrum penicillin (e.g., mezlocillin [not commercially available], piperacillin). Indifference generally occurs when ciprofloxacin is used in conjunction with an extended-spectrum penicillin against Enterobacteriaceae.

Ciprofloxacin used in conjunction with imipenem, cefoxitin, or a cephalosporin (e.g., cefotaxime, ceftazidime) has been reported to be additive or synergistic against some strains of *Ps. aeruginosa* or Enterobacteriaceae; however, these combinations generally are indifferent rather than additive or synergistic against these bacteria. Although the clinical importance has not been determined, ciprofloxacin used in conjunction with cefotaxime in vitro resulted in a synergistic effect against many strains of *Bacteroides fragilis* tested; antagonism did not occur.

● Lanthanum Carbonate

Concomitant administration of lanthanum carbonate may decrease GI absorption of ciprofloxacin and result in a substantial decrease in serum and urine concentrations of the anti-infective agent.

The manufacturers state that ciprofloxacin conventional tablets, extended-release tablets, or oral suspension should be administered at least 2 hours before or 6 hours after lanthanum carbonate.

● Lidocaine

Concomitant use of IV lidocaine hydrochloride (1.5 mg/kg) and ciprofloxacin (500 mg twice daily) increased the peak concentrations and AUC of lidocaine by 12 and 26%, respectively. Although lidocaine treatment was well tolerated at this elevated exposure, a possible interaction with ciprofloxacin and increase in lidocaine-associated adverse effects should be considered if the drugs are used concomitantly.

● Methotrexate

Concomitant use of ciprofloxacin and methotrexate may result in increased plasma concentrations of methotrexate (as the result of renal tubular transport inhibition) and may increase the risk of methotrexate-associated toxic reactions.

Methotrexate and ciprofloxacin should be used concomitantly with caution; patients should be carefully monitored.

● Metoclopramide

Although bioavailability of ciprofloxacin does not appear to be affected, concomitant use of metoclopramide reportedly accelerates the rate of GI absorption of ciprofloxacin resulting in a shorter time to peak plasma concentrations of the drug.

● Metronidazole

Concomitant use of metronidazole and ciprofloxacin does not affect serum concentrations of either drug.

● Nonsteroidal Anti-inflammatory Agents

Concomitant use of ciprofloxacin and a nonsteroidal anti-inflammatory agent (NSAIA) could increase the risk of CNS stimulation (e.g., seizures). In preclinical studies and during postmarketing experience, concomitant use of ciprofloxacin and very high doses of an NSAIA (except aspirin) provoked seizures. Animal studies suggest that the risk may vary depending on the specific NSAIA.

NSAIAs and ciprofloxacin should be used concomitantly with caution.

● Omeprazole

Concomitant administration of a single 500-mg conventional tablet of ciprofloxacin and omeprazole (20 mg once daily for 4 days) resulted in a 16% decrease in mean peak concentration and AUC of ciprofloxacin. Concomitant administration of ciprofloxacin extended-release tablets (single 1-g dose) and omeprazole (40 mg once daily for 3 days) in healthy individuals reduced peak plasma concentrations and AUC of ciprofloxacin by 23 and 20%, respectively. The clinical importance of this interaction has not been determined.

● Phenytoin

Concomitant use of ciprofloxacin and phenytoin has resulted in altered serum concentrations of phenytoin (increased or decreased).

Phenytoin and ciprofloxacin should be used concomitantly with caution. To avoid loss of seizure control and prevent adverse effects associated with phenytoin overdosage, phenytoin serum concentrations should be monitored during and shortly after concomitant therapy with ciprofloxacin.

● Phosphodiesterase Type 5 Inhibitors

Concomitant use of a single oral dose of sildenafil (50 mg) with ciprofloxacin (500 mg) in healthy individuals increased the mean peak concentration and AUC of sildenafil approximately twofold.

Sildenafil and ciprofloxacin should be used concomitantly with caution; patients should be monitored for sildenafil toxicity.

● Probenecid

Concomitant administration of probenecid interferes with renal tubular secretion of ciprofloxacin, resulting in a 50% decrease in renal clearance of ciprofloxacin, a 50% increase in systemic ciprofloxacin concentrations, and a prolonged serum half-life of the drug. This effect may potentiate ciprofloxacin toxicity.

Probenecid and ciprofloxacin should be used concomitantly with caution.

● Rifampin

Concomitant use of oral ciprofloxacin (750 mg twice daily) and oral rifampin (300 mg twice daily) does not appear to affect the pharmacokinetics of either drug.

In vitro, the combination of ciprofloxacin and rifampin generally is indifferent against S. aureus; however, antagonism also has been reported rarely.

● Ropinirole

Concomitant use of oral ciprofloxacin (500 mg twice daily) and oral ropinirole (6 mg daily) has resulted in 60 and 84% increases in peak concentrations and AUC of ropinirole, respectively.

Ropinirole and ciprofloxacin should be used concomitantly with caution; patients should be monitored for ropinirole-associated adverse effects during and shortly after concomitant therapy and ropinirole dosage adjustments should be made as necessary.

● Sevelamer

Concomitant administration of sevelamer may decrease GI absorption of ciprofloxacin and result in a substantial decrease in serum and urine concentrations of the anti-infective agent.

The manufacturers state that ciprofloxacin conventional tablets, extended-release tablets, or oral suspension should be administered at least 2 hours before or 6 hours after sevelamer.

● Sucralfate

Concomitant sucralfate, presumably because of its aluminum content, decreases GI absorption of ciprofloxacin and may result in a substantial (50–90%) decrease in serum concentrations of the anti-infective agent.

The manufacturers state that ciprofloxacin extended-release tablets, conventional tablets, or oral suspension should be administered at least 2 hours before or 6 hours after sucralfate.

● Tizanidine

Concomitant use of tizanidine (single dose of 4 mg) and ciprofloxacin (500 mg twice daily for 3 days) increased peak serum concentrations and AUC of tizanidine by sevenfold and tenfold, respectively.

Concomitant use of ciprofloxacin and tizanidine is contraindicated because the hypotensive and sedative effects of tizanidine are potentiated.

● Vancomycin

Synergism does not occur in vitro when ciprofloxacin is used in conjunction with vancomycin against Staphylococcus epidermidis, S. aureus (including methicillin-resistant S. aureus), Corynebacterium, or Listeria monocytogenes.

● Xanthine Derivatives

Theophyllines

Concomitant administration of ciprofloxacin in patients receiving a theophylline derivative may result in higher and prolonged serum theophylline concentrations

and may increase the risk of theophylline-related adverse effects. Alterations in theophylline pharmacokinetics have shown considerable interindividual variation, with serum theophylline concentrations reportedly increasing by 17–254% and theophylline clearance decreasing by 18–112% following initiation of ciprofloxacin. Generally, however, reductions in theophylline clearance induced by ciprofloxacin have averaged 20–35%. Alterations in theophylline pharmacokinetics may be related to inhibition of metabolism in the liver by the 4-oxo metabolites of these quinolones. However, the potential contribution of the 4-oxo metabolites to this interaction has not been fully elucidated, and there is some evidence that, while formation of these metabolites may correlate with inhibition of theophylline metabolism, the 4-oxo metabolites themselves may not be responsible for the observed inhibition. Theophyllines do not appear to affect the pharmacokinetics of quinolones. However, there is limited in vitro evidence that theophyllines may potentiate quinolone-induced inhibition of γ-aminobutyric acid (GABA), thus possibly potentiating CNS stimulation.

Serious and sometimes fatal reactions (e.g., cardiac arrest, seizures, status epilepticus, respiratory failure) have occurred in patients receiving ciprofloxacin and theophylline concomitantly. Death in at least one patient was associated with seizures and atrial fibrillation during concomitant therapy with the drugs. Other adverse reactions reported during concomitant therapy with the drugs include nausea, vomiting, dizziness, headache, tremor, restlessness, agitation, irritability, confusion, hallucinations, tachycardia, and palpitations. These adverse effects apparently occurred as the result of increased serum theophylline concentrations. While similar effects also have been reported in theophylline-treated patients who were not receiving ciprofloxacin concomitantly, the possibility that such toxicity may have been potentiated by ciprofloxacin cannot be excluded.

Concomitant use of ciprofloxacin and a theophylline derivative should be avoided, if possible, because of the risk of toxicity (e.g., CNS or other adverse effects) associated with increased plasma concentrations of theophylline. If concomitant use of theophylline and ciprofloxacin cannot be avoided, plasma theophylline concentrations should be monitored, the patient observed for manifestations of theophylline toxicity, and appropriate theophylline dosage adjustments made as needed, especially in geriatric patients. The need for theophylline dosage adjustment also should be considered when ciprofloxacin is discontinued since subtherapeutic concentrations may occur.

Caffeine

Ciprofloxacin inhibits formation of paraxanthine after caffeine administration, resulting in increased serum concentrations, reduced clearance, and prolonged elimination half-life of caffeine.

Caffeine and ciprofloxacin should be used concomitantly with caution. Patients receiving ciprofloxacin should be advised that regular consumption of large quantities of coffee, tea, or caffeine-containing soft drinks or drugs during therapy with the anti-infective may result in exaggerated or prolonged effects of caffeine. If excessive cardiac or CNS stimulation (e.g., nervousness, insomnia, anxiety, tachycardia) occurs, caffeine intake should be restricted. In addition, caffeine intake should be restricted during ciprofloxacin therapy in patients at risk of adverse effects from CNS or cardiac stimulation.

Pentoxifylline

Concomitant use of pentoxifylline and ciprofloxacin results in increased serum concentrations, reduced clearance, and prolonged elimination half-life of pentoxifylline. Ciprofloxacin and pentoxifylline should be used concomitantly with caution; patients should be monitored for xanthine toxicity and dosage adjusted as necessary.

● Zolpidem

Concomitant use of zolpidem and ciprofloxacin may increase serum concentrations of zolpidem and is not recommended.

LABORATORY TEST INTERFERENCES

● Tests for Urinary Glucose

Ciprofloxacin hydrochloride does not interfere with urinary glucose determinations using cupric sulfate solution (e.g., Benedict's solution, Clinitest®) or with glucose oxidase tests (e.g., Diastix®, Tes-Tape®).

ACUTE TOXICITY

The oral LD_{50} of the drug is greater than 5 g/kg in mice and rats and approximately 2.5 g/kg in rabbits. In mice, rats, rabbits, and dogs, substantial toxicity (including tonic/clonic convulsions) was observed with IV ciprofloxacin doses between 125 and 300 mg/kg.

Reversible renal toxicity has been reported in some cases of acute overdosage of ciprofloxacin. If acute oral overdosage of the drug occurs, the stomach should be emptied by inducing emesis or by gastric lavage; administration of antacids containing magnesium, aluminum, or calcium may reduce oral absorption of ciprofloxacin. If the patient is comatose, having seizures, or lacks the gag reflex, gastric lavage may be performed if an endotracheal tube with cuff inflated is in place to prevent aspiration of gastric contents. Supportive and symptomatic treatment should be initiated. The patient should be observed carefully; renal function and urinary pH should be monitored and the urine acidified if needed. Adequate hydration must be maintained to minimize the risk of crystalluria.

Only a small amount of ciprofloxacin (less than 10%) is removed by hemodialysis or peritoneal dialysis. Some clinicians suggest that the risks associated with hemodialysis or peritoneal dialysis do not justify their possible benefits in ciprofloxacin overdosage.

MECHANISM OF ACTION

Ciprofloxacin usually is bactericidal in action. Like other fluoroquinolone anti-infectives, ciprofloxacin inhibits DNA synthesis in susceptible organisms via inhibition of the enzymatic activities of 2 members of the DNA topoisomerase class of enzymes, DNA gyrase and topoisomerase IV. DNA gyrase and topoisomerase IV have distinct essential roles in bacterial DNA replication. DNA gyrase, a type II DNA topoisomerase, was the first identified quinolone target; DNA gyrase is a tetramer composed of 2 GyrA and 2 GyrB subunits. DNA gyrase introduces negative superhelical twists in DNA, an activity important for initiation of DNA replication. DNA gyrase also facilitates DNA replication by removing positive super helical twists. Topoisomerase IV, another type II DNA topoisomerase, is composed of 2 ParC and 2 ParE subunits. DNA gyrase and topoisomerase IV are structurally related; ParC is homologous to GyrA and ParE is homologous to GyrB. Topoisomerase IV acts at the terminal states of DNA replication by allowing for separation of interlinked daughter chromosomes so that segregation into daughter cells can occur. Fluoroquinolones inhibit these topoisomerase enzymes by stabilizing either the DNA—DNA gyrase complex or the DNA—topoisomerase IV complex; these stabilized complexes block movement of the DNA replication fork and thereby inhibit DNA replication resulting in cell death.

Although all fluoroquinolones generally are active against both DNA gyrase and topoisomerase IV, the drugs differ in their relative activities against these enzymes. For many gram-negative bacteria, DNA gyrase is the primary quinolone target and for many gram-positive bacteria, topoisomerase IV is the primary target; the other enzyme is the secondary target in both cases. However, there are exceptions to this pattern. For certain bacteria (e.g., *Streptococcus pneumoniae*), the principal target depends on the specific fluoroquinolone.

The mechanism by which ciprofloxacin's inhibition of DNA gyrase or topoisomerase IV results in death in susceptible organisms has not been fully determined. Unlike β-lactam anti-infectives, which are most active against susceptible bacteria when they are in the logarithmic phase of growth, studies using *Escherichia coli* and *Pseudomonas aeruginosa* indicate that ciprofloxacin can be bactericidal during both logarithmic and stationary phases of growth; this effect does not appear to occur with gram-positive bacteria (e.g., *Staphylococcus aureus*). In vitro studies indicate that ciprofloxacin concentrations that approximate the minimum inhibitory concentration (MIC) of the drug induce filamentation in susceptible organisms; high concentrations of the drug result in enlarged or elongated cells that may not be extensively filamented. Although the bactericidal effect of some fluoroquinolones evidently requires competent RNA and protein synthesis in the bacterial cell, and concurrent use of anti-infectives that affect protein synthesis (e.g., chloramphenicol, tetracyclines) or RNA synthesis (e.g., rifampin) inhibit the in vitro bactericidal activity of these drugs, the bactericidal effect of ciprofloxacin is only partially reduced in the presence of these anti-infectives. This suggests that ciprofloxacin has an additional mechanism of action that is independent of RNA and protein synthesis.

For most susceptible organisms, the minimum bactericidal concentration (MBC) of ciprofloxacin is 1–4 times higher than the minimum inhibitory concentration (MIC), although the MBC occasionally may be 8 times higher.

Mammalian cells contain type II topoisomerase similar to that contained in bacteria. At concentrations attained during therapy, quinolones do not appear to affect the mammalian enzyme, presumably because it functions differently than bacterial DNA gyrase and does not cause supercoiling of DNA.

Although the clinical importance has not been determined, ciprofloxacin appears to have a postantibiotic inhibitory effect against most susceptible aerobic organisms. The duration of the postantibiotic inhibitory effect and the ciprofloxacin concentration required to produce the effect vary depending on the organism; the duration of this effect also varies according to length of exposure to the drug, increasing with increased exposure. In vitro studies in Mueller-Hinton broth using *S. aureus*, Enterobacteriaceae, and *Ps. aeruginosa* exposed for 1–2 hours to ciprofloxacin concentrations several times higher than the MIC indicate that there is a recovery period of about 1–6 hours before these organisms resume growth after the drug is removed. Equivocal results have been observed following in vitro exposure of *Enterococcus faecalis* (formerly *Streptococcus faecalis*) to the drug, and it is unclear whether the drug exerts a postantibiotic inhibitory effect against this organism.

In vitro studies, particularly those involving in vitro susceptibility tests, indicate that the antibacterial activity of ciprofloxacin is decreased in the presence of urine, especially acidic urine. The clinical importance of this in vitro effect has not been determined to date; however, because ciprofloxacin concentrations attained in urine are usually substantially higher than ciprofloxacin MICs for most urinary tract pathogens, the effect probably is not clinically important. The antibacterial activity of ciprofloxacin also is decreased slightly in unbuffered peritoneal dialysis fluid with a pH of 5.5 compared with its activity in dialysis fluid buffered to a pH of 7.4.

SPECTRUM

Ciprofloxacin has a spectrum of activity similar to that of some other fluoroquinolones (e.g., ofloxacin). In vitro on a weight basis, the activity of ciprofloxacin is approximately equal to or slightly greater than that of ofloxacin against most susceptible organisms.

Ciprofloxacin is active in vitro against most gram-negative aerobic bacteria, including Enterobacteriaceae and *Pseudomonas aeruginosa*. Ciprofloxacin also is active in vitro against many gram-positive aerobic bacteria, including penicillinase-producing, nonpenicillinase-producing, and methicillin-resistant staphylococci (also known as oxacillin-resistant staphylococci), although many strains of streptococci are relatively resistant to the drug. The drug generally is less active against gram-positive than gram-negative bacteria. Ciprofloxacin has some activity in vitro against obligately anaerobic bacteria, but many of these organisms are considered resistant to the drug. The drug also has some activity in vitro against *Chlamydia*, *Mycoplasma*, *Mycobacterium*, *Plasmodium*, and *Rickettsia*. Ciprofloxacin is inactive against fungi.

● *In Vitro Susceptibility Testing*

Like those of other fluoroquinolones, results of ciprofloxacin in vitro susceptibility tests are affected by the pH of the media and the presence of certain cations (e.g., magnesium). There generally is little effect when the pH of the media is 6–8; however, minimum inhibitory concentrations (MICs) are at least 4–16 times greater when the pH of the media is less than 6. It has been suggested that ionization of the 7-piperazine group as pH decreases may interfere with access or binding to the drug's target enzyme.

Ciprofloxacin MICs also are increased when high concentrations of magnesium are present in the media. The mechanism by which magnesium interferes with the antibacterial activity of ciprofloxacin is unclear, but it has been suggested that this cation may form complexes with the drug which may prevent access or binding to its target enzyme. Presence of calcium or zinc does not appear to affect results of ciprofloxacin susceptibility tests.

Inoculum size generally does not affect in vitro susceptibility to ciprofloxacin. MICs for most organisms are only 2–4 times greater when the size of the inoculum is increased from 10^2 to 10^8 colony-forming units (CFU) per mL; however, in some studies, an inoculum effect did occur with some strains of

Enterobacteriaceae or *Pseudomonas aeruginosa* and MIC and minimum bactericidal concentration (MBC) of the drug appeared to be equally affected by increased inoculum size. Presence of serum generally has no effect on results of ciprofloxacin in vitro susceptibility tests, but reportedly may slightly decrease MICs of the drug for some organisms.

MICs of ciprofloxacin are higher when susceptibility tests are performed in pooled urine or urine agar rather than in nutrient broth or Mueller-Hinton media. The MIC of ciprofloxacin for *Escherichia coli* is less than 0.01 mcg/mL in Mueller-Hinton broth at pH 7.4, but is 1.6 mcg/mL in urine at pH 7.5 or 6.5 and 3.1 mcg/mL in urine at pH 5.5. The decreased antibacterial activity in the presence of urine probably occurs because of low pH and because urine contains a higher concentration of magnesium ions than nutrient broth or Mueller-Hinton media.

MICs of ciprofloxacin are increased when activated charcoal is present in the media.

When in vitro susceptibility testing is performed according to the standards of the Clinical and Laboratory Standards Institute (CLSI; formerly National Committee for Clinical Laboratory Standards [NCCLS]), clinical isolates identified as *susceptible* to ciprofloxacin are inhibited by drug concentrations usually achievable when the recommended dosage is used for the site of infection. Clinical isolates classified as *intermediate* have minimum inhibitory concentrations (MICs) that approach usually attainable blood and tissue concentrations and response rates may be lower than for strains identified as susceptible. Therefore, the intermediate category implies clinical applicability in body sites where the drug is physiologically concentrated or when a higher than usual dosage can be used. This intermediate category also includes a buffer zone that should prevent small, uncontrolled technical factors from causing major discrepancies in interpretation, especially for drugs with narrow pharmacotoxicity margins. If results of in vitro susceptibility testing indicate that a clinical isolate is *resistant* to ciprofloxacin, the strain is not inhibited by drug concentrations generally achievable with usual dosage schedules and/or MICs fall in the range where specific microbial resistance mechanisms are likely and clinical efficacy of the drug against the isolate has not been reliably demonstrated in clinical studies.

Results of ciprofloxacin susceptibility tests should not be used to predict susceptibility to other fluoroquinolones.

● Gram-positive Aerobic Bacteria

Gram-positive Aerobic Cocci

Ciprofloxacin is active in vitro against most strains of *Staphylococcus aureus*, *S. epidermidis*, *S. saprophyticus*, and *S. hemolyticus*. The drug is active against both penicillinase-producing and nonpenicillinase-producing staphylococci, and also is active in vitro against some methicillin-resistant strains, although to a lesser degree than against methicillin-susceptible strains. Ciprofloxacin is less active in vitro on a weight basis against streptococci than against staphylococci. *Streptococcus pneumoniae*, *S. pyogenes* (group A β-hemolytic streptococci), *S. agalactiae* (group B streptococci), and viridans streptococci generally are inhibited in vitro by ciprofloxacin concentrations of 4 mcg/mL or less. Groups C, F, and G streptococci and nonenterococcal group D streptococci are inhibited in vitro by ciprofloxacin concentrations of 16 mcg/mL or less. Ciprofloxacin is active in vitro against some strains of enterococci, including *Enterococcus faecalis* (formerly *S. faecalis*). The drug is more active in vitro against *E. faecalis* than against *E. faecium* or *E. durans* (formerly *S. faecium* and *S. durans*, respectively). Ciprofloxacin is bactericidal in vitro against enterococci and is active against some strains of *E. faecalis* resistant to penicillin combined with an aminoglycoside.

Gram-positive Aerobic Bacilli

Ciprofloxacin is active in vitro against *Bacillus anthracis*, and naturally occurring isolates have been inhibited in vitro by ciprofloxacin concentrations of 0.03–0.25 mcg/mL. The MIC of the drug reported for the strain of *B. anthracis* used in a study in the rhesus monkey model of inhalational anthrax was 0.08 mcg/mL. Results of in vitro susceptibility testing of 11 *B. anthracis* isolates that were associated with cases of inhalational or cutaneous anthrax that occurred in the US (Florida, New York, District of Columbia) during September and October 2001 in the context of an intentional release of anthrax spores (biologic warfare, bioterrorism) indicate that these strains had ciprofloxacin MICs of 0.06 mcg/mL or less. Based on interpretive criteria established for staphylococci, these strains are considered susceptible to ciprofloxacin. Anti-infectives are active against the germinated form of *B. anthracis* but are not active against the organism while it is still in the spore form. Strains of *B. anthracis* with naturally occurring resistance

to ciprofloxacin have not been reported to date. However, reduced susceptibility to ofloxacin (4-fold increase in MICs from baseline) has been produced in vitro following sequential subculture of the Sterne strain of *B. anthracis* in subinhibitory concentrations of the fluoroquinolone. There are published reports of *B. anthracis* strains that have been engineered to have tetracycline and penicillin resistance as well as resistance to other anti-infectives (e.g., macrolides, chloramphenicol, rifampin).

Ciprofloxacin is active in vitro against *Corynebacterium*. The MIC$_{90}$ of the drug reported for JK strains of *Corynebacterium* and *Corynebacterium* D2 is 0.5–1 mcg/mL.

Ciprofloxacin is active in vitro against *Listeria monocytogenes*, and the MIC$_{90}$ of the drug reported for this organism is 0.25–2 mcg/mL.

The MIC$_{90}$ of ciprofloxacin for *Nocardia asteroides* is 8–16 mcg/mL; these organisms generally are considered resistant to the drug.

● Gram-negative Aerobic Bacteria

Neisseria

Ciprofloxacin is active in vitro against some strains of penicillinase- and nonpenicillinase-producing *Neisseria gonorrhoeae* and *N. gonorrhoeae* with chromosomally mediated resistance to penicillin (CMRNG) or plasmid-mediated tetracycline resistance (TRNG). The MIC$_{90}$ of ciprofloxacin is 0.002–0.05 mcg/mL for most penicillinase- or nonpenicillinase-producing *N. gonorrhoeae*, CMRNG, and TRNG. However, strains of *N. gonorrhoeae* with decreased susceptibility to ciprofloxacin and other fluoroquinolones have been reported with increasing frequency.

Ciprofloxacin is active in vitro against *N. meningitidis*, and the MIC$_{90}$ of the drug for this organism usually is 0.004–0.06 mcg/mL.

Haemophilus

Ciprofloxacin is active in vitro against β-lactamase- and non-β-lactamase-producing *Haemophilus influenzae*, and the MIC$_{90}$ of the drug for these organisms is 0.008–0.05 mcg/mL. Ciprofloxacin is active in vitro against strains of β-lactamase-producing *H. influenzae* that are resistant to chloramphenicol. The MIC$_{90}$ of ciprofloxacin for *H. parainfluenzae* and *H. ducreyi* is 0.03 mcg/mL.

Moraxella catarrhalis

Ciprofloxacin is active in vitro against both β-lactamase- and non-β-lactamase-producing strains of *Moraxella catarrhalis*, and the MIC$_{90}$ of the drug reported for this organism is 0.015–0.64 mcg/mL.

Enterobacteriaceae

Ciprofloxacin is active in vitro against most clinically important Enterobacteriaceae, and the MIC$_{90}$ of the drug for most of these organisms is 1 mcg/mL or less. While ciprofloxacin is active against *Shigella dysenteriae* type 1, the MIC of the drug for this strain generally is several-fold higher than for other *Shigella* strains. Ciprofloxacin is active in vitro against some Enterobacteriaceae resistant to aminoglycosides and/or β-lactam antibiotics.

Pseudomonas

Ciprofloxacin is active in vitro against most strains of *Ps. aeruginosa* and also has some activity against some other *Pseudomonas*. The MIC$_{50}$ and MIC$_{90}$ of ciprofloxacin for *Ps. aeruginosa* are 0.06–1 and 0.03–4 mcg/mL, respectively. Ciprofloxacin is active in vitro against some strains of *Ps. aeruginosa* that are resistant to aminoglycosides, extended-spectrum penicillins, and cephalosporins. The MIC$_{90}$ of the drug for *Ps. fluorescens* and *Ps. putida* is 0.25–4 mcg/mL; however, the MIC$_{90}$ for *Ps. cepacia* (*Burkholderia cepacia*), *Stenotrophomonas maltophilia* (formerly *Xanthomonas* or *Ps. maltophilia*), and *Ps. pseudomallei* is 0.05–16 mcg/mL and many of these organisms are considered resistant to the drug.

Vibrio

Ciprofloxacin is active in vitro against *Vibrio cholerae* (*V. cholerae* 01 and 0139), *V. parahaemolyticus*, and *V. vulnificus*. The MIC$_{90}$ of the drug reported for *Vibrio* is 0.003–0.25 mcg/mL.

Other Gram-negative Aerobic Bacteria

The MIC$_{90}$ of ciprofloxacin for *Acinetobacter lwoffi* (*A. calcoaceticus* subsp. *lwoffi*) and *A. baumannii* (*A. calcoaceticus* subsp. *anitratus*) is 0.125–4 mcg/mL.

Aeromonas hydrophila, A. caviae, A. sobria, and *Plesiomonas shigelloides* generally are inhibited in vitro by ciprofloxacin concentrations of 0.1 mcg/mL or less. The MIC$_{90}$ of ciprofloxacin reported for *Alcaligenes,* including *A. faecalis,* is 1.4–12.5 mcg/mL.

Ciprofloxacin is active in vitro against strains of *Campylobacter coli, C. fetus,* and *Helicobacter pylori.* The MIC$_{90}$ of the drug for some strains of *Campylobacter fetus* subsp. *jejuni,* an organism that can be microaerophilic or anaerobic, is 0.12–0.62 mcg/mL. The MIC$_{90}$ of the drug reported for *H. pylori* is 0.25–0.5 mcg/mL, and the MIC$_{90}$ for *C. coli* is 0.39 mcg/mL. However, fluoroquinolone-resistant strains of *Campylobacter* have been reported in areas with widespread use or prolonged therapy with the drugs.

Brucella melitensis, Pasteurella multocida, Eikenella corrodens, and *Flavobacterium* generally are inhibited by ciprofloxacin concentrations of 0.01–1 mcg/mL.

Ciprofloxacin has in vitro activity against *Francisella tularensis.* In one study evaluating susceptibility of *F. tularensis* isolated from humans and animals, the MIC of ciprofloxacin for this organism was 0.016 mcg/mL.

Ciprofloxacin has in vitro activity against *Yersinia pestis.* In a study of *Y. pestis* isolates obtained from plague patients, rats, or fleas from Vietnam, the organism was inhibited in vitro by ciprofloxacin concentrations of 0.008–0.062 mcg/mL. In one in vitro study, the MBC of ciprofloxacin against intracellular *Y. pestis* was similar to or slightly higher than the MBC of the drug against extracellular *Y. pestis.* Ciprofloxacin has been shown to have in vivo activity against *Y. pestis* in murine plague infections. However, mutant strains of *Y. pestis* resistant to ciprofloxacin have been selected in vitro.

Some strains of *Gardnerella vaginalis* (formerly *Haemophilus vaginalis*) are inhibited in vitro by ciprofloxacin concentrations of 0.5–8 mcg/mL.

The MIC$_{90}$ of ciprofloxacin reported for *Legionella pneumophila, L. bozemanii, L. dumoffii, L. gormanii, L. jordanis, L. longbeachae, L. micdadei* (the Pittsburgh pneumonia agent), and *L. wadsworthii* is 0.01–0.5 mcg/mL.

● Anaerobic Bacteria

Ciprofloxacin has some activity against gram-positive and gram-negative anaerobic bacteria; however, high concentrations of the drug generally are required for in vitro inhibition and many of these organisms are considered resistant to the drug. The MIC$_{90}$ of ciprofloxacin for *Actinomyces, Bifidobacterium, Peptococcus,* and *Peptostreptococcus* is 0.5–8 mcg/mL. Some strains of *Clostridium perfringens* may be inhibited in vitro by ciprofloxacin concentrations of 0.5–1 mcg/mL, but most other *Clostridium* require ciprofloxacin concentrations of 4–32 mcg/mL or greater for in vitro inhibition and are considered resistant to the drug. The MIC$_{90}$ for *Eubacterium* is 1–16 mcg/mL.

The MIC$_{90}$ of ciprofloxacin for *Propionibacterium acnes* and *Veillonella* is 0.12–4 mcg/mL, and the MIC$_{90}$ for *Fusobacterium* is 2–16 mcg/mL. Although some strains of *Bacteroides* are susceptible to ciprofloxacin, most strains are considered resistant to the drug. The MIC$_{90}$ of ciprofloxacin for *Bacteroides fragilis* is 0.8–32 mcg/mL. The MIC$_{90}$ of ciprofloxacin for *B. melaninogenicus, B. ovatus, B. uniformis,* and *B. ureolyticus* is 0.25–16 mcg/mL and the MIC$_{90}$ of the drug for *B. distasonis, B. oralis* (*Prevotella oralis*), *B. thetaiotaomicron,* and *B. vulgatus* generally is 16–64 mcg/mL.

● Chlamydia and Mycoplasma

Ciprofloxacin has some in vitro activity against *Chlamydophila pneumoniae* (formerly *Chlamydia pneumoniae*), *Chlamydia trachomatis,* and *C. psittaci,* and these organisms generally are inhibited in vitro by concentrations of 0.5–5 mcg/mL. The MBC of ciprofloxacin reported for *C. trachomatis* is 1–10 mcg/mL.

The MIC$_{90}$ of ciprofloxacin reported for *Mycoplasma hominis* and *M. pneumoniae* is 0.5–2 mcg/mL. In some studies, the MIC$_{90}$ of ciprofloxacin for *Ureaplasma urealyticum* was 2–6.3 mcg/mL; however, in other studies, this organism was resistant to the drug since the MIC$_{90}$ was 32 mcg/mL and the MBC was greater than 64 mcg/mL.

● Mycobacterium

Ciprofloxacin is active in vitro against some *Mycobacterium.* In vitro on a weight basis, ciprofloxacin is less active than levofloxacin or moxifloxacin against these organisms. The MIC$_{90}$ of ciprofloxacin for *M. tuberculosis* is 0.1–3.1 mcg/mL.

Other mycobacteria usually are less susceptible to ciprofloxacin. The MIC$_{90}$ for *M. fortuitum, M. kansasii, M. smegmatis,* and *M. xenopi* is 0.05–8 mcg/mL.

The MIC$_{90}$ for *M. avium* complex, *M. abscessus,* and *M. chelonae* generally is 1–16 mcg/mL; most strains of *M. abscessus* and *M. chelonae* are considered resistant to ciprofloxacin.

Ciprofloxacin exhibited weak activity against *M. leprae* in an in vitro metabolic screen for potential antileprosy agents that measured intracellular ATP of the bacteria, and no more than a limited bacteriostatic effect in an in vivo mouse footpad study in mice receiving up to 150 mg/kg of the drug daily.

● Other Organisms

Ciprofloxacin has some activity in vitro against *Plasmodium falciparum.* In some studies, the drug appeared to be active against both chloroquine-susceptible and -resistant strains of the organism. However, in other studies, chloroquine-resistant strains required high concentrations of the drug for in vitro inhibition. When in vitro activity of ciprofloxacin was assessed using incorporation of radiolabeled hypoxanthine by the organism, the ID$_{50}$ (concentration of the drug required to inhibit hypoxanthine uptake by 50%) of ciprofloxacin for chloroquine-susceptible *P. falciparum* was 3.2 mcg/mL and the ID$_{50}$ of the drug for chloroquine-resistant strains was 6.6 mcg/mL.

Ciprofloxacin reportedly has some activity in vitro against *Rickettsia conorii,* the causative organism of Mediterranean spotted fever. In one study, the MIC of the drug for this organism was 0.5 mcg/mL.

Although further study is needed, results of one study indicate that ciprofloxacin may have some activity in vitro against *Leptospira interrogans.*

RESISTANCE

Resistance to ciprofloxacin can be produced in vitro in some organisms, including some strains of Enterobacteriaceae, *Pseudomonas aeruginosa, Staphylococcus aureus,* and *Enterococcus faecalis* (formerly *Streptococcus faecalis*), by serial passage in the presence of increasing concentrations of the drug. Ciprofloxacin resistance resulting from spontaneous mutation occurs rarely in vitro (i.e., with a frequency of 10^{-9} to 10^{-7}).

The mechanism(s) of resistance to fluoroquinolones, including ciprofloxacin, has not been fully elucidated but appears to involve mutations in the target DNA type II topoisomerase enzymes and mutations that result in alterations in membrane permeability and/or efflux pumps. Current evidence suggests that resistance to ciprofloxacin or other fluoroquinolones usually is chromosomally rather than plasmid mediated.

Resistant strains of *Ps. aeruginosa* have emerged occasionally during therapy with the drug.

Ciprofloxacin-resistant strains of *S. aureus,* including methicillin-resistant strains of *S. aureus* (MRSA; also known as oxacillin-resistant *S. aureus* or ORSA), and *S. epidermidis* also have emerged during therapy with the drug. Strains of *S. aureus,* especially oxacillin-resistant *S. aureus* resistant to ciprofloxacin and other fluoroquinolones have been reported with increasing frequency, and such strains can emerge at relatively rapid rates (e.g., increasing within an institution from 0% of isolates prior to introduction of the drug to 80% 1 year later for oxacillin-resistant *S. aureus*).

Rapid emergence of resistance to fluoroquinolones in *Campylobacter* also has been reported and appears to be associated with widespread use or prolonged therapy with the drugs. Over a 10- to 12-year period in Finland, fluoroquinolone-resistant strains of *C. jejuni* and *C. coli* increased from 0–4% to 9–11%. A similar increase was observed over a 7-year period in *Campylobacter* isolates obtained from poultry and humans in the Netherlands; this increase in resistance was attributed to use of enrofloxacin in the poultry industry. In the US, fluoroquinolone-resistant isolates of *Campylobacter* have been obtained from raw turkey or chicken products in the retail market.

S. typhi and *S. paratyphi* with reduced susceptibility to ciprofloxacin have been reported. *Salmonella* resistant to fluoroquinolones are common in India and southeast Asia.

● Resistance in Mycobacterium

Ciprofloxacin-resistant *Mycobacterium tuberculosis* have been reported and some multidrug-resistant strains (i.e., strains resistant to rifampin and isoniazid) also are resistant to ciprofloxacin or other fluoroquinolones. Extensively drug-resistant tuberculosis (XDR tuberculosis) caused by strains resistant to rifampin and isoniazid (multiple-drug resistant strains) and also resistant to a fluoroquinolone and at least one parenteral second-line antimycobacterial (capreomycin, kanamycin, amikacin) has been reported with increasing frequency.

Ciprofloxacin-resistant strains of initially susceptible *M. fortuitum* have developed in a few patients who received ciprofloxacin alone or in conjunction with amikacin. Many strains of *M. kansasii* are resistant to ciprofloxacin.

● Resistance in Neisseria gonorrhoeae

Neisseria gonorrhoeae with decreased susceptibility to ciprofloxacin and other fluoroquinolones (quinolone-resistant *N. gonorrhoeae*; QRNG) are widely disseminated throughout the world, including in the US. QRNG have ciprofloxacin MICs of 1 mcg/mL or greater; isolates with intermediate resistance to fluoroquinolones have ciprofloxacin MICs of 0.12–0.5 mcg/mL. Strains of *N. gonorrhoeae* with decreased susceptibility to ciprofloxacin also have decreased susceptibility to other fluoroquinolones (e.g., levofloxacin, ofloxacin), but may be susceptible to ceftriaxone, cefixime, and spectinomycin (currently not commercially available in the US). A few strains with decreased susceptibility to ciprofloxacin also were resistant to tetracycline.

Until 1992, virtually all strains of *N. gonorrhoeae* tested were susceptible to ciprofloxacin in vitro, but susceptibility of this organism to fluoroquinolones changed. QRNG are endemic in many Asian countries and have been reported sporadically in other parts of the world, including North America, Australia, Africa, Great Britain, and Israel. QRNG have been isolated from all regions of the US. The prevalence of these strains has been particularly high in Hawaii, Ohio, Oregon, California, and Washington and there have been substantial increases in QRNG prevalence reported over the last several years in some other areas of the US, including Philadelphia and Miami. In some cases, QRNG isolates appeared to have been introduced into the US by travelers returning from the Philippines; however, increases in QRNG in Hawaii and Ohio during 1992–1999 appeared to have been the result of endemic spread.

The prevalence of QRNG in the US is being monitored by the Centers for Disease Control and Prevention (CDC) Gonococcal Isolate Surveillance Project (GISP). During 1990–2001, QRNG prevalence in the US remained at less than 1%, but increased to 2.2% in 2002, 4.1% in 2003, 6.8% in 2004, and 9.4% in 2005. GISP data for the first 6 months of 2006 indicated that 13.3% of isolates collected by GISP were resistant to ciprofloxacin; when isolates from Hawaii and California were excluded (areas that discontinued use of fluoroquinolones for gonorrhea treatment in 2000 and 2002, respectively), 6.1 and 8.6% of GISP isolates were QRNG in 2005 and 2006, respectively. The prevalence of QRNG isolates decreased from 14.8% in 2007 to 9.6% in 2009 and then increased to 19.2% by 2014. The 2014 GISP data for the US indicated that QRNG were identified in 27.3% of isolates from the West, 21.4% of isolates from the Northeast, 14.3% from the South, and 10.2% from the Midwest.

QRNG strains are more common in men who have sex with men (MSM) than among heterosexual men, but prevalence has increased in both groups. QRNG prevalence in MSM was 1.6% in 2001, 7.2% in 2002, 15% in 2003, 23.8% in 2004, and 29% in 2005. QRNG prevalence increased more slowly in heterosexual men and was 0.6% in 2001, 0.9% in 2002, 1.5% in 2003, 2.9% in 2004, and 3.8% in 2005. The 2014 GISP data indicate that QRNG were identified in approximately 30% of isolates from MSM and men who have sex with both women and men and in 12.7% of isolates from men who have sex with women.

Beginning in April 2007, based on GISP data for the first 6 months of 2006 indicating that QRNG prevalence had increased among isolates obtained from MSM and heterosexual men and because QRNG was identified in all regions of the US, CDC recommended fluoroquinolones should no longer be used for the treatment of gonorrhea or any associated infections that may involve *N. gonorrhoeae* (e.g., pelvic inflammatory disease [PID], epididymitis).

● Resistance in Bacillus anthracis

Strains of *Bacillus anthracis* with natural resistance to ciprofloxacin have not been reported to date. There are published reports of *B. anthracis* strains that have been engineered to have tetracycline and penicillin resistance as well as resistance to other anti-infectives (e.g., macrolides, chloramphenicol, rifampin). In addition, reduced susceptibility to ofloxacin (4-fold increase in MICs from baseline) has been produced in vitro following sequential subculture of the Sterne strain of *B. anthracis* in subinhibitory concentrations of the fluoroquinolone.

● Cross-resistance

Cross-resistance can occur among the fluoroquinolones.

Cross-resistance generally does not occur between ciprofloxacin and other anti-infectives, including aminoglycosides, β-lactam antibiotics, sulfonamides (including co-trimoxazole), macrolides, and tetracyclines. However, rare strains of Enterobacteriaceae and *Ps. aeruginosa* resistant to ciprofloxacin have also been resistant to aminoglycosides, β-lactam antibiotics, chloramphenicol, trimethoprim, and/or tetracyclines. Resistance in these organisms appears to be related to decreased permeability of the organism to the drug, principally because of alterations in outer-membrane porin proteins; however, other mechanisms that affect permeability may also be involved.

PHARMACOKINETICS

In studies in the Pharmacokinetics section, ciprofloxacin was administered orally as conventional tablets containing the monohydrochloride monohydrate salt (i.e., ciprofloxacin hydrochloride), as extended-release tablets containing both ciprofloxacin hydrochloride and ciprofloxacin (base), or as an oral suspension containing the base; ciprofloxacin also was administered parenterally. Dosages and concentrations of the drug are expressed in terms of ciprofloxacin.

Body fluid and tissue concentrations of ciprofloxacin were measured with either a high-pressure liquid chromatographic (HPLC) assay or a microbiologic assay. HPLC assays are more specific for ciprofloxacin than microbiologic assays since the latter method measures the antibacterial activity of the parent drug as well as its microbiologically active metabolites. Controlled studies using HPLC and microbiologic assays indicate that there is good correlation between both methods for serum ciprofloxacin concentrations and pharmacokinetic parameters determined using these serum concentrations. However, mean ciprofloxacin concentrations in urine or bile generally are 30–40% higher when a microbiologic assay is used than when an HPLC assay is used.

The pharmacokinetics of ciprofloxacin after oral administration (as the hydrochloride) are best described by a 2-compartment model assuming zero-order absorption, and pharmacokinetics after IV administration are best described by an open, 3-compartment model.

The manufacturer states that a 500-mg dose of ciprofloxacin administered as ciprofloxacin oral suspension containing 250 mg/5 mL is bioequivalent to a 500-mg conventional tablet and that 10 mL of the ciprofloxacin oral suspension containing 250 mg/5 mL is bioequivalent to 5 mL of the oral suspension containing 500 mg/5 mL.

Ciprofloxacin conventional tablets are *not* bioequivalent to ciprofloxacin extended-release tablets.

● Absorption
Oral Administration

Ciprofloxacin hydrochloride is rapidly and well absorbed from the GI tract following oral administration, and undergoes minimal first-pass metabolism.

The oral bioavailability of ciprofloxacin administered as conventional tablets is 50–85% in healthy, fasting adults, and peak serum concentrations of the drug generally are attained within 0.5–2.3 hours. Peak serum concentrations and area under the serum concentration-time curve (AUC) increase in proportion to the dose over the oral dosage range of 250–1000 mg and are unaffected by gender. Following oral administration of a single 250-, 500-, 750-, or 1000-mg dose of ciprofloxacin as conventional tablets or oral suspension in healthy, fasting adults, peak serum concentrations average 0.76–1.5, 1.6–2.9, 2.5–4.3, or 3.4–5.4 mcg/mL, respectively; serum concentrations 12 hours after the dose average 0.1, 0.2, 0.4, or 0.6 mcg/mL, respectively. In adults, oral administration of 500 mg of ciprofloxacin as conventional tablets every 12 hours results in mean peak or trough serum concentrations at steady-state of 2.97 or 0.2 mcg/mL, respectively.

Following oral administration of extended-release tablets containing ciprofloxacin hydrochloride and base, peak plasma concentrations of ciprofloxacin are attained within 1–4 hours. Ciprofloxacin extended-release tablets contain approximately 35% of the dose within an immediate-release component; the remaining 65% of the dose is contained in a slow-release matrix. Oral administration of ciprofloxacin 500 mg once daily as ciprofloxacin extended-release tablets or 250 mg twice daily as conventional tablets results in steady-state mean peak plasma concentrations of 1.59 or 1.14 mcg/mL, respectively; however, the area under the concentration-time curve (AUC) is similar with both regimens. Oral administration of 1 g once daily as ciprofloxacin extended-release tablets or 500 mg twice daily as conventional tablets results in steady-state mean peak plasma concentrations of 3.11 or 2.06 mcg/mL, respectively; the AUC is similar with both regimens.

Data indicate that peak serum concentrations and AUCs of ciprofloxacin are slightly higher in geriatric patients than in younger adults; this may occur because of increased bioavailability, reduced volume of distribution, and/or reduced renal clearance in these patients. Single-dose oral studies using ciprofloxacin conventional tablets and single- and multiple-dose IV studies indicate that, compared with younger adults, peak plasma concentrations are 16–40% higher, mean AUC is approximately 30% higher, and elimination half-life is prolonged approximately 20% in individuals older than 65 years of age. These differences can be at least partially attributed to decreased renal clearance in this age group and are not clinically important.

Based on population pharmacokinetics, bioavailability of ciprofloxacin oral suspension in children is approximately 60%. Following a single oral dose of 10 mg/kg of ciprofloxacin given as the oral suspension to children 4 months to 7 years of age, the mean peak plasma concentration was 2.4 mcg/mL. There was no apparent age dependence and no increase in peak plasma concentrations following multiple doses.

In one study, GI absorption of ciprofloxacin was slower and the elimination half-life of the drug was shorter in cystic fibrosis patients 18 years of age or older than in healthy adults. Several other studies, however, indicate that the pharmacokinetics of ciprofloxacin are not appreciably altered in cystic fibrosis patients 18 years of age or older compared with healthy adults.

Although peak serum concentrations of ciprofloxacin and the AUC increased slightly after repeated oral doses in a few studies in fasting, healthy adults, most multiple-dose studies in fasting, healthy adults with normal renal function indicate that neither peak nor trough serum concentrations of ciprofloxacin increase after repeated oral doses and that the drug does not accumulate.

Magnesium-, aluminum-, and/or calcium-containing antacids or products containing calcium, iron, or zinc decrease the oral bioavailability of ciprofloxacin hydrochloride.

Food or Milk

The effect of food and/or milk on GI absorption of ciprofloxacin varies depending on the specific ciprofloxacin preparation (conventional tablets, extended-release tablets, oral solution) and situation.

When ciprofloxacin conventional tablets are administered concomitantly with food, there is a delay in absorption of the drug, but overall absorption is not substantially affected.

The manufacturer states that food does not affect the rate or extent of absorption of ciprofloxacin administered as the oral suspension.

The manufacturers state that, based on pharmacokinetic studies, ciprofloxacin extended-release tablets can be administered with or without food (e.g., with a high- or low-fat meal or under fasting conditions).

Concomitant administration of oral ciprofloxacin with dairy products (e.g., milk, yogurt) or calcium-fortified juices alone (i.e., without a meal) or with substantial calcium intake (greater than 800 mg) can reduce GI absorption of ciprofloxacin. In one study, administration of a 500-mg dose of ciprofloxacin (conventional tablet) with 300 mL of whole milk (360 mg calcium, 33 mg magnesium) or unflavored yogurt (450 mg calcium, 40 mg magnesium) decreased the AUC by 33 or 36%, respectively, and decreased peak plasma concentrations by 36 or 47%, respectively, compared with administration with water. The manufacturers state that oral ciprofloxacin can be taken with dairy products or calcium-fortified juices that are part of a meal.

Concomitant administration with nutritional supplements or enteral feedings may affect GI absorption of ciprofloxacin. When a 750-mg conventional ciprofloxacin tablet was crushed, mixed with 120 mL of enteral premixed liquid (Ensure), and swallowed, the AUC was 28% lower and peak plasma concentrations were 47% lower compared with results attained when the tablet was crushed and mixed with water before swallowing. In another crossover study in healthy adults, the AUC of the drug was 25% lower when a 750-mg conventional ciprofloxacin tablet was administered with 240 mL of a nutritional supplement containing calcium, magnesium, iron, and zinc (Resource) compared with administration with water.

● IV Administration

Following IV infusion over 60 minutes of a single 200- or 400-mg dose of ciprofloxacin in healthy adults, peak serum concentrations average 2.1 and 4.6 mcg/mL, respectively, immediately following the infusion; serum concentrations 6 hours after the start of infusion (i.e., 5 hours after completion) average 0.3 and 0.7 mcg/mL and those 12 hours after the start of infusion average 0.1 and 0.2 mcg/mL, respectively. In adults receiving 400 mg of ciprofloxacin IV every 12 hours, mean peak or trough serum concentrations at steady-state are 4.56 or 0.2 mcg/mL, respectively.

Following IV injection over 15 minutes of a single 100-mg dose of ciprofloxacin in healthy adults, serum concentrations of the drug average 2.8 mcg/mL immediately following the injection and 0.32, 0.14, and 0.07 mcg/mL at 1, 6, and 12 hours, respectively, after the dose. In healthy adults who receive a single 200-mg dose of ciprofloxacin by IV injection over 10 minutes, serum concentrations of the drug immediately following the injection average 6.3–6.5 mcg/mL and serum concentrations 1 and 12 hours later average 0.87 and 0.1 mcg/mL, respectively.

In a limited number of pediatric patients with severe sepsis who received ciprofloxacin 10 mg/kg given by IV infusion over 1 hour, mean peak plasma concentrations were 6.1 mcg/mL in those younger than 1 year of age and 7.2 mcg/mL in those 1–5 years of age.

● Distribution

Ciprofloxacin is widely distributed into body tissues and fluids following oral or IV administration. Highest concentrations of the drug generally are attained in bile, lungs, kidney, liver, gallbladder, uterus, seminal fluid, prostatic tissue and fluid, tonsils, endometrium, fallopian tubes, and ovaries. Concentrations of the drug achieved in most of these tissues and fluids substantially exceed those in serum. The drug also is distributed into adipose tissue, aqueous humor, bone, cartilage, heart tissue (heart valves, myocardia), muscle, nasal secretions, saliva, skin, sputum, and pleural, peritoneal, ascitic, blister, lymphatic, and renal cyst fluid. Ciprofloxacin is concentrated within neutrophils, achieving concentrations in these cells that may be 2–7 times greater than extracellular concentrations.

In healthy adults, the apparent volume of distribution of ciprofloxacin is 2–3.5 L/kg and the apparent volume of distribution at steady state is 1.7–2.7 L/kg. The apparent volume of distribution of ciprofloxacin in geriatric patients 64–91 years of age averages 3.5–3.6 L/kg.

Only low concentrations of ciprofloxacin are distributed into CSF; peak CSF concentrations may be 6–10% of peak serum concentrations. In adults with meningitis who received 200-mg doses of ciprofloxacin every 12 hours by IV infusion over 30 minutes, the ratio of CSF/serum concentrations in samples obtained 1–2 hours after a dose was 0.11–0.46 during the first 2–4 days of therapy when meninges were inflamed and 0.04–0.3 during days 10–14 when meninges were uninflamed. In one patient with meningitis caused by *Ps. aeruginosa* who received IV ciprofloxacin in a dosage of 400 mg every 8 hours, CSF concentrations of the drug were about 1 mg/mL and drug accumulation in CSF did not occur.

Following oral or IV administration of the drug, biliary ciprofloxacin concentrations are several fold higher than simultaneous serum concentrations of the drug. In adults undergoing cholecystectomy who received a single 750-mg oral dose of ciprofloxacin, peak concentrations of the drug and active metabolites ranged from 68–225 mcg/mL in gallbladder bile, 16–17 mcg/mL in common duct bile, 3.6–32.4 mcg/g in liver, 0.8–14.1 mcg/g in gallbladder, and 1.5–7.8 mcg/mL in serum.

Following oral administration, ciprofloxacin concentrations in prostatic tissue and fluid generally exceed concurrent serum concentrations of the drug. In a study in men undergoing transurethral resection for prostatic hyperplasia or cancer who received 500 mg of the drug orally every 12 hours, ciprofloxacin concentrations in prostatic tissue obtained 75–120 minutes after a dose averaged 3 mg/kg and the ratio of prostate/serum concentrations ranged from 1–7.

Ciprofloxacin is 16–43% bound to serum proteins in vitro.

Ciprofloxacin crosses the placenta and is distributed into amniotic fluid in humans.

Ciprofloxacin is distributed into milk. In lactating women who received 750 mg of ciprofloxacin every 12 hours for 3 doses, concentrations of the drug in milk obtained 2–4 hours after a dose averaged 2.26–3.79 mcg/mL; milk concentrations were higher than concomitant serum concentrations for up to 12 hours after a dose.

• Elimination

The serum elimination half-life of ciprofloxacin in adults with normal renal function is 3–7 hours. Following IV administration in healthy adults, the distribution half-life of ciprofloxacin averages 0.18–0.37 hours and the elimination half-life averages 3–4.8 hours.

The elimination half-life of the drug is slightly longer in geriatric adults than in younger adults, and ranges from 3.3–6.8 hours in adults 60–91 years of age with renal function normal for their age.

Based on population pharmacokinetic analysis of pediatric patients with various infections, the predicted mean half-life of ciprofloxacin in children is approximately 4–5 hours.

In patients with impaired renal function, serum concentrations of ciprofloxacin are higher and the half-life prolonged. In adults with creatinine clearances of 30 mL/minute or less, half-life of the drug ranges from 4.4–12.6 hours.

Further study is needed to evaluate that pharmacokinetics in patients with hepatic impairment. In one study in patients with stable chronic liver cirrhosis, there was no clinically important change in ciprofloxacin pharmacokinetics; however, slightly prolonged half-life has been reported in some other patients with hepatic impairment.

Ciprofloxacin is eliminated by renal and nonrenal mechanisms. The drug is partially metabolized in the liver by modification of the piperazinyl group to at least 4 metabolites. These metabolites, which have been identified as desethyleneciprofloxacin (M1), sulfociprofloxacin (M2), oxociprofloxacin (M3), and N-formylciprofloxacin (M4), have microbiologic activity that is less than that of the parent drug.

Ciprofloxacin and its metabolites are excreted in urine and feces. Unchanged ciprofloxacin is excreted in urine by both glomerular filtration and tubular secretion. Following oral administration of a single 250-, 500-, or 750-mg dose in adults with normal renal function, 15–50% of the dose is excreted in urine as unchanged drug and 10–15% as metabolites within 24 hours; 20–40% of the dose is excreted in feces as unchanged drug and metabolites within 5 days. Most, but not all, of unchanged ciprofloxacin in feces appears to result from biliary excretion.

Renal clearance of ciprofloxacin averages 300–479 mL/minute in adults with normal renal function. Urinary concentrations of ciprofloxacin generally exceed 200 mcg/mL during the first 2 hours and average about 30 mcg/mL 8–12 hours after a single 250-mg oral dose of the drug. Following oral administration of a single 500-mg dose in adults with normal renal function, urinary concentrations of ciprofloxacin and active metabolites average 350, 162, and 105 mcg/mL in urine collected over 1–3, 3–6, and 6–12 hours, respectively, after the dose.Concentrations of unchanged drug and active metabolites in feces range from 185–2220 mcg/g after 7 days of therapy with the drug in a dosage of 500 mg every 12 hours.

Small amounts of ciprofloxacin are removed by hemodialysis. The amount of the drug removed during hemodialysis depends on several factors (e.g., type of coil used, dialysis flow rate). In patients with end-stage renal disease undergoing hemodialysis, the serum half-life of ciprofloxacin averaged 3.2 hours during hemodialysis and 5.8 hours between dialysis sessions. A 4-hour period of hemodialysis generally removes into the dialysate 2–30% of a single 250- or 500-mg oral dose of the drug. Only small amounts of ciprofloxacin appear to be removed by peritoneal dialysis.

CHEMISTRY AND STABILITY

• Chemistry

Ciprofloxacin is a fluoroquinolone anti-infective agent. Like all other commercially available fluoroquinolones, ciprofloxacin contains a fluorine at the C-6 position of the quinolone nucleus. Like some other fluoroquinolones (levofloxacin, ofloxacin), ciprofloxacin contains a piperazinyl group at position 7 of the quinolone nucleus. The piperazinyl group in ciprofloxacin results in antipseudomonal activity. The drug also contains a cyclopropyl group at position 1, which enhances antimicrobial activity.

Ciprofloxacin is commercially available for oral administration as conventional tablets containing ciprofloxacin hydrochloride, which is the monohydrochloride monohydrate of the drug. Ciprofloxacin hydrochloride occurs as a faintly yellowish to yellow crystalline powder. Ciprofloxacin hydrochloride has a solubility of approximately 36 mg/mL in water at 25°C. The pK_as of the drug are 6 and 8.8.

Ciprofloxacin also is commercially available for oral administration as extended-release tablets containing ciprofloxacin hydrochloride and ciprofloxacin (base). Ciprofloxacin extended-release tablets contain approximately 35% of the dose within an immediate-release component; the remaining 65% of the dose is contained in a slow-release matrix. Ciprofloxacin (base) occurs as a pale yellowing to light yellow crystalline powder.

In addition, ciprofloxacin is commercially available for oral administration as microcapsules for oral suspension. Following mixture with the diluent provided by the manufacturer, ciprofloxacin oral suspensions containing 250 or 500 mg of the drug per 5 mL occur as a strawberry-flavored, white to slightly yellowish suspension and may contain yellow-orange droplets.

For IV administration, ciprofloxacin is commercially available as the base. Ciprofloxacin concentrate for IV infusion contains 10 mg of ciprofloxacin per mL in an aqueous solution and is provided in glass vials. The commercially available premixed injection for IV infusion contains 2 mg or ciprofloxacin per mL in 5% dextrose. The concentrate and premixed injection in 5% dextrose occur as clear, colorless to slightly yellow solutions. The concentrate for IV infusion has a pH of 3.3–3.9; the commercially available premixed injection in 5% dextrose has a pH of 3.5–4.6. The concentrate and commercially available premixed injection for IV infusion contain lactic acid as a solubilizing agent and may contain hydrochloric acid to adjust pH.

• Stability

Ciprofloxacin hydrochloride conventional tablets should be stored at 20–25°C, but may be exposed to temperatures ranging from 15–30°C.

Extended-release tablets containing ciprofloxacin hydrochloride and base should be stored at 20–25°C, in a tight, light-resistant container.

Ciprofloxacin microcapsules for oral suspension and the diluent provided by the manufacturer should be stored at less than 25°C, but may be exposed to temperatures ranging from 15–30°C. Following reconstitution with the diluent, ciprofloxacin oral suspension should be stored at 25°C, but may be exposed to temperatures ranging from 15–30°C, and is stable for 14 days. The microcapsules, diluent, and reconstituted oral suspension should be protected from freezing.

Ciprofloxacin concentrate for IV infusion (10 mg/mL) provided in vials should be stored at 5–30°C and protected from light, excessive heat, and freezing. Following dilution of the ciprofloxacin concentrate for IV infusion in sterile water for injection, 5% or 10% dextrose injection, 0.9% sodium chloride injection, 5% dextrose and 0.225 or 0.45% sodium chloride injection, or lactated Ringer's injection to a final concentration of 0.5–2 mg/mL, the resultant solutions are stable for up to 14 days when refrigerated or stored at room temperature.

The commercially available premixed injection for IV infusion containing 2 mg/mL in 5% dextrose should be stored at 5–25°C and protected from light, excessive heat, and freezing. The premixed injection for IV infusion is provided in single-dose flexible plastic containers. Solutions in contact with the plastic can leach out some of the chemical components in very small amounts (e.g., bis(2-ethylhexyl)phthalate [BEHP, DEHP] in up to 5 ppm) within the expiration period of the injection; however, safety of the plastic has been confirmed in tests in animals according to USP biological tests for plastic containers as well as by tissue culture toxicity studies.

PREPARATIONS

Excipients in commercially available drug preparations may have clinically important effects in some individuals; consult specific product labeling for details.

Ciprofloxacin

Oral

For suspension	250 mg/5 mL*	Cipro®, Bayer
		Ciprofloxacin for Oral Suspension
	500 mg/5 mL*	Cipro®, Bayer
		Ciprofloxacin for Oral Suspension

Parenteral

| For injection concentrate, for IV infusion | 10 mg (of ciprofloxacin) per mL (200 or 400 mg)* | Ciprofloxacin for Injection Concentrate |

* available from one or more manufacturer, distributor, and/or repackager by generic (nonproprietary) name

Ciprofloxacin and Ciprofloxacin Hydrochloride

Oral

Tablets, extended-release, film-coated	500 mg total ciprofloxacin (with ciprofloxacin 212.6 mg [of anhydrous ciprofloxacin] and ciprofloxacin hydrochloride 287.5 mg [of anhydrous ciprofloxacin])*	Ciprofloxacin Extended-release Tablets
	1 g total ciprofloxacin (with ciprofloxacin 425.2 mg [of anhydrous ciprofloxacin] and ciprofloxacin hydrochloride 574.9 mg [of anhydrous ciprofloxacin])*	Ciprofloxacin Extended-release Tablets

* available from one or more manufacturer, distributor, and/or repackager by generic (nonproprietary) name

Ciprofloxacin Hydrochloride

Oral

Tablets, film-coated	100 mg (of ciprofloxacin)*	Ciprofloxacin Tablets
	250 mg (of ciprofloxacin)*	Cipro®, Bayer
		Ciprofloxacin Tablets
	500 mg (of ciprofloxacin)*	Cipro®, Bayer
		Ciprofloxacin Tablets
	750 mg (of ciprofloxacin)*	Ciprofloxacin Tablets

* available from one or more manufacturer, distributor, and/or repackager by generic (nonproprietary) name

Ciprofloxacin in Dextrose

Parenteral

Injection, for IV infusion	2 mg (of ciprofloxacin) per mL (200 or 400 mg) in 5% dextrose*	Ciprofloxacin in 5% Dextrose Injection

* available from one or more manufacturer, distributor, and/or repackager by generic (nonproprietary) name

† Use is not currently included in the labeling approved by the US Food and Drug Administration.

Delafloxacin Meglumine

8:12.18 • QUINOLONES

■ Delafloxacin is a fluoroquinolone anti-infective agent.

USES

● Skin and Skin Structure Infections

Delafloxacin meglumine is used for the treatment of acute bacterial skin and skin structure infections (ABSSSI) caused by susceptible *Staphylococcus aureus* (including methicillin-resistant *S. aureus* [MRSA; also known as oxacillin-resistant *S. aureus* or ORSA] and methicillin-susceptible *S. aureus*), *S. haemolyticus*, *S. lugdunensis*, *Streptococcus pyogenes* (group A β-hemolytic streptococci, GAS), *S. agalactiae* (group B streptococci, GBS), *S. anginosus* group (includes *S. anginosus*, *S. intermedius*, and *S. constellatus*), *Enterococcus faecalis*, *Escherichia coli*, *Enterobacter cloacae*, *Klebsiella pneumoniae*, or *Pseudomonas aeruginosa*.

Clinical Experience

Efficacy and safety of delafloxacin were evaluated in 2 randomized, multicenter, multinational, double-blind, double-dummy, noninferiority, phase 3 studies in adults with acute bacterial skin and skin structure infections (e.g., cellulitis/erysipelas, wound infection, major cutaneous abscess, burn infection).

In the first study (Trial 1; NCT01811732), 660 patients (average age 46 years [range: 18–94 years of age], 63% male, 91% white, 9% with diabetes mellitus, 55% reported recent drug abuse [including IV drug abuse], 39% with cellulitis/erysipelas, 35% with wound infection, 25% with major cutaneous abscess, 1% with burn infection, 2% with documented bacteremia at baseline) were randomized to receive delafloxacin (300 mg IV every 12 hours) or a regimen of vancomycin (15 mg/kg IV every 12 hours) in conjunction with aztreonam (2 g IV every 12 hours) for a duration of 5–14 days. Aztreonam was discontinued if baseline cultures did not reveal gram-negative bacteria. Clinical response (i.e., at least 20% decrease in lesion size determined by digital planimetry of the leading edge of erythema) at 48–72 hours after initiation of treatment was achieved in 78.2% of those receiving delafloxacin and 80.9% of those receiving the vancomycin regimen. At a follow-up visit approximately 14 days (range: 13–15 days) after initiation of treatment, investigator-assessed treatment success (defined as complete resolution [cure] *or* clinical improvement with complete or nearly complete resolution of signs and symptoms with no further antibacterial treatment) was achieved by 81.6 or 83.3% of the intent-to-treat population receiving delafloxacin or the vancomycin regimen, respectively; in the subset of patients who were clinically evaluable at the 14-day follow-up visit, treatment success was achieved in 96.7 or 97.5% of patients, respectively.

In the second study (Trial 2; NCT01984684), 850 patients (average age 51 years [range: 18–93 years of age], 63% male, 83% white, 13% with diabetes mellitus, 30% reported recent drug abuse [including IV drug abuse], 48% with cellulitis/erysipelas, 26% with wound infection, 25% with major cutaneous abscess, 1% with burn infection, 2% with documented bacteremia at baseline) were randomized to receive delafloxacin (300 mg IV every 12 hours for 6 doses, then oral delafloxacin 450 mg every 12 hours) or a regimen of IV vancomycin (15 mg/kg every 12 hours) in conjunction with IV aztreonam (2 g every 12 hours) for a duration of 5–14 days. Aztreonam was discontinued if baseline cultures did not reveal gram-negative bacteria. Clinical response (i.e., at least 20% decrease in lesion size determined by digital planimetry of the leading edge of erythema) at 48–72 hours after initiation of treatment was achieved in 83.7% of those receiving delafloxacin and 80.6% of those receiving the vancomycin regimen. At a follow-up visit approximately 14 days (range: 13–15 days) after initiation of treatment, investigator-assessed treatment success (defined as complete resolution [cure] *or* nearly complete resolution of signs and symptoms with no further antibacterial treatment) was achieved in 87.2 or 84.8% of the intent-to-treat population receiving delafloxacin or the vancomycin regimen, respectively; in the subset of patients who were clinically evaluable at the 14-day follow-up visit, treatment success was achieved in 96 or 97% of patients, respectively.

In a pooled subset of microbiologically evaluable patients from both studies that were stratified according to the infecting pathogen, clinical response at 48–72 hours in those with infections caused by MRSA or methicillin-susceptible *S. aureus* was

86.8 or 84.2%%, respectively, in those treated with delafloxacin and 85.8 or 80.9%, respectively, in those treated with the vancomycin regimen. The clinical response in those with infections caused by *S. agalactiae*, *S. pyogenes*, or *S. anginosus* group was 71.4, 73.9, or 92.2%, respectively, in those treated with delafloxacin and 75, 50, or 90.2%, respectively, in those treated with the vancomycin regimen. The clinical response in those with infections caused by *S. haemolyticus*, *S. lugdunensis*, or *E. faecalis* was 73.3, 72.7, or 100%, respectively, in those treated with delafloxacin and 87.5, 66.7, or 75%, respectively, in those treated with the vancomycin regimen. The clinical response in those with infections caused by *E. coli*, *E. cloacae*, *K. pneumoniae*, or *Ps. aeruginosa* was 85.7, 71.4, 86.4, or 81.8%, respectively, in those treated with delafloxacin and 80, 72.7, 95.7, or 91.7%, respectively, in those treated with the vancomycin regimen.

DOSAGE AND ADMINISTRATION

● Administration

Delafloxacin meglumine is administered orally or by IV infusion.

Oral Administration

Delafloxacin tablets may be given without regard to food.

Delafloxacin tablets should be administered orally at least 2 hours before or 6 hours after antacids containing magnesium or aluminum, metal cations (e.g., iron), sucralfate, multivitamins or dietary supplements containing iron or zinc, or buffered didanosine preparations. These drugs may substantially interfere with oral absorption of delafloxacin, resulting in systemic concentrations lower than desired. (See Drug Interactions.)

IV Infusion

Delafloxacin solutions should *not* be infused simultaneously through the same tubing with other drugs and should *not* be administered with any solution containing multivalent cations (e.g., calcium, magnesium).

If a common IV line is used to administer delafloxacin and other drugs, the line should be flushed with 0.9% sodium chloride injection or 5% dextrose injection before and after each delafloxacin infusion.

Vials of delafloxacin lyophilized powder for injection are for single use only.

Reconstitution and Dilution

Delafloxacin meglumine for injection must be reconstituted and further diluted prior to IV infusion.

Vials labeled as containing 300 mg of delafloxacin should be reconstituted by adding 10.5 mL of 0.9% sodium chloride injection or 5% dextrose injection to provide a solution containing 25 mg/mL. The vial should be shaken vigorously until the contents are completely dissolved. The reconstituted solution should appear clear yellow to amber in color.

To prepare a 300-mg dose of delafloxacin in a 250-mL infusion bag containing 0.9% sodium chloride injection or 5% dextrose injection, 12 mL of the diluent should be removed from the infusion bag prior to injecting 12 mL of reconstituted delafloxacin solution into the bag; the concentration of the final infusion solution is 1.2 mg/mL.

To prepare a 200-mg dose of delafloxacin in a 250-mL infusion bag containing 0.9% sodium chloride injection or 5% dextrose injection, 8 mL of the diluent should be removed from the infusion bag prior to injecting 8 mL of reconstituted delafloxacin solution into the bag; the concentration of the final infusion solution is 0.8 mg/mL.

Reconstituted delafloxacin or reconstituted and further diluted solutions of delafloxacin may be stored under refrigeration (2–8°C) or at controlled room temperature (20–25°C) for up to 24 hours, but should not be frozen.

Delafloxacin solutions should be inspected visually for particulate matter and discoloration prior to administration.

Rate of Administration

IV infusions of delafloxacin should be given over 60 minutes.

● Dosage

Dosage of delafloxacin meglumine is expressed in terms of delafloxacin.

Adult Dosage
Skin and Skin Structure Infections

When delafloxacin tablets are used, the recommended dosage of the drug for the treatment of acute bacterial skin and skin structure infections (ABSSSI) in adults is 450 mg orally every 12 hours for a duration of 5–14 days.

When IV delafloxacin is used, the recommended dosage of the drug for the treatment of acute bacterial skin and skin structure infections in adults is 300 mg IV every 12 hours for a duration of 5–14 days.

Alternatively, when IV delafloxacin is used initially in a dosage of 300 mg every 12 hours, therapy may be switched at the discretion of the clinician to delafloxacin tablets given in a dosage of 450 mg orally every 12 hours. The total duration of therapy should be 5–14 days.

● Special Populations
Hepatic Impairment

Dosage adjustments are not necessary when delafloxacin is used in adults with mild, moderate, or severe hepatic impairment (Child-Pugh class A, B, or C).

Renal Impairment

Dosage adjustments are not necessary when delafloxacin is used in adults with mild or moderate renal impairment (estimated glomerular filtration rate [eGFR] of 30–89 mL/minute per 1.73 m²).

If delafloxacin tablets are used for the treatment of acute bacterial skin and skin structure infections in adults with severe renal impairment (eGFR of 15–29 mL/minute per 1.73 m²), dosage adjustments are not necessary.

If IV delafloxacin is used for the treatment of acute bacterial skin and skin structure infections in adults with severe renal impairment (eGFR of 15–29 mL/minute per 1.73 m²), the recommended dosage is 200 mg IV every 12 hours for a duration of 5–14 days. Alternatively, such patients may receive IV delafloxacin initially given in a dosage of 200 mg every 12 hours and therapy may then be switched to delafloxacin tablets given in a dosage of 450 mg orally every 12 hours. The total duration of therapy should be 5–14 days.

Delafloxacin (oral or IV) is *not* recommended in adults with end-stage renal disease (eGFR less than 15 mL/minute per 1.73 m²) since data are insufficient to provide dosage recommendations for such patients. (See Renal Impairment under Warnings/Precautions: Specific Populations, in Cautions.)

CAUTIONS

● Contraindications

Delafloxacin meglumine is contraindicated in patients with known hypersensitivity to delafloxacin, any component of the preparation, or other fluoroquinolones.

● Warnings/Precautions
Warnings
Disabling and Potentially Irreversible Serious Adverse Reactions

Systemic fluoroquinolones have been associated with disabling and potentially irreversible serious adverse reactions (e.g., tendinitis and tendon rupture, arthralgia, myalgia, peripheral neuropathy, CNS effects) that can occur together in the same patient. These serious reactions may occur within hours to weeks after a systemic fluoroquinolone is initiated and have occurred in all age groups and in patients without preexisting risk factors for such adverse reactions.

Delafloxacin should be discontinued immediately at the first signs or symptoms of any serious adverse reactions.

Systemic fluoroquinolones, including delafloxacin, should be avoided in patients who have experienced any of the serious adverse reactions associated with fluoroquinolones.

Tendinitis and Tendon Rupture

Systemic fluoroquinolones are associated with an increased risk of tendinitis and tendon rupture in all age groups.

The risk of developing fluoroquinolone-associated tendinitis and tendon rupture is increased in older adults (usually those older than 60 years of age),

individuals receiving concomitant corticosteroids, and kidney, heart, or lung transplant recipients. (See Geriatric Use under Warnings/Precautions: Specific Populations, in Cautions.)

Other factors that may independently increase the risk of tendon rupture include strenuous physical activity, renal failure, and previous tendon disorders such as rheumatoid arthritis. Tendinitis and tendon rupture have been reported in patients receiving fluoroquinolones who did not have any risk factors for such adverse effects.

Fluoroquinolone-associated tendinitis and tendon rupture most frequently involve the Achilles tendon and also have been reported in the rotator cuff (shoulder), hand, biceps, thumb, and other tendon sites. Tendinitis or tendon rupture can occur within hours or days after a fluoroquinolone is initiated or as long as several months after completion of therapy and can occur bilaterally.

Delafloxacin should be discontinued immediately if pain, swelling, inflammation, or rupture of a tendon occurs. (See Advice to Patients.)

Systemic fluoroquinolones, including delafloxacin, should be avoided in patients who have a history of tendon disorders or have experienced tendinitis or tendon rupture.

Peripheral Neuropathy

Systemic fluoroquinolones have been associated with an increased risk of peripheral neuropathy.

Sensory or sensorimotor axonal polyneuropathy affecting small and/or large axons resulting in paresthesias, hypoesthesias, dysesthesias, and weakness has been reported in patients receiving systemic fluoroquinolones, including delafloxacin. Symptoms may occur soon after initiation of a fluoroquinolone and, in some patients, may be irreversible.

Delafloxacin should be discontinued immediately if symptoms of peripheral neuropathy (e.g., pain, burning, tingling, numbness, and/or weakness) occur or if there are other alterations in sensations (e.g., light touch, pain, temperature, position sense, vibratory sensation, and/or motor strength). (See Advice to Patients.)

Systemic fluoroquinolones, including delafloxacin, should be avoided in patients who have experienced peripheral neuropathy.

CNS Effects

Systemic fluoroquinolones have been associated with an increased risk of adverse psychiatric effects, including toxic psychosis, hallucinations, paranoia, depression, suicidal thoughts or acts, delirium, disorientation, confusion, disturbances in attention, anxiety, agitation, nervousness, insomnia, nightmares, and memory impairment. These adverse effects may occur after the first dose.

Systemic fluoroquinolones have been associated with an increased risk of convulsions (seizures), increased intracranial pressure (including pseudotumor cerebri), dizziness, and tremors. Delafloxacin, like other fluoroquinolones, should be used in patients with known or suspected CNS disorders (e.g., severe cerebral arteriosclerosis, epilepsy) or other risk factors that predispose to seizures or lower seizure threshold *only* if potential benefits of the drug outweigh risks.

If psychiatric or other CNS effects occur, delafloxacin should be discontinued immediately and appropriate measures initiated. (See Advice to Patients.)

Exacerbation of Myasthenia Gravis

Fluoroquinolones have neuromuscular blocking activity and may exacerbate muscle weakness in individuals with myasthenia gravis. In postmarketing experience, use of fluoroquinolones in myasthenia gravis patients has resulted in requirements for ventilatory support and in death.

Delafloxacin should be avoided in patients with a known history of myasthenia gravis. Patients should be advised to immediately contact a clinician if they have any symptoms of muscle weakness, including respiratory difficulties. (See Advice to Patients.)

Sensitivity Reactions
Hypersensitivity Reactions

Serious and occasionally fatal hypersensitivity and/or anaphylactic reactions have been reported in patients receiving fluoroquinolones. These reactions may occur with the first dose or subsequent doses.

Some hypersensitivity reactions reported in patients receiving fluoroquinolones have been accompanied by cardiovascular collapse, loss of consciousness, tingling, edema (pharyngeal or facial), dyspnea, urticaria, or pruritus.

Hypersensitivity and urticaria have been reported in patients receiving delafloxacin.

Delafloxacin should be discontinued immediately at the first appearance of rash or any other sign of hypersensitivity. (See Advice to Patients.)

Photosensitivity Reactions

There was no evidence of phototoxic potential when oral delafloxacin (200 or 400 mg daily) was administered to healthy individuals exposed to ultraviolet (UVA and UVB) and visible radiation wavelengths ranging from 295–430 nm, including solar simulation.

Other Warnings and Precautions

Risk of Aortic Aneurysm and Dissection

Rupture or dissection of aortic aneurysms has been reported in patients receiving systemic fluoroquinolones. Epidemiologic studies indicate an increased risk of aortic aneurysm and dissection within 2 months following use of systemic fluoroquinolones, particularly in elderly patients. The cause for this increased risk has not been identified.

Unless there are no other treatment options, systemic fluoroquinolones, including delafloxacin, should not be used in patients who have an aortic aneurysm or are at increased risk for an aortic aneurysm. This includes elderly patients and patients with peripheral atherosclerotic vascular disease, hypertension, or certain genetic conditions (e.g., Marfan syndrome, Ehlers-Danlos syndrome).

If a patient reports adverse effects suggestive of aortic aneurysm or dissection, fluoroquinolone treatment should be discontinued immediately. (See Advice to Patients.)

Hypoglycemia or Hyperglycemia

Systemic fluoroquinolones have been associated with alterations in blood glucose concentrations, including symptomatic hypoglycemia and hyperglycemia. Blood glucose disturbances during fluoroquinolone therapy usually have occurred in patients with diabetes mellitus receiving an oral antidiabetic agent (e.g., glyburide) or insulin.

Severe cases of hypoglycemia resulting in coma or death have been reported with some systemic fluoroquinolones. Although most reported cases of hypoglycemic coma have involved patients with risk factors for hypoglycemia (e.g., older age, diabetes mellitus, renal insufficiency, concomitant use of antidiabetic agents [especially sulfonylureas]), some cases have occurred in patients receiving a fluoroquinolone who were not diabetic and were not reported to be receiving an oral antidiabetic agent or insulin.

Blood glucose concentrations should be carefully monitored when systemic fluoroquinolones, including delafloxacin, are used in patients with diabetes mellitus receiving antidiabetic agents.

If a hypoglycemic reaction occurs, fluoroquinolone treatment should be discontinued and appropriate therapy initiated immediately. (See Advice to Patients.)

C. difficile-associated Diarrhea and Colitis

Treatment with anti-infectives alters normal colon flora and may permit overgrowth of *Clostridioides difficile* (formerly known as *Clostridium difficile*). *C. difficile* infection (CDI) and *C. difficile*-associated diarrhea and colitis (CDAD; also known as antibiotic-associated diarrhea and colitis or pseudomembranous colitis) have been reported in patients receiving nearly all anti-infectives, including delafloxacin, and may range in severity from mild diarrhea to fatal colitis. *C. difficile* produces toxins A and B which contribute to development of CDAD; hypertoxin-producing strains of *C. difficile* are associated with increased morbidity and mortality since they may be refractory to anti-infectives and colectomy may be required.

CDAD should be considered in the differential diagnosis of patients who develop diarrhea during or after anti-infective therapy. Careful medical history is necessary since CDAD has been reported to occur as late as 2 months or longer after anti-infective therapy is discontinued.

If CDAD is suspected or confirmed, anti-infective therapy not directed against *C. difficile* should be discontinued as soon as possible. Patients should be managed with appropriate anti-infective therapy directed against *C. difficile* (e.g., vancomycin, fidaxomicin, metronidazole), supportive therapy (e.g., fluid and electrolyte management, protein supplementation), and surgical evaluation as clinically indicated.

Selection and Use of Anti-infectives

To reduce development of drug-resistant bacteria and maintain effectiveness of delafloxacin and other antibacterials, the drug should be used only for treatment of infections proven or strongly suspected to be caused by susceptible bacteria.

When selecting or modifying anti-infective therapy, results of culture and in vitro susceptibility testing should be used. In the absence of such data, local epidemiology and susceptibility patterns should be considered when selecting anti-infectives for empiric therapy.

Information on test methods and quality control standards for in vitro susceptibility testing of antibacterial agents and specific interpretive criteria for such testing recognized by FDA is available at https://www.fda.gov/STIC.

Specific Populations

Pregnancy

Available data regarding use of delafloxacin in pregnant women are insufficient to inform any drug-associated risk for miscarriages or major birth defects.

When delafloxacin (as the N-methyl glucamine salt) was administered orally to pregnant rats during organogenesis, no malformations or fetal deaths were observed at delafloxacin concentrations up to 7 times the estimated clinical exposure. Maternal toxicity and reduced fetal body weight were observed at the highest dosage (1.6 g/kg daily); fetal ossification delays were observed at all doses. When IV delafloxacin was administered to rats in late pregnancy through lactation, no adverse effects on offspring were observed at clinically relevant concentrations.

Lactation

It is not known whether delafloxacin is distributed into human milk, affects the breast-fed infant, or affects milk production. Delafloxacin is distributed into milk in lactating rats.

The developmental and health benefits of breast-feeding should be considered along with the mother's clinical need for delafloxacin and potential adverse effects on the breast-fed infant from the drug or from the underlying maternal condition.

Pediatric Use

Safety and efficacy of delafloxacin have not been established in pediatric patients younger than 18 years of age, and use of the drug in pediatric patients is not recommended.

Fluoroquinolones cause arthropathy in juvenile animals.

The manufacturer states that clinical trials evaluating delafloxacin for the treatment of bacterial skin and skin structure infections did not include patients younger than 18 years of age because the risks versus benefits of the drug do not support use for the treatment of such infections in this age group.

The American Academy of Pediatrics (AAP) states that use of a systemic fluoroquinolone may be justified in children younger than 18 years of age in certain specific circumstances when there are no safe and effective alternatives and the drug is known to be effective. For information regarding when fluoroquinolones may be a preferred option in children, see Cautions: Pediatric Precautions in Ciprofloxacin 8:12.18.

Geriatric Use

Approximately 15% of patients receiving delafloxacin in clinical studies were 65 years of age or older. The clinical response rate at 48–72 hours after initiation of delafloxacin was 75.7% in patients 65 years of age or older compared with 82.3% in those younger than 65 years of age. In the comparator group, the clinical response rate in patients 65 years of age or older was 71.3% compared with 82.1% in those younger than 65 years of age.

The risk of developing severe tendon disorders, including tendon rupture, is increased in older adults (usually those older than 60 years of age). This risk is further increased in those receiving concomitant corticosteroids. (See Tendinitis and Tendon Rupture under Warnings/Precautions: Warnings, in Cautions.) Caution is advised if delafloxacin is used in geriatric adults, especially those receiving concomitant corticosteroids.

The risk of aortic aneurysm and dissection may be increased in geriatric patients. (See Risk of Aortic Aneurysm and Dissection under Warnings/Precautions: Other Warnings and Precautions, in Cautions.)

Pharmacokinetic data indicate that mean peak plasma concentration and area under the plasma concentration-time curve (AUC) of delafloxacin reported in geriatric individuals 65 years of age or older are about 35% higher than those reported in younger adults (18–40 years of age); this difference is not considered clinically important.

Hepatic Impairment

Pharmacokinetics of delafloxacin in adults with mild, moderate, or severe hepatic impairment (Child-Pugh class A, B, or C) are similar to those in adults with normal hepatic function. Dosage adjustments are not necessary in patients with hepatic impairment.

Renal Impairment

Substantial accumulation of the IV delafloxacin vehicle, sulfobutylether-β-cyclodextrin (SBECD), occurs in patients with severe renal impairment (estimated glomerular filtration rate [eGFR] of 15–29 mL/minute per 1.73 m^2) or end-stage renal disease (eGFR less than 15 mL/minute per 1.73 m^2).

If IV delafloxacin is used in patients with severe renal impairment, dosage reduction is recommended (see Renal Impairment under Dosage and Administration: Special Populations) and serum creatinine concentrations and eGFR should be closely monitored. Consideration should be given to switching to oral delafloxacin if serum creatinine concentrations increase during treatment with IV delafloxacin. If eGFR decreases to less than 15 mL/minute per 1.73 m^2, delafloxacin should be discontinued.

Delafloxacin (oral or IV) is not recommended in patients with end-stage renal disease.

● Common Adverse Effects

Adverse effects occurring in 2% or more of patients receiving delafloxacin include GI effects (nausea, diarrhea, vomiting), headache, and elevated aminotransferase concentrations.

DRUG INTERACTIONS

● Drugs Metabolized by Hepatic Microsomal Enzymes

Delafloxacin meglumine does not inhibit cytochrome P-450 (CYP) isoenzymes 1A2, 2A6, 2B6, 2C8, 2C9, 2C19, 2D6, 2E1, or 3A4/5 in vitro at clinically relevant concentrations and shows no potential for induction of CYP1A2, 2B6, 2C19, or 2C8. In vitro, mild induction of CYP2C9 and 3A4 was observed.

● Drugs Affecting or Affected by Membrane Transporters

In vitro, delafloxacin is a substrate of P-glycoprotein (P-gp) transport and breast cancer resistance protein (BCRP); however, the clinical importance of concomitant use of delafloxacin and P-gp inhibitors and/or BCRP inhibitors is not known.

Delafloxacin does not inhibit multidrug-resistance gene (MDR) 1, BCRP, organic anion transporter (OAT) 1, OAT3, organic anion transporting polypeptide (OATP) 1B1, OATP1B3, bile salt export pump (BSEP), organic cation transporter (OCT) 1, or OCT2 at clinically relevant concentrations.

Delafloxacin is not a substrate of OAT1, OAT3, OCT1, OCT2, OATP1B1, or OATP1B3.

● Antacids

Pharmacokinetic interaction with delafloxacin tablets if administered concomitantly with aluminum- or magnesium-containing antacids (possible decreased absorption and decreased systemic concentrations of delafloxacin). Delafloxacin tablets should be administered at least 2 hours before or 6 hours after antacids containing aluminum or magnesium.

It is not known if an interaction exists between IV delafloxacin and oral antacids.

● Antibacterials

In vitro, there was no evidence of synergistic or antagonistic antibacterial effects when delafloxacin was used with aztreonam, ceftazidime, colistin (commercially available in the US as colistimethate sodium), co-trimoxazole, daptomycin, linezolid, meropenem, tigecycline, or vancomycin.

● Didanosine

Pharmacokinetic interaction if delafloxacin tablets are administered concomitantly with buffered didanosine (pediatric powder for oral solution) (possible decreased absorption and decreased systemic concentrations of delafloxacin). Delafloxacin tablets should be administered at least 2 hours before or 6 hours after buffered didanosine.

It is not known if an interaction exists between IV delafloxacin and buffered didanosine.

● Iron, Multivitamins, and Mineral Supplements

Pharmacokinetic interaction with delafloxacin tablets if administered concomitantly with oral iron preparations or multivitamins containing iron or zinc (possible decreased absorption and decreased systemic concentrations of delafloxacin). Delafloxacin tablets should be administered at least 2 hours before or 6 hours after such preparations.

It is not known if an interaction exists between IV delafloxacin and oral iron preparations or multivitamins containing iron or zinc. However, IV delafloxacin should not be administered through the same IV line with any solution containing multivalent cations.

● Midazolam

Concomitant use of delafloxacin tablets (450 mg every 12 hours for 5 days) and a single 5-mg dose of midazolam (a CYP3A substrate) in healthy individuals did not have a substantial effect on peak plasma concentrations or area under the plasma concentration-time curve (AUC) of midazolam or its metabolite, 1-hydroxymidazolam, compared with administration of midazolam alone.

● Sucralfate

Pharmacokinetic interaction if delafloxacin tablets are administered concomitantly with sucralfate (possible decreased absorption and decreased systemic concentrations of delafloxacin). Delafloxacin tablets should be taken at least 2 hours before or 6 hours after sucralfate.

It is not known if an interaction exists between IV delafloxacin and sucralfate.

PHARMACOKINETICS

● Absorption

Bioavailability

The absolute bioavailability of a single 450-mg oral dose of delafloxacin is 58.8%.

In adults receiving delafloxacin tablets in a dosage of 450 mg every 12 hours, peak plasma concentrations of the drug are attained 0.75 hours after a single dose and 1 hour after a dose at steady state. When delafloxacin is administered by IV infusion in a dosage of 300 mg every 12 hours, peak plasma concentrations are attained at the end of the 1-hour infusion after a single dose and at steady state.

Steady state is achieved within approximately 3 days after oral or IV administration of delafloxacin with accumulation of approximately 36 or 10%, respectively.

The area under the plasma concentration-time curve (AUC) of delafloxacin following a single 450-mg oral dose is comparable to the AUC following a single 300-mg IV dose. Although peak plasma concentrations following oral administration of 450 mg of delafloxacin are approximately 55% lower than peak plasma concentrations following IV administration of 300 mg of the drug, this is not considered clinically important.

Food

Food does not substantially affect oral bioavailability of delafloxacin tablets.

● Distribution

Extent

The steady-state volume of distribution of delafloxacin is 30–48 L, which approximates total body water.

Delafloxacin is distributed into breast milk in rats; it is not known whether the drug is distributed into human breast milk.

Plasma Protein Binding

Delafloxacin is 84% bound to plasma proteins, principally albumin.

Special Populations

Plasma protein binding is not substantially affected in patients with renal impairment.

● *Elimination*

Metabolism

Delafloxacin is metabolized primarily via glucuronidation by uridine diphosphate-glucuronosyltransferase (UGT) 1A1, 1A3, and 2B15; about 1% of a dose undergoes oxidative metabolism.

Elimination Route

Following a single oral dose of delafloxacin, 50% of the dose is excreted in urine as unchanged delafloxacin and glucuronide metabolites; 48% is excreted in feces as unchanged drug.

Following a single IV dose of delafloxacin, 65% of the dose is excreted in urine as unchanged delafloxacin and glucuronide metabolites; 28% is excreted in feces as unchanged drug.

Half-life

The mean half-life of delafloxacin following multiple oral doses of the drug is 4.2–8.5 hours.

The mean half-life of delafloxacin following a single IV dose of the drug is 3.7 hours.

Special Populations

In patients with mild, moderate, or severe hepatic impairment (Child-Pugh class A, B, or C), peak plasma concentrations and AUC of delafloxacin following a single 300-mg IV dose were not substantially affected compared with matched healthy control individuals.

In individuals with mild renal impairment (estimated glomerular filtration rate [eGFR] of 51–80 mL/minute per 1.73 m²) who received a single 400-mg oral dose of delafloxacin, mean total exposures of the drug were comparable to exposures in healthy individuals. Following a single 400-mg oral dose of delafloxacin in individuals with moderate or severe renal impairment (eGFR of 15–50 mL/minute per 1.73 m²), mean total exposures of the drug were increased about 1.5-fold compared with healthy individuals.

Following a single 300-mg IV dose of delafloxacin in individuals with mild, moderate, or severe renal impairment, mean total exposures of the drug were 1.3-, 1.6-, or 1.8-fold higher, respectively, than those observed in matched control individuals. In individuals with end-stage renal disease (ESRD) on hemodialysis who received a single 300-mg IV dose of delafloxacin 1 hour before and 1 hour after hemodialysis, mean total exposures of the drug were 2.1- and 2.6-fold higher, respectively, compared with exposures observed in matched control individuals. A 4-hour period of hemodialysis removed approximately 19% of the dose into the dialysate.

Accumulation of the IV vehicle, sulfobutylether-β-cyclodextrin (SBECD), occurs in patients with moderate or severe renal impairment and in those with ESRD on hemodialysis. Following IV administration of delafloxacin in individuals with moderate or severe renal impairment, mean systemic exposures of SBECD were twofold or fivefold higher, respectively, than those observed in matched control individuals. Following IV administration of delafloxacin 1 hour before and 1 hour after hemodialysis in individuals with ESRD, systemic exposures of SBECD were 7.5- and 27-fold higher, respectively, than those observed in matched control individuals. A 4-hour period of hemodialysis removed 56.1% of SBECD into the dialysate.

Pharmacokinetics of delafloxacin are not substantially affected by age, gender, race, weight, or body mass index.

DESCRIPTION

Delafloxacin meglumine is a fluoroquinolone anti-infective agent. Like other fluoroquinolones, delafloxacin contains a fluorine at the C-6 position of the quinolone nucleus. However, the molecular structure of delafloxacin differs from those of other commercially available fluoroquinolones in 3 notable areas: delafloxacin does not have a strong base at the C-7 position, which allows the drug to be anionic in neutral environments and uncharged in slightly acidic environments; it has a chlorine atom at the C-8 position, which acts as an electron-withdrawing group and reduces the reactivity of the heterocycle; and it has an aromatic ring attached to N1, which increases the molecular surface area compared with other fluoroquinolones. The anionic characteristics of delafloxacin appear to contribute to increased potency of the drug against susceptible bacteria compared with other fluoroquinolones, especially in environments with acidic pH.

Like other fluoroquinolone anti-infectives, the antibacterial activity of delafloxacin is due to inhibition of bacterial topoisomerase IV and DNA gyrase (i.e., topoisomerase II) enzymes, which are required for bacterial DNA replication, transcription, repair, and recombination. Delafloxacin demonstrates similar affinity for both topoisomerase IV and DNA gyrase.

In vitro, delafloxacin exhibits concentration-dependent bactericidal activity against gram-positive and gram-negative bacteria.

SPECTRUM

Delafloxacin is active in vitro and in clinical infections against many gram-positive aerobic bacteria, including *Staphylococcus aureus* (including methicillin-resistant *S. aureus* [MRSA; also known as oxacillin-resistant *S. aureus* or ORSA] and methicillin-susceptible *S. aureus*), *S. haemolyticus*, *S. lugdunensis*, *Streptococcus pyogenes* (group A β-hemolytic streptococci, GAS), *S. agalactiae* (group B streptococci, GBS), *S. anginosus* group (including *S. anginosus*, *S. intermedius*, and *S. constellatus*), and *Enterococcus faecalis*. Delafloxacin has been active in vitro against some staphylococci (including MRSA), streptococci, and enterococci that were resistant to some other fluoroquinolones.

Delafloxacin is active in vitro and in clinical infections against some gram-negative aerobic bacteria, including *Escherichia coli*, *Enterobacter cloacae*, *Klebsiella pneumoniae*, and *Pseudomonas aeruginosa*.

Although the clinical importance is unknown, delafloxacin also has in vitro activity against some other gram-positive aerobic bacteria, including *S. dysgalactiae*, *S. epidermidis*, *S. pneumoniae*, *E. faecium*, and *Listeria monocytogenes*, and some other gram-negative aerobic bacteria, including *Citrobacter freundii*, *C. koseri*, *Eikenella corrodens*, *E. aerogenes*, *Haemophilus influenzae*, *H. parainfluenzae*, *Helicobacter pylori*, *K. oxytoca*, *Legionella*, *Moraxella catarrhalis*, *Neisseria gonorrhoeae*, *Proteus mirabilis*, *Serratia marcescens*, *Salmonella*, and *Shigella*.

Delafloxacin has some in vitro activity against some anaerobic bacteria, including *Bacteroides fragilis*, *Clostridium perfringens*, and *Clostridioides difficile* (formerly known as *Clostridium difficile*); however, the clinical importance of these in vitro data is unknown.

RESISTANCE

Resistance to fluoroquinolones, including delafloxacin, can occur due to mutations in target regions of topoisomerase IV and/or DNA gyrase (i.e., quinolone-resistance determining regions [QRDRs]) or through altered efflux. In vitro, resistance to delafloxacin develops by multiple step mutations in QRDRs of gram-positive and gram-negative bacteria (e.g., double mutations in *gyr*A and *par*C).

Cross-resistance between delafloxacin and other fluoroquinolones has been observed; however, some gram-positive and gram-negative bacteria resistant to other fluoroquinolones may be susceptible to delafloxacin.

ADVICE TO PATIENTS

Advise patients to read the manufacturer's patient information (medication guide).

Advise patients that antibacterials (including delafloxacin) should only be used to treat bacterial infections and not used to treat viral infections (e.g., the common cold).

Advise patients that delafloxacin tablets may be taken without regard to food.

Importance of taking delafloxacin tablets at least 2 hours before or 6 hours after magnesium- or aluminum-containing antacids; sucralfate; multivitamins or dietary supplements containing iron or zinc; or buffered didanosine (pediatric powder for oral solution).

Importance of completing full course of therapy, even if feeling better after a few days. Advise patients that skipping doses or not completing the full course of therapy may decrease effectiveness and increase the likelihood that bacteria will develop resistance and will not be treatable with delafloxacin or other antibacterials in the future.

If a dose of delafloxacin is missed and remembered within 8 hours after the scheduled time, the dose should be taken as soon as possible and the next dose taken at the regularly scheduled time. If a dose is missed and remembered more than 8 hours after the scheduled time, the dose should be skipped and the next dose taken at the regularly scheduled time.

Inform patients that systemic fluoroquinolones have been associated with disabling and potentially irreversible serious adverse reactions (e.g., tendinitis and tendon rupture, peripheral neuropathy, CNS effects) that may occur together in the same patient. Advise patients to immediately discontinue delafloxacin and contact a clinician if they experience any signs or symptoms of serious adverse effects (e.g., unusual joint or tendon pain, muscle weakness, a "pins and needles" tingling or pricking sensation, numbness of the arms or legs, confusion, hallucinations) while taking the drug. Advise patients to talk with a clinician if they have any questions or concerns.

Inform patients that systemic fluoroquinolones are associated with an increased risk of tendinitis and tendon rupture in all age groups and that this risk is increased in adults older than 60 years of age, individuals receiving corticosteroids, and kidney, heart, or lung transplant recipients. Symptoms may be irreversible. Importance of resting and refraining from exercise at the first sign of tendinitis or tendon rupture (e.g., pain, swelling, or inflammation of a tendon or weakness or inability to use a joint) and importance of immediately discontinuing the drug and contacting a clinician. (See Tendinitis and Tendon Rupture under Warnings/Precautions: Warnings, in Cautions.)

Inform patients that peripheral neuropathies have been reported in patients receiving systemic fluoroquinolones and that symptoms may occur soon after initiation of the drug and may be irreversible. Importance of immediately discontinuing delafloxacin and contacting a clinician if symptoms of peripheral neuropathy (e.g., pain, burning, tingling, numbness, and/or weakness) occur.

Inform patients that systemic fluoroquinolones have been associated with CNS effects (e.g., convulsions, dizziness, lightheadedness, increased intracranial pressure). Importance of informing clinician of any history of convulsions before initiating therapy with the drug. Importance of contacting a clinician if persistent headache with or without blurred vision occurs.

Because fluoroquinolones may cause dizziness and lightheadedness, caution patients that they should not engage in activities requiring mental alertness and motor coordination (e.g., driving a vehicle, operating machinery) until the effects of delafloxacin on the individual are known.

Advise patients that systemic fluoroquinolones may worsen myasthenia gravis symptoms; importance of informing clinician of any history of myasthenia gravis. Importance of immediately contacting a clinician if any symptoms of muscle weakness, including respiratory difficulties, occur.

Inform patients that delafloxacin may be associated with hypersensitivity reactions (including anaphylactic reactions), even after the first dose. Importance of immediately discontinuing delafloxacin and contacting a clinician at first sign of rash, hives or other skin reaction, rapid heartbeat, difficulty swallowing or breathing, any swelling suggesting angioedema (e.g., swelling of lips, tongue, or face; throat tightness; hoarseness), jaundice, or any other sign of hypersensitivity.

Inform patients that systemic fluoroquinolones may increase the risk of aortic aneurysm and dissection; importance of informing clinician of any history of aneurysms, blockages or hardening of the arteries, high blood pressure, or genetic conditions such as Marfan syndrome or Ehlers-Danlos syndrome. Advise patients to seek immediate medical treatment if they experience sudden, severe, and constant pain in the stomach, chest, or back.

Inform patients that hypoglycemia has been reported when systemic fluoroquinolones were used in some patients receiving antidiabetic agents. Advise patients with diabetes mellitus receiving oral antidiabetic agents or insulin to discontinue fluoroquinolone treatment and contact a clinician if they experience hypoglycemia or symptoms of hypoglycemia.

Advise patients that diarrhea is a common problem caused by anti-infectives and usually ends when the drug is discontinued. Importance of contacting a clinician if watery and bloody stools (with or without stomach cramps and fever) occur during or as late as 2 months or longer after the last dose.

Importance of informing clinician of existing or contemplated concomitant therapy, including prescription and OTC drugs, as well as any concomitant illnesses.

Importance of women informing clinicians if they are or plan to become pregnant or plan to breast-feed.

Importance of advising patients of other important precautionary information. (See Cautions.)

PREPARATIONS

Excipients in commercially available drug preparations may have clinically important effects in some individuals; consult specific product labeling for details.

Delafloxacin Meglumine

Oral		
Tablets	450 mg (of delafloxacin)	Baxdela®, Melinta
Parenteral		
For injection, for IV infusion	300 mg (of delafloxacin)	Baxdela®, Melinta

Selected Revisions September 2, 2019, © Copyright, July 17, 2017, American Society of Health-System Pharmacists, Inc.

levoFLOXacin

8:12.18 • QUINOLONES

■ Levofloxacin is a fluoroquinolone anti-infective agent.

USES

● Respiratory Tract Infections

Acute Sinusitis

Levofloxacin is used for the treatment of acute bacterial sinusitis caused by susceptible *Streptococcus pneumoniae*, *Haemophilus influenzae*, or *Moraxella catarrhalis*.

Levofloxacin should be used for the treatment of acute bacterial sinusitis only when there are no other treatment options. Because systemic fluoroquinolones, including levofloxacin, have been associated with disabling and potentially irreversible serious adverse reactions (e.g., tendinitis and tendon rupture, peripheral neuropathy, CNS effects) that can occur together in the same patient (see Cautions) and because acute bacterial sinusitis may be self-limiting in some patients, the risks of serious adverse reactions outweigh the benefits of fluoroquinolones for patients with acute sinusitis.

Clinical Experience

In one open study in adults with acute bacterial sinusitis, therapy with oral levofloxacin (500 mg once daily) or oral amoxicillin and clavulanate potassium (500 mg of amoxicillin 3 times daily) resulted in success rates of 88 or 87%, respectively.

In a double-blind, prospective study in adults with acute bacterial sinusitis randomized to receive levofloxacin in a dosage of 500 mg once daily for 10 days or a dosage of 750 mg once daily for 5 days, safety and efficacy of both regimens were similar. The clinical success rate (defined as complete or partial resolution of pretreatment signs and symptoms of sinusitis to such an extent that no further anti-infective treatment was indicated) in the microbiologically evaluable patient population at the test-of-cure visit was 88.6% in those who received the 10-day regimen compared with 91.4% in those who received the 5-day regimen. When results were stratified according to pathogen, the clinical success rate was 96.3 or 92.6% in those with *S. pneumoniae*, 92.6 or 90.5% in those with *H. influenzae*, and 100 or 90.9% in those with *M. catarrhalis*.

Acute Exacerbations of Chronic Bronchitis

Levofloxacin is used for the treatment of acute bacterial exacerbations of chronic bronchitis caused by susceptible *Staphylococcus aureus* (methicillin-susceptible [oxacillin-susceptible] strains), *S. pneumoniae*, *H. influenzae*, *H. parainfluenzae*, or *M. catarrhalis*.

Levofloxacin should be used for the treatment of acute bacterial exacerbations of chronic bronchitis only when there are no other treatment options. Because systemic fluoroquinolones, including levofloxacin, have been associated with disabling and potentially irreversible serious adverse reactions (e.g., tendinitis and tendon rupture, peripheral neuropathy, CNS effects) that can occur together in the same patient (see Cautions) and because acute bacterial exacerbations of chronic bronchitis may be self-limiting is some patients, the risks of serious adverse reactions outweigh the benefits of fluoroquinolones for patients with these infections.

Clinical Experience

In controlled clinical studies in adults with acute bacterial exacerbations of chronic bronchitis, levofloxacin was as effective as therapy with cefaclor or cefuroxime. Levofloxacin therapy generally resulted in bacterial cure rates of 95–97% in patients with acute bacterial exacerbations of chronic bronchitis. The most prevalent pathogens in these studies were *H. influenzae*, *H. parainfluenzae*, *M. catarrhalis*, and *S. pneumoniae*.

Community-acquired Pneumonia

Levofloxacin is used for the treatment of community-acquired pneumonia (CAP) caused by susceptible *S. aureus* (methicillin-susceptible [oxacillin-susceptible] strains), *S. pneumoniae* (including multidrug-resistant *S. pneumoniae* [MDRSP]), *H. influenzae*, *H. parainfluenzae*, *Klebsiella pneumoniae*, *Legionella pneumophila*, *M. catarrhalis*, *Chlamydophila pneumoniae* (formerly *Chlamydia pneumoniae*), or *Mycoplasma pneumoniae*.

Initial treatment of CAP generally involves use of an empiric anti-infective regimen based on the most likely pathogens and local susceptibility patterns; treatment may then be changed (if possible) to provide a more specific regimen (pathogen-directed therapy) based on results of in vitro culture and susceptibility testing. The most appropriate empiric regimen varies depending on the severity of illness at the time of presentation, whether outpatient treatment or hospitalization in or out of an intensive care unit (ICU) is indicated, and the presence or absence of cardiopulmonary disease and other modifying factors that increase the risk of certain pathogens (e.g., methicillin-resistant *S. aureus* [MRSA; also known as oxacillin-resistant *S. aureus* or ORSA], penicillin-resistant *S. pneumoniae*, MDRSP, enteric gram-negative bacilli, *Ps. aeruginosa*).

For additional information on management of CAP, the current clinical practice guidelines from the Infectious Diseases Society of America (IDSA) available at http://www.idsociety.org should be consulted.

Clinical Experience

In one controlled clinical study in adults with CAP, a 7- to 14-day regimen that included IV and/or oral levofloxacin was as effective as a regimen that included IV ceftriaxone and/or oral cefuroxime. Levofloxacin generally resulted in clinical success (cure or improvement) 5–7 days following completion of therapy in 93–95% of adults with CAP. In a randomized study in CAP patients 65 years of age or older (mean age 77.9 years), the clinical cure rate at the test-of-cure visit (5–21 days after end of treatment) was 92.9% in those who received moxifloxacin and 87.9% in those who received levofloxacin; the bacteriologic success rate was 81% in those who received moxifloxacin and 75% in those who received levofloxacin.

In controlled clinical studies, presumptive bacteriologic eradication 5–7 days following completion of therapy was evident in 98% of patients with *H. influenzae* infection, 95% of those with *H. parainfluenzae* infection, 100% of those with *K. pneumoniae* infection, 94% of those with *M. catarrhalis* infection, 88% of those with *S. aureus* infection, and 95% of those with *S. pneumoniae* infection. Clinical success rate 5–7 days following completion of therapy in patients with atypical pneumonia caused by *C. pneumoniae*, *M. pneumoniae*, or *L. pneumoniae* was 96, 96, or 70%, respectively.

Safety and efficacy of a 5-day regimen of levofloxacin (750 mg IV or orally once daily for 5 days) was compared with that of a 10-day regimen of the drug (500 mg IV or orally once daily for 10 days) in a double-blind, randomized, prospective study in adults with clinically or radiologically confirmed mild to severe CAP. The clinical success rate (cure and improvement) was about 91% in both groups.

A clinical and bacteriologic success rate of 95% has been reported when levofloxacin was used in adults for the treatment of CAP caused by multidrug-resistant *S. pneumoniae*.

Nosocomial Pneumonia

Levofloxacin is used for the treatment of nosocomial pneumonia caused by susceptible *S. aureus* (methicillin-susceptible [oxacillin-susceptible] strains), *S. pneumoniae*, *H. influenzae*, *Escherichia coli*, *K. pneumoniae*, *Ps. aeruginosa*, or *Serratia marcescens*. Adjunctive therapy should be used as clinically indicated. If the infection is known or suspected of being caused by *Ps. aeruginosa*, concomitant therapy with an antipseudomonal β-lactam anti-infective is recommended.

Local susceptibility data should be used when selecting initial empiric regimens for the treatment of hospital-acquired pneumonia (HAP) not associated with mechanical ventilation or the treatment of ventilator-associated pneumonia (VAP).

For initial empiric treatment of HAP in adults who are not at high risk of mortality and have no factors that increase the likelihood of MRSA, IDSA and the American Thoracic Society (ATS) state that levofloxacin is one of several options that can be considered. However, these experts state that levofloxacin should be used in conjunction with an antibacterial active against MRSA (vancomycin, linezolid) if factors that increase the likelihood of MRSA are present or if the patient is at high risk of mortality or has received IV anti-infectives during the prior 90 days.

In adults with clinically suspected VAP, IDSA and ATS state that levofloxacin is one option that can be considered for initial empiric treatment in those not at increased risk for MRSA. However, in patients with factors that increase the risk of MRSA or multidrug-resistant gram-negative bacteria, these experts state that levofloxacin should be used in conjunction with an anti-infective active against MRSA (vancomycin, linezolid) plus an antipseudomonal β-lactam (fixed combination of piperacillin and tazobactam [piperacillin/tazobactam], cefepime, ceftazidime, imipenem, meropenem, aztreonam).

For additional information on management of nosocomial pneumonia, the current clinical practice guidelines from IDSA available at http://www.idsociety.org should be consulted.

Clinical Experience

In a multicenter, randomized, open-label study in adults with clinical and radiologically documented nosocomial pneumonia, patients were randomized to receive a 7- to 15-day regimen of IV levofloxacin (750 mg once daily) following by oral levofloxacin (750 mg once daily) or IV imipenem and cilastatin sodium (500–1000 mg every 6–8 hours) followed by oral ciprofloxacin (750 mg every 12 hours). Patients with documented *Ps. aeruginosa* infections received adjunctive therapy with ceftazidime or piperacillin and tazobactam sodium (for those receiving levofloxacin) or an aminoglycoside (for those receiving the comparator regimen); those with suspected MRSA received concomitant vancomycin. The overall clinical success rate 3–15 days after completion of therapy was 58.1% for those receiving levofloxacin and 60.6% for those receiving the comparator regimen; the overall microbiologic eradication rate was 66.7 and 60.6%, respectively.

● Skin and Skin Structure Infections

Levofloxacin is used for the treatment of mild to moderate uncomplicated skin and skin structure infections caused by susceptible *S. aureus* (methicillin-susceptible [oxacillin-susceptible] strains) or *S. pyogenes* (group A β-hemolytic streptococci) and for the treatment of complicated skin and skin structure infections caused by susceptible *S. aureus* (methicillin-susceptible [oxacillin-susceptible] strains), *Enterococcus faecalis*, *S. pyogenes*, or *Proteus mirabilis*.

For additional information on management of skin and skin structure infections, the current clinical practice guidelines from IDSA available at http://www.idsociety.org should be consulted.

Clinical Experience

Levofloxacin has been effective for the treatment of uncomplicated abscesses, cellulitis, erysipelas, furuncles, impetigo, pyoderma, and wound or surgical infections caused by susceptible bacteria. In 2 controlled studies, oral levofloxacin was as effective as oral ciprofloxacin in the treatment of mild to moderate skin infections caused by susceptible bacteria, mainly *S. aureus* and *S. pyogenes*. Levofloxacin resulted in a bacteriologic cure rate of 93–97.5% in patients with mild to moderate skin and skin structure infections.

In an open-label, randomized study in patients with complicated skin and skin structure infections, the overall success rate (improved or cured) in clinically evaluable patients at 2–5 days after completion of treatment was 84.1% in those randomized to receive levofloxacin (750 mg once daily for 7–14 days given IV and/or orally as indicated) and 80.3% in those randomized to the comparator regimen (fixed combination of IV ticarcillin and clavulanate [no longer commercially available in the US] followed by oral amoxicillin and clavulanate for a total duration of 7–14 days). Success rates varied depending on the diagnosis, ranging from 69% in those with infected diabetic ulcers to 90% in those with infected abscesses. In the microbiologically evaluable population, the overall rate of eradication was 83.7% in those who received levofloxacin and 71.4% in those who received the comparator regimen.

● Urinary Tract Infections and Prostatitis
Uncomplicated Urinary Tract Infections

Levofloxacin is used for the treatment of mild to moderate uncomplicated urinary tract infections (UTIs) caused by susceptible *E. coli*, *K. pneumoniae*, or *S. saprophyticus*.

Levofloxacin should be used for the treatment of uncomplicated UTIs only when there are no other treatment options. Because systemic fluoroquinolones, including levofloxacin, have been associated with disabling and potentially irreversible serious adverse reactions (e.g., tendinitis and tendon rupture, peripheral neuropathy, CNS effects) that can occur together in the same patient (see Cautions) and because uncomplicated UTIs may be self-limiting in some patients, the risks of serious adverse reactions outweigh the benefits of fluoroquinolones for patients with uncomplicated UTIs.

IDSA and other experts state that fluoroquinolones (ciprofloxacin, levofloxacin, ofloxacin) should be considered alternative agents for the treatment of uncomplicated UTIs (e.g., acute cystitis) and should be used in these infections *only* when other urinary anti-infectives are likely to be ineffective or are contraindicated or not tolerated.

Complicated Urinary Tract Infections

Levofloxacin is used for the treatment of mild to moderate complicated UTIs caused by susceptible *E. faecalis*, *Enterobacter cloacae*, *E. coli*, *K. pneumoniae*, *P. mirabilis*, or *Ps. aeruginosa* and acute pyelonephritis caused by susceptible *E. coli*, including cases with concurrent bacteremia.

In controlled clinical studies, levofloxacin therapy was as effective as ciprofloxacin in the treatment of complicated UTIs or pyelonephritis. In one study in adults with complicated UTIs, bacterial eradication 5–9 days following completion of therapy was evident in 93% of patients with *E. coli* infection, 97% of those with *K. pneumoniae* infection, and 90% of those with *P. mirabilis* infection.

Prostatitis

Levofloxacin is used for the treatment of chronic prostatitis caused by susceptible *E. coli*, *E. faecalis*, or *S. epidermidis* (methicillin-susceptible [oxacillin-susceptible] strains).

In one double-blind controlled study, adults with prostatitis were randomized to receive a 28-day regimen of oral levofloxacin (500 mg once daily) or ciprofloxacin (500 mg twice daily). The overall microbiologic eradication rate 5–18 days after completion of treatment was 75% in those who received levofloxacin and 76.8% in those who received ciprofloxacin. In those with infections caused by *E. coli*, *E. faecalis*, or *S. epidermidis*, the eradication rate was 93.3, 72.2, or 81.8%, respectively, in those who received levofloxacin and 81.8, 75, or 78.6%, respectively, in those who received ciprofloxacin.

● Endocarditis

Levofloxacin is used as an alternative for the treatment of endocarditis† (native or prosthetic valve or other prosthetic material) caused by fastidious gram-negative bacilli known as the HACEK group (*Haemophilus*, *Aggregatibacter*, *Cardiobacterium hominis*, *Eikenella corrodens*, *Kingella*).

The American Heart Association (AHA) and IDSA recommend ceftriaxone (or other third or fourth generation cephalosporin) for the treatment of endocarditis caused by the HACEK group, but state that a fluoroquinolone (ciprofloxacin, levofloxacin, moxifloxacin) may be considered in patients who cannot tolerate cephalosporins. Because only limited data are available regarding use of fluoroquinolones for the treatment of HACEK endocarditis, an infectious disease specialist should be consulted when treating such infections in patients who cannot tolerate cephalosporins.

● GI Infections
Campylobacter Infections

Levofloxacin has been recommended as an alternative for the treatment of campylobacteriosis† caused by susceptible *Campylobacter*.

Optimal treatment of campylobacteriosis in patients with human immunodeficiency virus (HIV) infection has not been identified. Some clinicians withhold anti-infective treatment in HIV-infected patients with CD4+ T-cell counts exceeding 200 cells/mm³ if they have only mild campylobacteriosis and initiate treatment if symptoms persist for more than several days. In HIV-infected patients with mild to moderate campylobacteriosis, treatment with a fluoroquinolone (preferably ciprofloxacin or, alternatively, levofloxacin or moxifloxacin) or azithromycin is reasonable. Anti-infective therapy should be modified based on results of in vitro susceptibility testing. In the US, resistance to fluoroquinolones has been reported in 22% of *C. jejuni* and 35% of *C. coli* isolates tested. To limit emergence of resistance, some clinicians suggest that it may be prudent to use an aminoglycoside concomitantly in patients with bacteremic infections.

Salmonella Gastroenteritis

Levofloxacin is used for the treatment of *Salmonella* gastroenteritis† (with or without bacteremia).

Anti-infective therapy is not usually indicated in otherwise healthy individuals with uncomplicated (noninvasive) gastroenteritis caused by *Salmonella* since such therapy may prolong the duration of fecal excretion of the organism and there is no evidence that it shortens the duration of the disease; however, the US Centers for Disease Control and Prevention (CDC), American Academy of Pediatrics (AAP), IDSA, and others recommend anti-infective therapy in individuals with severe *Salmonella* gastroenteritis and in those who are at increased risk of invasive disease. These individuals include infants younger than 3–6 months of age; individuals older than 50 years of age; individuals with hemoglobinopathies, severe atherosclerosis or valvular heart disease, prostheses, uremia, chronic GI disease, or severe colitis; and individuals who are immunocompromised because of malignancy, immunosuppressive therapy, HIV infection, or other immunosuppressive illness.

Because HIV-infected individuals with *Salmonella* gastroenteritis are at high risk for bacteremia, CDC, National Institutes of Health (NIH), and HIV Medicine Association of IDSA recommend that such patients receive anti-infective treatment. These experts state that the initial drug of choice for the treatment of salmonella gastroenteritis (with or without bacteremia) in HIV-infected adults is ciprofloxacin; other fluoroquinolones (levofloxacin, moxifloxacin) also are likely to be effective in these patients, but clinical data are limited. Depending on results of in vitro susceptibility testing of the causative organism, alternatives for treatment of *Salmonella* gastroenteritis in HIV-infected adults are co-trimoxazole or third generation cephalosporins (ceftriaxone, cefotaxime).

The role of long-term treatment (secondary prophylaxis) against *Salmonella* in HIV-infected individuals is not well established, and possible benefits of such prophylaxis should be weighed against the risks of long-term anti-infective exposure. CDC, NIH, and IDSA state that secondary prophylaxis should be considered in those with recurrent bacteremia and may also be considered in those with recurrent gastroenteritis (with or without bacteremia) and in those with CD4+ T-cell counts less than 200 cells/mm³ and severe diarrhea. These experts state that secondary prophylaxis should be discontinued if the *Salmonella* infection resolves and there has been a sustained response to antiretroviral therapy with CD4+ T-cell counts greater than 200 cells/mm³.

Shigella Infections

Levofloxacin is used as an alternative for the treatment of shigellosis† caused by susceptible *Shigella*.

Infections caused by *S. sonnei* usually are self-limited (48–72 hours), and mild cases may not require treatment with anti-infectives. However, because there is some evidence that anti-infectives may shorten the duration of diarrhea and the period of fecal excretion of *Shigella*, anti-infective treatment generally is recommended in addition to fluid and electrolyte replacement in patients with severe shigellosis, dysentery, or underlying immunosuppression. An empiric treatment regimen can be used initially, but in vitro susceptibility testing of clinical isolates is indicated since resistance is common. A fluoroquinolone (preferably ciprofloxacin or, alternatively, levofloxacin or moxifloxacin) generally has been recommended for the treatment of shigellosis. However, fluoroquinolone-resistant *Shigella* have been reported in the US, especially in international travelers, the homeless, and men who have sex with men (MSM). Depending on in vitro susceptibility, other drugs recommended for the treatment of shigellosis include co-trimoxazole, ceftriaxone, azithromycin (not recommended in those with bacteremia), or ampicillin.

Travelers' Diarrhea

Oral levofloxacin has been used for the short-term treatment of travelers' diarrhea† and has been used for the prevention of travelers' diarrhea† in adults traveling for relatively short periods of time to high-risk areas.

The most common cause of travelers' diarrhea worldwide is noninvasive enterotoxigenic strains of *E. coli* (ETEC), but travelers' diarrhea also can be caused by various other bacteria, including enteroaggregative and other *E. coli* pathotypes, *C. jejuni, Shigella, Salmonella, Aeromonas, Plesiomonas*, and, possibly, *Acrobacter, Larobacter*, and enterotoxigenic *Bacteroides fragilis*. In some cases, travelers' diarrhea is caused by parasitic enteric pathogens (e.g., *Giardia, Cryptosporidium, Entamoeba histolytica*) or viral enteric pathogens (e.g., norovirus, rotavirus, astrovirus).

Countries where travelers are at low risk of travelers' diarrhea include the US, Canada, Australia, New Zealand, Japan, and countries in Northern and Western Europe. Travelers are at intermediate risk for travelers' diarrhea in Eastern Europe, South Africa, and some of the Caribbean islands, but are at high risk in most of Asia, the Middle East, Africa, Mexico, and Central and South America.

Treatment

Travelers' diarrhea caused by bacteria may be self-limited and often resolves within 3–7 days without anti-infective treatment. CDC states that anti-infective treatment is *not* recommended in patients with mild travelers' diarrhea. However, CDC and other clinicians state that empiric short-term anti-infective treatment (single dose or up to 3 days) may be used if diarrhea is moderate or severe,

associated with fever or bloody stools, or extremely disruptive to travel plans. Since bacteria are the most common cause of travelers' diarrhea (80–90% of cases), an anti-infective directed against enteric bacterial pathogens usually is used. Fluoroquinolones (e.g., ciprofloxacin, levofloxacin) generally have been considered the anti-infectives of choice for empiric treatment, including self-treatment, of travelers' diarrhea in adults; alternatives include azithromycin and rifaximin.

If the causative pathogen is susceptible to the anti-infective chosen for empiric therapy, the duration of illness may be reduced by about a day. However, the increasing incidence of enteric bacteria resistant to fluoroquinolones and other anti-infectives may limit the usefulness of empiric treatment in individuals traveling in certain geographic areas, and the possible adverse effects of the anti-infective and adverse consequences of such treatment (e.g., development of resistance, effect on normal gut microflora) should be considered.

Prophylaxis

CDC and most experts do *not* recommend prophylactic use of anti-infectives to prevent travelers' diarrhea in most individuals traveling to areas of risk. However, anti-infective prophylaxis may be considered for short-term travelers who are high-risk individuals (e.g., HIV-infected or other immunocompromised individuals, travelers with poorly controlled diabetes mellitus or chronic renal failure) and those who are taking critical trips during which even a short period of diarrhea could adversely affect the purpose of the trip.

The use of anti-infective prophylaxis in travelers should be weighed against the use of prompt, early self-treatment with an empiric anti-infective if moderate to severe travelers' diarrhea occurs. If anti-infective prophylaxis is used, fluoroquinolones (e.g., ciprofloxacin, levofloxacin) usually have been recommended; alternatives include azithromycin and rifaximin. The increasing incidence of fluoroquinolone resistance in pathogens that cause travelers' diarrhea (e.g., *Campylobacter, Salmonella, Shigella*) should be considered and may limit their potential usefulness.

Helicobacter pylori Infection

Levofloxacin has been used as a component of various multiple-drug regimens for the treatment of infections caused by *Helicobacter pylori*†.

Although safety and efficacy of levofloxacin-containing regimens have not been established, a 3-drug regimen that includes a proton-pump inhibitor (PPI), levofloxacin, and amoxicillin has been suggested as a first-line option for the treatment of *H. pylori* infection. In addition, a 4-drug regimen that includes a PPI, levofloxacin, nitazoxanide, and doxycycline and a sequential regimen that includes initial treatment with a PPI and amoxicillin followed by treatment with a PPI, levofloxacin, and a nitroimidazole (either tinidazole or metronidazole) have been suggested as other possible first-line options. Levofloxacin-containing regimens also have been recommended for second-line or salvage therapy in patients with persistent *H. pylori* infection. Data are limited regarding the prevalence of fluoroquinolone-resistant *H. pylori* in the US; the possible impact of such resistance on the efficacy of fluoroquinolone-containing regimens used for the treatment of *H. pylori* infections is not known.

● Anthrax

Levofloxacin is used for inhalational anthrax (postexposure) to reduce the incidence or progression of disease following suspected or confirmed exposure to aerosolized *Bacillus anthracis* spores in adults and pediatric patients. Although efficacy of levofloxacin for postexposure prophylaxis to prevent inhalational anthrax has not been evaluated in human clinical trials, the drug is labeled by FDA for this indication based on a surrogate end point derived from a primate model of inhalational anthrax that predicts clinical benefit based on plasma levofloxacin concentrations achievable in humans with recommended oral or IV dosages.

CDC, AAP, US Working Group on Civilian Biodefense, and US Army Medical Research Institute of Infectious Diseases (USAMRIID) recommend oral ciprofloxacin and oral doxycycline as the initial drugs of choice for postexposure prophylaxis following exposure to aerosolized anthrax spores, including exposures that occur in the context of biologic warfare or bioterrorism. Other oral fluoroquinolones (levofloxacin, moxifloxacin, ofloxacin) are alternatives for postexposure prophylaxis when ciprofloxacin or doxycycline cannot be used.

Oral levofloxacin is one of several options recommended for the treatment of uncomplicated cutaneous anthrax† (without systemic involvement) that occurs in the context of biologic warfare or bioterrorism. CDC recommends that adults receive an oral regimen of ciprofloxacin, doxycycline, levofloxacin, or moxifloxacin for the treatment of such infections. AAP recommends that pediatric patients receive oral ciprofloxacin for the treatment of such infections and states that oral amoxicillin or penicillin V (if penicillin susceptibility is confirmed) or oral doxycycline, clindamycin, or levofloxacin are alternatives.

IV levofloxacin is recommended as an alternative to IV ciprofloxacin for use in multiple-drug parenteral regimens for initial treatment of systemic anthrax† (inhalational, GI, meningitis, or cutaneous with systemic involvement, extensive edema, or head or neck lesions) that occurs in the context of biologic warfare or bioterrorism. CDC, AAP, US Working Group on Civilian Biodefense, and USAMRIID recommend that treatment be initiated with a multiple-drug parenteral regimen that includes a fluoroquinolone (preferably ciprofloxacin) or doxycycline and 1 or 2 additional anti-infective agents predicted to be effective; after the patient is clinically stable, treatment can be changed to an oral anti-infective. For initial treatment of systemic anthrax with possible or confirmed meningitis, CDC and AAP recommend a regimen of IV ciprofloxacin in conjunction with another IV bactericidal anti-infective (preferably meropenem) and an IV protein synthesis inhibitor (preferably linezolid). If meningitis has been excluded, these experts recommend an initial regimen of IV ciprofloxacin in conjunction with an IV protein synthesis inhibitor (preferably clindamycin or linezolid).

Some experts suggest that oral ciprofloxacin or other oral fluoroquinolones (levofloxacin, moxifloxacin, ofloxacin) can be considered for the treatment of inhalational anthrax† when a parenteral regimen is not available. Although a multiple-drug parenteral regimen should be used for the treatment of inhalational anthrax, use of these parenteral regimens may not be possible if large numbers of individuals require treatment in a mass casualty setting and it may be necessary to use an oral regimen.

For additional information on postexposure prophylaxis and treatment of anthrax, see Uses: Anthrax in Ciprofloxacin 8:12.18.

● Chlamydial Infections

Levofloxacin is considered an alternative for the treatment of urogenital infections caused by Chlamydia trachomatis†. CDC states that a single oral dose of azithromycin or a 7-day regimen of oral doxycycline are the recommended regimens for the treatment of C. trachomatis urogenital infections in adults and adolescents; a 7-day regimen of oral erythromycin base or ethylsuccinate or a 7-day regimen of oral levofloxacin or ofloxacin are alternative regimens.

Individuals with HIV infection should receive the same treatment regimens recommended for other individuals with C. trachomatis urogenital infections.

Any individual who had sexual contact with a patient with C. trachomatis urogenital infection during the 60 days preceding the patient's onset of symptoms or diagnosis should be referred for evaluation, testing, and presumptive treatment with a regimen effective against Chlamydia. To minimize transmission and avoid reinfection, individuals treated for C. trachomatis urogenital infections should abstain from sexual intercourse until they and their partner(s) have been adequately treated (i.e., for 7 days after a single-dose regimen or after completion of a 7-day regimen) and symptoms have resolved.

● Gonorrhea and Associated Infections

Although levofloxacin was used in the past for the treatment of uncomplicated gonorrhea† caused by susceptible Neisseria gonorrhoeae, quinolone-resistant N. gonorrhoeae (QRNG) is widely disseminated throughout the world, including in the US. Therefore, CDC states that fluoroquinolones are no longer recommended for the treatment of gonorrhea and should not be used routinely for any associated infections that may involve N. gonorrhoeae (e.g., pelvic inflammatory disease [PID], epididymitis).

Levofloxacin is considered an alternative agent for the treatment of PID†. (See Uses: Pelvic Inflammatory Disease.)

Levofloxacin is considered an alternative agent for the treatment of acute epididymitis†. Although acute epididymitis in sexually active men younger than 35 years of age is most frequently caused by C. trachomatis or N. gonorrhoeae, epididymitis can also be caused by other organisms (e.g., sexually transmitted enteric bacteria, Mycoplasma, Ureaplasma, mycobacteria, fungi). Presumptive treatment is usually initiated prior to availability of all diagnostic laboratory test results, and the anti-infective regimen is selected based on the patient's risk for chlamydia, gonorrhea, and/or sexually transmitted enteric bacteria (e.g., E. coli). For treatment of acute epididymitis most likely caused by sexually transmitted chlamydia and gonorrhea, CDC recommends a single IM dose of ceftriaxone used

in conjunction with a 10-day regimen of oral doxycycline. For treatment of acute epididymitis most likely caused by sexually transmitted chlamydia and gonorrhea and enteric bacteria (e.g., in men who practice insertive anal sex), CDC recommends a single IM dose of ceftriaxone given in conjunction with a 10-day regimen of oral levofloxacin or ofloxacin. If acute epididymitis is most likely caused by enteric bacteria (e.g., in men who have undergone prostate biopsy, vasectomy, or other urinary tract instrumentation procedure) and gonorrhea has been ruled out (e.g., by gram, methylene blue, or gentian violet stain), CDC states that a 10-day regimen of oral levofloxacin or ofloxacin can be used alone.

For information on current recommendations for the treatment of gonorrhea and associated infections, see Uses: Gonorrhea and Associated Infections in Ceftriaxone 8:12.06.12. For additional information on quinolone-resistant N. gonorrhoeae (QRNG), see Uses: Gonorrhea and Associated Infections in Ciprofloxacin 8:12.18.

● Mycobacterial Infections
Treatment of Active Tuberculosis

Levofloxacin is used in multiple-drug regimens for the treatment of active tuberculosis† caused by Mycobacterium tuberculosis.

Although the potential role of fluoroquinolones and the optimal length of therapy have not been fully defined, ATS, CDC, IDSA, and others state that use of fluoroquinolones as alternative (second-line) agents can be considered for the treatment of active tuberculosis in patients intolerant of certain first-line agents and in those with relapse, treatment failure, or M. tuberculosis resistant to certain first-line agents. If a fluoroquinolone is used in multiple-drug regimens for the treatment of active tuberculosis, ATS, CDC, IDSA, and others recommend levofloxacin or moxifloxacin.

Although levofloxacin (or moxifloxacin) has been used instead of ethambutol during the intensive phase of treatment in adults who could not receive ethambutol and has been used instead of isoniazid throughout the course of treatment in adults who could not receive isoniazid, ATS, CDC, and IDSA state that there is no evidence that levofloxacin (or moxifloxacin) can be used to replace a rifamycin or pyrazinamide while maintaining a 6-month treatment regimen.

The fact that there are reports of fluoroquinolone-resistant M. tuberculosis and increasing reports of extensively drug-resistant tuberculosis (XDR tuberculosis) should be considered. XDR tuberculosis is caused by strains that are resistant to rifampin and isoniazid (multiple-drug resistant strains) and also are resistant to a fluoroquinolone and at least one parenteral second-line antimycobacterial (capreomycin, kanamycin, amikacin).

The most recent ATS, CDC, and IDSA recommendations for the treatment of tuberculosis should be consulted for more specific information.

Other Mycobacterial Infections

Levofloxacin has been used in multiple-drug regimens for the treatment of disseminated M. avium complex† (MAC) infections.

ATS and IDSA state that the role of fluoroquinolones in the treatment of MAC infections has not been established. If a fluoroquinolone is included in a multiple-drug treatment regimen (e.g., for macrolide-resistant MAC infections), levofloxacin or moxifloxacin may be preferred, although many strains are resistant in vitro.

The most recent ATS, CDC, and IDSA recommendations for the treatment of other mycobacterial infections should be consulted for more specific information.

● Nongonococcal Urethritis

Levofloxacin is considered as an alternative agent for the treatment of nongonococcal urethritis† (NGU). NGU can be caused by various organisms (e.g., Chlamydia, M. genitalium, Trichomonas vaginalis, Ureaplasma, enteric bacteria) and is treated presumptively at the time of diagnosis. CDC states that a single dose of oral azithromycin or a 7-day regimen of oral doxycycline are the recommended regimens for the treatment of NGU; a 7-day regimen of oral erythromycin base or ethylsuccinate or a 7-day regimen of oral levofloxacin or ofloxacin are alternative regimens.

CDC states that men with persistent or recurrent NGU who were not compliant with the treatment regimen or were reexposed to untreated sexual partner(s) can be retreated with the initial regimen. In other patients, symptoms alone (without documentation of signs or laboratory evidence of urethral inflammation) are not a sufficient basis for retreatment and an objective diagnosis of persistent or recurrent NGU should be made before considering additional treatment. Because there is some evidence that *M. genitalium* is the most frequent cause of persistent or recurrent NGU, CDC states that those initially treated with doxycycline should receive retreatment with a single dose of oral azithromycin and those initially treated with azithromycin should receive retreatment with a 7-day regimen of oral moxifloxacin. However, if the patient with persistent or recurrent urethritis has sex with women and is in an area where *T. vaginalis* is prevalent, CDC recommends presumptive retreatment with a single 2-g dose of oral metronidazole or tinidazole and referral of their partner(s) for evaluation and appropriate treatment.

NGU may facilitate transmission of HIV and men diagnosed with NGU should be tested for HIV. Individuals with HIV infection should receive the same treatment regimens recommended for other individuals with NGU.

Any individual who had sexual contact with a patient with NGU within the preceding 60 days should be referred for evaluation, testing, and presumptive treatment with a regimen effective against *Chlamydia*. To minimize transmission and avoid reinfection, men treated for NGU should abstain from sexual intercourse until they and their sexual partner(s) have been adequately treated.

● **Pelvic Inflammatory Disease**

Levofloxacin is considered an alternative agent for the treatment of acute pelvic inflammatory disease† (PID), but should *not* be used routinely for treatment of PID or any infections that may involve *N. gonorrhoeae*.

When a combined IM and oral regimen is used for the treatment of mild to moderately severe acute PID, CDC recommends a single IM dose of ceftriaxone, cefoxitin (with oral probenecid), or cefotaxime given in conjunction with a 14-day regimen of oral doxycycline (with or without a 14-day regimen of oral metronidazole). If parenteral cephalosporins are not feasible (e.g., because of cephalosporin allergy), CDC states that a 14-day regimen of oral levofloxacin, ofloxacin, or moxifloxacin given in conjunction with a 14-day regimen of oral metronidazole can be considered if the community prevalence and individual risk of gonorrhea are low and diagnostic testing for gonorrhea is performed. If culture results are positive for *N. gonorrhoeae*, the PID treatment regimen should be selected based on results of in vitro susceptibility testing. If QRNG are identified or if in vitro susceptibility cannot be determined (e.g., only nucleic acid amplification test [NAAT] for gonorrhea is available), consultation with an infectious disease specialist is recommended.

For further information on the treatment of PID, see Uses: Pelvic Inflammatory Disease in the Cephalosporins General Statement 8:12.06.

● **Plague**

Levofloxacin is used for the treatment of plague, including pneumonic and septicemic plague, caused by *Yersinia pestis* and for postexposure prophylaxis of plague in adults and children 6 months of age or older. Based on results of in vitro and animal testing, fluoroquinolones (ciprofloxacin, levofloxacin, moxifloxacin, ofloxacin) are recommended as alternatives for the treatment of plague and for postexposure prophylaxis following a high-risk exposure to *Y. pestis*, including exposures that occur in the context of biologic warfare or bioterrorism.

Efficacy of levofloxacin for treatment or prophylaxis of plague has not been evaluated in clinical trials in humans for ethical and feasibility reasons. The drug is labeled by FDA for this indication based on an efficacy study in animals that demonstrated a survival benefit. In a placebo-controlled study, African green monkeys were exposed to an inhaled dose of *Y. pestis* (mean dose of 65 LD$_{50}$ [range 3–145 LD$_{50}$]) and then randomized to receive a 10-day regimen of levofloxacin or placebo initiated within 6 hours after the onset of fever. In vitro testing indicated that the *Y. pestis* strain used in this study had a levofloxacin MIC of 0.03 mcg/mL. Pharmacokinetic data from the monkeys indicated that mean levofloxacin plasma concentrations at the end of a single 30-minute IV infusion of the drug ranged from 2.84–3.5 mcg/mL and trough concentrations 24 hours after the dose ranged from less than 0.03 to 0.06 mcg/mL. Study results indicated that mortality in the levofloxacin treatment group (1 out of 17) was significantly lower compared with mortality in the placebo group (7 out of 7). One of the levofloxacin-treated monkeys was euthanized on day 9 after exposure to *Y. pestis* because of a gastric complication; blood cultures in this monkey were positive for *Y. pestis* on day 3, but all subsequent daily blood cultures from days 4 through 7 were negative.

For the treatment of plague, IM streptomycin (or IM or IV gentamicin) historically has been considered the drug of choice. Alternatives recommended for

the treatment of plague when aminoglycosides are not used include an IV fluoroquinolone (ciprofloxacin [a drug of choice for plague meningitis], levofloxacin, moxifloxacin), IV doxycycline (or IV tetracycline), IV chloramphenicol (a drug of choice for plague meningitis), or co-trimoxazole (may be less effective than other alternatives).

Anti-infective regimens recommended for treatment of naturally occurring or endemic bubonic, septicemic, or pneumonic plague also are recommended for treatment of plague that occurs following exposure to *Y. pestis* in the context of biologic warfare or bioterrorism. Such exposures would most likely result in primary pneumonic plague, and prompt initiation of anti-infective therapy (within 18–24 hours of onset of symptoms) is essential in the treatment of pneumonic plague. Some experts (e.g., US Working Group on Civilian Biodefense, USAMRIID) recommend that treatment of plague in the context of biologic warfare or bioterrorism be initiated with a parenteral anti-infective regimen of streptomycin (or gentamicin) or, alternatively, a fluoroquinolone (ciprofloxacin, levofloxacin, moxifloxacin), doxycycline, or chloramphenicol. However, an oral regimen of doxycycline (or tetracycline) or a fluoroquinolone (ciprofloxacin, levofloxacin, moxifloxacin, ofloxacin) may be substituted when the patient's condition improves or when a parenteral regimen is unavailable (e.g., when there are supply or logistic problems because large numbers of individuals require treatment in a mass casualty setting).

In the context of biologic warfare or bioterrorism, some experts (e.g., US Working Group on Civilian Biodefense, USAMRIID) recommend that asymptomatic individuals with exposure to plague aerosol or asymptomatic individuals with household, hospital, or other close contact (within about 2 m) with an individual who has pneumonic plague receive an oral anti-infective regimen for postexposure prophylaxis; however, any exposed individual who develops a temperature of 38.5°C or higher or new cough should promptly receive a parenteral anti-infective for treatment of the disease. If postexposure prophylaxis is indicated, these experts recommend a regimen of oral doxycycline (or tetracycline) or an oral fluoroquinolone (ciprofloxacin, levofloxacin, moxifloxacin, ofloxacin).

For additional information on use of fluoroquinolones for treatment or prophylaxis of plague, see Uses: Plague in Ciprofloxacin 8:12.18.

● **Ophthalmic Infections**

For use of levofloxacin in the topical treatment of ophthalmic infections caused by susceptible organisms, see Levofloxacin 52:04.12.

DOSAGE AND ADMINISTRATION

● **Administration**

Levofloxacin is administered orally or by IV infusion. The drug should *not* be given IM, subcutaneously, intrathecally, or intraperitoneally.

IV administration of levofloxacin generally is reserved for patients who do not tolerate or are unable to take the drug orally and in other patients in whom the IV route offers a clinical advantage. Because the pharmacokinetics of levofloxacin are similar following oral and IV administration, these routes of administration are considered interchangeable.

Patients receiving oral or IV levofloxacin should be well hydrated and instructed to drink fluids liberally to prevent highly concentrated urine and formation of crystals in urine.

Oral Administration

Levofloxacin tablets and oral solution are bioequivalent.

Levofloxacin tablets may be given without regard to meals; however, levofloxacin oral solution should be given 1 hour before or 2 hours after meals.

When levofloxacin tablets are given with a standard high-fat breakfast (e.g., 2 eggs fried in butter, 2 strips of bacon, hash brown potatoes, 2 slices of toast with butter, 180 mL of milk), peak serum levofloxacin concentrations are decreased approximately 14% (not considered clinically important). When given with calcium-fortified orange juice, peak serum concentrations are decreased 18%; when given with a breakfast of calcium-fortified orange juice and whole grain, fortified, ready-to-eat cereal with skim milk, peak concentrations are decreased 24% and the time to peak concentrations is increased 46%. When levofloxacin is given as an oral solution, food decreases peak serum concentrations of the drug by approximately 25%.

Levofloxacin (tablets or oral solution) should be administered orally at least 2 hours before or 2 hours after antacids containing magnesium or aluminum, metal cations (e.g., iron), sucralfate, multivitamins or dietary supplements containing iron or zinc, or buffered didanosine (pediatric oral solution admixed with antacid). These drugs may interfere with oral absorption of levofloxacin, resulting in subtherapeutic systemic concentrations of the quinolone. (See Drug Interactions.)

The manufacturer states that levofloxacin tablets should not be used in pediatric patients weighing less than 30 kg.

IV Infusion

Commercially available levofloxacin premixed injection for IV infusion containing 5 mg/mL in 5% dextrose injection in single-use flexible containers is used without further dilution.

Alternatively, if commercially available levofloxacin concentrate for injection containing 25 mg/mL in single-use vials is used, the concentrate *must be diluted* prior to IV infusion with a compatible IV solution (e.g., 0.9% sodium chloride injection, 5% dextrose injection, 5% dextrose in lactated Ringer's injection or 0.9% sodium chloride injection, Plasma-Lyte 56 and 5% dextrose injection) to provide a solution containing 5 mg/mL.

Levofloxacin should not be admixed with other drugs or infused simultaneously through the same tubing with other drugs. Fluoroquinolones, including levofloxacin, should not be infused through the same tubing with any solution containing multivalent cations (e.g., magnesium). If the same administration set is used for sequential infusion of several different drugs, the tubing should be flushed before and after administration of levofloxacin with an IV solution that is compatible with both levofloxacin and the other drug(s).

Levofloxacin solutions should be inspected visually for particulate matter prior to administration whenever solution and container permit; the solutions should be discarded if they are cloudy or contain precipitates.

Levofloxacin premixed injection for IV infusion in 5% dextrose and levofloxacin concentrate for injection for IV infusion contain no preservatives; any unused portions of the solutions should be discarded.

Rate of Administration

Levofloxacin doses of 250 or 500 mg should be administered by IV infusion over a period of 60 minutes; doses of 750 mg should be administered by IV infusion over a period of 90 minutes.

Rapid IV infusion or injection has been associated with hypotension and must be avoided.

● Dosage

Dosage of oral and IV levofloxacin is identical.

When IV levofloxacin is used initially, therapy may be changed to oral levofloxacin (when appropriate) using the same dosage to complete therapy.

Safety of levofloxacin for treatment durations longer than 28 days in adults and longer than 14 days in pediatric patients has not been studied; therefore, the manufacturers state that the drug should be given for prolonged periods only when potential benefits outweigh risks.

Pediatric Dosage
Postexposure Prophylaxis of Anthrax

If levofloxacin is used for inhalational anthrax (postexposure) to reduce the incidence or progression of disease following suspected or confirmed exposure to aerosolized *Bacillus anthracis* spores, including exposures in the context of biologic warfare or bioterrorism, the manufacturers recommend that pediatric patients 6 months of age or older weighing less than 50 kg receive 8 mg/kg (up to 250 mg) every 12 hours and that pediatric patients 6 months of age or older weighing more than 50 kg receive a dosage of 500 mg once daily for 60 days.

If oral levofloxacin is used for postexposure prophylaxis of anthrax in the context of biologic warfare or bioterrorism, the American Academy of Pediatrics (AAP) suggests that pediatric patients as young as 1 month of age† can receive a dosage of 8 mg/kg (up to 250 mg) every 12 hours if they weigh less than 50 kg or 500 mg once daily if they weigh more than 50 kg.

Postexposure prophylaxis should be initiated as soon as possible following suspected or confirmed exposure to aerosolized *B. anthracis*.

Because of possible persistence of *B anthracis* spores in lung tissue following an aerosol exposure, the US Centers for Disease Control and Prevention (CDC), AAP, and others recommend that anti-infective postexposure prophylaxis be continued for 60 days following a confirmed exposure.

Treatment of Uncomplicated Cutaneous Anthrax

If oral levofloxacin is used for the treatment of uncomplicated cutaneous anthrax without systemic involvement† that occurs in the context of biologic warfare or bioterrorism, AAP recommends that pediatric patients 1 month of age or older† receive a dosage of 8 mg/kg (up to 250 mg) every 12 hours if they weigh less than 50 kg or 500 mg once daily if they weigh more than 50 kg.

If uncomplicated cutaneous anthrax occurred after exposure to aerosolized *B. anthracis* spores in the context of biologic warfare or bioterrorism, anti-infective treatment should be continued for 60 days after onset of the illness.

Treatment of Systemic Anthrax

If IV levofloxacin is used in a multiple-drug parenteral regimen for initial treatment of systemic anthrax† (inhalational, GI, meningitis, or cutaneous with systemic involvement, lesions on the head or neck, or extensive edema) that occurs in the context of biologic warfare or bioterrorism (see Uses: Anthrax), AAP recommends that pediatric patients 1 month of age or older† receive a dosage of 8 mg/kg (up to 250 mg) every 12 hours if they weigh less than 50 kg or 500 mg once daily if they weigh more than 50 kg. If meningitis has been excluded, these experts recommend that IV levofloxacin be given in a dosage of 10 mg/kg (up to 250 mg) every 12 hours in those weighing less than 50 kg or 500 mg once daily in those weighing more than 50 kg.

The multiple-drug parenteral regimen should be continued for at least 2–3 weeks until the patient is clinically stable and treatment can be switched to an appropriate oral anti-infective. If systemic anthrax occurred as the result of exposure to aerosolized *B. anthracis* spores in the context of biologic warfare or bioterrorism, the oral follow-up regimen should be continued until 60 days after onset of the illness.

If oral levofloxacin is used for follow-up therapy of systemic anthrax after completion of the initial multiple-drug parenteral regimen, AAP recommends that pediatric patients 1 month of age or older† receive a dosage of 8 mg/kg (up to 250 mg) every 12 hours if they weigh less than 50 kg or 500 mg once daily if they weigh 50 kg or more.

Plague

For the treatment or prophylaxis of plague caused by *Yersinia pestis* in pediatric patients 6 months of age or older weighing less than 50 kg, the manufacturers recommend a dosage of 8 mg/kg (up to 250 mg) every 12 hours for 10–14 days.

For the treatment or prophylaxis of plague in pediatric patients 6 months of age or older weighing more than 50 kg, the manufacturers recommend a dosage of 500 mg once daily for 10–14 days and state that these individuals can receive a higher dosage (i.e., 750 mg once daily) if clinically indicated.

The drug should be initiated as soon as possible after suspected or known exposure to *Y. pestis*.

Adult Dosage
Acute Sinusitis

If levofloxacin is used for the treatment of acute bacterial sinusitis, the usual adult dosage is 500 mg once every 24 hours for 10–14 days. Alternatively, adults can receive a dosage of 750 mg once every 24 hours for 5 days. (See Acute Sinusitis under Uses: Respiratory Tract Infections.)

Acute Exacerbations of Chronic Bronchitis

If levofloxacin is used for the treatment of acute bacterial exacerbations of chronic bronchitis, the usual adult dosage of levofloxacin is 500 mg once every 24 hours for 7 days. (See Acute Exacerbations of Chronic Bronchitis under Uses: Respiratory Tract Infections.)

Community-acquired Pneumonia

For the treatment of community-acquired pneumonia (CAP) caused by *Staphylococcus aureus*, *Streptococcus pneumoniae* (including multidrug-resistant *S. pneumoniae* [MDRSP]), *Haemophilus influenzae*, *H. parainfluenzae*, *Klebsiella pneumoniae*, *Legionella pneumophila*, *Moraxella catarrhalis*, *Chlamydophila pneumoniae*, or

Mycoplasma pneumoniae, the usual adult dosage of levofloxacin is 500 mg once every 24 hours for 7–14 days. Alternatively, adults with CAP caused by *S. pneumoniae* (except MDRSP), *H. influenzae*, *H. parainfluenzae*, *C. pneumoniae*, or *M. pneumoniae* can receive a dosage of 750 mg once every 24 hours for 5 days.

When used in empiric regimens for the treatment of CAP or for treatment of CAP caused by *Pseudomonas aeruginosa*, the Infectious Diseases Society of America (IDSA) and American Thoracic Society (ATS) recommend that levofloxacin be given in a dosage of 750 mg once daily.

IDSA and ATS state that CAP should be treated for a minimum of 5 days and patients should be afebrile for 48–72 hours before discontinuing anti-infective therapy.

Nosocomial Pneumonia

For the treatment of nosocomial pneumonia, the usual adult dosage of levofloxacin is 750 mg once every 24 hours for 7–14 days.

Skin and Skin Structure Infections

For the treatment of uncomplicated skin and skin structure infections, the usual adult dosage of levofloxacin is 500 mg once every 24 hours for 7–10 days.

For the treatment of complicated skin and skin structure infections, the usual adult dosage of levofloxacin is 750 mg once every 24 hours for 7–14 days.

Urinary Tract Infections and Prostatitis

If levofloxacin is used for the treatment of *uncomplicated* urinary tract infections (UTIs), the usual adult dosage is 250 mg once every 24 hours for 3 days. (See Uncomplicated Urinary Tract Infections under Uses: Urinary Tract Infections and Prostatitis.)

For the treatment of *complicated* UTIs caused by *Enterococcus faecalis*, *E. cloacae*, *Escherichia coli*, *K. pneumoniae*, *Proteus mirabilis*, or *Ps. aeruginosa* or the treatment of acute pyelonephritis caused by *E. coli*, the usual adult dosage of levofloxacin is 250 mg once every 24 hours for 10 days. Alternatively, adults with *complicated* UTIs caused by *E. coli*, *K. pneumoniae*, or *P. mirabilis* or acute pyelonephritis caused by *E. coli* can receive 750 mg once every 24 hours for 5 days.

The usual adult dosage of levofloxacin for the treatment of chronic prostatitis is 500 mg once every 24 hours for 28 days.

Campylobacter Infections

For the treatment of campylobacteriosis† caused by susceptible *Campylobacter* in adults with human immunodeficiency virus (HIV) infection, the recommended dosage of oral or IV levofloxacin is 750 mg once daily.

The recommended duration of fluoroquinolone treatment in HIV-infected patients is 7–10 days for gastroenteritis or at least 14 days for bacteremic infections. A duration of 2–6 weeks is recommended for recurrent infections.

Salmonella Gastroenteritis

For the treatment of *Salmonella* gastroenteritis† (with or without bacteremia) in HIV-infected adults, the recommended dosage of oral or IV levofloxacin is 750 mg once daily.

The recommended duration of treatment in HIV-infected adults is 7–14 days in those with CD4+ T-cell counts of 200 cells/mm³ or greater (14 days or longer if the patient is bacteremic or the infection is complicated) or 2–6 weeks in those with CD4+ T-cell counts less than 200 cells/mm³.

Shigella Infections

For the treatment of shigellosis† caused by susceptible *Shigella* in HIV-infected adults, the recommended dosage of oral or IV levofloxacin is 750 mg once daily.

The recommended duration of fluoroquinolone treatment in these patients is 7–10 days for gastroenteritis or at least 14 days for bacteremic infections. Recurrent infections, especially in patients with CD4+ T-cell counts less than 200 cells/mm³, may require up to 6 weeks of treatment.

Travelers' Diarrhea

If oral levofloxacin is used for the treatment of travelers' diarrhea† (see Travelers' Diarrhea under Uses: GI Infections), some clinicians recommend adults receive 500 mg once daily for 1–3 days.

Although the use of anti-infectives for prophylaxis of travelers' diarrhea† generally is discouraged (see Travelers' Diarrhea under Uses: GI Infections), if oral levofloxacin is used, the recommended adult dosage is 500 mg once daily during the period of risk (not exceeding 2–3 weeks) beginning the day of travel and continuing for 1 or 2 days after leaving the area of risk.

Helicobacter pylori Infection

When used as a component of various multiple-drug regimens for the treatment of infections caused by *Helicobacter pylori*† (see Helicobacter pylori Infection under Uses: GI Infections), levofloxacin usually has been given in a dosage of 500 mg once daily. A dosage of 250 mg once daily has been used in some regimens.

Postexposure Prophylaxis of Anthrax

If levofloxacin is used for inhalational anthrax (postexposure) to reduce the incidence or progression of disease following suspected or confirmed exposure to aerosolized *B. anthracis* spores, including exposures in the context of biologic warfare or bioterrorism, the manufacturers recommend that adults receive a dosage of 500 mg once daily.

CDC recommends that adults (including pregnant and postpartum women) receive oral levofloxacin in a dosage of 750 mg once daily for postexposure prophylaxis of anthrax in the context of biologic warfare or bioterrorism.

Anti-infective prophylaxis should be initiated as soon as possible following suspected or confirmed exposure to aerosolized *B. anthracis*.

Because of possible persistence of *B. anthracis* spores in lung tissue following an aerosol exposure, CDC and other experts recommend that anti-infective prophylaxis be continued for 60 days following a confirmed exposure.

Treatment of Uncomplicated Cutaneous Anthrax

If oral levofloxacin is used for the treatment of uncomplicated cutaneous anthrax without systemic involvement†, CDC recommends that adults (including pregnant and postpartum women) receive a dosage of 750 mg once daily.

If uncomplicated cutaneous anthrax occurred after exposure to aerosolized *B. anthracis* spores in the context of biologic warfare or bioterrorism, anti-infective treatment should be continued for 60 days after onset of illness.

Treatment of Systemic Anthrax

If IV levofloxacin is used as an alternative to IV ciprofloxacin in a multiple-drug parenteral regimen for initial treatment of systemic anthrax† (inhalational, GI, meningitis, or cutaneous with systemic involvement, lesions on the head or neck, or extensive edema) that occurs in the context of biologic warfare or bioterrorism, CDC recommends that adults (including pregnant and postpartum women) receive a dosage of 750 mg once daily.

The multiple-drug parenteral regimen should be continued for at least 2–3 weeks until the patient is clinically stable and treatment can be switched to an oral regimen. The oral follow-up regimen should be continued until 60 days after onset of the illness.

Chlamydial Infections

If oral levofloxacin is used as an alternative for the treatment of urogenital infections caused by *Chlamydia trachomatis*† in adults and adolescents, CDC recommends a dosage of 500 mg once daily for 7 days.

Epididymitis

For the treatment of acute epididymitis† most likely caused by sexually transmitted enteric bacteria (e.g., *E. coli*) and when *Neisseria gonorrhoeae* has been ruled out, CDC recommends that oral levofloxacin be given a dosage of 500 mg once daily for 10 days.

Levofloxacin should *not* be used alone for treatment of epididymitis unless *N. gonorrhoeae* has been ruled out. (See Uses: Gonorrhea and Associated Infections.)

Treatment of Active Tuberculosis

If levofloxacin is used as an alternative (second-line) agent in multiple-drug regimens for the treatment of active tuberculosis†, ATS, CDC, and IDSA recommend that adults receive 0.5–1 g daily. These experts state that data are insufficient to support intermittent regimens of levofloxacin for the treatment of tuberculosis.

Treatment of Other Mycobacterial Infections

If oral levofloxacin is used as an alternative in multiple-drug regimens for the treatment of disseminated infections caused by *Mycobacterium avium* complex† (MAC) in HIV-infected adults, CDC, National Institutes of Health (NIH), and IDSA recommend a dosage of 500 mg once daily.

Nongonococcal Urethritis

If oral levofloxacin is used as an alternative for the treatment of nongonococcal urethritis† (NGU), CDC recommends a dosage of 500 mg once daily for 7 days. (See Uses: Nongonococcal Urethritis.)

Pelvic Inflammatory Disease

If oral levofloxacin is used as an alternative for the treatment of mild to moderately severe acute pelvic inflammatory disease (PID), CDC recommends a dosage of 500 mg once daily for 14 days given in conjunction with oral metronidazole (500 mg twice daily for 14 days).

Levofloxacin should be used for the treatment of PID only when parenteral cephalosporins are not feasible, the community prevalence and individual risk of gonorrhea are low, and in vitro susceptibility has been confirmed. (See Uses: Pelvic Inflammatory Disease.)

Plague

If levofloxacin is used for the treatment or prophylaxis of plague caused by *Y. pestis* in adults, the manufacturers recommend a dosage of 500 mg once daily for 10–14 days and state that these individuals can receive a higher dosage (i.e., 750 mg once daily) if clinically indicated.

The drug should be initiated as soon as possible after suspected or known exposure to *Y. pestis*.

● Special Populations
Hepatic Impairment

Adjustment of levofloxacin dosage is not be expected to be necessary in patients with hepatic impairment because most of the drug is excreted unchanged in urine.

Renal Impairment

Dosage of levofloxacin should be modified according to the degree of renal impairment when the drug is used in adults with creatinine clearances less than 50 mL/minute. The only exception is when levofloxacin is used for the treatment of uncomplicated UTIs. (See Table 1.)

The manufacturers make no dosage recommendations for pediatric patients with renal insufficiency.

TABLE 1. Levofloxacin Dosage for Adults with Renal Impairment

Usual Daily Dosage for Normal Renal Function (Creatinine Clearance ≥50 mL/minute or greater)	Creatinine Clearance (mL/minute)	Dosage for Renal Impairment
250 mg	20–49	Dosage adjustment not required
250 mg	10–19	Uncomplicated UTIs: Dosage adjustment not required Other infections: 250 mg once every 48 hours
250 mg	Hemodialysis or CAPD patients	Information not available
500 mg	20–49	Initial 500-mg dose, then 250 mg once every 24 hours
500 mg	10–19	Initial 500-mg dose, then 250 mg once every 48 hours
500 mg	Hemodialysis or CAPD patients	Initial 500-mg dose, then 250 mg once every 48 hours; supplemental doses not required after dialysis
750 mg	20–49	750 mg once every 48 hours
750 mg	10–19	Initial 750-mg dose, then 500 mg once every 48 hours
750 mg	Hemodialysis or CAPD patients	Initial 750-mg dose, then 500 mg once every 48 hours; supplemental doses not required after dialysis

Geriatric Patients

Adjustment of levofloxacin dosage based solely on age is not necessary in geriatric patients. However, dosage of the drug should be selected carefully since geriatric patients are more likely to have decreased renal function than younger adults. (See Geriatric Use under Warnings/Precautions: Specific Populations, in Cautions.)

CAUTIONS

● Contraindications

Levofloxacin is contraindicated in patients with known hypersensitivity to levofloxacin or other quinolones.

● Warnings/Precautions
Warnings

Disabling and Potentially Irreversible Serious Adverse Reactions

Systemic fluoroquinolones, including levofloxacin, have been associated with disabling and potentially irreversible serious adverse reactions (e.g., tendinitis and tendon rupture, peripheral neuropathy, CNS effects) that can occur together in the same patient. These serious reactions may occur within hours to weeks after a systemic fluoroquinolone is initiated and have occurred in all age groups and in patients without preexisting risk factors for such adverse reactions.

Levofloxacin should be discontinued immediately at the first signs or symptoms of any serious adverse reactions.

Systemic fluoroquinolones, including levofloxacin, should be avoided in patients who have experienced any of the serious adverse reactions associated with fluoroquinolones.

Tendinitis and Tendon Rupture

Systemic fluoroquinolones, including levofloxacin, are associated with an increased risk of tendinitis and tendon rupture in all age groups.

The risk of developing fluoroquinolone-associated tendinitis and tendon rupture is increased in older adults (usually those over 60 years of age), individuals receiving concomitant corticosteroids, and kidney, heart, or lung transplant recipients. (See Geriatric Use under Warnings/Precautions: Specific Populations, in Cautions.)

Other factors that may independently increase the risk of tendon rupture include strenuous physical activity, renal failure, and previous tendon disorders such as rheumatoid arthritis. Tendinitis and tendon rupture have been reported in patients receiving fluoroquinolones who did not have any risk factors for such adverse reactions.

Fluoroquinolone-associated tendinitis and tendon rupture most frequently involve the Achilles tendon and have also been reported in the rotator cuff (shoulder), hand, biceps, thumb, and other tendon sites. Tendinitis or tendon rupture can occur within hours or days after levofloxacin is initiated or as long as several months after completion of therapy and can occur bilaterally.

Levofloxacin should be discontinued immediately if pain, swelling, inflammation, or rupture of a tendon occurs.

Systemic fluoroquinolones, including levofloxacin, should be avoided in patients who have a history of tendon disorders or have experienced tendinitis or tendon rupture.

Peripheral Neuropathy

Systemic fluoroquinolones, including levofloxacin, have been associated with an increased risk of peripheral neuropathy.

Sensory or sensorimotor axonal polyneuropathy affecting small and/or large axons resulting in paresthesias, hypoesthesias, dysesthesias, and weakness has been reported in patients receiving systemic fluoroquinolones, including levofloxacin. Symptoms may occur soon after initiation of levofloxacin and, in some patients, may be irreversible.

Levofloxacin should be discontinued immediately if symptoms of peripheral neuropathy (e.g., pain, burning, tingling, numbness, and/or weakness) occur or if there are other alterations in sensations (e.g., light touch, pain, temperature, position sense, vibratory sensation). (See Advice to Patients.)

Systemic fluoroquinolones, including levofloxacin, should be avoided in patients who have experienced peripheral neuropathy.

CNS Effects

Systemic fluoroquinolones, including levofloxacin, have been associated with an increased risk of psychiatric adverse effects, including toxic psychosis, hallucinations, paranoia, depression, suicidal thoughts or acts, anxiety, agitation, restlessness, nervousness, confusion, delirium, disorientation, disturbances in attention, insomnia, nightmares, and memory impairment. Attempted or completed suicides have been reported, especially in patients with a history of depression or an underlying risk factor for depression. These adverse effects may occur after the first dose.

System fluoroquinolones, including levofloxacin, have been associated with an increased risk of seizures (convulsions), increased intracranial pressure (including pseudotumor cerebri), dizziness, and tremors.

Levofloxacin, like other fluoroquinolones, should be used with caution in patients with known or suspected CNS disorders that predispose to seizures or lower the seizure threshold (e.g., severe cerebral arteriosclerosis, epilepsy) or with other risk factors that predispose to seizures or lower the seizure threshold (e.g., certain drugs, renal impairment).

If psychiatric or other CNS effects occur, levofloxacin should be discontinued immediately and appropriate measures initiated. (See Advice to Patients.)

Exacerbation of Myasthenia Gravis

Fluoroquinolones, including levofloxacin, have neuromuscular blocking activity and may exacerbate muscle weakness in individuals with myasthenia gravis. Use of fluoroquinolones in myasthenia gravis patients has resulted in requirements for ventilatory support and in death.

Levofloxacin should be avoided in patients with a known history myasthenia gravis. Patients should be advised to immediately contact a clinician if they experience any symptoms of muscle weakness, including respiratory difficulties. (See Advice to Patients.)

Sensitivity Reactions
Hypersensitivity Reactions

Serious and occasionally fatal hypersensitivity and/or anaphylactic reactions have been reported in patients receiving fluoroquinolones, including levofloxacin. These reactions often occur with the first dose.

Some hypersensitivity reactions have been accompanied by cardiovascular collapse, hypotension or shock, seizures, loss of consciousness, tingling, angioedema (e.g., edema or swelling of the tongue, larynx, throat, or face), airway obstruction (e.g., bronchospasm, shortness of breath, acute respiratory distress), dyspnea, urticaria, pruritus, and other severe skin reactions.

Other serious and sometimes fatal adverse reactions that have been reported with fluoroquinolones, including levofloxacin, and that may or may not be related to hypersensitivity reactions include one or more of the following: fever, rash or other severe dermatologic reactions (e.g., toxic epidermal necrolysis, Stevens-Johnson syndrome); vasculitis, arthralgia, myalgia, serum sickness; allergic pneumonitis; interstitial nephritis, acute renal insufficiency or failure; hepatitis, jaundice, acute hepatic necrosis or failure; anemia (including hemolytic and aplastic anemia), thrombocytopenia (including thrombotic thrombocytopenic purpura), leukopenia, agranulocytosis, pancytopenia and/or other hematologic effects.

Levofloxacin should be discontinued immediately at the first appearance of rash, jaundice, or any other sign of hypersensitivity. Appropriate therapy should be initiated as indicated. (See Advice to Patients.)

Photosensitivity Reactions

Moderate to severe photosensitivity/phototoxicity reactions have been reported with fluoroquinolones, including levofloxacin.

Phototoxicity may manifest as exaggerated sunburn reactions (e.g., burning, erythema, exudation, vesicles, blistering, edema) on areas exposed to sun or artificial ultraviolet (UV) light (usually the face, neck, extensor surfaces of forearms, dorsa of hands).

As with other fluoroquinolones, patients should be advised to avoid unnecessary or excessive exposure to sunlight or artificial UV light (e.g., tanning beds, UVA/UVB treatment) while receiving levofloxacin. If a patient needs to be outdoors, they should wear loose-fitting clothing that protects skin from sun exposure and use other sun protection measures (sunscreen).

Levofloxacin should be discontinued if photosensitivity or phototoxicity (sunburn-like reaction, skin eruption) occurs.

Other Warnings/Precautions
Hepatotoxicity

Severe hepatotoxicity, including acute hepatitis, has occurred in patients receiving levofloxacin and sometimes resulted in death. Most cases of severe hepatotoxicity occurred within 6–14 days of initiation of levofloxacin therapy and were not associated with hypersensitivity reactions. The majority of fatal cases of hepatotoxicity were in geriatric patients 65 years of age or older. (See Geriatric Use under Warnings/Precautions: Specific Populations, in Cautions.)

Levofloxacin should be discontinued immediately in any patient who develops signs or symptoms of hepatitis (e.g., loss of appetite, nausea, vomiting, fever, weakness, tiredness, right upper quadrant tenderness, itching, yellowing of the skin or eyes, light colored bowel movements, or dark colored urine).

Prolongation of QT Interval

Prolonged QT interval leading to ventricular arrhythmias, including torsades de pointes, has been reported with some fluoroquinolones, including levofloxacin.

Levofloxacin should be avoided in patients with a history of prolonged QT interval, in those with uncorrected electrolyte disorders (e.g., hypokalemia), and in those receiving class IA (e.g., quinidine, procainamide) or class III (e.g., amiodarone, sotalol) antiarrhythmic agents.

The risk of prolonged QT interval may be increased in geriatric patients. (See Geriatric Use under Warnings/Precautions: Specific Populations, in Cautions.)

Risk of Aortic Aneurysm and Dissection

Rupture or dissection of aortic aneurysms has been reported in patients receiving systemic fluoroquinolones. Epidemiologic studies indicate an increased risk of aortic aneurysm and dissection within 2 months following use of systemic fluoroquinolones, particularly in geriatric patients. The cause for this increased risk has not been identified.

Unless there are no other treatment options, systemic fluoroquinolones, including levofloxacin, should not be used in patients who have an aortic aneurysm or are at increased risk for an aortic aneurysm. This includes geriatric patients and patients with peripheral atherosclerotic vascular disease, hypertension, or certain genetic conditions (e.g., Marfan syndrome, Ehlers-Danlos syndrome).

If a patient reports adverse effects suggestive of aortic aneurysm or dissection, fluoroquinolone treatment should be discontinued immediately. (See Advice to Patients.)

Hypoglycemia or Hyperglycemia

Systemic fluoroquinolones, including levofloxacin, have been associated with alterations in blood glucose concentrations, including symptomatic hypoglycemia and hyperglycemia. Blood glucose disturbances during fluoroquinolone therapy usually have occurred in patients with diabetes mellitus receiving an oral antidiabetic agent (e.g., glyburide) or insulin.

Severe cases of hypoglycemia resulting in coma or death have been reported with some systemic fluoroquinolones. Although most reported cases of hypoglycemic coma have involved patients with risk factors for hypoglycemia (e.g., older age, diabetes mellitus, renal insufficiency, concomitant use of antidiabetic agents [especially sulfonylureas]), some cases have occurred in patients receiving a fluoroquinolone who were not diabetic and were not reported to be receiving an oral antidiabetic agent or insulin.

Blood glucose concentrations should be carefully monitored when systemic fluoroquinolones, including levofloxacin, are used in patients with diabetes mellitus receiving antidiabetic agents.

If a hypoglycemic reaction occurs, levofloxacin should be discontinued and appropriate therapy initiated immediately. (See Advice to Patients.)

Musculoskeletal Disorders

An increased incidence of musculoskeletal disorders (arthralgia, arthritis, tendinopathy, gait abnormality) has been reported in pediatric patients receiving levofloxacin. The manufacturers state that levofloxacin should be used in pediatric patients *only* for inhalational anthrax (postexposure) or treatment or prophylaxis of plague and *only* in those 6 months of age or older. (See Pediatric Use under Warnings/Precautions: Specific Populations, in Cautions.)

Fluoroquinolones, including levofloxacin, cause arthropathy and osteochondrosis in immature animals of various species. Persistent lesions in cartilage reported in levofloxacin studies in immature dogs; similar erosions in weight-bearing joints and other signs of arthropathy have been reported with other fluoroquinolones.

C. difficile-associated Diarrhea and Colitis

Treatment with anti-infectives alters normal colon flora and may permit overgrowth of Clostridioides difficile (formerly known as Clostridium difficile). C. difficile infection (CDI) and C. difficile-associated diarrhea and colitis (CDAD; also known as antibiotic-associated diarrhea and colitis or pseudomembranous colitis) have been reported with nearly all anti-infectives, including levofloxacin, and may range in severity from mild diarrhea to fatal colitis. C. difficile produces toxins A and B which contribute to development of CDAD; hypertoxin-producing strains of C. difficile are associated with increased morbidity and mortality since they may be refractory to anti-infectives and colectomy may be required.

CDAD should be considered if diarrhea develops during or after therapy and managed accordingly. Careful medical history is necessary since CDAD has been reported to occur as late as 2 months or longer after anti-infective therapy is discontinued.

If CDAD is suspected or confirmed, anti-infective therapy not directed against C. difficile should be discontinued as soon as possible. Patients should be managed with appropriate anti-infective therapy directed against C. difficile (e.g., vancomycin, fidaxomicin, metronidazole), supportive therapy (e.g., fluid and electrolyte management, protein supplementation), and surgical evaluation as clinically indicated.

Selection and Use of Anti-infectives

Levofloxacin should be used for the treatment of acute bacterial sinusitis, acute bacterial exacerbations of chronic bronchitis, or uncomplicated urinary tract infections (UTIs) *only* when no other treatment options are available. Because levofloxacin, like other systemic fluoroquinolones, has been associated with disabling and potentially irreversible serious adverse reactions (e.g., tendinitis and tendon rupture, peripheral neuropathy, CNS effects) that can occur together in the same patient, the risks of serious adverse reactions outweigh the benefits of levofloxacin for patients with these infections.

To reduce development of drug-resistant bacteria and maintain effectiveness of levofloxacin and other antibacterials, use only for treatment or prevention of infections proven or strongly suspected to be caused by susceptible bacteria.

When selecting or modifying anti-infective therapy, use results of culture and in vitro susceptibility testing. In the absence of such data, consider local epidemiology and susceptibility patterns when selecting anti-infectives for empiric therapy.

Information on test methods and quality control standards for in vitro susceptibility testing of antibacterial agents and specific interpretive criteria for such testing recognized by FDA is available at https://www.fda.gov/STIC.

Specific Populations

Pregnancy

There are no adequate and well-controlled studies of levofloxacin in pregnant women, and the drug should be used during pregnancy only if potential benefits justify potential risks to the fetus.

Reproduction studies in rats or rabbits have not revealed evidence of teratogenicity at oral doses 9.4 or 1.1 times the maximum recommended human dose, respectively, or IV doses 1.9 or 0.5 times the maximum human dose, respectively, based on relative body surface area.

Lactation

Levofloxacin is distributed into milk following oral or IV administration.

Because of the potential for serious adverse reactions in the infant, a decision should be made whether to discontinue nursing or the drug, taking into account the importance of the drug to the woman.

Pediatric Use

Safety and efficacy of levofloxacin have not been established for any indication in infants younger than 6 months of age.

Levofloxacin is labeled by FDA for inhalational anthrax (postexposure) or for treatment or prophylaxis of plague in adolescents and children 6 months of age or older. Safety and efficacy of the drug have not been established for any other indication in this age group.

Quinolones, including levofloxacin, cause arthropathy and osteochondrosis in juvenile animals of various species. (See Musculoskeletal Disorders under Warnings/Precautions: Other Warnings/Precautions, in Cautions.)

The American Academy of Pediatrics (AAP) states that use of a systemic fluoroquinolone may be justified in children younger than 18 years of age in certain specific circumstances when there are no safe and effective alternatives and the drug is known to be effective. For information regarding when fluoroquinolones may be a preferred option in children, see Cautions: Pediatric Precautions in Ciprofloxacin 8:12.18.

Geriatric Use

No overall differences in safety and efficacy were observed between geriatric patients and younger adults in clinical trials, but increased sensitivity in some older individuals cannot be ruled out.

The risk of fluoroquinolone-associated tendon disorders, including tendon rupture, is increased in older adults (usually those older than 60 years of age). This risk is further increased in those receiving concomitant corticosteroids. (See Tendinitis and Tendon Rupture under Warnings/Precautions: Warnings, in Cautions.) Caution is advised if levofloxacin is used in geriatric adults, especially those receiving concomitant corticosteroids.

Severe and sometimes fatal hepatotoxicity has been reported in patients receiving levofloxacin, and the majority of fatalities have occurred in geriatric patients 65 years of age or older. (See Hepatotoxicity under Warnings/Precautions: Other Warnings/Precautions, in Cautions.)

The risk of prolonged QT interval leading to ventricular arrhythmias may be increased in geriatric patients, especially those receiving concurrent therapy with other drugs that can prolong QT interval (e.g., class IA or III antiarrhythmic agents) or with risk factors for torsades de pointes (e.g., known QT prolongation, uncorrected hypokalemia). (See Prolongation of QT Interval under Warnings/Precautions: Other Warnings/Precautions, in Cautions.)

The risk of fluoroquinolone-associated aortic aneurysm and dissection may be increased in geriatric patients. (See Risk of Aortic Aneurysm and Dissection under Warnings/Precautions: Other Warnings/Precautions, in Cautions.)

Because levofloxacin is substantially eliminated by the kidneys, age-related decreases in renal function should be considered when selecting dosage for geriatric patients and it may be useful to monitor renal function. (See Geriatric Patients under Dosage and Administration: Special Populations.)

Hepatic Impairment

Pharmacokinetics of levofloxacin have not been studied in patients with hepatic impairment, but pharmacokinetic alterations are unlikely.

Renal Impairment

Levofloxacin clearance is substantially reduced and plasma elimination half-life of the drug is substantially prolonged in patients with impaired renal function (creatinine clearance less than 50 mL/minute).

Levofloxacin should be used with caution in patients with renal impairment. Appropriate renal function tests should be performed prior to and during levofloxacin therapy and dosage adjusted as needed. (See Renal Impairment under Dosage and Administration: Special Populations.)

● Common Adverse Effects

Adverse effected reported in 3% or more of patients receiving levofloxacin include GI effects (nausea, diarrhea, constipation), headache, insomnia, and dizziness.

DRUG INTERACTIONS

● Drugs That Prolong QT Interval

Potential pharmacologic interaction between levofloxacin and drugs that prolong the QT interval (additive effects on QT interval prolongation). Concomitant use of levofloxacin and class IA (e.g., quinidine, procainamide) or class III (e.g., amiodarone, sotalol) antiarrhythmic agents should be avoided. (See Prolongation of QT Interval under Warnings/Precautions: Other Warnings/Precautions, in Cautions.)

● Antacids

Potential pharmacokinetic interaction between levofloxacin (tablets or oral solution) and antacids containing magnesium or aluminum (decreased absorption of oral levofloxacin). Data are not available regarding concomitant use of IV levofloxacin and antacids.

Levofloxacin tablets or oral solution should be administered at least 2 hours before or 2 hours after such antacids.

● Antiarrhythmic Agents

Potential pharmacologic interaction between levofloxacin and antiarrhythmic agents (additive effect on QT interval prolongation). Levofloxacin should be avoided in patients receiving class IA (e.g., quinidine, procainamide) or class III (e.g., amiodarone, sotalol) antiarrhythmic agents. (See Prolongation of QT Interval under Warnings/Precautions: Other Warnings/Precautions, in Cautions.)

Pharmacokinetic interaction between levofloxacin and procainamide (increased half-life and decreased clearance of procainamide).

● Antidepressants

Potential pharmacologic interaction between levofloxacin and fluoxetine or imipramine (additive effect on QT interval prolongation).

● Antidiabetic Agents

Potential pharmacodynamic interaction (altered blood glucose concentrations and symptomatic hyperglycemia or hypoglycemia) in diabetic patients receiving levofloxacin concomitantly with antidiabetic agents (e.g., insulin, glyburide). (See Hypoglycemia or Hyperglycemia under Warnings/Precautions: Other Warnings/Precautions, in Cautions.)

Careful monitoring of blood glucose concentrations is recommended; levofloxacin should be discontinued if a hypoglycemic reaction occurs.

● Cimetidine

Pharmacokinetic interaction between levofloxacin and cimetidine (slightly increased levofloxacin area under the plasma concentration-time curve [AUC] and half-life). This interaction is not considered clinically important, and levofloxacin dosage adjustments are not warranted.

● Corticosteroids

Concomitant use of levofloxacin and corticosteroids increases the risk of severe tendon disorders (e.g., tendinitis, tendon rupture), especially in geriatric patients older than 60 years of age. Levofloxacin and corticosteroids should be used concomitantly with caution. (See Tendinitis and Tendon Rupture under Warnings/Precautions: Warnings, in Cautions.)

● Cyclosporine and Tacrolimus

Possible pharmacokinetic interactions between levofloxacin and cyclosporine or tacrolimus (increased AUC of the immunosuppressive agent).

The manufacturers of levofloxacin state that concomitant use of cyclosporine and levofloxacin did not have a clinically important effect on the pharmacokinetics of the immunosuppressive agent and dosage adjustments are not required for either drug. Some clinicians suggest that plasma concentrations of cyclosporine or tacrolimus should be monitored if used concomitantly with levofloxacin.

● Didanosine

Potential pharmacokinetic interaction between levofloxacin (tablets and oral solution) and buffered didanosine preparations (decreased GI absorption of oral levofloxacin). Data are not available regarding concomitant use of IV levofloxacin and buffered didanosine preparations.

Levofloxacin tablets or oral solution should be administered at least 2 hours before or 2 hours after buffered didanosine (pediatric oral solution admixed with antacid).

● Digoxin

Concomitant use of levofloxacin and digoxin did not result in any clinically important effects on the pharmacokinetics of either drug. Dosage adjustments are not necessary for either drug if levofloxacin and digoxin are used concomitantly.

● Iron, Multivitamins, and Mineral Supplements

Potential pharmacokinetic interaction between levofloxacin (tablets and oral solution) and iron, multivitamins, or mineral supplements (decreased absorption of oral levofloxacin). Data are not available regarding concomitant use of IV levofloxacin and such preparations.

Levofloxacin tablets or oral solution should be administered at least 2 hours before or 2 hours after iron preparations or multivitamins or dietary supplements containing zinc, calcium, magnesium, or iron.

● Nonsteroidal Anti-inflammatory Agents

Potential pharmacologic interaction between levofloxacin and nonsteroidal anti-inflammatory agents (NSAIAs) (possible increased risk of CNS stimulation and seizures). Animal studies suggest the risk may be less than that associated with some other fluoroquinolones and that risk varies depending on the specific NSAIA.

● Probenecid

Pharmacokinetic interaction between levofloxacin and probenecid (slightly increased levofloxacin AUC and half-life). This interaction is not considered clinically important; levofloxacin dosage adjustments are not warranted.

● Sucralfate

Potential pharmacokinetic interaction between levofloxacin (tablets or oral solution) and sucralfate (decreased absorption of oral levofloxacin); no pharmacokinetic interaction if given 2 hours apart. Data are not available regarding concomitant use of IV levofloxacin and sucralfate.

Levofloxacin tablets or oral solution should be administered at least 2 hours before or 2 hours after sucralfate.

● Theophylline

Concomitant use of levofloxacin and theophylline did not have a clinically important effect on the pharmacokinetics of either drug. However, pharmacokinetic interactions (increased theophylline half-life and increased risk of theophylline-related adverse effects) have been reported with some other quinolones.

If levofloxacin and theophylline are used concomitantly, serum theophylline concentrations should be closely monitored and theophylline dosage adjusted accordingly; clinicians should consider that adverse theophylline effects (e.g., seizures) may occur with or without elevated theophylline concentrations.

● Warfarin

Concomitant use of levofloxacin in patients receiving warfarin has resulted in increased prothrombin time (PT); clinical episodes of bleeding have been reported. Patients receiving the drugs concomitantly should be monitored for evidence of bleeding and PT and international normalized ratio (INR) should be monitored.

PHARMACOKINETICS

● *Absorption*

Bioavailability

Levofloxacin is rapidly absorbed from the GI tract. Following a 500- or 750-mg dose of levofloxacin given as tablets, absolute bioavailability of the drug is approximately 99%.

Peak plasma concentrations of levofloxacin usually are attained 1–2 hours after an oral dose; steady-state plasma concentrations are attained within 48 hours with once-daily regimens.

Levofloxacin tablets and oral solution are bioequivalent.

Plasma concentrations of levofloxacin and area under the plasma concentration-time curve (AUC) of the drug after oral administration of tablets are similar to those after IV administration.

Food

Food slightly prolongs the time to peak plasma concentration and decreases peak concentrations of levofloxacin. The effect varies depending on whether the drug is administered as tablets or oral solution.

Tablets: When a 500-mg tablet of levofloxacin is given with a standard high-fat breakfast (e.g., 2 fried eggs in butter, 2 strips of bacon, hash brown potatoes, 2 slices of toast with butter, 180 mL of milk), peak serum concentrations of the drug are decreased approximately 14% (not considered clinically important). When levofloxacin is given with calcium-fortified orange juice, peak serum concentrations of the drug are decreased 18%; when given with a breakfast of calcium-fortified orange juice and whole grain, fortified, ready-to-eat cereal with skim milk, peak concentrations are decreased 24% and time to peak concentrations is increased 46%.

Oral solution: When a 500-dose of levofloxacin is given as an oral solution with food, peak concentrations of the drug are decreased by approximately 25%.

● *Distribution*

Extent

Levofloxacin is widely distributed into body tissues and fluids, including skin, blister fluid, and lungs.

Levofloxacin is distributed into CSF. Following IV administration of 400 or 500 mg of levofloxacin twice daily, CSF concentrations have been reported to be up to 47% of concurrent plasma concentrations.

The drug is distributed into milk following oral or IV administration.

Plasma Protein Binding

Levofloxacin is 24–38% bound to serum proteins, principally albumin.

● *Elimination*

Metabolism

Levofloxacin undergoes limited metabolism to inactive metabolites.

Elimination Route

Levofloxacin is eliminated principally as unchanged drug in urine by glomerular filtration and active tubular secretion. Approximately 87% of an oral dose is eliminated in urine and less than 4% is eliminated in feces.

Levofloxacin is not removed by hemodialysis or continuous ambulatory peritoneal dialysis (CAPD).

Half-life

The terminal elimination half-life of levofloxacin is approximately 6–8 hours after oral or IV administration.

Special Populations

In pediatric patients 6 months to 16 years of age, clearance of levofloxacin is increased and plasma concentrations of the drug are decreased compared with adults.

Levofloxacin pharmacokinetics in geriatric individuals with normal renal function are similar to that reported in younger adults.

Levofloxacin pharmacokinetics have not been studied in patients with hepatic impairment, but pharmacokinetic alterations are unlikely.

In patients with impaired renal function, levofloxacin clearance is decreased and plasma half-life is prolonged. Mean plasma half-life of levofloxacin following a 500-mg dose given as a tablet is 27 hours in those with creatinine clearances of 20–49 mL/minute and 35 hours in those with creatinine clearances less than 20 mL/minute.

DESCRIPTION

Levofloxacin is a fluoroquinolone anti-infective agent. Like other commercially available fluoroquinolones, levofloxacin contains a fluorine at the C-6 position of the quinolone nucleus. Like some other fluoroquinolones (ciprofloxacin, ofloxacin), levofloxacin contains a piperazinyl group at C-7. The piperazinyl group in levofloxacin results in increased activity against gram-negative bacteria. Levofloxacin is the levorotatory isomer of ofloxacin and is 8–128 times as active against susceptible gram-positive and gram-negative bacteria as the dextrorotatory isomer and approximately twice as active as racemic ofloxacin.

Like other fluoroquinolone anti-infectives, levofloxacin inhibits DNA synthesis in susceptible organisms via inhibition of type II DNA topoisomerases (DNA gyrase, topoisomerase IV). In susceptible *S. pneumoniae*, levofloxacin principally targets topoisomerase IV.

SPECTRUM

Levofloxacin is more active in vitro against gram-positive bacteria (including *Streptococcus pneumoniae*) and anaerobes than some other currently available fluoroquinolones (e.g., ciprofloxacin, ofloxacin), but is less active in vitro than ciprofloxacin against *Pseudomonas aeruginosa*.

Levofloxacin is active in vitro and in clinical infections against *Staphylococcus aureus* (methicillin-susceptible [oxacillin-susceptible] strains only), *S. epidermidis* (oxacillin-susceptible strains only), *S. saprophyticus*, *S. pneumoniae* (including multidrug-resistant strains [MDRSP]), *S. pyogenes* (group A β-hemolytic streptococci, GAS), and *Enterococcus faecalis* (many strains only moderately susceptible). The drug also is active in vitro against some other gram-positive bacteria, including *S. haemolyticus*, *S. agalactiae* (group B streptococci, GBS), groups C, G, and F streptococci, *S. milleri*, and viridans streptococci. Levofloxacin is active against *Bacillus anthracis* in vitro and in a primate infection model.

Levofloxacin is active in vitro and in clinical infections against *Haemophilus influenzae*, *H. parainfluenzae*, *Klebsiella pneumoniae*, *Moraxella catarrhalis*, *Enterobacter cloacae*, *Escherichia coli*, *Proteus mirabilis*, *Serratia marcescens*, *Ps. aeruginosa* (some may develop resistance during therapy), and *Legionella pneumophila*. The drug also is active in vitro against some other gram-negative bacteria, including *Acinetobacter*, *Bordetella pertussis*, *Citrobacter koseri*, *C. freundii*, *E. aerogenes*, *E. sakazakii*, *K. oxytoca*, *Morganella morganii*, *Pantoea agglomerans*, *Proteus vulgaris*, *Providencia*, and *Ps. fluorescens*. Levofloxacin is active against *Yersinia pestis* in vitro and in a primate infection model.

Although levofloxacin has in vitro activity against *Helicobacter pylori*, resistance to the drug can occur and the prevalence of levofloxacin-resistant strains may be high in some geographic areas.

Levofloxacin also is active against some other organisms, including *Chlamydophila pneumoniae* (formerly *Chlamydia pneumoniae*), *Mycoplasma pneumoniae*, and *Clostridium perfringens*.

Levofloxacin is active in vitro against some mycobacteria, including *Mycobacterium tuberculosis*, and *M. fortuitum*. Although levofloxacin is active against some strains of *M. tuberculosis* resistant to isoniazid and/or rifampin, levofloxacin-resistant *M. tuberculosis* have been reported and some multidrug-resistant *M. tuberculosis* (i.e., strains resistant to rifampin and isoniazid) also are resistant to levofloxacin or other fluoroquinolones. Extensively drug-resistant tuberculosis (XDR tuberculosis) is caused by strains that are resistant to rifampin and isoniazid (multiple-drug resistant strains) and also resistant to a fluoroquinolone and at least one parenteral second-line antimycobacterial (capreomycin, kanamycin, amikacin).

RESISTANCE

Resistance to fluoroquinolones can occur as the result of mutations in defined regions of DNA gyrase or topoisomerase IV (i.e., quinolone-resistance determining regions [QRDRs]) or altered efflux.

Cross-resistance can occur between levofloxacin and other fluoroquinolones, but some bacteria resistant to other fluoroquinolones may be susceptible to levofloxacin.

ADVICE TO PATIENTS

Advise patients to read the manufacturer's patient information (medication guide) prior to initiating levofloxacin therapy and each time the prescription is refilled.

Advise patients that antibacterials (including levofloxacin) should only be used to treat bacterial infections and not used to treat viral infections (e.g., the common cold).

Importance of completing full course of therapy, even if feeling better after a few days.

Advise patients that skipping doses or not completing the full course of therapy may decrease effectiveness and increase the likelihood that bacteria will develop resistance and will not be treatable with levofloxacin or other antibacterials in the future.

Advise patients that the oral solution should be taken 1 hour before or 2 hours after meals; tablets may be taken without regard to meals.

Levofloxacin should be taken at the same time each day and with liberal amounts of fluids.

Importance of taking oral levofloxacin at least 2 hours before or 2 hours after aluminum- or magnesium-containing antacids, metal cations (e.g., iron), sucralfate, multivitamins containing iron or zinc, or buffered didanosine (pediatric oral solution prepared admixed with antacid).

Inform patients that systemic fluoroquinolones, including levofloxacin, have been associated with disabling and potentially irreversible serious adverse reactions (e.g., tendinitis and tendon rupture, peripheral neuropathy, CNS effects) that may occur together in the same patient. Advise patients to immediately discontinue levofloxacin and contact a clinician if they experience any signs or symptoms of serious adverse effects (e.g., unusual joint or tendon pain, muscle weakness, a "pins and needles" tingling or pricking sensation, numbness of the arms or legs, confusion, hallucinations) while taking the drug. Advise patients to talk with a clinician if they have any questions or concerns.

Inform patients that systemic fluoroquinolones, including levofloxacin, are associated with an increased risk of tendinitis and tendon rupture in all age groups and that this risk is increased in adults older than 60 years of age, individuals receiving corticosteroids, and kidney, heart, or lung transplant recipients. Symptoms may be irreversible. Importance of resting and refraining from exercise at the first sign of tendinitis or tendon rupture (e.g., pain, swelling, or inflammation of a tendon or weakness or inability to use a joint) and importance of immediately discontinuing the drug and contacting a clinician. (See Tendinitis and Tendon Rupture under Warnings/Precautions: Warnings, in Cautions.)

Inform patients that peripheral neuropathies have been reported in patients receiving systemic fluoroquinolones, including levofloxacin, and that symptoms may occur soon after initiation of the drug and may be irreversible. Importance of immediately discontinuing levofloxacin and contacting a clinician if symptoms of peripheral neuropathy (e.g., pain, burning, tingling, numbness, and/or weakness) occur.

Inform patients that systemic fluoroquinolones, including levofloxacin, have been associated with CNS effects (e.g., convulsions, dizziness, lightheadedness, increased intracranial pressure). Importance of informing clinician of any history of convulsions before initiating therapy with the drug. Importance of contacting a clinician if persistent headache with or without blurred vision occurs.

Advise patients that levofloxacin may cause dizziness and lightheadedness; caution patients that they should not engage in activities requiring mental alertness and motor coordination (e.g., driving a vehicle, operating machinery) until the effects of the drug on the individual are known.

Advise patients that systemic fluoroquinolones, including levofloxacin, may worsen myasthenia gravis symptoms; importance of informing clinician of any history of myasthenia gravis. Importance of immediately contacting a clinician if any symptoms of muscle weakness, including respiratory difficulties, occur.

Inform patients that levofloxacin may be associated with hypersensitivity reactions (including anaphylactic reactions), even after the first dose. Importance of immediately discontinuing levofloxacin and contacting a clinician at first sign of rash or any symptom of hypersensitivity (e.g., hives, other skin reaction, rapid heartbeat, difficulty swallowing or breathing, throat tightness, hoarseness, swelling of lips, tongue, or face).

Inform patients that photosensitivity/phototoxicity reactions have been reported following exposure to sun or UV light in patients receiving fluoroquinolones. Importance of avoiding or minimizing exposure to sunlight or artificial UV light (e.g., tanning beds, UVA/UVB treatment) and using protective measures (e.g., wearing loose-fitting clothes, sunscreen) if outdoors during levofloxacin therapy. Importance of discontinuing levofloxacin and contacting a clinician if a sunburn-like reaction or skin eruption occurs.

Importance of informing clinician of personal or family history of QT interval prolongation or proarrhythmic conditions (e.g., hypokalemia, bradycardia, recent myocardial ischemia) and of concurrent therapy with any drugs that may affect QT interval (e.g., class IA [quinidine, procainamide] or class III [e.g., amiodarone, sotalol] antiarrhythmic agents). Importance of contacting a clinician if symptoms of prolonged QT interval (e.g., prolonged heart palpitations, loss of consciousness) occur.

Inform patients that systemic fluoroquinolones may increase the risk of aortic aneurysm and dissection; importance of informing clinician of any history of aneurysms, blockages or hardening of the arteries, high blood pressure, or genetic conditions such as Marfan syndrome or Ehlers-Danlos syndrome. Advise patients to seek immediate medical treatment if they experience sudden, severe, and constant pain in the stomach, chest, or back.

Inform patients that hypoglycemia has been reported when systemic fluoroquinolones were used in some patients receiving antidiabetic agents. Advise patients with diabetes mellitus receiving an oral antidiabetic agent or insulin to discontinue levofloxacin and contact a clinician if they experience hypoglycemia or symptoms of hypoglycemia.

Inform patients that severe hepatotoxicity (including acute hepatitis and fatal events) has been reported in patients receiving levofloxacin. Importance of immediately discontinuing levofloxacin and informing clinician if any signs or symptoms of liver injury (e.g., loss of appetite, nausea, vomiting, fever, weakness, tiredness, right upper quadrant tenderness, itching, yellowing of the skin and eyes, light colored bowel movements, dark colored urine) occur.

Advise patients that diarrhea is a common problem caused by anti-infectives and usually ends when the drug is discontinued. Importance of contacting a clinician if watery and bloody stools (with or without stomach cramps and fever) occur during or as late as 2 months or longer after the last dose.

If considering levofloxacin for a pediatric patient (see Pediatric Use under Warnings/Precautions: Specific Populations, in Cautions), importance of parent informing clinician if the child has a history of joint-related problems. Importance of parent contacting a clinician if the child develops any joint-related problems during or following levofloxacin therapy.

Advise patients receiving levofloxacin for inhalational anthrax (postexposure) or for treatment or prophylaxis of plague that human efficacy studies have not been performed for ethical and feasibility reasons and that use in these conditions is based on animal efficacy studies.

Importance of informing clinician of existing or contemplated concomitant therapy, including prescription and OTC drugs (e.g., drugs that may affect QT interval, antidiabetic agents, warfarin), as well as any concomitant illnesses.

Importance of women informing clinicians if they are or plan to become pregnant or plan to breast-feed.

Importance of advising patients of other important precautionary information. (See Cautions.)

PREPARATIONS

Excipients in commercially available drug preparations may have clinically important effects in some individuals; consult specific product labeling for details.

levoFLOXacin

Oral		
Solution	125 mg/5 mL*	levoFLOXacin Solution
Tablets, film-coated	250 mg (of anhydrous levofloxacin)*	Levaquin®, Janssen levoFLOXacin Tablets
	500 mg (of anhydrous levofloxacin)*	Levaquin®, Janssen levoFLOXacin Tablets
	750 mg (of anhydrous levofloxacin)*	Levaquin®, Janssen levoFLOXacin Tablets

Parenteral		
For injection, concentrate, for IV infusion	equivalent to levofloxacin 25 mg/mL (500 mg)*	levoFLOXacin Concentrate, for IV Infusion

* available from one or more manufacturer, distributor, and/or repackager by generic (nonproprietary) name

levoFLOXacin in Dextrose

Parenteral		
Injection, for IV infusion	equivalent to levofloxacin 5 mg/mL (250, 500, or 750 mg) in 5% Dextrose*	levoFLOXacin in Dextrose Injection

* available from one or more manufacturer, distributor, and/or repackager by generic (nonproprietary) name

† Use is not currently included in the labeling approved by the US Food and Drug Administration.

Selected Revisions August 26, 2019, © Copyright, January 1, 1998, American Society of Health-System Pharmacists, Inc.

Moxifloxacin Hydrochloride

8:12.18 • QUINOLONES

■ Moxifloxacin is a fluoroquinolone anti-infective agent.

USES

● Respiratory Tract Infections

Acute Sinusitis

Moxifloxacin is used for the treatment of acute bacterial sinusitis caused by susceptible *Streptococcus pneumoniae*, *Haemophilus influenzae*, or *Moraxella catarrhalis*.

Moxifloxacin should be used for the treatment of acute bacterial sinusitis only when there are no other treatment options. Because systemic fluoroquinolones, including moxifloxacin, have been associated with disabling and potentially irreversible serious adverse reactions (e.g., tendinitis and tendon rupture, peripheral neuropathy, CNS effects) that can occur together in the same patient (see Cautions) and because acute bacterial sinusitis may be self-limiting in some patients, the risks of serious adverse reactions outweigh the benefits of fluoroquinolones for patients with acute sinusitis.

Clinical Experience

In a controlled, double-blind study in 457 patients with acute bacterial sinusitis, the clinical success rate (cure plus improvement) at the test-of-cure visit 7–21 days after treatment was 90% in those who received moxifloxacin (400 mg once daily for 10 days) and 89% in those who received cefuroxime axetil (250 mg twice daily for 10 days). In a noncomparative study, the clinical success and eradication/presumed eradication rate at 21–37 days after moxifloxacin treatment (400 mg once daily for 7 days) was 97, 83, or 80% for infections caused by *S. pneumoniae*, *M. catarrhalis*, or *H. influenzae*, respectively.

Acute Exacerbations of Chronic Bronchitis

Moxifloxacin is used for the treatment of acute bacterial exacerbations of chronic bronchitis caused by susceptible *S. pneumoniae*, *H. influenzae*, *H. parainfluenzae*, *Klebsiella pneumoniae*, *Staphylococcus aureus* (methicillin-susceptible [oxacillin-susceptible] strains), or *M. catarrhalis*.

Moxifloxacin should be used for the treatment of acute bacterial exacerbations of chronic bronchitis only when there are no other treatment options. Because systemic fluoroquinolones, including moxifloxacin, have been associated with disabling and potentially irreversible serious adverse reactions (e.g., tendinitis and tendon rupture, peripheral neuropathy, CNS effects) that can occur together in the same patient (see Cautions) and because acute bacterial exacerbations of chronic bronchitis may be self-limiting in some patients, the risks of serious adverse reactions outweigh the benefits of fluoroquinolones for patients with these infections.

Clinical Experience

In a randomized, double-blind, controlled trial in 629 patients with acute bacterial exacerbations of chronic bronchitis, the clinical success rate 7–17 days after treatment was 89% in those who received moxifloxacin (400 mg once daily for 5 days) and also was 89% in those who received clarithromycin (500 mg twice daily for 10 days). The microbiologic eradication rate (eradication plus presumed eradication) in those who received moxifloxacin was 100% for *S. pneumoniae*, 89% for *H. influenzae*, 100% for *H. parainfluenzae*, 85% for *M. catarrhalis*, 94% for *S. aureus*, and 85% for *K. pneumoniae*.

Community-acquired Pneumonia

Moxifloxacin is used for the treatment of community-acquired pneumonia (CAP) caused by susceptible *S. pneumoniae* (including multidrug-resistant strains [MDRSP]), *S. aureus* (methicillin-susceptible [oxacillin-susceptible] strains), *K. pneumoniae*, *H. influenzae*, *Mycoplasma pneumoniae*, *Chlamydophila pneumoniae* (formerly *Chlamydia pneumoniae*), or *M. catarrhalis*.

Initial treatment of CAP generally involves use of an empiric anti-infective regimen based on the most likely pathogens and local susceptibility patterns;

treatment may then be changed (if possible) to provide a more specific regimen (pathogen-directed therapy) based on results of in vitro culture and susceptibility testing. The most appropriate empiric regimen varies depending on the severity of illness at the time of presentation, whether outpatient treatment or hospitalization in or out of an intensive care unit (ICU) is indicated, and the presence or absence of cardiopulmonary disease and other modifying factors that increase the risk of certain pathogens (e.g., methicillin-resistant *S. aureus* [MRSA; also known as oxacillin-resistant *S. aureus* or ORSA], penicillin-resistant *S. pneumoniae*, MDRSP, enteric gram-negative bacilli, *Pseudomonas aeruginosa*).

For additional information on management of CAP, the current clinical practice guidelines from the Infectious Diseases Society of America (IDSA) available at http://www.idsociety.org should be consulted.

Clinical Experience

In randomized studies in patients with clinically and radiologically documented CAP, the rate of clinical success with a sequential regimen of IV moxifloxacin followed by oral moxifloxacin (400 mg daily for 7–14 days) was similar to that achieved with 7–14 days of therapy with similar regimens using other fluoroquinolones (levofloxacin) or a regimen of ceftriaxone with or without erythromycin. In a randomized study in CAP patients 65 years of age or older (mean age 77.9 years), the clinical cure rate at the test-of-cure visit (5–21 days after end of treatment) was 92.9% in those who received moxifloxacin and 87.9% in those who received levofloxacin; the bacteriologic success rate was 81% in those who received moxifloxacin and 75% in those who received levofloxacin.

Data on efficacy of moxifloxacin for the treatment of CAP caused by *S. pneumoniae* in adults have been obtained from various clinical studies. In these studies, moxifloxacin resulted in clinical cure in about 95% of patients with CAP caused by *S. pneumoniae*. In those patients with documented infections caused by penicillin-resistant *S. pneumoniae* (penicillin MICs of 2 mcg/mL or greater), the bacteriologic cure rate was 100%. In 37 patients with CAP caused by multidrug-resistant strains, the clinical cure rate with moxifloxacin was 95%. Moxifloxacin has been effective for the treatment of infections caused by *S. pneumoniae* resistant to penicillin, second generation cephalosporins (e.g., cefuroxime), macrolides, tetracyclines, and/or co-trimoxazole.

Nosocomial Pneumonia

Moxifloxacin has been used for the treatment of nosocomial pneumonia†.

Local susceptibility data should be used when selecting initial empiric regimens for the treatment of hospital-acquired pneumonia (HAP) not associated with mechanical ventilation or the treatment of ventilator-associated pneumonia (VAP). If a fluoroquinolone is used for initial empiric treatment of HAP or VAP, IDSA and the American Thoracic Society (ATS) recommend ciprofloxacin or levofloxacin.

For additional information on management of nosocomial pneumonia, the current clinical practice guidelines from IDSA available at http://www.idsociety.org should be consulted.

● Skin and Skin Structure Infections

Moxifloxacin is used for the treatment of uncomplicated skin and skin structure infections caused by susceptible *S. aureus* (methicillin-susceptible [oxacillin-susceptible] strains) or *Streptococcus pyogenes* (group A β-hemolytic streptococci) and for the treatment of complicated skin and skin structure infections caused by susceptible *S. aureus* (methicillin-susceptible [oxacillin-susceptible] strains), *Escherichia coli*, *K. pneumoniae*, or *Enterobacter cloacae*.

For additional information on management of skin and skin structure infections, the current clinical practice guidelines from IDSA available at http://www.idsociety.org should be consulted.

Clinical Experience

Moxifloxacin has been effective for the treatment of uncomplicated abscesses, furuncles, cellulitis, impetigo, and other skin infections. In a randomized double-blind study, moxifloxacin (400 mg once daily for 7 days) was as effective as cephalexin (500 mg 3 times daily for 7 days) in the treatment of uncomplicated skin and skin structure infections caused by susceptible bacteria; clinical success (resolution or improvement) occurred in 89 or 91% of those receiving moxifloxacin or cephalexin, respectively (intent-to-treat analysis).

In 2 randomized, comparator-controlled studies in adults with complicated skin and skin structure infections, the clinical success rate in those receiving a sequential regimen of IV moxifloxacin followed by oral moxifloxacin (400 mg once daily for 7–14 days) was similar to that in those who received a sequential IV then oral regimen of a fixed-combination preparation containing a β-lactam antibiotic and a β-lactamase inhibitor (77–81% for moxifloxacin versus 82–85% for the comparator agent). When data were stratified by the causative agent, the clinical success rate in patients who received moxifloxacin was about 82% in those with infections caused by *S. aureus* infections (methicillin-susceptible [oxacillin-susceptible] strains), *E. coli*, or *E. cloacae* and 92% in those with infections caused by *K. pneumoniae*.

● **Intra-abdominal Infections**

Moxifloxacin is used for the treatment of complicated intra-abdominal infections, including polymicrobial infections such as abscess caused by susceptible *Bacteroides fragilis*, *B. thetaiotaomicron*, *Clostridium perfringens*, *Enterococcus faecalis*, *E. coli*, *Proteus mirabilis*, *S. anginosus*, *S. constellatus*, or *Peptostreptococcus*.

Moxifloxacin has been recommended as one of several options for initial empiric treatment of mild to moderate, community-acquired intra-abdominal infections. IDSA states that use of moxifloxacin should be avoided in patients who received a quinolone within the past 3 months and are likely to harbor *B. fragilis* since such strains are likely to be resistant to the drug.

For additional information on management of intra-abdominal infections, the current clinical practice guidelines from IDSA available at http://www.idsociety.org should be consulted.

Clinical Experience

Safety and efficacy of moxifloxacin monotherapy for the treatment of surgically confirmed complicated intra-abdominal infections (including peritonitis, abscess, appendicitis with perforation, bowel perforation) were established in 2 randomized, active-controlled studies in adults. In one double-blind study, patients were randomized to receive a sequential regimen of IV moxifloxacin followed by oral moxifloxacin (400 mg once daily for 5–14 days) or a sequential regimen of the IV fixed-combination preparation of piperacillin and tazobactam followed by the oral fixed-combination preparation of amoxicillin and clavulanate potassium. At the test-of-cure visit (day 25–50 after initiation of study), the clinical cure rate in the efficacy-valid population was 80% in those who received moxifloxacin and 78% in those who received the comparator regimen. The bacteriologic success rate (eradication or presumed eradication) at the test-of-cure visit was 78% in those who received moxifloxacin (83% of those with hospital-acquired or 77% of those with community-acquired infections) and 77% in those who received the comparator regimen (55% of those with hospital-acquired or 82% of those with community-acquired infections). Similar results were obtained in an open-label study in which patients were randomized to receive 400 mg of moxifloxacin daily for 5–14 days or a sequential regimen of IV ceftriaxone in conjunction with IV metronidazole followed by the oral fixed-combination preparation of amoxicillin and clavulanate potassium. In this open-label study, the clinical success rate at the test-of-cure visit (day 25–50 after initiation of study) was 81% in those who received moxifloxacin and 82% in those who received the comparator regimen.

● **Endocarditis**

Moxifloxacin is used as an alternative for the treatment of endocarditis† (native or prosthetic valve or other prosthetic material) caused by fastidious gram-negative bacilli known as the HACEK group (*Haemophilus*, *Aggregatibacter*, *Cardiobacterium hominis*, *Eikenella corrodens*, *Kingella*).

The American Heart Association (AHA) and IDSA recommend ceftriaxone (or other third or fourth generation cephalosporin) for the treatment of endocarditis caused by the HACEK group, but state that a fluoroquinolone (ciprofloxacin, levofloxacin, moxifloxacin) may be considered in patients who cannot tolerate cephalosporins. Because only limited data are available regarding use of fluoroquinolones for the treatment of HACEK endocarditis, an infectious disease specialist should be consulted when treating such infections in patients who cannot tolerate cephalosporins.

● **GI Infections**
Campylobacter Infections

Moxifloxacin has been recommended as an alternative for the treatment of campylobacteriosis† caused by susceptible *Campylobacter*.

Optimal treatment of campylobacteriosis in patients with human immunodeficiency virus (HIV) infection has not been identified. Some clinicians withhold anti-infective treatment in HIV-infected patients with CD4+ T-cell counts

exceeding 200 cells/mm³ if they have only mild campylobacteriosis and initiate treatment if symptoms persist for more than several days. In HIV-infected patients with mild to moderate campylobacteriosis, treatment with a fluoroquinolone (preferably ciprofloxacin or, alternatively, levofloxacin or moxifloxacin) or azithromycin is reasonable. Anti-infective therapy should be modified based on results of in vitro susceptibility testing. In the US, resistance to fluoroquinolones has been reported in 22% of *C. jejuni* and 35% of *C. coli* isolates tested. To limit emergence of resistance, some clinicians suggest that it may be prudent to use an aminoglycoside concomitantly in patients with bacteremic infections.

Salmonella Gastroenteritis

Moxifloxacin is used for the treatment of *Salmonella* gastroenteritis† (with or without bacteremia).

Anti-infective therapy is not usually indicated in otherwise healthy individuals with uncomplicated (noninvasive) gastroenteritis caused by *Salmonella* since such therapy may prolong the duration of fecal excretion of the organism and there is no evidence that it shortens the duration of the disease; however, the US Centers for Disease Control and Prevention (CDC), American Academy of Pediatrics (AAP), IDSA, and others recommend anti-infective therapy in individuals with severe *Salmonella* gastroenteritis and in those who are at increased risk of invasive disease. These individuals include infants younger than 3–6 months of age; individuals older than 50 years of age; individuals with hemoglobinopathies, severe atherosclerosis or valvular heart disease, prostheses, uremia, chronic GI disease, or severe colitis; and individuals who are immunocompromised because of malignancy, immunosuppressive therapy, HIV infection, or other immunosuppressive illness.

Because HIV-infected individuals with *Salmonella* gastroenteritis are at high risk for bacteremia, CDC, National Institutes of Health (NIH), and HIV Medicine Association of IDSA recommend that such patients receive anti-infective treatment. These experts state that the initial drug of choice for the treatment of salmonella gastroenteritis (with or without bacteremia) in HIV-infected adults is ciprofloxacin; other fluoroquinolones (levofloxacin, moxifloxacin) also are likely to be effective in these patients, but clinical data are limited. Depending on results of in vitro susceptibility testing of the causative organism, alternatives for treatment of *Salmonella* gastroenteritis in HIV-infected adults are co-trimoxazole or third generation cephalosporins (ceftriaxone, cefotaxime).

The role of long-term treatment (secondary prophylaxis) against *Salmonella* in HIV-infected individuals is not well established, and possible benefits of such prophylaxis should be weighed against the risks of long-term anti-infective exposure. CDC, NIH, and IDSA state that secondary prophylaxis should be considered in those with recurrent bacteremia and may also be considered in those with recurrent gastroenteritis (with or without bacteremia) and in those with CD4+ T-cell counts less than 200 cells/mm³ and severe diarrhea. These experts state that secondary prophylaxis should be discontinued if the *Salmonella* infection resolves and there has been a sustained response to antiretroviral therapy with CD4+ T-cell counts greater than 200 cells/mm³.

Shigella Infections

Moxifloxacin is used as an alternative for the treatment of shigellosis† caused by susceptible *Shigella*.

Infections caused by *S. sonnei* usually are self-limited (48–72 hours), and mild cases may not require treatment with anti-infectives. However, because there is some evidence that anti-infectives may shorten the duration of diarrhea and the period of fecal excretion of *Shigella*, anti-infective treatment generally is recommended in addition to fluid and electrolyte replacement in patients with severe shigellosis, dysentery, or underlying immunosuppression. An empiric treatment regimen can be used initially, but in vitro susceptibility testing of clinical isolates is indicated since resistance is common. A fluoroquinolone (preferably ciprofloxacin or, alternatively, levofloxacin or moxifloxacin) generally has been recommended for the treatment of shigellosis. However, fluoroquinolone-resistant *Shigella* have been reported in the US, especially in international travelers, the homeless, and men who have sex with men (MSM). Depending on in vitro susceptibility, other drugs recommended for the treatment of shigellosis include co-trimoxazole, ceftriaxone, azithromycin (not recommended in those with bacteremia), or ampicillin.

● **Anthrax**

Oral moxifloxacin is recommended as an alternative for postexposure prophylaxis of anthrax† following suspected or confirmed exposure to aerosolized *Bacillus anthracis* spores (inhalational anthrax). CDC, AAP, US Working Group on

Civilian Biodefense, and US Army Medical Research Institute of Infectious Diseases (USAMRIID) recommend oral ciprofloxacin and oral doxycycline as the initial drugs of choice for postexposure prophylaxis following exposure to aerosolized anthrax spores, including exposures that occur in the context of biologic warfare or bioterrorism. Other oral fluoroquinolones (levofloxacin, moxifloxacin, ofloxacin) are alternatives for postexposure prophylaxis when ciprofloxacin or doxycycline cannot be used.

Oral moxifloxacin is one of several options recommended for the treatment of uncomplicated cutaneous anthrax† (without systemic involvement) that occurs in the context of biologic warfare or bioterrorism. CDC recommends that adults receive an oral regimen of ciprofloxacin, doxycycline, levofloxacin, or moxifloxacin for treatment of such infections.

IV moxifloxacin is recommended as an alternative to IV ciprofloxacin for use in multiple-drug parenteral regimens for initial treatment of systemic anthrax† (inhalational, GI, meningitis, or cutaneous with systemic involvement, extensive edema, or head or neck lesions) that occurs in the context of biologic warfare or bioterrorism. CDC, AAP, US Working Group on Civilian Biodefense, and USAMRIID recommend that treatment be initiated with a multiple-drug parenteral regimen that includes a fluoroquinolone (preferably ciprofloxacin) or doxycycline and 1 or 2 additional anti-infective agents predicted to be effective; after the patient is clinically stable, treatment can be changed to an oral anti-infective. For initial treatment of systemic anthrax with possible or confirmed meningitis, CDC and AAP recommend a regimen of IV ciprofloxacin in conjunction with another IV bactericidal anti-infective (preferably meropenem) and an IV protein synthesis inhibitor (preferably linezolid). If meningitis has been excluded, these experts recommend an initial regimen of IV ciprofloxacin in conjunction with an IV protein synthesis inhibitor (preferably clindamycin or linezolid).

Some experts suggest that oral ciprofloxacin or other oral fluoroquinolones (levofloxacin, moxifloxacin, ofloxacin) can be considered for the treatment of inhalational anthrax† when a parenteral regimen is not available. Although a multiple-drug parenteral regimen should be used for the treatment of inhalational anthrax, use of these parenteral regimens may not be possible if large numbers of individuals require treatment in a mass casualty setting and it may be necessary to use an oral regimen.

For additional information on postexposure prophylaxis or treatment of anthrax, see Uses: Anthrax in Ciprofloxacin 8:12.18.

● *Meningitis and Other CNS Infections*

Moxifloxacin is recommended as an alternative for the treatment of meningitis† caused by certain susceptible gram-positive bacteria (e.g., *S. pneumoniae*). Fluoroquinolones also have been recommended as alternatives for the treatment of meningitis† caused by some gram-negative bacteria (e.g., *Neisseria meningitidis*, *H. influenzae*, *E. coli*, *Ps. aeruginosa*).

Limited data from animal studies indicate that moxifloxacin is distributed into CSF to some extent, and the drug has been effective for the treatment of experimental meningitis caused by *S. pneumoniae* or *E. coli*. Some experts state that fluoroquinolones (e.g., ciprofloxacin, moxifloxacin) should be considered for the treatment of meningitis *only* when the infection is caused by susceptible bacteria and the usually recommended anti-infectives cannot be used or have been ineffective.

● *Mycobacterial Infections*

Treatment of Active Tuberculosis

Moxifloxacin is used in multiple-drug regimens for the treatment of active tuberculosis† caused by *Mycobacterium tuberculosis*.

Although the potential role of fluoroquinolones and the optimal length of therapy have not been fully defined, ATS, CDC, IDSA, and others state that use of fluoroquinolones as alternative (second-line) agents can be considered for the treatment of active tuberculosis in patients intolerant of certain first-line agents and in those with relapse, treatment failure, or *M. tuberculosis* resistant to certain first-line agents. If a fluoroquinolone is used in multiple-drug regimens for the treatment of active tuberculosis, ATS, CDC, IDSA, and others recommend levofloxacin or moxifloxacin.

Although levofloxacin (or moxifloxacin) has been used instead of ethambutol during the intensive phase of treatment in adults who could not receive ethambutol and has been used instead of isoniazid throughout the course of treatment in adults who could not receive isoniazid, ATS, CDC, and IDSA state that there is no evidence that levofloxacin (or moxifloxacin) can be used to replace a rifamycin or pyrazinamide while maintaining a 6-month treatment regimen.

The fact that there are reports of fluoroquinolone-resistant *M. tuberculosis* and increasing reports of extensively drug-resistant tuberculosis (XDR tuberculosis) should be considered. XDR tuberculosis is caused by strains of *M. tuberculosis* that are resistant to rifampin and isoniazid (multiple-drug resistant strains) and also are resistant to a fluoroquinolone and at least one parenteral second-line antimycobacterial (capreomycin, kanamycin, amikacin).

The most recent ATS, CDC, and IDSA recommendations for treatment of tuberculosis should be consulted for more specific information.

Other Mycobacterial Infections

Moxifloxacin is used in the treatment of *M. kansasii* infections† in conjunction with other antimycobacterials. ATS and IDSA recommend a multiple-drug regimen of isoniazid, rifampin, and ethambutol for treatment of pulmonary or disseminated infections caused by *M. kansasii*. If rifampin-resistant *M. kansasii* are involved, ATS and IDSA recommend a 3-drug regimen based on results of in vitro susceptibility testing, including clarithromycin (or azithromycin), moxifloxacin, ethambutol, sulfamethoxazole, or streptomycin.

Moxifloxacin has been used in multiple-drug regimens for the treatment of *M. avium* complex† (MAC) infections. ATS and IDSA state that the role of fluoroquinolones in the treatment of MAC infections has not been established. If a fluoroquinolone is included in a treatment regimen (e.g., for macrolide-resistant MAC infections), moxifloxacin or levofloxacin may be preferred, although many strains are resistant in vitro.

The most recent ATS, CDC, and IDSA recommendations for treatment of other mycobacterial infections should be consulted for more specific information.

● *Nongonococcal Urethritis*

Moxifloxacin is considered as an alternative agent for the treatment of nongonococcal urethritis† (NGU). NGU can be caused by various organisms (e.g., *Chlamydia*, *M. genitalium*, *Trichomonas vaginalis*, *Ureaplasma*, enteric bacteria) and is treated presumptively at the time of diagnosis. CDC states that a single dose of oral azithromycin or a 7-day regimen of oral doxycycline are the recommended regimens for the treatment of NGU; a 7-day regimen of oral erythromycin base or ethylsuccinate or a 7-day regimen of oral levofloxacin or ofloxacin are alternative regimens.

CDC states that men with persistent or recurrent NGU who were not compliant with the treatment regimen or were reexposed to untreated sexual partner(s) can be retreated with the initial regimen. In other patients, symptoms alone (without documentation of signs or laboratory evidence of urethral inflammation) are not a sufficient basis for retreatment and an objective diagnosis of persistent or recurrent NGU should be made before considering additional treatment. Because there is some evidence that *M. genitalium* is the most frequent cause of persistent or recurrent NGU, CDC states that those initially treated with doxycycline should receive retreatment with a single dose of oral azithromycin and those initially treated with azithromycin should receive retreatment with a 7-day regimen of oral moxifloxacin. However, if the patient with persistent or recurrent urethritis has sex with women and is in an area where *T. vaginalis* is prevalent, CDC recommends presumptive retreatment with a single 2-g dose of oral metronidazole or tinidazole and referral of their partner(s) for evaluation and appropriate treatment.

NGU may facilitate transmission of HIV and men diagnosed with NGU should be tested for HIV. Individuals with HIV infection should receive the same treatment regimens recommended for other individuals with NGU.

Any individual who had sexual contact with a patient with NGU within the preceding 60 days should be referred for evaluation, testing, and presumptive treatment with a regimen effective against *Chlamydia*. To minimize transmission and avoid reinfection, men treated for NGU should abstain from sexual intercourse until they and their sexual partner(s) have been adequately treated.

● *Plague*

Moxifloxacin is used for the treatment of plague, including pneumonic and septicemic plague, caused by susceptible *Yersinia pestis* and for prophylaxis of plague. Based on results of in vitro and animal testing, fluoroquinolones (e.g., ciprofloxacin, levofloxacin, moxifloxacin, ofloxacin) are recommended as alternatives for the treatment of plague and for postexposure prophylaxis following a high risk exposure to *Y. pestis*, including exposure in the context of biologic warfare or bioterrorism.

Efficacy of moxifloxacin for treatment or prophylaxis of plague has not been evaluated in clinical trials in humans for ethical and feasibility reasons. The drug is labeled by the FDA for this indication based on an efficacy study in animals that demonstrated a survival benefit and supportive animal and human pharmaco-kinetic data. In a randomized, blinded, placebo-controlled study, African green monkeys were exposed to an inhaled dose of *Y. pestis* (mean dose of 100 LD$_{50}$ [range 92–127 LD$_{50}$]) and then randomized to receive a 10-day regimen of moxi-floxacin or placebo initiated after fever developed and was sustained for at least 4 hours. All study monkeys were febrile and bacteremic with *Y. pestis* prior to initi-ation of study treatment. In vitro testing indicated that the *Y. pestis* strain (CO92 strain) used in this study had a moxifloxacin MIC of 0.06 mcg/mL. Pharmacoki-netic data indicated that mean plasma concentrations of moxifloxacin attained in the study monkeys (4.4 mcg/mL) were similar to mean peak plasma concentra-tions attained in adults receiving 400 mg of moxifloxacin IV (3.9 mcg/mL). Study results indicated that all monkeys in the moxifloxacin treatment group survived for the 30-day period after treatment (10 out of 10), but all monkeys in the placebo group succumbed to the disease within 83–139 hours (10 out of 10).

For the treatment of plague, IM streptomycin (or IM or IV gentamicin) his-torically has been considered the drug of choice. Alternatives recommended for the treatment of plague when aminoglycosides are not used include an IV fluo-roquinolone (ciprofloxacin [a drug of choice for plague meningitis], levofloxacin, moxifloxacin), IV doxycycline (or IV tetracycline), IV chloramphenicol (a drug of choice for plague meningitis), or co-trimoxazole (may be less effective than other alternatives).

Anti-infective regimens recommended for treatment of naturally occurring or endemic bubonic, septicemic, or pneumonic plague also are recommended for the treatment of plague that occurs following exposure to *Y. pestis* in the context of biologic warfare or bioterrorism. Such exposures would most likely result in pri-mary pneumonic plague, and prompt initiation of anti-infective therapy (within 18–24 hours of onset of symptoms) is essential in the treatment of pneumonic plague. Some experts (e.g., US Working Group on Civilian Biodefense, USAM-RIID) recommend that treatment of plague in the context of biologic warfare or bioterrorism be initiated with a parenteral anti-infective regimen of streptomy-cin (or gentamicin) or, alternatively, a fluoroquinolone (ciprofloxacin, levoflox-acin, moxifloxacin), doxycycline, or chloramphenicol. However, an oral regimen of doxycycline (or tetracycline) or a fluoroquinolone (ciprofloxacin, levoflox-acin, moxifloxacin, ofloxacin) may be substituted when the patient's condition improves or when a parenteral regimen is unavailable (e.g., when there are sup-ply or logistic problems because large numbers of individuals require treatment in a mass casualty setting).

In the context of biologic warfare or bioterrorism, some experts (e.g., US Working Group on Civilian Biodefense, USAMRIID) recommend that asymp-tomatic individuals with exposure to plague aerosol or asymptomatic individ-uals with household, hospital, or other close contact (within about 2 m) with an individual who has pneumonic plague receive an oral anti-infective regi-men for postexposure prophylaxis; however, any exposed individual who devel-ops a temperature of 38.5°C or higher or new cough should promptly receive a parenteral anti-infective for treatment of the disease. If postexposure prophy-laxis is indicated, these experts recommend a an oral regimen of doxycycline (or tetracycline) or a fluoroquinolone (ciprofloxacin, levofloxacin, moxifloxa-cin, ofloxacin).

For additional information on use of fluoroquinolones for treatment or prophylaxis of plague, see Uses: Plague in Ciprofloxacin 8:12.18.

● Ophthalmic Infections

For use of moxifloxacin in the topical treatment of ophthalmic infections caused by susceptible organisms, see Moxifloxacin Hydrochloride 52:04.12.

DOSAGE AND ADMINISTRATION

● Administration

Moxifloxacin hydrochloride is administered orally or by IV infusion. The drug should *not* be given IM, subcutaneously, intrathecally, or intraperitoneally.

IV administration of moxifloxacin is indicated in patients who do not tolerate or are unable to take the drug orally and in other patients in whom the IV route offers a clinical advantage.

Patients receiving oral or IV moxifloxacin should be well hydrated and instructed to drink fluids liberally.

Oral Administration

Moxifloxacin tablets may be given without regard to meals.

Administration of a 400-mg moxifloxacin tablet with a high-fat breakfast or with yogurt does not have a clinically important effect on absorption of the drug.

Moxifloxacin should be administered orally at least 4 hours before or 8 hours after antacids containing magnesium or aluminum, metal cations (e.g., iron), sucralfate, multivitamins or dietary supplements containing iron or zinc, or buff-ered didanosine (pediatric oral solution admixed with antacid). These drugs may substantially interfere with absorption of moxifloxacin, resulting in systemic con-centrations considerably lower than desired. (See Drug Interactions.)

IV Infusion

Commercially available injection for IV infusion containing 400 mg of moxiflox-acin in 0.8% sodium chloride injection in single-use flexible containers may be used without further dilution.

Moxifloxacin should not be admixed with other drugs or infused simultane-ously through the same tubing with other drugs. If the same IV line or a Y-type line is used for sequential infusion of other drugs or if the piggyback method of admin-istration is used, the tubing should be flushed before and after infusion of moxiflox-acin using an IV solution compatible with both moxifloxacin and the other drug(s).

Moxifloxacin IV solutions should be inspected visually for particulate matter prior to administration; the premixed solution should appear yellow.

Because commercially available moxifloxacin premixed injection for IV infu-sion contains no preservatives, any unused portions of the solution should be discarded.

Rate of Administration

Moxifloxacin solutions should be administered by IV infusion over 1 hour.

Rapid IV infusion of the drug should be avoided.

● Dosage

Dosage of moxifloxacin hydrochloride is expressed in terms of moxifloxacin.

Dosage of oral and IV moxifloxacin is identical.

When IV moxifloxacin is used initially, therapy may be changed to oral moxi-floxacin (when appropriate) using the same dosage to complete therapy.

Pediatric Dosage

Treatment of Systemic Anthrax

If IV moxifloxacin is used in a multiple-drug parenteral regimen for initial treatment of systemic anthrax† (inhalational, GI, meningitis, or cutaneous with systemic involvement, extensive edema, or head or neck lesions) that occurs in the context of biologic warfare or bioterrorism (see Uses: Anthrax), the American Academy of Pediatrics (AAP) recommends that preterm neo-nates† (gestational age 32–37 weeks) up to 4 weeks of age receive a dosage of 5 mg/kg once daily and that full-term neonates† up to 4 weeks of age receive a dosage of 10 mg/kg once daily.

If IV moxifloxacin is used in a multiple-drug parenteral regimen for initial treatment of systemic anthrax† (inhalational, GI, meningitis, or cutaneous with systemic involvement, lesions on the head or neck, or extensive edema) that occurs in the context of biologic warfare or bioterrorism (see Uses: Anthrax) in infants 3 months to less than 2 years of age†, AAP recommends a dosage of 6 mg/kg (up to 200 mg) every 12 hours. AAP recommends an IV dosage of 5 mg/kg (up to 200 mg) every 12 hours in children 2–5 years of age† and 4 mg/kg (up to 200 mg) every 12 hours in those 6–11 years of age†. In adolescents 12–17 years of age†, AAP recommends that those weighing less than 45 kg receive an IV moxi-floxacin dosage of 4 mg/kg (up to 200 mg) every 12 hours and that those weighing 45 kg or more receive a dosage of 400 mg once daily.

The multiple-drug parenteral regimen should be continued for at least 2–3 weeks until the patient is clinically stable and treatment can be switched to an appropriate oral anti-infective. If systemic anthrax occurred as the result of expo-sure to aerosolized *Bacillus anthracis* spores (e.g., in the context of biologic war-fare or bioterrorism), the oral follow-up regimen should be continued until 60 days after onset of the illness.

Adult Dosage

Acute Sinusitis

If moxifloxacin is used for the treatment of acute bacterial sinusitis, the usual adult dosage is 400 mg once daily for 10 days. (See Acute Sinusitis under Uses: Respiratory Tract Infections.)

Acute Exacerbations of Chronic Bronchitis

If moxifloxacin is used for the treatment of acute bacterial exacerbations of chronic bronchitis, the usual adult dosage is 400 mg once daily for 5 days. (See Acute Exacerbations of Chronic Bronchitis under Uses: Respiratory Tract Infections.)

Community-acquired Pneumonia

For the treatment of community-acquired pneumonia (CAP), the usual adult dosage of moxifloxacin is 400 mg once daily for 7–14 days.

Skin and Skin Structure Infections

For the treatment of uncomplicated skin and skin structure infections, the usual adult dosage of moxifloxacin is 400 mg once daily for 7 days.

For the treatment of complicated skin and skin structure infections, the usual adult dosage of moxifloxacin is 400 mg once daily for 7–21 days.

Intra-abdominal Infections

For the treatment of complicated intra-abdominal infections, the usual adult dosage of moxifloxacin is 400 mg once daily. The drug should be administered IV initially, but therapy may be changed to oral administration when clinically appropriate.

The manufacturer recommends a total duration of therapy of 5–14 days for the treatment of complicated intra-abdominal infections. The Infectious Diseases Society of America (IDSA) states that the usual duration of treatment for these infections is 4–7 day; a longer duration of treatment has not been associated with improved outcome and is not recommended unless adequate source control is difficult to achieve.

Campylobacter Infections

For the treatment of campylobacteriosis† caused by susceptible *Campylobacter* in adults with human immunodeficiency virus (HIV) infection, the recommended dosage of oral or IV moxifloxacin is 400 mg once daily.

The recommended duration of fluoroquinolone treatment in HIV-infected patients is 7–10 days for gastroenteritis or at least 14 days for bacteremic infections. A duration of 2–6 weeks is recommended for recurrent infections.

Salmonella Gastroenteritis

For the treatment of *Salmonella* gastroenteritis† (with or without bacteremia) in HIV-infected adults, the recommended dosage of oral or IV moxifloxacin is 400 mg once daily.

The recommended duration of treatment in HIV-infected patients is 7–14 days in those with CD4+ T-cell counts of 200 cells/mm³ or greater (14 days or longer if the patient is bacteremic or the infection is complicated) or 2–6 weeks in those with CD4+ T-cell counts less than 200 cells/mm³.

Shigella Infections

For the treatment of shigellosis† caused by susceptible *Shigella* in HIV-infected adults, the recommended dosage of oral or IV moxifloxacin is 400 mg once daily.

The recommended duration of fluoroquinolone treatment in HIV-infected patients is 7–10 days for gastroenteritis or at least 14 days for bacteremic infections. Recurrent infections, especially in those with CD4+ T-cell counts less than 200 cells/mm³, may require up to 6 weeks of treatment.

Postexposure Prophylaxis of Anthrax

If oral moxifloxacin is used as an alternative for postexposure prophylaxis of anthrax† following exposure to aerosolized *B. anthracis* spores in the context of biologic warfare or bioterrorism, CDC recommends that adults (including pregnant and postpartum women) receive a dosage of 400 mg once daily.

Anti-infective prophylaxis should be initiated as soon as possible following suspected or confirmed exposure to aerosolized *B. anthracis*.

Because of possible persistence of *B. anthracis* spores in lung tissue following an aerosol exposure, CDC and other experts recommend that anti-infective postexposure prophylaxis be continued for 60 days following a confirmed exposure.

Treatment of Uncomplicated Cutaneous Anthrax

If oral moxifloxacin is used for the treatment of uncomplicated cutaneous anthrax without systemic involvement†, CDC recommends that adults (including pregnant and postpartum women) receive a dosage of 400 mg once daily.

If uncomplicated cutaneous anthrax occurred after exposure to aerosolized *B. anthracis* spores in the context of biologic warfare or bioterrorism, anti-infective treatment should be continued for 60 days.

Treatment of Systemic Anthrax

If IV moxifloxacin is used as an alternative to IV ciprofloxacin in a multiple-drug parenteral regimen for initial treatment of systemic anthrax† (inhalational, GI, meningitis, or cutaneous with systemic involvement, lesions on the head or neck, or extensive edema) that occurs in the context of biologic warfare or bioterrorism, CDC recommends that adults (including pregnant and postpartum women) receive a dosage of 400 mg once daily.

The multiple-drug parenteral regimen should be continued for at least 2–3 weeks until the patient is clinically stable and treatment can be switched to an oral anti-infective. If systemic anthrax occurred as the result of exposure to aerosolized *B. anthracis* spores in the context of biologic warfare or bioterrorism, the oral follow-up regimen should be continued until 60 days after onset of the illness.

If oral moxifloxacin is used as an alternative for the treatment of inhalational anthrax† when a parenteral regimen is not available (see Uses: Anthrax), US Working Group on Civilian Biodefense suggests that adults can receive a dosage of 400 mg once daily for 60 days.

Treatment of Active Tuberculosis

If moxifloxacin is used as an alternative (second-line) agent in multiple-drug regimens for the treatment of active tuberculosis†, the American Thoracic Society (ATS), CDC, and IDSA recommend that adults receive 400 mg once daily. These experts state that data are insufficient to support intermittent regimens of moxifloxacin for the treatment of tuberculosis.

Other Mycobacterial Infections

If oral moxifloxacin is used as an alternative in multiple-drug regimens for the treatment of disseminated infections caused by *Mycobacterium avium* complex† (MAC) in HIV-infected adults, CDC, National Institutes of Health (NIH), and IDSA recommend a dosage of 400 mg once daily.

Nongonococcal Urethritis

If oral moxifloxacin is used as an alternative for the treatment of persistent or recurrent nongonococcal urethritis† (NGU) in patients initially treated with azithromycin (see Uses: Nongonococcal Urethritis), CDC recommends a dosage of 400 mg once daily for 7 days.

Plague

If moxifloxacin is used for the treatment or prophylaxis of plague caused by *Yersinia pestis* in adults, the manufacturer recommends a dosage of 400 mg once daily for 10–14 days. The drug should be initiated as soon as possible after suspected or known exposure to *Y. pestis*.

● Special Populations

Hepatic Impairment

Adjustment of moxifloxacin dosage is not necessary in adults with mild, moderate, or severe hepatic impairment (Child-Pugh class A, B, or C). However, moxifloxacin should be used with caution in patients with hepatic impairment. (See Hepatic Impairment under Warning/Precautions: Specific Populations, in Cautions.)

Renal Impairment

Adjustment of moxifloxacin dosage is not necessary in adults with renal impairment, including those receiving hemodialysis or continuous ambulatory peritoneal dialysis (CAPD).

Geriatric Patients

Adjustment of moxifloxacin dosage based solely on age is not necessary in geriatric patients 65 years of age and older.

CAUTIONS

● Contraindications

Moxifloxacin is contraindicated in patients with a history of hypersensitivity to moxifloxacin or other quinolones.

● Warnings/Precautions

Warnings

Disabling and Potentially Irreversible Serious Adverse Reactions

Systemic fluoroquinolones, including moxifloxacin, have been associated with disabling and potentially irreversible serious adverse reactions (e.g., tendinitis and tendon rupture, peripheral neuropathy, CNS effects) that can occur together in the same patient. These serious reactions may occur within hours to weeks after a systemic fluoroquinolone is initiated and have occurred in all age groups and in patients without preexisting risk factors for such adverse reactions.

Moxifloxacin should be discontinued immediately at the first signs or symptoms of any serious adverse reactions.

Systemic fluoroquinolones, including moxifloxacin, should be avoided in patients who have experienced any of the serious adverse reactions associated with fluoroquinolones.

Tendinitis and Tendon Rupture

Systemic fluoroquinolones, including moxifloxacin, are associated with an increased risk of tendinitis and tendon rupture in all age groups.

The risk of developing fluoroquinolone-associated tendinitis and tendon rupture is increased in older adults (usually those older than 60 years of age), individuals receiving concomitant corticosteroids, and kidney, heart, or lung transplant recipients. (See Geriatric Use under Warnings/Precautions: Specific Populations, in Cautions.)

Other factors that may independently increase the risk of tendon rupture include strenuous physical activity, renal failure, and previous tendon disorders such as rheumatoid arthritis. Tendinitis and tendon rupture have been reported in patients receiving fluoroquinolones who did not have any risk factors for such adverse effects.

Fluoroquinolone-associated tendinitis and tendon rupture most frequently involve the Achilles tendon and have also been reported in the rotator cuff (shoulder), hand, biceps, thumb, and other tendon sites. Tendinitis or tendon rupture can occur within hours or days after moxifloxacin is initiated or as long as several months after completion of therapy and can occur bilaterally.

Moxifloxacin should be discontinued immediately if pain, swelling, inflammation, or rupture of a tendon occurs. (See Advice to Patients.)

Systemic fluoroquinolones, including moxifloxacin, should be avoided in patients who have a history of tendon disorders or have experienced tendinitis or tendon rupture.

Peripheral Neuropathy

Systemic fluoroquinolones, including moxifloxacin, have been associated with an increased risk of peripheral neuropathy.

Sensory or sensorimotor axonal polyneuropathy affecting small and/or large axons resulting in paresthesias, hypoesthesias, dysesthesias, and weakness has been reported in patients receiving systemic fluoroquinolones, including moxifloxacin. Symptoms may occur soon after initiation of moxifloxacin and, in some patients, may be irreversible.

Moxifloxacin should be discontinued immediately if symptoms of peripheral neuropathy (e.g., pain, burning, tingling, numbness, and/or weakness) occur or if there are other alterations in sensations (e.g., light touch, pain, temperature, position sense, vibratory sensation). (See Advice to Patients.)

Systemic fluoroquinolones, including moxifloxacin, should be avoided in patients who have experienced peripheral neuropathy.

CNS Effects

Systemic fluoroquinolones, including moxifloxacin, have been associated with an increased risk of psychiatric adverse effects, including toxic psychosis, hallucinations, paranoia, depression, suicidal thoughts or acts, agitation, nervousness, confusion, delirium, disorientation, disturbances in attention, insomnia, nightmares, and memory impairment. These adverse effects may occur after the first dose.

System fluoroquinolones, including moxifloxacin, have been associated with an increased risk of seizures (convulsions), increased intracranial pressure (including pseudotumor cerebri), dizziness, and tremors. These CNS effects may occur after the first dose.

Moxifloxacin, like other fluoroquinolones, should be used with caution in patients with known or suspected CNS disorders (e.g., severe cerebral arteriosclerosis, epilepsy) or with other risk factors that predispose to seizures or lower seizure threshold.

If psychiatric or other CNS effects occur, moxifloxacin should be discontinued immediately and appropriate measures initiated. (See Advice to Patients.)

Exacerbation of Myasthenia Gravis

Fluoroquinolones, including moxifloxacin, have neuromuscular blocking activity and may exacerbate muscle weakness in individuals with myasthenia gravis. Use of fluoroquinolones in myasthenia gravis patients has resulted in requirements for ventilatory support and in death.

Moxifloxacin should be avoided in patients with a known history of myasthenia gravis. Patients should be advised to immediately contact a clinician if they have any symptoms of muscle weakness, including respiratory difficulties. (See Advice to Patients.)

Sensitivity Reactions

Hypersensitivity Reactions

Serious and occasionally fatal hypersensitivity and/or anaphylactic reactions have been reported in patients receiving fluoroquinolones, including moxifloxacin. Although generally reported after multiple doses, these reactions may occur with first dose.

Some hypersensitivity reactions have been accompanied by cardiovascular collapse, loss of consciousness, tingling, edema (pharyngeal or facial), dyspnea, urticaria, or pruritus.

Other serious and sometimes fatal adverse reactions that have been reported with fluoroquinolones, including moxifloxacin, and that may or may not be related to hypersensitivity reactions include one or more of the following: fever, rash or severe dermatologic reactions (e.g., toxic epidermal necrolysis, Stevens-Johnson syndrome); vasculitis, arthralgia, myalgia, serum sickness; allergic pneumonitis; interstitial nephritis, acute renal insufficiency or failure; hepatitis, jaundice, acute hepatic necrosis or failure; anemia (including hemolytic and aplastic), thrombocytopenia (including thrombotic thrombocytopenic purpura), leukopenia, agranulocytosis, pancytopenia, and/or other hematologic effects.

Moxifloxacin should be discontinued immediately at the first appearance of rash, jaundice, or any other sign of hypersensitivity. Appropriate therapy should be initiated as indicated (e.g., epinephrine, corticosteroids, maintenance of an adequate airway and oxygen). (See Advice to Patients.)

Photosensitivity Reactions

Moderate to severe photosensitivity/phototoxicity reactions have been reported with fluoroquinolones, including moxifloxacin.

Phototoxicity may manifest as exaggerated sunburn reactions (e.g., burning, erythema, exudation, vesicles, blistering, edema) on areas exposed to sun or artificial ultraviolet (UV) light (usually the face, neck, extensor surfaces of forearms, dorsa of hands).

As with other fluoroquinolones, patients should be advised to avoid unnecessary or excessive exposure to sunlight or artificial UV light (e.g., tanning beds, UVA/UVB treatment) while receiving moxifloxacin. If a patient needs to be outdoors, they should wear loose-fitting clothing that protects skin from sun exposure and use other sun protection measures (sunscreen).

Moxifloxacin should be discontinued if photosensitivity or phototoxicity (sunburn-like reaction, skin eruption) occurs.

Other Warnings/Precautions

Prolongation of QT Interval

Prolonged QT interval leading to ventricular arrhythmias, including torsades de pointes, has been reported with some fluoroquinolones, including moxifloxacin.

Following an oral dose of 400 mg of moxifloxacin, the mean change in QT interval corrected for rate (QT_c) from baseline was 6 msec. When moxifloxacin was given IV in a dosage of 400 mg once daily by IV infusion over 1 hour, the mean change in QT_c from baseline was 10 msec on day 1 and 7 msec on day 3.

The recommended moxifloxacin dosage and IV infusion rate should not be exceeded since this may increase the risk of QT interval prolongation.

Moxifloxacin should be avoided in patients with known prolongation of the QT interval, ventricular arrhythmias (including torsades de pointes), any ongoing proarrhythmic conditions (including clinically important bradycardia and acute myocardial ischemia), or uncorrected hypokalemia or hypomagnesemia.

Moxifloxacin also should be avoided in patients receiving class IA (e.g., quinidine, procainamide) or III (e.g., amiodarone, sotalol) antiarrhythmic agents or other drugs that prolong the QT interval (e.g., cisapride [commercially available under a limited-access protocol only], erythromycin, antipsychotic agents, tricyclic antidepressants). (See Drug Interactions: Drugs that Prolong QT Interval.)

In addition, moxifloxacin should be used with caution in patients with mild, moderate, or severe liver cirrhosis since metabolic disturbances associated with hepatic insufficiency may lead to QT prolongation. (See Hepatic Impairment under Warnings/Precautions: Specific Populations, in Cautions.)

The risk of prolonged QT interval may be increased in geriatric patients. (See Geriatric Use under Warnings/Precautions: Specific Populations, in Cautions.)

Risk of Aortic Aneurysm and Dissection

Rupture or dissection of aortic aneurysms has been reported in patients receiving systemic fluoroquinolones. Epidemiologic studies indicate an increased risk of aortic aneurysm and dissection within 2 months following use of systemic fluoroquinolones, particularly in geriatric patients. The cause for this increased risk has not been identified.

Unless there are no other treatment options, systemic fluoroquinolones, including moxifloxacin, should not be used in patients who have an aortic aneurysm or are at increased risk for an aortic aneurysm. This includes geriatric patients and patients with peripheral atherosclerotic vascular disease, hypertension, or certain genetic conditions (e.g., Marfan syndrome, Ehlers-Danlos syndrome).

If a patient reports adverse effects suggestive of aortic aneurysm or dissection, fluoroquinolone treatment should be discontinued immediately. (See Advice to Patients.)

Hypoglycemia or Hyperglycemia

Systemic fluoroquinolones, including moxifloxacin, have been associated with alterations in blood glucose concentrations, including symptomatic hypoglycemia and hyperglycemia. Blood glucose disturbances during fluoroquinolone therapy usually have occurred in patients with diabetes mellitus receiving an oral antidiabetic agent (e.g., glyburide) or insulin.

Severe cases of hypoglycemia resulting in coma or death have been reported with some systemic fluoroquinolones. Although most reported cases of hypoglycemic coma have involved patients with risk factors for hypoglycemia (e.g., older age, diabetes mellitus, renal insufficiency, concomitant use of antidiabetic agents [especially sulfonylureas]), some cases have occurred in patients receiving a fluoroquinolone who were not diabetic and were not reported to be receiving an oral antidiabetic agent or insulin.

Blood glucose concentrations should be carefully monitored when systemic fluoroquinolones, including moxifloxacin, are used in patients with diabetes mellitus receiving antidiabetic agents.

If a hypoglycemic reaction occurs, moxifloxacin should be discontinued and appropriate therapy initiated immediately. (See Advice to Patients.)

Hepatotoxicity

Severe hepatotoxicity, including acute hepatitis, has occurred in patients receiving moxifloxacin and sometimes resulted in death.

Musculoskeletal Effects

Fluoroquinolones, including moxifloxacin, cause arthropathy and osteochondrosis in immature animals of various species. The relevance of these adverse effects in immature animals to use in humans is unknown. Safety and efficacy of moxifloxacin have not been established in children younger than 18 years of age. (See Pediatric Use under Warnings/Precautions: Specific Populations, in Cautions.)

C. difficile-associated Diarrhea and Colitis

Treatment with anti-infectives alters normal colon flora and may permit overgrowth of *Clostridioides difficile* (formerly known as *Clostridium difficile*). C. difficile infection (CDI) and C. difficile-associated diarrhea and colitis (CDAD; also known as antibiotic-associated diarrhea and colitis or pseudomembranous colitis)

have been reported in patients receiving fluoroquinolones, including moxifloxacin, and may range in severity from mild diarrhea to fatal colitis. C. difficile produces toxins A and B which contribute to development of CDAD; hypertoxin-producing strains of C. difficile are associated with increased morbidity and mortality since they may be refractory to anti-infectives and colectomy may be required.

CDAD should be considered in the differential diagnosis of patients who develop diarrhea during or after anti-infective therapy. Careful medical history is necessary since CDAD has been reported to occur as late as 2 months or longer after anti-infective therapy is discontinued.

If CDAD is suspected or confirmed, anti-infective therapy not directed against C. difficile should be discontinued as soon as possible. Patients should be managed with appropriate anti-infective therapy directed against C. difficile (e.g., vancomycin, fidaxomicin, metronidazole), supportive therapy (e.g., fluid and electrolyte management, protein supplementation), and surgical evaluation as clinically indicated.

Selection and Use of Anti-infectives

Moxifloxacin should be used for the treatment of acute sinusitis or acute bacterial exacerbations of chronic bronchitis *only* when no other treatment options are available. Because moxifloxacin, like other systemic fluoroquinolones, has been associated with disabling and potentially irreversible serious adverse reactions (e.g., tendinitis and tendon rupture, peripheral neuropathy, CNS effects) that can occur together in the same patient, the risks of serious adverse reactions outweigh the benefits of moxifloxacin for patients with these infections.

To reduce development of drug-resistant bacteria and maintain effectiveness of moxifloxacin and other antibacterials, use only for treatment or prevention of infections proven or strongly suspected to be caused by susceptible bacteria.

When selecting or modifying anti-infective therapy, use results of culture and in vitro susceptibility testing. In the absence of such data, consider local epidemiology and susceptibility patterns when selecting anti-infectives for empiric therapy.

Information on test methods and quality control standards for in vitro susceptibility testing of antibacterial agents and specific interpretive criteria for such testing recognized by FDA is available at https://www.fda.gov/STIC.

Specific Populations
Pregnancy

Human data for moxifloxacin are insufficient to inform any drug-associated risk regarding use of the drug during pregnancy.

Based on animal studies, moxifloxacin may cause fetal harm. Although moxifloxacin was not teratogenic when administered to pregnant rats, rabbits, and monkeys at exposures up to 2.5 times higher than human exposures reported with the usual dosage of the drug, embryofetal toxicity (e.g., decreased neonatal body weights, increased incidence of skeletal variations [rib and vertebra combined], increased fetal loss) was observed when moxifloxacin was administered to pregnant rats or rabbits at dosages associated with maternal toxicity.

Pregnant women should be advised of the potential risk to the fetus.

Lactation

It is not known whether moxifloxacin is distributed into human milk; the drug is distributed into milk in rats.

The developmental and health benefits of breast-feeding should be considered along with the mother's clinical need for moxifloxacin and potential adverse effects on the breast-fed infant from the drug or from the underlying maternal condition.

Pediatric Use

Efficacy of moxifloxacin has not been established for any indication in pediatric patients younger than 18 years of age.

Limited data available from a clinical study in pediatric patients 3 months of age or older indicate that the overall safety profile of moxifloxacin in pediatric patients is comparable to that reported in adults. The most frequently reported adverse effects in pediatric patients were QT interval prolongation, vomiting, diarrhea, arthralgia, and phlebitis.

Fluoroquinolones, including moxifloxacin, cause arthropathy in juvenile animals. (See Musculoskeletal Effects under Warnings/Precautions: Warnings, in Cautions.)

The American Academy of Pediatrics (AAP) states that use of a systemic fluoroquinolone may be justified in children younger than 18 years of age in certain specific circumstances when there are no safe and effective alternatives and the drug is known to be effective. For information regarding when fluoroquinolones may be a preferred option in children, see Cautions: Pediatric Precautions in Ciprofloxacin 8:12.18.

Geriatric Use

Approximately 23 or 42% of patients were 65 years of age or older and 9 or 23% of patients were 75 years of age or older in clinical studies of oral or IV moxifloxacin, respectively. No overall differences in safety or efficacy were observed between geriatric individuals and younger adults.

The risk of developing severe tendon disorders, including tendon rupture, is increased in older adults (usually those older than 60 years of age). This risk is further increased in those receiving concomitant corticosteroids. (See Tendinitis and Tendon Rupture under Warnings/Precautions: Warnings, in Cautions.) Caution is advised if moxifloxacin is used in geriatric adults, especially those receiving concomitant corticosteroids.

The risk of QT interval prolongation may be increased in geriatric patients. Concomitant use of moxifloxacin and class IA (e.g., quinidine, procainamide) or class III (e.g., amiodarone, sotalol) antiarrhythmic agents and use in patients with risk factors for torsades de pointes (e.g., known QT prolongation, uncorrected hypokalemia) should be avoided. (See Prolongation of QT Interval under Warnings/Precautions: Warnings, in Cautions.)

The risk of aortic aneurysm and dissection may be increased in geriatric patients. (See Risk of Aortic Aneurysm and Dissection under Warnings/Precautions: Other Warnings/Precautions, in Cautions.)

Hepatic Impairment

Although dosage adjustments are not necessary in patients with mild, moderate, or severe hepatic impairment (Child-Pugh class A, B, or C), metabolic disturbances associated with hepatic insufficiency may lead to QT interval prolongation. Therefore, moxifloxacin should be used with caution in patients with any degree of hepatic impairment. ECGs should be monitored in patients with liver cirrhosis.

Renal Impairment

Pharmacokinetics of moxifloxacin are not substantially affected by mild, moderate, or severe renal impairment. Dosage adjustments are not necessary in patients with renal impairment.

● Common Adverse Effects

Adverse effects occurring in 3% or more of patients receiving moxifloxacin include nausea (7%), diarrhea (6%), headache (4%), and dizziness (3%).

DRUG INTERACTIONS

● Drugs That Prolong QT Interval

Potential pharmacologic interaction (additive effects on QT interval prolongation). Concomitant use of moxifloxacin and class IA (e.g., quinidine, procainamide) or class III (e.g., amiodarone, sotalol) antiarrhythmic agents should be avoided. Moxifloxacin should be used with caution in patients receiving other drugs that prolong the QT interval (e.g., cisapride [currently commercially available under a limited-access protocol only], erythromycin, antipsychotic agents, tricyclic antidepressants). (See Prolongation of QT Interval under Warnings/Precautions: Warnings, in Cautions.)

● Drugs Metabolized by Hepatic Microsomal Enzymes

Moxifloxacin is not metabolized by cytochrome P-450 (CYP) isoenzymes and does not inhibit CYP3A4, 2D6, 2C9, 2C19, or 1A2; pharmacokinetic interactions with drugs metabolized by CYP isoenzymes are unlikely.

● Antacids

Pharmacokinetic interaction with aluminum- or magnesium-containing antacids (decreased absorption and decreased bioavailability of oral moxifloxacin).

Oral moxifloxacin should be administered at least 4 hours before or 8 hours after antacids that contain aluminum or magnesium.

● Antidiabetic Agents

Concomitant use of moxifloxacin and oral antidiabetic agents (e.g., sulfonylurea agents) or insulin has resulted in alterations in blood glucose concentrations, including hypoglycemia and hyperglycemia. (See Hypoglycemia or Hyperglycemia under Warnings/Precautions: Other Warnings/Precautions, in Cautions.)

If moxifloxacin is used in patients with diabetes mellitus receiving an oral antidiabetic agent or insulin, blood glucose concentrations should be carefully monitored. If a hypoglycemic reaction occurs, moxifloxacin should be discontinued and appropriate therapy initiated immediately.

Glyburide

When moxifloxacin (40 mg once daily for 5 days) was used in patients with diabetes mellitus receiving glyburide (2.5 mg once daily beginning 2 weeks before initiation of moxifloxacin), mean peak plasma concentrations and area under the plasma concentration-time curve (AUC) of glyburide were decreased 21 and 12%, respectively. Although blood glucose concentrations were decreased slightly in patients receiving glyburide and moxifloxacin concurrently compared with glyburide alone, the manufacturer states that the pharmacokinetic interaction between the drugs was not considered clinically important and that interference by moxifloxacin on the activity of glyburide was not suggested.

● Antifungal Agents

No clinically important pharmacokinetic interactions between itraconazole and moxifloxacin.

● Atenolol

Moxifloxacin does not have a clinically important effect on the pharmacokinetics of atenolol.

● Corticosteroids

Concomitant use of corticosteroids increases the risk of severe tendon disorders (e.g., tendinitis, tendon rupture), especially in geriatric patients older than 60 years of age. (See Tendinitis and Tendon Rupture under Warnings/Precautions: Warnings, in Cautions.)

● Cyclosporine

No clinically important pharmacokinetic interactions between cyclosporine and moxifloxacin.

● Didanosine

Pharmacokinetic interaction (decreased absorption of oral moxifloxacin).

Oral moxifloxacin should be given at least 4 hours before or 8 hours after buffered didanosine (pediatric oral solution admixed with antacid).

● Digoxin

No clinically important pharmacokinetic interactions between digoxin and moxifloxacin. Although a transient increase in digoxin concentrations may occur, this is not considered clinically important. Dosage adjustments are not necessary for either drug.

● Estrogens and Progestins

Moxifloxacin does not have a clinically important effect on the pharmacokinetics of oral contraceptives containing ethinyl estradiol and levonorgestrel.

● Iron, Multivitamins, and Mineral Supplements

Pharmacokinetic interaction (decreased absorption and decreased bioavailability of oral moxifloxacin) if given concomitantly with iron preparations or multivitamins or dietary supplements containing iron or zinc. Oral moxifloxacin should be taken at least 4 hours before or 8 hours after these preparations.

Calcium dietary supplements do not have any clinically important effects on the pharmacokinetics of moxifloxacin.

● Morphine

Morphine does not have a clinically important effect on the pharmacokinetics of moxifloxacin.

● Nonsteroidal Anti-inflammatory Agents

Concomitant use of moxifloxacin and nonsteroidal anti-inflammatory agents (NSAIAs) may increase the risk of CNS stimulation and seizures. Animal studies using other fluoroquinolones suggest the risk varies depending on the specific NSAIA.

● *Probenecid*

Probenecid does not have a clinically important effect on the pharmacokinetics of moxifloxacin.

● *Ranitidine*

Ranitidine does not have a clinically important effect on the pharmacokinetics of moxifloxacin.

● *Sucralfate*

Pharmacokinetic interaction (decreased absorption of oral moxifloxacin). Oral moxifloxacin should be taken at least 4 hours before or 8 hours after sucralfate.

● *Theophylline*

No clinically important pharmacokinetic interactions between theophylline and moxifloxacin.

● *Warfarin*

Although clinically important pharmacokinetic interactions have not been reported when warfarin and moxifloxacin were used concomitantly, fluoroquinolones, including moxifloxacin, have been reported to enhance the anticoagulant effects of warfarin or its derivatives. In addition, infectious disease and its accompanying inflammatory process, age, and general status of the patient also are risk factors for increased anticoagulation activity. The prothrombin time (PT), international normalized ratio (INR), or other suitable coagulation tests should be monitored in patients receiving moxifloxacin concomitantly with warfarin.

PHARMACOKINETICS

● *Absorption*
Bioavailability

Moxifloxacin is well absorbed from the GI tract and absolute bioavailability is 86–92%.

Peak plasma concentrations are attained within 0.5–4 hours; steady state is attained after at least 3 days.

Food

Administration of a 400-mg moxifloxacin tablet with a high-fat breakfast or with yogurt does not have a clinically important effect on absorption of the drug.

● *Distribution*
Extent

Moxifloxacin is widely distributed into body tissues and fluids, including saliva, nasal and bronchial secretions, sinus mucosa, skin blister fluid, subcutaneous tissue, skeletal muscle, and abdominal tissues and fluids.

Moxifloxacin is distributed into CSF in rabbits.

The drug is distributed into milk in rats and may be distributed into human milk.

Plasma Protein Binding

Moxifloxacin is 30–50% bound to plasma proteins.

● *Elimination*
Metabolism

Approximately 52% of an oral or IV dose of moxifloxacin is metabolized via glucuronide and sulfate conjugation; the metabolites are not microbiologically active.

Moxifloxacin is not metabolized by cytochrome P-450 (CYP) isoenzymes.

Elimination Route

Moxifloxacin is eliminated in urine and by biliary excretion and metabolism.

Approximately 45% of an oral or IV dose of the drug is excreted unchanged (20% in urine and 25% in feces). A total of 96% of an oral dose is excreted as unchanged drug or metabolites.

Half-life

Adults with normal renal and hepatic function: Mean half-life of moxifloxacin is 11.5–15.6 hours following single or multiple oral doses and 8.2–15.4 hours following single or multiple IV doses.

Special Populations

Pharmacokinetics of moxifloxacin in geriatric patients are similar to that reported in younger adults.

Concentrations of the moxifloxacin sulfate and glucuronide conjugates are increased in patients with mild or moderate hepatic impairment (Child Pugh class A or B); the clinical importance of this finding has not been determined. A single-dose study indicates that plasma concentrations of moxifloxacin and its metabolites in patients with severe hepatic impairment (Child Pugh class C) are similar to those reported in patients with mild or moderate hepatic impairment.

Pharmacokinetics of moxifloxacin are not substantially affected by mild, moderate, or severe renal impairment. In patients with creatinine clearance less than 20 mL/minute undergoing hemodialysis or continuous ambulatory peritoneal dialysis (CAPD), moxifloxacin concentrations are not affected but concentrations of the sulfate and glucuronide conjugates are increased; the clinical importance of this finding has not be determined.

DESCRIPTION

Moxifloxacin is a fluoroquinolone anti-infective agent. Like other commercially available fluoroquinolones, moxifloxacin contains a fluorine at the C-6 position of the quinolone nucleus. Moxifloxacin, like gatifloxacin (no longer commercially available in the US), contains an 8-methoxy group and has been termed an 8-methoxy fluoroquinolone. The 8-methoxy and 7-diazabicyclo moieties on the quinolone nucleus of moxifloxacin appear to enhance activity against gram-positive bacteria and decrease selection of resistant mutants in gram-positive bacteria.

Like other fluoroquinolone anti-infectives, moxifloxacin inhibits DNA synthesis in susceptible organisms via inhibition of type II DNA topoisomerases (DNA gyrase, topoisomerase IV). In susceptible *S. pneumoniae*, moxifloxacin principally targets DNA gyrase.

Moxifloxacin is well absorbed following oral administration, and has an absolute bioavailability of approximately 90%. The drug has a mean serum elimination half-life of 11.5–15.6 or 8.2–15.4 hours following oral or IV administration, respectively, allowing once-daily dosing. Moxifloxacin is metabolized principally via sulfate and glucuronide conjugation; the drug is not metabolized by and does not appear to affect the cytochrome P-450 (CYP) enzyme system. (See Drug Interactions.)

● *Spectrum*

Moxifloxacin is active in vitro and in clinical infections against most strains of *Staphylococcus aureus* (methicillin-susceptible [oxacillin-susceptible] strains only), *Streptococcus pneumoniae* (including multidrug-resistant strains), *S. anginosus*, *S. constellatus*, *S. pyogenes* (group A β- hemolytic streptococci), *Haemophilus influenzae*, *H. parainfluenzae*, *Enterobacter cloacae*, *Escherichia coli*, *Klebsiella pneumoniae*, *Proteus mirabilis*, *Moraxella catarrhalis*, *Chlamydophila pneumoniae* (formerly *Chlamydia pneumoniae*), *Enterococcus faecalis*, *Bacteroides fragilis*, *B. thetaiotaomicron*, *Clostridium perfringens*, *Peptostreptococcus*, and *Mycoplasma pneumoniae*. Moxifloxacin is active against *Yersinia pestis* in vitro and in a primate infection model. The drug also has in vitro activity against *S. epidermidis* (methicillin-susceptible [oxacillin-susceptible] strains only), *S. agalactiae* (group B streptococci), viridans streptococci, *Citrobacter freundii*, *K. oxytoca*, *Legionella pneumophila*, *Actinomyces*, *Bilophila wadsworthia*, *Eubacterium*, *Fusobacterium* species, *Lactobacillus*, *Porphyromonas*, and *Prevotella* species; however, the clinical importance of this in vitro data is unknown.

Moxifloxacin is active in vitro against some mycobacteria, including *Mycobacterium tuberculosis*, *M. avium complex* (MAC), *M. kansasii*, and *M. fortuitum*. Although moxifloxacin is active against some strains of *M. tuberculosis* resistant to isoniazid, rifampin, or streptomycin, moxifloxacin-resistant *M. tuberculosis* have been reported and some multidrug-resistant strains (i.e., strains resistant to rifampin and isoniazid) also are resistant to moxifloxacin or other fluoroquinolones.

Moxifloxacin has greater activity in vitro against *S. pneumoniae* (including penicillin-resistant strains) than many other fluoroquinolones (e.g., ciprofloxacin, levofloxacin, ofloxacin) while generally retaining the in vitro activity of these drugs against gram-negative bacteria and etiologic agents of atypical pneumonia (e.g., *C. pneumoniae*, *M. pneumoniae*, *Legionella*). The relevance of these in vitro data to the treatment of clinical infections remains to be determined.

● *Resistance*

Resistance to fluoroquinolones can occur as the result of mutations in topoisomerase II (DNA gyrase) or topoisomerase IV genes, decreased outer membrane permeability, or drug efflux. In vitro, resistance to moxifloxacin develops slowly by multiple-step mutations.

Cross-resistance can occur between moxifloxacin and other fluoroquinolones, but some gram-positive bacteria resistant to other fluoroquinolones may be susceptible to moxifloxacin.

ADVICE TO PATIENTS

Advise patients to read the manufacturer's patient information (medication guide) prior to initiating moxifloxacin therapy and each time the prescription is refilled.

Advise patients that antibacterials (including moxifloxacin) should only be used to treat bacterial infections and not used to treat viral infections (e.g., the common cold).

Importance of completing full course of therapy, even if feeling better after a few days.

Advise patients that skipping doses or not completing the full course of therapy may decrease effectiveness and increase the likelihood that bacteria will develop resistance and will not be treatable with moxifloxacin or other antibacterials in the future.

Advise patients that moxifloxacin may be taken without regard to meals, but should be taken with liberal amounts of fluids.

Importance of taking moxifloxacin at least 4 hours before or 8 hours after multivitamins or dietary supplements containing iron or zinc; magnesium- or aluminum- containing antacids; sucralfate; or buffered didanosine (pediatric oral solution admixed with antacid).

Inform patients that systemic fluoroquinolones, including moxifloxacin, have been associated with disabling and potentially irreversible serious adverse reactions (e.g., tendinitis and tendon rupture, peripheral neuropathy, CNS effects) that may occur together in the same patient. Advise patients to immediately discontinue moxifloxacin and contact a clinician if they experience any signs or symptoms of serious adverse effects (e.g., unusual joint or tendon pain, muscle weakness, a "pins and needles" tingling or pricking sensation, numbness of the arms or legs, confusion, hallucinations) while taking the drug. Advise patients to talk with a clinician if they have any questions or concerns.

Inform patients that systemic fluoroquinolones, including moxifloxacin, are associated with an increased risk of tendinitis and tendon rupture in all age groups and that this risk is increased in adults older than 60 years of age, individuals receiving corticosteroids, and kidney, heart, or lung transplant recipients. Symptoms may be irreversible. Importance of resting and refraining from exercise at the first sign of tendinitis or tendon rupture (e.g., pain, swelling, or inflammation of a tendon or weakness or inability to use a joint) and importance of immediately discontinuing the drug and contacting a clinician. (See Tendinitis and Tendon Rupture under Warnings/Precautions: Warnings, in Cautions.)

Inform patients that peripheral neuropathies have been reported in patients receiving systemic fluoroquinolones, including moxifloxacin, and that symptoms may occur soon after initiation of the drug and may be irreversible. Importance of immediately discontinuing moxifloxacin and contacting a clinician if symptoms of peripheral neuropathy (e.g., pain, burning, tingling, numbness, and/or weakness) occur.

Inform patients that systemic fluoroquinolones, including moxifloxacin, have been associated with CNS effects (e.g., convulsions, dizziness, lightheadedness, increased intracranial pressure). Importance of informing clinician of any history of convulsions before initiating therapy with the drug. Importance of contacting a clinician if persistent headache with or without blurred vision occurs.

Advise patients that moxifloxacin may cause dizziness and lightheadedness; caution patients that they should not engage in activities requiring mental alertness and motor coordination (e.g., driving a vehicle, operating machinery) until the effects of the drug on the individual are known.

Advise patients that systemic fluoroquinolones, including moxifloxacin, may worsen myasthenia gravis symptoms; importance of informing clinician of any history of myasthenia gravis. Importance of immediately contacting a clinician if any symptoms of muscle weakness, including respiratory difficulties, occur.

Inform patients that moxifloxacin may be associated with hypersensitivity reactions (including anaphylactic reactions), even after the first dose. Importance of immediately discontinuing moxifloxacin and contacting a clinician at first sign of rash, hives or other skin reaction, rapid heartbeat, difficulty swallowing or breathing, any swelling suggesting angioedema (e.g., swelling of lips, tongue, or face; throat tightness; hoarseness), jaundice, or any other sign of hypersensitivity.

Inform patients that photosensitivity/phototoxicity reactions have been reported following exposure to sun or UV light in patients receiving fluoroquinolones. Importance of avoiding or minimizing exposure to sunlight or artificial UV light (e.g., tanning beds, UVA/UVB treatment) and using protective measures (e.g., wearing loose-fitting clothes, sunscreen) if outdoors during moxifloxacin therapy. Importance of discontinuing moxifloxacin and contacting a clinician if a sunburn-like reaction or skin eruption occurs.

Importance of informing clinician of personal or family history of QT interval prolongation or proarrhythmic conditions (e.g., hypokalemia, bradycardia, recent myocardial ischemia) and of concurrent therapy with any drugs that may affect QT interval (e.g., class IA [quinidine, procainamide] or class III [e.g., amiodarone, sotalol] antiarrhythmic agents). Importance of contacting clinician if symptoms of prolonged QT interval (e.g., prolonged heart palpitations, loss of consciousness) occur.

Inform patients that systemic fluoroquinolones may increase the risk of aortic aneurysm and dissection; importance of informing clinician of any history of aneurysms, blockages or hardening of the arteries, high blood pressure, or genetic conditions such as Marfan syndrome or Ehlers-Danlos syndrome. Advise patients to seek immediate medical treatment if they experience sudden, severe, and constant pain in the stomach, chest, or back.

Inform patients that hypoglycemia has been reported when systemic fluoroquinolones were used in some patients receiving antidiabetic agents. Advise patients with diabetes mellitus receiving an oral antidiabetic agent or insulin to discontinue moxifloxacin and contact a clinician if they experience hypoglycemia or symptoms of hypoglycemia.

Inform patients that severe hepatotoxicity (including acute hepatitis and fatal events) has been reported in patients receiving moxifloxacin. Importance of informing clinician if any signs or symptoms of liver injury (e.g., loss of appetite, nausea, vomiting, fever, weakness, tiredness, right upper quadrant tenderness, itching, yellowing of the skin and eyes, light colored bowel movements, dark colored urine) occur.

Advise patients that diarrhea is a common problem caused by anti-infectives and usually ends when the drug is discontinued. Importance of contacting a clinician if watery and bloody stools (with or without stomach cramps and fever) occur during or as late as 2 months or longer after the last dose.

Importance of informing clinician of existing or contemplated concomitant therapy, including prescription and OTC drugs (e.g., drugs that may affect QT interval), as well as any concomitant illnesses.

Importance of women informing clinicians if they are or plan to become pregnant or plan to breast-feed.

Importance of advising patients of other important precautionary information. (See Cautions.)

PREPARATIONS

Excipients in commercially available drug preparations may have clinically important effects in some individuals; consult specific product labeling for details.

Moxifloxacin Hydrochloride

Oral		
Tablets, film-coated	400 mg of (of moxifloxacin)*	Avelox®, Bayer
		Moxifloxacin Hydrochloride Tablets
Parenteral		
Injection, for IV infusion	400 mg (of moxifloxacin) in 0.8% sodium chloride*	Avelox®, Bayer
		Moxifloxacin Hydrochloride Injection for IV Infusion

* available from one or more manufacturer, distributor, and/or repackager by generic (nonproprietary) name

† Use is not currently included in the labeling approved by the US Food and Drug Administration.

Selected Revisions August 26, 2019, © Copyright, April 1, 2000, American Society of Health-System Pharmacists, Inc.

Ofloxacin

8:12.18 • QUINOLONES

■ Ofloxacin is a synthetic fluoroquinolone anti-infective agent.

USES

● Respiratory Tract Infections

Ofloxacin is used for the treatment of lower respiratory tract infections, including acute exacerbations of chronic bronchitis or community-acquired pneumonia (CAP) caused by susceptible *Haemophilus influenzae* or *Streptococcus pneumoniae*. Ofloxacin also has been used for the treatment of lower respiratory tract infections caused by susceptible *Moraxella catarrhalis*†, *S. aureus*†, viridans streptococci†, Enterobacteriaceae†, or *Ps. aeruginosa*†.

Ofloxacin should be used for the treatment of acute bacterial exacerbations of chronic bronchitis only when there are no other treatment options. Because systemic fluoroquinolones, including ofloxacin, have been associated with disabling and potentially irreversible serious adverse reactions (e.g., tendinitis and tendon rupture, peripheral neuropathy, CNS effects) that can occur together in the same patient (see Cautions) and because acute bacterial exacerbations of chronic bronchitis may be self-limiting in some patients, the risks of serious adverse reactions outweigh the benefits of fluoroquinolones for patients with these infections.

In controlled studies in adults with lower respiratory tract infections, oral ofloxacin therapy was at least as effective as oral therapy with amoxicillin, co-trimoxazole, erythromycin, cefazolin, or doxycycline, and more effective than cefaclor. For most susceptible bacteria, ofloxacin therapy resulted in clinical and bacteriologic cure rates of 60–100% in adults with lower respiratory tract infections. However, ofloxacin, like most fluoroquinolones, is less effective in the treatment of *S. pneumoniae* or *Ps. aeruginosa* infections; the bacteriologic cure rates in adults with infections caused by these bacteria were 55–79%.

● Skin and Skin Structure Infections

Ofloxacin is used for the treatment of mild to moderate skin and skin structure infections caused by susceptible *S. aureus* (oxacillin-susceptible [methicillin-susceptible] strains), *S. epidermidis*†, *S. pyogenes* (group A β-hemolytic streptococci; GAS), or *P. mirabilis*. However, the increasing emergence of strains of staphylococci resistant to fluoroquinolones limits the usefulness of the drugs in the treatment of these infections. Ofloxacin also has been effective when used in the treatment of skin and skin structure infections caused by other susceptible gram-negative bacteria, including *E. coli*† or *Ps. aeruginosa*†. The drug has been effective when used in the treatment of cellulitis, subcutaneous abscesses, surgical wound infections, furunculosis, and folliculitis, and has been used effectively for the treatment of skin and skin structure infections in patients with diabetes mellitus. Oral ofloxacin resulted in a clinical and bacteriologic cure rate of 76–96% in adults with skin and skin structure infections.

● Urinary Tract Infections and Prostatitis

Uncomplicated Urinary Tract Infections

Ofloxacin is used for the treatment of uncomplicated urinary tract infections (UTIs) (cystitis) caused by susceptible gram-negative bacteria, including *Citrobacter diversus*, *C. freundii*†, *Enterobacter aerogenes*, *E. cloacae*†, *Escherichia coli*, *Klebsiella pneumoniae*, *Morganella morganii*†, *Proteus mirabilis*, or *Pseudomonas aeruginosa*.

The drug also has been effective in a limited number of adults when used orally for the treatment of uncomplicated UTIs caused by susceptible gram-positive bacteria, including *Staphylococcus aureus*†, *S. epidermidis*†, *S. saprophyticus*†, *Enterococcus faecalis* (formerly *Streptococcus faecalis*)†, viridans streptococci†, or *Streptococcus agalactiae*† (group B streptococci; GBS). However, because of concerns about emergence of resistant strains of certain gram-positive bacteria (e.g., staphylococci) secondary to widespread use of fluoroquinolones, such use should be selective.

Ofloxacin should be used for the treatment of uncomplicated UTIs only when there are no other treatment options. Because systemic fluoroquinolones, including ofloxacin, have been associated with disabling and potentially irreversible serious adverse reactions (e.g., tendinitis and tendon rupture, peripheral neuropathy, CNS effects) that can occur together in the same patient (see Cautions) and because uncomplicated UTIs may be self-limiting in some patients, the risks of serious adverse reactions outweigh the benefits of fluoroquinolones for patients with uncomplicated UTIs.

In the treatment of uncomplicated UTIs in adults, the bacteriologic cure rate reported with 3–7 days of oral ofloxacin therapy has been 81–100%. In several controlled studies in men and women with uncomplicated UTIs, 3–7 days of oral ofloxacin therapy was as effective as 7 days of oral co-trimoxazole therapy. Although a single 100- or 400-mg oral dose† of ofloxacin has been effective in some adults for the treatment of acute cystitis caused by susceptible organisms, efficacy of a single dose of the drug for the treatment of these infections has not been established. In one controlled study, a single 400-mg oral dose of ofloxacin was less effective for the treatment of acute cystitis in women than 3 days of oral ofloxacin therapy (200 mg once daily) or 7 days of oral co-trimoxazole therapy; in another controlled study in adults with uncomplicated UTIs, a single 100-mg oral dose of ofloxacin was as effective as a 3-day regimen (100 mg twice daily) of the drug.

Complicated Urinary Tract Infections

Ofloxacin is used for the treatment of pyelonephritis and other complicated UTIs caused by susceptible gram-negative bacteria, including *C. diversus*, *C. freundii*†, *Enterobacter*†, *E. coli*, *K. pneumoniae*, *M. morganii*†, *P. mirabilis*, *P. rettgeri*†, or *Ps. aeruginosa*.

As with other anti-infectives, ofloxacin is more effective in the treatment of uncomplicated UTIs than in complicated infections. In adults with complicated UTIs caused by susceptible organisms, the bacteriologic cure rate reported for 7–10 days of oral ofloxacin therapy has been 63–100%. In controlled studies in adults with complicated UTIs, oral ofloxacin therapy was as effective as therapy with oral co-trimoxazole and slightly more effective than therapy with oral carbenicillin indanyl sodium. In controlled studies in adults with complicated UTIs, 7 days of oral ofloxacin (100 mg twice daily) was as effective as 7 days of oral ciprofloxacin (250 mg twice daily). Oral ofloxacin has been used effectively in renal transplant recipients for the treatment of complicated UTIs.

Prostatitis

Ofloxacin is used in men for the treatment of recurrent UTIs and chronic prostatitis caused by susceptible *E. coli*.

Oral ofloxacin therapy given for 6 weeks or longer reportedly has resulted in a bacteriologic cure of 79–100% in men with prostatitis.

● GI Infections

Shigella Infections

Oral ofloxacin has been used for the treatment of shigellosis† caused by susceptible *Shigella*.

Infections caused by *S. sonnei* usually are self-limited (48–72 hours), and mild cases may not require treatment with anti-infectives. However, because there is some evidence that anti-infectives may shorten the duration of diarrhea and the period of fecal excretion of *Shigella*, anti-infective treatment generally is recommended in addition to fluid and electrolyte replacement in patients with severe shigellosis, dysentery, or underlying immunosuppression. An empiric treatment regimen can be used initially, but in vitro susceptibility testing of clinical isolates is indicated since resistance is common. A fluoroquinolone (preferably ciprofloxacin or, alternatively, levofloxacin or moxifloxacin) generally has been recommended for the treatment of shigellosis. However, fluoroquinolone-resistant *Shigella* have been reported in the US, especially in international travelers, the homeless, and men who have sex with men (MSM). Depending on in vitro susceptibility, other drugs recommended for the treatment of shigellosis include co-trimoxazole, ceftriaxone, azithromycin (not recommended in those with bacteremia), or ampicillin.

Travelers' Diarrhea

Oral ofloxacin has been used for the short-term treatment of travelers' diarrhea† and has been used for the prevention of travelers' diarrhea† in adults traveling for relatively short periods of time to high-risk areas.

Treatment

Travelers' diarrhea caused by bacteria may be self-limited and often resolves within 3–7 days without anti-infective treatment. The US Centers for Disease Control and Prevention (CDC) states that anti-infective treatment is *not* recommended in patients with mild travelers' diarrhea. However, CDC and other clinicians state that empiric short-term anti-infective treatment (single dose or up to 3 days) may be used if diarrhea is moderate or severe, associated with fever or bloody stools, or extremely disruptive to travel plans. Since bacteria are the most common cause of travelers' diarrhea (80–90% of cases), an anti-infective directed against enteric bacterial pathogens usually is used. Fluoroquinolones (e.g., ciprofloxacin, levofloxacin) generally have been considered the anti-infectives of choice for empiric treatment, including self-treatment, of travelers' diarrhea in adults; alternatives include azithromycin and rifaximin.

If the causative pathogen is susceptible to the anti-infective chosen for empiric therapy, the duration of illness may be reduced by about a day. However, the increasing incidence of enteric bacteria resistant to fluoroquinolones and other anti-infectives may limit the usefulness of empiric treatment in individuals traveling in certain geographic areas, and the possible adverse effects of the anti-infective and adverse consequences of such treatment (e.g., development of resistance, effect on normal gut microflora) should be considered.

Prophylaxis

CDC and most experts do *not* recommend anti-infective prophylaxis to prevent travelers' diarrhea in most individuals traveling to areas of risk. However, anti-infective prophylaxis may be considered for short-term travelers who are high-risk individuals (e.g., human immunodeficiency virus [HIV]-infected or other immunocompromised individuals, travelers with poorly controlled diabetes mellitus or chronic renal failure) and those who are taking critical trips during which even a short period of diarrhea could adversely affect the purpose of the trip.

The use of anti-infective prophylaxis in travelers should be weighed against the use of prompt, early self-treatment with an empiric anti-infective if moderate to severe travelers' diarrhea occurs. If anti-infective prophylaxis is used, fluoroquinolones (e.g., ciprofloxacin, levofloxacin) usually have been recommended; alternatives include azithromycin and rifaximin. The increasing incidence of fluoroquinolone resistance in pathogens that cause travelers' diarrhea (e.g., *Campylobacter, Salmonella, Shigella*) should be considered and may limit their potential usefulness.

Helicobacter pylori Infection

Oral ofloxacin has been used in conjunction with other drugs for the treatment of infections caused by *Helicobacter pylori*†.

Multiple-drug regimens that include ofloxacin, azithromycin, omeprazole, and a bismuth salt or ofloxacin, tetracycline, metronidazole, omeprazole, and a bismuth salt have effectively eradicated *H. pylori* in some patients with infections that failed to respond to other treatment regimens. Levofloxacin usually is the fluoroquinolone included in multiple-drug regimens used for first- or second-line and salvage therapy of *H. pylori* infections. Data are limited regarding the prevalence of fluoroquinolone-resistant *H. pylori* in the US; the possible impact of such resistance on the efficacy of fluoroquinolone-containing regimens used for the treatment of *H. pylori* infection is not known.

● Anthrax

Oral ofloxacin has been recommended as an alternative for postexposure prophylaxis following suspected or confirmed exposure to aerosolized *Bacillus anthracis* spores (inhalational anthrax)† and for treatment of inhalational anthrax†.

CDC, American Academy of Pediatrics (AAP), US Working Group on Civilian Biodefense, and US Army Medical Research Institute of Infectious Diseases (USAMRIID) recommend oral ciprofloxacin and oral doxycycline as the initial drugs of choice for postexposure prophylaxis following exposure to aerosolized anthrax spores, including exposures that occur in the context of biologic warfare or bioterrorism. Other oral fluoroquinolones (levofloxacin, moxifloxacin, ofloxacin) are alternatives for postexposure prophylaxis when ciprofloxacin or doxycycline cannot be used.

Some experts suggest that oral ciprofloxacin or other oral fluoroquinolones (levofloxacin, moxifloxacin, ofloxacin) can be considered for the treatment of inhalational anthrax† when a parenteral regimen is not available. Although a multiple-drug parenteral regimen should be used for the treatment of inhalational anthrax that occurs as the result of exposure to anthrax spores in the context of biologic warfare or bioterrorism, use of these parenteral regimens may not be possible if large numbers of individuals require treatment in a mass casualty setting and it may be necessary to use an oral regimen.

For additional information on postexposure prophylaxis and treatment of anthrax, see Uses: Anthrax in Ciprofloxacin 8:12.18.

● Brucellosis

Ofloxacin has been used in conjunction with other anti-infectives for the treatment of brucellosis† caused by *Brucella melitensis*. Some experts recommend a multiple-drug regimen that includes a tetracycline (doxycycline) and streptomycin (or gentamicin) or a regimen that includes a tetracycline (doxycycline) and rifampin for the treatment of brucellosis; alternative regimens include co-trimoxazole with or without gentamicin or rifampin; ciprofloxacin (or ofloxacin) and rifampin; or chloramphenicol with or without streptomycin. Monotherapy with any drug usually is associated with a high relapse rate and is not recommended.

In one study in patients with brucellosis caused by *B. melitensis*, 6 weeks of a regimen of ofloxacin (400 mg once daily) given in conjunction with rifampin (600 mg once daily) was as effective as a regimen of doxycycline (200 mg once daily) given in conjunction with rifampin (600 mg once daily). The mean time to defervescence was 5.1 days for patients receiving doxycycline and rifampin and 6.3 days for those receiving ofloxacin and rifampin; the relapse rate 1 year after the drugs were discontinued was about 3% in both groups.

● Chlamydial Infections

Ofloxacin is used for the treatment of urethral and cervical infections caused by *Chlamydia trachomatis* and is considered an alternative for the treatment of these infections. A bacteriologic cure rate of 67–100% has been reported in men and women who received a 7–10 day regimen of oral ofloxacin (200- or 300-mg twice daily) for the treatment of urogenital chlamydial infections. In several controlled studies, a 7-day regimen of oral ofloxacin (300 mg twice daily) is at least as effective as a 7-day regimen of oral doxycycline (100 mg twice daily) for the treatment of these infections.

CDC states that a single oral dose of azithromycin or a 7-day regimen of oral doxycycline are the recommended regimens for the treatment of *C. trachomatis* urogenital infections in adults and adolescents; a 7-day regimen of oral erythromycin base or ethylsuccinate or a 7-day regimen of oral levofloxacin or ofloxacin are alternative regimens.

Individuals with HIV infection should receive the same treatment regimens recommended for other individuals with *C. trachomatis* urogenital infections.

Any individual who had sexual contact with a patient with *C. trachomatis* urogenital infection during the 60 days preceding the patient's onset of symptoms or diagnosis should be referred for evaluation, testing, and presumptive treatment with a regimen effective against *Chlamydia*. To minimize transmission and avoid reinfection, individuals treated for *C. trachomatis* urogenital infections should abstain from sexual intercourse until they and their partner(s) have been adequately treated (i.e., for 7 days after a single-dose regimen or after completion of a 7-day regimen) and symptoms have resolved.

Ofloxacin is considered an alternative for the treatment of acute epididymitis† that may involve *C. trachomatis*. (See Uses: Gonorrhea and Associated Infections.)

● Gonorrhea and Associated Infections

Although ofloxacin was used in the past for the treatment of uncomplicated gonorrhea caused by susceptible *Neisseria gonorrhoeae*, quinolone-resistant *N. gonorrhoeae* (QRNG) is widely disseminated throughout the world, including in the US. (See Resistance: Resistance in Neisseria gonorrhoeae.) Therefore, CDC states that fluoroquinolones are no longer recommended for the treatment of gonorrhea and should not be used routinely for any associated infections that may involve *N. gonorrhoeae* (e.g., pelvic inflammatory disease [PID], epididymitis).

Ofloxacin is considered an alternative for the treatment of acute PID. (See Uses: Pelvic Inflammatory Disease.)

Ofloxacin is considered an alternative for the treatment of acute epididymitis†. Although acute epididymitis in sexually active men younger than 35 years of age is most frequently caused by *C. trachomatis* or *N. gonorrhoeae*, epididymitis can also be caused by other organisms (e.g., sexually transmitted enteric bacteria, *Mycoplasma, Ureaplasma*, mycobacteria, fungi). Presumptive treatment is usually initiated prior to availability of all diagnostic laboratory test results, and the anti-infective regimen is selected based on the patient's risk for chlamydia, gonorrhea, and/or sexually transmitted enteric bacteria (e.g., *E. coli*). For treatment of acute epididymitis most likely caused by sexually transmitted chlamydia and gonorrhea, CDC recommends a single IM dose of ceftriaxone used in conjunction with a 10-day regimen of oral doxycycline. For treatment of acute epididymitis most likely caused by sexually transmitted chlamydia and gonorrhea and enteric bacteria (e.g., in men who practice insertive anal sex), CDC recommends a single IM dose of ceftriaxone given in conjunction with a 10-day regimen of oral levofloxacin or ofloxacin. If acute epididymitis is most likely caused by enteric bacteria (e.g., in men who have undergone prostate biopsy, vasectomy, or other urinary tract instrumentation procedure) and gonorrhea has been ruled out (e.g., by gram, methylene blue, or gentian violet stain), CDC states that a 10-day regimen of oral levofloxacin or ofloxacin can be used alone.

For information on current recommendations for the treatment of gonorrhea and associated infections, see Uses: Gonorrhea and Associated Infections in Ceftriaxone 8:12.06.12. For additional information on quinolone-resistant N. gonorrhoeae (QRNG), see Uses: Gonorrhea and Associated Infections in Ciprofloxacin 8:12.18.

• Mycobacterial Infections
Treatment of Active Tuberculosis

Ofloxacin has been used in multiple-drug regimens for the treatment of active tuberculosis† caused by *Mycobacterium tuberculosis*.

Although the potential role of fluoroquinolones and the optimal length of therapy have not been fully defined, the American Thoracic Society (ATS), CDC, Infectious Diseases Society of America (IDSA), and others state that use of fluoroquinolones as alternative (second-line) agents can be considered for the treatment of active tuberculosis in patients intolerant of certain first-line agents and in those with relapse, treatment failure, or *M. tuberculosis* resistant to certain first-line agents. If a fluoroquinolone is used in multiple-drug regimens for the treatment of active tuberculosis, ATS, CDC, IDSA, and others recommend levofloxacin or moxifloxacin.

The most recent ATS, CDC, and IDSA recommendations for the treatment of tuberculosis should be consulted for more specific information.

Leprosy

Ofloxacin is used as an alternative in multiple-drug therapy (MDT) for treatment of multibacillary leprosy† (Hansen's disease); the drug also is used as a component of a single-dose MDT regimen that has been used for treatment of single-lesion paucibacillary leprosy†.

The World Health Organization (WHO) and US National Hansen's Disease Program (NHDP) recommend that MDT regimens that include rifampin be used for the treatment of all forms of leprosy. MDT can rapidly kill *M. leprae* and render patients noninfectious after only a few days of treatment; however, clearance of dead *M. leprae* from the body may take several years. MDT regimens recommended by NHDP for US patients differ from those recommended by WHO.

For treatment of multibacillary leprosy (i.e., 6 or more lesions or skin smear positive) in adults, WHO recommends a 12-month MDT regimen of dapsone (once daily), rifampin (once monthly), and clofazimine (once daily and once monthly). For treatment of paucibacillary leprosy (i.e., 1–5 lesions) in adults, WHO recommends a 6-month MDT regimen of dapsone (once daily) and rifampin (once monthly). A single-dose rifampin-based MDT regimen that includes a single dose of rifampin, a single dose of ofloxacin, and a single dose of minocycline (ROM) has been used for treatment of paucibacillary leprosy in patients with only a single lesion (i.e., single-lesion paucibacillary leprosy).

For US patients, NHDP recommends more prolonged treatment. NHDP recommends that adults with multibacillary leprosy (i.e., those who are skin smear positive and/or have a biopsy indicating more advanced disease) receive a 24-month MDT regimen of dapsone (once daily), rifampin (once daily), and clofazimine (once daily); NHDP recommends that adults with paucibacillary leprosy (i.e., those who are skin smear negative without evidence of more advanced disease on biopsy) receive a 12-month MDT regimen of dapsone (once daily) and rifampin (once daily). Clofazimine is no longer commercially available in the US, but may be obtained from NHDP under an investigational new drug (IND) protocol for treatment of leprosy. (See Clofazimine 8:16.92.) Data indicate that leprosy is rare in the US (total of approximately 6500 living patients, about 3300 requiring active medical management), although about 150–200 new cases are reported each year.

Both WHO and NHDP recommend ofloxacin as an alternative that can be used instead of clofazimine in MDT regimens in adults who will not accept or cannot tolerate clofazimine.

Treatment of leprosy is complicated and should be undertaken in consultation with a specialist familiar with the disease. In the US, clinicians should contact NHDP at 800-642-2477 on weekdays from 9:00 a.m. to 5:30 p.m. Eastern Standard Time or via email at nhdped@hrsa.gov for assistance with diagnosis or treatment of leprosy or assistance obtaining clofazimine for treatment of leprosy.

Mycobacterium fortuitum Infections

Oral ofloxacin has been effective when used alone or in conjunction with amikacin for the treatment of postoperative sternotomy wound or soft tissue infections caused by *M. fortuitum†*. The drug also has been used effectively in a few patients for the treatment of *M. fortuitum* pulmonary or urinary tract infections.

Although optimum regimens have not been identified, ATS and IDSA recommend that *M. fortuitum* pulmonary infections be treated with a regimen consisting of at least 2 anti-infectives selected based on results of in vitro susceptibility testing and tolerability (e.g., amikacin, ciprofloxacin or ofloxacin, a sulfonamide, cefoxitin, imipenem, doxycycline).

• Nongonococcal Urethritis

Ofloxacin is used in adults for the treatment of nongonococcal urethritis (NGU). NGU can be caused by various organisms (e.g., *Chlamydia*, *M. genitalium*, *Trichomonas vaginalis*, *Ureaplasma*, enteric bacteria) and is treated presumptively at the time of diagnosis.

CDC states that a single dose of oral azithromycin or a 7-day regimen of oral doxycycline are the recommended regimens for the treatment of NGU; a 7-day regimen of oral erythromycin base or ethylsuccinate or a 7-day regimen of oral levofloxacin or ofloxacin are alternative regimens.

CDC states that men with persistent or recurrent NGU who were not compliant with the treatment regimen or were reexposed to untreated sexual partner(s) can be retreated with the initial regimen. In other patients, symptoms alone (without documentation of signs or laboratory evidence of urethral inflammation) are not a sufficient basis for retreatment and an objective diagnosis of persistent or recurrent NGU should be made before considering additional treatment. Because there is some evidence that *M. genitalium* is the most frequent cause of persistent or recurrent NGU, CDC states that those initially treated with doxycycline should receive retreatment with a single dose of oral azithromycin and those initially treated with azithromycin should receive retreatment with a 7-day regimen of oral moxifloxacin. However, if the patient with persistent or recurrent urethritis has sex with women and is in an area where *T. vaginalis* is prevalent, CDC recommends presumptive retreatment with a single dose of oral metronidazole or tinidazole and referral of their partner(s) for evaluation and appropriate treatment.

NGU may facilitate transmission of HIV and men diagnosed with NGU should be tested for HIV. Individuals with HIV infection should receive the same treatment regimens recommended for other individuals with NGU.

Any individual who had sexual contact with a patient with NGU within the preceding 60 days should be referred for evaluation, testing, and presumptive treatment with a regimen effective against *Chlamydia*. To minimize transmission and avoid reinfection, men treated for NGU should abstain from sexual intercourse until they and their sexual partner(s) have been adequately treated.

• Pelvic Inflammatory Disease

Ofloxacin has been used in the treatment of acute pelvic inflammatory disease (PID) caused by susceptible *C. trachomatis*. Ofloxacin is considered an alternative for the treatment of PID, but should *not* be used routinely for treatment of PID or any infections that may involve *N. gonorrhoeae*.

When a combined IM and oral regimen is used for the treatment of mild to moderately severe acute PID, CDC recommends a single IM dose of ceftriaxone, cefoxitin (with oral probenecid), or cefotaxime given in conjunction with a 14-day regimen of oral doxycycline (with or without a 14-day regimen of oral metronidazole). If parenteral cephalosporins are not feasible (e.g., because of cephalosporin allergy), CDC states that a 14-day regimen of oral levofloxacin, ofloxacin, or moxifloxacin given in conjunction with a 14-day regimen of oral metronidazole can be considered if the community prevalence and individual risk of gonorrhea are low and diagnostic testing for gonorrhea is performed. If culture results are positive for *N. gonorrhoeae*, the PID treatment regimen should be selected based on results of in vitro susceptibility testing. If QRNG are identified or if in vitro susceptibility cannot be determined (e.g., only nucleic acid amplification test [NAAT] for gonorrhea is available), consultation with an infectious disease specialist is recommended.

For further information on the treatment of PID, see Uses: Pelvic Inflammatory Disease in the Cephalosporins General Statement 8:12.06.

• Plague

Fluoroquinolones (e.g., ciprofloxacin, levofloxacin, moxifloxacin, ofloxacin) have been suggested as alternatives for the treatment of plague† caused by *Yersinia pestis* and also have been recommended for postexposure prophylaxis† following a high risk exposure to *Y. pestis*, including exposure in the context of biologic warfare or bioterrorism. The recommendation for use of fluoroquinolones for treatment or prophylaxis of plague is based on results of in vitro and animal testing. Although human studies are not available, results of in vitro studies indicate that ofloxacin is active against *Y. pestis* and the drug has been effective for the treatment of murine plague infections.

For the treatment of plague, IM streptomycin (or IM or IV gentamicin) historically has been considered the drug of choice. Alternatives recommended for the treatment of plague when aminoglycosides are not used include an IV fluoroquinolone (ciprofloxacin [a drug of choice for plague meningitis], levofloxacin, moxifloxacin), IV doxycycline (or IV tetracycline), IV chloramphenicol (drug of choice for plague meningitis), or co-trimoxazole (may be less effective than other alternatives).

Anti-infective regimens recommended for treatment of naturally occurring or endemic bubonic, septicemic, or pneumonic plague also are recommended for treatment of plague that occurs following exposure to *Y. pestis* in the context of biologic warfare or bioterrorism. Such exposures would most likely result in primary pneumonic plague, and prompt initiation of anti-infective therapy (within 18–24 hours of onset of symptoms) is essential in the treatment of pneumonic plague. Some experts (e.g., US Working Group on Civilian Biodefense, USAMRIID) recommend that treatment of plague in the context of biologic warfare or bioterrorism be initiated with a parenteral anti-infective regimen of streptomycin (or gentamicin) or, alternatively, a fluoroquinolone (ciprofloxacin, levofloxacin, moxifloxacin), doxycycline, or chloramphenicol. However, an oral regimen of doxycycline (or tetracycline) or a fluoroquinolone (e.g., ciprofloxacin, levofloxacin, moxifloxacin, ofloxacin) may be substituted when the patient's condition improves or if a parenteral regimen is unavailable (e.g., when there are supply or logistic problems because large numbers of individuals require treatment in a mass casualty setting).

In the context of biologic warfare or bioterrorism, some experts (e.g., the US Working Group on Civilian Biodefense, USAMRIID) recommend that asymptomatic individuals with exposure to plague aerosol or asymptomatic individuals with household, hospital, or other close contact (within about 2 m) with an individual who has pneumonic plague receive an oral anti-infective regimen for postexposure prophylaxis; however, any exposed individual who develops a temperature of 38.5°C or higher or new cough should promptly receive a parenteral anti-infective for treatment of the disease. If postexposure prophylaxis is indicated, these experts recommend a regimen of oral doxycycline (or tetracycline) or an oral fluoroquinolone (e.g., ciprofloxacin, levofloxacin, moxifloxacin, ofloxacin).

For additional information on use of fluoroquinolones for treatment or prophylaxis of plague, see Uses: Plague in Ciprofloxacin 8:12.18.

● Rickettsial Infections

Ofloxacin has been used in a limited number of patients for the treatment of various rickettsial infections†, including Mediterranean spotted fever† (boutonneuse fever) caused by *Rickettsia conorii*. CDC and other clinicians state that doxycycline is the drug of choice for the treatment of all tickborne rickettsial diseases. Although some fluoroquinolones have in vitro activity against Rickettsiae and some clinicians have suggested that fluoroquinolones (e.g., ciprofloxacin, ofloxacin) may be considered alternatives for the treatment of some rickettsial infections (e.g., Rocky Mountain spotted fever caused by *R. rickettsii*) when doxycycline cannot be used, CDC states that fluoroquinolones are *not* recommended for the treatment of Rocky Mountain spotted fever.

Ofloxacin has been used in a few patients for the treatment of acute Q fever pneumonia caused by *Coxiella burnetii*†; the drug produced apyrexia and clinical improvement within the first 2–4 days. However, Q fever pneumonia usually resolves within 15 days without treatment, and clinical evaluation of the efficacy of anti-infective regimens in the treatment of acute infections is difficult. Ofloxacin may be effective for the treatment of Q fever endocarditis†, and has been used in conjunction with doxycycline for the long-term treatment of Q fever endocarditis. However, in one limited study in patients with confirmed *C. burnetii* infection and chronic endocarditis, a regimen of doxycycline and ofloxacin was associated with a higher relapse rate than a regimen of doxycycline and hydroxychloroquine.

● Typhoid Fever

Oral ofloxacin has been used for the treatment of typhoid fever† (enteric fever) caused by susceptible *Salmonella enterica* serovar Typhi, including chloramphenicol-resistant strains. Although fluoroquinolones have been recommended for empiric treatment of *Salmonella* enteric fever in adults, resistance to fluoroquinolones has been reported in more than 80% of such infections in travelers to South and Southeast Asia and treatment failures will occur.

● Ophthalmic Infections

For use of ofloxacin in the topical treatment of ophthalmic infections caused by susceptible organisms, see Ofloxacin 52:04.12.

DOSAGE AND ADMINISTRATION

● Administration

Ofloxacin is administered orally. Although ofloxacin also has been administered IV, a parenteral preparation of the drug is no longer commercially available in the US.

While presence of food in the GI tract can decrease the rate and/or extent of absorption of ofloxacin, this is not usually considered clinically important and the manufacturer states that the drug can be given without regard to meals. Milk and yogurt do not appear to affect GI absorption of ofloxacin. (See Pharmacokinetics: Absorption.)

To minimize the possibility of interference with the GI absorption of ofloxacin, patients should be instructed not to ingest antacids containing calcium, magnesium, or aluminum, sucralfate, metal cations such as iron or zinc (including multivitamin preparations containing zinc), or buffered didanosine preparations concomitantly with or within 2 hours of an ofloxacin dose. (See Drug Interactions.)

Patients receiving ofloxacin should be well hydrated and should be instructed to drink fluids liberally. (See Cautions: Precautions and Contraindications.)

● Dosage

The usual adult oral dosage of ofloxacin is 200–400 mg every 12 hours.

Respiratory Tract Infections

If ofloxacin is used for the treatment of acute exacerbations of chronic bronchitis, the usual adult dosage is 400 mg every 12 hours given for 10 days. (See Uses: Respiratory Tract Infections.)

For the treatment of community-acquired pneumonia (CAP), the usual adult dosage of oral ofloxacin is 400 mg every 12 hours given for 10 days.

Skin and Skin Structure Infections

For the treatment of uncomplicated skin and skin structure infections, the usual adult dosage of oral ofloxacin is 400 mg every 12 hours given for 10 days.

Urinary Tract Infections and Prostatitis

If ofloxacin is used for the treatment of uncomplicated urinary tract infections (UTIs), the usual adult dosage is 200 mg every 12 hours. Although 3 days of ofloxacin therapy may be adequate for cystitis caused by susceptible *Escherichia coli* or *Klebsiella pneumoniae*, 7 days of therapy usually is required for the treatment of cystitis caused by other susceptible organisms. Various other oral dosage regimens have been used in the treatment of uncomplicated UTIs, including 100-mg doses given twice daily or 100- or 200-mg doses given once daily†; however, efficacy of these regimens has not been definitely established. (See Uncomplicated Urinary Tract Infections under Uses: Urinary Tract Infections and Prostatitis.)

For the treatment of complicated UTIs caused by susceptible organisms, the usual adult dosage of oral ofloxacin is 200 mg every 12 hours for 10 days. Some clinicians suggest that an oral dosage of 400 mg twice daily may be necessary for some complicated UTIs.

The usual adult dosage of oral ofloxacin for the treatment of prostatitis caused by *E. coli* is 300 mg every 12 hours given for 6 weeks or longer.

GI Infections
Travelers' Diarrhea

For the treatment of travelers' diarrhea†, ofloxacin has been given in a dosage of 300 mg twice daily. If anti-infectives are used in patients with travelers' diarrhea, a treatment duration of 1–3 days is recommended.

Although the use of anti-infectives for prophylaxis of travelers' diarrhea† generally is discouraged (see Travelers' Diarrhea under Uses: GI Infections), if oral ofloxacin is used for such prophylaxis, some clinicians recommend a dosage of 300 mg once daily. If anti-infective prophylaxis is used in travelers, it should be given during the period of risk (not exceeding 2–3 weeks) beginning the day of travel and continuing for 1 or 2 days after leaving the area of risk.

Helicobacter pylori Infection

When used as a component of multiple-drug regimens for the treatment of infections caused by *Helicobacter pylori*†, oral ofloxacin has been given in a dosage of 200 mg twice daily for 7–14 days.

Anthrax

Postexposure Prophylaxis of Anthrax

If oral ofloxacin is used as an alternative for postexposure prophylaxis following suspected or confirmed exposure to aerosolized *Bacillus anthracis* spores (inhalational anthrax)† (see Uses: Anthrax), the US Working Group on Civilian Biodefense suggests that adults can receive a dosage of 400 mg twice daily.

Anti-infective prophylaxis should be initiated as soon as possible following suspected or confirmed exposure to aerosolized *B. anthracis*.

Because of possible persistence of *B. anthracis* spores in lung tissue following an aerosol exposure, the US Centers for Disease Control and Prevention (CDC) and other experts recommend that anti-infective prophylaxis be continued for 60 days following a confirmed exposure.

Treatment of Anthrax

If oral ofloxacin is used as an alternative for treatment of inhalational anthrax† when a parenteral regimen is not available (see Uses: Anthrax), US Working Group on Civilian Biodefense suggests that adults can receive a dosage of 400 mg twice daily.

Because of possible persistence of *B. anthracis* spores in lung tissue following an aerosol exposure, the total duration of anti-infective therapy of inhalational anthrax that occurs as the result of exposure to *B. anthracis* in the context of biologic warfare or bioterrorism should be 60 days.

Brucellosis

For the treatment of brucellosis†, a 6-week regimen of oral ofloxacin in a dosage of 400 mg once daily in conjunction with oral rifampin (600 mg once daily) has been effective in some patients. Alternatively, an oral ofloxacin dosage of 400 mg twice daily for 6 weeks has been used in multiple-drug regimens for the treatment of brucellosis.

Chlamydial Infections

For the treatment of urethritis and/or cervicitis caused by *Chlamydia trachomatis* or uncomplicated urethral, endocervical, or rectal† chlamydial infections, the usual adult dosage of oral ofloxacin is 300 mg twice daily for 7 days.

Gonorrhea and Associated Infections

Although fluoroquinolones are no longer recommended for the treatment of gonorrhea or any associated infections that may involve *Neisseria gonorrhoeae* (see Uses: Gonorrhea and Associated Infections), the manufacturer recommends a single 400-mg oral dose of ofloxacin for the treatment of acute, uncomplicated urethral and cervical gonorrhea caused by susceptible *N. gonorrhoeae*.

Epididymitis

For the treatment of acute epididymitis† most likely caused by sexually transmitted enteric bacteria (e.g., *E. coli*) and when *N. gonorrhoeae* has been ruled out, CDC recommends that oral ofloxacin be given in a dosage of 300 mg twice daily for 10 days.

Ofloxacin should *not* be used alone for treatment of epididymitis unless *N. gonorrhoeae* has been ruled out. (See Uses: Gonorrhea and Associated Infections.)

Mycobacterial Infections

Leprosy

For the treatment of multibacillary leprosy† in adults who will not accept or cannot tolerate clofazimine, the World Health Organization (WHO) recommends a regimen of oral ofloxacin (400 mg once daily), oral rifampin (600 mg once monthly), and oral dapsone (100 mg once daily) given for 12 months. For US patients with multibacillary leprosy who will not accept or cannot tolerate clofazimine, the National Hansen's Disease Program (NHDP) recommends that adults receive oral ofloxacin (400 mg once daily), oral rifampin (600 mg once daily), and oral dapsone (100 mg once daily) given for 24 months.

For the treatment of single-lesion paucibacillary leprosy†, adults have received a single-dose multiple-drug regimen (ROM) that includes a single 600-mg dose of oral rifampin, a single 400-mg dose of oral ofloxacin, and a single 100-mg dose of oral minocycline.

Mycobacterium fortuitum Infections

For the treatment of postoperative sternotomy wound or soft tissue infections caused by *M. fortuitum*†, ofloxacin has been given in a dosage of 300 mg once daily or 1.2 g daily in 3 or 4 divided doses for 3–6 months in conjunction with amikacin (usually 250 mg IM or IV twice daily for 4–8 weeks).

For pulmonary infections, ATS and IDSA recommend that a regimen consisting of at least 2 anti-infectives be used (see Mycobacterium fortuitum Infections under Uses: Mycobacterial Infections) and that treatment be continued for at least 12 months after negative sputum cultures are attained. These experts also recommend that a regimen consisting of at least 2 anti-infectives be given for at least 4 months for the treatment of serious skin or soft tissue infections or for 6 months for bone infections.

Nongonococcal Urethritis

For the treatment of nongonococcal urethritis, the usual adult dosage of oral ofloxacin is 300 mg twice daily for 7 days. (See Uses: Nongonococcal Urethritis.)

Pelvic Inflammatory Disease

For the treatment of acute pelvic inflammatory disease (PID), the manufacturer recommends an oral ofloxacin dosage of 400 mg every 12 hours given for 10–14 days.

If oral ofloxacin is used as an alternative for the treatment of mild to moderately severe acute PID, CDC recommends a dosage of 400 mg twice daily for 14 days given in conjunction with oral metronidazole (500 mg twice daily for 14 days).

Ofloxacin should be used for the treatment of PID only when parenteral cephalosporins are not feasible, the community prevalence and individual risk of gonorrhea are low, and in vitro susceptibility has been confirmed. (See Uses: Pelvic Inflammatory Disease.)

Rickettsial Infections

Mediterranean Spotted Fever

For the treatment of Mediterranean spotted fever† (boutonneuse fever) caused by *Rickettsia conorii*, an oral ofloxacin dosage of 200 mg every 12 hours given for 7 days was effective in some patients.

Q Fever

For the treatment of acute Q fever† pneumonia caused by *Coxiella burnetii*, ofloxacin has been given in a dosage of 600 mg daily for up to 16 days. For the treatment of Q fever endocarditis, ofloxacin has been given in a dosage of 200 mg 3 times daily in conjunction with oral doxycycline (100 mg twice daily); long-term treatment (at least 4 years) may be required.

Typhoid Fever

For the treatment of typhoid fever† (enteric fever) caused by susceptible *Salmonella*, oral ofloxacin has been given to adults in a dosage of 200–400 mg every 12 hours for 7–14 days. (See Uses: Typhoid Fever.)

● Dosage in Renal and Hepatic Impairment

Renal Impairment

Modification of usual dosage of ofloxacin generally is unnecessary in patients with creatinine clearances greater than 50 mL/minute. In patients with creatinine clearances of 50 mL/minute or less, doses and/or frequency of administration of ofloxacin should be modified in response to the degree of renal impairment.

The manufacturer recommends that adults with creatinine clearances of 50 mL/minute or less receive an initial ofloxacin dose equal to the usually recommended dose and that subsequent dosage be modified according to creatinine clearance. Adults with creatinine clearances of 20–50 mL/minute should receive the usual oral dose of ofloxacin every 24 hours and those with creatinine clearances less than 20 mL/minute should receive half the usually recommended oral dose every 24 hours.

For adults undergoing hemodialysis, some clinicians recommend that a 200-mg loading dose of oral ofloxacin be given followed by 100-mg oral doses once daily. For most patients, additional supplemental doses of the drug are unnecessary following each hemodialysis procedure; however, some clinicians suggest that a single 100-mg supplemental oral dose of the drug be given after the first hemodialysis procedure.

Hepatic Impairment

Because excretion of ofloxacin may be reduced in patients with severe hepatic impairment (e.g., cirrhosis with or without ascites), the maximum ofloxacin dosage in these patients is 400 mg daily.

CAUTIONS

Adverse effects reported with ofloxacin are similar to those reported with other fluoroquinolone anti-infectives (e.g., ciprofloxacin). Adverse effects have been reported in 2–12% of patients receiving ofloxacin, and have been severe enough to require discontinuance in 1–4% of patients. The most frequent adverse effects of the drug involve the GI tract or CNS.

Systemic fluoroquinolones, including ofloxacin, have been associated with disabling and potentially irreversible serious adverse reactions (e.g., tendinitis and tendon rupture, peripheral neuropathy, CNS effects) that can occur together in the same patient. These serious reactions may occur within hours to weeks after a systemic fluoroquinolone is initiated and have occurred in all age groups and in patients without preexisting risk factors for such adverse reactions. (See Cautions: Precautions and Contraindications.)

● *Tendinitis and Tendon Rupture*

Systemic fluoroquinolones, including ofloxacin, are associated with an increased risk of tendinitis and tendon rupture in all age groups.

The risk of developing fluoroquinolone-associated tendinitis and tendon rupture is increased in older adults (usually those older than 60 years of age), individuals receiving concomitant corticosteroids, and kidney, heart, or lung transplant recipients. Other factors that may independently increase the risk of tendon rupture include strenuous physical activity, renal failure, and previous tendon disorders such as rheumatoid arthritis. However, tendinitis and tendon rupture have been reported in patients receiving fluoroquinolones who did not have any risk factors for such adverse reactions.

Fluoroquinolone-associated tendinitis and tendon rupture most frequently involve the Achilles tendon and have also been reported in the rotator cuff (shoulder), hand, biceps, thumb, and other tendon sites. Tendinitis or tendon rupture can occur within hours or days after ofloxacin is initiated or as long as several months after completion of therapy and can occur bilaterally.

Ofloxacin should be discontinued immediately if pain, swelling, inflammation, or rupture of a tendon occurs. (See Cautions: Precautions and Contraindications.)

● *Peripheral Neuropathy*

Systemic fluoroquinolones, including ofloxacin, have been associated with an increased risk of peripheral neuropathy.

Sensory or sensorimotor axonal polyneuropathy affecting small and/or large axons resulting in paresthesias, hypoesthesias, dysesthesias, and weakness has been reported in patients receiving systemic fluoroquinolones, including ofloxacin. Symptoms may occur soon after initiation of ofloxacin and, in some patients, may be irreversible.

Ofloxacin should be discontinued immediately if symptoms of peripheral neuropathy (e.g., pain, burning, tingling, numbness, and/or weakness) occur or if there are other alterations in sensations (e.g., light touch, pain, temperature, position sense, vibratory sensation). (See Cautions: Precautions and Contraindications.)

● *CNS Effects*

Systemic fluoroquinolones, including ofloxacin, have been associated with an increased risk of psychiatric adverse effects, including toxic psychosis, hallucinations, agitation, delirium, confusion, disorientation, disturbances in attention, nervousness, restlessness, and memory impairment. These adverse effects may occur after the first dose.

Systemic fluoroquinolones have been associated with an increased risk of convulsions (seizures), increased intracranial pressure (pseudotumor cerebri), lightheadedness, and tremors.

Headache, insomnia, and dizziness are the most frequently reported adverse CNS effects of ofloxacin. These effects have been reported in 1–9% of patients receiving the drug, generally become apparent during the first few days of therapy, and frequently subside during continued therapy with the drug. Fatigue, somnolence, sleep disorders, and nervousness have been reported in 1–3% and asthenia, malaise, anxiety, cognitive changes, depression, dream abnormality, euphoria, hallucinations, agitation, confusion, ataxia, tremor, paresthesia, seizures, myasthenia, syncope, and vertigo have been reported in less than 1% of patients receiving ofloxacin. Increased intracranial pressure, toxic psychosis, paranoia, and suicidal ideation or acts also have been reported. In most reported cases, hallucinations or psychotic reactions generally began within the first 3 days of therapy; these reactions subsided when the drug was discontinued.

Some adverse nervous system effects of ofloxacin may be related to the fact that the drug, like other fluoroquinolones, is an γ-aminobutyric acid (GABA) inhibitor. However, further study is needed to elucidate the mechanism(s) of these adverse CNS effects during fluoroquinolone therapy. In addition, while it also has been suggested that some CNS stimulant effects reported in patients receiving fluoroquinolones may result from quinolone-induced alterations in caffeine pharmacokinetics, ofloxacin is less likely than many other fluoroquinolones to induce such pharmacokinetic alterations. (See Drug Interactions: Xanthine Derivatives.)

If psychiatric or other CNS effects occur during ofloxacin therapy, the drug should be discontinued immediately and appropriate measures instituted. (See Cautions: Precautions and Contraindications.)

● *Exacerbation of Myasthenia Gravis*

Fluoroquinolones, including ofloxacin, have neuromuscular blocking activity and may exacerbate muscle weakness in individuals with myasthenia gravis. Use of fluoroquinolones in myasthenia gravis patients has resulted in requirements for ventilatory support and in death. (See Cautions: Precautions and Contraindications.)

● *Dermatologic and Sensitivity Reactions*

Rash and pruritus have been reported in 1–3% and eosinophilia, angioedema, urticaria, and vasculitis have been reported in up to 1% of patients receiving ofloxacin. Although a causal relationship was not definitely established, fatal vasculitis occurred in at least one patient receiving ofloxacin. Fever, chills, and diaphoresis have been reported in less than 3% of patients receiving the drug.

Hypersensitivity Reactions

Although most hypersensitivity reactions to ofloxacin are mild cutaneous reactions, serious and occasionally fatal hypersensitivity and/or anaphylactic reactions, sometimes occurring following the first dose, have been reported in patients receiving the drug. Severe hypersensitivity reactions, characterized by rash, fever, jaundice, and hepatic necrosis with a fatal outcome, also have been reported with other fluoroquinolones.

Some hypersensitivity reactions reported in patients receiving fluoroquinolones, including ofloxacin, have been accompanied by cardiovascular collapse, hypotension or shock, seizures, loss of consciousness, tingling, angioedema (including tongue, laryngeal, pharyngeal, or facial edema), airway obstruction (including bronchospasm, shortness of breath, and acute respiratory distress), dyspnea, urticaria, pruritus, and other serious skin reactions.

Other serious and sometimes fatal adverse reactions that have been reported with fluoroquinolones, including ofloxacin, and that may or may not be related to hypersensitivity reactions include one of more of the following: fever, rash or severe dermatologic reaction (e.g., toxic epidermal necrolysis, Stevens-Johnson syndrome); vasculitis, arthralgia, myalgia, serum sickness; allergic pneumonitis; interstitial nephritis, acute renal insufficiency or failure; hepatitis, jaundice, acute hepatic necrosis or failure; anemia (including hemolytic and aplastic anemia), thrombocytopenia (including thrombotic thrombocytopenic purpura), leukopenia, agranulocytosis, pancytopenia, and/or other hematologic abnormalities.

Ofloxacin should be discontinued immediately at the first appearance of rash, jaundice, or any other sign of hypersensitivity. Appropriate therapy (e.g., epinephrine, corticosteroids, maintenance of an adequate airway, oxygen, IV fluids, antihistamines, maintenance of blood pressure) should be initiated as indicated.

Because of a high percentage of false-positive results, skin testing with ofloxacin has not been useful in evaluating hypersensitivity to the drug and is not recommended.

Photosensitivity Reactions

Moderate to severe photosensitivity/phototoxicity reactions have been reported in patients receiving fluoroquinolones, including ofloxacin.

Phototoxicity may manifest as exaggerated sunburn reactions (e.g., burning, erythema, exudation, vesicles, blistering, edema) on areas exposed to sun or artificial ultraviolet (UV) light (usually the face, neck, extensor surfaces of fore-arms, dorsa of hands).

Although studies using topical ofloxacin in guinea pigs have not revealed evidence of phototoxicity, photoallergenicity, or contact allergy, in vitro studies indicate the drug is phototoxic.

Ofloxacin should be discontinued if photosensitivity or phototoxicity (sunburn-like reaction, skin eruption) occurs. (See Cautions: Precautions and Contraindications.)

● Aortic Aneurysm and Dissection

Rupture or dissection of aortic aneurysms has been reported in patients receiving systemic fluoroquinolones. Epidemiologic studies indicate an increased risk of aortic aneurysm and dissection within 2 months following use of systemic fluoroquinolones, particularly in geriatric patients. The cause for this increased risk has not been identified.

If a patient reports adverse effects suggestive of aortic aneurysm or dissection, fluoroquinolone treatment should be discontinued immediately. (See Cautions: Precautions and Contraindications.)

● Hypoglycemia or Hyperglycemia

Systemic fluoroquinolones, including ofloxacin, have been associated with alterations in blood glucose concentrations, including symptomatic hypoglycemia and hyperglycemia. Blood glucose disturbances during fluoroquinolone therapy usually have occurred in patients with diabetes mellitus receiving an oral antidiabetic agent (e.g., glyburide) or insulin.

Severe cases of hypoglycemia resulting in coma or death have been reported with some systemic fluoroquinolones. Although most reported cases of hypoglycemic coma have involved patients with risk factors for hypoglycemia (e.g., older age, diabetes mellitus, renal insufficiency, concomitant use of antidiabetic agents [especially sulfonylureas]), some cases have occurred in patients receiving a fluoroquinolone who were not diabetic and were not reported to be receiving an oral antidiabetic agent or insulin.

If a hypoglycemic reaction occurs, ofloxacin should be discontinued and appropriate therapy initiated immediately. (See Cautions: Precautions and Contraindications.)

● GI Effects

Nausea has been reported in 3–10% and diarrhea, vomiting, abdominal pain/discomfort, abdominal cramps, flatulence, constipation, dyspepsia, heartburn, dry mouth, dysgeusia, decreased appetite, and anorexia have been reported in 5% or less of patients receiving ofloxacin. Adverse GI effects generally are mild and transient and only rarely require discontinuance of ofloxacin.

Effects on GI Flora

Ofloxacin therapy has only a minimal effect on normal salivary flora. Following oral administration of a single 400-mg dose of ofloxacin, total bacterial counts of Branhamella in saliva were reduced and did not return to pretreatment levels until 4 weeks after the dose; total bacterial counts of salivary streptococci, micrococci, and corynebacteria were unaffected by the drug.

Ofloxacin exerts a selective effect on normal bowel flora. Total bacterial counts of normal anaerobic fecal flora generally are unaffected during or following ofloxacin therapy. However, ofloxacin therapy generally markedly reduces or completely eradicates normal fecal Enterobacteriaceae within 2–6 days and may reduce, but not eliminate, total bacterial counts of fecal aerobic gram-positive bacteria (e.g., Streptococcus faecalis). Total bacterial counts of normal fecal flora generally return to pretreatment levels within 1–4 weeks following discontinuance of ofloxacin. In studies evaluating the effects of ofloxacin on physiological and/or biochemical intestinal characteristics that depend on intestinal flora, the drug had no discernible effect on conversion of cholesterol to coprostanol, conversion of bilirubin to urobilinogen, breakdown of mucin, inactivation of tryptic activity, formation of short chain fatty acids, or presence of β-aspartylglycine.

C. difficile-associated Diarrhea and Colitis

Treatment with anti-infectives alters normal colon flora and may permit overgrowth of Clostridioides difficile (formerly known as Clostridium difficile).

C. difficile infection (CDI) and C. difficile-associated diarrhea and colitis (CDAD; also known as antibiotic-associated diarrhea and colitis or

pseudomembranous colitis) have been reported in patients receiving fluoroquinolones, including ofloxacin, and may range in severity from mild diarrhea to fatal colitis. C. difficile produces toxins A and B which contribute to development of CDAD; hypertoxin-producing strains of C. difficile are associated with increased morbidity and mortality since they may be refractory to anti-infectives and colectomy may be required. (See Superinfection/C. difficile-associated Diarrhea and Colitis under Cautions: Precautions and Contraindications.)

When fluoroquinolones were first marketed, there appeared to be a relative lack of association between use of the drugs and CDAD and the risk of CDAD appeared to be lower than that reported with some other anti-infectives. However, there now is some evidence that increasing use of the drugs may have resulted in emergence of C. difficile that are more resistant and/or more virulent than previous strains.

● Genitourinary Effects

In women receiving ofloxacin, external genital pruritus, candidal vaginitis, and vaginal discharge have been reported in 1–6% and burning, irritation, pain and rash of the genitalia, dysmenorrhea, menorrhagia, and metrorrhagia have been reported in less than 1%.

Ofloxacin does not appear to be nephrotoxic. Increased serum creatinine and BUN concentrations have been reported only rarely and dysuria, urinary retention, increased urinary frequency, and elevated urinary pH have been reported in less than 1% of patients receiving the drug. Glucosuria, proteinuria, hematuria, and pyuria, have been reported in at least 1% of patients receiving the drug. Although crystalluria and cylindruria have not been reported to date with ofloxacin, these adverse effects have been reported rarely in patients receiving some other fluoroquinolones (e.g., ciprofloxacin), generally occurring in patients with alkaline urine who received high dosages of the drugs; these effects were not associated with renal toxicity. Crystalluria, sometimes associated with nephropathy, has occurred in animals receiving other fluoroquinolones (e.g., ciprofloxacin) but has not been observed to date in animal studies using ofloxacin.

● Musculoskeletal Effects

Fluoroquinolones, including ofloxacin, cause arthropathies (arthrosis) in immature animals of various species. In various studies in immature animals, oral ofloxacin has caused blisters and/or erosions in articular cartilage and increased synovial fluid and lesion formation of diarthric joints; in one study in immature rats, adverse effects were detected as soon as 5 hours after a single 1- or 3-g/kg oral dose of the drug. The severity of these adverse effects appears to be species-specific, being more evident in dogs than in rats, rabbits, or mice, and also appears to depend on the age of the animal and dosage and duration of therapy. Morphologic changes observed in animals with quinolone-induced arthropathies include erosions in joint cartilage accompanied by noninflammatory, cell-free effusions of the joint space; the cartilage is incapable of regeneration and may serve as a site for the development of arthropathy deformans. Although arthropathies have been detected in adult dogs receiving some quinolones (e.g., pefloxacin [not commercially available in the US]), there has been no evidence of arthropathies in fully mature dogs or rats when ofloxacin was given in doses up to 5 times the usual human dosage. (See Cautions: Pediatric Precautions.)

Chest or trunk pain has been reported in 1–3% and transient arthralgia, myalgia, or pain in the extremities or body as a whole have been reported in less than 1% of patients receiving ofloxacin.

● Hepatic Effects

Transient, mild increases in serum concentrations of AST (SGOT) and/or ALT (SGPT) have been reported in 1–2% and increased serum concentrations of alkaline phosphatase, LDH, bilirubin, and γ-glutamyltransferase (γ-glutamyl transpeptidase, GGT, GGTP) have been reported in less than 1% of patients receiving ofloxacin.

Severe hepatotoxicity, including acute hepatitis and fatalities, has been reported in patients receiving ofloxacin. In some cases, substantial elevations in serum liver enzyme concentrations and other manifestations of hepatitis resolved following discontinuance of the drug.

● Hematologic Effects

Eosinophilia, lymphocytopenia, lymphocytosis, leukocytosis, neutropenia, neutrophilia, thrombocytosis, thrombocytopenia, leukopenia, anemia, and elevated erythrocyte sedimentation rate (ESR) have been reported in at least 1% of patients receiving ofloxacin; however, it is not clear in all cases whether these effects were caused by the drug or underlying conditions of the patients.

● Cardiovascular Effects

Prolonged QT interval leading to ventricular arrhythmias, including torsades de pointes, has been reported with some fluoroquinolones, including ofloxacin. Geriatric patients may be at increased risk for drug-associated effects on the QT interval. (See Cautions: Geriatric Precautions.)

Edema, hypertension, hypotension, palpitations, tachycardia, vasodilation, and cardiac arrest have been reported in less than 1% of patients receiving ofloxacin.

Rupture or dissection of aortic aneurysms has been reported in patients receiving systemic fluoroquinolones. (See Cautions: Aortic Aneurysm and Dissection.)

● Ocular Effects

Transient visual disturbances, including diplopia or changes in visual acuity or color perception, have been reported in 1–3% of patients receiving ofloxacin. Photophobia has been reported in less than 1% of patients receiving the drug. Although ophthalmologic abnormalities, including cataracts and multiple punctate lenticular opacities, have been reported with some other quinolones (e.g., pefloxacin [not commercially available in the US]) in both multiple-dose studies in humans and long-term, high dosage studies in animals, there has been no evidence of ofloxacin-induced ocular toxicity in humans or in animal studies. Although the clinical importance in unclear, in vitro studies using rabbit corneal epithelial cultures indicate that topical ofloxacin at concentrations exceeding 0.05 mg/mL delayed corneal epithelial wound healing.

● Other Adverse Effects

Cough, respiratory arrest, rhinorrhea, thirst, and weight loss have been reported in less than 1% of patients receiving ofloxacin.

Decreased hearing acuity and tinnitus have been reported in less than 1% of patients receiving ofloxacin.

● Precautions and Contraindications

Ofloxacin is contraindicated in patients with a history of hypersensitivity to the drug or to other quinolones.

Systemic fluoroquinolones, including ofloxacin, have been associated with disabling and potentially irreversible serious adverse reactions (e.g., tendinitis and tendon rupture, peripheral neuropathy, CNS effects) that can occur together in the same patient. These serious reactions may occur within hours to weeks after a systemic fluoroquinolone is initiated and have occurred in all age groups and in patients without preexisting risk factors for such adverse reactions. Patients receiving ofloxacin should be informed about these serious adverse reactions and advised to immediately discontinue ofloxacin and contact a clinician if they experience any signs or symptoms of serious adverse effects (e.g., unusual joint or tendon pain, muscle weakness, a "pins and needles" tingling or pricking sensation, numbness of the arms or legs, confusion, hallucinations) while taking the drug. Systemic fluoroquinolones, including ofloxacin, should be avoided in patients who have experienced any of the serious adverse reactions associated with fluoroquinolones.

Because fluoroquinolones, including ofloxacin, are associated with an increased risk of tendinitis and tendon rupture in all age groups (see Cautions: Tendinitis and Tendon Rupture), patients receiving ofloxacin should be informed of this potentially irreversible adverse effect and the drug should be discontinued immediately if pain, swelling, inflammation, or rupture of a tendon occurs. The risk of developing fluoroquinolone-associated tendinitis and tendon rupture is increased in adults older than 60 years of age, patients receiving concomitant corticosteroids, and kidney, heart, or lung transplant recipients. (See Cautions: Geriatric Precautions and see Drug Interactions: Corticosteroids.) Patients should be advised to rest and refrain from exercise at the first sign of tendinitis or tendon rupture (e.g., pain, swelling, or inflammation of a tendon or weakness or inability to use a joint) and advised to immediately discontinue the drug and contact a clinician. Systemic fluoroquinolones, including ofloxacin, should be avoided in patients who have a history of tendon disorders or have experienced tendinitis or tendon rupture.

Because fluoroquinolones, including ofloxacin, are associated with an increased risk of peripheral neuropathy (see Cautions: Peripheral Neuropathy), ofloxacin should be discontinued immediately if symptoms of peripheral neuropathy (e.g., pain, burning, tingling, numbness, and/or weakness) occur or if there are other alterations in sensations (e.g., light touch, pain, temperature, position sense, vibratory sensation). Patients receiving ofloxacin should be advised that peripheral neuropathies have been reported in patients receiving systemic fluoroquinolones, including ofloxacin, and that symptoms may

occur soon after initiation of the drug and, in some patients, may be irreversible. Patients should be advised of the importance of immediately discontinuing the drug and contacting a clinician if such symptoms occur. Systemic fluoroquinolones, including ofloxacin, should be avoided in patients who have experienced peripheral neuropathy.

Because fluoroquinolones, including ofloxacin, have been associated with an increased risk of adverse CNS effects (see Cautions: CNS Effects), ofloxacin should be used with caution in patients with known or suspected CNS disorders (e.g., severe cerebral arteriosclerosis, epilepsy) or other risk factors (e.g., certain drugs, renal impairment) that predispose to seizures or lower the seizure threshold. Patients should be informed that seizures have been reported in patients receiving ofloxacin and advised to inform their clinician of any history of seizures before initiating therapy with the drug. Patients receiving ofloxacin should be advised to notify their clinician if persistent headache (with or without blurred vision) occurs. Patients also should be cautioned not to operate a motor vehicle or machinery or engage in activities requiring mental alertness and coordination until they experience how the drug affects them. Systemic fluoroquinolones, including ofloxacin, should be avoided in patients who have experienced CNS effects associated with fluoroquinolones.

Ofloxacin should be avoided in patients with myasthenia gravis since fluoroquinolones, including ofloxacin, may exacerbate myasthenia gravis symptoms. Patients should be advised to immediately contact their clinician if they have any worsening muscle weakness or breathing problems.

Because an increased risk of aortic aneurysm and dissection has been reported with systemic fluoroquinolones, ofloxacin should not be used in patients who have an aortic aneurysm or are at increased risk for an aortic aneurysm unless there are no other treatment options. This includes geriatric patients and patients with peripheral atherosclerotic vascular disease, hypertension, or certain genetic conditions (e.g., Marfan syndrome, Ehlers-Danlos syndrome). Patients should be informed that systemic fluoroquinolones may increase the risk of aortic aneurysm and dissection and advised of the importance of informing their clinician of any history of aneurysms, blockages or hardening of the arteries, high blood pressure, or genetic conditions such as Marfan syndrome or Ehlers-Danlos syndrome. Patients receiving ofloxacin should be advised to seek immediate medical treatment if they experience sudden, severe, and constant pain in the stomach, chest, or back.

Blood glucose concentrations should be carefully monitored when systemic fluoroquinolones, including ofloxacin, are used in patients with diabetes mellitus receiving antidiabetic agents. Patients should be informed that hypoglycemia has been reported when systemic fluoroquinolones were used in some patients receiving antidiabetic agents. Patients with diabetes mellitus receiving oral antidiabetic agents or insulin should be advised to discontinue ofloxacin and contact a clinician if they experience hypoglycemia or symptoms of hypoglycemia. Appropriate therapy should be initiated immediately.

Because severe hepatotoxicity, including acute hepatitis and fatalities, has been reported in patients receiving ofloxacin, the drug should be discontinued immediately if any sign or symptom of hepatitis (e.g., anorexia, jaundice, dark urine, pruritus, tender abdomen) occurs. Patients should be advised to contact a clinician if any sign or symptom of hepatotoxicity (e.g., loss of appetite, nausea, vomiting, fever, weakness, tiredness, right upper quadrant tenderness, itching, yellowing of skin or eyes, light colored bowel movements, dark colored urine) occurs.

Use of ofloxacin should be avoided in patients with a history of QT interval prolongation, in those with uncorrected electrolyte disorders (e.g., hypokalemia), and in those receiving class IA (e.g., quinidine, procainamide) or class III (e.g., amiodarone, sotalol) antiarrhythmic agents. (See Drug Interactions.) The risk of drug-associated effects on the QT interval may be increased in geriatric patients. (See Cautions: Geriatric Precautions.)

Sensitivity Reactions

Ofloxacin, like other quinolones, can cause serious, potentially fatal hypersensitivity reactions, occasionally following the initial dose. (See Cautions: Dermatologic and Sensitivity Reactions.) Patients receiving ofloxacin should be advised of this possibility and instructed to immediately discontinue the drug and contact a clinician at the first sign of rash, urticaria, or other skin reactions, jaundice, or any other sign of hypersensitivity such as rapid heartbeat, difficulty in swallowing or breathing, or any swelling indicative of angioedema (e.g., swelling of the lips, tongue, face; tightness of the throat; hoarseness). Serious anaphylactic reactions require immediate emergency treatment with epinephrine and other resuscitation measures (e.g., oxygen, IV fluids, IV antihistamines, corticosteroids, pressor amines, airway management such as intubation) as indicated.

Because photosensitivity/phototoxicity reactions have been reported following exposure to direct sunlight in patients receiving fluoroquinolones, including ofloxacin, patients receiving ofloxacin should be cautioned to avoid excessive exposure to direct sunlight or artificial UV light (sunlamps, solariums) while receiving the drug. Ofloxacin should be discontinued if photosensitivity or phototoxicity (sunburn-like reaction, skin eruption) occurs.

Selection and Use of Anti-infectives

Ofloxacin should be used for the treatment of acute bacterial exacerbations of chronic bronchitis or uncomplicated urinary tract infections *only* when no other treatment options are available. Because ofloxacin, like other systemic fluoroquinolones, has been associated with disabling and potentially irreversible serious adverse reactions (e.g., tendinitis and tendon rupture, peripheral neuropathy, CNS effects) that can occur together in the same patient, the risks of serious adverse reactions outweigh the benefits of ofloxacin for patients with these infections.

To reduce development of drug-resistant bacteria and maintain effectiveness of ofloxacin and other antibacterials, the drug should be used only for the treatment or prevention of infections proven or strongly suspected to be caused by susceptible bacteria. When selecting or modifying anti-infective therapy, results of culture and in vitro susceptibility testing should be used. In the absence of such data, local epidemiology and susceptibility patterns should be considered when selecting anti-infectives for empiric therapy.

Patients should be advised that antibacterials (including ofloxacin) should only be used to treat bacterial infections and not used to treat viral infections (e.g., the common cold). Patients also should be advised about the importance of completing the full course of therapy, even if feeling better after a few days, and that skipping doses or not completing therapy may decrease effectiveness and increase the likelihood that bacteria will develop resistance and will not be treatable with ofloxacin or other antibacterials in the future.

Superinfection/C. difficile-associated Diarrhea and Colitis

As with other anti-infectives, use of ofloxacin may result in emergence and overgrowth of nonsusceptible bacteria or fungi, especially enterococci or *Candida*. Resistant strains of some organisms (e.g., *Pseudomonas aeruginosa*, staphylococci) have developed during ofloxacin therapy. Careful monitoring of the patient and periodic in vitro susceptibility tests are essential.

Because CDAD has been reported with the use of nearly all anti-infectives, including ofloxacin, it should be considered in the differential diagnosis in patients who develop diarrhea during or after ofloxacin therapy. Careful medical history is necessary since CDAD has been reported to occur as late as 2 months or longer after anti-infective therapy is discontinued.

If CDAD is suspected or confirmed, anti-infective therapy not directed against *C. difficile* should be discontinued as soon as possible. Patients should be managed with appropriate anti-infective therapy directed against *C. difficile* (e.g., vancomycin, fidaxomicin, metronidazole), supportive therapy (e.g., fluid and electrolyte management, protein supplementation), and surgical evaluation as clinically indicated.

Patients should be advised that diarrhea is a common problem caused by anti-infectives and usually ends when the drug is discontinued; however, it is important to contact a clinician if watery and bloody stools (with or without stomach cramps and fever) occur during or as late as 2 months or longer after the last dose.

Other Precautions and Contraindications

Renal, hepatic, and hematologic systems should be evaluated periodically during prolonged ofloxacin therapy.

Crystalluria, cylindruria, and hematuria have been reported with some other fluoroquinolones (e.g., ciprofloxacin). Although crystalluria is not expected to occur under usual conditions with the usual recommended dosages of ofloxacin, patients should be instructed to drink sufficient quantities of fluids to ensure proper hydration and adequate urinary output during therapy with the drug.

Ofloxacin should be used with caution in patients with impaired renal or hepatic function since elimination of the drug may be reduced in these patients. When ofloxacin is used in patients with known or suspected renal or hepatic impairment, the patient should be monitored carefully and appropriate laboratory studies should be performed prior to and during therapy with the drug.

Doses and/or frequency of administration of ofloxacin should be decreased in patients with creatinine clearances of 50 mL/minute or less. (See Dosage and Administration: Dosage in Renal and Hepatic Impairment.)

• Pediatric Precautions

Safety and efficacy of ofloxacin have not been established in children younger than 18 years of age. Because ofloxacin, like most other fluoroquinolones, causes arthropathy (arthrosis) in immature animals of several species, some clinicians state that the drug should not be used in children younger than 16–18 years of age. Other clinicians suggest that ofloxacin may be used cautiously in adolescents if skeletal growth is complete and suggest that the potential benefits of therapy with the drug may outweigh the possible risks in certain children 9–18 years of age with serious infections (e.g., cystic fibrosis patients) when the causative organism is resistant to other available anti-infectives.

The American Academy of Pediatrics (AAP) states that use of a systemic fluoroquinolone may be justified in children younger than 18 years of age in certain specific circumstances when there are no safe and effective alternatives and the drug is known to be effective. For information regarding when fluoroquinolones may be a preferred option in children, see Cautions: Pediatric Precautions in Ciprofloxacin 8:12.18.

In immature rats, oral ofloxacin in dosages 5–16 times the usual human oral dosage increased the incidence and severity of osteochondrosis; the lesions were still present and had not regressed 13 weeks after the drug was discontinued. Ofloxacin and most other fluoroquinolones (e.g., ciprofloxacin,) have caused erosions of the cartilage in weight-bearing joints and other signs of arthropathies (arthrosis) in immature animals of various species. (See Cautions: Musculoskeletal Effects.)

• Geriatric Precautions

When the total number of patients studied in phase II/III clinical studies of ofloxacin is considered, 14.2 % (688 patients) were 65 years of age or older, while 5.2% (252 patients) were 75 years of age and older. Ofloxacin generally is well tolerated in geriatric patients; the frequency and severity of adverse effects reported in patients older than 65 years of age generally are similar to those reported in younger adults.

Pharmacokinetic parameters in geriatric patients receiving ofloxacin generally are similar to those in younger adults. Results of pharmacokinetic studies in geriatric individuals 65–81 years of age indicate that the rate of absorption, volume of distribution, and route of elimination of ofloxacin in geriatric individuals are similar to those reported in younger adults. However, mean peak plasma concentrations of ofloxacin are 9–21% higher and the plasma elimination half-life more prolonged in geriatric individuals compared with younger adults. (See Pharmacokinetics.) The slower elimination of ofloxacin in geriatric individuals presumably is secondary to reduced renal function and clearance observed in geriatric individuals. Because ofloxacin is excreted by the kidneys and geriatric individuals are more likely to have decreased renal function than younger individuals, dosage adjustment may be necessary in geriatric patients with renal impairment as recommended for all patients with renal impairment. Dosage of ofloxacin does not need to be modified in geriatric patients with creatinine clearances greater than 50 mL/minute. (See Dosage and Administration: Dosage in Renal and Hepatic Impairment.)

The risk of fluoroquinolone-associated tendon disorders, including tendon rupture, is increased in geriatric adults older than 60 years of age. This risk is further increased in those receiving concomitant corticosteroids. (See Cautions: Precautions and Contraindications.) Ofloxacin should be used with caution in geriatric adults, especially those receiving concomitant corticosteroids.

The risk of QT interval prolongation, leading to ventricular arrhythmias may be increased in geriatric patients, especially those receiving concurrent therapy with other drugs that can prolong QT interval (e.g., class IA or III antiarrhythmic agents) or with risk factors for torsades de pointes (e.g., known QT prolongation, uncorrected hypokalemia). (See Cautions: Cardiovascular Effects.)

The risk of fluoroquinolone-associated aortic aneurysm and dissection may be increased in geriatric patients. (See Cautions: Aortic Aneurysm and Dissection.)

• Mutagenicity and Carcinogenicity

Ofloxacin was not mutagenic in the Ames microbial (*Salmonella*) mutagen test or in in vitro and in vivo cytogenic assays, including the sister chromatid exchange (Chinese hamster and human cell lines) assay, unscheduled DNA repair assay using human fibroblasts, dominant lethal assay, or mouse micronucleus assay. When ofloxacin was tested in the in vitro rat hepatocyte DNA repair assay, mouse lymphoma assay, and Rec-assay for DNA repair, results were positive, which may indicate a potential for primary DNA damage. However, other more sensitive tests, such as the V-79 mammalian cell assay, have not shown evidence of mutagenicity.

Studies have not been performed to date to evaluate the carcinogenic potential of ofloxacin.

● Pregnancy, Fertility, and Lactation

Pregnancy

There are no adequate and controlled studies to date using ofloxacin in pregnant women. Since the drug, like most other fluoroquinolones, causes arthropathy in immature animals, ofloxacin should not be used in pregnant women unless the potential benefits justify the possible risks to the fetus.

Reproduction studies in rats and rabbits using oral ofloxacin in dosages up to 810 and 160 mg/kg daily, respectively, have not revealed evidence of teratogenicity. However, fetotoxicity (decreased fetal body weight and increased fetal mortality) did occur in rats and rabbits receiving oral ofloxacin dosages equivalent to 50 and 10 times the usual human dosage, respectively. In rats receiving ofloxacin dosages of 810 mg/kg daily (more than 50 times the maximum human dosage), retardation in the degree of ossification and minor skeletal variations such as cervical ribs and shortened or absent 13th ribs occurred. Perinatal and postnatal studies in rats using oral dosages up to 360 mg/kg daily revealed a decrease in food intake during gestation and an increase in food and water intake during lactation, but did not reveal evidence of adverse effects on late fetal development, labor, delivery, lactation, neonatal viability, or growth of the offspring.

Fertility

Studies in male and female rats using ofloxacin doses up to 360 mg/kg indicate that the drug does not have an appreciable effect on fertility or reproductive performance. Although administration of high dosages of some other quinolones (e.g., norfloxacin [no longer commercially available in the US]) has been associated with impaired spermatogenesis and/or testicular damage (atrophy in rats and dogs) in chronic (for 3 months or longer) toxicity studies, similar studies using ofloxacin have not revealed evidence of these adverse effects.

Lactation

Ofloxacin is distributed into milk. Because of the potential for serious adverse effects of ofloxacin in nursing infants, a decision should be made whether to discontinue nursing or the drug, taking into account the importance of the drug to the woman.

DRUG INTERACTIONS

● Drugs That Prolong QT Interval

Ofloxacin, like some other fluoroquinolones, can prolong the QT interval and should be avoided in patients receiving class IA (e.g., quinidine, procainamide) or class III (e.g., amiodarone, sotalol) antiarrhythmic agents.

● Antacids

Antacids containing magnesium, aluminum, or calcium may decrease absorption of oral quinolones resulting in decreased serum and urine concentrations of the anti-infectives. The extent of this interaction appears to vary depending on the specific quinolone and antacid involved. In patients receiving ofloxacin and an antacid concomitantly, peak serum ofloxacin concentrations may be decreased by 20-77% and areas under the plasma concentration-time curve (AUCs) decreased by 60-70%. The mechanism of this interaction has not been fully elucidated to date, but magnesium and aluminum ions may bind to and form insoluble complexes with quinolones. To minimize the possibility of an interaction, patients should be instructed not to ingest antacids concomitantly with or within 2 hours of an ofloxacin dose.

● Antiarrhythmic Agents

Concomitant use of antiarrhythmic agents may increase the risk of QT interval prolongation during ofloxacin therapy. Concomitant use of class IA (e.g., quinidine, procainamide) or class III (e.g., amiodarone, sotalol) antiarrhythmic agents should be avoided.

● Aminoglycosides

The antibacterial activities of ofloxacin and aminoglycosides (e.g., amikacin, gentamicin, tobramycin) may be additive or partially synergistic in vitro against susceptible strains of *Pseudomonas aeruginosa* or *Escherichia coli*. However, synergism between the drugs appears to be unpredictable, and indifference or antagonism has been reported more frequently.

● Antimycobacterial Agents

In vitro, the combination of ofloxacin and aminosalicylic acid, ethambutol, ethionamide, isoniazid, kanamycin, rifampin, or streptomycin is neither synergistic nor antagonistic against *Mycobacterium tuberculosis*. Although the clinical importance has not been determined, ofloxacin used in conjunction with ethambutol results in a synergistic effect in vitro against *M. avium* complex (MAC).

Adverse neurologic effects, including insomnia and seizures, have been reported in a few patients with multidrug-resistant pulmonary tuberculosis† who received concomitant oral ofloxacin (600 or 800 mg once daily) and cycloserine (500 or 750 mg once daily or a 2-dose regimen of 500 mg in the morning and 250 mg in the evening). Some clinicians suggest that, pending accumulation of additional information on this possible drug interaction, ofloxacin and cycloserine should be used concomitantly with caution.

In vitro, the combination of ofloxacin and rifampin generally is indifferent or antagonistic against *S. aureus*.

● β-Lactam Antibiotics

An additive or synergistic effect has occurred in vitro against some strains of *Staphylococcus epidermidis* and methicillin-resistant *Staphylococcus aureus* (MRSA; also known as oxacillin-resistant *S. aureus* or ORSA) when ofloxacin was used concomitantly with oxacillin; this combination generally was indifferent against ORSA. Synergism was demonstrated more readily at 30°C than at 35°C and did not appear to depend on the ofloxacin susceptibility of the organisms since it occurred in some cases even when the strain was resistant to ofloxacin alone. The clinical importance of this in vitro effect is unclear since many strains of staphylococci, principally ORSA, are resistant to ofloxacin.

Indifference generally occurred in vitro when ofloxacin was used in combination with ampicillin or nafcillin against Enterobacteriaceae or *Ps. aeruginosa*.

In vitro, the combination of ofloxacin and cefotaxime was neither synergistic nor antagonistic against Enterobacteriaceae, including *Klebsiella pneumoniae* and *E. coli* that were slightly susceptible or resistant to cefotaxime.

Ofloxacin used in conjunction with imipenem has been additive or synergistic in vitro against some strains of staphylococci, streptococci, *Ps. aeruginosa*, and Enterobacteriaceae; however, synergism appears to be unpredictable and this combination may be indifferent or antagonistic against these organisms.

● Antiretroviral Agents

Didanosine

Buffered didanosine preparations (pediatric oral solution admixed with antacid) may interfere with oral absorption of ofloxacin. To minimize the possibility of interaction, patients should be instructed not to ingest buffered didanosine preparations concomitantly with or within 2 hours of an ofloxacin dose.

Zidovudine

In vitro studies using ofloxacin and zidovudine indicate that the antiviral agent does not antagonize ofloxacin's antibacterial activity against susceptible *S. aureus*, *S. epidermidis*, *E. coli*, *Salmonella typhimurium*, or *Ps. aeruginosa*. Although the clinical importance in unclear, the combination of ofloxacin and zidovudine resulted in a slightly additive antibacterial effect in vitro against *E. coli* and *S. typhimurium*.

● Other Anti-infectives

In one in vitro study, the combination of ofloxacin and bismuth subcitrate was not synergistic against *Helicobacter pylori*.

In vitro, the antibacterial activity of ofloxacin and metronidazole is additive or indifferent against anaerobic bacteria; neither synergism nor antagonism occurs with this combination.

● Antidiabetic Agents

Alterations in blood glucose concentrations resulting in hypoglycemia have been reported in diabetic patients receiving ofloxacin and concomitant antidiabetic agents (e.g., insulin, glyburide). If ofloxacin is used in a diabetic patient receiving insulin or an oral antidiabetic agent, blood glucose and concentrations should be monitored carefully. Ofloxacin should be discontinued immediately and a clinician consulted if a hypoglycemic reaction occurs.

● Cimetidine, Ranitidine, and Sucralfate

Concomitant administration of cimetidine reportedly may interfere with the elimination of some quinolones resulting in prolonged serum half-lives and AUCs of the drugs. It is not known if this occurs with ofloxacin.

Concomitant administration of ranitidine does not appear to alter oral absorption of ofloxacin.

Concomitant administration of sucralfate reportedly may interfere with GI absorption of ofloxacin, and some clinicians state that concomitant use of ofloxacin with sucralfate is not recommended. If concomitant use of ofloxacin and sucralfate is necessary, the manufacturer and some clinicians recommend that patients be instructed not to ingest sucralfate concomitantly with or within 2 hours of an ofloxacin dose.

● Corticosteroids

Concomitant use of corticosteroids increases the risk of severe tendon disorders (e.g., tendinitis, tendon rupture), especially in geriatric patients older than 60 years of age. (See Cautions: Tendinitis and Tendon Rupture.)

● Coumarin Anticoagulants

In some patients stabilized on warfarin, prolongation of the prothrombin time occurred following initiation of ofloxacin therapy. Concomitant administration of some other quinolones (e.g., ciprofloxacin) in patients receiving coumarin anticoagulants also has resulted in increased prothrombin times. The mechanism of this interaction has not been determined to date; these drugs may displace the anticoagulants from serum albumin binding sites or may suppress vitamin K production by intestinal bacteria. Ofloxacin should be administered with caution in patients receiving a coumarin anticoagulant, and prothrombin times should be monitored in patients receiving concomitant therapy.

● Cyclosporine

Concomitant use of some quinolones in patients receiving cyclosporine reportedly may result in increased cyclosporine serum concentrations. It is not known if this occurs with ofloxacin.

● Iron, Multivitamins, and Mineral Supplements

Oral multivitamin and mineral supplements containing divalent or trivalent cations such as iron or zinc may decrease oral absorption of ofloxacin resulting in decreased serum concentrations of the quinolone; therefore, these multivitamins and/or mineral supplements should not be ingested concomitantly with or within 2 hours of an ofloxacin dose.

In a crossover study, concomitant administration of a single dose of oral ferrous sulfate complex and ofloxacin decreased the AUC of the anti-infective by 36%.

● Nonsteroidal Anti-inflammatory Agents

Concomitant administration of a fluoroquinolone (i.e., ofloxacin) and fenbufen (a nonsteroidal anti-inflammatory agent [NSAIA]) reportedly resulted in an increased incidence of seizures. Concomitant use of a fluoroquinolone with an NSAIA could increase the risk of CNS stimulation (e.g., seizures). Animal studies using other fluoroquinolones suggest that the risk may vary depending on the specific NSAIA.

● Probenecid

Studies using other fluoroquinolones (e.g., ciprofloxacin) indicate that concomitant administration of probenecid interferes with renal tubular secretion of the drugs. The effect of concomitant administration of probenecid and ofloxacin has not been studied to date.

● Xanthine Derivatives

Concomitant administration of some fluoroquinolone anti-infectives (e.g., ciprofloxacin, ofloxacin) in patients receiving theophylline has resulted in higher and prolonged serum theophylline concentrations and may increase the risk of theophylline-related adverse effects. The extent of this interaction varies considerably among the commercially available fluoroquinolones; the effect is less pronounced

with ofloxacin than with ciprofloxacin. While it has been suggested that the 4-oxo metabolites of these quinolones may inhibit metabolism of theophylline in the liver, and there is some evidence that the degree to which the various quinolones are metabolized to 4-oxo metabolites may correlate with the extent of alteration in theophylline pharmacokinetics when the drugs are administered concomitantly, the potential contribution, if any, of the 4-oxo metabolites to this interaction has not been fully elucidated. In addition, other evidence indicates that, while formation of these metabolites may correlate with inhibition of theophylline metabolism, the 4-oxo metabolites themselves are not responsible for the observed effect.

In some controlled studies in patients receiving ofloxacin and theophylline concomitantly, the pharmacokinetics of theophylline were not altered substantially; in other studies, serum theophylline concentrations were increased by 9-10%, the AUC of the drug increased by 10–13%, and theophylline clearance decreased by 0–16%. Concomitant theophylline does not affect the pharmacokinetics of ofloxacin.

Although the risk of serious adverse effects resulting from theophylline toxicity appears to be low when usual dosages of ofloxacin are used, most studies to date evaluating concomitant therapy have been done in healthy adults; experience with concomitant use of the drugs in patients considered at higher risk for adverse effects (e.g., geriatric patients with chronic obstructive pulmonary disease, patients with impaired renal or hepatic function) is limited. Therefore, the manufacturer and some clinicians recommend that plasma theophylline concentrations be monitored and the patient observed for manifestations of theophylline toxicity whenever ofloxacin is given concomitantly; appropriate theophylline dosage adjustments should be made if needed.

Although some quinolones (e.g., ciprofloxacin) have been reported to alter the pharmacokinetics of caffeine, results of several studies in healthy adults indicate that ofloxacin does not have a clinically important effect on the elimination half-life, total body clearance, or volume of distribution of caffeine. Therefore, although precautions relating to caffeine intake may be necessary in patients receiving these other quinolones, these precautions do not appear to be necessary in patients receiving ofloxacin.

LABORATORY TEST INTERFERENCES

● Tests for Opiates

Some quinolones, including ofloxacin, may cause false-positive results for opiates when commercially available immunoassay kits for urine screening are used. It may be necessary to confirm positive opiate screening test results using more specific methods.

ACUTE TOXICITY

The oral LD$_{50}$ of ofloxacin is 3.6–5.5 g/kg in mice and rats and exceeds 200 mg/kg in dogs. The IV LD$_{50}$ of the drug is 208–276 mg/kg in mice and rats and exceeds 70 mg/kg in dogs.

● Manifestations

In animals receiving oral ofloxacin, acute toxicity is manifested as ptosis, hypoactivity, sedation, prostration, hypopnea, dyspnea, and seizures. Limited information is available on the acute toxicity of ofloxacin in humans. Overdosage of ofloxacin would be expected to produce manifestations that principally are extensions of the adverse reactions reported with the drug, and may include nausea, vomiting, seizures, vertigo, dysgeusia, and psychosis.

A 23-year-old woman who inadvertently received approximately 3 g of ofloxacin IV over 45 minutes (a parenteral preparation is no longer commercially available in the US) developed drowsiness, nausea, hot and cold flashes, facial flushing and edema, slurred speech, dizziness, and disorientation during the infusion; all manifestations except dizziness, which was exacerbated on standing, and nausea resolved within 1 hour after discontinuance of the infusion, with the latter effects resolving several hours later. Serum ofloxacin concentration 15 minutes after completion of the infusion in this woman was approximately 40 mcg/mL. In a 14-year-old who ingested an unknown quantity of ofloxacin along with therapeutic doses of diphenhydramine and chlormezanone (no longer commercially available in the US), confusion, delirium, agitation, hallucinations, extreme mydriasis, and dry and warm skin occurred within a few hours; plasma concentrations of ofloxacin 12 hours after ingestion were

15 mcg/mL. Although activated charcoal was administered and forced diuresis was initiated, symptoms persisted for the next several days until IV physostigmine salicylate was given. It was suggested that the anticholinergic and psychotic manifestations observed in this patient may have resulted from a drug interaction between ofloxacin and diphenhydramine and/or chlormezanone.

● Treatment

If acute overdosage of ofloxacin occurs, the stomach should be emptied by inducing emesis or by gastric lavage. Supportive and symptomatic treatment should be initiated, and the patient should be observed carefully; adequate hydration should be maintained. Because ofloxacin is not efficiently removed by hemodialysis or peritoneal dialysis, these procedures should not be relied on to enhance elimination of the drug from the body.

MECHANISM OF ACTION

Ofloxacin usually is bactericidal in action. Like other fluoroquinolone anti-infectives, ofloxacin inhibits DNA synthesis in susceptible organisms via inhibition of the enzymatic activities of 2 members of the DNA topoisomerase class of enzymes, DNA gyrase and topoisomerase IV. DNA gyrase and topoisomerase IV have distinct essential roles in bacterial DNA replication. DNA gyrase, a type II DNA topoisomerase, was the first identified quinolone target; DNA gyrase is a tetramer composed of 2 GyrA and 2 GyrB subunits. DNA gyrase introduces negative superhelical twists in DNA, an activity important for initiation of DNA replication. DNA gyrase also facilitates DNA replication by removing positive super helical twists. Topoisomerase IV, another type II DNA topoisomerase, is composed of 2 ParC and 2 ParE subunits. DNA gyrase and topoisomerase IV are structurally related; ParC is homologous to GyrA and ParE is homologous to GyrB. Topoisomerase IV acts at the terminal states of DNA replication by allowing for separation of interlinked daughter chromosomes so that segregation into daughter cells can occur. Fluoroquinolones inhibit these topoisomerase enzymes by stabilizing either the DNA–DNA gyrase complex or the DNA–topoismerase IV complex; these stabilized complexes block movement of the DNA replication fork and thereby inhibit DNA replication resulting in cell death.

Although all fluoroquinolones generally are active against both DNA gyrase and topoisomerase IV, the drugs differ in their relative activities against these enzymes. For many gram-negative bacteria, DNA gyrase is the primary quinolone target and for many gram-positive bacteria, topoisomerase IV is the primary target. The other enzyme is the secondary target in both cases. However, there are exceptions to this pattern. For certain bacteria (e.g., *Streptococcus pneumoniae*), the principal target depends on the specific fluoroquinolone.

The mechanism by which ofloxacin's inhibition of DNA gyrase or topoisomerase IV results in death in susceptible organisms has not been fully determined. Unlike β-lactam anti-infectives, which are most active against susceptible bacteria when they are in the logarithmic phase of growth, studies using *Escherichia coli* and *Pseudomonas aeruginosa* indicate that ofloxacin can be bactericidal during both logarithmic and stationary phases of growth. In vitro studies indicate that ofloxacin concentrations that approximate the minimum inhibitory concentration (MIC) of the drug induce filamentation in susceptible organisms and lysis; high concentrations of the drug result in enlarged or elongated cells that may not be extensively filamented and may not lyse. Although the bactericidal effect of some fluoroquinolones evidently requires competent RNA and protein synthesis in the bacterial cell, and concurrent use of anti-infectives that affect protein synthesis (e.g., chloramphenicol, tetracyclines) or RNA synthesis (e.g., rifampin) inhibit the in vitro bactericidal activity of these drugs, the bactericidal effect of ofloxacin, like that of ciprofloxacin, is only partially reduced in the presence of these anti-infectives. This suggests that ofloxacin, like ciprofloxacin, has an additional mechanism of action that is independent of RNA and protein synthesis.

For most susceptible organisms, the minimum bactericidal concentration (MBC) of ofloxacin is 1–4 times higher than the MIC.

Mammalian cells contain type II topoisomerase similar to that contained in bacteria. At concentrations attained during therapy, quinolones do not appear to appreciably affect the mammalian enzyme.

Results of in vitro studies indicate that exposure of some plasmid-containing bacteria (e.g., *E. coli*) to ofloxacin or other fluoroquinolones may result in loss of plasmid DNA. This effect is unpredictable and depends on the specific plasmid and concentration of drug. It is unclear whether this effect is related to inhibition of DNA gyrase or some other mechanism of action of the drugs.

In vitro studies, particularly those involving in vitro susceptibility tests, indicate that the antibacterial activity of ofloxacin, like that of ciprofloxacin, is decreased in the presence of urine, especially acidic urine. The clinical importance of this in vitro effect has not been determined to date; however, because ofloxacin concentrations attained in urine are usually substantially higher than ofloxacin MICs for most urinary tract pathogens, the effect probably is not clinically important.

SPECTRUM

Ofloxacin has a spectrum of activity similar to that of some other fluoroquinolones (e.g., ciprofloxacin). In vitro on a weight basis, the activity of ofloxacin against susceptible gram-positive bacteria is approximately equal to that of ciprofloxacin. The activity of ofloxacin against susceptible gram-negative bacteria is slightly less than that of ciprofloxacin.

Ofloxacin is active in vitro against many gram-positive aerobic bacteria, including penicillinase-producing, nonpenicillinase-producing, and some oxacillin-resistant staphylococci (previously known as methicillin-resistant staphylococci). Ofloxacin is active in vitro against most gram-negative aerobic bacteria, including Enterobacteriaceae and *Pseudomonas aeruginosa*. Like other fluoroquinolones, ofloxacin generally is less active against gram-positive than gram-negative bacteria. Ofloxacin has some activity in vitro against obligately anaerobic bacteria, but most of these organisms, including *Bacteroides fragilis*, are considered resistant to the drug. The drug also has some activity in vitro against *Chlamydia*, *Mycoplasma*, *Mycobacterium*, *Plasmodium*, and *Rickettsia*. Ofloxacin is inactive against fungi.

● Gram-positive Aerobic Bacteria
Gram-positive Aerobic Cocci

Ofloxacin is active in vitro against most strains of *Staphylococcus aureus*, *S. epidermidis*, and *S. saprophyticus*. The drug is active against both penicillinase-producing and nonpenicillinase-producing staphylococci and also is active in vitro against some oxacillin-resistant *S. aureus* (ORSA). However, *S. aureus*, including ORSA, that are resistant to ofloxacin and other fluoroquinolones have been reported with increasing frequency. (See: Resistance.)

Ofloxacin is less active in vitro on a weight basis against streptococci than against staphylococci. *Streptococcus pneumoniae*, *S. pyogenes* (group A β-hemolytic streptococci; GAS), and group B streptococci (*S. agalactiae*; GBS), viridans streptococci (e.g., *S. mitis*), Groups C, F, and G streptococci, and nonenterococcal group D streptococci (e.g., *S. bovis*) generally are inhibited in vitro by ofloxacin concentrations of 4 mcg/mL or less. Ofloxacin is equally active against both penicillin-susceptible and -resistant strains of *S. pneumoniae*. Ofloxacin is active in vitro against some strains of enterococci, including *Enterococcus faecalis* (formerly *S. faecalis*).

Table 1 includes MIC$_{50}$s (minimum inhibitory concentrations of the drug at which 50% of strains tested are inhibited) and MIC$_{90}$s (minimum inhibitory concentrations of the drug at which 90% of strains tested are inhibited) of ofloxacin reported for gram-positive aerobic cocci:

TABLE 1.

Organism	MIC$_{50}$ (mcg/mL)	MIC$_{90}$ (mcg/mL)
Staphylococcus aureus	0.2–0.5	0.2–1.6
S. epidermidis	0.2–0.5	0.125–1
S. saprophyticus	0.5–2	0.5–2
Oxacillin-resistant *S. aureus*	0.25–2	0.25–4
Streptococcus pneumoniae	1–3.1	1–6.25
Group A streptococci	1–2	1–4
Group B streptococci	1–4	1–6.3
Groups C, F, and G streptococci	1–2	2–4
Viridans streptococci	1–2	2–4
Nonenterococcal group D streptococci	1.2–2	2.5–4
Enterococci	0.8–4	1.6–6.3

Gram-positive Aerobic Bacilli

Ofloxacin is active against *Bacillus anthracis* in vitro. In several in vitro studies, *B. anthracis* isolates had ofloxacin MICs of 0.03–0.25 mcg/mL. Anti-infectives are active against the germinated form of *B. anthracis*, but are not active against the organism when it is still in the spore form. Strains of *B. anthracis* with naturally occurring resistance to fluoroquinolones have not been reported to date. However, reduced susceptibility to ofloxacin (fourfold increase in MICs from baseline) was produced in vitro following sequential subculture of the Sterne strain of *B. anthracis* in subinhibitory concentrations of the fluoroquinolone.

Ofloxacin is active in vitro against *Corynebacterium*. The MIC_{90} of the drug reported for *C. diphtheria*, JK strains of *Corynebacterium*, *Corynebacterium* D2, and *C. jeikeium* is 0.5–1 mcg/mL.

Ofloxacin is active in vitro against *Listeria monocytogenes*, and the MIC_{90} of the drug reported for this organism is 1–8 mcg/mL.

Although some strains of *Nocardia asteroides* are inhibited in vitro by ofloxacin concentrations of 4–8 mcg/mL, this organism generally is considered resistant to the drug.

● *Gram-negative Aerobic Bacteria*

Neisseria

Ofloxacin is active in vitro against some strains of penicillinase- and nonpenicillinase-producing *Neisseria gonorrhoeae* and *N. gonorrhoeae* with chromosomally mediated resistance to penicillin (CMRNG) or plasmid-mediated tetracycline resistance (TRNG). The MIC_{90} of ofloxacin is 0.007–0.1 mcg/mL for most penicillinase- or nonpenicillinase-producing *N. gonorrhoeae*, CMRNG, and TRNG. However, *N. gonorrhoeae* with decreased susceptibility to fluoroquinolones (quinolone-resistant *N. gonorrhoeae*; QRNG) have been reported with increasing frequency. To date, most strains of *N. gonorrhoeae* with reduced susceptibility have ofloxacin MICs of 0.13–0.5 mcg/mL; however, strains with ofloxacin MICs of 2 mcg/mL also have been reported. (See Resistance: Resistance in Neisseria gonorrhoeae.)

Ofloxacin is active in vitro against *N. meningitidis*, and the MIC_{90} of the drug for this organisms usually is 0.015–0.03 mcg/mL.

Haemophilus

Ofloxacin is active in vitro against β-lactamase- and non-β-lactamase-producing *Haemophilus influenzae*, and the MIC_{90} of the drug for these organisms is 0.02–0.13. *H. parainfluenzae* generally are inhibited in vitro by ofloxacin concentrations of 0.25 mcg/mL. The MIC_{90} of ofloxacin for *H. ducreyi* is 0.03–2 mcg/mL. Ofloxacin is active against β-lactamase-producing *H. ducreyi* and is active against strains resistant to tetracycline, ampicillin, and sulfamethoxazole.

Moraxella catarrhalis

Ofloxacin is active in vitro against both β-lactamase- and non-β-lactamase-producing strains of *Moraxella catarrhalis* (formerly *Branhamella catarrhalis*), and the MIC_{90} of the drug reported for this organism is 0.06–1 mcg/mL.

Enterobacteriaceae

Ofloxacin is active in vitro against most clinically important Enterobacteriaceae. With the exception of *Providencia* and *Serratia*, the MIC_{90} of ofloxacin for Enterobacteriaceae generally is 2.5 mcg/mL or less. Ofloxacin is active against some Enterobacteriaceae resistant to aminoglycosides and/or β-lactam antibiotics.

Table 2 includes MIC_{50}s and MIC_{90}s of ofloxacin reported for Enterobacteriaceae:

TABLE 2.

Organism	MIC₅₀ (mcg/mL)	MIC₉₀ (mcg/mL)
Citrobacter spp.	0.03–0.1	0.06–0.6
C. diversus	0.03–0.13	0.06–1
C. freundii	0.06–0.4	0.12–0.8
Enterobacter spp.	0.03–0.1	0.06–2.5
E. aerogenes	0.06–0.13	0.125–1.6
E. agglomerans	0.06–0.2	0.25–2

Organism	MIC₅₀ (mcg/mL)	MIC₉₀ (mcg/mL)
E. cloacae	0.05–0.13	0.25–3.1
Escherichia coli	0.015–0.06	0.05–0.2
Hafnia alvei	0.03–0.125	0.06–0.25
Klebsiella spp.	0.03–0.125	0.06–0.25
K. oxytoca	0.06–0.25	0.06–0.5
K. pneumoniae	0.06–0.25	0.12–0.5
Morganella morganii	0.03–0.15	0.06–0.5
Proteus mirabilis	0.06–0.3	0.12–0.5
P. vulgaris	0.03–0.125	0.06–1.6
Providencia rettgeri	0.12–1	0.5–8
P. stuartii	0.12–1	0.25–6.25
Serratia spp.	0.25–0.3	0.5–2.5
S. marcescens	0.25–1.6	0.5–6.3
Salmonella spp.	0.04–0.13	0.06–0.25
S. enteritidis	0.06	0.125
S. typhi	0.03	0.06–0.12
Shigella spp.	0.03–0.125	0.03–0.25
Yersinia enterocolitica	0.06–0.125	0.06–0.25

Ofloxacin is active in vitro against most strains of *Ps. aeruginosa* and also has some activity against other *Pseudomonas*. The MIC_{50} and MIC_{90} of ofloxacin for *Ps. aeruginosa* are 0.25–3.2 and 1–6.3 mcg/mL, respectively. The MIC_{90} of the drug for *Ps. acidovorans*, *Ps. fluorescens*, and *Ps. putida* is 0.4–1.6 mcg/mL and the MIC_{90} for *Xanthomonas maltophilia* (*Ps. maltophilia*) is 1.6–8 mcg/mL. Although some strains of *Burkholderia cepacia* (formerly *Ps. cepacia*), *Brevundimonas diminuta* (formerly *Ps. diminuta*, *Ps. paucimobilis*, and *B. pseudomallei* (formerly *Ps. pseudomallei*) are inhibited by ofloxacin concentrations of 8 mcg/mL or less, many of these organisms require concentrations of 16–32 mcg/mL for in vitro inhibition and are considered resistant to the drug.

Vibrio

Ofloxacin is active in vitro against *Vibrio cholerae* and *V. parahaemolyticus*, and the MIC_{90} of the drug reported for these organisms is 0.008–0.13 mcg/mL.

Other Gram-negative Aerobic Bacteria

The MIC_{90} of ofloxacin for *Acinetobacter lwoffi* (*A. calcoaceticus* subsp. *lwoffi*) and *A. baumannii* (*A. calcoaceticus* subsp. *anitratus*) is 0.25–2 mcg/mL.

Aeromonas hydrophila, *A. caviae*, and *A. sobria* generally are inhibited in vitro by ofloxacin concentrations of 0.03–0.1 mcg/mL. The MIC_{90} of ofloxacin reported for *Plesiomonas shigelloides* is 0.015–0.06 mcg/mL. *Alcaligenes xylosoxidans* (*Achromobacter xylosoxidans*) and *Alcaligenes faecalis* may require ofloxacin concentrations of 1.6–32 mcg/mL for in vitro inhibition.

Ofloxacin is active in vitro against some strains of *Campylobacter fetus* subsp. *jejuni*, and the MIC_{90} of the drug for this organism is 0.25–1.25 mcg/mL. The MIC_{90} of ofloxacin reported for *Helicobacter pylori* is 0.25 mcg/mL. However, emergence of strains of *Campylobacter* resistant to fluoroquinolones has been reported in areas with widespread use of the drugs. (See Resistance.)

Bordetella pertussis and *B. parapertussis* generally are inhibited by ofloxacin concentrations of 0.03–0.125 mcg/mL. *B. bronchiseptica* may be inhibited by ofloxacin concentrations of 1.6–8 mcg/mL.

The MIC_{90} of ofloxacin reported for *Brucella melitensis*, *B. abortus*, and *Flavobacterium* is 0.5–4 mcg/mL, and the MIC_{90} reported for *Pasteurella multocida* and *Eikenella corrodens* is 0.03–0.125 mcg/mL.

Ofloxacin has in vitro activity against *Francisella tularensis*.

Ofloxacin has in vitro activity against *Yersinia pestis*. In a study evaluating in vitro susceptibility of 100 *Y. pestis* isolates obtained from plague patients in Africa, all isolates were inhibited by ofloxacin concentrations of 0.12 mcg/mL or less. In another study, isolates obtained from plague patients, rats, or fleas from Vietnam were inhibited by ofloxacin concentrations of 0.03–0.25 mcg/mL. Ofloxacin also has been shown to have in vivo activity against *Y. pestis* in murine plague infections. However, mutant strains of *Y. pestis* resistant to fluoroquinolones (e.g., ciprofloxacin) have been selected in vitro.

Some strains of *Gardnerella vaginalis* (formerly *Haemophilus vaginalis*) are inhibited in vitro by ofloxacin concentrations of 1–2 mcg/mL; other strains require concentrations of 16–32 mcg/mL for in vitro inhibition and are considered resistant to the drug.

Ofloxacin is active in vitro against *Legionella pneumophila*, *L. bozemanii*, *L. dumoffii*, *L. gormanii*, *L. jordanis*, *L. longbeachae*, *L. micdadei* (the Pittsburgh pneumonia agent), and *L. wadsworthii*, and the MIC of the drug reported for these organisms is 0.03–0.25 mcg/mL.

● Anaerobic Bacteria

Ofloxacin has some activity against gram-positive and -negative anaerobic bacteria; however, high concentrations of the drug generally are required for in vitro inhibition and most of these organisms are considered resistant to the drug. The MIC$_{90}$ of ofloxacin for *Peptococcus* and *Peptostreptococcus* is 2–8 mcg/mL. Some strains of *Clostridium perfringens* and *C. welchii* may be inhibited in vitro by ofloxacin concentrations of 0.5–1 mcg/mL, but most clostridia require ofloxacin concentrations of 8 mcg/mL or greater for in vitro inhibition and are considered resistant to the drug.

The MIC$_{90}$ of ofloxacin reported for *Bacteroides fragilis* is 2–8 mcg/mL. Ofloxacin concentrations of 0.02–2 mcg/mL may inhibit some strains of *Prevotella melaninogenica* and *B. ureolyticus*. The MIC$_{90}$ of ofloxacin for *B. distasonis*, *B. ovatus*, *B. thetaiotaomicron*, *B. uniformis*, and *B. vulgatus* is 8–32 mcg/mL, and these organisms are considered resistant to the drug. Some strains of *Eubacterium*, *Fusobacterium*, and *Veillonella* may be inhibited in vitro by ofloxacin concentrations of 0.5–4 mcg/mL.

● Chlamydia and Mycoplasma

Ofloxacin is active in vitro against *Chlamydia trachomatis*, *C. pneumoniae*, and *C. psittaci*, and these organisms generally are inhibited in vitro by concentrations of 0.5–4 mcg/mL. The minimum lethal concentration (MLC) of ofloxacin reported for *C. trachomatis* is similar to the MIC and ranges from 0.5–8 mcg/mL. Both urogenital and ocular isolates of *C. trachomatis* are inhibited in vitro by ofloxacin.

Ofloxacin also is active in vitro against *Mycoplasma hominis*, *M. pneumoniae*, and *Ureaplasma urealyticum*. The MIC$_{90}$ of ofloxacin reported for *M. hominis* and *M. pneumoniae* is 1–2 mcg/mL and the MIC$_{90}$ for *U. urealyticum* is 1.6–8 mcg/mL.

● Mycobacterium

Ofloxacin is active in vitro against some *Mycobacterium*. In vitro on a weight basis, ofloxacin is slightly less active than ciprofloxacin or levofloxacin against these organisms. The MIC$_{90}$ of ofloxacin for *M. tuberculosis* and *M. kansasii* is 0.6–2.4 mcg/mL. The MIC$_{90}$ for *M. bovis*, *M. fortuitum*, *M. gordonae*, and *M. xenopi* is 0.03–2.5 mcg/mL. The MIC$_{90}$ of the drug for *M. avium* complex generally is 2–16 mcg/mL; ofloxacin concentrations greater than 8 mcg/mL are required for in vitro inhibition of *M. chelonae* and *M. scrofulaceum*.

Ofloxacin is active in vitro against *M. leprae* and is bactericidal in vivo against *M. leprae* in mouse footpad studies.

● Other Organisms

Although the clinical importance in unclear, ofloxacin has some activity in vitro against *Plasmodium falciparum*. Results of in vitro tests indicate that ofloxacin is active against both chloroquine-susceptible and -resistant *P. falciparum*, but is less active against these organisms than ciprofloxacin.

Ofloxacin has some activity in vitro against *Rickettsia conorii*, the causative organism of Mediterranean spotted fever, and *Coxiella burnetii*, the causative organism of Q fever.

Although the clinical importance has not been determined, ofloxacin has some activity against the Lister strain of vaccinia virus in vitro in mammalian cell cultures and in vivo in mice. In similar tests, the drug had only weak antiviral effects against herpes simplex virus (HSV) and no appreciable effects against influenza virus.

Ofloxacin has some activity against *Trypanosoma cruzi*, the causative organism of Chagas' disease. The drug is inactive against *Treponema pallidum*. Ofloxacin also is inactive against *Trichomonas vaginalis*.

RESISTANCE

Resistance to ofloxacin can be produced easily in vitro in some strains of Enterobacteriaceae, *Pseudomonas aeruginosa*, streptococci, and *Staphylococcus aureus*, including methicillin-resistant *Staphylococcus aureus* (MRSA; also known as oxacillin-resistant *S. aureus* or ORSA), by serial passage in the presence of increasing concentrations of the drug. Ofloxacin resistance resulting from spontaneous mutation occurs only rarely in vitro (i.e., with a frequency of 10^{-11} to 10^{-9}). Spontaneous mutation occurs in a single step and results in low-level resistance to the drug.

Resistant strains of *Ps. aeruginosa* have emerged rarely during therapy with the drug, especially in patients with cystic fibrosis; in some cases, the development of resistance was not associated with clinical failure of ofloxacin therapy. Resistant strains of *Escherichia coli* also have emerged rarely during therapy with the drug. Although the clinical importance is unclear, ofloxacin-resistant strains of *Ps. aeruginosa* and *Bacteroides fragilis* have been reported with increasing frequency since the drug was introduced.

Strains of *S. aureus*, especially ORSA resistant to fluoroquinolones, have been reported with increasing frequency. Emergence of fluoroquinolone resistance in staphylococci has been alarmingly rapid. In one hospital in Georgia, high-level resistance to ciprofloxacin (MIC$_{90}$ 64 mcg/mL or greater) was apparent within 3 months of availability of the drug and increased from a baseline of 0% to 79% of ORSA isolates over a 1-year period; such resistance also increased to 14% of isolates in oxacillin-susceptible strains over the same period. In some countries (e.g., Israel, France, Canada), approximately 30–90% of clinical isolates of ORSA reportedly are resistant to fluoroquinolones; less than 10% of oxacillin-susceptible strains in these countries are resistant to the drugs. Results of resistance surveys indicate that fluoroquinolone resistance has emerged in multiple strains of ORSA; however, at some institutions, resistance occurred principally in a single ORSA strain which was then nosocomially transmitted to other patients.

Rapid emergence of resistance to fluoroquinolones in *Campylobacter* also has been reported and appears to be associated with widespread use or prolonged therapy with the drugs. In several patients with chronic active gastritis and duodenal ulcers, MICs of ofloxacin for *H. pylori* (formerly *C. pylori*) increased from 0.25–1 mcg/mL prior to ofloxacin therapy to 16–32 mcg/mL after 4 weeks of therapy. Over a 10- to 12-year period in Finland, fluoroquinolone-resistant strains of *C. jejuni* and *C. coli* increased from 0–4% to 9–11%. A similar increase was observed over a 7-year period in *Campylobacter* isolates obtained from poultry and humans in the Netherlands; this increase in resistance was attributed to use of enrofloxacin in the poultry industry. In the US, fluoroquinolone-resistant isolates of *Campylobacter* have been obtained from raw turkey or chicken products in the retail market.

● Resistance in Neisseria gonorrhoeae

Neisseria gonorrhoeae with decreased susceptibility to ofloxacin and other fluoroquinolones (quinolone-resistant *N. gonorrhoeae*; QRNG) are widely disseminated throughout the world, including in the US. *N. gonorrhoeae* with decreased susceptibility to one fluoroquinolone also have decreased susceptibility to other fluoroquinolones (e.g., ciprofloxacin, ofloxacin), but may be susceptible to ceftriaxone, cefixime, and spectinomycin (currently not commercially available in the US).

● Resistance in Mycobacterium

Ofloxacin-resistant strains of *Mycobacterium tuberculosis* have been reported. Resistance has developed in initially susceptible *M. tuberculosis* in some patients with pulmonary tuberculosis receiving ofloxacin in conjunction with antituberculosis agents. Some multidrug-resistant strains of *M. tuberculosis* (i.e., strains resistant to rifampin and isoniazid) also are resistant to ofloxacin or other fluoroquinolones. Extensively drug-resistant tuberculosis (XDR tuberculosis) caused by strains resistant to rifampin and isoniazid (multiple-drug resistant strains) and also resistant to a fluoroquinolone and at least one parenteral second-line antimycobacterial (capreomycin, kanamycin, amikacin) has been reported with increasing frequency.

Some strains of *M. kansasii* are resistant to ofloxacin.

● Mechanisms of Fluoroquinolone Resistance

The mechanism(s) of resistance to fluoroquinolones, including ofloxacin, has not been fully elucidated but appears to involve mutations in the target DNA type II topoisomerase enzymes and mutations that result in alterations in membrane permeability and/or efflux pumps.

Resistance to fluoroquinolones generally occurs as a result of mutational amino acid substitutions in the subunits (i.e., Gyr A, Gyr B, Par C, Par E) of the more sensitive (i.e., the primary target) topoisomerase enzyme (i.e., DNA gyrase or topoisomerase IV). Mutations in the primary target precede those in the secondary target, in a stepwise selection for resistance; mutations in both targets produce high level resistance. A single mutational event in the more sensitive primary target can result in an increase in the MIC of the drug. If the altered primary-target enzyme remains more sensitive to the quinolone than does the secondary target, the altered primary target will continue to determine the MIC. If the altered primary target becomes less sensitive than the secondary target, the MIC will be determined by the inhibitory activity of the quinolone against the secondary target. If both DNA gyrase and topoisomerase IV are equally sensitive to the quinolone, a single mutational alteration in either enzyme will not result in an increase in MIC.

Resistance to ofloxacin in gram-negative organisms (e.g., Enterobacteriaceae, *Ps. aeruginosa*) appears to result from mutations that alter the A subunits. Resistance in some gram-negative organisms also may be related to alterations in outer-membrane porin proteins and/or other factors that affect permeability of the organism to the drug. The mechanism of resistance in gram-positive bacteria has not been studied as extensively, but results of in vitro studies using *S. aureus* indicate that resistance to fluoroquinolones in some gram-positive bacteria also results from alterations in one of the subunits of topoisomerase IV and DNA gyrase. In addition, resistance in some *S. aureus* appears to be related to the *norA* gene located in the D fragment of the organism's chromosome. The *norA* gene apparently encodes a hydrophobic membrane protein that results in decreased membrane permeability by hydrophilic quinolones such as ofloxacin. A third possible mechanism of resistance in *S. aureus* also has been suggested and appears to be related to mutations(s) in the *flq* locus of the A fragment of the chromosome; further study is needed to determine whether mutation(s) in this fragment alters a second topoisomerase or another gene controlling supercoiling or whether it affects permeability. Although further study is needed, it appears that *S. aureus* can have either low-level or high-level resistance to fluoroquinolones that results from one or more alterations in topoisomerase IV and DNA gyrase. Current evidence suggests that resistance to ofloxacin or other fluoroquinolones in either gram-negative or -positive bacteria is chromosomally rather than plasmid mediated.

● **Cross-resistance**

Cross-resistance can occurs between ofloxacin and other fluoroquinolones.

Cross-resistance generally does not occur between ofloxacin and other anti-infectives, including aminoglycosides, β-lactam antibiotics, sulfonamides (including co-trimoxazole), macrolides, and tetracyclines. However, rare strains of Enterobacteriaceae and *Ps. aeruginosa* resistant to fluoroquinolones also are resistant to aminoglycosides, β-lactam antibiotics, chloramphenicol, trimethoprim, and/or tetracyclines. Resistance in these organisms appears to be related to alterations in outer-membrane porin proteins. Rarely, strains of *E. coli* or *Ps. aeruginosa* that were originally susceptible to fluoroquinolones and resistant to aminoglycosides and β-lactam antibiotics developed resistance to fluoroquinolones and reverted to being susceptible to aminoglycosides and β-lactams. It has been suggested that this may occur because exposure of some plasmid-containing bacteria to ofloxacin and other fluoroquinolones can result in loss of plasmid DNA in these organisms. (See Mechanism of Action.) In addition, fluoroquinolone-resistant ORSA frequently also are resistant to aminoglycosides.

PHARMACOKINETICS

In studies described in the Pharmacokinetics section, body fluid and tissue concentrations of ofloxacin were measured with either a high-pressure liquid chromatographic (HPLC) assay or a microbiologic assay. HPLC assays presumably would be more specific for ofloxacin than microbiologic assays since the latter method measures the antibacterial activity of the parent drug as well as its microbiologically active metabolite(s). However, controlled studies comparing results obtained using HPLC and microbiologic assays indicate that these methods provide essentially equivalent results for serum, urine, and CSF ofloxacin concentrations and pharmacokinetic parameters determined using these concentrations. This apparently occurs because ofloxacin is not extensively metabolized and only low concentrations of active ofloxacin metabolite(s) are attained in serum or urine.

The pharmacokinetics of ofloxacin after oral administration are best described by a 2-compartment open model. There is some evidence that disposition of the commercially available racemic mixture of ofloxacin (see Chemistry and Stability: Chemistry) is stereoselective principally as a result of differences in renal excretion of the enantiomers; however, such differences appear to be small.

● **Absorption**

Ofloxacin is rapidly and almost completely absorbed from the GI tract following oral administration. The drug does not undergo appreciable first-pass metabolism.

Although presence of food in the GI tract can decrease the rate and/or extent of absorption of ofloxacin to some extent, this effect is not usually considered clinically important. In an open, randomized, cross-over study in healthy adult men receiving a single 300-mg oral dose of ofloxacin with or without a standard breakfast, maximum serum concentrations and area under the concentration-time curves (AUCs) were slightly lower when the dose was given with food, but the time to peak serum concentrations, terminal elimination half-life, and urinary concentrations of the drug did not differ substantially between fasted and nonfasting conditions. When a 400-mg ofloxacin tablet was crushed and mixed with 120 mL of enteral premixed liquid (Ensure) and swallowed, the AUC was 10% lower and peak plasma concentrations were 36% lower compared with results attained when the tablet was crushed and mixed with water before swallowing. Milk and yogurt do not appear to affect GI absorption of ofloxacin.

Antacids may decrease the oral bioavailability of ofloxacin. (See Drug Interactions: Antacids.)

The oral bioavailability of ofloxacin is 85–100% in healthy, fasting adults, and peak serum concentrations of the drug generally are attained within 0.5–2 hours. In patients with normal renal and hepatic function, peak serum concentrations and AUCs increase in proportion to the dose over the oral dosage range of 100–600 mg and generally are unaffected by age.

Following oral administration of a single 100-, 200-, 300-, or 400-mg dose of ofloxacin in healthy, fasting adults, peak serum concentrations average 1–1.3, 1.5–2.7, 2.4–4.6, or 2.9–5.6 mcg/mL, respectively. Some accumulation occurs following multiple doses. Steady-state serum concentrations of ofloxacin are achieved after 4 doses of the drug and are approximately 40% higher than concentrations achieved following single oral doses.

Pharmacokinetic parameters in geriatric patients receiving ofloxacin generally are similar to those in younger adults. Although results of pharmacokinetic studies in geriatric individuals 65–81 years of age indicate that the rate of absorption, volume of distribution, and route of excretion in geriatric individuals are similar to those in younger adults, peak serum concentrations are slightly higher (9–21% higher) and half-life more prolonged in geriatric patients than in younger adults. There also is evidence that peak plasma concentration are higher in geriatric women than geriatric men (114% higher following single doses or 54% higher following multiple doses).

Following oral administration of usual dosage of ofloxacin in patients with cystic fibrosis, peak serum concentrations and AUCs are similar to those reported in healthy adults.

● **Distribution**

Ofloxacin is widely distributed into body tissues and fluids following oral administration. In healthy adults, the apparent volume of distribution of ofloxacin averages 1–2.5 L/kg. Impaired renal function does not appear to affect the volume of distribution of ofloxacin; the apparent volume of distribution of the drug averages 1.1–2 L/kg in patients with impaired renal function, including those with severe renal failure undergoing hemodialysis.

Ofloxacin is distributed into bone, cartilage, bile, skin, sputum, bronchial secretions, pleural effusions, tonsils,saliva, gingival mucosa, nasal secretions, aqueous humor, tears, sweat, lung, blister fluid, pancreatic fluid, ascitic fluid, peritoneal fluid, gynecologic tissue, vaginal fluid, cervix, ovary, semen, prostatic fluid, and prostatic tissue. For most of these tissues and fluids, ofloxacin concentrations are approximately 0.5–1.7 times concurrent serum concentrations. Ofloxacin is concentrated within neutrophils, achieving concentrations in these cells that may be up to 8 times greater than extracellular concentrations.

In cholecystectomy patients who received oral ofloxacin in a dosage of 200 mg every 12 hours, concentrations of the drug in samples obtained during surgery (6 hours after the 7th dose) ranged from 1.7–9.9 mcg/g in gallbladder wall, 2.1–79.2 mcg/mL in gallbladder bile, and 3.2–19.6 mcg/mL in common duct bile; concomitant serum concentrations ranged from 1–4.2 mcg/mL.

Following a single 400-mg oral dose of ofloxacin in geriatric men 65–81 years of age, prostatic fluid concentrations ranged from 2.5–5.6 mcg/mL and prostatic adenoma tissue concentrations ranged from 2.4–5.6 mcg/g.

Ofloxacin is distributed into CSF following oral administration. Peak concentrations of ofloxacin in CSF generally are attained within 2–6 hours and exhibit considerable interindividual variation, depending in part on the degree of meningeal inflammation. Peak CSF concentrations may be 28–87% of concurrent serum concentrations. In adults with meningitis, a single 300-mg oral dose of ofloxacin resulted in CSF concentrations ranging from 0.1–2.8 or 0.1–2.2 mcg/mL in samples obtained 3 or 6 hours, respectively, after the dose.

Ofloxacin is 20–32% bound to serum proteins.

Ofloxacin crosses the placenta and is distributed into cord blood and amniotic fluid. The drug is distributed into milk following oral administration. In one study in lactating women who received 400-mg oral doses of ofloxacin every 12 hours, drug concentrations averaged 0.29–2.4 mcg/mL in milk and 0.26–2.5 mcg/mL in serum 2–12 hours after a dose; the drug still was detectable in milk 24 hours after a dose.

● Elimination

In healthy adults with normal renal function, the elimination half-life of ofloxacin in the distribution phase ($t_{1/2}\alpha$) averages 0.5–0.6 hours and the elimination half-life in the terminal phase ($t_{1/2}\beta$) averages 4–8 hours. In healthy geriatric adults 64–86 years of age with renal function normal for their age, half-life of the drug averages 6.4–8.5 hours. The slower elimination of ofloxacin in geriatric individuals presumably is due to reduced renal function and clearance observed in geriatric individuals.

In adults with impaired renal function, serum concentrations of ofloxacin are higher and the half-life prolonged. In adults with creatinine clearances of 10–50 mL/minute, half-life of the drug averages 16.4 hours (range: 11–33.5 hours); in adults with creatinine clearances less than 10 mL/minute, half-life averages 21.7 hours (range: 16.9–28.4 hours). In patients with end-stage renal failure, half-life of the drug may range from 25–48 hours. Further study is needed to determine whether hepatic impairment effects the pharmacokinetics of ofloxacin. In one study in cirrhotic adults with ascites and creatinine clearances of 47–123 mL/minute who received a single 200-mg oral dose of ofloxacin, peak serum concentrations of the drug averaged 3.6 mcg/mL and half-life averaged 11.6 hours; however, these alterations in pharmacokinetics appeared to result from renal (tubular) rather than hepatic effects.

Less than 10% of a single dose of ofloxacin is metabolized; approximately 3–6% of the dose is metabolized to desmethyl ofloxacin and 1–5% is metabolized to ofloxacin N-oxide. Desmethyl ofloxacin is microbiologically active, but is less active against susceptible organisms than is ofloxacin; ofloxacin N-oxide has only minimal antibacterial activity. Ofloxacin and its metabolites are excreted in both urine and feces. Following a single 100- to 600-mg oral dose of ofloxacin, 65–90% of the dose is excreted unchanged in urine within 48 hours; less than 5% of the dose is excreted in urine as metabolites. Approximately 4–8% of the dose is excreted in feces. Following oral administration of a single 200-mg oral dose of ofloxacin, urine concentrations average 220 mcg/mL in urine collected over 0–6 hours after the dose; concentrations in urine collected over 12–24 hours after the dose average 34 mcg/mL. In healthy adults receiving 200-mg oral doses of ofloxacin every 12 hours, fecal concentrations of the drug have been reported to average 38–44 mcg/g (range: 30–65 mcg/g). However, other limited data suggest that this dosage produces fecal concentrations of approximately 300 mcg/g.

Renal clearance of ofloxacin averages 133–200 mL/minute in adults with normal renal function.

Small amounts of ofloxacin and desmethyl ofloxacin are removed by hemodialysis. The amount of drug removed during hemodialysis depends on several factors (e.g., type of coil used, dialysis flow rate). In patients with end-stage renal disease undergoing hemodialysis, the serum half-life of ofloxacin averages 8–12 hours during hemodialysis and 13–48 hours between dialysis sessions. Approximately 10–21% of a single 100- or 200-mg oral dose of ofloxacin is removed by hemodialysis, and approximately 10% of a single 200-mg oral dose is removed by peritoneal dialysis. In a study in patients with end-stage renal failure who were maintained on continuous ambulatory peritoneal dialysis (CAPD), less than 2% of a 400-mg oral dose of ofloxacin was removed by the procedure.

CHEMISTRY AND STABILITY

● Chemistry

Ofloxacin is a fluoroquinolone anti-infective agent. Like all other commercially available fluoroquinolones, ofloxacin contains a fluorine at the C-6 position of the quinolone nucleus. Like some other fluoroquinolones (ciprofloxacin, levofloxacin), ofloxacin contains a piperazinyl group at position 7 of the quinolone nucleus. The piperazinyl group in ofloxacin results in antipseudomonal activity. The piperazinyl group contained in ofloxacin is methylated, unlike the piperazinyl group contained in ciprofloxacin, and this may contribute to the greater oral bioavailability of ofloxacin compared with that of these other fluoroquinolones. Ofloxacin also contains an oxazine ring linking the nitrogen at position 1 and the carbon at position 8 of the quinolone nucleus. This fused ring results in increased activity against gram-positive and anaerobic bacteria and also contributes to ofloxacin's low degree of in vivo metabolism. The methyl group at the C-3 position in the oxazine ring results in the formation of isoenantiomers; ofloxacin occurs as a racemic mixture of the two isomers. The S-(-)isomer is 8–128 times as active against susceptible gram-positive and gram-negative organisms as the R-(+)isomer and approximately twice as active as racemic ofloxacin.

Ofloxacin occurs as an off-white to pale yellow crystalline powder. At room temperature, ofloxacin is soluble in aqueous solutions with pH 2–5, sparingly to slightly soluble (4 mg/mL) in aqueous solutions with pH 7, and freely soluble in aqueous solutions with pH greater than 9. The pK_as of the drug are 5.74 and 7.9.

● Stability

Ofloxacin tablets should be stored at 20–25°C in tight, light-resistant containers.

PREPARATIONS

Excipients in commercially available drug preparations may have clinically important effects in some individuals; consult specific product labeling for details.

Ofloxacin

Oral		
Tablets, film-coated	200 mg*	Ofloxacin Tablets
	300 mg*	Ofloxacin Tablets
	400 mg*	Ofloxacin Tablets

* available from one or more manufacturer, distributor, and/or repackager by generic (nonproprietary) name

† Use is not currently included in the labeling approved by the US Food and Drug Administration.

Selected Revisions September 9, 2019, © Copyright, December 1, 1991, American Society of Health-System Pharmacists, Inc.

Co-trimoxazole

8:12.20 • SULFONAMIDES

■ Co-trimoxazole is a synergistic fixed combination of sulfamethoxazole (an intermediate-acting antibacterial sulfonamide), and trimethoprim; both sulfamethoxazole and trimethoprim are synthetic folate-antagonist anti-infectives.

USES

● Acute Otitis Media

Co-trimoxazole is used in adults† and children for the treatment of acute otitis media (AOM) caused by susceptible strains of *Streptococcus pneumoniae* or *Haemophilus influenzae* when the clinician makes the judgment that the drug offers some advantage over use of a single anti-infective. Data are limited to date regarding safety of repeated use of co-trimoxazole in pediatric patients younger than 2 years of age; the drug should not be administered prophylactically or for prolonged periods for the treatment of otitis media in any age group.

Various anti-infectives, including oral amoxicillin, oral amoxicillin and clavulanate potassium, various oral cephalosporins (cefaclor, cefdinir, cefixime, cefpodoxime proxetil, cefprozil, ceftibuten, cefuroxime axetil, cephalexin), IM ceftriaxone, oral co-trimoxazole, oral erythromycin-sulfisoxazole, oral azithromycin, oral clarithromycin, and oral loracarbef, have been used in the treatment of AOM. The AAP, CDC, and other clinicians state that, despite the increasing prevalence of multidrug-resistant *S. pneumoniae* and presence of β-lactamase-producing *H. influenzae* or *M. catarrhalis* in many communities, amoxicillin remains the anti-infective of first choice for treatment of uncomplicated AOM since amoxicillin is highly effective, has a narrow spectrum of activity, is well distributed into middle ear fluid, and is well tolerated and inexpensive.

Co-trimoxazole is not considered a first-line agent for treatment of AOM, but is recommended as an alternative for individuals with type I penicillin hypersensitivity. Because *S. pneumoniae* resistant to amoxicillin also frequently are resistant to co-trimoxazole, clarithromycin, and azithromycin, these drugs may not be effective in patients with AOM who fail to respond to amoxicillin. For additional information regarding treatment of AOM and information regarding prophylaxis of recurrent AOM, treatment of persistent or recurrent AOM, and treatment of otitis media with effusion (OME), see Uses: Otitis Media in the Aminopenicillins General Statement 8:12.16.08.

● GI Infections

Travelers' Diarrhea

Oral co-trimoxazole is used in adults and children† for the treatment of enteritis caused by enterotoxigenic *Escherichia coli* that occurs during or soon after travel to developing countries or other areas where hygiene is poor (travelers' diarrhea). Travelers' diarrhea is a condition characterized by a twofold or greater increase in the frequency of unformed bowel movements; other manifestations may include abdominal cramps, nausea, bloating, urgency, fever, and malaise. The principal cause of travelers' diarrhea is infection with enterotoxigenic *E. coli*, but other infectious agents (e.g., *Shigella*, *Salmonella*, *Campylobacter* spp.) have also been associated with the disease.

Treatment of the condition depends on severity of the illness; travelers' diarrhea is usually a mild, self-limited disorder. In individuals with mild to moderate disease, replacement therapy with oral fluids and electrolytes may be sufficient, although therapy with nonspecific or antimotility agents (e.g., bismuth subsalicylate, loperamide) may be useful for temporary relief of associated symptoms (e.g., abdominal cramps and diarrhea). Travelers who develop diarrhea with at least 3 loose stools in an 8-hour period, especially if associated with nausea, vomiting, abdominal cramps, fever, or blood in the stools, may benefit from short-term treatment with an anti-infective agent. Fluoroquinolones (ciprofloxacin, levofloxacin, norfloxacin ofloxacin) usually are considered the drugs of choice when treatment of travelers' diarrhea is indicated. Co-trimoxazole can be used as an alternative in children who cannot receive fluoroquinolones; however, resistance to co-trimoxazole has been reported in many areas.

Efficacy of anti-infective therapy may depend on the etiologic agent and its susceptibility to antibiotics. In several controlled studies, therapy for 3–5 days with oral co-trimoxazole or trimethoprim alone substantially reduced the duration of abdominal pain and nausea and the number of unformed stools in individuals with the disease; mild rash occurred infrequently with both therapies. In another controlled study, concomitant therapy with co-trimoxazole and loperamide for 3 days provided more rapid relief of travelers' diarrhea than therapy with either drug alone, and co-trimoxazole given alone as a single dose† (320 mg of trimethoprim given as co-trimoxazole) was also more effective than placebo in treating the condition. However, because of the development of resistance to co-trimoxazole in many areas, other anti-infective agents (e.g., ciprofloxacin, levofloxacin, ofloxacin), which also have been used with success in the treatment of travelers' diarrhea, may be considered first. Nausea and vomiting without diarrhea should not be treated with anti-infectives. Individuals with persistent diarrhea and severe fluid loss, fever, and blood or mucus in the stools should seek medical attention.

Oral co-trimoxazole also has been used effectively to prevent travelers' diarrhea† in individuals traveling for relatively short periods to areas where enterotoxigenic *E. coli* and other causative bacterial pathogens (e.g., *Shigella*) are known to be susceptible to the drug. Because travelers' diarrhea is a relatively nonthreatening illness that is usually mild and self-limiting and can be effectively treated and because of the risks of widespread use of anti-infective agents prophylactically (i.e., potential adverse drug reactions, selection of resistant organisms and increased susceptibility to infections caused by these or other organisms), the US Centers for Disease Control and Prevention (CDC) and most experts recommend that anti-infectives *not* be used prophylactically by most individuals traveling to areas of risk. In addition, although controlled studies have indicated that various anti-infectives when taken prophylactically have been 52–95% effective in preventing travelers' diarrhea in several developing areas of the world, efficacy depends on resistance patterns of pathogenic bacteria in each travel area, and such information seldom is available. While fluoroquinolone resistance for bacteria causing travelers' diarrhea currently is least common, this could change as use of these drugs increases worldwide. The CDC states that although use of anti-infective agents for prophylaxis of travelers' diarrhea in certain high-risk groups, such as travelers with immunosuppression or immunodeficiency, may seem reasonable, there currently are no specific data to support such prevention in these populations. (For information on prophylaxis of travelers' diarrhea in HIV-infected individuals, see Travelers' Diarrhea under Uses: GI Infections, in Ciprofloxacin 8:12.18.) Anti-infectives that have been used for prophylaxis of travelers' diarrhea are not effective in preventing diarrhea caused by viral or parasitic infections, and use of such prophylaxis may give a false sense of security to the traveler about the risk associated with consuming certain local foods and beverages. The principal preventive measure is prudent dietary practices. If prophylaxis is used, ciprofloxacin, levofloxacin, ofloxacin, or norfloxacin can be given for a maximum of 3 weeks.

Shigella Infections

Co-trimoxazole is used IV or orally for the treatment of enteritis caused by susceptible strains of *Shigella flexneri* or *S. sonnei*. Choice of anti-infective therapy should be based on drug susceptibility of the isolated organism. Although therapy may be initiated based on local susceptibility patterns pending results of susceptibility testing, some clinicians currently state that, when the susceptibility of the isolate is unknown, fluoroquinolones are the anti-infectives of choice with co-trimoxazole as an alternate, especially in areas where ampicillin-resistant strains of *Shigella* have been reported. Fluoroquinolones are the drugs of choice and co-trimoxazole an alternate for the treatment of shigellosis when the organism is resistant to ampicillin or the patient is allergic to ampicillin.

Escherichia coli Infections

Co-trimoxazole has been used in the treatment of GI infections caused by *Escherichia coli*†.

Optimal therapy for diarrhea caused by enterotoxigenic *E. coli*† (ETEC) is not established and resistance is common. AAP states that if diarrhea caused by ETEC is suspected in a traveler to a resource-limited country, use of co-trimoxazole, azithromycin, or ciprofloxacin should be considered if diarrhea is severe or intractable and if in vitro testing indicates that the causative organism is susceptible. A parenteral regimen should be used if systemic infection is suspected.

For the treatment of dysentery caused by enteroinvasive *E. coli*† (EIEC), the AAP suggests than an oral anti-infective (e.g., co-trimoxazole, azithromycin, ciprofloxacin) can be used if in vitro tests indicate the causative organism is susceptible.

The role of anti-infectives in patients with hemorrhagic colitis caused by shiga toxin-producing *Escherichia coli* (STEC; formerly known as enterohemorrhagic *E. coli*†) is unclear and most experts do not recommend use of anti-infectives for treatment of children with enteritis caused by *E. coli* 0157:H7.

● Respiratory Infections

Co-trimoxazole is used in adults for treatment of acute exacerbation of chronic bronchitis caused by susceptible strains of *Streptococcus pneumoniae* or *Haemophilus influenzae* when the clinician makes the judgment that the drug offers some advantage over use of a single anti-infective. Co-trimoxazole is considered by many clinicians to be the drug of choice for the treatment of upper respiratory tract infections and bronchitis caused by *H. influenzae*. The drug also is used as an alternative to penicillin G or penicillin V for the treatment of respiratory tract infections caused by *Streptococcus pneumoniae*. Co-trimoxazole is as effective as amoxicillin, ampicillin, erythromycin, or tetracycline in the treatment of acute exacerbations of chronic bronchitis.

Many clinicians consider co-trimoxazole an alternative for the treatment of infections caused by *Legionella micdadei*† (*L. pittsburgensis*) or *L. pneumophila*†.

Co-trimoxazole should *not* be used in the treatment of pharyngitis caused by *S. pyogenes* (group A β-hemolytic streptococci); results of clinical studies indicate that co-trimoxazole therapy is associated with a higher bacteriologic failure rate (as evidenced by failure to eradicate *S. pyogenes* from the tonsillopharyngeal area) than penicillin therapy.

● Urinary Tract Infections

Co-trimoxazole is used for the treatment of urinary tract infections (UTIs) caused by susceptible strains of *E. coli*, *Proteus* (indole-positive or -negative), *Klebsiella*, *Morganella morganii*, or *Enterobacter*.

Co-trimoxazole, given in single doses, as 3-day therapy, or for 7–10 days, is effective in the treatment of acute uncomplicated UTIs. Some clinicians consider a 3-day regimen of co-trimoxazole the treatment of choice for the empiric treatment of acute uncomplicated UTIs. Co-trimoxazole also is used for the treatment of acute complicated UTIs (e.g., UTIs associated with abnormalities of the urinary tract or neurogenic bladder), but other anti-infectives are preferred by most clinicians. For the treatment of acute pyelonephritis, some clinicians recommend anti-infective treatment for 7–14 days. Mild cases of pyelonephritis in women can be treated with an oral fluoroquinolone or with co-trimoxazole (if the causative organism is known to be susceptible). If the infection is likely to be caused by gram-positive bacteria, amoxicillin or amoxicillin and clavulanate potassium may be used. Patients with more severe infections should be hospitalized and therapy should be initiated using a parenteral regimen. Some clinicians recommend that acute pyelonephritis be treated with a parenteral fluoroquinolone or, alternatively, an aminoglycoside with or without ampicillin or an extended-spectrum cephalosporin; an aminoglycoside with or without ampicillin sodium and sulbactam sodium is recommended if the infection is likely to be caused by gram-positive bacteria. When treating acute uncomplicated UTI, the causative organism should be cultured and susceptibility tests conducted prior to initiation of co-trimoxazole therapy; co-trimoxazole may be initiated, however, before obtaining the results of these tests. Some clinicians also recommend obtaining follow-up urine cultures after discontinuance of anti-infective therapy to determine whether the bacteria have been eliminated.

Most clinicians reserve co-trimoxazole for the treatment of chronic or recurrent UTIs. In chronic or recurrent UTIs, the drug suppresses fecal and vaginal flora and usually does not select out resistant coliforms. For the treatment of chronic or recurrent UTIs resulting from reinfection or relapse in women, low doses of co-trimoxazole (e.g., 40 mg of trimethoprim and 200 mg of sulfamethoxazole given nightly or 3 times weekly) are as effective as other anti-infectives (e.g., methenamine mandelate, nalidixic acid, nitrofurantoin) and are preferred by many clinicians. Men with prostatitis-associated recurrent UTIs usually respond poorly to anti-infectives. Although 14-day courses of co-trimoxazole in such patients reportedly are associated with failure rates of greater than 60%, efficacy of the drug appears to be increased markedly with treatment courses of 3–6 months.

● Brucellosis

Oral co-trimoxazole is considered an alternative to tetracyclines for the treatment of brucellosis† when tetracyclines are contraindicated, including brucellosis in pediatric patients. To decrease the incidence of relapse, many clinicians recommend that rifampin be used in conjunction with co-trimoxazole or a tetracycline.

For treatment of serious brucellosis or when there are complications, including endocarditis, meningitis, or osteomyelitis, some clinicians recommend that an aminoglycoside (streptomycin or gentamicin) be used concomitantly with co-trimoxazole or a tetracycline for the first 7–14 days of therapy; rifampin can also be included in the regimen to reduce the risk of relapse.

● Burkholderia Infections

Co-trimoxazole is used for the treatment of infections caused by *Burkholderia cepacia*†. Co-trimoxazole is considered the drug of choice and ceftazidime, chloramphenicol, or imipenem are alternatives for these infections.

Co-trimoxaozle is used for the treatment of melioidosis† caused by susceptible *B. pseudomallei*, usually in a multiple-drug regimen with chloramphenicol and doxycycline. Ceftazidime or imipenem monotherapy is recommended as the drug of choice for these infections. *B. pseudomallei* is difficult to eradicate and relapse of melioidosis is common.

● Cholera

Co-trimoxazole is used in the treatment of cholera† when anti-infective therapy is indicated as an adjunct to fluid and electrolyte replacement. Tetracyclines usually are considered the drugs of choice for the treatment of cholera, and co-trimoxazole, a fluoroquinolone, erythromycin, or furazolidone (no longer commercially available in the US) is recommended when tetracyclines are contraindicated or when the infection is caused by tetracycline-resistant *Vibrio cholerae*. *V. cholerae* serogroup 0139 Bengal may not be susceptible to co-trimoxazole or furazolidone.

● Cyclospora Infections

The CDC and others consider co-trimoxazole the treatment of choice for cyclosporiasis infection† caused by *Cyclospora cayetanensis*, a coccidian parasite that causes severe, generally self-limiting, diarrhea.

● Granuloma Inguinale (Donovanosis)

Co-trimoxazole is used for the treatment of granuloma inguinale (donovanosis) caused by *Calymmatobacterium granulomatis*†. The CDC recommends that donovanosis be treated with a regimen of oral co-trimoxazole or oral doxycycline or, alternatively, a regimen of oral ciprofloxacin, oral erythromycin, or oral azithromycin. Anti-infective treatment of donovanosis should be continued until all lesions have healed completely; a minimum of 3 weeks of treatment usually is necessary. If lesions do not respond within the first few days of therapy, the CDC recommends that addition of a parenteral aminoglycoside (e.g., 1 mg/kg of gentamicin IV every 8 hours) to the regimen be considered. Erythromycin should be used to treat donovanosis in pregnant and lactating women; addition of a parenteral aminoglycoside (e.g., gentamicin) to the regimen should be strongly considered in these women. Anti-infective treatment appears to halt progressive destruction of tissue, although prolonged duration of therapy often is required to enable granulation and reepithelialization of ulcers. Despite effective anti-infective therapy, donovanosis may relapse 6–18 months later.

Individuals with HIV infection should receive the same treatment regimens recommended for other individuals with donovanosis; however, the CDC suggests that addition of a parenteral aminoglycoside (e.g., gentamicin) to the regimen should be strongly considered in HIV-infected patients.

Any individual who had sexual contact with a patient with donovanosis should be examined and treated if they had sexual contact with the patient during the 60 days preceding the onset of symptoms in the patient and they have clinical signs and symptoms of the disease.

● Isosporiasis

Many clinicians consider co-trimoxazole the drug of choice for the treatment of isosporiasis† caused by *Isospora belli*.

● Listeria Infections

Co-trimoxazole has been used successfully in the treatment of meningitis caused by *Listeria monocytogenes*†, and some clinicians consider the drug the preferred alternative for the treatment of listeria infections (except endocarditis) in penicillin-allergic patients.

● Mycobacterial Infections

Co-trimoxazole has been used in the treatment of cutaneous infections caused by *Mycobacterium marinum*† and is considered an alternative to minocycline.

• Nocardia Infections

Co-trimoxazole has been used in the treatment of infections caused by Nocardia†, including *N. asteroides*, *N. brasiliensis*, and *N. caviae*.Co-trimoxazole or a sulfonamide alone (e.g., sulfisoxazole, sulfamethoxazole) are considered drugs of choice for the treatment of nocardiosis. Alternative anti-infectives for the treatment of nocardiosis include a tetracycline (should not be used in pregnant women or children younger than 8 years of age), amoxicillin and clavulanate potassium, imipenem, meropenem, amikacin, cycloserine, or linezolid. Amikacin and cycloserine generally should be reserved for use in the treatment of severe infections when other drugs are ineffective. Some clinicians suggest that in patients with nocardiosis involving the CNS or when the infection is disseminated or overwhelming, amikacin be included during the first 4–12 weeks of therapy or until there is clinical improvement. In vitro susceptibility testing, if available, is recommended to guide selection of an anti-infective agent for the treatment of severe nocardiosis or for the treatment of patients unable to tolerate a sulfonamide.

Nocardiosis in immunocompetent patients with lymphocutaneous disease usually responds after 6–12 weeks of appropriate anti-infective therapy. Immunocompromised patients and those with invasive disease require 6–12 months of anti-infective therapy and, because of the possibility of relapse, therapy should be continued for at least 3 months after apparent cure; nocardiosis in patients with human immunodeficiency virus (HIV) infection may require even longer therapy. Drainage of abscesses may be beneficial, especially in immunocompromised patients.

• Pertussis

Although efficacy of the drug remains to be fully determined, the CDC and other experts currently consider co-trimoxazole an alternative to erythromycin for the treatment of the catarrhal stage of pertussis† to potentially ameliorate the disease and reduce its communicability. Co-trimoxazole also is considered an alternative to erythromycin for the prevention of pertussis† in household and other close contacts (e.g., day-care facility attendees) of patients with the disease.

• Plague

Co-trimoxazole has been used for *postexposure prophylaxis* of plague†. Although recommended by the CDC and other clinicians as an alternative agent for such prophylaxis in infants and children younger than 8 years of age, efficacy of the drug for prevention of plague is unknown. Most experts (e.g., CDC, AAP, US Working Group on Civilian Biodefense, US Army Medical Research Institute of Infectious Diseases) recommend oral ciprofloxacin or doxycycline for postexposure prophylaxis in adults and most children. Postexposure prophylaxis with anti-infectives is recommended after high-risk exposures to plague, including close exposure to individuals with naturally occurring plague, during unprotected travel in active epizootic or epidemic areas, or laboratory exposure to viable *Yersinia pestis*.

Co-trimoxazole also has been used in the *treatment* of plague†, but appears to be less effective than other anti-infectives used for treatment of the disease (e.g., streptomycin, gentamicin). Because of lack of efficacy, some experts state that co-trimoxazole should not be used for the treatment of pneumonic plague.

For more information on the management of plague exposure, see Uses: Plague, in Streptomycin 8:12.02.

• Pneumocystis jiroveci (Pneumocystis carinii) Pneumonia

Treatment

Co-trimoxazole is used for the treatment of *Pneumocystis jiroveci* (formerly *Pneumocystis carinii*) pneumonia (PCP). When given IV or orally, the drug has a cure rate of 70–80% in patients with PCP. Because co-trimoxazole has excellent tissue penetration and therapy with the agent is associated with rapid clinical response (i.e., 3–5 days in patients with mild to moderate infection), co-trimoxazole currently is considered the initial drug of choice for most patients with this infection. Co-trimoxazole also is considered the drug of choice for the treatment of PCP in patients with acquired immunodeficiency syndrome (AIDS); however, in patients with AIDS, co-trimoxazole is associated with an increased incidence of adverse reactions (especially fever and adverse dermatologic and hematologic reactions). In patients who are intolerant of co-trimoxazole, treatment alternatives include pentamidine isethionate (IV), trimetrexate glucuronate, trimethoprim and dapsone, clindamycin and primaquine, or atovaquone.

Prevention

Co-trimoxazole is used for the prophylaxis of PCP, both for the prevention of initial episodes (*primary prevention*) and for the prevention of recurrence (*secondary prevention* or chronic maintenance therapy) following an initial episode, in immunosuppressed individuals considered to be at increased risk of developing PCP. Some clinicians consider HIV-infected patients, patients with cancer (especially children with acute lymphocytic leukemia receiving maintenance chemotherapy), or renal transplant recipients with active cytomegalovirus infections to be candidates for co-trimoxazole prophylaxis.

Co-trimoxazole is used for prophylaxis of PCP in patients with HIV infection, although an increased risk of toxicity in these patients has been reported. Some evidence indicates that co-trimoxazole may be better tolerated in HIV-infected children than adults. In addition, patients receiving the drug for prophylaxis of PCP appear to tolerate the drug better than those patients receiving it for treatment of PCP. In a placebo-controlled study in adults with AIDS and newly diagnosed Kaposi's sarcoma but no history of opportunistic infections, no cases of PCP were observed in patients receiving co-trimoxazole (*primary prevention*) for a mean survival period of about 2 years; such pneumonia occurred in 53% of patients receiving placebo and developed within 5 months in 80% of patients who discontinued co-trimoxazole because of toxicity.

Data from a study of 2 cohorts of HIV-positive men whose cases were followed for more than 9 years demonstrated that the largest increase in survival time from the development of a helper/inducer ($CD4^+$, $T4^+$) T-cell count of 200 cells/ mm^3 was in patients diagnosed with PCP, suggesting that the combination of prophylaxis and antiretroviral therapy was a more important factor than antiretroviral therapy alone in prolonging survival. In another cohort of HIV-infected men, such prophylaxis was associated with a decreased incidence of PCP as the initial AIDS-related illness and, because of this beneficial effect and resultant delays in the onset of initial AIDS-related illness, was associated with increases in the rates of other less common opportunistic infections as the initial AIDS-related illness, including *Mycobacterium avium*complex, wasting syndrome, esophageal candidiasis, and cytomegalovirus infection. It was suggested that PCP prophylaxis may delay the development of the first AIDS-defining illness by 6–12 months. Although the generalizability of these data to other HIV-positive populations (e.g., women) is unclear, they suggest that PCP prophylaxis may have a role in prolonging survival and/or in delaying the development of AIDS-related illness in HIV-infected patients.

Primary Prophylaxis

The Prevention of Opportunistic Working Group of the US Public Health Service and the Infectious Diseases Society of America (USPHS/IDSA) recommends primary prophylaxis against PCP in HIV-infected adults and adolescents with $CD4^+$ T-cell counts less than 200/ mm^3 or a history of oropharyngeal candidiasis. HIV-infected adults and adolescents with a $CD4^+$ T-cell percentage of less than 14% or a history of an AIDS-defining illness who do not otherwise qualify for prophylaxis also should be considered for primary prophylaxis. If $CD4^+$ T-cell counts are monitored less frequently than every 3 months, individuals with $CD4^+$ T-cell counts of greater than 200 but less than 250/ mm^3 also should be considered for primary prophylaxis.

The USPHS/IDSA recommends oral co-trimoxazole as the drug of choice for primary prophylaxis of PCP in HIV-infected individuals. When co-trimoxazole is used for the primary prevention of PCP in adults and adolescents, the preferred dosage regimen is 160 mg of trimethoprim (as co-trimoxazole) daily. This regimen also provides prophylaxis against *Toxoplasma gondii* and some common respiratory bacterial infections. Alternatively, 80 mg of trimethoprim (as co-trimoxazole) daily or 160 mg of trimethoprim (as co-trimoxazole) 3 times a week can be used. For individuals who experience an adverse reaction to co-trimoxazole that is not life-threatening, the USPHS/IDSA recommends that the drug be continued if feasible; for individuals who have discontinued the drug because of an adverse effect, reinstitution of co-trimoxazole should be considered once the adverse effect has resolved. Patients who have experienced adverse effects, especially fever and rash, may tolerate reintroduction of co-trimoxazole better with a gradual increase in dose (desensitization) or reintroduction of the drug at a reduced dose or frequency of administration. Alternative regimens that can be used in patients who cannot tolerate co-trimoxazole include dapsone, dapsone with pyrimethamine and leucovorin, aerosolized pentamidine, or atovaquone.

Current evidence indicates that primary PCP prophylaxis can be discontinued in adults and adolescents responding to potent antiretroviral therapy who have a sustained (3 months or longer) increase in $CD4^+$ T-cell counts from less than 200/ mm^3 to greater than 200/ mm^3. Patients included in studies evaluating discontinuance of prophylaxis generally were receiving primary prophylaxis and antiretroviral regimens that included HIV protease inhibitors; median follow-up ranged from 6–16 months and median CD4$^+$ T-cell count at the time prophylaxis was discontinued exceeded 300/ mm^3. In addition, at the time prophylaxis was discontinued, most patients had CD4$^+$ T-cell counts exceeding 200/ mm^3 for at least 3 months and many patients had sustained plasma HIV-1 RNA levels below the detection limits of the available assays. The USPHS/IDSA states that discontinuance of primary PCP prophylaxis is recommended in patients who have sustained a CD4$^+$ T-cell count exceeding 200/ mm^3 for at least 3 months because such prophylaxis appears to add little benefit in terms of disease prevention (PCP, toxoplasmosis, bacterial infections) and discontinuance reduces the medication burden, the potential for toxicity, drug interactions, selection of drug-resistant pathogens, and cost. However, the USPHS/IDSA states that primary PCP prophylaxis should be restarted if the CD4$^+$ T-cell count decreases to less than 200/ mm^3.

Prevention of Recurrence

The USPHS/IDSA recommends long-term suppressive therapy or chronic maintenance therapy (secondary prophylaxis) in HIV-infected adults and adolescents who have a history of PCP to prevent recurrence. The same regimens recommended for primary prophylaxis are used for suppressive therapy. Secondary prophylaxis generally is administered for life, unless immune recovery has occurred as a result of potent antiretroviral therapy.

Current evidence indicates that secondary PCP prophylaxis can be discontinued in HIV-infected adults and adolescents responding to potent antiretroviral therapy who have a sustained (3 months or longer) increase in CD4$^+$ T-cell counts from less than 200/ mm^3 to greater than 200/ mm^3. Patients in studies evaluating discontinuance of secondary prophylaxis had responded to potent antiretroviral therapy with an increase in CD4$^+$ T-cell count to greater than 200/ mm^3 for at least 3 months. Most patients were receiving an antiretroviral regimen that included HIV protease inhibitors; the median CD4$^+$ T-cell count at the time prophylaxis was discontinued was greater than 300/ mm^3 and most patients had sustained plasma HIV-1 RNA levels below the detection limits of the available assays. The longest follow-up was 13 months. The USPHS/IDSA states that discontinuance of secondary PCP prophylaxis in adults and adolescents who have a sustained (3 months or longer) increase in CD4$^+$ T-cell counts to greater than 200/ mm^3 is recommended because such prophylaxis appears to add little benefit in terms of disease prevention (PCP, toxoplasmosis, bacterial infections) and discontinuance reduces the medication burden, the potential for toxicity, drug interactions, selection of drug-resistant pathogens, and cost. However, in patients who had PCP episodes when they had CD4$^+$ T-cell counts exceeding 200/ mm^3, it probably is prudent to continue secondary PCP prophylaxis for life regardless of how high the CD4$^+$ T-cell count increases in response to potent antiretroviral therapy.

If secondary PCP prophylaxis is discontinued in HIV-infected adults or adolescents meeting the recommended criteria, the USPHS/IDSA recommends that it be restarted if the CD4$^+$ T-cell count decreases to less than 200/ mm^3 or if PCP recurs at a CD4$^+$ T-cell count exceeding 200/ mm^3.

Prophylaxis in HIV-Infected Children

The CDC, American Academy of Pediatrics (AAP), USPHS/IDSA, and most clinicians recommend antimicrobial prophylaxis for PCP in selected HIV-infected children. This recommendation is based on the high mortality rate associated with PCP in infants and children and the established efficacy of prophylaxis in HIV-infected adults; it is unlikely that placebo-controlled studies will ever be performed in HIV-infected children. PCP is the most common serious HIV-associated opportunistic infection among children, occurring in more than 50% of those with perinatally acquired HIV infection that progresses to AIDS within the first year of life, and in about 40% of pediatric AIDS cases overall. In children with perinatally acquired HIV infection, PCP occurs most often at 3–6 months of age. Despite the availability of effective anti-infectives for the treatment of *P. jiroveci* infections, the median survival from the first episode in infants and children is 1–4 months; among AIDS cases reported to CDC, 35% of children with PCP died within 2 months of diagnosis. Overall, about 90% of children with PCP died and 70% survived for less than 6 months in one retrospective study despite active treatment with co-trimoxazole and/or pentamidine. Therefore, current strategies should be aimed at preventing initial and subsequent infection with the protozoa in children at high risk for HIV infection by initiating early prophylactic therapy.

The CDC, USPHS/IDSA, AAP, and other experts recommend that all infants born to HIV-infected women receive primary PCP prophylaxis starting at 4–6 weeks of age, regardless of their CD4$^+$ T-cell count. Infants who are first identified as being HIV-exposed after 6 weeks of age should receive prophylaxis beginning at the time of identification. Because of the potential for adverse drug effects in neonates and the low incidence of *P. jiroveci* infection in this age group, *primary* but not *secondary* prophylaxis should be delayed until 1 month of age. Prophylaxis can be discontinued in children who are found not to be infected with HIV. All HIV-infected infants and infants whose infection status has not yet been determined should continue prophylaxis until 12 months of age.

The need for subsequent prophylaxis should be based on age-specific CD4$^+$ T-cell count thresholds. In HIV-infected children 1–5 years of age, primary prophylaxis against PCP should be initiated if CD4$^+$ T-cell counts are less than 500/ mm^3 or the CD4$^+$ percentage is less than 15%. In HIV-infected children 6–12 years of age, primary prophylaxis against PCP should be initiated if CD4$^+$ T-cell counts are less than 200/ mm^3 or the CD4$^+$ percentage is less than 15%.

The USPHS/IDSA recommends oral co-trimoxazole as the drug of choice for the primary and secondary (suppressive or chronic maintenance therapy) prevention of PCP in HIV-infected infants and children. When co-trimoxazole is used for the primary or secondary prevention of PCP, the preferred dosage regimen is 150 mg/m^2 of trimethoprim (as co-trimoxazole) daily in 2 divided doses for 3 consecutive days each week. Alternatively, this dose can be administered as a single dose for 3 consecutive days each week, in 2 divided doses daily, or in 2 divided doses 3 times a week on alternate days. Alternative regimens that can be used in HIV-infected infants and children include dapsone, aerosolized pentamidine, or atovaquone.

The safety of discontinuing primary or secondary PCP prophylaxis in HIV-infected children receiving potent antiretroviral therapy has not been extensively studied. Children who have a history PCP should receive life-long suppressive therapy to prevent recurrence.

● Toxoplasmosis
Prevention
Primary Prophylaxis

The USPHS/IDSA recommends that, shortly after being diagnosed with HIV infection, all HIV-infected individuals be tested for IgG antibody to *Toxoplasma* to detect latent infection with *T. gondii*. HIV-infected individuals (particularly those seronegative for *Toxoplasma* antibody) should be counseled concerning the various sources of toxoplasmic infection and how best to avoid these sources, including avoiding raw or undercooked meat, washing raw vegetables, hand washing after contact with raw meat or soil, and hand washing after changing cat litter boxes. The USPHS/IDSA recommends that all HIV-infected adults and adolescents who are seropositive for *Toxoplasma* IgG antibody and who have CD4$^+$ T-cell counts less than 100/ mm^3 receive *primary* prophylaxis against toxoplasmic encephalitis. Primary prophylaxis against toxoplasmosis encephalitis generally is recommended for HIV-infected infants and children with severe immunosuppression who are seropositive for *Toxoplasma* IgG antibody. Co-trimoxazole is the drug of choice for primary prophylaxis against toxoplasmosis encephalitis and dosages of the drug recommended for prophylaxis against PCP appear to be effective against toxoplasmosis encephalitis. When co-trimoxazole is used for primary prevention of toxoplasmosis encephalitis in adults and adolescents, the preferred dosage regimen is 160 mg of trimethoprim (as co-trimoxazole) daily. In patients who cannot tolerate co-trimoxazole, regimens used for primary prophylaxis of PCP that consist of dapsone with pyrimethamine and leucovorin also provide protection against toxoplasmosis encephalitis. Atovaquone with or without pyrimethamine and leucovorin also can be used for primary prophylaxis against toxoplasmosisencephalitis. However, aerosolized pentamidine does not provide protection against toxoplasmosis encephalitis and regimens consisting of dapsone, pyrimethamine, azithromycin, or clarithromycin used alone cannot be recommended for prophylaxis against toxoplasmosis encephalitis based on current data.

HIV-infected individuals who are seronegative for *Toxoplasma* antibody and who are not currently receiving primary PCP prophylaxis with a regimen known to be active against toxoplasmosis encephalitis should be retested for *Toxoplasma* antibody if their CD4$^+$ T-cell count falls below 100/ mm^3 to determine whether they have seroconverted, are now at risk for toxoplasmosis encephalitis, and have become candidates for primary prophylaxis against the infection.

Current evidence indicates that primary prophylaxis can be discontinued with minimal risk of developing toxoplasmic encephalitis in HIV-infected adults and adolescents responding to potent antiretroviral therapy who have a sustained (3 months or longer) increase in CD4$^+$ T-cell counts from less than 200/ mm^3 to greater than 200/ mm^3. Patients included in these studies generally were receiving primary prophylaxis and antiretroviral regimens that included HIV-protease inhibitors; median follow-up ranged from 7–22 months and median CD4⁺ T-cell count at the time prophylaxis was discontinued exceeded 300/ mm³. At the time prophylaxis was discontinued, many patients had sustained plasma HIV-1 RNA levels below the detection limits of the available assays. While patients with CD4⁺ T-cell counts below 100/ mm³ are at greatest risk for toxoplasmic encephalitis, the risk in patients whose CD4⁺ T-cell counts have increased to 100–200/ mm³ has not been studied as extensively as in those whose CD4⁺ T-cell counts have increased to greater than 200/ mm³. Therefore, the recommendation to discontinue primary toxoplasmosis prophylaxis specifies that prophylaxis can be discontinued when the CD4⁺ T-cell count exceeds 200/ mm³. The USPHS/IDSA states that discontinuation of primary toxoplasmosis prophylaxis is recommended in adults and adolescents who have a sustained (3 months or longer) increase in CD4⁺ T-cell counts to greater than 200/ mm³ because such prophylaxis appears to add little benefit in terms of disease prevention for toxoplasmosis, and discontinuance reduces the pill burden, the potential for toxicity, drug interactions, selection of drug-resistant pathogens, and cost.

If primary toxoplasmosis prophylaxis is discontinued in adults and adolescents meeting the recommended criteria, the USPHS/IDSA states that it should be restarted if the CD4⁺ T-cell count decreases to less than 100–200/ mm³.

The safety of discontinuing primary toxoplasmosis prophylaxis in HIV-infected children receiving potent antiretroviral therapy has not been extensively studied.

Prevention of Recurrence

The USPHS/IDSA recommends that HIV-infected individuals who have had toxoplasmic encephalitis receive long-term suppressive or chronic maintenance therapy (secondary prophylaxis) to prevent relapse. Secondary toxoplasmosis prophylaxis generally is administered for life, unless immune recovery has occurred as a result of potent antiretroviral therapy.

The USPHS/IDSA states that the regimen of choice for secondary prophylaxis to prevent relapse of toxoplasmosis in HIV-infected adults, adolescents, infants, and children is a regimen of sulfadiazine and pyrimethamine (with leucovorin). In patients who cannot tolerate sulfonamides, a regimen of clindamycin and pyrimethamine (with leucovorin) is recommended; a regimen of atovaquone with or without pyrimethamine (with leucovorin) also is an alternative in adults and adolescents; Co-trimoxazole is not recommended for secondary toxoplasmosis prophylaxis.

For information on USPHS/IDSA recommendations regarding secondary prophylaxis of toxoplasmosis in HIV-infected individuals, including when to initiate or discontinue such prophylaxis, see Uses: Toxoplasmosis, in Pyrimethamine 8:30.08.

● Wegener's Granulomatosis

Co-trimoxazole has reportedly produced beneficial responses in a limited number of patients with Wegener's granulomatosis†, but further study is needed. Prolonged remissions have been observed in many of these patients, including some whose disease relapsed while receiving conventional therapy (e.g., cyclophosphamide), and co-trimoxazole therapy may reduce or eliminate the need for cytotoxic (e.g., cyclophosphamide) and corticosteroid therapy. Relapse has occurred occasionally during co-trimoxazole therapy but may respond to supplemental dosages of trimethoprim or the addition of small dosages of cytotoxic therapy. The precise role of co-trimoxazole in the management of Wegener's granulomatosis and the drug's effect on long-term morbidity and mortality remain to be determined, but the drug appears to be a useful alternative to more toxic drugs (e.g., cyclophosphamide) in some patients.

● Whipple's Disease

Co-trimoxazole is used in the treatment of Whipple's disease† caused by *Tropheryma whippelii*.

DOSAGE AND ADMINISTRATION

● Reconstitution and Administration

Co-trimoxazole is administered orally or by IV infusion. When oral therapy is not feasible or for severe infections, the drug may be administered IV. The drug should *not* be injected IM.

Co-trimoxazole for injection concentrate *must* be diluted prior to IV infusion. For IV infusion, each 5 mL of the concentrate for injection containing 80 mg of trimethoprim is usually diluted with 125 mL of 5% dextrose. In patients in whom fluid intake is restricted, each 5 mL of the concentrate may be diluted in 75 mL of 5% dextrose.

● Dosage

Dosage of co-trimoxazole is expressed in terms of the trimethoprim content of the fixed combination containing 5 mg of sulfamethoxazole to 1 mg of trimethoprim.

Acute Otitis Media

For the treatment of acute otitis media in children 2 months of age or older, the usual oral dosage of co-trimoxazole is 8 mg/kg of trimethoprim (as co-trimoxazole) daily in 2 divided doses every 12 hours. The usual duration of treatment is 10 days.

GI Infections
Shigella Infections

For the treatment of enteritis caused by *S. flexneri* or *S. sonnei*, the usual adult oral dosage of co-trimoxazole is 160 mg of trimethoprim (as co-trimoxazole) administered every 12 hours. The usual oral dosage for children 2 months of age or older is 8 mg/kg daily of trimethoprim (as co-trimoxazole), administered in 2 divided doses every 12 hours for 5 days.

For enteritis caused by *S. flexneri* or *S. sonnei* in children 2 months of age or older and in adults, the usual IV dosage of co-trimoxazole is 8–10 mg/kg of trimethoprim (as co-trimoxazole) daily, administered in 2–4 equally divided doses every 6, 8, or 12 hours for 5 days.

Travelers' Diarrhea

For the treatment of travelers' diarrhea in adults, co-trimoxazole has been given in a dosage of 160 mg of trimethoprim (as co-trimoxazole) every 12 hours for 3–5 days. A single oral dose of 320 mg of trimethoprim (as co-trimoxazole) has also been used for the treatment of travelers' diarrhea.

Although the use of anti-infectives for prophylaxis of travelers' diarrhea† generally is discouraged, an adult oral dosage of trimethoprim 160 mg (as co-trimoxazole) once daily during the period of risk has been used.

Respiratory Tract Infections

For the treatment of bronchitis, the usual adult oral dosage of co-trimoxazole is 160 mg of trimethoprim (as co-trimoxazole) administered every 12 hours for 14 days.

Urinary Tract Infections

For the treatment of chronic or recurrent urinary tract infections (UTIs) or prostatitis†, the usual adult oral dosage of co-trimoxazole is 160 mg of trimethoprim (as co-trimoxazole) administered every 12 hours. Most clinicians recommend continuing co-trimoxazole treatment for 10–14 days for chronic or recurrent UTIs or for 3–6 months in men with prostatitis†. For the prophylaxis† of chronic or recurrent UTIs, co-trimoxazole doses of 40–80 mg of trimethoprim (as co-trimoxazole) have been administered daily or 3 times weekly for 3–6 months. For the treatment of chronic or recurrent UTIs in children 2 months of age or older, the usual oral dosage is 8 mg/kg daily of trimethoprim (as co-trimoxazole), administered in 2 divided doses every 12 hour for 10 days.

For severe UTIs in children 2 months of age or older and in adults, the usual IV dosage of trimethoprim is 8–10 mg/kg (as co-trimoxazole) daily, administered in 2–4 equally divided doses every 6, 8, or 12 hours for up to 14 days.

Brucellosis

For the treatment of brucellosis†, some clinicians recommend that pediatric patients receive a dosage of oral trimethoprim (as co-trimoxazole) of 10 mg/kg daily (maximum 480 mg/daily) in 2 divided doses for 4–6 weeks.

Cholera

For the treatment of cholera†, the usual oral dosage of trimethoprim (as co-trimoxazole) is 4–5 mg/kg twice daily for 3 days in children or 160 mg twice daily for 3 days in adults, in conjunction with fluid and electrolyte replacement.

Cyclospora Infections

For the treatment of cyclosporiasis†, the usual oral dosage of co-trimoxazole is 160 mg of trimethoprim (as co-trimoxazole) twice daily for 7–10 days in adults or 5 mg/kg twice daily for 7–10 days in children. However, HIV-infected patients may require higher dosage and more prolonged therapy.

Granuloma Inguinale (Donovanosis)

For the treatment of granuloma inguinale (donovanosis) caused by *Calymmatobacterium granulomatis†*, the CDC recommends that oral trimethoprim (as co-trimoxazole) be given in a dosage of 160 mg twice daily for at least 3 weeks. If lesions do not respond within the first few days, addition of a parenteral aminoglycoside (1 mg/kg of gentamicin IV every 8 hours) to the regimen should be considered; addition of the aminoglycoside should be strongly considered when treating donovanosis in patients with human immunodeficiency virus (HIV) infection and in pregnant and lactating women. Despite effective anti-infective therapy, donovanosis may relapse 6–18 months later.

Isosporiasis

For the treatment of isosporiasis†, some clinicians recommend that adults receive an oral co-trimoxazole dosage of 160 mg of trimethoprim (as co-trimoxazole) twice daily for 10 days and that children receive an oral co-trimoxazole dosage of trimethoprim (as co-trimoxazole) of 5 mg/kg twice daily for 10 days. However, immunocompromised patients may require higher dosage and more prolonged therapy.

Nocardia Infections

For the treatment of nfections caused by Nocardia†, an average adult oral dosage of trimethoprim (as co-trimoxazole) of 640 mg daily has been administered for an average of 7 months.

Pertussis

Although the optimum dosage and duration of co-trimoxazole for the treatment or prevention of pertussis† have not been established, an oral dosage of 8 mg/kg of trimethoprim and 40 mg/kg of sulfamethoxazole daily in 2 divided doses has been recommended for children and a dosage of 320 mg daily in 2 divided doses has been recommended for adults. Because of reports of prophylaxis failures and delays or failure in eradication with shorter courses of anti-infective therapy in this infection, the US Public Health Service Advisory Committee on Immunization Practices (ACIP), American Academy of Pediatrics (AAP), and some clinicians recommend that a 14-day course of therapy be employed for the treatment or prevention of pertussis.

Plague

For anti-infective prophylaxis of individuals with close exposure to pneumonic plague or an exceptionally high risk of exposure to plague, the CDC recommends an oral trimethoprim (as co-trimoxazole) dosage of 320–640 mg daily in 2 equally divided doses for 7 days or a dosage of 8 mg/kg daily in 2 equally divided doses for 7 days in children at least 2 months of age.

Pneumocystis jiroveci (Pneumocystis carinii) Pneumonia

For the *treatment* of *Pneumocystis jiroveci* (formerly *Pneumocystis carinii*) pneumonia (PCP) in adults and children older than 2 months of age, the usual oral or IV dosage of trimethoprim (as co-trimoxazole) is 15–20 mg/kg daily, given in 3 or 4 equally divided doses. An IV dosage of 10–15 mg/kg daily has also been suggested for the treatment of PCP in adults with normal renal function. The usual duration of co-trimoxazole for treatment of PCP is 14–21 days.

For both *primary* and *secondary* prevention of PCP in HIV-infected adults and adolescents, the Prevention and Opportunistic Infections Working Group of the US Public Health Service and the Infectious Disease Society of America (USPHS/IDSA) and other experts recommend an oral trimethoprim (as co-trimoxazole) dosage of 160 mg once daily; alternatively, an oral trimethoprim (as co-trimoxazole) dosage of 80 mg once daily also is recommended. In patients with acute lymphocytic leukemia undergoing induction and maintenance chemotherapy, co-trimoxazole therapy given on 3 consecutive days (e.g., Monday, Tuesday, and Wednesday) weekly appears to be as effective as daily therapy for the prevention of PCP and may be associated with a lower frequency of systemic fungal infections.

For primary or secondary prophylaxis of PCP in children, including HIV-infected children, the USPHS/IDSA and other clinicians recommend an intermittent regimen of trimethoprim 150 mg/m^2 daily (as co-trimoxazole) in 2 divided doses for 3 consecutive days each week is recommended. Alternatively, the USPHS/IDSA and AAP state that 150 mg/m^2 can be administered as a single daily dose for 3 consecutive days each week, in 2 divided doses daily 7 days each week, or in 2 divided daily doses given 3 times each week on alternate days. AAP states that these dosages can be used in children 4 weeks of age† or older.

Toxoplasmosis

For primary prophylaxis against toxoplasmosis† in HIV-infected adults and adolescents, the USPHS/IDSA recommends an oral trimethoprim dosage of 160 mg (as co-trimoxazole) once daily. Alternatively, an oral dosage of trimethoprim of 80 mg once daily (as co-trimoxazole) may be used. For primary prophylaxis against toxoplasmosis in HIV-infected children, the dosage recommended by USPHS/IDSA is trimethoprim 150 mg/m^2 (as co-trimoxazole) daily in 2 divided doses.

● Dosage in Renal Impairment

In patients with impaired renal function, doses and/or frequency of administration of co-trimoxazole must be modified in response to the degree of renal impairment, severity of the infection, susceptibility of the causative organism, and serum concentrations of the drug. The manufacturers recommend that the usual adult daily dosage of co-trimoxazole be reduced 50% in patients with creatinine clearances of 15–30 mL/minute. Although the manufacturers recommend not using the drug in patients with creatinine clearances less than 15 mL/minute, some clinicians suggest using the drug in reduced dosages in these patients.

CAUTIONS

The most frequent adverse effects of co-trimoxazole are adverse GI effects (nausea, vomiting, anorexia) and sensitivity skin reactions (e.g., rash, urticaria), each reportedly occurring in about 3.5% of patients. The incidence and severity of these adverse reactions are generally dose related, and adverse reactions may occasionally be obviated by a reduction in dosage. Hypersensitivity and hematologic reactions are the most serious adverse effects of co-trimoxazole, reportedly occurring in less than 0.5% of patients. Fatal hypersensitivity reactions, including Stevens-Johnson syndrome and erythema multiforme, have occurred in several children who received co-trimoxazole. Deaths associated with hypersensitivity reactions, fulminant hepatocellular necrosis, agranulocytosis, aplastic anemia, and other blood dyscrasias have occurred with the administration of sulfonamides.

The frequency of some co-trimoxazole-induced adverse effects, including rash (usually diffuse, erythematous, and maculopapular), fever, leukopenia (neutropenia), thrombocytopenia, hyperkalemia, hyponatremia, and increased serum aminotransferase concentrations, is substantially higher in patients with acquired immunodeficiency syndrome (AIDS) than in other patients. Such adverse effects have occurred in up to 80% of AIDS patients receiving the drug, usually during the second week of therapy, but generally have been reversible following discontinuance of co-trimoxazole therapy. The exact mechanism(s) of this increased risk of co-trimoxazole toxicity has not been determined, but may be immunologically based. While it has been suggested that glutathione deficiency in HIV-infected patients and resultant accumulation of reactive hydroxylamine metabolites of sulfamethoxazole may be involved in this increased risk, this hypothesis requires confirmation. These adverse effects usually recur following rechallenge with the drug, although cautious desensitization has been performed successfully in some patients in whom continued co-trimoxazole therapy was considered necessary. Limited evidence suggests that white AIDS patients may be at greater risk of these adverse effects than black AIDS patients, indicating that genetic factors may also be important. Some evidence also indicates that co-trimoxazole may be better tolerated in HIV-infected children than adults. Adverse effects usually are less severe in patients receiving the drug for prophylaxis of *Pneumocystis jiroveci* (formerly *Pneumocystis carinii*) pneumonia compared with those receiving co-trimoxazole for treatment of the disease.

● Sensitivity Reactions

Epidermal necrolysis, exfoliative dermatitis, Stevens-Johnson syndrome, serum sickness, and allergic myocarditis are the most severe allergic reactions reported with sulfonamides alone or co-trimoxazole. Other reported allergic and anaphylactoid reactions include anaphylaxis, arthralgia, erythema multiforme, Schönlein-Henoch purpura, pruritus, urticaria, periorbital edema, corneal ring infiltrates, conjunctival and scleral injection, and photosensitivity. Mild to moderate rashes, when they occur, usually appear within 7–14 days after initiation of co-trimoxazole. Rashes are generally erythematous, maculopapular, morbilliform, and/or pruritic. Generalized pustular dermatosis and fixed drug eruption also have been reported. Patients with AIDS appear to be at particular risk of developing rash (usually diffuse, erythematous, and maculopapular) during co-trimoxazole therapy. (See the opening discussion in Cautions.)

● Hematologic Effects

Co-trimoxazole-induced hematologic toxicity has resulted rarely in aplastic anemia, agranulocytosis, leukopenia, neutropenia, thrombocytopenia, eosinophilia, megaloblastic and/or hemolytic anemia, methemoglobinemia, pancytopenia, hypoprothrombinemia, and/or purpura. Hematologic toxicity may occur with increased frequency in folate-depleted patients including geriatric, malnourished, alcoholic, pregnant, or debilitated patients; in patients receiving folate antimetabolites (e.g., phenytoin) or diuretics; in patients with hemolysis or impaired renal function; and in patients receiving co-trimoxazole in high dosages and/or for prolonged periods (e.g., longer than 6 months). In geriatric patients receiving some diuretics (principally thiazides) and co-trimoxazole concomitantly, an increased incidence of thrombocytopenia with purpura has been reported. The risk of leukopenia, neutropenia, and thrombocytopenia also appear to be increased in patients with AIDS.

Folic acid may be administered during co-trimoxazole therapy and will not interfere with the drug's antibacterial effect. Megaloblastic anemia and occasionally neutropenia and thrombocytopenia can be reversed by administration of leucovorin (folinic acid). If signs of bone marrow suppression occur in patients receiving co-trimoxazole, leucovorin should be administered; some clinicians recommend a leucovorin dosage of 5–15 mg daily until normal hematopoiesis is restored.

● GI Effects

Nausea, vomiting, and anorexia are the most frequent GI reactions to co-trimoxazole, but glossitis, stomatitis, abdominal pain, pancreatitis (sometimes fatal), pseudomembranous enterocolitis, and diarrhea also have been reported.

● Local Effects

Pain, local irritation, inflammation, and rarely thrombophlebitis may occur with IV co-trimoxazole, especially if extravascular infiltration of the drug occurs.

● Nervous System Effects

Adverse nervous system effects of co-trimoxazole include headache, insomnia, fatigue, apathy, nervousness, muscle weakness, ataxia, vertigo, tinnitus, peripheral neuritis, mental depression, aseptic meningitis, seizures, and hallucinations. Tremor and other neurologic manifestations (e.g., ataxia, ankle clonus, apathy) developed during co-trimoxazole therapy in several patients with AIDS; although such manifestations also have been associated with the underlying disease process, they resolved in these patients within 2–3 days after discontinuing the drug.

● Other Adverse Effects

Other adverse effects reported with co-trimoxazole therapy include drug fever, chills, myalgia, hepatitis (including cholestatic jaundice and hepatic necrosis), increased serum aminotransferase and bilirubin concentrations, renal failure, interstitial nephritis, increased BUN and serum creatinine concentrations, crystalluria and stone formation, toxic nephrosis with oliguria and anuria, pulmonary infiltrates, cough, shortness of breath, hypotension, periarteritis nodosa, and a positive lupus erythematosus phenomenon. Rhabdomyolysis has been reported rarely in patients receiving co-trimoxazole, mainly in HIV-infected patients. Sulfonamides chemically resemble some goitrogens, diuretics (acetazolamide, thiazides), and oral hypoglycemic agents, and cross-sensitivity may exist with these agents. Diuresis and hypoglycemia have been reported rarely in patients receiving sulfonamides.

● Precautions and Contraindications

Co-trimoxazole shares the toxic potentials of sulfonamides and trimethoprim, and the usual precautions associated with therapy with these drugs should be observed. (See Cautions in the Sulfonamides General Statement 8:12.20 and see Cautions in Trimethoprim 8:36.) Fatalities, although rare, have occurred in patients receiving sulfonamides, secondary to severe reactions induced by the drugs, including Stevens-Johnson syndrome, toxic epidermal necrolysis, fulminant hepatic necrosis, agranulocytosis, aplastic anemia, and other blood dyscrasias. Such fatal reactions also have been reported when sulfonamides were used in fixed combination with other drugs (e.g., with trimethoprim or erythromycin). Although probably rare, the precise incidence of severe dermatologic, hematologic, and hepatic effects with these combinations, including co-trimoxazole, is not known. Patients receiving co-trimoxazole should be monitored appropriately for the possible occurrence of such potentially severe reactions, and the drug should be discontinued at the first sign of such a reaction. The development of rash, sore throat, fever, pallor, arthralgia, cough, shortness of breath, purpura, or jaundice may be an early sign of a serious adverse reaction.

Co-trimoxazole should be used with caution in patients with impaired renal or hepatic function, possible folate deficiency (e.g., geriatric individuals, chronic alcoholics, patients receiving anticonvulsants, malnourished patients, those with malabsorption syndrome), with severe allergy or bronchial asthma,

or with possible folate or glucose-6-phosphate-dehydrogenase (G-6-PD) deficiency. Patients should be warned to report any early signs and symptoms of a serious hematologic disorder, including fever, sore throat, pallor, jaundice, or purpura. The manufacturers recommend that a complete blood count be obtained frequently in patients receiving co-trimoxazole, especially if signs and symptoms of blood disorders occur. The drug should be discontinued at the first appearance of rash or if any reduction in formed blood elements occurs. Leucovorin (folinic acid) should be administered if bone marrow depression occurs, especially if megaloblastic anemia, neutropenia, or thrombocytopenia occurs. Patients with acquired immunodeficiency syndrome (AIDS) who receive co-trimoxazole should be carefully monitored, since they appear to have a particularly high incidence of adverse reactions to the drug (especially fever and adverse dermatologic and hematologic reactions).

Urinalysis and careful microscopic examination of the urine should be performed in patients receiving co-trimoxazole, especially patients with impaired renal function. Patients receiving co-trimoxazole should be cautioned to maintain adequate fluid intake to prevent crystalluria and stone formation.

Co-trimoxazole should be used with caution in geriatric patients, particularly when complicating conditions (e.g., impaired renal and/or hepatic function, concomitant use of other drugs) are present, since these patients may have an increased risk of severe adverse reactions to the drug. Severe adverse dermatologic reactions, generalized bone marrow suppression, and a specific decrease in platelets (with or without purpura) are the most frequently reported severe adverse effects of the drug in geriatric patients. Co-trimoxazole also should be used with caution in patients with a history of hypersensitivity to sulfonamide-derivative drugs (e.g., acetazolamide, thiazides, tolbutamide), since cross-sensitivity may exist with these agents.

Commercially available formulations of co-trimoxazole for injection concentrate contain sodium metabisulfite, a sulfite that may cause allergic-type reactions, including anaphylaxis and life-threatening or less severe asthmatic episodes, in certain susceptible individuals. The overall prevalence of sulfite sensitivity in the general population is unknown and probably low; such sensitivity appears to occur more frequently in asthmatic than in nonasthmatic individuals.

Co-trimoxazole is contraindicated in patients with known hypersensitivity to trimethoprim or sulfonamides, with marked hepatic damage or severe renal impairment when renal function status cannot be monitored, or with documented megaloblastic anemia secondary to folate deficiency. However, cautious desensitization has been performed in some hypersensitive patients in whom co-trimoxazole therapy was considered necessary. The manufacturers recommend that the drug not be used in patients with creatinine clearances less than 15 mL/minute.

● Pediatric Precautions

The manufacturers of co-trimoxazole recommend that the drug *not* be used in infants younger than 2 months of age. Commercially available co-trimoxazole injections contain benzyl alcohol as a preservative. Although a causal relationship has not been established, administration of injections preserved with benzyl alcohol has been associated with toxicity in neonates. Toxicity appears to have resulted from administration of large amounts (i.e., about 100-400 mg/kg daily) of benzyl alcohol in these neonates. Safety and efficacy of repeated courses of co-trimoxazole therapy in children younger than 2 years of age, except those with documented *Pneumocystis* infections, have not been fully evaluated. Co-trimoxazole should be used with caution in children who have the fragile X chromosome associated with mental retardation, because folate depletion may worsen the psychomotor regression associated with the disorder.

● Mutagenicity and Carcinogenicity

Bacterial mutagenic studies have not been performed with co-trimoxazole. Trimethoprim did not exhibit mutagenic activity in the Ames test. No chromosomal damage was observed in cultured Chinese hamster ovary cells at concentrations approximately 500 times human plasma concentrations, but a low level of chromosomal damage was observed in some studies at concentrations approximately 1000 times human plasma concentrations. No chromosomal abnormalities were observed in human leukocytes cultured in vitro at trimethoprim concentrations up to 20 times human steady-state plasma concentrations. In addition, no chromosomal abnormalities were found in peripheral lymphocytes of patients receiving 320 mg of trimethoprim in combination with up to 1600 mg of sulfamethoxazole daily for as long as 112 weeks.

Long-term studies in animals to evaluate the carcinogenic potential of co-trimoxazole have not been performed.

Pregnancy, Fertility, and Lactation

Pregnancy

Trimethoprim and sulfamethoxazole, alone and in combination, have produced teratogenic effects, manifested principally as cleft palate, in some (but not all) studies in rats receiving dosages exceeding the usual human dosages. In addition, in some rabbit studies, an overall increase in fetal loss was associated with trimethoprim doses 6 times the usual human dose. Although there are no adequate and controlled studies to date in humans, studies in pregnant women suggest that the incidence of congenital abnormalities in those who received co-trimoxazole was similar to that in those who received a placebo; there were no abnormalities in 10 children whose mothers had received the drug during the first trimester. In one report, there were no congenital abnormalities in 35 children whose mothers had received co-trimoxazole at the time of conception or shortly thereafter. Because co-trimoxazole crosses the placenta and may interfere with folic acid metabolism, the drug should be used during pregnancy only when the potential benefits justify the possible risks to the fetus. Because sulfonamides may cause kernicterus in neonates, the manufacturers state that use of co-trimoxazole in pregnant women is contraindicated.

Fertility

The effect of co-trimoxazole on fertility in humans is not known. Reproduction studies in rats using oral trimethoprim (as co-trimoxazole) dosages up to 70 mg/kg daily have not revealed evidence of impaired fertility.

Lactation

Co-trimoxazole is distributed into milk. Because co-trimoxazole may interfere with folic acid metabolism, the drug should be used in nursing women only if the potential benefits justify the possible risks to the infant. Because sulfonamides may cause kernicterus in infants younger than 2 months of age, a decision should be made whether to discontinue nursing or co-trimoxazole or to use an alternative drug, taking into account the importance of co-trimoxazole to the woman.

DRUG INTERACTIONS

Warfarin

Co-trimoxazole may prolong the prothrombin time (PT) of patients receiving concomitant warfarin by inhibiting metabolic clearance of warfarin. If co-trimoxazole is used with warfarin, dosage of warfarin and PT must be monitored carefully.

Other Drugs

Because co-trimoxazole possesses anti-folate properties, the drug could theoretically increase the incidence of folate deficiencies induced by other drugs such as phenytoin when used concomitantly. Co-trimoxazole inhibits the metabolism of phenytoin. Concomitant administration of usual dosages of co-trimoxazole and phenytoin can increase the half-life of phenytoin by 39% and decrease metabolic clearance rate of phenytoin by 27%. If the drugs are administered concomitantly, the possibility of an increase in effects associated with phenytoin should be considered.

Co-trimoxazole should be used with caution in patients receiving methotrexate, since sulfonamides can displace methotrexate from plasma protein-binding sites resulting in increased free methotrexate concentrations.

Marked but reversible nephrotoxicity has been reported in renal transplant recipients receiving co-trimoxazole together with cyclosporine.

Increases in serum digoxin concentrations can occur in patients receiving co-trimoxazole; this interaction is more likely to occur in geriatric patients. Serum digoxin concentrations should be monitored in patients receiving digoxin and co-trimoxazole.

Increased plasma sulfamethoxazole concentration may occur in patients receiving indomethacin.

Megaloblastic anemia has been reported in patients receiving co-trimoxazole and pyrimethamine dosages exceeding 25 mg weekly (for malaria prophylaxis).

Concomitant administration of tricyclic antidepressants and co-trimoxazole may decrease the efficacy of the antidepressant.

Like other sulfonamides, co-trimoxazole potentiates the effect of oral hypoglycemic agents.

Toxic delirium has been reported in one individual following administration of co-trimoxazole and amantadine.

ACUTE TOXICITY

Manifestations

Overdosage with co-trimoxazole may produce symptoms of nausea, vomiting, diarrhea, mental depression, confusion, facial swelling, headache, bone marrow depression, and slight elevations of serum aminotransferases (transaminases).

Treatment

In acute overdosage with oral co-trimoxazole, the stomach should be emptied immediately by inducing emesis or by lavage. Supportive and symptomatic treatment should be initiated. Patients should be monitored with blood counts and other appropriate laboratory studies (e.g., serum electrolyte concentrations). Hemodialysis may remove only moderate amounts of the drug; peritoneal dialysis is not effective in enhancing the elimination of co-trimoxazole.

MECHANISM OF ACTION

Co-trimoxazole usually is bactericidal. Of its components, sulfamethoxazole is bacteriostatic and trimethoprim usually is bactericidal. Co-trimoxazole acts by sequentially inhibiting enzymes of the folic acid pathway; sulfamethoxazole inhibits the formation of dihydrofolic acid from p-aminobenzoic acid and, by inhibiting dihydrofolate reductase, trimethoprim inhibits the formation of tetrahydrofolic acid from dihydrofolic acid. By inhibiting synthesis of tetrahydrofolic acid, the metabolically active form of folic acid, co-trimoxazole inhibits bacterial thymidine synthesis.

Sequential inhibition by co-trimoxazole of two steps in the folic acid pathway appears to be responsible for the antibacterial synergism of the trimethoprim-sulfamethoxazole combination. For most organisms, optimum synergistic antibacterial action occurs in vitro at a trimethoprim:sulfamethoxazole ratio of about 1:20, which is also the approximate peak serum concentration ratio of the 2 drugs achieved following oral or IV administration of co-trimoxazole. Synergistic activity also has been observed in vitro at trimethoprim:sulfamethoxazole ratios of 1:1–1:40.

Susceptibility of organisms to trimethoprim usually is more critical to the efficacy of co-trimoxazole than is susceptibility to sulfamethoxazole. Many organisms that are resistant to sulfamethoxazole but susceptible or only moderately susceptible to trimethoprim will show synergistic antibacterial response to co-trimoxazole. However, for Neisseria gonorrhoeae, susceptibility to sulfamethoxazole is required for antibacterial response to co-trimoxazole.

SPECTRUM

In Vitro Susceptibility Testing

For most organisms, inoculum size may influence the result of in vitro co-trimoxazole susceptibility tests. Accurate in vitro susceptibility testing requires that thymidine *not* be present in the growth medium or that the medium be supplemented with thymidine phosphorylase to inactivate any thymidine that might be present.

The Clinical and Laboratory Standards Institute (CLSI; formerly National Committee for Clinical Laboratory Standards [NCCLS]) states that, if results of in vitro susceptibility testing indicate that a clinical isolate is *susceptible* to co-trimoxazole, then an infection caused by this strain may be appropriately treated with the dosage of the drug recommended for that type of infection and infecting species, unless otherwise contraindicated. If results indicate that a clinical isolate has *intermediate susceptibility* to co-trimoxazole, then the strain has a minimum inhibitory concentration (MIC) that approaches usually attainable blood and tissue concentrations and response rates may be lower than for strains identified as susceptible. Therefore, the intermediate category implies clinical applicability in body sites where the drug is physiologically concentrated or when a high dosage of the drug can be used. This intermediate category also includes a buffer zone which should prevent small, uncontrolled technical factors from causing major discrepancies in interpretation, especially for drugs with narrow pharmacotoxicity margins. If results of in vitro susceptibility testing indicate that a clinical isolate is *resistant* to co-trimoxazole, the strain is not inhibited by systemic concentrations of the drug achievable with normal dosage schedules and/or MICs fall in the range where specific microbial resistance mechanisms are likely and efficacy has not been reliable in clinical studies.

Disk Susceptibility Tests

When the disk-diffusion procedure is used for susceptibility testing, a 1.25-mcg trimethoprim/23.75-mcg sulfamethoxazole disk should be used.

When the disk-diffusion susceptibility test is performed according to CLSI standardized procedures, Enterobacteriaceae, *Pseudomonas aeruginosa, Acinetobacter,* or *Staphylococci* with growth inhibition zones of 16 mm or greater are susceptible to co-trimoxazole, those with zones of 11–15 mm have intermediate susceptibility, and those with zones of 10 mm or less are resistant to the drug.

When disk-diffusion susceptibility testing is performed according to CLSI standardized procedures using *Haemophilus* test medium (HTM), *Haemophilus* with growth inhibition zones of 16 mm or greater are susceptible to co-trimoxazole, those with zones of 11–15 mm have intermediate susceptibility, and those with zones of 10 mm or less are resistant to the drug.

When testing susceptibility of *S. pneumoniae* according to CLSI standardized procedures using Mueller-Hinton agar (supplemented with 5% defibrinated sheep blood), *S. pneumoniae* with growth inhibition zones of 19 mm or greater are susceptible to co-trimoxazole, those with zones of 16–18 mm have intermediate susceptibility, and those with zones of 15 mm or less are resistant to the drug.

When the disk diffusion procedure is performed according to CLSI standardized procedures, *Vibrio cholerae* with growth inhibition zones of 16 mm or greater are susceptible to co-trimoxazole, those with zones of 11–15 mm have intermediate susceptibility, and those with zones of 10 mm or less are resistant to the drug.

Dilution Susceptibility Tests

When dilution susceptibility testing (agar or broth dilution) is performed according to CLSI standardized procedures, Enterobacteriaceae, *Ps. aeruginosa,* other non-Enterobacteriaceae gram-negative bacilli (e.g., *Acinetobacter, Stenotrophomonas maltophilia,* other *Pseudomonas* spp), or *Staphylococcus* with MICs equal to or less than 2 mcg/mL of trimethoprim and 38 mcg/mL of sulfamethoxazole are susceptible to co-trimoxazole and those with MICs equal to or greater than 4 mcg/mL of trimethoprim and 76 mcg/mL of sulfamethoxazole are resistant to the drug.

When dilution susceptibility testing for *Haemophilus* is performed according to CLSI standardized procedures using HTM, *Haemophilus* with MICs equal to or less than 0.5 mcg/mL of trimethoprim and 9.5 mcg/mL of sulfamethoxazole are susceptible to co-trimoxazole and those with MICs equal to or greater than 4 mcg/mL of trimethoprim and 76 mcg/mL of sulfamethoxazole are resistant to the drug. *Haemophilus* with an MIC of 1–2 mcg/mL of trimethoprim and 19–38 mcg/mL of sulfamethoxazole have intermediate susceptibility to co-trimoxazole. These same interpretive criteria are used when dilution susceptibility testing for *S. pneumoniae* is performed according to CLSI standardized procedures using cation-adjusted Mueller-Hinton broth (with 2–5% lysed horse blood).

When dilution susceptibility testing is performed according to CLSI standardized procedures, *V. cholerae* with MICs equal to or less than 2 mcg/mL of trimethoprim and 38 mcg/mL of sulfamethoxazole are susceptible to co-trimoxazole and those with MICs of 4 mcg/mL or greater of trimethoprim and 76 mcg/mL or greater are resistant to the drug.

● Gram-positive Aerobic Bacteria

In vitro, when the optimum 1:20 synergistic ratio of trimethoprim:sulfamethoxazole is used, trimethoprim concentrations of 0.05–0.15 mcg/mL and sulfamethoxazole concentrations of 0.95–2.85 mcg/mL inhibit most strains of *Streptococcus pneumoniae.* Many strains of *Staphylococcus aureus,* group A β-hemolytic streptococci (*Streptococcus pyogenes*), and *Nocardia* also are susceptible to co-trimoxazole. Some strains of enterococci, including some *E. faecalis* (formerly *Streptococcus faecalis*), are not susceptible to the drug; to accurately determine susceptibility of enterococci to co-trimoxazole, the growth medium must be free of thymidine and other sources of exogenous folate. Some group A β-hemolytic streptococci may not respond to co-trimoxazole in tonsillopharyngeal infections, possibly because of inadequate concentrations of the drug in this area.

Bacillus anthracis strains with in vitro resistance to sulfamethoxazole or trimethoprim have been reported, and these anti-infectives should not be used in the treatment of *B. anthracis* infections (i.e., anthrax).

● Gram-negative Aerobic Bacteria

Co-trimoxazole is active in vitro against common gram-negative bacteria associated with urinary tract infections, including most Enterobacteriaceae. The drug is not active against *Pseudomonas aeruginosa.*

Generally, co-trimoxazole is active in vitro against most of the following Enterobacteriaceae: *Acinetobacter, Enterobacter, Escherichia coli, Klebsiella pneumoniae,*

Proteus mirabilis, Salmonella, and *Shigella.* When the optimum 1:20 synergistic ratio of trimethoprim:sulfamethoxazole is used in vitro, the MIC for most of these organisms is 1.5 mcg/mL or less of trimethoprim; for sulfamethoxazole, MICs for *P. mirabilis, Shigella,* and *Salmonella* generally are 2.85 mcg/mL or less, for *E. coli* are 9.5 mcg/mL or less, and for *Klebsiella* and *Enterobacter* are 28.5 mcg/mL or less. Co-trimoxazole also is active in vitro against *Haemophilus influenzae* (including ampicillin-resistant strains), *H. ducreyi,* and *Neisseria gonorrhoeae.* Approximately 70% of indole-positive *Proteus* and 50% of *Providencia* and *Serratia* strains are susceptible to co-trimoxazole.

● Anaerobic Bacteria

Co-trimoxazole generally is considered inactive against most strains of *Bacteroides,* and appears to have no activity against strict anaerobes (e.g., *Clostridium*).

● Protozoa

Co-trimoxazole is active in vitro and in vivo against *Pneumocystis jiroveci* (formerly *Pneumocystis carinii*).

RESISTANCE

In vitro, resistance develops more slowly to co-trimoxazole than to trimethoprim or sulfamethoxazole alone.

Use of sulfamethoxazole alone results in rapid selection of sulfonamide-resistant fecal coliforms. As many as 50% of hospital-isolated and 20% of community-isolated *Escherichia coli* are resistant to sulfonamides, including sulfamethoxazole. Resistance to sulfamethoxazole in gram-negative bacteria is usually plasmid mediated. In many organisms (e.g., *E. coli, Neisseria meningitis, Streptococcus pneumoniae, Plasmodium falciparum*), point mutations in conserved regions of dihydropteroate synthase (DHPS), an essential enzyme for folate biosynthesis, confer sulfonamide resistance. Mutations in DHPS also have been identified in *Pneumocystis carinii* isolates obtained from HIV-infected patients, including some patients who had not previously received a sulfonamide, and these mutations are being reported with increasing frequency in this organism. It is unclear whether DHPS mutations in *P. carinii* are associated with resistance to co-trimoxazole since *P. carinii* pneumonia has been effectively treated with co-trimoxazole in some patients despite the presence of DHPS mutants. However, there is some evidence from a study in HIV-infected patients with *P. carinii* pneumonia that presence of strains with DHPS mutations may be associated with decreased survival. Resistance to trimethoprim has been shown to occur by several mechanisms, most often chromosomally mediated, but also rarely involving mutation of bacteria to thymidine-dependent strains or plasmid-mediated resistance involving altered production or sensitivity of bacterial dihydrofolate reductase. Plasmid-mediated resistance to trimethoprim has been shown to be transferable among some bacterial strains; plasmid-mediated resistance to trimethoprim usually results in concomitant coding for sulfonamide resistance. Thymidine-dependent strains account for less than 1% of trimethoprim resistance, and chromosomal- and plasmid-mediated resistance accounts for approximately 90% and 10% of reported resistant strains, respectively.

Resistant strains of Enterobacteriaceae, especially *E. coli, Klebsiella,* and *Proteus,* have occurred during therapy with co-trimoxazole. Strains of *Klebsiella* and *Proteus* that are only moderately susceptible to co-trimoxazole in vitro at the beginning of therapy appear to be especially likely to develop resistance during therapy. The incidence of trimethoprim resistance among Enterobacteriaceae in fecal flora and associated with urinary tract infections has been reported to range from 8–38% in some hospitals and to range from 30–100% among fecal Enterobacteriaceae following 2 weeks of co-trimoxazole therapy. In a study in Mexico, more than 95% of fecal *E. coli* resistant to trimethoprim also were resistant to sulfamethoxazole, but the resistant strains were not associated with clinical infection. Strains of Enterobacteriaceae and *S. pneumoniae* resistant to trimethoprim, but sensitive to sulfonamides and penicillin, respectively, have been reported.

Although co-trimoxazole previously was considered nearly uniformly active against *H. influenzae,* resistant strains have been reported rarely. In a national collaborative study of *H. influenzae* isolates from 1986, the incidence of co-trimoxazole resistance was about 1%, including several strains that also were resistant to ampicillin (β-lactamase mediated), chloramphenicol, and tetracycline.

PHARMACOKINETICS

● Absorption

The fixed-combination preparation containing trimethoprim and sulfamethoxazole (co-trimoxazole) is rapidly and well absorbed from the GI tract. Peak serum concentrations of 1–2 mcg/mL of trimethoprim and 40–60 mcg/mL of unbound sulfamethoxazole are reached 1–4 hours after a single oral dose of co-trimoxazole containing 160 mg of trimethoprim and 800 mg of sulfamethoxazole. Following multiple-dose oral administration, steady-state peak serum concentrations usually are 50% greater than those obtained after single-dose administration of the drug. Following oral administration of the fixed-ratio combination preparation, the trimethoprim:sulfamethoxazole ratio of mean steady-state serum concentrations usually is about 1:20.

Mean peak steady-state serum concentrations of approximately 9 and 105 mcg/mL of trimethoprim and sulfamethoxazole, respectively, are reached after IV infusion of 160 mg of trimethoprim and 800 mg of sulfamethoxazole every 8 hours in adults with normal renal function. Steady-state trough concentrations reached with this IV dose are approximately 6 mcg/mL of trimethoprim and 70 mcg/mL of sulfamethoxazole.

● Distribution

Both trimethoprim and sulfamethoxazole are widely distributed into body tissues and fluids, including sputum, aqueous humor, middle ear fluid, prostatic fluid, vaginal fluid, bile, and CSF; trimethoprim also distributes into bronchial secretions. Trimethoprim has a larger volume of distribution (V_d) than does sulfamethoxazole. In adults, apparent V_ds of 100–120 and 12–18 L have been reported for trimethoprim and sulfamethoxazole, respectively. In patients with uninflamed meninges, trimethoprim and sulfamethoxazole concentrations in CSF are about 50 and 40%, respectively, of concurrent serum concentrations of the drugs. Trimethoprim and sulfamethoxazole concentrations in middle ear fluid are approximately 75 and 20%, respectively, and in prostatic fluid are approximately 200 and 35%, respectively, of concurrent serum concentrations of the drugs.

Trimethoprim is approximately 44% and sulfamethoxazole is approximately 70% bound to plasma proteins.

Both trimethoprim and sulfamethoxazole readily crosses the placenta. Amniotic fluid concentrations of trimethoprim and sulfamethoxazole are reported to be 80 and 50%, respectively, of concurrent maternal serum concentrations. Both trimethoprim and sulfamethoxazole is distributed into milk. Trimethoprim and sulfamethoxazole concentrations in milk are approximately 125 and 10%, respectively, of concurrent maternal serum concentrations.

● Elimination

Trimethoprim and sulfamethoxazole have serum half-lives of approximately 8–11 and 10–13 hours, respectively, in adults with normal renal function. In adults with creatinine clearances of 10–30 and 0–10 mL/minute, serum half-life of trimethoprim may increase to 15 and greater than 26 hours, respectively. In adults with chronic renal failure, sulfamethoxazole half-life may be 3 times that in patients with normal renal function. Trimethoprim serum half-lives of about 7.7 and 5.5 hours have been reported in children less than 1 year of age and between 1 and 10 years of age, respectively.

Both trimethoprim and sulfamethoxazole are metabolized in the liver. Trimethoprim is metabolized to oxide and hydroxylated metabolites and sulfamethoxazole is principally N-acetylated and also conjugated with glucuronic acid. Both drugs are rapidly excreted in urine via glomerular filtration and tubular secretion. In adults with normal renal function, approximately 50–60% of a trimethoprim and 45–70% of a sulfamethoxazole oral dose are excreted in urine within 24 hours. Approximately 80% of the amount of trimethoprim and 20% of the amount of sulfamethoxazole recovered in urine are unchanged drug. In adults with normal renal function, urinary concentrations of active trimethoprim are approximately equal to those of active sulfamethoxazole. Urinary concentrations of both active drugs are decreased in patients with impaired renal function.

Only small amounts of trimethoprim are excreted in feces via biliary elimination. Trimethoprim and active sulfamethoxazole are moderately removed by hemodialysis.

CHEMISTRY AND STABILITY

● Chemistry

Co-trimoxazole is a fixed combination of sulfamethoxazole and trimethoprim. Sulfamethoxazole is an intermediate-acting antibacterial sulfonamide. Both sulfamethoxazole and trimethoprim are synthetic folate-antagonist anti-infectives. Co-trimoxazole contains a 5:1 ratio of sulfamethoxazole to trimethoprim. Potency of co-trimoxazole is expressed in terms of the trimethoprim content.

Trimethoprim occurs as white to cream-colored, bitter-tasting, odorless crystals or crystalline powder and sulfamethoxazole occurs as a white to off-white, practically odorless, crystalline powder. Sodium hydroxide is added during manufacture of co-trimoxazole for injection concentrate to adjust pH to 10. Co-trimoxazole oral suspension has a pH of 5–6.5.

● Stability

Co-trimoxazole for injection concentrate should be stored at 15–25°C or 15–30°C, depending on the formulation (the manufacturers' recommendations should be followed) and should *not* be refrigerated. Oral suspensions of the drug should be stored in tight, light-resistant containers at 15–25 or 15–30°C, depending on the formulation (the manufacturers' recommendations should be followed), and the tablets should be stored in well-closed, light-resistant containers at 15–30°C.

Co-trimoxazole for injection concentrate is physically and chemically compatible with IV solutions of 5% dextrose; admixed solutions of co-trimoxazole in 5% dextrose that are cloudy or contain a precipitate should be discarded. Because of the potential for incompatibility, the manufacturers state that co-trimoxazole IV solutions should not be admixed with other drugs or solutions other than 5% dextrose. Specialized references should be consulted for specific compatibility information.

Co-trimoxazole solutions containing 0.64 mg of trimethoprim and 3.2 mg of sulfamethoxazole per mL of 5% dextrose (1:25 dilution) are stable for 6 hours at room temperature. Co-trimoxazole solutions containing 0.64–0.8 mg of trimethoprim and 3.2–4 mg of sulfamethoxazole per mL of 5% dextrose (1:20 dilution) are stable for 4 hours at room temperature. Co-trimoxazole solutions containing 0.8–1.1 mg of trimethoprim and 4–5.3 mg of sulfamethoxazole per mL of 5% dextrose (1:15 dilution) are stable for 2 hours at room temperature. Co-trimoxazole solutions in 5% dextrose should not be refrigerated. Prior to infusion, solutions of the drug should be inspected visually and discarded if there is evidence of crystallization or cloudiness.

Following initial entry into a multiple-dose vial of co-trimoxazole for injection concentrate, the manufacturers recommend that the contents be used within 48 hours.

PREPARATIONS

Excipients in commercially available drug preparations may have clinically important effects in some individuals; consult specific product labeling for details.

Co-trimoxazole

Oral

Suspension	Trimethoprim 40 mg/5 mL and Sulfamethoxazole 200 mg/5 mL*	**Septra® Suspension**, Monarch **Septra® Grape Suspension**, Monarch **Sulfatrim® Pediatric Suspension**, Actavis **Sulfatrim® Suspension**, Actavis, United Research
Tablets	Trimethoprim 80 mg and Sulfamethoxazole 400 mg*	**Bactrim®** (scored), Women First HealthCare **Septra®**, Monarch **Sulfamethoxazole and Trimethoprim Tablets**
	Trimethoprim 160 mg and Sulfamethoxazole 800 mg*	**Bactrim® DS**, Women First HealthCare **Septra® DS**, Monarch

Parenteral

For injection concentrate, for IV infusion	Trimethoprim 16 mg/mL and Sulfamethoxazole 80 mg/mL	**Sulfamethoxazole and Trimethoprim Concentrate for Injection**

* available from one or more manufacturer, distributor, and/or repackager by generic (nonproprietary) name

† Use is not currently included in the labeling approved by the US Food and Drug Administration.

Selected Revisions January 1, 2009, © Copyright, January 1, 1984, American Society of Health-System Pharmacists, Inc.

Omadacycline Tosylate

8:12.24.04 • AMINOMETHYLCYCLINES

■ Omadacycline tosylate, a semisynthetic aminomethylcycline, is a tetracycline anti-infective.

USES

● Community-acquired Pneumonia

Omadacycline tosylate is used for the treatment of community-acquired bacterial pneumonia (CABP) caused by *Streptococcus pneumoniae*, *Staphylococcus aureus* (methicillin-susceptible strains), *Haemophilus influenzae*, *H. parainfluenzae*, *Klebsiella pneumoniae*, *Legionella pneumophila*, *Mycoplasma pneumoniae*, and *Chlamydophila pneumoniae* (formerly *Chlamydia pneumoniae*).

Clinical Experience

Efficacy and safety of omadacycline were evaluated in a randomized, double-blind, double-dummy, phase 3, noninferiority trial (OPTIC; NCT02531438) that included 774 adults with community-acquired bacterial pneumonia (i.e., patients with at least 3 of the following symptoms: cough, purulent sputum production, dyspnea, or pleuritic chest pain; or with at least 2 abnormal vital signs, at least 1 clinical sign or laboratory finding associated with community-acquired bacterial pneumonia, radiologically confirmed pneumonia, and a pneumonia severity index [PSI] risk class of II, III, or IV). Results of this study indicated that omadacycline was noninferior to moxifloxacin for the treatment of community-acquired pneumonia.

Patients in the OPTIC trial were randomized in a 1:1 ratio to receive 7–14 days of treatment with omadacycline (100 mg IV every 12 hours for 2 doses on day 1 followed by 100 mg IV once daily with the option to switch to oral omadacycline 300 mg once daily after at least 3 days of IV therapy) or moxifloxacin (400 mg IV once daily with the option to switch to oral moxifloxacin 400 mg once daily after at least 3 days of IV therapy). The primary efficacy end point was clinical success (i.e., survival with improvement of at least 2 out of 4 symptoms of community-acquired pneumonia [cough, sputum production, chest pain, dyspnea] without deterioration in any of the 4 symptoms) at the early clinical response time point (72–120 hours after the first dose). Patient characteristics were balanced between groups (55% male, 92% white, median age 62 years, 86% with PSI risk class III or IV). In the intent-to-treat (ITT) population at the early clinical response time point, the clinical success rate in the omadacycline group was noninferior to that of the moxifloxacin group (81 and 83%, respectively). At 5–10 days after the last dose of study drug, the clinical response rate (i.e., survival and improvement in signs and symptoms of community-acquired pneumonia to the extent that further antibacterial therapy was not needed) in the ITT population was 87% in the omadacycline group and 85% in the moxifloxacin group.

In the subset of patients in the OPTIC trial who were microbiologically evaluable and stratified according to the infecting pathogen, clinical response on day 5–10 in those with infections caused by *S. pneumoniae* or methicillin-susceptible *S. aureus* was 86 or 73%, respectively, in those treated with omadacycline and 91 or 80%, respectively, in those treated with moxifloxacin. The clinical response in those with infections caused by *H. influenzae*, *H. parainfluenzae*, or *K. pneumoniae* was 81, 83, or 77%, respectively, in those treated with omadacycline and 100, 77, or 85%, respectively, in those treated with moxifloxacin. The clinical response in those with infections caused by *L. pneumophila*, *M. pneumoniae*, or *C. pneumoniae* was 93, 89, or 93%, respectively, in those treated with omadacycline and 96, 86, or 93%, respectively, in those treated with moxifloxacin.

● Skin and Skin Structure Infections

Omadacycline is used for the treatment of acute bacterial skin and skin structure infections (ABSSSI) caused by *S. aureus* (including methicillin-resistant S. aureus [MRSA; also known as oxacillin-resistant *S. aureus* or ORSA] and methicillin-susceptible S. aureus), *S. lugdunensis*, *S. pyogenes*, *S. anginosus* group (*S. anginosus*, *S. intermedius*, *S. constellatus*), *Enterococcus faecalis*, *Enterobacter cloacae*, and *K. pneumoniae*.

Clinical Experience

Efficacy and safety of omadacycline were evaluated in 2 randomized, double-blind, double-dummy, phase 3 studies (OASIS-1; NCT02378480 and OASIS-2; NCT02877927) that included 1390 adults with acute bacterial skin and skin structure infections (e.g., cellulitis or erysipelas, major abscess, wound infection). In both studies, patients were randomized in a 1:1 ratio to receive omadacycline or linezolid for 7–14 days and efficacy was determined by clinical success at the early clinical response time point (i.e., at least 20% decreased lesion size at 48–72 hours after the first dose of study drug). Results of these studies indicated that omadacycline is noninferior to linezolid for the treatment of acute bacterial skin infections.

In OASIS-1, 38% of patients had cellulitis, 33% had a wound infection, and 29% had a major abscess; the mean surface area of the infected lesion was 455 cm^2 in patients receiving omadacycline and 498 cm^2 in those receiving linezolid. Baseline characteristics were balanced between treatment groups (mean age 47 years, 65% male, 92% white, 60% enrolled in the US, 54% with comorbid drug abuse, 29% with hepatitis C virus [HCV] infection). Patients in the omadacycline group received 100 mg of omadacycline IV every 12 hours for 2 doses followed by 100 mg IV once daily with the option to switch to oral omadacycline 300 mg once daily after at least 3 days of IV therapy; patients in the linezolid group received 600 mg of linezolid IV every 12 hours with the option to switch to oral linezolid 600 mg every 12 hours after at least 3 days of IV therapy. The total treatment duration was 7–14 days. In the modified ITT (mITT) population, clinical success at 48–72 hours was achieved by 84.8% of patients receiving omadacycline and 85.5% of patients receiving linezolid. Clinical response (i.e., survival after completion of treatment without use of any alternative anti-infectives, no unplanned major surgical interventions, and sufficient resolution of infection without need for additional treatment at the post-therapy evaluation 7–14 days after the last dose) in the mITT population who had at least 1 gram-positive causative pathogen at baseline was achieved by 86.1% of patients in the omadacycline group and 83.6% of patients in the linezolid group.

In OASIS-2, 24% of patients had cellulitis, 58% had a wound infection, and 18% had a major abscess; the mean surface area of the infected lesion was 424 cm^2 in patients receiving omadacycline and 399 cm^2 in those receiving linezolid. Patients had a mean age of 44 years, 63% were male, 91% were white, 100% were enrolled in the US, 73% had comorbid drug abuse, and 32% had HCV infection. Patients were randomized to receive omadacycline (450 mg orally once daily on days 1 and 2 followed by 300 mg orally once daily) or linezolid (600 mg orally every 12 hours) for a total treatment duration of 7–14 days. Clinical success at 48–72 hours was achieved by 87.3% of patients receiving omadacycline and 82.2% of patients receiving linezolid. Clinical response (i.e., survival after completion of treatment without use of any alternative anti-infectives, without unplanned major surgical intervention, and with sufficient resolution of infection without need for additional treatment at the post-therapy evaluation 7–14 days after the last dose) in the mITT population who had at least 1 gram-positive causative pathogen at baseline was achieved by 83.9% of patients in the omadacycline group and 80.5% of patients in the linezolid group.

In a pooled subset of microbiologically evaluable patients from OASIS-1 and OASIS-2 who were stratified according to the infecting pathogen, clinical response at 7–14 days after the last dose in those with infections caused by MRSA or methicillin-susceptible *S. aureus* was 84 or 82%, respectively, in those treated with omadacycline and 82 or 80%, respectively, in those treated with linezolid. The clinical response in those with infections caused by *S. lugdunensis*, *S. pyogenes*, or *S. anginosus* group was 91, 70, or 81%, respectively, in those treated with omadacycline and 67, 74, or 72%, respectively, in those treated with linezolid. The clinical response in those with infections caused by *E. cloacae*, *E. faecalis*, or *K. pneumoniae* was 79, 94, or 73%, respectively, in those treated with omadacycline and 82, 84, or 55%, respectively, in those treated with linezolid.

DOSAGE AND ADMINISTRATION

● Administration

Omadacycline tosylate is administered orally or by IV infusion.

Oral Administration

Omadacycline tablets should be taken orally with water under fasting conditions.

The patient should fast for at least 4 hours before taking omadacycline tablets and should *not* consume any food or drink (except water) for 2 hours after receiving the drug. The patient also should *not* consume dairy products, antacids, iron-containing preparations, or multivitamins for 4 hours after receiving omadacycline tablets.

IV Administration

Omadacycline powder for injection must be reconstituted and further diluted prior to IV infusion.

IV solutions of omadacycline should be administered IV through a dedicated line or a Y-site. IV solutions of omadacycline should *not* be infused simultaneously through the same IV line with any solution containing multivalent cations (e.g., calcium, magnesium). Infusion of omadacycline using the same IV line as other drugs has not been studied.

If the same IV line is used for sequential infusion of several drugs, the line should be flushed with 0.9% sodium chloride injection or 5% dextrose injection before and after infusion of omadacycline.

Reconstitution and Dilution

The appropriate number of single-dose vials labeled as containing 100 mg of omadacycline should be reconstituted by adding 5 mL of sterile water for injection, 0.9% sodium chloride injection, or 5% dextrose injection to each vial and swirling gently. The vials should be left to stand until the cake completely dissolves and any foam disperses; the vials should not be shaken. If necessary, vials should be inverted to dissolve any remaining powder; to avoid foaming, the vials should be swirled gently. Reconstituted solutions should be yellow to dark orange; the solution should be discarded if it is not the correct color.

To prepare a 100- or 200-mg dose of IV omadacycline, 5 or 10 mL of reconstituted solution, respectively, should be withdrawn from the vial(s) immediately (within 1 hour of reconstitution) and added to 100 mL of 0.9% sodium chloride injection or 5% dextrose injection. The final concentration of the diluted solution will be 1 mg/mL for a 100-mg dose or 2 mg/mL for a 200-mg dose. Any unused portions of the reconstituted solution should be discarded.

Following reconstitution and dilution, omadacycline solutions may be stored for up to 24 hours at room temperature (not exceeding 25°C) or for up to 7 days under refrigeration (2–8°C), but should not be frozen. If stored under refrigeration, solutions should be allowed to reach room temperature prior to administration.

Omadacycline solutions should be inspected visually for particulate matter and discoloration prior to administration.

Rate of Administration

IV doses of 100 or 200 mg of omadacycline should be given by IV infusion over 30 or 60 minutes, respectively.

● Dosage

Dosage of omadacycline tosylate is expressed in terms of omadacycline.

Community-acquired Pneumonia

For the treatment of community-acquired pneumonia in adults, either IV or oral omadacycline may be used for *initial* treatment.

When omadacycline tablets are used for the treatment of community-acquired pneumonia, adults should receive an initial loading dose of 300 mg orally twice on day 1, followed by a maintenance dosage of 300 mg orally once daily for a total treatment duration of 7–14 days.

When IV omadacycline is used for the treatment of community-acquired pneumonia, adults should receive an initial loading dose of 200 mg on day 1 (single 200-mg dose by IV infusion over 60 minutes or two 100-mg doses by IV infusion over 30 minutes given 12 hours apart) followed by a maintenance dosage of 100 mg once daily given by IV infusion over 30 minutes for a total treatment duration of 7–14 days.

Alternatively, when IV omadacycline is used initially, therapy may be switched at the discretion of the clinician to omadacycline tablets given in a dosage of 300 mg orally once daily. The total treatment duration (IV and oral) should be 7–14 days.

Skin and Skin Structure Infections

For the treatment of acute bacterial skin and skin structure infections (ABSSSI) in adults, either IV omadacycline or oral omadacycline may be used for *initial* treatment.

When omadacycline tablets are used for the treatment of acute bacterial skin and skin structure infections, adults should receive an initial loading dose of 450 mg orally once daily on days 1 *and* 2, followed by a maintenance dosage of 300 mg orally once daily for a total treatment duration of 7–14 days.

When IV omadacycline is used for the treatment of acute bacterial skin and skin structure infections, adults should receive an initial loading dose of 200 mg on day 1 (single 200-mg dose by IV infusion over 60 minutes *or* two 100-mg doses by IV infusion over 30 minutes given 12 hours apart) followed by a maintenance dosage of 100 mg once daily given by IV infusion over 30 minutes for a total treatment duration of 7–14 days.

Alternatively, when IV omadacycline is used initially, therapy may be switched at the discretion of the clinician to omadacycline tablets given in a dosage of 300 mg orally once daily. The total treatment duration (IV and oral) should be 7–14 days.

● Special Populations

Hepatic Impairment

Dosage adjustments are not necessary in adults with hepatic impairment (Child-Pugh class A, B, or C).

Renal Impairment

Dosage adjustments are not necessary in adults with renal impairment, including those with end-stage renal disease receiving hemodialysis.

Geriatric Patients

Dosage adjustments based on age are not necessary.

CAUTIONS

● Contraindications

Omadacycline tosylate is contraindicated in patients with known hypersensitivity to omadacycline, other tetracyclines, or any excipients in the preparation.

● Warnings/Precautions

Sensitivity Reactions

Hypersensitivity Reactions

Hypersensitivity reactions have been reported with omadacycline. Life-threatening hypersensitivity (anaphylactic) reactions have been reported with other tetracyclines. Because omadacycline is structurally similar to other tetracyclines, it is contraindicated in patients with known hypersensitivity to any tetracycline.

Omadacycline should be discontinued if an allergic reaction occurs.

Increased Mortality

Mortality imbalance was observed in a clinical trial evaluating omadacycline in patients with community-acquired bacterial pneumonia; 8 deaths (2%) occurred in patients receiving omadacycline compared with 4 deaths (1%) in patients receiving the comparator drug (moxifloxacin). The cause of the difference in mortality rates between treatment groups has not been established. All deaths in both treatment groups occurred in patients older than 65 years of age and most patients had multiple comorbid conditions. Causes of death varied and included complications of and/or worsening of the infection and underlying conditions.

When omadacycline is used for the treatment of community-acquired bacterial pneumonia, clinical response to treatment should be closely monitored, particularly in those at higher risk of mortality.

Tooth Discoloration and Enamel Hypoplasia

The use of tetracyclines, including omadacycline, during tooth development (i.e., last half of pregnancy, infancy, childhood up to 8 years of age) may cause permanent discoloration of the teeth (yellow-gray-brown). Tooth discoloration is more common during long-term use of tetracyclines, but has been observed following repeated short-term use of the drugs. Enamel hypoplasia also has been reported with tetracyclines.

Inhibition of Bone Growth

The use of tetracyclines, including omadacycline, during the second or third trimester of pregnancy, infancy, or childhood up to 8 years of age may cause reversible inhibition of bone growth. Tetracyclines form a stable calcium complex in any bone-forming tissue. Decreased fibula growth rate has been observed in premature infants receiving oral tetracycline in a dosage of 25 mg/kg every 6 hours; this effect was shown to be reversible when the drug was discontinued.

Tetracycline-class Effects

Because omadacycline is structurally similar to conventional tetracyclines, adverse effects reported with tetracyclines (e.g., photosensitivity, pseudotumor cerebri, anti-anabolic action leading to increased BUN, azotemia, acidosis, hyperphosphatemia, pancreatitis, abnormal liver function tests) may occur with omadacycline. Omadacycline should be discontinued if any of these adverse effects are suspected.

C. difficile-associated Diarrhea and Colitis

Treatment with anti-infectives alters normal colon flora and may permit overgrowth of *Clostridioides difficile* (formerly known as *Clostridium difficile*). *C. difficile* infection (CDI) and *C. difficile*-associated diarrhea and colitis (CDAD; also known as antibiotic-associated diarrhea and colitis or pseudomembranous colitis) have been reported in patients receiving nearly all anti-infectives, including omadacycline, and may range in severity from mild diarrhea to fatal colitis. *C. difficile* produces toxins A and B which contribute to development of CDAD; hypertoxin-producing strains of *C. difficile* are associated with increased morbidity and mortality since they may be refractory to anti-infectives and colectomy may be required.

CDAD should be considered in the differential diagnosis of patients who develop diarrhea during or after anti-infective therapy. Careful medical history is necessary since CDAD has been reported to occur as late as 2 months or longer after anti-infective therapy is discontinued.

If CDAD is suspected or confirmed, anti-infective therapy not directed against *C. difficile* should be discontinued as soon as possible. Patients should be managed with appropriate anti-infective therapy directed against *C. difficile* (e.g., vancomycin, fidaxomicin, metronidazole), supportive therapy (e.g., fluid and electrolyte management, protein supplementation), and surgical evaluation as clinically indicated.

Selection and Use of Anti-infectives

To reduce development of drug-resistant bacteria and maintain effectiveness of omadacycline and other antibacterials, the drug should be used only for treatment of infections proven or strongly suspected to be caused by susceptible bacteria. Prescribing omadacycline in the absence of a proven or strongly suspected bacterial infection is unlikely to provide benefit to the patient and increases the risk of development of drug-resistant bacteria.

When selecting or modifying anti-infective therapy, results of culture and in vitro susceptibility testing should be used. In the absence of such data, local epidemiology and susceptibility patterns should be considered when selecting anti-infectives for empiric therapy.

Information on test methods and quality control standards for in vitro susceptibility testing of antibacterial agents and specific interpretive criteria for such testing recognized by FDA is available at https://www.fda.gov/STIC.

Specific Populations

Pregnancy

The manufacturer recommends that women of childbearing potential use an effective form of contraception while receiving omadacycline.

Omadacycline, like other tetracyclines, may cause permanent discoloration of deciduous teeth and reversible inhibition of bone growth if administered during the second or third trimester of pregnancy.

There are insufficient data on the use of omadacycline in pregnant women to inform a drug-associated risk of major birth defects and miscarriages.

Results of animal studies indicate that tetracyclines cross the placenta, are found in fetal tissues, and may have toxic effects on the developing fetus (often related to retardation of skeletal development). Evidence of embryotoxicity also has been noted in animals that received tetracyclines early in pregnancy.

In rats and rabbits, use of omadacycline during the period of organogenesis resulted in fetal loss and/or congenital malformations at dosages resulting in area under the plasma concentration-time curve (AUC) exposures 7 and 3 times higher, respectively, than clinical exposures reported with IV doses of 100 mg or oral doses of 300 mg. Reduced fetal weight occurred in rats at all administered doses. In a fertility study in rats, use of omadacycline during mating and early pregnancy resulted in embryo loss at a dosage of 20 mg/kg daily and systemic exposures approximately equal to clinical exposures. Omadacycline has caused tooth discoloration in rats.

Patients should be advised of potential risks to the fetus if omadacycline is used during the second or third trimester of pregnancy.

Lactation

It is not known if omadacycline is distributed into human milk, affects the breast-fed infant, or affects milk production.

Tetracyclines are distributed into human milk; however, the extent of absorption of tetracyclines, including omadacycline, by the breast-fed infant is not known.

Because other antibacterial options are available to treat community-acquired pneumonia and skin and skin structure infections in lactating women and because of the potential for serious adverse effects in the breast-fed infant, breast-feeding is *not* recommended during omadacycline treatment and for 4 days after the last dose of the drug.

Fertility

Although human data are not available, there is evidence from animal studies that omadacycline can affect fertility.

In fertility studies in male rats, omadacycline caused injury to the testis and reduced sperm counts and sperm motility at doses resulting in exposures approximately 1.3 times higher than human exposures, but had no effect on fertility parameters. In general toxicity studies in rats, inhibition of spermatogenesis occurred after administration of omadacycline for 37 days or longer at doses resulting in exposures 6–8 times higher than human exposures; such effects did not occur when lower doses or shorter treatment periods (4 weeks or less) were used.

In fertility studies in female rats, reduced ovulation and increased embryonic loss were reported with doses resulting in exposures similar to human exposures.

Pediatric Use

Safety and efficacy of omadacycline have not been established in patients younger than 18 years of age.

Use of omadacycline in pediatric patients younger than 8 years of age is *not* recommended because of the adverse effects of tetracyclines on tooth development and bone growth.

Geriatric Use

Of the total number of patients who received omadacycline in phase 3 clinical trials, 18.6% were 65 years of age or older, including 8.6% who were 75 years of age or older.

In the clinical trial evaluating omadacycline in adults with community-acquired bacterial pneumonia, the clinical success rate at the early clinical response time point in patients 65 years of age or older (75.5 or 78.7% in those treated with omadacycline or moxifloxacin, respectively) was lower than that reported in patients younger than 65 years of age (85.2 or 86.3%, respectively). All deaths in this study occurred in patients older than 65 years of age.

No substantial difference in omadacycline exposures were observed between healthy geriatric individuals and younger adults following a single 100-mg IV dose of omadacycline. Dosage adjustments based on age are not necessary.

Hepatic Impairment

Omadacycline exposures, peak plasma concentrations, and clearance in individuals with mild, moderate, or severe hepatic impairment (Child-Pugh class A, B, or C) were similar to those observed in healthy individuals. Hepatic impairment did not affect omadacycline elimination.

Dosage adjustments of omadacycline are not needed in patients with mild, moderate, or severe hepatic impairment.

Renal Impairment

Omadacycline exposures, peak plasma concentrations, and clearance in adults with end-stage renal disease receiving hemodialysis were similar to those observed in healthy individuals. During dialysis, approximately 8% of omadacycline was recovered in the dialysate. Renal impairment does not affect omadacycline elimination.

Dosage adjustments of omadacycline are not needed in patients with mild, moderate, or severe renal impairment, including patients with end-stage renal disease receiving hemodialysis.

● Common Adverse Effects

Adverse effects reported in 1% or more of patients receiving omadacycline include infusion site reactions, increased AST and ALT, increased γ-glutamyltransferase (GGT, γ-glutamyltranspeptidase, GGTP), hypertension, insomnia, GI effects (diarrhea, vomiting, constipation, nausea), and headache.

DRUG INTERACTIONS

● Drugs Metabolized by Hepatic Microsomal Enzymes

In vitro, omadacycline tosylate does not inhibit or induce cytochrome P-450 (CYP) isoenzymes 1A1, 1A2, 2A6, 2B6, 2C8, 2C9, 2C19, 2D6, or 3A4/5.

Omadacycline is not expected to affect the pharmacokinetics of drugs metabolized by CYP isoenzymes.

● Drugs Metabolized by Uridine Diphosphate-glucuronosyltransferase 1A1

In vitro, omadacycline does not inhibit or induce uridine diphosphate-glucuronosyltransferase (UGT) 1A1.

Omadacycline is not expected to affect the pharmacokinetics of drugs metabolized by UGT1A1.

● Drugs Affecting or Affected by Membrane Transporters

Omadacycline is a low-affinity substrate of the P-glycoprotein (P-gp) transport system. The drug is not a substrate of breast cancer resistance protein (BCRP), organic anion transporter (OAT) 1, OAT3, or multidrug resistance-associated protein (MRP) 2. At supratherapeutic concentrations (5–13 times higher than clinically relevant concentrations), omadacycline is not a substrate of organic anion transporting polypeptide (OATP) 1B1 or 1B3.

Omadacycline does not inhibit P-gp, BCRP, OATP1B1, OATP1B3, OAT1, OAT3, or MRP2. It is unlikely that omadacycline induces P-gp or MRP2 expression.

● Antacids

Antacids containing aluminum, bismuth, calcium, or magnesium impair absorption of oral omadacycline.

Antacids should not be administered until 4 hours after oral omadacycline tablets.

● Antibacterial Agents

There is no in vitro evidence of antagonistic antibacterial effects between omadacycline and other commonly used antibacterials (e.g., ampicillin, ceftazidime, ceftriaxone, daptomycin, gentamicin, imipenem, linezolid, fixed combination of piperacillin and tazobactam, vancomycin).

● Anticoagulants

Because tetracyclines have been shown to decrease plasma prothrombin activity, patients receiving anticoagulant therapy concomitantly with omadacycline may require a decreased dosage of the anticoagulant.

● Iron and Multivitamins

Iron-containing preparations and multivitamins impair absorption of oral omadacycline.

Iron-containing preparations and multivitamins should not be administered until 4 hours after oral omadacycline tablets.

● Verapamil

Administration of oral verapamil (P-gp inhibitor) 2 hours before oral omadacycline (single 300-mg dose) increased omadacycline area under the plasma concentration-time curve (AUC) by approximately 25% and increased peak plasma concentrations of omadacycline by approximately 9%.

DESCRIPTION

Omadacycline tosylate is an aminomethylcycline and is a semisynthetic tetracycline derived from minocycline. Omadacycline differs structurally from other commercially available tetracyclines since it contains an aminomethyl group at position C-9 of the tetracycline core D-ring. This and other structural differences result in an expanded spectrum of activity compared with conventional tetracyclines (doxycycline, minocycline, tetracycline) since omadacycline is active in vitro against some bacteria that possess certain tetracycline-specific resistance mechanisms that can inactivate conventional tetracyclines. In addition, omadacycline generally is more potent in vitro against some susceptible bacteria than conventional tetracyclines.

Like other tetracyclines, omadacycline inhibits bacterial protein synthesis in susceptible organisms by binding to the 30S ribosomal subunit, which prevents incorporation of amino acid residues into peptide chains.

Omadacycline usually is bacteriostatic in action; however, the drug has been bactericidal against some isolates of Streptococcus pneumoniae and Haemophilus influenzae.

Following oral administration, omadacycline has an absolute bioavailability of 34.5%. Compared with administration in the fasted state, peak plasma concentrations were decreased 40 or 59% when a single 300-mg dose of oral omadacycline was administered 2 hours after a high-fat nondairy meal or a high-fat dairy-containing meal, respectively. No substantial effect on absorption was observed when oral omadacycline was administered 4 hours after a high-fat nondairy meal. Additionally, no substantial effect on peak plasma concentrations or area under the plasma concentration-time curve (AUC) was observed when oral omadacycline was administered 2 hours before a light non-fat meal, a standard low-fat meal, or a standard high-fat meal. In healthy adults, systemic omadacycline exposure is similar following a 300-mg oral dose (in the fasted state) or a 100-mg IV dose. Peak plasma concentrations of omadacycline are achieved approximately 2.5 hours after oral doses or at the end of a 30-minute IV infusion. Peak plasma concentrations and AUC increase in a dose-proportional manner following single 300- and 450-mg oral doses. Steady-state concentrations of omadacycline are achieved within 5 days; the accumulation ratio is 1.5. Omadacycline is distributed into alveolar cells and epithelial lining fluid at concentrations exceeding those in plasma by 25.8- and 1.5-fold, respectively. The drug is 20% bound to plasma proteins. Omadacycline is not metabolized. Following a single 300-mg oral dose, omadacycline is eliminated in feces (78–84%) and urine (approximately 14%) as unchanged drug; following a single 100-mg IV dose, 27% is eliminated in urine as unchanged drug. The mean elimination half-life of omadacycline following a single 100-mg IV dose, a single 300-mg oral dose, or a single 450-mg oral dose is approximately 16, 15, or 13.5 hours, respectively. Approximately 8% of a dose is removed by dialysis.

● Spectrum

Omadacycline has a broad spectrum of activity and is active against various gram-positive and gram-negative aerobic and anaerobic bacteria.

Omadacycline is active in vitro and in clinical community-acquired pneumonia infections against many gram-positive aerobic bacteria, including *S. pneumoniae* and methicillin-susceptible *Staphylococcus aureus*; the drug also is active in vitro and in clinical acute bacterial skin and skin structure infections against *Enterococcus faecalis*, *S. aureus* (methicillin-resistant *S. aureus* [MRSA; also known as oxacillin-resistant *S. aureus* or ORSA] and methicillin-susceptible *S. aureus*), *S. lugdunensis*, *S. anginosus* group (*S. anginosus*, *S. intermedius*, *S. constellatus*), and *S. pyogenes*. Omadacycline also is active in vitro against *E. faecium* (vancomycin-susceptible and -resistant isolates), *S. pseudintermedius*, *S. agalactiae*, *Bacillus anthracis*, and *Pasteurella canis*; however, the clinical importance of this in vitro activity is not known and efficacy of the drug for the treatment of clinical infections caused by these gram-positive bacteria has not been established.

Omadacycline is active in vitro and in clinical community-acquired pneumonia infections against many gram-negative aerobic bacteria, including *H. influenzae*, *H. parainfluenzae*, and *Klebsiella pneumoniae*; the drug also is active in vitro and in clinical skin and skin structure infections against *Enterobacter cloacae* and *K. pneumoniae*. Omadacycline also is active in vitro against *Citrobacter freundii*, *C. koseri*, *E. aerogenes*, *Escherichia coli*, *K. oxytoca*, *Moraxella catarrhalis*, *Serratia marcescens*, *Salmonella*, *Shigella*, *Stenotrophomonas maltophilia*, *Bergeyella zoohelcum*, *Neisseria weaveri*, *N. zoodegmatis*, and *Yersinia pestis*; however, the clinical importance of this in vitro activity is not known and efficacy of the drug for the treatment of clinical infections caused by these gram-negative bacteria has not been established.

Omadacycline is active in vitro and in clinical community-acquired pneumonia infections against other bacteria, including *Chlamydophila pneumoniae* (formerly *Chlamydia pneumoniae*), *Legionella pneumophila*, and *Mycoplasma pneumoniae*.

Although the clinical importance is not known, omadacycline is active in vitro against some gram-positive anaerobic bacteria, including *Clostridium perfringens* and *Peptostreptococcus*, and some gram-negative anaerobic bacteria, including *Bacteroides* (*B. fragilis*, *B. thetaiotaomicron*, *B. vulgatus*, *B. ovatus*, *B. pyogenes*), *Fusobacterium*, *Pasteurella multocida*, *Prevotella asaccharolytica*, *P. heparinolytica*, and *Porphyromonas*.

Omadacycline is not active in vitro against *Pseudomonas*, *Proteus*, *Providencia*, or *Morganella*.

● Resistance

Resistance to tetracyclines usually occurs as the result of tetracycline-specific resistance mechanisms such as efflux pumps, ribosomal protection proteins (RPPs), tetracycline degradation, and mutations in the rRNA target.

Because of its chemical structure, omadacycline has in vitro activity against some gram-positive and gram-negative bacteria that are resistant to conventional tetracyclines. Omadacycline is not affected by common tetracycline-specific efflux pumps (e.g., *tet*[B,] *tet*[K], *tet*[L]) and RPPs (e.g., *tet*[M], *tet*[O], *tet*[S]). However, resistance to omadacycline has been reported in some bacteria (e.g., *E. coli*) with tetracycline-specific mutations in 16S rRNA.

Based on surveillance data, omadacycline retains activity against tetracycline-resistant strains of *S. aureus*, *E. faecalis*, and *S. pneumoniae*. The drug also has been active in vitro against *S. aureus*, *S. pneumoniae*, and *H. influenzae* strains with macrolide resistance genes (*erm*A, B, and/or C) or ciprofloxacin resistance genes (*gyr*A, *par*C) and against β-lactamase-producing *H. influenzae*.

ADVICE TO PATIENTS

Advise patients that antibacterials, including omadacycline, should only be used to treat bacterial infections and not used to treat viral infections (e.g., the common cold).

Importance of completing the full course of therapy, even if feeling better after a few days.

Advise patients that skipping doses or not completing the full course of therapy may decrease effectiveness and increase the likelihood that bacteria will develop resistance and will not be treatable with omadacycline or other antibacterials in the future.

Instruct patients to fast for 4 hours before *and* 2 hours after taking omadacycline tablets; advise patients not to consume dairy products, antacids, iron-containing preparations, or multivitamins until 4 hours after taking omadacycline tablets.

Advise patients that allergic reactions, including serious allergic reactions, could occur and that serious reactions require immediate treatment. Inquire about any previous hypersensitivity reactions to omadacycline or other tetracyclines.

Advise patients that nausea and vomiting can occur with omadacycline therapy and that these adverse GI effects have been reported most frequently with the initial oral loading dosage of omadacycline used for treatment of acute bacterial skin and skin structure infection.

Advise patients that diarrhea is a common problem caused by anti-infectives and usually ends when the drug is discontinued. Importance of contacting a clinician if watery and bloody stools (with or without stomach cramps and fever) occur during or as late as 2 months or longer after the last dose.

Advise patients that omadacycline is similar to other tetracyclines and may have similar adverse effects.

Importance of women informing their clinician if they are or plan to become pregnant. Advise patients that omadacycline, like other tetracyclines, may cause permanent tooth discoloration of deciduous teeth and reversible inhibition of bone growth if administered during the second or third trimester of pregnancy.

Importance of women informing their clinician if they plan to breast-feed. Advise women not to breast-feed during omadacycline treatment and for 4 days after the last dose of the drug.

Importance of informing clinicians of existing or contemplated concomitant therapy, including prescription and OTC drugs and dietary or herbal supplements, as well as any concomitant illnesses.

Importance of informing patients of other important precautionary information. (See Cautions.)

PREPARATIONS

Excipients in commercially available drug preparations may have clinically important effects in some individuals; consult specific product labeling for details.

Omadacycline Tosylate

Oral		
Tablets, film-coated	150 mg (of omadacycline)	Nuzyra®, Paratek
Parenteral		
For injection, for IV infusion	100 mg (of omadacycline)	Nuzyra®, Paratek

Selected Revisions August 28, 2023, © Copyright, October 29, 2018, American Society of Health-System Pharmacists, Inc.

Eravacycline Dihydrochloride

8:12.24.08 • FLUOROCYCLINES

■ Eravacycline dihydrochloride, a synthetic fluorocycline, is a tetracycline anti-infective.

USES

● Intra-abdominal Infections

Eravacycline dihydrochloride is used for the treatment of complicated intra-abdominal infections caused by susceptible *Escherichia coli*, *Klebsiella pneumoniae*, *Citrobacter freundii*, *Enterobacter cloacae*, *K. oxytoca*, *Enterococcus faecalis*, *E. faecium*, *Staphylococcus aureus*, *Streptococcus anginosus* group, *Clostridium perfringens*, *Bacteroides*, and *Parabacteroides distasonis*.

Clinical Experience

Efficacy and safety of eravacycline for the treatment of complicated intra-abdominal infections were evaluated in 2 randomized, double-blind, active-controlled, phase 3 studies (IGNITE1; NCT01844856 and IGNITE4; NCT02784704). Results of these studies indicated that clinical cure rates in patients receiving eravacycline were noninferior to those in patients receiving ertapenem or meropenem.

IGNITE1 and IGNITE4 included a total of 1041 hospitalized adults with complicated intra-abdominal infections (e.g., appendicitis, cholecystitis, diverticulitis, gastric/duodenal perforation, intra-abdominal abscess, intestinal perforation, peritonitis) who were randomized to receive eravacycline (1 mg/kg IV every 12 hours) or a carbapenem (ertapenem 1 g every 24 hours [IGNITE1] or meropenem 1 g every 8 hours [IGNITE4]) for a duration of 4–14 days. There were a total of 846 patients in the microbiologic intent-to-treat (ITT) population (i.e., patients with at least 1 baseline intra-abdominal pathogen); characteristics of patients in IGNITE1 and IGNITE4 were similar (median age 56 years, 56% male, 95% from Europe, 5% from the US, 60% diagnosed with intra-abdominal abscess, 8% with bacteremia at baseline). In the microbiologic ITT population, clinical cure (i.e., complete resolution or substantial improvement of signs or symptoms of the index infection at the test-of-cure visit occurring 25–31 days after randomization) was achieved by 86.8 or 87.6% of patients in IGNITE1 receiving eravacycline or ertapenem, respectively; clinical cure was achieved by 90.8 or 91.2% of patients in IGNITE4 receiving eravacycline or meropenem, respectively.

When results of IGNITE1 and IGNITE4 were stratified according to causative organism, clinical cure rates in patients treated with eravacycline or a comparator (i.e., ertapenem, meropenem) were 86 or 80% for *C. freundii*, 81 or 96% for *E. cloacae*, 87 or 89% for *E. coli*, 93 or 84% for *K. oxytoca*, 95 or 84% for *K. pneumoniae*, 83 or 87% for *E. faecalis*, 84 or 91% for *E. faecium*, 100 or 86% for *S. aureus*, 86 or 85% for *S. anginosus* group, and 87 or 91% for anaerobes (e.g., *B. caccae*, *B. fragilis*, *B. ovatus*, *B. thetaiotaomicron*, *B. uniformis*, *B. vulgatus*, *C. perfringens*, *P. distasonis*), respectively.

● Urinary Tract Infections

Eravacycline is *not* labeled by FDA for the treatment of complicated urinary tract infections. Results from 2 randomized, double-blind, active-controlled, phase 3 clinical studies evaluating use of eravacycline for the treatment of complicated urinary tract infections† did not demonstrate efficacy of a once-daily IV regimen of the drug for the treatment of such infections based on the combined end points of clinical cure and microbiologic success in the microbiologic ITT population at the test-of-cure visit.

DOSAGE AND ADMINISTRATION

● Administration

Eravacycline dihydrochloride is administered by IV infusion.

IV Administration

Eravacycline powder for injection must be reconstituted and further diluted prior to IV infusion.

IV solutions of eravacycline should *not* be admixed with or added to solutions containing other drugs. Eravacycline is compatible with 0.9% sodium chloride injection, but compatibility with other drugs or other infusion solutions has not been established.

Eravacycline may be administered IV through a dedicated line or a Y-site. If the same IV line is used for sequential infusion of several drugs, the line should be flushed with 0.9% sodium chloride injection before and after the eravacycline infusion.

Reconstitution and Dilution

The appropriate number of single-dose vials labeled as containing 50 mg of eravacycline should be reconstituted by adding 5 mL of sterile water for injection or 0.9% sodium chloride injection to each vial and swirling gently until the contents are dissolved. To avoid foaming, the vials should not be shaken or moved rapidly. The reconstituted solution contains 10 mg of eravacycline per mL.

Prior to IV infusion, reconstituted eravacycline solutions *must* be further diluted. To prepare the indicated dose, the appropriate volume of reconstituted solution should be withdrawn from the vial(s) and added to 0.9% sodium chloride to achieve a target concentration of 0.3 mg/mL (range 0.2–0.6 mg/mL). Diluted eravacycline solutions should not be shaken.

Reconstituted eravacycline solutions containing 10 mg/mL are stable for 1 hour at room temperature (not exceeding 25°C) and should be discarded if not further diluted within 1 hour after reconstitution. Following reconstitution *and* dilution, eravacycline solutions must be infused within 24 hours if stored at room temperature (not exceeding 25°C) or within 7 days if stored under refrigeration (2–8°C). Eravacycline solutions should not be frozen. Unused portions of the reconstituted and diluted solution should be discarded.

Reconstituted and diluted eravacycline solutions should be inspected visually for particulate matter and discoloration prior to administration. The solution should appear clear and light yellow to orange in color and should not be used if it is cloudy or contains particulates.

Rate of Administration

IV solutions of eravacycline should be given by IV infusion over approximately 60 minutes.

● Dosage

Dosage of eravacycline dihydrochloride is expressed in terms of eravacycline.

Intra-abdominal Infections

The recommended dosage of eravacycline for the treatment of complicated intra-abdominal infections in adults is 1 mg/kg every 12 hours for 4–14 days. The duration of therapy should be guided by the severity and location of the infection and the patient's clinical response.

Concomitant Use with CYP3A Inducers

If eravacycline is used concomitantly with a potent inducer of cytochrome P-450 (CYP) isoenzyme 3A, the dosage of eravacycline should be increased to 1.5 mg/kg every 12 hours for 4–14 days. (See Drug Interactions.)

Eravacycline dosage adjustments are not needed if the drug is used concomitantly with a weak or moderate inducer of CYP3A.

● Special Populations

Hepatic Impairment

Mild or moderate hepatic impairment (Child-Pugh class A or B): Dosage adjustments are not needed.

Severe hepatic impairment (Child-Pugh class C): The manufacturer recommends that eravacycline be given in a dosage of 1 mg/kg every 12 hours on day 1, followed by 1 mg/kg once every 24 hours starting on day 2 of treatment and continued for a total treatment duration of 4–14 days.

Renal Impairment

Dosage adjustments are not needed in patients with renal impairment.

CAUTIONS

● Contraindications

Eravacycline dihydrochloride is contraindicated in patients with known hypersensitivity to eravacycline, other tetracyclines, or any excipients in the preparation.

● Warnings/Precautions

Sensitivity Reactions

Hypersensitivity Reactions

Life-threatening hypersensitivity reactions, including anaphylactic reactions, have been reported in patients receiving eravacycline. Because eravacycline is structurally similar to other tetracyclines, it is contraindicated in patients with known hypersensitivity to any tetracycline.

Eravacycline should be discontinued if an allergic reaction occurs.

Tooth Discoloration and Enamel Hypoplasia

The use of tetracyclines, including eravacycline, during tooth development (i.e., last half of pregnancy, infancy, childhood up to 8 years of age) may cause permanent discoloration of the teeth (yellow-grey-brown). Tooth discoloration is more common during long-term use of tetracyclines, but has been observed following repeated short-term use of the drugs. Enamel hypoplasia also has been reported with tetracyclines.

Inhibition of Bone Growth

The use of tetracyclines, including eravacycline, during the second or third trimester of pregnancy, infancy, or childhood up to 8 years of age may cause reversible inhibition of bone growth. Tetracyclines form a stable calcium complex in any bone-forming tissue. Decreased fibula growth rate has been observed in premature infants given oral tetracycline in a dosage of 25 mg/kg every 6 hours; this effect was shown to be reversible when the drug was discontinued.

Tetracycline-class Effects

Because eravacycline is structurally similar to conventional tetracyclines, adverse effects reported with tetracyclines (e.g., photosensitivity, pseudotumor cerebri, anti-anabolic action leading to increased BUN, azotemia, acidosis, hyperphosphatemia, pancreatitis, abnormal liver function tests) may occur with eravacycline. Eravacycline should be discontinued if any of these adverse effects are suspected.

For further information on tetracycline-class effects, see Cautions in the Tetracyclines General Statement 8:12.24.

Superinfection/C. difficile-associated Diarrhea and Colitis

Use of eravacycline may result in emergence and overgrowth of nonsusceptible bacteria or fungi. If such infections occur, eravacycline should be discontinued and appropriate therapy instituted.

Treatment with anti-infectives alters normal colon flora and may permit overgrowth of *Clostridioides difficile* (formerly known as *Clostridium difficile*). *C. difficile* infection (CDI) and *C. difficile*-associated diarrhea and colitis (CDAD; also known as antibiotic-associated diarrhea and colitis or pseudomembranous colitis) have been reported in patients receiving nearly all anti-infectives, including eravacycline, and may range in severity from mild diarrhea to fatal colitis. *C. difficile* produces toxins A and B which contribute to development of CDAD; hypertoxin-producing strains of *C. difficile* are associated with increased morbidity and mortality since they may be refractory to anti-infectives and colectomy may be required.

CDAD should be considered in the differential diagnosis of patients who develop diarrhea during or after anti-infective therapy. Careful medical history is necessary since CDAD has been reported to occur as late as 2 months or longer after anti-infective therapy is discontinued.

If CDAD is suspected or confirmed, anti-infective therapy not directed against *C. difficile* should be discontinued as soon as possible. Patients should be managed with appropriate anti-infective therapy directed against *C. difficile*

(e.g., vancomycin, fidaxomicin, metronidazole), supportive therapy (e.g., fluid and electrolyte management, protein supplementation), and surgical evaluation as clinically indicated.

Selection and Use of Anti-infectives

To reduce development of drug-resistant bacteria and maintain effectiveness of eravacycline and other antibacterials, the drug should be used only for the treatment of infections proven or strongly suspected to be caused by susceptible bacteria. Prescribing eravacycline in the absence of a proven or strongly suspected bacterial infection is unlikely to provide benefit to the patient and increases the risk of development of drug-resistant bacteria.

When selecting or modifying anti-infective therapy, results of culture and in vitro susceptibility testing should be used. In the absence of such data, local epidemiology and susceptibility patterns should be considered when selecting anti-infectives for empiric therapy.

Information on test methods and quality control standards for in vitro susceptibility testing of antibacterial agents and specific interpretive criteria for such testing recognized by FDA is available at https://www.fda.gov/STIC.

Specific Populations

Pregnancy

Eravacycline, like other tetracyclines, may cause permanent discoloration of deciduous teeth and reversible inhibition of bone growth if administered during the second or third trimester of pregnancy. (See Tooth Discoloration and Enamel Hypoplasia and see Inhibition of Bone Growth under Cautions: Warnings/Precautions.)

There are insufficient data regarding use of eravacycline in pregnant women to inform a drug-associated risk of major birth defects and miscarriages.

Results of animal studies indicate that tetracyclines, including eravacycline, cross the placenta, are found in fetal plasma, and can have toxic effects on the developing fetus. Evidence of embryotoxicity has been noted in animals that received tetracyclines early in pregnancy.

In rats, eravacycline crosses the placenta and is found in fetal plasma following IV administration to the dams. In rats and rabbits, eravacycline administered during the period of organogenesis at doses approximately 8.6 and 6.3 times higher, respectively, than clinical exposures based on area under the plasma concentration-time curve (AUC) was associated with decreased ossification, decreased fetal body weight, and/or increased post-implantation loss.

Patients should be advised of the potential risks to the fetus if eravacycline is used during the second or third trimester of pregnancy. (See Advice to Patients.)

Lactation

Eravacycline and its metabolites are distributed into milk in lactating rats. It is not known if the drug is distributed into milk in humans, affects the breast-fed infant, or affects milk production.

Because other antibacterial options are available to treat complicated intra-abdominal infections in lactating women and because of the potential for serious adverse effects in the breast-fed infant (see Tooth Discoloration and Enamel Hypoplasia and see Inhibition of Bone Growth under Cautions: Warnings/Precautions), breast-feeding is *not* recommended during eravacycline treatment and for 4 days after the last dose of the drug.

Fertility

Although human data are not available, there is evidence from animal studies that eravacycline can lead to impaired spermiation and sperm maturation resulting in abnormal sperm morphology and poor motility.

In fertility studies in male rats, eravacycline did not affect mating or fertility at IV dosages resulting in exposures approximately 1.5 times higher than human exposures; however, higher doses were associated with adverse effects on fertility and spermatogenesis (impaired spermiation and sperm maturation, decreased sperm counts, abnormal sperm morphology, reduced sperm motility). These effects on male rats appeared to be reversible.

Fertility studies in female rats have not revealed evidence of adverse effects on mating or fertility.

Pediatric Use

Safety and efficacy of eravacycline have not been established in patients younger than 18 years of age.

Use of eravacycline in pediatric patients younger than 8 years of age is *not* recommended because of the adverse effects of tetracyclines on tooth development and bone growth. (see Tooth Discoloration and Enamel Hypoplasia and see Inhibition of Bone Growth under Cautions: Warnings/Precautions)

Geriatric Use

In phase 3 clinical studies evaluating eravacycline for the treatment of complicated intra-abdominal infections, 30% of patients were 65 years of age or older and 11% were 75 years of age or older. No overall differences in safety or efficacy were observed between geriatric and younger adults.

Based on population pharmacokinetic analysis, no clinically relevant age-related differences in eravacycline pharmacokinetics were observed in adults 18–86 years of age.

Hepatic Impairment

Peak plasma concentrations of eravacycline were approximately 14, 16, or 20% higher in individuals with mild (Child-Pugh class A), moderate (Child-Pugh class B), or severe (Child-Pugh class C) hepatic impairment, respectively, compared with healthy individuals. Eravacycline AUC was approximately 23, 38, or 110% higher in individuals with mild, moderate, or severe hepatic impairment, respectively, compared with healthy individuals.

Dosage adjustments are not needed in patients with mild or moderate hepatic impairment. Eravacycline dosage should be adjusted in patients with severe hepatic impairment. (See Hepatic Impairment under Dosage and Administration: Special Populations.)

Renal Impairment

In individuals with end-stage renal disease, peak plasma concentrations of eravacycline were increased by 8.8% and the AUC was decreased by 4% compared with healthy individuals.

Dosage adjustments are not needed in patients with renal impairment.

● Common Adverse Effects

Adverse effects reported in 1% or more of patients receiving eravacycline include infusion site reactions, nausea, vomiting, diarrhea, hypotension, wound dehiscence, and anemia.

DRUG INTERACTIONS

● Drugs Affecting or Metabolized by Hepatic Microsomal Enzymes

Eravacycline dihydrochloride is metabolized by cytochrome P-450 (CYP) isoenzyme 3A4.

Concomitant use of eravacycline and potent inducers of CYP3A (e.g., rifampin, phenytoin) decreases eravacycline exposures and may reduce eravacycline efficacy. Eravacycline dosage should be increased if the drug is used concomitantly with a potent inducer of CYP3A. (See Concomitant Use with CYP3A Inducers under Dosage: Intra-abdominal Infections, in Dosage and Administration.)

In vitro, eravacycline does not inhibit CYP1A2, 2B6, 2C8, 2C9, 2C19, 2D6, or 3A4/5 and does not induce CYP1A2, 2B6, or 3A4.

● Drugs Affecting or Affected by Membrane Transporters

Eravacycline is not a substrate of P-glycoprotein (P-gp) transport system, breast cancer resistance protein (BCRP), bile salt export pump (BSEP), organic anion transport polypeptide (OATP) 1B1, OATP1B3, organic anion transporter (OAT) 1, OAT3, organic cation transporter (OCT) 1, OCT2, multidrug and toxin extrusion transporter (MATE) 1, or MATE2-K transporters.

Eravacycline does not inhibit BCRP, BSEP, OATP1B1, OATP1B3, OAT1, OAT3, OCT1, OCT2, MATE1, or MATE2-K.

● Antibacterial Agents

There is no in vitro evidence of antagonistic antibacterial effects between eravacycline and other antibacterials commonly used for eravacycline's labeled indications and pathogens.

● Anticoagulants

Because tetracyclines have been shown to decrease plasma prothrombin activity, patients receiving anticoagulant therapy concomitantly with eravacycline may require a decreased dosage of the anticoagulant.

● Anticonvulsants

Phenytoin

If eravacycline is used concomitantly with phenytoin (potent CYP3A inducer), the dosage of eravacycline should be increased to 1.5 mg/kg every 12 hours.

● Antifungal Agents

Itraconazole

Concomitant use of eravacycline and itraconazole (potent CYP3A inhibitor) increases eravacycline peak plasma concentrations by 5% and area under the plasma concentration-time curve (AUC) by 32%; eravacycline clearance is decreased by 32%.

● Antimycobacterial Agents

Rifampin

Concomitant use of eravacycline and rifampin (potent CYP3A4/5 inducer) decreases eravacycline AUC by 35% and increases eravacycline clearance by 54%.

If eravacycline is used concomitantly with rifampin, the dosage of eravacycline should be increased to 1.5 mg/kg every 12 hours.

DESCRIPTION

Eravacycline dihydrochloride is a fluorocycline. Eravacycline differs structurally from other commercially available tetracyclines since it contains a fluorine atom at position C-7 and a pyrrolidinoacetamido group at position C-9 of the tetracycline core D-ring. These structural differences result in an expanded spectrum of activity compared with conventional tetracyclines (doxycycline, minocycline, tetracycline) since eravacycline is active in vitro against some bacteria that possess certain tetracycline-specific resistance mechanisms that can inactivate conventional tetracyclines. In addition, eravacycline generally is more potent in vitro against some susceptible bacteria than conventional tetracyclines or tigecycline (a glycylcycline).

Like other tetracyclines, eravacycline disrupts bacterial protein synthesis in susceptible organisms by binding to the 30S ribosomal subunit, which prevents incorporation of amino acid residues into peptide chains.

Eravacycline usually is bacteriostatic in action against susceptible gram-positive bacteria (e.g., *Staphylococcus aureus*, *Enterococcus faecalis*); the drug has been bactericidal in vitro against certain strains of *Escherichia coli* and *Klebsiella pneumoniae*.

Following single IV doses of eravacycline ranging from 1–3 mg/kg, the area under the plasma concentration-time curve (AUC) and peak plasma concentrations increase in an approximately dose-proportional manner. Peak plasma concentrations are attained by the end of a 60-minute IV infusion. When an eravacycline dosage of 1 mg/kg IV every 12 hours is used, there is approximately 45% accumulation and steady-state concentrations are attained on day 5. The volume of distribution of eravacycline at steady state is approximately 4 L/kg, which suggests extensive tissue distribution; the drug is distributed into bone and lungs following IV administration. Plasma protein binding of eravacycline is concentration dependent and increases from 79–90% with increasing plasma concentrations ranging from 100–10,000 ng/mL. Eravacycline is primarily metabolized by cytochrome P-450 (CYP) isoenzyme 3A4 and flavin-containing monooxygenase (FMO). Following a single 60-mg IV dose of eravacycline, approximately 34% of the dose is eliminated in urine and 47% is eliminated in feces as unchanged eravacycline and metabolites (20% in urine and 17% in feces as unchanged drug). The mean elimination half-life of eravacycline following IV administration is 20 hours.

SPECTRUM

Eravacycline has a broad spectrum of activity and is active against various gram-positive and gram-negative aerobic and anaerobic bacteria.

Eravacycline is active in vitro and in clinical infections against many gram-positive aerobic bacteria, including *S. aureus* (including methicillin-resistant *S. aureus* [MRSA; also known as oxacillin-resistant *S. aureus* or ORSA] and methicillin-susceptible *S. aureus*), Streptococcus anginosus group, *E. faecalis*, and *E. faecium*. Eravacycline also is active in vitro against *S. epidermidis, S. agalactiae, S. pneumoniae, S. pyogenes, S. salivarius* group, and *Bacillus anthracis*; however, the clinical importance of this in vitro activity is not known, and efficacy of eravacycline for the treatment of clinical infections caused by these gram-positive bacteria has not been established.

Eravacycline is active in vitro and in clinical infections against many gram-negative aerobic bacteria, including *Citrobacter freundii, Enterobacter cloacae, E. coli, K. oxytoca,* and *K. pneumoniae*. Eravacycline also is active in vitro against *Acinetobacter baumannii, C. koseri, E. aerogenes, Francisella tularensis, Haemophilus influenzae, Moraxella catarrhalis, Neisseria gonorrhoeae, Proteus vulgaris, Salmonella, Shigella, Strenotrophomonas maltophilia,* and *Yersinia pestis*; however, the clinical importance of this in vitro activity is not known, and efficacy of eravacycline for the treatment of clinical infections caused by these gram-negative bacteria has not been established.

Eravacycline is active in vitro and in clinical infections against some gram-positive anaerobic bacteria, including *Clostridium perfringens*. The drug also is active in vitro and in clinical infections against some gram-negative anaerobic bacteria, including *Bacteroides (B. caccae, B. fragilis, B. ovatus, B. thetaiotaomicron, B. uniformis, B. vulgatus)* and *Parabacteroides distasonis*.

Eravacycline is not active against *Pseudomonas aeruginosa*. Although some *Burkholderia mallei* and *B. pseudomallei* may be susceptible to eravacycline in vitro, *B. cenocepacia* are resistant.

RESISTANCE

Resistance to tetracyclines usually occurs as the result of tetracycline-specific resistance mechanisms such as efflux pumps, ribosomal protection proteins (RPPs), tetracycline degradation, and mutations in the rRNA target.

The C-7 and C-9 substitutions in the chemical structure of eravacycline enhance its in vitro activity against some gram-positive and gram-negative bacteria that are resistant to conventional tetracyclines. Eravacycline is not affected, or is only minimally affected, by common tetracycline-specific resistance mechanisms that involve efflux pumps mediated by *tet*(A), *tet*(B), *tet*(L), and *tet*(K) and RPPs encoded by *tet*(M) and *tet*(Q).

Eravacycline is active in vitro against some Enterobacteriaceae that produce certain β-lactamases, including extended-spectrum β-lactamases (ESBLs) and AmpC. However, some β-lactamase-producing isolates may be resistant to eravacycline because of other resistance mechanisms. Resistance to eravacycline has been demonstrated in some bacteria with upregulated, nonspecific, intrinsic,

multidrug-resistant (MDR) efflux or target-site modifications (e.g., 16s rRNA or certain 30S ribosomal proteins [S10]).

ADVICE TO PATIENTS

Advise patients that antibacterials, including eravacycline, should only be used to treat bacterial infections and not used to treat viral infections (e.g., the common cold).

Importance of completing the full course of therapy, even if feeling better after a few days.

Advise patients that skipping doses or not completing the full course of therapy may decrease effectiveness and increase the likelihood that bacteria will develop resistance and will not be treatable with eravacycline or other antibacterials in the future.

Advise patients that allergic reactions, including serious allergic reactions, could occur and that serious reactions require immediate treatment. Inquire about any previous hypersensitivity reactions to tetracyclines, other antibiotics, or other allergens.

Advise patients that diarrhea is a common problem caused by anti-infectives, including eravacycline, and usually ends when the drug is discontinued. Importance of contacting a clinician if watery and bloody stools (with or without stomach cramps and fever) occur during or as late as 2 months or longer after the last dose.

Advise patients that eravacycline is similar to other tetracyclines and may have similar adverse effects.

Importance of women informing their clinician if they are or plan to become pregnant. Advise patients that eravacycline, like other tetracyclines, may cause permanent tooth discoloration of deciduous teeth and reversible inhibition of bone growth if administered during the second or third trimester of pregnancy.

Importance of women informing their clinician if they plan to breast-feed. Advise women not to breast-feed during eravacycline treatment and for 4 days after the last dose of the drug.

Importance of informing clinicians of existing or contemplated concomitant therapy, including prescription and OTC drugs and dietary or herbal supplements, as well as any concomitant illnesses.

Importance of informing patients of other important precautionary information. (See Cautions.)

PREPARATIONS

Excipients in commercially available drug preparations may have clinically important effects in some individuals; consult specific product labeling for details.

Eravacycline Dihydrochloride

Parenteral

For injection, for IV infusion	50 mg (of eravacycline)	Xerava®, Tetraphase

† Use is not currently included in the labeling approved by the US Food and Drug Administration.

Selected Revisions February 3, 2020, © Copyright, September 17, 2018, American Society of Health-System Pharmacists, Inc.

Tigecycline

8:12.24.12 • GLYCYLCYCLINES

■ Tigecycline, a synthetic derivative of minocycline, is a glycylcycline antibiotic.

USES

Tigecycline is used for the treatment of complicated intra-abdominal infections, community-acquired pneumonia, and complicated skin and skin structure infections caused by certain susceptible gram-positive and gram-negative bacteria.

Because a higher incidence of all-cause mortality has been reported in patients receiving tigecycline compared with those receiving comparator anti-infectives, tigecycline should be reserved for use in situations when alternative anti-infectives are not suitable. (See Increased Mortality under Warnings/Precautions: Warnings, in Cautions.)

Prior to initiation of tigecycline, appropriate specimens should be obtained for identification of the causative organism and in vitro susceptibility testing. Tigecycline may be initiated as empiric monotherapy pending results of these tests.

● Intra-abdominal Infections

Tigecycline is used for the treatment of complicated intra-abdominal infections caused by *Citrobacter freundii*, *Enterobacter cloacae*, *Escherichia coli*, *Klebsiella oxytoca*, *K. pneumoniae*, *Enterococcus faecalis* (vancomycin-susceptible strains only), *Staphylococcus aureus* (including methicillin-resistant *S. aureus* [MRSA; also known as oxacillin-resistant *S. aureus* or ORSA]), *Streptococcus anginosus* group (*S. anginosus*, *S. intermedius*, *S. constellatus*), *Bacteroides fragilis*, *B. thetaiotaomicron*, *B. uniformis*, *B. vulgatus*, *Clostridium perfringens*, or *Peptostreptococcus micros*.

For initial empiric treatment of mild to moderate community-acquired, extrabiliary, complicated intra-abdominal infections in adults (e.g., perforated or abscessed appendicitis), the Infectious Diseases Society of America (IDSA) recommends either monotherapy with cefoxitin, ertapenem, moxifloxacin, tigecycline, or the fixed combination of ticarcillin and clavulanic acid, or a combination regimen that includes either a cephalosporin (cefazolin, ceftriaxone, cefotaxime, cefuroxime) or fluoroquinolone (ciprofloxacin, levofloxacin) in conjunction with metronidazole.

For additional information regarding management of intra-abdominal infections, the current IDSA clinical practice guidelines available at http://www.idsociety.org should be consulted.

Clinical Experience

Safety and efficacy of tigecycline were established in 2 randomized, double-blind, active-controlled phase 3 studies in adults with complicated intra-abdominal infections, including appendicitis, cholecystitis, diverticulitis, gastric/duodenal perforation, intra-abdominal abscess, intestinal perforation, and peritonitis. In these studies, patients were randomized to receive tigecycline (100 mg IV initially, followed by 50 mg IV every 12 hours) or imipenem and cilastatin sodium (500 mg of imipenem IV every 6 hours) for 5–14 days. In a pooled analysis of both studies, the clinical cure rate in the clinically evaluable population was similar in patients treated with tigecycline (87%) and in those treated with imipenem and cilastatin (87%). In the subset of microbiologically evaluable patients from these clinical studies and 2 additional resistant-pathogen studies, the clinical cure rate in those who received tigecycline ranged from 71–95%, depending on the pathogen. When stratified according to causative organism, the clinical cure rate was 85% in infections caused by *E. coli*, 85% in infections caused by *S. anginosus*, 89% in infections caused by *K. pneumoniae*, and 77% in infections caused by the *B. fragilis* group.

In 2 randomized, open-label, multicenter, phase 3b/4 studies, tigecycline was compared with a combination regimen of ceftriaxone in conjunction with metronidazole for the treatment of complicated intra-abdominal infections in adults. In both studies, patients were randomized to receive either tigecycline (100 mg IV initially, followed by 50 mg IV every 12 hours) or a 2-drug regimen of ceftriaxone (2 g IV once daily) and metronidazole (1–2 g daily in divided doses) for 4–14 days. In the first open-label study, demographic characteristics were balanced between groups (mean age 48 years, 64.7% male, 65.3% Caucasian, 52% with primary diagnosis of complicated appendicitis). Clinical cure rate in the clinically evaluable

population (376 patients) was 70% in the tigecycline group compared with 74% in the ceftriaxone and metronidazole group. In the subset of microbiologically evaluable patients (275 patients), the clinical cure rate in those who received tigecycline was 66% compared with 70% in the ceftriaxone and metronidazole group. When stratified according to causative organism, the clinical cure rate in the tigecycline group was 70% for infections caused by *E. coli*, 79% for infections caused by *S. anginosus*, 40% for infections caused by *Klebsiella*, and 64% for infections caused by the *B. fragilis* group.

In the second open-label study, demographic characteristics were balanced between groups (mean age 47–49 years, 66–69% male, 38–47% with primary diagnosis of complicated appendicitis). The mean Acute Physiological Assessment and Chronic Health Evaluation (APACHE) II score was 6–7 and the mean duration of treatment was 7 days in both groups. Clinical cure rate in the clinically evaluable population (387 patients) was 82% in the tigecycline group compared with 79% in the ceftriaxone and metronidazole group. In the subset of microbiologically evaluable patients (227 patients), the clinical cure rate in those who received tigecycline was 82% compared with 80% in the ceftriaxone and metronidazole group. When stratified according to causative organism, the clinical cure rate in the tigecycline group was 83% for infections caused by *E. coli*, 94% for infections caused by the *S. anginosus* group, 77% for infections caused by *K. pneumoniae*, and 67% for infections caused by the *B. fragilis* group.

● Respiratory Tract Infections

Community-acquired Pneumonia

Tigecycline is used for the treatment of community-acquired pneumonia caused by *S. pneumoniae* (penicillin-susceptible strains only), including cases with concurrent bacteremia, or caused by *Haemophilus influenzae* (β-lactamase-negative strains only) or *Legionella pneumophila*.

Clinical Experience

Safety and efficacy of tigecycline were established in 2 randomized, double-blind, active-controlled studies in adults with community-acquired pneumonia requiring hospitalization. Patients were randomized to receive tigecycline (100 mg IV initially, followed by 50 mg IV every 12 hours) or levofloxacin (500 mg IV every 12 or 24 hours) for 7–14 days. Clinical cure rates in the clinically evaluable population from the first study were similar in tigecycline-treated patients (89%) and levofloxacin-treated patients (85%). In the second study, patients in both treatment arms could be switched to oral levofloxacin (500 mg daily) after at least 3 days of IV treatment, and the clinical cure rates in the clinically evaluable population were 91% for tigecycline-treated patients and 87% for levofloxacin-treated patients. In the subset of microbiologically evaluable patients from both studies, the clinical cure rate in patients who received tigecycline was 96% in infections caused by *S. pneumoniae* (penicillin-susceptible strains only), 82% in infections caused by *H. influenzae*, and 100% in infections caused by *L. pneumophila*.

Hospital-acquired Pneumonia

Tigecycline has *not* been shown to be effective and is *not* labeled by the US Food and Drug Administration (FDA) for the treatment of hospital-acquired pneumonia†, including ventilator-associated pneumonia†. Results of a randomized, comparator-controlled trial evaluating tigecycline in patients with hospital-acquired pneumonia† failed to show efficacy. The subgroup of patients with ventilator-associated pneumonia† who received tigecycline demonstrated lower cure rates (47.9% in those treated with tigecycline versus 70.1% in those treated with a comparator anti-infective) and a higher incidence of death (19.1% in those treated with tigecycline versus 12.3% in those treated with a comparator anti-infective). (See Increased Mortality under Warnings/Precautions: Warnings, in Cautions.)

● Skin and Skin Structure Infections

Tigecycline is used for the treatment of complicated skin and skin structure infections caused by *S. aureus* (including MRSA), *Streptococcus agalactiae* (group B streptococci), *S. anginosus* group (*S. anginosus*, *S. intermedius*, *S. constellatus*), *S. pyogenes* (group A β-hemolytic streptococci), *E. faecalis* (vancomycin-susceptible strains only), *E. cloacae*, *E. coli*, *K. pneumoniae*, or *B. fragilis*.

Tigecycline has *not* been shown to be effective and is *not* labeled by FDA for the treatment of diabetic foot infections†. In a phase 3, randomized, double-blind study that included 813 clinically evaluable adults with diabetic foot infection, tigecycline (150 mg IV once daily) did not meet the primary end point of noninferiority to ertapenem (1g IV once daily with or without vancomycin). In addition, a higher incidence of death has been observed in patients with diabetic foot infections receiving tigecycline (1.3%) compared with those receiving comparator anti-infectives (0.6%). (See Increased Mortality under Warnings/Precautions: Warnings, in Cautions.)

Clinical Experience

Safety and efficacy of tigecycline were established in 2 randomized, double-blind, active-controlled studies in adults with complicated deep soft tissue infections, including wound infections and cellulitis (10 cm or larger, requiring surgery or drainage, or with complicated underlying disease), major abscesses, infected ulcers, and burns. In these studies, patients were randomized to receive tigecycline (100 mg IV initially, followed by 50 mg IV every 12 hours) or a combination regimen of vancomycin (1 g IV every 12 hours) and aztreonam (2 g IV every 12 hours) for 5–14 days. In a pooled analysis of both studies, the clinical cure rate in the clinically evaluable population was 87% in patients treated with tigecycline and 89% in those treated with the 2-drug regimen of vancomycin and aztreonam. In the subset of microbiologically evaluable patients from these clinical studies and 2 additional resistant-pathogen studies, clinical cure rates ranged from 71–100%, depending on the pathogen. This included clinical cure rates of 91% in those with infections caused by methicillin-susceptible (oxacillin-susceptible) S. aureus, 83% in those with infections caused by MRSA, 97% in those with infections caused by S. pyogenes, and 81% in those with infections caused by E. coli.

In a phase 3b/4 randomized, open-label, multicenter study, the safety and efficacy of tigecycline for the treatment of complicated skin and skin structure infections (e.g., deep soft tissue infection, major abscess, infected ulcers, burns covering less than 5% of body surface area) were evaluated in 405 adults. Patients were randomized to receive tigecycline (100 mg IV initially, followed by 50 mg IV every 12 hours) or a comparator anti-infective regimen (i.e., fixed combination of ampicillin and sulbactam [1.5–3 g IV every 6 hours] or fixed combination of amoxicillin and clavulanate [1.2 g IV every 6–8 hours]) for 4–14 days. Baseline characteristics were balanced between groups (mean age 51–52 years, 61–64% male, 53–56% white). Clinical cure was achieved in 77.5% of patients in the tigecycline group compared with 77.6% of patients in the comparator group. In the subset of microbiologically evaluable patients (219 patients), the eradication rate at the test-of-cure assessment was 79 and 77% in the tigecycline and comparator groups, respectively. When stratified according to causative organism, the clinical cure rate in the tigecycline group was 83% in those with infections caused by methicillin-susceptible (oxacillin-susceptible) S. aureus, 69% in those with infections caused by MRSA, 73% in those with infections caused by S. pyogenes, and 77% in those with infections caused by E. coli.

DOSAGE AND ADMINISTRATION

● Administration

Tigecycline is administered by IV infusion.

Tigecycline may be administered through a dedicated line or through a Y-site. If the same IV line is used for sequential infusion of several drugs, the line should be flushed before and after infusion of tigecycline with 0.9% sodium chloride, 5% dextrose, or lactated Ringer's injection. Tigecycline should not be administered simultaneously through the same Y-site with amphotericin B, amphotericin B lipid complex, diazepam, esomeprazole, or omeprazole.

Reconstitution and Dilution

Tigecycline powder for injection must be reconstituted and diluted before IV infusion. The final tigecycline solution should have a maximum concentration of 1 mg/mL.

Tigecycline powder for injection should be reconstituted by adding 5.3 mL of 0.9% sodium chloride, 5% dextrose, or lactated Ringer's injection to the vial labeled as containing 50 mg of tigecycline to provide a solution containing 10 mg/mL. The vial should be swirled gently until the drug dissolves. The reconstituted solution should be yellow or orange in color; if not, the solution should be discarded.

For preparation of a 50-mg dose, 5 mL of the reconstituted solution should be withdrawn from the vial and diluted in 100 mL of 0.9% sodium chloride or 5% dextrose injection. For preparation of a 100-mg dose, two 50-mg vials of tigecycline should be reconstituted, and 10 mL of the reconstituted solution should be diluted in 100 mL of 0.9% sodium chloride or 5% dextrose injection.

Following reconstitution with 0.9% sodium chloride injection, 5% dextrose injection, or lactated Ringer's injection, tigecycline solutions may be stored at room temperature (not to exceed 25°C) for up to a total of 24 hours (up to 6 hours in original vial, remaining time after dose is diluted in an IV bag containing 0.9% sodium chloride or 5% dextrose injection). If storage conditions after reconstitution exceed 25°C, tigecycline should be used immediately. Alternatively, if the dose of reconstituted tigecycline is immediately diluted in an IV bag containing 0.9% sodium chloride or 5% dextrose, the solution may be stored at 2–8°C for up to 48 hours.

Parenteral tigecycline solutions should be inspected visually for particulate matter and discoloration (e.g., green, black) prior to administration.

Rate of Administration

Tigecycline should be administered by IV infusion over approximately 30–60 minutes.

● Dosage

Adult Dosage

Intra-abdominal Infections

The recommended dosage of tigecycline for the treatment of complicated intra-abdominal infections in adults 18 years of age and older is an initial dose of 100 mg, followed by 50 mg every 12 hours. Duration of therapy should be guided by the severity and site of infection and the patient's clinical and bacteriologic progress; the usual duration of therapy is 5–14 days.

Community-acquired Pneumonia

The recommended dosage of tigecycline for the treatment of community-acquired pneumonia in adults 18 years of age and older is an initial dose of 100 mg, followed by 50 mg every 12 hours. Duration of therapy should be guided by the severity and site of infection and the patient's clinical and bacteriologic progress; the usual duration of therapy is 7–14 days.

Skin and Skin Structure Infections

The recommended dosage of tigecycline for the treatment of complicated skin and skin structure infections in adults 18 years of age and older is an initial dose of 100 mg, followed by 50 mg every 12 hours. Duration of therapy should be guided by the severity and site of infection and the patient's clinical and bacteriologic progress; the usual duration of therapy is 5–14 days.

Pediatric Dosage

General Pediatric Dosage

Safety and efficacy of tigecycline have not been established in pediatric patients and the drug should not be used in patients younger than 18 years of age unless no alternative anti-infectives are available. If no alternative anti-infectives are available, the manufacturer recommends the following tigecycline dosage for patients 8 years of age or older based on pharmacokinetic studies that included limited numbers of pediatric patients. (See Pediatric Use under Warnings/Precautions: Specific Populations, in Cautions.)

When use of the drug is considered necessary, the manufacturer states that children 8–11 years of age can receive tigecycline in a dosage of 1.2 mg/kg IV every 12 hours (maximum 50 mg IV every 12 hours) and children and adolescents 12–17 years of age can receive a dosage of 50 mg IV every 12 hours.

● Special Populations

Dosage adjustments are not required in patients with mild to moderate hepatic impairment (Child-Pugh class A or B). If tigecycline is used in adults with severe hepatic impairment (Child-Pugh class C), an initial dose of 100 mg should be given followed by a maintenance dosage of 25 mg every 12 hours. (See Hepatic Impairment under Warnings/Precautions: Specific Populations, in Cautions.)

Dosage adjustments are not necessary in patients with renal impairment or in those undergoing hemodialysis.

Dosage adjustments based on age are not necessary in geriatric patients.

Dosage adjustments based on gender or race are not necessary.

CAUTIONS

• Contraindications

Known hypersensitivity to tigecycline or any ingredient in the formulation.

• Warnings/Precautions

Warnings

Increased Mortality

Meta-analyses of phase 3 and 4 clinical trials indicate that all-cause mortality was higher in patients treated with tigecycline than in those treated with comparator anti-infectives. Tigecycline should be reserved for use in situations when alternative treatments are not suitable.

Based on meta-analyses of data from clinical trials, there was an increased risk of death when tigecycline was used for FDA-labeled or unlabeled uses. The reason for the increased mortality risk has not been established. In general, deaths resulted from worsening infections, complications of infection, or other underlying medical conditions.

In a pooled analysis of over 7400 patients from 13 phase 3 and 4, active-controlled clinical trials evaluating tigecycline for the treatment of serious infections, the mortality rate was 4% in tigecycline-treated patients versus 3% in patients treated with comparator anti-infectives. Overall, the adjusted risk difference in all-cause mortality between patients receiving tigecycline and those receiving comparator anti-infectives was 0.6%.

Data from 10 clinical trials evaluating tigecycline for FDA-labeled indications (i.e., complicated skin and skin structure infections, complicated intra-abdominal infections, community-acquired pneumonia) indicate an adjusted mortality rate of 2.5% for tigecycline-treated patients versus 1.8% for patients treated with comparator anti-infectives. The adjusted risk difference in mortality stratified by trial weight was 0.6%.

Data indicate that the mortality risk has been greatest when tigecycline was used for the treatment of hospital-acquired pneumonia†, particularly ventilator-associated pneumonia†, a use not included in FDA-approved labeling. (See Patients with Hospital-acquired Pneumonia under Warnings/Precautions: Other Warnings/Precautions, in Cautions.)

Sensitivity Reactions

Hypersensitivity Reactions

Potentially life-threatening anaphylaxis/anaphylactoid reactions have been reported with tigecycline.

There have been postmarketing reports of severe skin reactions, including Stevens-Johnson syndrome.

Tigecycline should be used with caution in patients with known hypersensitivity to tetracyclines.

Other Warnings/Precautions

Hepatic Effects

Elevated total bilirubin and aminotransferase concentrations and prolonged prothrombin time have been reported in tigecycline-treated patients. Clinically important hepatic dysfunction and hepatic failure have been reported rarely, and there have been postmarketing reports of hepatic cholestasis and jaundice in patients receiving tigecycline. Adverse hepatic effects may occur after the drug is discontinued.

Patients who develop abnormal liver function tests during tigecycline therapy should be monitored for evidence of worsening hepatic function, and the risks and benefits of continuing tigecycline treatment should be evaluated.

Patients with Hospital-acquired Pneumonia

Tigecycline has *not* been shown to be effective and is *not* labeled by FDA for the treatment of hospital-acquired pneumonia†, including ventilator-associated pneumonia†.

Results of a randomized, comparator-controlled trial evaluating tigecycline in patients with hospital-acquired pneumonia† failed to show efficacy. In the subgroup of patients with ventilator-associated pneumonia†, the mortality rate was 19.1% in those treated with tigecycline compared with 12.3% in those treated with comparator anti-infectives. Mortality was particularly high in tigecycline-treated patients with ventilator-associated pneumonia† who had bacteremia at baseline (mortality rate 50% in those treated with tigecycline versus 7.7% in those treated with a comparator anti-infective). (See Increased Mortality under Warnings/Precautions: Warnings, in Cautions.)

Pancreatitis

Acute pancreatitis, including fatalities, has been reported in patients receiving tigecycline. Some cases have been reported in patients with no known risk factors for pancreatitis. Improvement usually occurs after the drug is discontinued.

A diagnosis of pancreatitis should be considered in any patient receiving tigecycline who develops symptoms, signs, or laboratory abnormalities suggestive of acute pancreatitis. In suspected cases of pancreatitis, consideration should be given to discontinuing tigecycline.

Fetal/Neonatal Morbidity and Mortality

Tigecycline may cause fetal harm; teratogenicity and embryolethality have been demonstrated in animals. Pregnancy should be avoided during tigecycline therapy. If a patient becomes pregnant while receiving tigecycline, she should be apprised of the potential fetal hazard.

Superinfection/Clostridium difficile-associated Diarrhea and Colitis (CDAD)

Use of tigecycline may result in emergence and overgrowth of nonsusceptible bacteria or fungi. The patient should be carefully monitored and appropriate therapy instituted if a superinfection occurs.

Treatment with anti-infectives alters normal colon flora and may permit overgrowth of *Clostridium difficile*. C. difficile infection (CDI) and C. difficile-associated diarrhea and colitis (CDAD; also known as antibiotic-associated diarrhea and colitis or pseudomembranous colitis) have been reported with nearly all anti-infectives, including tigecycline, and may range in severity from mild diarrhea to fatal colitis. C. difficile produces toxins A and B which contribute to development of CDAD; hypertoxin-producing strains of C. difficile are associated with increased morbidity and mortality since these infections may be refractory to anti-infectives and colectomy may be required.

CDAD should be considered in the differential diagnosis of patients who develop diarrhea during or after anti-infective therapy. Careful medical history is necessary since CDAD has been reported to occur as late as 2 months or longer after anti-infective therapy is discontinued.

If CDAD is suspected or confirmed, anti-infective therapy not directed against C. difficile should be discontinued whenever possible. Patients should be managed with appropriate supportive therapy (e.g., fluid and electrolyte management, protein supplementation), anti-infective therapy directed against C. difficile (e.g., metronidazole, vancomycin), and surgical evaluation as clinically indicated.

Patients with Intestinal Perforation

Tigecycline should be used with caution in patients with complicated intra-abdominal infections secondary to clinically apparent intestinal perforation. Although a causal relationship has not been established, sepsis or septic shock has been reported in several patients who received tigecycline for the treatment of complicated intra-abdominal infections secondary to intestinal perforation.

Tetracycline-class Effects

Because tigecycline is structurally related to conventional tetracyclines, adverse effects reported with tetracyclines (e.g., photosensitivity, pseudotumor cerebri, antianabolic activity that may result in increased BUN, azotemia, acidosis, and hypophosphatemia) may occur. (See Cautions in the Tetracyclines General Statement 8:12.24.) Pancreatitis has been associated with conventional tetracyclines and has been reported in patients receiving tigecycline. (See Pancreatitis under Warnings/Precautions: Other Warnings/Precautions, in Cautions.)

Endocrine Effects

Symptomatic hypoglycemia has been reported during postmarketing experience in patients with and without diabetes receiving tigecycline.

Selection and Use of Anti-infectives

To reduce development of drug-resistant bacteria and maintain effectiveness of tigecycline and other antibacterials, the drug should be used only for treatment of infections proven or strongly suspected to be caused by susceptible bacteria.

When selecting or modifying anti-infective therapy, results of culture and in vitro susceptibility testing should be used. In the absence of such data, local epidemiology and susceptibility patterns should be considered when selecting anti-infectives for empiric therapy.

Specific Populations

Pregnancy

Category D. (See Users Guide.) Tigecycline crosses the placenta and is found in fetal tissues. (See Fetal/Neonatal Morbidity and Mortality under Warnings/Precautions: Other Warnings/Precautions, in Cautions.)

Use of tigecycline during tooth development (last half of pregnancy) may cause permanent discoloration (yellow-gray-brown) of the teeth. (See Cautions: Pediatric Precautions in the Tetracyclines General Statement 8:12.24.)

Lactation

Tigecycline is distributed into milk in rats. It is not known whether tigecycline is distributed into human milk; caution is advised if the drug is administered in nursing women.

Pediatric Use

Safety and efficacy of tigecycline have *not* been established in patients younger than 18 years of age and use in this age group is *not* recommended. Because of the increased mortality observed in adults receiving tigecycline, clinical trials evaluating safety and efficacy of tigecycline in pediatric patients have not been conducted.

For circumstances when there are no alternative anti-infectives, pediatric dosage has been proposed based on data from pharmacokinetic studies that included limited numbers of pediatric patients. For children 8–11 years of age, a pharmacokinetic simulation showed that a tigecycline dosage of 1.2 mg/kg in this age group would likely result in an area under the plasma concentration-time curve (AUC) similar to that reported in adults receiving the recommended adult dosage. For children and adolescents 12–16 years of age, a tigecycline dosage of 50 mg twice daily would likely result in exposures comparable to those observed in adults receiving the recommended adult dosage. (See Pediatric Dosage under Dosage and Administration: Dosage.)

Because use of tigecycline during tooth development (i.e., in infants and children younger than 8 years of age) may cause permanent discoloration (yellow-gray-brown) of the teeth, the drug should not be used in this age group unless other anti-infectives cannot be used. (See Cautions: Pediatric Precautions in the Tetracyclines General Statement 8:12.24.)

Geriatric Use

There are no substantial differences in safety and efficacy in patients 65 years of age or older relative to younger adults, but increased sensitivity cannot be ruled out.

Hepatic Impairment

Tigecycline should be used with caution and at a reduced dosage in patients with severe hepatic impairment (Child-Pugh class C); such patients should be monitored for treatment response. (See Dosage and Administration: Special Populations.)

In adults with mild hepatic impairment (Child-Pugh class A), tigecycline pharmacokinetics were similar to those in healthy adults. In those with moderate hepatic impairment (Child-Pugh class B), systemic clearance of tigecycline was reduced by 25%, AUC was increased by 50%, and half-life was prolonged by 23%. In those with severe hepatic impairment (Child-Pugh class C), systemic clearance was reduced by 55%, AUC was increased by 105%, and half-life was prolonged by 43%.

Renal Impairment

In a small study, the pharmacokinetic profile of tigecycline in adults with severe renal impairment (creatinine clearance less than 30 mL/minute) or end-stage renal impairment was not substantially altered. Tigecycline is not removed by hemodialysis. Dosage adjustments are not necessary in patients with renal impairment or in those undergoing hemodialysis.

Obese Patients

In otherwise healthy adults with class III obesity (body mass index [BMI] 40 kg/m^2 or higher), a single 100-mg IV dose of tigecycline resulted in serum and urine concentrations of the drug that were similar to concentrations in healthy adults with normal weight (BMI 18.5–24.99 kg/m^2).

● Common Adverse Effects

Nausea, vomiting, and diarrhea are the most common adverse effects reported with tigecycline and have been reported in up to 35% of patients in clinical studies.

Adverse effects reported in 2–8% of patients receiving tigecycline include abdominal pain, abnormal healing, abscess, anemia, asthenia, bilirubinemia, dizziness, dyspepsia, headache, hypoproteinemia, increased ALT or AST concentrations, increased alkaline phosphatase concentrations, increased amylase concentrations, increased BUN, infection, phlebitis, and rash.

DRUG INTERACTIONS

● Drugs Affecting or Metabolized by Hepatic Microsomal Enzymes

Pharmacokinetic interactions are unlikely with drugs metabolized by or affecting cytochrome P-450 (CYP) isoenzymes 1A2, 2C8, 2C9, 2C19, 2D6, or 3A4. Tigecycline is not metabolized by these CYP isoenzymes and does not inhibit these isoenzymes in vitro.

● Antibacterials

Although the clinical importance is unknown, in vitro studies indicate that tigecycline and colistin (commercially available as colistimethate sodium) are synergistic against some strains of *Escherichia coli*, *Klebsiella pneumoniae*, *Enterobacter*, and *Acinetobacter baumannii*, including some carbapenem-resistant strains; however, indifference or only an additive effect has also been reported. There also is some evidence of in vitro synergism between tigecycline and levofloxacin, amikacin, or imipenem against some multidrug-resistant (MDR) *A. baumanii*.

Although in vitro antagonism between tigecycline and colistin against *Serratia marcescens* was reported in one study, in vitro antagonism between tigecycline and other commonly used anti-infectives has not been confirmed.

● Digoxin

Potential pharmacokinetic interaction (slight decrease in peak plasma concentrations of digoxin, but no change in area under the concentration time curve [AUC]); no effect on digoxin pharmacodynamics (as measured by changes in ECG parameters). No effect on tigecycline pharmacokinetics. Dosage adjustment are not needed for either drug.

● Oral Contraceptives

Potential pharmacologic interaction (decreased effectiveness of oral contraceptives).

● Warfarin

Potential pharmacokinetic interaction (decreased clearance of warfarin, resulting in increased warfarin concentrations and AUC); pharmacologic interaction (altered international normalized ratio [INR]) unlikely. No effect on tigecycline pharmacokinetics. Monitor prothrombin time (PT) or other suitable coagulation tests if tigecycline is used concomitantly with warfarin.

DESCRIPTION

Tigecycline, a synthetic derivative of minocycline, is a glycylcycline antibiotic. Tigecycline is structurally related to tetracyclines, differing mainly in the addition of a glycylamido moiety at position 9 of the tetracycline nucleus. Like tetracyclines, tigecycline inhibits protein synthesis in susceptible organisms mainly by reversibly binding to 30S ribosomal subunits, thereby inhibiting binding of aminoacyl transfer-RNA to those ribosomes.

Tigecycline has a broad spectrum of antibacterial activity and usually is bacteriostatic in action. Tigecycline is active in vitro and in clinical infections against various gram-positive aerobic and facultatively aerobic bacteria, including *Staphylococcus aureus* (including methicillin-resistant [oxacillin-resistant] strains), *Streptococcus agalactiae* (group B streptococci), *S. anginosus* group (*S. anginosus*, *S. intermedius*, *S. constellatus*), *S. pneumoniae* (penicillin-susceptible strains), *S. pyogenes* (group A β-hemolytic streptococci), and *Enterococcus faecalis* (vancomycin-susceptible strains only). The drug also is active in vitro and in clinical infections against various gram-negative aerobic and facultatively aerobic bacteria, including *Citrobacter freundii*, *Enterobacter cloacae*, *Escherichia coli*, *Haemophilus influenzae* (β-lactamase-negative strains), *Klebsiella oxytoca*, *K. pneumoniae*, and *Legionella pneumophila*, and some anaerobic bacteria, including *Bacteroides fragilis*, *B. thetaiotaomicron*, *B. uniformis*, *B. vulgatus*, *Clostridium perfringens*, and *Peptostreptococcus micros*.

Tigecycline may be active against some bacteria resistant to conventional tetracyclines since susceptibility to the drug is not affected by the 2 major tetracycline resistance mechanisms (i.e., ribosomal protection, efflux). In addition, susceptibility to tigecycline is not affected by many other common resistance mechanisms, including β-lactamases (e.g., extended-spectrum β-lactamases [ESBLs]), target site modifications, macrolide efflux pumps, or enzyme target (e.g., gyrase, topoisomerase) changes. Tigecycline resistance in some bacteria (e.g., *Acinetobacter calcoaceticus-baumannii* complex) is attributed to multidrug-resistant (MDR) efflux pumps. In vitro studies have demonstrated synergism between tigecycline and some other antibacterials (e.g., colistin) against some Enterobacteriaceae. (See Drug Interactions: Antibacterials.)

Tigecycline is extensively distributed into various tissues, including alveolar cells, epithelial lining fluid, skin blister fluid, gall bladder, lung, colon, synovial fluid, and bone. Tigecycline concentrations in certain tissues (i.e., alveolar cells, gallbladder, lung, colon, epithelial fluid) are substantially higher than concentrations in serum. Animal studies indicate that tigecycline crosses the placenta and is found in fetal tissues. The drug is approximately 71–89% bound to plasma proteins. Tigecycline is not extensively metabolized; each of the recovered metabolites (a glucuronide, an N-acetyl metabolite, and a tigecycline epimer) constitutes less than 10% of the administered dose. The half-life of tigecycline is 27.1 or 42.4 hours following single or multiple dosing, respectively. Tigecycline is principally eliminated by biliary and fecal excretion as unchanged tigecycline and metabolites. About 59% of a dose is eliminated by biliary and fecal excretion; 33% is eliminated in urine (22% as unchanged drug).

ADVICE TO PATIENTS

Advise patients that antibacterials (including tigecycline) should only be used to treat bacterial infections and not used to treat viral infections (e.g., the common cold).

Importance of completing full course of therapy, even if feeling better after a few days.

Advise patients that skipping doses or not completing the full course of therapy may decrease effectiveness and increase the likelihood that bacteria will develop resistance and will not be treatable with tigecycline or other antibacterials in the future.

Advise patients that diarrhea is a common problem caused by anti-infectives and usually ends when the drug is discontinued. Importance of contacting a clinician if watery and bloody stools (with or without stomach cramps and fever) occur during or as late as 2 months or longer after the last dose.

Importance of informing clinicians of existing or contemplated concomitant therapy, including prescription and OTC drugs, as well as any concomitant illnesses.

Importance of women informing clinicians if they are or plan to become pregnant or plan to breast-feed. Advise pregnant women of risk to the fetus.

Importance of informing patients of other important precautionary information. (See Cautions.)

PREPARATIONS

Excipients in commercially available drug preparations may have clinically important effects in some individuals; consult specific product labeling for details.

Tigecycline

Parenteral

For injection, for IV infusion	50 mg	Tygacil®, Pfizer

† Use is not currently included in the labeling approved by the US Food and Drug Administration.

Selected Revisions August 4, 2014, © Copyright, November 1, 2005, American Society of Health-System Pharmacists, Inc.

Daptomycin

8:12.28.12 • CYCLIC LIPOPEPTIDES

■ Daptomycin is a cyclic lipopeptide antibiotic.

USES

Daptomycin is used for the treatment of complicated skin and skin structure infections or bacteremia caused by certain susceptible gram-positive bacteria. The drug should *not* be used in the treatment of pneumonia.

● Skin and Skin Structure Infections

Daptomycin is used for the treatment of complicated skin and skin structure infections caused by susceptible *Staphylococcus aureus* (including methicillin-resistant *S. aureus* [MRSA; also known as oxacillin-resistant *S. aureus* or ORSA]), *Streptococcus pyogenes* (group A β-hemolytic streptococci, GAS), *S. agalactiae* (group B streptococci, GBS), *S. dysgalactiae* subsp. *equisimilis*, and *Enterococcus faecalis* (vancomycin-susceptible strains only).

For information on management of skin and skin structure infections, the current clinical practice guidelines from the Infectious Diseases Society of America (IDSA) available at http://www.idsociety.org should be consulted.

Clinical Experience

In 2 randomized, multicenter, comparative studies in adults with complicated skin and skin structure infections (e.g., wound infection, major abscess, ulcer infection, complicated cellulitis), clinical success rates reported with daptomycin (4 mg/kg IV once every 24 hours) were similar to those reported with vancomycin (1 g IV every 12 hours) or a penicillinase-resistant penicillin (4–12 g IV daily of nafcillin, oxacillin, or cloxacillin [no longer commercially available in the US], or flucloxacillin [not commercially available in the US]). After a minimum of 4 days of IV treatment, patients could be switched to oral anti-infective therapy if clinical improvement was observed; however, most patients (approximately 90%) received IV therapy exclusively. In the intent-to-treat population, clinical success was achieved in 63–80% of patients receiving daptomycin and 61–81% of those receiving comparator anti-infectives.

In a subset of patients who were microbiologically evaluable and stratified according to the infecting pathogen, the daptomycin clinical success rate was 73% in those with infections caused by *E. faecalis* (vancomycin-susceptible strains only), 75% in those with MRSA, 86% in those with methicillin-susceptible *S. aureus*, 85% in those with *S. agalactiae*, 94% in those with *S. pyogenes*, and 100% in those with *S. dysgalactiae* subsp. *equisimilis*.

● Bacteremia and Endocarditis

Daptomycin is used for the treatment of bacteremia (blood stream infection) caused by susceptible *S. aureus* (including MRSA).

Daptomycin also is used for the treatment of *S. aureus* bacteremia in patients with right-sided infective endocarditis. However, efficacy of the drug has not been established in patients with left-sided infective endocarditis caused by *S. aureus*; limited data suggest that such patients have a poor outcome despite daptomycin treatment.

Safety and efficacy of daptomycin have not been studied in patients with prosthetic valve endocarditis.

Infective endocarditis usually is treated empirically until results of blood cultures are available and a pathogen is identified. The empiric regimen is selected based on various patient characteristics (e.g., history of injection drug use, presence of indwelling cardiovascular devices, immunocompromising medical conditions, prior infections and anti-infective treatment); consultation with an infectious disease specialist is recommended for assistance in selecting the optimal regimen. For the treatment of native valve infective endocarditis caused by methicillin-susceptible *S. aureus*, the American Heart Association (AHA) recommends a parenteral β-lactam (nafcillin or oxacillin; cefazolin for those with nonanaphylactoid reactions to penicillins) and states that daptomycin is a reasonable alternative to vancomycin for the treatment of these infections in patients with anaphylactoid-type hypersensitivity to β-lactams. Although these experts also state that daptomycin may be a reasonable alternative to vancomycin for the treatment of left-sided native valve infective endocarditis† caused by MRSA,

optimal daptomycin dosage for these infections has not been identified and consultation with an infectious disease expert is recommended.

For information on diagnosis and management of infective endocarditis and its complications, including anti-infective treatment of staphylococcal bacteremia and endocarditis, the current AHA guidelines available at http://my.american-heart.org/statements should be consulted.

Clinical Experience

Efficacy of daptomycin for the treatment of *S. aureus* bacteremia with or without endocarditis was evaluated in a randomized, multicenter, controlled, open-label study in 246 adults with at least one positive blood culture for *S. aureus* (obtained within 2 days prior to the first dose of the study drug). At study entry, 16% of patients had a definite diagnosis of endocarditis and 61% had a possible diagnosis of endocarditis based on the modified Duke criteria. Patients were randomized to receive daptomycin (6 mg/kg IV once every 24 hours) or a comparator anti-infective regimen of vancomycin (1 g IV every 12 hours) or a penicillinase-resistant penicillin (2 g IV every 4 hours of nafcillin, oxacillin, or flucloxacillin [not commercially available in the US]). Less than 1% of patients in the daptomycin group also received gentamicin (1 mg/kg IV every 8 hours for the first 4 days of treatment), whereas 93% of those in the comparator group also received gentamicin. Patients with prosthetic heart valves, intravascular foreign material that was not planned for removal within 4 days after the first anti-infective dose, severe neutropenia, known osteomyelitis, polymicrobial bloodstream infections, creatinine clearance less than 30 mL/minute, and pneumonia were excluded from the study.

The clinical success rate in the intent-to-treat population 6 weeks after the last treatment dose was 44% in patients who received daptomycin and 42% in those who received a comparator anti-infective. There was no overall difference in time to clearance of *S. aureus* bacteremia between the 2 groups; the median time to clearance of methicillin-susceptible *S. aureus* was 4 days and the median time to clearance of MRSA was 8 days.

There were some persisting or relapsing infections, including some deaths, during the study. Most patients who failed treatment due to persisting or relapsing *S. aureus* infection had deep-seated infections and did not receive necessary surgical intervention. Among patients with persisting or relapsing *S. aureus* infections, there were 8 deaths in those who had been randomized to receive daptomycin and 7 deaths in those randomized to receive a comparator anti-infective. (See Persisting or Relapsing Staphylococcus aureus Bacteremia/Endocarditis under Cautions: Warnings/Precautions.)

DOSAGE AND ADMINISTRATION

● Reconstitution and Administration

Daptomycin is administered by IV injection or infusion.

Daptomycin is commercially available for IV use as 2 different formulations: a lyophilized powder for solution that does not contain sucrose (Cubicin® or generics) and a lyophilized powder for solution that contains 713 mg of sucrose per vial (Cubicin® RF). Instructions for storage, reconstitution, and dilution differ for the 2 daptomycin formulations and recommendations for the specific formulation used should be followed.

Additives and other drugs should not be added to daptomycin solutions or infused simultaneously through the same IV line. If the same IV line is used for sequential infusion of different drugs, the line should be flushed with a compatible infusion solution before and after infusion of daptomycin. Daptomycin is *not* compatible with dextrose-containing diluents (e.g., 5% dextrose injection).

Daptomycin should not be used in conjunction with ReadyMed® elastomeric infusion pumps since stability studies identified an impurity (i.e., 2-mercaptobenzothiazole) leaching from this pump system into the daptomycin solution.

Strict aseptic technique must be observed in preparing daptomycin solutions since the drug contains no preservative. Daptomycin solutions should be inspected visually for particulate matter prior to administration. Reconstituted daptomycin solutions range in color from pale yellow to light brown.

Daptomycin (Cubicin® or generics): The lyophilized powder should be stored at 2–8°C. The reconstituted daptomycin solution (in the original vial) and reconstituted and further diluted solutions (in an IV infusion bag) are stable for 12 hours at room temperature or up to 48 hours when refrigerated at 2–8°C; the combined storage time (vial and infusion bag) at room temperature or under refrigeration should not exceed 12 or 48 hours, respectively.

Daptomycin (Cubicin® RF): The lyophilized powder should be stored at 20–25°C, but may be exposed to 15–30°C. The stability of reconstituted daptomycin solution and reconstituted and further diluted solutions varies based on the specific diluent and container used. (See Table 1.)

TABLE 1. Stability of Daptomycin (Cubicin® RF) After Reconstitution

Container	Diluent	°	Stability at 20–25°C	Stability at 2–8°C
Vial	Sterile water for injection		1 day	3 days
	Bacteriostatic water for injection		2 days	3 days
Syringe ª	Sterile water for injection		1 day	3 days
	Bacteriostatic water for injection		2 days	5 days
Infusion bag	Reconstituted with sterile water for injection and immediate dilution in 0.9% sodium chloride injection		19 hours	3 days
	Reconstituted with bacteriostatic water for injection and immediate dilution in 0.9% sodium chloride injection		2 days	5 days

ª Polypropylene syringe with elastomeric plunger stopper.

IV Injection

Reconstitution

Daptomycin (Cubicin® or generics): Single-dose vials labeled as containing 500 mg of daptomycin should be reconstituted by slowly adding 10 mL of 0.9% sodium chloride injection to provide a solution containing 50 mg/mL. The diluent should be added to the vial using a beveled sterile transfer needle (21 gauge or smaller) or a needleless device, and the diluent should be directed toward the wall of the vial. The vial should be gently rotated to ensure that the entire lyophilized powder is wetted. The vial should be allowed to remain undisturbed for 10 minutes, and then should be rotated or swirled for a few minutes (as needed) to obtain a completely reconstituted solution. To minimize foaming, vigorous agitation or shaking of the vial should be avoided during and after reconstitution. For IV injection, the appropriate volume of reconstituted daptomycin solution containing 50 mg/mL should be slowly removed from the vial using a beveled sterile needle (21 gauge or smaller) and administered without further dilution. Any unused portion of the reconstituted solution should be discarded.

Daptomycin (Cubicin® RF): Sodium chloride solutions should *not* be used for reconstitution of this formulation since this would result in a hyperosmotic solution. Single-dose vials labeled as containing 500 mg of daptomycin should be reconstituted by slowly adding 10 mL of sterile water for injection or bacteriostatic water for injection to provide a solution containing 50 mg/mL. The diluent should be added to the vial using a beveled sterile transfer needle (21 gauge or smaller), and the diluent should be directed toward the wall of the vial. The vial should be rotated or swirled for a few minutes (as needed) to obtain a completely reconstituted solution. For IV injection, the appropriate volume of reconstituted daptomycin solution containing 50 mg/mL should be slowly removed from the vial using a beveled sterile needle (21 gauge or smaller) and administered without further dilution. Any unused portion of the reconstituted solution should be discarded.

Rate of Administration

IV injections of daptomycin (Cubicin® or generics; Cubicin® RF) should be given over 2 minutes.

IV Infusion

Reconstitution and Dilution

Daptomycin (Cubicin® or generics): Single-dose vials labeled as containing 500 mg of daptomycin should be reconstituted by slowly adding 10 mL of 0.9% sodium chloride injection to provide a solution containing 50 mg/mL. The diluent should be added to the vial using a beveled sterile transfer needle (21 gauge or smaller) or a needleless device, and the diluent should be directed toward the wall of the vial. The vial should be gently rotated to ensure that the entire lyophilized powder is wetted. The vial should be allowed to remain undisturbed for 10 minutes, and then should be rotated or swirled for a few minutes (as needed) to obtain a completely reconstituted solution. To minimize foaming, vigorous agitation or shaking of the vial should be avoided during and after reconstitution. For IV infusion, the appropriate volume of reconstituted daptomycin solution containing 50 mg/mL should be slowly removed from the vial using a beveled sterile needle (21 gauge or smaller) and added to 50 mL of 0.9% sodium chloride injection in an IV infusion bag. The final concentration of the diluted solution should not exceed 20 mg/mL. Any unused portion of the reconstituted solution should be discarded.

Daptomycin (Cubicin® RF): Sodium chloride solutions should *not* be used for reconstitution of this formulation since this would result in a hyperosmotic solution. Single-dose vials labeled as containing 500 mg of daptomycin should be reconstituted by slowly adding 10 mL of sterile water for injection or bacteriostatic water for injection to provide a solution containing 50 mg/mL. The diluent should be added to the vial using a beveled sterile transfer needle (21 gauge or smaller), and the diluent should be directed toward the wall of the vial. The vial should be rotated or swirled for a few minutes (as needed) to obtain a completely reconstituted solution. For IV infusion, the appropriate volume of reconstituted daptomycin solution containing 50 mg/mL should be slowly removed from the vial using a beveled sterile needle (21 gauge or smaller) and added to 50 mL of 0.9% sodium chloride injection in an IV infusion bag. Any unused portion of the reconstituted solution should be discarded.

Rate of Administration

IV infusions of daptomycin (Cubicin® or generics; Cubicin® RF) should be given over 30 minutes.

● Dosage

Skin and Skin Structure Infections

For the treatment of complicated skin and skin structure infections in adults, the usual dosage of daptomycin is 4 mg/kg IV once every 24 hours for 7–14 days.

Daptomycin should not be administered more frequently than once daily. (See Musculoskeletal Effects under Cautions: Warnings/Precautions.)

Bacteremia and Endocarditis

For the treatment of bacteremia (blood stream infections) and right-sided infective endocarditis in adults, the usual dosage of daptomycin is 6 mg/kg IV once every 24 hours for 2–6 weeks. Limited safety data are available regarding use of daptomycin for longer than 28 days; in a phase 3 clinical study, only 14 patients received daptomycin for more than 28 days.

Daptomycin should not be administered more frequently than once daily. (See Musculoskeletal Effects under Cautions: Warnings/Precautions.)

● Special Populations

Because daptomycin is eliminated principally by renal excretion, patients with creatinine clearances less than 30 mL/minute, including those requiring hemodialysis or continuous ambulatory peritoneal dialysis (CAPD), should receive reduced daptomycin dosage. The recommended dosage of daptomycin for adults with creatinine clearances less than 30 mL/minute is 4 mg/kg IV once every 48 hours for the treatment of complicated skin and skin structure infections or 6 mg/kg IV once every 48 hours for the treatment of bacteremia and right-sided infective endocarditis. In hemodialysis patients, dosing of the drug should be timed so that the daily dose given on hemodialysis days is administered following the procedure, whenever possible.

Dosage adjustments are not necessary when daptomycin is used in patients with mild to moderate hepatic impairment; pharmacokinetics of the drug have not been evaluated in patients with severe hepatic impairment.

Dosage adjustments based solely on age are not necessary when daptomycin is used in geriatric patients, but dosage adjustments are indicated in those with renal impairment.

Dosage adjustments are not necessary based on gender or weight.

CAUTIONS

● *Contraindications*

Daptomycin is contraindicated in patients with known hypersensitivity to the drug.

● *Warnings/Precautions*

Sensitivity Reactions

Hypersensitivity reactions, including anaphylaxis and other reactions that may be life-threatening, have been reported in patients receiving daptomycin.

Angioedema, drug rash with eosinophilia and systemic symptoms (DRESS), pruritus, urticaria, shortness of breath, difficulty swallowing, truncal erythema, and pulmonary eosinophilia (see Eosinophilic Pneumonia under Cautions: Warnings/Precautions) have been reported during postmarketing experience in patients receiving daptomycin.

If a hypersensitivity reaction occurs, daptomycin should be discontinued and appropriate therapy initiated.

Musculoskeletal Effects

Myopathy, defined as muscle aching or muscle weakness, in conjunction with serum creatine kinase (CK, creatine phosphokinase, CPK) concentrations increased up to 10 times the upper limit of normal (ULN) have been reported in patients receiving daptomycin. Rhabdomyolysis, with or without renal failure, also has been reported.

In a phase 3 study evaluating daptomycin (4 mg/kg IV once daily) for the treatment of complicated skin and skin structure infections, elevated CK concentrations were reported in 2.8% of patients receiving daptomycin and 1.8% of those receiving a comparator anti-infective. In a study evaluating daptomycin (6 mg/kg IV once daily) for the treatment of bacteremia, elevated CK concentrations were reported in 9.2% of those receiving daptomycin and less than 1% of those receiving a comparator anti-infective. Some patients who developed increased CK concentrations were previously or concomitantly treated with an hydroxymethylglutaryl-CoA (HMG-CoA) reductase inhibitor (statin).

Because there is evidence from phase 1 and 2 studies that elevated serum CK concentrations occurred more frequently when daptomycin was given more than once daily, the drug should not be administered more frequently than once daily.

Patients receiving daptomycin should be monitored for the development of muscle pain or weakness, particularly of the distal extremities. Serum CK concentrations should be monitored weekly in patients receiving daptomycin; however, these concentrations should be monitored more frequently than once weekly in patients who develop increases in serum CK concentrations during daptomycin therapy and in those who recently received or are currently receiving treatment with an HMG-CoA reductase inhibitor. Serum CK concentrations and renal function also should be monitored more frequently than once weekly in patients with renal insufficiency.

Daptomycin should be discontinued in patients with unexplained signs and symptoms of myopathy in conjunction with increases in CK greater than 1000 U/L (i.e., approximately 5 times the ULN) or in patients without reported symptoms who have substantial increases in serum CK concentrations (i.e., at least 2000 U/L [10 times the ULN]).

Consideration should be given to temporarily discontinuing drugs associated with rhabdomyolysis (e.g., HMG-CoA reductase inhibitors) in patients receiving daptomycin. (See Drug Interactions: HMG-CoA Reductase Inhibitors.)

Eosinophilic Pneumonia

Eosinophilic pneumonia has been reported in some patients receiving daptomycin. In most reported cases, patients developed fever, dyspnea with hypoxic respiratory insufficiency, and diffuse pulmonary infiltrates, usually 2–4 weeks after daptomycin therapy was initiated. Improvement or resolution of symptoms generally occurred following discontinuance of the drug; most patient received treatment with systemic corticosteroids. When daptomycin was reinitiated in a few of these patients, eosinophilic pneumonia recurred.

Based on a review of postmarketing reports of possible cases of eosinophilic pneumonia in patients who received daptomycin, FDA determined that there appears to be a temporal association between use of the drug and the development of eosinophilic pneumonia. Some cases were reported in patients receiving daptomycin for uses that are not FDA labeled. Clinicians should consider that eosinophilic pneumonia can progress to respiratory failure and is potentially fatal if not recognized quickly and managed appropriately.

Patients receiving daptomycin should be closely monitored for signs and symptoms of eosinophilic pneumonia (e.g., new onset or worsening fever, dyspnea, difficulty breathing, new pulmonary infiltrates).

Daptomycin should be discontinued immediately if there are any signs or symptoms of eosinophilic pneumonia. Prompt medical evaluation is indicated, and treatment with systemic corticosteroids is recommended.

Nervous System Effects

There have been postmarketing reports of peripheral neuropathy in patients receiving daptomycin. Clinicians should be alert to possible manifestations of neuropathy in patients receiving daptomycin.

Persisting or Relapsing Staphylococcus aureus Bacteremia/Endocarditis

Treatment failure due to persisting or relapsing *Staphylococcus aureus* infection can occur. *S. aureus* with reduced susceptibility or resistance to daptomycin have been reported and have emerged during treatment with the drug.

In a clinical study evaluating daptomycin for the treatment of bacteremia, 16% of daptomycin-treated patients and 10% of patients treated with a comparator anti-infective (vancomycin or a penicillinase-resistant penicillin) had persisting or relapsing *S. aureus* infections; some fatalities occurred. In vitro studies indicated that isolates from some of these patients developed reduced susceptibility to the anti-infective during or following treatment. Most patients with persistent or relapsing infections had deep-seated infections and did not receive necessary surgical intervention.

Repeat blood cultures should be performed in patients with persisting or relapsing infection or with poor clinical response. If cultures are positive for *S. aureus*, in vitro susceptibility testing of the isolate should be performed using standardized MIC procedures. In addition, a diagnostic evaluation should be performed to rule out sequestered foci of infection. Surgical intervention (e.g., debridement, removal of prosthetic devices, valve replacement surgery) and/or a change in anti-infective regimen may be required.

Reduced Efficacy in Patients with Moderate Renal Impairment

Results of a subgroup analysis of a phase 3 study in patients with *S. aureus* bacteremia/endocarditis indicated that the clinical success rate in daptomycin-treated patients with baseline creatinine clearances of 30 to less than 50 mL/minute was only 14% and was lower than clinical success rates observed in those with baseline creatinine clearances of 50–80 mL/minute or greater than 80 mL/minute (46 or 60%, respectively). Decreased clinical success rates to this extent were not observed in patients receiving comparator anti-infectives.

Although only limited data are available from phase 3 studies in patients with complicated skin and skin structure infections, the clinical success rate in daptomycin-treated patients with creatinine clearances of 30 to less than 50 mL/minute was 47% compared with a clinical success rate of 66% in those with creatinine clearances of 50–70 mL/minute.

Clinicians should consider these data regarding reduced efficacy when selecting anti-infective treatment for patients with baseline moderate to severe renal impairment.

Tests Used to Monitor Coagulation

Daptomycin causes concentration-dependent false prolongation of the prothrombin time (PT) and elevated international normalized ratio (INR) if certain recombinant thromboplastin reagents are used for these tests. Interference with PT/INR testing may be minimized by drawing blood specimens for coagulation tests near the time of trough plasma daptomycin concentrations; however, the possibility that trough plasma concentrations still may be high enough to interfere with such tests should be considered.

If abnormally elevated PT/INR tests are reported in a patient receiving daptomycin, coagulation testing should be repeated using blood specimens drawn just prior to the next daptomycin dose (i.e., at trough concentrations). If results using these blood specimens remain substantially elevated over what would otherwise be expected, alternative methods of measuring PT/INR should be considered. In addition, the patient should be evaluated for other causes of abnormally elevated PT/INR.

Superinfection/Clostridium difficile-associated Diarrhea and Colitis (CDAD)

Use of daptomycin may result in emergence and overgrowth of nonsusceptible bacteria or fungi. The patient should be carefully monitored and appropriate therapy instituted if superinfection occurs.

Treatment with anti-infectives alters normal colon flora and may permit overgrowth of *Clostridium difficile*. *C. difficile* infection (CDI) and *C. difficile*-associated diarrhea and colitis (CDAD; also known as antibiotic-associated diarrhea and colitis or pseudomembranous colitis) have been reported with nearly all anti-infectives, including daptomycin, and may range in severity from mild diarrhea to fatal colitis. *C. difficile* produces toxins A and B which contribute to development of CDAD; hypertoxin-producing strains of *C. difficile* are associated with increased morbidity and mortality since they may be refractory to anti-infectives and colectomy may be required.

CDAD should be considered in the differential diagnosis of patients who develop diarrhea during or after anti-infective therapy. Careful medical history is necessary since CDAD has been reported to occur as late as 2 months or longer after anti-infective therapy is discontinued.

If CDAD is suspected or confirmed, anti-infective therapy not directed against *C. difficile* should be discontinued whenever possible. Patients should be managed with appropriate supportive therapy (e.g., fluid and electrolyte management, protein supplementation), anti-infective therapy directed against *C. difficile* (e.g., metronidazole, vancomycin), and surgical evaluation as clinically indicated.

Selection and Use of Anti-infectives

To reduce development of drug-resistant bacteria and maintain effectiveness of daptomycin and other antibacterials, the drug should be used only for the treatment of infections proven or strongly suspected to be caused by susceptible bacteria.

When selecting or modifying anti-infective therapy, results of culture and in vitro susceptibility testing should be used. In the absence of such data, local epidemiology and susceptibility patterns should be considered when selecting anti-infectives for empiric therapy.

Daptomycin should not be used for the treatment of pneumonia.

Safety and efficacy of daptomycin have not been studied in patients with prosthetic valve endocarditis .

Specific Populations

Pregnancy

Category B. (See Users Guide.)

There are no adequate and well-controlled studies evaluating daptomycin in pregnant women. Daptomycin should be used during pregnancy only if potential benefits to the woman outweigh possible risks to the fetus.

Lactation

Daptomycin is distributed into human milk, but has poor oral bioavailability. In a case study involving a nursing woman receiving daptomycin (6.7 mg/kg IV once daily for 28 days), the highest daptomycin concentration measured in breast milk was 45 ng/mL and the calculated maximum daily daptomycin dose for a nursing infant (assuming mean milk consumption of 150 mL/kg daily) was 0.1% of the maternal dose.

Daptomycin should be used with caution in nursing women.

Pediatric Use

Safety and efficacy of daptomycin have not been established in pediatric patients.

Use of daptomycin should be avoided in children younger than 12 months of age because of the potential risk of adverse muscular, neuromuscular, peripheral nervous system, and CNS effects; such adverse effects have been observed in neonatal dogs receiving IV daptomycin.

Geriatric Use

When the total number of patients studied in phase 3 clinical trials of daptomycin for the treatment of complicated skin and skin structure infections are considered, 27% were 65 years of age or older and 12% were 75 years of age or older. In a phase 3 clinical trial of daptomycin for the treatment of bacteremia and endocarditis, 25% of patients were 65 years of age or older and 16% were 75 years of age or older. There was some evidence from these studies that clinical success rates were lower and treatment-emergent adverse effects were more common in geriatric patients 65 years of age or older compared with younger adults.

Although daptomycin exposures are higher in healthy geriatric adults than in healthy young adults, adjustment of daptomycin dosage is not necessary in geriatric patients based solely on age. However, age-related decreases in renal function should be considered when selecting dosage in geriatric patients. (See Dosage and Administration: Special Populations.)

Hepatic Impairment

The pharmacokinetics of daptomycin were not altered in patients with moderate hepatic impairment (Child-Pugh class B) compared with healthy individuals without liver disease. Daptomycin has not been studied in patients with severe hepatic impairment.

Renal Impairment

Daptomycin is eliminated principally by the kidneys, and plasma clearance of the drug is decreased and area under the concentration-time curve (AUC) and half-life are increased in patients with impaired renal function.

Renal function and serum CK concentrations should be monitored more frequently than once weekly in patients with renal impairment.

Dosage adjustments are recommended in adults with creatinine clearances less than 30 mL/minute. (See Dosage and Administration: Special Populations and also see Musculoskeletal Effects under Cautions: Warnings/Precautions.)

• Common Adverse Effects

Adverse effects occurring in 2% or more of patients receiving daptomycin for the treatment of complicated skin and skin structure infections in clinical trials and reported as frequently or more frequently than with comparator anti-infectives include diarrhea, nervous system effects (headache, dizziness), rash, abnormal liver function test results, elevated serum creatine kinase (CK, creatine phosphokinase, CPK) concentrations, urinary tract infections, hypotension, and dyspnea.

Adverse effects occurring in 5% or more of patients receiving daptomycin for the treatment of bacteremia and endocarditis in a clinical trial and reported as frequently or more frequently than with comparator anti-infectives include abdominal pain, insomnia, pharyngolaryngeal pain, infections (sepsis, bacteremia), chest pain, edema, pruritus, increased sweating, elevated CK concentrations, and hypertension.

DRUG INTERACTIONS

• Drugs Metabolized by Hepatic Microsomal Enzymes

Daptomycin does not inhibit or induce cytochrome P-450 (CYP) isoenzymes 1A2, 2A6, 2C9, 2C19, 2D6, 2E1, and 3A4; pharmacokinetic interactions with drugs metabolized by these isoenzymes is unlikely.

• Aminoglycosides

In vitro studies using gentamicin and tobramycin indicate that daptomycin and aminoglycosides may exert synergistic antibacterial effects against staphylococci and enterococci. Additive or indifferent antibacterial effects also were reported, but antagonism did not occur.

Tobramycin

Concomitant use of tobramycin (1 mg/kg IV) and daptomycin (2 mg/kg IV) increased the mean peak plasma concentration and area under the plasma concentration-time curve (AUC) of daptomycin by approximately 13 and 9%, respectively, and decreased the mean peak plasma concentration and AUC of tobramycin by approximately 11 and 7%, respectively. These differences were not statistically significant; however, the extent of possible interaction between daptomycin and tobramycin when the recommended daptomycin dosages are used is not known.

• β-Lactam Anti-infectives

In vitro studies using penicillins (ampicillin, oxacillin, ampicillin and sulbactam, piperacillin and tazobactam, ticarcillin and clavulanate), cephalosporins (cefepime, ceftriaxone), aztreonam, or imipenem indicate that daptomycin and β-lactam anti-infectives may exert synergistic antibacterial effects against staphylococci and enterococci. Additive or indifferent antibacterial effects also were reported, but antagonism generally did not occur.

Aztreonam

Concomitant use of daptomycin (6 mg/kg IV) and aztreonam (1 g IV) did not have a clinically important effect on the mean peak plasma concentration and AUC of daptomycin.

● *HMG-CoA Reductase Inhibitors*

Concomitant use of hydroxymethylglutaryl-CoA (HMG-CoA) reductase inhibitors (statins) and daptomycin may increase the risk of myopathy, manifested as muscle pain or weakness in association with increased serum creatine kinase (CK, creatine phosphokinase, CPK). In a phase 3 study evaluating daptomycin in adults with *Staphylococcus aureus* bacteremia/endocarditis, elevated serum CK concentrations were reported in some patients who received prior or concurrent treatment with an HMG-CoA reductase inhibitor.

In a study in healthy adults receiving a stable simvastatin dosage of 40 mg daily, concurrent use of daptomycin (4 mg/kg IV once daily for 14 days) did not affect plasma trough concentrations of simvastatin and was not associated with a higher incidence of adverse effects (including skeletal myopathy) compared with patients receiving placebo.

The manufacturer of daptomycin states that experience with concurrent use of HMG-CoA reductase inhibitors and daptomycin is limited, and temporary discontinuance of HMG-CoA reductase inhibitors should be considered in patients receiving daptomycin. (See Musculoskeletal Effects under Cautions: Warnings/Precautions.)

● *Probenecid*

Concurrent use of probenecid (500 mg 4 times daily) and a single daptomycin dose (4 mg/kg IV) did not substantially alter the peak plasma concentration or AUC of daptomycin.

● *Rifampin*

In vitro studies indicate that daptomycin and rifampin may exert synergistic antibacterial effects against staphylococci and enterococci, including vancomycin-resistant enterococci. Additive or indifferent antibacterial effects also were reported, but antagonism did not occur.

● *Warfarin*

Concurrent use of daptomycin (6 mg/kg IV once every 24 hours for 5 days) and warfarin (single 25-mg oral dose) did not result in substantial effects on the pharmacokinetics of either drug or substantial alterations of the international normalized ratio (INR). However, if warfarin and daptomycin are used concomitantly, the possibility that daptomycin may cause concentration-dependent false prolongation of the prothrombin time (PT) and elevated INR when certain testing methods are used should be considered. (See Tests Used to Monitor Coagulation under Cautions: Warnings/Precautions.)

DESCRIPTION

Daptomycin is a cyclic lipopeptide antibiotic produced by fermentation of *Streptomyces roseosporus*. The drug differs structurally and pharmacologically from other currently available anti-infective agents. In vitro studies indicate that daptomycin exhibits rapid concentration-dependent bactericidal effects against susceptible gram-positive bacteria. Daptomycin binds to bacterial cell membranes and causes rapid membrane depolarization in susceptible bacteria, which leads to inhibition of protein, DNA, and RNA synthesis and results in cell death.

Daptomycin is active against many gram-positive bacteria, but is inactive against gram-negative bacteria. The drug is active in vitro and in clinical infections against *Staphylococcus aureus* (including methicillin-resistant *S. aureus* [MRSA; also known as oxacillin-resistant *S. aureus* or ORSA]), *Streptococcus pyogenes* (group A β-hemolytic streptococci, GAS), *S. agalactiae* (group B streptococci, GBS), *S. dysgalactiae* subsp. *equisimilis*, and *Enterococcus faecalis* (vancomycin-susceptible strains only). Daptomycin also has in vitro activity against some strains of *Corynebacterium jeikeium*, *E. faecalis* (vancomycin-resistant strains), *E. faecium* (including vancomycin-resistant strains), *S. epidermidis* (including methicillin-resistant strains), and *S. haemolyticus*; however, the safety and efficacy of daptomycin in treating clinical infections caused by these bacteria have not been established in adequate and well-controlled studies to date.

S. aureus and *E. faecalis* with reduced susceptibility or resistance to daptomycin have been reported. The mechanism of resistance or transferable elements that might confer resistance to daptomycin have not been identified to date. Reduced susceptibility to daptomycin (8- to 32-fold increase in MIC) has been produced in vitro by serial passage of *S. aureus* in the presence of increasing concentrations of the drug. In addition, daptomycin-resistant strains of *S. aureus* have emerged in patients treated with the drug. In a clinical study in patients with complicated skin and skin structure infections, *S. aureus* resistant to daptomycin was isolated from a patient who received the drug at less than the protocol-specified dosage during the first 5 days of therapy.

Although further study is needed, there is evidence that cross-resistance can occur between daptomycin and vancomycin. Some strains of MRSA that develop resistance to daptomycin also may develop resistance or reduced susceptibility to vancomycin and daptomycin-resistant MRSA may emerge during daptomycin therapy in some patients with prior exposure to vancomycin.

Daptomycin exhibits nearly linear and time-independent pharmacokinetics at dosages up to 4–12 mg/kg once daily administered by IV infusion over 30 minutes. Steady-state concentrations are achieved by the third daily dose. Daptomycin has a mean elimination half-life of 7.7–8.3 hours at steady state in adults. The drug is eliminated principally by renal excretion, with approximately 78 and 6% of an administered dose recovered in urine and feces, respectively. In vitro studies indicate that daptomycin is not metabolized by cytochrome P-450 (CYP) isoenzymes. In vitro studies using human hepatocytes indicate that daptomycin does not inhibit or induce CYP1A2, 2A6, 2C9, 2C19, 2D6, 2E1, or 3A4.

ADVICE TO PATIENTS

Advise patients that antibacterials (including daptomycin) should only be used to treat bacterial infections and not used to treat viral infections (e.g., the common cold).

Importance of completing full course of therapy, even if feeling better after a few days.

Advise patients that skipping doses or not completing the full course of therapy may decrease effectiveness and increase the likelihood that bacteria will develop resistance and will not be treatable with daptomycin or other antibacterials in the future.

Advise patients that allergic reactions, including serious allergic reactions, could occur and that serious reactions require immediate treatment. Importance of informing clinician of any previous allergic reactions to daptomycin.

Importance of patients immediately informing their clinician if they develop new or worsening fever, cough, shortness of breath, or difficulty breathing.

Importance of contacting a clinician if muscle pain, weakness, tingling, or numbness occurs, particularly in the forearms or lower legs.

Advise patients that diarrhea is a common problem caused by anti-infectives and usually ends when the drug is discontinued. Importance of contacting a clinician if watery and bloody stools (with or without stomach cramps and fever) occur during or as late as 2 months or longer after the last dose.

Importance of women informing clinicians if they are or plan to become pregnant or plan to breast-feed.

Importance of informing clinicians of existing or contemplated concomitant therapy, including prescription and OTC drugs.

Importance of informing patients of other important precautionary information. (See Cautions.)

PREPARATIONS

Excipients in commercially available drug preparations may have clinically important effects in some individuals; consult specific product labeling for details.

Daptomycin

Parenteral		
For injection	500 mg*	Cubicin®, Merck
		Cubicin® RF, Merck
		Daptomycin for Injection

* available from one or more manufacturer, distributor, and/or repackager by generic (nonproprietary) name

† Use is not currently included in the labeling approved by the US Food and Drug Administration.

Selected Revisions March 20, 2017, © Copyright, December 1, 2003, American Society of Health-System Pharmacists, Inc.

Dalbavancin Hydrochloride

8:12.28.16 • GLYCOPEPTIDES

■ Dalbavancin hydrochloride, a lipoglycopeptide antibacterial, is a semi-synthetic derivative of a naturally occurring glycopeptide.

USES

● Skin and Skin Structure Infections

Dalbavancin hydrochloride is used for the treatment of acute bacterial skin and skin structure infections (ABSSSI) caused by susceptible *Staphylococcus aureus* (including methicillin-resistant *S. aureus* [MRSA; also known as oxacillin-resistant *S. aureus* or ORSA] and methicillin-susceptible *S. aureus*), *Streptococcus pyogenes* (group A β-hemolytic streptococci, GAS), *S. agalactiae* (group B streptococci, GBS), or *S. anginosus* group (includes *S. anginosus, S. intermedius*, and *S. constellatus*).

Clinical Experience

Efficacy and safety of dalbavancin were evaluated in 2 randomized, multicenter, double-blind, noninferiority, phase 3 studies (DISCOVER 1 and DISCOVER 2) in adults with acute bacterial skin and skin structure infections (e.g., cellulitis, major abscess, or wound infection, each associated with at least 75 cm² of erythema). Patients had at least 2 local signs of infection (e.g., purulent drainage or discharge, fluctuance, localized warmth, tenderness, swelling or induration) and were thought to require at least 3 days of IV therapy or had at least 1 sign of systemic infection at baseline (e.g., temperature 38°C or higher, leukocyte count greater than 12,000 cells/mm³, 10% or more band forms on leukocyte differential). Over 1300 patients (mean age 50 years, 57–60% male, 12–14% with diabetes mellitus, 14–16% IV drug users, 53–54% with cellulitis, 25–27% with major abscess, 20–21% with wound or surgical site infection, median baseline lesion area 341 cm²) were randomized to receive a 2-dose regimen of dalbavancin (1 g IV on day 1 followed by 500 mg IV on day 8; those with creatinine clearance less than 30 mL/minute received 750 mg IV on day 1 followed by 375 mg on day 8) or a 10–14 day regimen of vancomycin (1 g or 15 mg/kg IV every 12 hours) with the option to switch to oral linezolid (600 mg every 12 hours) after 3 days of vancomycin. Protocol-specified empiric gram-negative coverage with aztreonam could be used concomitantly. In a pooled analysis of both studies using data at 48–72 hours after initiation of treatment, the dalbavancin regimen was noninferior to the vancomycin regimen. Clinical response (i.e., no increase in lesion area from baseline, temperature consistently 37.6°C or less) was achieved in 79.7% of those receiving dalbavancin and 79.8% of those receiving the vancomycin regimen. A similar proportion of patients receiving dalbavancin or the vancomycin regimen (88.6 or 88.1%, respectively) achieved a 20% or greater reduction in lesion area from baseline at 48–72 hours. In the subset of patients who were microbiologically evaluable and stratified according to the infecting pathogen, the clinical success rate (defined as decrease in lesion size, temperature of 37.6° C or less, and meeting pre-specified criteria for local signs of infection) on day 26–30 in those with infections caused by MRSA or methicillin-susceptible *S. aureus* was 83 or 85%, respectively, in those treated with dalbavancin and 85 or 91%, respectively, in those treated with the vancomycin regimen. The clinical success rate in those with infections caused by *S. agalactiae, S. pyogenes*, or *S. anginosus* group was 83, 89, or 96%, respectively, in those treated with dalbavancin and 79, 89, or 92%, respectively, in those treated with the vancomycin regimen.

Dalbavancin was evaluated in a randomized, double-blind, phase 3 study in 854 adults with complicated skin and skin structure infections (e.g., major abscess, major burn, traumatic or surgical wound infection, extensive or ulcerating cellulitis, infection suspected to be caused by MRSA) with at least 2 signs of local infection and at least 1 sign of systemic infection. Patients were randomized in a 2:1 ratio to receive dalbavancin (1 g IV on day 1 followed by 500 mg IV on day 8) or a 14-day regimen of linezolid (600 mg IV every 12 hours) with the option to switch to oral linezolid. Empiric coverage with aztreonam and/or metronidazole could be used concomitantly. Baseline characteristics were balanced between groups (61–62% male, 30–33% major abscess, 27–30% cellulitis); however, there was a higher proportion of patients with vascular disease in the dalbavancin group than in the linezolid group (11 and 6%, respectively). Of the clinically evaluable patients at the test-of-cure visit (approximately 14 days after completion of treatment), 88.9% of patients in the dalbavancin group and 91.2% of patients in the linezolid group achieved clinical success (i.e., improvement of signs and symptoms of infection such that no further antibacterial therapy was needed). In the subset of patients who were microbiologically evaluable, the microbiologic success rate at the test-of-cure visit was 90% in those treated with dalbavancin and 88% in those treated with linezolid; MRSA eradication rates at the test-of-cure visit were 91 or 89% in the dalbavancin or linezolid groups, respectively.

DOSAGE AND ADMINISTRATION

● Administration

Dalbavancin hydrochloride is administered by IV infusion.

IV Administration

If the same IV line is used for sequential infusion of dalbavancin and other drugs, the IV line should be flushed with 5% dextrose injection before and after the dalbavancin infusion.

Dalbavancin solutions should *not* be infused with other drugs or electrolytes. Dalbavancin solutions are compatible with 5% dextrose injection, but compatibility with other IV solutions, drugs, additives, or substances has not been established.

Vials of dalbavancin lyophilized powder for injection contain no preservatives and are intended for single use only.

Reconstitution and Dilution

Dalbavancin hydrochloride for injection must be reconstituted and further diluted prior to IV infusion. Strict aseptic technique must be observed when preparing IV solutions of the drug.

Vials labeled as containing 500 mg of dalbavancin should be reconstituted by adding 25 mL of sterile water for injection to provide a solution containing 20 mg/mL. To avoid foaming, the vial should be alternately swirled and inverted until vial contents are completely dissolved; the vial should not be shaken. The reconstituted solution should appear clear and colorless to yellow.

Reconstituted dalbavancin must then be further diluted by withdrawing the correct dose of the drug from the reconstituted vial(s) and adding it to an IV bag or bottle containing 5% dextrose injection. The final diluted solution *must* have a dalbavancin concentration of 1–5 mg/mL. Any unused portion of reconstituted solution should be discarded.

Reconstituted or further diluted solutions of dalbavancin may be stored under refrigeration (2–8°C) or at controlled room temperature (i.e., 20–25°C), but should not be frozen. Total storage time from the time of reconstitution to administration should not exceed 48 hours whether refrigerated at 2–8°C or stored at room temperature.

Dalbavancin solutions should be inspected visually for particulate matter prior to administration.

Rate of Administration

Dalbavancin solutions should be administered by IV infusion over 30 minutes.

● Dosage

Dosage of dalbavancin hydrochloride is expressed in terms of dalbavancin.

Adult Dosage
Skin and Skin Structure Infections

The recommended dosage of dalbavancin for the treatment of acute bacterial skin and skin structure infections (ABSSSI) in adults is a 2-dose regimen of 1 g given by IV infusion followed 1 week later by 500 mg given by IV infusion.

● Special Populations
Renal Impairment

Dosage adjustments are not needed in adults with mild (creatinine clearance 50–79 mL/minute) or moderate (creatinine clearance 30–49 mL/minute) renal impairment.

Adults with severe renal impairment (creatinine clearances less than 30 mL/minute) *not* receiving regularly scheduled hemodialysis should receive a 2-dose regimen of 750 mg of dalbavancin given by IV infusion followed 1 week later by 375 mg given by IV infusion.

Dosage adjustments are not recommended for adults with renal impairment receiving regularly scheduled hemodialysis; dalbavancin may be administered in such patients without regard to hemodialysis timing. (See Renal Impairment under Warnings/Precautions: Specific Populations, in Cautions.)

Hepatic Impairment

Dosage adjustments are not needed in adults with mild hepatic impairment (Child-Pugh class A).

Dosage recommendations for those with moderate or severe hepatic impairment (Child-Pugh class B or C) are not available; the drug should be used with caution in such individuals. (See Hepatic Impairment under Warnings/Precautions: Specific Populations, in Cautions.)

Geriatric Patients

Dosage adjustments are not needed in geriatric patients based solely on age. Dosage should be selected with caution since geriatric patients are more likely to have decreased renal function than younger adults. (See Geriatric Use under Warnings/Precautions: Specific Populations, in Cautions.)

CAUTIONS

● Contraindications

Dalbavancin is contraindicated in patients with known hypersensitivity to the drug.

● Warnings/Precautions

Sensitivity Reactions

Serious hypersensitivity (anaphylactic) and skin reactions have been reported in patients receiving dalbavancin.

Data are not available to date regarding cross-reactivity between dalbavancin and other glycopeptides (e.g., oritavancin, telavancin, vancomycin). Because of the possibility of cross-sensitivity, patients should be questioned about previous hypersensitivity reactions to glycopeptides and dalbavancin should be used with caution in those with a history of glycopeptide allergy.

If an allergic reaction occurs, dalbavancin should be discontinued.

Infusion Reactions

Rapid IV infusion of dalbavancin can cause a reaction referred to as "red-man syndrome" (i.e., flushing of the upper body, urticaria, pruritus, rash).

To reduce the risk of infusion-related reactions, IV infusions of dalbavancin should be given over 30 minutes. If an infusion-related reaction occurs, stopping or decreasing the infusion rate may result in cessation of symptoms.

Hepatic Effects

In patients with normal baseline aminotransferase concentrations in phase 2 and phase 3 clinical trials, more dalbavancin-treated patients developed ALT elevations greater than 3 times the upper limit of normal (ULN) compared with patients receiving a comparator treatment (0.8 or 0.2%, respectively). Overall, the frequency of liver laboratory test abnormalities (e.g., ALT, AST, bilirubin) was similar in patients receiving dalbavancin or a comparator treatment.

Superinfection/Clostridium difficile-associated Diarrhea and Colitis (CDAD)

Use of dalbavancin may result in emergence and overgrowth of nonsusceptible bacteria or fungi. The patient should be carefully monitored and appropriate therapy instituted if superinfection occurs.

Treatment with anti-infectives alters normal colon flora and may permit overgrowth of *Clostridium difficile*. *C. difficile* infection (CDI) and *C. difficile*-associated diarrhea and colitis (CDAD; also known as antibiotic-associated diarrhea and colitis or pseudomembranous colitis) have been reported in patients receiving nearly all anti-infectives, including dalbavancin, and may range in severity from mild diarrhea to fatal colitis. *C. difficile* produces toxins A and B which contribute to development of CDAD; hypertoxin-producing strains of *C. difficile* are associated with increased morbidity and mortality since they may be refractory to anti-infectives and colectomy may be required.

CDAD should be considered in the differential diagnosis of patients who develop diarrhea during or after anti-infective therapy. Careful medical history is necessary since CDAD has been reported to occur as late as 2 months or longer after anti-infective therapy is discontinued.

If CDAD is suspected or confirmed, anti-infective therapy not directed against *C. difficile* should be discontinued whenever possible. Patients should be managed with appropriate supportive therapy (e.g., fluid and electrolyte management, protein supplementation), anti-infective therapy directed against *C. difficile* (e.g., metronidazole, vancomycin), and surgical evaluation as clinically indicated.

Selection and Use of Anti-infectives

To reduce development of drug-resistant bacteria and maintain effectiveness of dalbavancin and other antibacterials, the drug should be used only for treatment of infections proven or strongly suspected to be caused by susceptible bacteria.

When selecting or modifying anti-infective therapy, results of culture and in vitro susceptibility testing should be used. In the absence of such data, local epidemiology and susceptibility patterns should be considered when selecting anti-infectives for empiric therapy.

Specific Populations

Pregnancy

Category C. (See Users Guide.)

There are no adequate and well-controlled studies of dalbavancin in pregnant women, and the drug should be used during pregnancy only if potential benefits justify potential risks to the fetus.

In an embryofetal study in rats, delayed fetal maturation was observed at a dosage of 45 mg/kg daily (3.5 times the human dosage on an exposure basis). In a prenatal and postnatal development study in rats, increased embryolethality and increased offspring deaths during the first week postpartum were observed at a dosage of 45 mg/kg daily.

Lactation

Dalbavancin is distributed into milk in lactating rats; it is not known whether the drug is distributed into human milk.

Dalbavancin should be used with caution in nursing women.

Pediatric Use

Safety and efficacy of dalbavancin have not been established in pediatric patients.

Geriatric Use

In clinical studies evaluating dalbavancin for the treatment of acute bacterial skin and skin structure infections, efficacy and tolerability were similar to comparator treatments regardless of age.

There were no substantial differences in the pharmacokinetics of dalbavancin according to age; therefore, dosage adjustments are not needed based solely on age.

Dalbavancin is substantially eliminated by the kidneys; the risk of adverse effects may be greater in patients with impaired renal function. Dosage should be selected with caution since geriatric patients are more likely to have decreased renal function.

Hepatic Impairment

Dalbavancin should be used with caution in patients with moderate or severe hepatic impairment (Child-Pugh class B or C); there are no data available to determine an appropriate dosage of the drug in such patients. The mean area under the plasma concentration-time curve (AUC) of dalbavancin is decreased by 28 or 31% in patients with moderate or severe hepatic impairment (Child-Pugh class B or C); however, the clinical importance of decreased AUC in such patients has not been established.

Dalbavancin pharmacokinetics are not altered in patients with mild hepatic impairment (Child-Pugh class A).

Renal Impairment

In patients with mild, moderate, or severe renal impairment, mean plasma clearance of dalbavancin is decreased by 11, 35, or 47%, respectively, and AUC is increased compared with patients with normal renal function. Dalbavancin pharmacokinetics in patients with end-stage renal disease receiving regularly scheduled hemodialysis are similar to those in patients with mild to moderate renal impairment.

Patients with creatinine clearance less than 30 mL/minute who are *not* receiving regularly scheduled hemodialysis should receive reduced dalbavancin dosage. (See Renal Impairment under Dosage and Administration: Special Populations.)

● **Common Adverse Effects**

Adverse effects reported in 2% or more of patients receiving dalbavancin include nausea, vomiting, diarrhea, headache, rash, and pruritus.

DRUG INTERACTIONS

Formal drug interaction studies have not been conducted with dalbavancin to date.

● **Drugs Affecting or Metabolized by Hepatic Microsomal Enzymes**

Based on in vitro studies, dalbavancin is not a substrate, inhibitor, or inducer of cytochrome P-450 (CYP) isoenzymes, and there is minimal potential that the drug will interact with substrates, inhibitors, or inducers of CYP isoenzymes. Results of a population pharmacokinetic analysis indicate that dalbavancin pharmacokinetics are not affected when the drug is used concomitantly with known CYP isoenzyme substrates, inducers, inhibitors, or other tested drugs (e.g., acetaminophen, aztreonam, fentanyl, metronidazole, furosemide, proton-pump inhibitors [omeprazole, esomeprazole, pantoprazole, lansoprazole], midazolam, simvastatin).

● **Antibacterial Agents**

Dalbavancin pharmacokinetics do not appear to be affected by concomitant use of aztreonam or metronidazole.

In vitro studies indicate that the antibacterial effects of dalbavancin and oxacillin are synergistic against some gram-positive bacteria (methicillin-resistant *Staphylococcus aureus* [MRSA; also known as oxacillin-resistant *S. aureus* or ORSA]).

In vitro studies indicate that the antibacterial effects of dalbavancin and aztreonam, clindamycin, daptomycin, gentamicin, levofloxacin, linezolid, quinupristin and dalfopristin, rifampin, or vancomycin are not synergistic or antagonistic.

DESCRIPTION

Dalbavancin hydrochloride is a semisynthetic lipoglycopeptide antibacterial derived from a naturally occurring glycopeptide produced by *Nonomuraea*, an actinomycete. The drug is a teicoplanin-type lipoglycopeptide and contains a heptapeptide core structure that differs from that of vancomycin. Dalbavancin is a mixture of 5 closely related homologs (i.e., A_0, A_1, B_0, B_1, B_2), each sharing the same core structure. Of the 5 homologs, B_0 is the major component of dalbavancin.

The mechanism of action of dalbavancin is similar to that of other glycopeptides (e.g., oritavancin, telavancin, vancomycin). Dalbavancin binds to the D-alanyl-D-alanine terminus of growing peptidoglycan chains, thereby inhibiting bacterial cell wall synthesis. The drug also appears to dimerize and anchor in the bacterial membranes.

In vitro, dalbavancin is bactericidal in action against certain gram-positive bacteria, including staphylococci, streptococci, and enterococci. The drug is active in vitro and in clinical infections against *S. aureus* (including methicillin-resistant *S. aureus* [MRSA; also known as oxacillin-resistant *S. aureus* or ORSA]), *S. pyogenes* (group A β-hemolytic streptococci, GAS), *S. agalactiae* (group B streptococci, GBS), and *S. anginosus* group (includes *S. anginosus*, *S. intermedius*, and *S. constellatus*). Dalbavancin also is active in vitro against some vancomycin-susceptible *Enterococcus faecium* and *E. faecalis*; however, safety and efficacy of the drug in treating clinical infections caused by these bacteria have not been established. Dalbavancin is active in vitro against some vancomycin-intermediate *S. aureus* (VISA) and VanB and VanC phenotypes of vancomycin-resistant enterococci (VRE), but VRE with the VanA phenotype have reduced in vitro susceptibility or resistance to dalbavancin.

Reduced susceptibility or resistance to dalbavancin was not produced in vitro by serial passage of *S. aureus* in the presence of increasing concentrations of the drug. Certain intrinsically glycopeptide-resistant bacteria and those expressing the VanA phenotype of acquired resistance to vancomycin also may be resistant to dalbavancin. Cross-resistance between dalbavancin and nonglycopeptide anti-infectives is unlikely.

Dalbavancin exhibits linear, dose-dependent pharmacokinetics following IV administration, and there is no apparent accumulation following multiple IV doses of the drug. In adults with skin and skin structure infections, a single 1-g IV dose of dalbavancin given on day 1 followed by a single 500-mg IV dose on day 8 resulted in mean plasma dalbavancin concentrations of 30 mg/L immediately before the second dose and mean plasma concentrations of 21 mg/mL (range 8–40 mg/L) 20 days after the initial dose. Dalbavancin is distributed into skin blister fluid following IV administration, and mean blister fluid concentrations are at least 30 mg/L for up to 7 days following a single 1-g IV dose. The drug is approximately 93% bound to plasma proteins, mainly albumin. Dalbavancin is not a substrate, inhibitor, or inducer of cytochrome P-450 (CYP) isoenzymes; a minor metabolite, hydroxydalbavancin, has been detected in urine. Based on population pharmacokinetic analyses, the effective half-life of dalbavancin is approximately 8.5 days (204 hours). Following a single 1-g dose of dalbavancin, 20% of a dose is eliminated in feces by day 70 after the dose. An average of 33% of the dose is eliminated in urine as unchanged drug and approximately 12% is eliminated in urine as the metabolite by day 42 after the dose. Less than 6% of an administered dose of dalbavancin is removed after 3 hours of hemodialysis.

ADVICE TO PATIENTS

Advise patients that antibacterials (including dalbavancin) should only be used to treat bacterial infections and not used to treat viral infections (e.g., the common cold).

Importance of completing full course of therapy, even if feeling better after a few days.

Advise patients that skipping doses or not completing the full course of therapy may decrease effectiveness and increase the likelihood that bacteria will develop resistance and will not be treatable with dalbavancin or other antibacterials in the future.

Advise patients that allergic reactions, including serious allergic reactions, could occur and require immediate treatment. Importance of informing clinician about any previous hypersensitivity reactions to dalbavancin or other glycopeptides (e.g., oritavancin, telavancin, vancomycin).

Advise patients that diarrhea is a common problem caused by anti-infectives and usually ends when the drug is discontinued. Importance of contacting a clinician if watery and bloody stools (with or without stomach cramps and fever) occur during or as late as 2 months or longer after the last dose.

Importance of informing clinicians of existing or contemplated concomitant therapy, including prescription and OTC drugs and dietary or herbal supplements, as well as any concomitant illnesses.

Importance of women informing clinicians if they are or plan to become pregnant or plan to breast-feed.

Importance of informing patients of other important precautionary information. (See Cautions.)

PREPARATIONS

Excipients in commercially available drug preparations may have clinically important effects in some individuals; consult specific product labeling for details.

Dalbavancin Hydrochloride

Parenteral		
For injection, for IV infusion	500 mg (of dalbavancin)	**Dalvance®**, Durata Therapeutics

© Copyright, April 7, 2015, American Society of Health-System Pharmacists, Inc.

Oritavancin Diphosphate

8:12.28.16 • GLYCOPEPTIDES

■ Oritavancin diphosphate, a lipoglycopeptide antibacterial, is a semisynthetic derivative of a naturally occurring glycopeptide.

USES

● Skin and Skin Structure Infections

Oritavancin diphosphate is used for the treatment of acute bacterial skin and skin structure infections (ABSSSI) caused by susceptible *Staphylococcus aureus* (including methicillin-resistant *S. aureus* [MRSA; also known as oxacillin-resistant *S. aureus* or ORSA] and methicillin-susceptible *S. aureus*), *Streptococcus pyogenes* (group A β-hemolytic streptococci, GAS), *S. agalactiae* (group B streptococci, GBS), *S. dysgalactiae, S. anginosus* group (includes *S. anginosus, S. intermedius,* and *S. constellatus*), or vancomycin-susceptible *Enterococcus faecalis.*

Clinical Experience

Efficacy and safety of oritavancin were evaluated in 2 randomized, multicenter, double-blind, noninferiority, phase 3 studies (SOLO I and SOLO II) in 1987 adults with acute bacterial skin and skin structure infections (e.g., cellulitis, major abscess, wound infection, erysipelas) suspected or proven to be caused by a gram-positive pathogen. Eligible patients exhibited at least 2 local signs of infection (e.g., purulent drainage or discharge, fluctuance, localized warmth, tenderness, swelling or induration), at least 1 sign of systemic inflammation at baseline (e.g., proximal lymph node swelling, temperature 38°C or higher or less than 36°C, leukocyte count greater than 10,000 cells/mm³, greater than 10% bandemia, increased C-reactive protein), and were thought to require at least 7 days of IV therapy. Patients were randomized in a 1:1 ratio to receive oritavancin (single 1.2-g IV dose) or vancomycin (1 g or 15 mg/kg IV every 12 hours for 7–10 days). Aztreonam or metronidazole could be used concomitantly for gram-negative or anaerobic coverage, respectively.

In SOLO I, baseline demographic characteristics were similar between groups (mean age 44–46 years, 63% male, 20% with diabetes mellitus, 49–51% with cellulitis, 29–30% with abscess, 19–22% with wound infection, median baseline lesion area 226–248 cm²). At 48–72 hours after initiation of treatment, 82.3% of patients receiving oritavancin and 78.9% of patients receiving vancomycin achieved the primary efficacy end point of early clinical response (i.e., no increase in lesion area from baseline, absence of fever, and no rescue antibacterial drugs needed). Decrease in lesion size of 20% or more at 48–72 hours after initiation of treatment was achieved by 86.9 or 82.9% of patients receiving oritavancin or vancomycin, respectively, and investigator-assessed clinical success at 7–14 days after the end of therapy was achieved by 79.6 or 80% of patients, respectively.

In SOLO II, baseline demographic characteristics were similar between groups (mean age 44–45 years, 67–68% male, 9% with diabetes mellitus, 29–33% with cellulitis, 32–33% with abscess, 35–38% with wound infection, median baseline lesion area 288–309 cm²). At 48–72 hours after initiation of treatment, 80.1% of patients receiving oritavancin and 82.9% of patients receiving vancomycin achieved the primary efficacy end point of early clinical response (i.e., no increase in lesion area from baseline, absence of fever, and no rescue antibacterial drugs needed). Decrease in lesion size of 20% or more at 48–72 hours after initiation of treatment was achieved by 85.9 or 85.3% of patients receiving oritavancin or vancomycin, respectively, and investigator-assessed clinical success at 7–10 days after the end of therapy was achieved by 82.7 or 80.5% of patients, respectively.

In a pooled analysis (SOLO I and SOLO II) of the subset of patients who were microbiologically evaluable and stratified according to the infecting pathogen, the clinical success rate (defined as complete or nearly complete resolution of baseline signs and symptoms) on day 14–24 in those with infections caused by MRSA or methicillin-susceptible *S. aureus* was 83 or 82%, respectively, in those treated with oritavancin and 84 or 84%, respectively, in those treated with vancomycin. The clinical success rate in those with infections caused by *S. agalactiae, S. pyogenes, S. anginosus* group, *S. dysgalactiae,* or *E. faecalis* was 88, 81, 76, 78, or 62%, respectively, in those treated with oritavancin and 92, 72, 84, 50, or 75%, respectively, in those treated with vancomycin.

DOSAGE AND ADMINISTRATION

● Administration

Oritavancin diphosphate is administered by IV infusion.

IV Administration

Oritavancin should *not* be administered simultaneously with commonly used IV drugs through a common port.

If the same IV line or port is used for sequential infusion of oritavancin and other drugs, the IV line should be flushed with 5% dextrose injection before and after the oritavancin infusion.

Sodium chloride 0.9% is incompatible with oritavancin diphosphate and may cause precipitation. Sodium chloride 0.9% should *not* be used to dilute oritavancin. Other IV solutions, additives, or drugs mixed in 0.9% sodium chloride injection should *not* be added to oritavancin vials or infused simultaneously through the same IV line or port.

Drugs formulated at an alkaline or neutral pH may be incompatible with oritavancin.

Vials of oritavancin lyophilized powder for injection contain no preservatives and are intended for single use only.

Reconstitution and Dilution

Oritavancin diphosphate for injection must be reconstituted and further diluted prior to IV infusion. Strict aseptic technique must be observed when preparing IV solutions of the drug.

Vials labeled as containing 400 mg of oritavancin should be reconstituted by adding 40 mL of sterile water for injection to provide a solution containing 10 mg/mL. A total of 3 vials is required to prepare a single 1.2-g dose. To avoid foaming, vials should be gently swirled until contents are completely dissolved. The reconstituted solution should appear clear and colorless to pale yellow.

Reconstituted oritavancin must then be further diluted in 5% dextrose injection. Before adding oritavancin to a 1-L IV bag of 5% dextrose injection, 120 mL of the dextrose injection should be withdrawn and discarded. Then, 40 mL of reconstituted oritavancin should be withdrawn from each of the 3 reconstituted vials and added to the 5% dextrose IV bag bringing the bag volume to 1 L. The final diluted oritavancin solution has a concentration of 1.2 mg/mL.

Following reconstitution and further dilution, oritavancin solutions should be used within 6 hours when stored at room temperature or within 12 hours when refrigerated at 2–8°C. The combined total storage time and 3-hour infusion time should not exceed 6 hours at room temperature or 12 hours at 2–8°C.

Oritavancin solutions should be inspected visually for particulate matter prior to administration.

Rate of Administration

Oritavancin solutions should be administered by IV infusion over 3 hours.

● Dosage

Dosage of oritavancin diphosphate is expressed in terms of oritavancin.

Adult Dosage
Skin and Skin Structure Infections

The recommended dosage of oritavancin for the treatment of acute bacterial skin and skin structure infections (ABSSSI) in adults is a single 1.2-g dose given by IV infusion.

● Special Populations
Renal Impairment

Dosage adjustments are not needed in patients with mild or moderate renal impairment. Pharmacokinetics of oritavancin have not been studied in patients with severe renal impairment. (See Renal Impairment under Warnings/Precautions: Specific Populations, in Cautions.)

Hepatic Impairment

Dosage adjustments are not needed in patients with mild or moderate hepatic impairment. Pharmacokinetics of oritavancin have not been studied in patients with severe hepatic impairment. (See Hepatic Impairment under Warning/Precautions: Specific Populations, in Cautions.)

CAUTIONS

● Contraindications

Oritavancin is contraindicated in patients with known hypersensitivity to the drug.

Unfractionated heparin sodium is contraindicated for 48 hours after oritavancin because activated partial thromboplastin time (aPTT) is expected to remain falsely elevated for this period of time after administration of the anti-infective. (See Tests Used to Monitor Coagulation under Cautions: Warnings/Precautions.)

● Warnings/Precautions

Sensitivity Reactions

Serious hypersensitivity reactions have been reported in patients receiving oritavancin. In phase 3 clinical trials, the median onset of hypersensitivity reactions in patients receiving oritavancin was 1.2 days and the median duration of the reactions was 2.4 days.

Because of the possibility of cross-sensitivity, patients should be questioned about previous hypersensitivity reactions to glycopeptides (e.g., dalbavancin, telavancin, vancomycin). Individuals with a history of glycopeptide allergy should be carefully monitored for signs of hypersensitivity during oritavancin infusion.

If an acute hypersensitivity reaction occurs during the oritavancin infusion, the drug should be discontinued immediately and appropriate supportive care initiated.

Infusion Reactions

Infusion-related reactions (e.g., pruritus, urticaria, flushing) have been reported in patients receiving oritavancin.

If an infusion-related reaction occurs, slowing or interrupting the oritavancin infusion should be considered.

Tests Used to Monitor Coagulation

Oritavancin has been shown to artificially prolong certain tests used to monitor coagulation, including prothrombin time (PT), international normalized ratio (INR), and aPTT, and also is expected to prolong activated clotting time (ACT). This occurs because oritavancin binds to phospholipid reagents and prevents activation of coagulation in commonly used laboratory coagulation tests. Oritavancin does *not* have an effect on the coagulation system.

PT and INR have been shown to be artificially prolonged for 24 hours after oritavancin administration and aPTT has been shown to be artificially prolonged for 48 hours after oritavancin administration. These effects may complicate laboratory monitoring in patients receiving certain anticoagulants (e.g., heparin, warfarin).

For patients requiring aPTT monitoring within 48 hours of oritavancin administration, a non-phospholipid-dependent coagulation test (e.g., factor Xa [chromogenic] assay) should be used or an alternative anticoagulant not requiring aPTT monitoring considered.

Concomitant Use with Warfarin

Concomitant use of oritavancin and warfarin may increase warfarin exposure and may increase the risk of bleeding. (See Drug Interactions: Warfarin.)

Oritavancin and chronic warfarin therapy should be used concomitantly *only* when the benefits are expected to outweigh the risk of bleeding. If the drugs are used concomitantly, the patient should be frequently monitored for signs of bleeding. Clinicians should consider that laboratory monitoring of the anticoagulant effects of warfarin is unreliable for 24 hours after oritavancin administration because the anti-infective artificially prolongs certain coagulation tests. (See Tests Used to Monitor Coagulation under Cautions: Warnings/Precautions.)

Osteomyelitis

In clinical trials, osteomyelitis was reported more frequently in patients receiving oritavancin than in those receiving vancomycin.

Patients receiving oritavancin should be monitored for signs and symptoms of osteomyelitis. If osteomyelitis is suspected or diagnosed, appropriate alternative antibacterial therapy should be initiated.

Superinfection/Clostridium difficile-associated Diarrhea and Colitis (CDAD)

Use of oritavancin may result in emergence and overgrowth of nonsusceptible bacteria or fungi. The patient should be carefully monitored and appropriate therapy instituted if superinfection occurs.

Treatment with anti-infectives alters normal colon flora and may permit overgrowth of *Clostridium difficile*. *C. difficile* infection (CDI) and *C. difficile*-associated diarrhea and colitis (CDAD; also known as antibiotic-associated diarrhea and colitis or pseudomembranous colitis) have been reported in patients receiving nearly all anti-infectives, including oritavancin, and may range in severity from mild diarrhea to fatal colitis. *C. difficile* produces toxins A and B which contribute to development of CDAD; hypertoxin-producing strains of *C. difficile* are associated with increased morbidity and mortality since they may be refractory to anti-infectives and colectomy may be required.

CDAD should be considered in the differential diagnosis of patients who develop diarrhea during or after anti-infective therapy. Careful medical history is necessary since CDAD has been reported to occur as late as 2 months or longer after anti-infective therapy is discontinued.

If CDAD is suspected or confirmed, anti-infective therapy not directed against *C. difficile* should be discontinued whenever possible. Patients should be managed with appropriate supportive therapy (e.g., fluid and electrolyte management, protein supplementation), anti-infective therapy directed against *C. difficile* (e.g., metronidazole, vancomycin), and surgical evaluation as clinically indicated.

Selection and Use of Anti-infectives

To reduce development of drug-resistant bacteria and maintain effectiveness of oritavancin and other antibacterials, the drug should be used only for treatment of infections proven or strongly suspected to be caused by susceptible bacteria.

When selecting or modifying anti-infective therapy, results of culture and in vitro susceptibility testing should be used. In the absence of such data, local epidemiology and susceptibility patterns should be considered when selecting anti-infectives for empiric therapy.

Specific Populations

Pregnancy

Category C. (See Users Guide.)

There are no adequate and well-controlled studies of oritavancin in pregnant women, and the drug should be used during pregnancy only if potential benefits justify potential risks to the fetus.

Reproduction studies in rats or rabbits have not revealed evidence of harm to the fetus at dosages equivalent to a human dose of 300 mg (25% of the recommend 1.2-g single dose); higher doses have not been evaluated.

Lactation

Oritavancin is distributed into milk in lactating rats; it is not known whether the drug is distributed into human milk.

Oritavancin should be used with caution in nursing women.

Pediatric Use

Safety and efficacy of oritavancin have not been established in pediatric patients younger than 18 years of age.

Geriatric Use

Clinical trials of oritavancin did not include sufficient numbers of patients 65 years of age and older to determine whether they respond differently than younger adults. Other clinical experience has not revealed age-related differences in response, but the possibility of greater sensitivity in some older patients cannot be ruled out.

Hepatic Impairment

The pharmacokinetics of oritavancin have not been studied in patients with severe hepatic impairment. There were no clinically important differences in pharmacokinetics of oritavancin in patients with moderate hepatic impairment (Child-Pugh class B) compared with healthy adults.

Renal Impairment

The pharmacokinetics of oritavancin have not been studied in patients with severe renal impairment or in those receiving dialysis. There were no clinically important differences in pharmacokinetics of oritavancin in patients with mild or moderate renal impairment compared with those with normal renal function.

● Common Adverse Effects

Adverse effects reported in 1.5% or more of patients receiving oritavancin include GI effects (i.e., diarrhea, nausea, vomiting, constipation), dizziness, headache, infusion site reactions (including phlebitis and extravasation), pruritus, urticaria, pyrexia, chills, abscess (limb or subcutaneous), cellulitis, increased AST and ALT concentrations, tachycardia, insomnia, and fatigue.

DRUG INTERACTIONS

● Drugs Affecting or Metabolized by Hepatic Microsomal Enzymes

Oritavancin is a weak inhibitor of cytochrome P-450 (CYP) 2C9 and CYP2C19 and a weak inducer of CYP3A4 and CYP2D6. Oritavancin and drugs that are metabolized by these CYP isoenzymes and have a narrow therapeutic index should be used concomitantly with caution and patients closely monitored for signs of toxicity or lack of efficacy.

● Drugs Affecting or Affected by P-glycoprotein Transport System

Oritavancin is not a substrate or inhibitor of the P-glycoprotein (P-gp) efflux transporter.

● Antibacterial Agents

In vitro, the antibacterial effects of oritavancin and gentamicin, moxifloxacin, or rifampin are synergistic against methicillin-susceptible Staphylococcus aureus. In vitro studies indicate that the antibacterial effects of oritavancin and gentamicin or linezolid are synergistic against vancomycin-intermediate S. aureus (VISA), heterogeneous VISA (hVISA), and vancomycin-resistant S. aureus (VRSA). In addition, the antibacterial effects of oritavancin and rifampin are synergistic in vitro against VRSA.

In vitro, the antibacterial effects of oritavancin and ciprofloxacin or gentamicin are synergistic against some vancomycin-resistant enterococci (VRE).

There is no in vitro evidence of antagonistic antibacterial effects between oritavancin and ciprofloxacin, gentamicin, moxifloxacin, linezolid, or rifampin.

● Dextromethorphan

Concomitant use of oritavancin (single 1.2-g dose) and dextromethorphan results in a 31% decrease in the ratio of dextromethorphan to dextrorphan concentrations in urine.

● Heparin

Because the activated partial thromboplastin time (aPTT) is expected to be falsely elevated for approximately 48 hours after oritavancin administration, unfractionated heparin sodium is contraindicated for 48 hours after oritavancin. (See Tests Used to Monitor Coagulation under Cautions: Warnings/Precautions.)

● Midazolam

Concomitant use of oritavancin (single 1.2-g dose) and midazolam results in an 18% decrease in the mean area under the plasma concentration-time curve (AUC) of midazolam.

● Omeprazole

Concomitant use of oritavancin (single 1.2-g dose) and omeprazole results in a 15% increase in the ratio of omeprazole to 5-hydroxyomeprazole concentrations in plasma.

● Warfarin

Concomitant use of oritavancin (single 1.2-g dose) and warfarin results in a 31% increase in the mean AUC of warfarin and may increase the risk of bleeding.

Oritavancin and chronic warfarin therapy should be used concomitantly *only* when the benefits are expected to outweigh the risk of bleeding.

If oritavancin and warfarin are used concomitantly, the patient should be frequently monitored for signs of bleeding. Because prothrombin time (PT) and international normalized ratio (INR) are expected to be falsely elevated for approximately 24 hours after oritavancin administration, monitoring the anticoagulation effects of warfarin is unreliable for 24 hours after oritavancin. (See Tests Used to Monitor Coagulation under Cautions: Warnings/Precautions.)

DESCRIPTION

Oritavancin diphosphate is a semisynthetic lipoglycopeptide antibacterial derived from chloroeremomycin, a naturally occurring glycopeptide. Oritavancin contains a heptapeptide core structure similar to that of vancomycin, but has side chains that enhance antibacterial activity.

The mechanism of action of oritavancin is similar to that of other glycopeptides (e.g., dalbavancin, vancomycin). Oritavancin binds to the D-alanyl-D-alanine terminus of growing peptidoglycan chains, thereby inhibiting bacterial cell wall, synthesis. In addition, the drug binds to the peptide bridging segments of the cell wall, thereby inhibiting the transpeptidation (crosslinking) step of cell wall biosynthesis, and can dimerize and anchor into the bacterial cell membrane, which improves its ability to bind to its target.

In vitro, oritavancin is bactericidal in action against certain gram-positive bacteria, including staphylococci, streptococci, and enterococci. In vitro and in clinical studies, oritavancin is active against Staphylococcus aureus (including methicillin-resistant S. aureus [MRSA; also known as oxacillin-resistant S. aureus or ORSA]), Streptococcus pyogenes (group A β-hemolytic streptococci, GAS), S. agalactiae (group B streptococci, GBS), S. dysgalactiae, S. anginosus group (includes S. anginosus, S. intermedius, and S. constellatus), and vancomycin-susceptible Enterococcus faecalis.

Oritavancin also is active in vitro against vancomycin-susceptible E. faecium, Clostridium perfringens, C. difficile, Peptostreptococcus, Propionibacterium acnes, S. pneumoniae, vancomycin-intermediate S. aureus (VISA), vancomycin-resistant S. aureus (VRSA), and daptomycin-nonsusceptible S. aureus (DNSSA). However, safety and efficacy of oritavancin in treating clinical infections caused by these bacteria have not been established.

Reduced susceptibility or resistance to oritavancin has been produced in vitro by serial passage of S. aureus or E. faecalis in the presence of increasing concentrations of the drug.

Oritavancin exhibits linear, dose-dependent pharmacokinetics following IV administration. Oritavancin is extensively distributed into tissues, including skin blister fluid, extracellular lung fluid, and alveolar macrophages. Mean oritavancin concentrations in skin blister fluid are approximately 20% of those in plasma after a single 800-mg dose in healthy individuals. The drug is approximately 85% bound to plasma proteins. Oritavancin is not metabolized. Based on population pharmacokinetic analyses, the terminal half-life of oritavancin is approximately 10 days (245 hours). The drug is slowly eliminated unchanged in feces and urine; less than 1 and 5% of a single IV dose is recovered in feces and urine, respectively, by 2 weeks after the dose. The drug is not removed by hemodialysis or continuous renal replacement therapy (CRRT).

ADVICE TO PATIENTS

Advise patients that antibacterials (including oritavancin) should only be used to treat bacterial infections and not used to treat viral infections (e.g., the common cold).

Importance of completing full course of therapy, even if feeling better after a few days.

Advise patients that skipping doses or not completing the full course of therapy may decrease effectiveness and increase the likelihood that bacteria will develop resistance and will not be treatable with oritavancin or other antibacterials in the future.

Advise patients that allergic reactions, including serious allergic reactions, could occur and require immediate treatment. Importance of informing clinician about any previous hypersensitivity reactions to oritavancin or other glycopeptides (e.g., dalbavancin, telavancin, vancomycin).

Advise patients that diarrhea is a common problem caused by anti-infectives and usually ends when the drug is discontinued. Importance of contacting a clinician if watery and bloody stools (with or without stomach cramps and fever) occur during or as late as 2 months or longer after the last dose.

Importance of informing clinicians of existing or contemplated concomitant therapy, including prescription and OTC drugs and dietary or herbal supplements, as well as any concomitant illnesses.

Importance of women informing clinicians if they are or plan to become pregnant or plan to breast-feed.

Importance of informing patients of other important precautionary information. (See Cautions.)

PREPARATIONS

Excipients in commercially available drug preparations may have clinically important effects in some individuals; consult specific product labeling for details.

Oritavancin Diphosphate

Parenteral

| For injection, for IV infusion | 400 mg (of oritavancin) | Orbactiv®, Medicines Company |

Selected Revisions © Copyright, April 7, 2015, American Society of Health-System Pharmacists, Inc.

Telavancin Hydrochloride

8:12.28.16 • GLYCOPEPTIDES

■ Telavancin, a lipoglycopeptide antibacterial, is a semisynthetic derivative of vancomycin.

USES

● Respiratory Tract Infections

Nosocomial Pneumonia

Telavancin hydrochloride is used for the treatment of nosocomial pneumonia, including hospital-acquired and ventilator-associated pneumonia, caused by susceptible *Staphylococcus aureus* (including methicillin-resistant *S. aureus* [MRSA; also known as oxacillin-resistant *S. aureus* or ORSA]). If documented or presumed pathogens also include gram-negative or anaerobic bacteria, concomitant use of an anti-infective active against such bacteria may be clinically indicated.

The manufacturer states that telavancin should be reserved for use when alternative treatments for hospital-acquired or ventilator-associated bacterial pneumonia are not suitable.

Clinical Experience

Telavancin was evaluated in 2 identical, randomized, double-blind, parallel-group, phase 3 studies in adults with hospital-acquired or ventilator-associated pneumonia known or suspected to be caused by *S. aureus*. The mean age of study patients was 63 years, 64% were male, 70% were white, more than 50% were admitted to an intensive care unit, 23% had chronic obstructive pulmonary disease, 29% had ventilator-associated pneumonia, and 6% had bacteremia. Patients were randomized to receive 7–21 days of treatment with telavancin (10 mg/kg IV once every 24 hours) or vancomycin (1 g IV every 12 hours with dosage individualized and adjusted according to standard practices at the site). Other appropriate anti-infectives (e.g., aztreonam and/or metronidazole) were used concomitantly if documented or presumed pathogens also included gram-negative or anaerobic bacteria; the fixed combination of piperacillin sodium and tazobactam sodium could be used concomitantly for gram-negative coverage if aztreonam resistance was confirmed or suspected. The primary end point was clinical response (i.e., resolution of signs and symptoms, no further antibacterial therapy after completion of treatment, improvement or no progression of baseline radiographic findings) at the test-of-cure visit 7–14 days after completion of treatment; 28-day all-cause mortality was a prespecified secondary end point. In both studies, clinical response rates in telavancin-treated patients were similar to those reported in vancomycin-treated patients. In clinically evaluable patients (CE population), clinical response was achieved in 83.7 or 81.3% of those who received telavancin and in 80 or 81% of those who received vancomycin. In a subset of patients who were microbiologically evaluable and stratified according to the infecting pathogen, the clinical cure rate in those with infections caused by methicillin-susceptible *S. aureus* or MRSA was 78% in those treated with telavancin and 75% in those treated with vancomycin. The overall 28-day all-cause mortality in patients with at least one baseline gram-positive respiratory pathogen was 29 or 24% in telavancin-treated patients and 24 or 22% in vancomycin-treated patients. All-cause mortality in patients treated with telavancin was higher in those with baseline creatinine clearances of 50 mL/minute or lower (41 or 44%) compared with those with baseline creatinine clearances exceeding 50 mL/minute (22 or 18%).

● Skin and Skin Structure Infections

Telavancin hydrochloride is used for the treatment of complicated skin and skin structure infections caused by susceptible *S. aureus* (including MRSA), *Streptococcus pyogenes* (group A β-hemolytic streptococci, GAS), *S. agalactiae* (group B streptococci, GBS), *S. anginosus* group (includes *S. anginosus*, *S. intermedius*, and *S. constellatus*), or *Enterococcus faecalis* (vancomycin-susceptible strains only). If documented or presumed pathogens also include gram-negative or anaerobic bacteria, concomitant use of an anti-infective active against such bacteria may be clinically indicated.

For information on diagnosis and management of skin and skin structure infections, the current clinical practice guidelines from the Infectious Diseases Society of America (IDSA) available at http://www.idsociety.org should be consulted.

Clinical Experience

Telavancin was evaluated in 2 randomized, multicenter, active-controlled phase 3 studies in adults with complicated skin and skin structure infections (e.g., major abscess, deep/extensive cellulitis, wound infection, infected ulcer, infected burn) with MRSA as the suspected or confirmed primary cause of infection (studies 0017 and 0018; ATLAS 1 and 2). Patients were randomized to receive 7–14 days of treatment with telavancin (10 mg/kg IV once every 24 hours) or vancomycin (1 g IV every 12 hours with dosage individualized and adjusted according to standard practices at the site). Other appropriate anti-infectives (e.g., aztreonam and/or metronidazole) were used concomitantly if documented or presumptive pathogens also included gram-negative or anaerobic bacteria. The primary end point was clinical cure rates 7–14 days after completion of treatment. Clinical cure rates reported with telavancin were similar to those reported with vancomycin. In clinically evaluable patients (CE population), clinical cure was achieved in 84.3 or 83.9% of those who received telavancin and 82.8 or 87.7% of those who received vancomycin. In a subset of patients who were microbiologically evaluable and stratified according to the infecting pathogen, the clinical cure rate in those with infections caused by methicillin-susceptible *S. aureus* or MRSA was 82 or 87%, respectively, in those treated with telavancin and 85.1 or 85.9%, respectively, in those treated with vancomycin. The clinical cure rate in those with infections caused by *S. pyogenes*, *S. agalactiae*, *S. anginosus* group, or *E. faecalis* was 84.2, 73.7, 76.5, or 95.6%, respectively, in those treated with telavancin and 90.5, 86.7, 100, or 80%, respectively, in those treated with vancomycin. There was evidence that the clinical cure rate with telavancin was lower in patients in the CE population who were 65 years of age or older (72%) compared with those younger than 65 years of age (87%). In addition, the clinical cure rate with telavancin was lower in those with baseline creatinine clearances of 50 mL/minute or lower compared with those with baseline creatinine clearances exceeding 50 mL/minute.

DOSAGE AND ADMINISTRATION

● Administration

Telavancin hydrochloride is administered by IV infusion.

Telavancin solutions should not be admixed or added to solutions containing other drugs.

If the same IV line is used for sequential infusion of other drugs, the IV line should be flushed with 0.9% sodium chloride injection, 5% dextrose injection, or lactated Ringer's injection before and after the telavancin infusion.

IV Infusion

Reconstitution and Dilution

Commercially available telavancin hydrochloride for injection must be reconstituted and then further diluted prior to IV infusion. Strict aseptic technique must be observed when preparing IV solutions of telavancin since the drug contains no preservative.

Single-dose vials labeled as containing 250 or 750 mg of telavancin should be reconstituted by adding 15 or 45 mL, respectively, of 5% dextrose injection, sterile water for injection, or 0.9% sodium chloride injection to provide a solution containing 15 mg/mL. To minimize foaming during reconstitution, the vial vacuum should be allowed to pull the diluent from the syringe into the vial; the diluent should not be forcefully injected into the vial. The vial should be discarded if the vacuum is insufficient to pull the diluent into the vial. The reconstituted solution should be mixed thoroughly without forcefully shaking the vial and inspected to ensure complete dissolution. Reconstitution usually takes less than 2 minutes, but may take up to 20 minutes.

For telavancin doses of 150–800 mg, the correct dose should be withdrawn from the reconstituted vial and added to 100–250 mL of appropriate IV infusion solution (i.e., 0.9% sodium chloride injection, 5% dextrose injection, lactated Ringer's injection).

For telavancin doses less than 150 mg or greater than 800 mg, the correct dose should be withdrawn from the reconstituted vial and added to a volume of appropriate IV infusion solution (i.e., 0.9% sodium chloride injection, 5% dextrose injection, or lactated Ringer's injection) that results in a final concentration of 0.6–8 mg/mL.

Reconstituted telavancin solutions (in the original vial) and reconstituted and diluted telavancin solutions (in an IV infusion bag) are stable for 12 hours at room temperature or 7 days when refrigerated at 2–8°C. The total storage time (vial plus IV infusion bag) should not exceed 12 hours at room temperature or 7 days at 2–8°C. Final telavancin IV infusion solutions also can be stored in the infusion bag for up to 32 days at –30 to –10°C.

IV infusion solutions of telavancin should not be shaken. Telavancin solutions should be inspected visually for particulate matter prior to administration.

Rate of Administration

Telavancin solutions should be administered by IV infusion over 1 hour.

Rapid IV infusions should be avoided. (See Infusion Reactions under Warnings/Precautions: Other Warnings/Precautions, in Cautions.)

● Dosage

Dosage of telavancin hydrochloride is expressed in terms of telavancin.

Respiratory Tract Infections

Nosocomial Pneumonia

The recommended dosage of telavancin for the treatment of hospital-acquired or ventilator-associated bacterial pneumonia in adults 18 years of age or older is 10 mg/kg given by IV infusion once every 24 hours for 7–21 days.

The duration of therapy should be guided by the severity of the infection and the patient's clinical response.

Skin and Skin Structure Infections

The recommended dosage of telavancin for the treatment of complicated skin and skin structure infections in adults 18 years of age or older is 10 mg/kg given by IV infusion once every 24 hours for 7–14 days.

The duration of therapy should be guided by the severity and location of the infection and the patient's clinical response.

● Special Populations

Renal Impairment

Because telavancin is eliminated principally by renal excretion, dosage of the drug should be reduced in adults with creatinine clearances of 10–50 mL/minute. (See Table 1.)

Data are insufficient to make dosage recommendations for adults with end-stage renal disease (creatinine clearance less than 10 mL/minute), including those undergoing hemodialysis.

Use of telavancin in patients with preexisting moderate or severe renal impairment (creatinine clearances of 50 mL/minute or lower) should be considered only when anticipated benefits outweigh potential risks. (See Increased Mortality in Patients with Renal Impairment under Warnings/Precautions: Warnings, in Cautions.)

TABLE 1. Telavancin Dosage for Adults with Renal Impairment

Creatinine Clearance (mL/minute) [a]	Telavancin Dosage
>50	10 mg/kg once every 24 hours
30–50	7.5 mg/kg once every 24 hours
10–<30	10 mg/kg once every 48 hours

[a] Calculate using Cockcroft-Gault formula and ideal body weight; use actual body weight if it is less than ideal body weight.

Hepatic Impairment

Dosage adjustments are not needed in adults with mild or moderate hepatic impairment. Pharmacokinetics of telavancin have not been studied in adults with severe hepatic impairment. (See Hepatic Impairment under Warnings/Precautions: Specific Populations, in Cautions.)

Geriatric Patients

Dosage adjustments based solely on age are not needed when telavancin is used in geriatric patients, but dosage should be adjusted based on renal function.

Because geriatric patients are more likely to have decreased renal function than younger adults, dosage should be selected with caution. (See Geriatric Use under Warnings/Precautions: Specific Populations, in Cautions.)

CAUTIONS

● Contraindications

Telavancin is contraindicated in patients with known hypersensitivity to the drug.

IV unfractionated heparin sodium is contraindicated in patients receiving telavancin. Activated partial thromboplastin time (aPTT) is expected to be artificially prolonged for up to 18 hours after telavancin administration. (See Tests Used to Monitor Coagulation under Cautions: Other Warnings/Precautions.)

● Warnings/Precautions

Warnings

Increased Mortality in Patients with Renal Impairment

Increased mortality was observed in patients with preexisting moderate or severe renal impairment (creatinine clearances of 50 mL/minute or lower) receiving telavancin for the treatment of hospital-acquired or ventilator-associated bacterial pneumonia compared with those receiving vancomycin. In an analysis of 2 phase 3 clinical studies evaluating telavancin for the treatment of hospital-acquired or ventilator-associated bacterial pneumonia, all-cause mortality within 28 days of starting treatment in patients with baseline moderate or severe renal impairment was 39% in those treated with telavancin compared with 30% in those treated with vancomycin. In patients with baseline creatinine clearances exceeding 50 mL/minute, all-cause mortality was 17% in those treated with telavancin and 18% in those treated with vancomycin.

Use of telavancin in patients with preexisting moderate or severe renal impairment (creatinine clearances of 50 mL/minute or lower) should be considered only when anticipated benefits outweigh potential risks.

Nephrotoxicity

New-onset or worsening renal impairment has been reported in patients receiving telavancin for the treatment of hospital-acquired or ventilator-associated bacterial pneumonia or complicated skin and skin structure infections. In patients with normal baseline serum creatinine concentrations in clinical studies, increased serum creatinine (1.5 times baseline) was reported more frequently in telavancin-treated patients than in vancomycin-treated patients.

Adverse renal effects are more likely to occur in patients with conditions known to increase the risk of renal impairment (e.g., preexisting renal disease, diabetes mellitus, congestive heart failure, hypertension) and in those receiving concomitant therapy with a drug that affects renal function (e.g., nonsteroidal anti-inflammatory agents [NSAIAs], certain diuretics, angiotensin-converting enzyme [ACE] inhibitors).

Renal function (i.e., serum creatinine, creatinine clearance) should be monitored in all patients receiving telavancin. Renal function tests should be performed prior to initiation of telavancin, every 48–72 hours during treatment (more frequently if indicated), and at the end of treatment.

If renal function decreases, the benefits of continuing telavancin treatment should be weighed against discontinuing the drug and initiating an alternative anti-infective.

Fetal/Neonatal Morbidity

Adverse developmental outcomes have been observed in 3 animal species given telavancin at clinically relevant doses during the period of organogenesis. Because these animal studies have raised concerns about potential adverse developmental outcomes in humans, telavancin should be avoided during pregnancy unless the potential benefits to the woman outweigh potential risks to the fetus. (See Pregnancy under Warnings/Precautions: Specific Populations, in Cautions.)

Women of childbearing potential (i.e., those who have not had complete absence of menses for at least 24 months, medically confirmed menopause or primary ovarian failure, history of hysterectomy, bilateral oophorectomy, or tubal ligation) should have a serum pregnancy test to exclude pregnancy before initiating telavancin. In addition, women of childbearing potential should use effective contraception to prevent pregnancy while receiving telavancin.

Sensitivity Reactions

Serious and potentially fatal hypersensitivity reactions, including anaphylactic reactions, have been reported after the first dose or subsequent doses of telavancin.

Telavancin should be discontinued at the first sign of rash or any other sign of hypersensitivity.

Telavancin is a semisynthetic derivative of vancomycin; however, it is not known if patients with hypersensitivity reactions to vancomycin will experience cross-reactivity to telavancin. Telavancin should be used with caution in patients with known hypersensitivity to vancomycin.

Although data are not available regarding cross-reactivity with other glycopeptides (e.g., dalbavancin, oritavancin), the possibility of cross-sensitivity among the glycopeptides should be considered.

Other Warnings/Precautions

Infusion Reactions

Rapid IV infusion of glycopeptide anti-infectives (including telavancin) can result in a reaction referred to as the "red-man syndrome". Flushing of the upper body, urticaria, pruritus, or rash may occur.

To reduce the risk of infusion-related reactions, IV infusions of telavancin should be given over 1 hour. If an infusion reaction occurs, such reactions may cease if the infusion is discontinued or the rate of infusion slowed.

Cardiovascular Effects

Prolongation of the corrected QT (QT_c) interval has been reported in individuals receiving telavancin.

Caution is advised if telavancin is used concomitantly with drugs known to prolong the QT interval.

Telavancin should be avoided in patients with congenital long QT syndrome, known prolongation of the QT_c interval, uncompensated heart failure, or severe left ventricular hypertrophy since such individuals were not included in telavancin clinical trials.

Hematologic Effects

Telavancin does not interfere with coagulation and has no effect on platelet aggregation. Increased risk of bleeding was not observed in clinical trials of the drug. Evidence of hypercoagulability has not been observed, and healthy adults receiving telavancin have normal levels of D-dimer and fibrin degradation products.

Reduced Efficacy in Patients with Moderate or Severe Renal Impairment

Results of a subgroup analysis of phase 3 clinical trials in patients with skin and skin structure infections indicated that the clinical cure rate in telavancin-treated patients with baseline moderate or severe renal impairment (creatinine clearances of 50 mL/minute or lower) was 67% and was lower than the clinical cure rate in those with baseline creatinine clearances exceeding 50 mL/minute (87%). Reductions in clinical cure rates of this magnitude were not observed in patients receiving the comparator anti-infective (vancomycin).

Clinicians should consider such data regarding reduced efficacy when selecting anti-infectives for treatment of complicated skin and skin structure infections in patients with baseline moderate or severe renal impairment (creatinine clearances of 50 mL/minute or lower).

Tests Used to Monitor Coagulation

Telavancin interferes with certain tests used to monitor coagulation, including prothrombin time (PT), international normalized ratio (INR), activated partial thromboplastin time (aPTT), activated clotting time, and tests based on factor X activity assay, if blood for these tests is drawn 0–18 hours after a telavancin dose. This occurs because telavancin binds to the artificial phospholipid surfaces added to the anticoagulation tests and interferes with the ability of the coagulation complexes to assemble on the surface of the phospholipids and promote in vitro clotting. The manufacturer recommends that blood specimens for such tests be drawn just before a dose of telavancin.

Telavancin does not affect the results of other coagulation tests, including thrombin time, whole blood (Lee-White) clotting time, platelet aggregation study, chromogenic anti-factor Xa assay, functional (chromogenic) factor X activity assay, bleeding time, and tests for D-dimer and fibrin degradation products. Blood specimens for these coagulation tests may be collected at any time in patients receiving telavancin.

In patients requiring aPTT monitoring while receiving telavancin, a non-phospholipid-dependent coagulation test (e.g., factor Xa chromogenic assay) should be used or an alternative anticoagulant not requiring aPTT monitoring may be considered.

Tests Used to Monitor Urine Protein

Telavancin interferes with urine qualitative dipstick protein assays and quantitative dye methods (e.g., pyrogallol red-molybdate) used to measure urine protein. Microalbumin assays are not affected by telavancin and can be used to monitor urinary protein excretion in patients receiving telavancin.

Superinfection/Clostridium difficile-associated Diarrhea and Colitis (CDAD)

Use of telavancin may result in overgrowth of nonsusceptible organisms, including fungi. The patient should be carefully monitored and appropriate therapy should be instituted if a superinfection occurs.

Treatment with anti-infectives alters normal colon flora and may permit overgrowth of Clostridium difficile. C. difficile infection (CDI) and C. difficile-associated diarrhea and colitis (CDAD; also known as antibiotic-associated diarrhea and colitis or pseudomembranous colitis) have been reported with nearly all anti-infectives and may range in severity from mild diarrhea to fatal colitis. C. difficile produces toxins A and B which contribute to development of CDAD; hypertoxin-producing strains of C. difficile are associated with increased morbidity and mortality since these infections may be refractory to anti-infective therapy and may require colectomy.

CDAD should be considered in the differential diagnosis of patients who develop diarrhea during or after anti-infective therapy. Careful medical history is necessary since CDAD has been reported to occur as late as 2 months or longer after anti-infective therapy is discontinued.

If CDAD is suspected or confirmed, anti-infective therapy not directed against C. difficile should be discontinued whenever possible. Patients should be managed with appropriate supportive therapy (fluid and electrolyte management, protein supplementation), anti-infective therapy directed against C. difficile (e.g., metronidazole, vancomycin), and surgical evaluation as clinically indicated.

Selection and Use of Anti-infectives

To reduce development of drug-resistant bacteria and maintain effectiveness of telavancin and other antibacterials, the drug should be used only for treatment of infections proven or strongly suspected to be caused by susceptible bacteria.

When selecting or modifying anti-infective therapy, results of culture and in vitro susceptibility testing should be used. In the absence of such data, local epidemiology and susceptibility patterns should be considered when selecting anti-infectives for empiric therapy.

If documented or presumed pathogens include gram-negative or anaerobic bacteria, concomitant use of an anti-infective active against such bacteria may be clinically indicated. (See Uses.)

Specific Populations

Pregnancy

Category C. (See Users Guide.)

A pregnancy registry has been established to monitor maternal-fetal outcomes in pregnant women exposed to telavancin. Clinicians are encouraged to contact the registry at 855-633-8479 to report cases of prenatal exposure to telavancin; alternatively, pregnant women may enroll.

In reproduction studies in rats, rabbits, and minipigs that received telavancin during the period of organogenesis at doses that resulted in exposure levels approximately onefold to twofold the human exposure (area under the plasma concentration-time curve [AUC]) at the maximum recommended human dosage, there was evidence that telavancin has the potential to cause limb and skeletal malformations and reduced fetal weight. Malformations included brachymelia (rats, rabbits), syndactyly (rats, minipigs), adactyly (rabbits), and polydactyly (minipigs).

Although telavancin has not been evaluated in pregnant women, the animal data raise concerns about potential adverse developmental outcomes in humans. Telavancin should be avoided during pregnancy unless the potential benefits to the woman outweigh the potential risks to the fetus. (See Fetal/Neonatal Morbidity under Warnings/Precautions: Warnings, in Cautions.)

Lactation

Not known whether telavancin is distributed into milk in humans. Telavancin should be used with caution in nursing women.

Pediatric Use

Safety and efficacy of telavancin have not been evaluated in patients younger than 18 years of age.

Geriatric Use

In clinical studies evaluating telavancin for the treatment of complicated skin and skin structure infections, the drug appeared to be less effective in adults 65 years of age or older relative to adults younger than 65 years of age. Although there were no overall differences in frequency of treatment-emergent adverse events in geriatric adults compared with younger adults in these studies, the incidence of adverse events indicating renal impairment was higher in geriatric adults treated with telavancin than in younger adults treated with the drug.

In clinical studies evaluating telavancin for the treatment of hospital-acquired or ventilator-associated bacterial pneumonia, treatment-emergent adverse events as well as deaths and other serious adverse events occurred more often in patients 65 years of age or older than in those younger than 65 years of age in both the telavancin treatment group and comparator treatment group.

Telavancin is substantially eliminated by the kidneys, and the risk of adverse effects may be greater in patients with impaired renal function. Dosage should be selected with caution since geriatric patients are more likely to have decreased renal function. Dosage adjustments in geriatric patients should be based on renal function.

Hepatic Impairment

Telavancin pharmacokinetics are not altered in adults with moderate hepatic impairment (Child-Pugh class B); pharmacokinetics of the drug have not been evaluated in those with severe hepatic impairment (Child-Pugh class C). Dosage adjustment is not needed in adults with mild or moderate hepatic impairment.

Renal Impairment

In clinical studies evaluating telavancin for the treatment of hospital-acquired or ventilator-associated bacterial pneumonia, mortality rates in adults with creatinine clearances of 50 mL/minute or lower were higher in telavancin-treated patients compared with those receiving the comparator anti-infective (vancomycin). In clinical studies evaluating telavancin for the treatment of complicated skin and skin structure infections, the clinical cure rate with telavancin was lower in adults with creatinine clearances of 50 mL/minute or lower compared with those with creatinine clearances exceeding 50 mL/minute. Such data should be considered when selecting an anti-infective for adults with baseline moderate or severe renal impairment (creatinine clearances of 50 mL/minute or lower), and telavancin should be considered for such patients only when the anticipated benefits outweigh the potential risks.

Patients with preexisting renal impairment or risk factors for renal dysfunction may be at greater risk for adverse renal effects during telavancin therapy than individuals with normal renal function. (See Nephrotoxicity under Warnings/Precautions: Other Warnings/Precautions, in Cautions.)

Patients with creatinine clearances of 10–50 mL/minute should receive a reduced telavancin dosage. (See Dosage and Administration: Special Populations.)

Hydroxypropyl-β-cyclodextrin (an inactive ingredient in the formulation) may accumulate in individuals with renal impairment. If renal toxicity is suspected, an alternative anti-infective should be considered.

● Common Adverse Effects

Adverse effects reported in 5% or more of patients receiving telavancin for the treatment of hospital-acquired or ventilator-associated bacterial

pneumonia include GI effects (nausea, vomiting, diarrhea, constipation), anemia, hypokalemia, hypotension, decubitus ulcer, insomnia, peripheral edema, and renal effects (renal impairment or insufficiency, acute renal failure, chronic renal failure, increased serum creatinine).

Adverse effects reported in 7% or more of patients receiving telavancin for the treatment of complicated skin and skin structure infections include GI effects (taste disturbance, nausea, vomiting, diarrhea, constipation), headache, insomnia, and foamy urine.

DRUG INTERACTIONS

● Drugs Affecting or Metabolized by Hepatic Microsomal Enzymes

In vitro studies indicate that telavancin inhibits the cytochrome P-450 (CYP) isoenzyme 3A4/5.

● Anti-infective Agents

In vitro, the antibacterial effects of telavancin and cefepime, ceftriaxone, ciprofloxacin, gentamicin, meropenem, or rifampin are synergistic against methicillin-resistant *Staphylococcus aureus* (MRSA; also known as oxacillin-resistant *S. aureus* or ORSA).

In vitro studies indicate that the antibacterial effects of telavancin and amikacin, aztreonam, cefepime, ceftriaxone, ciprofloxacin, co-trimoxazole, gentamicin, imipenem, meropenem, oxacillin, fixed combination of piperacillin sodium and tazobactam sodium (piperacillin and tazobactam), or rifampin are not antagonistic against telavancin-susceptible staphylococci, streptococci, or enterococci.

Aztreonam

Concomitant use of aztreonam and telavancin does not affect the pharmacokinetics of either drug.

Dosage adjustments are not needed if aztreonam and telavancin are used concomitantly.

Piperacillin and Tazobactam

Concomitant use of piperacillin and tazobactam and telavancin does not affect the pharmacokinetics of either drug.

Dosage adjustments are not needed if piperacillin and tazobactam is used concomitantly with telavancin.

● Heparin

Because activated partial thromboplastin time (aPTT) is expected to be artificially prolonged for up to 18 hours after telavancin administration, IV unfractionated heparin sodium is contraindicated in patients receiving telavancin. (See Tests Used to Monitor Coagulation under Warnings/Precautions: Other Warnings/Precautions, in Cautions.)

● Midazolam

Concomitant use of midazolam and telavancin does not affect the pharmacokinetics of either drug.

DESCRIPTION

Telavancin is a lipoglycopeptide antibacterial and is a semisynthetic derivative of vancomycin.

In vitro, telavancin is bactericidal in action against susceptible gram-positive bacteria. Telavancin inhibits bacterial cell wall synthesis by inhibiting peptidoglycan synthesis and blocking the transglycosylation step. Telavancin binds to the bacterial membrane and disrupts membrane barrier function.

Telavancin is active in vitro and in clinical infections against *Staphylococcus aureus* (including methicillin-resistant *S. aureus* [MRSA; also known as oxacillin-resistant *S. aureus* or ORSA]), *Streptococcus pyogenes* (group A β-hemolytic streptococci, GAS), *S. agalactiae* (group B streptococci, GBS), *S. anginosus* group (includes *S. anginosus*, *S. intermedius*, and *S. constellatus*), and *Enterococcus faecalis* (vancomycin-susceptible strains only).

Telavancin also is active in vitro against *E. faecium* (vancomycin-susceptible strains only), *S. haemolyticus*, *S. dysgalactiae* subsp. *equisimilis*, and *S. epidermidis*;

however, safety and efficacy of the drug in treating clinical infections caused by these bacteria have not been established.

Some vancomycin-resistant enterococci have reduced susceptibility to telavancin. Cross-resistance between telavancin and other anti-infectives has not been reported to date.

ADVICE TO PATIENTS

Telavancin medication guide must be provided to the patient each time the drug is dispensed; importance of patient reading the medication guide prior to initiating telavancin therapy and each time the prescription is refilled.

Advise patients that antibacterials (including telavancin) should only be used to treat bacterial infections and not used to treat viral infections (e.g., the common cold).

Importance of completing full course of therapy, even if feeling better after a few days.

Advise patients that skipping doses or not completing the full course of therapy may decrease effectiveness and increase the likelihood that bacteria will develop resistance and will not be treatable with telavancin or other antibacterials in the future.

Advise patients that diarrhea is a common problem caused by anti-infectives and usually ends when the drug is discontinued. Importance of contacting a clinician if watery and bloody stools (with or without stomach cramps and fever) occur during or as late as 2 months or longer after the last dose.

Advise patients about the common adverse effects reported with telavancin (e.g., taste disturbance, nausea, vomiting, headache, foamy urine) and importance of informing a clinician if they develop any unusual symptom or if any known symptom persists or worsens.

Importance of informing clinicians of existing or contemplated concomitant therapy, including prescription and OTC drugs, and any concomitant illnesses.

Importance of women informing clinicians if they are or plan to become pregnant or plan to breast-feed. Advise women of childbearing potential about potential risk of fetal harm if telavancin is used during pregnancy. (See Pregnancy under Warnings/Precautions: Specific Populations, in Cautions.)

Importance of excluding pregnancy with a serum pregnancy test before starting telavancin. Advise women of childbearing potential to use effective contraception to prevent pregnancy during telavancin therapy and to notify a clinician if pregnancy occurs during telavancin therapy. (See Pregnancy under Warnings/Precautions: Specific Populations, in Cautions.)

Importance of informing patients of other important precautionary information. (See Cautions.)

PREPARATIONS

Excipients in commercially available drug preparations may have clinically important effects in some individuals; consult specific product labeling for details.

Telavancin Hydrochloride

Parenteral

For injection, for IV infusion	250 mg (of telavancin)	**Vibativ®**, Theravance
	750 mg (of telavancin)	**Vibativ®**, Theravance

September 25, 2017, © Copyright, September 1, 2010, American Society of Health-System Pharmacists, Inc.

Vancomycin Hydrochloride

8:12.28.16 • GLYCOPEPTIDES

■ Vancomycin is a tricyclic glycopeptide antibiotic.

USES

● Gram-Positive Bacterial Infections

Vancomycin is used orally for the treatment of diarrhea caused by *Clostridioides difficile* (formerly known as *Clostridium difficile*) infection (CDI; *C. difficile*-associated diarrhea [CDAD]). Oral vancomycin is also used for the treatment of enterocolitis caused by *Staphylococcus aureus (S. aureus)*, including methicillin-resistant *S. aureus* (MRSA), The parenteral form of vancomycin hydrochloride may be administered orally for the treatment of antibiotic-associated pseudomembranous colitis produced by *C. difficile* and for staphylococcal enterocolitis. Orally administered vancomycin is *not* effective for the treatment of other types of infections.

IV vancomycin is used for the treatment of infections caused by susceptible bacteria when other anti-infectives cannot be used or would be ineffective. IV vancomycin is used principally in the treatment of severe infections caused by gram-positive bacteria in patients who cannot receive or who have failed to respond to penicillins or cephalosporins or for the treatment of gram-positive bacterial infections that are resistant to β-lactams and other anti-infectives.

The effectiveness of IV vancomycin has been documented in infections due to staphylococci, including staphylococcal endocarditis, septicemia, bone infections, lower respiratory tract infections, skin and skin structure infections. When staphylococcal infections are localized and purulent, antibiotics are used as adjuncts to appropriate surgical measures. IV vancomycin is used for initial therapy when MRSA is suspected; after susceptibility data are available, therapy should be adjusted accordingly.

IV vancomycin also is used alone or in conjunction with an aminoglycoside for the treatment of endocarditis caused by enterococci (e.g., *Enterococcus faecalis*), viridans streptococci, or *Staphylococcus bovis* (also known as *S. gallolyticus*).

See individual sections below in Uses for additional details on the use of vancomycin for specific gram-positive infections.

● C. difficile-associated Diarrhea

Vancomycin is used *orally* for the treatment of diarrhea caused by *Clostridioides difficile* (formerly known as *Clostridium difficile*) infection in adults and pediatric patients.

Efficacy and safety of oral vancomycin (125 mg 4 times daily for 10 days) for the treatment of *C. difficile*-associated diarrhea (CDAD) were evaluated in 2 clinical trials. The studies included a total of 266 adults with *C. difficile*-associated diarrhea, defined as ≥3 loose or watery bowel movements within 24 hours prior to study enrollment, and the presence of either *C. difficile* toxin A or B, or pseudomembranes on endoscopy within 72 hours preceding enrollment. Patients with fulminant CDAD, sepsis with hypotension, ileus, peritoneal signs, or severe hepatic disease were excluded. The median age of patients was 67 years, 93% were white, and 52% were male. CDAD was classified as severe (defined as ≥10 unformed bowel movements per day or white blood cell counts ≥15,000/mm^3) in 25% of patients; 47% of patients were previously treated for CDAD. The rate of clinical success with vancomycin (defined as resolution of diarrhea and absence of severe abdominal discomfort due to CDAD) on day 10 was 81% in both trials. The median time to resolution of diarrhea was 5 days in one trial and 4 days in the other trial.

Results of 2 randomized controlled studies that compared oral vancomycin to fidaxomicin for the treatment of CDAD found that resolution of diarrhea was similar between the 2 agents; however, fidaxomicin was superior to vancomycin for sustained clinical response (defined as resolution of diarrhea at the end of treatment without recurrence 25 days after treatment).

Clinical Perspective

C. difficile can cause asymptomatic colonization in the intestinal tract or symptomatic intestinal *C. difficile* infection (CDI) that can range in severity from mild to moderate diarrhea to more severe complications. *C. difficile* is the most commonly recognized cause of infectious diarrhea in healthcare settings. Risk factors include advanced age, duration of hospitalization, immunosuppression as the result of disease or drug therapy, exposure to antibiotic agents, cancer chemotherapy, and GI surgery or manipulation of the GI tract. The most important modifiable risk factor for development of CDI is exposure to antibiotic agents. Antibiotics can alter the normal intestinal flora, providing an environment for overgrowth of *C. difficile*. CDI has been reported with nearly all systemic antibiotic agents and should be considered in the differential diagnosis in patients who develop diarrhea during or after anti-infective therapy. The risk of CDI from disruption of intestinal flora is increased during antibiotic therapy and for 3 months after such therapy is discontinued. Discontinuance of the inciting antibiotic is recommended as soon as possible to prevent recurrence of CDI.

The Infectious Diseases Society of America (IDSA) and Society for Healthcare Epidemiology of America (SHEA) have published guidelines on the management of CDI. The guidelines state that either oral vancomycin (125 mg 4 times daily for 10 days) or fidaxomicin (200 mg twice daily for 10 days) may be used for the initial treatment of CDI. When both agents are available, fidaxomicin may be preferred because of its favorable efficacy and safety profile; however, this recommendation is based on a moderate certainty of evidence and vancomycin remains an acceptable alternative. When vancomycin and fidaxomicin are not available, metronidazole (500 mg 3 times daily orally for 10–14 days) may be used for treatment of an initial CDI episode.

For treatment of the first recurrent CDI episode, IDSA/SHEA states that fidaxomicin (standard or extended-pulsed regimen) is preferred; however, oral vancomycin (in a tapered and pulsed regimen or standard 10-day course) is an acceptable alternative. For patients with multiple recurrences, oral vancomycin (in a tapered and pulsed regimen), oral vancomycin followed by rifaximin, and fecal microbiota transplantation are options in addition to fidaxomicin.

Vancomycin is the treatment of choice for fulminant CDI (characterized by hypotension or shock, ileus, or megacolon) in adults; a regimen that includes vancomycin (given orally, by nasogastric tube, and/or rectally as clinically indicated) in conjunction with IV metronidazole is recommended for the treatment of such infections, especially if ileus is present.

● Enterocolitis Caused by S. aureus

Vancomycin is used *orally* for the treatment of enterocolitis caused by *S. aureus* (including MRSA) in adults and pediatric patients.

Clinical Perspective

Enterocolitis caused by *S. aureus* is rare, but several cases have been described in the literature. Patients often present with high fever, abdominal distension, and watery and/or bloody diarrhea that may lead to dehydration, shock, or multi-organ failure. In the reported cases, patient characteristics often included recent gastric surgery, underlying disease of the colon, recent antibiotic use, advanced age, immunocompromised state, decreased gastric acid production, or colonization with MRSA. Usually, patients were successfully treated with oral vancomycin, but in some cases required other antibiotic therapy or surgical intervention.

● Endocarditis

IV vancomycin is used for the treatment of endocarditis caused by staphylococci (e.g., *S. aureus* or *S. epidermidis*, including methicillin-resistant strains [MRSA]), streptococci (e.g., viridans streptococci, *S. bovis* [currently known as *S. gallolyticus*]), or enterococci (e.g., *E. faecalis*). Vancomycin also has been reported to be effective for the treatment of diphtheroid endocarditis.

Clinical Experience

The American Heart Association (AHA) has published guidelines on the management of infective endocarditis in adults. A separate guideline is available for the treatment of infective endocarditis in children. Initial therapy of infective endocarditis is generally empiric; selection of an appropriate empiric antibiotic regimen is based on patient characteristics, prior antimicrobial exposures, microbiological findings, and other factors that help predict the presumed causative microorganism (e.g., injection drug use, indwelling cardiovascular medical devices, genitourinary disorders, chronic skin disorders, prosthetic valve replacement). Consultation with an infectious diseases specialist is recommended to define an appropriate empiric regimen. Once cultures are available and a pathogen is defined, the antimicrobial regimen should be adjusted accordingly. *S. aureus* is the most common cause of infective endocarditis in much of the developed world. Infective endocarditis also may be caused by coagulase negative staphylococci (e.g., *S. epidermidis*). It is important to consider both pathogen groups in a patient with suspected staphylococci infection.

Vancomycin is generally recommended for the treatment of endocarditis caused by MRSA. While a regimen of vancomycin administered alone is recommended for MRSA endocarditis in patients with native cardiac valves, adults with a prosthetic valve should receive a combination regimen (e.g., IV vancomycin, oral or IV rifampin, and IV or IM gentamicin) because of the high mortality rate associated with *S. aureus*-associated prosthetic-valve endocarditis. Those with native-valve endocarditis caused by methicillin-susceptible staphylococci generally should receive a regimen containing a β-lactam antibiotic (e.g., IV nafcillin, IV oxacillin, or IV cefazolin for penicillin-allergic patients); additional agents (e.g., oral or IV rifampin and IV or IM gentamicin) should be considered in patients with a prosthetic valve.

Vancomycin has been effective alone or in combination with an aminoglycoside for the treatment of endocarditis caused by *S. viridans* or *S. bovis (currently known as S. gallolyticus)*. While a regimen of IV penicillin G (with or without IM or IV gentamicin) or IV or IM ceftriaxone (with or without IM or IV gentamicin) usually is recommended for the treatment of endocarditis caused by viridans streptococci or *S. bovis* (*S. gallolyticus)*, IV vancomycin is a reasonable alternative for adults who cannot tolerate penicillin or ceftriaxone therapy.

For endocarditis caused by enterococci (e.g., *E. faecalis*), vancomycin has been reported to be effective only in combination with an aminoglycoside. For the treatment of enterococcal endocarditis, AHA guidelines state that a regimen of either IV penicillin G or IV ampicillin with IM or IV gentamicin is preferred for most adults; a regimen of IV vancomycin *and* IM or IV gentamicin is recommended for the treatment of enterococcal endocarditis only when the patient is unable to tolerate penicillin or ampicillin or in cases of endocarditis caused by *E. faecalis* resistant to penicillin.

For information on management of endocarditis in pediatric patients, consult the most recent guidelines from AHA.

● *Respiratory Tract Infections*

Community-acquired Pneumonia

IV vancomycin has been used in the treatment of lower respiratory tract infections due to staphylococci.

The American Thoracic Society (ATS) and Infectious Diseases Society of America (IDSA) have published guidelines on the management of adults with community-acquired pneumonia (CAP). Although not considered a drug of choice for empiric treatment of CAP, there are some instances when IV vancomycin is included in anti-infective regimens for CAP treatment.

The guidelines recommend empiric coverage for MRSA (e.g., vancomycin or linezolid) in hospitalized adults with CAP *only* if locally validated risk factors for MRSA are present (e.g., prior isolation of MRSA from the respiratory tract). Appropriate blood cultures, sputum cultures, and/or nasal polymerase chain reaction (PCR) should be obtained to allow de-escalation or confirmation of the need for continued MRSA coverage.

Nosocomial Pneumonia

IV vancomycin also has been used for empiric coverage against MRSA in patients with nosocomial pneumonia.

For empiric treatment of ventilator-associated pneumonia or hospital-acquired pneumonia (*non*-ventilator-associated), ATS and IDSA recommend use of anti-infectives that have a broad spectrum of activity against gram-positive (e.g., *S. aureus*) and gram-negative (e.g., *Pseudomonas aeruginosa*) bacteria. For the treatment of ventilator-associated pneumonia, an antibiotic active against MRSA (e.g., vancomycin, linezolid) should be included in the initial empiric regimen in patients with certain risk factors (i.e., risk of antimicrobial resistance, treatment in units where 10–20% of *S. aureus* isolates are methicillin-resistant, treatment in units where the prevalence of MRSA is not known). For the treatment of hospital-acquired pneumonia, an anti-infective active against MRSA should be included in the initial empiric regimen in patients with certain risk factors for MRSA infection (i.e., IV antibiotic use in the previous 90 days,

hospitalization in units where over 20% of *S. aureus* isolates are methicillin-resistant, hospitalization in units where the prevalence of MRSA is not known, high risk of mortality).

● *Skin and Skin Structure Infections*

IV vancomycin is used in the treatment of various skin and skin structure infections due to staphylococci.

The Infectious Diseases Society of America (IDSA) has published guidelines on the management of skin and skin structure infections. Such infections include purulent skin and soft tissue infections (e.g., cutaneous abscesses, furuncles, carbuncles, inflamed epidermoid cysts); an antibiotic that is active against MRSA is recommended in patients with these infections who have failed initial antibiotic treatment, have markedly impaired host defenses, or have systemic inflammatory response syndrome (SIRS) and hypotension.

For patients with cellulitis associated with penetrating trauma, evidence of MRSA infection in another location, nasal colonization with MRSA, injection drug use, purulent drainage, or SIRS, vancomycin or another antibiotic effective against both MRSA and streptococci is recommended.

Vancomycin is recommended for MRSA coverage in surgical site infections where risk factors for MRSA are high (e.g., nasal colonization with MRSA, prior MRSA infection, recent hospitalization, recent antibiotic use, high local prevalence of MRSA).

Vancomycin also is recommended for broad-spectrum coverage in the treatment of necrotizing fasciitis.

IDSA recommends use of vancomycin for initial empiric treatment of pyomyositis. For immunocompromised patients or in those with open trauma to the muscles, empiric treatment should also include an antibiotic active against gram-negative bacilli.

Broad spectrum coverage with vancomycin plus either ampicillin/sulbactam, piperacillin/tazobactam, or a carbapenem is recommended in the treatment of clostridial gas gangrene or myonecrosis in the absence of definitive etiologic diagnosis.

● *Antimicrobial Prophylaxis in Surgery*

IV vancomycin (usually administered as a single preoperative dose) has been used for the prevention of surgical site infections. However, *routine* use of vancomycin for antimicrobial surgical prophylaxis is *not* recommended since such use may promote emergence of vancomycin-resistant enterococci or staphylococci.

The American Society of Health-System Pharmacists (ASHP), Infectious Diseases Society of America (IDSA), Surgical Infection Society (SIS), and Society for Healthcare Epidemiology of America (SHEA) have published a joint guideline on antimicrobial prophylaxis in surgery. The guideline states that routine use of vancomycin is not recommended for any procedure; however, vancomycin may be included in the regimen of choice when a cluster of MRSA cases (e.g., mediastinitis after cardiac procedures) or methicillin-resistant coagulase negative staphylococci surgical site infections has been observed at a particular institution or in patients with known MRSA colonization or at high risk for MRSA colonization in the absence of surveillance data (e.g., recent hospitalization, nursing-home residents, patients receiving hemodialysis). Each institution is encouraged to develop guidelines for the proper use of vancomycin.

● *Meningitis and Other CNS Infections*

Vancomycin has been used for the empiric treatment of healthcare-associated ventriculitis and meningitis† in conjunction with an anti-pseudomonal β-lactam (e.g., cefepime, ceftazidime, meropenem).

For the treatment of healthcare-associated ventriculitis and meningitis caused by MRSA, IDSA states that IV vancomycin is considered the drug of choice. However, if the vancomycin MIC is ≥1 mcg/mL, an alternative anti-infective agent (e.g., linezolid, daptomycin, trimethoprim/sulfamethoxazole) should be considered.

● Corynebacterium *Infections*

Vancomycin has been used for the treatment of infections caused by *Corynebacterium*†, including pulmonary infections, central venous catheter-related infections, osteomyelitis, endophthalmitis, and orthopedic infections. There also are case reports of intravitreal injection† of vancomycin to treat ocular infections caused by *Corynebacterium*; however, safety and efficacy of this method of administration have not been established.

● *Prevention of Perinatal Group B Streptococcal Disease*

IV vancomycin has been used for prevention of perinatal group B streptococcal (GBS) disease† in certain women with a high-risk penicillin allergy and whose GBS isolate is not susceptible to clindamycin. Pregnant women who are colonized with GBS in the genital or rectal areas can transmit GBS infection to their infants during labor and delivery resulting in invasive neonatal infection that can be associated with substantial morbidity and mortality. Intrapartum anti-infective prophylaxis for prevention of early-onset neonatal GBS disease is administered *selectively* to women at high risk for transmitting GBS infection to their neonates.

● *Febrile Neutropenia*

Although IV vancomycin is generally *not* recommended as a standard part of the initial antibiotic regimen for empiric anti-infective therapy in patients with febrile neutropenia†, consideration may be given to adding vancomycin to recommended empiric anti-infective therapy for other specific clinical conditions (e.g., suspected catheter-related infection, skin or soft-tissue infection, pneumonia, hemodynamic instability).

DOSAGE AND ADMINISTRATION

● *General*

Patient Monitoring

● Monitor renal function, especially in patients with underlying renal impairment, patients with risk factors for renal impairment, and patients receiving concomitant therapy with nephrotoxic drugs. Nephrotoxicity has been reported following both oral and IV administration of vancomycin and can occur during or after completion of therapy.

● Therapeutic drug monitoring of vancomycin is recommended in certain patients and situations (e.g., serious methicillin-resistant *S. aureus* [MRSA] infections, pediatric patients).

● Monitor patient's blood pressure during IV infusion of vancomycin.

● *Administration*

Vancomycin hydrochloride is administered by IV infusion for the treatment of systemic infections.

Vancomycin hydrochloride is administered orally as capsules or solution for the treatment of *Clostridioides difficile (formerly known as Clostridium difficile)*-associated diarrhea or enterocolitis caused by *Staphylococcus aureus* (including MRSA). If necessary, the parenteral form of vancomycin hydrochloride may be diluted and administered orally by mouth or nasogastric tube for these indications. Orally administered vancomycin is *not* effective for and should *not* be used for the treatment of systemic infections.

Vancomycin has been administered rectally† in the treatment of fulminant CDI in adults.

Safety and efficacy of intrathecal (intralumbar or intraventricular), intracameral, intravitreal, or intraperitoneal administration of vancomycin have not been established.

Oral Administration

Commercially available vancomycin hydrochloride capsules, powder for oral solution, or the powder for IV administration can be used for oral administration.

Preparation of Oral Solution Using Commercially Available Powder for Oral Solution

Each bottle of commercially available vancomycin hydrochloride powder for oral solution must be reconstituted by a healthcare professional. The manufacturer-supplied premeasured diluent should be used to reconstitute the powder. Prior to reconstitution, tap the bottle on a hard surface to loosen the powder. Shake the bottle of diluent and then add approximately half of the diluent to the powder. Shake the mixture for approximately 45 seconds. Then, add the remaining diluent

and shake the bottle for approximately 30 seconds. The final concentration of the solution is 25 or 50 mg/mL.

Preparation of Oral Solution Using Parenteral Form of Vancomycin

When necessary, a solution for oral administration can be prepared by diluting the appropriate dose of the parental form of vancomycin hydrochloride lyophilized powder in 30 mL of water. Common flavoring syrups may be added to the solution to improve the taste. The 500-mg single-use vial should be used to prepare these oral solutions; ADD-Vantage® vials should *not* be used to prepare such oral solutions, and premixed solutions of vancomycin hydrochloride injection should *not* be administered orally.

IV Administration

Vancomycin hydrochloride usually is administered by intermittent IV infusion, but has been administered by continuous IV infusion. Various commercial IV preparations of the drug are available.

Commercially available lyophilized powder in single-dose vials must be reconstituted and further diluted prior to administration. Each 250 mg of vancomycin hydrochloride powder for injection should be reconstituted with 5 mL of sterile water for injection to provide a solution containing 50 mg/mL. The reconstituted solution must be further diluted in at least 100 mL of a compatible diluent to a achieve a final vancomycin concentration of 5 mg/mL.

Alternatively, ADD-Vantage® vials labeled as containing 500 mg, 750 mg, or 1 g of vancomycin may be reconstituted according to the manufacturer's directions using 5% dextrose injection or 0.9% sodium chloride injection. ADD-Vantage® vials of the drug should be used only when actual doses of 500 mg, 750 mg, or 1 g are appropriate and should *not* be used in neonates, infants, or young children who require doses less than 500 mg.

Vancomycin hydrochloride is also available as a pharmacy bulk package; reconstitution of the lyophilized powder contained in the bag and further dilution are required prior to administration. Consult the manufacturer's prescribing information for detailed instructions on preparation of this dosage form.

Vancomycin hydrochloride is also commercially available as a frozen premixed solution containing 500 mg/100 mL, 750 mg/150 mL, or 1 g/200 mL in 5% dextrose injection or 0.9% sodium chloride injection in single-dose Galaxy plastic containers. The premixed solution should be thawed at room temperature (25°C) or under refrigeration (5°C) and should *not* be thawed by immersion in a water bath or by exposure to microwave radiation. A precipitate may form in the frozen state; however, this will usually dissolve with little or no agitation upon reaching room temperature, and the potency of the drug is not affected. The thawed injection should not be used in series connections with other plastic containers, since such use could result in air embolism from residual air being drawn from the primary container before administration of fluid from the secondary container is complete.

Vancomycin injection is also commercially available in premixed single-dose flexible bags containing 500 mg, 750 mg, 1 g, 1.25 g, 1.5 g, 1.75 g, and 2 g vancomycin in 100 mL, 150 mL, 200 mL, 250 mL, 300 mL, 350 mL, and 400 mL, respectively, of liquid (consisting of water and PEG together with the excipients NADA and lysine). This formulation of vancomycin should only be used in patients who require the entire dose of the drug contained in the bags and not any fraction thereof.

Rate of Administration

Vancomycin should be administered as intermittent IV infusions. IV infusion should be given over a period of at least 1 hour to reduce the risk of infusion reactions.

Avoid rapid IV infusion (e.g., over several minutes) which can cause exaggerated hypotension, including shock and rarely cardiac arrest. To minimize adverse effects, IV vancomycin should be administered at a rate not exceeding 10 mg/minute.

Therapeutic Drug Monitoring

To achieve optimal serum vancomycin concentrations while minimizing toxicity in the treatment of serious infections, therapeutic drug monitoring of IV vancomycin is recommended in certain clinical situations. A consensus guideline on therapeutic monitoring of vancomycin for serious MRSA infections (e.g., bacteremia, sepsis, infective endocarditis, pneumonia, osteomyelitis, meningitis) has been published by the American Society of Health-System Pharmacists (ASHP), the Infectious Diseases Society of America (IDSA), the Pediatric Infectious Diseases Society (PIDS), and the Society of Infectious Diseases Pharmacists (SIDP).

The primary predictive pharmacokinetic/pharmacodynamic parameter for vancomycin efficacy is the AUC/minimum inhibitory concentration (MIC) ratio. Based on in vitro, animal, and human data, an AUC/MIC ratio ≥400 mg×h/L (MIC determined by broth dilution [BMD]) has been established as the current accepted critical target for optimum vancomycin activity. Because of difficulty in estimating AUC in clinical practice, previous guidelines recommended monitoring trough concentrations as a surrogate marker for the AUC/MIC ratio. In this method of monitoring, an initial trough vancomycin level is evaluated after steady state has been reached (i.e., after approximately 4 doses). Then, the vancomycin dosage may be adjusted, if needed, to achieve the desired therapeutic trough concentration by calculating an optimized dose based on patient specific parameters (e.g., creatinine clearance, body weight). The risk of acute kidney injury with vancomycin increases as a function of the trough concentration, especially when the concentration exceeds 15–20 mg/L. Therefore, therapeutic monitoring has traditionally focused on maintaining trough concentrations between 15 and 20 mg/L for serious infections due to MRSA.

The utility of trough vancomycin concentration monitoring is limited, and therefore this method may be insufficient to guide vancomycin dosing in all patients. Trough concentrations of 15–20 mg/L do not guarantee optimal exposures in patients with infections due to MRSA with a vancomycin MIC >1 mg/L and, conversely, trough concentrations of 15–20 mg/L may lead to AUCs associated with an increased risk of nephrotoxicity. Additionally, in some instances when trough vancomycin concentrations are considered to be subtherapeutic (i.e., <10 mg/L), the AUC may be in the therapeutic range. Therefore, trough-only monitoring, with a target of 15–20 mg/L, is no longer recommended based on efficacy and nephrotoxicity data in patients with serious infections due to MRSA. Current guidelines recommend AUC-guided therapeutic monitoring of vancomycin in both adults and pediatric patients with serious MRSA infections. There is insufficient evidence to provide recommendations on vancomycin therapeutic drug monitoring for patients with MSSA, noninvasive MRSA, or other infections.

AUC-based monitoring targets a vancomycin AUC/MIC ratio of ≥400 mg×h/L while limiting high exposures associated with nephrotoxicity (i.e., vancomycin AUC/MIC ratio ≥ 600 mg×h/L). Two AUC-based therapeutic monitoring methods have been described. The first is the Bayesian method in which population pharmacokinetic modeling is done by software programs to optimize the dosage of vancomycin based on the collection of a single vancomycin serum concentration. The second method utilizes first-order pharmacokinetic equations based on the collection of 2 timed steady-state serum vancomycin concentrations to estimate the AUC. Although AUC-based therapeutic drug monitoring methods present logistical and clinical challenges, they may be emerging as preferred dosing strategies because of their potential to increase the proportion of patients who obtain vancomycin AUC/MIC ratios within therapeutic range, decreasing unnecessary high exposures to vancomycin and preventing associated toxicities.

The current consensus guideline issued by ASHP, IDSA, PIDS, and SIDP recommends vancomycin monitoring to achieve sustained targeted AUC values for patients with serious MRSA infections. Vancomycin monitoring is also recommended for all patients at high risk for nephrotoxicity, patients with unstable renal function, and those receiving prolonged courses of therapy (more than 3 to 5 days) regardless of whether they have a MRSA infection. Given the narrow vancomycin AUC range for therapeutic effect and minimal risk of acute kidney injury, the most accurate and optimal way to manage vancomycin dosing should be through AUC-guided dosing and monitoring. The guideline states that in patients with suspected or definitive serious MRSA infections, an individualized target AUC/MIC$_{BMD}$ ratio of 400–600 mg×h/L (assuming a vancomycin MIC$_{BMD}$ of 1 mg/L) should be advocated to achieve clinical efficacy while improving patient safety. When transitioning to AUC/MIC monitoring, clinicians should conservatively target AUC values for patients with suspected or documented serious infections due to MRSA assuming a vancomycin MIC$_{BMD}$ ≤1 mg/L at most institutions. Given the importance of early appropriate therapy in patients with suspected or documented serious infections due to MRSA, vancomycin targeted

exposure should be achieved early during the course of therapy, preferably within the first 24–8 hours. In such cases, use of the Bayesian method may be prudent since vancomycin concentrations can be collected more rapidly (within the first 24–48 hours rather than at steady state) to allow for early assessment of AUC target attainment.

For additional information, consult the guideline document at https://www.ashp.org/-/media/assets/policy-guidelines/docs/therapeutic-guidelines/therapeutic-guidelines-monitoring-vancomycin-ASHP-IDSA-PIDS.pdf.

● Dosage

Dosage of vancomycin hydrochloride is expressed in terms of vancomycin.

Oral Vancomycin

Clostridioides difficile (formerly known as Clostridium difficile) Infection (CDI)

For the treatment of diarrhea caused by CDI, the usual adult oral dosage of vancomycin is 125 mg 4 times daily for 10 days.

For the treatment of a first recurrence of CDI in adults, vancomycin in a tapered and pulsed regimen or vancomycin as a standard course may be given. An example of a tapered and pulsed regimen is as follows: vancomycin 125 mg 4 times daily for 10–14 days; followed by 125 mg twice daily for 7 days; then, 125 mg once daily for 7 days; then, 125 mg once every 2–3 days for 2–8 weeks.

For the treatment of diarrhea caused by CDI in children, the usual oral dosage of vancomycin is 40 mg/kg daily given in 3 or 4 divided doses for 7–10 days. Dosage of oral vancomycin in children should not exceed 2 g daily.

Enterocolitis Caused by S. aureus

For the treatment of enterocolitis caused by S. aureus (including MRSA), the usual adult oral dosage of vancomycin is 0.5–2 g daily given in 3 or 4 divided doses for 7–10 days.

For the treatment of staphylococcal enterocolitis in pediatric patients, the usual oral dosage of vancomycin is 40 mg/kg daily given in 3 or 4 divided doses for 7–10 days. The total daily dosage should not exceed 2 g.

IV Vancomycin

General Adult Dosage

For the treatment of serious or severe infections in adults with normal renal function, the usual IV dosage of vancomycin is 500 mg every 6 hours or 1 g every 12 hours.

A consensus guideline published by the American Society of Health-System Pharmacists (ASHP), the Infectious Diseases Society of America (IDSA), the Pediatric Infectious Diseases Society (PIDS), and the Society of Infectious Diseases Pharmacists (SIDP) provides recommendations for vancomycin dosing and monitoring in the treatment of serious MRSA infections (e.g., bacteremia, sepsis, infective endocarditis, pneumonia, osteomyelitis, meningitis). In critically ill patients with suspected or documented serious MRSA infections, a vancomycin loading dose of 20–35 mg/kg (based on actual body weight with a maximum dose of 3 g) can be considered for intermittent-infusion administration. A vancomycin loading dose of 20–25 mg/kg using actual body weight, with a maximum dose of 3 g, may be considered in obese adult patients with serious infections. Consult the guidelines for additional information (https://www.ashp.org/-/media/assets/policy-guidelines/docs/therapeutic-guidelines/therapeutic-guidelines-monitoring-vancomycin-ASHP-IDSA-PIDS.pdf)

General Pediatric Dosage

For neonates, the manufacturers suggest an initial IV vancomycin dose of 15 mg/kg, followed by 10 mg/kg either every 12 hours (in neonates <1 week of age) or every 8 hours (in infants 1 week to 1 month of age); close monitoring of serum vancomycin concentrations is recommended in these patients. Longer dosing intervals may be necessary in premature infants.

The American Academy of Pediatrics (AAP) provides recommendations for vancomycin dosing in neonates based on serum creatinine concentrations. An initial IV loading dose of 20 mg/kg is recommended followed by a maintenance dosage in Table 1.

TABLE 1. AAP Recommended General Dosage of Vancomycin in Neonates Following an Initial Loading Dose of 20 mg/kg.[a, b]

Gestational Age	Serum Creatinine (mg/dL)	Dosage
28 weeks or less	Less than 0.5	15 mg/kg every 12 hours
	0.5–0.7	20 mg/kg every 24 hours
	0.8–1	15 mg/kg every 24 hours
	1.1–1.4	10 mg/kg every 24 hours
	Greater than 1.4	15 mg/kg every 48 hours
Greater than 28 weeks	Less than 0.7	15 mg/kg every 12 hours
	0.7–0.9	20 mg/kg every 24 hours
	1–1.2	15 mg/kg every 24 hours
	1.3–1.6	10 mg/kg every 24 hours
	Greater than 1.6	15 mg/kg every 48 hours

[a] The maintenance dosage should begin at the same number of hours after the loading dose as the interval in the recommended dosage regimen.

[b] For invasive MRSA infections, a 24-hour AUC/MIC ratio ≥400 mg×h/L is recommended based on adult studies.

For older infants and children with normal renal function, manufacturers recommend an IV vancomycin dosage of 10 mg/kg every 6 hours. AAP suggests that children ≥1 month of age receive IV vancomycin in a dosage of 45–60 mg/kg daily given in 3–4 divided doses.

For children with normal renal function and suspected serious MRSA infections (e.g., pneumonia, pyomyositis, multifocal osteomyelitis, complicated bacteremia, necrotizing fasciitis), the consensus guideline published by ASHP, IDSA, PIDS, and SIDP recommends an initial IV vancomycin dosage of 60–80 mg/kg per day, in divided doses given every 6 hours for children 3 months to <12 years of age, or an initial vancomycin dosage of 60–70 mg/kg per day, in divided doses given every 6 to 8 hours, for pediatric patients ≥12 years of age. The consensus guideline states that the maximum empiric daily dose of IV vancomycin is usually 3.6 g in children with adequate renal function. Consult the guidelines for additional information (https://www.ashp.org/-/media/assets/policy-guidelines/docs/therapeutic-guidelines/therapeutic-guidelines-monitoring-vancomycin-ASHP-IDSA-PIDS.pdf)

Prevention of Neonatal Group B Streptococcal Disease

If IV vancomycin is used for intrapartum anti-infective prophylaxis of perinatal group B streptococcal (GBS) disease† in women with penicillin hypersensitivity who cannot receive clindamycin, the American College of Obstetrics and Gynecologists (ACOG) recommends an IV dosage of 20 mg/kg (not exceeding 2 g) administered every 8 hours until delivery. When indicated, such prophylaxis is initiated at the time of labor or rupture of membranes.

Antimicrobial Prophylaxis in Surgery

For antimicrobial prophylaxis† in adults undergoing certain cardiac, neurosurgical, orthopedic, thoracic (noncardiac), or vascular surgical procedures when use of vancomycin is considered necessary, a single 15-mg/kg dose of IV vancomycin should be given.

Because vancomycin should be administered by IV infusion over 1–2 hours, the infusion should be started within 120 minutes prior to the time of incision.

● Special Populations

Hepatic Impairment

Limited data suggest dosage adjustments of vancomycin are not necessary based on hepatic impairment.

Renal Impairment

In patients with impaired renal function, doses and/or frequency of administration of vancomycin must be modified.

The consensus guideline published by ASHP, IDSA, PIDS, and SIDP recommends vancomycin loading and maintenance doses for patients with serious MRSA infections who are receiving hemodialysis (see Table 2).

TABLE 2. ASHP, IDSA, PIDS, and SIDP Recommended Loading and Maintenance Doses of IV Vancomycin in Patients Receiving Hemodialysis.

Timing	Dialyzer Permeability	IV Vancomycin Dosage
After dialysis ends	Low permeability	Loading Dose: 25 mg/kg
		Maintenance Dosage: 7.5 mg/kg three times a week
	High permeability	Loading Dose: 25 mg/kg
		Maintenance Dosage: 10 mg/kg three times a week
Intradialytic	Low permeability	Loading Dose: 30 mg/kg
		Maintenance Dosage: 7.5–10 mg/kg three times a week
	High permeability	Loading Dose: 35 mg/kg
		Maintenance Dosage: 10–15 mg/kg three times a week

The guideline recommends an IV loading dose of 20–25 mg/kg based on actual body weight in patients with serious MRSA infections who are receiving continuous renal replacement therapy (CRRT) at conventional, KDIGO-recommended effluent rates. The initial vancomycin maintenance dosage for such patients should be 7.5–10 mg/kg every 12 hours. Consult the guidelines for additional information (https://www.ashp.org/-/media/assets/policy-guidelines/docs/therapeutic-guidelines/therapeutic-guidelines-monitoring-vancomycin-ASHP-IDSA-PIDS.pdf)

Geriatric Patients

Vancomycin dosage should be adjusted accordingly in geriatric patients; consider the greater frequency of renal impairment in this age group.

Obese Patients

The consensus guideline published by ASHP, IDSA, PIDS, and SIDP recommends an IV vancomycin loading dose of 20–25 mg/kg (up to a maximum dose of 3 g) based on actual body weight in obese adult patients with serious infections. Initial maintenance doses of vancomycin can be calculated using a population pharmacokinetic estimate of vancomycin clearance and the target AUC in obese patients. Empiric maintenance doses for most obese patients usually do not exceed 4.5 g/day, depending on renal function. Early and frequent monitoring of AUC exposure is recommended for dosage adjustment, especially when empiric doses exceed 4 g/day. Consult the guidelines for additional information (https://www.ashp.org/-/media/assets/policy-guidelines/docs/therapeutic-guidelines/therapeutic-guidelines-monitoring-vancomycin-ASHP-IDSA-PIDS.pdf)

CAUTIONS

● Contraindications

- Hypersensitivity to vancomycin.
- Commercially available frozen vancomycin hydrochloride injection in 5% dextrose may be contraindicated in patients with known allergy to corn or corn products.

● Warnings/Precautions

Warnings

Risk of Embryo-Fetal Toxicity Due to PEG 400 and NADA Excipients

Certain formulations of vancomycin injection contain the excipients polyethylene glycol (PEG 400) and N-acetyl D-alanine (NADA), which may cause fetal malformations. A boxed warning about this risk is included in the prescribing information for these formulations. Formulations of vancomycin containing PEG 400 and NADA should be avoided in pregnant patients.

Other Warnings and Precautions

Nephrotoxicity

Nephrotoxicity has occurred during parenteral vancomycin therapy; such toxicity rarely has been observed during oral vancomycin therapy.

Vancomycin-induced nephrotoxicity (i.e., acute kidney injury) may be manifested by transient elevations in BUN or serum creatinine concentrations, and the presence of hyaline and granular casts and albumin in the urine. Rarely, the drug has been associated with acute tubular necrosis and acute interstitial nephritis. In clinical studies, the reported rate of nephrotoxicity associated with vancomycin is highly variable ranging from 0 (when the drug is *not* used concomitantly with other nephrotoxic drugs) up to 40% (when vancomycin is used concomitantly with other nephrotoxic drugs). Patient characteristics that increase the risk of vancomycin-associated nephrotoxic adverse effects include advanced age, reduced kidney function, dehydration, reduced renal mass, female sex, obesity, hypoalbuminemia, and sepsis. An increased risk of acute kidney injury is associated with increased duration of therapy and increased exposures or serum concentrations of vancomycin. Although there is conflicting data regarding the causal relationship between vancomycin exposures and nephrotoxicity, many studies have demonstrated an increased risk of nephrotoxicity in patients with trough serum vancomycin concentrations ≥15 mg/L when compared with those with trough concentrations <15 mg/L. With regard to vancomycin AUC, limited data indicate that an AUC ≥600 mg×h/L may be associated with increased risk of nephrotoxicity.

Because vancomycin may cause nephrotoxic effects, the drug should be used with caution in patients with impaired renal function. Renal function should be monitored in all patients receiving vancomycin.

Ototoxicity

Ototoxicity has occurred during parenteral vancomycin therapy; such toxicity rarely has been observed during oral vancomycin therapy. Reported ototoxicity included damage to the auditory branch of the eighth cranial nerve and permanent deafness, vertigo, dizziness, and tinnitus.

Ototoxicity may be transient or permanent. It has been reported mostly in patients who receive excessive doses or prolonged IV therapy, patients with underlying hearing loss, or those receiving concomitant therapy with another ototoxic agent, such as an aminoglycoside. The incidence of ototoxicity associated with vancomycin use has been variable between 1–9%. Ototoxicity usually has been associated with serum or blood vancomycin concentrations of 80–100 mcg/mL, but has occurred with concentrations as low as 25 mcg/mL. Serial auditory function tests may be used to minimize the risk of ototoxicity.

Local Effects

Vancomycin is very irritating to tissue and causes necrosis when given IM; therefore, it must be administered IV and care must be taken to avoid extravasation. Pain and thrombophlebitis may occur after IV administration; to minimize this, it is recommended that the drug be administered slowly as a dilute solution (2.5 to 5 g/L) and that venous access sites be rotated.

Infusion-related Reactions

Rapid IV administration of vancomycin has resulted in a hypotensive reaction known as vancomycin flushing syndrome (previously referred to as "red man syndrome"). The reaction is characterized by a sudden decrease in blood pressure which can be severe and may be accompanied by flushing and/or a maculopapular or erythematous rash on the face, neck, chest, and upper extremities; the latter manifestations may also occur in the absence of hypotension. Wheezing, dyspnea, angioedema, urticaria, pruritus, and shock may also occur; rarely, cardiac arrest or seizures have occurred.

Vancomycin-induced hypotension appears to result from a negative inotropic and vasodilating action produced in part by a release of histamine, which is directly related to the rate of infusion; the release of histamine also appears to be responsible for the usual manifestations (e.g., erythema, rash, pruritus) of the "red" characterization. The reaction usually begins a few minutes after the vancomycin infusion is started, but may not occur until after the infusion is completed, and usually resolves spontaneously over one to several hours after discontinuance

of the infusion. If the hypotensive reaction is severe, the use of antihistamines, corticosteroids, or IV fluids may be necessary. The hypotensive reaction is related to the rate of infusion of vancomycin and has been reported most frequently when the drug was administered over a period of 10 minutes or less; however, the reaction may also occur rarely when the drug is infused over a period of ≥1 hour.

To minimize the risk of a hypotensive reaction, vancomycin should be infused over a period of at least 1 hour at a rate ≤10 mg/minute, and the patient's blood pressure should be monitored during the infusion. In patients who have had the reaction, subsequent doses of vancomycin can usually be given without adverse effect if administered at a slow rate (e.g., over several hours). Pretreatment with antihistamines may be of benefit. If attempts to minimize the reaction fail, use of another anti-infective agent may be necessary. The reaction reportedly has occurred in more than 50% of healthy individuals given vancomycin but less frequently when the drug is used therapeutically.

In one study, intradermal skin tests with vancomycin were used to assess the possibility of predicting the *severity* of vancomycin-associated anaphylactoid reactions. Although the intradermal tests were positive (wheal and flare) in all patients and all patients subsequently experienced anaphylactoid reactions following an IV dose of the drug, the magnitude of cutaneous response was of little value in predicting the severity of the reaction. Desensitization, employing sequential incremental concentration and dose increases (in a manner typical for drug desensitization procedures) and pretreatment with an antihistamine and corticosteroid, has been performed successfully in a few patients in whom vancomycin therapy was considered necessary.

Concomitant administration of vancomycin and anesthetic agents has been associated with an increased frequency of infusion-related events (e.g., hypotension, flushing, erythema, urticaria, pruritus). Infusion-related events may be minimized by the administration of vancomycin as a 60-minute infusion prior to anesthetic induction.

In at least one patient, *oral* administration of vancomycin resulted in the vancomycin flushing syndrome. This reaction was characterized by intense pruritus on the arms, scalp, and face; flushing on the face and neck; and erythema on the face, neck, chest, and arms. Administration of a parenteral antihistamine provided some relief.

The possibility that infusion reactions, including potentially severe hypotension, may occur with IV vancomycin should be considered. Rapid IV administration (e.g., over several minutes) of the drug should be avoided since it may be associated with exaggerated hypotension, including shock, and may rarely be with associated with cardiac arrest.

Other Dermatologic and Sensitivity Reactions

Urticaria, exfoliative dermatitis, macular rashes, eosinophilia, vasculitis, a shock-like state, transient anaphylaxis, linear IgA bullous dermatosis, toxic epidermal necrolysis, vasculitis associated with IV administration, inflammation at the injection site, and, occasionally, vascular collapse have been reported in patients receiving vancomycin. The drug also has been associated with Stevens-Johnson syndrome. Skin and subcutaneous disorders and drug rash with eosinophilia and systemic symptoms (DRESS) have been observed in postmarketing experience.

Hypersensitivity reactions reportedly occur in 5–10% of patients receiving vancomycin. Successful desensitization was reported in some patients who had experienced severe systemic allergic reactions to vancomycin but required further therapy with the drug.

Ocular Effects

Hemorrhagic occlusive retinal vasculitis (HORV), including permanent blindness, has occurred in patients receiving vancomycin by intracameral or intravitreal injection during or after cataract surgery. Safety and efficacy of vancomycin administered by the intracameral or intravitreal route have not been established by adequate and well-controlled trials, and vancomycin is not indicated for prophylaxis of endophthalmitis.

Hematologic Effects

Adverse hematologic effects reported in patients receiving vancomycin include neutropenia, eosinophilia, and thrombocytopenia. Neutropenia, which appears to be rapidly reversible following discontinuance of the drug, usually has occurred 7 or more days after initiation of vancomycin therapy or after a total dose of more than 25 g of the drug.

Although a causal relationship to vancomycin has not been established, reversible agranulocytosis (granulocytes <500/mm^3) has been reported rarely in patients receiving the drug.

Leukocyte counts should be monitored periodically in patients receiving prolonged vancomycin therapy and in those who are receiving concomitant therapy with drugs that may cause neutropenia.

C. difficile-associated Diarrhea and Colitis

Treatment with anti-infectives alters normal colon flora and may permit overgrowth of *Clostridioides difficile* (formerly known as *Clostridium difficile*).

C. difficile infection (CDI) and *C. difficile*-associated diarrhea and colitis (CDAD; also known as antibiotic-associated diarrhea and colitis or pseudomembranous colitis) have been reported with the use of nearly all anti-infectives, including IV vancomycin, and may range in severity from mild diarrhea to fatal colitis.

Selection and Use of Anti-infectives

To reduce development of drug-resistant bacteria and maintain effectiveness of vancomycin and other antibacterials, the drug should be used only for the treatment or prevention of infections proven or strongly suspected to be caused by susceptible bacteria. When selecting or modifying anti-infective therapy, use results of culture and in vitro susceptibility testing. In the absence of such data, consider local epidemiology and susceptibility patterns when selecting anti-infectives for empiric therapy. Patients should be advised that antibacterials (including vancomycin) should only be used to treat bacterial infections and not used to treat viral infections (e.g., the common cold). Patients also should be advised about the importance of completing the full course of therapy, even if feeling better after a few days, and that skipping doses or not completing therapy may decrease effectiveness and increase the likelihood that bacteria will develop resistance and will not be treatable with vancomycin or other antibacterials in the future.

Information on test methods and quality control standards for in vitro susceptibility testing of antibacterial agents and specific interpretive criteria for such testing recognized by the FDA is available at https://www.fda.gov/drugs/development-resources/antibacterial-susceptibility-test-interpretive-criteria. For most antibacterial agents, FDA recognizes the standards published by the Clinical and Laboratory Standards Institute (CLSI).

Prolonged use of vancomycin may result in overgrowth of nonsusceptible organisms. The patient should be carefully monitored and appropriate therapy should be instituted if a superinfection occurs. Because antibiotic-associated CDI has been reported with the use of anti-infective agents, including IV vancomycin, it should be considered in the differential diagnosis of patients who develop diarrhea during therapy with the drug.

Use of, and exposure to, anti-infectives are major risk factors for the emergence of anti-infective–resistant pathogens, and anti-infective resistance results in increased morbidity, mortality, and healthcare costs. Prevention of the emergence of drug resistance, its dissemination among pathogens, and the spread of such pathogens has become an increasingly important public health problem. Medical, pharmacy, and other staff and individuals responsible for drug-use policy and formulary decisions should review and restrict the use of certain anti-infectives, including vancomycin, and ensure that their use is appropriate. Clinicians should recognize that unnecessary and inappropriate use of anti-infectives has important, far-reaching implications for human health globally.

Subsequently, other updated guidance regarding implementation of antibiotic stewardship programs, therapeutic vancomycin monitoring, and treatment of specific infections has been published to aid in the appropriate use of antibiotics, including vancomycin. For additional information, the current IDSA clinical practice guidelines available at https://www.idsociety.org/ should be consulted.

Warning and Precautions Related to Oral Formulations

Orally administered vancomycin capsules or solution *must* be used for the treatment of *Clostridioides difficile* (formerly known as *Clostridium difficile*) infection (CDI; *C. difficile*-associated diarrhea [CDAD]) and enterocolitis caused by *S. aureus*. Parenterally administered vancomycin does *not* effectively treat such infections. Because vancomycin is not systemically absorbed following oral administration, vancomycin capsules and oral solution are *not* effective for other types of infections.

Following oral administration of vancomycin for diarrhea caused by CDI, clinically important vancomycin serum concentrations have been reported. Systemic absorption of vancomycin following oral administration may occur in patients with inflammatory disorders of the intestinal mucosa. Such patients receiving high doses of oral vancomycin may be at risk for experiencing systemic adverse effects and serum concentration monitoring may be warranted in certain situations (i.e., patients with renal insufficiency and/or colitis, concomitant use with an aminoglycoside antibiotic).

● Other Adverse Effects

A throbbing pain in the muscles of the back and neck has been reported with vancomycin and can usually be minimized or avoided by slower administration of the drug. In patients undergoing continuous ambulatory peritoneal dialysis (CAPD), intraperitoneal administration of vancomycin has been associated with chemical peritonitis, a syndrome consisting of a cloudy dialysate, which may be accompanied by abdominal pain and fever. Chemical peritonitis usually disappears shortly after discontinuance of intraperitoneal vancomycin.

Other adverse effects of vancomycin include chills and fever. Priapism after a second IV dose of vancomycin, with recurrence on inadvertent rechallenge, occurred in a 37-year-old man with severe underlying diabetes mellitus; bilateral phlebotomy of the corpus cavernosum resulted in resolution of the priapism.

Specific Populations

Pregnancy

There was no evidence of teratogenicity when vancomycin was administered IV to rats in dosages up to 200 mg/kg daily (1180 mg/m^2 or equivalent to the recommended maximum human dosage based on mg/m^2) or to rabbits in dosages up to 120 mg/kg daily (1320 mg/m^2 or 1.1 times the recommended maximum human dosage based on mg/m^2). There were no effects on fetal weight or development in rats at the highest dosage tested or in rabbits given 80 mg/kg daily (880 mg/m^2 or 0.74 times the maximum recommended human dosage based on mg/m^2).

In one study, no sensorineural hearing loss or nephrotoxicity was reported in neonates born to women who received IV vancomycin for severe staphylococcal infections associated with injection drug abuse- during pregnancy. In one infant whose mother received IV vancomycin in the third trimester of pregnancy, conductive hearing loss was reported; however, a causal relationship to vancomycin has not been established. Because the number of pregnant women in this study was limited and vancomycin was only administered during the second and third trimester of pregnancy, it is not known whether the drug can cause fetal harm when administered to pregnant women.

In a prospective study, no major adverse effects were observed in mothers or their newborns when IV vancomycin was administered at the time of delivery. This study included 55 pregnant women with positive group B *Streptococcus* culture with resistance to clindamycin or unknown sensitivity and a high-risk penicillin allergy. Vancomycin dosage ranged from 1 g every 12 hours to 20 mg/kg (maximum individual dose 2 g) every 8 hours. None of the newborns had sensorineural hearing loss; although renal function of the neonates was not assessed, all neonates were discharged in good condition.

Vancomycin should be used during pregnancy only when clearly needed.

Lactation

Vancomycin is distributed into milk following IV administration. Systemic absorption of oral vancomycin is very low and it is not known whether the drug distributes into human milk following oral administration. However, IV and oral vancomycin should be used with caution in nursing women. Because of the potential for serious adverse reactions from the drug in nursing infants, a decision should be made whether to discontinue nursing or the drug, taking into account the importance of vancomycin to the woman.

Pediatric Use

Safety and efficacy of oral vancomycin have not been established in pediatric patients.

IV vancomycin should be used with caution in premature neonates and young infants because of the renal immaturity of these patients and the potential for increased serum concentrations of the drug. Close monitoring of serum vancomycin concentrations may be warranted in pediatric patients, especially neonates and young infants.

Safety of the chemical components that may leach out of the plastic containers of commercially available frozen vancomycin injections has not been established in children.

Geriatric Use

In clinical studies of oral vancomycin, 54% of patients were >65 years of age; of these, 40% were >65–75 years of age and 60% were >75 years of age. In these studies, geriatric patients treated with oral vancomycin capsules for diarrhea associated with CDI were more likely to develop nephrotoxicity during or after completion of therapy. Renal function should be monitored during and after treatment with oral vancomycin in all geriatric patients, including those with normal renal function.

Geriatric patients >65 years of age may take longer to respond to oral vancomycin therapy compared with younger patients. Clinicians should be aware of the appropriate duration of oral vancomycin treatment in geriatric patients and therapy should not be prematurely discontinued or prematurely switched to an alternate therapy.

IV vancomycin dosage in geriatric patients should be adjusted based on the degree of renal impairment. Because geriatric patients may have decreasing glomerular filtration with increasing age, increased serum vancomycin concentrations may occur if dosage is not adjusted in these patients.

Renal Impairment

Vancomycin is only minimally removed by hemodialysis when a low-flux capillary is used (e.g., cuprophan) or peritoneal dialysis, including continuous ambulatory peritoneal dialysis. Hemodialysis using a high-flux capillary (e.g., polysulfone, polyacrylonitrile, polymethylmethacrylate) results in removal of approximately 30–46% of the drug with a subsequent rebound effect of 16–36% after completion of hemodialysis due to recirculation of vancomycin from protein binding sites over a 3–6 hour period. The drug is substantially removed by hemodiafiltration.

• Common Adverse Effects

IV: Local effects (pain and thrombophlebitis); infusion reactions; hypersensitivity reactions.

Oral solution: Nausea, abdominal pain, and hypokalemia.

DRUG INTERACTIONS

• Ototoxic and Nephrotoxic Drugs

Because of the possibility of additive toxicities, the concurrent or sequential systemic or topical use of other ototoxic and/or nephrotoxic drugs (e.g., aminoglycosides, amphotericin B, bacitracin, cisplatin, colistin, polymyxin B) and vancomycin requires careful serial monitoring of renal and auditory function. These drugs should be used with caution in patients receiving vancomycin therapy.

Aminoglycosides

In vitro, the antibacterial effects of vancomycin and aminoglycosides are synergistic against many strains of *Staphylococcus aureus*, *Streptococcus bovis (also known as S. gallolyticus)*, enterococci (*Enterococcus faecalis*), and viridans streptococci.

Anesthetics

Concomitant use of vancomycin and anesthetic agents has been associated with anaphylactoid reactions and an increased frequency of infusion reactions (e.g., hypotension, flushing, erythema, urticaria, pruritus). Erythema and histamine-like flushing has occurred in pediatric patients receiving vancomycin and anesthetic agents concomitantly. Infusion-related events may be minimized by the administration of vancomycin as a 60-minute infusion prior to anesthetic induction.

DESCRIPTION

Vancomycin is bactericidal and binds to the bacterial cell wall causing blockage of glycopeptide polymerization. This effect, which occurs at a site different from that affected by the penicillins, produces immediate inhibition of cell wall synthesis

and secondary damage to the cytoplasmic membrane. Magnesium, manganese, calcium, and ferrous ions reduce the degree of adsorption of vancomycin to the cell wall, but the in vivo importance of this interaction is unknown.

• Spectrum

Vancomycin is active in vitro and in vivo against many gram-positive bacteria, including *Staphylococcus aureus* (including methicillin-resistant *S. aureus* [MRSA]), *S. epidermidis* (including methicillin-resistant strains), nonenterococcal group D streptococci (*Streptococcus bovis* [also known as *S. gallolyticus*]), enterococci (*Enterococcus faecalis*), viridans streptococci, *Corynebacterium*, and *Clostridioides* (including *C. difficile*). The drug also is active in vitro against *S. pyogenes* (group A β-hemolytic streptococci), *S. agalactiae* (group B streptococci), *S. pneumoniae* (including penicillin-resistant strains), *Listeria monocytogenes*, *Actinomyces*, and *Lactobacillus*.

Vancomycin is not active against gram-negative bacteria, mycobacteria, or fungi.

• Resistance

Resistance in Enterococci

Resistance to vancomycin has been reported in *Enterococcus faecalis*, *E. faecium* (VREF), *E. gallinarum*, *E. casseliflavus*, and *E. flavescens* and strains of enterococci resistant to vancomycin have been reported with increasing frequency.

Several different forms of vancomycin resistance have been identified in enterococci, including high-level resistance and low-level resistance. Strains of enterococci with high-level resistance generally require vancomycin concentrations of 128 mcg/mL or more and strains with low-level resistance generally require concentrations of 16–64 mcg/mL for in vitro inhibition. High-level vancomycin resistance has been reported in *E. faecium* and *E. faecalis*, appears to be plasmid mediated, and can be induced by exposure to vancomycin and, to a lesser extent, exposure to teicoplanin. Low-level vancomycin resistance has been reported in *E. faecium*, *E. faecalis*, *E. gallinarum*, *E. casseliflavus*, and *E. flavescens* and may also be induced by exposure to vancomycin, but may or may not be induced by exposure to teicoplanin.

High-level vancomycin resistance most frequently has been associated with the presence of a certain protein and a phenotype, VanA; high- to variable-level resistance usually has been associated with the presence VanB. Other phenotypes, (i.e., VanC, D, E, G, L, M, N) also have been identified. VanA, VanB, and VanD are associated with synthesis of the altered D-ala D-lac target; VanC, VanE, VanG, and VanL are associated with the altered D-ala D-ser target. In general, VanA resistance is high level, transferable (i.e., acquired resistance), and accompanied by high-level teicoplanin resistance. VanB resistance is variable in level, transferable, and *not* accompanied by teicoplanin resistance; VanC resistance is low level, *not* transferable (i.e., intrinsic resistance), and *not* associated with teicoplanin resistance; and VanD is associated with low- to high-level resistance to vancomycin and teicoplanin. Transferable genes (e.g., VanA, VanB) can be spread from organism to organism whereas non-transferable genes (e.g., VanC) are less likely to cause serious infections and have not been associated with outbreaks.

Some strains of *E. faecium* or *E. faecalis* resistant to vancomycin may be susceptible in vitro to linezolid, daptomycin, or tigecycline. Strains of vancomycin-resistant enterococci may also be resistant to other drugs (e.g., aminoglycosides, ampicillin, penicillin G, imipenem, tetracyclines, synergistic combinations of β-lactam anti-infectives). Enterococci resistant to linezolid also has been observed. These multidrug-resistant strains of enterococci have been reported with increasing frequency. Although telavancin and dalbavancin are inactive against VanA enterococci, oritavancin retains activity against VanA-type vancomycin-resistant enterococci. Newer oxazolidinones (e.g., tedizolid) also have demonstrated efficacy against multi-drug resistant gram-positive isolates, including vancomycin-resistant enterococci.

• Resistance in Staphylococci

In vitro exposure of staphylococci to increasing concentrations of glycopeptide anti-infectives can produce strains with decreased susceptibility and emergence of vancomycin-resistant strains of *S. haemolyticus* and *S. epidermidis* have been reported in patients receiving the drug. The first vancomycin-resistant *S. aureus* isolate in the United States was reported in 2002 and other isolates have been subsequently reported.

Although the mechanisms of vancomycin intermediate-resistant *S. aureus* have not been fully elucidated, several mutations are known to contribute to the development of these resistant isolates including genes encoding 2 component regulatory systems controlling transcription of genes in cell wall synthesis (e.g., graRS, vraSR, walKR) and genes encoding DNA-dependent RNA polymerase β–subunit (e.g., rpoB). Isolates with intermediate resistance to vancomycin have thicker cell walls containing subunits that are able to bind vancomycin extracellularly and have several altered metabolic pathways. Vancomycin-resistant *S. aureus* (i.e., MIC ≥16 mcg/mL) is conferred by VanA encoded on transposing Tn1546, which was originally a part of a vancomycin-resistant enterococci conjugative plasmid. Oritavancin retains activity against vancomycin-resistant *S. aureus*.

● *Pharmacokinetics*

Absorption

Vancomycin hydrochloride is not appreciably absorbed from the GI tract in most patients and must be given parenterally for the treatment of systemic infections. Oral bioavailability usually is less than 5%; however, limited data suggest that clinically important serum concentrations may occur following enteral or oral administration of vancomycin in some patients with colitis and/or in those with renal impairment.

In adults with normal renal function who received multiple 1-g doses of vancomycin (15 mg/kg) given by IV infusion over 1 hour, mean plasma concentrations immediately after completion of the infusion are approximately 63 mcg/mL and mean plasma concentrations 2 and 11 hours later are approximately 23 or 8 mcg/mL, respectively. When multiple 500-mg doses are given by IV infusion over 30 minutes, mean plasma concentrations are about 49 mcg/mL immediately following the infusion and about 10 mcg/mL 6 hours after infusion.

Serum vancomycin concentrations are higher in patients with renal dysfunction than in those with normal renal function, and toxic serum concentrations may result.

● *Distribution*

Following IV administration, vancomycin is widely distributed in body tissues and diffuses readily into pericardial, pleural, ascitic, and synovial fluids. Small amounts of the drug are distributed into bile.

Vancomycin does *not* readily distribute into CSF in the absence of inflammation unless serum concentrations are exceedingly high. Low concentrations of the drug may be present in CSF if meninges are inflamed, but negligible amounts are detected in the CSF of most patients with uninflamed meninges. In a limited number of adults and children with meningitis who received IV vancomycin in a dosage of 10–15 mg/kg daily, average CSF concentrations 1–3 hours after a dose were 3.3–3.8 mcg/mL and were 21–22% of concurrent serum concentrations. However, the relationship between CSF concentrations and clinical efficacy of vancomycin in the treatment of meningitis is unclear.

Vancomycin is 30–60% bound to serum proteins. Protein binding may be lower (19–29%) in patients with hypoalbuminemia (e.g., burn patients, those with end-stage renal disease).

Vancomycin readily crosses the placenta and is distributed into cord blood. Vancomycin is distributed into milk.

● *Elimination*

The serum elimination half-life of vancomycin in adults with normal renal function has been reported to average 4–7 hours; accumulation tends to occur after 2–3 days of IV administration at 6- or 12-hour intervals. In geriatric adults 65 years of age older, the mean half-life of the drug has been reported to be 12.1 hours.

The mean half-life of vancomycin is 6.7 hours in full-term neonates and 4.1 hours in infants 1 month of age or older but younger than 1 year of age. In children 2.5–11 years of age, half-life of the drug is reported to be 5.6 hours.

The serum elimination half-life of vancomycin is increased in patients with renal dysfunction. In one study, the elimination half-life averaged 32.3 hours (range: 10.1–75.1 hours) in patients with creatinine clearances of 10–60 mL/minute and 146.7 hours (range: 44.1–406.4 hours) in those with creatinine clearances less than 10 mL/minute. However, because of increased clearance, half-life of vancomycin averages 4 hours in burn patients.

Vancomycin does not appear to be metabolized. Following oral administration, the drug is excreted mainly in feces. Following IV administration, about 75–90% of a dose is eliminated unchanged in urine by glomerular filtration and only small amounts are excreted in bile.

ADVICE TO PATIENTS

- Advise patients that vancomycin should only be used to treat bacterial infections and not used to treat viral infections (e.g., the common cold).
- Importance of completing full course of therapy, even if feeling better after a few days.
- Advise patients that skipping doses or not completing the full course of therapy may decrease effectiveness and increase the likelihood that bacteria will develop resistance and will not be treatable with vancomycin or other antibacterials in the future.
- Importance of reporting possible manifestations of adverse effects to the clinician, including ototoxicity, nephrotoxicity, infusion site reactions, and hypersensitivity.
- Risk of diarrhea; usually ends when vancomycin is discontinued. If watery and bloody stools (with or without stomach cramps and fever) occur as late as two or more months after having taken the last dose of the drug, advise patient to contact their physician as soon as possible.
- Importance of informing clinicians of existing or contemplated concomitant therapy, including prescription and OTC drugs, and any concomitant illnesses.
- Importance of women informing clinicians if they are or plan to become pregnant or plan to breast-feed.
- Importance of advising patients of other important precautionary information. (See Cautions.)

PREPARATIONS

Excipients in commercially available drug preparations may have clinically important effects in some individuals; consult specific product labeling for details.

Vancomycin Hydrochloride

Oral			
Capsules	125 mg (of vancomycin)*	**Vancocin®**, Ani Vancomycin Hydrochloride Capsule	
	250 mg (of vancomycin)*	**Vancocin®**, Ani Vancomycin Hydrochloride Capsule	
Powder for Oral Solution	3.75 g (of vancomycin)*	**Firvanq®** Azurity, supplied with flavored diluent	
	7.5 g (of vancomycin)*	**Firvanq®** Azurity, supplied with flavored diluent	
	15 g*	**Firvanq®** Azurity, supplied with flavored diluent	
Parenteral			
For injection	5 g (of vancomycin) pharmacy bulk package*	**Vancomycin Hydrochloride for Injection**	
	10 g (of vancomycin) pharmacy bulk package*	**Vancomycin Hydrochloride for Injection**	
	100 g (of vancomycin) pharmacy bulk package*	**Vancomycin Hydrochloride for Injection**	

For injection, for IV infusion	250 mg (of vancomycin)*	Vancomycin Hydrochloride for Injection
		Vancomycin Hydrochloride for Injection
	500 mg (of vancomycin)*	Vancomycin Hydrochloride for Injection
		Vancomycin Hydrochloride for Injection ADD-Vantage®
	750 mg (of vancomycin)*	Vancomycin Hydrochloride for Injection
		Vancomycin Hydrochloride for Injection ADD-Vantage®
	1 g (of vancomycin)*	Vancomycin Hydrochloride for Injection, Vancomycin Hydrochloride for Injection ADD-Vantage®
	1.25 g (of vancomycin)*	Vancomycin Hydrochloride for Injection
	1.5 g (of vancomycin)*	Vancomycin Hydrochloride for Injection

Vancomycin Hydrochloride in Dextrose

Parenteral		
Injection (frozen), for IV infusion	5 mg (of vancomycin) per mL (500 mg, 750 mg, 1 g) in 5% dextrose*	Vancomycin Injection in 5% Dextrose

Vancomycin Hydrochloride in Sodium Chloride

Parenteral		
Injection (frozen), for IV infusion	5 mg (of vancomycin) per mL (500 mg, 750 mg, 1 g) in 0.9% sodium chloride*	Vancomycin Injection in 0.9% Sodium Chloride

Vancomycin Hydrochloride in Water and PEG

Parenteral		
Injection, for IV infusion	5 mg (of vancomycin) per mL (500 mg, 750, mg, 1 g, 1.25 g, 1.5 g, 2 g) in diluent consisting of water and PEG, and excipients NADA and lysine*	Vancomycin Injection

† Use is not currently included in the labeling approved by the US Food and Drug Administration.

*available from one or more manufacturer, distributor, and/or repackager by generic (nonproprietary) name

Selected Revisions October 13, 2022, © Copyright, May 1, 1976, American Society of Health-System Pharmacists, Inc.

Clindamycin Hydrochloride Clindamycin Palmitate Hydrochloride Clindamycin Phosphate

8:12.28.20 • LINCOMYCINS

■ Clindamycin, a lincosamide antibiotic, is a derivative of lincomycin.

USES

Clindamycin is used for the treatment of certain serious infections caused by susceptible aerobic gram-positive bacteria (staphylococci, streptococci, pneumococci) and for the treatment of certain serious infections caused by susceptible anaerobic bacteria. Use of clindamycin generally should be reserved for the treatment of serious infections when less toxic anti-infectives cannot be used (e.g., penicillin-allergic patients or other patients for whom a penicillin is inappropriate). Because clindamycin has been associated with potentially fatal colitis (see Cautions: GI Effects), the manufacturer recommends that clinicians consider the nature of the infection and the suitability of less toxic alternatives (e.g., erythromycin).

Certain infections may require incision and drainage or other indicated surgical procedures in addition to anti-infective treatment. Use of clindamycin does not eliminate the need for surgical procedures when indicated.

Because clindamycin does not distribute adequately into the CNS, the drug should *not* be used for the treatment of meningitis.

● Gram-positive Aerobic Bacterial Infections

Clindamycin is used orally or parenterally for the treatment of serious respiratory tract infections caused by susceptible staphylococci, *Streptococcus pneumoniae*, or other streptococci or serious skin and skin structure infections caused by susceptible staphylococci, *S. pneumoniae*, or *S. pyogenes* (group A β-hemolytic streptococci; GAS). Clindamycin also is used parenterally for the treatment of septicemia caused by susceptible *Staphylococcus aureus* or streptococci, treatment of serious bone and joint infections (including acute hematogenous osteomyelitis) caused by susceptible *S. aureus*, and as adjunctive therapy in the surgical treatment of chronic bone and joint infections caused by susceptible bacteria. However, clindamycin generally should be reserved for use in penicillin-allergic or other patients when less toxic alternatives cannot be used.

● Anaerobic Bacterial Infections

Clindamycin is used orally or parenterally for the treatment of serious lower respiratory tract infections (e.g., empyema, pneumonia, lung abscess), serious skin and skin structure infections, septicemia, intra-abdominal infections (e.g., peritonitis, intra-abdominal abscess), and gynecologic infections (e.g., endometritis, nongonococcal tubo-ovarian abscess, pelvic cellulitis, postsurgical vaginal cuff infections) caused by susceptible anaerobic bacteria. Parenteral clindamycin also is used for the treatment of serious bone and joint infections (including acute hematogenous osteomyelitis) caused by susceptible anaerobes and as adjunctive therapy in the surgical treatment of chronic bone and joint infections caused by susceptible bacteria. Although previously considered a drug of choice for the treatment of infections caused by *Bacteroides*, clindamycin is no longer *routinely* recommended for the treatment of intra-abdominal infections because of the increasing incidence of *B. fragilis* resistant to the drug. In the treatment of mixed aerobic-anaerobic bacterial infections (e.g., pelvic inflammatory disease), clindamycin has been used in conjunction with an IM or IV aminoglycoside.

● Acute Otitis Media

Oral clindamycin is used as an alternative for the treatment of acute otitis media† (AOM).

When anti-infective therapy is indicated for the treatment of AOM, the American Academy of Pediatrics (AAP) recommends high-dose amoxicillin or amoxicillin and clavulanate as the drug of first choice for initial treatment. These experts

recommend certain cephalosporins (cefdinir, cefpodoxime, cefuroxime, ceftriaxone) as alternatives for initial treatment in penicillin-allergic patients who do not have a history of severe and/or recent penicillin-allergic reactions.

AAP states that clindamycin (with or without a third generation cephalosporin) is a possible alternative for the treatment of AOM in patients who fail to respond to initial treatment with first-line or preferred alternatives. When retreatment of AOM is indicated after failure of initial treatment, high-dose amoxicillin and clavulanate or IM ceftriaxone usually is recommended. Although clindamycin may be effective in infections caused by penicillin-resistant *S. pneumoniae*, the drug may not be effective against multidrug-resistant *S. pneumoniae* and usually is inactive against *Haemophilus influenzae*. If clindamycin is used for retreatment of AOM, concomitant use of an anti-infective active against *H. influenzae* and *Moraxella catarrhalis* (e.g., cefdinir, cefixime, cefuroxime) should be considered.

For additional information regarding treatment of AOM, including information on diagnosis and management strategies, anti-infectives for initial treatment, duration of initial treatment, and anti-infectives after initial treatment failure, see Acute Otitis Media under Uses: Otitis Media, in the Cephalosporins General Statement 8:12.06.

● Pharyngitis and Tonsillitis

Oral clindamycin is used as an alternative for the treatment of pharyngitis and tonsillitis† caused by *S. pyogenes* (group A β-hemolytic streptococci; GAS). Although clindamycin usually is effective in eradicating *S. pyogenes* from the nasopharynx, it is reserved for use as an alternative in patients who cannot receive β-lactam anti-infectives. In addition, clindamycin is recommended as one of several possible alternatives for the treatment of symptomatic patients who failed to respond to initial penicillin treatment or have multiple, recurrent episodes of pharyngitis known to be caused by *S. pyogenes*.

Selection of an anti-infective for the treatment of *S. pyogenes* pharyngitis and tonsillitis should be based on the drug's spectrum of activity, bacteriologic and clinical efficacy, potential adverse effects, ease of administration, patient compliance, and cost. No regimen has been found to date that effectively eradicates group A β-hemolytic streptococci in 100% of patients.

Because the drugs have a narrow spectrum of activity, are inexpensive, and generally are effective with a low frequency of adverse effects, AAP, Infectious Diseases Society of America (IDSA), and American Heart Association (AHA) recommend a penicillin regimen (i.e., 10 days of oral penicillin V or oral amoxicillin or a single dose of IM penicillin G benzathine) as the treatment of choice for *S. pyogenes* pharyngitis and tonsillitis and prevention of initial attacks (primary prevention) of rheumatic fever. Other anti-infectives (e.g., oral cephalosporins, oral macrolides, oral clindamycin) are recommended as alternatives in penicillin-allergic patients.

● Respiratory Tract Infections

Clindamycin is used for the treatment of serious respiratory tract infections (e.g., pneumonia, empyema, lung abscess) caused by susceptible *S. aureus*, *S. pneumoniae*, other streptococci, or anaerobes.

IDSA and American Thoracic Society (ATS) consider clindamycin an alternative agent for the treatment of community-acquired pneumonia (CAP) caused by *S. pneumoniae* or *S. aureus* (methicillin-susceptible strains) in adults. IDSA also considers clindamycin an alternative for the treatment of CAP caused by *S. pneumoniae*, *S. pyogenes*, or *S. aureus* in pediatric patients. For the treatment of pneumonia caused by methicillin-resistant *S. aureus* (MRSA; also known as oxacillin-resistant *S. aureus* or ORSA), IDSA states that clindamycin is one of several options, unless the strain is resistant to clindamycin.

For information regarding the treatment of CAP, including infections caused by MRSA, the current clinical practice guidelines from IDSA available at http://www.idsociety.org should be consulted.

● Skin and Skin Structure Infections

Clindamycin is used for the treatment of serious skin and skin structure infections caused by susceptible staphylococci, *S. pneumoniae*, other streptococci, or anaerobes. Clindamycin is recommended as one of several options for the treatment of staphylococcal and streptococcal skin and skin structure infections, including those known or suspected to be caused by susceptible MRSA.

Clindamycin is used in conjunction with or as an alternative to penicillin G for the treatment of clostridial myonecrosis† (gas gangrene) caused by *Clostridium perfringens* or other *Clostridium*.

Although the fixed combination of amoxicillin and clavulanate usually is the drug of choice for the treatment of infected human or animal (e.g., dog, cat, reptile) bite wounds, alternative regimens include clindamycin in conjunction with either an extended-spectrum cephalosporin or co-trimoxazole. Purulent bite wounds usually are polymicrobial and broad-spectrum anti-infective coverage is recommended. Nonpurulent infected bite wounds usually are caused by staphylococci and streptococci, but can be polymicrobial.

For information regarding the treatment of skin and skin structure infections, including infections caused by MRSA, the current clinical practice guidelines from IDSA available at http://www.idsociety.org should be consulted.

● Actinomycosis

Clindamycin has been recommended as an alternative to penicillin G or ampicillin for the treatment of actinomycosis†, including infections caused by *Actinomyces israelii*.

● Anthrax

Although limited clinical data are available regarding use of clindamycin in the treatment of anthrax†, clindamycin was included in a multiple-drug regimen that was effective for the treatment of several patients in the US who developed anthrax during September and October 2001 following exposure to an intentional release of anthrax spores (biologic warfare, bioterrorism). At least 2 patients were treated with a parenteral regimen of ciprofloxacin (400 mg every 8 hours), rifampin (300 mg every 12 hours), and clindamycin (900 mg every 8 hours).

Because of the rapid course of symptomatic inhalational anthrax and high mortality rate, prompt recognition of symptoms and early initiation of anti-infective therapy is essential. The US Centers for Disease Control and Prevention (CDC) and other experts (e.g., US Working Group on Civilian Biodefense) recommend that treatment of inhalational anthrax that occurs as the result of exposure to anthrax spores in the context of biologic warfare or bioterrorism should be initiated with a multiple-drug parenteral regimen that includes ciprofloxacin or doxycycline and 1 or 2 additional anti-infective agents predicted to be effective. Multiple-drug parenteral regimens also are recommended for the treatment of cutaneous anthrax if there are signs of systemic involvement, extensive edema, or lesions on the head and neck. Based on in vitro data, drugs that have been suggested as possibilities to augment ciprofloxacin or doxycycline in such multiple-drug regimens include chloramphenicol, clindamycin, rifampin, vancomycin, clarithromycin, imipenem, penicillin, or ampicillin. Strains of *Bacillus anthracis* that were associated with cases of inhalational or cutaneous anthrax† that occurred in the US (Florida, New York, District of Columbia) during September and October 2001 following bioterrorism-related anthrax exposures were susceptible to clindamycin in vitro.

Based on in vitro data, clindamycin also has been suggested as a possible alternative for postexposure prophylaxis following a suspected or confirmed exposure to aerosolized anthrax spores† (inhalational anthrax) when the drugs of choice (ciprofloxacin, doxycycline) are not tolerated or cannot be used.

For information on treatment of anthrax and recommendations for prophylaxis following exposure to anthrax spores, see Uses: Anthrax, in Ciprofloxacin 8:12.18.

● Babesiosis

Oral or IV clindamycin is used in conjunction with oral quinine sulfate for the treatment of babesiosis† caused by *Babesia microti* or other *Babesia*.

Although several species of *Babesia* can infect humans (e.g., *B. microti*, *B. divergens*, *B. duncani*, *B. venatorum*), *B. microti* is the most common cause of babesiosis in the US. *B. microti* is transmitted by *Ixodes scapularis* ticks, which also may be simultaneously infected with and transmit *Borrelia burgdorferi* (causative agent of Lyme disease) and *Anaplasma phagocytophilum* (causative agent of human granulocytotropic anaplasmosis [HGA, formerly known as human granulocytic ehrlichiosis]). Therefore, the possibility of coinfection with *B. burgdorferi* and/or *A. phagocytophilum* should be considered in patients who have severe or persistent symptoms despite appropriate anti-infective treatment for babesiosis.

IDSA states that all patients with active babesiosis (i.e., symptoms of viral-like infection and identification of babesial parasites in blood smears or by polymerase chain reaction [PCR] amplification of babesial DNA) should receive anti-infective treatment because of the risk of complications; however, symptomatic patients whose serum contains antibody to babesia but whose blood lacks identifiable babesial parasites on smear or babesial DNA by PCR should not receive treatment. In addition, these experts state that treatment is not generally

recommended initially for asymptomatic individuals, regardless of the results of serologic examination, blood smears, or PCR, but should be considered if parasitemia persists for longer than 3 months.

When anti-infective treatment of babesiosis is indicated, IDSA and other clinicians recommend that either a regimen of clindamycin and quinine or a regimen of atovaquone and azithromycin be used. There is some evidence that, in patients with mild or moderate illness, the atovaquone and azithromycin regimen may be as effective and better tolerated than the clindamycin and quinine regimen. However, the clindamycin and quinine regimen generally is preferred for the treatment of severe babesiosis caused by *M. microti* and infections caused by *M. divergens*, *B. duncani*, *B. divergens*-like organisms, or *B. venatorum*. Patients with moderate to severe babesiosis should be monitored closely during treatment to ensure clinical improvement. Exchange transfusions have been used successfully in asplenic patients with life-threatening babesiosis and should be considered, especially in severely ill patients with high levels of parasitemia (10% or more), significant hemolysis, or compromised renal, hepatic, or pulmonary function.

● Bacterial Vaginosis

Oral clindamycin is used in the treatment of bacterial vaginosis† (formerly called *Haemophilus* vaginitis, *Gardnerella* vaginitis, nonspecific vaginitis, *Corynebacterium* vaginitis, or anaerobic vaginosis). The drug also is used intravaginally as a vaginal cream or vaginal suppository for the treatment of bacterial vaginosis (see Clindamycin Phosphate 84:04.04).

Bacterial vaginosis is a polymicrobial syndrome that can occur when normal hydrogen peroxide-producing *Lactobacillus* in the vagina are replaced by overgrowth of various anaerobic bacteria (e.g., *Prevotella*, *Mobiluncus*), *Gardnerella vaginalis*, *Ureaplasma urealyticum*, *Mycoplasma hominis*, *Atopobium vaginae*, or other bacteria. Treatment of bacterial vaginosis usually is recommended to relieve signs and symptoms of infection, regardless of pregnancy status.

For the treatment of bacterial vaginosis, CDC and other experts recommend a 7-day regimen of oral metronidazole (500 mg twice daily); a 5-day regimen of intravaginal metronidazole 0.75% gel; or a 7-day regimen of intravaginal clindamycin 2% cream. Alternative regimens include a 2-day regimen of oral tinidazole (2 g once daily); a 5-day regimen of oral tinidazole (1 g once daily); a 7-day regimen of oral clindamycin (300 mg twice daily); or a 3-day regimen of intravaginal clindamycin 100-mg suppositories. CDC and other clinicians state that the oral or intravaginal metronidazole or clindamycin regimens can be used to treat symptomatic bacterial vaginosis in pregnant women.

Regardless of the treatment regimen used, relapse or recurrence of bacterial vaginosis is common. Retreatment with the same regimen or an alternative regimen (e.g., oral therapy when topical therapy was used initially) can be effective for treating persistent or recurrent bacterial vaginosis after the first occurrence. Maintenance suppressive therapy with intravaginal metronidazole (0.75% gel twice weekly for 4–6 months) may reduce recurrences, but this benefit may not persist after suppressive therapy is discontinued.

● Malaria

Treatment of Uncomplicated Malaria

Oral clindamycin is used in conjunction with oral quinine sulfate for the *treatment* of uncomplicated chloroquine-resistant *Plasmodium falciparum* malaria† or when the plasmodial species has not been identified. Clindamycin is *not* effective when used alone for the treatment of malaria.

For the treatment of uncomplicated malaria caused by chloroquine-resistant *P. falciparum* or the treatment of uncomplicated malaria when the plasmodial species has not been identified, CDC and other clinicians recommend the fixed combination of atovaquone and proguanil hydrochloride (atovaquone/proguanil), the fixed combination of artemether and lumefantrine (artemether/lumefantrine), or a regimen that includes quinine sulfate in conjunction with doxycycline, tetracycline, or clindamycin. Although mefloquine is another option for treatment in these patients, CDC states that mefloquine should only be considered when other options cannot be used and is not recommended if malaria was acquired in Southeast Asia.

When a quinine sulfate regimen is used, concomitant doxycycline or tetracycline generally is preferable to concomitant clindamycin because more efficacy data exist regarding regimens that include tetracyclines. However, for pregnant women with uncomplicated malaria caused by chloroquine-resistant *P. falciparum*, a regimen of quinine sulfate and clindamycin is recommended. Although tetracyclines generally are contraindicated in pregnant women, in rare circumstances (e.g., if other treatment options are not available or are not tolerated) quinine sulfate may be used in conjunction with doxycycline or tetracycline if the benefits outweigh the risks.

Pediatric patients with uncomplicated malaria generally can receive the same treatment regimens recommended for adults using age- and weight-appropriate drugs and dosages. However, because doxycycline and tetracycline generally are contraindicated in children younger than 8 years of age, children in this age group with uncomplicated chloroquine-resistant *P. falciparum* malaria or when the plasmodial species has not been identified may receive a regimen of oral quinine sulfate *alone* for a full 7 days (regardless of geographic area where infection was acquired) or atovaquone/proguanil, artemether/lumefantrine, or a regimen of oral quinine sulfate in conjunction with oral clindamycin. Mefloquine should only be considered in these children when other options cannot be used and is not recommended if malaria was acquired in Southeast Asia. In rare circumstances when other treatment options are unavailable or are not tolerated, CDC states that doxycycline or tetracycline may be used in conjunction with quinine sulfate in children younger than 8 years of age if the benefits of tetracycline therapy outweigh the risks.

Treatment of Severe Malaria

Oral or IV clindamycin is used in conjunction with IV quinidine gluconate for the *treatment* of severe *P. falciparum* malaria† in adults and children.

Patients with severe malaria require aggressive antimalarial treatment initiated as soon as possible after the diagnosis using a parenteral regimen. CDC recommends that severe malaria be treated with IV quinidine gluconate therapy in conjunction with a 7-day course of doxycycline, tetracycline, or clindamycin administered orally or IV as tolerated. After parasitemia is reduced to less than 1% and the patient can tolerate oral therapy, IV quinidine gluconate can be discontinued and oral quinine sulfate initiated to complete 3 or 7 days of total quinidine and quinine therapy as determined by the geographic origin of the infecting parasite (7 days if acquired in Southeast Asia or 3 days if acquired elsewhere).

Assistance with diagnosis or treatment of malaria is available by contacting the CDC Malaria Hotline at 770-488-7788 or 855-856-4713 from 9:00 a.m. to 5:00 p.m. Eastern Standard Time or the CDC Emergency Operation Center at 770-488-7100 after hours and on weekends and holidays.

● Pelvic Inflammatory Disease

IV clindamycin used in conjunction with IV or IM gentamicin is one of several possible parenteral regimens for the treatment of acute pelvic inflammatory disease (PID) in adults and adolescents. PID is a polymicrobial infection most frequently caused by *Neisseria gonorrhoeae* and/or *Chlamydia trachomatis*; however, organisms that can be part of the normal vaginal flora (e.g., anaerobic bacteria, *G. vaginalis*, *H. influenzae*, enteric gram-negative bacilli, *S. agalactiae*) or mycoplasma (e.g., *M. hominis*, *U. urealyticum*) also may be involved. PID is treated with an empiric regimen that provides broad-spectrum coverage. The regimen should be effective against *N. gonorrhoeae* and *C. trachomatis* and also probably should be effective against anaerobes. In addition, women with PID often have bacterial vaginosis concurrently, a polymicrobial infection that can include anaerobes. (See Uses: Bacterial Vaginosis.)

The optimum regimen for the treatment of PID has not been identified. A variety of parenteral and oral regimens have been recommended by CDC and other clinicians. When a parenteral regimen is used, these experts recommend a regimen of IV cefotetan in conjunction with oral or IV doxycycline; IV cefoxitin in conjunction with oral or IV doxycycline; or IV clindamycin in conjunction with IM or IV gentamicin. The parenteral regimen should be continued until 24–48 hours after the patient improves clinically and then an oral regimen of either doxycycline (100 mg twice daily) or clindamycin (450 mg 4 times daily) is used to complete 14 days of therapy. If tubo-ovarian abscess is present, at least 24 hours of inpatient observation is recommended and use of oral clindamycin or oral metronidazole in addition to oral doxycycline is preferred for follow-up oral therapy since this provides more effective coverage against anaerobes than doxycycline alone.

● Pneumocystis jirovecii Pneumonia
Treatment of Pneumocystis jirovecii Pneumonia

Clindamycin is used in conjunction with primaquine for the treatment of *Pneumocystis jirovecii* (formerly *Pneumocystis carinii*) pneumonia† (PCP) in individuals with human immunodeficiency virus (HIV) infection. Clindamycin is designated an orphan drug by FDA for the treatment of PCP associated with acquired immunodeficiency syndrome (AIDS).

Co-trimoxazole is the drug of choice for the treatment of mild, moderate, or severe PCP, including PCP in HIV-infected adults, adolescents, and children. CDC, National Institutes of Health (NIH), and IDSA state that a regimen of primaquine and clindamycin is an alternative for the treatment of mild, moderate, or severe PCP in HIV-infected adults and adolescents who have had an inadequate response to co-trimoxazole or when co-trimoxazole is contraindicated or not tolerated. Although data are not available regarding use in children, CDC, NIH, IDSA, and AAP state that a regimen of primaquine and clindamycin also can be considered an alternative to co-trimoxazole for the treatment of PCP in HIV-infected children based on data in adults.

Results of clinical studies indicate that clindamycin administered IV (1.8–3.6 g given in 3 or 4 divided doses daily) or orally (1.2–3.6 g in 3 or 4 divided doses daily [in some cases oral clindamycin was administered after initial IV administration]) in conjunction with oral primaquine (15 or 30 mg daily) for a total 21 days of therapy is effective for the treatment of PCP in HIV-infected adults. Most patients exhibit clinical improvement within 2–7 days, and the combination generally appears to be well tolerated.

Prevention of Pneumocystis jirovecii Pneumonia

Co-trimoxazole is the drug of choice for prevention of initial episodes (primary prophylaxis) of PCP in HIV-infected adults, adolescents, and children. CDC, NIH, and IDSA state that a regimen of primaquine and clindamycin is *not* recommended for primary PCP prophylaxis because data are insufficient to determine efficacy of the regimen for such prophylaxis.

Although a regimen of clindamycin and primaquine has been used as an alternative to co-trimoxazole for long-term suppressive or chronic maintenance therapy (secondary prophylaxis) of PCP† in a limited number of AIDS patients, this regimen is *not* included in CDC, NIH, IDSA, and AAP recommendations for secondary prophylaxis of PCP in HIV-infected adults, adolescents, or children. Co-trimoxazole is the drug of choice for secondary PCP prophylaxis in HIV-infected adults, adolescents, and children.

● Toxoplasmosis
Treatment of Toxoplasmosis

Clindamycin is used in conjunction with pyrimethamine (and leucovorin) as an alternative for the treatment of toxoplasmosis caused by *Toxoplasma gondii*.

Pyrimethamine (and leucovorin) in conjunction with sulfadiazine is the regimen of choice for initial treatment of toxoplasmosis, including toxoplasmic encephalitis in HIV-infected adults, adolescents, and children. A regimen of pyrimethamine (and leucovorin) in conjunction with clindamycin is the preferred alternative in HIV-infected adults and adolescents who are unable to tolerate sulfadiazine or who failed to respond to an initial regimen of pyrimethamine and sulfadiazine. When a parenteral regimen is required for initial treatment of toxoplasmosis in severely ill adults or adolescents, some experts suggest parenteral co-trimoxazole or a regimen of oral pyrimethamine (and leucovorin) in conjunction with parenteral clindamycin.

Pyrimethamine (and leucovorin) in conjunction with sulfadiazine also is the regimen of choice for the treatment of congenital toxoplasmosis and the treatment of acquired CNS, ocular, or systemic toxoplasmosis in HIV-infected children. The preferred alternative for the treatment of toxoplasmosis in neonates or HIV-infected children with sulfonamide sensitivity is pyrimethamine (and leucovorin) in conjunction with clindamycin. Empiric treatment of congenital toxoplasmosis should be strongly considered in infants born to HIV-infected women who had symptomatic or asymptomatic toxoplasmosis during pregnancy, regardless of whether the mother received toxoplasmosis treatment during the pregnancy. Pregnant women with suspected or confirmed primary toxoplasmosis and neonates with possible or documented congenital toxoplasmosis should be managed in consultation with an appropriate infectious disease specialist.

Prevention of Recurrence of Toxoplasmosis

CDC, NIH, IDSA, and AAP state that HIV-infected adults, adolescents, and children who have completed initial treatment of *T. gondii* encephalitis should receive chronic maintenance therapy (secondary prophylaxis) to prevent relapse.

Pyrimethamine (and leucovorin) in conjunction with sulfadiazine is the regimen of choice for long-term suppressive or chronic maintenance therapy (secondary prophylaxis) of toxoplasmosis in HIV-infected adults, adolescents, and children. A regimen of pyrimethamine (and leucovorin) in conjunction with clindamycin is one of several alternatives for secondary prophylaxis of toxoplasmosis in HIV-infected adults, adolescents, and children who cannot tolerate sulfonamides.

CDC, NIH, and IDSA state that secondary prophylaxis against toxoplasmosis generally can be discontinued in HIV-infected adults and adolescents who have successfully completed initial therapy for toxoplasmic encephalitis, remain asymptomatic with respect to toxoplasmic encephalitis, and have CD4+ T-cell counts that have remained greater than 200/mm³ for more than 6 months in response to antiretroviral therapy. Some experts recommend obtaining a magnetic resonance image (MRI) of the brain as part of the evaluation to determine whether discontinuance of secondary prophylaxis is appropriate. Secondary prophylaxis against toxoplasmosis should be reinitiated in HIV-infected adults and adolescents if CD4+ T-cell counts decrease to less than 200/mm³, regardless of plasma HIV viral load.

The safety of discontinuing secondary toxoplasmosis prophylaxis in HIV-infected children receiving potent antiretroviral therapy has not been extensively studied. However, based on data from adults, CDC, NIH, IDSA, and AAP state that discontinuance of secondary prophylaxis against toxoplasmosis can be considered in HIV-infected children 1 to less than 6 years of age who have completed toxoplasmosis treatment, have received more than 6 months of stable antiretroviral therapy, are asymptomatic with respect to toxoplasmosis, and have CD4+ T-cell percentages that have remained greater than 15% for more than 6 consecutive months. In HIV-infected children 6 years of age or older who have received more than 6 months of antiretroviral therapy, consideration can be given to discontinuing secondary prophylaxis against toxoplasmosis if CD4+ T-cell counts have remained greater than 200/mm³ for more than 6 consecutive months. Prophylaxis should be reinitiated in HIV-infected children if these parameters are not met.

● Perioperative Prophylaxis

IV clindamycin is recommended as an alternative for perioperative prophylaxis† to reduce the incidence of infections in patients undergoing certain clean, contaminated surgeries when the drugs of choice (e.g., cefazolin, cefuroxime, cefoxitin, cefotetan) cannot be used because the patient is hypersensitive to β-lactam anti-infectives.

Some experts state that clindamycin or vancomycin is a reasonable alternative for perioperative prophylaxis in patients allergic to β-lactam anti-infectives who are undergoing cardiac surgery (e.g., coronary artery bypass grafting, valve repairs, cardiac device implantation), neurosurgery (e.g., craniotomy, spinal and CSF-shunting procedures, intrathecal pump placement), orthopedic surgery (e.g., spinal procedures, hip fracture, internal fixation, total joint replacement), non-cardiac thoracic surgery (e.g., lobectomy, pneumonectomy, lung resection, thoracotomy), vascular surgery (e.g., arterial procedures involving a prosthesis, the abdominal aorta, or a groin incision), lower extremity amputation for ischemia, or certain transplant procedures (e.g., heart and/or lung). These experts state that clindamycin also is a reasonable alternative for perioperative prophylaxis in patients allergic to β-lactam anti-infectives who are undergoing head and neck surgery (e.g., incisions through oral or pharyngeal mucosa).

For procedures that might involve exposure to enteric gram-negative bacteria, some experts state that clindamycin or vancomycin used in conjunction with an aminoglycoside (e.g., amikacin, gentamicin, tobramycin), aztreonam, or a fluoroquinolone is a reasonable alternative in patients allergic to β-lactam anti-infectives. These procedures include certain GI and biliary tract procedures (e.g., esophageal or gastroduodenal procedures, appendectomy for uncomplicated appendicitis, surgery involving unobstructed small intestine, colorectal procedures), gynecologic and obstetric surgery (e.g., cesarean section, hysterectomy), urologic procedures involving an implanted prosthesis, and certain transplant procedures (e.g., liver, pancreas and/or kidney).

● Prevention of Bacterial Endocarditis

Clindamycin is used as an alternative to amoxicillin or ampicillin for prevention of α-hemolytic (viridans group) streptococcal bacterial endocarditis† in penicillin-allergic adults and children undergoing certain dental or upper respiratory tract procedures who have cardiac conditions that put them at highest risk of adverse outcomes from endocarditis.

The cardiac conditions identified by AHA as those associated with highest risk and for which endocarditis prophylaxis is reasonable are prosthetic cardiac valves or prosthetic material used for cardiac valve repair, previous infective endocarditis, cardiac valvulopathy after cardiac transplantation, and certain forms of congenital heart disease (i.e., unrepaired

cyanotic congenital heart disease including palliative shunts and conduits; a completely repaired congenital heart defect where prosthetic material or device was placed by surgery or catheter intervention within the last 6 months; repaired congenital heart disease with residual defects at the site or adjacent to the site of a prosthetic patch or prosthetic device that inhibit endothelialization).

AHA states that anti-infective prophylaxis for prevention of α-hemolytic (viridans group) streptococcal bacterial endocarditis is reasonable for patients with the above cardiac risk factors if they are undergoing any dental procedures that involve manipulation of gingival tissue or the periapical region of teeth or perforation of the oral mucosa (e.g., biopsies, suture removal, placement of orthodontic bands). AHA states that anti-infective prophylaxis is not needed for routine anesthetic injections through noninfected tissue, dental radiographs, placement of removable prosthodontic or orthodontic appliances, adjustment of orthodontic appliances, placement of orthodontic brackets, shedding of deciduous teeth, or bleeding from trauma to the lips or oral mucosa.

AHA states that anti-infective prophylaxis for prevention of bacterial endocarditis also is reasonable for patients with these cardiac risk factors if they are undergoing invasive procedures of the respiratory tract that involve incision or biopsy of respiratory mucosa (e.g., tonsillectomy, adenoidectomy) and may be reasonable for such patients if they are undergoing surgical procedures that involve infected skin, skin structure, or musculoskeletal tissue. However, anti-infective prophylaxis solely to prevent infective endocarditis is no longer recommended by AHA for GI or genitourinary tract procedures.

For additional information on which cardiac conditions are associated with the highest risk of adverse outcomes from endocarditis and more specific information regarding use of prophylaxis to prevent endocarditis in these patients, the current recommendations published by AHA should be consulted.

● Prevention of Perinatal Group B Streptococcal Disease

IV clindamycin is used as an alternative to parenteral penicillin G or ampicillin for prevention of perinatal group B streptococcal (GBS) disease† in certain women who are hypersensitive to penicillins.

Pregnant women who are colonized with GBS in the genital or rectal areas can transmit GBS infection to their infants during labor and delivery, resulting in invasive neonatal infection that can be associated with substantial morbidity and mortality. Intrapartum anti-infective prophylaxis for prevention of early-onset neonatal GBS disease is administered *selectively* to women at high risk for transmitting GBS infection to their neonates. CDC and AAP recommend *routine* universal prenatal screening for GBS colonization (e.g., vaginal and rectal cultures) in *all* pregnant women at 35–37 weeks of gestation, unless GBS bacteriuria is known to be present during the current pregnancy or the woman had a previous infant with invasive GBS disease. Intrapartum anti-infective prophylaxis for prevention of perinatal GBS is indicated in pregnant women identified as GBS carriers during the routine prenatal GBS screening performed at 35–37 weeks during the current pregnancy, in women with GBS bacteriuria identified at any time during the current pregnancy, and in women who had a previous infant diagnosed with invasive GBS disease. Intrapartum anti-infective prophylaxis also is indicated in women with unknown GBS status at the time of onset of labor (i.e., culture not done, incomplete, or results unknown), if delivery is at less than 37 weeks of gestation, the duration of amniotic membrane rupture is 18 hours or longer, intrapartum temperature is 38°C or higher, or an intrapartum nucleic acid amplification test (NAAT) was positive for GBS.

When intrapartum anti-infective prophylaxis is indicated in the mother for prevention of GBS in the neonate, it should be initiated at the onset of labor or rupture of membranes. CDC, AAP, and others recommend penicillin G as the drug of choice and ampicillin as the preferred alternative for such prophylaxis. If intrapartum prophylaxis is indicated in a penicillin-allergic woman who is *not* at high risk for anaphylaxis (i.e., does not have a history of anaphylaxis, angioedema, respiratory distress, or urticaria after receiving a penicillin or cephalosporin), CDC, AAP, and others recommend IV cefazolin. If intrapartum prophylaxis is indicated in a penicillin-allergic woman who is at high risk for anaphylaxis (e.g., history of anaphylaxis, angioedema, respiratory distress, or urticaria after receiving a penicillin or cephalosporin), IV clindamycin is recommended if the GBS isolate is tested and found to be susceptible to clindamycin *and* erythromycin. GBS isolates susceptible to clindamycin but resistant to erythromycin in vitro should be evaluated for inducible clindamycin resistance. IV vancomycin can be used as an alternative in penicillin-allergic women if the GBS isolate is intrinsically resistant to clindamycin, demonstrates inducible resistance to clindamycin, or if susceptibility to clindamycin and erythromycin is unknown.

For additional information regarding prevention of perinatal group B streptococcal disease, the current guidelines from CDC or AAP should be consulted.

● Topical Uses

For topical uses of clindamycin, see Clindamycin Phosphate 84:04.04.

DOSAGE AND ADMINISTRATION

● Reconstitution and Administration

Clindamycin hydrochloride and clindamycin palmitate hydrochloride are administered orally.

Clindamycin phosphate is administered by IM injection or by intermittent or continuous IV infusion. Clindamycin phosphate should *not* be administered by rapid IV injection.

In the treatment of serious anaerobic infections, the parenteral route is usually used initially but may be switched to the oral route when warranted by the patient's condition. In clinically appropriate circumstances, the oral route may be used initially.

Oral Administration

Clindamycin hydrochloride capsules and clindamycin palmitate hydrochloride oral solution can be administered without regard to food.

Capsules

Clindamycin hydrochloride capsules should be administered orally with a full glass of water to avoid the possibility of esophageal irritation.

The capsules should be swallowed whole and are not suitable for use in pediatric patients who are unable to swallow capsules.

Oral Solution

Clindamycin palmitate hydrochloride powder (granules) for oral solution must be reconstituted by adding 75 mL of water to the 100-mL bottle. A large portion of the 75 mL should be added initially and the bottle shaken vigorously; the remainder of the water should then be added and the bottle shaken until the solution is uniform.

The reconstituted oral solution contains 75 mg of clindamycin per 5 mL.

IM Injection

For IM injection, commercially available clindamycin phosphate solution containing 150 mg of clindamycin per mL is administered undiluted.

Single IM doses should not exceed 600 mg.

IV Infusion

Prior to IV infusion, commercially available clindamycin phosphate solution (including solutions provided in ADD-Vantage® vials) must be diluted with a compatible IV solution to a concentration not exceeding 18 mg/mL.

Clindamycin phosphate usually is administered by intermittent IV infusion. As an alternative, clindamycin phosphate may be given by continuous IV infusion *after* the first dose of the drug has been given by rapid IV infusion. (See Table 1.)

Commercially available premixed solutions of clindamycin phosphate in 5% dextrose are administered *only* by IV infusion. Clindamycin phosphate in 5% dextrose injection should be inspected visually for particulate matter and discoloration before administration whenever solution and container permit. Premixed solutions provided in flexible containers should be checked for minute leaks by firmly squeezing the bag. Premixed solutions should be discarded if the container seal is not intact or leaks are found or if the solution is not clear. Additives should not be introduced into containers of premixed solutions of clindamycin phosphate in 5% dextrose. Flexible containers should not be used in series connections with other plastic containers, since such use could result in air embolism from residual air being drawn from the primary container before administration of the fluid from the secondary container is complete.

Dilution

When commercially available clindamycin phosphate solution containing 150 mg of clindamycin per mL is used for IV infusion, the appropriate dose should be diluted in a compatible IV infusion solution and administered using the recommended rate of administration. (See Rate of Administration under Reconstitution and Administration: IV Infusion, in Dosage and Administration.)

Clindamycin phosphate solution provided in ADD-Vantage® vials must be diluted prior to IV infusion according to the directions provided by the manufacturer. The ADD-Vantage® vials are for IV infusion only.

Commercially available clindamycin phosphate pharmacy bulk packages are *not* intended for direct IV infusion; doses of the drug from the bulk package must be further diluted in a compatible IV infusion solution. The bulk package is intended for use only in a laminar flow hood. Entry into the bulk pharmacy vial should be made using a sterile transfer set or other sterile dispensing device, and the contents dispensed in aliquots using appropriate technique; multiple entries with a syringe and needle are not recommended. After entry into a pharmacy bulk package vial, the entire contents of the vial should be used promptly; any unused portion should be discarded within 24 hours after initial entry into the pharmacy bulk package vial.

Rate of Administration

Intermittent IV infusions of clindamycin phosphate solutions should be given over a period of at least 10–60 minutes and at a rate less than 30 mg/minute. No more than 1.2 g should be given by IV infusion in a single 1-hour period.

The manufacturer recommends that 300-mg doses should be diluted in 50 mL of compatible diluent and infused over 10 minutes; 600-mg doses should be diluted in 50 mL of diluent and infused over 20 minutes; 900-mg doses should be diluted in 50–100 mL of diluent and infused over 30 minutes; and 1.2-g doses should be diluted in 100 mL of diluent and infused over 40 minutes.

As an alternative to intermittent IV infusions, the manufacturer states that the drug can be given by continuous IV infusion in adults *after* an initial dose is given by IV infusion over 30 minutes. (See Table 1.)

TABLE 1. Infusion Rates for Continuous IV Infusion of Clindamycin Phosphate in Adults

Target Serum Clindamycin Concentrations	Infusion Rate for Initial Dose	Maintenance Infusion Rate
Greater than 4 mcg/mL	10 mg/minute for 30 minutes	0.75 mg/minute
Greater than 5 mcg/mL	15 mg/minute for 30 minutes	1 mg/minute
Greater than 6 mcg/mL	20 mg/minute for 30 minutes	1.25 mg/minute

● Dosage

Dosage of clindamycin hydrochloride, clindamycin palmitate hydrochloride, and clindamycin phosphate is expressed in terms of clindamycin.

Dosage and duration of treatment depend on the severity of the infection. If clindamycin is used in infections caused by *Streptococcus pyogenes* (group A β-hemolytic streptococci; GAS), therapy should be continued for at least 10 days. At least 6 weeks of therapy may be required for certain serious infections (e.g., osteomyelitis).

Oral Dosage

General Dosage for Neonates

When clindamycin oral solution is used in pediatric patients, the manufacturer recommends 8–12 mg/kg daily for the treatment of serious infections, 13–16 mg/kg daily for severe infections, and 17–25 mg/kg daily for more severe infections; daily dosage is given in 3 or 4 equally divided doses. In pediatric patients weighing 10 kg or less, the manufacturer recommends a minimum clindamycin dosage of 37.5 mg 3 times daily.

When oral clindamycin is used in neonates 7 days of age or younger, the American Academy of Pediatrics (AAP) recommends a dosage of 5 mg/kg every

12 hours in those weighing 2 kg or less or 5 mg/kg every 8 hours in those weighing more than 2 kg.

In neonates 8–28 days of age, AAP recommends an oral clindamycin dosage of 5 mg/kg every 8 hours in those weighing 2 kg or less or 5 mg/kg every 6 hours in those weighing more than 2 kg. In extremely low-birthweight neonates (less than 1 kg), a dosage of 5 mg/kg every 12 hours can be considered until 2 weeks of age.

General Dosage for Infants and Children

When clindamycin capsules are used in pediatric patients able to swallow capsules, the manufacturer recommends 8–16 mg/kg daily given in 3 or 4 equally divided doses for the treatment of serious infections or 16–20 mg/kg daily given in 3 or 4 equally divided doses for more severe infections.

When the oral solution is used in pediatric patients, the manufacturer recommends 8–12 mg/kg daily for the treatment of serious infections, 13–16 mg/kg daily for severe infections, and 17–25 mg/kg daily for more severe infections; daily dosage is given in 3 or 4 equally divided doses. In pediatric patients weighing 10 kg or less, the manufacturer recommends a minimum dosage of 37.5 mg 3 times daily.

When oral clindamycin is used in pediatric patients beyond the neonatal period, AAP recommends a dosage of 10–25 mg/kg daily given in 3 equally divided doses for the treatment of mild to moderate infections or 30–40 mg/kg daily given in 3 or 4 divided doses for the treatment of severe infections.

General Adult Dosage

The usual adult dosage of oral clindamycin is 150–300 mg every 6 hours for the treatment of serious infections or 300–450 mg every 6 hours for the treatment of more severe infections.

Acute Otitis Media

If oral clindamycin is used as an alternative for the treatment of acute otitis media† (AOM) in children 6 months through 12 years of age, AAP recommends a dosage of 30–40 mg/kg daily given in 3 divided doses (with or without a third generation cephalosporin). (See Uses: Acute Otitis Media.)

Pharyngitis and Tonsillitis

If oral clindamycin is used as an alternative for the treatment of pharyngitis and tonsillitis caused by S. pyogenes† (group A β-hemolytic streptococci; GAS) (see Uses: Pharyngitis and Tonsillitis), AAP recommends a dosage of 10 mg/kg 3 times daily (up to 900 mg daily) for 10 days. The Infectious Diseases Society of America (IDSA) recommends a dosage of 7 mg/kg (up to 300 mg) 3 times daily for 10 days. The American Heart Association (AHA) recommends a dosage of 20 mg/kg daily (up to 1.8 g daily) given in 3 divided doses for 10 days.

Although anti-infective treatment is not recommended for most individuals identified as chronic pharyngeal GAS carriers, AAP and IDSA state that oral clindamycin can be given in a dosage of 20–30 mg/kg daily in 3 equally divided doses (up to 300 mg per dose or up to 900 mg daily) for 10 days when treatment is indicated in such patients.

Respiratory Tract Infections

If oral clindamycin is used in adults for the treatment of healthcare-associated or community-acquired pneumonia (CAP) caused by susceptible methicillin-resistant Staphylococcus aureus (MRSA; also known as oxacillin-resistant S. aureus or ORSA), IDSA recommends a dosage of 600 mg 3 times daily for 7–21 days.

If oral clindamycin is used for the treatment of CAP caused by susceptible gram-positive bacteria (e.g., S. pneumoniae, S. pyogenes, S. aureus) in children older than 3 months of age, IDSA recommends a dosage of 30–40 mg/kg daily given in 3 or 4 divided doses.

Babesiosis

For the treatment of babesiosis† caused by Babesia microti or other Babesia species, IDSA and other experts recommend that adults receive clindamycin in a dosage of 600 mg orally every 8 hours (or 300–600 mg IV every 6 hours) in conjunction with oral quinine sulfate (650 mg every 6 or 8 hours) given for 7–10 days.

For the treatment of babesiosis in pediatric patients, IDSA recommends an oral (or IV) clindamycin dosage of 7–10 mg/kg (up to 600 mg) every 6–8 hours in conjunction with oral quinine sulfate (8 mg/kg [up to 650 mg] every 8 hours)

given for 7–10 days. Other clinicians recommend an oral (or IV) clindamycin dosage of 20–40 mg/kg (up to 600 mg) daily given in 3 or 4 divided doses for 7–10 days in conjunction with oral quinine sulfate (24 mg/kg daily given in 3 divided doses for 7–10 days).

Patients with mild to moderate babesiosis should have clinical improvement within 48 hours after treatment is initiated; symptoms should resolve completely within 3 months. Patients with severe babesiosis should receive IV clindamycin rather than oral clindamycin. Some patients may have persistent low-grade parasitemia for months after anti-infective treatment. Some experts suggest that anti-infective treatment in immunosuppressed patients should be continued for a minimum of 6 weeks and at least 2 weeks after the last positive smear. Regardless of the presence or absence of symptoms, IDSA suggests that retreatment be considered if babesial parasites or amplifiable babesial DNA is detected in blood 3 months or longer after initial treatment.

Bacterial Vaginosis

When oral clindamycin is used as an alternative for the treatment of bacterial vaginosis† in symptomatic women, the US Centers for Disease Control and Prevention (CDC) and other clinicians recommend a dosage of 300 mg twice daily for 7 days.

Malaria

If clindamycin is used in conjunction with quinine sulfate for the treatment of uncomplicated malaria caused by chloroquine-resistant Plasmodium falciparum† or when the plasmodial species has not been identified, CDC and other clinicians recommend that adults receive oral clindamycin in a dosage of 20 mg/kg daily in 3 equally divided doses given for 7 days in conjunction with oral quinine sulfate (650 mg 3 times daily given for 7 days if acquired in Southeast Asia or for 3 days if acquired elsewhere). Children with uncomplicated chloroquine-resistant P. falciparum malaria can receive oral clindamycin in a dosage of 20 mg/kg daily in 3 equally divided doses given for 7 days in conjunction with oral quinine sulfate (10 mg/kg 3 times daily given for 7 days if acquired in Southeast Asia or 3 days if acquired elsewhere).

If clindamycin is used in conjunction with IV quinidine gluconate (followed by oral quinine sulfate) for the treatment of severe malaria caused by P. falciparum† and if the patient is intolerant of oral therapy, treatment may be initiated in adults and children with a 10-mg/kg loading dose of IV clindamycin followed by 5 mg/kg IV every 8 hours continued until treatment can be switched to oral clindamycin (given in dosages recommended for uncomplicated malaria). The total duration of clindamycin therapy should be 7 days.

Pneumocystis jirovecii Pneumonia

If a regimen of oral clindamycin and primaquine is used as an alternative for the treatment of mild to moderate Pneumocystis jirovecii pneumonia† (PCP), CDC, National Institutes of Health (NIH), and IDSA recommend that adults and adolescents receive oral clindamycin in a dosage of 450 mg every 6 hours or 600 mg every 8 hours for 21 days in conjunction with oral primaquine (30 mg once daily for 21 days).

If a regimen of oral clindamycin and primaquine is used as an alternative for the treatment of moderate to severe PCP†, CDC, NIH, and IDSA recommend that adults and adolescents receive oral clindamycin in a dosage of 450 mg every 6 hours or 600 mg every 8 hours for 21 days in conjunction with oral primaquine (30 mg once daily for 21 days).

Although data regarding use in children are not available, if a regimen of oral clindamycin and primaquine is used as an alternative for the treatment of PCP in pediatric patients, some clinicians recommend that oral clindamycin be given in a dosage of 10 mg/kg (up to 300–450 mg) every 6 hours for 21 days in conjunction with oral primaquine (0.3 mg/kg once daily [up to 30 mg daily] for 21 days).

Toxoplasmosis

For the treatment of toxoplasmosis† caused by Toxoplasma gondii in HIV-infected adults and adolescents who cannot receive sulfadiazine or did not respond to an initial regimen, CDC, NIH, and IDSA recommend an oral (or IV) clindamycin dosage of 600 mg every 6 hours in conjunction with oral pyrimethamine (200-mg loading dose followed by 50 mg once daily in those weighing less than 60 kg or 75 mg once daily in those weighing 60 kg or more) and oral leucovorin (10–25 mg once daily; may be increased to 50 mg once or twice daily). Treatment should be continued for at least 6 weeks; a longer duration may be appropriate if disease is extensive or there is an incomplete response at 6 weeks.

For the treatment of congenital toxoplasmosis† or the treatment of acquired CNS, ocular, or systemic toxoplasmosis† in HIV-infected children who cannot receive sulfadiazine, CDC, NIH, and IDSA recommend an oral (or IV) clindamycin dosage of 5–7.5 mg/kg (up to 600 mg) 4 times daily in conjunction with oral pyrimethamine (2 mg/kg once daily for 2 days followed by 1 mg/kg once daily) and oral or IM leucovorin (10 mg with each pyrimethamine dose). Although optimal duration of treatment of congenital toxoplasmosis has not been determined, some clinicians recommend that the treatment regimen be continued for 12 months. In HIV-infected children with acquired CNS, ocular, or systemic toxoplasmosis, the treatment regimen should be continued for at least 6 weeks; a longer duration may be appropriate if disease is extensive or there is an incomplete response at 6 weeks.

For long-term suppressive therapy or chronic maintenance therapy† (secondary prophylaxis) to prevent relapse of toxoplasmosis in HIV-infected patients when the regimen of first choice (pyrimethamine and sulfadiazine) cannot be used, CDC, NIH, and IDSA recommend that adults and adolescents receive oral clindamycin in a dosage of 600 mg every 8 hours with pyrimethamine (25–50 mg once daily) and leucovorin (10–25 mg once daily). For secondary prophylaxis in HIV-infected infants and children, CDC, NIH, IDSA, and AAP recommend an oral clindamycin dosage of 7–10 mg/kg 3 times daily with oral pyrimethamine (1 mg/kg or 15 mg/m² [up to 25 mg] once daily) and oral leucovorin (5 mg once every 3 days). Long-term suppressive therapy for prophylaxis against relapse of toxoplasmosis in HIV-infected individuals generally can be discontinued if immune recovery has occurred as the result of potent antiretroviral therapy. (See Prevention of Recurrence of Toxoplasmosis under Uses: Toxoplasmosis.)

Prevention of Bacterial Endocarditis

When oral clindamycin is used as an alternative for prevention of bacterial endocarditis† in penicillin-allergic patients with certain cardiac conditions who are undergoing certain dental procedures or certain other procedures (see Uses: Prevention of Bacterial Endocarditis), AHA recommends that adults receive a single 600-mg dose and that children receive a single 20-mg/kg dose of the drug 30–60 minutes before the procedure.

Parenteral Dosage
General Dosage for Neonates

The manufacturer recommends that neonates younger than 1 month of age receive IM or IV clindamycin in a dosage of 15–20 mg/kg daily given in 3 or 4 equally divided doses. The lower dosage may be adequate for small, premature neonates.

When IM or IV clindamycin is used in neonates 7 days of age or younger, AAP recommends 5 mg/kg every 12 hours in those weighing 2 kg or less or 5 mg/kg every 8 hours in those weighing more than 2 kg.

In neonates 8–28 days of age, AAP recommends an IM or IV clindamycin dosage of 5 mg/kg every 8 hours in those weighing 2 kg or less or 5 mg/kg every 6 hours in those weighing more than 2 kg. In extremely low-birthweight neonates (less than 1 kg), a dosage of 5 mg/kg every 12 hours can be considered until 2 weeks of age.

General Dosage for Infants and Children

The IM or IV dosage of clindamycin recommended by the manufacturer for infants and children 1 month of age or older is 20–40 mg/kg daily administered in 3 or 4 equally divided doses; the higher dosage should be used for more severe infections. Alternatively, the manufacturer states that these infants and children may receive 350 mg/m² daily for the treatment of serious infections or 450 mg/m² daily for the treatment of more severe infections.

In pediatric patients beyond the neonatal period, AAP recommends an IM or IV clindamycin dosage of 20–30 mg/kg daily given in 3 equally divided doses for the treatment of mild to moderate infections or 40 mg/kg daily given in 3 or 4 equally divided doses for the treatment of severe infections.

General Adult Dosage

The recommended adult dosage of IM or IV clindamycin is 600 mg to 1.2 g daily given in 2–4 equally divided doses for the treatment of serious infections or 1.2–2.7 g daily given in 2–4 equally divided doses for the treatment of more severe infections. In the treatment of life-threatening infections, adult IV dosage may be increased to a maximum of 4.8 g daily.

If continuous IV infusion of clindamycin is used to maintain serum clindamycin concentrations above 4–6 mcg/mL in adults, an initial dose is given by rapid IV infusion prior to continuous IV infusion. (See Table 1.)

Respiratory Tract Infections

If IV clindamycin is used in adults for the treatment of healthcare-associated pneumonia or CAP caused by susceptible methicillin-resistant *S. aureus* (MRSA), IDSA recommends a dosage of 600 mg 3 times daily for 7–21 days.

If parenteral clindamycin is used for the treatment of CAP caused by susceptible gram-positive bacteria (e.g., *S. pneumoniae*, *S. pyogenes*, *S. aureus*) in children older than 3 months of age, IDSA recommends a dosage of 40 mg/kg daily given in divided doses every 6–8 hours.

Anthrax

Although the optimum regimen for the treatment of inhalational anthrax† remains to be established, several patients who developed inhalational anthrax in the context of an intentional release of anthrax spores (biologic warfare, bioterrorism) were treated successfully with a multiple-drug regimen that included IV clindamycin (900 mg every 8 hours), IV ciprofloxacin (400 mg every 8 hours), and IV rifampin (300 mg every 12 hours). (See Uses: Anthrax.)

Duration of treatment is 60 days if anthrax occurred as the result of exposure to anthrax spores in the context of biologic warfare or bioterrorism.

Babesiosis

For the treatment of babesiosis† caused by *B. microti* or other *Babesia* species, IDSA and other experts recommend that adults receive clindamycin in a dosage of 300–600 mg IV every 6 hours (or 600 mg orally every 8 hours) in conjunction with oral quinine sulfate (650 mg every 6 or 8 hours) given for 7–10 days.

For the treatment of babesiosis in pediatric patients, IDSA recommends an IV (or oral) clindamycin dosage of 7–10 mg/kg (up to 600 mg) every 6–8 hours in conjunction with oral quinine sulfate (8 mg/kg [up to 650 mg] every 8 hours) given for 7–10 days. Other clinicians recommend an IV (or oral) clindamycin dosage of 20–40 mg/kg (up to 600 mg) daily given in 3 or 4 divided doses for 7–10 days in conjunction with oral quinine sulfate (24 mg/kg daily given in 3 divided doses for 7–10 days).

Patients with mild to moderate babesiosis should have clinical improvement within 48 hours after treatment is initiated; symptoms should resolve completely within 3 months. Patients with severe babesiosis should receive IV clindamycin rather than oral clindamycin. Some patients may have persistent low-grade parasitemia for months after anti-infective treatment. Some experts suggest that anti-infective treatment in immunosuppressed patients should be continued for a minimum of 6 weeks and at least 2 weeks after the last positive smear. Regardless of the presence or absence of symptoms, IDSA suggests that retreatment be considered if babesial parasites or amplifiable babesial DNA is detected in blood 3 months or longer after initial treatment.

Pelvic Inflammatory Disease

For the treatment of acute pelvic inflammatory disease (PID) when a parenteral regimen is indicated, adults and adolescents may receive 900 mg of clindamycin IV every 8 hours. Gentamicin sulfate should be administered concomitantly (initial IM or IV gentamicin dose of 2 mg/kg followed by 1.5 mg/kg every 8 hours; alternatively, 3–5 mg/kg of gentamicin can be given as a single daily dose). Both parenteral drugs can be discontinued 24–48 hours after there is clinical improvement and therapy continued with oral clindamycin in a dosage of 450 mg 4 times daily to complete 14 days of therapy. Alternatively, oral doxycycline (100 mg twice daily) can be given to complete 14 days of therapy. (See Uses: Pelvic Inflammatory Disease.)

Patients with PID who do not demonstrate substantial clinical improvement (e.g., defervescence; reduction in direct or rebound abdominal tenderness; reduction in uterine, adnexal, and cervical motion tenderness) within 72 hours of initiating parenteral or oral therapy usually require additional diagnostic tests and/or surgical intervention.

Pneumocystis jirovecii Pneumonia

If a regimen of IV clindamycin and oral primaquine is used as an alternative for the treatment of moderate to severe PCP†, CDC, NIH, and IDSA recommend that adults and adolescents receive IV clindamycin in a dosage of 600 mg every 6 hours or 900 mg every 8 hours for 21 days in conjunction with oral primaquine (30 mg once daily for 21 days).

Although data regarding use in children are not available, if a regimen of IV clindamycin and oral primaquine is used as an alternative for the treatment of PCP in pediatric patients, some clinicians recommend that IV clindamycin be given in a dosage of 10 mg/kg (up to 600 mg) every 6 hours for 21 days in conjunction with oral primaquine (0.3 mg/kg once daily [up to 30 mg daily] for 21 days).

Toxoplasmosis

For the treatment of toxoplasmosis† in HIV-infected adults and adolescents who cannot receive sulfadiazine or did not respond to an initial regimen, CDC, NIH, and IDSA recommend that adults and adolescents receive IV (or oral) clindamycin in a dosage of 600 mg every 6 hours in conjunction with oral pyrimethamine (200-mg loading dose followed by 50 mg once daily in those weighing less than 60 kg or 75 mg once daily in those weighing 60 kg or more) and oral leucovorin (10–25 mg once daily; may be increased to 50 mg once or twice daily).

For the treatment of congenital toxoplasmosis† or the treatment of acquired CNS, ocular, or systemic toxoplasmosis† in HIV-infected children, CDC, NIH, and IDSA recommend an IV (or oral) clindamycin dosage of 5–7.5 mg/kg (up to 600 mg) 4 times daily in conjunction with oral pyrimethamine (2 mg/kg once daily for 2 days followed by 1 mg/kg once daily) and oral or IM leucovorin (10 mg with each pyrimethamine dose). Although optimal duration of treatment has not been determined, some experts recommend that treatment of congenital toxoplasmosis be continued for 12 months. The treatment regimen should be continued for at least 6 weeks in HIV-infected children with acquired CNS, ocular, or systemic toxoplasmosis; a longer duration may be appropriate for extensive disease or if there is an incomplete response at 6 weeks.

Perioperative Prophylaxis

If clindamycin is used alone or in conjunction with another anti-infective for perioperative prophylaxis in patients undergoing certain surgeries when the drugs of choice cannot be used (see Uses: Perioperative Prophylaxis), some clinicians recommend that adults receive 900 mg of the drug and that pediatric patients receive 10 mg/kg of the drug given IV within 60 minutes prior to the initial incision.

During prolonged procedures, some clinicians suggest that additional intraoperative doses of clindamycin can be given every 6 hours for the duration of the procedure in patients with normal renal function. Postoperative doses of prophylactic anti-infectives generally are not recommended.

Prevention of Bacterial Endocarditis

When IM or IV clindamycin is used as an alternative for prevention of bacterial endocarditis† in penicillin-allergic patients (or patients unable to take oral medication) with certain cardiac conditions who are undergoing certain dental procedures or certain other procedures (see Uses: Prevention of Bacterial Endocarditis), AHA recommends that adults receive a single 600-mg dose and that children receive a single 20-mg/kg dose of the drug given 30–60 minutes before the procedure.

Prevention of Perinatal Group B Streptococcal Disease

If clindamycin is used for intrapartum anti-infective prophylaxis for prevention of perinatal group B streptococcal (GBS) disease† in women with penicillin hypersensitivity who should not receive a β-lactam anti-infective, CDC and AAP recommend that 900 mg of clindamycin be given IV at the time of onset of labor or rupture of membranes followed by 900 mg IV every 8 hours until delivery. Because *S. agalactiae* (group B streptococci; GBS) with resistance to clindamycin has been reported with increasing frequency, clinical isolates obtained during GBS prenatal screening should be tested for in vitro susceptibility to clindamycin whenever use of the drug is being considered for prevention of perinatal GBS disease. (See Uses: Prevention of Perinatal Group B Streptococcal Disease.)

● Dosage in Renal and Hepatic Impairment
Renal Impairment

Dosage adjustments are not usually necessary in patients with renal impairment.

Hepatic Impairment

Dosage adjustments are not usually necessary in patients with hepatic impairment. However, because the plasma half-life of clindamycin may be prolonged, hepatic function should be monitored if the drug is used in those with severe hepatic impairment.

CAUTIONS

● GI Effects

Adverse GI effects frequently occur with oral, IM, or IV clindamycin and may be severe enough to necessitate discontinuance of the drug. Adverse GI effects reported in patients receiving clindamycin include nausea, vomiting, diarrhea, abdominal pain, and esophagitis. In addition, tenesmus, flatulence, bloating, anorexia, and weight loss have been reported.

An unpleasant or metallic taste has been reported in patients receiving oral clindamycin and also has been reported following IV administration of high doses of the drug.

Clostridium difficile-associated Diarrhea and Colitis

Treatment with anti-infectives alters normal colon flora and may permit overgrowth of *Clostridium difficile*.

C. difficile infection (CDI) and *C. difficile*-associated diarrhea and colitis (CDAD; also known as antibiotic-associated diarrhea and colitis or pseudomembranous colitis) have been reported with nearly all anti-infectives, including clindamycin, and may range in severity from mild diarrhea to fatal colitis. *C. difficile* produces toxins A and B, which contribute to the development of CDAD; hypertoxin-producing strains of *C. difficile* are associated with increased morbidity and mortality since they may be refractory to anti-infectives and colectomy may be required. (See Superinfection/Clostridium difficile-associated Diarrhea and Colitis under Cautions: Precautions and Contraindications.)

● Sensitivity and Dermatologic Reactions

Anaphylactic shock and anaphylactoid reactions with hypersensitivity have been reported in patients receiving clindamycin.

Other severe hypersensitivity reactions, including severe skin reactions such as toxic epidermal necrolysis, drug reaction with eosinophilia and systemic symptoms (DRESS), and Stevens-Johnson syndrome, have been reported and have been fatal in some cases. Acute generalized exanthematous pustulosis and erythema multiforme also have been reported.

Generalized mild to moderate morbilliform-like (maculopapular) rash is the most frequently reported adverse reaction to clindamycin. Vesiculobullous rash, urticaria, pruritus, angioedema, and rare instances of exfoliative dermatitis also have been reported.

● Local Effects

Thrombophlebitis, erythema, pain, and swelling have occurred with IV administration of clindamycin.

IM administration of clindamycin has caused pain, induration, and sterile abscess at the injection site. Reversible increases in serum creatine kinase (CK, creatine phosphokinase, CPK) concentrations have been reported.

Local reactions can be minimized by giving deep IM injections or avoiding prolonged use of indwelling IV catheters.

● Other Adverse Effects

Cardiopulmonary arrest and hypotension have been reported when IV clindamycin was administered too rapidly.

Although renal damage has not been directly attributed to clindamycin, renal dysfunction manifested as azotemia, oliguria, and/or proteinuria has been observed in patients receiving clindamycin.

Transient neutropenia (leukopenia) and eosinophilia, agranulocytosis, and thrombocytopenia have been reported in patients receiving clindamycin; however, a causal relationship was not established.

Jaundice, abnormal liver function tests, polyarthritis, and vaginitis also have been reported.

● Precautions and Contraindications

Clindamycin is contraindicated in patients hypersensitive to clindamycin or lincomycin.

Prior to initiation of clindamycin, the patient should be questioned regarding prior hypersensitivity to drugs and other allergens. Clindamycin should be used with caution in atopic individuals.

If an anaphylactic or severe hypersensitivity reaction occurs during clindamycin therapy, the drug should be permanently discontinued and appropriate therapy instituted as necessary.

Superinfection/Clostridium difficile-associated Diarrhea and Colitis

As with other anti-infectives, use of clindamycin may result in overgrowth of nonsusceptible organisms, especially yeasts. If superinfection occurs, appropriate therapy should be instituted.

Because CDAD has been reported with the use of nearly all anti-infectives, including clindamycin, it should be considered in the differential diagnosis in patients who develop diarrhea during or after clindamycin therapy. Careful medical history is necessary since CDAD has been reported to occur as late as 2 months or longer after anti-infective therapy is discontinued. If CDAD is suspected or confirmed, anti-infective therapy not directed against *C. difficile* should be discontinued whenever possible. Patients should be managed with appropriate supportive therapy (e.g., fluid and electrolyte management, protein supplementation), anti-infective therapy directed against *C. difficile* (e.g., metronidazole, vancomycin), and surgical evaluation as clinically indicated.

Patients should be advised that diarrhea is a common problem caused by anti-infectives and usually ends when the drug is discontinued; however, it is important to contact a clinician if watery and bloody stools (with or without stomach cramps and fever) occur during or as late as 2 months or longer after the last dose.

Clindamycin should always be discontinued if clinically important diarrhea occurs. The drug should be used with caution in patients with a history of GI disease, particularly colitis.

Selection and Use of Anti-infectives

To reduce development of drug-resistant bacteria and maintain effectiveness of clindamycin and other antibacterials, the drug should be used only for the treatment or prevention of infections proven or strongly suspected to be caused by susceptible bacteria. When selecting or modifying anti-infective therapy, results of culture and in vitro susceptibility testing should be used. In the absence of such data, local epidemiology and susceptibility patterns should be considered when selecting anti-infectives for empiric therapy. Culture and susceptibility testing performed periodically during therapy provides information on the therapeutic effect of the anti-infective agent and the possible emergence of bacterial resistance.

Patients should be advised that antibacterials (including clindamycin) should only be used to treat bacterial infections and not used to treat viral infections (e.g., the common cold). Patients also should be advised about the importance of completing the full course of therapy, even if feeling better after a few days, and that skipping doses or not completing therapy may decrease effectiveness and increase the likelihood that bacteria will develop resistance and will not be treatable with clindamycin or other antibacterials in the future.

Other Precautions and Contraindications

Some commercially available capsules of clindamycin hydrochloride (e.g., Cleocin HCl® 75- and 150-mg capsules) contain the dye tartrazine (FD&C yellow No. 5), which may cause allergic reactions, including bronchial asthma, in susceptible individuals. Although the incidence of tartrazine sensitivity is low, it frequently occurs in patients who are sensitive to aspirin.

Because clindamycin does not distribute adequately into the CNS, the drug should *not* be used for the treatment of CNS infections.

During prolonged clindamycin therapy, liver and renal function tests and blood cell counts should be performed periodically.

If clindamycin is used in patients with hepatic impairment, dosage adjustments may not be necessary; however, liver enzymes should be monitored periodically when the drug is used in those with severe hepatic impairment.

● *Pediatric Precautions*

When clindamycin is used in pediatric patients (birth to 16 years of age), organ system functions should be monitored.

Each mL of clindamycin phosphate injection contains 9.45 mg of benzyl alcohol. Although a causal relationship has not been established, administration of injections preserved with benzyl alcohol has been associated with toxicity in neonates, including potentially fatal "gasping syndrome." Toxicity appears to have

resulted from administration of large amounts (i.e., about 100–400 mg/kg daily) of benzyl alcohol in these neonates. Although the amounts of benzyl alcohol in recommended dosages of IM or IV clindamycin are substantially lower than amounts reported in association with "gasping syndrome," the minimum amount of benzyl alcohol at which toxicity may occur is unknown. The risk of benzyl alcohol toxicity depends on the quantity administered and capacity of the liver and kidneys to detoxify the chemical. Premature and low-birthweight infants may be more likely to develop toxicity. Although use of drugs preserved with benzyl alcohol should be avoided in neonates whenever possible, the American Academy of Pediatrics (AAP) states that the presence of small amounts of the preservative in a commercially available injection should not proscribe its use when indicated in an infant.

● *Geriatric Precautions*

Clinical studies of clindamycin did not include sufficient numbers of patients 65 years of age or older to determine whether geriatric patients respond differently than younger patients. Clinical experience indicates that *C. difficile*-associated diarrhea and colitis (see Cautions: GI Effects) seen in association with most anti-infectives may occur more frequently and be more severe in patients older than 60 years of age. Therefore, geriatric patients receiving clindamycin should be carefully monitored for the development of diarrhea (e.g., changes in bowel frequency).

Studies to date have not revealed any clinically important differences in the pharmacokinetics of oral or parenteral clindamycin between younger adults and geriatric patients with normal hepatic function and normal (age-adjusted) renal function. Dosage adjustments are not usually necessary if clindamycin is used in geriatric patients with normal hepatic function and normal (age-adjusted) renal function.

● *Mutagenicity and Carcinogenicity*

Clindamycin was not mutagenic in a rat micronucleus test or the Ames *Salmonella* reversion test.

Long-term studies in animals have not been performed to date to evaluate the carcinogenic potential of clindamycin.

● *Pregnancy, Fertility, and Lactation*
Pregnancy

Reproduction studies in rats and mice using oral or parenteral dosages of clindamycin up to 600 mg/kg daily (3.2 and 1.6 times, respectively, the maximum recommended human oral dosage or 2.1 and 1.1 times, respectively, the maximum recommended human parenteral dosage on a mg/m^2 basis) have not revealed evidence of teratogenicity.

In clinical trials that included pregnant women, systemic clindamycin administered during the second and third trimesters was not associated with an increased frequency of congenital abnormalities. There are no adequate and well-controlled studies to date using clindamycin in pregnant women during the first trimester of pregnancy. Because animal reproduction studies are not always predictive of human response, clindamycin should be used during pregnancy only when clearly needed.

Clindamycin phosphate injection contains benzyl alcohol as a preservative; benzyl alcohol can cross the placenta. (See Cautions: Pediatric Precautions.)

Fertility

Fertility studies in rats treated with oral clindamycin doses up to 300 mg/kg daily (about 1.1–1.6 times the maximum recommended human dose on a mg/m^2 basis) have not revealed evidence of impaired fertility or mating ability.

Lactation

Clindamycin is distributed into milk (see Pharmacokinetics: Distribution), and has the potential to cause adverse effects on the GI flora of breast-fed infants.

The manufacturer states that use of oral or IV clindamycin in the mother is not a reason to discontinue breast-feeding; however, it may be preferable to use an alternate anti-infective. If clindamycin is used in a breast-feeding mother, the infant should be monitored for possible adverse effects on GI flora, including diarrhea and candidiasis (thrush, diaper rash) or, rarely, blood in the stool indicating possible antibiotic-associated colitis. The benefits of breast-feeding and the importance of clindamycin to the woman should be considered along with potential adverse effects on the breast-fed child from the drug or from the underlying maternal condition.

DRUG INTERACTIONS

● Drugs Affecting or Metabolized by Hepatic Microsomal Enzymes

In vitro studies indicate that clindamycin is a moderate inhibitor of cytochrome P-450 (CYP) isoenzyme 3A4 and does not inhibit CYP1A2, 2C9, 2C19, 2E1, or 2D6.

Clindamycin is a substrate of CYP3A4 and, to a lesser extent, CYP3A5. Concomitant use with CYP3A4 or 3A5 inhibitors may result in increased plasma concentrations of clindamycin, and concomitant use with CYP3A4 or 3A5 inducers may result in decreased plasma concentrations of clindamycin. If clindamycin is used concomitantly with a potent CYP3A4 inhibitor, the patient should be monitored for adverse effects. If clindamycin is used concomitantly with a potent CYP3A4 inducer (e.g., rifampin), the patient should be monitored for loss of clindamycin effectiveness.

● Neuromuscular Blocking Agents

Clindamycin has been shown to have neuromuscular blocking properties that may enhance the neuromuscular blocking action of other agents (e.g., ether, tubocurarine, pancuronium). Clindamycin should be used with caution in patients receiving such agents, and such patients should be observed for prolongation of neuromuscular blockade.

ACUTE TOXICITY

Convulsions, depression, and death have been reported in mice receiving IV clindamycin doses of 855 mg/kg; death has been reported in rats receiving oral or subcutaneous clindamycin doses of 2.6 mg/kg.

Clindamycin is not removed by hemodialysis or peritoneal dialysis.

MECHANISM OF ACTION

Clindamycin palmitate hydrochloride and clindamycin phosphate are inactive until hydrolyzed to free clindamycin. This hydrolysis occurs rapidly in vivo.

Clindamycin usually is bacteriostatic in action, but may be bactericidal depending on the concentration of the drug attained at the site of infection and the susceptibility of the infecting organism.

Clindamycin inhibits protein synthesis in susceptible bacteria by binding to the 23S RNA of the 50S ribosomal subunits; the primary effect is inhibition of peptide bond formation. The site of action appears to be the same as that of erythromycin, chloramphenicol, and lincomycin.

SPECTRUM

Clindamycin is active in vitro against many gram-positive aerobic and anaerobic bacteria and some gram-negative anaerobic bacteria. Clindamycin generally is inactive against most gram-negative aerobic bacteria.

Clindamycin is active in vitro against *Staphylococcus aureus* (methicillin-susceptible strains), *S. epidermidis* (methicillin-susceptible strains), *Streptococcus pneumoniae* (penicillin-susceptible strains), *S. pyogenes* (group A β-hemolytic streptococci; GAS), *S. agalactiae* (group B streptococci; GBS), *S. anginosus, S. mitis,* and *S. oralis.* The drug is not active against *Enterococcus faecalis* or *E. faecium.*

Clindamycin is active in vitro against some anaerobic and microaerophilic organisms including *Actinomyces israelii, Clostridium clostridioforme, C. perfringens, Eggerthella lenta* (previously known as *Eubacterium lentum*), *Finegoldia anaerobius, Finegoldia magna, Fusobacterium necrophorum, F. nucleatum, Micromonas micros, Mobiluncus, Prevotella* (*P. disiens, P. intermedia, P. melaninogenica, P. vivia*), *Porphyromonas,* and *Propionibacterium acnes.*

Clindamycin is active in vitro and in vivo against *Gardnerella vaginalis.*

Clindamycin has in vitro activity against *Toxoplasma gondii* in infected human fibroblasts. The drug has been reported to have some activity against *Plasmodium falciparum* in vitro.

Clindamycin generally is inactive against gram-negative aerobic bacteria, including Enterobacteriaceae, *Pseudomonas, Acinetobacter,* and most strains of *Haemophilus influenzae* and *Neisseria.*

● In Vitro Susceptibility Testing

When in vitro susceptibility testing is performed according to the standards of the Clinical and Laboratory Standards Institute (CLSI; formerly National Committee for Clinical Laboratory Standards [NCCLS]), clinical isolates identified as *susceptible* to clindamycin are inhibited by drug concentrations usually achievable when the recommended dosage is used for the site of infection. Clinical isolates classified as *intermediate* have minimum inhibitory concentrations (MICs) that approach usually attainable blood and tissue concentrations and response rates may be lower than for strains identified as susceptible. Therefore, the intermediate category implies clinical applicability in body sites where the drug is physiologically concentrated or when a higher than usual dosage can be used. This intermediate category also includes a buffer zone which should prevent small, uncontrolled technical factors from causing major discrepancies in interpretation, especially for drugs with narrow pharmacotoxicity margins. If results of in vitro susceptibility testing indicate that a clinical isolate is *resistant* to clindamycin, the strain is not inhibited by drug concentrations generally achievable with usual dosage schedules and/or MICs fall in the range where specific microbial resistance mechanisms are likely and clinical efficacy of the drug against the isolate has not been reliably demonstrated in clinical studies.

Disk Susceptibility Tests

When the disk-diffusion procedure is used to test susceptibility to clindamycin, a disk containing 2 mcg of the drug should be used.

When disk susceptibility testing is performed according to CLSI standardized procedures, *Staphylococcus* with growth inhibition zones of 21 mm or greater are susceptible to clindamycin, those with zones of 15–20 mm have intermediate susceptibility, and those with zones of 14 mm or less are resistant to the drug.

When susceptibility of *Streptococcus* is evaluated according to CLSI standardized procedures, *Streptococcus* (including *S. pneumoniae*) with growth inhibition zones of 19 mm or greater are susceptible to clindamycin, those with zones of 16–18 mm have intermediate susceptibility, and those with zones of 15 mm or less are resistant to the drug.

Dilution Susceptibility Tests

When dilution susceptibility testing (agar or broth dilution) is performed according to CLSI standardized procedures, *Staphylococcus* with MICs of 0.5 mcg/mL or less are susceptible to clindamycin, those with MICs of 1–2 mcg/mL have intermediate susceptibility, and those with MICs of 4 mcg/mL or greater are resistant to the drug.

When broth dilution susceptibility testing is performed according to CLSI standardized procedures, *Streptococcus* (including *S. pneumoniae*) with MICs of 0.25 mcg/mL or less are susceptible to clindamycin, those with MICs of 0.5 mcg/mL have intermediate susceptibility, and those with MICs of 1 mcg/mL or greater are resistant to the drug.

When broth dilution susceptibility testing is performed according to CLSI standardized procedures, anaerobic bacteria with MICs of 2 mcg/mL or less are susceptible to clindamycin, those with MICs of 4 mcg/mL have intermediate susceptibility, and those with MICs of 8 mcg/mL or greater are resistant to the drug.

RESISTANCE

Resistance to clindamycin has been induced in vitro in staphylococci and has been shown to be acquired in a stepwise manner. Clindamycin resistance has been reported in clinical isolates of *Staphylococcus aureus,* especially methicillin-resistant *S. aureus* (MRSA; also known as oxacillin-resistant *S. aureus* or ORSA).

S. agalactiae (group B streptococci; GBS) clinical isolates resistant to clindamycin have been reported with increasing frequency. Data from 2006–2011 indicated that 13–30% of GBS clinical isolates in the US were resistant to clindamycin. Because GBS isolates that appear susceptible to clindamycin but resistant to erythromycin in vitro may have inducible resistance to clindamycin, appropriate in vitro susceptibility testing methods should be used whenever in vitro susceptibility of GBS to clindamycin is being evaluated.

Clinical isolates of *Bacteroides fragilis* with resistance or reduced susceptibility to clindamycin have been reported with increasing frequency.

Resistance to clindamycin is most frequently caused by modification of specific bases of the 23S ribosomal RNA.

Complete cross-resistance occurs between clindamycin and lincomycin. Because of overlapping binding sites, partial cross-resistance has been reported between clindamycin and macrolides (e.g., erythromycin) and streptogramin B. In vitro, bacteria resistant to erythromycin and susceptible to clindamycin may exhibit a dissociated type of resistance to clindamycin during susceptibility testing if erythromycin is also present. This phenomenon may be the result of competition between erythromycin and clindamycin for the ribosomal binding site.

PHARMACOKINETICS

● Absorption

Following oral administration of clindamycin hydrochloride, approximately 90% of the dose is rapidly absorbed from the GI tract. Following oral administration of a single 150-mg dose of clindamycin hydrochloride to healthy fasting adults, peak serum concentrations of clindamycin average 1.9–3.9 mcg/mL and are attained within 45–60 minutes; serum concentrations of clindamycin average 1.5 mcg/mL at 3 hours and 0.7 mcg/mL at 6 hours. Serum concentrations of clindamycin appear to be predictable, increasing linearly with increased doses.

Following oral administration of clindamycin palmitate hydrochloride oral solution, the drug is rapidly hydrolyzed in the GI tract to active clindamycin. Oral doses of clindamycin palmitate hydrochloride produce serum concentrations of clindamycin similar to those achieved with oral clindamycin hydrochloride. In a study in healthy children receiving 2, 3, or 4 mg/kg of clindamycin every 6 hours as the clindamycin palmitate hydrochloride oral solution, mean peak serum clindamycin concentrations were 1.24, 2.25, or 2.44 mcg/mL, respectively, 1 hour after the first dose. After the fifth dose, peak serum concentrations of the drug averaged 2.46, 2.98, or 3.79 mcg/mL, respectively.

Clindamycin is not inactivated by gastric acidity. Administration of clindamycin hydrochloride capsules or clindamycin palmitate hydrochloride oral solution with food does not appreciably affect absorption or serum concentrations of the drug. Accumulation in plasma does not occur following multiple oral doses, including in neonates and infants up to 6 months of age.

Following IM or IV administration, clindamycin phosphate is rapidly hydrolyzed in plasma to active clindamycin. Following IM administration of clindamycin phosphate, peak serum concentrations occur within 3 hours in adults and 1 hour in children. In healthy adult males, IM doses of 600 mg of clindamycin every 12 hours resulted in average peak serum clindamycin concentrations of 9 mcg/mL. IV doses of 600 mg of clindamycin infused over 30 minutes every 6 or 8 hours in healthy adult males resulted in average peak serum clindamycin concentrations of 11 mcg/mL and IV doses of 900 mg infused over 30 minutes every 8 hours resulted in average peak serum clindamycin concentrations of 14 mcg/mL. In a study in pediatric patients with infections, a single IM dose of 3–5 mg/kg resulted in average peak serum clindamycin concentrations of 4 mcg/mL and single IV or IM doses of 5–7 mg/kg resulted in average peak serum clindamycin concentrations of 10 or 8 mcg/mL, respectively.

● Distribution

Clindamycin is widely distributed into body tissues and fluids, including saliva, ascites fluid, peritoneal fluid, pleural fluid, synovial fluid, bone, and bile. The concentration of clindamycin in synovial fluid and bone is reported to be 60–80% of concurrent serum concentrations of the drug; the degree of penetration does not appear to be affected by joint inflammation.

Clinically important concentrations of clindamycin are not attained in CSF, even in the presence of inflamed meninges.

Clindamycin readily crosses the placenta, and cord blood concentrations of the drug have been reported to be up to 50% of concurrent maternal blood concentrations.

Clindamycin is distributed into milk. Breast milk concentrations of 0.7–3.8 mcg/mL have been reported following clindamycin dosages of 150 mg orally to 600 mg IV. In one study in women who received oral clindamycin in a dosage of 150 mg 3 times daily, breast milk concentrations of the drug ranged from less than 0.5 to 3.1 mcg/mL.

At a concentration of 1 mcg/mL, clindamycin is approximately 93% bound to serum proteins.

● Elimination

Clindamycin is partially metabolized to bioactive and inactive metabolites. In vitro studies indicate that clindamycin is predominantly metabolized by cytochrome P-450 (CYP) isoenzyme 3A4 and, to a lesser extent, by CYP3A5 to the major bioactive metabolite clindamycin sulfoxide and minor metabolite N-desmethylclindamycin.

The serum half-life of clindamycin is 2–3 hours in adults and children. In neonates, the serum half-life of clindamycin depends on gestational and chronologic age and body weight. Half-life of the drug reportedly averages 8.7 or 3.6 hours in premature or full-term neonates, respectively, and about 3 hours in infants 4 weeks to 1 year of age; serum half-life was longer in infants weighing less than 3.5 kg than in heavier infants.

Pharmacokinetic studies using IV clindamycin phosphate in healthy older adults (61–79 years of age) and younger adults (18–39 years of age) indicate that age alone does not alter clindamycin pharmacokinetics (clearance, elimination half-life, volume of distribution, area under the serum concentration-time curve [AUC]). Following oral administration of clindamycin hydrochloride, elimination half-life increased to approximately 4 hours (range: 3.4–5.1 hours) in geriatric patients compared with 3.2 hours (range: 2.1–4.2 hours) in younger adults. Following oral administration of clindamycin palmitate, the elimination half-life in geriatric adults was 4.5 hours.

The serum half-life of clindamycin is increased slightly in patients with markedly reduced renal or hepatic function.

Clindamycin sulfoxide and N-desmethylclindamycin are excreted in urine, bile, and feces. Approximately 10% of an oral dose of clindamycin is excreted in urine and 3.6% is excreted in feces as active drug and metabolites; the remainder is excreted as inactive metabolites.

Clindamycin is not appreciably removed by hemodialysis or peritoneal dialysis.

CHEMISTRY AND STABILITY

● Chemistry

Clindamycin is a semisynthetic derivative of lincomycin that differs structurally from lincomycin by the presence of a methoxy group instead of the hydroxyl group at position 7 on the molecule.

Clindamycin is commercially available as the hydrochloride hydrate, the palmitate hydrochloride, and the phosphate ester. Potency of clindamycin hydrochloride, clindamycin palmitate hydrochloride, and clindamycin phosphate is expressed in terms of clindamycin. Each mg of the hydrochloride hydrate, palmitate hydrochloride, or phosphate has a potency of not less than 800, 540, or 758 mcg of clindamycin, respectively; potency of the phosphate is calculated on the anhydrous basis. The hydrochloride, palmitate hydrochloride, and phosphate occur as a white or practically white crystalline powder, a white to off-white amorphous powder, and a white to off-white hygroscopic crystalline powder, respectively, which may have faint, characteristic odors and are freely soluble in water. Clindamycin phosphate reportedly has a solubility of about 400 mg/mL in water at 25°C. The pK_a of clindamycin is 7.45.

Clindamycin hydrochloride is commercially available for oral administration as capsules. Clindamycin palmitate hydrochloride is commercially available as a powder (granules) for oral solution; when reconstituted as directed, each 5 mL of oral solution contains 75 mg of clindamycin.

Clindamycin phosphate is commercially available as a sterile solution containing 150 mg of clindamycin that must be diluted prior to IV administration; each mL of the solution also contains 0.5 mg of disodium edetate per mL and 9.45 mg of benzyl alcohol as a preservative. Clindamycin phosphate also is commercially available as a premixed solution for IV infusion containing 300, 600, or 900 mg of clindamycin in 5% dextrose. The premixed solutions contain 0.04 mg of disodium edetate per mL and sodium hydroxide and/or hydrochloric acid may have been added to adjust pH.

● Stability

Clindamycin hydrochloride capsules should be stored at 20–25°C.

Clindamycin palmitate hydrochloride powder (granules) for oral solution should be stored at 20–25°C. Following reconstitution with water, clindamycin palmitate hydrochloride oral solution is stable for 2 weeks at room temperature. The reconstituted oral solution should *not* be refrigerated since it will thicken if chilled and become difficult to pour.

Clindamycin phosphate solutions containing 150 mg of clindamycin per mL (including ADD-Vantage® vials) should be stored at a controlled room temperature of 20–25°C.

Premixed solutions containing clindamycin phosphate in 5% dextrose injection should be stored at room temperature (25°C), and exposure to temperatures warmer than 30°C should be avoided. Some premixed solutions of clindamycin phosphate in 5% dextrose are provided in plastic containers fabricated from specially formulated multilayered plastic PL 2501. Solutions in contact with the plastic can leach out some of the chemical components in very small amounts within the expiration period of the injection; however, safety of the plastic has been confirmed in tests in animals as well as by tissue culture studies.

At a concentration of 6, 9, or 12 mg of clindamycin per mL, clindamycin phosphate is physically and chemically compatible for at least 16 days at 25°C or at least 32 days when refrigerated at 4°C in glass or polyvinyl chloride (PVC) containers, or for at least 8 weeks when frozen at –10°C in PVC containers of the following IV solutions: 5% dextrose, 0.9% sodium chloride, or lactated Ringer's. At a concentration of 18 mg of clindamycin per mL, clindamycin phosphate is physically and chemically compatible for at least 16 days at 25°C in PVC containers of 5% dextrose.

Clindamycin phosphate is physically and microbiologically compatible for 24 hours at room temperature in IV solutions containing sodium chloride, dextrose, potassium, or vitamin B complex in concentrations used clinically. However, certain concentrations or admixtures of calcium salts may result in physical incompatibility. Clindamycin phosphate has been reported to be incompatible with various drugs (e.g., aminophylline, barbiturates, ceftriaxone, ciprofloxacin, magnesium sulfate, phenytoin sodium); however, the compatibility depends on several factors (e.g., concentration of the drugs, specific diluents used, resulting pH, temperature). Specialized references should be consulted for specific compatibility information.

PREPARATIONS

Excipients in commercially available drug preparations may have clinically important effects in some individuals; consult specific product labeling for details.

Clindamycin Hydrochloride

Oral

Capsules	75 mg (of clindamycin)*	Cleocin HCl®, Pfizer
		Clindamycin Hydrochloride Capsules
	150 mg (of clindamycin)*	Cleocin HCl®, Pfizer
		Clindamycin Hydrochloride Capsules
	300 mg (of clindamycin)*	Cleocin HCl®, Pfizer
		Clindamycin Hydrochloride Capsules

* available from one or more manufacturer, distributor, and/or repackager by generic (nonproprietary) name

Clindamycin Palmitate Hydrochloride

Oral

| For solution | 75 mg (of clindamycin) per 5 mL* | Cleocin Pediatric®, Pfizer |
| | | Clindamycin Palmitate Hydrochloride for Oral Solution |

* available from one or more manufacturer, distributor, and/or repackager by generic (nonproprietary) name

Clindamycin Phosphate

Parenteral

Injection	150 mg (of clindamycin) per mL*	Cleocin Phosphate®, Pfizer
		Clindamycin Phosphate Injection
	9 g (150 mg/mL) (of clindamycin) pharmacy bulk package	Cleocin Phosphate®, Pfizer
Injection, for IV infusion only	150 mg (of clindamycin) per mL (300 mg)*	Cleocin Phosphate® ADD-Vantage®, Pfizer
		Clindamycin Phosphate ADD-Vantage®
	150 mg (of clindamycin) per mL (600 and 900 mg)*	Cleocin Phosphate® ADD-Vantage®, Pfizer
		Clindamycin Phosphate ADD-Vantage®

* available from one or more manufacturer, distributor, and/or repackager by generic (nonproprietary) name

Clindamycin Phosphate in Dextrose

Parenteral

Injection, for IV infusion	6 mg (of clindamycin) per mL (300 mg) in 5% Dextrose*	Cleocin Phosphate® IV, Pfizer
		Clindamycin Phosphate in 5% Dextrose
	12 mg (of clindamycin) per mL (600 mg) in 5% Dextrose*	Cleocin Phosphate® IV, Pfizer
		Clindamycin Phosphate in 5% Dextrose
	18 mg (of clindamycin) per mL (900 mg) in 5% Dextrose*	Cleocin Phosphate® IV, Pfizer
		Clindamycin Phosphate in 5% Dextrose

* available from one or more manufacturer, distributor, and/or repackager by generic (nonproprietary) name

† Use is not currently included in the labeling approved by the US Food and Drug Administration.

Selected Revisions July 9, 2018, © Copyright, May 1, 1980, American Society of Health-System Pharmacists, Inc.

Linezolid

8:12.28.24 • OXAZOLIDINONES

■ Linezolid is an oxazolidinone anti-infective agent.

USES

Linezolid is used for the treatment of community-acquired pneumonia, nosocomial pneumonia, and uncomplicated or complicated skin and skin structure infections caused by certain susceptible staphylococci or streptococci. Linezolid also is used for the treatment of infections caused by vancomycin-resistant *Enterococcus faecium*.

Linezolid is *not* indicated for the treatment of infections caused by gram-negative bacteria. It is critical that an anti-infective active against gram-negative bacteria be used concomitantly if documented or presumed pathogens include gram-negative bacteria.

● *Respiratory Tract Infections*

Community-acquired Pneumonia

Linezolid is used for the treatment of community-acquired pneumonia (CAP), including infections associated with concurrent bacteremia, caused by susceptible *Staphylococcus aureus* (methicillin-susceptible [oxacillin-susceptible] strains only) or *Streptococcus pneumoniae*). Although not labeled by FDA for the treatment of CAP caused by methicillin-resistant *S. aureus*† (MRSA; also known as oxacillin-resistant *S. aureus* or ORSA), linezolid is one of several anti-infectives that have been recommended for the treatment of these infections.

Initial treatment of CAP generally involves use of an empiric anti-infective regimen based on the most likely pathogens and local susceptibility patterns; treatment may then be changed (if possible) to provide a more specific regimen (pathogen-directed therapy) based on results of in vitro culture and susceptibility testing. The most appropriate empiric regimen varies depending on the severity of illness at the time of presentation, whether outpatient treatment or hospitalization in or out of an intensive care unit (ICU) is indicated, and the presence or absence of cardiopulmonary disease and other modifying factors that increase the risk of certain pathogens (e.g., MRSA, penicillin-resistant *S. pneumoniae*, multidrug-resistant *S. pneumoniae* [MDRSP], enteric gram-negative bacilli, *Pseudomonas aeruginosa*).

For information regarding the treatment of CAP, current clinical practice guidelines from the Infectious Diseases Society of America (IDSA) available at http://www.idsociety.org should be consulted.

Clinical Experience

In 2 randomized clinical studies in patients 13 years of age or older with CAP, cure rates with linezolid (600 mg every 12 hours for 7–14 days given IV or orally initially, then orally) were approximately 90% and were similar to those achieved with oral cefpodoxime proxetil (200 mg every 12 hours for 10–14 days) or IV ceftriaxone (1 g every 12 hours) followed by oral cefpodoxime proxetil (200 mg every 12 hours) for 7–14 days. In a subset of hospitalized patients with CAP and associated *S. pneumoniae* bacteremia, linezolid was substantially more effective than a regimen of IV ceftriaxone (cure rate of 93 versus 70%, respectively).

Efficacy and safety of linezolid for the treatment of CAP in pediatric patients is supported by evidence from adequate and well-controlled studies in adults, pharmacokinetic studies in pediatric patients, an uncontrolled study in pediatric patients 8 months through 12 years of age, and additional data from a randomized, open-label, comparator-controlled study of documented or suspected gram-positive bacterial infections in neonates and pediatric patients through 11 years of age.

Nosocomial Pneumonia

Linezolid is used for the treatment of nosocomial pneumonia caused by susceptible *S. aureus* (including MRSA) or *S. pneumoniae*.

For empiric treatment of hospital-acquired bacterial pneumonia, including healthcare-associated and ventilator-associated pneumonia in patients with risk factors for multidrug-resistant bacteria, the American Thoracic Society (ATS) and IDSA recommend use of anti-infectives that have a broad spectrum of activity against gram-positive, gram-negative, and anaerobic bacteria. An anti-infective active against MRSA (e.g., vancomycin, linezolid) should be included in the initial empiric regimen in hospitals where MRSA is common or if there are other factors that increase the risk for these strains.

For information regarding the diagnosis and management of nosocomial pneumonia, current IDSA clinical practice guidelines available at http://www.idsociety.org should be consulted.

Clinical Experience

In a randomized, double-blind study in adults with nosocomial bacterial pneumonia, the cure rate in clinically evaluable patients was 57% in those treated with linezolid (600 mg every 12 hours IV for 7–21 days) compared with 60% in those treated with vancomycin (1 g every 12 hours IV for 7–21 days). Both treatment groups also received concomitant therapy with aztreonam (1–2 g every 8 hours IV) for gram-negative coverage. In clinically evaluable patients with ventilator-associated pneumonia, the cure rate was 47% in those who received linezolid and 40% in those who received vancomycin. When results were stratified according to causative organism, linezolid was effective in 59% of infections caused by MRSA and 100% of infections caused by *S. pneumoniae*.

Efficacy and safety of linezolid for the treatment of nosocomial bacterial pneumonia in pediatric patients is supported by evidence from adequate and well-controlled studies in adults, pharmacokinetic studies in pediatric patients, and additional data from a randomized, open-label, comparator-controlled study of documented or suspected gram-positive bacterial infections in neonates and pediatric patients through 11 years of age. In the comparator-controlled study in pediatric patients with documented or suspected gram-positive infections, the cure rate in pediatric patients with nosocomial pneumonia (intent-to-treat analysis) was 72% in those treated with linezolid and 92% in those treated with vancomycin; the cure rate in clinically evaluable pediatric patients with nosocomial pneumonia was 100% in both groups.

● *Skin and Skin Structure Infections*

Linezolid is used for the treatment of uncomplicated skin and skin structure infections caused by susceptible *S. aureus* (methicillin-susceptible strains only) or *S. pyogenes* (group A β-hemolytic streptococci, GAS). The drug also is used for the treatment of complicated skin and skin structure infections (including diabetic foot infections), without concurrent osteomyelitis, caused by susceptible *S. aureus* (including MRSA), *S. pyogenes*, or *S. agalactiae* (group B streptococci, GBS). The use of linezolid in the treatment of decubitus ulcers has not been studied.

For information regarding the treatment of skin and skin structure infections, current IDSA clinical practice guidelines available at http://www.idsociety.org should be consulted.

Clinical Experience

In a randomized, double-blind clinical study in adults with complicated skin and skin structure infections, the efficacy rates (clinical, microbiologic, and overall outcomes) were similar for linezolid (600 mg every 12 hours IV initially, with an option to convert to oral administration) or oxacillin (2 g every 6 hours IV) with an option to switch to oral dicloxacillin (500 mg every 6 hours) for 10–21 days. Patients in both treatment groups received concomitant aztreonam (1–2 g every 6–8 hours IV) if empiric gram-negative coverage was considered necessary. The cure rate in clinically evaluable patients was 90% in those treated with linezolid and 85% in those treated with oxacillin. When results for treatment of these complicated skin and skin structure infections were stratified according to causative organism, linezolid was effective in 88% of infections caused by *S. aureus*, 67% of infections caused by MRSA, 69% of infections caused by *S. pyogenes*, and 100% of infections caused by *S. agalactiae*.

In a randomized clinical study in patients 13 years of age or older with known or suspected MRSA skin and skin structure infections, efficacy (clinical, microbiologic, and overall outcomes) was similar for therapy with linezolid (600 mg every 12 hours IV initially, with an option to convert to oral administration) or vancomycin (1 g every 12 hours IV) for 14–28 days. In an open-label, randomized study in hospitalized adults with documented or suspected MRSA skin and skin structure infections who received 7–28 days of treatment with linezolid (600 mg every 12 hours given IV initially, then orally) or vancomycin (1 g every 12 hours

IV) given with or without concomitant aztreonam or gentamicin if clinically indicated, the cure rate in microbiologically evaluable patients was 79% in those treated with linezolid and 73% in those treated with vancomycin.

In a randomized, multicenter open-label comparative study in adults with diabetic foot infections, efficacy rates (clinical and microbiologic outcomes) were similar in patients receiving linezolid (600 mg every 12 hours IV or orally) or an aminopenicillin (ampicillin sodium and sulbactam sodium 1.5–3 g every 6 hours IV, amoxicillin and clavulanate potassium 500–875 mg every 8–12 hours orally, or amoxicillin and clavulanate potassium 0.5–2 g every 6 hours IV [IV preparation not commercially available in the US]) for 14–28 days. Patients in both treatment groups received concomitant aztreonam (1–2 g every 8–12 hours IV) if gram-negative pathogens were isolated from the infection site and patients receiving an aminopenicillin also were treated with vancomycin (1 g every 12 hours IV) if MRSA was isolated from the foot infection. Most patients also received appropriate adjunctive treatment usually required for the treatment of diabetic foot infections (e.g., debridement). When results for treatment of these diabetic foot infections were stratified according to causative organism, linezolid was effective in 78% of infections caused by *S. aureus*, 71% of infections caused by MRSA, and 86% of infections caused by *S. agalactiae*.

Efficacy and safety of linezolid for the treatment of complicated skin and skin structure infections in pediatric patients is supported by evidence from adequate and well-controlled studies in adults, pharmacokinetic studies in pediatric patients, and additional data from a randomized, comparator-controlled study of documented or suspected gram-positive bacterial infections in neonates and pediatric patients through 11 years of age. In the comparator-controlled study in pediatric patients with documented or suspected gram-positive infections, the cure rate in pediatric patients with complicated skin and skin structure infections (intent-to-treat analysis) was 85% in those treated with linezolid and 91% in those treated with vancomycin; the cure rate in clinically evaluable pediatric patients with complicated skin and skin structure infections was 94 and 96%, respectively.

Efficacy and safety of linezolid for the treatment of uncomplicated skin and skin structure infections in pediatric patients caused by *S. aureus* (methicillin-susceptible [oxacillin-susceptible] strains only) or *S. pyogenes* is supported by data from a comparator-controlled study in pediatric patients 5–17 years of age.

● Vancomycin-resistant *Enterococcus faecium* Infections

Linezolid is used for the treatment of vancomycin-resistant *E. faecium* infections, including infections associated with concurrent bacteremia.

Linezolid has been used in some patients for the treatment of native valve or prosthetic valve infective endocarditis† caused by vancomycin-resistant or multidrug-resistant *E. faecium*. The American Heart Association (AHA) states that patients with infective endocarditis attributable to enterococci resistant to penicillins, aminoglycosides, and vancomycin should be managed by a team of specialists in infectious disease, cardiology, cardiovascular surgery, clinical pharmacy, and, if necessary, pediatrics.

For information on diagnosis and management of infective endocarditis and its complications, including anti-infective treatment of enterococcal endocarditis, the current AHA guidelines available at http://my.americanheart.org/statements should be consulted.

Clinical Experience

In a randomized, double-blind study in adults comparing high-dose linezolid (600 mg every 12 hours IV or orally) with low-dose linezolid (200 mg every 12 hours IV or orally) for 7–28 days, cure rates for patients with documented vancomycin-resistant *E. faecium* at any infection site were 67 or 52% for those treated with high- or low-dose linezolid, respectively, based on intent-to-treat analysis. Some patients received concomitant therapy with aztreonam or aminoglycosides. Compared with patients in the high-dose group, there were more adverse events and more deaths among patients in the low-dose group.

Efficacy and safety of linezolid for the treatment of vancomycin-resistant *E. faecium* infections in pediatric patients is supported by evidence from adequate and well-controlled studies in adults, pharmacokinetic studies in pediatric patients, and additional data from a randomized, open-label, comparator-controlled study of documented or suspected gram-positive bacterial infections in neonates and pediatric patients through 11 years of age. Data from the open-label, comparator-controlled study indicate that the cure rate was 75% in the 8 microbiologically

evaluable pediatric patients with vancomycin-resistant *E. faecium* infections who received linezolid.

● Catheter-related Bloodstream Infections

Although linezolid has been investigated for the treatment of intravascular catheter-related bloodstream infections†, linezolid is *not* labeled by FDA for the treatment of catheter-related bacteremia or catheter-site infections and is *not* indicated for the treatment of gram-negative bacterial infections.

Data from an open-label, randomized study in patients with intravascular catheter-related bloodstream infections indicated that mortality was higher in patients receiving linezolid than in patients receiving comparator anti-infectives. In this study, seriously ill patients with intravascular catheter-related bloodstream infections were randomized to receive linezolid or vancomycin (patients randomized to vancomycin were switched to dicloxacillin or oxacillin if the pathogen was oxacillin-susceptible); patients could receive concomitant therapy for gram-negative infection. Although there was no difference in mortality between linezolid and the comparator regimens in patients with only gram-positive bacteria identified in the baseline culture, mortality was higher in linezolid-treated patients who had gram-negative bacterial infections, mixed gram-negative and gram-positive bacterial infections, or no pathogen identified at baseline.

● Mycobacterial Infections

Treatment of Active Tuberculosis

Linezolid is used in multiple-drug regimens for the treatment of multidrug-resistant (MDR) pulmonary tuberculosis† (i.e., caused by *Mycobacterium tuberculosis* resistant to isoniazid and rifampin). ATS, US Centers for Disease Control and Prevention (CDC), and IDSA state that linezolid is one of various options that can be considered for inclusion in multiple-drug regimens used for the treatment of pulmonary MDR tuberculosis. The World Health Organization (WHO) recommends that linezolid be included in multiple-drug regimens used for longer-term treatment (i.e., 18 months or longer) of multidrug- or rifampin-resistant (MDR/RR) tuberculosis.

Linezolid is used in a 3-drug combination regimen that includes bedaquiline and pretomanid for the treatment of extensively drug resistant (XDR) pulmonary tuberculosis (i.e., caused by *M. tuberculosis* resistant to isoniazid, rifampin, any fluoroquinolone, and at least one injectable antituberculosis agent) or treatment-intolerant or non-responsive MDR pulmonary tuberculosis. WHO states that the 3-drug regimen of pretomanid, bedaquiline, and linezolid (also known as BPaL) may be used for treatment of MDR tuberculosis in patients who have not previously received either bedaquiline or linezolid (or received the drugs for no more than 2 weeks) and have documented evidence that the MDR strain also is resistant to a fluoroquinolone.

Patients with MDR or XDR tuberculosis are at high risk for treatment failure and acquisition of further drug resistance. ATS, CDC, IDSA, and other experts recommend that such patients be referred to or that consultation be obtained from a specialized treatment center as identified by local or state health departments or the CDC.

For additional information on the treatment of MDR and XDR tuberculosis, current guidelines from ATS/CDC/IDSA and WHO should be consulted.

DOSAGE AND ADMINISTRATION

● Administration

Linezolid is administered orally or by IV infusion.

Oral Administration

Orally administered linezolid may be given without regard to meals. However, large quantities of foods or beverages with high tyramine content should be avoided during linezolid treatment. (See Monoamine Oxidase Inhibition under Cautions.)

Linezolid powder for oral suspension should be reconstituted at the time of dispensing with the amount of water specified on the bottle to provide a suspension containing 100 mg/5 mL. After tapping the bottle gently to loosen the powder, the water should be added in 2 portions and the suspension agitated well after each addition.

The reconstituted oral suspension should be stored at room temperature and used within 21 days. Prior to administration of each dose, the suspension should be *gently* mixed by inverting the bottle 3–5 times but should not be shaken.

IV Administration

Linezolid premixed injection for IV administration in single-use flexible containers is administered by IV infusion without further dilution.

Linezolid premixed solutions should be inspected visually for particulate matter prior to administration and should not be used if visible particles are evident. The solution may exhibit a yellow color that can intensify over time without adversely affecting potency. The bags should be squeezed firmly to check for minute leaks. If leaks are detected, the solution should be discarded since sterility may be impaired.

Linezolid premixed injection for IV administration in single-use flexible infusion bags should not be used in series connections, and additives should not be introduced into the solution.

Linezolid is compatible with 5% dextrose, 0.9% sodium chloride, and lactated Ringer's injection.

During simulated Y-site administration, linezolid was physically incompatible with amphotericin B, chlorpromazine hydrochloride, co-trimoxazole, diazepam, erythromycin lactobionate, pentamidine isethionate, and phenytoin sodium. In addition, linezolid is chemically incompatible with ceftriaxone sodium.

Rate of Administration

Linezolid premixed injection for IV administration in single-use flexible containers should be administered by IV infusion over 30–120 minutes.

● Dosage

When clinically appropriate, patients treated initially with IV linezolid may be switched to oral linezolid without dosage adjustment.

The manufacturer states that safety and efficacy of more than 28 days of linezolid treatment have not been evaluated in controlled clinical trials. Linezolid is administered for longer durations when used in multiple-drug regimens for the treatment of multidrug-resistant (MDR) tuberculosis.

Adult Dosage

Respiratory Tract Infections

The usual adult oral or IV dosage of linezolid for the treatment of community-acquired pneumonia (CAP) caused by susceptible *Staphylococcus aureus* (methicillin-susceptible [oxacillin-susceptible] strains only) or *Streptococcus pneumoniae* is 600 mg every 12 hours for 10–14 days.

The usual adult oral or IV dosage of linezolid for the treatment of nosocomial pneumonia caused by susceptible *S. aureus* (including MRSA) or *S. pneumoniae* is 600 mg every 12 hours for 10–14 days.

Skin and Skin Structure Infections

For the treatment of uncomplicated skin and skin structure infections caused by susceptible *S. aureus* (methicillin-susceptible [oxacillin-susceptible] strains only) or *S. pyogenes* (group A β-hemolytic streptococci, GAS), the usual adult oral dosage of linezolid is 400 mg every 12 hours for 10–14 days.

The usual adult oral or IV dosage of linezolid for the treatment of complicated skin and skin structure infections, including diabetic foot infections, without concomitant osteomyelitis, caused by susceptible *S. aureus* (including MRSA), *S. pyogenes* (group A β-hemolytic streptococci), or *S. agalactiae* (group B streptococci, GBS) is 600 mg every 12 hours for 10–14 days.

Vancomycin-resistant Enterococcus faecium Infections

The usual adult oral or IV dosage of linezolid for the treatment of vancomycin-resistant *Enterococcus faecium* infections, including infections with concurrent bacteremia, is 600 mg every 12 hours for 14–28 days.

Treatment of XDR Tuberculosis or Treatment-intolerant or Non-responsive MDR Tuberculosis

When oral linezolid is used in conjunction with pretomanid and bedaquiline for the treatment of XDR pulmonary tuberculosis or treatment-intolerant or non-responsive MDR pulmonary tuberculosis in adults, the recommended dosage of the drug is 1.2 g daily for 26 weeks. Adjustment of linezolid dosage to 600 mg daily with further reductions to 300 mg daily or interruption of linezolid therapy may be required if myelosuppression, peripheral neuropathy, or optic neuropathy occurs.

This recommended linezolid dosage must be administered in conjunction with oral pretomanid (200 mg once daily for 26 weeks) and oral bedaquiline (400 mg once daily for 2 weeks followed by 200 mg 3 times weekly [with at least 48 hours between doses] for 24 weeks).

The 3-drug combination regimen of pretomanid, bedaquiline, and linezolid should be continued for 26 weeks, but may be extended beyond 26 weeks if necessary.

Pediatric Dosage

General Dosage for Neonates

In premature neonates younger than 7 days of age, the manufacturer recommends an initial linezolid dosage of 10 mg/kg every 12 hours; a dosage of 10 mg/kg every 8 hours may be considered in those with an inadequate response to the lower dosage. The manufacturer recommends that all neonates 7 days of age or older receive a linezolid dosage of 10 mg/kg every 8 hours.

When linezolid is used in neonates 7 days of age or younger, the American Academy of Pediatrics (AAP) recommends an IV dosage of 10 mg/kg every 12 hours in those with gestational age less than 34 weeks and 10 mg/kg every 8 hours in those with gestational age of 24 weeks or more. For neonates 8–28 days of age, AAP recommends an IV dosage of 10 mg/kg every 8 hours, regardless of gestational age.

Respiratory Tract Infections

The usual oral or IV dosage of linezolid for the treatment of CAP caused by susceptible *S. aureus* (methicillin-susceptible [oxacillin-susceptible] strains only) or *S. pneumoniae* is 10 mg/kg every 8 hours in pediatric patients 7 days of age through 11 years of age and 600 mg every 12 hours in adolescents 12 years of age or older. The recommended duration of treatment is 10–14 days.

The usual oral or IV dosage of linezolid for the treatment of nosocomial pneumonia caused by susceptible *S. aureus* (including MRSA) or *S. pneumoniae* is 10 mg/kg every 8 hours in pediatric patients 7 days through 11 years of age and 600 mg every 12 hours in adolescents 12 years of age or older. The recommended duration of treatment is 10–14 days.

Skin and Skin Structure Infections

For the treatment of uncomplicated skin and skin structure infections caused by susceptible *S. aureus* (methicillin-susceptible [oxacillin-susceptible] strains only) or *S. pyogenes* in pediatric patients, the usual oral dosage of linezolid is 10 mg/kg every 8 hours in those younger than 5 years of age, 10 mg/kg every 12 hours in those 5 through 11 years of age, and 600 mg every 12 hours in adolescents 12 years of age or older. The recommended duration of treatment is 10–14 days.

The usual oral or IV dosage of linezolid for the treatment of complicated skin and skin structure infections caused by susceptible *S. aureus* (including MRSA), *S. pyogenes*, or *S. agalactiae* is 10 mg/kg every 8 hours in pediatric patients 7 days of age through 11 years of age and 600 mg every 12 hours in adolescents 12 years of age or older. The recommended duration of treatment is 10–14 days.

Vancomycin-resistant Enterococcus faecium Infections

The usual oral or IV dosage of linezolid for the treatment of vancomycin-resistant *E. faecium* infections is 10 mg/kg every 8 hours in pediatric patients 7 days of age through 11 years of age and 600 mg every 12 hours in adolescents 12 years of age or older. The recommended duration of treatment is 14–28 days.

● Special Populations

Hepatic Impairment

Dosage adjustments are not necessary in patients with mild to moderate hepatic impairment (Child-Pugh class A or B). Data are not available regarding the pharmacokinetics of linezolid in patients with severe hepatic impairment.

Renal Impairment

Dosage adjustments are not necessary in patients with renal impairment. However, the 2 principal metabolites of linezolid may accumulate in patients with renal impairment and the clinical importance of accumulation of these metabolites has not been determined.

Because linezolid is removed by hemodialysis, patients undergoing hemodialysis should receive linezolid doses after the dialysis session.

Geriatric Patients

Dosage adjustments are not necessary in geriatric patients.

CAUTIONS

● Contraindications

Linezolid is contraindicated in patients with known hypersensitivity to linezolid or any ingredient in the formulation.

Linezolid should not be used in patients who are receiving (or have received within the last 2 weeks) drugs that inhibit monoamine oxidase (MAO) A or B, including MAO inhibitor antidepressants (e.g., isocarboxazid, phenelzine). (See Monoamine Oxidase Inhibitors under Drug Interactions.)

● Warnings/Precautions

Hematologic Effects

Myelosuppression (e.g., anemia, leukopenia, pancytopenia, thrombocytopenia) has been reported in patients receiving linezolid.

Toxicity studies in adult and juvenile dogs and rats indicate myelosuppression (bone marrow hypocellularity/decreased hematopoiesis; decreased extramedullary hematopoiesis in spleen and liver; decreased levels of circulating erythrocytes, leukocytes, and platelets) and lymphoid depletion in thymus, lymph nodes, and spleen.

Complete blood cell counts (CBCs) should be monitored weekly during linezolid treatment, especially in patients receiving the drug for more than 2 weeks and in those who have preexisting myelosuppression, are receiving concomitant drugs that produce bone marrow suppression, or have a chronic infection that was or is being treated with concomitant anti-infective therapy.

Discontinuance of linezolid should be considered if myelosuppression develops or worsens. Hematologic parameters generally have increased toward pretreatment values following discontinuance of the drug.

Peripheral and Optic Neuropathy

Peripheral and optic neuropathies have been reported in adults and children receiving linezolid; these events have occurred principally in patients receiving the drug for longer than the maximum recommended duration of treatment (28 days). Optic neuropathy sometimes progressed to loss of vision when linezolid was used for longer than 28 days. Blurred vision has been reported in some patients who received the drug for less than 28 days.

If a patient experiences symptoms of visual impairment (e.g., changes in visual acuity or color vision, blurred vision, or visual field defect), an ophthalmic evaluation should be performed promptly. All patients receiving linezolid for extended periods of time (i.e., 3 months or longer) should have their visual function monitored. In addition, all patients reporting a new visual symptom, regardless of the length of linezolid treatment, should have their visual function monitored.

If peripheral or optic neuropathy occurs, the potential benefits of linezolid should be weighed against the potential risks of continued treatment with the drug.

Serotonin Syndrome

Serotonin syndrome (including some fatalities) has been reported in patients receiving linezolid concomitantly with serotonergic drugs. Signs and symptoms of serotonin syndrome include mental changes (confusion, hyperactivity, memory problems), muscle twitching, excessive sweating, shivering, shaking, diarrhea, loss of coordination, and/or fever.

Most reported cases of serotonin syndrome have occurred in patients receiving linezolid concomitantly with selective serotonin-reuptake inhibitors (SSRIs)

or selective serotonin- and norepinephrine-reuptake inhibitors (SNRIs). FDA has not concluded whether concomitant use of linezolid and other drugs with lesser degrees of serotonergic activity (e.g., tricyclic antidepressants, MAO inhibitors) is associated with a risk comparable to that reported with concomitant use of linezolid and SSRIs or SNRIs.

Linezolid should not be used in patients with carcinoid syndrome or in patients receiving SSRIs, tricyclic antidepressants, serotonin 5-HT$_1$ receptor agonists (triptans), meperidine, bupropion, or buspirone unless concomitant therapy is considered clinically appropriate and patients can be carefully monitored for signs and/or symptoms of serotonin syndrome or neuroleptic malignant syndrome-like (NMS-like) reactions. (See Drug Interactions.)

Mortality

In a study in seriously ill patients with intravascular catheter-related infections†, mortality was higher in linezolid-treated patients than in those treated with a comparator anti-infective (vancomycin, dicloxacillin, oxacillin). (See Catheter-related Bloodstream Infections under Uses.)

Monoamine Oxidase Inhibition

Linezolid is a weak, nonselective, reversible inhibitor of monoamine oxidase (MAO). The drug potentially may interact with MAO inhibitors and adrenergic and serotonergic agents. (See Drug Interactions.)

A significant pressor response has been reported when tyramine doses exceeding 100 mg were used in adults receiving linezolid. Patients should be instructed to avoid large quantities of foods or beverages with high tyramine content during linezolid treatment. Foods high in tyramine include those that may have undergone protein changes by aging, fermentation, pickling, or smoking to improve flavor (e.g., aged cheeses, fermented or air-dried meat, sauerkraut, soy sauce, tap beer, red wine). Tyramine content of any protein-rich food may be increased if stored for long periods or improperly refrigerated. For additional information on interactions in patients receiving MAO inhibitors and foods containing large amounts of tyramine, see Food under Drug Interactions, in the Monoamine Oxidase Inhibitors General Statement 28:16.04.12.

Risk of Hypertension

Unless patients are monitored for potential increases in blood pressure, linezolid should not be used in patients with uncontrolled hypertension, pheochromocytoma, or thyrotoxicosis or in patients receiving direct- or indirect-acting sympathomimetic agents (e.g., pseudoephedrine), vasopressor agents (e.g., epinephrine, norepinephrine), or dopaminergic agents (e.g., dopamine, dobutamine). (See Sympathomimetic Agents under Drug Interactions.)

Lactic Acidosis

Lactic acidosis, characterized by recurrent nausea and vomiting, has been reported in patients receiving linezolid. Patients who develop recurrent nausea and vomiting, unexplained acidosis, or a low bicarbonate concentration while receiving linezolid should undergo immediate medical evaluation.

Seizures

Seizures have been reported in patients receiving linezolid. Some cases were reported in patients with a history of seizures or risk factors for seizures.

Hypoglycemia

Symptomatic hypoglycemia has been reported in patients with diabetes mellitus receiving linezolid concomitantly with insulin or oral antidiabetic agents. (See Antidiabetic Agents under Drug Interactions.)

Although a causal relationship between linezolid and hypoglycemia has not been established, patients with diabetes mellitus should be cautioned about the potential for hypoglycemia during linezolid treatment.

If hypoglycemia occurs, dosage reduction of insulin or oral antidiabetic agents or discontinuance of linezolid, insulin, or oral antidiabetic agents may be necessary.

Sensitivity Reactions

Anaphylaxis, angioedema, and bullous skin disorders, including severe cutaneous adverse reactions (SCAR) such as toxic epidermal necrolysis and Stevens-Johnson syndrome, reported.

Tooth Discoloration

Superficial tooth discoloration and tongue discoloration have been reported in patients receiving linezolid. In cases with known outcome, tooth discoloration was removable with professional dental cleaning (manual descaling).

Phenylketonuria

Individuals who must restrict their intake of phenylalanine should be warned that linezolid for oral suspension contains aspartame, which is metabolized in the GI tract following oral administration, to provide 20 mg of phenylalanine per 5 mL of suspension.

Linezolid tablets do not contain aspartame and should be used in individuals with phenylketonuria (i.e., homozygous genetic deficiency of phenylalanine hydroxylase) and other individuals who must restrict their intake of phenylalanine.

Superinfection/Clostridioides difficile-associated Diarrhea and Colitis

Use of linezolid may result in emergence and overgrowth of nonsusceptible organisms. Appropriate therapy should be instituted if superinfection occurs.

Treatment with anti-infectives alters normal colon flora and may permit overgrowth of *Clostridioides difficile* (formerly *Clostridium difficile*). *C. difficile* infection (CDI) and *C. difficile*-associated diarrhea and colitis (CDAD; also known as antibiotic-associated diarrhea and colitis or pseudomembranous colitis) have been reported with nearly all anti-infectives, including linezolid, and may range in severity from mild diarrhea to fatal colitis. *C. difficile* produces toxins A and B which contribute to the development of CDAD; hypertoxin-producing strains of *C. difficile* are associated with increased morbidity and mortality since they may be refractory to anti-infectives and colectomy may be required.

CDAD should be considered in the differential diagnosis of patients who develop diarrhea during or after anti-infective therapy. Careful medical history is necessary since CDAD has been reported to occur as late as 2 months or longer after anti-infective therapy is discontinued.

If CDAD is suspected or confirmed, anti-infective therapy not directed against *C. difficile* should be discontinued whenever possible. Patients should be managed with appropriate anti-infective therapy directed against *C. difficile* (e.g., fidaxomicin, vancomycin, metronidazole), supportive therapy (e.g., fluid and electrolyte management, protein supplementation), and surgical evaluation as clinically indicated.

Selection and Use of Anti-infectives

Linezolid is indicated only for the treatment of certain infections caused by certain gram-positive bacteria. The drug has no clinical activity against gram-negative bacteria and is *not* indicated for the treatment of infections caused by gram-negative bacteria.

It is imperative that an anti-infective active against gram-negative bacteria be used concomitantly if documented or presumed pathogens include gram-negative bacteria. (See Uses.)

Safety and efficacy of linezolid given for longer than 28 days have not been evaluated in controlled clinical trials.

To reduce development of drug-resistant bacteria and maintain effectiveness of linezolid and other antibacterials, the drug should be used only for treatment of infections proven or strongly suspected to be caused by susceptible bacteria.

When selecting or modifying anti-infective therapy, results of culture and in vitro susceptibility testing should be used. In the absence of such data, local epidemiology and susceptibility patterns should be considered when selecting anti-infectives for empiric therapy.

Information on test methods and quality control standards for in vitro susceptibility testing of antibacterials and specific interpretive criteria for such testing recognized by FDA is available at https://www.fda.gov/STIC. For most antibacterials, including linezolid, FDA recognizes the standards published by the Clinical and Laboratory Standards Institute (CLSI).

Specific Populations

Pregnancy

Available data from published and postmarketing case reports regarding use of linezolid in pregnant women have not identified a drug-associated risk of major birth defects, miscarriage, or adverse maternal or fetal outcomes.

In studies in mice, rats, and rabbits, linezolid was not teratogenic; however, embryofetal toxicities were reported. These nonteratogenic effects included increased post-implantational embryo death, decreased fetal body weights, and increased incidence of costal cartilage fusion in mice; decreased fetal body weights, reduced ossification of sternebrae, and decreased survival of pups in rats; and reduced fetal body weight in rabbits.

Lactation

Linezolid is distributed into human milk. It is not known whether the drug affects the breast-fed infant or affects milk production. Available data suggest that a breast-fed infant would receive approximately 6–9% of the recommended daily therapeutic infant dose (10 mg/kg every 8 hours).

The benefits of breast-feeding and the importance of linezolid to the woman should be considered along with the potential adverse effects on the breast-fed child from the drug or from the underlying maternal condition.

If linezolid is used in a nursing woman, the manufacturer recommends that the breast-fed infant be monitored for diarrhea and vomiting since these are the most common adverse reactions reported in infants being treated with linezolid.

Males of Reproductive Potential

Based on findings from animal studies, linezolid may reversibly impair fertility in males.

In adult male rats receiving linezolid dosages of at least 50 mg/kg daily resulting in exposures approximately equal to or greater than human exposures (based on AUC), a reversible decrease in fertility and reproductive performance was reported. The effects on fertility were mediated through altered spermatogenesis; affected spermatids contained abnormally formed and oriented mitochondria and were nonviable. Epithelial cell hypertrophy and hyperplasia in the epididymis was observed in conjunction with decreased fertility. Similar epididymal changes were not seen in dogs.

Pediatric Use

Safety and efficacy of linezolid for the treatment of community-acquired pneumonia (CAP), nosocomial pneumonia, complicated skin and skin structure infections, and vancomycin-resistant *Enterococcus faecium* infections in pediatric patients are supported by adequate and well-controlled studies in adults, pharmacokinetic studies in pediatric patients, and additional data from a comparator-controlled study of gram-positive infections in neonates and children through 11 years of age. Safety and efficacy of the drug for the treatment of CAP in pediatric patients also is supported by evidence from an uncontrolled study in patients 8 months through 12 years of age.

Safety and efficacy of linezolid for the treatment of uncomplicated skin and skin structure infections in pediatric patients have been established in a comparator-controlled study in pediatric patients 5–17 years of age.

While some pharmacokinetic parameters (i.e., peak plasma concentration, volume of distribution) are similar in children of all ages, linezolid clearance varies with age. Excluding neonates younger than 1 week of age, clearance is most rapid in the youngest age groups (i.e., those 7 days to 11 years of age); as children age, the clearance of linezolid decreases and clearance values in adolescents approach those observed in adults. Systemic exposure (mean daily area under the plasma concentration-time curve [AUC]) in pediatric patients younger than 12 years of age receiving linezolid every 8 hours generally is similar to that in adults and adolescents receiving the drug every 12 hours. There is wider intraindividual variability in linezolid clearance and in systemic drug exposure in all pediatric age groups relative to adults.

The manufacturer states that linezolid is not recommended for empiric treatment of CNS infections in pediatric patients; therapeutic concentrations of the drug were not consistently achieved or maintained in CSF of pediatric patients with ventriculoperitoneal shunts.

Inadequate systemic exposure, site and severity of infection, and underlying medical conditions should be considered in children with a suboptimal response to linezolid, especially those with infections caused by gram-positive bacteria that have minimum inhibitory concentrations (MICs) of 4 mcg/mL.

Geriatric Use

No overall differences in safety, efficacy, or pharmacokinetics have been observed in geriatric adults 65 years of age or older compared with younger adults. Other clinical experience has not revealed age-related differences in response, but the possibility of greater sensitivity in some older patients cannot be ruled out.

Renal Impairment

Linezolid pharmacokinetics are not altered in patients with renal impairment. However, the 2 principal metabolites of linezolid may accumulate in patients with impaired renal function and the amount of accumulation increases with the severity of renal impairment. Because the clinical importance of accumulation of linezolid metabolites has not been determined, the potential benefits of linezolid in patients with renal impairment should be weighed against the potential risks of accumulation of the metabolites. (See Renal Impairment under Dosage and Administration.)

Hepatic Impairment

Linezolid pharmacokinetics are not altered in patients with mild or moderate hepatic impairment (Child-Pugh class A or B); pharmacokinetics of the drug have not been evaluated in patients with severe hepatic impairment.

● Common Adverse Effects

Adverse effects occurring in 2% or more of adults receiving linezolid include GI effects (diarrhea, nausea, vomiting), headache, anemia, rash, and dizziness. Adverse effects reported in 2% or more of pediatric patients receiving linezolid in clinical studies include GI effects (diarrhea, nausea, vomiting, localized or generalized abdominal pain, loose stools), headache, anemia, and thrombocytopenia.

DRUG INTERACTIONS

● Drugs Affecting or Metabolized by Hepatic Microsomal Enzymes

Linezolid is minimally metabolized (possibly mediated by cytochrome P-450 [CYP] enzymes), does not induce CYP enzymes, and does not inhibit CYP isoenzymes 1A2, 2C9, 2C19, 2D6, 2E1, or 3A4.

Linezolid is not expected to affect the pharmacokinetics of other drugs metabolized by CYP isoenzymes.

Although the mechanism of the interaction is unknown and may be related to induction of hepatic enzymes, concomitant use of rifampin and linezolid has resulted in decreased linezolid concentrations. It is possible that concomitant use of other potent inducers of hepatic enzymes (e.g., carbamazepine, phenytoin, phenobarbital) could result in decreased linezolid exposures.

● Antidiabetic Agents

Hypoglycemia has been reported in patients with diabetes mellitus receiving linezolid concomitantly with insulin or oral antidiabetic agents. Although a causal relationship has not been established, linezolid is a nonselective, reversible monoamine oxidase (MAO) inhibitor and some MAO inhibitors have been associated with hypoglycemic episodes in patients with diabetes mellitus who were also receiving insulin or oral antidiabetic agents. Patients should be warned of the potential for hypoglycemia. If hypoglycemia occurs, dosage reduction of the antidiabetic agent or discontinuance of linezolid or the antidiabetic agent may be necessary.

● Anti-infective Agents

Aminoglycosides

Concomitant use of linezolid and gentamicin does not affect the pharmacokinetics of either drug.

In vitro studies indicate the antibacterial effects of linezolid and gentamicin or streptomycin may be additive or indifferent.

Ampicillin

In vitro studies indicate the antibacterial effects of linezolid and ampicillin may be additive or indifferent.

Aztreonam

Concomitant use of linezolid and aztreonam does not result in clinically important effects on the pharmacokinetics of either drug.

In vitro studies indicate the antibacterial effects of linezolid and aztreonam may be additive or indifferent.

Carbapenems

In vitro studies indicate the antibacterial effects of linezolid and imipenem may be additive or indifferent.

Rifampin

Concomitant use of linezolid (600 mg twice daily for 2.5 days) and rifampin (600 mg once daily for 8 days) resulted in a 21% decrease in peak plasma concentrations of linezolid and a 32% decrease in the area under the plasma concentration-time curve (AUC) of linezolid. The mechanism and clinical importance of this pharmacokinetic interaction are unknown, although the interaction may be related to induction of hepatic enzymes.

In vitro studies indicate the antibacterial effects of linezolid and rifampin may be additive or indifferent.

Vancomycin

In vitro studies indicate the antibacterial effects of linezolid and vancomycin may be additive or indifferent.

● Monoamine Oxidase Inhibitors

Linezolid is a weak, nonselective, reversible MAO inhibitor and there is potential for pharmacologic interactions with other MAO inhibitors. Because of the potential for interaction, linezolid should not be used in patients who are receiving (or have received within the last 2 weeks) a drug that inhibits MAO-A or MAO-B (e.g., isocarboxazid, phenelzine, selegiline, tranylcypromine).

Although FDA has not concluded whether the risk of serotonin syndrome associated with concomitant use of linezolid and MAO inhibitors is comparable to that reported when linezolid is used concomitantly with selective serotonin-reuptake inhibitors (SSRIs) or selective serotonin- and norepinephrine-reuptake inhibitors (SNRIs), linezolid generally should not be used in patients receiving serotonergic drugs, including MAO inhibitors (e.g., isocarboxazid, phenelzine, selegiline, tranylcypromine). (See Serotonergic Drugs under Drug Interactions.)

● Phenytoin

Concomitant use of linezolid and phenytoin is not expected to affect the pharmacokinetics of phenytoin, but may possibly result in decreased linezolid exposures. Dosage adjustments are not required if linezolid and phenytoin are used concomitantly.

● Serotonergic Drugs

Concomitant use of linezolid and serotonergic drugs is associated with a risk of serotonin syndrome. There have been postmarketing reports of serotonin syndrome, including some fatalities, in patients who received linezolid concurrently with or shortly after discontinuance of serotonergic agents, particularly SSRIs (e.g., citalopram, escitalopram, fluoxetine, fluvoxamine, paroxetine, sertraline) or SNRIs (e.g., desvenlafaxine, duloxetine, venlafaxine). While FDA has not received reports of serotonin syndrome with concomitant use of linezolid and vilazodone, the risk is considered comparable to that with SSRIs. It is unclear whether concomitant use of linezolid and other drugs with lesser degrees of serotonergic activity, including tricyclic antidepressants (amitriptyline, clomipramine, desipramine, doxepin, imipramine, nortriptyline, protriptyline, trimipramine), MAO inhibitors (isocarboxazid, phenelzine, transdermal selegiline, tranylcypromine), amoxapine, bupropion, buspirone, maprotiline, mirtazapine, nefazodone, and trazodone, is associated with a risk of serotonin syndrome comparable to that reported when linezolid is used concomitantly with SSRIs or SNRIs.

Because of the risk of serotonin syndrome, linezolid should not be used in patients receiving serotonergic drugs, including SSRIs, tricyclic antidepressants, serotonin 5-HT$_1$ receptor agonists (triptans), meperidine, bupropion, or buspirone, unless concomitant therapy is considered clinically appropriate and patients can be carefully monitored for signs and/or symptoms of serotonin syndrome or neuroleptic malignant syndrome-like (NMS-like) reactions.

There may be some cases when a patient is already receiving a serotonergic antidepressant or buspirone and requires urgent treatment with linezolid (e.g., life-threatening infections caused by methicillin-resistant *Staphylococcus aureus*

[MRSA; also known as oxacillin-resistant *S. aureus* or ORSA] or vancomycin-resistant *Enterococcus faecium*). In these situations, if alternatives to linezolid are not available and the potential benefits of linezolid outweigh the risks of serotonin syndrome or NMS-like reactions, the serotonergic antidepressant should be stopped promptly and linezolid administered. The patient should be monitored for manifestations of serotonin syndrome or NMS-like reactions (e.g., hyperthermia, rigidity, myoclonus, autonomic instability, mental status changes that include extreme agitation progressing to delirium and coma) for 2 weeks (5 weeks if fluoxetine was taken) or until 24 hours after the last dose of linezolid, whichever comes first. The patient also should be monitored for symptoms associated with discontinuance of the antidepressant.

Treatment with serotonergic drugs should not be initiated in a patient receiving linezolid; when necessary, the serotonergic drug may be started or reinitiated 24 hours after the last linezolid dose.

For further information on serotonin syndrome, including manifestations and treatment, see Drug Interactions: Serotonergic Drugs, in Fluoxetine Hydrochloride 28:16.04.20.

● Sympathomimetic Agents

Concomitant use of linezolid and indirect-acting sympathomimetic agents (e.g., phenylpropanolamine, pseudoephedrine), vasopressor agents (e.g., epinephrine, norepinephrine), or dopaminergic agents (e.g., dopamine, dobutamine) may result in a reversible enhancement of the pressor response to these agents.

Unless patients are monitored for potential increases in blood pressure, linezolid should not be used in patients receiving direct- or indirect-acting sympathomimetic agents (e.g., pseudoephedrine), vasopressor agents (e.g., epinephrine, norepinephrine), or dopaminergic agents (e.g., dopamine, dobutamine).

If an adrenergic agent (e.g., dopamine, epinephrine) is initiated in a patient receiving linezolid, lower initial doses of the adrenergic agent should be used and dosage titrated to achieve the desired response.

● Vitamins

Concomitant use of linezolid (600 mg orally on day 1 and day 8) and ascorbic acid (1 g daily on days 2–9) or vitamin E (800 units daily on days 2–9) increased the AUC of linezolid by 2.3 or 10.9%, respectively.

Adjustment of linezolid dosage is not needed if the drug is used concomitantly with ascorbic acid or vitamin E.

● Warfarin

Linezolid does not have a substantial effect on the pharmacokinetics of warfarin; dosage adjustments are not required if linezolid and warfarin are used concomitantly.

PHARMACOKINETICS

● Absorption

Elimination Bioavailability

Linezolid is rapidly and extensively absorbed after oral administration; absolute oral bioavailability of the drug is approximately 100%.

Peak plasma concentrations of linezolid are attained within 1–2 hours following oral administration.

Elimination Food

The time to peak concentrations is delayed and peak concentrations are decreased when linezolid is administered with a high-fat meal, but the extent of absorption is not affected. This effect is not considered clinically important.

● Distribution

Elimination Extent

Linezolid is readily distributed into well-perfused tissues.

In adults with CNS infections, IV administration of linezolid (600 mg twice daily) resulted in steady-state mean peak CSF concentrations that were 36–58% of mean peak plasma concentrations; the time to peak CSF concentrations was approximately 3–4 hours after a dose.

In pediatric patients with ventriculoperitoneal shunts receiving single or multiple doses of linezolid, therapeutic concentrations of the drug were not consistently achieved or maintained in CSF.

Linezolid is distributed into human milk.

Plasma Protein Binding

Linezolid is approximately 31% bound to plasma proteins.

● Elimination

Metabolism

Linezolid is metabolized principally by oxidation of the morpholine ring to 2 inactive metabolites, an aminoethoxyacetic acid metabolite (A) and a hydroxyethyl glycine metabolite (B). Although metabolite A is presumed to be formed via an enzymatic pathway, in vitro studies indicate metabolite B is formed by nonenzymatic chemical oxidation. In vitro studies indicate linezolid is minimally metabolized and this may be mediated by the cytochrome P-450 (CYP) enzyme system.

Elimination Route

Approximately 65% of a linezolid dose is eliminated via nonrenal clearance. Under steady-state conditions, approximately 30% of a linezolid dose is eliminated in urine as unchanged drug, 10% is eliminated as metabolite A, and 40% is eliminated as metabolite B. Mean renal clearance of linezolid is 40 mL/minute, suggesting net tubular reabsorption.

Almost no linezolid is found in feces as unchanged drug; approximately 3 and 6% of a dose is eliminated in feces as metabolite A and metabolite B, respectively.

Linezolid and its metabolites are removed by hemodialysis. Approximately 30% of a linezolid dose is removed by a 3-hour hemodialysis session started 3 hours after the dose.

It is not known whether linezolid and its metabolites are removed by peritoneal dialysis.

Half-life

The mean elimination half-life of linezolid is 4.3–6.4 hours in adults.

In neonates, the mean elimination half-life of linezolid is 5.6 hours in preterm neonates younger than 1 week of age, 3 hours in full-term neonates younger than 1 week of age, and 1.5 hours in neonates 1 week to 28 days of age.

In infants and children, the mean elimination half-life of linezolid is 1.8 hours in infants older than 28 days through 2 months of age and 2.9 hours in infants and children 3 months through 11 years of age.

In adolescents 12 through 17 years of age, the mean elimination half-life of linezolid is 4.1 hours.

Special Populations

Linezolid pharmacokinetics in patients 65 years of age or older are similar to the pharmacokinetics in younger adults.

In pediatric patients, clearance of linezolid varies with age and there is wide intraindividual variability. Excluding neonates younger than 7 days of age, clearance is most rapid in the youngest age groups (i.e., those 7 days to 11 years of age); as children age, clearance of linezolid decreases and clearance in adolescents is similar to that observed in adults.

Linezolid pharmacokinetics are not affected by mild to moderate hepatic impairment (Child-Pugh class A or B); pharmacokinetics of the drug have not been studied in patients with severe hepatic impairment.

Pharmacokinetics of linezolid are not affected by renal impairment. However, the 2 principal metabolites of the drug accumulate in patients with impaired renal function and the amount of accumulation increases with the severity of renal impairment.

DESCRIPTION

Linezolid is an oxazolidinone anti-infective agent. The mechanism of action of linezolid involves binding to a site on the bacterial 23S ribosomal RNA of the 50S subunit and prevention of formation of a functional 70S initiation complex, which is an essential component of the bacterial translation process.

In vitro, linezolid is bacteriostatic against susceptible enterococci and staphylococci and bactericidal against susceptible streptococci. Linezolid is active in vitro against most strains of *Staphylococcus aureus* (including methicillin-resistant *S. aureus* [MRSA; also known as oxacillin-resistant *S. aureus* or ORSA]), *Streptococcus agalactiae* (group B streptococci, GBS), *S. pneumoniae*, *S. pyogenes* (group A β-hemolytic streptococci, GAS), and vancomycin-resistant *Enterococcus faecium*. Linezolid also has in vitro activity against *E. faecalis* (including vancomycin-resistant strains), *E. faecium* (vancomycin-susceptible strains), *S. epidermidis* (including methicillin-resistant strains [oxacillin-resistant strains]), *S. haemolyticus*, viridans group streptococci, group G streptococci, *Corynebacterium*, and *Pasteurella multocida*; however, safety and efficacy of linezolid in treating clinical infections caused by these bacteria have not been established in adequate and well-controlled clinical studies to date.

Linezolid is active in vitro against *Mycobacterium tuberculosis*, including some multiple-drug resistant (MDR) and extensively drug-resistant (XDR) strains. Linezolid also has activity in vitro against some strains of *M. chelonaei*, *M. fortuitum*, *M. gilvum*, *M. gordonae*, *M. kansasii*, *M. mucgenicum*, and *M. simiae*.

Resistance to linezolid has been produced in vitro by serial passage of MRSA or enterococci (i.e., *E. faecalis*, *E. faecium*) in the presence of increasing concentrations of the drug, and resistance to linezolid has emerged in patients receiving the drug for the treatment of infections caused by MRSA or enterococci. Linezolid resistance generally is associated with point mutations in the 23S rRNA gene. However, linezolid resistance in staphylococci mediated by the chloramphenicol-florfenicol (*cfr*) gene located on a plasmid has been reported and such resistance is transferable between staphylococci.

Cross-resistance between linezolid and other oxazolidinones (e.g., tedizolid) has been reported. Bacteria resistant to linezolid because of mutations in chromosomal genes encoding the 23S rRNA or ribosomal proteins (L3 and L4) usually are cross-resistant to other oxazolidinones (e.g., tedizolid) and vice versa. However, in vitro data indicate that the presence of the *cfr* gene in *S. aureus* that results in resistance to linezolid does not necessarily result in cross-resistance to tedizolid in the absence of chromosomal mutations. Cross-resistance between linezolid and non-oxazolidinone anti-infectives is unlikely.

Linezolid is well absorbed following oral administration (absolute bioavailability approximately 100%) and is readily distributed to well-perfused tissues. The drug is metabolized principally via oxidation to 2 inactive metabolites: an aminoethoxyacetic acid metabolite and a hydroxyethyl glycine metabolite. Linezolid is minimally metabolized and metabolism may be mediated by the cytochrome P-450 (CYP) enzyme system. Linezolid does not inhibit CYP isoenzymes 1A2, 2C9, 2C19, 2D6, 2E1, or 3A4 and is not an enzyme inducer, suggesting that the drug is unlikely to alter the pharmacokinetics of drugs metabolized by these enzymes.

ADVICE TO PATIENTS

Advise patients that antibacterials (including linezolid) should only be used to treat bacterial infections and not used to treat viral infections (e.g., the common cold).

Importance of completing full course of treatment, even if feeling better after a few days.

Advise patients that skipping doses or not completing the full course of treatment may decrease effectiveness and increase the likelihood that bacteria will develop resistance and will not be treatable with linezolid or other antibacterials in the future.

Advise patients that linezolid may be taken orally without regard to meals.

If using the oral suspension, importance of not shaking the bottle vigorously and gently inverting the bottle 3–5 times to resuspend the drug prior to administration of each dose.

Advise patients of the potential risk of serotonin syndrome, particularly if linezolid is used concomitantly with monoamine oxidase (MAO) inhibitors, selective serotonin-reuptake inhibitors (SSRIs), selective serotonin- and norepinephrine-reuptake inhibitors (SNRIs), tricyclic antidepressants, or other serotonergic drugs. Importance of immediately contacting clinician if signs and symptoms of serotonin syndrome develop (e.g., confusion, hyperactivity, memory problems, muscle twitching, excessive sweating, shivering, shaking, diarrhea, loss of coordination, fever). Importance of not discontinuing serotonergic drugs without first consulting clinician.

Advise patients, particularly those with diabetes mellitus, that hypoglycemic reactions (diaphoresis and tremulousness) and low blood glucose concentrations may occur during linezolid treatment. Importance of contacting a clinician to obtain proper treatment if such reactions occur.

Importance of avoiding large quantities of foods or beverages with high tyramine content during linezolid treatment; this includes foods or beverages that have been aged, fermented, pickled, or smoked to improve flavor (e.g., aged cheeses, fermented or air-dried meats, sauerkraut, soy sauce, tap beer, red wine). Consider that tyramine content of any protein-rich food may be increased if stored for long periods or improperly refrigerated.

Advise individuals with phenylketonuria that the oral suspension contains aspartame, which is metabolized in the GI tract to provide 20 mg of phenylalanine per 5 mL of suspension.

Importance of notifying clinicians of any history of hypertension or seizures.

Importance of notifying clinicians if recurrent nausea and vomiting occurs.

Importance of notifying clinician if any change in vision occurs.

Advise patients that diarrhea is a common problem caused by anti-infectives and usually ends when the drug is discontinued. Importance of contacting a clinician if watery and bloody stools (with or without stomach cramps and fever) occur during or as late as 2 months or longer after the last dose.

Importance of informing clinicians of existing or contemplated concomitant therapy, including prescription drugs (e.g., antidepressants) and OTC drugs (e.g., pseudoephedrine), as well as any concomitant illnesses.

Importance of women informing clinicians if they are or plan to become pregnant or plan to breast-feed. Advise nursing women to monitor the breast-fed infant for diarrhea and vomiting.

Importance of informing patients of other important precautionary information. (See Cautions.)

PREPARATIONS

Excipients in commercially available drug preparations may have clinically important effects in some individuals; consult specific product labeling for details.

Linezolid

Oral		
For suspension	100 mg/5 mL*	**Linezolid for Suspension** Zyvox®, Pfizer
Tablets, film-coated	600 mg*	**Linezolid Tablets** Zyvox®, Pfizer
Parenteral		
Injection, for IV infusion	2 mg/mL (200 and 600 mg) in sterile isotonic solution*	**Linezolid Injection** Zyvox® Injection (in flexible containers), Pfizer

† Use is not currently included in the labeling approved by the US Food and Drug Administration.

* available from one or more manufacturer, distributor, and/or repackager by generic (nonproprietary) name

Tedizolid Phosphate

8:12.28.24 • OXAZOLIDINONES

■ Tedizolid phosphate is an oxazolidinone antibacterial agent.

USES

● *Skin and Skin Structure Infections*

Tedizolid phosphate is used for the treatment of acute bacterial skin and skin structure infections (ABSSSI) caused by susceptible *Staphylococcus aureus* (including methicillin-resistant *S. aureus* [MRSA; also known as oxacillin-resistant *S. aureus* or ORSA] and methicillin-susceptible *S. aureus*), *Streptococcus pyogenes* (group A β-hemolytic streptococci, GAS), *S. agalactiae* (group B streptococci, GBS), *S. anginosus* group (includes *S. anginosus*, *S. intermedius*, and *S. constellatus*), or *Enterococcus faecalis*.

Clinical Experience

Efficacy and safety of tedizolid were evaluated in 2 randomized, multicenter, double-blind, noninferiority, phase 3 studies (ESTABLISH-1 and ESTABLISH-2) in adults with acute bacterial skin and skin structure infections (e.g., cellulitis, erysipelas, major cutaneous abscess, wound infection) with local signs and symptoms of infection and at least 1 regional or systemic sign of infection at baseline (i.e., lymphadenopathy, temperature 38°C or greater, leukocyte count greater than 10,000 cells/mm^3 or less than 4000 cells/mm^3, or 10% or greater band forms on leukocyte differential).

In ESTABLISH-1, 649 patients (median age 43 years, 61% male, 7% with diabetes mellitus, 36% current or recent IV drug users, 40% with cellulitis/erysipelas, 30% with major cutaneous abscess, 30% with wound infection, overall median baseline lesion surface area 190 cm^2) were randomized to receive oral tedizolid (200 mg of tedizolid phosphate once daily for 6 days) or oral linezolid (600 mg twice daily for 10 days). In patients with wound infections, adjunctive use of aztreonam and/or metronidazole for coverage against gram-negative bacteria was permitted. After 48–72 hours of treatment, 79.3 or 79.1% of patients in the intent-to-treat (ITT) population who received tedizolid or linezolid, respectively, achieved early clinical response (i.e., no increase in lesion surface area from baseline, oral temperature 37.6°C or less), and 78 or 75.5%, respectively, achieved a 20% or greater reduction in lesion surface area from baseline. At 7–14 days after the end of treatment, 85.8% of patients receiving tedizolid and 85.6% of patients receiving linezolid achieved clinical success (i.e., resolution or near resolution of most disease-specific signs and symptoms, absence or near resolution of systemic signs of infection, and no new signs, symptoms, or complications attributable to the infection requiring further treatment of the primary lesion).

In ESTABLISH-2, 666 patients (median age 46 years, 68% male, 10% with diabetes mellitus, 20% current or recent IV drug users, 50% with cellulitis/erysipelas, 20% with major cutaneous abscess, 30% with wound infection, overall median baseline lesion surface area 231 cm^2) were randomized to receive tedizolid (200 mg of tedizolid phosphate IV once daily for 6 days) or linezolid (600 mg IV twice daily for 10 days). All patients received at least 2 IV doses with the option to switch to oral therapy if the patient met study criteria. In patients with wound infections, adjunctive use of aztreonam and/or metronidazole for coverage against gram-negative bacteria was permitted. After 48–72 hours of treatment, 86.1 or 84.1% of patients in the ITT population who received tedizolid or linezolid, respectively, achieved early clinical response (i.e., no increase in lesion surface area from baseline, oral temperature 37.6°C or less), and 85.2 or 82.6%, respectively, achieved a 20% or greater reduction in lesion surface area from baseline. At 7–14 days after the end of treatment, 88% of patients receiving tedizolid and 87.7% of patients receiving linezolid achieved clinical success (i.e., resolution or near resolution of most disease-specific signs and symptoms, absence or near resolution of systemic signs of infection, and no new signs, symptoms, or complications attributable to the infection requiring further treatment of the primary lesion).

In a pooled analysis of the subset of patients who were microbiologically evaluable and stratified according to the infecting pathogen (ESTABLISH-1 and ESTABLISH-2), the clinical success rate on day 7–14 in those with infections caused by MRSA or methicillin-susceptible *S. aureus* was 84 or 92%, respectively, in those treated with tedizolid and 81 or 94%, respectively, in those treated with

linezolid. The clinical success rate in those with infections caused by *S. agalactiae*, *S. pyogenes*, *S. anginosus* group, or *E. faecalis* was 89, 91, 70, or 70%, respectively, in those treated with tedizolid and 80, 95, 89, or 100%, respectively, in those treated with linezolid.

DOSAGE AND ADMINISTRATION

● *Administration*

Tedizolid phosphate is administered orally or by IV infusion.

Oral Administration

Tedizolid phosphate tablets may be given orally without regard to meals.

IV Administration

Tedizolid phosphate for injection should be administered *only* by IV infusion. The drug should *not* be administered by rapid or direct IV injection, and is *not* intended for IM, intra-arterial, intrathecal, intraperitoneal, or subcutaneous administration.

Other IV substances, additives, or drugs should *not* be added to tedizolid phosphate vials or infused simultaneously.

If the same IV line is used for sequential infusion of several different drugs, the line should be flushed with 0.9% sodium chloride injection before and after infusion of tedizolid phosphate.

Tedizolid phosphate is incompatible with solutions containing divalent cations (e.g., calcium, magnesium), including lactated Ringer's injection and Hartmann's solution.

Vials of tedizolid phosphate lyophilized powder for injection contain no preservatives and are intended for single use only.

Reconstitution and Dilution

Tedizolid phosphate for injection must be reconstituted and further diluted prior to IV infusion. Strict aseptic technique must be observed when preparing IV solutions of the drug.

Vials labeled as containing 200 mg of tedizolid phosphate should be reconstituted by adding 4 mL of sterile water for injection. The vial should be gently swirled, then left standing until the lyophilized powder or cake dissolves and foam disperses; vigorous agitation or shaking of the vial should be avoided to minimize foaming. Reconstituted solutions should be inspected to ensure that no particulate matter, powder, or cake is attached to the sides of the vial. If needed, the vial may be inverted and gently swirled to dissolve any remaining powder. The reconstituted solution should appear clear and colorless to pale yellow in color.

Reconstituted tedizolid phosphate must then be further diluted in 250 mL of 0.9% sodium chloride injection. The vial containing the reconstituted solution should be tilted and 4 mL of the solution withdrawn from the bottom corner of the vial using a syringe; inverting the vial while withdrawing the solution should be avoided. The 4 mL of reconstituted solution should be slowly added to an infusion bag containing 250 mL of 0.9% sodium chloride injection; the bag should be gently inverted to mix and should not be shaken. The reconstituted and diluted IV solution should appear clear and colorless to pale yellow in color. The solution should be inspected visually for particulate matter prior to administration and should be discarded if particles are observed.

Reconstituted or further diluted solutions of tedizolid phosphate may be stored under refrigeration (2–8°C) or at room temperature. Total storage time from reconstitution to administration should not exceed 24 hours whether stored at 2–8°C or room temperature.

Rate of Administration

Tedizolid phosphate solutions should be administered by IV infusion over 1 hour.

● *Dosage*

Tedizolid phosphate is a prodrug that is inactive until metabolized in vivo to tedizolid (see Description); dosage of the drug is expressed in terms of the prodrug (i.e., tedizolid phosphate).

Dosage adjustments of tedizolid phosphate are not needed when switching from IV to oral administration.

Adult Dosage

Skin and Skin Structure Infections

The recommended oral or IV dosage of tedizolid phosphate for the treatment of acute bacterial skin and skin structure infections (ABSSSI) in adults is 200 mg once daily for 6 days.

● **Special Populations**

Dosage adjustments are not needed in adults with hepatic impairment or renal impairment, including those undergoing hemodialysis.

Dosage adjustments are not needed based on age, gender, race, body weight, or body mass index (BMI).

CAUTIONS

● **Contraindications**

The manufacturer states there are no contraindications to use of tedizolid phosphate.

● **Warnings/Precautions**

Patients with Neutropenia

Safety and efficacy of tedizolid in patients with neutropenia (i.e., neutrophil counts less than 1000 cells/mm^3) have not been evaluated. In an animal model of infection, the antibacterial activity of tedizolid was reduced in the absence of granulocytes.

Alternative therapies should be considered for the treatment of acute bacterial skin and skin structure infections in patients with neutropenia.

Hematologic Effects

In phase 1 studies in healthy adults who received tedizolid for 21 days, there was evidence of a possible dose and duration effect on hematologic parameters after day 6. In phase 3 studies in patients with acute bacterial skin and skin structure infections, the rate of clinically important changes in neutrophil count, platelet count, and hemoglobin concentration generally were similar in those treated with a 6-day regimen of tedizolid or a 10-day regimen of linezolid.

Neuropathy

Peripheral and optic neuropathies have been reported in patients who received more than 28 days of treatment with an oxazolidinone anti-infective (not tedizolid). In phase 3 studies evaluating tedizolid in patients with acute bacterial skin and skin structure infections, peripheral neuropathy or optic nerve disorders were reported in 1.2 or 0.3%, respectively, of patients receiving tedizolid compared with 0.6 or 0.2%, respectively, of patients receiving linezolid. Data are not available for patients exposed to tedizolid for longer than 6 days.

Superinfection/Clostridium difficile-associated Diarrhea and Colitis (CDAD)

Use of tedizolid may result in emergence and overgrowth of nonsusceptible bacteria or fungi. The patient should be carefully monitored and appropriate therapy instituted if superinfection occurs.

Treatment with anti-infectives alters normal colon flora and may permit overgrowth of *Clostridium difficile*. *C. difficile* infection (CDI) and *C. difficile*-associated diarrhea and colitis (CDAD; also known as antibiotic-associated diarrhea and colitis or pseudomembranous colitis) have been reported in patients receiving nearly all anti-infectives, including tedizolid, and may range in severity from mild diarrhea to fatal colitis. *C. difficile* produces toxins A and B which contribute to development of CDAD; hypertoxin-producing strains of *C. difficile* are associated with increased morbidity and mortality since they may be refractory to anti-infectives and colectomy may be required.

CDAD should be considered in the differential diagnosis of patients who develop diarrhea during or after anti-infective therapy. Careful medical history is necessary since CDAD has been reported to occur as late as 2 months or longer after anti-infective therapy is discontinued.

If CDAD is suspected or confirmed, anti-infective therapy not directed against *C. difficile* should be discontinued whenever possible. Patients should be managed with appropriate supportive therapy (e.g., fluid and electrolyte management, protein supplementation), anti-infective therapy directed against *C. difficile* (e.g., metronidazole, vancomycin), and surgical evaluation as clinically indicated.

Selection and Use of Anti-infectives

To reduce development of drug-resistant bacteria and maintain effectiveness of tedizolid and other antibacterials, the drug should be used only for treatment of infections proven or strongly suspected to be caused by susceptible bacteria.

When selecting or modifying anti-infective therapy, results of culture and in vitro susceptibility testing should be used. In the absence of such data, local epidemiology and susceptibility patterns should be considered when selecting anti-infectives for empiric therapy.

Specific Populations

Pregnancy

Category C. (See Users Guide.)

There are no adequate and well-controlled studies of tedizolid in pregnant women, and the drug should be used during pregnancy only if potential benefits justify potential risks to the fetus.

In embryofetal studies, tedizolid was shown to produce fetal developmental toxicities in mice, rats, and rabbits. In mice, reduced fetal weight and increased incidence of costal cartilage anomalies were observed at a dosage of 25 mg/kg daily (4 times the estimated human exposure level based on area under the plasma concentration-time curve [AUC]). In rats, decreased fetal weight and increased skeletal variations (e.g., reduced ossification of the sternebrae, vertebrae, and skull) were observed at a dosage of 15 mg/kg daily (6 times the estimated human exposure based on AUC) and were associated with maternal toxicity (reduced maternal body weight). In rabbits, reduced fetal weights, but no malformations or variations, were observed at dosages associated with maternal toxicity.

Lactation

Tedizolid is distributed into milk in rats; it is not known whether the drug is distributed into human milk.

Tedizolid phosphate should be used with caution in nursing women.

Pediatric Use

Safety and efficacy of tedizolid phosphate have not been established in pediatric patients younger than 18 years of age.

Geriatric Use

Clinical studies did not include sufficient numbers of patients 65 years of age or older to determine whether they respond differently than younger adults. Differences in tedizolid pharmacokinetics were not observed between geriatric and younger patients. Dosage adjustments are not needed in geriatric patients.

Hepatic Impairment

Clinically important changes in tedizolid pharmacokinetics (peak plasma concentrations, AUC) were not observed in adults with moderate or severe hepatic impairment (Child-Pugh class B or C); dosage adjustments are not needed.

Renal Impairment

Clinically important changes in tedizolid pharmacokinetics (peak plasma concentrations, AUC) were not observed in adults with severe renal impairment (creatinine clearance less than 30 mL/minute per 1.73 m^2). Hemodialysis does not result in clinically important removal of tedizolid from systemic circulation. Dosage adjustments are not needed in patients with renal impairment or undergoing hemodialysis.

● **Common Adverse Effects**

Adverse effects reported in 2% or more of patients receiving tedizolid phosphate include nausea, headache, diarrhea, vomiting, dizziness, and fatigue.

DRUG INTERACTIONS

● **Drugs Affecting or Metabolized by Hepatic Microsomal Enzymes**

In vitro, tedizolid phosphate and tedizolid do not appear to be substrates for and do not inhibit or induce cytochrome P-450 (CYP) isoenzymes, including CYP1A2, 2B6, 2D6, 2C8, 2C9, 2C19, and 3A4. Drug interactions involving oxidative metabolism and CYP isoenzymes are unlikely.

● Drugs Affecting or Affected by Membrane Transporters

In vitro, tedizolid phosphate and tedizolid do not have clinically important effects on drug uptake or drug efflux membrane transporters (e.g., organic anion transporter [OAT] 1, OAT3, organic anion transporting polypeptide [OATP] 1B1, OATP1B3, organic cation transporter [OCT] 1, OCT2, P-glycoprotein [P-gp], breast cancer resistance protein [BCRP]).

● Antibacterial Agents

In vitro studies indicate that the antibacterial effects of tedizolid and aztreonam, ceftazidime, ceftriaxone, ciprofloxacin, clindamycin, co-trimoxazole, daptomycin, gentamicin, imipenem, minocycline, rifampin, or vancomycin are not synergistic or antagonistic against gram-positive bacteria (methicillin-resistant *Staphylococcus aureus*, *Streptococcus pneumoniae*, *S. pyogenes*, *Enterococcus faecalis*) or gram-negative bacteria (*Escherichia coli*).

● Antifungal Agents

In vitro studies indicate that tedizolid and amphotericin B, ketoconazole, or terbinafine are not synergistic or antagonistic against gram-positive bacteria (methicillin-resistant *S. aureus*, *S. pneumoniae*, *S. pyogenes*, *E. faecalis*).

● Monoamine Oxidase Inhibitors

In vitro, tedizolid is a weak reversible inhibitor of monoamine oxidase (MAO). Patients receiving MAO inhibitors were excluded during phase 2 and 3 clinical trials evaluating tedizolid phosphate; interactions between tedizolid and MAO inhibitors have not been evaluated.

● Pseudoephedrine

Concomitant use of oral tedizolid (200 mg of tedizolid phosphate once daily for 5 days) and pseudoephedrine (single 60-mg dose on day 5) in healthy adults did not result in substantial increases in maximum blood pressure or heart rate when compared with increases observed in those receiving pseudoephedrine concomitantly with placebo. Concomitant use of tedizolid and pseudoephedrine did not affect the pharmacokinetics of either drug.

● Serotonergic Drugs

When studied in a mouse model that predicts serotonergic activity, the serotonergic effects of tedizolid phosphate dosages up to 30-fold higher than the equivalent human dosages were similar to those seen with a vehicle control. Patients receiving serotonergic agents (e.g., selective serotonin-reuptake inhibitors [SSRIs], tricyclic antidepressants, serotonin type 1 [5-hydroxytryptamine type 1; 5-HT$_1$] receptor agonists ["triptans"], meperidine, buspirone) were excluded from phase 3 trials evaluating tedizolid phosphate.

● Tyramine-containing Foods

In healthy adults receiving tedizolid (200 mg of tedizolid phosphate once daily), the median tyramine dose required to increase systolic blood pressure by 30 mm Hg or more from baseline within 2 hours of tyramine administration was 325 mg compared with a dose of 425 mg when tyramine was used concomitantly with placebo. Palpitations were reported in 72.4% of those receiving tedizolid concomitantly with tyramine compared with 46.4% of those receiving tyramine and placebo.

Recommended dosage of tedizolid phosphate (200 mg daily) is not expected to exert a clinically important pressor response in patients receiving a tyramine-rich meal; restriction of foods with high tyramine content is not necessary.

DESCRIPTION

Tedizolid phosphate is an oxazolidinone anti-infective agent. Tedizolid phosphate is a prodrug that is inactive until hydrolyzed in vivo to tedizolid. The phosphate prodrug is highly water soluble, which facilitates oral absorption and enhances bioavailability of tedizolid. The mechanism of activity of tedizolid is mediated by binding to the 50S subunit of bacterial ribosomes resulting in inhibition of bacterial translation and inhibition of protein synthesis. Although the binding site for tedizolid is similar to the binding site for other oxazolidinones (e.g., linezolid), tedizolid may engage additional ribosomal sites compared with linezolid.

In vitro, tedizolid is bacteriostatic against certain gram-positive bacteria, including staphylococci, streptococci, and enterococci. The drug is active in vitro and in clinical infections against *Staphylococcus aureus* (including methicillin-resistant *S. aureus* [MRSA; also known as oxacillin-resistant *S. aureus*]), *S. pyogenes* (group A β-hemolytic streptococci, GAS), *Streptococcus agalactiae* (group B streptococci, GBS), *S. anginosus* group (includes *S. anginosus*, *S. intermedius*, and *S. constellatus*), and *Enterococcus faecalis*. There is some evidence from in vitro studies that tedizolid may be more potent than linezolid against susceptible bacteria, and tedizolid has been active against some strains of *S. aureus* resistant to linezolid. Tedizolid also has in vitro activity against *E. faecium*, *S. epidermidis* (including methicillin-resistant strains [oxacillin-resistant strains]), *S. haemolyticus*, and *S. lugdunensis*; however, safety and efficacy of the drug in treating clinical infections caused by these bacteria have not been established in adequate and well-controlled clinical studies to date. Although further study is needed, there is some in vitro evidence that tedizolid has activity against *Mycobacterium tuberculosis*.

Reduced susceptibility or resistance to tedizolid has been produced in vitro by serial passage of *S. aureus* or *E. faecium* in the presence of increasing concentrations of the drug. In vitro, spontaneous mutations conferring reduced susceptibility to tedizolid have occurred at a frequency rate of approximately 10^{-10}.

Cross-resistance between tedizolid and linezolid has been reported. Bacteria resistant to oxazolidinones (e.g., linezolid) because of mutations in chromosomal genes encoding the 23S rRNA or ribosomal proteins (L3 and L4) usually are cross-resistant to tedizolid. However, in vitro date indicate that the presence of the chloramphenicol-florfenicol resistance (*cfr*) gene in *S. aureus* that results in resistance to linezolid may not result in resistance to tedizolid in the absence of chromosomal mutations. Cross-resistance between tedizolid and non-oxazolidinone anti-infectives is unlikely.

Tedizolid phosphate is rapidly converted in vivo by phosphatases to the active moiety, tedizolid. The drug is well absorbed following oral administration (absolute bioavailability approximately 91%); systemic exposure is similar whether the drug is given orally in the fasted state or with a high-fat, high-calorie meal. Peak plasma concentrations of tedizolid are achieved approximately 3 hours after oral administration of tedizolid phosphate in the fasted state or at the end of a 1-hour IV infusion. Steady-state concentrations are achieved within approximately 3 days with oral or IV administration; accumulation is approximately 30% after 7 or more days of once-daily dosing. Tedizolid has a half-life of approximately 12 hours. The drug is distributed into the interstitial space fluid of adipose and skeletal muscle tissue at concentrations similar to plasma concentrations; the drug also has been shown to distribute into epithelial lining fluid of pulmonary tissue in concentrations higher than those found in plasma. Tedizolid is 70–90% bound to plasma proteins. Tedizolid phosphate and tedizolid do not appear to be substrates of cytochrome P-450 (CYP) enzymes. A major metabolite (tedizolid sulfate) and several minor metabolites have been identified in feces and urine. Following a single oral dose of tedizolid phosphate, tedizolid is excreted in feces (82%) and urine (18%), principally as the noncirculating sulfate conjugate; less than 3% of the tedizolid phosphate dose is eliminated in feces and urine as unchanged tedizolid. Approximately 10% of a dose is removed by hemodialysis.

ADVICE TO PATIENTS

Advise patients that antibacterials (including tedizolid) should only be used to treat bacterial infections and not used to treat viral infections (e.g., the common cold).

Importance of completing full course of therapy, even if feeling better after a few days.

Advise patients that skipping doses or not completing the full course of therapy may decrease effectiveness and increase the likelihood that bacteria will develop resistance and will not be treatable with tedizolid or other antibacterials in the future.

Advise patients that tedizolid may be taken orally without regard to meals and without any dietary restriction.

Importance of informing patients that if they miss a dose and it is remembered within 8 hours after the scheduled time, they should take the dose as soon as possible and then take their next scheduled dose at the usual time. If less than 8 hours remain before the next scheduled dose, the patient should skip the dose and wait until their next scheduled dose.

Advise patients that diarrhea is a common problem caused by anti-infectives and usually ends when the drug is discontinued. Importance of contacting a clinician if watery and bloody stools (with or without stomach cramps and fever) occur during or as late as 2 months or longer after the last dose.

Importance of informing clinicians of existing or contemplated concomitant therapy, including prescription and OTC drugs and dietary or herbal supplements, as well as any concomitant illnesses.

Importance of women informing clinicians if they are or plan to become pregnant or plan to breast-feed.

Importance of informing patients of other important precautionary information. (See Cautions.)

PREPARATIONS

Excipients in commercially available drug preparations may have clinically important effects in some individuals; consult specific product labeling for details.

Tedizolid Phosphate

Oral		
Tablets, film-coated	200 mg	**Sivextro®**, Cubist
Parenteral		
For injection, for IV infusion only	200 mg	**Sivextro®**, Cubist

Colistimethate Sodium

8:12.28.28 • POLYMYXINS

■ Colistimethate sodium is a prodrug of colistin. Colistin (also known as polymyxin E) is a polymyxin antibiotic structurally and pharmacologically related to polymyxin B.

USES

● Gram-negative Aerobic Bacterial Infections

Colistimethate sodium is used parenterally for the treatment of acute or chronic infections caused by certain susceptible gram-negative bacteria (e.g., *Enterobacter aerogenes, Escherichia coli, Klebsiella pneumoniae, Pseudomonas aeruginosa*). Other more effective and less toxic anti-infectives (e.g., fluoroquinolones, aminoglycosides, third generation cephalosporins, extended-spectrum penicillins, carbapenems) usually are drugs of choice for most gram-negative bacterial infections. Colistimethate sodium should be used in the treatment of infections caused by susceptible gram-negative bacteria only when other more effective and less toxic anti-infectives are contraindicated or are ineffective. However, colistimethate sodium may be useful alone or in conjunction with other anti-infectives for the treatment of infections caused by multiple-drug resistant gram-negative bacteria, such as respiratory tract infections in cystic fibrosis patients caused by multiple-drug resistant *Ps. aeruginosa*. Colistimethate sodium is not indicated for infections caused by *Proteus* or *Neisseria*.

Colistin sulfate (no longer commercially available in the US) has been used orally for the treatment of gastroenteritis caused by susceptible *Shigella*; however, substantial evidence of effectiveness is lacking and other anti-infectives (e.g., fluoroquinolones, azithromycin, ampicillin, co-trimoxazole) generally are preferred if anti-infective therapy is indicated in the treatment of these infections. Colistin sulfate also has been used orally for the treatment of diarrhea caused by susceptible strains of enteropathogenic *E. coli*; however, use of anti-infectives for treatment of diarrhea caused by enteropathogenic *E. coli* is controversial and management usually involves replacement of fluids and electrolytes.

● Respiratory Tract Infections

Cystic Fibrosis Patients

Oral Inhalation

Colistimethate sodium has been administered by oral inhalation via nebulization† for early treatment of *Ps. aeruginosa* respiratory tract infections in adult and pediatric cystic fibrosis patients and for suppressive therapy in cystic fibrosis patients colonized with *Ps. aeruginosa*. Safety and efficacy of such treatment have not been established, and colistimethate sodium is not labeled by the US Food and Drug Administration (FDA) for administration via nebulization. Adverse respiratory effects (e.g., bronchoconstriction) have occurred with this route, and there has been at least one fatality in a patient who self-administered a nebulizer treatment using a premixed solution of the drug. (See Cautions: Respiratory Effects.)

There is some evidence from a randomized study and observational studies that early initiation of a treatment regimen that includes colistimethate sodium administered by oral inhalation† (usually given in conjunction with oral ciprofloxacin) in addition to standard therapy for cystic fibrosis may prevent or delay chronic colonization in some adult and pediatric cystic fibrosis patients with *Ps. aeruginosa* respiratory tract infections. A review of anti-infective strategies for eradicating *Ps. aeruginosa* in patients with cystic fibrosis that analyzed results of studies involving tobramycin or colistimethate sodium administered by oral inhalation concluded that there is some evidence that such anti-infective treatment of early *Ps. aeruginosa* infection in cystic fibrosis patients results in short-term eradication, but it remains uncertain whether there is an associated clinical benefit.

Results of a randomized study of colistimethate sodium or tobramycin administered by oral inhalation in adult and pediatric cystic fibrosis patients chronically infected with *Ps. aeruginosa* indicate that either treatment reduced the bacterial load, but only nebulized tobramycin significantly improved lung function as measured by FEV₁. Results of a randomized study

of colistimethate sodium administered by oral inhalation in adult and pediatric cystic fibrosis patients with chronic *Ps. aeruginosa* lung infections indicate that such therapy may be a useful supplement to IV antipseudomonal anti-infectives. A review of use of nebulized antipseudomonal anti-infectives in patients with cystic fibrosis concluded that such treatment may have a beneficial effect on lung function and may reduce exacerbations of respiratory infections, but that more research is needed to determine the duration of benefit, risk of emergence of resistant *Ps. aeruginosa*, and optimal drug and dosage regimens.

DOSAGE AND ADMINISTRATION

● Reconstitution and Administration

Colistimethate sodium is administered by IM injection, IV injection, or continuous IV infusion. The drug also has been administered by oral inhalation via nebulization†.

Dispensing and Dosage and Administration Precautions

The Institute for Safe Medication Practices (ISMP) alerted healthcare professionals about the risk of serious and potentially fatal medication errors related to dosage of colistimethate sodium.

Colistimethate sodium is a prodrug of colistin and is inactive until hydrolyzed in vivo to colistin. In the US, vials and carton packaging of colistimethate sulfate are labeled as colistimethate for injection; however, strength and dosage of the drug are expressed in terms of colistin base activity (colistin). This dosage convention *must* be considered when prescribing, preparing, and dispensing colistimethate sodium.

Healthcare professionals should be aware that, in the US, colistimethate sodium must *only* be prescribed in terms of colistin. If the drug is prescribed as colistimethate or colistimethate sodium, the prescriber should be contacted to verify the dosage in terms of colistin. At least 1 fatality related to acute renal failure and other complications occurred when colistimethate sodium was prescribed in terms of the prodrug (instead of colistin), resulting in administration of a dosage approximately 2.5 times greater than it should have been.

Healthcare professionals also should be aware that strength and dosage of colistimethate sodium preparations commercially available in some other countries may be expressed in terms of colistimethate sodium, in terms of colistin, or as international units. (See Dosage and Administration: Dosage.)

Any medication errors involving colistimethate sodium should be reported to the ISMP National Medication Error Reporting Program and the FDA MedWatch program.

Parenteral Administration

Colistimethate sodium sterile powder is reconstituted by adding 2 mL of sterile water for injection to a vial labeled as containing 150 mg of colistin; the vial should be swirled gently to avoid frothing. The resultant solution contains 75 mg of colistin per mL.

Reconstituted solutions of colistimethate sodium should be used within 7 days, but final solutions for continuous IV infusion should be freshly prepared and used within 24 hours. (See Chemistry and Stability: Stability)

IM Administration

For IM injection, the appropriate dose (as reconstituted solution) should be given by deep IM injection into a large muscle mass (e.g., gluteal muscle or lateral part of the thigh).

IV Injection

For direct intermittent IV administration, one-half of the total daily dose (as reconstituted solution) should be injected directly into a vein over a 3- to 5-minute period every 12 hours.

IV Infusion

For continuous IV infusion, one-half of the total daily dose (as reconstituted solution) should be injected directly into a vein over a 3- to 5-minute period; the remaining one-half of the total daily dose (as reconstituted solution) should be added to a compatible IV solution (see Chemistry and Stability: Stability) and administered 1–2 hours later (over the next 22–23 hours) by slow IV infusion.

The specific IV solution and volume of the solution used should be based on the patient's fluid and electrolyte requirements.

Oral Inhalation

For oral inhalation via nebulization†, an isotonic solution of colistimethate sodium has been prepared by diluting the appropriate dose in 2–4 mL of preservative-free 0.9% sodium chloride injection, sterile water, or a mixture of 0.9% sodium chloride injection and sterile water.

Solutions of colistimethate sodium for oral inhalation via nebulization† should be used promptly after being prepared. A fatality has been reported in a cystic fibrosis patient who self-administered a nebulizer treatment using a premixed solution of the drug. (See Cautions: Respiratory Effects.)

● Dosage

Dosage of colistimethate sodium commercially available in the US is expressed in terms of colistin.

Dosage of colistimethate sodium preparations commercially available in some other countries (e.g., United Kingdom, Greece) may be expressed in terms of colistimethate sodium, in terms of colistin, or as international units. *The fact that dosages reported in published clinical studies or case reports may vary depending on the country of origin and the preparation used should be considered.*

Although not the dosage convention in the US, it has been suggested that dosage of colistimethate sodium should preferably be expressed in terms of international units to avoid confusion. When expressed in terms of international units, each mg of colistin base has a potency of 30,000 international units and each mg of colistimethate sodium has a potency of 12,500 international units.

Parenteral Dosage

The usual IM or IV dosage of colistimethate sodium for adults and children with normal renal function is 2.5–5 mg/kg of colistin daily given in 2–4 divided doses, depending on the severity of the infection.

The maximum IM or IV dosage of colistimethate sodium recommended by the manufacturer for patients with normal renal function is 5 mg/kg of colistin daily.

The manufacturer recommends that dosage for obese patients should be based on an estimate of ideal body weight.

Oral Inhalation Dosage

For early treatment of *Pseudomonas aeruginosa* respiratory tract infections in adult and pediatric cystic fibrosis patients or for suppressive therapy in adult or pediatric cystic fibrosis patients colonized with *Ps. aeruginosa*, colistimethate sodium has been given by oral inhalation via nebulization† in a dosage of 33.33–66.66 mg of colistin 2 or 3 times daily. This corresponds to a dosage of 1–2 million international units 2 or 3 times daily.

● Dosage in Renal Impairment

In patients with renal impairment, dosage of colistimethate sodium should be decreased in proportion to the degree of renal impairment.

DOSAGE FOR ADULTS WITH RENAL IMPAIRMENT

Creatinine Clearance (mL/minute)	IM or IV Dosage (of Colistin)
80 or greater	2.5–5 mg/kg daily given in 2–4 divided doses
50–79	2.5–3.8 mg/kg daily given in 2 divided doses
30–49	2.5 mg/kg daily given as a single dose or in 2 divided doses
10–29	1.5 mg/kg given once every 36 hours

CAUTIONS

Adverse effects reported with colistimethate sodium are similar to those reported with polymyxin B sulfate. Nephrotoxicity and neurotoxicity are the most serious adverse effects of colistimethate sodium and are most likely to occur when the drug is used in higher than recommended dosages or in patients with impaired renal function.

● Renal Effects

Nephrotoxicity, manifested as decreased urine output, increased serum concentrations of BUN and creatinine, proteinuria, hematuria, and casts in the urine, has been reported in patients receiving usual dosage of colistimethate sodium. Acute tubular necrosis has been reported with colistimethate sodium and was not necessarily preceded by progressive renal impairment.

Nephrotoxicity is generally reversible when colistimethate sodium is discontinued; however, additional increases in concentrations of serum creatinine have frequently occurred for 1–2 weeks following discontinuance of the drug. Administration of colistimethate sodium in doses that exceed the renal excretory capacity will lead to high serum concentrations of the drug which can result in further impairment of renal function. (See Cautions: Precautions and Contraindications.)

● GI Effects

GI disturbance has been reported in patients receiving colistimethate sodium.

Clostridium difficile-associated diarrhea and colitis (CDAD; also known as antibiotic-associated diarrhea and colitis or pseudomembranous colitis) has been reported with nearly all anti-infectives, including colistimethate sodium, and may range in severity from mild diarrhea to fatal colitis. CDAD should be considered in the differential diagnosis of patients who develop diarrhea during or after anti-infective therapy. Mild cases of colitis may respond to discontinuance of the drug alone, but management of moderate to severe cases should include treatment with fluid, electrolyte, protein supplementation, appropriate anti-infective therapy (e.g., oral metronidazole or vancomycin), and surgical evaluation when clinically indicated. Careful medical history is necessary since CDAD has been reported to occur as late as 2 months or longer after anti-infective therapy is discontinued.

● Nervous System Effects

Transient nervous system effects, including circumoral or peripheral paresthesia or numbness, tingling or formication of the extremities or tongue, dizziness, vertigo, giddiness, ataxia, blurred vision, and slurred speech, have been reported in patients receiving colistimethate sodium. If these adverse nervous system effects occur, they generally appear within the first 4 days of therapy and disappear when the drug is discontinued. If adverse nervous system effects occur, colistimethate sodium therapy does not necessarily have to be discontinued, but the patient should be monitored closely; some of these adverse nervous system effects may be alleviated by reducing dosage of the drug.

More severe neurotoxic effects including mental confusion, coma, psychosis, and seizures also have been reported with colistimethate sodium, especially in patients receiving high dosage or in patients with renal impairment.

Neuromuscular blockade, which may result in respiratory arrest, can occur in patients receiving colistimethate sodium, especially when the drug is used in patients with neuromuscular disease such as myasthenia gravis or in patients who are receiving neuromuscular blocking agents, general anesthetics, or other drugs with neuromuscular blocking potential. (See Drug Interactions.) Apnea and neuromuscular blockade have been reported most frequently when colistimethate sodium was used in patients with impaired renal function and dosage of the drug was not reduced in proportion to the degree of renal impairment. If apnea occurs during therapy with colistimethate sodium, respiration should be assisted and calcium chloride injections and oxygen should be administered if appropriate. Neuromuscular blockade induced by colistimethate sodium is noncompetitive and is not reversed by neostigmine.

● Respiratory Effects

Bronchoconstriction has been reported in adult and pediatric cystic fibrosis patients who received colistimethate sodium by oral inhalation via nebulization†. Bronchoconstriction has occurred almost immediately after initiation of nebulization and can last for more than 30 minutes in some patients. It has been suggested that premedication with bronchodilators may reduce the potential for development of bronchoconstriction in patients receiving the drug by nebulization. Pre- and post-treatment pulmonary function tests have been recommended to identify patients who may be predisposed to bronchoconstriction. In young children who are unable to perform pulmonary function tests, bronchodilator premedication has been recommended.

Respiratory distress that progressed over several days to acute respiratory failure, multi-organ system failure, and death has been reported in a patient who received colistimethate sodium by oral inhalation via nebulization†. This patient self-administered the nebulizer treatment using a solution of colistimethate sodium that had been prepared by a pharmacy and dispensed in premixed unit dose ready-to-use vials. The patient developed respiratory distress within hours of the nebulization treatment and died about 19 days later. It has been suggested that this fatality may have been related to the fact that a premixed solution of colistimethate sodium was used in the nebulizer. After colistimethate sodium is mixed with water and buffer, it undergoes spontaneous hydrolysis to colistin. A component of colistin (polymyxin E1) has been shown to cause pulmonary inflammatory reactions in animals and may contribute to such local toxicity in humans. (See Cautions: Precautions and Contraindications.)

● **Other Adverse Effects**

Generalized pruritus, urticaria, rash, and fever have been reported in patients receiving colistimethate sodium. Anaphylaxis has also been reported.

Although a causal relationship has not been definitely established, leukopenia, granulocytopenia, and hepatotoxicity have been reported rarely with colistimethate sodium.

● **Precautions and Contraindications**

Colistimethate sodium is contraindicated in individuals who are hypersensitive to the drug or any ingredient in its formulation.

Because transient neurologic disturbances may occur during therapy with colistimethate sodium (see Cautions: Nervous System Effects), patients should be warned that the drug may impair their ability to perform hazardous activities requiring mental alertness or physical coordination (e.g., operating machinery, driving a motor vehicle).

Renal function should be monitored in patients receiving colistimethate sodium, since adverse renal effects may occur regardless of the dosage of the drug. If diminishing urine output or increasing concentrations of BUN or serum creatinine occur, colistimethate sodium should be discontinued immediately.

Colistimethate sodium should be used with caution in patients in whom the possibility of renal impairment exists (e.g., geriatric patients). Administration of colistimethate sodium in dosages in excess of renal excretory capacity will lead to high serum concentrations of the drug which can result in further impairment of renal function and possibly acute renal insufficiency, renal shutdown, and neuromuscular blockade. If colistimethate sodium is used in patients with renal impairment, extreme caution should be exercised and dosage and frequency of administration reduced in proportion to the degree of impairment.

Adults and children who receive colistimethate sodium by oral inhalation via nebulization† may be at risk of bronchoconstriction. Premedication with bronchodilators may reduce the potential for development of bronchoconstriction in patients receiving the drug by nebulization. The FDA states that healthcare providers who choose to prescribe colistimethate sodium for administration by oral inhalation via nebulization† should be familiar with the chemistry of the drug and aware of the potential for serious and life-threatening side effects from inhalation of premixed, ready-to-use liquid preparations of the drug. If colistimethate sodium is administered via a nebulizer, the solution should be used promptly after being mixed. Premixing colistimethate sodium into an aqueous solution and storing it for longer than 24 hours results in increased concentrations of colistin in the solution and increases the potential for lung toxicity if the premixed solution is administered via nebulization. Patients should be advised not to use any premixed, ready-to-use liquid preparations of colistimethate sodium for nebulization and to discard any unused vials of premixed, ready-to-use liquid preparations of the drug that they may have in their possession.

Prolonged use of colistimethate sodium may result in overgrowth of nonsusceptible organisms (e.g., *Proteus*). If suprainfection or superinfection occurs during therapy with colistimethate sodium, appropriate anti-infective therapy should be instituted.

To reduce development of drug-resistant bacteria and maintain effectiveness of colistimethate sodium and other antibacterials, the drug should be used only for the treatment or prevention of infections proven or strongly suspected to be caused by susceptible bacteria. When selecting or modifying anti-infective therapy, use results of culture and in vitro susceptibility testing. In the absence of such data, consider local epidemiology and susceptibility patterns when selecting anti-infectives for empiric therapy.

Because *Clostridium difficile*-associated diarrhea and colitis has been reported with colistimethate sodium, it should be considered in the differential diagnosis of patients who develop diarrhea during or after therapy. Patients should be advised that diarrhea is a common problem caused by anti-infectives and usually ends when the drug is discontinued; however, they should contact a clinician if watery and bloody stools (with or without stomach cramps and fever) occur during or as late as 2 months or longer after the last dose.

Patients should be advised that antibacterials (including colistimethate sodium) should only be used to treat bacterial infections and not used to treat viral infections (e.g., the common cold). Patients also should be advised about the importance of completing the full course of therapy, even if feeling better after a few days, and that skipping doses or not completing therapy may decrease effectiveness and increase the likelihood that bacteria will develop resistance and will not be treatable with colistimethate or other antibacterials in the future.

● **Pediatric Precautions**

Colistimethate sodium has been used in neonates, infants, children, and adolescents. The adverse effect profile in pediatric patients appears to be similar to that in adults; however, subjective symptoms of toxicity may not be reported by pediatric patients and close monitoring of these patients is recommended.

● **Geriatric Precautions**

Clinical studies of colistimethate sodium did not include sufficient numbers of patients 65 years of age and older to determine whether geriatric patients respond differently than younger patients. While other clinical experience has not revealed age-related differences in response, dosage generally should be selected carefully for geriatric patients, usually initiating therapy at the low end of the dosage range. The greater frequency of decreased hepatic, renal, and/or cardiac function and of concomitant disease and drug therapy observed in the elderly also should be considered.

Since the drug is substantially eliminated by the kidney, the risk of adverse effects may be greater in patient with impaired renal function. The greater frequency of decreased renal function observed in the elderly should be considered and dosage should be selected carefully in geriatric patients; monitoring renal function may be useful in these patients.

● **Mutagenicity and Carcinogenicity**

Long-term studies in animals have not been performed to date to evaluate the carcinogenic potential of colistimethate sodium.

● **Pregnancy, Fertility, and Lactation**

Pregnancy

Safe use of colistimethate sodium during pregnancy has not been established. When colistimethate sodium was given to rabbits during organogenesis in an IM dosage of 4.15 or 9.3 mg/kg (0.25 or 0.55 times, respectively, the maximum daily human dosage based on mg/m^2), talipes varus occurred in 2.6 or 2.9% of fetuses, respectively. In addition, increased resorption occurred at the 9.3 mg/kg dosage. The drug was not teratogenic when the same dosages were used in rats (0.13 or 0.3 times the maximum daily human dosage, respectively, based on mg/mm^2). There are no adequate and controlled studies to date using colistimethate sodium in pregnant women, and the drug should be used during pregnancy only when the potential benefits justify the possible risks to the fetus.

Fertility

There was no evidence of adverse effects on fertility or reproduction when colistimethate sodium was given to rats at dosages of 9.3 mg/kg daily (0.3 times the maximum daily dosage based on mg/m^2).

Lactation

It is not known whether colistimethate sodium is distributed into milk, but colistin sulfate has been detected in milk. Therefore, colistimethate sodium should be used with caution in nursing women.

DRUG INTERACTIONS

Since nephrotoxic and/or neurotoxic effects may be additive, concurrent or sequential use of colistimethate sodium and other drugs with similar toxic potentials (e.g., aminoglycosides, amphotericin B, capreomycin, methoxyflurane [no longer commercially available in the US], polymyxin B sulfate, vancomycin) should be avoided, if possible.

Neuromuscular blocking agents (e.g., tubocurarine, succinylcholine, ether, decamethonium [no longer commercially available in the US], gallamine [no longer commercially available in the US], decamethonium) and other drugs (e.g., sodium citrate) potentiate neuromuscular blockade induced by colistimethate sodium and these drugs should be used with extreme caution in patients receiving colistimethate sodium.

ACUTE TOXICITY

Overdosage of colistimethate sodium can cause neuromuscular blockade characterized by paresthesia, lethargy, confusion, dizziness, ataxia, nystagmus, disorders of speech, and apnea. Respiratory muscle paralysis may lead to apnea, respiratory arrest, and death. Overdosage of the drug may also cause acute renal failure, manifested as decreased urine output and increases in serum concentrations of BUN and creatinine.

If overdosage of colistimethate sodium occurs, the drug should be discontinued and general supportive measures initiated. Colistimethate sodium may be removed by hemodialysis and, to a lesser extent, by peritoneal dialysis.

MECHANISM OF ACTION

Colistimethate sodium is a prodrug and is inactive until hydrolyzed to colistin; this hydrolysis occurs in vivo and in vitro in aqueous solutions of the drug.

Colistin is usually bactericidal in action. The mechanism of action of colistin is similar to that of polymyxin B. Colistin acts like a cationic detergent and binds to and damages the bacterial cytoplasmic membrane of susceptible bacteria. Damage to the bacterial cytoplasmic membrane alters the osmotic barrier of the membrane and causes leakage of essential intracellular metabolites and nucleosides.

SPECTRUM

Colistin (the active metabolite of colistimethate sodium) has a spectrum of activity that is similar to that of polymyxin B. Colistin is active in vitro against many gram-negative bacteria; however, the drug is inactive against gram-positive bacteria, fungi, and viruses.

● Gram-negative Bacteria

Colistin is active in vitro against many strains of *Acinetobacter*, *Citrobacter*, *Escherichia coli*, *Enterobacter*, *Haemophilus influenzae*, *Klebsiella pneumoniae*, *Pseudomonas aeruginosa*, *Salmonella*, *Shigella*, and some strains of *Bordetella* and *Vibrio*. Most strains of *Proteus*, *Providencia*, *Serratia*, *Neisseria gonorrhoeae*, *N. meningitidis*, and *Bacteroides fragilis* are resistant to colistin.

In vitro, colistin concentrations of 0.01–4 mcg/mL inhibit most susceptible strains of *E. coli*, *E. aerogenes*, *H. influenzae*, *K. pneumoniae*, *Salmonella*, and *Shigella* and concentrations of 0.8–8 mcg/mL inhibit most susceptible strains of *Ps. aeruginosa*.

RESISTANCE

Resistance to colistin (the active metabolite of colistimethate sodium) has been induced in vitro in strains originally susceptible to the drug; in some cases, resistance may be reversible when the antibiotic is withdrawn. Resistance to colistin has developed rarely during therapy with colistimethate sodium or colistin sulfate.

Pseudomonas aeruginosa resistant to colistin have been reported rarely, including in some patients who received long-term treatment with colistimethate sodium administered by oral inhalation via nebulization†. *Acinetobacter baumannii Enterobacter cloacae*, and *Klebsiella pneumoniae* resistant to colistin also have been reported rarely.

Complete cross-resistance occurs between colistin and polymyxin B; however, cross-resistance with other anti-infectives has not been reported to date.

PHARMACOKINETICS

● Absorption

Colistimethate sodium, a prodrug of colistin, is not absorbed from the GI tract and must be given parenterally. Colistimethate sodium does not appear to be absorbed from mucous membranes or intact or denuded skin.

Following IM administration of colistimethate sodium in a dosage of 150 mg of colistin, peak serum concentrations of antimicrobial activity are attained within 2 hours and average 5–7.5 mcg/mL; serum concentrations of antimicrobial activity may be detectable 12 hours after the dose.

Following IV administration of colistimethate sodium in a dosage of 5–7 mg/kg of colistin daily given in 3 equally divided doses (maximum 70–100 mg every 8 hours) in cystic fibrosis patients 14–53 years of age, mean peak serum concentrations were 21.4 mcg/mL after the first dose and 23 mcg/mL at steady state. Mean 8-hour trough concentrations were 2.8 mcg/mL after the first dose and 4.5 mcg/mL at steady state. Peak serum concentrations of antimicrobial activity are higher, but decline more rapidly than those achieved with IM administration of the drug.

Following oral inhalation via nebulization† of colistimethate sodium in a dosage of 66.66 mg of colistin (2 million international units) in cystic fibrosis patients 12–48 years of age, mean peak serum concentrations were 0.17 mcg/mL and were attained in 1.5 hours.

● Distribution

Following IM or IV administration of colistimethate sodium, the drug is widely distributed into body tissues, but only negligible concentrations of antimicrobial activity are attained in synovial, pleural, or pericardial fluids. Animal studies indicate that colistin, like polymyxin B sulfate, reversibly binds to and persists in body tissues such as the liver, kidneys, lung, heart, and muscle.

In cystic fibrosis patients 14–53 years of age receiving IV colistimethate sodium in a dosage of 5–7 mg/kg of colistin daily given in 3 equally divided doses, the volume of distribution at steady state was 0.09 L/kg.

Following oral inhalation via nebulization† of colistimethate sodium in a dosage of 66.66 mg of colistin (2 million international units) in cystic fibrosis patients 12–48 years of age, sputum concentrations peaked 1 hour after inhalation and remained greater than 4 mcg/mL for up to 12 hours in most patients.

Colistin is reportedly more than 50% bound to serum proteins.

Only minimal concentrations of antimicrobial activity are attained in CSF following IM or IV administration of colistimethate sodium in patients with normal or inflamed meninges.

Colistin crosses the placenta and is distributed into milk.

● Elimination

Colistimethate sodium is hydrolyzed in vivo to colistin and possibly other metabolites with fewer substituted amino groups. The rate and extent of hydrolysis as well as the specific metabolites and their antibacterial activities have not been determined to date.

The plasma half-life of antimicrobial activity following IM or IV administration of colistimethate sodium is 1.5–8 hours in adults with normal renal function. Serum concentrations of antimicrobial activity following administration of colistimethate sodium appear to decline more rapidly in children than in adults.

Serum concentrations are higher and the half-life is prolonged in patients with impaired renal function. In patients with creatinine clearances less than 20 mL/minute, the half-life of colistin ranges from 10–20 hours. Following administration of colistimethate sodium in a few anuric patients, half-life of antimicrobial activity reportedly ranged up to 2–3 days.

The mean plasma half-life in cystic fibrosis patients 14–53 years of age who received IV colistimethate sodium in a dosage of 5–7 mg/kg of colistin daily given in 3 equally divided doses was 3.4 hours after the first dose and 3.5 hours at steady state.

The plasma half-life following oral inhalation via nebulization† of colistimethate sodium in a dosage of 66.66 mg of colistin (2 million international units) in cystic fibrosis patients 12–48 years of age was 4.1–4.5 hours.

Colistimethate sodium and metabolites of the drug are excreted mainly by the kidneys via glomerular filtration. Antimicrobial activity in urine is generally higher than antimicrobial activity in serum. Following IM or IV administration of a single 150-mg dose of colistin as colistimethate sodium in patients with normal renal function, antimicrobial concentrations in urine are 200–270 mcg/mL at 2 hours after the dose and 15–25 mcg/mL at 8 hours after the dose.

Colistimethate sodium may be removed by hemodialysis and, to a lesser extent, by peritoneal dialysis.

CHEMISTRY AND STABILITY

● Chemistry

Colistimethate sodium is the sulfamethyl derivative (methane sulfonate) of colistin. Colistimethate sodium is a prodrug that is inactive until hydrolyzed in vivo and in vitro to colistin. Colistin (also known as polymyxin E) is a polymyxin antibiotic obtained from cultures of *Bacillus polymyxa* var. *colistinus* and is structurally and pharmacologically related to polymyxin B.

Colistin may be commercially available as colistin sulfate for oral administration in other countries; however, oral colistin sulfate is no longer commercially available in the US.

Colistimethate sodium occurs as a white to slightly yellow, fine powder and is freely soluble in water. Following reconstitution with sterile water for injection, colistimethate sodium solutions have a pH of 7–8.

● Stability

Colistimethate sodium powder for injection should be stored at 20–25°C.

Following reconstitution with sterile water for injection, colistimethate sodium solutions containing 75 mg of colistin per mL should be stored at 2–8°C or 20–25°C and used within 7 days. However, reconstituted solutions that have been further diluted with a compatible IV solution should be used within 24 hours.

Solutions of colistimethate sodium prepared extemporaneously for oral inhalation via nebulization† should be used promptly after being mixed. (See Cautions: Respiratory Effects.)

Colistimethate sodium is physically and chemically compatible with the following IV solutions: 0.9% sodium chloride, 5% dextrose, 5% dextrose and 0.225%, 0.45%, or 0.9% sodium chloride, lactated Ringer's, or 10% invert sugar.

Colistimethate sodium is potentially physically and/or chemically incompatible with some drugs, but the compatibility depends on several factors (e.g., concentrations of the drugs, specific diluents used, resulting pH, temperature). Specialized references should be consulted for specific compatibility information.

PREPARATIONS

Excipients in commercially available drug preparations may have clinically important effects in some individuals; consult specific product labeling for details.

Colistimethate Sodium

Parenteral		
For injection	150 mg (of colistin)*	Colistimethate Sodium for Injection
		Coly-Mycin® M Parenteral, Par

* available from one or more manufacturer, distributor, and/or repackager by generic (nonproprietary) name

† Use is not currently included in the labeling approved by the US Food and Drug Administration.

Selected Revisions March 31, 2017, © Copyright, April 1, 1971, American Society of Health-System Pharmacists, Inc.

Polymyxin B Sulfate

8:12.28.28 • POLYMYXINS

■ Polymyxin B is a polymyxin antibiotic that is structurally and pharmacologically related to colistin.

USES

Polymyxin B sulfate is used for the treatment of serious infections, including infections of the urinary tract, meninges, or bloodstream, caused by susceptible gram-negative bacteria (e.g., *Pseudomonas aeruginosa*, *Escherichia coli*, *Enterobacter aerogenes*, *Klebsiella pneumoniae*, *Haemophilus influenzae*). The drug also is used in the treatment of respiratory tract infections† caused by susceptible gram-negative bacteria (e.g., *Ps. aeruginosa*, *Acinetobacter baumannii*†). Although other less toxic anti-infectives (e.g., fluoroquinolones, aminoglycosides, third generation cephalosporins, extended-spectrum penicillins, carbapenems) usually are the drugs of choice for most gram-negative bacterial infections, polymyxin B may be indicated when these drugs are ineffective or contraindicated, especially for serious infections caused by multidrug-resistant *Ps. aeruginosa* or *A. baumannii*.

● Meningitis and Other CNS Infections

Polymyxin B sulfate is used intrathecally or intraventricularly† for the treatment of meningeal infections caused by susceptible gram-negative bacteria, including *Ps. aeruginosa*, *E. coli*†, *K. pneumoniae*†, and *H. influenzae*. In some cases, intrathecal polymyxin B has been effective when used alone for the treatment of these infections; however, intrathecal or intraventricular polymyxin B usually has been used in conjunction with a parenteral anti-infective (e.g., IV or IM polymyxin B, IV meropenem, IV penicillin, IV cephalosporin). Because polymyxin B penetrates poorly into CSF following IM or IV administration, parenteral therapy with the drug should not be used alone for the treatment of meningitis or other CNS infections.

Treatment of meningitis caused by *Ps. aeruginosa* should be guided by results of in vitro susceptibility tests. The usual regimen of choice for these infections is parenteral therapy with an antipseudomonal cephalosporin (ceftazidime, cefepime) or carbapenem (meropenem) with or without an aminoglycoside (amikacin, gentamicin, tobramycin). Intrathecal or intraventricular polymyxin B may be indicated for infections caused by multidrug-resistant *Ps. aeruginosa* that are resistant to or do not respond to the usual regimens of choice.

Polymyxin B has been used intraventricularly† in conjunction with IV meropenem for the treatment of ventriculitis caused by ceftazidime-resistant *K. pneumoniae*†.

Intrathecal polymyxin B is considered an alternative for the treatment of meningitis caused by susceptible *H. influenzae*. The usual drug of choice for the treatment of these infections is a parenteral third-generation cephalosporin (e.g., cefotaxime, ceftriaxone), although parenteral ampicillin can be used if the infection is caused by β-lactamase-negative strains.

● Respiratory Tract Infections

IV polymyxin B sulfate is used as an alternative for the treatment of respiratory tract infections†, including nosocomial pneumonia, ventilator-associated pneumonia, or healthcare-associated pneumonia, caused by multidrug-resistant gram-negative bacteria (e.g., *Ps. aeruginosa*, *A. baumannii*). Polymyxin B is not usually considered a drug of choice for *initial* empiric therapy of respiratory tract infections, and generally is used in these infections only when other less toxic anti-infectives are ineffective or contraindicated.

In some patients, IV polymyxin B has been used alone or in conjunction with IV aztreonam for the treatment of nosocomial pneumonia caused by multidrug-resistant *Ps. aeruginosa* that produce metallo-β-lactamases. Nosocomial infections caused by metallo-β-lactamase-producing *Ps. aeruginosa* have a high mortality rate and fatalities may occur despite appropriate anti-infective therapy. Optimal regimens for treatment of these infections have not been identified to date.

Polymyxin B has been administered by oral inhalation via nebulization† for the treatment of respiratory tract infections† caused by susceptible gram-negative bacteria (e.g., *Ps. aeruginosa*, *A. baumannii*). In patients with pneumonia, polymyxin B administered by oral inhalation generally has been used in conjunction with a parenteral anti-infective (e.g., IV polymyxin B); however, the drug has been effective when given by oral inhalation alone in some patients with infections caused by susceptible gram-negative bacteria. Although safety and efficacy have not been established and additional study is needed, the American Thoracic Society (ATS) and the Infectious Diseases Society of America (IDSA) and other clinicians suggest that adjunctive use of aerosolized polymyxin B can be considered for the treatment of serious respiratory tract infections (e.g., ventilator-associated pneumonia) caused by multidrug-resistant gram-negative bacteria that have not responded to treatment with parenteral anti-infectives alone.

Polymyxin B also has been administered by oral inhalation for prophylaxis in an attempt to prevent nosocomial pneumonia† in seriously ill patients; however, such prophylaxis appears to promote development of polymyxin B-resistant bacteria.

● Septicemia

IV or IM polymyxin B sulfate is used for the treatment of septicemia or bacteremia caused by susceptible *Ps. aeruginosa*, *E. aerogenes*, or *K. pneumoniae*. The drug also has been used IV for the treatment of bloodstream infections caused by multidrug-resistant *A. baumannii*†. Polymyxin B generally is used in the treatment of septicemia or bacteremia only when other less toxic anti-infectives are ineffective or contraindicated.

Polymyxin B may be a drug of choice for the treatment of septicemia or bacteremia caused by *Ps. aeruginosa* and has been used alone or in conjunction with other anti-infectives (e.g., aztreonam) for infections caused by multidrug-resistant *Ps. aeruginosa*, including those that produce metallo-β-lactamases. Nosocomial blood stream infections caused by metallo-β-lactamase-producing *Ps. aeruginosa* have a high mortality rate, and fatalities may occur despite appropriate anti-infective therapy. Optimal regimens for treatment of these infections have not been identified to date.

● Urinary Tract Infections

IV or IM polymyxin B sulfate is used for the treatment of serious urinary tract infections caused by susceptible *Ps. aeruginosa* or *E. coli*. Polymyxin B generally is used in these infections only when other less toxic anti-infectives are ineffective or contraindicated.

● Bacteriuria and Bacteremia Associated with Indwelling Catheters

The fixed-combination solution for irrigation containing polymyxin B sulfate and neomycin sulfate is used in abacteriuric patients for short-term (up to 10 days) irrigation or rinse of the urinary bladder to help prevent bacteriuria and gram-negative rod septicemia associated with the use of indwelling catheters.

Bacteria can gain entrance to the bladder by way of, through, and around indwelling catheters and clinically significant bacteriuria may be induced by bacterial multiplication in bladder urine, the mucoid film that may be present between the catheter and urethra, and in other sites. Urinary tract infection may result from the repeated presence of large numbers of pathogenic bacteria in the urine, and the use of closed systems with indwelling catheters has been shown to reduce the risk of infection. The manufacturers state that use of a 3-way closed catheter system and bladder rinse with the fixed-combination solution for irrigation containing polymyxin B sulfate and neomycin sulfate may help prevent development of infection in patients with indwelling catheters. However, some clinicians state that irrigation or rinse of the urinary bladder with anti-infective solutions is unlikely to be of benefit while the catheter is in place and such a strategy is not recommended.

In a randomized, double-blind study in adults 19–82 years of age with spinal cord injury and neurogenic bladder dysfunction who had indwelling urinary catheters and existing bacteriuria (at least 100,000 colony-forming units per mL [cfu/mL]), bladder irrigation (30 mL twice daily for 8 weeks) with neomycin sulfate and polymyxin B sulfate solution for irrigation, 0.25% acetic acid, or normal saline did not reduce the degree of bacteriuria or inflammation. Culture data obtained prior to, during, and after the 8-week irrigation regimen indicated no substantial change in colony count (counts remained at least 100,000 cfu/mL in almost all individuals). Although there was an increase in the number of patients harboring *Enterococcus*, the variety of other bacteria present in the urine generally remained the same. In addition, there was no evidence of an increased incidence of resistant bacteria, including multidrug-resistant strains.

For information on use of topical fixed-combination preparations containing polymyxin B sulfate and other anti-infectives for the prevention or treatment of superficial skin infections, see Bacitracin 84:04.04 and see Neomycin Sulfate 84:04.04.

For information on use of topical or subconjunctival polymyxin B sulfate for the treatment of ophthalmic infections or use of topical fixed-combination preparations containing polymyxin B sulfate and other anti-infectives for the treatment of ophthalmic or otic infections, see Polymyxin B Sulfate 52:04.04.

DOSAGE AND ADMINISTRATION

● Reconstitution and Administration

Polymyxin B sulfate usually is administered IV. Although polymyxin B sulfate may also be given by IM injection, IM administration of the drug is not routinely recommended because severe pain occurs at the injection site, especially in infants and children.

For the treatment of meningitis, polymyxin B sulfate is administered intrathecally or intraventricularly†. Polymyxin B should *not* be given IV or IM alone for the treatment of meningitis or other CNS infections since distribution of the drug into CNS is expected to be low following these routes.

Although safety and efficacy have not been established, polymyxin B sulfate has been administered by oral inhalation via nebulization† for the adjunctive treatment of respiratory tract infections†. (See Uses: Respiratory Tract Infections.)

The fixed-combination solution for irrigation containing polymyxin B sulfate and neomycin sulfate is administered by continuous irrigation of the urinary bladder.

IV Administration

For IV administration, polymyxin B sulfate powder for injection is reconstituted by dissolving 500,000 units of the drug in 300–500 mL of 5% dextrose injection to provide solutions containing approximately 1000–1667 units/mL.

IV infusions of polymyxin B usually are given over a period of 60–90 minutes. An infusion period less than 30 minutes should *not* be used. Because of the risk of neuromuscular blockade, rapid IV injections should be avoided.

IM Administration

For IM administration, polymyxin B sulfate powder for injection is reconstituted by adding 2 mL of sterile water for injection, 0.9% sodium chloride injection, or 1% procaine hydrochloride injection to a vial labeled as containing 500,000 units of polymyxin B to provide a solution containing approximately 250,000 units/mL.

IM injections should be given deeply into the upper outer quadrant of the gluteal muscle and injection sites should be alternated. The fact that IM injections may cause severe injection site pain should be considered.

Intrathecal Administration

For intrathecal administration, polymyxin B sulfate powder for injection is reconstituted by adding 10 mL of 0.9% sodium chloride injection to a vial labeled as containing 500,000 units of the drug to provide a solution containing approximately 50,000 units/mL. Procaine hydrochloride solutions should *not* be used to prepare intrathecal injections of polymyxin B.

Oral Inhalation

For oral inhalation via nebulization†, 0.5% solutions of polymyxin B sulfate have been prepared using 0.9% sodium chloride. Polymyxin B concentrations higher than 10 mg/mL should not be used for administration by oral inhalation since the drug may cause bronchial irritation.

Urinary Bladder Irrigation

For continuous irrigation of the urinary bladder, the commercially available fixed-combination solution for irrigation containing 200,000 units of polymyxin B and 40 mg of neomycin should be diluted by adding the contents of the 1-mL ampul containing the irrigation solution to 1 L of 0.9% sodium chloride solution.

The diluted solution for irrigation should be administered via a 3-way catheter at a rate of 1 L every 24 hours (approximately 40 mL/hour). If the patient's urine output exceeds 2 L/day, the inflow rate should be adjusted to deliver 2 L every 24 hours. If not used immediately, the diluted solution should be stored at 4°C and used within 48 hours.

It is important that the bladder irrigation be given continuously for up to 10 days; the inflow or rinse solution should not be interrupted for more than a few minutes.

● Dosage

Dosage of polymyxin B sulfate usually is expressed in terms of polymyxin B activity (units of polymyxin B). Dosage of the drug also may be expressed as mg of polymyxin B base. Each mg of polymyxin B is equivalent to 10,000 units of polymyxin B.

Adult Dosage
Meningitis and Other CNS Infections

For the treatment of meningitis caused by susceptible gram-negative bacteria, the manufacturers recommend that adults receive an intrathecal dosage of polymyxin B of 50,000 units once daily for 3 or 4 days, followed by 50,000 units once every other day given for at least 2 weeks after CSF cultures are negative and CSF glucose content is normal.

For the treatment of ventriculitis† in an adult caused by ceftazidime-resistant *Klebsiella pneumoniae*, polymyxin B has been given intraventricularly† in a dosage of 50,000 units once daily for 7 days in conjunction with IV meropenem continued for 21 days after the first negative CSF culture.

Although safety and efficacy have not been established, a variety of other dosage regimens of intrathecal or intraventricular† polymyxin B (with or without concomitant parenteral therapy with IV or IM polymyxin B or other anti-infectives) have been used for the treatment of meningitis caused by susceptible gram-negative bacteria.

Respiratory Tract Infections

Although safety and efficacy of polymyxin B administered by oral inhalation via nebulization† have not been established, adults have received the drug by oral inhalation in a dosage of 2.5 mg/kg daily in divided doses every 6 hours for adjunctive treatment of respiratory tract infections caused by susceptible *Pseudomonas aeruginosa*.' If a 0.5% solution of the drug is prepared using 0.9% sodium chloride and this dosage regimen is used, the average 70-kg patient would receive 6 mL of solution per dose.

In a study in adults who had respiratory tract infections caused by multidrug-resistant gram-negative bacilli that had not responded to parenteral anti-infectives alone, polymyxin B was given by oral inhalation in a dosage of 500,000 units twice daily given approximately 20 minutes after an oral inhalation dose of a β_2-adrenergic agonist. Patients with pneumonia received polymyxin B administered by oral inhalation in conjunction with IV polymyxin B therapy; those with tracheobronchitis caused by *Ps. adrenergic* received the drug by oral inhalation alone. Treatment was continued for an average of 14 days (range: 4–25 days).

The total daily dosage administered by oral inhalation should not exceed that recommended for parenteral administration.

Septicemia or Urinary Tract Infections

The usual IV dosage of polymyxin B for the treatment of septicemia or urinary tract infections caused by susceptible gram-negative bacteria in adults with normal renal function is 15,000–25,000 units/kg daily (1.5–2.5 mg/kg daily). Daily dosage may be given in 2 divided doses every 12 hours. The total daily IV dosage in these patients should not exceed 25,000 units/kg.

The usual IM dosage of polymyxin B for the treatment of septicemia or urinary tract infections caused by susceptible gram-negative bacteria in adults with normal renal function is 25,000–30,000 units/kg daily (2.5–3 mg/kg daily); the daily dosage may be divided and given at 4- to 6-hour intervals. The total daily IM dosage in these patients should not exceed 30,000 units/kg.

Bacteriuria and Bacteremia Associated with Indwelling Catheters

For continuous irrigation of the urinary bladder, the diluted solution of neomycin sulfate and polymyxin B sulfate irrigation solution should be administered via a 3-way catheter at a rate of 1 L every 24 hours (approximately 40 mL/hour). The solution should be administered at a rate of 2 L every 24 hours if the patient's urine output exceeds 2 L/day.

The duration of irrigation therapy should not exceed 10 days.

Pediatric Dosage
Meningitis and Other CNS Infections

For the treatment of meningitis caused by susceptible gram-negative bacteria in children younger than 2 years of age, the manufacturers recommend an initial intrathecal dosage of polymyxin B of 20,000 units once daily for 3 or 4 days or

25,000 units once every other day. With either regimen, treatment should be continued with 25,000 units once every other day given for at least 2 weeks after CSF cultures are negative and CSF glucose content is normal.

For the treatment of meningitis caused by susceptible gram-negative bacteria in children older than 2 years of age, the manufacturers recommend an intrathecal dosage of polymyxin B of 50,000 units once daily for 3 or 4 days, followed by 50,000 units once every other day given for at least 2 weeks after CSF cultures are negative and CSF glucose content is normal.

Although safety and efficacy have not been established, a variety of other dosage regimens of intrathecal or intraventricular† polymyxin B (with or without concomitant parenteral therapy with IV or IM polymyxin B or other anti-infectives) have been used for the treatment of meningitis caused by susceptible gram-negative bacteria.

Septicemia or Urinary Tract Infections

The usual IV dosage of polymyxin B for the treatment of septicemia or urinary tract infections caused by susceptible gram-negative bacteria in children with normal renal function is 15,000–25,000 units/kg daily (1.5–2.5 mg/kg daily). Daily dosage may be administered in 2 divided doses every 12 hours. The manufacturers state that the total daily IV dosage in children should not exceed 25,000 units/kg, but that infants with normal renal function may receive an IV dosage of up to 40,000 units/kg daily (4 mg/kg daily) without adverse effects.

Clinicians should consider that IM administration of polymyxin B is not routinely recommended in children and infants because severe pain occurs at the injection site. If the drug is given IM for the treatment of septicemia or urinary tract infections caused by susceptible gram-negative bacteria in children with normal renal function, the usual IM dosage is 25,000–30,000 units/kg daily (2.5–3 mg/kg daily); daily dosage may be divided and given at 4- to 6-hour intervals. The manufacturers state that the total daily IM dosage in children should not exceed 30,000 units/kg, but that infants with normal renal function may receive an IM dosage of up to 40,000 units/kg daily (4 mg/kg daily) without adverse effects. A dosage as high as 45,000 units/kg daily (4.5 mg/kg daily) has been used in limited clinical studies in premature and full-term neonates for the treatment of sepsis caused by *Ps. aeruginosa*.

● Dosage in Renal Impairment

Dosage of polymyxin B should be decreased in patients with renal impairment. Serum polymyxin B concentrations should be monitored and IV or IM dosage adjusted to maintain desired serum concentrations of the drug.

Various dosage regimens have been recommended for use of polymyxin B in patients with renal impairment; however, these regimens are *not* well established and are *not* based on pharmacokinetic data from patients with renal impairment.

It has been recommended that patients with creatinine clearances of 30–80 mL/minute receive an IV loading dose of polymyxin B of 2.5 mg/kg on the first day of treatment followed by 1–1.5 mg/kg daily and that those with creatinine clearances less than 25–30 mL/minute receive these doses once every 2–3 days. For anuric patients, some clinicians have recommended an IV loading dose of 2.5 mg/kg followed by 1–1.5 mg/kg given once every 5–7 days.

Alternatively, it has been suggested that patients with creatinine clearances greater than 20 mL/minute receive 75–100% of the usual daily dose in 2 divided doses every 12 hours, those with creatinine clearances of 5–20 mL/minute receive 50% of the usual daily dose in 2 divided doses every 12 hours, and those with creatinine clearances less than 5 mL/minute receive 30% of the usual daily dose every 12–18 hours. Some clinicians have used 75% of the usual daily dose in those with creatinine clearances 20–50 mL/minute and 33% of the usual daily dose in those with creatinine clearances less than 20 mL/minute.

CAUTIONS

Adverse effects reported with polymyxin B sulfate are similar to those reported with colistimethate sodium and colistin sulfate (not commercially available in the US). Nephrotoxicity and neurotoxicity are the most serious adverse effects of polymyxin B and are most likely to occur when the drug is used in higher than recommended dosages or in patients with renal impairment.

● Nephrotoxicity

Polymyxin B can cause nephrotoxicity. Polymyxin B-associated nephrotoxicity is considered to be dose-dependent and has been reported in 6–25% of patients receiving usual dosages of the drug. Nephrotoxicity generally is reversible after the drug is discontinued.

Nephrotoxicity usually is manifested by albuminuria or proteinuria, cylindruria, azotemia, increasing blood concentrations of the drug (not related to an increase in dosage), and an increase in serum creatinine concentration and decrease in creatinine clearance. Acute tubular necrosis, oliguria, hematuria, leukocyturia, and excessive excretion of electrolytes may occur.

Renal function should be assessed prior to initiation of polymyxin B therapy and monitored frequently during therapy. If signs of renal impairment develop, the drug should be discontinued. (See Cautions: Precautions and Contraindications.)

● Neurotoxicity

Polymyxin B can cause neurotoxicity. Neurotoxicity is considered to be dose-dependent and may manifest as facial flushing, dizziness that may progress to ataxia, altered mental status or mental confusion, irritability, nystagmus, muscle weakness, drowsiness, giddiness, and peripheral paresthesia (circumoral and stocking glove). Numbness, blurring of vision or vision disturbances, slurred speech, coma, or seizures also can occur. These adverse effects generally subside after the drug is discontinued.

Respiratory paralysis resulting in respiratory failure or apnea may occur as a result of neuromuscular blockade, especially in patients with neuromuscular disease such as myasthenia gravis or in patients who are receiving neuromuscular blocking agents or general anesthetics. (See Drug Interactions.) Polymyxin B-induced neuromuscular blockade is not easily reversed and is resistant to neostigmine and edrophonium; calcium chloride has been used successfully in some cases. Neuromuscular blockade usually improves within 24 hours after polymyxin B is discontinued.

Intrathecal administration of polymyxin B sulfate may cause meningeal irritation, such as headache, fever, stiff neck, and increased leukocytes and protein in the CSF. In addition, nerve root irritation may occur causing neuritic pain and urine retention. High doses given intrathecally or intraventricularly† may lead to seizures and signs of meningismus.

● Other Adverse Effects

Fever, rash, pruritus, urticaria, skin exanthemata, eosinophilia, and anaphylactoid reactions with dyspnea and tachycardia have been reported rarely during parenteral polymyxin B therapy.

Cough, bronchospasm, and acute airway obstruction have been reported when polymyxin B was administered by oral inhalation via nebulization†. Bronchospasm may have been the result of an allergic reaction or bronchial irritation.

Severe pain may occur at IM injection sites, especially in infants and children. Thrombophlebitis has been reported at IV injection sites.

● Precautions and Contraindications

Polymyxin B sulfate is contraindicated in individuals with a history of hypersensitivity to polymyxins.

Polymyxin B can cause potentially serious nephrotoxicity and/or neurotoxicity. The drug should be given IV, IM, and/or intrathecally only to hospitalized patients who are under constant supervision by a clinician.

Baseline renal function should be determined prior to initiation of polymyxin B therapy and renal function should be monitored frequently during therapy using blood tests and urinalysis. The manufacturers also recommend that serum concentrations of the drug be monitored frequently during therapy. Dosage of polymyxin B should be reduced in patients with impaired renal function or renal damage and nitrogen retention. (See Dosage and Administration: Dosage in Renal Impairment.) If urine output diminishes or BUN concentration increases during polymyxin B therapy, the drug should be discontinued.

Polymyxin B-associated neurotoxicity may be manifested by irritability, weakness, drowsiness, ataxia, perioral paresthesia, numbness of the extremities, and blurred vision. These symptoms usually are associated with high serum polymyxin B concentrations found in patients with impaired renal function and/or nephrotoxicity. Neurotoxicity can result in respiratory paralysis from neuromuscular blockade, especially if polymyxin B is given soon after anesthesia and/or muscle relaxants. (See Drug Interactions.) If signs of respiratory paralysis occur, respiration should be assisted as required and the drug discontinued.

Concurrent or sequential use of other nephrotoxic and/or neurotoxic drugs should be avoided. (See Drug Interactions.)

To reduce development of drug-resistant bacteria and maintain effectiveness of polymyxin B and other antibacterials, the drug should be used only for the treatment or prevention of infections proven or strongly suspected to be caused by susceptible bacteria. When selecting or modifying anti-infective therapy, results of culture and in vitro susceptibility testing should be used. In the absence of such data, local epidemiology and susceptibility patterns should be considered when selecting anti-infectives for empiric therapy.

Patients should be advised that antibacterials (including polymyxin B) should only be used to treat bacterial infections and not used to treat viral infections (e.g., the common cold). Patients also should be advised about the importance of completing the full course of therapy, even if feeling better after a few days, and that skipping doses or not completing therapy may decrease effectiveness and increase the likelihood that bacteria will develop resistance and will not be treatable with polymyxin B or other antibacterials in the future.

As with other anti-infectives, use of polymyxin B may result in overgrowth of nonsusceptible organisms, including fungi. Appropriate therapy should be instituted if superinfection occurs.

Precautions Related to Fixed-combination Solution for Bladder Irrigation

When the fixed-combination solution for bladder irrigation containing polymyxin B sulfate and neomycin sulfate solution is used, the precautions and contraindications related to both polymyxin B and neomycin should be considered.

The fixed-combination solution for irrigation is contraindicated in individuals hypersensitive to polymyxins, neomycin, or any ingredient in the solution. Because cross-sensitivity can occur among aminoglycosides, a history of hypersensitivity or serious toxic reaction to an aminoglycoside may also contraindicate use of any other aminoglycoside.

The fixed-combination solution for irrigation should be used *only* for irrigation of the bladder and should *not* be used for irrigation of other areas.

The fixed-combination solution for irrigation should not be used for prophylactic bladder care if there is a possibility of systemic absorption. The likelihood of toxicity following topical irrigation of the intact urinary bladder with the fixed-combination solution is low since appreciable amounts of polymyxin B or neomycin do not enter systemic circulation if the duration of irrigation does not exceed 10 days. However, absorption of neomycin from the denuded bladder surface has been reported. Systemic absorption after topical application of neomycin to open wounds, burns, and granulating surfaces is clinically significant, and serum concentrations comparable to and often higher than those attained following oral and parenteral therapy have been reported.

The fixed-combination solution for irrigation is intended for continuous prophylactic irrigation (maximum of 10 days) of the lumen of the intact urinary bladder of patients with indwelling catheters who are under constant supervision by a clinician. Because of the risk of toxicity due to systemic absorption following diffusion into absorptive tissues and spaces, irrigation should be avoided in patients with defects in bladder mucosa or bladder wall, such as vesical rupture, or in association with operative procedures on the bladder wall.

If absorption occurs, the fact that both polymyxin B and neomycin are nephrotoxic and neurotoxic and that the effects of these drugs may be additive should be considered.

Irrigation of the bladder with the fixed-combination solution containing polymyxin B and neomycin may result in overgrowth of nonsusceptible organisms, including fungi, and appropriate measures should be taken if this occurs.

Urine specimens for urinalysis, culture, and susceptibility testing should be collected during prophylactic bladder care. Positive cultures suggest the presence of organisms resistant to polymyxin B and neomycin.

● Pediatric Precautions

IV polymyxin B sulfate is used in infants and children. IM polymyxin B sulfate is not routinely recommended in infants and children because severe pain occurs at the injection site, especially in this age group.

Safety and efficacy of the fixed-combination solution for irrigation containing polymyxin B sulfate and neomycin sulfate have not been established in children.

● Pregnancy, Fertility, and Lactation
Pregnancy

The safety of polymyxin B sulfate in pregnant women has not been established.

Some clinicians state that polymyxin B should not be used during pregnancy, except in rare situations when other appropriate anti-infectives cannot be used.

If use of the fixed-combination solution for irrigation containing polymyxin B sulfate and neomycin sulfate is being considered for a pregnant woman, the woman should be informed of the potential hazard to the fetus. Aminoglycosides cross the placenta and there have been reports of complete, irreversible, bilateral congenital deafness in children whose mothers received an aminoglycoside (i.e., streptomycin) during pregnancy.

DRUG INTERACTIONS

● Nephrotoxic and Neurotoxic Drugs

Since nephrotoxic and neurotoxic effects may be additive, concurrent or sequential use of polymyxin B sulfate and other nephrotoxic and/or neurotoxic drugs, particularly aminoglycosides (amikacin, gentamicin, kanamycin, neomycin, paromomycin, streptomycin, tobramycin), bacitracin, colistimethate/colistin, and viomycin (not commercially available in the US) should be avoided.

● Anti-infectives
Carbapenems

In vitro, the antibacterial effects of polymyxin B and imipenem have been synergistic against some strains of *Pseudomonas aeruginosa*, but were indifferent against other strains. In one study, the combination of polymyxin B and meropenem was indifferent against *Ps. aeruginosa*.

In vitro studies evaluating the antibacterial effects of combinations of polymyxin B and imipenem or meropenem against *Acinetobacter baumannii* have provided conflicting results. In some in vitro studies, these combinations had synergistic, partially synergistic, or additive antibacterial effects against *A. baumannii*; however, there was no evidence of synergism in other in vitro studies.

The clinical importance of in vitro studies evaluating combinations of polymyxin B and carbapenems against gram-negative bacteria is unclear.

Rifampin

In an in vitro study, the antibacterial effects of polymyxin B and rifampin were synergistic against only 1 out of 10 strains of multidrug-resistant *Ps. aeruginosa*; however, a 3-drug combination of polymyxin B, rifampin, and imipenem was bactericidal against all strains.

In some in vitro studies, the combination of polymyxin B and rifampin (with or without imipenem) was synergistic or additive against *A. baumannii*.

The combination of polymyxin B and rifampin has been synergistic in vitro against *Klebsiella pneumoniae*.

The clinical importance of in vitro studies evaluating combinations of polymyxin B and rifampin against gram-negative bacteria is unclear.

Other Anti-infectives

A synergistic antibacterial effect has been reported between polymyxin B and some other anti-infectives (e.g., tetracyclines, chloramphenicol, azithromycin, erythromycin, sulfonamides).

In an in vitro study, the antibacterial effects of polymyxin B and azithromycin were synergistic against 6 out of 10 strains of multidrug-resistant *Ps. aeruginosa*; the combination was bactericidal against some strains, but bacteriostatic against other strains. The clinical importance of in vitro studies evaluating combinations of polymyxin B and azithromycin against gram-negative bacteria is unclear.

● Neuromuscular Blocking Agents and Anesthetics

Polymyxin B can cause respiratory paralysis from neuromuscular blockade, especially if the drug is given soon after anesthesia and/or muscle relaxants. Concurrent use of polymyxin B and neuromuscular blocking agents (e.g., succinylcholine, ether, gallamine [not commercially available in the US], tubocurarine [not commercially available in the US], decamethonium [not commercially available in the US]) and other neurotoxic drugs (e.g., sodium citrate) should be avoided since these agents may precipitate respiratory paralysis. If signs of respiratory paralysis occur, respiration should be assisted as required and the drug discontinued.

MECHANISM OF ACTION

Polymyxin B usually is bactericidal in action. The bactericidal activity of the drug is concentration dependent.

Polymyxin B binds to phosphate groups in the lipids of the bacterial cytoplasmic membrane of susceptible bacteria and acts as a cationic detergent, thereby altering the osmotic barrier of the membrane and causing leakage of essential intracellular components.

SPECTRUM

Polymyxin B has a spectrum of activity that is similar to that of colistin. Polymyxin B is active in vitro against many gram-negative aerobic bacteria; however, the drug is inactive against gram-positive bacteria, anaerobic bacteria, fungi, and viruses.

● Gram-negative Bacteria

Polymyxin B generally is active in vitro against *Pseudomonas aeruginosa* and is active against many multidrug-resistant strains, including metallo-β-lactamase-producing *Ps. aeruginosa*. The drug also is active against many strains of *Acinetobacter baumannii*, including multidrug-resistant strains. Although polymyxin B is active against some strains of *Stenotrophomonas maltophilia*, it is inactive against *Burkholderia cepacia* (formerly *Ps. cepacia*).

Polymyxin B is active in vitro against most Enterobacteriaceae, including most strains of *Citrobacter, Escherichia coli, Klebsiella pneumoniae, Salmonella,* and *Shigella,* and some strains of *Enterobacter*. Polymyxin B generally is inactive against *Proteus, Providencia, Morganella,* and *Serratia marcescens*.

Polymyxin B has some activity against *Haemophilus influenzae, Bordetella pertussis,* and *Legionella pneumophila,* but is inactive against *Moraxella catarrhalis, Neisseria,* and *Brucella*.

● In Vitro Susceptibility Tests

When broth or agar dilution susceptibility tests are used to test in vitro susceptibility of *Ps. aeruginosa* to polymyxin B, the Clinical and Laboratory Standards Institute (CLSI; formerly National Committee for Clinical Laboratory Standards [NCCLS]) states that strains with minimum inhibitory concentrations (MICs) of 2 mcg/mL or less are susceptible to polymyxin B, those with MICs of 4 mcg/mL have intermediate susceptibility, and those with MICs of 8 mcg/mL or greater are resistant to the drug.

When broth or agar dilution susceptibility tests are used to test in vitro susceptibility of *Acinetobacter* to polymyxin B, CLSI states that strains with MICs of 2 mcg/mL or less are susceptible to polymyxin B and those with MICs of 4 mcg/mL or greater are resistant to the drug.

If a disk diffusion procedure is used to test susceptibility to polymyxin B, a 300-unit polymyxin B disk is used and organisms with growth inhibition zones 12 mm or greater are considered susceptible to polymyxin B. However, the disk diffusion method usually is not recommended for testing susceptibility to polymyxin B since the drug diffuses poorly in agar and false-susceptible results may occur. If a disk diffusion procedure is used, results indicating susceptibility to polymyxin B should be confirmed using a broth or agar dilution method.

RESISTANCE

Resistance to polymyxin B has been reported rarely in *Pseudomonas aeruginosa* and *Acinetobacter baumannii*. Surveillance data based on clinical isolates obtained from North America, Latin America, Europe, and the Asia-Pacific region during 2001–2004 indicated that 1.1–2.9% of *Ps. aeruginosa* isolates and 1.7–2.7% of *Acinetobacter* isolates were resistant to polymyxin B.

Two types of resistance to polymyxin B have been identified in *Ps. aeruginosa,* including low-level, transmissible mutations and high-level, stepwise resistance.

Complete cross-resistance occurs between polymyxin B and colistin, but there is no evidence to date of cross-resistance between these polymyxins and other anti-infectives.

PHARMACOKINETICS

● Absorption

Polymyxin B sulfate is not absorbed from the GI tract.

After IM administration of a single polymyxin B dose of 20,000–40,000 units/kg (2–4 mg/kg) in adults, peak serum concentrations of 1–8 mcg/mL are obtained within approximately 2 hours. Serum concentrations are higher in infants and children. Following IM administration of polymyxin B to adults with normal renal function, detectable amounts of the drug are present in serum for up to 12 hours.

In a study in critically ill adults who received polymyxin B doses of 0.5–1.5 mg/kg by IV infusion over 60 minutes, peak plasma concentrations at completion of the infusion ranged from 2.38–13.9 mcg/mL, and concentrations of polymyxin B_1 were fourfold higher than concentrations of polymyxin B_2. (See Chemistry.)

Serum concentrations are higher and more prolonged in patients with renal impairment.

Polymyxin B does not appear to be absorbed to an appreciable extent from mucous membranes or intact or denuded skin.

● Distribution

In a study in critically ill adults, the volume of distribution of polymyxin B ranged from 71–194 mL/kg.

Polymyxin B diffuses poorly in tissues.

Following IV or IM administration, polymyxin B is not distributed into CSF (even when meninges are inflamed) or synovial fluid. Systemically administered polymyxin B does not penetrate into the aqueous humor of the eye, even in the presence of inflammation.

Polymyxin B does not cross the placenta.

Animal studies indicate that following IV or IM administration, approximately 50% of a dose is reversibly bound to phospholipids of cell membranes in the liver, kidneys, heart, muscle, brain, and probably other tissues.

In an in vitro study using plasma from critically ill adults receiving polymyxin B, the drug was 78.5–92.4% bound to plasma proteins; however, mean protein binding was only 55.9% when testing was done using pooled plasma from healthy individuals.

● Elimination

The serum half-life of polymyxin B is reported to be 4.3–6 hours in adults with normal renal function. In patients with creatinine clearances less than 10 mL/minute, the serum half-life of polymyxin B has been reported to be 2–3 days.

Polymyxin B is eliminated in urine principally by glomerular filtration. Some studies indicate only low amounts of the dose are eliminated in urine within the first 12 hours after a dose, but eventually approximately 60% of a dose of polymyxin B is excreted in urine. Other studies suggest that less than 1% of a dose is eliminated unchanged in urine over 3 days. In adults, there is a 12- to 24-hour time lag following the initial dose during which very little polymyxin B appears in the urine, possibly as a result of binding of the drug to phospholipids of kidney cell membranes. Excretion continues for 24–72 hours after the final dose is administered. In adults with normal renal function, urinary drug concentrations have averaged 20–100 mcg/mL following usual IM doses at 6-hour intervals over a period of a few days. Infants excrete polymyxin B faster than do adults; 40–60% of an administered dose is excreted within 8 hours in the urine.

In a study in critically ill adults who received polymyxin B doses by IV infusion over 60 minutes, total body clearance ranged from 0.27–0.81 mL/minute per kg and less than 1% of a dose was eliminated unchanged in urine.

Polymyxin B is not removed to an appreciable extent by hemodialysis or peritoneal dialysis.

CHEMISTRY AND STABILITY

● Chemistry

Polymyxin B is a polymyxin antibiotic derived from *Bacillus polymyxa*. Polymyxin B is structurally and pharmacologically related to colistin. Commercially available polymyxin B sulfate is a mixture of the sulfate salts of polymyxins B_1 and B_2.

Polymyxin B sulfate occurs as a white to buff-colored, hygroscopic powder that is odorless or has a faint odor. The drug is freely soluble in water and in 0.9% sodium chloride injection and slightly soluble in alcohol. Each mg of pure polymyxin B is equivalent to 10,000 units of polymyxin B activity. Aqueous solutions of polymyxin B sulfate have a pH of 5–7.5.

● *Stability*

Polymyxin B sulfate powder for injection should be stored at 15–30°C or 20–25°C, depending on the manufacturer, and should be protected from light. Following reconstitution, polymyxin B solutions should be stored at 2–8°C; any unused portions should be discarded after 72 hours.

The commercially available fixed-combination solution for irrigation containing polymyxin B sulfate and neomycin sulfate should be stored at 2–8°C. Following dilution in 0.9% sodium chloride solution, the solution for irrigation should be stored at 4°C and used within 48 hours.

Polymyxin B is inactivated by strong acidic or alkaline solutions. The drug is chemically incompatible with many drugs including amphotericin B, ampicillin, cefazolin, chloramphenicol sodium succinate, chlorothiazide sodium, and heparin sodium. Polymyxin B in solution is also incompatible with the salts of calcium and magnesium.

PREPARATIONS

Excipients in commercially available drug preparations may have clinically important effects in some individuals; consult specific product labeling for details.

Polymyxin B Sulfate		
Powder	100 million units (of polymyxin B)*	Poly-Rx®, X-Gen
Parenteral		
For injection	500,000 units (of polymyxin B)*	**Polymyxin B Sulfate For Injection**

* available from one or more manufacturer, distributor, and/or repackager by generic (nonproprietary) name

Neomycin and Polymyxin B Sulfates		
Urogenital		
Solution, for irrigation	Neosporin Sulfate (40 mg of neomycin) per mL and Polymyxin B Sulfate 200,000 units (of polymyxin B) per mL	**Neomycin and Polymyxin B Sulfates Solution for Irrigation**
		Neosporin® G.U. Irrigant, Monarch

† Use is not currently included in the labeling approved by the US Food and Drug Administration.

Selected Revisions November 1, 2009, © Copyright, March 1, 1976, American Society of Health-System Pharmacists, Inc.

rifAXIMin

8:12.28.30 • RIFAMYCINS

■ Rifaximin, a structural analog of rifampin, is a rifamycin antibiotic.

USES

● Hepatic Encephalopathy—Reduction in Risk of Recurrence

Rifaximin is used for reduction of risk of recurrence of overt hepatic encephalopathy in adults.

In clinical trials, rifaximin was used in conjunction with lactulose in 91% of patients, and differences compared to patients without lactulose could not be determined. Rifaximin has not been studied for reduction of risk of recurrence of overt hepatic encephalopathy in patients with scores exceeding 25 on the model for end-stage liver disease (MELD); there were only 8.6% of patients with MELD scores >19 in clinical studies. Guidelines generally recommend rifaximin be used as an adjunct to lactulose for prevention of hepatic encephalopathy recurrence in patients who have had at least 1 episode of overt hepatic encephalopathy while receiving lactulose alone.

Clinical Experience

Efficacy of rifaximin for reduction of risk of recurrence of overt hepatic encephalopathy was evaluated in a randomized, placebo-controlled, double-blind study in adults who were in remission from hepatic encephalopathy (Conn score of 0 or 1) after having 2 or more episodes associated with chronic liver disease during the previous 6 months. A total of 299 adults (mean age 56 years [81% <65 years of age], 61% male, 86% white, 67% with Conn score of 0, 68% with asterixis grade 0, 27% with MELD score ≤10, 64% with MELD score 11–18, 9% Child-Pugh class C) were randomized to receive rifaximin 550 mg or placebo twice daily for 6 months or until the drug was discontinued because of a breakthrough episode of hepatic encephalopathy or another reason (e.g., adverse effects, request to withdraw). Concomitant use of lactulose was permitted (91.4% of those receiving rifaximin and 91.2% of those receiving placebo also received lactulose). The primary end point was time to first breakthrough episode of overt hepatic encephalopathy (defined as a marked deterioration in neurologic function and an increase from a baseline Conn score of 0 or 1 to a score of 2 or more, or an increase from a baseline Conn score of 0 to a score of 1 plus a 1-unit increase in asterixis grade). Comparison of Kaplan-Meier estimates of event-free curves showed that rifaximin reduced the risk of hepatic encephalopathy episodes by 58% compared with placebo during the 6-month treatment period; 22% of patients in the rifaximin treatment group and 46% of patients in the placebo group experienced breakthrough episodes of overt hepatic encephalopathy. Efficacy of rifaximin was consistent regardless of gender, baseline Conn score, duration of current remission, and presence or absence of diabetes mellitus. During the 6-month treatment period, rifaximin also reduced the risk of hepatic encephalopathy-associated hospitalizations by 50% compared with placebo; hepatic encephalopathy-associated hospitalizations were reported in 14 and 23% of patients in the rifaximin and placebo groups, respectively.

Clinical Perspective

Guidelines from the American Association for the Study of Liver Diseases (AASLD) and European Association for the Study of the Liver (EASL) generally recommend lactulose for prevention of recurrent hepatic encephalopathy. The guidelines recommend that rifaximin be used as an adjunct to lactulose for prevention of hepatic encephalopathy recurrence in patients who have had at least 1 episode of overt hepatic encephalopathy while receiving lactulose alone.

● Hepatic Encephalopathy—Treatment

Although safety and efficacy have not been established, rifaximin also has been used for the treatment of hepatic encephalopathy† and is designated an orphan drug by FDA for treatment of this condition.

Efficacy of rifaximin for the treatment of hepatic encephalopathy has been evaluated in several controlled studies and adjunctive use of the drug appears to be effective in reducing blood ammonia concentrations and decreasing the severity of neurologic manifestations. In one double-blind, dose-ranging study, 54 adults with cirrhosis and mild to moderate hepatic encephalopathy were randomized to receive 600, 1200, or 2400 mg of rifaximin daily in 3 divided doses for 7 days. Rifaximin treatment at the 2 higher dosages (1200 or 2400 mg daily) was associated with an improvement in the portal-systemic encephalopathy index (based on mental state, asterixis grade, number connection test time, EEG mean cycle frequency, and blood ammonia concentrations). In another double-blind study, 58 adults with cirrhosis and portosystemic encephalopathy were randomized to receive 1200 mg of rifaximin daily for 15 days or 30 g of lactulose daily for 15 days. Although clinical improvement in manifestations of portosystemic encephalopathy was reported for both drugs and correlated with reductions in serum ammonia concentrations, data suggest that rifaximin may be better tolerated than lactulose. Clinical improvement was also reported in a study of 55 adults with cirrhosis and grade 1, 2, and 3 portosystemic encephalopathy treated with rifaximin (1200 mg daily in 3 divided doses) in conjunction with lactulose therapy at a dosage sufficient to induce 2 or 3 evacuations daily.

A meta-analysis of 12 randomized, controlled trials comparing rifaximin to nonabsorbable disaccharides (e.g., lactulose, lactitol) or to other oral anti-infectives (e.g., neomycin, paromomycin) was conducted to assess the efficacy and safety of rifaximin for the treatment of hepatic encephalopathy in adults. Results from an analysis of the 7 studies that compared rifaximin to nonabsorbable disaccharides indicated that resolution or clinical improvement of hepatic encephalopathy occurred with both types of treatment; analysis of the 5 studies that compared rifaximin to other anti-infectives indicated that efficacy of rifaximin was similar to that of neomycin or paromomycin. A combined analysis of all 12 studies indicated that rifaximin was associated with fewer adverse effects than the other treatments. Another meta-analysis of 6 randomized, controlled trials found that rifaximin alone did not improve mental status or blood ammonia compared to lactulose or lactitol alone.

Information from the AASLD and EASL regarding management of hepatic encephalopathy, including recommendations for treatment and prevention of recurrence, is available at http://www.aasld.org.

● Irritable Bowel Syndrome with Diarrhea

Rifaximin is used for the treatment of irritable bowel syndrome (IBS) with diarrhea in adults. Guidelines for diarrhea-predominant IBS generally include use of rifaximin for treating global symptoms. Rifaximin is also recommended for retreatment in those who had a response and develop recurrent symptoms.

Clinical Experience

Efficacy of rifaximin for the treatment of IBS with diarrhea has been evaluated in 3 randomized, double-blind, placebo-controlled, phase 3 studies.

TARGET 1 (NCT00731679) and TARGET 2 (NCT00724126) were identically designed studies that included a total of 1258 adults who met Rome II criteria for diarrhea-predominant IBS (mean age: 46 years, 24–30% male, 89–94% white, 4–10% Black); patients with constipation-predominant IBS (according to Rome II criteria) were excluded. After a screening phase of 7–13 days, patients were randomized in a 1:1 ratio to receive rifaximin 550 mg or placebo 3 times daily for 14 days followed by a 10-week treatment-free evaluation period. The primary end point was the proportion of patients who had adequate relief of global IBS symptoms for at least 2 of the 4 weeks during the first month of the treatment-free evaluation period (primary evaluation period). This end point (adequate relief) was defined as a "yes" by the patient to a once-weekly subject global assessment question: "In regard to all your symptoms of IBS, as compared with the way you felt before you started the study medication, have you, in the past 7 days, had adequate relief of your IBS symptoms?". During the primary evaluation period, adequate relief was experienced by 41% of patients treated with rifaximin and 31–32% of patients treated with placebo. Substantially more patients in the rifaximin group experienced continued relief through 3 months compared with those in the placebo group. In addition, an exploratory, composite end point (defined as at least 30% improvement from baseline in abdominal pain *and* weekly mean stool consistency score less than 4 for at least 2 of the 4 weeks during the primary evaluation period) was achieved in 47% of patients treated with rifaximin compared with 36–39% of those treated with placebo.

TARGET 3 evaluated efficacy of repeat courses of rifaximin for the treatment of diarrhea-predominant IBS. A total of 2579 adults received open-label rifaximin for 14 days followed by a 4-week treatment-free evaluation period. Of the 2438 evaluable patients, 1074 (44%) responded to initial rifaximin treatment (defined as the composite end point of at least a 30% improvement from baseline in abdominal pain *and* at least a 50% reduction in the number of days per week with a daily stool consistency of Bristol Stool Scale type 6 or 7). These responders were then followed for recurrence for up to an additional 20-week treatment-free period. A total of 636 initial responders subsequently had recurrence of IBS symptoms (return of abdominal pain or lack of stool consistency for at least 3 weeks during a 4-week follow-up period); the median time to recurrence was 10 weeks (range 6–24 weeks). Patients who experienced recurrence were then enrolled in a double-blind, placebo-controlled, repeat treatment phase and randomized in a 1:1 ratio to receive rifaximin 550 mg or placebo 3 times daily for 2 additional 14-day repeat treatment courses separated by 10 weeks. The primary end point of this randomized portion of the study was the proportion of patients who were responders to repeat treatment in the composite outcome of at least a 30% improvement from baseline in IBS-related abdominal pain *and* at least a 50% reduction in the number of days per week with a daily stool consistency of Bristol Stool Scale type 6 or 7 during the 4 weeks following the first 14-day repeat treatment course. Response at 4 weeks after completion of the first repeat treatment course was achieved by 38% of patients treated with rifaximin and 31% of those treated with placebo. During the 10-week treatment free follow up period, 17.1 or 11.7% of patients treated with rifaximin or placebo, respectively, had no recurrence of signs and symptoms of IBS.

A meta-analysis including TARGET 1 and TARGET 2 did not find rifaximin effective compared to placebo for global IBS symptom response in patients with diarrhea-predominant IBS. However, a separate meta-analysis of 5 studies primarily in patients with diarrhea-predominant IBS (including TARGET 1 and TARGET 2) found rifaximin more effective than placebo for improving IBS symptoms.

Clinical Perspective

All patients with IBS are recommended to try dietary changes for global symptoms. Guideline recommendations for diarrhea-predominant IBS include use of rifaximin for treating global symptoms. Rifaximin is also recommended for retreatment in those who had a response to rifaximin and develop recurrent symptoms.

● Travelers' Diarrhea

Rifaximin is used for the treatment of travelers' diarrhea caused by noninvasive strains of *Escherichia coli* (*E. coli*) in adults and adolescents 12 years of age and older.

Rifaximin is *not* effective in and should *not* be used for the treatment of diarrhea complicated by fever or bloody stools or for the treatment of diarrhea caused by pathogens other than *E. coli*. Guidelines generally consider rifaximin an alternative to fluoroquinolones or azithromycin for noninvasive moderate-to-severe travelers' diarrhea.

Clinical Experience

In a multicenter, randomized, double-blind, placebo-controlled study in 380 adults with travelers' diarrhea, including 43 cases caused by enteroaggregative *E. coli*, treatment with rifaximin (200 mg three times daily for 3 days) was associated with a more rapid resolution of diarrhea and an increased rate of clinical cure (defined as 48 hours without unformed stools and without fever or 24 hours without watery stools, no more than 2 soft stools, and absence of other clinical symptoms) compared with placebo. The primary study end point was the median elapsed time after initiating therapy to the passage of the last unformed stool (time to the last unformed stool [TLUS]) and was 32.5 hours in patients treated with rifaximin and 59–60 hours in those treated with placebo. The rate of clinical cure within 5 days (120 hours) of initiating therapy was 79% in those treated with rifaximin and 60–61% in those treated with placebo. Treatment with a higher rifaximin dosage (400 mg 3 times daily) did not provide additional clinical benefit. The overall rate of microbiological cure (i.e., the absence of *E. coli* or other pathogen in stool cultured after 72 hours of therapy) in those treated with rifaximin (69%) was similar to the microbiologic cure rate in those treated with placebo (67%).

A randomized controlled trial compared rifaximin to monotherapy with either levofloxacin or azithromycin for travelers' diarrhea. Although noninferiority

could not be shown with rifaximin, the efficacy at 48 and 72 hours was equivalent, median TLUS did not differ, treatment failures were not common, and there was no difference in adverse events between treatment arms. Therefore, the authors considered rifaximin to be similar to levofloxacin and azithromycin.

Although safety and efficacy have not been established, rifaximin has been used in some adults for prevention of travelers' diarrhea†. Because travelers' diarrhea is a relatively nonthreatening illness that usually is mild and self-limiting and because of the risks of widespread use of prophylactic anti-infectives (i.e., potential adverse drug reactions, selection of resistant organisms, increased susceptibility to infections caused by these or other organisms), the US Centers for Disease Control and Prevention (CDC) and other experts state that anti-infective prophylaxis for prevention of travelers' diarrhea is not recommended for most travelers.

Clinical Perspective

Travelers' diarrhea caused by bacteria may be self-limited and often resolves within 3–7 days without anti-infective treatment. If diarrhea is moderate or severe, associated with fever or bloody stools, persisting longer than 3 days, or extremely disruptive to travel plans, short-term (1–3 days) treatment with an anti-infective usually is recommended. Since bacteria are the most common cause of travelers' diarrhea (80–90% of cases), an anti-infective directed against enteric bacterial pathogens is used for empiric treatment. The CDC and other experts previously recommended a fluoroquinolone (e.g., ciprofloxacin, levofloxacin) as the anti-infective of choice for empiric treatment of travelers' diarrhea in adults. However, due to potential resistance, azithromycin is now also considered an agent of choice, especially for individuals who should not receive fluoroquinolones (e.g., children, pregnant women) and for travelers in areas with a high prevalence of fluoroquinolone-resistant Campylobacter (e.g., South and Southeast Asia). Rifaximin or rifamycin can be considered an alternative when the causative organism is a noninvasive pathogen. However, because it may be difficult for travelers to distinguish between invasive and noninvasive diarrhea, the overall usefulness of anti-infective agents for empiric self-treatment of travelers' diarrhea remains to be determined.

● Other Uses

Although safety and efficacy have not been established, rifaximin has been used in some adults as treatment for *Clostridioides difficile* (*C. difficile*) infection in patients with multiple recurrences†; however, not all guidelines recommend its use as an alternative to other recommended treatments.

Although safety and efficacy have not been established, rifaximin has been used in combination therapy for patients with refractory acute pouchitis†.

Although safety and efficacy have not been established, rifaximin may also be an effective anti-infective for treatment of small intestinal overgrowth†.

DOSAGE AND ADMINISTRATION

● General

Patient Monitoring

- Monitor for signs and symptoms of hypersensitivity reactions to rifaximin.
- Monitor for worsening or persistence of travelers' diarrhea for more than 24–48 hours after initiation of rifaximin. Discontinue rifaximin if either occurs, and consider treatment with an alternative anti-infective.

● Administration

Rifaximin is administered orally without regard to meals.

Store at 20–25°C (excursions permitted between 15–30°C).

● Dosage

Pediatric Patients

Travelers' Diarrhea

For the treatment of travelers' diarrhea caused by noninvasive strains of *E. coli* in adolescents 12 years of age or older, the recommended dosage of rifaximin is 200 mg three times daily for 3 days.

If diarrhea worsens or persists for more than 24–48 hours after initiating rifaximin, discontinue the drug and consider an alternative anti-infective.

Adults

Hepatic Encephalopathy

For reduction of risk of recurrence of overt hepatic encephalopathy in adults, the recommended dosage of rifaximin is 550 mg twice daily.

For the treatment of hepatic encephalopathy† in adults, the recommended dosage of rifaximin is 600–1200 mg daily (usually in 3 divided doses) for 7–21 days.

Irritable Bowel Syndrome with Diarrhea

For the treatment of irritable bowel syndrome (IBS) with diarrhea in adults, the recommended dosage of rifaximin is 550 mg three times daily for 14 days. If symptoms recur, up to 2 additional courses of rifaximin may be given using the same 14-day regimen.

Travelers' Diarrhea

For the treatment of travelers' diarrhea caused by noninvasive strains of *E.coli* in adults, the recommended dosage of rifaximin is 200 mg three times daily for 3 days. If diarrhea worsens or persists for more than 24–48 hours after initiating rifaximin, the drug should be discontinued and an alternative anti-infective considered.

For the prevention of travelers' diarrhea†, the recommended dosage of rifaximin is 200–1100 mg daily (divided in 1–3 doses).

Clostridioides difficile *Infection—Patients With Multiple Recurrences*

For the treatment of *C. difficile* infection in patients with multiple recurrences†, dosages of rifaximin have included 400 mg three times daily for 20 days or 400 mg three times daily for 14 days, followed by 200 mg three times daily for an additional 14 days.

Refractory Acute Pouchitis

For the treatment of refractory acute pouchitis†, dosages of rifaximin have included 400 mg three times daily for 4 weeks or 1 gram twice daily for 15 days.

Small Intestinal Bacterial Overgrowth

For the treatment of small intestinal bacterial overgrowth†, dosages of rifaximin have included 400 mg three times daily for 10 days.

● Special Populations

Hepatic Impairment

Rifaximin dosage adjustment is not necessary in patients with hepatic impairment; however, the drug should be used with caution in patients with severe hepatic impairment (Child-Pugh class C) as increased systemic exposure is observed.

Renal Impairment

The manufacturer makes no specific dosage recommendations for patients with renal impairment.

Geriatric Use

The pharmacokinetics of rifaximin have not been specifically studied in geriatric patients 65 years of age or older. Other reported clinical experience has not identified differences in responses between the elderly and younger patients, but greater sensitivity of some older individuals cannot be ruled out.

CAUTIONS

● Contraindications

● Hypersensitivity to rifaximin, other rifamycin anti-infectives, or any ingredient in the formulation. Hypersensitivity reactions such as exfoliative dermatitis, angioedema, and anaphylaxis have been reported, some occurring within 15 minutes of a dose of rifaximin.

● Warnings/Precautions

Travelers' Diarrhea Not Caused by *Escherichia Coli*

Rifaximin should *not* be used for the treatment of diarrhea complicated by fever or bloody stools or for the treatment of diarrhea known or suspected to be caused by pathogens other than *E. coli* (e.g., *Campylobacter jejuni, Salmonella, Shigella*). Rifaximin was not found to be effective in patients with diarrhea due to pathogens other than *E. coli*.

If diarrhea worsens or persists for more than 24–48 hours after initiating rifaximin, discontinue the drug and consider treatment with another anti-infective.

Clostridium difficile-associated Diarrhea (CDAD)

Treatment with anti-infectives alters normal colon flora and may permit overgrowth of *C. difficile*. *C. difficile* infection (CDI) and *C. difficile*-associated diarrhea (CDAD; also known as antibiotic-associated diarrhea and colitis or pseudomembranous colitis) have been reported in patients receiving nearly all anti-infectives, including rifaximin, and may range in severity from mild diarrhea to fatal colitis.

C. difficile produces toxins A and B, which contribute to development of CDAD; hypertoxin-producing strains of *C. difficile* are associated with increased morbidity and mortality since they may be refractory to anti-infectives and colectomy may be required.

Consider CDAD in the differential diagnosis of patients who develop diarrhea during or after anti-infective therapy. Careful medical history is necessary since CDAD has been reported to occur as late as 2 months or longer after anti-infective therapy is discontinued.

If CDAD is suspected or confirmed, discontinue anti-infective therapy not directed against *C. difficile* whenever possible. Patients should be managed with appropriate supportive therapy (e.g., fluid and electrolyte management, protein supplementation), anti-infective therapy directed against *C. difficile*, and surgical evaluation as clinically indicated.

Development of Drug-Resistant Bacteria

Prescribing rifaximin for travelers' diarrhea in the absence of a proven or strongly suspected bacterial infection or a prophylactic indication is unlikely to provide benefit to the patient and increases the risk of the development of drug-resistant bacteria.

Severe (Child-Pugh Class C) Hepatic Impairment

Increased systemic exposure to rifaximin occurs in patients with severe hepatic impairment. Clinical trials were limited to patients with Model for End-Stage Liver Disease (MELD) scores ≤25. Therefore, exercise caution when administering rifaximin to patients with severe hepatic impairment (Child-Pugh Class C).

Concomitant Use With P-Glycoprotein Inhibitors

Concomitant use of rifaximin with drugs that are P-glycoprotein (P-gp) transport inhibitors (e.g., cyclosporine) may substantially increase rifaximin systemic exposure. In patients with hepatic impairment, a potential additive effect of reduced hepatic metabolism and concomitant use with P-gp inhibitors may further increase rifaximin exposure. Exercise caution when concomitant use of rifaximin and a P-gp inhibitor is necessary.

Specific Populations

Pregnancy

Data are not available regarding the use of rifaximin in pregnant females. In animal reproduction studies, teratogenic effects (e.g., ocular, oral and maxillofacial, cardiac, and lumbar spine malformations) were observed in rats and rabbits at rifaximin dosages approximately 0.9–5 times and 0.7–33 times, the recommended human dosage (600–1650 mg daily), respectively. Advise pregnant females of the potential risk to the fetus.

Lactation

It is not known whether rifaximin is distributed into human milk, affects human milk production, or affects the breast-fed infant.

Consider the benefits of breast-feeding and the importance of rifaximin to the female along with the potential adverse effects on the breast-fed child from the drug or from the underlying maternal condition.

Pediatric Use

Hepatic encephalopathy: Safety and efficacy of rifaximin have not been established in children and adolescents younger than 18 years of age.

Irritable bowel syndrome (IBS) with diarrhea: Safety and efficacy of rifaximin have not been established in children and adolescents younger than 18 years of age.

Travelers' diarrhea: Safety and efficacy of rifaximin have not been established in children younger than 12 years of age.

Geriatric Use

Hepatic encephalopathy: There were no overall differences in safety or efficacy between patients 65 years of age and older and younger adults in clinical studies (19% of patients were 65 years of age or older); other reported clinical experience has not identified differences in response between geriatric and younger patients, but greater sensitivity in some older individuals cannot be ruled out.

IBS with diarrhea: There were no overall differences in safety or efficacy between patients 65 years of age and older and younger adults in clinical studies (11% of patients were 65 years of age or older) or other reported clinical experience, but greater sensitivity in some older individuals cannot be ruled out.

Travelers' diarrhea: Experience in those 65 years of age or older is insufficient to determine whether they respond differently than younger patients.

Hepatic Impairment

Use rifaximin with caution in patients with severe hepatic impairment (Child-Pugh class C). Although dosage adjustments are not necessary in patients with hepatic impairment, severe hepatic impairment results in increased rifaximin systemic exposure.

In patients with a history of hepatic encephalopathy, mean rifaximin exposure (based on area under the plasma concentration-time curve [AUC]) is higher than that reported in healthy individuals. When rifaximin dosage of 550 mg twice daily was evaluated in patients with a history of hepatic encephalopathy, mean systemic exposure in those with mild, moderate, or severe hepatic impairment was approximately 10-, 14-, or 21-fold higher, respectively, than systemic exposure reported in healthy individuals. Clinical trials evaluating rifaximin in patients with a history of hepatic encephalopathy did not include patients with scores exceeding 25 on the MELD.

Renal Impairment

The pharmacokinetics of rifaximin have not been specifically studied in patients with renal impairment.

● Common Adverse Effects

Hepatic encephalopathy: Adverse effects occurring in ≥10% of patients receiving rifaximin include peripheral edema, nausea, constipation, dizziness, fatigue, urinary tract infection, insomnia, anemia, pruritus, and ascites.

IBS with diarrhea: Adverse effects occurring in ≥2% of patients receiving rifaximin include nausea and increased ALT concentrations.

Travelers' diarrhea: Adverse effects occurring in ≥2% of patients receiving rifaximin include headache.

DRUG INTERACTIONS

Rifaximin is a substrate of cytochrome P-450 (CYP) isoenzyme 3A4. Based on in vitro studies, rifaximin is not expected to inhibit CYP1A2, 2A6, 2B6, 2C9, 2C19, 2D6, 2E1, or 3A4. In vitro, rifaximin is a substrate of organic anion transporting polypeptides (OATP) 1A2, 1B1, and 1B3; the drug is not a substrate of OATP2B1.

Although in vitro studies indicate that rifaximin inhibits OATP1B1, 1A2, and 1B3, the effect of the drug on these transporters in vivo is unknown.

● Drugs Affected by Hepatic Microsomal Enzymes

Although in vitro studies indicate that rifaximin induces CYP3A4, drug interaction studies with midazolam (a CYP3A4 substrate) indicate that therapeutic dosages of rifaximin do not have clinically important effects on the activity of intestinal or hepatic CYP3A4. In patients with normal hepatic function, pharmacokinetic interactions between rifaximin and drugs metabolized by CYP3A4 are not expected. However, it is not known whether rifaximin can have a clinically important effect on the pharmacokinetics of such drugs in patients with hepatic impairment who have increased plasma concentrations of rifaximin.

● Drugs Affecting or Affected by Transport Systems

Rifaximin is a substrate of P-glycoprotein (P-gp) transport in vitro. Concomitant use of rifaximin and cyclosporine, an inhibitor of P-gp and OATPs substantially increased rifaximin exposures. Exercise caution when a P-gp inhibitor and rifaximin are used concomitantly. In patients with impaired hepatic function and concomitant P-gp inhibitor use, additive effects of reduced metabolism and concomitant P-gp inhibitors may further increase exposure to rifaximin.

Although in vitro studies indicate that rifaximin inhibits P-gp transport, the effect of the drug on P-gp transport in vivo is unknown.

● Cyclosporine

In healthy individuals, concomitant use of rifaximin (single 550-mg dose) and cyclosporine (single 600-mg dose) results in an 83- and 124-fold increase in rifaximin peak plasma concentrations and AUC, respectively. In patients with impaired hepatic function and concomitant cyclosporine use, additive effects of reduced metabolism and concomitant cyclosporine may further increase exposure to rifaximin.

Because cyclosporine inhibits P-gp and OATPs and is a weak inhibitor of CYP3A4, the relative contributions of these effects on rifaximin pharmacokinetics are unknown. In addition, the clinical importance of increased rifaximin systemic exposures in patients receiving cyclosporine is unknown.

● Midazolam

Concurrent use of rifaximin (200 mg orally 3 times daily for 3 or 7 days) and a single dose of midazolam (2 mg IV or 6 mg orally) did not substantially alter systemic exposure or elimination of midazolam or its major metabolite (1′-hydroxymidazolam). Concurrent use of rifaximin (550 mg orally three times daily for 7 or 14 days) and midazolam (single 2-mg IV dose) resulted in slightly decreased midazolam peak plasma concentrations and AUC; this effect is not considered clinically important.

● Hormonal Contraceptives

Concurrent use of rifaximin (200 mg orally three times daily for 3 days) and a single dose of an oral estrogen-progestin combination contraceptive (ethinyl estradiol 70 mcg in fixed combination with norgestimate 500 mcg) did not substantially alter the disposition of ethinyl estradiol and norgestimate. Concurrent use of rifaximin (550 mg three times daily for 7 days) and a single dose of an oral estrogen-progestin combination contraceptive (ethinyl estradiol 25 mcg in fixed combination with norgestimate 250 mcg) resulted in a 25 and 13% decrease in peak plasma concentrations of ethinyl estradiol and norgestimate, respectively; the mean AUCs of norgestimate metabolites were decreased by 7–11% but the AUC of ethinyl estradiol was not affected. The clinical importance of these effects on estrogen-progestin combination contraceptives is not known.

● Warfarin

Changes in the international normalized ratio (INR) have been identified in postmarketing reports of concomitant warfarin and rifaximin use. Monitor the INR and prothrombin time. Dosage adjustments of warfarin may be necessary to maintain a therapeutic INR range.

DESCRIPTION

Rifaximin is a semisynthetic derivative of rifampin. Like other rifamycins, rifaximin inhibits RNA synthesis in susceptible bacteria by binding to the β subunit of bacterial DNA-dependent RNA polymerase.

Due to limited and variable systemic absorption, rifaximin is not suitable for the treatment of systemic bacterial infections. Rifaximin systemic exposure is dose-proportional over a dosage range of 200–400 mg, and systemic exposure is less than dose-proportional over a dosage range of 400–600 mg. Following oral administration of rifaximin (single or multiple doses of 550 mg) in healthy individuals, mean peak plasma concentrations are attained about 1 hour after dosing and range from 2.4–4 ng/mL. In patients treated with oral rifaximin (200 mg three times daily for 3 days), plasma concentrations and systemic exposure (area under the plasma concentration-time curve [AUC]) are low and variable and accumulation of the drug does not occur. In patients with a history of hepatic encephalopathy receiving rifaximin (550 mg twice daily), the mean AUC of rifaximin is approximately 12-fold higher than that reported in healthy individuals. In patients with irritable bowel syndrome (IBS) with diarrhea receiving rifaximin (550 mg three times daily for 14 days), the time to peak plasma concentrations, mean peak plasma concentrations, and AUC of rifaximin are similar to those reported in healthy individuals. When rifaximin was administered 30 minutes after a high-fat meal in healthy individuals, peak plasma concentrations of the drug were not affected; however, the time to peak plasma concentrations was delayed from 0.75 to 1.5 hours after the dose and AUC was increased twofold. Rifaximin is moderately bound to human plasma proteins (67.5 or 62% in healthy individuals or patients with hepatic impairment, respectively). Systemically absorbed rifaximin undergoes extensive metabolism, principally by cytochrome P-450 (CYP) isoenzyme 3A4. Following a 400-mg oral dose of rifaximin, 96.6% of the dose is excreted in feces (mostly as unchanged drug) and 0.3% is excreted in urine (mostly as metabolites). The mean half-life of rifaximin at steady-state is 5.6 hours in healthy individuals and 6 hours in patients with IBS with diarrhea.

Rifaximin is active in vitro and in clinical infections (i.e., infectious diarrhea) against most isolates of enterotoxigenic *Escherichia coli* (ETEC) and enteroaggregative *Escherichia coli* (EAEC).

Rifaximin should not be used to treat diarrhea accompanied by fever or blood in the stool, or due to pathogens other than *E. coli*. Do not use rifaximin in patients where *Campylobacter jejuni* (*C. jejuni*), *Shigella*, and *Salmonella* are suspected as causative organisms. Rifaximin is not effective against *C. jejuni*, and has not been proven effective against *Shigella* and *Salmonella*.

When selecting or modifying anti-infective therapy, results of culture and in vitro susceptibility testing should be used. In the absence of such data, local epidemiology and susceptibility patterns should be considered when selecting anti-infectives for empiric therapy.

Resistance to rifaximin generally is associated with mutations in the *rpoB* gene that change the binding site on DNA-dependent RNA polymerase and decrease rifaximin binding affinity. Cross-resistance between rifaximin and other classes of anti-infectives has not been observed.

ADVICE TO PATIENTS

- Advise patients that antibacterials (including rifaximin) should only be used to treat bacterial infections and not used to treat viral infections (e.g., the common cold).
- Advise patients that rifaximin may be taken with or without food.
- If used for the treatment of travelers' diarrhea, advise patients of the importance of discontinuing rifaximin and seeking medical care if diarrhea worsens or persists for more than 24–48 hours after the drug is initiated or if fever and/or bloody diarrhea develop.
- Advise patients that diarrhea is a common problem caused by anti-infectives and usually ends when the drug is discontinued. Importance of contacting a clinician if watery and bloody stools (with or without stomach cramps and fever) occur during or as late as 2 months or longer after the last dose as this may be related to CDAD.
- Importance of informing clinicians of existing or contemplated concomitant therapy, including prescription and OTC drugs, as well as any concomitant illnesses.
- Advise females of child bearing potential to inform clinicians if they are or plan to become pregnant or plan to breast-feed.
- Inform patients of other important precautionary information.

PREPARATIONS

Excipients in commercially available drug preparations may have clinically important effects in some individuals; consult specific product labeling for details.

rifAXIMin

Oral

Tablets	200 mg	Xifaxan®, Salix
	550 mg	Xifaxan®, Salix

† Use is not currently included in the labeling approved by the US Food and Drug Administration.

Quinupristin and Dalfopristin

8:12.28.32 • STREPTOGRAMINS

■ Quinupristin and dalfopristin (quinupristin/dalfopristin) is a fixed combination containing 2 semisynthetic streptogramin antibiotics; quinupristin and dalfopristin act synergistically against susceptible bacteria, resulting in increased antibacterial activity compared with either drug alone.

USES

● Skin and Skin Structure Infections

Quinupristin and dalfopristin (quinupristin/dalfopristin) is used IV for the treatment of complicated skin and skin structure infections caused by *Staphylococcus aureus* (methicillin-susceptible [oxacillin-susceptible] strains) or *Streptococcus pyogenes* (group A β-hemolytic streptococci, GAS).

In 2 randomized, open-label, phase 3, comparator-controlled studies in adults with complicated skin and skin structure infections (e.g., erysipelas, postoperative infections, traumatic wound infections), efficacy and safety of quinupristin/dalfopristin (7.5 mg/kg given IV every 12 hours) was compared with oxacillin (2 g given IV every 6 hours) or cefazolin (1 g given IV every 8 hours). In the comparator groups, vancomycin (1 g given IV every 12 hours) could be substituted for the comparator drug if necessary (e.g., β-lactam hypersensitivity, suspected or confirmed methicillin-resistant *S. aureus* [MRSA; also known as oxacillin-resistant *S. aureus* or ORSA]). The clinical success rate (defined as cure or improvement) in the clinically evaluable population in these 2 studies was 50 or 66% in those treated with quinupristin/dalfopristin versus 52 or 64% in those treated with the comparator anti-infective. Drug discontinuance because of adverse effects occurred more than 4 times as often in the quinupristin/dalfopristin treatment groups than in the comparator treatment groups; approximately 50% of those who discontinued quinupristin/dalfopristin did so because of adverse effects at the IV infusion site. (See Administration Precautions under Warnings/Precautions: Other Warnings and Precautions, in Cautions.)

For information on diagnosis and management of skin and skin structure infections, the current clinical practice guidelines from the Infectious Diseases Society of America (IDSA) available at http://www.idsociety.org should be consulted.

● Methicillin-resistant Staphylococcus aureus Infections

Quinupristin/dalfopristin has been used IV as salvage therapy in critically ill patients for the treatment of severe infections (e.g., bacteremia, infective endocarditis) caused by methicillin-resistant *S. aureus*† (MRSA; also known as oxacillin-resistant *S. aureus* or ORSA) when vancomycin was ineffective.

Although safety and efficacy of quinupristin/dalfopristin for the treatment of MRSA infections has not been established, some clinicians state that the drug is one of several options for the treatment of persistent MRSA bacteremia in adults who fail to respond to vancomycin or when the infection is known to be caused by MRSA with reduced susceptibility to vancomycin and daptomycin.

For information regarding the treatment of infections caused by MRSA, the current clinical practice guidelines from IDSA available at http://www.idsociety.org should be consulted. For information on diagnosis and management of infective endocarditis caused by MRSA, the current AHA guidelines available at http://my.americanheart.org/statements should be consulted.

● Vancomycin-resistant Enterococcus faecium Infections

Quinupristin/dalfopristin has been used IV for the treatment of serious or life-threatening infections caused by susceptible vancomycin-resistant *Enterococcus faecium*†, including bacteremia, infective endocarditis, intra-abdominal infections, skin and skin structure infections, and urinary tract infections. Although quinupristin/dalfopristin has been effective in some patients for the treatment of infections caused by vancomycin-resistant *E. faecium*, this indication is no longer included in FDA-approved labeling for the drug because data submitted to FDA failed to confirm clinical benefit. Some clinicians suggest that use of quinupristin/dalfopristin for the treatment of infections caused by vancomycin-resistant *E. faecium* should be reserved for refractory infections that fail to respond to other anti-infectives.

Efficacy of quinupristin/dalfopristin for the treatment of serious infections caused by vancomycin-resistant *S. faecium* varies depending on the site of infection. Data from 2 prospective emergency-use studies indicated lower success rates when the drug was used for the treatment of bacteremia of unknown origin (52%) or intra-abdominal infections (59%) caused by vancomycin-resistant *S. faecium* and higher success rates when the drug was used for the treatment of skin and skin structure infections (72%), central catheter-related bacteremia (83%), or urinary tract infections (89%) caused by vancomycin-resistant *S. faecium*.

DOSAGE AND ADMINISTRATION

● Administration

Quinupristin and dalfopristin (quinupristin/dalfopristin) is administered by IV infusion over 60 minutes.

Quinupristin/dalfopristin should *not* be given by rapid IV infusion or injection. An infusion pump or device may be used to control the rate of infusion.

Following completion of peripheral infusions of quinupristin/dalfopristin, the vein should be flushed with 5% dextrose injection to decrease the incidence of venous irritation. If necessary, a peripherally inserted central catheter (PICC) or central venous catheter can be used to administer quinupristin/dalfopristin. (See Administration Precautions under Warnings/Precautions: Other Warnings and Precautions, in Cautions.)

Other drugs should not be added to quinupristin/dalfopristin solutions.

If the same IV line is used for sequential infusion of different drugs, the IV line should be flushed with 5% dextrose injection before and after infusion of quinupristin/dalfopristin. Because of incompatibilities, sodium chloride injections or heparin solutions should *not* be used to flush the IV line.

IV Infusion

Reconstitution and Dilution

Quinupristin/dalfopristin powder for injection must be reconstituted and then further diluted prior to IV infusion. Strict aseptic technique must be observed when preparing IV solutions of quinupristin/dalfopristin since the drug contains no preservatives.

The manufacturer states that *only* 5% dextrose injection or sterile water for injection should be used to reconstitute quinupristin/dalfopristin powder for injection and *only* 5% dextrose injection should be used to dilute the reconstituted drug. Because of incompatibility, sodium chloride injections should *not* be used.

Single-dose vials labeled as containing 500 mg (150 mg of quinupristin and 350 mg of dalfopristin) should be reconstituted by slowly adding 5 mL of 5% dextrose injection or sterile water for injection to provide a solution containing 100 mg/mL. The vial should be gently swirled by manual rotation to ensure dissolution; shaking should be avoided to limit foaming. The vial should then be allowed to sit for a few minutes until all the foam has disappeared; the resulting solution should be clear.

Reconstituted solutions of quinupristin/dalfopristin *must* be further diluted in 5% dextrose injection within 30 minutes. The appropriate dose of reconstituted solution should be diluted in 250 mL of 5% dextrose injection. For infusion via a central line, the appropriate dose of reconstituted solution may be diluted in 100 mL of 5% dextrose injection.

If moderate or severe venous irritation occurs (see Administration Precautions under Warnings/Precautions: Other Warnings and Precautions, in Cautions), consideration should be given to increasing the infusion volume to 500 or 750 mL, changing the infusion site, or infusing the drug via a PICC or central venous catheter.

Reconstituted and diluted solutions of quinupristin/dalfopristin should be used as soon as possible. The manufacturer states that diluted solutions of the drug are stable for up to 5 hours at room temperature or up to 54 hours when refrigerated at 2–8°C. Quinupristin/dalfopristin solutions should not be frozen.

Reconstituted and diluted solutions of quinupristin/dalfopristin should be inspected visually for particulate matter prior to administration.

Rate of Administration

Quinupristin/dalfopristin solutions should be administered by IV infusion over 60 minutes.

Rapid IV infusion should be avoided. (See Administration Precautions under Warnings/Precautions: Other Warnings and Precautions, in Cautions.)

● *Dosage*

Quinupristin/dalfopristin is a fixed combination containing a 30:70 (w/w) ratio of quinupristin to dalfopristin.

Dosage of the fixed combination quinupristin/dalfopristin is expressed in terms of the total dosage of the 2 components (i.e., dosage of quinupristin plus dosage of dalfopristin).

Each single-dose vial of quinupristin/dalfopristin contains a total of 500 mg (i.e., 150 mg of quinupristin and 350 mg of dalfopristin).

Skin and Skin Structure Infections

The recommended dosage of quinupristin/dalfopristin for the treatment of complicated skin and skin structure infections caused by susceptible *Staphylococcus aureus* (methicillin-susceptible [oxacillin-susceptible] strains) or *Streptococcus pyogenes* (group A β-hemolytic streptococci, GAS) in adults is 7.5 mg/kg every 12 hours. The minimum recommended treatment duration for complicated skin and skin structure infections is 7 days.

Although safety and efficacy of quinupristin/dalfopristin have not been established in pediatric patients younger than 16 years of age (see Pediatric Use under Warnings/Precautions: Specific Populations, in Cautions), the manufacturer states that the recommended dosage of the drug for children 12 years of age or older is 7.5 mg/kg every 12 hours. Dosage recommendations are not available for pediatric patients younger than 12 years of age.

Methicillin-resistant Staphylococcus aureus Infections

Quinupristin/dalfopristin has been given in a dosage of 7.5 mg/kg every 8 hours for salvage therapy in the treatment of severe infections caused by methicillin-resistant *S. aureus*† (MRSA; also known as oxacillin-resistant *S. aureus* or ORSA) when vancomycin was ineffective.

Vancomycin-resistant Enterococcus faecium Infections

Quinupristin/dalfopristin has been given in a dosage of 7.5 mg/kg every 8 hours for the treatment of vancomycin-resistant *Enterococcus faecium* infections†.

● *Special Populations*

Hepatic Impairment

Although quinupristin/dalfopristin pharmacokinetic data in patients with hepatic cirrhosis (Child-Pugh class A and B) suggest that dosage reductions may be necessary in patients with hepatic impairment, the manufacturer states that data are insufficient to make specific recommendations for dosage modifications in such patients. (See Hepatic Impairment under Warnings/Precautions: Specific Populations, in Cautions.)

Renal Impairment

Dosage adjustments are not necessary when quinupristin/dalfopristin is used in patients with renal impairment or in those undergoing peritoneal dialysis. (See Renal Impairment under Warnings/Precautions: Specific Populations, in Cautions.)

Geriatric Patients

Dosage adjustments are not necessary when quinupristin/dalfopristin is used in geriatric patients.

CAUTIONS

● *Contraindications*

Quinupristin and dalfopristin (quinupristin/dalfopristin) is contraindicated in patients with known hypersensitivity to quinupristin/dalfopristin or other streptogramins (e.g., pristinamycin, virginiamycin).

● *Warnings/Precautions*

Warnings

Interactions

Concomitant use of quinupristin/dalfopristin and drugs that are metabolized by cytochrome P-450 (CYP) 3A4 and have a narrow therapeutic index requires caution and monitoring (e.g., cyclosporine) or should be avoided (e.g., drugs that prolong the QT interval corrected for rate [QT_c]). (See Drug Interactions.)

Sensitivity Reactions

Anaphylactic shock and angioedema have been reported in patients receiving quinupristin/dalfopristin.

Rash, urticaria, and pruritus also have been reported.

Other Warnings and Precautions

Administration Precautions

Adverse effects at the quinupristin/dalfopristin IV infusion site often occur, especially with peripheral infusions. In comparative clinical trials, inflammation or pain was reported in 38–45%, edema in 17–18%, and thrombophlebitis in 2% of patients receiving quinupristin/dalfopristin. Concomitant use of hydrocortisone or diphenhydramine in clinical trials did not appear to alleviate venous inflammation or pain associated with quinupristin/dalfopristin.

To minimize venous irritation, IV infusion lines should be flushed with 5% dextrose injection following completion of peripheral infusions of quinupristin/dalfopristin. Because of possible incompatibilities, IV infusion lines should *not* be flushed with sodium chloride injections or heparin solutions.

If moderate to severe venous irritation occurs following IV infusion of quinupristin/dalfopristin that has been diluted in 250 mL of 5% dextrose injection, consideration should be given to increasing the infusion volume to 500 or 750 mL, changing the infusion site, or establishing central venous access.

Rapid IV administration of quinupristin/dalfopristin in animals was associated with greater toxicity than slow IV infusion of the drug. Because safety of rapid IV injection of the drug has not been studied in humans and because clinical trial experience has exclusively involved IV infusion over 60 minutes, the manufacturer states that more rapid IV infusion rates cannot be recommended.

Musculoskeletal Effects

Arthralgia and myalgia, severe in some cases, have been reported in patients receiving quinupristin/dalfopristin. In some patients receiving the drug every 8 hours, symptoms improved when frequency was changed to every 12 hours. In those available for follow-up, symptoms resolved after the drug was discontinued. The etiology of these myalgias and arthralgias is unknown.

Hepatic Effects

Hyperbilirubinemia, with total bilirubin concentrations exceeding 5 times the upper limit of normal, occurred in approximately 25% of patients receiving quinupristin/dalfopristin in noncomparative clinical studies. In some patients, isolated hyperbilirubinemia (principally increased conjugated bilirubin) can occur during treatment, possibly as the result of competition between bilirubin and quinupristin/dalfopristin for excretion.

In comparative clinical studies, AST and ALT elevations occurred with similar frequency in those receiving quinupristin/dalfopristin or comparator therapy.

Precautions Related to Use of Fixed Combinations

When quinupristin/dalfopristin is used, the cautions, precautions, contraindications, and drug interactions associated with both drugs in the fixed combination must be considered. Cautionary information applicable to specific populations (e.g., pregnant or nursing women, individuals with hepatic or renal impairment, geriatric patients) should be considered for each drug.

When prescribing, preparing, and dispensing quinupristin/dalfopristin, healthcare professionals should consider that dosage of the fixed combination is expressed as the total (sum) of the dosage of each of the 2 active components (i.e., dosage of quinupristin plus dosage of dalfopristin). (See Dosage and Administration: Dosage.)

Superinfection/Clostridium difficile-associated Diarrhea and Colitis

Use of quinupristin/dalfopristin may result in overgrowth of nonsusceptible organisms. If superinfection occurs, appropriate therapy should be instituted.

Treatment with anti-infectives alters normal colon flora and may permit overgrowth of *Clostridium difficile*. *C. difficile* infection (CDI) and *C. difficile*-associated diarrhea and colitis (CDAD; also known as antibiotic-associated diarrhea and colitis or pseudomembranous colitis) have been reported with nearly all anti-infectives, including quinupristin/dalfopristin, and may range in severity from mild diarrhea to fatal colitis. *C. difficile* produces toxins A and B which contribute to the development of CDAD; hypertoxin-producing strains of *C. difficile* are associated with increased morbidity and mortality since they may be refractory to anti-infectives and colectomy may be required.

CDAD should be considered in the differential diagnosis of patients who develop diarrhea during or after anti-infective therapy. Careful medical history is necessary since CDAD has been reported to occur as late as 2 months or longer after anti-infective therapy is discontinued.

If CDAD is suspected or confirmed, anti-infective therapy not directed against *C. difficile* should be discontinued whenever possible. Patients should be managed with appropriate supportive therapy (e.g., fluid and electrolyte management, protein supplementation), anti-infective therapy directed against *C. difficile* (e.g., metronidazole, vancomycin), and surgical evaluation as clinically indicated.

Specific Populations

Pregnancy

Category B. (See Users Guide.)

There are no adequate and well-controlled studies evaluating quinupristin/dalfopristin in pregnant women; the drug should be used during pregnancy only if clearly needed.

Lactation

Quinupristin and dalfopristin are distributed into milk in rats; it is not known whether the drugs are distributed into human milk.

Quinupristin/dalfopristin should be used with caution in nursing women.

Pediatric Use

Safety and efficacy of quinupristin/dalfopristin have not been established in pediatric patients younger than 16 years of age. In addition, pharmacokinetics of the drug have not been studied in pediatric patients younger than 16 years of age. Quinupristin/dalfopristin has been given in a dosage of 7.5 mg/kg every 8 or 12 hours in a limited number of pediatric patients under emergency-use conditions. (See Skin and Skin Structure Infections under Dosage and Administration: Dosage.)

Geriatric Use

No overall differences in frequency, type, or severity of adverse effects, including cardiovascular effects, have been observed in geriatric adults 65 years of age or older compared with younger adults. Results of a study in adults 69–74 years of age indicate that the pharmacokinetics of quinupristin/dalfopristin in geriatric adults are similar to pharmacokinetics reported in younger adults.

Hepatic Impairment

In patients with hepatic impairment (Child-Pugh class A and B), the areas under the plasma concentration-time curves (AUCs) of quinupristin and dalfopristin and their major metabolites are increased. However, because the effect of reducing the dose or increasing the dosing interval on the pharmacokinetics of quinupristin and dalfopristin has not been studied, the manufacturer states that specific recommendations for dosage modifications in patients with hepatic impairment cannot be made.

Clinical studies suggest that the incidence of adverse effects in patients with chronic hepatic disease or cirrhosis is comparable to that in patients without hepatic impairment.

Renal Impairment

Although the AUCs of quinupristin and dalfopristin and their major metabolites are increased in patients with creatinine clearances of 6–28 mL/minute, the manufacturer states that dosage adjustments are not necessary in patients with renal impairment or in those undergoing peritoneal dialysis.

Only negligible amounts of quinupristin, dalfopristin, and their metabolites are removed by continuous ambulatory peritoneal dialysis (CAPD); it is unlikely that the drugs would be removed by hemodialysis.

Common Adverse Effects

Adverse effects at the IV infusion site (pain, burning, inflammation, edema) occur in a large percentage of patients, particularly when quinupristin/dalfopristin is given by peripheral infusion. (See Administration Precautions under Warnings/Precautions: Other Warnings and Precautions, in Cautions.) Other adverse effects occurring in 1% or more of patients include GI effects (nausea, vomiting, diarrhea, anorexia), arthralgia and myalgia, hyperbilirubinemia, headache, thrombophlebitis, pain, asthenia, rash, or pruritus.

DRUG INTERACTIONS

Drugs Metabolized by Hepatic Microsomal Enzymes

Quinupristin and dalfopristin (quinupristin/dalfopristin) inhibits cytochrome P-450 (CYP) isoenzyme 3A4 and may increase plasma concentrations of drugs metabolized by this hepatic enzyme, resulting in increased or prolonged therapeutic effects and/or increased adverse effects associated with the drugs. Caution is advised if quinupristin/dalfopristin is used concomitantly with drugs that are CYP3A4 substrates and have a narrow therapeutic index.

Quinupristin/dalfopristin does not have a clinically important effect on CYP isoenzymes 1A2, 2A6, 2C9, 2C19, 2D6, or 2E1; drug interactions with drugs metabolized by these CYP isoenzymes are not expected.

Drugs That Prolong QT Interval

Concomitant use with drugs that are CYP3A4 substrates and are known to prolong the QT interval corrected for rate (QT$_c$) should be avoided.

Antiarrhythmic Agents

Possible pharmacokinetic interactions between antiarrhythmic agents metabolized by CYP3A4 (e.g., disopyramide, lidocaine, quinidine) and quinupristin/dalfopristin (increased plasma concentrations of the antiarrhythmic agent). Caution is advised if quinupristin/dalfopristin is used concomitantly with an antiarrhythmic agent metabolized by CYP3A4.

Antibacterial Agents

There is some in vitro evidence that the antibacterial effects of vancomycin and quinupristin/dalfopristin are synergistic against vancomycin-resistant *Enterococcus faecium*.

In vitro studies indicate that the antibacterial effects of quinupristin/dalfopristin and certain aminoglycosides (gentamicin), β-lactams (amoxicillin, ampicillin, cefepime), glycopeptides (vancomycin), quinolones (ciprofloxacin), tetracyclines (doxycycline), or chloramphenicol are not antagonistic against staphylococci or enterococci.

In vitro studies indicate that the antibacterial effects of quinupristin/dalfopristin and certain aminoglycosides (gentamicin), β-lactams (aztreonam, cefotaxime), or quinolones (ciprofloxacin) are not antagonistic against Enterobacteriaceae or *Pseudomonas aeruginosa*.

Antineoplastic Agents

Possible pharmacokinetic interactions between vinca alkaloids (e.g., vinblastine), docetaxel, or paclitaxel and quinupristin/dalfopristin (increased plasma concentrations of the antineoplastic agent). Caution is advised if quinupristin/dalfopristin is used concomitantly with any of these antineoplastic agents.

Antiretroviral Agents

Possible pharmacokinetic interactions between quinupristin/dalfopristin and certain antiretrovirals metabolized by CYP3A4, including some HIV nonnucleoside reverse transcriptase inhibitors such as delavirdine and nevirapine and some HIV protease inhibitors such as indinavir and ritonavir (increased plasma concentrations of the antiretroviral). Caution is advised if quinupristin/dalfopristin is used concomitantly with antiretroviral agents metabolized by CYP3A4.

Benzodiazepines

Concomitant use of midazolam (single dose) and quinupristin/dalfopristin in healthy individuals increased the peak plasma concentration and area under the plasma concentration-time curve (AUC) of midazolam by 14 and 33%, respectively.

Possible pharmacokinetic interactions between other benzodiazepines metabolized by CYP3A4 (e.g., diazepam) and quinupristin/dalfopristin (increased plasma concentrations of the benzodiazepine).

Caution is advised if quinupristin/dalfopristin is used concomitantly with benzodiazepines metabolized by CYP3A4.

● Calcium-channel Blocking Agents

Concomitant use of nifedipine and quinupristin/dalfopristin in healthy individuals increased the peak plasma concentration and AUC of nifedipine by 18 and 44%, respectively.

Possible pharmacokinetic interactions between other calcium-channel blocking agents metabolized by CYP3A4 (e.g., diltiazem, verapamil) and quinupristin/dalfopristin (increased plasma concentrations of the calcium-channel blocker).

Caution is advised if quinupristin/dalfopristin is used concomitantly with calcium-channel blocking agents metabolized by CYP3A4.

● Carbamazepine

Possible pharmacokinetic interactions between carbamazepine and quinupristin/dalfopristin (increased plasma concentrations of the anticonvulsant). Caution is advised if carbamazepine and quinupristin/dalfopristin are used concomitantly.

● Cisapride

Possible pharmacokinetic interactions between cisapride and quinupristin/dalfopristin (increased plasma concentrations of cisapride). Caution is advised if cisapride and quinupristin/dalfopristin are used concomitantly.

● Corticosteroids

Possible pharmacokinetic interactions between methylprednisolone and quinupristin/dalfopristin (increased plasma concentrations of the corticosteroid). Caution is advised if methylprednisolone and quinupristin/dalfopristin are used concomitantly.

● Digoxin

Pharmacokinetic interactions between digoxin and quinupristin/dalfopristin based on CYP3A4 inhibition are unlikely. However, in vitro data indicate that quinupristin/dalfopristin inhibits *Eubacterium lentum*; therefore, the drug possibly may interfere with GI metabolism of digoxin that occurs via intestinal bacteria.

● HMG-CoA Reductase Inhibitors

Possible pharmacokinetic interactions between HMG-CoA reductase inhibitors (statins) metabolized by CYP3A4 (e.g., lovastatin) and quinupristin/dalfopristin (increased plasma concentrations of the statin). Caution is advised if quinupristin/dalfopristin is used concomitantly with statins metabolized by CYP3A4.

● Immunosuppressive Agents

Cyclosporine

Concomitant use of cyclosporine and quinupristin/dalfopristin affects the pharmacokinetics of cyclosporine and has resulted in a 30% increase in peak plasma concentrations, 63% increase in AUC, 77% increase in plasma half-life, and 34% decrease in clearance of the immunosuppressive agent.

If cyclosporine and quinupristin/dalfopristin must be used concomitantly, caution is advised and cyclosporine plasma concentrations should be monitored.

Tacrolimus

Possible pharmacokinetic interactions between tacrolimus and quinupristin/dalfopristin (increased plasma concentrations of tacrolimus). Tacrolimus and quinupristin/dalfopristin should be used concomitantly with caution.

DESCRIPTION

Quinupristin and dalfopristin (quinupristin/dalfopristin) is a fixed combination containing 2 semisynthetic streptogramin antibiotics. Naturally occurring streptogramin antibiotics (e.g., pristinamycin, virginiamycin) are produced by certain *Streptomyces* bacteria and contain 2 macrocyclic lactone peptolide components (i.e., streptogramin type A and streptogramin type B) that act synergistically

against susceptible bacteria. Quinupristin is derived from pristinamycin I and is a type B streptogramin; dalfopristin is derived from pristinamycin II$_A$ and is a type A streptogramin.

Quinupristin/dalfopristin is commercially available as a lyophilized powder containing a 30:70 (w/w) ratio of quinupristin to dalfopristin. Unlike pristinamycin, quinupristin and dalfopristin are both water-soluble and therefore suitable for IV administration. In vitro studies indicate that metabolism of quinupristin and dalfopristin is not dependent on cytochrome P-450 (CYP) isoenzymes or glutathione transferase enzymes.

Quinupristin and dalfopristin act synergistically against susceptible bacteria, and the in vitro activity of the fixed combination is greater than that of each individual component. In addition, quinupristin is partially converted in vivo to 2 major active metabolites (a glutathione conjugate and a cysteine conjugate) and quinupristin is partially converted in vivo to a major active metabolite formed by hydrolysis. These major active metabolites contribute to the antibacterial activity of quinupristin/dalfopristin since they have antibacterial activity and act synergistically with the parent drugs.

The mechanism of action of quinupristin/dalfopristin, like other streptogramins, involves inhibition of protein synthesis. The 2 components of quinupristin/dalfopristin bind to different sites on the 50S subunit of the bacterial ribosome. Dalfopristin (a type A streptogramin) affects an early phase of protein synthesis and inhibits peptidyl transferase activity; quinupristin (a type B streptogramin) affects a later phase of protein synthesis and inhibits peptide chain elongation. Synergy results in part because quinupristin's affinity for the 50S subunit is enhanced by the conformational change produced when dalfopristin binds to the 50S subunit.

Quinupristin/dalfopristin usually is bactericidal against susceptible staphylococci and streptococci, but bacteriostatic against susceptible enterococci.

● Spectrum

Quinupristin/dalfopristin is active in vitro and in clinical infections caused by methicillin-susceptible (oxacillin-susceptible) *Staphylococcus aureus* and *Streptococcus pyogenes* (group A β-hemolytic streptococci, GAS). Although the clinical importance in unknown, quinupristin also has in vitro activity against methicillin-resistant *S. aureus* (MRSA; also known as oxacillin-resistant *S. aureus* or ORSA), *S. epidermidis* (including methicillin-resistant strains), *S. pneumoniae*, *S. agalactiae* (group B streptococci, GBS), groups C and G streptococci, viridans streptococci, *Listeria monocytogenes*, and *Corynebacterium jeikeium*. The MIC$_{90}$ of quinupristin/dalfopristin for most susceptible staphylococci and streptococci is 1 mcg/mL or less.

Quinupristin/dalfopristin is active in vitro against *Enterococcus faecium*, including vancomycin-resistant *E. faecium* and multidrug-resistant *E. faecium*. The drug appears to be equally active in vitro against VanA and VanB phenotypes of vancomycin-resistant *E. faecium*. Susceptible *E. faecium*, including vancomycin-resistant strains, are usually inhibited in vitro by quinupristin/dalfopristin concentrations of 2 mcg/mL or less. However, *E. faecalis* generally require high concentrations of quinupristin/dalfopristin for in vitro inhibition and most strains are intrinsically resistant to the drug.

Although the clinical importance is unclear, quinupristin/dalfopristin has in vitro activity against some aerobic gram-negative bacteria, including *Haemophilus influenzae*, *Legionella*, *Moraxella catarrhalis*, and *Neisseria*, and some anaerobic bacteria, including *Clostridium* and *Lactobacillus*. Quinupristin/dalfopristin is inactive against Enterobacteriaceae, *Pseudomonas aeruginosa*, and *Acinetobacter*.

● Resistance

Resistance to quinupristin/dalfopristin has been reported and has emerged during treatment with the drug. Resistance to streptogramins, including quinupristin/dalfopristin, can occur as the result of alterations in the ribosomal target site, enzymatic inactivation, or efflux systems that actively transport the drugs out of the bacterial cell.

Resistance to quinupristin/dalfopristin has been reported only rarely in staphylococci or *S. pyogenes*.

Reduced susceptibility or resistance to quinupristin/dalfopristin has emerged in vancomycin-resistant *E. faecium* during treatment with quinupristin/dalfopristin.

The manufacturer states that cross-resistance between quinupristin/dalfopristin and aminoglycosides, β-lactams, glycopeptides, quinolones, macrolides, lincomycins, and tetracyclines has not been reported.

ADVICE TO PATIENTS

Advise patients that diarrhea is a common problem caused by anti-infectives and usually ends when the drug is discontinued. Importance of contacting a clinician if watery and bloody stools (with or without stomach cramps and fever) occur during or as late as 2 months or longer after the last dose.

Importance of informing clinicians of existing or contemplated concomitant therapy, including prescription and OTC drugs, as well as any concomitant illnesses.

Importance of women informing clinicians if they are or plan to become pregnant or plan to breast-feed.

Importance of informing patients of other important precautionary information. (See Cautions.)

PREPARATIONS

Excipients in commercially available drug preparations may have clinically important effects in some individuals; consult specific product labeling for details.

Quinupristin and Dalfopristin

Parenteral

For injection, for IV infusion	500 mg (150 mg of quinupristin and 350 mg of dalfopristin)	**Synercid®**, Pfizer

† Use is not currently included in the labeling approved by the US Food and Drug Administration.

Selected Revisions June 1, 2016, © Copyright, October 1, 1999, American Society of Health-System Pharmacists, Inc.

Fluconazole

8:14.08 · AZOLES

■ Fluconazole, a synthetic triazole derivative, is an azole antifungal agent.

USES

Fluconazole is used in the treatment of various infections caused by *Candida*, including candidemia and disseminated candidiasis, oropharyngeal candidiasis, esophageal candidiasis, and vulvovaginal candidiasis.

Fluconazole also is used for the treatment of cryptococcal meningitis and for the treatment of blastomycosis†, coccidioidomycosis†, and histoplasmosis†. Fluconazole has been used for the treatment of superficial fungal infections, dermatophytoses†, onychomycosis†, and pityriasis (tinea) versicolor. In addition, the drug is used for prevention of serious fungal infections (e.g., coccidioidomycosis, cryptococcosis, mucocutaneous candidiasis) in patients with human immunodeficiency virus (HIV) infection†, and for prevention of *Candida* infections in other immunocompromised individuals (e.g., cancer patients and bone marrow, hematopoietic stem cell†, and solid organ transplant recipients†).

Prior to initiation of fluconazole therapy, appropriate specimens for fungal culture and other relevant laboratory studies (e.g., serology, histopathology) should be obtained in order to isolate and identify the causative organism(s). Fluconazole therapy may be started pending results of these in vitro tests; however, once results are available, therapy should be adjusted accordingly. If fluconazole in vitro susceptibility tests are performed, results should be interpreted cautiously since in vitro tests may not accurately reflect fluconazole's in vivo activity.

● Candida Infections

Candidemia and Disseminated Candida Infections

Fluconazole is used for the treatment of candidemia, disseminated candidiasis (e.g., chronic disseminated hepatosplenic infections), and other serious *Candida* infections, including urinary tract infections, peritonitis, meningitis, osteoarticular infections (e.g., osteomyelitis, septic arthritis), intravascular infections (e.g., endocarditis, implantable cardiac device infections), pneumonia, endophthalmitis, and neonatal candidiasis† (including CNS infections). The drug has been effective in the treatment of some *Candida* infections that did not respond to IV amphotericin B.

While fluconazole may be better tolerated and easier to administer than IV amphotericin B, fluconazole-resistant strains of *C. albicans* are being isolated with increasing frequency from patients who have received prior fluconazole therapy (especially in HIV-infected patients) and some *Candida* infections (e.g., candidemia) are increasingly caused by strains that are intrinsically resistant to fluconazole (e.g., *C. krusei*) or likely to be resistant or have reduced susceptibility to fluconazole (e.g., *C. glabrata*). The choice of an antifungal for the treatment of candidemia or invasive *Candida* infections should take into consideration any history of recent exposure to azole or echinocandin antifungals or intolerance to antifungals, local and/or institutional epidemiologic data regarding prevalence of the various *Candida* strains and their patterns of resistance, severity of illness, relevant comorbidities, presence and duration of neutropenia or immunosuppression, and evidence of involvement of the CNS, cardiac valves, and/or visceral organs.

For the treatment of candidemia in *nonneutropenic* patients or for empiric treatment of suspected invasive candidiasis† in *nonneutropenic* patients in intensive care units (ICUs), the Infectious Diseases Society of America (IDSA) recommends an IV echinocandin (anidulafungin, caspofungin, micafungin) for *initial* therapy. IDSA states that fluconazole (IV or oral) is an acceptable alternative for *initial* therapy in selected patients, including those who are not critically ill and are unlikely to have infections caused by fluconazole-resistant *Candida*. If echinocandin- and azole-resistant *Candida* are suspected, IV amphotericin B is recommended; IV amphotericin B also is a reasonable alternative when echinocandins and fluconazole cannot be used because of intolerance, limited availability, or resistance. IDSA states that transition from the echinocandin (or amphotericin B) to fluconazole can be considered (usually within 5–7 days) in patients who are clinically stable, have isolates susceptible to fluconazole (e.g., *C. albicans*), and have negative repeat blood cultures after initial antifungal treatment. Although

fluconazole has been considered the drug of choice for the treatment of infections caused by *C. parapsilosis* in nonneutropenic patients (based in part on concerns related to decreased in vitro susceptibility and resistance to echinocandins), IDSA states that there are no clinical studies to date indicating superiority of fluconazole over echinocandins for the treatment of *C. parapsilosis* infections.

For the treatment of candidemia in *neutropenic* patients, IDSA recommends an IV echinocandin (anidulafungin, caspofungin, micafungin) or, alternatively, IV amphotericin B for *initial* therapy. Fluconazole is an alternative for *initial* therapy in those who are not critically ill and have had no prior exposure to azole antifungals and also can be used for step-down therapy during neutropenia in clinically stable patients who have fluconazole-susceptible isolates and documented bloodstream clearance. Voriconazole can be used as an alternative for *initial* therapy when broader antifungal coverage is required and also can be used as step-down therapy during neutropenia in clinically stable patients who have voriconazole-susceptible isolates and documented bloodstream clearance. For infections known to be caused by *C. krusei*, an echinocandin, amphotericin B, or voriconazole is recommended.

For the treatment of disseminated candidiasis in neonates† (neonatal candidiasis), IV amphotericin B usually is the drug of choice. IDSA states that fluconazole is a reasonable alternative in those who have not been receiving fluconazole prophylaxis, and the American Academy of Pediatrics (AAP) states that fluconazole can be considered for step-down treatment after an initial response has been obtained with IV amphotericin B. Fluconazole also has been used for prophylaxis to reduce the incidence of invasive candidiasis in low birthweight neonates at high risk†. (See Uses: Prevention of Candidiasis in Transplant Recipients, Cancer Patients, or Other Patients at High Risk.)

For the treatment of CNS candidiasis, IDSA recommends initial treatment with IV amphotericin B (with or without oral flucytosine) and follow-up (step-down) treatment with fluconazole.

IDSA states that antifungal treatment is not recommended in patients with asymptomatic candiduria, unless there is a high risk of disseminated candidiasis (e.g., neutropenic patients, low birthweight infants [less than 1.5 kg], patients who will undergo urologic manipulations). These experts state that asymptomatic candiduria in neutropenic patients and low birthweight infants should be treated using regimens recommended for patients with candidemia and that patients undergoing urologic procedures who have asymptomatic candiduria should be treated with oral fluconazole or IV amphotericin B for several days before and after the procedures. For the treatment of symptomatic candiduria (e.g., cystitis, pyelonephritis, fungus balls) caused by fluconazole-susceptible *Candida*, fluconazole is the drug of choice. When fluconazole-resistant *Candida* (e.g., *C. glabrata, C. krusei*) are likely, IV amphotericin B or oral flucytosine is recommended for symptomatic cystitis, and IV amphotericin B (with or without oral flucytosine) or oral flucytosine alone is recommended for pyelonephritis and fungus balls.

For the treatment of osteoarticular infections (e.g., osteomyelitis, septic arthritis) caused by *Candida*, IDSA recommends *initial* treatment with fluconazole or an IV echinocandin (anidulafungin, caspofungin, micafungin) and follow-up treatment with fluconazole. If septic arthritis involved a prosthetic device that cannot be removed, long-term suppressive or maintenance therapy (secondary prophylaxis)† with fluconazole is recommended if the isolate is susceptible.

For the treatment of endocarditis (native or prosthetic valve) or implantable cardiac device infections caused by *Candida*, IDSA recommends *initial* treatment with IV amphotericin B (with or without oral flucytosine) or an IV echinocandin (anidulafungin, caspofungin, micafungin) and follow-up treatment with fluconazole. If the isolate is susceptible, long-term suppressive or maintenance therapy (secondary prophylaxis)† with fluconazole is recommended to prevent recurrence in those with native valve endocarditis who cannot undergo valve replacement and in those with prosthetic valve endocarditis.

Fluconazole has been used with good results in some patients with endophthalmitis† caused by *Candida*, but treatment failures have been reported. Studies in rabbits indicate that fluconazole is distributed into the eye and that the drug inhibits growth of *C. albicans* in rabbit choroid-retina tissue and vitreous body when IV therapy is initiated within 24 hours postinoculation; the drug did not effectively inhibit growth of the organism when IV therapy was initiated 7 days postinoculation when the infection was well established. For the treatment of chorioretinitis (with or without vitritis) caused by *Candida*, IDSA recommends fluconazole or voriconazole when isolates are susceptible and amphotericin B (with or without oral flucytosine) when isolates are resistant to fluconazole and voriconazole; intravitreal amphotericin B or voriconazole may also be indicated.

Fluconazole is used prophylactically to reduce the incidence of candidiasis in bone marrow or hematopoietic stem cell transplant recipients† who are receiving chemotherapy or radiation therapy. The drug also has been used for primary prophylaxis of candidiasis in other patients considered at high risk for developing such infections (e.g., high-risk patients undergoing urologic procedures†, solid organ transplant recipients†, high-risk patients in ICUs†). (See Uses: Prevention of Candidiasis in Transplant Recipients, Cancer Patients, or Other Patients at High Risk.)

For additional information on management of candidemia and disseminated candidiasis, the current clinical practice guidelines from IDSA available at http://www.idsociety.org should be consulted.

Oropharyngeal Candidiasis

Oral or IV fluconazole is used for the treatment of oropharyngeal candidiasis in immunocompromised adults with acquired immunodeficiency syndrome (AIDS), advanced AIDS-related complex (ARC), malignancy, or other serious underlying disease.

Fluconazole appears to be at least as effective as and, in some cases, more effective than other antifungals used for initial treatment of oropharyngeal *Candida* infections and is considered a drug of choice for the treatment of moderate to severe disease. Fluconazole has produced clinical resolution of signs and symptoms of the infection in 79–100% of patients with oropharyngeal candidiasis; however, microbiologic cures generally have been obtained in 44–87% of patients and the rate of relapse may be high, especially in neutropenic patients. In a study in HIV-infected adults with oropharyngeal candidiasis, the response rate and mycologic eradication rate after 14 days of therapy were 100 and 75%, respectively, in those who received oral fluconazole (100 mg once daily) and were 65 and 20%, respectively, in those who received topical clotrimazole (10-mg oral lozenge 5 times daily). In another study, 14 days of therapy with oral fluconazole (100 mg once daily as an oral suspension) was more effective than 14 days of therapy with topical nystatin (500,000 units as an oral suspension 4 times daily). The mycologic cure rate was 60% in the fluconazole group and 6% in the nystatin group and the rate of relapse at day 42 was 27 and 11%, respectively.

For the treatment of mild oropharyngeal candidiasis, IDSA recommends topical treatment with clotrimazole lozenges or miconazole buccal tablets; nystatin (oral suspension or tablets) is the recommended alternative. For moderate to severe disease, IDSA recommends oral fluconazole. For fluconazole-refractory oropharyngeal candidiasis, IDSA recommends itraconazole oral solution or posaconazole oral suspension; oral voriconazole or amphotericin B oral suspension (not commercially available in US) are recommended as alternatives. Other alternatives for refractory oropharyngeal candidiasis are IV echinocandins (anidulafungin, caspofungin, micafungin) or IV amphotericin B.

For the treatment of oropharyngeal candidiasis in HIV-infected adults and adolescents, the US Centers for Disease Control and Prevention (CDC), National Institutes of Health (NIH), and IDSA recommend oral fluconazole as the preferred drug of choice for initial episodes. If topical therapy is used for the treatment of oropharyngeal candidiasis (e.g., mild to moderate episodes), these experts recommend clotrimazole lozenges or miconazole buccal tablets. Alternatives for systemic treatment of oropharyngeal candidiasis in HIV-infected adults and adolescents are itraconazole oral solution or posaconazole oral suspension; nystatin oral suspension is an alternative if topical treatment is used. For fluconazole-refractory oropharyngeal infections in HIV-infected adults and adolescents, posaconazole oral suspension is preferred; itraconazole oral solution is an alternative.

Routine long-term suppressive or maintenance therapy (secondary prophylaxis)† to prevent relapse or recurrence is not usually recommended in patients adequately treated for oropharyngeal candidiasis (including HIV-infected individuals), unless the patient has frequent or severe recurrences of oropharyngeal candidiasis. If secondary prophylaxis of oropharyngeal candidiasis is indicated, oral fluconazole is recommended; however, the potential for development of azole resistance should be considered.

For additional information on management of oropharyngeal candidiasis, the current clinical practice guidelines from IDSA available at http://www.idsociety.org and the current clinical practice guidelines from CDC, NIH, and IDSA on prevention and treatment of opportunistic infections in HIV-infected individuals available at http://www.aidsinfo.nih.gov should be consulted.

Esophageal Candidiasis

Oral or IV fluconazole is used for the treatment of esophageal candidiasis in adults with AIDS, malignancy, or other serious underlying disease, including progressive

systemic sclerosis. Fluconazole appears to be at least as effective as and, in some cases, more effective than other antifungals used for initial treatment of esophageal *Candida* infections and is considered a drug of choice.

In adults with esophageal candidiasis documented by endoscopy, fluconazole has produced clinical resolution of signs and symptoms of the infection in about 61–93% of patients. In one study in adults with esophageal candidiasis and progressive systemic sclerosis, fluconazole therapy produced mycologic cures in about 93% of patients within 2–4 weeks, but the relapse rate was almost 100% within 3 months after fluconazole therapy was discontinued.

Esophageal candidiasis requires treatment with a systemic antifungal (not a topical antifungal).

IDSA recommends oral fluconazole as the preferred drug of choice for the treatment of esophageal candidiasis; if oral therapy is not tolerated, IV fluconazole or an IV echinocandin (anidulafungin, caspofungin, micafungin) is recommended; IV amphotericin B is another alternative. For fluconazole-refractory esophageal candidiasis, IDSA recommends itraconazole oral solution or oral or IV voriconazole; alternatives for fluconazole-refractory disease are IV echinocandins (anidulafungin, caspofungin, micafungin) or IV amphotericin B. IDSA states that oral posaconazole (oral suspension or delayed-release tablets) could be considered another alternative for the treatment of fluconazole-refractory esophageal candidiasis.

For the treatment of esophageal candidiasis in HIV-infected adults and adolescents, CDC, NIH, and IDSA recommend oral or IV fluconazole or itraconazole oral solution. Alternatives include oral or IV voriconazole, an IV echinocandin (anidulafungin, caspofungin, micafungin), or IV amphotericin B. For refractory esophageal candidiasis in HIV-infected adults and adolescents, including fluconazole-refractory infections, these experts recommend posaconazole oral suspension or itraconazole oral solution; alternatives include an IV echinocandin (anidulafungin, caspofungin, micafungin), oral or IV voriconazole, or IV amphotericin B.

Routine long-term suppressive or maintenance therapy (secondary prophylaxis)† to prevent relapse or recurrence is not usually recommended in patients adequately treated for esophageal candidiasis (including HIV-infected individuals) unless the patient has frequent or severe recurrences of esophageal candidiasis. If secondary prophylaxis of esophageal candidiasis is indicated, oral fluconazole is recommended and posaconazole oral suspension is a possible alternative; however, the potential for development of azole resistance should be considered.

For additional information on management of esophageal candidiasis, the current clinical practice guidelines from IDSA available at http://www.idsociety.org and the current clinical practice guidelines from CDC, NIH, and IDSA on the prevention and treatment of opportunistic infections in HIV-infected individuals available at http://www.aidsinfo.nih.gov should be consulted.

Vulvovaginal Candidiasis

Oral fluconazole is used for the treatment of uncomplicated vulvovaginal candidiasis and for the treatment of complicated vulvovaginal candidiasis† in *nonpregnant* women.

Vulvovaginal candidiasis frequently occurs during pregnancy. CDC states that topical (intravaginal) azole antifungals (not oral fluconazole) should be used for the treatment of vulvovaginal candidiasis during pregnancy. (See Pregnancy under Cautions: Pregnancy, Fertility, and Lactation.)

Uncomplicated Vulvovaginal Candidiasis

Oral fluconazole is effective for the treatment of uncomplicated vulvovaginal candidiasis when given as a single dose. A single 150-mg oral dose of fluconazole produces clinical cures (i.e., absence of vulvovaginal burning, itching, swelling, erythema, excoriation, dyspareunia, and/or ulceration and substantial decreases in vaginal discharge) 5–16 days after the dose in approximately 90–100% and mycologic cures in approximately 77–100% of *nonpregnant* women with uncomplicated vulvovaginal candidiasis. At 27–62 days after the single dose, clinical and mycologic cure rates are 61–90%, and the rate of relapse, reinfection, or recolonization is about 23%. Results of several studies in patients with uncomplicated vulvovaginal candidiasis suggest that a single 150-mg dose of oral fluconazole is as effective for this condition as multiple dose regimens of intravaginal clotrimazole, econazole, miconazole, or terconazole. In addition, the single-dose oral fluconazole regimen appears to be as effective for uncomplicated vulvovaginal candidiasis as oral itraconazole or oral ketoconazole.

In controlled studies in patients with vulvovaginal candidiasis, clinical and mycologic cure rates at 14 and 30–35 days were similar in patients receiving oral fluconazole (given as a single 150-mg dose) compared with patients receiving intravaginal clotrimazole (given as a 100-mg vaginal tablet once daily for 7 days) or miconazole (given as a 100-mg vaginal cream once daily for 7 days). At 14 days, the clinical cure rate was reported to be about 95–96% with fluconazole and 95–97% with intravaginal clotrimazole or miconazole and the mycologic cure rate was reported to be 77–80% with fluconazole and 72–82% with intravaginal clotrimazole or miconazole. At 30–35 days, the clinical cure rate was reported to be about 69–75% with fluconazole and 72–80% with intravaginal clotrimazole or miconazole and the mycologic cure rate was reported to be 61–63% with fluconazole and 57–63% with intravaginal clotrimazole or miconazole.

CDC, IDSA, and other clinicians recommend that uncomplicated vulvovaginal candidiasis (defined as vulvovaginal candidiasis that is mild to moderate, sporadic or infrequent, most likely caused by C. albicans, and occurring in immunocompetent women) in nonpregnant women should be treated with a topical (intravaginal) azole antifungal (e.g., butoconazole, clotrimazole, miconazole, terconazole, tioconazole) given in appropriate single-dose or short-course (1–3 days) regimens or, alternatively, oral fluconazole given in a single-dose regimen. These regimens generally have been associated with clinical and mycologic cure rates of 80–90% in otherwise healthy, nonpregnant women with uncomplicated infections. Some clinicians suggest that a single oral dose of fluconazole may offer some advantage over conventional intravaginal antifungal therapy since it ensures compliance and may reduce or eliminate concurrent rectal infections that may serve as a source of reinfection. In weighing the potential risks and benefits of oral versus intravaginal therapy, the potential for toxicity (e.g., hepatotoxicity) and drug interactions (see Drug Interactions) associated with oral therapy should be considered. The incidence of adverse effects is higher in patients receiving single oral doses of fluconazole compared with those receiving intravaginal antifungal therapy; and this also should be weighed carefully.

Complicated and Recurrent Vulvovaginal Candidiasis

Oral fluconazole is used for the treatment of complicated vulvovaginal candidiasis†, including recurrent and severe infections. Complicated vulvovaginal candidiasis is defined as infections that are recurrent or severe, caused by Candida other than C. albicans, or occurring in women with underlying disease such as diabetes mellitus, debilitation, or immunocompromising conditions (e.g., HIV infection), or those receiving immunosuppressive therapy (e.g., corticosteroids). CDC recommends that vaginal cultures be obtained from women with complicated vulvovaginal candidiasis to confirm the clinical diagnosis and identify unusual species (e.g., C. glabrata).

Recurrent vulvovaginal candidiasis (usually defined as 4 or more episodes of symptomatic vulvovaginal candidiasis within a year) affects a small percentage of women (less than 5%). Although each individual episode caused by C. albicans may respond to a short course of intravaginal azole antifungal or oral fluconazole, some experts recommend a longer duration of initial therapy (e.g., 7–14 days of an intravaginal azole antifungal or a 3-dose regimen of oral fluconazole [100, 150, or 200 mg given every third day for a total of 3 doses]) to attempt mycologic remission before initiating a maintenance antifungal regimen. For the maintenance regimen, CDC and IDSA recommend oral fluconazole (100, 150, or 200 mg once weekly) for 6 months. If this regimen cannot be used, intermittent use of intravaginal treatments can be considered. These maintenance regimens can be effective in reducing recurrent infections; however, 30–50% of women will have recurrent disease once maintenance therapy is discontinued. Women with recurrent infections who are symptomatic and remain culture-positive despite maintenance antifungal therapy should be managed in consultation with a specialist.

Severe vulvovaginal candidiasis (i.e., extensive vulvar erythema, edema, excoriation, and fissure formation) usually has a lower clinical response rate to short courses of intravaginal or oral antifungal therapy. CDC and IDSA recommend that severe vulvovaginal candidiasis be treated with either 7–14 days of an intravaginal azole antifungal or a 2-dose regimen of oral fluconazole (150 mg repeated 3 days later).

HIV-infected women have higher rates of vaginal Candida colonization, and symptomatic vulvovaginal candidiasis may occur more frequently and be more severe than in women without HIV infection. However, because there is no evidence to date that HIV-infected women have a lower response rate to intravaginal or oral antifungal regimens than other women, CDC, IDSA, and other clinicians recommend that treatment of vulvovaginal candidiasis in HIV-infected women should be the same as that in women without HIV infection. Routine long-term suppressive or maintenance therapy (secondary prophylaxis) to prevent relapse or recurrence of vulvovaginal candidiasis is not usually recommended in HIV-infected or other women unless the patient has recurrent or severe infections. If secondary prophylaxis or maintenance therapy of vulvovaginal candidiasis is indicated, oral fluconazole (150 or 200 mg once weekly or 100 mg 3 times weekly) is recommended.

Recurrent vulvovaginal candidiasis rarely may be caused by resistant strains of C. albicans or, more commonly, by other Candida with reduced susceptibility to azole antifungals (e.g., C. glabrata). It has been suggested that repeated treatment of recurrent vulvovaginal candidiasis with intravaginal azole antifungals and widespread and/or injudicious use of these agents for self-medication of vulvovaginal candidiasis may favor the selection of Candida that are resistant to azole antifungals. Optimum therapy for the treatment of vulvovaginal candidiasis caused by Candida other than C. albicans has not been determined. CDC recommends 7–14 days of therapy with an antifungal (oral or intravaginal) other than fluconazole. If recurrence occurs, alternatives include topical (intravaginal) boric acid (600-mg gelatin capsule once daily for 14 days; no FDA-labeled preparation commercially available in the US). Referral to a specialist is advised.

For additional information on management of vulvovaginal candidiasis, the current CDC guidelines available at http://www.cdc.gov/std, the current clinical practice guidelines from IDSA available at http://www.idsociety.org, and the current clinical practice guidelines from CDC, NIH, and IDSA on the prevention and treatment of opportunistic infections in HIV-infected individuals available at http://www.aidsinfo.nih.gov should be consulted.

• Coccidioidomycosis

Oral fluconazole is used for the treatment and prevention of coccidioidomycosis† caused by Coccidioides immitis or C. posadasii.

Treatment of Coccidioidomycosis

Fluconazole is used for the treatment of coccidioidal pulmonary infections, meningitis, and disseminated (extrapulmonary) infections involving soft tissue or bones and joints.

Antifungal treatment may not be necessary in patients with mild, uncomplicated coccidioidal pneumonia since such infections often are self-limited and may resolve spontaneously. However, antifungal treatment is recommended for patients with more severe or rapidly progressing coccidioidal infections, those with chronic pulmonary or disseminated infections, and immunocompromised or debilitated individuals (e.g., HIV-infected individuals, organ transplant recipients, those receiving immunosuppressive therapy, those with diabetes or cardiopulmonary disease).

IDSA and others state that an oral azole (fluconazole or itraconazole) usually is recommended for initial treatment of symptomatic pulmonary coccidioidomycosis and chronic fibrocavitary or disseminated (extrapulmonary) coccidioidomycosis. However, IV amphotericin B is recommended as an alternative and is preferred for initial treatment of severely ill patients (e.g., those with hypoxia or rapidly progressing disease), for immunocompromised individuals, or when azole antifungals cannot be used (e.g., pregnant women).

For the treatment of clinically mild coccidioidomycosis (e.g., focal pneumonia) in HIV-infected adults and adolescents, CDC, NIH, and IDSA recommend initial therapy with oral fluconazole or oral itraconazole. For the treatment of diffuse pulmonary or extrathoracic disseminated coccidioidomycosis (nonmeningeal) in HIV-infected adults and adolescents, CDC, NIH, and IDSA recommend initial therapy with IV amphotericin B followed by oral azole therapy. Alternatively, some experts recommend initial therapy with IV amphotericin B used in conjunction with an oral azole (e.g., fluconazole or itraconazole) followed by an oral azole alone.

For the treatment of diffuse pulmonary or disseminated coccidioidomycosis (nonmeningeal) in HIV-infected infants and children, CDC, NIH, and IDSA recommend initial treatment with IV amphotericin B followed by oral fluconazole or oral itraconazole. In those with severe disseminated coccidioidomycosis, some experts recommend initial therapy with IV amphotericin B used in conjunction with an oral azole (e.g., fluconazole) followed by an oral azole alone. Use of fluconazole or itraconazole alone may be sufficient for the treatment of coccidioidomycosis in HIV-infected infants and children with only mild disease (e.g., focal pneumonia) and also can be considered an alternative for those with stable pulmonary or disseminated coccidioidomycosis (nonmeningeal).

For the treatment of coccidioidal meningitis in HIV-infected adults, adolescents, and children or other individuals, IV or oral fluconazole (with or without intrathecal amphotericin B) is considered the regimen of choice. Oral itraconazole, oral posaconazole, and oral voriconazole are recommended as alternatives for the treatment of coccidioidal meningitis in adults and adolescents. Patients who do not respond to an azole antifungal alone may be candidates for intrathecal amphotericin B (with or without continued azole therapy) or IV amphotericin B used in conjunction with intrathecal amphotericin B; however, consultation with an expert who has experience in treating coccidioidal meningitis is recommended. Fluconazole has produced clinical and/or laboratory evidence of improvement when used alone or in conjunction with IV amphotericin B in adults with coccidioidal meningitis and has been used for the treatment of coccidioidal meningitis in both HIV-infected and HIV-negative individuals. Because fluconazole generally is well tolerated and exhibits favorable pharmacokinetics (e.g., is distributed into CSF in high concentrations following oral or IV administration), the drug is considered a good option for the treatment of coccidioidal meningitis.

Primary Prophylaxis to Prevent First Episode of Coccidioidomycosis

Oral fluconazole is used in certain HIV-infected adults and adolescents for primary prophylaxis against coccidioidomycosis†.

CDC, NIH, and IDSA recommend that HIV-infected adults and adolescents living in areas in the US where coccidioidomycosis is endemic (e.g., lower San Joaquin Valley in California, much of Arizona, southern regions of Utah, Nevada, and New Mexico, western Texas) be tested annually for the disease using IgM or IgG serologic tests. Those with a newly positive IgM or IgG serologic test and CD4+ T-cell counts less than 250/mm³ should receive oral fluconazole for primary prophylaxis against coccidioidomycosis† (preemptive antifungal therapy) since they are at increased risk of developing active coccidioidomycosis. Routine primary prophylaxis against coccidioidomycosis is not recommended in other HIV-infected adults and adolescents (e.g., those who reside in coccidioidomycosis endemic areas but do not have positive IgM or IgG serologic tests, those who reside in areas where the disease is not endemic) and is not recommended in HIV-infected infants and children.

Prevention of Recurrence (Secondary Prophylaxis) of Coccidioidomycosis

Oral fluconazole is used for long-term suppressive or maintenance therapy (secondary prophylaxis) to prevent recurrence or relapse of coccidioidomycosis†.

Because of the risk of relapse, individuals who were treated for coccidioidal meningitis generally should receive long-term (life-long) secondary prophylaxis with oral fluconazole or oral itraconazole.

CDC, NIH, and IDSA recommend that all HIV-infected adults, adolescents, and children who have been adequately treated for coccidioidomycosis should receive long-term secondary prophylaxis with oral fluconazole or oral itraconazole to prevent recurrence or relapse. Because HIV-infected adults and adolescents who had focal coccidioidal pneumonia and responded clinically to antifungal treatment may be at low risk for recurrence if their CD4+ T-cell count increases to greater than 250/mm³ in response to antiretroviral therapy, it may be reasonable to consider discontinuing secondary prophylaxis against coccidioidomycosis after 12 months, provided such individuals are monitored for recurrence (e.g., serial chest radiographs, coccidioidal serology). However, secondary prophylaxis should be continued indefinitely in HIV-infected adults and adolescents who were treated for more extensive coccidioidomycosis and in all HIV-infected children, regardless of the immune response to antiretroviral therapy. Consultation with an expert is recommended when making decisions regarding discontinuance of secondary prophylaxis against coccidioidomycosis.

For additional information on management of coccidioidomycosis, the current clinical practice guidelines from IDSA available at http://www.idsociety.org and the current clinical practice guidelines from CDC, NIH, and IDSA on the prevention and treatment of opportunistic infections in HIV-infected individuals available at http://www.aidsinfo.nih.gov should be consulted.

● Cryptococcosis

Treatment of Cryptococcosis

Oral or IV fluconazole is used in immunocompetent or immunocompromised adults for the treatment of meningitis caused by *Cryptococcus neoformans*.

Fluconazole is considered an alternative for initial (induction) therapy of cryptococcal infections involving the CNS, but is the drug of choice for follow-up (consolidation) therapy of these infections. Fluconazole also is used for the treatment of pulmonary cryptococcosis†, cryptococcemia†, and disseminated cryptococcal infections†.

For the treatment of cryptococcal meningitis in HIV-infected adults, adolescents, and children, CDC, NIH, IDSA, and other clinicians state that the preferred regimen is initial (induction) therapy with IV amphotericin B (conventional or lipid formulation) given in conjunction with oral flucytosine for at least 2 weeks until there is evidence of clinical improvement and negative CSF culture after repeat lumbar puncture, then follow-up (consolidation) therapy with oral fluconazole administered for at least 8 weeks.

If an alternative regimen is necessary for the treatment of cryptococcal meningitis in HIV-infected adults, adolescents, and children who cannot receive the preferred regimen, some experts recommend initial (induction) and follow-up (consolidation) therapy with IV amphotericin B (conventional or lipid formulation) alone; induction therapy with IV amphotericin B (conventional or lipid formulation) given in conjunction with oral fluconazole, then consolidation therapy with oral fluconazole; induction therapy with oral or IV fluconazole used in conjunction with oral flucytosine, then consolidation therapy with oral fluconazole; or induction and consolidation therapy with oral fluconazole given alone. These alternative regimens may be less effective and are recommended only in patients who cannot tolerate or have not responded to the preferred regimen.

For the treatment of cryptococcal CNS infections in organ transplant recipients, IDSA recommends initial (induction) therapy with IV amphotericin B liposomal or amphotericin B lipid complex given in conjunction with oral flucytosine for at least 2 weeks, then follow-up (consolidation) therapy with oral fluconazole given for 8 weeks. If the induction regimen does not include flucytosine, it should be continued for at least 4–6 weeks. For organ transplant recipients with mild to moderate pulmonary cryptococcosis (without diffuse pulmonary infiltrates) or other mild to moderate cryptococcal infections not involving the CNS, IDSA recommends fluconazole given for 6–12 months.

In adults and children who do not have HIV infection and are not transplant recipients, IDSA states that the preferred regimen for the treatment of cryptococcal meningitis is initial (induction) therapy with IV amphotericin B (conventional formulation) given in conjunction with oral flucytosine for at least 4 weeks (a 2-week period of induction therapy can be considered in those who are immunocompetent, are without uncontrolled underlying disease, and are at low risk for therapeutic failure), then follow-up (consolidation) therapy with oral fluconazole administered for an additional 8 weeks or longer. IDSA states that data are insufficient to date to recommend fluconazole used alone or in conjunction with flucytosine for induction therapy in non-HIV-infected individuals with cryptococcal meningitis.

For the treatment of mild to moderate pulmonary cryptococcosis† (nonmeningeal) in immunocompetent or immunosuppressed adults or children, IDSA states that the regimen of choice is oral fluconazole given for 6–12 months. A regimen of oral fluconazole given for 6–12 months also can be considered for the treatment of nonmeningeal, nonpulmonary cryptococcosis† in immunocompetent individuals if the infection occurs at a single site and fungemia is not present.

Severe pulmonary cryptococcosis†, cryptococcemia†, and disseminated cryptococcal infections† in immunocompetent or immunosuppressed individuals should be treated using regimens recommended for cryptococcal meningitis.

Clinical Experience

The relative efficacy of initial therapy with conventional IV amphotericin B (0.7 mg/kg daily) given with oral flucytosine (100 mg/kg daily) or placebo for 2 weeks followed by oral fluconazole (800 mg daily for 2 days, then 400 mg daily for 8 weeks) or oral itraconazole (600 mg daily for 3 days, then 400 mg daily for 8 weeks) has been evaluated in a double-blind multicenter trial in patients with AIDS-associated cryptococcal meningitis. At 2 weeks, CSF cultures were negative in 60% of those who received amphotericin B with flucytosine compared with 51% of those who received amphotericin B alone. The clinical response to oral fluconazole or oral itraconazole for follow-up therapy was similar, but the rate of CSF sterilization at 10 weeks was higher in those who received fluconazole (72%) compared with those who received itraconazole (60%).

Fluconazole has been effective in the treatment of acute cryptococcal meningitis in some patients who failed to respond to amphotericin B therapy. However, there is some evidence that fluconazole may be less effective than amphotericin B during early therapy of acute cryptococcal meningitis in patients with AIDS and may produce slower sterilization of CSF. In a randomized, multicenter study comparing IV amphotericin B (mean dosage of 0.4–0.5 mg/kg daily for 10 weeks with or without concomitant oral flucytosine) with oral fluconazole (400 mg in the first day and 200–400 mg thereafter for 10 weeks) in AIDS patients with cryptococcal meningitis, therapy was effective in 40% of patients receiving amphotericin B and in 34% of those receiving fluconazole. Although overall mortality between patients receiving amphotericin B and patients receiving fluconazole was similar (14% in patients receiving amphotericin B versus 18% in patients receiving fluconazole), mortality was higher during the first 2 weeks of therapy in patients receiving fluconazole (15% versus 8% in those receiving amphotericin B). CSF cultures were positive for an average of about 42 or 64 days in patients receiving amphotericin B or fluconazole, respectively. In another study comparing amphotericin B (0.7 mg/kg daily for 1 week, followed by this dose 3 times weekly for 9 weeks combined with flucytosine 150 mg/kg daily) with oral fluconazole (400 mg daily for 10 weeks) in a limited number of AIDS patients with cryptococcal meningitis, initial therapy was effective in all patients receiving amphotericin B but in only 43% of patients receiving fluconazole; CSF cultures were positive for an average of about 16 and 41 days in patients receiving these respective therapies. While patient groups in this study were similar with respect to severity of cryptococcal infection, the helper/inducer (CD4+, T4+) T-cell count was lower in the fluconazole group, confounding interpretation.

Primary Prophylaxis to Prevent First Episode of Cryptococcosis

Although there is some evidence that primary prophylaxis with fluconazole or itraconazole can reduce the frequency of cryptococcal disease in HIV-infected adults who have CD4+ T-cell counts less than 100/mm³, primary prophylaxis against cryptococcal disease in HIV-infected adults, adolescents, and children is not recommended in the US because of the relative infrequency of cryptococcal disease, lack of survival benefits associated with such prophylaxis, possibility of drug interactions, potential antifungal resistance, and cost.

Some experts recommend routine testing for cryptococcal antigen (CrAg) in all newly diagnosed HIV-infected individuals if they have CD4+ T-cell counts of 100/mm³ or lower.

Prevention of Recurrence (Secondary Prophylaxis) of Cryptococcosis

Oral fluconazole is used for long-term suppressive or maintenance therapy (secondary prophylaxis) to prevent recurrence or relapse of cryptococcosis†.

CDC, NIH, and IDSA recommend that all HIV-infected adults, adolescents, and children who have been adequately treated for cryptococcus should receive secondary prophylaxis to prevent recurrence. Oral fluconazole is the drug of choice for secondary prophylaxis of cryptococcosis in HIV-infected adults, adolescents, and children; some experts suggest that oral itraconazole is an alternative in those who cannot tolerate fluconazole, but the drug may be less effective than fluconazole in preventing relapse of cryptococcosis. Conventional IV amphotericin B can be used for secondary prophylaxis if necessary in individuals who cannot receive azole antifungals, but is less effective and not generally recommended.

There is some evidence that the risk for recurrence of cryptococcosis is low in HIV-infected individuals who have been treated successfully with antifungal therapy, remain asymptomatic with regard to signs and symptoms of cryptococcosis, and have a sustained increase in CD4+ T-cell counts in response to antiretroviral therapy. CDC, NIH, and IDSA state that consideration can be given to discontinuing secondary prophylaxis against cryptococcosis in HIV-infected adults, adolescents, and children 6 years of age or older who are asymptomatic for cryptococcosis and have received secondary antifungal prophylaxis (maintenance therapy) for at least 1 year, are receiving antiretroviral therapy, have had undetectable or low plasma HIV RNA levels for at least 3 months, and have CD4+ T-cell counts of 100/mm³ or greater. If secondary prophylaxis against cryptococcosis is discontinued, the patient should be followed closely and serial cryptococcal serum antigen tests performed. These experts state that secondary prophylaxis against cryptococcosis should be reinitiated if the CD4+ T-cell count decreases to less than 100/mm³ and/or the serum cryptococcal antigen titer increases.

Maintenance therapy (secondary prophylaxis) with oral fluconazole also is recommended in non-HIV-infected adults and children who have been adequately treated for cryptococcal meningitis, including organ transplant recipients who have been adequately treated for CNS cryptococcosis.

For additional information on management of cryptococcosis, the current clinical practice guidelines from IDSA available at http://www.idsociety.org and the current clinical practice guidelines from CDC, NIH, and IDSA on the prevention and treatment of opportunistic infections in HIV-infected individuals available at http://www.aidsinfo.nih.gov should be consulted.

Cryptococcus gattii Infections

Although data are limited, CDC, NIH, and IDSA state that recommendations for the treatment of CNS, pulmonary, or disseminated infections caused by *Cryptococcus gattii* and recommendations for maintenance therapy (secondary prophylaxis) of *C. gattii* infections are the same as the recommendations for *C. neoformans* infections. IDSA states that single, small cryptococcoma may be treated with oral fluconazole; however, induction therapy with a regimen of IV amphotericin B (conventional formulation) and oral flucytosine given for 4–6 weeks, followed by consolidation therapy with fluconazole given for 6–18 months should be considered for very large or multiple cryptococcomas caused by *C. gattii*. Regimens that include IV amphotericin B (conventional or liposomal formulations), oral flucytosine, and fluconazole have been effective in a few patients with CNS infections known to be caused by *C. gattii*.

There is some in vitro evidence that fluconazole may be less active against *C. gattii* than some other azole antifungals (e.g., itraconazole, posaconazole, voriconazole). (See Spectrum.)

● *Blastomycosis*

Oral fluconazole has been used in the treatment of blastomycosis† caused by *Blastomyces dermatitidis*. Oral itraconazole and IV amphotericin B are the drugs of choice for the treatment of blastomycosis. Although oral fluconazole is considered an alternative for the treatment of blastomycosis, it may be less effective and should be used only when the drugs of choice are contraindicated or cannot be used.

IV amphotericin B generally is the drug of choice for initial treatment of severe blastomycosis, especially infections involving the CNS, and for initial treatment of presumptive blastomycosis in immunocompromised patients, including HIV-infected individuals. Oral itraconazole is the preferred azole antifungal for the treatment of mild to moderate pulmonary blastomycosis or mild to moderate disseminated blastomycosis (without CNS involvement) and also is the preferred azole antifungal for follow-up therapy in patients with more severe infections after an initial response has been obtained with IV amphotericin B.

For the treatment of CNS blastomycosis, IDSA recommends initial treatment with IV amphotericin B, followed by an oral azole antifungal. Although oral fluconazole, oral itraconazole, or oral voriconazole can be used for follow-up treatment of CNS blastomycosis, the most appropriate azole for such treatment is unclear. Azole antifungals should not be relied on for initial treatment of CNS blastomycosis. The fact that treatment failures have been reported when an oral antifungal (e.g., ketoconazole) was used in the treatment of cutaneous or pulmonary blastomycosis in patients who had asymptomatic or subclinical CNS involvement at the time of the initial diagnosis should be considered when selecting an antifungal for patients with blastomycosis.

For additional information on management of blastomycosis, the current clinical practice guidelines from IDSA available at http://www.idsociety.org should be consulted.

● *Histoplasmosis*

Although oral fluconazole has been used with some success for the treatment of histoplasmosis† caused by *Histoplasma capsulatum*, it may be less effective than itraconazole and fluconazole-resistant *H. capsulatum* have developed in some HIV-infected patients who failed to respond to the drug.

The drugs of choice for the treatment of histoplasmosis, including histoplasmosis in HIV-infected individuals, are IV amphotericin B or oral itraconazole. IV amphotericin B is preferred for initial treatment of severe, life-threatening histoplasmosis, especially in immunocompromised patients such as those with HIV infection. Oral itraconazole generally is used for initial treatment of less severe disease (e.g., mild to moderate acute pulmonary histoplasmosis, chronic cavitary pulmonary histoplasmosis) and as follow-up therapy in the treatment of severe infections after a response has been obtained with IV amphotericin B. Other azole antifungals (fluconazole, ketoconazole, posaconazole, voriconazole) are considered second-line alternatives to itraconazole, but can be considered in patients who have less severe disease and cannot tolerate itraconazole.

In HIV-infected adults and adolescents, oral itraconazole is the drug of choice when primary prophylaxis is indicated to prevent initial episodes of histoplasmosis and also is the drug of choice for long-term suppressive or maintenance therapy (secondary prophylaxis) to prevent recurrence or relapse of histoplasmosis in HIV-infected adults, adolescents, and children. Although fluconazole may be less effective, some experts state that it can be considered an alternative for secondary prophylaxis against histoplasmosis in HIV-infected adults, adolescents, and children when itraconazole cannot be used.

For additional information on management of histoplasmosis, the current clinical practice guidelines from IDSA available at http://www.idsociety.org and the current clinical practice guidelines from CDC, NIH, and IDSA on the prevention and treatment of opportunistic infections in HIV-infected individuals available at http://www.aidsinfo.nih.gov should be consulted.

● *Sporotrichosis*

Fluconazole has been used as an alternative agent for the treatment of lymphocutaneous and cutaneous sporotrichosis† caused by *Sporothrix schenckii*.

IV amphotericin B usually is the drug of choice for initial treatment of severe, life-threatening sporotrichosis and whenever sporotrichosis is disseminated or has CNS involvement. Oral itraconazole is the drug of choice for the treatment of cutaneous, lymphocutaneous, or mild pulmonary or osteoarticular sporotrichosis and for follow-up treatment of severe infections after a response has been obtained with IV amphotericin B.

Although fluconazole can be used as an alternative for the treatment of cutaneous and lymphocutaneous sporotrichosis, it may be less effective than itraconazole and should be used only if the patient cannot tolerate itraconazole or other alternatives (oral terbinafine, oral potassium iodide, local hyperthermia).

Fluconazole should *not* be used for the treatment of pulmonary, osteoarticular, or meningeal sporotrichosis.

For additional information on management of sporotrichosis, the current clinical practice guidelines from IDSA available at http://www.idsociety.org should be consulted.

● *Dermatophytoses*

Oral fluconazole has been used in the treatment of certain dermatophytoses† (e.g., tinea capitis, tinea corporis, tinea cruris, tinea pedis) caused by *Epidermophyton*, *Microsporum*, or *Trichophyton*.

Oral fluconazole (3–6 mg/kg daily for 2–6 weeks) has been effective for the treatment of tinea capitis† in children 1.5–16 years of age, and has resulted in a clinical and mycologic cure in about 88–90% of patients. For the treatment of tinea corporis†, tinea cruris†, or tinea pedis† in adults, oral fluconazole has been effective when given in a once-weekly regimen (150 mg once weekly for 2–6 weeks), and there is evidence that this once-weekly regimen is as effective as a once-daily regimen of the drug (50 mg once daily) for the treatment of these infections. Results of a randomized study indicate that the eradication rate at the end of treatment in patients with tinea corporis or tinea cruris is 82–88% in those receiving the once-weekly regimen or 94–100% in those receiving the once-daily regimen; at 1-month follow-up, the overall eradication rates were 91–100 or 91–94%, respectively.

Tinea corporis and tinea cruris generally can be effectively treated using a topical antifungal; however, an oral antifungal regimen may be necessary if the disease is extensive, dermatophyte folliculitis is present, the infection is chronic or does not respond to topical therapy, or the patient is immunocompromised or has coexisting disease. Tinea capitis and tinea barbae generally are treated using an oral antifungal regimen. While topical antifungals usually are effective for the treatment of uncomplicated tinea manuum and tinea pedis, an oral antifungal usually is necessary for treatment of severe, chronic, or recalcitrant tinea pedis and for treatment of chronic moccasin-type (dry-type) tinea pedis.

● *Onychomycosis*

Oral fluconazole has been used for the treatment of onychomycosis†.

Selection of the most appropriate regimen for treatment of onychomycosis depends on the severity and extent of nail involvement, organisms involved, reported cure rates, adverse effects, drug interactions, cost, and patient and clinician preference. Onychomycosis generally is treated using an oral antifungal (e.g., terbinafine, itraconazole, fluconazole) and adjunctive physical modalities (nail trimming, aggressive debridement, nail avulsion) with or without a topical antifungal. Oral fluconazole has been recommended as an alternative in patients

those who cannot tolerate terbinafine or itraconazole, but may be less effective than the other oral antifungals.

● *Pityriasis (Tinea) Versicolor*

Oral fluconazole has been used in the treatment of pityriasis (tinea) versicolor† caused by *Malassezia furfur* (*Pityrosporum orbiculare* or *P. ovale*).

Pityriasis (tinea) versicolor generally can be treated topically with an azole antifungal (e.g., clotrimazole, econazole, ketoconazole, miconazole, oxiconazole, sulconazole), an allylamine antifungal (e.g., naftifine, terbinafine), ciclopirox olamine, or certain other topical therapies (e.g., selenium sulfide 2.5%). An oral antifungal (e.g., fluconazole, itraconazole, ketoconazole) may be indicated, with or without a topical agent, in patients who have extensive or severe infections or who fail to respond to or have frequent relapses with topical therapy.

● *Prevention of Candidiasis in Transplant Recipients, Cancer Patients, or Other Patients at High Risk*

Fluconazole is used prophylactically to reduce the incidence of candidiasis in patients at high risk, including those undergoing bone marrow transplantation (BMT), hematopoietic stem cell transplantation† (HSCT), or solid organ transplantation† and neutropenic patients undergoing chemotherapy or radiation therapy†. Fluconazole also is used to prevent *Candida* infections in high-risk patients undergoing urologic procedures† and for prevention of invasive candidiasis in high-risk patients in ICUs† and in low birthweight neonates† at high risk.

There is some evidence that fluconazole prophylaxis in transplant and cancer patients can reduce the frequency of oropharyngeal and/or systemic candidiasis during the period prior to neutrophil recovery. In addition, fluconazole prophylaxis may reduce the need for empiric antifungal therapy in such patients. Efficacy of oral fluconazole (400 mg once daily) for prophylaxis against fungal infections in neutropenic patients has been evaluated in a randomized, placebo-controlled study involving 274 cancer patients 18–80 years of age receiving cytotoxic chemotherapy or conditioning therapy for BMT. While the percentage of patients not requiring empiric therapy with IV amphotericin B therapy was similar in both groups (57% of those receiving fluconazole and 50% of those receiving placebo required no such therapy), complete success without fungal colonization was achieved in 37% of those receiving fluconazole and 20% of those receiving placebo. In addition, there was a lower incidence of superficial fungal infections in those receiving fluconazole (7%) than in those receiving placebo (18%), and only 3% of those receiving fluconazole developed definite invasive fungal infections compared with 17% of those receiving placebo. While fluconazole prophylaxis did not affect the overall mortality rate, intent-to-treat analysis indicates that the number of deaths attributable to definite invasive fungal infection was lower in the fluconazole group (1 of 15) than in the placebo group (6 of 15).

Use of primary antifungal prophylaxis in cancer patients undergoing myelosuppressive therapy or patients undergoing BMT or solid organ transplantation has been controversial, particularly since such prophylaxis may predispose the patient to colonization with resistant fungi and/or result in the emergence of highly resistant organisms. Some retrospective studies have shown an increased risk of colonization with *C. krusei* in BMT recipients and in neutropenic patients who received fluconazole prophylaxis; in one study, about 41% of patients receiving fluconazole had colonization with *C. krusei* compared with 17% of those not receiving fluconazole.

IDSA and other experts recommend primary prophylaxis against *Candida* infections in neutropenic patients when the risk of invasive candida infection is substantial (e.g., allogeneic HSCT recipients, patients with acute leukemia undergoing intensive remission-induction or salvage-induction chemotherapy) and states that an azole antifungal (fluconazole, itraconazole, posaconazole, voriconazole) or IV echinocandin (caspofungin or micafungin) can be used. These experts state that antifungal prophylaxis is not recommended if the anticipated duration of neutropenia is less than 7 days. If primary prophylaxis is used to prevent invasive candidiasis in high-risk adults in ICUs, IDSA recommends fluconazole as the drug of choice and IV echinocandins (anidulafungin, caspofungin, micafungin) as alternatives.

Fluconazole has been used for prophylaxis to reduce the incidence of invasive candidiasis in low birthweight neonates† at high risk. Although such prophylaxis has been controversial since there is concern that it may be associated with emergence of resistant fungi or increased colonization with fluconazole-resistant *Candida*, there is some evidence from retrospective and randomized controlled trials that fluconazole prophylaxis in low birthweight neonates can prevent colonization and reduce the incidence of invasive candidiasis. IDSA and AAP state that use of fluconazole prophylaxis can be considered for very low birthweight neonates (less than 1 kg) in nurseries that have high rates of neonatal invasive candidiasis.

For additional information on prevention of fungal infections in neutropenic patients, the current clinical practice guidelines from IDSA available at http://www.idsociety.org should be consulted.

DOSAGE AND ADMINISTRATION

● Administration

Fluconazole is administered orally or by IV infusion.

Since absorption of fluconazole from the GI tract is rapid and almost complete, IV therapy with the drug generally is reserved for patients who do not tolerate or are unable to take the drug orally.

Oral Administration

Fluconazole may be given orally without regard to meals.

Fluconazole powder for oral suspension should be reconstituted at the time of dispensing by adding 24 mL of distilled or purified water to the container labeled as containing 0.35 or 1.4 g of the drug to provide a suspension containing 50 or 200 mg/5 mL, respectively. The bottle should be shaken vigorously to suspend the powder; in addition, the suspension should be shaken well just prior to administration.

IV Administration

IV infusions of fluconazole should be administered once daily at a rate not exceeding 200 mg/hour. Fluconazole injections for IV infusion should be inspected visually for discoloration and particulate matter prior to administration whenever solution and container permit. The injection for IV infusion should be discarded if the solution is cloudy or precipitated or if the seal is not intact.

Viaflex® Plus containers of fluconazole should be checked for minute leaks by firmly squeezing the bag. The injection should be discarded if the container seal is not intact or leaks are found or if the solution is cloudy or contains a precipitate. Additives should not be introduced into the plastic injection container. The injection in plastic containers should not be used in series connections with other plastic containers, since such use could result in air embolism from residual air being drawn from the primary container before administration from the secondary container is complete.

● Dosage

Oral and IV dosage of fluconazole are identical.

Use of a fluconazole loading dose that is twice the daily dosage generally is recommended on the first day of treatment since this results in fluconazole plasma concentrations on the second day of treatment that are close to steady-state concentrations.

Dosage of the drug should be based on the type and severity of the infection, identity of the causative organism, and the patient's renal function and response to therapy. Fluconazole therapy should be continued until clinical parameters and/or laboratory tests indicate that active fungal infection has subsided; an inadequate period of treatment may lead to recurrence of active infection.

Adult Dosage
Candidemia and Disseminated Candida Infections

For the treatment of systemic candidiasis (candidemia, disseminated candidiasis, pneumonia), the manufacturer states that adults have received fluconazole in a dosage of 400 mg daily.

For the treatment of urinary tract infections or peritonitis, the manufacturer states that fluconazole has been given in a dosage of 50–200 mg daily.

For the treatment of candidemia in nonneutropenic or neutropenic adults, the Infectious Diseases Society of America (IDSA) recommends a loading dose of 800 mg (12 mg/kg) of fluconazole on the first day of therapy, followed by 400 mg (6 mg/kg) daily with treatment continued for 2 weeks after documented clearance of Candida from the bloodstream, resolution of candidemia symptoms, and resolution of neutropenia.

For the treatment of chronic disseminated candidiasis (hepatosplenic) in adults who are clinically stable, IDSA recommends that fluconazole be given in a dosage of 400 mg (6 mg/kg) daily. These experts recommend that severely ill patients receive IV amphotericin B initially for several weeks, then follow-up therapy with fluconazole in a dosage of 400 mg (6 mg/kg) daily. Antifungal treatment should be continued until lesions resolve (usually several months) and should be continued through periods of immunosuppression.

For the treatment of CNS candidiasis, IDSA recommends an initial regimen of IV amphotericin B (with or without oral flucytosine) for several weeks, then follow-up therapy with fluconazole in a dosage of 400–800 mg (6–12 mg/kg) daily. Antifungal treatment should be continued until signs and symptoms, CSF abnormalities, and radiologic abnormalities have resolved.

When fluconazole is used for the treatment of urinary tract infections caused by fluconazole-susceptible Candida, IDSA recommends that adults receive fluconazole in a dosage of 200 mg (3 mg/kg) daily for 2 weeks for the treatment of symptomatic cystitis or 200–400 mg (3–6 mg/kg) daily for 2 weeks for the treatment of pyelonephritis.

For the treatment of osteoarticular infections caused by Candida, IDSA recommends that adults receive fluconazole in a dosage of 400 mg (6 mg/kg) daily given for 6–12 months in those with osteomyelitis or for 6 weeks in those with septic arthritis. If septic arthritis involved a prosthetic device that cannot be removed, long-term suppressive or maintenance therapy (secondary prophylaxis)† with fluconazole given in a dosage of 400 mg (6 mg/kg) daily is recommended to prevent recurrence.

For the treatment of endocarditis (native or prosthetic valve) or implantable cardiac device infections caused by Candida, IDSA recommends an initial regimen of IV amphotericin B (with or without oral flucytosine) or an IV echinocandin (anidulafungin, caspofungin, micafungin), then follow-up treatment with fluconazole in a dosage of 400–800 mg (6–12 mg/kg) daily. Antifungal treatment should be continued for at least 6 weeks after valve replacement surgery. Long-term suppressive or maintenance therapy (secondary prophylaxis)† with fluconazole given in dosage of 400–800 mg (6–12 mg/kg) daily is recommended to prevent recurrence in those with native valve endocarditis who cannot undergo valve replacement and in those with prosthetic valve endocarditis.

For the treatment of chorioretinitis (with or without vitritis) caused by Candida, IDSA recommends a loading dose of 800 mg (12 mg/kg) of fluconazole on the first day of therapy, followed by 400–800 mg (6–12 mg/kg) daily for at least 4–6 weeks. If there is macular involvement, intravitreal amphotericin B or voriconazole may also be indicated.

Oropharyngeal Candidiasis

For the treatment of oropharyngeal candidiasis, the manufacturer recommends that fluconazole be given in a dosage of 200 mg as a single dose on day 1, then 100 mg once daily. Although clinical evidence of oropharyngeal candidiasis generally resolves within several days following initiation of fluconazole therapy, the manufacturer recommends that the drug be continued for at least 2 weeks to decrease the likelihood of relapse.

For the treatment of moderate to severe oropharyngeal candidiasis, IDSA recommends that adults receive fluconazole in a dosage of 100–200 mg daily for 7–14 days.

For the treatment of oropharyngeal candidiasis in adults and adolescents with human immunodeficiency virus (HIV) infection, the US Centers for Disease Control and Prevention (CDC), National Institutes of Health (NIH), and IDSA recommend that fluconazole be given in a dosage of 100 mg daily for 7–14 days.

If long-term suppressive or maintenance therapy (secondary prophylaxis)† with fluconazole is used in HIV-infected adults and adolescents with frequent or severe recurrences of oropharyngeal candidiasis, a dosage of 100 mg once daily or 3 times weekly is recommended. Although only limited data are available regarding the safety of discontinuing secondary prophylaxis against oropharyngeal candidiasis in HIV-infected individuals, consideration can be given to discontinuing such prophylaxis in HIV-infected adults if the CD4+ T-cell count increases to greater than 200/mm³ in response to antiretroviral therapy.

Esophageal Candidiasis

For the treatment of esophageal candidiasis, the manufacturer recommends that adults receive fluconazole in a dosage of 200 mg as a single dose on day 1, followed by 100 mg once daily. Dosages up to 400 mg once daily may be used depending on the patient's response. The manufacturer recommends that fluconazole therapy be continued for a minimum of 3 weeks and for at least 2 weeks after symptoms have resolved.

For the treatment of esophageal candidiasis, IDSA recommends that adults receive fluconazole in a dosage of 200–400 mg (3–6 mg/kg) daily for 14–21 days.

For the treatment of esophageal candidiasis in HIV-infected adults and adolescents, CDC, NIH, and IDSA recommend that adults receive fluconazole in a dosage of 100 mg (up to 400 mg) once daily for 14–21 days.

If long-term suppressive or maintenance therapy (secondary prophylaxis)† with fluconazole is used in HIV-infected adults and adolescents with frequent or severe recurrences of esophageal candidiasis, a dosage of 100–200 mg daily or, alternatively, 100–200 mg 3 times weekly is recommended. Although only limited data are available regarding the safety of discontinuing secondary prophylaxis against esophageal candidiasis in HIV-infected individuals, consideration can be given to discontinuing such prophylaxis in these HIV-infected adults if the CD4+ T-cell count increases to greater than 200/mm³ in response to antiretroviral therapy.

Vulvovaginal Candidiasis

For the treatment of uncomplicated vulvovaginal candidiasis in *nonpregnant* women, the usual dosage of oral fluconazole is a single (1 day only) 150-mg oral dose.

For the treatment of recurrent vulvovaginal candidiasis† in *nonpregnant* women, CDC recommends that 100, 150, or 200 mg of oral fluconazole be given every third day for 3 doses (i.e., days 1, 4, and 7) to attempt mycologic remission. Then, to prevent recurrence, a maintenance regimen of 100, 150, or 200 mg of oral fluconazole should be given once weekly for 6 months. IDSA recommends a maintenance regimen of 150 mg of oral fluconazole given once weekly for 6 months.

For the treatment of severe vulvovaginal candidiasis† in *nonpregnant* women, CDC recommends a 2-dose regimen of oral fluconazole (two 150-mg doses given 72 hours [3 days] apart). IDSA recommends that 150 mg of oral fluconazole be given once every 72 hours for a total of 2 or 3 doses.

For the treatment of uncomplicated vulvovaginal candidiasis or recurrent or severe vulvovaginal candidiasis† in *nonpregnant* HIV-infected women, CDC, NIH, and IDSA recommend the same regimens used for the treatment of these infections in women without HIV infection.

Blastomycosis

If oral fluconazole is used as an alternative for the treatment of mild to moderate pulmonary or mild to moderate disseminated blastomycosis† without CNS involvement in adults, IDSA recommends a dosage of 400–800 mg daily.

If oral fluconazole is used for follow-up therapy in the treatment of CNS blastomycosis† in adults after an initial regimen of IV amphotericin B given for 4–6 weeks, IDSA recommends that fluconazole be given in a dosage of 800 mg daily for at least 12 months and until CSF abnormalities have resolved.

Coccidioidomycosis

For the treatment of coccidioidomycosis†, IDSA and others recommend that adults receive oral or IV fluconazole in a dosage of 400–800 mg once daily. For diffuse pneumonia or disseminated coccidioidomycosis (nonmeningeal), fluconazole usually is used in conjunction with IV amphotericin B or as follow-up after an initial regimen of IV amphotericin B. The duration of treatment for uncomplicated coccidioidal pneumonia usually is 3–6 months; the total duration of treatment for diffuse pneumonia and chronic progressive fibrocavitary pneumonia usually is at least 1 year.

For the treatment of mild coccidioidomycosis (e.g., focal pneumonia) in HIV-infected adults and adolescents, CDC, NIH, and IDSA recommend that oral fluconazole be given in a dosage of 400 mg once daily. This dosage also is recommended for the treatment of severe, nonmeningeal coccidioidomycosis (e.g., diffuse pulmonary infection) in HIV-infected adults and adolescents, but the drug usually is used in conjunction with IV amphotericin B or as follow-up after an initial regimen of IV amphotericin B.

For the treatment of coccidioidal meningitis† in HIV-infected adults and adolescents or other individuals, a fluconazole dosage of 400–800 mg once daily has been recommended. Concomitant intracisternal, intraventricular, or intrathecal amphotericin B therapy has been used in some patients. Consultation with an expert who has experience in treating coccidioidal meningitis is recommended.

When primary prophylaxis against coccidioidomycosis† is indicated in HIV-infected adults and adolescents who live in areas endemic for coccidioidomycosis, have a newly positive IgM or IgG serologic test suggesting imminent active disease, and have CD4+ T-cell counts less than 250/mm³, CDC, NIH, and IDSA recommend that fluconazole be given in a dosage of 400 mg once daily.

For long-term suppressive or maintenance therapy (secondary prophylaxis) to prevent recurrence or relapse of coccidioidomycosis† in HIV-infected adults and adolescents who have been adequately treated for the disease, CDC, NIH, and IDSA recommend that fluconazole be given in a dosage of 400 mg once daily. In HIV-infected adults and adolescents with a history of adequately treated focal coccidioidal pneumonia, discontinuance of secondary prophylaxis against coccidioidomycosis can be considered after 12 months if they are receiving antiretroviral therapy and have CD4+ T-cell counts of 250/mm³ or greater. Such patients should be monitored for recurrence (e.g., serial chest radiographs, coccidioidal serology). In HIV-infected adults and adolescents with a history of adequately treated diffuse pulmonary or disseminated coccidioidomycosis (including meningeal infections), secondary prophylaxis against coccidioidomycosis should be continued lifelong, regardless of antiretroviral therapy or immune reconstitution.

Cryptococcosis

For the treatment of cryptococcal meningitis, the manufacturer recommends that adults receive fluconazole in a dosage of 400 mg as a single dose on day 1, followed by 200–400 mg once daily for 10–12 weeks after the CSF is sterile. Some evidence suggests that the 400-mg dosage is more effective than lower dosage in the treatment of this infection.

For the treatment of cryptococcal meningitis in HIV-infected adults and adolescents, CDC, NIH, and IDSA recommend a regimen than includes initial (induction) therapy with IV amphotericin B and oral flucytosine given for at least 2 weeks, then follow-up (consolidation) therapy with oral fluconazole given in a dosage of 400 mg (6 mg/kg) once daily and continued for at least 8 weeks.

For the treatment of cryptococcal meningitis in HIV-infected adults who cannot receive flucytosine, IDSA recommends induction therapy with IV amphotericin B given in conjunction with oral or IV fluconazole 800 mg daily for at least 2 weeks, then consolidation therapy with oral fluconazole given in a dosage of 800 mg daily and continued for at least 8 weeks. For the treatment of cryptococcal meningitis in HIV-infected adults who cannot receive IV amphotericin B or oral flucytosine, IDSA states that fluconazole can be given as monotherapy in a dosage of 800 mg daily or higher (preferably 1.2 g daily or higher) and continued for 10–12 weeks. Although fluconazole dosage as high as 2 g daily has been used, this dosage may be associated with toxicity. If high fluconazole dosage is used, the daily dosage should be given in divided doses to minimize GI toxicity.

For the treatment of cryptococcal meningitis in HIV-infected adults and adolescents who cannot receive amphotericin B, CDC, NIH, and IDSA recommend induction therapy with oral or IV fluconazole given in a dosage of 400 or 800 mg daily in conjunction with oral flucytosine for at least 2 weeks, then consolidation therapy with oral fluconazole given in a dosage of 400 mg daily and continued for at least 8 weeks. Alternatively, if oral or IV fluconazole is used alone for induction therapy, these experts recommend that the drug be given in a dosage of 1.2 g daily for at least 2 weeks, then consolidation therapy with oral fluconazole be given in a dosage of 400 mg daily and continued for at least 8 weeks.

For the treatment of CNS cryptococcosis in adult organ transplant recipients, IDSA recommends induction therapy with IV amphotericin B liposomal or IV amphotericin B lipid complex and oral flucytosine given for at least 2 weeks, then consolidation therapy with oral fluconazole 400–800 mg (6–12 mg/kg) daily given for 8 weeks. For the treatment of mild to moderate pulmonary cryptococcosis (without pulmonary infiltrates) or other mild to moderate non-CNS disease, IDSA recommends fluconazole in a dosage of 400 mg (6 mg/kg) daily for 6–12 months.

For the treatment of cryptococcal meningitis in immunocompetent adults *without* HIV infection who are not transplant recipients, IDSA recommends induction therapy with IV amphotericin B in conjunction with oral flucytosine given for at least 4 weeks, then consolidation therapy with oral fluconazole given in a dosage of 400 mg daily and continued for 8 weeks. If the patient is immunocompetent without uncontrolled, underlying disease and is at low risk for therapeutic failure, IDSA states that this induction regimen can be given for only 2 weeks, then consolidation therapy with oral fluconazole administered in a dosage of 800 mg (12 mg/kg) daily should be given for 8 weeks.

For the treatment of mild to moderate pulmonary cryptococcosis† (nonmeningeal) in immunocompetent or immunocompromised adults, IDSA recommends that fluconazole be given in a dosage of 400 mg (6 mg/kg) daily for 6–12 months. This same dosage can be used for the treatment of nonpulmonary cryptococcosis at a single site† (nonmeningeal).

Severe pulmonary cryptococcosis†, cryptococcemia†, or disseminated cryptococcosis† in immunocompetent or immunocompromised adults should be treated using a regimen recommended for adults with cryptococcal meningitis.

For long-term suppressive or maintenance therapy (secondary prophylaxis) to prevent recurrence or relapse of cryptococcosis† in adult organ transplant recipients or immunocompetent adults *without* HIV infection who are not transplant recipients who have been adequately treated for CNS cryptococcosis, the usual dosage of oral fluconazole is 200–400 mg once daily for 6–12 months.

For long-term suppressive or maintenance therapy (secondary prophylaxis) to prevent recurrence or relapse of cryptococcosis† in HIV-infected adults and adolescents or other adults and adolescents who have had documented, adequately treated cryptococcal meningitis, the usual dosage of oral fluconazole is 200 mg once daily. Secondary prophylaxis should be initiated after the primary infection has been adequately treated and usually is continued for at least 1 year. Consideration can be given to discontinuing secondary prophylaxis against cryptococcosis in HIV-infected adults who are asymptomatic for cryptococcosis and have received secondary antifungal prophylaxis for at least 1 year, are receiving antiretroviral therapy, have had undetectable or low plasma HIV RNA levels for at least 3 months, and have CD4+ T-cell counts of 100/mm³ or greater. Secondary prophylaxis against cryptococcosis should be reinitiated if the CD4+ T-cell count decreases to less than 100/mm³ and/or the serum cryptococcal antigen titer increases.

Histoplasmosis

If fluconazole is used for the treatment of histoplasmosis†, a dosage of 400–800 mg once daily is recommended. A fluconazole regimen of 800 mg daily given for 12 weeks, then 400 mg daily has been used.

If fluconazole is used as an alternative for treatment of less severe histoplasmosis† in HIV-infected adults and adolescents, CDC, NIH, and IDSA recommend a dosage of 800 mg daily.

If fluconazole is used as an alternative for long-term suppressive or maintenance therapy (secondary prophylaxis) to prevent recurrence or relapse of histoplasmosis† in HIV-infected adults and adolescents, CDC, NIH, and IDSA recommend a dosage of 400 mg daily. Consideration can be given to discontinuing secondary prophylaxis against histoplasmosis in HIV-infected adults and adolescents who have received secondary antifungal prophylaxis for at least 1 year, have negative fungal blood cultures and serum histoplasma antigen levels less than 2 ng/mL, have been receiving antiretroviral therapy for at least 6 months, and have CD4+ T-cell counts of 150/mm³ or greater. Secondary prophylaxis against histoplasmosis should be reinitiated if the CD4+ T-cell count decreases to less than 150/mm³.

Sporotrichosis

If oral fluconazole is used for the treatment of lymphocutaneous and cutaneous sporotrichosis†, a dosage of 400–800 mg once daily is recommended in adults when other drugs cannot be used.

Dermatophytoses

For the treatment of dermatophytoses†, oral fluconazole has been given in a dosage of 150 mg once weekly for 2–6 weeks. For the treatment of tinea corporis that involves small, well-defined lesions, some clinicians recommend that oral fluconazole be given in a dosage of 250 mg once weekly for 2–4 weeks.

For the treatment of tinea pedis†, some clinicians recommend that oral fluconazole be given in a dosage of 150–200 mg once weekly for 1–8 weeks.

Onychomycosis

For the treatment of onychomycosis†, oral fluconazole has been given in a dosage of 100–450 mg once weekly for 2–12 months. Some clinicians recommend that oral fluconazole be given in a dosage of 150–300 mg once weekly for 3–6 months for fingernail infections or for 6–12 months for toenail infections.

Pityriasis (Tinea) Versicolor

For the treatment of pityriasis (tinea) versicolor†, adults have received oral fluconazole as a single 400-mg dose. Alternatively, 150 mg has been given once weekly for 2 or 4 weeks or 300 mg has been given once weekly for 2 weeks.

Prevention of Candidiasis in Transplant Recipients, Cancer Patients, or Other Patients at High Risk

For the prevention of candidiasis in bone marrow transplant (BMT) recipients, the recommended dosage of fluconazole is 400 mg once daily. In patients in whom severe granulocytopenia (neutrophil count less than 500/ mm³) is anticipated, fluconazole therapy should be initiated several days before expected onset of neutropenia and should be continued for 7 days after the neutrophil count exceeds 1000/ mm³. Antifungal prophylaxis is not usually recommended if the anticipated duration of neutropenia is less than 7 days.

For the prevention of *Candida* infections in hematopoietic stem cell transplant (HSCT) recipients†, adults and adolescents should receive oral or IV fluconazole in a dosage of 400 mg once daily. Fluconazole prophylaxis should be initiated on the day of transplantation (i.e., day 0) and continued until engraftment occurs (i.e., approximately 30 days after HSCT) or until 7 days after the neutrophil count exceeds 1000/mm³.

If fluconazole is used for prophylaxis against candidiasis in high-risk patients in intensive care units (ICUs)† with a known high incidence of invasive candidiasis, IDSA states that the drug should be given in a dosage of 400 mg (6 mg/kg) once daily.

Pediatric Dosage

The usual oral or IV dosage of fluconazole in pediatric patients ranges from 3–12 mg/kg once daily; dosages exceeding 600 mg daily are not recommended. The manufacturer states that a dosage of 3, 6, or 12 mg/kg daily in pediatric patients is equivalent to a dosage of 100, 200, or 400 mg daily, respectively, in adults. Some older children may have clearances similar to those of adults.

Based on limited pharmacokinetic data, the manufacturer recommends that premature neonates (gestational age 26–29 weeks) receive the usual pediatric dosage once every 72 hours during the first 2 weeks of life and then the usual pediatric dosage once daily thereafter.

Candidemia and Disseminated Candida Infections

The usual dosage of fluconazole for the treatment of systemic *Candida* infections in pediatric patients is 6–12 mg/kg daily.

For the treatment of meningitis or septicemia caused by susceptible *Candida*, neonates and infants 3 months of age or younger† have received fluconazole in a dosage of 5–6 mg/kg once daily given orally or by IV infusion over 1 hour. In some neonates and infants with septicemia, an initial loading dose of 10 mg/kg was administered followed by 5 mg/kg once daily.

If fluconazole is used as an alternative for the treatment of neonatal candidiasis†, IDSA and the American Academy of Pediatrics (AAP) recommend a dosage of 12 mg/kg daily for at least 3 weeks.

Oropharyngeal Candidiasis

For the treatment of oropharyngeal candidiasis in pediatric patients, the recommended dosage of fluconazole is 6 mg/kg on day 1, followed by 3 mg/kg once daily. The manufacturer recommends that treatment be continued for a minimum of 2 weeks to decrease the likelihood of relapse.

For the treatment of oropharyngeal candidiasis in HIV-infected infants and children, CDC, NIH, and IDSA recommend that fluconazole be given in a dosage of 6–12 mg/kg (up to 400 mg) once daily for 7–14 days.

If long-term suppressive or maintenance therapy (secondary prophylaxis)† with fluconazole is used in HIV-infected infants and children with frequent or severe recurrences of oropharyngeal candidiasis, a dosage of 3–6 mg/kg (up to 200 mg) once daily is recommended. Limited data are available regarding the safety of discontinuing secondary prophylaxis against oropharyngeal candidiasis in HIV-infected individuals. In HIV-infected infants and children, consideration can be given to discontinuing such prophylaxis when the CD4+ T-cell count or percentage increases to CDC immunologic category 2 or 1.

Esophageal Candidiasis

For the treatment of esophageal candidiasis in pediatric patients, the manufacturer recommends 6 mg/kg of fluconazole on day 1, followed by 3 mg/kg once daily. Dosage may be increased up to 12 mg/kg daily if necessary, based on the condition of the patient and the response to the drug. The manufacturer recommends that treatment be continued for a minimum of 3 weeks and for at least 2 weeks after symptoms have resolved.

For the treatment of esophageal candidiasis in HIV-infected children, CDC, NIH, and IDSA recommend that fluconazole be given in a dosage of 6–12 mg/kg (up to 600 mg) once daily for a minimum of 3 weeks and for at least 2 weeks after symptoms resolve.

If long-term suppressive or maintenance therapy (secondary prophylaxis)† with fluconazole is used in HIV-infected infants and children with frequent or severe recurrences of esophageal candidiasis, a dosage of 3–6 mg/kg (up to 200 mg) once daily is recommended. Limited data are available regarding the safety of discontinuing secondary prophylaxis against esophageal candidiasis in HIV-infected individuals. In HIV-infected infants and children, consideration can be given to discontinuing such prophylaxis when the CD4+ T-cell count or percentage increases to CDC immunologic category 2 or 1.

Coccidioidomycosis

For the treatment of mild to moderate coccidioidomycosis (nonmeningeal)† (e.g., focal pneumonia) in HIV-infected infants and children, CDC, NIH, and IDSA recommend that oral or IV fluconazole be given in a dosage of 6–12 mg/kg (up to 400 mg) once daily. If oral or IV fluconazole is used for the treatment of diffuse pulmonary or disseminated coccidioidomycosis (nonmeningeal)† in HIV-infected infants and children who cannot receive IV amphotericin B, these experts recommend a dosage of 12 mg/kg (up to 800 mg) once daily.

For the treatment of coccidioidal meningitis† in HIV-infected infants and children, CDC, NIH, and IDSA recommend that oral or IV fluconazole be given in a dosage of 12 mg/kg (up to 800 mg) once daily. Consultation with an expert in treating coccidioidal meningitis is recommended.

For prevention of recurrence (secondary prophylaxis) of coccidioidomycosis† in HIV-infected infants and children, CDC, NIH, and IDSA recommend that fluconazole be given in a dosage of 6 mg/kg (up to 400 mg) once daily. Secondary prophylaxis should be initiated after the primary infection has been adequately treated and continued indefinitely in HIV-infected infants and children, regardless of antiretroviral therapy or immune reconstitution.

Cryptococcosis

The manufacturer recommends that cryptococcal meningitis in pediatric patients be treated with an initial 12-mg/kg dose on day 1, followed by 6 mg/kg once daily for 10–12 weeks after the CSF becomes culture negative. Dosage may be increased to 12 mg/kg daily if necessary based on the condition of the patient and the response to the drug.

For the treatment of cryptococcal meningitis in HIV-infected infants and children, CDC, NIH, and IDSA recommend a regimen that includes induction therapy with IV amphotericin B given in conjunction with oral flucytosine for at least 2 weeks, then consolidation therapy with oral or IV fluconazole given in a dosage of 12 mg/kg on day 1 and then 10–12 mg/kg (up to 800 mg) once daily for at least 8 weeks.

For the treatment of cryptococcal meningitis in HIV-infected infants and children who cannot receive IV amphotericin B, CDC, NIH, and IDSA recommend induction therapy with oral or IV fluconazole given in a dosage of 12 mg/kg on day 1 and then 10–12 mg/kg (up to 800 mg) once daily given in conjunction with oral flucytosine (25 mg/kg 4 times daily) for at least 2 weeks, then consolidation therapy with oral or IV fluconazole given in a dosage of 10–12 mg/kg (up to 800 mg) once daily for at least 8 weeks.

For the treatment of localized cryptococcosis without CNS involvement† (e.g., isolated pulmonary disease), CDC, NIH, and IDSA recommend that HIV-infected infants and children receive fluconazole in a dosage of 12 mg/kg on day 1 and then 6–12 mg/kg (up to 600 mg) once daily. The duration of treatment depends on the clinical response and site and severity of infection. A duration of 6–12 months has been recommended.

For the treatment of disseminated or severe pulmonary cryptococcosis without CNS involvement† in HIV-infected infants and children who cannot receive amphotericin B, CDC, NIH, and IDSA recommend that fluconazole be given in a dosage of 12 mg/kg on day 1 and then 6–12 mg/kg (up to 600 mg) once daily. The duration of treatment depends on the clinical response and site and severity of infection. A duration of 6–12 months has been recommended.

For long-term suppressive or maintenance therapy (secondary prophylaxis) to prevent recurrence or relapse of cryptococcosis† in HIV-infected infants and children who have been treated for cryptococcal meningitis, fluconazole is given in a dosage of 6 mg/kg (up to 200 mg) once daily. Secondary prophylaxis should be initiated after the primary infection has been adequately treated and usually is continued for at least 1 year. Consideration can be given to discontinuing secondary prophylaxis against cryptococcosis in HIV-infected children 6 years of age or older who are asymptomatic for cryptococcosis, have received secondary prophylaxis for at least 1 year, are receiving antiretroviral therapy, have had undetectable or low plasma HIV RNA levels for at least 3 months, and have CD4+ T-cell counts of 100/mm³ or higher. Secondary prophylaxis against cryptococcosis should be reinitiated if the CD4+ T-cell count decreases to less than 100/mm³.

Histoplasmosis

If oral fluconazole is used as an alternative for treatment of less severe histoplasmosis† in HIV-infected infants and children, CDC, NIH, and IDSA recommend a dosage of 3–6 mg/kg (up to 200 mg) once daily for acute primary pulmonary histoplasmosis.

If oral fluconazole is used as an alternative for long-term suppressive or maintenance therapy (secondary prophylaxis) to prevent recurrence or relapse of histoplasmosis† in HIV-infected infants and children, CDC, NIH, and IDSA recommend a dosage of 3–6 mg/kg (up to 200 mg) once daily. Consideration can be given to discontinuing secondary prophylaxis against histoplasmosis in HIV-infected infants and children who have received secondary prophylaxis for at least 1 year, have negative fungal blood cultures and serum histoplasma antigen levels less than 2 ng/mL, have been receiving antiretroviral therapy for at least 6 months, and have CD4+ T-cell percentage greater than 15% (CD4+ T-cell counts exceeding 150/mm³ in those 6 years of age or older). Secondary prophylaxis against histoplasmosis should be reinitiated if these parameters are not met.

Dermatophytoses

For the treatment of tinea capitis† in children 1.5–16 years of age, oral fluconazole has been given in a dosage of 3–6 mg/kg daily for 2–6 weeks. AAP recommends a dosage of 6 mg/kg daily for 3–6 weeks.

For the treatment of tinea corporis† or tinea cruris† in children, some clinicians recommend that oral fluconazole be given in a dosage of 150 mg once weekly for 2–6 weeks.

For the treatment of tinea manuum† or tinea pedis† in children, some clinicians recommend that oral fluconazole be given in a dosage of 150 mg once weekly for 4–6 weeks.

Onychomycosis

For the treatment of onychomycosis† in children, some clinicians recommend that oral fluconazole be given in a dosage of 3–6 mg/kg once weekly for 12–16 weeks for fingernail infections or 3–6 mg/kg once weekly for 18–26 weeks for toenail infections. Others recommend 150 mg once weekly for 4–6 months for fingernail infections or 150 mg once weekly for 9–12 months for toenail infections.

Pityriasis (Tinea) Versicolor

For the treatment of pityriasis (tinea) versicolor†, children 11 years of age or older have received oral fluconazole as a single 400-mg dose. Alternatively, 150 mg has been given once weekly for 4 weeks.

Prevention of Candida Infections in Hematopoietic Stem Cell Transplant Recipients

For the prevention of *Candida* infections in HSCT recipients†, children 6 months to 13 years of age should receive oral or IV fluconazole in a dosage of 3–6 mg/kg daily (maximum 600 mg daily). Fluconazole prophylaxis should be initiated on the day of transplantation (i.e., day 0) and continued until engraftment occurs (i.e., approximately 30 days after HSCT) or until 7 days after the neutrophil count exceeds 1000/mm³.

Prevention of Candida Infections in Low Birthweight Neonates

For prophylaxis to reduce the incidence of invasive candidiasis in low birthweight neonates† at high risk, oral or IV fluconazole has been given in a variety of dosage regimens. If fluconazole prophylaxis is used in neonates at high risk, antifungal resistance, toxicity, and neurodevelopmental outcomes should be monitored.

IDSA states that fluconazole given in a dosage of 3 or 6 mg/kg twice weekly reduces the rate of invasive candidiasis in premature neonates in nurseries that have a high incidence of *Candida* infections.

For prophylaxis in low birthweight neonates (less than 1 kg) at high risk, AAP recommends that fluconazole be initiated with a dose of 3 mg/kg given IV during the first 48–72 hours after birth, followed by 3 mg/kg IV twice weekly for 4–6 weeks or until IV access is no longer required for care.

● Dosage in Renal Impairment

In patients with impaired renal function receiving multiple doses, fluconazole dosage must be modified in response to the degree of impairment and should be based on the patient's measured or estimated creatinine clearance. The patient's creatinine clearance (Cl$_{cr}$) can be estimated by using the following formula:

$$Ccr \; male = \frac{(140 \; - \; age) \times weight}{72 \times serum \; creatinine}$$

$$Ccr \; female = 0.85 \times Ccr \; male$$

where age is in years, weight is in kg, and serum creatinine is in mg/dL.

The manufacturer recommends that adults with impaired renal function receive an initial loading dose of 50–400 mg of fluconazole (based on the type of infection being treated), then patients with creatinine clearances exceeding 50 mL/minute should receive 100% of the usual daily dose and those with creatinine clearances of 50 mL/minute or less should receive 50% of the usual daily dose. Patients who are undergoing regular dialysis should receive 100% of the usual daily dose after each dialysis period; on days the patient is not receiving dialysis, reduced dosage based on creatinine clearance should be used. These dosage recommendations are based on the pharmacokinetics of the drug following multiple doses; further dosage adjustments may be necessary depending on the condition of the patient.

The manufacturer states that modification of the recommended single-dose regimen of oral fluconazole for the treatment of vulvovaginal candidiasis is not necessary in patients with impaired renal function.

The manufacturer states that the pharmacokinetics of fluconazole have not been studied in children with impaired renal function; recommendations for dosage reduction in such children should parallel those recommended for adults.

CAUTIONS

Although fluconazole generally is well tolerated, there have been rare reports of serious hepatotoxicity (including some fatalities) in patients receiving the drug. Adverse effects have been reported in about 5–30% of patients receiving fluconazole for 7 days or longer and have been severe enough to require discontinuance of the drug in about 1–2.8% of patients. In addition, adverse effects have been reported in 26–31% of women receiving a single 150-mg oral dose of fluconazole for the treatment of vulvovaginal candidiasis.

Evaluation of some adverse effects and establishment of a causal relationship to fluconazole have been difficult since the drug has been used in many patients with serious underlying diseases, including leukemia, cancer, and acquired immunodeficiency syndrome (AIDS), who were receiving multiple drugs concomitantly. In some cases, the underlying fungal infection being treated (e.g., meningitis) may have caused or contributed to the reported effect (e.g., nervous system effects). In some patients, particularly those with serious underlying diseases such as AIDS and cancer, changes in renal and hematologic function and hepatic abnormalities have been observed during treatment with fluconazole or comparative agents, but the clinical importance and relation to treatment is uncertain. The manufacturer states that adverse effects have been reported more frequently in patients with human immunodeficiency virus (HIV) infection than in patients without HIV infection; however, the proportion of patients requiring discontinuance of fluconazole because of severe adverse effects is similar in both groups.

● GI Effects

Mild to moderate nausea, vomiting, abdominal pain, and diarrhea have been reported in about 1.5–8.5% of patients receiving fluconazole. Only rarely were such adverse GI effects severe enough to require discontinuance of the drug. Flatus, bloating, dry mouth, hiccups, heartburn, and anorexia have been reported rarely. Adverse GI effects have been reported in about 15% of women receiving a single dose of fluconazole for the treatment of vulvovaginal candidiasis; abdominal pain, nausea, diarrhea, dyspepsia, and dysgeusia occurred in about 6, 7, 3, 1, and 1% of such women, respectively.

● Dermatologic and Sensitivity Reactions

Rash, including diffuse rash accompanied by eosinophilia, and pruritus have been reported in up to about 5% of patients receiving fluconazole. Exfoliative skin disorders have been reported rarely in patients with serious underlying disease (principally AIDS or malignancy) receiving fluconazole; fatalities have been reported. Stevens-Johnson syndrome, which can be fatal, also has been reported in patients receiving fluconazole. However, a definite causal relationship between exfoliative skin eruptions and the drug has not been established, since most patients were receiving multiple drugs concomitantly with fluconazole. Acute generalized exanthematous pustulosis and increased sweating also have been reported during postmarketing experience.

Anaphylaxis has been reported rarely in patients receiving fluconazole. Angioedema and anaphylactic reactions have been reported rarely in women who received a single 150-mg oral dose of fluconazole for the treatment of vulvovaginal candidiasis.

● Hepatic Effects

Serious hepatic reactions (e.g., necrosis, clinical hepatitis, cholestasis, fulminant hepatic failure) have been reported rarely in patients receiving fluconazole therapy. The manufacturer states that a clear relationship between these hepatic effects and daily dosage, duration of therapy, gender, or age has not been demonstrated. While hepatotoxicity usually has been reversible, fatalities have been reported. Fatalities principally have occurred in patients with serious underlying disease (e.g., AIDS, malignancy) who were receiving fluconazole concomitantly with other drugs; however, at least one fatality involved an immunocompetent geriatric individual with renal impairment who developed fulminant hepatic necrosis within 10 days after fluconazole therapy was initiated.

Mild, transient increases (1.5–3 times the upper limit of normal) in serum concentrations of AST (SGOT), ALT (SGPT), alkaline phosphatase, γ-glutamyltransferase (GGT, γ-glutamyl transpeptidase, GGTP), and bilirubin have been reported in about 5–7% of patients receiving fluconazole. In most reported cases, concentrations returned to pretreatment levels either during or after fluconazole therapy and were not associated with hepatotoxicity. However, higher increases in serum transaminase concentrations (8 or more times the upper limit of normal), which required discontinuance of the drug, have been reported in about 1% of patients receiving fluconazole. Any patient who develops abnormal liver function test results while receiving fluconazole should be closely monitored for the development of more severe hepatic injury. (See Cautions: Precautions and Contraindications.)

● Cardiovascular Effects

Prolonged QT interval has occurred in patients receiving azole antifungals. Prolonged QT interval and torsades de pointes have been reported rarely during postmarketing surveillance in patients receiving fluconazole. Most reported cases involved seriously ill patients with multiple confounding risk factors (e.g., structural heart disease, electrolyte abnormalities, concomitant drugs) that may have contributed to these events.

● Nervous System Effects

Dizziness and headache have been reported in up to about 2% of patients receiving fluconazole. Somnolence, insomnia, delirium/coma, dysesthesia, psychiatric disturbances, malaise, asthenia, paresthesia of hands and feet, tremor, and fatigue have been reported rarely. Seizures also have been reported and have occurred in at least one AIDS patient immediately following administration of a single 100-mg oral dose of the drug. Adverse nervous system effects have been reported in about 14–20% of women receiving a single dose of fluconazole for the treatment of vulvovaginal candidiasis; headache and dizziness occurred in about 13 and 1% of such women, respectively.

● Hematologic Effects

Eosinophilia has been reported in some patients receiving fluconazole. Anemia, leukopenia, neutropenia, and thrombocytopenia also have been reported. In at least one AIDS patient, thrombocytopenia occurred during fluconazole therapy and resolved following discontinuance of the drug. Severe thrombocytopenia that required treatment and necessitated discontinuance of fluconazole therapy also has been reported.

● Endocrine Effects

Studies using usual dosages of fluconazole have not shown evidence of adverse effects related to possible inhibition of testosterone or steroid synthesis. In one study in healthy premenopausal women receiving fluconazole, there was no effect on serum estradiol concentrations or on serum cortisol stimulation response. Results of studies in men receiving oral fluconazole dosages of 25–400 mg once daily for up to 30 days indicate that serum testosterone concentrations are unaffected by the drug. The manufacturer states that in healthy adults who receive fluconazole dosages of 200–400 mg once daily for up to 14 days, there are only small and inconsistent effects on testosterone concentrations, endogenous corticosteroid concentrations, or ACTH-stimulated cortisol response.

● Other Adverse Effects

Fever, edema, pleural effusion, oliguria, hypotension, arthralgia/myalgia, and finger stiffness have been reported rarely in patients receiving fluconazole.

Hypokalemia, which required potassium replacement therapy and/or discontinuance of fluconazole, has occurred occasionally, including in several neutropenic patients with acute myeloid leukemia. Increased serum creatinine and BUN concentrations also have been reported. Mild (1.5–2 times the upper limit of normal) increases in serum concentrations of creatine kinase (CK, creatine phosphokinase, CPK) have been reported in at least one patient with coccidioidal meningitis who received fluconazole concomitantly with intrathecal amphotericin B.

Alopecia has been reported in patients receiving fluconazole. In a retrospective study of patients who received fluconazole (100–800 mg daily) for the treatment of systemic fungal infections, alopecia was reported in up to 20% of patients. Alopecia occurred in both men and women, usually was evident at about 3 months (range: 2 weeks to 7 months) after initiation of fluconazole therapy, and resolved in most patients within about 6 months after discontinuance of the drug or dosage reduction. Alopecia involved varying degrees of loss of scalp hair in all patients, but about 30% of patients also reported substantial loss of facial, axillary, pubic, leg, or chest hair.

● Precautions and Contraindications

Fluconazole is contraindicated in patients with known hypersensitivity to the drug or any ingredient in the formulation. Although information concerning cross-sensitivity between fluconazole and other triazole or imidazole antifungals is not available, the manufacturer states that fluconazole should be used with caution in individuals hypersensitive to other azoles.

Fluconazole should be used with caution in patients with hepatic impairment. Although serious adverse hepatic effects have been reported only rarely with fluconazole, the possibility that these effects may occur during fluconazole therapy should be considered. (See Cautions: Hepatic Effects.) Fluconazole should be discontinued if signs and symptoms consistent with liver disease develop. If abnormal liver function test results occur during fluconazole therapy, the patient should be monitored for the development of more severe hepatic injury.

Fluconazole should be used with caution in patients with renal impairment. (See Dosage and Administration: Dosage in Renal Impairment.)

Patients receiving fluconazole who drive or operative machinery should be cautioned to take into account that dizziness or seizures may occur occasionally.

Diflucan® powder for oral suspension contains sucrose and should not be used in patients with hereditary fructose, glucose-galactose malabsorption, and sucrase-isomaltase deficiency.

Use of fluconazole may result in overgrowth of nonsusceptible strains of Candida other than C. albicans, including C. krusei. Superinfection caused by nonsusceptible strains of Candida has been reported in some patients receiving fluconazole; these patients may require alternative antifungal therapy.

Because prolonged QT interval and torsades de pointes have occurred in patients receiving fluconazole, the drug should be used with caution in patients with potentially proarrhythmic conditions and risk factors for QT prolongation. (See Cautions: Cardiovascular Effects.) Concomitant use of fluconazole and drugs that are metabolized by the cytochrome P450 (CYP) isoenzyme 3A4 and are known to prolong the QT interval (e.g., astemizole [no longer commercially available in the US], cisapride, pimozide, quinidine) is contraindicated. (See Drug Interactions: Drugs that Prolong the QT Interval.)

Because potentially fatal exfoliative skin disorders have been reported rarely in patients with a serious underlying disease receiving fluconazole, the possibility that these effects can occur should be considered. (See Cautions: Dermatologic and Sensitivity Reactions.) If a patient with deep-seated fungal infection develops rash during fluconazole therapy, the patient should be monitored closely and the drug discontinued if the lesions progress. If rash that may be attributable to fluconazole develops in a patient with superficial fungal infections, the drug should be discontinued.

● Pediatric Precautions

The manufacturer states that efficacy of fluconazole in children younger than 6 months has not been established; however, the drug has been used safely and effectively in neonates and children younger than 6 months of age (including neonates as young as 1 day of age).

Adverse effects reported in children receiving fluconazole generally have been similar to those reported in adults. In phase II/III trials in pediatric patients 1 day to 17 years of age who received fluconazole in dosages up to 15 mg/kg daily, adverse effects occurred in 13% and were severe enough to require discontinuance of the drug in 2.3% of patients. GI effect, including vomiting, abdominal pain, nausea, and diarrhea, occurred in 2–5% of these pediatric patients. Adverse effects reported when oral or IV fluconazole has been used in neonates and infants (3–6 mg/kg daily) have included transient increases in serum transaminase concentrations, vomiting, and eosinophilia; severe thrombophlebitis was reported in at least one neonate.

● Geriatric Precautions

Rash, vomiting, and diarrhea have been reported more frequently in geriatric adults than in younger adults. Although anemia and acute renal failure occurred more frequently in patients 65 years of age and older than in those 12–65 years of age during postmarketing surveillance, the relationship of these events to fluconazole is unknown.

Clinical studies of fluconazole did not include a sufficient number of patients 65 years of age or older to determine whether geriatric patients respond differently for each indication than younger individuals. Other reported clinical experience has not identified differences in response between geriatric and younger patients.

Fluconazole is primarily excreted by the kidneys as unchanged drug. Because geriatric patients may have decreased renal function, careful dosage selection and monitoring of renal function are advised.

● Mutagenicity and Carcinogenicity

There was no evidence of mutagenicity when fluconazole was tested with or without metabolic inactivation in 4 strains of Salmonella typhimurium or in the mouse lymphoma L5178Y system. In addition, there was no evidence of chromosomal mutations in vivo on murine bone marrow cells following administration of fluconazole or in vitro on human lymphocytes exposed to fluconazole concentrations of 1 mg/mL.

There was no evidence of carcinogenicity in studies in mice and rats receiving oral fluconazole dosages of 2.5–10 mg/kg daily (approximately 2–7 times the usual human dosage) for 24 months. However, there was an increased incidence of hepatocellular adenomas in male rats receiving an oral fluconazole dosage of 5 or 10 mg/kg daily.

● Pregnancy, Fertility, and Lactation
Pregnancy

FDA alerted clinicians in April 2016 that it is reviewing safety data regarding use of oral fluconazole during pregnancy and advised cautious prescribing of the drug until the review is completed.

There are no adequate and controlled studies to date using fluconazole in pregnant women.

Congenital abnormalities have been reported in infants born to women who received high-dose fluconazole (400–800 mg daily) for the treatment of serious, life-threatening fungal infections during most or all of the first trimester. These reports have involved a rare and distinct pattern of birth defects that includes brachycephaly, abnormal facies, abnormal calvarial development, cleft palate, femoral bowing, thin ribs and long bones, arthrogryposis, and congenital heart disease and are similar to those reported in animal reproduction studies. Based on these data, FDA reclassified high-dose fluconazole (400–800 mg daily) as pregnancy category D (i.e., there is positive evidence of human fetal risk based on human data, but potential benefits of the drug in pregnant women with serious or life-threatening conditions may be acceptable despite its risks).

Because human data available at that time did not identify an increased risk of congenital anomalies with the use of fluconazole administered as a single 150-mg oral dose for the treatment of vulvovaginal candidiasis, the single-dose oral fluconazole regimen was classified by FDA as pregnancy category C (see Users Guide). Data from a recent Danish study designed to assess the association between use of oral fluconazole during pregnancy and risk of spontaneous abortion and stillbirth indicate an increased risk of spontaneous abortion (i.e., miscarriage during gestational weeks 7 through 22) in pregnant women treated with oral fluconazole (most women received a total cumulative dose of 150–300 mg) compared with matched control pregnancies not exposed to oral fluconazole. Therefore, FDA alerted clinicians that it is reviewing data from the Danish study and additional data and, after completing the review, will communicate its conclusions and updated recommendations regarding use of the single-dose 150-mg oral fluconazole regimen during pregnancy.

The US Centers for Disease Control and Prevention (CDC) states that topical (intravaginal) azole antifungals (not oral fluconazole) should be used for the treatment of vulvovaginal candidiasis during pregnancy.

The Infectious Diseases Society of America (IDSA) states that use of fluconazole for the treatment of serious fungal infections (e.g., blastomycosis†, candidiasis, histoplasmosis†, coccidioidomycosis†, cryptococcosis) should be avoided during pregnancy.

Patients who are pregnant or actively trying to become pregnant should talk to their clinician about alternatives for treatment of vulvovaginal candidiasis.

If fluconazole is used during pregnancy or if the patient becomes pregnant while receiving the drug, the patient should be informed of the potential hazard to the fetus.

In several reproduction studies in pregnant rabbits receiving oral fluconazole dosages of 5, 10, 20, 25, or 75 mg/kg once daily during organogenesis, maternal weight gain was impaired at all dosage levels and abortions occurred with the 75-mg/kg dosage (approximately 20–60 times the usual human dosage); no adverse fetal effects were detected. In studies in pregnant rats receiving oral fluconazole during organogenesis, maternal weight gain was impaired and placental weights were increased at dosages of 25 mg/kg once daily. Although there were no fetal effects in rats receiving oral fluconazole in a dosage of 5 or 10 mg/kg once daily, increases in fetal anatomical variants (supernumerary ribs, renal pelvis dilation) and delays in ossification occurred in those receiving oral dosages of 25 mg/kg or greater once daily. When oral fluconazole dosages of 80 mg/kg once daily (approximately 20–60 times the usual human dosage) to 320 mg/kg once daily were used in these rats, there was an increase in embryolethality and fetal abnormalities (i.e., wavy ribs, cleft palate, abnormal craniofacial ossification). These adverse effects in rats may be attributed to a species-specific effect of fluconazole on estrogen synthesis since lowered estrogen is known to cause effects on pregnancy, organogenesis, and parturition. There is no evidence to date that estrogen concentrations are decreased in women receiving fluconazole. (See Cautions: Other Adverse Effects.)

Fertility

Reproduction studies in male and female rats receiving fluconazole in an oral dosage of 5, 10, or 20 mg/kg once daily or an IV dosage of 5, 25, or 75 mg/kg once daily did not reveal evidence of impaired fertility; however, onset of parturition was delayed slightly with the 20-mg/kg oral dosage. In one study in rats receiving an IV fluconazole dosage of 5, 20, or 40 mg/kg once daily, dystocia and prolongation of parturition occurred in a few dams with the 20-mg/kg (approximately 5–15 times the usual human dosage) and 40-mg/kg dosages but not with the 5-mg/kg dosage. Disturbances in parturition in rats were reflected by a slight increase in the number of stillborn pups and a decrease in neonatal survival; these effects presumably are related to a species-specific estrogen-lowering effect caused by high doses of fluconazole.

Lactation

Fluconazole is distributed into human milk in concentrations similar to those achieved in plasma. Administration of a single 150-mg oral dose to several nursing women resulted in peak plasma fluconazole concentrations of 2.61 mcg/mL (range: 1.57–3.65 mcg/mL). Fluconazole should be used with caution in nursing woman.

DRUG INTERACTIONS

While fluconazole can alter the pharmacokinetics of certain drugs that undergo hepatic metabolism, the magnitude of such alterations appears to be less than those associated with ketoconazole; however, comparative studies have not been performed to date. In addition, the possibility that the risk of developing such interactions may be increased at relatively high fluconazole dosages (e.g., 200 mg daily or more) should be considered.

● Drugs Metabolized by Hepatic Microsomal Enzymes

Fluconazole is a potent inhibitor of cytochrome P450 (CYP) isoenzyme 2C9 and a moderate inhibitor of CYP3A4. Because fluconazole has a long half-life, its enzyme-inhibiting effects persist for 4–5 days following discontinuance. Concomitant use of fluconazole and drugs metabolized by CYP2C9 or 3A4 may result in increased plasma concentrations of the concomitant drug. When fluconazole is used concomitantly with drugs metabolized by these enzymes, caution should be used and the patient carefully monitored.

● Drugs Affecting Gastric Acidity

Studies in fasting, healthy adults indicate that GI absorption of fluconazole is not affected substantially by concomitant use of drugs that decrease gastric acid output or increase gastric pH. When a single 100-mg oral dose of fluconazole was administered 2 hours after a single 400-mg oral dose of cimetidine, the area under the plasma concentration-time curve (AUC) of fluconazole was decreased 13% and peak plasma fluconazole concentrations were decreased by 21%; these effects were *not* considered clinically important. Administration of antacids containing aluminum hydroxide or magnesium hydroxide either with or immediately prior to a single 100-mg oral dose of fluconazole had no effect on absorption or elimination of the antifungal.

● Drugs that Prolong the QT Interval

Concomitant use of fluconazole with drugs that are metabolized by CYP3A4 and known to prolong the QT interval (e.g., cisapride, astemizole, pimozide, quinidine) is contraindicated. Concomitant use with erythromycin should be avoided (see Erythromycin under Drugs Interactions: Macrolides).

Prolongation of the QT interval and QT interval corrected for rate (QT_c) and, rarely, serious cardiovascular effects, including arrhythmias (e.g., ventricular tachycardia, atypical ventricular tachycardia [torsades de pointes, ventricular fibrillation]), cardiac arrest, palpitations, hypotension, dizziness, syncope, and death, have been reported in patients receiving recommended dosages of terfenadine or astemizole (neither antihistamine currently is commercially available in the US) concomitantly with another azole antifungal, ketoconazole. Ketoconazole can markedly inhibit the metabolism of astemizole or terfenadine, probably via inhibition of the cytochrome P-450 microsomal enzyme system, resulting in increased plasma concentrations of unchanged drug (to measurable levels) and reduced clearance of the active desmethyl or carboxylic acid metabolite, respectively. Such alterations in the pharmacokinetics of these antihistamines may be associated with prolongation of the QT and QT_c intervals. Similar alterations in the pharmacokinetics of these antihistamines and/or adverse cardiac effects also have been reported in patients receiving the drugs concomitantly with itraconazole, although in vitro data suggest that itraconazole may have a less pronounced effect than ketoconazole on the pharmacokinetics of astemizole. Studies have been performed to determine whether similar interactions occur with concomitant use of terfenadine and fluconazole. In one study, concomitant use of terfenadine and fluconazole (at a dosage of 200 mg daily) did not result in prolongation of QT interval; however, use of higher fluconazole dosages (400 or 800 mg daily) in another study resulted in increased plasma concentrations of terfenadine. The manufacturer of fluconazole has stated that concomitant use of terfenadine and fluconazole in a daily dosage of 400 mg or greater has been contraindicated and it was recommended that patients be carefully monitored if lower fluconazole dosages (i.e., less than 400 mg daily) were administered in patients receiving terfenadine.

Concomitant use of fluconazole and cisapride (currently commercially available in the US only under a limited-access protocol) may result in increased plasma cisapride concentrations and has rarely been associated with adverse cardiac events including torsades de pointes. In a placebo-controlled, randomized, multiple-dose study in individuals receiving fluconazole (200 mg daily), initiation of cisapride (20 mg 4 times daily) after 7 days of fluconazole therapy resulted in a 102–192% increase in the AUC and a 92–153% increase in peak plasma concentrations of cisapride. In addition, administration of fluconazole to individuals receiving cisapride (20 mg 4 times daily for 5 days) resulted in a significant increase in the QT interval corrected for rate. The manufacturer of fluconazole states that concomitant use of fluconazole and cisapride is contraindicated.

Concomitant use of erythromycin and fluconazole may increase the risk of QT interval prolongation and torsades de pointes and subsequent sudden cardiac death. Concomitant use of erythromycin and fluconazole should be avoided.

● Anticoagulants

Increased prothrombin time has been reported in patients receiving fluconazole concomitantly with a coumarin anticoagulant (e.g., warfarin). In one study in healthy adults receiving 200 mg of fluconazole daily or placebo, area under the prothrombin time versus time (for a 7-day post-warfarin period) curve for a single 15-mg warfarin dose increased by about 12% when concomitant fluconazole versus placebo were compared. Increased prothrombin times also have been reported when lower dosages of fluconazole (100 mg once daily) were administered concomitantly with warfarin sodium. Concomitant use of fluconazole with nicoumalone (a coumarin anticoagulant not commercially available in the US) resulted in increased prothrombin time and intracranial hemorrhage in at least one patient. Prothrombin times should be monitored carefully when fluconazole is used concomitantly with a coumarin anticoagulant.

● Antidiabetic Agents

Administration of fluconazole in individuals receiving tolbutamide, glyburide, or glipizide has resulted in increased AUCs and peak plasma concentrations and reduced metabolism of the antidiabetic agent. The mean increase in AUC or peak plasma concentrations of tolbutamide, glyburide, or glipizide reported in healthy adults receiving concomitant fluconazole is 26–49 or 11–19%, respectively. Clinically important hypoglycemia may be precipitated by concomitant use of oral hypoglycemic agents and fluconazole, and at least one fatality has been reported from hypoglycemia in a patient receiving glyburide and fluconazole concomitantly. In several individuals, symptoms consistent with hypoglycemia occurred; oral glucose therapy was necessary in a few cases.

If fluconazole is used concomitantly with tolbutamide, glyburide, glipizide, or any other oral sulfonylurea antidiabetic agent, blood glucose concentrations should be monitored carefully and dosage of the antidiabetic agent adjusted as necessary.

● Antifungal Agents

Amphotericin B

Although the clinical importance is unclear, results of in vitro studies evaluating the antifungal effects of amphotericin B used concomitantly with fluconazole or other azole antifungals (e.g., clotrimazole, itraconazole, ketoconazole) against *Candida albicans, C. pseudotropicalis, C. glabrata,* or *Aspergillus fumigatus* indicate that antagonism can occur with these combinations. Since amphotericin B exerts its antifungal activity by binding to sterols in the fungal cell membrane and azole antifungals act by altering the cell membrane, antagonism is theoretically possible; however, it is unclear whether such antagonism actually would occur in vivo. Results of studies evaluating combined use of fluconazole and amphotericin B in animal models of aspergillosis, candidiasis, or cryptococcosis have been conflicting. While antagonism occurred in some models (*A. fumigatus* infection in mice, rabbits, or rats treated with amphotericin B and fluconazole), the combination resulted in additive or indifferent effects in other models (e.g., *C. albicans* or *Cryptococcus neoformans* infection in mice or rabbits treated with amphotericin B and fluconazole). In a few studies evaluating the drugs in murine cryptococcosis or candidiasis, sequential use of an initial large dose of amphotericin B followed by an azole antifungal (e.g., fluconazole) was uniformly effective in prolonging survival and decreasing fungal burden. Because further study is needed regarding the interaction between azole antifungals and amphotericin B, it has been suggested that fluconazole and amphotericin B be used concomitantly with caution and close monitoring, particularly in immunocompromised patients.

Results of an in vitro study indicate that the combination of amphotericin B and fluconazole may be synergistic, additive, or indifferent against *Pseudallescheria boydii;* there was no evidence of antagonism.

Flucytosine

In an in vitro study, the combination of fluconazole and flucytosine was synergistic, additive, or indifferent against *Cryptococcus neoformans;* there was no evidence of antagonism. Synergism generally did not occur if the *C. neoformans* isolates had fluconazole MICs of 8 mcg/mL or greater. It has been suggested that synergism between the drugs may occur because fluconazole damages the fungal cell membrane allowing greater intracellular penetration of flucytosine.

Voriconazole

In healthy men, concomitant use of oral voriconazole (400 mg every 12 hours for 1 day, then 200 mg every 12 hours for 2.5 days) and oral fluconazole (400 mg on day 1, then 200 mg once daily for 4 days) resulted in a 79 and 57% increase in AUC and

peak plasma concentration of voriconazole, respectively. Reduced dosage or dosing frequency of voriconazole and fluconazole did not overcome this pharmacokinetic interaction. Concomitant use of voriconazole and fluconazole is not recommended and should be avoided. If voriconazole is used sequentially after fluconazole, the patient should be monitored closely for voriconazole-associated adverse events, particularly during the first 24 hours after the last fluconazole dose.

● Antimycobacterial Agents

Rifabutin

Concomitant use of fluconazole (200 mg daily) and rifabutin (300 mg daily) in individuals with human immunodeficiency virus (HIV) infection results in substantially increased plasma concentrations and AUCs of rifabutin and its major metabolite (LM565). This effect presumably occurs via inhibition of CYP isoenzymes involved in metabolism of rifabutin and may account in part for the increased incidence of certain adverse effects (e.g., uveitis) reported with concomitant rifabutin and fluconazole therapy.

Rifabutin and fluconazole should be used concomitantly with caution and close monitoring.

Rifampin

Concomitant use of fluconazole and rifampin may affect the pharmacokinetics of both drugs. Administration of a single 200-mg oral dose of fluconazole in healthy adults receiving rifampin (600 mg daily) resulted in approximately a 25% decrease in the AUC and a 20% decrease in the plasma half-life of fluconazole. There also is some evidence that concomitant use of fluconazole and rifampin results in increased rifampin plasma concentrations compared with administration of rifampin alone. The clinical importance of this possible pharmacokinetic interaction between fluconazole and rifampin is unclear; however, it has been suggested that such an interaction may have contributed to relapse of cryptococcal meningitis in a few patients who were receiving fluconazole concomitantly with rifampin.

Rifampin and fluconazole should be used concomitantly with caution and close monitoring. The manufacturer of fluconazole states that, depending on clinical circumstances, consideration can be given to increasing fluconazole dosage when the drug is administered concomitantly with rifampin.

● Antiretroviral Agents

HIV Nonnucleoside Reverse Transcriptase Inhibitors (NNRTIs)

Delavirdine

Concomitant use of delavirdine (300 mg every 8 hours) and fluconazole (400 mg daily) for 2 weeks in HIV-infected patients was well tolerated and did not appear to affect the pharmacokinetics of either drug. Dosage adjustments are not necessary in patients receiving delavirdine and fluconazole concomitantly.

Efavirenz

Concomitant use of efavirenz (400 mg daily) and fluconazole (200 mg daily) for 7 days in healthy individuals did not result in clinically important changes in the pharmacokinetics of either drug; dosage adjustments are not necessary in patients receiving the drugs concomitantly.

Etravirine

Concomitant use of etravirine and fluconazole results in substantial increases in etravirine plasma concentrations and AUC, but does not have a clinically important effect on fluconazole concentrations. Although dosage adjustments are not needed for either drug if etravirine is used concomitantly with fluconazole, these drugs should be used concomitantly with caution because only limited data are available regarding the safety of increased etravirine concentrations.

Nevirapine

Concomitant use of nevirapine and fluconazole may result in increased nevirapine concentrations, but has no effect on fluconazole concentrations. If nevirapine and fluconazole are used concomitantly, the patient should be monitored for nevirapine toxicity since the risk of hepatotoxicity may be increased. Alternatively, a different antiretroviral agent can be used.

Rilpivirine

Concomitant use of fluconazole and rilpivirine may result in increased rilpivirine plasma concentrations. If rilpivirine is used concomitantly with fluconazole, rilpivirine dosage adjustments are not needed; however, the patient should be monitored for breakthrough fungal infections.

HIV Nucleoside Reverse Transcriptase Inhibitors (NRTIs)

Concomitant use of fluconazole appears to interfere with the metabolism and clearance of zidovudine. In one study in men with HIV infection who received zidovudine (200 mg every 8 hours) alone or in conjunction with fluconazole (400 mg daily), the AUC of zidovudine was increased 74% (range: 20–173%), peak serum zidovudine concentrations were increased 84% (range: –1 to 227%), and the terminal elimination half-life of the drug was increased 128% (range: –4 to 189%) in patients receiving concomitant fluconazole. Zidovudine and fluconazole should be used concomitantly with caution and close monitoring. Patients should be monitored closely for zidovudine-associated adverse effects, and zidovudine dosage reductions may be considered.

In one limited study in patients with HIV infection receiving oral didanosine (3.2–7.8 mg/kg daily), concomitant use of oral fluconazole (200 mg every 12 hours for 2 doses, then 200 mg once daily for 6 days) did not result in any clinically important differences in the AUC of didanosine, peak serum didanosine concentrations, or time to peak concentrations.

Concomitant use of fluconazole and stavudine does not result in a clinically important alteration in the pharmacokinetics of either drug.

HIV Protease Inhibitors (PIs)

Atazanavir

Pharmacokinetic interactions have not been observed and are unlikely if atazanavir (unboosted, *ritonavir-boosted*, or *cobicistat-boosted*) is used concomitantly with fluconazole. Dosage adjustments are not necessary if *ritonavir-boosted* or *cobicistat-boosted* atazanavir is used concomitantly with fluconazole.

Indinavir

Concomitant use of indinavir (1 g every 8 hours) and fluconazole (400 mg once daily) for 1 week resulted in a slight decrease in the AUC of indinavir and no change in the AUC of fluconazole. This pharmacokinetic interaction is not considered clinically important; dosage adjustments are not necessary in patients receiving indinavir concomitantly with fluconazole.

Lopinavir

Clinically important pharmacokinetic interactions between the fixed combination of lopinavir and ritonavir (lopinavir/ritonavir) and fluconazole are not expected.

Ritonavir

Concomitant use of ritonavir (200 mg every 6 hours for 4 days) and fluconazole (400 mg on day 1, then 200 mg daily for 4 days) resulted in a 12 and 15% increase in the AUC and peak plasma concentration of ritonavir, respectively. Dosage adjustments are not needed.

Saquinavir

Concomitant use of saquinavir (1200 mg as Invirase® 3 times daily) and fluconazole (single 400-mg dose on day 2, then 200 mg daily) has resulted in approximate increases of 50 and 56% in saquinavir AUC and peak plasma concentrations, respectively. This interaction is a result of inhibition of CYP3A4 with decreased metabolism of saquinavir and inhibition of P-glycoprotein. Saquinavir and fluconazole should be used concomitantly with caution and close monitoring; saquinavir dosage may need to be adjusted.

Data are not available regarding concomitant use of *ritonavir-boosted* saquinavir and fluconazole; some experts state that dosage adjustments are not needed.

Tipranavir

Concomitant use of *ritonavir-boosted* tipranavir and fluconazole results in increased tipranavir peak plasma concentrations and AUC, but does not affect the pharmacokinetics of fluconazole.

Although dosage adjustments are not needed, fluconazole dosage should not exceed 200 mg daily in patients receiving *ritonavir-boosted* tipranavir. If high-dose fluconazole is indicated, an alternative antiretroviral should be considered.

● Calcium-channel Blocking Agents

Fluconazole has the potential to increase systemic exposure to certain dihydropyridine calcium channel blocking agents (amlodipine, felodipine, isradipine,

nifedipine, verapamil) that are metabolized by CYP3A4. Calcium channel blocking agents and fluconazole should be used concomitantly with caution and close monitoring; patients should be monitored frequently for adverse events.

● CNS Agents

Anticonvulsants

Concomitant use of carbamazepine and fluconazole has resulted in a 30% increase in carbamazepine concentrations and has increased carbamazepine-associated toxicity, presumably as the result of fluconazole inhibiting CYP isoenzymes involved in metabolism of the anticonvulsant. Carbamazepine and fluconazole should be used concomitantly with caution and close monitoring; carbamazepine dosage adjustment may be necessary based on plasma carbamazepine concentrations and clinical effect.

Concomitant use of fluconazole and phenytoin has resulted in increased plasma phenytoin concentrations and AUC and has resulted in phenytoin toxicity. In one study in healthy adults, minimum plasma phenytoin concentrations increased 128% and the AUC of the drug increased 75% during concomitant fluconazole administration; fluconazole pharmacokinetics were not affected. It has been suggested that such alterations in phenytoin pharmacokinetics result from fluconazole-induced inhibition of metabolism of the anticonvulsant. Phenytoin and fluconazole should be used concomitantly with caution and close monitoring. Plasma phenytoin concentrations should be monitored carefully, and dosage of the anticonvulsant adjusted as needed whenever fluconazole is initiated or discontinued.

Antipsychotics

Although data are lacking, concomitant use of fluconazole and pimozide may result in increased plasma pimozide concentrations with the potential for QT interval prolongation and, rarely, torsades de pointes. Concomitant use of fluconazole and pimozide is contraindicated.

Benzodiazepines

Concomitant use of oral or IV fluconazole and midazolam results in substantial increases in the peak plasma concentration and AUC of midazolam (AUC increased 244–272%) and can increase the psychomotor effects of the benzodiazepine; peak plasma concentration and AUC of fluconazole are not affected. This pharmacokinetic interaction appears to be more pronounced with oral fluconazole than with IV fluconazole. In mechanically ventilated patients sedated with IV midazolam, concomitant use of IV fluconazole resulted in a 20–300% increase in plasma midazolam concentrations in some patients within 18–48 hours after the first dose of fluconazole. In addition, administration of oral fluconazole to healthy individuals receiving IV midazolam reportedly results in a 50% decrease in clearance of the benzodiazepine. Administration of fluconazole to healthy individuals receiving oral midazolam resulted in a 3.5-fold increase in midazolam AUC, a 2.5-fold increase in peak plasma midazolam concentrations, and prolonged midazolam half-life. If a short-acting benzodiazepine metabolized by CYP isoenzymes is used in a patient receiving fluconazole, the patient should be carefully monitored and a decrease in benzodiazepine dosage considered. Because of concerns that prolonged sedation may occur if fluconazole is administered to patients sedated with IV midazolam, some clinicians suggest that a decrease in the midazolam dosage be considered if there is evidence of increased sedation during concomitant fluconazole therapy.

Concomitant use of fluconazole and a single dose of triazolam has resulted in a 50% increase in the AUC of triazolam and a 20–32% increase in peak plasma triazolam concentrations and has prolonged the half-life of triazolam by 25–50%. Triazolam and fluconazole should be used concomitantly with caution and close monitoring; adjustment of triazolam dosage may be necessary.

Nonsteroidal Anti-inflammatory Agents

Concomitant use of fluconazole (200 mg daily) and celecoxib (200 mg) has increased the peak plasma concentration and AUC of celecoxib by 68 and 134%, respectively.

Concomitant use of flurbiprofen and fluconazole has increased the peak plasma concentration and AUC of flurbiprofen by 23 and 81%, respectively.

When ibuprofen (single 400-mg dose) was administered to healthy individuals receiving oral fluconazole (400 mg on day 1 and 200 mg on day 2), the peak plasma concentration and AUC of the pharmacologically active S-isomer of ibuprofen were increased by about 15 and 82%, respectively.

Although data are lacking, fluconazole has the potential to increase systemic exposure to other nonsteroidal anti-inflammatory agents (NSAIAs) that are metabolized by CYP2C9 (e.g., diclofenac, lornoxicam [not commercially available in the US], meloxicam, naproxen).

NSAIAs and fluconazole should be used concomitantly with caution and close monitoring. Patients should be monitored frequently for NSAIA-associated adverse events; NSAIA dosage adjustment may be needed.

Opiate Agonists

Concomitant use of alfentanil and oral or IV fluconazole in healthy individuals reduced alfentanil clearance by 55%, reduced alfentanil volume of distribution by 19%, and nearly doubled the mean elimination half-life of the drug. This interaction may be a result of inhibition of CYP3A4 by fluconazole. Alfentanil and fluconazole should be used concomitantly with caution and close monitoring; adjustment of alfentanil dosage may be necessary.

Concomitant use of a single IV dose of fentanyl in healthy adults receiving oral fluconazole resulted in substantially delayed fentanyl elimination. Elevated fentanyl concentrations may lead to respiratory depression. A fatality possibly related to fentanyl intoxication has been reported in a patient who received concomitant fluconazole and transdermal fentanyl. Fentanyl and fluconazole should be used concomitantly with caution and close monitoring.

When fluconazole (200 mg daily) was administered for 14 days to individuals receiving stable doses of methadone, mean methadone AUC and peak plasma concentration were increased 35 and 27%, respectively, and methadone clearance was reduced 24%. Methadone and fluconazole should be used concomitantly with caution and close monitoring; methadone dosage adjustment may be necessary.

Tricyclic Antidepressants

Concomitant use of amitriptyline or nortriptyline and fluconazole has resulted in increased serum concentrations of the tricyclic antidepressant and may increase adverse effects of the antidepressants. CNS toxicity has been reported in a few patients receiving amitriptyline and fluconazole concomitantly. It has been suggested that fluconazole may interfere with metabolism of amitriptyline by inhibition of CYP isoenzymes involved in metabolism of the antidepressant. Fluconazole and amitriptyline or nortriptyline should be used concomitantly with caution and close monitoring. The manufacturer of fluconazole states that S-amitriptyline and/or 5-nortriptyline may be measured when concomitant therapy is initiated and after 1 week of concomitant use; dosage of amitriptyline or nortriptyline should be adjusted if necessary.

● Corticosteroids

In a liver transplant recipient receiving prednisone who received a 3-month course of fluconazole, acute adrenal cortex insufficiency occurred when fluconazole was discontinued. This may be a consequence of increased CYP3A4 activity and enhanced metabolism of prednisone as a result of fluconazole discontinuance. Prednisone and fluconazole should be used concomitantly with caution and close monitoring; if the drugs are used concomitantly for a prolonged period of time, the patient should be monitored carefully for adrenal cortex insufficiency when fluconazole is discontinued.

● Cyclophosphamide

Concomitant use of cyclophosphamide and fluconazole results in increased concentrations of serum bilirubin and serum creatinine. Cyclophosphamide and fluconazole should be used concomitantly with caution and close monitoring; the risk of increased serum bilirubin and serum creatinine should be considered.

● Estrogens and Progestins

Concomitant use of oral fluconazole and oral estrogen-progestin contraceptives may affect the pharmacokinetics of the contraceptives. Although limited data indicate that fluconazole may inhibit metabolism of ethinyl estradiol, levonorgestrel, and norethindrone, there is no evidence that fluconazole induces metabolism of these hormones. When fluconazole is used in the dosage range of 50–200 mg daily concomitantly with combined oral contraceptives, interference with oral contraceptive efficacy is unlikely.

In healthy premenopausal women who received a single dose of oral contraceptive before and after receiving oral fluconazole given in a low dosage (50

mg once daily for 10 days), the mean increase in AUCs of ethinyl estradiol and levonorgestrel were 6% (range: –47 to 108%) and 17% (range: –33 to 141%), respectively. Although some women had ethinyl estradiol and levonorgestrel concentrations that were decreased 47 and 33%, respectively, the manufacturer suggests that this may have been the result of random variation. In a controlled study in healthy women who received a single dose of oral contraceptive following a 10-day regimen of placebo or oral fluconazole (200 mg once daily), AUCs of both levonorgestrel and ethinyl estradiol were increased substantially in those who received oral fluconazole compared with placebo; mean increases in AUCs of ethinyl estradiol and levonorgestrel were 38% (range: –11 to 101%) and 25% (range: –12 to 82%), respectively.

In another placebo-controlled study, women who had received a full cycle of an oral contraceptive preparation containing ethinyl estradiol and norethindrone received a once-weekly fluconazole regimen (300 mg once weekly) or placebo during the second and third cycles of contraceptive use. During fluconazole treatment, the mean AUCs of ethinyl estradiol and norethindrone were increased by 24 and 13%, respectively, compared with placebo. Fluconazole did not cause a decrease in the ethinyl estradiol AUC in any individual and caused only a slight (less than 5%) decrease in the AUC of norethindrone.

● Halofantrine

Concomitant use of fluconazole and halofantrine (not commercially available in the US) may result in increased halofantrine concentrations because of CYP3A4 inhibition by fluconazole. Halofantrine and fluconazole should be used concomitantly with caution and close monitoring.

● HCV Antivirals

HCV Protease Inhibitor
Simeprevir

Concomitant use of simeprevir and fluconazole may result in increased plasma concentrations of simeprevir.

Concomitant use of fluconazole and simeprevir is not recommended.

HCV Replication Complex Inhibitor
Daclatasvir

If fluconazole and daclatasvir are used concomitantly, daclatasvir dosage adjustments are not needed.

● HMG-CoA Reductase Inhibitors

When fluconazole is used concomitantly with a hydroxymethylglutaryl-CoA (HMG-CoA) reductase inhibitor (i.e., statin) that is metabolized by CYP3A4 (e.g., atorvastatin, simvastatin) or 2C9 (e.g., fluvastatin), the risk of myopathy and rhabdomyolysis is increased. If concomitant therapy is necessary, creatinine kinase (CK, creatine phosphokinase, CPK) should be monitored and the patient assessed for symptoms of myopathy and rhabdomyolysis. If a substantial increase in CK occurs or myopathy or rhabdomyolysis is diagnosed or suspected, the statin should be discontinued.

In a placebo-controlled crossover study, a single dose of fluvastatin (40 mg on day 4) administered to healthy individuals receiving oral fluconazole (400 mg on day 1, then 200 mg daily on days 2-4) resulted in an 84% increase in fluvastatin AUC, a 44% increase in fluvastatin peak plasma concentration, and an 80% prolongation of fluvastatin half-life, but did not affect the AUC of fluconazole.

Fluconazole had no clinically important effect on pravastatin pharmacokinetics in a placebo-controlled crossover study in healthy individuals.

● Immunosuppressive Agents

Cyclosporine

Concomitant use of fluconazole and cyclosporine may result in increased plasma cyclosporine concentrations, especially when the drugs are used in renal transplant recipients. In several studies in bone marrow transplant recipients receiving cyclosporine maintenance therapy, administration of 100- or 200-mg oral doses of fluconazole once daily for 14 days resulted in only slight increases in plasma cyclosporine concentrations, which were not considered clinically important. However, administration of usual oral dosages of fluconazole to renal transplant recipients (with or without impaired renal function) receiving cyclosporine has resulted in increases in the AUC and peak plasma concentrations of the immu-nosuppressive agent. In one study in renal transplant patients who had received at least 6 months of cyclosporine therapy and had been receiving a stable cyclosporine dosage for at least 6 weeks, administration of fluconazole 200 mg daily for 14 days resulted in a mean increase of 60 or 157% in peak or minimum cyclosporine plasma concentrations, respectively, and a mean decrease of 45% in the apparent oral clearance of the drug. In addition, increased serum creatinine concentrations, which returned to pretreatment levels with dosage reduction of both drugs, have been reported in patients receiving fluconazole and cyclosporine concomitantly. While the mechanism of this possible interaction is not known, displacement of cyclosporine from protein-binding sites is unlikely since fluconazole is only minimally protein bound.

Fluconazole and cyclosporine should be used concomitantly with caution and close monitoring. Plasma cyclosporine concentrations and serum creatinine should be monitored carefully; cyclosporine dosage should be decreased based on plasma concentrations of the immunosuppressive agent.

Tacrolimus

Concomitant use of oral tacrolimus and fluconazole has resulted in a fivefold increase in serum concentrations of tacrolimus as the result of inhibition of intestinal CYP3A4; clinically important alterations in pharmacokinetics were not observed with IV tacrolimus. Increased tacrolimus concentrations have been associated with nephrotoxicity.

Tacrolimus and fluconazole should be used concomitantly with caution and close monitoring. Tacrolimus dosage should be decreased based on tacrolimus concentrations.

Sirolimus

Concomitant use of sirolimus and fluconazole results in increased plasma concentrations of the immunosuppressive agent, probably as a result of decreased sirolimus metabolism secondary to inhibition of CYP3A4 and P-glycoprotein.

Sirolimus and fluconazole should be used concomitantly with caution and close monitoring. Sirolimus dosage should be adjusted based on sirolimus concentrations and clinical effects.

● Losartan

When a single dose of losartan (50 mg on day 4) was administered to healthy individuals receiving fluconazole (400 mg on day 1, then 200 mg on days 2-4), the AUC and mean peak plasma concentration of the active losartan metabolite (E-3174) were decreased 30 and 47%, respectively, and the half-life of E-3174 was increased by 167%.

Losartan and fluconazole should be used concomitantly with caution and close monitoring. Because fluconazole inhibits metabolism of losartan to its active metabolite (E-3174) and the metabolite is principally responsible for angiotensin II receptor antagonism during losartan therapy, the possibility of decreased therapeutic effect should be considered and blood pressure closely monitored.

● Macrolides

Azithromycin

Concomitant use of a single 1.2-g dose of azithromycin and a single 800-mg dose of fluconazole did not alter the pharmacokinetics of either drug.

Erythromycin

Concomitant use of erythromycin and fluconazole should be avoided because of the potential for an increased risk of adverse cardiovascular effects (prolonged QT interval, torsades de pointes) and subsequent sudden cardiac death.

● Quinidine

Concomitant use of quinidine and fluconazole may result in inhibition of quinidine metabolism. Quinidine has been associated with QT interval prolongation and rare occurrences of torsades de pointes. (See Drug Interactions: Drugs that Prolong the QT Interval.)

Concomitant use of quinidine and fluconazole is contraindicated.

● Theophylline

Concomitant use of theophylline and fluconazole increases serum theophylline concentrations. In a study in healthy adults, administration of a single dose of IV

aminophylline (6 mg/kg) after 14 days of oral fluconazole (200 mg daily) resulted in a 21 or 13% increase in the mean AUC or peak plasma concentration of theophylline, respectively, and a mean decrease of 16% in theophylline clearance; the half-life of theophylline increased from 6.6 to 7.9 hours.

Theophylline and fluconazole should be used concomitantly with caution and close monitoring. Serum theophylline concentrations should be monitored carefully in patients receiving fluconazole.

● Thiazide Diuretics

In healthy adults receiving 100-mg doses of fluconazole, concomitant administration of 50-mg doses of hydrochlorothiazide resulted in a 43% increase in peak plasma fluconazole concentrations and a 45% increase in the AUC of fluconazole compared with results obtained when the antifungal was given alone. These changes are attributed to a 30% decrease in renal clearance of fluconazole. Fluconazole and hydrochlorothiazide should be used concomitantly with caution and close monitoring; adjustment of fluconazole dosage probably is not necessary.

● Tofacitinib

Concomitant use of fluconazole (400 mg on day 1, then 200 mg once daily for 6 days) and tofacitinib (single 30-mg dose on day 5) in healthy individuals increased the mean peak plasma concentration and AUC of tofacitinib by 27 and 79%, respectively, compared with administration of tofacitinib alone.

If tofacitinib and fluconazole are used concomitantly, tofacitinib dosage should be reduced from 5 mg twice daily to 5 mg once daily.

● Tretinoin

Pseudotumor cerebri has been reported in a patient who received tretinoin (all-trans retinoic acid) and fluconazole concomitantly; this adverse CNS effect resolved after discontinuance of fluconazole. Tretinoin and fluconazole should be used concomitantly with caution and close monitoring; the possibility of adverse CNS effects should be considered.

● Vinca Alkaloids

Although data are not available, inhibition of CYP3A4 by fluconazole may result in increased plasma levels of concomitant vinca alkaloids (e.g., vinblastine, vincristine) and possible neurotoxicity. Vinca alkaloids and fluconazole should be used concomitantly with caution and close monitoring.

ACUTE TOXICITY

● Manifestations

Limited information is available on the acute toxicity of fluconazole in humans. In mice and rats receiving very high dosages of fluconazole, decreased motility and respiration, ptosis, lacrimation, salivation, urinary incontinence, loss of righting reflex, and cyanosis occurred. There were no fatalities in mice and rats receiving fluconazole doses of 1 g/kg or less. At higher doses (1–2 g/kg), death occurred 1.5 hours to 3 days after the dose; in some cases, death was preceded by clonic seizures. There have been reports of fluconazole overdosage accompanied by hallucination and paranoid behavior in humans.

● Treatment

If acute overdosage of fluconazole occurs, supportive and symptomatic treatment should be initiated. If indicated, the stomach should be emptied by gastric lavage. Elimination of fluconazole can be facilitated by hemodialysis; plasma concentrations of the drug generally are decreased 50% by a 3-hour period of hemodialysis.

MECHANISM OF ACTION

Fluconazole usually is fungistatic in action. Fluconazole and other triazole-derivative antifungals (e.g., itraconazole, terconazole) appear to have a mechanism of action similar to that of the imidazole-derivative antifungals (e.g., butoconazole, clotrimazole, econazole, ketoconazole, miconazole, oxiconazole). Like imidazoles, fluconazole presumably exerts its antifungal activity by altering cellular membranes resulting in increased membrane permeability, leakage of essential elements (e.g., amino acids, potassium), and impaired uptake of precursor molecules (e.g., purine and pyrimidine precursors to DNA). Although the exact mechanism of action of fluconazole and other triazoles has not been fully determined, the drugs inhibit cytochrome P-450 14-α-desmethylase in susceptible fungi, which leads to accumulation of C-14 methylated sterols (e.g., lanosterol) and decreased concentrations of ergosterol. It appears that this may occur because a nitrogen atom (−4) in the triazole molecule binds to the heme iron of cytochrome P-450 14-α-desmethylase in susceptible fungi. Unlike some imidazoles (e.g., clotrimazole, econazole, miconazole, oxiconazole) that suppress ATP concentrations in intact cells and spheroplasts of *C. albicans*, fluconazole does not appear to have an appreciable effect on ATP concentrations in the organism. It is unclear whether this effect is related to the in vivo antifungal effects of the drugs. Fluconazole generally is fungistatic against *Candida albicans* when the organism is in either the stationary or early logarithmic phase of growth.

Fluconazole and other triazoles (e.g., itraconazole) have a high affinity for fungal P-450 enzymes and only a weak affinity for mammalian P-450 enzymes and are more specific inhibitors of fungal cytochrome P-450 systems than many imidazoles (e.g., ketoconazole). The drug does not appear to have any effect on cholesterol synthesis in mammalian liver homogenates. In an in vitro study using rat Leydig cells, fluconazole concentrations of 10 mcg/mL caused less than a 30% inhibition of basal testosterone production whereas the same concentration of ketoconazole caused a 95% inhibition. Further study is needed to fully evaluate whether fluconazole affects P-450 enzyme systems and steroid synthesis in humans. While there is some evidence that fluconazole has only a minimal inhibitory effect on microsomal cytochrome P-450 systems, other evidence suggests that the drug may have a potent inhibitory effect. Results of an in vitro study using rat liver indicate that fluconazole may act as a potent inducer of some hepatic cytochrome P-450 enzymes systems involved in drug metabolism, acting as an enzyme inhibitor at low concentrations and an inducer at high concentrations. Unlike most imidazoles (e.g., ketoconazole), fluconazole appears to have only minimal, if any, effects on human steroid synthesis, including production of cholesterol, testosterone, and estrogen in dosages up to 400 mg daily.

Results of in vitro studies using human polymorphonuclear leukocytes (PMNs) obtained from healthy individuals indicate that exposure of PMNs to fluconazole concentrations of 1–50 mcg/mL does not appreciably affect PMN function, including chemotaxis, phagocytosis, and oxidative metabolism, and does not interfere with intracellular killing of *C. albicans* blastoconidia. The drug also does not affect lymphocyte proliferation in vitro.

SPECTRUM

Fluconazole is active against many fungi, including yeasts and dermatophytes. Fluconazole does not appear to have antibacterial activity.

• *In Vitro Susceptibility Testing*

Like imidazole derivatives and other triazole derivatives, results of in vitro fluconazole susceptibility tests are method dependent, and MIC values vary depending on the culture medium used, incubation temperature, pH, and inoculum size. In addition, currently available in vitro tests do not necessarily reflect the in vivo susceptibility of many fungi (especially *Candida*). Consequently, in vivo animal models of fungal infections may provide a more accurate assessment of the antifungal effectiveness of fluconazole than currently available in vitro susceptibility tests. While fluconazole is less active on a weight basis in vitro than many other antifungals (e.g., itraconazole, ketoconazole, miconazole), the drug often is as or more active than these agents in vivo. The reasons for the current lack of correlation between results of in vitro and in vivo tests are unclear. It has been suggested that substances contained in media used for in vitro susceptibility testing, especially complex media, may antagonize fluconazole. Other factors also probably contribute to the apparent poor correlation between in vitro and in vivo results.

• *Fungi*

When results of in vitro susceptibility tests are compared, fluconazole appears to be less active than ketoconazole against most susceptible organisms since MICs of fluconazole reported for *C. albicans*, *C. neoformans*, and *H. capsulatum* generally are 4–16 times higher than those reported for ketoconazole. However, results of studies using the drugs in various animal models of fungal infections indicate that, despite higher MIC values in vitro, the in vivo effectiveness of fluconazole is equal to or, in many cases, greater than the in vivo effectiveness of ketoconazole. This difference may occur because results of fluconazole in vitro susceptibility tests are affected to a greater extent than those of ketoconazole and/or because pharmacologic differences between the drugs (e.g., fluconazole's higher oral bioavailability and lower protein binding) affect the in vivo effectiveness of the drugs.

Candida

In vitro, fluconazole is active against some strains of *Candida*, including some strains of *C. albicans*, *C. dubliniensis*, *C. guilliermondii*, *C. kefyr*, *C. glabrata*, *C. parapsilosis*, *C. lusitaniae*, and *C. tropicalis*. In vitro, susceptible strains of *C. albicans*, *C. guilliermondii*, *C. parapsilosis*, and *C. tropicalis* usually are inhibited by fluconazole concentrations of 0.03–8 mcg/mL. In one study evaluating in vitro susceptibility of clinical isolates of *C. dubliniensis* obtained from patients with or without human immunodeficiency virus (HIV) infection, most strains were inhibited by fluconazole concentrations of 0.125–1 mcg/mL, but some strains had reduced susceptibility to the drug and required fluconazole concentrations of 8–32 mcg/mL for in vitro inhibition.

C. krusei are intrinsically resistant to fluconazole and many strains of *C. glabrata* also are resistant or have reduced susceptibility to the drug. (See Resistance.)

In vitro, some strains of *C. duobushaemulonii* have been inhibited by fluconazole concentrations of 1–16 mcg/mL. *C. haemulonii* and *C. auris* (often misidentified as *C. haemulonii*, *C. famata*, or *Rhodotorula glutinis*) generally are resistant to fluconazole in vitro.

Other Fungi

Fluconazole has in vitro activity against some strains of *Cryptococcus neoformans*. In vitro, some strains of *C. neoformans* are inhibited by fluconazole concentrations of 0.125–12.8 mcg/mL. Although fluconazole may be active in vitro against some strains of *C. gattii*, there is in vitro evidence that fluconazole may be less active against *C. gattii* than some other azoles (e.g., itraconazole, posaconazole, voriconazole).

Coccidioides immitis and *C. posadasii* are inhibited in vitro by fluconazole. In one study, the mean MIC of fluconazole for these organisms was 8 mcg/mL.

Fluconazole is active in vitro against some strains of *Histoplasma capsulatum*. A wide range of fluconazole MICs has been reported for this organism. In some in vitro studies, MICs of fluconazole reported for *H. capsulatum* were 0.125–4 mcg/mL; however, in other studies, MICs ranged from 16–250 mcg/mL. In addition, some amphotericin B-susceptible strains of *H. capsulatum* with fluconazole MICs exceeding 1000 mcg/mL have been reported.

Some strains of *Blastomyces dermatitidis* are inhibited in vitro by fluconazole concentrations of 2.5–10 mcg/mL, but other strains require concentrations of 20–80 mcg/mL for in vitro inhibition.

Fluconazole is inactive against *Malassezia pachydermatis* in vitro. The drug generally is inactive against *Aspergillus* in vitro.

Although a few strains of *Penicillium marneffei* may be inhibited in vitro by fluconazole concentrations of 4–8 mcg/mL, most strains tested are resistant to the drug. In vitro, fluconazole is considerably less active than itraconazole or ketoconazole against *P. marneffei*.

Scopulariopsis, including *S. acremonium* and *S. brevicaulis*, generally are resistant to fluconazole in vitro.

• *In Vivo Susceptibility Testing*

In vivo studies using various animal models (e.g., mice, rats, rabbits) and standard laboratory strains of fungi indicate that oral or IV fluconazole has fungistatic activity against a variety of fungal infections. Activity of the drug against fungi in these in vivo studies was generally evaluated based on increased survival rate and reduction of fungal burden in the animals' organs. Fluconazole has been active in vivo in both normal and immunosuppressed mice, rats, and rabbits against systemic and local infections caused by *C. albicans*, including endophthalmitis, endocarditis, pyelonephritis, and intestinal, vaginal, and disseminated candidiasis; in several studies, fluconazole was at least as effective as amphotericin B (alone or combined with flucytosine) and more effective than ketoconazole in vivo against these infections. Fluconazole also has been effective in vivo in animals against systemic *C. parapsilosis* infections. Although fluconazole was active in vivo in mice against infections caused by *C. tropicalis* or *C. glabrata*, the drug was less effective against these infections than amphotericin B; neither fluconazole nor amphotericin B were effective in reducing tissue concentrations of *C. krusei* in these mice.

Fluconazole has been effective in vivo in mice and rabbits against infections caused by *C. neoformans*, including meningitis and pulmonary infections. The drug generally has been effective against systemic infections, including pulmonary infections, caused by *H. capsulatum* in normal and immunosuppressed mice, and was as effective as or less effective than amphotericin B. Fluconazole also generally has been effective in mice against systemic infections, including intracranial infections, caused by *C. immitis*; pulmonary infections in mice caused by

Blastomyces dermatitidis; and infections in mice caused by *Paracoccidioides brasiliensis.* Results of in vivo testing of fluconazole activity against *Aspergillus* have been conflicting. In some in vivo studies in normal or immunosuppressed mice or rabbits, high dosages of the drug (60–120 mg/kg daily) were effective against infections caused by *A. flavus* and *A. fumigatus.* However, in at least one in vivo study in mice, fluconazole was ineffective against experimental aspergillosis.

In in vivo models of dermatomycoses, fluconazole has been effective against pityriasis (tinea) versicolor caused by *Malassezia furfur* (*Pityrosporum orbiculare* or *P. ovale*) and infections caused by *Trichophyton* or *Microsporum canis.*

RESISTANCE

Resistance to fluconazole can be produced in vitro by serial passage of *Candida albicans* in the presence of increasing concentrations of the drug. Some *Candida* species are intrinsically resistant to fluconazole (e.g., *C. krusei*), and many strains of *C. glabrata* are resistant or have reduced susceptibility to the drug. In addition, strains of *Candida* with decreased in vitro susceptibility to fluconazole have been isolated with increasing frequency. Fluconazole-resistant strains of *C. albicans, C. glabrata, C. lusitaniae, C. norvegensis, C. parapsilosis,* and *C. tropicalis* have been isolated from patients receiving fluconazole. Strains of *Cryptococcus neoformans* with decreased susceptibility to fluconazole also have been isolated from patients receiving the drug. Prolonged or intermittent use of oral fluconazole in immunocompromised patients has been suggested as a major contributing factor to the emergence of fluconazole resistance in *Candida.* In one study evaluating the in vitro susceptibility of *Candida* isolates obtained from patients with candidemia, 72% of the isolates obtained from patients who had received prior fluconazole therapy had decreased in vitro susceptibility to fluconazole (MIC greater than 8 mcg/mL) compared with only 12% of isolates obtained from patients who had not previously received fluconazole. There is evidence that decreased in vitro susceptibility to fluconazole may correlate with clinical failure in the treatment of *Candida* infections (e.g., esophageal candidiasis) in HIV-infected patients. Emergence of fluconazole-resistant strains of *C. albicans* also have been reported rarely in immunocompetent patients receiving the drug.

Several mechanisms for decreased susceptibility to fluconazole have been suggested, including reduced intracellular accumulation of the drug as the result of defective lipids or sterols in the fungal cell membrane or active efflux of the drug or mutation of fungal 14-α-desmethylase leading to diminished affinity for the enzyme. In one in vitro study, fluconazole-resistant strains of *C. albicans* reverted to susceptible phenotypes when grown without the presence of fluconazole.

Fluconazole-resistant fungi also may be cross-resistant to other azole antifungals (e.g., itraconazole, ketoconazole, posaconazole, voriconazole).

While the clinical importance is unclear, fluconazole-resistant strains of *C. albicans* that were cross-resistant to amphotericin B have been isolated from a few immunocompromised individuals, including leukemia patients and HIV-infected individuals. In addition, a few isolates of *Cryptococcus neoformans* with decreased susceptibility to fluconazole have shown cross resistance to amphotericin B.

PHARMACOKINETICS

● *Absorption*

The pharmacokinetics of fluconazole are similar following IV or oral administration. The drug is rapidly and almost completely absorbed from the GI tract, and there is no evidence of first-pass metabolism.

Oral bioavailability of fluconazole exceeds 90% in healthy, fasting adults; peak plasma concentrations of the drug generally are attained within 1–2 hours after oral administration. Results of a few limited studies indicate that oral bioavailability of fluconazole in adults with human immunodeficiency virus (HIV) infection appears to be similar to that reported for healthy adults.

The manufacturer states that the commercially available fluconazole suspensions are bioequivalent to the 100-mg fluconazole tablets.

Unlike some imidazole-derivative antifungals (e.g., ketoconazole), GI absorption of fluconazole does not appear to be affected by gastric pH. In one patient with achlorhydria who received 100-mg oral doses of fluconazole once daily, plasma concentrations of the drug 2 hours after a dose were similar to those reported at the same time interval in healthy adults. Studies in healthy, fasting adults indicate that peak plasma concentrations, areas under the concentration-time curves (AUCs), time to peak plasma concentrations, and elimination half-life of fluconazole are not affected substantially by concurrent administration of drugs that increase gastric pH. (See Drug Interactions: Drugs Affecting Gastric Acidity.)

Peak plasma fluconazole concentrations and AUCs increase in proportion to the dose over the oral dosage range of 50–400 mg. Steady-state plasma concentrations of fluconazole are attained within 5–10 days following oral doses of 50–400 mg given once daily. The manufacturer states that when fluconazole therapy is initiated with a single loading dose equal to twice the usual daily dosage and followed by the usual dosage given once daily thereafter, plasma concentrations of the drug reportedly approach steady state by the second day of therapy.

In healthy, fasting adults who received a single 1-mg/kg oral dose of fluconazole, peak plasma concentrations of the drug averaged 1.4 mcg/mL. Following oral administration of a single 400-mg dose of fluconazole in healthy, fasting adults, peak plasma concentrations average 6.72 mcg/mL (range: 4.12–8.1 mcg/mL). In adults with coccidioidal meningitis who received oral fluconazole in a dosage of 50 or 100 mg daily, peak serum concentrations of the drug ranged from 2.5–3.5 or 4.5–8 mcg/mL, respectively, and were attained in 2–6 hours; serum concentrations averaged 1.2 or 3.1 mcg/mL, respectively, at 24–27 hours after a dose.

In healthy adults receiving 50- or 100-mg doses of fluconazole given once daily by IV infusion over 30 minutes, serum concentrations of the drug 1 hour after dosing on the sixth or seventh day of therapy ranged from 2.14–2.81 or 3.86–4.96 mcg/mL, respectively.

In children 9 months to 13 years of age, oral administration of a single 2- or 8-mg/kg dose of fluconazole resulted in mean peak plasma concentrations of 2.9 or 9.8 mcg/mL, respectively. In a multiple-dose study in children 5–15 years of age, IV administration of 2-, 4-, or 8-mg/kg doses of fluconazole resulted in mean peak plasma concentrations of 5.5, 11.4, or 14.1 mcg/mL, respectively. In a limited study in premature neonates who received 6-mg/kg doses of fluconazole IV every 72 hours, peak serum concentrations of the drug ranged from 3.7–10.2 mcg/mL after the first dose and from 6–17.8 mcg/mL after the third dose (day 7).

Food

Data from a pharmacokinetic study in healthy individuals indicate that administration with a high-fat meal does not affect peak plasma concentrations or AUC of fluconazole compared with administration in the fasting state.

● *Distribution*

Fluconazole is widely distributed into body tissues and fluids following oral or IV administration. Studies in mice using IV doses of radiolabeled fluconazole indicate that the drug is evenly distributed throughout body tissues. In adult humans with normal renal function, concentrations of the drug attained in urine and skin may be 10 times higher than concurrent plasma concentrations; concentrations attained in saliva, sputum, nails, blister fluid, blister skin, and vaginal tissue are approximately equal to concurrent plasma concentrations. Concentrations attained in vaginal secretions following administration of a single 150-mg oral dose reportedly are about 40–86% of concurrent plasma concentrations. Fluconazole concentrations in prostatic tissue reportedly average about 30% of concurrent plasma concentrations. In adults with bronchiectasis who received a single 150-mg oral dose of fluconazole, sputum concentrations of the drug in samples obtained at 4 and 24 hours after the dose averaged 3.7 and 2.23 mcg/mL, respectively, and were approximately equal to concurrent plasma concentrations. Studies in rabbits indicate that high concentrations of fluconazole are attained in the cornea, aqueous humor, and vitreous body following IV administration; these concentrations were higher in inflamed than uninflamed eyes.

Fluconazole, unlike some azole-derivative antifungals (e.g., itraconazole, ketoconazole), distributes readily into CSF following oral or IV administration; CSF concentrations of fluconazole may be 50–94% of concurrent plasma concentrations regardless of the degree of meningeal inflammation. In adults with coccidioidal meningitis who received an oral fluconazole dosage of 50 or 100 mg daily, CSF concentrations of the drug in samples obtained 0.5–8 hours after a dose averaged 0.7–2.1 or 3.5–5.3 mcg/mL, respectively.

The apparent volume of distribution of fluconazole approximates that of total body water and has been reported to be 0.7–1 L/kg. In a limited study, the estimated volume of distribution at steady state of fluconazole was slightly lower in HIV-infected adults than in healthy adults.

Unlike some azole-derivative antifungals (e.g., itraconazole, ketoconazole, miconazole), which are highly protein bound, fluconazole is only 11–12% bound to plasma proteins.

It is not known whether fluconazole crosses the placenta in humans. The drug crosses the placenta in rats, and concentrations in amniotic fluid, placenta, fetus, and fetal liver are approximately equal to maternal plasma concentrations. Fluconazole is distributed into human milk in concentrations similar to those attained in plasma. Following administration of a single 150-mg oral dose in nursing women, peak plasma fluconazole concentrations were 2.61 mcg/mL (range: 1.57–3.65 mcg/mL).

● Elimination

The plasma elimination half-life of fluconazole in adults with normal renal function is approximately 30 hours (range: 20–50 hours). In one study, plasma elimination half-life of the drug was 22 hours after the first day of therapy and 23.8 and 28.6 hours after 7 and 26 days of therapy, respectively. In a limited, single-dose study in HIV-infected adults, the plasma elimination half-life of fluconazole averaged 32 hours (range: 25–42 hours) in those with absolute helper/inducer ($CD4^+$, $T4^+$) T-cell counts greater than $200mm^3$ and 50 hours (range: 32–69 hours) in those with $CD4^+$ T-cell counts less than $200mm^3$. In other single-dose studies in a limited number of HIV-infected adults with $CD4^+$ T-cell counts less than $200mm^3$, the plasma elimination half-life of the drug averaged 35–40 hours (range 22–75 hours).

The mean plasma half-life of fluconazole in children 9 months to 15 years of age has ranged from about 15–25 hours. In a limited study in premature neonates who received IV fluconazole once every 72 hours, the plasma half-life decreased over time, averaging 88 hours after the first dose and 55 hours after the fifth dose (day 13).

In patients with impaired renal function, plasma concentrations of fluconazole are higher and the half-life prolonged; elimination half-life of the drug is inversely proportional to the patient's creatinine clearance. In addition, elimination of the drug may be impaired in geriatric patients because of decreased kidney function in this age group. The elimination half-life of fluconazole reportedly is not affected by impaired hepatic function.

In healthy adults, fluconazole is eliminated principally by renal excretion. Renal clearance of the drug averages 0.27 mL/minute per kg in adults with normal renal function. In a limited, single-dose study, renal clearance of fluconazole averaged 0.79 L/hour in healthy adults, 0.58 L/hour in HIV-infected adults with $CD4^+$ T-cell counts greater than $200mm^3$, and 0.2 L/hour in those with $CD4^+$ T-cell counts less than $200mm^3$. Approximately 60–80% of a single oral or IV dose of fluconazole is excreted in urine unchanged, and about 11% is excreted in urine as metabolites. Small amounts of the drug are excreted in feces.

Fluconazole is removed by hemodialysis and peritoneal dialysis. The amount of the drug removed during hemodialysis depends on several factors (e.g., type of coil used, dialysis flow rate). A 3-hour period of hemodialysis generally decreases plasma concentrations of the drug by 50%. In 2 adults with fungal peritonitis undergoing continuous ambulatory peritoneal dialysis (CAPD) and receiving an oral fluconazole dosage of 100 mg/kg daily, concentrations of the drug in peritoneal dialysis fluid ranged from 2.3–9 mcg/mL and concurrent plasma concentrations ranged from 3.2–9 mcg/mL.

CHEMISTRY AND STABILITY

● Chemistry

Fluconazole, a synthetic triazole derivative, is an azole antifungal agent. The drug is structurally related to imidazole-derivative azole antifungals (e.g., butoconazole, clotrimazole, econazole, ketoconazole, miconazole, oxiconazole) since it contains a 5-membered azole ring attached by a carbon-nitrogen bond to other aromatic rings. However, imidazoles have 2 nitrogens in the azole ring (imidazole ring) and fluconazole and other triazoles (e.g., itraconazole, terconazole) have 3 nitrogens in the ring (triazole ring).

Replacement of the imidazole ring with a triazole ring apparently results in increased antifungal activity and an expanded antifungal spectrum of activity. In addition to this triazole ring, fluconazole contains a second triazole ring and thus is a bistriazole derivative. Presence of these triazole rings may contribute to fluconazole's resistance to first-pass metabolism and the drug's low lipophilicity and protein binding. However, other structural modifications to bistriazole derivatives also affect these characteristics since itraconazole, which also is a bistriazole, is highly lipophilic and protein bound and undergoes extensive hepatic metabolism. Presence of a halogenated phenyl ring increases antifungal activity of bistriazole derivatives and the 2,4-difluorophenyl derivative (fluconazole) has an aqueous solubility suitable for IV formulation.

Fluconazole occurs as a white crystalline powder and is slightly soluble in water, having an aqueous solubility of 8 mg/mL at 37°C. The drug has a solubility of 25 mg/mL in alcohol at room temperature. Fluconazole has a pK_a of 1.76 at 24°C in 0.1 M sodium chloride. Fluconazole injections are sterile, iso-osmotic solutions of the drug in a sodium chloride or dextrose diluent; each mL contains 2 mg of fluconazole and either 9 mg of sodium chloride or 56 mg of dextrose. The

injections have an osmolarity of 300–315 mOsm/L; the pH ranges from 4–8 in the sodium chloride diluent and from 3.5–6.5 in the dextrose diluent.

● Stability

Fluconazole tablets should be stored in tight containers at a temperature less than 30°C; fluconazole powder for oral suspension should be stored at a temperature less than 30°C. After reconstitution, refrigeration of fluconazole oral suspension is not necessary and freezing of the suspension should be avoided. The manufacturer states that the reconstituted suspension is stable for 14 days when stored at 5–30°C and any unused suspension should be discarded after this period.

Commercially available fluconazole injection provided in glass bottles should be stored at 5–30°C and protected from freezing. Fluconazole injection provided in Viaflex® Plus plastic containers should be stored at 5–25°C and protected from freezing; brief exposure of the drug in Viaflex® Plus containers to temperatures up to 40°C will not adversely affect the injection. Commercially available fluconazole injection in glass or plastic containers is stable for 24 or 18 months, respectively, following the date of manufacture. The Viaflex® Plus plastic containers are fabricated from specially formulated polyvinyl chloride (PVC). The amount of water that can permeate from inside the container into the overwrap is insufficient to substantially affect the solution. Solutions in contact with the plastic can leach out some of its chemical components in very small amounts (e.g., bis(2-ethylhexyl)phthalate BEHP, DEHP in up to 5 ppm) within the expiration period of the injection; however, safety of the plastic has been confirmed in tests in animals according to USP biological tests for plastic containers as well as by tissue culture toxicity studies. Additives should not be introduced into the glass or Viaflex® Plus containers of commercially available fluconazole injection.

PREPARATIONS

Excipients in commercially available drug preparations may have clinically important effects in some individuals; consult specific product labeling for details.

Fluconazole

Oral		
For suspension	50 mg/5 mL*	Diflucan®, Pfizer
		Fluconazole for Oral Suspension
	200 mg/5 mL	Diflucan®, Pfizer
		Fluconazole for Oral Suspension
Tablets	50 mg*	Diflucan®, Pfizer
		Fluconazole Tablets
	100 mg*	Diflucan®
		Fluconazole Tablets
	150 mg*	Diflucan®, Pfizer
		Fluconazole Tablets
	200 mg*	Diflucan®, Pfizer
		Fluconazole Tablets

* available from one or more manufacturer, distributor, and/or repackager by generic (nonproprietary) name

Fluconazole in Dextrose

Parenteral		
Injection, for IV infusion only	2 mg/mL (200 or 400 mg) in 5.6% Dextrose*	Diflucan® in Iso-osmotic Dextrose Injection (in Viaflex® Plus [Baxter]), Pfizer
		Fluconazole in Iso-osmotic Dextrose Injection

* available from one or more manufacturer, distributor, and/or repackager by generic (nonproprietary) name

Fluconazole in Sodium Chloride

Parenteral		
Injection, for IV infusion only	2 mg/mL (200 or 400 mg) in 0.9% Sodium Chloride*	Diflucan® in Iso-osmotic Sodium Chloride Injection (in glass and Viaflex® Plus [Baxter]), Pfizer
		Fluconazole in Iso-osmotic Sodium Chloride Injection

* available from one or more manufacturer, distributor, and/or repackager by generic (nonproprietary) name

† Use is not currently included in the labeling approved by the US Food and Drug Administration.

Selected Revisions October 3, 2016, © Copyright, July 1, 1990, American Society of Health-System Pharmacists, Inc.

Isavuconazonium Sulfate

8:14.08 • AZOLES

■ Isavuconazonium sulfate, a prodrug of isavuconazole, is a triazole antifungal agent; isavuconazole is active against certain fungi.

USES

● Aspergillosis

Isavuconazonium sulfate is used for the treatment of invasive aspergillosis, and has been designated an orphan drug by FDA for this indication. Isavuconazonium for injection is indicated for use in adults and pediatric patients 1 year of age and older; the capsules are indicated for use in adults and pediatric patients 6 years of age and older who weigh ≥16 kg.

Clinical Experience

Safety and efficacy of isavuconazonium sulfate were evaluated in a randomized, double-blind, active-controlled, noninferiority, phase 3 trial (SECURE) in 516 adults (mean age 51 years, 60% male, 78% white, 66% neutropenic, 84% with hematologic malignancy, 95% with pulmonary involvement) with proven, probable, or possible primary invasive fungal disease caused by Aspergillus or other filamentous fungi. Patients were randomized to receive IV isavuconazonium sulfate (loading dosage of 372 mg [equivalent to 200 mg of isavuconazole] every 8 hours for the first 48 hours) or IV voriconazole (loading dosage of 6 mg/kg every 12 hours for the first 24 hours, followed by 4 mg/kg every 12 hours for the next 24 hours). After 48 hours, patients in the isavuconazonium group received IV or oral isavuconazonium sulfate (maintenance dosage of 372 mg [equivalent to 200 mg of isavuconazole] once every 24 hours) and patients in the voriconazole group continued IV therapy (maintenance dosage of 4 mg/kg every 12 hours) or were switched to oral voriconazole (maintenance dose of 200 mg every 12 hours) for a maximum total treatment duration of 84 days. At least one Aspergillus species was identified in 30% of patients; the most commonly identified pathogens were A. fumigatus and A. flavus.

The all-cause mortality rate through day 42 in the intent-to-treat population (the primary end point) was 19% in the isavuconazonium group and 20% in the voriconazole group; similar results were observed in the subgroup of patients with proven or probable invasive aspergillosis confirmed by serology, culture, or histology. Based on prespecified clinical, mycologic, and radiologic criteria in this subgroup, overall success rate at the end of treatment was 35% in the isavuconazonium group and 38.9% in the voriconazole group. These data indicate that isavuconazonium sulfate is noninferior to voriconazole for the treatment of invasive aspergillosis.

Clinical Perspective

The Infectious Diseases Society of America (IDSA) considers IV voriconazole the drug of choice for primary treatment of invasive aspergillosis; liposomal amphotericin B and isavuconazonium sulfate are the recommended alternatives for primary treatment of such infections. For salvage therapy in patients refractory to or intolerant of primary antifungal therapy, IDSA recommends IV liposomal amphotericin B, an IV echinocandin (caspofungin, micafungin), oral or IV posaconazole, or itraconazole oral suspension.

● Mucormycosis

Isavuconazonium sulfate is used for the treatment of invasive mucormycosis, and has been designated an orphan drug by FDA for this indication. Isavuconazonium for injection is indicated for use in adults and pediatric patients 1 year of age and older; the capsules are indicated for use in adults and pediatric patients 6 years of age and older who weigh ≥16 kg.

Clinical Experience

Safety and efficacy of isavuconazonium sulfate for the treatment of mucormycosis were evaluated in a single-arm, open-label, phase 3 trial in a subset of 37 adults (mean age 49 years, 81% male, 68% white, 27% neutropenic, 60% with hematologic malignancy, 59% with pulmonary involvement) with proven or probable invasive mucormycosis (VITAL). Patients received IV or oral isavuconazonium sulfate (loading dosage of 372 mg [equivalent to 200 mg of isavuconazole] every 8 hours for the first 48 hours followed by a maintenance dosage of 372 mg [equivalent to 200 mg of isavuconazole] once every 24 hours). Patients were stratified by treatment status into 3 groups: those receiving isavuconazonium for initial treatment (primary treatment group), those with disease refractory to other antifungal therapy (refractory treatment group), and those with intolerance to other antifungal therapy (intolerant treatment group). The most commonly identified pathogens were Rhizopus oryzae, Mucor, and Mucormycetes (not otherwise specified).

The all-cause mortality rate through day 42 (the primary end point) was 38% overall and 33, 45–46, and 40% in the primary, refractory, and intolerant treatment groups, respectively. Median treatment duration in these treatment groups was 102, 33, and 85 days, respectively. The response success rate at the end of treatment was 31% overall and 32, 36, and 20% in the primary, refractory, and intolerant treatment groups, respectively. These data provide evidence that isavuconazonium sulfate is effective for the treatment of mucormycosis when historical data for untreated mucormycosis are used as the basis for comparison; invasive mucormycosis has a mortality rate approaching 100% if left untreated. Efficacy of isavuconazonium sulfate for the treatment of invasive mucormycosis has not been evaluated to date in controlled, comparative clinical trials.

Clinical Perspective

The European Confederation of Medical Mycology in cooperation with the Mycoses Study Group Education and Research Consortium published a global guideline for the diagnosis and management of mucormycosis in 2019. The guideline strongly recommends liposomal amphotericin as first-line treatment of mucormycosis across all patterns of organ involvement. IV isavuconazonium or IV or oral posaconazole (delayed-release tablets) are moderately recommended as first-line treatments. In the salvage setting, both isavuconazonium and posaconazole are strongly recommended treatment options.

● Candida Infections

Esophageal Candidiasis

Isavuconazonium sulfate has been used for the treatment of esophageal candidiasis†, and is recommended as an alternative for the treatment of such infections.

Esophageal candidiasis requires treatment with a systemic antifungal (not a topical antifungal).

IDSA published guidelines for the management of candidiasis in 2016. The guidelines recommend oral fluconazole as the preferred drug of choice for the treatment of esophageal candidiasis; if oral therapy is not tolerated, these experts recommend IV fluconazole or an IV echinocandin (anidulafungin, caspofungin, micafungin) and state that IV amphotericin B is another alternative. For fluconazole-refractory esophageal candidiasis, IDSA recommends itraconazole oral solution or oral or IV voriconazole; alternatives include an IV echinocandin (anidulafungin, caspofungin, micafungin), IV amphotericin B, or oral posaconazole (oral suspension or delayed-release tablets). Isavuconazonium was recently approved when the IDSA guideline was published, and therefore there is no discussion regarding place of therapy in the guideline.

For the treatment of esophageal candidiasis in adults with human immunodeficiency virus (HIV) infection, joint guidelines published by the US Centers for Disease Control and Prevention (CDC), National Institutes of Health (NIH), and IDSA recommend IV or oral fluconazole or itraconazole oral solution. Alternatives recommended for such patients include oral or IV voriconazole, oral isavuconazonium sulfate, an IV echinocandin (anidulafungin, caspofungin, micafungin), or IV amphotericin B.

Clinical Experience

Safety and efficacy of isavuconazonium sulfate for the treatment of uncomplicated esophageal candidiasis† were evaluated in a phase 2, randomized, double-blind, parallel-group, noninferiority trial in adults that compared 3 different dosage regimens of oral isavuconazonium sulfate with a regimen of oral fluconazole. A total of 160 eligible adults 18–65 years of age (37% had HIV infection) were randomized to receive 372 mg of oral isavuconazonium sulfate (equivalent to 200 mg of isavuconazole) on day 1 followed by 93 mg of oral isavuconazonium sulfate (equivalent to 50 mg of isavuconazole) once daily (arm A); 744 mg of oral isavuconazonium sulfate (equivalent to 400 mg of isavuconazole) on day 1 followed by 744 mg of oral isavuconazonium sulfate (equivalent to 400 mg of isavuconazole) once weekly given on days 7, 14, and 21 (arm B); 744 mg of oral isavuconazonium sulfate (equivalent to 400 mg of isavuconazole) on day 1 followed by 186 mg of oral isavuconazonium sulfate (equivalent to 100 mg of isavuconazole) once daily (arm C); or 200 mg of oral fluconazole on day 1 followed by 100 mg of oral fluconazole once daily (arm D). The duration of treatment was based on disease severity and clinical response with a minimum duration of 14 days and a maximum duration of 21 days. The primary efficacy end point was endoscopically confirmed clinical response at the end of treatment. Overall, 95.4% of patients in the per-protocol population achieved endoscopically confirmed clinical success at the end of treatment and each of the oral isavuconazonium sulfate regimens (arms A, B, and C) were noninferior to the oral fluconazole regimen (arm D). The oral isavuconazonium sulfate regimens were generally well tolerated; however, adverse GI effects (diarrhea, nausea, vomiting, gastritis) occurred more frequently in patients in arm C than in those treated with the other isavuconazonium sulfate regimens or the fluconazole regimen.

Candidemia and Other Invasive Candida Infections

Isavuconazonium sulfate has been used in some patients for the treatment of candidemia and other invasive infections caused by *Candida*†, and has been designated an orphan drug by FDA for the treatment of invasive candidiasis/candidemia. IDSA provides recommendations for the treatment of candidemia and invasive candidiasis; isavuconazonium was recently approved when the guidelines were published.

Clinical Experience

Safety and efficacy of isavuconazonium sulfate for the treatment of candidemia and other invasive *Candida* infections were evaluated in a phase 3, randomized, double-blind, noninferiority trial (ACTIVE). A total of 450 adults were randomized to receive treatment with IV isavuconazonium sulfate (loading dosage of 372 mg of isavuconazonium sulfate [equivalent to 200 mg of isavuconazole] 3 times daily on days 1 and 2 followed by a maintenance dosage of 372 mg of isavuconazonium sulfate [equivalent to 200 mg of isavuconazole] once daily) or IV caspofungin (single dose of 70 mg on day 1 followed by 50 mg [70 mg in those weighing more than 80 kg] once daily). After 10 days of the IV regimen, patients who were not neutropenic could be switched to an oral regimen at the discretion of the investigator; those receiving IV isavuconazonium sulfate could be switched to 372 mg of oral isavuconazonium sulfate (equivalent to 200 mg of isavuconazole) once daily and those receiving IV caspofungin could be switched to oral voriconazole (400 mg twice daily on day 1 of oral dosing followed by 200 mg twice daily). Treatment was continued until at least 14 days after the last positive blood culture (up to a maximum total duration of 56 days). Results for the primary end point of overall response at the end of IV therapy (EOIVT) failed to demonstrate noninferiority of isavuconazonium sulfate relative to caspofungin based on the prespecified noninferiority margin; the overall response at EOIVT in the modified intent-to-treat population was 60.3% in patients treated with isavuconazonium sulfate and 71.1% in those treated with caspofungin. The overall response rates at the secondary end point (2 weeks after the end of treatment) were similar in both treatment groups (54.8% in the isavuconazonium sulfate group and 57.2% in the caspofungin group) and all-cause mortality rates on days 14 and 56 were comparable in both treatment groups.

● Coccidioidomycoses

Isavuconazonium sulfate has been used for the treatment of coccidioidomycosis,† more commmonly known as Valley Fever, which is an invasive fungal infection caused by *Coccidioides immitis* and *Coccidioides posadasii*. The majority of coccidioidomycosis infections are asymptomatic in nature; however, the most common clinical presentation in diagnosed cases is acute or subacute pneumonic illness. Extrapulmonary dissemination may occur at virtually any body site with the most frequently involved being the skin, skeletal system, and meninges.

IDSA released clinical practice guidelines for the treatment of coccidioidomycosis in 2016. The guideline states that for patients with newly diagnosed, uncomplicated coccidioidal pneumonia, an orally absorbed azole antifungal should be initiated in select patients (e.g., those with significantly debilitating illness, extensive pulmonary involvement, concurrent diabetes, or otherwise frail due to age or comorbidities). Oral azole antifungal therapy is also recommended in cases of extrapulmonary soft tissue coccidioidomycosis, bone and joint coccidioidomycosis (except severe disease), and coccidioidal meningitis. For patients with coccidioidal meningitis, azole antifungal treatment is recommended for life.

For the treatment of coccidioidal meningitis in adults and adolescents with HIV infection, joint guidelines published by CDC, NIH, and IDSA recommend IV or oral fluconazole therapy. Isavuconazonium is among one of several antifungal agents that may be used as an alternative treatment.

There are limited published data on the use of isavuconazonium for the treatment of coccidioidomycosis; however, this azole antifungal therapy may be a treatment option for select patients. A retrospective review evaluated the efficacy of isavuconazonium in the treatment of coccidioidal meningitis in 9 patients (median age: 46 years; 8 men). All patients were administered fluconazole as an initial therapy, and 8 were subsequently transitioned to voriconazole therapy. All 9 patients were eventually administered isavuconazonium due to treatment failure or the presence of treatment-related adverse effects. At the last assessment, the mean time on isavuconazonium therapy was 504 days (range: 274-810 days) per patient. Three patients had a successful response and 6 had stable disease per Mycosis Study Group (MSG) scoring criteria. No isavuconazonium treatment failures were noted; however, a single patient was transitioned back to voriconazole due to worsening dyspepsia with isavuconazole.

In another retrospective review, the experience of 2 high-volume centers treating 82 patients with chronic forms of coccidioidomycosis with isavuconazonium was detailed. The median age of included patients was 52.5 years (range: 22-86 years) and 71% were male. The majority of patients had pulmonary disease (55%) with 17%, 39%, and 9% having joint/bone, meningitis, and skin/soft tissue involvement, respectively. Prior antifungal therapy included liposomal amphotericin B, fluconazole, itraconazole, voriconazole, and posaconazole. Medication intolerance and disease refractory to prior antifungal therapy were the most common reasons for a therapeutic change to isavuconazonium. Disease improvement was noted in 57 (70%) of the 82 patients following a change to isavuconazonium; no change and worsening of disease status was documented in 17 (21%) and 8 (10%) patients, respectively. The median treatment duration for isavuconazonium in all patients was 897 days (interquartile range: 416-1308) and therapeutic responses were seen across all patient groups including those with meningitis. Three patients discontinued isavuconazonium due to potential adverse events (palpitations, transaminitis, and hot flashes). Five patients with meningitis experienced treatment failure.

DOSAGE AND ADMINISTRATION

● General

Pretreatment Screening

- Obtain specimens for fungal culture and other relevant laboratory studies (including histopathology) to isolate and identify causative organism(s) prior to initiating isavuconazonium therapy.

- Evaluate liver-related laboratory tests at the initiation of isavuconazonium therapy.

Patient Monitoring

- Evaluate liver-related laboratory tests during therapy and monitor patients who have abnormal test results for the development of more severe hepatic injury.

- Monitor for signs and symptoms of hypersensitivity reactions.

● Administration

Isavuconazonium sulfate is administered orally or by IV infusion.

The injection formulation may also be administered via a nasogastric (NG) tube. Do not administer the capsules through a nasogastric tube.

Oral Administration

The capsule formulation is intended for use in patients 6 years of age or older who weigh 16 kg or greater.

Isavuconazonium sulfate capsules may be given orally without regard to meals.

Capsules should be swallowed whole and should *not* be chewed, crushed, dissolved, or opened.

The capsules should be stored at 20-25°C (excursions permitted beteween 15-30°C) in the original packaging to protect from moisture.

Nasogastric Administration

Isavuconazonium sulfate for injection may be administered via NG tube in patients 6 years of age and older weighing ≥16 kg. The drug must be reconstituted prior to NG administration. A vial containing 372 mg of isavuconazonium sulfate lyophilized powder should be reconstituted by adding 5 mL of sterile water for injection; the resultant solution contains 74.4 mg/mL of isavuconazonium sulfate.

The appropriate volume of the reconstituted solution (based on the adult or pediatric dosage) should be withdrawn from the vial using an appropriate syringe and needle. The needle should be discarded and the syringe capped. For administration, the cap from the syringe should be removed and the syringe should be connected to the NG tube to deliver the dose. After dose delivery, three 5 mL water rinses should be administered to the NG tube.

For NG tube administration, the reconstituted solution should be stored between 5-25°C and administered within 1 hour of reconstitution.

IV Administration

Isavuconazonium sulfate for injection should be administered *only* by IV infusion. The drug should *not* be administered by rapid or direct IV injection.

Other IV drugs should not be infused simultaneously with isavuconazonium sulfate.

The IV line to be used for infusion of isavuconazonium sulfate solutions should be flushed with 0.9% sodium chloride injection or 5% dextrose injection before and after infusion of the drug.

Reconstituted and diluted isavuconazonium sulfate solutions *must* be administered using an IV infusion set with an inline membrane filter that has a pore size of 0.2-1.2 µm.

Vials of isavuconazonium sulfate lyophilized powder for injection contain no preservatives and are intended for single use only.

Unreconstituted vials should be stored at 2-8°C in a refrigerator.

Reconstitution and Dilution

Isavuconazonium sulfate for injection must be reconstituted and further diluted prior to IV infusion. Strict aseptic technique must be observed when preparing IV solutions of the drug.

Vials labeled as containing 372 mg of isavuconazonium sulfate should be reconstituted by adding 5 mL of sterile water for injection; the resultant solution contains 74.4 mg/mL of isavuconazonium sulfate. The vial should be gently shaken to completely dissolve the lyophilized powder. Reconstituted solutions should be visually inspected for particulate matter and discoloration; the reconstituted solution should appear clear and free of visible particulates. The reconstituted solution should be immediately diluted, but may be stored between 5-25°C for a maximum of 1 hour prior to dilution.

Reconstituted isavuconazonium sulfate must then be further diluted by removing the appropriate volume of the reconstituted solution (based on the adult or pediatric dosage) from the vial and adding it to an IV infusion bag containing 250 mL of 0.9% sodium chloride injection or 5% dextrose injection to yield a solution containing approximately 1.5 mg of isavuconazonium sulfate per mL. A smaller volume infusion bag of compatible diluent may be used as long as the final concentration does not exceed approximately 1.5 mg/mL. Translucent to white particulates of isavuconazole may be visible in the diluted solution; the IV bag should be gently mixed or rolled to minimize the formation of particulates. Any unnecessary vibration or vigorous shaking of the solution should be avoided; a pneumatic transport system should *not* be used to transport the diluted solution.

Because reconstituted and diluted isavuconazonium sulfate solutions *must* be administered using an infusion set with an inline membrane filter that has a pore size of 0.2-1.2 µm, a reminder sticker for the use of the inline filter should be applied to the IV bag.

IV infusion of isavuconazonium sulfate solutions should be completed within 6 hours after dilution when stored at room temperature. Alternatively, the solution

may be refrigerated at 2-8°C immediately after dilution and the IV infusion completed within 24 hours after dilution. The solution should *not* be frozen.

Rate of Administration

Isavuconazonium sulfate solutions should be administered by IV infusion over at least 1 hour.

● Dosage

Isavuconazonium sulfate is a prodrug that is inactive until metabolized in vivo to isavuconazole. Dosage of the drug usually is expressed in terms of the prodrug (i.e., isavuconazonium sulfate), but also has been expressed in terms of isavuconazole.

Each 186 mg of isavuconazonium sulfate is equivalent to 100 mg of isavuconazole.

Oral and IV dosages of isavuconazonium sulfate are identical; bioequivalence has been demonstrated between the dosage forms. Switching between the oral and IV routes is acceptable; a loading dosage is not needed when switching between the oral and IV preparations.

Adult Dosage

Aspergillosis

For the treatment of invasive aspergillosis in adults, an oral or IV loading dosage of 372 mg of isavuconazonium sulfate (equivalent to 200 mg of isavuconazole) should be given every 8 hours for 6 doses; beginning 12–24 hours after the final loading dose, therapy should be continued using a maintenance dosage of 372 mg of isavuconazonium sulfate (equivalent to 200 mg of isavuconazole) once every 24 hours. Table 1 summarizes the recommended loading and maintenance doses for oral and IV dosage forms.

TABLE 1. Recommended Dosage of Isavuconazonium Sulfate in Adults.

Dosage Form	Loading Dose	Maintenance Dose
Injection (372 mg/vial)	One reconstituted vial (372 mg) every 8 hours for 6 doses	One reconstituted vial (372 mg) once daily
Capsules (186 mg)	Two 186 mg capsules (372 mg) every 8 hours for 6 doses	Two 186 mg capsules (372 mg) once daily
Capsules (74.5 mg)	Five 74.5 mg capsules (372 mg) every 8 hours for 6 doses	Five 74.5 mg capsules (372 mg) once daily

The total duration of IV and oral therapy should be based on the severity of the patient's underlying disease, recovery from immunosuppression, and response to the drug. In a clinical study in adults with invasive aspergillosis, the mean duration of isavuconazonium sulfate therapy was 45 days and the protocol-defined maximum treatment duration was 84 days. The Infectious Diseases Society of America (IDSA) recommends that treatment of invasive pulmonary aspergillosis be continued for at least 6–12 weeks.

Mucormycosis

For the treatment of invasive mucormycosis in adults, an oral or IV loading dosage of 372 mg of isavuconazonium sulfate (equivalent to 200 mg of isavuconazole) should be given every 8 hours for 6 doses; beginning 12–24 hours after the final loading dose, therapy should be continued using a maintenance dosage of 372 mg of isavuconazonium sulfate (equivalent to 200 mg of isavuconazole) once daily. See Table 1 for recommended loading and maintenance doses for oral and IV dosage forms.

The total duration of IV and oral therapy should be based on the severity of the patient's underlying disease, recovery from immunosuppression, and response to the drug. In a clinical study in adults with invasive mucormycosis, the median treatment duration of isavuconazonium sulfate therapy was 102, 33, or 85 days in those receiving the drug for initial treatment (primary treatment), disease refractory to other antifungal therapy, or intolerance to other antifungal therapy, respectively.

Esophageal Candidiasis

If oral isavuconazonium sulfate is used as an alternative for the treatment of esophageal candidiasis† in adults with human immunodeficiency virus (HIV) infection, the US Centers for Disease Control and Prevention (CDC), National Institutes of Health (NIH), and IDSA state that 3 different dosage regimens of the drug can be considered. A loading dose of 372 mg of isavuconazonium sulfate (equivalent to 200 mg of isavuconazole) can be given followed by 93 mg of isavuconazonium sulfate (equivalent to 50 mg of isavuconazole) once daily or a loading dose of 744 mg of isavuconazonium sulfate (equivalent to 400 mg of isavuconazole) can be given followed by 186 mg of isavuconazonium sulfate (equivalent to 100 mg of isavuconazole) once daily. Alternatively, a once-weekly regimen of 744 mg of isavuconazonium sulfate (equivalent to 400 mg of isavuconazole) can be used.

CDC, NIH, and IDSA recommend that treatment of esophageal candidiasis be continued for 14–21 days.

Pediatric Patients

Aspergillosis

For the treatment of invasive aspergillosis, the dosage of isavuconazonium sulfate in pediatric patients is based on dosage form, age, and body weight. Table 2 summarizes the recommended loading and maintenance doses of isavuconazonium sulfate in pediatric patients.

TABLE 2. Recommended Dosage of Isavuconazonium Sulfate in Pediatric Patients

Dosage Form	Age	Body Weight (kg)	Loading Dose	Maintenance Dose [a]
Injection (372 mg/vial)	1 to <3 years	<18	15 mg/kg every 8 hours for 6 doses	15 mg/kg once daily
	3 to <18 years	<37	10 mg/kg every 8 hours for 6 doses	10 mg/kg once daily
		≥37	One reconstituted vial (372 mg) every 8 hours for 6 doses	One reconstituted vial (372 mg) once daily
Capsules 74.5 mg	6 to <18 years	16 to <18	Two capsules (149 mg) every 8 hours for 6 doses	Two capsules (149 mg) once daily
		18 to <25	Three capsules (223.5 mg) every 8 hours for 6 doses	Three capsules (223.5 mg) once daily
		25 to <32	Four capsules (298 mg) every 8 hours for 6 doses	Four capsules (298 mg) once daily
		≥32	Five capsules (372 mg) every 8 hours for 6 doses	Five capsules (372 mg) once daily

[a] Start maintenance doses 12 to 24 hours after the last loading dose.

Mucormycosis

For the treatment of invasive mucormycosis, the dosage of isavuconazonium sulfate in pediatric patients is based on dosage form, age, and body weight (see Table 2).

● Special Populations

Hepatic Impairment

The manufacturer states that dosage adjustments are not needed when isavuconazonium sulfate is used in adults with mild or moderate hepatic impairment (Child-Pugh class A or B). Some clinicians suggest that reduced dosage should be considered in such patients.

Dosage recommendations for those with severe hepatic impairment (Child-Pugh class C) are not available. The drug has not been studied in patients with severe hepatic impairment and should be used in such patients only when benefits outweigh risks.

Renal Impairment

Dosage adjustments are not needed when isavuconazonium sulfate is used in adults with mild, moderate, or severe renal impairment, including those with end-stage renal disease.

Geriatric Patients

Dosage adjustments based on age are not needed when isavuconazonium sulfate is used in geriatric patients.

CAUTIONS

● Contraindications

- Known hypersensitivity to isavuconazole (active metabolite of isavuconazonium sulfate).
- Familial short QT syndrome.
- Concomitant use with strong cytochrome P-450 (CYP) 3A4 inhibitors (e.g., ketoconazole, high-dose ritonavir) or inducers (e.g., rifampin, carbamazepine, St. John's wort [Hypericum perforatum], long-acting barbiturates).

● Warnings/Precautions

Hepatic Adverse Drug Reactions

Serious hepatic effects, including hepatitis, cholestasis, and hepatic failure (sometimes fatal), have been reported in patients with serious underlying medical conditions (e.g., hematologic malignancy) receiving an azole antifungal, including isavuconazonium sulfate.

Less severe hepatic effects (e.g., increased ALT, AST, alkaline phosphatase, total bilirubin concentrations) have been reported in clinical trials of isavuconazonium sulfate. Liver function test elevations generally were reversible and discontinuance of isavuconazonium was not required.

Liver function should be evaluated prior to and monitored during isavuconazonium sulfate therapy. If abnormal liver function test results occur during therapy with the drug, the patient should be monitored for the development of more severe hepatic injury. If signs and symptoms consistent with liver disease develop, isavuconazonium sulfate should be discontinued.

Infusion-related Reactions

Infusion-related reactions, including hypotension, dyspnea, chills, dizziness, paresthesia, and hypoesthesia, have occurred during IV infusion of isavuconazonium sulfate. If an infusion-related reaction occurs, the IV infusion should be discontinued.

Hypersensitivity Reactions

Serious hypersensitivity reactions (e.g., anaphylaxis, including with fatal outcome) have occurred with isavuconazonium sulfate therapy. Symptoms including dyspnea, hypotension, generalized erythema with flushing, and urticaria have been reported; these have often occurred soon after therapy initiation.

Severe skin reactions (e.g., Stevens-Johnson syndrome) have occurred in patients receiving other azole antifungals.

If an anaphylactic or severe adverse cutaneous reaction occurs during isavuconazonium therapy, the drug should be discontinued and supportive treatment initiated if necessary.

No information is available regarding cross-sensitivity of isavuconazonium sulfate and other azole antifungals; however, cross-sensitivity between other triazole agents has been reported. Patients with hypersensitivity to other azoles should be monitored for signs and symptoms of hypersensitivity reactions when administered isavuconazonium sulfate.

Embryo-fetal Toxicity

Isavuconazonium sulfate may cause fetal harm if administered to pregnant women based on animal reproduction study findings. Advise pregnant women of the potential fetal risk.

Isavuconazonium has been shown to cause increased perinatal mortality and skeletal abnormalities when given orally to pregnant rats and rabbits.

Females of reproductive potential should be advised to use an effective contraceptive method during treatment and for 28 days after the last dose.

Drug Interactions

Concomitant use of isavuconazonium sulfate with drugs that are strong cytochrome P-450 (CYP) 3A4 inhibitors (e.g., ketoconazole, high-dose ritonavir) or inducers (e.g., rifampin, carbamazepine, St. John's wort, long-acting barbiturates) is contraindicated.

Drug Particulates

Following dilution, the IV formulation of isavuconazonium sulfate may form a precipitate. Isavuconazonium sulfate should be administered IV through an in-line filter.

Specific Populations

Pregnancy

There are no human data on the use of isavuconazonium sulfate in pregnant women to evaluate for a drug-associated risk of major birth defects, miscarriage, or adverse maternal or fetal outcomes. Based on data from animal reproduction studies, isavuconazonium sulfate may cause fetal harm.

Increased perinatal mortality occurred in rats given oral isavuconazonium sulfate at doses up to 90 mg/kg/day during pregnancy through the weaning period. In addition, increases in the incidences of skeletal abnormalities, including rudimentary cervical ribs and fused zygomatic arches, were observed in the offspring of pregnant rats and rabbits.

Lactation

Isavuconazole is distributed into milk in rats; there are no data on the presence of the drug in human milk, the effects on the breastfed infant, or the effects on milk production. Women receiving isavuconazonium sulfate should not breast-feed.

Females and Males of Reproductive Potential

Isavuconazonium sulfate may cause embryo-fetal harm when administered to pregnant women. Advise female patients of reproductive potential to use effective contraception during treatment and for 28 days after the final dose.

Pediatric Use

For the treatment of invasive aspergillosis, the safety and efficacy of isavuconazonium sulfate for *injection* have been established in pediatric patients ≥1 year of age and for *capsules* in pediatric patients ≥6 years of age weighing ≥16 kg. Use of isavuconazonium sulfate in this age group for treatment of invasive aspergillosis is supported by evidence from one adequate and well-controlled trial in adult patients and additional pharmacokinetic and safety data in pediatric patients ≥1 year of age.

For the treatment of invasive mucormycosis, the safety and efficacy of isavuconazonium sulfate for *injection* have been established in pediatric patients ≥1 year of age and for *capsules* in pediatric patients ≥6 years of age weighing ≥16 kg. Use of isavuconazonium sulfate in this age group for treatment of invasive mucormycosis is supported by one open-label trial in adult patients, a retrospective review of survival data for adult patients, and additional pharmacokinetic and safety data in pediatric patients ≥1 year of age.

Geriatric Use

In phase 2 and 3 trials of isavuconazonium sulfate, 16% of patients were older than 65 years of age and 4% were older than 75 years of age. No substantial differences in pharmacokinetics were observed between geriatric and younger adults. No overall differences in efficacy or safety were seen between geriatric and younger patients; however, greater sensitivity of some older individuals cannot be ruled out.

Hepatic Impairment

Isavuconazonium sulfate has not been studied in patients with severe hepatic impairment (Child-Pugh class C). The drug should be used in patients with severe hepatic impairment only if benefits outweigh risks; if the drug is used in such patients, they should be monitored for adverse effects.

Although hepatic impairment does not affect the extent of in vivo conversion of isavuconazonium sulfate to isavuconazole (the active drug), increased peak plasma concentrations and AUC, reduced clearance, and increased half-life of isavuconazole have been reported in individuals with hepatic impairment. Data from patients with mild or moderate hepatic impairment (Child-Pugh class A or B) indicate that mean peak plasma concentrations of isavuconazole are decreased by 2 or 30%, respectively, and mean AUC of isavuconazole is increased by 64 or 84%, respectively, relative to healthy individuals with normal hepatic function. After IV administration, systemic clearance is decreased by 29 or 48% in individuals with mild or moderate hepatic impairment, respectively, relative to healthy individuals and elimination half-life is increased to 224 or 302 hours, respectively, compared with 123 hours in healthy individuals. Similarly, in a population pharmacokinetic evaluation, isavuconazole clearance was decreased by 40 or 48% in those with mild or moderate hepatic impairment, respectively, relative to the healthy population. The clinical importance of such effects is unknown. The manufacturer states that dosage adjustments are not necessary in patients with mild or moderate hepatic impairment.

Renal Impairment

Clinically important changes in isavuconazole pharmacokinetics (peak plasma concentrations, AUC) were not observed in adults with mild, moderate, or severe renal impairment. Hemodialysis does not remove isavuconazole from the circulation. Dosage adjustments are not needed in patients with renal impairment or in those with end-stage renal disease.

● Common Adverse Effects

The most common adverse reactions in adults include nausea, vomiting, diarrhea, headache, elevated liver chemistry tests, hypokalemia, constipation, dyspnea, cough, peripheral edema, and back pain.

The most common adverse reactions in pediatric patients include diarrhea, abdominal pain, vomiting, elevated liver chemistry tests, rash, nausea, pruritus, and headache.

DRUG INTERACTIONS

Because isavuconazonium sulfate is rapidly metabolized to isavuconazole in vivo, drug interactions are reported for isavuconazole.

● Drugs Affecting or Metabolized by Hepatic Microsomal Enzymes

Isavuconazole is a substrate of cytochrome P-450 (CYP) 3A4, and inhibitors or inducers of CYP3A4 may increase or decrease plasma concentrations of isavuconazole, respectively. Concomitant use of isavuconazonium with potent CYP3A4 inhibitors (e.g., ketoconazole, high-dose ritonavir) or inducers (e.g., rifampin, carbamazepine, St. John's wort [*Hypericum perforatum*], long-acting barbiturates) is contraindicated.

Isavuconazole also is a substrate of CYP3A5. Isavuconazole is a moderate inhibitor of CYP3A4. In vitro, isavuconazole inhibits CYP isoenzymes 2C8, 2C9, 2C19, and 2D6 and induces CYP isoenzymes 3A4, 2B6, 2C8, and 2C9.

● Drugs Affecting or Affected by Transport Proteins

Isavuconazole is a weak inhibitor of the P-glycoprotein (P-gp) transport system. Concomitant use of isavuconazonium sulfate with P-gp substrates that have a narrow therapeutic index (e.g., digoxin) may require dosage adjustment of the P-gp substrate.

Isavuconazole is a weak inhibitor of organic cation transporter (OCT) 2. The drug also is an inhibitor of breast cancer resistance protein (BCRP).

Isavuconazole does not inhibit organic anion transporting polypeptide (OATP) 1B1 or OATP1B3.

● Drugs that Shorten the QT Interval

Concomitant use of isavuconazonium sulfate with other drugs that shorten the corrected QT (QT$_c$) interval has not been evaluated in formal ECG studies; the additive effects of such use are unknown.

● Anticonvulsants

Carbamazepine

Potential pharmacokinetic interactions with carbamazepine (decreased isavuconazole concentrations).

Concomitant use of carbamazepine and isavuconazonium sulfate is contraindicated.

● Antifungal Agents

Ketoconazole

Pharmacokinetic interactions with ketoconazole (9% increase in isavuconazole peak plasma concentration and greater than fivefold increase in isavuconazole area under the concentration-time curve [AUC]).

Concomitant use of ketoconazole and isavuconazonium sulfate is contraindicated.

● Antimycobacterial Agents

Rifampin

Pharmacokinetic interactions with rifampin (75% decrease in isavuconazole peak plasma concentration and 97% decrease in isavuconazole AUC).

Concomitant use of rifampin and isavuconazonium sulfate is contraindicated.

● Barbiturates

Potential pharmacokinetic interactions with long-acting barbiturates (decreased isavuconazole concentrations).

Concomitant use of long-acting barbiturates and isavuconazonium sulfate is contraindicated.

● Bupropion

Pharmacokinetic interactions with bupropion (decreased bupropion exposure).

Bupropion and isavuconazonium sulfate should be used concomitantly with caution; increased bupropion dosage may be necessary but dosage should not exceed the maximum recommended dosage.

● Caffeine

No clinically important effects on caffeine pharmacokinetics.

● Corticosteroids

No clinically important effects on prednisone pharmacokinetics.

● Cyclophosphamide

Cyclophosphamide and isavuconazonium sulfate should be used concomitantly with caution.

● Dextromethorphan

No clinically important effects on dextromethorphan pharmacokinetics.

● Digoxin

Pharmacokinetic interactions with digoxin (increased digoxin exposure).

Digoxin and isavuconazonium sulfate should be used concomitantly with caution; digoxin serum concentrations should be monitored and digoxin dosage adjusted accordingly.

● Estrogens and Progestins

No clinically important effects on the pharmacokinetics of oral contraceptives containing ethinyl estradiol or norethindrone.

● HMG-CoA Reductase Inhibitors

Atorvastatin

Potential pharmacokinetic interactions with atorvastatin (increased atorvastatin exposure).

Atorvastatin and isavuconazonium sulfate should be used concomitantly with caution and patients monitored for atorvastatin-related adverse effects.

● Immunosuppressive Agents

Cyclosporine

Pharmacokinetic interactions with cyclosporine (increased cyclosporine exposure).

Isavuconazonium sulfate and cyclosporine should be used concomitantly with caution; cyclosporine concentrations should be monitored and cyclosporine dosage adjusted accordingly.

Mycophenolate Mofetil

Pharmacokinetic interactions with mycophenolate mofetil (increased mycophenolic acid exposure).

Mycophenolate mofetil and isavuconazonium sulfate should be used concomitantly with caution; patients should be monitored for mycophenolic acid-related toxicities.

Sirolimus

Pharmacokinetic interactions with sirolimus (approximately twofold increase in sirolimus exposure).

Sirolimus and isavuconazonium sulfate should be used concomitantly with caution; sirolimus plasma concentrations should be monitored and sirolimus dosage adjusted accordingly.

Tacrolimus

Pharmacokinetic interactions with tacrolimus (approximately twofold increase in tacrolimus exposure).

Tacrolimus and isavuconazonium sulfate should be used concomitantly with caution; tacrolimus concentrations should be monitored and tacrolimus dosage adjusted accordingly.

● Metformin

No clinically important effects on metformin pharmacokinetics.

● Methadone

No clinically important effects on methadone pharmacokinetics.

● Methotrexate

No clinically important effects on methotrexate pharmacokinetics.

● Midazolam

Pharmacokinetic interactions with midazolam (approximately twofold increase in midazolam exposure).

Midazolam and isavuconazonium sulfate should be used concomitantly with caution; consideration should be given to reducing midazolam dosage.

● Proton-pump Inhibitors

Esomeprazole

No clinically important effects on isavuconazole pharmacokinetics.

Omeprazole

No clinically important effects on omeprazole pharmacokinetics.

● Repaglinide

No clinically important effects on repaglinide pharmacokinetics.

● St. John's Wort

Potential pharmacokinetic interactions with St. John's wort (*Hypericum perforatum*) (decreased isavuconazole concentrations).

Concomitant use of St. John's wort and isavuconazonium sulfate is contraindicated.

● Vincristine

Avoid concomitant use; may increase exposure to vincristine and the risk of vincristine-related adverse reactions.

• *Warfarin*

No clinically important effects on warfarin pharmacokinetics.

DESCRIPTION

Isavuconazonium sulfate, a prodrug of isavuconazole, is a triazole antifungal agent structurally similar to fluconazole and voriconazole. Isavuconazonium is inactive until converted in vivo to isavuconazole.

Like other triazole antifungals, isavuconazole inhibits 14-α-demethylase, which leads to accumulation of methylated sterols (e.g., 14-α-methylated lanosterol, 4,14-dimethylzymosterol, 24-methylenedihydrolanosterol) and decreased concentrations of ergosterol in fungal cell membranes. Depletion of ergosterol affects cell membrane integrity and function and can lead to fungal cell death.

Following oral or IV administration of isavuconazonium sulfate, the drug is rapidly and almost completely (greater than 98%) hydrolyzed by esterases (principally butylcholinesterase) in the blood to yield the active moiety, isavuconazole, and an inactive cleavage product. Peak plasma concentrations of isavuconazole are achieved in approximately 2–4 hours after oral administration and 0.7–1 hour after the start of IV infusion of isavuconazonium sulfate. It has been estimated that steady-state concentrations of isavuconazole are not achieved until after 2 weeks. The absolute bioavailability of isavuconazole following oral administration of isavuconazonium sulfate is 98%. Oral administration of a 744-mg dose of isavuconazonium sulfate with a high-fat meal resulted in a 9% decrease in isavuconazole peak plasma concentrations and a 9% increase in isavuconazole area under the plasma concentration-time curve (AUC); these effects were not considered clinically important. Isavuconazonium sulfate given orally as an IV solution administered via a nasogastric tube provides systemic isavuconazole exposure that is similar to the oral capsule. Isavuconazole is greater than 99% bound to plasma proteins, mainly albumin. In vivo studies indicate that isavuconazole is metabolized by cytochrome P-450 (CYP) isoenzymes 3A4 and 3A5 and, subsequently, by uridine diphosphate-glucuronosyltransferase (UGT). In a single-dose study in adults using oral or IV isavuconazonium sulfate, the mean distribution half-life of isavuconazole was 1.7–2.1 or 0.42–1.6 hours, respectively, and the mean terminal elimination half-life of isavuconazole was 56–77 or 76–104 hours, respectively. Following oral administration of radiolabeled isavuconazonium sulfate, 46% of the total radioactive dose was recovered in feces (approximately 33% as isavuconazole) and 46% was recovered in urine (principally as metabolites of isavuconazole and metabolites of the inactive cleavage product). Less than 1% of a dose of isavuconazonium sulfate is eliminated in urine as active isavuconazole.

• *Spectrum*

Isavuconazole is active in vitro and in clinical infections against *Aspergillus flavus*, *A. fumigatus*, and *A. niger*, and also has in vitro activity against *A. lentulus*, *A. nidulans*, *A. sydowii*, *A. terreus*, *A. versicolor*, and *A. welsitschiae*.

Isavuconazole is active in vitro and in clinical infections against fungi in the order Mucorales, including *Rhizopus* (*R. oryzae*, *R. azygosporus*, *R. microsporus*), *Mucor* (*M. amphibiorum*, *M. circinelloides*), *Lichtheimia* (*L. corymbifera*; formerly *Absidia corymbifera*), and *Rhizomucor* (*R. pusillus*). In vitro studies indicate that isavuconazole is less active against Mucorales compared with *Aspergillus*.

Isavuconazole is active in vitro against *Candida*, including *C. albicans*, *C. dubliniensis*, *C. glabrata*, *C. guilliermondii*, *C. kefyr*, *C. krusei*, *C. lusitaniae*, *C. orthopsilosis*, *C. parapsilosis*, and *C. tropicalis*. Some strains of *C. auris* (often misidentified as *C. haemulonii*, *C. famata*, or *Rhodotorula glutinis*) have been inhibited in vitro by isavuconazole concentrations of 0.004–0.25 mcg/mL. Isavuconazole has in vitro activity against some *Candida* that have reduced susceptibility or resistance to fluconazole.

Although the clinical importance is unclear, isavuconazole also has in vitro activity against *Blastomyces dermatitidis*, *Coccidioides posadasii*, *Cryptococcus gattii*, *C. neoformans*, *Geotrichum capitatum*, *Histoplasma capsulatum*, *Penicillium*, *Pichia*, *Rhodotorula*, *Saccharomyces cerevisiae*, *Scedosporium*, *Trichosporon*, and dermatophytes (*Trichophyton rubrum*, *T. mentagrophytes*, *T. tonsurans*, *Epidermophyton floccosum*, *Microsporum canis*).

• *Resistance*

Resistance or reduced susceptibility to isavuconazole may occur. *Aspergillus* and *Candida* with reduced susceptibility or resistance to isavuconazole have been reported.

Like other azole antifungals, resistance to isavuconazole is likely conferred by multiple mechanisms involving substitutions in the target gene. Resistance to azole antifungals can result from altered cellular accumulation of the drug, increased levels of and/or decreased affinity for the target enzyme, and modifications of the ergosterol biosynthesis pathway. Changes in sterol profile and elevated efflux pump activity have been observed; however, the clinical relevance of such findings is unclear.

Cross-resistance can occur between isavuconazole and other azoles (e.g., itraconazole, voriconazole). Although the relevance of cross-resistance to clinical outcomes has not been fully characterized, alternative antifungal therapy may be required in patients in whom prior azole therapy has failed.

ADVICE TO PATIENTS

- Advise patients that isavuconazonium sulfate can be taken with or without food.

- Inform patients to swallow capsules whole, without crushing, chewing, dissolving, or opening.

- Inform patients that infusion-related reactions, including hypotension, dyspnea, chills, dizziness, paresthesia, and hypoesthesia, have occurred with IV administration.

- Advise patients to inform their physician immediately if they have ever had an allergic reaction to isavuconazole or other antifungal medicines (e.g., ketoconazole, fluconazole, itraconazole, posaconazole, or voriconazole). Advise patients to discontinue therapy and seek immediate medical attention if any signs or symptoms of severe allergic reaction occur.

- Advise patients to inform their clinicians of existing or contemplated concomitant therapy, including prescription and OTC drugs and dietary or herbal supplements, as well as any concomitant illnesses.

- Advise women to inform their clinicians if they are or plan to become pregnant or plan to breastfeed. Advise female patients of reproductive potential to use effective contraception during treatment and for 28 days after the final dose.

- Inform patients of other important precautionary information.

PREPARATIONS

Excipients in commercially available drug preparations may have clinically important effects in some individuals; consult specific product labeling for details.

Isavuconazonium Sulfate

Oral

Capsules	74.5 mg (equivalent to 40 mg isavuconazole)	Cresemba®, Astellas
	186 mg (equivalent to 100 mg isavuconazole)	Cresemba®, Astellas

Parenteral

For injection, for IV infusion	372 mg (equivalent to 200 mg isavuconazole)	Cresemba®, Astellas

† Use is not currently included in the labeling approved by the US Food and Drug Administration.

Selected Revisions July 10, 2024, © Copyright, September 25, 2015, American Society of Health-System Pharmacists, Inc.

Posaconazole

8:14.08 • AZOLES

■ Posaconazole, a synthetic triazole derivative, is an azole antifungal agent.

USES

● Prevention of Invasive Aspergillus and Candida Infections in Immunocompromised Individuals

Oral posaconazole (delayed-release tablets, oral suspension) is used for prophylaxis of invasive *Aspergillus* and *Candida* infections in severely immunocompromised adults and adolescents 13 years of age and older at high risk of developing these infections, including hematopoietic stem cell transplant (HSCT) recipients with graft-versus-host disease (GVHD) or patients with hematologic malignancies and prolonged chemotherapy-associated neutropenia. Alternatively, IV posaconazole is used for such prophylaxis in adults 18 years of age or older.

For primary prophylaxis to prevent invasive aspergillosis in immunocompromised individuals at high risk for such infections (i.e., neutropenic patients with acute myelogenous leukemia [AML] or myelodysplastic syndrome [MDS], HSCT recipients with GVHD), the Infectious Diseases Society of America (IDSA) recommends posaconazole as the drug of choice; itraconazole and micafungin are recommended as alternatives.

IDSA recommends primary prophylaxis against *Candida* infections in neutropenic patients when the risk of invasive candida infection is substantial (e.g., allogeneic HSCT recipients, patients with acute leukemia undergoing intensive remission-induction or salvage-induction chemotherapy) and states that an azole antifungal (fluconazole, itraconazole, posaconazole, voriconazole) or IV echinocandin (caspofungin or micafungin) can be used. These experts state that antifungal prophylaxis is not recommended if the anticipated duration of neutropenia is less than 7 days. If primary prophylaxis is used to prevent invasive candidiasis in high-risk adults in intensive care settings, IDSA recommends fluconazole as the drug of choice and IV echinocandins (anidulafungin, caspofungin, micafungin) as alternatives.

Posaconazole is used for secondary prophylaxis to prevent relapse or recurrence of esophageal candidiasis† in HIV-infected adults and adolescents who have been adequately treated. (See Esophageal Candidiasis under Uses: Candida Infections.)

For additional information on prevention of fungal infections in immunocompromised patients, the current clinical practice guidelines from IDSA available at http://www.idsociety.org should be consulted.

Clinical Experience

Safety and efficacy of posaconazole oral suspension for prophylaxis of invasive *Aspergillus* and *Candida* infections in adults and adolescents 13 years of age or older have been evaluated in a randomized, double-blind comparative study in HSCT recipients with GVHD and in a randomized, open-label comparative study in neutropenic patients receiving cytotoxic chemotherapy for acute myelogenous leukemia or myelodysplastic syndrome.

In the study in HSCT recipients 13 years of age or older with GVHD, patients were randomized to receive posaconazole oral suspension (200 mg 3 times daily) or fluconazole capsules (400 mg once daily) for up to 112 days. The mean duration of prophylaxis with posaconazole or fluconazole was 80 or 77 days, respectively. Results indicate that posaconazole and fluconazole prophylaxis produced similar rates of clinical failure (based on a composite endpoint of proven or probable invasive fungal infections, death, and/or treatment with systemic antifungals) at 16 weeks (33 versus 37%). Breakthrough infections caused by *Aspergillus* were reported in 2% of patients receiving posaconazole compared with 7% of patients receiving fluconazole during the fixed treatment period; the rate of breakthrough infections caused by *Candida* was similar with both drugs.

In the study in neutropenic patients receiving cytotoxic chemotherapy for acute myelogenous leukemia or myelodysplastic syndrome (study NCT00044486), patients were randomized to receive posaconazole oral suspension (200 mg 3 times daily) or either fluconazole oral suspension (400 mg once daily) or itraconazole oral solution (200 mg twice daily); the mean duration of prophylaxis was 29 days with posaconazole and 25 days with fluconazole or itraconazole. Clinical

failure assessed up to 1 week after prophylaxis ended was lower in those receiving posaconazole (27%) than in those receiving fluconazole or itraconazole (42%); at 100 days after randomization, the clinical failure rate was 52 or 64%, respectively. Fewer breakthrough infections caused by *Aspergillus* were reported in patients receiving posaconazole than in those receiving fluconazole or itraconazole; the rates of breakthrough infections caused by *Candida* were similar.

Use of posaconazole delayed-release tablets for prophylaxis of invasive *Aspergillus* and *Candida* infections in adults and adolescents 13 years of age or older is supported by a phase 1/3b safety, tolerability, and pharmacokinetic study evaluating the delayed-release tablets in patients with hematologic malignancies at risk for these infections.

● Candida Infections
Oropharyngeal Candidiasis

Oral posaconazole (oral suspension) is used for the treatment of oropharyngeal candidiasis in adults, including oropharyngeal candidiasis refractory to fluconazole and/or itraconazole.

For the treatment of mild oropharyngeal candidiasis, IDSA recommends topical treatment with clotrimazole lozenges or miconazole buccal tablets; nystatin (oral suspension or tablets) is the recommended alternative. For moderate to severe disease, IDSA recommends oral fluconazole. For fluconazole-refractory oropharyngeal candidiasis, IDSA recommends itraconazole oral solution or posaconazole oral suspension; oral voriconazole or amphotericin B oral suspension (not commercially available in US) are recommended as alternatives. Other alternatives for refractory oropharyngeal candidiasis are IV echinocandins (anidulafungin, caspofungin, micafungin) or IV amphotericin B.

For the treatment of oropharyngeal candidiasis in adults and adolescents with human immunodeficiency virus (HIV) infection, the US Centers for Disease Control and Prevention (CDC), National Institutes of Health (NIH), and IDSA recommend oral fluconazole as the preferred drug of choice for initial episodes. If topical therapy is used for the treatment of mild to moderate episodes, these experts recommend clotrimazole lozenges or miconazole buccal tablets. Alternatives for systemic treatment of oropharyngeal candidiasis in HIV-infected adults and adolescents are itraconazole oral solution or posaconazole oral suspension; nystatin oral suspension is an alternative if topical treatment is used. For fluconazole-refractory oropharyngeal infections in HIV-infected adults and adolescents, posaconazole oral suspension is preferred; itraconazole oral solution is an alternative.

Routine long-term suppressive or maintenance therapy (secondary prophylaxis) to prevent relapse or recurrence is not usually recommended in patients adequately treated for oropharyngeal candidiasis (including HIV-infected individuals) unless the patient has frequent or severe recurrences of oropharyngeal candidiasis. If secondary prophylaxis of oropharyngeal candidiasis is indicated, oral fluconazole is recommended; however, the potential for development of azole resistance should be considered.

For additional information on prophylaxis and treatment of oropharyngeal candidiasis, the current clinical practice guidelines from IDSA available at http://www.idsociety.org and current clinical practice guidelines from CDC, NIH, and IDSA on the prevention and treatment of opportunistic infections in HIV-infected individuals available at http://www.aidsinfo.nih.gov should be consulted.

Clinical Experience

In a randomized, evaluator-blinded study of posaconazole for the treatment of oropharyngeal candidiasis, HIV-infected adults 18 years of age or older with oropharyngeal candidiasis were randomized to receive posaconazole oral suspension (100 mg twice daily for 1 day, followed by 100 mg once daily for 13 days) or fluconazole oral suspension (100 mg twice daily for 1 day, followed by 100 mg once daily for 13 days). Patients evaluated for efficacy included those who received at least one dose of posaconazole or fluconazole and had a baseline oral swish culture positive for *Candida* (*C. albicans* was isolated from most patients). The clinical and mycologic cure rates after 14 days of antifungal therapy and clinical and mycologic relapse rates at 4 weeks posttreatment were similar for posaconazole and fluconazole. Clinical cure (defined as complete or partial resolution of all ulcers and/or plaques and symptoms) at day 14 was attained in 92 or 93% of those receiving posaconazole or fluconazole, respectively. The mycologic cure rate (defined as the absence of colony-forming units in quantitative culture at the end of the 14-day regimen) was 52 or 50% in those receiving posaconazole or fluconazole, respectively. At 4 weeks posttreatment, the rate of clinical relapse (defined as recurrence of signs or symptoms after initial cure or improvement) was 29 or 35% and the rate of mycologic relapse was 56 or 64% in patients receiving posaconazole or fluconazole, respectively.

Efficacy of posaconazole oral suspension for the treatment of oropharyngeal candidiasis refractory to fluconazole or itraconazole was evaluated in a phase 3, open-label, noncomparative study in HIV-infected adults 18 years of age or older. Oropharyngeal candidiasis was considered refractory to fluconazole or itraconazole if the infection failed to improve or worsened after the usual regimen of oral fluconazole (at least 100 mg daily for at least 10 consecutive days) or oral itraconazole (200 mg daily for at least 10 consecutive days) and treatment with these drugs had not been discontinued for more than 14 days prior to initiation of posaconazole. Of 199 adults enrolled in the study, 89 met these criteria for refractory oropharyngeal candidiasis. Forty-five adults with refractory oropharyngeal candidiasis received posaconazole oral suspension (400 mg twice daily for 3 days, followed by 400 mg once daily for 25 days); patients also received optional suppressive or maintenance therapy with the drug (400 mg twice daily 3 times weekly) for 3 additional months. As the result of a protocol amendment to simplify the regimen, the remaining 44 adults with refractory oropharyngeal candidiasis received oral posaconazole (400 mg twice daily for 28 days). Clinical cure or improvement was attained in 74% of patients overall; similar rates of clinical cure or improvement were attained in patients receiving the initial and increased dosage regimens (73 and 75%, respectively).

Esophageal Candidiasis

Although safety and efficacy have not been established, oral posaconazole (oral suspension) has been effective for the treatment of esophageal candidiasist refractory to oral fluconazole and/or itraconazole in HIV-infected adults and has been recommended as an alternative for the treatment of esophageal candidiasis.

Esophageal candidiasis requires treatment with a systemic antifungal (not a topical antifungal).

IDSA recommends oral fluconazole as the preferred drug of choice for the treatment of esophageal candidiasis; if oral therapy is not tolerated, IV fluconazole or an IV echinocandin (anidulafungin, caspofungin, micafungin) usually is recommended and IV amphotericin B is another alternative. For fluconazole-refractory esophageal candidiasis, IDSA recommends itraconazole oral solution or oral or IV voriconazole; alternatives for fluconazole-refractory disease are IV echinocandins (anidulafungin, caspofungin, micafungin) or IV amphotericin B. IDSA states that oral posaconazole (oral suspension or delayed-release tablets) could be considered as another alternative for the treatment of fluconazole-refractory esophageal candidiasis.

For the treatment of esophageal candidiasis in HIV-infected adults and adolescents, CDC, NIH, and IDSA recommend oral or IV fluconazole or itraconazole oral solution. Alternatives include oral or IV voriconazole, an IV echinocandin (caspofungin, micafungin, anidulafungin), or IV amphotericin B. For refractory esophageal candidiasis in HIV-infected adults and adolescents, including fluconazole-refractory infections, these experts recommend posaconazole oral suspension or itraconazole oral solution; alternatives include an IV echinocandin (anidulafungin, caspofungin, micafungin), oral or IV voriconazole, or IV amphotericin B.

Routine long-term suppressive or maintenance therapy (secondary prophylaxis) to prevent relapse or recurrence is not usually recommended in patients adequately treated for esophageal candidiasis (including HIV-infected individuals) unless the patient has frequent or severe recurrences of esophageal candidiasis. If secondary prophylaxis of esophageal candidiasis is indicated, oral fluconazole is recommended and posaconazole oral suspension is a possible alternative; however, the potential for development of azole resistance should be considered.

For additional information on prophylaxis and treatment of esophageal candidiasis, the current clinical practice guidelines from IDSA available at http://www.idsociety.org and current clinical practice guidelines from CDC, NIH, and IDSA on the prevention and treatment of opportunistic infections in HIV-infected individuals available at http://www.aidsinfo.nih.gov should be consulted.

● Aspergillosis

Although safety and efficacy have not been established, posaconazole has been effective in some patients when used as salvage therapy for the treatment of invasive aspergillosist when other antifungals (e.g., voriconazole, amphotericin B, itraconazole) were ineffective or could not be used. In a limited study evaluating posaconazole salvage therapy, the overall success rate was 42% (median duration of treatment was 56 days); 39% of those with pulmonary aspergillosis and 53% of those with extrapulmonary aspergillosis responded to the posaconazole salvage regimen.

IDSA considers IV or oral voriconazole the drug of choice for primary treatment of invasive aspergillosis in most patients and IV amphotericin B the preferred alternative. For salvage therapy in patients refractory to or intolerant of primary antifungal therapy, IDSA recommends IV amphotericin B, an echinocandin (caspofungin or micafungin), posaconazole, or itraconazole. For empiric or preemptive therapy of presumed aspergillosis, IDSA recommends amphotericin B, caspofungin, itraconazole, or voriconazole.

For the treatment of invasive aspergillosis in HIV-infected adults and adolescents, CDC, NIH, and IDSA recommend voriconazole as the drug of choice; alternatives are IV amphotericin B, an IV echinocandin (anidulafungin, caspofungin, micafungin), and oral posaconazole.

Posaconazole is used for primary prophylaxis against invasive aspergillosis in immunocompromised individuals at high risk. (See Uses: Prevention of Invasive Aspergillus and Candida Infections in Immunocompromised Individuals.)

For additional information on prophylaxis and treatment of aspergillosis, the current clinical practice guidelines from IDSA available at http://www.idsociety. org and current clinical practice guidelines from CDC, NIH, and IDSA on the prevention and treatment of opportunistic infections in HIV-infected individuals available at http://www.aidsinfo.nih.gov should be consulted.

● Coccidioidomycosis

Although safety and efficacy have not been established, posaconazole has been used in some adults for the treatment of coccidioidomycosist caused by *Coccidioides immitis*, and is recommended as an alternative for the treatment or prevention of these infections in HIV-infected individuals.

Antifungal treatment may not be necessary in patients with mild, uncomplicated coccidioidal pneumonia since such infections often are self-limited and may resolve spontaneously. However, antifungal treatment is recommended for patients with more severe or rapidly progressing coccidioidal infections, those with chronic pulmonary or disseminated infections, and immunocompromised or debilitated individuals (e.g., HIV-infected individuals, organ transplant recipients, those receiving immunosuppressive therapy, those with diabetes mellitus or cardiopulmonary disease).

IDSA and others state that an oral azole (fluconazole or itraconazole) usually is recommended for initial treatment of symptomatic pulmonary coccidioidomycosis and chronic fibrocavitary or disseminated (extrapulmonary) coccidioidomycosis. However, IV amphotericin B is recommended as an alternative and is preferred for initial treatment of severely ill patients who have hypoxia or rapidly progressing disease, for immunocompromised individuals, or when azole antifungals have been ineffective or cannot be used (e.g., pregnant women).

For the treatment of clinically mild coccidioidomycosis (e.g., focal pneumonia) in HIV-infected adults and adolescents, CDC, NIH, and IDSA recommend initial therapy with oral fluconazole or oral itraconazole. These experts state that, although clinical data are limited, oral voriconazole or posaconazole oral suspension may be used as an alternative for the treatment of clinically mild coccidioidomycosist that has not responded to fluconazole or itraconazole.

HIV-infected individuals who have been adequately treated for coccidioidomycosis should receive long-term (usually life-long) secondary prophylaxis to prevent recurrence or relapse. Although oral fluconazole or oral itraconazole are the drugs of choice recommended by CDC, NIH, and IDSA for secondary prophylaxis to prevent recurrence or relapse of coccidioidomycosis in HIV-infected adults and adolescents, these experts state that oral voriconazole or posaconazole oral suspension can be used as an alternative for secondary prophylaxis of coccidioidomycosist in patients who did not initially respond to fluconazole or itraconazole treatment.

For additional information on prophylaxis and treatment of coccidioidomycosis, the current clinical practice guidelines from IDSA available at http://www. idsociety.org and current clinical practice guidelines from CDC, NIH, and IDSA on the prevention and treatment of opportunistic infections in HIV-infected individuals available at http://www.aidsinfo.nih.gov should be consulted.

● Fusarium Infections

Although safety and efficacy have not been established, posaconazole has been effective in some patients for the treatment of infections caused by *Fusarium*t, including salvage therapy when other antifungals were ineffective or could not be used.

Amphotericin B and/or voriconazole has been recommended for the treatment of *Fusarium* infections in immunocompromised individuals; amphotericin B may be preferred for infections caused by *F. solani* or *F. verticillioides*. Some clinicians suggest that posaconazole may be an alternative for treatment of fusariosis in patients who fail to respond to or cannot tolerate other antifungals.

In an open-label, retrospective analysis of 21 patients with invasive fusariosis who received salvage therapy with posaconazole oral suspension, the overall response rate (complete or partial) was 48%; the response rate was 57–75% in those with localized infections (e.g., pulmonary infections), but was only 29–33% in those with disseminated infections (with or without pulmonary involvement). Most patients (95%) had received initial therapy with IV amphotericin B given for a median duration of 8 days (range: 2–38 days) and 81% met a criteria for refractory infection with or without intolerance to standard antifungal therapy.

● Histoplasmosis

Although safety and efficacy have not been established, posaconazole has been used in some patients for the treatment of histoplasmosis† caused by *Histoplasma capsulatum*, including salvage therapy, and is recommended as an alternative for the treatment of these infections.

The drugs of choice for the treatment of histoplasmosis are IV amphotericin B or oral itraconazole. IV amphotericin B is preferred for initial treatment of severe, life-threatening histoplasmosis, especially in immunocompromised patients such as those with HIV infection. Oral itraconazole generally is used for initial treatment of less severe disease (e.g., mild to moderate acute pulmonary histoplasmosis, chronic cavitary pulmonary histoplasmosis) and as follow-up therapy in the treatment of severe infections after a response has been obtained with IV amphotericin B. Other azole antifungals (fluconazole, ketoconazole, posaconazole, voriconazole) are considered second-line alternatives to itraconazole.

For the treatment of less severe disseminated histoplasmosis† in HIV-infected adults and adolescents, CDC, NIH, and IDSA recommend initial treatment with oral itraconazole. These experts state that, although clinical data are limited, oral voriconazole, oral posaconazole, or oral fluconazole may be used as an alternative for the treatment of less severe disseminated histoplasmosis in patients intolerant of itraconazole who are only moderately ill.

HIV-infected individuals who have been adequately treated for histoplasmosis should receive long-term suppressive or maintenance therapy (secondary prophylaxis) to prevent recurrence or relapse if they had severe disseminated or CNS infections or had to be retreated for a relapse after appropriate initial treatment. Oral itraconazole is the drug of choice for secondary prophylaxis of histoplasmosis in HIV-infected adults and adolescents. The role of posaconazole for secondary prophylaxis of histoplasmosis in HIV-infected patients has not been evaluated to date.

For additional information on prophylaxis and treatment of histoplasmosis, the current clinical practice guidelines from IDSA available at http://www.idsociety.org and current clinical practice guidelines from CDC, NIH, and IDSA on the prevention and treatment of opportunistic infections in HIV-infected individuals available at http://www.aidsinfo.nih.gov should be consulted.

● Mucormycosis

Although safety and efficacy have not been established, posaconazole has been effective in some patients when used as salvage therapy for the treatment of mucormycosis†, including infections caused by *Mucor* or *Rhizopus*, when other antifungals were ineffective or could not be used.

In a retrospective analysis of 91 patients with proven or probable zygomycosis who received salvage therapy with posaconazole, the overall response rate (complete or partial) was 60%. In another open-label analysis of 24 patients with zygomycosis, the overall response rate to posaconazole therapy was 79% (11 patients had a complete response, 8 patients had a partial response, 5 patients failed to respond).

IV amphotericin B usually is recommended as the drug of first choice for the treatment of mucormycosis (with or without surgical intervention). Some clinicians suggest that posaconazole is a possible alternative for the treatment of mucormycosis (e.g., when IV amphotericin B is ineffective or cannot be used) and may be useful for oral follow-up therapy in patients who have an initial response to IV amphotericin B and can tolerate an oral regimen.

DOSAGE AND ADMINISTRATION

● Administration

Posaconazole is administered orally or by slow IV infusion.

Oral Administration

Posaconazole is administered orally as an oral suspension or delayed-release tablets.

Posaconazole oral suspension and delayed-release tablets are not interchangeable because they require different dosages and frequencies of administration. The oral suspension and delayed-release tablets cannot be substituted for each other without a change in dosage. (See Dispensing and Dosage and Administration Precautions under Administration: Oral Administration, in Dosage and Administration.)

Posaconazole delayed-release tablets are labeled by FDA *only* for prophylaxis of invasive *Aspergillus* and *Candida* infections. Because the delayed-release tablets generally provide higher posaconazole exposures than the oral suspension under both fed and fasting conditions, the manufacturer states that the delayed-release tablets are the preferred preparation when oral posaconazole is used for such prophylaxis.

Patients with severe diarrhea or vomiting receiving posaconazole oral suspension or delayed-release tablets should be monitored closely for breakthrough fungal infections since plasma concentrations of the drug may be affected.

Dispensing and Dosage and Administration Precautions

FDA alerted healthcare professionals about the risk of medication errors with oral preparations of posaconazole. Because of differences in oral bioavailability, posaconazole oral suspension and posaconazole delayed-release tablets *cannot* be substituted for each other without a change in dosage and frequency of administration. There have been reports of errors occurring when the wrong oral preparation was prescribed and/or dispensed to patients without consideration for the different dosage and frequency of administration required for the other preparation. At least 1 fatality occurred in a patient who received incorrect dosage (underdosage) of posaconazole as the result of being provided with posaconazole oral suspension (instead of posaconazole delayed-release tablets) without consideration for the dosage and frequency of administration required for the oral suspension. In other cases, clinicians switched patients from posaconazole oral suspension to the delayed-release tablets and the delayed-release tablets were prescribed and/or dispensed without adjusting the dosage to that required for the delayed-release tablets. Adverse effects (e.g., nausea, vomiting, low serum potassium concentrations) were reported in some of these patients, possibly as the result of the incorrect dosage and higher posaconazole exposures.

To avoid medication errors, healthcare professionals should be aware that dosage recommendations for posaconazole oral suspension and posaconazole delayed-release tablets are *not* the same and that dosage recommendations for the specific oral preparation must be followed. (See Dosage and Administration: Dosage.) Prescribers should write posaconazole prescriptions that specify the dosage form, strength, and frequency of administration and pharmacists should request clarification from prescribers when the dosage form, strength, or frequency is not specified. In addition, patients should talk to their healthcare provider before they switch from one oral preparation to the other.

Oral Suspension

Posaconazole oral suspension should be administered during or immediately (i.e., within 20 minutes) following a full meal to enhance oral absorption and optimize plasma concentrations of the drug. Alternatively, if the patient cannot eat a full meal and if posaconazole delayed-release tablets and IV posaconazole are not options, each dose of posaconazole oral suspension should be administered with a liquid nutritional supplement or an acidic carbonated beverage (e.g., ginger ale).

If oral posaconazole is indicated for prophylaxis of invasive *Aspergillus* and *Candida* infections and the patient cannot eat a full meal, posaconazole delayed-release tablets should be used.

If the patient cannot eat a full meal and cannot tolerate an oral nutritional supplement or acidic carbonated beverage (e.g., ginger ale) and if posaconazole delayed-release tablets and IV posaconazole are not options, alternative antifungal therapy should be considered or the patient should be monitored closely for breakthrough fungal infections.

Posaconazole oral suspension should be shaken well prior to each dose. The oral suspension contains 40 mg of posaconazole per mL. Posaconazole oral suspension should be administered using the calibrated measuring spoon provided by the manufacturer that is designed to measure 2.5- and 5-mL doses. The calibrated spoon should be rinsed with water after each dose and before storage.

Although posaconazole oral suspension has been administered via nasogastric tube† with a liquid nutritional supplement, patients receiving the drug via a nasogastric tube should be monitored closely for breakthrough fungal infections since this route is associated with lower posaconazole concentrations than the oral route and may be associated with an increased risk of treatment failure.

Delayed-release Tablets

Posaconazole delayed-release tablets must be swallowed whole and should not be divided, crushed, or chewed.

The delayed-release tablets should be administered with food to enhance oral absorption and optimize posaconazole plasma concentrations.

Posaconazole delayed-release tablets are labeled by FDA *only* for prophylaxis of invasive *Aspergillus* and *Candida* infections in adults and adolescents 13 years of age or older.

IV Infusion

IV posaconazole is administered by slow IV infusion; the drug should *not* be administered by rapid IV infusion or injection.

Posaconazole injection concentrate *must* be diluted in a compatible diluent prior to IV infusion.

Diluted posaconazole IV solutions *must* be administered through a 0.22-μm polyethersulfone (PES) or polyvinylidene difluoride (PVDF) filter.

Diluted posaconazole IV solutions should be administered by slow IV infusion into a central venous line (e.g., central venous catheter or peripherally inserted central catheter [PICC]). If a central venous line is not available (i.e., prior to placement of a central venous line, to bridge the period during which a central venous line is replaced, when the central venous line is in use for other treatment), a *single* dose of diluted posaconazole IV solution may be administered through a peripheral venous catheter.

Dilution

A single-dose vial of posaconazole injection concentrate containing 300 mg of the drug should be removed from the refrigerator and allowed to reach room temperature. Using proper aseptic technique, the contents of the 300-mg vial (16.7 mL) should be transferred to an IV bag or bottle containing a compatible diluent (i.e., 0.45 or 0.9% sodium chloride, 5% dextrose, 5% dextrose and 0.45 or 0.9% sodium chloride, potassium chloride 20 mEq in 5% dextrose). The resultant IV solution should contain a final posaconazole concentration of 1–2 mg/mL. Posaconazole should *not* be diluted using any other diluents since particulate formation may occur.

Posaconazole IV solutions should be used immediately after dilution; however, if not used immediately, diluted IV solutions may be refrigerated at 2–8° C for up to 24 hours.

Posaconazole IV solutions should be visually inspected for particulate matter prior to administration whenever solution and container permit. The IV solution should appear colorless to yellow; variations of color within this range do not affect the quality of the drug.

Any unused portion of the diluted IV solution should be discarded.

Rate of Administration

IV infusions of posaconazole should be given over 90 minutes into a central venous line (e.g., central venous catheter or PICC).

If a peripheral venous catheter must be used because a central venous catheter is not available (i.e., prior to placement of a central venous line, to bridge the period during which a central venous line is being replaced, when the central venous line is in use for other treatment), a *single* posaconazole dose may be given by slow IV infusion over 30 minutes through a peripheral venous catheter.

● Dosage

Posaconazole oral suspension and delayed-release tablets are *not* interchangeable and cannot be substituted for each other without a change in dosage and frequency of administration. (See Dispensing and Dosage and Administration Precautions under Administration: Oral Administration, in Dosage and Administration.)

Dosage recommendations for the specific posaconazole preparation must be followed.

Prevention of Invasive Aspergillus and Candida Infections in Immunocompromised Individuals

The recommended dosage of posaconazole oral suspension for prevention of invasive *Aspergillus* or *Candida* infections in adults and children 13 years of age or older is 200 mg (5 mL of oral suspension containing 40 mg/mL) 3 times daily.

The recommended dosage of posaconazole delayed-release tablets for prevention of invasive *Aspergillus* or *Candida* infections in adults and children 13 years of age or older is 300 mg (three 100-mg delayed-release tablets) twice daily on day 1 (loading dosage), followed by 300 mg (three 100-mg delayed-release tablets) once daily thereafter (maintenance dosage).

If IV posaconazole is used for prevention of invasive *Aspergillus* or *Candida* infections in adults 18 years of age or older, the recommended dosage is 300 mg IV twice daily on day 1 (loading dosage), followed by 300 mg IV once daily thereafter (maintenance dosage).

The duration of antifungal prophylaxis is based on the patient's recovery from immunosuppression or neutropenia. Posaconazole prophylaxis has been continued for up to 12–16 weeks in clinical studies.

Candida Infections

Treatment of Oropharyngeal Candidiasis

The recommended dosage of posaconazole oral suspension for the treatment of oropharyngeal candidiasis in adults is 100 mg (2.5 mL of oral suspension containing 40 mg/mL) twice daily on day 1 (loading dosage), followed by 100 mg (2.5 mL of oral suspension containing 40 mg/mL) once daily for 13 days (maintenance dosage).

If posaconazole oral suspension is used for the treatment of oropharyngeal candidiasis refractory to fluconazole and/or itraconazole, the manufacturer recommends that adults receive 400 mg (10 mL of oral suspension containing 40 mg/mL) twice daily and states that the duration of treatment should be based on clinical response and the severity of underlying disease. For the treatment of fluconazole-refractory oropharyngeal candidiasis, the Infectious Diseases Society of America (IDSA) recommends that posaconazole oral suspension be given in a dosage of 400 mg twice daily for 3 days, followed by 400 mg once daily for up to 28 days.

If posaconazole oral suspension is used as an alternative for the treatment of oropharyngeal candidiasis in adults and adolescents with human immunodeficiency virus (HIV) infection, the US Centers for Disease Control and Prevention (CDC), National Institutes of Health (NIH), and IDSA recommend a dosage of 400 mg twice daily on day 1, followed by 400 mg once daily for 7–14 days. For the treatment of fluconazole-refractory oropharyngeal candidiasis in HIV-infected adults and adolescents, these experts state that posaconazole oral suspension given in a dosage of 400 mg twice daily for 28 days has been effective in some patients. CDC, NIH, IDSA, and the American Academy of Pediatrics (AAP) state that data are insufficient to recommend use of posaconazole for the treatment of oropharyngeal candidiasis in HIV-infected children.

Treatment of Esophageal Candidiasis

If posaconazole oral suspension is used for the treatment of fluconazole-refractory esophageal candidiasis†, IDSA recommends a dosage of 400 mg twice daily. Alternatively, if posaconazole delayed-release tablets are used for the treatment of fluconazole-refractory esophageal candidiasis†, IDSA recommends a dosage of 300 mg once daily.

For the treatment of fluconazole-refractory esophageal candidiasis† in HIV-infected adults and adolescents, CDC, NIH, and IDSA state that posaconazole oral suspension given in a dosage of 400 mg twice daily for 28 days has been effective in some patients. CDC, NIH, IDSA, and AAP state that data are insufficient to recommend use of posaconazole for the treatment of esophageal candidiasis in HIV-infected children.

Prevention of Recurrence (Secondary Prophylaxis) of Esophageal Candidiasis

If long-term suppressive or maintenance therapy (secondary prophylaxis)† with oral posaconazole is used in HIV-infected adults and adolescents with frequent or severe recurrences of esophageal candidiasis, CDC, NIH, and IDSA recommend that posaconazole oral suspension be given in a dosage of 400 mg twice daily.

Although only limited data are available regarding the safety of discontinuing secondary prophylaxis against esophageal candidiasis in HIV-infected individuals, consideration can be given to discontinuing such prophylaxis when CD4+ T-cell counts increase to greater than 200/mm³ in response to antiretroviral therapy.

Aspergillosis

If posaconazole oral suspension is used in adults for salvage therapy for the treatment of invasive aspergillosis† when other antifungals are ineffective or cannot be used, IDSA recommends an initial dosage of 200 mg 4 times daily until the disease stabilizes, followed by 400 mg twice daily thereafter. For salvage therapy in a clinical trial, posaconazole oral suspension has been given in a dosage of 400 mg twice daily or 200 mg 4 times daily for up to approximately 12 months.

If posaconazole oral suspension is used as an alternative for the treatment of invasive aspergillosis† in HIV-infected adults and adolescents, CDC, NIH, and IDSA recommend a dosage of 200 mg 4 times daily; after improvement occurs, dosage can be changed to 400 mg twice daily. The optimal duration of therapy in these patients has not been established, but antifungal therapy should be continued at least until the CD4+ T-cell count increases to greater than 200/mm³ as a result of potent antiretroviral therapy and there is evidence that the infection has resolved.

Coccidioidomycosis

If posaconazole oral suspension is used as an alternative for the treatment of clinically mild coccidioidomycosis† (e.g., focal pneumonia) in HIV-infected adults and adolescents, a dosage of 200–400 mg twice daily is recommended by CDC, NIH, and IDSA.

If posaconazole oral suspension is used as an alternative for long-term suppressive or maintenance therapy (secondary prophylaxis)† to prevent relapse or recurrence of coccidioidomycosis in HIV-infected adults and adolescents who have completed initial treatment of the disease, a dosage of 200 mg twice daily is recommended by CDC, NIH, and IDSA. In HIV-infected patients who were treated for focal coccidioidal pneumonia and are receiving effective antiretroviral therapy, consideration can be given to discontinuing secondary prophylaxis against coccidioidomycosis after 12 months if CD4+ T-cell counts are 250/mm³ or higher, provided the patient is monitored for recurrence (e.g., serial chest radiographs, coccidioidal serology). HIV-infected patients who were treated for diffuse pulmonary, disseminated, or meningeal coccidioidomycosis usually require lifelong secondary prophylaxis.

Fusarium Infections

For salvage therapy in adults for the treatment of infections caused by Fusarium† when other antifungals were ineffective or could not be used, posaconazole oral suspension has been given in a dosage of 400 mg twice daily or 200 mg 4 times daily for up to 12 months or longer.

Histoplasmosis

If posaconazole oral suspension is used as an alternative for the treatment of less severe disseminated histoplasmosis† in HIV-infected adults and adolescents who are only moderately ill, CDC, NIH, and IDSA recommend a dosage of 400 mg twice daily.

Mucormycosis

For salvage therapy in adults for the treatment of mucormycosis† when other antifungals were ineffective or could not be used, posaconazole oral suspension has been given in a dosage of 400 mg twice daily or 200 mg 4 times daily.

In the treatment of mucormycosis† after a response has been obtained with an initial regimen of IV amphotericin B, some clinicians suggest that posaconazole oral suspension can be given for follow-up therapy in a dosage of 200 mg 3 or 4 times daily.

● Special Populations
Hepatic Impairment

Dosage adjustments are not necessary if posaconazole oral suspension is used in patients with hepatic impairment† (Child-Pugh class A, B, or C). However, discontinuance of the drug must be considered if clinical signs and symptoms consistent with liver disease develop that may be attributable to posaconazole. (See Hepatic Effects under Cautions: Warnings/Precautions.)

Dosage adjustments are not necessary if posaconazole delayed-release tablets or IV posaconazole is used in patients with hepatic impairment. However, specific studies have not been conducted to evaluate these posaconazole preparations in patients with hepatic impairment.

Renal Impairment

Dosage adjustments are not necessary if posaconazole oral suspension or posaconazole delayed-release tablets are used in patients with mild, moderate, or severe renal impairment. However, because the area under the plasma

concentration-time curve (AUC) is highly variable in patients with severe renal impairment receiving posaconazole oral suspension or delayed-release tablets, such patients should be monitored closely for breakthrough fungal infections. (See Renal Impairment under Warnings/Precautions: Specific Populations, in Cautions.)

IV posaconazole should be avoided in patients with moderate or severe renal impairment (estimated glomerular filtration rate [eGFR] less than 50 mL/minute) unless benefits of the IV preparation outweigh risks in such patients. The IV vehicle (betadex sulfobutyl ether sodium [SBECD]) contained in the posaconazole IV preparation is expected to accumulate in patients with moderate or severe renal impairment. If IV posaconazole is used in such patients, serum creatinine concentrations should be closely monitored and consideration given to switching to oral posaconazole if serum creatinine concentrations increase. (See Renal Impairment under Warnings/Precautions: Specific Populations, in Cautions.)

Because posaconazole is not dialyzable, the drug may be administered without regard to the timing of hemodialysis.

Geriatric Patients

Dosage adjustments are not necessary when oral or IV posaconazole is used in geriatric adults 65 years of age or older.

Obese Patients

Because pharmacokinetic modeling suggests that patients weighing more than 120 kg may have lower posaconazole exposures, such patients should be closely monitored for breakthrough fungal infections.

Other Special Populations

Dosage adjustments are not necessary based on gender or race.

CAUTIONS

● Contraindications

Posaconazole is contraindicated in patients with known hypersensitivity to posaconazole or other azole antifungals.

Concomitant use with sirolimus is contraindicated. (See Drug Interactions: Immunosuppressive Agents.)

Concomitant use with ergot alkaloids (e.g., ergotamine, dihydroergotamine) is contraindicated. (See Drug Interactions: Ergot Alkaloids.)

Concomitant use with drugs that are substrates for cytochrome P-450 (CYP) 3A4 and for which elevated plasma concentrations may be associated with prolonged QT interval corrected for rate (QTc) and rare occurrences of torsades de pointes (e.g., pimozide, quinidine) is contraindicated. (See Drug Interactions: Drugs that Prolong the QT Interval.)

Concomitant use with HMG-CoA reductase inhibitors (statins) principally metabolized by CYP3A4 (e.g., atorvastatin, lovastatin, simvastatin) is contraindicated. (See Drug Interactions: HMG-CoA Reductase Inhibitors.)

● Warnings/Precautions
Sensitivity Reactions

Allergic and/or hypersensitivity reactions, including rash and pruritus, have been reported in patients receiving posaconazole.

Data regarding cross-sensitivity among azole antifungals (e.g., fluconazole, isavuconazole [active metabolite of isavuconazonium], itraconazole, posaconazole, voriconazole) are not available. Posaconazole is contraindicated in patients hypersensitive to other azole antifungals.

Cardiovascular Effects

Similar to some other azole antifungals (e.g., fluconazole, voriconazole), posaconazole has been associated with prolongation of the QT interval. Torsades de pointes has been reported during posaconazole therapy in some patients; one case occurred in a patient who was seriously ill and had multiple confounding risk factors (e.g., prior cardiotoxic chemotherapy, hypokalemia, concomitant drugs) that may have been contributory.

In a multiple time-matched ECG analysis in 173 healthy adults 18–85 years of age, administration of posaconazole oral suspension (400 mg twice daily with a high-fat meal) did not increase mean QT_c intervals. Multiple, time-matched ECGs were collected over a 12-hour period at baseline and at steady state. In a pooled analysis, the mean QT_c interval change from baseline was –5 msec following administration of the recommended posaconazole dose. Decreased QT_c interval (–3 msec) also was observed in a small number of individuals receiving placebo. The placebo-adjusted mean maximum QT_c interval change from baseline was –8 msec. No healthy individuals receiving posaconazole had a QT_c interval of 500 msec or higher or had an increase of 60 msec or more in their QT_c interval from baseline.

Posaconazole should be used with caution in patients with potentially proarrhythmic conditions and should not be used concomitantly with drugs that are metabolized by CYP3A4 and known to prolong the QT_c interval. (See Drug Interactions: Drugs that Prolong the QT Interval.)

Rigorous attempts should be made to correct electrolyte imbalances (i.e., potassium, magnesium, calcium) before initiating posaconazole therapy.

Hepatic Effects

Serious hepatic effects, including cholestasis or hepatic failure (sometimes fatal), have been reported rarely during posaconazole therapy in patients with serious underlying medical conditions (e.g., hematologic malignancy). These severe hepatic effects generally have occurred in patients receiving posaconazole oral suspension in a dosage of 800 mg daily (400 mg twice daily or 200 mg 4 times daily) in clinical trials.

Less severe hepatic effects, including mild to moderate elevations in ALT, AST, alkaline phosphatase, total bilirubin, and/or clinical hepatitis, have been reported infrequently in clinical trials. Liver function test elevations generally were reversible following discontinuance of posaconazole and did not appear to be associated with increased plasma posaconazole concentrations; in some cases, test results returned to normal levels without interrupting posaconazole therapy and only rarely required discontinuance of the drug.

Liver function should be monitored (liver function tests, bilirubin) prior to and during posaconazole therapy. If abnormal liver function test results occur during posaconazole therapy, the patient should be monitored for the development of more severe hepatic injury using appropriate laboratory tests. Discontinuance of posaconazole must be considered if signs and symptoms consistent with liver disease develop that may be attributable to the drug.

Interactions

Concomitant use of posaconazole and certain drugs may result in serious and/or life-threatening adverse effects as the result of higher exposures of the concomitant drug. Concomitant use of posaconazole and some drugs is contraindicated (e.g., sirolimus, drugs that are CYP3A4 substrates and are known to prolong the QT interval, HMG-CoA reductase inhibitors metabolized by CYP3A4, ergot alkaloids) or requires particular caution (e.g., cyclosporine, tacrolimus, midazolam). (See Cautions: Contraindications and see Drug Interactions.)

Specific Populations

Pregnancy

There are no adequate and well-controlled studies in pregnant women. Posaconazole should be used during pregnancy only when potential benefits outweigh possible risks to the fetus.

The Infectious Diseases Society of America (IDSA) states that use of posaconazole should be avoided during pregnancy, especially during the first trimester.

Posaconazole has been shown to cause skeletal malformations (cranial malformations and missing ribs) when given to rats at dosages at least 1.4 times greater than a human dosage of the oral suspension of 400 mg twice daily (based on steady-state plasma concentrations). No malformations were seen in rabbits given a posaconazole dosage of 80 mg/kg (exposure levels 5.2 times higher than human exposures achieved with a dosage of the oral suspension of 400 mg twice daily); however, this dosage was associated with an increase in resorptions, reduction in body weight gain of females, and reduction in litter size.

Lactation

Posaconazole is distributed into milk in rats; it is not known whether the drug is distributed into milk in humans.

Because of the potential for serious adverse reactions in nursing infants, a decision should be made whether to discontinue nursing or posaconazole, taking into account the importance of the drug to the woman.

Pediatric Use

Safety and efficacy of posaconazole oral suspension and delayed-release tablets have not been established in children younger than 13 years of age.

Safety and efficacy of IV posaconazole have not been established in patients younger than 18 years of age.

The manufacturer states that use of posaconazole oral suspension or delayed-release tablets in pediatric patients 13–17 years of age is supported by evidence from adequate and well-controlled studies in adults.

Data from a limited number of pediatric patients 13–17 years of age who received posaconazole oral suspension (200 mg 3 times daily) for prophylaxis of invasive fungal infections indicate that the safety profile and mean steady-state plasma posaconazole concentrations in this age group are similar to those reported in adults 18 years of age or older.

Comparison of pharmacokinetic data from a limited number of pediatric patients 8–17 years of age who received posaconazole oral suspension (400 mg 2 times or 200 mg 4 times daily) for the treatment of invasive fungal infections† with pharmacokinetic data from adults 18 years of age or older indicates that mean steady-state plasma posaconazole concentrations in pediatric patients and adults are similar.

Posaconazole oral suspension has been used in a limited number of children 7 years of age† or older without unusual adverse effects.

The US Centers for Disease Control and Prevention (CDC), National Institutes of Health (NIH), IDSA, and American Academy of Pediatrics (AAP) state that data are insufficient to date to make recommendations regarding use of posaconazole in HIV-infected infants and children.

Geriatric Use

Although no overall differences in safety and pharmacokinetics were observed between geriatric and younger adults in clinical studies evaluating posaconazole oral suspension, posaconazole delayed-release tablets, or IV posaconazole, the possibility that some older patients may exhibit increased sensitivity to the drug cannot be ruled out.

Hepatic Impairment

Patients who develop evidence of hepatic impairment during posaconazole therapy (i.e., abnormal liver function test results) should be carefully monitored for the development of more severe hepatic injury. (See Hepatic Effects under Cautions: Warnings/Precautions.)

Although there are some differences in posaconazole pharmacokinetics in individuals with hepatic impairment compared with those with normal hepatic function, the manufacturer states that dosage adjustments are not considered necessary in patients with mild, moderate, or severe hepatic impairment. (See Hepatic Impairment under Dosage and Administration: Special Populations.)

Renal Impairment

Patients with severe renal impairment receiving posaconazole oral suspension or delayed-release tablets should be closely monitored for breakthrough fungal infections since the area under the plasma concentration-time curve (AUC) of posaconazole is highly variable in these patients.

IV posaconazole should not be used in patients with moderate or severe renal impairment (estimated glomerular filtration rate [eGFR] less than 50 mL/minute) unless potential benefits of the IV route justify the risks in such patients. Accumulation of the IV vehicle (SBECD) contained in the posaconazole IV preparation is expected in patients with moderate or severe renal impairment. If IV posaconazole is used in such patients, serum creatinine concentrations should be closely monitored. If serum creatinine concentrations increase, consideration should be given to switching to oral posaconazole.

● Common Adverse Effects

Adverse effects reported in 5% or more of patients receiving posaconazole include GI effects (nausea, vomiting, diarrhea, abdominal pain, anorexia, constipation, dry mouth, dyspepsia, flatulence, decreased appetite), fever, headache, increased sweating, rigors, chills, mucosal inflammation, dizziness, fatigue, edema (legs), asthenia, weakness, decreased weight, dehydration, hypertension, and hypotension. Vaginal hemorrhage, tachycardia, bacteremia, pneumonia, herpes simplex infection, cytomegalovirus infection, oral candidiasis, pharyngitis, musculoskeletal pain, arthralgia, back pain, petechiae, insomnia, coughing, dyspnea, epistaxis, rash, and pruritus also were reported in 5% or more of patients. Anemia, neutropenia, thrombocytopenia, hypocalcemia, hypokalemia, hypomagnesemia, hyperglycemia, increased AST, increased ALT, increased γ-glutamyltransferase (GGT, γ-glutamyl transpeptidase, GGPT), increased alkaline phosphatase, and bilirubinemia were reported in 2% or more of patients. Serious adverse effects, including fever and neutropenia, were reported more frequently when the drug was used in patients with refractory oropharyngeal candidiasis (especially in those severely immunocompromised by advanced HIV infection) than when used for prophylaxis.

DRUG INTERACTIONS

● Drugs Metabolized by Hepatic Microsomal Enzymes

Posaconazole inhibits the metabolic activity of cytochrome P-450 (CYP) isoenzyme 3A4 (CYP3A4) and may increase plasma concentrations of other drugs metabolized by this hepatic enzyme.

Posaconazole does not appear to inhibit CYP isoenzymes 1A2, 2C8/9, 2D6, or 2E1.

● Drugs that Prolong the QT Interval

Potential pharmacokinetic interactions with drugs that are CYP3A4 substrates and prolong the QT interval corrected for rate (QT_c) (e.g., pimozide, quinidine). Potential increased plasma concentrations of the concomitantly used CYP3A4 substrate, which can result in QT interval prolongation and, rarely, torsades de pointes. Concomitant use of posaconazole and these drugs that prolong the QT_c interval is contraindicated.

● Drugs Affecting P-glycoprotein Transport

Because posaconazole is a substrate of P-glycoprotein (P-gp), inhibitors or inducers of the P-gp transport system may increase or decrease plasma posaconazole concentrations, respectively.

● Drugs Affecting Uridine Diphosphate-glucuronosyltransferase

Because posaconazole is principally metabolized via uridine diphosphate (UDP)-glucuronosyltransferase glucuronidation (UGT; phase 2 enzymes), inhibitors or inducers of UGT may increase or decrease posaconazole plasma concentrations, respectively.

● Antifungal Agents

Amphotericin B

Although the clinical importance is unclear, the antifungal effects of posaconazole and amphotericin B usually have been synergistic in vitro against *Aspergillus* hyphae, but indifferent against *Aspergillus* conidia.

In vitro, the antifungal effects of posaconazole and amphotericin B were indifferent against *Rhizopus oryzae*; there was no evidence of synergism or antagonism.

● Antimycobacterial Agents

Rifabutin

Concomitant use of rifabutin (300 mg once daily for 17 days) and posaconazole (200 mg once daily for 10 days) results in decreased peak plasma concentration and area under the plasma concentration-time curve (AUC) of posaconazole and increased peak plasma concentration and AUC of rifabutin; possible increased risk of rifabutin-associated adverse effects.

Concomitant use of rifabutin and posaconazole should be avoided unless benefits outweigh risks. If concomitant use is considered necessary, the patient should be closely monitored for breakthrough fungal infections. In addition, the patient should be monitored for adverse effects associated with increased rifabutin concentrations (e.g., uveitis, leukopenia) and complete blood counts should be assessed frequently.

● Antiretroviral Agents

HIV Integrase Inhibitors

Elvitegravir

Possible pharmacokinetic interactions if posaconazole is used concomitantly with elvitegravir and a *ritonavir-boosted* HIV protease inhibitor (increased elvitegravir concentrations).

Possible pharmacokinetic interaction if posaconazole is used concomitantly with the fixed combination of elvitegravir, cobicistat, emtricitabine, and tenofovir disoproxil fumarate (EVG/c/FTC/TDF) (increased posaconazole, elvitegravir, and cobicistat concentrations). If posaconazole is used concomitantly with EVG/c/FTC/TDF, some experts state that posaconazole concentrations should be monitored.

HIV Nonnucleoside Reverse Transcriptase Inhibitors (NNRTIs)

Efavirenz

Pharmacokinetic interaction (decreased posaconazole peak plasma concentrations and AUC) with efavirenz.

Concomitant use of efavirenz and posaconazole should be avoided unless benefits outweigh risks; if concomitant use is necessary, posaconazole plasma concentrations should be monitored and dosage adjusted accordingly.

Etravirine

Possible pharmacokinetic interaction if posaconazole is used concomitantly with etravirine (increased etravirine plasma concentrations, no change in posaconazole concentrations).

Some experts state that dosage adjustments are not needed when etravirine is used concomitantly with posaconazole; the manufacturer of etravirine states that dosage adjustment of posaconazole may be needed depending on other concomitantly administered drugs.

Rilpivirine

Possible pharmacokinetic interaction if posaconazole is used concomitantly with rilpivirine (increased rilpivirine concentrations).

Some experts state that dosage adjustments are not needed if rilpivirine is used concomitantly with posaconazole; however, because rilpivirine reduces ketoconazole exposure and effects of rilpivirine on posaconazole exposure have not been established, the patient should be monitored for breakthrough fungal infections.

HIV Nucleoside Reverse Transcriptase Inhibitors (NRTIs)

Lamivudine

No clinically important pharmacokinetic interactions when posaconazole is used concomitantly with lamivudine; dosage adjustments are not needed if lamivudine is used with posaconazole 200 mg daily.

Zidovudine

No clinically important pharmacokinetic interactions when posaconazole is used concomitantly with zidovudine; dosage adjustments are not needed if zidovudine is used with posaconazole 200 mg daily.

HIV Protease Inhibitors (PIs)

Atazanavir

Pharmacokinetic interactions if posaconazole is used concomitantly with *ritonavir-boosted* or unboosted atazanavir (increased plasma concentrations and AUC of atazanavir); possible pharmacokinetic interactions if used concomitantly with *cobicistat-boosted* atazanavir (increased atazanavir concentrations).

If posaconazole is used concomitantly with *ritonavir-boosted*, *cobicistat-boosted*, or unboosted atazanavir, the patient should be frequently monitored for atazanavir-associated adverse effects and toxicity.

Darunavir

Possible pharmacokinetic interactions if posaconazole is used concomitantly with *ritonavir-boosted* or *cobicistat-boosted* darunavir (increased posaconazole, darunavir, and ritonavir or cobicistat concentrations).

If posaconazole and *ritonavir-boosted* or *cobicistat-boosted* darunavir are used concomitantly, patients should be monitored for increased posaconazole-, darunavir-, and ritonavir- or cobicistat-associated adverse effects and posaconazole plasma concentration monitoring should be considered.

Fosamprenavir

Pharmacokinetic interactions when posaconazole is used concomitantly with fosamprenavir (decreased posaconazole concentrations). Possible pharmacokinetic interactions if used concomitantly with *ritonavir-boosted* fosamprenavir (increased amprenavir [active metabolite of fosamprenavir] and posaconazole concentrations).

If posaconazole is used concomitantly with unboosted fosamprenavir, the patient should be closely monitored for breakthrough fungal infections; some experts state that posaconazole concentrations should be monitored.

If posaconazole is used concomitantly with *ritonavir-boosted* fosamprenavir, some experts state that posaconazole concentration monitoring should be considered and the patient should be monitored for amprenavir adverse effects.

Indinavir

No clinically important pharmacokinetic interactions when posaconazole is used concomitantly with indinavir; dosage adjustments are not needed if indinavir is used with posaconazole 200 mg daily.

Lopinavir

Possible pharmacokinetic interaction if posaconazole is used concomitantly with the fixed combination of lopinavir and ritonavir (lopinavir/ritonavir) (increased lopinavir and posaconazole concentrations). If posaconazole is used concomitantly with lopinavir/ritonavir, some experts state that posaconazole concentration monitoring should be considered and the patient should be monitored for lopinavir adverse effects.

Ritonavir

Pharmacokinetic interaction (increased ritonavir peak plasma concentrations and AUC) when used with low-dose ritonavir (100 mg once daily).

If ritonavir is used concomitantly with posaconazole, the patient should be frequently monitored for ritonavir adverse effects and toxicity.

Saquinavir

Possible pharmacokinetic interaction if posaconazole is used concomitantly with *ritonavir-boosted* saquinavir (increased saquinavir and posaconazole concentrations). If posaconazole is used concomitantly with *ritonavir-boosted* saquinavir, some experts state that posaconazole concentration monitoring should be considered and the patient should be monitored for saquinavir adverse effects.

Tipranavir

Possible pharmacokinetic interaction if posaconazole is used concomitantly with *ritonavir-boosted* tipranavir (increased tipranavir and posaconazole concentrations). If posaconazole is used concomitantly with *ritonavir-boosted* tipranavir, some experts state that posaconazole concentration monitoring should be considered and the patient should be monitored for tipranavir adverse effects.

● Benzodiazepines

Pharmacokinetic interaction if posaconazole is used concomitantly with midazolam (substantially increased peak plasma concentrations, AUC, and mean terminal half-life of midazolam), which may potentiate and prolong hypnotic and sedative effects of midazolam. Potential pharmacokinetic interaction (increased benzodiazepine plasma concentrations) with other benzodiazepines that are metabolized by CYP3A4 isoenzyme (e.g., alprazolam, triazolam).

If posaconazole is used in patients receiving midazolam or other benzodiazepines metabolized by CYP3A4 (e.g., alprazolam, triazolam), the patient must be closely monitored for adverse effects associated with high benzodiazepine concentrations and a benzodiazepine receptor antagonist must be available to reverse possible adverse effects.

● Caffeine

No clinically important pharmacokinetic interactions when posaconazole is used concomitantly with caffeine; dosage adjustments are not needed if caffeine is used concomitantly with posaconazole 200 mg daily.

● Calcium-channel Blocking Agents

Potential pharmacokinetic interaction (increased plasma concentrations of the calcium-channel blocker) if posaconazole is used concomitantly with calcium-channel blocking agents that are metabolized by CYP3A4 (e.g., diltiazem, felodipine, nicardipine, nifedipine, verapamil).

If posaconazole is used concomitantly with calcium-channel blocking agents metabolized by CYP3A4, the patient should be frequently monitored for adverse effects and toxicity associated with calcium-channel blockers; reduction of the calcium-channel blocker dosage may be needed.

● Digoxin

Pharmacokinetic interaction if posaconazole is used concomitantly with digoxin (increased digoxin plasma concentrations).

If digoxin is used concomitantly with posaconazole, digoxin plasma concentrations should be monitored.

● Ergot Alkaloids

Potential pharmacokinetic interactions if posaconazole is used concomitantly with ergot alkaloids (increased plasma concentrations of ergot alkaloids resulting in ergotism).

Concomitant use of ergot alkaloids (e.g., ergotamine, dihydroergotamine) and posaconazole is contraindicated.

● GI Drugs

Antacids

No clinically important pharmacokinetic interactions have been reported when antacids were used concomitantly with posaconazole oral suspension or delayed-release tablets.

Dosage adjustments are not needed if posaconazole oral suspension or delayed-release tablets are used concomitantly with antacids.

Antidiarrhea Agents
Loperamide

No clinically important pharmacokinetic interactions have been reported when loperamide was used concomitantly with posaconazole oral suspension; dosage adjustments are not needed when loperamide and posaconazole are used concomitantly.

Histamine H$_2$-receptor Antagonists

Concomitant use of cimetidine and posaconazole oral suspension results in decreased peak plasma concentrations and AUC of posaconazole. Concomitant use of cimetidine and posaconazole oral suspension should be avoided unless benefits outweigh risks; if concomitant use is necessary, the patient should be closely monitored for breakthrough fungal infections.

No clinically important pharmacokinetic interactions have been reported when posaconazole oral suspension or delayed-release tablets were used concomitantly with other histamine H$_2$-receptor antagonists (e.g., ranitidine); dosage adjustments are not needed if posaconazole oral suspension or delayed-release tablets are used concomitantly with these drugs.

Metoclopramide

Concomitant use of metoclopramide and posaconazole oral suspension results in decreased posaconazole mean peak plasma concentrations and AUC. If metoclopramide is used concomitantly with posaconazole oral suspension, the patient should be closely monitored for breakthrough fungal infections.

No clinically important pharmacokinetic interactions occurred when metoclopramide was used concomitantly with posaconazole delayed-release tablets. Dosage adjustments are not needed if metoclopramide is used concomitantly with posaconazole delayed-release tablets.

Proton-pump Inhibitors
Esomeprazole

Concomitant use of esomeprazole and posaconazole oral suspension results in decreased posaconazole mean peak plasma concentrations and AUC. Concomitant use of esomeprazole and posaconazole oral suspension should be avoided unless benefits outweigh risks; if esomeprazole is used concomitantly with posaconazole oral suspension, the patient should be monitored closely for breakthrough fungal infections.

No clinically important pharmacokinetic interactions occurred when esomeprazole and posaconazole delayed-release tablets were used concomitantly; dosage adjustments are not necessary if posaconazole delayed-release tablets are used concomitantly with proton-pump inhibitors.

Omeprazole

Concomitant use of omeprazole and posaconazole oral suspension results in decreased posaconazole trough concentrations. If omeprazole is used concomitantly with posaconazole oral suspension, plasma posaconazole concentrations should be monitored or consideration given to switching to an alternative antifungal.

● Glipizide

Concomitant use of posaconazole and glipizide does not result in clinically important pharmacokinetic interactions; however, decreased blood glucose concentrations have been reported in healthy adults following concomitant use of glipizide and posaconazole.

Dosage adjustments are not needed if posaconazole and glipizide are used concomitantly, but blood glucose concentrations should be monitored.

● HCV Antivirals

HCV Replication Complex Inhibitors

Daclatasvir

Possible pharmacokinetic interaction if posaconazole is used concomitantly with daclatasvir (increased daclatasvir concentrations).

If daclatasvir and posaconazole are used concomitantly, a daclatasvir dosage of 30 mg once daily should be used.

HCV Protease Inhibitors

Simeprevir

Possible pharmacokinetic interaction if posaconazole is used concomitantly with simeprevir (substantially increased simeprevir concentrations).

Concomitant use of simeprevir and posaconazole is not recommended.

● HMG-CoA Reductase Inhibitors

Concomitant use of posaconazole oral suspension (100 or 200 mg once daily for 13 days) and simvastatin (single 40-mg dose) results in substantially increased simvastatin concentrations and AUC. Similar pharmacokinetic interactions are likely if posaconazole is used concomitantly with other HMG-CoA reductase inhibitors (statins) metabolized by CYP3A4.

Because increased plasma concentrations of HMG-CoA reductase inhibitors can lead to rhabdomyolysis, concomitant use of posaconazole and HMG-CoA reductase inhibitors metabolized by CYP3A4 (e.g., atorvastatin, lovastatin, simvastatin) is contraindicated.

● Immunosuppressive Agents

Cyclosporine

Pharmacokinetic interaction if cyclosporine is used concomitantly with posaconazole (increased cyclosporine concentrations, no change in posaconazole concentrations); elevated cyclosporine concentrations have been associated with serious adverse effects (e.g., nephrotoxicity, leukoencephalopathy, death).

If posaconazole is initiated in a patient receiving cyclosporine, the cyclosporine dosage should be reduced by approximately 25%. Trough cyclosporine concentrations should be monitored frequently during and following discontinuance of posaconazole therapy and cyclosporine dosage should be adjusted as required.

Sirolimus

Pharmacokinetic interaction if sirolimus and posaconazole are used concomitantly (substantially increased sirolimus peak concentrations and AUC); possible sirolimus toxicity.

Concomitant use of sirolimus and posaconazole is contraindicated.

Tacrolimus

Pharmacokinetic interaction if tacrolimus and posaconazole are used concomitantly (increased tacrolimus peak concentrations and AUC).

If posaconazole is initiated in a patient receiving tacrolimus, the tacrolimus dosage should be reduced by approximately 66%. Trough tacrolimus concentrations should be monitored frequently during and following discontinuance of posaconazole therapy and tacrolimus dosage should be adjusted as required.

● Phenytoin

Concomitant use of phenytoin (200 mg once daily for 10 days) and posaconazole (200 mg once daily for 10 days) results in decreased peak plasma concentrations and AUC of posaconazole and increased peak plasma concentrations and AUC of phenytoin.

Concomitant use of phenytoin and posaconazole should be avoided unless benefits outweigh risks. If concomitant use is necessary, the patient should be closely monitored for breakthrough fungal infections. In addition, plasma phenytoin concentrations should be assessed frequently and reduced phenytoin dosage considered.

● Pimozide

Possible pharmacokinetic interaction and potential for serious or life-threatening reactions (e.g., prolonged QT interval, torsades de pointes) if pimozide and posaconazole are used concomitantly.

Concomitant use of pimozide and posaconazole is contraindicated.

● Quinidine

Possible pharmacokinetic interaction and potential for serious or life-threatening reactions (e.g., prolonged QT interval, torsades de pointes) if quinidine and posaconazole are used concomitantly.

Concomitant use of quinidine and posaconazole is contraindicated.

● Vinca Alkaloids

Potential pharmacokinetic interaction if vinca alkaloids (e.g., vincristine, vinblastine) are used concomitantly with posaconazole (increased plasma concentrations of vinca alkaloids); possible increased risk of neurotoxicity.

If vinca alkaloids and posaconazole are used concomitantly, the patient should be monitored for manifestations of vinca alkaloid toxicity (i.e., neurotoxicity) and adjustment of the vinca alkaloid dosage should be considered.

PHARMACOKINETICS

● Absorption

When posaconazole oral suspension is administered over a dosage range of 50 mg twice daily to 400 mg twice daily, posaconazole exhibits dose-proportional increases in the area under the plasma concentration-time curve (AUC). In febrile neutropenic patients or those with refractory invasive fungal infections, no further increases in posaconazole exposure occur if dosage is increased from 400 mg twice daily to 600 mg twice daily. Following administration of posaconazole oral suspension, the median time to peak plasma concentrations of posaconazole is approximately 3–8 hours. Steady-state posaconazole concentrations are achieved at 7–10 days in patients receiving the oral suspension.

Posaconazole delayed-release tablets contain posaconazole mixed with a pH-sensitive polymer (hypromellose acetate succinate) that enhances oral bioavailability of the drug. The pH-sensitive polymer contained in the tablets limits release of posaconazole in the acidic pH of the stomach, allowing release of the drug in the elevated pH environment of the intestines. The polymer may also inhibit recrystallization of posaconazole in intestinal fluid, resulting in a greater portion of the drug being available for absorption. Several studies in solid organ transplant recipients or patients with hematologic malignancies indicate that posaconazole delayed-release tablets (300 mg once daily or 300 mg twice daily on day 1 followed by 300 mg once daily) result in consistently higher posaconazole plasma concentrations than posaconazole oral suspension (400 mg twice daily or 200 mg 3 or 4 times daily).

When posaconazole delayed-release tablets are administered in single or multiple doses up to 300 mg, posaconazole exhibits dose-proportional pharmacokinetics. Following administration of posaconazole delayed-release tablets, the median time to peak plasma concentrations is 4–5 hours. When posaconazole delayed-release tablets are given in a dosage of 300 mg twice daily on day 1 (loading dosage) followed by 300 mg once daily thereafter (maintenance dosage), steady-state posaconazole concentrations are achieved by day 6. The absolute bioavailability of posaconazole delayed-release tablets is approximately 54% under fasting conditions.

When IV posaconazole is given in single doses of 200–300 mg, posaconazole exhibits dose-proportional pharmacokinetics. The median time to peak plasma concentrations following IV administration of posaconazole is 1.5 hours.

In a crossover study in healthy adults who received a single 400-mg dose of posaconazole oral suspension orally or via a nasogastric tube† after a liquid nutritional supplement (Boost® Plus), the mean time to peak plasma concentrations of posaconazole was similar (4 hours) but mean peak plasma concentrations and AUC were 19 and 23% lower, respectively, when the dose was administered using a nasogastric tube. In some patients, posaconazole peak plasma concentrations and AUC were reduced substantially (up to approximately 50%) when the drug was administered via a nasogastric tube compared to when it was administered orally.

Data from a limited number of pediatric patients 13–17 years of age receiving posaconazole oral suspension (200 mg 3 times daily) for prophylaxis of invasive fungal infections indicate that mean steady-state posaconazole plasma concentrations in this age group are similar to those reported in adults.

Comparison of data from a limited number of pediatric patients 8–17 years of age who received posaconazole oral suspension (400 mg twice daily or 200 mg 4 times daily) for treatment of invasive fungal infections with data from adults indicates that mean steady-state posaconazole plasma concentrations in pediatric patients and adults are similar.

In individuals with mild, moderate, or severe hepatic impairment, the mean AUC of posaconazole following a single 400-mg dose of posaconazole oral suspension given after a high-fat meal was 43, 27, or 21% higher, respectively, and the mean peak plasma concentration was 1% higher, 40% higher, or 34% lower, respectively, compared with individuals with normal hepatic function.

Specific studies have not been performed to date to evaluate posaconazole pharmacokinetics following administration of the delayed-release tablets in individuals with hepatic impairment.

In individuals with mild or moderate renal impairment (estimated glomerular filtration rate [eGFR] 20–80 mL/minute per 1.73 m²), posaconazole pharmacokinetics following a single dose of the oral suspension is similar to that reported in individuals with normal renal function. In individuals with severe renal insufficiency (eGFR less than 20 mL/minute per 1.73 m²), the mean AUC of posaconazole following a single dose of posaconazole oral suspension is similar to that reported in individuals with normal renal function; however, the range of AUC estimates is highly variable compared with that in individuals with mild or moderate renal impairment.

The manufacturer states that renal impairment does not have a clinically important effect on the pharmacokinetics of posaconazole delayed-release tablets. However, although specific studies have not been performed to date using the delayed-release tablets, posaconazole exposures in patients with severe renal impairment receiving the tablets are expected to be highly variable.

Pharmacokinetic modeling suggests that posaconazole plasma concentrations may be lower in patients weighing more than 120 kg than in other patients. (See Other Special Populations under Dosage and Administration: Specific Populations.)

Food

Food or a liquid nutritional supplement increases posaconazole plasma concentrations and AUC.

Following oral administration of a single 200-mg dose of posaconazole oral suspension with a nonfat or high-fat meal (approximately 50 g of fat), both the mean peak plasma concentration and AUC of the drug were approximately threefold or fourfold higher, respectively, compared with those observed following administration in the fasted state.

In a crossover study in healthy adults who received a single 400-mg dose of posaconazole oral suspension during or 20 minutes following a high-fat meal, mean peak plasma posaconazole concentrations and AUC were approximately threefold or fourfold higher, respectively, compared with those observed

following administration in the fasted state. When the dose was administered 5 minutes prior to the high-fat meal, mean peak plasma posaconazole concentrations and AUC were similar to those observed when the drug is administered in the fasted state.

Following oral administration of a single 400-mg dose of posaconazole oral suspension with 240 mL of liquid nutritional supplement (Boost® Plus; 360 calories, 14 g fat), both the mean peak plasma concentration and AUC were approximately threefold higher than following administration in the fasted state. Bioavailability of posaconazole is lower if the posaconazole dose is administered with less than 240 mL of the liquid nutritional supplement; posaconazole bioavailability is about 20% lower if only 120 mL of the liquid nutritional supplement is used instead of 240 mL.

Following oral administration of a single 400-mg dose of posaconazole oral suspension with an acidic beverage (i.e., ginger ale) in healthy adults in the fasted state, mean peak plasma concentrations and AUC were increased by 92 and 70%, respectively, compared with those reported following administration of posaconazole alone in the fasted state.

Following oral administration of a single 300-mg dose of posaconazole as delayed-release tablets given with a high-fat meal, peak plasma concentrations and AUC were increased by 16 and 51%, respectively, compared with administration in the fasted state.

● **Distribution**

The mean volume of distribution of posaconazole is 261 L following IV administration.

Following oral administration of posaconazole oral suspension, the drug has been detected in skin and in pulmonary epithelial lining fluid and alveolar cell tissue.

Posaconazole is distributed into milk in rats; it is not known whether the drug is distributed into milk in humans.

Posaconazole is more than 98% bound to plasma proteins (primarily albumin).

● **Elimination**

Posaconazole is principally metabolized via uridine diphosphate (UDP)-glucuronosyltransferase UDP glucuronidation (UGT; phase 2 enzymes). Posaconazole circulates in plasma principally as the parent drug; the majority of circulating metabolites are glucuronide conjugates formed via UDP glucuronidation.

No major circulating posaconazole metabolites are formed via cytochrome P-450 (CYP) isoenzymes.

Following administration of posaconazole oral suspension, 71% of a posaconazole dose is recovered in feces (66% as the parent drug) over 120 hours; 13% of a dose is recovered in urine over 120 hours (less than 0.2% as the parent drug). Metabolites recovered in urine and feces represent approximately 17% of a dose.

The mean elimination half-life of posaconazole is 35 hours (range: 20–66 hours) following administration of the oral suspension and 26–31 hours following administration of the delayed-release tablets. Following IV infusion, the mean terminal elimination half-life of posaconazole is 27 hours.

In individuals with mild, moderate, or severe hepatic impairment, the mean apparent oral clearance following a single 400-mg dose of posaconazole oral suspension is decreased 18, 36, or 28%, respectively, compared with individuals with normal hepatic function. The elimination half-life of the drug is 39, 27, or 43 hours in those with mild, moderate, or severe hepatic impairment, respectively.

In patients with moderate or severe renal impairment (eGFR less than 50 mL/minute) receiving IV posaconazole, accumulation of the IV vehicle contained in the preparation (betadex sulfobutyl ether sodium [SBECD]) is expected to occur. (See Renal Impairment under Warnings/Precautions: Specific Populations, in Cautions.)

DESCRIPTION

Posaconazole, a triazole antifungal agent, is structurally similar to itraconazole. The drug inhibits the cytochrome P-450 (CYP)-dependent enzyme lanosterol 14-α-demethylase, thus inhibiting an essential step in fungal ergosterol biosynthesis and weakening the structure and function of the fungal cell membrane. Posaconazole may be fungicidal or fungistatic in action.

Posaconazole is commercially available for oral administration as an oral suspension or delayed-release tablets; a parenteral preparation also is available for IV administration. The oral suspension and delayed-release tablets are *not* interchangeable and cannot be directly substituted for each other since they have different pharmacokinetics and require different dosages and frequencies of administration. (See Dispensing and Dosage and Administration Precautions under Administration: Oral Administration, in Dosage and Administration.) The delayed-release tablets contain posaconazole mixed with a pH-sensitive polymer (hypromellose acetate succinate) that enhances oral bioavailability and results in higher plasma concentrations of the drug compared with the oral suspension. The pH-sensitive polymer in the tablets limits release of posaconazole in the acidic pH of the stomach, allowing release of the drug in the elevated pH environment of the intestines. The polymer may also inhibit recrystallization of posaconazole in intestinal fluid, resulting in a greater portion of the drug being available for absorption. (See Pharmacokinetics.)

Posaconazole is principally metabolized via uridine diphosphate (UDP)-glucuronosyltransferase-glucuronidation (UGT; phase 2 enzymes) and is a substrate for the P-glycoprotein transport system. Therefore, inhibitors or inducers of these metabolic pathways (e.g., rifabutin, phenytoin) may affect posaconazole plasma concentrations. Posaconazole is an inhibitor of CYP3A4; therefore, plasma concentrations of drugs predominantly metabolized by this isoenzyme (e.g., cyclosporine, tacrolimus, rifabutin, midazolam, phenytoin) may be increased by posaconazole. (See Drug Interactions.)

SPECTRUM

Posaconazole is active in vitro against *Candida*, including *C. albicans, C. dubliniensis, C. fumata, C. glabrata, C. guilliermondii, C. kefyr, C. krusei, C. lipolytica, C. lusitaniae, C. metapsilosis, C. orthopsilosis, C. parapsilosis, C. pelliculosa, C. rugosa,* and *C. tropicalis.* Posaconazole is active in vitro against some fluconazole-resistant *Candida,* and has been active in vitro against some *C. albicans* isolates obtained from patients with infections refractory to fluconazole and/or itraconazole therapy.

Posaconazole has in vitro activity against *Aspergillus,* including *A. fumigatus, A. flavus, A. niger,* and *A. terreus.*

Posaconazole also has in vitro activity against *Blastomyces, Coccidioides immitis, C. posadasii, Cryptococcus neoformans, C. gattii, Histoplasma capsulatum,* and some strains of *Fusarium oxysporum* and *F. moniliforme.* The drug is active in vitro against some fungi in the order Mucorales, including *Rhizopus* (*R. arrhizus, R. microsporus, R. oryzae*), *Mucor* (*M. circinelloides*), *Lichtheimia* (formerly *Absidia*), *Cunninghamella* (*C. bertholletiae*), *Rhizomucor pusillus, Saksenaea, Syncephalastrum racemosum,* and *Apophysomyces* (*A. elegans*).

RESISTANCE

C. albicans and *C. glabrata* with decreased in vitro susceptibility to posaconazole have been reported. Such strains reportedly have developed in some patients receiving the drug for prophylaxis of fungal infections.

Posaconazole-resistant fungi may be cross-resistant to other azole antifungals (e.g., fluconazole, itraconazole).

ADVICE TO PATIENTS

Advise patients of the importance of taking posaconazole as directed by their healthcare provider and importance of reading the patient information provided by the manufacturer.

Advise patients that posaconazole oral suspension and posaconazole delayed-release tablets are *not* interchangeable and cannot be directly substituted for each other since they require different dosages and frequencies of administration. Importance of consulting their healthcare provider before switching from delayed-release tablets to oral suspension or vice versa.

If using posaconazole oral suspension, importance of taking each dose during or immediately (i.e., within 20 minutes) following a full meal or liquid nutritional supplement to ensure adequate GI absorption of the drug. Alternatively, the oral suspension may be taken with an acidic carbonated beverage (e.g., ginger ale). Advise patients to inform clinicians if they are unable to eat full meals or drink nutritional supplements.

If using posaconazole oral suspension, advise patients that if they miss a dose it should be taken as soon as it is remembered and the next dose should be taken at the usual time. If a missed dose is remembered near the time of the next dose, advise patients to skip the missed dose. The dose should not be doubled to replace a missed dose.

If using posaconazole delayed-release tablets, importance of taking each dose with food. Advise patients that the delayed-release tablets must be swallowed whole and should not be divided, crushed, or chewed.

If using posaconazole delayed-release tablets, advise patients that if they a miss a dose and it is remembered within 12 hours after the scheduled time, the missed dose should be taken with food and the next dose should be taken at the usual time. If a missed dose is remembered more than 12 hours after the scheduled time, advise patients to skip the missed dose and resume the usual schedule. The dose should not be doubled to replace a missed dose.

Importance of informing clinicians of a history of allergic reactions to other antifungals (e.g., fluconazole, itraconazole, ketoconazole, voriconazole).

Importance of informing clinicians if currently taking drugs known to prolong QT interval corrected for rate (QT_c) that are metabolized by cytochrome P-450 (CYP) 3A4 (e.g., pimozide, quinidine).

Importance of informing clinicians if currently taking cyclosporine or tacrolimus.

Importance of immediately informing clinicians if a change in heart rate or heart rhythm occurs and informing clinicians of existing heart conditions or circulatory diseases. Posaconazole can be used with caution in patients with potentially proarrhythmic conditions.

Importance of immediately informing clinicians if itching, nausea or vomiting, yellowing of skin or eyes, extreme fatigue or flu-like symptoms, swelling in an arm or leg, or shortness of breath occurs.

Importance of informing clinicians of existing or contemplated concomitant therapy, including prescription and OTC drugs, and any concomitant illnesses (e.g., liver, kidney, or heart disease).

Importance of women informing clinicians if they are or plan to become pregnant or plan to breast-feed.

Importance of informing patients of other important precautionary information. (See Cautions.)

PREPARATIONS

Excipients in commercially available drug preparations may have clinically important effects in some individuals; consult specific product labeling for details.

Posaconazole

Oral		
Suspension	40 mg/mL	Noxafil®, Merck
Tablets, delayed-release	100 mg	Noxafil®, Merck
Parenteral		
Injection, for IV infusion only	18 mg/mL (300 mg)	Noxafil®, Merck

† Use is not currently included in the labeling approved by the US Food and Drug Administration.

Selected Revisions June 1, 2016, © Copyright, November 1, 2006, American Society of Health-System Pharmacists, Inc.

Voriconazole

8:14.08 • AZOLES

■ Voriconazole, a triazole antifungal agent, is a synthetic derivative of fluconazole.

USES

● Aspergillosis

Voriconazole is used for the treatment of invasive aspergillosis. Voriconazole has been evaluated in clinical studies for primary and salvage therapy of invasive aspergillosis, including treatment of invasive aspergillosis in patients intolerant of, or whose disease was refractory to, other antifungals. In these studies, the majority of isolates were *Aspergillus fumigatus.*

The Infectious Diseases Society of America (IDSA) considers voriconazole the drug of choice for primary treatment of invasive aspergillosis in most patients and IV amphotericin B the preferred alternative. For salvage therapy in patients refractory to or intolerant of primary antifungal therapy, IDSA recommends amphotericin B, caspofungin, micafungin, posaconazole, or itraconazole. For empiric or preemptive therapy of presumed aspergillosis, IDSA recommends amphotericin B, caspofungin, itraconazole, or voriconazole.

For the treatment of invasive aspergillosis in adults and adolescents with human immunodeficiency virus (HIV) infection, the US Centers for Disease Control and Prevention (CDC), National Institutes of Health (NIH), and IDSA recommend voriconazole as the drug of choice; IV amphotericin B, IV echinocandins (caspofungin, micafungin, anidulafungin), and oral posaconazole are recommended as alternatives. Voriconazole also is considered the drug of choice for treatment of invasive aspergillosis in HIV-infected children†; IV amphotericin B and IV caspofungin are alternatives.

Clinical Experience

Efficacy of voriconazole as primary or salvage therapy for invasive aspergillosis was evaluated in an open-label, noncomparative study in 116 patients 18–79 years of age with definite or probable invasive aspergillosis. A complete or partial response was achieved in 48% of patients in this study, but lower response rates observed in patients with definite disease (38%) than in those with probable disease (58%).

In a randomized, nonblinded study of voriconazole as primary therapy for invasive aspergillosis, 277 patients 12–79 years of age with definite or probable invasive aspergillosis received voriconazole (6 mg/kg IV twice daily for 2 doses and then 4 mg/kg IV twice daily for at least 7 days followed by oral voriconazole 200 mg twice daily) or amphotericin B (1–1.5 mg/kg IV once daily) for up to 12 weeks. At the end of the study, a complete or partial response was achieved in 53% of patients randomized to receive voriconazole compared with 32% of those randomized to receive amphotericin B and the survival rate at the end of the study was 71 or 58%, respectively. Pooled analysis of data from this study and an additional study in patients intolerant of, or whose disease was refractory to, other antifungals indicate a response rate of 44 or 40% in patients with invasive infections caused by *A. fumigatus* or other *Aspergillus* species, respectively,

● Candidemia and Disseminated Candida Infections

Voriconazole is used for the treatment of candidemia in nonneutropenic patients and for the treatment of disseminated *Candida* infections involving the skin, abdomen, kidney, bladder wall, or wounds. The drug has been effective in *Candida albicans, C. tropicalis, C. parapsilosis, C. glabrata,* and *C. krusei* infections.

For the treatment of candidemia in *nonneutropenic* patients or for empiric treatment of suspected invasive candidiasis in such patients, the IDSA recommends fluconazole or an echinocandin (caspofungin, micafungin, anidulafungin) for initial therapy; amphotericin B is the preferred alternative. These experts state that voriconazole offers little advantage over fluconazole and generally has been reserved for step-down oral therapy for treatment of *C. krusei* candidiasis or for treatment of fluconazole-resistant, voriconazole-susceptible *C. glabrata* infections. Although an echinocandin is preferred for initial treatment of *C. glabrata* infections, if the patient initially received fluconazole or voriconazole, continuation of the azole antifungal until treatment completion is reasonable if the patient is clinically improved and follow-up culture results are negative.

For the treatment of candidemia in *neutropenic*† patients, the IDSA recommends an echinocandin (caspofungin, micafungin, anidulafungin) or amphotericin B for initial therapy; fluconazole is a reasonable alternative in those who are less critically ill or have not recently received an azole; voriconazole can be used as an alternative when broader antifungal coverage is required. An echinocandin is preferred for *C. glabrata* infections; fluconazole or amphotericin B is preferred for *C. parapsilosis* infections; an echinocandin, amphotericin B, or voriconazole is recommended for *C. krusei* infections. Although an echinocandin is preferred for initial treatment of *C. glabrata* infections, if the patient initially received fluconazole or voriconazole, continuation of the azole antifungal until treatment completion is reasonable if the patient is clinically improved and follow-up culture results are negative. For initial empiric treatment of suspected invasive candidiasis in *neutropenic*† patients, amphotericin B, caspofungin, or voriconazole is recommended; alternatives are fluconazole or itraconazole.

Voriconazole has been used prophylactically to reduce the incidence of candidiasis in patients at risk, including hematopoietic stem cell transplant recipients†.

Clinical Experience

Efficacy of voriconazole for the treatment of candidemia and other disseminated or invasive infections caused by *Candida* was evaluated in an open-label comparative study in nonneutropenic patients with candidemia associated with clinical signs of infection. Patients were randomized to receive IV voriconazole (followed by oral voriconazole) or IV amphotericin B (followed by oral fluconazole); antifungal therapy was continued for a median of 15 days. In patients evaluated for efficacy, most infections were caused by *C. albicans* (46%), followed by *C. tropicalis* (19%), *C. parapsilosis* (17%), *C. glabrata* (15%), and *C. krusei* (1%). Analysis at 12 weeks after the end of therapy indicates that voriconazole is as effective as IV amphotericin B followed by oral fluconazole. A successful response (defined as resolution or improvement in all clinical signs and symptoms of infection, blood cultures negative for *Candida,* or infected deep tissue sites negative for *Candida* or resolution of all local signs of infection, and no systemic antifungal therapy other than study drugs) was observed in 41% of patients in each group.

Voriconazole has resulted in a favorable response in patients with invasive fungal infections (intra-abdominal infection, kidney and bladder wall infection, deep tissue abscess or wound infection, pneumonia/pleural space infection, skin lesions, suppurative phlebitis, hepatosplenic infection) caused by *Candida* whose disease was refractory to, or who were intolerant of, other antifungals.

● Oropharyngeal Candidiasis

Voriconazole has been used for the treatment of oropharyngeal candidiasis† refractory to other antifungals.

For the treatment of mild oropharyngeal candidiasis, the IDSA recommends topical treatment with clotrimazole lozenges or nystatin oral suspension; oral fluconazole is recommended for moderate to severe disease. For refractory oropharyngeal candidiasis, including fluconazole-refractory infections, itraconazole oral solution, oral posaconazole, or oral voriconazole is recommended. An IV echinocandin (caspofungin, micafungin, anidulafungin) or IV amphotericin B also are recommended as alternatives for refractory infections.

For the treatment of oropharyngeal candidiasis in HIV-infected adults and adolescents, the CDC, NIH, and IDSA recommend oral fluconazole as the drug of choice for initial episodes; if topical therapy is used for the treatment of mild to moderate episodes, the drugs of choice are miconazole buccal tablets or clotrimazole lozenges. Alternatives for systemic treatment of oropharyngeal candidiasis in HIV-infected adults and adolescents are itraconazole oral solution or oral posaconazole; nystatin oral suspension is an alternative if topical treatment is used. For fluconazole-refractory oropharyngeal infections in HIV-infected adults and adolescents, oral posaconazole is preferred; itraconazole oral solution is an alternative.

Although routine long-term suppressive or maintenance therapy (secondary prophylaxis) to prevent relapse or recurrence is not usually recommended in patients adequately treated for oropharyngeal candidiasis, patients with frequent or severe recurrences (including HIV-infected adults, adolescents, and children) may benefit from secondary prophylaxis with oral fluconazole or itraconazole oral solution; however, the potential for azole resistance should be considered.

● Esophageal Candidiasis

Voriconazole is used for the treatment of esophageal candidiasis. The drug has been effective in immunocompromised patients with esophageal candidiasis caused by *C. albicans, C. glabrata,* or *C. krusei.*

Esophageal candidiasis requires treatment with a systemic antifungal (not a topical antifungal).

The IDSA recommends oral fluconazole as the preferred drug of choice for the treatment of esophageal candidiasis; if oral therapy is not tolerated, IV fluconazole, IV amphotericin B, or an IV echinocandin (caspofungin, micafungin, anidulafungin) is recommended. For fluconazole-refractory infections, preferred alternatives are itraconazole oral solution, oral posaconazole, or oral or IV voriconazole; other alternatives are an IV echinocandin or IV amphotericin B.

For the treatment of esophageal candidiasis in HIV-infected adults and adolescents, the CDC, NIH, and IDSA recommend oral or IV fluconazole as the drug of choice and itraconazole oral solution as the preferred alternative. Other alternatives include oral or IV voriconazole, oral posaconazole, IV echinocandins (caspofungin, micafungin, anidulafungin), or IV amphotericin B. For refractory esophageal candidiasis, including fluconazole-refractory infections, in HIV-infected adults and adolescents, oral posaconazole is preferred; alternatives include itraconazole oral solution, IV amphotericin B, IV echinocandins (caspofungin, micafungin, anidulafungin), or oral or IV voriconazole.

Although routine long-term suppressive or maintenance therapy (secondary prophylaxis) to prevent relapse or recurrence is not usually recommended in patients adequately treated for esophageal candidiasis, patients with frequent or severe recurrences (including HIV-infected adults, adolescents, and children) may benefit from secondary prophylaxis with oral fluconazole or oral posaconazole; however, the potential for azole resistance should be considered.

Clinical Experience

Efficacy of voriconazole has been evaluated in a comparative study in immunocompromised patients with esophageal candidiasis documented by endoscopy. Patients were randomized to receive oral voriconazole (200 mg twice daily) or oral fluconazole (200 mg once daily); antifungals were given for a median of 15 days. A successful response (defined as normal endoscopy at end of treatment or at least a 1 grade improvement over baseline endoscopic score) occurred in 98% of those who received voriconazole and in 95% of those who received fluconazole. In voriconazole-treated patients, mycologic eradication was achieved in 84% of those with *C. albicans* infection, in 57% of those with *C. glabrata* infection, and in the single patient with *C. krusei* infection.

● Coccidioidomycosis

Voriconazole has been used for the treatment of coccidioidomycosis† caused by *Coccidioides immitis* or *C. posadasii*, and is recommended as an alternative for the treatment or prevention of these infections.

Antifungal treatment may not be necessary in patients with mild, uncomplicated coccidioidal pneumonia since such infections often are self-limited and may resolve spontaneously. However, antifungal treatment is recommended for patients with more severe or rapidly progressing coccidioidal infections, those with chronic pulmonary or disseminated infections, and immunocompromised or debilitated individuals (e.g., HIV-infected individuals, organ transplant recipients, those receiving immunosuppressive therapy, those with diabetes or cardiopulmonary disease).

The IDSA and others state that an oral azole (fluconazole or itraconazole) usually is recommended for initial treatment of symptomatic pulmonary coccidioidomycosis and chronic fibrocavitary or disseminated (extrapulmonary) coccidioidomycosis. However, IV amphotericin B is recommended as an alternative and is preferred for initial treatment of severely ill patients who have hypoxia or rapidly progressing disease, for immunocompromised individuals, or when azole antifungals have been ineffective or cannot be used (e.g., pregnant women).

For the treatment of clinically mild coccidioidomycosis (e.g., focal pneumonia) in HIV-infected adults and adolescents, the CDC, NIH, and IDSA recommend initial therapy with oral fluconazole or oral itraconazole. These experts state that, although clinical data are limited, oral voriconazole or oral posaconazole may be used as an alternative for the treatment of clinically mild coccidioidomycosis† that has not responded to fluconazole or itraconazole.

HIV-infected individuals who have been adequately treated for coccidioidomycosis should receive long-term (usually life-long) secondary prophylaxis to prevent recurrence or relapse. Although oral fluconazole or oral itraconazole are the drugs of choice recommended by the CDC, NIH, and IDSA for secondary prophylaxis to prevent recurrence or relapse of coccidioidomycosis in HIV-infected adults and adolescents, these experts state that oral voriconazole or oral posaconazole can be used as an alternative for secondary prophylaxis of

coccidioidomycosis† if the patient did not initially respond to fluconazole or itraconazole.

● Exserohilum Infections

Amphotericin B has been used for the treatment of infections known or suspected to be caused by *Exserohilum rostratum*†.

Exserohilum is a common mold found in soil and on plants, especially grasses, and thrives in warm and humid climates. *E. rostratum* is considered an opportunistic human pathogen and rarely has been involved in human infections, including cutaneous and subcutaneous infections or keratitis, typically as the result of skin or eye trauma. More invasive infections (e.g., infections involving the sinuses, heart, lungs, or bones) and life-threatening infections also have been reported rarely, usually in immunocompromised individuals. In addition, *E. rostratum* was identified as the predominant pathogen in the 2012–2013 multistate outbreak of fungal meningitis and other fungal infections that occurred in the US in patients who received contaminated preservative-free methylprednisolone acetate injections prepared by a compounding pharmacy. *Exserohilum* infections cannot be transmitted person-to-person.

Although data are limited and the clinical relevance of in vitro testing remains uncertain, in vitro studies indicate that *Exserohilum* is inhibited by some triazole antifungals (e.g., voriconazole, itraconazole, posaconazole) and amphotericin B. Echinocandins (e.g., caspofungin, micafungin) have variable in vitro activity and fluconazole has poor in vitro activity against the fungus.

Exserohilum Infections Related to Contaminated Injections

In September 2012, the CDC and US Food and Drug Administration (FDA) initiated investigations in response to fungal CNS infections (including some fatalities) reported in patients who received epidural injections of contaminated extemporaneously prepared methylprednisolone acetate injections from the New England Compounding Center (NECC). Subsequently, there were reports of joint infections and osteomyelitis in some patients who received intra-articular injections of methylprednisolone acetate from NECC, as well as infections possibly related to other NECC products.

Out of an abundance of caution at that time, the FDA recommended that health-care professionals and consumers not use any product that was produced by NECC, and the company recalled all products that were compounded at and distributed from its facility in Framingham, Massachusetts. Recall information is available at http://www.neccrx.com.

The predominant pathogen identified in samples taken from patients who received contaminated products from NECC has been *E. rostratum*; *Aspergillus* also was identified in an index patient and *Cladosporium cladosporioides* was recovered from several other patients. The presence of *E. rostratum* was confirmed in recalled lots of the contaminated products. Other organisms identified in unopened vials from these recalled lots were *C. cladosporioides*, *Bacillus subtilis*, *B. pumilus*, *Paecilomyces formosus*, *Rhodotorula laryngis*, and *Rhizopus stolonifer*; *Rhodotorula* and *Rhizopus* are not known to cause human disease and do not grow at human body temperature.

CDC data indicate that, as of September 6, 2013, there were a total of 750 cases of fungal infections (including 64 deaths) reported in 20 states that have been linked to 3 specific lots of contaminated methylprednisolone acetate injections. Although the majority of initial cases involved fungal meningitis (some with stroke), subsequent reports involved localized spinal or paraspinal infections (e.g., epidural abscess). More than 6 months after the outbreak related to contaminated products was first identified, the CDC continued to receive reports of patients presenting with localized spinal and paraspinal infections (e.g., epidural abscess, phlegmon, discitis, vertebral osteomyelitis, arachnoiditis, or other complications at or near the site of injection). These localized infections have occurred in patients with or without a diagnosis of fungal meningitis. In some patients being treated for fungal meningitis who had no previous evidence of localized infections, such infections were found at the site of injection using magnetic resonance imaging (MRI) studies. Some cases have occurred in patients without any previous evidence of infection or in those with persistent, worsening, or new symptoms.

Patients with meningitis generally presented 1–4 weeks or longer after receiving contaminated methylprednisolone acetate injections; the greatest risk for development of fungal meningitis appeared to be during the first 6 weeks after an epidural or paraspinal injection. Data from one group of patients indicate that the median time from the last injection with contaminated product to the date of the first MRI finding indicative of infection was 50 days (range 12–121 days) for all patients with a spinal or paraspinal infection, and the median time from the first positive lumbar puncture finding to the first positive MRI finding was 21 days for those with meningitis and spinal or paraspinal infections.

Clinicians treating fungal infections in patients who received contaminated methylprednisolone acetate injections from NECC should consult an infectious disease expert to assist with diagnosis, management, and follow-up, which may be complex and prolonged. A clinical consultant network for clinicians can be reached by calling CDC at 800-232-4636. Because of evidence of latent disease, the CDC cautions clinicians to maintain a high index of suspicion and remain vigilant for fungal infections in patients who received the contaminated methylprednisolone acetate injections, especially in those who have mild or baseline symptoms, and to consider MRI evaluation if clinically warranted.

In October 2012, the CDC released interim treatment guidance documents containing recommendations for empiric antifungal treatment of CNS and parameningeal infections and osteoarticular infections associated with the contaminated methylprednisolone acetate products. As additional information became available, these treatment guidance documents were updated and revised several times. Although the following information regarding the CDC recommendations for treatment of these fungal infections was current at the time the voriconazole monograph was finalized for publication, these recommendations may change and the most recent CDC guidance documents at http://www.cdc.gov/hai/outbreaks/meningitis.html should be consulted for the most current recommendations for selection of antifungal agents and the appropriate dosages and duration of treatment.

For the treatment of CNS infections (including meningitis, stroke, and arachnoiditis) and/or parameningeal infections (epidural or paraspinal abscess, discitis or osteomyelitis, and sacroiliac infection) in adults who received the contaminated methylprednisolone acetate injections, the CDC recommends voriconazole. In most patients with these CNS or parameningeal infections, voriconazole should be given IV initially and a transition to oral voriconazole considered only after the patient is clinically stable or improving. Initial treatment with oral voriconazole should be considered only in patients with mild disease who can be monitored closely. Use of IV amphotericin B liposomal *in addition* to IV voriconazole should be strongly considered in patients who present with severe disease and in patients who do not improve or experience clinical deterioration or manifest new sites of disease activity while receiving voriconazole monotherapy. IV amphotericin B liposomal also is an alternative in patients who are unable to tolerate voriconazole. IV amphotericin B liposomal is preferred over other lipid formulations of amphotericin B because of better CNS penetration. Because of limited data and associated toxicities, routine use of intrathecal amphotericin B is not recommended. Although posaconazole or itraconazole has been used in some patients who could not tolerate voriconazole or amphotericin B, efficacy of these drugs for the treatment of infections associated with the contaminated methylprednisolone acetate injections has not been established. Expert consultation is advised when making decisions regarding alternative regimens.

For the treatment of osteoarticular infections (discitis, vertebral osteomyelitis, and epidural abscess or osteoarticular infections not involving the spine) in adults who received intra-articular injections of contaminated methylprednisolone acetate, the CDC recommends voriconazole. Voriconazole should be given IV initially in those with more severe osteoarticular infections, clinical instability, discitis, vertebral osteomyelitis, or epidural abscess; a transition to oral voriconazole should be considered only after the patient is clinically stable or improving. Initial treatment with oral voriconazole should be considered only in patients with mild osteoarticular infections not involving the spine who can be monitored closely. Use of a lipid formulation of IV amphotericin B *in addition* to IV voriconazole should be considered in patients with severe osteoarticular infection and/or clinical instability. A lipid formulation of IV amphotericin B, posaconazole, or itraconazole are alternatives in patients who cannot tolerate voriconazole. Expert consultation is advised when making decisions regarding alternative regimens.

Adequate duration of antifungal treatment for *Exserohilum* infections associated with contaminated methylprednisolone acetate injections is unknown, but prolonged therapy is required. (See Exserohilum Infections under Dosage and Administration: Dosage.) In addition, close follow-up monitoring after completion of treatment is essential in all patients to detect potential relapse.

The CDC website at http://www.cdc.gov/hai/outbreaks/meningitis.html and FDA website at http://www.fda.gov/Drugs/DrugSafety/ucm322734.htm should be consulted for the most recent information regarding the contaminated NECC products and associated infections. The CDC website includes specific information regarding case definitions and diagnostic testing as well as management and treatment of these infections.

● *Fusarium and Scedosporium Infections*

Voriconazole is used for the treatment of serious fungal infections caused by *Fusarium* (including *F. solani*) or *Scedosporium apiospermum* (asexual form of *Pseudallescheria boydii*) in patients intolerant of, or whose disease is refractory to, other antifungals.

For the treatment of fusariosis, the most appropriate antifungal should be selected based on in vitro susceptibility testing. Amphotericin B may be preferred for infections caused by *F. solani* or *F. verticillioides*; either voriconazole or amphotericin B are recommended for infections caused by other *Fusarium*.

For the treatment of scedosporiosis, some clinicians consider voriconazole the drug of choice and posaconazole the preferred alternative.

● *Histoplasmosis*

Voriconazole has been used for the treatment of histoplasmosis† caused by *Histoplasma capsulatum*.

The drugs of choice for the treatment of histoplasmosis are IV amphotericin B or oral itraconazole. IV amphotericin B is preferred for initial treatment of severe, life-threatening histoplasmosis, especially in immunocompromised patients such as those with HIV infection. Oral itraconazole generally is used for initial treatment of less severe disease (e.g., mild to moderate acute pulmonary histoplasmosis, chronic cavitary pulmonary histoplasmosis) and as follow-up therapy in the treatment of severe infections after a response has been obtained with IV amphotericin B. Other azole antifungals (fluconazole, ketoconazole, posaconazole, voriconazole) are considered second-line alternatives to oral itraconazole.

For the treatment of less severe disseminated histoplasmosis† in HIV-infected adults and adolescents, the CDC, NIH, and IDSA recommend initial treatment with oral itraconazole. These experts state that, although clinical data are limited, oral voriconazole or oral posaconazole may be used as an alternative for the treatment of less severe disseminated histoplasmosis in patients intolerant of itraconazole who are only moderately ill.

HIV-infected individuals who have been adequately treated for histoplasmosis should receive long-term suppressive or maintenance therapy (secondary prophylaxis) to prevent recurrence or relapse. Oral itraconazole is the drug of choice for secondary prophylaxis of histoplasmosis in HIV-infected adults and adolescents. The role of voriconazole for secondary prophylaxis of histoplasmosis in HIV-infected patients has not been evaluated to date.

● *Penicilliosis*

Voriconazole is used for treatment of penicilliosis† caused by *Penicillium marneffei*.

For the treatment of severe acute penicilliosis in HIV-infected adults and adolescents, the CDC, NIH, and IDSA recommend an initial regimen of IV amphotericin B liposomal followed by oral itraconazole. These experts state that a voriconazole regimen (IV initially, then oral) can be used as an alternative in patients with severe penicilliosis, including those who fail to respond to a regimen of amphotericin B followed by itraconazole.

For the treatment of mild penicilliosis† in HIV-infected adults and adolescents, the CDC, NIH, and IDSA recommend oral itraconazole as the drug of choice and oral voriconazole as an alternative.

HIV-infected patients who have been treated for penicilliosis should receive long-term suppressive or maintenance therapy (secondary prophylaxis) with oral itraconazole to prevent recurrence or relapse. (See Uses: Penicilliosis, in Itraconazole 8:14.08.) An optimal voriconazole regimen for secondary prophylaxis of penicilliosis has not been identified to date.

● *Empiric Therapy in Febrile Neutropenic Patients*

Voriconazole also has been used for empiric therapy of presumed fungal infections in febrile neutropenic patients†.

Clinical Experience

Efficacy of voriconazole for empiric therapy in febrile neutropenic patients has been evaluated in an open-label, randomized, multicenter study in patients 12–82 years of age who were neutropenic following chemotherapy or stem cell transplantation. In this study, patients received voriconazole or amphotericin B liposomal for up to 3 days following neutrophil recovery, or for a maximum of 12 weeks. A response (based on a composite assessment including no breakthrough infections within 7 days of the completion of therapy, survival for 7 days following completion of therapy, discontinuance of the drug because of toxicity or lack of efficacy prior to recovery from neutropenia, resolution of fever during neutropenia, and complete or partial response in patients with baseline fungal infections by the completion of therapy) was obtained in 26 or 31% of patients receiving voriconazole or amphotericin B liposomal, respectively. The composite results failed to meet protocol-defined statistical criteria for concluding that voriconazole was not inferior to amphotericin B liposomal. Exploratory analyses of the individual elements of the composite measure suggested that breakthrough infections occurred in a smaller proportion of patients receiving voriconazole (1.9%) compared with amphotericin B liposomal (5%); exploratory analyses of the other individual elements of the composite measure failed to identify other substantial differences between the 2 regimens.

DOSAGE AND ADMINISTRATION

● Administration

Voriconazole is administered orally or by slow IV infusion.

The IV route usually is used for initial treatment of systemic fungal infections, but may be switched to oral treatment when clinically indicated.

Electrolyte disturbances (e.g., hypokalemia, hypomagnesemia, hypocalcemia) should be corrected prior to initiation of voriconazole. (See IV Infusion under Dosage and Administration: Administration and see Cardiovascular Effects under Warnings/Precautions: General Precautions, in Cautions.)

Oral Administration

Voriconazole film-coated tablets or oral suspension should be given at least 1 hour before or 1 hour after meals.

Reconstituted voriconazole oral suspension should be administered using the oral dispenser provided by the manufacturer and should not be mixed with other drugs or flavoring agents. Prior to withdrawal of each dose, the reconstituted oral suspension should be shaken for 10 seconds.

If a dose is missed, the missed dose should be taken as soon as possible; however, if it has been more than 6 hours since the missed dose, the next scheduled dose should be taken at the appropriate time. A double dose should not be taken.

Reconstitution

Voriconazole powder for oral suspension is reconstituted by adding 46 mL of water to the bottle containing 45 g of voriconazole to provide a suspension containing 40 mg/mL. The bottle should be shaken vigorously for about 1 minute.

The oral suspension should not be mixed with other drugs or additional flavoring agents. The reconstituted oral suspension should *not* be further diluted with water or any other vehicle and is stable for 14 days at 15–30°C.

IV Infusion

Voriconazole IV solutions should *not* be administered concomitantly with short-term infusions of *concentrated* electrolytes, even if the 2 infusions are running in separate IV lines or cannulas. Voriconazole IV solutions may be administered at the same time as other IV solutions containing *nonconcentrated* electrolytes; however, the drug must be infused through a separate line.

Voriconazole IV solutions should *not* be administered concomitantly with any blood product, even if the 2 infusions are running in separate IV lines or cannulas.

Voriconazole IV solutions may be administered at the same time as total parenteral nutrition (TPN); however, the drug must be infused through a separate IV line. If infused through a multiple-lumen catheter, TPN must be administered using a different port from the one used for voriconazole.

Reconstitution and Dilution

For IV infusion, the contents of a single-use vial labeled as containing 200 mg of voriconazole should be reconstituted with exactly 19 mL of sterile water for injection to prepare a solution containing 10 mg/mL of the drug. The vial should be shaken until all the powder is dissolved. Reconstituted voriconazole solutions must be further diluted in a compatible IV infusion solution prior to administration. The reconstituted solutions should be used immediately since they contain no preservative; if not used immediately, reconstituted solutions should be stored for no longer than 24 hours at 2–8°C before being diluted and used.

To dilute reconstituted voriconazole solutions, calculate the volume of reconstituted solution required to administer the appropriate weight-based dose and then withdraw and discard a volume of diluent from the final infusion container that equals or exceeds that volume. The volume of diluent remaining in the container should be such that a final concentration of at least 0.5 mg/mL but not greater than 5 mg/mL will be achieved following addition of the reconstituted solution. The appropriate dose should then be withdrawn from the required number of reconstituted vials and added to the infusion container. Any unused portion of reconstituted solution should be discarded.

Rate of Administration

IV infusions of voriconazole should be given over 1–2 hours at a maximum rate of 3 mg/kg per hour. The drug should not be administered by rapid IV infusion.

● Dosage

In adults, the voriconazole 200-mg tablet and 40-mg/mL oral suspension are bioequivalent when administered using a loading dose regimen (400 mg every 12 hours) followed by maintenance dosage (200 mg every 12 hours).

In adults, an oral voriconazole dosage of 200 mg every 12 hours results in an area under the plasma-concentration time curve (AUC) similar to that achieved with an IV dosage of 3 mg/kg every 12 hours; an oral dosage of 300 mg every 12 hours results in an AUC similar to that reported with an IV dosage of 4 mg/kg every 12 hours.

Aspergillosis
Adult Dosage

For the treatment of invasive aspergillosis, adults should receive an initial loading dose regimen of 6 mg/kg of voriconazole by IV infusion every 12 hours for 2 doses, followed by a maintenance dosage of 4 mg/kg by IV infusion every 12 hours for at least 7 days until the patient is clinically improved and can be switched to oral voriconazole. If this IV maintenance dosage cannot be tolerated, the maintenance dosage can be decreased to 3 mg/kg IV every 12 hours.

After an initial IV regimen, the recommended oral maintenance dosage of voriconazole in patients with invasive aspergillosis is 200 mg every 12 hours in patients weighing 40 kg or more or 100 mg every 12 hours in adults weighing less than 40 kg; if the therapeutic response is not adequate, the dosage may be increased to 300 mg every 12 hours in patients weighing 40 kg or more or 150 mg every 12 hours in those weighing less than 40 kg. If this dosage cannot be tolerated, the dosage may be decreased by increments of 50 mg to a minimum of 200 mg every 12 hours in those weighing 40 kg or more or 100 mg every 12 hours in adults weighing less than 40 kg.

The total duration of IV and oral therapy should be based on the severity of the patient's underlying disease, recovery from immunosuppression, and response to the drug. The optimal duration of therapy for aspergillosis is uncertain. In a clinical study in patients with invasive aspergillosis, the median duration of initial IV therapy was 10 days (range 2–90 days) and the median duration of maintenance oral therapy was 76 days (range 2–232 days). The Infectious Diseases Society of America (IDSA) recommends that treatment of invasive pulmonary aspergillosis be continued for at least 6–12 weeks and continued throughout the period of immunosuppression.

For the treatment of invasive aspergillosis in adults with human immunodeficiency virus (HIV) infection, the US Centers for Disease Control and Prevention (CDC), National Institutes of Health (NIH), and IDSA recommend an initial loading dose regimen of 6 mg/kg by IV infusion every 12 hours on day 1, followed by a maintenance dosage of 4 mg/kg by IV infusion every 12 hours. After clinical improvement, an oral dosage of 200 mg every 12 hours is recommended. The optimal duration of therapy in these patients has not been established, but antifungal therapy should be continued at least until the CD4$^+$ T-cell count increases to 200/mm^3 as a result of potent antiretroviral therapy and there is evidence that aspergillosis has resolved.

Pediatric Dosage

In children 12 years of age or older, an IV regimen of voriconazole that consists of a loading dose regimen of 6 mg/kg every 12 hours for 2 doses, followed by an IV maintenance regimen of 4 mg/kg every 12 hours has been recommended; the IV maintenance dosage should be decreased to 3 mg/kg every 12 hours if higher dosage is not tolerated.

In children 12 years of age or older weighing less than 40 kg, an oral regimen of voriconazole that consists of a loading dose regimen of 200 mg every 12 hours for 2 doses, followed by a maintenance dosage of 100 mg every 12 hours has been recommended; if the response is inadequate, the dosage may be increased to 150 mg every 12 hours. In children 12 years of age or older weighing 40 kg or more, an oral regimen of 400 mg every 12 hours for 2 doses, followed by a maintenance dosage of 200 mg every 12 hours has been recommended; if the response is inadequate, the dosage may be increased to 300 mg every 12 hours.

The IDSA recommends that pediatric patients receive 5–7 mg/kg IV every 12 hours for the treatment of invasive aspergillosis.

For the treatment of invasive aspergillosis in HIV-infected adolescents, some clinicians recommend an initial loading dose regimen of 6 mg/kg by IV infusion twice daily on day 1, followed by a maintenance dosage of 4 mg/kg by IV infusion twice daily. After clinical improvement, an oral dosage of 200 mg twice daily is recommended. The optimal duration of therapy in these patients has not been established, but antifungal therapy should be continued at least until the CD4+ T-cell count increases to 200/mm³ as a result of potent antiretroviral therapy and there is evidence of clinical response.

For the treatment of invasive aspergillosis in HIV-infected children†, some clinicians recommend an initial loading dose regimen of 8 mg/kg (maximum 400 mg) orally twice daily on day 1, followed by a maintenance dosage of 7 mg/kg (maximum 200 mg) orally twice daily. Alternatively, an initial loading dose regimen of 6–8 mg/kg given by IV infusion twice daily on day 1, followed by a maintenance dosage of 7 mg/kg (maximum 200 mg) given by IV infusion twice daily has been recommended. Treatment should be continued for at least 12 weeks; however, treatment duration should be individualized according to clinical response.

Candidemia and Disseminated Candida Infections
Adult Dosage
The usual initial dosage of voriconazole for the treatment of candidemia and disseminated *Candida* infections in *nonneutropenic* adults is 6 mg/kg by IV infusion every 12 hours for 2 doses, followed by a maintenance dosage of 3–4 mg/kg by IV infusion every 12 hours until the patient can be switched to oral voriconazole. In clinical studies, patients with candidemia received 3 mg/kg every 12 hours and those with deep tissue infections received 4 mg/kg every 12 hours as salvage therapy. Dosage generally should be based on the nature and severity of the infection. If the patient cannot tolerate a dosage of 4 mg/kg, the dosage can be decreased to 3 mg/kg every 12 hours.

After an initial IV regimen, the usual oral dosage of voriconazole in *nonneutropenic* adults with candidemia and disseminated *Candida* infections is 200 mg every 12 hours in patients weighing 40 kg or more or 100 mg every 12 hours in those weighing less than 40 kg; if the therapeutic response is not adequate, the dosage may be increased to 300 mg every 12 hours in patients weighing 40 kg or more or 150 mg every 12 hours in adults weighing less than 40 kg. If this dosage is not tolerated, the dosage may be decreased by increments of 50 mg to a minimum of 200 mg every 12 hours in patients weighing 40 kg or more or 100 mg every 12 hours in adults weighing less than 40 kg.

If voriconazole is used for the treatment of candidemia in *neutropenic*† adults, the IDSA recommends an initial dosage of 6 mg/kg by IV infusion every 12 hours for 2 doses, followed by a maintenance dosage of 3 mg/kg by IV infusion every 12 hours.

The manufacturer recommends that treatment of candidemia be continued for at least 14 days after symptoms have resolved or the last positive culture, whichever is longer. The IDSA and others recommend that antifungal treatment for candidemia (without persistent fungemia or metastatic complications) be continued for 14 days after the first negative blood culture and resolution of signs and symptoms of candidemia.

Pediatric Dosage
In children 12 years of age or older, an IV regimen that consists of a loading dose regimen of 6 mg/kg every 12 hours for 2 doses, followed by an IV maintenance regimen of 4 mg/kg every 12 hours has been recommended; the IV maintenance dosage should be decreased to 3 mg/kg every 12 hours if higher dosage is not tolerated.

In children 12 years of age or older weighing less than 40 kg, an oral regimen of 200 mg every 12 hours for 2 doses, followed by a maintenance dosage of 100 mg every 12 hours has been recommended; if the response is inadequate, the dosage may be increased to 150 mg every 12 hours. In children 12 years of age or older weighing 40 kg or more, an oral regimen of 400 mg every 12 hours for 2 doses, followed by a maintenance dosage of 200 mg every 12 hours has been recommended; if the response is inadequate, the dosage may be increased to 300 mg every 12 hours.

The manufacturer recommends that treatment of candidemia be continued for at least 14 days after symptoms have resolved or the last positive culture, whichever is longer. The IDSA and others recommend that antifungal treatment for candidemia (without persistent fungemia or metastatic complications) be continued for 14 days after the first negative blood culture and resolution of signs and symptoms of candidemia.

Oropharyngeal Candidiasis
Adult Dosage
For the treatment of oropharyngeal candidiasis† refractory to other antifungals, the IDSA and others recommend an oral voriconazole dosage of 200 mg twice daily.

The IDSA and others recommend that antifungal treatment for oropharyngeal candidiasis be continued for 7–14 days.

Esophageal Candidiasis
Adult Dosage
The usual adult oral dosage of voriconazole for the treatment of esophageal candidiasis is 200 mg every 12 hours in patients weighing 40 kg or more or 100 mg every 12 hours in adults weighing less than 40 kg; if the therapeutic response is not adequate, the dosage may be increased to 300 mg every 12 hours in patients weighing 40 kg or more or 150 mg every 12 hours in adults weighing less than 40 kg. If this dosage is not tolerated, the dosage may be decreased by increments of 50 mg to a minimum of 200 mg every 12 hours in patients weighing 40 kg or more or 100 mg every 12 hours in adults weighing less than 40 kg.

For the treatment of esophageal candidiasis in HIV-infected adults, some clinicians recommend a voriconazole dosage of 200 mg twice daily given orally or by IV infusion.

The manufacturer recommends that treatment of esophageal candidiasis be continued for at least 14 days and for at least 7 days after symptoms resolve. The IDSA and others recommend that antifungal treatment of esophageal candidiasis be continued for 14–21 days after clinical improvement.

Pediatric Dosage
For the treatment of esophageal candidiasis in children 12 years of age or older weighing less than 40 kg, an oral regimen of 100 mg every 12 hours has been recommended. For children 12 years of age or older weighing 40 kg or more, an oral regimen of 200 mg every 12 hours has been recommended.

For the treatment of esophageal candidiasis in HIV-infected adolescents, some clinicians recommend a voriconazole dosage of 200 mg twice daily given orally or by IV infusion.

The manufacturer recommends that treatment of esophageal candidiasis be continued for at least 14 days and for at least 7 days after symptoms resolve. The IDSA and others recommend that antifungal treatment of esophageal candidiasis be continued for 14–21 days after clinical improvement.

Coccidioidomycosis
If oral voriconazole is used as an alternative for the treatment of clinically mild coccidioidomycosis† (e.g., focal pneumonia) in HIV-infected adults and adolescents, a dosage of 200 mg twice daily is recommended by the CDC, NIH, and IDSA.

If oral voriconazole is used as an alternative for long-term suppressive or maintenance therapy (secondary prophylaxis)† to prevent relapse or recurrence of coccidioidomycosis in HIV-infected adults and adolescents who have completed initial treatment of the disease, a dosage of 200 mg twice daily is recommended by the CDC, NIH, and IDSA. In HIV-infected patients who were treated for focal coccidioidal pneumonia and are receiving effective antiretroviral therapy, consideration can be given to discontinuing secondary prophylaxis against coccidioidomycosis after 12 months if CD4+ T-cell counts are 250/mm³ or higher, provided the patient is monitored for recurrence (e.g., serial chest radiographs, coccidioidal serology). HIV-infected patients who were treated for diffuse pulmonary, disseminated, or meningeal coccidioidomycosis usually require life-long secondary prophylaxis.

Exserohilum Infections
Adult Dosage
For the treatment of CNS and/or parameningeal infections known or suspected to be caused by *Exserohilum rostratum*† in adults who received injections of contaminated methylprednisolone acetate (see Uses: Exserohilum Infections), the CDC recommends that voriconazole be given in a dosage of 6 mg/kg every 12 hours. In most

patients with these CNS or parameningeal infections, voriconazole should be given IV initially and a transition to oral voriconazole should be considered only after the patient is clinically stable or improving. Initial treatment with oral voriconazole should be considered only in those with mild disease who can be monitored closely.

For the treatment of osteoarticular infections known or suspected to be caused by *E. rostratum†* in adults who received intra-articular injections of contaminated methylprednisolone acetate (see Uses: Exserohilum Infections), the CDC recommends that voriconazole be given in a dosage of 6 mg/kg every 12 hours. For osteoarticular infections that do not involve the spine, voriconazole can be given in a dosage of 6 mg/kg every 12 hours for 2 doses, followed by 4 mg/kg every 12 hours. In most patients with osteoarticular infections, voriconazole should be given IV initially and a transition to oral voriconazole should be considered only after the patient is clinically stable or improving. Initial treatment with oral voriconazole should be considered only in those with mild infections who can be monitored closely.

Serum voriconazole concentrations should be measured in all patients on treatment day 5 and dosage adjusted if needed, aiming for trough concentrations of 2–5 mcg/mL. Serum concentrations should be monitored once weekly during the initial 4–6 weeks of treatment and whenever dosage changes are made, maintaining trough voriconazole concentrations of 2–5 mcg/mL. Voriconazole serum concentrations greater than 5 mcg/mL should be avoided because of the risk of neurotoxicity and other adverse effects.

Adequate duration of antifungal treatment for these *E. rostratum* infections is unknown, but prolonged treatment is required and should be based on disease severity and clinical response. A treatment duration of 6–12 months is probably necessary in patients who have severe CNS disease with complications (arachnoiditis, stroke), persistent CSF abnormalities, or underlying immunosuppression. In those with parameningeal infection, a minimum treatment duration of 3–6 months should be considered, and at least 6 months or longer probably is required for more severe disease (e.g., discitis, osteomyelitis) and in those with underlying immunosuppression or complications not amenable to surgical treatment. In those with osteoarticular infections, a minimum treatment duration of 3 months should be considered, and longer than 3 months is probably necessary in those with severe disease, bone infections, or underlying immunosuppression. After completion of treatment, close follow-up monitoring is essential in all patients to detect potential relapse.

An infectious disease expert and the most recent guidelines from the CDC should be consulted for information regarding the management of fungal infections in patients who received injections of potentially contaminated products. Clinicians should consult the CDC website at http://www.cdc.gov/hai/outbreaks/meningitis.html for the most recent recommendations regarding the drugs of choice, dosage, and duration of treatment of these infections.

Fusarium and Scedosporium Infections
Adult Dosage

The recommended initial adult IV dosage of voriconazole for the treatment of infections caused by *Fusarium* or *Scedosporium apiospermum* is 6 mg/kg by IV infusion every 12 hours for 2 doses, followed by a maintenance dosage of 4 mg/kg by IV infusion every 12 hours until the patient can be switched to oral voriconazole. If this dosage is not tolerated, the IV maintenance dosage can be decreased to 3 mg/kg every 12 hours.

After an initial IV regimen, the usual oral dosage of voriconazole in patients with infections caused by *Fusarium* or *Scedosporium apiospermum* is 200 mg every 12 hours in those weighing 40 kg or more or 100 mg every 12 hours in adults weighing less than 40 kg; if the therapeutic response is not adequate, the dosage may be increased to 300 mg every 12 hours in those weighing 40 kg or more or 150 mg every 12 hours in adults weighing less than 40 kg. If this dosage cannot be tolerated, the dosage may be decreased by increments of 50 mg to a minimum of 200 mg every 12 hours in those weighing 40 kg or more or 100 mg every 12 hours in adults weighing less than 40 kg.

Total duration of therapy should be based on the severity of the patient's underlying disease, recovery from immunosuppression, and response to the drug.

Pediatric Dosage

In children 12 years of age of older, an IV regimen of voriconazole that consists of a loading dose regimen of 6 mg/kg every 12 hours for 2 doses, followed by an IV maintenance regimen of 4 mg/kg every 12 hours has been recommended the IV maintenance dosage should be decreased to 3 mg/kg every 12 hours if higher dosage is not tolerated.

In children 12 years of age or older weighing less than 40 kg, an oral regimen of voriconazole that consists of a loading dose regimen of 200 mg every 12 hours for 2 doses, followed by a maintenance dosage of 100 mg every 12 hours has been recommended; if the response is inadequate, the dosage may be increased to 150 mg every 12 hours. In children 12 years of age or older weighing 40 kg or more, an oral regimen of 400 mg every 12 hours for 2 doses, followed by a maintenance dosage of 200 mg every 12 hours has been recommended; if the response is inadequate, the dosage may be increased to 300 mg every 12 hours.

Total duration of therapy should be based on the severity of the patient's underlying disease, recovery from immunosuppression, and response to the drug.

Histoplasmosis

If oral voriconazole is used as an alternative for the treatment of less severe disseminated histoplasmosis† in HIV-infected adults and adolescents who are only moderately ill (see Uses: Histoplasmosis), the CDC, NIH, and IDSA recommend a dosage of 400 mg twice daily for 2 doses followed by 200 mg twice daily.

Penicilliosis

If voriconazole is used as an alternative for the treatment of severe acute penicilliosis in HIV-infected adults and adolescents, the CDC, NIH, and IDSA recommend an initial IV regimen of 6 mg/kg every 12 hours for 2 doses, followed by 4 mg/kg IV every 12 hours for at least 3 days, then an oral regimen of 200 mg twice daily for a maximum of 12 weeks.

If oral voriconazole is used as an alternative for the treatment of mild penicilliosis in HIV-infected adults and adolescents, the CDC, NIH, and IDSA recommend a dosage of 400 mg twice daily for 2 doses, followed by 200 mg twice daily for a maximum of 12 weeks.

● Special Populations
Hepatic Impairment

In adults with mild-to-moderate hepatic cirrhosis (Child-Pugh class A or B), usual IV or oral loading dosages of voriconazole should be used, but IV or oral maintenance dosages should be decreased by 50%.

Voriconazole should be used in patients with severe hepatic impairment only if benefits outweigh risks; the drug has not been studied in patients with severe hepatic cirrhosis (Child-Pugh class C) or with chronic hepatitis B virus (HBV) or hepatitis C virus (HCV) infection. (See Hepatic Effects under Cautions: Warnings/Precautions.)

Renal Impairment

Adjustment of oral voriconazole dosage is not necessary in patients with mild to severe renal impairment.

Because of potential accumulation of the IV vehicle (sulfobutyl ether β-cyclodextrin sodium [SBECD]), IV voriconazole should be avoided in patients with moderate or severe renal impairment (creatinine clearance less than 50 mL/minute); voriconazole should be administered orally in these patients unless potential benefits of the IV route outweigh risks. If IV voriconazole is used in patients with creatinine clearance less than 50 mL/minute, serum creatinine should be monitored closely; if increases occur, switching to oral voriconazole should be considered.

Geriatric Patients

Dosage adjustment based on age is not necessary in geriatric adults.

CAUTIONS

● Contraindications

Known hypersensitivity to voriconazole or any ingredient in the formulation.

Concomitant use with astemizole or terfenadine (drugs no longer commercially available in the US), carbamazepine, cisapride (currently commercially available in the US only under a limited-access protocol), ergot alkaloids (e.g., ergotamine, dihydroergotamine), pimozide, quinidine, rifabutin, rifampin, sirolimus, St. John's wort (*Hypericum perforatum*), or long-acting barbiturates (e.g., phenobarbital, mephobarbital). (See Drug Interactions.)

Concomitant use with ritonavir (400 mg every 12 hours) is contraindicated. Concomitant use with low-dose ritonavir (100 mg every 12 hours) should be avoided, unless potential benefits outweigh risks. (See HIV Protease Inhibitors under Drug Interactions: Antiretroviral Agents.)

● *Warnings/Precautions*

Sensitivity Reactions

Anaphylactoid reactions (e.g., flushing, fever, sweating, tachycardia, chest tightness, dyspnea, faintness, nausea, pruritus, rash) occurring immediately after initiation of voriconazole IV infusions have been reported rarely. Clinician should consider stopping the infusion if these reactions occur.

Serious cutaneous reactions (e.g., Stevens-Johnson syndrome, erythema multiforme, toxic epidermal necrolysis) and photosensitivity reactions have been reported rarely in patients receiving voriconazole. (See Dermatologic Effects under Warnings/Precautions: General Precautions, in Cautions.)

Data regarding cross-sensitivity with other azole antifungals are not available. Voriconazole should be used with caution in patients hypersensitive to other azoles.

Hepatic Effects

Serious hepatic effects, including hepatitis, cholestasis, and fulminant hepatic failure, have been reported rarely in clinical trials. Hepatic effects (including hepatitis and jaundice) have occurred in patients with no identifiable risk factors.

Hepatic effects usually are reversible when voriconazole is discontinued; however, fatalities have occurred.

If abnormal liver function test results occur during voriconazole therapy, the patient should be monitored for the development of more severe hepatic injury using appropriate laboratory evaluations (particularly liver function tests and bilirubin). Discontinuance of voriconazole must be considered if signs and symptoms consistent with liver disease develop.

Ocular Effects

Visual disturbances (e.g., abnormal vision, blurred vision, color vision change, photophobia) have been reported and may be related to high dosage and high plasma voriconazole concentrations.

There have been postmarketing reports of prolonged visual disturbances, including optic neuritis and papilledema, in patients receiving voriconazole.

Effect of voriconazole on visual function is unknown if duration of therapy exceeds 28 days. Monitor visual function (visual acuity, visual field, and color perception) if duration of therapy exceeds 28 days.

Fetal/Neonatal Morbidity and Mortality

Voriconazole can cause fetal harm. Teratogenicity, embryotoxicity, and embryomortality have been demonstrated in animals.

If voriconazole is used during pregnancy or if the patient becomes pregnant while receiving voriconazole, clinicians should advise the patient of the potential hazard to the fetus. (See Pregnancy under Warnings/Precautions: Specific Populations, in Cautions.)

Pregnancy should be avoided. Women of childbearing potential should use effective contraception during voriconazole treatment. (See Drug Interactions: Estrogens and Progestins.)

Fructose or Galactose Intolerance

Patients with a history of galactose intolerance, Lapp lactase deficiency, or glucose-galactose malabsorption should not be given voriconazole tablets since lactose is used in the manufacture of the tablets.

Patients with fructose intolerance, sucrase-isomaltase deficiency, or glucose-galactose malabsorption should not be given voriconazole oral suspension since the suspension contains sucrose.

Cardiovascular Effects

Similar to other azole antifungals, voriconazole has been associated with prolongation of the QT interval. Arrhythmias (e.g., torsades de pointes), cardiac arrest, and sudden death have occurred rarely in patients receiving voriconazole. Most reported cases involved patients with multiple confounding risk factors (e.g., prior cardiotoxic chemotherapy, cardiomyopathy, hypokalemia, concomitant drugs) that may have been contributory.

Voriconazole should be used with caution in patients with potentially proarrhythmic conditions. Rigorous attempts should be made to correct electrolyte imbalances (i.e., potassium, magnesium, calcium) before initiating voriconazole therapy.

Laboratory Monitoring

Hepatic function (liver function tests and bilirubin) should be evaluated prior to and during voriconazole therapy.

Serum electrolytes (i.e., potassium, magnesium, calcium) should be evaluated and any electrolyte abnormalities corrected prior to initiation of voriconazole therapy.

Renal function (e.g., serum creatinine concentrations) should be monitored in patients receiving voriconazole.

Patients with risk factors for acute pancreatitis (e.g., recent chemotherapy, hematopoietic stem cell transplantation [HSCT]) should be monitored for the development of pancreatitis during voriconazole therapy.

Dermatologic Effects

Serious exfoliative cutaneous reactions (e.g., Stevens-Johnson syndrome, erythema multiforme, toxic epidermal necrolysis) have occurred rarely in patients receiving voriconazole. If an exfoliative cutaneous reaction occurs, voriconazole should be discontinued.

Photosensitivity skin reactions have been reported in patients receiving voriconazole. Patients receiving the drug should avoid intense or prolonged exposure to direct sunlight.

Squamous cell carcinoma of the skin and melanoma have been reported during long-term voriconazole therapy in patients with photosensitivity reactions. If a skin lesion consistent with squamous cell carcinoma or melanoma develops, voriconazole should be discontinued.

Renal Effects

Acute renal failure has been reported in severely ill patients with other factors predisposing to impaired renal function (e.g., underlying conditions, concomitant nephrotoxic drugs).

Skeletal Effects

Fluorosis and periostitis have been reported during long-term voriconazole therapy. If a patient develops skeletal pain and radiologic findings compatible with fluorosis or periostitis, voriconazole should be discontinued.

Specific Populations

Pregnancy

Category D. (See Users Guide.)

Because voriconazole can cause fetal harm, it should not be used during pregnancy except when benefits for the mother clearly outweigh potential risks for the fetus.

In rats, voriconazole was teratogenic (cleft palates, hydronephrosis/hydroureter) at a dosage of 10 mg/kg (0.3 times the recommended human maintenance dosage [RMD] based on mg/m²). Other effects in rats included reduced ossification of sacral and caudal vertebrae, skull, and pubic and hyoid bone; supernumerary ribs; anomalies of sternebrae; and dilatation of the ureter/renal pelvis. Reduced plasma estradiol concentrations in pregnant rats, increased gestational length, and dystocia (associated with increased perinatal pup mortality at a dosage of 10 mg/kg) also were reported. In rabbits, voriconazole was embryotoxic at a dosage of 100 mg/kg (6 times the RMD); increased embryomortality, reduced fetal weight, and increased incidence of skeletal variations, cervical ribs, and extrasternebral ossification sites also were reported.

Lactation

It is not known whether voriconazole is distributed into milk.

Because many drugs are distributed into human milk and because of the potential for serious adverse reactions to voriconazole in nursing infants, a decision should be made whether to discontinue nursing or the drug, taking into account the importance of the drug to the mother.

Pediatric Use

Safety and efficacy of voriconazole have not been established in children younger than 12 years of age.

Voriconazole has been recommended for the treatment of fungal infections in children. Some clinicians consider voriconazole the drug of choice for the treatment of invasive aspergillosis in HIV-infected children†, but state that data are insufficient to recommend use of the drug for the treatment of candidemia or esophageal candidiasis in these children.

In one study, a limited number of pediatric patients 9 months to 15 years of age whose disease was refractory to, or who were intolerant of, other antifungals have received voriconazole for the treatment of aspergillosis, candidiasis, infections caused by *Scedosporium*, or other invasive fungal infections. At the completion of therapy, 45% of pediatric patients receiving voriconazole had a complete or partial response. Adverse effects in children receiving voriconazole were similar to those reported in adults.

There have been postmarketing reports of pancreatitis in pediatric patients receiving voriconazole. Children with risk factors for acute pancreatitis (e.g., recent chemotherapy, HSCT) should be monitored for the development of pancreatitis during voriconazole therapy.

In a population pharmacokinetic analysis of voriconazole concentrations in children 2 through 12 years of age who received various dosage regimens, systemic exposures of the drug (areas under the concentration-time curve [AUCs]) achieved with an IV dosage of 7 mg/kg twice daily or an oral dosage of 200 mg twice daily (oral suspension) were comparable to values observed in adults receiving usual dosages of the drug. Data from this study also indicated that loading doses do not appear to reduce the length of time required to reach steady-state in children 2 through 11 years of age and appear to offer little benefit in this age group. Based on a comparison of pharmacokinetic data from pediatric patients (2 years to less than 12 years of age) with data from adults, the manufacturer states that the predicted steady-state plasma voriconazole concentrations were similar in pediatric patients or adults (median concentration of 1.19 or 1.16 mcg/mL, respectively) at a maintenance IV dosage of 4 mg/kg every 12 hours in children or 3 mg/kg every 12 hours in adults.

Geriatric Use

Clinical experience with voriconazole in geriatric patients is limited. Plasma voriconazole concentrations are increased, but overall safety profile is similar to that in younger adults.

Hepatic Impairment

Patients with hepatic impairment should be monitored carefully for voriconazole toxicity, including hepatic effects. (See Hepatic Effects under Warnings/Precautions: Warnings, in Cautions.)

Voriconazole has not been evaluated in patients with severe hepatic cirrhosis (Child-Pugh class C) or with chronic hepatitis B virus (HBV) or hepatitis C virus (HCV) infection.

Voriconazole should be used in patients with severe hepatic impairment only if benefits outweigh risks. (See Dosage and Administration: Special Populations.)

Renal Impairment

IV voriconazole contains sulfobutyl ether β-cyclodextrin sodium (SBECD) which may accumulate in patients with moderate or severe renal impairment (creatinine clearance less than 50 mL/minute).

IV voriconazole should not be used in patients with creatinine clearance less than 50 mL/minute unless potential benefits outweigh risks. If IV voriconazole is used in these patients, serum creatinine concentrations should be monitored closely; if increases occur, consideration should be given to switching to oral voriconazole. (See Dosage and Administration: Special Populations.)

● Common Adverse Effects

Common adverse effects include visual disturbances (e.g., abnormal vision, blurred vision, color vision change, photophobia), GI effects (nausea, vomiting, diarrhea, abdominal pain), fever, rash, chills, headache, abnormalities in liver function test results, tachycardia, and hallucinations. The most commonly reported adverse effects resulting in discontinuance of voriconazole therapy include elevated liver function test results, rash, and visual disturbances.

DRUG INTERACTIONS

● Drugs Affecting or Metabolized by Hepatic Microsomal Enzymes

Inhibitors or inducers of cytochrome P-450 (CYP) isoenzymes 2C9, 2C19, or 3A4 may increase or decrease plasma voriconazole concentrations, respectively.

Voriconazole and its major metabolite inhibit the metabolic activity of CYP2C9, 2C19, and 3A4 and may increase plasma concentrations of other drugs metabolized by these hepatic enzymes. Voriconazole appears to be a less potent inhibitor of CYP3A4 than some other azoles (e.g., itraconazole, ketoconazole).

Because carbamazepine, long-acting barbiturates (e.g., phenobarbital, mephobarbital), ergot alkaloids, rifabutin, rifampin, ritonavir (400 mg every 12 hours), sirolimus, and St. John's wort *(Hypericum perforatum)* are inducers, inhibitors, and/or substrates of CYP isoenzymes, concomitant use with voriconazole is contraindicated.

● Drugs that Prolong the QT Interval

Potential pharmacokinetic interaction with CYP3A4 substrates that prolong the QT interval (e.g., cisapride [currently commercially available in the US only under a limited-access protocol], pimozide, quinidine, terfenadine [no longer commercially available in the US], astemizole [no longer commercially available in the US]). Potential increased plasma concentrations of the concomitantly administered CYP3A4 substrate, which can result in QT interval prolongation and rarely, torsades de pointes. Concomitant use of these drugs that prolong the QT interval and voriconazole is contraindicated.

● Alfentanil

Pharmacokinetic interaction (6- and 4-fold increase in mean area under the plasma concentration-time curve [AUC] and elimination half-life, respectively, of alfentanil) when voriconazole was administered concomitantly with alfentanil (patients also received and naloxone). Concomitant administration also resulted in an increased incidence of delayed and persistent alfentanil-induced nausea and vomiting.

If voriconazole is administered concomitantly with alfentanil or other opiate agonists metabolized by CYP3A4 (e.g., sufentanil), decreased dosage of the opiate agonist and extended close monitoring for opiate-related adverse events (e.g., respiratory depression) may be necessary.

● Antifungal Agents

Fluconazole

Pharmacokinetic interaction with fluconazole (substantially increased plasma concentrations and AUC of voriconazole).

Concomitant use of fluconazole and voriconazole should be avoided. Patients should be monitored for voriconazole-related adverse effects if the drug is initiated within 24 hours after the last dose of fluconazole.

● Antiretroviral Agents

HIV Entry Inhibitors

Possible pharmacokinetic interaction with maraviroc (increased maraviroc plasma concentrations). If used concomitantly, consider reducing the maraviroc dosage to 150 mg twice daily.

HIV Integrase Inhibitor

Elvitegravir

Potential pharmacokinetic interaction with the fixed combination of elvitegravir, cobicistat, emtricitabine, and tenofovir disoproxil fumarate (increased concentrations of voriconazole, elvitegravir, and/or cobicistat).

Voriconazole and the fixed combination of elvitegravir, cobicistat, emtricitabine, and tenofovir disoproxil fumarate should not be used concomitantly unless potential benefits outweigh risks. If used concomitantly, consideration should be given to monitoring voriconazole concentrations and adjusting voriconazole dosage accordingly.

Raltegravir

Pharmacokinetic interaction with raltegravir unlikely; dosage adjustments not needed.

HIV Protease Inhibitors

Pharmacokinetic interactions are likely if voriconazole is used in patients receiving HIV protease inhibitors (PIs) (e.g., atazanavir, darunavir, fosamprenavir, indinavir, lopinavir, nelfinavir, ritonavir, saquinavir, tipranavir), especially if *ritonavir-boosted* PI regimens are used. Concomitant use may result in altered serum concentrations of the PIs and/or the antifungal.

Atazanavir

Possible pharmacokinetic interaction with atazanavir (increased plasma concentrations of voriconazole and atazanavir); possible pharmacokinetic interaction with *ritonavir-boosted* atazanavir (decreased voriconazole concentrations).

If voriconazole is used concomitantly with atazanavir (without low-dose ritonavir), monitor for toxicities. Concomitant use with *ritonavir-boosted* atazanavir should be avoided unless benefits outweigh risks; if used concomitantly, consideration should be given to monitoring voriconazole concentrations and adjusting voriconazole dosage accordingly.

Darunavir

Possible pharmacokinetic interaction with *ritonavir-boosted* darunavir (decreased voriconazole concentrations).

Concomitant use with *ritonavir-boosted* darunavir should be avoided unless benefits outweigh risks; if used concomitantly, consideration should be given to monitoring voriconazole concentrations and adjusting voriconazole dosage accordingly.

Fosamprenavir

Possible pharmacokinetics interaction with fosamprenavir (increased fosamprenavir concentrations and/or increased voriconazole concentrations); possible pharmacokinetic interaction with *ritonavir-boosted* fosamprenavir (decreased voriconazole concentrations).

If voriconazole is used concomitantly with fosamprenavir (without low-dose ritonavir), monitor for toxicities. Concomitant use with *ritonavir-boosted* fosamprenavir should be avoided unless benefits outweigh risks; if used concomitantly, consideration should be given to monitoring voriconazole concentrations and adjusting voriconazole dosage accordingly.

Indinavir

Concomitant use of multiple doses of indinavir and voriconazole does not affect pharmacokinetics of either drug; dosage adjustments are not needed for either drug.

Possible pharmacokinetic interactions with *ritonavir-boosted* indinavir (decreased voriconazole concentrations). Concomitant use with *ritonavir-boosted* indinavir should be avoided unless benefits outweigh risks; if used concomitantly, consideration should be given to monitoring voriconazole concentrations and adjusting voriconazole dosage accordingly.

Lopinavir

Possible pharmacokinetic interaction with lopinavir/ritonavir (decreased voriconazole concentrations). Concomitant use should be avoided unless benefits outweigh risks; if used concomitantly, consideration should be given to monitoring voriconazole concentrations and adjusting voriconazole dosage accordingly.

Nelfinavir

Possible pharmacokinetic interaction with nelfinavir (increased nelfinavir concentrations and/or increased voriconazole concentrations) (without low-dose ritonavir); possible pharmacokinetic interactions with *ritonavir-boosted* nelfinavir (decreased voriconazole concentrations).

If voriconazole is used concomitantly with nelfinavir (without low-dose ritonavir), monitor for toxicities. Concomitant use with *ritonavir-boosted* nelfinavir should be avoided unless benefits outweigh risks; if used concomitantly, consideration should be given to monitoring voriconazole concentrations and adjusting voriconazole dosage accordingly.

Ritonavir

Pharmacokinetic interaction with full-dose ritonavir (400 mg every 12 hours) (mean 66% decrease in steady-state peak plasma voriconazole concentrations and mean 82% decrease in voriconazole AUC; no clinically important effect on ritonavir pharmacokinetics). Concomitant use of voriconazole and full-dose ritonavir (400 mg every 12 hours) is contraindicated.

Pharmacokinetic interaction with low-dose ritonavir (100 mg every 12 hours) (mean 24% decrease in steady-state peak plasma voriconazole concentrations and mean 39% decrease in voriconazole AUC; 24% decrease in steady-state peak ritonavir concentrations and 14% decrease in ritonavir AUC). Concomitant use of voriconazole and low-dose ritonavir (100 mg every 12 hours) should be avoided unless benefits of such therapy outweigh risks; if used concomitantly,

consideration should be given to monitoring voriconazole concentrations and adjusting voriconazole dosage accordingly.

Saquinavir

Possible pharmacokinetic interactions with saquinavir (increased saquinavir concentrations and/or increased voriconazole concentrations); possible pharmacokinetic interaction with *ritonavir-boosted* saquinavir (decreased voriconazole concentrations).

If voriconazole is used concomitantly with saquinavir (without low-dose ritonavir), monitor for toxicities. Concomitant use with *ritonavir-boosted* saquinavir should be avoided unless benefits outweigh risks; if used concomitantly, consideration should be given to monitoring voriconazole concentrations and adjusting voriconazole dosage accordingly.

Tipranavir

Possible pharmacokinetic interaction with *ritonavir-boosted* tipranavir (decreased voriconazole concentrations). Concomitant use with *ritonavir-boosted* tipranavir should be avoided unless benefits outweigh risks; if used concomitantly, consideration should be given to monitoring voriconazole concentrations and adjusting voriconazole dosage accordingly.

Nonnucleoside Reverse Transcriptase Inhibitors

Delavirdine

Potential pharmacokinetic interaction with delavirdine (increased voriconazole concentrations). Monitor patients for voriconazole toxicities and clinical response.

Efavirenz

Concomitant use of voriconazole (400 mg every 12 hours for 1 day, then 200 mg every 12 hours for 8 days) and usual dosage of efavirenz (400 mg once daily for 9 days) reduced voriconazole peak plasma concentrations and AUC by 61 and 77%, respectively, and increased efavirenz peak plasma concentrations and AUC by 38 and 44%, respectively. When a lower dosage of voriconazole (400 mg once daily) was used concomitantly with a lower dosage of efavirenz (300 mg once daily), voriconazole peak plasma concentration was increased 23%, voriconazole AUC was decreased 7%, and efavirenz AUC was increased by 17%.

If concomitant use of efavirenz and voriconazole is necessary, voriconazole maintenance dosage should be increased to 400 mg every 12 hours and efavirenz dosage decreased to 300 mg once daily. After voriconazole therapy is discontinued, the initial dosage of efavirenz should be restored.

Etravirine

Possible pharmacokinetic interaction with etravirine (substantially increased etravirine plasma concentrations, increased voriconazole plasma concentrations). Because of limited data regarding the safety of increased etravirine concentrations, the manufacturer of etravirine states that caution is advised when the drug is administered concomitantly with voriconazole.

Although dosage adjustment is not needed for either drug, some experts state that consideration should be given to monitoring plasma concentrations of voriconazole.

Nevirapine

Potential pharmacokinetic interaction with nevirapine (decreased voriconazole concentrations, increased nevirapine concentrations). Monitor patients for nevirapine toxicity and monitor clinical response to voriconazole and/or voriconazole plasma concentrations.

Rilpivirine

Potential pharmacokinetic interaction (increased rilpivirine concentrations, unknown effect on voriconazole concentrations). Rilpivirine dosage adjustments are not needed; however, patients should be monitored for breakthrough fungal infections.

● Barbiturates

Potential pharmacokinetic interaction (decreased plasma voriconazole concentrations) with long-acting barbiturates (e.g., phenobarbital, mephobarbital) and risk of prolonged sedative effects. Concomitant use of long-acting barbiturates and voriconazole is contraindicated.

● Benzodiazepines

Potential pharmacokinetic interaction (increased plasma benzodiazepine concentrations and AUC) with benzodiazepines that are metabolized by CYP3A4 isoenzyme (e.g., diazepam, midazolam, triazolam, alprazolam). Monitor patient for manifestations of benzodiazepine toxicity and adjust benzodiazepine dosage as necessary.

● Calcium-channel Blocking Agents

Potential pharmacokinetic interaction (increased plasma concentrations of calcium-channel blocker) with calcium-channel blocking agents that are metabolized by CYP3A4 isoenzyme (e.g., felodipine). Monitor patient for manifestations of calcium-channel blocker toxicity and adjust dosage of the calcium-channel blocker as necessary.

● Carbamazepine

Potential pharmacokinetic interaction (decreased plasma voriconazole concentrations) with carbamazepine. Concomitant use of carbamazepine and voriconazole is contraindicated.

● Cimetidine

Pharmacokinetic interaction (increased voriconazole concentrations and AUC) with cimetidine; not considered clinically important and dosage adjustments not needed.

● Clopidogrel

Possible pharmacokinetic interaction (decreased plasma concentrations of the active metabolite of clopidogrel) and reduced antiplatelet effects of clopidogrel.

Concomitant use of clopidogrel and CYP2C19 inhibitors should be avoided since clopidogrel is metabolized to its active metabolite by CYP2C19; in vitro studies indicate voriconazole inhibits CYP2C19.

● Coumarin Anticoagulants

Pharmacokinetic interaction (increased prothrombin time) with coumarin anticoagulant. Monitor prothrombin time or other appropriate tests closely if a coumarin anticoagulant (e.g., warfarin) is used concomitantly with voriconazole; reduction of anticoagulant dosage may be necessary.

● Digoxin

No clinically important pharmacokinetic interaction; no dosage adjustments needed.

● Ergot Alkaloids

Potential pharmacokinetic interaction (increased plasma concentrations of ergot alkaloid). Concomitant use of ergot alkaloids (e.g., ergotamine, dihydroergotamine) and voriconazole is contraindicated.

● Estrogens and Progestins

Pharmacokinetic interaction with oral contraceptives containing ethinyl estradiol and norethindrone (increased peak plasma concentrations and AUC of ethinyl estradiol and norethindrone; increased peak plasma concentrations and AUC of voriconazole).

The manufacturer of voriconazole states that this pharmacokinetic interaction is unlikely to affect efficacy of the oral contraceptive. If concomitant therapy is necessary, monitor for oral contraceptive-related and voriconazole-related adverse events.

● Fentanyl

Pharmacokinetic interaction with IV fentanyl (decreased mean plasma fentanyl clearance and increased fentanyl AUC). If voriconazole is used concomitantly with IV, oral, or transdermal fentanyl, extended and frequent monitoring for respiratory depression and other fentanyl-associated adverse effects is recommended and fentanyl dosage should be reduced if warranted.

● HCV Protease Inhibitors

Boceprevir

Potential pharmacokinetic interaction with boceprevir (increased voriconazole plasma concentrations).

Telaprevir

Potential pharmacokinetic interaction with telaprevir (altered voriconazole plasma concentrations, increased telaprevir plasma concentrations). Although clinically important changes in the QT interval corrected for rate (QT$_c$) have not been reported with telaprevir, QT interval prolongation and torsades de pointes have been reported with voriconazole.

Voriconazole should be used in patients receiving telaprevir only if potential benefits outweigh risks. If the drugs are used concomitantly, caution is warranted and patients should be monitored clinically.

● HMG-CoA Reductase Inhibitors

Potential pharmacokinetic interaction (increased plasma concentrations of antilipemic agent) with HMG-CoA reductase inhibitors (i.e., statins) that are metabolized by CYP3A4 isoenzyme (e.g., lovastatin). Monitor patient for toxicities associated with HMG-CoA reductase inhibitors and adjust dosage of the antilipemic agent as necessary.

● Immunosuppressive Agents

Cyclosporine

Pharmacokinetic interaction (increased plasma concentrations and AUC of cyclosporine).

When initiating voriconazole therapy in patients currently receiving cyclosporine, dosage of cyclosporine should be reduced by 50%. When voriconazole is discontinued, plasma concentrations of cyclosporine should be monitored frequently and dosage of the immunosuppressive agent adjusted as necessary.

Sirolimus

Pharmacokinetic interaction (increased plasma concentrations and AUC of sirolimus).

Concomitant use of sirolimus and voriconazole is contraindicated.

Tacrolimus

Pharmacokinetic interaction (increased plasma concentrations of tacrolimus).

When initiating voriconazole therapy in patients currently receiving tacrolimus, dosage of tacrolimus should be reduced to 33% of the original dose; plasma concentrations of tacrolimus should be monitored frequently. When voriconazole is discontinued, plasma concentrations of tacrolimus should be monitored frequently and dosage of the immunosuppressive agent adjusted as necessary.

● Macrolides

Concomitant use of voriconazole and azithromycin or erythromycin does not have a clinically important effect on voriconazole pharmacokinetics; effects on macrolide pharmacokinetics are not known. Dosage adjustments not needed.

● Methadone

Pharmacokinetic interaction (increased AUC and peak plasma concentrations of pharmacologically active R-methadone) and risk of toxicity (e.g., QT prolongation). Monitor patient for manifestation of methadone toxicity; adjust methadone dosage if necessary.

● Mycophenolic Acid

No clinically important effect on pharmacokinetics of mycophenolic acid or its major metabolite (mycophenolic acid glucuronide); dosage adjustments not needed.

● Nonsteroidal Anti-inflammatory Agents

If voriconazole is used concomitantly with a nonsteroidal anti-inflammatory agent (NSAIA) that is metabolized by CYP2C9 (e.g., celecoxib, diclofenac, ibuprofen, naproxen, lornoxicam [not commercially available in the US], meloxicam), increased plasma concentrations of the NSAIA are possible. Patients receiving voriconazole concomitantly with an NSAIA should be monitored closely for NSAIA-related adverse effects and toxicity and dosage of the NSAIA reduced if warranted.

Diclofenac

Pharmacokinetic interaction with diclofenac (114% increase in peak plasma diclofenac concentrations and 78% increase in diclofenac AUC). If voriconazole is used concomitantly, reduced dosage of diclofenac may be necessary; patients should be monitored closely for NSAIA-related adverse effects and toxicity.

Ibuprofen

Pharmacokinetic interaction (20% increase in peak plasma concentrations and 100% increase in AUC of the pharmacologically active isomer of ibuprofen). If voriconazole is used concomitantly, reduced dosage of ibuprofen may be necessary; patients should be monitored closely for NSAIA-related adverse effects and toxicity.

● Oxycodone

Pharmacokinetic interaction (increased peak plasma concentration, AUC, and elimination half-life of oxycodone); increased oxycodone-associated adverse visual effects (heterophoria, miosis). If voriconazole is used concomitantly with oxycodone, extended and frequent monitoring for oxycodone-associated adverse effects is recommended and reduced oxycodone dosage may be necessary to avoid opiate-related adverse effects.

● Phenytoin

Pharmacokinetic interaction (substantially decreased plasma voriconazole concentrations) with voriconazole 200 mg every 12 hours. Increasing the voriconazole dosage to 400 mg every 12 hours in patients receiving concomitant phenytoin results in plasma voriconazole concentrations that are essentially the same as those in patients receiving usual dosages of voriconazole (200 mg every 12 hours) without phenytoin. Pharmacokinetic interaction (increased plasma phenytoin concentrations) with voriconazole 400 mg every 12 hours.

When phenytoin and voriconazole are used concomitantly, increase IV maintenance dosage of voriconazole to 5 mg/kg every 12 hours and increase oral maintenance dosage of the drug to 400 mg every 12 hours in patients weighing 40 kg or more or 200 mg every 12 hours in those weighing less than 40 kg. Plasma phenytoin concentrations should be monitored frequently and the patient observed for potential phenytoin adverse effects.

● Pimozide

Possible pharmacokinetic interaction and potential for serious or life-threatening reactions (e.g., cardiac arrhythmias). Concomitant use of pimozide and voriconazole is contraindicated.

● Prednisolone

Pharmacokinetic interaction (increased concentration and AUC of prednisolone); no dosage adjustments needed.

● Proton-pump Inhibitors

Pharmacokinetic interaction (substantially increased plasma omeprazole concentrations and AUC, clinically unimportant increases in plasma voriconazole concentrations, GI absorption of voriconazole not affected) with omeprazole. In patients currently receiving omeprazole in dosages of 40 mg or more daily, reduce omeprazole dosage by one-half when voriconazole therapy is initiated. Adjustment of voriconazole dosage not needed.

Potential increased plasma concentrations of other proton-pump inhibitors that are metabolized by CYP2C19 isoenzyme.

● Quinidine

Possible pharmacokinetic interaction and potential for serious or life-threatening reactions (e.g., cardiac arrhythmias). Concomitant use of quinidine and voriconazole is contraindicated.

● Ranitidine

No pharmacokinetic interaction with ranitidine; dosage adjustments not needed.

● Rifampin and Rifabutin

Pharmacokinetic interaction with rifampin (substantially decreased plasma voriconazole concentrations and AUC). Pharmacokinetic interaction with rifabutin (clinically important decreased plasma voriconazole concentrations and decreased AUC of voriconazole, substantially increased plasma rifabutin concentrations and AUC).

Concomitant use of rifampin or rifabutin and voriconazole is contraindicated.

● St. John's Wort

Pharmacokinetic interaction (59% decrease in mean voriconazole AUC) following multiple doses of St. John's wort (Hypericum perforatum); no clinically important effect on voriconazole AUC when a single dose of St. John's wort and a single dose of voriconazole are used concomitantly. Because long-term use of St.

John's wort could result in decreased voriconazole exposure, concomitant use of voriconazole and St. John's wort is contraindicated.

● Sulfonylurea Antidiabetic Agents

Potential pharmacokinetic interaction (increased plasma concentrations of antidiabetic agent) with sulfonylurea antidiabetic agents (e.g., tolbutamide, glipizide, glyburide). Monitor blood glucose concentrations and monitor patient for signs and symptoms of hypoglycemia; adjust dosage of antidiabetic agent as necessary.

● Venlafaxine

Pharmacokinetic interaction (increased venlafaxine AUC); if used concomitantly, monitor for venlafaxine-associated toxicity.

● Vinca Alkaloids

Potential pharmacokinetic interaction (increased plasma concentrations of vinca alkaloid). Monitor patient for manifestations of vinca alkaloid toxicity (i.e., neurotoxicity) and adjust dosage as necessary.

● Zolpidem

Pharmacokinetic interaction (increased peak plasma concentration and AUC of zolpidem and prolonged zolpidem half-life); monitor for zolpidem-associated toxicity and adjust dosage as necessary.

DESCRIPTION

Voriconazole, a triazole antifungal agent, is a synthetic derivative of fluconazole. Like other azole antifungals, voriconazole presumably exerts its antifungal activity by altering cellular membranes, resulting in increased permeability, secondary metabolic effects, and growth inhibition. Although the exact mechanism of action of voriconazole has not been fully determined, the drug inhibits cytochrome P-450-dependent sterol 14-α-demethylase in susceptible fungi, which leads to accumulation of C-14-methylated sterols (e.g., lanosterol) and decreased concentrations of ergosterol.

Voriconazole is active in vitro against *Aspergillus*, including *A. fumigatus*, *A. flavus*, *A. niger*, and *A. terreus*, and *Candida*, including *C. albicans*, *C. dubliniensis*, *C. fumata*, *C. glabrata*, *C. guilliermondii*, *C. kefyr*, *C. krusei*, *C. lipolytica*, *C. lusitaniae*, *C. metapsilosis*, *C. orthopsilosis*, *C. parapsilosis*, *C. pelliculosa*, *C. rugosa*, and *C. tropicalis*. Voriconazole is active in vitro against *Exserohilum rostratum*. The drug has variable activity in vitro against *Fusarium* (including *F. solani*) and *Scedosporium apiospermum*. Voriconazole is active in vitro against *Cryptococcus neoformans* and *C. gattii*. Fungi with reduced susceptibility to other azoles (e.g., fluconazole, itraconazole) may also have reduced susceptibility to voriconazole.

The pharmacokinetics of voriconazole are similar following IV or oral administration. Absorption of the drug is rapid and almost complete (oral bioavailability of 96%) when given in the fasting state. Peak plasma voriconazole concentrations are achieved 1–2 hours following a dose. In adults, steady-state concentrations are achieved within 24 hours if a loading dose is administered or after 5–7 days if a loading dose is not administered. Loading doses do not appear to reduce the length of time required to reach steady-state in children 2 through 11 years of age† and appear to offer little benefit in this age group. (See Pediatric Use under Warnings/Precautions: Specific Populations, in Cautions.) Voriconazole exhibits nonlinear, dose-dependent pharmacokinetics, apparently because of saturable first-pass metabolism or systemic clearance. In vitro studies indicate that voriconazole is extensively metabolized in the liver by cytochrome P-450 (CYP) isoenzymes 2C9, 2C19, and 3A4. (See Drug Interactions: Drugs Affecting or Metabolized by Hepatic Microsomal Enzymes.) The drug is primarily eliminated by hepatic metabolism with less than 2% of a dose eliminated as unchanged drug in the urine.

ADVICE TO PATIENTS

Importance of taking oral voriconazole at least 1 hour before or 1 hour after meals.

Advise patients that tablets contain lactose and should not be used in patients with galactose intolerance, Lapp lactase deficiency, or glucose-galactose malabsorption and that the oral suspension contains sucrose and is not recommended for those with fructose intolerance, sucrase-isomaltase deficiency, or glucose-galactose malabsorption.

Possibility of visual changes, including blurred vision and photophobia. Avoid driving, operating machinery, or performing hazardous tasks if visual changes occur; importance of not driving at night while taking voriconazole.

Possibility of photosensitivity reactions; importance of avoiding exposure to strong, direct sunlight during voriconazole therapy.

Importance of informing clinicians if any of the following symptoms develop during voriconazole therapy: changes in heart rate or rhythm, chest tightness, itching, yellowing of skin or eyes, extreme fatigue or flu-like symptoms, nausea or vomiting, visual changes, loss of appetite, changes in thinking, difficulty breathing, or seizures.

Importance of informing clinicians and discontinuing voriconazole if serious skin reactions (e.g., rash, hives, mouth sores, blisters, peeling skin) occur.

Importance of informing clinicians of existing or contemplated concomitant therapy, including prescription and OTC drugs, and any concomitant illnesses (e.g., liver disease, heart disease).

Importance of women informing clinicians if they are or plan to become pregnant or to breast-feed. Importance of contraceptive measures during voriconazole therapy.

Importance of advising patients of other important precautionary information. (See Cautions.)

PREPARATIONS

Excipients in commercially available drug preparations may have clinically important effects in some individuals; consult specific product labeling for details.

Voriconazole

Oral

For suspension	200 mg/5 mL*	Vfend®, Pfizer
		Voriconazole for Suspension
Tablets, film-coated	50 mg*	Vfend®, Pfizer
		Voriconazole Tablets
	200 mg*	Vfend®, Pfizer
		Voriconazole Tablets

Parenteral

For injection, for IV infusion only	200 mg*	Vfend®, Pfizer
		Voriconazole for Injection

* available from one or more manufacturer, distributor, and/or repackager by generic (nonproprietary) name

† Use is not currently included in the labeling approved by the US Food and Drug Administration.

Selected Revisions October 18, 2013, © Copyright, November 1, 2002, American Society of Health-System Pharmacists, Inc.

Anidulafungin

8:14.16 • ECHINOCANDINS

■ Anidulafungin is a semisynthetic, echinocandin antifungal agent.

USES

● Candida Infections

Candidemia and Other Invasive Candida Infections

Anidulafungin is used for the treatment of candidemia and certain other invasive *Candida* infections (intra-abdominal abscess, peritonitis). The manufacturer states that safety and efficacy of anidulafungin have not been established for the treatment of endocarditis, osteomyelitis, or meningitis caused by *Candida*. In addition, the manufacturer states that data are insufficient to date to evaluate efficacy of anidulafungin for the treatment of candidemia or other invasive *Candida* infections in neutropenic patients.

For the treatment of candidemia in *nonneutropenic* patients or for empiric treatment of suspected invasive candidiasis in *nonneutropenic* patients in intensive care units (ICUs), the Infectious Diseases Society of America (IDSA) recommends an IV echinocandin (anidulafungin, caspofungin, micafungin) for *initial* therapy. IDSA states that fluconazole (IV or oral) is an acceptable alternative for *initial* therapy in selected patients, including those who are not critically ill and are unlikely to have infections caused by fluconazole-resistant *Candida*. If echinocandin- and azole-resistant *Candida* are suspected, IV amphotericin B is recommended; IV amphotericin B also is a reasonable alternative when echinocandins and fluconazole cannot be used because of intolerance, limited availability, or resistance. IDSA states that transition from the echinocandin (or amphotericin B) to fluconazole can be considered (usually within 5–7 days) in patients who are clinically stable, have isolates susceptible to fluconazole (e.g., *C. albicans*), and have negative repeat blood cultures after initial antifungal treatment. Although fluconazole has been considered the drug of choice for the treatment of infections caused by *C. parapsilosis* in nonneutropenic patients (based in part on concerns related to decreased in vitro susceptibility and resistance to echinocandins), IDSA states that there are no clinical studies to date indicating superiority of fluconazole over echinocandins for the treatment of *C. parapsilosis* infections.

For the treatment of candidemia in *neutropenic* patients†, IDSA recommends an IV echinocandin (anidulafungin, caspofungin, micafungin) or, alternatively, IV amphotericin B for *initial* therapy. Fluconazole is an alternative for *initial* therapy in those who are not critically ill and have had no prior exposure to azole antifungals and also can be used for step-down therapy during neutropenia in clinically stable patients who have fluconazole-susceptible isolates and documented bloodstream clearance. Voriconazole can be used as an alternative for *initial* therapy when broader antifungal coverage is required and also can be used as step-down therapy during neutropenia in clinically stable patients who have voriconazole-susceptible isolates and documented bloodstream clearance. For infections known to be caused by *C. krusei*, an echinocandin, amphotericin B, or voriconazole is recommended.

For the treatment of osteoarticular infections† (e.g., osteomyelitis, septic arthritis) caused by *Candida*, IDSA recommends *initial* treatment with fluconazole or an IV echinocandin (anidulafungin, caspofungin, micafungin) and follow-up treatment with fluconazole. If septic arthritis involves a prosthetic device that cannot be removed, long-term suppressive or maintenance therapy (secondary prophylaxis) with fluconazole is recommended if the isolate is susceptible.

For the treatment of endocarditis† (native or prosthetic valve) or implantable cardiac device infections† caused by *Candida*, IDSA recommends *initial* treatment with IV amphotericin B (with or without oral flucytosine) or an IV echinocandin (anidulafungin, caspofungin, micafungin) and follow-up treatment with fluconazole. If the isolate is susceptible, long-term suppressive or maintenance therapy (secondary prophylaxis) with fluconazole is recommended to prevent recurrence in those with native valve endocarditis who cannot undergo valve replacement and in those with prosthetic valve endocarditis.

For additional information on management of candidemia and disseminated candidiasis, the current clinical practice guidelines from IDSA available at http://www.idsociety.org should be consulted.

Clinical Experience

Safety and efficacy of anidulafungin for the treatment of candidemia or other forms of invasive candidiasis were evaluated in a phase 3, randomized, double-blind study in adults (97% were nonneutropenic, 61.6% had *C. albicans* infections). Patients were randomized to receive initial therapy with either IV anidulafungin (200-mg loading dose followed by 100 mg once daily) or IV fluconazole (800-mg loading dose followed by 400 mg once daily). After a minimum of 10 days of IV therapy, patients in both treatment groups were permitted to switch to oral fluconazole if they were afebrile for at least 24 hours, had blood cultures negative for *Candida*, and were able to tolerate oral therapy. The total duration of antifungal treatment was at least 14 days (maximum 42 days); 26% of those receiving IV anidulafungin and 28% of those receiving IV fluconazole switched to oral fluconazole. When data analysis was done using the modified intent-to-treat population, a successful global response consisting of clinical cure or improvement (defined as substantial but incomplete resolution of signs and symptoms of *Candida* infection without additional antifungal treatment) with documented or presumed microbiological eradication was observed in 74% of those in the anidulafungin group (median duration of 14 days of IV anidulafungin and 7 days of oral fluconazole) and in 56.8% of those in the fluconazole group (median duration of 11 days of IV fluconazole and 5 days of oral fluconazole). At 2 or 6 weeks posttreatment, a successful global response was maintained in 64.6 or 55.9%, respectively, of patients randomized to anidulafungin and 49.2 or 44.1%, respectively, of patients randomized to fluconazole.

Esophageal Candidiasis

Anidulafungin is used for the treatment of esophageal candidiasis.

Esophageal candidiasis requires treatment with a systemic antifungal (not a topical antifungal).

IDSA recommends oral fluconazole as the preferred drug of choice for the treatment of esophageal candidiasis; if oral therapy is not tolerated, IV fluconazole or an IV echinocandin (anidulafungin, caspofungin, micafungin) usually is recommended and IV amphotericin B is another alternative. For fluconazole-refractory esophageal candidiasis, IDSA recommends itraconazole oral solution or oral or IV voriconazole; alternatives for fluconazole-refractory disease are IV echinocandins (anidulafungin, caspofungin, micafungin) or IV amphotericin B. IDSA states that oral posaconazole (oral suspension or delayed-release tablets) could be considered another alternative for the treatment of fluconazole-refractory esophageal candidiasis.

For the treatment of esophageal candidiasis in adults and adolescents with human immunodeficiency virus (HIV) infection, the Centers for Disease Control and Prevention (CDC), National Institutes of Health (NIH), and IDSA recommend IV or oral fluconazole or itraconazole oral solution. Alternatives include oral or IV voriconazole, an IV echinocandin (anidulafungin, caspofungin, micafungin), or IV amphotericin B. For refractory esophageal candidiasis in HIV-infected adults and adolescents, including fluconazole-refractory infections, these experts recommend posaconazole oral suspension or itraconazole oral solution; alternatives include an IV echinocandin (anidulafungin, caspofungin, micafungin), oral or IV voriconazole, or IV amphotericin B. Although data are limited, some experts state that an IV echinocandin (anidulafungin, caspofungin, micafungin) can be considered an alternative for the treatment of azole-refractory esophageal candidiasis in HIV-infected children†.

Routine long-term suppressive or maintenance therapy (secondary prophylaxis) to prevent relapse or recurrence is not usually recommended in patients adequately treated for esophageal candidiasis (including HIV-infected individuals) unless the patient has frequent or severe recurrences of esophageal candidiasis. If secondary prophylaxis of esophageal candidiasis is indicated, oral fluconazole or posaconazole oral suspension is recommended; however, the potential for development of azole resistance should be considered.

For additional information on management of esophageal candidiasis, the current clinical practice guidelines from IDSA available at http://www.idsociety.org and the current clinical practice guidelines from CDC, NIH, and IDSA on the prevention and treatment of opportunistic infections in HIV-infected individuals available at http://www.aidsinfo.nih.gov should be consulted.

Clinical Experience

There is some evidence that IV anidulafungin may be at least as effective as oral fluconazole for the treatment of esophageal candidiasis, but further study is needed since there also is some evidence that the relapse rate may be higher with anidulafungin.

In a phase 3, randomized, double-blind study designed to establish noninferiority of anidulafungin for the treatment of endoscopically and microbiologically confirmed esophageal candidiasis, adults received either IV anidulafungin (100-mg loading dose followed by 50 mg once daily) or oral fluconazole (200-mg loading dose followed by 100 mg once daily). Most patients who were tested for HIV were HIV-positive (85%) and most patients with culture-confirmed esophageal candidiasis had *C. albicans* infections (91%). Treatment groups were similar in demographic and other baseline characteristics. In the group of anidulafungin-treated patients, the age range was 16–69 years, the gender distribution was 42% male and 58% female, and the race distribution was 15% white, 49% black/African American, 15% Asian, 0.3% Hispanic, and 21% other races. Antifungal treatment was continued for 7 days after resolution of clinical symptoms (minimum duration of 14 days, maximum duration of 21 days). Efficacy was assessed by endoscopic examination at the end of treatment, and endoscopic success (cure or improvement) was similar following treatment with IV anidulafungin (97.4%) or oral fluconazole (98.7%); however, at 2 weeks posttreatment, the relapse rate based on recurrence of endoscopic lesions was higher with IV anidulafungin (53.3%) than with oral fluconazole (19.3%).

Oropharyngeal Candidiasis

Anidulafungin is used as an alternative for the treatment of oropharyngeal candidiasis†.

For the treatment of mild oropharyngeal candidiasis, IDSA recommends topical treatment with clotrimazole lozenges or miconazole buccal tablets; nystatin (oral suspension or tablets) is the recommended alternative. For moderate to severe disease, IDSA recommends oral fluconazole. For fluconazole-refractory oropharyngeal candidiasis, IDSA recommends itraconazole oral solution or posaconazole oral suspension; oral voriconazole or amphotericin B oral suspension (not commercially available in the US) are recommended as alternatives. Other alternatives for refractory oropharyngeal candidiasis are an IV echinocandin (anidulafungin, caspofungin, micafungin) or IV amphotericin B.

For the treatment of oropharyngeal candidiasis in HIV-infected adults and adolescents, CDC, NIH, and IDSA recommend oral fluconazole as the preferred drug of choice for initial episodes. If topical therapy is used for the treatment of oropharyngeal candidiasis (e.g., mild to moderate episodes), these experts recommend clotrimazole lozenges or miconazole buccal tablets. Alternatives for systemic treatment of oropharyngeal candidiasis in HIV-infected adults and adolescents are itraconazole oral solution or posaconazole oral suspension; nystatin oral suspension is an alternative if topical treatment is used. For fluconazole-refractory oropharyngeal infections in HIV-infected adults and adolescents, posaconazole oral suspension is preferred; itraconazole oral solution is an alternative.

Routine long-term suppressive or maintenance therapy (secondary prophylaxis) to prevent relapse or recurrence is not usually recommended in patients adequately treated for oropharyngeal candidiasis (including HIV-infected individuals) unless the patient has frequent or severe recurrences of oropharyngeal candidiasis. If secondary prophylaxis of oropharyngeal candidiasis is indicated, oral fluconazole is recommended; however, the potential for development of azole resistance should be considered.

For additional information on management of oropharyngeal candidiasis, the current clinical practice guidelines from IDSA available at http://www.idsociety.org and the current clinical practice guidelines from CDC, NIH, and IDSA on the prevention and treatment of opportunistic infections in HIV-infected individuals available at http://www.aidsinfo.nih.gov should be consulted.

Clinical Experience

Efficacy of anidulafungin in the treatment of oropharyngeal candidiasis† was evaluated in a limited open-label, noncomparative study in 19 adults with confirmed azole-refractory oropharyngeal and/or esophageal candidiasis who received IV anidulafungin (100-mg loading dose on day 1 followed by 50 mg once daily) alone for 13–21 days. A total of 18 patients completed the study and were included in the modified intention to treat analysis. An overall clinical response was achieved in 94% of patients with oropharyngeal candidiasis; 61% (11/18) were considered cured and 33% (6/18) demonstrated improvement. At the follow-up visit 10–14 days after study completion, clinical success was maintained in 44% (8/18) of patients treated for oropharyngeal candidiasis. In one HIV-infected patient who had multiple prior episodes of oropharyngeal candidiasis and 2 prior episodes of esophageal candidiasis, treatment was considered a clinical and endoscopic failure.

Candida auris Infections

Anidulafungin is used for the treatment of infections caused by *C. auris*, an emerging pathogen that has been associated with potentially fatal candidemia or other invasive infections.

C. auris, first identified in 2009, has now been reported as the cause of serious invasive infections (including fatalities) in multiple countries worldwide (e.g., Japan, South Korea, India, Kuwait, South Africa, Pakistan, United Kingdom, Venezuela, Colombia, US). As of May 2017, a total of 77 clinical cases of *C. auris* had been reported to CDC from 7 different states in the US. *C. auris* may be difficult to identify using standard in vitro methods and has been misidentified as *C. haemulonii*, *C. famata*, or *Rhodotorula glutinis*. A large percentage of *C. auris* clinical isolates are resistant to fluconazole and multidrug-resistant isolates with reduced susceptibility or resistance to all 3 major classes of antifungal agents (azoles, polyenes, echinocandins) have been reported.

Pending further accumulation of data, CDC has issued interim recommendations regarding laboratory diagnosis, treatment, and infection control measures for suspected or known *C. auris* infections. Based on limited data available to date, CDC recommends that an IV echinocandin (anidulafungin, caspofungin, micafungin) be used for initial treatment of invasive *C. auris* infections (e.g., bloodstream or intra-abdominal infections) in adults. CDC states that a switch to IV amphotericin B (lipid formulation) could be considered if the patient is clinically unresponsive to the echinocandin or fungemia persists longer than 5 days. Consultation with an infectious disease specialist is highly recommended.

Unless there is evidence of infection, CDC does not currently recommend antifungal treatment when *C. auris* is isolated only from noninvasive body sites (e.g., urine, external ear, wounds, respiratory secretions). Some individuals are colonized with *C. auris* in the axilla, groin, nose, external ear canal, oropharynx, urine, wounds, rectum, and stool; however, data are limited and the duration of *C. auris* colonization is unclear. Therefore, CDC recommends that infection control measures be observed for all patients with cultures yielding *C. auris*, including those with positive cultures only from noninvasive body sites.

Whenever *C. auris* infection is suspected, clinicians should immediately contact state or local public health authorities and the CDC (candidaauris@cdc.gov) for guidance. For additional information on diagnosis and management of *C. auris* infections, the interim recommendations and most recent information from CDC available at https://www.cdc.gov/fungal/diseases/candidiasis/candida-auris.html should be consulted.

● Aspergillosis

Safety and efficacy of anidulafungin for the treatment of invasive aspergillosis† have not been established, and only limited data are available regarding use of the drug for the treatment of such infections.

IDSA and other clinicians consider IV voriconazole the drug of choice for primary treatment of invasive aspergillosis in adult and pediatric patients, including those with HIV infection; IV amphotericin B or isavuconazonium sulfate (prodrug of isavuconazole) is usually recommended as an alternative for primary treatment. For salvage therapy in patients refractory to or intolerant of primary antifungal therapy, IDSA recommends IV amphotericin B, an IV echinocandin (caspofungin, micafungin), oral or IV posaconazole, or itraconazole oral suspension. IDSA states that echinocandins (either alone or in conjunction with other antifungals) may be effective for salvage therapy of invasive aspergillosis; however, routine use of echinocandin monotherapy is not recommended for primary treatment of invasive aspergillosis.

For additional information on management of aspergillosis, the current clinical practice guidelines from IDSA available at http://www.idsociety.org and the current clinical practice guidelines from CDC, NIH, and IDSA on the prevention and treatment of opportunistic infections in HIV-infected individuals available at http://www.aidsinfo.nih.gov should be consulted.

DOSAGE AND ADMINISTRATION

● Administration

Anidulafungin is administered by slow IV infusion. The drug should *not* be given by rapid IV injection.

IV Infusion

Anidulafungin should not be admixed or infused concomitantly with other drugs.

Strict aseptic technique should be observed when preparing anidulafungin solutions. since the drug contains no preservatives. Anidulafungin solutions should be inspected visually for particulate matter and discoloration and should not be used if discolored or if particulates are present.

Reconstitution and Dilution

Commercially available anidulafungin lyophilized powder for injection must be reconstituted and then further diluted prior to IV infusion.

Based on the indicated anidulafungin dosage, the appropriate number of vials labeled as containing 50 or 100 mg of anidulafungin should be reconstituted with 15 or 30 mL, respectively, of sterile water for injection to provide a solution containing 3.33 mg/mL.

The contents of the appropriate number of reconstituted vials should then be diluted in 50, 100, or 200 mL of 5% dextrose injection or 0.9% sodium chloride injection to provide an IV infusion solution containing 0.77 mg/mL. (See Table 1.)

TABLE 1. Instructions for Diluting Reconstituted Vials of Anidulafungin

Anidulafungin Dose Indicated	Number of Reconstituted Vials Required	Required Volume of Diluent (5% Dextrose Injection or 0.9% Sodium Chloride Injection)	Total Infusion Volume of 0.77-mg/mL Solution	Minimum Duration of Infusion (minutes)
50 mg	One 50-mg vial	50 mL	65 mL	45
100 mg	Two 50-mg vials or one 100-mg vial	100 mL	130 mL	90
200 mg	Four 50-mg vials or two 100-mg vials	200 mL	260 mL	180

Vials of lyophilized anidulafungin should be stored at 2–8°C, but may be exposed to temperatures up to 25°C for 96 hours and then returned to 2–8°C; the vials should not be frozen. Following reconstitution, anidulafungin solutions may be stored at temperatures up to 25°C for up to 24 hours. Reconstituted anidulafungin solutions that have been further diluted in 5% dextrose injection or 0.9% sodium chloride injection to a concentration of 0.77 mg/mL may be stored at temperatures up to 25°C for up to 48 hours or, alternatively, may be stored frozen for at least 72 hours.

Rate of Administration

IV infusions of anidulafungin should be given at a rate not exceeding 1.1 mg/minute (1.4 mL/minute). More rapid infusion may increase the risk of a histamine-mediated reaction. (See Sensitivity Reactions under Cautions: Warnings/Precautions.)

● Dosage
Adult Dosage
Candidemia and Other Invasive Candida Infections

The recommended dosage of anidulafungin for the treatment of candidemia and certain other invasive *Candida* infections (intra-abdominal abscess, peritonitis) in *nonneutropenic* adults or *neutropenic†* adults is a single 200-mg loading dose on day 1, followed by 100 mg once daily.

When anidulafungin is used for initial treatment of candidemia or other invasive *Candida* infections, the Infectious Diseases Society of America (IDSA) states that a transition from the echinocandin to fluconazole can be considered (usually within 5–7 days) in patients who are clinically stable, have isolates susceptible to fluconazole (e.g., *C. albicans*), and have negative repeat blood cultures after initial antifungal treatment.

The duration of treatment should be based on the clinical response of the patient. The manufacturer recommends that anidulafungin therapy in patients with candidemia or other invasive *Candida* infections should be continued for at least 14 days after the last positive culture. IDSA recommends that antifungal treatment for candidemia (without persistent fungemia or metastatic complications) be continued for 2 weeks after documented clearance of *Candida* from the bloodstream, resolution of candidemia symptoms, and resolution of neutropenia.

If anidulafungin is used for *initial* treatment of osteoarticular infections† (e.g., osteomyelitis, septic arthritis) caused by *Candida*, IDSA recommends a dosage of 100 mg once daily in adults. After at least 2 weeks, treatment can be switched to fluconazole.

If anidulafungin is used for *initial* treatment of endocarditis† (native or prosthetic valve) or implantable cardiac device infections† caused by *Candida*, IDSA recommends a dosage of 200 mg once daily in adults. If the infection is caused by fluconazole-susceptible *Candida*, treatment can be switched to fluconazole after the patient is stabilized and *Candida* has been cleared from the bloodstream.

Esophageal Candidiasis

For the treatment of esophageal candidiasis in adults, the manufacturer recommends that a single 100-mg loading dose of anidulafungin be given on day 1, followed by 50 mg once daily.

If anidulafungin is used for the treatment of esophageal candidiasis, including fluconazole-refractory disease (see Esophageal Candidiasis under Uses: Candida Infections), IDSA recommends that adults receive anidulafungin in a dosage of 200 mg once daily.

If anidulafungin is used for the treatment of esophageal candidiasis in adults with human immunodeficiency virus (HIV) infection, the US Centers for Disease Control and Prevention (CDC), National Institutes of Health (NIH), and IDSA recommend a single 100-mg loading dose of anidulafungin on day 1, followed by 50 mg once daily.

The duration of treatment should be based on the clinical response of the patient. The manufacturer states that anidulafungin therapy in patients with esophageal candidiasis should be continued for at least 14 days and for at least 7 days following resolution of symptoms. CDC, NIH, and IDSA recommend that antifungal treatment of esophageal candidiasis be continued for 14–21 days.

Oropharyngeal Candidiasis

If anidulafungin is used for the treatment of oropharyngeal candidiasis†, IDSA recommends that adults receive a single 200-mg loading dose on day 1, followed by 100 mg once daily for 7–14 days.

Candida auris Infections

If anidulafungin is used for initial treatment of invasive *C. auris* infections (e.g., bloodstream or intra-abdominal infections), CDC recommends that adults receive a single 200-mg loading dose, followed by 100 mg once daily.

Aspergillosis

If anidulafungin is used for the treatment of invasive aspergillosis†, some experts recommend that adults receive a single 200-mg loading dose, followed by 100 mg daily.

The duration of treatment is based on the degree and duration of immunosuppression, disease site, and clinical response. IDSA recommends that antifungal treatment of invasive pulmonary aspergillosis be continued for at least 6–12 weeks.

Pediatric Dosage
General Dosing for Pediatric Patients

If anidulafungin is used in children†, the American Academy of Pediatrics (AAP) recommends a loading dose of 1.5–3 mg/kg, followed by 0.75–1.5 mg/kg once daily.

Candidemia and Other Invasive Candida Infections

If anidulafungin is used as for the treatment of invasive candidiasis in HIV-infected children 2 years of age or older†, some experts recommend an initial loading dose of 3 mg/kg on day 1, followed by 1.5 mg/kg once daily.

IDSA recommends that antifungal treatment for candidemia (without persistent fungemia or metastatic complications) be continued for 2 weeks after documented clearance of *Candida* from the bloodstream, resolution of candidemia symptoms, and resolution of neutropenia.

Esophageal Candidiasis

If anidulafungin is used as an alternative for the treatment of esophageal candidiasis in HIV-infected children 2 years of age or older†, some experts recommend an initial loading dose of 3 mg/kg on day 1, followed by 1.5 mg/kg (up to 100 mg) once daily.

For the treatment of esophageal candidiasis in HIV-infected adolescents†, CDC, NIH, and IDSA recommend a single 100-mg loading dose of anidulafungin on day 1, followed by 50 mg once daily.

CDC, NIH, and IDSA recommend that antifungal treatment of esophageal candidiasis be continued for 14–21 days.

● Special Populations
Hepatic Impairment

Dosage adjustments are not necessary in patients with hepatic impairment (Child-Pugh class A, B, or C).

Renal Impairment

Dosage adjustments are not necessary in patients with renal impairment (including those receiving hemodialysis).

Because anidulafungin is not dialyzable, the drug may be administered without regard to the timing of hemodialysis.

Geriatric Patients

Dosage adjustments are not necessary in patients 65 years of age or older.

CAUTIONS

● Contraindications

Anidulafungin is contraindicated in patients with known hypersensitivity to the drug, other echinocandin antifungals (e.g., caspofungin, micafungin), or any ingredient in the formulation.

● Warnings/Precautions
Sensitivity Reactions
Hypersensitivity Reactions

Anaphylactic reactions, including anaphylactic shock, have been reported in patients receiving anidulafungin. If such reactions occur, the drug should be discontinued and appropriate treatment administered.

Possible histamine-mediated symptoms (e.g., rash, urticaria, flushing, pruritus, dyspnea, hypotension) have occurred in patients receiving anidulafungin. These symptoms are infrequent when the infusion rate does not exceed 1.1 mg/minute.

Infusion-related adverse reactions (e.g., rash, urticaria, flushing, pruritus, bronchospasm, dyspnea, hypotension) have occurred in patients receiving anidulafungin and possibly may be histamine-mediated reactions. To reduce the occurrence of infusion-related adverse reactions, the infusion rate should not exceed 1.1 mg/minute.

Hepatic Effects

Abnormal liver function test results have been reported in healthy individuals and patients receiving anidulafungin. Hepatic abnormalities, including hepatic dysfunction, hepatitis, or worsening hepatic failure, have been reported in patients with serious underlying conditions receiving anidulafungin and multiple other drugs. A causal relationship to anidulafungin has not been established to date.

If abnormal liver function test results occur during anidulafungin therapy, the patient should be monitored for evidence of worsening hepatic function and the risks of continued anidulafungin therapy should be weighed against potential benefits.

Selection and Use of Antifungals

Prior to initiation of anidulafungin therapy, appropriate specimens for fungal cultures and other relevant laboratory studies (e.g., histopathology) should be obtained to isolate and identify causative organisms. The drug may be started pending availability of results, but antifungal therapy should be adjusted as needed when results become available.

Specific Populations
Pregnancy

Category B. (See Users Guide.)

There are no adequate and well-controlled studies of anidulafungin in pregnant women, and the manufacturer states that the drug should be used during pregnancy only if clearly needed.

In rats, anidulafungin crosses the placenta, is detected in fetal plasma, and has been associated with incomplete ossification of several bones.

Lactation

Anidulafungin is distributed into milk in rats; it is not known whether the drug is distributed into milk in humans.

Anidulafungin should be used with caution in nursing women.

Pediatric Use

Safety and efficacy of anidulafungin have not been established in pediatric patients 16 years of age or younger.

Anidulafungin has been used in a limited number of neutropenic children 2–17 years of age† without unusual adverse effects.

Although data are limited, some experts state that anidulafungin can be considered for first-line treatment of invasive candidiasis or for alternative treatment of esophageal candidiasis in children 2–17 years of age† with human immunodeficiency virus (HIV) infection.

Geriatric Use

Of the total number of patients treated with anidulafungin in clinical trials, 35% were 65 years of age or older and 18% were 75 years of age and older. Although no overall differences in safety and efficacy were observed between geriatric adults 65 years of age or older and younger adults in clinical trials and other clinical experience has not revealed any evidence of age-related differences, the possibility that some older patients may have increased sensitivity to the drug cannot be ruled out.

Dosage adjustments are not necessary when anidulafungin is used in geriatric patients.

Hepatic Impairment

Anidulafungin pharmacokinetics are not altered in adults with mild, moderate, or severe hepatic impairment (Child-Pugh class A, B, or C). Although the area under the concentration-time curve (AUC) of anidulafungin may be slightly decreased in those with Child-Pugh class C hepatic impairment, this is not considered clinically important.

Dosage adjustments are not necessary if anidulafungin is used in adults with mild, moderate, or severe hepatic impairment.

Renal Impairment

Anidulafungin pharmacokinetics are not altered in adults with mild, moderate, or severe renal impairment.

Dosage adjustments are not necessary if anidulafungin is used in adults with mild, moderate, or severe renal impairment.

● Common Adverse Effects

Adverse effects reported in 5% or more of patients receiving anidulafungin include GI effects (nausea, diarrhea, vomiting, dyspepsia), phlebitis/thrombophlebitis, hypokalemia, increased ALT, increased alkaline phosphatase, increased γ-glutamyltransferase (GGT, γ-glutamyl transpeptidase, GGPT), pyrexia, headache, rash, insomnia, anemia, and neutropenia.

DRUG INTERACTIONS

● Drugs Affecting or Metabolized by Hepatic Microsomal Enzymes

Pharmacokinetic interactions unlikely. In vitro studies indicate that anidulafungin does not inhibit cytochrome P-450 (CYP) isoenzymes 1A2, 2B6, 2C8, 2C9, 2C19, 2D6, or 3A at clinically relevant concentrations. Anidulafungin is not a clinically important substrate, inducer, or inhibitor of CYP isoenzymes.

● Drugs Affecting or Affected by P-glycoprotein Transport

Anidulafungin is not an inhibitor or substrate of the P-glycoprotein transport system; pharmacokinetic interactions unlikely.

● Antifungal Agents
Amphotericin B

No clinically important pharmacokinetic interactions if IV amphotericin B liposomal (AmBisome®) is used concomitantly with IV anidulafungin. Dosage of anidulafungin does not need to be adjusted if the drug is used concomitantly with IV amphotericin B liposomal.

In vitro, the antifungal effects of anidulafungin and amphotericin B usually have been additive against Candida, including C. albicans, C. glabrata, C. krusei, C. parapsilosis, and C. tropicalis. Although the combination usually has been indifferent against Aspergillus or Fusarium, antagonism occurred against some strains of A. flavus and A. terreus and synergism occurred against some strains of A. fumigatus. Clinical importance of these in vitro studies is unclear.

Fluconazole

In vitro, the antifungal effects of anidulafungin and fluconazole have been additive or indifferent against C. albicans and C. glabrata and indifferent against C. krusei, C. parapsilosis, and C. tropicalis. Clinical importance of these in vitro studies is unclear.

Flucytosine

In vitro, the antifungal effects of anidulafungin and flucytosine have been additive or indifferent against *C. albicans*, *C. glabrata*, *C. krusei*, *C. parapsilosis*, and *C. tropicalis*. Clinical importance of these in vitro studies is unclear.

Itraconazole

In vitro, the antifungal effects of anidulafungin and itraconazole have been additive or indifferent against *Candida*, including *C. albicans*, *C. glabrata*, *C. krusei*, *C. parapsilosis*, and *C. tropicalis*. Although the antifungal effects of anidulafungin and itraconazole usually have been synergistic or indifferent against *Aspergillus*, the combination has been indifferent against *Fusarium*. Clinical importance of these in vitro studies is unclear.

Ketoconazole

In vitro, the antifungal effects of anidulafungin and ketoconazole have been additive or indifferent against *C. albicans*, *C. glabrata*, *C. krusei*, and *C. parapsilosis*, but have been antagonistic against *C. tropicalis*. Clinical importance of these in vitro studies is unclear.

Voriconazole

No clinically important pharmacokinetic interactions were reported when oral voriconazole was used concomitantly with IV anidulafungin in healthy adults.

If voriconazole and anidulafungin are used concomitantly, dosage adjustment not necessary for either drug.

● *Immunosuppressive Agents*

Cyclosporine

Pharmacokinetic interaction with cyclosporine (22% increase in steady-state area under the concentration-time curve [AUC] of anidulafungin; no clinically important effect on steady-state peak anidulafungin plasma concentrations). Results of an in vitro study indicate that anidulafungin has no effect on cyclosporine metabolism.

If cyclosporine and anidulafungin are used concomitantly, dosage adjustments are not necessary for either drug.

Tacrolimus

No clinically important pharmacokinetic interactions were reported when oral tacrolimus was used concomitantly with IV anidulafungin in healthy adults.

If tacrolimus and anidulafungin are used concomitantly, dosage adjustments are not necessary for either drug.

● *Rifampin*

No clinically important pharmacokinetic interactions when rifampin is used concomitantly with IV anidulafungin.

Dosage of anidulafungin does not need to be adjusted if the drug is used concomitantly with rifampin.

DESCRIPTION

Anidulafungin, a semisynthetic lipopeptide synthesized from a fermentation product of *Aspergillus nidulans*, is an echinocandin antifungal agent. Echinocandins (e.g., anidulafungin, caspofungin, micafungin) are glucan synthesis inhibitors and differ structurally and pharmacologically from other currently available antifungal agents.

Like other echinocandins, anidulafungin inhibits the synthesis of β(1,3)-D-glucan, an integral component of the fungal cell wall that is not present in mammalian cells. The drug may be fungistatic and fungicidal in action.

Anidulafungin undergoes slow chemical degradation at physiologic temperature and pH to a ring-opened peptide that lacks antifungal activity. The drug does not appear to undergo hepatic metabolism. Anidulafungin is not a clinically important substrate for and does not inhibit or induce cytochrome P-450 (CYP) isoenzymes and does not appear to have clinically important effects on the metabolism of drugs metabolized by these hepatic isoenzymes. The drug is more than 99% bound to plasma proteins. The elimination half-life of anidulafungin at steady state is approximately 27–52 hours. Steady-state concentrations are achieved within 24 hours of administration of the initial loading dose (twice the daily maintenance dosage); the estimated plasma accumulation factor during steady state is approximately 2. Anidulafungin is eliminated principally in feces via the biliary tract, mostly as degradation products of the drug. In healthy individuals, about 30% of a single IV dose of radiolabeled anidulafungin was recovered in feces over 9 days (less than 10% was unchanged drug); less than 1% of the dose is eliminated in urine.

● *Spectrum*

Anidulafungin is active in vitro against many *Candida*, including *C. albicans*, *C. dubliniensis*, *C. glabrata*, *C. guilliermondii*, *C. keyfri*, *C. krusei*, *C. lusitaniae*, *C. metapsilosis*, *C. orthopsilosis*, *C. parapsilosis*, and *C. tropicalis*. The drug has been active against some fluconazole-resistant strains of *C. albicans*, *C. glabrata*, and *C. krusei*.

Clinical isolates of *C. auris* (often misidentified as *C. haemulonii*, *C. famata*, or *Rhodotorula glutinis*) generally have been inhibited in vitro by anidulafungin concentrations of 0.125–1 mcg/mL.

Anidulafungin has in vitro activity against *Aspergillus*, including *A. flavus*, *A. fumigatus*, *A. niger*, and *A. terreus*.

Like other echinocandins, anidulafungin is not active against *Cryptococcus neoformans*, *Trichosporon*, *Fusarium*, or zygomycetes.

● *Resistance*

Although the clinical importance is unclear, *Candida* (e.g., *C. glabrata*) with reduced susceptibility to echinocandins have been reported. Some clinical isolates of *C. auris* have reduced susceptibility or resistance to anidulafungin in vitro (i.e., MICs 4 mcg/mL or greater).

Resistance to echinocandins usually is due to point mutations within the genes (FKS1 and FKS2) encoding for subunits in the glucan synthase enzyme complex.

The potential for development of resistance to anidulafungin or for cross-resistance with other echinocandins (caspofungin, micafungin) is not known. Anidulafungin has been active against some strains of *C. glabrata* resistant to caspofungin and *C. parapsilosis* resistant to caspofungin and micafungin.

ADVICE TO PATIENTS

Inform patients about the risk of developing abnormal liver function tests and/or hepatic dysfunction. Advise patients that liver function tests may be monitored during anidulafungin treatment.

Inform patients that anaphylactic reactions, including shock, have been reported in patients receiving anidulafungin. Advise patients that the drug may be discontinued and appropriate treatment administered if such reactions occur.

Inform patients that infusion-related adverse reactions, possibly histamine mediated, may occur and advise them of the importance of reporting symptoms (e.g., rash, urticaria, flushing, pruritus, dyspnea, hypotension) to their clinician.

Importance of informing clinicians of existing or contemplated concomitant therapy, including prescription and OTC drugs, and any concomitant illnesses.

Importance of women informing clinicians if they are or plan to become pregnant or plan to breast-feed.

Importance of informing patients of other important precautionary information. (See Cautions.)

PREPARATIONS

Excipients in commercially available drug preparations may have clinically important effects in some individuals; consult specific product labeling for details.

Anidulafungin

Parenteral

For injection, for IV infusion	50 mg		Eraxis®, Pfizer
	100 mg		Eraxis®, Pfizer

† Use is not currently included in the labeling approved by the US Food and Drug Administration.

Caspofungin Acetate

8:14.16 • ECHINOCANDINS

■ Caspofungin acetate is a semisynthetic, echinocandin antifungal agent.

USES

● Aspergillosis

Caspofungin acetate is used for the treatment of invasive aspergillosis in adults, adolescents, and children 3 months of age and older whose disease is refractory to, or who are intolerant of, other antifungal agents. The drug has not been evaluated for initial therapy of invasive aspergillosis.

The Infectious Diseases Society of America (IDSA) and other clinicians consider IV voriconazole the drug of choice for primary treatment of invasive aspergillosis in adult and pediatric patients, including those with human immunodeficiency virus (HIV) infection; IV amphotericin B or isavuconazonium sulfate (prodrug of isavuconazole) is usually recommended as an alternative for primary treatment. For salvage therapy in patients refractory to or intolerant of primary antifungal therapy, IDSA recommends IV amphotericin B, an IV echinocandin (caspofungin, micafungin), oral or IV posaconazole, or itraconazole oral suspension. IDSA states that echinocandins (either alone or in conjunction with other antifungals) may be effective for salvage therapy of invasive aspergillosis; however, routine use of echinocandin monotherapy is not recommended for primary treatment of invasive aspergillosis.

For additional information on management of aspergillosis, the current clinical practice guidelines from IDSA available at http://www.idsociety.org and the current clinical practice guidelines from the Centers for Disease Control and Prevention (CDC), National Institutes of Health (NIH), and IDSA on the prevention and treatment of opportunistic infections in HIV-infected individuals available at http://www.aidsinfo.nih.gov should be consulted.

Clinical Experience

Safety and efficacy of caspofungin for the treatment of invasive aspergillosis in adults whose disease is refractory to, or who are intolerant of, other antifungal agents (i.e., conventional amphotericin B, lipid-based amphotericin B, itraconazole) have been evaluated in an open-label, noncomparative study in 69 adults 18–80 years of age with definite or probable invasive aspergillosis who received a 70-mg loading dose followed by 50 mg once daily for a mean duration of 33.7 days (range: 1–162 days). Study patients consisted of those with infections categorized as refractory (i.e., disease progression or no improvement despite at least 7 days of therapy with amphotericin B [conventional or lipid-based formulation], itraconazole, or an investigational azole antifungal with activity against *Aspergillus*) or those who were intolerant of other antifungals (i.e., previous therapy associated with doubling of serum creatinine concentration or serum creatinine 2.5 mg/dL or greater, infusion-related toxicities, other acute reactions). A favorable response (defined as complete resolution or clinically meaningful improvement of all signs and symptoms of the infection and related radiographic findings) was observed in 41% of patients after at least 1 dose of caspofungin and in 50% of patients who received more than 7 days of treatment with the drug. Caspofungin therapy was associated with a favorable response rate in 36% of patients refractory to prior antifungal therapy and 70% of patients intolerant of prior antifungal therapy.

● Candida Infections

Candidemia and Other Invasive Candida Infections

Caspofungin acetate is used for the treatment of candidemia and certain other invasive *Candida* infections (intra-abdominal abscess, peritonitis, pleural space infections) in adults, adolescents, and children 3 months of age and older. The drug has been effective in *C. albicans*, *C. glabrata*, *C. krusei*, *C. parapsilosis*, and *C. tropicalis* infections, principally in nonneutropenic patients. The manufacturer states that safety and efficacy of caspofungin have not been established for the treatment of endocarditis, osteomyelitis, or meningitis caused by *Candida*.

For the treatment of candidemia in *nonneutropenic* patients or for empiric treatment of suspected invasive candidiasis in *nonneutropenic* patients in intensive

care units (ICUs), IDSA recommends an IV echinocandin (anidulafungin, caspofungin, micafungin) for *initial* therapy. IDSA states that fluconazole (IV or oral) is an acceptable alternative for *initial* therapy in selected patients, including those who are not critically ill and are unlikely to have infections caused by fluconazole-resistant *Candida*. If echinocandin- and azole-resistant *Candida* are suspected, IV amphotericin B is recommended; IV amphotericin B also is a reasonable alternative when echinocandins and fluconazole cannot be used because of intolerance, limited availability, or resistance. IDSA states that transition from the echinocandin (or amphotericin B) to fluconazole can be considered (usually within 5–7 days) in patients who are clinically stable, have isolates susceptible to fluconazole (e.g., *C. albicans*), and have negative repeat blood cultures after initial antifungal treatment. Although fluconazole has been considered the drug of choice for the treatment of infections caused by *C. parapsilosis* in nonneutropenic patients (based in part on concerns related to decreased in vitro susceptibility and resistance to echinocandins), IDSA states that there are no clinical studies to date indicating superiority of fluconazole over echinocandins for the treatment of *C. parapsilosis* infections.

For the treatment of candidemia in *neutropenic* patients, IDSA recommends an IV echinocandin (anidulafungin, caspofungin, micafungin) or, alternatively, IV amphotericin B for *initial* therapy. Fluconazole is an alternative in *initial* therapy in those who are not critically ill or have had no prior exposure to azole antifungals and also can be used for step-down therapy during neutropenia in clinically stable patients who have fluconazole-susceptible isolates and documented bloodstream clearance. Voriconazole can be used as an alternative for *initial* therapy when broader antifungal coverage is required and also can be used as step-down therapy during neutropenia in clinically stable patients who have voriconazole-susceptible isolates and documented bloodstream clearance. For infections known to be caused by *C. krusei*, an echinocandin, amphotericin B, or voriconazole is recommended.

For the treatment of osteoarticular infections† (e.g., osteomyelitis, septic arthritis) caused by *Candida*, IDSA recommends *initial* treatment with fluconazole or an IV echinocandin (anidulafungin, caspofungin, micafungin) and follow-up treatment with fluconazole. If septic arthritis involves a prosthetic device that cannot be removed, long-term suppressive or maintenance therapy (secondary prophylaxis) with fluconazole is recommended if the isolate is susceptible.

For the treatment of endocarditis† (native or prosthetic valve) or implantable cardiac device infections† caused by *Candida*, IDSA recommends *initial* treatment with IV amphotericin B (with or without oral flucytosine) or an IV echinocandin (anidulafungin, caspofungin, micafungin) and follow-up treatment with fluconazole. If the isolate is susceptible, long-term suppressive or maintenance therapy (secondary prophylaxis) with fluconazole is recommended to prevent recurrence in those with native valve endocarditis who cannot undergo valve replacement and in those with prosthetic valve endocarditis.

For additional information on management of candidemia and disseminated candidiasis, the current clinical practice guidelines from IDSA available at http://www.idsociety.org should be consulted.

Clinical Experience

Safety and efficacy of caspofungin for the treatment of candidemia or other invasive *Candida* infections were evaluated in a randomized, double-blind study in adults (87% were nonneutropenic). Patients were randomized to receive initial therapy with either IV caspofungin (70-mg loading dose on day 1 followed by 50 mg once daily) or IV amphotericin B deoxycholate (0.6–0.7 mg/kg daily for nonneutropenic patients; 0.7–1 mg/kg daily for neutropenic patients) for 14 days following the most recent positive *Candida* culture. After a minimum of 10 days of IV therapy, patients in both treatment groups were permitted to switch to oral fluconazole (400 mg daily) if they had a baseline *Candida* isolate susceptible to fluconazole and were nonneutropenic, were clinically improved, and had blood cultures negative for *Candida* for 48 hours; those with *C. krusei* or *C. glabrata* infections were not switched to oral fluconazole. A greater proportion of patients receiving amphotericin B deoxycholate compared with those receiving caspofungin switched to oral fluconazole (34.8 versus 24.8%, respectively). When data analysis was done using the modified intent-to-treat population, a favorable response (defined as complete resolution of signs and symptoms of *Candida* infection with documented or presumed microbiological eradication) was observed in 73.4% of those in the caspofungin group (mean duration of 12.1 days of IV caspofungin) and in 61.7% of those in the amphotericin B deoxycholate group (mean duration of 11.7 days of IV amphotericin B deoxycholate). The efficacy of caspofungin was comparable to that of amphotericin B deoxycholate at all time points evaluated (i.e., day 10 of IV therapy, completion of antifungal treatment, 2 weeks and 6–8 weeks after treatment) and at all sites of infection included in the study.

Results of a randomized, double-blind study in adults with invasive candidiasis that was designed to compare the safety and efficacy of a high dosage regimen of caspofungin (150 mg daily) and a dosage regimen that included a 70-mg loading dose on day 1 followed by 50 mg daily indicate that the higher dosage did not result in significant improvement in efficacy.

Esophageal Candidiasis

Caspofungin acetate is used for the treatment of esophageal candidiasis in adults, adolescents, and children 3 months of age and older.

Esophageal candidiasis requires treatment with a systemic antifungal (not a topical antifungal).

IDSA recommends oral fluconazole as the preferred drug of choice for the treatment of esophageal candidiasis; if oral therapy is not tolerated, IV fluconazole or an IV echinocandin (anidulafungin, caspofungin, micafungin) usually is recommended and IV amphotericin B is another alternative. For fluconazole-refractory esophageal candidiasis, IDSA recommends itraconazole oral solution or IV or oral voriconazole; alternatives for fluconazole-refractory disease are an IV echinocandin (anidulafungin, caspofungin, micafungin) or IV amphotericin B. IDSA states that oral posaconazole (oral suspension or delayed-release tablets) could be considered another alternative for the treatment of fluconazole-refractory esophageal candidiasis.

For the treatment of esophageal candidiasis in HIV-infected adults and adolescents, CDC, NIH, and IDSA recommend IV or oral fluconazole or itraconazole oral solution. Alternatives include oral or IV voriconazole, an IV echinocandin (anidulafungin, caspofungin, micafungin), or IV amphotericin B. For refractory esophageal candidiasis in HIV-infected adults and adolescents, including fluconazole-refractory infections, these experts recommend posaconazole oral suspension or itraconazole oral solution; alternatives include an IV echinocandin (anidulafungin, caspofungin, micafungin), oral or IV voriconazole, or IV amphotericin B. Although data are limited, some experts state that an IV echinocandin (anidulafungin, caspofungin, micafungin) can be considered an alternative for treatment of azole-refractory esophageal candidiasis in HIV-infected children.

Routine long-term suppressive or maintenance therapy (secondary prophylaxis) to prevent relapse or recurrence is not usually recommended in patients adequately treated for esophageal candidiasis (including HIV-infected individuals) unless the patient has frequent or severe recurrences of esophageal candidiasis. If secondary prophylaxis of esophageal candidiasis is indicated, oral fluconazole or posaconazole oral suspension is recommended; however, the potential for development of azole resistance should be considered.

For additional information on management of esophageal candidiasis, the current clinical practice guidelines from IDSA available at http://www.idsociety.org and the current clinical practice guidelines from CDC, NIH, and IDSA on the prevention and treatment of opportunistic infections in HIV-infected individuals available at http://www.aidsinfo.nih.gov should be consulted.

Clinical Experience

Safety and efficacy of caspofungin for the treatment of esophageal candidiasis have been evaluated in a multicenter, noninferiority clinical study and in 2 smaller dose-ranging studies in adults with symptoms and microbiological documentation of esophageal candidiasis. The majority of patients in all 3 studies had advanced HIV infection (CD4+ T-cell counts less than 50/mm³). Patients in the multicenter, double-blind, noninferiority clinical study were randomized to receive either IV caspofungin (50 mg once daily) or IV fluconazole (200 mg once daily) for 7–21 days. Most patients in this study had both esophageal and oropharyngeal candidiasis at baseline. A favorable overall response (defined as complete resolution of clinical symptoms, with either total clearing of esophageal lesions [mucosal grade of 0] or a reduction in endoscopy score by at least 2 grade levels) at 5–7 days after completion of treatment was attained in 81.5 and 85.1% of patients in the caspofungin and fluconazole groups, respectively. The median time to symptom resolution in both groups was 4–5 days. The rate of relapse (defined as recurrence of clinical symptoms within 1 month after completion of treatment) at 2 and 4 weeks posttreatment was similar in those who received caspofungin (10.6 and 28.1%, respectively) or fluconazole (7.9 and 16.7%, respectively). The results from the 2 smaller dose-ranging studies corroborate the efficacy of caspofungin demonstrated in this study.

Oropharyngeal Candidiasis

Although safety and efficacy of caspofungin for the treatment of oropharyngeal candidiasis have not been established, the drug has been recommended as an alternative for the treatment of oropharyngeal candidiasis†.

For the treatment of mild oropharyngeal candidiasis, IDSA recommends topical treatment with clotrimazole lozenges or miconazole buccal tablets; nystatin (oral suspension or tablets) is the recommended alternative. For moderate to severe disease, IDSA recommends oral fluconazole. For fluconazole-refractory oropharyngeal candidiasis, IDSA recommends itraconazole oral solution or posaconazole oral suspension; oral voriconazole or amphotericin B oral suspension (not commercially available in the US) are recommended as alternatives. Other alternatives for refractory oropharyngeal candidiasis are an IV echinocandin (anidulafungin, caspofungin, micafungin) or IV amphotericin B.

For the treatment of oropharyngeal candidiasis in HIV-infected adults and adolescents, CDC, NIH, and IDSA recommend oral fluconazole as the preferred drug of choice for initial episodes. If topical therapy is used for the treatment of oropharyngeal candidiasis (e.g., mild to moderate episodes), these experts recommend clotrimazole lozenges or miconazole buccal tablets. Alternatives for systemic treatment of oropharyngeal candidiasis in HIV-infected adults and adolescents are itraconazole oral solution or posaconazole oral suspension; nystatin oral suspension is an alternative if topical treatment is used. For fluconazole-refractory oropharyngeal infections in HIV-infected adults and adolescents, posaconazole oral suspension is preferred; itraconazole oral solution is an alternative.

Routine long-term suppressive or maintenance therapy (secondary prophylaxis) to prevent relapse or recurrence is not usually recommended in patients adequately treated for oropharyngeal candidiasis (including HIV-infected individuals) unless the patient has frequent or severe recurrences of oropharyngeal candidiasis. If secondary prophylaxis of oropharyngeal candidiasis is indicated, oral fluconazole is recommended; however, the potential for development of azole resistance should be considered.

For additional information on management of oropharyngeal candidiasis, the current clinical practice guidelines from IDSA available at http://www.idsociety.org and the current clinical practice guidelines from CDC, NIH, and IDSA on the prevention and treatment of opportunistic infections in HIV-infected individuals available at http://www.aidsinfo.nih.gov should be consulted.

Clinical Experience

In a randomized, double-blind study evaluating caspofungin for the treatment of endoscopically and microbiologically confirmed esophageal candidiasis, the majority of patients also had oropharyngeal candidiasis† in addition to esophageal candidiasis. Patients were randomized to receive either IV caspofungin (50 mg once daily) or IV fluconazole (200 mg once daily) for 7–21 days. Data for those with oropharyngeal infections indicate that a favorable response (based on resolution of symptoms and oropharyngeal lesions) 5–7 days after completion of treatment was achieved in 71.4% of those who received caspofungin and 83.3% of those who received fluconazole. However, the rate of relapse of oropharyngeal candidiasis (defined as recurrence of symptoms within 1 month of completion of treatment) was higher at 2 and 4 weeks posttreatment in those who received caspofungin (42.5 and 59%, respectively) than in those who received fluconazole (13.2 and 35.3%, respectively).

Safety and efficacy of caspofungin for the treatment of oropharyngeal candidiasis† and/or esophageal candidiasis in adults also have been evaluated in a phase 2 randomized, double-blind, dose-ranging study (98% had HIV infection, 79% had C. albicans infection). Patients were randomized to receive IV caspofungin (35, 50, or 70 mg once daily) or IV amphotericin B (0.5 mg/kg once daily) for 7–14 days. When data analysis was done using the modified intent-to-treat population, a favorable response (defined as complete resolution of symptoms and quantifiable improvement of mucosal lesions 3–4 days after completion of treatment) was achieved in a greater proportion of patients with oropharyngeal candidiasis who received caspofungin (84–93%) than in those who received amphotericin B (67%).

Candida auris Infections

Caspofungin is used for the treatment of infections caused by C. auris, an emerging pathogen that has been associated with potentially fatal candidemia or other invasive infections.

C. auris, first identified in 2009, has now been reported as the cause of serious invasive infections (including fatalities) in multiple countries worldwide (e.g., Japan, South Korea, India, Kuwait, South Africa, Pakistan, United Kingdom, Venezuela, Colombia, US). As of May 2017, a total of 77 clinical cases of *C. auris* had been reported to CDC from 7 different states in the US. *C. auris* may be difficult to identify using standard in vitro methods and has been misidentified as *C. haemulonii, C. famata,* or *Rhodotorula glutinis*. A large percentage of *C. auris* clinical isolates are resistant to fluconazole and multidrug-resistant isolates with reduced susceptibility or resistance to all 3 major classes of antifungal agents (azoles, polyenes, echinocandins) have been reported.

Pending further accumulation of data, CDC has issued interim recommendations regarding laboratory diagnosis, treatment, and infection control measures for suspected or known *C. auris* infections. Based on limited data available to date, CDC recommends that an IV echinocandin (anidulafungin, caspofungin, micafungin) be used for initial treatment of invasive *C. auris* infections (e.g., bloodstream or intra-abdominal infections) in adults. CDC states that a switch to IV amphotericin B (lipid formulation) could be considered if the patient is clinically unresponsive to the echinocandin or fungemia persists longer than 5 days. Consultation with an infectious disease specialist is highly recommended.

Unless there is evidence of infection, CDC does not currently recommend antifungal treatment when *C. auris* is isolated only from noninvasive body sites (e.g., urine, external ear, wounds, respiratory secretions). Some individuals are colonized with *C. auris* in the axilla, groin, nose, external ear canal, oropharynx, urine, wounds, rectum, and stool; however, data are limited and the duration of *C. auris* colonization is unclear. Therefore, CDC recommends that infection control measures be observed for all patients with cultures yielding *C. auris*, including those with positive cultures only from noninvasive body sites.

Whenever *C. auris* infection is suspected, clinicians should immediately contact state or local public health authorities and the CDC (candidaauris@cdc.gov) for guidance. For additional information on diagnosis and management of *C. auris* infections, the interim recommendations and most recent information from CDC available at https://www.cdc.gov/fungal/diseases/candidiasis/candida-auris.html should be consulted.

● *Empiric Therapy in Febrile Neutropenic Patients*

Caspofungin acetate is used for empiric treatment of presumed fungal infections in febrile, neutropenic adults, adolescents, and children 3 months of age and older.

Clinical Experience

Safety and efficacy of caspofungin for empiric therapy of presumed fungal infections in febrile neutropenic patients have been evaluated in a randomized, double-blind, noninferiority study in patients 16 years of age and older. In this study, patients received IV caspofungin (70-mg loading dose on day 1 followed by 50 mg once daily) or IV amphotericin B liposomal (3 mg/kg daily) until resolution of neutropenia or up to a maximum of 28 days (unless a fungal infection was documented). After 5 days of IV therapy, patients who remained febrile and clinically deteriorated could receive caspofungin 70 mg daily or amphotericin B liposomal 5 mg/kg daily. When data analysis was done using the modified intent-to-treat population, an overall favorable response (defined as resolution of fever during the neutropenic period, successful treatment of any baseline fungal infections, absence of emergent fungal infections up to 7 days after completion of study drug, patient survival for 7 days after empiric therapy, and use of study drug without premature discontinuance because of toxicity or lack of efficacy) was attained in 33.9 or 33.7% of those receiving caspofungin or amphotericin B liposomal, respectively.

Safety and efficacy of caspofungin for empiric treatment of presumed fungal infections in pediatric patients have been evaluated in a randomized, double-blind study comparing IV caspofungin (70-mg/m^2 loading dose on day 1 [up to 70 mg daily] followed by 50 mg/m^2 once daily) with IV amphotericin B liposomal (3 mg/kg daily) in patients 2–17 years of age with persistent fever and neutropenia. An overall favorable response was attained in 46.4 or 32% of those receiving caspofungin or amphotericin B liposomal, respectively.

DOSAGE AND ADMINISTRATION

● *Administration*

Caspofungin acetate is administered by slow IV infusion. The drug should *not* be given by rapid IV injection.

Caspofungin acetate should not be admixed or infused concomitantly with other drugs. Dextrose-containing diluents (e.g., 5% dextrose injection) should *not* be used.

IV Infusion
Reconstitution and Dilution

Commercially available caspofungin acetate lyophilized powder for injection must be reconstituted and then further diluted prior to IV infusion.

Vials of lyophilized caspofungin acetate should be stored at 2–8 °C and should be allowed to reach room temperature prior to reconstitution.

The 50- or 70-mg vial of caspofungin acetate should be reconstituted by adding 10.8 mL of 0.9% sodium chloride injection, sterile water for injection, bacteriostatic water for injection (with methylparaben and propylparaben), or bacteriostatic water for injection (with 0.9% benzyl alcohol) to provide a solution containing 5 or 7 mg/mL, respectively. The vial should be mixed gently until the drug is dissolved completely and a clear solution is obtained. The 50- and 70-mg vials are formulated to provide a slight overfill when reconstituted as directed, yielding 54.6 and 75.6 mg of caspofungin, respectively.

The reconstituted solution should be inspected for evidence of particulate matter or discoloration and should not be used if cloudy or if a precipitate has formed. After reconstitution and before dilution, the vial may be stored at a temperature of 25°C or less for up to 1 hour. After the reconstituted solution is diluted for IV administration, it may be stored at a temperature of 25°C or less for 24 hours or at a temperature of 2–8°C for 48 hours. Caspofungin vials are for single-use only, partially used vials of reconstituted solution should be discarded.

The appropriate volume of reconstituted solution (mL equivalent to the indicated loading or maintenance dose) should be withdrawn from the vial and added to 250 mL of 0.225%, 0.45%, or 0.9% sodium chloride injection or lactated Ringer's injection. Alternatively, the appropriate volume of reconstituted drug may be added to a reduced volume of 0.225%, 0.45%, or 0.9% sodium chloride injection or lactated Ringer's injection, provided the final concentration does not exceed 0.5 mg/mL.

For pediatric patients 3 months to 17 years of age, caspofungin vials should be reconstituted the same as for adults. After reconstitution, the appropriate volume of reconstituted solution equivalent to the calculated loading or maintenance dose based on a concentration of 5 mg/mL (if using the 50 mg vial) or 7 mg/mL (if using the 70 mg vial) should be withdrawn from the vial and added to 0.225%, 0.45%, or 0.9% sodium chloride injection or lactated Ringer's injection. The manufacturer recommends that the 50-mg vial (concentration of 5 mg/mL) be used for pediatric doses less than 50 mg and that the 70-mg vial (concentration of 7 mg/mL) be used for pediatric doses greater than 50 mg.

Rate of Administration

IV infusions of caspofungin acetate should be given over approximately 1 hour.

● *Dosage*

Dosage of caspofungin acetate is expressed in terms of the salt.

Adult Dosage
Aspergillosis

The recommended dosage of caspofungin acetate for the treatment of invasive aspergillosis in adults whose disease is refractory to, or who are intolerant of, other antifungal therapy is a single loading dose of 70 mg on day 1, followed by 50 mg once daily thereafter.

The duration of treatment is based on the severity of the patient's underlying disease, recovery from immunosuppression, and clinical response. The Infectious Diseases Society of America (IDSA) recommends that antifungal treatment of invasive pulmonary aspergillosis be continued for at least 6–12 weeks.

Candidemia and Other Invasive Candida Infections

The recommended dosage of caspofungin acetate for the treatment of candidemia or certain other invasive *Candida* infections (intra-abdominal abscess, peritonitis, pleural space infections) in *nonneutropenic* or *neutropenic* adults is a single loading dose of 70 mg given on day 1, followed by 50 mg once daily thereafter.

When caspofungin acetate is used for initial treatment of candidemia or other invasive *Candida* infections, IDSA states that a transition from the echinocandin to fluconazole can be considered (usually within 5–7 days) in patients who are clinically stable, have isolates susceptible to fluconazole (e.g., *C. albicans*), and have negative repeat blood cultures after initial antifungal treatment.

The duration of treatment should be based on clinical and microbiological response. The manufacturer recommends that treatment be continued for at least

14 days after the last positive culture and states that those who remain persistently neutropenic may require a longer course of therapy pending resolution of neutropenia. IDSA recommends that antifungal treatment for candidemia (without persistent fungemia or metastatic complications) be continued for 2 weeks after documented clearance of *Candida* from the bloodstream, resolution of candidemia symptoms, and resolution of neutropenia.

If caspofungin acetate is used for *initial* treatment of osteoarticular infections† (e.g., osteomyelitis, septic arthritis) caused by *Candida*, IDSA recommends a dosage of 50–70 mg once daily in adults. After at least 2 weeks, treatment can be switched to fluconazole.

If caspofungin acetate is used for *initial* treatment of endocarditis† (native or prosthetic valve) or implantable cardiac device infections† caused by *Candida*, IDSA recommends a dosage of 150 mg once daily in adults. If the infection is caused by fluconazole-susceptible *Candida*, treatment can be switched to fluconazole after the patient is stabilized and *Candida* has been cleared from the bloodstream.

Esophageal Candidiasis

The manufacturer recommends that caspofungin acetate be given in a dosage of 50 mg once daily for the treatment of esophageal candidiasis in adults.

Although the manufacturer states that use of a 70-mg loading dose has not been evaluated for the treatment of esophageal candidiasis, IDSA recommends a single 70-mg loading dose on day 1, followed by 50 mg once daily for the treatment of esophageal candidiasis in adults.

For the treatment of esophageal candidiasis in adults with human immunodeficiency virus (HIV) infection, some experts recommend that caspofungin acetate be given in a dosage of 50 mg once daily.

The manufacturer recommends that treatment of esophageal candidiasis be continued for 7–14 days after resolution of symptoms. The Centers for Disease Control and Prevention (CDC), National Institutes of Health (NIH), and IDSA recommend that antifungal treatment of esophageal candidiasis be continued for 14–21 days.

Oropharyngeal Candidiasis

If caspofungin acetate is used for the treatment of oropharyngeal candidiasis†, IDSA recommends that adults receive a single 70-mg loading dose on day 1, followed by 50 mg once daily for 7–14 days.

Candida auris Infections

If caspofungin acetate is used for initial treatment of invasive *C. auris* infections (e.g., bloodstream or intra-abdominal infections), CDC recommends that adults receive a single 70-mg loading dose on day 1, followed by 50 mg once daily.

Empiric Therapy in Febrile Neutropenic Patients

The recommended dosage of caspofungin acetate for empiric therapy of presumed fungal infections in febrile neutropenic adults is a single loading dose of 70 mg given on day 1, followed by 50 mg once daily thereafter. If 50 mg once daily is well tolerated but does not provide an adequate clinical response, the manufacturer states that the dosage may be increased to 70 mg once daily.

The duration of empiric treatment should be based on clinical response and should be continued until neutropenia resolves. If a fungal infection is identified, the drug should be continued for at least 14 days after the last positive culture and for at least 7 days after both neutropenia and clinical symptoms resolve.

Pediatric Dosage

General Dosing for Pediatric Patients

Caspofungin acetate dosage for pediatric patients 3 months to 17 years of age is based on body surface area (BSA) calculated using the Mosteller Formula. The loading dose (in mg) should be calculated as BSA (m^2) x 70 mg/m^2 and the maintenance dose (in mg) should be calculated as BSA (m^2) x 50 mg/m^2.

Regardless of the patient's calculated dose, the maximum loading dose and maximum daily maintenance dosage in pediatric patients should not exceed 70 mg.

Aspergillosis

The recommended dosage of caspofungin acetate for pediatric patients 3 months to 17 years of age with invasive aspergillosis whose disease is refractory to, or who are intolerant of, other antifungal therapy is a single loading dose of 70 mg/m^2 given on day 1, followed by 50 mg/m^2 once daily thereafter. If 50 mg/m^2 once daily is well tolerated but does not provide an adequate clinical response, dosage may be increased to 70 mg/m^2 once daily.

The duration of treatment is based on the severity of the patient's underlying disease, recovery from immunosuppression, and clinical response. IDSA recommends that antifungal treatment of invasive pulmonary aspergillosis be continued for at least 6–12 weeks.

Candidemia and Other Invasive Candida Infections

The recommended dosage of caspofungin acetate for the treatment of candidemia or certain other invasive *Candida* infections (intra-abdominal abscess, peritonitis, pleural space infections) in pediatric patients 3 months to 17 years of age is a single loading dose of 70 mg/m^2 given on day 1, followed by 50 mg/m^2 once daily thereafter. If 50 mg/m^2 once daily is well tolerated but does not provide an adequate clinical response, dosage may be increased to 70 mg/m^2 once daily.

The duration of treatment should be based on clinical and microbiological response. The manufacturer recommends that treatment be continued for at least 14 days after the last positive culture and states that those who remain persistently neutropenic may require a longer course of therapy pending resolution of neutropenia. IDSA recommends that antifungal treatment for candidemia (without persistent fungemia or metastatic complications) be continued for 2 weeks after documented clearance of *Candida* from the bloodstream, resolution of candidemia symptoms, and resolution of neutropenia.

Esophageal Candidiasis

The recommended dosage of caspofungin acetate for the treatment of esophageal candidiasis in pediatric patients 3 months to 17 years of age is a single loading dose of 70 mg/m^2 given on day 1, followed by 50 mg/m^2 once daily thereafter. If 50 mg/m^2 once daily is well tolerated but does not provide an adequate clinical response, dosage may be increased to 70 mg/m^2 once daily.

For the treatment of esophageal candidiasis in HIV-infected adolescents, some experts recommend that caspofungin acetate be given in a dosage of 50 mg once daily.

The manufacturer recommends that treatment of esophageal candidiasis be continued for 7–14 days after resolution of symptoms. CDC, NIH, and IDSA recommend that antifungal treatment of esophageal candidiasis be continued for 14–21 days.

Empiric Therapy in Febrile Neutropenic Patients

The recommended dosage of caspofungin acetate for empiric treatment of presumed fungal infections in febrile neutropenic pediatric patients 3 months to 17 years of age is a single loading dose of 70 mg/m^2 given on day 1, followed by 50 mg/m^2 once daily thereafter. If 50 mg/m^2 once daily is well tolerated but does not provide an adequate clinical response, dosage may be increased to 70 mg/m^2 once daily.

The duration of empiric treatment should be based on clinical response and should be continued until neutropenia resolves. If a fungal infection is identified, the drug should be continued for at least 14 days after the last positive culture and for at least 7 days after neutropenia and clinical symptoms resolve.

● Special Populations

Hepatic Impairment

Dosage adjustments are not necessary in adults with mild hepatic impairment (Child-Pugh score 5–6). When caspofungin acetate is used in adults with moderate hepatic impairment (Child-Pugh score 7–9), a dosage of 35 mg once daily following the initial 70-mg loading dose (if usually indicated) is recommended.

Data are not available regarding use of caspofungin acetate in adults with severe hepatic impairment (Child-Pugh score exceeding 9) or in pediatric patients with any degree of hepatic impairment.

Renal Impairment

Dosage adjustments are not necessary in patients with renal impairment.

Because caspofungin is not dialyzable, supplementary doses are not required following hemodialysis.

Geriatric Patients

Dosage adjustments are not necessary in patients 65 years of age or older.

CAUTIONS

● Contraindications

Caspofungin acetate is contraindicated in patients with known hypersensitivity (e.g., anaphylaxis) to the drug or any ingredient in the formulation.

• *Warnings/Precautions*

Sensitivity Reactions

Hypersensitivity Reactions

Anaphylaxis has been reported in patients receiving caspofungin. If such reactions occur, the drug should be discontinued and appropriate treatment administered.

Possible histamine-mediated symptoms (e.g., rash, facial swelling, pruritus, sensation of warmth, bronchospasm) have been reported in patients receiving caspofungin and may require discontinuance of the drug and/or administration of appropriate treatment.

There have been postmarketing reports of Stevens-Johnson syndrome (SJS) and toxic epidermal necrolysis (TEN) in patients receiving caspofungin. The drug should be used with caution in patients with a history of allergic skin reactions.

Hepatic Effects

Abnormal liver function test results have been reported in healthy individuals and adult and pediatric patients receiving caspofungin. Hepatic abnormalities, including hepatic dysfunction, hepatitis, and hepatic failure, have been reported in some adult and pediatric patients with serious underlying conditions receiving caspofungin and multiple other drugs. A causal relationship to caspofungin has not been established to date.

Transient elevations in liver enzymes have been reported in patients receiving caspofungin and cyclosporine concomitantly. (See Cyclosporine under Drug Interactions: Immunosuppressive Agents.)

If abnormal liver function test results occur during caspofungin therapy, the patient should be monitored for evidence of worsening hepatic function and the risks of continued caspofungin therapy should be weighed against potential benefits.

Specific Populations

Pregnancy

Category C. (See Users Guide.)

There are no adequate and well-controlled studies of caspofungin acetate in pregnant women, and the manufacturer states that the drug should be used during pregnancy only if potential benefits justify potential risks to the fetus.

In animals, embryofetal toxicity (increased resorptions, increased peri-implantation loss, incomplete ossification at multiple fetal sites) has been reported with caspofungin dosages about 2 times the recommended human dosage (based on body surface area comparisons).

Lactation

Caspofungin is distributed into milk in rats; it is not known whether the drug is distributed into milk in humans.

Caspofungin should be used with caution in nursing women.

Pediatric Use

Safety and efficacy of caspofungin have not been established in neonates and infants younger than 3 months of age. Although limited pharmacokinetic data are available for this age group, the manufacturer states that data are insufficient to date to establish a safe and effective dosage for treatment of neonatal candidiasis. In addition, invasive candidiasis in neonates has a higher rate of CNS and multi-organ involvement than do such infections in older patients, and data are insufficient to date regarding distribution of caspofungin into the CNS or regarding efficacy in the treatment of meningitis and endocarditis.

Caspofungin has not been evaluated in pediatric patients for the treatment of endocarditis, osteomyelitis, or meningitis caused by *Candida* or for initial therapy of invasive aspergillosis. The drug also has not been evaluated for use in pediatric patients with hepatic impairment.

Safety and efficacy of caspofungin for use in infants and children 3 months to 17 years of age for treatment of invasive aspergillosis in those refractory to or intolerant of other antifungals; for treatment of candidemia and certain other invasive *Candida* infections (intra-abdominal abscesses, peritonitis, pleural space infections) or esophageal candidiasis; and for empiric treatment of presumed fungal infections in febrile neutropenic patients is based on adequate and well-controlled studies in adults, pharmacokinetic data in pediatric patients, and additional data from prospective studies in this age group.

The manufacturer states that the overall safety profile of caspofungin in pediatric patients is comparable to that in adults. Adverse effects reported in 7% or more of pediatric patients receiving caspofungin include pyrexia, rash, decreased potassium, increased AST, diarrhea, increased ALT, chills, hypotension, vomiting, tachycardia, mucosal inflammation, hypertension, headache, erythema, central line infection, cough, respiratory distress, hypokalemia, abdominal pain, and pruritus.

Although data are limited, some experts state that caspofungin can be considered for first-line treatment of invasive candidiasis or for alternative treatment of esophageal candidiasis in children with human immunodeficiency virus (HIV) infection.

Geriatric Use

Clinical studies of caspofungin did not include a sufficient number of patients 65 years of age or older to determine whether they respond differently than younger individuals. Although no overall differences in efficacy or safety were observed between geriatric and younger adults, the possibility that some older patients may have increased sensitivity to the drug cannot be ruled out.

Although caspofungin plasma concentrations are increased slightly in men and women 65 years of age and older compared with young healthy males, dosage adjustments are not necessary in geriatric patients.

Hepatic Impairment

Although the area under the concentration-time curve (AUC) of caspofungin is increased slightly in adults with mild hepatic impairment (Child-Pugh score 5–6) compared with healthy adults, dosage adjustments are not necessary. A greater increase in AUC occurs in adults with moderate hepatic impairment (Child-Pugh score 7–9), and a dosage reduction is recommended in these patients. (See Hepatic Impairment under Dosage and Administration: Special Populations.)

Data are not available regarding use of caspofungin in adults with severe hepatic impairment or in pediatric patients with any degree of hepatic impairment.

Renal Impairment

Renal impairment does not have a clinically important effect on the pharmacokinetics of caspofungin. Dosage adjustments are not necessary in patients with renal impairment.

• *Common Adverse Effects*

Adverse effects reported in 5% or more of patients receiving caspofungin include pyrexia, diarrhea, chills, decreased potassium, increased alkaline phosphatase, decreased hemoglobin, hypotension, respiratory failure, increased ALT, fever, decreased hematocrit, phlebitis, vomiting, rash, increased AST, nausea, headache, increased bilirubin, septic shock, decreased leukocyte count, peripheral edema, cough, pneumonia, increased creatinine, anemia, abdominal pain, dyspnea, increased blood urea, pleural effusion, increased conjugated bilirubin, tachycardia, decreased albumin, decreased magnesium, rales, and sepsis.

DRUG INTERACTIONS

• *Drugs Affecting Or Metabolized by Hepatic Microsomal Enzymes*

In vitro studies indicate that caspofungin does not inhibit and is a poor substrate for cytochrome P-450 (CYP) isoenzymes. The drug does not induce CYP3A4.

Concomitant use of caspofungin and drugs that induce CYP isoenzymes may result in clinically important decreases in plasma concentrations of caspofungin. It is not known which mechanism involved in caspofungin clearance may be inducible.

• *Drugs Affecting or Affected by P-glycoprotein Transport*

Caspofungin is not a substrate of the P-glycoprotein transport system; pharmacokinetic interactions unlikely.

• *Antifungal Agents*

Amphotericin B

No evidence of pharmacokinetic interactions if caspofungin is used concomitantly with amphotericin B.

In vitro, the antifungal effects of caspofungin and amphotericin B have been synergistic or additive against some *Aspergillus*, including *A. fumigatus*, and some *Fusarium* species. In vitro, caspofungin and amphotericin B have shown indifferent or additive antifungal effects against *Candida glabrata*. Although the clinical importance is not known, the combination of caspofungin and amphotericin B has not demonstrated antagonistic antifungal effects against *A. fumigatus*, *C. albicans* (including azole-resistant strains), or other *Candida*.

Fluconazole

In vitro, the antifungal effects of caspofungin and fluconazole have been synergistic against *C. glabrata*. No in vitro evidence of antagonistic antifungal effects against *C. albicans* (including azole-resistant strains) or against various other *Candida*.

Itraconazole

No evidence of pharmacokinetic interactions if caspofungin is used concomitantly with itraconazole.

In vitro, the antifungal effects of caspofungin and itraconazole usually have been synergistic or additive against *Aspergillus*, including *A. fumigatus*.

Posaconazole

In vitro, the antifungal effects of caspofungin and posaconazole usually have been synergistic against *Aspergillus* and *C. glabrata*.

Voriconazole

In vitro, the antifungal effects of caspofungin and voriconazole have been additive against *C. glabrata*. In vitro, the antifungal effects of caspofungin and voriconazole have been indifferent, additive, or synergistic against some *Aspergillus*, including *A. fumigatus*. There was no in vitro evidence of antagonistic antifungal effects against *Aspergillus*.

● *Antiretroviral Agents*
Efavirenz

Possible pharmacokinetic interaction (decreased caspofungin concentrations).

If caspofungin is used concomitantly with efavirenz, caspofungin dosage should be 70 mg once daily in adults and a dosage of 70 mg/m² (maximum 70 mg) once daily should be considered in pediatric patients.

Nelfinavir

Pharmacokinetics of caspofungin are not affected by concomitant nelfinavir.

Nevirapine

Possible pharmacokinetic interaction (decreased caspofungin concentrations).

If caspofungin is used concomitantly with nevirapine, caspofungin dosage should be 70 mg once daily in adults and a dosage of 70 mg/m² (maximum 70 mg) once daily should be considered in pediatric patients.

● *Carbamazepine*

Possible pharmacokinetic interaction (decreased caspofungin concentrations).

If caspofungin is used concomitantly with carbamazepine, caspofungin dosage should be 70 mg once daily in adults and a dosage of 70 mg/m² (maximum 70 mg) once daily should be considered in pediatric patients.

● *Dexamethasone*

Possible pharmacokinetic interaction (decreased caspofungin concentrations).

If caspofungin is used concomitantly with dexamethasone, caspofungin dosage should be 70 mg once daily in adults and a dosage of 70 mg/m² (maximum 70 mg) once daily should be considered in pediatric patients.

● *Immunosuppressive Agents*
Cyclosporine

Concomitant use of caspofungin and cyclosporine increases the area under the concentration-time curve (AUC) of caspofungin by about 35%, but does not affect plasma concentrations of cyclosporine.

Transient elevations in ALT (SGPT) and AST (SGOT) have been reported when caspofungin and cyclosporine were used concomitantly in healthy adults and immunocompromised patients.

Caspofungin and cyclosporine should be used concomitantly with caution and only when potential benefits outweigh risks. If the drugs are used concomitantly, the patient should be monitored closely. If abnormal liver function test results occur, the risks and benefits of continuing concomitant therapy should be evaluated.

Mycophenolate

No evidence of pharmacokinetic interactions if caspofungin is used concomitantly with mycophenolate.

Tacrolimus

Concomitant use of caspofungin and tacrolimus reduces peak plasma concentrations and AUC of tacrolimus by 16 and 20%, respectively, but does not affect the pharmacokinetics of caspofungin.

Tacrolimus concentrations should be monitored in patients receiving concomitant caspofungin; tacrolimus dosage should be adjusted if appropriate.

● *Phenytoin*

Possible pharmacokinetic interaction (decreased caspofungin concentrations).

If caspofungin is used concomitantly with phenytoin, caspofungin dosage should be 70 mg once daily in adults and a dosage of 70 mg/m² (maximum 70 mg) once daily should be considered in pediatric patients.

● *Rifampin*

Concomitant use of caspofungin and rifampin results in a 30% decrease in trough plasma concentrations of caspofungin.

If caspofungin is used concomitantly with rifampin, caspofungin dosage should be 70 mg once daily in adults or 70 mg/m² (maximum 70 mg) once daily in pediatric patients.

DESCRIPTION

Caspofungin acetate, a semisynthetic lipopeptide synthesized from a fermentation product of *Glarea lozoyensis*, is an echinocandin antifungal agent. Echinocandins (e.g., anidulafungin, caspofungin, micafungin) are glucan synthesis inhibitors and differ structurally and pharmacologically from other currently available antifungal agents.

Like other echinocandins, caspofungin inhibits the synthesis of $\beta(1,3)$-D-glucan, an integral component of the fungal cell wall that is not present in mammalian cells. Depending on the concentration, the drug may be fungicidal against *Candida*, but usually is fungistatic against *Aspergillus*.

Following IV infusion of caspofungin acetate over 1 hour, plasma concentrations of caspofungin decline in a polyphasic manner. The drug is extensively (about 97%) protein bound (to albumin), with distribution (rather than excretion or biotransformation) being the predominant mechanism influencing plasma clearance. Caspofungin acetate is slowly metabolized in the liver via hydrolysis and *N*-acetylation. Following a single IV dose, 35 and 41% of the dose is eliminated in feces and urine, respectively, as the parent drug and metabolites.

SPECTRUM

Caspofungin is active in vitro against *C. albicans*, *C. glabrata*, *C. guilliermondii*, *C. krusei*, *C. parapsilosis*, and *C. tropicalis*. The drug also is active in vitro against *C. dubliniensis*, *C. kefyr*, *C. lusitaniae*, *C. metapsilosis*, *C. orthopsilosis*, and *C. pseudotropicalis*. Caspofungin has been active against some *Candida*, including *C. glabrata* and *C. krusei*, resistant to fluconazole.

Clinical isolates of *C. auris* (often misidentified as *C. haemulonii*, *C. famata*, or *Rhodotorula glutinis*) generally have been inhibited in vitro by caspofungin concentrations of 0.06–1 mcg/mL.

Caspofungin is active in vitro against *Aspergillus*, including *A. fumigatus*, *A. flavus*, and *A. terreus*. The drug also is active in vitro against *A. niger*, *A. strictum*, and *A. versicolor*.

Like other echinocandins, caspofungin is not active against *Cryptococcus neoformans*, *Fusarium*, *Trichosporon*, or zygomycetes.

RESISTANCE

Strains of *Candida*, including *C. albicans*, *C. glabrata*, *C. krusei*, and *C. parapsilosis*, with reduced susceptibility or resistance to caspofungin have emerged in some patients who received the drug for treatment and, in some cases, were associated with clinical failures. Some clinical isolates of *C. auris* have reduced susceptibility or resistance to caspofungin in vitro (i.e., MICs 2 mcg/mL or greater).

Resistance to caspofungin has been associated with specific mutations in the FKS subunits of the glucan synthase enzyme. These mutations are associated with higher MICs and breakthrough infection. *Candida* with reduced susceptibility to caspofungin as a result of an increase in the chitin content of the fungal cell wall have also been identified, although the clinical importance of this phenomenon is unknown.

Some strains of *C. albicans* with reduced susceptibility to caspofungin may also have reduced susceptibility to micafungin.

ADVICE TO PATIENTS

Inform patients that anaphylactic reactions have been reported in patients receiving caspofungin acetate. Advise patients the drug can cause hypersensitivity reactions (e.g., rash, facial swelling, angioedema, pruritus, sensation of warmth, bronchospasm) and of the importance of contacting clinicians if any of these signs or symptoms occur.

Advise patients about isolated reports of serious hepatic effects (e.g., hepatitis, hepatic failure) associated with caspofungin and the importance of clinicians assessing the benefits versus risks of caspofungin therapy if abnormal liver function tests occur.

Importance of informing clinicians of existing or contemplated concomitant therapy, including prescription and OTC drugs, and any concomitant illnesses.

Importance of women informing clinicians if they are or plan to become pregnant or plan to breast-feed.

Importance of informing patients of other important precautionary information. (See Cautions.)

PREPARATIONS

Excipients in commercially available drug preparations may have clinically important effects in some individuals; consult specific product labeling for details.

Caspofungin Acetate

Parenteral

For injection, for IV infusion	50 mg*	Cancidas®, Merck **Caspofungin Acetate for Injection**
	70 mg*	Cancidas®, Merck **Caspofungin Acetate for Injection**

* available from one or more manufacturer, distributor, and/or repackager by generic (nonproprietary) name

† Use is not currently included in the labeling approved by the US Food and Drug Administration.

Selected Revisions September 4, 2017, © Copyright, June 1, 2001, American Society of Health-System Pharmacists, Inc.

Micafungin Sodium

8:14.16 • ECHINOCANDINS

■ Micafungin sodium is a semisynthetic, echinocandin antifungal agent.

USES

● Candida Infections

Candidemia and Other Invasive Candida Infections

Micafungin sodium is used for the treatment of candidemia, acute disseminated candidiasis, and certain other invasive *Candida* infections (peritonitis,
abscesses). The manufacturer states that safety and efficacy of micafungin have
not been established for the treatment of endocarditis, osteomyelitis, or meningitis caused by *Candida*.

For the treatment of candidemia in *nonneutropenic* patients or for empiric
treatment of suspected invasive candidiasis in *nonneutropenic* patients in intensive care units (ICUs), the Infectious Diseases Society of America (IDSA) recommends an IV echinocandin (anidulafungin, caspofungin, micafungin) for
initial therapy. IDSA states that fluconazole (IV or oral) is an acceptable alternative for *initial* therapy in selected patients, including those who are not critically
ill and are unlikely to have infections caused by fluconazole-resistant *Candida*.
If echinocandin- and azole-resistant *Candida* are suspected, IV amphotericin
B is recommended; IV amphotericin B also is a reasonable alternative when
echinocandins and fluconazole cannot be used because of intolerance, limited
availability, or resistance. IDSA states that transition from the echinocandin (or
amphotericin B) to fluconazole can be considered (usually within 5–7 days) in
patients who are clinically stable, have isolates susceptible to fluconazole (e.g.,
C. albicans), and have negative repeat blood cultures after initial antifungal
treatment. Although fluconazole has been considered the drug of choice for
the treatment of infections caused by *C. parapsilosis* in nonneutropenic patients
(based in part on concerns related to decreased in vitro susceptibility and resistance to echinocandins), IDSA states that there are no clinical studies to date
indicating superiority of fluconazole over echinocandins for the treatment of
C. parapsilosis infections.

For the treatment of candidemia in *neutropenic* patients, IDSA recommends an IV echinocandin (anidulafungin, caspofungin, micafungin) or, alternatively, IV amphotericin B for *initial* therapy. Fluconazole is an alternative for
initial therapy in those who are not critically ill or have had no prior exposure to
azole antifungals and also can be used for step-down therapy during neutropenia
in clinically stable patients who have fluconazole-susceptible isolates and documented bloodstream clearance. Voriconazole can be used as an alternative for *initial* therapy when broader antifungal coverage is required and also can be used
as step-down therapy during neutropenia in clinically stable patients who have
voriconazole-susceptible isolates and documented bloodstream clearance. For
infections known to be caused by *C. krusei*, an echinocandin, amphotericin B, or
voriconazole is recommended.

For the treatment of osteoarticular infections† (e.g., osteomyelitis, septic
arthritis) caused by *Candida*, IDSA recommends *initial* treatment with fluconazole or an IV echinocandin (anidulafungin, caspofungin, micafungin) and follow-up treatment with fluconazole. If septic arthritis involves a prosthetic device
that cannot be removed, long-term suppressive or maintenance therapy (secondary prophylaxis) with fluconazole is recommended if the isolate is susceptible.

For the treatment of endocarditis† (native or prosthetic valve) or implantable
cardiac device infections† caused by *Candida*, IDSA recommends *initial* treatment with IV amphotericin B (with or without oral flucytosine) or an IV echinocandin (anidulafungin, caspofungin, micafungin) and follow-up treatment
with fluconazole. If the isolate is susceptible, long-term suppressive or maintenance therapy (secondary prophylaxis) with fluconazole is recommended to prevent recurrence in those with native valve endocarditis who cannot undergo valve
replacement and in those with prosthetic valve endocarditis.

For additional information on management of candidemia and disseminated
candidiasis, the current clinical practice guidelines from IDSA available at http://
www.idsociety.org should be consulted.

Clinical Experience

Safety and efficacy of micafungin for the treatment of candidemia or other
forms of invasive candidiasis were evaluated in a phase 3, randomized, double-blind, noninferiority study in 578 adults (8.7% were neutropenic, 48% had
C. albicans infections). Patients were randomized to receive initial therapy with
either IV micafungin (100 or 150 mg once daily) or IV caspofungin acetate
(70-mg loading dose followed by 50 mg once daily). After a minimum of 10 days
of IV therapy, patients were permitted to switch to oral fluconazole if the *Candida* isolate at baseline was susceptible to fluconazole and was not *C. krusei* or *C.
glabrata* and if the patient was nonneutropenic, had improvement or resolution
of clinical signs and symptoms, and had 2 blood cultures drawn at least 24 hours
apart that were now negative for *Candida*. Patients with proven or suspected
endocarditis, osteomyelitis, or meningitis due to *Candida* were excluded from
the study. The median total duration of antifungal treatment (including switch
to oral fluconazole) was 14 days (maximum 61 days); 20.9% of those receiving
IV micafungin (100-mg regimen) and 21.2% of those receiving IV caspofungin
acetate switched to oral fluconazole. At study completion, IV micafungin (100-
and 150-mg regimens) was found to be noninferior to IV caspofungin acetate
(50 mg daily), and the 100-mg micafungin regimen was as effective as the 150-
mg micafungin regimen. Overall treatment success based on clinical response
(defined as complete resolution or improvement in signs and symptoms and
radiographic abnormalities of *Candida* infection without additional antifungal
treatment) and mycologic response (documented or presumed microbiological
eradication) at the end of the IV regimen was observed in 76.4% of those in the
micafungin 100-mg group, 71.4% of those in the micafungin 150-mg group, and
72.3% of those in the caspofungin acetate 50-mg group. At 6 weeks posttreatment, the overall relapse rate was 36.3% in those who received micafungin (100-
mg regimen) and 37% in those who received caspofungin.

In a multicenter, randomized, double-blind trial in 106 pediatric patients
under 16 years of age with candidemia or other invasive candidiasis who received
micafungin (2–4 mg/kg daily for those weighing up to 40 kg; 100–200 mg daily for
those weighing over 40 kg) for a median duration of 15 days (range: 3–42 days),
the overall treatment response rate (both clinical and mycologic response) was
73% and was similar to the 76% response rate in children who received amphotericin B liposomal (3–5 mg/kg daily); treatment success was independent of neutropenic status.

Esophageal Candidiasis

Micafungin sodium is used for the treatment of esophageal candidiasis.

Esophageal candidiasis requires treatment with a systemic antifungal (not a
topical antifungal).

IDSA recommends oral fluconazole as the preferred drug of choice for the
treatment of esophageal candidiasis; if oral therapy is not tolerated, IV fluconazole or an IV echinocandin (anidulafungin, caspofungin, micafungin)
usually is recommended and IV amphotericin B is another alternative. For fluconazole-refractory esophageal candidiasis, IDSA recommends itraconazole
oral solution or oral or IV voriconazole; alternatives for fluconazole-refractory disease are an IV echinocandin (anidulafungin, caspofungin, micafungin)
or IV amphotericin B. IDSA states that oral posaconazole (oral suspension or
delayed-release tablets) could be considered another alternative for the treatment of fluconazole-refractory esophageal candidiasis.

For the treatment of esophageal candidiasis in adults and adolescents with
human immunodeficiency virus (HIV) infection, the Centers for Disease Control and Prevention (CDC), National Institutes of Health (NIH), and IDSA recommend IV or oral fluconazole or itraconazole oral solution. Alternatives include
oral or IV voriconazole, an IV echinocandin (anidulafungin, caspofungin, micafungin), or IV amphotericin B. For refractory esophageal candidiasis in HIV-infected adults and adolescents, including fluconazole-refractory infections, these
experts recommend posaconazole oral suspension or itraconazole oral solution; alternatives include an IV echinocandin (anidulafungin, caspofungin, micafungin), oral or IV voriconazole, or IV amphotericin B. Although data are limited,
some experts state that an IV echinocandin (anidulafungin, caspofungin, micafungin) can be considered an alternative for treatment of azole-refractory esophageal candidiasis in HIV-infected children†.

Routine long-term suppressive or maintenance therapy (secondary prophylaxis) to prevent relapse or recurrence is not usually recommended in patients adequately treated for esophageal candidiasis (including HIV-infected individuals)
unless the patient has frequent or severe recurrences of esophageal candidiasis. If

secondary prophylaxis of esophageal candidiasis is indicated, oral fluconazole or posaconazole oral suspension is recommended; however, the potential for development of azole resistance should be considered.

For additional information on management of esophageal candidiasis, the current clinical practice guidelines from IDSA available at http://www.idsociety.org and the current clinical practice guidelines from CDC, NIH, and IDSA on the prevention and treatment of opportunistic infections in HIV-infected individuals available at http://www.aidsinfo.nih.gov should be consulted.

Clinical Experience

In a randomized, double-blind study of micafungin sodium for the treatment of endoscopically confirmed esophageal candidiasis, adults received either micafungin (150 mg IV once daily) or fluconazole (200 mg IV once daily) for a median duration of 14 days (range: 1–33 days). Most patients in this study had both esophageal and oropharyngeal candidiasis at baseline (C. albicans was isolated from 96% of patients) and most patients had HIV infection (CD4+ T-cell counts less than 100/mm³). An endoscopic cure (defined as normal endoscopy [mucosal grade of 0] at end of treatment) was attained in 87.7% of those who received micafungin and 88% of those who received fluconazole. Clinical cure (defined as complete resolution of clinical symptoms including dysphagia, odynophagia, and retrosternal pain) was attained in 91.9% of patients in each group. The mycologic eradication rate (determined by culture and histologic or cytologic evaluation of esophageal biopsy/brushings obtained endoscopically at the end of treatment) was 74.6% in those who received micafungin and 77.6% in those who received fluconazole. The rate of relapse (defined as recurrence of clinical symptoms or endoscopic lesions) at 2 and 4 weeks posttreatment was similar in those who received micafungin (17.9 and 32.7%, respectively) or fluconazole (13.6 and 28.2%, respectively).

Oropharyngeal Candidiasis

Although safety and efficacy of micafungin for the treatment of oropharyngeal candidiasis† have not been established, the drug has been recommended as an alternative for the treatment of oropharyngeal candidiasis.

For the treatment of mild oropharyngeal candidiasis, IDSA recommends topical treatment with clotrimazole lozenges or miconazole buccal tablets; nystatin (oral suspension or tablets) is the recommended alternative. For moderate to severe disease, IDSA recommends oral fluconazole. For fluconazole-refractory oropharyngeal candidiasis, IDSA recommends itraconazole oral solution or posaconazole oral suspension; oral voriconazole or amphotericin B oral suspension (not commercially available in the US) are recommended as alternatives. Other alternatives for refractory oropharyngeal candidiasis are an IV echinocandin (anidulafungin, caspofungin, micafungin) or IV amphotericin B.

For the treatment of oropharyngeal candidiasis in HIV-infected adults and adolescents, CDC, NIH, and IDSA recommend oral fluconazole as the preferred drug of choice for initial episodes. If topical therapy is used for the treatment of oropharyngeal candidiasis (e.g., mild to moderate episodes), these experts recommend clotrimazole lozenges or miconazole buccal tablets. Alternatives for systemic treatment of oropharyngeal candidiasis in HIV-infected adults and adolescents are itraconazole oral solution or posaconazole oral suspension; nystatin oral suspension is an alternative if topical treatment is used. For fluconazole-refractory oropharyngeal infections in HIV-infected adults and adolescents, posaconazole oral suspension is preferred; itraconazole oral solution is an alternative.

Routine long-term suppressive or maintenance therapy (secondary prophylaxis) to prevent relapse or recurrence is not usually recommended in patients adequately treated for oropharyngeal candidiasis (including HIV-infected individuals) unless the patient has frequent or severe recurrences of oropharyngeal candidiasis. If secondary prophylaxis of oropharyngeal candidiasis is indicated, oral fluconazole is recommended; however, the potential for development of azole resistance should be considered.

For additional information on management of oropharyngeal candidiasis, the current clinical practice guidelines from IDSA available at http://www.idsociety.org and the current clinical practice guidelines from CDC, NIH, and IDSA on the prevention and treatment of opportunistic infections in HIV-infected individuals available at http://www.aidsinfo.nih.gov should be consulted.

Clinical Experience

In a randomized, double-blind study in adults with endoscopically confirmed esophageal candidiasis who also had oropharyngeal candidiasis† and were treated with micafungin (150 mg IV once daily) or fluconazole (200 mg IV once daily),

the clinical response rates for the oropharyngeal infections (based on resolution of signs and symptoms) were 83.5% in those treated with micafungin and 82.1% in those treated with fluconazole. However, the rate of relapse (defined as recurrence of symptoms and/or requirement of posttreatment systemic antifungal therapy) was higher at 2 and 4 weeks posttreatment in those who received micafungin (32.3 and 52.1%, respectively) than in those who received fluconazole (18.1 and 39.4%, respectively).

Candida auris Infections

Micafungin is used for the treatment of infections caused by C. auris, an emerging pathogen that has been associated with potentially fatal candidemia or other invasive infections.

C. auris, first identified in 2009, has now been reported as the cause of serious invasive infections (including fatalities) in multiple countries worldwide (e.g., Japan, South Korea, India, Kuwait, South Africa, Pakistan, United Kingdom, Venezuela, Colombia, US). As of May 2017, a total of 77 clinical cases of C. auris had been reported to CDC from 7 different states in the US. C. auris may be difficult to identify using standard in vitro methods and has been misidentified as C. haemulonii, C. famata, or Rhodotorula glutinis. A large percentage of C. auris clinical isolates are resistant to fluconazole and multidrug-resistant isolates with reduced susceptibility or resistance to all 3 major classes of antifungal agents (azoles, polyenes, echinocandins) have been reported.

Pending further accumulation of data, CDC has issued interim recommendations regarding laboratory diagnosis, treatment, and infection control measures for suspected or known C. auris infections. Based on limited data available to date, CDC recommends that an IV echinocandin (anidulafungin, caspofungin, micafungin) be used for initial treatment of invasive C. auris infections (e.g., bloodstream or intra-abdominal infections) in adults. CDC states that a switch to IV amphotericin B (lipid formulation) could be considered if the patient is clinically unresponsive to the echinocandin or fungemia persists longer than 5 days. Consultation with an infectious disease specialist is highly recommended.

Unless there is evidence of infection, CDC does not currently recommend antifungal treatment when C. auris is isolated only from noninvasive body sites (e.g., urine, external ear, wounds, respiratory secretions). Some individuals are colonized with C. auris in the axilla, groin, nose, external ear canal, oropharynx, urine, wounds, rectum, and stool; however, data are limited and the duration of C. auris colonization is unclear. Therefore, CDC recommends that infection control measures be observed for all patients with cultures yielding C. auris, including those with positive cultures only from noninvasive body sites.

Whenever C. auris infection is suspected, clinicians should immediately contact state or local public health authorities and the CDC (candidaauris@cdc.gov) for guidance. For additional information on diagnosis and management of C. auris infections, the interim recommendations and most recent information from CDC available at https://www.cdc.gov/fungal/diseases/candidiasis/candida-auris.html should be consulted.

Prevention of Candida Infections in Hematopoietic Stem Cell Transplant Recipients

Micafungin sodium is used for prophylaxis of Candida infections in hematopoietic stem cell transplant (HSCT) recipients.

Clinical Experience

Safety and efficacy of micafungin sodium compared with fluconazole for prophylaxis of Candida infections in HSCT recipients were evaluated in a randomized, double-blind study in adults and pediatric patients† undergoing autologous or syngeneic (46%) or allogeneic (54%) stem cell transplant. The autologous and syngeneic transplant recipients had underlying diseases that included multiple myeloma, non-Hodgkin's lymphoma, and Hodgkin's disease; the allogeneic transplant recipients had underlying diseases that included chronic myelogenous leukemia, acute myelogenous leukemia, acute lymphocytic leukemia, and non-Hodgkin's lymphoma. During the study, 22.4% of patients had proven graft-versus-host disease (GVHD) and 53.9% received immunosuppressive medications for treatment or prophylaxis of GVHD.

Patients were randomized to receive micafungin (50 mg IV once daily) or fluconazole (400 mg IV once daily) until neutrophil recovery (defined as an absolute neutrophil count [ANC] of 500/mm³ or greater) up to a maximum of 42 days after transplant. The average duration of antifungal prophylaxis was 18 days (range: 1–51 days). Successful antifungal prophylaxis (defined as the absence of a proven, probable, or suspected systemic fungal infection during the period of prophylactic therapy and the absence of a proven or probable systemic fungal infection during the 4-week posttherapy period) was achieved in 80.7 or 73.7% of patients receiving micafungin or fluconazole, respectively. Systemic antifungal treatment was required after prophylaxis in 42% of those who received micafungin or fluconazole.

• Aspergillosis

Micafungin sodium, alone or in conjunction with other antifungals, has been used with some success as primary or salvage therapy for the treatment of invasive aspergillosis†.

IDSA and other clinicians consider IV voriconazole the drug of choice for primary treatment of invasive aspergillosis in adult and pediatric patients, including those with HIV infection; IV amphotericin B or isavuconazonium sulfate (prodrug of isavuconazole) is usually recommended as an alternative for primary treatment. For salvage therapy in patients refractory to or intolerant of primary antifungal therapy, IDSA recommends IV amphotericin B, an IV echinocandin (caspofungin, micafungin), oral or IV posaconazole, or itraconazole oral suspension. IDSA states that echinocandins (either alone or in conjunction with other antifungals) may be effective for salvage therapy of invasive aspergillosis; however, routine use of echinocandin monotherapy is not recommended for primary treatment of invasive aspergillosis.

For additional information on management of aspergillosis, the current clinical practice guidelines from IDSA available at http://www.idsociety.org and the current clinical practice guidelines from CDC, NIH, and IDSA on the prevention and treatment of opportunistic infections in HIV-infected individuals available at http://www.aidsinfo.nih.gov should be consulted.

Clinical Experience

Efficacy of micafungin sodium in the treatment of invasive aspergillosis† was evaluated in an open-label, noncomparative study in 70 adults with confirmed or presumed invasive fungal infections who received IV micafungin (12.5–150 mg daily; dosage escalation permitted after 4–7 days at the same dosage) alone for 7–56 days. An overall clinical response was achieved in 60% (6/10) of patients with invasive pulmonary aspergillosis, 67% (6/9) of those with chronic necrotizing pulmonary aspergillosis, 55% (12/22) of those with pulmonary aspergilloma, 100% (6/6) of those with candidemia, and 71% (5/7) of those with esophageal candidiasis. The overall clinical response was lower in those with invasive aspergillosis (57%) than in those with candidiasis (79%).

DOSAGE AND ADMINISTRATION

• Administration

Micafungin sodium is administered by slow IV infusion. The drug should *not* be given by rapid IV injection.

IV Infusion

Micafungin should not be admixed or infused concomitantly with other drugs.

Strict aseptic technique must be observed when preparing micafungin solutions because the drug contains no preservatives.

If micafungin is administered via an existing IV line, the line should be flushed with 0.9% sodium chloride injection before the drug is infused.

To minimize the risk of infusion reactions, micafungin solutions with a concentration greater than 1.5 mg/mL should be administered IV via a central catheter.

Reconstitution and Dilution

Commercially available micafungin sodium lyophilized powder for injection must be reconstituted and then further diluted prior to administration.

Based on the indicated micafungin dosage, the appropriate number of vials labeled as containing 50 or 100 mg of micafungin should be reconstituted with 5 mL of 0.9% sodium chloride injection or 5% dextrose injection to provide a solution containing approximately 10 or 20 mg/mL, respectively. After the diluent has been added to the powder, the vial should be gently swirled; to minimize excessive foaming, the vial should not be shaken vigorously.

The appropriate volume of reconstituted micafungin solution should then be withdrawn from the vials and added to 100 mL of 0.9% sodium chloride injection or 5% dextrose injection.

The final solution for IV infusion should have a concentration of 0.5–4 mg/mL.

Vials of lyophilized micafungin must be stored at 25°C, but may be exposed to temperatures ranging from 15–30°C. Following reconstitution, micafungin solutions may be stored in the original vial at 25°C for up to 24 hours. Reconstituted micafungin solutions that have been further diluted in 0.9% sodium chloride injection or 5% dextrose injection may be stored at 25°C for up to 24 hours and should be protected from light; covering the infusion drip chamber or the IV tubing is not necessary during IV infusion of the drug.

Rate of Administration

IV infusions of micafungin should be given over 1 hour. More rapid infusion may increase the risk of a histamine-mediated reaction. (See Sensitivity Reactions under Cautions: Warnings/Precautions.)

• Dosage

Dosage of micafungin sodium is expressed in terms of micafungin.

A loading dose of micafungin is not required.

Adult Dosage
Candidemia and Other Invasive Candida Infections

The recommended dosage of micafungin for the treatment of candidemia, acute disseminated candidiasis, and certain other invasive *Candida* infections (peritonitis, abscesses) in *nonneutropenic* or *neutropenic* adults is 100 mg once daily.

When micafungin is used for initial treatment of candidemia or other invasive *Candida* infections, the Infectious Diseases Society of America (IDSA) states that a transition from the echinocandin to fluconazole can be considered (usually within 5–7 days) in patients who are clinically stable, have isolates susceptible to fluconazole (e.g., *C. albicans*), and have negative repeat blood cultures after initial antifungal treatment.

IDSA recommends that antifungal treatment for candidemia (without persistent fungemia or metastatic complications) be continued for 2 weeks after documented clearance of *Candida* from the bloodstream, resolution of candidemia symptoms, and resolution of neutropenia. The mean duration of micafungin therapy in patients treated successfully in clinical trials was 15 days (range: 10–47 days).

If micafungin is used for *initial* treatment of osteoarticular infections† (e.g., osteomyelitis, septic arthritis) caused by *Candida*, IDSA recommends a dosage of 100 mg once daily in adults. After at least 2 weeks, treatment can be switched to fluconazole.

If micafungin is used for *initial* treatment of endocarditis† (native or prosthetic valve) or implantable cardiac device infections† caused by *Candida*, IDSA recommends a dosage of 150 mg once daily in adults. If the infection is caused by fluconazole-susceptible *Candida*, treatment can be switched to fluconazole after the patient is stabilized and *Candida* has been cleared from the bloodstream.

Esophageal Candidiasis

The recommended dosage of micafungin for the treatment of esophageal candidiasis in adults is 150 mg once daily.

If micafungin is used for the treatment of esophageal candidiasis in adults with human immunodeficiency virus (HIV) infection, the US Centers for Disease Control and Prevention (CDC), National Institutes of Health (NIH), and IDSA recommend a dosage of 150 mg daily.

CDC, NIH, and IDSA recommend that antifungal treatment of esophageal candidiasis be continued for 14–21 days. The mean duration of micafungin therapy in patients treated successfully in clinical trials was 15 days (range: 10–30 days).

Oropharyngeal Candidiasis

If micafungin is used for the treatment of oropharyngeal candidiasis†, IDSA recommends that adults receive 100 mg once daily for 7–14 days.

Candida auris Infections

If micafungin is used for initial treatment of invasive *C. auris* infections (e.g., bloodstream or intra-abdominal infections), CDC recommends that adults receive 100 mg once daily.

Prevention of Candida Infections in Hematopoietic Stem Cell Transplant Recipients

The recommended dosage of micafungin for the prevention of *Candida* infections in adult hematopoietic stem cell transplant (HSCT) recipients is 50 mg once daily.

Micafungin dosage adjustments are not required. Monitor for nifedipine toxicity and reduce nifedipine dosage if necessary.

● *Prednisolone*

No evidence of pharmacokinetic interactions when micafungin was used with prednisolone; micafungin dosage adjustments are not required.

● *Rifampin*

Pharmacokinetics of micafungin were not affected by concomitant rifampin; micafungin dosage adjustments are not required.

● *Ritonavir*

Pharmacokinetics of micafungin were not affected by concomitant ritonavir; micafungin dosage adjustments are not required.

DESCRIPTION

Micafungin sodium, a semisynthetic lipopeptide synthesized from a fermentation product of *Coleophoma empetri* F-11899, is an echinocandin antifungal agent. Echinocandins (e.g., anidulafungin, caspofungin, micafungin) are glucan synthesis inhibitors and differ structurally and pharmacologically from other currently available antifungal agents.

Like other echinocandins, micafungin inhibits the synthesis of $\beta(1,3)$-D-glucan, an essential component of the fungal cell wall that is not present in mammalian cells. The drug may be fungistatic or fungicidal in action. Depending on concentration, micafungin may be fungicidal against some *Candida*, but usually is fungistatic against *Aspergillus*.

Micafungin appears to be metabolized slowly in the liver, principally via arylsulfatase with further metabolism by catechol-*O*-methyltransferase. Hydroxylation of micafungin by the cytochrome P-450 (CYP) 3A isoenzyme appears to be only a minor metabolic pathway. The drug is about 99% protein bound (primarily albumin and to a lesser extent α_1-acid glycoprotein). The elimination half-life of micafungin at steady state is approximately 13.4–17.2 hours in adults. Typically, 85% of the steady-state concentration is achieved after 3 days of once-daily IV micafungin. Micafungin is eliminated principally in feces. In healthy individuals, about 71% of a single IV dose of radiolabeled micafungin sodium was recovered in feces over 28 days.

● *Spectrum*

Micafungin is active in vitro against *Candida*, including *C. albicans, C. dubliniensis, C. glabrata, C. guilliermondii, C. krusei, C. lusitaniae, C. metapsilosis, C. orthopsilosis, C. parapsilosis,* and *C. tropicalis.*

Clinical isolates of *C. auris* (often misidentified as *C. haemulonii, C. famata,* or *Rhodotorula glutinis*) generally have been inhibited in vitro by micafungin concentrations of 0.03–2 mcg/mL.

Micafungin is active in vitro against *Aspergillus,* including *A. fumigatus, A. flavus, A. niger,* and *A. terreus.*

Like other echinocandins, micafungin is not active against *Cryptococcus neoformans, Trichosporon,* or zygomycetes.

● *Resistance*

Resistance to micafungin has been reported. *C. albicans* with reduced susceptibility or resistance to micafungin have been reported after long-term treatment with the drug. Resistance also has developed in *C. parapsilosis.* Some clinical isolates of *C. auris* have reduced susceptibility or resistance to micafungin in vitro (i.e., MICs 4 mcg/mL or greater).

Resistance to micafungin may be related to specific mutations in the FKS protein component of the glucan synthase enzyme.

Some *C. albicans* with reduced susceptibility to micafungin also have reduced susceptibility to caspofungin.

ADVICE TO PATIENTS

Inform patients about the possible benefits and risks associated with micafungin.

Inform patients about potential adverse effects associated with micafungin, including hypersensitivity reactions (anaphylaxis and anaphylactoid reactions including shock), hematologic effects (acute intravascular hemolysis, hemolytic anemia, hemoglobinuria), hepatic effects (abnormal liver function tests, hepatic impairment, hepatitis or worsening hepatic failure), and renal effects (elevated BUN and creatinine concentrations, renal impairment or acute renal failure). (See Cautions: Warnings/Precautions.)

Importance of informing clinicians if any unusual symptoms develop or if any known symptoms persist or worsen.

Importance of informing clinicians of existing or contemplated concomitant therapy, including prescription and OTC drugs, and any concomitant illnesses.

Importance of women informing clinicians if they are or plan to become pregnant or plan to breast-feed.

Importance of informing patients of other important precautionary information. (See Cautions.)

PREPARATIONS

Excipients in commercially available drug preparations may have clinically important effects in some individuals; consult specific product labeling for details.

Micafungin Sodium

Parenteral		
For injection, for IV infusion	50 mg (of micafungin)	**Mycamine®**, Astellas
	100 mg (of micafungin)	**Mycamine®**, Astellas

† Use is not currently included in the labeling approved by the US Food and Drug Administration.

Geri.

Dosage adju

Amphotericin B

8:14.28 • POLYENES

■ Amphotericin B, a macrocyclic polyene, is an antifungal agent.

USES

Conventional IV amphotericin B (formulated with sodium desoxycholate) is used for the treatment of potentially life-threatening fungal infections including aspergillosis, blastomycosis, systemic candidiasis, coccidioidomycosis, cryptococcosis, histoplasmosis, paracoccidioidomycosis†, sporotrichosis, and zygomycosis. The drug also has been used IV for empiric antifungal therapy in febrile neutropenic patients† or for prevention of fungal infections in other immunocompromised individuals† (e.g., cancer patients, bone marrow or solid organ transplant recipients). In addition, conventional IV amphotericin B is used for the treatment of certain protozoal infections, including leishmaniasis and primary amebic meningoencephalitis caused by *Naegleria fowleri*†.

Conventional IV amphotericin B should be used principally in patients with progressive, potentially life-threatening fungal infections and should not be used to treat noninvasive fungal infections (e.g., oral thrush, vaginal candidiasis, esophageal candidiasis) in immunocompetent patients with normal neutrophil counts. When necessary, conventional amphotericin B has been administered intrathecally† or intraventricularly† (either alone or in conjunction with systemic antifungal therapy) for the treatment of CNS infections caused by susceptible fungi. Conventional amphotericin B also has been administered by bladder irrigation† for the treatment of *Candida* cystitis, administered intraperitoneally† for the treatment of fungal peritonitis, and given intrabronchially† or by nebulization† for the treatment or prophylaxis of pulmonary fungal infections.

Amphotericin B lipid complex (Abelcet®) is labeled for the treatment of invasive fungal infections in patients who are refractory to or intolerant of conventional IV amphotericin B.

Amphotericin B liposomal (AmBisome®) is labeled for the treatment of infections caused by *Aspergillus*, *Candida*, or *Cryptococcus* that are refractory to conventional IV amphotericin B and for the treatment of these infections in patients who cannot receive conventional amphotericin B because of renal impairment or unacceptable toxicity. Amphotericin B liposomal also is labeled for the treatment of cryptococcal meningitis in patients with human immunodeficiency virus (HIV) infection, for empiric therapy of presumed fungal infections in febrile, neutropenic patients, and for the treatment of visceral leishmaniasis.

IV amphotericin B is considered a drug of choice for the treatment of many systemic infections caused by susceptible fungi, especially for initial treatment in patients with severe infections. Although clinical experience with lipid formulations of amphotericin B (amphotericin B lipid complex, amphotericin B liposomal) has been obtained principally from small, open-label studies and case reports, the lipid formulations of amphotericin B generally appear to be better tolerated (e.g., lower incidence of acute infusion reactions and adverse hematologic and renal effects) and may be preferred for some infections. Additional study is needed to determine the relative efficacy of these lipid formulations of amphotericin B compared with conventional IV amphotericin B for the treatment of severe, potentially life-threatening fungal infections.

● Aspergillosis

Conventional IV amphotericin B, amphotericin B lipid complex, and amphotericin B liposomal are used for the treatment of invasive aspergillosis caused by *Aspergillosis*.

The Infectious Diseases Society of America (IDSA) and other clinicians consider voriconazole the drug of choice for primary treatment of invasive aspergillosis in most patients, including HIV-infected patients. These experts state that IV amphotericin B liposomal or isavuconazonium sulfate (prodrug of isavuconazole) are the preferred alternatives for primary treatment of aspergillosis; IV amphotericin B lipid complex is another alternative. For salvage therapy in patients refractory to or intolerant of primary antifungal therapy, IV amphotericin B (a lipid formulation), an IV echinocandin (caspofungin, micafungin), oral or IV posaconazole, or itraconazole oral suspension are recommended. IDSA states that conventional IV amphotericin B and lipid formulations of amphotericin B are appropriate options

for initial and salvage treatment of invasive aspergillosis when voriconazole cannot be used; however, conventional IV amphotericin B should be reserved for use in resource-limited settings when no alternative agents are available.

For the treatment of invasive aspergillosis in HIV-infected adults and adolescents, the US Centers for Disease Control and Prevention (CDC), National Institutes of Health (NIH), and IDSA recommend voriconazole as the drug of choice; IV amphotericin B (conventional or lipid formulation), IV echinocandins (anidulafungin, caspofungin, micafungin), and oral posaconazole are recommended as alternatives.

Clinical Experience

Invasive aspergillosis (especially in immunocompromised patients) is difficult to diagnose and treat, and the overall response rate of invasive aspergillosis to conventional IV amphotericin B has been highly variable ranging from 14–83%. In a controlled study in immunocompromised adults and adolescents 12 years of age or older with invasive aspergillosis, patients were randomized to receive voriconazole (6 mg/kg IV twice daily on day 1, then 4 mg/kg IV twice daily for at least 7 days, followed by oral voriconazole 200 mg twice daily) or conventional amphotericin B (1–1.5 mg/kg IV once daily). A successful outcome (complete and partial responses) at week 12 in the modified intention-to-treat population (ITT) was achieved in 53% of those treated with voriconazole compared with 32% of those treated with amphotericin B. In addition, the survival rate at 12 weeks was 71% in the voriconazole group compared with 58% in the amphotericin B group.

In several studies involving patients with invasive aspergillosis, the response rates to amphotericin B lipid complex or amphotericin B liposomal have ranged from 32–69%.

Although conventional IV amphotericin B has been used in conjunction with other antifungals (e.g., flucytosine) for salvage therapy in some patients with invasive aspergillosis (e.g., CNS, endocarditis) that did not respond to conventional IV amphotericin B alone, it is unclear whether these combination regimens offer any benefit over use of IV amphotericin B alone and there are concerns related to possible drug interactions between amphotericin B and flucytosine. (See Flucytosine under Drug Interactions: Anti-infective Agents.)

For additional information on management of aspergillosis, the current clinical practice guidelines from IDSA available at http://www.idsociety.org and the current clinical practice guidelines from CDC, NIH, and IDSA on the prevention and treatment of opportunistic infections in HIV-infected individuals available at http://www.aidsinfo.nih.gov should be consulted.

● Blastomycosis

IV amphotericin B is used for the treatment of pulmonary and extrapulmonary blastomycosis caused by *Blastomyces dermatitidis*.

While both oral itraconazole and IV amphotericin B are considered drugs of choice for the treatment of blastomycosis, IV amphotericin B is preferred for initial treatment of severe blastomycosis, especially infections involving the CNS, and for initial treatment of presumptive blastomycosis in immunocompromised patients, including HIV-infected individuals. Oral itraconazole is the drug of choice for the treatment of nonmeningeal, non-life-threatening blastomycosis, including mild to moderate pulmonary blastomycosis or mild to moderate disseminated blastomycosis (without CNS involvement) and also is recommended for follow-up therapy in patients with more severe infections after an initial response has been obtained with IV amphotericin B.

When amphotericin B is used for the treatment of blastomycosis, conventional IV amphotericin B or a lipid formulation of amphotericin B can be used. However, IDSA and others state that a lipid formulation of amphotericin B (e.g., amphotericin B liposomal) may be preferred for the treatment of CNS blastomycosis since higher CSF concentrations may be obtained.

For additional information on management of blastomycosis, the current clinical practice guidelines from IDSA available at http://www.idsociety.org should be consulted.

● Candida Infections

IV amphotericin B is used for the treatment of disseminated or invasive infections caused by *Candida*, including candidemia, cardiovascular infections (endocarditis, pericarditis, myocarditis), and meningitis, and for the treatment of other serious infections caused by *Candida*, including osteoarticular infections (osteomyelitis, septic arthritis), peritonitis, intra-abdominal abscesses, urinary tract infections (symptomatic cystitis, pyelonephritis, urinary fungus balls), and endophthalmitis. The drug also is used for the treatment of certain severe or refractory mucocutaneous *Candida* infections (e.g., esophageal candidiasis†, oropharyngeal candidiasis†).

Amphotericin B generally is effective against infections caused by *C. albicans*, *C. glabrata*, *C. krusei*, *C. parapsilosis*, or *C. tropicalis*, and is a drug of choice for many infections caused by fluconazole-resistant *Candida*. Fluconazole-resistant *C. albicans* are being isolated with increasing frequency from patients who have received prior fluconazole therapy (especially in HIV-infected patients) and some *Candida* infections (e.g., candidemia) are increasingly caused by strains that are intrinsically resistant to fluconazole (e.g., *C. krusei*) or likely to have resistance or reduced susceptibility to fluconazole (e.g., *C. glabrata*).

For the treatment of candidemia in *nonneutropenic* patients or for empiric treatment of suspected invasive candidiasis† in *nonneutropenic* patients in intensive care units (ICUs), IDSA recommends an IV echinocandin (anidulafungin, caspofungin, micafungin) for *initial* therapy. IDSA states that fluconazole (IV or oral) is an acceptable alternative for *initial* therapy in selected patients, including those who are not critically ill and are unlikely to have infections caused by fluconazole-resistant *Candida*. If echinocandin- and azole-resistant *Candida* are suspected, IV amphotericin B (a lipid formulation) is recommended; IV amphotericin B (a lipid formulation) also is a reasonable alternative when echinocandins and fluconazole cannot be used because of intolerance, limited availability, or resistance. IDSA states that transition from the echinocandin (or amphotericin B) to fluconazole can be considered (usually within 5–7 days) in patients who are clinically stable, have isolates susceptible to fluconazole (e.g., *C. albicans*), and have negative repeat blood cultures after initial antifungal treatment.

For the treatment of candidemia in *neutropenic* patients, IDSA recommends an IV echinocandin (anidulafungin, caspofungin, micafungin) or, alternatively, IV amphotericin B (a lipid formulation) for *initial* therapy. Fluconazole is an alternative for *initial* therapy in those who are not critically ill or have had no prior exposure to azole antifungals and also can be used for step-down therapy during neutropenia in clinically stable patients who have fluconazole-susceptible isolates and documented bloodstream clearance. Voriconazole can be used as an alternative for *initial* therapy when broader antifungal coverage is required and also can be used as step-down therapy during neutropenia in clinically stable patients who have voriconazole-susceptible isolates and documented bloodstream clearance. For infections known to be caused by *C. krusei*, an echinocandin, amphotericin B (a lipid formulation), or voriconazole is recommended.

For the treatment of chronic disseminated (hepatosplenic) candidiasis, IDSA recommends initial treatment with IV amphotericin B (a lipid formulation) or an IV echinocandin (anidulafungin, caspofungin, micafungin) followed by oral fluconazole therapy.

For the treatment of CNS candidiasis, IDSA recommends initial treatment with IV amphotericin B liposomal (with or without oral flucytosine) and step-down treatment with fluconazole. Infected CNS devices (e.g., ventriculostomy drains, shunts, stimulators, prosthetic reconstructive devices, biopolymer wafers that deliver chemotherapy) should be removed if possible. If a ventricular device cannot be removed, IDSA states that conventional amphotericin B can be administered through the device. Conventional amphotericin B has been administered intrathecally† as an adjunct to systemic antifungal treatment in patients with *Candida* meningitis.

For the treatment of neonatal candidiasis, including CNS infections, conventional IV amphotericin B usually is the drug of choice for *initial* treatment. Although not routinely recommended in neonates, concomitant use of flucytosine can be considered as salvage therapy if CNS infections do not respond to initial therapy with IV amphotericin B alone. The IDSA and American Academy of Pediatrics (AAP) state that fluconazole can be considered for step-down treatment after an initial response has been obtained with IV amphotericin B. Fluconazole also is a reasonable alternative for initial treatment of neonatal candidiasis (without CNS involvement), provided the patient had not been receiving fluconazole prophylaxis and the causative agent is susceptible. Although lipid formulations of IV amphotericin B can be considered as alternatives for the treatment of neonatal candidiasis, these formulations should be used with caution in this age group, particularly in the presence of urinary tract involvement.

For the treatment of endocarditis (native or prosthetic valve) or implantable cardiac device infections caused by *Candida*, IDSA recommends *initial* treatment with a lipid formulation of IV amphotericin B (with or without oral flucytosine) or an IV echinocandin (anidulafungin, caspofungin, micafungin) and step-down treatment with fluconazole. If the isolate is susceptible, long-term suppressive or maintenance therapy (secondary prophylaxis) with fluconazole is recommended

to prevent recurrence in those with native valve endocarditis who cannot undergo valve replacement and in those with prosthetic valve endocarditis.

Mucocutaneous or noninvasive *Candida* infections, such as esophageal, oropharyngeal, or vaginal candidiasis, usually can be adequately treated with an appropriate oral or topical antifungal; however, severe or refractory mucocutaneous infections (e.g., esophageal candidiasis†, oropharyngeal candidiasis†) caused by azole-resistant *Candida* or infections that fail to respond to such therapy may require IV amphotericin B therapy. In addition, IV amphotericin B has been recommended as an alternative for the treatment of esophageal candidiasis† in patients who cannot tolerate oral therapy.

Amphotericin B has been used for the treatment of urinary tract infections caused by *Candida*. IDSA states that antifungal treatment is not usually indicated in patients with asymptomatic cystitis, unless there is a high risk of disseminated candidiasis (e.g., neutropenic patients, low birthweight infants [less than 1.5 kg], patients undergoing urologic manipulations). For the treatment of symptomatic cystitis, pyelonephritis, or fungus balls likely to be caused by fluconazole-susceptible *Candida*, fluconazole is the drug of choice. If symptomatic cystitis is caused by fluconazole-resistant *Candida*, IDSA recommends conventional IV amphotericin B or oral flucytosine for infections caused by *C. glabrata* and conventional IV amphotericin B for infections caused by *C. krusei*. If pyelonephritis is caused by fluconazole-resistant *Candida*, conventional IV amphotericin B (with or without oral flucytosine) is recommended for *C. glabrata* and conventional IV amphotericin B is recommended for *C. krusei*. Although conventional amphotericin B has been administered by bladder irrigation† for the treatment of candiduria (funguria), such therapy has been controversial since candiduria may be self-limited in some patients (e.g., after changing or removing indwelling catheters) and the risks and benefits of bladder irrigation versus systemic antifungal treatment have not been clearly identified. IDSA states that bladder irrigation† with conventional amphotericin B is not generally recommended, but may be useful for patients with refractory, symptomatic cystitis caused by fluconazole-resistant *Candida* (e.g., *C. glabrata*, *C. krusei*) or as an adjunct to systemic antifungal therapy for the treatment of urinary fungus balls.

IDSA states that IV amphotericin B liposomal (with or without oral flucytosine) is the regimen of choice for the treatment of endophthalmitis caused by fluconazole- and voriconazole-resistant *Candida*. In patients with macular involvement, intravitreal† administration of conventional amphotericin B also is recommended to ensure prompt high levels of antifungal activity. Decisions regarding antifungal treatment and surgical intervention should be made jointly by an ophthalmologist and an infectious disease clinician.

Amphotericin B lipid complex has been effective when used in pediatric cancer patients with chronic disseminated candidiasis or other *Candida* infections. Liposomal amphotericin B has been used effectively for the treatment of disseminated *Candida* infections, and the overall response rate in patients with candidiasis who received the lipid formulation has been reported to be 56–70%.

Candida auris Infections

IV amphotericin B has been used for the treatment of infections caused by *C. auris*, an emerging pathogen that has been associated with potentially fatal candidemia or other invasive infections.

C. auris, first identified in 2009, has now been reported as the cause of serious invasive infections (including fatalities) in multiple countries worldwide (e.g., Japan, South Korea, India, Kuwait, South Africa, Pakistan, United Kingdom, Venezuela, Columbia, US). As of May 2017, a total of 77 clinical cases of *C. auris* had been reported to CDC from 7 different states in the US. *C. auris* may be difficult to identify using standard in vitro methods and has been misidentified as *C. haemulonii*, *C. famata*, or *Rhodotorula glutinis*. A large percentage of *C. auris* clinical isolates are resistant to fluconazole and multidrug-resistant isolates with reduced susceptibility or resistance to all 3 major classes of antifungal agents (azoles, polyenes, echinocandins) have been reported.

Pending further accumulation of data, CDC has issued interim recommendations regarding laboratory diagnosis, treatment, and infection control measures for suspected or known *C. auris* infections. Based on limited data available to date, CDC recommends that an IV echinocandin (anidulafungin, caspofungin, micafungin) be used for initial treatment of invasive *C. auris* infections (e.g., bloodstream or intra-abdominal infections) in adults. CDC states that a switch to IV amphotericin B (a lipid formulation) could be considered if the patient is clinically unresponsive to the echinocandin or fungemia persists longer than 5 days. Consultation with an infectious disease specialist is highly recommended.

Unless there is evidence of infection, CDC does not currently recommend antifungal treatment when *C. auris* is isolated only from noninvasive body sites (e.g., urine, external ear, wounds, respiratory secretions). Some individuals are colonized with *C. auris* in the axilla, groin, nose, external ear canal, oropharynx, urine, wounds, rectum, and stool; however, data are limited and the duration of *C. auris* colonization is unclear. Therefore, CDC recommends that infection control measures be observed for all patients with cultures yielding *C. auris*, including those with positive cultures only from noninvasive body sites.

Whenever *C. auris* infection is suspected, clinicians should immediately contact state or local public health authorities and the CDC (candidaauris@cdc.gov) for guidance. For additional information on diagnosis and management of *C. auris* infections, the interim recommendations and most recent information from CDC available at https://www.cdc.gov/fungal/diseases/candidiasis/candida-auris.html should be consulted.

● *Coccidioidomycosis*

IV amphotericin B is used for the treatment of coccidioidomycosis caused by *Coccidioides immitis* or *C. posadasii*.

IDSA states that antifungal treatment is not considered necessary in patients with newly diagnosed, uncomplicated coccidioidal pneumonia who have mild or nondebilitating symptoms, including those with an asymptomatic pulmonary nodule or cavity due to coccidioidomycosis and no overt immunocompromising conditions. However, antifungal treatment is recommended for patients with symptomatic chronic cavitary coccidioidal pneumonia, ruptured coccidioidal cavities, extrapulmonary soft tissue coccidioidomycosis, bone and joint coccidioidomycosis, or coccidioidal meningitis. Antifungal treatment of coccidioidomycosis also is usually recommended for patients who are immunocompromised or debilitated (e.g., HIV-infected individuals, organ transplant recipients, those receiving immunosuppressive therapy, those with diabetes or cardiopulmonary disease).

IDSA and others state that an oral azole (fluconazole or itraconazole) usually is recommended for initial treatment of symptomatic pulmonary coccidioidomycosis and chronic fibrocavitary or disseminated (extrapulmonary) coccidioidomycosis. However, IV amphotericin B is recommended as an alternative and is preferred for initial treatment of severely ill patients who have rapidly progressing or extrathoracic disseminated disease, for immunocompromised individuals, or when azole antifungals cannot be used (e.g., pregnant women).

For the treatment of clinically mild coccidioidomycosis (e.g., focal pneumonia) in HIV-infected adults, adolescents, or children, CDC, NIH, and IDSA recommend initial therapy with oral fluconazole or oral itraconazole. Although clinical data are limited, oral voriconazole or oral posaconazole may be used as alternatives in HIV-infected adults or adolescents for the treatment of clinically mild coccidioidomycosis† that has not responded to fluconazole or itraconazole.

For the treatment of severe (nonmeningeal) coccidioidomycosis (e.g., diffuse pulmonary or extrathoracic disseminated infections) in HIV-infected adults, adolescents, or children, CDC, NIH, and IDSA recommend initial therapy with IV amphotericin B (conventional or lipid formulation) followed by oral azole therapy. Alternatively, some experts recommend initial therapy with IV amphotericin B used in conjunction with an oral azole (fluconazole or itraconazole) followed by the oral azole alone.

For the treatment of coccidioidal meningitis, the regimen of choice in HIV-infected adults, adolescents, or children or other individuals is IV or oral fluconazole (with or without intrathecal† conventional amphotericin B). Other oral azoles (itraconazole, posaconazole, voriconazole) are considered alternatives for the treatment of coccidioidal meningitis in adults and adolescents. Patients who do not respond to fluconazole or itraconazole alone may be candidates for intrathecal† conventional amphotericin B (with or without continued azole therapy) or IV amphotericin B used in conjunction with intrathecal† conventional amphotericin B. Consultation with an expert who has experience in treating coccidioidal meningitis is recommended.

HIV-infected adults, adolescents, or children who have been adequately treated for coccidioidomycosis should receive long-term (usually life-long) secondary prophylaxis to prevent recurrence or relapse. Although oral fluconazole or oral itraconazole are the drugs of choice recommended by CDC, NIH, and IDSA for secondary prophylaxis to prevent recurrence or relapse of coccidioidomycosis in HIV-infected adults, adolescents, or children, these experts state that oral posaconazole or oral voriconazole can be used as an alternative for secondary prophylaxis of coccidioidomycosis in HIV-infected adults or adolescents who did not initially respond to fluconazole or itraconazole.

While data regarding use of lipid formulations of amphotericin B in the treatment of coccidioidomycosis are limited to date, amphotericin B lipid complex has been used with some success in a limited number of patients for the treatment of this infection. Some experts state that there is no evidence that lipid formulations of IV amphotericin B are more effective than conventional IV amphotericin B for the treatment of coccidioidomycosis.

For additional information on management of coccidioidomycosis, the current clinical practice guidelines from IDSA available at http://www.idsociety.org and the current clinical practice guidelines from CDC, NIH, and IDSA on the prevention and treatment of opportunistic infections in HIV-infected individuals available at http://www.aidsinfo.nih.gov should be consulted.

● *Cryptococcosis*

Treatment of Cryptococcosis

IV amphotericin B is used for the treatment of infections caused by *Cryptococcus neoformans*, and generally is considered a drug of choice, especially for the treatment of cryptococcal meningitis. Because of reported in vitro and in vivo synergism, IDSA and other clinicians recommend concomitant use of amphotericin B and flucytosine for initial treatment of cryptococcal infections, especially in HIV-infected patients. Addition of flucytosine to the regimen appears to reduce the time required for sterilization of the CSF in those with CNS involvement and may decrease the risk of subsequent relapse and improve survival.

Conventional IV amphotericin had been the preferred amphotericin B formulation for the treatment of cryptococcosis, but IV amphotericin B liposomal may now be preferred, especially in patients who have or are predisposed to renal dysfunction. Conventional IV amphotericin B can be used if cost is an issue and the risk of renal dysfunction is low. Although data are limited, IV amphotericin B lipid complex is considered an alternative to IV amphotericin B liposomal or conventional IV amphotericin B for the treatment of cryptococcosis.

For the treatment of cryptococcal meningitis in HIV-infected adults, adolescents, and children, CDC, NIH, IDSA, and other clinicians state that the preferred regimen is initial (induction) therapy with IV amphotericin B (liposomal or conventional formulation) given in conjunction with flucytosine for at least 2 weeks until there is evidence of clinical improvement and negative CSF culture after repeat lumbar puncture, then follow-up (consolidation) therapy with oral fluconazole given for at least 8 weeks, followed by long-term suppressive or maintenance therapy (secondary prophylaxis) with oral fluconazole to complete at least 1 year of azole therapy.

For the initial (induction) phase of treatment of cryptococcal meningitis in HIV-infected adults and adolescents, IV amphotericin B (liposomal or conventional formulation) in conjunction with oral flucytosine is the preferred regimen. Alternative regimens for initial (induction) treatment of cryptococcal meningitis in HIV-infected adults and adolescents who cannot receive the preferred regimen are IV amphotericin B lipid complex given in conjunction with oral flucytosine; IV amphotericin B (liposomal or conventional formulation) given in conjunction with oral or IV fluconazole; IV amphotericin B (liposomal or conventional formulation) alone; oral or IV fluconazole given in conjunction with oral flucytosine; or oral or IV fluconazole alone. Alternative regimens may be less effective and are recommended only in patients who cannot tolerate or have not responded to the preferred regimen. IDSA states that use of intrathecal† or intraventricular† conventional amphotericin B in the treatment of cryptococcal meningitis generally is discouraged and is rarely necessary.

For the treatment of cryptococcal CNS infections in organ transplant recipients, IDSA recommends initial (induction) therapy with IV amphotericin B liposomal or IV amphotericin B lipid complex given in conjunction with oral flucytosine for at least 2 weeks, then follow-up (consolidation) therapy with oral fluconazole given for 8 weeks. If the induction regimen does not include flucytosine, it should be continued for at least 4–6 weeks. Conventional IV amphotericin B is not usually recommended for first-line treatment of cryptococcosis in transplant recipients because of the risk of nephrotoxicity. For organ transplant recipients with mild to moderate pulmonary cryptococcosis (without diffuse pulmonary infiltrates) or other mild to moderate cryptococcal infections not involving the CNS, IDSA recommends fluconazole given for 6–12 months.

In adults and children who do not have HIV infection and are not transplant recipients, IDSA states that the preferred regimen for the treatment of cryptococcal meningitis is initial (induction) therapy with conventional IV amphotericin B given in conjunction with oral flucytosine for at least 4 weeks (a 2-week period of induction therapy can be considered in those who are immunocompetent, are without uncontrolled underlying disease, and are at low risk for therapeutic failure), then follow-up (consolidation) therapy with oral fluconazole administered for an additional 8 weeks or longer.

For the treatment of mild to moderate pulmonary cryptococcosis (nonmeningeal) in immunocompetent or immunosuppressed adults or children, IDSA states that the regimen of choice is oral fluconazole given for 6–12 months. However, severe pulmonary cryptococcosis, cryptococcemia, and disseminated cryptococcal infections in immunocompetent or immunosuppressed adults, adolescents, or children should be treated using regimens recommended for cryptococcal meningitis.

Clinical Experience

In a randomized, multicenter study comparing conventional IV amphotericin B (mean dose of 0.4–0.5 mg/kg daily for 10 weeks with or without concomitant flucytosine) with oral fluconazole (400 mg on day 1 followed by 200–400 mg daily for 10 weeks) in HIV-infected patients with cryptococcal meningitis, therapy was effective in 40% of patients receiving amphotericin B and in 34% of those receiving fluconazole. Although overall mortality between patients receiving conventional amphotericin B and patients receiving fluconazole was similar (14% in patients receiving amphotericin B versus 18% in patients receiving fluconazole), mortality was higher during the first 2 weeks of therapy in patients receiving fluconazole (15% versus 8% in those receiving amphotericin B). CSF cultures were positive for an average of about 42 or 64 days in patients receiving conventional amphotericin B or fluconazole, respectively. In a double-blind multicenter trial in patients with AIDS-associated cryptococcal meningitis, the relative efficacy of initial therapy with conventional IV amphotericin B (0.7 mg/kg daily) given with flucytosine (100 mg/kg daily) or placebo for 2 weeks followed by oral fluconazole (800 mg daily for 2 days, then 400 mg daily for 8 weeks) or oral itraconazole (600 mg daily for 3 days, then 400 mg daily for 8 weeks) was evaluated. At 2 weeks, CSF cultures were negative in 60% of those who received amphotericin B with concomitant flucytosine compared with 51% of those who received amphotericin B alone. The clinical response to oral fluconazole or oral itraconazole for follow-up therapy was similar, but the rate of CSF sterilization at 10 weeks was higher in those who received fluconazole (72%) compared with those who received itraconazole (60%).

In a study evaluating safety and efficacy of IV amphotericin B lipid complex for the treatment of cryptococcal meningitis in HIV- infected patients, the lipid formulation was at least as effective as conventional IV amphotericin B for initial therapy in these patients and was associated with less hematologic and renal toxicity than the conventional formulation. An initial clinical response was obtained in 86% of patients who received amphotericin B lipid complex (5 mg/kg once daily during weeks 1 and 2, and 3 times weekly during weeks 3–6) and in 65% of those who received conventional IV amphotericin (0.7 mg/kg during weeks 1 and 2, and 1.2 mg/kg 3 times weekly during weeks 3–6); all patients received follow-up therapy with oral fluconazole for an additional 12 weeks). The overall response rate (resolution of all signs and symptoms and conversion of CNS, blood, and urine cultures to negative) was 38% in those who received amphotericin B lipid complex and 41% in those who received conventional IV amphotericin B.

Amphotericin B liposomal was compared with conventional amphotericin B for empiric treatment of cryptococcal meningitis in HIV-infected patients in a randomized, double-blind study in 267 patients (study 94-0-013). Patients were randomized to receive 11–21 days of IV amphotericin B liposomal (3 or 6 mg/kg daily) or conventional IV amphotericin B (0.7 mg/kg daily); this induction regimen was followed by oral fluconazole (400 mg daily for adults and 200 mg daily in a pediatric patient younger than 13 years of age) given to complete 10 weeks of protocol-directed therapy. At 2 weeks, the success rate (defined as CSF culture conversion) for mycologically evaluable patients (defined as all randomized patients who received at least 1 dose of study drug, had positive baseline CSF culture, and at least 1 follow-up culture) was 47.5% in those who received conventional amphotericin B and 58.3 or 48% in those who received amphotericin B liposomal in a dosage of 3 or 6 mg/kg daily, respectively. At 10 weeks, the success rate (defined as clinical success at week 10 plus CSF culture conversion at or prior to week 10) in those with documented cryptococcal meningitis at baseline was 53% in those who received conventional amphotericin B and 49% in those who received amphotericin B liposomal in a dosage of 6 mg/kg daily; the success rate was only 37% in those who received the lower dosage of amphotericin B liposomal. The survival rate at 10 weeks was similar in those receiving conventional amphotericin B (89%) or the higher dosage of amphotericin B liposomal (90%); the incidence of adverse effects (infusion reactions or adverse cardiovascular or renal effects) was lower in those receiving amphotericin B liposomal than in those receiving conventional amphotericin B. In another randomized study in HIV-infected patients with cryptococcal meningitis who received a 3-week course of liposomal amphotericin B (4 mg/kg daily) or a 3-week course of conventional IV amphotericin B (0.7 mg/kg daily) followed by a 7-week course of oral fluconazole (400 mg daily), the median time to negative CSF cultures was 7–14 days in those receiving amphotericin B liposomal compared with more than 21 days in those receiving conventional IV amphotericin B.

Prevention of Recurrence (Secondary Prophylaxis) of Cryptococcosis

HIV-infected adults, adolescents, or children who have been adequately treated for cryptococcosis should receive long-term suppressive or maintenance therapy (secondary prophylaxis) to prevent recurrence. Oral fluconazole is the drug of choice for secondary prophylaxis of cryptococcosis in HIV-infected patients and other individuals who have had documented, adequately treated cryptococcal meningitis; some experts suggest that oral itraconazole is an alternative in those who cannot tolerate fluconazole, but the drug may be less effective than fluconazole in preventing relapse of cryptococcosis.

Although conventional IV amphotericin B has been used or recommended as an alternative for secondary prophylaxis to prevent relapse of cryptococcal meningitis† (e.g., in patients who could not receive azole antifungals), it is less effective and is associated with IV catheter-related infections. Results of a multicenter study comparing safety and efficacy of conventional IV amphotericin B (1 mg/kg once weekly) or oral fluconazole (200 mg once daily) for prevention of relapse of the disease in HIV-infected patients with negative cryptococcal cultures after initial adequate amphotericin B therapy indicate that the fluconazole regimen is more effective (in terms of preventing relapse of culture-positive meningitis) and better tolerated than the amphotericin B regimen for maintenance therapy in these patients.

Cryptococcus gattii Infections

Although data are limited, CDC, NIH, and IDSA state that recommendations for the treatment of CNS, pulmonary, or disseminated infections caused by *Cryptococcus gattii* and recommendations for long-term suppressive or maintenance therapy (secondary prophylaxis) of *C. gattii* infections are the same as the recommendations for *C. neoformans* infections. IDSA states that single, small cryptococcoma may be treated with oral fluconazole; however, induction therapy with a regimen of conventional IV amphotericin B and flucytosine given for 4–6 weeks, followed by consolidation therapy with fluconazole given for 6–18 months should be considered for very large or multiple cryptococcomas caused by *C. gattii*. Regimens that include amphotericin B (conventional or liposomal formulations), flucytosine, and fluconazole have been effective in a few patients with CNS infections known to be caused by *C. gattii*.

For additional information on management of cryptococcosis, the current clinical practice guidelines from IDSA available at http://www.idsociety.org and the current clinical practice guidelines from CDC, NIH, and IDSA on the prevention and treatment of opportunistic infections in HIV-infected individuals available at http://www.aidsinfo.nih.gov should be consulted.

● Histoplasmosis

IV amphotericin B is used for the treatment of histoplasmosis caused by *Histoplasma capsulatum*.

The drugs of choice for the treatment of histoplasmosis, including histoplasmosis in HIV-infected individuals, are IV amphotericin B and oral itraconazole. IV amphotericin B is preferred for initial treatment of severe, life-threatening histoplasmosis, especially in immunocompromised patients such as those with HIV infection. Oral itraconazole generally is used for initial treatment of less severe disease (e.g., mild to moderate acute pulmonary histoplasmosis, chronic cavitary pulmonary histoplasmosis) and as follow-up therapy in the treatment of severe infections after a response has been obtained with IV amphotericin B. Other azole antifungals (fluconazole, posaconazole, voriconazole) are considered second-line alternatives to itraconazole, but can be considered in patients who have less severe disease and cannot tolerate itraconazole.

For the treatment of moderately severe to severe acute pulmonary histoplasmosis in HIV-infected adults and adolescents, CDC, NIH, and IDSA recommend initial (induction) treatment with IV amphotericin B liposomal and follow-up treatment with oral itraconazole. Alternatively, if necessary because of cost or tolerability, IV amphotericin B lipid complex can be used.

For the treatment of progressive disseminated histoplasmosis in children, IDSA states that conventional IV amphotericin B or an initial regimen of conventional IV amphotericin B and follow-up treatment with oral itraconazole can be used. IDSA states that conventional amphotericin B usually is well tolerated in children, but a lipid formulation may be substituted if necessary.

For the treatment of moderately severe to severe disseminated histoplasmosis in HIV-infected infants and children, CDC, NIH, and IDSA recommend initial treatment with IV amphotericin B liposomal and follow-up treatment with oral itraconazole; conventional IV amphotericin B can be used as an alternative to the lipid formulation for initial treatment in these children. Although oral itraconazole may be used alone for the treatment of mild to moderate progressive disseminated histoplasmosis in children, including HIV-infected infants and children, this regimen is not recommended for more severe infections.

For the treatment of meningitis caused by *H. capsulatum* in HIV-infected adults, adolescents, or children and other individuals, CDC, NIH, and IDSA recommend initial (induction) treatment with IV amphotericin B liposomal and follow-up treatment with oral itraconazole. The liposomal formulation of amphotericin B generally is preferred for the treatment of CNS histoplasmosis since CSF concentrations may be higher with the liposomal formulation than with some other formulations. Conventional IV amphotericin B has been administered alone or in conjunction with intrathecal† administration of the drug for the treatment of meningitis caused by *H. capsulatum.*

HIV-infected adults, adolescents, or children who have been adequately treated for histoplasmosis should receive long-term suppressive or maintenance therapy (secondary prophylaxis) to prevent recurrence or relapse of histoplasmosis. Oral itraconazole is the drug of choice for secondary prophylaxis of histoplasmosis in HIV-infected patients.

For additional information on management of histoplasmosis, the current clinical practice guidelines from IDSA available at http://www.idsociety.org and the current clinical practice guidelines from CDC, NIH, and IDSA on the prevention and treatment of opportunistic infections in HIV-infected individuals available at http://www.aidsinfo.nih.gov should be consulted.

● **Paracoccidioidomycosis**

IV amphotericin B is used for the treatment of paracoccidioidomycosis† (South American blastomycosis) caused by *Paracoccidioides brasiliensis.*

IV amphotericin B is the drug of choice for initial treatment of severe paracoccidioidomycosis. Oral itraconazole is the drug of choice for the treatment of less severe or localized paracoccidioidomycosis and for follow-up therapy in more severe infections after initial treatment with IV amphotericin B.

● **Penicilliosis**

IV amphotericin B is used in the treatment of penicilliosis† caused by *Penicillium marneffei.*

Although oral itraconazole can be used alone for the treatment of mild penicilliosis, an initial regimen of IV amphotericin B is recommended for the treatment of severe or disseminated *P. marneffei* infections†.

For the treatment of severe, acute penicilliosis† in HIV-infected adults and adolescents, CDC, NIH, and IDSA recommend an initial regimen of IV amphotericin B liposomal followed by oral itraconazole. These experts state that a voriconazole regimen (IV initially, then oral) can be used as an alternative in patients with severe penicilliosis, including those who fail to respond to a regimen of IV amphotericin B followed by itraconazole.

HIV-infected patients who have been treated for penicilliosis should receive long-term suppressive or maintenance therapy (secondary prophylaxis) with oral itraconazole to prevent recurrence or relapse.

For additional information on management of penicilliosis, the current clinical practice guidelines from CDC, NIH, and IDSA on the prevention and treatment of opportunistic infections in HIV-infected individuals available at http://www.aidsinfo.nih.gov should be consulted.

● **Sporotrichosis**

IV amphotericin B is used in the treatment of disseminated, pulmonary, osteoarticular, and meningeal sporotrichosis caused by *Sporothrix schenckii.*

IV amphotericin B is the drug of choice for initial treatment of severe, life-threatening sporotrichosis and whenever sporotrichosis is disseminated or has CNS involvement. Oral itraconazole is the drug of choice for the treatment of cutaneous, lymphocutaneous, or mild pulmonary or osteoarticular sporotrichosis and for follow-up treatment of severe infections after a response has been obtained with IV amphotericin B.

Since sporotrichosis in immunocompromised patients (e.g., HIV-infected individuals) is particularly aggressive and difficult to treat, IV amphotericin B usually is the drug of choice for initial therapy in these patients; however, treatment failures occur. IDSA and other clinicians state that a lipid formulation of

amphotericin B is preferred for the treatment of sporotrichosis since the lipid formulations generally are associated with fewer adverse effects.

For additional information on management of sporotrichosis, the current clinical practice guidelines from IDSA available at http://www.idsociety.org should be consulted.

● **Exserohilum Infections**

Amphotericin B has been used for the treatment of infections known or suspected to be caused by *Exserohilum rostratum*†.

Exserohilum is a common mold found in soil and on plants, especially grasses, and thrives in warm and humid climates. *E. rostratum* is considered an opportunistic human pathogen and rarely has been involved in human infections, including cutaneous and subcutaneous infections or keratitis, typically as the result of skin or eye trauma. More invasive infections (e.g., infections involving the sinuses, heart, lungs, or bones) and life-threatening infections also have been reported rarely, usually in immunocompromised individuals. In addition, *E. rostratum* was identified as the predominant pathogen in the 2012–2013 multistate outbreak of fungal meningitis and other fungal infections that occurred in the US in patients who received contaminated preservative-free methylprednisolone acetate injections prepared by a compounding pharmacy. *Exserohilum* infections cannot be transmitted person-to-person.

Although data are limited and the clinical relevance of in vitro testing remains uncertain, in vitro studies indicate that *Exserohilum* is inhibited by some triazole antifungals (e.g., voriconazole, itraconazole, posaconazole) and amphotericin B. Echinocandins (e.g., caspofungin, micafungin) have variable in vitro activity and fluconazole has poor in vitro activity against the fungus.

Exserohilum Infections Related to Contaminated Injections

In September 2012, the CDC and US Food and Drug Administration (FDA) initiated investigations in response to fungal CNS infections (including some fatalities) reported in patients who received epidural injections of contaminated extemporaneously prepared methylprednisolone acetate injections from the New England Compounding Center (NECC). Subsequently, there were reports of joint infections and osteomyelitis in some patients who received intra-articular injections of methylprednisolone acetate from NECC, as well as infections possibly related to other NECC products.

Out of an abundance of caution at that time, the FDA recommended that health-care professionals and consumers not use any product that was produced by NECC, and the company recalled all products that were compounded at and distributed from its facility in Framingham, Massachusetts.

E. rostratum was one of the predominant pathogen identified in samples taken from patients who received contaminated products from NECC; *Aspergillus* also was identified in an index patient and *Cladosporium cladosporioides* was recovered from several other patients. The presence of *E. rostratum* was confirmed in recalled lots of the contaminated products. Other organisms identified in unopened vials from recalled lots of corticosteroid products were *A. fumigatus, A. tubingensis,* various *Bacillus* species (including *Bacillus subtilis*), *Cladosporium, Paenibacillus,* and *Penicillium.*

CDC data indicate that, as of October 30, 2015, there were a total of 753 cases of fungal infections (including 64 deaths) reported in 20 states that have been linked to specific lots of contaminated methylprednisolone acetate injections. Although the majority of initial cases involved fungal meningitis (some with stroke), subsequent reports involved localized spinal or paraspinal infections (e.g., epidural abscess). More than 6 months after the outbreak related to contaminated products was first identified, CDC continued to receive reports of patients presenting with localized spinal and paraspinal infections (e.g., epidural abscess, phlegmon, discitis, vertebral osteomyelitis, arachnoiditis, or other complications at or near the site of injection). These localized infections occurred in patients with or without a diagnosis of fungal meningitis. In some patients being treated for fungal meningitis who had no previous evidence of localized infections, such infections were found at the site of injection using magnetic resonance imaging (MRI) studies. Some cases occurred in patients without any previous evidence of infection or in those with persistent, worsening, or new symptoms.

Patients with meningitis generally presented 1–4 weeks or longer after receiving contaminated methylprednisolone acetate injections; the greatest risk for development of fungal meningitis appeared to be during the first 6 weeks after an epidural or paraspinal injection. Data from one group of patients indicated that the median time from the last injection with contaminated product to the date of the first MRI finding indicative of infection was 50 days (range 12–121 days) for all patients with a spinal or paraspinal infection, and the median time from the first positive lumbar puncture finding to the first positive MRI finding was 21 days for those with meningitis and spinal or paraspinal infections.

Clinicians treating fungal infections in patients who received contaminated methylprednisolone acetate injections from NECC should consult an infectious disease expert to assist with diagnosis, management, and follow-up, which may be complex and prolonged. A clinical consultant network for clinicians can be reached by calling CDC at 800-232-4636.

Because of evidence of latent disease, CDC cautions clinicians to continue to remain vigilant for the possibility of infections in patients who received injections of NECC products and to consider such infections in the differential diagnosis when evaluating symptomatic patients who received such products. CDC recommends routine laboratory and microbiologic tests, including bacterial and fungal cultures, as necessary; MRI evaluations should be considered if clinically warranted.

CDC released interim treatment guidance documents containing recommendations for empiric antifungal treatment of CNS and parameningeal infections and osteoarticular infections associated with the contaminated methylprednisolone acetate products. These recommendations were based on evidence that *E. rostratum* was the predominant pathogen in the outbreak and consultation with experts.

For the treatment of CNS infections (including meningitis, stroke, and arachnoiditis) and/or parameningeal infections (epidural or paraspinal abscess, discitis or osteomyelitis, and sacroiliac infection) in adults who received contaminated corticosteroid injections, CDC recommends voriconazole. Use of IV amphotericin B liposomal *in addition* to voriconazole should be strongly considered in patients who present with severe disease and in patients who do not improve or experience clinical deterioration or manifest new sites of disease activity while receiving voriconazole monotherapy. IV amphotericin B liposomal also is recommended as an alternative in patients who unable to tolerate voriconazole. IV amphotericin B liposomal is preferred over other lipid formulations of amphotericin B because of better CNS penetration. Because of limited data and associated toxicities, routine use of intrathecal conventional amphotericin B is not recommended in these patients.

For the treatment of osteoarticular infections (discitis, vertebral osteomyelitis, and epidural abscess or osteoarticular infections not involving the spine) in adults who received intra-articular injections of contaminated corticosteroid products, CDC recommends voriconazole. Use of a lipid formulation of IV amphotericin B *in addition* to IV voriconazole should be considered in patients with severe osteoarticular infection and/or clinical instability. A lipid formulation of IV amphotericin B, posaconazole, or itraconazole are recommended as alternatives in patients who cannot tolerate voriconazole. Expert consultation is advised when making decisions regarding alternative regimens.

Adequate duration of antifungal treatment for infections associated with the contaminated corticosteroid injections is unknown, but prolonged therapy is required. (See Exserohilum Infections under Dosage: Amphotericin B Liposomal (AmBisome®), in Dosage and Administration.) In addition, close follow-up monitoring after completion of treatment is essential in all patients to detect potential relapse.

The CDC website at https://www.cdc.gov/hai/outbreaks/meningitis.html should be consulted for the most recent information regarding the contaminated NECC products and associated infections, including specific information regarding diagnosis and treatment of these infections.

● *Fusarium Infections*

Amphotericin B has been used for the treatment of serious fungal infections caused by *Fusarium*, and a lipid formulation of amphotericin B is recommended as a drug of choice for the treatment of these fungal infections.

For the treatment of fusariosis, the most appropriate antifungal should be selected based on in vitro susceptibility testing. Amphotericin B may be preferred for infections caused by *F. solani* or *F. verticillioides*; either voriconazole or amphotericin B are recommended for infections caused by other *Fusarium*. Some clinicians suggest that concomitant use of amphotericin B and voriconazole should be considered in patients with severe infections or immunosuppression.

● *Zygomycosis*

IV amphotericin B is used for the treatment of zygomycosis, including mucormycosis, caused by susceptible species of *Lichtheimia* (formerly *Absidia*), *Mucor*, or *Rhizopus* and for the treatment of infections caused by susceptible species of *Conidiobolus* or *Basidiobolus*. IV amphotericin B generally has been considered the drug of choice for these infections. However, in several cases of GI basidiobolomycosis caused by *Basidiobolus ranarum*, the response to amphotericin B

(e.g., amphotericin B liposomal) was poor. Most cases of GI basidiobolomycosis reported to date have been successfully treated with oral itraconazole after partial surgical resection of the GI tract.

While most experience to date in treating zygomycosis has involved use of conventional IV amphotericin B, lipid formulations (amphotericin B lipid complex, amphotericin B liposomal) also have been used to treat these infections, including rhinocerebral and pulmonary mucormycosis in some patients who did not respond to conventional amphotericin B or had to discontinue conventional amphotericin B because of adverse renal effects.

● *Empiric Therapy in Febrile Neutropenic Patients*

Conventional IV amphotericin B†, amphotericin B lipid complex†, and amphotericin B liposomal are used for empiric therapy of presumed fungal infections in febrile, neutropenic patients who have not responded to empiric treatment with broad-spectrum antibacterial agents.

Because systemic fungal infections (e.g., *Candida*, *Aspergillus*) are present in up to one-third of neutropenic patients who remain febrile after a 7-day course of empiric broad-spectrum anti-infective therapy, IDSA and other clinicians recommend that consideration be given to administering empiric antifungal therapy (with or without a change in the antibacterial regimen) to neutropenic patients who have persistent or recurrent fever after 4–7 days of antibacterial therapy. Conventional IV amphotericin B historically has been considered the drug of choice for empiric antifungal treatment in such patients; however, lipid formulations of amphotericin B or other antifungals (e.g., caspofungin, voriconazole) also have been used.

Empiric therapy with conventional IV amphotericin B has been used in patients undergoing bone marrow transplantation (BMT) who have persistent fever despite 3–7 days of broad-spectrum antibacterial therapy, and such therapy was included in the Eastern Cooperative Oncology Group (ECOG) guidelines for the management of autologous and allogeneic BMT patients. If conventional IV amphotericin B is used for empiric antifungal therapy in febrile, neutropenic allogeneic BMT patients who are receiving cyclosporine, the potential for additive nephrotoxic effects should be considered before initiating such therapy. (See Drug Interactions: Nephrotoxic Drugs.)

Published protocols for the treatment of infections in febrile neutropenic patients should be consulted for specific recommendations regarding selection of the initial empiric anti-infective regimen, when to change the initial regimen, possible subsequent regimens, and duration of therapy in these patients. In addition, consultation with an infectious disease expert knowledgeable about infections in immunocompromised patients is advised.

Clinical Experience

The relative efficacy of conventional IV amphotericin B and amphotericin B liposomal for empiric therapy in febrile, neutropenic patients has been evaluated in a randomized, double-blind, multicenter study that involved 687 adult and pediatric cancer patients 2–80 years of age who were febrile despite having received at least 5 days of empiric therapy with broad spectrum anti-infectives. The overall therapeutic success rate (defined as resolution of fever during the neutropenic period, successful treatment of any baseline fungal infections, absence of emergent fungal infections during therapy or within 7 days after completion of study drug, patient survival for at least 7 days after empiric therapy, and use of study drug without premature discontinuance because of toxicity or lack of efficacy) was 50.1% for amphotericin B liposomal and 49.4% for conventional amphotericin B. Emergent fungal infections were mycologically confirmed in 3.2% of those receiving amphotericin B liposomal and in 7.8% of those receiving conventional amphotericin B. While the overall success rate was similar in both groups, the group receiving amphotericin B liposomal had a lower incidence of documented emergent fungal infections and also had a lower incidence of acute infusion reactions and adverse renal effects than those receiving conventional amphotericin B. Amphotericin B liposomal also appeared to be as effective as conventional IV amphotericin B for empiric therapy of presumed fungal infections in several randomized, open label, multicenter studies that involved febrile neutropenic adults and pediatric patients undergoing chemotherapy for hematologic malignancy or as part of bone marrow transplantation.

● *Prevention of Fungal Infections in Transplant Recipients, Cancer Patients, or Other Patients at High Risk*

Conventional IV amphotericin B† and amphotericin B liposomal† have been used prophylactically in an attempt to reduce the incidence of fungal infections (e.g., aspergillosis, candidiasis) in neutropenic cancer patients† or patients undergoing

BMT† or solid organ transplantation†. IV amphotericin B also has been used to prevent *Candida* infections in patients undergoing urologic procedures†.

Use of primary antifungal prophylaxis in cancer patients undergoing myelosuppressive therapy or patients undergoing BMT or solid organ transplantation has been controversial, particularly since such prophylaxis may predispose the patient to colonization with resistant fungi and/or result in the emergence of highly resistant organisms. Some clinicians discourage primary prophylaxis with antifungals except in certain carefully selected high-risk patients in whom potential benefits are expected to justify possible risks (e.g., patients in institutions that have a high incidence of fungal infections or circumstances where the frequency of systemic *Candida* infections is high). When primary antifungal prophylaxis is warranted in cancer patients or BMT or solid organ transplant recipients, IDSA and other clinicians generally prefer use of an oral azole antifungal.

For postoperative antifungal prophylaxis in recipients of solid organ transplants† at high risk for invasive candidiasis (i.e., liver, pancreas, or small bowel transplant recipients), IDSA recommends fluconazole or IV amphotericin B liposomal. IDSA states that the risk of invasive candidiasis in recipients of other solid organ transplants (e.g., kidney, heart) appears to be too low to warrant routine antifungal prophylaxis.

For high-risk patients undergoing urologic procedures†, IDSA states that fluconazole or conventional IV amphotericin B can be used for several days before and after the procedure to prevent *Candida* infections.

Conventional amphotericin B, amphotericin B lipid complex, and amphotericin B liposomal have been administered by nasal instillation† or nebulization† in an attempt to prevent aspergillosis in immunocompromised patients, including solid organ transplant recipients† (e.g., lung transplant recipients) and neutropenic chemotherapy patients†.

For additional information on prevention of fungal infections in neutropenic patients, the current clinical practice guidelines from IDSA available at http://www.idsociety.org should be consulted.

Clinical Experience

When used for antifungal prophylaxis in cancer patients or patients undergoing BMT, conventional amphotericin B has been administered in usual IV dosages or, more frequently, as low-dose IV therapy (i.e., 0.1–0.25 mg/kg daily). Safety and efficacy of low-dose conventional IV amphotericin B for prophylaxis in neutropenic patients undergoing BMT have been evaluated in a prospective, randomized, placebo-controlled study. Patients undergoing autologous BMT were randomized to receive low-dose conventional IV amphotericin B (0.1 mg/kg daily) or placebo; any patient with persistent neutropenia and fever despite prophylaxis with low-dose amphotericin B and broad-spectrum antibacterial agent therapy was withdrawn from the study and given empiric therapy with a higher dosage of conventional IV amphotericin B (0.6 mg/kg daily). During the study, 8.8% of those receiving low-dose amphotericin B and 14.3% of those receiving placebo had mycologically confirmed fungal infections (*Candida, Aspergillus*); 6-week mortality was higher in those receiving placebo (11 deaths in those receiving placebo compared with 3 deaths in those receiving amphotericin B), but this difference did not appear to be related to fungal infections. Because there is some evidence that administration of low-dose conventional IV amphotericin B therapy to BMT patients can decrease the incidence posttransplant fungal infections, some clinicians suggest that secondary prophylaxis with low-dose conventional IV amphotericin B be considered for all transplant patients with a history of documented invasive aspergillosis since these patients are at risk for reactivation of the disease. However, there is evidence that prophylaxis with low-dose conventional IV amphotericin B may be ineffective in preventing posttransplant fungal infections in liver transplant patients since candidemia and invasive aspergillosis have been reported in liver transplant recipients receiving prophylaxis with conventional IV amphotericin B (0.5 mg/kg daily).

Data are accumulating regarding use of amphotericin B liposomal for antifungal prophylaxis in neutropenic cancer patients or BMT or transplant patients. Safety and efficacy of amphotericin B liposomal (2 mg/kg 3 times weekly) for antifungal prophylaxis in patients undergoing chemotherapy or BMT have been evaluated in a double-blind, placebo-controlled study. Systemic or superficial fungal infections were suspected in 42 or 46% of those receiving amphotericin B liposomal or placebo, respectively; however, while there were mycologically confirmed fungal infections in 3.4% of those receiving placebo, there were none in those receiving amphotericin B liposomal prophylaxis. There was fungal colonization of at least one site (fungal pathogen isolated but not associated with clinical or

other evidence of disease) in 20 or 40% of those receiving amphotericin B liposomal or placebo, respectively. The mortality rate was similar in both groups (14–15%). In a limited placebo-controlled study in liver transplant recipients, there was no evidence of posttransplant fungal infections in those who received 5 days of amphotericin B liposomal prophylaxis (1 mg/kg daily initiated at the time of transplantation); 16% of patients who received placebo developed *C. albicans* infections posttransplant. However, in another study in liver transplant recipients who received amphotericin B liposomal for antifungal prophylaxis (1 mg/kg daily initiated after transplant and continued for 7 days), the regimen appeared to effectively prevent *Candida* infections but several patients developed posttransplant *Aspergillus* infections that were fatal.

• *Protozoal Infections*

Leishmaniasis

Conventional IV amphotericin B, amphotericin B lipid complex†, and amphotericin B liposomal have been used for the treatment of leishmaniasis.

Leishmaniasis is caused by more than 15–20 different species of *Leishmania* that are transmitted to humans by the bite of infected sand flies. *Leishmania* also can be transmitted via blood (e.g., blood transfusions, needles shared by IV drug abusers) and transmitted perinatally from mother to infant. In the Eastern Hemisphere, leishmaniasis is found most frequently in parts of Asia, the Middle East, Africa, and southern Europe; in the Western Hemisphere, the disease is found most frequently in Mexico and Central and South America and has been reported occasionally in Texas and Oklahoma. Leishmaniasis has been reported in short-term travelers to endemic areas and in immigrants and expatriates from such areas, and also has been reported in US military personnel and contract workers serving or working in endemic areas (e.g., Iraq, Afghanistan).

Leishmania infection in humans may cause uncomplicated cutaneous leishmaniasis, diffuse cutaneous leishmaniasis, mucosal leishmaniasis, visceral leishmaniasis, or post-kala-azar leishmaniasis and may be termed Old World (Eastern Hemisphere) or New World (Western Hemisphere). The specific form of leishmaniasis and disease severity depend on the *Leishmania* species involved, geographic area of origin, location of sand fly bite, and patient factors (e.g., nutritional and immune status). Treatment of leishmaniasis (e.g., drug, dosage, duration of treatment) must be individualized based on the region where the disease was acquired, likely infecting species, drug susceptibilities reported in the area of origin, form of the disease, and patient factors (e.g., age, pregnancy, immune status). No single treatment approach is appropriate for all possible clinical presentations. Consultation with clinicians experienced in management of leishmaniasis is recommended.

For assistance with diagnosis or treatment of leishmaniasis in the US, clinicians can contact CDC Parasitic Diseases Hotline at 404-718-4745 from 8:00 a.m. to 4:00 p.m. Eastern Standard Time or CDC Emergency Operation Center at 770-488-7100 after business hours and on weekends and holidays. CDC Drug Service should be contacted at 404-639-3670 for information on how to obtain antiparasitic drugs not commercially available in the US.

Cutaneous and Mucocutaneous Leishmaniasis

Conventional IV amphotericin B is used for the treatment of American cutaneous leishmaniasis, including infections caused by *Leishmania braziliensis* or *L. mexicana*, and for mucocutaneous leishmaniasis, including infections caused by *L. braziliensis*.

Although some cases of cutaneous leishmaniasis (usually Old World) may subside or resolve spontaneously over months or years, treatment of cutaneous leishmaniasis is recommended if there are multiple or large lesions, lesions are disabling or disfiguring or fail to heal within 6 months, the patient is immunocompromised, or dissemination to mucosal leishmaniasis is likely (e.g., New World disease caused by *L. braziliensis* or *L. panamensis*). Local treatment (e.g., topical paromomycin [not commercially available in the US], thermotherapy, intralesional pentavalent antimonials [not commercially available in the US], cryotherapy) may be appropriate in selected cases. For systemic treatment of cutaneous leishmaniasis, pentavalent antimonials (i.e., sodium stibogluconate or meglumine antimonate [drugs not commercially available in the US, but may be available from CDC]) usually are used. Other treatment options for cutaneous leishmaniasis include amphotericin B, miltefosine, pentamidine, and ketoconazole, especially when antimonials cannot be used because of tolerance or resistance.

Data are limited regarding use of lipid formulations of amphotericin B in the treatment of cutaneous leishmaniasis, but amphotericin B lipid complex† and amphotericin B liposomal† have been used in a limited number of patients for the treatment of cutaneous leishmaniasis. At least one patient with cutaneous leishmaniasis unresponsive to meglumine antimonate therapy was successfully treated with a 2-week regimen of IV amphotericin B liposomal (1.5 mg/kg daily) followed by a 4-week regimen of conventional IV amphotericin B (3 mg/kg once weekly).

Visceral Leishmaniasis

IV amphotericin B liposomal is used in the treatment of visceral leishmaniasis (also known as kala-azar) and is recommended by some clinicians as a drug of choice, especially for immunocompromised patients. Conventional IV amphotericin B† and amphotericin B lipid complex† also have been used for the treatment of visceral leishmaniasis.

Pentavalent antimonials (i.e., sodium stibogluconate or meglumine antimonate [drugs not commercially available in the US, but may available from CDC]) have historically been considered the drugs of first choice for initial treatment of visceral leishmaniasis; however, drug resistance and treatment failures have become a major concern in some areas (e.g., India, Nepal). Other treatment options for visceral leishmaniasis include amphotericin B, miltefosine, or paromomycin. Relapse of visceral leishmaniasis is common in immunocompromised patients (e.g., HIV-infected patients), regardless of the treatment regimen.

In a group of patients with visceral leishmaniasis who were infected in the Mediterranean basin with documented or presumed *L. infantum*, amphotericin B liposomal was associated with an overall success rate (clearance with no relapse during a follow-up period of 6 months or longer) of 96.5% in immunocompetent patients. In patients who were immunocompromised, amphotericin B liposomal therapy was able to initially clear the infection in 94.7% of patients; however, the overall success rate was only 11.8% and there was a high rate of relapse in these patients. The manufacturer states that data are inconclusive regarding efficacy of IV amphotericin B liposomal for the treatment of infections caused by *L. donovani* or *L. chagasi*.

Leishmaniasis in HIV-infected Individuals

Based on data from individuals who are not infected with HIV, CDC, NIH, and IDSA state that the drugs of choice for the treatment of cutaneous leishmaniasis in HIV-infected adults or adolescents are amphotericin B liposomal† or sodium stibogluconate (not commercially available in the US, but may be available from CDC). Possible alternatives are miltefosine, topical paromomycin (not commercially available in the US), intralesional pentavalent antimony (not commercially available in the US), or local heat therapy.

For the treatment of visceral leishmaniasis in HIV-infected adults and adolescents, CDC, NIH, and IDSA recommend amphotericin B liposomal as the drug of choice since the drug appears to have similar efficacy but is better tolerated in these patients than conventional amphotericin B or pentavalent antimony compounds. Alternatives for the treatment of visceral leishmaniasis in HIV-infected adults and adolescents include amphotericin B lipid complex†, conventional amphotericin B†, sodium stibogluconate (not commercially available in the US, but may be available from CDC), or miltefosine.

CDC, NIH, and IDSA recommend long-term suppressive or maintenance therapy (secondary prophylaxis)† to decrease the risk of relapse in HIV-infected adults and adolescents who have been treated for visceral leishmaniasis and have CD4⁺ T-cell counts less than 200/mm³. Although data are limited, these experts state that long-term suppressive or maintenance therapy (secondary prophylaxis) also should be offered to those who have been adequately treated for cutaneous leishmaniasis but are immunocompromised and have had multiple relapses. If secondary prophylaxis against leishmaniasis is indicated in HIV-infected adults and adolescents, CDC, NIH, and IDSA recommend use of amphotericin B liposomal† or amphotericin B lipid complex†; the alternative is sodium stibogluconate (not commercially available in the US, but may be available from CDC). The manufacturer of amphotericin B liposomal states that, while the drug may have a role for long-term suppressive therapy to prevent relapse of visceral leishmaniasis in HIV-infected individuals, the efficacy and safety of repeated courses of amphotericin B liposomal or maintenance therapy with the drug in immunocompromised individuals have not been evaluated to date.

If secondary prophylaxis against leishmaniasis is initiated in HIV-infected adults and adolescents, some experts state that consideration can be given to discontinuing such prophylaxis if CD4⁺ T-cell counts remain greater than 200–350/mm³ for at least 3–6 months in response to antiretroviral therapy. However, others suggest that such prophylaxis should be continued indefinitely.

Primary Amebic Meningoencephalitis

Conventional IV amphotericin B has been used for the treatment of primary amebic meningoencephalitis caused by *Naegleria fowleri*†, a free-living ameba.

CNS infections caused by free-living ameba have a high mortality rate, and only a very limited number of cases have been successfully treated. Early diagnosis and aggressive treatment of these infections may increase the chance of survival. Although data are limited, most reported cases of *N. fowleri* have been treated empirically with multiple-drug regimens. Treatment regimens used or recommended for the treatment of *N. fowleri* infections include several anti-infectives (e.g., amphotericin B, azole antifungals [fluconazole], flucytosine, macrolides [azithromycin, clarithromycin], miltefosine, rifampin) and other therapies (e.g., dexamethasone, phenytoin, therapeutic hypothermia).

Based on multiple-drug regimens used to date in documented survivors, CDC recommends an anti-infective regimen that includes conventional amphotericin B (administered IV and intrathecally†), azithromycin, fluconazole, miltefosine, and rifampin for treatment of primary amebic meningoencephalitis caused by *N. fowleri*. Because there is some evidence that amphotericin B liposomal may be less effective than conventional amphotericin B in mice for the treatment of primary amebic meningoencephalitis caused by *N. fowleri*, the conventional formulation is preferred if amphotericin B is used for the treatment of primary amebic meningoencephalitis.

For assistance with diagnosis or treatment of patients with suspected free-living ameba infections, clinicians should contact the CDC Emergency Operation Center at 770-488-7100.

DOSAGE AND ADMINISTRATION

● Reconstitution and Administration

Conventional Amphotericin B

Conventional amphotericin B is administered by IV infusion. The drug also has been given intra-articularly†, intrapleurally†, intrathecally†, by nasal instillation† or nebulization†, and by bladder irrigation†.

Commercially available conventional amphotericin B for IV infusion must be reconstituted and diluted prior to administration. *The drug must not be prepared with any diluents other than those specified below since precipitation may occur. Strict aseptic technique must be observed.*

Conventional amphotericin B should be reconstituted to a concentration of 5 mg/mL by rapidly adding 10 mL of sterile water for injection *without bacteriostatic agent* to a vial labeled as containing 50 mg of drug. The sterile water diluent should be added to the vial using a sterile syringe (minimum needle size of 20 gauge) and the vial should be immediately shaken until the colloidal dispersion is clear. For IV infusion, the colloidal dispersion is further diluted, usually to a concentration of 0.1 mg/mL, with 500 mL of 5% dextrose injection (the dextrose injection must have a pH exceeding 4.2). Although the pH of commercially available 5% dextrose injection usually exceeds 4.2, the pH of each container of 5% dextrose injection should be determined and, if the pH is low, it may be adjusted with 1 or 2 mL of sterile buffer solution in accordance with the instructions provided by the manufacturers of conventional amphotericin B.

Reconstituted conventional amphotericin B or dilutions of the drug must not be used if precipitation or foreign matter is evident. An inline membrane filter may be used during IV administration of conventional amphotericin B; however, the mean pore diameter of the filter should *not* be less than 1 μm to ensure passage of the amphotericin B colloidal dispersion. IV infusions of conventional amphotericin B containing a drug concentration of 0.1 mg/mL or less should be used promptly after preparation.

Rate of Administration

IV infusions of conventional amphotericin B are given *slowly* over a period of approximately 2–6 hours, depending on the dose being administered.

Although IV infusions of conventional amphotericin B have been well tolerated in some patients when given over 1–2 hours, the manufacturers and many clinicians state that rapid IV infusions of conventional amphotericin B should be avoided since potentially serious adverse effects (e.g., hypotension, hypokalemia, arrhythmias, shock) may occur.

Amphotericin B Lipid Complex (Abelcet®)

Amphotericin B lipid complex is administered by IV infusion. The drug also has been administered by nasal inhalation† or nebulization†.

Commercially available amphotericin B lipid complex injectable suspension concentrate must be diluted prior to IV infusion. The injectable suspension concentrate must be diluted in 5% dextrose injection to a concentration of 1 mg/mL; a concentration of 2 mg/mL may be appropriate for pediatric patients and patients with cardiovascular disease. Solutions containing sodium chloride or bacteriostatic agents should *not* be used to dilute amphotericin B lipid complex, and the drug should *not* be mixed with other drugs or with electrolytes.

To prepare IV infusions of amphotericin B lipid complex, vials labeled as containing 5 mg/mL should be shaken gently until there is no evidence of yellow sediment on the bottom of the vial. The appropriate dose should be withdrawn from the required number of vials into one or more sterile 20-mL syringes using an 18-gauge needle. The needle should be removed from the filled syringe and replaced with the 5-μm filter needle provided by the manufacturer; each filter needle may be used to filter the contents of up to four 100-mg vials of the drug. The filter needle should then be inserted into an IV container of 5% dextrose injection and the contents of the syringe injected into the container.

Prior to initiation of the infusion, the IV container of diluted drug should be shaken until the contents are thoroughly mixed; the infusion container should then be shaken every 2 hours if the infusion time exceeds 2 hours. Amphotericin B lipid complex diluted in 5% dextrose injection should not be used if there is any evidence of foreign matter in the solution.

The drug should be administered using a separate infusion line; if an existing IV line is used, it should be flushed with 5% dextrose injection before amphotericin B lipid complex is infused. An inline membrane filter should *not* be used during administration of amphotericin B lipid complex.

Rate of Administration

IV infusions of diluted amphotericin B lipid complex should be infused at a rate of 2.5 mg/kg per hour.

Amphotericin B Liposomal (AmBisome®)

Amphotericin B liposomal is administered by IV infusion. The drug also has been administered by nasal inhalation† or nebulization†.

Amphotericin B liposomal must be reconstituted by adding 12 mL of sterile water for injection to a vial labeled as containing 50 mg of amphotericin B to provide a solution containing 4 mg/mL. Other diluents (e.g., diluents containing sodium chloride or a bacteriostatic agent) should *not* be used to reconstitute amphotericin B liposomal, and reconstituted solutions should *not* be admixed with other drugs. The appropriate amount of reconstituted amphotericin B liposomal should be withdrawn into a sterile syringe. The 5-μm sterile, disposable filter provided by the manufacturer should then be attached to the syringe and the syringe contents injected through the filter into the appropriate volume of 5% dextrose injection to provide a final concentration of 1–2 mg/mL. Lower concentrations (0.2–0.5 mg/mL) may be appropriate for infants and small children.

Amphotericin B liposomal may be infused through an in-line membrane filter provided the mean pore diameter of the filter is not less than 1 μm. The drug may be administered through an existing IV line; however, the line must be flushed with 5% dextrose injection prior to infusion of the antifungal. If this is not feasible, amphotericin B liposomal must be administered through a separate line.

Rate of Administration

IV infusions of amphotericin B liposomal should be given over a period of approximately 2 hours using a controlled infusion device. If the infusion is well tolerated, infusion time may be reduced to approximately 1 hour; however, the duration of infusion should be increased in patients who experience discomfort during infusion.

● Dosage

Dosage of amphotericin B varies depending on whether the drug is administered as conventional amphotericin B (formulated with sodium desoxycholate), amphotericin B lipid complex, or amphotericin B liposomal. Dosage recommendations for the specific formulation being administered should be followed.

Conventional Amphotericin B

Dosage of conventional amphotericin B must be individualized and adjusted according to the patient's tolerance and clinical status (e.g., site and severity of infection, etiologic agent, cardiopulmonary and renal function status).

The manufacturers caution that under no circumstances should the total daily dose of conventional amphotericin B exceed 1.5 mg/kg. Overdosage can result in potentially fatal cardiac or cardiopulmonary arrest. (See Acute Toxicity.)

Prior to initiation of conventional IV amphotericin B therapy, a single test dose of the drug (1 mg in 20 mL of 5% dextrose injection) should be administered IV over 20–30 minutes and the patient carefully monitored (i.e., pulse and

respiration rate, temperature, blood pressure) every 30 minutes for 2–4 hours. In patients with good cardiorenal function who tolerate the test dose, the manufacturers recommend that therapy be initiated with a daily dosage of 0.25 mg/kg (0.3 mg/kg in those with severe or rapidly progressing fungal infections) given as a single daily dose. In patients with impaired cardiorenal function and in patients who have severe reactions to the test dose, the manufacturers recommend that therapy be initiated with a smaller daily dosage (i.e., 5–10 mg). Depending on the patient's cardiorenal status, dosage may gradually be increased by 5–10 mg daily to a final daily dosage of 0.5–0.7 mg/kg.

The manufacturers state that the optimal dosage of conventional amphotericin B is unknown and data are insufficient to define total dosage and duration of treatment for eradication of specific fungal infections. Dosage up to 1 mg/kg daily or up to 1.5 mg/kg when given on alternate days is recommended by the manufacturers. When converting a daily IV dosage schedule to alternate-day therapy, dosage must be increased gradually every other day until it is twice the previous daily dosage.

If conventional amphotericin B therapy is discontinued for longer than 1 week, the manufacturers recommend that administration of the drug be resumed at the usual initial dosage of 0.25 mg/kg daily, and dosage should again be gradually increased.

Aspergillosis

For the treatment of invasive aspergillosis, conventional IV amphotericin B has been administered in a dosage of 0.5–1.5 mg/kg daily. The duration of treatment is based on the degree and duration of immunosuppression, disease site, and clinical response. The Infectious Diseases Society of America (IDSA) recommends that antifungal treatment of invasive pulmonary aspergillosis be continued for at least 6–12 weeks.

If conventional IV amphotericin B is used as an alternative for the treatment of invasive aspergillosis in HIV-infected adults or adolescents, the US Centers for Disease Control and Prevention (CDC), National Institutes of Health (NIH), and IDSA recommend a dosage of 1 mg/kg daily. The optimal duration of therapy in these patients has not been established, but antifungal therapy should be continued at least until CD4+ T-cell counts exceed 200/mm³ and there is evidence of resolution of aspergillosis.

Blastomycosis

For the treatment of blastomycosis, the usual dosage of conventional IV amphotericin B is 0.7–1 mg/kg once daily.

For the treatment of moderately severe to severe pulmonary or disseminated extrapulmonary blastomycosis (without CNS involvement), IDSA recommends that adults (including immunocompromised individuals) receive initial therapy with conventional IV amphotericin B in a dosage of 0.7–1 mg/kg once daily for 1–2 weeks or until improvement occurs, followed by oral itraconazole therapy. The total treatment duration should be 6–12 months for pulmonary blastomycosis or at least 12 months for disseminated extrapulmonary blastomycosis or for immunocompromised individuals.

For the treatment of severe blastomycosis in children, IDSA recommends initial therapy with conventional IV amphotericin B in a dosage of 0.7–1 mg/kg once daily, followed by oral itraconazole therapy for a total treatment duration of 12 months.

Candida Infections

For the treatment of disseminated or invasive *Candida* infections, the usual dosage of conventional IV amphotericin B in adults or pediatric patients is 0.5–1 mg/kg daily. The recommended duration of antifungal treatment for candidemia (without persistent fungemia or metastatic complications) is 2 weeks after documented clearance of *Candida* from the bloodstream, resolution of candidemia symptoms, and resolution of neutropenia.

For the treatment of neonatal candidiasis, including CNS infections, IDSA recommends that conventional IV amphotericin B be given in a dosage of 1 mg/kg daily. The recommended duration of antifungal treatment for uncomplicated neonatal candidiasis is 2 weeks after documented clearance of *Candida* from the bloodstream and resolution of candidemia symptoms. If neonatal candidiasis involves the CNS, antifungal treatment should be continued until resolution of all signs, symptoms, and CSF and radiologic abnormalities (if present).

If conventional IV amphotericin B is used as an alternative for the treatment of esophageal candidiasis† in adults who cannot tolerate oral therapy or have fluconazole-refractory infections, IDSA recommends a dosage of 0.3–0.7 mg/kg daily for 21 days. If conventional IV amphotericin B is used as an alternative for the treatment of esophageal candidiasis†, including fluconazole-refractory infections, in HIV-infected adults and adolescents, CDC, NIH, and IDSA recommend a dosage of 0.6 mg/kg daily for 14–21 days. If used as an alternative for the treatment of esophageal candidiasis† in HIV-infected infants and children, CDC, NIH, and IDSA recommend that conventional IV amphotericin B be given in a dosage of 0.3–0.7 mg/kg once daily for at least 3 weeks and for at least 2 weeks after resolution of symptoms.

If conventional IV amphotericin B is used as an alternative for the treatment of severe or refractory oropharyngeal candidiasis† (e.g., caused by fluconazole-resistant strains), IDSA recommends a dosage of 0.3 mg/kg daily.

For the treatment of symptomatic cystitis caused by fluconazole-resistant *Candida* (e.g., *C. glabrata*, *C. krusei*), IDSA recommends that conventional IV amphotericin B be given in a dosage of 0.3–0.6 mg/kg daily for 1–7 days. For the treatment of pyelonephritis caused by fluconazole-resistant *Candida*, conventional IV amphotericin B should be given in a dosage of 0.3–0.6 mg/kg daily (with or without oral flucytosine) for 1–7 days. The same regimen can be used for the treatment of urinary tract infections associated with fungus balls.

For the treatment of candiduria, conventional amphotericin B has been administered by bladder irrigation†. The optimal concentration of conventional amphotericin B for bladder irrigation†, method of irrigation (continuous or intermittent), and duration of therapy have not been established. For use as a continuous bladder irrigant†, conventional amphotericin B for injection has been reconstituted with sterile water for injection to a concentration of 50 mg/L and administered at a rate of 42 mL/hour for up to 15 days. Some clinicians suggest that lower concentrations (5–10 mg/L) may be acceptable based on usual susceptibilities of *Candida* and potential toxicity. IDSA states that a 5-day regimen of conventional amphotericin B administered by bladder irrigation† as a 50-mg/L solution in sterile water may be useful for treatment of symptomatic cystitis caused by fluconazole-resistant *Candida* (e.g., *C. glabrata*, *C. krusei*). For treatment of *Candida* urinary tract infections associated with fungus balls, IDSA states that 25–50 mg of conventional amphotericin B in 200–500 mL of sterile water administered by irrigation† through nephrostomy tubes (if present) is recommended.

Coccidioidomycosis

For the treatment of coccidioidomycosis, the usual dosage of conventional IV amphotericin B is 0.5–1.5 mg/kg daily. For the treatment of severe and/or rapidly progressive acute pulmonary or disseminated coccidioidomycosis (nonmeningeal), IV amphotericin B usually is used initially with follow-up therapy with oral fluconazole or oral itraconazole. The total duration of treatment usually is at least 1 year.

For the treatment of diffuse pulmonary or extrathoracic disseminated coccidioidomycosis (nonmeningeal) in HIV-infected adults and adolescents, CDC, NIH, and IDSA recommend initial therapy with conventional IV amphotericin B given in a dosage of 0.7–1 mg/kg daily until improvement occurs, then follow-up treatment with oral fluconazole or oral itraconazole.

For the treatment of diffuse pulmonary or disseminated coccidioidomycosis (nonmeningeal) in HIV-infected infants and children, CDC, NIH, and IDSA recommend initial therapy with conventional IV amphotericin B given in a dosage of 0.5–1 mg/kg once daily until improvement occurs, then follow-up treatment with oral fluconazole or oral itraconazole. The total duration of treatment should be 1 year.

HIV-infected adults, adolescents, or children who have been adequately treated for coccidioidomycosis should receive long-term suppressive or maintenance therapy (secondary prophylaxis) with oral fluconazole or oral itraconazole to prevent recurrence or relapse.

Cryptococcosis

If conventional IV amphotericin B is used for initial (induction) therapy in HIV-infected adults or adolescents with cryptococcal meningitis, CDC, NIH, and IDSA recommend a dosage of 0.7–1 mg/kg daily in conjunction with oral flucytosine (25 mg/kg 4 times daily) given for at least 2 weeks and until there is evidence of clinical improvement and negative CSF culture after repeat lumbar puncture, then follow-up (consolidation) therapy with oral or IV fluconazole alone given for at least 8 weeks.

If conventional IV amphotericin B is used for the treatment of cryptococcal meningitis in HIV-infected adults and adolescents who cannot receive flucytosine, CDC, NIH, and IDSA recommend initial (induction) therapy with a dosage of 0.7–1 mg/kg daily in conjunction with oral or IV fluconazole (800 mg daily) given for at least 2 weeks and until there is evidence of clinical improvement and negative CSF culture after repeat lumbar puncture, then follow-up

(consolidation) therapy with oral or IV fluconazole alone given for at least 8 weeks. Alternatively, if necessary, IDSA states that conventional IV amphotericin B can be given alone in a dosage of 0.7–1 mg/kg daily for 4–6 weeks for initial (induction) therapy followed by the usual consolidation therapy.

For the treatment of cryptococcal meningitis in immunocompetent adults without HIV infection who are not transplant recipients, IDSA recommends a regimen than includes induction therapy with conventional IV amphotericin B in a dosage of 0.7–1 mg/kg daily and oral flucytosine (25 mg/kg 4 times daily) given for at least 4 weeks (6 weeks in those with neurologic complications), then consolidation therapy with oral fluconazole alone given for 8 weeks. If the patient is immunocompetent without uncontrolled, underlying disease and is at low risk for therapeutic failure, IDSA states that the induction regimen can be given for only 2 weeks, followed by consolidation therapy with oral fluconazole alone for 8 weeks. In those who cannot receive flucytosine, induction therapy with IV amphotericin B can be given in a dosage of 0.7–1 mg/kg daily alone for at least 6 weeks, then consolidation therapy with oral fluconazole alone given for 8 weeks.

For the treatment of CNS and disseminated cryptococcal infections in children, IDSA recommends a regimen that includes induction therapy with conventional IV amphotericin B in a dosage of 1 mg/kg daily and oral flucytosine (25 mg/kg daily 4 divided doses) given for 2 weeks, then consolidation therapy with oral fluconazole alone given for at least 8 weeks. In children without HIV infection who are not transplant recipients, the induction phase should be continued for at least 4 weeks (6 weeks in those with neurologic complications) before initiating the consolidation regimen.

For the treatment of cryptococcal meningitis in HIV-infected infants and children, CDC, NIH, and IDSA recommend a regimen that includes induction therapy with conventional IV amphotericin B in a dosage of 1 mg/kg once daily in conjunction with oral flucytosine (25 mg/kg 4 times daily) given for at least 2 weeks until there is evidence of clinical improvement and negative CSF culture after repeat lumbar puncture, then consolidation therapy with IV or oral fluconazole given alone for at least 8 weeks. In HIV-infected infants and children who cannot receive flucytosine, CDC, NIH, and IDSA recommend induction therapy with conventional IV amphotericin B in a dosage of 1–1.5 mg/kg once daily alone or in conjunction with fluconazole for at least 2 weeks until there is evidence of clinical improvement and negative CSF culture after repeat lumbar puncture, then consolidation therapy with IV or oral fluconazole alone for at least 8 weeks.

For the treatment of severe pulmonary or disseminated cryptococcosis (nonmeningeal) in HIV-infected infants and children, CDC, NIH, and IDSA recommend that conventional IV amphotericin B be given in a dosage of 0.7–1 mg/kg daily (with or without oral flucytosine). The same dosage can be used without flucytosine for localized disease (e.g., isolated pulmonary disease). The treatment duration depends on the patient's response and the site and severity of infection.

Severe pulmonary cryptococcosis, cryptococcemia, or disseminated cryptococcosis in immunocompetent or immunocompromised adults, adolescents, or children should be treated using a regimen recommended for cryptococcal meningitis.

HIV-infected adults, adolescents, or children who have been adequately treated for cryptococcosis should receive long-term suppressive or maintenance therapy (secondary prophylaxis) with oral fluconazole to prevent recurrence or relapse.

If conventional IV amphotericin B is used as an alternative to oral fluconazole for long-term suppressive or maintenance therapy (secondary prophylaxis)† to prevent recurrence or relapse of cryptococcosis in HIV-infected adults and adolescents or other adults and adolescents who were adequately treated for cryptococcal meningitis, IDSA recommends a dosage of 1 mg/kg once weekly.

Histoplasmosis

If conventional IV amphotericin B is used for the treatment of moderately severe to severe acute pulmonary histoplasmosis or progressive disseminated histoplasmosis, IDSA recommends that adults receive an initial regimen of 0.7–1 mg/kg daily for 1–2 weeks, followed by oral itraconazole. The total duration of treatment should be 12 weeks in those with acute pulmonary disease or at least 12 months in those with progressive disseminated disease.

For the treatment of progressive disseminated histoplasmosis in children, IDSA states that conventional IV amphotericin B can be given in a dosage of 1 mg/kg daily for 4–6 weeks or, alternatively, an initial regimen of 1 mg/kg daily can be given for 2–4 weeks followed by oral itraconazole for a total treatment duration of 3 months.

If conventional IV amphotericin B is used as an alternative for the treatment of moderately severe to severe disseminated histoplasmosis in HIV-infected infants or children, CDC, NIH, and IDSA recommend an initial regimen of 0.7–1 mg/kg once daily for at least 2 weeks or until a response is obtained, then follow-up treatment with oral itraconazole for 12 months.

HIV-infected adults, adolescents, or children and other immunosuppressed individuals who have been adequately treated for histoplasmosis should receive long-term suppressive or maintenance therapy (secondary prophylaxis) with oral itraconazole to prevent recurrence or relapse.

Paracoccidioidomycosis

For the treatment of paracoccidioidomycosis†, conventional IV amphotericin B has been given in a dosage of 0.4–0.5 mg/kg daily, although higher dosages (i.e., 1 mg/kg daily or, rarely, 1.5 mg/kg daily) have been used for the treatment of rapidly progressing, potentially fatal infections. Prolonged therapy usually is required. In severely ill patients, some clinicians recommend that conventional IV amphotericin B be given in a dosage of 0.7–1 mg/kg daily for initial treatment followed by oral itraconazole therapy.

Sporotrichosis

For the treatment of sporotrichosis, the manufacturers state that conventional IV amphotericin B has been given for up to 9 months with a total dose of up to 2.5 g.

For the treatment of osteoarticular sporotrichosis, severe or life-threatening pulmonary sporotrichosis, or disseminated sporotrichosis, IDSA recommends that adults receive conventional IV amphotericin B in a dosage of 0.7–1 mg/kg daily until a response is obtained, followed by oral itraconazole (200 mg twice daily) given for a total treatment duration of at least 12 months. IDSA and other clinicians state that a lipid formulation of amphotericin B may be preferred for the treatment of disseminated sporotrichosis.

For the treatment of meningeal sporotrichosis, IDSA recommends that adults receive conventional IV amphotericin B in a dosage of 0.7–1 mg/kg daily for at least 4–6 weeks, followed by oral itraconazole (200 mg twice daily) for a total treatment duration of at least 12 months. IDSA and other clinicians state that a lipid formulation of amphotericin B may be preferred (rather than conventional amphotericin B) for the treatment of meningeal sporotrichosis.

For the treatment of disseminated sporotrichosis in children, IDSA recommends that conventional IV amphotericin B be given in a dosage of 0.7 mg/kg daily until a response is obtained, followed by oral itraconazole for a total treatment duration of at least 12 months.

Zygomycosis

For the treatment of zygomycosis, including mucormycosis, the usual dosage of conventional IV amphotericin B is 1–1.5 mg/kg daily for 2–3 months. For the treatment of rhinocerebral phycomycosis, the manufacturer recommends a total treatment dose of at least 3 g. Although a total treatment dose of 3–4 g can cause lasting renal impairment, the manufacturer states that this is a reasonable minimum dosage if there is clinical evidence of invasion of deep tissue since such infections usually are rapidly fatal and an aggressive therapeutic approach is necessary.

Adjunctive Therapy in CNS Fungal Infections

For the treatment of CNS fungal infections (e.g., candidal, coccidioidal, or cryptococcal meningitis), intracisternal†, intraventricular†, or intrathecal† injection of conventional amphotericin B has been used in conjunction with IV administration. For intrathecal† administration, amphotericin B has been reconstituted with sterile water for injection to a concentration of 0.25 mg/mL. The usual initial dose is 0.025 mg (0.1 mL of the reconstituted injection diluted with 10–20 mL of CSF and administered by barbotage) 2 or 3 times per week. The dose is gradually increased until the maximum dose is reached that can be given without causing severe discomfort. This dose usually is 0.5–1 mg, although 0.2–0.3 mg may be effective in some infections and others (e.g., coccidioidal meningitis) may require up 1.5 mg; corticosteroids (10–15 mg of hydrocortisone in adults) usually are added to relieve headache. (See Drug Interactions: Corticosteroids.)

Empiric Therapy in Febrile Neutropenic Patients

For the empiric treatment of presumed fungal infections in febrile neutropenic patients†, conventional IV amphotericin B has been given in a dosage of 0.5–1 mg/kg daily.

Empiric antifungal therapy should be discontinued when neutropenia resolves. In those with prolonged neutropenia, IDSA suggests that such therapy may be discontinued after 2 weeks if the patient is clinically well and no discernible lesions are found by clinical evaluation, chest radiographs, or CT scans of abdominal organs. If the patient appears ill or is at high risk, consideration can be given to continuing empiric antifungal treatment throughout the neutropenic episode.

Prevention of Fungal Infections in Transplant Recipients, Cancer Patients, or Other Individuals at High Risk

For prophylaxis of fungal infections in neutropenic cancer patients† or patients undergoing bone marrow transplantation† (BMT), conventional IV amphotericin B has been administered in a dosage of 0.1 mg/kg daily.

For high-risk patients undergoing urologic procedures†, IDSA states that conventional IV amphotericin B can be given in a dosage of 0.3–0.6 mg/kg daily for several days before and after the procedure.

Leishmaniasis

For the treatment of American cutaneous leishmaniasis caused by *Leishmania braziliensis* or *L. mexicana* or the treatment of mucocutaneous leishmaniasis caused by *L. braziliensis*, conventional IV amphotericin B has been given in a dosage of 0.25–0.5 mg/kg daily, with dosage gradually increased until 0.5–1 mg/kg daily was reached, at which time the drug was given on alternate days. Duration of therapy depends on the severity of disease and response to the drug, but is generally 3–12 weeks and the total dose generally ranges from 1–3 g.

For the treatment of mucosal disease, some clinicians recommend that conventional IV amphotericin B be given in a dosage 0.5–1 mg/kg daily or every other day for 4–8 weeks.

Visceral leishmaniasis (also known as kala-azar) in adults and children has been treated with 0.5–1 mg/kg of conventional IV amphotericin B† administered on alternate days for 14–20 doses. Some clinicians recommend that adults and children with visceral leishmaniasis receive a total treatment dosage of 15–20 mg/kg of conventional IV amphotericin B† given as 1 mg/kg daily for 15–20 days or 1 mg/kg every second day for 4–8 weeks.

If conventional IV amphotericin B† is used as an alternative to amphotericin B liposomal in HIV-infected adults and adolescents with visceral leishmaniasis, CDC, NIH, and IDSA recommend a dosage of 0.5–1 mg/kg daily for a total treatment dosage of 1.5–2 g. Long-term suppressive or maintenance therapy (secondary prophylaxis) with amphotericin B liposomal may be indicated. (See Leishmaniasis under Dosage: Amphotericin B Liposomal [Ambisome®], in Dosage and Administration.)

Primary Amebic Meningoencephalitis

If conventional IV amphotericin B is used for the treatment of primary amebic meningoencephalitis caused by *Naegleria fowleri*†, a dosage of 1.5 mg/kg daily in 2 divided doses for 3 consecutive days, then 1 mg/kg IV once daily for 11 consecutive days, has been recommended. If conventional amphotericin B is administered intrathecally† for the treatment of primary amebic meningoencephalitis, a dosage of 1.5 mg once daily for 2 days, then 1 mg every other day for 8 days, has been recommended. If conventional amphotericin B is administered by both routes in the same patient, some clinicians state that the maximum total dosage in adults and children is 1.5 mg/kg daily. Amphotericin B should be used in conjunction with other anti-infectives. Consultation with a specialist at CDC is recommended. (See Primary Amebic Meningoencephalitis under Uses: Protozoal Infections.)

Amphotericin B Lipid Complex (Abelcet®)

For the treatment of invasive fungal infections in adults and children, the manufacturer of amphotericin B lipid complex recommends a dosage of 5 mg/kg IV once daily.

Aspergillosis

If IV amphotericin B lipid complex is used as an alternative for the treatment of invasive aspergillosis, IDSA recommends a dosage of 5 mg/kg daily. The duration of treatment is based on the degree and duration of immunosuppression, disease site, and clinical response. IDSA recommends that antifungal treatment of invasive pulmonary aspergillosis be continued for at least 6–12 weeks.

If a lipid formulation of amphotericin B is used as an alternative for the treatment of invasive aspergillosis in HIV-infected adults and adolescents, CDC, NIH, and IDSA recommend a dosage of 5 mg/kg IV once daily. The optimal duration of therapy in these patients has not been established, but antifungal therapy should be continued at least until CD4+ T-cell counts exceed 200/mm³ and there is evidence of resolution of aspergillosis.

Blastomycosis

If a lipid formulation of IV amphotericin B is used for the treatment of moderate to severe pulmonary or disseminated extrapulmonary blastomycosis (without CNS involvement), IDSA recommends that adults (including immunocompromised individuals) receive initial therapy with a dosage of 3–5 mg/kg once daily for 1–2 weeks or until improvement occurs, followed by oral itraconazole therapy. Total treatment duration should be 6–12 months for pulmonary blastomycosis or at least 12 months for disseminated extrapulmonary blastomycosis or for immunocompromised individuals.

If a lipid formulation of IV amphotericin B is used for the treatment of severe blastomycosis in children, IDSA recommends initial therapy with a dosage of 3–5 mg/kg daily, followed by oral itraconazole therapy for a total treatment duration of 12 months.

For the treatment of CNS blastomycosis, IDSA recommends that adults receive initial therapy with a lipid formulation of IV amphotericin B given in a dosage of 5 mg/kg daily for 4–6 weeks, followed by an oral azole (fluconazole, itraconazole, voriconazole) given for at least 12 months and until resolution of CSF abnormalities.

Candida Infections

If a lipid formulation of amphotericin B is used for initial treatment of candidemia or other invasive *Candida* infections in nonneutropenic or neutropenic adults, IDSA recommends a dosage of 3–5 mg/kg daily. These experts state that a transition to fluconazole can be considered (usually within 5–7 days) in nonneutropenic patients who are clinically stable, have isolates susceptible to fluconazole (e.g., *C. albicans*), and have negative repeat blood cultures after initial antifungal treatment. IDSA recommends that antifungal treatment for candidemia (without persistent fungemia or metastatic complications) be continued for 2 weeks after documented clearance of *Candida* from the bloodstream, resolution of candidemia symptoms, and resolution of neutropenia.

If a lipid formulation of amphotericin B is used for the treatment of chronic disseminated (hepatosplenic) candidiasis, IDSA recommends initial treatment with a dosage of 3–5 mg/kg daily for several weeks followed by oral fluconazole. Antifungal treatment should be continued until lesions resolve on repeat imaging (usually several months).

If a lipid formulation of amphotericin B is used for initial treatment of endocarditis (native or prosthetic valve) or implantable cardiac device infections caused by *Candida*, IDSA recommends a dosage of 3–5 mg/kg daily given with or without oral flucytosine. If the infection is caused by fluconazole-susceptible *Candida*, treatment can be transitioned to fluconazole after the patient is stabilized and *Candida* has been cleared from the bloodstream.

If a lipid formulation of amphotericin B is used as an alternative for the treatment of esophageal candidiasis†, including fluconazole-refractory infections, in HIV-infected adults and adolescents, CDC, NIH, and IDSA recommend a dosage of 3–4 mg/kg IV once daily for 14–21 days.

If a lipid formulation of amphotericin B is used for the treatment of invasive *C. auris* infections (e.g., bloodstream or intra-abdominal infections) in adults (see Candida auris Infections under Uses: Candida Infections), CDC recommends a dosage of 3–5 mg/kg IV daily.

Coccidioidomycosis

If a lipid formulation of IV amphotericin B is used for the treatment of diffuse pulmonary or extrathoracic disseminated coccidioidomycosis (nonmeningeal) in HIV-infected adults of adolescents, CDC, NIH, and IDSA recommend a dosage of 4–6 mg/kg daily until improvement occurs, then follow-up treatment with oral fluconazole or oral itraconazole.

If a lipid formulation of IV amphotericin B is used for the treatment of diffuse pulmonary or disseminated coccidioidomycosis (nonmeningeal) in HIV-infected infants and children, CDC, NIH, and IDSA recommend a dosage of 5 mg/kg once daily until improvement occurs, then follow-up treatment with oral fluconazole or oral itraconazole. The total duration of treatment should be 1 year.

HIV-infected adults, adolescents, or children who have been adequately treated for coccidioidomycosis should receive long-term suppressive or maintenance therapy (secondary prophylaxis) with oral fluconazole or oral itraconazole to prevent recurrence or relapse.

Cryptococcosis

If amphotericin B lipid complex is used for initial (induction) therapy in HIV-infected adults and adolescents with cryptococcal meningitis, CDC, NIH, and IDSA recommend a dosage of 5 mg/kg daily in conjunction with oral flucytosine (25 mg/kg 4 times daily) given for at least 2 weeks and until there is evidence of clinical improvement and negative CSF culture after repeat lumbar puncture, then follow-up (consolidation) therapy with oral or IV fluconazole given for at least 8 weeks. Alternatively, if necessary, IDSA states that IV amphotericin B lipid complex can be given alone in a dosage of 5 mg/kg daily for 4–6 weeks for initial (induction) therapy followed by the usual consolidation therapy.

For the treatment of CNS cryptococcosis in adult organ transplant recipients, IDSA recommends induction therapy with IV amphotericin B lipid complex in a dosage of 5 mg/kg daily and oral flucytosine (100 mg/kg daily in 4 divided doses) given for at least 2 weeks, then consolidation therapy with oral fluconazole given for 8 weeks followed by a maintenance regimen of oral fluconazole given for 6–12 months. If flucytosine cannot be used in the induction regimen, consideration should be given to continuing induction therapy with IV amphotericin B lipid complex for at least 4–6 weeks before initiating consolidation therapy with oral fluconazole.

For the treatment of cryptococcal meningitis in immunocompetent adults without HIV infection who are not transplant recipients and when conventional IV amphotericin B cannot be used (e.g., patients who have or are predisposed to renal dysfunction), IDSA recommends a regimen than includes induction therapy with IV amphotericin B lipid complex in a dosage of 5 mg/kg daily given with oral flucytosine (100 mg/kg daily in 4 divided doses) for at least 4 weeks (6 weeks in those with neurologic complications), then consolidation therapy with oral fluconazole given for 8 weeks. If the patient is immunocompetent without uncontrolled, underlying disease and is at low risk for therapeutic failure, IDSA states that the induction regimen can be given for only 2 weeks, followed by consolidation therapy with oral fluconazole for 8 weeks. In those who cannot receive flucytosine, induction therapy with IV amphotericin B lipid complex can be given in a dosage of 5 mg/kg daily alone for at least 6 weeks, then consolidation therapy with oral fluconazole given for 8 weeks.

If amphotericin B lipid complex is used for the treatment of cryptococcal meningitis in HIV-infected infants and children, CDC, NIH, and IDSA recommend induction therapy with 5 mg/kg once daily given with oral flucytosine for at least 2 weeks until there is evidence of clinical improvement and negative CSF culture after repeat lumbar puncture, then consolidation therapy with oral or IV fluconazole alone for at least 8 weeks.

For the treatment of CNS and disseminated cryptococcal infections in children who cannot receive conventional IV amphotericin B, IDSA recommends a regimen that includes induction therapy with IV amphotericin B lipid complex in a dosage of 5 mg/kg daily given with oral flucytosine (100 mg/kg daily in 4 divided doses) for 2 weeks, then consolidation therapy with oral fluconazole given for at least 8 weeks. In children without HIV infection who are not transplant recipients, the induction phase should be continued for at least 4 weeks (6 weeks in those with neurologic complications) before initiating the consolidation regimen.

If amphotericin B lipid complex is used in HIV-infected infants and children with severe pulmonary or disseminated cryptococcosis (nonmeningeal), CDC, NIH, and IDSA recommend a dosage of 5 mg/kg once daily (with or without oral flucytosine). The same dosage can be used without flucytosine for localized disease (e.g., isolated pulmonary disease). The treatment duration depends on the patient's response and site and severity of infection.

HIV-infected adults, adolescents, or children who have been adequately treated for cryptococcosis should receive long-term suppressive or maintenance therapy (secondary prophylaxis) with oral fluconazole to prevent recurrence or relapse.

Histoplasmosis

If IV amphotericin B lipid complex is used for the treatment of moderately severe to severe disseminated histoplasmosis in HIV-infected adults and adolescents, CDC, NIH, and IDSA recommend an initial (induction) regimen of 3 mg/kg daily given for at least 2 weeks or until a response is obtained, then follow-up treatment with oral itraconazole for at least 12 months.

HIV-infected adults, adolescents, or children and other immunosuppressed individuals who have been adequately treated for histoplasmosis should receive long-term suppressive or maintenance therapy (secondary prophylaxis) with oral itraconazole to prevent recurrence or relapse.

Empiric Therapy in Febrile Neutropenic Patients

For the empiric treatment of presumed fungal infections in febrile neutropenic patients†, amphotericin B lipid complex has been given in a dosage of 3–5 mg/kg daily.

Empiric antifungal therapy should be discontinued when neutropenia resolves. In those with prolonged neutropenia, IDSA suggests that such therapy may be discontinued after 2 weeks if the patient is clinically well and no discernible lesions are found by clinical evaluation, chest radiographs, or CT scans of abdominal organs. If the patient appears ill or is at high risk, consideration can be given to continuing empiric antifungal treatment throughout the neutropenic episode.

Leishmaniasis

For the treatment of visceral leishmaniasis† (kala-azar), amphotericin B lipid complex has been given in a dosage of 1–3 mg/kg once daily for 5–10 days.

If amphotericin B lipid complex is used for the treatment of cutaneous leishmaniasis† in HIV-infected adults and adolescents, CDC, NIH, and IDSA recommend a dosage of 2–4 mg/kg daily for a total treatment dosage of 20–60 mg/kg. Alternatively, a dosage of 4 mg/kg daily on days 1–5, 10, 17, 24, 31, and 38 for a total treatment dosage of 20–60 mg/kg can be used.

If amphotericin B lipid complex is used for long-term suppressive or maintenance therapy (secondary prophylaxis)† in HIV-infected adults and adolescents who have been adequately treated for visceral leishmaniasis, CDC, NIH, and IDSA recommend a dosage of 3 mg/kg once every 21 days. Some experts state that consideration can be given to discontinuing secondary prophylaxis against leishmaniasis in HIV-infected individuals who have CD4+ T-cell counts that have remained greater than 200–350/mm^3 for 3–6 months or longer. Other clinicians suggest that secondary prophylaxis against leishmaniasis should be continued indefinitely in HIV-infected individuals.

Amphotericin B Liposomal (AmBisome®)

For the treatment of systemic fungal infections, the usual dosage of IV amphotericin B liposomal for adults or children 1 month of age or older is 3–5 mg/kg once daily.

Aspergillosis

For the treatment of aspergillosis, the usual dosage of IV amphotericin B liposomal for adults or children 1 month of age or older is 3–5 mg/kg once daily. In the treatment of invasive aspergillosis, use of higher dosage (10 mg/kg daily) does not result in improved efficacy and is associated with an increased incidence of adverse effects (e.g., nephrotoxicity).

The duration of treatment is based on the degree and duration of immunosuppression, disease site, and clinical response. IDSA recommends that antifungal treatment of invasive pulmonary aspergillosis be continued for at least 6–12 weeks. In published studies, the median duration of amphotericin B liposomal therapy for the effective treatment of aspergillosis has ranged from 15–29 days.

If a lipid formulation of IV amphotericin B is used as an alternative for the treatment of invasive aspergillosis in HIV-infected adults, CDC, NIH, and IDSA recommend 5 mg/kg IV once daily. The optimal duration of therapy in these patients has not been established, but antifungal therapy should be continued at least until CD4+ T-cell counts exceed 200/mm^3 and there is evidence of resolution of aspergillosis.

Blastomycosis

If a lipid formulation of IV amphotericin B is used for the treatment of moderate to severe pulmonary or disseminated extrapulmonary blastomycosis (without CNS involvement), IDSA recommends that adults (including immunocompromised individuals) receive initial therapy with a dosage of 3–5 mg/kg once daily for 1–2 weeks or until improvement occurs, followed by oral itraconazole therapy. The total treatment duration should be 6–12 months for pulmonary blastomycosis or at least 12 months for disseminated extrapulmonary blastomycosis or for immunocompromised individuals.

If a lipid formulation of IV amphotericin B is used for the treatment of severe blastomycosis in children, IDSA recommends initial therapy with a dosage of 3–5 mg/kg once daily, followed by oral itraconazole therapy for a total treatment duration of 12 months.

For the treatment of CNS blastomycosis, IDSA recommends that adults receive initial therapy with a lipid formulation of IV amphotericin B given in a dosage of 5 mg/kg once daily for 4–6 weeks, followed by oral azole therapy (fluconazole, itraconazole, voriconazole). The total duration of treatment should be at least 12 months and until CSF abnormalities resolve.

Candida Infections

For the treatment of systemic *Candida* infections, the usual dosage of IV amphotericin B liposomal for adults and children 1 month of age or older is 3–5 mg/kg once daily. In published studies, the median duration of amphotericin B liposomal therapy for the effective treatment of candidiasis has ranged from 15–29 days, although some *Candida* infections were effectively treated with a median duration of therapy of 5–7 days.

If a lipid formulation of IV amphotericin B is used for initial treatment of candidemia or other invasive *Candida* infections in nonneutropenic or neutropenic adults, IDSA recommends a dosage of 3–5 mg/kg daily. These experts state that a transition to fluconazole can be considered (usually within 5–7 days) in nonneutropenic patients who are clinically stable, have isolates susceptible to fluconazole (e.g., *C. albicans*), and have negative repeat blood cultures after initial antifungal treatment. IDSA recommends that antifungal treatment for candidemia (without persistent fungemia or metastatic complications) be continued for 2 weeks after documented clearance of *Candida* from the bloodstream, resolution of candidemia symptoms, and resolution of neutropenia.

If a lipid formulation of amphotericin B is used for the treatment of chronic disseminated (hepatosplenic) candidiasis, IDSA recommends initial treatment with a dosage of 3–5 mg/kg daily for several weeks followed by oral fluconazole. Antifungal treatment should be continued until lesions resolve on repeat imaging (usually several months).

If IV amphotericin B liposomal is used for treatment of CNS candidiasis, IDSA recommends a dosage of 5 mg/kg daily (with or without oral flucytosine). After a response is attained, transition to fluconazole can be considered. Antifungal treatment should be continued until signs and symptoms, CSF abnormalities, and radiologic abnormalities have resolved.

If a lipid formulation of IV amphotericin B is used for initial treatment of endocarditis (native or prosthetic valve) or implantable cardiac device infections caused by *Candida*, IDSA recommends a dosage of 3–5 mg/kg daily given with or without oral flucytosine. If the infection is caused by fluconazole-susceptible *Candida*, treatment can be transitioned to fluconazole after the patient is stabilized and *Candida* has been cleared from the bloodstream.

If a lipid formulation of IV amphotericin B is used as an alternative for the treatment of esophageal candidiasis†, including fluconazole-refractory infections, in HIV-infected adults and adolescents, CDC, NIH, and IDSA recommend a dosage of 3–4 mg/kg IV once daily for 14–21 days.

If IV amphotericin B liposomal is used for treatment of endophthalmitis caused by fluconazole- and voriconazole-resistant *Candida*, IDSA recommends a dosage of 3–5 mg/kg daily (with or without oral flucytosine). In patients with macular involvement, intravitreal administration of *conventional* IV amphotericin B† also is recommended to ensure prompt high levels of antifungal activity.

If a lipid formulation of IV amphotericin B is used for the treatment of invasive *C. auris* infections (e.g., bloodstream or intra-abdominal infections) in adults (see Candida auris Infections under Uses: Candida Infections), CDC recommends a dosage of 3–5 mg/kg IV daily.

Coccidioidomycosis

If a lipid formulation of IV amphotericin B is used for the treatment of diffuse pulmonary or extrathoracic disseminated coccidioidomycosis (nonmeningeal) in HIV-infected adults of adolescents, CDC, NIH, and IDSA recommend a dosage of 4–6 mg/kg daily until improvement occurs, then follow-up treatment with oral fluconazole or oral itraconazole.

If a lipid formulation of IV amphotericin B is used for the treatment of diffuse pulmonary or disseminated coccidioidomycosis (nonmeningeal) in HIV-infected infants and children, CDC, NIH, and IDSA recommend a dosage of 5 mg/kg daily until improvement occurs, then follow-up treatment with oral fluconazole or oral itraconazole. The total duration of treatment should be 1 year.

HIV-infected adults, adolescents, or children who have been adequately treated for coccidioidomycosis should receive long-term suppressive or maintenance therapy (secondary prophylaxis) with oral fluconazole or oral itraconazole to prevent recurrence or relapse.

Cryptococcosis

For empiric treatment of cryptococcosis in adults and children 1 month of age or older, the manufacturer recommends that IV amphotericin B liposomal be given in a dosage of 3–5 mg/kg daily. For the treatment of cryptococcal meningitis in HIV-infected adults and children 1 month of age or older, the manufacturer recommends that IV amphotericin B liposomal be given in a dosage of 6 mg/kg daily.

For the treatment of cryptococcal meningitis in HIV-infected adults and adolescents, CDC, NIH, and IDSA recommend a regimen than includes initial (induction) therapy with IV amphotericin B liposomal in a dosage of 3–4 mg/kg daily in conjunction with oral flucytosine (25 mg/kg 4 times daily) given for at least 2 weeks and until there is evidence of clinical improvement and negative CSF culture after repeat lumbar puncture, then follow-up (consolidation) therapy with oral or IV fluconazole given for at least 8 weeks.

For the treatment of cryptococcal meningitis in HIV-infected adults and adolescents who cannot receive flucytosine, CDC, NIH, and IDSA recommend initial (induction) therapy with IV amphotericin B liposomal given in a dosage of 3–4 mg/kg once daily in conjunction with oral or IV fluconazole (800 mg daily) for at least 2 weeks and until there is evidence of clinical improvement and negative CSF culture after repeat lumbar puncture, then follow-up (consolidation) therapy with oral or IV fluconazole alone given for at least 8 weeks. Alternatively, if necessary, a regimen of IV amphotericin B liposomal alone given in a dosage of 3–4 mg/kg once daily can be used for initial (induction) therapy followed by the usual consolidation therapy.

For the treatment of CNS cryptococcosis in adult organ transplant recipients, IDSA recommends induction therapy with IV amphotericin B liposomal in a dosage of 3–4 mg/kg daily and oral flucytosine (100 mg/kg daily in 4 divided doses) given for at least 2 weeks, then consolidation therapy with oral fluconazole given for 8 weeks followed by a maintenance regimen of oral fluconazole given for 6–12 months. Alternatively, if flucytosine cannot be used in the induction regimen, consideration should be given to using a regimen of IV amphotericin B liposomal in a dosage of 6 mg/kg daily given for at least 4–6 weeks followed by the usual consolidation therapy with oral fluconazole.

For the treatment of cryptococcal meningitis in immunocompetent adults without HIV infection who are not transplant recipients and when conventional IV amphotericin B cannot be used (e.g., patients who have or are predisposed to renal dysfunction), IDSA recommends a regimen than includes induction therapy with IV amphotericin B liposomal in a dosage of 3–4 mg/kg daily with oral flucytosine (100 mg/kg daily in 4 divided doses) given for at least 4 weeks (6 weeks in those with neurologic complications), then consolidation therapy with oral fluconazole given for 8 weeks. If the patient is immunocompetent without uncontrolled, underlying disease and is at low risk for therapeutic failure, IDSA states that the induction regimen can be given for only 2 weeks, followed by consolidation therapy with oral fluconazole for 8 weeks. In those who cannot receive flucytosine, induction therapy with IV amphotericin B liposomal alone given in a dosage of 3–4 mg/kg daily for at least 6 weeks can be used, followed by consolidation therapy with oral fluconazole given for 8 weeks.

For the treatment of CNS and disseminated cryptococcal infections in children who cannot receive conventional IV amphotericin B, IDSA recommends a regimen that includes induction therapy with IV amphotericin B liposomal in a dosage of 5 mg/kg daily with oral flucytosine (100 mg/kg daily in 4 divided doses) given for 2 weeks, then consolidation therapy with oral fluconazole given for at least 8 weeks. In children without HIV infection who are not transplant recipients, the induction phase should be continued for at least 4 weeks (6 weeks in those with neurologic complications) before initiating the consolidation regimen.

For the treatment of cryptococcal meningitis in HIV-infected infants and children, CDC, NIH, and IDSA recommend a regimen that includes induction therapy with IV amphotericin B liposomal in a dosage of 6 mg/kg once daily in conjunction with oral flucytosine (25 mg/kg 4 times daily) given for at least 2 weeks until there is evidence of clinical improvement and negative CSF culture after repeat lumbar puncture, then consolidation therapy with IV or oral fluconazole given alone for at least 8 weeks. In HIV-infected infants and children who cannot receive flucytosine, CDC, NIH, and IDSA recommend induction therapy with IV amphotericin B liposomal in a dosage of 6 mg/kg once daily alone or in conjunction with IV fluconazole for at least 2 weeks until there is evidence of clinical improvement and negative CSF culture after repeat lumbar puncture, then consolidation therapy with IV or oral fluconazole alone for at least 8 weeks.

If amphotericin B liposomal is used in HIV-infected infants and children with severe pulmonary or disseminated cryptococcosis (nonmeningeal), CDC, NIH, and IDSA recommend a dosage of 3–5 mg/kg once daily (with or without oral flucytosine). The same dosage can be used without flucytosine for localized disease (e.g., isolated pulmonary disease). The treatment duration depends on the patient's response and site and severity of infection.

HIV-infected adults, adolescents, or children who have been adequately treated for cryptococcosis should receive long-term suppressive or maintenance therapy (secondary prophylaxis) with oral fluconazole to prevent recurrence or relapse.

Histoplasmosis

For the treatment of moderately severe to severe acute pulmonary histoplasmosis, IDSA recommends that adults receive an initial regimen of IV amphotericin B liposomal given in a dosage of 3–5 mg/kg daily for 1–2 weeks, followed by oral itraconazole for a total treatment duration of 12 weeks. For the treatment of moderately severe to severe progressive disseminated histoplasmosis, IDSA recommends that adults receive an initial regimen of IV amphotericin B liposomal

given in a dosage of 3 mg/kg daily for 1–2 weeks, followed by oral itraconazole for a total treatment duration of at least 12 months.

For the treatment of moderately severe to severe disseminated histoplasmosis in HIV-infected adults or adolescents, CDC, NIH, and IDSA recommend an initial (induction) regimen of IV amphotericin B liposomal in a dosage of 3 mg/kg once daily given for at least 2 weeks or until a response is obtained, then follow-up treatment with oral itraconazole for at least 12 months. In HIV-infected infants or children, CDC, NIH, and IDSA recommend an initial (induction) regimen of IV amphotericin B liposomal in a dosage of 3–5 mg/kg once daily given for at least 2 weeks or until a response is obtained, then follow-up treatment with oral itraconazole for 12 months.

For the treatment of CNS histoplasmosis in HIV-infected adults, adolescents, or children or other adults, CDC, NIH, and IDSA recommend an initial regimen of IV amphotericin B liposomal given in a dosage of 5 mg/kg once daily for 4–6 weeks and follow-up treatment with oral itraconazole given for a total treatment duration of at least 12 months and until abnormal CSF findings resolve and histoplasmal antigen is undetectable.

HIV-infected adults, adolescents, or children and other immunosuppressed individuals who have been adequately treated for histoplasmosis should receive long-term suppressive or maintenance therapy (secondary prophylaxis) with oral itraconazole to prevent recurrence or relapse.

Exserohilum Infections

If IV amphotericin B liposomal is used for the treatment of CNS and/or parameningeal infections known or suspected to be caused by *Exserohilum rostratum*† in adults who received injections of a contaminated corticosteroid product (see Uses: Exserohilum Infections), CDC recommends a dosage of 5–6 mg/kg daily. Higher dosage (7.5 mg/kg daily) may be considered in patients who are not improving, but the increased risk of nephrotoxicity should be considered. Administration of 1 L of 0.9% sodium chloride injection prior to IV infusion of amphotericin B liposomal may be considered to minimize risk of nephrotoxicity.

If IV amphotericin B liposomal is used for the treatment of osteoarticular infections known or suspected to be caused by *E. rostratum*† in adults who received intra-articular injections of a contaminated corticosteroid product (see Uses: Exserohilum Infections), CDC recommends a dosage of 5 mg/kg daily.

Adequate duration of antifungal treatment for infections related to contaminated corticosteroid products is unknown, but prolonged treatment is required and should be based on disease severity and clinical response. A treatment duration of 6–12 months is probably necessary in patients who have severe CNS disease with complications (arachnoiditis, stroke), persistent CSF abnormalities, or underlying immunosuppression. In those with parameningeal infection, a minimum treatment duration of 3–6 months should be considered, and at least 6 months or longer probably is required for more severe disease (e.g., discitis, osteomyelitis) and in those with underlying immunosuppression or complications not amenable to surgical treatment. In those with osteoarticular infections, a minimum treatment duration of 3 months should be considered, and longer than 3 months is probably necessary in those with severe disease, bone infections, or underlying immunosuppression. After completion of treatment, close follow-up monitoring is essential in all patients to detect potential relapse.

An infectious disease expert and the most recent guidelines from CDC should be consulted for information regarding the management of infections in patients who received injections of potentially contaminated products. Clinicians should consult the CDC website at https://www.cdc.gov/hai/outbreaks/meningitis.html for the most recent recommendations regarding the drugs of choice, dosage, and duration of treatment of these infections.

Penicilliosis

For the treatment of severe, acute penicilliosis† in HIV-infected adults and adolescents, CDC, NIH, and IDSA recommend that IV amphotericin B liposomal be given in a dosage of 3–5 mg/kg daily for 2 weeks, followed by oral itraconazole (200 mg twice daily) for 10 weeks.

After the patient has been adequately treated, long-term suppressive or maintenance therapy (secondary prophylaxis) with oral itraconazole is recommended to prevent recurrence or relapse.

Empiric Therapy in Febrile Neutropenic Patients

For the empiric treatment of presumed fungal infections in febrile neutropenic patients 1 month of age or older, the usual dosage of amphotericin B liposomal is 3 mg/kg once daily. In one limited study, the median duration of empiric therapy was 10.8 days.

Empiric antifungal therapy should be discontinued when neutropenia resolves. In those with prolonged neutropenia, IDSA suggests that such therapy may be discontinued after 2 weeks if the patient is clinically well and no discernible lesions are found by clinical evaluation, chest radiographs, or CT scans of abdominal organs. If the patient appears ill or is at high risk, consideration can be given to continuing empiric antifungal treatment throughout the neutropenic episode.

Prevention of Fungal Infections in Transplant Recipients, Cancer Patients, or Other Individuals at High Risk

For postoperative prophylaxis in liver, pancreas, or small bowel transplant recipients† at high risk of candidiasis, IDSA states that IV amphotericin B liposomal can be given in a dosage of 1–2 mg/kg daily for at least 7–14 days.

Leishmaniasis

For the treatment of visceral leishmaniasis (also known as kala-azar) in immunocompetent adults and children 1 month of age or older, the manufacturer recommends that amphotericin B liposomal be given in a dosage of 3 mg/kg once daily on days 1–5, then 3 mg/kg should be given once daily on days 14 and 21; a second course of the drug may be useful if the parasitic infection is not completely cleared with a single course. For the treatment of visceral leishmaniasis in immunocompromised adults and children 1 month of age or older, the manufacturer recommends that amphotericin B liposomal be given in a dosage of 4 mg/kg once daily on days 1–5, then 4 mg/kg once daily on days 10, 17, 24, 31, and 38; however, if the parasitic infection is not completely cleared after the first course or if relapses occur, an expert should be consulted regarding further treatment. Various other dosage regimens have been used, including 5–7.5 mg/kg or 10 mg/kg once daily for 2 consecutive days.

If amphotericin B liposomal is used for the treatment of cutaneous leishmaniasis† in HIV-infected adults and adolescents, CDC, NIH, and IDSA recommend a dosage of 2–4 mg/kg daily for a total treatment dosage of 20–60 mg/kg. Alternatively, a dosage of 4 mg/kg daily on days 1–5, 10, 17, 24, 31, and 38 for a total treatment dosage of 20–60 mg/kg can be used.

If amphotericin B liposomal is used for the treatment of visceral leishmaniasis in HIV-infected adults and adolescents, CDC, NIH, and IDSA recommend a dosage of 2–4 mg/kg daily for a total treatment dosage of 20–60 mg/kg. Alternatively, a dosage of 4 mg/kg daily on days 1–5, 10, 17, 24, 31, and 38 for a total treatment dosage of 20–60 mg/kg can be used.

If amphotericin B liposomal is used for long-term suppressive or maintenance therapy (secondary prophylaxis)† in HIV-infected adults and adolescents who have been adequately treated for visceral leishmaniasis and have CD4+ T-cell counts less than 200/mm³, CDC, NIH, and IDSA recommend a dosage of 4 mg/kg once every 2–4 weeks. Some experts state that consideration can be given to discontinuing secondary prophylaxis against leishmaniasis in HIV-infected adults and adolescents who have CD4+ T-cell counts that have remained greater than 200–350/mm³ for 3–6 months or longer. Other clinicians suggest that secondary prophylaxis against leishmaniasis should be continued indefinitely in HIV-infected individuals.

CAUTIONS

Conventional IV amphotericin B is associated with a high incidence of adverse effects, and most patients who receive the drug experience potentially severe adverse effects at some time during the course of therapy. Acute infusion reactions (e.g., fever, shaking chills, hypotension, headache, anorexia, nausea, vomiting, tachypnea) and nephrotoxicity are common adverse reactions to conventional IV amphotericin B.

Although clinical experience with amphotericin B lipid complex (Abelcet®) and amphotericin B liposomal (AmBisome®) is limited to date, these drugs appear to be better tolerated than conventional IV amphotericin B. As with conventional IV amphotericin B, the most frequent adverse reactions to amphotericin B lipid complex or amphotericin B liposomal are acute infusion reactions; however, data accumulated to date indicate that lipid formulations of amphotericin B may be associated with a lower overall incidence of adverse effects and a lower incidence of hematologic and renal toxicity than the conventional formulation of the drug.

● Acute Infusion Reactions

Acute infusion reactions consisting of fever, shaking chills, hypotension, anorexia, nausea, vomiting, headache, dyspnea, and tachypnea may occur 1–3 hours after initiation of IV infusions of conventional amphotericin B, amphotericin B lipid complex, or amphotericin B liposomal. These reactions are most severe and occur most frequently with initial doses and usually lessen with subsequent doses. Fever (with or without shaking chills) usually occurs within 15–20 minutes after IV infusions of conventional amphotericin B are started. The majority of patients receiving conventional IV amphotericin B (50–90%) exhibit some degree of intolerance to initial doses of the drug, even when therapy is initiated with low doses.

In a study designed to evaluate the incidence of infusion reactions occurring in patients receiving conventional IV amphotericin B, 71% of patients had at least one infusion-related reaction during the first 7 days of therapy; fever and chills occurred in 28–51% and nausea and headache occurred in 9–18% of patients. In patients receiving amphotericin B lipid complex, chills and fever have been reported in 14–18% of patients and nausea, vomiting, and hypotension have been reported in 8–9% of patients. In a large, double-blind study in adults and pediatric febrile neutropenic patients, infusion reactions (i.e., fever, chills/rigors, nausea, vomiting) occurred in 4–20% of those receiving the first dose of amphotericin B liposomal and 7–56% of those receiving the first dose of conventional IV amphotericin B. In a randomized study in HIV-infected patients with cryptococcal meningitis, infusion reactions (i.e., fever, chills/rigors, nausea, vomiting) occurred in 6–16% of those receiving amphotericin B liposomal (3 or 6 mg/kg daily) and 18–48% of those receiving conventional amphotericin B. There have been reports of flushing, back pain (with or without chest tightness), and chest pain occurring within a few minutes after initiation of IV infusions of amphotericin B liposomal; these reactions occasionally were severe but disappeared when the infusion was stopped. These symptoms do not occur with every dose and usually do not recur with subsequent doses given at a slower IV infusion rate.

Although the precise mechanism for these infusion reactions is not known, limited evidence indicates that amphotericin-induced increases in prostaglandin (e.g., PGE_2) synthesis may be involved. Aspirin, antipyretics (e.g., acetaminophen), antiemetics, meperidine, antihistamines (e.g., diphenhydramine), or corticosteroids have been used for the treatment or prevention of acute infusion reactions in patients receiving conventional IV amphotericin or other formulations of the drug. It has been suggested that meperidine (25–50 mg IV) may decrease the duration of shaking chills and fever occurring in association with IV infusion of amphotericin B. There is some evidence that IV administration of small doses of corticosteroids just prior to or during IV infusion of conventional amphotericin B may help decrease the severity of febrile and other systemic reactions; however, corticosteroids should be used only when necessary using minimal dosage for as short a period as possible. (See Drug Interactions: Corticosteroids.) Use of a premedication regimen (e.g., acetaminophen and diphenhydramine; acetaminophen, corticosteroid, and diphenhydramine) is not routinely recommended prior to the initial dose of any amphotericin B formulation, but can be administered promptly to treat a reaction if it occurs and then as pretreatment prior to subsequent doses.

Rapid IV infusion of conventional IV amphotericin B has been associated with a more severe reaction consisting of hypotension, hypokalemia, arrhythmias, and shock. Some of these adverse effects also have been reported rarely with amphotericin B lipid complex or amphotericin B liposomal. It may be difficult to determine whether these severe reactions indicate intolerance or hypersensitivity to the drug.

● Renal and Electrolyte Effects

Nephrotoxicity is the major dose-limiting toxicity reported with conventional IV amphotericin B, and nephrotoxicity occurs to some degree in the majority of patients receiving the drug. Adverse renal effects in patients receiving conventional IV amphotericin B include decreased renal function and renal function abnormalities such as azotemia, hypokalemia, hyposthenuria, renal tubular acidosis, and nephrocalcinosis. Increased BUN and serum creatinine concentrations have been reported. Hypokalemia and hypomagnesemia develop in a large proportion of patients, and hypocalcemia has been reported. Uric acid excretion is increased and nephrocalcinosis can occur. Renal tubular acidosis may be present without concurrent systemic acidosis. It has been suggested that hydration and sodium repletion prior to administration of IV amphotericin B may decrease the risk of nephrotoxicity, and supplemental alkali therapy may decrease complications related to renal tubular acidosis. Nephrotoxicity associated with conventional IV amphotericin B appears to involve several mechanisms, including a direct vasoconstrictive effect on renal arterioles that reduces glomerular and renal tubular blood flow and a lytic action on cholesterol-rich lysosomal membranes of renal tubular cells. On biopsy, juxtamedullary glomerulitis and intratubular and interstitial calcium deposits in the distal nephron are found. Although renal function usually improves within a few months after discontinuance of conventional amphotericin B therapy, some degree of permanent impairment may remain in some patients, especially in patients who received a large cumulative dose of the drug (exceeding 5 g) or concomitant therapy with other nephrotoxic drugs. Patients with higher serum low-density lipoprotein (LDL) concentrations appear to be more susceptible to amphotericin B-induced renal toxicity than those with lower concentrations.

Increased BUN and/or serum creatinine, hypokalemia, hypomagnesemia, and hypocalcemia also have been reported in patients receiving amphotericin B lipid complex or amphotericin B liposomal. While these formulations appear to be associated with a lower risk of nephrotoxicity than conventional IV amphotericin B and have been used in patients with preexisting renal impairment (in most cases resulting from prior therapy with conventional IV amphotericin B), additional experience with the drugs is necessary to more accurately determine the extent of nephrotoxicity that occurs with these formulations. In several studies when amphotericin B lipid complex was substituted for conventional IV amphotericin B in patients who developed nephrotoxicity while receiving the conventional formulation and had baseline serum creatinine concentrations of 2 mg/dL or greater, serum creatinine concentrations generally declined during therapy with the lipid formulations. In a randomized, double-blind study comparing safety and efficacy of amphotericin B liposomal or conventional IV amphotericin B for antifungal prophylaxis in febrile, neutropenic patients, nephrotoxicity occurred in about 19 or 34% of patients, respectively. In a randomized study in HIV-infected patients with cryptococcal meningitis, serum creatinine concentrations twofold higher than baseline concentrations were reported in 14–21% of those receiving amphotericin B liposomal (3 or 6 mg/kg daily) and in 33% of those receiving conventional amphotericin B.

Other adverse renal effects that have been reported in patients receiving conventional IV amphotericin B, amphotericin B lipid complex, or amphotericin B liposomal include anuria, oliguria, dysuria, decreased renal function, hematuria, urinary incontinence, renal tubular acidosis, and acute renal failure. Nephrogenic diabetes insipidus has been reported in patients receiving conventional IV amphotericin B.

● **Hematologic Effects**

Patients receiving conventional IV amphotericin B may develop normocytic, normochromic anemia. The anemia develops gradually and may not occur until after 10 weeks of therapy; it may be related either to a direct inhibition of erythrocytes or erythropoietin production or may be secondary to renal toxicity. The hematocrit rarely decreases below 20–25% and generally returns to baseline within several months following discontinuance of the drug. Anemia also has been reported rarely in patients receiving amphotericin B lipid complex or amphotericin B liposomal.

Other hematologic effects, including agranulocytosis, coagulation disorders, decreased or increased prothrombin, thrombocytopenia, leukopenia, eosinophilia, or leukocytosis, have been reported rarely in patients receiving conventional IV amphotericin B, amphotericin B lipid complex, or amphotericin B liposomal.

● **Cardiopulmonary and Sensitivity Reactions**

Various adverse cardiopulmonary effects, including hypotension, tachypnea, cardiac failure, cardiac arrest, cardiomyopathy, shock, pulmonary edema, hypersensitivity pneumonitis, arrhythmias (including ventricular fibrillation), dyspnea, and hypertension, have been reported in individuals receiving conventional IV amphotericin B.

Bronchospasm, wheezing, angioedema, and anaphylaxis or anaphylactoid reactions have been reported in patients receiving conventional IV amphotericin B or the lipid formulations of amphotericin B. If severe respiratory distress, anaphylaxis, or an anaphylactoid reaction occurs in a patient receiving amphotericin B, the drug should be discontinued immediately and the patient given appropriate therapy (e.g., epinephrine, corticosteroids, maintenance of an adequate airway, oxygen) as indicated. The manufacturer of amphotericin B lipid complex states that the drug is contraindicated in patients who have experienced severe respiratory distress after receiving a prior dose of the drug.

Cardiac enlargement with congestive heart failure occurred in a few patients receiving conventional IV amphotericin B with 20–40 mg of hydrocortisone sodium succinate added to each infusion. Congestive heart failure was considered to be due to amphotericin B-induced hypokalemic cardiopathy and corticosteroid-induced salt and fluid retention. (See Drug Interactions: Corticosteroids.) Following discontinuance of hydrocortisone and administration of oral potassium supplements, cardiac status returned to normal although conventional amphotericin B therapy was continued.

● **GI Effects**

In addition to the nausea and vomiting reported as part of acute infusion reactions to the drugs, other adverse GI effects have been reported in patients receiving conventional IV amphotericin B, amphotericin B lipid complex, or amphotericin B liposomal. These adverse effects include anorexia and weight loss, diarrhea, dyspepsia, cramping, epigastric pain, hemorrhagic gastroenteritis, GI hemorrhage, and melena. Alternate-day therapy may decrease the incidence of anorexia.

● **Local Reactions**

IV administration of conventional amphotericin B, amphotericin B lipid complex, or amphotericin B liposomal may cause erythema, pain, or inflammation at the injection site. Phlebitis or thrombophlebitis has been reported with conventional IV amphotericin B. The manufacturers of conventional IV amphotericin B and some clinicians suggest that the addition of 500–1000 units of heparin to the amphotericin B infusion, the use of a pediatric scalp-vein needle, or alternate-day therapy may decrease the incidence of thrombophlebitis. Extravasation of the drug causes local irritation.

● **Nervous System Effects**

Adverse neurologic effects that have been reported in patients receiving conventional IV amphotericin B, amphotericin B lipid complex, or amphotericin B liposomal include malaise, depression, confusion, dizziness, insomnia, somnolence, coma, anxiety, agitation, nervousness, abnormal thinking, hallucinations, tremor, seizures, myasthenia, hearing loss, tinnitus, transient vertigo, visual impairment, diplopia, peripheral neuropathy, encephalopathy, cerebrovascular accident, and extrapyramidal syndrome. Leukoencephalopathy has been reported following use of amphotericin B; literature reports suggest that total body irradiation may be a predisposition.

● **Other Adverse Effects**

Adverse musculoskeletal effects, including generalized pain, dystonia, and muscle, bone, or joint pain, have been reported in patients receiving conventional IV amphotericin B, amphotericin B lipid complex, or amphotericin B liposomal.

Rash (including maculopapular or vesiculobullous rash), purpura, pruritus, urticaria, sweating, exfoliative dermatitis, erythema multiforme, toxic epidermal necrolysis, Stevens-Johnson syndrome, alopecia, dry skin, skin discoloration, and ulcer have been reported in patients receiving amphotericin B.

Increased serum concentrations of AST (SGOT), ALT (SGPT), alkaline phosphatase, bilirubin, γ-glutamyltransferase (GGT, γ-glutamyltranspeptidase, GGTP), and LDH have been reported in patients receiving conventional IV amphotericin B, amphotericin B lipid complex, or amphotericin B liposomal. Acute liver failure, hepatotoxicity, hepatitis, jaundice, hyperglycemia, and hypoglycemia have been reported rarely.

Intrathecal† administration of conventional amphotericin B has produced headache, nausea and vomiting, urinary retention, pain along lumbar nerves, paresthesia, vision changes, and arachnoiditis.

● **Precautions and Contraindications**

Initial doses of conventional IV amphotericin B, amphotericin B lipid complex, or amphotericin B liposomal should be administered under close clinical observation by medically trained personnel. The fact that acute infusion reactions (e.g., fever, chills, hypotension, nausea, vomiting, headache, dyspnea, and tachypnea) often occur 1–3 hours after initiation of amphotericin B IV infusions (especially after the first few doses) and that severe reactions including anaphylaxis have been reported rarely should be considered. Conventional IV amphotericin B is associated with a high incidence of adverse effects and should be reserved principally for the treatment of progressive, potentially life-threatening fungal infections caused by susceptible organisms when the potential benefits of the drug outweigh its untoward and dangerous side effects.

Renal, hepatic, and hematologic function should be monitored in patients receiving conventional IV amphotericin B, amphotericin B lipid complex, or amphotericin B liposomal. Some clinicians suggest that renal function be monitored at least 2–3 times weekly during initial amphotericin B therapy and that hepatic and hematologic function be monitored 1–2 times weekly. Serum electrolytes (especially potassium and magnesium) and complete blood cell counts (CBCs) also should be monitored in patients receiving any of these drugs. Because of the drug's nephrotoxic potential, conventional IV amphotericin B should be used with caution in patients with reduced renal function and patients receiving any amphotericin B formulation concomitantly with a nephrotoxic drug should be closely monitored. (See Drug Interactions: Nephrotoxic Drugs.)

Conventional amphotericin B, amphotericin B lipid complex, and amphotericin B liposomal are contraindicated in patients who are hypersensitive to amphotericin B or any other component in the respective formulation. The manufacturers of conventional amphotericin B and amphotericin B liposomal suggest that use of these drugs can be considered in patients with hypersensitivity if the clinician determines that the benefits of such therapy outweigh the risks; however, they are contraindicated in patients who have had severe respiratory distress or a severe anaphylactic reaction while receiving the drugs.

● Pediatric Precautions

Although safety and efficacy of conventional IV amphotericin B in pediatric patients have not been established through adequate and well-controlled studies, the drug has been used effectively to treat systemic fungal infections in pediatric patients without unusual adverse effects. The manufacturers state that the lowest effective dosage of the drug should be employed whenever conventional IV amphotericin B is used in pediatric patients.

IV amphotericin B lipid complex generally is well tolerated in pediatric patients, and has been used for the treatment of invasive fungal infections in children 3 weeks to 16 years of age without unusual adverse effects. Acute infusion reactions (fever, chills, rigors) and anaphylaxis have been reported in pediatric patients receiving amphotericin B lipid complex and have necessitated discontinuance of the drug in these patients.

IV amphotericin B liposomal has been administered to pediatric patients 1 month to 16 years of age without any unusual adverse effects. Although safety and efficacy of the drug in neonates younger than 1 month of age have not been established to date, amphotericin B liposomal has been used in a limited number of neonates† for the treatment of severe fungal infections without any unusual adverse effects. Transient hypokalemia that responded to potassium supplementation was the only adverse effect reported in a group of neonates who received amphotericin B liposomal in a dosage of 1–5 mg/kg given by IV infusion over 0.5–1 hours. In a large, double-blind study comparing the safety and efficacy of amphotericin B liposomal and conventional IV amphotericin B, the incidence of chills, vomiting, hypokalemia, or hypertension in patients 16 years of age or younger ranged from 10–37% in those receiving amphotericin B liposomal and from 21–68% in those receiving the conventional formulation of the drug.

● Geriatric Precautions

While safety and efficacy of conventional IV amphotericin B, amphotericin B lipid complex, and amphotericin B liposomal have not been studied specifically in geriatric patients, no unusual age-related adverse effects have been reported when the drugs were used in patients 65 years of age or older.

Although clinical experience to date indicates that dosage modification is unnecessary when amphotericin B liposomal is used in geriatric patients, the manufacturer recommends that these patients be carefully monitored while receiving the drug.

● Mutagenicity and Carcinogenicity

There have been no long-term studies to date to evaluate the carcinogenic potential of conventional amphotericin B, amphotericin B lipid complex, or amphotericin B liposomal.

The mutagenic potential of conventional amphotericin B or amphotericin B liposomal has not been evaluated to date. There was no evidence of mutagenicity when amphotericin B lipid complex was evaluated using in vitro studies (e.g., bacterial reverse mutation assay, mouse lymphoma forward mutation assay, CHO chromosomal aberration assay) or in vivo studies (e.g., mouse bone marrow micronucleus assay) with or without metabolic activation.

● Pregnancy, Fertility, and Lactation
Pregnancy

Safe use of amphotericin B during pregnancy has not been established. Conventional IV amphotericin B has been used to treat systemic fungal infections or visceral leishmaniasis in a limited number of pregnant women without obvious adverse effects to the fetus. While reproduction studies in rats and rabbits using conventional amphotericin B, amphotericin B lipid complex, or amphotericin B liposomal have not revealed evidence of harm to the fetus, rabbits receiving amphotericin B liposomal dosages equivalent to 0.5–2 times the usual human

dosage experienced a higher rate of spontaneous abortions than the control group. However, animal reproduction studies are not always predictive of human response. There are no adequate or controlled studies to date using any amphotericin B formulation in pregnant women, and these drugs should be used during pregnancy only when clearly needed.

Fertility

There have been no studies to date to determine whether conventional amphotericin B affects fertility. Studies in male and female rats using amphotericin B lipid complex at doses up to 0.32 times the usual human dose (based on body surface area) indicate that the drug does not affect fertility. When liposomal amphotericin was administered to rats in 10- or 15-mg/kg doses (equivalent to human doses of 1.6 or 2.4 mg/kg based on body surface area), there was evidence of an abnormal estrous cycle (prolonged diestrus) and decreased number of corpora lutea in female rats receiving the higher dosage but no effect on fertility or days to copulation; there were no effects on male reproductive function.

Lactation

It is not known whether amphotericin B is distributed into human milk. Because many drugs are distributed into human milk and because of the potential for serious adverse reactions to amphotericin B in nursing infants if it were distributed, a decision should be made whether to discontinue nursing or the drug, taking into account the importance of the drug to the woman.

DRUG INTERACTIONS

Systematic drug interaction studies have not been performed to date using amphotericin B lipid complex or amphotericin B liposomal. The fact that drug interactions reported with conventional IV amphotericin B could also occur with these lipid formulations of the drug should be considered.

● Nephrotoxic Drugs

Since nephrotoxic effects may be additive, the concurrent or sequential use of IV amphotericin B and other drugs with similar toxic potentials (e.g., aminoglycosides, cyclosporine, pentamidine) should be avoided, if possible. Great caution and intensive monitoring of renal function is recommended if any amphotericin B formulation is used concomitantly with a nephrotoxic agent.

Cyclosporine

There is evidence from a prospective study in patients undergoing bone marrow transplantation (BMT) that concurrent initiation of cyclosporine and amphotericin B lipid complex therapy may be associated with increased nephrotoxicity. In a renal transplant recipient who was receiving cyclosporine and had stable whole blood cyclosporine concentrations, blood cyclosporine concentrations in the days after initiation of amphotericin B lipid complex therapy were more than twice those reported prior to initiation of antifungal therapy; however, this increase was transient and did not necessitate adjustment of cyclosporine dosage.

Pentamidine

Acute, reversible renal failure occurred in at least 4 patients with human immunodeficiency virus (HIV) infection who received IV amphotericin B concomitantly with IV or IM pentamidine; there was no evidence of adverse renal effects in patients who received IV amphotericin B concomitantly with pentamidine administered by oral inhalation.

● Drugs Affected by Potassium Depletion

Because amphotericin B may induce hypokalemia, the drug may predispose patients receiving cardiac glycosides to glycoside-induced cardiotoxicity and may enhance the effects of skeletal muscle relaxants (e.g., tubocurarine). Serum potassium concentrations should be monitored closely in patients receiving any amphotericin B formulation concomitantly with a cardiac glycoside or skeletal muscle relaxant.

● Anti-infective Agents
Flucytosine

In some in vitro studies, the combination of flucytosine and amphotericin B resulted in synergistic inhibition of strains of Cryptococcus neoformans, Candida albicans, and C. tropicalis. The suggested mechanism of the synergism is that the binding of amphotericin B to sterols in cell membranes increases the permeability of the cytoplasmic membrane, thus allowing greater penetration of flucytosine into the fungal cell. However, in a study evaluating the antifungal effects of the drugs in the presence of serum, the combination of amphotericin B and flucytosine was not additive or synergistic against *C. albicans*.

There is some evidence that concomitant use of amphotericin B and flucytosine may increase the toxicity of flucytosine, possibly by increasing cellular uptake and/or by decreasing renal excretion of the drug. Flucytosine and amphotericin B should be used concomitantly with caution. If flucytosine is used in conjunction with amphotericin B, especially in HIV-infected patients, serum flucytosine concentrations and blood cell counts should be monitored carefully. In addition, it has been suggested that flucytosine be initiated at a low dosage (i.e., 75–100 mg/kg daily) and subsequent dosage adjusted based on serum flucytosine concentrations.

Imidazole and Triazole Antifungal Agents

Although the clinical importance is unclear, results of in vitro studies evaluating the antifungal effects of amphotericin B used concomitantly with imidazole- or triazole-derivative antifungals (e.g., clotrimazole, fluconazole, itraconazole, ketoconazole) against *C. albicans*, *C. pseudotropicalis*, *C. glabrata*, or *Aspergillus fumigatus* indicate that antagonism can occur with these combinations. Since amphotericin B exerts its antifungal activity by binding to sterols in the fungal cell membrane and imidazoles and triazoles act by altering the cell membrane, antagonism is theoretically possible; however, it is unclear whether such antagonism actually would occur in vivo. Results of studies evaluating combined use of amphotericin B and fluconazole, ketoconazole, or itraconazole in animal models of aspergillosis, candidiasis, or cryptococcosis have been conflicting. While antagonism occurred in some models (*A. fumigatus* infection in mice, rabbits, or rats treated with amphotericin B and fluconazole or itraconazole), these combinations resulted in additive or indifferent effects in other models (e.g., *C. albicans* or *C. neoformans* infection in mice or rabbits treated with amphotericin B and fluconazole). In a few studies evaluating the drugs in murine cryptococcosis or candidiasis, sequential use of an initial large dose of amphotericin B followed by an azole antifungal (e.g., fluconazole) was uniformly effective in prolonging survival and decreasing fungal burden. Because further study is needed regarding the interaction between amphotericin B and imidazole- or triazole-derivative antifungals (e.g., fluconazole, itraconazole, or ketoconazole), such combination therapy should be used with caution, particularly in immunocompromised patients.

Results of an in vitro study indicate that the combination of amphotericin B and fluconazole or itraconazole may be synergistic, additive, or indifferent against *Pseudallescheria boydii*; there was no evidence of antagonism.

Quinolones

Norfloxacin may enhance the antifungal activity of some antifungals (e.g., amphotericin B, flucytosine, ketoconazole, nystatin). There are conflicting reports on this interaction, however, and in at least one in vitro study norfloxacin had no effect on the antifungal activity of amphotericin B. Further study is needed to evaluate the antifungal effect when norfloxacin is used in conjunction with an antifungal.

Rifabutin

Results of an in vitro study indicate that the combination of rifabutin and amphotericin B may be additive or synergistic against *Aspergillus fumigatus*, *A. flavus*, *Fusarium solani*, *F. moniliforme*, *F. pallidoroseum* (formerly *F. semitectum*), and *F. proliferatum*; there was no evidence of antagonism with this combination. While rifabutin has no in vitro antifungal activity against *Aspergillus* or *Fusarium* when used alone, an antifungal effect was evident when the drug was used in combination with amphotericin B.

Zidovudine

Results of a study in dogs indicate that concomitant administration of zidovudine and conventional amphotericin B (at 0.5 times the recommended human dosage) or amphotericin B lipid complex (at 0.16 or 0.5 times the recommended human dosage) for 30 days was associated with increased myelotoxicity and nephrotoxicity. Although the clinical importance of this animal study is unclear, renal and hematologic function should be closely monitored in patients receiving zidovudine concomitantly with amphotericin B.

● *Antineoplastic Agents*

The manufacturers state that antineoplastic agents (e.g., mechlorethamine) may enhance the potential for renal toxicity, bronchospasm, and hypotension in patients receiving amphotericin B and such concomitant therapy should be used only with great caution.

● *Corticosteroids*

Corticosteroids reportedly may enhance the potassium depletion caused by conventional amphotericin B. The manufacturers state that concomitant use of corticosteroids should be avoided, unless necessary to control adverse effects of conventional amphotericin B. In such cases, the corticosteroid should be administered using minimal dosage for as short a duration as possible.

If corticosteroids are used concomitantly with any amphotericin B formulation, serum electrolytes and cardiac function should be monitored closely.

● *Leukocyte Transfusions*

IV infusion of conventional amphotericin B during or shortly after leukocyte transfusions has rarely been associated with acute pulmonary reactions characterized by acute dyspnea, tachypnea, hypoxemia, hemoptysis, and diffuse interstitial infiltrates. The most severe pulmonary reactions have been reported when amphotericin B was administered within the first 4 hours after a leukocyte transfusion; respiratory deterioration appeared to contribute to death in at least 5 patients with such reactions.

It has been recommended that amphotericin B be used with caution in patients receiving leukocyte transfusions, especially in those with gram-negative septicemia. The manufacturer of amphotericin B lipid complex states that the drug should not be used concurrently with leukocyte transfusions. The manufacturers of conventional amphotericin B recommend that doses of the drug be separated in time as much as possible from leukocyte transfusions and that pulmonary function be monitored in patients receiving both therapies.

ACUTE TOXICITY

● *Manifestations*

Acute overdosage of conventional amphotericin B may result in potentially fatal cardiac or cardiorespiratory arrest. Adverse cardiovascular effects, including hypotension, bradycardia, and cardiac arrest, have been reported in several pediatric patients who inadvertently received overdosage of conventional amphotericin B. One child who received conventional amphotericin B in a dosage of 4.6 mg/kg given by IV infusion over 2 hours experienced vomiting, followed by seizures, and cardiac arrest immediately after the infusion.

In patients who received 1 or more amphotericin B lipid complex doses of 7–13 mg/kg., serious acute reactions did not occur.

Information on acute toxicity of amphotericin B liposomal is not available. There was no reported dose-related toxicity following repeated daily doses up to 15 mg/kg in adult patients or up to 10 mg/kg in pediatric patients.

● *Treatment*

In the event of overdosage with any amphotericin B formulation, therapy with the drug should be discontinued and the patient's clinical status (e.g., cardiorespiratory, renal, and liver function, hematologic status, serum electrolytes) monitored. Supportive therapy should be administered as required. Amphotericin B is not removed by hemodialysis. The manufacturers of conventional amphoteric B state that the patient's condition should be stabilized, including correction of electrolyte abnormalities, prior to reinstituting the drug.

MECHANISM OF ACTION

Amphotericin B usually is fungistatic in action at concentrations obtained clinically, but may be fungicidal in high concentrations or against very susceptible organisms. Amphotericin B exerts its antifungal activity principally by binding to sterols (e.g., ergosterol) in the fungal cell membrane. As a result of this binding, the cell membrane is no longer able to function as a selective barrier and leakage of intracellular contents occurs. Cell death occurs in part as a result of permeability changes, but other mechanisms also may contribute to the in vivo antifungal effects of amphotericin B against some fungi. Amphotericin B is not active in vitro against organisms that do not contain sterols in their cell membranes (e.g., bacteria).

Binding to sterols in mammalian cells (such as certain kidney cells and erythrocytes) may account for some of the toxicities reported with conventional amphotericin B therapy. At usual therapeutic concentrations of amphotericin B, the drug does not appear to hemolyze mature erythrocytes, and the anemia seen with conventional IV amphotericin B therapy may result from the action of the drug on actively metabolizing and dividing erythropoietic cells.

SPECTRUM

Amphotericin B is active against most pathogenic fungi, including yeasts, and also is active against some protozoa. Amphotericin B is inactive against bacteria, rickettsiae, or viruses.

• Fungi

In vitro, amphotericin B concentrations of 0.03–1.0 mcg/mL usually inhibit *Aspergillus fumigatus*, *A. flavus*, *Coccidioides immitis*, *C. posadasii*, *Cryptococcus neoformans*, *C. gattii*, *Exophiala castellanii*, *E. spinifera*, *Histoplasma capsulatum*, *Rhodotorula*, and *Sporothrix schenckii*. *Blastomyces dermatitidis* may require slightly higher drug concentrations for inhibition.

Amphotericin B is active in vitro against most strains of *Candida*. In vitro, *C. albicans*, *C. dubliniensis*, *C. glabrata* (formerly *Torulopsis glabrata*), *C. krusei*, *C. parapsilosis*, and *C. tropicalis* usually are inhibited by amphotericin B concentrations of 0.03–1 mcg/mL. In a study evaluating in vitro susceptibility of clinical isolates of *C. dubliniensis* obtained from patients with or without human immunodeficiency virus (HIV) infection, these strains were inhibited by amphotericin B concentrations of 0.03–0.125 mcg/mL. While some strains of *C. lusitaniae* are inhibited in vitro by amphotericin B concentrations of 0.06–0.5 mcg/mL, other strains appear to be resistant to the drug. Clinical isolates of *C. auris* (often misidentified as *C. haemulonii*, *C. famata*, or *Rhodotorula glutinis*) generally have been inhibited in vitro by amphotericin B concentrations of 0.5–1 mcg/mL.

Some *Penicillium marneffei* isolates have been inhibited in vitro by amphotericin B concentrations of 0.002–4 mcg/mL, but other strains required concentrations as high as 32 mcg/mL for in vitro inhibition.

Many zygomycetes, including *Lichtheimia* (formerly *Absidia*), *Mucor*, *Rhizopus*, *Rhizomucor*, *Apophysomyces elegans*, and *Cunninghamella*, are inhibited in vitro by amphotericin B concentrations of 0.003–2 mcg/mL. Some clinical isolates of *Basidiobolus*, including *B. ranarum*, have amphotericin B MICs of 0.5–4 mcg/mL; however, other isolates are resistant to the drug. *Conidiobolus coronatus* has been inhibited in vitro by amphotericin B concentrations of 0.5–4 mcg/mL.

While some strains of *Pseudallescheria boydii* are inhibited in vitro by amphotericin B concentrations of 0.5 mcg/mL or less, most strains are resistant to the drug. Amphotericin B concentrations of 1–16 mcg/mL were necessary for in vitro inhibition of clinical isolates of *Scedosporium apiospermum* or *S. prolificans*, and these filamentous fungi probably are resistant to the drug.

Amphotericin B is active against *Exserohilum*, and *E. rostratum* has been inhibited in vitro by amphotericin B concentrations of 0.03–0.5 mcg/mL. In vitro studies of *E. rostratum* obtained from patients with infections related to injections of contaminated methylprednisolone acetate preparations (see Uses: Exserohilum Infections) indicate that the MIC of amphotericin B was 0.032–2 mcg/mL for these strains. However, the clinical relevance of MIC testing for *E. rostratum* remains uncertain, and MIC values indicating susceptibility have not been identified.

While many strains of *Fusarium* are resistant to amphotericin B, some strains of *F. solani*, *F. oxysporum*, and *F. verticillioides* have been inhibited in vitro by amphotericin B concentrations of 2–8 mcg/mL. Some strains of *Scopulariopsis*, including some strains of *S. acremonium* and *S. brevicaulis*, are inhibited in vitro by amphotericin B concentrations of 1–4 mcg/mL; other strains are resistant to the drug.

In one in vitro study, MICs of conventional amphotericin B reported for *B. dermatitidis*, *C. immitis*, *H. capsulatum*, *P. brasiliensis*, *C. albicans*, *C. tropicalis*, *C. parapsilosis*, and *C. neoformans* ranged from 0.125–2 mcg/mL. *C. glabrata* or *A. fumigatus* were inhibited in vitro by conventional amphotericin B concentrations of 1–2 mcg/mL; *A. flavus* was inhibited in vitro by conventional amphotericin B concentrations of 4 mcg/mL. In a study that evaluated the in vitro susceptibility of *C. albicans*, *C. parapsilosis*, *C. tropicalis*, and *C. glabrata* to several different amphotericin B formulations, MICs reported for conventional amphotericin B, amphotericin B lipid complex, or amphotericin B liposomal were 0.1–0.78, 0.2–0.78, or 0.2–6.25 mcg/mL, respectively. When *C. krusei* was tested, the MICs of conventional amphotericin B or amphotericin B lipid complex were 0.78–1.56 or 3.13–6.25 mcg/mL, respectively; however, MICs of amphotericin B liposomal reported for this organism were greater than 50 mcg/mL.

• Protozoa

Amphotericin B is active in vitro and in vivo against *Leishmania braziliensis*. The drug also is active in vitro and in vivo against *L. mexicana* and *L. donovani*, including antimony-resistant strains of the organisms. In vitro, amphotericin B concentrations of 1 mcg/mL result in complete elimination of *L. donovani* amastigotes in human monocyte-derived macrophages and *L. donovani* promastigotes in cell-free media. The drug also is active in vitro against *L. tropica*.

Amphotericin B is active in vitro and apparently in vivo against *Naegleria* spp., particularly *N. fowleri*. The drug has variable and limited activity in vitro against *Acanthamoeba castellanii* and *A. polyphaga*.

RESISTANCE

Resistance to amphotericin B has been produced in vitro by serial passage of fungi in the presence of increasing concentrations of the drug, and resistant strains of some fungi (e.g., *Candida*) have been isolated from patients who received long-term therapy with conventional amphotericin B. Amphotericin B-resistant *Candida* are reported relatively infrequently; however, primary resistance to the drug occurs in some strains of *C. lusitaniae* and also occurs in *C. guilliermondii*. Some clinical isolates of *C. auris* have reduced susceptibility or resistance to amphotericin B in vitro (i.e., MIC 2 mcg/mL or greater).

While the clinical importance is unclear, fluconazole-resistant strains of *C. albicans* that were cross-resistant to amphotericin B have been isolated from a few immunocompromised individuals, including leukemia patients and patients with human immunodeficiency virus (HIV) infection. In addition, a few isolates of *Cryptococcus neoformans* resistant to fluconazole also have been resistant to amphotericin B.

Fungi resistant to conventional amphotericin B also may be resistant to amphotericin B lipid complex and amphotericin B liposomal.

PHARMACOKINETICS

The pharmacokinetics of amphotericin B vary substantially depending on whether the drug is administered as conventional amphotericin B (formulated with sodium desoxycholate), amphotericin B lipid complex, or amphotericin B liposomal, and pharmacokinetic parameters reported for one amphotericin B formulation should not be used to predict the pharmacokinetics of any other amphotericin B formulation.

In general, usual dosages of amphotericin B lipid complex result in lower serum concentrations of amphotericin B and greater volumes of distribution than those reported for the conventional formulation of the drug. Plasma drug concentrations attained after administration of amphotericin B liposomal generally are higher and the volume of distribution is lower than those reported for similar doses of conventional amphotericin B. The clinical importance of differences in pharmacokinetics of the various amphotericin B formulations has not been elucidated, and interpretation of serum or tissue concentrations of amphotericin B reported in published studies is complicated by the fact that many assays used to measure the drug do not differentiate between free amphotericin B and amphotericin B that is lipid-complexed, liposome-encapsulated, or protein-bound. It has been suggested that differences in the distribution and clearance of amphotericin B following administration of lipid-complexed or liposomal-encapsulated formulations relative to those reported following administration of conventional amphotericin B (i.e., increased uptake by the liver and spleen and decreased kidney concentrations) are one of several factors that may contribute to the improved toxicity profiles reported for these formulations; however, how these pharmacokinetic differences affect the therapeutic efficacy of the various formulations is unclear. The manufacturers' literature and specialized references should be consulted for information regarding the absorption, distribution, or elimination of amphotericin B administered as amphotericin B lipid complex or amphotericin B liposomal.

• Absorption

After an initial IV infusion of 1–5 mg of amphotericin B daily, with dosage gradually increased to 0.4–0.6 mg/kg daily, plasma concentrations ranging from approximately 0.5–2 mcg/mL were reported. Following a rapid initial decrease, plasma concentrations plateau at about 0.5 mcg/mL.

In one study, immediately after completion of IV infusion of 30 mg of amphotericin B (administered as conventional amphotericin B over a period of several hours), average peak serum concentrations were about 1 mcg/mL; when the dose was 50 mg, average peak serum concentrations were approximately 2 mcg/mL. Immediately after infusion, no more than 10% of the amphotericin B dose can be accounted for in serum. Average minimum serum concentrations (recorded just prior to the next drug infusion) of approximately 0.4 mcg/mL have been reported when 30-mg doses of conventional amphotericin B were given once daily or 60-mg doses were given every other day.

● Distribution

Information on the distribution of amphotericin B is limited.

The volume of distribution of the drug following administration of conventional amphotericin B has been reported to be 4 L/kg.

Amphotericin B concentrations attained in inflamed pleura, peritoneum, synovium, and aqueous humor following IV administration of conventional amphotericin B reportedly are about 60% of concurrent plasma concentrations. Penetration into vitreous humor is low.

Following IV administration of conventional amphotericin B, CSF concentrations of the drug rarely exceed 2.5% of concurrent serum concentrations. To achieve fungistatic CSF concentrations, the drug must usually be administered intrathecally†. In patients with meningitis, intrathecal† administration of 0.2–0.3 mg of conventional amphotericin B via a subcutaneous reservoir has produced peak CSF concentrations of 0.5–0.8 mcg/mL; 24 hours after the dose, CSF concentrations were 0.11–0.29 mcg/mL. Amphotericin B is removed from the CSF by arachnoid villi and appears to be stored in the extracellular compartment of the brain, which may act as a reservoir for the drug.

Low concentrations of amphotericin B are attained in amniotic fluid.

It is not known whether amphotericin B is distributed into milk.

Amphotericin B is more than 90% bound to plasma proteins.

● Elimination

The metabolic fate of amphotericin B in humans has not been fully elucidated.

Following IV administration of conventional amphotericin B in patients whose renal function is normal prior to therapy, the initial plasma half-life is approximately 24 hours. After the first 24 hours, the rate at which amphotericin B is eliminated decreases and an elimination half-life of approximately 15 days has been reported.

Conventional amphotericin B is eliminated very slowly (over weeks to months) by the kidneys; slow release of the drug from the peripheral compartment may account for the long elimination half-life. Over a 7-day period, the cumulative urinary excretion of a single dose of conventional amphotericin B is about 40% of the administered drug. It has been estimated that only about 2–5% of a total dose of amphotericin B is excreted in urine unchanged. When conventional IV amphotericin B therapy is discontinued, the drug can be detected in blood for up to 4 weeks and in urine for up to 4–8 weeks.

Amphotericin B is not hemodialyzable.

CHEMISTRY AND STABILITY

● Chemistry

Amphotericin B is an antifungal antibiotic produced by *Streptomyces nodosus*. The drug is an amphoteric polyene macrolide which occurs as a yellow to orange, odorless or practically odorless powder and is insoluble in water and in anhydrous alcohol. Each mg of amphotericin B contains not less than 750 mcg of anhydrous drug, and amphotericin A (a contaminant of amphotericin B) may be present in a concentration of not more than 5%. Because amphotericin B is amphoteric, it can form salts in acidic or basic media. Although the salts are more water soluble, they have less antifungal activity.

Various amphotericin B preparations are commercially available for parenteral administration. Amphotericin B formulated with sodium desoxycholate (conventional amphotericin B) was the first parenteral amphotericin B preparation to become commercially available. Because conventional amphotericin B is associated with certain dose-limiting toxicities (principally nephrotoxicity), various other formulations have been investigated with the goal of increasing the tolerability of amphotericin B without compromising the antifungal effects of the drug. As a result, amphotericin B now also is commercially available as amphotericin B lipid complex and amphotericin B liposomal. These formulations contain novel lipid-based drug delivery systems that may affect the pharmacokinetics and functional properties of amphotericin B and improve the toxicity profile of the drug.

Conventional Amphotericin B

Conventional amphotericin B for injection contains amphotericin B and sodium desoxycholate. Amphotericin B is insoluble in water; presence of sodium desoxycholate in the formulation solubilizes amphotericin B during reconstitution with sterile water providing a colloidal dispersion of the drug. Commercially available conventional amphotericin B occurs as a sterile, yellow to orange lyophilized cake which may partially reduce to powder following manufacture. Each vial labeled as containing 50 mg of amphotericin B contains 41 mg of sodium desoxycholate and is buffered with 20.2 mg of sodium phosphates; at the time of manufacture, air in the vial is replaced with nitrogen.

Extemporaneous lipid emulsions of conventional IV amphotericin B have been prepared by diluting the drug in 20% fat emulsion (Intralipid®) in an attempt to provide a vehicle for amphotericin B that would decrease the nephrotoxicity of the drug; however, because of limited information on the safety and efficacy of these admixtures, lack of standardization, and the commercial availability of lipid formulations of amphotericin B, these extemporaneous lipid emulsions are not recommended.

Amphotericin B Lipid Complex

Amphotericin B lipid complex (ABLC; Abelcet®) consists of a 1:1 molar ratio of amphotericin B complexed to a phospholipid vehicle composed of a 7:3 molar ratio of L-α-dimyristoylphosphatidylcholine (DMPC) to L-α-dimyristoylphosphatidylglycerol (DMPG). The amphotericin B-phospholipid complex has a microscopic, ribbon-like structure with a diameter of about 2–11 μm. Each mL of commercially available amphotericin B lipid complex suspension contains 5 mg of amphotericin B, 3.4 mg of DMPC, 1.5 mg of DMPG, and 9 mg of sodium chloride. The suspension occurs as a yellow, opaque liquid with a pH of 5–7.

Amphotericin B Liposomal

Commercially available amphotericin B liposomal (L-AmB; AmBisome®) is a lyophilized powder containing amphotericin B intercalated into a unilamellar bilayer liposomal membrane. Liposomes are microscopic vesicles composed of a phospholipid bilayer capable of encapsulating drugs; the lipid bilayer separates the internal aqueous core from the external environment. The liposomal membranes used in commercially available amphotericin B liposomal have a diameter of less than 100 nm and consist of hydrogenated soy phosphatidylcholine (HSPC), cholesterol, distearoylphosphatidylglycerol, and alpha tocopherol. Commercially available amphotericin B liposomal also contains sucrose for isotonicity and disodium succinate hexahydrate as a buffer. Because of the amphophilic substances used in the membrane and the lipophilic nature of amphotericin B, the drug is an integral part of the overall structure of the liposomes. Reconstitution of commercially available amphotericin B liposomal with sterile water for injection results in a yellow, translucent suspension with a pH of 5–6.

● Stability
Conventional Amphotericin B

Conventional amphotericin B powder for injection should be stored at 2–8°C and protected from light.

Following reconstitution with sterile water for injection, colloidal solutions of conventional amphotericin B containing 5 mg/mL should be protected from light and are stable for 24 hours at room temperature or 1 week when refrigerated.

Reconstituted colloidal solutions of conventional amphotericin B must be diluted *only* with 5% dextrose in water having a pH greater than 4.2 since the colloidal particles of the drug tend to coagulate quickly at pH less than 5. (See Reconstitution and Administration: Conventional Amphotericin B, in Dosage and Administration.) IV solutions of the drug containing 0.1 mg/mL or less should be used promptly after dilution. Although the manufacturers state that IV infusions of amphotericin B should be protected from light during administration, potency is unaffected if reconstituted dispersions or IV infusions of the drug are exposed to light for less than 8–24 hours.

Dilutions of amphotericin B apparently are compatible with limited amounts of heparin sodium and hydrocortisone sodium succinate or methylprednisolone sodium succinate. Specialized references should be consulted for specific compatibility information.

Amphotericin B Lipid Complex

Commercially available amphotericin B lipid complex (Abelcet®) suspension for IV infusion should be refrigerated at 2–8°C and protected from light. Following dilution in 5% dextrose injection, amphotericin B lipid complex is stable for up to 48 hours at 2–8°C and for an additional 6 hours at room temperature. Amphotericin B lipid complex suspension and dilutions of the drug should not be frozen; any unused solutions of the drug should be discarded.

Amphotericin B Liposomal

Commercially available lyophilized amphotericin B liposomal (AmBisome®) should be stored at 25°C or lower. Following reconstitution with sterile water for injection, liposomal amphotericin B solutions containing 4 mg/mL may be stored for up to 24 hours at 2–8°C and should not be frozen. IV infusions of amphotericin B liposomal should be initiated within 6 hours after dilution in 5% dextrose injection. Any partially used vials of the drug should be discarded.

PREPARATIONS

Excipients in commercially available drug preparations may have clinically important effects in some individuals; consult specific product labeling for details.

Amphotericin B

Parenteral		
For injection, for IV infusion	50 mg*	Amphotericin B for Injection

* available from one or more manufacturer, distributor, and/or repackager by generic (nonproprietary) name

Amphotericin B Lipid Complex

Parenteral		
Injectable suspension concentrate, for IV infusion	5 mg (of amphotericin B) per mL (100 mg)	Abelcet®, Sigma Tau

Amphotericin B Liposomal

Parenteral		
For injection, for IV infusion	50 mg (of amphotericin B)	AmBisome®, Astellas (also promoted by Gilead Sciences)

† Use is not currently included in the labeling approved by the US Food and Drug Administration.

Selected Revisions October 9, 2017, © Copyright, March 1, 1975, American Society of Health-System Pharmacists, Inc.

Flucytosine

8:14.32 • PYRIMIDINES

■ Flucytosine, a fluorinated pyrimidine analog, is a synthetic antifungal agent.

USES

Flucytosine is used for the treatment of serious infections caused by susceptible *Candida* or *Cryptococcus neoformans*.

Flucytosine usually is used as an adjunct to IV amphotericin B, and should *not* be used alone in the treatment of systemic candidiasis and cryptococcosis. Use of flucytosine alone may be ineffective and may result in emergence of flucytosine resistance. Although concomitant use of flucytosine and amphotericin B is based on reported in vitro and in vivo synergistic effects, there is some evidence that combined use of the drugs may be associated with an increased risk of serious adverse effects, especially in immunocompromised patients such as those with human immunodeficiency virus (HIV) infection.

To optimize efficacy and reduce the risk of toxicity when flucytosine is used concomitantly with another antifungal, flucytosine dosage should be carefully adjusted based on serum concentrations of the drug and patients receiving such therapy should be monitored closely for adverse effects. (See Dosage and Administration: Dosage.) In addition, because of concerns related to intrinsic resistance or emergence of resistance to flucytosine, it has been recommended that in vitro susceptibility tests be performed prior to and during flucytosine therapy, whenever available.

● Candida Infections

Oral flucytosine is used in conjunction with IV amphotericin B for the treatment of serious *Candida* infections, including urinary tract or pulmonary infections, candidemia, endocarditis, meningitis, and endophthalmitis.

For the treatment of CNS candidiasis in adults, the Infectious Diseases Society of America (IDSA) recommends initial treatment with IV amphotericin B (with or without oral flucytosine) followed by step-down treatment with fluconazole.

For initial treatment of CNS candidiasis in neonates, IDSA and the American Academy of Pediatrics (AAP) recommend monotherapy with IV amphotericin B. Although oral flucytosine has been used in conjunction with IV amphotericin B for the treatment of severe invasive candidiasis, including CNS candidiasis, in pediatric patients†, this combination regimen is not usually recommended for the treatment of candidiasis in children, including HIV-infected children. AAP and other clinicians state that routine use of flucytosine for the treatment of meningitis in neonates† is not recommended because of concerns regarding toxicity. IDSA states that salvage therapy with a regimen of flucytosine and amphotericin B should be considered in neonates† *only* if there is no response to amphotericin B alone.

For the treatment of endocarditis (native or prosthetic valve) or implantable cardiac device infections caused by *Candida*, IDSA recommends initial treatment with a lipid formulation of IV amphotericin B (with or without oral flucytosine) or an IV echinocandin (anidulafungin, caspofungin, micafungin) followed by step-down treatment with fluconazole.

Oral flucytosine is used alone or in conjunction with IV amphotericin B for the treatment of certain urinary tract infections caused by *Candida*, especially fluconazole-resistant strains. IDSA states that antifungal treatment is not usually indicated in patients with asymptomatic cystitis, unless there is a high risk of disseminated candidiasis (e.g., neutropenic patients, low-birthweight infants [less than 1.5 kg], patients undergoing urologic manipulations). Fluconazole is the drug of choice for the treatment of symptomatic cystitis, pyelonephritis, or fungus balls likely to be caused by fluconazole-susceptible *Candida*. When fluconazole-resistant *C. glabrata* are likely, IV amphotericin B or oral flucytosine is recommended for symptomatic cystitis and IV amphotericin B (with or without oral flucytosine) or oral flucytosine alone is recommended for pyelonephritis.

For the treatment of endophthalmitis caused by fluconazole- and voriconazole-resistant *Candida*, IDSA states that IV amphotericin B liposomal (with or without oral flucytosine) is the regimen of choice. In patients with macular involvement, intravitreal administration of conventional amphotericin B also is recommended to ensure prompt high intraocular levels of antifungal activity. Decisions regarding antifungal treatment and surgical intervention should be made jointly by an ophthalmologist and an infectious disease clinician.

● Cryptococcosis

Oral flucytosine usually is used in conjunction with IV amphotericin B for the treatment of serious cryptococcal infections, including pulmonary infections, septicemia, and meningitis caused by *C. neoformans*. Concomitant use of amphotericin B and flucytosine for initial treatment of cryptococcosis appears to reduce the time required for sterilization of CSF in those with CNS involvement and may decrease the risk of subsequent relapse and improve survival. Oral flucytosine also has been used in conjunction with fluconazole for the treatment of cryptococcal meningitis in HIV-infected individuals. Flucytosine should *not* be used alone for the treatment of cryptococcosis.

For the treatment of cryptococcal meningitis in HIV-infected adults, adolescents, and children, the US Centers for Disease Control and Prevention (CDC), National Institutes of Health (NIH), IDSA, and other clinicians state that the preferred regimen is initial (induction) therapy with IV amphotericin B (liposomal or conventional formulation) given in conjunction with oral flucytosine for at least 2 weeks until there is evidence of clinical improvement and negative CSF cultures after repeat lumbar puncture, then follow-up (consolidation) therapy with oral or IV fluconazole given for at least 8 weeks, followed by long-term suppressive or maintenance therapy (secondary prophylaxis) with oral fluconazole to complete at least 1 year of azole therapy.

One alternative regimen for initial (induction) treatment of cryptococcal meningitis in HIV-infected adults, adolescents, and children who cannot receive the preferred regimen is oral or IV fluconazole used in conjunction with oral flucytosine. Alternative regimens may be less effective and are recommended only in patients who cannot tolerate or have not responded to the preferred regimen.

Although data are limited, CDC, NIH, and IDSA state that recommendations for the treatment of CNS, pulmonary, or disseminated infections caused by *C. gattii* and recommendations for long-term suppressive or maintenance therapy (secondary prophylaxis) of *C. gattii* infections are the same as the recommendations for *C. neoformans* infections. IDSA states that single, small cryptococcoma may be treated with oral fluconazole, but induction therapy with a regimen of IV amphotericin B and oral flucytosine given for 4–6 weeks, followed by consolidation therapy with fluconazole given for 6–18 months should be considered for very large or multiple cryptococcomas caused by *C. gattii*. Regimens that include IV amphotericin B (conventional or liposomal formulations), flucytosine, and fluconazole have been effective in a few patients with CNS infections known to be caused by *C. gattii*.

● Chromoblastomycosis

Oral flucytosine has been used alone or in conjunction with other antifungals for the treatment of chromoblastomycosis† (chromomycosis) caused by various dematiaceous fungi (e.g., *Cladosporium*, *Exophiala*, *Phialophora*). Optimum treatment of chromoblastomycosis has not been identified. Azole antifungals (usually itraconazole) or terbinafine have been effective and may be the preferred antifungals for the treatment of chromoblastomycosis; surgery and/or adjunctive use of other therapies (e.g., heat therapy, laser therapy, photodynamic therapy) may be indicated.

A regimen of itraconazole and flucytosine has been effective for the treatment of chromoblastomycosis in some patients and a regimen of posaconazole and flucytosine has been suggested as a possible alternative in refractory cases. Although amphotericin B has been used in conjunction with flucytosine for the treatment of chromoblastomycosis, this regimen is no longer recommended for such infections.

● Aspergillosis

Oral flucytosine has been used concomitantly with IV amphotericin B for the treatment of invasive aspergillosis† or other infections caused by *Aspergillus* (e.g., osteomyelitis and joint infections); however, it is unclear whether concomitant use of amphotericin B and flucytosine offers any benefit over use of amphotericin B alone for the treatment of invasive aspergillosis and there are concerns related to a possible increased incidence of adverse effects with concomitant therapy.

Voriconazole is considered the drug of choice for initial treatment of invasive aspergillosis in most patients and IV amphotericin B (a lipid formulation) is the preferred alternative.

● Free-living Ameba Infections

Flucytosine has been used in conjunction with other anti-infectives in a few patients for the treatment of free-living ameba infections†, including granulomatous amebic encephalitis or other infections caused by *Acanthamoeba*† or *Balamuthia mandrillaris*†.

CNS infections caused by free-living ameba have a high mortality rate, and only a very limited number of cases have been successfully treated. Early diagnosis and treatment with a multiple-drug regimen may increase the chance of survival. Although data are limited, most reported cases of *Acanthamoeba* and *B. mandrillaris* infection have been treated empirically with regimens that included a variety of anti-infectives (e.g., albendazole, amphotericin B, azole antifungals [fluconazole, itraconazole, ketoconazole], flucytosine, macrolides [azithromycin or clarithromycin], miltefosine, rifampin, pentamidine, sulfonamides [co-trimoxazole or sulfadiazine]).

For assistance with diagnosis or treatment of suspected free-living ameba infections, clinicians can contact the CDC Emergency Operations Center at 770-488-7100.

DOSAGE AND ADMINISTRATION

● Administration

Flucytosine is administered orally. The manufacturer suggests that nausea and vomiting associated with oral flucytosine may be reduced or avoided if each dose is administered by ingesting the capsules a few at a time over a 15-minute period.

Flucytosine has been administered IV; however, a parenteral dosage form of the drug is not commercially available in the US. Flucytosine also has been administered topically as a cream, but topical preparations of the drug are not commercially available in the US.

Extemporaneously Compounded Oral Liquid Formulations

For patients unable to swallow capsules, oral suspensions containing 10 or 50 mg/mL have been prepared extemporaneously using the commercially available capsules of the drug.

Standardize 4 Safety

Standardized concentrations for an extemporaneously compounded oral suspension of flucytosine have been established through Standardize 4 Safety (S4S), a national patient safety initiative to reduce medication errors, especially during transitions of care. Multidisciplinary expert panels were convened to determine recommended standard concentrations. Because recommendations from the S4S panels may differ from the manufacturer's prescribing information, caution is advised when using concentrations that differ from labeling, particularly when using rate information from the label. For additional information on S4S (including updates that may be available), see https://www.ashp.org/pharmacy-practice/standardize-4-safety-initiative.

TABLE 1: Standardize 4 Safety Compounded Oral Liquid Standards for Flucytosine

Concentration Standards
50 mg/mL

● Dosage

Because prolonged serum flucytosine concentrations exceeding 100 mcg/mL may be associated with an increased risk of toxicity (e.g., adverse hematologic, GI, and hepatic effects), flucytosine dosage usually should be adjusted to ensure that peak serum concentrations of the drug remain below 100 mcg/mL. However, optimal target serum concentrations have not been identified, and a variety of target ranges have been recommended. The American Academy of Pediatrics (AAP), US Centers for Disease Control and Prevention (CDC), National Institutes of Health (NIH), Infectious Diseases Society of America (IDSA), and others generally recommend target serum flucytosine concentrations of 30–80 mcg/mL.

Some clinicians suggest that serum flucytosine concentrations should be measured beginning 3–5 days after initiation of the drug (or beginning after 3–5 doses) and then once or twice weekly during treatment and whenever there is evidence of toxicity or a change in renal function. Peak serum concentrations usually are measured using blood samples taken 2 hours after an oral dose.

Adult Dosage

General Adult Dosage

The usual adult dosage of oral flucytosine recommended by the manufacturer is 50–150 mg/kg daily given in divided doses at 6-hour intervals. The manufacturer recommends that the lower dosage be used initially in patients with elevated BUN or serum creatinine concentrations.

To reduce the risk of toxicity in patients receiving flucytosine concomitantly with IV amphotericin B, some clinicians suggest that flucytosine therapy be initiated using a low dosage (i.e., 75 mg/kg daily given in 4 divided doses). Dosage can then be adjusted based on serum concentrations of flucytosine and the presence or absence of amphotericin B-associated renal toxicity.

Candida Infections

When used alone or in conjunction with IV amphotericin B for the treatment of *Candida* infections, IDSA recommends that oral flucytosine be given in a dosage of 25 mg/kg 4 times daily.

For the treatment of CNS candidiasis, IDSA recommends that flucytosine be given in a dosage of 25 mg/kg 4 times daily in conjunction with IV amphotericin B. After several weeks of concomitant therapy and when a response is attained, treatment can be transitioned to fluconazole step-down therapy. Antifungal treatment should be continued until all signs and symptoms, CSF abnormalities, and radiologic abnormalities resolve.

For the treatment of endocarditis (native or prosthetic valve) or implantable cardiac device infections caused by *Candida*, IDSA recommends that flucytosine be given in a dosage of 25 mg/kg 4 times daily in conjunction with IV amphotericin B. If the infection is caused by fluconazole-susceptible strains, treatment can be transitioned to fluconazole step-down therapy after the patient is clinically stable and *Candida* have been cleared from the bloodstream.

If flucytosine is used as an alternative for the treatment of symptomatic cystitis caused by fluconazole-resistant *C. glabrata*, IDSA recommends that the drug be given in a dosage of 25 mg/kg 4 times daily for 7–10 days.

For the treatment of pyelonephritis caused by fluconazole-resistant *C. glabrata*, IDSA recommends that flucytosine be given in a dosage of 25 mg/kg 4 times daily in conjunction with IV amphotericin B for up to 7 days. Alternatively, if flucytosine monotherapy is used, a dosage of 25 mg/kg 4 times daily for 2 weeks is recommended. These same regimens can be used for the treatment of *Candida* urinary tract infections associated with fungus balls.

For the treatment of *Candida* endophthalmitis caused by fluconazole- and voriconazole-resistant *Candida*, flucytosine should be given in a dosage of 25 mg/kg 4 times daily in conjunction with IV amphotericin B liposomal. The duration of treatment should be at least 4–6 weeks as determined by repeated examinations to verify resolution.

Cryptococcosis

When flucytosine is used in conjunction with another antifungal (e.g., IV amphotericin B, fluconazole) for the treatment of severe cryptococcal infections, a dosage of 100–150 mg/kg daily is recommended.

For the treatment of cryptococcal meningitis in HIV-infected adults and adolescents, CDC, NIH, and IDSA recommend a regimen than includes initial (induction) therapy with oral flucytosine in a dosage of 25 mg/kg 4 times daily in conjunction with IV amphotericin B (liposomal or conventional formulation) given for at least 2 weeks until there is evidence of clinical improvement and negative CSF cultures after repeat lumbar puncture, then follow-up (consolidation) therapy with oral or IV fluconazole alone.

As an alternative for the treatment of cryptococcal meningitis in HIV-infected adults and adolescents who cannot receive amphotericin B, CDC, NIH, and IDSA recommend initial (induction) therapy with oral flucytosine in a dosage of 25 mg/kg 4 times daily in conjunction with oral or IV fluconazole.

Free-living Ameba Infections

If flucytosine is used in conjunction with other anti-infectives for the treatment of free-living ameba infections†, including granulomatous amebic encephalitis or other infections caused by *Acanthamoeba*† or *Balamuthia mandrillaris*† (see Uses: Free-living Ameba Infections), some clinicians recommend a dosage of 37.5 mg/kg every 6 hours (up to 150 mg/kg daily). Higher dosage has been used in some patients.

Pediatric Dosage

General Pediatric Dosage

If flucytosine is used in pediatric patients†, AAP recommends a dosage of 100 mg/kg daily given in divided doses every 6 hours.

Candidiasis

For salvage therapy of CNS candidiasis in neonates† who have not responded to initial treatment with IV amphotericin B alone, IDSA states that oral flucytosine can be given in a dosage of 25 mg/kg 4 times daily in conjunction with IV amphotericin B. After several weeks and when a response is attained, transition to fluconazole step-down therapy is recommended. Antifungal treatment should be continued until all signs, symptoms, CSF abnormalities, and radiologic abnormalities (if present) have resolved.

Cryptococcosis

For the treatment of CNS or disseminated cryptococcosis in children†, IDSA recommends an initial (induction) regimen of oral flucytosine given in a dosage of 100 mg/kg daily in 4 divided doses in conjunction with IV amphotericin B given for at least 2 weeks, then follow-up (consolidation) therapy with oral fluconazole alone for at least 8 weeks.

For the treatment of cryptococcal meningitis in HIV-infected infants and children†, CDC, NIH, IDSA, and other clinicians recommend a regimen than includes initial (induction) therapy with oral flucytosine in a dosage of 25 mg/kg 4 times daily in conjunction with IV amphotericin B given for at least 2 weeks until there is evidence of clinical improvement and negative CSF cultures after repeat lumbar puncture, then follow-up (consolidation) therapy with oral or IV fluconazole alone.

For the treatment of cryptococcal meningitis in HIV-infected infants and children† who cannot receive amphotericin B, CDC, NIH, IDSA, and other clinicians recommend initial (induction) therapy with oral flucytosine in a dosage of 25 mg/kg 4 times daily in conjunction with oral or IV fluconazole.

For the treatment of severe pulmonary or disseminated (non-CNS) cryptococcosis in HIV-infected infants and children†, CDC, NIH, IDSA, and other clinicians recommend that flucytosine be given in a dosage of 25 mg/kg 4 times daily in conjunction with IV amphotericin B. Treatment duration depends on the response and site and severity of infection.

● Dosage in Renal Impairment

In patients with impaired renal function, doses and/or frequency of administration of flucytosine must be modified in response to the degree of impairment and serum concentrations of the drug. Several methods of calculating flucytosine dosage for patients with impaired renal function have been proposed; however, for greater accuracy, dosage in these patients should be based on actual serum concentrations of the drug. Precise dosing is limited, since flucytosine is commercially available only as 250- and 500-mg capsules.

Some clinicians recommend that adults with creatinine clearances of 20–40 mL/minute receive 25 mg/kg of flucytosine every 12 hours and that those with creatinine clearances of 10–20 mL/minute receive 25 mg/kg once daily. In those with creatinine clearances less than 10 mL/minute, these clinicians recommend a flucytosine dosage of 25 mg/kg once every 48 hours.

Other clinicians recommend that the usual individual dose of flucytosine (12.5–37.5 mg/kg) be administered every 12 hours in patients with creatinine clearances of 20–40 mL/minute, every 24 hours in those with creatinine clearances of 10–20 mL/minute, and every 24–48 hours or longer (as determined by serum drug concentrations) in those with creatinine clearances less than 10 mL/minute. Alternatively, other clinicians have recommended that flucytosine doses of 12–35 mg/kg be administered at intervals equal to twice the half-life of the drug.

In patients undergoing hemodialysis, some clinicians recommend that flucytosine doses of 20–50 mg/kg be given once every 48–72 hours and that the doses be administered after dialysis.

CAUTIONS

● Hematologic Effects

The most frequent adverse effects of flucytosine therapy appear to be related to the drug's effect on rapidly proliferating tissues, particularly the bone marrow. Anemia, leukopenia, pancytopenia, thrombocytopenia, eosinophilia, agranulocytosis, and aplastic anemia have been reported in patients receiving flucytosine.

Fatal bone marrow aplasia has been reported in some patients receiving flucytosine. Bone marrow toxicity can be irreversible and may lead to death in immunosuppressed patients.

The risk of bone marrow toxicity appears to be increased in patients who have hematologic disease and in those who are receiving or previously received radiation or drug therapy that depresses the bone marrow. The risk of adverse hematologic effects also may be increased in patients who have prolonged, high serum flucytosine concentrations (i.e., greater than 100 mcg/mL), particularly in those with renal dysfunction or during concomitant therapy with amphotericin B.

● GI Effects

Adverse GI effects, which are sometimes severe, have been reported in patients receiving flucytosine and have included anorexia, abdominal bloating, abdominal pain, diarrhea, dry mouth, duodenal ulcer, GI hemorrhage, nausea, vomiting, ulcerative colitis, and enterocolitis.

● Hepatic Effects

Increased hepatic enzyme concentrations (serum alkaline phosphatase, AST [SGOT], ALT [SGPT]) and increased serum bilirubin concentrations have been reported in patients receiving flucytosine. Hepatic dysfunction and jaundice have been reported.

Increased serum hepatic enzyme concentrations generally appear to be dose related and reversible. However, acute hepatic injury with possible fatal outcome has been reported in debilitated patients receiving flucytosine. In one patient, abnormal lactic dehydrogenase concentrations and sulfobromophthalein retention were attributed to hepatic necrosis, possibly resulting from flucytosine therapy.

● Renal Effects

Increased concentrations of BUN and serum creatinine have been reported in patients receiving flucytosine. Azotemia, crystalluria, and renal failure also have been reported.

● Nervous System Effects

Adverse nervous system effects that have been reported with flucytosine include ataxia, hearing loss, headache, paresthesia, parkinsonism, seizures, peripheral neuropathy, vertigo, and sedation. Confusion, hallucinations, and psychosis also have been reported.

An acute cerebellar syndrome with dysmetria and ataxia occurred in a patient receiving flucytosine concomitantly with amphotericin B. The syndrome resolved over the next 4 weeks following discontinuance of flucytosine, although mild dysmetria persisted.

● *Dermatologic and Sensitivity Reactions*

Rash, pruritus, urticaria, and photosensitivity have been reported with flucytosine. Allergic reactions and toxic epidermal necrolysis (Lyell syndrome) also have been reported.

Anaphylaxis, manifested as diffuse erythema, pruritus, conjunctival injection, fever, abdominal pain, edema, tachycardia, and hypotension, has been reported in at least one patient with acquired immunodeficiency syndrome (AIDS) receiving flucytosine therapy. Anaphylaxis recurred following rechallenge with the drug.

● *Other Adverse Effects*

Other adverse effects that have been reported with flucytosine include fatigue, pyrexia, hypoglycemia, hypokalemia, weakness, cardiac arrest, myocardial toxicity, ventricular dysfunction, chest pain, dyspnea, and respiratory arrest.

● *Precautions and Contraindications*

Flucytosine is contraindicated in patients hypersensitive to the drug.

Flucytosine should be used with extreme caution in patients with bone marrow depression and in patients with impaired renal function. Flucytosine is eliminated mainly by the kidneys and renal impairment may lead to accumulation of the drug and increase the risk of toxicity. Dosage of the drug should be adjusted in patients with renal impairment to prevent accumulation of the drug. (See Dosage and Administration: Dosage in Renal Impairment.)

Hematologic, renal, and hepatic status must be monitored closely during flucytosine therapy. Hematologic status (leucocyte and thrombocyte counts), renal function, hepatic function (serum alkaline phosphatase, AST, ALT), and electrolytes should be evaluated prior to initiation of flucytosine and at frequent intervals during therapy with the drug.

Because serum flucytosine concentrations exceeding 100 mcg/mL may be associated with an increased incidence of toxicity, especially GI effects (diarrhea, nausea, vomiting), hematologic effects (leukopenia, thrombocytopenia), and hepatic effects (hepatitis), flucytosine serum concentrations should be monitored and dosage adjusted to ensure that serum concentrations of the drug remain below 100 mcg/mL. (See Dosage and Administration: Dosage.)

● *Pediatric Precautions*

Safety and efficacy of flucytosine have not been systematically studied in children.

If flucytosine is used in neonates and infants†, serum concentrations of the drug should be closely monitored. Limited data regarding the pharmacokinetics of flucytosine in neonates indicate considerable interindividual variation in plasma concentrations attained, which does not correlate with gestational age. High plasma concentrations of the drug may accumulate in very low-birthweight infants because of immature renal function.

Some clinicians state that flucytosine should be avoided in children† with severe renal impairment.

The manufacturer states that no unexpected adverse effects were reported when flucytosine was given to some neonates† in a dosage of 25–200 mg/kg daily (with or without concomitant amphotericin B). Hypokalemia and acidemia occurred in one neonate receiving flucytosine and amphotericin B concomitantly, and anemia was reported in another who received flucytosine monotherapy. Transient thrombocytopenia also has been reported in pediatric patients receiving flucytosine (with or without amphotericin B).

● *Geriatric Precautions*

Flucytosine dosage adjustment may be required in geriatric patients based on renal function. (See Dosage and Administration: Dosage in Renal Impairment.)

● *Mutagenicity and Carcinogenicity*

Flucytosine was not mutagenic in various in vitro studies using microbial (e.g., *Salmonella typhimurium*) test systems in the presence or absence of activating enzymes. In addition, there was no evidence of mutagenicity in repair assay systems.

The carcinogenic potential of flucytosine has not been adequately studied to date.

● *Pregnancy, Fertility, and Lactation*

Pregnancy

Flucytosine was shown to be teratogenic in rats. When flucytosine was given to rats in a dosage of 40 mg/kg daily (0.051 times the human dosage) on days 7–13 of gestation, vertebral fusions occurred; at a dosage of 700 mg/kg daily (0.89 times the human dosage) on days 9–12 of gestation, cleft lip and palate and micrognathia were reported. In mice, flucytosine dosage of 400 mg/kg daily (0.236 times the human dosage) on days 7–13 of gestation was associated with a low incidence of cleft palate that was not statistically significant. Flucytosine was not teratogenic in rabbits when given in dosages up to 100 mg/kg daily (0.243 times the human dosage) on days 6–18 of gestation.

There are no adequate or controlled studies to date using flucytosine in pregnant women, and the drug should be used during pregnancy only when potential benefits justify possible risks to the fetus.

Fertility

The effects of flucytosine on fertility or reproductive performance have not been adequately studied in animals.

Lactation

It is not known whether flucytosine is distributed into human milk.

Because many drugs are distributed into human milk and because of the potential for serious adverse effects in nursing infants, a decision should be made whether to discontinue nursing or the drug, taking into account the importance of the drug to the mother.

DRUG INTERACTIONS

● *Drugs that Affect Renal Function*

Because flucytosine is principally excreted by glomerular filtration, concomitant use of drugs that impair glomerular filtration may prolong the elimination half-life of flucytosine and increase the risk of toxicity. Flucytosine serum concentrations should be closely monitored if drugs that reduce glomerular filtration are used concomitantly.

● *Myelosuppressive Agents*

The risk of bone marrow toxicity may be increased if flucytosine is used concomitantly with other agents that depress the bone marrow. Because of potential additive effects on bone marrow, caution is advised if flucytosine is used concomitantly with other myelosuppressive drugs (e.g., zidovudine).

● *Antifungal Agents*

Amphotericin B

In some in vitro studies, the combination of flucytosine and amphotericin B resulted in synergistic inhibition of *Cryptococcus neoformans*, *Candida albicans*, and *C. tropicalis*. The suggested mechanism of this synergism is that the binding of amphotericin B to sterols in cell membranes increases the permeability of the cytoplasmic membrane, thus allowing greater penetration of flucytosine into the fungal cell. However, in a study evaluating the antifungal effects of the drugs in the presence of serum, the combination of amphotericin B and flucytosine was not additive or synergistic against *C. albicans*.

There is some evidence that concomitant use of amphotericin B and flucytosine may increase the toxicity of flucytosine, possibly by increasing cellular uptake and/or by decreasing renal excretion of the drug.

If flucytosine is used in conjunction with amphotericin B, especially in patients with human immunodeficiency virus (HIV) infection, some clinicians suggest using a low initial dosage of flucytosine. In addition, serum flucytosine concentrations and blood cell counts should be carefully monitored and flucytosine dosage adjusted if needed. (See Dosage and Administration: Dosage.)

Azole Antifungal Agents

The combination of flucytosine and fluconazole or itraconazole was synergistic, additive, or indifferent in vitro against *C. neoformans*; there was no evidence of antagonism. The combination of fluconazole and flucytosine generally did not exert a synergistic effect against *C. neoformans* isolates that had fluconazole MICs of 8 mcg/mL or greater. Synergism also has been demonstrated when the combination of fluconazole and flucytosine was evaluated in vivo in a murine model of cryptococcal meningitis. It has been suggested that synergism between the drugs may occur because fluconazole damages the fungal cell membrane allowing greater intracellular penetration of flucytosine.

● *Cytarabine*

Cytarabine (cytosine arabinoside) reportedly antagonizes the antifungal activity of flucytosine, possibly by competitive inhibition. Concomitant use of cytarabine and flucytosine is not recommended.

LABORATORY TEST INTERFERENCES

● *Tests for Creatinine*

There have been reports that flucytosine can cause markedly false elevations in serum creatinine values when certain test methods are used. Because flucytosine does not affect serum creatinine values when the Jaffé reaction or other alkaline picrate methods are used, such methods should be used to evaluate serum creatinine concentrations in patients receiving flucytosine.

ACUTE TOXICITY

Limited information is available on the acute toxicity of flucytosine. Although there have been no reports to date of intentional overdosage of flucytosine, overdosage would be expected to produce pronounced manifestations of the known adverse effects of the drug. Prolonged serum flucytosine concentrations greater than 100 mcg/mL may be associated with an increased incidence of toxicity, especially GI effects (diarrhea, nausea, vomiting), hematologic effects (leukopenia, thrombocytopenia), and hepatic effects (hepatitis).

In the event of flucytosine overdosage, the manufacturer recommends prompt use of gastric lavage or an emetic. Because flucytosine is eliminated essentially unchanged in urine, adequate fluid intake should be maintained and IV fluids given if necessary. Hematologic parameters should be assessed frequently and liver and kidney function carefully monitored. Appropriate symptomatic therapy should be instituted if indicated. The manufacturer suggests that consideration be given to the use of hemodialysis in the management of flucytosine overdosage since the procedure readily removes the drug in anuric patients.

MECHANISM OF ACTION

Flucytosine may be fungistatic or fungicidal in action depending on the concentration of the drug. Two possible mechanisms of action have been identified for flucytosine. Flucytosine appears to enter fungal cells via the action of fungal-specific cytosine permease. Inside the cell, flucytosine is converted to fluorouracil (5-FU) by cytosine deaminase and then after several intermediate steps is converted to 5-fluorouridine triphosphate (FUTP). FUTP is incorporated into fungal RNA and interferes with protein synthesis. Flucytosine also appears to be converted to 5-fluorodeoxyuridine monophosphate, which noncompetitively inhibits thymidylate synthetase and interferes with DNA synthesis. Flucytosine does not appear to have antineoplastic activity.

SPECTRUM

Flucytosine is active in vitro and in clinical infections against *Candida albicans* and *Cryptococcus neoformans*.

Flucytosine is inactive against *Blastomyces dermatitidis*, *Coccidioides immitis*, *Histoplasma capsulatum*, *Paracoccidioides brasiliensis*, *Madurella*, dermatophytes (*Microsporum*, *Trichophyton*, *Epidermophyton*), and bacteria.

● *Fungi*

Flucytosine is active in vitro against most strains of *C. albicans*, *C. glabrata*, *C. guilliermondii*, *C. parapsilosis*, and *C. tropicalis*. In vitro, susceptible strains of *Candida* generally are inhibited by flucytosine concentrations of 4 mcg/mL or less.

Although some strains of *C. krusei* and *C. lusitaniae* may be susceptible to flucytosine in vitro, other strains are inhibited only by high concentrations of the drug and are considered resistant. Some clinical isolates of *C. auris* (often misidentified as *C. haemulonii*, *C. famata*, or *Rhodotorula glutinis*) have been susceptible to flucytosine in vitro; however, a wide range of minimum inhibitory concentrations (MICs) has been reported and reduced susceptibility or resistance to flucytosine occurs. *C. kefyr* usually is resistant to flucytosine.

Susceptible strains of *C. neoformans* generally are inhibited in vitro by flucytosine concentrations of 0.03–8 mcg/mL. Flucytosine concentrations of 0.25–2 mcg/mL inhibit some strains of *C. gattii*. However, some strains of *C. neoformans* and *C. gattii* are resistant to flucytosine.

There is some in vitro evidence that flucytosine has activity against some of the causative agents of chromoblastomycosis and phaeohyphomycosis, including some strains of *Cladophialophora*, *Phialophora verrucosa*, *Exophiala* (*E. castellanii*, *E. dermatitidis*, *E. spinifera*), and *Cladosporium*. Although some strains of *Fonsecaea* have been susceptible to flucytosine in vitro, the drug reportedly has limited or no activity against the organism.

Although *Sporothrix schenckii* usually is resistant to flucytosine, some strains may be inhibited in vitro by flucytosine concentrations of 0.6–2 mcg/mL. Some strains of *Penicillium marneffei* are inhibited in vitro by flucytosine concentrations of 0.002–0.25 mcg/mL.

Aspergillus generally are resistant to flucytosine, but rare strains may be inhibited in vitro by flucytosine concentrations of 4 mcg/mL or less.

RESISTANCE

Resistance to flucytosine can be readily induced in vitro in *Candida* and *Cryptococcus neoformans*. Strains of *Candida* or *Cryptococcus* resistant to flucytosine have been isolated from patients who have never received the drug, and resistant strains of *Candida* and *C. neoformans* have emerged in patients receiving oral flucytosine alone or in conjunction with IV amphotericin B. Resistance to flucytosine can develop during monotherapy with the drug.

Resistance to flucytosine may be related to mutations that affect the production of fungal enzymes (e.g., uridine monophosphate pyrophosphorylase, cytosine permease, cytosine deaminase) important to the mechanism of action of the drug. Resistance also may result from mutations that result in increased production of pyrimidines.

Cross-resistance does not occur between flucytosine and amphotericin B.

PHARMACOKINETICS

● *Absorption*

Flucytosine is rapidly and almost completed absorbed from the GI tract. Bioavailability is 78–90% following oral administration. Food decreases the rate, but not the extent, of absorption.

In patients with normal renal function, peak serum flucytosine concentrations of 30–40 mcg/mL are reached within 2 hours following a single 2-g oral dose. In other studies in patients with normal renal function receiving a 6-week regimen of oral flucytosine (150 mg/kg daily given in divided doses every 6 hours) and concomitant IV amphotericin B, mean serum concentrations of flucytosine 1–2 hours after a dose were approximately 70–80 mcg/mL.

In a limited number of neonates† receiving oral flucytosine in a dosage of 25, 50, or 100 mg/kg daily for the treatment of systemic candidiasis, median peak serum concentrations after 5 days of treatment were 19.6, 27.7, and 83.9 mcg/mL, respectively, and the mean time to peak concentrations was 2.5 hours. There was considerable interindividual variation in serum concentrations, which did not correlate with gestational age, and some neonates had serum flucytosine concentrations greater than 100 mcg/mL.

Peak serum concentrations of flucytosine are higher, more prolonged, and reached more slowly in patients with impaired renal function. In anephric patients, peak serum concentrations may be 50% higher than those in patients with normal renal function. It has been recommended that steady-state serum flucytosine concentrations should not exceed 100 mcg/mL to avoid toxic effects.

● Distribution

Flucytosine is widely distributed into body tissues and fluids including liver, kidney, spleen, heart, bronchial secretions, joints, peritoneal fluid, brain, bile, bone, and aqueous humor.

Flucytosine is distributed into CSF following oral administration, and CSF concentrations may range from 60–100% of serum concentrations of the drug. In an infant† who received a 25-mg oral dose of flucytosine, CSF concentrations of the drug were 43 mcg/mL 3 hours after the dose. In a neonate† receiving oral flucytosine in a dosage of 120–150 mg/kg daily, CSF concentrations ranged from 20–67 mcg/mL.

Studies in pregnant rats indicate that flucytosine administered intraperitoneally crosses the placenta.

It is not known if flucytosine is distributed into milk.

The apparent volume of distribution of flucytosine is about 0.68 L/kg in healthy adults and has ranged from 0.4–0.7 L/kg in patients with renal failure.

In vitro studies indicate that flucytosine is approximately 2.9–4% bound to serum proteins over the range of therapeutic concentrations found in blood.

● Elimination

Only minimal amounts of flucytosine are metabolized in humans. The drug is deaminated (probably by gut bacteria) to fluorouracil. The area under the concentration-time curve (AUC) ratio of fluorouracil to flucytosine is 4%.

The elimination half-life of flucytosine in patients with normal renal function has been reported to range from 2.4–4.8. Half-life of the drug is prolonged in patients with renal impairment and has been reported to be 6–14 hours in those with creatinine clearances of 40 mL/minute, 12–15 hours in those with creatinine clearances of 20 mL/minute, 21–27 hours in those with creatinine clearances of 10 mL/minute, and 30–250 hours in those with creatinine clearances less than 10 mL/minute. Half-lives up to 1160 hours have been reported in a few patients with creatinine clearances less than 2 mL/minute. Some clinicians have suggested that the half-life of flucytosine in hours is approximately 5 or 6 times the serum creatinine concentration in mg/dL.

In a limited number of neonates and infants†, the median half-life of flucytosine was 7.4 hours.

Flucytosine is eliminated by the kidneys, principally by glomerular filtration without substantial tubular reabsorption. More than 90% of an oral dose of flucytosine is excreted unchanged in the urine. Urinary concentrations of flucytosine are generally 10–100 times greater than serum concentrations, although urinary drug concentrations are much lower in patients with impaired renal function. In one study, patients with flucytosine serum half-lives of 40–83 hours achieved urinary flucytosine concentrations of 42–500 mcg/mL within 24 hours after a single 2-g oral dose. Unabsorbed flucytosine is excreted unchanged in the feces.

Hepatic impairment does not affect the pharmacokinetics of flucytosine.

Flucytosine is readily removed by peritoneal dialysis and hemodialysis.

CHEMISTRY AND STABILITY

● Chemistry

Flucytosine, a synthetic antifungal agent, is a fluorinated pyrimidine analog structurally related to fluorouracil and floxuridine. Flucytosine occurs as a white to off-white, crystalline powder that is odorless or has a slight odor; the drug is sparingly soluble in water and slightly soluble in alcohol. The drug has pK$_a$s of 2.9 and 10.71.

● Stability

Flucytosine capsules should be stored at 25°C, but may be exposed to temperatures ranging from 15–30°C.

PREPARATIONS

Excipients in commercially available drug preparations may have clinically important effects in some individuals; consult specific product labeling for details.

Flucytosine

Oral		
Capsules	250 mg*	Ancobon®, Valeant
		Flucytosine Capsules
	500 mg*	Ancobon®, Valeant
		Flucytosine Capsules

* available from one or more manufacturer, distributor, and/or repackager by generic (nonproprietary) name

† Use is not currently included in the labeling approved by the US Food and Drug Administration.

Selected Revisions June 10, 2024, © Copyright, November 1, 1976, American Society of Health-System Pharmacists, Inc.

Bictegravir Sodium, Emtricitabine, and Tenofovir Alafenamide Fumarate

8:18.08.12 · HIV INTEGRASE INHIBITORS

■ Bictegravir sodium, emtricitabine, and tenofovir alafenamide fumarate (BIC/FTC/TAF) is a fixed-combination antiretroviral agent containing bictegravir (human immunodeficiency virus type 1 [HIV-1] integrase strand transfer inhibitor), emtricitabine (HIV-1 nucleoside reverse transcriptase inhibitor), and tenofovir alafenamide (HIV-1 nucleotide reverse transcriptase inhibitor).

USES

● Treatment of HIV Infection

The fixed combination of bictegravir sodium, emtricitabine, and tenofovir alafenamide fumarate (BIC/FTC/TAF) is used as a complete regimen for the treatment of HIV-1 infection in adults and pediatric patients weighing ≥14 kg who are antiretroviral-naïve (have not previously received antiretroviral therapy) or to replace the current antiretroviral regimen in those who are virologically suppressed (HIV-1 RNA <50 copies/mL) on a stable antiretroviral regimen with no known or suspected substitutions associated with resistance to bictegravir or tenofovir.

Clinical Experience
Antiretroviral-naïve Adults

Efficacy of BIC/FTC/TAF in antiretroviral-naïve, HIV-infected adults was evaluated in 2 randomized, double blind, active-control, noninferiority phase 3 studies (study 1489; NCT02607930 and study 1490; NCT02607956). These studies indicated that BIC/FTC/TAF was noninferior to the fixed combination of abacavir, dolutegravir, and lamivudine (ABC/DTG/3TC) at 48, 96, and 144 weeks (study 1489) and was noninferior to a regimen of dolutegravir in conjunction with the fixed combination of emtricitabine and tenofovir alafenamide fumarate (FTC/TAF) at 48, 96, and 144 weeks (study 1490).

In study 1489, 629 antiretroviral-naïve adults (mean age 34 years, 90% male, 57% white, 36% Black, 3% Asian, 22% Hispanic/Latino, mean baseline plasma HIV-1 RNA level 4.4 $\log_{10}$ copies/mL, mean baseline CD4+ T-cell count 464 cells/mm^3) were randomized in a 1:1 ratio to receive BIC/FTC/TAF (bictegravir 50 mg, emtricitabine 200 mg, tenofovir alafenamide 25 mg) once daily or ABC/DTG/3TC (abacavir 600 mg, dolutegravir 50 mg, lamivudine 300 mg) once daily. The primary end point was virologic response (defined as a plasma HIV-1 RNA level <50 copies/mL) at 48 weeks. Results at 48 weeks indicated that BIC/FTC/TAF is noninferior to ABC/DTG/3TC in the proportion of patients achieving virologic response (92.4 and 93%, respectively). The mean increase in CD4+ T-cell count from baseline was 233 cells/mm^3 in those receiving BIC/FTC/TAF compared with 229 cells/mm^3 in those receiving ABC/DTG/3TC. Treatment outcomes were similar across subgroups (i.e., age, sex, race, baseline viral load, and baseline CD4+ T-cell count). At 96 weeks, 88% of patients receiving BIC/FTC/TAF and 90% of patients receiving ABC/DTG/3TC were still virologically suppressed (i.e., plasma HIV-1 RNA level <50 copies/mL); treatment-emergent resistance was not reported in any patient in either treatment group. At 144 weeks, 82% of patients receiving BIC/FTC/TAF and 84% of patients receiving ABC/DTG/3TC remained virologically suppressed with a plasma HIV-1 RNA level <50 copies/mL. The mean increase in CD4+ T-cell count from baseline to week 144 was 299 cells/mm^3 in those receiving BIC/FTC/TAF compared with 317 cells/mm^3 in those receiving ABC/DTG/3TC. No treatment-emergent resistance was reported in either treatment group.

In study 1490, 645 antiretroviral-naïve adults (mean age 37 years, 88% male, 59% white, 31% Black, 3% Asian, 25% Hispanic/Latino, mean baseline plasma HIV-1 RNA level 4.4 $\log_{10}$ copies/mL, mean baseline CD4+ T-cell count 456 cells/mm^3) were randomized to receive BIC/FTC/TAF (bictegravir 50 mg, emtricitabine 200 mg, tenofovir alafenamide 25 mg) once daily or a regimen of dolutegravir 50 mg in conjunction with FTC/TAF (emtricitabine 200 mg and tenofovir alafenamide 25 mg) once daily. The primary end point was virologic response (defined as a plasma HIV-1 RNA level <50 copies/mL) at 48 weeks. Results at 48 weeks indicated that BIC/FTC/TAF is noninferior to a regimen of dolutegravir and FTC/TAF in the proportion of patients achieving virologic response (89.4% and 92.9%, respectively). The mean increase in CD4+ T-cell count from baseline was 180 cells/mm^3 in those receiving BIC/FTC/TAF compared with 201 cells/mm^3 in those receiving the regimen of dolutegravir and FTC/TAF. Treatment outcomes were similar across subgroups (i.e., age, sex, race, baseline viral load, and baseline CD4+ T-cell count). At 96 weeks, 84% of patients receiving BIC/FTC/TAF and 86% of patients receiving dolutegravir and FTC/TAF were still virologically suppressed (i.e., plasma HIV-1 RNA level <50 copies/mL); treatment-emergent resistance was not reported in any patient in either treatment group. At 144 weeks, 82% of patients receiving BIC/FTC/TAF and 84% of patients receiving dolutegravir and FTC/TAF remained virologically suppressed with a plasma HIV-1 RNA level <50 copies/mL. The mean increase in CD4+ T-cell count from baseline to week 144 was 278 cells/mm^3 in those receiving BIC/FTC/TAF compared with 289 cells/mm^3 in those receiving dolutegravir and FTC/TAF. No treatment-emergent resistance was reported in either treatment group.

Antiretroviral-experienced Adults

Efficacy of BIC/FTC/TAF in antiretroviral-experienced adults was primarily evaluated in a randomized, double-blind, active-control, noninferiority, phase 3 study (trial 1844; NCT02603120) and a randomized, open-label, active-control, noninferiority, phase 3 study (trial 1878; NCT02603107).

In trial 1844, 563 previously treated adults with baseline plasma HIV-1 RNA levels <50 copies/mL for at least 3 months and no history of treatment failure (mean age 45 years, 89% male, 73% white, 22% Black, 17% Hispanic/Latino, mean baseline CD4+ T-cell count 723 cells/mm^3) were randomized to either switch to BIC/FTC/TAF (bictegravir 50 mg, emtricitabine 200 mg, tenofovir alafenamide 25 mg) once daily or continue their baseline antiretroviral regimen of ABC/DTG/3TC. At 48 weeks, 94% of those receiving BIC/FTC/TAF had a plasma HIV-1 RNA level <50 copies/mL compared with 95% of those who continued to receive ABC/DTG/3TC. The mean change in CD4+ T-cell count from baseline was -31 cells/mm^3 in those receiving BIC/FTC/TAF compared with 4 cells/mm^3 in those who continued to receive ABC/DTG/3TC.

In trial 1878, 577 previously treated adults with baseline plasma HIV-1 RNA levels <50 copies/mL for at least 6 months, no previous treatment with an INSTI, and no history of treatment failure (mean age 46 years, 83% male, 66% white, 26% Black, 19% Hispanic/Latino, mean baseline CD4+ T-cell count 663 cells/mm^3) were randomized to either switch to BIC/FTC/TAF (bictegravir 50 mg, emtricitabine 200 mg, tenofovir alafenamide 25 mg) once daily or continue their baseline antiretroviral regimen (at baseline, 15% were receiving *cobicistat-* or *ritonavir-boosted* atazanavir or darunavir concomitantly with the fixed combination of abacavir and lamivudine [abacavir/lamivudine], 85% were receiving *cobicistat-* or *ritonavir-boosted* atazanavir or darunavir concomitantly with the fixed combination of emtricitabine and tenofovir disoproxil fumarate [emtricitabine/TDF]). At 48 weeks, 92% of those receiving BIC/FTC/TAF had plasma HIV-1 RNA levels <50 copies/mL compared with 89% of those who continued to receive their baseline regimen. The mean change in CD4+ T-cell count from baseline was 25 cells/mm^3 in those receiving BIC/FTC/TAF compared with 0 cells/mm^3 in those who continued to receive their baseline regimen. Treatment outcomes in trial 1844 and trial 1878 were similar across subgroups (i.e., age, sex, race, and region).

An additional randomized, double-blind, active-control, noninferiority, phase 3 study examined the safety and efficacy of switching to BIC/FTC/TAF in 565 adults with baseline plasma HIV-1 RNA levels <50 copies/mL on a stable regimen of dolutegravir plus either emtricitabine/tenofovir alafenamide (FTC/TAF) or emtricitabine/tenofovir disoproxil fumarate (FTC/TDF). Patients were randomized 1:1 to receive BIC/FTC/TAF (bictegravir 50 mg, emtricitabine 200 mg, tenofovir alafenamide 25 mg) once daily or dolutegravir 50 mg plus FTC/TAF (emtricitabine 200 mg, tenofovir alafenamide 25 mg) once daily. The primary endpoint was the proportion of patients with virologic failure (plasma HIV-1 RNA ≥50 copies/mL) at week 48. The median age was 51 years in the BIC/FTC/TAF group and 50 years in the dolutegravir plus FTC/TAF group; the majority of participants were white and male. Virologic failure at 48 weeks occurred in 0.4% of patients treated with BIC/FTC/TAF and 1.1% of patients treated with dolutegravir plus FTC/TAF, demonstrating noninferiority of BIC/FTC/TAF. At week 48, plasma HIV-1 RNA levels <50 copies/mL were documented in 93.3% of patients treated with BIC/FTC/TAF and 91.1% of patients treated with dolutegravir plus FTC/TAF.

Additional studies have examined the efficacy and safety of BIC/FTC/TAF in various subgroups of patients, including elderly, women, and Black patients, and are described below.

An open-label single-arm trial (trial 4449) evaluated the efficacy and safety of switching from a stable antiretroviral regimen to BIC/FTC/TAF (bictegravir 50 mg, emtricitabine 200 mg, tenofovir alafenamide 25 mg) in 86 virologically-suppressed HIV-1 infected adults ≥65 years of age. The mean age of patients treated with BIC/FTC/TAF was 70 years. The primary endpoint was the proportion of patients with HIV-1 RNA >50 copies/mL at week 48; no patient had HIV-1 RNA >50 copies/mL at week 48, and 91% of patients remained virologically suppressed at week 48 (defined as HIV-1 RNA <50 copies/mL). At week 96, no patients had HIV-1 RNA ≥50 copies/mL; the rate of virologic suppression at week 96 was 74.4%; however, virologic data were missing for 22 patients largely due to the impact of the COVID-19 pandemic.

An open-label, randomized, active-controlled noninferiority trial evaluated the efficacy and safety of BIC/FTC/TAF in 470 women with HIV-1 who were virologically suppressed (plasma HIV-1 RNA levels <50 copies/mL) on their current antiretroviral regimen containing either TAF or TDF. Patients were randomly assigned (1:1) to switch to BIC/FTC/TAF (bictegravir 50 mg, emtricitabine 200 mg, tenofovir alafenamide 25 mg) once daily or stay on their baseline antiretroviral regimen. The primary outcome was the proportion of patients with virologic failure (plasma HIV-1 RNA ≥50 copies/mL) at week 48. The median age of patients was 39 years in the BIC/FTC/TAF group and 40 years in the group continuing baseline ART. Switching to BIC/FTC/TAF was noninferior to continuing the baseline antiretroviral regimen in terms of virologic failure rates at week 48; virologic failure was observed in 1.7% of patients in both treatment groups. The proportion of patients with documented plasma HIV-1 RNA <50 copies/mL at week 48 was 95.7% in the BIC/FTC/TAF group and 95.3% in the group continuing baseline ART.

An additional randomized, open-label, active-controlled noninferiority trial (BRAAVE) evaluated the efficacy and safety of BIC/FTC/TAF in 495 Black or African American adults with HIV-1 who were virologically suppressed (plasma HIV-1 RNA levels <50 copies/mL) on their current antiretroviral regimen of 2 NRTIs plus a third agent. Patients were randomized 2:1 to switch to BIC/FTC/TAF (bictegravir 50 mg, emtricitabine 200 mg, tenofovir alafenamide 25 mg) once daily or stay on their baseline antiretroviral regimen. The primary outcome was the proportion of patients with virologic failure (plasma HIV-1 RNA ≥50 copies/mL) at week 24. The median age of patients was 49 years; 32% of participants were ciswomen, 2% were transwomen, and 10% had documented baseline M184V/I mutation. Switching to BIC/FTC/TAF was noninferior to continuing the baseline antiretroviral regimen in terms of virologic failure rates at week 24; virologic failure was observed in 0.6% of patients who switched to BIC/FTC/TAF and 1.8% of patients who continued baseline ART. Virologic suppression (plasma HIV-1 RNA <50 copies/mL) at week 24 was confirmed in 96.3% of patients who switched to BIC/FTC/TAF and 94.5% of patients who continued baseline ART.

Pediatric Patients

Efficacy of BIC/FTC/TAF in pediatric patients was evaluated in an open-label, single-arm trial (trial 1474; NCT02881320) that included 50 virologically suppressed adolescents 12 to <18 years of age weighing ≥35 kg (cohort 1), 50 virologically suppressed children 6 to <12 years of age weighing ≥25 kg (cohort 2), and 22 virologically suppressed children ≥2 years of age weighing 14 to <25 kg (cohort 3).

Patients in cohort 1 of trial 1474 (mean age 14 years, mean baseline weight 51.7 kg, 64% female, 27% Asian, 65% Black, baseline median CD4+ T-cell count 750 cells/mm³, median CD4+ T-cell percentage 33%) were switched from their existing regimen to 1 tablet of BIC/FTC/TAF (bictegravir 50 mg, emtricitabine 200 mg, tenofovir alafenamide 25 mg) once daily. At week 48 after switching to BIC/FTC/TAF, 98% of these pediatric patients remained virologically suppressed (i.e., plasma HIV-1 RNA levels <50 copies/mL).

Patients in cohort 2 of trial 1474 (mean age 10 years, mean baseline weight 31.9 kg, 54% female, 22% Asian, 72% Black, baseline median CD4+ T-cell count 898 cells/mm³, median CD4+ T-cell percentage 37%) were switched from their existing regimen to 1 tablet of BIC/FTC/TAF (bictegravir 50 mg, emtricitabine 200 mg, tenofovir alafenamide 25 mg) once daily. At week 24 after switching to BIC/FTC/TAF, 100% of these pediatric patients remained virologically suppressed (i.e., plasma HIV-1 RNA levels <50 copies/mL).

Patients in cohort 3 of trial 1474 (mean age 5 years, mean baseline weight 18.8 kg, 50% female, 23% Asian, 73% Black, baseline mean CD4+ T-cell count 1104 cells/mm³, mean CD4+ T-cell percentage 33.4%) were switched from their existing regimen to BIC/FTC/TAF (bictegravir 30 mg, emtricitabine 120 mg, tenofovir alafenamide 15 mg) once daily. At week 24 after switching to BIC/FTC/TAF, 91% of these pediatric patients remained virologically suppressed (i.e., plasma HIV-1 RNA levels <50 copies/mL).

Clinical Perspective

Therapeutic options for the treatment and prevention of HIV infection and recommendations concerning the use of antiretrovirals are continuously evolving. Antiretroviral therapy is recommended for all individuals with HIV regardless of CD4 counts, and should be initiated as soon as possible after diagnosis of HIV and continued indefinitely. The primary goals of antiretroviral therapy are to achieve and maintain durable suppression of HIV viral load (as measured by plasma HIV-1 RNA levels) to a level below which drug-resistance mutations cannot emerge (i.e., below detectable limits), restore and preserve immunologic function, reduce HIV-related morbidity and mortality, improve quality of life, and prevent transmission of HIV. While the most appropriate antiretroviral regimen cannot be defined for each clinical scenario, the US Department of Health and Human Services (HHS) Panel on Antiretroviral Guidelines for Adults and Adolescents, HHS Panel on Antiretroviral Therapy and Medical Management of Children Living with HIV, and HHS Panel on Treatment of Pregnant Women with HIV Infection and Prevention of Perinatal Transmission, have developed comprehensive guidelines that provide information on selection and use of antiretrovirals for the treatment or prevention of HIV infection. Because of the complexity of managing patients with HIV, it is recommended that clinicians with HIV expertise be consulted when needed.

The use of combination antiretroviral regimens that generally include 3 drugs from 2 or more drug classes is currently recommended to achieve viral suppression. In both treatment-naïve adults and children, an initial antiretroviral regimen generally consists of 2 NRTIs administered in combination with a third active antiretroviral drug from 1 of 3 drug classes: an INSTI, a non-nucleoside reverse transcriptase inhibitor (NNRTI), or a protease inhibitor (PI) with a pharmacokinetic enhancer (also known as a booster; the 2 drugs used for this purpose are cobicistat and ritonavir). Selection of an initial antiretroviral regimen should be individualized based on factors such as virologic efficacy, toxicity, pill burden, dosing frequency, drug–drug interaction potential, resistance-test results, comorbid conditions, access, and cost. In patients with comorbid infections (e.g., hepatitis B, tuberculosis), antiretroviral regimen selection should also consider the potential for activity against other present infections and timing of initiation relative to other anti-infective regimens.

Bictegravir, emtricitabine, and tenofovir alafenamide (BIC/FTC/TAF) is a coformulation of 2 NRTIs (tenofovir alafenamide and emtricitabine) and an INSTI (bictegravir). In the HHS adult and adolescent HIV treatment guideline, BIC/FTC/TAF is listed as a recommended regimen for most people with HIV.

In the HHS pediatric HIV treatment guideline, BIC/FTC/TAF is recommended as a preferred regimen for children ≥2 years of age weighing ≥14 kg.

In the HHS perinatal HIV treatment guideline, BIC/FTC/TAF is listed as an alternative regimen for use in pregnancy as safety, pharmacokinetic, and efficacy data in pregnancy are more limited than data for preferred regimens.

DOSAGE AND ADMINISTRATION

● General

Pretreatment Screening

- Determine serum creatinine, estimated creatinine clearance, urine glucose, and urine protein prior to initiation of the fixed combination of bictegravir sodium, emtricitabine, and tenofovir alafenamide fumarate (BIC/FTC/TAF). In patients with chronic kidney disease, also assess serum phosphorus.

- Test for hepatitis B virus (HBV) infection prior to initiation of BIC/FTC/TAF.

Patient Monitoring

- Monitor serum creatinine, estimated creatinine clearance, urine glucose, and urine protein during treatment in all patients as clinically appropriate. In patients with chronic kidney disease, serum phosphorus also should be assessed.

- For several months after discontinuation of BIC/FTC/TAF, closely follow hepatic laboratory and clinical monitoring for signs of acute exacerbation of hepatitis B in patients coinfected with HBV infection.

Dispensing and Administration Precautions

- The Institute for Safe Medication Practices (ISMP) list of error-prone abbreviations, symbols, and dose designations states that the use of abbreviations for antiretroviral medications (e.g., DOR, TAF, TDF) during the medication use process should be avoided as their use has been associated with serious medication errors.

● Administration

The fixed combination BIC/FTC/TAF is administered orally once daily without regard to food.

In children unable to swallow the whole fixed combination tablet of BIC/FTC/TAF, the tablet can be split, and each part swallowed separately; the full dose must be consumed within approximately 10 minutes.

Store bottles below 30°C. Store blister packs at 25°C (excursions permitted between 15–30°C).

● Dosage

Fixed combination tablets of BIC/FTC/TAF contain bictegravir sodium, emtricitabine, and tenofovir alafenamide fumarate; dosage of bictegravir sodium is expressed in terms of bictegravir and dosage of tenofovir alafenamide fumarate is expressed in terms of tenofovir alafenamide.

Fixed-combination tablets of BIC/FTC/TAF are available in 2 different strengths: bictegravir 50 mg, emtricitabine 200 mg, and tenofovir alafenamide 25 mg, and bictegravir 30 mg, emtricitabine 120 mg, and tenofovir alafenamide 15 mg.

Pediatric Dosage

HIV-1 Infection

For the treatment of human immunodeficiency virus type 1 (HIV-1) infection in pediatric patients weighing ≥25 kg, the usual dosage of BIC/FTC/TAF is 1 tablet containing 50 mg of bictegravir, 200 mg of emtricitabine, and 25 mg of tenofovir alafenamide once daily.

For the treatment of HIV-1 infection in pediatric patients weighing ≥14 kg to <25 kg, the usual dosage of BIC/FTC/TAF is 1 tablet containing 30 mg of bictegravir, 120 mg of emtricitabine, and 15 mg of tenofovir alafenamide once daily.

Adults

HIV-1 Infection

For the treatment of HIV-1 infection, the usual adult dosage of BIC/FTC/TAF is 1 tablet containing 50 mg of bictegravir, 200 mg of emtricitabine, and 25 mg of tenofovir alafenamide once daily.

● Special Populations

Hepatic Impairment

Dosage adjustments are not necessary if BIC/FTC/TAF is used in patients with mild or moderate hepatic impairment (Child-Pugh class A or B).

BIC/FTC/TAF is not recommended in patients with severe hepatic impairment (Child-Pugh class C).

Renal Impairment

Dosage adjustments are not necessary if BIC/FTC/TAF is used in patients with an estimated creatinine clearance of ≥30 mL/minute, or in virologically-suppressed adult patients with end-stage renal disease (ESRD; estimated creatinine clearance <15 mL/min) who are receiving hemodialysis. On hemodialysis days, the dose of BIC/FTC/TAF should be administered after dialysis treatment. BIC/FTC/TAF has not been studied in pediatric patients with a creatinine clearance of <30 mL/minute.

BIC/FTC/TAF is not recommended in patients with an estimated creatinine clearance 15 to <30 mL/minute, in patients with ESRD (estimated creatinine clearance <15 mL/minute) who are not receiving chronic hemodialysis, and in antiretroviral naïve patients with ESRD (estimated creatinine clearance <15 mL/minute) who are receiving chronic hemodialysis.

Geriatric Use

The manufacturer does not provide recommendations on dosage adjustments in geriatric patients; however, increased sensitivity to BIC/FTC/TAF in some older individuals cannot be ruled out.

Pregnancy

In pregnant individuals who are virologically suppressed (HIV-1 RNA <50 copies/mL) on a stable antiretroviral regimen with no known substitutions associated with resistance to the individual components of the drug, the recommended dosage of BIC/FTC/TAF is 1 tablet containing 50 mg of bictegravir, 200 mg of emtricitabine, and 25 mg of tenofovir alafenamide once daily. Reduced drug exposures have been observed with use of BIC/FTC/TAF in pregnancy. Viral load should be monitored closely.

CAUTIONS

● Contraindications

- Concomitant use of dofetilide since serious and/or life-threatening adverse effects due to possible increased dofetilide plasma concentrations may occur.

- Concomitant use of rifampin since substantially decreased plasma bictegravir concentrations may occur and result in loss of virologic response and development of resistance.

● Warnings/Precautions

Warnings

Severe Acute Exacerbation of Hepatitis B in Patients Coinfected with HIV and HBV

A boxed warning regarding the risk of hepatitis B virus (HBV) infection exacerbation in HIV-infected patients is included in the prescribing information of BIC/FTC/TAF. HIV-infected patients should be tested for HBV infection before antiretroviral therapy is initiated.

In HIV-infected patients with HBV coinfection, severe acute exacerbations of HBV infection, including liver decompensation and liver failure, have occurred following discontinuance of preparations containing emtricitabine and/or tenofovir disoproxil fumarate (TDF; tenofovir DF). Such reactions could occur following discontinuance of BIC/FTC/TAF.

Hepatic function should be closely monitored with clinical and laboratory follow-up for at least several months after BIC/FTC/TAF is discontinued in patients coinfected with HIV-1 and HBV. If appropriate, initiation of HBV treatment may be warranted, especially in patients with advanced liver disease or cirrhosis.

Other Warnings and Precautions

Risk of Adverse Reactions or Loss of Virologic Response Due to Drug Interactions

Concomitant use of BIC/FTC/TAF with certain drugs may result in substantial drug interactions, which may lead to loss of therapeutic effect of BIC/FTC/TAF and possible development of resistance or possible adverse effects from increased exposures of concomitant drugs.

The potential for drug interactions should be considered prior to and during treatment with BIC/FTC/TAF and the patient should be monitored for adverse effects associated with concomitant drugs.

New Onset or Worsening Renal Impairment

Renal impairment, including acute renal failure, proximal renal tubulopathy, and Fanconi syndrome, has been reported during postmarketing experience in patients receiving products that contained tenofovir alafenamide. While other confounding variables were present in most cases that may have contributed to the development of renal toxicity, it is also possible that these factors helped precipitate the adverse event.

Serum creatinine, estimated creatinine clearance, urine glucose, and urine protein should be determined prior to initiating BIC/FTC/TAF and monitored during treatment in all patients as clinically appropriate. In patients with chronic kidney disease, serum phosphorus also should be assessed.

BIC/FTC/TAF is not recommended in adult or pediatric patients with severe renal impairment (estimated creatinine clearance 15 to <30 mL/minute), in adult patients with ESRD (estimated creatinine clearance <15 mL/minute) not receiving chronic hemodialysis, and in treatment-naïve patients with ESRD who are receiving chronic hemodialysis.

Patients receiving a tenofovir prodrug who have impaired renal function or are receiving a nephrotoxic agent (e.g., nonsteroidal anti-inflammatory agents [NSAIAs]) are at increased risk of developing adverse renal effects.

BIC/FTC/TAF should be discontinued in patients who develop clinically important decreases in renal function or evidence of Fanconi syndrome.

Lactic Acidosis and Severe Hepatomegaly with Steatosis

Lactic acidosis and severe hepatomegaly with steatosis, including fatalities, have been reported in patients receiving HIV nucleoside reverse transcriptase inhibitors (NRTIs), including emtricitabine and the tenofovir prodrug TDF, alone or in conjunction with other antiretrovirals.

BIC/FTC/TAF treatment should be interrupted in any patient who develops clinical or laboratory findings suggestive of lactic acidosis or pronounced hepatotoxicity (signs of hepatotoxicity may include hepatomegaly and steatosis even in the absence of marked increases in serum aminotransferase concentrations).

Immune Reconstitution Syndrome

Immune reconstitution syndrome has been reported in HIV-infected patients receiving multiple-drug antiretroviral therapy. During the initial phase of treatment, HIV-infected patients whose immune systems respond to antiretroviral therapy may develop an inflammatory response to indolent or residual opportunistic infections (e.g., *Mycobacterium avium*, *M. tuberculosis*, cytomegalovirus [CMV], *Pneumocystis jirovecii* [formerly *P. carinii*]); such response may necessitate further evaluation and treatment.

Autoimmune disorders (e.g., Graves' disease, polymyositis, Guillain-Barré syndrome, autoimmune hepatitis) also have been reported to occur in the setting of immune reconstitution; however, the time to onset is more variable and can occur many months after initiation of antiretroviral therapy.

Use of Fixed Combinations

The usual cautions, precautions, contraindications, and interactions associated with each component of BIC/FTC/TAF should be considered. Cautionary information applicable to specific populations (e.g., pregnant or nursing women, individuals with hepatic or renal impairment, geriatric patients) should be considered for each drug in the fixed combination.

BIC/FTC/TAF is used alone as a complete regimen for the treatment of HIV-1 infection and use in conjunction with other antiretrovirals is not recommended.

Specific Populations

Pregnancy

The Antiretroviral Pregnancy Registry (APR) monitors pregnancy outcomes in women exposed to BIC/FTC/TAF during pregnancy. Clinicians are encouraged to register patients in the APR by calling 800-258-4263 or visiting https://www.apregistry.com/.

The manufacturer states that data regarding use of BIC, FTC, and TAF in pregnant women have not established a drug-associated risk of birth defects, miscarriage, or other adverse maternal or fetal outcomes. Prospective reports to the APR reveal that of over 500 BIC exposures during pregnancy resulting in live births, the prevalence of birth defects was 4.3% following first trimester exposure and 1.8% following second-/third-trimester exposure. Of over 6500 FTC exposures during pregnancy resulting in live births, the prevalence of birth defects was 2.9% following first trimester exposure and 2.8% following second-/third-trimester exposure. Of over 1200 TAF exposures during pregnancy resulting in live births, the prevalence of birth defects was 3.9% following first trimester exposure and 4.8% following second-/third-trimester exposure.

In an open-label, multicenter, single-arm, phase 1b study, the pharmacokinetics, safety, and efficacy of BIC/FTC/TAF during pregnancy were evaluated. The trial included 33 virologically suppressed (HIV-1 RNA <50 copies/mL) pregnant adult women with no known substitutions associated with resistance to BIC, FTC, or TAF. The patients were administered BIC/FTC/TAF (containing 50 mg of bictegravir, 200 mg of emtricitabine, and 25 mg of tenofovir alafenamide) once daily from the second or third trimester through postpartum. Of the 32 patients who completed the study, 100% maintained viral suppression during pregnancy, at delivery, and through Week 18 postpartum. The baseline median CD4$^+$ cell count for evaluable patients was 558 cells/μL; median change in CD4$^+$ cell count from baseline to Week 12 postpartum was 159 cells/μL. Of the 29 neonates assessed, all had a negative/nondetectable HIV-1 polymerase chain reaction result at birth and/or at 4 to 8 weeks post-birth. Safety findings were consistent with those observed in other adult trials involving BIC/FTC/TAF.

Lactation

Published literature demonstrate that BIC, FTC, and TAF are present in human milk.

There are no reported adverse effects of FTC or TAF on the breastfed child; no data exist on the effects of BIC on breastfed children. It is not known whether BIC/FTC/TAF affects human milk production.

The HHS perinatal HIV transmission guideline provides updated recommendations on infant feeding. The guideline states that patients with HIV should receive evidence-based, patient-centered counseling to support shared decision making about infant feeding. During counseling, patients should be informed that feeding with appropriate formula or pasteurized donor human milk from a milk bank eliminates the risk of postnatal HIV transmission to the infant. Additionally, achieving and maintaining viral suppression with antiretroviral therapy during pregnancy and postpartum reduces the risk of breastfeeding HIV transmission to <1%, but does not completely eliminate the risk. Replacement feeding with formula or banked pasteurized donor milk is recommended when patients with HIV are *not* on antiretroviral therapy and/or do *not* have a suppressed viral load during pregnancy (at a minimum throughout the third trimester), as well as at delivery.

Pediatric Use

Safety and efficacy of BIC/FTC/TAF have not been established in pediatric patients weighing <14 kg.

Safety and efficacy of BIC/FTC/TAF have been established for the treatment of HIV-1 infection in pediatric patients weighing 14 kg or more. Use of BIC/FTC/TAF in pediatric patients 2 to <18 years of age weighing at least 14 kg is supported by results of clinical trials in adults, and by results of an open-label study in 3 age-based cohorts of pediatric patients. Patients in these cohorts were virologically suppressed, and received BIC/FTC/TAF for a treatment duration of 24 or 48 weeks. No patients 2 years of age were enrolled in these clinical studies of BIC/FTC/TAF; the youngest patient was 3 years of age at enrollment and weighed at least 14 kg. Safety and efficacy of BIC/FTC/TAF in these pediatric patients were similar to that in adults, and there was no clinically important difference in exposures of the components of BIC/FTC/TAF in these pediatric patients compared with adults.

Adverse effects reported in pediatric patients receiving BIC/FTC/TAF are similar to those reported in adults receiving the drug.

Geriatric Use

In studies of virologically-suppressed patients 65 years of age and older receiving BIC/FTC/TAF, 90% of 111 subjects were 65–74 years of age, and 10% were 75–84 years of age. These studies identified no overall differences in response based on safety or efficacy between older adults and younger adult subjects, although greater sensitivity of some older individuals cannot be ruled out.

Hepatic Impairment

Mild hepatic impairment (Child-Pugh class A) does not have a clinically important effect on the pharmacokinetics of tenofovir alafenamide. Moderate hepatic impairment (Child-Pugh class B) does not have a clinically important effect on the pharmacokinetics of bictegravir or tenofovir alafenamide. Hepatic impairment is not expected to affect the pharmacokinetics of emtricitabine.

BIC/FTC/TAF is *not* recommended in patients with severe hepatic impairment (Child-Pugh class C). Data are not available to date regarding the pharmacokinetics or safety of BIC/FTC/TAF in such patients.

Renal Impairment

Serum creatinine, estimated creatinine clearance, urine glucose, and urine protein should be determined prior to initiating BIC/FTC/TAF and routinely monitored during treatment in all patients as clinically appropriate. In patients with chronic kidney disease, serum phosphorus also should be determined.

There are no clinically important differences in the pharmacokinetics of bictegravir, tenofovir alafenamide, or tenofovir in individuals with severe renal impairment compared with healthy individuals.

● Common Adverse Effects

The most common adverse effects (≥5% incidence) in patients receiving BIC/FTC/TAF include diarrhea, nausea, and headache.

DRUG INTERACTIONS

The following drug interactions are based on studies that used bictegravir sodium, emtricitabine, or tenofovir alafenamide fumarate alone or the fixed combination of bictegravir, emtricitabine, and tenofovir alafenamide fumarate (BIC/FTC/TAF) or are predicted to occur.

Potential drug interactions associated with each drug in the fixed combination should be considered.

● Drugs Affecting or Metabolized by Hepatic Microsomal Enzymes

Bictegravir is a substrate of cytochrome P-450 (CYP) isoenzyme 3A. The drug does not inhibit CYP isoenzymes (including CYP3A) at clinically relevant concentrations.

Emtricitabine is not a substrate of CYP isoenzymes; emtricitabine does not inhibit CYP1A2, 2A6, 2B6, 2C9, 2C19, 2D6, or 3A4.

Tenofovir alafenamide does not inhibit CYP isoenzymes (including CYP3A) at clinically relevant concentrations.

Potential pharmacokinetic interactions if BIC/FTC/TAF is used concomitantly with drugs that are potent inducers of CYP3A *and* also are inducers of uridine diphosphate-glucuronosyltransferase (UGT) 1A1 enzyme (decreased plasma concentrations of bictegravir; possible decreased antiretroviral efficacy and development of resistance).

Potential pharmacokinetic interactions if BIC/FTC/TAF is used concomitantly with drugs that are potent inhibitors of CYP3A *and* also are inhibitors of UGT1A1 (increased plasma concentrations of bictegravir).

● Drugs Affecting or Metabolized by Uridine Diphosphate-glucuronosyltransferase

Bictegravir is a substrate of UGT1A1. Bictegravir and tenofovir alafenamide do not inhibit UGT1A1.

Potential pharmacokinetic interactions if BIC/FTC/TAF is used concomitantly with drugs that are potent inducers of CYP3A *and* also are inducers of UGT1A1 (decreased plasma concentrations of bictegravir; possible decreased antiretroviral efficacy and development of resistance).

Potential pharmacokinetic interactions if BIC/FTC/TAF is used concomitantly with drugs that are potent inhibitors of CYP3A *and* also are inhibitors of UGT1A1 (increased plasma concentrations of bictegravir).

● Drugs Affecting or Affected by P-glycoprotein Transport

Tenofovir alafenamide is a substrate of P-glycoprotein (P-gp) transport. The drug does not inhibit P-gp.

Potential pharmacokinetic interactions if BIC/FTC/TAF is used concomitantly with drugs that induce P-gp (decreased absorption and decreased plasma concentrations of tenofovir alafenamide; possible decreased antiretroviral efficacy and development of resistance).

Potential pharmacokinetic interactions if BIC/FTC/TAF is used concomitantly with drugs that inhibit P-gp *and* breast cancer resistance protein (BCRP) (increased absorption and increased plasma concentrations of tenofovir alafenamide).

● Drugs Affecting or Affected by Breast Cancer Resistance Protein

Tenofovir alafenamide is a substrate of BCRP. The drug does not inhibit BCRP.

Potential pharmacokinetic interactions if BIC/FTC/TAF is used concomitantly with drugs that inhibit P-gp *and* BCRP (increased absorption and increased plasma concentrations of tenofovir alafenamide).

● Drugs Affecting or Affected by Multidrug and Toxin Extrusion Transporter

Bictegravir inhibits multidrug and toxin extrusion transporter (MATE) 1. Therefore, bictegravir may increase plasma concentrations of drugs eliminated by MATE1 (e.g., dofetilide).

Tenofovir alafenamide does not inhibit MATE1.

● Drugs Affecting or Affected by Renal Organic Anion Transporters

Bictegravir and tenofovir alafenamide do not inhibit renal organic anion transporter (OAT) 1 or OAT3.

Bictegravir and tenofovir alafenamide do not inhibit hepatic organic anion transporter polypeptide (OATP) 1B1 or OATP1B3.

● Drugs Affecting or Affected by Renal Organic Cation Transporters

Bictegravir inhibits renal organic cation transporter (OCT) 2. Therefore, bictegravir may increase plasma concentrations of drugs eliminated by OCT2 (e.g., dofetilide).

Bictegravir and tenofovir alafenamide do not inhibit OCT1. Tenofovir alafenamide does not inhibit OCT2.

● Drugs Affecting or Affected by Bile Salt Export Pump

Bictegravir and tenofovir alafenamide do not inhibit bile salt export pump (BSEP).

● Drugs Affecting Renal Function

The emtricitabine and tenofovir components of BIC/FTC/TAF are principally excreted by the kidneys by a combination of glomerular filtration and active tubular secretion.

Potential pharmacokinetic interactions if BIC/FTC/TAF is used concomitantly with drugs that reduce renal function or compete for active tubular secretion (e.g., acyclovir, aminoglycosides [gentamicin], cidofovir, ganciclovir, valacyclovir, valganciclovir, high-dose or multiple nonsteroidal anti-inflammatory agents [NSAIAs]); may result in increased concentrations of emtricitabine, tenofovir, and/or the concomitant drug and may increase the risk of adverse effects. Concomitant use of BIC/FTC/TAF and nephrotoxic drugs should be avoided.

● Anticonvulsants

Concomitant use of carbamazepine or oxcarbazepine with BIC/FTC/TAF may result in decreased bictegravir and tenofovir concentrations. Concomitant use of carbamazepine (300 mg twice daily) and tenofovir alafenamide (single 25-mg dose) in fixed combination with emtricitabine results in decreased peak plasma concentrations and AUC of tenofovir.

Concomitant use of BIC/FTC/TAF and phenobarbital or phenytoin is expected to decrease plasma concentrations of bictegravir and tenofovir alafenamide.

Concomitant use of BIC/FTC/TAF with carbamazepine, oxcarbazepine, phenobarbital, or phenytoin is not recommended; an alternative anticonvulsant should be considered.

● Antimycobacterial Agents

Rifabutin

Concomitant use of rifabutin (300 mg once daily) and bictegravir (75 mg once daily) under fasting conditions decreases bictegravir peak plasma concentrations by 20%, AUC by 38%, and trough plasma concentrations by 56%. Concomitant use of rifabutin with BIC/FTC/TAF may decrease plasma concentrations of tenofovir alafenamide.

Concomitant use of rifabutin and BIC/FTC/TAF is not recommended.

Rifampin

Concomitant use of rifampin (600 mg once daily) and bictegravir (single 75-mg dose) under fed conditions decreases bictegravir peak plasma concentrations by 28% and AUC by 75%. Concomitant use of rifampin and BIC/FTC/TAF may decrease plasma concentrations of tenofovir alafenamide.

Concomitant use of rifampin and BIC/FTC/TAF is contraindicated.

Rifapentine

Pharmacokinetic interactions with rifapentine are expected (decreased bictegravir and tenofovir alafenamide plasma concentrations).

Concomitant use of rifapentine and BIC/FTC/TAF is not recommended.

● *Antiretroviral Agents*

Fixed-combination BIC/FTC/TAF should not be used in conjunction with any other antiretrovirals.

● *Calcium, Iron, Multivitamins, and Other Preparations Containing Polyvalent Cations*

Pharmacokinetic interactions reported when a single 1.2-g dose of calcium carbonate was administered simultaneously with a single 50-mg dose of bictegravir in the fasting state (decreased peak plasma concentrations and AUC of bictegravir). No clinically important pharmacokinetic interactions were observed when a single 1.2-g dose of calcium carbonate was administered simultaneously with a single 50-mg dose of bictegravir under fed conditions.

Pharmacokinetic interactions reported when a single 324-mg dose of ferrous fumarate was administered simultaneously with a single 50-mg dose of bictegravir in the fasting state (decreased peak plasma concentrations and AUC of bictegravir). No clinically important pharmacokinetic interactions were observed when a single 324-mg dose of ferrous fumarate was administered simultaneously with a single 50-mg dose of bictegravir under fed conditions.

Concomitant use of BIC/FTC/TAF with laxatives, buffered preparations, or other preparations containing polyvalent cations may decrease plasma concentrations of bictegravir.

BIC/FTC/TAF and supplements containing calcium or iron can be administered simultaneously with food.

Administration of BIC/FTC/TAF in the *fasting* state simultaneously with or 2 hours *after* supplements containing calcium or iron is *not* recommended.

● *Dofetilide*

Concomitant use of dofetilide and BIC/FTC/TAF may increase dofetilide plasma concentrations and increase the risk of serious and/or life-threatening adverse effects.

Concomitant use of dofetilide and BIC/FTC/TAF is contraindicated.

● *Ethinyl Estradiol and Norgestimate*

Concomitant use of the fixed combination of norgestimate and ethinyl estradiol with bictegravir or tenofovir alafenamide does not have a clinically important effect on ethinyl estradiol, norelgestromin, or norgestrel concentrations.

Clinically important pharmacokinetic interactions are not expected if BIC/FTC/TAF is used concomitantly with oral contraceptives containing ethinyl estradiol or norgestimate.

● *GI Drugs*
Antacids

Pharmacokinetic interactions were reported when a single dose of antacid containing aluminum, magnesium, and simethicone was administered simultaneously with a single 50-mg dose of bictegravir in the fasting or fed state (decreased peak plasma concentrations and AUC of bictegravir). Similarly, decreased peak plasma concentrations and AUC of bictegravir were observed when a single 50-mg dose of the drug was administered in the fasting state 2 hours *after* the antacid. No clinically important pharmacokinetic interactions were observed when a single 50-mg dose of bictegravir was administered in the fasting state 2 hours *before* the antacid.

BIC/FTC/TAF should be administered in the fasting state at least 2 hours *before* or 6 hours *after* antacids containing aluminum or magnesium. Administration of BIC/FTC/TAF simultaneously with or 2 hours *after* an antacid containing aluminum or magnesium is *not* recommended.

BIC/FTC/TAF and antacids containing calcium carbonate may be administered simultaneously with food. Administration of BIC/FTC/TAF in the *fasting* state simultaneously with or 2 hours *after* antacids containing calcium carbonate is *not* recommended.

Sucralfate

Concomitant use of sucralfate and BIC/FTC/TAF may decrease plasma concentrations of bictegravir.

● *HCV Antivirals*
HCV Polymerase Inhibitors
Sofosbuvir

Clinically important pharmacokinetic interactions are not expected if sofosbuvir is used concomitantly with BIC/FTC/TAF.

Sofosbuvir and Velpatasvir

Clinically important pharmacokinetic interactions are not expected if the fixed combination of sofosbuvir and velpatasvir (sofosbuvir/velpatasvir) is used concomitantly with BIC/FTC/TAF.

Sofosbuvir, Velpatasvir, and Voxilaprevir

Concomitant use of the fixed combination of sofosbuvir, velpatasvir, and voxilaprevir (sofosbuvir/velpatasvir/voxilaprevir) with bictegravir or tenofovir alafenamide does not have a clinically important effect on sofosbuvir, velpatasvir, voxilaprevir, bictegravir, or tenofovir alafenamide concentrations.

Clinically important pharmacokinetic interactions are not expected if sofosbuvir/velpatasvir/voxilaprevir is used concomitantly with BIC/FTC/TAF.

HCV Replication Complex Inhibitors
Ledipasvir and Sofosbuvir

Concomitant use of the fixed combination of ledipasvir and sofosbuvir (ledipasvir/sofosbuvir) with bictegravir or with tenofovir alafenamide does not have a clinically important effect on ledipasvir, sofosbuvir, bictegravir, or tenofovir alafenamide concentrations.

Clinically important pharmacokinetic interactions are not expected if BIC/FTC/TAF is used concomitantly with ledipasvir/sofosbuvir.

Metformin

Concomitant use of metformin hydrochloride (500 mg twice daily), bictegravir (50 mg once daily), and tenofovir alafenamide (25 mg once daily) increases metformin peak plasma concentrations by 1.3-fold, trough plasma concentrations by 1.4-fold, and AUC by 1.4-fold.

If BIC/FTC/TAF and metformin are used concomitantly, refer to the prescribing information for metformin. The benefits and risks of concomitant use should be considered.

Midazolam

Concomitant use of midazolam with bictegravir and tenofovir alafenamide does not have a clinically important effect on midazolam concentrations.

Sertraline

Concomitant use of sertraline with tenofovir alafenamide does not have a clinically important effect on sertraline concentrations.

● *St. John's Wort*

Pharmacokinetic interactions are possible if St. John's wort (*Hypericum perforatum*) is used concomitantly with BIC/FTC/TAF (decreased concentrations of bictegravir and tenofovir alafenamide).

Concomitant use of St. John's wort and BIC/FTC/TAF is not recommended.

• *Voriconazole*

Concomitant use of voriconazole (300 mg twice daily) and bictegravir (single 75-mg dose) under fasting conditions increases AUC of bictegravir, but does not substantially affect peak plasma concentrations of bictegravir.

DESCRIPTION

The fixed combination of bictegravir sodium, emtricitabine, and tenofovir alafenamide fumarate (BIC/FTC/TAF) contains a human immunodeficiency virus (HIV) integrase strand transfer inhibitor (INSTI) antiretroviral (bictegravir; BIC), an HIV nucleoside reverse transcriptase inhibitor (NRTI) antiretroviral (emtricitabine; FTC), and a nucleotide reverse transcriptase inhibitor antiretroviral classified as an HIV NRTI (tenofovir alafenamide; TAF).

Bictegravir inhibits the activity of HIV-1 integrase, an enzyme that integrates HIV DNA into the host cell genome. Integration is required for viral replication; therefore, inhibition of integration prevents propagation of viral infection. Bictegravir is active against HIV-1 and also has some in vitro activity against HIV type 2 (HIV-2).

Emtricitabine is inactive until converted intracellularly to an active 5′-triphosphate metabolite. After conversion to the pharmacologically active metabolite, the drug acts as a reverse transcriptase inhibitor antiretroviral. Emtricitabine is active against HIV-1 and also has some in vitro activity against HIV-2.

Tenofovir alafenamide is a tenofovir prodrug and is inactive until hydrolyzed intracellularly by cathepsin A to form tenofovir and subsequently metabolized by cellular kinases to the active metabolite (tenofovir diphosphate). After conversion to the pharmacologically active metabolite, the drug acts as a reverse transcriptase inhibitor antiretroviral. Tenofovir is active against HIV-1 and has some in vitro activity against HIV-2.

HIV-1 resistant to bictegravir, emtricitabine, or tenofovir has been produced in vitro. In clinical trials evaluating BIC/FTC/TAF, no specific bictegravir or NRTI resistance-associated substitutions emerged in patients receiving BIC/FTC/TAF who were considered to be virologic treatment failures. Cross-resistance between bictegravir and other HIV INSTIs (e.g., dolutegravir, elvitegravir, raltegravir) has been reported. Cross-resistance also occurs among HIV NRTIs.

Following oral administration of the components of BIC/FTC/TAF, peak plasma concentrations of bictegravir, emtricitabine, and tenofovir occur at 2–4, 1.5–2, and 0.5–2 hours, respectively. Administration of BIC/FTC/TAF components with a high-fat meal (approximately 800 kcal, 50% fat) increases mean systemic exposures of bictegravir and tenofovir by 24 and 63%, respectively, compared with administration in the fasting state; mean systemic exposures of emtricitabine are comparable to those observed with administration in the fasting state. Bictegravir is over 99%, emtricitabine is <4%, and tenofovir alafenamide is approximately 80% bound to plasma proteins. Bictegravir is metabolized by cytochrome P-450 (CYP) isoenzyme 3A and uridine diphosphate-glucuronsyltransferase (UGT) 1A1. Emtricitabine is converted intracellularly to the active 5′-triphosphate metabolite, but is not substantially metabolized further. Tenofovir alafenamide is hydrolyzed intracellularly in peripheral blood mononuclear cells (PBMCs) and macrophages by cathepsin A to form tenofovir (the major metabolite), which is then phosphorylated to the active metabolite tenofovir diphosphate; in vitro studies indicate tenofovir alafenamide also is converted to tenofovir by carboxylesterase 1 (CES1) in hepatocytes. Following a single dose of bictegravir, 60% is excreted in feces and 35% in urine. Emtricitabine is principally excreted in urine (70% of a dose) and to a lesser extent in feces (14% of a dose). Following a single dose of tenofovir alafenamide, 32% is excreted in feces and <1% is eliminated in urine. The median terminal plasma half-lives of bictegravir, emtricitabine, and tenofovir alafenamide are 17.3, 10.4, and 0.5 hours, respectively. The half-life of tenofovir diphosphate, the active metabolite of tenofovir alafenamide, is 150–180 hours within PBMCs. There are no clinically important differences in the pharmacokinetics of the components of BIC/FTC/TAF in pediatric patients 6 years of age or older weighing 25 kg or more compared with pharmacokinetics of the drugs reported in adults.

ADVICE TO PATIENTS

• Advise patients of the critical need for compliance with HIV therapy and importance of remaining under the care of a clinician. Advise patients of the importance of taking the fixed combination of bictegravir sodium, emtricitabine, and tenofovir alafenamide (BIC/FTC/TAF) as prescribed; do not alter or discontinue antiretroviral regimen without consulting clinician.

• Advise patients that BIC/FTC/TAF is a complete regimen for treatment of HIV-1 infection and should *not* be used in conjunction with other antiretrovirals.

• Inform patients that testing for hepatitis B virus (HBV) infection is recommended before antiretroviral therapy is initiated. Also advise patients that severe acute exacerbations of HBV infection have been reported following discontinuance of emtricitabine and/or tenofovir disoproxil fumarate (TDF; tenofovir DF) in HIV-infected patients coinfected with HBV and may occur with BIC/FTC/TAF.

• Advise patients that renal impairment, including cases of acute renal failure or Fanconi syndrome, has occurred in patients receiving tenofovir prodrugs. Advise patients to not use BIC/FTC/TAF concomitantly with or shortly after nephrotoxic agents (e.g., high-dose or multiple nonsteroidal anti-inflammatory agents [NSAIAs]).

• Advise patients that lactic acidosis and severe hepatomegaly with steatosis, including fatalities, have occurred in patients receiving HIV nucleoside reverse transcriptase inhibitors (NRTIs), including emtricitabine and/or TDF, in conjunction with other antiretrovirals. Advise patients to contact a clinician if symptoms suggestive of lactic acidosis or pronounced hepatotoxicity (e.g., unusual muscle pain, shortness of breath or fast breathing, cold or blue hands and feet, dizziness or lightheadedness, fast or abnormal heartbeat, nausea, vomiting, unusual/unexpected stomach discomfort, weakness or unusual tiredness) occur.

• Advise patients that signs and symptoms of inflammation from previous infections may occur soon after initiation of antiretroviral therapy in some individuals with advanced HIV infection. These symptoms may be due to an improvement in immune response, enabling the body to fight infections that may have been present with no obvious symptoms. Advise patients to immediately inform a healthcare provider if any symptoms of infection occur.

• Inform caregivers that the BIC/FTC/TAF tablet may be split for children with difficulty swallowing the whole tablet. If the tablet is split, the portions must all be taken within approximately 10 minutes.

• Advise patients to inform their clinicians of existing or contemplated concomitant therapy, including prescription and OTC drugs and herbal supplements (e.g., St. John's wort), as well as any concomitant illnesses.

• Advise women to inform their clinicians if they are or plan to become pregnant or plan to breast-feed. Inform patients that there is a registry that monitors fetal outcomes of women exposed to BIC/FTC/TAF during pregnancy.

• Inform patients of other important precautionary information.

PREPARATIONS

Excipients in commercially available drug preparations may have clinically important effects in some individuals; consult specific product labeling for details.

Bictegravir Sodium, Emtricitabine, and Tenofovir Alafenamide Fumarate

Oral

Tablets, film-coated	Bictegravir Sodium 30 mg (of bictegravir), Emtricitabine 120 mg, and Tenofovir Alafenamide Fumarate 15 mg (of tenofovir alafenamide)	Biktarvy®, Gilead
	Bictegravir Sodium 50 mg (of bictegravir), Emtricitabine 200 mg, and Tenofovir Alafenamide Fumarate 25 mg (of tenofovir alafenamide)	Biktarvy®, Gilead

† Use is not currently included in the labeling approved by the US Food and Drug Administration.

Selected Revisions October 10, 2024, © Copyright, March 5, 2018, American Society of Health-System Pharmacists, Inc.

Cabotegravir Sodium

8:18.08.12 • HIV INTEGRASE INHIBITORS

■ Cabotegravir, an antiretroviral agent, is a human immunodeficiency virus (HIV) integrase strand transfer inhibitor (INSTI).

USES

Cabotegravir sodium tablets are used orally in combination with rilpivirine for the short-term treatment of HIV-1 infection and as short-term preexposure prophylaxis (PrEP) to reduce the risk of sexually-acquired HIV-1 infection in HIV-1-negative individuals.

Cabotegravir extended-release injectable suspension is used as pre-exposure prophylaxis (PrEP) to reduce the risk of sexually acquired HIV-1 infection in HIV-1-negative individuals.

● Treatment of HIV Infection

Cabotegravir sodium tablets (Vocabria®) are used in combination with rilpivirine for short-term treatment of HIV-1 infection in adults and adolescents ≥12 years of age, weighing ≥35 kg, and who are virologically suppressed (HIV-1 RNA<50 copies/mL) on a stable antiretroviral regimen, have no history of treatment failure, and have no known or suspected resistance to either cabotegravir or rilpivirine. The tablet preparation of cabotegravir can be used as an oral lead-in therapy to assess the tolerability of the drug prior to administration of cabotegravir injection, a component of cabotegravir and rilpivirine combination injectable therapy (cabotegravir/rilpivirine; Cabenuva®). Cabotegravir also can be used as oral therapy for patients who will miss planned doses of cabotegravir/rilpivirine injections.

Clinical Experience

Efficacy of oral cabotegravir sodium in combination with rilpivirine in HIV-1-infected patients as short-term treatment including oral lead-in therapy was established in 3 clinical studies (FLAIR, ATLAS, ATLAS-2M).

FLAIR was a phase 3, randomized, active-controlled, parallel-arm, open-label, non-inferiority study in antiretroviral-naive HIV-1-infected adults with baseline plasma HIV-1 RNA levels ≥50 copies/mL. Patients received a dolutegravir INSTI-containing regimen for 20 weeks (either dolutegravir/abacavir/lamivudine or dolutegravir plus 2 other NRTIs if subjects were HLA-B*5701 positive). Patients who were virologically suppressed (HIV-1 RNA <50 copies/mL) were then randomized (1:1) to receive either cabotegravir plus rilpivirine or remain on their current antiretroviral regimen. Patients randomized to receive cabotegravir plus rilpivirine initiated treatment with daily oral lead-in dosing with one 30-mg cabotegravir tablet plus one 25-mg rilpivirine tablet for at least 4 weeks followed by monthly injections with cabotegravir and rilpivirine extended-release injections for an additional 44 weeks. At week 48, an HIV-1 RNA level ≥50 copies/mL was found in 2% of patients who received cabotegravir/rilpivirine injection and in 2% of patients who received a current antiretroviral regimen, meeting the criteria for non-inferiority. At 96 weeks, the proportion of subjects with HIV-1 RNA ≥50 copies/mL was 3.2% for both the cabotegravir plus rilpivirine and current antiretroviral regimen treatment arms. In the extension phase of the FLAIR study (week 100 to 124), the efficacy of long-acting injectable cabotegravir and rilpivirine was evaluated in patients who switched at week 100 from their current antiretroviral regimen to injectable cabotegravir and rilpivirine, with or without oral cabotegravir lead-in therapy. At 124 weeks, 0.8% of patients who received oral cabotegravir lead-in therapy and 0.9% of patients who switched directly to the injectable therapy had plasma HIV-1 RNA levels ≥50 copies/mL, meeting the criteria for non-inferiority. In addition, the rates of virologic suppression (HIV-1 RNA levels <50 copies/mL) were similar in patients who received oral cabotegravir lead-in therapy compared with those that switched directly to the injections.

In the ATLAS study, antiretroviral-experienced HIV-1 infected, virologically suppressed adults with plasma HIV-1 RNA levels <50 copies/mL were randomly assigned to receive cabotegravir/rilpivirine injections or remain on their current antiretroviral regimen. Patients randomized to cabotegravir/rilpivirine initiated treatment with daily oral lead-in dosing with cabotegravir 30 mg plus one rilpivirine 25 mg for at least 4 weeks followed by monthly injections with cabotegravir/rilpivirine for an additional 44 weeks. At week 48, 1.6% of patients who received cabotegravir/rilpivirine and 1% of patients who received current antiretroviral therapy achieved an HIV-1 RNA level ≥50 copies/mL, meeting the criteria for non-inferiority.

An additional phase 3b, randomized, multicenter, parallel-arm, open-label, non-inferiority trial (ATLAS 2M) was conducted to evaluate the efficacy of long-acting injectable cabotegravir and rilpivirine dosed every 2 months. In this study, HIV-1–infected, antiretroviral-experienced, virologically suppressed patients were randomized to receive a cabotegravir plus rilpivirine regimen (administered in injection doses of cabotegravir 400 mg plus rilpivirine 600 mg monthly or cabotegravir 600 mg plus rilpivirine 900 mg every 2 months). Patients without prior exposure to cabotegravir plus rilpivirine initiated treatment with daily oral lead-in dosing with cabotegravir 30 mg and rilpivirine 25 mg for at least 4 weeks followed by monthly or every 2 month injections of cabotegravir/rilpivirine for an additional 44 weeks. The primary endpoint of this study was the proportion of subjects with a plasma HIV-1 RNA ≥50 copies/mL at 48 weeks. At 48 weeks, 2% of patients who received every 2 months dosing had plasma HIV-1 RNA levels ≥50 copies/mL compared with 1% of patients receiving monthly dosing, meeting the criteria for non-inferiority. In addition, the rates of virologic suppression (HIV-1 RNA levels <50 copies/mL) were similar (94%) in patients who received every 2 months therapy compared with those receiving monthly injections.

Clinical Perspective

Therapeutic options for the treatment and prevention of HIV infection and recommendations concerning the use of antiretrovirals are continuously evolving. Antiretroviral therapy (ART) is recommended for all individuals with HIV regardless of CD4 counts, and should be initiated as soon as possible after diagnosis of HIV and continued indefinitely. The primary goals of ART are to achieve and maintain durable suppression of HIV viral load (as measured by plasma HIV-1 RNA levels) to a level below which drug-resistance mutations cannot emerge (i.e., below detectable limits), restore and preserve immunologic function, reduce HIV-related morbidity and mortality, improve quality of life, and prevent transmission of HIV. While the most appropriate antiretroviral regimen cannot be defined for each clinical scenario, the US Department of Health and Human Services (HHS) Panel on Antiretroviral Guidelines for Adults and Adolescents, HHS Panel on Antiretroviral Therapy and Medical Management of Children Living with HIV, and HHS Panel on Treatment of Pregnant Women with HIV Infection and Prevention of Perinatal Transmission, have developed comprehensive guidelines that provide information on selection and use of antiretrovirals for the treatment or prevention of HIV infection. Because of the complexity of managing patients with HIV, it is recommended that clinicians with HIV expertise be consulted when needed.

The HHS Panel on Antiretroviral Guidelines for Adults and Adolescents does not recommend use of long acting cabotegravir plus rilpivirine as initial therapy for people with HIV because of the lack of data supporting the efficacy of this combination in antiretroviral therapy-naïve patients. Patients desiring to use long-acting injectable cabotegravir plus rilpivirine early in their treatment history should first attain viral suppression on a recommended regimen, then transition to a month of oral cabotegravir and rilpivirine with maintenance of suppression before transitioning to long-acting injectable cabotegravir plus rilpivirine. The long-acting antiretroviral therapy combination of injectable cabotegravir and rilpivirine is not currently recommended for patients with virologic failure.

The HHS Panel on Antiretroviral Therapy and Medical Management of Children Living with HIV states the data on use of cabotegravir and rilpivirine are limited to safety, pharmacokinetics, and acceptability; data are not yet available on potential use of this antiretroviral therapy in adolescents with adherence concerns.

● Pre-exposure Prophylaxis for Prevention of HIV-1 Infection

Cabotegravir extended-release injectable suspension (Apretude®) is used in at-risk adults and adolescents weighing ≥35 kg for PrEP to reduce the risk of sexually acquired HIV-1 infection. Cabotegravir sodium tablets (Vocabria®) are used for at-risk adults and adolescents weighing at least 35 kg for short-term PrEP to reduce the risk of sexually acquired HIV-1 infection. Cabotegravir is used orally to determine the tolerability of the drug prior to administration of parenteral cabotegravir. Cabotegravir is also used orally in patients who will miss planned doses of cabotegravir injection.

Clinical Experience

Efficacy of injectable cabotegravir for PreEP was evaluated in 2 randomized, double-blind, controlled, multinational trials; one of the studies was conducted in HIV-1 uninfected men and transgender women who have sex with men and have evidence of high-risk behavior for HIV-1 infection and the other study was conducted in HIV-1 uninfected cisgender women at risk of acquiring HIV-1.

Both studies compared injectable cabotegravir to oral tenofovir disoproxil fumarate–emtricitabine for PreEP. Patients randomized to receive injectable cabotegravir initiated oral lead-in dosing with one oral cabotegravir 30-mg tablet and a placebo daily for up to 5 weeks, followed by cabotegravir 600 mg IM injections at months 1 and 2 and every 2 months thereafter and a daily placebo tablet. Patients randomized to receive oral tenofovir disoproxil fumarate–emtricitabine initiated the oral regimen and placebo daily for up to 5 weeks, followed by oral tenofovir disoproxil fumarate–emtricitabine daily and placebo IM injections at months 1 and 2 and every 2 months thereafter.

In the HPTN 083 trial, 4,566 cisgender men and transgender women who have sex with men were randomized to receive injectable cabotegravir or oral tenofovir disoproxil fumarate–emtricitabine as blinded study medication up to 153 weeks. The primary endpoint was the rate of incident HIV-1 infections among participants randomized to injectable cabotegravir every 2 months compared with oral tenofovir disoproxil fumarate–emtricitabine (corrected for early stopping). Compared with oral tenofovir disoproxil fumarate–emtricitabine, treatment with cabotegravir resulted in a 66% reduction in the risk of acquiring HIV-1 infection.

In the HPTN 084 trial, 3,224 cisgender women were randomized 1:1 to receive injectable cabotegravir or oral tenofovir disoproxil fumarate–emtricitabine as blinded study medication up to 153 weeks. The primary endpoint was the rate of incident HIV-1 infections among participants randomized to cabotegravir injection compared with oral tenofovir disoproxil fumarate–emtricitabine (corrected for early stopping). Cabotegravir therapy reduced the risk of acquiring incident HIV-1 infection by 88% compared with oral tenofovir disoproxil fumarate–emtricitabine.

Clinical Perspective

The CDC clinical practice guideline, Preexposure Prophylaxis for the Prevention of HIV infection in the United States—2021 Update, states that cabotegravir extended-release injection is recommended for PrEP in adults and adolescents weighing at least 35 kg at risk of acquiring HIV. Use of oral cabotegravir is optional for a 4-week lead-in prior to initiation of the injections. The guideline also states that cabotegravir injections may be especially appropriate for patients with significant renal disease, those who have had difficulty with adherent use of oral PrEP, and those who prefer injections every 2 months to an oral PrEP dosing schedule.

In 2023, the US Preventive Services Task Force (USPSTF) released a recommendation statement on PrEP to prevent acquisition of HIV. The statement recommends PrEP with effective antiretroviral therapy to decrease the risk of acquiring HIV in adults and adolescents weighing at least 35 kg at increased risk of HIV acquisition. Injectable cabotegravir is listed as an effective PrEP option for this patient population.

The Department of Health and Human Services Panel on Antiretroviral Guidelines for Adults and Adolescents also recommends resistance testing (including testing for resistance to INSTIs) in all persons who have acquired HIV after receiving long-acting injectable cabotegravir as PrEP, regardless of the amount of time since drug discontinuation.

DOSAGE AND ADMINISTRATION

● General

Pretreatment Screening

- Review concomitant medications and consider potential drug interactions.
- A negative HIV-1 test should be confirmed immediately prior to initiation of cabotegravir for HIV-1 PrEP.

Patient Monitoring

- Perform screening for HIV-1 infection prior to each IM injection for HIV-1 PrEP. Negative results from an antigen/antibody-specific test should be confirmed using an RNA-specific assay.
- Periodically monitor liver function tests (i.e., AST, ALT).
- Monitor for drug interactions and adverse effects that may result from interactions.
- Assess patient adherence to the prescribed therapy during scheduled dosing visits for PrEP.

● Administration

Cabotegravir sodium (Vocabria®) is administered orally as tablets. Cabotegravir extended-release injectable suspension (Apretude®) is administered by IM injection.

Oral Administration

Cabotegravir sodium (Vocabria®) is administered orally once daily in combination with rilpivirine (Edurant®). Take cabotegravir and rilpivirine at the same time each day with food.

Oral lead-in dosing to assess the tolerability of cabotegravir may be used for approximately 1 month (≥28 days) prior to the initiation of cabotegravir extended-release injectable suspension (Apretude®) or the combined regimen of cabotegravir and rilpivirine extended-release injectable suspension (Cabenuva®).

Oral therapy with cabotegravir sodium tablets can be considered for patients planning to miss a monthly or every 2 month scheduled injection of cabotegravir extended-release injectable suspension (Apretude®) or the combined regimen of cabotegravir and rilpivirine extended-release injectable suspension (Cabenuva®) by more than 7 days. For patients missing a monthly scheduled injection by more than 7 days, oral cabotegravir in combination with oral rilpivirine should be initiated approximately 1 month (+/- 7 days) after the last IM injection and continued until the day that IM extended-release injection is restarted. Oral replacement therapy with cabotegravir and rilpivirine may be continued for up to 2 months to replace missed monthly IM extended-release injections. For patients missing an every 2 month scheduled injection by more than 7 days, oral therapy with cabotegravir and rilpivirine should be initiated approximately 2 months after the last IM injection and continued until the day that IM extended-release injection is restarted.

IM Injection

Cabotegravir extended-release injectable suspension must be administered by a healthcare provider by gluteal IM injection. The ventrogluteal site is recommended; however, a dorsogluteal approach is acceptable, if preferred by the healthcare provider. Consider the body mass index (BMI) of the patient to ensure appropriate needle length to reach the gluteus muscle. Longer needle lengths, which are not present in the available dosing kit, may be required for patients with higher BMI (e.g., >30 kg/m²) to ensure IM administration.

Cabotegravir extended-release injectable suspension should be visually inspected for particulate matter and discoloration prior to administration; discard the vial if particulate matter or discoloration are present. The drug vial has a brown tint that may limit visual inspection.

Shake the drug vial vigorously prior to injection so that the suspension looks uniform. Small air bubbles may be present and are acceptable.

If the drug is stored in the refrigerator, the vial should be brought to room temperature prior to administration (not to exceed 30°C). Once the suspension has been drawn into the syringe, administer the injection as soon as possible. The suspension may remain in the syringe for up to 2 hours, but the filled syringes should not be placed in the refrigerator. If the medicine remains in the syringe for more than 2 hours, discard the filled syringe and needle.

Therapy with cabotegravir may be initiated with the oral form of the drug prior to beginning the IM injections or the patient may proceed directly to injection therapy without an oral lead-in. If oral cabotegravir lead-in therapy is used, administer initiation injections of cabotegravir on the last day of oral lead-in or within 3 days thereafter. The recommended initiation injection doses of cabotegravir extended-release injectable suspension is a single IM injection given one month apart for 2 consecutive months. Individuals may be given the second cabotegravir injection up to 7 days before or after the date the individual is scheduled to receive the injections.

After the 2 initial injections are given consecutively one month apart, the recommended continuation dose of cabotegravir injection is a single IM injection every 2 months. Cabotegravir continuation injections may be given up to 7 days before or after the date the patient is scheduled to receive the injections.

● Dosage

Available orally as cabotegravir sodium; dosage expressed in terms of cabotegravir.

Adult Dosage

Treatment of HIV Infection

Oral Lead-in Dosing to Assess Tolerability: The recommended daily dose of cabotegravir for the treatment of HIV infection is cabotegravir 30 mg in combination with rilpivirine 25 mg for approximately 1 month (at least 28 days).

Oral Dosing to Replace Planned Missed Injections (Monthly Schedule): If a patient plans to miss a monthly scheduled dose of cabotegravir and rilpivirine extended-release injectable suspensions by more than 7 days, take oral cabotegravir 30 mg with oral rilpivirine 25 mg daily for up to 2 months to replace missed injection visits. For oral therapy with cabotegravir and rilpivirine of durations greater than 2 months, an alternative oral regimen is recommended.

Oral Dosing to Replace Planned Missed Injections (2 Month Schedule): If a patient plans to miss a scheduled every 2 month injection of cabotegravir and rilpivirine extended-release injectable suspension by more than 7 days, take oral cabotegravir 30 mg with oral rilpivirine 25 mg daily for up to 2 months to replace 1 missed scheduled every 2 month injection.. Refer to the Vocabria® prescribing information for further information related to the dosing of oral cabotegravir in this setting.

Pre-exposure Prophylaxis (PrEP) for Prevention of HIV-1 Infection

Oral Lead-in Dosing to Assess Tolerability: The recommended daily dose of cabotegravir for the prevention of HIV infection is cabotegravir 30 mg for approximately 1 month (at least 28 days). Following oral lead-in, start initiation injection of cabotegravir extended-release injectable suspension on the last day of oral lead-in or within 3 days.

Initiation and Continuation Injections: Initially administer a single IM dose of cabotegravir extended-release injection 600 mg injection given 1 month apart for 2 consecutive months on the last day or within 3 days of an oral lead-in (if used) and then continue with the injections every 2 months thereafter.

Oral Dosing to Replace Planned Missed Injections (2 month schedule): If a patient plans to miss a scheduled dose of cabotegravir and rilpivirine extended-release injectable suspensions by more than 7 days, take oral cabotegravir 30 mg for up to 2 months to replace 1 missed scheduled every 2 month injection.

Unplanned Missed Injections: If a scheduled injection visit is missed or delayed by more than 7 days and oral dosing has not been taken in the interim, clinically reassess the individual to determine if resumption of injection dosing remains appropriate. If the injection dosing schedule will be continued, see the following dosing recommendations in Table 1.

TABLE 1. Cabotegravir Injection Dosing Recommendations after Missed Injections

Time since last injection	Recommendation
Second injection is missed and time since first injection is ≤2 months	Administer 600 mg gluteal IM injection of cabotegravir extended-release injection as soon as possible, then continue to follow the every 2 month injection dosing schedule.
Second injection is missed and time since first injection is >2 months	Restart with 600 mg gluteal IM injection of cabotegravir extended-release injection, followed by a second 600 mg initiation injection dose 1 month later. Then continue to follow the every 2 month injection dosing schedule thereafter.

TABLE 1. Continued

Time since last injection	Recommendation
Third or subsequent injection is missed and time since prior injection is ≤3 months	Administer 600 mg IM injection of cabotegravir extended-release injection as soon as possible, then continue with the every 2-month injection dosing schedule.
Third or subsequent injection is missed and time since prior injection is >3 months	Restart with 600 mg gluteal IM injection of cabotegravir extended-release injection, followed by the second 600 mg initiation injection dose 1 month later. Then continue with the every 2 month injection dosing schedule thereafter.

Pediatric Dosage

Treatment of HIV Infection

Oral Lead-in Dosing to Assess Tolerability: The recommended daily dose of cabotegravir for the treatment of HIV infection in pediatric patients ≥12 years of age who weigh ≥35 kg is cabotegravir 30 mg in combination with rilpivirine 25 mg for approximately 1 month (at least 28 days).

Oral Dosing to Replace Planned Missed Injections (Monthly Schedule): If a pediatric patient ≥12 years of age who weighs ≥35 kg plans to miss a monthly scheduled dose of cabotegravir and rilpivirine extended-release injectable suspensions by more than 7 days, take oral cabotegravir 30 mg with oral rilpivirine 25 mg daily for up to 2 months to replace missed injection visits. For oral therapy durations greater than 2 months, an alternative oral regimen is recommended.

Oral Dosing to Replace Planned Missed Injections (2-Month Schedule): If a patient ≥12 years of age who weighs ≥35 kg plans to miss a scheduled dose of cabotegravir and rilpivirine extended-release injectable suspensions by more than 7 days, take oral cabotegravir 30 mg with oral rilpivirine 25 mg daily for up to 2 months to replace 1 missed scheduled every 2 month injection. Refer to the Vocabria® prescribing information for further information related to the dosing of oral cabotegravir in this setting.

Pre-exposure Prophylaxis (PrEP) for Prevention of HIV-1 Infection

Oral Lead-in Dosing to Assess Tolerability: The recommended daily dose of cabotegravir for the prevention of HIV infection in at risk adolescents who weigh ≥35 kg is cabotegravir 30 mg for approximately 1 month (at least 28 days). Following oral lead-in, start initiation injection of cabotegravir extended-release injectable suspension on the last day of oral lead-in or within 3 days.

Initiation and Continuation Injections: Initially, for at risk adolescents weighing at least 35 kg, administer a single IM injection of cabotegravir 600 mg given 1 month apart for 2 consecutive months on the last day or within 3 days of an oral lead-in (if used) and then continue with the injections every 2 months thereafter.

Oral Dosing to Replace Planned Missed Injections (2-month schedule): If an at risk adolescent who weighs ≥35 kg plans to miss a scheduled dose of cabotegravir and rilpivirine extended-release injectable suspensions by more than 7 days, take oral cabotegravir 30 mg to replace the every 2 month injection.

Unplanned Missed Injections: If a scheduled injection visit is missed or delayed by more than 7 days and oral dosing has not been taken in the interim, clinically reassess the individual to determine if resumption of injection dosing remains appropriate. If the injection dosing schedule will be continued, see the following dosing recommendations in Table 1.

● Special Populations

Hepatic Impairment

No dosage adjustment of IV or oral cabotegravir is necessary in patients with mild or moderate hepatic impairment (Child-Pugh A or B) based on clinical studies with oral cabotegravir. The effect of severe hepatic impairment (Child-Pugh C) on the pharmacokinetics of cabotegravir is unknown.

Renal Impairment

No dosage adjustment of oral cabotegravir is necessary for patients with mild to moderate (creatinine clearance 30 to <90 mL/minute) or severe renal impairment (creatinine clearance <30 mL/minute).

The effect of end-stage renal disease (creatinine clearance <15 mL/minute) on the pharmacokinetics of oral cabotegravir is unknown.

Based on studies with oral cabotegravir, no dosage adjustment of cabotegravir extended-release injection is necessary for individuals with mild (creatinine clearance 60 to <90 mL/minute) or moderate renal impairment (creatinine clearance 30 to <60 mL/minute).

In individuals with severe renal impairment (creatinine clearance 15 to <30 mL/minute) or end-stage renal disease (creatinine clearance <15 mL/minute), increased monitoring for adverse effects is recommended.

Geriatric Use

Use caution when administering cabotegravir in geriatric patients.

CAUTIONS

● Contraindications

- Previous hypersensitivity reaction to cabotegravir.
- Coadministration with carbamazepine, oxcarbazepine, phenobarbital, phenytoin, rifampin, or rifapentine; significant decreases in cabotegravir plasma concentrations may occur due to uridine diphosphate (UDP)-glucuronosyl transferase (UGT)1A1 enzyme induction, which may result in loss of virologic response.
- For HIV-1 pre-exposure prophylaxis: Unknown or positive HIV-1 status.

● Warnings/Precautions

Warnings

Potential Risk of Resistance with Cabotegravir PrEP in Undiagnosed HIV-1 Infection

A boxed warning about the risk of drug resistance with use of cabotegravir PrEP in undiagnosed HIV-1 infection is included in the prescribing information for the drug.

There is a potential risk of developing resistance to cabotegravir extended-release injection if an individual acquires HIV-1 either before or while receiving the drug or following discontinuation. Drug-resistant HIV-1 variants have been identified with use of cabotegravir extended-release injection by individuals with undiagnosed HIV-1 infection. To minimize this risk, test patients for HIV-1 infection prior to initiating cabotegravir extended-release injection or oral cabotegravir, and with each subsequent injection of cabotegravir extended-release, using a test approved or cleared by the FDA for the diagnosis of acute or primary HIV-1 infection. Do not initiate cabotegravir extended-release injection for HIV-1 PrEP unless a negative infection status is confirmed. Individuals who become infected with HIV-1 while receiving cabotegravir extended-release injection for PrEP must transition to a complete HIV-1 treatment regimen. Alternative forms of PrEP should be considered following discontinuation of cabotegravir extended-release injection for those individuals at continuing risk of HIV-1 acquisition and initiated within 2 months of the final injection of cabotegravir extended-release.

Other Warnings and Precautions

Hypersensitivity Reactions

Serious or severe hypersensitivity reactions have been reported in association with other integrase inhibitors and could occur with cabotegravir extended-release injection or oral cabotegravir. Remain vigilant and discontinue cabotegravir if a hypersensitivity reaction is suspected.

Discontinue cabotegravir extended-release injection or oral cabotegravir immediately if signs or symptoms of hypersensitivity reactions develop (including, but not limited to, severe rash, or rash accompanied by fever, general malaise, fatigue, muscle or joint aches, blisters, mucosal involvement [oral blisters or lesions], conjunctivitis, facial edema, hepatitis, eosinophilia, angioedema, difficulty breathing). Clinical status, including liver aminotransferases, should be monitored and appropriate therapy initiated.

Comprehensive Management to Reduce the Risk of HIV-1 Infection When Cabotegravir is Used for HIV-1 PrEP

Use cabotegravir for HIV-1 PrEP to reduce the risk of HIV-1 infection as part of a comprehensive prevention strategy including adherence to the administration schedule and safer sex practices, including condoms, to reduce the risk of sexually transmitted infections (STIs). Counsel patients on the use of other prevention measures (e.g., consistent and correct condom use; knowledge of partner(s)' HIV-1 status, including viral suppression status; regular testing for STIs that can facilitate HIV-1 transmission). Treatment with cabotegravir is not always effective in preventing HIV-1 acquisition. The time from initiation of cabotegravir for HIV-1 PrEP to maximal protection against HIV-1 infection is unknown.

Counsel HIV-1–uninfected patients to strictly adhere to the recommended dosing and testing schedule for cabotegravir extended-release injection or oral cabotegravir in order to reduce the risk of HIV-1 acquisition and the potential development of resistance. Some patients, such as adolescents, may benefit from frequent visits and counseling to support adherence to the dosing and testing schedule.

Long-Acting Properties and Potential Associated Risks with Cabotegravir Extended-release Injection

Residual concentrations of cabotegravir may remain in the systemic circulation of individuals for prolonged periods (up to 12 months or longer) after receiving cabotegravir extended-release injection. Carefully select patients who agree to the required every 2 month injection dosing schedule because non-adherence could lead to HIV-1 acquisition and development of resistance. Consider the prolonged-release characteristics of cabotegravir when cabotegravir extended-release injection is prescribed.

Hepatotoxicity

Hepatotoxicity has been reported in patients receiving cabotegravir with or without known pre-existing hepatic disease or identifiable risk factors.

Patients with underlying liver disease or marked elevations in transaminases prior to treatment may be at increased risk for worsening or development of transaminase elevations when cabotegravir is used for treatment of HIV-1 infection.

Monitor liver chemistries and discontinue treatment with cabotegravir if hepatotoxicity is suspected.

Depressive Disorders

Depressive disorders (including depressed mood, depression, mood altered, mood swings, persistent depressive disorder, suicidal ideation/suicide attempt) have been reported with the use of cabotegravir for treatment of HIV-1 infection or HIV-1 PrEP. Promptly evaluate patients with depressive symptoms to assess whether the symptoms are related to cabotegravir and to determine whether the risks of continued therapy outweigh the benefits.

Risk of Adverse Reactions or Loss of Virologic Response Due to Drug Interactions

The concomitant use of cabotegravir or cabotegravir sodium and other drugs may result in known or potentially significant drug interactions, some of which may lead to adverse events, loss of virologic response of cabotegravir, and possible development of viral resistance.

See manufacturer's labeling for steps to prevent or manage these possible and known significant drug interactions, including dosing recommendations. Consider the potential for drug interactions prior to and during therapy with cabotegravir; review concomitant medications during therapy with cabotegravir.

Risks Associated with Rilpivirine Treatment

Cabotegravir sodium is indicated for use in combination with rilpivirine. Review the prescribing information for rilpivirine for information on rilpivirine prior to initiation of combination therapy with cabotegravir sodium and rilpivirine.

Specific Populations

Pregnancy

Antiretroviral Pregnancy Registry at 800-258-4263 or http://www.apregistry.com.

The manufacturer states that data are insufficient regarding use of oral cabotegravir or extended-release cabotegravir injection in pregnant females to inform a drug-associated risk of birth defects or miscarriage. In animal reproduction studies, there was evidence of adverse embryofetal or pre- and post-natal development with oral cabotegravir at systemic exposures approximately 28 times higher (rats) than human exposures at the maximum recommended human dosage. There was no evidence of adverse development with oral cabotegravir given during organogenesis at systemic exposures approximately 28 times higher (rats or rabbits) than or similar to human exposures at the maximum recommended human dosage. The manufacturers state that the use of oral cabotegravir or extended-release cabotegravir should only be used if the expected benefit justifies the potential risk to the fetus.

Data from an observational birth outcome surveillance study in Botswana showed an increased risk of neural tube defects associated with use of dolutegravir (another integrase inhibitor) at the time of conception and during early pregnancy compared with use of antiretroviral regimens that did not contain dolutegravir. Data from clinical trials are insufficient to address this risk with cabotegravir.

The Health and Human Services Panel on Treatment of Pregnant Women with HIV Infection and Prevention of Perinatal Transmission states that data are not available regarding use of cabotegravir for the treatment of HIV-1 infection during pregnancy and, therefore, cabotegravir is not recommended as a complete treatment regimen in pregnant females or females of reproductive potential trying to conceive. The Panel recommends that pregnant individuals who present to care on this regimen should be switched to an appropriate three-drug antiretroviral regimen recommended for use in pregnancy.

The Health and Human Services Panel on Treatment of Pregnant Women with HIV Infection and Prevention of Perinatal Transmission states that although cabotegravir has been approved by the FDA for use in PrEP, safety data are limited regarding use of the drug during conception and breastfeeding.

Lactation

It is not known whether cabotegravir is distributed into human milk; however, the drug is distributed into animal milk. When a drug is present in animal milk, it is likely present in human milk.

It is not known whether cabotegravir affects human milk production or affects the breast-fed infant. However, because detectable concentrations of cabotegravir remain in systemic circulation for up to 12 months after discontinuing cabotegravir extended-release injection, it is recommended that women receiving this treatment breastfeed only if the expected benefit justifies the potential risk to the infant.

Because of the risk of adverse effects in the infant and the risk of HIV transmission, HIV-infected women should not breast-feed infants. For uninfected mothers receiving oral cabotegravir for HIV-1 PrEP, assess the benefit-risk of using this medication to the infant while breastfeeding.

Pediatric Use

Safety, efficacy, and pharmacokinetics of cabotegravir and cabotegravir sodium have not been established in pediatric patients younger than 12 years of age or weighing <35 kg.

Safety, efficacy, and pharmacokinetics of oral and injectable cabotegravir were evaluated in 8 HIV-1-infected pediatric patients 12 to <18 years of age weighing ≥35 kg in an ongoing, open-label, non-comparative clinical trial (MOCHA; IMPAACT 2017). Safety of cabotegravir observed in pediatric patients in this trial is expected to be similar to that reported in adults receiving the drug. In addition, drug exposure to cabotegravir was similar to that in adults.

Safety and efficacy of oral cabotegravir for HIV-1 PrEP in pediatric patients ≥12 years of age weighing ≥35 kg who are at-risk of HIV-1 infection is supported by data from 2 controlled clinical trials in adults. Safety and efficacy of injectable cabotegravir is being evaluated in 54 pediatric patients 12 to <18 years of age years who are at-risk of HIV-1 infection in 2 ongoing, open-label, multicenter clinical trials. Safety of cabotegravir observed in pediatric patients in these trials is similar to that reported in adults receiving the drug.

When cabotegravir is used for HIV-1 PrEP in pediatric patients, HIV-1 testing should be conducted prior to initiating therapy and prior to each scheduled injection of cabotegravir extended-release injectable suspension. Adolescents may benefit from more frequent visits and counseling to support adherence to the dosing schedule.

Geriatric Use

Experience in patients ≥65 years of age is insufficient to determine whether these patients respond differently to cabotegravir than younger adults.

Cabotegravir products should be used with caution in geriatric patients because of age-related decreases in hepatic, renal, and/or cardiac function and potential for concomitant disease and drug therapy.

Renal Impairment

Based on studies with oral cabotegravir, no dosage adjustment of oral or injectable cabotegravir is necessary for patients with mild or moderate (creatinine clearance 30 to <90 mL/minute) renal impairment. In patients with severe renal impairment (creatinine clearance <30 mL/minute), no dosage changes are recommended for patients receiving oral cabotegravir; however, in patients receiving injectable extended-release cabotegravir with severe renal impairment (creatinine clearance 15 to <30 mL/minute) or end-stage renal disease (creatinine clearance <15 mL/minute), increased monitoring for adverse effects is recommended. The effect of end-stage renal disease (creatinine clearance <15 mL/minute) on the pharmacokinetics of cabotegravir is unknown. As cabotegravir is >99% protein bound, dialysis is not expected to alter exposures of the drug.

Hepatic Impairment

Based on studies with oral cabotegravir, no dosage adjustment is necessary for individuals with mild or moderate hepatic impairment (Child-Pugh A or B). The effect of severe hepatic impairment (Child-Pugh C) on the pharmacokinetics of cabotegravir is unknown.

● Common Adverse Effects

The most common adverse reactions reported in at least 3 HIV-infected patients receiving oral cabotegravir include fatigue, headache, diarrhea, nausea, dizziness, abnormal dreams, anxiety, insomnia, abdominal discomfort, abdominal distension, and asthenia.

The most common adverse reactions reported in ≥1% of HIV-uninfected patients receiving oral cabotegravir include headache, diarrhea, nausea, dizziness, upper respiratory tract infection, somnolence, fatigue, abnormal dreams, and abdominal pain.

The most common adverse reactions reported in ≥1% of patients receiving cabotegravir extended-release injection include injection site reactions, diarrhea, headache, pyrexia, fatigue, sleep disorders, nausea, dizziness, flatulence, abdominal pain, vomiting, myalgia, rash, decreased appetite, somnolence, back pain, and upper respiratory infection.

DRUG INTERACTIONS

● Drugs Affecting or Metabolized by Uridine Diphosphate-glucuronosyltransferases

Cabotegravir is primarily metabolized by uridine diphosphate-glucuronosyltransferase (UGT) 1A1 with some contribution from UGT1A9. Drugs that are strong inducers of UGT1A1 or UGT1A9 are expected to decrease cabotegravir plasma concentrations and may result in loss of efficacy; therefore, coadministration of cabotegravir with these drugs is contraindicated.

● Concomitant Use with Other Antiretroviral Medicines

Cabotegravir in combination with rilpivirine is a recommended complete regimen for the treatment of HIV-1 infection; coadministration of cabotegravir with other antiretroviral medications for PrEP is not recommended.

● Use of Other Antiretroviral Drugs after Discontinuation of Cabotegravir extended-release injection

Residual concentrations of cabotegravir may remain in the systemic circulation of individuals for prolonged periods (up to 12 months or longer); however, these residual concentrations are not expected to affect the exposures of antiretroviral drugs that are initiated after discontinuation of cabotegravir extended-release injection.

• *Antacids*

Coadministration of oral cabotegravir with antacid preparations containing polyvalent cations (e.g., aluminum or magnesium hydroxide, calcium carbonate) may lead to decreased absorption of cabotegravir.

The manufacturer recommends administration of drugs or preparations containing polyvalent cations at least 2 hours before or 4 hours after taking oral cabotegravir.

• *Anticonvulsants*

Coadministration of oral cabotegravir with carbamazepine, oxcarbazepine, phenobarbital, or phenytoin may cause significant decreases in cabotegravir plasma concentrations due to UGT1A1 enzyme induction, which may result in loss of cabotegravir efficacy. Coadministration of cabotegravir with these drugs is contraindicated.

• *Antimycobacterials*

Coadministration of oral cabotegravir with rifampin or rifapentine may cause significant decreases in cabotegravir plasma concentrations due to UGT1A1 enzyme induction, which may result in loss of cabotegravir efficacy. Coadministration of cabotegravir with these drugs is contraindicated.

Rifabutin can be coadministered with cabotegravir; however, it is contraindicated with cabotegravir and rilpivirine extended release injection (Cabenuva®) for HIV-1 treatment. The following dosage modification is recommended with cabotegravir injection for HIV-1 PrEP. When rifabutin is started before or concomitantly with the first initiation injection of cabotegravir, the recommended dosage of cabotegravir is one 600-mg injection, followed 2 weeks later by a second 600-mg initiation injection and monthly thereafter while on rifabutin. When rifabutin is started at the time of the second cabotegravir initiation injection or later, the recommended dosage of cabotegravir is 600 mg monthly while on rifabutin; after stopping rifabutin, the recommended dosage of cabotegravir is 600 mg every 2 months.

• *Hormonal Contraceptives*

Use of oral contraceptives was associated with lower concentrations of cabotegravir extended-release injection compared with women not receiving any hormonal contraception; however, the association is not likely to be clinically significant. No adjustments are needed for oral contraceptives containing levonorgestrel and ethinyl estradiol. The HHS Panel on Treatment of Pregnant Women with HIV Infection and Prevention of Perinatal Transmission states that no additional contraceptive protection is necessary.

DESCRIPTION

Cabotegravir, an an antiretroviral agent, is a human immunodeficiency virus (HIV) integrase strand transfer inhibitor (INSTI). Cabotegravir inhibits HIV integrase by binding to the integrase active site and blocking the strand transfer step of retroviral deoxyribonucleic acid (DNA) integration, which is essential for the HIV replication cycle.

Cabotegravir-resistant HIV-1 has been produced in vitro and has also emerged during cabotegravir therapy. In clinical studies of cabotegravir for treatment of HIV-1 infection, there were virologic failures on the cabotegravir plus rilpivirine regimen, including treatment-emergent INSTI resistance-associated substitutions and reduced phenotypic susceptibility to cabotegravir. In clinical studies of cabotegravir for HIV-1 pre-exposure prophylaxis, INSTI resistance-associated substitutions were detected in viruses from patients who achieved target plasma concentrations of cabotegravir. Infection was also reported in those with cabotegravir exposures below the target; although, no variants expressing INSTI resistance-associated substitutions were detected. Cross-resistance between cabotegravir and other INSTIs (e.g., elvitegravir, raltegravir) has been reported.

Following oral administration of cabotegravir sodium, peak plasma concentrations of cabotegravir are attained approximately 3 hours after dosing.

Following parenteral administration of cabotegravir extended-release suspension, peak plasma concentrations of cabotegravir are attained approximately 7 days after dosing. Cabotegravir and cabotegravir sodium are approximately 99.8% bound to plasma protein. Cabotegravir and cabotegravir sodium are metabolized primarily by uridine diphosphate-glucuronosyltransferase (UGT) 1A1. Following an oral dose of cabotegravir sodium or injection of cabotegravir extended-release suspension, approximately 59% of the dose is eliminated in feces (as cabotegravir) and 27% is eliminated in urine (as cabotegravir). Cabotegravir sodium has an apparent terminal half-life of approximately 41 hours; cabotegravir extended-release suspension has a terminal half-life of approximately 5.6 to 11.5 weeks.

ADVICE TO PATIENTS

- For patients receiving cabotegravir for HIV-1 PrEP: Advise patients to adhere to the dosing schedule and safer sex practices, including use of condoms, to reduce the risk of STIs.

- For patients receiving cabotegravir for HIV-1 PrEP: Advise patients that use of cabotegravir as part of a HIV-1 PrEP regimen is not always effective in prevention of HIV-1 and time from initiation of treatment to maximal protection is not known.

- For patients receiving cabotegravir for HIV-1 PrEP: Inform individuals about and support their efforts in reducing sexual risk behavior and the use of other prevention measures (e.g., knowledge of partner HIV-1 status, testing for STIs, condom use).

- For patients receiving cabotegravir for HIV-1 PrEP: Inform patients that cabotegravir is to be used to reduce the risk of acquiring HIV-1 only in individuals confirmed to be HIV-1 negative as HIV-1 resistance substitutions may emerge in individuals with undiagnosed HIV-1 infection who are taking only cabotegravir; cabotegravir alone does not constitute a complete regimen for HIV-1 treatment.

- For patients receiving cabotegravir for HIV-1 PrEP: Inform patients that if an HIV-1 test indicates possible HIV-1 infection, or if symptoms consistent with acute HIV-1 infection develop following an exposure event, additional HIV testing to determine HIV status is needed. If an HIV-1 infection is confirmed, then transition the individual to a complete HIV-1 treatment regimen.

- Advise patients to immediately contact their healthcare provider if they develop a rash. Instruct patients to immediately stop taking cabotegravir sodium and seek medical attention if they develop a rash associated with any of the following symptoms: fever; generally ill feeling; extreme tiredness; muscle or joint aches; blisters; oral blisters or lesions; eye inflammation; facial swelling; swelling of the eyes, lips, tongue, or mouth; difficulty breathing; and/or signs and symptoms of liver problems (e.g., yellowing of the skin or whites of the eyes; dark or tea-colored urine; pale-colored stools or bowel movements; nausea; vomiting; loss of appetite; or pain, aching, or sensitivity on the right side below the ribs).

- Inform patients that hepatotoxicity has been reported with cabotegravir. Instruct patients that monitoring for liver transaminases is recommended.

- Inform patients that depressive disorders (including depressed mood, depression, mood altered, mood swings, persistent depressive disorder, suicide ideation or attempt) have been reported with cabotegravir. Promptly evaluate patients with severe depressive symptoms to assess whether the symptoms are related to cabotegravir and to determine whether the risks of continued therapy outweigh the benefits.

- Advise patients to inform their clinicians of existing or contemplated concomitant therapy, including prescription and OTC drugs, as well as any concomitant illnesses.

- Inform patients that it is important to take oral cabotegravir once daily on a regular dosing schedule with a meal at the same time as rilpivirine and to avoid missing doses, as this can result in development of resistance. Instruct patients that if they miss a dose of cabotegravir sodium, to take it as soon as they remember.

- Advise women to inform their clinician if they are or plan to become pregnant. Inform patients of the antiretroviral pregnancy registry to monitor fetal outcomes in those exposed to cabotegravir during pregnancy.

- Instruct mothers with HIV-1 infection not to breastfeed because HIV-1 can be passed to the baby in the breast milk.

- Inform patients of other important precautionary information.

PREPARATIONS

Excipients in commercially available drug preparations may have clinically important effects in some individuals; consult specific product labeling for details.

Cabotegravir

Parenteral		
Injection, extended-release suspension for IM administration	600 mg/3mL (200 mg/mL)	**Apretude®**, ViiV Healthcare

Cabotegravir Sodium

Oral		
Tablets, film-coated	30 mg (of cabotegravir)	**Vocabria®**, ViiV Healthcare

† Use is not currently included in the labeling approved by the US Food and Drug Administration.

Selected Revisions April 10, 2024, © Copyright, February 8, 2021, American Society of Health-System Pharmacists, Inc.

Cabotegravir and Rilpivirine

8:18.08.12 • HIV INTEGRASE INHIBITORS

■ Cabotegravir, an HIV integrase strand transfer inhibitor (INSTI), and rilpivirine, an HIV non-nucleoside reverse transcriptase inhibitor (NNRTI), are used in combination as an antiretroviral agent.

USES

● Treatment of HIV Infection

Cabotegravir, a human immunodeficiency virus type 1 (HIV-1) integrase strand transfer inhibitor (INSTI), and rilpivirine, an HIV-1 non-nucleoside reverse transcriptase inhibitor (NNRTI) are indicated as a complete regimen for the treatment of HIV-1 infection in adults and pediatric patients ≥12 years of age weighing at least 35 kg to replace the current antiretroviral regimen in those who are virologically suppressed (HIV-1 RNA <50 copies/mL) on a stable antiretroviral regimen with no history of treatment failure and with no known or suspected resistance to either cabotegravir or rilpivirine. The combination regimen (cabotegravir/rilpivirine [Cabenuva®]) is commercially available as a copackaged product containing cabotegravir extended-release injectable suspension and rilpivirine extended-release injectable suspension.

Clinical Experience

The efficacy of cabotegravir in combination with rilpivirine has been evaluated in 2 phase 3 randomized, multicenter, active-controlled, parallel-arm, open-label, non-inferiority trials (FLAIR and ATLAS). The primary endpoint of these studies was the proportion of patients with plasma HIV-1 RNA ≥50 copies/mL at week 48 who received cabotegravir/rilpivirine combination therapy compared to those who remained on their current antiretroviral regimen.

The FLAIR study was conducted in antiretroviral-naïve HIV-1-infected adults with baseline plasma HIV-1 RNA levels ≥50 copies/mL. Patients received a dolutegravir INSTI-containing regimen for 20 weeks (either dolutegravir/abacavir/lamivudine or dolutegravir plus 2 other NRTIs if subjects were HLA-B*5701 positive). Patients who were virologically suppressed (HIV-1 RNA <50 copies/mL) were then randomized (1:1) to receive either cabotegravir plus rilpivirine or remain on their current antiretroviral regimen. Subjects randomized to receive cabotegravir plus rilpivirine initiated treatment with daily oral lead-in dosing with cabotegravir 30 mg and rilpivirine 25 mg for at least 4 weeks followed by monthly injections with cabotegravir/rilpivirine for an additional 44 weeks. At week 48, an HIV-1 RNA level ≥50 copies/mL was found in 2% of patients who received cabotegravir/rilpivirine and in 2% of patients who received a current antiretroviral regimen, meeting the criteria for non-inferiority. At 96 weeks, the proportion of subjects with HIV-1 RNA ≥50 copies/mL was 3.2% for both the cabotegravir plus rilpivirine and current antiretroviral regimen treatment arms. In the extension phase of the FLAIR study (week 100 to 124), the efficacy of long-acting injectable cabotegravir and rilpivirine was evaluated in patients who switched at week 100 from their current antiretroviral regimen to injectable cabotegravir and rilpivirine, with or without oral cabotegravir lead-in therapy. At 124 weeks, 0.8% of patients who received oral cabotegravir lead-in therapy and 0.9% of patients who switched directly to the injectable therapy had plasma HIV-1 RNA levels ≥50 copies/mL, meeting the criteria for non-inferiority. In addition, the rates of virologic suppression (HIV-1 RNA levels <50 copies/mL) were similar in patients who received oral cabotegravir lead-in therapy compared with those who switched directly to the injections.

In the ATLAS study, antiretroviral-experienced HIV-1 infected, virologically suppressed adults with plasma HIV-1 RNA levels <50 copies/mL were randomly assigned (1:1) to receive cabotegravir/rilpivirine or remain on their current antiretroviral regimen. Patients randomized to cabotegravir/rilpivirine initiated treatment with daily oral lead-in dosing with cabotegravir 30 mg and rilpivirine

25 mg for at least 4 weeks followed by monthly injections with cabotegravir/rilpivirine for an additional 44 weeks. At week 48, 2% of patients who received cabotegravir/rilpivirine and 1% of patients who received current antiretroviral therapy achieved an HIV-1 RNA level ≥50 copies/mL, meeting the criteria for non-inferiority. Patients who completed 52 weeks of therapy were given the option to withdraw from the study, transition to the ATLAS 2M study, or enter an extension phase; in the extension phase, patients either continued long-acting cabotegravir/rilpivirine therapy or switched from a current antiretroviral regimen to long-acting therapy. Among 52 patients who entered the extension phase, 100% who continued long-acting therapy and 97% who switched from their current regimen to long-acting therapy had plasma HIV-1 RNA levels <50 copies/mL.

An additional phase 3b, randomized, multicenter, parallel-arm, open-label, non-inferiority trial (ATLAS 2M) was conducted to evaluate the efficacy of long-acting injectable cabotegravir and rilpivirine dosed every 2 months. In this study, HIV-1–infected, antiretroviral-experienced, virologically suppressed patients were randomized to receive a cabotegravir plus rilpivirine regimen (administered in injection doses of cabotegravir 400 mg plus rilpivirine 600 mg monthly or cabotegravir 600 mg plus rilpivirine 900 mg every 2 months). Patients without prior exposure to cabotegravir plus rilpivirine initiated treatment with daily oral lead-in dosing with cabotegravir 30 mg and rilpivirine 25 mg for at least 4 weeks followed by monthly or every 2 month injections of cabotegravir/rilpivirine for an additional 44 weeks. The primary endpoint of this study was the proportion of subjects with a plasma HIV-1 RNA ≥50 copies/mL at 48 weeks. At 48 weeks, 2% of patients who received every 2 months dosing had plasma HIV-1 RNA levels ≥50 copies/mL compared with 1% of patients receiving monthly dosing, meeting the criteria for non-inferiority. In addition, the rates of virologic suppression (HIV-1 RNA levels <50 copies/mL) were similar (94%) in patients who received every 2 months therapy compared with those receiving monthly injections.

Clinical Perspective

Therapeutic options for the treatment and prevention of HIV infection and recommendations concerning the use of antiretrovirals are continuously evolving. Antiretroviral therapy (ART) is recommended for all individuals with HIV regardless of CD4 counts, and should be initiated as soon as possible after diagnosis of HIV and continued indefinitely. The primary goals of ART are to achieve and maintain durable suppression of HIV viral load (as measured by plasma HIV-1 RNA levels) to a level below which drug-resistance mutations cannot emerge (i.e., below detectable limits), restore and preserve immunologic function, reduce HIV-related morbidity and mortality, improve quality of life, and prevent transmission of HIV. While the most appropriate antiretroviral regimen cannot be defined for each clinical scenario, the US Department of Health and Human Services (HHS) Panel on Antiretroviral Guidelines for Adults and Adolescents, HHS Panel on Antiretroviral Therapy and Medical Management of Children Living with HIV, and HHS Panel on Treatment of Pregnant Women with HIV Infection and Prevention of Perinatal Transmission, have developed comprehensive guidelines that provide information on selection and use of antiretrovirals for the treatment or prevention of HIV infection. Because of the complexity of managing patients with HIV, it is recommended that clinicians with HIV expertise be consulted when needed.

The HHS Panel on Antiretroviral Guidelines for Adults and Adolescents does not recommend use of long acting cabotegravir plus rilpivirine as initial therapy for people with HIV because of the lack of data supporting the efficacy of this combination in antiretroviral therapy-naïve patients. Patients desiring to use long-acting injectable cabotegravir plus rilpivirine early in their treatment history should first attain viral suppression on a recommended regimen, then transition to a month of oral cabotegravir and rilpivirine with maintenance of suppression before transitioning to long-acting injectable cabotegravir plus rilpivirine. The long-acting antiretroviral therapy combination of injectable cabotegravir and rilpivirine is not currently recommended for patients with virologic failure.

The HHS Panel on Antiretroviral Therapy and Medical Management of Children Living with HIV states that the data on use of cabotegravir plus rilpivirine in adolescents are limited to safety, pharmacokinetics, and acceptability; data are not yet available on potential use of this ART in adolescents with adherence concerns.

DOSAGE AND ADMINISTRATION

● General

Pretreatment Screening

- Consider the potential for drug interactions and review concomitant medications.

- Carefully select patients who agree to the required monthly or every-2-month IM injection dosing and testing schedules.

Patient Monitoring

- Periodically monitor liver function tests (i.e., AST, ALT).

- Monitor for the potential for drug interactions and adverse effects that may result from interactions.

- Assess patient adherence to the prescribed therapy during scheduled dosing visits.

● Administration

Cabotegravir/rilpivirine is commercially available as cabotegravir extended-release injectable suspension in a single-dose vial and rilpivirine extended-release injectable suspension in a single-dose vial copackaged for coadministration by IM administration. The injections *must* be administered by a healthcare provider by gluteal IM injection only; administer the IM injections at separate gluteal sites (on opposite sides or at least 2 cm apart) during the same visit. The ventrogluteal site is recommended, but a dorsogluteal approach (upper outer quadrant) is acceptable, if preferred by the healthcare professional. Do not administer by any other route or anatomical site. Consider the body mass index (BMI) of the patient to ensure that the needle length is sufficient to reach the gluteus muscle. Longer needle lengths (not included in the dosing kit) may be required for patients with higher BMI (e.g., >30 kg/m^2) to ensure that injections are administered intramuscularly as opposed to subcutaneously. The administration order of cabotegravir and rilpivirine extended-release injections is not important.

Cabotegravir and rilpivirine combination therapy may be initiated with oral forms of the drugs (oral lead-in daily dose is cabotegravir 30 mg and rilpivirine 25 mg with a meal for approximately 1 month [at least 28 days]) prior to beginning the IM injections to assess tolerability or the combination therapy may be initiated directly with the injectable forms without an oral lead-in. Cabotegravir and rilpivirine extended-release suspensions can be injected monthly or every 2 months. Discuss these 2 dosing options with the patient prior to starting treatment to determine which dosing frequency is more appropriate.

Store the co-packaged cabotegravir/rilpivirine extended-release suspensions at 2–8°C in their original carton; do not freeze.

IM Injection

Prior to preparing the injections, remove the vials from the refrigerator and wait at least 15 minutes to allow them to come to room temperature. The vials may remain in the carton at room temperature for up to 6 hours; do not place the vials back into the refrigerator. Discard the drugs if not used within 6 hours.

Inspect the vial contents visually for particulate matter and discoloration prior to administration. The cabotegravir vial has a brown tint to the glass that may limit visual inspection of the suspension. Discard if either vial exhibits particulate matter or discoloration.

Shake each vial vigorously until the suspensions are uniform before injecting; small air bubbles are expected and acceptable.

Once the injections are drawn into their respective syringes, administer the drugs as soon as possible. Do not store filled syringes in the refrigerator. Discard the syringes and needles if the suspension remains in the syringes for more than 2 hours.

● Dosage

Adult Dosage

Treatment of HIV Infection

Prior to initiating treatment with cabotegravir/rilpivirine injections, an oral lead-in dosing regimen may be used for approximately 1 month (at least 28 days) to assess patient tolerability to the drug.

Monthly Schedule: The recommended initial injection doses for adults are a single 600 mg IM injection of cabotegravir and a single 900 mg IM injection of rilpivirine, given on the last day of current antiretroviral therapy or oral lead-in. After the initiation injections, the recommended monthly continuation injection doses are a single 400 mg IM injection of cabotegravir and a single 600 mg IM injection of rilpivirine at each visit (see Table 1). Patients may be given these injections up to 7 days before or after the date the patient is scheduled to receive monthly injections.

TABLE 1. Recommended Dosing Schedule with Optional Oral Lead-in or Direct to Injection for Monthly Injection

Drug	Oral lead-in for at least 28 days prior to starting injections (Optional)	IM (Gluteal) Initiation Injections (One-Time Dosing) at Month 1	IM (Gluteal) Continuation Injections (Once-Monthly Dosing) after Initiation Injection
Cabotegravir	30 mg once daily with a meal	600 mg	400 mg
Rilpivirine	25 mg once daily with a meal	900 mg	600 mg

Every 2 Months Schedule: Initiate injections on the last day of current antiretroviral therapy or oral lead-in, if used. The recommended initiation injection doses are a single 600 mg IM injection of cabotegravir and a single 900 mg IM injection of rilpivirine 1 month apart for 2 consecutive months. Patients may be given these injections up to 7 days before or after the date the patient is scheduled to receive the second initiation injections.

After the 2 initiation doses given consecutively 1 month apart (Months 1 and 2), the recommended continuation injection doses (Month 4 and onwards) are a single 600 mg IM injection of cabotegravir and a single 900 mg IM injection of rilpivirine administered every 2 months (See Table 2). Patients may be given these injections up to 7 days before or after the date the patient is scheduled to receive the injections.

TABLE 2. Recommended Dosing Schedule with Optional Oral Lead-in or Direct to Injection for Every-2-Month Injection

Drug	Oral lead-in for at least 28 days prior to starting injections (Optional)	IM (Gluteal) Continuation Injections at Month 1, Month 2, and then Every 2 Months Onwards (starting at Month 4)
Cabotegravir	30 mg once daily with a meal	600 mg
Rilpivirine	25 mg once daily with a meal	900 mg

Pediatric Dosage

Treatment of HIV Infection

Prior to initiating treatment with cabotegravir/rilpivirine injections, an oral lead-in dosing regimen may be used for approximately 1 month (at least 28 days) to assess patient tolerability to the drugs.

Monthly Schedule: The recommended initial injection doses for adolescents ≥12 years of age weighing at least 35 kg are a single 600 mg IM injection of cabotegravir and a single 900 mg IM injection of rilpivirine, given on the last day of current antiretroviral therapy or oral lead-in. After the initiation injections, the recommended monthly continuation injection doses are a single 400 mg IM injection of cabotegravir and a single 600 mg IM injection of rilpivirine at each visit (see Table 1). Patients may be given these injections up to 7 days before or after the date the patient is scheduled to receive monthly injections.

Every 2 Months Schedule: Initiate injections on the last day of current antiretroviral therapy or oral lead-in, if used. The recommended initiation injection doses for adolescents ≥12 years of age weighing at least 35 kg are a single 600 mg IM injection of cabotegravir and a single 900 mg IM injection of rilpivirine 1 month apart for 2 consecutive months. Patients may be given these injections up to 7 days before or after the date the patient is scheduled to receive the second initiation injections.

After the 2 initiation doses given consecutively 1 month apart (Months 1 and 2), the recommended continuation injection doses (Month 4 and onwards) are a single 600-mg IM injection of cabotegravir and a single 900-mg IM injection of rilpivirine administered every 2 months (See Table 2). Patients may be given these injections up to 7 days before or after the date the patient is scheduled to receive the injections.

Recommended Dosing Schedule for Missed Injections

Monthly Dosing Schedule (Planned Missed Injections): If a patient plans to miss a scheduled injection visit by >7 days, oral cabotegravir in combination with oral rilpivirine may be given once daily for up to 2 months to replace missed injection visits or any other fully suppressive oral antiretroviral regimen until injections are resumed. Recommended oral daily dose is cabotegravir 30 mg and rilpivirine 25 mg taken at approximately the same time each day with a meal. The first dose of oral therapy should be taken 1 month (+/-7 days) after the last injection dose of cabotegravir/rilpivirine and continued until the day injection dosing is restarted. If the duration of oral therapy with cabotegravir and rilpivirine is >2 months, an alternative oral regimen is recommended.

Monthly Dosing Schedule (Unplanned Missed Injections): If monthly injections are missed or delayed by >7 days and oral therapy has not been taken in the interim, clinically reassess the patient to determine if resumption of injection dosing remains appropriate. If injection dosing will be continued, see Table 3 for dosing recommendations.

TABLE 3. Injection Dosing Recommendations after Missed Injections for Patients on the Monthly Dosing Schedule

Time since Last Injection	Recommendation
≤2 months	Resume with 400 mg cabotegravir and 600 mg rilpivirine IM monthly injections as soon as possible.
>2 months	Re-initiate the patient with 600 mg cabotegravir and 900 mg rilpivirine IM injections then continue to follow the 400 mg cabotegravir and 600 mg rilpivirine IM monthly injection dosing schedule.

Every 2 Months Schedule (Planned Missed Injections): If a patient plans to miss a scheduled injection visit by more than 7 days, oral cabotegravir in combination with oral rilpivirine once daily may be administered for up to 2 months to replace 1 missed injection visit, or any other fully suppressive oral antiretroviral regimen may be used until injections are resumed. The recommended oral daily dose is cabotegravir 30 mg and rilpivirine 25 mg. Take cabotegravir in combination with rilpivirine at approximately the same time each day with a meal. The first dose of oral therapy should be taken approximately 2 months after the last injection dose of cabotegravir plus rilpivirine and continued until the day injection dosing is restarted (see Table 4 for injection dosing recommendations). If the duration of oral therapy with cabotegravir and rilpivirine is more than 2 months, an alternative oral regimen is recommended.

Every 2 Months Schedule (Unplanned Missed Injections): If a scheduled every 2 month injection visit is missed or delayed by >7 days and oral therapy has not been taken in the interim, clinically reassess the patient to determine if resumption of injection dosing remains appropriate. If the every 2 month dosing schedule will be continued, see Table 4 for dosing recommendations.

TABLE 4. Injection Dosing Recommendations after Missed Injections for Patients on the Every 2 Month Dosing Schedule

Missed Injection (Visit)	Time since Last Injection	Recommendation
Injection 2 (Month 2)	≤2 months	Resume with 600 mg cabotegravir and 900 mg rilpivirine IM injections as soon as possible, then continue to follow the every 2 month injection dosing schedule.
Injection 2 (Month 2)	>2 months	Re-initiate the patient with 600 mg cabotegravir and 900 mg rilpivirine IM injections, followed by the second initiation injection dose 1 month later; then continue to follow the every 2 month injection dosing schedule thereafter.
Injection 3 or later (Month 4 onwards)	≤3 months	Resume with 600 mg cabotegravir and 900 mg rilpivirine IM injections as soon as possible and continue with the every 2 month injection dosing schedule.
Injection 3 or later (Month 4 onwards)	>3 months	Re-initiate the patient with 600-mg cabotegravir and 900-mg rilpivirine IM injections, followed by the second initiation injection dose 1 month later; then continue with the every 2 month injection dosing schedule thereafter.

Transitioning between Monthly and Every 2 Month Schedules

Patients switching from a monthly continuation injection schedule to an every 2 months continuation injection dosing schedule should receive a single 600 mg IM injection of cabotegravir and a single 900 mg IM injection of rilpivirine administered 1 month after the last monthly continuation injections and then every 2 months thereafter.

Patients switching from an every 2 months continuation injection schedule to a monthly continuation dosing schedule should receive a single 400 mg IM injection of cabotegravir and a single 600 mg IM injection of rilpivirine 2 months after the last every 2 month continuation injection and then monthly thereafter.

● Special Populations

Hepatic Impairment

Dosage adjustment of cabotegravir/rilpivirine is not necessary for patients with mild or moderate hepatic impairment (Child-Pugh A or B). The effect of cabotegravir/rilpivirine on severe hepatic impairment (Child-Pugh C) is unknown.

Renal Impairment

Dosage adjustment of cabotegravir/rilpivirine is not necessary for patients with mild (creatinine clearance 60 to <90 mL/minute) or moderate renal impairment (creatinine clearance 30 to <60 mL/minute). In patients with severe (creatinine clearance 15 to <30 mL/minute) or end stage renal impairment (creatinine clearance <15 mL/minute), increase monitoring for adverse effects. In patients with end-stage renal disease not on dialysis, the effects on pharmacokinetics are unknown. Dialysis is not expected to alter exposures of cabotegravir or rilpivirine.

Geriatric Use

Use caution when administering cabotegravir/rilpivirine in elderly patients.

CAUTIONS

● Contraindications

- Previous hypersensitivity reaction to cabotegravir or rilpivirine.
- Coadministration with drugs for which significant decreases in cabotegravir plasma concentrations may occur due to uridine diphosphate glucuronosyl

transferase (UGT)1A1 enzyme induction and/or cytochrome P-450 (CYP) 3A enzyme induction, which may result in loss of virologic response (e.g., anticonvulsants [carbamazepine, oxcarbazepine, phenobarbital, phenytoin], antimycobacterials [rifampin, rifabutin, rifapentine], systemic glucocorticoids [dexamethasone; more than a single dose treatment], and herbal products [St John's wort]).

● *Warnings/Precautions*

Sensitivity Reactions

Hypersensitivity Reactions

Hypersensitivity reactions have been reported in association with rilpivirine-containing regimens, including cases of drug reaction with eosinophilia and systemic symptoms (DRESS). While some skin reactions were accompanied by constitutional symptoms such as fever, other skin reactions were associated with organ dysfunctions, including elevations in hepatic serum biochemistries.

Serious or severe hypersensitivity reactions have been reported in association with other integrase inhibitors and could occur with cabotegravir extended-release injection. Administration of cabotegravir and rilpivirine oral lead-in dosing was used in clinical studies to help identify patients who may be at risk of a hypersensitivity reaction.

Discontinue cabotegravir/rilpivirine immediately if signs or symptoms of hypersensitivity reactions develop (including, but not limited to, severe rash, or rash accompanied by fever, general malaise, fatigue, muscle or joint aches, blisters, mucosal involvement [oral blisters or lesions], conjunctivitis, facial edema, hepatitis, eosinophilia, angioedema, difficulty breathing). Monitor clinical status and perform hepatic function tests as clinically indicated; initiate appropriate therapy as indicated. Administer cabotegravir and rilpivirine oral lead-in dosing prior to use of extended-release injections to help identify patients who may be at risk of a hypersensitivity reaction.

Post-Injection Reactions

Serious post-injection reactions were reported in clinical studies within minutes after the injection of rilpivirine suspension. These events included symptoms such as dyspnea, bronchospasm, agitation, abdominal cramping, rash/urticaria, dizziness, flushing, sweating, oral numbness, changes in blood pressure, and pain (e.g., back and chest). These events were reported in <1% of subjects and began to resolve within minutes after the injection, with some patients receiving supportive care. These events may have been associated with accidental IV administration during the IM injection procedure.

Carefully follow the administration instructions when preparing and administering cabotegravir/rilpivirine. The suspensions should be injected slowly via IM injection, and care should be taken to avoid accidental IV administration. Observe patients briefly (approximately 10 minutes) after the injection. If a patient experiences a post-injection reaction, monitor and treat as clinically indicated.

Hepatotoxicity

Hepatotoxicity has been reported in patients receiving cabotegravir or rilpivirine with or without known pre-existing hepatic disease or identifiable risk factors.

Patients with underlying liver disease or marked elevations in transaminases prior to treatment may be at increased risk for worsening or development of transaminase elevations.

Monitoring of liver chemistries is recommended and treatment with cabotegravir/rilpivirine should be discontinued if hepatotoxicity is suspected.

Depressive Disorders

Depressive disorders (including depressed mood, depression, mood altered, mood swings, dysphoria, negative thoughts, suicidal ideation or attempt) have been reported with the use of cabotegravir/rilpivirine or the individual medications. Promptly evaluate patients with depressive symptoms to assess whether the symptoms are related to cabotegravir and to determine whether the risks of continued therapy outweigh the benefits.

Risk of Adverse Reactions or Loss of Virologic Response Due to Drug Interactions

The concomitant use of cabotegravir/rilpivirine and other drugs may result in known or potentially significant drug interactions, some of which may lead to adverse events, loss of virologic response of cabotegravir and rilpivirine extended-release injection, and possible development of viral resistance.

Rilpivirine 75-mg and 300-mg once-daily oral doses (3 and 12 times, respectively, the recommended oral dosage) in healthy adults prolonged the QTc interval with mean steady-state peak plasma concentrations values 4.4- and 11.6-fold, respectively, higher than peak serum concentrations associated with the recommended 600-mg monthly dose of rilpivirine injection, and 4.1- and 10.7-fold, respectively, higher than peak serum concentrations associated with the recommended 900-mg every 2 month dose of rilpivirine injection. Cabotegravir/rilpivirine should be used with caution in combination with drugs with a known risk of torsade de pointes.

Long-Acting Properties and Potential Associated Risks

Residual concentrations of both cabotegravir and rilpivirine may remain in the systemic circulation of patients for prolonged periods (up to 12 months or longer) after administration of cabotegravir/rilpivirine. It is important to carefully select patients who agree to the required monthly or every 2 month injection dosing schedule because non-adherence to monthly or every month injections or missed doses could lead to loss of virologic response and development of resistance.

To minimize the potential risk of developing viral resistance, it is essential to initiate an alternative, fully suppressive antiretroviral regimen no later than 1 month after the final injections of cabotegravir/rilpivirine when dosed monthly and no later than 2 months after the final injections of cabotegravir/rilpivirine when dosed every 2 months. If virologic failure is suspected, switch the patient to an alternative regimen as soon as possible.

Specific Populations

Pregnancy

Antiretroviral Pregnancy Registry at 800-258-4263 or http://www.apregistry.com.

The manufacturer states that data are insufficient on the use of cabotegravir/rilpivirine during pregnancy to adequately assess a drug-associated risk of birth defects and miscarriage. While there are insufficient human data to assess the risk of neural tube defects (NTDs) with exposure to cabotegravir and rilpivirine extended-release injection during pregnancy, NTDs were associated with dolutegravir, another integrase inhibitor. Healthcare professionals should discuss the risks and benefits of using cabotegravir and rilpivirine extended-release injection with individuals of childbearing potential or during pregnancy.

The Health and Human Services Panel on Treatment of Pregnant Women with HIV Infection and Prevention of Perinatal Transmission states that data are not available regarding use of cabotegravir for the treatment of HIV-1 infection during pregnancy and, therefore is not recommended as a complete treatment regimen in pregnant females or females of reproductive potential trying to conceive. The Panel recommends that pregnant individuals who present to care on this regimen should be switched to an appropriate 3-drug antiretroviral regimen recommended for use in pregnancy.

Lower exposures with oral rilpivirine were observed during pregnancy. Viral load should be monitored closely if the patient remains on cabotegravir and rilpivirine extended-release injection during pregnancy. Cabotegravir and rilpivirine are detected in systemic circulation for up to ≥12 months after discontinuing injections of cabotegravir and rilpivirine injection; therefore, consideration should be given to the potential for fetal exposure during pregnancy.

Lactation

Rilpivirine is present in human milk. There are no data on the presence of cabotegravir in human milk; however, cabotegravir is present in animal milk. When a drug is present in animal milk, it is likely present in human milk. If cabotegravir and/or rilpivirine are present in human milk, residual exposures may remain for ≥12 months after the last injections have been administered. It is unknown if cabotegravir and rilpivirine affect milk production or have effects on the breastfed infant.

Because of the potential for HIV-1 transmission (in HIV-1 negative infants), development of viral resistance (in HIV-1 positive infants), adverse reactions in a breastfed infant similar to those seen in adults, and detectable cabotegravir and rilpivirine concentrations in systemic circulation for up to ≥12 months after discontinuing administration of cabotegravir/rilpivirine, instruct mothers not to breastfeed if they are receiving the combined regimen.

Pediatric Use

Safety and effectiveness of cabotegravir/rilpivirine have been established in pediatric patients 12 to younger than 18 years of age and weighing at least 35 kg.

Efficacy and safety of cabotegravir/rilpivirine in HIV-1-infected patients as a complete regimen including oral lead-in therapy were established in 3 adult clinical studies (FLAIR, ATLAS, ATLAS-2M) and an adolescent clinical study (MOCHA).

Safety, tolerability, and pharmacokinetics of oral and injectable cabotegravir and oral and injectable rilpivirine in adolescent patients are being assessed in an ongoing Phase 1/2, open-label, non-comparative study (MOCHA). The primary objective of this study at week 16 was to confirm the use of the adult dose, through the evaluation of safety and pharmacokinetics, for oral and injectable cabotegravir and injectable rilpivirine in 23 HIV-1–infected virologically suppressed patients 12 to younger than 18 years of age and weighing at least 35 kg. Patients were assigned to 1 of 2 cohorts, 1C or 1R, based on their background antiretroviral regimen. In cohort 1C, 8 patients received cabotegravir 30 mg daily for 1 month, followed by monthly cabotegravir injections (Month 1: 600 mg injection, Months 2 and 3: 400 mg injection) for an additional 3 months, while continuing background antiretroviral therapy. In cohort 1R, 15 patients received rilpivirine 25 mg daily for 1 month, followed by monthly rilpivirine injections (Month 1: 900 mg injection, Months 2 and 3: 600 mg injection) for an additional 3 months, while continuing background antiretroviral therapy. The safety of cabotegravir and rilpivirine injections in patients 12 to younger than 18 years of age and weighing at least 35 kg is expected to be similar to adults, as there was no clinically significant difference in drug exposure for the components of cabotegravir and rilpivirine extended-release injection. The efficacy of cabotegravir and rilpivirine injections in patients 12 to younger than 18 years of age and weighing at least 35 kg is extrapolated from adults with support from pharmacokinetic analyses showing similar drug exposure.

The safety, efficacy, and pharmacokinetics of the combined regimen of cabotegravir and rilpivirine extended-release injection have not been established in pediatric patients <12 years of age or weighing <35 kg.

Geriatric Use

Experience in patients ≥65 years of age is insufficient to determine whether they respond differently to cabotegravir/rilpivirine than younger adults.

Cabotegravir/rilpivirine should be used with caution in geriatric patients because of age-related decreases in hepatic, renal, and/or cardiac function and potential for concomitant disease and drug therapy.

Hepatic Impairment

Based on separate studies with oral cabotegravir and oral rilpivirine, no dosage adjustment of the combined regimen of cabotegravir and rilpivirine extended-release injection is necessary for patients with mild or moderate hepatic impairment (Child-Pugh A or B). The effect of severe hepatic impairment (Child-Pugh C) on the pharmacokinetics of cabotegravir or rilpivirine is unknown.

Renal Impairment

Based on studies with oral cabotegravir and population pharmacokinetic analyses of oral rilpivirine, no dosage adjustment of cabotegravir/rilpivirine is necessary for patients with mild (creatinine clearance 60 to <90 mL/minute) or moderate (creatinine clearance 30 to <60 mL/minute) renal impairment. In patients with severe renal impairment (creatinine clearance 15 to <30 mL/minute) or end-stage renal disease (creatinine clearance <15 mL/min), increased monitoring for adverse effects is recommended. In patients with end-stage renal disease not on dialysis, effects on the pharmacokinetics of cabotegravir or rilpivirine are unknown. As cabotegravir and rilpivirine are >99% protein bound, dialysis is not expected to alter exposures of the drugs.

● Common Adverse Effects

The most common adverse reactions observed in ≥2% of subjects receiving cabotegravir/rilpivirine were injection site reactions, pyrexia, fatigue, headache, musculoskeletal pain, nausea, sleep disorders, dizziness, and rash.

DRUG INTERACTIONS

Rilpivirine is primarily metabolized by cytochrome P-450 (CYP) 3A and cabotegravir is primarily metabolized by uridine diphosphate-glucuronosyltransferases (UGT) 1A1 with some contribution from UGT1A9.

● Concomitant Use with Other Antiretroviral Medicines

Because cabotegravir/rilpivirine is a complete regimen, coadministration with other antiretroviral medications for the treatment of HIV-1 infection is not recommended.

● Use of Other Antiretroviral Drugs after Discontinuation

Residual concentrations of cabotegravir and rilpivirine may remain in the systemic circulation of patients for up to ≥12 months. These residual concentrations are not expected to affect the exposures of antiretroviral drugs that are initiated after discontinuation of cabotegravir/rilpivirine.

● Drugs Affecting or Metabolized by Uridine Diphosphate-glucuronosyltransferases

Cabotegravir is primarily metabolized by UGT1A1 with some contribution from UGT1A9. Drugs that are strong inducers of UGT1A1 or UGT1A9 are expected to decrease cabotegravir plasma concentrations and may result in loss of virologic response; therefore, coadministration of cabotegravir/rilpivirine with these drugs is contraindicated.

● Drugs Affecting or Metabolized by CYP3A

Rilpivirine is primarily metabolized by CYP3A. Coadministration of cabotegravir/rilpivirine and drugs that induce CYP3A may result in decreased plasma concentrations of rilpivirine and loss of virologic response and possible resistance to rilpivirine or to the class of NNRTIs. Coadministration of cabotegravir/rilpivirine and drugs that inhibit CYP3A may result in increased plasma concentrations of rilpivirine. Coadministration of cabotegravir/rilpivirine with these drugs is contraindicated.

● QT-Prolonging Drugs

At mean steady-state peak concentrations 4.4- and 11.6-fold higher than those with the recommended 600 mg dose of rilpivirine extended-release injectable suspension, rilpivirine may prolong the QTc interval. Cabotegravir/rilpivirine should be used with caution in combination with drugs with a known risk of torsade de pointes.

● Anticonvulsants

Coadministration of cabotegravir/rilpivirine with carbamazepine, oxcarbazepine, phenobarbital, or phenytoin may cause significant decreases in cabotegravir and rilpivirine plasma concentrations due to UGT1A1 and CYP3A enzyme induction, which may result in loss of virologic response. Concomitant use of these anticonvulsants and cabotegravir/rilpivirine is contraindicated.

● Antimycobacterials

Coadministration of cabotegravir/rilpivirine with rifampin, rifabutin, or rifapentine may cause significant decreases in cabotegravir and rilpivirine plasma concentrations due to UGT1A1 and CYP3A enzyme induction, which may result in loss of virologic response. Concomitant use of these medications and cabotegravir/rilpivirine is contraindicated.

● Glucocorticoid

Coadministration of cabotegravir/rilpivirine with systemic glucocorticoids such as dexamethasone for more than a single-dose treatment may cause a significant decrease in rilpivirine plasma concentrations due to CYP3A enzyme induction, which may result in loss of virologic response. Concomitant use of dexamethasone for more than a single-dose treatment and cabotegravir/rilpivirine is contraindicated.

● **Macrolide Antibiotics**

Coadministration of cabotegravir/rilpivirine with macrolides (clarithromycin, erythromycin) is expected to increase concentrations of rilpivirine and is associated with a risk of torsade de pointes. Consider therapeutic alternatives, such as azithromycin, which increase rilpivirine concentrations less than other macrolides.

● **Methadone**

Coadministration of cabotegravir/rilpivirine with the opiate agonist methadone may decrease methadone concentrations. No dose adjustment of methadone is required when starting coadministration of methadone with cabotegravir/rilpivirine, but clinical monitoring is recommended as methadone maintenance therapy may need to be adjusted in some patients.

● **St. John's Wort**

Concomitant use of St. John's wort (*Hypericum perforatum*) and cabotegravir/rilpivirine may result in substantially decreased rilpivirine concentrations due to potent CYP3A induction by St. John's wort, which may lead to loss of virologic response and possible resistance to rilpivirine or to the class of NNRTIs.

Concomitant use of St. John's wort and cabotegravir/rilpivirine is contraindicated.

DESCRIPTION

Cabotegravir extended-release injectable suspension and rilpivirine extended-release injectable suspension (cabotegravir/rilpivirine) is a 2-drug co-packaged product containing long-acting HIV-1 antivirals. Cabotegravir, an antiretroviral agent, is a HIV integrase strand transfer inhibitor (INSTI). Cabotegravir inhibits HIV integrase by binding to the integrase active site and blocking the strand transfer step of retroviral deoxyribonucleic acid (DNA) integration, which is essential for the HIV replication cycle. Rilpivirine, a diarylpyrimidine HIV non-nucleoside reverse transcriptase inhibitor (NNRTI), inhibits replication of HIV type 1 (HIV-1) by interfering with viral RNA- and DNA-directed polymerase activities of reverse transcriptase.

Cabotegravir- and rilpivirine-resistant HIV-1 has been produced in vitro and has also emerged during combined cabotegravir and rilpivirine therapy. There were virologic failures in clinical studies of the combined regimen of cabotegravir and rilpivirine for treatment of HIV-1 infection. These failures included treatment-emergent INSTI resistance-associated substitutions and reduced phenotypic susceptibility to cabotegravir and rilpivirine in patients treated with both oral and injectable cabotegravir and rilpivirine treatments. An increased risk of cabotegravir plus rilpivirine confirmed virologic failure is associated with baseline virological factors: HIV-1 subtype A1, the presence of baseline integrase L74I polymorphism, and archived NNRTI resistance-associated substitutions.

Cross-resistance between cabotegravir plus rilpivirine to other INSTIs and NNRTIs has been reported in clinical trials (FLAIR, ATLAS, and ATLAS-2M). All confirmed virologic isolates with genotypic evidence of cabotegravir resistance had cross-resistance to elvitegravir and raltegravir but retained phenotypic susceptibility to dolutegravir and, when tested, bictegravir. Virologic failure isolates with rilpivirine resistance had cross resistance with NNRTIs delavirdine, doravirine, efavirenz, etravirine, and nevirapine.

Following injection of cabotegravir/rilpivirine, peak plasma concentrations of cabotegravir and rilpivirine occur approximately 7 and 3-4 days, respectively, after the dose. Peak plasma concentrations of cabotegravir and rilpivirine are similar between the monthly and every 2 month injection schedules.

Cabotegravir is metabolized primarily by uridine diphosphate-glucuronosyl-transferase (UGT) 1A1, with some minor metabolism by UGT1A9. Rilpivirine is metabolized principally by cytochrome P-450 (CYP) 3A enzymes. The half life of cabotegravir and rilpivirine is 5.6–11.5 weeks and 13–28 weeks, respectively; elimination half-life of the drugs is driven by slow absorption rate from the IM injection site.

ADVICE TO PATIENTS

● Advise patients to immediately contact their healthcare provider if they develop a rash after receiving the combined regimen. Instruct patients to not receive further doses and to immediately seek medical attention if they develop a rash associated with any of the following symptoms, as it may be a sign of a more serious reaction such as DRESS or severe hypersensitivity: fever; generally ill feeling; extreme tiredness; muscle or joint aches; blisters; oral blisters or lesions; eye inflammation; facial swelling; swelling of the eyes, lips, tongue, or mouth; difficulty breathing; and/or signs and symptoms of liver problems (e.g., yellowing of the skin or whites of the eyes; dark or tea-colored urine; pale-colored stools or bowel movements; nausea; vomiting; loss of appetite; or pain, aching, or sensitivity on the right side below the ribs).

● Advise patients that injection site reactions have been reported in the majority of patients receiving the combined regimen. These reactions typically consist of one or more of the following: pain, erythema, tenderness, pruritus, and local swelling. Systemic reactions have also been reported, such as fever, musculoskeletal pain, and sciatica pain. Serious post-injection reactions also were reported within minutes after the injection of rilpivirine, including dyspnea, bronchospasm, agitation, abdominal cramping, rash/urticaria, dizziness, flushing, sweating, oral numbness, changes in blood pressure, and back pain (e.g., back and chest). Advise patients that they will be observed briefly (approximately 10 minutes) after the injection.

● Inform patients that hepatotoxicity has been reported. Inform patients that monitoring for liver transaminases is recommended.

● Advise patients that depressive disorders (including depressed mood, depression, major depression, mood altered, mood swings, unusual mood, feeling tense, negative thoughts, suicidal ideation or attempt) have been reported with at least one of the components of the combined regimen. Instruct patients to seek prompt medical evaluation if they experience depressive symptoms.

● Instruct patients about the importance of continued medication adherence and scheduled visits to help maintain viral suppression and to reduce risk of loss of virologic response and development of resistance.

● Advise patients that the combined regimen can be injected monthly or every 2 months after oral lead-in with cabotegravir and rilpivirine to assess tolerability. Discuss the two injection dosing frequency options with patients prior to starting this medication regimen and decide which injection dosing frequency would be the most appropriate option.

● Inform patients that cabotegravir and rilpivirine can remain in the body for up to >12 months after receiving the last extended-release injections. Advise patients that they should contact their healthcare provider if they miss or plan to miss a scheduled injection visit and that oral therapy with cabotegravir and rilpivirine may be used up to 2 months to replace missed injection visits, or any other fully suppressive oral antiretroviral regimen may be used until injections are resumed. Advise patients that if they stop treatment with the combined regimen of cabotegravir and rilpivirine extended-release injection, they will need to take other medicines to treat their HIV-1 infection.

● Advise patients to inform their clinicians of existing or contemplated concomitant therapy, including prescription and OTC drugs and dietary or herbal supplements (e.g., St. John's wort), as well as any concomitant illnesses. The combined regimen of cabotegravir and rilpivirine extended-release injection may be systemically present for ≥12 months. These residual concentrations are not expected to affect the exposures of other antiretroviral drugs that are initiated after discontinuation of this medication.

● Advise women to inform clinicians if they are or plan to become pregnant. Inform patients that there is an antiretroviral pregnancy registry to monitor fetal outcomes in those exposed to the combined regimen of cabotegravir and rilpivirine extended-release injection during pregnancy. Patients who are of reproductive potential should be informed of the long duration of exposure of the combined regimen of cabotegravir and rilpivirine extended-release injection and that there is very limited clinical experience in human pregnancy.

● Instruct mothers with HIV-1 infection not to breastfeed because HIV-1 can be passed to the baby in the breast milk.

● Inform patients of other important precautionary information.

PREPARATIONS

Excipients in commercially available drug preparations may have clinically important effects in some individuals; consult specific product labeling for details.

Cabotegravir and Rilpivirine

Parenteral

Kit	Cabotegravir 200 mg/mL (400 mg) and rilpivirine 300 mg/mL (600 mg)	**Cabenuva® 400 mg/600 mg,** ViiV Healthcare Company
	Each kit contains 1 single-dose vial of cabotegravir extended-release injectable suspension and 1 single-dose vial of rilpivirine extended-release injectable suspension	
	Cabotegravir 200 mg/mL (600 mg) and rilpivirine 300 mg/mL (900 mg)	**Cabenuva® 600 mg/900 mg,** ViiV Healthcare Company
	Each kit contains 1 single-dose vial of cabotegravir extended-release injectable suspension and 1 single-dose vial of rilpivirine extended-release injectable suspension	

† Use is not currently included in the labeling approved by the US Food and Drug Administration.

Selected Revisions April 10, 2024, © Copyright, February 8, 2021, American Society of Health-System Pharmacists, Inc.

Dolutegravir Sodium

8:18.08.12 • HIV INTEGRASE INHIBITORS

■ Dolutegravir sodium, an antiretroviral agent, is a human immunodeficiency virus (HIV) integrase strand transfer inhibitor (INSTI).

USES

● Treatment of HIV Infection

Dolutegravir sodium is used in conjunction with other antiretroviral agents for the treatment of human immunodeficiency virus type 1 (HIV-1) infection in adults who are antiretroviral-naïve (have not previously received antiretroviral therapy) or antiretroviral-experienced (previously treated) and in pediatric patients ≥4 weeks of age weighing ≥3 kg who are antiretroviral-naïve or antiretroviral-experienced but have not previously received an HIV integrase strand transfer inhibitor (INSTI-naïve).

Dolutegravir is commercially available as a single entity and in various fixed-combination preparations that contain additional antiretrovirals; refer to separate combination product monographs for information related to the specific uses of these products.

The single entity dolutegravir preparation is used in conjunction with rilpivirine as a complete regimen for the treatment of HIV-1 infection in adults to replace the current antiretroviral regimen in those who are virologically suppressed (HIV-1 RNA <50 copies/mL) on a stable antiretroviral regimen for ≥6 months with no history of treatment failure and no known substitutions associated with resistance to either agent; for more information on dolutegravir/rilpivirine as a complete regimen, refer to the monograph for the fixed-combination dolutegravir/rilpivirine preparation.

Dolutegravir is commonly used as part of a fully suppressive antiretroviral regimen in conjunction with 1 or 2 nucleotide/nucleoside reverse transcriptase inhibitors (NRTIs); consult guidelines for the most current information on recommended regimens. Selection of an initial antiretroviral regimen should be individualized based on factors such as virologic efficacy, toxicity, pill burden, dosing frequency, drug-drug interaction potential, resistance test results, comorbid conditions, access, and cost.

Clinical Experience

Antiretroviral-naïve Adults

Efficacy and safety of dolutegravir in antiretroviral-naïve HIV-1-infected adults have been evaluated in phase 3 randomized studies (SPRING-2, SINGLE, FLAMINGO).

SPRING-2 is a phase 3, randomized, active-controlled, double-placebo, non-inferiority study in antiretroviral-naïve HIV-1-infected adults with baseline plasma HIV-1 RNA levels of 1000 copies/mL or higher. Patients were randomized to receive dolutegravir 50 mg once daily or raltegravir 400 mg twice daily in conjunction with an investigator-selected dual NRTI regimen of either the fixed-combination preparation containing emtricitabine and tenofovir disoproxil fumarate (emtricitabine/tenofovir DF) or fixed-combination preparation containing abacavir and lamivudine (abacavir/lamivudine). Baseline characteristics of the 822 study patients were similar in both treatment groups (median age 36 years, 87% male, 15% non-white, 11% with hepatitis B virus [HBV] and/or hepatitis C virus [HCV] coinfection, 2% Centers for Disease Control and Prevention [CDC] Class C, median baseline plasma HIV-1 RNA level 4.52 or 4.58 $\log_{10}$ copies/mL, median baseline CD4$^+$ T-cell count 359 or 362 cells/mm³). At 96 weeks, 82% of patients in the dolutegravir group and 78% of those in the raltegravir group had plasma HIV-1 RNA levels <50 copies/mL; the median increase in CD4$^+$ T-cell count was 276 cells/mm³ in the dolutegravir group and 264 cells/mm³ in the raltegravir group.

SINGLE is a 96-week randomized, double-blind, active-controlled study in antiretroviral-naïve HIV-1-infected adults evaluating the efficacy and safety of dolutegravir 50 mg once daily in conjunction with abacavir/lamivudine compared with the fixed-combination preparation containing efavirenz, emtricitabine,

and tenofovir DF (efavirenz/emtricitabine/tenofovir DF) followed by an open-label phase through week 144. Baseline characteristics of the 833 study patients were similar in both treatment groups (median age 35 years, 16% female, 32% non-white, 7% with HCV coinfection, 4% CDC Class C, 32% with HIV-1 RNA >100,000 copies/mL, 53% with CD4$^+$ T-cell count <350 cells/mm³). At 144 weeks, 71% of patients receiving dolutegravir with abacavir/lamivudine and 63% of those receiving efavirenz/emtricitabine/tenofovir DF achieved plasma HIV-1 RNA levels <50 copies/mL. The adjusted mean increase in CD4$^+$ T-cell count was 378 cells/mm³ in those receiving dolutegravir and abacavir/lamivudine compared with 332 cells/mm³ in those receiving efavirenz/emtricitabine/tenofovir DF.

FLAMINGO was an open-label, randomized, noninferiority study in antiretroviral-naïve HIV-1-infected adults that compared the efficacy and safety of dolutegravir 50 mg once daily with that of *ritonavir-boosted* darunavir when the drugs were given in conjunction with an investigator-selected dual NRTI regimen of abacavir/lamivudine or emtricitabine/tenofovir DF. At baseline, the 484 study patients had a median age of 34 years, 15% were female, 28% were non-white, 25% had plasma HIV-1 RNA levels >100,000 copies/mL, and 35% had CD4$^+$ T-cell counts <350 cells/mm³. At 96 weeks, 80% of patients in the dolutegravir group achieved plasma HIV-1 RNA levels <50 copies/mL compared with 68% in the *ritonavir-boosted* darunavir group.

Antiretroviral-experienced Adults

The comparative efficacy and safety of dolutegravir in 715 antiretroviral-experienced, INSTI-naïve HIV-1-infected adults was studied in a phase 3, randomized, double-blind, active-controlled, double-placebo study (SAILING). All enrolled patients had previously received antiretroviral therapy (average duration 77 months of prior therapy) and had infections resistant to at least 2 classes of antiretrovirals (49% had HIV-1 resistant to at least 3 classes of antiretrovirals). Patients were randomized to receive dolutegravir 50 mg once daily or raltegravir 400 mg twice daily, each in conjunction with an investigator-selected optimized background antiretroviral regimen (OBR) consisting of ≥1 fully active antiretroviral. Baseline characteristics were similar in both treatment groups (median age 43 years, 32% female, 50% non-white, 16% with HBV and/or HCV coinfection, 46% CDC Class C, 20% with plasma HIV-1 RNA levels >100,000 copies/mL, 72% with CD4$^+$ T-cell counts <350 cells/mm³). At 48 weeks, 71% of patients in the dolutegravir group and 64% of those in the raltegravir group had plasma HIV-1 RNA levels <50 copies/mL; CD4$^+$ T-cell counts were increased from baseline in both groups (mean change 162 cells/mm³ in the dolutegravir group and 153 cells/mm³ in the raltegravir group)

An open-label, single-arm, phase 3 study (VIKING-3) evaluated use of dolutegravir and an OBR in 183 antiretroviral-experienced adults with current or prior virologic failure on another INSTI-containing regimen (elvitegravir, raltegravir) and current or historical evidence of resistance to these other INSTIs. At baseline, most patients had HIV-1 resistant to other antiretroviral classes (79% with resistance to ≥2 NRTIs, 75% with resistance to ≥1 HIV nonnucleoside reverse transcriptase inhibitor [NNRTI], 71% with resistance to ≥2 HIV protease inhibitors [PIs]). At baseline, the median age of study patients was 48 years, 23% were female, 29% were non-white, 20% had HBV and/or HCV coinfection, median plasma HIV-1 RNA level was 4.38 $\log_{10}$ copies/mL, median CD4$^+$ T-cell count was 140 cells/mm³, and median duration of prior antiretroviral therapy was 13–14 years. Patients received dolutegravir 50 mg twice daily with their current failing background regimen for 7 days; on day 8, dolutegravir was continued and the background regimen was further optimized if possible. The mean reduction in plasma HIV-1 RNA level on day 8 (primary efficacy end point) was 1.4 $\log_{10}$ copies/mL. At 48 weeks after initiation of dolutegravir, 63% of study patients had plasma HIV-1 RNA levels <50 copies/mL and the median increase in CD4$^+$ T-cell count was 80 cells/mm³. The presence of INSTI-resistance substitutions at baseline affected the 48-week response rate. The response rate to the dolutegravir regimen was 74% in those who had HIV-1 without the Q148 resistance substitution present at baseline, but was 61% if the Q148H/R and G140S/A/C substitutions were present at baseline and 29% if the Q148H/R substitution plus 2 or more additional INSTI-resistance substitutions (T66A, L74I/M, E138A/K/T, G140S/A/C, Y143R/C/H, E157Q, G163S/E/K/Q, or G193E/R) were present at baseline.

In a randomized, double-blind, placebo-controlled, phase 3 study (VIKING-4), antiretroviral-experienced, dolutegravir-naïve adults receiving a failing INSTI-based regimen that included elvitegravir or raltegravir were randomized to receive dolutegravir (50 mg twice daily) or placebo with their previous failing antiretroviral regimen for 7 days, followed by a single-arm, open-label regimen of dolutegravir (50 mg twice daily) in conjunction with an optimized antiretroviral regimen containing ≥1 fully active antiretroviral selected based on baseline resistance data. At baseline, all patients had plasma HIV-1 RNA levels of 1000 copies/mL or greater and HIV-1 with INSTI genotypic resistance. In addition, most patients had HIV-1 resistant to other antiretroviral classes (63% with resistance to ≥3 NRTIs, 53% with resistance to ≥2 NNRTIs, 67% with resistance to ≥2 PIs). The mean reduction in plasma HIV-1 RNA level on day 8 (primary efficacy end point) in those initially randomized to dolutegravir was 1.06 $\log_{10}$ copies/mL. At 48 weeks, 40% of all study patients had plasma HIV-1 RNA levels <50 copies/mL and the median increase in CD4+ T-cell count was 125 cells/mm³. The response rate at 48 weeks was 57% in those with HIV-1 without the Q148 resistance substitution present at baseline, but was only 25% if the Q148 substitution plus ≥1 additional INSTI-resistance substitutions were present at baseline.

Pediatric Patients

The safety, efficacy, and pharmacokinetic profile of dolutegravir in HIV-1-infected pediatric patients ≥4 weeks of age were evaluated in a phase 1/phase 2, open-label, noncomparative study (IMPAACT P1093). Patients were stratified by age into cohort 1 (12 to <18 years of age), cohort 2A (6 to <12 years of age), cohort 3 (2 to <6 years of age), cohort 4 (6 months to <2 years of age), and cohort 5 (4 weeks to <6 months of age).

Seventy-five pediatric patients received the recommended dolutegravir dosage (based on weight and age) administered either as conventional tablets (Tivicay®) or tablets for oral suspension (Tivicay® PD) in conjunction with other antiretrovirals. The median age of these patients was 27 months (range: 1 to 214 months), 59% were female, and 68% were Black or African American. At baseline, mean plasma HIV-1 RNA level was 4.4 $\log_{10}$ copies/mL, median CD4+ T-cell count was 1225 cells/mm³ (range: 1–8255), and median CD4+ T-cell percentage was 23% (range: 0.3–49%). Overall, 33% of these pediatric patients had baseline plasma HIV-1 RNA levels >50,000 copies/mL and 12% had a CDC HIV clinical classification of category C. The majority (80%) were treatment-experienced, but all were INSTI-naïve; 44% had previously received at least 1 HIV NNRTI and 76% had previously received at least 1 HIV PI (76%).

Virologic outcomes are available for the pediatric patients who received the recommended weight-based dolutegravir dosage through week 24 (58 patients) or week 48 (42 patients). At week 24, 62% of patients achieved plasma HIV-1 RNA levels <50 copies/mL and 86% achieved plasma HIV-1 RNA levels <400 copies/mL (snapshot algorithm); the median CD4+ T-count increase from baseline was 105 cells/mm³. At week 48, 69% of patients achieved plasma HIV-1 RNA levels <50 copies/mL and 79% achieved plasma HIV-1 RNA levels <400 copies/mL (snapshot algorithm); the median CD4+ T-count increase from baseline was 141 cells/mm³.

Clinical Perspective

Therapeutic options for the treatment and prevention of HIV infection and recommendations concerning the use of antiretrovirals are continuously evolving. Antiretroviral therapy is recommended for all individuals with HIV regardless of CD4 counts, and should be initiated as soon as possible after diagnosis of HIV and continued indefinitely. The primary goals of antiretroviral therapy are to achieve and maintain durable suppression of HIV viral load (as measured by plasma HIV-1 RNA levels) to a level below which drug-resistance mutations cannot emerge (i.e., below detectable limits), restore and preserve immunologic function, reduce HIV-related morbidity and mortality, improve quality of life, and prevent transmission of HIV. While the most appropriate antiretroviral regimen cannot be defined for each clinical scenario, the US Department of Health and Human Services (HHS) Panel on Antiretroviral Guidelines for Adults and Adolescents, HHS Panel on Antiretroviral Therapy and Medical Management of Children Living with HIV, and HHS Panel on Treatment of Pregnant Women with HIV Infection and Prevention of Perinatal Transmission, have developed comprehensive guidelines that provide information on selection and use of antiretrovirals for the treatment or prevention of HIV infection. Because of the complexity of managing patients with HIV, it is recommended that clinicians with HIV expertise be consulted when needed.

The use of combination antiretroviral regimens that generally include 3 drugs from 2 or more drug classes is currently recommended to achieve viral suppression. In both treatment-naïve adults and children, an initial antiretroviral regimen generally consists of 2 NRTIs administered in combination with a third active

antiretroviral drug from 1 of 3 drug classes: an INSTI, an NNRTI, or a PI with a pharmacokinetic enhancer (also known as a booster; the 2 drugs used for this purpose are cobicistat and ritonavir). Selection of an initial antiretroviral regimen should be individualized based on factors such as virologic efficacy, toxicity, pill burden, dosing frequency, drug–drug interaction potential, resistance-test results, comorbid conditions, access, and cost. In patients with comorbid infections (e.g., hepatitis B, tuberculosis), antiretroviral regimen selection should also consider the potential for activity against other present infections and timing of initiation relative to other anti-infective regimens.

Dolutegravir, an INSTI, is commonly used as part of a fully suppressive regimen in conjunction with 1 or 2 NRTIs. In the HHS adult and adolescent HIV treatment guideline, dolutegravir is included in various antiretroviral regimens. Some of these dolutegravir-containing regimens are listed among recommended initial regimens for most people with HIV, and include the following: dolutegravir/abacavir/lamivudine (only in patients who are negative for human leukocyte antigen (HLA)-B*5701); dolutegravir plus tenofovir DF or tenofovir alafenamide plus lamivudine or emtricitabine; dolutegravir/lamivudine (except in individuals with HIV RNA >500,000 copies/mL, HBV coinfection, or in whom antiretroviral therapy is to be started before the results of HIV genotypic resistance testing for reverse transcriptase or HBV testing are available). The 2-drug regimen of dolutegravir/rilpivirine is not recommended for initial therapy because it has not been studied for use in this setting.

In the HHS pediatric HIV treatment guideline, dolutegravir is included in various antiretroviral regimens. Dolutegravir plus 2 NRTIs is a preferred initial regimen for infants and children ≥4 weeks of age weighing ≥3 kg.

In the HHS perinatal HIV treatment guideline, dolutegravir is included in various antiretroviral regimens. Some of these dolutegravir-containing regimens are listed among preferred options, and include the following: dolutegravir/abacavir/lamivudine or dolutegravir plus a preferred dual-NRTI backbone.

• Postexposure Prophylaxis following Nonoccupational Exposure to HIV

Dolutegravir is used in conjunction with other antiretrovirals for postexposure prophylaxis of HIV infection following nonoccupational exposure† (nPEP) in individuals exposed to blood, genital secretions, or other potentially infectious body fluids that might contain HIV when the exposure represents a substantial risk for HIV transmission.

Clinical Perspective

When nPEP is indicated following a nonoccupational exposure to HIV, the US Centers for Disease Control and Prevention (CDC) states that the preferred regimen in adults and adolescents 13 years of age or older with normal renal function is either raltegravir or dolutegravir used in conjunction with emtricitabine and tenofovir DF (administered as the fixed combination emtricitabine/tenofovir DF; e.g., Truvada®). The alternative nPEP regimen recommended in these patients is *ritonavir-boosted* darunavir used in conjunction with emtricitabine/tenofovir DF (e.g., Truvada®).

Consultation with an infectious disease specialist, clinician with expertise in administration of antiretroviral agents, and/or the National Clinicians' Postexposure Prophylaxis Hotline (PEPline at 888-448-4911) is recommended if nPEP is indicated in certain exposed individuals (e.g., pregnant women, children, those with medical conditions such as renal impairment) or if an antiretroviral regimen not included in the CDC guidelines is being considered, the source virus is known or likely to be resistant to antiretrovirals, or the healthcare provider is inexperienced in prescribing antiretrovirals. However, initiation of nPEP should not be delayed while waiting for expert consultation.

DOSAGE AND ADMINISTRATION

• General

Pretreatment Screening

- Perform testing for hepatitis B virus (HBV) infection and hepatitis C virus (HCV) infection in all patients with human immunodeficiency virus (HIV) infection prior to initiation of antiretroviral therapy.

Patient Monitoring

- Monitor for signs and symptoms of hepatotoxicity during treatment with dolutegravir.

Dispensing and Administration Precautions

- Dolutegravir is commercially available as a single entity and in various fixed-combination preparations that contain additional antiretrovirals. Refer to the full prescribing information for information on specific uses, cautions, precautions, contraindications, and drug interactions of the combination products.

- Dolutegravir tablets and dolutegravir tablets for oral suspension are *not* bioequivalent and are *not* interchangeable on a mg-per-mg basis.

• Administration

Single-entity dolutegravir is commercially available as conventional tablets (Tivicay®) and as tablets for oral suspension (Tivicay® PD). The single-entity tablets and tablets for oral suspension must be used in conjunction with other antiretrovirals.

Administer dolutegravir sodium orally once or twice daily without regard to food.

Do not chew, cut, or crush the tablets for oral suspension. Dolutegravir tablets for oral suspension may be either swallowed whole (1 tablet at time if more than a single tablet is required for the dose, to reduce the risk of choking), or dispersed in drinking water to provide an oral suspension.

To prepare an oral suspension, add the indicated number of 5-mg tablets for oral suspension to the appropriate volume of clean drinking water in the plastic cup provided by the manufacturer. To prepare a 5- or 15-mg dose of dolutegravir, place 5 mL of drinking water into the cup and add 1 or 3 tablets for oral suspension, respectively, to the water. To prepare a 20-, 25-, or 30-mg dose, place 10 mL of drinking water into the cup and add 4, 5, or 6 tablets for oral suspension, respectively, to the water. Gently swirl the cup for 1–2 minutes until there are no remaining lumps. After full dispersion, administer the oral suspension within 30 minutes of mixing For infants who cannot drink from the plastic cup, administer the oral suspension using the oral syringe provided by the manufacturer. To ensure that the child receives the full dose, place an additional 5 mL of drinking water into the cup, swirl the cup, and administer to the child directly from the cup or using the oral syringe. For more specific instructions on preparation and administration of dolutegravir oral suspension, consult the manufacturer's instructions for use and labeling.

Store the conventional tablets at controlled room temperature of 25°C (excursions permitted to 15–30°C).

Store the tablets for oral suspension below 30°C. Store and dispense in the original bottle, protect from moisture, and keep the bottle tightly closed; do not remove the desiccant.

Fixed Combinations Containing Dolutegravir

Dolutegravir is also commercially available in the following fixed-combination tablets: abacavir, dolutegravir, and lamivudine (Triumeq®); dolutegravir and lamivudine (Dovato®); and dolutegravir and rilpivirine (Juluca®). See the full prescribing information for administration of each of these combination products.

• Dosage

Dolutegravir conventional tablets and tablets for oral suspension contain dolutegravir sodium; dosage is expressed in terms of dolutegravir.

Dolutegravir tablets and dolutegravir tablets for oral suspension are *not* bioequivalent and are *not* interchangeable on a mg-per-mg basis. The relative bioavailability of dolutegravir tablets for oral suspension is approximately 1.6-fold higher than that of dolutegravir conventional tablets. If a patient is switched from one tablet formulation to the other, adjust the dosage to that recommended for the specific formulation now being used.

Adult Dosage

Treatment of HIV-1 Infection

For the treatment of HIV-1 infection in treatment-naïve, or treatment-experienced but integrase strand transfer inhibitor (INSTI)-naïve individuals, the recommended dosage of dolutegravir is 50 mg once daily.

For the treatment of HIV-1 infection in treatment-naïve, or treatment-experienced but INSTI-naïve individuals, if dolutegravir is coadministered with certain uridine diphosphate-glucuronosyltransferase (UGT) 1A or cytochrome P-450 (CYP) 3A inducers (i.e., efavirenz, *ritonavir-boosted* fosamprenavir, *ritonavir-boosted* tipranavir, carbamazepine, rifampin), the recommended dosage of dolutegravir is 50 mg twice daily. Whenever possible, consider alternative regimens that do not contain these inducers.

For the treatment of HIV-1 infection in virologically suppressed (HIV-1 RNA <50 copies/mL) adults switching to dolutegravir plus rilpivirine, the recommended dosage of dolutegravir is 50 mg once daily. Rilpivirine dosage is 25 mg once daily for those switching to dolutegravir plus rilpivirine.

For the treatment of HIV-1 infection in INSTI-experienced adults who have certain INSTI-associated resistance substitutions or clinically suspected INSTI resistance, the recommended dosage of dolutegravir is 50 mg twice daily.

Fixed-dose combinations containing abacavir, dolutegravir, and lamivudine (Triumeq®); dolutegravir and lamivudine (Dovato®); and dolutegravir and rilpivirine (Juluca®) are used in the treatment of HIV-1 infection in adults. The usual dosage of dolutegravir is 50 mg in conjunction with other antiretrovirals for treatment of HIV-1 infection; consult the full prescribing information for specific dosage of each of the combination products.

Postexposure Prophylaxis following Nonoccupational Exposure to HIV

For postexposure prophylaxis of HIV infection following nonoccupational exposure (nPEP)† when the exposure represents a substantial risk for HIV transmission, the usual adult dosage of dolutegravir is 50 mg once daily in conjunction with 2 HIV nucleoside reverse transcriptase inhibitors (NRTIs).

Initiate the nPEP regimen as soon as possible (within 72 hours) following nonoccupational exposure to HIV, and continue the regimen for 28 days. If the exposed individual seeks care >72 hours after the exposure, nPEP is not recommended.

Pediatric Dosage

Dosage is based on weight. The tablets for oral suspension are labeled for pediatric patients ≥4 weeks of age weighing ≥3 kg; conventional tablets are labeled for use in pediatric patients ≥4 weeks of age weighing ≥14 kg.

Treatment of HIV-1 Infection in Pediatric Patients 4 Weeks of Age or Older

Do not use dolutegravir conventional tablets in pediatric patients weighing 3–14 kg.

For the recommended dosage of dolutegravir tablets for oral suspension for the treatment of HIV-1 infection in pediatric patients 4 weeks of age or older weighing ≥3 kg, who are treatment-naïve or treatment-experienced but INSTI-naïve, see Table 1. Dolutegravir tablets for oral suspension are preferred for pediatric patients weighing <20 kg.

TABLE 1. Recommended Dosage of Dolutegravir Tablets for Oral Suspension in Pediatric Patients 4 Weeks of Age or Older Weighing ≥3 kg

Weight (kg)	Daily Dose[a]	Number of 5-mg Tablets for Oral Suspension
3 to <6	5 mg once daily	1
6 to <10	15 mg once daily	3
10 to <14	20 mg once daily	4
14 to <20	25 mg once daily	5
≥20	30 mg once daily	6

[a] If dolutegravir is used concomitantly with certain UGT1A or CYP3A inducers (i.e., efavirenz, *ritonavir-boosted* fosamprenavir, *ritonavir-boosted* tipranavir, carbamazepine, rifampin), administer the recommended weight-based dose twice daily.

For the recommended dosage of dolutegravir conventional tablets for the treatment of HIV-1 infection in pediatric patients 4 weeks of age or older weighing ≥14 kg, see Table 2.

TABLE 2. Recommended Dosage of Dolutegravir Tablets in Pediatric Patients 4 Weeks of Age or Older Weighing ≥14 kg

Weight (kg)	Daily Dose[a]	Number of 10- or 50-mg Tablets
14 to <20	40 mg once daily	Four 10-mg tablets
≥20	50 mg once daily	One 50-mg tablet

[a] If dolutegravir is used concomitantly with certain UGT1A or CYP3A inducers (i.e., efavirenz, *ritonavir-boosted* fosamprenavir, *ritonavir-boosted* tipranavir, carbamazepine, rifampin), administer the recommended weight-based dose twice daily.

The fixed-dose combination containing abacavir, dolutegravir, and lamivudine (Triumeq®) is used in the treatment of HIV-1 infection in pediatric patients; consult the full prescribing information for specific dosage of this combination product.

• Special Populations

Hepatic Impairment

Dosage adjustment of dolutegravir is not necessary in patients with mild or moderate hepatic impairment (Child-Pugh class A or B). Do not use dolutegravir in those with severe hepatic impairment (Child-Pugh class C).

Renal Impairment

Dosage adjustment of dolutegravir is not necessary in antiretroviral-naïve, or antiretroviral-experienced but INSTI-naïve, patients with mild, moderate, or severe renal impairment.

Dosage adjustment of dolutegravir is not necessary in INSTI-experienced patients (with certain INSTI-associated resistance substitutions or clinically suspected INSTI resistance) with mild or moderate renal impairment. However, use dolutegravir with caution in INSTI-experienced patients (with certain INSTI-associated resistance substitutions or clinically suspected INSTI resistance) with severe renal impairment

The manufacturer states that data are insufficient to make specific dolutegravir dosage recommendations for use in patients requiring dialysis; it is unlikely that the drug would be removed by dialysis to any clinically important extent.

Geriatric Patients

The manufacturer makes no specific dosage recommendations in geriatric patients, but recommends caution because of possible age-related decreases in hepatic, renal, and/or cardiac function and concomitant disease and drug therapy.

CAUTIONS

• Contraindications

- Previous hypersensitivity reaction to dolutegravir.
- Concomitant use with dofetilide.

• Warnings/Precautions

Hypersensitivity Reactions

Hypersensitivity reactions were reported in <1% of patients receiving dolutegravir in phase 3 clinical trials. Reactions were manifested by rash and constitutional findings and, occasionally, organ dysfunction including liver toxicity.

If signs or symptoms of hypersensitivity reactions occur, discontinue dolutegravir and any other suspect agents immediately. These signs or symptoms include, but are not limited to, severe rash or rash accompanied by fever, general malaise, fatigue, muscle or joint aches, blisters or peeling skin, oral blisters or lesions, conjunctivitis, facial edema, hepatitis, eosinophilia, angioedema, or difficulty breathing. Monitor clinical status, including liver aminotransferases, and initiate appropriate therapy.

A life-threatening reaction could occur if there is a delay in discontinuing dolutegravir or any other suspect agents after the onset of a hypersensitivity reaction.

Hepatotoxicity

Adverse hepatic effects have been reported in patients receiving dolutegravir-containing regimens.

Patients with human immunodeficiency virus (HIV) infection and with hepatitis B virus (HBV) or hepatitis C virus (HCV) coinfection may be at increased risk for development or worsening of aminotransferase elevations. In some patients receiving a dolutegravir-containing regimen, serum aminotransferase elevations were consistent with immune reconstitution syndrome or HBV reactivation, particularly in the setting where HBV therapy had been discontinued.

Cases of hepatic toxicity, including elevated serum liver biochemistries, hepatitis, and acute liver failure, also have been reported in patients receiving a dolutegravir-containing regimen who had no preexisting hepatic disease or other identifiable risk factors. Drug-induced liver injury leading to liver transplant has been reported with abacavir/dolutegravir/lamivudine. Monitor for hepatoxicity in patients receiving dolutegravir.

Immune Reconstitution Syndrome

Immune reconstitution syndrome has been reported in HIV-infected patients receiving multiple-drug antiretroviral therapy, including dolutegravir. During the initial phase of treatment, HIV-infected patients whose immune systems respond to antiretroviral therapy may develop an inflammatory response to indolent or residual opportunistic infections (e.g., *Mycobacterium avium*, *M. tuberculosis*, cytomegalovirus, *Pneumocystis jirovecii*); such responses may necessitate further evaluation and treatment.

Autoimmune disorders (e.g., Graves' disease, polymyositis, Guillain-Barré syndrome) have also been reported to occur in the setting of immune reconstitution; however, the time to onset is more variable and can occur many months after initiation of antiretroviral therapy.

Different Formulations Are Not Interchangeable

Dolutegravir conventional tablets and dolutegravir tablets for oral suspension are *not* bioequivalent and are *not* interchangeable on a mg-per-mg basis. If a pediatric patient is switched from one tablet formulation to the other, adjust the dosage to that recommended for the specific formulation now being used. Incorrect dosage of a given formulation may result in under-dosing and loss of therapeutic effect and possible development of resistance or may result in clinically important adverse effects from greater dolutegravir exposure.

Specific Populations

Pregnancy

The Antiretroviral Pregnancy Registry (APR) monitors pregnancy outcomes in women exposed to dolutegravir during pregnancy. Clinicians are encouraged to register patients in the APR by calling 800-258-4263 or visiting https://www.apregistry.com/.

Data regarding the use of dolutegravir in pregnant women are insufficient to date to definitively assess a drug-associated risk for birth defects and miscarriage; however, human data from the APR do not indicate an increased birth defect risk. Of 1,377 dolutegravir exposures during pregnancy resulting in live births, the prevalence of birth defects was 3.3% following first trimester exposure and 5% following second-/third-trimester exposure.

There has been a concern regarding the development of neural tube defects in infants exposed to dolutegravir during pregnancy. The first interim analysis from an ongoing birth outcome surveillance study in Botswana identified an association between dolutegravir and an increased risk of neural tube defects when dolutegravir was administered at the time of conception and in early pregnancy. In a larger subsequent analysis, the prevalence of neural tube defects in infants delivered to individuals taking dolutegravir at conception was 0.11%, which did not differ significantly from that of infants delivered to HIV-positive individuals not administered dolutegravir (0.11%) or to HIV-negative individuals (0.06%).

Results from an Eswatini birth outcome surveillance study revealed similar outcomes; the prevalence of neural tube defects in infants delivered to individuals taking dolutegravir at conception was 0.08%, which did not differ significantly from that of infants delivered to individuals taking non-dolutegravir-containing regimens (0.22%) or to HIV-negative individuals (0.08%).

Lactation

Dolutegravir is distributed into human milk. It is not known whether dolutegravir affects human milk production or affects the breast-fed infant.

The HHS perinatal HIV transmission guideline provides updated recommendations on infant feeding. The guideline states that patients with HIV should receive evidence-based, patient-centered counseling to support shared decision making about infant feeding. During counseling, patients should be informed that feeding with appropriate formula or pasteurized donor human milk from a milk bank eliminates the risk of postnatal HIV transmission to the infant. Additionally, achieving and maintaining viral suppression with antiretroviral therapy during pregnancy and postpartum reduces the risk of breastfeeding HIV transmission to <1%, but does not completely eliminate the risk. Replacement feeding with formula or banked pasteurized donor milk is recommended when patients with HIV are *not* on antiretroviral therapy and/or do *not* have a suppressed viral load during pregnancy (at a minimum throughout the third trimester), as well as at delivery.

Pediatric Use

Safety and efficacy of dolutegravir have not been established in pediatric patients younger than 4 weeks of age or weighing <3 kg. In addition, safety and efficacy of the drug have not been established in pediatric patients who previously received another HIV integrase strand inhibitor (INSTI-experienced) and have HIV-1 with documented or suspected resistance to other HIV INSTIs (e.g., elvitegravir, raltegravir)

Safety, efficacy, and pharmacokinetics of dolutegravir were evaluated in 75 HIV-1-infected, treatment-naïve or treatment-experienced INSTI-naïve pediatric patients 4 weeks to less than 18 years of age weighing at least 3 kg in an ongoing, open-label, multicenter, dose-finding clinical trial (IMPAACT P1093). In addition, pharmacokinetic data were evaluated in 2 weight-based pharmacokinetic substudies in an ongoing open-label, randomized, noninferiority trial evaluating safety, efficacy, and pharmacokinetics of dolutegravir in conjunction with 2 HIV NRTIs in HIV-1-infected pediatric patients younger than 18 years of age (ODYSSEY).

Effectiveness of dolutegravir observed in pediatric patients in the IMPAACT P1093 trial is comparable to that reported in treatment-experienced adults receiving the drug. Overall, safety data for dolutegravir in 75 pediatric patients 4 weeks to less than 18 years of age in the IMPAACT P1093 trial were comparable to those observed in adults receiving the drug. Pharmacokinetic parameters for dolutegravir reported in pediatric patients in the IMPAACT P1093 and ODYSSEY trials receiving weight-based dosages of the drug indicate that peak plasma concentrations and AUC are comparable to those in adults receiving 50 mg of dolutegravir once or twice daily. Although mean peak plasma concentrations of dolutegravir are higher in pediatric patients, the increase is not considered clinically important since the safety profiles are similar in adult and pediatric patients.

Geriatric Use

Experience in patients ≥65 years of age is insufficient to determine whether they respond differently to dolutegravir than younger adults. Use dolutegravir with caution in geriatric patients because of age-related decreases in hepatic, renal, and/or cardiac function and potential for concomitant disease and drug therapy.

Hepatic Impairment

Do not use dolutegravir in patients with severe hepatic impairment (Child-Pugh class C); pharmacokinetics of the drug have not been evaluated in such patients.

Pharmacokinetics of dolutegravir in patients with moderate hepatic impairment are similar to those in healthy individuals, and dosage adjustments are not needed when the drug is used in those with mild or moderate hepatic insufficiency (Child-Pugh class A or B).

In phase 3 trials, the safety profile of dolutegravir in patients with HBV or HCV coinfection was similar to that in patients without HBV or HCV; however, rates of AST and ALT abnormalities were increased in this subset of patients. Population analyses using pooled pharmacokinetic data from adult trials indicated no

clinically relevant effect of HCV coinfection on the pharmacokinetics of dolutegravir. There were limited data on HBV coinfection.

Renal Impairment

Use dolutegravir with caution in patients with severe renal impairment who are INSTI-experienced and have certain INSTI-associated resistance mutations or clinically suspected INSTI resistance. Plasma concentrations of dolutegravir are decreased in patients with severe renal impairment, which may result in loss of therapeutic effects and development of resistance to the drug or other antiretrovirals.

Mild or moderate renal impairment does not have a clinically important effect on the pharmacokinetics of dolutegravir. Therefore, dosage adjustments are not needed when dolutegravir is used in antiretroviral-naïve or antiretroviral-experienced, INSTI-naïve patients with mild, moderate, or severe renal impairment. Dosage adjustments also are not needed when the drug is used in INSTI-experienced patients with mild or moderate renal impairment.

Data are insufficient to make specific dosage recommendations for use of dolutegravir in patients requiring dialysis. It is unlikely that dialysis would have a clinically important effect on the pharmacokinetics of dolutegravir since the drug is highly bound to plasma proteins.

Dolutegravir has been shown to increase serum creatinine concentrations; however, it does not cause a clinically important change in glomerular filtration rate or renal plasma flow. In vivo, dolutegravir inhibits tubular secretion of creatinine by inhibiting renal organic cation transporter (OCT) 2 and, possibly, multidrug and toxin extrusion transporter (MATE) 1.

● Common Adverse Effects

In patients receiving dolutegravir in an adult clinical trial, the most common adverse effects of moderate to severe intensity and incidence ≥2% were insomnia, headache, and fatigue.

DRUG INTERACTIONS

The following drug interactions are based on studies using dolutegravir; refer to the full prescribing information for further details. Additional drug interactions exist for fixed-combinations containing abacavir, dolutegravir, and lamivudine (Triumeq®); dolutegravir and lamivudine (Dovato®); and dolutegravir and rilpivirine (Juluca®). When a fixed combination is used, consider the interactions associated with each drug in the fixed combination; see the full prescribing information for drug interactions of each combination product.

● Drugs Affecting or Metabolized by Hepatic Microsomal Enzymes

Cytochrome P-450 (CYP) isoenzyme 3A plays a minor role in the metabolism of dolutegravir.

In vitro studies indicate that dolutegravir does not inhibit CYP isoenzymes 1A2, 2A6, 2B6, 2C8, 2C9, 2C19, 2D6, or 3A and does not induce CYP1A2, 2B6, or 3A4.

Concomitant use of dolutegravir and drugs that induce CYP3A may decrease dolutegravir plasma concentrations and decrease therapeutic effects of the drug. Concomitant use with drugs that inhibit CYP3A may increase dolutegravir plasma concentrations.

● Drugs Affecting or Metabolized by Uridine Diphosphate-glucuronosyltransferases

Dolutegravir is metabolized by uridine diphosphate-glucuronosyltransferase (UGT) 1A1. In vitro studies indicate the drug also is a substrate for UGT1A3 and UGT1A9.

Dolutegravir does not inhibit UGT1A1 or UGT2B7 in vitro.

Pharmacokinetic interactions are possible if dolutegravir is used with inducers of UGT1A1, 1A3, or 1A9 (decreased plasma concentrations of dolutegravir and decreased therapeutic effects of the drug) or with inhibitors of these enzymes (increased plasma concentrations of dolutegravir).

● Drugs Affecting or Affected by P-glycoprotein Transport

Dolutegravir is a substrate of the P-glycoprotein (P-gp) transport system in vitro; dolutegravir does not inhibit P-gp-mediated transport in vitro.

Pharmacokinetic interactions are possible if dolutegravir is used with inducers of P-gp (decreased plasma concentrations of dolutegravir and decreased therapeutic effects of the drug) or with inhibitors of P-gp (increased plasma concentrations of dolutegravir).

● Drugs Affecting or Affected by Bile Salt Export Pump

Dolutegravir does not inhibit the bile salt export pump (BSEP) in vitro; pharmacokinetic interactions with drugs that are substrates of BSEP are not expected.

● Drugs Affecting or Affected by Breast Cancer Resistance Protein

Dolutegravir is a substrate of breast cancer resistance protein (BCRP) in vitro.

Pharmacokinetic interactions are possible if dolutegravir is used with inducers of BCRP (decreased plasma concentrations of dolutegravir and decreased therapeutic effects of the drug) or with inhibitors of BCRP (increased plasma concentrations of dolutegravir).

Dolutegravir does not inhibit BCRP in vitro; pharmacokinetic interactions with drugs that are substrates for BCRP are not expected.

● Drugs Affecting or Affected by Multidrug and Toxin Extrusion Transporter

Dolutegravir inhibits multidrug and toxin extrusion transporter (MATE) 1 in vitro.

Concomitant use of dolutegravir may increase plasma concentrations of drugs eliminated by MATE1 (e.g., dofetilide, metformin).

● Drugs Affecting or Affected by Multidrug Resistance Protein

Dolutegravir does not inhibit multidrug resistance protein (MRP) 2 or MRP4 in vitro; pharmacokinetic interactions with drugs that are substrates for these transporters are not expected.

● Drugs Affecting or Affected by Organic Anion Transporters

In vitro, dolutegravir inhibits renal organic anion transporter (OAT) 1 and OAT3. In vivo, dolutegravir does not alter plasma concentrations of OAT1 or OAT3 substrates (e.g., tenofovir, aminohippurate).

Dolutegravir does not inhibit organic anion transporter polypeptide (OATP) 1B1 or OATP1B3 in vitro; pharmacokinetic interactions with drugs that are substrates for these transporters are not expected. Dolutegravir is not a substrate of OATP1B1 or 1B3 in vitro.

● Drugs Affecting or Affected by Organic Cation Transporters

In vitro, dolutegravir inhibits renal organic cation transporter (OCT) 2. Therefore, dolutegravir may increase plasma concentrations of drugs eliminated by OCT2 (e.g., dalfampridine, dofetilide, metformin).

Dolutegravir does not inhibit OCT1 in vitro; pharmacokinetic interactions with drugs that are substrates for this transporter are not expected.

● Anticonvulsants

Carbamazepine

Concomitant use of carbamazepine (300 mg twice daily) and dolutegravir (50 mg once daily) decreases peak plasma concentrations and AUC of dolutegravir.

If carbamazepine is used concomitantly with dolutegravir in adults who are antiretroviral-naïve or antiretroviral-experienced but have not previously received an HIV integrase strand transfer inhibitor (INSTI-naïve), administer the recommended dolutegravir dose twice daily. If carbamazepine is used concomitantly with dolutegravir in antiretroviral-naïve or antiretroviral-experienced pediatric patients, administer the recommended weight-based dolutegravir dose twice

daily. Whenever possible, use an alternative anticonvulsant in patients receiving dolutegravir who are INSTI-experienced and have HIV-1 with documented or suspected INSTI resistance.

Oxcarbazepine, Phenobarbital, and Phenytoin

Oxcarbazepine, phenobarbital, and phenytoin induce metabolism of dolutegravir and may cause decreased plasma concentrations of dolutegravir.

Avoid concomitant use of oxcarbazepine, phenobarbital, or phenytoin and dolutegravir since data are insufficient to make dosage recommendations.

● Antidiabetic Agents

Metformin

Concomitant use of metformin hydrochloride (500 mg twice daily) and dolutegravir (50 mg once or twice daily) increases peak plasma concentrations and AUC of metformin.

If concomitant use of metformin and dolutegravir is being considered, assess the benefits and risks. Some experts state that, if metformin is initiated in patients receiving dolutegravir, the lowest metformin dosage should be used initially and dosage of the antidiabetic agent should be titrated to achieve glycemic control while monitoring for metformin-associated adverse effects. Metformin dosage may need to be adjusted when initiating or discontinuing dolutegravir.

● Antimycobacterial Agents

Rifampin

Concomitant use of rifampin and dolutegravir decreases plasma concentrations and AUC of dolutegravir.

If rifampin is used concurrently with dolutegravir in adults who are antiretroviral-naïve or antiretroviral-experienced but INSTI-naïve, administer the recommended dolutegravir dose twice daily. If rifampin is used concurrently with dolutegravir in antiretroviral-naïve or antiretroviral-experienced pediatric patients, administer the recommended weight-based dolutegravir dose twice daily. Whenever possible, consider an alternative to rifampin in patients receiving dolutegravir who are INSTI-experienced and have HIV-1 with documented or suspected INSTI resistance.

● Antiretroviral Agents

Efavirenz

Concomitant use of efavirenz and dolutegravir decreases plasma concentrations and AUC of dolutegravir.

If efavirenz is used concurrently with dolutegravir in adults who are antiretroviral-naïve or antiretroviral-experienced but INSTI-naïve, increase dolutegravir dosage to 50 mg twice daily. If efavirenz is used concurrently with dolutegravir in antiretroviral-naïve or antiretroviral-experienced pediatric patients, increase dolutegravir dosage by giving the recommended weight-based dolutegravir dosage twice daily. Whenever possible, consider an alternative to efavirenz that is not a metabolic inducer in patients receiving dolutegravir who are INSTI-experienced and have HIV-1 with documented or suspected INSTI resistance.

Etravirine

Concomitant use of etravirine and dolutegravir results in substantially decreased plasma concentrations and AUC of dolutegravir. The effect on dolutegravir pharmacokinetics is mitigated if *ritonavir-boosted* darunavir or the fixed combination of lopinavir and ritonavir (lopinavir/ritonavir) is used concomitantly with etravirine and dolutegravir and is expected to be mitigated if *ritonavir-boosted* atazanavir is used concomitantly with etravirine and dolutegravir.

Do not use etravirine concomitantly with dolutegravir unless *ritonavir-boosted* atazanavir, *ritonavir-boosted* darunavir, or lopinavir/ritonavir is included in the regimen.

If etravirine is used concomitantly with dolutegravir in adults who are antiretroviral-naïve or antiretroviral-experienced without INSTI resistance, some experts state that dolutegravir should be given in a dosage of 50 mg once daily and *ritonavir-boosted* atazanavir, *ritonavir-boosted* darunavir, or lopinavir/ritonavir should also be included in the regimen. If etravirine is used concomitantly with dolutegravir in adults with known or suspected INSTI resistance, these experts state that dolutegravir should be given in a dosage of 50 mg twice daily and *ritonavir-boosted* atazanavir, *ritonavir-boosted* darunavir, or lopinavir/ritonavir should also be included in the regimen.

Nevirapine

Concomitant use of nevirapine and dolutegravir may decrease dolutegravir plasma concentrations and AUC.

The manufacturer states that concomitant use of nevirapine and dolutegravir should be avoided since data are insufficient to make dosage recommendations.

Rilpivirine

Concomitant use of rilpivirine and dolutegravir does not have a clinically important effect on the pharmacokinetics of either drug.

Dosage adjustments are not needed if rilpivirine and dolutegravir are used concomitantly.

● HIV Nucleoside and Nucleotide Reverse Transcriptase Inhibitors (NRTIs)

There is no in vitro evidence of antagonistic antiretroviral effects between dolutegravir and abacavir.

Tenofovir

Concomitant use of tenofovir alafenamide fumarate (TAF) or tenofovir disoproxil fumarate (tenofovir DF) and dolutegravir does not have a clinically important effect on the pharmacokinetics of the tenofovir prodrug or dolutegravir. Dosage adjustments are not needed if TAF or TDF is used concomitantly with dolutegravir.

● HIV Protease Inhibitors (PIs)

There is no in vitro evidence of antagonistic antiretroviral effects between dolutegravir and amprenavir (active metabolite of fosamprenavir) or lopinavir.

Darunavir

Concomitant use of dolutegravir and *ritonavir-boosted* darunavir decreases peak plasma concentrations and AUC of dolutegravir, but does not appear to affect the pharmacokinetics of darunavir. Clinically important drug interactions are not expected if *cobicistat-boosted* darunavir is used concomitantly with once-daily dolutegravir.

Dosage adjustments are not needed if dolutegravir is used concomitantly with *cobicistat-boosted* or *ritonavir-boosted* darunavir.

Fosamprenavir

Concomitant use of *ritonavir-boosted* fosamprenavir and dolutegravir decreases plasma concentrations and AUC of dolutegravir, but does not appear to affect the pharmacokinetics of fosamprenavir or ritonavir.

If *ritonavir-boosted* fosamprenavir is used concomitantly with dolutegravir in adults who are antiretroviral-naïve or antiretroviral-experienced but INSTI-naïve, administer the recommended dose of dolutegravir twice daily. If *ritonavir-boosted* fosamprenavir is used concomitantly with dolutegravir in antiretroviral-naïve or antiretroviral-experienced pediatric patients, administer the recommended weight-based dolutegravir dose twice daily. Whenever possible, use an alternative to *ritonavir-boosted* fosamprenavir that is not a metabolic inducer in patients receiving dolutegravir who are INSTI-experienced and have HIV-1 with documented or suspected INSTI resistance.

Lopinavir

Concomitant use of lopinavir/ritonavir (lopinavir 400 mg/ritonavir 100 mg twice daily) and dolutegravir (30 mg once daily) does not have a clinically important effect on the pharmacokinetics of dolutegravir.

Tipranavir

Concomitant use of *ritonavir-boosted* tipranavir and dolutegravir decreases peak plasma concentrations and AUC of dolutegravir.

If *ritonavir-boosted* tipranavir is used concomitantly with dolutegravir in adults who are antiretroviral-naïve or antiretroviral-experienced but INSTI-naïve, administer the recommended dose of dolutegravir twice daily. If *ritonavir-boosted* tipranavir is used concomitantly with dolutegravir in antiretroviral-naïve or antiretroviral-experienced pediatric patients, administer the recommended weight-based dolutegravir dose twice daily. Whenever possible, use an alternative to *ritonavir-boosted* tipranavir that is not a metabolic inducer in patients receiving dolutegravir who are INSTI-experienced and have HIV-1 with documented or suspected INSTI resistance.

● Benzodiazepines

Dolutegravir does not have a clinically important effect on the AUC of midazolam. Concomitant use of dolutegravir with other benzodiazepines (e.g., clonazepam, clorazepate, diazepam, estazolam, flurazepam) is not expected to affect concentrations of the benzodiazepine. Dosage adjustments are not needed if dolutegravir is used concomitantly with any of these benzodiazepines.

● Calcium, Iron, Multivitamins, and Other Preparations Containing Polyvalent Cations

Calcium, Iron, and Multivitamins

Oral calcium supplements, oral iron preparations, or other oral supplements containing calcium or iron (e.g., multivitamins) may decrease plasma concentrations of dolutegravir when used concomitantly in the fasted state.

Under fasting conditions, administer dolutegravir at least 2 hours before or 6 hours after oral supplements containing calcium or iron. If dolutegravir is administered with food, the drugs can be taken concomitantly with oral supplements containing calcium or iron.

Preparations Containing Polyvalent Cations

Concomitant use of dolutegravir and drugs containing polyvalent cations (e.g., magnesium, aluminum, laxatives, buffered preparations) may decrease absorption and plasma concentrations of dolutegravir when used concomitantly in the fasted state.

Administer dolutegravir at least 2 hours before or 6 hours after drugs or preparations containing polyvalent cations.

● Cardiac Drugs

Antiarrhythmic Agents

Dofetilide

Concomitant use of dofetilide and dolutegravir may increase dofetilide plasma concentrations and increase the risk of serious and/or life-threatening adverse effects.

Concomitant use of dofetilide and dolutegravir is contraindicated.

● Corticosteroids

Prednisone

Concomitant use of prednisone (60 mg once daily with taper) and dolutegravir (50 mg once daily) does not have a clinically important effect on the pharmacokinetics of dolutegravir.

● Dalfampridine

Concomitant use of dalfampridine and dolutegravir may result in increased dalfampridine concentrations and may increase the risk of seizures. Weigh the potential benefits of concomitant use of dalfampridine and dolutegravir against the risk of seizures.

● Estrogens and Progestins

Ethinyl Estradiol and Norgestimate

Dolutegravir does not have a clinically important effect on the pharmacokinetics of hormonal contraceptives containing ethinyl estradiol or norgestimate.

Dosage adjustments are not needed if oral contraceptives containing ethinyl estradiol and norgestimate are used in patients receiving dolutegravir.

• GI Drugs

Antacids

Antacids containing aluminum, calcium, or magnesium decrease peak plasma concentrations and AUC of dolutegravir.

Administer dolutegravir at least 2 hours before or 6 hours after antacids containing polyvalent cations (e.g., aluminum, calcium, magnesium).

Proton-pump Inhibitors

Concomitant use of omeprazole (40 mg once daily) and dolutegravir (single 50-mg dose) does not have a clinically important effect on the pharmacokinetics of dolutegravir.

Sucralfate

Sucralfate may decrease plasma concentrations of dolutegravir.

Administer dolutegravir at least 2 hours before or 6 hours after sucralfate.

• HCV Antivirals

HCV Polymerase Inhibitors

Sofosbuvir and Velpatasvir

No clinically important pharmacokinetic interactions were observed when the fixed combination of sofosbuvir and velpatasvir (sofosbuvir/velpatasvir) was used concomitantly with dolutegravir.

Dosage adjustments are not needed if sofosbuvir/velpatasvir and dolutegravir are used concomitantly.

HCV Replication Complex Inhibitors

Elbasvir and Grazoprevir

Concomitant use of dolutegravir and the fixed combination of elbasvir and grazoprevir (elbasvir/grazoprevir) does not result in clinically important changes in the pharmacokinetics of dolutegravir.

Dosage adjustments are not needed if elbasvir/grazoprevir and dolutegravir are used concomitantly.

Nucleoside and Nucleotide Antivirals

There is no in vitro evidence of antagonistic antiviral effects between dolutegravir and adefovir or ribavirin.

• Opiate Agonists and Partial Agonists

Methadone

Dolutegravir does not have a clinically important effect on the pharmacokinetics of methadone; dosage adjustments are not needed if methadone and dolutegravir are used concomitantly.

• St. John's Wort

St. John's wort (*Hypericum perforatum*) induces metabolism of dolutegravir and may cause decreased plasma concentrations of dolutegravir.

Avoid concomitant use of St. John's wort with dolutegravir.

DESCRIPTION

Dolutegravir sodium, an antiretroviral agent, is a human immunodeficiency virus (HIV) integrase strand transfer inhibitor (INSTI). Dolutegravir binds to the active site of HIV integrase and blocks the strand transfer step of retroviral DNA integration, which is essential for HIV replication. The drug is active against HIV type 1 (HIV-1) and also has in vitro activity against HIV type 2 (HIV-2). Dolutegravir is not active against hepatitis C virus (HCV).

Dolutegravir-resistant HIV-1 has been produced in vitro and has emerged during dolutegravir therapy. In initial clinical studies in antiretroviral-naïve patients, dolutegravir treatment was not associated with emergence of INSTI resistance. Treatment-emergent INSTI resistance has been reported when dolutegravir was used in clinical studies in antiretroviral-experienced patients who had not previously received an INSTI (INSTI-naïve) or patients who had previously received an INSTI (INSTI-experienced), including some patients with historical genotypic evidence of INSTI-resistance substitutions or phenotypic evidence of resistance to other INSTIs (elvitegravir, raltegravir). In some studies, treatment-emergent INSTI resistance was reported less frequently in those who received dolutegravir than those who received raltegravir, and it has been suggested that dolutegravir may possess a higher barrier to resistance than elvitegravir and raltegravir. Evidence of dolutegravir resistance substitutions has been reported in clinical studies of patients with confirmed virologic failure.

Although there is some evidence that dolutegravir has a different resistance profile than other HIV INSTIs and has been active in vitro against some HIV-1 strains resistant to other INSTIs (e.g., elvitegravir, raltegravir), cross-resistance between dolutegravir and other INSTIs (e.g., elvitegravir and/or raltegravir) has been reported. Dolutegravir has been active against HIV-1 resistant to HIV nucleoside reverse transcriptase inhibitors (NRTIs), HIV nonnucleoside reverse transcriptase inhibitors (NNRTIs), or HIV protease inhibitors (PIs).

Following oral administration of 50 mg of dolutegravir as conventional tablets once or twice daily, peak plasma concentrations of the drug are attained 1–3 hours after a dose; steady state is achieved within approximately 5 days when a once-daily regimen is used. Although studies using dolutegravir tablets indicate that food increases the extent and decreases the rate of oral absorption of the drug, dolutegravir may be taken with or without food. Dolutegravir tablets and dolutegravir tablets for oral suspension are not bioequivalent; the relative bioavailability of dolutegravir tablets for oral suspension is approximately 1.6-fold higher than that of dolutegravir conventional tablets. Studies in HIV-1-infected pediatric patients 4 weeks to less than 18 years of age indicate that peak plasma concentrations and AUC reported with weight-based dolutegravir dosages of the tablets for oral suspension or conventional tablets are comparable to those in adults receiving 50 mg of the drug once or twice daily.

In vitro studies indicate that dolutegravir is approximately 99% bound to plasma proteins. Dolutegravir is distributed into cerebrospinal fluid; the clinical importance of this is unknown. Dolutegravir is metabolized primarily by uridine diphosphate-glucuronosyltransferase (UGT) 1A1; cytochrome P-450 (CYP) isoenzyme 3A plays only a minor role in metabolism of the drug. Results of a meta-analysis of healthy individuals indicate that those with UGT1A1 genotypes that confer poor dolutegravir metabolism have a 32% lower clearance of dolutegravir and a 46% higher area under the plasma concentration-time curve (AUC) of the drug compared with those with genotypes associated with normal metabolism via UGT1A1. Following a single oral dose, 53% is excreted as unchanged drug in the feces and 31% is eliminated in urine (<1% as unchanged drug). Dolutegravir has a terminal half-life of approximately 14 hours.

ADVICE TO PATIENTS

- Inform patients of the critical nature of compliance with HIV therapy and importance of remaining under the care of a clinician. Advise patients that it is important to take the antiretroviral regimen as prescribed, and to not alter or discontinue the antiretroviral regimen without consulting clinician.

- Inform patients and/or caregivers that dolutegravir tablets and dolutegravir tablets for oral suspension are not bioequivalent and are not interchangeable on a mg-per-mg basis and that dosage must be adjusted if a switch is made from one formulation to the other. To avoid dosage errors from using the wrong formulation of dolutegravir, strongly advise patients and/or caregivers to visually inspect the tablets to verify that they were given the correct formulation each time the prescription is filled.

- If the tablets for oral suspension are used, inform patients and/or caregivers that the tablets may be swallowed whole or dispersed in drinking water and should not be chewed, cut, or crushed. Inform patients that the amount of water needed to disperse the tablets depends on the dose (i.e., required number of tablets). Instruct patients to refer to the instructions for use regarding preparation and administration of the tablets for oral suspension.

- Advise patients and/or caregivers that if a dose of dolutegravir is missed, it should be taken as soon as it is remembered and the next dose taken at the regularly scheduled time. Advise patients that a double dose should not be taken to make up for a missed dose.

- Advise patients to immediately discontinue dolutegravir and other suspect agents and seek medical attention if rash occurs and is associated with fever, generally ill feeling, extreme tiredness, muscle or joint aches, breathing difficulty, blisters or peeling skin, oral blisters or lesions, eye inflammation, swelling of the face, eyes, lips, or mouth, and/or signs and symptoms of liver problems (e.g., yellowing of skin or whites of the eyes, dark or tea-colored urine, pale stools/bowel movements, nausea, vomiting, loss of appetite, or pain, aching, or sensitivity on right side below ribs).

- Advise patients that hepatotoxicity has been reported in patients receiving dolutegravir and that monitoring for hepatotoxicity is recommended.

- Advise patients that signs and symptoms of inflammation from previous infections may occur soon after initiation of antiretroviral therapy in some individuals. Advise patients to immediately inform their clinician if any signs or symptoms of infection occur.

- Advise women to inform their clinician if they plan to become or are pregnant. Advise patients that there is a pregnancy registry to monitor fetal outcomes in those exposed to dolutegravir during pregnancy.

- Advise women to inform their clinician if they plan to breast-feed.

- Advise patients to inform their clinician of existing or contemplated concomitant therapy, including prescription and OTC drugs and herbal supplements (e.g., St. John's wort), as well as any concomitant illnesses.

- Advise patients of other important precautionary information.

PREPARATIONS

Excipients in commercially available drug preparations may have clinically important effects in some individuals; consult specific product labeling for details.

Dolutegravir Sodium

Oral

Tablets, Film-Coated	10 mg	**Tivicay®**, ViiV Healthcare
	25 mg	**Tivicay®**, ViiV Healthcare
	50 mg	**Tivicay®**, ViiV Healthcare
Tablets, for oral suspension	5 mg	**Tivicay® PD**, ViiV Healthcare

† Use is not currently included in the labeling approved by the US Food and Drug Administration.

Selected Revisions September 10, 2024, © Copyright, February 1, 2014, American Society of Health-System Pharmacists, Inc.

Dolutegravir Sodium and Lamivudine

8:18.08.12 • HIV INTEGRASE INHIBITORS

■ Dolutegravir sodium and lamivudine (dolutegravir/lamivudine) is a fixed-combination antiretroviral agent containing dolutegravir (human immunodeficiency virus integrase strand transfer inhibitor [INSTI]) and lamivudine (HIV nucleoside reverse transcriptase inhibitor [NRTI]).

USES

● Treatment of HIV Infection

The fixed combination of dolutegravir sodium and lamivudine (dolutegravir/lamivudine) is used for the treatment of human immunodeficiency virus type 1 (HIV-1) infection in antiretroviral-naive (have not previously received antiretroviral therapy) adults who have no known substitutions associated with resistance to dolutegravir or lamivudine.

Dolutegravir/lamivudine is used alone as a complete regimen for the treatment of HIV-1 infection; the manufacturer states that concomitant use with other antiretrovirals is not recommended.

The most appropriate antiretroviral regimen cannot be defined for every clinical scenario, and selection of specific antiretroviral regimens should be individualized based on information regarding antiretroviral potency, potential rate of development of resistance, known toxicities, and potential for pharmacokinetic interactions as well as virologic, immunologic, and clinical characteristics of the patient. For some additional information on the general principles and guidelines for use of antiretroviral therapy, see the Antiretroviral Agents General Statement 8:18.08. Guidelines for the management of HIV infection, including specific recommendations for initial treatment in antiretroviral-naive patients and recommendations for changing antiretroviral regimens, are available at http://www.aidsinfo.nih.gov.

Antiretroviral-naive Adults

The HHS Panel on Antiretroviral Guidelines for Adults and Adolescents states that a 2-drug regimen of dolutegravir and lamivudine is a recommended HIV integrase strand transfer inhibitor-based (INSTI-based) regimen for *initial* treatment in most antiretroviral-naive HIV-infected adults and also is a recommended regimen for *initial* treatment in adults when abacavir, tenofovir alafenamide fumarate (TAF), and tenofovir disoproxil fumarate (TDF) cannot be used or are not optimal. However, these experts state that the 2-drug regimen of dolutegravir/lamivudine should *not* be used for initial treatment in patients with plasma HIV-1 RNA levels greater than 500,000 copies/mL or with hepatitis B virus (HBV) coinfection and should *not* be used if results of HIV genotypic resistance testing for reverse transcriptase or results of HBV testing are not available.

Clinical Experience

Efficacy and safety of dolutegravir/lamivudine for the treatment of HIV-1 infection in antiretroviral-naive adults is supported by data from 2 identically designed, randomized, double-blind, phase 3 noninferiority trials (GEMINI-1; NCT02831673 and GEMINI-2; NCT02831764). Pooled 48-week data from these studies indicated that a 2-drug regimen of dolutegravir and lamivudine is noninferior to a 3-drug regimen of dolutegravir, emtricitabine, and TDF in antiretroviral-naive adults. Pooled 96-week data from GEMINI-1 and GEMINI-2 confirmed these results and indicated long-term noninferiority of the 2-drug regimen of dolutegravir and lamivudine compared with the 3-drug regimen.

GEMINI-1 and GEMINI-2 included a total of 1433 adults with HIV-1 infection who had received no prior antiretroviral treatment and had plasma HIV-1 RNA levels of 1000–500,000 copies/mL, no evidence of HBV infection, and no major HIV mutations associated with resistance to HIV nucleoside reverse transcriptase inhibitors (NRTIs), HIV nonnucleoside reverse transcriptase inhibitors (NNRTIs), or HIV protease inhibitors (PIs) at initial screening. Patients were randomized 1:1 to receive a 2-drug regimen of single-entity dolutegravir and single-entity lamivudine (dolutegravir 50 mg and lamivudine 300 mg) once daily or a 3-drug regimen of single-entity dolutegravir and the fixed combination of emtricitabine and TDF (dolutegravir 50 mg, emtricitabine 200 mg, and TDF 300 mg) once daily. The primary efficacy end point in both trials was the proportion of patients in the intention-to-treat (ITT) population with plasma HIV-1 RNA levels less than 50 copies/mL at 48 weeks. Pooled analysis of the ITT populations indicated that study participants had a median age of 33 years, 15% were female, 68% were white, 9% were CDC stage 3 (acquired immunodeficiency syndrome [AIDS]), 20% had baseline plasma HIV-1 RNA levels greater than 100,000 copies/mL, and the median CD4$^+$ T-cell count was 432 cells/mm^3 (8% had CD4$^+$ T-cell counts of 200 cells/mm^3 or lower); patient characteristics were similar in both studies.

At 48 weeks, pooled data for the ITT populations in GEMINI-1 and GEMINI-2 indicated that 91% of patients receiving the 2-drug regimen and 93% of those receiving the 3-drug regimen had plasma HIV-1 RNA levels less than 50 copies/mL. The adjusted mean change in CD4$^+$ T-cell count from baseline at week 48 was 224 cells/mm^3 in those receiving dolutegravir and lamivudine and 217 cells/mm^3 in those receiving dolutegravir and the fixed combination of emtricitabine and TDF. When results were stratified by baseline CD4$^+$ T-cell count, the response rate (i.e., plasma HIV-1 RNA levels less than 50 copies/mL) was lower in patients with baseline CD4$^+$ T-cell counts of 200 cells/mm^3 or lower (pooled response rate was 79% in those receiving the 2-drug regimen and 93% in those receiving the 3-drug regimen) compared with the response rate in patients with higher baseline CD4$^+$ T-cell counts (pooled response rate was 93% in both treatment groups); the lower response in patients with baseline CD4$^+$ T-cell counts of 200 cells/mm^3 or lower was observed irrespective of baseline plasma HIV-1 RNA levels. At week 48, treatment-emergent substitutions associated with resistance to dolutegravir or NRTIs were not detected in any patients in either treatment arm.

Pooled data from a prespecified secondary analysis of GEMINI-1 and GEMINI-2 performed at 96 weeks indicated that the 2-drug regimen of dolutegravir and lamivudine remained noninferior to the 3-drug regimen of dolutegravir and the fixed combination of emtricitabine and TDF and indicated that the 2-drug regimen was not associated with an increased risk of treatment-emergent resistance. At 96 weeks, 86% of patients receiving the 2-drug regimen of dolutegravir and lamivudine and 89.5% of those receiving the 3-drug regimen of dolutegravir and the fixed combination of emtricitabine and TDF still had plasma HIV-1 RNA levels less than 50 copies/mL. These results met the criteria for noninferiority of the 2-drug regimen at 96 weeks; treatment-emergent resistance was not reported in any patients in either treatment arm.

Antiretroviral-experienced Adults

A 2-drug regimen of dolutegravir and lamivudine has been used for the treatment of HIV-1 infection in antiretroviral-experienced† (previously treated) adults to replace the current antiretroviral regimen in those who were virologically suppressed (i.e., plasma HIV-1 RNA levels less than 50 copies/mL) on a stable antiretroviral regimen.

The HHS Panel on Antiretroviral Guidelines for Adults and Adolescents states that there is growing evidence that some 2-drug antiretroviral regimens are effective in maintaining virologic control in patients who initiated therapy and achieved virologic suppression with a 3-drug regimen; however, these experts state that a 2-drug regimen of dolutegravir and lamivudine should *not* be used in antiretroviral-experienced adults with HBV coinfection.

Clinical Experience

Efficacy of a switch to a 2-drug antiretroviral regimen of dolutegravir and lamivudine in antiretroviral-experienced† adults has been evaluated in several clinical trials and observational studies.

In one open-label, single-arm, phase 2 study (LAMIDOL; NCT02527096), a 2-drug regimen of dolutegravir and lamivudine (dolutegravir 50 mg and lamivudine 300 mg once daily) was evaluated as a possible switch strategy in 104 previously treated HIV-infected adults who were virologically suppressed for at least 2 years on a 3-drug regimen (i.e., 2 NRTIs in conjunction with an HIV INSTI, NNRTI, or boosted PI) and had no evidence of resistance to NRTIs, NNRTIs, or PIs and, when data were available, no evidence of resistance to INSTIs. After 48 weeks of the 2-drug regimen, 97% of patients remained virologically suppressed; therapeutic failure was reported in 3 patients (only 1 failure was related to virologic failure).

In an open-label, randomized, phase 3 study (ASPIRE; NCT02263326), 89 previously treated HIV-infected adults who were virologically suppressed on a 3-drug antiretroviral regimen for at least 48 weeks and had no history of virologic failure and no evidence of resistance to NRTIs or INSTIs were randomized 1:1 to switch to a 2-drug regimen of dolutegravir and lamivudine (dolutegravir 50 mg and lamivudine 300 mg once daily) or continue their current 3-drug regimen. At 24 weeks, 93% of patients receiving dolutegravir and lamivudine and 91% of patients receiving a 3-drug regimen remained virologically suppressed (i.e., plasma HIV-1 RNA levels less than 50 copies/mL); at 48 weeks, 91% of those receiving the 2-drug regimen and 89% of those receiving a 3-drug regimen remained virologically suppressed.

In an ongoing open-label, randomized, phase 3 study (TANGO; NCT03446573), 743 previously treated HIV-infected adults who were virologically suppressed for more than 6 months on a 3-drug antiretroviral regimen that included TAF (i.e., TAF and emtricitabine in conjunction with an HIV INSTI, NNRTI, or boosted PI) and had no history of virologic failure and no evidence of resistance to INSTIs or NRTIs were randomized 1:1 to switch to a 2-drug regimen of dolutegravir and lamivudine (fixed-combination tablet containing dolutegravir 50 mg/lamivudine 300 mg once daily) or continue their current TAF-based regimen. Patients with HBV coinfection were excluded. The 48-week data indicated that a switch to a 2-drug regimen of dolutegravir/lamivudine in virologically suppressed patients was noninferior to continued treatment with a 3-drug TAF-based regimen. In the ITT population, 1 patient receiving dolutegravir/lamivudine (0.3%) and 2 patients receiving a TAF-based regimen (0.5%) had plasma HIV-1 RNA levels of 50 copies/mL or greater at 48 weeks; treatment-emergent resistance was not reported in either treatment group.

DOSAGE AND ADMINISTRATION

● General

Patients should be tested for hepatitis B virus (HBV) infection prior to initiation of the fixed combination of dolutegravir sodium and lamivudine (dolutegravir/lamivudine). (See HIV-infected Individuals Coinfected with Hepatitis B Virus under Warnings/Precautions: Warnings, in Cautions.)

Women of childbearing potential should be tested for pregnancy prior to initiation of dolutegravir/lamivudine. (See Fetal/Neonatal Morbidity and Mortality under Warnings/Precautions: Other Warnings and Precautions, in Cautions.)

● Administration

The fixed combination dolutegravir/lamivudine is administered orally once daily with or without food.

● Dosage

Fixed-combination tablets of dolutegravir/lamivudine contain dolutegravir sodium and lamivudine; dosages are expressed in terms of dolutegravir and lamivudine, respectively.

Each fixed-combination tablet of dolutegravir/lamivudine contains 50 mg of dolutegravir and 300 mg of lamivudine.

Adult Dosage

Treatment of HIV-1 Infection in Antiretroviral-naive Adults

For the treatment of human immunodeficiency virus type 1 (HIV-1) infection in antiretroviral-naive adults (see Uses: Treatment of HIV Infection), the recommended dosage of dolutegravir/lamivudine is 1 tablet (50 mg of dolutegravir and 300 mg of lamivudine) once daily.

Treatment of HIV-1 Infection in Antiretroviral-naive Adults Receiving Carbamazepine or Rifampin

If dolutegravir/lamivudine is used for the treatment of HIV-1 infection in antiretroviral-naive adults (see Uses: Treatment of HIV Infection) receiving carbamazepine or rifampin, patients should receive 1 tablet of the fixed combination (50 mg of dolutegravir and 300 mg of lamivudine) once daily and a 50-mg tablet of single-entity dolutegravir once daily given 12 hours after the fixed-combination tablet. (See Drug Interactions.)

● Special Populations

Hepatic Impairment

Dosage adjustment of dolutegravir/lamivudine is not necessary in adults with mild or moderate hepatic impairment (Child-Pugh class A or B).

Dolutegravir/lamivudine is not recommended in patients with severe hepatic impairment (Child-Pugh class C). (See Hepatic Impairment under Warnings/Precautions: Specific Populations, in Cautions.)

Renal Impairment

Dolutegravir/lamivudine is not recommended in patients with creatinine clearances less than 50 mL/minute. (See Renal Impairment under Warnings/Precautions: Specific Populations, in Cautions.)

Geriatric Patients

The manufacturer makes no specific dosage recommendations for dolutegravir/lamivudine in geriatric patients, but recommends caution because of possible age-related decreases in hepatic, renal, and/or cardiac function and concomitant disease and drug therapy. (See Geriatric Use under Warnings/Precautions: Specific Populations, in Cautions.)

CAUTIONS

● Contraindications

The fixed combination of dolutegravir sodium and lamivudine (dolutegravir/lamivudine) is contraindicated in patients hypersensitive to dolutegravir or lamivudine.

Concomitant use of dolutegravir/lamivudine with dofetilide is contraindicated since concomitant use may result in serious and/or life-threatening adverse effects due to possible increased dofetilide plasma concentrations. (See Drug Interactions.)

● Warnings/Precautions

Warnings

HIV-infected Individuals Coinfected with Hepatitis B Virus

Patients with human immunodeficiency virus (HIV) infection should be tested for hepatitis B virus (HBV) before antiretroviral therapy is initiated.

Lamivudine-resistant strains of HBV have emerged in HIV-infected patients coinfected with HBV who were receiving lamivudine-containing antiretroviral regimens.

In HIV-infected patients with HBV coinfection, severe acute exacerbations of HBV infection, including liver decompensation and liver failure, have occurred following discontinuance of lamivudine-containing regimens. Such reactions could occur following discontinuance of dolutegravir/lamivudine.

Some experts state that a 2-drug antiretroviral regimen of dolutegravir and lamivudine should *not* be used in patients coinfected with HBV.

The manufacturer states that if a decision is made to use dolutegravir/lamivudine in patients coinfected with HIV-1 and HBV, appropriate additional treatment for chronic HBV infection should be considered; alternatively, a different antiretroviral regimen should be considered.

Hepatic function should be closely monitored with clinical and laboratory follow-up for at least several months after dolutegravir/lamivudine is discontinued in patients coinfected with HIV-1 and HBV. If appropriate, initiation of HBV treatment may be warranted, especially in patients with advanced liver disease or cirrhosis.

Sensitivity Reactions

Hypersensitivity reactions (e.g., rash, constitutional findings, and, sometimes, organ dysfunction including liver injury) have been reported in patients receiving dolutegravir. These adverse effects were reported in less than 1% of patients receiving dolutegravir in phase 3 clinical trials.

Dolutegravir/lamivudine should be immediately discontinued if signs or symptoms of hypersensitivity reactions occur (including, but not limited to, severe rash or rash accompanied by fever, general malaise, fatigue, muscle or joint aches, blisters or peeling of the skin, oral blisters or lesions, conjunctivitis, facial edema, hepatitis, eosinophilia, angioedema, difficulty breathing). Clinical status, including liver aminotransferase concentrations, should be monitored and appropriate therapy initiated.

Delay in stopping dolutegravir/lamivudine treatment or other suspect agents after onset of a hypersensitivity reaction may result in a life-threatening reaction.

Other Warnings and Precautions

Hepatotoxicity

Adverse hepatic effects have been reported in patients receiving dolutegravir-containing regimens.

HIV-infected patients with HBV or hepatitis C virus (HCV) coinfection may be at increased risk for development or worsening of serum aminotransferase elevations. In some patients receiving a dolutegravir-containing regimen, serum aminotransferase elevations were consistent with immune reconstitution syndrome or HBV reactivation, particularly in the setting where HBV treatment had been discontinued.

Cases of hepatic toxicity, including elevated serum liver biochemistries, hepatitis, and acute liver failure, also have been reported in patients receiving dolutegravir-containing regimens who had no preexisting hepatic disease or other identifiable risk factors. Drug-induced liver injury leading to liver transplantation has been reported with the fixed combination of abacavir, dolutegravir, and lamivudine (abacavir/dolutegravir/lamivudine).

Patients receiving dolutegravir/lamivudine should be monitored for hepatotoxicity.

Fetal/Neonatal Morbidity and Mortality

Data from an observational study in Botswana showed an association between dolutegravir and an increased risk of neural tube defects when the drug is administered at the time of conception and during early pregnancy.

Because there is only a limited understanding of reported types of neural tube defects associated with dolutegravir use and because the date of conception may not be determined with precision, the manufacturer states that an alternative to dolutegravir/lamivudine should be considered for women at the time of conception through the first trimester of pregnancy. In addition, the manufacturer states that initiation of dolutegravir/lamivudine is not recommended in women actively trying to become pregnant, unless there is no suitable alternative. (See Pregnancy under Warnings/Precautions: Specific Populations, in Cautions.)

Lactic Acidosis and Severe Hepatomegaly with Steatosis

Lactic acidosis and severe hepatomegaly with steatosis (sometimes fatal) have been reported in patients receiving nucleoside analogs, including lamivudine. These cases were reported most frequently in women; obesity also may be a risk factor.

If dolutegravir/lamivudine is used in patients with known risk factors for liver disease, such patients should be closely monitored.

Dolutegravir/lamivudine should be discontinued in patients who develop clinical or laboratory findings suggestive of lactic acidosis or pronounced hepatotoxicity (e.g., hepatomegaly and steatosis even in the absence of markedly increased serum aminotransferase concentrations).

Interactions

Concomitant use of dolutegravir/lamivudine and certain other drugs may result in known or potentially clinically important drug interactions, some of which may lead to loss of therapeutic effect of dolutegravir/lamivudine and possible development of resistance or result in greater exposures of the concomitant drug.

The potential for drug interactions should be considered prior to and during dolutegravir/lamivudine therapy; concomitant drugs should be reviewed during dolutegravir/lamivudine therapy and the patient should be monitored for adverse effects. (See Drug Interactions.)

Immune Reconstitution Syndrome

Immune reconstitution syndrome has been reported in patients treated with multiple-drug antiretroviral therapy, including dolutegravir/lamivudine. During the initial phase of treatment, HIV-infected patients whose immune systems respond to antiretroviral therapy may develop an inflammatory response to indolent or residual opportunistic infections (e.g., *Mycobacterium avium* infection, cytomegalovirus [CMV], *Pneumocystis jirovecii*, tuberculosis); such responses may necessitate further evaluation and treatment.

Autoimmune disorders (e.g., Graves' disease, polymyositis, Guillain-Barré syndrome) have also been reported to occur in the setting of immune reconstitution; however, the time to onset is more variable, and can occur many months after initiation of antiretroviral therapy.

Use of Fixed Combinations

When dolutegravir/lamivudine is used, the cautions, precautions, contraindications, and drug interactions associated with both drugs in the fixed combination must be considered.

Cautionary information applicable to specific populations (e.g., pregnant or nursing women, individuals with hepatic or renal impairment, geriatric patients) should be considered for each drug. For cautionary information related to

dolutegravir and lamivudine, see Cautions in Dolutegravir Sodium 8:18.08.12 and in Lamivudine 8:18.08.20.

Specific Populations

Pregnancy

Antiretroviral Pregnancy Registry (APR) at 800-258-4263 or http://www.apregistry.com/.

Dolutegravir crosses the placenta and results of an ex vivo perfusion model indicate a high fetal-to-maternal ratio for the drug (0.6). Lamivudine readily crosses the placenta.

Data from an observational birth outcome surveillance study in Botswana (Tsepamo study) showed an increased risk of neural tube defects associated with use of dolutegravir-containing regimens at the time of conception and during early pregnancy compared with use of antiretroviral regimens that did not contain dolutegravir. From August 2014 through March 2019, 5 cases of neural tube defects were identified out of 1683 deliveries (0.3%) to women exposed to dolutegravir-containing regimens at the time of conception. In comparison, the prevalence rate of neural tube defects was 0.1% (15/14,792 deliveries) when the mother was receiving an antiretroviral regimen that did not contain dolutegravir at the time of conception and 0.08% (70/89,372 deliveries) when the mother did not have HIV infection. The 5 cases of neural tube defects reported with dolutegravir included 2 cases of myelomeningocele and 1 case each of encephalocele, anencephaly, and iniencephaly. In the same study, one infant out of 3840 deliveries (0.03%) to women who started dolutegravir during pregnancy had a neural tube defect, compared with 3 infants out of 5952 deliveries (0.05%) to women who started non-dolutegravir antiretroviral regimens during pregnancy.

Defects related to closure of the neural tube occur from conception through the first 6 weeks of gestation and embryos exposed to dolutegravir from the time of conception through the first 6 weeks of gestation are at potential risk. In addition, 2 of the 5 birth defects (encephalocele and iniencephaly) that have been observed with dolutegravir use, although often termed neural tube defects, may occur post-neural tube closure, a time period that may be later than 6 weeks of gestation, but within the first trimester.

To date, data from the birth outcome surveillance study in Botswana and postmarketing sources including more than 1000 pregnancy outcomes have not shown evidence of an increased risk of adverse birth outcomes from dolutegravir exposures occurring during the second and third trimesters of pregnancy.

Human data regarding use of dolutegravir/lamivudine in pregnant women are insufficient to definitively assess a drug-associated risk for birth defects and miscarriage associated with the fixed combination. Based on prospective reports to the APR of over 12,000 exposures to lamivudine during pregnancy resulting in live births (including over 5000 exposures in the first trimester), there was no difference between the overall risk of birth defects for lamivudine compared with the background birth defect rate of 2.7% in the US reference population.

Pregnancy testing should be performed in all women of childbearing potential before initiation of dolutegravir/lamivudine.

The manufacturer states that dolutegravir/lamivudine should not be used during the first trimester of pregnancy, but use of the drug may be considered during the second and third trimesters of pregnancy if expected benefits justify potential risks to the pregnant woman and fetus. The manufacturer also states that initiation of dolutegravir/lamivudine is not recommended in women actively trying to become pregnant, unless there is no suitable alternative.

The HHS Panel on Treatment of Pregnant Women with HIV Infection and Prevention of Perinatal Transmission states that data are not available regarding use of 2-drug regimens for the treatment of HIV-1 infection during pregnancy and, therefore, a 2-drug regimen of dolutegravir/lamivudine is not recommended as a complete treatment regimen in antiretroviral-naive or antiretroviral-experienced pregnant women or women of childbearing potential trying to conceive.

Women of childbearing potential should be advised to consistently use effective contraception during dolutegravir/lamivudine therapy. If a woman is currently receiving dolutegravir/lamivudine and is actively trying to become pregnant or if pregnancy is confirmed in the first trimester, the risks and benefits of continuing the drug versus switching to a different antiretroviral regimen should be assessed and consideration given to switching to a regimen that does not contain dolutegravir. Pregnant women should be advised of the potential risk to an embryo exposed to dolutegravir/lamivudine from the time of conception through the first trimester of pregnancy. A benefit-risk assessment should consider factors such as the feasibility of switching to a different regimen, tolerability, ability to maintain viral suppression, and risk of HIV transmission to the infant versus the risk of neural tube defects.

Lactation

There are some reports that dolutegravir is distributed into human milk in low concentrations. The drug is distributed into milk in rats (milk concentrations of up to approximately 1.3 times those of maternal plasma concentrations have been reported in rats at 8 hours after an oral dose on lactation day 10).

Lamivudine is distributed into human milk.

It is not known whether dolutegravir/lamivudine or its components affect human milk production or affect the breast-fed infant.

Because of the risk of adverse effects in the infant and the risk of HIV transmission, HIV-infected women should not breast-feed infants.

Pediatric Use

The safety and efficacy of dolutegravir/lamivudine have not been established in pediatric patients.

Geriatric Use

Clinical trials of dolutegravir/lamivudine did not include a sufficient number of patients 65 years of age or older to determine whether they respond differently compared with younger patients.

Dolutegravir/lamivudine should be used with caution in geriatric patients because of age-related decreases in hepatic, renal, and/or cardiac function and potential for concomitant disease and drug therapy.

Hepatic Impairment

Dosage adjustment of dolutegravir/lamivudine is not necessary in patients with mild or moderate hepatic impairment (Child-Pugh class A or B).

Dolutegravir has not been studied in patients with severe hepatic impairment (Child-Pugh class C); therefore, dolutegravir/lamivudine is not recommended in those with severe hepatic impairment.

Renal Impairment

Dolutegravir/lamivudine is not recommended in patients with creatinine clearances less than 50 mL/minute because dolutegravir/lamivudine is a fixed-dose combination preparation and dosage of its components cannot be adjusted individually. Single-entity dolutegravir and single-entity lamivudine should be used in patients with creatinine clearances less than 50 mL/minute since reduction of lamivudine dosage is required in such patients.

● Common Adverse Effects

Adverse effects reported in 2% or more of patients receiving dolutegravir/lamivudine include headache, diarrhea, nausea, insomnia, and fatigue.

DRUG INTERACTIONS

The following drug interactions are based on studies using the individual components of the fixed combination of dolutegravir and lamivudine (dolutegravir/lamivudine) or are predicted to occur with the fixed combination. When dolutegravir/lamivudine is used, interactions associated with both drugs in the fixed combination should be considered.

● Drugs Affecting or Metabolized by Hepatic Microsomal Enzymes

Cytochrome P-450 (CYP) isoenzyme 3A plays a minor role in the metabolism of dolutegravir; lamivudine is not metabolized by CYP isoenzymes to any clinically important extent.

In vitro studies indicate that dolutegravir does not inhibit CYP isoenzymes 1A2, 2A6, 2B6, 2C8, 2C9, 2C19, 2D6, or 3A and does not induce CYP1A2, 2B6, or 3A4.

Concomitant use of dolutegravir and drugs that induce CYP3A may decrease dolutegravir plasma concentrations and decrease therapeutic effects of the drug.

Concomitant use with drugs that inhibit CYP3A may increase dolutegravir plasma concentrations.

● Drugs Affecting or Metabolized by Uridine Diphosphate-glucuronosyltransferases

Dolutegravir is metabolized by uridine diphosphate-glucuronosyltransferase (UGT) 1A1 and in vitro studies indicate the drug also is a substrate for UGT1A3 and UGT1A9.

Dolutegravir does not inhibit UGT1A1 or UGT2B7 in vitro.

Pharmacokinetic interactions are possible if dolutegravir is used with inducers of UGT1A1, 1A3, or 1A9 (decreased plasma concentrations of dolutegravir and decreased therapeutic effects of the drug) or with inhibitors of these enzymes (increased plasma concentrations of dolutegravir).

● Drugs Affecting or Affected by P-glycoprotein Transport

Dolutegravir is a substrate of the P-glycoprotein (P-gp) transport system in vitro; dolutegravir does not inhibit P-gp-mediated transport in vitro.

Pharmacokinetic interactions are possible if dolutegravir is used with inducers of P-gp (decreased plasma concentrations of dolutegravir and decreased therapeutic effects of the drug) or with inhibitors of P-gp (increased plasma concentrations of dolutegravir).

Although lamivudine is a substrate of P-gp, concomitant use with P-gp inhibitors is unlikely to affect lamivudine concentrations. Lamivudine does not inhibit P-gp in vitro and is not expected to affect the pharmacokinetics of drugs that are P-gp substrates.

● Drugs Affecting or Affected by Bile Salt Export Pump

Dolutegravir does not inhibit the bile salt export pump (BSEP) in vitro.

● Drugs Affecting or Affected by Breast Cancer Resistance Protein

Dolutegravir is a substrate of breast cancer resistance protein (BCRP) in vitro; dolutegravir does not inhibit BCRP in vitro.

Pharmacokinetic interactions are possible if dolutegravir is used with inducers of BCRP (decreased plasma concentrations of dolutegravir and decreased therapeutic effects of the drug) or with inhibitors of BCRP (increased plasma concentrations of dolutegravir).

Although lamivudine is a substrate of BCRP, concomitant use with BCRP inhibitors is unlikely to affect lamivudine concentrations. Lamivudine does not inhibit BCRP in vitro and is not expected to affect the pharmacokinetics of drugs that are BCRP substrates.

● Drugs Affecting or Affected by Multidrug and Toxin Extrusion Transporter

Dolutegravir inhibits multidrug and toxin extrusion transporter (MATE) 1 in vitro.

Concomitant use of dolutegravir may increase plasma concentrations of drugs eliminated by MATE1 (e.g., dofetilide, metformin).

Lamivudine is a substrate of MATE1 and MATE2-K in vitro. Although inhibitors of MATE1 or MATE2-K may increase lamivudine concentrations, this effect is not considered clinically important. Lamivudine does not inhibit MATE1 or MATE2-K in vitro and is not expected to affect the pharmacokinetics of drugs that are MATE-1 or MATE2-K substrates.

● Drugs Affecting or Affected by Multidrug Resistance Protein

Dolutegravir does not inhibit multidrug resistance protein (MRP) 2 or MRP4 in vitro.

● Drugs Affecting or Affected by Organic Anion Transporters

In vitro, dolutegravir inhibits renal organic anion transporter (OAT) 1 and OAT3. In vivo, dolutegravir does not alter plasma concentrations of OAT1 or OAT3 substrates (e.g., tenofovir, aminohippurate).

Dolutegravir does not inhibit hepatic organic anion transporter polypeptide (OATP) 1B1 or OATP1B3 in vitro; dolutegravir is not a substrate of OATP1B1 or 1B3 in vitro.

Lamivudine does not inhibit OATP1B1/3 in vitro and is not expected to affect the pharmacokinetics of drugs that are OATP1B1/3 substrates.

● *Drugs Affecting or Affected by Organic Cation Transporters*

In vitro, dolutegravir inhibits renal organic cation transporter (OCT) 2; dolutegravir does not inhibit OCT1 in vitro.

Dolutegravir may increase plasma concentrations of drugs eliminated by OCT2 (e.g., dalfampridine, dofetilide, metformin).

Lamivudine is a substrate of OCT2 in vitro. Although inhibitors of OCT2 may increase lamivudine concentrations, this effect is not considered clinically important. Lamivudine does not inhibit OCT1, OCT2, or OCT3 in vitro and is not expected to affect the pharmacokinetics of drugs that are OCT1, OCT2, or OCT3 substrates.

● *α₁-Adrenergic Blocking Agents*

Concomitant use of dolutegravir with certain α₁-adrenergic blocking agents (alfuzosin, doxazosin, silodosin, tamsulosin, terazosin) is not expected to affect concentrations of the α₁-adrenergic blocking agent; dosage adjustments are not needed if dolutegravir is used concomitantly with any of these drugs.

● *Anticoagulants*

Apixaban, Betrixaban, Dabigatran, Edoxaban, and Rivaroxaban

Concomitant use of dolutegravir with certain anticoagulants (e.g., apixaban, betrixaban, dabigatran, edoxaban, rivaroxaban) is not expected to affect concentrations of the anticoagulant; dosage adjustments are not needed if dolutegravir is used concomitantly with any of these anticoagulants.

Warfarin

Concomitant use of dolutegravir and warfarin is not expected to affect warfarin concentrations; dosage adjustments are not needed if warfarin and dolutegravir are used concomitantly.

● *Anticonvulsants*

Carbamazepine

Concomitant use of carbamazepine (300 mg twice daily) and dolutegravir (50 mg once daily) decreases peak plasma concentrations and area under the plasma concentration-time curve (AUC) of dolutegravir.

If carbamazepine and dolutegravir/lamivudine are used concomitantly, patients should receive a 50-mg dose of single-entity dolutegravir once daily given 12 hours after the usual daily dose of dolutegravir/lamivudine.

Eslicarbazepine

Possible pharmacokinetic interactions if eslicarbazepine is used concomitantly with dolutegravir (decreased dolutegravir concentrations). Some experts recommend that an alternative anticonvulsant or alternative antiretroviral should be considered.

Ethosuximide and Lamotrigine

Concomitant use of dolutegravir and ethosuximide or lamotrigine is not expected to affect concentrations of the anticonvulsant; dosage adjustments are not needed if dolutegravir is used concomitantly with ethosuximide or lamotrigine.

Oxcarbazepine, Phenobarbital, and Phenytoin

Possible pharmacokinetic interactions if oxcarbazepine, phenobarbital, or phenytoin is used concomitantly with dolutegravir (decreased dolutegravir concentrations).

Concomitant use of oxcarbazepine, phenobarbital, or phenytoin and dolutegravir/lamivudine should be avoided since data are insufficient to make dosage recommendations.

Valproic Acid

Data are not available regarding concomitant use of valproic acid and dolutegravir; some experts recommend that valproic acid concentrations and virologic response should be monitored if valproic acid is used concomitantly with dolutegravir.

● *Antidepressants*

Selective Serotonin-reuptake Inhibitors

Pharmacokinetic interactions are not expected if dolutegravir is used concomitantly with selective serotonin-reuptake inhibitors (SSRIs) (e.g., citalopram, escitalopram, fluoxetine, fluvoxamine, paroxetine, sertraline); dosage adjustments are not needed if dolutegravir is used concomitantly with any of these SSRIs.

Serotonin Modulators

Nefazodone

Concomitant use of nefazodone and dolutegravir is not expected to affect nefazodone concentrations; dosage adjustments are not needed if nefazodone and dolutegravir are used concomitantly.

Trazodone

Concomitant use of dolutegravir and trazodone is not expected to affect trazodone concentrations; dosage adjustments are not needed if trazodone and dolutegravir are used concomitantly.

Tricyclic Antidepressants

Concomitant use of dolutegravir with tricyclic antidepressants (e.g., amitriptyline, desipramine, doxepin, imipramine, nortriptyline) is not expected to affect concentrations of the tricyclic antidepressant; dosage adjustments are not needed if dolutegravir is used concomitantly with any of these tricyclic antidepressants.

Other Antidepressants

Bupropion

Concomitant use of bupropion and dolutegravir is not expected to affect bupropion concentrations; dosage adjustments are not needed if bupropion and dolutegravir are used concomitantly.

● *Antidiabetic Agents*

Dapagliflozin and Saxagliptin

Concomitant use of dolutegravir and saxagliptin or the fixed combination of dapagliflozin and saxagliptin (dapagliflozin/saxagliptin) is not expected to affect concentrations of the antidiabetic agent(s); dosage adjustments are not needed if dolutegravir is used concomitantly with saxagliptin or dapagliflozin/saxagliptin.

Metformin

Concomitant use of metformin hydrochloride (500 mg twice daily) and dolutegravir (50 mg once or twice daily) increases peak plasma concentrations and AUC of metformin.

If concomitant use of metformin and dolutegravir/lamivudine is being considered, the benefits and risks should be considered. Some experts recommend that if metformin is initiated in a patient receiving dolutegravir, the lowest metformin dosage should be used and dosage should be titrated based on glycemic control while monitoring for metformin-associated adverse effects. When initiating or discontinuing dolutegravir in patients receiving metformin, dosage of the antidiabetic agent may need to be adjusted to maintain optimal glycemic control and/or minimize metformin-associated adverse effects.

● *Antifungal Agents*

Itraconazole, Posaconazole, and Voriconazole

Pharmacokinetic interactions are not expected if dolutegravir is used concomitantly with itraconazole, posaconazole, or voriconazole; dosage adjustments are not needed if dolutegravir is used concomitantly with any of these antifungals.

● *Antilipemic Agents*

HMG-CoA Reductase Inhibitors

Concomitant use of dolutegravir with hydroxymethylglutaryl-CoA (HMG-CoA) reductase inhibitors (statins) (e.g., atorvastatin, lovastatin, pitavastatin, pravastatin, rosuvastatin, simvastatin) is not expected to affect concentrations of the statin; dosage adjustments are not needed if dolutegravir is used concomitantly with any of these statins.

Lomitapide

Concomitant use of lomitapide and dolutegravir is not expected to affect lomitapide concentrations; dosage adjustments are not needed if lomitapide and dolutegravir are used concomitantly.

● **Antimycobacterial Agents**

Rifabutin

Rifabutin does not have a clinically important effect on the pharmacokinetics of dolutegravir.

Dosage adjustments are not needed if rifabutin and dolutegravir are used concomitantly.

Rifampin

Concomitant use of rifampin and dolutegravir decreases plasma concentrations and AUC of dolutegravir.

If rifampin and dolutegravir/lamivudine are used concomitantly, patients should receive a 50-mg dose of single-entity dolutegravir once daily given 12 hours after the usual daily dose of dolutegravir/lamivudine.

Rifapentine

Clinically important decreases in dolutegravir plasma concentrations are expected if rifapentine and dolutegravir are used concomitantly.

Rifapentine and dolutegravir should not be used concomitantly.

● **Antiplatelet Agents**

Concomitant use of dolutegravir with certain antiplatelet agents (e.g., clopidogrel, prasugrel, ticagrelor, vorapaxar) is not expected to affect concentrations of the antiplatelet agent; dosage adjustments are not needed if dolutegravir is used concomitantly with any of these antiplatelet agents.

● **Antipsychotic Agents**

Concomitant use of dolutegravir with certain antipsychotic agents (e.g., aripiprazole, brexpiprazole, cariprazine, iloperidone, lurasidone, pimavanserin, pimozide, quetiapine, ziprasidone) is not expected to affect concentrations of the antipsychotic agent; dosage adjustments are not needed if dolutegravir is used concomitantly with any of these antipsychotic agents.

● **Antiretroviral Agents**

Dolutegravir/lamivudine is a complete regimen for the treatment of human immunodeficiency virus type 1 (HIV-1) infection in certain adults (see Uses: Treatment of HIV Infection), and the manufacturer states that concomitant use with other antiretroviral agents is not recommended.

There is no in vitro evidence of antagonistic antiretroviral effects between dolutegravir and lamivudine.

● **Benzodiazepines**

Dolutegravir does not have a clinically important effect on the AUC of midazolam. Concomitant use of dolutegravir with other benzodiazepines (e.g., clonazepam, clorazepate, diazepam, estazolam, flurazepam) is not expected to affect concentrations of the benzodiazepine. Dosage adjustments are not needed if dolutegravir is used concomitantly with any of these benzodiazepines.

● **Buspirone**

Concomitant use of buspirone and dolutegravir is not expected to affect buspirone concentrations; dosage adjustments are not needed if buspirone and dolutegravir are used concomitantly.

● **Calcifediol**

Concomitant use of calcifediol and dolutegravir is not expected to affect calcifediol concentrations; dosage adjustments are not needed if calcifediol and dolutegravir are used concomitantly.

● **Calcium, Iron, Multivitamins, and Other Preparations Containing Polyvalent Cations**

Calcium, Iron, and Multivitamins

Concomitant administration of oral calcium supplements, oral iron preparations, or other oral supplements containing calcium or iron (e.g., multivitamins) and dolutegravir in the fasted state may decrease absorption of dolutegravir resulting in decreased plasma concentrations and AUC of the drug.

Dolutegravir/lamivudine should be administered at least 2 hours before or 6 hours after oral supplements containing calcium or iron. Alternatively, if dolutegravir/lamivudine is administered with food, the drug can be used concomitantly with oral supplements containing calcium or iron.

Preparations Containing Polyvalent Cations

Concomitant administration of drugs containing polyvalent cations (e.g., magnesium, aluminum, laxatives, buffered medications, cation-containing products) with dolutegravir in the fasted state may decrease absorption of dolutegravir resulting in decreased plasma concentrations of the drug.

Dolutegravir/lamivudine should be administered at least 2 hours before or 6 hours after drugs or preparations containing polyvalent cations.

● **Cardiac Drugs**

Antiarrhythmic Agents

Amiodarone

Concomitant use of amiodarone and dolutegravir is not expected to affect concentrations of either drug; dosage adjustments are not needed if amiodarone and dolutegravir are used concomitantly.

Disopyramide

Pharmacokinetic interactions are possible if disopyramide is used with dolutegravir (increased disopyramide concentrations).

Some experts state that patients should be monitored for disopyramide-associated adverse effects if the drug is used concomitantly with dolutegravir.

Dofetilide

Concomitant use of dofetilide and dolutegravir/lamivudine may increase dofetilide plasma concentrations and increase the risk of serious and/or life-threatening adverse effects.

Concomitant use of dofetilide and dolutegravir/lamivudine is contraindicated.

Other Antiarrhythmic Agents

Concomitant use of dolutegravir and digoxin, dronedarone, flecainide, systemic lidocaine, mexiletine, propafenone, or quinidine is not expected to affect concentrations of the antiarrhythmic agent; dosage adjustments are not needed if dolutegravir is used concomitantly with any of these antiarrhythmic agents.

β-Adrenergic Blocking Agents

Concomitant use of dolutegravir and β-adrenergic blocking agents (e.g., metoprolol, timolol) is not expected to affect concentrations of the β-adrenergic blocking agent; dosage adjustments are not needed if dolutegravir is used concomitantly with these drugs.

Bosentan

Pharmacokinetic interactions are possible if dolutegravir is used concomitantly with bosentan (decreased dolutegravir concentrations); some experts state that dosage adjustments are not needed if bosentan and dolutegravir are used concomitantly.

Calcium-channel Blocking Agents

Pharmacokinetic interactions are not expected if dolutegravir is used concomitantly with calcium-channel blocking agents; dosage adjustments are not needed if dolutegravir is used concomitantly with calcium-channel blocking agents.

Eplerenone, Ivabradine, and Ranolazine

Concomitant use of dolutegravir and eplerenone, ivabradine, or ranolazine is not expected to affect concentrations of the cardiac drug; dosage adjustments are not needed if dolutegravir is used concomitantly with eplerenone, ivabradine, or ranolazine.

● **Colchicine**

Concomitant use of colchicine and dolutegravir is not expected to affect colchicine concentrations; dosage adjustments are not needed if colchicine and dolutegravir are used concomitantly.

● Corticosteroids

Systemic Corticosteroids

Betamethasone, Budesonide, Dexamethasone

Pharmacokinetic interactions are not expected if dolutegravir is used concomitantly with systemic betamethasone, budesonide, or dexamethasone; dosage adjustments are not needed if dolutegravir is used concomitantly with any of these systemic corticosteroids.

Prednisone and Prednisolone

Concomitant use of prednisone (60 mg once daily with taper) and dolutegravir (50 mg once daily) does not have a clinically important effect on the pharmacokinetics of dolutegravir. Concomitant use of dolutegravir is not expected to affect prednisone or prednisolone concentrations.

Dosage adjustments are not needed if dolutegravir is used concomitantly with prednisone or prednisolone.

Orally Inhaled or Intranasal Corticosteroids

Concomitant use of dolutegravir with orally inhaled or intranasal beclomethasone, budesonide, ciclesonide, fluticasone, or mometasone is not expected to affect concentrations of the corticosteroid; dosage adjustments are not needed if dolutegravir is used concomitantly with any of these orally inhaled or intranasal corticosteroids.

Local Injections of Corticosteroids

Concomitant use of dolutegravir with local injections (e.g., intra-articular, epidural, intraorbital) of betamethasone, methylprednisolone, prednisolone, or triamcinolone is not expected to affect concentrations of the corticosteroid; dosage adjustments are not needed if dolutegravir is used concomitantly with local injections of any of these corticosteroids.

● Co-trimoxazole

Concomitant use of co-trimoxazole (fixed combination of trimethoprim and sulfamethoxazole) and lamivudine doses not have clinically important effects on the pharmacokinetics of lamivudine.

● Dalfampridine

Concomitant use of dalfampridine and dolutegravir/lamivudine may result in increased dalfampridine concentrations and may increase the risk of seizures. The potential benefits of concomitant use of dalfampridine and dolutegravir/lamivudine should be weighed against the risk of seizures.

● Dronabinol

Concomitant use of dronabinol and dolutegravir is not expected to affect dronabinol concentrations; dosage adjustments are not needed if dronabinol and dolutegravir are used concomitantly.

● Ergot Alkaloids and Derivatives

Concomitant use of dolutegravir and ergot alkaloids (e.g., dihydroergotamine, ergotamine, methylergonovine) is not expected to affect concentrations of the ergot alkaloid; dosage adjustments are not needed if dolutegravir is used concomitantly with ergot alkaloids.

● Estrogens and Progestins

Estradiol, Estrogen, and Conjugated Estrogens

Concomitant use of dolutegravir and estradiol, estrogen, or conjugated estrogens (equine or synthetic) is not expected to affect estrogen concentrations.

Dosage adjustments are not needed if dolutegravir is used concomitantly with estradiol, estrogen, or conjugated estrogens.

Ethinyl Estradiol and Norgestimate

Dolutegravir does not have a clinically important effect on the pharmacokinetics of hormonal contraceptives containing ethinyl estradiol or norgestimate.

Dosage adjustments are not needed if oral contraceptives containing ethinyl estradiol and norgestimate are used in patients receiving dolutegravir.

Drospirenone, Medroxyprogesterone, and Progesterone

Concomitant use of dolutegravir and drospirenone, medroxyprogesterone, or micronized progesterone is not expected to affect concentrations of these hormones.

Dosage adjustments are not needed if dolutegravir is used concomitantly with drospirenone, medroxyprogesterone, or micronized progesterone.

● Flibanserin

Concomitant use of flibanserin and dolutegravir is not expected to affect flibanserin concentrations; dosage adjustments are not needed if flibanserin and dolutegravir are used concomitantly.

● GI Drugs

Antacids

Antacids containing aluminum, calcium, or magnesium decrease plasma concentrations and AUC of dolutegravir.

Dolutegravir/lamivudine should be administered at least 2 hours before or 6 hours after antacids containing aluminum, calcium, or magnesium.

Eluxadoline

Concomitant use of eluxadoline and dolutegravir is not expected to affect eluxadoline concentrations; dosage adjustments are not needed if eluxadoline and dolutegravir are used concomitantly.

Histamine H$_2$-receptor Antagonists

Concomitant use of histamine H$_2$-receptor antagonists and dolutegravir is not expected to affect dolutegravir exposures; dosage adjustments are not needed if dolutegravir is used concomitantly with histamine H$_2$-receptor antagonists.

Proton-pump Inhibitors

Concomitant use of omeprazole (40 mg once daily) and dolutegravir (single 50-mg dose) does not have a clinically important effect on the pharmacokinetics of dolutegravir.

Dosage adjustments are not needed if dolutegravir is used concomitantly with omeprazole or other proton-pump inhibitors.

Sucralfate

Sucralfate may decrease plasma concentrations of dolutegravir.

Dolutegravir/lamivudine should be administered at least 2 hours before or 6 hours after sucralfate.

● Goserelin

Concomitant use of goserelin and dolutegravir is not expected to affect goserelin concentrations; dosage adjustments are not needed if goserelin and dolutegravir are used concomitantly.

● HCV Antivirals

HCV Polymerase Inhibitors

Sofosbuvir

Concomitant use of sofosbuvir (400 mg once daily) and dolutegravir (50 mg once daily) does not have a clinically important effect on sofosbuvir pharmacokinetics and is not expected to effect dolutegravir pharmacokinetics.

Dosage adjustments are not needed if sofosbuvir and dolutegravir are used concomitantly.

Sofosbuvir and Velpatasvir

Concomitant use of velpatasvir (100 mg once daily) and dolutegravir (50 mg once daily) does not have a clinically important effect on velpatasvir pharmacokinetics. The fixed combination of sofosbuvir and velpatasvir (sofosbuvir/velpatasvir) does not have a clinically important effect on the pharmacokinetics of dolutegravir.

Dosage adjustments are not needed if sofosbuvir/velpatasvir and dolutegravir are used concomitantly.

Sofosbuvir, Velpatasvir, and Voxilaprevir

No clinically important pharmacokinetic interactions are expected if the fixed combination of sofosbuvir, velpatasvir, and voxilaprevir (sofosbuvir/velpatasvir/voxilaprevir) is used concomitantly with dolutegravir.

Dosage adjustments are not needed if sofosbuvir/velpatasvir/voxilaprevir and dolutegravir are used concomitantly.

HCV Protease Inhibitors

Glecaprevir and Pibrentasvir

Concomitant use of dolutegravir and the fixed combination of glecaprevir and pibrentasvir (glecaprevir/pibrentasvir) does not result in clinically important interactions.

Dosage adjustments are not needed if glecaprevir/pibrentasvir and dolutegravir are used concomitantly.

HCV Replication Complex Inhibitors

Elbasvir and Grazoprevir

Concomitant use of grazoprevir (200 mg once daily) and dolutegravir (single 50-mg dose) does not have a clinically important effect on the pharmacokinetics of grazoprevir. Concomitant use of elbasvir (50 mg once daily), grazoprevir (200 mg once daily), and dolutegravir (single 50-mg dose) does not have a clinically important effect on the pharmacokinetics of elbasvir, grazoprevir, or dolutegravir.

Dosage adjustments are not needed if the fixed combination of elbasvir and grazoprevir (elbasvir/grazoprevir) is used concomitantly with dolutegravir.

Ledipasvir and Sofosbuvir

Concomitant use of the fixed combination of ledipasvir and sofosbuvir (ledipasvir/sofosbuvir) and dolutegravir does not have a clinically important effect on the pharmacokinetics of dolutegravir, ledipasvir, or sofosbuvir.

Dosage adjustments are not needed if ledipasvir/sofosbuvir and dolutegravir are used concomitantly.

● Immunosuppressive Agents

Concomitant use of dolutegravir and immunosuppressive agents (e.g., cyclosporine, everolimus, sirolimus, tacrolimus) is not expected to affect concentrations of the immunosuppressive agent; dosage adjustments are not needed if dolutegravir is used concomitantly with any of these immunosuppressive agents.

● Interferon Alfa

Concomitant use of interferon alfa and lamivudine does not have any clinically important effects on the pharmacokinetics of lamivudine.

● Leuprolide

Concomitant use of leuprolide and dolutegravir is not expected to affect leuprolide concentrations; dosage adjustments are not needed if leuprolide and dolutegravir are used concomitantly.

● Lofexidine

Concomitant use of lofexidine and dolutegravir is not expected to affect lofexidine concentrations; dosage adjustments are not needed if lofexidine and dolutegravir are used concomitantly.

● Macrolides

Concomitant use of dolutegravir and azithromycin, clarithromycin, or erythromycin is not expected to affect concentrations of the macrolide; dosage adjustments are not needed if dolutegravir is used concomitantly with any of these macrolides.

● Opiate Agonists and Partial Agonists

Buprenorphine

Concomitant use of buprenorphine (buccal, sublingual, subdermal implant) and dolutegravir is not expected to affect concentrations of buprenorphine or its active metabolite (norbuprenorphine); dosage adjustments are not needed if buprenorphine and dolutegravir are used concomitantly.

Fentanyl

Concomitant use of fentanyl and dolutegravir is not expected to affect fentanyl concentrations; dosage adjustments are not needed if fentanyl and dolutegravir are used concomitantly.

Methadone

Dolutegravir does not have a clinically important effect on the pharmacokinetics of methadone; dosage adjustments are not needed if methadone and dolutegravir are used concomitantly.

Tramadol

Concomitant use of tramadol and dolutegravir is not expected to affect concentrations of tramadol or its active metabolite; dosage adjustments are not needed if tramadol and dolutegravir are used concomitantly.

● Phosphodiesterase Type 5 Inhibitors

Concomitant use of dolutegravir with selective phosphodiesterase type 5 (PDE5) inhibitors (e.g., avanafil, sildenafil, tadalafil, vardenafil) is not expected to affect concentrations of the PDE5 inhibitor; dosage adjustments are not needed if dolutegravir is used concomitantly with PDE5 inhibitors.

● Ribavirin

Concomitant use of ribavirin and lamivudine does not have any clinically important effects on the pharmacokinetics of lamivudine.

● Selective β-adrenergic Agonists

Concomitant use of dolutegravir and certain orally inhaled selective β-adrenergic agonists (e.g., arformoterol, formoterol, indacaterol, olodaterol, salmeterol) is not expected to affect concentrations of the β-adrenergic agonist; dosage adjustments are not needed if dolutegravir is used concomitantly with any of these β-adrenergic agonists.

● Sorbitol

Concomitant use of lamivudine and sorbitol decreases plasma concentrations and AUC of lamivudine.

Concomitant use of dolutegravir/lamivudine and sorbitol-containing drugs should be avoided.

● Spironolactone

Concomitant use of spironolactone and dolutegravir is not expected to affect spironolactone concentrations; dosage adjustments are not needed if spironolactone and dolutegravir are used concomitantly.

● St. John's Wort

Concomitant use of St. John's wort (*Hypericum perforatum*) and dolutegravir may decrease dolutegravir plasma concentrations.

Concomitant use of St. John's wort and dolutegravir/lamivudine should be avoided; data are insufficient to make dosage recommendations.

● Suvorexant

Concomitant use of suvorexant and dolutegravir is not expected to affect suvorexant concentrations; dosage adjustments are not needed if suvorexant and dolutegravir are used concomitantly.

● Testosterone

Concomitant use of testosterone and dolutegravir is not expected to affect testosterone concentrations; dosage adjustments are not needed if testosterone and dolutegravir are used concomitantly.

● Zolpidem

Concomitant use of zolpidem and dolutegravir is not expected to affect zolpidem concentrations; dosage adjustments are not needed if zolpidem and dolutegravir are used concomitantly.

DESCRIPTION

Dolutegravir sodium and lamivudine (dolutegravir/lamivudine) is a fixed combination containing 2 human immunodeficiency virus (HIV) antiretrovirals. Dolutegravir is an HIV integrase strand transfer inhibitor (INSTI) and lamivudine is an HIV nucleoside reverse transcriptase inhibitor (NRTI). There is no in vitro evidence of antagonistic anti-HIV effects between dolutegravir and lamivudine.

Dolutegravir binds to the active site of HIV integrase and blocks the strand transfer step of retroviral DNA integration, which is essential for HIV replication. Dolutegravir is active against HIV type 1 (HIV-1) and also has in vitro activity against HIV type 2 (HIV-2).

Lamivudine is a prodrug that is phosphorylated intracellularly to the active 5′-triphosphate metabolite (lamivudine triphosphate). After conversion to the pharmacologically active metabolite, the drug acts as a reverse transcriptase inhibitor via DNA chain termination after incorporation of the nucleotide analogue. Lamivudine is active against HIV-1 and also is active against hepatitis B virus (HBV).

Strains of HIV-1 resistant to dolutegravir have been produced in vitro and have emerged in HIV-infected patients receiving the drug; amino acid substitution G118R confers a tenfold decrease in in vitro susceptibility to dolutegravir. Strains of HIV-1 resistant to lamivudine have been produced in vitro and have emerged in HIV-infected patients receiving lamivudine-containing regimens; HIV-1 resistance to lamivudine often involves amino acid substitutions M184V or M184I. In a phase 3 clinical study evaluating a 2-drug regimen of dolutegravir and lamivudine in antiretroviral-naive adults, treatment-emergent INSTI- or NRTI-resistance substitutions were not reported in any patients at 48 or 96 weeks. In preliminary studies evaluating a 2-drug regimen of dolutegravir and lamivudine for switch therapy in previously treated HIV-1-infected adults, emergence of dolutegravir resistance-associated mutations was not reported and presence of the M184V lamivudine resistance-associated mutation was not a predictor of virological failure. Cross-resistance occurs among HIV INSTIs (e.g., dolutegravir, elvitegravir, raltegravir). Cross-resistance also occurs among HIV NRTIs (e.g., abacavir, emtricitabine, lamivudine, zidovudine).

Following oral administration of dolutegravir in the fasted state, peak plasma concentrations of the drug are attained 2–3 hours after a dose; absolute oral bioavailability has not been established. Dolutegravir is metabolized primarily by uridine diphosphate-glucuronosyltransferase (UGT) 1A1; cytochrome P-450 (CYP) isoenzyme 3A plays only a minor role in metabolism of the drug. Following an oral dose of dolutegravir, 64% of the dose is eliminated in feces (53% as unchanged drug) and 31% is eliminated in urine (less than 1% as unchanged drug). Dolutegravir has a plasma elimination half-life of approximately 14 hours. In vitro studies indicate that dolutegravir is approximately 99% bound to plasma proteins.

Following oral administration of lamivudine as a tablet, peak plasma concentrations of the drug are attained 1 hour after a dose and absolute oral bioavailability is 86%. Lamivudine is principally eliminated in urine by active cationic secretion; approximately 71% of a dose is eliminated in urine. Lamivudine is not metabolized by CYP isoenzymes to any clinically important extent. The mean elimination half-life of lamivudine has been reported to be 5–7 hours following a single oral dose. Lamivudine is 36% bound to plasma proteins.

Administration with a high-fat meal does not have a clinically important effect on the pharmacokinetics of dolutegravir or lamivudine or a fixed combination containing both drugs.

ADVICE TO PATIENTS

Critical nature of compliance with human immunodeficiency virus (HIV) therapy and importance of remaining under the care of a clinician. Importance of taking as prescribed; do not alter or discontinue antiretroviral regimen without consulting clinician.

Antiretroviral therapy is not a cure for HIV infection; opportunistic infections and other complications associated with HIV disease may still occur.

Advise patients that early initiation of antiretroviral therapy and sustained decreases in plasma HIV RNA have been associated with reduced risk of progression to acquired immunodeficiency syndrome (AIDS) and death.

Advise patients that effective antiretroviral regimens can decrease HIV levels in blood and genital secretions and strict adherence to such regimens in conjunction with risk-reduction measures may decrease, but cannot absolutely eliminate, the risk of secondary transmission of HIV to others. Importance of continuing to practice safer sex (e.g., using latex or polyurethane condoms to minimize sexual contact with body fluids) and reducing high-risk behaviors (e.g., reusing or sharing needles).

Importance of reading patient information provided by the manufacturer.

Advise patients to take dolutegravir/lamivudine once every day at a regularly scheduled time with or without food. Dolutegravir/lamivudine is used alone as a complete regimen for the treatment of HIV-1 infection.

If a dose of dolutegravir/lamivudine is missed, it should be taken as soon as it is remembered. Advise patients not to double their next dose and not to take more than the prescribed dose.

Inform patients that testing for hepatitis B virus (HBV) infection is recommended before antiretroviral therapy is initiated. Advise patients that emergence of HBV resistant to lamivudine has been reported in HIV-infected patients coinfected with HBV who have received lamivudine-containing antiretroviral regimens. Also advise patients that severe acute exacerbations of HBV infection have been reported following discontinuance of lamivudine in HIV-infected patients coinfected with HBV and may occur with dolutegravir/lamivudine. Importance of patients with HIV and HBV coinfection discussing with their healthcare provider whether additional treatment for chronic HBV is warranted.

Importance of immediately discontinuing dolutegravir/lamivudine and seeking medical attention if rash occurs and is associated with fever, generally ill feeling, extreme tiredness, muscle or joint aches, breathing difficulty, blisters or peeling skin, oral blisters or lesions, eye inflammation, swelling of the face, eyes, lips, or mouth, and/or signs and symptoms of liver problems (e.g., yellowing of skin or whites of the eyes, dark or tea-colored urine, pale stools/bowel movements, nausea, vomiting, loss of appetite, or pain, aching, or sensitivity on right side below ribs). Advise patients that close monitoring and appropriate laboratory testing and treatment may be required if a hypersensitivity reaction occurs.

Inform patients that hepatotoxicity has been reported in patients receiving the components of dolutegravir/lamivudine, and that monitoring for hepatotoxicity is recommended.

Inform patients that some HIV drugs, including dolutegravir/lamivudine, can cause a rare, but serious condition called lactic acidosis with liver enlargement (hepatomegaly).

Advise patients that signs and symptoms of inflammation from other previous infections may occur soon after initiation of antiretroviral therapy in some HIV-infected individuals. Importance of immediately informing clinicians if any signs or symptoms of infection occur.

Importance of informing clinicians of existing or contemplated concomitant therapy, including prescription and OTC drugs and herbal supplements (e.g., St. John's wort), as well as any concomitant illnesses.

Importance of women informing their clinicians if they plan to become pregnant, become pregnant, or if pregnancy is suspected during treatment with dolutegravir/lamivudine. Advise women of childbearing potential of the risks to the fetus if dolutegravir/lamivudine is used at the time of conception through the first trimester. Inform women of childbearing potential about the need for pregnancy testing before initiation of dolutegravir/lamivudine and counsel them that alternative antiretroviral regimens should be considered at the time of conception through the first trimester. Advise women of childbearing potential taking dolutegravir/lamivudine to consistently use effective contraception during dolutegravir/lamivudine treatment. (See Pregnancy under Warnings/Precautions: Specific Populations, in Cautions.)

Importance of women informing clinicians if they plan to breast-feed. Advise HIV-infected women not to breast-feed.

Importance of advising patients of other important precautionary information. (See Cautions.)

PREPARATIONS

Excipients in commercially available drug preparations may have clinically important effects in some individuals; consult specific product labeling for details.

Dolutegravir Sodium and Lamivudine

Oral

Tablets, film-coated	50 mg (of dolutegravir) and Lamivudine 300 mg	Dovato®, ViiV

† Use is not currently included in the labeling approved by the US Food and Drug Administration.

Selected Revisions July 6, 2020, © Copyright, April 22, 2019, American Society of Health-System Pharmacists, Inc.

Dolutegravir Sodium and Rilpivirine Hydrochloride

8:18.08.12 • HIV INTEGRASE INHIBITORS

■ Dolutegravir sodium and rilpivirine hydrochloride (dolutegravir/rilpivirine) is a fixed-combination antiretroviral agent containing dolutegravir (human immunodeficiency virus [HIV] integrase strand transfer inhibitor [INSTI]) and rilpivirine (HIV nonnucleoside reverse transcriptase inhibitor [NNRTI]).

USES

● Treatment of HIV Infection

The fixed combination of dolutegravir sodium and rilpivirine hydrochloride (dolutegravir/rilpivirine) is used as a complete regimen for the treatment of human immunodeficiency virus type 1 (HIV-1) infection in antiretroviral-experienced (previously treated) adults to replace the current antiretroviral regimen in those who are virologically suppressed (i.e., plasma HIV-1 RNA levels <50 copies/mL) on a stable antiretroviral regimen for ≥6 months, have no known history of treatment failure, and are infected with HIV-1 with no known substitutions associated with resistance to dolutegravir or rilpivirine.

Dolutegravir and rilpivirine are available as a fixed-combination preparation (dolutegravir/rilpivirine) and as separate single-entity products. Refer to the full prescribing information of the single-entity products for information on specific uses.

Clinical Experience

Antiretroviral-experienced Adults

Efficacy of a 2-drug antiretroviral regimen of dolutegravir and rilpivirine in antiretroviral-experienced adults was evaluated in 2 identically designed, randomized, open-label, active-control, phase 3, noninferiority studies (SWORD-1; NCT02429791 and SWORD-2; NCT02422797). Patients enrolled in these studies were adults with plasma HIV-1 RNA levels <50 copies/mL for ≥6 months (median age 43 years, 22% female, 20% non-white, 11% with baseline CD4+ T-cell count <350 cells/mm³). At initial screening, all patients were on a stable suppressive antiretroviral regimen (i.e., an INSTI, NNRTI, or PI in conjunction with 2 HIV nucleoside reverse transcriptase inhibitors [NRTIs]) for ≥6 months and had no known history of resistance to dolutegravir or rilpivirine. Patients were randomized in a 1:1 ratio to either switch to the 2-drug regimen of dolutegravir and rilpivirine (dolutegravir 50 mg and rilpivirine 25 mg) once daily (early-switch group) or stay on their current antiretroviral regimen for 52 weeks before switching to the 2-drug regimen (late-switch group). The primary end point was virologic response (defined as plasma HIV-1 RNA levels <50 copies/mL) at 48 weeks. Pooled virologic outcomes at 48 weeks (95% of patients in each treatment group had plasma HIV-1 RNA levels <50 copies/mL) indicated that the switch to a 2-drug regimen of dolutegravir and rilpivirine was noninferior to continuing the 3-drug antiretroviral regimen. At week 52, all 513 study participants in the early-switch group continued with the 2-drug regimen of dolutegravir and rilpivirine and 477 of the 511 patients in the late-switch group changed to the 2-drug regimen. At week 100, 89% of patients in the early-switch group and 93% of patients in the late-switch group were still virologically suppressed (i.e., plasma HIV-1 RNA levels <50 copies/mL). At week 148, 84% of patients in the early-switch group and 90% of patients in the late-switch group were still virologically suppressed (i.e., plasma HIV-1 RNA levels <50 copies/mL).

Clinical Perspective

Therapeutic options for the treatment and prevention of HIV infection and recommendations concerning the use of antiretrovirals are continuously evolving. Antiretroviral therapy is recommended for all individuals with HIV regardless of CD4 counts, and should be initiated as soon as possible after diagnosis of HIV and continued indefinitely. The primary goals of antiretroviral therapy are to achieve and maintain durable suppression of HIV viral load (as measured by plasma HIV-1 RNA levels) to a level below which drug-resistance mutations cannot emerge (i.e., below detectable limits), restore and preserve immunologic function, reduce HIV-related morbidity and mortality, improve quality of life, and prevent transmission of HIV. While the most appropriate antiretroviral regimen cannot be defined for each clinical scenario, the US Department of Health and Human Services (HHS) Panel on Antiretroviral Guidelines for Adults and Adolescents, HHS Panel on Antiretroviral Therapy and Medical Management of Children Living with HIV, and HHS Panel on Treatment of Pregnant Women with HIV Infection and Prevention of Perinatal Transmission, have developed comprehensive guidelines that provide information on selection and use of antiretrovirals for the treatment or prevention of HIV infection. Because of the complexity of managing patients with HIV, it is recommended that clinicians with HIV expertise be consulted when needed.

The use of combination antiretroviral regimens that generally include 3 drugs from 2 or more drug classes is currently recommended to achieve viral suppression. In both treatment-naïve adults and children, an initial antiretroviral regimen generally consists of 2 NRTIs administered in combination with a third active antiretroviral drug from 1 of 3 drug classes: an INSTI, an NNRTI, or a PI with a pharmacokinetic enhancer (also known as a booster; the 2 drugs used for this purpose are cobicistat and ritonavir). Selection of an initial antiretroviral regimen should be individualized based on factors such as virologic efficacy, toxicity, pill burden, dosing frequency, drug–drug interaction potential, resistance-test results, comorbid conditions, access, and cost. In patients with comorbid infections (e.g., hepatitis B, tuberculosis), antiretroviral regimen selection should also consider the potential for activity against other present infections and timing of initiation relative to other anti-infective regimens.

Dolutegravir/rilpivirine is a co-formulation of an INSTI (dolutegravir) and an NNRTI (rilpivirine). In the HHS adult and adolescent HIV treatment guideline, the 2-drug regimen of dolutegravir/rilpivirine is not recommended for initial therapy because it has not been studied for use in this setting. Growing evidence suggests that some 2-drug regimens are effective in maintaining virologic control in patients who have initiated therapy and achieved sustained virologic suppression; however, 2-drug regimens are not recommended for patients with hepatitis B virus (HBV) coinfection, unless the patient is also on a specific anti-HBV active regimen.

In the HHS pediatric HIV treatment guideline, dolutegravir/rilpivirine is not a recommended regimen for children with HIV; data are insufficient to support the use of 2-drug regimens in children at this time.

In the HHS perinatal HIV treatment guideline, dolutegravir is included in various antiretroviral regimens. The 2-drug regimen of dolutegravir/rilpivirine is not recommended for use in pregnant patients due to a lack of data in this patient population. However, if a pregnant patient presents to care on dolutegravir/rilpivirine and demonstrates successful maintenance of viral suppression, they can continue the 2-drug regimen with more frequent viral load monitoring (every 1–2 months throughout pregnancy).

DOSAGE AND ADMINISTRATION

● General

Pretreatment Screening

- Perform testing for hepatitis B virus (HBV) infection prior to initiation of dolutegravir/rilpivirine.

Patient Monitoring

- Monitor for hepatotoxicity during treatment with dolutegravir/rilpivirine.

- Monitor for signs or symptoms of severe skin or hypersensitivity reactions based on clinical status and laboratory parameters; discontinue dolutegravir/rilpivirine immediately if signs or symptoms develop.

- Evaluate patients with severe depressive symptoms to determine relationship to treatment with dolutegravir/rilpivirine and whether continued treatment is warranted.

- Monitor more frequently for adverse effects in patients with severe renal impairment (creatinine clearance <30 mL/minute) or end-stage renal disease.

● *Administration*

The fixed combination dolutegravir/rilpivirine is administered orally once daily with a meal. The manufacturer states that a protein drink alone does not constitute a meal.

Store dolutegravir/rilpivirine at room temperature of 20–25°C (excursions permitted to 15–30°C). Store and dispense in the original package, protect from moisture, and keep the bottle tightly closed; do not remove the desiccant.

● *Dosage*

Fixed-combination tablets of dolutegravir/rilpivirine contain dolutegravir sodium and rilpivirine hydrochloride; dosages are expressed in terms of dolutegravir and rilpivirine, respectively.

Each fixed-combination tablet of dolutegravir/rilpivirine contains 50 mg of dolutegravir and 25 mg of rilpivirine.

Adult Dosage

Treatment of HIV-1 Infection in Antiretroviral-experienced Adults

For the treatment of human immunodeficiency virus type 1 (HIV-1) infection in certain antiretroviral-experienced adults, the usual dosage of dolutegravir/rilpivirine is 1 tablet (50 mg of dolutegravir and 25 mg of rilpivirine) once daily with a meal.

Treatment of HIV-1 Infection in Antiretroviral-experienced Adults Receiving Rifabutin

If dolutegravir/rilpivirine is used for the treatment of HIV-1 infection in certain antiretroviral-experienced adults receiving rifabutin, patients should receive 1 tablet of the fixed combination (50 mg of dolutegravir and 25 mg of rilpivirine) *and* a 25-mg tablet of single-entity rilpivirine once daily with a meal to provide a total rilpivirine dosage of 50 mg daily for the duration of rifabutin coadministration.

● *Special Populations*

Hepatic Impairment

Dosage adjustment of dolutegravir/rilpivirine is not necessary in adults with mild or moderate hepatic impairment (Child-Pugh class A or B).

The effect of severe hepatic impairment (Child-Pugh class C) on the pharmacokinetics of dolutegravir/rilpivirine is not known and the manufacturer makes no specific dosage recommendations for such patients.

Renal Impairment

Dosage adjustment of dolutegravir/rilpivirine is not necessary in adults with mild or moderate renal impairment (creatinine clearance ≥30 mL/minute).

The manufacturer makes no specific dosage recommendations for those with severe renal impairment (creatinine clearance <30 mL/minute) or end-stage renal disease; increased monitoring for adverse effects is recommended in such individuals.

Geriatric Patients

The manufacturer makes no specific dosage recommendations for dolutegravir/rilpivirine in geriatric patients, but recommends caution because of possible age-related decreases in hepatic, renal, and/or cardiac function and concomitant disease and drug therapy.

CAUTIONS

● *Contraindications*

- Previous hypersensitivity reaction to dolutegravir or rilpivirine.
- Concomitant use with dofetilide due to potential for serious and/or life-threatening adverse effects resulting from increased dofetilide plasma concentrations.
- Concomitant use with drugs that induce cytochrome P-450 (CYP) isoenzyme 3A or drugs that elevate gastric pH since substantially decreased plasma rilpivirine concentrations may occur and may result in loss of

virologic response; these drugs include certain anticonvulsants (carbamazepine, oxcarbazepine, phenobarbital, phenytoin), certain antimycobacterials (rifampin, rifapentine), systemic dexamethasone (given in multiple doses), proton-pump inhibitors (e.g., esomeprazole, lansoprazole, omeprazole, pantoprazole, rabeprazole), and St. John's wort (*Hypericum perforatum*).

● *Warnings/Precautions*

Skin and Hypersensitivity Reactions

Hypersensitivity reactions (e.g., rash, constitutional findings, and sometimes organ dysfunction, including liver injury) have been reported in patients receiving dolutegravir. These adverse effects were reported in <1% of patients receiving dolutegravir in phase 3 clinical trials.

Severe skin and hypersensitivity reactions, including cases of Drug Reaction with Eosinophilia and Systemic Symptoms (DRESS), have been reported during postmarketing experience with rilpivirine-containing regimens. Some skin reactions were accompanied by constitutional symptoms such as fever; other skin reactions were associated with organ dysfunction, including elevated hepatic enzyme concentrations. During phase 3 clinical trials evaluating rilpivirine, treatment-associated rash with at least grade 2 severity was reported in 3% of patients.

Discontinue dolutegravir/rilpivirine immediately if signs or symptoms of severe skin or hypersensitivity reactions occur (including, but not limited to, severe rash or rash accompanied by fever, general malaise, fatigue, muscle or joint aches, blisters or peeling of the skin, mucosal involvement [oral blisters or lesions], conjunctivitis, facial edema, hepatitis, eosinophilia, angioedema, difficulty breathing). Monitor the patient's clinical status, including laboratory parameters with liver aminotransferases, and initiate appropriate therapy. Delay in stopping dolutegravir/rilpivirine treatment after onset of a hypersensitivity reaction may result in a life-threatening reaction.

Hepatotoxicity

Adverse hepatic effects have been reported in patients receiving dolutegravir- or rilpivirine-containing regimens.

Patients with human immunodeficiency virus (HIV) infection and with hepatitis B virus (HBV) or hepatitis C virus (HCV) coinfection or markedly elevated serum aminotransferase concentrations prior to initiation of dolutegravir/rilpivirine may be at increased risk for development or worsening of aminotransferase elevations. In some patients receiving a dolutegravir-containing regimen, serum aminotransferase elevations were consistent with immune reconstitution syndrome or HBV reactivation, particularly in the setting where HBV therapy had been discontinued.

Cases of hepatic toxicity, including elevated serum liver biochemistries and hepatitis, also have been reported in patients receiving dolutegravir- or rilpivirine-containing regimens who had no preexisting hepatic disease or other identifiable risk factors. Drug-induced liver injury leading to acute liver failure has been reported with dolutegravir-containing regimens; drug-induced liver injury leading to liver transplant has been reported with the fixed combination of abacavir, dolutegravir, and lamivudine (abacavir/dolutegravir/lamivudine).

Monitor for hepatotoxicity in patients receiving dolutegravir/rilpivirine.

Depressive Disorders

Depressive disorders (depressed mood, depression, dysphoria, major depression, altered mood, negative thoughts, suicide attempt, suicidal ideation) have been reported in patients receiving dolutegravir and/or rilpivirine.

Promptly evaluate patients experiencing severe depressive symptoms to determine the likelihood that symptoms are related to dolutegravir/rilpivirine and to determine if the benefits of continued therapy outweigh the risks.

Drug Interactions

Concomitant use of dolutegravir/rilpivirine and certain other drugs may result in known or potentially clinically important drug interactions, some of which may lead to loss of therapeutic effect of dolutegravir/rilpivirine and possible development of resistance or result in possible adverse effects from increased exposures of concomitant drugs.

Consider the potential for drug interactions prior to and during treatment; review concomitant drugs during dolutegravir/rilpivirine therapy and monitor the patient for adverse effects associated with concomitant drugs.

Because prolongation of the QT interval corrected for rate (QT_c) has been reported in healthy individuals receiving rilpivirine in a dosage of 75 or 300 mg once daily (3 or 12 times higher, respectively, than the rilpivirine dose in dolutegravir/rilpivirine), consider use of alternative antiretrovirals in patients receiving a drug with a known risk of torsades de pointes.

Use of Fixed Combinations

When dolutegravir/rilpivirine is used, consider the cautions, precautions, contraindications, and drug interactions associated with both drugs in the fixed combination.

Consider cautionary information applicable to specific populations (e.g., pregnant or nursing women, individuals with hepatic or renal impairment, geriatric patients) for each drug.

Specific Populations

Pregnancy

The Antiretroviral Pregnancy Registry (APR) monitors pregnancy outcomes in women exposed to dolutegravir/rilpivirine during pregnancy. Clinicians are encouraged to register patients in the APR by calling 800-258-4263 or visiting https://www.apregistry.com/.

Data regarding the use of dolutegravir/rilpivirine in pregnant women are insufficient to date to definitively assess a drug-associated risk for birth defects and miscarriage; however, human data from the APR do not indicate an increased birth defect risk. Of 1,377 dolutegravir exposures during pregnancy resulting in live births, the prevalence of birth defects was 3.3% following first trimester exposure and 5% following second-/third-trimester exposure. Of 870 rilpivirine exposures during pregnancy resulting in live births, the prevalence of birth defects was 2.1% following first trimester exposure and 0.9% following second-/third-trimester exposure.

There has been a concern regarding the development of neural tube defects in infants exposed to dolutegravir during pregnancy. The first interim analysis from an ongoing birth outcome surveillance study in Botswana identified an association between dolutegravir and an increased risk of neural tube defects when dolutegravir was administered at the time of conception and in early pregnancy. In a larger subsequent analysis, the prevalence of neural tube defects in infants delivered to individuals taking dolutegravir at conception was 0.11%, which did not differ significantly from that of infants delivered to HIV-positive individuals not administered dolutegravir (0.11%) or to HIV-negative individuals (0.06%).

Results from an Eswatini birth outcome surveillance study revealed similar outcomes; the prevalence of neural tube defects in infants delivered to individuals taking dolutegravir at conception was 0.08%, which did not differ significantly from that of infants delivered to individuals taking non-dolutegravir-containing regimens (0.22%) or to HIV-negative individuals (0.08%).

Lactation

Dolutegravir is distributed into human milk. It is not known whether rilpivirine is distributed into human milk; the drug was present in milk when administered to lactating rats.

It is not known whether dolutegravir or rilpivirine affects human milk production or the breastfed infant.

The HHS perinatal HIV transmission guideline provides updated recommendations on infant feeding. The guideline states that patients with HIV should receive evidence-based, patient-centered counseling to support shared decision making about infant feeding. During counseling, patients should be informed that feeding with appropriate formula or pasteurized donor human milk from a milk bank eliminates the risk of postnatal HIV transmission to the infant. Additionally, achieving and maintaining viral suppression with antiretroviral therapy during pregnancy and postpartum reduces the risk of breastfeeding HIV transmission to <1%, but does not completely eliminate the risk. Replacement feeding with formula or banked pasteurized donor milk is recommended when patients with HIV are *not* on antiretroviral therapy and/or do *not* have a suppressed viral load during pregnancy (at a minimum throughout the third trimester), as well as at delivery.

Pediatric Use

Safety and efficacy of dolutegravir/rilpivirine have not been established in pediatric patients. Pharmacokinetics of the drug have not been evaluated in pediatric patients.

Geriatric Use

Clinical studies of dolutegravir/rilpivirine did not include a sufficient number of patients ≥65 years of age to determine whether they respond differently compared with younger patients. Population pharmacokinetic analyses indicate that age has no clinically important effect on the pharmacokinetics of dolutegravir or rilpivirine.

Use dolutegravir/rilpivirine with caution in geriatric patients because of age-related decreases in hepatic, renal, and/or cardiac function and potential for concomitant disease and drug therapy.

Hepatic Impairment

Dosage adjustments are not necessary if dolutegravir/rilpivirine is used in patients with mild or moderate hepatic impairment (Child-Pugh class A or B).

Dolutegravir exposures in individuals with moderate hepatic impairment (Child-Pugh class B) were similar to those observed in healthy individuals. The effect of severe hepatic impairment (Child-Pugh class C) on dolutegravir exposures has not been evaluated.

Rilpivirine exposures were 47 or 5% higher in individuals with mild or moderate hepatic impairment (Child-Pugh class A or B), respectively, compared with healthy individuals. The effect of severe hepatic impairment (Child-Pugh class C) on rilpivirine exposures has not been evaluated.

Renal Impairment

Dosage adjustments are not necessary if dolutegravir/rilpivirine is used in patients with mild or moderate renal impairment (creatinine clearance ≥30 mL/minute). Increased monitoring for adverse effects is recommended if dolutegravir/rilpivirine is used in patients with severe renal impairment (creatinine clearance <30 mL/minute) or end-stage renal disease.

Population pharmacokinetic analyses indicate that mild and moderate renal impairment do not have a clinically important effect on dolutegravir pharmacokinetics. In individuals with severe renal impairment, dolutegravir AUC, peak plasma concentrations, and plasma concentrations measured 24 hours after dosing were 40, 23, and 43% lower, respectively, compared with healthy individuals. The pharmacokinetics of dolutegravir have not been evaluated in individuals requiring dialysis.

Population pharmacokinetic analyses indicate that mild renal impairment does not have a clinically important effect on rilpivirine pharmacokinetics. The pharmacokinetics of rilpivirine have not been evaluated in individuals with moderate or severe renal impairment, end-stage renal disease, or renal disease requiring dialysis.

● Common Adverse Effects

Adverse effects reported in ≥2% of patients receiving dolutegravir/rilpivirine include diarrhea, headache, and nausea.

DRUG INTERACTIONS

The following drug interactions are based on studies using the individual components of the fixed combination of dolutegravir and rilpivirine (dolutegravir/rilpivirine) or are predicted to occur with the fixed combination. When dolutegravir/rilpivirine is used, consider interactions associated with both drugs in the fixed combination.

● Drugs Affecting or Metabolized by Hepatic Microsomal Enzymes

Cytochrome P-450 (CYP) isoenzyme 3A plays a minor role in the metabolism of dolutegravir; rilpivirine is primarily metabolized by CYP3A4. Concomitant use with drugs that induce CYP3A may decrease dolutegravir and rilpivirine plasma concentrations, decrease therapeutic effect of the drugs, and may lead to resistance to rilpivirine or other HIV nonnucleoside reverse transcriptase inhibitors (NNRTIs). Concomitant use with drugs that inhibit CYP3A may increase dolutegravir and rilpivirine plasma concentrations.

In vitro studies indicate that dolutegravir does not inhibit CYP isoenzymes 1A2, 2A6, 2B6, 2C8, 2C9, 2C19, 2D6, or 3A and does not induce CYP1A2, 2B6, or 3A4. Rilpivirine is not likely to have a clinically important effect on exposures of drugs metabolized by CYP isoenzymes.

● **Drugs Affecting or Metabolized by Uridine Diphosphate-glucuronosyltransferases**

Dolutegravir is metabolized by uridine diphosphate-glucuronosyltransferase (UGT) 1A1, and in vitro studies indicate the drug also is a substrate for UGT1A3 and UGT1A9. Pharmacokinetic interactions are possible with inducers of these enzymes (decreased plasma concentrations of dolutegravir and decreased therapeutic effect of the drug) or with inhibitors of these enzymes (increased plasma concentrations of dolutegravir).

Dolutegravir does not inhibit UGT1A1 or UGT2B7 in vitro.

● **Drugs Affecting or Affected by P-glycoprotein Transport**

Dolutegravir is a substrate of the P-glycoprotein (P-gp) transport system in vitro; dolutegravir does not inhibit P-gp-mediated transport in vitro.

Pharmacokinetic interactions are possible with inducers of P-gp (decreased plasma concentrations of dolutegravir and decreased therapeutic effect of the drug) or with inhibitors of P-gp (increased plasma concentrations of dolutegravir).

● **Drugs Affecting or Affected by Bile Salt Export Pump**

Dolutegravir does not inhibit the bile salt export pump (BSEP) in vitro.

● **Drugs Affecting or Affected by Breast Cancer Resistance Protein**

Dolutegravir is a substrate of breast cancer resistance protein (BCRP) in vitro; dolutegravir does not inhibit BCRP in vitro.

Pharmacokinetic interactions are possible with inducers of BCRP (decreased plasma concentrations of dolutegravir and decreased therapeutic effects of the drug) or with inhibitors of BCRP (increased plasma concentrations of dolutegravir).

● **Drugs Affecting or Affected by Multidrug and Toxin Extrusion Transporter**

Dolutegravir inhibits multidrug and toxin extrusion transporter (MATE) 1 in vitro. Therefore, dolutegravir may increase plasma concentrations of drugs eliminated by MATE1 (e.g., dalfampridine, dofetilide, metformin).

● **Drugs Affecting or Affected by Multidrug Resistance Protein**

Dolutegravir does not inhibit multidrug resistance protein (MRP) 2 or MRP4 in vitro.

● **Drugs Affecting or Affected by Organic Anion Transporters**

In vitro, dolutegravir inhibits renal organic anion transporter (OAT) 1 and OAT3. In vivo, dolutegravir does not alter plasma concentrations of OAT1 or OAT3 substrates (e.g., tenofovir, aminohippurate).

Dolutegravir does not inhibit organic anion transporter polypeptide (OATP) 1B1 or OATP1B3 in vitro; dolutegravir is not a substrate of OATP1B1 or 1B3 in vitro.

● **Drugs Affecting or Affected by Organic Cation Transporters**

In vitro, dolutegravir inhibits renal organic cation transporter (OCT) 2; dolutegravir does not inhibit OCT1 in vitro.

Dolutegravir may increase plasma concentrations of drugs eliminated by OCT2 (e.g., dalfampridine, dofetilide, metformin).

● **Drugs that Prolong the QT Interval**

Because rilpivirine can prolong the QT interval corrected for rate (QT$_c$), consider an alternative to dolutegravir/rilpivirine in patients receiving drugs with a known risk of torsades de pointes.

● **Acetaminophen**

Concomitant use of rilpivirine and acetaminophen does not have a clinically important effect on the pharmacokinetics of either drug.

● **Anticonvulsants**
Carbamazepine

Concomitant use of carbamazepine (300 mg twice daily) and dolutegravir (50 mg once daily) decreases peak plasma concentrations and AUC of dolutegravir. Concomitant use of carbamazepine and rilpivirine is expected to substantially decrease rilpivirine exposures, which may lead to loss of virologic response.

Concomitant use of carbamazepine and dolutegravir/rilpivirine is contraindicated.

Oxcarbazepine, Phenobarbital, and Phenytoin

Oxcarbazepine, phenobarbital, and phenytoin are expected to decrease dolutegravir and rilpivirine exposures, which may lead to loss of virologic response.

Concomitant use of oxcarbazepine, phenobarbital, or phenytoin and dolutegravir/rilpivirine is contraindicated.

● **Antilipemic Agents**
HMG-CoA Reductase Inhibitors

Concomitant use of rilpivirine and atorvastatin does not have a clinically important effect on the pharmacokinetics of either drug. Concomitant use of rilpivirine and other statins (e.g., fluvastatin, lovastatin, pitavastatin, pravastatin, rosuvastatin, simvastatin) is not expected to affect concentrations of the statin. Dosage adjustments are not needed if rilpivirine is used concomitantly with any of these statins.

● **Antimycobacterial Agents**
Rifabutin

Rifabutin does not have a clinically important effect on the pharmacokinetics of dolutegravir. Concomitant use of rilpivirine and rifabutin results in decreased rilpivirine plasma concentrations and AUC.

If dolutegravir/rilpivirine is used concomitantly with rifabutin, the manufacturer recommends that patients receive 1 tablet of the fixed combination (50 mg of dolutegravir and 25 mg of rilpivirine) *and* a 25-mg tablet of single-entity rilpivirine once daily with a meal to provide a total rilpivirine dosage of 50 mg daily.

Rifampin

Concomitant use of dolutegravir and rifampin decreases plasma concentrations and AUC of dolutegravir. Concomitant use of rilpivirine and rifampin decreases plasma concentrations and AUC of rilpivirine and may result in loss of virologic response.

Concomitant use of rifampin and dolutegravir/rilpivirine is contraindicated.

Rifapentine

Concomitant use of rifapentine and dolutegravir/rilpivirine is expected to result in clinically important decreases in rilpivirine plasma concentrations and may lead to loss of virologic response; clinically important decreases in dolutegravir plasma concentrations also are expected.

Concomitant use of rifapentine and dolutegravir/rilpivirine is contraindicated.

● **Antiretroviral Agents**

Dolutegravir/rilpivirine is a complete regimen for the treatment of human immunodeficiency virus type 1 (HIV-1) infection in certain antiretroviral-experienced adults, and the manufacturer states that concomitant use with other antiretroviral agents is not recommended.

There is no in vitro evidence of antagonistic antiretroviral effects between dolutegravir and rilpivirine.

● Calcium, Iron, Multivitamins, and Other Preparations Containing Polyvalent Cations

Calcium, Iron, and Multivitamins

Oral calcium supplements, oral iron preparations, or other oral supplements containing calcium or iron (e.g., multivitamins) may decrease plasma concentrations of dolutegravir when used concomitantly with dolutegravir/rilpivirine in the fasted state.

Administer dolutegravir/rilpivirine at least 4 hours before or 6 hours after oral supplements containing calcium or iron. Alternatively, if dolutegravir/rilpivirine is administered with food, the drug can be used concomitantly with oral supplements containing calcium or iron.

Preparations Containing Polyvalent Cations

Concomitant use of dolutegravir/rilpivirine and drugs containing polyvalent cations (e.g., magnesium, aluminum, laxatives, buffered medications, cation-containing products) may decrease absorption of dolutegravir resulting in decreased plasma concentrations of the drug.

Administer dolutegravir/rilpivirine at least 4 hours before or 6 hours after drugs or preparations containing polyvalent cations.

● Cardiac Drugs

Antiarrhythmic Agents

Dofetilide

Concomitant use of dofetilide and dolutegravir/rilpivirine may increase dofetilide plasma concentrations and increase the risk of serious and/or life-threatening adverse effects.

Concomitant use of dofetilide and dolutegravir/rilpivirine is contraindicated.

● Corticosteroids

Dexamethasone

Concomitant use of systemic dexamethasone (multiple doses) with dolutegravir/rilpivirine may result in decreased plasma concentrations of rilpivirine and may lead to loss of virologic response.

Concomitant use of more than a single dose of dexamethasone with dolutegravir/rilpivirine is contraindicated.

Prednisone

Prednisone does not have a clinically important effect on the pharmacokinetics of dolutegravir.

● Dalfampridine

Concomitant use of dolutegravir and dalfampridine may result in increased dalfampridine concentrations and may increase the risk of seizures. Weigh the potential benefits of concomitant use of dalfampridine and dolutegravir against the risk of seizures.

● Estrogens and Progestins

Ethinyl Estradiol and Norethindrone or Norgestimate

Dolutegravir does not have a clinically important effect on the pharmacokinetics of hormonal contraceptives containing ethinyl estradiol or norgestimate. Dosage adjustments are not needed if oral contraceptives containing ethinyl estradiol and norgestimate are used in patients receiving dolutegravir.

Concomitant use of rilpivirine with ethinyl estradiol and norethindrone does not have a clinically important effect on rilpivirine, ethinyl estradiol, or norethindrone pharmacokinetics.

● GI Drugs

Antacids

Antacids containing aluminum, calcium, or magnesium are expected to decrease plasma concentrations of rilpivirine and may result in loss of therapeutic response

and lead to resistance to rilpivirine or other HIV NNRTIs. Antacids also decrease plasma concentrations and AUC of dolutegravir.

Administer dolutegravir/rilpivirine at least 4 hours before or 6 hours after antacids containing aluminum, calcium, or magnesium.

Histamine H₂-receptor Antagonists

Concomitant use of rilpivirine (single dose) and famotidine (single dose taken 2 hours before rilpivirine) results in decreased rilpivirine plasma concentrations and AUC. Concomitant use of other histamine H_2-receptor antagonists (e.g., cimetidine, nizatidine) also may result in decreased rilpivirine plasma concentrations and loss of therapeutic response and may lead to resistance to rilpivirine or other HIV NNRTIs. Concomitant use of histamine H_2-receptor antagonists and dolutegravir is not expected to affect dolutegravir exposures.

Administer dolutegravir/rilpivirine at least 4 hours before or 12 hours after a histamine H_2-receptor antagonist.

Proton-pump Inhibitors

Concomitant use of omeprazole and rilpivirine results in decreased rilpivirine plasma concentrations and AUC. Concomitant use of other proton-pump inhibitors (e.g., esomeprazole, lansoprazole, pantoprazole, rabeprazole) also may result in decreased rilpivirine plasma concentrations and loss of therapeutic response and may lead to resistance to rilpivirine or other HIV NNRTIs. Concomitant use of omeprazole and dolutegravir does not have a clinically important effect on the pharmacokinetics of dolutegravir.

Concomitant use of dolutegravir/rilpivirine and proton-pump inhibitors (e.g., esomeprazole, lansoprazole, omeprazole, pantoprazole, rabeprazole) is contraindicated.

Sucralfate

Sucralfate may decrease plasma concentrations of dolutegravir.

Administer dolutegravir/rilpivirine at least 4 hours before or 6 hours after sucralfate.

● HCV Antivirals

HCV Polymerase Inhibitors

Sofosbuvir

In cirrhotic patients with HIV and hepatitis C virus (HCV) coinfection receiving dolutegravir and rilpivirine (with or without HIV nucleoside reverse transcriptase inhibitors [NRTIs]) concomitantly with simeprevir (no longer commercially available in the US) and sofosbuvir (with or without ribavirin), no clinically important drug interactions were observed.

● Macrolides

Concomitant use of dolutegravir/rilpivirine and clarithromycin or erythromycin may result in increased rilpivirine plasma concentrations, but is not expected to affect dolutegravir concentrations. Consider an alternative to these macrolides (e.g., azithromycin) whenever possible in patients receiving dolutegravir/rilpivirine.

● Metformin

Concomitant use of metformin hydrochloride (500 mg twice daily) and dolutegravir (50 mg once or twice daily) increases peak plasma concentrations and AUC of metformin.

Assess the benefit and risk of concomitant use of dolutegravir/rilpivirine and metformin.

Some experts state that the lowest metformin dosage should be used initially and dosage of the antidiabetic agent should be titrated to achieve glycemic control while monitoring for metformin-associated adverse effects in patients receiving dolutegravir. Metformin dosage may need to be adjusted when initiating or discontinuing dolutegravir.

Concomitant use of rilpivirine and metformin is not expected to affect metformin concentrations; dosage adjustments are not needed if rilpivirine and metformin are used concomitantly.

● *Methadone*

Dolutegravir does not have a clinically important effect on the pharmacokinetics of methadone. Concomitant use of methadone and rilpivirine results in decreased methadone concentrations, but does not have a clinically important effect on rilpivirine concentrations or AUC.

Although adjustment of initial methadone dosage is not needed when methadone and dolutegravir/rilpivirine are used concomitantly, close clinical monitoring is recommended and adjustment of methadone maintenance dosage may be required in some patients.

● *St. John's Wort*

Concomitant use of St. John's wort (*Hypericum perforatum*) and dolutegravir/rilpivirine may result in clinically important decreases in rilpivirine plasma concentrations and may lead to loss of virologic response to the drug; dolutegravir plasma concentrations also may be decreased.

Concomitant use of St. John's wort and dolutegravir/rilpivirine is contraindicated.

DESCRIPTION

Dolutegravir sodium and rilpivirine hydrochloride (dolutegravir/rilpivirine) is a fixed combination containing 2 human immunodeficiency virus (HIV) antiretrovirals. Dolutegravir is an HIV integrase strand transfer inhibitor (INSTI) and rilpivirine is a diarylpyrimidine HIV nonnucleoside reverse transcriptase inhibitor (NNRTI). There is no in vitro evidence of antagonistic anti-HIV effects between dolutegravir and rilpivirine.

Dolutegravir binds to the active site of HIV integrase and blocks the strand transfer step of retroviral DNA integration, which is essential for HIV replication. Dolutegravir is active against HIV type 1 (HIV-1) and also has in vitro activity against HIV type 2 (HIV-2).

Rilpivirine noncompetitively inhibits HIV-1 reverse transcriptase. HIV-2 is intrinsically resistant to NNRTIs.

Strains of HIV-1 resistant to dolutegravir or rilpivirine have been produced in vitro and have emerged during clinical use. In clinical studies evaluating a 2-drug regimen of dolutegravir and rilpivirine in antiretroviral-experienced adults, virologic failure during treatment with the regimen was reported in 12 patients, of which 10 had post-baseline resistance data. Six isolates showed genotypic and/or phenotypic resistance to rilpivirine with emergent NNRTI resistance substitutions E138E/A, M230M/L, L100L/I, K101Q, E138A, K101K/E, M230M/L, L100L/V/M, and M230M/L. In addition, 1 patient had NNRTI-resistance substitutions K103N and V179I with rilpivirine phenotypic fold change of 5.2 but had no baseline sample. Two isolates showed evidence of dolutegravir resistance substitutions. One isolate had emergent INSTI-resistance substitution V151V/I present post-baseline with baseline INSTI-resistance substitutions N155N/H and G163G/R, but no integrase phenotypic data were available at virologic failure. The other patient had the dolutegravir-resistance substitution G193E at baseline and virologic failure, but no detectable phenotypic resistance. Cross-resistance occurs among HIV NNRTIs. Cross-resistance to efavirenz, etravirine, and/or nevirapine is likely after virologic failure and development of resistance to rilpivirine.

The effect of dolutegravir/rilpivirine on the QT interval has not been studied. Following oral administration of dolutegravir, peak plasma concentrations of the drug are attained 3 hours after a dose. Administration with a moderate- or high-fat meal increases the AUC of dolutegravir by approximately 1.9-fold; this effect is not considered clinically important. Dolutegravir is metabolized primarily by uridine diphosphate-glucuronosyltransferase (UGT) 1A1; cytochrome P-450 (CYP) isoenzyme 3A plays only a minor role in metabolism of the drug. Following an oral dose of dolutegravir, 64% of the dose is eliminated in feces (53% as unchanged drug) and 31% is eliminated in urine as metabolites (<1% as unchanged drug). Dolutegravir has a plasma elimination half-life of 14 hours. In vitro studies indicate that dolutegravir is approximately 99% bound to plasma proteins.

Following oral administration of rilpivirine, peak plasma concentrations of the drug are generally attained 4 hours after a dose. Administration with a moderate- or high-fat meal increases the AUC of rilpivirine by approximately 1.6- or 1.7-fold, respectively. If taken with only a protein-rich nutritional drink, rilpivirine exposures are 50% lower than when taken with a meal. Rilpivirine is primarily metabolized by CYP3A. Following an oral dose, 85% of the dose is eliminated in feces (25% as unchanged drug) and 6.5% is eliminated in urine (<1% as

unchanged drug). The half-life of rilpivirine is 50 hours. In vitro studies indicate that rilpivirine is approximately 99% bound to plasma proteins.

Population pharmacokinetic analyses from studies with the individual components of dolutegravir/rilpivirine have found that gender and race have no clinically important effect on the pharmacokinetics of either drug. Population pharmacokinetic analyses have not shown any clinically important effects on dolutegravir or rilpivirine exposures in HIV-infected individuals with HCV coinfection. Individuals with HBV coinfection were excluded from clinical studies evaluating dolutegravir/rilpivirine.

ADVICE TO PATIENTS

- Inform patients about the critical nature of compliance with HIV therapy and importance of remaining under the care of a clinician. Inform patients to take the antiretroviral regimen as prescribed, and to not alter or discontinue the antiretroviral regimen without consulting a clinician.

- Advise patients to take dolutegravir/rilpivirine once daily with a meal; a protein drink alone does not constitute a meal.

- If a dose of dolutegravir/rilpivirine is missed, inform patients to take the dose with a meal as soon as it is remembered. Inform patients not to double their next dose to make up for a missed dose.

- Advise patients to immediately discontinue dolutegravir/rilpivirine and seek medical attention if rash occurs and is associated with fever, generally ill feeling, extreme tiredness, muscle or joint aches, breathing difficulty, blisters or peeling skin, oral blisters or lesions, eye inflammation or redness, swelling of the face, eyes, lips, or mouth, and/or signs and symptoms of liver problems (e.g., yellowing of skin or whites of the eyes, dark or tea-colored urine, pale stools/bowel movements, nausea, vomiting, loss of appetite, or pain, aching, or sensitivity on right side of the abdomen below ribs). Advise patients that close monitoring and appropriate laboratory testing or treatment may be required if a hypersensitivity reaction occurs.

- Advise patients that depressive disorders (depressed mood, depression, dysphoria, major depression, altered mood, negative thoughts, suicide attempt, suicidal ideation) have been reported in patients receiving the components of dolutegravir/rilpivirine. Inform patients to immediately contact their clinician if depressive symptoms (e.g., feeling sad, hopeless, anxious, or restless; hurting oneself; having thoughts of hurting oneself) occur.

- Advise patients that hepatotoxicity has been reported in patients receiving the components of dolutegravir/rilpivirine and that monitoring for hepatotoxicity is recommended.

- Advise women to inform their clinician if they plan to become pregnant, or if pregnancy is confirmed, during treatment with dolutegravir/rilpivirine. Inform patients that a registry exists that monitors outcomes in women exposed to dolutegravir/rilpivirine during pregnancy.

- Advise women to inform their clinician if they plan to breastfeed.

- Advise patients of the potential for serious drug interactions and to inform their clinician of existing or contemplated concomitant therapy, including prescription and OTC drugs and herbal products, and any concomitant illnesses.

- Advise patients of other important precautionary information.

PREPARATIONS

Excipients in commercially available drug preparations may have clinically important effects in some individuals; consult specific product labeling for details.

Dolutegravir Sodium and Rilpivirine Hydrochloride

Oral

Tablets, film-coated	Dolutegravir Sodium 50 mg (of dolutegravir) and Rilpivirine Hydrochloride 25 mg (of rilpivirine)	Juluca®, ViiV

† Use is not currently included in the labeling approved by the US Food and Drug Administration.

Elvitegravir, Cobicistat, Emtricitabine, and Tenofovir Alafenamide Fumarate

8:18.08.12 · HIV INTEGRASE INHIBITORS

■ Elvitegravir, cobicistat, emtricitabine, and tenofovir alafenamide fumarate (EVG/c/FTC/TAF) is a fixed-combination antiretroviral agent containing elvitegravir (human immunodeficiency virus type 1 [HIV-1] integrase strand transfer inhibitor [INSTI]), cobicistat (pharmacokinetic enhancer), emtricitabine (HIV-1 nucleoside reverse transcriptase inhibitor [NRTI]), and tenofovir alafenamide (HIV-1 nucleotide reverse transcriptase inhibitor). Cobicistat, a mechanism-based cytochrome P-450 (CYP) 3A inhibitor, is included in the fixed combination to increase plasma concentrations of elvitegravir (cobicistat-boosted elvitegravir) and is not active against HIV.

USES

● Treatment of HIV Infection

The fixed combination of elvitegravir, cobicistat, emtricitabine, and tenofovir alafenamide fumarate (EVG/c/FTC/TAF) is used as a complete regimen for the treatment of HIV-1 infection in adult and pediatric patients weighing ≥25 kg who have no antiretroviral treatment history or to replace the current antiretroviral regimen in patients who are virologically suppressed (HIV-1 RNA <50 copies/mL) on a stable antiretroviral regimen for at least 6 months with no history of treatment failure and no known substitutions associated with resistance to the individual components of EVG/c/FTC/TAF.

EVG/c/FTC/TAF is a co-formulation of 2 nucleotide/nucleoside reverse transcriptase inhibitors (NRTIs; tenofovir alafenamide fumarate and emtricitabine), an integrase strand transfer inhibitor (INSTI; elvitegravir), and a pharmacokinetic enhancer (cobicistat); consult guidelines for the most current information on the place in therapy for this regimen. Selection of an initial antiretroviral regimen should be individualized based on factors such as virologic efficacy, toxicity, pill burden, dosing frequency, drug-drug interaction potential, resistance test results, comorbid conditions, access, and cost.

Clinical Experience

Antiretroviral-naïve Adults

The comparative efficacy of EVG/c/FTC/TAF and the fixed combination of elvitegravir, cobicistat, emtricitabine, and tenofovir disoproxil fumarate (tenofovir DF) (EVG/c/FTC/TDF) was evaluated in 2 identical randomized, double blind, active-control, phase 3, noninferiority studies in antiretroviral-naïve HIV-infected adults (study 104 and study 111). Patients enrolled in these studies were adults (mean age 36 years, 85% male, 57% white, 25% Black, 10% Asian, 19% Hispanic, mean baseline plasma HIV-1 RNA level 4.5 $\log_{10}$ copies/mL, mean baseline CD4+ T-cell count 427 cells/mm³). Patients were randomized in a 1:1 ratio to receive EVG/c/FTC/TAF (elvitegravir 150 mg, cobicistat 150 mg, emtricitabine 200 mg, tenofovir alafenamide 10 mg) or EVG/c/FTC/TDF (elvitegravir 150 mg, cobicistat 150 mg, emtricitabine 200 mg, tenofovir DF 300 mg) once daily. The primary end point was virologic response (defined as HIV-1 RNA <50 copies/mL). Pooled data from both studies at 144 weeks indicated that 84% of those receiving EVG/c/FTC/TAF had plasma HIV-1 RNA <50 copies/mL compared with 80% of those receiving EVG/c/FTC/TDF. The mean increase in CD4+ T-cell count from baseline to week 144 was 326 cells/mm³ in those receiving EVG/c/FTC/TAF compared with 305 cells/mm³ in those receiving EVG/c/FTC/TDF. Treatment outcomes were similar across subgroups (age, sex, race, baseline viral load, and baseline CD4+ T-cell count).

Antiretroviral-experienced Adults

The efficacy of EVG/c/FTC/TAF in antiretroviral-experienced, virologically suppressed adults was evaluated in a randomized, open-label, active-control, phase 3 noninferiority study (study 109; NCT01815736). Patients enrolled in the study were adults with baseline plasma HIV-1 RNA <50 copies/mL for at least 6 months (mean age 41 years, 90% male, 67% white, 21% Black, mean baseline CD4+ T-cell count 705 cells/mm³). At initial screening, all patients were on a suppressive antiretroviral regimen (ritonavir-boosted or cobicistat-boosted atazanavir in conjunction with the fixed combination of emtricitabine and tenofovir DF [42%], EVG/c/FTC/TDF [32%], or fixed combination of efavirenz, emtricitabine, and tenofovir DF [26%]) for at least 6 months with no known history of resistance to the antiretroviral components of EVG/c/FTC/TAF. Patients were randomized in a 2:1 ratio to either switch to EVG/c/FTC/TAF (elvitegravir 150 mg, cobicistat 150 mg, emtricitabine 200 mg, tenofovir alafenamide 10 mg) or stay on their baseline antiretroviral regimen. The primary end point was virologic response (defined as HIV-1 RNA <50 copies/mL). At 96 weeks, 93% of those receiving EVG/c/FTC/TAF had plasma HIV-1 RNA <50 copies/mL compared with 89% of those who continued to receive their baseline antiretroviral regimen. The mean increase in CD4+ T-cell count from baseline was 60 cells/mm³ in those receiving EVG/c/FTC/TAF compared with 42 cells/mm³ in those who continued to receive their baseline antiretroviral regimen.

The efficacy of EVG/c/FTC/TAF in antiretroviral-experienced, virologically suppressed adults with mild to moderate renal impairment (estimated glomerular filtration rate [eGFR] 30–69 mL/minute) was evaluated in a single-arm, open-label study (study 112; NCT01818596). The study included 242 patients (mean age 58 years [26% 65 years of age or older], 79% male, 18% Black, median baseline CD4+ T-cell count 632 cells/mm³) with plasma HIV-1 RNA <50 copies/mL for at least 6 months on their existing antiretroviral regimen (65% had been receiving a regimen that included tenofovir DF) and also included 6 treatment-naive patients. All patients then received EVG/c/FTC/TAF (elvitegravir 150 mg, cobicistat 150 mg, emtricitabine 200 mg, tenofovir alafenamide 10 mg) once daily with food. The primary end point was the change in eGFR from baseline to 24 weeks; a secondary end point was the proportion of patients maintaining virologic control. In the previously treated patients, eGFR (using the Cockcroft-Gault equation) was reduced by 0.4 mL/minute at 24 weeks after switching to EVG/c/FTC/TAF and there was no appreciable change in estimated creatinine clearance from baseline through 48 weeks. At 144 weeks after switching to EVG/c/FTC/TAF, 81% of previously treated patients had maintained plasma HIV-1 RNA <50 copies/mL; 5 patients experienced virologic failure.

A similar open-label, single-arm study evaluated the efficacy and safety of switching to EVG/c/FTC/TAF in 55 antiretroviral-experienced, virologically suppressed adults with end-stage renal disease (eGFR <15 mL/minute; study 1825). Enrollees had, for at least 6 months, both an HIV-1 RNA <50 copies/mL with their previous antiretroviral regimen and were receiving chronic hemodialysis, and switched therapy to EVG/c/FTC/TAF once daily for up to 96 weeks. The primary endpoint was treatment-emergent grade 3 or higher adverse events up to week 48, with the proportion of patients with HIV-1 RNA <50 copies/mL as a secondary endpoint. At week 48, 45 patients (82%) maintained HIV-1 RNA <50 copies/mL, 7 of whom had discontinued EVG/c/FTC/TAF due to adverse events or other reasons while virologically suppressed; 2 patients had HIV-1 RNA ≥50 copies/mL.

Two randomized noninferiority trials evaluated the efficacy of switching from other regimens to EVG/c/FTC/TAF in antiretroviral-experienced, virologically suppressed adults. The first study initially randomized treatment-naïve women to receive EVG/c/FTC/TDF or ritonavir-boosted atazanavir plus emtricitabine and tenofovir DF (ATV/RTV/FTC/TDF); patients in the ATV/RTV/FTC/TDF arm who achieved virologic suppression at 48 weeks were rerandomized (3:1) to switch to EVG/c/FTC/TAF or continue on ATV/RTV/FTC/TDF. The second study randomized virologically suppressed adults who were receiving abacavir plus lamivudine and a third antiretroviral 2:1 to switch to EVG/c/FTC/TAF or continue on their current regimen. Among 212 women who underwent re-randomization in the first study, similar rates of maintained virologic suppression were noted at 48 weeks in those who switched to EVG/c/FTC/TAF (94%) and those who continued on ATV/RTV/FTC/TDF (87%). Among 274 patients randomized and analyzed in the second study, similar rates of maintained virologic suppression were noted at 24 weeks in those who switched to EVG/c/FTC/TAF (93.4%) and those who continued on their current regimen (97.8%).

Pediatric Patients

The efficacy of EVG/c/FTC/TAF in pediatric patients was evaluated in a 2-cohort, open-label study enrolling treatment-naïve adolescents (12 to <18 years of age, weighing ≥35 kg; cohort 1) and antiretroviral-experienced, virologically suppressed children (6 to <12 years of age, weighing ≥25 kg; cohort 2) (study 106). Cohort 1 included 50 patients (mean age 15 years, 44% male, 88% Black, 12% Asian, mean baseline CD4+ T-cell count 471 cells/mm³, mean CD4+ percentage 23.6%, mean baseline HIV-1 RNA 4.6 $\log_{10}$ copies/mL). Cohort 2 included 52 patients (mean age 10 years, 42% male, 71% Black, 25% Asian, mean baseline CD4+ T-cell count 961 cells/mm³, mean CD4+ percentage 38.2%). All patients received EVG/c/FTC/TAF once daily. In cohort 1, 92% had achieved plasma HIV-1 RNA <50 copies/mL at 48 weeks; the mean increase in CD4+ T-cell count from baseline was 224 cells/mm³. Virologic failure was observed in 3 adolescents; there was no evidence of treatment-emergent resistance to EVG/c/FTC/TAF. In cohort 2, 98% remained virologically suppressed 48 weeks after switching to EVG/c/FTC/TAF; all patients maintained CD4+ T-cell counts above 400 cells/mm³ and none qualified for resistance analysis.

Clinical Perspective

Therapeutic options for the treatment and prevention of HIV infection and recommendations concerning the use of antiretrovirals are continuously evolving. Antiretroviral therapy (ART) is recommended for all individuals with HIV regardless of CD4 counts, and should be initiated as soon as possible after diagnosis of HIV and continued indefinitely. The primary goals of ART are to achieve and maintain durable suppression of HIV viral load (as measured by plasma HIV-1 RNA levels) to a level below which drug-resistance mutations cannot emerge (i.e., below detectable limits), restore and preserve immunologic function, reduce HIV-related morbidity and mortality, improve quality of life, and prevent transmission of HIV. While the most appropriate antiretroviral regimen cannot be defined for each clinical scenario, the US Department of Health and Human Services (HHS) Panel on Antiretroviral Guidelines for Adults and Adolescents, HHS Panel on Antiretroviral Therapy and Medical Management of Children Living with HIV, and HHS Panel on Treatment of Pregnant Women with HIV Infection and Prevention of Perinatal Transmission, have developed comprehensive guidelines that provide information on selection and use of antiretrovirals for the treatment or prevention of HIV infection. Because of the complexity of managing patients with HIV, it is recommended that clinicians with HIV expertise be consulted when needed.

The use of combination antiretroviral regimens that generally include 3 drugs from 2 or more drug classes is currently recommended to achieve viral suppression. In both treatment-naïve adults and children, an initial anti-retroviral regimen generally consists of 2 nucleoside reverse transcriptase inhibitors (NRTIs) administered in combination with a third active antiretroviral from 1 of 3 drug classes: an integrase strand transfer inhibitor (INSTI), a non-nucleoside reverse transcriptase inhibitor (NNRTI), or a protease inhibitor (PI) with a pharmacokinetic enhancer (also known as a booster; the 2 drugs used for this purpose are cobicistat and ritonavir). Selection of an initial regimen should be individualized based on factors such as virologic efficacy, toxicity, pill burden, dosing frequency, drug–drug interaction potential, resistance-test results, comorbid conditions, access, and cost. In patients with comorbid infections (e.g., hepatitis B, tuberculosis), antiretroviral regimen selection should also consider the potential for activity against other present infections and timing of initiation relative to other anti-infective regimens.

The fixed-dose combination of EVG/c/FTC/TAF is commonly used as a complete antiretroviral regimen. In the 2023 HHS adult and adolescent HIV treatment guideline, EVG/c/FTC/TAF is listed among initial regimens recommended in certain clinical situations.

In the 2023 HHS pediatric HIV treatment guideline, EVG/c/FTC/TAF is listed among alternative initial regimens for children and adolescents weighing ≥25 kg.

In the 2023 HHS perinatal HIV treatment guideline, EVG/c/FTC/TAF is not recommended as an initial antiretroviral regimen in pregnancy due to data suggesting insufficient levels of cobicistat and elvitegravir in the second and third trimesters and risk of viral breakthrough at delivery. In patients who become pregnant while virologically suppressed on EVG/c/FTC/TAF, HHS recommends continuing therapy with frequent viral load monitoring or considering switching therapy.

DOSAGE AND ADMINISTRATION

● General

Pretreatment Screening

- Test patients for hepatitis B virus (HBV) infection prior to initiation of elvitegravir, cobicistat, emtricitabine, and tenofovir alafenamide (EVG/c/FTC/TAF).
- Assess serum creatinine, estimated creatinine clearance, urine glucose, and urine protein prior to initiation of EVG/c/FTC/TAF.
- In patients with chronic kidney disease (CKD), determine serum phosphorus prior to initiation of EVG/c/FTC/TAF.

Patient Monitoring

- Routinely monitor serum creatinine, estimated creatinine clearance, urine glucose, and urine protein during treatment in all patients.
- Routinely monitor serum phosphorus during treatment in patients with CKD.

● Administration

The fixed combination of EVG/c/FTC/TAF is administered orally once daily with food.

● Dosage

Each fixed-combination tablet of EVG/c/FTC/TAF contains elvitegravir 150 mg, cobicistat 150 mg, emtricitabine 200 mg, and tenofovir alafenamide 10 mg.

Although tenofovir alafenamide is provided in the fixed combination as tenofovir alafenamide fumarate, dosage of this tenofovir component is expressed in terms of tenofovir alafenamide.

Store tablets below 30°C in the original container and keep container tightly closed.

Adult Dosage

Treatment of HIV Infection

For the treatment of HIV-1 infection in antiretroviral naïve or experienced adults, the usual dosage of EVG/c/FTC/TAF is 1 tablet (150 mg of elvitegravir, 150 mg of cobicistat, 200 mg of emtricitabine, and 10 mg of tenofovir alafenamide) once daily.

Pediatric Dosage

Treatment of HIV Infection

For the treatment of HIV-1 infection in antiretroviral naïve or experienced pediatric patients weighing at least 25 kg, the usual dosage of EVG/c/FTC/TAF is 1 tablet (150 mg of elvitegravir, 150 mg of cobicistat, 200 mg of emtricitabine, and 10 mg of tenofovir alafenamide) once daily.

● Special Populations

Hepatic Impairment

Dosage adjustments are not necessary if EVG/c/FTC/TAF is used in patients with mild or moderate hepatic impairment (Child-Pugh class A or B).

EVG/c/FTC/TAF has not been studied and use is therefore not recommended in patients with severe hepatic impairment (Child-Pugh class C).

Renal Impairment

Dosage adjustments are not necessary if EVG/c/FTC/TAF is used in patients with estimated creatinine clearance of 30 mL/minute or greater.

In adults with an estimated creatinine clearance <15 mL/minute who are receiving chronic hemodialysis, on days of hemodialysis, administer EVG/c/FTC/TAF after completion of hemodialysis treatment.

EVG/c/FTC/TAF is not recommended in patients with severe renal impairment (estimated creatinine clearance of 15–29 mL/minute), or in patients with end-stage renal disease (ESRD) (estimated creatinine clearance <15 mL/minute) who are not receiving chronic hemodialysis.

Geriatric Use

The manufacturer makes no specific dosage recommendations in geriatric patients.

CAUTIONS

• Contraindications

• Concomitant use with drugs highly dependent on cytochrome P-450 (CYP) 3A for clearance and for which elevated plasma concentrations are associated with serious and/or life-threatening events. These drugs and other contraindicated drugs, which may lead to reduced efficacy of the fixed combination of elvitegravir, cobicistat, emtricitabine, and tenofovir alafenamide fumarate (EVG/c/FTC/TAF) and possible resistance include alfuzosin, carbamazepine, phenobarbital, phenytoin, rifampin, lurasidone, pimozide, ergot derivatives, St. John's wort, lomitapide, lovastatin, simvastatin, sildenafil (when given for pulmonary arterial hypertension), triazolam, and orally administered midazolam.

• Warnings/Precautions

Warnings

HIV-infected Individuals Coinfected with Hepatitis B Virus

A boxed warning is included in the prescribing information for EVG/c/FTC/TAF regarding the risk of severe acute exacerbations of hepatitis B virus (HBV) infection following discontinuance of preparations containing emtricitabine and/or tenofovir disoproxil fumarate (tenofovir DF). In some patients receiving emtricitabine, exacerbations of HBV have been associated with hepatic decompensation and hepatic failure. Such reactions could occur with EVG/c/FTC/TAF.

HIV-infected patients should be tested for HBV before or when antiretroviral therapy is initiated.

EVG/c/FTC/TAF is not indicated for treatment of chronic HBV infection, and safety and efficacy of EVG/c/FTC/TAF have not been established in HIV-infected patients coinfected with HBV.

Hepatic function should be closely monitored with clinical and laboratory follow-up for at least several months after EVG/c/FTC/TAF is discontinued in patients coinfected with HIV and HBV. If appropriate, initiation of HBV treatment may be warranted, especially in patients with advanced liver disease or cirrhosis.

Other Warnings/Precautions

New Onset or Worsening Renal Impairment

Post marketing cases of renal impairment, including acute renal failure and Fanconi syndrome (renal tubular injury with severe hypophosphatemia), have been reported in patients receiving TAF-containing products. Although the majority of these cases had potential confounding factors that may have contributed to the development of renal impairment, these confounding factors may have predisposed patients to tenofovir-related adverse events.

EVG/c/FTC/TAF is not recommended in patients with estimated creatinine clearance of 15 to <30 mL/minute, or in patients with estimated creatinine clearance <15 mL/minute who are not receiving chronic hemodialysis.

Cobicistat (a component of EVG/c/FTC/TAF) may cause a modest increase in serum creatinine and modest decrease in estimated creatinine clearance because of inhibition of tubular secretion of creatinine; there is a corresponding decrease in serum creatinine-based eGFR, but renal glomerular function is not affected. Elevated serum creatinine concentrations typically occurred within 2 weeks after the drug was initiated and generally were reversible after the drug was discontinued.

Assess serum creatinine, estimated creatinine clearance, urine glucose, and urine protein prior to initiating EVG/c/FTC/TAF and monitor routinely during treatment in all patients. In patients with chronic kidney disease, also assess serum phosphorus.

Patients with a confirmed increase in serum creatinine of greater than 0.4 mg/dL from baseline while receiving EVG/c/FTC/TAF should be closely monitored for renal toxicity. EVG/c/FTC/TAF should be discontinued in patients who develop clinically important decreases in renal function or evidence of Fanconi syndrome.

Patients receiving a tenofovir prodrug who have impaired renal function or are receiving a nephrotoxic agent (e.g., nonsteroidal anti-inflammatory agents [NSAIAs]) are at increased risk of developing adverse renal effects.

Lactic Acidosis and Severe Hepatomegaly with Steatosis

Lactic acidosis and severe hepatomegaly with steatosis, including fatalities, have been reported in patients receiving HIV nucleoside reverse transcriptase inhibitors (NRTIs), including emtricitabine and the tenofovir prodrug tenofovir DF, in conjunction with other antiretroviral agents.

EVG/c/FTC/TAF treatment should be interrupted in any patient who develops clinical or laboratory findings suggestive of lactic acidosis or pronounced hepatotoxicity (signs of hepatotoxicity may include hepatomegaly and steatosis even in the absence of marked increases in serum aminotransferase concentrations).

Use of Fixed Combinations

The usual cautions, precautions, contraindications, and interactions associated with each component of EVG/c/FTC/TAF should be considered. Cautionary information applicable to specific populations (e.g., pregnant or nursing women, individuals with hepatic or renal impairment, geriatric patients) should be considered for each drug in the fixed combination.

EVG/c/FTC/TAF is used alone as a complete regimen for the treatment of HIV-1 infection and should not be used in conjunction with other antiretroviral agents.

EVG/c/FTC/TAF should not be used concomitantly with any preparation that contains any of its components (elvitegravir, cobicistat, emtricitabine, tenofovir alafenamide). In addition, EVG/c/FTC/TAF should not be used concomitantly with any preparation containing tenofovir DF, lamivudine, adefovir dipivoxil, or ritonavir.

Immune Reconstitution Syndrome

Immune reconstitution syndrome has been reported in HIV-infected patients receiving multiple-drug antiretroviral therapy, including emtricitabine (a component of EVG/c/FTC/TAF). During the initial phase of treatment, HIV-infected patients whose immune systems respond to antiretroviral therapy may develop an inflammatory response to indolent or residual opportunistic infections (e.g., *Mycobacterium avium*, *M. tuberculosis*, cytomegalovirus [CMV], *Pneumocystis jirovecii* [formerly *P. carinii*]); such response may necessitate further evaluation and treatment.

Autoimmune disorders (e.g., Graves' disease, polymyositis, Guillain-Barré syndrome, autoimmune hepatitis) have also been reported to occur in the setting of immune reconstitution; however, the time to onset is more variable and can occur many months after initiation of antiretroviral therapy.

Specific Populations

Pregnancy

The use of EVG/c/FTC/TAF is not recommended during pregnancy due to substantially lower exposures of elvitegravir and cobicistat in the second and third trimesters.

The Antiretroviral Pregnancy Registry (APR) monitors pregnancy outcomes in women exposed to EVG/c/FTC/TAF during pregnancy. Clinicians are encouraged to register patients in the APR by calling 800-258-4263 or visiting https://www.apregistry.com/.

The overall risk of birth defects with EVG/c/FTC/TAF use in pregnancy was not markedly different compared to the background rate for major birth defects of 2.7% in the United States reference population of the Metropolitan Atlanta Congenital Defects Program (MACDP). Limitations of using an external comparator (the MACDP) includes differences in populations and methodology, and confounding due to the underlying disease. The rate of miscarriage is not reported in the APR.

Lactation

Elvitegravir and cobicistat are distributed into milk in rats. Tenofovir is distributed into milk in rats and rhesus monkey following administration of tenofovir DF; it is not known whether tenofovir alafenamide is distributed into animal milk. It is not known whether elvitegravir, cobicistat, or tenofovir alafenamide are distributed into human milk. Emtricitabine is distributed into human milk.

It is not known whether EVG/c/FTC/TAF affects human milk production or the breast-fed infant.

Because of the risk of adverse effects in the infant and the risk of HIV transmission, HIV-infected women should not breast-feed infants.

Pediatric Use

Safety and efficacy of EVG/c/FTC/TAF have not been established in pediatric patients weighing <25 kg.

Use of EVG/c/FTC/TAF in pediatric patients <18 years of age and weighing at least 25 kg is supported by studies in adults and by an open-label study in antiretroviral treatment-naïve HIV-1 infected pediatric patients 12 to <18 years of age weighing at least 35 kg and in virologically-suppressed pediatric patients 6 to <12 years of age weighing at least 25 kg.

Clinical trial data indicate that the safety and efficacy of EVG/c/FTC/TAF in HIV-1-infected, treatment-naïve pediatric patients 6 to <12 years of age weighing at least 25 kg is similar to that reported in antiretroviral naïve adults and adolescents with the exception of a decrease in baseline CD4+ count.

Geriatric Use

No differences in safety or efficacy of EVG/c/FTC/TAF have been observed between individuals 65 years of age and older and individuals 18 to less than 65 years of age.

Pharmacokinetics of EVG/c/FTC/TAF have not been fully evaluated in adults 65 years of age and older. Population pharmacokinetic analysis of EVG/c/FTC/TAF in HIV-infected individuals showed that age does not have a clinically important effect on tenofovir alafenamide exposures in adults up to 75 years of age.

Hepatic Impairment

Mild hepatic impairment (Child-Pugh class A) does not have a clinically important effect on the pharmacokinetics of tenofovir alafenamide. Moderate hepatic impairment (Child-Pugh class B) does not have a clinically important effect on the pharmacokinetics of elvitegravir, cobicistat, or tenofovir alafenamide and is not expected to affect the pharmacokinetics of emtricitabine.

EVG/c/FTC/TAF is *not* recommended in patients with severe hepatic impairment (Child-Pugh class C). Data are not available to date regarding the pharmacokinetics or safety of EVG/c/FTC/TAF in such patients.

Renal Impairment

The pharmacokinetics of EVG/c/FTC/TAF were evaluated in HIV-1 infected patients with mild to moderate renal impairment (estimated creatinine clearance of 30–69 mL/minute) and in HIV-1 infected patients with ESRD (estimated creatinine clearance of <15 mL/minute) receiving chronic hemodialysis. The pharmacokinetics of elvitegravir, cobicistat, and tenofovir alafenamide in these patients were similar to those in healthy subjects. Increased emtricitabine and tenofovir exposures in patients with renal impairment were not considered clinically relevant.

Not recommended in patients with severe renal impairment (estimated creatinine clearance of 15–29 mL/minute), or in patients with end-stage renal disease (ESRD) (estimated creatinine clearance <15 mL/minute) who are not receiving chronic hemodialysis.

● Common Adverse Effects

The most common adverse reaction (≥10%, all grades) is nausea.

DRUG INTERACTIONS

The following drug interactions are based on studies that used elvitegravir, elvitegravir administered with cobicistat (*cobicistat-boosted* elvitegravir), elvitegravir administered with low-dose ritonavir (*ritonavir-boosted* elvitegravir), cobicistat alone, or the fixed combination of elvitegravir, cobicistat, emtricitabine, and tenofovir alafenamide (EVG/c/FTC/TAF) or are predicted to occur.

Potential drug interactions associated with each drug in the fixed combination should be considered.

● Drugs Affecting or Metabolized by Hepatic Microsomal Enzymes

Elvitegravir is a substrate of cytochrome P-450 (CYP) 3A and a weak inducer and weak inhibitor of CYP3A; elvitegravir is an inducer of CYP2C9. The drug does not inhibit CYP1A, 2A6, 2C9, 2C19, 2D6, or 2E1 in vitro.

Cobicistat is a substrate of CYP3A and, to a minor extent, CYP2D6; cobicistat also is an inhibitor of CYP3A and 2D6.

Emtricitabine is not a substrate of CYP enzymes; emtricitabine does not inhibit CYP1A2, 2A6, 2B6, 2C9, 2C19, 2D6, or 3A4.

Tenofovir alafenamide is a weak inhibitor of CYP3A in vitro, but is not an inhibitor or inducer of CYP3A in vivo. Tenofovir alafenamide does not induce or inhibit other CYP enzymes, including CYP1A2, 2B6, 2C8, 2C9, 2C19, or 2D6.

Potential pharmacokinetic interactions if EVG/c/FTC/TAF is used concomitantly with drugs that are principally metabolized by CYP3A or 2D6 (increased plasma concentrations of the concomitant drug). Concomitant use of EVG/c/FTC/TAF with some drugs that are CYP3A substrates and for which elevated plasma concentrations are associated with serious and/or life-threatening events is contraindicated.

Potential pharmacokinetic interactions if EVG/c/FTC/TAF is used concomitantly with drugs that induce CYP3A (decreased plasma concentrations of elvitegravir, cobicistat, and tenofovir alafenamide; possible decreased antiretroviral efficacy and development of resistance). Concomitant use of EVG/c/FTC/TAF with some drugs that are potent inducers of CYP3A is contraindicated.

Potential pharmacokinetic interactions if EVG/c/FTC/TAF is used concomitantly with drugs that inhibit CYP3A (increased plasma concentrations of cobicistat).

● Drugs Affected by P-glycoprotein Transport

Cobicistat is an inhibitor of P-glycoprotein (P-gp) transport; tenofovir alafenamide is a substrate of P-gp.

Potential pharmacokinetic interactions if EVG/c/FTC/TAF is used concomitantly with drugs that are P-gp substrates (increased plasma concentrations of the concomitant drug).

Drugs that inhibit P-gp may increase absorption of tenofovir alafenamide. Cobicistat (a P-gp inhibitor) increases tenofovir alafenamide concentrations when the drugs are administered as the fixed combination EVG/c/FTC/TAF; further increases in tenofovir alafenamide concentrations are not expected if an additional P-gp inhibitor is used concomitantly with EVG/c/FTC/TAF.

Drugs that induce P-gp are expected to decrease absorption of tenofovir alafenamide, resulting in decreased plasma concentrations of tenofovir alafenamide.

● Drugs Affected by Breast Cancer Resistance Protein

Cobicistat is an inhibitor of breast cancer resistance protein (BCRP); tenofovir alafenamide is a substrate of BCRP.

Potential pharmacokinetic interactions if EVG/c/FTC/TAF is used concomitantly with drugs that are substrates for BCRP (increased plasma concentrations of the concomitant drug).

Drugs that inhibit BCRP may increase absorption of tenofovir alafenamide. Cobicistat (a BCRP inhibitor) increases tenofovir alafenamide concentrations when the drugs are administered as the fixed combination EVG/c/FTC/TAF; further increases in tenofovir alafenamide concentrations are not expected if an additional BCRP inhibitor is used concomitantly with EVG/c/FTC/TAF.

● Drugs Affected by Organic Anion Transport Polypeptides

Elvitegravir and cobicistat are inhibitors of organic anion transport polypeptides (OATP) 1B1 and 1B3; tenofovir alafenamide is a substrate of OATP1B1 and 1B3.

Potential pharmacokinetic interactions if EVG/c/FTC/TAF is used concomitantly with drugs that are substrates for OATP1B1 or 1B3 (increased plasma concentrations of the concomitant drug).

● *Drugs Metabolized by Uridine Diphosphate-glucuronosyltransferase*

Elvitegravir is partially metabolized by uridine diphosphate-glucuronosyltransferase (UGT) 1A1/3 enzymes. Tenofovir alafenamide does not inhibit UGT1A1.

● *Drugs Affecting Renal Function*

The emtricitabine and tenofovir components of EVG/c/FTC/TAF are principally excreted by the kidneys by a combination of glomerular filtration and active tubular secretion.

Potential pharmacokinetic interactions if EVG/c/FTC/TAF is used concomitantly with drugs that reduce renal function or compete for active tubular secretion (e.g., acyclovir, aminoglycosides [gentamicin], cidofovir, ganciclovir, valacyclovir, valganciclovir, high-dose or multiple nonsteroidal anti-inflammatory agents [NSAIAs]); may result in increased concentrations of emtricitabine, tenofovir, and/or the concomitant drug and may increase the risk of adverse effects.

● *Alfuzosin*

Potential pharmacokinetic interaction with alfuzosin (increased plasma concentrations of alfuzosin); may result in hypotension.

Concomitant use of alfuzosin and EVG/c/FTC/TAF is contraindicated.

● *Anticoagulants*

Apixaban, Dabigatran, Edoxaban, Rivaroxaban

Pharmacokinetic interactions are expected if apixaban, dabigatran, edoxaban, or rivaroxaban is used concomitantly with EVG/c/FTC/TAF (increased anticoagulant concentrations).

Due to an increased risk of bleeding, recommendations for the concomitant use of apixaban with EVG/c/FTC/TAF depend on the dosage of apixaban. Refer to apixaban prescribing information for dosing instructions on the concomitant use of apixaban with strong CYP3A and P-gp inhibitors.

Due to an increased risk of bleeding, dosing recommendations for the concomitant use of dabigatran and edoxaban with a P-gp inhibitor such as EVG/c/FTC/TAF are dependent upon underlying renal function and the indication for anticoagulant use. Refer to the prescribing information for the direct oral anticoagulant (DOAC) in use for dosage recommendations with a P-gp inhibitor.

Concomitant use of rivaroxaban with EVG/c/FTC/TAF is not recommended.

Warfarin

The effect of concomitant use of warfarin and EVG/c/FTC/TAF on the pharmacokinetics of warfarin is unknown.

If warfarin is used concomitantly with EVG/c/FTC/TAF, monitor the international normalized ratio (INR).

● *Anticonvulsants*

Carbamazepine, Phenobarbital, Phenytoin

Concomitant use of carbamazepine and *cobicistat-boosted* elvitegravir results in decreased elvitegravir plasma concentrations and area under the plasma concentration-time curve (AUC); increased carbamazepine plasma concentrations and AUC also occur. Potential pharmacokinetic interactions if carbamazepine, phenobarbital, or phenytoin is used concomitantly with EVG/c/FTC/TAF (decreased elvitegravir, cobicistat, and tenofovir alafenamide plasma concentrations with possible decreased antiretroviral efficacy and development of resistance).

Concomitant use of EVG/c/FTC/TAF and carbamazepine, phenobarbital, or phenytoin is contraindicated.

Ethosuximide

Potential pharmacokinetic interaction if ethosuximide is used concomitantly with EVG/c/FTC/TAF (increased ethosuximide plasma concentrations and decreased elvitegravir, cobicistat, and tenofovir alafenamide plasma concentrations).

If ethosuximide and EVG/c/FTC/TAF are used concomitantly, the patient should be monitored clinically.

Oxcarbazepine

Potential pharmacokinetic interaction if oxcarbazepine is used concomitantly with EVG/c/FTC/TAF (decreased elvitegravir, cobicistat, and tenofovir alafenamide plasma concentrations). An alternative anticonvulsant should be considered.

● *Antifungal Agents*

Itraconazole

Potential pharmacokinetic interactions with itraconazole (increased plasma concentrations of itraconazole, elvitegravir, and cobicistat).

If itraconazole and EVG/c/FTC/TAF are used concomitantly, itraconazole dosage should not exceed 200 mg daily.

Ketoconazole

Pharmacokinetic interactions with ketoconazole (increased plasma concentrations of ketoconazole, elvitegravir, and cobicistat).

If ketoconazole and EVG/c/FTC/TAF are used concomitantly, ketoconazole dosage should not exceed 200 mg daily.

Voriconazole

Potential pharmacokinetic interactions with voriconazole (increased plasma concentrations of voriconazole, elvitegravir, and cobicistat).

Voriconazole and EVG/c/FTC/TAF should not be used concomitantly unless potential benefits outweigh risks.

● *Antimycobacterial Agents*

Rifabutin

Pharmacokinetic interactions when *cobicistat-boosted* elvitegravir (elvitegravir 150 mg and cobicistat 150 mg once daily) was used concomitantly with rifabutin 150 mg once every other day (decreased elvitegravir plasma concentrations and AUC, increased 25-O-desacetyl-rifabutin concentrations and AUC relative to those achieved with rifabutin 300 mg once daily without concomitant *cobicistat-boosted* elvitegravir). Concomitant use of EVG/c/FTC/TAF also may decrease plasma concentrations of tenofovir alafenamide. Possible decreased antiretroviral efficacy and development of resistance.

Concomitant use of rifabutin and EVG/c/FTC/TAF is not recommended.

Rifampin

Potential pharmacokinetic interactions with rifampin (decreased elvitegravir, cobicistat, and tenofovir alafenamide plasma concentrations); possible decreased antiretroviral efficacy and development of resistance.

Concomitant use of rifampin and EVG/c/FTC/TAF is contraindicated.

Rifapentine

Potential pharmacokinetic interactions with rifapentine (decreased elvitegravir, cobicistat, and tenofovir alafenamide plasma concentrations); possible decreased antiretroviral efficacy and development of resistance.

Concomitant use of rifapentine and EVG/c/FTC/TAF is not recommended.

● *Antiplatelet Agents*

Clopidogrel, Prasugrel, Ticagrelor

Pharmacokinetic interactions are expected if clopidogrel or ticagrelor are used concomitantly with EVG/c/FTC/TAF (increased ticagrelor concentrations, decreased clopidogrel active metabolite concentrations).

Concomitant use of EVG/c/FTC/TAF and clopidogrel is not recommended due to the potential for decreased antiplatelet activity with clopidogrel.

Concomitant use of EVG/c/FTC/TAF and ticagrelor is not recommended.

Concomitant use of EVG/c/FTC/TAF and prasugrel is not expected to result in clinically important drug interactions.

● *Antipsychotic Agents*

Lurasidone

Concomitant use of lurasidone and EVG/c/FTC/TAF may result in serious and/or life-threatening reactions.

Concomitant use of lurasidone and EVG/c/FTC/TAF is contraindicated.

Perphenazine, Risperidone, Thioridazine

Potential pharmacokinetic interactions with antipsychotics, including perphenazine, risperidone, and thioridazine (increased antipsychotic plasma concentrations).

If EVG/c/FTC/TAF is used concomitantly with certain antipsychotics (e.g., perphenazine, risperidone, thioridazine), decreased dosage of the antipsychotic may be necessary.

Pimozide

Potential pharmacokinetic interaction with pimozide (increased pimozide plasma concentrations); potential for serious and/or life-threatening adverse effects (e.g., cardiac arrhythmias).

Concomitant use of pimozide and EVG/c/FTC/TAF is contraindicated.

Quetiapine

Pharmacokinetic interaction with quetiapine (increased quetiapine plasma concentrations expected).

Alternative antiretroviral therapy should be considered. If EVG/c/FTC/TAF is necessary in a patient receiving quetiapine, the quetiapine dosage should be reduced to one-sixth of the original dosage and the patient monitored for quetiapine-associated adverse effects.

● *Antiretroviral Agents*

EVG/c/FTC/TAF should not be used in conjunction with any other antiretroviral agents.

HIV Integrase Inhibitors (INSTIs)

EVG/c/FTC/TAF contains elvitegravir and should not be used concomitantly with any preparation containing elvitegravir.

HIV Nucleoside and Nucleotide Reverse Transcriptase Inhibitors (NRTIs)

Emtricitabine

EVG/c/FTC/TAF contains emtricitabine and should not be used concomitantly with any preparation containing emtricitabine.

Lamivudine

EVG/c/FTC/TAF and lamivudine (or preparations containing lamivudine) should not be used concomitantly.

Tenofovir Disoproxil Fumarate

EVG/c/FTC/TAF and tenofovir disoproxil fumarate (tenofovir DF) (or preparations containing tenofovir DF) should not be used concomitantly.

HIV Protease Inhibitors (PIs)

Ritonavir

EVG/c/FTC/TAF and ritonavir (or preparations containing ritonavir) should not be used concomitantly.

● *β-Adrenergic Blocking Agents*

Potential pharmacokinetic interactions with β-adrenergic blocking agents, including metoprolol and timolol (increased β-adrenergic blocking agent plasma concentrations).

If EVG/c/FTC/TAF is used concomitantly with a β-adrenergic blocking agent, patients should be monitored clinically and decreased dosage of the β-adrenergic blocking agent may be necessary.

● *Benzodiazepines*

Diazepam

Potential pharmacokinetic interaction with diazepam (increased diazepam plasma concentrations).

Concomitant use of diazepam and EVG/c/FTC/TAF should be undertaken in a monitored setting where respiratory depression and/or prolonged sedation can be managed.

Midazolam or Triazolam

Potential pharmacokinetic interaction with midazolam or triazolam (increased benzodiazepine plasma concentrations); potential for serious and/or life-threatening adverse effects (e.g., prolonged or increased sedation or respiratory depression).

Concomitant use of oral midazolam or triazolam with EVG/c/FTC/TAF is contraindicated.

Concomitant use of parenteral midazolam and EVG/c/FTC/TAF should be undertaken in a monitored setting where respiratory depression and/or prolonged sedation can be managed. In addition, use of a reduced midazolam dosage should be considered, especially if more than a single dose of the drug will be administered.

Other Benzodiazepines

Potential pharmacokinetic interactions with clorazepate, estazolam, or flurazepam (increased benzodiazepine plasma concentrations).

● *Bosentan*

Potential pharmacokinetic interaction with bosentan (increased bosentan plasma concentrations).

In patients who have already been receiving EVG/c/FTC/TAF for at least 10 days, bosentan should be initiated using a dosage of 62.5 mg once daily or every other day based on individual tolerability.

In patients who have already been receiving bosentan, bosentan should be discontinued for at least 36 hours prior to initiating EVG/c/FTC/TAF; after at least 10 days of EVG/c/FTC/TAF therapy, bosentan can be resumed using a dosage of 62.5 mg once daily or every other day based on individual tolerability.

● *Bupropion*

Potential pharmacokinetic interaction with bupropion (increased bupropion plasma concentrations).

If bupropion is used concomitantly with EVG/c/FTC/TAF, dosage of the antidepressant should be titrated carefully while monitoring for antidepressant response.

● *Buspirone*

Potential pharmacokinetic interaction with buspirone (increased buspirone plasma concentrations).

If buspirone is used concomitantly with EVG/c/FTC/TAF, patients should be monitored clinically; reduced buspirone dosage may be necessary.

● *Calcium-channel Blocking Agents*

Potential pharmacokinetic interactions with calcium-channel blocking agents, including amlodipine, diltiazem, felodipine, nicardipine, nifedipine, and verapamil (increased plasma concentrations of the calcium-channel blocking agent).

Calcium-channel blocking agents and EVG/c/FTC/TAF should be used concomitantly with caution; the patient should be clinically monitored.

● *Calcium, Iron, Multivitamins, and Other Preparations Containing Polyvalent Cations*

Oral calcium supplements, oral iron preparations, other oral supplements containing calcium, iron, aluminum, magnesium, or zinc (e.g., multivitamins), and laxatives, buffered medications, sucralfate, or other preparations containing polyvalent cations may decrease plasma concentrations of elvitegravir when used concomitantly. Separate administration of medications, antacids, and oral supplements containing polyvalent cations from EVG/c/FTC/TAF administration by at least 2 hours.

● *Cardiac Drugs*
Antiarrhythmic Agents
Potential pharmacokinetic interactions if EVG/c/FTC/TAF is used with certain antiarrhythmic agents (e.g., amiodarone, bepridil [no longer commercially available in the US], disopyramide, dronedarone, flecainide, lidocaine [systemic], mexiletine, propafenone, quinidine) (increased plasma concentrations of the antiarrhythmic agent). Concomitant use of digoxin (single 0.5-mg dose) and cobicistat (150 mg once daily) has resulted in increased plasma concentrations of digoxin.

EVG/c/FTC/TAF and antiarrhythmic agents or digoxin should be used concomitantly with caution; plasma concentrations of the antiarrhythmic agents or cardiac glycoside should be monitored, if possible.

● *Cisapride*
Potential pharmacokinetic interaction with cisapride (increased cisapride plasma concentrations); potential for serious and/or life-threatening adverse effects (e.g., cardiac arrhythmias).

Concomitant use of cisapride and EVG/c/FTC/TAF is contraindicated.

● *Cobicistat*
Pharmacokinetic interaction with elvitegravir (increased plasma concentrations and AUC of elvitegravir); occurs because cobicistat inhibits CYP3A. Cobicistat acts as a pharmacokinetic enhancer when used concomitantly with elvitegravir (*cobicistat-boosted* elvitegravir) and is used to therapeutic advantage in the EVG/c/FTC/TAF fixed combination.

Pharmacokinetic interaction with tenofovir alafenamide (increased tenofovir alafenamide plasma concentrations and AUC).

Cobicistat does not antagonize the antiretroviral effects of elvitegravir, emtricitabine, or tenofovir.

● *Colchicine*
Potential pharmacokinetic interaction with colchicine (increased colchicine plasma concentrations).

Colchicine and EVG/c/FTC/TAF should not be used concomitantly in patients with renal or hepatic impairment.

When colchicine is used for *treatment* of gout flares in patients receiving EVG/c/FTC/TAF, an initial colchicine dose of 0.6 mg should be given followed by 0.3 mg 1 hour later; the colchicine course should be repeated no earlier than 3 days later.

When colchicine is used for *prophylaxis* of gout flares in patients receiving EVG/c/FTC/TAF, colchicine dosage should be reduced to 0.3 mg once daily in those originally receiving 0.6 mg twice daily or decreased to 0.3 mg once every other day in those originally receiving 0.6 mg once daily.

When colchicine is used for treatment of familial Mediterranean fever (FMF) in patients receiving EVG/c/FTC/TAF, a maximum colchicine dosage of 0.6 mg daily (may be given as 0.3 mg twice daily) should be used.

● *Corticosteroids*
Corticosteroids Affected by Potent CYP3A Inhibition
Concomitant use of EVG/c/FTC/TAF and corticosteroids via all routes of administration whose exposures are substantially affected by potent CYP3A inhibitors (e.g., betamethasone, budesonide, ciclesonide, fluticasone, methylprednisolone, mometasone, triamcinolone) may increase plasma concentrations of the corticosteroid, which may result in adrenal insufficiency or Cushing syndrome. Alternative corticosteroids (e.g., beclomethasone, prednisone, prednisolone) less affected by CYP3A inhibition relative to other corticosteroids should be considered in patients receiving EVG/c/FTC/TAF, particularly if long-term corticosteroid therapy is required.

Dexamethasone
Concomitant use of systemic dexamethasone or other systemic corticosteroids that induce CYP3A may decrease elvitegravir and cobicistat plasma concentrations and may lead to decreased antiretroviral efficacy and development of resistance to elvitegravir.

An alternative corticosteroid should be considered in patients receiving EVG/c/FTC/TAF.

● *Ergot Alkaloids*
Potential for serious and/or life-threatening adverse effects (e.g., peripheral vasospasm, ischemia of the extremities and other tissues) if EVG/c/FTC/TAF is used concomitantly with ergot alkaloids (e.g., dihydroergotamine, ergotamine, methylergonovine).

Concomitant use of ergot alkaloids and EVG/c/FTC/TAF is contraindicated.

● *Estrogens and Progestins*
Pharmacokinetic interactions are possible with oral contraceptives containing ethinyl estradiol and norgestimate (decreased ethinyl estradiol plasma concentrations and increased norgestimate plasma concentrations).

Effects of increased norgestimate plasma concentrations are not established, but may include increased risk of insulin resistance, dyslipidemia, acne, and venous thrombosis. The potential risks and benefits of concomitant use of EVG/c/FTC/TAF and oral contraceptives containing ethinyl estradiol and norgestimate should be considered, particularly in women with risk factors for these effects.

Pharmacokinetic interactions are possible with oral contraceptives containing ethinyl estradiol and drospirenone (decreased ethinyl estradiol plasma concentrations and increased drospirenone plasma concentrations). Clinical monitoring is recommended due to an increased risk for hyperkalemia.

Pharmacokinetic interactions are possible with contraceptives containing levonorgestrel (increased plasma concentrations of levonorgestrel).

Concomitant use of EVG/c/FTC/TAF with oral contraceptives containing progestins other than drosperinone, levonorgestrel, and norgestimate or with other hormonal contraceptives (e.g., transdermal contraceptive systems, vaginal ring, injections) have not been studied; alternative nonhormonal methods of contraception should be considered when estrogen-based contraceptives are used.

Additional or nonhormonal methods of contraception should be used when estrogen-based contraceptives are used concomitantly with EVG/c/FTC/TAF.

● *GI Drugs*
Antacids
Antacids containing aluminum, calcium, and/or magnesium decrease plasma concentrations and AUC of elvitegravir.

EVG/c/FTC/TAF should be given at least 2 hours before or at least 2 hours after antacids containing aluminum, calcium, or magnesium.

Histamine H$_2$-receptor Antagonists
Concomitant use of famotidine and *cobicistat-boosted* elvitegravir did not have a clinically important effect on elvitegravir plasma concentrations or AUC.

Concomitant use of EVG/c/FTC/TAF and famotidine is not expected to result in clinically important drug interactions.

Proton-pump Inhibitors
Concomitant use of omeprazole and *cobicistat-boosted* elvitegravir did not result in clinically important alterations in elvitegravir pharmacokinetics.

Concomitant use of EVG/c/FTC/TAF and proton-pump inhibitors is not expected to result in clinically important drug interactions.

● *HCV Antivirals*
HCV Polymerase Inhibitors
Sofosbuvir
Clinically important pharmacokinetic interactions are not expected if EVG/c/FTC/TAF is used concomitantly with sofosbuvir.

Sofosbuvir and Velpatasvir
No clinically important pharmacokinetic interactions were observed when EVG/c/FTC/TAF was used concomitantly with sofosbuvir or velpatasvir.

Concomitant use of the fixed combination of sofosbuvir and velpatasvir (sofosbuvir/velpatasvir) with *cobicistat-boosted* elvitegravir or with tenofovir alafenamide did not have a clinically important effect on elvitegravir or tenofovir alafenamide concentrations.

Sofosbuvir, Velpatasvir, and Voxilaprevir

Clinically important pharmacokinetic interactions are not expected if EVG/c/FTC/TAF is used concomitantly with the fixed combination of sofosbuvir/velpatasvir/voxilaprevir.

HCV Replication Complex Inhibitors
Ledipasvir, Sofosbuvir, and Voxilaprevir

Concomitant use of the fixed combination of ledipasvir, sofosbuvir, and voxilaprevir (ledipasvir/sofosbuvir/voxilaprevir) with *cobicistat-boosted* elvitegravir or with tenofovir alafenamide does not have a clinically important effect on elvitegravir or tenofovir alafenamide concentrations.

Clinically important pharmacokinetic interactions are not expected if EVG/c/FTC/TAF is used concomitantly with ledipasvir, sofosbuvir, or voxilaprevir.

● HMG-CoA Reductase Inhibitors

Concomitant use of certain hydroxymethylglutaryl-CoA (HMG-CoA) reductase inhibitors (statins) metabolized by CYP3A (e.g., atorvastatin, lovastatin, simvastatin) and EVG/c/FTC/TAF may increase plasma concentrations of the HMG-CoA reductase inhibitor resulting in increased effects and increased risk of statin-associated adverse effects, including myopathy and rhabdomyolysis.

Atorvastatin

If atorvastatin is used concomitantly with EVG/c/FTC/TAF, the statin should be initiated at the lowest dosage and titrated carefully while monitoring for atorvastatin-associated adverse effects. Do not exceed a dosage of atorvastatin 20 mg daily with concomitant EVG/c/FTC/TAF therapy.

Lovastatin

Concomitant use of lovastatin and EVG/c/FTC/TAF is contraindicated.

Rosuvastatin

Pharmacokinetic interaction when rosuvastatin is used concomitantly with *cobicistat-boosted* elvitegravir (increased rosuvastatin plasma concentrations and AUC; no clinically important effect on elvitegravir pharmacokinetics).

Simvastatin

Concomitant use of simvastatin and EVG/c/FTC/TAF is contraindicated.

● Immunosuppressive Agents
Cyclosporine

Potential pharmacokinetic interactions with cyclosporine (increased plasma concentrations of cyclosporine, elvitegravir, and cobicistat).

If EVG/c/FTC/TAF is used concomitantly with cyclosporine, plasma concentrations of the immunosuppressive agent should be monitored and the patient monitored for adverse effects associated with EVG/c/FTC/TAF.

Everolimus, Sirolimus, or Tacrolimus

Potential pharmacokinetic interactions with everolimus, sirolimus, or tacrolimus (increased plasma concentrations of the immunosuppressant agent).

If EVG/c/FTC/TAF is used concomitantly with everolimus, sirolimus or tacrolimus, plasma concentrations of the immunosuppressive agent should be monitored.

● Lomitapide

Concomitant use of lomitapide and EVG/c/FTC/TAF is contraindicated due to the potential for marked increases in transaminase levels.

● Macrolides
Clarithromycin

Potential pharmacokinetic interactions if EVG/c/FTC/TAF is used concomitantly with clarithromycin (increased plasma concentrations of the macrolide and cobicistat).

Modification of the usual dosage of clarithromycin is not necessary in those with creatinine clearances of 60 mL/minute or greater; however, clarithromycin dosage should be reduced by 50% in those with creatinine clearances of 50–60 mL/minute.

● Nucleoside and Nucleotide Antivirals

Potential pharmacokinetic interactions if EVG/c/FTC/TAF is used concomitantly with drugs that compete for active tubular secretion, including acyclovir, cidofovir, ganciclovir, valacyclovir, and valganciclovir; increased plasma concentrations of certain components of EVG/c/FTC/TAF (i.e., emtricitabine, tenofovir) or the concomitant drug may occur and increase the risk of adverse effects.

Adefovir

EVG/c/FTC/TAF should not be used concomitantly with adefovir dipivoxil.

Entecavir or Famciclovir

Clinically important interactions are not expected if EVG/c/FTC/TAF is used concomitantly with entecavir or famciclovir.

Ribavirin

Clinically important interactions are not expected if EVG/c/FTC/TAF is used concomitantly with ribavirin.

● Opiate Agonists, Opiate Partial Agonists, and Opiate Antagonists
Buprenorphine

Concomitant use of the fixed combination of buprenorphine and naloxone (buprenorphine/naloxone) with *cobicistat-boosted* elvitegravir increased plasma concentrations and AUC of buprenorphine and norbuprenorphine and decreased peak plasma concentrations and AUC of naloxone.

If buprenorphine/naloxone is used concomitantly with EVG/c/FTC/TAF, dosage adjustments are not necessary; however, patients should be monitored closely for sedation and adverse cognitive effects.

Fentanyl

Potential pharmacokinetics interactions with fentanyl (increased fentanyl plasma concentrations. If fentanyl and EVG/c/FTC/TAF are used concomitantly, carefully monitor for therapeutic and adverse effects of fentanyl.

Methadone

Concomitant use of methadone and *cobicistat-boosted* elvitegravir did not result in clinically important alterations in methadone pharmacokinetics.

Concomitant use of methadone and EVG/c/FTC/TAF is not expected to result in clinically important drug interactions.

Tramadol

Potential pharmacokinetics interactions with tramadol (increased tramadol plasma concentrations). A dose decrease of tramadol may be necessary if used concomitantly with EVG/c/FTC/TAF.

● Phosphodiesterase Type 5 Inhibitors

Concomitant use of EVG/c/FTC/TAF and selective phosphodiesterase type 5 (PDE5) inhibitors (e.g., sildenafil, tadalafil, vardenafil) is expected to result in increased plasma concentrations of the PDE5 inhibitor and increase the risk of adverse effects (e.g., hypotension, syncope, visual disturbances, priapism) associated with these agents.

Sildenafil

Concomitant use of EVG/c/FTC/TAF is contraindicated in patients receiving sildenafil for treatment of pulmonary arterial hypertension (PAH).

If sildenafil is used for treatment of erectile dysfunction in a patient receiving EVG/c/FTC/TAF, sildenafil dosage should not exceed 25 mg once every 48 hours and the patient should be monitored for sildenafil-related adverse effects.

Tadalafil

If tadalafil is used for treatment of PAH in a patient who has been receiving EVG/c/FTC/TAF for at least 1 week, tadalafil should be initiated at a dosage of 20 mg once daily and, if tolerated, dosage may be increased to 40 mg once daily. EVG/c/FTC/TAF should not be initiated in patients receiving tadalafil for treatment of PAH; tadalafil should be discontinued for at least 24 hours prior to initiating EVG/c/FTC/TAF. After at least 1 week, tadalafil may be resumed at a dosage of 20 mg once daily and, if tolerated, dosage may be increased to 40 mg once daily.

If tadalafil is used for treatment of erectile dysfunction in a patient receiving EVG/c/FTC/TAF, tadalafil dosage should not exceed 10 mg once every 72 hours and the patient should be monitored for tadalafil-related adverse effects.

Vardenafil

If vardenafil is used for treatment of erectile dysfunction in a patient receiving EVG/c/FTC/TAF, vardenafil dosage should not exceed 2.5 mg once every 72 hours and the patient should be monitored for vardenafil-related adverse effects.

● Salmeterol

Potential pharmacokinetic interaction with salmeterol (increased salmeterol plasma concentrations); may result in increased risk of salmeterol-associated adverse cardiovascular effects, including QT interval prolongation, palpitations, and sinus tachycardia.

Concomitant use of salmeterol and EVG/c/FTC/TAF is not recommended.

● Selective Serotonin-reuptake Inhibitors (SSRIs)

Potential pharmacokinetic interaction with SSRIs (increased SSRI plasma concentrations). However, clinically important interactions are not expected if EVG/c/FTC/TAF is used concomitantly with sertraline.

If an SSRI is used concomitantly with EVG/c/FTC/TAF, dosage of the SSRI should be carefully titrated and antidepressant response monitored.

● Trazodone

Potential pharmacokinetic interaction with trazodone (increased trazodone plasma concentrations).

If trazodone is used concomitantly with EVG/c/FTC/TAF, dosage of trazodone should be carefully titrated and antidepressant response monitored.

● Tricyclic Antidepressants

Potential pharmacokinetic interactions if EVG/c/FTC/TAF is used concomitantly with tricyclic antidepressants, including amitriptyline, desipramine, doxepin, imipramine, and nortriptyline (increased tricyclic antidepressant plasma concentrations). Increased desipramine plasma concentrations and AUC reported when used concomitantly with *cobicistat-boosted* elvitegravir.

If a tricyclic antidepressant is used concomitantly with EVG/c/FTC/TAF, the lowest initial dosage of the tricyclic antidepressant should be used and dosage of the antidepressant should be carefully titrated according to clinical response.

● Zolpidem

Possible pharmacokinetic interaction with zolpidem (increased zolpidem plasma concentrations).

If zolpidem is used concomitantly with EVG/c/FTC/TAF, patients should be monitored clinically; reduced zolpidem dosage may be necessary.

● Dietary and Herbal Supplements

St. John's Wort

Potential pharmacokinetic interactions with St. John's wort (*Hypericum perforatum*) (decreased elvitegravir, cobicistat, and tenofovir alafenamide plasma concentrations); possible decreased antiretroviral efficacy and development of resistance.

Concomitant use of St. John's wort and EVG/c/FTC/TAF is contraindicated.

DESCRIPTION

The fixed combination of elvitegravir, cobicistat, emtricitabine, and tenofovir alafenamide (EVG/c/FTC/TAF) contains a human immunodeficiency virus (HIV) integrase strand transfer inhibitor (INSTI) antiretroviral (elvitegravir; EVG), a pharmacokinetic enhancer (cobicistat), an HIV nucleoside reverse transcriptase inhibitor (NRTI) antiretroviral (emtricitabine; FTC), and a nucleotide reverse transcriptase inhibitor antiretroviral classified as an HIV NRTI (tenofovir alafenamide; TAF). Cobicistat, a potent cytochrome P-450 (CYP) 3A inhibitor, is included in the fixed combination to increase plasma concentrations of elvitegravir (*cobicistat-boosted* elvitegravir).

Elvitegravir inhibits the activity of HIV-1 integrase, an enzyme that integrates HIV DNA into the host cell genome. Integration is required for viral replication. Inhibition of integration prevents propagation of viral infection. Elvitegravir is active against HIV-1 and also has some in vitro activity against HIV type 2 (HIV-2); the drug does not have activity against hepatitis B virus (HBV) or hepatitis C virus (HCV).

Cobicistat is a mechanism-based inhibitor of CYP3A and decreases metabolism and increases plasma concentrations of CYP3A substrates; cobicistat also is a weak inhibitor of CYP2D6, but does not inhibit CYP1A2, 2C9, or 2C19. Cobicistat is included in EVG/c/FTC/TAF for therapeutic advantage and acts as a pharmacokinetic enhancer to decrease elvitegravir metabolism and increase plasma concentrations of the drug (*cobicistat-boosted* elvitegravir). Cobicistat does not have any antiretroviral or antiviral activity and is not active against HIV-1, HBV, or HCV; cobicistat does not antagonize the antiretroviral activity of elvitegravir, emtricitabine, or tenofovir.

Emtricitabine is inactive until converted intracellularly to an active 5′-triphosphate metabolite. After conversion to the pharmacologically active metabolite, the drug acts as a reverse transcriptase inhibitor antiretroviral. Emtricitabine is active against HIV-1 and also has some in vitro activity against HIV-2.

Tenofovir alafenamide is a tenofovir prodrug and is inactive until hydrolyzed intracellularly by cathepsin A to form tenofovir and subsequently metabolized by cellular kinases to the active metabolite (tenofovir diphosphate). After conversion to the pharmacologically active metabolite, the drug acts as a reverse transcriptase inhibitor antiretroviral. Tenofovir alafenamide is more stable in blood and plasma and more efficiently converted intracellularly to tenofovir diphosphate than the tenofovir prodrug tenofovir disoproxil fumarate (tenofovir DF; TDF), resulting in higher concentrations of the active metabolite within HIV target cells and lower circulating concentrations of tenofovir than those reported with tenofovir DF. Tenofovir is active against HIV-1 and also has some in vitro activity against HIV-2; the drug also is active against HBV.

HIV-1 resistant to elvitegravir, emtricitabine, or tenofovir have been produced in vitro and has emerged during EVG/c/FTC/TAF therapy. In clinical trials evaluating EVG/c/FTC/TAF in antiretroviral-naïve patients, genotypic resistance to elvitegravir, emtricitabine, and/or tenofovir was identified in patients who received EVG/c/FTC/TAF and were considered to be virologic treatment failures. Cross-resistance between elvitegravir and other HIV INSTIs (e.g., dolutegravir, raltegravir) has been reported. Cross-resistance also occurs among the HIV NRTIs.

Following an oral dose of EVG/c/FTC/TAF, peak plasma concentrations of elvitegravir and cobicistat occur at 4 and 3 hours, respectively, and peak plasma concentrations of emtricitabine and tenofovir occur at 3 and 1 hours, respectively. Administration of EVG/c/FTC/TAF with a high-fat meal (approximately 800 kcal, 50% fat) increases mean systemic exposures of elvitegravir by 87% compared with administration in the fasting state; changes in mean systemic exposures of cobicistat, emtricitabine, and tenofovir alafenamide are not clinically important compared with administration in the fasting state. Elvitegravir and cobicistat are approximately 99 and 98% bound to plasma proteins, respectively; emtricitabine and tenofovir alafenamide are less than 4% and approximately 80% bound to plasma proteins, respectively. Elvitegravir is metabolized principally by CYP3A isoenzymes, but also undergoes glucuronidation via uridine diphosphate-glucuronsyltransferase (UGT) 1A1/3 enzymes. Cobicistat is metabolized by CYP3A and, to a minor extent, by CYP2D6. Emtricitabine is not substantially metabolized. Tenofovir alafenamide is hydrolyzed intracellularly in peripheral blood mononuclear cells and macrophages by cathepsin A to form tenofovir (the major metabolite); in vitro, tenofovir alafenamide also is converted to tenofovir by carboxylesterase 1 in hepatocytes. Tenofovir alafenamide is metabolized by CYP3A to a minor extent. Elvitegravir and cobicistat are principally excreted in feces (94.8 and 86.2% of a dose, respectively) and to a lesser extent in urine (6.7 and 8.2% of a dose, respectively). Emtricitabine is principally excreted in urine (70% of a dose) and to a lesser extent in feces (13.7% of a dose). Following a single dose of tenofovir alafenamide, 31.7% is excreted in feces and less than 1% is excreted in urine. The median terminal plasma half-lives of elvitegravir, cobicistat, emtricitabine, and tenofovir alafenamide are 12.9, 3.5, 10, and 0.51 hours, respectively. The half-life of tenofovir diphosphate, the active metabolite of tenofovir alafenamide, is 150–180 hours within peripheral blood mononuclear cells.

ADVICE TO PATIENTS

- Advise patients of the critical nature of compliance with HIV therapy and importance of remaining under the care of a clinician. Importance of taking the fixed combination of elvitegravir, cobicistat, emtricitabine, and tenofovir alafenamide (EVG/c/FTC/TAF) as prescribed; do not alter or discontinue antiretroviral regimen without consulting clinician.

- Advise patients that EVG/c/FTC/TAF is a complete regimen for treatment of HIV-1 infection and should not be used in conjunction with other antiretroviral agents.

- Advise patients of the importance of taking EVG/c/FTC/TAF with food.

- Inform patients that testing for hepatitis B virus (HBV) infection is recommended before antiretroviral therapy is initiated. Also advise patients that severe acute exacerbations of HBV infection have been reported following discontinuance of emtricitabine and/or tenofovir DF in HIV-infected patients coinfected with HBV and may occur with EVG/c/FTC/TAF.

- Advise patients that renal impairment, including cases of acute renal failure or Fanconi syndrome, has occurred. Importance of not using EVG/c/FTC/TAF concomitantly with or shortly after nephrotoxic agents (e.g., high-dose or multiple nonsteroidal anti-inflammatory agents [NSAIAs]).

- Advise patients of reproductive potential that additional or nonhormonal methods of contraception should be used when estrogen-based contraceptives are used concomitantly with EVG/c/FTC/TDF.

- Advise patients that lactic acidosis and severe hepatomegaly with steatosis, including fatalities, have occurred in patients receiving HIV nucleoside reverse transcriptase inhibitors (NRTIs), including emtricitabine and/or tenofovir disoproxil fumarate (tenofovir DF), in conjunction with other antiretrovirals. Importance of contacting clinician if symptoms suggestive of lactic acidosis or pronounced hepatotoxicity (e.g., nausea, vomiting, unusual/unexpected stomach discomfort, weakness) occur.

- Advise patients that signs and symptoms of inflammation from previous infections may occur soon after initiation of antiretroviral therapy in some individuals with advanced HIV infection (AIDS). These symptoms may be due to an improvement in immune response, enabling the body to fight infections that may have been present with no obvious symptoms. Importance of immediately informing a healthcare provider if any symptoms of infection occur.

- Advise patients to inform their clinician of existing or contemplated concomitant therapy, including prescription and OTC drugs and dietary or herbal supplements, as well as any concomitant illnesses.

- Advise women to inform clinicians if they are or plan to become pregnant or plan to breast-feed. Advise HIV-infected women not to breast-feed.

- Advise patients of other important precautionary information.

PREPARATIONS

Excipients in commercially available drug preparations may have clinically important effects in some individuals; consult specific product labeling for details.

Elvitegravir, Cobicistat, Emtricitabine, and Tenofovir Alafenamide Fumarate

Oral

Tablets, film-coated	Elvitegravir 150 mg, Cobicistat 150 mg, Emtricitabine 200 mg, and Tenofovir Alafenamide Fumarate 10 mg (of tenofovir alafenamide)	Genvoya®, Gilead

† Use is not currently included in the labeling approved by the US Food and Drug Administration.

Elvitegravir, Cobicistat, Emtricitabine, and Tenofovir Disoproxil Fumarate

8:18.08.12 · HIV INTEGRASE INHIBITORS

■ Elvitegravir, cobicistat, emtricitabine, and tenofovir disoproxil fumarate (EVG/c/FTC/TDF) is a fixed-combination antiretroviral agent containing elvitegravir (human immunodeficiency virus [HIV] integrase strand transfer inhibitor [INSTI]), cobicistat (pharmacokinetic enhancer), emtricitabine (HIV nucleoside reverse transcriptase inhibitor), and tenofovir disoproxil fumarate (HIV nucleotide reverse transcriptase inhibitor). Cobicistat, a mechanism-based cytochrome P-450 (CYP) 3A inhibitor, is included in the fixed combination to increase plasma concentrations of elvitegravir (*cobicistat-boosted* elvitegravir) and is not active against HIV.

USES

● **Treatment of HIV Infection**

The fixed combination of elvitegravir, cobicistat, emtricitabine, and tenofovir disoproxil fumarate (tenofovir DF) (EVG/c/FTC/TDF) is used as a complete regimen for the treatment of human immunodeficiency virus type 1 (HIV-1) infection in adults and pediatric patients 12 years of age and older weighing ≥35 kg who have no antiretroviral treatment history or to replace the current antiretroviral regimen in patients who are virologically suppressed (HIV-1 RNA <50 copies/mL) on a stable antiretroviral regimen for at least 6 months with no history of treatment failure and no known substitutions associated with resistance to the individual components of EVG/c/FTC/TDF. The fixed-dose combination of EVG/c/FTC/TDF is among alternative regimens recommended in guidelines for treatment of HIV in adults and sexually mature adolescent patients, but is *not* recommended in pregnant patients. Selection of an initial antiretroviral regimen should be individualized based on factors such as virologic efficacy, toxicity, pill burden, dosing frequency, drug-drug interaction potential, resistance test results, comorbid conditions, access, and cost.

Clinical Experience

Antiretroviral-naïve Adults

The comparative efficacy and safety of EVG/c/FTC/TDF and the fixed combination of efavirenz, emtricitabine, and tenofovir DF (EFV/FTC/TDF) were evaluated in a randomized, active-control, phase 3 study in antiretroviral-naïve HIV-infected adults (study 102). All patients had baseline HIV-1 RNA ≥5000 copies/mL, baseline creatinine clearance ≥70 mL/minute, and were randomized to receive EVG/c/FTC/TDF (elvitegravir 150 mg, cobicistat 150 mg, emtricitabine 200 mg, tenofovir DF 300 mg) once daily with food or EFV/FTC/TDF (efavirenz 600 mg, emtricitabine 200 mg, tenofovir DF 300 mg) once daily in the fasting state. Among 700 patients enrolled in study 102, the mean age was 38 years, 89% were male, 63% were white, 28% were Black, 2% were Asian, 24% were Hispanic; mean baseline HIV-1 RNA was 4.8 $\log_{10}$ copies/mL, and mean baseline CD4+ T-cell count was 386 cells/mm³. At 144 weeks, 80% of those receiving EVG/c/FTC/TDF had HIV-1 RNA <50 copies/mL compared with 75% of those receiving EFV/FTC/TDF. The mean increase in CD4+ T-cell count from baseline was 298 cells/mm³ in those receiving EVG/c/FTC/TDF compared with 272 cells/mm³ in those receiving EFV/FTC/TDF.

In a similarly designed phase 3 study, the comparative efficacy and safety of EVG/c/FTC/TDF and a regimen of ritonavir-boosted atazanavir in conjunction with tenofovir DF and emtricitabine was evaluated in antiretroviral-naïve HIV-infected adults (study 103). All patients had baseline HIV-1 RNA ≥5000 copies/mL, baseline creatinine clearance ≥70 mL/minute, and were randomized to receive EVG/c/FTC/TDF (elvitegravir 150 mg, cobicistat 150 mg, emtricitabine 200 mg,

tenofovir DF 300 mg) once daily with food or atazanavir 300 mg and ritonavir 100 mg in conjunction with the fixed combination of emtricitabine 200 mg and tenofovir DF 300 mg (FTC/TDF) once daily with food. Among 708 patients enrolled in study 103, the mean age was 38 years, 90% were male, 74% were white, 17% were Black, 5% were Asian, 16% were Hispanic, mean baseline HIV-1 RNA was 4.8 $\log_{10}$ copies/mL, and mean baseline CD4+ T-cell count was 370 cells/mm³. At 144 weeks, 78% of those receiving EVG/c/FTC/TDF had HIV-1 RNA <50 copies/mL compared with 75% of those receiving ritonavir-boosted atazanavir with FTC/TDF. The mean increase in CD4+ T-cell count from baseline was 261 cells/mm³ in those receiving EVG/c/FTC/TDF compared with 269 cells/mm³ in those receiving ritonavir-boosted atazanavir with FTC/TDF.

Antiretroviral-experienced Adults

The comparative efficacy and safety of EVG/c/FTC/TDF and an HIV protease inhibitor (PI)-based regimen in antiretroviral-experienced, virologically suppressed (HIV-1 RNA <50 copies/mL) adults were evaluated in a randomized, open-label, phase 3b noninferiority study (study 115; STRATEGY-PI). Among 433 patients enrolled in study 115, the mean age was 41 years, 86% were male, 80% were white, 15% were Black, and mean baseline CD4+ T-cell count was 610 cells/mm³. At initial screening, all patients were receiving either their first or second antiretroviral regimen with no history of virologic failure, had no current evidence or history of resistance to the antiretroviral components of EVG/c/FTC/TDF, and had been receiving a ritonavir-boosted HIV PI (40% atazanavir, 40% darunavir, 17% lopinavir, 3% fosamprenavir, <1% saquinavir) in conjunction with the fixed combination of emtricitabine 200 mg and tenofovir DF 300 mg (FTC/TDF) for at least 6 months. Patients were randomized in a 2:1 ratio to either switch to EVG/c/FTC/TDF (elvitegravir 150 mg, cobicistat 150 mg, emtricitabine 200 mg, tenofovir DF 300 mg) or continue receiving their baseline HIV PI-based antiretroviral regimen. At 48 weeks, 94% of those receiving EVG/c/FTC/TDF had plasma HIV-1 RNA levels <50 copies/mL compared with 87% of those receiving a ritonavir-boosted HIV PI with FTC/TDF.

In a similarly designed study, the comparative efficacy and safety of EVG/c/FTC/TDF and an HIV nonnucleoside reverse transcriptase inhibitor-based (NNRTI-based) regimen in antiretroviral-experienced, virologically suppressed (HIV-1 RNA <50 copies/mL) adults were evaluated in a randomized, open-label, phase 3b noninferiority study (study 121; STRATEGY-NNRTI). Among 434 patients enrolled in study 121, the mean age was 41 years, 93% were male, 78% were white, 17% were Black, and mean baseline CD4+ T-cell count was 588 cells/mm³. At initial screening, all patients were receiving either their first or second antiretroviral regimen with no history of virologic failure, had no current evidence or history of resistance to the antiretroviral components of EVG/c/FTC/TDF, and had been receiving an HIV NNRTI in conjunction with the fixed combination of emtricitabine 200 mg and tenofovir DF 300 mg (FTC/TDF) for at least 6 months. Patients were randomized in a 2:1 ratio to either switch to EVG/c/FTC/TDF (elvitegravir 150 mg, cobicistat 150 mg, emtricitabine 200 mg, tenofovir DF 300 mg) or continue receiving their baseline NNRTI-based antiretroviral regimen. Randomization was stratified by use of efavirenz in the NNRTI-based regimen (78% were receiving efavirenz [74% as EFV/FTC/TDF]); 17% were receiving nevirapine, 4% were receiving rilpivirine (as emtricitabine/rilpivirine/tenofovir DF), and 1% were receiving etravirine. At 48 weeks, 93% of those receiving EVG/c/FTC/TDF had HIV-1 RNA <50 copies/mL compared with 88% of those receiving an HIV NNRTI with FTC/TDF.

Pediatric Patients

The efficacy and safety of EVG/c/FTC/TDF in antiretroviral-naïve HIV-infected children 12 to <18 years of age weighing at least 35 kg were evaluated in an uncontrolled, open-label study (Study 112). The study included 50 patients (mean age 15 years, 70% male, 68% black, 28% Asian, mean baseline HIV-1 RNA level 4.6 $\log_{10}$ copies/mL, mean baseline CD4+ T-cell count 399 cells/mm³, mean CD4+ percentage 20.9%) and all patients received EVG/c/FTC/TDF. At 48 weeks, 88% had HIV-1 RNA <50 copies/mL; the mean increase in CD4+ T-cell count from baseline was 229 cells/mm³.

Clinical Perspective

Therapeutic options for the treatment and prevention of HIV infection and recommendations concerning the use of antiretrovirals are continuously evolving. Antiretroviral therapy (ART) is recommended for all individuals with HIV regardless of CD4 counts, and should be initiated as soon as possible after diagnosis of HIV and continued indefinitely. The primary goals of ART are to achieve and maintain durable suppression of HIV viral load (as measured by plasma HIV-1 RNA levels) to a level below which drug-resistance mutations cannot emerge (i.e., below detectable limits), restore and preserve immunologic function, reduce HIV-related morbidity and mortality, improve quality of life, and prevent transmission of HIV. While the most appropriate antiretroviral regimen cannot be defined for each clinical scenario, the US Department of Health and Human Services (HHS) Panel on Antiretroviral Guidelines for Adults and Adolescents, HHS Panel on Antiretroviral Therapy and Medical Management of Children Living with HIV, and HHS Panel on Treatment of Pregnant Women with HIV Infection and Prevention of Perinatal Transmission, have developed comprehensive guidelines that provide information on selection and use of antiretrovirals for the treatment or prevention of HIV infection. Because of the complexity of managing patients with HIV, it is recommended that clinicians with HIV expertise be consulted when needed.

The use of combination antiretroviral regimens that generally include 3 drugs from 2 or more drug classes is currently recommended to achieve viral suppression. In both treatment-naïve adults and children, an initial antiretroviral regimen generally consists of 2 nucleoside reverse transcriptase inhibitors (NRTIs) administered in combination with a third active antiretroviral drug from 1 of 3 drug classes: an integrase strand transfer inhibitor (INSTI), a non-nucleoside reverse transcriptase inhibitor (NNRTI), or a protease inhibitor (PI) with a pharmacokinetic enhancer (also known as a booster; the 2 drugs used for this purpose are cobicistat and ritonavir). Selection of an initial regimen should be individualized based on factors such as virologic efficacy, toxicity, pill burden, dosing frequency, drug-drug interaction potential, resistance-test results, comorbid conditions, access, and cost. In patients with comorbid infections (e.g., hepatitis B, tuberculosis), antiretroviral regimen selection should also consider the potential for activity against other present infections and timing of initiation relative to other antiinfective regimens.

The fixed-dose combination of EVG/c/FTC/TDF is commonly used as a complete antiretroviral regimen. In the 2023 HHS adult and adolescent HIV treatment guideline, EVG/c/FTC/TDF is listed among initial regimens recommended in certain clinical situations.

In the 2023 HHS pediatric HIV treatment guideline, HHS recommends limiting use of EVG/c/FTC/TDF to sexually mature adolescents (according to recommendations in the HHS adult and adolescent HIV treatment guideline) due to concerns related to decreased bone mineral density with tenofovir DF use in pre-pubertal patients.

In the 2023 HHS perinatal HIV treatment guideline, EVG/c/FTC/TDF is *not* recommended as an initial regimen in pregnancy due to data suggesting insufficient levels of cobicistat and elvitegravir in the second and third trimesters and risk of viral breakthrough at delivery. In patients who become pregnant while virologically suppressed on EVG/c/FTC/TDF, HHS recommends continuing therapy with frequent viral load monitoring or considering switching therapy.

• Postexposure Prophylaxis following Nonoccupational Exposure to HIV

EVG/c/FTC/TDF is used as a complete regimen for postexposure prophylaxis of HIV infection following nonoccupational exposure †(nPEP) in individuals exposed to blood, genital secretions, or other potentially infectious body fluids that might contain HIV when the exposure represents a substantial risk for HIV transmission. EVG/c/FTC/TDF is listed among alternative regimen options in guidelines for nPEP.

Clinical Experience

The fixed-dose combination of EVG/c/FTC/TDF was evaluated as nPEP in adults presenting to an emergency department following suspected sexual exposure to HIV in the open-label, randomized STRIBPEP study. Patients were randomized 3:1 to EVG/c/FTC/TDF (n=119) or tenofovir DF plus emtricitabine and ritonavir-boosted lopinavir (TDF/FTC + LPV/RTV, n=38), both administered for 28 days. A higher proportion of patients in the TDF/FTC + LPV/RTV arm had not completed their assigned treatment at 28 days compared to those in the EVG/c/FTC/TDF arm (47% and 33%, respectively), and a substantially higher proportion in the TDF/FTC + LPV/RTV arm reported <94% adherence to the regimen (47% vs 9%, respectively). HIV infection was detected in 2 patients (1 in each arm) on the day 1 follow-up visit. HIV infection was detected in 1 patient assigned to EVG/c/FTC/TDF at day 90 follow-up; this patient reported multiple high-risk exposures prior to and after initiating study treatment.

Clinical Perspective

When nPEP is indicated following a nonoccupational exposure to HIV, the US Centers for Disease Control and Prevention (CDC) states that the preferred regimen in adults and adolescents 13 years of age or older with normal renal function is either raltegravir or dolutegravir used in conjunction with emtricitabine and tenofovir DF (administered as the fixed combination emtricitabine/tenofovir DF; Truvada®). The alternative nPEP regimen recommended in these patients is ritonavir-boosted darunavir used in conjunction with emtricitabine/tenofovir DF (Truvada®). EVG/c/FTC/TDF is one of several other alternative regimens recommended by CDC for nPEP.

Consultation with an infectious disease specialist, clinician with expertise in administration of antiretroviral agents, and/or the National Clinicians' Postexposure Prophylaxis Hotline (PEPline at 888-448-4911) is recommended if nPEP is indicated in certain exposed individuals (e.g., pregnant women, children, those with medical conditions such as renal impairment) or if an antiretroviral regimen not included in the CDC guidelines is being considered, the source virus is known or likely to be resistant to antiretrovirals, or the healthcare provider is inexperienced in prescribing antiretrovirals. However, initiation of nPEP should not be delayed while waiting for expert consultation.

• Postexposure Prophylaxis following Occupational Exposure to HIV

EVG/c/FTC/TDF is used as a complete regimen for postexposure prophylaxis of HIV infection following occupational exposure† (PEP) in health-care personnel and other individuals exposed via percutaneous injury (e.g., needlestick, cut with sharp object) or mucous membrane or nonintact skin (e.g., chapped, abraded, dermatitis) contact with blood, tissue, or other body fluids that might contain HIV.

The US Public Health Service (USPHS) states that the preferred regimen for PEP following an occupational exposure to HIV is a 3-drug regimen of raltegravir used in conjunction with emtricitabine and tenofovir DF (may be administered as the fixed combination emtricitabine/tenofovir DF; Truvada®) for 28 days. These experts recommend several alternative regimens that include an INSTI, NNRTI, or PI and 2 NRTIs (dual NRTIs). The preferred dual NRTI option for use in PEP regimens is emtricitabine and tenofovir DF (may be administered as the fixed combination emtricitabine/tenofovir DF; Truvada®); alternative dual NRTIs are tenofovir DF and lamivudine, lamivudine and zidovudine (may be administered as the fixed combination lamivudine/zidovudine; Combivir®), or zidovudine and emtricitabine. EVG/c/FTC/TDF is also recommended as an alternative complete PEP regimen.

Because management of occupational exposures to HIV is complex and evolving, consultation with an infectious disease specialist, clinician with expertise in administration of antiretroviral agents, and/or the National Clinicians' Postexposure Prophylaxis Hotline (PEPline at 888-448-4911) is recommended whenever possible. However, initiation of PEP should not be delayed while waiting for expert consultation.

DOSAGE AND ADMINISTRATION

• General

Pretreatment Screening

- Patients should be tested for hepatitis B virus (HBV) infection prior to initiation of elvitegravir, cobicistat, emtricitabine, and tenofovir disoproxil fumarate (tenofovir DF) (EVG/c/FTC/TDF).

- Serum creatinine, estimated creatinine clearance, urine glucose, and urine protein should be determined prior to initiation of EVG/c/FTC/TDF.

- In patients with chronic kidney disease (CKD), serum phosphorus should be determined prior to initiation of EVG/c/FTC/TDF.

Patient Monitoring

- Routinely monitor serum creatinine, estimated creatinine clearance, urine glucose, and urine protein during treatment in all patients.

- Routinely monitor serum phosphorus during treatment in patients with CKD.

● Administration

The fixed combination of EVG/c/FTC/TDF is administered orally once daily with food.

Store below 30°C in the original container and keep container tightly closed.

● Dosage

Each fixed-combination tablet of EVG/c/FTC/TDF contains elvitegravir 150 mg, cobicistat 150 mg, emtricitabine 200 mg, and tenofovir DF 300 mg.

Adult Dosage

Treatment of HIV Infection

For the treatment of HIV-1 infection in antiretroviral-naïve or -experienced adults, the usual dosage of EVG/c/FTC/TDF is 1 tablet (150 mg of elvitegravir, 150 mg of cobicistat, 200 mg of emtricitabine, and 300 mg of tenofovir DF) once daily.

Postexposure Prophylaxis following Nonoccupational Exposure to HIV

For postexposure prophylaxis of HIV infection following nonoccupational exposure† (nPEP) when the exposure represents a substantial risk for HIV transmission, the recommended dosage of EVG/c/FTC/TDF is 1 tablet (150 mg of elvitegravir, 150 mg of cobicistat, 200 mg of emtricitabine, and 300 mg of tenofovir DF) once daily.

Initiate nPEP as soon as possible (within 72 hours) following nonoccupational exposure associated with a substantial risk for HIV transmission and continue for 28 days. If the exposed individual seeks care more than 72 hours after the exposure, nPEP is not recommended.

Postexposure Prophylaxis following Occupational Exposure to HIV

For postexposure prophylaxis of HIV infection following occupational exposure† (PEP) in health-care personnel or other individuals, the recommended dosage of EVG/c/FTC/TDF is 1 tablet (150 mg of elvitegravir, 150 mg of cobicistat, 200 mg of emtricitabine, and 300 mg of tenofovir DF) once daily.

PEP should be initiated as soon as possible following occupational exposure to HIV (preferably within hours) and continued for 4 weeks, if tolerated.

Pediatric Dosage

Treatment of HIV Infection

For the treatment of HIV-1 infection in antiretroviral-naïve or -experienced adolescents 12 years of age or older weighing at least 35 kg, the usual dosage of EVG/c/FTC/TDF is 1 tablet (150 mg of elvitegravir, 150 mg of cobicistat, 200 mg of emtricitabine, and 300 mg of tenofovir DF) once daily.

● Special Populations

Hepatic Impairment

Dosage adjustments are not necessary if EVG/c/FTC/TDF is used in adults with mild or moderate hepatic impairment (Child-Pugh class A or B).

EVG/c/FTC/TDF should not be used in patients with severe hepatic impairment (Child-Pugh class C).

Renal Impairment

EVG/c/FTC/TDF should *not* be initiated in adults with estimated creatinine clearance <70 mL/minute.

If estimated creatinine clearance decreases to <50 mL/minute, or if clinically significant renal dysfunction or evidence of Fanconi syndrome develop during EVG/c/FTC/TDF treatment, the drug should be discontinued.

Data are insufficient to make dosage recommendations for pediatric patients with renal impairment.

Geriatric Use

No dosage adjustments are necessary in geriatric patients; however, EVG/c/FTC/TDF should be used with caution.

CAUTIONS

● Contraindications

● Concomitant use of the fixed combination of elvitegravir, cobicistat, emtricitabine, and tenofovir disoproxil fumarate (tenofovir DF) (EVG/c/FTC/TDF) with drugs highly dependent on cytochrome P-450 isoenzyme 3A (CYP3A) for metabolism and for which elevated plasma concentrations are associated with serious and/or life-threatening events (e.g., alfuzosin, cisapride, ergot alkaloids, lovastatin, lurasidone, oral midazolam, pimozide, sildenafil used for treatment of pulmonary arterial hypertension [PAH], simvastatin, triazolam) is contraindicated.

● Concomitant use of EVG/c/FTC/TDF with drugs that are potent inducers of CYP3A and which may decrease elvitegravir and/or cobicistat concentrations resulting in possible decreased antiretroviral efficacy and development of resistance (e.g., carbamazepine, phenobarbital, phenytoin, rifampin, St. John's wort [*Hypericum perforatum*]) is contraindicated.

● Warnings/Precautions

Warnings

Severe Acute Exacerbation of Hepatitis B in Patients Coinfected with HIV and HBV

The prescribing information of EVG/c/FTC/TDF includes a boxed warning regarding the risk of severe acute exacerbations of HBV in patients coinfected with HIV-1 and HBV who have discontinued emtricitabine or tenofovir DF, two of the components of EVG/c/FTC/TDF. In some patients, post-treatment exacerbations of HBV have been associated with hepatic decompensation and hepatic failure. HIV-infected patients should be tested for HBV before antiretroviral therapy is initiated. EVG/c/FTC/TDF is not indicated for treatment of chronic HBV infection, and safety and efficacy of EVG/c/FTC/TDF have not been established in HIV-infected patients coinfected with HIV-1. Hepatic function should be closely monitored with clinical and laboratory follow-up for at least several months after EVG/c/FTC/TDF is discontinued in patients coinfected with HIV and HBV. If appropriate, initiation of HBV treatment may be warranted.

Other Warnings/Precautions

Renal Toxicity

Renal impairment, including cases of acute renal failure and Fanconi syndrome (renal tubular injury with severe hypophosphatemia), have been reported in patients receiving tenofovir DF (a component of EVG/c/FTC/TDF).

In clinical trials, 1.9% of patients receiving EVG/c/FTC/TDF and up to 2.3% of patients receiving an active comparator discontinued treatment by 144 weeks because of adverse renal effects. Laboratory findings consistent with proximal renal tubular dysfunction resulting in discontinuance of the drugs occurred in 4 (0.6%) patients receiving EVG/c/FTC/TDF during the first 48 weeks of treatment; estimated creatinine clearances <70 mL/minute were reported at baseline in 2 of the 4 patients receiving EVG/c/FTC/TDF. Laboratory findings improved after EVG/c/FTC/TDF was discontinued, but did not completely resolve in all patients; no patient required renal replacement therapy.

Cobicistat (a component of EVG/c/FTC/TDF) may cause a modest increase in serum creatinine and modest decrease in estimated creatinine clearance due to inhibition of tubular secretion of creatinine; there is a corresponding decrease in serum creatinine-based estimated glomerular filtration rate (eGFR), but renal glomerular function is not affected. Elevated serum creatinine concentrations generally were reversible when the drug was discontinued.

Serum creatinine, estimated creatinine clearance, urine glucose, and urine protein should be determined prior to initiation of EVG/c/FTC/TDF and routinely monitored during treatment in all patients. Assess serum phosphorus in patients with CKD. Discontinue EVG/c/FTC/TDF if clinically significant renal dysfunction develops or there is evidence of Fanconi syndrome.

EVG/c/FTC/TDF should *not* be initiated in patients with estimated creatinine clearances <70 mL/minute, and the drug should be discontinued if estimated creatinine clearance decreases to <50 mL/minute during treatment.

Patients who experience a confirmed increase in serum creatinine of greater than 0.4 mg/dL from baseline while receiving EVG/c/FTC/TDF should be closely monitored for renal toxicity.

Because persistent or worsening bone pain, pain in extremities, fractures, and/or muscular pain or weakness may be manifestations of proximal renal tubulopathy, renal function should be promptly evaluated in patients at risk for renal dysfunction who present with such symptoms.

EVG/c/FTC/TDF should be avoided in patients who are receiving or have recently received a nephrotoxic agent (e.g., high-dose or multiple nonsteroidal anti-inflammatory agents [NSAIAs]). Acute renal failure has been reported after initiation of high-dose or multiple NSAIA therapy in HIV-infected patients at risk for renal dysfunction who appeared stable while receiving tenofovir DF. Hospitalization and renal replacement therapy were required in some patients. Alternatives to NSAIAs should be considered if such therapy is needed in patients at risks for renal dysfunction.

Lactic Acidosis and Severe Hepatomegaly with Steatosis

Lactic acidosis and severe hepatomegaly with steatosis, including fatalities, have been reported in patients receiving HIV nucleoside reverse transcriptase inhibitors (NRTIs), including emtricitabine and tenofovir DF, in conjunction with other antiretroviral agents.

EVG/c/FTC/TDF treatment should be interrupted in any patient who develops clinical or laboratory findings suggestive of lactic acidosis or pronounced hepatotoxicity (signs of hepatotoxicity may include hepatomegaly and steatosis even in the absence of marked increases in serum aminotransferase concentrations).

Bone Effects

Decreases in bone mineral density (BMD) from baseline at lumbar spine and hip, increases in several biochemical markers of bone metabolism, and increased serum parathyroid hormone levels and 1,25 vitamin D levels have been reported during clinical trials of tenofovir DF (a component of EVG/c/FTC/TDF). The effects of tenofovir-associated changes in BMD on long-term bone health and future fracture risk are unknown.

Osteomalacia associated with proximal renal tubulopathy, which manifested as bone pain or pain in extremities and may contribute to fractures, has been reported in patients receiving tenofovir DF. Arthralgias and muscle pain or weakness also have been reported in patients with proximal renal tubulopathy. Hypophosphatemia and osteomalacia secondary to proximal renal tubulopathy should be considered in patients at risk for renal dysfunction who present with persistent or worsening bone or muscle symptoms while receiving preparations containing tenofovir DF.

In a clinical study evaluating safety and efficacy of EVG/c/FTC/TDF (study 103), the mean percentage decrease in BMD from baseline to week 144 in patients receiving EVG/c/FTC/TDF was similar to that in patients receiving a regimen of *ritonavir-boosted* atazanavir and the fixed combination of emtricitabine and tenofovir DF (FTC/TDF). The mean change from baseline in BMD at the lumbar spine or hip was -1.4 or -2.8%, respectively, in those receiving EVG/c/FTC/TDF and -3.7 or -3.8%, respectively, in those receiving *ritonavir-boosted* atazanavir with FTC/TDF. Data from clinical studies 102 and 103 indicate that 3.9% of those receiving EVG/c/FTC/TDF experienced bone fractures compared with 2.3% of those receiving a fixed combination containing efavirenz, emtricitabine, tenofovir DF (EFV/FTC/TDF) and 5.4% of those receiving *ritonavir-boosted* atazanavir and FTC/TDF. In clinical studies evaluating tenofovir DF in pediatric and adolescent patients, bone effects were similar to those reported in adults.

BMD monitoring should be considered for adult and pediatric patients who have a history of pathologic bone fracture or other risk factors for osteoporosis or bone loss. Although the effect of calcium and vitamin D supplementation was not studied, such supplementation may be beneficial for all patients. If bone abnormalities are suspected, appropriate consultation should be obtained.

Interactions

Concomitant use of EVG/c/FTC/TDF with certain drugs may result in clinically important interactions, including some that may decrease plasma concentrations of the antiretroviral agents leading to loss of therapeutic effect and possible development of resistance and some that may increase plasma concentrations of the antiretroviral agents and/or concomitant drugs leading to clinically important adverse reactions, including potentially severe, life-threatening, or fatal events. Loss of therapeutic effect of concomitant drugs that utilize CYP3A to form active metabolites may also occur.

The potential for drug interactions should be considered prior to and during EVG/c/FTC/TDF therapy. Drugs used concomitantly should be reviewed during EVG/c/FTC/TDF therapy and the patient should be monitored for adverse reactions associated with the concomitant drugs.

Use of Fixed Combinations

The usual cautions, precautions, contraindications, and interactions associated with each component of EVG/c/FTC/TDF should be considered. Cautionary information applicable to specific populations (e.g., pregnant or nursing women, individuals with hepatic or renal impairment, geriatric patients) should be considered for each drug in the fixed combination. For cautionary information related to emtricitabine or tenofovir disoproxil fumarate, see Cautions in Emtricitabine 8:18.08.20 and in Tenofovir Disoproxil Fumarate 8:18.08.20.

EVG/c/FTC/TDF is used alone as a complete regimen for the treatment of HIV-1 infection and should not be used in conjunction with other antiretroviral agents.

EVG/c/FTC/TDF should not be used concomitantly with any preparation that contains any of its components (elvitegravir, cobicistat, emtricitabine, tenofovir DF). In addition, EVG/c/FTC/TDF should not be used concomitantly with any preparation containing lamivudine, adefovir dipivoxil, or ritonavir.

Immune Reconstitution Syndrome

Immune reconstitution syndrome has been reported in HIV-infected patients receiving multiple-drug antiretroviral therapy, including EVG/c/FTC/TDF. During the initial phase of treatment, HIV-infected patients whose immune systems respond to antiretroviral therapy may develop an inflammatory response to indolent or residual opportunistic infections (e.g., *Mycobacterium avium*, *M. tuberculosis*, cytomegalovirus [CMV], *Pneumocystis jirovecii* [formerly *P. carinii*]); such response may necessitate further evaluation and treatment.

Autoimmune disorders (e.g., Graves' disease, polymyositis, Guillain-Barré syndrome, autoimmune hepatitis) have also been reported to occur in the setting of immune reconstitution; however, the time to onset is more variable and can occur many months after initiation of antiretroviral therapy.

Specific Populations

Pregnancy

Use of EVG/c/FTC/TDF is *not* recommended during pregnancy, and should not be initiated during pregnancy due to substantially lower elvitegravir and cobicistat exposures in the second and third trimesters. An alternative regimen is recommended for individuals who become pregnant during treatment with EVG/c/FTC/TDF.

The Antiretroviral Pregnancy Registry (APR) monitors pregnancy outcomes in women exposed to EVG/c/FTC/TDF during pregnancy. Clinicians are encouraged to register patients in the APR by calling 800-258-4263 or visiting https://www.apregistry.com/.

The overall risk of birth defects with EVG/c/FTC/TDF use in pregnancy was not markedly different compared to the background rate for major birth defects of 2.7% in the United States reference population of the Metropolitan Atlanta Congenital Defects Program (MACDP). Limitations of using an external comparator (the MACDP) includes differences in populations and methodology, and confounding due to the underlying disease. The rate of miscarriage is not reported in the APR.

Lactation

Elvitegravir and cobicistat are distributed into milk in rats; it is not known whether these drugs are distributed into human milk. The emtricitabine and tenofovir components of EVG/c/FTC/TDF are distributed into human milk.

It is not known whether EVG/c/FTC/TDF affects human milk production or affects the breast-fed infant.

Because of the risk of adverse effects in the infant and the risk of HIV transmission, HIV-infected women should not breast-feed infants.

Pediatric Use

Safety and efficacy of EVG/c/FTC/TDF have not been established in pediatric patients younger than 12 years of age or in those weighing less than 35 kg.

Clinical trial data indicate that the safety profile of EVG/c/FTC/TDF in HIV-1-infected, treatment-naïve pediatric patients 12 to less than 18 years of age is similar to that reported in adults.

Bone effects reported when tenofovir DF is used in pediatric and adolescent patients are similar to those reported in adults. In clinical studies, total body BMD gain in tenofovir DF-treated pediatric patients was less than that reported in control groups; skeletal growth appeared to be unaffected. Effects of tenofovir DF-associated changes in BMD and biochemical markers on long-term bone health and future fracture risk are unknown.

Following oral administration of EVG/c/FTC/TDF, elvitegravir and tenofovir exposures in children and adolescents 12 to less than 18 years of age were 30 and 37% higher, respectively, than those reported in adults; this difference is not considered clinically important based on exposure-response relationships. Cobicistat and emtricitabine exposures in children and adolescents 12 to less than 18 years of age were similar to those reported in adults.

Geriatric Use

Experience in adults 65 years of age and older is insufficient to determine whether they respond differently than younger adults.

EVG/c/FTC/TDF should be used with caution in geriatric patients because of age-related decreases in hepatic, renal, and/or cardiac function and potential for concomitant disease and drug therapy.

Hepatic Impairment

Moderate hepatic impairment (Child-Pugh class B) does not have a clinically important effect on the pharmacokinetics of elvitegravir, cobicistat, or tenofovir DF and is not expected to affect the pharmacokinetics of emtricitabine.

EVG/c/FTC/TDF is *not* recommended in patients with severe hepatic impairment (Child-Pugh class C). Data are not available to date regarding the pharmacokinetics or safety of EVG/c/FTC/TDF in such patients.

Renal Impairment

Serum creatinine, estimated creatinine clearance, serum phosphorus, urine glucose, and urine protein should be determined prior to initiating EVG/c/FTC/TDF and routinely monitored during treatment in all patients.

EVG/c/FTC/TDF should *not* be initiated in adults with estimated creatinine clearances <70 mL/minute. If estimated creatinine clearance decreases to <50 mL/minute, clinically significant decreases in renal function, or evidence of Fanconi syndrome develop during EVG/c/FTC/TDF treatment, the fixed-combination drug should be discontinued.

Data are insufficient to make dosage recommendations for pediatric patients with renal impairment.

● Common Adverse Effects

The most common (incidence ≥10%) adverse effects in patients receiving EVG/c/FTC/TDF are nausea and diarrhea.

DRUG INTERACTIONS

The following drug interactions are based on studies that used elvitegravir, elvitegravir administered with cobicistat (*cobicistat-boosted* elvitegravir), elvitegravir administered with low-dose ritonavir (*ritonavir-boosted* elvitegravir), cobicistat alone, or the fixed combination of elvitegravir, cobicistat, emtricitabine, and tenofovir disoproxil fumarate (tenofovir DF) (EVG/c/FTC/TDF) or are predicted to occur.

Potential drug interactions associated with each drug in the fixed combination should be considered.

● Drugs Affecting or Metabolized by Hepatic Microsomal Enzymes

Elvitegravir is a substrate of cytochrome P-450 (CYP) 3A and a weak inducer and weak inhibitor of CYP3A; elvitegravir is an inducer of CYP2C9. The drug does not inhibit CYP1A, 2A6, 2C9, 2C19, 2D6, or 2E1 in vitro.

Cobicistat is a substrate of CYP3A and, to a minor extent, CYP2D6; cobicistat also is an inhibitor of CYP3A and 2D6.

Emtricitabine is not a substrate of CYP enzymes and does not inhibit CYP1A2, 2A6, 2B6, 2C9, 2C19, 2D6, or 3A4.

Tenofovir DF and tenofovir are not substrates of CYP enzymes; tenofovir does not inhibit CYP3A4, 2D6, 2C9, or 2E1, but may have a slight inhibitory effect on CYP1A.

Potential pharmacokinetic interactions if EVG/c/FTC/TDF is used concomitantly with drugs that are principally metabolized by CYP3A or 2D6 (increased plasma concentrations of the concomitant drug). Concomitant use of EVG/c/FTC/TDF with some drugs that are CYP3A substrates and for which elevated plasma concentrations are associated with serious and/or life-threatening events is contraindicated.

Potential pharmacokinetic interactions if EVG/c/FTC/TDF is used concomitantly with drugs that induce CYP3A (decreased plasma concentrations of elvitegravir and cobicistat and possible decreased antiretroviral efficacy and development of resistance). Concomitant use of EVG/c/FTC/TDF with some drugs that are potent inducers of CYP3A is contraindicated.

Potential pharmacokinetic interactions if EVG/c/FTC/TDF is used concomitantly with drugs that inhibit CYP3A (increased plasma concentrations of cobicistat).

● Drugs Affected by P-glycoprotein Transport

Cobicistat is an inhibitor of P-glycoprotein (P-gp) transport.

Potential pharmacokinetic interactions if EVG/c/FTC/TDF is used concomitantly with drugs that are P-gp substrates (increased plasma concentrations of the concomitant drug).

● Drugs Affected by Breast Cancer Resistance Protein

Cobicistat is an inhibitor of breast cancer resistance protein (BCRP).

Potential pharmacokinetic interactions if EVG/c/FTC/TDF is used concomitantly with drugs that are substrates for BCRP (increased plasma concentrations of the concomitant drug).

● Drugs Affected by Organic Anion Transport Polypeptides

Elvitegravir and cobicistat are inhibitors of organic anion transport polypeptides (OATP) 1B1 and 1B3.

Potential pharmacokinetic interactions if EVG/c/FTC/TDF is used concomitantly with drugs that are substrates for OATP1B1 or 1B3 (increased plasma concentrations of the concomitant drug).

● Drugs Affecting Renal Function

The emtricitabine and tenofovir components of EVG/c/FTC/TDF are principally excreted by the kidneys by a combination of glomerular filtration and active tubular secretion.

Potential pharmacokinetic interactions if EVG/c/FTC/TDF is used concomitantly with drugs that reduce renal function or compete for active tubular secretion (e.g., acyclovir, aminoglycosides [gentamicin], cidofovir, ganciclovir, valacyclovir, valganciclovir, high-dose or multiple nonsteroidal anti-inflammatory agents [NSAIAs]); may result in increased concentrations of emtricitabine, tenofovir, and/or the concomitant drug and may increase the risk of adverse effects.

● Alfuzosin

Potential pharmacokinetic interaction with alfuzosin (increased plasma concentrations of alfuzosin) may result in hypotension.

Concomitant use of alfuzosin and EVG/c/FTC/TDF is contraindicated.

● Anticoagulants

Apixaban, Dabigatran, Edoxaban, Rivaroxaban

Due to an increased risk of bleeding, dosing recommendations for the concomitant use of apixaban with EVG/c/FTC/TDF depend on the dosage of apixaban. Refer to apixaban prescribing information for dosing instructions on the concomitant use of apixaban with strong CYP3A and P-gp inhibitors.

Due to an increased risk of bleeding, dosing recommendations for the concomitant use of dabigatran and edoxaban with a P-gp inhibitor such as EVG/c/FTC/TDF are dependent upon underlying renal function and the indication for anticoagulant use. Refer to the prescribing information for the direct oral anticoagulant (DOAC) in use for dosage recommendations with a concomitant P-gp inhibitor.

Concomitant use of rivaroxaban with EVG/c/FTC/TDF is not recommended due to an increased risk of bleeding.

Warfarin

The effect of concomitant use of warfarin and EVG/c/FTC/TDF on the pharmacokinetics of warfarin is unknown.

If warfarin is used concomitantly with EVG/c/FTC/TDF, monitor the international normalized ratio (INR).

● Anticonvulsants
Carbamazepine, Phenobarbital, Phenytoin

Concomitant use of carbamazepine and cobicistat-boosted elvitegravir results in decreased elvitegravir plasma concentrations and area under the plasma concentration-time curve (AUC) and may lead to loss of antiretroviral efficacy and development of resistance; increased carbamazepine plasma concentrations and AUC also occur. Potential pharmacokinetic interactions if phenobarbital or phenytoin is used concomitantly with EVG/c/FTC/TDF (decreased elvitegravir and cobicistat plasma concentrations with possible decreased antiretroviral efficacy and development of resistance).

Concomitant use of EVG/c/FTC/TDF and carbamazepine, phenobarbital, or phenytoin is contraindicated.

Ethosuximide

Potential pharmacokinetic interaction if ethosuximide is used concomitantly with EVG/c/FTC/TDF (increased ethosuximide plasma concentrations).

If ethosuximide and EVG/c/FTC/TDF are used concomitantly, the patient should be monitored clinically for ethosuximide-related adverse effects.

Oxcarbazepine

Potential pharmacokinetic interaction if oxcarbazepine is used concomitantly with EVG/c/FTC/TDF (decreased elvitegravir and cobicistat plasma concentrations). An alternative anticonvulsant should be considered.

● Antifungal Agents
Itraconazole

Potential pharmacokinetic interactions with itraconazole (increased itraconazole plasma concentrations expected, increased elvitegravir and cobicistat plasma concentrations possible).

If itraconazole and EVG/c/FTC/TDF are used concomitantly, itraconazole dosage should not exceed 200 mg daily.

Ketoconazole

Pharmacokinetic interactions with ketoconazole (increased plasma concentrations of ketoconazole, elvitegravir, and cobicistat).

If ketoconazole and EVG/c/FTC/TDF are used concomitantly, ketoconazole dosage should not exceed 200 mg daily.

Voriconazole

Potential pharmacokinetic interactions with voriconazole (increased voriconazole plasma concentrations expected, increased elvitegravir and cobicistat plasma concentrations possible).

Voriconazole and EVG/c/FTC/TDF should not be used concomitantly unless potential benefits outweigh risks.

● Antimycobacterial Agents
Rifabutin

Pharmacokinetic interactions when cobicistat-boosted elvitegravir (elvitegravir 150 mg and cobicistat 150 mg once daily) was used concomitantly with rifabutin 150 mg once every other day (decreased elvitegravir plasma concentrations and AUC, increased 25-O-desacetyl-rifabutin concentrations and AUC relative to those achieved with rifabutin 300 mg once daily without concomitant cobicistat-boosted elvitegravir); possible decreased antiretroviral efficacy and development of resistance.

Concomitant use of rifabutin and EVG/c/FTC/TDF is not recommended.

Rifampin

Potential pharmacokinetic interactions with rifampin (decreased elvitegravir and cobicistat plasma concentrations); possible decreased antiretroviral efficacy and development of resistance.

Concomitant use of rifampin and EVG/c/FTC/TDF is contraindicated.

Rifapentine

Potential pharmacokinetic interactions with rifapentine (decreased elvitegravir and cobicistat plasma concentrations); possible decreased antiretroviral efficacy and development of resistance.

Concomitant use of rifapentine and EVG/c/FTC/TDF is not recommended.

● Antiplatelet Agents
Clopidogrel, Prasugrel, Ticagrelor

Pharmacokinetic interactions are expected if clopidogrel or ticagrelor is used concomitantly with EVG/c/FTC/TDF (decreased clopidogrel concentrations; increased ticagrelor concentrations).

Concomitant use of EVG/c/FTC/TDF and clopidogrel or ticagrelor is not recommended.

Clinically relevant interactions are not expected with the active metabolite of prasugrel and EVG/c/FTC/TDF.

● Antipsychotic Agents
Lurasidone

Concomitant use of lurasidone and EVG/c/FTC/TDF may result in serious and/or life-threatening adverse effects.

Concomitant use of lurasidone and EVG/c/FTC/TDF is contraindicated.

Perphenazine, Risperidone, Thioridazine

Potential pharmacokinetic interactions with antipsychotics, including perphenazine, risperidone, and thioridazine (increased antipsychotic plasma concentrations).

If EVG/c/FTC/TDF is used concomitantly with perphenazine, risperidone, or thioridazine, decreased dosage of the antipsychotic may be necessary.

Pimozide

Potential pharmacokinetic interaction with pimozide (increased pimozide plasma concentrations); potential for serious and/or life-threatening adverse effects (e.g., cardiac arrhythmias).

Concomitant use of pimozide and EVG/c/FTC/TDF is contraindicated.

Quetiapine

Pharmacokinetic interaction with quetiapine expected (increased quetiapine plasma concentrations).

Alternative antiretroviral therapy should be considered. If EVG/c/FTC/TDF is necessary in a patient receiving a stable dosage of quetiapine, the quetiapine dosage should be reduced to one-sixth of the original dosage. Refer to the prescribing information for quetiapine for recommendations on monitoring for adverse events. Patients receiving quetiapine and EVG/c/FTC/TDF concomitantly should be closely monitored for quetiapine efficacy and adverse effects.

● Antiretroviral Agents

EVG/c/FTC/TDF should not be used in conjunction with any other antiretroviral agents.

HIV Integrase Inhibitors (INSTIs)

Raltegravir

Raltegravir and EVG/c/FTC/TDF should not be used concomitantly.

HIV Nucleoside and Nucleotide Reverse Transcriptase Inhibitors (NRTIs)

EVG/c/FTC/TDF contains emtricitabine and tenofovir DF and should not be used concomitantly with any preparation containing these or any other NRTIs.

HIV Protease Inhibitors (PIs)

EVG/c/FTC/TDF should not be used concomitantly with HIV PIs.

Ritonavir

EVG/c/FTC/TDF and ritonavir (or preparations containing ritonavir) should not be used concomitantly.

• β-Adrenergic Blocking Agents

Potential pharmacokinetic interactions with β-adrenergic blocking agents, including metoprolol and timolol (increased β-adrenergic blocking agent plasma concentrations).

If EVG/c/FTC/TDF is used concomitantly with a β-adrenergic blocking agent, patients should be monitored clinically and decreased dosage of the β-adrenergic blocking agent may be necessary.

• Benzodiazepines

Midazolam or Triazolam

Pharmacokinetic interaction with midazolam or triazolam (increased benzodiazepine plasma concentrations); potential for serious and/or life-threatening adverse effects (e.g., prolonged or increased sedation or respiratory depression).

Concomitant use of oral midazolam or triazolam with EVG/c/FTC/TDF is contraindicated.

Concomitant use of parenteral midazolam and EVG/c/FTC/TDF should be undertaken in a monitored setting where respiratory depression and/or prolonged sedation can be managed. In addition, use of a reduced midazolam dosage should be considered, especially if more than a single dose of the drug will be administered.

Other Benzodiazepines

Potential pharmacokinetic interactions with clorazepate, diazepam, estazolam, or flurazepam (increased benzodiazepine plasma concentrations).

If clorazepate, diazepam, estazolam, or flurazepam is used concomitantly with EVG/c/FTC/TDF, patients should be monitored clinically.

• Bosentan

Potential pharmacokinetic interaction with bosentan (increased bosentan plasma concentrations).

In patients who have already been receiving EVG/c/FTC/TDF for at least 10 days, bosentan should be initiated using a dosage of 62.5 mg once daily or every other day based on individual tolerability.

In patients who have already been receiving bosentan, bosentan should be discontinued for at least 36 hours prior to initiating EVG/c/FTC/TDF; after at least 10 days of EVG/c/FTC/TDF therapy, bosentan can be resumed using a dosage of 62.5 mg once daily or every other day based on individual tolerability.

• Bupropion

Potential pharmacokinetic interaction with bupropion (increased or decreased bupropion plasma concentrations).

If bupropion is used concomitantly with EVG/c/FTC/TDF, dosage of the antidepressant should be titrated carefully based on clinical response.

• Buspirone

Potential pharmacokinetic interaction with buspirone (increased buspirone plasma concentrations).

If buspirone is used concomitantly with EVG/c/FTC/TDF, patients should be monitored clinically; reduced buspirone dosage may be necessary.

• Calcium-channel Blocking Agents

Potential pharmacokinetic interactions with calcium-channel blocking agents, including amlodipine, diltiazem, felodipine, nicardipine, nifedipine, and verapamil (increased plasma concentrations of the calcium-channel blocking agent).

The patient should be monitored for efficacy and adverse effects if calcium-channel blocking agents and EVG/c/FTC/TDF are used concomitantly.

• Calcium, Iron, Multivitamins, and Other Preparations Containing Polyvalent Cations

Oral calcium supplements, oral iron preparations, other oral supplements containing calcium, iron, aluminum, magnesium, or zinc (e.g., multivitamins), cation-containing antacids or laxatives, buffered medications, or other preparations containing polyvalent cations may decrease plasma concentrations of elvitegravir when used concomitantly.

EVG/c/FTC/TDF should be administered at least 2 hours before or at least 2 hours after medications, antacids, and oral supplements containing calcium, iron, aluminum, magnesium, or zinc.

• Cardiac Drugs

Antiarrhythmic Agents

Potential pharmacokinetic interactions if EVG/c/FTC/TDF is used with amiodarone, digoxin, disopyramide, dronedarone, flecainide, lidocaine (systemic), mexiletine, propafenone, or quinidine (increased plasma concentrations of the antiarrhythmic agent or cardiac glycoside). Concomitant use of digoxin (single 0.5-mg dose) and cobicistat (single 150-mg dose) has resulted in increased plasma concentrations of digoxin.

Plasma concentrations of the antiarrhythmic agents or cardiac glycoside should be monitored, if possible.

• Cisapride

Potential pharmacokinetic interaction with cisapride (increased cisapride plasma concentrations); potential for serious and/or life-threatening adverse effects (e.g., cardiac arrhythmias).

Concomitant use of cisapride and EVG/c/FTC/TDF is contraindicated.

• Cobicistat

Pharmacokinetic interaction with elvitegravir (increased plasma concentrations and AUC of elvitegravir); occurs because cobicistat inhibits CYP3A. Cobicistat acts as a pharmacokinetic enhancer when used concomitantly with elvitegravir (cobicistat-boosted elvitegravir) and this effect is used to therapeutic advantage in the EVG/c/FTC/TDF fixed combination.

Cobicistat does not antagonize the antiretroviral effects of elvitegravir, emtricitabine, or tenofovir.

• Colchicine

Potential pharmacokinetic interaction (increased colchicine plasma concentrations expected).

Colchicine and EVG/c/FTC/TDF should not be used concomitantly in patients with renal or hepatic impairment.

When colchicine is used for treatment of gout flares in patients receiving EVG/c/FTC/TDF, an initial colchicine dose of 0.6 mg should be given followed by 0.3 mg 1 hour later; the colchicine course should be repeated no earlier than 3 days later.

When colchicine is used for prophylaxis of gout flares in patients receiving EVG/c/FTC/TDF, colchicine dosage should be reduced to 0.3 mg once daily in those originally receiving 0.6 mg twice daily or decreased to 0.3 mg once every other day in those originally receiving 0.6 mg once daily.

When colchicine is used for treatment of familial Mediterranean fever (FMF) in patients receiving EVG/c/FTC/TDF, a maximum colchicine dosage of 0.6 mg daily (may be given as 0.3 mg twice daily) should be used.

● Corticosteroids

Corticosteroids Affected by Potent CYP3A Inhibition

Concomitant use of EVG/c/FTC/TDF and corticosteroids via all routes of administration whose exposures are substantially affected by potent CYP3A inhibitors (e.g., betamethasone, budesonide, ciclesonide, fluticasone, methylprednisolone, mometasone, triamcinolone) may increase plasma concentrations of the corticosteroid, which may result in adrenal insufficiency or Cushing's syndrome. Alternative corticosteroids (e.g., beclomethasone, prednisone, prednisolone) less affected by CYP3A inhibition relative to other corticosteroids should be considered in patients receiving EVG/c/FTC/TDF, particularly if long-term corticosteroid therapy is required.

Dexamethasone

Concomitant use of systemic dexamethasone may decrease elvitegravir and cobicistat plasma concentrations and may lead to decreased antiretroviral efficacy and development of resistance.

An alternative corticosteroid should be considered in patients receiving EVG/c/FTC/TDF.

● Ergot Alkaloids

Potential for serious and/or life-threatening adverse effects (e.g., peripheral vasospasm, ischemia of the extremities and other tissues) if EVG/c/FTC/TDF is used concomitantly with ergot alkaloids (e.g., dihydroergotamine, ergotamine, methylergonovine).

Concomitant use of ergot alkaloids and EVG/c/FTC/TDF is contraindicated.

● Estrogens and Progestins

Pharmacokinetic interactions with oral contraceptives containing ethinyl estradiol and norgestimate or drospirenone (decreased ethinyl estradiol plasma concentrations and AUC and increased norgestimate plasma concentrations and AUC).

Possible effects of increased norgestimate plasma concentrations are not established, but may include increased risk of insulin resistance, dyslipidemia, acne, and venous thrombosis. The potential risks and benefits of concomitant use of EVG/c/FTC/TDF and oral contraceptives containing ethinyl estradiol and norgestimate should be considered, particularly in women with risk factors for these effects.

If ethinyl estradiol and drospirenone are given concomitantly with EVG/c/FTC/TDF, clinical monitoring for hyperkalemia is recommended.

Concomitant use of EVG/c/FTC/TDF with oral contraceptives containing progestins other than drospirenone, levonorgestrel, or norgestimate or with other hormonal contraceptives (e.g., patch, vaginal ring, injections) has not been studied; alternative nonhormonal methods of contraception should be considered.

Additional or nonhormonal methods of contraception should be used when estrogen-based contraceptives are used concomitantly with EVG/c/FTC/TDF.

● GI Drugs

Antacids

Pharmacokinetic interaction with antacids containing aluminum, calcium, and/or magnesium hydroxide (decreased plasma concentrations and AUC of elvitegravir).

EVG/c/FTC/TDF should be given at least 2 hours before or at least 2 hours after antacids containing aluminum, calcium, or magnesium.

Histamine H₂-receptor Antagonists

Concomitant use of famotidine and *cobicistat-boosted* elvitegravir did not have a clinically important effect on elvitegravir plasma concentrations or AUC.

Concomitant use of EVG/c/FTC/TDF and famotidine is not expected to result in clinically important drug interactions.

Proton-pump Inhibitors

Concomitant use of omeprazole and *cobicistat-boosted* elvitegravir did not result in clinically important alterations in elvitegravir pharmacokinetics.

Concomitant use of EVG/c/FTC/TDF and proton-pump inhibitors is not expected to result in clinically important drug interactions.

Sucralfate

Sucralfate may decrease plasma concentrations of elvitegravir if used concomitantly with EVG/c/FTC/TDF.

EVG/c/FTC/TDF should be administered at least 2 hours before or at least 2 hours after sucralfate.

● HCV Antivirals

HCV Polymerase Inhibitors

Sofosbuvir and Velpatasvir

Concomitant use of the fixed combination of sofosbuvir and velpatasvir (sofosbuvir/velpatasvir) with EVG/c/FTC/TDF results in increased tenofovir exposures.

If sofosbuvir/velpatasvir and EVG/c/FTC/TDF are used concomitantly, the patient should be monitored for tenofovir-associated adverse effects.

Sofosbuvir, Velpatasvir, and Voxilaprevir

Concomitant use of the fixed combination of sofosbuvir, velpatasvir and voxilaprevir (sofosbuvir/velpatasvir/voxilaprevir) with EVG/c/FTC/TDF results in increased tenofovir exposures. If sofosbuvir/velpatasvir/voxilaprevir and EVG/c/FTC/TDF are used concomitantly, the patient should be monitored for tenofovir-associated adverse effects.

HCV Replication Complex Inhibitors

Ledipasvir and Sofosbuvir

Concomitant use of the fixed combination of ledipasvir and sofosbuvir (ledipasvir/sofosbuvir) and EVG/c/FTC/TDF results in increased ledipasvir plasma concentrations and is expected to result in increased tenofovir plasma concentrations. Safety of increased tenofovir plasma concentrations in patients receiving ledipasvir/sofosbuvir and EVG/c/FTC/TDF concomitantly has not been established.

Ledipasvir/sofosbuvir and EVG/c/FTC/TDF should not be used concomitantly.

● HMG-CoA Reductase Inhibitors

Concomitant use of certain hydroxymethylglutaryl-CoA (HMG-CoA) reductase inhibitors (statins) metabolized by CYP3A (e.g., atorvastatin, lovastatin, simvastatin) and EVG/c/FTC/TDF may increase plasma concentrations of the HMG-CoA reductase inhibitor resulting in increased effects and increased risk of statin-associated adverse effects, including myopathy and rhabdomyolysis.

Atorvastatin

If atorvastatin is used concomitantly with EVG/c/FTC/TDF, the statin should be initiated at the lowest dosage and titrated carefully while monitoring for atorvastatin-associated adverse effects. Do not exceed a dosage of atorvastatin 20 mg daily with concomitant EVG/c/FTC/TDF therapy.

Lovastatin

Concomitant use of lovastatin and EVG/c/FTC/TDF is contraindicated.

Rosuvastatin

Pharmacokinetic interaction when rosuvastatin is used concomitantly with *cobicistat-boosted* elvitegravir (increased rosuvastatin plasma concentrations and AUC; no clinically important effect on elvitegravir pharmacokinetics).

Simvastatin

Concomitant use of simvastatin and EVG/c/FTC/TDF is contraindicated.

● Immunosuppressive Agents

Potential pharmacokinetic interactions with cyclosporine, everolimus, sirolimus, or tacrolimus (increased plasma concentrations of the immunosuppressive agent).

If EVG/c/FTC/TDF is used concomitantly with cyclosporine, sirolimus, or tacrolimus, plasma concentrations of the immunosuppressive agent should be monitored and the patient monitored for toxicities.

● *Lomitapide*

Concomitant use of lomitapide and EVG/c/FTC/TDF is contraindicated due to the potential for marked increases in transaminase levels.

● *Macrolides*

Clarithromycin

Potential pharmacokinetic interactions (increased plasma concentrations of clarithromycin and cobicistat).

Modification of the usual dosage of clarithromycin is not necessary in those with a creatinine clearance of 60 mL/minute or greater; however, clarithromycin dosage should be reduced by 50% in those with a creatinine clearance of 50–60 mL/minute. EVG/c/FTC/TDF should not be used in those with a creatinine clearance less than 50 mL/minute.

● *Nucleoside and Nucleotide Antivirals*

Potential pharmacokinetic interactions if EVG/c/FTC/TDF is used concomitantly with drugs that compete for active tubular secretion, including acyclovir, cidofovir, ganciclovir, valacyclovir, and valganciclovir; increased plasma concentrations of some of the components of EVG/c/FTC/TDF (i.e., emtricitabine, tenofovir) or the concomitant drug may occur and increase the risk of adverse effects.

Adefovir

EVG/c/FTC/TDF should not be used concomitantly with adefovir.

Entecavir or Famciclovir

Clinically important interactions are not expected if EVG/c/FTC/TDF is used concomitantly with entecavir or famciclovir.

Ribavirin

Clinically important interactions are not expected if EVG/c/FTC/TDF is used concomitantly with ribavirin.

● *Opiates Agonists, Opiate Partial Agonists, and Opiate Antagonists*

Buprenorphine

Concomitant use of the fixed combination of buprenorphine and naloxone (buprenorphine/naloxone) with *cobicistat-boosted* elvitegravir increased plasma concentrations and AUC of buprenorphine and norbuprenorphine and decreased peak plasma concentrations and AUC of naloxone.

If buprenorphine/naloxone is used concomitantly with EVG/c/FTC/TDF, dosage adjustments are not necessary; however, patients should be monitored closely for sedation and adverse cognitive effects.

Fentanyl

Potential pharmacokinetic interactions with fentanyl (increased fentanyl plasma concentrations). If fentanyl and EVG/c/FTC/TDF are used concomitantly, carefully monitor for therapeutic and adverse effects of fentanyl.

Methadone

Concomitant use of methadone and *cobicistat-boosted* elvitegravir did not result in clinically important alterations in methadone pharmacokinetics.

Concomitant use of methadone and EVG/c/FTC/TDF is not expected to result in clinically important drug interactions.

Tramadol

Potential pharmacokinetic interactions with tramadol (increased tramadol plasma concentrations). Decreased doses of tramadol may be necessary if used concomitantly with EVG/c/FTC/TDF.

● *Phosphodiesterase Type 5 Inhibitors*

Concomitant use of EVG/c/FTC/TDF and selective phosphodiesterase type 5 (PDE5) inhibitors (e.g., sildenafil, tadalafil, vardenafil) is expected to result in increased plasma concentrations of the PDE5 inhibitor and increase the risk of adverse effects (e.g., hypotension, syncope, visual disturbances, priapism) associated with these agents.

Sildenafil

Concomitant use of EVG/c/FTC/TDF is contraindicated in patients receiving sildenafil for treatment of pulmonary arterial hypertension (PAH).

If sildenafil is used for treatment of erectile dysfunction in a patient receiving EVG/c/FTC/TDF, sildenafil dosage should not exceed 25 mg once every 48 hours and the patient should be monitored for sildenafil-related adverse effects.

Tadalafil

If tadalafil is used for treatment of PAH in a patient who has been receiving EVG/c/FTC/TDF for at least 1 week, tadalafil should be initiated at a dosage of 20 mg once daily and, if tolerated, dosage may be increased to 40 mg once daily. EVG/c/FTC/TDF should not be initiated in patients receiving tadalafil for treatment of PAH; tadalafil should be discontinued for at least 24 hours prior to initiating EVG/c/FTC/TDF. After at least 1 week, tadalafil may be resumed at a dosage of 20 mg once daily and, if tolerated, dosage may be increased to 40 mg once daily.

If tadalafil is used for treatment of erectile dysfunction in a patient receiving EVG/c/FTC/TDF, tadalafil dosage should not exceed 10 mg once every 72 hours and the patient should be monitored for tadalafil-related adverse effects.

Vardenafil

If vardenafil is used for treatment of erectile dysfunction in a patient receiving EVG/c/FTC/TDF, vardenafil dosage should not exceed 2.5 mg once every 72 hours and the patient should be monitored for vardenafil-related adverse effects.

● *Salmeterol*

Potential pharmacokinetic interaction with salmeterol (increased salmeterol plasma concentrations) may result in increased risk of salmeterol-associated adverse cardiovascular effects, including QT interval prolongation, palpitations, and sinus tachycardia.

Concomitant use of salmeterol and EVG/c/FTC/TDF is not recommended.

● *Selective Serotonin-reuptake Inhibitors*

Potential pharmacokinetic interactions with certain selective serotonin-reuptake inhibitors (SSRIs), including citalopram, escitalopram, fluoxetine, and paroxetine (increased SSRI plasma concentrations).

If citalopram, escitalopram, fluoxetine, or paroxetine is used concomitantly with EVG/c/FTC/TDF, the lowest initial dosage of the SSRI should be used and dosage carefully titrated based on clinical response.

● *Trazodone*

Potential pharmacokinetic interaction with trazodone (increased trazodone plasma concentrations).

If trazodone is initiated in a patient receiving EVG/c/FTC/TDF, the lowest initial dosage of the antidepressant should be used and dosage carefully titrated according to response.

● *Tricyclic Antidepressants*

Potential pharmacokinetic interactions with tricyclic antidepressants, including amitriptyline, desipramine, imipramine, and nortriptyline (increased tricyclic antidepressant plasma concentrations and AUC). Increased desipramine plasma concentrations and AUC reported when used concomitantly with cobicistat or EVG/c/FTC/TDF.

If a tricyclic antidepressant is initiated in a patient receiving EVG/c/FTC/TDF, the lowest initial dosage of the antidepressant should be used and dosage carefully titrated based on clinical response and/or plasma concentrations of the antidepressant.

● *Zolpidem*

Pharmacokinetic interaction with zolpidem expected (increased zolpidem plasma concentrations).

If zolpidem is used concomitantly with EVG/c/FTC/TDF, patients should be monitored clinically; reduced zolpidem dosage may be necessary.

● **Dietary and Herbal Supplements**

St. John's Wort

Potential pharmacokinetic interactions with St. John's wort (*Hypericum perforatum*) (decreased elvitegravir and/or cobicistat plasma concentrations); possible decreased antiretroviral efficacy and development of resistance.

Concomitant use of St. John's wort and EVG/c/FTC/TDF is contraindicated.

DESCRIPTION

The fixed-dose combination of elvitegravir, cobicistat, emtricitabine, and tenofovir disoproxil fumarate (EVG/c/FTC/TDF) contains elvitegravir (a human immunodeficiency virus [HIV] integrase strand transfer inhibitor [INSTI]), cobicistat (a pharmacokinetic enhancer), emtricitabine (an HIV nucleoside reverse transcriptase inhibitor [NRTI]), and tenofovir disoproxil fumarate (an HIV nucleotide reverse transcriptase inhibitor). Cobicistat, a potent cytochrome P-450 (CYP) 3A inhibitor, is included in the fixed combination to increase plasma concentrations of elvitegravir (*cobicistat-boosted* elvitegravir).

Elvitegravir inhibits the activity of HIV-1 integrase, an enzyme that is required for viral replication. This results in the inhibition of integration of HIV-1 DNA into host genomic DNA, which is required for maintenance of the viral genome and for efficient viral gene expression and replication. Inhibition of integration prevents propagation of viral infection. Elvitegravir is active against HIV-1 and also has some in vitro activity against HIV type 2 (HIV-2); the drug does not have activity against hepatitis B virus (HBV) or hepatitis C virus (HCV).

Cobicistat is a selective mechanism-based inhibitor of CYP3A that decreases metabolism and increases plasma concentrations of CYP3A substrates; cobicistat also is a weak inhibitor of CYP2D6, but does not inhibit CYP1A2, 2C9, or 2C19. Cobicistat is included in EVG/c/FTC/TDF for therapeutic advantage and acts as a pharmacokinetic enhancer (also known as a booster) to increase systemic exposure of elvitegravir sufficient to allow for once-daily dosing (*cobicistat-boosted* elvitegravir). Cobicistat does not have any antiretroviral or antiviral activity and is not active against HIV-1, HBV, or HCV; cobicistat does not antagonize the antiretroviral activity of elvitegravir, emtricitabine, or tenofovir.

Emtricitabine, a synthetic nucleoside analog of cytidine, is a prodrug that is inactive until converted intracellularly to an active 5′-triphosphate metabolite. After conversion to the pharmacologically active metabolite, the drug acts as a reverse transcriptase inhibitor antiretroviral. Emtricitabine is active against HIV-1 and also has some in vitro activity against HIV-2.

Tenofovir DF is a tenofovir prodrug and is inactive until it undergoes diester hydrolysis in vivo to tenofovir and is subsequently metabolized to the active metabolite (tenofovir diphosphate). After conversion to the pharmacologically active metabolite, the drug act as a reverse transcriptase inhibitor antiretroviral. Tenofovir is active against HIV-1 and also has some in vitro activity against HIV-2; the drug also is active against HBV.

HIV-1 resistant to elvitegravir, emtricitabine, or tenofovir has been produced in vitro and has emerged during EVG/c/FTC/TDF therapy. In clinical trials evaluating EVG/c/FTC/TDF in antiretroviral-naïve patients, 1 or more primary mutations associated with resistance to elvitegravir, emtricitabine, and/or tenofovir were identified in HIV-1 isolates from 51% of patients who received EVG/c/FTC/TDF and were considered to be virologic treatment failures. Cross-resistance between elvitegravir and other HIV INSTIs (e.g., dolutegravir, raltegravir) has been reported. Cross-resistance also occurs among the HIV NRTIs.

Following an oral dose of EVG/c/FTC/TDF given with food, peak plasma concentrations of elvitegravir and cobicistat occur at 4 and 3 hours, respectively, and peak plasma concentrations of emtricitabine and tenofovir occur at 3 and 2 hours, respectively. Administration of EVG/c/FTC/TDF with a high-fat meal (approximately 800 kcal, 50% fat) increases mean systemic exposures of elvitegravir and tenofovir by 87 and 23%, respectively, compared with administration in the fasting state; mean systemic exposures of cobicistat and emtricitabine are decreased by 17 and 4%, respectively, compared with administration in the

fasting state. Elvitegravir is approximately 99% and cobicistat is approximately 98% bound to plasma proteins; emtricitabine is less than 4% and tenofovir is less than 1% bound to plasma proteins. Elvitegravir is metabolized principally by CYP3A isoenzymes, but also undergoes glucuronidation via uridine diphosphate-glucuronsyltransferase (UGT) 1A1/3 enzymes. Cobicistat is metabolized by CYP3A and to a minor extent by CYP2D6. Although the cobicistat component of EVG/c/FTC/TDF acts as a pharmacokinetic enhancer for elvitegravir, cobicistat does not have any clinically important effects on the pharmacokinetics of emtricitabine or tenofovir DF. Elvitegravir and cobicistat are principally excreted in feces (94.8 and 86.2% of a dose, respectively) and to a lesser extent in urine (6.7 and 8.2% of a dose, respectively). Emtricitabine is principally excreted in urine (70% of a dose) and to a lesser extent in feces (13.7% of a dose); approximately 70–80% of a dose of TDF is excreted in urine. The median terminal plasma half-lives of elvitegravir, cobicistat, emtricitabine, and tenofovir are 12.9, 3.5, 10, and 12–18 hours, respectively. No clinically significant differences in the pharmacokinetics of EVG/c/FTC/TDF have been identified based on race or gender.

ADVICE TO PATIENTS

- Advise patients of the critical nature of compliance with HIV therapy and the importance of remaining under the care of a clinician. Importance of taking EVG/c/FTC/TDF as prescribed; do not alter or discontinue antiretroviral regimen without consulting clinician.

- Advise patients that EVG/c/FTC/TDF is a complete regimen for treatment of HIV-1 infection and should *not* be used in conjunction with other antiretroviral agents.

- Advise patients on the importance of taking EVG/c/FTC/TDF with food.

- If a dose is missed, take the dose as soon as it is remembered and take next dose at regularly scheduled time. If a dose is skipped, do not take a double dose to make up for the missed dose.

- Inform patients that testing for hepatitis B virus (HBV) infection is recommended before antiretroviral therapy is initiated. Also advise patients that severe acute exacerbations of HBV infection have been reported following discontinuance of emtricitabine or tenofovir DF in HIV-infected patients coinfected with HBV.

- Advise patients that renal impairment, including cases of acute renal failure or Fanconi syndrome, has occurred. Advise patients on the importance of not using EVG/c/FTC/TDF concomitantly with or shortly after nephrotoxic agents (e.g., high-dose or multiple nonsteroidal anti-inflammatory agents [NSAIAs]).

- Advise patients of reproductive potential that additional or nonhormonal methods of contraception should be used when estrogen-based contraceptives are used concomitantly with EVG/c/FTC/TDF.

- Advise patients that lactic acidosis and severe hepatomegaly with steatosis, including fatalities, have occurred with emtricitabine and tenofovir (components of EVG/c/FTC/TDF). Advise patients on the importance of contacting a clinician if symptoms suggestive of lactic acidosis or hepatotoxicity (e.g., nausea, vomiting, unusual/unexpected stomach discomfort, weakness) occur.

- Advise patients that decreased bone mineral density (BMD) has occurred and that assessment of BMD should be considered in those with a history of pathologic bone fracture or other risk factors for osteoporosis or bone loss.

- Advise patients that signs and symptoms of inflammation from previous infections may occur soon after initiation of antiretroviral therapy in some individuals with advanced HIV infection (AIDS). These symptoms may be due to an improvement in immune response, enabling the body to fight infections that may have been present with no obvious symptoms. Advise patients on the importance of immediately informing a healthcare provider if any symptoms of infection occur.

- Advise patients to inform their clinician of existing or contemplated concomitant therapy, including prescription and OTC drugs and herbal products (e.g., St. John's wort), as well as any concomitant illnesses.

- Advise women to inform clinician if they are or plan to become pregnant or plan to breast-feed. Due to the risk of HIV transmission, HIV-infected women should not breast-feed infants.
- Advise patients of other important precautionary information.

PREPARATIONS

Excipients in commercially available drug preparations may have clinically important effects in some individuals; consult specific product labeling for details.

Elvitegravir, Cobicistat, Emtricitabine, and Tenofovir Disoproxil Fumarate

Oral

Tablets, film-coated	Elvitegravir 150 mg, Cobicistat 150 mg, Emtricitabine 200 mg, and Tenofovir Disoproxil Fumarate 300 mg	**Stribild®**, Gilead

† Use is not currently included in the labeling approved by the US Food and Drug Administration.

Selected Revisions February 10, 2024, © Copyright, October 22, 2013, American Society of Health-System Pharmacists, Inc.

Raltegravir Potassium

8:18.08.12 • HIV INTEGRASE INHIBITORS

■ Raltegravir potassium, an antiretroviral agent, is a human immunodeficiency virus (HIV) integrase strand transfer inhibitor (INSTI).

USES

● Treatment of HIV Infection

Raltegravir is used in conjunction with other antiretroviral agents for the treatment of human immunodeficiency virus type 1 (HIV-1) infection in adults and pediatric patients weighing ≥2 kg (Isentress®) or pediatric patients weighing ≥40 kg (Isentress® HD).

Raltegravir is commonly used as part of a fully suppressive antiretroviral regimen; consult guidelines for the most current information on recommended regimens. Selection of an initial antiretroviral regimen should be individualized based on factors such as virologic efficacy, toxicity, pill burden, dosing frequency, drug-drug interaction potential, resistance test results, comorbid conditions, access, and cost.

Clinical Experience

Antiretroviral-naïve Adults

The comparative efficacy of raltegravir (twice daily) and efavirenz (once daily) for the treatment of HIV-1 infection in antiretroviral-naïve adults was evaluated in a phase 3, randomized, active-control study (STARTMRK). The comparative efficacy of raltegravir (twice daily) and raltegravir (once daily) in antiretroviral-naïve, HIV-infected adults was evaluated in a phase 3, randomized, double-blind, parallel-group, noninferiority study (ONCEMRK).

In STARTMRK, 563 antiretroviral-naïve adults with baseline plasma HIV-1 RNA levels >5000 copies/mL were randomized to receive raltegravir (400-mg tablet twice daily) or efavirenz (600 mg once daily) in conjunction with the fixed combination of emtricitabine and tenofovir disoproxil fumarate (emtricitabine/tenofovir DF). At baseline, enrolled patients had a median age of 37 years (range: 19–71 years), 81% were male, 58% were non-white, 53% had baseline plasma HIV-1 RNA levels exceeding 100,000 copies/mL, 47% had baseline CD4+ T-cell counts <200 cells/mm³, and 6% had hepatitis B virus (HBV) or hepatitis C virus (HCV) coinfection. At 240 weeks, 66% of those receiving the twice-daily raltegravir regimen had plasma HIV-1 RNA levels <50 copies/mL compared with 60% of those receiving once-daily efavirenz.

In ONCEMRK, 797 antiretroviral-naïve adults with baseline plasma HIV-1 RNA levels of ≥1000 copies/mL were randomized to receive 1.2 g of raltegravir once daily (two 600-mg tablets once daily) or 400 mg of raltegravir twice daily (400-mg tablet twice daily) in conjunction with the fixed combination emtricitabine/tenofovir DF. At baseline, enrolled patients had a median age of 34 years (range: 18–84 years), 85% were male, 41% were non-white, 28% had baseline plasma HIV-1 RNA levels exceeding 100,000 copies/mL, 13% had baseline CD4+ T-cell counts <200 cells/mm³, and 3% had HBV and/or HCV coinfection. At 96 weeks, 82% of the patients randomized to the once-daily raltegravir regimen (433/531 patients) and 80% of those randomized to the twice-daily raltegravir regimen (213/266 patients) had plasma HIV-1 RNA levels <40 copies/mL and the mean change in CD4+ T-cell count from baseline was 262 cells/mm³ in both treatment groups. These results indicate that the once-daily raltegravir regimen is noninferior to the twice-daily raltegravir regimen in antiretroviral-naïve adults.

Efficacy of a 2-drug antiretroviral regimen of *ritonavir-boosted* darunavir and raltegravir for the treatment of HIV-1 infection in antiretroviral-naïve adults was evaluated in a randomized, open-label, noninferiority trial (NEAT/ANRS 143). In this study, 805 antiretroviral-naïve adults with plasma HIV-1 RNA levels >1000 copies/mL were randomized 1:1 to receive a 2-drug regimen of *ritonavir-boosted* darunavir (800 mg of darunavir and 100 mg of ritonavir once daily) in conjunction with raltegravir (400 mg twice daily) or a 3-drug regimen of *ritonavir-boosted* darunavir (800 mg of darunavir and 100 mg of ritonavir once daily) in conjunction with the fixed combination emtricitabine/tenofovir DF. Baseline characteristics were similar in both treatment groups. At 96 weeks, the 2-drug regimen was noninferior to the 3-drug regimen based on the primary end point of proportion of patients with virologic or clinical failure (19% patients receiving the 2-drug regimen and 15% of those receiving the 3-drug regimen experienced treatment failure). However, among those with baseline CD4+ T-cell counts <200 cells/mm³, there were more virologic failures in the 2-drug arm than in the 3-drug arm and a trend towards more virologic failures was observed among those with baseline plasma HIV-1 RNA levels of ≥100,000 copies/mL. In a smaller open-label, randomized study in antiretroviral-naïve adults, a 2-drug regimen of *ritonavir-boosted* darunavir and raltegravir was associated with high rates of virologic failure in the subgroup of patients with baseline plasma HIV-1 RNA levels exceeding 100,000 copies/mL.

Raltegravir (400 mg twice daily) was compared to efavirenz (600 mg nightly), both in combination with lamivudine (150 mg twice daily) and zidovudine (300 mg twice daily) or an alternate nucleoside reverse transcriptase inhibitor (NRTI) backbone, in pregnant women living with HIV in a randomized, multicenter, open-label, Phase 4 trial (NICHD P1081). Participants were antiretroviral-naïve with gestational age between 20 and 36 weeks. The primary efficacy outcome was maternal virologic response, defined as a plasma HIV-1 viral load <200 copies/mL, within 21 days prior to delivery. Among 408 patients who were randomized, median age was 27 years and median gestational age was 27 weeks; most patients were Hispanic (52%) or non-Hispanic Black (36%). In the primary analysis, patients receiving raltegravir-based therapy experienced a significantly higher rate of virologic suppression at delivery than those receiving efavirenz-based therapy (94 and 84%, respectively). Subgroup analysis indicated differences in response rate were associated with gestational age at study entry. In patients who entered the study at a gestational age between 20 and 27 weeks, rates of virologic suppression at delivery were similar between treatment arms. However, in patients who entered the study at a gestational age between 28 and 36 weeks, those assigned to raltegravir-based treatment achieved substantially greater virologic suppression at delivery compared to patients assigned to efavirenz-based treatment.

Antiretroviral-experienced Adults

Raltegravir has been evaluated in 2 phase 3, randomized, double-blind, placebo-controlled, multicenter studies (BENCHMRK 1, BENCHMRK 2) in antiretroviral-experienced adults with documented resistance to at least one HIV NRTI, HIV nonnucleoside reverse transcriptase inhibitor (NNRTI), and HIV protease inhibitor (PI). Patients enrolled in these studies were adults 16 years of age or older (mean age 45 years, 88–89% male, 65–73% white, 11–14% Black, 3% Asian, 8–11% Hispanic, median baseline plasma HIV-1 RNA level 4.7–4.8 log₁₀ copies/mL, median baseline CD4+ T-cell count 119–123 cells/mm³) who had previously received various antiretrovirals (median number of previous antiretrovirals was 12) for a median duration of 10 years. All patients received an optimized background antiretroviral regimen (OBR; selected on the basis of the individual's prior antiretroviral treatment and results of genotypic/phenotypic viral resistance testing; median number of antiretrovirals in the OBR was 4). A total of 699 patients were randomized to receive raltegravir 400 mg twice daily or placebo in conjunction with an OBR. Random assignment was stratified by degree of resistance to PIs at study entry (i.e., resistant to one PI or more than one PI [95–97% were resistant to more than one PI]) and use of enfuvirtide in the OBR (38% received enfuvirtide). At 96 weeks, pooled analysis of these 699 patients indicated that 55% of those randomized to raltegravir in conjunction with an OBR had plasma HIV-1 RNA levels <50 copies/mL compared with 27% of those randomized to placebo and an OBR; the mean increase in CD4+ T-cell count was 118 and 47 cells/mm³, respectively. At 156 weeks (after completion of the double-blind treatment period), 251 patients from the raltegravir group and 47 patients from the placebo group received open-label treatment with raltegravir (400 mg twice daily) in conjunction with an OBR. At 240 weeks (after 84 weeks of open-label treatment), 77% of patients originally enrolled in the raltegravir group had plasma HIV-1 RNA levels <50 copies/mL compared with 81% of patients originally enrolled in the placebo group; the mean increase in CD4+ T-cell count from baseline was 293 and 267 cells/mm³, respectively.

Two phase 3 studies designed to evaluate the use of raltegravir and 2 NRTIs in patients who had been receiving a suppressive regimen of the fixed combination of lopinavir and ritonavir (lopinavir/ritonavir) and 2 NRTIs were terminated early based on 24-week data that failed to demonstrate non-inferiority of switching to raltegravir versus continuing the lopinavir/ritonavir regimen (SWITCHMRK 1 and 2). In these studies, a total of 352 HIV-1-infected patients who had been receiving a regimen of lopinavir/ritonavir and at least 2 NRTIs for longer than 3 months and had plasma HIV-1 RNA levels <50 copies/mL were randomized to either continue the lopinavir/ritonavir regimen or be switched to raltegravir (400 mg twice daily) with the NRTIs. At 24 weeks, combined analysis of the studies indicated that plasma HIV-1 RNA levels <50 copies/mL were maintained in 90% of those who continued the lopinavir/ritonavir regimen compared with 82% of those who were switched to the raltegravir regimen.

Pediatric Patients

Efficacy of raltegravir in conjunction with other antiretrovirals in pediatric patients have been evaluated in a phase 1/phase 2 open-label study (IMPAACT P1066) that included 126 antiretroviral-experienced HIV-infected children and adolescents 2–18 years of age. These pediatric patients were enrolled into the following cohorts based on age and received raltegravir in conjunction with an OBR: cohort I (12 to <18 years of age; 400 mg film-coated tablets), cohort IIa (6 to <12 years of age; 400 mg film-coated tablets), cohort IIb (6 to <12 years old; chewable tablets), and cohort III (2 to <6 years of age; chewable tablets). In the initial dose-finding stage, raltegravir dosage was selected to achieve raltegravir plasma exposures and trough concentrations similar to those reported in adults and acceptable short-term safety. After dose selection, additional patients were enrolled for evaluation of long-term safety, tolerability, and efficacy. Of the initial 126 patients in cohorts I, IIa, IIb, and III, 96 received the recommended dosage of raltegravir (median age 13 years, 51% female, 34% white, 59% Black, mean baseline plasma HIV-1 RNA level 4.3 $\log_{10}$ copies/mL, median baseline CD4+ T-cell count 481 cells/mm³, median CD4 percentage 23%). A total of 93 of these patients completed 24 weeks of treatment and 91 completed 48 weeks of treatment. At week 24, 66 and 54% had achieved plasma HIV-1 RNA levels <400 and 50 copies/mL, respectively; the mean increase in CD4+ T-cell count from baseline was 119 cells/mm³, and the mean increase in CD4+ T-cell percentage from baseline was 3.8%. At week 48, 74 and 57% had achieved plasma HIV-1 RNA levels <400 and 50 copies/mL, respectively; the mean increase in CD4+ T-cell count from baseline was 156 cells/mm³, and the mean increase in CD4+ T-cell percentage from baseline was 4.6%.

IMPAACT P1066 also evaluated the safety and efficacy of raltegravir oral suspension in conjunction with an OBR in children 4 weeks to <2 years of age (cohorts IV and V). The 26 patients enrolled in cohorts IV and V (median age 28 weeks, 35% female, 8% white, 85% Black, mean baseline plasma HIV-1 RNA level 5.7 $\log_{10}$ copies/mL, median baseline CD4+ T-cell count 1400 cells/mm³, median CD4 percentage 18.6%) had previously received antiretroviral therapy as prophylaxis for prevention of perinatal HIV transmission and/or as combination antiretroviral therapy for treatment of HIV infection. Twenty-three patients were included in the 24-week and 48-week efficacy analyses. At week 24, 61 and 39% had achieved plasma HIV-1 RNA levels <400 and 50 copies/mL, respectively; the mean increase in CD4+ T-cell count from baseline was 500 cells/mm³, and the mean increase in CD4+ T-cell percentage from baseline was 7.5%. At week 48, 61 and 44% had achieved plasma HIV-1 RNA levels <400 and 50 copies/mL, respectively; the mean increase in CD4+ T-cell count from baseline was 492 cells/mm³, and the mean increase in CD4+ T-cell percentage from baseline was 7.8%.

Clinical Perspective

Therapeutic options for the treatment and prevention of HIV infection and recommendations concerning the use of antiretrovirals are continuously evolving. Antiretroviral therapy (ART) is recommended for all individuals with HIV regardless of CD4 counts, and should be initiated as soon as possible after diagnosis of HIV and continued indefinitely. The primary goals of ART are to achieve and maintain durable suppression of HIV viral load (as measured by plasma HIV-1 RNA levels) to a level below which drug-resistance mutations cannot emerge (i.e., below detectable limits), restore and preserve immunologic function, reduce HIV-related morbidity and mortality, improve quality of life, and prevent transmission of HIV. While the most appropriate antiretroviral regimen cannot be defined for each clinical scenario, the US Department of Health and Human Services (HHS) Panel on Antiretroviral Guidelines for Adults and Adolescents, HHS Panel on Antiretroviral Therapy and Medical Management of Children Living with HIV, and HHS Panel on Treatment of Pregnant Women with HIV Infection and Prevention of Perinatal Transmission, have developed comprehensive guidelines that provide information on selection and use of antiretrovirals for the treatment or prevention of HIV infection. Because of the complexity of managing patients with HIV, it is recommended that clinicians with HIV expertise be consulted when needed.

The use of combination antiretroviral regimens that generally include 3 drugs from 2 or more drug classes is currently recommended to achieve viral suppression. In both treatment-naïve adults and children, an initial antiretroviral regimen generally consists of 2 NRTIs administered in combination with a third active antiretroviral drug from 1 of 3 drug classes: an INSTI, a NNRTI, or a PI with a pharmacokinetic enhancer (also known as a booster; the 2 drugs used for this purpose are cobicistat and ritonavir). Selection of an initial antiretroviral regimen should be individualized based on factors such as virologic efficacy, toxicity, pill burden, dosing frequency, drug–drug interaction potential, resistance-test results, comorbid conditions, access, and cost. In patients with comorbid infections (e.g., hepatitis B, tuberculosis), regimen selection should also consider the potential for activity against other present infections and timing of initiation relative to other anti-infective regimens.

In the 2023 HHS adult and adolescent HIV treatment guideline, raltegravir, an INSTI, is included in various antiretroviral regimens. Some of these raltegravir-containing regimens are listed among recommended or alternative initial regimens in certain clinical situations, and include the following regimens: raltegravir plus tenofovir alafenamide or tenofovir DF plus emtricitabine or lamivudine, or, when abacavir, tenofovir alafenamide, and tenofovir DF cannot be used or are not optimal, *ritonavir-boosted* darunavir plus raltegravir twice a day (*only* in patients with CD4 count >200 cells/mm³ and HIV viral load <100,000 copies/mL).

In the 2023 HHS pediatric HIV treatment guideline, raltegravir is included in various regimens. Raltegravir plus 2 NRTIs is a preferred initial regimen from birth to <4 weeks of age (*only* in patients weighing ≥2 kg) and is recommended as an alternative initial regimen in patients ≥4 weeks of age (*only* in patients weighing ≥2 kg).

In the 2023 HHS perinatal HIV treatment guideline, raltegravir is included in various antiretroviral regimens. Raltegravir plus a preferred dual-NRTI backbone is listed as an alternative initial option for pregnant patients.

● Postexposure Prophylaxis following Occupational Exposure to HIV

Raltegravir is used in conjunction with 2 NRTIs for postexposure prophylaxis of HIV infection following occupational exposure (PEP)† in health-care personnel and other individuals exposed via percutaneous injury (e.g., needlestick, cut with sharp object) or mucous membrane or nonintact skin (e.g., chapped, abraded, dermatitis) contact with blood, tissue, or other body fluids that might contain HIV.

The US Public Health Service (USPHS) states that the preferred regimen for PEP following an occupational exposure to HIV is a 3-drug regimen of raltegravir used in conjunction with emtricitabine and tenofovir DF (may be administered as the fixed combination emtricitabine/tenofovir DF; Truvada®). These experts recommend several alternative regimens that include an INSTI (such as raltegravir), NNRTI, or PI and 2 NRTIs (dual NRTIs). The preferred dual NRTI option for use in PEP regimens is emtricitabine and tenofovir DF (may be administered as the fixed combination emtricitabine/tenofovir DF; Truvada®); alternative dual NRTIs are tenofovir DF and lamivudine, lamivudine and zidovudine (may be administered as the fixed combination lamivudine/zidovudine; Combivir®), or zidovudine and emtricitabine.

Because management of occupational exposures to HIV is complex and evolving, consultation with an infectious diseases specialist, clinician with expertise in administration of antiretroviral agents, and/or the National Clinicians' Postexposure Prophylaxis Hotline (PEPline at 888-448-4911) is recommended whenever possible. However, initiation of PEP should not be delayed while waiting for expert consultation.

● Postexposure Prophylaxis following Nonoccupational Exposure to HIV

Raltegravir is used in conjunction with other antiretrovirals for postexposure prophylaxis of HIV infection following nonoccupational exposure (nPEP)† in individuals exposed to blood, genital secretions, or other potentially infectious body fluids that might contain HIV when the exposure represents a substantial risk for HIV transmission. Raltegravir in combination with emtricitabine and tenofovir DF is a preferred regimen in guidelines for nPEP, and several raltegravir-containing combinations are listed as alternative regimens.

Clinical Experience

Raltegravir in combination with tenofovir DF and emtricitabine has been evaluated as nPEP† in 2 non-comparative clinical trials. In the first study, 86 HIV-negative men who have sex with men received raltegravir in combination with tenofovir DF and emtricitabine for 28 days following potential sexual exposure to HIV. In the second study, 100 HIV-negative adults received raltegravir in combination with tenofovir DF and emtricitabine for 28 days following potential sexual exposure to HIV. Regimen completion rates were 92% and 57%, respectively; no patients in either study had developed HIV infection at 3-month follow-up.

Clinical Perspective

When nPEP is indicated following a nonoccupational exposure to HIV, the US Centers for Disease Control and Prevention (CDC) states that the preferred regimen in adults and adolescents 13 years of age or older with normal renal function is either raltegravir or dolutegravir used in conjunction with emtricitabine and tenofovir DF (administered as the fixed combination emtricitabine/tenofovir DF; Truvada®). The alternative nPEP regimen recommended in these patients is *ritonavir-boosted* darunavir used in conjunction with emtricitabine/tenofovir DF (Truvada®). Raltegravir in combination with 2 other NRTIs is one of several other alterative regimens recommended by CDC for nPEP.

Consultation with an infectious diseases specialist, clinician with expertise in administration of antiretroviral agents, and/or the National Clinicians' Postexposure Prophylaxis Hotline (PEPline at 888-448-4911) is recommended if nPEP is indicated in certain exposed individuals (e.g., pregnant women, children, those with medical conditions such as renal impairment) or if an antiretroviral regimen not included in the CDC guidelines is being considered, the source virus is known or likely to be resistant to antiretrovirals, or the healthcare provider is inexperienced in prescribing antiretrovirals. However, initiation of nPEP should not be delayed while waiting for expert consultation.

DOSAGE AND ADMINISTRATION

● *General*

Pretreatment Screening

- Evaluate patients for history of phenylketonuria.
- Evaluate patients for history of rhabdomyolysis, myopathy, or increased creatine kinase.
- Evaluate use of concomitant medications including statins, fenofibrate, gemfibrozil, or zidovudine.

Patient Monitoring

- Monitor for symptoms of infection.
- Monitor for rash associated with severe symptoms such as fever, extreme fatigue, hypersensitivity, and hepatotoxicity.

● *Administration*

Raltegravir potassium is available for oral administration as 400-mg and 600-mg (Isentress® HD) film-coated tablets, 25-mg and 100-mg chewable tablets, and a 100-mg powder for oral suspension. Raltegravir is administered orally once or twice daily without regard to food. Use the drug in conjunction with other antiretrovirals.

Chewable Tablets

Raltegravir chewable tablets may be chewed or swallowed whole. If necessary, the 100-mg chewable tablet can be divided into equal halves. For children who have difficulty chewing, the 25 mg chewable tablet can be crushed. To administer, place the chewable tablet in a small, clean cup and add a teaspoonful (5 mL) of a liquid such as water, juice, or breast milk. Within 2 minutes, the tablet(s) will absorb the liquid and fall apart. Crush any remaining pieces with a spoon and immediately administer the entire dose orally. For any remaining portion of the dose, add another teaspoonful of liquid, swirl, and administer immediately.

The chewable tablets are used in pediatric patients 4 weeks of age or older weighing at least 3 kg to less than 25 kg. If necessary, the chewable tablets may be used as an alternative in pediatric patients weighing 25 kg or more who are not able to swallow the film-coated tablets; however, the film-coated tablets are the preferred formulation in pediatric patients weighing 25 kg or more if they can swallow a tablet.

Store raltegravir chewable tablets at 20–25°C (excursions permitted between 15–30°C). Keep bottle tightly closed; do not remove desiccant.

Film-coated Tablets

Raltegravir film-coated tablets must be swallowed whole. Raltegravir (Isentress®) 400-mg film-coated tablets are used in adults and pediatric patients weighing 25 kg or more. Raltegravir (Isentress® HD) 600-mg film-coated tablets are used in adults and pediatric patients weighing 40 kg or more.

Store raltegravir film-coated tablets at 20–25°C (excursions permitted between 15–30°C). Keep bottle tightly closed; do not remove desiccant.

Powder for Oral Suspension

Raltegravir powder for oral suspension is provided in single-use packets containing 100 mg of raltegravir and is used in pediatric patients weighing 2 kg to less than 20 kg. When the oral suspension is used, the maximum dosage is 100 mg twice daily. To prepare the oral suspension, use the proper syringe provided by the manufacturer to measure and add 10 mL of water to the mixing cup provided by the manufacturer. Add the entire contents of a single-use packet of raltegravir for oral suspension to the water in the mixing cup and tightly close the mixing cup and gently swirl in a circular motion for 45 seconds. If the powder is not completely mixed, gently swirl the mixing cup some more. Do not shake the mixing cup; the oral suspension will appear cloudy. Withdraw the recommended dosage of the oral suspension into the correct dosing syringe provided by the manufacturer and administer orally. After each use, handwash the dosing syringe and mixing cup with warm water and dish soap, rinse with water, and air dry.

Do not open the foil packets containing the powder for oral suspension until ready to use. After the contents of the packet are suspended in water, use the oral suspension within 30 minutes and discard any unused portion.

Store raltegravir powder for oral suspension at 20–25°C (excursions permitted between 15–30°C).

● *Dosage*

Raltegravir chewable tablets, film-coated tablets, and powder for oral suspension contain raltegravir potassium; dosage is expressed in terms of raltegravir.

Because the formulations have different pharmacokinetic profiles, raltegravir chewable tablets and oral suspension are not bioequivalent to raltegravir film-coated tablets. Do not substitute the chewable tablets or oral suspension for the 400- or 600-mg film-coated tablets.

Adults

Treatment of HIV-1 Infection in Antiretroviral-naïve Adults

For the initial treatment of human immunodeficiency virus type 1 (HIV-1) infection in antiretroviral-naïve adults, the recommended dosage of raltegravir is 400 mg twice daily (one 400-mg film-coated tablet twice daily). Alternatively, 1.2 g of raltegravir can be given once daily (two 600-mg film-coated tablets once daily).

When raltegravir is used in antiretroviral-naïve adults receiving rifampin, the drug should be given in a dosage of 800 mg twice daily (two 400-mg film-coated tablets twice daily).

Treatment of HIV-1 Infection in Antiretroviral-experienced Adults

For the treatment of HIV-1 infection in antiretroviral-experienced adults, the recommended dosage of raltegravir is 400 mg twice daily (one 400-mg film-coated tablet twice daily). In adults who are virologically suppressed on an initial regimen of raltegravir 400 mg twice daily, the same twice-daily raltegravir regimen can be continued or the patient may be switched to a regimen of 1.2 g of raltegravir once daily (two 600-mg film-coated tablets once daily).

When raltegravir is used in antiretroviral-experienced adults receiving rifampin, the drug should be given in a dosage of 800 mg twice daily (two 400-mg film-coated tablets twice daily).

Postexposure Prophylaxis following Occupational Exposure to HIV

For postexposure prophylaxis of HIV infection following occupational exposure (PEP)† in health-care personnel or other individuals, the recommended dosage of raltegravir is 400 mg twice daily. Raltegravir usually is used in conjunction with emtricitabine and tenofovir disoproxil fumarate (DF). PEP should be initiated as soon as possible following occupational exposure to HIV (preferably within hours) and continued for 4 weeks, if tolerated.

Postexposure Prophylaxis following Nonoccupational Exposure to HIV

For postexposure prophylaxis of HIV infection following nonoccupational exposure (nPEP)† when the exposure represents a substantial risk for HIV transmission, the usual adult dosage of raltegravir is 400 mg twice daily in conjunction with 2 HIV nucleoside reverse transcriptase inhibitors (NRTIs).

The nPEP regimen should be initiated as soon as possible (within 72 hours) following nonoccupational exposure to HIV and continued for 28 days. If the exposed individual seeks care more than 72 hours after the exposure, nPEP is not recommended.

Pediatric Dosage

Treatment of HIV-1 Infection

When raltegravir is used for the treatment of HIV-1 infection in full-term neonates (birth through 4 weeks [28 days] of age) weighing at least 2 kg, the powder for oral suspension should be used and dosage is based on weight. A once-daily raltegravir regimen is recommended in neonates up to 1 week of age and a twice-daily regimen is recommended in those 1–4 weeks of age. (See Table 1.)

TABLE 1. Recommended Dosage of Raltegravir Oral Suspension (Isentress®) in Full-term Neonates (Birth to 4 Weeks of Age)[a]

Weight (kg)	Volume (Dose) of Oral Suspension Containing 10 mg/mL
Birth to 1 Week of Age (Once-daily Regimen)[b]	
2 to <3	0.4 mL (4 mg) once daily
3 to <4	0.5 mL (5 mg) once daily
4 to <5	0.7 mL (7 mg) once daily
1–4 Weeks of Age (Twice-daily Regimen)[c]	
2 to <3	0.8 mL (8 mg) twice daily
3 to <4	1 mL (10 mg) twice daily
4 to <5	1.5 mL (15 mg) twice daily

[a] If the mother received a dose of raltegravir (Isentress® or Isentress® HD) within 2–24 hours before delivery, the first raltegravir dose in the neonate should be given 24–48 hours after birth.

[b] Recommended dosage of raltegravir oral suspension in neonates from birth to 1 week of age is based on approximately 1.5 mg/kg per dose.

[c] Recommended dosage of raltegravir oral suspension in neonates 1–4 weeks of age is based on approximately 3 mg/kg per dose.

When raltegravir is used for the treatment of HIV-1 infection in pediatric patients 4 weeks of age or older weighing 3 to less than 20 kg, the powder for oral suspension or chewable tablets can be used. For patients weighing less than 14 kg, the chewable tablets can be crushed. The chewable tablets should be used in pediatric patients weighing 20 to less than 25 kg. Dosage is based on weight and depends on whether the powder for oral suspension or chewable tablets are used. A twice-daily raltegravir regimen is used in these pediatric patients. (See Table 2.)

TABLE 2. Recommended Dosage of Raltegravir Oral Suspension or Chewable Tablets (Isentress®) in Pediatric Patients 4 Weeks of Age Weighing 3 to less than 25 kg[a]

Weight (kg)	Volume (Dose) of Oral Suspension Containing 10 mg/mL	Number of 25- or 100-mg Chewable Tablets
3 to <4	2.5 mL (25 mg) twice daily	1 x 25 mg twice daily[b]
4 to <6	3 mL (30 mg) twice daily	1 x 25 mg twice daily[b]
6 to <8	4 mL (40 mg) twice daily	2 x 25 mg twice daily[b]
8 to <10	6 mL (60 mg) twice daily	2 x 25 mg twice daily[b]
10 to <14	8 mL (80 mg) twice daily	3 x 25 mg twice daily[b]
14 to <20	10 mL (100 mg) twice daily	1 x 100 mg twice daily
20 to <25	Do not use	1.5 x 100 mg twice daily[c]

[a] Recommended weight-based dosage of raltegravir oral suspension or chewable tablets in pediatric patients 4 weeks of age or older weighing 3 to less than 25 kg is based on approximately 6 mg/kg/dose twice daily.

[b] May be administered as a crushed tablet(s).

[c] The 100-mg chewable tablets can be divided into equal halves.

For the treatment of HIV-1 infection in pediatric patients weighing 25 kg or more, raltegravir film-coated tablets are preferred, but the chewable tablets can be used in those unable to swallow the film-coated tablets. When the chewable tablets are used in pediatric patients weighing 25 kg or more, dosage is based on weight and a twice-daily raltegravir regimen is used. (See Table 3.)

TABLE 3. Recommended Dosage of Raltegravir Chewable Tablets (Isentress®) In Pediatric Patients Weighing 25 kg or More and Unable to Swallow the Film- coated Tablets[a]

Weight (kg)	Dosage	Number of 100-mg Chewable Tablets
25 to <28	150 mg twice daily	One and one-half 100-mg tablets twice daily[b]
28 to <40	200 mg twice daily	Two 100-mg tablets twice daily
≥40	300 mg twice daily	Three 100-mg tablets twice daily

[a] Recommended weight-based dosage of raltegravir chewable tablets in pediatric patients weighing 25 kg or more is based on approximately 6 mg/kg per dose twice daily.

[b] The 100-mg chewable tablets can be divided into equal halves.

For the treatment of HIV-1 infection in pediatric patients weighing 25 to less than 40 kg who can swallow the film-coated tablets, the recommended raltegravir dosage is 400 mg twice daily (one 400-mg film-coated tablet twice daily).

For the treatment of HIV-1 infection in antiretroviral-naïve pediatric patients weighing 40 kg or more, the recommended dosage of raltegravir is 400 mg twice daily (one 400-mg film-coated tablet twice daily). Alternatively, antiretroviral-naïve pediatric patients weighing 40 kg or more can receive 1.2 g of raltegravir once daily (two 600-mg film-coated tablets once daily). For those who are virologically suppressed on an initial regimen of raltegravir 400 mg twice daily, the same twice-daily raltegravir regimen can be continued or the patient may be switched to a regimen of 1.2 g of raltegravir once daily (two 600-mg film-coated tablets once daily).

• Special Populations

Hepatic Impairment

Dosage adjustment of raltegravir (twice daily) is not needed in patients with mild to moderate hepatic impairment. Pharmacokinetics of raltegravir have not been studied in those with severe hepatic impairment.

Raltegravir (once daily) has not been studied in patients with hepatic impairment and is not recommended in patients with hepatic impairment.

Renal Impairment

Dosage adjustment of raltegravir (once or twice daily) is not needed in patients with renal impairment.

Because the extent to which raltegravir is removed by dialysis is not known, administering the drug before a dialysis session should be avoided.

Geriatric Use

The manufacturer makes no specific dosage recommendations for raltegravir in geriatric patients, but recommends careful dosage selection because of possible age-related decreases in hepatic, renal, and/or cardiac function and concomitant disease and drug therapy.

CAUTIONS

• Contraindications

• None.

• Warnings/Precautions

Severe Skin and Hypersensitivity Reactions

Severe, potentially life-threatening skin reactions, including some fatalities, have been reported in patients receiving raltegravir. Such reactions have included Stevens-Johnson syndrome, toxic epidermal necrolysis, and hypersensitivity reactions characterized by rash, constitutional findings, and, occasionally, organ dysfunction including hepatic failure.

Discontinue raltegravir immediately if signs or symptoms of severe skin or hypersensitivity reactions occur, including (but not limited to) severe rash or rash accompanied by fever, general malaise, fatigue, muscle or joint aches, blisters, oral lesions, conjunctivitis, facial edema, hepatitis, eosinophilia, or angioedema. Monitor clinical status, including liver aminotransferases, and initiate appropriate therapy.

A life-threatening reaction could occur if there is a delay in discontinuing raltegravir and any other suspect agents after the onset of severe rash.

Immune Reconstitution Syndrome

Immune reconstitution syndrome has been reported in patients receiving multiple-drug antiretroviral therapy, including raltegravir. During the initial phase of treatment, patients whose immune systems respond to antiretroviral therapy may develop an inflammatory response to indolent or residual opportunistic infections (e.g., Mycobacterium avium, M. tuberculosis, cytomegalovirus [CMV], Pneumocystis jirovecii); such responses may necessitate further evaluation and treatment.

Autoimmune disorders (e.g., Graves' disease, polymyositis, Guillain-Barré syndrome) have also been reported to occur in the setting of immune reconstitution; however, the time to onset is more variable and can occur many months after initiation of antiretroviral therapy.

Phenylketonurics

Each 25- or 100-mg raltegravir chewable tablet contains approximately 0.05 or 0.1 mg of phenylalanine, respectively. Phenylalanine can be harmful to patients with phenylketonuria.

Specific Populations

Pregnancy

The Antiretroviral Pregnancy Registry (APR) monitors pregnancy outcomes in females. Healthcare providers should register patients at 800-258-4263.

Available data from the APR show no difference in the rate of overall birth defects in infants of pregnant females receiving raltegravir compared with the background rate of major birth defects of 2.7% in the US reference population of the Metropolitan Atlanta Congenital Defects Program (MACDP).

Based on prospective reports from the APR of over 850 exposures to raltegravir during pregnancy resulting in live births (including over 450 exposures in the first trimester), the prevalence of defects in live births was 3.1% following first trimester exposure to raltegravir-containing regimens and 3.7% following second and third trimester exposure to raltegravir-containing regimens.

In animal reproduction studies (rats and rabbits), there was no evidence of adverse developmental outcomes when raltegravir was given orally during organogenesis at doses producing exposures approximately 4 times those reported with the maximum recommended human dose of 1.2 g.

In animal studies, raltegravir has been shown to cross the placenta with fetal plasma concentrations 1.5–2.5 times greater than in maternal plasma in rats and 2% of maternal plasma concentrations in rabbits on gestation day 20.

There are limited data on the use of raltegravir 1.2 g (two 600-mg film-coated tablets) once daily in pregnant females.

Lactation

There are no data available regarding the presence of raltegravir in human milk, the effects on the breastfed infant, or the effects on milk production. The drug is distributed into milk in rats; milk concentrations approximately 3 times higher than maternal plasma concentrations were reported at 2 hours after a dose on lactation day 14 in rats receiving oral raltegravir from gestation day 6 to lactation day 14.

Because of both the potential for HIV-1 transmission (in HIV-negative infants), developing viral resistance (in infants who are HIV-positive), and adverse reactions in breastfed infants similar to those seen in adults, instruct mothers not to breastfeed if they are taking raltegravir. The Centers for Disease Control and Prevention recommend that mothers with HIV-1 infection not breastfeed their infants to avoid risking postnatal transmission of HIV-1 infection.

Pediatric Use

Raltegravir (Isentress®; 400-mg film-coated tablets) is indicated for use in pediatric patients weighing 2 kg or more and is not recommended in preterm neonates or pediatric patients weighing less than 2 kg.

Raltegravir (Isentress® HD; 600-mg film-coated tablets) is indicated for use in pediatric patients weighing 40 kg or more. Although this formulation has not been studied in pediatric patients, the manufacturer states that population pharmacokinetic modeling and simulation support the use of the once-daily regimen (two 600-mg film-coated tablets once daily) in those weighing 40 kg or more.

Safety and pharmacokinetics of raltegravir for oral suspension were evaluated in 42 full-term HIV-1 exposed neonates at high risk of acquiring HIV-1 infection in a phase 1, open-label, multicenter, clinical trial (IMPAACT P1110). The safety profile of the drug in these neonates was comparable to that observed in adults receiving the drug.

Safety, efficacy, and pharmacokinetics of twice-daily raltegravir were evaluated in HIV-1 infected pediatric patients 4 weeks to 18 years of age in an open-label, multicenter, clinical trial (IMPAACT P1066). The safety profile of the drug in these pediatric patients was comparable to that observed in adults receiving the drug.

Geriatric Use

Experience in adults 65 years of age and older is insufficient to determine whether they respond differently to raltegravir than younger adults. Reported clinical experience has not identified differences in response between elderly and younger subjects.

Raltegravir should be used with caution in geriatric patients because of age-related decreases in hepatic, renal, and/or cardiac function and potential for concomitant disease and drug therapy.

Hepatic Impairment

Pharmacokinetics of a single 400-mg dose of raltegravir are not altered in adults with moderate hepatic impairment (Child-Pugh score 7–9). Pharmacokinetics of the drug have not been studied in patients with severe hepatic impairment.

Dosage adjustment in patients with mild to moderate hepatic impairment is not required.

A once-daily raltegravir regimen is not recommended in patients with hepatic impairment since the pharmacokinetics of the once-daily regimen (two 600-mg film-coated tablets once daily) have not been studied in such patients.

Patients with chronic hepatitis B virus (HBV) or hepatitis C virus (HCV) infection may be at increased risk for further elevations in hepatic enzyme concentrations.

Renal Impairment

Pharmacokinetics of a single 400-mg dose of raltegravir are not altered in adults with severe renal impairment (creatinine clearance less than 30 mL/minute per 1.73 m^2).

Pharmacokinetics of a once-daily raltegravir regimen (two 600-mg film-coated tablets once daily) have not been evaluated in patients with renal impairment.

Because renal clearance is a minor elimination pathway for unchanged raltegravir, dosage of raltegravir (once or twice daily) does not need to be adjusted in patients with any degree of renal impairment.

The extent to which raltegravir is removed by dialysis is not known; administration of the drug before a dialysis session should be avoided.

● Common Adverse Effects

Adverse effects reported in 2% or more of patients receiving raltegravir in conjunction with other antiretrovirals include insomnia, headache, dizziness, nausea, and fatigue. Creatine kinase elevations, myopathy, and rhabdomyolysis have been reported.

DRUG INTERACTIONS

● Drugs Affecting or Metabolized by Hepatic Microsomal Enzymes

Raltegravir is not a substrate for cytochrome P-450 (CYP) isoenzymes.

In vitro studies indicate that raltegravir does not inhibit CYP isoenzymes 1A2, 2B6, 2C8, 2C9, 2C19, 2D6, or 3A4 and does not induce CYP1A2, 2B6, or 3A4.

Pharmacokinetic interactions are unlikely with drugs that are substrates for these isoenzymes.

● Drugs Affecting or Metabolized by Uridine Diphosphate-glucuronosyltransferases

Raltegravir is primarily metabolized by uridine diphosphate-glucuronosyltransferase (UGT) 1A1

Pharmacokinetic interactions are possible with drugs that are potent inducers of UGT1A1 (decreased plasma concentrations of raltegravir) or with inhibitors of UGT1A1 (increased plasma concentrations of raltegravir).

In vitro studies indicate that raltegravir does not inhibit UGT1A1 or 2B7.

● Drugs Affected by P-glycoprotein Transport

Raltegravir does not inhibit P-glycoprotein (P-gp).

● Anticonvulsants

Carbamazepine

The effects of carbamazepine on the pharmacokinetics of raltegravir are not known. Concomitant use of carbamazepine and raltegravir is not recommended.

Phenobarbital or Phenytoin

The effects of phenobarbital or phenytoin on raltegravir are unknown. Concomitant use with these anticonvulsants is not recommended.

● Antilipemic Agents

Myopathy, increased creatine kinase, and rhabdomyolysis have been reported with raltegravir use. Interactions between antilipemic agents such as statins or fibrates and raltegravir have not been evaluated. However, the manufacturer advises caution with concomitant use of raltegravir and agents known to cause these conditions.

● Antimycobacterial Agents

Rifampin

There is a pharmacokinetic interaction between rifampin and raltegravir (decreased raltegravir plasma concentrations and area under the plasma concentration-time curve [AUC]); rifampin is a potent inducer of UGT1A1.

If raltegravir (twice daily) is used in adults receiving rifampin, raltegravir dosage should be increased to 800 mg twice daily. Data are insufficient to make dosage recommendations for concomitant use of raltegravir and rifampin in patients younger than 18 years of age.

Concomitant use of raltegravir (once daily) and rifampin is not recommended.

● Antiretroviral Agents

HIV Entry and Fusion Inhibitors

Enfuvirtide

There is no in vitro evidence of antagonistic antiretroviral effects between raltegravir and enfuvirtide.

HIV Nonnucleoside Reverse Transcriptase Inhibitors (NNRTIs)

There is no in vitro evidence of antagonistic antiretroviral effects between raltegravir and NNRTIs.

Efavirenz

Pharmacokinetic interactions between efavirenz and raltegravir (decreased plasma concentrations and AUC of raltegravir); not considered clinically meaningful.

Dosage adjustments are not needed if raltegravir is used concomitantly with efavirenz.

Etravirine

In a pharmacokinetic evaluation, etravirine decreased raltegravir plasma concentrations and AUC; however, the interaction is not considered clinically important. Raltegravir does not have a clinically important effect on etravirine pharmacokinetics.

Dosage adjustments are not needed if etravirine is used concomitantly with raltegravir (twice daily).

Concomitant use of etravirine and raltegravir (once daily) is not recommended.

HIV Nucleoside and Nucleotide Reverse Transcriptase Inhibitors (NRTIs)

There is no in vitro evidence of antagonistic antiretroviral effects between raltegravir and NRTIs.

Lamivudine

Raltegravir does not have a clinically important effect on the pharmacokinetics of lamivudine. Dosage adjustments are not needed if lamivudine and raltegravir are used concomitantly.

Tenofovir

In a pharmacokinetic evaluation, tenofovir disoproxil fumarate (DF) increased raltegravir plasma concentrations and AUC; however, the interaction is not considered clinically important. Raltegravir does not have a clinically important effect on tenofovir DF pharmacokinetics. Dosage adjustments are not needed if raltegravir is used concomitantly with tenofovir DF.

Pharmacokinetic interactions between raltegravir and tenofovir alafenamide fumarate are not expected.

HIV Protease Inhibitors (PIs)

There is no in vitro evidence of antagonistic antiretroviral effects between raltegravir and HIV PIs.

Atazanavir

Pharmacokinetic interactions between raltegravir and *ritonavir-boosted* atazanavir or unboosted atazanavir (increased raltegravir plasma concentrations and AUC) are not considered clinically important.

Dosage adjustments are not needed if raltegravir is used concomitantly with *ritonavir-boosted* atazanavir, or unboosted atazanavir.

Darunavir

No clinically important pharmacokinetic effects occurred in studies of coadministration of raltegravir with *ritonavir-boosted* darunavir. Raltegravir has no clinically important effect on pharmacokinetics of *ritonavir-boosted* darunavir.

Dosage adjustments are not needed if raltegravir is used concomitantly with *ritonavir-boosted* darunavir.

Tipranavir

The pharmacokinetic interaction between raltegravir and *ritonavir-boosted* tipranavir (decreased raltegravir plasma concentrations and AUC) is not considered clinically important.

Dosage adjustments are not needed if raltegravir (twice daily) is used concomitantly with *ritonavir-boosted* tipranavir.

Concomitant use of raltegravir (once daily) and *ritonavir-boosted* tipranavir is not recommended.

● Benzodiazepines

Raltegravir does not have a clinically important effect on the pharmacokinetics of midazolam.

● Estrogens and Progestins

Ethinyl Estradiol and Norgestimate

Raltegravir does not have a clinically important effect on the pharmacokinetics of hormonal contraceptives containing ethinyl estradiol or norgestimate.

Dosage adjustments are not needed if oral contraceptives containing ethinyl estradiol and norgestimate are used in patients receiving raltegravir.

● GI Drugs

Antacids

Antacids containing aluminum and/or magnesium administered concomitantly with or 2, 4, or 6 hours before or after a 400-mg raltegravir dose in individuals receiving a twice-daily raltegravir regimen resulted in decreased raltegravir peak plasma concentrations and AUC. Similar effects on raltegravir peak plasma concentrations and AUC were reported when antacids containing aluminum and/or magnesium were administered 12 hours after a single 1.2-g raltegravir dose. Aluminum- and/or magnesium-containing antacids should not be used in patients receiving raltegravir.

Concomitant use of antacids containing calcium carbonate in individuals receiving raltegravir (twice daily) resulted in decreased raltegravir peak plasma concentrations and AUC. Dosage adjustments are not needed if calcium carbonate-containing antacids are used concomitantly with raltegravir (twice daily). Concomitant use of calcium carbonate antacids and raltegravir (once daily) is not recommended.

Proton Pump Inhibitors

Pharmacokinetic interactions between omeprazole and raltegravir (increased raltegravir peak plasma concentrations and AUC) is not considered clinically important.

Dosage adjustments are not needed if raltegravir is used concomitantly with omeprazole.

● Opiates and Opiate Partial Agonists

Methadone

Raltegravir does not have a clinically important effect on the pharmacokinetics of methadone; dosage adjustments are not needed if raltegravir is used concomitantly with methadone.

DESCRIPTION

Raltegravir potassium, an antiretroviral agent, is a human immunodeficiency virus (HIV) integrase strand transfer inhibitor (INSTI). Raltegravir inhibits the activity of HIV integrase, an enzyme that integrates HIV DNA into the host cell genome. Integration is required for maintenance of the viral genome and for efficient viral gene expression and replication. Inhibition of integration prevents propagation of viral infection. Raltegravir is active against HIV type 1 (HIV-1) and also has some in vitro activity against HIV type 2 (HIV-2).

Raltegravir-resistant HIV-1 have been produced in vitro and have emerged during raltegravir therapy. Amino acid substitutions in HIV-1 integrase conferring resistance to raltegravir generally also confer resistance to elvitegravir. Substitutions at amino acid Y143 confer greater reductions in susceptibility to raltegravir than to elvitegravir, and the E92Q substitution confers greater reductions in susceptibility to elvitegravir than to raltegravir. Viruses harboring a substitution at amino acid Q148, along with one or more other raltegravir resistance substitutions, may also have clinically significant resistance to dolutegravir.

Following oral administration of 400 mg of raltegravir as film-coated tablets in fasting adults, peak plasma concentrations of the drug are attained approximately 3 hours after dosing. Following oral administration of raltegravir in a dosage of 1.2 g once daily (two 600-mg film-coated tablets once daily) in fasting individuals, peak plasma concentrations of the drug are attained approximately 1.5–2 hours after a dose. Although absolute bioavailability of raltegravir has not been established, oral bioavailability is higher with raltegravir chewable tablets or oral suspension compared with the 400-mg film-coated tablets and oral bioavailability of raltegravir 600-mg film-coated tablets is higher than that of the 400-mg film-coated tablets. When raltegravir film-coated tablets are used, steady state is attained in 2 days with the twice-daily regimen (400 mg twice daily) or the once-daily regimen (1.2 g once daily), with little or no accumulation with multiple doses. Studies using the 400- or 600-mg film-coated tablets and the chewable tablets indicate that food affects peak plasma concentrations and area under the plasma concentration-time curve (AUC) of raltegravir; however, all formulations of the drug may be administered with or without food. Raltegravir is approximately 83% bound to plasma protein. Raltegravir is metabolized primarily by uridine diphosphate-glucuronosyltransferase (UGT) 1A1. Following an oral dose of raltegravir, approximately 51% of the dose is eliminated in feces (as raltegravir) and 32% is eliminated in urine (as raltegravir and raltegravir glucuronide). Raltegravir has an apparent terminal half-life of approximately 9 hours.

Raltegravir is metabolized primarily by UGT1A. However, common UGT1A1 polymorphisms do not appear to alter the pharmacokinetics of raltegravir to any clinically important extent.

In one study in adults, the AUC of raltegravir in those with UGT1A1*28/*28 genotype (associated with reduced activity of UGT1A1) was compared to the AUC of the drug in those with wild-type UGT1A1 genotype and the geometric mean AUC ratio was 1.41.

In a neonatal clinical trial (IMPAACT P1110), there was no association between apparent clearance of raltegravir and UGT1A1 polymorphisms. Dosage recommendations for raltegravir in neonates younger than 4 weeks of age take into consideration the rapidly increasing UGT1A1 activity and drug clearance that occurs from birth to 4 weeks of age; UGT1A1 catalytic activity is negligible at birth and matures after birth.

ADVICE TO PATIENTS

- Inform patients of the critical nature of compliance with HIV therapy and importance of remaining under the care of a clinician.
- Advise patients of the importance of using raltegravir in conjunction with other antiretrovirals—not for monotherapy.

- If using raltegravir film-coated tablets, advise patients of the importance of swallowing whole; raltegravir chewable tablets can be chewed or swallowed whole.

- Advise patients to not switch between the film-coated tablet, the chewable tablet, or the oral suspension without first consulting a healthcare professional.

- Inform patients with phenylketonuria that the chewable tablets contain phenylalanine.

- If using raltegravir for oral suspension, advise parents and/or caregivers of the importance of reading the manufacturer's instructions for use before preparing and administering the drug. Instruct parents and/or caregivers that the oral suspension should be administered within 30 minutes of mixing.

- If a dose of raltegravir is missed, take the dose as soon as it is remembered and the next dose at the regularly scheduled time. If a dose is skipped, do not take a double dose to make up for the missed dose.

- Advise patients that a severe and potentially life-threatening rash has been reported with use. Importance of immediately discontinuing raltegravir and other suspect agents and seeking medical attention if rash occurs and is associated with fever, generally ill feeling, extreme tiredness, muscle or joint aches, breathing difficulty, blisters, oral lesions, eye inflammation, swelling of the face, eyes, lips, or mouth, and/or signs and symptoms of liver problems (e.g., yellowing of skin or whites of the eyes, dark or tea-colored urine, pale stools/bowel movements, nausea, vomiting, loss of appetite, or pain, aching, or sensitivity on the right side below ribs).

- Advise patients to inform clinician if patient has a history of rhabdomyolysis, myopathy, or increased serum creatine kinase concentrations or is receiving drugs known to cause these conditions (e.g., hydroxymethylglutaryl-CoA [HMG-CoA] reductase inhibitors [statins], fenofibrate, gemfibrozil). Instruct patients to immediately inform their clinician if unexplained muscle pain, tenderness, or weakness occurs while receiving raltegravir.

- Advise patients that signs and symptoms of inflammation from previous infections may occur soon after initiation of antiretroviral therapy in some individuals. Advise patients of the importance of immediately informing clinicians if any signs or symptoms of infection occur.

- Advise patients that raltegravir may interact with some drugs and to inform clinicians of existing or contemplated concomitant therapy, including prescription and OTC drugs and herbal products, as well as any concomitant illnesses.

- Advise females of child bearing age to inform clinicians if they are or plan to become pregnant. Inform females of child bearing age that there is a pregnancy registry that monitors pregnancy outcomes in females exposed to raltegravir during pregnancy.

- Advise HIV-infected females not to breast-feed.

- Advise patients of other important precautionary information.

PREPARATIONS

Excipients in commercially available drug preparations may have clinically important effects in some individuals; consult specific product labeling for details.

Raltegravir Potassium

Oral		
For Suspension	100 mg	**Isentress®** single-use packet
Tablets, Chewable	25 mg	**Isentress®**
	100 mg	**Isentress®**
Tablets, film coated	400 mg	**Isentress®**
	600 mg	**Isentress HD®**, Merck

† Use is not currently included in the labeling approved by the US Food and Drug Administration.

Selected Revisions February 10, 2024, © Copyright, November 1, 2007, American Society of Health-System Pharmacists, Inc.

Doravirine, Lamivudine, and Tenofovir Disoproxil Fumarate

8:18.08.16 • HIV NONNUCLEOSIDE REVERSE TRANSCRIPTASE INHIBITORS

■ Doravirine, lamivudine, and tenofovir disoproxil fumarate (doravirine/lamivudine/tenofovir DF) is a fixed-combination antiretroviral agent containing doravirine (human immunodeficiency virus [HIV] nonnucleoside reverse transcriptase inhibitor [NNRTI]), lamivudine (HIV nucleoside reverse transcriptase inhibitor [NRTI]), and tenofovir DF (HIV nucleotide reverse transcriptase inhibitor classified as an NRTI).

USES

● Treatment of HIV Infection

The fixed combination of doravirine, lamivudine, and tenofovir disoproxil fumarate (doravirine/lamivudine/tenofovir DF) is used for the treatment of human immunodeficiency virus type 1 (HIV-1) infection in adults and pediatric patients weighing ≥35 kg who are antiretroviral-naïve or to replace a current antiretroviral regimen in patients who are virologically suppressed (HIV-1 RNA levels <50 copies/mL) on a stable antiretroviral regimen with no history of treatment failure and no known resistance to any of the individual components of the fixed combination.

Doravirine/lamivudine/tenofovir DF is used as a single-tablet antiretroviral regimen; consult guidelines for the most current information on recommended regimens. Selection of an initial antiretroviral regimen should be individualized based on factors such as virologic efficacy, toxicity, pill burden, dosing frequency, drug-drug interaction potential, resistance test results, comorbid conditions, access, and cost.

Clinical Experience

Antiretroviral-naïve Adults

Efficacy and safety of doravirine/lamivudine/tenofovir DF in antiretroviral-naïve HIV-1-infected adults were evaluated in a phase 3 randomized study (DRIVE-AHEAD). Results indicated that doravirine/lamivudine/tenofovir DF was noninferior to a regimen of efavirenz in conjunction with 2 NRTIs for initial treatment in antiretroviral-naïve adults.

In DRIVE-AHEAD, 728 patients (median age 31 years, median baseline HIV-1 RNA level of 4.4 $\log_{10}$ copies/mL, median baseline CD4+ T-cell count of 397 cells/mm^3) were randomized in a 1:1 ratio to receive either the fixed combination of doravirine 100 mg, lamivudine 300 mg, and tenofovir DF 300 mg (doravirine/lamivudine/tenofovir DF) once daily or the fixed combination of efavirenz 600 mg, emtricitabine 200 mg, and tenofovir DF 300 mg (efavirenz/emtricitabine/tenofovir DF) once daily.

At 48 weeks, 84.3% of patients in the doravirine/lamivudine/tenofovir DF group achieved an HIV-1 RNA level <50 copies/mL, compared with 80.8% of patients in the efavirenz/emtricitabine/tenofovir DF group, showing noninferiority of the doravirine-containing regimen. At 96 weeks, 77.5% of patients in the doravirine/lamivudine/tenofovir DF group and 73.6% of those in the efavirenz/emtricitabine/tenofovir DF group had plasma HIV-1 RNA levels <50 copies/mL, which again demonstrated noninferiority of doravirine/lamivudine/tenofovir DF to efavirenz/emtricitabine/tenofovir DF in antiretroviral-naïve adults. The mean increase in CD4+ T-cell count was 238 cells/mm^3 in the doravirine/lamivudine/tenofovir DF group and 223 cells/mm^3 in the efavirenz/emtricitabine/tenofovir DF group.

Antiretroviral-experienced Adults

Efficacy of switching antiretroviral-experienced HIV-1-infected adults from a stable baseline regimen to doravirine/lamivudine/tenofovir DF was evaluated in a phase 3, open-label, active-controlled, noninferiority trial (DRIVE-SHIFT). Results indicated that switching to doravirine/lamivudine/tenofovir DF in virologically suppressed HIV-1-infected adults was noninferior to continuing treatment on a stable baseline antiretroviral regimen.

Patients enrolled in DRIVE-SHIFT had to be virologically suppressed (plasma HIV-1 RNA levels <50 copies/mL) on their baseline regimen for at least 6 months prior to trial entry and have no history of virologic failure. Stable baseline regimens consisted of 2 NRTIs in conjunction with a *cobicistat-boosted* or *ritonavir-boosted* HIV protease inhibitor (PI; atazanavir, darunavir, lopinavir), *cobicistat-boosted* elvitegravir, or a nonnucleoside reverse transcriptase inhibitor (NNRTI; efavirenz, nevirapine, or rilpivirine). Patients were randomized 2:1 to switch to doravirine/lamivudine/tenofovir DF on day 1 (immediate-switch group; 447 patients) or stay on their baseline regimen and switch to doravirine/lamivudine/tenofovir DF at week 24 (delayed-switch group; 223 patients). The primary efficacy end point was the proportion of participants with plasma HIV-1 RNA levels <50 copies/mL at 48 weeks (immediate-switch group) or 24 weeks (delayed-switch group).

Patient characteristics were similar between treatment groups (median age 43 years, median baseline CD4+ T-cell count of 628 cells/mm^3). At 24 or 48 weeks, 94 or 91%, respectively, of patients in the immediate-switch group had plasma HIV-1 RNA levels <50 copies/mL. In the delayed-switch group, 95% had plasma HIV-1 RNA levels <50 copies/mL at 24 weeks (baseline regimen) and at 48 weeks (24 weeks after switching to doravirine/lamivudine/tenofovir DF). At week 144, virologic suppression (HIV-1 RNA levels <50 copies/mL) was maintained in 80.1 and 83.7% of patients in the immediate- and delayed-switch groups, respectively.

Antiretroviral-experienced or -naïve Pediatric Patients

The combination of doravirine/lamivudine/tenofovir DF was evaluated in a phase 1/2 open-label trial (IMPAACT 2014) enrolling pediatric patients (12 to <18 years of age weighing ≥35 kg). Cohort 1 evaluated the pharmacokinetics of a single dose of doravirine in virologically-suppressed pediatric patients. Cohort 2 enrolled patients (median age 15 years, median baseline CD4+ T-cell count of 713 cells/mm^3) who were either naïve to antiretroviral therapy (2 patients) or virologically suppressed on a stable regimen (43 patients). All patients in cohort 2 were started on or switched to doravirine/lamivudine/tenofovir DF.

At week 24, 95% of virologically-suppressed patients maintained HIV-1 RNA levels <50 copies/mL. Of the 2 antiretroviral-naïve patients, 1 achieved an HIV-1 RNA level <50 copies/mL at week 24; the second patient met the criteria for virologic failure (HIV-1 RNA levels ≥200 copies/mL at week 24), due to nonadherence to treatment.

Clinical Perspective

Therapeutic options for the treatment of HIV infection and recommendations concerning the use of antiretrovirals are continuously evolving. Antiretroviral therapy is recommended for all individuals with HIV regardless of CD4 counts, and should be initiated as soon as possible after diagnosis of HIV and continued indefinitely. The primary goals of antiretroviral therapy are to achieve and maintain durable suppression of HIV viral load (as measured by plasma HIV-1 RNA levels) to a level below which drug-resistance mutations cannot emerge (i.e., below detectable limits), restore and preserve immunologic function, reduce HIV-related morbidity and mortality, improve quality of life, and prevent transmission of HIV. While the most appropriate antiretroviral regimen cannot be defined for each clinical scenario, the US Department of Health and Human Services (HHS) Panel on Antiretroviral Guidelines for Adults and Adolescents, HHS Panel on Antiretroviral Therapy and Medical Management of Children Living with HIV, and HHS Panel on Treatment of Pregnant Women with HIV Infection and Prevention of Perinatal Transmission, have developed comprehensive guidelines that provide information on selection and use of antiretrovirals for the treatment of HIV infection. Because of the complexity of managing patients with HIV, it is recommended that clinicians with HIV expertise be consulted when needed.

The use of combination antiretroviral regimens that generally include 3 drugs from 2 or more drug classes is currently recommended to achieve viral suppression. In both treatment-naïve adults and children, an initial antiretroviral regimen generally consists of 2 NRTIs administered in combination with a third active antiretroviral drug from 1 of 3 drug classes: an integrase strand transfer inhibitor (INSTI), an NNRTI, or a PI with a pharmacokinetic enhancer (also known as a booster; the 2 drugs used for this purpose are cobicistat and ritonavir). Selection of an initial antiretroviral regimen should be individualized based on factors such as virologic efficacy, toxicity, pill burden, dosing frequency, drug–drug interaction potential, resistance-test results, comorbid conditions, access, and cost. In patients with comorbid infections (e.g., hepatitis B, tuberculosis), antiretroviral regimen selection should also consider the potential for activity against other present infections, drug-drug interactions, and timing of initiation relative to other anti-infective regimens.

Doravirine/lamivudine/tenofovir DF is used as a single-tablet antiretroviral regimen; the tablet contains an NNRTI (doravirine) plus 2 NRTIs (lamivudine and tenofovir DF). The regimen of doravirine/lamivudine/tenofovir DF is listed among recommended initial regimens in certain clinical situations (e.g., in situations where a one-pill, once-daily regimen is desired).

In the 2024 HHS pediatric HIV treatment guideline, doravirine/lamivudine/tenofovir DF is included as an alternative NNRTI-based regimen for initial treatment of HIV in children and adolescents weighing ≥35 kg.

In the 2024 HHS perinatal HIV treatment guideline, doravirine/lamivudine/tenofovir DF is described as having insufficient data for use as an initial regimen before or during pregnancy, primarily due to a lack of data on the doravirine component. For patients already receiving doravirine/lamivudine/tenofovir DF who have achieved viral suppression and who become pregnant, the regimen may be continued, with frequent monitoring of viral load. Alternatively, it may be appropriate to consider switching to a different regimen due to insufficient data on the use of doravirine during pregnancy.

DOSAGE AND ADMINISTRATION

• General

Pretreatment Screening

- Test patients for hepatitis B virus (HBV) infection prior to or when initiating doravirine/lamivudine/tenofovir DF.

- Evaluate serum creatinine, estimated creatinine clearance, urine glucose, and urine protein in all patients prior to or when initiating doravirine/lamivudine/tenofovir DF. In patients with chronic kidney disease, additionally assess serum phosphorus.

Patient Monitoring

- Monitor serum creatinine, estimated creatinine clearance, urine glucose, and urine protein periodically in all patients during treatment with doravirine/lamivudine/tenofovir DF. In patients with chronic kidney disease, additionally monitor serum phosphorus.

- Consider monitoring bone mineral density (BMD) in adults and pediatric patients who have a history of pathologic bone fracture or other risk factors for osteoporosis or bone loss.

Other General Considerations

- Avoid doravirine/lamivudine/tenofovir DF in patients who are receiving or have recently received a nephrotoxic agent (e.g., high-dose or multiple nonsteroidal anti-inflammatory agents [NSAIAs]). Consider alternatives to NSAIAs if such therapy is needed in patients at risk for renal dysfunction.

• Administration

The fixed combination of doravirine, lamivudine, and tenofovir disoproxil fumarate (doravirine/lamivudine/tenofovir DF) is administered orally once daily without regard to food.

Doravirine/lamivudine/tenofovir DF is used alone as a complete antiretroviral regimen for the treatment of HIV-1 infection.

If a dose is missed, the missed dose should be taken as soon as possible, unless it is almost time for the next dose; the patient should not take 2 doses at one time.

Store doravirine/lamivudine/tenofovir DF at 20-25°C (excursions permitted between 15-30°C).

Store in original bottle. Protect from moisture; do not remove desiccant and keep bottle tightly closed.

• Dosage

Each fixed-combination tablet of doravirine/lamivudine/tenofovir DF contains doravirine 100 mg, lamivudine 300 mg, and tenofovir DF 300 mg.

Adults

Treatment of HIV Infection

For the treatment of HIV-1 infection in adults, the recommended dosage of doravirine/lamivudine/tenofovir DF is 1 tablet (100 mg of doravirine, 300 mg of lamivudine, and 300 mg of tenofovir DF) once daily.

Pediatric Patients

Treatment of HIV Infection

For the treatment of HIV-1 infection in pediatric patients weighing ≥35 kg, the recommended dosage of doravirine/lamivudine/tenofovir DF is 1 tablet (100 mg of doravirine, 300 mg of lamivudine, and 300 mg of tenofovir DF) once daily.

Dosage Modification for Concomitant Use with Rifabutin

If doravirine/lamivudine/tenofovir DF is used for the treatment of HIV-1 infection in pediatric or adult patients receiving concomitant therapy with rifabutin, patients should receive 1 tablet of the fixed combination (100 mg of doravirine, 300 mg of lamivudine, and 300 mg of tenofovir DF) once daily and a 100-mg tablet of single-entity doravirine once daily given approximately 12 hours after the fixed-combination tablet.

• Special Populations

Hepatic Impairment

Dosage adjustments are not necessary if doravirine/lamivudine/tenofovir DF is used in patients with mild or moderate hepatic impairment (Child-Pugh class A or B).

Doravirine/lamivudine/tenofovir DF has not been studied in patients with severe hepatic impairment (Child-Pugh class C).

Renal Impairment

Doravirine/lamivudine/tenofovir DF is not recommended in patients with an estimated creatinine clearance <50 mL/minute.

Geriatric Patients

The manufacturer makes no specific dosage recommendations for doravirine/lamivudine/tenofovir DF in geriatric patients, but recommends caution because of possible age-related decreases in hepatic, renal, and/or cardiac function and potential for concomitant disease and drug therapy.

CAUTIONS

• Contraindications

- Concomitant use with potent inducers of cytochrome P-450 (CYP) isoenzyme 3A (e.g., carbamazepine, oxcarbazepine, phenobarbital, phenytoin, enzalutamide, rifampin, rifapentine, mitotane, St. John's wort [*Hypericum perforatum*]).

- History of hypersensitivity reaction to lamivudine.

• Warnings/Precautions

Warnings

Post-treatment Acute Exacerbations of Hepatitis B

A boxed warning is included in the prescribing information for doravirine/lamivudine/tenofovir DF regarding the risk of severe post-treatment acute exacerbations of hepatitis B virus (HBV) infection in human immunodeficiency virus type 1 (HIV-1) patients coinfected with HBV who discontinue products containing lamivudine and/or tenofovir DF.

In HIV-infected patients with HBV coinfection, severe acute exacerbations of HBV infection, including liver decompensation and liver failure, have occurred following discontinuance of preparations containing lamivudine and/or tenofovir DF (components of doravirine/lamivudine/tenofovir DF).

All patients with HIV infection should be tested for HBV before antiretroviral therapy is initiated. Hepatic function should be closely monitored with clinical and laboratory follow-up for at least several months after doravirine/lamivudine/tenofovir DF is discontinued in patients coinfected with HIV and HBV. If appropriate, initiation of HBV treatment may be warranted, especially in patients with advanced liver disease or cirrhosis.

Other Warnings and Precautions

New Onset or Worsening Renal Impairment

Renal impairment, including cases of acute renal failure and Fanconi syndrome (renal tubular injury with severe hypophosphatemia), has been reported in patients receiving tenofovir DF (a component of doravirine/lamivudine/tenofovir DF).

Serum creatinine, estimated creatinine clearance, urine glucose, and urine protein should be determined prior to initiation of doravirine/lamivudine/tenofovir DF and routinely monitored during treatment with the drug in all patients as clinically appropriate. In patients with chronic kidney disease, serum phosphorus also should be monitored.

Doravirine/lamivudine/tenofovir DF should be discontinued if clinically important decreases in renal function or evidence of Fanconi syndrome occur. The fixed combination also should be discontinued if estimated creatinine clearance decreases to <50 mL/minute.

Because persistent or worsening bone pain, pain in extremities, fractures, and/or muscular pain or weakness may be manifestations of proximal renal tubulopathy, renal function should be promptly evaluated in patients at risk for renal dysfunction who present with such symptoms.

Doravirine/lamivudine/tenofovir DF should be avoided in patients who are receiving or have recently received a nephrotoxic agent (e.g., high-dose or multiple nonsteroidal anti-inflammatory agents [NSAIAs]). Acute renal failure has been reported after initiation of high-dose or multiple NSAIA therapy in HIV-infected patients at risk for renal dysfunction who appeared stable while receiving tenofovir DF; hospitalization and renal replacement therapy were required in some patients. Alternatives to NSAIAs should be considered if such therapy is needed in patients at risk for renal dysfunction.

Bone Loss and Mineralization Defects

Decreases in bone mineral density (BMD) from baseline, increases in several biochemical markers of bone metabolism, and increased serum parathyroid hormone levels and 1,25 vitamin D levels have been reported during adult clinical trials of tenofovir DF (a component of doravirine/lamivudine/tenofovir DF). The effects of tenofovir-associated changes in BMD on long-term bone health and future fracture risk are unknown.

Clinical studies of tenofovir DF in pediatric patients 2 to <18 years of age found similar bone effects with tenofovir DF to those observed in adults, suggesting increased bone turnover. Typically, BMD undergoes rapid increases in pediatric patients; however, total body increases in BMD were shown to be reduced in HIV-1 infected pediatric patients receiving tenofovir DF compared to controls. Similar trends have been observed in pediatric patients 2 to <18 years of age with chronic HBV infection. Across pediatric clinical studies, normal skeletal growth (height) was observed for the duration of the studies.

Osteomalacia associated with proximal renal tubulopathy, which manifested as bone pain or pain in extremities and may contribute to fractures, has been reported in patients receiving tenofovir DF. Arthralgia and muscle pain or weakness also have been reported in patients with proximal renal tubulopathy. Hypophosphatemia and osteomalacia secondary to proximal renal tubulopathy should be considered in patients at risk for renal dysfunction who present with persistent or worsening bone or muscle symptoms while receiving preparations containing tenofovir DF.

Bone mineral density monitoring should be considered in HIV-1-infected adults and pediatric patients who have a history of pathologic bone fracture or other risk factors for osteoporosis or bone loss. Although the effect of calcium and vitamin D supplementation was not studied, such supplementation may be beneficial for all patients. If bone abnormalities are suspected, appropriate consultation should be obtained.

Interactions

Concomitant use of doravirine/lamivudine/tenofovir DF with certain drugs may result in clinically important interactions, including decreased plasma concentrations of the antiretroviral agents leading to loss of therapeutic effect and possible development of resistance; other interactions may increase plasma concentrations of the antiretroviral agents and/or concomitant drugs leading to clinically important adverse reactions.

The potential for drug interactions should be considered prior to and during doravirine/lamivudine/tenofovir DF therapy; concomitant drugs should be reviewed during doravirine/lamivudine/tenofovir DF therapy and the patient should be monitored for adverse effects.

Immune Reconstitution Syndrome

Immune reconstitution syndrome has been reported in HIV-infected patients receiving multiple-drug antiretroviral therapy. During the initial phase of treatment, HIV-infected patients whose immune systems respond to antiretroviral therapy may develop an inflammatory response to indolent or residual opportunistic infections (e.g., *Mycobacterium avium*, cytomegalovirus [CMV], *Pneumocystis jirovecii* [formerly *P. carinii*], tuberculosis); such responses may necessitate further evaluation and treatment.

Autoimmune disorders (e.g., Graves' disease, polymyositis, Guillain-Barré syndrome, autoimmune hepatitis) have also been reported to occur in the setting of immune reconstitution; however, the time to onset is more variable and can occur many months after initiation of antiretroviral therapy.

Use of Fixed Combinations

The usual cautions, precautions, contraindications, and interactions associated with each component of doravirine/lamivudine/tenofovir DF should be considered. Cautionary information applicable to specific populations (e.g., pregnant or nursing women, individuals with hepatic or renal impairment, geriatric patients) should be considered for each drug in the fixed combination.

Specific Populations

Pregnancy

An Antiretroviral Pregnancy Registry is available at 800-258-4263 or http://www.apregistry.com/.

There are insufficient prospective data in pregnant women to assess the risk of birth defects and miscarriage in those receiving doravirine/lamivudine/tenofovir DF. Human data are not available to establish whether or not doravirine poses a risk to pregnancy outcomes. In animal reproduction studies, no adverse developmental effects were observed when doravirine was administered to rabbits or rats at exposures that were 8 or 9 times higher, respectively, than human exposures at the recommended human dosage. Available data from the antiretroviral pregnancy registry show no differences in the overall risk of major birth defects for lamivudine and tenofovir DF.

Lactation

It is not known whether doravirine is distributed into human milk. Doravirine was distributed into the milk of lactating rats following oral administration (milk concentrations were approximately 1.5 times higher than maternal plasma concentrations at 2 hours after a dose on lactation day 14). Lamivudine and tenofovir DF are distributed into milk in humans. It is not known whether doravirine/lamivudine/tenofovir DF or the individual drug components affect human milk production or the breast-fed infant.

The HHS perinatal HIV transmission guideline provides updated recommmendations on infant feeding. The guideline states that patients with HIV should receive evidence-based, patient-centered counseling to support shared decision-making about infant feeding. During counseling, patients should be informed that feeding with appropriate formula or pasteurized donor human milk from a milk bank eliminates the risk of postnatal HIV transmission to the infant. Additionally, achieving and maintaining viral suppression with antiretroviral therapy during pregnancy and postpartum reduces the risk of breastfeeding HIV transmission to <1%, but does not eliminate the risk. Replacement feeding with formula or banked pasteurized donor milk is recommended when patients with HIV are *not* on antiretroviral therapy and/or do *not* have a suppressed viral load during pregnancy (at a minimum throughout the third trimester), as well as at delivery.

Pediatric Use

Safety and efficacy of doravirine/lamivudine/tenofovir DF have been established in pediatric patients weighing at least 35 kg.

Use of doravirine/lamivudine/tenofovir DF in this population is supported by data from randomized studies in adults, with additional pharmacokinetic, safety, and efficacy data from a 24-week, open-label study conducted in 54 antiretroviral naïve or antiretroviral experienced pediatric patients 12 to <18 years of age. Doravirine/lamivudine/tenofovir DF demonstrated similar safety and efficacy in this population compared to adult patients, with no clinically important differences detected in exposures for the individual components of doravirine/lamivudine/tenofovir DF.

Safety and efficacy of doravirine/lamivudine/tenofovir DF have not been established in pediatric patients weighing <35 kg.

Geriatric Use

Experience in patients 65 years of age and older is insufficient to determine whether they respond differently to doravirine, lamivudine, or tenofovir DF than younger patients.

Doravirine/lamivudine/tenofovir DF should be used with caution in geriatric patients because of age-related decreases in hepatic, renal, and/or cardiac function and potential for concomitant disease and drug therapy.

Hepatic Impairment

Doravirine pharmacokinetics are not substantially affected in individuals with moderate hepatic impairment (Child-Pugh class B) compared with those without hepatic impairment. Doravirine has not been studied in patients with severe hepatic impairment (Child-Pugh class C).

Lamivudine pharmacokinetics are not substantially affected by diminishing hepatic function. Safety and efficacy of lamivudine have not been established in patients with decompensated liver disease.

Tenofovir pharmacokinetics are not substantially affected by any degree of hepatic impairment.

No dosage adjustment of doravirine/lamivudine/tenofovir DF is required in patients with mild or moderate (Child-Pugh class A or B) hepatic impairment; no studies have been conducted in patients with severe (Child-Pugh class C) hepatic impairment.

Renal Impairment

Because doravirine/lamivudine/tenofovir DF is a fixed-combination tablet and the dosage of lamivudine and tenofovir DF (components of doravirine/lamivudine/tenofovir DF) cannot be adjusted, doravirine/lamivudine/tenofovir DF is not recommended in patients with estimated creatinine clearance <50 mL/minute.

The pharmacokinetics of doravirine were not significantly impacted in patients with mild to severe renal impairment (creatinine clearance >15 mL/minute). Doravirine has not been studied in patients with end-stage renal disease or in patients undergoing dialysis.

Lamivudine exposures, peak plasma concentrations, and half-life are increased and clearance of the drug is decreased to a clinically important extent by diminishing renal function (creatinine clearances 111 to <10 mL/minute).

Tenofovir exposures and peak plasma concentrations are substantially increased in individuals with creatinine clearances <50 mL/minute or with end-stage renal disease requiring dialysis.

● Common Adverse Effects

Adverse effects reported in ≥5% of patients receiving doravirine/lamivudine/tenofovir DF include dizziness, nausea, and abnormal dreams.

DRUG INTERACTIONS

The following drug interactions are based on studies using the individual components of the fixed combination of doravirine, lamivudine, and tenofovir disoproxil fumarate (doravirine/lamivudine/tenofovir DF).

When doravirine/lamivudine/tenofovir DF is used, interactions associated with each drug in the fixed combination should be considered.

● Drugs Affecting or Metabolized by Microsomal Enzymes

Doravirine is primarily metabolized by cytochrome P-450 (CYP) isoenzyme 3A. Concomitant use of doravirine and CYP3A inducers may result in decreased doravirine plasma concentrations and may reduce the efficacy of doravirine. Concomitant use of doravirine and CYP3A inhibitors may result in increased plasma concentrations of doravirine. In vitro, doravirine does not inhibit CYP1A2, 2B6, 2C8, 2C9, 2C19, 2D6, or 3A4 and is not likely to induce CYP1A2, 2B6, or 3A4. Doravirine is not likely to have a clinically important effect on the exposure of drugs metabolized by CYP isoenzymes.

Lamivudine is not substantially metabolized by CYP isoenzymes and does not inhibit or induce CYP isoenzymes. It is unlikely that clinically important CYP-mediated drug interactions with lamivudine will occur.

Pharmacokinetic interactions between tenofovir and drugs that are inhibitors or substrates of CYP isoenzymes are unlikely.

● Drugs Affecting or Metabolized by Uridine Diphosphate-gluuronosyltransferases

In vitro, doravirine does not inhibit uridine diphosphate-glucuronosyltransferase (UGT) 1A1.

● Drugs Affecting or Affected by Other Transporters

Based on in vitro studies, doravirine is not likely to inhibit the P-glycoprotein (P-gp) transport system, organic anion transport polypeptide (OATP) 1B1, OATP1B3, bile salt export pump (BSEP), organic anion transporter (OAT) 1, OAT3, organic cation transporter (OCT) 2, multidrug and toxin extrusion transporter (MATE) 1, or MATE2K.

● Drugs Affecting Renal Function

There is potential for pharmacokinetic interactions with drugs that reduce renal function or that may compete with lamivudine or tenofovir for active renal tubular secretion (e.g., acyclovir, aminoglycosides [e.g., gentamicin], cidofovir, ganciclovir, valacyclovir, valganciclovir, high-dose or multiple nonsteroidal anti-inflammatory agents [NSAIAs]); increased plasma concentrations of lamivudine, tenofovir, and/or the concomitantly administered drug may occur.

● Drugs Affecting Gastric Acidity

Antacids

No clinically important effect on doravirine concentrations when doravirine was used concomitantly with an antacid containing aluminum hydroxide, magnesium hydroxide and simethicone.

Proton pump Inhibitors

No clinically important effect on doravirine concentrations were observed when the drug was used concomitantly with pantoprazole.

● Anticonvulsants

Carbamazepine, Oxcarbazepine, Phenobarbital, and Phenytoin

Pharmacokinetic interactions with certain anticonvulsants that are CYP3A inducers (e.g., carbamazepine, oxcarbazepine, phenobarbital, phenytoin) are expected (decreased doravirine concentrations; possible decreased efficacy of doravirine).

Concomitant use of doravirine/lamivudine/tenofovir DF and carbamazepine, oxcarbazepine, phenobarbital, or phenytoin is contraindicated. Doravirine/lamivudine/tenofovir DF should not be initiated until at least 4 weeks after such anticonvulsants are discontinued.

● Antimycobacterial Agents

Rifabutin

When doravirine (single 100-mg dose) was used with rifabutin (300 mg once daily), doravirine area under the plasma concentration-time curve (AUC) and trough plasma concentrations were decreased by 50 and 68%, respectively, but peak plasma concentrations were not affected. When doravirine (100 mg twice daily) was used with rifabutin (300 mg once daily), doravirine AUC, peak plasma concentrations, and trough plasma concentrations were not affected, and were similar to concentrations observed without concomitant rifabutin.

If doravirine/lamivudine/tenofovir DF is used concomitantly with rifabutin, the patient should receive 1 tablet of the fixed combination (100 mg of doravirine, 300 mg of lamivudine, and 300 mg of tenofovir DF) and 100 mg of single-entity doravirine once daily (the single-entity tablet should be given approximately 12 hours after the fixed-combination tablet).

Rifampin

When doravirine (single 100-mg dose) was used with rifampin (600 mg once daily), doravirine AUC, peak plasma concentrations, and trough plasma concentrations were decreased by 88, 57, and 97%, respectively;1, decreased doravirine exposures may decrease efficacy of the drug.

Concomitant use of doravirine/lamivudine/tenofovir DF and rifampin is contraindicated. Doravirine/lamivudine/tenofovir DF should not be initiated until at least 4 weeks after rifampin is discontinued.

Rifapentine

Pharmacokinetic interactions with rifapentine expected (decreased doravirine concentrations; possible decreased efficacy of doravirine).

Concomitant use of doravirine/lamivudine/tenofovir DF and rifapentine is contraindicated. Doravirine/lamivudine/tenofovir DF should not be initiated until at least 4 weeks after rifapentine is discontinued.

● Antiretroviral Agents

Doravirine/lamivudine/tenofovir DF is a complete regimen for the treatment of human immunodeficiency virus type 1 (HIV-1) infection in antiretroviral-naïve adults, and concomitant use with other antiretroviral agents is not recommended.

No clinically important pharmacokinetic interactions have been reported between the components of the fixed combination (i.e., doravirine, lamivudine, tenofovir DF). There is no in vitro evidence of antagonistic antiretroviral effects between doravirine and lamivudine or tenofovir DF.

● Atorvastatin

Concomitant use of atorvastatin and doravirine did not result in clinically important interactions.

● Co-trimoxazole

Concomitant use of co-trimoxazole and lamivudine resulted in a 43% increase in lamivudine AUC and a 30% decrease in lamivudine renal clearance, but did not affect the pharmacokinetics of trimethoprim or sulfamethoxazole.

● Entecavir

No clinically important pharmacokinetic interactions between entecavir and tenofovir DF.

● Enzalutamide

Pharmacokinetic interactions with enzalutamide are expected (decreased doravirine concentrations; possible decreased efficacy of doravirine).

Concomitant use of doravirine/lamivudine/tenofovir DF and enzalutamide is contraindicated. Doravirine/lamivudine/tenofovir DF should not be initiated until at least 4 weeks after enzalutamide is discontinued.

● Estrogens and Progestins

No clinically important effects on the pharmacokinetics of ethinyl estradiol or levonorgestrel when doravirine was used concomitantly with an oral contraceptive containing ethinyl estradiol and levonorgestrel. No clinically important pharmacokinetic interactions between tenofovir DF and oral contraceptives containing ethinyl estradiol and norgestimate.

● HCV Antivirals

HCV Polymerase Inhibitors

Sofosbuvir

No clinically important pharmacokinetic interactions between sofosbuvir and tenofovir DF.

Sofosbuvir and Velpatasvir

Possible pharmacokinetic interactions with the fixed combination of sofosbuvir and velpatasvir (sofosbuvir/velpatasvir) (increased tenofovir concentrations and AUC).

If doravirine/lamivudine/tenofovir DF is used concomitantly with sofosbuvir/velpatasvir, the patient should be monitored for tenofovir-associated adverse effects.

HCV Replication Complex Inhibitors

Elbasvir and Grazoprevir

No clinically important pharmacokinetic interactions when doravirine was used concomitantly with elbasvir and grazoprevir.

Ledipasvir and Sofosbuvir

No clinically important pharmacokinetic interactions when doravirine was used concomitantly with the fixed combination of ledipasvir and sofosbuvir. Concomitant use of ledipasvir/sofosbuvir and tenofovir DF results in increased tenofovir exposures.

If doravirine/lamivudine/tenofovir DF is used concomitantly with ledipasvir/sofosbuvir, the patient should be monitored for tenofovir-associated adverse effects.

● Ketoconazole

When doravirine (single 100-mg dose) was used with ketoconazole (400 mg once daily), doravirine exposures increased by approximately threefold and peak plasma concentrations increased by 25%. However, these changes are not considered clinically important.

● Metformin

No clinically important interactions observed when metformin was used concomitantly with doravirine.

● Methadone

No clinically important effects on the pharmacokinetics of either drug when doravirine was used concomitantly with methadone. No clinically important pharmacokinetic interactions between methadone and tenofovir DF.

● Midazolam

Concomitant use of midazolam and doravirine did not result in clinically important pharmacokinetic interactions.

● Mitotane

Pharmacokinetic interactions with mitotane are expected (decreased doravirine concentrations; possible decreased efficacy of doravirine).

Concomitant use of doravirine/lamivudine/tenofovir DF and mitotane is contraindicated. Doravirine/lamivudine/tenofovir DF should not be initiated until at least 4 weeks after mitotane is discontinued.

● St. John's Wort

Pharmacokinetic interactions with St. John's wort (Hypericum perforatum) are expected (decreased doravirine concentrations; possible decreased efficacy of doravirine).

Concomitant use of doravirine/lamivudine/tenofovir DF and St. John's wort is contraindicated. Doravirine/lamivudine/tenofovir DF should not be initiated until at least 4 weeks after St. John's wort is discontinued.

● Sorbitol

Concomitant use of a single dose of lamivudine with a single 3.2-, 10.2-, or 13.4-g dose of sorbitol results in a 14, 32, or 36% decrease in lamivudine AUC, respectively, and a 28, 52, or 55% decrease in lamivudine peak plasma concentrations, respectively.

Concomitant use of sorbitol-containing drugs and lamivudine-containing drugs, including doravirine/lamivudine/tenofovir DF, should be avoided.

● Tacrolimus

No clinically important pharmacokinetic interactions between tacrolimus and tenofovir DF.

DESCRIPTION

The fixed combination of doravirine, lamivudine, and tenofovir disoproxil fumarate (doravirine/lamivudine/tenofovir DF) contains a human immunodeficiency virus (HIV) nonnucleoside reverse transcriptase inhibitor (NNRTI) antiretroviral (doravirine), an HIV nucleoside reverse transcriptase inhibitor (NRTI) antiretroviral (lamivudine), and a nucleotide reverse transcriptase inhibitor antiretroviral classified as an HIV NRTI (tenofovir disoproxil fumarate; tenofovir DF).

Doravirine is a pyridinone NNRTI and inhibits replication of HIV type 1 (HIV-1) by interfering with viral polymerase activities of reverse transcriptase. Doravirine is active against HIV-1, including certain strains resistant to some other NNRTIs (i.e., those with K103N and/or Y181C substitutions).

Lamivudine is a synthetic nucleoside analog that is phosphorylated intracellularly to the active 5'-triphosphate metabolite (lamivudine triphosphate). After conversion to the pharmacologically active metabolite, the drug acts as a reverse transcriptase inhibitor via DNA chain termination after incorporation of the nucleotide analogue. Lamivudine is active against HIV-1.

Tenofovir DF is a tenofovir prodrug and is inactive until it undergoes diester hydrolysis in vivo to tenofovir and is subsequently metabolized to the active metabolite (tenofovir diphosphate). Tenofovir is active against HIV-1.

HIV-1 strains resistant to doravirine, lamivudine, or tenofovir have been produced in vitro and have emerged during doravirine/lamivudine/tenofovir DF therapy. In the clinical trial evaluating doravirine/lamivudine/tenofovir DF in antiretroviral-naive patients, one or more primary mutations associated with resistance to doravirine were identified in HIV-1 isolates from 10 of 24 patients in the resistance analysis subset (i.e., those with plasma HIV-1 RNA levels exceeding 400 copies/mL at virologic failure or early study discontinuation with resistance data); genotypic resistance against lamivudine and tenofovir DF developed in 7 patients. Cross-resistance occurs among HIV NNRTIs (e.g., efavirenz, etravirine, nevirapine, rilpivirine). Treatment-emergent doravirine resistance-associated substitutions can confer cross-resistance to other NNRTIs; however, the treatment-emergent doravirine resistance-associated substitution Y318F does not appear to confer reduced susceptibility to efavirenz, etravirine, or rilpivirine. Cross-resistance also occurs among the HIV NRTIs.

A fixed-combination tablet containing doravirine 100 mg, lamivudine 300 mg, and tenofovir DF 300 mg is bioequivalent to a 100-mg tablet of doravirine, 300-mg tablet of lamivudine, and 300-mg tablet of tenofovir DF given simultaneously. The absolute oral bioavailability of doravirine, lamivudine, and tenofovir DF is 64, 86, and 25%, respectively; peak plasma concentrations of doravirine and tenofovir occur 2 hours and 1 hour, respectively, after administration. Administration of doravirine, lamivudine, and tenofovir DF with a high-fat meal increases the area under the plasma concentration-time curve (AUC) of doravirine and tenofovir by 10 and 27%, respectively, and decreases the AUC of lamivudine by 7% compared with administration in the fasted state; this effect of food is not considered clinically important. Doravirine is primarily metabolized in the liver by cytochrome P-450 (CYP) isoenzyme 3A; lamivudine is metabolized by CYP isoenzymes only to a minor extent and tenofovir does not undergo hepatic metabolism. Approximately 6% of an oral dose of doravirine is eliminated in urine as unchanged drug; unchanged doravirine also is eliminated to a minor extent by biliary and/or fecal routes. Lamivudine and tenofovir are eliminated by glomerular filtration and active tubular secretion. The elimination half-life of doravirine, lamivudine, and tenofovir is 15, 5–7, and 17 hours, respectively. Doravirine, lamivudine, and tenofovir are 76, <35, and <0.7% bound to plasma proteins, respectively.

There are no clinically relevant differences in pharmacokinetics based on age in adults (doravirine), race (doravirine, lamivudine), body mass index (BMI) (doravirine), or sex (doravirine, lamivudine, tenofovir DF). Doravirine, lamivudine, and tenofovir DF exposures in pediatric patients 12 to <18 years of age weighing ≥35 kg are similar to those in adults following administration.

ADVICE TO PATIENTS

- Stress the importance of taking as prescribed; do not alter or discontinue antiretroviral regimen without consulting clinician.

- Advise the patient to read the patient information provided by the manufacturer.

- Advise patients to take doravirine/lamivudine/tenofovir DF once every day at a regularly scheduled time with or without food.

- Advise patients not to miss or skip doses since this can result in development of resistance. If a patient forgets to take doravirine/lamivudine/tenofovir DF, tell the patient to take the missed dose right away, unless it is almost time for the next dose. Advise the patient not to take 2 doses at one time and to take the next dose at the regularly scheduled time.

- Inform patients that testing for hepatitis B virus (HBV) infection is recommended before antiretroviral therapy is initiated. Also advise patients that severe acute exacerbations of HBV infection have been reported following discontinuance of lamivudine or tenofovir DF (components of doravirine/lamivudine/tenofovir DF) in HIV-infected patients coinfected with HBV. Stress importance of not discontinuing doravirine/lamivudine/tenofovir DF without consulting a clinician.

- Inform patients that renal impairment, including cases of acute renal failure or Fanconi syndrome, has occurred in association with use of tenofovir DF (a component of doravirine/lamivudine/tenofovir DF). Stress importance of not using doravirine/lamivudine/tenofovir DF concomitantly with or shortly after nephrotoxic agents (e.g., high-dose or multiple nonsteroidal anti-inflammatory agents [NSAIAs]).

- Inform patients that decreased bone mineral density (BMD) has occurred with the use of tenofovir DF (a component of doravirine/lamivudine/tenofovir DF) and that assessment of BMD should be considered in those with a history of pathologic bone fracture or other risk factors for osteoporosis or bone loss.

- Advise patients that doravirine/lamivudine/tenofovir DF may interact with certain other drugs. For patients receiving rifabutin, stress importance of taking one 100-mg tablet of single-entity doravirine each day approximately 12 hours after taking doravirine/lamivudine/tenofovir DF.

- Stress importance of informing clinicians of existing or contemplated concomitant therapy, including prescription and OTC drugs and herbal supplements (e.g., St. John's wort), as well as any concomitant illnesses.

- Inform patients that signs and symptoms of inflammation from other previous infections may occur soon after initiation of antiretroviral therapy in some patients with advanced HIV infection. These symptoms may be due to an improvement in immune response, enabling the body to fight infections that may have been present with no obvious symptoms. Stress importance of immediately informing a clinician if any symptoms of infection occur.

- Stress importance of women informing clinicians if they are or plan to become pregnant or plan to breast-feed.

- Inform patients of other important precautionary information.

PREPARATIONS

Excipients in commercially available drug preparations may have clinically important effects in some individuals; consult specific product labeling for details.

Doravirine, Lamivudine, and Tenofovir Disoproxil Fumarate

Oral

Tablets, film-coated	Doravirine 100 mg, Lamivudine 300 mg, and Tenofovir Disoproxil Fumarate 300 mg	Delstrigo®, Merck

† Use is not currently included in the labeling approved by the US Food and Drug Administration.

Selected Revisions August 10, 2024, © Copyright, September 17, 2018, American Society of Health-System Pharmacists, Inc.

Rilpivirine Hydrochloride

8:18.08.16 • HIV NONNUCLEOSIDE REVERSE TRANSCRIPTASE INHIBITORS

■ Rilpivirine, an antiretroviral agent, is a human immunodeficiency virus (HIV) nonnucleoside reverse transcriptase inhibitor (NNRTI).

USES

● Treatment of HIV Infection

Rilpivirine is used in conjunction with other antiretroviral (ARV) agents for the treatment of human immunodeficiency virus type 1 (HIV-1) infection in treatment-naïve and previously treated† adults and adolescents ≥12 years of age and weighing ≥35 kg with baseline HIV-1 RNA levels ≤100,000 copies/mL. Rilpivirine is included in various ARV regimens recommended in guidelines for treatment of HIV in adults and adolescents, pediatric patients, and pregnant patients (only in patients aged ≥12 years and weighing ≥35 kg with HIV viral load <100,000 copies/mL). Fixed dose combinations containing rilpivirine and dolutegravir (Juluca®); rilpivirine and cabotegravir (Cabenuva®); rilpivirine, emtricitabine, and tenofovir disoproxil fumarate (DF, Complera®); and rilpivirine, emtricitabine, and tenofovir alafenamide (Odefsey®) are also used in the treatment of HIV infection. See the full prescribing information for use of each of these combination products.

Rilpivirine is also indicated in combination with cabotegravir for short-term treatment of HIV-1 infection in adults and adolescents ≥12 years of age and weighing ≥35 kg who are virologically suppressed (HIV-1 RNA <50 copies/mL) on a stable regimen with no history of treatment failure and with no known or suspected resistance to either cabotegravir or rilpivirine.

Clinical Experience in Antiretroviral Naïve Adults

Rilpivirine has been evaluated in two phase 3, randomized, double-blind, multicenter, noninferiority studies (studies TMC278-C209 [ECHO], TMC278-C215 [THRIVE]) in antiretroviral-naïve adults with baseline plasma HIV-1 RNA levels of at least 5000 copies/mL. Patients enrolled in these studies were screened to ensure they had HIV-1 that did not have specific non-nucleoside reverse transcriptase inhibitor (NNRTI) resistance-associated substitutions and were susceptible to nucleoside reverse transcriptase inhibitors (NRTIs). All patients received a background regimen of 2 NRTIs (dual NRTIs); patients enrolled in the ECHO study received a fixed combination of emtricitabine and tenofovir DF (emtricitabine/tenofovir DF) and patients enrolled in the THRIVE study received an investigator-selected dual NRTI option of emtricitabine and tenofovir DF, zidovudine and lamivudine, or abacavir and lamivudine. Over 1300 patients (median age, 36 years [range 18-78], 76% male, 60-61% white, 23-24% Black, 11-14% Asian, median baseline plasma HIV-1 RNA level 5.0 $\log_{10}$ copies/mL, median baseline CD4+ T-cell count 249–260 cells/mm³) were randomized to receive rilpivirine 25 mg once daily or efavirenz 600 mg once daily. At 48 weeks, rilpivirine was noninferior to efavirenz in both studies. Based on pooled results at 48 weeks, 84% of those receiving rilpivirine and 2 NRTIs and 82% of those receiving efavirenz and 2 NRTIs had plasma HIV-1 RNA levels below 50 copies/mL. In addition, the mean increase in CD4+ T-cell count from baseline at week 48 was 192 cells/mm³ in patients receiving a rilpivirine regimen and 176 cells/mm³ in those receiving an efavirenz regimen. Pooled results at week 96 showed that 76% of those receiving rilpivirine and 2 NRTIs and 77% of those receiving efavirenz and 2 NRTIs had plasma HIV-1 RNA levels below 50 copies/mL. The mean increase in CD4+ T-cell count from baseline at week 96 was 228 cells/mm³ in patients receiving a rilpivirine regimen and 219 cells/mm³ in those receiving an efavirenz regimen.

Pooled data from the ECHO and THRIVE studies indicated that the virologic failure rate at week 96 (plasma HIV-1 RNA levels 50 copies/mL or greater) was 16 or 10% in those randomized to rilpivirine or efavirenz, respectively, and 2 NRTIs; most virologic failures occurred in the first 48 weeks. When results were stratified by baseline plasma HIV-1 RNA levels among patients randomized to receive rilpivirine, virologic failure occurred in 9% of patients with baseline plasma HIV-1 RNA levels of 100,000 copies/mL or less and in 24% of those with baseline levels exceeding 100,000 copies/mL.

Rilpivirine also has been evaluated in a randomized, active-controlled, phase 2b, dose-comparison study (TMC278-C204) in 368 antiretroviral-naïve HIV-infected adults (median age, 35 years, 67% male, 45% white, 24% Black, 18% Asian) with baseline plasma HIV-1 RNA levels of at least 5000 copies/mL. Patients enrolled in this study had previously received no more than 2 weeks of treatment with NRTIs or HIV protease inhibitors (PIs), had not previously received any NNRTIs, and were screened to ensure they had HIV-1 that did not have specific NNRTI resistance-associated mutations and were susceptible to NRTIs. Patients received an investigator-selected background regimen of 2 NRTIs (lamivudine and zidovudine or emtricitabine and tenofovir DF; administered as fixed-combination preparations whenever possible) and were randomized (1:1:1:1) to receive open-label efavirenz (600 mg once daily) or 1 of 3 blinded rilpivirine dosage regimens (25, 75, or 150 mg once daily) for 96 weeks. At 96 weeks, 76% of patients receiving a regimen of rilpivirine 25 mg and 2 NRTIs and 71% of patients receiving a regimen of efavirenz and 2 NRTIs had plasma HIV-1 RNA levels below 50 copies/mL. The mean increase in CD4+ T-cell count from baseline was 146 cells/mm³ in those receiving rilpivirine 25 mg and 160 cells/mm³ in those receiving efavirenz. At 96 weeks, patients originally randomized to any dose of rilpivirine were switched to an open label rilpivirine regimen of 25 mg once daily and 2 NRTIs for long-term follow-up. At 240 weeks, virologic suppression (plasma HIV-1 RNA levels below 50 copies/mL) was achieved in 60% of patients originally randomized to rilpivirine 25 mg and 57% of those randomized to efavirenz.

Clinical Experience in Antiretroviral-Experienced Adults

Use of rilpivirine in combination with dolutegravir for maintenance of HIV virological suppression in previously-treated adults† was compared to continuation of current ARV therapy in the identical, phase 3, randomized, open-label, multicenter, non-inferiority, SWORD-1 and SWORD-2 trials. Patients receiving first- or second-line ARV regimens with sustained virological suppression (HIV viral load <50 copies/mL) for at least 6 months were randomized to switch to rilpivirine with dolutegravir or continue their current regimen. Patients randomized to continuation were switched to rilpivirine with dolutegravir after 52 weeks. Among 1024 patients who were randomized and included in the primary analysis, no difference in virological suppression was identified between groups at 48 weeks (95% in each group), demonstrating non-inferiority of rilpivirine with dolutegravir. In an updated analysis at 148 weeks from randomization, 84% of patients initially randomized to rilpivirine with dolutegravir and 90% of patients who switched to rilpivirine and dolutegravir after 52 weeks maintained virologic suppression.

Rilpivirine has also been studied in combination with cobicistat-boosted darunavir for maintenance of HIV virological suppression in previously-treated adults† in the phase 3, randomized, open-label, non-inferiority, PROBE 2 trial. Patients receiving ARV therapy with stable virological suppression (HIV viral load <50 copies/mL) for at least 6 months were randomized to switch to rilpivirine with cobicistat-boosted darunavir or continue their current regimen. Patients randomized to continuation were switched to rilpivirine with cobicistat-boosted darunavir after 24 weeks. Among 160 randomized patients, no difference in virological suppression was identified between groups at 24 weeks (90% of patients randomized to rilpivirine with cobicistat-boosted darunavir and 94% of patients randomized to continuation). In an updated analysis at 48 weeks from randomization, 88% of patients initially randomized to rilpivirine with cobicistat-boosted darunavir and 95% of patients who switched to rilpivirine with cobicistat-boosted darunavir at 24 weeks maintained virologic suppression.

Clinical Experience in Virologically-Suppressed Adults in Combination With Cabotegravir

Use of oral rilpivirine in combination with oral cabotegravir has been evaluated in clinical trials as a short-term lead-in to assess tolerability of rilpivirine prior to use of the fixed dose extended-release injectable suspension combination of rilpivirine and cabotegravir (Cabenuva®) and as short-term therapy in patients who miss planned injections of Cabenuva®. See full prescribing information for oral cabotegravir and Cabenuva® for details of clinical experience with these regimens.

Clinical Experience in Antiretroviral-Naïve Pediatric Patients

The efficacy and safety of rilpivirine in conjunction with 2 NRTIs were evaluated in the single-arm, open-label, phase 2, PAINT trial (TMC278-C213) in 36 treatment-naïve pediatric patients 12 to <18 years of age weighing at least 32 kg (median age, 14.5 years, 56% female, 89% Black, 11% Asian, median baseline plasma HIV-1 RNA level 49,550 copies/mL, median baseline CD4+ T-cell count

438 cells/mm³). Of the 36 patients, 24 received rilpivirine in conjunction with emtricitabine and tenofovir DF. At week 48, virologic response (plasma HIV-1 RNA levels <50 copies/mL) was achieved in 79% of patients with baseline plasma HIV-1 RNA levels of 100,000 copies/mL or less compared with 50% of those with baseline HIV-1 RNA levels greater than 100,000 copies/mL. The mean increase in CD4⁺ T-cell count from baseline was 201 cells/mm³. In a subgroup of patients receiving rilpivirine in conjunction with emtricitabine and tenofovir DF who had baseline plasma HIV-1 RNA levels of 100,000 copies/mL or less, virologic response (plasma HIV-1 RNA levels <50 copies/mL) was achieved by 80% at 48 weeks and the mean increase in CD4⁺ T-cell count from baseline was 225 cells/mm³ at 48 weeks. In 32 patients included in a post-48 week efficacy analysis of PAINT, 24 of whom continued treatment with rilpivirine and 2 NRTIs after week 48 (up to 240 weeks), virologic response was observed in 44% of patients at week 240. Among patients with baseline HIV-1 RNA of 100,000 copies/mL or less, virologic response was observed in 48% at week 240, whereas virologic response was observed in 29% at week 240 in patients with baseline HIV-1 RNA levels greater than 100,000 copies/mL.

Clinical Experience in Antiretroviral-Experienced Pediatric Patients

Use of fixed-dose combination rilpivirine with emtricitabine and tenofovir DF (Complera®) for treatment of HIV in previously-treated pediatric patients† has been described in a multicenter case series from the Cohort of the Spanish Pediatric HIV Network (CoRISpe) database. See full prescribing information for Complera® for details of clinical experience with this regimen.

Clinical Perspective in Adult and Pediatric Patients

Therapeutic options for the treatment and prevention of HIV infection and recommendations concerning the use of antiretrovirals are continuously evolving. Antiretroviral therapy is recommended for all individuals with HIV regardless of CD4 counts, and should be initiated as soon as possible after diagnosis of HIV and continued indefinitely. The primary goals of ART are to achieve and maintain durable suppression of HIV viral load (as measured by plasma HIV-1 RNA levels) to a level below which drug-resistance mutations cannot emerge (i.e., below detectable limits), restore and preserve immunologic function, reduce HIV-related morbidity and mortality, improve quality of life, and prevent transmission of HIV. While the most appropriate ARV regimen cannot be defined for each clinical scenario, the US Department of Health and Human Services (HHS) Panel on Antiretroviral Guidelines for Adults and Adolescents, HHS Panel on Antiretroviral Therapy and Medical Management of Children Living with HIV, and HHS Panel on Treatment of Pregnant Women with HIV Infection and Prevention of Perinatal Transmission, have developed comprehensive guidelines that provide information on selection and use of ARVs for the treatment or prevention of HIV infection. Because of the complexity of managing patients with HIV, it is recommended that clinicians with HIV expertise be consulted when needed.

The use of combination ARV regimens that generally include 3 drugs from 2 or more drug classes is currently recommended to achieve viral suppression. In both treatment-naïve adults and children, an initial ARV regimen generally consists of 2 NRTIs administered in combination with a third active ARV drug from 1 of 3 drug classes: an integrase strand transfer inhibitor (INSTI), a NNRTI, or a PI with a pharmacokinetic enhancer (also known as a booster; the 2 drugs used for this purpose are cobicistat and ritonavir). Selection of an initial ARV regimen should be individualized based on factors such as virologic efficacy, toxicity, pill burden, dosing frequency, drug–drug interaction potential, resistance-test results, comorbid conditions, access, and cost. In patients with comorbid infections (e.g., hepatitis B, tuberculosis), regimen selection should also consider the potential for activity against other present infections and timing of initiation relative to other anti-infective regimens.

In the 2022 HHS Adult and Adolescent HIV treatment guideline, rilpivirine, an NNRTI, is included in various ARV regimens. One of these rilpivirine-containing regimens is listed among alternative initial regimens recommended in certain clinical situations: rilpivirine/tenofovir alafenamide/emtricitabine or rilpivirine/tenofovir DF/emtricitabine (only in patients with <200 cells/mm³, HIV viral load <100,000 copies/mL, and who have drug resistance testing results available).

In the 2022 HHS Pediatric HIV treatment guideline, rilpivirine is included in various ARV regimens. Rilpivirine in combination with 2 NRTIs is recommended as an alternative initial regimen in certain clinical situations (only in patients aged

≥12 years and weighing ≥35 kg with HIV viral load <100,000 copies/mL), based primarily on evidence in adults.

In the 2022 HHS Perinatal HIV treatment guideline, rilpivirine is included in various ARV regimens. Some of these rilpivirine-containing regimens are listed among alternative initial options for pregnant patients, and include the following: rilpivirine/tenofovir alafenamide/emtricitabine, rilpivirine/tenofovir DF/emtricitabine, and rilpivirine in combination with a preferred dual-NRTI backbone (rilpivirine regimens are recommended only in patients with HIV viral load <100,000 copies/mL).

● Postexposure Prophylaxis following Occupational Exposure to HIV

Rilpivirine has been used in conjunction with 2 NRTIs for postexposure prophylaxis of HIV infection following occupational exposure† (PEP) in health-care personnel and other individuals exposed via percutaneous injury (e.g., needlestick, cut with sharp object) or mucous membrane or nonintact skin (e.g., chapped, abraded, dermatitis) contact with blood, tissue, or other body fluids that might contain HIV. Rilpivirine in combination with 2 NRTIs is one of several alternative regimens recommended in guidelines for PEP when the preferred regimen cannot be used.

The US Public Health Service (USPHS) states that the preferred regimen for PEP following an occupational exposure to HIV is a 3-drug regimen of raltegravir used in conjunction with emtricitabine and tenofovir DF (may be administered as the fixed combination emtricitabine/tenofovir DF; Truvada®). These experts recommend several alternative regimens that include an INSTI, NNRTI, or PI and 2 NRTIs (dual NRTIs). These alternatives include use of rilpivirine and 2 NRTIs when the preferred regimen cannot be used. The preferred dual NRTI option for use in PEP regimens is emtricitabine and tenofovir DF (may be administered as the fixed combination emtricitabine/tenofovir DF; Truvada®); alternative dual NRTIs are tenofovir DF and lamivudine, lamivudine and zidovudine (may be administered as the fixed combination lamivudine/zidovudine; Combivir®), or zidovudine and emtricitabine.

Because management of occupational exposures to HIV is complex and evolving, consultation with an infectious disease specialist, clinician with expertise in administration of ARV agents, and/or the National Clinicians' Postexposure Prophylaxis Hotline (PEPline at 888-448-4911) is recommended whenever possible. However, initiation of PEP should not be delayed while waiting for expert consultation.

● Postexposure Prophylaxis following Nonoccupational Exposure to HIV

Rilpivirine has been used in conjunction with 2 NRTIs for postexposure prophylaxis of HIV infection following nonoccupational exposure† (nPEP) in individuals exposed to blood, genital secretions, or other potentially infectious body fluids that might contain HIV, when that exposure represents a substantial risk for HIV transmission. Rilpivirine in combination with 2 NRTIs is one of several alternative regimens recommended in guidelines for nPEP. A fixed dose combination containing rilpivirine, emtricitabine, and tenofovir DF (Complera®) has been used for nPEP† in this setting. See the full prescribing information for use of Complera®.

Clinical Experience

Use of fixed dose combination rilpivirine with emtricitabine and tenofovir DF (Complera®) as nPEP† has been described in an open-label, non-randomized trial and a prospective, observational study. See full prescribing information for Complera® for details of clinical experience with this regimen.

Clinical Perspective

When nPEP is indicated following a nonoccupational exposure to HIV, the US Centers for Disease Control and Prevention (CDC) states that the preferred regimen in adults and adolescents 13 years of age or older with normal renal function is either raltegravir or dolutegravir used in conjunction with emtricitabine and tenofovir DF (administered as the fixed combination emtricitabine/tenofovir DF; Truvada®). The alternative nPEP regimen recommended in these patients is ritonavir-boosted darunavir used in conjunction with emtricitabine/tenofovir DF (Truvada®). Rilpivirine in combination with 2 NRTIs is one of several other alternative regimens recommended by CDC for nPEP.

Consultation with an infectious disease specialist, clinician with expertise in administration of ARV agents, and/or the National Clinicians' Postexposure Prophylaxis Hotline (PEPline at 888-448-4911) is recommended if nPEP is indicated in certain exposed individuals (e.g., pregnant women, children, those with medical conditions such as renal impairment) or if an ARV regimen not included in the CDC guidelines is being considered, the source virus is known or likely to be resistant to ARVs, or the healthcare provider is inexperienced in prescribing ARVs. However, initiation of nPEP should not be delayed while waiting for expert consultation.

DOSAGE AND ADMINISTRATION

● General

Pretreatment Screening

- Assess liver function tests prior to therapy initiation in patients with underlying hepatic disease such as hepatitis B and/or C co-infection or marked elevations in transaminase.
- Review concomitant medications for potential drug interactions prior to initiation of rilpivirine to avoid potential loss of virologic response.

Patient Monitoring

- Monitor liver function tests during therapy in patients with underlying hepatic disease such as hepatitis B virus and/or C co-infection, or marked elevations in transaminase. Consider monitoring liver function tests if no underlying hepatic dysfunction or risk factors.
- Review concomitant medications during therapy and consider potential for drug interactions with rilpivirine to avoid potential loss of virologic response.

Dispensing and Administration Precautions

- Rilpivirine is commercially available as a single entity and in various fixed-combination preparations containing additional ARV agents. Refer to the full prescribing information for specific, distinct uses of the combination products. Since the ARV agents contained in the fixed combination preparations also may be available in single-entity or other fixed-combination preparations, exercise care to ensure that therapy is not duplicated if a fixed combination is used in conjunction with other ARVs.

● Administration

Rilpivirine hydrochloride is available as oral tablets and is administered orally once daily with a meal.

Food enhances rilpivirine bioavailability. Systemic exposure is 40 or 50% lower if rilpivirine is administered under fasting conditions or with only a protein-rich nutritional drink, respectively, compared with following a standard meal (533 kcal) or high-caloric meal (928 kcal).

If a dose of rilpivirine is missed within 12 hours of the time it is usually taken, take the missed dose as soon as possible with a meal. If a dose of rilpivirine is missed by more than 12 hours, then skip the missed dose and resume the normal dosing schedule.

Rilpivirine must be used in conjunction with other ARVs. Single-entity rilpivirine should not be used concomitantly with emtricitabine/rilpivirine/tenofovir alafenamide or cabotegravir/rilpivirine injeciton. Single-entity rilpivirine should not be used concomitantly with emtricitabine/rilpivirine/tenofovir DF, unless needed for adjustment of rilpivirine dosage (e.g., when the fixed combination is used concomitantly with rifabutin).

Store rilpivirine tablets at 25°C; (excursions permitted between 15–30°C).

Fixed Combinations Containing Rilpivirine

Rilpivirine hydrochloride is commercially available in fixed-combination tablets containing dolutegravir sodium and rilpivirine (Juluca®); emtricitabine, rilpivirine, and tenofovir alafenamide (Odefsey®) and emtricitabine, rilpivirine, and tenofovir DF (Complera®). Rilpivirine is also commercially available as an extended-release injectable suspension kit containing copackaged cabotegravir and rilpivirine (Cabenuva®). See the full prescribing information for administration of each of these combination products.

● Dosage

Rilpivirine is commercially available as rilpivirine hydrochloride; dosage is expressed in terms of rilpivirine.

Pediatric Dosage

Treatment of HIV Infection in Antiretroviral-naïve Pediatric Patients

For the treatment of HIV-1 infection in antiretroviral-naïve adolescents 12 years of age or older weighing at least 35 kg with plasma RNA levels ≤100,000 copies/mL at therapy initiation, the usual dosage of rilpivirine (Edurant®) is 25 mg once daily.

Treatment of HIV Infection in Antiretroviral-experienced Pediatric Patients in Combination with Cabotegravir

For the treatment of HIV-1 infection in previously treated adolescents 12 years of age and older weighing at least 35 kg who are virologically suppressed (HIV-1 RNA levels <50 copies/mL) in combination with cabotegravir oral tablets (Vocabria®), the usual dosage of rilpivirine (Edurant®) is 25 mg once daily. Single-entity rilpivirine is indicated in combination with cabotegravir (Vocabria®) for short-term treatment to assess the tolerability of rilpivirine prior to cabotegravir/rilpivirine (Cabenuva®) initiation, and as a dosing bridge when missed injections of cabotegravir/rilpivirine (Cabenuva®) are planned; consult the prescribing information of these products before initiating rilpivirine oral tablets.

Oral lead-in therapy should be used for approximately 1 month (at least 28 days) to assess rilpivirine tolerability prior to initiation of cabotegravir/rilpivirine (Cabenuva®) . The last oral dose of rilpivirine (Edurant®) and cabotegravir (Vocabria®) should be administered on the same day that cabotegravir/rilpivirine (Cabenuva®) is initiated.

If a scheduled monthly injection of cabotegravir/rilpivirine (Cabenuva®) is planned to be missed by more than 7 days, daily oral rilpivirine (Edurant®) and cabotegravir (Vocabria®) can be taken together for up to 2 months to replace missed injection visits. The recommended oral daily dose is one 25-mg tablet of rilpivirine and one 30-mg tablet of cabotegravir. The first dose of oral therapy should be initiated at approximately the same time as the planned missed injection and continued until the day injection dosing is restarted. For durations longer than 2 months, use an alternative oral regimen.

If a scheduled every-2-month injection of cabotegravir/rilpivirine (Cabenuva®) is planned to be missed by more than 7 days, daily oral rilpivirine (Edurant®) and cabotegravir (Vocabria®) can be taken together for up to 2 months to replace 1 missed scheduled every-2-month injection. The recommended oral daily dose is one 25-mg tablet of rilpivirine and one 30-mg tablet of cabotegravir. The first dose of oral therapy should be initiated at approximately the same time as the planned missed injection and continued until the day injection dosing is restarted. For durations longer than 2 months, use an alternative oral regimen.

Treatment of HIV Infection in Pediatric Patients Receiving Rifabutin

If single-entity rilpivirine is used in conjunction with other ARVs for the treatment of HIV-1 infection in pediatric patients weighing at least 35 kg receiving rifabutin, an increased rilpivirine dosage of 50 mg daily should be used. When rifabutin coadministration is stopped, the rilpivirine dose should be decreased to 25 mg once daily.

Adult Dosage

Treatment of HIV Infection in Antiretroviral-naïve Adults

For the treatment of human immunodeficiency virus type 1 (HIV-1) infection in antiretroviral-naïve adults, the usual dosage of rilpivirine (Edurant®) is 25 mg once daily.

Treatment of HIV Infection in Antiretroviral-experienced Adults in Combination with Cabotegravir

For the treatment of HIV-1 infection in previously treated adults who are virologically suppressed (HIV-1 RNA <50 copies/mL), the usual dosage of rilpivirine (Edurant®) is 25 mg once daily. Single-entity rilpivirine is indicated in combination with cabotegravir (Vocabria®) for short-term treatment to assess the tolerability of rilpivirine prior to cabotegravir/rilpivirine (Cabenuva®) initiation, and as a dosing bridge when missed injections of Cabenuva® are planned; consult the prescribing information of these products before initiating rilpivirine oral tablets.

Oral lead-in therapy should be used for approximately 1 month (at least 28 days) to assess rilpivirine tolerability prior to initiation of cabotegravir/rilpivirine (Cabenuva®) . The last oral dose of rilpivirine (Edurant®) and cabotegravir (Vocabria®) should be administered on the same day that cabotegravir/rilpivirine (Cabenuva®) is initiated.

If a scheduled monthly injection of cabotegravir/rilpivirine (Cabenuva®) is planned to be missed by more than 7 days, daily oral rilpivirine (Edurant®) and cabotegravir (Vocabria®) can be taken together for up to 2 months to replace missed injection visits. The recommended oral daily dose is one 25-mg tablet of rilpivirine and one 30-mg tablet of cabotegravir. The first dose of oral therapy should be initiated at approximately the same time as the planned missed injection and continued until the day injection dosing is restarted. For durations longer than 2 months, use an alternative oral regimen.

If a scheduled every-2-month injection of cabotegravir/rilpivirine (Cabenuva®) is planned to be missed by more than 7 days, daily oral rilpivirine (Edurant®) and cabotegravir (Vocabria®) can be taken together for up to 2 months to replace 1 missed scheduled every-2-month injection. The recommended oral daily dose is one 25-mg tablet of rilpivirine and one 30-mg tablet of cabotegravir. The first dose of oral therapy should be initiated at approximately the same time as the planned missed injection and continued until the day injection dosing is restarted. For durations longer than 2 months, use an alternative oral regimen.

Treatment of HIV Infection in Adults Receiving Rifabutin

If single-entity rilpivirine is used in conjunction with other ARVs for the treatment of HIV-1 infection in adults receiving rifabutin, an increased rilpivirine dosage of 50 mg daily should be used. When rifabutin coadministration is stopped, the rilpivirine dose should be decreased to 25 mg once daily.

Postexposure Prophylaxis following Occupational Exposure to HIV

For postexposure prophylaxis of HIV infection following occupational exposure† (PEP) in health-care personnel or other individuals, rilpivirine is administered in a dosage of 25 mg once daily in conjunction with 2 HIV NRTIs.

The PEP regimen should be initiated as soon as possible following occupational exposure to HIV (preferably within hours) and continued for 4 weeks, if tolerated.

Postexposure Prophylaxis following Nonoccupational Exposure to HIV

When emtricitabine/rilpivirine/tenofovir DF (Complera®) is used as a complete regimen for postexposure prophylaxis of HIV infection following nonoccupational exposure† (nPEP), adults should receive 1 tablet (200 mg of emtricitabine, 25 mg of rilpivirine, and 300 mg of tenofovir DF) once daily.

The nPEP regimen should be initiated as soon as possible (within 72 hours) following nonoccupational exposure to HIV and continued for 28 days. If the exposed individual seeks care more than 72 hours after the exposure, nPEP is not recommended.

● *Special Populations*

Hepatic Impairment

Dosage adjustment of rilpivirine (Edurant®) is not necessary for the treatment of HIV-1 infection in patients with mild or moderate hepatic impairment (Child-Pugh class A or B). Rilpivirine has not been studied in those with severe hepatic impairment (Child-Pugh class C).

Consult the product labeling of commercially available fixed-combination products containing rilpivirine for specific dosage adjustments of each component in hepatic impairment.

Renal Impairment

Dosage adjustment of rilpivirine (Edurant®) is not necessary for the treatment of HIV-1 infection in patients with mild or moderate renal impairment. The manufacturer makes no specific dosage recommendations for those with severe renal impairment or end-stage renal disease; rilpivirine should be used with caution in such individuals.

Consult the product labeling of commercially available fixed-combination products containing rilpivirine for specific dosage adjustments of each component in renal impairment.

Geriatric Use

The manufacturer makes no specific dosage recommendations for geriatric patients.

Consult the product labeling of commercially available fixed-combination products containing rilpivirine for specific dosage adjustments of each component in geriatric patients.

CAUTIONS

● *Contraindications*

Concomitant use of rilpivirine with drugs that induce cytochrome P-450 isoenzyme 3A (CYP3A) or drugs that elevate gastric pH is contraindicated since substantially decreased plasma rilpivirine concentrations may occur and may result in loss of virologic response and development of resistance to rilpivirine and/or class resistance to HIV NNRTIs.

● *Warnings/Precautions*

Skin and Hypersensitivity Reactions

Severe skin and hypersensitivity reactions, including cases of drug reaction with eosinophilia and systemic symptoms (DRESS), have been reported during postmarketing experience in patients receiving rilpivirine-containing antiretroviral (ARV) regimens. While some skin reactions were accompanied by constitutional symptoms such as fever, other skin reactions were associated with organ dysfunction, including elevated serum concentrations of hepatic enzymes. During phase 3 studies of rilpivirine-containing ARV regimens, treatment-associated rash with at least grade 2 severity was reported in 1-3% of patients. Most rashes were grade 1 or 2 and occurred in the first 4-6 weeks of therapy.

Rilpivirine should be discontinued immediately if signs or symptoms of severe skin or hypersensitivity reactions develop (e.g., severe rash or rash accompanied by fever, blisters, mucosal involvement, conjunctivitis, facial edema, angioedema, hepatitis, or eosinophilia). Clinical status, including laboratory parameters, should be monitored and appropriate therapy initiated.

Hepatotoxicity

Adverse hepatic effects have been reported in patients receiving rilpivirine in conjunction with other ARVs. Hepatotoxicity has been reported in patients receiving rilpivirine who had no preexisting hepatic disease or other risk factors.

HIV-infected patients with hepatitis B virus (HBV) or hepatitis C virus (HCV) coinfection or markedly elevated serum aminotransferase concentrations prior to initiation of rilpivirine may be at increased risk for development or worsening of transaminase elevations. If rilpivirine is used in patients with underlying hepatic disease (e.g., HBV or HCV infection, markedly elevated aminotransferase concentrations), laboratory tests should be performed to evaluate hepatic function prior to and during rilpivirine treatment. Liver enzyme monitoring also should be considered in patients without preexisting hepatic disease or other risk factors.

Depressive Disorders

Depressive disorders (e.g., depressed mood, depression, dysphoria, major depression, altered mood, negative thoughts, suicide attempt, suicidal ideation) have been reported in patients receiving rilpivirine. During phase 3 studies, 9% of adults receiving rilpivirine reported depressive disorders compared with 8% of patients receiving efavirenz. While most depressive events were reported to be mild or moderate in severity, 1% of adults in each treatment group reported a grade 3 or 4 depressive disorder and 1% in each treatment group discontinued therapy as a result of a depressive disorder. Suicidal ideation was reported in 4 adults in each treatment group and suicide attempt was reported in 2 adults receiving rilpivirine.

During a phase 2 study evaluating rilpivirine in pediatric patients 12 to <18 years of age, the incidence of depressive disorders was 19.4%. While most depressive events were reported to be mild or moderate in severity, 5.6% of pediatric patients reported a grade 3 or 4 depressive disorder. Suicidal ideation and suicide attempt were reported in a single pediatric patient.

Patients experiencing severe depressive symptoms should seek immediate medical evaluation to determine the likelihood that symptoms are related to rilpivirine and to determine if the benefits of continued rilpivirine therapy outweigh the risks.

Risk of Adverse Reactions or Loss of Virologic Response Due to Drug Interactions

Concomitant use of rilpivirine with certain drugs (e.g., drugs that may reduce rilpivirine concentrations, drugs known to increase the risk of torsade de pointes) is contraindicated or requires particular caution. Some drug interactions may lead to loss of virologic effect of rilpivirine and the possible development of resistance. Consider the potential for drug interactions with concomitant medications prior to and during treatment with rilpivirine.

Immune Reconstitution Syndrome

During the initial phase of treatment, HIV-infected patients whose immune systems respond to antiretroviral therapy may develop an inflammatory response to indolent or residual opportunistic infections (e.g., *Mycobacterium avium*, *M. tuberculosis*, cytomegalovirus [CMV], *Pneumocystis jirovecii* [formerly *P. carinii*]); such responses may necessitate further evaluation and treatment.

Autoimmune disorders (e.g., Graves' disease, polymyositis, Guillain-Barré syndrome, autoimmune hepatitis) have also been reported to occur in the setting of immune reconstitution; however, the time to onset is more variable and can occur many months after initiation of ARV therapy.

Specific Populations

Pregnancy

The Antiretroviral Pregnancy Registry (APR) monitors pregnancy outcomes in women exposed to rilpivirine during pregnancy. Clinicians are encouraged to register patients in the APR by calling 800-258-4263 or visiting https://www.apregistry.com/.

The overall risk of birth defects with first-trimester exposure for rilpivirine was not markedly different compared to the background rate for major birth defects of 2.7% in the United States reference population of the Metropolitan Atlanta Congenital Defects Program (MACDP). Limitations of using an external comparator (the MACDP) includes differences in populations and methodology, and confounding due to the underlying disease. The rate of miscarriage is not reported in the APR.

In a small study of 19 HIV-1 infected women on a rilpivirine-based regimen, protein binding was similar during the second and third trimesters and the postpartum period; however, total exposure of rilpivirine was approximately 30–40% lower during pregnancy when compared to the postpartum period. Of the 12 virologically suppressed patients at baseline (<50 copies/mL), virologic suppression with a rilpivirine-based regimen was maintained through the third trimester in 10 patients, and was well-tolerated. Among 10 infants born to HIV-1 infected women, all were HIV-1 negative at delivery and for 16 weeks post-partum. All infants received prophylactic zidovudine treatment at delivery.

Animal data have shown no increases in embryo-fetal toxicity at rilpivirine exposures 15–70 -times the equivalent human exposure.

No dosage adjustments are necessary in pregnancy for females who are stable on a rilpivirine-containing regimen prior to pregnancy and who are virologically suppressed (<50 copies/mL). The recommended dosage in pregnancy is 25 mg once daily. Monitor viral load closely in pregnant women; lower rilpivirine exposures have been observed in pregnant individuals.

Lactation

It is not known whether rilpivirine is distributed into human milk or the effects on a breastfed infant or milk production; however, the drug is distributed into milk in rats.

Because of the risk of adverse effects in the infant and the risk of HIV transmission, HIV-infected females should not breast-feed infants.

Pediatric Use

Safety and efficacy of single-entity rilpivirine (Edurant®) have *not* been established in pediatric patients younger than 12 years of age or weighing <35 kg.

Depressive disorders have been reported in pediatric patients 12 to <18 years of age receiving rilpivirine-containing regimens.

Geriatric Use

Experience in those 65 years of age and older is insufficient to determine whether they respond differently to rilpivirine than younger adults. Dosage should be selected with caution because of age-related decreases in hepatic, renal, and/or cardiac function and potential for concomitant disease and drug therapy.

Hepatic Impairment

Rilpivirine (Edurant®) has not been studied in patients with severe hepatic impairment (Child-Pugh class C).

During phase 3 clinical trials evaluating rilpivirine, HIV-infected patients coinfected with HBV and/or HCV had a higher incidence of increased serum aminotransferase concentrations compared with those without coinfection.

Renal Impairment

Rilpivirine (Edurant®) should be used with caution, and with increased monitoring for adverse effects, in patients with severe renal impairment or end-stage renal disease since concentrations of the drug may be increased due to alterations in absorption, distribution, or metabolism.

● Common Adverse Effects

Adverse effects of at least moderate to severe intensity reported in 2% or more of patients in clinical trials include depressive disorders, insomnia, headache, and rash.

DRUG INTERACTIONS

Most rilpivirine drug interaction studies reported to date used rilpivirine dosages of 75 or 150 mg once daily; these dosages are considerably higher than the usually recommended rilpivirine dosage (25 mg once daily). Rilpivirine is primarily metabolized by cytochrome P-450 isoenzyme 3A (CYP3A).

The following drug interactions are based on studies using single-entity rilpivirine. When rilpivirine fixed combinations are used, interactions associated with each drug in the fixed combination should be considered.

● Drugs Affecting or Metabolized by Hepatic Microsomal Enzymes

Rilpivirine is metabolized by CYP3A. Concomitant use with drugs that induce CYP3A may result in decreased plasma rilpivirine concentrations and may result in possible loss of virologic response and development of resistance to rilpivirine or the HIV NNRTI class. Concomitant use with drugs that inhibit CYP3A may result in increased plasma rilpivirine concentrations.

When the recommended rilpivirine dosage (25 mg once daily) is used, it is unlikely to have clinically important effects on the pharmacokinetics of drugs that are metabolized by CYP isoenzymes.

● Drugs that Increase Gastric pH

Concomitant use of rilpivirine and drugs that increase gastric pH may result in decreased plasma rilpivirine concentrations and may result in loss of virologic response and development of resistance to rilpivirine or the NNRTI class.

Antacids

Potential pharmacokinetic interaction if antacids such as aluminum hydroxide, calcium carbonate, or magnesium hydroxide are used concomitantly with rilpivirine (decreased plasma rilpivirine concentrations).

Antacids and rilpivirine should be used concomitantly with caution; antacids should be administered at least 2 hours before or at least 4 hours after rilpivirine.

Histamine H₂-receptor Antagonists

Concomitant use of famotidine and rilpivirine has resulted in decreased rilpivirine plasma concentrations and area under the concentration-time curve (AUC). Concomitant use of other histamine H₂-receptor antagonists may result in decreased rilpivirine plasma concentrations.

Histamine H$_2$-receptor antagonists and rilpivirine should be used concomitantly with caution; histamine H$_2$-receptor antagonists should be administered at least 12 hours before or at least 4 hours after rilpivirine.

Proton-pump Inhibitors

Concomitant use of omeprazole and rilpivirine has resulted in decreased rilpivirine plasma concentrations and AUC. Concomitant use of other proton-pump inhibitors (e.g., esomeprazole, lansoprazole, pantoprazole, rabeprazole) also may result in decreased rilpivirine plasma concentrations.

Concomitant use of proton-pump inhibitors and rilpivirine is contraindicated.

● *Drugs that Prolong the QT Interval*

Only limited data are available to date regarding the potential for pharmacodynamic interactions if rilpivirine is used concomitantly with drugs known to prolong the QT interval and increase the risk of torsade de pointes. Data from healthy individuals indicate that the recommended rilpivirine dosage (25 mg once daily) can result in increases in the corrected QT (QT$_c$) interval that are not considered clinically important; however, higher rilpivirine dosage (75 or 300 mg once daily) results in clinically important prolongation of the QT$_c$ interval.

● *Anticonvulsants*

Potential pharmacokinetic interactions when rilpivirine is used concomitantly with carbamazepine, oxcarbazepine, phenobarbital, or phenytoin may result in decreased virologic response.

Concomitant use of anticonvulsants (e.g., carbamazepine, oxcarbazepine, phenobarbital, phenytoin) and rilpivirine is contraindicated.

● *Antifungal Agents*

Concomitant use of ketoconazole and rilpivirine has resulted in increased rilpivirine plasma concentrations and AUC and decreased ketoconazole plasma concentrations and AUC. Concomitant use of other azole antifungals (e.g., fluconazole, itraconazole, posaconazole, voriconazole) and rilpivirine also may result in increased rilpivirine plasma concentrations and decreased antifungal plasma concentrations.

When rilpivirine is used concomitantly with an azole antifungal (e.g., fluconazole, itraconazole, ketoconazole, posaconazole, voriconazole), dosage adjustments are not needed; however, patients should be monitored for breakthrough fungal infections.

● *Antimycobacterial Agents*
Rifampin and Rifapentine

Concomitant use of rilpivirine and rifampin or rifapentine results in decreased rilpivirine plasma concentrations and AUC and potential loss of virologic response.

Concomitant use of rifampin or rifapentine with rilpivirine is contraindicated.

Rifabutin

Concomitant use of rifabutin and rilpivirine results in decreased rilpivirine plasma concentrations and AUC.

If single-entity rilpivirine is used concomitantly with rifabutin, rilpivirine dosage should be increased to 50 mg once daily; if rifabutin is discontinued, the usual dosage of single-entity rilpivirine (25 mg once daily) should be resumed.

● *Antiretroviral Agents*
HIV Entry and Fusion Inhibitors
Enfuvirtide

No in vitro evidence of antagonistic antiretroviral effects between rilpivirine and enfuvirtide.

Maraviroc

No in vitro evidence of antagonistic antiretroviral effects between rilpivirine and maraviroc.

Clinically important pharmacokinetic interactions are not expected.

HIV Integrase Inhibitors (INSTIs)
Cabotegravir

Concomitant use of cabotegravir and rilpivirine does not have a clinically important effect on rilpivirine plasma concentrations or AUC. No dosage adjustments necessary.

Raltegravir

No in vitro evidence of antagonistic antiretroviral effects between rilpivirine and raltegravir.

Concomitant use of raltegravir and rilpivirine does not have a clinically important effect on plasma concentrations or AUC of raltegravir or rilpivirine. Dosage adjustments are not needed for either drug.

HIV Nonnucleoside Reverse Transcriptase Inhibitors (NNRTIs)

No in vitro evidence of antagonistic antiretroviral effects between rilpivirine and NNRTIs (efavirenz, etravirine, nevirapine).

Concomitant use of delavirdine and rilpivirine may result in increased rilpivirine plasma concentrations; concomitant use of efavirenz, etravirine, or nevirapine may result in decreased rilpivirine plasma concentrations.

Concomitant use of rilpivirine and other NNRTIs (delavirdine, efavirenz, etravirine, nevirapine) is not recommended.

HIV Nucleoside and Nucleotide Reverse Transcriptase Inhibitors (NRTIs)

No in vitro evidence of antagonistic antiretroviral effects between rilpivirine and NRTIs (abacavir, didanosine, emtricitabine, lamivudine, tenofovir, zidovudine).

Although not specifically studied, clinically important pharmacokinetic interactions are not expected if rilpivirine is used concomitantly with abacavir, emtricitabine, lamivudine, or zidovudine.

Didanosine

Pharmacokinetic interactions were not observed when didanosine delayed-release capsules were administered 2 hours before rilpivirine. Although dosage adjustments are not needed if rilpivirine and didanosine are used concomitantly, didanosine should be administered (without food) at least 2 hours before or 4 hours after rilpivirine (with food).

Tenofovir

Concomitant use of tenofovir DF and rilpivirine has resulted in increased tenofovir plasma concentrations and AUC, but did not have a clinically important effect on rilpivirine plasma concentrations or AUC.

Dosage adjustments are not needed if tenofovir DF and rilpivirine are used concomitantly.

HIV Protease Inhibitors (PIs)

No in vitro evidence of antagonistic antiretroviral effects between rilpivirine and PIs (amprenavir [commercially available as fosamprenavir], atazanavir, darunavir, indinavir, lopinavir, nelfinavir, ritonavir, saquinavir, tipranavir).

Atazanavir

Concomitant use of rilpivirine and *ritonavir-boosted* atazanavir or unboosted atazanavir may result in increased rilpivirine plasma concentrations, but is not expected to affect atazanavir concentrations.

Dosage adjustments are not needed if rilpivirine is used concomitantly with *ritonavir-boosted* or unboosted atazanavir.

Darunavir

Concomitant use of rilpivirine and *ritonavir-boosted* darunavir resulted in increased rilpivirine plasma concentrations and AUC, but did not have a clinically important effect on darunavir concentrations or AUC.

Dosage adjustments are not needed if rilpivirine is used concomitantly with *ritonavir-boosted* darunavir.

Fosamprenavir

Concomitant use of rilpivirine and fosamprenavir or *ritonavir-boosted* fosamprenavir may result in increased rilpivirine plasma concentrations, but is not expected to affect amprenavir concentrations (active metabolite of fosamprenavir).

Dosage adjustments are not needed if fosamprenavir (with or without low-dose ritonavir) and rilpivirine are used concomitantly.

Indinavir

Concomitant use of rilpivirine and indinavir may result in increased rilpivirine plasma concentrations, but is not expected to affect indinavir concentrations. Dosage adjustments are not necessary if rilpivirine and indinavir are used concomitantly.

Lopinavir

Concomitant use of rilpivirine and the fixed combination of lopinavir and ritonavir (lopinavir/ritonavir) increased rilpivirine plasma concentrations and AUC, but did not have a clinically important effect on lopinavir plasma concentrations or AUC.

Dosage adjustments are not needed if lopinavir/ritonavir and rilpivirine are used concomitantly.

Nelfinavir

Concomitant use of nelfinavir may result in increased rilpivirine plasma concentrations, but is not expected to affect nelfinavir concentrations. Dosage adjustments are not necessary if nelfinavir and rilpivirine are used concomitantly.

Saquinavir

Concomitant use of rilpivirine and *ritonavir-boosted* saquinavir may result in increased rilpivirine plasma concentrations, but is not expected to affect saquinavir concentrations.

Dosage adjustments are not needed if *ritonavir-boosted* saquinavir and rilpivirine are used concomitantly.

Tipranavir

Concomitant use of rilpivirine and *ritonavir-boosted* tipranavir may result in increased rilpivirine plasma concentrations, but is not expected to affect tipranavir concentrations.

Dosage adjustments are not needed if *ritonavir-boosted* tipranavir and rilpivirine are used concomitantly.

● Atorvastatin

Clinically important pharmacokinetic interactions have not been observed when atorvastatin and rilpivirine were used concomitantly; dosage adjustments are not needed.

● Chlorzoxazone

Clinically important pharmacokinetic interactions between rilpivirine and chlorzoxazone have not been observed; dosage adjustments are not needed.

● Dexamethasone

Potential pharmacokinetic interaction if multiple doses of systemic dexamethasone are used concomitantly with rilpivirine (decreased plasma rilpivirine concentrations). Concomitant use of more than a single dose of dexamethasone with rilpivirine is contraindicated.

● Digoxin

Rilpivirine does not have a clinically important effect on digoxin pharmacokinetics.

● Estrogens and Progestins

Clinically important pharmacokinetic interactions have not been observed when usual rilpivirine dosage was used concomitantly with hormonal contraceptives containing ethinyl estradiol and norethindrone; dosage adjustments are not needed.

● Macrolides or Ketolide Antibiotics

Concomitant use of rilpivirine and clarithromycin or erythromycin may result in increased rilpivirine plasma concentrations and is associated with an increased risk of torsade de points, but is not expected to affect plasma concentrations of the macrolide. When possible, an alternative agent, or a macrolide such as azithromycin should be considered since azithromycin has less effect on rilpivirine concentrations in comparison to other macrolides.

● Metformin

Rilpivirine does not have a clinically important effect on metformin pharmacokinetics.

● Methadone

Concomitant use of methadone and usual rilpivirine dosage resulted in decreased concentrations of the R-enantiomer of methadone and increased concentrations of the S-enantiomer of methadone in a clinical study, but did not have a clinically important effect on rilpivirine concentrations or AUC.

Although adjustment of initial methadone dosage is not needed when methadone and rilpivirine are used concomitantly, close monitoring is recommended and methadone maintenance dosage may need to be adjusted in some patients.

● Sildenafil

Clinically important pharmacokinetic interactions have not been observed when sildenafil and rilpivirine were used concomitantly; dosage adjustments are not needed.

● Simeprevir

Concomitant use of simeprevir and rilpivirine does not have a clinically important effect on simeprevir or rilpivirine pharmacokinetics; dosage adjustments are not needed.

● Ribavirin

Clinically important pharmacokinetic interactions between rilpivirine and ribavirin are not expected.

● St. John's Wort

Potential pharmacokinetic interaction if St. John's wort (*Hypericum perforatum*) is used concomitantly with rilpivirine (decreased plasma rilpivirine concentrations); may result in loss of therapeutic effect and development of resistance. Concomitant use of St. John's wort and rilpivirine is contraindicated.

DESCRIPTION

Rilpivirine, a diarylpyrimidine human immunodeficiency virus (HIV) nonnucleoside reverse transcriptase inhibitor (NNRTI), inhibits replication of HIV type 1 (HIV-1) by interfering with viral RNA- and DNA-directed polymerase activities of reverse transcriptase. Diarylpyrimidine NNRTIs (e.g., rilpivirine, etravirine) are capable of adapting to mutations in HIV-1 reverse transcriptase because of structural flexibility that allows for binding to the allosteric NNRTI binding pocket in a variety of conformations. Unlike other currently available NNRTIs, rilpivirine contains a cyanovinyl group that contributes to potency and maintains the drug's binding ability, despite the emergence of some resistance mutations. In vitro, rilpivirine is highly active against wild-type HIV-1, but has limited activity against HIV type 2 (HIV-2). Rilpivirine has been active against some clinical HIV-1 isolates resistant to other commercially available NNRTIs (delavirdine, efavirenz, nevirapine). However rilpivirine-resistant strains have been selected in cell culture and have emerged during clinical use.

Cross-resistance can occur between rilpivirine and other commercially available NNRTIs, and is expected in patients who have virologic failure while receiving a regimen that contains rilpivirine. Considerable cross-resistance occurs between rilpivirine and etravirine; up to 90% of rilpivirine-resistant isolates that developed in patients receiving rilpivirine in phase 3 clinical studies also were resistant to etravirine. In addition, patients experiencing virologic failure while receiving a rilpivirine regimen in phase 3 clinical studies were more likely to have developed NNRTI-class resistance and treatment-emergent resistance to nucleoside and HIV nucleotide reverse transcriptase inhibitors (NRTIs) than patients experiencing virologic failure while receiving an efavirenz regimen.

After oral administration, peak rilpivirine plasma concentrations are generally attained within 4–5 hours. Rilpivirine is primarily metabolized in the liver by cytochrome (CYP) P-450 isoenzyme 3A. After a single oral dose, an average of 85% of the dose is eliminated in feces (75% as metabolites) and 6% is eliminated in urine (only trace amounts as unchanged rilpivirine). The terminal elimination half-life of rilpivirine is approximately 50 hours. In individuals with mild (Child-Pugh class A) or moderate (Child-Pugh class B) hepatic impairment receiving multiple doses of rilpivirine, exposure to the drug was 47 or 5% higher, respectively, compared to healthy individuals. Coinfection with HIV and hepatitis B virus (HBV) and/or hepatitis C virus (HCV) does not appear to have a clinically important effect on exposure to the drug. Mild renal impairment does not have a clinically important effect on rilpivirine pharmacokinetics. Only limited data are available regarding pharmacokinetics of the drug in patients with moderate or severe renal impairment or end-stage renal disease, but rilpivirine concentrations may be increased as a result of altered absorption, distribution, or elimination. In vitro studies indicate that rilpivirine is approximately 99.7% bound to plasma proteins, primarily albumin. Because rilpivirine is highly bound to plasma proteins, peritoneal dialysis and hemodialysis are unlikely to result in clinically important removal of the drug. Total exposure to rilpivirine dosage of 25 mg once daily is 30–40% lower during pregnancy when compared to the postpartum period; however, based on the exposure-response relationship of rilpivirine, this is not considered clinically relevant in patients who are virologically suppressed (<50 copies/mL). Protein binding of rilpivirine is approximately 99% during the second and third trimesters, and the postpartum period. Clinically relevant differences in pharmacokinetics based on gender, race, or hepatitis B and/or C coinfection have not been observed. Pharmacokinetics in treatment-naïve HIV-1-infected pediatric patients 12 to less than 18 years of age receiving rilpivirine 25 mg once daily are similar to those observed in treatment-naïve adult patients. In clinical trials, body weight in pediatric patients (ranging from 33–93 kg) did not have a clinically important effect on rilpivirine pharmacokinetics.

ADVICE TO PATIENTS

- Advise patients of the critical nature of compliance with human immunodeficiency virus (HIV) therapy and importance of remaining under the care of a clinician. Importance of taking as prescribed; do not alter or discontinue antiretroviral regimen without consulting clinician.

- Counsel patients on the importance of using single-entity rilpivirine in conjunction with other antiretrovirals ot for monotherapy.

- Antiretroviral therapy is not a cure for HIV infection; opportunistic infections and other complications associated with HIV disease may still occur.

- Advise patients that sustained decreases in plasma HIV RNA have been associated with reduced risk of progression to acquired immunodeficiency syndrome (AIDS) and death.

- Advise patients that effective antiretroviral regimens can decrease HIV concentrations in blood and genital secretions and strict adherence to such regimens in conjunction with risk-reduction measures may decrease, but cannot absolutely eliminate, the risk of secondary transmission of HIV

to others. Importance of continuing to practice safer sex (e.g., using latex or polyurethane condoms to minimize sexual contact with body fluids), never sharing personal items that can have blood or body fluids on them (e.g., toothbrushes, razor blades), and never reusing or sharing needles.

- Advise patients of the importance of taking once daily with a meal; a protein drink alone does not constitute a meal. Food enhances absorption of rilpivirine.

- Counsel patients that if a missed dose of rilpivirine is remembered within 12 hours, it should be taken with a meal as soon as possible and the next dose taken at the regularly scheduled time. If the missed dose is remembered more than 12 hours after the scheduled time, the dose should be omitted and the next dose taken at the regularly scheduled time. Advise patients that doses that are larger or smaller than the prescribed dosage should not be taken at any time.

- Advise patients that skin reactions ranging from mild to severe, including drug reaction with eosinophilia and systemic symptoms (DRESS), have been reported with rilpivirine-containing antiretroviral regimens. Instruct patients to immediately stop taking rilpivirine (single-entity or fixed-combination preparations) and contact a clinician if rash develops and is also associated with fever, blisters, mucosal involvement, eye inflammation (conjunctivitis), swelling of the face, eyes, lips, mouth, tongue, or throat which may lead to difficulty swallowing or breathing, or any signs and symptoms of liver problems.

- Advise patients that depressive disorders (e.g., depressed mood, depression, dysphoria, major depression, altered mood, negative thoughts, suicide attempt, suicidal ideation) have been reported. Importance of immediately contacting clinician if depressive symptoms (e.g., feeling sad, hopeless, anxious, or restless; hurting oneself; having thoughts of hurting oneself) occur.

- Advise patients that hepatotoxicity has been reported in patients receiving rilpivirine.

- Advise patients to inform their clinician of existing or contemplated concomitant therapy, including prescription and OTC drugs and herbal supplements (e.g., St. John's wort), and any concomitant illnesses.

- Importance of females informing clinicians if they are or plan to become pregnant or plan to breast-feed.

- Importance of advising patients of other important precautionary information.

PREPARATIONS

Excipients in commercially available drug preparations may have clinically important effects in some individuals; consult specific product labeling for details.

Rilpivirine Hydrochloride

Oral

Tablets, film-coated	25 mg (of rilpivirine)	Edurant®, Janssen

† Use is not currently included in the labeling approved by the US Food and Drug Administration.

Selected Revisions October 27, 2023, © Copyright, October 20, 2011, American Society of Health-System Pharmacists, Inc.

Emtricitabine

8:18.08.20 • HIV NUCLEOSIDE AND NUCLEOTIDE REVERSE TRANSCRIPTASE INHIBITORS

■ Emtricitabine, an antiretroviral agent, is a human immunodeficiency virus (HIV) nucleoside reverse transcriptase inhibitor (NRTI).

USES

● Treatment of HIV Infection

Emtricitabine is used in conjunction with other antiretroviral agents for the treatment of human immunodeficiency virus type 1 (HIV-1) infection.

Emtricitabine is commercially available as a single-entity preparation and in various fixed-combination preparations that contain 2 or 3 additional antiretrovirals; refer to separate combination product monographs for information related to the specific uses of these products.

Emtricitabine is commonly used as part of a dual-nucleoside reverse transcriptase inhibitor (NRTI) "backbone" of a fully suppressive antiretroviral regimen; consult guidelines for the most current information on recommended regimens. Selection of an initial antiretroviral regimen should be individualized based on factors such as virologic efficacy, toxicity, pill burden, dosing frequency, drug-drug interaction potential, resistance test results, comorbid conditions, access, and cost.

Clinical Experience
Antiretroviral-naïve Adults

Safety and efficacy of a regimen of efavirenz, emtricitabine, and tenofovir disoproxil fumarate (DF) are based on results of a randomized, open-label study designed to demonstrate noninferiority of this regimen compared with a regimen of efavirenz, zidovudine, and lamivudine (study 934). In this study, 511 antiretroviral-naïve HIV-infected patients (mean age 38 years, 86% male, 59% white, 23% Black, median baseline plasma HIV-1 RNA level 5.01 $\log_{10}$ copies/mL [range: 3.56–6.54 $\log_{10}$ copies/mL], mean baseline CD4+ T-cell count 245 cells/mm³) were randomized to receive a once-daily regimen of efavirenz, emtricitabine, and tenofovir DF or a regimen of efavirenz once daily with the fixed combination of lamivudine and zidovudine (lamivudine/zidovudine; Combivir®) twice daily. The primary measure used to assess noninferiority of the regimen of efavirenz, emtricitabine, and tenofovir DF to the regimen of efavirenz and lamivudine/zidovudine was plasma HIV-1 RNA levels at week 48, specifically, the number of patients with HIV-1 RNA levels <400 copies/mL. The 487 patients without baseline resistance to efavirenz who underwent randomization and received treatment were the predefined population used for the primary endpoint analysis.

Through week 48, the regimen of efavirenz, emtricitabine, and tenofovir DF met the criteria for noninferiority to the regimen of efavirenz and lamivudine/zidovudine. At week 48, 84 or 80% of adults receiving the efavirenz, tenofovir DF, and emtricitabine regimen and 73 or 70% of adults receiving the efavirenz and lamivudine/zidovudine regimen had plasma HIV-1 RNA levels <400 or 50 copies/mL, respectively. At week 48, increases in CD4+ T-cell counts were greater in patients receiving the efavirenz, emtricitabine, and tenofovir DF regimen (mean increase of 190 cells/mm³) than in those receiving the efavirenz and lamivudine/zidovudine regimen (mean increase of 158 cells/mm³). Virologic failure (i.e., individuals who failed to achieve virologic suppression or experienced rebound after achieving virologic suppression) was reported in 2% of those receiving efavirenz, emtricitabine, and tenofovir DF and in 4% of those receiving efavirenz and lamivudine/zidovudine at week 48.

At 144 weeks, 64% of adults receiving the efavirenz, emtricitabine, and tenofovir DF regimen and 56% of those receiving the efavirenz and lamivudine/zidovudine regimen had plasma HIV-1 RNA levels <50 copies/mL. The mean increase in CD4+ T-cell count from baseline in these groups was 312 and 271 cells/mm³, respectively, at 144 weeks.

Trial 301A was a 48-week, double-blind, active-control study evaluating emtricitabine versus stavudine, both in combination with a background regimen containing didanosine and efavirenz, in 571 antiretroviral-naïve adults (mean CD4+ T-cell count of 318 cells/mm³ and median HIV-1 RNA levels of 4.9 $\log_{10}$ copies/mL). The primary outcome was persistent virologic response, considered an HIV1-RNA level <400 or 50 copies/mL. At 48 weeks, a persistent virologic response (<400 copies/mL) was seen in 81 or 68% of patients given emtricitabine or stavudine, respectively. An HIV-1 RNA level <50 copies/mL was achieved in 78 or 59% of patients given emtricitabine or stavudine, respectively. Virologic failure (i.e., individuals who failed to achieve virologic suppression or experienced rebound after achieving virologic suppression) was reported in 3% of those receiving the emtricitabine-containing regimen and in 11% of those receiving the stavudine-containing regimen at week 48. Administration of the emtricitabine-containing regimen resulted in a mean increase in CD4+ T-cell counts of 168 cells/mm³ ; administration of the stavudine-containing regimen resulted in a mean increase in CD4+ T-cell counts of 134 cells/mm³.

Antiretroviral-experienced Adults

Emtricitabine has been evaluated in a randomized, open-label, multicenter study (Trial 303) in 440 previously treated adults (mean age 42 years, 86% male, 64% white, 13% Hispanic, 21% African American, median baseline plasma HIV-1 RNA level 1.7 $\log_{10}$ copies/mL, mean baseline CD4+ T-cell count 527 cells/mm³) who received a lamivudine-containing regimen that also included 2 other antiretrovirals (background regimen) for at least 12 weeks prior to study entry and had plasma HIV-1 levels of <400 copies/mL. Patients in this study were randomized to receive emtricitabine in conjunction with stavudine or zidovudine and a protease inhibitor (PI) or non-nucleoside reverse transcriptase inhibitor (NNRTI) or to continue their lamivudine-containing background regimen (i.e., lamivudine in conjunction with stavudine or zidovudine and a PI or NNRTI).

At week 48, 77 or 67% of adults receiving the regimen that included emtricitabine and 82 or 72% of those receiving the regimen that included lamivudine had plasma HIV-1 RNA levels <400 or 50 copies/mL, respectively. Virologic failure was reported in 7% of those receiving the emtricitabine-containing regimen and in 8% of those receiving the lamivudine-containing regimen at week 48. Administration of the emtricitabine-containing regimen resulted in a mean increase in CD4+ T-cell counts of 29 cells/mm³; administration of the lamivudine-containing regimen resulted in a mean increase in CD4+ T-cell counts of 61 cells/mm³.

Pediatric Patients

Safety and efficacy of emtricitabine in conjunction with other antiretrovirals have been evaluated in 3 open-label, nonrandomized studies in patients 3 months to 21 years of age (mean age 7.9 years, 49% male, 15% white, 24% Hispanic, 61% Black, median baseline plasma HIV-1 RNA level 4.6 $\log_{10}$ copies/mL, mean baseline CD4+ T-cell count 745 cells/mm³) who were treatment naïve or treatment experienced (i.e., virologic suppression on a lamivudine-containing regimen; emtricitabine substituted for lamivudine). At week 48, 86 or 73% of these patients had plasma HIV-1 RNA levels <400 or 50 copies/mL, respectively. The mean increase in CD4+ T-cell counts was 232 cells/mm³.

Clinical Perspective

Therapeutic options for the treatment and prevention of human immunodeficiency virus (HIV) infection and recommendations concerning the use of antiretrovirals are continuously evolving. Antiretroviral therapy is recommended for all individuals with HIV regardless of CD4+ T-cell counts, and should be initiated as soon as possible after diagnosis of HIV and continued indefinitely. The primary goals of antiretroviral therapy are to achieve and maintain durable suppression of HIV viral load (as measured by plasma HIV-1 RNA levels) to a level below which drug-resistance mutations cannot emerge (i.e., below detectable limits), restore and preserve immunologic function, reduce HIV-related morbidity and mortality, improve quality of life, and prevent transmission of HIV. While the most appropriate antiretroviral regimen cannot be defined for each clinical scenario, the US Department of Health and Human Services (HHS) Panel on Antiretroviral Guidelines for Adults and Adolescents, HHS Panel on Antiretroviral Therapy and Medical Management of Children Living with HIV, and HHS Panel on Treatment of Pregnant Women with HIV Infection and Prevention of Perinatal Transmission, have developed comprehensive guidelines that provide information on selection and use of antiretrovirals for the treatment or prevention of HIV infection. Because of the complexity of managing patients with HIV, it is recommended that clinicians with HIV expertise be consulted when needed.

The use of combination antiretroviral regimens that generally include 3 drugs from 2 or more drug classes is currently recommended to achieve viral suppression. In both treatment-naïve adults and children, an initial antiretroviral regimen generally consists of 2 NRTIs administered in combination with a third active antiretroviral drug from 1 of 3 drug classes: an integrase strand transfer inhibitor (INSTI), a NNRTI, or a PI with a pharmacokinetic enhancer (also known as a booster; the 2 drugs used for this purpose are cobicistat and ritonavir). Selection of an initial antiretroviral regimen should be individualized based on factors such as virologic efficacy, toxicity, pill burden, dosing frequency, drug–drug interaction potential, resistance-test results, comorbid conditions, access, and cost. In patients with comorbid infections (e.g., hepatitis B, tuberculosis), regimen selection should also consider the potential for activity against other present infections and timing of initiation relative to other anti-infective regimens.

Emtricitabine, an NRTI, is commonly used as part of a dual-NRTI "backbone" of a fully suppressive antiretroviral regimen. In the 2023 HHS adult and adolescent HIV treatment guideline, emtricitabine is included in various antiretroviral regimens. Some of these emtricitabine-containing regimens are listed among recommended initial regimens in certain clinical situations, and include the following: bictegravir/tenofovir alafenamide/emtricitabine or dolutegravir/tenofovir (alafenamide or DF)/emtricitabine (for patients who do not have a history of using long-acting cabotegravir as preexposure prophylaxis); boosted darunavir/tenofovir (alafenamide or DF)/emtricitabine (for individuals with prior exposure to cabotegravir pending results of INSTI genotypic testing); and rilpivirine/tenofovir (alafenamide or DF)/emtricitabine (if HIV-1 RNA <100,000 copies/mL and CD4$^+$ T-cell count >200 cells/mm^3).

In the 2023 HHS pediatric HIV treatment guideline, emtricitabine is included in various antiretroviral regimens. Emtricitabine/tenofovir alafenamide/bictegravir is recommended as a preferred INSTI-based regimen for children ≥2 years of age and weighing ≥14 kg. Emtricitabine/tenofovir alafenamide is recommended as a preferred dual NRTI-combination in children and adolescents weighing ≥14 kg when used with an INSTI or an NNRTI. Abacavir/emtricitabine is recommended as a preferred dual-NRTI combination in children ≥3 months and for full-term infants from birth to <3 months of age.

In the 2023 HHS perinatal HIV treatment guideline, emtricitabine is included as a preferred NRTI for initial antiretroviral treatment during pregnancy, restarting antiretroviral treatment during pregnancy, as a new treatment regimen if an existing regimen is not well tolerated or not fully suppressive, or prior to pregnancy. Emtricitabine/tenofovir DF started as preexposure prophylaxis prior to pregnancy can be continued throughout pregnancy.

● *Preexposure Prophylaxis for Prevention of HIV-1 Infection*

Emtricitabine is used in combination with tenofovir DF or alafenamide for preexposure prophylaxis (PrEP) to reduce the risk of sexually acquired HIV-1 infection in at-risk HIV-negative adults and adolescents; refer to the fixed-combination product monograph for detailed information on this use.

Clinical Perspective

In the 2021 CDC HIV preexposure prophylaxis guideline, several PrEP regimens are recommended based on an individual patient's characteristics to reflect the populations evaluated in pivotal clinical studies. Options for PrEP include oral emtricitabine/tenofovir DF in sexually active adults and adolescents and men and women who inject drugs, oral emtricitabine/tenofovir alafenamide in men and transgender women who have sex with men, and intramuscular cabotegravir in adults and adolescents.

● *Postexposure Prophylaxis following Occupational Exposure to HIV*

Emtricitabine is used in conjunction with other antiretrovirals as part of preferred and alternative regimens for postexposure prophylaxis of HIV infection following occupational exposure† (PEP) in health-care personnel and other individuals exposed via percutaneous injury (e.g., needlestick, cut with sharp object) or mucous membrane or nonintact skin (e.g., chapped, abraded, dermatitis) contact with blood, tissue, or other body fluids that might contain HIV.

Clinical Perspective

The US Public Health Service (USPHS) states that the preferred regimen for PEP following an occupational exposure to HIV is a 3-drug regimen of raltegravir used in conjunction with emtricitabine and tenofovir DF (may be administered as the fixed combination emtricitabine/tenofovir DF; Truvada®). These experts recommend several alternative regimens that include an INSTI, NNRTI, or PI and 2 NRTIs (dual NRTIs). The preferred dual NRTI option for use in PEP regimens is emtricitabine and tenofovir DF (may be administered as the fixed combination emtricitabine/tenofovir DF; Truvada®); alternative dual NRTIs are tenofovir DF and lamivudine, lamivudine and zidovudine (may be administered as the fixed combination lamivudine/zidovudine; Combivir®), or zidovudine and emtricitabine.

Because management of occupational exposures to HIV is complex and evolving, consultation with an infectious diseases specialist, clinician with expertise in administration of antiretroviral agents, and/or the National Clinicians' Postexposure Prophylaxis Hotline (PEPline at 888-448-4911) is recommended whenever possible. However, initiation of PEP should not be delayed while waiting for expert consultation.

● *Postexposure Prophylaxis following Nonoccupational Exposure to HIV*

Emtricitabine is used in conjunction with other antiretrovirals as part of preferred and alternative regimens for postexposure prophylaxis of HIV infection following nonoccupational exposure† (nPEP) in individuals exposed to blood, genital secretions, or other potentially infectious body fluids that might contain HIV when that exposure represents a substantial risk for HIV transmission.

Clinical Perspective

When nPEP is indicated following a nonoccupational exposure to HIV, the US Centers for Disease Control and Prevention (CDC) states that the preferred regimen in adults and adolescents 13 years of age or older with normal renal function is either raltegravir or dolutegravir used in conjunction with emtricitabine and tenofovir DF (administered as the fixed combination emtricitabine/tenofovir DF; Truvada®). The alternative nPEP regimen recommended in these patients is *ritonavir-boosted* darunavir used in conjunction with emtricitabine/tenofovir DF (Truvada®).

Consultation with an infectious diseases specialist, clinician with expertise in administration of antiretroviral agents, and/or the National Clinicians' Postexposure Prophylaxis Hotline (PEPline at 888-448-4911) is recommended if nPEP is indicated in certain exposed individuals (e.g., pregnant women, children, those with medical conditions such as renal impairment) or if an antiretroviral regimen not included in the CDC guidelines is being considered, the source virus is known or likely to be resistant to antiretrovirals, or the healthcare provider is inexperienced in prescribing antiretrovirals. However, initiation of nPEP should not be delayed while waiting for expert consultation.

DOSAGE AND ADMINISTRATION

● *General*

Pretreatment Screening

● Test for hepatitis B virus (HBV) infection prior to or upon initiation of emtricitabine (single entity or fixed combinations).

Patient Monitoring

● If emtricitabine (single entity or fixed combinations) is used in patients coinfected with human immunodeficiency virus (HIV) and HBV, closely monitor hepatic function (using both clinical and laboratory follow-up) for at least several months after discontinuation of therapy.

● *Administration*

Emtricitabine is administered orally once daily without regard to meals.

Single-entity emtricitabine is commercially available as 200-mg capsules or an oral solution containing 10 mg/mL.

Emtricitabine is also commercially available in the following fixed-combination tablets for oral use: emtricitabine/tenofovir DF (Truvada®), efavirenz/emtricitabine/tenofovir DF (Atripla®), emtricitabine/rilpivirine/tenofovir DF (Complera®), elvitegravir/cobicistat/emtricitabine/tenofovir DF (Stribild®), elvitegravir/cobicistat/emtricitabine/tenofovir alafenamide (Genvoya®), emtricitabine/rilpivirine/tenofovir alafenamide (Odefsey®), emtricitabine/tenofovir alafenamide (Descovy®), and bictegravir/emtricitabine/tenofovir alafenamide (Biktarvy®). See the full prescribing information for administration of each of these combination products.

Emtricitabine is used in conjunction with other antiretrovirals. Single-entity emtricitabine should not be used concomitantly with any other emtricitabine-containing preparations.

Store capsules at 25°C (excursions permitted to 15–30°C).

Store oral solution at 2–8°C. For patient use, store at 25°C (excursions permitted to 15–30°C); use within 3 months.

● Dosage

Emtricitabine capsules and oral solution are not bioequivalent. Bioavailability of the oral solution is 80% relative to that of the capsule.

Pediatric Dosage

Treatment of HIV Infection

The usual dosage of emtricitabine for the treatment of HIV-1 infection in infants 0–3 months of age is 3 mg/kg (as the oral solution containing 10 mg/mL) once daily.

For the treatment of HIV-1 infection in pediatric patients 3 months to 17 years of age, the usual dosage of emtricitabine is 6 mg/kg (as the oral solution containing 10 mg/mL) once daily (maximum 240 mg daily). Alternatively, children weighing more than 33 kg who can swallow an intact capsule may receive one 200-mg capsule once daily.

Adult Dosage

Treatment of HIV Infection

For the treatment of HIV-1 infection in adults 18 years of age or older, the usual dosage of emtricitabine is 200 mg (as the capsule) once daily. Alternatively, when the oral solution containing 10 mg/mL is used, the usual dosage of emtricitabine is 240 mg (24 mL) once daily.

Preexposure Prophylaxis for Prevention of HIV-1 Infection

The fixed dose combination containing emtricitabine/tenofovir DF (Truvada®) is used for preexposure prophylaxis (PrEP) for prevention of HIV-1 infection. For PrEP, the usual dosage of emtricitabine is 200 mg once daily in conjunction with other antiretrovirals; see the full prescribing information for specific dosage of emtricitabine/tenofovir DF (Truvada®).

Postexposure Prophylaxis following Occupational Exposure to HIV

For postexposure prophylaxis of HIV infection following occupational exposure† (PEP) in health-care personnel or other individuals, the recommended dosage of emtricitabine is 200 mg (as the capsule) once daily. Emtricitabine usually is used with tenofovir DF or zidovudine in conjunction with a recommended HIV integrase strand transferase inhibitor (INSTI), nonnucleoside reverse transcriptase inhibitor (NNRTI), or HIV protease inhibitor (PI).

The preferred dual nucleoside transcriptase inhibitor (NRTI) backbone option for use in PEP† regimens is emtricitabine and tenofovir DF commonly administered as the fixed-dose combination of emtricitabine/tenofovir DF (Truvada®). See the full prescribing information for specific dosage of emtricitabine/tenofovir DF (Truvada®).

Postexposure Prophylaxis following Nonoccupational Exposure to HIV

For postexposure prophylaxis of HIV infection following nonoccupational exposure† (nPEP) when the exposure represents a substantial risk for HIV transmission, the usual adult dosage of emtricitabine is 200 mg once daily in conjunction with other antiretrovirals. Emtricitabine usually is used in conjunction with tenofovir DF and a recommended or alternative INSTI, PI, or NNRTI.

The preferred dual NRTI backbone option for use in nPEP† regimens is emtricitabine/tenofovir DF, commonly administered as the fixed-dose combination of emtricitabine/tenofovir DF (Truvada®). See the full prescribing information for specific dosage of emtricitabine/tenofovir DF (Truvada®).

● Special Populations

Hepatic Impairment

While the pharmacokinetics of emtricitabine have not been specifically studied in patients with hepatic impairment, the drug is not metabolized by liver enzymes and clinically important changes in emtricitabine metabolism are not expected if the drug is used in patients with hepatic impairment.

Renal Impairment

When emtricitabine is used for the treatment of HIV-1 infection in adults, dosage should be adjusted in those with a creatinine clearance less than 50 mL/minute (see Table 1). The manufacturer states that data are insufficient to make emtricitabine dosage recommendations for treatment of HIV-1 infection in pediatric patients with renal impairment.

TABLE 1. Emtricitabine Dosage for Treatment of HIV-1 Infection in Adults with Renal Impairment

Creatinine Clearance (mL/minute)	Dosage of Capsules	Dosage of Oral Solution
30–49	200 mg every 48 hours	120 mg every 24 hours
15–29	200 mg every 72 hours	80 mg every 24 hours
Less than 15	200 mg every 96 hours	60 mg every 24 hours
Hemodialysis patients	200 mg every 96 hours; on day of dialysis, give dose after the procedure	60 mg every 24 hours; on day of dialysis, give dose after the procedure

Geriatric Patients

The manufacturer makes no specific dosage recommendations for geriatric patients, but recommends cautious dosage selection due to the greater frequency of decreased hepatic, renal, and/or cardiac function, and of concomitant disease and drug therapy.

CAUTIONS

● Contraindications

- Known hypersensitivity to the drug or any ingredient in the formulation.

● Warnings/Precautions

Warnings

Severe Acute Exacerbation of Hepatitis B in Patients Coinfected with Human Immunodeficiency Virus Type 1 (HIV-1) and Hepatitis B Virus (HBV)

A boxed warning regarding the risk of acute exacerbations of HBV infection after emtricitabine discontinuation in patients coinfected with HIV-1 and HBV is included in the prescribing information for emtricitabine. Prior to initiating emtricitabine (single-entity or fixed-combination preparations) for treatment of HIV-1 infection, the patient should be tested for chronic HBV.

Severe acute exacerbations of HBV infection have been reported in patients coinfected with HIV-1 and HBV following discontinuance of emtricitabine. In some of these patients, exacerbations of HBV have been associated with hepatic decompensation and hepatic failure. Hepatic function should be closely monitored with clinical and laboratory follow-up for at least several months after stopping emtricitabine therapy (single-entity or fixed-combination preparations) in HIV-infected patients coinfected with HBV. If appropriate, initiation of treatment for HBV infection may be warranted.

Other Warnings/Precautions

Immune Reconstitution Syndrome

Immune reconstitution syndrome has been reported in HIV-infected patients receiving multiple-drug antiretroviral therapy, including emtricitabine. During the initial phase of treatment, HIV-infected patients whose immune systems respond to antiretroviral therapy may develop an inflammatory response to indolent or residual opportunistic infections (e.g., *Mycobacterium avium* complex [MAC], *M. tuberculosis*, cytomegalovirus [CMV], *Pneumocystis jirovecii* [formerly *P. carinii*]); such response may necessitate further evaluation and treatment.

Autoimmune disorders (e.g., Graves' disease, polymyositis, Guillain-Barré syndrome) have also been reported to occur in the setting of immune reconstitution; however, the time to onset is more variable and can occur many months after initiation of antiretroviral therapy.

Lactic Acidosis and Severe Hepatomegaly with Steatosis

Lactic acidosis and severe hepatomegaly with steatosis, including fatalities, have been reported in patients receiving HIV nucleoside reverse transcriptase inhibitors (NRTIs), including emtricitabine with or without other antiretroviral agents.

Emtricitabine (single-entity or fixed-combination preparations) should be discontinued in any patient with clinical or laboratory findings suggestive of lactic acidosis or pronounced hepatotoxicity (signs of hepatotoxicity include hepatomegaly and steatosis even in the absence of marked increases in serum aminotransferase concentrations).

Precautions Related to Use of Fixed Combinations

When emtricitabine is used in fixed combination with other drugs, the cautions, precautions, contraindications, and drug interactions associated with each drug in the fixed combination must be considered.

Dosage Adjustment in Patients with New Onset or Worsening Renal Impairment

Reduce dosage in patients with renal impairment; emtricitabine is principally eliminated by the kidney.

Specific Populations

Pregnancy

The Antiretroviral Pregnancy Registry (APR) monitors pregnancy outcomes in women exposed to emtricitabine during pregnancy. Clinicians are encouraged to register patients in the APR by calling 800-258-4263 or visiting http://www .APRegistry.com.

Based on prospective reports to the APR, the overall risk of birth defects among live births with first-trimester exposure to emtricitabine was 2.4%, and 2.3% with second/third trimester exposure, compared to the background rate for major birth defects of 2.7% in the United States reference population of the Metropolitan Atlanta Congenital Defects Program (MACDP). Limitations of using an external comparator (i.e., MACDP) include differences in populations and methodology, and confounding due to the underlying disease. The rate of miscarriage for individual drugs is not reported in the APR.

Additional observational data have not shown an increase in major malformations with emtricitabine exposure in pregnancy.

Lactation

Based on published data, emtricitabine is distributed into human milk. It is not known whether emtricitabine affects milk production or has effects on the breast-fed infant.

Because of the risk of adverse effects in the infant and the risk of HIV transmission, HIV-infected women should not breast-feed infants.

Pediatric Use

Safety and efficacy of emtricitabine have been established for treatment of HIV-1 infection in children 3 months of age and older.

The pharmacokinetics and safety of emtricitabine were evaluated in a dose-finding study in 20 neonates born to HIV-infected mothers. These neonates received zidovudine prophylaxis for 6 weeks. In addition, these neonates received 2 short courses of emtricitabine (3 mg/kg daily for 4 days per course) during the first 12 weeks of life. This dosage was not associated with any safety issues. Systemic exposure (AUC) in infants 0–3 months of age receiving emtricitabine 3 mg/kg daily was similar to that reported in children 3 months to 17 years of age receiving emtricitabine 6 mg/kg daily. All neonates were HIV-1 negative at the end of the study (6 months postpartum); the efficacy of emtricitabine for the prevention or treatment of HIV was not determined.

Geriatric Use

Experience in those 65 years of age or older is insufficient to determine whether they respond differently to emtricitabine than younger adults. Dosage should be selected with caution because of age-related decreases in hepatic, renal, and/or cardiac function and potential for concomitant disease and drug therapy.

Hepatic Impairment

Emtricitabine has not been studied in patients with hepatic impairment; impact of hepatic impairment is expected to be minimal.

Renal Impairment

Emtricitabine is principally eliminated by the kidney and the pharmacokinetics of the drug are altered in patients with renal impairment. Maximum serum concentration and AUC were increased in adults with creatinine clearance less than 50 mL/minute or in those with end-stage renal disease requiring dialysis. The effects of renal impairment on the pharmacokinetics of emtricitabine in pediatric patients are not known. If renal function is impaired, dosage of single-entity emtricitabine must be adjusted based on creatinine clearance.

● Common Adverse Effects

The most common adverse reactions experienced in at least 10% of adult patients with HIV-1 treated with emtricitabine include headache, GI effects (diarrhea, nausea), fatigue, dizziness, depression, insomnia, abnormal dreams, rash, abdominal pain, asthenia, increased cough, and rhinitis. Adverse effects reported in pediatric patients 3 months of age and older receiving emtricitabine in clinical studies have been similar to those in adults, with the exception of a higher frequency of hyperpigmentation.

DRUG INTERACTIONS

In vitro studies indicate that emtricitabine does not inhibit cytochrome P-450 (CYP) isoenzymes 1A2, 2A6, 2B6, 2C9, 2C19, 2D6, or 3A4. Emtricitabine does not inhibit uridine-5′-disphosphoglucuronyl transferase. The following drug interactions are based on studies using emtricitabine. When a fixed combination containing emtricitabine is used, interactions associated with each drug in the fixed combination should be considered.

● Drugs Metabolized by Hepatic Microsomal Enzymes

Pharmacokinetic interactions between emtricitabine and drugs metabolized by hepatic microsomal enzymes are unlikely.

● Drugs Metabolized by Uridine Diphosphate-glucuronosyltransferase

Pharmacokinetic interactions between emtricitabine and drugs metabolized by uridine diphosphate-glucuronosyltransferase are unlikely. Emtricitabine does not inhibit uridine-5′-disphosphoglucuronyl transferase, an enzyme responsible for glucuronidation.

● Antiretroviral Agents

HIV Nonnucleoside Reverse Transcriptase Inhibitors (NNRTIs)

No in vitro evidence of antagonistic antiretroviral effects between emtricitabine and NNRTIs (e.g., delavirdine, efavirenz, nevirapine).

HIV Nucleoside and Nucleotide Reverse Transcriptase Inhibitors (NRTIs)

No in vitro evidence of antagonistic antiretroviral effects between emtricitabine and nucleoside and HIV nucleotide reverse transcriptase inhibitors (NRTIs) (e.g., abacavir, lamivudine, tenofovir disoproxil fumarate [DF], zidovudine).

Tenofovir

No clinically important pharmacokinetic interactions between emtricitabine and tenofovir DF.

Zidovudine

Although not considered clinically important, concomitant use of emtricitabine (200 mg once daily for 7 days) and zidovudine (300 mg twice day for 7 days) increased zidovudine peak plasma concentrations and area under the concentration-time curve (AUC) by 17 and 13%, respectively, but did not affect emtricitabine peak plasma concentrations or AUC.

HIV Protease Inhibitors (PIs)

No in vitro evidence of antagonistic antiretroviral effects between emtricitabine and HIV PIs (e.g., nelfinavir, ritonavir, saquinavir).

• *Famciclovir*

No clinically important pharmacokinetic interactions between emtricitabine and famciclovir.

DESCRIPTION

Emtricitabine, a synthetic antiretroviral agent, is a human immunodeficiency virus (HIV) nucleoside reverse transcriptase inhibitor (NRTI). Emtricitabine is inactive until converted intracellularly to an active 5′-triphosphate metabolite. Following conversion to the pharmacologically active metabolite, the drug inhibits replication of human retroviruses by interfering with viral RNA-directed DNA polymerase (reverse transcriptase).

The pharmacokinetics of emtricitabine in healthy individuals are similar to that in individuals with human immunodeficiency virus type 1 (HIV-1) infection. Following oral administration, emtricitabine is rapidly and extensively absorbed; peak plasma concentrations of the drug are attained within 1–2 hours. The mean absolute oral bioavailability of emtricitabine capsules is 93%. The mean absolute oral bioavailability of emtricitabine oral solution is 75%. Food does not appear to have a clinically important effect on emtricitabine absorption. Administration of emtricitabine capsules with food (approximately 1000 kcal high-fat meal) did not affect the area under the concentration-time curve (AUC) of emtricitabine, but resulted in a 29% decrease in peak plasma concentrations of the drug. Administration of emtricitabine oral solution with a high-fat or low-fat meal did not affect the AUC or peak plasma concentrations of emtricitabine. Pharmacokinetics in pediatric patients 3 months to 17 years of age receiving recommended emtricitabine dosage (6 mg/kg daily [up to 240 mg daily] as the oral solution or 200-mg capsule once daily) is similar to that reported in adults receiving 200 mg daily. The AUC reported in neonates receiving emtricitabine 3 mg/kg daily for 4 days is similar to that reported in children 3 months to 17 years of age receiving the recommended dosage. Emtricitabine is less than 4% bound to plasma proteins; binding is independent of drug concentrations over the range of 0.01–200 mcg/mL. Emtricitabine is distributed into human milk in low concentrations. Emtricitabine undergoes oxidation and conjugation with glucuronic acid. Intracellularly, emtricitabine is phosphorylated and converted by cellular enzymes to the active metabolite, emtricitabine 5′-triphosphate. Emtricitabine is eliminated in urine (86%) and feces (14%). The drug is eliminated in urine by glomerular filtration and active tubular secretion; 13% of a dose is recovered in urine as 3 metabolites. Emtricitabine is removed by hemodialysis; it is not known whether the drug is removed by peritoneal dialysis. The plasma elimination half-life of emtricitabine is approximately 10 hours.

Peak plasma concentrations and AUC of emtricitabine are increased in adults with renal impairment (creatinine clearance less than 50 mL/minute or end-stage renal disease requiring dialysis) due to reduced renal clearance of the drug. Dosage adjustments are needed. The pharmacokinetics of emtricitabine are not affected by race or gender.

Emtricitabine is active against HIV type 1 (HIV-1) and also has some in vitro activity against HIV type 2 (HIV-2). HIV-1 strains with reduced susceptibility to emtricitabine can be produced in vitro and strains with reduced susceptibility to the drug have emerged during emtricitabine therapy. These strains have contained a M184V/I mutation. HIV-1 strains with the M184V/I mutation have been resistant to lamivudine but retained susceptibility to didanosine, tenofovir, zidovudine, delavirdine, efavirenz, and nevirapine.

ADVICE TO PATIENTS

- Inform patients of the importance of reading patient information provided by the manufacturer.

- Advise patients that lactic acidosis and severe hepatomegaly with steatosis, including fatalities, have occurred in patients receiving emtricitabine or other NRTIs, in conjunction with other antiretrovirals. Advise patients to inform their clinician if symptoms suggestive of lactic acidosis or hepatotoxicity (e.g., nausea, vomiting, unusual/unexpected stomach discomfort, weakness) occur.

- Inform patients that testing for hepatitis B virus (HBV) infection is recommended before antiretroviral therapy is initiated, and that all patients with HBV will require close medical follow-up for several months following emtricitabine discontinuation to monitor for hepatitis exacerbations. Advise patients to not discontinue emtricitabine without first informing their clinician. Also advise patients that severe acute exacerbations of HBV infection have been reported following discontinuance of emtricitabine (single-entity or fixed-combination preparations) in HIV-infected patients coinfected with HBV.

- Inform patients that in those with advanced HIV infection, after anti-HIV treatment is initiated, signs and symptoms of inflammation from prior infections can occur, most likely due to an improvement in the body's immune response. Also advise patients to inform their clinician if symptoms of infection develop.

- Advise patients to inform their clinicians of existing or contemplated concomitant therapy, including prescription and OTC drugs and dietary and herbal products, as well as concomitant medical problems such as renal impairment.

- Advise women to inform their clinicians if they are or plan to become pregnant or plan to breast-feed. Inform patients that an antiretroviral pregnancy registry is available to monitor outcomes of babies born to women taking emtricitabine during pregnancy. Advise HIV-infected women not to breast-feed due to the risk of passing the HIV-1 virus to the baby.

- Inform patients of other precautionary information.

PREPARATIONS

Excipients in commercially available drug preparations may have clinically important effects in some individuals; consult specific product labeling for details.

Emtricitabine

Oral		
Capsules	200 mg	Emtriva®, Gilead
Solution	10 mg/mL	Emtriva®, Gilead

† Use is not currently included in the labeling approved by the US Food and Drug Administration.

Selected Revisions June 10, 2024, © Copyright, December 1, 2003, American Society of Health-System Pharmacists, Inc.

Emtricitabine and Tenofovir Alafenamide Fumarate

8:18.08.20 • HIV NUCLEOSIDE AND NUCLEOTIDE REVERSE TRANSCRIPTASE INHIBITORS

■ Emtricitabine and tenofovir alafenamide fumarate (emtricitabine/tenofovir alafenamide fumarate; FTC/TAF) is a fixed-combination antiretroviral agent containing emtricitabine (a human immunodeficiency virus [HIV] nucleoside reverse transcriptase inhibitor [NRTI]) and tenofovir alafenamide fumarate (a HIV nucleotide reverse transcriptase inhibitor).

USES

● Treatment of HIV Infection

The fixed combination of emtricitabine and tenofovir alafenamide fumarate (FTC/TAF) is used in combination with other antiretroviral agents for the treatment of human immunodeficiency virus type 1 (HIV-1) infection in adults and pediatric patients weighing ≥35 kg. FTC/TAF also is used in combination with other antiretroviral agents, excluding protease inhibitors that require a CYP3A inhibitor, for the treatment of HIV-1 infection in pediatric patients weighing ≥14 kg and <35 kg. FTC/TAF must be used in conjunction with other antiretrovirals for treatment of HIV-1.

Clinical Experience

Adults

Efficacy and safety of FTC/TAF in combination with other antiretroviral agents for the treatment of HIV-1 infection in adults were investigated in clinical trials of FTC/TAF with elvitegravir and cobicistat in HIV-1-infected adults as initial treatment (866 patients) or to replace a stable antiretroviral regimen in those who were virologically suppressed for at least 6 months with no known resistance substitutions (799 patients). HIV-1 RNA of <50 copies/mL at week 48 of treatment was achieved in 92% of patients receiving FTC/TAF with elvitegravir and cobicistat as initial treatment and in 96% of patients receiving FTC/TAF with elvitegravir and cobicistat as a replacement regimen.

Pediatric Patients

Efficacy and safety of FTC/TAF in combination with other antiretroviral agents were studied in an open-label, single-arm trial of FTC/TAF with elvitegravir and cobicistat in 50 treatment-naïve, HIV-1 infected, adolescents 12 to <18 years of age weighing ≥35 kg (cohort 1) and 52 virologically suppressed children 6 to <12 years of age weighing ≥25 kg (cohort 2). In cohort 1, the virologic response rate (i.e., HIV-1 RNA less than 50 copies/mL) was 92%, and the mean increase from baseline in $CD4^+$ cell count was 224 cells/mm³ at week 48. In cohort 2, 98% of subjects remained virologically suppressed at week 48. A mean decrease of 66 cells/mm³ from a baseline $CD4^+$ cell count of 961 cells/mm³ was observed at week 48. All subjects maintained CD4+ cell counts >400 cells/mm³.

In a separate open-label, single-arm trial of FTC/TAF with bictegravir in 24 virologically suppressed children <2 years of age and weighing 14 to <25 kg (cohort 3), 91% of subjects remained virologically suppressed at week 24. A mean decrease in $CD4^+$ cell count of 126 cells/mm³ from a baseline mean $CD4^+$ cell count of 1104 cells/mm³ was observed at week 24.

Clinical Perspective

Therapeutic options for the treatment and prevention of HIV infection and recommendations concerning the use of antiretrovirals are continuously evolving. Antiretroviral therapy is recommended for all individuals with HIV regardless of $CD4^+$ T-cell counts, and should be initiated as soon as possible after diagnosis of HIV and continued indefinitely. The primary goals of antiretroviral therapy are to achieve and maintain durable suppression of HIV viral load (as measured by plasma HIV-1 RNA levels) to a level below which drug-resistance mutations cannot emerge (i.e., below detectable limits), restore and preserve immunologic function, reduce HIV-related morbidity and mortality, improve quality of life, and prevent transmission of HIV. While the most appropriate antiretroviral regimen cannot be defined for each clinical scenario, the US Department of Health and Human Services (HHS) Panel on Antiretroviral Guidelines for Adults and Adolescents, HHS Panel on Antiretroviral Therapy and Medical Management of Children Living with HIV, and HHS Panel on Treatment of Pregnant Women with HIV Infection and Prevention of Perinatal Transmission, have developed comprehensive guidelines that provide information on selection and use of antiretrovirals for the treatment or prevention of HIV infection. Because of the complexity of managing patients with HIV, it is recommended that clinicians with HIV expertise be consulted when needed.

The use of combination antiretroviral regimens that generally include 3 drugs from 2 or more drug classes is currently recommended to achieve viral suppression. In both treatment-naïve adults and children, an initial antiretroviral regimen generally consists of 2 NRTIs administered in combination with a third active antiretroviral drug from 1 of 3 drug classes: an integrase strand transfer inhibitor (INSTI), NNRTI, or a protease inhibitor (PI) with a pharmacokinetic enhancer (also known as a booster; the 2 drugs used for this purpose are cobicistat and ritonavir). Selection of an initial regimen should be individualized based on factors such as virologic efficacy, toxicity, pill burden, dosing frequency, drug–drug interaction potential, resistance-test results, comorbid conditions, access, and cost. In patients with comorbid infections (e.g., hepatitis B, tuberculosis), antiretroviral regimen selection should also consider the potential for activity against other present infections and timing of initiation relative to other anti-infective regimens.

In the 2024 HHS adult and adolescent HIV treatment guideline, the combination of emtricitabine and tenofovir alafenamide is recommended as a component of various initial therapeutic regimens for HIV infection.

In the 2024 HHS pediatric HIV treatment guideline, the combination of emtricitabine and tenofovir alafenamide is recommended as a component of several preferred and alternative regimens for pediatric patients in various age groups.

In the 2024 HHS perinatal HIV treatment guideline, the combination of emtricitabine and tenofovir alafenamide is recommended as a component of various preferred and alternative initial regimens during pregnancy for patients who are antiretroviral-naïve.

● Preexposure Prophylaxis for Prevention of HIV-1 Infection

The fixed combination of FTC/TAF is used in at risk adults and adolescents weighing ≥35 kg for preexposure prophylaxis (PrEP) to reduce the risk of HIV-1 infection from sexual acquisition, excluding individuals at risk from receptive vaginal sex. Individuals must have a negative HIV-1 test immediately prior to initiating FTC/TAF for PrEP.

Clinical Experience

Adults

The comparative efficacy and safety of a once-daily regimen of FTC/TAF (single tablet containing 200 mg of emtricitabine and 25 mg of TAF once daily) and a once-daily regimen of emtricitabine/tenofovir disoproxil fumarate (FTC/TDF; single tablet containing 200 mg of emtricitabine and 300 mg of TDF once daily) for HIV-1 PrEP were evaluated in a multinational, randomized, double-blind, noninferiority trial (DISCOVER) that included 5262 HIV-seronegative men and 73 HIV-seronegative transgender women who have sex with men and have evidence of high-risk behavior for HIV-1 infection. The primary outcome was the incidence of documented HIV-1 infection per 100 person-years in individuals randomized to FTC/TAF and FTC/TDF (with a minimum follow-up of 48 weeks and at least 50% of participants having 96 weeks of follow-up). Results indicate that FTC/TAF is noninferior to FTC/TDF in reducing the risk of acquiring HIV-1 infection. The rate of HIV-1 infection per 100 person-years was 0.16 in those receiving FTC/TAF (4370 person-years of follow-up) and 0.34 in those receiving FTC/TDF (4386 person-years of follow-up). Results were similar across the subgroups of age, race, and gender identity, and efficacy for both regimens was strongly correlated with adherence.

Pediatric Patients

The safety and efficacy of FTC/TAF for HIV-1 PrEP in at-risk adolescents weighing ≥35 kg, excluding individuals at risk from receptive vaginal sex, is supported by data from an adequate and well-controlled trial of FTC/TAF for HIV-1 PrEP in adults with additional data from safety and pharmacokinetic studies in previously conducted trials with the individual drug products, emtricitabine and tenofovir alafenamide, with elvitegravir and cobicistat, in HIV-1 infected adults and pediatric subjects.

Clinical Perspective

According to the 2021 United States Public Health Service clinical practice guideline on PrEP for the prevention of HIV infection, the ultimate goal of PrEP care is to prevent HIV transmission and thereby reduce associated morbidity, mortality, and costs. In order to achieve this goal, the clinician should only prescribe PrEP regimens that have been proven to be clinically effective and safe for at risk HIV-negative patients; instruct patients regarding the appropriate use of the PrEP regimen in order to maximize safety; provide medication adherence support to maintain protective antiretroviral levels; offer HIV risk-reduction and prevention services or referrals to minimize exposure to HIV and other sexually transmitted infections; recommend effective contraception to people of childbearing potential who are taking PrEP and who do not wish to become pregnant; and continually monitor all patients for their HIV status, potential drug toxicities, and levels of risk behavior in order to alter the PrEP care plan if necessary. A significant change in the updated 2021 Public Health Service PrEP guideline is a new recommendation for clinicians to inform all sexually active adults and adolescents about PrEP. This is intended to increase awareness of PrEP more broadly versus the historical use of a risk-based approach to PrEP education only.

The fixed combination of FTC/TAF is one of three FDA-approved PrEP medications. The other approved medications include the combination of emtricitabine with tenofovir disoproxil fumarate and single-agent cabotegravir injection. When taken as prescribed, all 3 approved PrEP medications reduce the risk of HIV acquisition from sexual intercourse by approximately 99%.

DOSAGE AND ADMINISTRATION

● General

Pretreatment Screening

- Prior to or when initiating emtricitabine/tenofovir alafenamide fumarate (FTC/TAF), test patients for hepatitis B virus (HBV) infection.

- Prior to initiation of FTC/TAF, assess serum creatinine, estimated creatinine clearance, urine glucose, and urine protein in all patients; in patients with chronic kidney disease, also assess serum phosphorus.

- Immediately prior to initiating FTC/TAF for HIV-1 preexposure prophylaxis (PrEP), screen for HIV-1 infection. If recent (<1 month) exposures to HIV-1 are suspected or clinical symptoms consistent with acute HIV-1 infection are present, use a test approved or cleared by the FDA as an aid in the diagnosis of acute or primary HIV-1 infection.

Patient Monitoring

- Monitor hepatic function closely with clinical and laboratory follow-up for at least several months after discontinuance of FTC/TAF in patients infected with HBV.

- On a clinically appropriate schedule, assess serum creatinine, estimated creatinine clearance, urine glucose, and urine protein in all patients; in patients with chronic kidney disease, also assess serum phosphorus.

- In patients receiving FTC/TAF for PrEP, screen for HIV-1 infection at least once every 3 months and upon diagnosis of any other sexually transmitted infections.

Dispensing and Administration Precautions

- The Institute for Safe Medication Practices (ISMP) list of error-prone abbreviations, symbols, and dose designations states that the use of abbreviations for antiretroviral medications (e.g., DOR, TAF, TDF) during the medication use process should be avoided as their use has been associated with serious medication errors.

● Administration

The fixed combination FTC/TAF is administered orally once daily without regard to food.

For the treatment of human immunodeficiency virus type 1 (HIV-1) infection, FTC/TAF is used in conjunction with other antiretrovirals. For preexposure prophylaxis (PrEP) for prevention of HIV-1 infection, FTC/TAF is used alone without any other antiretrovirals.

● Dosage

Fixed-combination tablets of FTC/TAF contain emtricitabine and tenofovir alafenamide fumarate; dosage of tenofovir alafenamide fumarate is expressed in terms of tenofovir alafenamide.

Fixed-combination tablets of FTC/TAF contain emtricitabine 200 mg and tenofovir alafenamide 25 mg or emtricitabine 120 mg and tenofovir alafenamide 15 mg.

Adults

Treatment of HIV Infection

When FTC/TAF is used in conjunction with other antiretrovirals for the treatment of HIV-1 infection in adults, the recommended dosage is 1 tablet containing 200 mg of emtricitabine and 25 mg of tenofovir alafenamide once daily. This dosage recommendation is applicable to adults weighing ≥35 kg who have an estimated creatinine clearance ≥30 mL/minute or who have creatinine clearance <15 mL/minute and are receiving chronic hemodialysis.

Preexposure Prophylaxis for Prevention of HIV-1 Infection

When FTC/TAF is used for preexposure prophylaxis (PrEP) for prevention of HIV-1 infection in HIV-1-negative adults at risk, the recommended dosage is 1 tablet containing 200 mg of emtricitabine and 25 mg of tenofovir alafenamide once daily.

Pediatric Patients

Treatment of HIV Infection

When FTC/TAF is used in conjunction with other antiretrovirals for the treatment of HIV-1 infection in children weighing ≥35 kg, the recommended dosage is 1 tablet containing 200 mg of emtricitabine and 25 mg of tenofovir alafenamide once daily. When FTC/TAF is used in conjunction with other antiretrovirals for the treatment of HIV-1 infection in children weighing 14 to <35 kg, the recommended dosage is based on weight; a low-strength fixed-combination tablet of the drug (containing emtricitabine 120 mg and tenofovir alafenamide 15 mg) should be used in children weighing <25 kg. (See Table 1.) This dosing information is applicable to pediatric patients with estimated creatinine clearance ≥30 mL/minute who are not receiving an HIV protease inhibitor that is administered with either ritonavir or cobicistat.

TABLE 1. Emtricitabine/tenofovir alafenamide Dosage for Treatment of HIV-1 Infection in Children Weighing ≥14 kg

Weight (kg)	Dosage of Emtricitabine/Tenofovir Alafenamide given Once Daily
14 to <25 kg	1 tablet (emtricitabine 120 mg and tenofovir alafenamide 15 mg)
25 to <35 kg	1 tablet (emtricitabine 200 mg and tenofovir alafenamide 25 mg)
≥35 kg	1 tablet (emtricitabine 200 mg and tenofovir alafenamide 25 mg)

The safety and efficacy of concomitant use of FTC/TAF with an HIV-1 protease inhibitor that is administered with either ritonavir or cobicistat have not been established in pediatric patients weighing <35 kg.

Preexposure Prophylaxis for Prevention of HIV-1 Infection

When FTC/TAF is used for preexposure prophylaxis (PrEP) for prevention of HIV-1 infection in at-risk HIV-1-negative adolescents weighing ≥35 kg, the recommended dosage is 1 tablet containing 200 mg of emtricitabine and 25 mg of tenofovir alafenamide once daily. This dosing information is applicable to pediatric patients with estimated creatinine clearance ≥30 mL/minute.

● *Special Populations*

Renal Impairment

Dosage adjustments are not necessary if FTC/TAF is used in patients with creatinine clearance ≥30 mL/minute.

Dosage adjustments are not necessary if FTC/TAF is used in adults with estimated creatinine clearance <15 mL/minute (end-stage renal disease) who are receiving chronic hemodialysis. On days of hemodialysis, administer the daily dose of FTC/TAF after completion of hemodialysis treatment.

FTC/TAF is *not* recommended in patients with severe renal impairment (estimated creatinine clearance of 15 to <30 mL/minute) or in patients with end-state renal disease (estimated creatinine clearance <15 mL/minute) who are not receiving hemodialysis.

The safety and efficacy of concomitant use of FTC/TAF with an HIV-1 protease inhibitor that is administered with either ritonavir or cobicistat have not been established in adults with creatinine clearance <15 mL/ minute, with or without hemodialysis.

Hepatic Impairment

Dosage adjustments are not necessary if FTC/TAF is used in patients with mild (Child-Pugh class A) or moderate (Child-Pugh class B) hepatic impairment.

FTC/TAF has not been studied in patients with severe hepatic impairment (Child-Pugh class C).

Geriatric Patients

The manufacturer makes no specific dosage recommendations for geriatric patients.

CAUTIONS

● *Contraindications*

● Do not use the fixed combination of emtricitabine and tenofovir alafenamide fumarate (FTC/TAF) for preexposure prophylaxis (PrEP) of HIV-1 infection in individuals with unknown or positive HIV-1 status.

● *Warnings/Precautions*

Warnings

Severe Acute Exacerbation of Hepatitis B in Individuals with Hepatitis B Virus Infection

Prior to or when initiating FTC/TAF, test all patients for chronic hepatitis B virus (HBV) infection. The prescribing information contains a boxed warning regarding the risk of post-treatment acute exacerbation of hepatitis B. Severe acute exacerbations of HBV infection, including liver decompensation and liver failure, have been reported in HBV-infected patients following discontinuance of preparations containing emtricitabine and/or tenofovir disoproxil fumarate; such reactions also may occur following discontinuance of FTC/TAF.

Monitor hepatic function closely with both clinical and laboratory follow-up for at least several months after FTC/TAF is discontinued in HBV-infected patients. If appropriate, initiation of HBV treatment may be warranted, especially in individuals with advanced liver disease or cirrhosis. Offer HBV vaccination to HBV-uninfected individuals.

Although emtricitabine and tenofovir alafenamide fumarate have some activity against HBV, FTC/TAF is *not* indicated for treatment of chronic HBV infection.

Precautions Related to HIV-1 Preexposure Prophylaxis

Use FTC/TAF for HIV-1 PrEP *only* for at-risk individuals confirmed to be HIV-1-negative immediately prior to initiation of PrEP; confirm HIV-1-negative status periodically (at least every 3 months and upon diagnosis of any other sexually transmitted infection) during PrEP.

Drug-resistant HIV-1 variants have been identified when FTC/TDF PrEP was used following undetected acute HIV-1 infection. The prescribing information contains a boxed warning regarding the risk of drug resistance with use of FTC/TDF for HIV-1 PrEP in undiagnosed early HIV-1 infection. Do *not* initiate FTC/TAF PrEP if signs or symptoms of acute HIV-1 infection are present, unless negative infection status is confirmed.

Clinicians should consider that some HIV-1 tests only detect anti-HIV antibodies and may not identify HIV-1 during the acute stage of infection. Prior to initiating FTC/TAF PrEP, clinicians should evaluate HIV-seronegative individuals for current or recent signs or symptoms consistent with acute viral infection (e.g., fever, fatigue, myalgia, rash) and ask about any potential exposure events that may have occurred within the last month (e.g., unprotected sex, condom broke during sex with a partner of unknown HIV-1 status or unknown viremic status, a recent sexually transmitted infection).

If recent (<1 month) exposures to HIV-1 are suspected or clinical symptoms consistent with acute HIV-1 infection are present, use a test approved or cleared by the FDA as an aid in the diagnosis of acute or primary HIV-1 infection.

Uninfected individuals should be counseled to strictly adhere to the recommended FTC/TAF dosage schedule. Effectiveness of the fixed combination in reducing the risk of acquiring HIV-1 is strongly correlated with adherence as demonstrated by measurable drug concentrations in clinical trials. Some individuals (e.g., adolescents) may benefit from more frequent visits and counseling to support adherence.

Adverse effects reported in HIV-negative adults receiving FTC/TAF PrEP are similar to those reported in HIV-infected patients receiving the drugs for treatment of HIV-1 infection.

Other Warnings/Precautions

Immune Reconstitution Syndrome

Immune reconstitution syndrome has been reported in HIV-infected patients receiving multiple-drug antiretroviral therapy, including regimens containing emtricitabine, a component of FTC/TAF. During the initial phase of treatment, HIV-infected patients whose immune systems respond to antiretroviral therapy may develop an inflammatory response to indolent or residual opportunistic infections (e.g., *Mycobacterium avium* complex [MAC], *M. tuberculosis*, cytomegalovirus [CMV], *Pneumocystis jirovecii* [formerly *P. carinii*]); such response may necessitate further evaluation and treatment.

Autoimmune disorders (e.g., Graves' disease, polymyositis, Guillain-Barré syndrome, autoimmune hepatitis) have also been reported to occur in the setting of immune reconstitution; however, the time to onset is more variable and can occur many months after initiation of antiretroviral therapy.

Renal Impairment

Renal impairment, including cases of acute renal failure, proximal renal tubulopathy, and Fanconi syndrome (renal tubular injury with severe hypophosphatemia), has been reported with the use of preparations containing tenofovir alafenamide, a component of FTC/TAF. Most of these cases were characterized by potential confounding factors that may have contributed to the reported renal events; however, these factors may have predisposed patients to tenofovir-related renal toxicity.

Individuals with impaired renal function and those receiving nephrotoxic agents (e.g., nonsteroidal anti-inflammatory agents [NSAIAs]) are at increased risk of developing renal-related adverse reactions.

Assess serum creatinine, estimated creatinine clearance, urine glucose, and urine protein prior to initiating FTC/TAF and monitor during treatment as clinically appropriate. In patients with chronic kidney disease, also assess serum phosphorus at baseline and during treatment as clinically appropriate.

Discontinue FTC/TAF in individuals who develop a clinically important decrease in renal function or evidence of Fanconi syndrome.

Use of FTC/TAF is *not* recommended in patients with estimated creatinine clearance of 15 to <30 mL/minute or in patients with an estimated creatinine clearance <15 mL/minute who are not receiving chronic hemodialysis.

Lactic Acidosis and Severe Hepatomegaly with Steatosis

Lactic acidosis and severe hepatomegaly with steatosis, including fatalities, have been reported in patients receiving HIV nucleoside reverse transcriptase inhibitors (NRTIs), including emtricitabine and tenofovir disoproxil fumarate, alone or in combination with other antiretroviral agents.

FTC/TAF treatment should be interrupted in any patient who develops clinical or laboratory findings suggestive of lactic acidosis or pronounced hepatotoxicity (signs of hepatotoxicity may include hepatomegaly and steatosis even in the absence of marked increases in serum aminotransferase concentrations).

Use of Fixed Combinations

The usual cautions, precautions, contraindications, and interactions associated with each component of FTC/TAF should be considered. Cautionary information applicable to specific populations (e.g., pregnant or nursing women, individuals with hepatic or renal impairment, geriatric patients) should be considered for each drug in the fixed combination.

For the treatment of HIV-1 infection, FTC/TAF is used in conjunction with other antiretrovirals. For PrEP for prevention of HIV-1 infection, FTC/TAF is used alone without any other antiretrovirals.

Specific Populations

Pregnancy

Antiretroviral Pregnancy Registry (APR) at 800-258-4263 or https://www.APRegistry.com.

Available data from the APR show no difference in the overall risk of major birth defects for emtricitabine or tenofovir alafenamide compared with the background rate of 2.7% for major birth defects in a US reference population of the Metropolitan Atlanta Congenital Defects Program. Available data from the APR show an incidence of major birth defects with first-trimester exposure of 2.6 or 4.2%, and with second- or third-trimester exposure of 2.7 or 3%, for emtricitabine or tenofovir alafenamide, respectively. No congenital abnormalities were reported among 117 infants exposed to TAF after 24 weeks' gestation in mothers with hepatitis B.

In animal studies, no adverse developmental effects were observed when the components of FTC/TAF were administered separately during the period of organogenesis at exposures 60 and 108 times (mice and rabbits, respectively) the FTC exposure and at exposures 1 and 53 times (rats and rabbits, respectively) the TAF exposure at the recommended daily dose of FTC/TAF. In addition, no adverse developmental effects were observed when FTC was administered to mice through lactation at exposures up to approximately 60 times the exposure at the recommended daily dose of FTC/TAF. No adverse effects were observed in the offspring when TDF was administered through lactation at tenofovir exposures of approximately 14 times the exposure at the recommended daily dosage of FTC/TAF.

FTC/TAF has not been demonstrated to be effective for preexposure prophylaxis (PrEP) for prevention of HIV-1 infection in people with receptive vaginal exposure to HIV-1.

Lactation

Emtricitabine is distributed into human milk; it is not known whether tenofovir alafenamide is distributed into human milk. Tenofovir is distributed into milk in animals following administration of tenofovir disoproxil fumarate. It is not known whether FTC/TAF affects human milk production or affects the breast-fed infant.

The HHS perinatal HIV transmission guideline provides updated recommendations on infant feeding. The guideline states that patients with HIV should receive evidence-based, patient-centered counseling to support shared decision making about infant feeding. During counseling, patients should be informed that feeding with appropriate formula or pasteurized donor human milk from a milk bank eliminates the risk of postnatal HIV transmission to the infant. Additionally, achieving and maintaining viral suppression with antiretroviral therapy during pregnancy and postpartum reduces the risk of breastfeeding HIV transmission to <1%, but does not completely eliminate the risk. Replacement feeding with formula or banked pasteurized donor milk is recommended when patients with HIV are *not* on antiretroviral therapy and/or do *not* have a suppressed viral load during pregnancy (at a minimum throughout the third trimester), as well as at delivery.

Pediatric Use

Safety and efficacy of FTC/TAF for treatment of HIV-1 infection have *not* been established in pediatric patients weighing <14 kg; safety and efficacy of this fixed combination for HIV-1 PrEP have *not* been established in pediatric patients weighing <35 kg.

Safety and efficacy of concomitant use of FTC/TAF with an HIV-1 protease inhibitor that is administered with either ritonavir or cobicistat have not been established in pediatric patients weighing <35 kg.

Adverse effects reported in children 6 to <18 years of age weighing ≥25 kg receiving FTC/TAF in combination with elvitegravir and cobicistat in clinical studies for the treatment of HIV-1 infection were similar to those in adults and adolescents, with the exception of a decrease from baseline in mean CD4$^+$ cell count observed in virologically suppressed subjects between 6 to <12 years of age.

Waning adherence to a daily oral PrEP regimen following a switch from monthly to quarterly clinic visits has been reported in at-risk adolescents; therefore, adolescents receiving FTC/TAF for PrEP may benefit from more frequent visits and counseling.

Geriatric Use

No differences in safety or efficacy of FTC/TAF in combination with other antiretrovirals for the treatment of HIV-1 infection have been observed between patients ≥65 years of age and younger adults.

Hepatic Impairment

FTC/TAF has not been studied in patients with severe hepatic impairment.

No dosage adjustment of FTC/TAF is required in patients with mild or moderate hepatic impairment.

Renal Impairment

Assess serum creatinine, estimated creatinine clearance, urine glucose, and urine protein prior to initiating FTC/TAF and routinely monitor during treatment in all patients as clinically appropriate. In patients with chronic kidney disease, also assess serum phosphorus at baseline and during treatment as clinically appropriate.

No dosage adjustment of FTC/TAF is required in patients with creatinine clearance ≥30 mL/minute.

No dosage adjustment of FTC/TAF is required in adults with estimated creatinine clearance <15 mL/minute (end-stage renal disease) who are receiving chronic hemodialysis. On days of hemodialysis, administer the daily dose of FTC/TAF after completion of hemodialysis treatment.

Use of FTC/TAF is not recommended in patients with severe renal impairment (estimated creatinine clearance of 15 to <30 mL/minute) or in patients with end-state renal disease (estimated creatinine clearance <15 mL/minute) who are not receiving hemodialysis.

The safety and efficacy of concomitant use of FTC/TAF with an HIV-1 protease inhibitor that is administered with either ritonavir or cobicistat have not been established in adults with creatinine clearance <15 mL/ minute, with or without hemodialysis.

● Common Adverse Effects

Nausea was reported in ≥10% of HIV-infected patients receiving FTC/TAF in conjunction with other antiretrovirals. Diarrhea was reported in ≥5% of patients receiving FTC/TAF for PrEP for prevention of HIV-1 infection.

DRUG INTERACTIONS

The following drug interactions are based on studies that used emtricitabine or tenofovir alafenamide fumarate alone or the fixed combination of emtricitabine and tenofovir alafenamide fumarate (FTC/TAF) or are predicted to occur.

Potential drug interactions associated with each drug in the fixed combination should be considered.

● Drugs Affecting or Metabolized by Hepatic Microsomal Enzymes

Emtricitabine is not a substrate of CYP isoenzymes; emtricitabine does not inhibit CYP1A2, 2A6, 2B6, 2C9, 2C19, 2D6, or 3A4.

Tenofovir alafenamide is minimally metabolized by CYP3A. Tenofovir alafenamide is not an inhibitor of CYP1A2, CYP2B6, CYP2C8, CYP2C9, CYP2C19, CYP2D6, or UGT1A1. Tenofovir alafenamide is a weak inhibitor of CYP3A in vitro but is not an inhibitor or inducer of CYP3A in vivo.

Pharmacokinetic interactions between FTC/TAF and drugs affecting or metabolized by hepatic microsomal enzymes are considered unlikely.

● Drugs Affecting or Affected by P-glycoprotein Transport

Tenofovir alafenamide is a substrate of P-glycoprotein (P-gp). When tenofovir alafenamide is used concomitantly with drugs that strongly affect P-gp, changes in absorption of tenofovir may be observed. Concomitant use of FTC/TAF with drugs that inhibit P-gp may increase the absorption and plasma concentration of tenofovir. Drugs that induce P-gp activity are expected to decrease the absorption of TAF, resulting in decreased plasma concentration of TAF, which may lead to loss of therapeutic effect of FTC/TAF and development of resistance.

● Drugs Affecting Breast Cancer Resistance Protein

Tenofovir alafenamide is a substrate of breast cancer resistance protein (BCRP). When TAF is used concomitantly with drugs that strongly affect BCRP, changes in absorption of tenofovir may be observed. Concomitant use of FTC/TAF with drugs that inhibit BCRP may increase the absorption and plasma concentration of tenofovir.

● Drugs Affecting Organic Anion-transporting Polypeptide 1B1 or 1B3

Tenofovir alafenamide is a substrate of organic anion transport proteins (OATP) 1B1 and OATP1B3.

● Drugs Affecting Renal Function

Emtricitabine and tenofovir are principally excreted by the kidneys by a combination of glomerular filtration and active tubular secretion.

Pharmacokinetic interactions may occur if FTC/TAF is used concomitantly with drugs that reduce renal function or compete for active tubular secretion (e.g., acyclovir, aminoglycosides [e.g., gentamicin], cidofovir, ganciclovir, valacyclovir, valganciclovir, high-dose or multiple nonsteroidal anti-inflammatory agents [NSAIAs]); may result in increased concentrations of emtricitabine, tenofovir, and/or the concomitant drug and may increase the risk of adverse effects. Concomitant use of FTC/TAF and nephrotoxic drugs should be avoided.

● Anticonvulsants

Concomitant use of carbamazepine, oxcarbazepine, phenobarbital, or phenytoin with FTC/TAF results in decreased tenofovir concentrations. Use of alternative anticonvulsants should be considered.

● Antifungal Agents

No clinically important drug interactions are expected when FTC/TAF is used concomitantly with itraconazole or ketoconazole.

● Antimycobacterial Agents

Concomitant use of rifabutin, rifampin, or rifapentine with FTC/TAF results in decreased tenofovir concentrations. Concomitant use of rifabutin, rifampin, or rifapentine with FTC/TAF is not recommended.

● Antiretroviral Agents

HIV Entry and Fusion Inhibitors

Maraviroc

No clinically important drug interactions are expected when FTC/TAF is used concomitantly with maraviroc.

HIV Integrase Strand Transfer Inhibitors (INSTIs)

Dolutegravir

No clinically important drug interactions are expected when FTC/TAF is used concomitantly with dolutegravir.

Raltegravir

No clinically important drug interactions are expected when FTC/TAF is used concomitantly with raltegravir.

HIV Nonnucleoside Reverse Transcriptase Inhibitors (NNRTIs)

Efavirenz

No clinically important drug interactions are expected when FTC/TAF is used concomitantly with efavirenz.

Nevirapine

No clinically important drug interactions are expected when FTC/TAF is used concomitantly with nevirapine.

Rilpivirine

No clinically important drug interactions are expected when FTC/TAF is used concomitantly with rilpivirine.

HIV Nucleoside and Nucleotide Reverse Transcriptase Inhibitors (NRTIs)

Lamivudine

Emtricitabine and lamivudine should not be used concomitantly. Because emtricitabine is an analog of lamivudine, the drugs have similar resistance profiles and concomitant use provides no additional benefit.

HIV Protease Inhibitors (PIs)

Atazanavir

No clinically important drug interactions are expected when FTC/TAF is used concomitantly with atazanavir and ritonavir or cobicistat.

Darunavir

No clinically important drug interactions are expected when FTC/TAF is used concomitantly with darunavir and ritonavir or cobicistat.

Lopinavir/Ritonavir

No clinically important drug interactions are expected when FTC/TAF is used concomitantly with lopinavir and ritonavir.

Tipranavir/Ritonavir

Concomitant use of tipranavir/ritonavir and FTC/TAF results in a decrease in tenofovir concentrations. Concomitant use of tipranavir/ritonavir and FTC/TAF is *not* recommended.

● Nucleoside and Nucleotide Antivirals

Pharmacokinetic interaction (increased concentrations of emtricitabine, tenofovir, and/or the other antiviral) may occur with concomitant use of FTC/TAF with antiviral agents eliminated by active tubular secretion (e.g., acyclovir, cidofovir, ganciclovir, valacyclovir, valganciclovir).

● Benzodiazepines

No clinically important drug interactions are expected when FTC/TAF is used concomitantly with lorazepam or midazolam.

● Estrogens and Progestins

No clinically important drug interactions are expected when FTC/TAF is used concomitantly with norgestimate/ethinyl estradiol.

● HCV Antivirals

HCV Polymerase Inhibitors

Sofosbuvir

No clinically important drug interactions are expected when FTC/TAF is used concomitantly with sofosbuvir.

HCV Replication Complex Inhibitors

Ledipasvir

No clinically important drug interactions are expected when FTC/TAF is used concomitantly with ledipasvir.

● Opiate Agonists, Opiate Partial Agonists, and Opiate Antagonists

Buprenorphine

No clinically important drug interactions are expected when FTC/TAF is used concomitantly with buprenorphine.

Methadone

No clinically important drug interactions are expected when FTC/TAF is used concomitantly with methadone.

Naloxone

No clinically important drug interactions are expected when FTC/TAF is used concomitantly with naloxone.

● *Sertraline*

No clinically important drug interactions are expected when FTC/TAF is used concomitantly with sertraline.

● *St. John's Wort*

Concomitant use of St. John's wort (*Hypericum perforatum*) with FTC/TAF results in decreased tenofovir concentrations. Concomitant use of St. John's wort with FTC/TAF is *not* recommended.

DESCRIPTION

The fixed combination of emtricitabine, and tenofovir alafenamide fumarate (emtricitabine/tenofovir alafenamide fumarate; FTC/TAF) contains two antiretroviral agents: emtricitabine (an HIV nucleoside reverse transcriptase inhibitor [NRTI]) and tenofovir alafenamide fumarate (an HIV nucleotide reverse transcriptase inhibitor).

Emtricitabine is inactive until converted intracellularly to an active 5′-triphosphate metabolite. Following conversion to the pharmacologically active metabolite, the drug inhibits replication of human retroviruses by interfering with viral RNA-directed DNA polymerase (reverse transcriptase). Emtricitabine is active against HIV type 1 (HIV-1) and also has some in vitro activity against HIV type 2 (HIV-2). The drug also has some activity against hepatitis B virus (HBV).

Tenofovir alafenamide fumarate is a tenofovir prodrug and is inactive until it undergoes diester hydrolysis in vivo to tenofovir and is subsequently metabolized to the active metabolite (tenofovir diphosphate). After conversion to the pharmacologically active metabolite, the drug acts as a reverse transcriptase inhibitor antiretroviral. Tenofovir is active against HIV-1 and has some in vitro activity against HIV-2; the drug also is active against HBV.

HIV-1 isolates with reduced susceptibility to emtricitabine and tenofovir have been selected in cell culture. Genotypic analysis of these isolates identified the M184V/I, K65R, or K70E amino acid substitutions in the viral RT.

Cross-resistance among certain NRTIs has been recognized. HIV resistant to emtricitabine or tenofovir may be cross-resistant to some other NRTIs (e.g., lamivudine, abacavir, didanosine).

Peak plasma concentrations of emtricitabine and tenofovir occur 3 hours and 1 hour, respectively, after oral administration. Food does not have a clinically important effect on the pharmacokinetics of emtricitabine or tenofovir. Administration of FTC/TAF components with a high-fat meal (approximately 800 kcal, 50% fat) decreased peak concentration and AUC of emtricitabine by 26 and 9%, respectively, compared with administration in the fasting state; for tenofovir, a 15% decrease in peak concentration and a 75% increase in AUC were observed. Plasma protein binding is less than 4 or approximately 80% for emtricitabine or tenofovir alafenamide, respectively. Emtricitabine is distributed into human milk. Emtricitabine is phosphorylated intracellularly and converted by cellular enzymes to the active metabolite, emtricitabine 5′-triphosphate. Metabolites of emtricitabine include 3′-sulfoxide diastereomers and their glucuronic acid conjugate. Tenofovir alafenamide undergoes hydrolysis in vivo to tenofovir and is subsequently metabolized to the active metabolite, tenofovir diphosphate. In vitro studies indicate that tenofovir alafenamide is metabolized to tenofovir by cathepsin A in peripheral blood mononuclear cells (PBMCs) and macrophages and by carboxylesterase 1 (CES1) in hepatocytes. Metabolism accounts for >80% of tenofovir alafenamide elimination following oral administration; the drug is minimally metabolized via CYP3A. Emtricitabine is excreted in urine (70%) and feces (13.7%). Elimination of emtricitabine occurs by glomerular filtration and active tubular secretion. Emtricitabine is removed by hemodialysis; it is not known whether the drug is removed by peritoneal dialysis. Tenofovir alafenamide is excreted in feces (31.7%) and minimally in urine (<1%). Tenofovir is eliminated by glomerular filtration and active tubular secretion. Tenofovir is removed by hemodialysis. The median terminal plasma half-lives of emtricitabine, and tenofovir alafenamide are 10 and 0.51 hours, respectively. The half-life of tenofovir diphosphate, the active metabolite of tenofovir alafenamide, is 150–180 hours within PBMCs. Exposure of emtricitabine and tenofovir is increased in patients with severe renal impairment and in patients with end-stage renal impairment not receiving chronic hemodialysis. There are no clinically important differences in the pharmacokinetics of the components of FTC/TAF in pediatric patients ≥6 years of age weighing ≥25 kg compared with pharmacokinetics of the drugs reported in adults.

ADVICE TO PATIENTS

- Advise patients to read the FDA-approved patient labeling (medication guide).

- Critical nature of compliance with therapy for HIV-1 infection and importance of remaining under the care of a clinician. Stress importance of taking as prescribed; do not alter or discontinue antiretroviral regimen without consulting clinician. Advise patients that missing doses may result in development of resistance.

- Advise HIV-negative individuals taking FTC/TAF for HIV-1 PrEP of the importance of confirming that they are HIV-1-negative before starting PrEP, importance of regular HIV-1 testing (at least every 3 months or more frequently for some individuals [e.g., adolescents]) during PrEP, importance of strictly adhering to recommended dosage schedule and not missing any doses, and importance of using a complete prevention strategy that also includes other measures (e.g., consistent condom use, testing for other sexually transmitted infections such as syphilis, chlamydia, and gonorrhea that may facilitate HIV-1 transmission, reducing sexual risk behavior). Advise uninfected individuals that PrEP does not protect all individuals from acquiring HIV-1 and to report any symptoms of acute HIV-1 infection (e.g., fever, headache, fatigue, arthralgia, vomiting, myalgia, diarrhea, pharyngitis, rash, night sweats, cervical and inguinal adenopathy) immediately to a clinician. Advise patients that HIV-1 resistance substitutions may emerge in individuals with undetected HIV-1 infection who are taking FTC/TAF, because FTC/TAF alone does not constitute a complete regimen for HIV-1 treatment.

- Inform patients that testing for HBV infection is recommended before antiretroviral therapy is initiated. Also advise patients that severe acute exacerbations of HBV infection have been reported following discontinuance of emtricitabine and/or tenofovir disoproxil fumarate in HIV-infected patients coinfected with HBV and may occur with discontinuance of FTC/TAF. Advise patients with HBV not to discontinue FTC/TAF without consulting their clinician.

- Inform patients that in some patients with advanced HIV infection, signs and symptoms of inflammation from previous infections may occur soon after antiretroviral therapy is initiated. These symptoms may be due to an improvement in immune response, enabling the body to fight infections that may have been present with no obvious symptoms. Advise patients with HIV-1 infection to inform their clinician immediately if symptoms of possible infection occur.

- Advise patients that cases of renal impairment, including acute renal failure, have been reported. Advise patients to avoid FTC/TAF with concurrent or recent use of nephrotoxic agents (e.g., high-dose or multiple NSAIAs).

- Advise patients that cases of lactic acidosis and severe hepatomegaly with steatosis, including fatal cases, have been reported with the use of drugs similar to FTC/TAF. Stress importance of contacting clinician and suspending treatment if recommended if symptoms suggestive of lactic acidosis or pronounced hepatotoxicity (e.g., unusual muscle pain, shortness of breath or fast breathing, cold or blue hands and feet, dizziness or lightheadedness, fast or abnormal heartbeat, nausea, vomiting, unusual/unexpected stomach discomfort, weakness or unusual tiredness) occur.

- Stress importance of informing clinician of existing or contemplated concomitant therapy, including prescription (e.g., other antiviral agents) and OTC drugs and dietary or herbal products (e.g., St. John's wort).

- Stress importance of women informing clinicians if they are or plan to become pregnant or plan to breast-feed. Advise patients of pregnancy registry.

- Advise patients of other important precautionary information.

PREPARATIONS

Excipients in commercially available drug preparations may have clinically important effects in some individuals; consult specific product labeling for details.

Emtricitabine and Tenofovir Alafenamide Fumarate

Oral

Tablets, film-coated	Emtricitabine 120 mg and Tenofovir Alafenamide 15 mg	**Descovy®**, Gilead
	Emtricitabine 200 mg and Tenofovir Alafenamide 25 mg	**Descovy®**, Gilead

† Use is not currently included in the labeling approved by the US Food and Drug Administration.

Selected Revisions October 10, 2024, © Copyright, November 28, 2022, American Society of Health-System Pharmacists, Inc.

Emtricitabine and Tenofovir Disoproxil Fumarate

8:18.08.20 • HIV NUCLEOSIDE AND NUCLEOTIDE REVERSE TRANSCRIPTASE INHIBITORS

- Emtricitabine and tenofovir disoproxil fumarate (emtricitabine/tenofovir disoproxil fumarate; FTC/TDF) is a fixed-combination antiretroviral agent containing emtricitabine (a human immunodeficiency virus [HIV] nucleoside reverse transcriptase inhibitor [NRTI]) and tenofovir disoproxil fumarate (an HIV nucleotide reverse transcriptase inhibitor).

USES

• Treatment of HIV Infection

The fixed combination of emtricitabine and tenofovir disoproxil fumarate (FTC/TDF) is used in combination with other antiretroviral agents for the treatment of HIV-1 infection in adults and pediatric patients weighing ≥17 kg. FTC/TDF must be used in conjunction with other antiretrovirals for treatment of HIV-1.

Clinical Experience

Adults and Adolescents

Efficacy of a regimen of emtricitabine and tenofovir DF in combination with efavirenz is based on results of a randomized, open-label study designed to demonstrate noninferiority of this regimen compared with a regimen of efavirenz, zidovudine, and lamivudine (study 934; NCT0112047). In this study, 511 antiretroviral-naïve HIV-infected adult patients (mean age 38 years, 86% male, 59% white, 23% Black, median baseline plasma HIV-1 RNA level 5.01 $\log_{10}$ copies/mL [range: 3.56–6.54 $\log_{10}$ copies/mL], mean baseline CD4+ T-cell count 245 cells/mm³) were randomized to receive a once-daily regimen of efavirenz, emtricitabine, and tenofovir DF or a regimen of efavirenz once daily with the fixed combination of lamivudine and zidovudine (lamivudine/zidovudine; Combivir®) twice daily. The primary endpoint was the proportion of patients with HIV-1 RNA levels <400 copies/mL at week 48. The 487 patients without baseline resistance to efavirenz who underwent randomization and received treatment were the predefined population used for the primary endpoint analysis.

Through week 48, the regimen of efavirenz, emtricitabine, and tenofovir DF met the criteria for noninferiority to the regimen of efavirenz and lamivudine/zidovudine. At week 48, 84 or 80% of adults receiving the efavirenz, tenofovir DF, and emtricitabine regimen and 73 or 70% of adults receiving the efavirenz and lamivudine/zidovudine regimen had plasma HIV-1 RNA levels <400 or 50 copies/mL, respectively. At week 48, increases in CD4+ T-cell counts were greater in patients receiving the efavirenz, emtricitabine, and tenofovir DF regimen (mean increase of 190 cells/mm³) than in those receiving the efavirenz and lamivudine/zidovudine regimen (mean increase of 158 cells/mm³). Virologic failure (i.e., individuals who failed to achieve virologic suppression or experienced rebound after achieving virologic suppression) was reported in 2% of those receiving efavirenz, emtricitabine, and tenofovir DF and in 4% of those receiving efavirenz and lamivudine/zidovudine at week 48.

At 144 weeks, 64% of adults receiving the efavirenz, emtricitabine, and tenofovir DF regimen and 56% of those receiving the efavirenz and lamivudine/zidovudine regimen had plasma HIV-1 RNA levels less than 50 copies/mL. The mean increase in CD4+ T-cell count from baseline in these groups was 312 and 271 cells/mm³, respectively, at 144 weeks.

Pediatric Patients

Clinical trials to evaluate the safety and efficacy of the fixed combination of emtricitabine and tenofovir DF (FTC/TDF) in pediatric patients with HIV-1 infection have not been performed to date. Data from previously conducted trials with the individual drugs in the fixed combination were relied upon to support pediatric dosage recommendations for FTC/TDF.

Clinical Perspective

Therapeutic options for the treatment and prevention of HIV infection and recommendations concerning the use of antiretrovirals are continuously evolving. Antiretroviral therapy is recommended for all individuals with HIV regardless of CD4+ T-cell counts, and should be initiated as soon as possible after diagnosis of HIV and continued indefinitely. The primary goals of antiretroviral therapy are to achieve and maintain durable suppression of HIV viral load (as measured by plasma HIV-1 RNA levels) to a level below which drug-resistance mutations cannot emerge (i.e., below detectable limits), restore and preserve immunologic function, reduce HIV-related morbidity and mortality, improve quality of life, and prevent transmission of HIV. While the most appropriate antiretroviral regimen cannot be defined for each clinical scenario, the US Department of Health and Human Services (HHS) Panel on Antiretroviral Guidelines for Adults and Adolescents, HHS Panel on Antiretroviral Therapy and Medical Management of Children Living with HIV, and HHS Panel on Treatment of Pregnant Women with HIV Infection and Prevention of Perinatal Transmission, have developed comprehensive guidelines that provide information on selection and use of antiretrovirals for the treatment or prevention of HIV infection. Because of the complexity of managing patients with HIV, it is recommended that clinicians with HIV expertise be consulted when needed.

The use of combination antiretroval regimens that generally include 3 drugs from 2 or more drug classes is currently recommended to achieve viral suppression. In both treatment-naïve adults and children, an initial antiretroviral regimen generally consists of 2 NRTIs administered in combination with a third active antiretroviral drug from 1 of 3 drug classes: an integrase strand transfer inhibitor (INSTI), NNRTI, or a protease inhibitor (PI) with a pharmacokinetic enhancer (also known as a booster; the 2 drugs used for this purpose are cobicistat and ritonavir). Selection of an initial regimen should be individualized based on factors such as virologic efficacy, toxicity, pill burden, dosing frequency, drug–drug interaction potential, resistance-test results, comorbid conditions, access, and cost. In patients with comorbid infections (e.g., hepatitis B, tuberculosis), regimen selection should also consider the potential for activity against other present infections and timing of initiation relative to other anti-infective regimens.

In the 2024 HHS adult and adolescent treatment guideline, the combination of emtricitabine and tenofovir disoproxil fumarate is recommended as a component of various initial therapeutic regimens for HIV infection.

In the 2024 HHS pediatric HIV treatment guideline, the combination of emtricitabine and tenofovir disoproxil fumarate is recommended as a component of an alternative regimen for adolescents weighing ≥40 kg and may also be considered as a component of an alternative regimen in adolescents with special concerns (e.g., weight gain, increased risk for obesity, or high-risk lipid profile).

In the 2024 HHS perinatal HIV treatment guideline, the combination of emtricitabine and tenofovir disoproxil fumarate is recommended as a component of various preferred and alternative initial regimens during pregancy for patients who are antiretroviral-naïve.

• Preexposure Prophylaxis for Prevention of HIV-1 Infection

The fixed combination containing emtricitabine and tenofovir DF (FTC/TDF) is used for preexposure prophylaxis (PrEP) to reduce the risk of sexually-acquired HIV infection in HIV-1-negative adults and adolescents weighing ≥35 kg who are at risk.

Adults and adolescents at risk for HIV-1 infection include those with partner(s) known to be infected with HIV-1 or those engaging in sexual activity within a high prevalence area or social network and with 1 or more of the following factors: inconsistent or no condom use, past or current sexually transmitted infections, use of illicit drugs, alcohol dependence, or partner(s) of unknown HIV-1 status.

PrEP with FTC/TDF is *not* always effective in preventing acquisition of HIV-1 infection and *must* be used as part of a comprehensive prevention strategy that includes safer sex practices.

Clinical Experience in Adults

Efficacy and safety of a once-daily regimen of FTC/TDF for HIV-1 PrEP were evaluated in a multinational, randomized, double-blind, placebo-controlled, phase 3 trial (Preexposure Prophylaxis Initiative [iPrEx trial]; NCT00458393) that included 2499 HIV-seronegative men or transgender women (male at birth) who have sex with men and have evidence of high-risk behavior for HIV-1 infection. Study participants (mean age 27 years [range 18–67 years], 5% Asian, 9% Black, 18% white, 72% Hispanic/Latino) were randomized to receive FTC/TDF (a fixed-combination tablet containing 200 mg of emtricitabine and 300 mg of tenofovir DF once daily) or placebo in conjunction with usual prevention strategies (i.e., monthly HIV-1 testing, risk-reduction counseling, condoms, diagnosis and management of sexually transmitted infections) and were followed for 4237 person-years. The primary outcome measure was the incidence of documented HIV seroconversion. There was a 42% reduction in the risk of HIV-1 seroconversion in the group receiving FTC/TDF (48 individuals receiving FTC/TDF and 83 individuals receiving placebo seroconverted). Results of a post-hoc case-control study of plasma and intracellular drug concentrations in about 10% of study participants indicated that efficacy of FTC/TDF PrEP is strongly correlated with adherence since risk reduction appeared to be greatest in those with detectable intracellular TDF.

Efficacy and safety of FTC/TDF for PrEP in HIV-1-seronegative partners of serodiscordant heterosexual couples were evaluated in a randomized, double-blind, placebo-controlled, 3-arm trial (Partners Preexposure Prophylaxis [Partners PrEP] trial; NCT00557245) that included 4758 serodiscordant couples in Kenya and Uganda. The infected partners had median plasma HIV-1 RNA levels of 3.9 $\log_{10}$ copies/mL and median CD4+ T-cell counts of 495 cells/mm³ (80% had CD4+ T-cell counts of 350 cells/mm³ or higher). The uninfected partners (mean age 33–34 years, 61–64% male) were randomized to receive FTC/TDF (a fixed-combination tablet containing 200 mg of FTC and 300 mg of TDF once daily), TDF (300 mg of TDF once daily), or placebo (once daily). Study participants received monthly HIV-1 testing, adherence evaluations, sexual behavior assessments, and safety evaluations. Women received monthly pregnancy tests; if pregnancy occurred, the study drug was interrupted during pregnancy and breast-feeding. After 7827 person-years of follow-up, there were a total of 82 emergent HIV-1 seroconversions (overall observed seroincidence rate of 1.05 per 100 person-years). The risk reduction for the FTC/TDF group relative to the placebo group was 75%. There were 13 seroconversions in partners randomized to FTC/TDF and 52 seroconversions in partners randomized to placebo (2 and 3 seroconversions, respectively, occurred during interruption of PrEP for pregnancy). Results of a post-hoc case-control study of plasma and drug concentrations in about 10% of study participants indicated that efficacy of FTC/TDF PrEP is strongly correlated with adherence since risk reduction appeared to be greatest in those with detectable plasma tenofovir.

Clinical Experience in Pediatric Patients

The safety and efficacy of FTC/TDF for HIV-1 PrEP in at-risk adolescents weighing ≥35 kg are supported by data from adequate and well-controlled studies of FTC/TDF for HIV-1 PrEP in adults with additional data from safety and pharmacokinetic studies in previously conducted trials with the individual drugs, FTC and TDF, in HIV-1 infected adults and pediatric subjects.

Safety, adherence, and resistance were evaluated in a single-arm, open-label clinical trial (ATN113) in 67 HIV-1 uninfected at-risk adolescent men who have sex with men who received FTC/TDF once daily for HIV-1 PrEP. The mean age of subjects was 17 years (range 15–18 years); patients were 46% Hispanic, 52% Black, and 37% white. The safety profile of FTC/TDF in ATN113 was similar to that observed in HIV-1 PrEP trials in adults. HIV-1 seroconversion occurred in 3 subjects. Tenofovir diphosphate levels in dried blood spot assays indicated that these subjects had poor adherence. No tenofovir- or FTC-associated HIV-1 resistance substitutions were detected in virus isolated from the 3 subjects who experienced seroconversion. A marked decline in adherence to study drug, as demonstrated by tenofovir diphosphate levels in dried blood spot assays, was observed after week 12, when subjects switched from monthly to quarterly visits, suggesting that adolescents may benefit from more frequent visits and counseling.

● Postexposure Prophylaxis following Occupational Exposure to HIV

FTC/TDF has been used in conjunction with other antiretrovirals for postexposure prophylaxis of HIV infection following occupational exposure† (PEP) in health-care personnel and other individuals exposed via percutaneous injury (e.g., needlestick, cut with sharp object) or mucous membrane or nonintact skin (e.g., chapped, abraded, dermatitis) contact with blood, tissue, or other body fluids that might contain HIV.

The US Public Health Service (USPHS) states that the preferred regimen for PEP following an occupational exposure to HIV is a 3-drug regimen of raltegravir used in conjunction with FTC and tenofovir DF (may be administered as the fixed combination FTC/TDF). These experts recommend several alternative regimens that include an INSTI, NNRTI, or PI and 2 NRTIs (dual NRTIs). The preferred dual NRTI option for use in PEP regimens is emtricitabine and tenofovir DF (may be administered as the fixed combination FTC/TDF); alternative dual NRTIs are tenofovir DF and lamivudine, lamivudine and zidovudine (may be administered as the fixed combination lamivudine/zidovudine; Combivir®), or zidovudine and emtricitabine.

Because management of occupational exposures to HIV is complex and evolving, consultation with an infectious disease specialist, clinician with expertise in administration of antiretroviral agents, and/or the National Clinicians' Postexposure Prophylaxis Hotline (PEPline at 888-448-4911) is recommended whenever possible. However, initiation of PEP should not be delayed while waiting for expert consultation.

● Postexposure Prophylaxis following Nonoccupational Exposure to HIV

FTC/TDF has been used in conjunction with other antiretrovirals for postexposure prophylaxis of HIV infection following nonoccupational exposure† (nPEP) in individuals exposed to blood, genital secretions, or other potentially infectious body fluids that might contain HIV when that exposure represents a substantial risk for HIV transmission.

When nPEP is indicated following a nonoccupational exposure to HIV, the US Centers for Disease Control and Prevention (CDC) states that the preferred regimen in adults and adolescents ≥13 years of age with normal renal function is either raltegravir or dolutegravir used in conjunction with FTC/TDF. The alternative nPEP regimen recommended in these patients is *ritonavir-boosted* darunavir used in conjunction with FTC/TDF.

Consultation with an infectious disease specialist, clinician with expertise in administration of antiretroviral agents, and/or the National Clinicians' Postexposure Prophylaxis Hotline (PEPline at 888-448-4911) is recommended if nPEP is indicated in certain exposed individuals (e.g., pregnant women, children, those with medical conditions such as renal impairment) or if an antiretroviral regimen not included in the CDC guidelines is being considered, the source virus is known or likely to be resistant to antiretrovirals, or the healthcare provider is inexperienced in prescribing antiretrovirals. However, initiation of nPEP should not be delayed while waiting for expert consultation.

DOSAGE AND ADMINISTRATION

● General

Pretreatment Screening

- Prior to or when initiating the fixed combination of emtricitabine and tenofovir disoproxil fumarate (FTC/TDF), test patients for hepatitis B virus (HBV) infection.

- Prior to initiation of FTC/TDF, assess S_{cr}, estimated Cl_{cr}, urine glucose, and urine protein in all patients; in patients with chronic kidney disease, also assess serum phosphorus.

- Immediately prior to initiating FTC/TDF for human immunodeficiency virus type 1 (HIV-1) preexposure prophylaxis (PrEP), screen for HIV-1 infection. If recent (<1 month) exposures to HIV-1 are suspected or clinical symptoms consistent with acute HIV-1 infection are present, use a test approved or cleared by the FDA as an aid in the diagnosis of acute or primary HIV-1 infection.

Patient Monitoring

- Monitor hepatic function closely with clinical and laboratory follow-up for at least several months after discontinuance of FTC/TDF in patients infected with HBV.

- On a clinically appropriate schedule, assess S_{cr}, estimated Cl_{cr}, urine glucose, and urine protein in all patients; in patients with chronic kidney disease, also assess serum phosphorus.

- In patients receiving FTC/TDF for PrEP, screen for HIV-1 infection at least once every 3 months and upon diagnosis of any other sexually transmitted infections.
- Consider bone mineral density (BMD) monitoring in adult and pediatric patients who have a history of pathologic bone fracture or other risk factors for osteoporosis or bone loss.

● Administration

Emtricitabine/tenofovir disoproxil fumarate (FTC/TDF) tablets are administered orally once daily without regard to food. A fixed-combination tablet containing 200 mg of emtricitabine and 300 mg of tenofovir DF is bioequivalent to a 200-mg capsule of FTC and a 300-mg tablet of tenofovir DF given simultaneously.

For the treatment of HIV-1 infection, FTC/TDF is used in conjunction with other antiretrovirals. For preexposure prophylaxis (PrEP) for prevention of HIV-1 infection, FTC/TDF is used alone without any other antiretrovirals.

Tablets should be stored at 25°C; excursions permitted to 15-30°C.

● Dosage

Fixed-combination tablets of FTC/TDF contain emtricitabine and tenofovir DF; dosage of tenofovir DF is expressed in terms of tenofovir DF.

Adult Dosage

Treatment of HIV Infection

When FTC/TDF is used in conjunction with other antiretrovirals for the treatment of HIV-1 infection, adults should receive 1 tablet containing 200 mg of emtricitabine and 300 mg of tenofovir DF once daily.

Preexposure Prophylaxis for Prevention of HIV-1 Infection

When FTC/TDF is used for preexposure prophylaxis (PrEP) for prevention of HIV-1 infection in HIV-1-negative adults at risk, the recommended dosage is 1 tablet containing 200 mg of emtricitabine and 300 mg of tenofovir DF once daily.

Postexposure Prophylaxis following Occupational Exposure to HIV

When FTC/TDF is used as the dual NRTI option in postexposure prophylaxis of HIV infection following occupational exposure† (PEP) regimens, adults should receive 1 tablet containing 200 mg of emtricitabine and 300 mg of tenofovir DF once daily in conjunction with a recommended HIV integrase strand transfer inhibitor (INSTI), nonnucleoside reverse transcriptase inhibitor (NNRTI), or HIV protease inhibitor (PI).

The PEP regimen should be initiated as soon as possible following occupational exposure to HIV (preferably within hours) and continued for 4 weeks, if tolerated.

Postexposure Prophylaxis following Nonoccupational Exposure to HIV

When FTC/TDF is used as the dual NRTI option in postexposure prophylaxis of HIV infection following nonoccupational exposure† (nPEP) regimens, adults should receive 1 tablet containing 200 mg of emtricitabine and 300 mg of tenofovir DF once daily in conjunction with a preferred or alternative INSTI, PI, or NNRTI.

The nPEP regimen should be initiated as soon as possible (within 72 hours) following nonoccupational exposure to HIV and continued for 28 days. If the exposed individual seeks care more than 72 hours after the exposure, nPEP is not recommended.

Pediatric Dosage

Treatment of HIV Infection

When FTC/TDF is used in conjunction with other antiretrovirals for the treatment of HIV-1 infection in children weighing ≥35 kg, the recommended dosage is 1 tablet containing 200 mg of emtricitabine and 300 mg of tenofovir DF once daily. When FTC/TDF is used in conjunction with other antiretrovirals for the treatment of HIV-1 infection in children weighing 17 to <35 kg who are able to swallow a tablet, the recommended dosage is based on weight; a low-strength fixed-combination tablet of the drug should be used. (See Table 1.) Monitor weight periodically and adjust dosage of FTC/TDF accordingly.

TABLE 1. Emtricitabine/tenofovir DF Dosage for Treatment of HIV-1 Infection in Children Weighing ≥17 kg

Weight (kg)	Dosage of Emtricitabine/tenofovir DF given Once Daily
17 to <22 kg	1 tablet (100 mg of emtricitabine and 150 mg of tenofovir DF)
22 to <28 kg	1 tablet (133 mg of emtricitabine and 200 mg of tenofovir DF)
28 to <35 kg	1 tablet (167 mg of emtricitabine and 250 mg of tenofovir DF)
≥35 kg	1 tablet (200 mg of emtricitabine and 300 mg of tenofovir DF)

Preexposure Prophylaxis for Prevention of HIV-1 Infection

When FTC/TDF is used for preexposure prophylaxis (PrEP) for prevention of HIV-1 infection in at-risk HIV-1-negative adolescents weighing ≥35 kg, the recommended dosage is 1 tablet containing 200 mg of emtricitabine and 300 mg of tenofovir DF once daily.

● Special Populations

Hepatic Impairment

While the pharmacokinetics of emtricitabine have not been specifically studied in patients with hepatic impairment, the drug is not substantially metabolized by liver enzymes and clinically important changes in emtricitabine metabolism are not expected if the drug is used in patients with hepatic impairment.

No changes in tenofovir pharmacokinetics were observed in patients with moderate to severe hepatic impairment receiving a 300-mg dose of tenofovir DF.

Emtricitabine/tenofovir DF (FTC/TDF) has not been studied in patients with hepatic impairment.

Renal Impairment

When FTC/TDF is used for the treatment of HIV-1 infection in adults, the usual dosage can be used in those with mild renal impairment (creatinine clearance of 50–80 mL/minute). If the fixed combination is used in adults with creatinine clearance of 30–49 mL/minute, dosage should be reduced to 1 tablet containing 200 mg of emtricitabine and 300 mg of tenofovir DF once every 48 hours; clinical response and renal function should be closely monitored since this dosage has not been evaluated clinically. FTC/TDF should *not* be used for treatment of HIV-1 infection in adults with creatinine clearances <30 mL/minute (including hemodialysis patients). Data are insufficient to make dosage recommendations for the fixed combination for pediatric patients with renal impairment.

When FTC/TDF is used for PrEP for prevention of HIV-1 infection in HIV-1-negative adults at risk, the usual dosage can be used in those with creatinine clearances of ≥60 mL/minute. If creatinine clearance decreases while FTC/TDF is being used for PrEP, potential causes should be evaluated and potential risks and benefits of continued use should be reassessed. FTC/TDF should *not* be used for PrEP in adults with creatinine clearances <60 mL/minute.

Geriatric Patients

The manufacturer makes no specific dosage recommendations for geriatric patients.

CAUTIONS

● Contraindications

- Do not use for preexposure prophylaxis (PrEP) of HIV-1 infection in individuals with unknown or positive HIV-1 status.

● Warnings/Precautions

Warnings

Severe Acute Exacerbations of Hepatitis B

The prescribing information contains a boxed warning regarding the risk of severe acute exacerbations of hepatitis B in patients with hepatitis B virus (HBV) infection. Prior to or when initiating FTC/TDF, test all patients for chronic HBV infection. Severe acute exacerbations of HBV infection, including liver decompensation and liver failure, have been reported in HBV-infected patients following discontinuance of FTC/TDF.

Monitor hepatic function closely with both clinical and laboratory follow-up for at least several months after FTC/TDF is discontinued in HBV-infected patients. If appropriate, initiation of HBV treatment may be warranted, especially in individuals with advanced liver disease or cirrhosis. Offer HBV vaccination to HBV-uninfected individuals.

Although emtricitabine and tenofovir DF have some activity against HBV, FTC/TDF is *not* indicated for treatment of chronic HBV infection.

Precautions Related to HIV-1 Preexposure Prophylaxis

The prescribing information contains a boxed warning regarding the risk of drug resistance with use of FTC/TDF for PrEP in undiagnosed early HIV-1 infection. Use FTC/TDF for HIV-1 PrEP *only* for individuals confirmed to be HIV-1-negative immediately prior to initiation of PrEP; confirm HIV-1-negative status periodically (at least every 3 months and upon diagnosis of any other sexually transmitted infection) during PrEP.

Drug-resistant HIV-1 variants have been identified when FTC/TDF PrEP was used following undetected acute HIV-1 infection. Do *not* initiate PrEP if signs or symptoms of acute HIV-1 infection are present, unless negative infection status is confirmed.

Clinicians should consider that some HIV-1 tests only detect anti-HIV antibodies and may not identify HIV-1 during the acute stage of infection. Prior to initiating FTC/TDF PrEP, clinicians should evaluate HIV-negative individuals for current or recent signs or symptoms consistent with acute viral infection (e.g., fever, fatigue, myalgia, rash) and ask about any potential exposure events that may have occurred within the last month (e.g., unprotected sex, condom broke during sex with a partner of unknown HIV-1 status or unknown viremic status or a recent sexually transmitted infection).

If recent (<1 month) exposures to HIV-1 are suspected or clinical symptoms consistent with acute HIV-1 infection are present, use a test approved or cleared by the FDA as an aid in the diagnosis of acute or primary HIV-1 infection.

Uninfected individuals should be counseled to strictly adhere to the recommended FTC/TDF dosage schedule. Effectiveness of the fixed combination in reducing the risk of acquiring HIV-1 is strongly correlated with adherence as demonstrated by measurable drug concentrations in clinical trials. Some individuals (e.g., adolescents) may benefit from more frequent visits and counseling to support adherence.

Adverse effects reported in HIV-negative adults receiving FTC/TDF PrEP are similar to those reported in HIV-infected patients receiving the drugs for treatment of HIV-1 infection.

Other Warnings/Precautions
Renal Impairment

Renal impairment, including cases of acute renal failure and Fanconi syndrome (renal tubular injury with severe hypophosphatemia), has been reported with the use of tenofovir DF, a component of FTC/TDF.

Serum creatinine, estimated creatinine clearance, urine glucose, and urine protein should be determined prior to initiating FTC/TDF and monitored during treatment in all patients as clinically appropriate. In patients with chronic kidney disease, serum phosphorus also should be assessed.

In individuals at risk for renal dysfunction, evaluate renal function if possible manifestations of proximal renal tubulopathy (e.g., persistent or worsening bone pain, pain in extremities, fractures, and/or muscular pain or weakness) occur.

When used for the treatment of HIV-1 infection, dosing interval adjustment of FTC/TDF and close monitoring of renal function are recommended in all patients with estimated creatinine clearance 30–49 mL/minute. No safety or efficacy data are available in patients with renal impairment who received FTC/TDF using these dosing guidelines, so the potential benefit of FTC/TDF therapy should be assessed against the potential risk of renal toxicity. Use of FTC/TDF for treatment of HIV-1 infection is not recommended in patients with estimated creatinine clearance below 30 mL/min or patients disquiring hemodialysis.

Use of FTC/TDF for PrEP is not recommended in patients with estimated creatinine clearance <60 mL/minute. If a decrease in estimated creatinine clearance

is observed while using FTC/TDF for HIV-1 PrEP, evaluate potential causes and reassess potential risks and benefits of continued use.

Avoid FTC/TDF in patients with concurrent or recent use of a nephrotoxic agent (e.g., high-dose or multiple nonsteroidal anti-inflammatory agents [NSAIAs]). Cases of acute renal failure after initiation of high-dose or multiple NSAIAs have been reported in HIV-infected patients with risk factors for renal dysfunction who appeared stable on tenofovir DF; some patients required hospitalization and renal replacement therapy. Consider alternatives to NSAIAs, if needed, in patients at risk for renal dysfunction.

Immune Reconstitution Syndrome

Immune reconstitution syndrome has been reported in HIV-infected patients receiving multiple-drug antiretroviral therapy, including FTC/TDF. During the initial phase of treatment, HIV-infected patients whose immune systems respond to antiretroviral therapy may develop an inflammatory response to indolent or residual opportunistic infections (e.g., *Mycobacterium avium* complex [MAC], *M. tuberculosis*, cytomegalovirus [CMV], *Pneumocystis jirovecii* [formerly *P. carinii*]); such response may necessitate further evaluation and treatment.

Autoimmune disorders (e.g., Graves' disease, polymyositis, Guillain-Barré syndrome, autoimmune hepatitis) have also been reported to occur in the setting of immune reconstitution; however, the time to onset is more variable and can occur many months after initiation of antiretroviral therapy.

Bone Loss and Mineralization Defects

Decreases in bone mineral density (BMD) from baseline, increases in several biochemical markers of bone metabolism, and increased serum parathyroid hormone levels and 1,25-vitamin D levels have been reported during clinical trials of tenofovir DF (a component of emtricitabine/tenofovir DF [FTC/TDF]). The effects of tenofovir-associated changes in BMD on long-term bone health and future fracture risk are unknown.

In clinical trials in HIV-1 infected subjects 2 years of age to less than 18 years of age, bone effects in pediatric and adolescent subjects receiving tenofovir DF were similar to those observed in adult subjects, suggesting increased bone turnover. Total body BMD gain was less in the tenofovir DF-treated HIV-1-infected pediatric subjects compared with control groups. Similar trends were observed in adolescent subjects 12 years of age to <18 years of age treated for chronic hepatitis B infection. Skeletal growth (height) appeared to be unaffected in all pediatric trials.

Osteomalacia associated with proximal renal tubulopathy, which manifested as bone pain or pain in extremities and may contribute to fractures, has been reported in patients receiving tenofovir DF. Arthralgia and muscle pain or weakness also have been reported in patients with proximal renal tubulopathy. Hypophosphatemia and osteomalacia secondary to proximal renal tubulopathy should be considered in patients at risk for renal dysfunction who present with persistent or worsening bone or muscle symptoms while receiving preparations containing tenofovir DF.

BMD monitoring should be considered in adult and pediatric patients who have a history of pathologic bone fracture or other risk factors for osteoporosis or bone loss. Although the effect of calcium and vitamin D supplementation was not studied, such supplementation may be beneficial. If bone abnormalities are suspected, appropriate consultation should be obtained.

Lactic Acidosis and Severe Hepatomegaly with Steatosis

Lactic acidosis and severe hepatomegaly with steatosis, including fatalities, have been reported in patients receiving HIV nucleoside reverse transcriptase inhibitors (NRTIs), including emtricitabine and tenofovir DF, alone or in combination with other antiretroviral agents.

FTC/TDF treatment should be interrupted in any patient who develops clinical or laboratory findings suggestive of lactic acidosis or pronounced hepatotoxicity (signs of hepatotoxicity may include hepatomegaly and steatosis even in the absence of marked increases in serum aminotransferase concentrations).

Interactions

Concomitant use of emtricitabine/tenofovir DF (FTC/TDF) with certain drugs may result in known or potentially clinically important drug interactions, some of which may increase plasma concentrations of concomitant drugs leading to clinically important adverse reactions.

Consider potential for drug interactions prior to and during FTC/TDF therapy; review concomitant drugs during FTC/TDF therapy and monitor for adverse effects.

Specific Populations

Pregnancy

Antiretroviral Pregnancy Registry (APR) at 800-258-4263 or https://www.APRegistry.com.

Available data from the APR show an incidence of major birth defects with first-trimester exposure of 2.3 or 2.1% for emtricitabine or tenofovir DF, respectively, compared with a background rate for major birth defects of 2.7% in a US reference population of the Metropolitan Atlanta Congenital Defects Program. In animal reproduction studies, no adverse developmental effects were observed when the components of emtricitabine/tenofovir DF (FTC/TDF) were administered separately at doses/exposures ≥60 (emtricitabine), ≥14 (tenofovir DF), and 2.7 (tenofovir) times those of the recommended daily dose of FTC/TDF.

In HIV-1-negative women at risk of acquiring HIV-1, consideration should be given to methods to prevent HIV-1, including initiating or continuing FTC/TDF PrEP, taking into account the potential increased risk of HIV-1 infection during pregnancy and the increased risk of mother-to-child transmission during acute HIV-1 infection.

Lactation

Emtricitabine and tenofovir DF are distributed into human milk in low concentrations. It is not known whether emtricitabine/tenofovir DF (FTC/TDF) affects human milk production or affects the breast-fed infant.

The HHS perinatal HIV transmission guideline provides updated recommendations on infant feeding. The guideline states that patients with HIV should receive evidence-based, patient-centered counseling to support shared decision making about infant feeding. During counseling, patients should be informed that feeding with appropriate formula or pasteurized donor human milk from a milk bank eliminates the risk of postnatal HIV transmission to the infant. Additionally, achieving and maintaining viral suppression with antiretroviral therapy during pregnancy and postpartum reduces the risk of breastfeeding HIV transmission to <1%, but does not completely eliminate the risk. Replacement feeding with formula or banked pasteurized donor milk is recommended when patients with HIV are *not* on antiretroviral therapy and/or do *not* have a suppressed viral load during pregnancy (at a minimum throughout the third trimester), as well as at delivery.

Pediatric Use

Safety and efficacy of FTC/TDF for treatment of HIV-1 infection have *not* been established in pediatric patients weighing <17 kg; safety and efficacy of this fixed combination for HIV-1 PrEP have *not* been established in pediatric patients weighing <35 kg.

Adverse effects reported in pediatric patients 3 months to <18 years of age receiving emtricitabine in clinical studies have been similar to those in adults, with the exception of a higher frequency of anemia and hyperpigmentation. Adverse effects reported in pediatric patients 2 to <18 years of age receiving tenofovir DF in clinical studies have been similar to those in adults.

Adverse effects reported in adolescents 15–18 years of age receiving FTC/TDF in clinical trials for HIV-1 PrEP were similar to those in adults.

In clinical trials in HIV-1 infected subjects 2 to <18 years of age, bone effects in pediatric and adolescent subjects receiving tenofovir DF were similar to those observed in adult subjects, suggesting increased bone turnover. Total body bone mineral density (BMD) gain was less in the tenofovir DF-treated HIV-1 infected pediatric subjects compared with control groups. Similar trends were observed in adolescent subjects 12 to <18 years of age treated for chronic hepatitis B infection. Skeletal growth (height) appeared to be unaffected in all pediatric trials.

BMD monitoring should be considered in pediatric patients who have a history of pathologic bone fracture or other risk factors for osteoporosis or bone loss. Although the effect of calcium and vitamin D supplementation was not studied, such supplementation may be beneficial. If bone abnormalities are suspected, appropriate consultation should be obtained.

Geriatric Use

Experience in patients ≥65 years of age is insufficient to determine whether they respond differently to FTC/TDF than younger adults.

Hepatic Impairment

FTC/TDF has not been studied in patients with hepatic impairment. Hepatic impairment does not have a substantial effect on tenofovir DF pharmacokinetics and is expected to have a minimal impact on emtricitabine pharmacokinetics.

Renal Impairment

Assess serum creatinine, estimated creatinine clearance, urine glucose, and urine protein prior to initiating FTC/TDF and routinely monitor during treatment in all patients as clinically appropriate. In patients with chronic kidney disease, also assess serum phosphorus at baseline and during treatment as clinically appropriate.

FTC/TDF should *not* be used for treatment of HIV-1 infection in patients with creatinine clearance <30 mL/minute or in those with end-stage renal disease requiring dialysis; dosage adjustments are necessary when the drug is used for treatment of HIV-1 infection in those with creatinine clearance 30–49 mL/minute.

FTC/TDF should *not* be used for PrEP in HIV-1 uninfected adults with creatinine clearance <60 mL/minute. If creatinine clearance decreases while FTC/TDF is being used for PrEP, potential causes should be evaluated and potential risks and benefits of continued use should be reassessed.

● Common Adverse Effects

Adverse effects reported in ≥10% of HIV-infected patients receiving FTC/TDF in conjunction with other antiretrovirals are diarrhea, nausea, fatigue, headache, dizziness, depression, insomnia, abnormal dreams, and rash.

Adverse effects reported in ≥2% of patients receiving FTC/TDF for preexposure prophylaxis of HIV-1 infection (PrEP) and more frequently than in patients receiving placebo include headache, abdominal pain, and decrease in weight.

DRUG INTERACTIONS

The following drug interactions are based on studies that used emtricitabine or tenofovir disoproxil fumarate alone or the fixed combination of emtricitabine and tenofovir disoproxil fumarate (FTC/TDF) or are predicted to occur.

Potential drug interactions associated with each drug in the fixed combination should be considered.

● Drugs Affecting or Metabolized by Hepatic Microsomal Enzymes

Emtricitabine is not a substrate of CYP isoenzymes; emtricitabine does not inhibit CYP1A2, 2A6, 2B6, 2C9, 2C19, 2D6, or 3A4.

Tenofovir is not a substrate of CYP isoenzymes; in vitro studies indicate tenofovir does not inhibit CYP isoenzymes 3A4, 2D6, 2C9, or 2E1, but may have a slight inhibitory effect on CYP1A.

Based on in vitro studies and clinical pharmacokinetic drug-drug interaction trials, pharmacokinetic interactions between FTC/TDF and drugs affecting or metabolized by hepatic microsomal enzymes are considered unlikely.

● Drugs Affecting or Affected by P-glycoprotein Transport

Tenofovir DF is a substrate of P-glycoprotein (P-gp). When tenofovir DF is used concomitantly with an inhibitor of P-gp, an increase in tenofovir absorption may be observed.

● Drugs Affecting or Affected by Breast Cancer Resistance Protein

Tenofovir DF is a substrate of breast cancer resistance protein (BCRP). When tenofovir DF is used concomitantly with an inhibitor of BCRP, an increase in tenofovir absorption may be observed.

● Drugs Affecting Renal Function

Emtricitabine and tenofovir are principally excreted by the kidneys by a combination of glomerular filtration and active tubular secretion.

No drug-drug interactions due to competition for renal excretion have been observed; however, potential pharmacokinetic interactions if FTC/TDF is used concomitantly with drugs that reduce renal function or compete for active tubular secretion (e.g., acyclovir, adefovir dipivoxil, aminoglycosides [e.g., gentamicin], cidofovir, ganciclovir, valacyclovir, valganciclovir, high-dose or multiple nonsteroidal anti-inflammatory agents [NSAIAs]); may result in increased concentrations of emtricitabine, tenofovir, and/or the concomitant drug and may increase the risk of adverse effects. Concomitant use of FTC/TDF and nephrotoxic drugs should be avoided.

● Antiretroviral Agents

HIV Entry and Fusion Inhibitors

Maraviroc

No in vitro evidence of antagonistic antiretroviral effects between maraviroc and emtricitabine.

HIV Nonnucleoside Reverse Transcriptase Inhibitors (NNRTIs)

No antagonism was observed in drug combination studies of emtricitabine or tenofovir DF with efavirenz or nevirapine. In addition, no in vitro evidence of antagonistic antiviral effects was observed in drug combination studies of emtricitabine with etravirine or rilpivirine.

Efavirenz

No clinically important pharmacokinetic interactions have been observed between tenofovir DF and efavirenz.

Rilpivirine

Although not specifically studied, clinically important pharmacokinetic interactions between rilpivirine and emtricitabine are unlikely.

HIV Nucleoside and Nucleotide Reverse Transcriptase Inhibitors (NRTIs)

No pharmacokinetic interactions have been reported between the components of the fixed combination (i.e., emtricitabine, tenofovir DF). Administration of emtricitabine 200 mg once daily with tenofovir DF 300 mg once daily for 7 days in healthy subjects had no effect on the pharmacokinetics of tenofovir; a 20% increase in emtricitabine minimum concentration and no change in emtricitabine peak concentration or AUC were observed.

No antagonism was observed in drug combination studies of emtricitabine with abacavir, lamivudine, tenofovir, or zidovudine. No antagonism was observed in drug combination studies of tenofovir DF with abacavir, didanosine, lamivudine, or zidovudine.

Abacavir

FTC/TDF does not affect the pharmacokinetics of abacavir.

Administration of tenofovir DF 300 mg once daily concomitantly with a single 300-mg dose of abacavir resulted in a 12% increase in maximum concentrations of abacavir and no change in AUC of abacavir.

Didanosine

Tenofovir DF increases didanosine concentrations. Higher didanosine concentrations could potentiate didanosine-associated adverse reactions (e.g., pancreatitis, neuropathy). Suppression of CD4+ cell counts has been observed in patients receiving tenofovir DF with didanosine 400 mg daily.

In patients weighing greater than 60 kg, reduce didanosine dosage to 250 mg when it is used concomitantly with FTC/TDF. Data are not available to recommend an adjusted dosage of didanosine for adult or pediatric patients weighing less than 60 kg who are receiving FTC/TDF. When used concomitantly, FTC/TDF and delayed-release didanosine capsules (Videx® EC) may be taken under fasted conditions or with a light meal (less than 400 kcal, 20% fat).

Patients receiving FTC/TDF and didanosine should be monitored closely for didanosine-associated adverse reactions. Discontinue didanosine in patients who develop didanosine-associated adverse reactions.

Lamivudine

Emtricitabine and lamivudine should not be used concomitantly. Because emtricitabine is an analog of lamivudine, the drugs have similar resistance profiles and concomitant use provides no additional benefit.

Tenofovir

No clinically important pharmacokinetic interactions between emtricitabine and tenofovir DF have been observed.

Zidovudine

No clinically important pharmacokinetic interactions between emtricitabine and zidovudine have been observed.

Although not considered clinically important, concomitant use of emtricitabine (200 mg once daily for 7 days) and zidovudine (300 mg twice daily for 7 days) increased zidovudine peak plasma concentrations and AUC by 17 and 13%, respectively, but did not affect emtricitabine peak plasma concentrations or AUC.

HIV Protease Inhibitors (PIs)

No antagonism was observed in drug combination studies of emtricitabine with amprenavir, atazanavir, nelfinavir, or ritonavir. No antagonism was observed in drug combination studies of tenofovir DF with amprenavir, nelfinavir, or ritonavir.

Atazanavir

Tenofovir DF decreases atazanavir concentrations. Administration of tenofovir DF 300 mg once daily with atazanavir 400 mg once daily for 14 days resulted in decreases in atazanavir maximum concentration, AUC, and minimum concentration of 21, 25, and 40%, respectively. Administration of tenofovir DF 300 mg once daily with atazanavir/ritonavir 300 mg/100 mg once daily for 42 days resulted in decreases in atazanavir maximum concentration, AUC, and minimum concentration of 28, 25, and 23%, respectively. In HIV-infected subjects, addition of tenofovir DF to atazanavir 300 mg plus ritonavir 100 mg resulted in AUC and minimum concentration values of atazanavir that were 2.3-fold and 4-fold higher than the respective values observed for atazanavir 400 mg when given alone.

Atazanavir also may increase tenofovir concentrations. Concomitant administration of atazanavir 400 mg once daily for 14 days with tenofovir DF 300 mg once daily resulted in increases in tenofovir peak concentration, AUC, and minimum concentration of 14, 24, and 22%, respectively. Administration of atazanavir/ritonavir 300 mg/100 mg once daily with tenofovir DF 300 mg once daily resulted in increases in tenofovir peak concentration, AUC, and minimum concentration of 34, 37, and 29%, respectively.

When used concomitantly with FTC/TDF, use atazanavir (300 mg) given with ritonavir (100 mg). Monitor patients receiving FTC/TDF concomitantly with ritonavir-boosted atazanavir for tenofovir-associated adverse reactions. Discontinue FTC/TDF in patients who develop tenofovir-associated adverse reactions.

Darunavir/Ritonavir

Ritonavir-boosted darunavir increases tenofovir concentrations. Administration of darunavir/ritonavir 300 mg/100 mg twice daily with tenofovir DF 300 mg once daily resulted in increases in tenofovir peak concentration, AUC, and minimum concentration of 24, 22, and 37%, respectively; increases in darunavir peak concentration, AUC, and minimum concentration of 16, 21, and 24%, respectively, also were observed.

Monitor patients receiving FTC/TDF concomitantly with ritonavir-boosted darunavir for tenofovir-associated adverse reactions. Discontinue FTC/TDF in patients who develop tenofovir-associated adverse reactions.

Lopinavir/Ritonavir

Lopinavir/ritonavir increases tenofovir concentrations. Administration of lopinavir/ritonavir 400 mg/100 mg twice daily for 14 days with tenofovir DF 300 mg once daily resulted in increases in tenofovir AUC and minimum concentration of 32 and 51%, respectively, and no change in tenofovir peak concentration; no changes in peak concentration, AUC, or minimum concentration of lopinavir or ritonavir were observed.

Monitor patients receiving FTC/TDF concomitantly with lopinavir/ritonavir for tenofovir-associated adverse reactions. Discontinue FTC/TDF in patients who develop tenofovir-associated adverse reactions.

Nelfinavir

No clinically important pharmacokinetic interactions between tenofovir DF and nelfinavir have been observed.

Tipranavir/Ritonavir

Potential pharmacokinetic interaction. Administration of tipranavir/ritonavir 500 mg/100 mg twice daily with tenofovir DF 300 mg once daily resulted in decreases in tenofovir peak concentration and AUC of 23 and 2%, respectively, and an increase in tenofovir minimum concentration of 7%; decreases in tipranavir peak concentration, AUC, and minimum concentration of 17, 18, and 21%, respectively, also were observed. Administration of tipranavir/ritonavir 750 mg/200 mg twice daily for 23 doses with tenofovir DF 300 mg once daily resulted in a decrease in tenofovir peak concentration of 38% and an increase in tenofovir AUC and minimum concentration of 2 and 14%, respectively; decreases in tipranavir peak concentration, AUC, and minimum concentration of 11, 9, and 12%, respectively, also were observed.

In vitro evidence of additive antiretroviral effects between emtricitabine and tipranavir has been observed.

• Nucleoside and Nucleotide Antiviral Agents

Possible pharmacokinetic interaction (increased concentrations of emtricitabine, tenofovir, and/or the other antiviral) with antiviral agents eliminated by active tubular secretion (e.g., acyclovir, cidofovir dipivoxil, ganciclovir, valacyclovir, valganciclovir).

Famciclovir

No clinically important pharmacokinetic interactions between emtricitabine and famciclovir have been reported. Administration of a single 500-mg dose of famciclovir with a single 200-mg dose of emtricitabine resulted in no change in maximum concentrations or AUC of emtricitabine or famciclovir.

Ribavirin

No clinically important pharmacokinetic interactions between tenofovir DF and ribavirin have been reported.

• HBV Antivirals

Adefovir Dipivoxil

Possible pharmacokinetic interaction (increased concentrations of emtricitabine, tenofovir, and/or adefovir dipivoxil) due to competition for active tubular secretion.

Entecavir

Clinically important interaction between emtricitabine/tenofovir DF and entecavir unlikely. Administration of tenofovir DF 300 mg once daily with entecavir 1 mg once daily for 10 days resulted in a 13% increase in entecavir AUC and no change in entecavir peak or minimum concentrations.

• HCV Antivirals

HCV Polymerase Inhibitors

Sofosbuvir

No clinically important pharmacokinetic interactions between tenofovir DF and sofosbuvir have been observed. Administration of a single 400-mg dose of sofosbuvir with tenofovir DF resulted in an increase in tenofovir peak concentration of 25% and no change in tenofovir AUC or minimum concentration. Concomitant use of emtricitabine and sofosbuvir does not have a clinically important effect on the pharmacokinetics of either drug.

Sofosbuvir/Velpatasvir

Sofosbuvir/velpatasvir (Epclusa®) increases tenofovir concentrations. Administration of sofosbuvir/velpatasvir 400 mg/100 mg once daily with tenofovir DF resulted in increases in tenofovir peak concentration, AUC, and minimum concentration of 44–46, 40, and 70–84%, respectively.

Monitor patients receiving FTC/TDF concomitantly with sofosbuvir/velpatasvir for adverse reactions associated with tenofovir.

Sofosbuvir/Velpatasvir/Voxilaprevir

Sofosbuvir/velpatasvir/voxilaprevir (Vosevi®) increases tenofovir concentrations. Administration of sofosbuvir/velpatasvir/voxilaprevir 400 mg/100 mg/100 mg and voxilaprevir 100 mg once daily with tenofovir DF resulted in increases in tenofovir peak concentration, AUC, and minimum concentration of 48, 39, and 47%, respectively.

Monitor patients receiving FTC/TDF concomitantly with sofosbuvir/velpatasvir/voxilaprevir for adverse reactions associated with tenofovir.

HCV Replication Complex Inhibitors

Elbasvir and Grazoprevir

Clinically important pharmacokinetic interactions are not expected if emtricitabine is used concomitantly with the fixed combination of elbasvir and grazoprevir (elbasvir/grazoprevir).

Ledipasvir/Sofosbuvir

Ledipasvir/sofosbuvir (Harvoni®) increases tenofovir concentrations. Administration of ledipasvir/sofosbuvir 90 mg/400 mg once daily for 10–14 days with tenofovir DF 300 mg once daily resulted in increases in tenofovir peak concentration, AUC, and minimum concentration of 32–79, 35–98, and 47–163%, respectively.

Monitor patients receiving FTC/TDF concomitantly with ledipasvir/sofosbuvir without an HIV-1 protease inhibitor/ritonavir or HIV-1 protease inhibitor/cobicistat combination for adverse reactions associated with tenofovir. In patients receiving FTC/TDF concomitantly with ledipasvir/sofosbuvir and an HIV-1 protease inhibitor/ritonavir or an HIV-1 protease inhibitor/cobicistat combination, consider an alternative HCV or antiretroviral therapy, as the safety of increased tenofovir concentrations in this setting has not been established. If coadministration is necessary, monitor for adverse reactions associated with tenofovir.

• Methadone

No clinically important interactions have been observed between tenofovir DF and methadone.

• Nonsteroidal Anti-inflammatory Agents (NSAIAs)

Possible pharmacokinetic interaction (increased concentrations of emtricitabine, tenofovir, and/or the NSAIA), particularly with high-dose or multiple NSAIA use, due to competition for active tubular secretion. Consider alternatives to NSAIAs, if needed, in patients at risk for renal dysfunction.

• Oral Contraceptives

No clinically important interactions have been observed between tenofovir DF and oral contraceptives.

• Tacrolimus

Clinically important interactions between tacrolimus and FTC/TDF unlikely. Administration of tacrolimus 0.05 mg/kg twice daily for 7 days with tenofovir DF 300 mg once daily resulted in an increase in tenofovir peak concentration of 13% and no change in tenofovir AUC or minimum concentration; no changes in tacrolimus peak concentration, AUC, or minimum concentration were observed.

DESCRIPTION

The fixed combination of emtricitabine, and tenofovir disoproxil fumarate (emtricitabine/tenofovir DF; FTC/TDF) contains emtricitabine, an HIV nucleoside reverse transcriptase inhibitor (NRTI), and tenofovir DF, an HIV nucleotide reverse transcriptase inhibitor.

Emtricitabine is inactive until converted intracellularly to an active 5′-triphosphate metabolite. Following conversion to the pharmacologically active metabolite, the drug apparently inhibits replication of human retroviruses by interfering with viral RNA-directed DNA polymerase (reverse transcriptase). Emtricitabine is active against HIV type 1 (HIV-1) and also has some in vitro activity against HIV type 2 (HIV-2). The drug also has some activity against hepatitis B virus (HBV).

Tenofovir DF is a tenofovir prodrug and is inactive until it undergoes diester hydrolysis in vivo to tenofovir and is subsequently metabolized to the active metabolite (tenofovir diphosphate). After conversion to the pharmacologically active metabolite, the drug acts as a reverse transcriptase inhibitor antiretroviral. Tenofovir is active against HIV-1 and has some in vitro activity against HIV-2; the drug also is active against HBV.

HIV-1 isolates with reduced susceptibility to the combination of emtricitabine and tenofovir have been selected in cell culture. Genotypic analysis of these isolates identified the M184V/I and/or K65R amino acid substitutions in the viral reverse transcriptase. In addition, a K70E substitution in the HIV-1 reverse transcriptase has been selected by tenofovir and results in reduced susceptibility to tenofovir.

Cross-resistance among certain NRTIs has been recognized. The M184V/I and/or K65R substitutions selected in cell culture by the combination of emtricitabine and tenofovir are also observed in some HIV-1 isolates from subjects failing treatment with tenofovir in combination with either emtricitabine or lamivudine, and either abacavir or didanosine. Therefore, cross-resistance among these drugs may occur in patients whose virus harbors either or both of these amino acid substitutions.

A fixed-combination tablet containing emtricitabine 200 mg and tenofovir DF 300 mg is bioequivalent to a 200-mg capsule of emtricitabine and 300-mg tablet of tenofovir DF. The absolute oral bioavailability of emtricitabine and tenofovir DF is 92 and 25%, respectively; peak plasma concentrations of emtricitabine and tenofovir occur 1–2 hours and 1 hour, respectively, after administration. Food does not have a clinically important effect on the pharmacokinetics of emtricitabine or tenofovir. Administration of FTC/TDF with a high-fat meal (784 kcal, 49 g fat) or a light meal (373 kcal, 8 g fat) delayed time to peak tenofovir concentration by approximately 0.75 hours and increased tenofovir AUC and peak plasma concentration by 35 and 15%, respectively, compared with administration in the fasting state; emtricitabine exposure was not affected by administration with either a high fat or light meal. Plasma protein binding is less than 4 or 0.7% for emtricitabine or tenofovir, respectively. Emtricitabine and tenofovir DF are distributed into human milk in low concentrations. Emtricitabine is phosphorylated intracellularly and converted by cellular enzymes to the active metabolite, emtricitabine 5'-triphosphate. Metabolites of emtricitabine include 3'-sulfoxide diastereomers and their glucuronic acid conjugate. Tenofovir DF undergoes diester hydrolysis in vivo to tenofovir and is subsequently metabolized to the active metabolite, tenofovir diphosphate. Tenofovir does not undergo hepatic metabolism. Emtricitabine is excreted in urine (86%; 13% as metabolites). Elimination of emtricitabine occurs by glomerular filtration and active tubular secretion. Emtricitabine is removed by hemodialysis; it is not known whether the drug is removed by peritoneal dialysis. Tenofovir is also eliminated by glomerular filtration and active tubular secretion; following an IV dose of tenofovir, 70–80% is eliminated in urine as unchanged drug. Tenofovir is removed by hemodialysis. The median terminal plasma half-lives of emtricitabine, and tenofovir DF are 10 and 17 hours, respectively. Exposure of emtricitabine and tenofovir is increased in patients with renal impairment. Emtricitabine/tenofovir DF has not been studied in patients with hepatic impairment.

ADVICE TO PATIENTS

- Advise patients to read the FDA-approved patient labeling (medication guide).

- Critical nature of compliance with HIV therapy and importance of remaining under the care of a clinician. Stress importance of taking as prescribed; do not alter or discontinue antiretroviral regimen without consulting clinician. Advise patients that missing doses may result in development of resistance.

- Advise HIV-negative individuals taking FTC/TDF for HIV-1 PrEP of the importance of confirming that they are HIV-1-negative before starting PrEP, importance of regular HIV-1 testing during PrEP, importance of strictly adhering to recommended dosage schedule and not missing any doses, and importance of using a complete prevention strategy that also includes other measures (e.g., consistent condom use, testing [self and partners] for other sexually transmitted infections such as syphilis, chlamydia, and gonorrhea that may facilitate HIV-1 transmission).

- Advise uninfected individuals that PrEP does not protect all individuals from acquiring HIV-1 and to report any symptoms of acute HIV-1 infection (e.g., fever, headache, fatigue, arthralgia, vomiting, myalgia, diarrhea, pharyngitis, rash, night sweats, cervical and inguinal adenopathy) immediately to a clinician. Advise patients that HIV-1 resistance substitutions may emerge in individuals with undetected HIV-1 infection who are taking FTC/TDF, because FTC/TDF alone does not constitute a complete regimen for HIV-1 treatment.

- Inform patients that testing for HBV infection is recommended before antiretroviral therapy is initiated. Also advise patients that severe acute exacerbations of HBV infection have been reported following discontinuance of FTC/TDF in patients infected with HBV. Advise patients with HBV not to discontinue FTC/TDF without consulting their clinician.

- Advise patients that renal impairment, including cases of acute renal failure and Fanconi syndrome, has been reported in association with the use of TDF, a component of FTC/TDF. Advise patients to avoid FTC/TDF with concurrent or recent use of a nephrotoxic agent (e.g., high-dose or multiple nonsteroidal anti-inflammatory agents [NSAIAs]).

- Inform patients that in some patients with advanced HIV infection, signs and symptoms of inflammation from previous infections may occur soon after anti-HIV treatment is initiated. Advise patients to inform their clinician immediately of any symptoms of possible infection.

- Inform patients that decreases in bone mineral density have been observed with the use of TDF or FTC/TDF. Bone monitoring may be recommended in those with a history of pathologic bone fracture or at risk for osteopenia.

- Advise patients of risk of lactic acidosis and severe hepatomegaly with steatosis, including fatal cases. Stress importance of contacting clinician and suspending treatment if recommended if symptoms suggestive of lactic acidosis or pronounced hepatotoxicity (e.g., unusual muscle pain, shortness of breath or fast breathing, cold or blue hands and feet, dizziness or lightheadedness, fast or abnormal heartbeat, nausea, vomiting, unusual/unexpected stomach discomfort, weakness or unusual tiredness) occur.

- Stress importance of women informing clinicians if they are or plan to become pregnant or plan to breast-feed. Advise patients of pregnancy registry.

- Stress importance of informing clinician of existing or contemplated concomitant therapy, including prescription (e.g., other antiviral agents) and OTC drugs and dietary or herbal products. Advise patients that FTC/TDF may interact with many other drugs.

- Inform patients of other important precautionary information.

PREPARATIONS

Excipients in commercially available drug preparations may have clinically important effects in some individuals; consult specific product labeling for details.

Emtricitabine and Tenofovir Disoproxil Fumarate

Oral		
Tablets, film-coated	Emtricitabine 100 mg and Tenofovir Disoproxil Fumarate 150 mg*	**Emtricitabine and Tenofovir Disoproxil Fumarate Tablets**
		Truvada®, Gilead
	Emtricitabine 133 mg and Tenofovir Disoproxil Fumarate 200 mg*	**Emtricitabine and Tenofovir Disoproxil Fumarate Tablets**
		Truvada®, Gilead
	Emtricitabine 167 mg and Tenofovir Disoproxil Fumarate 250 mg*	**Emtricitabine and Tenofovir Disoproxil Fumarate Tablets**
		Truvada®, Gilead
	Emtricitabine 200 mg and Tenofovir Disoproxil Fumarate 300 mg*	**Emtricitabine and Tenofovir Disoproxil Fumarate Tablets**
		Truvada®, Gilead

* available from one or more manufacturer, distributor, and/or repackager by generic (nonproprietary) name

† Use is not currently included in the labeling approved by the US Food and Drug Administration.

Selected Revisions September 10, 2024, © Copyright, November 28, 2022, American Society of Health-System Pharmacists, Inc.

lamiVUDine

8:18.08.20 • HIV NUCLEOSIDE AND NUCLEOTIDE REVERSE TRANSCRIPTASE INHIBITORS

■ Lamivudine, an antiretroviral agent, is a human immunodeficiency virus (HIV) nucleoside reverse transcriptase inhibitor (NRTI) that is active against human immunodeficiency virus (HIV) and hepatitis B virus (HBV).

USES

● Treatment of HIV Infection

Lamivudine is used in conjunction with other antiretroviral agents for the treatment of human immunodeficiency virus type 1 (HIV-1) infection in adult and pediatric patients.

Lamivudine is commonly used as part of a dual-nucleoside reverse transcriptase inhibitor (NRTI) "backbone" of a fully suppressive antiretroviral regimen; consult guidelines for the most current information on recommended regimens. Selection of an initial antiretroviral regimen should be individualized based on factors such as virologic efficacy, toxicity, pill burden, dosing frequency, drug-drug interaction potential, resistance test results, comorbid conditions, access, and cost.

Clinical Experience

Antiretroviral-naïve Adults and Adolescents

Lamivudine has been used in dual or triple NRTI regimens that include lamivudine plus zidovudine, abacavir, and/or tenofovir.

A Cochrane review of 4 randomized clinical trials (N=2247) comparing a co-formulation of lamivudine-abacavir-zidovudine to non-nucleoside reverse transcriptase inhibitors (NNRTI)- or protease inhibitor (PI)-based regimens (including efavirenz, nelfinavir, atazanavir, and ritonavir-boosted lopinavir) as initial treatment for HIV infection found no significant differences in viral suppression between lamivudine and the NNRTI- or PI-based regimens.

Study ESS30009 was a randomized, open-label trial comparing lamivudine plus abacavir in combination with either tenofovir disoproxil fumarate (DF) or efavirenz in treatment-naïve patients. A total of 340 patients with a median baseline HIV-1 RNA level of 4.7 $\log_{10}$ copies/mL and CD4+ T-cell count of 251 cells/mm^3 were enrolled. An unplanned interim analysis of data from 194 patients with ≥8 weeks of treatment indicated a high rate of early virologic nonresponse in those receiving the triple NRTI regimen (almost 50%) versus 5% among patients given an efavirenz-containing regimen. After 48 weeks, 71% of patients in the efavirenz arm had HIV-1 RNA levels below 50 copies/mL. Based on these results, the abacavir, lamivudine, and tenofovir DF arm of the study was terminated; the ESS30009 investigators suggested that this 3-drug combination not be used. The most likely cause of this high rate of nonresponse was a low genetic barrier to resistance because of synergistic selection from all 3 NRTIs for 2 specific resistance mutations (M184V and K65R).

In an open-label, pilot study, a quadruple NRTI regimen was compared with an NNRTI-based regimen of efavirenz with lamivudine and zidovudine; both regimens had similar efficacy and tolerability.

Once-daily Versus Twice-daily Lamivudine Regimen

The comparative efficacy of a once- or twice-daily lamivudine regimen used in conjunction with zidovudine and efavirenz in an NNRTI-based regimen was evaluated in a 48-week, double-blind, double-dummy, randomized study (EPV20001) in 554 antiretroviral-naïve adults (median age 35 years, median baseline CD4+ T-cell count 362 cells/mm^3 [range 69–1089/mm^3], median baseline plasma HIV-1 RNA level 4.66 $\log_{10}$ copies/mL). Patients were randomized (in a 1:1 ratio) to receive lamivudine 300 mg once daily or lamivudine 150 mg twice daily, both with matching placebos. All patients also received efavirenz 600 mg once daily and zidovudine 300 mg twice daily. The primary outcome was the proportion of patients achieving an HIV-1 RNA level <400 copies/mL at week 48; additional outcomes included HIV-1 RNA levels <50 copies/mL, changes in CD4+ T-cell counts, and disease progression or death.

At 48 weeks, 67% of patients given lamivudine once daily and 65% given lamivudine twice daily achieved HIV-1 RNA levels <400 copies/mL. Plasma HIV-1 RNA levels were <50 copies/mL through week 48 in 61% of patients receiving the once-daily lamivudine regimen and in 63% of those receiving the twice-daily lamivudine regimen. At week 48, the median increase in CD4+ T-cell count was 144 cells/mm^3 in those receiving the once-daily lamivudine regimen and 146 cells/mm^3 in those receiving the twice-daily lamivudine regimen. The virologic failure rate was 8% in both groups. Disease progression was seen in 6 and 8% of patients in the once-daily and twice-daily lamivudine regimens, respectively.

Antiretroviral-experienced Adults and Adolescents

Although monotherapy or 2-drug regimens that include only NRTIs are no longer recommended for treatment of HIV infection, early studies evaluating the safety and efficacy of lamivudine in antiretroviral-experienced (previously-treated) patients used such regimens. These studies showed that patients who received lamivudine (150 or 300 mg every 12 hours) in conjunction with zidovudine (200 mg 3 times daily) for 24 weeks experienced greater increases in CD4+ T-cell counts than those who received zidovudine monotherapy (200 mg 3 times daily) or zidovudine (200 mg 3 times daily) in conjunction with zalcitabine (0.75 mg 3 times daily; no longer commercially available in the US).

Lamivudine was evaluated in a randomized, double-blind study (study NUCB3007; CAESAR) in 1816 HIV-infected patients (median age 36 years, median baseline CD4+ T-cell count 122 cells/mm^3, 84% nucleoside-experienced, 16% treatment-naïve). Patients were randomized to lamivudine (with or without an NNRTI) or placebo added to an existing regimen (i.e., monotherapy with zidovudine [62%] or a 2-drug regimen of zidovudine plus either didanosine or zalcitabine [38%]). Efficacy was assessed by disease progression (a new AIDS-defining event) or death over the following 12 months.

The 12-month cumulative incidence of disease progression or death was 8.9–9.6% in patients randomized to receive lamivudine (with or without an NNRTI) in conjunction with their existing regimen and 19.6% in patients randomized to receive placebo in conjunction with their existing regimen. The 12-month cumulative mortality was 2.6–3% in patients randomized to receive lamivudine (with or without an NNRTI) and 5.9% in patients given placebo in conjunction with their existing regimen.

Pediatric Patients

Lamivudine is used in conjunction with other antiretrovirals, including zidovudine, abacavir, and/or dolutegravir, for the treatment of HIV-1 infection in children 3 months of age or older and weighing at least 10–40 kg.

ACTG 300 was a randomized, double-blind trial comparing lamivudine plus zidovudine to didanosine (alone or in combination with zidovudine) in treatment-naïve HIV-1 infected pediatric patients. A total of 471 patients (median age 2.7 years [range 6 weeks to 14 years]) with a mean baseline HIV-1 RNA level of 5.0 $\log_{10}$ copies/mL and a mean CD4+ T-cell count of 868 cells/mm^3 were enrolled. The primary outcome was time to progression of HIV disease or death. Disease progression or death was seen in 6.4% of patients given lamivudine/zidovudine compared to 15.7% given didanosine at a mean duration of treatment of 9–10 months.

The ARROW study (COL105677) was a 5-year study enrolling 1206 treatment-naïve pediatric patients (aged 3 months to 17 years) initially randomized to treatment with either lamivudine plus abacavir with an NNRTI (Group A); lamivudine, abacavir, and zidovudine plus an NNRTI for 36 weeks followed by abacavir, lamivudine and an NNRTI (Group B); or lamivudine, abacavir, and zidovudine plus an NNRTI for 36 weeks followed by lamivudine, abacavir, and zidovudine (Group C). After at least 36 weeks of treatment, eligible patients (n=669) could then be randomized to either once- or twice-daily lamivudine plus abacavir, in combination with a third antiretroviral agent. At 96 weeks, HIV-1 RNA levels <80 copies/mL were seen in 70 and 67% of patients in the twice- and once-daily dosing regimens, respectively.

Clinical Perspective

Therapeutic options for the treatment and prevention of HIV infection and recommendations concerning the use of antiretrovirals are continuously evolving. Antiretroviral therapy (ART) is recommended for all individuals with HIV regardless of CD4 counts and should be initiated as soon as possible after diagnosis of HIV and continued indefinitely. The primary goals of ART are to achieve and maintain durable suppression of HIV viral load (as measured by plasma

HIV-1 RNA levels) to a level below which drug-resistance mutations cannot emerge (i.e., below detectable limits), restore and preserve immunologic function, reduce HIV-related morbidity and mortality, improve quality of life, and prevent transmission of HIV. While the most appropriate antiretroviral regimen cannot be defined for each clinical scenario, the US Department of Health and Human Services (HHS) Panel on Antiretroviral Guidelines for Adults and Adolescents, HHS Panel on Antiretroviral Therapy and Medical Management of Children Living with HIV, and HHS Panel on Treatment of Pregnant Women with HIV Infection and Prevention of Perinatal Transmission, have developed comprehensive guidelines that provide information on selection and use of antiretrovirals for the treatment or prevention of HIV infection. Because of the complexity of managing patients with HIV, it is recommended that clinicians with HIV expertise be consulted when needed.

The use of combination antiretroviral regimens that generally include 3 drugs from 2 or more drug classes is currently recommended to achieve viral suppression. In both treatment-naïve adults and children, an initial antiretroviral regimen generally consists of 2 nucleoside reverse transcriptase inhibitors (NRTIs) administered in combination with a third active antiretroviral drug from 1 of 3 drug classes: an integrase strand transfer inhibitor (INSTI), a non-nucleoside reverse transcriptase inhibitor (NNRTI), or a protease inhibitor (PI) with a pharmacokinetic enhancer (also known as a booster; the 2 drugs used for this purpose are cobicistat and ritonavir). Selection of an initial antiretroviral regimen should be individualized based on factors such as virologic efficacy, toxicity, pill burden, dosing frequency, drug–drug interaction potential, resistance test results, comorbid conditions, access, and cost. In patients with comorbid infections (e.g., hepatitis B, tuberculosis), antiretroviral regimen selection should also consider the potential for activity against other present infections and timing of initiation relative to other anti-infective regimens.

Lamivudine, an NRTI, is commonly used as part of a dual-NRTI "backbone" of a fully suppressive antiretroviral regimen. In the 2023 HHS adult and adolescent HIV treatment guideline, lamivudine is included in various regimens. Some of these lamivudine-containing regimens are listed among recommended initial regimens in certain clinical situations, and include the following: dolutegravir/lamivudine (except for HIV-1 RNA >500,000 copies/mL, chronic HBV coinfection, or before HIV genotypic resistance testing results are available), dolutegravir/abacavir/lamivudine (only in patients who are negative for human leukocyte antigen [HLA-B*5701] and without HBV coinfection), dolutegravir/tenofovir (alafenamide [TAF] or disoproxil fumarate [TDF])/lamivudine, and boosted darunavir/tenofovir (TAF or TDF)/lamivudine for individuals with prior exposure to cabotegravir pending results of INSTI genotypic testing.

In the 2023 HHS pediatric HIV treatment guideline, lamivudine is included in various antiretroviral regimens. Lamivudine is recommended as part of a preferred dual-NRTI combination for initial therapy in neonates aged birth to 1 month and includes the following regimens: abacavir/lamivudine and zidovudine/lamivudine. For pediatric patients aged >1 month to <2 years, abacavir/lamivudine is a preferred regimen as initial therapy. For patients ≥2 years of age, preferred regimens include abacavir/lamivudine. Lamivudine is also included in alternative dual-NRTI "backbone" regimens for pediatric patients (infants ≥1 month to children aged 12 years).

● *Prevention of Perinatal HIV Transmission*

Clinical Experience

Lamivudine is used in conjunction with other antiretrovirals for empiric HIV+ therapy†in neonates for prevention of perinatal HIV transmission† Lamivudine in combination with zidovudine for prevention of maternal-infant HIV-1 transmission was evaluated in an open-label, nonrandomized trial. Lamivudine was initiated at 32 weeks gestation in 445 HIV+ pregnant women, along with standard zidovudine. The HIV-1 maternal-infant transmission rate with lamivudine plus zidovudine was 1.6%, a 5-fold lower rate compared to zidovudine alone.

Clinical Perspective

In the 2023 HHS perinatal HIV treatment guideline, lamivudine is included in various antiretroviral regimens as part of a dual-NRTI "backbone." Some of these lamivudine-containing regimens are listed among preferred options for antiretroviral-naïve patients during pregnancy and include the following: lamivudine plus abacavir; tenofovir alafenamide plus either emtricitabine or lamivudine; and tenofovir DF plus lamivudine. Additionally, lamivudine is included as part of

a preferred INSTI regimen and a preferred PI regimen for initial therapy during pregnancy and as part of alternate NRTI and NNRTI regimens. For treatment-experienced patients during and prior to pregnancy, lamivudine is included as a preferred agent in various regimens.

The choice of a neonatal antiretroviral prophylaxis regimen or a neonatal empiric HIV therapy† regimen should be based on an assessment of the likelihood of perinatal HIV transmission. In the 2023 HHS perinatal HIV treatment guideline, lamivudine is included in a 3-drug regimen for neonates at high risk for perinatal HIV acquisition: zidovudine (for 6 weeks), lamivudine, and either nevirapine or raltegravir (each for 2–6 weeks).

● *Postexposure Prophylaxis following Occupational Exposure to HIV*

Lamivudine is used as an alternative regimen in conjunction with other antiretrovirals for postexposure prophylaxis of HIV infection following occupational exposure† (PEP) in healthcare personnel and other individuals.

Clinical Perspective

The US Public Health Service (USPHS) states that the preferred regimen for PEP following occupational exposure to HIV is a 3-drug regimen of raltegravir used in conjunction with emtricitabine and tenofovir DF (may be administered as the fixed combination emtricitabine/tenofovir DF; Truvada®). These experts recommend several alternative regimens that include an INSTI, NNRTI, or PI and 2 NRTIs (dual NRTIs). The preferred dual NRTI option for use in PEP regimens is emtricitabine and tenofovir DF (may be administered as the fixed combination emtricitabine/tenofovir DF; Truvada®); alternative dual NRTIs are tenofovir DF and lamivudine, lamivudine and zidovudine (may be administered as the fixed combination lamivudine/zidovudine; Combivir®), or zidovudine and emtricitabine.

Because management of occupational exposures to HIV is complex and evolving, consultation with an infectious disease specialist, a clinician with expertise in the administration of antiretroviral agents, and/or the National Clinicians' Postexposure Prophylaxis Hotline (PEPline at 888-448-4911) is recommended whenever possible. However, initiation of PEP should not be delayed while waiting for expert consultation.

● *Postexposure Prophylaxis following Nonoccupational Exposure to HIV*

Lamivudine is used in conjunction with other antiretrovirals for postexposure prophylaxis of HIV infection following nonoccupational exposure† (nPEP) after sexual, injection drug use, or other nonoccupational exposures.

Clinical Perspective

When nPEP is indicated following a nonoccupational exposure to HIV, the US Centers for Disease Control and Prevention (CDC) states that the preferred regimen in adults and adolescents 13 years of age or older with normal renal function is either raltegravir or dolutegravir used in conjunction with emtricitabine and tenofovir DF (administered as the fixed combination emtricitabine/tenofovir DF; Truvada®). Lamivudine is included as an alternative agent in conjunction with other antiretroviral agents for patients aged ≥13 years with renal dysfunction and in pediatric patients aged 2–12 years.

Consultation with an infectious disease specialist, clinician with expertise in the administration of antiretroviral agents, and/or the National Clinicians' Postexposure Prophylaxis Hotline (PEPline at 888-448-4911) is recommended if nPEP is indicated in certain exposed individuals (e.g., pregnant women, children, those with medical conditions such as renal impairment), or if an antiretroviral regimen not included in the CDC guidelines is being considered, the source virus is known or likely to be resistant to antiretrovirals, or the healthcare provider is inexperienced in prescribing antiretrovirals. However, initiation of nPEP should not be delayed while waiting for expert consultation.

● *Chronic Hepatitis B Virus Infection*

Lamivudine is used for the treatment of chronic hepatitis B virus (HBV) infection associated with evidence of HBV replication and active liver inflammation.

Guidelines from the American Association for the Study of Liver Diseases (AASLD) state that lamivudine is *not* considered a preferred antiviral for treatment of chronic HBV infection because a high rate of lamivudine-resistant HBV has been reported. The manufacturer states that lamivudine should be considered for the treatment of chronic HBV infection only when alternative antiviral agents associated with a higher genetic barrier to resistance are not available or appropriate.

Clinical Experience

Adults

Safety and efficacy of lamivudine for treatment of HBV infection were evaluated in 3 controlled studies in patients 16 years of age or older with compensated chronic HBV infection (serum HBsAg positive for at least 6 months) accompanied by evidence of HBV replication (positive for serum HBeAg and positive for serum HBV DNA as measured by a research solution hybridization assay) and persistently elevated serum ALT concentrations and/or chronic inflammation on liver biopsy compatible with a diagnosis of chronic viral hepatitis.

Trial 1 was a randomized, double-blind, placebo-controlled trial enrolling 143 previously untreated adult patients with chronic HBV. Patients were treated with lamivudine 100 mg or placebo for 52 weeks, with a primary outcome of improvement in Histologic Activity Index (HAI) score of at least 2 points. Secondary outcomes included the appearance of antibodies to HBeAg (seroconversion). Histologic improvement occurred in 55% of patients given lamivudine and in 25% of placebo-treated patients. Seroconversion occurred in 17 and 6% of patients in the lamivudine and placebo groups, respectively. Histologic response was seen in 56 and 25% of patients treated with lamivudine 100 mg and placebo, respectively.

Trial 2, a randomized, double-blind trial, enrolled 358 adults in China with chronic HBV who were randomized to treatment with lamivudine 25 mg, lamivudine 100 mg, or placebo once daily for 12 months. The primary endpoint was a reduction in Knodell necroinflammatory score by at least 2 points (histologic response); secondary endpoints included HBeAg seroconversion. Hepatic necroinflammatory activity improved in 56, 49, and 25% and deteriorated in 7, 8, and 26% of patients in the lamivudine 100 mg, 25 mg, and placebo groups, respectively. Therapy with lamivudine 100 mg daily was associated with a reduction in the progression of hepatic fibrosis compared with placebo. At 12 months, HBeAg seroconversion occurred in 16, 13, and 4% of patients receiving lamivudine 100 mg daily, 25 mg daily, and placebo, respectively. Therapy with lamivudine 100 mg daily was associated with a rapid and sustained reduction in HBV DNA (97% reduction at week 2, 98% reduction at week 52 compared with baseline) and sustained serum ALT response in 72% of patients; therapy with lamivudine 25 mg daily or placebo was associated with a 93 or 54% reduction in HBV DNA at week 52 and sustained ALT response in 65 or 24% of patients, respectively. In this study, therapy with lamivudine 100 mg daily was more effective than lamivudine 25 mg daily or placebo.

Trial 3 was a randomized, partially blinded trial with 238 adult patients randomly assigned to treatment with lamivudine 100 mg once daily for 52 weeks, placebo once daily for 52 weeks, or a regimen with lamivudine and interferon alpha-2b for 24 weeks. Histologic response, based on a reduction in HAI scores of ≥2 was the primary outcome; seroconversion was included in the secondary outcomes. Histologic response occurred in 52 or 25% of patients treated with lamivudine for 52 weeks or placebo, respectively. Seroconversion at 68 weeks occurred in 15 or 13% of patients treated with lamivudine or placebo, respectively. For the combination group, histologic response and seroconversion occurred in 32 and 9% of patients treated with lamivudine or placebo, respectively.

While therapy with lamivudine is associated with histologic improvement in most patients and is well tolerated, the optimum duration of therapy, the durability of HBeAg seroconversions occurring during treatment, and the relationship between treatment response and long-term outcomes such as hepatocellular carcinoma or decompensated cirrhosis remain to be determined. There is some evidence that the efficacy of lamivudine may not be sustained during continued therapy. Results from 52-week studies in adults indicate that HBV DNA levels decrease to below the limits of detection in the majority of lamivudine-treated patients early in the course of treatment; however, assay-detectable HBV DNA reappears during treatment in approximately one-third of those who had an initial response. Strains of HBV with resistance to lamivudine have emerged during therapy with the drug, especially during long-term treatment. Development of lamivudine-resistant HBV during treatment with the drug has been associated with decreased treatment responses evidenced by lower rates of HBeAg

seroconversion and HBeAg loss and more frequent increases in HBV DNA levels and serum ALT concentrations after an initial response. Progression of HBV infection, including death, has been reported in some patients with lamivudine-resistant HBV.

Pediatric Patients

Lamivudine is used for the treatment of chronic HBV infection in children 2 years of age or older. Safety and efficacy of lamivudine were evaluated in a randomized, placebo-controlled, double-blind clinical study in 286 children and adolescents 2–17 years of age with compensated chronic HBV infection accompanied by evidence of HBV replication (positive serum HBeAg and positive for serum HBV DNA as measured by a research branched DNA [bDNA] assay) and persistently elevated serum ALT concentrations. Loss of HBeAg and reduction of HBV DNA to below the limits of detection of the research assay (evaluated at week 52) occurred in 23% of children who received 52 weeks of lamivudine (3 mg/kg once daily; maximum 100 mg once daily) compared with 13% of those who received placebo. In addition, normalization of serum ALT concentrations was achieved and maintained to week 52 more frequently in patients treated with lamivudine (55%) compared with placebo (12%). As in the controlled studies in adults, most lamivudine-treated pediatric patients had decreases in serum HBV DNA concentrations below the limits of detection early in treatment, but about one-third of subjects with this initial response had reappearance of detectable HBV DNA during treatment. Adolescents (13–17 years of age) showed less evidence of this treatment effect than younger children.

HIV-infected Patients

Safety and efficacy of lamivudine for treatment of chronic HBV infection in patients coinfected with HIV † have not been established.

HIV-infected patients coinfected with HBV often have higher HBV viral loads and are more likely to have detectable HBeAg, lower rates of HBeAg seroconversion, and an increased risk for and more rapid progression to cirrhosis, end-stage liver disease, and/or hepatocellular carcinoma compared with individuals not infected with HIV. Decisions to initiate HBV treatment in patients coinfected with HIV and HBV and the most appropriate drugs for HBV treatment in such patients depend on various factors, including the possible effects on replication of both HIV and HBV and whether the patient is currently receiving antiretroviral therapy.

Although lamivudine is active against both HBV and HIV, it should not be used for treatment of chronic HBV infection in HIV-infected individuals who are not currently receiving antiretroviral therapy since dosages used for treatment of HBV infection are lower than those recommended for treatment of HIV infection and use of suboptimal dosages in HIV-infected individuals may allow for the selection of lamivudine-resistant HIV. In addition, the emergence of lamivudine-resistant HBV has been reported in HIV-infected individuals who were coinfected with HBV and receiving lamivudine-containing antiretroviral regimens. Although a high rate of emergence of lamivudine-resistant HBV has been reported with long-term lamivudine therapy in HBV-infected patients without HIV infection, there is some evidence to suggest that the rate of emergence of HBV resistance may be even higher in HIV-infected individuals who receive the drug. Reactivation of chronic HBV has been reported in HIV-infected patients who received long-term lamivudine therapy, and fulminant and fatal reactivation of chronic HBV infection as the result of emergence of lamivudine-resistant HBV has been reported.

Clinical Perspective

The 2018 Hepatitis B Practice Guidance from AASLD identifies preferred approaches to the diagnosis and treatment of chronic HBV. Patients testing positive on screening tests require additional testing and management of HBV. Antiviral therapies for HBV include a number of agents; preferred agents include interferons, entecavir, tenofovir DF, and tenofovir alafenamide. Lamivudine, adefovir, and telbivudine are nonpreferred agents for HBV. Treatment of patients who are HBsAg-positive depends on a number of factors, including ALT levels, hepatitis B e-antigen (HBeAg) status, and HBV DNA viral load.

Patients with HBV and HIV coinfection should be treated with antiretroviral therapy, with the regimen including 2 drugs with activity against HBV (a "backbone" regimen of TDF or TAF plus lamivudine or emtricitabine).

DOSAGE AND ADMINISTRATION

• General

Pretreatment Screening

- When lamivudine is used for treatment of hepatitis B virus (HBV), offer human immunodeficiency virus (HIV) testing prior to starting therapy.

Patient Monitoring

- When lamivudine is used for treatment of HBV, offer HIV testing periodically during therapy.
- Closely monitor for exacerbation of hepatitis in patients with HBV and HIV-1 coinfection for at least several months after stopping lamivudine treatment.
- Consider more frequent monitoring of HBV viral load when chronic coadministration of sorbitol-containing products cannot be avoided.

Dispensing and Administration Precautions

- Lamivudine is commercially available as a single entity and in various fixed-combination preparations containing additional antiretroviral agents. Refer to the full prescribing information for specific, distinct uses of the combination products. Since the antiretroviral agents contained in the fixed combination preparations also may be available in single-entity or other fixed-combination preparations, exercise care to ensure that therapy is not duplicated if a fixed combination is used in conjunction with other antiretrovirals.

• Administration

Lamivudine is administered orally once or twice daily without regard to meals.

For the treatment of HIV-1 infection, lamivudine is commercially available as an oral solution containing 10 mg/mL or tablets containing 150 or 300 mg of the drug (Epivir®, generic). The 150-mg scored tablets are the preferred preparation in pediatric patients who weigh 14 kg or more and can swallow tablets. The oral solution should be used in those unable to safely and reliably swallow tablets. Lamivudine is used in conjunction with other antiretrovirals for the treatment of HIV-1 infection.

For the treatment of chronic HBV infection, lamivudine is commercially available as an oral solution containing 5 mg/mL or film-coated tablets containing 100 mg of the drug (Epivir-HBV®, generic). The 5-mg/mL oral solution should be used in patients requiring a dosage less than 100 mg and in children unable to reliably swallow tablets.

Lamivudine preparations labeled by FDA for treatment of chronic HBV infection should not be used in HIV-infected patients because they contain a lower dosage of the drug than that required for treatment of HIV-1 infection. If such preparations are used for the management of chronic HBV infection in a patient with unrecognized or untreated HIV infection, rapid emergence of HIV resistance is likely to result because of the subtherapeutic dose and the inappropriateness of monotherapy for HIV-infected individuals.

Store lamivudine 100-mg, 150-mg, and 300-mg tablets at 25°C (excursions permitted between 15–30°C). Store lamivudine 5-mg/mL oral solution at 20–25°C and store lamivudine 10-mg/mL oral solution at 25°C.

Fixed Combinations Containing Lamivuidine

Lamivudine is also commercially available in the following fixed-combination preparations for oral use: lamivudine/zidovudine (Combivir®, generic), abacavir/lamivudine (Epzicom®, generic), abacavir/lamivudine/zidovudine (Trizivir®, generic), lamivudine/tenofovir disoproxil fumarate (Cimduo®), doravirine/lamivudine/tenofovir disoproxil fumarate (Delstrigo®), dolutegravir/lamivudine (Dovato®), efavirenz/lamivudine/tenofovir disoproxil fumarate (Symfi®; Symfi® Lo), and abacavir/dolutegravir/lamivudine (Triumeq®; Triumeq PD®). See the full prescribing information for administration of each of these combination products.

• Dosage

Treatment of HIV Infection

Adult Dosage

The usual dosage of lamivudine for the treatment of HIV-1 infection in adults is 150 mg twice daily or 300 mg once daily.

Pediatric Dosage

When lamivudine oral solution containing 10 mg/mL is used for the treatment of HIV-1 infection in pediatric patients 3 months of age or older, the recommended dosage is 5 mg/kg twice daily or 10 mg/kg once daily (up to 300 mg maximum daily dosage). Consider HIV-1 viral load and CD4+ cell count/percentage when selecting the dosing interval for patients initiating treatment with oral solution.

When lamivudine 150-mg scored tablets are used in pediatric patients 3 months of age or older who weigh 14 kg or more and are able to swallow tablets, the recommended dosage is based on weight (see Table 1 and Table 2). Data regarding efficacy of the once-daily regimen of lamivudine given as 150-mg scored tablets in pediatric patients 3 months of age or older is limited to those who transitioned from a twice-daily regimen to a once-daily regimen after 36 weeks of treatment.

TABLE 1. Twice-daily Lamivudine for Treatment of HIV-1 Infection in Pediatric Patients Weighing at least 14 kg (150-mg Tablets)

Weight (kg)	AM Dose	PM Dose
14 to <20	75 mg (half of 150-mg tablet)	75 mg (half of 150-mg tablet)
20 to <25	75 mg (half of 150-mg tablet)	150 mg (one 150-mg tablet)
≥25	150 mg (one 150-mg tablet)	150 mg (one 150-mg tablet)

TABLE 2. Once-daily Lamivudine for Treatment of HIV-1 Infection in Pediatric Patients Weighing at least 14 kg (150-mg Tablets)

Weight (kg)	Once-daily Dose
14 to <20	150 mg (one 150-mg tablet)
20 to <25	225 mg (one and one-half 150-mg tablets)
≥25	300 mg (two 150-mg tablets or one 300-mg tablet)

Although safety and efficacy of lamivudine in infants younger than 3 months of age have not been established, some experts suggest that neonates younger than 4 weeks of age† can receive lamivudine in a dosage of 2 mg/kg twice daily and infants 4 weeks of age or older† can receive a dosage of 4 mg/kg (up to 150 mg) twice daily.

Prevention of Perinatal Transmission

Pediatric Dosage

When empiric HIV therapy† is used for prevention of perinatal HIV transmission † in neonates at highest risk of HIV acquisition, a 3-drug antiretroviral regimen of zidovudine, lamivudine, and nevirapine is recommended and should be initiated as soon as possible after birth (within 6–12 hours).

For empiric HIV therapy† in HIV-exposed neonates, experts recommend that lamivudine be given in a dosage of 2 mg/kg twice daily from birth to 4 weeks of age followed by 4 mg/kg twice daily from 4–6 weeks of age.

The optimal duration of empiric HIV therapy† in HIV-exposed neonates at highest risk of HIV acquisition is unknown. Many experts recommend that the 3-drug regimen be continued for 6 weeks; others discontinue nevirapine and/or lamivudine if the result of the neonate's HIV nucleic acid amplification test (NAAT) is negative, but recommend continuing zidovudine for 6 weeks.

Clinicians can consult the National Perinatal HIV Hotline at 888-448-8765 for information regarding selection of antiretrovirals, including dosage considerations, for the prevention of perinatal HIV transmission.

Postexposure Prophylaxis following Occupational Exposure to HIV

For postexposure prophylaxis of HIV infection following occupational exposure† (PEP) in health-care personnel or other individuals, the preferred dosage of lamivudine is 300 mg once daily. Alternatively, lamivudine can be given in a dosage of 150 mg twice daily. Lamivudine is usually used with tenofovir DF or zidovudine in conjunction with a recommended HIV integrase strand transferase inhibitor (INSTI), HIV nonnucleoside reverse transcriptase inhibitor (NNRTI), or HIV protease inhibitor (PI).

PEP should be initiated as soon as possible following occupational exposure to HIV (preferably within hours) and continued for 4 weeks if tolerated.

Postexposure Prophylaxis following Nonoccupational Exposure to HIV

For postexposure prophylaxis of HIV infection following nonoccupational exposure† (nPEP) in adults and adolescents ≥13 years of age with impaired renal function (creatinine clearance 59 mL/minute or less), lamivudine is usually used in conjunction with another HIV nucleoside reverse transcriptase inhibitor (NRTI; zidovudine) in addition to another recommended agent (either an INSTI, PI, or NNRTI). Lamivudine dosage should be adjusted based on the degree of renal impairment.

The nPEP regimen should be initiated as soon as possible (within 72 hours) following nonoccupational exposure to HIV and continued for 28 days. If it has been more than 72 hours since the exposure, nPEP is not recommended.

Chronic Hepatitis B Virus Infection

Prior to and periodically during lamivudine therapy for the treatment of chronic HBV infection, the HIV status of the patient should be determined since the dosage of the drug used for the treatment of HBV infection is lower than the dosage used for the treatment of HIV infection and use of suboptimal dosages in HIV-infected individuals may allow for the selection of lamivudine-resistant HIV isolates.

The optimum duration of lamivudine therapy for the treatment of chronic HBV infection is not known.

Patients receiving lamivudine for the treatment of chronic HBV infection should be monitored regularly by a clinician experienced in the management of chronic HBV infection. During lamivudine therapy, events that may be considered as potentially reflecting loss of therapeutic response include combinations of such events as return of persistently elevated serum ALT concentrations, increasing levels of HBV DNA over time after an initial decline below the limits of detection of the assay, progression of clinical signs or symptoms of hepatic disease, and/or worsening of hepatic necroinflammatory findings. Such events should be taken into consideration when determining the advisability of continuing lamivudine therapy.

Adult Dosage

When lamivudine (100-mg tablets or oral solution containing 5 mg/mL) is used for the treatment of chronic HBV infection in adults, the recommended dosage is 100 mg once daily.

Pediatric Dosage

The recommended oral dosage of lamivudine for pediatric patients 2–17 years of age is 3 mg/kg once daily up to a maximum daily dosage of 100 mg. The oral solution formulation should be prescribed for patients requiring a dosage less than 100 mg or if unable to swallow tablets.

Hepatic Impairment

Because lamivudine pharmacokinetics are not affected by hepatic impairment, dosage adjustments are not necessary. However, safety and efficacy have not been established in those with decompensated liver disease.

Renal Impairment

Because the elimination of lamivudine may be reduced in patients with renal impairment, dosage of the drug should be decreased in those with a creatinine clearance less than 50 mL/minute. If lamivudine is used for the treatment of HIV infection in adults and adolescents weighing 25 kg or more with impaired renal function, dosage of the drug should be adjusted based on creatinine clearance (See Table 3). The manufacturer states that data are insufficient to make dosage recommendations for HIV-infected pediatric patients with renal impairment; however, a reduction in the dose and/or an increase in the dosing interval should be considered.

TABLE 3. Lamivudine Dosage for Treatment of HIV-1 Infection in Adults and Adolescents with Renal Impairment Weighing 25 kg or More

Creatinine Clearance (mL/minute)	Dosage
30-49	150 mg once daily
15-29	150 mg initial dose, then 100 mg once daily
5-14	150 mg initial dose, then 50 mg once daily
<5	50 mg initial dose, then 25 mg once daily
Hemodialysis patients	Supplemental doses unnecessary after routine (4-hour) hemodialysis
Peritoneal dialysis patients	Supplemental doses unnecessary after peritoneal dialysis

If lamivudine is used for treatment of chronic HBV infection in adults with impaired renal function, dosage of the drug should be adjusted based on creatinine clearance (See Table 4). The manufacturer states that data are insufficient to make specific dosage recommendations for pediatric patients with renal impairment.

TABLE 4. Lamivudine Dosage for Treatment of Chronic HBV Infection in Adults with Renal Impairment

Creatinine Clearance (mL/minute)	Dosage
30-49	100 mg initial dose, then 50 mg once daily
15-29	100 mg initial dose, then 25 mg once daily
5-14	35 mg initial dose, then 15 mg once daily
<5	35 mg initial dose, then 10 mg once daily
Hemodialysis patients	Supplemental doses unnecessary after routine (4-hour) hemodialysis
Peritoneal dialysis patients	Supplemental doses unnecessary after peritoneal dialysis

Geriatric Patients

Use with caution in geriatric patients because of age-related decreases in hepatic, renal, and/or cardiac function and concomitant disease and drug therapy.

CAUTIONS

● Contraindications

- Previous hypersensitivity to lamivudine.

● Warnings/Precautions

Warnings

Patients with Hepatitis B Virus and HIV-1 Coinfection

The prescribing information of lamivudine contains a boxed warning regarding the risk of severe acute exacerbations of hepatitis B in patients who are coinfected with hepatitis B virus (HBV) and HIV-1 and have discontinued lamivudine. Monitor hepatic function closely in these patients, and if appropriate, initiate anti-hepatitis B treatment. Clinical and laboratory evidence of exacerbations of hepatitis have occurred after discontinuation of lamivudine. These exacerbations have been detected primarily by serum ALT elevations in addition to the re-emergence of HBV DNA. Although most events appear to have been self-limited, fatalities have been reported. Similar events have been reported from postmarketing experience after changes from lamivudine-containing HIV-1 treatment regimens to non-lamivudine-containing regimens in patients infected with both HIV-1 and HBV. The causal relationship to discontinuation of lamivudine treatment is unknown. Monitor patients closely with both clinical and laboratory follow-up for at least several months after stopping treatment.Safety and efficacy of lamivudine have not been established for the treatment of chronic hepatitis B in subjects dually infected with HIV-1 and HBV. Emergence of HBV variants associated with resistance to lamivudine has also been reported in HIV-1-infected subjects who have received lamivudine-containing antiretroviral regimens in the presence of concurrent infection with HBV.

Differences Between Lamivudine Preparations and Risk of HIV-1 Resistance in Patients with Unrecognized or Untreated HIV-1 Infection

Boxed warnings about the different formulations of lamivudine and the risk of HIV-1 resistance in patients with unrecognized or untreated HIV-1 infection are included in the prescribing information for lamivudine. Epivir-HBV® tablets and oral solution contain a lower lamivudine dose than the lamivudine dosage used to treat HIV-1 infection with Epivir® tablets and oral solution or with lamivudine-containing antiretroviral fixed-dose combination products. Epivir-HBV® is not appropriate for patients co-infected with HBV and HIV-1. If a patient with unrecognized or untreated HIV-1 infection is prescribed Epivir-HBV® for the treatment of HBV, rapid emergence of HIV-1 resistance is likely to result because of the subtherapeutic dose and the inappropriate use of monotherapy for HIV-1 treatment. Offer HIV counseling and testing to all patients before beginning treatment with Epivir-HBV® and periodically during treatment because of the risk of rapid emergence of resistant HIV-1 and the limitation of treatment options if Epivir-HBV® is prescribed to treat chronic hepatitis B in a patient who has unrecognized or untreated HIV-1 infection or who acquires HIV-1 infection during treatment.

Other Warnings/Precautions

Lactic Acidosis and Severe Hepatomegaly with Steatosis

Lactic acidosis and severe hepatomegaly with steatosis, including fatal cases, have been reported with the use of nucleoside analogues, including lamivudine. A majority of these cases have been in women; female sex and obesity may be risk factors in patients treated with antiretroviral nucleoside analogues. Most of these reports have described patients receiving nucleoside analogues for treatment of HIV infection, but there have been reports of lactic acidosis in patients receiving lamivudine for hepatitis B. Suspend treatment with lamivudine in any patient who develops clinical or laboratory findings suggestive of lactic acidosis or pronounced hepatotoxicity, which may include hepatomegaly and steatosis, even in the absence of marked transaminase elevations.

Pancreatitis

Use lamivudine with caution in pediatric patients with a history of prior antiretroviral nucleoside exposure, a history of pancreatitis, or other significant risk factors for the development of pancreatitis. Discontinue treatment with lamivudine immediately if clinical signs, symptoms, or laboratory abnormalities suggestive of pancreatitis occur.

Immune Reconstitution Syndrome

Immune reconstitution syndrome has been reported in patients treated with combination antiretroviral therapy, including lamivudine. During the initial phase of combination antiretroviral treatment, patients whose immune systems respond may develop an inflammatory response to indolent or residual opportunistic infections (e.g., *Mycobacterium avium* complex infection, cytomegalovirus, *Pneumocystis jirovecii* pneumonia [PCP], or tuberculosis); this may necessitate further evaluation and treatment. Autoimmune disorders (e.g., Graves' disease, polymyositis, Guillain-Barré syndrome) have also been reported in the setting of immune reconstitution; however, the time to onset is more variable and can occur many months after initiation of treatment.

Lower Virologic Suppression Rates and Increased Risk of Viral Resistance with Oral Solution

Pediatric subjects who received lamivudine oral solution (Epivir®; at weight band-based doses approximating 8 mg/kg per day) along with other antiretroviral oral solutions at any time during the ARROW trial had lower rates of virologic suppression, lower plasma lamivudine exposure, and developed viral resistance more frequently than those receiving Epivir® tablets. Epivir® scored tablet is the preferred formulation for HIV-1-infected pediatric patients who weigh at least 14 kg and for whom a solid dosage form is appropriate. An all-tablet regimen should be used when possible to avoid a potential interaction with sorbitol. Consider more frequent monitoring of HIV-1 viral load when using Epivir® oral solution.

Emergence of Resistance-Associated HBV Substitutions

In controlled clinical trials, YMDD-mutant HBV was detected in subjects with on–Epivir-HBV® re-appearance of HBV DNA after an initial decline below the assay limit. Adult and pediatric subjects treated with Epivir-HBV® with YMDD-mutant HBV at 52 weeks showed decreased treatment responses in comparison with those treated with Epivir-HBV® without evidence of YMDD substitutions, including the following: lower rates of HBeAg seroconversion and HBeAg loss (no greater than placebo recipients), more frequent return of positive HBV DNA, and more frequent ALT elevations. In the controlled trials, when subjects developed YMDD-mutant HBV, they had a rise in HBV DNA and ALT from their previous on-treatment levels. Progression of hepatitis B, including death, has been reported in some subjects with YMDD-mutant HBV, including patients in a liver transplant setting and from other clinical trials. To decrease the risk of resistance in patients receiving Epivir-HBV® alone, switching to an alternative regimen should be considered if serum HBV DNA remains detectable after 24 weeks of therapy. Optimal treatment should be guided by resistance testing.

Specific Populations

Pregnancy

Lamivudine crosses the placenta and is distributed into cord blood in concentrations similar to maternal serum concentrations.

To monitor maternal-fetal outcomes of pregnant women exposed to antiretroviral agents, including lamivudine, the Antiretroviral Pregnancy Registry was established. Clinicians are encouraged to contact the registry at 800-258-4263 or https://www.apregistry.com/ to report cases of prenatal exposure to antiretroviral agents.

Data from the Antiretroviral Pregnancy Registry show no difference in the risk of overall major birth defects for lamivudine compared with the background rate for major birth defects in the US reference population of the Metropolitan Atlanta Congenital Defects Program (MACDP). Reproduction studies in rats or rabbits using oral lamivudine dosages that resulted in plasma concentrations up to approximately 35 times higher than plasma concentrations attained with the recommended human dosage used for the treatment of HIV infection in adults have not revealed evidence of teratogenicity. Although there was evidence of early embryolethality in rabbits at exposure levels similar to those observed in humans, this effect was not seen in rats at exposure levels up to 35 times higher than those in humans.

Lactation

Lamivudine is distributed into milk in humans. It is not known whether the drug affects human milk production or affects the breast-fed infant.

Because of the risk of transmission of HIV to an uninfected infant through breast milk, the HHS Panel and the US Centers for Disease Control and Prevention (CDC) recommend that HIV-infected women not breast-feed infants, regardless of antiretroviral therapy. Therefore, because of the potential for HIV transmission and the potential for serious adverse effects from lamivudine in nursing infants, women should be instructed not to breast-feed while they are receiving lamivudine.

If lamivudine is being used for treatment of chronic HBV infection, the benefits of breast-feeding and the importance of lamivudine to the woman should be considered along with the potential adverse effects on the breast-fed infant from the drug or from the underlying maternal condition.

Females and Males of Reproductive Potential

In animal studies involving lamivudine administration producing plasma levels 47–104 times those in humans, no evidence of impaired fertility and no effect on survival, growth, and development to weaning of the offspring were detected.

Pediatric Use

The safety and efficacy of lamivudine for HIV-1 (Epivir®) have been established in pediatric patients 3 months of age and older. The scored tablet is the preferred formulation for HIV-1-infected pediatric patients weighing at least 14 kg for whom a solid dosage form is appropriate; in the ARROW trial, pediatric patients who received the oral solution had lower rates of virologic suppression, lower plasma lamivudine exposure, and developed viral resistance more frequently.

The safety and efficacy of lamivudine for chronic HBV (Epivir-HBV®) in pediatric patients younger than 2 years have not been established.

Geriatric Use

Clinical trials of lamivudine (Epivir® and Epivir-HBV®) did not include sufficient numbers of subjects 65 years of age or older to determine whether they respond differently from younger subjects. Use caution when administering lamivudine to elderly patients, reflecting the greater frequency of decreased hepatic, renal, or cardiac function, and of concomitant disease or other drug therapy.

Hepatic Impairment

Pharmacokinetic parameters of lamivudine were not altered by diminishing hepatic function. Safety and efficacy of lamivudine have not been established in the presence of decompensated liver disease.

Renal Impairment

The dosage of lamivudine should be reduced in patients with renal impairment (see Tables 3 and 4). Time to maximum concentration is not significantly affected by renal function. In a trial including otherwise healthy subjects with impaired renal function, hemodialysis increased lamivudine clearance; however, the length of time of hemodialysis (4 hours) was insufficient to significantly alter mean lamivudine exposure after a single-dose administration. Continuous ambulatory peritoneal dialysis and automated peritoneal dialysis have negligible effects on lamivudine clearance. Therefore, it is recommended, following correction of dose for creatinine clearance, that no additional dose modification be made after routine hemodialysis or peritoneal dialysis. The effects of renal impairment on lamivudine pharmacokinetics in pediatric patients are not known.

● Common Adverse Effects

In the treatment of HIV infection in adults, the most common reported adverse reactions (incidence ≥15%) were headache, nausea, malaise and fatigue, nasal signs and symptoms, diarrhea, and cough. In the treatment of HIV infection in pediatric patients, the most common reported adverse reactions (incidence ≥15%) were fever and cough.

In the treatment of HBV infection, the most common reported adverse reactions (incidence ≥10% and reported at a rate greater than placebo) were ear, nose, and throat infections; sore throat; and diarrhea.

DRUG INTERACTIONS

The following drug interactions are based on studies using lamivudine. Additional drug interactions may exist for fixed-dose combination products containing lamivudine/zidovudine (Combivir®, generic), abacavir/lamivudine (Epzicom®, generic), abacavir/lamivudine/zidovudine (Trizivir®, generic), lamivudine/tenofovir disoproxil fumarate (Cimduo®), doravirine/lamivudine/tenofovir disoproxil fumarate (Delstrigo®), dolutegravir/lamivudine (Dovato®), efavirenz/lamivudine/tenofovir disoproxil fumarate (Symfi®; Symfi Lo), and abacavir/dolutegravir/lamivudine (Triumeq®; Triumeq PD®). See the full prescribing information for information on each of these combination products.

● Drugs Affecting or Affected by Membrane Transporters

Based on in vitro studies, lamivudine at clinically important concentrations is not expected to affect the pharmacokinetics of drugs that are substrates of organic anion transporter polypeptide 1B1/3 (OATP1B1/3), breast cancer resistance protein (BCRP), P-glycoprotein (P-gp), multidrug and toxin extrusion protein (MATE) 1 or MATE2-K, organic cation transporter (OCT) 1, OCT2, or OCT3.

Lamivudine is predominantly eliminated in the urine by active organic cationic secretion. Consider the possibility of interactions with other drugs administered concurrently, particularly when their main route of elimination is active renal secretion via the OCT system (e.g., trimethoprim). No data are available regarding interactions with other drugs that have renal clearance mechanisms similar to that of lamivudine.

Lamivudine is a substrate of P-gp and BCRP; however, it is unlikely that these transporters play a clinically important role in the absorption of lamivudine. Therefore, concomitant use of drugs that are inhibitors of these efflux transporters is unlikely to affect the disposition and elimination of lamivudine.

Lamivudine is a substrate of MATE1, MATE2-K, and OCT2 in vitro.

● Interferon Alfa and Peginterferon Alfa

Concomitant use of interferon alfa and lamivudine does not result in clinically important pharmacokinetic interactions.

● Ribavirin

Concomitant use of ribavirin and lamivudine does not result in clinically important pharmacokinetic interactions.

● Sorbitol

Concomitant use of sorbitol and lamivudine results in a sorbitol dose-dependent decrease in lamivudine exposures. When healthy adults received a single 300-mg dose of lamivudine oral solution alone or in conjunction with a single 3.2-, 10.2-, or 13.4-g dose of sorbitol in solution, peak plasma concentrations of lamivudine were decreased 28, 52, or 55%, respectively, and the AUC of lamivudine was decreased 20, 39, or 44%, respectively.

Concomitant use of lamivudine and sorbitol-containing preparations should be avoided whenever possible. If chronic concomitant use of sorbitol cannot be avoided in patients receiving lamivudine for the treatment of chronic HBV infection, more frequent monitoring of HBV viral load should be considered.

● Trimethoprim

Trimethoprim has been shown to increase lamivudine plasma concentrations. However, this interaction is not considered clinically important and lamivudine dosage adjustments are not needed.

DESCRIPTION

Lamivudine, an antiretroviral agent, is a human immunodeficiency virus (HIV) nucleoside reverse transcriptase inhibitor (NRTI). Following conversion to a pharmacologically active metabolite, lamivudine apparently inhibits replication of human retroviruses by interfering with viral RNA-directed DNA polymerase (reverse transcriptase). Lamivudine, therefore, exerts a virustatic effect against retroviruses by acting as a reverse transcriptase inhibitor.

Like other HIV nucleoside reverse transcriptase agents and other nucleoside antiviral agents, the antiviral activity of lamivudine appears to depend on intracellular conversion of the drug to a 5′-triphosphate metabolite; thus, 2′,3′-dideoxy,3′-thiacytidine-5′-triphosphate (3TC-TP) and not unchanged lamivudine appears to be the pharmacologically active form of the drug. 3TC-TP is a structural analog of deoxycytidine triphosphate (dC-TP), the natural substrate for reverse transcriptase (viral RNA-directed DNA polymerase). Although other mechanisms may be involved in the antiretroviral activity of the drug, 3TC-TP appears to compete with naturally occurring dC-TP for incorporation into viral DNA by reverse transcriptase. Following incorporation of 3TC-TP into the viral DNA chain instead of dC-TP, viral DNA synthesis is terminated prematurely because the absence of a 3′-hydroxy group on the oxathiolane ring prevents further 5′ to 3′ phosphodiester linkages.

Lamivudine is rapidly absorbed from the GI tract in patients with HIV or hepatitis B virus (HBV) infection. In HIV-infected patients or healthy individuals, peak plasma concentrations are achieved within 0.5–2 hours after a single dose. The absolute bioavailability of lamivudine 150-mg scored tablets and oral solution in adults is similar (86 and 87%, respectively). In a crossover study in healthy adults evaluating the steady-state pharmacokinetics of lamivudine administered in a once-daily regimen (300-mg tablet once daily) or twice-daily regimen (150-mg tablet twice daily), AUC was similar with both regimens; however, peak plasma concentrations were 66% higher and trough concentrations were 53% lower with the once-daily regimen compared with the twice-daily regimen.

The absolute bioavailability of lamivudine tablets and lamivudine oral solution is lower in children than in adults. In addition, the relative bioavailability of the oral solution is approximately 40% lower than that of the tablets in children, despite no difference between the preparations in adults. It has been suggested that lower lamivudine exposures reported in pediatric patients receiving lamivudine oral solution are likely due to an interaction between lamivudine and concomitant solutions containing sorbitol (e.g., abacavir oral solution). Data from pharmacokinetic studies evaluating once- and twice-daily lamivudine regimens in HIV-1-infected pediatric patients 3 months through 12 years of age indicate that AUCs attained with once-daily regimens were similar to those attained with twice-daily regimens when comparing the dosage regimens within the same formulation (i.e., either tablets or the oral solution). However, mean peak plasma concentrations were approximately 80–90% higher with once-daily lamivudine regimens compared with twice-daily lamivudine regimens.

Pharmacokinetics of lamivudine in pregnant women are similar to those reported in nonpregnant adults and postpartum women. Food does not appear to affect the AUC of lamivudine. In a small study in HIV-infected patients, peak plasma concentrations of lamivudine were decreased 40% and the rate of absorption was reduced when lamivudine was administered with food, but clinically important decreases in systemic availability of the drug (AUC) were not observed.

Lamivudine is distributed into CSF. In HIV-infected children who received oral lamivudine in a dosage of 8 mg/kg daily, CSF concentrations ranged from 0.04–0.3 mcg/mL and were 5.6–30.9% of concurrent serum concentrations. Lamivudine crosses the placenta and is distributed into cord blood and amniotic fluid. Lamivudine concentrations in amniotic fluid are typically twofold higher than maternal serum concentrations and have ranged from 1.2–2.5 mcg/mL or 2.1–5.2 mcg/mL when lamivudine dosage in the mother was 150 or 300 mg twice daily, respectively. Lamivudine is distributed into milk. Lamivudine is less than 36% bound to plasma proteins.

Intracellularly, lamivudine is phosphorylated and converted by cellular enzymes to the active 5′-triphosphate metabolite. Lamivudine is not substantially metabolized by cytochrome P-450 (CYP) isoenzymes. Metabolism is a minor route of elimination of lamivudine; the only known metabolite is the trans-sulfoxide metabolite. The majority of a lamivudine dose is eliminated unchanged in urine by active organic cationic secretion. Within 12 hours after an oral dose, approximately 5% is excreted in urine as the trans-sulfoxide metabolite. In single-dose studies in healthy individuals or patients with HIV or HBV infection, the mean plasma half-life of lamivudine was 5–7 hours. The plasma half-life in HIV-infected children 4 months to 14 years of age is 2 hours.

The pharmacokinetics of lamivudine are not altered in patients with hepatic impairment. In patients with impaired renal function, peak plasma concentrations, AUC, and plasma half-life of lamivudine are increased. Hemodialysis increases lamivudine clearance; however, the length of time of hemodialysis (4 hours) is insufficient to substantially alter mean lamivudine exposure after a single dose of the drug. Continuous ambulatory peritoneal dialysis and automated peritoneal dialysis have negligible effects on lamivudine clearance. There are no significant or clinically relevant racial or gender differences in lamivudine pharmacokinetics.

● Spectrum

Lamivudine is an antiviral agent that possesses in vitro virustatic activity against HIV-1 and HIV-2. The drug is also active against human HBV but appears to be inactive against other common human viruses (e.g., cytomegalovirus, Epstein-Barr virus, influenza virus, herpes simplex virus types 1 and 2, respiratory syncytial virus, varicella-zoster virus).

● Resistance

Resistance to lamivudine can be produced in vitro in cell culture by serial passage of HIV-1 in the presence of increasing concentrations of the drug, and strains of HIV-1 with in vitro resistance to lamivudine have emerged during therapy with the drug.

Cross-resistance occurs among the HIV NRTIs. HIV isolates resistant to didanosine, lamivudine, stavudine, and zidovudine have been isolated from patients who received zidovudine in conjunction with didanosine for up to 2 years.

Evidence of diminished treatment response has been reported in adult and pediatric patients with HBV infection following 52 weeks of lamivudine therapy. Lamivudine-resistant HBV develops M204V/I substitutions in the YMDD motif of the catalytic domain of HBV reverse transcriptase. These substitutions are frequently accompanied by other substitutions (V173L, L180M) that enhance lamivudine resistance or act as compensatory mutations improving replication efficiency. L80I and A181T substitutions also have been detected in lamivudine-resistant HBV.

In controlled clinical trials, YMDD-mutant HBV were detected in 19% of pediatric patients and in 24% (range: 16–32%) of adults who received lamivudine for 52 weeks. In follow-up studies of patients who continued to receive lamivudine therapy, the prevalence of YMDD mutations in pediatric patients increased from 24% at 12 months to 59% at 24 months and 64% at 36 months of lamivudine treatment. Similarly, in a follow-up study in adults, the prevalence of YMDD mutations was 18% at 1 year and 41, 53, and 69% at 2, 3, and 4 years, respectively.

Some lamivudine-resistant HBV remain susceptible to adefovir dipivoxil but have reduced susceptibility to entecavir and telbivudine. Other lamivudine-resistant HBV have reduced susceptibility to telbivudine and/or tenofovir.

ADVICE TO PATIENTS

- When used for treatment of chronic HBV infection, advise patients that the long-term benefits of the drug are unknown and that the relationship between treatment response and outcomes, such as hepatocellular carcinoma and decompensated cirrhosis, is also unknown. Explain importance of reporting any new symptoms to a clinician.

- Advise patients that lactic acidosis and severe hepatomegaly with steatosis have been reported with use of nucleoside analogs and other antiretrovirals. Explain importance of discontinuing lamivudine and notifying a clinician if symptoms suggestive of lactic acidosis or pronounced hepatotoxicity develop.

- Advise patients that an all-tablet regimen should be used when possible due to an increased rate of treatment failure among pediatric subjects who received lamivudine (Epivir®) oral solution concomitantly with other antiretroviral oral solutions.

- Advise diabetic patients receiving lamivudine oral solutions that each mL contains 200 mg of sucrose.

- Advise patients to immediately contact a clinician if they have any signs or symptoms of infection since inflammation from previous infections may occur soon after antiretroviral therapy is initiated.

- Explain that redistribution/accumulation of body fat may occur, with as yet unknown long-term health effects.

- Explain the possibility for pancreatitis in pediatric patients; advise parents or guardians to monitor pediatric patients for signs and symptoms.

- Advise patients to inform their clinician of existing or contemplated concomitant therapy, including prescription and OTC drugs and dietary or herbal supplements, as well as any concomitant illnesses.

- Advise women to inform their clinician if they are or plan to become pregnant or plan to breast-feed. Instruct HIV-infected women not to breast-feed due to risk of HIV transmission and adverse effects in the infant.

- Advise patients of other important precautionary information.

PREPARATIONS

Excipients in commercially available drug preparations may have clinically important effects in some individuals; consult specific product labeling for details.

lamiVUDine

Oral		
Solution	5 mg/mL	**Epivir-HBV®**, GlaxoSmithKline
	10 mg/mL*	**Epivir®**, ViiV
		Lamivudine Oral Solution
Tablets, film-coated	100 mg*	**Epivir-HBV®**, GlaxoSmithKline
		Lamivudine Tablets
	150 mg*	**Epivir®** (scored), ViiV
		Lamivudine Tablets (scored),
	300 mg*	**Epivir®**, ViiV
		Lamivudine Tablets

* available from one or more manufacturer, distributor, and/or repackager by generic (nonproprietary) name

† Use is not currently included in the labeling approved by the US Food and Drug Administration.

Selected Revisions April 10, 2024, © Copyright, June 1, 1996, American Society of Health-System Pharmacists, Inc.

Zidovudine

8:18.08.20 • HIV NUCLEOSIDE AND NUCLEOTIDE REVERSE TRANSCRIPTASE INHIBITORS

- Zidovudine, an antiretroviral agent, is a human immunodeficiency virus (HIV) nucleoside reverse transcriptase inhibitor (NRTI).

USES

● Treatment of HIV Infection

Oral and IV zidovudine are used in conjunction with other antiretroviral agents for the treatment of human immunodeficiency virus type 1 (HIV-1) infection in adult and pediatric patients >4 weeks of age.

Although the drug was used more commonly in the past, zidovudine is currently not recommended for clinical use to treat HIV-1 infection in most adults and adolescents due to its high risk for serious toxicities. In pediatric patients, zidovudine is a preferred component of a dual-nucleoside reverse transcriptase inhibitor (NRTI) backbone in infants ≤1 month of age and an alternative component of a dual-NRTI backbone in pediatric patients ≥1 month of age. Selection of an initial antiretroviral regimen should be individualized based on factors such as virologic efficacy, toxicity, pill burden, dosing frequency, drug-drug interaction potential, resistance test results, comorbid conditions, access, and cost. Consult guidelines for the most current information on recommended regimens.

Clinical Experience

Monotherapy

Although monotherapy and 2-drug regimens that include only NRTIs are no longer recommended for the treatment of HIV infection, early studies evaluating safety and efficacy of zidovudine for initial antiretroviral therapy in antiretroviral-naïve HIV-infected adults used zidovudine monotherapy or 2-drug regimens of zidovudine and didanosine, lamivudine, or zalcitabine (no longer commercially available in the US).

Efficacy of zidovudine as monotherapy was demonstrated in several early clinical trials, including BW 002, ACTG 016, and ACTG 019. Compared to placebo, zidovudine was more effective in reducing the risk of HIV-1 disease progression; however, ACTG 016 and ACTG 019 did not find a survival benefit associated with zidovudine monotherapy. Later trials found that the clinical efficacy of monotherapy with zidovudine was time limited.

Combination Therapy

Efficacy and safety of combination therapy with zidovudine were established in the ACTG Study 320, a multicenter, double-blind, placebo-controlled trial. A total of 1156 treatment-naïve adult patients were given zidovudine as part of a 2-drug or 3-drug regimen. The primary endpoint (development of an AIDS-defining event or death) was lower with the 3-drug regimen versus a 2-drug regimen (6.1 versus 10.9%, respectively).

Pediatric Patients

ACTG 300 was a multicenter, randomized, double-blind trial comparing zidovudine plus lamivudine to didanosine monotherapy. A total of 471 treatment-naïve pediatric patients (median age 2.7 years; mean baseline CD4+ cell count 868 cells/mm³; mean baseline HIV-1 RNA level 5.0 log₁₀ copies/mL) were enrolled. Disease progression occurred in 6.4% of patients who received zidovudine plus lamivudine versus 15.7% who received didanosine monotherapy. The risk of death was also lower in the combination therapy group compared with the didanosine monotherapy group (0.8 versus 4.7%, respectively).

Clinical Perspective

Therapeutic options for the treatment and prevention of HIV infection and recommendations concerning the use of antiretrovirals are continuously evolving. Antiretroviral therapy is recommended for all individuals with HIV regardless of CD4 counts, and should be initiated as soon as possible after diagnosis of HIV and continued indefinitely. The primary goals of antiretroviral therapy are to achieve and maintain durable suppression of HIV viral load (as measured by plasma HIV-1 RNA levels) to a level below which drug-resistance mutations cannot emerge (i.e., below detectable limits), restore and preserve immunologic function, reduce HIV-related morbidity and mortality, improve quality of life, and prevent transmission of HIV. While the most appropriate antiretroviral regimen cannot be defined for each clinical scenario, the US Department of Health and Human Services (HHS) Panel on Antiretroviral Guidelines for Adults and Adolescents, HHS Panel on Antiretroviral Therapy and Medical Management of Children Living with HIV, and HHS Panel on Treatment of Pregnant Women with HIV Infection and Prevention of Perinatal Transmission, have developed comprehensive guidelines that provide information on selection and use of antiretrovirals for the treatment or prevention of HIV infection. Because of the complexity of managing patients with HIV, it is recommended that clinicians with HIV expertise be consulted when needed.

The use of combination antiretroviral regimens that generally include 3 drugs from 2 or more drug classes is currently recommended to achieve viral suppression. In both treatment-naïve adults and children, an initial antiretroviral regimen generally consists of 2 NRTIs administered in combination with a third active antiretroviral drug from 1 of 3 drug classes: an integrase strand transfer inhibitor (INSTI), a non-nucleoside reverse transcriptase inhibitor (NNRTI), or a protease inhibitor (PI) with a pharmacokinetic enhancer (also known as a booster; the 2 drugs used for this purpose are cobicistat and ritonavir). Selection of an initial antiretroviral regimen should be individualized based on factors such as virologic efficacy, toxicity, pill burden, dosing frequency, drug-drug interaction potential, resistance-test results, comorbid conditions, access, and cost. In patients with comorbid infections (e.g., hepatitis B, tuberculosis), regimen selection should also consider the potential for activity against other present infections and timing of initiation relative to other anti-infective regimens.

Zidovudine, an NRTI, was commonly used as part of a dual-NRTI "backbone" of a fully suppressive antiretroviral regimen. In the 2023 HHS adult and adolescent HIV treatment guideline, zidovudine is no longer recommended for use in clinical practice due to its high risk for serious toxicities.

In the 2023 HHS pediatric HIV treatment guideline, zidovudine is included in various antiretroviral regimens. Zidovudine plus lamivudine or emtricitabine is recommended as a preferred dual-NRTI backbone combination for children from birth to 1 month of age. Zidovudine plus lamivudine or emtricitabine, or plus abacavir is recommended as an alternative dual-NRTI backbone combination with other drugs for infants and children ≥1 month to <6 years, and for children and adolescents ≥6 years who are not sexually mature.

● Prevention of Perinatal HIV Transmission

Oral and IV zidovudine are used for prevention of maternal-fetal HIV-1 transmission, including maternal antepartum and intrapartum therapy and post-partum therapy of an HIV-1 exposed neonate. Guidelines generally recommend zidovudine as a preferred or non-preferred alternative treatment option for these indications; consult guidelines for the most current information on recommended regimens.

Clinical Experience

Efficacy of zidovudine for the prevention of maternal-infant transmission of HIV-1 was demonstrated in ACTG 076, a placebo-controlled, double-blind, randomized trial. A total of 477 primarily treatment-naïve pregnant women infected with HIV-1 (median CD4+ cell count of 560 cells/mm³) were randomized to treatment with zidovudine or placebo; treatment was initiated orally between 14 to 34 weeks gestation (median duration 11 weeks), administered IV during labor and delivery, and administered to the newborn orally for 6 weeks following delivery. Based on evaluation of 363 infants, the risk of HIV-1 infection was 7.8% in the group that received zidovudine compared with 24.9% in the placebo group, for a relative risk reduction of 68.7%.

Clinical Perspective

In the 2023 HHS perinatal HIV treatment guideline, zidovudine/lamivudine is included as a non-preferred alternative dual-NRTI backbone component for antiretroviral-naïve patients during pregnancy. Zidovudine is also listed as a non-preferred alternative dual-NRTI backbone component for pregnant patients who are restarting antiretroviral therapy, if a current regimen is not well-tolerated or fully suppressive, or prior to pregnancy. Additionally, intrapartum IV zidovudine is recommended for pregnant patients with HIV-1 RNA levels >1000 copies/mL, unknown HIV-1 RNA levels, adherence concerns, those who are not receiving ART, and those who are diagnosed with HIV while in labor. For newborns at low-risk for perinatal HIV acquisition, a 2 to 6 week zidovudine regimen is recommended, with duration of treatment dependent on maternal HIV-1 and antiretroviral treatment status and infant age at birth. For newborns at high-risk for perinatal HIV acquisition, zidovudine is recommended as part of a 3-drug regimen, with either lamivudine plus nevirapine or lamivudine plus raltegravir for 2 to 6 weeks; zidovudine should be given for a total of 6 weeks.

● **Postexposure Prophylaxis following Occupational Exposure to HIV**

Oral zidovudine is used in conjunction with other antiretrovirals for postexposure prophylaxis of HIV infection following occupational exposure† (PEP) in healthcare personnel and other individuals.

The US Public Health Service (USPHS) states that the preferred regimen for PEP following an occupational exposure to HIV is a 3-drug regimen of raltegravir used in conjunction with emtricitabine and tenofovir DF (may be administered as the fixed combination emtricitabine/tenofovir DF; Truvada®). These experts recommend several alternative regimens that include an INSTI, NNRTI, or PI and 2 NRTIs (dual NRTIs). The preferred dual NRTI option for use in PEP regimens is emtricitabine and tenofovir DF (may be administered as emtricitabine/tenofovir DF; Truvada®); alternative dual NRTIs are tenofovir DF and lamivudine, lamivudine and zidovudine (may be administered as the fixed combination lamivudine/zidovudine), or zidovudine and emtricitabine.

Because management of occupational exposures to HIV is complex and evolving, consultation with an infectious disease specialist, clinician with expertise in administration of antiretroviral agents, and/or the National Clinicians' Postexposure Prophylaxis Hotline (PEPline at 888-448-4911) is recommended whenever possible. However, initiation of PEP should not be delayed while waiting for expert consultation.

● **Postexposure Prophylaxis following Nonoccupational Exposure to HIV**

Zidovudine is used in conjunction with other antiretrovirals as a part of preferred and alternative regimens for adult and adolescent patients with renal dysfunction, as a part of an alternative regimen for children aged 2 to 12 years, and as part of preferred and alternative regimens for children 4 weeks to <2 years of age for postexposure prophylaxis of HIV infection following nonoccupational exposure† (nPEP) after sexual, injection drug use, or other nonoccupational exposures in individuals.

When nPEP is indicated following a nonoccupational exposure to HIV, the US Centers for Disease Control and Prevention (CDC) states that the preferred regimen in adults and adolescents 13 years of age or older with normal renal function is either raltegravir or dolutegravir used in conjunction with emtricitabine and tenofovir DF (administered as the fixed combination emtricitabine/tenofovir DF; Truvada®). In adults and adolescents 13 years of age or older with impaired renal function (creatinine clearance 59 mL/minute or less), CDC recommends a regimen of either raltegravir or dolutegravir used in conjunction with zidovudine and lamivudine.

Consultation with an infectious disease specialist, clinician with expertise in administration of antiretroviral agents, and/or the National Clinicians' Postexposure Prophylaxis Hotline (PEPline at 888-448-4911) is recommended if nPEP is indicated in certain exposed individuals (e.g., pregnant women, children, those with medical conditions such as renal impairment) or if an antiretroviral regimen not included in the CDC guidelines is being considered, the source virus is known or likely to be resistant to antiretrovirals, or the healthcare provider is inexperienced in prescribing antiretrovirals. However, initiation of nPEP should not be delayed while waiting for expert consultation.

DOSAGE AND ADMINISTRATION

● **General**

Patient Monitoring

- Frequently monitor complete blood counts (CBC) to detect severe anemia and neutropenia, particularly in patients with advanced human immunodeficiency virus (HIV)-1 infection receiving zidovudine. Periodically monitor CBC in asymptomatic or early HIV-1 infection.

- Frequently monitor for hematologic toxicities in patients with hepatic impairment or liver cirrhosis.

- Closely monitor for treatment toxicities such as hepatic decompensation, neutropenia, and anemia in patients coinfected with HIV and hepatitis C who receive concomitant zidovudine and interferon alfa with or without ribavirin.

● **Reconstitution and Administration**

Zidovudine is administered orally or by intermittent or continuous IV infusion. Do *not* administer zidovudine by rapid IV infusion or injection and do *not* give IM.

When used for the treatment of HIV infection, administer zidovudine by intermittent IV infusion only until oral therapy can be substituted.

Store commercially available zidovudine capsules and oral solution at 15–25°C. Store zidovudine film-coated tablets at 20–25°C. Store commercially available zidovudine for injection concentrate for IV infusion at 15–25°C and protect from light. Following dilution in 5% dextrose injection, solutions containing 4 mg or less of zidovudine per mL are physically and chemically stable for 24 hours at room temperature or 48 hours when refrigerated at 2–8°C. However, because zidovudine for injection concentrate for IV infusion contains no preservatives, the manufacturer recommends that diluted solutions of the concentrate be administered within 8 hours if stored at 25°C or within 24 hours if refrigerated at 2–8°C to minimize the potential administration of a microbiologically contaminated solution.

Oral Administration

Administer zidovudine capsules, tablets, or oral solution without regard to meals.

Administer zidovudine oral solution to children who cannot reliably swallow an intact capsule or tablet.

IV Administration

Commercially available zidovudine concentrate for IV infusion containing 10 mg of the drug per mL *must* be diluted prior to administration. Withdraw the appropriate dose of zidovudine from the vial and dilute in 5% dextrose injection to provide a solution containing no more than 4 mg of the drug per mL.

Rate of Administration

In adults, administer intermittent IV infusions of zidovudine over 60 minutes.

In neonates, administer intermittent IV infusions of zidovudine over 30 minutes.

When used for intrapartum IV prophylaxis in pregnant HIV-infected women, administer an initial zidovudine dose by IV infusion over 60 minutes followed by continuous IV infusion at a rate of 1 mg/kg per hour.

Fixed Combinations Containing Zidovudine

For treatment of HIV infection, zidovudine is commercially available in fixed-combination tablets containing lamivudine and zidovudine (lamivudine/zidovudine; Combivir®, generic) and fixed-combination tablets containing abacavir, lamivudine, and zidovudine (abacavir/lamivudine/zidovudine; Trizivir®, generic). See the full prescribing information for dosage of each of these combination products.

● **Dosage**

Pediatric Dosage

Dosage of zidovudine in pediatric patients usually is based on body weight or, alternatively, body surface area. To avoid medication errors, use extra care in calculating the dose, transcribing the medication order, dispensing the prescription, and providing dosage instructions. Use a graduated oral syringe with 0.1 mL measurement increments to ensure accurate dosing of zidovudine oral solution in neonates. Zidovudine dosage in pediatric patients should not exceed adult dosage.

Treatment of HIV Infection in Infants and Children

For recommended weight-based dosage of oral zidovudine for the treatment of HIV-1 infection in infants and children 4 weeks of age or older weighing at least 4 kg, see Table 1.

TABLE 1. Oral Zidovudine Dosage Recommended for Treatment of HIV-1 Infection in Pediatric Patients 4 Weeks of Age or Older Weighing 4 kg or More

Body Weight (kg)	Twice-daily Dosage Regimen	Three-times-daily Dosage Regimen
4 to less than 9	12 mg/kg	8 mg/kg
9 to less than 30	9 mg/kg	6 mg/kg
30 or more	300 mg	200 mg

Alternatively, if body surface area is used to calculate dosage of oral zidovudine for the treatment of HIV-1 infection in pediatric patients 4 weeks of age or older, the manufacturer recommends 240 mg/m^2 twice daily or 160 mg/m^2 3 times daily.

Prevention of Perinatal HIV Transmission

For prevention of perinatal HIV transmission in HIV-exposed neonates, zidovudine can be used alone for prophylaxis in neonates at low risk of perinatal HIV acquisition, but is used in conjunction with other antiretrovirals for prophylaxis or empiric HIV therapy† in neonates at higher risk of perinatal HIV acquisition.

When used for prophylaxis of perinatal HIV transmission in premature neonates (gestational age less than 30 weeks), experts recommend an oral zidovudine dosage of 2 mg/kg twice daily or an IV dosage of 1.5 mg/kg twice daily initiated as soon as possible after birth (within 6 hours). At 4 weeks of age, dosage should be increased to 3 mg/kg orally twice daily or 2.3 mg/kg IV twice daily. If HIV infection is confirmed in the infant, at 8 weeks of age, dosage should be increased to 12 mg/kg orally twice daily or 9 mg/kg IV twice daily.

When used for prophylaxis of perinatal HIV transmission in premature neonates (gestational age of 30 weeks to less than 35 weeks), experts recommend an oral zidovudine dosage of 2 mg/kg twice daily or an IV dosage of 1.5 mg/kg twice daily initiated as soon as possible after birth (within 6 hours). At 2 weeks of age, dosage should be increased to 3 mg/kg orally twice daily or 2.3 mg/kg IV twice daily. If HIV infection is confirmed in the infant, at 6 weeks of age, dosage should be increased to 12 mg/kg orally twice daily or 9 mg/kg IV twice daily.

When used for prophylaxis of perinatal HIV transmission in full-term neonates (gestational age 35 weeks or more), experts recommend an oral zidovudine dosage of 4 mg/kg twice daily or an IV dosage of 3 mg/kg twice daily, initiated as soon as possible after birth (within 6 hours). If HIV infection is confirmed in the infant, at 4 weeks of age, dosage should be increased to 12 mg/kg twice daily orally or 9 mg/kg IV twice daily. Alternatively, when a simplified weight-based dosage of zidovudine oral solution containing 10 mg/mL is used in full-term neonates (gestational age 35 weeks or more), experts recommend that those weighing 2 to less than 3 kg receive 10 mg (1 mL) twice daily, those weighing 3 to less than 4 kg receive 15 mg (1.5 mL) twice daily, and those weighing 4 to less than 5 kg receive 20 mg (2 mL) twice daily.

When full-term neonates (gestational age ≥37 weeks) meet criteria for low risk of HIV acquisition (i.e., infants born to mothers who received ≥10 weeks of antiretroviral therapy during pregnancy with sustained viral suppression near delivery, did not have acute HIV infection during pregnancy, and no concerns related to maternal adherence to the treatment regimen), a 2-week zidovudine prophylaxis regimen may be used alone.

The manufacturer recommends that HIV-exposed neonates receive oral zidovudine in a dosage of 2 mg/kg every 6 hours, initiated within 12 hours of birth

and continued through 6 weeks of age for prevention of perinatal HIV transmission. The manufacturer states that neonates unable to receive oral therapy should receive IV zidovudine in a dosage of 1.5 mg/kg every 6 hours (given by IV infusion over 30 minutes) initiated within 12 hours of birth and continued through 6 weeks of age.

When empiric HIV therapy† is used for prevention of perinatal HIV transmission in neonates at highest risk of HIV acquisition, a 3-drug regimen of zidovudine, lamivudine, and nevirapine, or zidovudine, lamivudine, and raltegravir is recommended and should be initiated as soon as possible after birth (within 6 hours). Zidovudine dosage recommended for empiric HIV therapy† in neonates for prevention of perinatal HIV transmission is identical to that recommended for prophylaxis. Optimal duration of empiric HIV therapy in HIV-exposed neonates at highest risk of HIV acquisition is unknown. The lamivudine and nevirapine or lamivudine and raltegravir components of the 3-drug regimens may be administered for 2–6 weeks; recommended duration is dependent on HIV nucleic acid tests (NAT), maternal viral load at delivery, and additional risk factors for HIV transmission. If either regimen duration is shorter than 6 weeks, experts recommend continuing zidovudine alone for a total prophylaxis regimen length of 6 weeks in high-risk patients.

Clinicians can consult the National Perinatal HIV Hotline at 888-448-8765 for information regarding selection of antiretrovirals, including dosage considerations, for prevention of perinatal HIV transmission.

Adult Dosage
Treatment of HIV Infection

The recommended oral dosage of zidovudine for the treatment of HIV-1 infection in adults is 300 mg twice daily in combination with other antiretroviral agents.

The recommended IV dosage of zidovudine for the treatment of HIV-1 infection in adults is 1 mg/kg every 4 hours.

Prevention of Perinatal HIV Transmission

When the intrapartum IV zidovudine prophylaxis regimen is indicated for prevention of perinatal HIV transmission in pregnant HIV-infected women based on plasma HIV-1 RNA levels near the time of delivery, the IV prophylaxis regimen should be initiated at the start of labor (or 3 hours before scheduled cesarean delivery), regardless of the woman's current antiretroviral treatment regimen.

If the intrapartum IV zidovudine prophylaxis regimen is indicated in pregnant HIV-infected women, an initial zidovudine dose of 2 mg/kg should be given by IV infusion over 60 minutes followed by 1 mg/kg per hour for 2 hours (at least 3 hours total) given by continuous IV infusion. If an urgent, unscheduled cesarean delivery is indicated, some experts recommend administering the 2 mg/kg loading dose, then proceeding to delivery. Intrapartum IV zidovudine is indicated in pregnant HIV-infected women, regardless of the the antepartum antiretroviral regimen; if the peripartum antiretroviral regimen must be temporarily stopped for less than 24 hours, stop and restart all drugs simultaneously to minimize the development of resistance.

Postexposure Prophylaxis following Occupational Exposure to HIV

For postexposure prophylaxis of HIV infection following occupational exposure† (PEP) in health-care personnel or other individuals, the recommended dosage of oral zidovudine is 300 mg twice daily. Zidovudine usually is used with lamivudine or emtricitabine in conjunction with a recommended HIV integrase strand transferase inhibitor (INSTI), HIV nonnucleoside reverse transcriptase inhibitor (NNRTI), or HIV protease inhibitor (PI).

When lamivudine/zidovudine is used as the dual NRTI option in PEP† regimens, adults should receive 1 tablet (150 mg of lamivudine and 300 mg of zidovudine) twice daily in conjunction with a recommended INSTI, NNRTI, or PI.

PEP should be initiated as soon as possible following occupational exposure to HIV (preferably within hours) and continued for 4 weeks, if tolerated.

Postexposure Prophylaxis following Nonoccupational Exposure to HIV

For postexposure prophylaxis of HIV infection following nonoccupational exposure† (nPEP) in individuals with impaired renal function (creatinine clearance 59 mL/minute or less), oral zidovudine in conjunction with lamivudine and either raltegravir or dolutegravir is a preferred regimen. Zidovudine dosage should be adjusted based on the degree of renal impairment.

The nPEP regimen should be initiated as soon as possible (within 72 hours) following nonoccupational exposure to HIV and continued for 28 days. If it has been more than 72 hours since the exposure, nPEP may not be recommended.

Dosage Modification for Toxicity

Dosage interruption of zidovudine may be required in patients that develop significant anemia (hemoglobin levels of less than 7.5 g/dL or a reduction of over 25% from baseline) and/or neutropenia (granulocyte count less than 750 cells/mm³ or a reduction of over 50% from baseline) until bone marrow recovery is evident. In patients who develop significant anemia, dosage interruption does not necessarily eliminate the need for blood transfusions.

If marrow recovery occurs following dosage interruption, reinitiation of zidovudine therapy may be appropriate using adjunctive measures (e.g., epoetin alfa), depending on hematologic indices such as serum erythropoetin level and patient tolerance.

• Special Populations

Hepatic Impairment

Data are insufficient to recommend zidovudine dosage adjustments for patients with impaired hepatic function or liver cirrhosis. However, because plasma concentrations of zidovudine appear to be increased in patients with hepatic impairment and may increase the risk of adverse hematologic effects, frequent monitoring for hematologic toxicities is advised.

Renal Impairment

Zidovudine dosage should be reduced in patients with severe renal impairment (i.e., creatinine clearance less than 15 mL/minute). Adults maintained on hemodialysis or peritoneal dialysis or with creatinine clearance less than 15 mL/minute should receive an oral zidovudine dosage of 100 mg every 6–8 hours or an IV dosage of 1 mg/kg every 6–8 hours for treatment of HIV infection.

Geriatric Patients

The manufacturer provides no specific dosage recommendations in geriatric patients. The manufacturer states that in general, the dosage of zidovudine should be selected with caution in geriatric patients because these individuals frequently have decreased hepatic, renal, and/or cardiac function and concomitant disease and drug therapy.

CAUTIONS

• Contraindications

- History of potentially life-threatening hypersensitivity reaction (e.g., anaphylaxis, Stevens-Johnson syndrome) to the drug or any ingredient in the formulation.

• Warnings/Precautions

Warnings

Hematologic Toxicity

A boxed warning regarding the risk of hematologic toxicity is included in the prescribing information for zidovudine. Zidovudine therapy has been associated with hematologic toxicity, including neutropenia and/or severe anemia, especially in patients with advanced human immunodeficiency virus (HIV) disease. Zidovudine should be used with caution in patients who have bone marrow compromise evidenced by a granulocyte count less than 1000 cells/mm³ or hemoglobin concentrations less than 9.5 g/dL. Hematologic toxicity is related to bone marrow reserve at baseline, and to dosage and duration of therapy with zidovudine.

A decrease in hemoglobin concentration may occur as early as 2–4 weeks after initiation of zidovudine therapy. Neutropenia occurs most commonly after 6–8 weeks of therapy. Pancytopenia has also been reported, which is usually reversible after discontinuation of zidovudine.

Frequent monitoring of blood cell counts (CBCs) and indices of anemia (e.g., hemoglobin, mean corpuscular volume) are recommended during treatment with zidovudine to detect severe anemia and neutropenia, particularly in those with advanced HIV disease. Periodic monitoring of the CBC is recommended in patients with early or asymptomatic HIV infection.

Dose interruption of zidovudine, and potential transfusion, may be required in patients that develop significant anemia (hemoglobin levels of less than 7.5 g/dL or a reduction of over 25% from baseline) or neutropenia (granulocyte count less than 750 cells/mm³ or reduction of over 50% from baseline) until bone marrow recovery is evident. In patients who develop significant anemia, dosage interruption does not necessarily eliminate the need for blood transfusions. If marrow recovery occurs following dosage interruption, reinitiation of zidovudine therapy may be appropriate using adjunctive measures (e.g., epoetin alfa), depending on hematologic indices such as serum erythropoetin level and patient tolerance.

Musculoskeletal Effects

A boxed warning regarding the risk of musculoskeletal effects is included in the prescribing information for zidovudine. Myopathy and myositis with pathologic changes, similar to that produced by HIV infection, have been associated with prolonged use of zidovudine.

Lactic Acidosis and Severe Hepatomegaly with Steatosis

A boxed warning regarding the risk of lactic acidosis and severe hepatomegaly with steatosis is included in the prescribing information for zidovudine. Lactic acidosis and severe hepatomegaly with steatosis, including some fatalities, have been reported in patients receiving nucleoside analogs, including zidovudine. Most reported cases have involved female patients; obesity also may be a risk factor.

Suspend treatment with zidovudine if there are clinical or laboratory findings suggestive of lactic acidosis or pronounced hepatotoxicity (e.g., hepatomegaly and steatosis even in the absence of markedly increased serum aminotransferase concentrations).

Other Warnings and Precautions

Allergic Reaction to Latex

The vial stoppers of zidovudine concentrate for IV infusion contain dry natural rubber, which may cause allergic reactions in latex-sensitive individuals.

Use with Interferon- and Ribavirin-Based Regimens in HIV-1/ Hepatitis C Virus (HCV) Coinfected Patients

Exacerbation of anemia has been reported in patients coinfected with HIV and HCV receiving zidovudine, interferon alfa, and ribavirin concomitantly. Hepatic decompensation, sometimes fatal, has also been reported in HIV-infected patients coinfected with HCV who received antiretroviral therapy concomitantly with interferon alfa with or without ribavirin. Closely monitor for signs of toxicity (e.g., hepatic decompensation, neutropenia, anemia) in patients receiving concomitant zidovudine and interferon alfa with or without ribavirin.

Concomitant use of ribavirin and zidovudine is not recommended. Consider replacing zidovudine in established HIV-1/HCV regimens, particularly in those patients with a known history of anemia caused by zidovudine.

Discontinue zidovudine as medically necessary. Also consider dosage reduction or discontinuation of interferon alfa, ribavirin, or both agents, if worsening toxicity, including hepatic decompensation (e.g., Child Pugh score of over 6) occurs.

Immune Reconstitution Syndrome

During initial treatment, patients who respond to antiretroviral therapy may develop an inflammatory response to indolent or residual opportunistic infections (e.g., Mycobacterium avium complex [MAC], M. tuberculosis, cytomegalovirus [CMV], Pneumocystis jirovecii [formerly P. carinii]); this may necessitate further evaluation and treatment.

Autoimmune disorders (e.g., Graves' disease, polymyositis, Guillain-Barré syndrome) have also been reported to occur in the setting of immune reconstitution; however, the time to onset is more variable and can occur many months after initiation of antiretroviral therapy.

Lipodystrophy

Zidovudine treatment has been associated with lipoatrophy (loss of subcutaneous fat); the incidence and severity of this effect are related to cumulative exposure to the drug. Fat loss, which is most evident in the face, limbs, and buttocks, may be only partially reversible and improvement may take months to years after switching to an antiretroviral regimen that does not contain zidovudine. Patients receiving zidovudine should be regularly assessed for signs of lipoatrophy. If fat loss is suspected, therapy should be switched to an alternative antiretroviral regimen if feasible.

Specific Populations

Pregnancy

Zidovudine crosses the human placenta and concentrations in neonatal plasma at birth were equivalent to maternal plasma concentrations. In neonates and infants exposed to zidovudine in utero, cases of mild and transient serum lactate elevations, possibly due to mitochondrial dysfunction, have been reported; the clinical significance of these elevations is unknown. There have also been few reports of seizures, developmental delays, and other neurological disorders; however, a causal relationship of zidovudine exposure in utero or during the peri-partum phase with these events has not been established.

To monitor maternal-fetal outcomes of pregnant women exposed to antiretroviral agents, including zidovudine, the Antiretroviral Pregnancy Registry was established. Clinicians are encouraged to contact the registry at 800-258-4263 or http://www.APRegistry.com to enroll such women.

Data from the Antiretroviral Pregnancy Registry show no difference in the overall risk of birth defects for zidovudine compared with the background rate for birth defects in the US reference population of the Metropolitan Atlanta Congenital Defects Program (MACDP). Registry data include over 13,000 prospective reports of zidovudine exposures during pregnancy resulting in live births, including over 4000 first trimester exposures to the drug.

Lactation

Zidovudine is distributed into human milk. The effects of zidovudine on milk production, or on the breast-fed infant are not known.

Because of the risk of transmission of HIV to an uninfected infant through breast milk, the US Centers for Disease Control and Prevention (CDC) recommend that HIV-infected women *not* breast-feed infants.

Pediatric Use

Pharmacokinetics of zidovudine in pediatric patients older than 3 months of age are similar to those reported in adults. Zidovudine pharmacokinetics in neonates 2 weeks of age and younger are substantially different from neonates over 2 weeks of age

Geriatric Use

While clinical experience to date has not revealed age-related differences in response to zidovudine, clinical studies evaluating zidovudine have not included sufficient numbers of adults 65 years of age or older to determine whether geriatric patients respond differently than younger adults.

Zidovudine should be used with caution in geriatric patients because these individuals frequently have decreased hepatic, renal, and/or cardiac function and concomitant disease and drug therapy.

Hepatic Impairment

Zidovudine is primarily eliminated via hepatic metabolism. Because plasma concentrations of zidovudine appear to be increased in patients with hepatic impairment and may increase the risk of adverse hematologic effects, frequent monitoring for hematologic toxicities is advised.

Renal Impairment

Unchanged zidovudine and its glucuronide metabolite primarily undergo renal excretion. In patients with severe renal impairment (creatinine clearance less than 15 mL/minute), zidovudine exposure based on AUC and the elimination half-life are increased in comparison to normal renal function. The elimination half-life of zidovudine in severe renal impairment averages approximately 1.4 hours.

• Common Adverse Effects

Adverse reactions occurring in 15% or more of adult patients receiving zidovudine for HIV-1 in clinical trials include headache, malaise, nausea, vomiting, and anorexia. In pediatric patients receiving zidovudine for HIV-1 in clinical trials, fever and cough were the most commonly reported adverse reactions, occurring in 15% or more of patients. In neonates who received zidovudine for the prevention of maternal-fetal transmission of HIV-1, the most common adverse reaction was anemia (incidence of 15% or greater).

Adverse systemic effects reported with IV zidovudine are similar to those reported with oral zidovudine. However, long-term IV zidovudine therapy (i.e., longer than 2–4 weeks) has not been evaluated in adults and may enhance adverse hematologic effects.

DRUG INTERACTIONS

The following drug interactions are based on studies using single-entity zidovudine. When a fixed combination containing zidovudine is used, interactions associated with each drug in the fixed combination should be considered.

• Atovaquone

Concomitant use of zidovudine (200 mg every 8 hours) and atovaquone (750 mg every 12 hours with food) in 14 human immunodeficiency virus (HIV)-infected adults increased the AUC of zidovudine by about 31% (range 23–78% increase), and did not affect the pharmacokinetics of atovaquone.

Routine zidovudine dosage adjustments are not warranted in patients receiving zidovudine concomitantly with atovaquone.

• Clarithromycin

Concomitant use of clarithromycin (500 mg twice daily) and zidovudine (100 mg every 4 hours for 7 days) decreased the AUC of zidovudine by 12% (range 34% decrease to 14% increase).

Routine zidovudine dosage adjustments are not warranted in patients receiving zidovudine and clarithromycin concomitantly.

• Doxorubicin

Because there is in vitro evidence that doxorubicin antagonizes the antiretroviral activity of zidovudine, concomitant use of doxorubicin and zidovudine should be avoided.

• Fluconazole

Concomitant use of zidovudine (200 mg every 8 hours) and fluconazole (400 mg daily) increased the AUC of zidovudine by 74% (range 54–98% increase).

The manufacturer of zidovudine states that routine zidovudine dosage adjustments are not warranted in patients receiving concomitant fluconazole.

• HIV Protease Inhibitors

Concomitant use of zidovudine (single 200-mg dose) and nelfinavir (750 mg every 8 hours for 7–10 days) resulted in a 35% decrease in the AUC of zidovudine (range 28–41% decrease); concentrations of nelfinavir were not affected by concomitant zidovudine.

Routine zidovudine dosage adjustments are not warranted in patients receiving zidovudine and nelfinavir concomitantly.

Concomitant use of oral zidovudine (200 mg every 8 hours) and oral ritonavir (300 mg every 6 hours) for 4 days decreased the AUC of zidovudine by 25% (range 15–34% decrease), but did not affect the pharmacokinetics of ritonavir.

Dosage adjustments are not necessary in patients receiving zidovudine and ritonavir concomitantly.

• Ganciclovir

Concomitant use of zidovudine and ganciclovir may increase the hematologic toxicity of zidovudine.

● **Interferon Alfa**

Concomitant use of interferon alfa and zidovudine can increase the risk of hematologic (e.g., neutropenia, thrombocytopenia) and hepatic toxicity. Potentially fatal hepatic decompensation has been reported in HIV-infected patients coinfected with hepatitis C virus (HCV) who received antiretroviral therapy concomitantly with interferon alfa with or without ribavirin. Patients receiving zidovudine with interferon alfa with or without ribavirin should be closely monitored for toxicities, especially hepatic decompensation, neutropenia, and anemia. Consider discontinuation of zidovudine as medically appropriate. If worsening toxicities (e.g., hepatic decompensation with Child-Pugh scores greater than 6) occur, consider immediate discontinuation or dosage reduction of interferon alfa and/or ribavirin.

● **Lamivudine**

Concomitant use of lamuvidine (300 mg every 12 hours) and oral zidovudine (single 200-mg dose) resulted in a 13% increase in the AUC of zidovudine (range 2–27% increase), but did not affect concentrations of lamivudine.

The manufacturer of zidovudine states that routine zidovudine dosage adjustments are not warranted in patients receiving concomitant lamivudine.

● **Methadone**

Concomitant use of methadone (30–90 mg daily) and oral zidovudine (200 mg every 4 hours) resulted in an 43% increase in the AUC of zidovudine (range 16-64% increase), but did not affect the pharmacokinetics of methadone.

The manufacturer of zidovudine states that routine zidovudine dosage adjustments are not warranted in patients receiving concomitant methadone.

● **Myelosuppressive Agents**

Drugs that are cytotoxic or myelosuppressive (e.g., ganciclovir, interferon alfa, ribavirin) may increase the risk of hematologic toxicity of zidovudine.

● **Phenytoin**

Decreased plasma phenytoin concentrations have been reported in some patients receiving concomitant zidovudine and, in at least one patient, an increased phenytoin concentration was reported.

In one study in adults with HIV infection receiving oral zidovudine therapy (200 mg every 4 hours), administration of a single 300-mg dose of phenytoin resulted in a 30% decrease in clearance of zidovudine; pharmacokinetics of phenytoin were not affected.

● **Probenecid**

Concomitant use of probenecid (500 mg every 6 hours for 2 days) and zidovudine (2 mg/kg every 8 hours for 3 days) increased the AUC of zidovudine by 106% (range 100–170% increase).

The manufacturer of zidovudine states that routine zidovudine dosage adjustments are not warranted if probenecid and zidovudine are used concomitantly.

● **Rifampin**

Concomitant use of zidovudine (200 mg every 8 hours) and rifampin (600 mg once daily) for 14 days resulted in a 47% decrease in zidovudine AUC (range 41–53% decrease).

The manufacturer of zidovudine states that routine dosage adjustments are not necessary if rifampin and zidovudine are used concomitantly.

● **Ribavirin**

The manufacturers of zidovudine state that the concomitant use of zidovudine and ribavirin is not recommended and should be avoided. If zidovudine and ribavirin are used concomitantly, closely monitor for virologic response and toxicities such as hepatic decompensation, neutropenia, and anemia.

In vitro, ribavirin antagonizes the antiviral activity of zidovudine against HIV. This antagonism appears to result from the inhibition of zidovudine phosphorylation. Despite this antagonism, no evidence of pharmacokinetic or pharmacodynamic (e.g., loss of virologic suppression of HIV or HCV) interactions were observed when ribavirin and zidovudine were given concomitantly to HIV-1 and HCV-coinfected patients, although exacerbation of anemia from ribavirin has been reported when zidovudine is used concomitantly.

● **Valproic Acid**

Concomitant use of valproic acid (250 or 500 mg every 8 hours) and oral zidovudine (100 mg every 8 hours) for 4 days in 6 HIV-infected adults resulted in an 80% increase in the AUC of zidovudine. The effect of concomitant zidovudine on the pharmacokinetics of valproic acid was not evaluated. Severe anemia has been reported following initiation of valproic acid therapy (500 mg twice daily) in an HIV-infected adult who was receiving an antiretroviral regimen that contained zidovudine, lamivudine, and abacavir; the patient had stable hematologic status at the time valproic acid was started.

The manufacturer of zidovudine states that routine zidovudine dosage adjustments are not warranted in patients receiving zidovudine and valproic acid concomitantly.

DESCRIPTION

Zidovudine is a human immunodeficiency virus (HIV) nucleoside reverse transcriptase inhibitor (NRTI). Following conversion to a pharmacologically active metabolite, zidovudine inhibits replication of HIV by interfering with viral RNA-directed DNA polymerase (reverse transcriptase). Like other HIV NRTIs, the antiviral activity of zidovudine appears to depend on intracellular conversion of the drug to a triphosphate metabolite. Zidovudine 5'-triphosphate and not unchanged zidovudine appears to be the pharmacologically active form of the drug.

Zidovudine has a limited spectrum of antiviral activity. Following intracellular conversion to a pharmacologically active metabolite, the drug is active in vitro against HIV type 1. The antiretroviral activity of zidovudine has been evaluated in vitro in cell culture systems, including monocytes and human blood lymphocytes.

HIV type 1 strains with reduced susceptibility or resistance to zidovudine have been selected in vitro in cell culture and also have emerged during therapy with the drug. Genotypic analyses of isolates selected in cell culture and recovered from zidovudine-treated patients showed thymidine analog mutations (TAMs) in the HIV-1 reverse transcriptase that include M41L, D67N, K70R, L210W, T215Y or F, and K219E/R/H/Q/N/Q. The degree of zidovudine resistance appears to depend on the number and combination of these mutations. Cross-resistance has been reported among the HIV NRTIs. TAM substitutions in HIV-1 reverse transcriptase selected by zidovudine can confer cross-resistance to abacavir, didanosine, and tenofovir.

Following IV infusion of zidovudine, dose-independent pharmacokinetics are observed over the dosage range of 1–5 mg/kg. Zidovudine is rapidly absorbed from the GI tract, with peak serum concentrations generally occurring within 0.5–1.5 hours after an oral dose of the drug. In fasting adults, mean oral bioavailability of zidovudine is 64%. In pediatric patients, mean oral bioavailability is 61% in infants 14 days to 3 months of age and 65% in pediatric patients 3 months to 12 years of age. Bioavailability is greater in neonates 14 days old or younger and is reported to be 89%. Systemic exposure of zidovudine following administration of zidovudine tablets or oral solution is equivalent to that following administration of the capsules. In children 3 months to 12 years of age, zidovudine appears to have dose-dependent increases in plasma concentrations after administration of an oral solution over the dosage range of 90–240 mg/m^2 every 6 hours. Zidovudine is distributed into CSF following oral or IV administration. The drug is less than 38% bound to plasma proteins. Zidovudine primarily undergoes elimination via hepatic metabolism. Following oral administration of zidovudine, 14% of the total dose is excreted in urine as unchanged zidovudine and 74% as the major metabolite, 3'-azido-3'-deoxy-5'- O -β- D -glucopyranuronosylthymidine (GZDV). Following IV administration, 18% of the total dose is excreted in the urine as unchanged zidovudine, and 60% as GZDV. The plasma half-life of zidovudine in adults averages approximately 0.5–3 hours following oral or IV administration. The plasma half-life of zidovudine in neonates and infants averages approximately 3.1 hours in neonates up to 14 days of age, 1.9 hours in infants 14 days to 3 months of age, and 1.5 hours in pediatric patients 3 months to 12 years of age. Zidovudine clearance is decreased and plasma concentrations are increased in patients with hepatic impairment. Hemodialysis and peritoneal dialysis appear to have a negligible effect on removal of zidovudine, but may enhance elimination of GZDV. Results of a limited single-dose study indicate that sex does not affect the pharmacokinetics of zidovudine.

ADVICE TO PATIENTS

- Inform patients that neutropenia and/or anemia are the major toxicities reported with zidovudine and that the frequency and severity are greater in patients with more advanced HIV disease and in those who initiate therapy later in the course of their infection. Importance of CBC monitoring, especially in patients with advanced symptomatic HIV disease. Advise patients that if hematologic toxicity develops, transfusions or discontinuance of the drug may be required.

- Inform patients that potentially life-threatening hypersensitivity reactions (e.g., anaphylaxis, Stevens-Johnson syndrome) have been reported in patients receiving zidovudine. Importance of immediately contacting a clinician if rash develops since this may be a sign of a more serious reaction.

- Advise latex-sensitive patients that vial stoppers of zidovudine concentrate for IV infusion contain dry natural rubber (a latex derivative), which may cause allergic reactions in individuals sensitive to latex.

- Inform patients that myopathy and myositis with pathological changes, similar to that produced by HIV-1 disease, have been associated with prolonged use of zidovudine.

- Advise patients that lactic acidosis and severe hepatomegaly with steatosis have been reported with use of nucleoside analogs and other antiretrovirals. Importance of discontinuing zidovudine and notifying a clinician if symptoms suggestive of lactic acidosis or pronounced hepatotoxicity develop.

- Inform HIV-infected patients coinfected with HCV that hepatic decompensation (sometimes fatal) has been reported when antiretrovirals were used for treatment of HIV infection in patients receiving interferon alfa with or without ribavirin.

- Inform patients that myopathy and myositis with pathologic changes have been reported in individuals who received long-term zidovudine therapy.

- Advise patients to immediately contact a clinician if they have any signs or symptoms of infection since inflammation from previous infections may occur soon after antiretroviral therapy is initiated.

- Inform patients that loss of subcutaneous fat may occur in patients receiving zidovudine and that they will be regularly assessed for this effect during therapy.

- Advise caregivers to use an appropriate-sized oral syringe with 0.1 mL graduations in neonates to ensure the accurate dosing of zidovudine oral solution.

- Instruct patients that if they miss a dose of zidovudine, to take it as soon as they remember. Advise patients not to double their next dose or take more than the prescribed dose.

- Importance of informing clinician of existing or contemplated concomitant therapy, including prescription (e.g., ganciclovir, interferon alfa, ribavirin) and OTC drugs and dietary or herbal products, and any concomitant illnesses.

- Importance of women informing clinicians if they are or plan to become pregnant or plan to breast-feed. Inform pregnant women considering the use of zidovudine during pregnancy for prevention of HIV transmission to their infants that transmission may still occur in some cases despite therapy. Advise patients that there is a pregnancy exposure registry that monitors pregnancy outcomes in women exposed to zidovudine during pregnancy. Advise HIV-infected women not to breast-feed because HIV can be passed to the baby in the breast milk.

- Inform patients of other important precautionary information.

PREPARATIONS

Excipients in commercially available drug preparations may have clinically important effects in some individuals; consult specific product labeling for details.

Zidovudine

Oral		
Capsules	100 mg*	Retrovir®, ViiV
		Zidovudine Capsules
Solution	10 mg/mL*	Retrovir® Oral Solution, ViiV
		Zidovudine Oral Solution
Tablets, film-coated	300 mg*	Zidovudine Tablets
Parenteral		
For injection concentrate, for IV infusion only	10 mg/mL*	Retrovir® Injection, ViiV
		Zidovudine for Injection
		Concentrate

* available from one or more manufacturer, distributor, and/or repackager by generic (nonproprietary) name

† Use is not currently included in the labeling approved by the US Food and Drug Administration.

Selected Revisions June 10, 2024, © Copyright, June 1, 1987, American Society of Health-System Pharmacists, Inc.

Oseltamivir Phosphate

8:18.28 • NEURAMINIDASE INHIBITORS

■ Oseltamivir phosphate is a prodrug of oseltamivir carboxylate, a sialic acid analog and neuraminidase inhibitor antiviral that is pharmacologically related to zanamivir and active against influenza A and B viruses.

USES

● *Treatment of Seasonal Influenza A and B Virus Infections*

Oseltamivir is used for the *treatment* of acute, uncomplicated illness caused by influenza A or B viruses in adults, adolescents, and pediatric patients 2 weeks of age or older. Although safety and efficacy have not been established in neonates younger than 2 weeks of age†, oseltamivir also is recommended when *treatment* of influenza is necessary in this age group.

For the treatment of suspected or confirmed acute, uncomplicated seasonal influenza in otherwise healthy outpatients, the US Centers for Disease Control and Prevention (CDC), Infectious Diseases Society of America (IDSA), and other experts state that any age-appropriate influenza antiviral (oral oseltamivir, inhaled zanamivir, oral baloxavir marboxil, IV peramivir) can be used if not contraindicated. CDC states that early empiric antiviral treatment can be considered in outpatients with suspected influenza (e.g., influenza-like illness such as fever with either cough or sore throat) based on clinical judgement if such treatment can be initiated within 48 hours of illness onset.

For the treatment of suspected or confirmed seasonal influenza in hospitalized patients or outpatients with severe, complicated, or progressive illness (e.g., pneumonia, exacerbation of underlying chronic medical conditions), CDC states that oseltamivir is the preferred influenza antiviral and should be initiated as soon as possible, ideally within 48 hours, without waiting for laboratory confirmation. Oseltamivir is the preferred influenza antiviral in hospitalized patients or outpatients with severe, complicated, or progressive influenza because of the lack of data regarding use of other influenza antivirals in such patients. Although controlled clinical trials evaluating oseltamivir for the treatment of influenza generally only included patients with acute, uncomplicated influenza illness, observational studies indicate that oseltamivir reduces severe clinical outcomes in patients hospitalized with influenza. Limited data suggest that oral oseltamivir usually is well absorbed in critically ill influenza patients, including patients in intensive care units and those requiring continuous renal replacement therapy and/or extracorporeal membrane oxygenation, but there have been reports of suspected decreased oral absorption of the drug in patients with decreased gastric motility or GI bleeding. In patients with severe influenza who cannot tolerate or absorb oseltamivir administered orally or enterically (e.g., because of suspected or known gastric stasis, malabsorption, or GI bleeding), CDC states that use of IV peramivir may be considered.

CDC and American Academy of Pediatrics (AAP) recommend antiviral treatment of seasonal influenza illness as soon as possible in all individuals with suspected or confirmed influenza if they require hospitalization or have severe, complicated, or progressive illness (regardless of vaccination status or underlying illness). These experts also recommend early empiric antiviral treatment in individuals with suspected or confirmed influenza of any severity who are at high risk for influenza-related complications because of age or underlying medical conditions (regardless of vaccination status). Individuals at increased risk for influenza-related complications include children younger than 2 years of age; adults 65 years of age or older; individuals of any age with chronic pulmonary (including asthma), cardiovascular (except hypertension alone), renal, hepatic, hematologic (including sickle cell disease), or metabolic disorders (including diabetes mellitus); individuals with neurologic and neurodevelopmental conditions (including disorders of the brain, spinal cord, peripheral nerve, and muscle such as cerebral palsy, epilepsy [seizure disorders], stroke, intellectual disability [mental retardation], moderate to severe developmental delay, muscular dystrophy, or spinal cord injury); individuals with immunosuppression (including that caused by medications or human immunodeficiency virus [HIV] infection); women who are pregnant or up to 2 weeks postpartum; individuals younger than 19 years of age

receiving long-term aspirin therapy; American Indians or Alaskan natives; morbidly obese individuals with a body mass index (BMI) of 40 or greater; and residents of any age in nursing homes or other long-term care facilities.

When treatment of seasonal influenza is indicated, an appropriate antiviral should be initiated as soon as possible after illness onset (ideally within 48 hours), and should *not* be delayed while waiting for laboratory confirmation. The manufacturer states that oseltamivir should be used for the treatment of influenza only in patients who have been symptomatic for no more than 48 hours. However, although clinical benefit is greatest when oseltamivir is initiated within 48 hours of onset of influenza symptoms, there is some evidence from observational studies of hospitalized patients that antiviral treatment may still be beneficial when initiated up to 4 or 5 days after illness onset. Therefore, CDC and AAP recommend that antiviral treatment be initiated in all patients with severe, complicated, or progressive illness attributable to influenza and all hospitalized patients and patients at increased risk of influenza complications (either hospitalized or outpatient) who have suspected or confirmed influenza, even if it has been more than 48 hours after illness onset. Decisions regarding use of empiric antiviral treatment in outpatients, especially high-risk patients, should be based on disease severity and progression, age, underlying medical conditions, likelihood of influenza, and time since onset of symptoms.

Influenza and coronavirus disease 2019 (COVID-19) caused by severe acute respiratory syndrome coronavirus 2 (SARS-CoV-2) have overlapping signs and symptoms and coinfection with influenza A or B viruses and SARS-CoV-2 can occur and should be considered, particularly in hospitalized patients with severe respiratory disease. Although laboratory testing can help distinguish between influenza virus infection and SARS-CoV-2 infection, CDC recommends that empiric influenza treatment should be initiated in patients with suspected influenza who are hospitalized, have severe, complicated, or progressive illness, or are at high risk for influenza complication without waiting for results of influenza testing, SARS-CoV-2 testing, or multiplex molecular assays that detect influenza A and B viruses and SARS-CoV-2.

Viral surveillance data available from local and state health departments and CDC should be considered when selecting an antiviral for treatment of seasonal influenza. Strains of circulating influenza viruses and the antiviral susceptibility of these strains constantly evolve, and emergence of resistant strains may decrease effectiveness of influenza antivirals. Although circulating influenza A and B viruses during recent years generally have been susceptible to oseltamivir, clinicians should consult the most recent information on susceptibility of circulating viruses when selecting an antiviral for the treatment of influenza.

CDC issues recommendations concerning the use of antivirals for the treatment of influenza, and these recommendations are updated as needed during each influenza season. Information regarding influenza surveillance and updated recommendations for treatment of seasonal influenza are available from CDC at http://www.cdc.gov/flu.

Clinical Trials and Experience

Adults and Adolescents

Efficacy of oseltamivir for the treatment of seasonal influenza in adults 18 years of age or older has been established in randomized placebo-controlled studies in which the predominant influenza infection was influenza A; only a limited number of adults in studies to date have been infected with influenza B. When initiated within 40 hours of onset of symptoms in otherwise healthy adults 18–65 years of age with uncomplicated influenza, the drug has decreased the severity of influenza symptoms (i.e., nasal congestion, sore throat, cough, aches, fatigue, headache, chills/sweats) and shortened the average duration of these symptoms by about 1.3 days. When used in geriatric patients 65 years of age or older, oseltamivir has reduced the time to symptom improvement by 1 day.

Analysis of data from several studies indicated that adults who received oseltamivir for seasonal influenza had a lower incidence of respiratory complications requiring anti-infective therapy and hospitalization. Individuals who initiate therapy sooner (i.e., no later than 24 hours after symptom onset) exhibit greater benefit (e.g., a 2-day decrease in symptom duration). Oseltamivir therapy also has reduced the magnitude and duration of viral replication.

Efficacy and safety of oseltamivir for the treatment of seasonal influenza in adolescents 13–17 years of age are supported by data from adequate and well-controlled trials in adults, adolescents, and younger pediatric patients and safety data in adolescents.

Children 1–12 Years of Age

Efficacy and safety of oseltamivir for the treatment of seasonal influenza in children 1–12 years of age was established in a double-blind, placebo-controlled study in children infected with influenza A (67%) or influenza B (33%). When used in these children within 48 hours of symptom onset, the drug reduced influenza symptoms (i.e., cough, coryza, duration of fever) and shortened the average duration of illness by about 1.5 days. Data from this study also indicate that children who received oseltamivir had a lower incidence of newly diagnosed otitis media (a common secondary complication of influenza) than those who received placebo.

The manufacturer states that efficacy could not be established in pediatric patients with asthma. In a study in children 6–12 years of age with asthma who received oseltamivir or placebo for the treatment of acute influenza virus infection, use of oseltamivir improved pulmonary function and reduced the risk of influenza-induced asthma exacerbations. When initiated within 48 hours of symptom onset, oseltamivir shortened the duration of illness in these children by about 24 hours; however, if initiated within 24 hours of symptom onset, oseltamivir shortened the duration of illness by about 40 hours.

Infants Younger than 1 Year of Age

Efficacy and safety of oseltamivir for the treatment of seasonal influenza in infants 2 weeks to less than 1 year of age are supported by adequate and well-controlled studies in adults and older pediatric patients and 2 open-label studies in 136 pediatric patients 2 weeks to less than 1 year of age. In addition, data from these 2 studies indicate that plasma concentrations of oseltamivir in pediatric patient 2 weeks to less than 1 year of age are similar to or greater than plasma concentrations observed in older pediatric patients and adults.

Immunocompromised Individuals

Although the manufacturer states that efficacy of oseltamivir for the *treatment* of influenza in immunocompromised patients has not been established, oseltamivir has been used to treat seasonal influenza A or B virus infections in bone marrow transplant (BMT) recipients† in a prospective, uncontrolled study. This study provides some evidence that oseltamivir treatment (75 mg twice daily for 5 days) may prevent influenza complications and is not associated with any unusual adverse effects in these patients. Oseltamivir also has been used for the treatment of influenza infections in hematopoietic stem cell transplant (HSCT) recipients†. Treatment with oseltamivir prevented progression to pneumonia in influenza-infected HSCT recipients in a small study.

● Prevention of Seasonal Influenza A and B Virus Infections

Oseltamivir is used for *prophylaxis* of influenza A or B virus infections in adults, adolescents, and children 1 year of age or older.

Annual vaccination with seasonal influenza virus vaccine, as recommended by CDC's Advisory Committee on Immunization Practices (ACIP), is the primary means of preventing seasonal influenza and its severe complications. Prophylaxis with an appropriate antiviral active against circulating influenza strains is considered an adjunct to vaccination for the control and prevention of influenza in certain individuals.

Decisions regarding use of antivirals for prophylaxis of seasonal influenza should be based on the risk of influenza-related complications in the exposed individual, the type and duration of contact, recommendations from local or public health authorities, and clinical judgment. In general, antiviral postexposure prophylaxis should be used only if it can be initiated within 48 hours of the most recent exposure.

CDC and others do not recommend *routine* use of influenza antivirals for postexposure prophylaxis of seasonal influenza in exposed individuals; however, such prophylaxis can be considered in certain situations in exposed individuals at high risk for influenza-related complications for whom influenza vaccine is contraindicated, unavailable, or expected to have low efficacy (e.g., immunocompromised individuals). Other possible candidates for antiviral postexposure prophylaxis include unvaccinated health care personnel, public health workers, and first responders with unprotected, close-contact exposure to a patient with confirmed, probable, or suspected influenza during the time when the patient was infectious. Antiviral prophylaxis also can be considered for controlling influenza outbreaks in nursing and long-term care facilities or other closed or semi-closed settings with large numbers of individuals at high risk for influenza complications. In individuals at high risk of influenza complications who receive influenza

virus vaccine inactivated or influenza vaccine recombinant, use of prophylaxis can be considered during the 2 weeks after vaccination to provide protection until an adequate immune response develops. (See Influenza Vaccines under Drug Interactions.)

CDC issues recommendations concerning the use of antivirals for prophylaxis of influenza, and these recommendations are updated as needed during each influenza season. Information regarding influenza surveillance and updated recommendations for prevention of seasonal influenza are available from CDC at http://www.cdc.gov/flu.

Clinical Trials and Experience

Adults and Adolescents

Results of community studies in healthy, unvaccinated adults indicate that oseltamivir is about 82% effective in preventing febrile, laboratory-confirmed influenza illness. Efficacy of oseltamivir in preventing naturally occurring influenza illness has been demonstrated in seasonal prophylaxis studies and in postexposure prophylaxis studies in household contacts. The efficacy end point for these studies was the incidence of laboratory-confirmed clinical influenza, which was defined as oral temperature exceeding 37.2°C with at least one respiratory symptom (cough, sore throat, nasal congestion) and at least one constitutional symptom (aches and pain, fatigue, headache, chills/sweats) all occurring within a single 24-hour period and either a positive virus isolation or a fourfold increase in virus antibody titer from baseline.

In 2 seasonal prophylaxis studies in healthy, unvaccinated adults 18–65 years of age who received oseltamivir (75 mg once daily) or placebo for 42 days during a community outbreak, pooled analysis indicates that the incidence of laboratory-confirmed clinical influenza was 1 or 5% in those receiving oseltamivir or placebo, respectively. In a seasonal prophylaxis study in geriatric residents of skilled nursing facilities (80% vaccinated, 14% with chronic airway obstructive disorders, 43% with cardiac disorders) who received oseltamivir (75 mg once daily) or placebo for 42 days, the incidence of laboratory-confirmed clinical influenza was less than 1 or 4% of those receiving oseltamivir or placebo, respectively.

In a postexposure prophylaxis study in household contacts (13 years of age or older) of influenza-infected index cases (not treated with antivirals) who received oseltamivir (75 mg once daily) or placebo for 7 days within 48 hours of onset of symptoms in the index case, the incidence of laboratory-confirmed clinical influenza was 1 or 12% of those receiving oseltamivir or placebo, respectively. In another postexposure prophylaxis study, there was evidence that oseltamivir prophylaxis effectively reduced the secondary spread of influenza within households when given to household contacts of index patients who were receiving the drug for treatment.

Children 1–12 Years of Age

Efficacy of oseltamivir in preventing naturally occurring influenza illness in children 1–12 years of age was evaluated in a randomized, open-label, postexposure prophylaxis study. In this study, oseltamivir prophylaxis was used during a documented community influenza outbreak and was given to adults and children 1 year of age or older residing in households that had an index patient with an influenza-like illness who was receiving oseltamivir for treatment. The efficacy parameter for this study was the incidence of laboratory-confirmed clinical influenza (defined as oral temperature 37.8°C or higher with cough and/or coryza occurring within a single 48-hour period and either a positive virus isolation or a fourfold or greater increase in virus antibody titer from baseline). In household contacts 1–12 years of age not shedding virus at baseline, the incidence of laboratory-confirmed clinical influenza was 3 or 17% in those receiving oseltamivir or placebo, respectively. The overall incidence of influenza illness in children who received oseltamivir prophylaxis was higher than that in adults and adolescents 13 years of age or older who received such prophylaxis.

Immunocompromised Individuals

Although the manufacturer states that efficacy of oseltamivir for prevention of influenza in immunocompromised patients has not been established, the drug has been used for prophylaxis of influenza in some immunocompromised individuals†, including cancer patients, BMT recipients, HSCT recipients, and solid organ transplant recipients.

In a prospective, uncontrolled study, oseltamivir was used for prophylaxis of influenza in cancer patients† 6.3–23.4 years of age who were immunocompromised because of current or recent chemotherapy or BMT. There were no laboratory-confirmed cases of influenza in the study participants; however, a few patients withdrew from the study because of adverse GI effects.

Safety and efficacy of oseltamivir for prevention of seasonal influenza in immunocompromised patients were evaluated in a double-blind, placebo-controlled study that included 475 immunocompromised adults, adolescents, and pediatric patients 1–12 years of age who had received solid organ transplants (liver, kidney, liver and kidney) or HSCT. The median time since solid organ transplant was 1105 days in those randomized to placebo and 1379 days in those randomized to oseltamivir prophylaxis; the median time since HSCT transplant was 424 days in those randomized to placebo and 367 days in those randomized to oseltamivir. Approximately 40% of patients had received influenza vaccine prior to study entry. The primary efficacy endpoint was the incidence of confirmed clinical influenza, defined as oral temperature exceeding 37.2°C plus cough and/or coryza (all recorded within 24 hours) plus either a positive virus culture or a fourfold increase in virus antibody titers from baseline. The incidence of confirmed clinical influenza was 3% in the placebo group and 2% in the oseltamivir group; this difference was not statistically significant. The safety profile of oseltamivir reported in these immunocompromised patients (up to 12 weeks of prophylaxis) was similar to that reported in other clinical trials evaluating oseltamivir prophylaxis.

● Avian Influenza A Virus Infections

Oseltamivir is used for the treatment or prevention of infections caused by susceptible avian influenza A viruses† (e.g., H5N1, H7N3, H7N7, H7N9).

Risk of Exposure and Infection

Worldwide, most avian influenza A viruses isolated in wild birds, water fowl, or poultry have been designated as low pathogenic strains; however, highly pathogenic avian influenza (HPAI) strains are occasionally detected. Since December 2014, HPAI viruses (H5N1, H5N2, H5N8) have been reported in wild birds, water fowl, and/or domestic poultry (commercial or backyard flocks) in the US (e.g., Arkansas, California, Idaho, Iowa, Minnesota, Missouri, Nebraska, North Dakota, Oregon, South Dakota, Utah, Washington, Wisconsin). Although CDC states that the risk of human infection with these HPAI H5 viruses is considered low in the US, human infection is possible since other closely related HPAI H5 viruses in Asia and other countries have caused sporadic cases of human respiratory illness. The HPAI (H5N1) strain reported in poultry outbreaks in the US is a new reassortant virus that is genetically different from the highly pathogenic Asian strain of influenza A (H5N1) that has caused human infections in Asia and other countries and has been associated with a high mortality rate.

Since 2003, avian influenza A (H5N1) infection in poultry or wild birds has been reported in parts of Asia, Africa, the Pacific, Eastern Europe, and the Middle East. World Health Organization (WHO) data indicate that there were 863 confirmed human cases of highly pathogenic avian influenza A (H5N1) infection (including 456 fatalities; case fatality rate of 53%) reported in 17 countries from January 2003 to August 2021. These human cases occurred in Azerbaijan, Bangladesh, Cambodia, Canada, China, Djibouti, Egypt, Indonesia, Iraq, Laos, Myanmar, Nepal, Nigeria, Pakistan, Thailand, Turkey, and Vietnam.

In March 2013, a novel avian influenza A (H7N9) virus causing human infection was identified in China. By June 2013, 132 human cases had been confirmed in mainland China and Taiwan. From early 2013 to August 2021, WHO had received reports of 1568 human cases of avian influenza A (H7N9) infection (including 616 fatalities; case fatality rate of 39%). To date, no cases have been reported in animals or humans in the US. Most reported cases of avian influenza A (H7N9) infection have involved severe respiratory illness, including pneumonia and acute respiratory distress syndrome (ARDS). Many of the infected individuals had close contact with poultry (chickens or ducks) and the source of infection is assumed to be infected poultry or contaminated environments. Preliminary investigations of patients and close contacts have not revealed evidence of sustained human-to-human transmission of influenza A (H7N9), but limited non-sustained human-to-human transmission of the virus could not be excluded in a few family clusters.

In addition, confirmed human cases of H5N6, H7N2, H7N3, H7N7, and H9N2 avian influenza A infection and illness have been reported, including a few cases in Australia, Canada, Italy, Mexico, the Netherlands, the United Kingdom, and the US. Most of these infections occurred in association with poultry outbreaks and mainly resulted in conjunctivitis and mild upper respiratory symptoms. There was a large outbreak of avian influenza A (H7N7) in commercial poultry farms in the Netherlands in 2003 that resulted in large numbers of human cases of H7N7 infection (principally conjunctivitis and influenza-like illnesses). Human infection with avian influenza A (H10N8) also has been reported rarely in China.

Experience to date indicates that human cases of avian influenza infection are rare and that these viruses do not transmit easily from wild or domestic birds, water fowl, or poultry to humans. Most, but not all, human cases reported to date have been linked to direct contact with infected poultry, uncooked poultry products, or surfaces contaminated with infected poultry feces or respiratory secretions. Sustained person-to-person transmission of avian influenza viruses has not been reported to date, but clustering and limited person-to-person transmission of H5N1 and H7N9 viruses has been reported. Most clusters of human infection with avian influenza A (H5N1) reported to date have included documented exposure to birds. Person-to-person transmission of H7N7 has occurred among household contacts during the outbreak of that virus that occurred in the Netherlands.

In humans, avian influenza A viruses can cause typical influenza illness (fever, cough, sore throat, muscle aches), conjunctivitis, or respiratory disease; however, severe illness can occur, especially with highly pathogenic avian influenza (H5N1) and avian influenza A (H7N9). The fatality rate in patients hospitalized with H5N1 infection has been high (exceeding 50%). In one group of patients in Vietnam with severe H5N1 infections, the median time to death was 9 days (range 6–17 days) with or without treatment.

Although most avian influenza A virus strains (e.g., H5N1, H7N7, H7N9, H9N2) tested have been susceptible to oseltamivir and zanamivir in vitro, avian influenza A (H5N1) and avian influenza A (H7N9) isolates with reduced susceptibility or resistance to oseltamivir in vitro have been reported. (See Spectrum and see Resistance.) Avian influenza A virus strains (including H5N1 and H7N9 strains causing human illness) generally have been resistant to adamantanes (amantadine, rimantadine).

Treatment and Prevention of Avian Influenza A Infections

Although safety and efficacy have not been established, neuraminidase inhibitors (oseltamivir, peramivir, zanamivir) have been used or are recommended for the treatment or prophylaxis of infections caused by susceptible avian influenza A viruses†.

Appropriate use of a neuraminidase inhibitor antivirals is an important component of response and control measures to treat avian influenza A virus infections and help reduce the risk of additional human infections.

For the treatment of uncomplicated avian influenza A infections in outpatients, CDC states that oral oseltamivir, IV peramivir, or inhaled zanamivir may be used. For the treatment of severe, complicated, or progressive avian influenza A infections in hospitalized patients or outpatients, including infections caused by avian influenza A (H7N9), avian influenza A (H5N1), or novel avian influenza A H5 viruses, oseltamivir is considered the antiviral of choice. In those with severe avian influenza A infections who cannot tolerate or absorb oseltamivir administered orally or enterically (e.g., because of suspected or known gastric stasis, malabsorption, or GI bleeding), CDC states that use of IV peramivir may be considered. Because of limited data, inhaled zanamivir is not recommended for the treatment of severe avian influenza A infections in hospitalized patients or outpatients.

When antiviral prophylaxis is indicated in close contacts of individuals with confirmed or probable infection with avian influenza A viruses that have caused or potentially may cause severe disease or indicated in individuals who have been exposed to birds infected with such avian influenza A viruses, CDC recommends oral oseltamivir or inhaled zanamivir.

Information regarding treatment and prevention of avian influenza A infections is available from CDC at http://www.cdc.gov/flu/avianflu/ and WHO at https://www.who.int/teams/global-influenza-programme/avian-influenza.

● Variant Influenza Virus Infections

Oseltamivir is used for the treatment of infections cause by variant influenza viruses†.

Influenza viruses that circulate in swine are called swine influenza viruses when isolated from swine, but are called variant influenza viruses when isolated from humans. Human infection with influenza A (H1N1) variant (H1N1v), influenza A (H1N2) variant (H1N2v), and influenza A (H3N2) variant (H3N2v) have been detected in the US. Limited data to date indicate that variant influenza viruses are susceptible to neuraminidase inhibitor antivirals (oseltamivir, peramivir, zanamivir).

CDC states that management of infections caused by variant influenza viruses is similar to management of seasonal influenza virus infections. CDC recommends early initiation of oseltamivir for treatment of hospitalized patients, those with severe and progressive illness, and any high-risk patient with suspected or confirmed variant influenza virus infection. Antiviral treatment with a neuraminidase inhibitor also is recommended for outpatients with suspected influenza, including variant influenza virus infection, if the individual is considered at high risk for influenza complications. CDC states that antiviral treatment also can be considered for any previously healthy, symptomatic outpatient not at high risk who has confirmed or suspected variant virus infection on the basis of clinical judgment, if treatment can be initiated within 48 hours of illness onset.

Information regarding variant influenza virus infections is available from CDC at https://www.cdc.gov/flu/swineflu/variant.htm.

● Pandemic Influenza

Oseltamivir is used for the treatment or prevention of pandemic influenza† caused by susceptible strains of influenza virus.

Influenza viruses can cause seasonal epidemics and, occasionally, pandemics during which rates of illness and death from influenza-related complications can increase dramatically worldwide. The most recent influenza pandemic occurred during 2009 and was related to a novel influenza A (H1N1) strain, influenza A (H1N1)pdm09. Influenza A strains also were involved in prior influenza pandemics occurring in 1918 (H1N1), 1957 (H2N2; originated in China), and 1968 (H3N2; originated in Hong Kong).

On June 11, 2009, the WHO declared that the first global influenza pandemic in 41 years was occurring and issued a pandemic alert regarding influenza A (H1N1)pdm09, previously referred to as the novel 2009 influenza A (H1N1) virus or swine-origin influenza A (H1N1) virus. Influenza outbreaks caused by the influenza A (H1N1)pdm09 virus were reported in several countries, including the US, beginning in March and April 2009. The virus is a triple-reassortant swine influenza virus with genes from human, swine, and avian influenza A viruses and contained a unique combination of gene segments not previously reported among human or swine influenza A in the US or elsewhere. The influenza A (H1N1)pdm09 virus was antigenically distinct from previous human influenza A (H1N1) viruses that had been in circulation since 1977, and widespread transmission of the virus occurred since most individuals had no preexisting antibody to the strain. In the US, the 2009 influenza A (H1N1)pdm09 pandemic was characterized by a substantial increase in influenza activity that peaked in late October and early November 2009 and returned to seasonal baseline levels by January 2010. During the pandemic, more than 99% of influenza viruses circulating in the US were the influenza A (H1N1)pdm09 virus; more than 60 million Americans become ill with the virus and more than 270,000 hospitalizations and 12,500 deaths were reported. After the pandemic, influenza A (H1N1)pdm09 became a seasonal influenza virus and continues to circulate with other seasonal influenza viruses.

The spread of the highly pathogenic H5N1 strain of avian influenza A in poultry in Asia and other countries that has been occurring since 2003 may represent a future pandemic threat. In addition, the novel avian influenza A (H7N9) virus that was first identified in China in March 2013 and has been causing sporadic human infections has pandemic potential. (See Avian Influenza A Virus Infections under Uses.)

Information on pandemic influenza, including planning and preparedness resources if an influenza pandemic occurs, is available from CDC at https://www.cdc.gov/flu/pandemic-resources/index.htm and WHO at https://www.who.int/initiatives/pandemic-influenza-preparedness-framework.

DOSAGE AND ADMINISTRATION

● Administration

Oseltamivir phosphate is administered orally without regard to meals, although administration with meals may improve GI tolerability.

Oseltamivir phosphate is commercially available as 30-, 45-, and 75-mg capsules and as a powder for oral suspension that is reconstituted to provide an oral suspension containing 6 mg of oseltamivir per mL.

Reconstituted oseltamivir phosphate oral suspension is preferred for patients who cannot swallow capsules. Alternatively, if the powder for oral suspension is not available from the manufacturer or wholesaler, the appropriate strength of commercially available oseltamivir capsules can be administered by opening the capsules and mixing the contents with a sweet liquid (e.g., regular or sugar-free chocolate syrup, corn syrup, caramel topping, light brown sugar dissolved in water).

During emergency situations if the powder for oral suspension is not available *and* the appropriate strength of oseltamivir capsules is not available to mix with sweetened liquids, an emergency supply of oseltamivir phosphate oral suspension can be prepared extemporaneously by a pharmacist using the commercially available 75-mg capsules of the drug. (See Extemporaneous Oral Suspensions under Dosage and Administration.)

Reconstitution

The commercially available oseltamivir phosphate powder for oral suspension should be reconstituted at the time of dispensing. The bottle should be tapped to thoroughly loosen the white powder and then the amount of water specified on the bottle should be added; the bottle should be shaken for 15 seconds.

The reconstituted oral suspension contains 6 mg/mL; each 12.5 mL of the suspension contains 75 mg of oseltamivir. An oral dosing device that can accurately measure the appropriate volume in mL should be provided with the reconstituted suspension. Patients and/or caregivers should be counseled on how to use the oral dosing dispenser to correctly measure and administer the appropriate dose.

The suspension should be shaken well prior to each dose.

Extemporaneous Oral Suspensions

If necessary for use during emergency situations, an oral suspension containing 6 mg/mL can be prepared extemporaneously by a pharmacist using 75-mg capsules and simple syrup, cherry syrup vehicle (Humco®), or Ora-Sweet® SF (Paddock).

Extemporaneous oral suspensions should be used *only* if the commercially available powder for oral suspension *and* appropriate strength of commercially available oseltamivir capsules are not available from the manufacturer or wholesalers. The manufacturer's information should be consulted for specific directions on how to prepare extemporaneous oral suspensions of the drug.

● Dosage

Dosage of oseltamivir phosphate is expressed in terms of oseltamivir.

Treatment of Seasonal Influenza A and B Virus Infections

When indicated for the *treatment* of seasonal influenza, oseltamivir should be initiated as soon as possible (preferably within 48 hours of symptom onset). Although efficacy has only been established when oseltamivir treatment is initiated no more than 48 hours after onset of symptoms, there is some evidence from observational studies in hospitalized patients that antiviral treatment may still be beneficial when initiated up to 4 or 5 days after illness onset. (See Treatment of Seasonal Influenza A and B Virus Infections under Uses.)

Oseltamivir usually is given for 5 days for the *treatment* of seasonal influenza. However, hospitalized patients with severe or prolonged infections or individuals with immunosuppression may require more than 5 days of treatment.

Adults and Adolescents 13 Years of Age or Older

For the *treatment* of influenza in adults (including geriatric adults) and adolescents 13 years of age and older, the recommended dosage of oseltamivir is 75 mg twice daily for 5 days. Each dose can be given as a single 75-mg capsule or 12.5 mL of oral suspension containing 6 mg/mL.

Children 1–12 Years of Age

Dosage of oseltamivir for the *treatment* of influenza in children 1–12 years of age is based on weight. (See Table 1.)

TABLE 1. Oseltamivir Dosage for Treatment of Seasonal Influenza A and B in Children 1–12 Years of Age

Weight (kg)	Daily Dosage (mg)	Daily Dosage (Volume of Reconstituted Oral Suspension Containing 6 mg/mL)	Daily Dosage (Capsules)
≤15	30 mg twice daily for 5 days	5 mL twice daily for 5 days	One 30-mg capsule twice daily for 5 days
15.1–23	45 mg twice daily for 5 days	7.5 mL twice daily for 5 days	One 45-mg capsule twice daily for 5 days
23.1–40	60 mg twice daily for 5 days	10 mL twice daily for 5 days	Two 30-mg capsules twice daily for 5 days
≥40.1	75 mg twice daily for 5 days	12.5 mL twice daily for 5 days	One 75-mg capsule twice daily for 5 days

Infants Younger than 1 Year of Age

For the *treatment* of influenza in infants 2 weeks to less than 1 year of age, the manufacturer recommends that oseltamivir be given in a dosage of 3 mg/kg twice daily for 5 days.

For the *treatment* of influenza in neonates and infants younger than 1 year of age, AAP recommends that oseltamivir be given in a dosage of 3.5 mg/kg twice daily for 5 days in infants 9 through 11 months of age and 3 mg/kg twice daily for 5 days in *full-term* neonates and infants through 8 months of age. Although safety and efficacy have not been established in neonates younger than 2 weeks of age† (see Pediatric Precautions under Cautions), AAP states that, because of the known safety profile of the drug, oseltamivir can be used for the *treatment* of influenza in neonates from birth† if indicated.

Weight-based oseltamivir dosage recommended for *full-term* infants may be excessive in *preterm* neonates since clearance of the drug is slower in those with immature renal function. Limited data suggest that, if oseltamivir is considered necessary for *treatment* of influenza in *preterm* neonates†, dosage should be based on postmenstrual age (i.e., gestational age plus chronological age). AAP and CDC recommend an oseltamivir dosage of 1 mg/kg twice daily in *preterm* neonates with postmenstrual age less than 38 weeks, 1.5 mg/kg twice daily in those with postmenstrual age of 38 through 40 weeks, and 3 mg/kg twice daily in those with postmenstrual age exceeding 40 weeks. For *treatment* of influenza in extremely premature neonates (postmenstrual age less than 28 weeks), a pediatric infectious disease expert should be consulted.

Prevention of Seasonal Influenza A and B Virus Infections

When indicated for *prophylaxis* of influenza following close contact with an infected individual, oseltamivir should be initiated within 48 hours of exposure. Protection lasts as long as oseltamivir is continued.

CDC recommends that oseltamivir *prophylaxis* be continued for 7 days after the most recent exposure. For *prophylaxis* of influenza when an outbreak is occurring in institutional settings (e.g., long-term care facilities for elderly individuals and children), CDC recommends that oseltamivir *prophylaxis* be given for a minimum of 2 weeks and continued for up to 1 week after the last known case of influenza is identified.

Adults and Adolescents 13 Years of Age or Older

For *prophylaxis* of influenza in adults (including geriatric adults) and adolescents 13 years of age or older following close contact with an infected individual or during community outbreaks, the recommended dosage of oseltamivir is 75 mg once daily. The manufacturer states that oseltamivir *prophylaxis* should be continued for at least 10 days following close contact with an infected individual; during community outbreaks, the manufacturer states that prophylaxis may be continued for up to 6 weeks in immunocompetent individuals and for up to 12 weeks in immunocompromised individuals.

Children 1–12 Years of Age

Dosage of oseltamivir for *prophylaxis* of influenza in children 1–12 years of age following close contact with an infected individual or during community outbreaks is based on weight. (See Table 2.)

TABLE 2. Oseltamivir Dosage for Prevention of Seasonal Influenza A and B in Children 1–12 Years of Age

Weight (kg)	Daily Dosage (mg)	Daily Dosage (Volume of Reconstituted Oral Suspension Containing 6 mg/mL) [a]	Daily Dosage (Capsules) [a]
≤15	30 mg once daily for 10 days	5 mL once daily for 10 days	One 30-mg capsule once daily for 10 days
15.1–23	45 mg once daily for 10 days	7.5 mL once daily for 10 days	One 45-mg capsule once daily for 10 days
23.1–40	60 mg once daily for 10 days	10 mL once daily for 10 days	Two 30-mg capsules once daily for 10 days
≥40.1	75 mg once daily for 10 days	12.5 mL once daily for 10 days	One 75-mg capsule once daily for 10 days

[a] The manufacturer states that oseltamivir *prophylaxis* in pediatric patients should be continued for 10 days following close contact with an infected individual; during community outbreaks, manufacturer states *prophylaxis* may be continued for up to 6 weeks in immunocompetent individuals and for up to 12 weeks in immunocompromised individuals.

Infants Younger than 1 Year of Age

Although safety and efficacy have not been established for *prophylaxis* of influenza in infants younger than 1 year of age† (see Pediatric Precautions under Cautions), CDC states that infants 3 months to less than 1 year of age† can receive oseltamivir in a dosage of 3 mg/kg once daily for 7 days if considered necessary for prevention of influenza. For *prophylaxis* of influenza, AAP recommends a dosage of 3.5 mg/kg once daily for 10 days in infants 9 through 11 months of age† and 3 mg/kg once daily for 10 days in infants 3 through 8 months of age†.

Because of limited safety and efficacy data, CDC and AAP state that oseltamivir should *not* be used for *prophylaxis* of influenza in *full-term* or *preterm* infants younger than 3 months of age† unless the situation is judged critical.

Avian Influenza A Virus Infections

Treatment

Only limited data are available to date regarding *treatment* of infections caused by avian influenza A (H1N1) or avian influenza A (H7N9)†, and the optimum dosage and duration of oseltamivir for treatment of these infections, especially severe or complicated infections, are unknown.

Some clinicians suggest that the twice-daily oseltamivir dosage usually recommended for the *treatment* of seasonal influenza A and B virus infection can be used for the *treatment* of avian influenza A virus infections† in adults and pediatric patients. (See Treatment of Seasonal Influenza A and B Virus Infections under Dosage and Administration.) Although some experts have suggested a higher oseltamivir dosage (i.e., 150 mg twice daily in adults with normal renal function) be considered for severely ill or immunocompromised patients, oral oseltamivir is adequately absorbed in critically ill patients and limited data from those with severe influenza, including some with avian influenza A (H1N1) infection, suggest that higher dosage may not provide additional clinical benefit.

Although 5 days of treatment may be adequate for uncomplicated illness, a longer duration of treatment (i.e., 7–10 days) should be considered in severely ill hospitalized patients and may be necessary in immunosuppressed individuals.

Treatment should be initiated as early as possible and may be most beneficial if initiated within 2 days of symptom onset. However, because the viruses continue to replicate for prolonged periods of time, treatment with oseltamivir is warranted even if initiated more than 48 hours after onset of illness or in patients who present for care in the later stages of illness.

Prevention

If oseltamivir is used for *prophylaxis* of avian influenza A infection† in close contacts of individuals with confirmed or probable infection or in individuals who have been exposed to birds infected with such viruses, CDC and WHO state that the twice-daily oseltamivir dosage usually recommended for *treatment* of seasonal influenza A and B virus infections can be used in adults and pediatric patients. (See Treatment of Seasonal Influenza A and B Virus Infections under Dosage and Administration.)

Antiviral prophylaxis for avian influenza A virus infection should be continued for 5–10 days after the last known exposure. If exposure was time-limited and not ongoing, CDC states that prophylaxis should be continued for 5 days after the last known exposure.

● Dosage in Renal and Hepatic Impairment

Hepatic Impairment

Dosage adjustments are not needed in patients with mild to moderate hepatic impairment (Child-Pugh score 9 or less). The safety and pharmacokinetics of the drug have not been evaluated in those with severe hepatic impairment.

Renal Impairment

Dosage of oseltamivir for the treatment or prevention of influenza should be adjusted in adults with creatinine clearance of 10–60 mL/minute and in those with end-stage renal disease (ESRD; creatinine clearance 10 mL/minute or less) undergoing hemodialysis or continuous peritoneal dialysis. (See Table 3 and Table 4.)

Oseltamivir is *not* recommended in adults with ESRD who are *not* undergoing dialysis.

Although dosage recommendations are not available for pediatric patients with renal impairment, CDC states that oseltamivir dosage recommendations for adults with renal impairment may be useful for treatment or prevention of influenza in children with renal impairment who weigh more than 40 kg.

TABLE 3. Oseltamivir Dosage for Treatment of Influenza in Adults with Renal Impairment

Creatinine Clearance (mL/minute)	Dosage
>30 to 60	30 mg twice daily for 5 days
>10 to 30	30 mg once daily for 5 days
≤10 (ESRD receiving hemodialysis)	30 mg given immediately and then 30 mg after each hemodialysis cycle for maximum of 5 days [a]
≤10 (ESRD receiving continuous peritoneal dialysis)	Single 30-mg dose given immediately [b]
ESRD not receiving dialysis	Not recommended

[a] Dosage assumes 3 hemodialysis sessions in the 5-day period. If influenza symptoms developed during the 48 hours between hemodialysis sessions, give initial oseltamivir dose immediately and give the posthemodialysis dose regardless of when initial dose was given.

[b] Data derived from studies in patients undergoing continuous ambulatory peritoneal dialysis (CAPD).

TABLE 4. Oseltamivir Dosage for Prevention of Influenza in Adults with Renal Impairment [a]

Creatinine Clearance (mL/minute)	Dosage
>30 to 60	30 mg once daily for ≥10 days
>10 to 30	30 mg once every other day for ≥10 days
≤10 (ESRD receiving hemodialysis)	30 mg given immediately and then 30 mg after alternate hemodialysis cycles
≤10 (ESRD receiving continuous peritoneal dialysis)	30 mg given immediately and then 30 mg once weekly [b]
ESRD not receiving dialysis	Not recommended

[a] The manufacturer states that *prophylaxis* with oseltamivir during community outbreaks may be continued for up to 6 weeks in immunocompetent individuals and for up to 12 weeks in immunocompromised individuals.

[b] Data derived from studies in patients undergoing CAPD.

Geriatric Patients

Dosage adjustments are not needed in geriatric patients. (See Geriatric Precautions under Cautions.)

CAUTIONS

Oseltamivir generally is well tolerated. Adverse effects occurring in 1% or more of adults and at an incidence greater than that with placebo include GI effects (nausea, vomiting, diarrhea, abdominal pain), headache, bronchitis, insomnia, and vertigo. In one study in frail older individuals residing in residential homes or sheltered accommodations, the incidence of adverse effects reported in those receiving oseltamivir was similar to that reported in those receiving placebo.

Safety data from dose-ranging studies indicate that a 5-day course of oseltamivir 150 mg twice daily or a 6-week course of oseltamivir 75 mg twice daily are tolerated as well as the usual recommended dosage for treatment or prophylaxis of influenza.

Adverse effects occurring in 1% or more of children receiving oseltamivir for the treatment of influenza include vomiting, abdominal pain, epistaxis, otic disorder, and conjunctivitis. GI effects, especially vomiting, were the most frequently reported adverse effects in children receiving the drug for prophylaxis of influenza.

● Dermatologic and Hypersensitivity Reactions

Anaphylaxis and serious dermatologic reactions (toxic epidermal necrolysis, Stevens-Johnson syndrome, erythema multiforme) have been reported in patients receiving oseltamivir, including pediatric patients.

Rash, swelling of the face or tongue, allergy, dermatitis, eczema, or urticaria has been reported during postmarketing experience.

● Nervous System Effects

Headache has occurred in about 2% of adults receiving oseltamivir for treatment of influenza and in about 18% of adults receiving the drug for prophylaxis of influenza.

Neuropsychiatric Events

Adverse neuropsychiatric events (e.g., agitation, anxiety, self-injury, delirium, hallucinations, altered level of consciousness, confusion, nightmares, delusions, abnormal behavior, seizures), which occasionally were fatal, have been reported in patients receiving oseltamivir. Cases generally had an abrupt onset and rapid resolution. The contribution of oseltamivir to these events has not been established. (See Pediatric Precautions under Cautions.)

Influenza itself can be associated with a variety of neurologic and behavioral symptoms (e.g., hallucinations, delirium, abnormal behavior) and fatalities can occur. Although such events may occur in the setting of encephalitis or encephalopathy, they can occur without obvious severe disease.

● GI Effects

Nausea, with or without vomiting, has been reported in up to 10% of adults and adolescents 13 years of age or older receiving oseltamivir. Nausea usually occurs after the initial dose and resolves within 1–2 days; administration of the drug with food improves GI tolerance. In pediatric patients in clinical studies, vomiting was reported in 16% of children 1–12 years of age and diarrhea or vomiting was reported in up to 7 or 9%, respectively, of pediatric patients 2 weeks to less than 1 year of age.

GI bleeding and hemorrhagic colitis have been reported during postmarketing experience.

● Other Adverse Effects

Hepatitis or abnormal liver function test values have been reported during postmarketing experience.

Arrhythmia, hypothermia, or metabolic events (e.g., deterioration in diabetes control) has been reported during postmarketing experience.

● Precautions and Contraindications

Oseltamivir is contraindicated in patients with known hypersensitivity to the drug or any ingredient in the formulation. If an allergic reaction occurs or is suspected, oseltamivir should be discontinued and appropriate treatment initiated. Patients and/or their caregivers should be advised of the risk of severe allergic reactions (including anaphylaxis) or serious skin reactions and should be instructed to discontinue oseltamivir and immediately contact a clinician if an allergic-like reaction occurs or is suspected.

Because there have been postmarketing reports of neuropsychiatric events (e.g., self-injury, delirium) in influenza patients receiving oseltamivir (see Neuropsychiatric Events under Cautions), patients with influenza (especially children) should be closely monitored for signs of abnormal behavior during oseltamivir treatment. Patients and/or their caregivers should be instructed to contact a clinician if there are any signs of unusual behavior during oseltamivir treatment. If neuropsychiatric symptoms develop, the risks and benefits of continued therapy with oseltamivir should be evaluated.

Efficacy of oseltamivir has not been established in patients with chronic cardiac disease and/or pulmonary disease; however, no difference in incidence of complications between drug and placebo has been observed in these populations. Safety and efficacy have not been established in those with any medical condition severe or unstable enough to require inpatient care.

Although efficacy of oseltamivir for treatment or prevention of influenza in immunocompromised patients† has not been established, safety of oseltamivir prophylaxis has been demonstrated for up to 12 weeks in immunocompromised patients. The drug has been used for treatment or prevention of influenza in some immunocompromised individuals, including bone marrow transplant (BMT) recipients, hematopoietic stem cell transplant (HSCT) recipients, solid organ transplant recipients, and chemotherapy patients. (See Uses.)

There is no evidence that oseltamivir is effective for illness caused by any organisms other than influenza viruses. Serious bacterial infections may begin with influenza-like symptoms or may coexist with or occur as complications of influenza. There is no evidence that oseltamivir prevents such complications. Clinicians should consider the potential for secondary bacterial infections; if such infections occur, they should be treated appropriately.

Influenza antivirals, including oseltamivir, are important adjuncts to vaccination in the control of influenza but are not a substitute for annual vaccination with a seasonal influenza vaccine (influenza virus vaccine inactivated, influenza vaccine recombinant, influenza vaccine live intranasal). Although influenza antivirals used for treatment or prevention of influenza, including oseltamivir, may be used concomitantly with or at any time before or after influenza virus vaccine inactivated or influenza vaccine recombinant, influenza antivirals may inhibit the vaccine virus contained in influenza vaccine live intranasal and decrease efficacy of the live vaccine. (See Influenza Vaccines under Drug Interactions.)

When the commercially available oral suspension containing 6 mg/mL is used, each 75-mg dose of oseltamivir contains 2 g of sorbitol. Patients with hereditary fructose intolerance should be informed that this amount of sorbitol exceeds the maximum daily limit of sorbitol for such individuals and may result in dyspepsia and diarrhea.

Safety and pharmacokinetics of oseltamivir have not been evaluated in patients with severe hepatic impairment.

Patients with renal impairment (i.e., creatinine clearance of 60 mL/minute or less) may be at increased risk of adverse effects during oseltamivir therapy because of decreased clearance of the drug; dosage adjustments are recommended when oseltamivir is used in adults with creatinine clearance of 10–60 mL/minute or adults with end-stage renal disease (ESRD; creatinine clearance 10 mL/minute or less) undergoing hemodialysis or continuous peritoneal dialysis. Oseltamivir is *not* recommended in adults with ESRD who are *not* undergoing dialysis. (See Renal Impairment under Dosage and Administration:.)

● Pediatric Precautions

Safety and efficacy of oseltamivir for the *treatment* of influenza have not been established in infants younger than 2 weeks of age.

Safety and efficacy of oseltamivir for *prophylaxis* of influenza have not been established in infants younger than 1 year of age.

When used for the *treatment* of influenza, the safety profile of oseltamivir observed in neonates and infants 2 weeks to less than 1 year of age has been consistent with the safety profile for the drug established in adults and pediatric patients older than 1 year of age. Data from open-label studies evaluating oseltamivir for *treatment* of influenza in infants 2 weeks to less than 1 year of age (including some premature infants with a postconceptional age of at least 36 weeks) indicated that the safety profile was similar across this young age range, and that vomiting, diarrhea, and diaper rash were the most frequently reported adverse effects. In addition, serum concentrations of oseltamivir in these infants were similar to or greater than those observed in older children and adults.

Young children, especially those younger than 2 years of age, are at increased risk of influenza infection, hospitalization, and complications. During the 2009 influenza A (H1N1)pdm09 pandemic, the US Food and Drug Administration (FDA) issued an Emergency Use Authorization (EUA) that temporarily allowed use of oseltamivir for emergency treatment or prevention of these infections in infants younger than 1 year of age†. Although the EUA expired in June 2010, the AAP states that, because of the known safety profile of the drug, use of oseltamivir for the *treatment* of influenza in *full-term* or *preterm* neonates from birth† or for *prevention* of influenza in infants 3 months of age or older† is appropriate if indicated. However, because of limited safety and efficacy data, CDC and AAP state that oseltamivir is not recommended for *prevention* of influenza in infants younger than 3 months of age† unless the situation is judged critical. (See Dosage under Dosage and Administration.)

Unusual adverse neurologic and/or psychiatric effects, including self-injury, delirium, hallucinations, mental confusion, abnormal behavior, seizures, and encephalitis, have been reported in pediatric patient receiving oseltamivir. Adverse neurologic and psychiatric events, including some fatalities, have been reported principally in children in Japan. A relationship to oseltamivir was difficult to assess because of concomitantly used drugs, comorbid conditions, and/or lack of adequate detail in reports. After reviewing available data, FDA concluded that the increased reports of neuropsychiatric events in Japanese children receiving oseltamivir were most likely related to an increased awareness of influenza-related encephalopathy, increased access to the drug in the Japanese population, and a coincident period of intensive monitoring for potential adverse effects. Therefore, based on available information, FDA stated that it was unable to conclude that a causal relationship exists between oseltamivir and the reported pediatric deaths.

● Geriatric Precautions

Safety of oseltamivir for the treatment of influenza in geriatric individuals has been established in clinical studies. In addition, safety and efficacy were demonstrated in geriatric individuals (many with cardiac and/or respiratory disease) residing in nursing homes who received oseltamivir for up to 42 days for the prevention of influenza.

When the total number of patients studied in oseltamivir clinical trials is considered, 20% of those in studies evaluating the drug for the treatment of influenza were 65 years of age or older (7% were 75 years of age or older) and 23% of those in studies evaluating the drug for the prevention of influenza were 65 years or older

(16% were 75 years of age or older). No overall differences in efficacy or safety were observed between geriatric and younger adults, and other clinical experience revealed no evidence of age-related differences.

Oseltamivir dosage adjustments based solely on age are not necessary for geriatric patients older than 65 years of age.

● Mutagenicity and Carcinogenicity

Oseltamivir was not mutagenic in the Ames microbial test, the human lymphocyte chromosome assay, or the mouse micronucleus test; oseltamivir was mutagenic in the Syrian hamster embryo cell transformation assay. Oseltamivir carboxylate was not mutagenic in the Ames microbial test, the L5178Y mouse lymphoma assay, or the Syrian hamster embryo cell transformation assay.

Oseltamivir was not carcinogenic in studies in rats or mice.

● Pregnancy, Fertility, and Lactation

Pregnancy

There are no adequate and well-controlled studies using oseltamivir in pregnant women to inform a drug-associated risk of adverse developmental outcomes. Available published epidemiological data suggest that oseltamivir administered during any trimester of pregnancy is not associated with an increased risk of birth defects; however, these studies had various limitations (e.g., small sample sizes, use of different comparison groups, lack of dosage information) which preclude a definitive assessment of the risk. Although data are insufficient to make a definitive assessment of the risk, prospective and retrospective observational studies that included approximately 5000 women exposed to oseltamivir during pregnancy (including approximately 1000 women exposed during the first trimester) suggest that the observed rate of congenital malformations following oseltamivir exposures during any trimester was not greater than that reported in the general population.

In animal reproduction studies, no adverse embryofetal effects were observed in pregnant rats and rabbits treated with oral oseltamivir at dosages resulting in clinically relevant exposures. There was a dose-dependent increase in the incidence rates of a variety of minor skeletal abnormalities and variants in offspring of rats and rabbits exposed to maternally toxic dosages (approximately 190 and at least 8 times usual human exposure, respectively). No adverse maternal or embryofetal effects were observed in rats exposed to maternally toxic dosages (approximately 44 times usual human exposure).

Pregnant women are at increased risk for severe complications from influenza, which may lead to adverse pregnancy and/or fetal outcomes including maternal death, still births, birth defects, preterm delivery, low birthweight, and small size for gestational age.

Oseltamivir is the preferred antiviral for the treatment of suspected or confirmed influenza or prevention of influenza in women who are pregnant or up to 2 weeks postpartum.

Fertility

No effects on fertility, mating performance, or early embryonic development were observed in rats given oseltamivir at doses up to 100 times the human systemic exposure of oseltamivir carboxylate.

Lactation

Limited data indicate that oseltamivir and its active metabolite, oseltamivir carboxylate, are distributed into human milk in low concentrations that are considered unlikely to cause toxicity in nursing infants.

The benefits of breast-feeding and the importance of oseltamivir to the woman should be considered along with potential adverse effects on the breast-fed child from the drug or from the underlying maternal condition.

DRUG INTERACTIONS

● Drugs Affected or Metabolized by Hepatic Microsomal Enzymes

Oseltamivir phosphate and its active metabolite, oseltamivir carboxylate, are not metabolized by and do not inhibit cytochrome P-450 (CYP) isoenzymes; interactions with drugs that are substrates for or inhibitors of these enzymes are unlikely.

● Acetaminophen

Concomitant use of acetaminophen and oseltamivir does not result in clinically important pharmacokinetic interactions; dosage adjustments are not needed.

● Amantadine and Rimantadine

Concomitant use of oseltamivir and amantadine or rimantadine does not result in clinically important pharmacokinetic interactions; dosage adjustments are not needed if oseltamivir is used concomitantly with amantadine or rimantadine.

● Amoxicillin

Concomitant use of amoxicillin and oseltamivir does not result in clinically important pharmacokinetic interactions; dosage adjustments are not needed.

● Antacids

Concomitant use of oseltamivir and antacids containing magnesium hydroxide, aluminum hydroxide, or calcium carbonate does not result in clinically important pharmacokinetic interactions; dosage adjustments are not needed.

● Anticoagulants

Concomitant use of oseltamivir and warfarin does not result in clinically important pharmacokinetic interactions; dosage adjustments are not needed.

● Aspirin

Concomitant use of aspirin and oseltamivir does not result in clinically important pharmacokinetic interactions; dosage adjustments are not needed.

● Cimetidine

Concomitant use of cimetidine and oseltamivir does not affect plasma concentrations of oseltamivir or oseltamivir carboxylate. Dosage adjustments are not needed.

● Influenza Vaccines

Influenza virus vaccine inactivated (IIV) and influenza vaccine recombinant (RIV) may be administered concomitantly with or at any time before or after oseltamivir. Although drug interaction studies have not been conducted to evaluate the immune response to inactivated influenza vaccines in patients receiving oseltamivir, oseltamivir therapy does not appear to impair normal humoral antibody response to infection in patients with naturally or experimentally acquired influenza.

Safety and efficacy of concomitant use of oseltamivir and influenza vaccine live intranasal (LAIV) have not been evaluated. Because influenza antivirals, including oseltamivir, inhibit replication of influenza viruses and may inhibit the vaccine virus, these antivirals potentially could decrease the immune response to LAIV and decrease efficacy of the live vaccine. LAIV should not be administered until at least 48 hours after oseltamivir is discontinued and oseltamivir should not be administered until at least 2 weeks after administration of LAIV. ACIP recommends that individuals who received oseltamivir 48 hours before to 14 days after LAIV should be revaccinated using age-appropriate IIV or RIV.

● Peramivir

There was no evidence of drug interactions when IV peramivir was used concomitantly with oral oseltamivir.

● Probenecid

Concomitant use of oseltamivir with probenecid results in a twofold increase in systemic exposure to oseltamivir carboxylate because of decreased renal tubular secretion. However, this pharmacokinetic interaction is not expected to be clinically important and the usual oseltamivir dosage can be used in patients receiving probenecid.

MECHANISM OF ACTION

Oseltamivir phosphate is a prodrug and has little, if any, pharmacologic activity until hydrolyzed in vivo to oseltamivir carboxylate. Oseltamivir is pharmacologically related to other neuraminidase inhibitors (e.g., zanamivir, peramivir).

Oseltamivir carboxylate is a potent selective competitive inhibitor of the influenza virus neuraminidase, an enzyme essential for viral replication in vivo. Neuraminidase cleaves terminal sialic acid residues from glycoconjugates to enable the release of virus from infected cells, prevents the formation of viral aggregates after release from host cells, and possibly facilitates viral invasion of the upper airways.

Neuraminidase inhibitors interfere with the release of progeny influenza virus from infected host cells, thus preventing infection of new host cells and halting the spread of infection. Because replication of influenza virus in the respiratory tract reaches its peak between 24 and 72 hours after the onset of illness, neuraminidase inhibitors must be administered as early as possible.

SPECTRUM

Oseltamivir (as oseltamivir carboxylate, the active metabolite of oseltamivir phosphate) exhibits potent antiviral activity in vitro against both influenza A and B viruses. Oseltamivir appears to be a potent and selective inhibitor of all influenza A neuraminidase subtypes (i.e., N1–N9) tested to date.

Viral surveillance data indicate that the majority of seasonal influenza A (H1N1)pdm09, influenza A (H3N2), and influenza B viruses circulating during recent influenza seasons, including in the US, have been susceptible to oseltamivir in vitro.

In vitro studies indicate that oseltamivir is active against avian influenza A (H5N1) and some other avian influenza A viruses (e.g., H7N7, H7N9, H9N2, H10N8). However, avian influenza A (H5N1) and avian influenza A (H7N9) with reduced in vitro susceptibility or resistance to oseltamivir have been reported rarely. (See Resistance.)

RESISTANCE

The major mechanisms of resistance to neuraminidase inhibitors (i.e., oseltamivir, zanamivir) that have been identified in vitro are viral neuraminidase (NA) mutations that affect the ability of the drugs to inhibit the enzyme and hemagglutinin (HA) mutations that reduce viral dependence on neuraminidase activity.

Influenza A and B viruses with decreased susceptibility to oseltamivir have been produced in vitro by serial passage of virus in cell culture in the presence of increasing concentrations of oseltamivir carboxylate and reduced in vitro susceptibility have been observed in clinical isolates.

HA substitutions selected in cell culture and associated with reduced susceptibility to oseltamivir include A11T, K173E, and R453M in influenza A (H3N2) and H99Q in influenza B (Yamagata lineage). In some cases, HA substitutions were selected in conjunction with known NA resistance substitutions and may contribute to reduced susceptibility to oseltamivir; however, the impact of HA substitutions on antiviral activity of oseltamivir in humans is unknown and likely depends on the influenza strain.

Influenza A virus variants with reduced susceptibility to oseltamivir include substitutions in neuraminidase N1 (i.e., I117V, E119V, R152K, Y155H, F174V, D199G/N, I223K/R/T/V, S247G/N, G249R+I267V, H275Y, N295S, Q313R+I427T, N325K, R368K) and in neuraminidase N2 (i.e., E41G, E119I/V, D151V, I222L/V, N294S, Q226H, R292K, SASG245–248 deletion, S247P). Influenza B virus variants with reduced susceptibility to oseltamivir recovered from patients receiving the drug or identified during viral surveillance include E117A, P139S, G140R, R150K, I221L/T/V, D197E/N/Y, A245D/S/T, H273Y, N294S, R374K, and G407S. The H275Y substitution in influenza A (H1N1) has been the major substitution associated with resistance to oseltamivir. In the event of an H5N1 pandemic, the N1 mutation at position 274 would be important because this is associated with a greater than 600-fold increase in inhibitory concentrations for oseltamivir in enzyme inhibition assays. Viruses that have neuraminidase mutations generally have reduced virulence. Although it has been suggested that these mutant viruses may have some degree of compromised infectivity and transmissibility compared with wild-type viruses, person-to-person transmission of oseltamivir-resistant variants of influenza A (H1N1) has been documented.

Strains of seasonal influenza with reduced in vitro susceptibility to oseltamivir have emerged in posttreatment isolates obtained from 1.3% of adults and adolescents and 8.6% of pediatric patients 1–12 years of age who received the drug in clinical studies of naturally acquired influenza infection. In pediatric treatment studies, the rate of treatment-emergent resistance to oseltamivir was

27–37% in children with influenza A (H1N1) and 3–18% in children with influenza A (H3N2). In one group of Japanese children who received oseltamivir for the treatment of seasonal influenza, oseltamivir-resistant mutants were detected in 18% of patients posttreatment. Resistant strains of influenza A and influenza B viruses have emerged in immunocompromised patients who received oseltamivir therapy, and there is evidence that influenza viruses resistant to oseltamivir may be selected at higher frequencies in immunocompromised adults and pediatric patients than in otherwise healthy individuals. In a study evaluating oseltamivir for treatment of influenza in immunocompromised patients, the rate of treatment-emergent resistance to oseltamivir was 27% in immunocompromised patients infected with influenza A (H1N1) and 12% in those infected with influenza A (H3N2); the rate of treatment-emergent resistance to oseltamivir was 32% in hematopoietic stem cell transplant (HSCT) recipients.

The frequency of resistance selection to oseltamivir and the prevalence of such resistant virus vary seasonally and geographically. Viral surveillance data from recent influenza seasons indicate that reduced in vitro susceptibility or resistance to oseltamivir was reported rarely in circulating strains of influenza A (H1N1) pdm09, influenza A (H3N2), influenza B (Yamagata lineage), and influenza B (Victoria lineage).

Avian influenza A (H5N1) and avian influenza A (H7N9) isolates with reduced in vitro susceptibility or resistance to oseltamivir have been reported. In a patient with influenza A (H5N1) infection who received prophylaxis with oseltamivir (75 mg once daily for 3 days) immediately followed by oseltamivir treatment (75 mg twice daily for 7 days), isolates obtained on the third day of oseltamivir prophylaxis had mutations associated with oseltamivir resistance (these isolates remained susceptible to zanamivir). In 2 patients in Vietnam who received oseltamivir for treatment of avian influenza A (H5N1) infection, isolates had an amino acid substitution (H274Y) associated with high-level oseltamivir resistance; both patients subsequently died. In a few patients with avian influenza A (H7N9) infection who were receiving oseltamivir for treatment, oseltamivir resistance emerged and was associated with treatment failure and adverse clinical outcomes. Genetic analyses of isolates from an ongoing epidemic of avian influenza A (H7N9) that has been occurring in China since October 2016 indicate that approximately 7–9% of isolates tested (many may have been collected after antiviral treatment was started) have known or suspected markers for reduced susceptibility to one or more neuraminidase inhibitor antivirals.

● Cross-resistance

Cross-resistance between oseltamivir and other neuraminidase inhibitors (e.g., peramivir, zanamivir) has been reported in influenza A and B viruses. However, because oseltamivir, peramivir, and zanamivir bind to different sites on the neuraminidase enzyme or interact differently with the binding sites, cross-resistance among the drugs is variable.

Some influenza A strains may have reduced susceptibility to oseltamivir and/or peramivir, but are susceptible to zanamivir; other strains may have reduced susceptibility to zanamivir, but are susceptible to oseltamivir and/or peramivir. Circulating influenza B (Victoria lineage) with reduced susceptibility to both oseltamivir and peramivir have been reported. Avian influenza A (H5N1) with the H274Y mutation that are resistant to oseltamivir have been susceptible to zanamivir in vitro.

Reduced in vitro susceptibility to all 3 drugs (oseltamivir, peramivir, zanamivir) has been observed in some circulating seasonal influenza A and influenza B viruses. Cross-resistance to both oseltamivir and zanamivir has been reported in vitro in influenza B with I222T, D198E/N, R371K, or G402S resistance-associated neuraminidase substitutions. The H275Y (N1 numbering) or N294S (N2 numbering) oseltamivir resistance-associated substitutions observed in the N1 neuraminidase subtype and the E119V or N294S oseltamivir resistance-associated substitutions observed in the N2 subtype (N2 numbering) are associated with reduced in vitro susceptibility to oseltamivir, but not zanamivir. The Q136K and K150T zanamivir resistance-associated substitutions observed in N1 neuraminidase or the S250G zanamivir resistance-associated substitutions observed in influenza B virus neuraminidase confer reduced in vitro susceptibility to zanamivir, but not oseltamivir. Influenza A (H1N1)pdm09 with the H275Y N1 amino acid substitution are cross-resistant to oseltamivir and peramivir, but susceptible to zanamivir in vitro. Avian influenza A (H5N1) isolates with the H274Y mutation that are resistant to oseltamivir have been susceptible to zanamivir in vitro.

An amino acid substitution that confers cross-resistance between neuraminidase inhibitors (oseltamivir, peramivir, zanamivir) and adamantane derivatives (M2 ion channel inhibitors; amantadine, rimantadine) has not been identified.

However, influenza strains that have a neuraminidase substitution that confers resistance to neuraminidase inhibitors and also have an M2 substitution that confers resistance to M2 ion channel inhibitors may be resistant to both classes of influenza antivirals. The clinical relevance of phenotypic cross-resistance evaluations has not been established.

PHARMACOKINETICS

● Absorption

Oseltamivir phosphate is readily absorbed following oral administration and then extensively converted by hepatic esterases to the active metabolite, oseltamivir carboxylate. Following oral administration of oseltamivir 75 mg twice daily for multiple days in healthy adults, peak plasma concentrations of oseltamivir or oseltamivir carboxylate were 65 or 348 ng/mL, respectively. Following oral administration of oseltamivir phosphate, oseltamivir carboxylate is detectable in plasma within 30 minutes; peak concentrations of oseltamivir carboxylate are attained within 3–4 hours. The absolute bioavailability of oseltamivir carboxylate is 80% following oral administration of oseltamivir phosphate. Plasma concentrations of oseltamivir carboxylate are proportional to dosage up to an oseltamivir dosage of 500 mg twice daily.

Administration of oseltamivir phosphate with food has no effect on peak plasma concentrations or area under the plasma concentration-time curve (AUC) of oseltamivir carboxylate.

Pharmacokinetic data indicate that a dosage of 3 mg/kg twice daily in neonates and infants 2 weeks to less than 1 year of age result in oseltamivir concentrations similar to or higher than those reported in adults and children 1 year of age or older receiving usual dosage of the drug.

Following oral administration of oseltamivir phosphate in geriatric individuals (65–78 years of age), systemic exposure to oseltamivir carboxylate at steady-state is about 25–35% higher compared with younger adults receiving the same dosage.

In individuals with varying degrees of renal impairment receiving 100 mg of oseltamivir phosphate twice daily (about 1.3 times the maximum recommended dosage) for 5 days, oseltamivir carboxylate exposure increases with declining renal function. In patients undergoing continuous ambulatory peritoneal dialysis (CAPD), peak concentrations of oseltamivir carboxylate following a single 30-mg dose of oseltamivir or once-weekly oseltamivir was approximately threefold higher than peak concentrations in patients with normal renal function receiving 75 mg twice daily.

Limited data in patients with cirrhosis indicate that hepatic carboxylesterase activity in patients with moderate hepatic impairment is sufficient to metabolize oseltamivir phosphate to oseltamivir carboxylate. Systemic exposure to oseltamivir carboxylate in individuals with mild or moderate hepatic impairment is comparable to that in individuals without hepatic impairment.

● Distribution

Following oral administration of oseltamivir phosphate, oseltamivir carboxylate is distributed throughout the body, including into the upper and lower respiratory tract.

It is not known whether oseltamivir or oseltamivir carboxylate crosses the placenta in humans; placental transfer of oseltamivir carboxylate has been demonstrated in rats and rabbits.

Oseltamivir and oseltamivir carboxylate are distributed into milk.

Oseltamivir phosphate is 42% bound to plasma proteins; oseltamivir carboxylate is 3% bound to plasma proteins.

● Elimination

Oseltamivir phosphate is extensively (greater than 90%) converted to oseltamivir carboxylate (the active metabolite), principally by hepatic esterases. Oseltamivir carboxylate is not further metabolized.

Oseltamivir phosphate and oseltamivir carboxylate are not metabolized by cytochrome P-450 (CYP) enzymes.

Oseltamivir carboxylate is eliminated (greater than 99%) by renal excretion; less than 20% of an oral radiolabeled dose of oseltamivir phosphate is eliminated in feces.

The plasma half-life of oseltamivir phosphate is 1–3 hours; half-life of oseltamivir carboxylate is 6–10 hours. Half-lives observed in geriatric individuals are similar to those observed in younger adults.

Clearance of both oseltamivir phosphate and oseltamivir carboxylate is increased in younger pediatric patients compared with adults. Total clearance of oseltamivir carboxylate decreases linearly with increasing age (up to 12 years of age); pharmacokinetics in those 12 years of age or older is similar to that in adults.

Renal clearance of oseltamivir carboxylate decreases linearly with creatinine clearance.

CHEMISTRY AND STABILITY

● Chemistry

Oseltamivir phosphate is a carbocyclic transition state sialic acid analog. Oseltamivir differs structurally from zanamivir (another sialic acid analog) by the absence of glycerol and guanidino groups. These structural modifications in oseltamivir result in a compound with substantially improved oral bioavailability compared with that of zanamivir.

Oseltamivir phosphate occurs as a white, crystalline solid with a bitter taste. Oseltamivir phosphate has an aqueous solubility of 588 mg/mL at 25°C.

● Stability

Oseltamivir phosphate capsules should be stored at 25°C, but may be exposed to temperatures ranging from 15–30°C.

Oseltamivir phosphate powder for oral suspension should be stored at 25°C, but may be exposed to temperatures ranging from 15–30°C. The reconstituted oral suspension should be stored at 2–8°C for up to 17 days. Alternatively, the reconstituted suspension may be stored for up to 10 days at 25°C and may be exposed to temperatures ranging from 15–30°C during this time. The reconstituted oral suspension should not be frozen.

Extemporaneous oral suspensions of oseltamivir phosphate prepared according to the manufacturer's directions using commercially available 75-mg capsules of the drug are stable for 5 weeks when refrigerated at 2–8°C or for 5 days when stored at room temperature (25°C).

PREPARATIONS

Excipients in commercially available drug preparations may have clinically important effects in some individuals; consult specific product labeling for details.

Oseltamivir Phosphate

Oral

Capsules	30 mg* (of oseltamivir)	**Tamiflu®**, Genentech
	45 mg* (of oseltamivir)	**Tamiflu®**, Genentech
	75 mg* (of oseltamivir)	**Tamiflu®**, Genentech
For suspension	6 mg* (of oseltamivir) per mL	**Tamiflu®**, Genentech

* available from one or more manufacturer, distributor, and/or repackager by generic (nonproprietary) name

† Use is not currently included in the labeling approved by the US Food and Drug Administration.

Selected Revisions October 4, 2021, © Copyright, November 1, 1999, American Society of Health-System Pharmacists, Inc.

Peramivir

8:18.28 • NEURAMINIDASE INHIBITORS

■ Peramivir is a neuraminidase inhibitor antiviral active against influenza A and B viruses.

USES

● **Treatment of Seasonal Influenza A and B Virus Infections**

Peramivir is used for the *treatment* of acute, uncomplicated illness caused by influenza A or B viruses in adults, adolescents, and children 6 months of age or older who have been symptomatic for no longer than 2 days.

Although peramivir has been used for the treatment of serious influenza† in some patients, efficacy of the drug has not been established in patients with serious influenza requiring hospitalization.

Safety and efficacy of peramivir have not been established for prevention of influenza virus infection†, and use of the drug for prophylaxis of influenza is not recommended.

For the treatment of suspected or confirmed acute, uncomplicated seasonal influenza in otherwise healthy outpatients, the US Centers for Disease Control and Prevention (CDC), Infectious Diseases Society of America (IDSA), and other experts state that any age-appropriate influenza antiviral (oral oseltamivir, inhaled zanamivir, oral baloxavir marboxil, IV peramivir) can be used if not contraindicated. CDC states that early empiric antiviral treatment can be considered in outpatients with suspected influenza (e.g., influenza-like illness such as fever with either cough or sore throat) based on clinical judgement if such treatment can be initiated within 48 hours of illness onset.

For the treatment of suspected or confirmed seasonal influenza in hospitalized patients or outpatients with severe, complicated, or progressive illness (e.g., pneumonia, exacerbation of underlying chronic medical conditions), CDC states that oseltamivir is the preferred influenza antiviral and should be initiated as soon as possible, ideally within 48 hours, without waiting for laboratory confirmation. Oseltamivir is the preferred influenza antiviral in hospitalized patients or outpatients with severe, complicated, or progressive influenza because of the lack of data regarding use of other influenza antivirals in such patients. Although data are insufficient regarding use of IV peramivir for the treatment of severe influenza in hospitalized patients or outpatients†, CDC states that use of the drug should be considered in patients who cannot tolerate or absorb oseltamivir administered orally or enterically (e.g., because of suspected or known gastric stasis, malabsorption, or GI bleeding).

Influenza and coronavirus disease 2019 (COVID-19) caused by severe acute respiratory syndrome coronavirus 2 (SARS-CoV-2) have overlapping signs and symptoms and coinfection with influenza A or B viruses and SARS-CoV-2 can occur and should be considered, particularly in hospitalized patients with severe respiratory disease. Although laboratory testing can help distinguish between influenza virus infection and SARS-CoV-2 infection, CDC recommends that empiric influenza treatment should be initiated in patients with suspected influenza who are hospitalized, have severe, complicated, or progressive illness, or are at high risk for influenza complication without waiting for results of influenza testing, SARS-CoV-2 testing, or multiplex molecular assays that detect influenza A and B viruses and SARS-CoV-2.

Viral surveillance data available from local and state health departments and CDC should be considered when selecting an antiviral for the treatment of seasonal influenza. Strains of circulating influenza viruses and the antiviral susceptibility of these strains constantly evolve, and the possibility that emergence of resistant strains may decrease effectiveness of influenza antivirals should be considered. Although circulating influenza A and B viruses during recent years generally have been susceptible to peramivir, clinicians should consult the most recent information on susceptibility of circulating viruses when selecting an antiviral for the treatment of influenza.

CDC issues recommendations concerning the use of antivirals for the treatment of influenza, and these recommendations are updated as needed during each influenza season. Information regarding influenza surveillance and updated recommendations for treatment of seasonal influenza are available from CDC at http://www.cdc.gov/flu.

Clinical Trials and Experience

Acute, Uncomplicated Influenza in Adults

Efficacy and safety of peramivir for the treatment of acute, uncomplicated influenza in adults were evaluated in randomized, controlled studies in otherwise healthy adults with documented influenza infection (study 621). The majority of patients enrolled in these studies had infections caused by seasonal influenza A; only a limited number of patients had infections caused by seasonal influenza B. In a placebo-controlled study in adults 20–65 years of age with documented influenza infection, peramivir (single 600-mg IV dose) initiated in an outpatient setting within 48 hours of onset of symptoms decreased the median duration of influenza symptoms (i.e., nasal congestion, sore throat, cough, aches or pains in muscles or joints, fatigue, headache, feverishness) by approximately 21 hours and decreased the median time to recovery of normal temperature (oral temperature less than 37°C) by approximately 12 hours compared with placebo. In a phase 3, double-blind, randomized study in adults 20 years of age or older with documented influenza infection who received treatment in an outpatient setting within 48 hours of onset of symptoms, peramivir (single 600-mg IV dose) was noninferior to oseltamivir (75 mg orally twice daily for 5 days) based on median time to alleviation of influenza symptoms.

Acute, Uncomplicated Influenza in Pediatric Patients 6 months to 17 years of Age

Efficacy and safety of peramivir for the treatment of acute, uncomplicated influenza in pediatric patients 6 months to 17 years of age were evaluated in a randomized, multicenter, open-label, active-controlled trial (study 305). At study entry, patients had fever (oral temperature 37.8°C or greater) with at least one respiratory symptom (cough or rhinitis) or a positive influenza rapid antigen test and were randomized to receive a single dose of IV peramivir (12 mg/kg [up to 600 mg] in those 6 months to 12 years of age or 600 mg in those 13–17 years of age) or a 5-day regimen of oral oseltamivir (twice daily). Antiviral treatment was initiated within 48 hours of onset of symptoms and adjunctive use of fever-reducing medications was allowed. The primary end point was the safety of peramivir compared to oseltamivir as measured by adverse events, laboratory analysis, vital signs, and physical examination. Secondary end points included efficacy outcomes such as time to resolution of influenza symptoms and time to resolution of fever; however, the trial was not powered to detect statistically significant differences in the secondary end points. A total of 81 pediatric patients received IV peramivir (median age 7.5 years, 52% male, 60% infected with influenza A virus, 33% infected with influenza B virus, 6% coinfected with both influenza A and B viruses). The median time to alleviation of combined influenza symptoms was 79 hours in those treated with peramivir and 100 hours in those treated with oseltamivir; the median time to recovery to normal temperature (less than 37°C) was 40 and 35 hours, respectively.

Serious Influenza Requiring Hospitalization

Efficacy and safety of peramivir for the treatment of influenza in patients requiring hospitalization† were evaluated in a phase 3, randomized, double-blind, placebo-controlled study that included adults and children 6 years of age or older. Patients who were hospitalized with influenza and had been symptomatic for less than 72 hours were randomized to receive the usual standard of care in conjunction with a 5-day regimen of peramivir (600 mg IV once daily in adults; 10 mg/kg IV once daily [up to 600 mg daily] in children and adolescents) or placebo. The primary end point was time to clinical resolution (defined as time from initiation of study treatment until at least 4 of 5 vital sign abnormalities, including body temperature and oxygen saturation, had been resolved for at least 24 hours). A preplanned interim analysis indicated that there was no clinically important difference in the median time to clinical resolution in those treated with peramivir (41.8 hours) or placebo (48.9 hours), although there was some evidence that peramivir provided some benefit in time to clinical resolution in those who had been symptomatic for less than 48 hours prior to treatment and in those who required treatment in an intensive care unit (ICU). The study was terminated after the interim analysis because of practical considerations regarding the ability to obtain a sample size adequate for further evaluation.

● **Avian Influenza A Virus Infections**

Although safety and efficacy have not been established, neuraminidase inhibitors (oseltamivir, peramivir, zanamivir) have been used or are recommended for the treatment or prevention of infections caused by susceptible avian influenza A viruses†.

Experience to date indicates that avian influenza A viruses do not easily transmit from wild or domestic birds, water fowl, or poultry to humans, but human infections may rarely occur and have been linked to contact with live or dead infected birds or poultry, uncooked poultry products, or surfaces contaminated with infected poultry feces or respiratory secretions. Human cases generally have involved a highly pathogenic Asian strain of avian influenza A (H5N1) that has been circulating since 2003 in poultry in Asia, Africa, the Pacific, Eastern Europe, and the Middle East or a novel avian influenza A (H7N9) virus that was first identified in China in March 2013.

Worldwide, most avian influenza A viruses isolated in wild birds, water fowl, or poultry have been designated as low pathogenic strains; however, highly pathogenic avian influenza (HPAI) strains are occasionally detected. Since December 2014, HPAI viruses (H5N1, H5N2, H5N8) have been reported in wild birds, water fowl, and/or domestic poultry (commercial or backyard flocks) in the US (e.g., Arkansas, California, Idaho, Iowa, Minnesota, Missouri, Nebraska, North Dakota, Oregon, South Dakota, Utah, Washington, Wisconsin). Although CDC states that the risk of human infection with these HPAI H5 viruses is considered low in the US, human infection is possible since other closely related HPAI H5 viruses in Asia and other countries have caused sporadic cases of human respiratory illness. The HPAI (H5N1) strain reported in poultry outbreaks in the US is a new reassortant virus that is genetically different from the highly pathogenic Asian strain of influenza A (H5N1) that has caused human infections in Asia and other countries and has been associated with a high mortality rate.

Appropriate use of a neuraminidase inhibitor antivirals is an important component of response and control measures to treat avian influenza A virus infections and help reduce the risk of additional human infections.

For the treatment of uncomplicated avian influenza A infections in outpatients, CDC states that oral oseltamivir, IV peramivir, or inhaled zanamivir may be used. For the treatment of severe, complicated, or progressive avian influenza A infections in hospitalized patients or outpatients, including infections caused by avian influenza A (H7N9), avian influenza A (H5N1), or novel avian influenza A H5 viruses, CDC recommends oseltamivir as the antiviral of choice. In those with severe avian influenza A infections who cannot tolerate or absorb oseltamivir administered orally or enterically (e.g., because of suspected or known gastric stasis, malabsorption, or GI bleeding), CDC states that use of IV peramivir may be considered.

When antiviral prophylaxis is indicated in close contacts of individuals with confirmed or probable infection with avian influenza A viruses associated with severe disease or with potential to cause severe disease or is indicated in individuals who have been exposed to birds infected with such avian influenza A viruses, CDC recommends oral oseltamivir or inhaled zanamivir.

Information regarding treatment and prevention of avian influenza A infections is available from CDC at http://www.cdc.gov/flu/avianflu/ and WHO at https://www.who.int/teams/global-influenza-programme/avian-influenza.

● **Pandemic Influenza**

Peramivir is recommended as an alternative for the treatment of pandemic influenza† caused by susceptible strains of influenza virus.

Influenza viruses can cause seasonal epidemics and, occasionally, pandemics during which rates of illness and death from influenza-related complications can increase dramatically worldwide. The most recent influenza pandemic occurred during 2009 and was related to a novel influenza A (H1N1) strain, influenza A (H1N1)pdm09.

Influenza outbreaks caused by influenza A (H1N1)pdm09 virus were reported in several countries, including the US, beginning in March and April 2009. The virus is a triple-reassortant swine influenza virus with genes from human, swine, and avian influenza A viruses and contained a unique combination of gene segments that had not been previously reported among human or swine influenza A in the US or elsewhere. The influenza A (H1N1)pdm09 virus was antigenically distinct from previous human influenza A (H1N1) viruses that had been in circulation since 1977, and widespread transmission of the virus occurred since most individuals had no preexisting antibody to the strain. In the US, the 2009 influenza A (H1N1)pdm09 pandemic was characterized by a substantial increase in influenza activity that peaked in late October and early November 2009 and returned to seasonal baseline levels by January 2010. At that time, more than 99% of influenza viruses circulating in the US were the influenza A (H1N1)pdm09 virus; more than 60 million Americans become ill with the virus and more than 270,000 hospitalizations and 12,500 deaths were reported. After the pandemic, influenza A (H1N1)pdm09 became a seasonal influenza virus and continues to circulate with other seasonal influenza viruses.

The spread of the highly pathogenic Asian strain of influenza A (H5N1) in poultry in Asia, Africa, the Pacific, Eastern Europe, and the Middle East that has been occurring since 2003 and has caused human infections (including fatalities) represents a potential future pandemic threat. In addition, the novel avian

influenza A (H7N9) virus that was first identified in China in March 2013 and has been causing sporadic human infections has pandemic potential.

Information on pandemic influenza, including planning and preparedness resources if an influenza pandemic occurs, is available from CDC at https://www.cdc.gov/flu/pandemic-resources/index.htm and WHO at https://www.who.int/initiatives/pandemic-influenza-preparedness-framework.

DOSAGE AND ADMINISTRATION

● Administration

Peramivir is administered by IV infusion.

IV Administration

Peramivir injection concentrate for IV use containing 10 mg of the drug per mL must be diluted prior to IV infusion.

Peramivir is compatible with 0.9% or 0.45% sodium chloride, 5% dextrose, or lactated Ringer's injection. Solutions of the drug are compatible with materials commonly used for administration (e.g., polyvinyl chloride and polyvinyl chloride-free infusion bags, polypropylene syringes, polyethylene tubing).

Peramivir solutions should *not* be mixed with or administered simultaneously with other drugs.

Vials of peramivir injection concentrate for IV use contain no preservatives or bacteriostatic agents and are intended for single use only.

Dilution

The appropriate dose of peramivir injection concentrate for IV use containing 10 mg/mL should be withdrawn from the vial and diluted in 0.9% sodium chloride injection, 0.45% sodium chloride injection, 5% dextrose injection, or lactated Ringer's injection to provide a solution for IV infusion containing 1–6 mg/mL of the drug. The maximum recommended total infusion volume depends on the patient's age and weight. (See Table 1.)

TABLE 1. Maximum Total Infusion Volume of Diluted Peramivir

Age	Weight	Maximum Volume of Diluted Peramivir Solution Containing 1–6 mg/mL
Infants 6 months to 1 year of age	Any	25 mL
Adults and pediatric patients ≥1 year of age	5 kg to <10 kg	25 mL
	10 kg to <15 kg	50 mL
	15 kg to <20 kg	75 mL
	≥20 kg	100 mL

Following dilution, peramivir solutions should be administered immediately. Alternatively, diluted peramivir solutions may be stored for up to 24 hours at 2–8°C. Refrigerated solutions should be allowed to reach room temperature and then administered immediately. Unused portions should be discarded 24 hours after dilution.

Peramivir solutions should appear clear and colorless and should be inspected visually for particulate matter and discoloration prior to administration.

Rate of Administration

Peramivir solutions should be administered by IV infusion over 15–30 minutes.

● Dosage

Adult Dosage

Treatment of Seasonal Influenza A and B Virus Infections

For the *treatment* of acute, uncomplicated influenza in adults 18 years of age or older, the recommended dosage of peramivir is a single 600-mg dose given by IV infusion within 2 days of symptom onset.

Treatment of Avian Influenza A Virus Infections

If peramivir is used for the *treatment* of avian influenza virus infections†, including avian influenza A (H7N9), avian influenza A (H5N1), and novel avian influenza A H5 viruses, CDC recommends that adults receive a dosage of 600 mg given IV once daily for 5 days or longer. Only limited data are available regarding use of peramivir for the treatment of these infections; a single-dose regimen is not recommended.

Pediatric Dosage

Treatment of Seasonal Influenza A and B Virus Infections

For the *treatment* of acute, uncomplicated influenza in children 6 months to 12 years of age, the recommended dosage of peramivir is a single dose of 12 mg/kg (up to 600 mg) given by IV infusion within 2 days of symptom onset.

For the *treatment* of acute, uncomplicated influenza in adolescents 13 years of age or older, the recommended dosage of peramivir is a single 600-mg dose given by IV infusion within 2 days of symptom onset.

Treatment of Avian Influenza A Virus Infections

If peramivir is used for the *treatment* of avian influenza virus infections†, including avian influenza A (H7N9), avian influenza A (H5N1), and novel avian influenza A H5 viruses, CDC recommends that children receive a dosage of 10 mg/kg (up to 600 mg) given IV once daily for 5 days or longer. Only limited data are available regarding use of peramivir for the treatment of these infections; a single-dose regimen is not recommended.

● Special Populations

Hepatic Impairment

Peramivir has not been studied in patients with hepatic impairment; clinically important alterations in peramivir pharmacokinetics are not expected in such patients.

Renal Impairment

Dosage of peramivir should be decreased in adults and pediatric patients 2 years of age or older with creatinine clearances less than 50 mL/minute. (See Table 2.)

TABLE 2. Recommended Peramivir Dosage for Treatment of Seasonal Influenza in Adult and Pediatric Patients with Renal Impairment

Age	Creatinine Clearance (mL/minute)	Dosage (Single Dose)
≥13 years of age	30–49	200 mg
	10–20	100 mg
2–12 years of age	30–49	4 mg/kg
	10–20	2 mg/kg

Data are not available to inform a recommendation for dosage adjustment of peramivir in pediatric patients 6 months to less than 2 years of age with creatinine clearances less than 50 mL/minute.

If peramivir is used in patients with chronic renal impairment maintained on hemodialysis, dosage should be adjusted based on renal function and the drug should be administered after hemodialysis. (See Renal Impairment under Cautions.)

Geriatric Adults

Dosage adjustments based solely on age are not necessary in geriatric patients.

CAUTIONS

● Contraindications

Known serious hypersensitivity (e.g., anaphylaxis, erythema multiforme, Stevens-Johnson syndrome) to peramivir or any ingredient in the formulation.

● Warnings/Precautions

Sensitivity Reactions

Hypersensitivity Reactions

Serious dermatologic reactions (erythema multiforme, Stevens-Johnson syndrome) have been reported in patients receiving peramivir. Anaphylactic/anaphylactoid reactions, exfoliative dermatitis, and rash also have been reported during postmarketing experience.

If anaphylaxis or a serious skin reaction occurs or is suspected, peramivir should be discontinued and appropriate treatment initiated.

Neuropsychiatric and CNS Effects

Delirium and abnormal behavior leading to injury have been reported during postmarketing experience in patients with influenza receiving neuraminidase inhibitors, including peramivir. Most cases involved pediatric patients and generally had an abrupt onset and rapid resolution. The role of peramivir in these events has not been established.

Influenza itself can be associated with a variety of neurologic and behavioral symptoms (e.g., hallucinations, delirium, abnormal behavior) that sometimes result in fatalities. Although such events may occur in the setting of encephalitis or encephalopathy, they can occur in patients with uncomplicated influenza.

Patients with influenza should be closely monitored for signs of abnormal behavior.

Differential Diagnosis

When making treatment decisions in patients with suspected influenza, clinicians should consider the possibility of primary or concomitant bacterial infections for which peramivir would be ineffective.

Serious bacterial infections may begin with influenza-like symptoms or may coexist with or occur as complications of influenza. There is no evidence that peramivir prevents such complications.

There is no evidence that peramivir is effective for illness caused by any organisms other than influenza A or B.

Influenza Vaccination

Influenza antivirals, including peramivir, are important adjuncts to vaccination in the control of influenza but are not a substitute for annual vaccination with a seasonal influenza vaccine (influenza virus vaccine inactivated, influenza vaccine recombinant, influenza vaccine live).

Although influenza antivirals, including peramivir, may be used concomitantly with or at any time before or after influenza virus vaccine inactivated or influenza vaccine recombinant, influenza antivirals may inhibit the vaccine virus contained in influenza vaccine live intranasal and decrease efficacy of the live vaccine. (See Influenza Vaccines under Drug Interactions.)

Specific Populations

Pregnancy

Data regarding use of peramivir in pregnant women are insufficient to determine whether the drug is associated with a risk of adverse developmental outcomes.

In animal reproduction studies, no adverse embryofetal effects were observed in pregnant rats when peramivir was administered by IV injection once daily at the maximum feasible dosage, resulting in systemic drug exposures approximately 8 times those in humans at the recommended dosage. However, when peramivir was administered to pregnant rats by continuous IV infusion, fetal abnormalities (reduced renal papilla, dilated ureters) were observed. In rabbits, peramivir administered by IV injection once daily during organogenesis at exposures 8 times those in humans at the recommended dosage resulted in developmental toxicity (abortion or premature delivery) at maternally toxic doses.

Pregnant women are at increased risk for severe complications from influenza, which may lead to adverse pregnancy and/or fetal outcomes including maternal death, stillbirths, birth defects, preterm delivery, low birthweight, and small size for gestational age.

CDC states that only limited data are available regarding use of peramivir for the treatment of influenza in pregnant women. Oseltamivir is the preferred antiviral for the treatment of suspected or confirmed influenza in women who are pregnant or up to 2 weeks postpartum.

Lactation

It is not known whether peramivir is distributed into human milk, affects milk production, or has any effects on breast-fed infants. Peramivir is distributed into milk in rats. (See Distribution under Pharmacokinetics.)

The benefits of breast-feeding and the importance of peramivir to the woman should be considered along with potential adverse effects on the breast-fed child from the drug or from the underlying maternal condition.

Pediatric Use

Safety and efficacy of peramivir have not been established in pediatric patients younger than 6 months of age.

Safety and efficacy of peramivir for the treatment of acute, uncomplicated influenza in pediatric patients 6 months to 17 years of age have been established and are supported by evidence from adequate and well-controlled trials of the drug in adults and additional data from a randomized, open-label, active-controlled trial in pediatric patients in this age group (86 patients 6 months to 12 years of age and 21 patients 13–17 years of age received peramivir). Data from the open-label pediatric study indicated that the safety profile of the drug in pediatric patients 6 months to 17 years of age generally is similar to that reported in adults. The only adverse effects reported in 2% or more of pediatric patients treated with peramivir and not reported in adults were vomiting and proteinuria.

Geriatric Use

Clinical studies of peramivir did not include sufficient numbers of patients 65 years of age and older to determine whether geriatric patients respond differently than younger adults. Other reported clinical experience has not identified differences in responses between geriatric and younger adults.

Peramivir pharmacokinetics in geriatric adults are similar to the pharmacokinetics of the drug reported in younger adults; therefore, dosage adjustments based solely on age are not necessary in adults 65 years of age and older.

Hepatic Impairment

The pharmacokinetics of peramivir have not been studied in patients with hepatic impairment; however, hepatic function is not expected to substantially affect pharmacokinetics of peramivir since the drug does not undergo clinically important metabolism.

Renal Impairment

The mean AUC of peramivir in adults following IV administration of a single 2-mg/kg dose was increased by 28, 302, or 412% in those with creatinine clearances of 50–79, 30–49, or 10–29 mL/minute, respectively, compared with AUCs reported in adults with normal renal function. Pharmacokinetics of peramivir have not been evaluated in pediatric patients with renal impairment.

Dosage of peramivir should be adjusted in adults and pediatric patients 2 years of age or older with creatinine clearances less than 50 mL/minute. Data are not available to inform a recommendation for dosage adjustment in pediatric patients 6 months to less than 2 years of age with creatinine clearances less than 50 mL/minute. (See Renal Impairment under Dosage and Administration.)

● *Common Adverse Effects*

Adverse effects occurring in 2% or more of adults or pediatric patients receiving peramivir include diarrhea, vomiting, constipation, insomnia, and hypertension.

DRUG INTERACTIONS

● *Drugs Affected or Metabolized by Hepatic Microsomal Enzymes*

Peramivir is not metabolized by and does not induce or inhibit cytochrome P-450 (CYP) isoenzymes. Drug interactions with drugs that are substrates or inhibitors of these enzymes are unlikely.

● *Drugs Affecting or Affected by P-glycoprotein Transport System*

Peramivir is not a substrate for and is not an inhibitor of the P-glycoprotein (P-gp) transport system.

● *Antivirals*

Oseltamivir

There was no evidence of pharmacokinetic interactions when oseltamivir (single 75-mg oral dose) was used concomitantly with peramivir (single 600-mg IV dose).

There was no in vitro evidence of antagonistic antiviral effects between oseltamivir and peramivir when the combination was evaluated in cell cultures infected with influenza A (H1N1).

Rimantadine

There was no evidence of pharmacokinetic interactions when rimantadine (single 100-mg oral dose) was used concomitantly with peramivir (single 600-mg IV dose).

There was no in vitro evidence of antagonistic antiviral effects between rimantadine and peramivir when the combination was evaluated in cell cultures infected with influenza A (H1N1) or influenza A (H3N2).

Zanamivir

Concomitant use of zanamivir and peramivir is not recommended.

● *Estrogens and Progestins*

There was no evidence of pharmacokinetic interactions when oral contraceptives containing ethinyl estradiol and levonorgestrel were used concomitantly with peramivir.

● *Probenecid*

There was no evidence of pharmacokinetic interactions when probenecid was used concomitantly with peramivir.

● *Vaccines*

Influenza Vaccines

Although concomitant use of peramivir and influenza virus vaccine inactivated (IIV) or influenza vaccine recombinant (RIV) has not been evaluated, CDC's Advisory Committee on Immunization Practices (ACIP) states that antivirals used for the treatment of influenza have no effect on the immune response to inactivated IIV or RIV and these inactivated vaccines may be administered simultaneously with or at any time before or after influenza antivirals, including peramivir.

Safety and efficacy of concomitant use of peramivir and influenza vaccine live intranasal (LAIV) have not been studied. Because influenza antivirals, including peramivir, inhibit replication of influenza viruses and may inhibit the vaccine virus, these antivirals potentially could decrease the immune response to LAIV and efficacy of the live vaccine. Although the manufacturer of peramivir states that LAIV should not be administered until at least 48 hours after administration of peramivir and that peramivir should be avoided until at least 14 days after administration of LAIV unless medically indicated, the optimal interval between administration of influenza antivirals and LAIV is not known. Based on the long half-life of peramivir, ACIP states that it is reasonable to assume that peramivir might interfere with LAIV if given from 5 days before through 2 weeks after vaccination. This interval for potential interference might be further prolonged in patients with medical conditions that delay drug clearance (e.g., renal insufficiency). ACIP states that individuals who received peramivir from 5 days before to 2 weeks after LAIV should be revaccinated using age-appropriate IIV or RIV.

PHARMACOKINETICS

● *Absorption*

Bioavailability

Following IV infusion over 30 minutes, peak serum concentrations of peramivir are attained at the end of the infusion. Accumulation of the drug is negligible following multiple doses for up to 10 days.

There is a linear relationship between the dose of peramivir and exposure parameters (peak plasma concentrations, area under the plasma concentration-time curve [AUC]) of the drug.

● *Distribution*

Extent

Following IV administration, peramivir is well distributed within extracellular fluid spaces, including the nose and throat.

It is not known whether peramivir is distributed into human milk. Peramivir is distributed into milk in rats; peak milk concentrations are attained 0.75 hours after an IV dose in rats and the milk to plasma AUC ratio is approximately 0.5.

Plasma Protein Binding

Peramivir is less than 30% bound to plasma proteins.

● *Elimination*

Metabolism

Peramivir does not undergo clinically important metabolism.

The drug is not a substrate for and does not affect cytochrome P-450 (CYP) isoenzymes.

Elimination Route

Following IV administration of peramivir, approximately 90% of the dose is eliminated unchanged in urine, principally by glomerular filtration.

Peramivir is removed by hemodialysis; systemic exposure is decreased 73–81% in patients undergoing hemodialysis.

Half-life

The plasma half-life of peramivir following a single 600-mg IV dose in healthy adults is approximately 20 hours.

Special Populations

In pediatric patients 2–12 years of age, the pharmacokinetics of peramivir following a single 12-mg/kg IV dose of the drug are similar to the pharmacokinetics reported in adults following a single 600-mg IV dose of the drug. Peramivir pharmacokinetics following a single 600-mg IV dose in adolescents 13–17 years of age are similar to the pharmacokinetics reported in adults following a single 600-mg IV dose. Although geometric mean peak plasma concentrations and AUCs of peramivir in pediatric patients 6 months to less than 2 years of age are lower than those reported in healthy adults, the difference in exposure is not considered clinically important.

In adults with creatinine clearances of 50–79, 30–49, or less than 30 mL/minute, the AUC of peramivir was increased by 28, 302, or 412%, respectively, compared with those with normal renal function. Pharmacokinetics of peramivir have not been evaluated in pediatric patients with renal impairment.

Although the pharmacokinetics of peramivir have not been studied in patients with hepatic impairment, substantial alterations in peramivir pharmacokinetics are not expected in such patients since the drug does not undergo clinically important metabolism.

Peramivir pharmacokinetics in geriatric individuals are similar to the pharmacokinetics in younger adults.

DESCRIPTION

Peramivir is a neuraminidase inhibitor antiviral and is pharmacologically related to other neuraminidase inhibitors (e.g., oseltamivir, zanamivir).

Peramivir is a potent selective competitive inhibitor of the influenza virus neuraminidase, an enzyme essential for viral replication. Neuraminidase cleaves terminal sialic acid residues from glycoconjugates to enable the release of virus from infected cells, prevents the formation of viral aggregates after release from host cells, and possibly facilitates viral invasion of the upper airways.

● *Spectrum*

Peramivir is active in vitro in cell culture against both influenza A and B viruses.

Viral surveillance data indicate that the majority of seasonal influenza A (H1N1)pdm09, influenza A (H3N2), and influenza B viruses circulating worldwide, including in the US, during recent influenza seasons have been susceptible to peramivir in vitro; reduced in vitro susceptibility or resistance to peramivir has been reported rarely.

Peramivir has been active in vitro in cell culture against some avian influenza A viruses, including some strains of avian influenza A (H5N1) and (H7N9).

● *Resistance*

The major mechanisms of resistance to neuraminidase inhibitors that have been identified in vitro are viral neuraminidase mutations that affect the ability of the drugs to inhibit the enzyme and hemagglutinin mutations that reduce viral dependence on neuraminidase activity.

Resistance to peramivir has been produced in vitro by serial passage of influenza A and B viruses in the presence of increasing concentrations of the drug. In addition, reduced in vitro susceptibility or resistance to peramivir due to mutations in viral neuraminidase or hemagglutinin have been observed rarely in clinical isolates of seasonal influenza A and B viruses. The clinical importance of reduced in vitro susceptibility to peramivir in these strains is unknown.

Influenza A virus variants with reduced in vitro susceptibility to peramivir have included those with substitutions in neuraminidase N1 (i.e., N58D, I211T,

I223R/V, G147R, S247N, H275Y) or neuraminidase N2 (i.e., E119V, Q136K, D151A/E/G/N/V, K249E, R292K, N294S, Q391K). Influenza B virus variants with reduced in vitro susceptibility to peramivir have included those with E105K, D197N, I221T/V, H134Y, P139S, D197E/N/Y, A200T, H273Y, H275Y, R374K, H431Y, or T146I substitutions. Hemagglutinin mutations associated with reduced susceptibility to peramivir include D125S and R208K (influenza A H1N1); N63K, G78D, N145D, and K189E (influenza A H3N2); and T139N, G141E, R162M, D195N, T198N, and Y319H (influenza B).

Some clinical isolates of avian influenza A (H5N1) and (H7N9) have had amino acid substitutions that conferred reduced susceptibility to peramivir. The clinical importance of reduced in vitro susceptibility to peramivir in these avian influenza A viruses is unknown; the effects of specific substitutions on susceptibility may be strain-dependent.

Cross-resistance between peramivir and other neuraminidase inhibitors (e.g., oseltamivir, zanamivir) has been reported in influenza A and B viruses. However, because oseltamivir, peramivir, and zanamivir bind to different sites on the neuraminidase enzyme or interact differently with the binding sites, cross-resistance among the drugs is variable.

Cross-resistance between peramivir and baloxavir, a polymerase acidic (PA) endonuclease inhibitor antiviral, is not expected since neuraminidase inhibitors and baloxavir have different mechanisms of action against influenza viruses. However, influenza viruses with substitutions that confer resistance to neuraminidase inhibitors may also have amino acid substitutions in the PA protein that confer resistance to baloxavir. The clinical relevance of phenotypic cross-resistance evaluations has not been established.

Amino acid substitutions that confer cross-resistance between neuraminidase inhibitors (oseltamivir, peramivir, zanamivir) and adamantane derivatives (M2 ion channel inhibitors; amantadine, rimantadine) have not been identified. However, influenza strains that have a neuraminidase substitution that confers resistance to neuraminidase inhibitors and also have an M2 substitution that confers resistance to M2 ion channel inhibitors may be resistant to both classes of influenza antivirals.

ADVICE TO PATIENTS

Advise patients of the risk of severe allergic reactions (including anaphylaxis) or serious skin reactions with peramivir and the importance of immediately seeking medical attention if an allergic-like reaction occurs or is suspected.

Advise patients of the risk of neuropsychiatric reactions in patients with influenza and the importance of immediately contacting a clinician if they experience signs of abnormal behavior after receiving peramivir.

Importance of informing clinicians of existing or contemplated concomitant therapy, including prescription and OTC drugs, as well as any concomitant illnesses.

Importance of women informing clinicians if they are or plan to become pregnant or plan to breast-feed.

Importance of informing patients of other important precautionary information. (See Cautions.)

PREPARATIONS

Excipients in commercially available drug preparations may have clinically important effects in some individuals; consult specific product labeling for details.

Peramivir

Parenteral

Concentrate, for injection, for IV use	10 mg/mL	Rapivab®, Biocryst

† Use is not currently included in the labeling approved by the US Food and Drug Administration

Zanamivir

8:18.28 • NEURAMINIDASE INHIBITORS

■ Zanamivir, a sialic acid derivative, is a neuraminidase inhibitor antiviral that is pharmacologically related to oseltamivir and active against influenza A and B viruses.

USES

● Treatment of Seasonal Influenza A and B Virus Infections

Zanamivir is used for the symptomatic *treatment* of acute, uncomplicated influenza caused by influenza A or B viruses in adults, adolescents, and children 7 years of age or older who have been symptomatic for no longer than 2 days.

Efficacy of zanamivir for the treatment of influenza is *not* established in patients with underlying airways disease (e.g., asthma, chronic obstructive pulmonary disease [COPD]). The drug is *not* recommended in patients with underlying airways disease because of the risk of serious bronchospasm. (See Individuals with Asthma or COPD under Cautions.) Treatment with zanamivir has not been shown to reduce the risk of transmission of influenza to others.

For the treatment of suspected or confirmed acute, uncomplicated seasonal influenza in otherwise healthy outpatients, the US Centers for Disease Control and Prevention (CDC), Infectious Diseases Society of America (IDSA), and other experts state that any age-appropriate influenza antiviral (oral oseltamivir, inhaled zanamivir, oral baloxavir marboxil, IV peramivir) can be used if not contraindicated. CDC states that early empiric antiviral treatment can be considered in outpatients with suspected influenza (e.g., influenza-like illness such as fever with either cough or sore throat) based on clinical judgement if such treatment can be initiated within 48 hours of illness onset.

For the treatment of suspected or confirmed seasonal influenza in hospitalized patients or outpatients with severe, complicated, or progressive illness (e.g., pneumonia, exacerbation of underlying chronic medical conditions), CDC states that oseltamivir is the preferred influenza antiviral and should be initiated as soon as possible, ideally within 48 hours, without waiting for laboratory confirmation. Oseltamivir is the preferred influenza antiviral in hospitalized patients or outpatients with severe, complicated, or progressive influenza because of the lack of data regarding use of other influenza antivirals in such patients. CDC states that use of IV peramivir should be considered in patients who cannot tolerate or absorb oseltamivir administered orally or enterically (e.g., because of suspected or known gastric stasis, malabsorption, or GI bleeding); inhaled zanamivir is not recommended for the treatment of influenza in hospitalized patients.

Influenza and coronavirus disease 2019 (COVID-19) caused by severe acute respiratory syndrome coronavirus 2 (SARS-CoV-2) have overlapping signs and symptoms and coinfection with influenza A or B viruses and SARS-CoV-2 can occur and should be considered, particularly in hospitalized patients with severe respiratory disease. Although laboratory testing can help distinguish between influenza virus infection and SARS-CoV-2 infection, CDC recommends that empiric influenza treatment should be initiated in patients with suspected influenza who are hospitalized, have severe, complicated, or progressive illness, or are at high risk for influenza complication without waiting for results of influenza testing, SARS-CoV-2 testing, or multiplex molecular assays that detect influenza A and B viruses and SARS-CoV-2.

Viral surveillance data available from local and state health departments and CDC should be considered when selecting an antiviral for the treatment of seasonal influenza. Strains of circulating influenza viruses and the antiviral susceptibility of these strains constantly evolve, and emergence of resistant strains may decrease effectiveness of influenza antivirals. Although circulating influenza A and B viruses during recent years generally have been susceptible to zanamivir, clinicians should consult the most recent information on susceptibility of circulating viruses when selecting an antiviral for the treatment of influenza.

CDC issues recommendations concerning the use of antivirals for the treatment of influenza, and these recommendations are updated as needed during each influenza season. Information regarding influenza surveillance and updated recommendations for the treatment of seasonal influenza are available from CDC at http://www.cdc.gov/flu.

Clinical Trials and Experience

Acute, Uncomplicated Influenza

Efficacy of zanamivir for the treatment of influenza has been established in randomized placebo-controlled studies in which the predominant influenza infection was seasonal influenza A; a smaller number of patients in these studies were infected with seasonal influenza B. When used within 2 days of onset of symptoms in otherwise healthy adults, adolescents, and children with uncomplicated influenza, the drug has decreased viral shedding in adults and adolescents and reduced the degree and duration of fever, headache, myalgia, cough, and sore throat in adults, adolescents, and children. Zanamivir therapy generally has been associated with a median 1- to 1.5-day decrease in the duration of symptoms, although those who initiate therapy sooner (i.e., no later than 30 hours after symptom onset) and those with more pronounced illness may exhibit greater benefit (e.g., a 3-day decrease in symptom duration).

● Prevention of Seasonal Influenza A and B Virus Infections

Zanamivir is used for *prophylaxis* of influenza A or B virus infection in adults, adolescents, and children 5 years of age and older.

Safety and efficacy of zanamivir have been established for prophylaxis of seasonal influenza in household settings and during community outbreaks; the manufacturer states that efficacy of the drug has *not* been established for prophylaxis of seasonal influenza in nursing home settings.

Annual vaccination with seasonal influenza virus vaccine, as recommended by CDC's Advisory Committee on Immunization Practices (ACIP), is the primary means of preventing seasonal influenza and its severe complications. Prophylaxis with an appropriate antiviral active against circulating influenza strains is considered an adjunct to vaccination for the control and prevention of influenza in certain individuals.

Decisions regarding use of antivirals for prophylaxis of seasonal influenza should be based on the risk of influenza-related complications in the exposed individual, the type and duration of contact, recommendations from local or public health authorities, and clinical judgment. In general, antiviral postexposure prophylaxis should be used only if it can be initiated within 48 hours of the most recent exposure.

CDC and others do not recommend *routine* use of influenza antivirals for postexposure prophylaxis of seasonal influenza in exposed individuals; however, such prophylaxis can be considered in certain situations in exposed individuals at high risk for influenza-related complications for whom influenza vaccine is contraindicated, unavailable, or expected to have low efficacy (e.g., immunocompromised individuals). Other possible candidates for antiviral prophylaxis include unvaccinated health care personnel, public health workers, and first responders with unprotected, close-contact exposure to a patient with confirmed, probable, or suspected influenza during the time when the patient was infectious. Antiviral prophylaxis also may be considered for controlling influenza outbreaks in nursing and long-term care facilities or other closed or semi-closed settings with large numbers of individuals at high risk for influenza-related complications. In individuals at high risk of influenza complications who receive influenza virus vaccine inactivated or influenza vaccine recombinant, use of prophylaxis can be considered during the 2 weeks after vaccination to provide protection until an adequate immune response develops. (See Influenza Vaccines under Drug Interactions.)

CDC issues recommendations concerning the use of antivirals for prophylaxis of influenza, and these recommendations are updated as needed during each influenza season. Information regarding influenza surveillance and updated recommendations for prevention of seasonal influenza are available from CDC at http://www.cdc.gov/flu.

Clinical Trials and Experience

Efficacy of zanamivir for prevention of seasonal influenza was demonstrated in postexposure prophylaxis studies in households and seasonal prophylaxis studies during community outbreaks of influenza. The primary efficacy end point in these studies was the incidence of symptomatic, laboratory-confirmed influenza, which was defined as the presence of at least 2 symptoms (oral temperature 37.8°C or higher, feverishness, cough, headache, sore throat, myalgia) and laboratory confirmation by culture, polymerase chain reaction (PCR), or seroconversion.

In the placebo-controlled studies evaluating zanamivir for postexposure prophylaxis in household contacts of an index case, each household (including all household members 5 years of age or older) was randomized to receive zanamivir (10 mg once daily for 10 days) or placebo initiated within 1.5 days of symptom onset in the index cases. The proportion of households with at least 1 new case of symptomatic, laboratory-confirmed influenza was 4.1% in the groups that received zanamivir and 19% in the groups that received placebo.

In a placebo-controlled seasonal prophylaxis study in university students (86% were unvaccinated), the incidence of symptomatic, laboratory-confirmed influenza was 2% in those who received zanamivir (10 mg once daily for 28 days) and 6.1% in those who received placebo during a community outbreak. In another seasonal prophylaxis study in adults and children 12–94 years of age (33% were unvaccinated), the incidence of symptomatic, laboratory-confirmed influenza was 0.2% in those who received zanamivir and 1.4% in those who received placebo during a community outbreak.

● Avian Influenza A Virus Infections

Although safety and efficacy have not been established, neuraminidase inhibitors (oseltamivir, peramivir, zanamivir) have been used or are recommended for the treatment or prevention of infections caused by susceptible avian influenza A viruses†.

Experience to date indicates that avian influenza A viruses do not easily transmit from wild or domestic birds, water fowl, or poultry to humans, but human infections may rarely occur and have been linked to contact with live or dead infected birds or poultry, uncooked poultry products, or surfaces contaminated with infected poultry feces or respiratory secretions. Human cases generally have involved a highly pathogenic Asian strain of avian influenza A (H5N1) that has been circulating since 2003 in poultry in Asia, Africa, the Pacific, Eastern Europe, and the Middle East or a novel avian influenza A (H7N9) virus that was first identified in China in March 2013.

Worldwide, most avian influenza A viruses isolated in wild birds, water fowl, or poultry have been designated as low pathogenic strains; however, highly pathogenic avian influenza (HPAI) strains are occasionally detected. Since December 2014, HPAI viruses (H5N1, H5N2, H5N8) have been reported in wild birds, water fowl, and/or domestic poultry (commercial or backyard flocks) in the US (e.g., Arkansas, California, Idaho, Iowa, Minnesota, Missouri, Nebraska, North Dakota, Oregon, South Dakota, Utah, Washington, Wisconsin). Although CDC states that the risk of human infection with these HPAI H5 viruses is considered low in the US, human infection is possible since other closely related HPAI H5 viruses in Asia and other countries have caused sporadic cases of human respiratory illness. The HPAI (H5N1) strain reported in poultry outbreaks in the US is a new reassortant virus that is genetically different from the highly pathogenic Asian strain of influenza A (H5N1) that has caused human infections in Asia and other countries and has been associated with a high mortality rate.

Appropriate use of a neuraminidase inhibitor antivirals is an important component of response and control measures to treat avian influenza A virus infections and help reduce the risk of additional human infections.

For the treatment of uncomplicated avian influenza A infections in outpatients, CDC states that oral oseltamivir, IV peramivir, or inhaled zanamivir may be used. For the treatment of severe, complicated, or progressive avian influenza A infections in hospitalized patients or outpatients, including infections caused by avian influenza A (H7N9), avian influenza A (H5N1), or novel avian influenza A H5 viruses, CDC recommends oseltamivir as the antiviral of choice. In those with severe avian influenza A infections who cannot tolerate or absorb oseltamivir administered orally or enterically (e.g., because of suspected or known gastric stasis, malabsorption, or GI bleeding), CDC states that use of IV peramivir may be considered. Inhaled zanamivir is not recommended because data are insufficient regarding use for treatment of severe avian influenza A infections in hospitalized patients or outpatients.

When antiviral prophylaxis is indicated in close contacts of individuals with confirmed or probable infection with avian influenza A viruses that have caused or potentially may cause severe disease or indicated in individuals who have been exposed to birds infected with such avian influenza A viruses, CDC recommends oral oseltamivir or inhaled zanamivir.

Information regarding treatment and prevention of avian influenza A infections is available from CDC at http://www.cdc.gov/flu/avianflu/ and WHO at https://www.who.int/teams/global-influenza-programme/avian-influenza.

● Pandemic Influenza

Zanamivir is used for the treatment or prevention of pandemic influenza† caused by susceptible strains of influenza virus.

Influenza viruses can cause seasonal epidemics and, occasionally, pandemics during which rates of illness and death from influenza-related complications can increase dramatically worldwide. The most recent influenza pandemic occurred during 2009 and was related to a novel influenza A (H1N1) strain, influenza A (H1N1)pdm09.

Influenza outbreaks caused by influenza A (H1N1)pdm09 virus were reported in several countries, including the US, beginning in March and April 2009. The virus is a triple-reassortant swine influenza virus with genes from human, swine, and avian influenza A viruses and contained a unique combination of gene segments that had not been previously reported in the US or elsewhere. The influenza A (H1N1)pdm09 virus was antigenically distinct from seasonal human influenza A (H1N1) viruses that had been in circulation since 1977, and widespread transmission of the virus occurred since most individuals had no pre-existing antibody to the strain. In the US, the 2009 influenza A (H1N1)pdm09 pandemic was characterized by a substantial increase in influenza activity that peaked in late October and early November 2009 and returned to seasonal baseline levels by January 2010. At that time, more than 99% of influenza viruses circulating in the US were the influenza A (H1N1)pdm09 virus; more than 60 million Americans become ill with the virus and more than 270,000 hospitalizations and 12,500 deaths were reported. After the pandemic, influenza A (H1N1)pdm09 became a seasonal influenza virus and continues to circulate with other seasonal viruses.

The spread of the highly pathogenic H5N1 strain of avian influenza A in poultry in Asia and other countries that has been occurring since 2003 may represent a potential future pandemic threat. In addition, the novel avian influenza A (H7N9) virus that was first identified in China in March 2013 and has been causing sporadic human infections has pandemic potential.

Information on pandemic influenza, including planning and preparedness resources if an influenza pandemic occurs, is available from CDC at https://www.cdc.gov/flu/pandemic-resources/index.htm and WHO at https://www.who.int/initiatives/pandemic-influenza-preparedness-framework.

DOSAGE AND ADMINISTRATION

● Administration

Zanamivir powder for inhalation is administered *only* by oral inhalation using the inhaler (Diskhaler®) provided by the manufacturer.

Zanamivir has been administered IV†, but a parenteral dosage form of the drug is not available in the US.

*Zanamivir powder for inhalation must **not** be used to prepare an extemporaneous solution and must **not** be administered using a nebulizer or mechanical ventilator.* (See Administration Precautions under Cautions.)

Oral Inhalation

Zanamivir powder for inhalation is commercially available in a disk containing 4 foil blisters of the drug (Rotadisk®) and is provided with an inhaler (Diskhaler®) that is used to deliver the drug to the respiratory tract.

The commercially available powder for inhalation should *not* be removed from its foil blister packaging.

The manufacturer's instructions should be consulted for information on how to load the Rotadisk® onto the drug delivery system (Diskhaler®) and how to use the Diskhaler® to administer the drug.

Patients should be instructed in the safe and effective use of the Diskhaler®, and instructions should include a demonstration whenever possible.

Patients scheduled to use an inhaled bronchodilator at the same time as zanamivir should use the bronchodilator before zanamivir.

● Dosage

Treatment of Seasonal Influenza A and B Virus Infections

For the *treatment* of influenza infection in adults, adolescents, and children 7 years of age or older, the usual dosage of zanamivir is 2 inhalations (one 5-mg blister per inhalation for a total dose of 10 mg) twice daily (about 12 hours apart) for 5 days. Two doses should be administered the first day provided there is an interval of at least 2 hours between doses. On subsequent days, zanamivir doses should be administered about 12 hours apart (e.g., morning and evening) at about the same time each day.

Zanamivir treatment should be initiated within 2 days after the onset of symptoms. Although efficacy has not been established if treatment is initiated more than 2 days after onset of symptoms, there is some evidence that antiviral treatment initiated up to 4 or 5 days after onset of symptoms may still be beneficial in reducing morbidity and mortality in hospitalized patients and in those with severe, complicated, or progressive influenza.

Zanamivir usually is given for 5 days for the *treatment* of seasonal influenza. However, hospitalized patients with severe or prolonged infections or individuals with immunosuppression may require more than 5 days of antiviral treatment.

Prevention of Seasonal Influenza A and B Virus Infections

Household Setting

For *prophylaxis* of influenza in adults, adolescents, and children 5 years of age or older in household settings, the usual dosage of zanamivir is 2 inhalations (one 5-mg blister per inhalation for a total dose of 10 mg) once daily for 10 days. The daily dose should be administered at approximately the same time each day. CDC recommends that zanamivir be continued for 7 days after the last known exposure.

Efficacy of zanamivir for prophylaxis in household settings is not established if the drug is initiated more than 1.5 days after the onset of symptoms in the index case.

Community Outbreaks

For *prophylaxis* of influenza in adults and adolescents in community settings, the usual dosage of zanamivir is 2 inhalations (one 5-mg blister per inhalation for a total dose of 10 mg) once daily for 28 days. The daily dose should be administered at approximately the same time each day. CDC recommends that zanamivir be continued for 7 days after the last known exposure.

Efficacy of zanamivir for prophylaxis in community outbreaks is not established if the drug is initiated more than 5 days after the outbreak is identified in the community. The safety and efficacy of zanamivir prophylaxis given for longer than 28 days have not been evaluated.

Outbreaks in Institutional Settings

Although the manufacturer states that efficacy of zanamivir for prophylaxis of influenza in nursing home settings† has not been established, CDC states that adults, adolescents, and children 5 years of age or older may receive zanamivir *prophylaxis* in a dosage of 2 inhalations (one 5-mg blister per inhalation for a total dose of 10 mg) once daily for control of influenza outbreaks in institutional settings (e.g., long-term care facilities for elderly individuals and children). In such situations, CDC recommends that zanamivir be given for a minimum of 2 weeks and continued for up to 1 week after the last known case of influenza is identified.

Avian Influenza A Virus Infections

Treatment

If zanamivir is used for the *treatment* of uncomplicated infections caused by avian influenza A viruses† in adults and pediatric patients, the twice-daily zanamivir dosage usually recommended for the *treatment* of seasonal influenza A and B virus infections should be given for 5 days. (See Treatment of Seasonal Influenza A and B Virus Infections under Dosage and Administration.)

Zanamivir administered by oral inhalation is not recommended for the treatment of severe avian influenza virus A virus infections.

Prophylaxis

If zanamivir is used for *prophylaxis* of avian influenza virus A virus infection† in close contacts of individuals with confirmed or probable infection or in individuals who have been exposed to birds infected with such viruses, CDC and WHO state that the twice-daily zanamivir dosage usually recommended for *treatment* of seasonal influenza A and B virus infections can be used in adults and pediatric patients. (See Treatment of Seasonal Influenza A and B Virus Infections under Dosage and Administration.)

Antiviral prophylaxis for avian influenza A virus infection should be continued for 5–10. If the exposure was time-limited and not ongoing, CDC states that antiviral prophylaxis should be continued for 5 days after the last known exposure.

● Special Populations

Dosage adjustment is not needed in patients with renal impairment, but the potential for drug accumulation should be considered. (See Renal Impairment under Cautions.)

CAUTIONS

● Contraindications

History of hypersensitivity reaction to zanamivir or any ingredient in the formulation (e.g., milk protein contained in the lactose vehicle).

● Warnings/Precautions

Respiratory Effects

Serious bronchospasm, including fatalities, have been reported in patients receiving zanamivir; some (but not all) of these patients had chronic underlying pulmonary disease (e.g., asthma, chronic obstructive pulmonary disease [COPD]). (See Individuals with Asthma or COPD under Cautions.) Many of these cases were reported during postmarketing surveillance and causality to the drug is difficult to assess.

Some patients without prior respiratory disease also may have respiratory abnormalities from acute respiratory infection that could resemble adverse drug reactions or increase vulnerability to adverse drug reactions.

Zanamivir should be discontinued in any patient who experiences bronchospasm or decline in respiratory function; immediate treatment and hospitalization may be required.

Individuals with Asthma or COPD

Zanamivir is not recommended for the treatment or prophylaxis of influenza in individuals with underlying airways disease (e.g., asthma, COPD) because of the risk of serious bronchospasm.

Bronchospasm has occurred when zanamivir was used in patients with mild or moderate asthma (but without acute influenza-like illness). When used in patients with acute influenza-like illness superimposed on underlying asthma or COPD, a greater than 20% decline in the forced expiratory volume in 1 second (FEV_1) occurred in more patients receiving the drug than in those receiving placebo.

The benefits and risks should be considered carefully if use of zanamivir is considered for a patient with underlying respiratory disease. If a decision is made to use the drug in such patients, monitor respiratory function carefully and have appropriate supportive care available, including short-acting β-adrenergic bronchodilators.

Sensitivity Reactions

Hypersensitivity Reactions

Allergic-like reactions (e.g., oropharyngeal edema, serious skin rash, anaphylaxis) have been reported in patients receiving zanamivir.

If an allergic reaction occurs or is suspected, zanamivir should be discontinued immediately and appropriate treatment initiated.

Neuropsychiatric and CNS Effects

There have been postmarketing reports of delirium and abnormal behavior leading to self-injury, principally involving children. The contribution of zanamivir to these events has not been established.

Influenza itself can be associated with a variety of neurologic and behavioral symptoms (e.g., seizures, hallucinations, delirium, abnormal behavior) and fatalities can occur. Although such events may occur in the setting of encephalitis or encephalopathy, they can occur without obvious severe disease.

Patients should be closely monitored for signs of abnormal behavior. If neuropsychiatric symptoms develop, the risks and benefits of continued therapy with zanamivir should be evaluated.

There have been postmarketing reports of vasovagal-like episodes shortly after oral inhalation of zanamivir.

Concomitant Illness

Safety and efficacy for treatment or prophylaxis of influenza have not established in patients with high-risk underlying medical conditions. (see Individuals with Asthma or COPD under Cautions)

No data are available regarding use of zanamivir in patients with severe or unstable medical conditions that may require inpatient care.

Differential Diagnosis

When making treatment decisions in patients with suspected influenza, consider the possibility of primary or concomitant bacterial infection for which zanamivir would be ineffective.

Serious bacterial infections may begin with influenza-like symptoms or may coexist with or occur as complications of influenza. There is no evidence that zanamivir prevents such complications.

There is no evidence that zanamivir is effective for illness caused by any organisms other than influenza A or B.

Administration Precautions

Zanamivir powder for inhalation *must* be administered using *only* the inhaler (Diskhaler®) provided by the manufacturer. The powder should *not* be removed from its foil blister packaging (Rotadisk®).

Zanamivir powder for inhalation must **not** *be made into an extemporaneous solution for administration by nebulization or mechanical ventilation.* **No** *attempt should be made to reconstitute or solubilize the powder in liquid;* **no** *attempt should be made to administer the drug in a nebulizer or mechanical ventilator.*

Safety and efficacy have *not* been established for administration by nebulization. Lactose in the formulation may obstruct or interfere with proper functioning of mechanical ventilator equipment. There have been reports of hospitalized patients with influenza who received extemporaneous solutions made with the powder and administered by nebulization or mechanical ventilation; at least 1 death occurred when lactose in the formulation apparently obstructed the proper functioning of the equipment.

Patients should be instructed in the safe and effective use of the drug delivery system (Diskhaler®) provided by the manufacturer. Instructions on use of the inhaler should include a demonstration whenever possible.

Some geriatric patients may need assistance with the inhaler.

Children should be under adult supervision with close attention to use of the inhaler. (See Pediatric Use under Cautions.)

Prior Use

No data are available regarding safety and efficacy of repeated courses of zanamivir for treatment of influenza.

Influenza Vaccination

Influenza antivirals, including zanamivir, are important adjuncts to vaccination in the control of influenza but are not a substitute for annual vaccination with a seasonal influenza vaccine (influenza virus vaccine inactivated, influenza vaccine recombinant, influenza vaccine live intranasal).

Although influenza antivirals, including zanamivir, may be used concomitantly with or at any time before or after influenza virus vaccine inactivated or influenza vaccine recombinant, influenza antivirals may inhibit the vaccine virus contained in influenza vaccine live intranasal and decrease efficacy of the live vaccine. (See Influenza Vaccines under Drug Interactions.)

Specific Populations

Pregnancy

Available data from published studies suggest that the use of zanamivir during pregnancy is not associated with an increased risk of birth defects or adverse maternal or fetal outcomes; however, these studies had several limitations (e.g., lack of specific analyses for zanamivir, possible exposure and outcome misclassifications, small sample sizes) which preclude a definitive assessment of the risk.

In animal reproduction studies, no adverse maternal or embryofetal effects were observed in rats or rabbits treated with IV zanamivir at dosages that resulted in systemic exposures approximately 300 times those in humans receiving 10 mg of the drug twice daily by oral inhalation.

Pregnant women are at increased risk for severe complications from influenza, which may lead to adverse pregnancy and/or fetal outcomes including maternal death, stillbirths, birth defects, preterm delivery, low birthweight, and small size for gestational age.

Oseltamivir is the preferred antiviral for the treatment of suspected or confirmed influenza or prevention of influenza in women who are pregnant or up to 2 weeks postpartum.

Lactation

It is not known whether zanamivir is distributed into human milk, affects milk production, or has any effects on breast-fed infants. Zanamivir is distributed into milk in rats.

The benefits of breast-feeding and the importance of zanamivir to the woman should be considered along with potential adverse effects on the breast-fed child from the drug or from the underlying maternal condition.

Pediatric Use

Safety and efficacy for *treatment* of influenza have not been established in children younger than 7 years of age. Some clinical studies evaluating zanamivir have included children 5–6 years of age†; however, there is some evidence that the drug is not as effective in these children as in older children and adults.

Safety and efficacy for *prophylaxis* of influenza have not been established in children younger than 5 years of age. Safety and efficacy in adolescents and children 5 years of age or older for *prophylaxis* of influenza are similar to adults.

Some young children may have suboptimal inspiratory flow rates through the drug delivery system (Diskhaler®). When considering use of zanamivir in pediatric patients, clinicians should carefully evaluate the ability of the child to use the inhaler.

Children should receive zanamivir only under adult supervision and with close attention to proper use of the inhaler. The supervising adult should be instructed on proper use of the inhaler.

Geriatric Use

Safety and efficacy for *treatment* of influenza in geriatric adults 65 years of age or older is similar to that reported in younger adults.

Safety and efficacy for *prophylaxis* of influenza in geriatric adults 65 years of age or older in household or community settings are similar to that reported in younger adults. Efficacy has *not* been established for *prophylaxis* of influenza in geriatric individuals in nursing home settings.

The possibility exists of greater sensitivity to the drug in some older individuals.

Some geriatric patients may need assistance with the drug delivery system (Diskhaler®).

Hepatic Impairment

The pharmacokinetics of zanamivir have not been studied in patients with hepatic impairment.

Renal Impairment

Safety and efficacy of zanamivir have not been documented in patients with severe renal impairment. Although zanamivir systemic exposure is limited after oral inhalation, the potential for drug accumulation should be considered.

● *Common Adverse Effects*

Adverse effects occurring in 1–3% or more of adults and children 12 years of age or older include diarrhea; nausea; vomiting; nasal signs and symptoms; bronchitis; sinusitis; cough; ear, nose, and throat infections; headache; and dizziness. Adverse effects occurring in up to 5% of children 5–12 years of age include ear, nose, and throat infections; vomiting; nausea; and diarrhea. Bronchospasm and allergic-like reactions, including oropharyngeal edema and serious rash, have been reported. Some adverse effects may be related to the lactose vehicle (contains milk proteins) used in the powder for oral inhalation formulation.

DRUG INTERACTIONS

Zanamivir not metabolized by and does not affect cytochrome P-450 (CYP) enzymes, including CYP1A1, 1A2, 2A6, 2C9, 2C19, 2D6, 2E1, or 3A4. Drug interactions with drugs that are substrates or inhibitors of these enzymes unlikely.

Zanamivir is not a substrate of P-glycoprotein (P-gp).

Zanamivir does not inhibit organic anion transporter (OAT) 1, OAT2, OAT3, OAT4, organic cation transporter (OCT) 1, OCT2, OCT3, or urate transporter (URAT) 1.

● *Influenza Vaccines*

Zanamivir does not interfere with the antibody response to influenza virus vaccine inactivated (IIV) and is not expected to interfere with the antibody response to influenza vaccine recombinant (RIV). These inactivated influenza vaccines may be administered concomitantly with or at any time before or after zanamivir.

Safety and efficacy of concomitant use of zanamivir and influenza vaccine live intranasal (LAIV) have not been studied. Because influenza antivirals, including zanamivir, reduce replication of influenza viruses and may inhibit the vaccine virus, these antivirals potentially could decrease the immune response to LAIV and efficacy of the live vaccine. LAIV should not be administered until at least 48 hours after zanamivir is discontinued and zanamivir should not be administered until at least 2 weeks after administration of LAIV unless medically indicated. ACIP recommends that individuals who received zanamivir 48 hours before to 14 days after LAIV should be revaccinated using age-appropriate IIV or RIV.

PHARMACOKINETICS

● *Absorption*

Bioavailability

Following oral inhalation of zanamivir, approximately 4–17% of the inhaled dose is absorbed systemically.

Absolute bioavailability averages 2% following oral inhalation; peak serum concentrations are attained within 1–2 hours.

Special Populations

In pediatric patients younger than 12 years of age with signs and symptoms of respiratory illness, zanamivir serum concentrations may be low or undetectable following oral inhalation because of inadequate or absent inspiratory flow rates. (See Pediatric Use under Cautions.)

In a study that included a limited number of individuals with renal impairment who received a single dose of IV zanamivir, systemic exposure was increased in those with creatinine clearances of 70 mL/minute or less.

● *Distribution*

Extent

Zanamivir is delivered to the epithelial lining of the respiratory tract following oral inhalation. The amount of the drug in the respiratory tract depends on patient factors such as inspiratory flow rate; it may be present in sputum and nasal washings for at least 12 hours after a dose.

Zanamivir crosses the placenta in animals.

Zanamivir is distributed into milk in rats; it is not known whether the drug is distributed into human milk.

Plasma Protein Binding

Zanamivir is less than 10% bound to plasma proteins.

● *Elimination*

Metabolism

Zanamivir is not metabolized.

The drug is not a substrate for and does not affect cytochrome P-450 (CYP) isoenzymes.

Elimination Route

Following oral inhalation, absorbed zanamivir is excreted in urine within 24 hours; unabsorbed drug is excreted in feces.

Half-life

The serum half-life of zanamivir following oral inhalation is 2.5–5.1 hours.

Special Populations

The pharmacokinetics of zanamivir have not been studied in patients with impaired hepatic function.

DESCRIPTION

Zanamivir, a sialic acid derivative, is a neuraminidase inhibitor antiviral. Zanamivir is pharmacologically related to other neuraminidase inhibitors (e.g., oseltamivir, peramivir).

Zanamivir is a potent selective competitive inhibitor of the influenza virus neuraminidase, an enzyme essential for viral replication. Neuraminidase cleaves terminal sialic acid residues from glycoconjugates to enable the release of virus from infected cells, prevent the formation of viral aggregates after release from host cells, and possibly decrease viral inactivation by respiratory mucus.

● *Spectrum*

Zanamivir is active in vitro in cell culture against both influenza A and B viruses.

Viral surveillance data indicate that the majority of seasonal influenza A (H1N1)pdm09, influenza A (H3N2), and influenza B viruses circulating during recent influenza seasons, including in the US, have been susceptible to zanamivir in vitro; reduced in vitro susceptibility or resistance to zanamivir has been reported rarely. Zanamivir may be active in vitro against some influenza strains, including some influenza A (H1N1)pdm09 strains, resistant to oseltamivir.

Zanamivir has been active in vitro against some avian influenza A viruses, including avian influenza A H5N1, H6N1, H7N7, H7N9, and H9N2.

● *Resistance*

The major mechanisms of resistance to neuraminidase inhibitors that have been identified in vitro are viral neuraminidase (NA) mutations that affect the ability of the drugs to inhibit the enzyme and hemagglutinin (HA) mutations that reduce viral dependence on neuraminidase activity. The clinical importance of decreased in vitro susceptibility to zanamivir is not known.

Resistance to zanamivir has been produced in vitro by serial passage of influenza A and B viruses in the presence of increasing concentrations of the drug. In addition, reduced in vitro susceptibility or resistance to zanamivir due to NA or HA mutations have been observed in some clinical isolates of seasonal influenza A and B viruses. The clinical importance of reduced in vitro susceptibility to zanamivir in these strains is unknown.

Avian influenza A (H5N1) virus variants with reduced susceptibility to zanamivir include V96A , E99A/G, Q116L, V129A, and D179G. Avian influenza A (H7N9) virus variants with reduced susceptibility to zanamivir include E115V, R148K, I219K/R, R289K. The clinical importance of reduced in vitro susceptibility to zanamivir in these avian influenza A viruses is unknown; the effects of specific substitutions on susceptibility may be strain-dependent.

Cross-resistance between zanamivir and other neuraminidase inhibitors (e.g., oseltamivir, peramivir) has been reported in influenza A and B viruses in cell culture and neuraminidase inhibition assays. However, because oseltamivir, peramivir, and zanamivir bind to different sites on the neuraminidase enzyme or interact differently with the binding sites, cross-resistance among the drugs is variable.

ADVICE TO PATIENTS

Importance of understanding proper inhalation technique and use of the drug delivery system (Diskhaler®); importance of reading the patient instructions for use.

Instruct patients that if they miss a dose, to take it as soon as they remember. If it is ≤2 hours before their next dose, instruct patients to skip the dose and take the next dose at the next scheduled time. Advise patients not to double their next dose or take more than the prescribed dose.

Advise patients of the possible risk of bronchospasm, especially in those with chronic underlying respiratory disease (e.g., asthma, chronic obstructive pulmonary disease [COPD]); importance of patients with asthma or COPD having a short-acting inhaled β-adrenergic bronchodilator readily available.

Importance of discontinuing zanamivir and promptly contacting a clinician if there is an increase in respiratory symptoms (e.g., wheezing, dyspnea, signs or symptoms of bronchospasm) or if symptoms of an allergic reaction occur.

Advise patients using an inhaled bronchodilators at the same time as zanamivir of the importance of using the bronchodilator first.

Importance of immediately contacting a clinician if patient demonstrates signs of unusual behavior. Influenza patients, particularly children and adolescents, may be at increased risk of seizures, confusion, or abnormal behavior early in their illness and should be closely observed for signs of unusual behavior. Such events are uncommon, but may occur after starting zanamivir treatment or when influenza is not treated and can result in accidental injury to the patient.

Advise patients that zanamivir treatment does not reduce the risk of transmission of influenza virus to others.

Importance of informing clinicians of existing or contemplated concomitant therapy, including prescription and OTC drugs, as well as any concomitant illnesses.

Importance of women informing clinicians if they are or plan to become pregnant or plan to breast-feed.

Importance of informing patients of other important precautionary information. (See Cautions.)

PREPARATIONS

Excipients in commercially available drug preparations may have clinically important effects in some individuals; consult specific product labeling for details.

Zanamivir

Oral inhalation

Powder for inhalation (contained in Rotadisk® foil pack)	5 mg per inhalation	Relenza®, (with Diskhaler®), GlaxoSmithKline

† Use is not currently included in the labeling approved by the US Food and Drug Administration.

Baloxavir Marboxil

8:18.30 • ENDONUCLEASE INHIBITORS

- Baloxavir marboxil is a prodrug of baloxavir, a polymerase acidic (PA) endonuclease inhibitor antiviral active against influenza A and B viruses.

USES

● Treatment of Seasonal Influenza A and B Virus Infections

Baloxavir marboxil is used for the *treatment* of acute, uncomplicated influenza caused by influenza A or B viruses in adults and adolescents 12 years of age or older who have been symptomatic for no longer than 48 hours, including those who are otherwise healthy and those who are at high risk for influenza-related complications. Efficacy of baloxavir marboxil administered more than 48 hours after onset of influenza symptoms has not been evaluated.

Data are not available to date regarding use of baloxavir marboxil for the treatment of severe or complicated influenza in hospitalized patients or outpatients.

For the treatment of suspected or confirmed acute, uncomplicated seasonal influenza in otherwise healthy outpatients, the US Centers for Disease Control and Prevention (CDC), Infectious Diseases Society of America (IDSA), and other experts state that any age-appropriate influenza antiviral (oral oseltamivir, inhaled zanamivir, oral baloxavir marboxil, IV peramivir) can be used if not contraindicated. CDC states that early empiric antiviral treatment can be considered in outpatients with suspected influenza (e.g., influenza-like illness such as fever with either cough or sore throat) based on clinical judgement if such treatment can be initiated within 48 hours of illness onset.

For the treatment of suspected or confirmed seasonal influenza in hospitalized patients or outpatients with severe, complicated, or progressive illness (e.g., pneumonia, exacerbation of underlying chronic medical conditions), CDC states that oseltamivir is the preferred influenza antiviral and should be initiated as soon as possible, ideally within 48 hours, without waiting for laboratory confirmation. Oseltamivir is the preferred influenza antiviral in hospitalized patients or outpatients with severe, complicated, or progressive influenza because of the lack of data regarding use of other influenza antivirals in such patients. CDC states that baloxavir marboxil is not recommended for the treatment of influenza in hospitalized patients.

Influenza and coronavirus disease 2019 (COVID-19) caused by severe acute respiratory syndrome coronavirus 2 (SARS-CoV-2) have overlapping signs and symptoms and coinfection with influenza A or B viruses and SARS-CoV-2 can occur and should be considered, particularly in hospitalized patients with severe respiratory disease. Although laboratory testing can help distinguish between influenza virus infection and SARS-CoV-2 infection, CDC recommends that empiric influenza treatment should be initiated in patients with suspected influenza who are hospitalized, have severe, complicated, or progressive illness, or are at high risk for influenza complication without waiting for results of influenza testing, SARS-CoV-2 testing, or multiplex molecular assays that detect influenza A and B viruses and SARS-CoV-2.

Viral surveillance data available from local and state health departments and CDC should be considered when selecting an antiviral for the treatment of seasonal influenza. Strains of circulating influenza viruses and the antiviral susceptibility of these strains constantly evolve, and the possibility that emergence of resistant strains may decrease effectiveness of influenza antivirals should be considered. Although circulating influenza A and B viruses during recent years have been susceptible to baloxavir, clinicians should consult the most recent information on susceptibility of circulating viruses when selecting an antiviral for the treatment of influenza.

CDC issues recommendations concerning the use of antivirals for the treatment of influenza, and these recommendations are updated as needed during each influenza season. Information regarding influenza surveillance and updated recommendations for the treatment of seasonal influenza are available from CDC at https://www.cdc.gov/flu/.

Clinical Trials and Experience

Acute, Uncomplicated Influenza in Otherwise Healthy Adults and Adolescents 12 Years of Age or Older

Efficacy and safety of a single dose of baloxavir marboxil for the treatment of acute, uncomplicated influenza have been evaluated in 2 randomized, double-blinded trials that included otherwise healthy individuals 12–64 years of age and were conducted during 2 different influenza seasons. For both studies, enrollment criteria included an axillary temperature of at least 38°C, at least one moderate or severe respiratory symptom (cough, nasal congestion, or sore throat), and at least one moderate or severe systemic symptom (headache, feverishness or chills, muscle or joint pain, or fatigue); patients with severe illness requiring hospitalization, those weighing less than 40 kg, those older than 65 years of age, and pregnant women were excluded. The primary efficacy population was defined as those with a positive rapid influenza diagnostic test (study 1) or with reverse transcriptase-polymerase chain reaction (RT-PCR)-confirmed influenza (study 2). Patients were treated within 48 hours of symptom onset and were required to self-assess the severity of 7 influenza symptoms (cough, sore throat, headache, nasal congestion, feverishness or chills, muscle or joint pain, and fatigue) twice daily on days 1–9 and once daily on days 10–14 and to rate these symptoms as none, mild, moderate, or severe. The primary end point was the time to alleviation of influenza symptoms and was defined as the time when all 7 influenza symptoms were assessed by the study participant as absent or mild for a duration of at least 21.5 hours. The majority of patients enrolled in these studies had infections caused by seasonal influenza A; a smaller number of patients had infections caused by seasonal influenza B.

Trial 1 was a phase 2, placebo-controlled, dose-ranging study conducted in Japan that included 400 adults 20–64 years of age (mean age 38 years, 100% Asian) with acute, uncomplicated influenza infection who were randomized in a 1:1:1:1 ratio to receive oral baloxavir marboxil (single 10-, 20-, or 40-mg dose) or placebo administered in an outpatient setting and initiated within 48 hours of onset of symptoms. The median time to alleviation of influenza symptoms was 50 hours in those who received a single 40-mg dose of baloxavir marboxil compared with a duration of 78 hours in those who received placebo. Among study 1 participants treated with baloxavir marboxil who had their influenza strains typed, 63% had influenza A (H1N1), 25% had influenza B, and 12% had influenza A (H3N2). In the subset of patients with influenza B infections, the median time to alleviation of influenza symptoms was 63 hours in those treated with baloxavir marboxil compared with 83 hours in those who received placebo.

Trial 2 (NCT02954354; CAPSTONE-1) was a phase 3, double-blind, randomized study conducted in the US and Japan that included 1436 otherwise healthy adults and adolescents 12–64 years of age (mean age 34 years, 78% Asian, 17% White, 4% Black) with acute, uncomplicated influenza infection. Study participants 20–64 years of age were randomized in a 2:2:1 ratio to receive oral baloxavir marboxil (single 40-mg dose in those weighing less than 80 kg or single 80-mg dose in those weighing 80 kg or more), oral oseltamivir (75 mg twice daily for 5 days), or placebo administered in an outpatient setting and initiated within 48 hours of onset of symptoms. Adolescents 12–19 years of age were randomized in a 2:1 ratio to receive baloxavir marboxil (single 40-mg oral dose in those weighing less than 80 kg or single 80-mg oral dose in those weighing 80 kg or more) or placebo administered in an outpatient setting and initiated within 48 hours of onset of symptoms. The efficacy analysis population included 1062 patients with RT-PCR-confirmed influenza (455 received baloxavir marboxil, 230 received placebo, and 377 received oseltamivir). The median time to alleviation of influenza symptoms in those 12–64 years of age treated with baloxavir marboxil or placebo was 54 or 80 hours, respectively. In the subset of patients 12–17 years of age, the median time to alleviation of influenza symptoms was 54 hours in those treated with baloxavir marboxil and 93 hours in those who received placebo. In addition, data from study participants 20–64 years of age indicated that the median time to alleviation of influenza symptoms in patients who received a single weight-based dose of baloxavir marboxil was the same as that reported in patients receiving a 5-day regimen of oseltamivir (54 hours in both groups). Among study 2 participants treated with baloxavir marboxil who had their influenza strains typed, 90% had influenza A (H3N2), 9% had influenza B, and 2% had influenza A (H1N1). In the subset of patients with influenza B infections, the median time to alleviation of influenza symptoms was 93 hours in those treated with baloxavir marboxil compared with 77 hours in those who received placebo; these results may have been affected by the low number of study participants with influenza B infections who received baloxavir marboxil.

Acute, Uncomplicated Influenza in Adults and Adolescents 12 Years of Age or Older at High Risk

Efficacy and safety of a single dose of baloxavir marboxil for the treatment of acute, uncomplicated influenza in adults and adolescents 12 years of age or older at high risk for influenza-related complications were evaluated in a phase 3, multicenter, randomized, double-blind, placebo- and active-controlled trial (NCT02949011; CAPSTONE-2; trial 3). A total of 2182 patients with signs and symptoms of influenza (mean age 52 years; 28% Asian, 59% White, 10% Black or African American) were randomized 1:1:1 to receive baloxavir marboxil (single 40-mg dose in those weighing less than 80 kg or single 80-mg dose in those weighing 80 kg or more), oral oseltamivir (75 mg twice daily for 5 days), or placebo within 48 hours after symptom onset. High-risk factors for influenza-related complications were those defined by CDC; the majority of enrolled patients had underlying asthma or chronic lung disease, diabetes mellitus, heart disease, morbid obesity, or were 65 years of age or older. Enrollment criteria included an axillary temperature of at least 38°C, at least one moderate or severe respiratory symptom (cough, nasal congestion, or sore throat), and at least one moderate or severe systemic symptom (headache, feverishness or chills, muscle or joint pain, or fatigue). Trial participants were required to self-assess the severity of influenza symptoms twice daily as none, mild, moderate, or severe; 19% of trial participants had preexisting symptoms (cough, muscle or joint pain, or fatigue) associated with their underlying high-risk condition that worsened as a result of influenza infection. The efficacy analysis population included 1158 patients with RT-PCR-confirmed influenza and, among those infected with only a single influenza type, 50% had influenza A (H3N2), 43% had influenza type B, and 7% had influenza A (H1N1). The primary efficacy end point was time to improvement of influenza symptoms (cough, sore throat, headache, nasal congestion, feverishness or chills, muscle or joint pain, and fatigue) and included alleviation of new symptoms and improvement of any preexisting symptoms that had worsened due to influenza. Results indicated that treatment with a single dose of baloxavir marboxil shortened the time to improvement of influenza symptoms in patients at high risk for influenza-related complications compared with placebo (median of 73 or 102 hours, respectively). The median time to improvement of influenza symptoms was 73 hours in patients treated with a single dose of baloxavir marboxil compared with 81 hours in those treated with a 5-day regimen of oseltamivir. The trial included only a limited number of adolescents 12–17 years of age at high risk for influenza-related complications, and results indicated that the median time to improvement of influenza symptoms was similar in the 13 adolescents treated with baloxavir marboxil and the 12 adolescents who received placebo (median of 188 or 191 hours, respectively).

● Prevention of Seasonal Influenza A and B Virus Infections

Baloxavir marboxil is used for *postexposure prophylaxis* of influenza A or B virus infection in adults and adolescents 12 years of age or older who are contacts of an individual with influenza.

Annual vaccination with seasonal influenza virus vaccine, as recommended by CDC's Advisory Committee on Immunization Practices (ACIP), is the primary means of preventing seasonal influenza and its severe complications. Prophylaxis with an appropriate antiviral active against circulating influenza strains is considered an adjunct to vaccination for the control and prevention of influenza in certain individuals.

Decisions regarding use of antivirals for prophylaxis of seasonal influenza should be based on the risk of influenza-related complications in the exposed individual, the type and duration of contact, recommendations from local or public health authorities, and clinical judgment. CDC and others do not recommend *routine* use of influenza antivirals for postexposure prophylaxis in individuals exposed to influenza; however, such prophylaxis can be considered for prevention of influenza in certain situations in exposed individuals at high risk for influenza-related complications for whom influenza vaccine is contraindicated, unavailable, or expected to have low efficacy (e.g., immunocompromised individuals). In general, antiviral postexposure prophylaxis should be used only if it can be initiated within 48 hours after the most recent exposure.

CDC issues recommendations concerning the use of antivirals for prophylaxis of influenza, and these recommendations are updated as needed during each influenza season. Information regarding influenza surveillance and updated recommendations for prevention of seasonal influenza are available from CDC at https://www.cdc.gov/flu/.

Clinical Trials and Experience
Adults and Adolescents 12 Years of Age or Older

Efficacy and safety of a single dose of baloxavir marboxil for postexposure prophylaxis of influenza were evaluated in a phase 3, multicenter, randomized, double-blind, placebo-controlled trial in Japan. A total of 607 individuals 12 years of age or older who were household contacts of someone with influenza were randomized 1:1 to receive a single dose of baloxavir marboxil (single 40-mg oral dose in those weighing less than 80 kg or single 80-mg oral dose in those weighing 80 kg or more) or placebo. Influenza-infected index patients were required to have onset of symptoms within the last 48 hours (49% of index patients had influenza A [H3N2], 46% had influenza A [H1N1], 1% had influenza B) and household contacts were required to have been living with the influenza-infected index patient for at least 48 hours (91% of household contacts were 18 to less than 65 years of age, 5% were 12–17 years of age, 4% were 65 years of age or older). The primary efficacy end point was the proportion of household contacts with RT-PCR-confirmed influenza and with fever (axillary temperature 37.5°C or higher) and at least one respiratory symptom (cough or nasal congestion assessed as moderate or severe) on days 1–10 after the dose. Results indicated that 1% of household contacts who received postexposure prophylaxis with a single dose of baloxavir marboxil developed RT-PCR-confirmed symptomatic influenza compared with 13% of those who received placebo.

DOSAGE AND ADMINISTRATION

● Administration

Baloxavir marboxil is administered orally without regard to meals. However, concomitant administration with dairy products; calcium-fortified beverages; or antacids, laxatives, or oral supplements containing polyvalent cations (aluminum, calcium, iron, magnesium, selenium, or zinc) should be avoided. (See Antacids and Other Preparations Containing Polyvalent Cations under Drug Interactions.)

Baloxavir marboxil is commercially available as tablets or as granules for oral suspension that must be suspended in water prior to administration.

Granules for Oral Suspension

Baloxavir marboxil granules for oral suspension are intended for use in patients unable to easily swallow tablets or those requiring enteral administration.

Prior to dispensing, 20 mL of drinking or sterile water should be added to a bottle containing baloxavir marboxil granules and the bottle swirled to ensure that the granules are evenly suspended; the bottle should not be shaken. Each bottle provides an oral suspension containing 40 mg/20 mL (2 mg/mL) of the drug. Depending on the required dosage, 1 or 2 bottles of oral suspension should be prepared.

Baloxavir marboxil oral suspension does not contain preservatives and must be administered within 10 hours following preparation. The oral suspension may be stored at room temperature (20–25°C) for up to 10 hours after preparation and must be discarded if not used within 10 hours or if stored at a temperature greater than 25°C. The expiration date and time must be marked on the bottle at the time of preparation.

A measuring device (e.g., oral syringe, measuring cup) should be provided with the oral suspension.

For enteral administration (i.e., feeding tube), the oral suspension should be drawn up into an enteral syringe; the feeding tube should be flushed with 1 mL of water before and after enteral administration of the dose of oral suspension.

● Dosage
Adult Dosage
Treatment of Seasonal Influenza A and B Virus Infections

For the treatment of acute, uncomplicated influenza infection in adults, the recommended dosage of oral baloxavir marboxil is a single 40-mg dose in those weighing less than 80 kg or a single 80-mg dose in those weighing 80 kg or more.

The dose should be given as soon as possible and within 48 hours after onset of influenza symptoms.

Prevention of Seasonal Influenza A and B Virus Infections

For postexposure prophylaxis of influenza in adults who have had contact with an individual with influenza, the recommended dosage of oral baloxavir marboxil is a single 40-mg dose in those weighing less than 80 kg or a single 80-mg dose in those weighing 80 kg or more.

The dose should be given as soon as possible and within 48 hours after contact with an individual with influenza.

Pediatric Dosage

Treatment of Seasonal Influenza A and B Virus Infections

For the treatment of acute, uncomplicated influenza infection in adolescents 12 years of age or older, the recommended dosage of oral baloxavir marboxil is a single 40-mg dose in those weighing less than 80 kg or a single 80-mg dose in those weighing 80 kg or more.

The dose should be given as soon as possible and within 48 hours after onset of influenza symptoms.

Prevention of Seasonal Influenza A and B Virus Infections

For postexposure prophylaxis of influenza in adolescents 12 years of age or older who have had contact with an individual with influenza, the recommended dosage of oral baloxavir marboxil is a single 40-mg dose in those weighing less than 80 kg or a single 80-mg dose in those weighing 80 kg or more.

The dose should be given as soon as possible and within 48 hours after contact with an individual with influenza.

● Special Populations

The manufacturer makes no special population dosage recommendations for geriatric individuals or patients with impaired hepatic or renal function.

CAUTIONS

● Contraindications

- History of hypersensitivity to baloxavir marboxil or any ingredient in the formulation.

● Warnings/Precautions

Sensitivity Reactions

Serious allergic reactions, including anaphylaxis, anaphylactic or anaphylactoid reactions, angioedema (face, eyelids, tongue, lips), urticaria, and erythema multiforme, have been reported during postmarketing experience in individuals who received baloxavir marboxil. Rash also has been reported.

If an allergic-like reaction occurs or is suspected, appropriate treatment should be initiated.

Bacterial Infections

When making treatment decisions in patients with suspected influenza, the possibility of primary or concomitant bacterial infection should be considered.

Serious bacterial infections may begin with influenza-like symptoms or may coexist with or occur as complications of influenza. There is no evidence that baloxavir marboxil prevents such complications. If a bacterial infection occurs, it should be treated as appropriate.

There is no evidence that baloxavir marboxil is effective for illness caused by any organisms other than influenza viruses.

Immunocompromised Individuals

Data are not available regarding efficacy and safety of baloxavir marboxil for the treatment of influenza in individuals with severe immunosuppression. Emergence of resistance to baloxavir may be a concern because the duration of influenza virus replication may be prolonged in such patients.

CDC does not recommend use of baloxavir marboxil monotherapy for the treatment of influenza in individuals with severe immunosuppression.

Influenza Vaccination

Influenza antivirals, including baloxavir marboxil, are important adjuncts to vaccination in the control of influenza, but are not a substitute for annual vaccination with a seasonal influenza vaccine (influenza virus vaccine inactivated, influenza vaccine recombinant, influenza vaccine live intranasal).

Although influenza antivirals, including baloxavir marboxil, may be used concomitantly with or at any time before or after influenza vaccine inactivated or influenza vaccine recombinant, influenza antivirals may inhibit the vaccine virus contained in influenza vaccine live intranasal and decrease efficacy of the live vaccine. (See Influenza Vaccines under Drug Interactions.)

Specific Populations

Pregnancy

There are no adequate and well-controlled studies using baloxavir marboxil in pregnant women to inform a drug-associated risk of adverse developmental outcomes.

In animal reproduction studies, no adverse embryofetal effects were observed in rats or rabbits receiving oral baloxavir marboxil in dosages resulting in baloxavir exposures approximately 5 or 7 times, respectively, the systemic baloxavir exposures achieved in humans with the maximum recommended human dosage.

Pregnant women are at increased risk for severe complications from influenza, which may lead to adverse pregnancy and/or fetal outcomes including maternal death, stillbirths, birth defects, preterm delivery, low birthweight, and small size for gestational age.

CDC states that baloxavir marboxil is not recommended for the treatment of influenza in pregnant women because of the lack of safety and efficacy data in such patients. Oseltamivir is the preferred antiviral for the treatment of suspected or confirmed influenza and prevention of influenza in women who are pregnant or up to 2 weeks postpartum.

Lactation

It is not known whether baloxavir marboxil is distributed into human milk, affects milk production, or has any effects on breast-fed infants. Baloxavir and its metabolites are distributed into milk in rats.

The manufacturer states that the benefits of breast-feeding and the importance of baloxavir marboxil to the woman should be considered along with the potential adverse effects on the breast-fed child from the drug or from the underlying maternal condition.

CDC states that baloxavir marboxil is not recommended for the treatment of influenza in nursing women because of the lack of safety data in such patients.

Pediatric Use

Safety and efficacy of baloxavir marboxil have not been established in pediatric patients younger than 12 years of age.

Safety and efficacy of baloxavir marboxil for the treatment of influenza in adolescents 12 years of age or older weighing 40 kg or more were established in a phase 3, randomized, double-blind, placebo-controlled study. Data from this study indicated that the safety profile of the drug in adolescent patients 12 years of age or older is similar to that reported in adults.

Safety and efficacy of baloxavir marboxil for postexposure prophylaxis of influenza in adolescents 12 years of age or older weighing 40 kg or more is supported by a randomized, double-blind, placebo-controlled trial conducted in Japan that included 12 individuals 12–17 years of age who received the drug for postexposure prophylaxis. Adverse effects reported in these adolescents were similar to those reported in adults in the trial who received the drug.

Geriatric Use

Safety and efficacy of baloxavir marboxil for the treatment of acute, uncomplicated influenza in adults 65 years of age or older have been established and are supported by a randomized, double-blind, controlled trial that included 209 adults in this age group at high risk of influenza-related complications who were treated with the drug. The median time to improvement of influenza symptoms in patients 65 years of age or older was 70 hours in those treated with baloxavir marboxil compared with 88 hours in those who received placebo. The safety profile of the drug in patients 65 years of age or older was similar to that reported in the overall trial population, with the exception of nausea (reported in 6% of adults 65 years of age or older compared with 1% of those 18–64 years of age).

Hepatic Impairment

Baloxavir marboxil has not been evaluated in patients with severe hepatic impairment (Child-Pugh class C).

Population pharmacokinetic analysis indicates there are no clinically important differences in the pharmacokinetics of baloxavir marboxil in individuals with moderate hepatic impairment (Child-Pugh class B) compared with individuals with normal hepatic function.

Renal Impairment

Baloxavir marboxil has not been evaluated in patients with severe renal impairment.

Population pharmacokinetic analysis indicates that there are no clinically important differences in the pharmacokinetics of baloxavir marboxil in individuals with creatinine clearances of 50 mL/minute or greater compared with individuals with normal renal function.

• Common Adverse Effects

Adverse effects reported in 1% or more of patients receiving baloxavir marboxil in clinical studies include GI effects (nausea, diarrhea), bronchitis, sinusitis, and headache.

DRUG INTERACTIONS

After baloxavir marboxil is converted in vivo to baloxavir, the active metabolite, baloxavir is metabolized principally by uridine diphosphate-glucuronosyltransferase (UGT) 1A3 and, to a minor extent, by cytochrome P-450 (CYP) isoenzyme 3A4.

In vitro studies indicate that baloxavir marboxil and baloxavir do not inhibit CYP isoenzymes 1A2, 2B6, 2C8, 2C9, 2C19, or 2D6 and do not induce CYP isoenzymes 1A2, 2B6, or 3A4.

Baloxavir marboxil and baloxavir are both substrates of P-glycoprotein (P-gp).

In vitro studies indicate that baloxavir marboxil and baloxavir do not inhibit UGT1A1, 1A3, 1A4, 1A6, 1A9, 2B7, or 2B15. In addition, baloxavir does not inhibit organic anion transport polypeptide (OATP) 1B1, OATP1B3, organic cation transporter (OCT) 1, OCT2, organic anion transporter (OAT) 1, OAT3, multidrug and toxin extrusion (MATE) 1, or MATE2K.

• Drugs Affecting or Metabolized by Hepatic Microsomal Enzymes

The pharmacokinetics of baloxavir marboxil and baloxavir were not affected when baloxavir marboxil was used concomitantly with a potent CYP3A inhibitor (itraconazole).

Concomitant use of baloxavir marboxil and a CYP3A substrate (midazolam) did not affect the pharmacokinetics of the CYP3A substrate.

• Drugs Affecting or Affected by the P-glycoprotein Transport System

The pharmacokinetics of baloxavir marboxil and baloxavir were not affected when baloxavir marboxil was used concomitantly with a P-gp inhibitor (itraconazole).

Concomitant use of baloxavir marboxil and a P-gp substrate (digoxin) did not affect the pharmacokinetics of the P-gp substrate.

• Drugs Affected by Other Membrane Transporters

The pharmacokinetics of baloxavir marboxil and baloxavir were not affected when baloxavir marboxil was used concomitantly with a UGT inhibitor (probenecid).

Concomitant use of baloxavir marboxil and a breast cancer resistance protein (BCRP) substrate (rosuvastatin) did not affect the pharmacokinetics of the BCRP substrate.

• Antacids and Other Preparations Containing Polyvalent Cations

Baloxavir may form a chelate with polyvalent cations (e.g., aluminum, calcium, iron, magnesium). Although specific drug interaction studies have not been performed to evaluate concomitant administration of baloxavir marboxil and food, beverages, drugs, or other preparations containing polyvalent cations, results of a study in monkeys indicated that baloxavir exposures were decreased 48–63% when baloxavir marboxil was administered concomitantly with aluminum, calcium, iron, or magnesium.

Antacids

Concomitant use of baloxavir marboxil and antacids containing aluminum, calcium, or magnesium may decrease baloxavir concentrations and decrease efficacy of baloxavir marboxil.

Concomitant administration of baloxavir marboxil and antacids containing polyvalent cations (e.g., aluminum, calcium, magnesium) should be avoided

Calcium, Iron, and Multivitamins

Concomitant use of baloxavir marboxil and calcium-containing foods or drinks (dairy products, calcium-fortified beverages), calcium supplements, iron preparations, or other oral supplements containing calcium, iron, magnesium, selenium, or zinc (e.g., multivitamins) may decrease baloxavir concentrations and decrease efficacy of baloxavir marboxil.

Concomitant administration of baloxavir marboxil and oral supplements containing polyvalent cations (e.g., calcium, iron, magnesium, selenium, or zinc) should be avoided.

Other Preparations Containing Polyvalent Cations

Concomitant use of baloxavir marboxil and drugs containing polyvalent cations (e.g., laxatives) may decrease baloxavir concentrations and decrease efficacy of baloxavir marboxil.

Concomitant administration of baloxavir marboxil and drugs or preparations containing polyvalent cations should be avoided.

• Oseltamivir

There was no evidence of pharmacokinetic interactions when baloxavir marboxil (single 40-mg dose) was used concomitantly with oseltamivir (75 mg twice daily for 5 days).

• Vaccines
Influenza Vaccines

Although concomitant use of baloxavir marboxil and influenza virus vaccine inactivated (IIV) or influenza vaccine recombinant (RIV) has not been evaluated, ACIP states that antivirals used for the treatment of influenza have no effect on the immune response to IIV and RIV and these inactivated influenza vaccines may be administered concomitantly with or at any time before or after influenza antivirals, including baloxavir marboxil.

Concomitant use of baloxavir marboxil and influenza vaccine live intranasal (LAIV) has not been evaluated. Because influenza antivirals, including baloxavir, inhibit replication of influenza viruses and may inhibit the vaccine virus, these antivirals potentially could decrease the immune response to LAIV and efficacy of the live vaccine. Based on the long half-life of baloxavir, ACIP states that it is reasonable to assume that baloxavir marboxil might interfere with LAIV if given from 17 days before through 2 weeks after vaccination. This interval for potential interference might be further prolonged in patients with medical conditions that delay drug clearance (e.g., renal insufficiency). ACIP states that individuals who received baloxavir marboxil from 17 days before to 2 weeks after LAIV should be revaccinated using age-appropriate IIV or RIV.

PHARMACOKINETICS

• Absorption
Bioavailability

Following oral administration of baloxavir marboxil, the drug is rapidly and almost completely converted to the active metabolite, baloxavir, by esterases in the GI lumen, liver, and blood.

The median time to peak plasma concentrations of baloxavir after oral administration of baloxavir marboxil is 4 hours.

Following a single 40- or 80-mg dose of baloxavir marboxil, mean peak plasma concentrations of baloxavir are 68.9 or 82.5 ng/mL, respectively.

Baloxavir exposure decreases as body weight increases. No clinically important difference in exposures are observed between body weight groups when the recommended weight-based dosage of baloxavir marboxil is used (40-mg dose in those weighing less than 80 kg or 80-mg dose in those weighing 80 kg or more).

Food

Administration of oral baloxavir marboxil with a meal (approximately 400–500 kcal including 150 kcal from fat) decreases the peak plasma concentration and area under the plasma concentration-time curve (AUC) of baloxavir by approximately 48 and 36%, respectively.

Although specific studies have not been performed, baloxavir may form chelates with polyvalent cations (e.g., aluminum, calcium, iron, magnesium, selenium, zinc). Systemic baloxavir exposures may be decreased if oral baloxavir marboxil is administered with dairy products, calcium-fortified beverages, or other foods, drugs, or preparations containing polyvalent cations. (See Antacids and Other Preparations Containing Polyvalent Cations under Drug Interactions.)

● Distribution

Extent

Baloxavir and its related metabolites are distributed into milk in rats following oral administration of baloxavir marboxil; it is not known whether the drug is distributed into human milk.

Plasma Protein Binding

Baloxavir is approximately 93–94% bound to serum proteins in vitro.

● Elimination

Metabolism

Following oral administration, baloxavir marboxil is rapidly hydrolyzed by esterases to the active metabolite, baloxavir. Baloxavir is then metabolized principally by uridine diphosphate-glucuronosyltransferase (UGT) 1A3 and, to a minor extent, by cytochrome P-450 (CYP) isoenzyme 3A4.

Elimination Route

Approximately 80% of an oral dose of baloxavir marboxil is eliminated in feces as baloxavir and less than 15% is eliminated in urine.

Half-life

The mean apparent terminal elimination half-life of baloxavir is 79.1 hours.

Special Populations

Based on a population pharmacokinetic analysis, baloxavir exposure is approximately 35% lower in non-Asians compared with Asians; this difference is not considered clinically important when the recommended dosage of baloxavir marboxil is used.

No clinically important differences in the pharmacokinetics of baloxavir were observed based on age, sex, creatinine clearance (50 mL/minute or greater), or moderate hepatic impairment (Child-Pugh class B). The effects of severe renal or hepatic impairment on baloxavir pharmacokinetics have not been evaluated.

DESCRIPTION

Baloxavir marboxil is a prodrug of baloxavir, a polymerase acidic (PA) endonuclease inhibitor antiviral. Baloxavir marboxil exhibits no antiviral activity until hydrolyzed in vivo to baloxavir, its active metabolite. Baloxavir has a mechanism of action against influenza viruses that differs from that of the neuraminidase inhibitor antivirals (oseltamivir, peramivir, zanamivir) and adamantane derivative antivirals (amantadine, rimantadine).

Baloxavir selectively inhibits the cap-dependent endonuclease activity of the PA subunit of the viral RNA polymerase complex, which is essential for viral replication. Inhibition of the cap-dependent endonuclease activity of the PA subunit prevents transcription of influenza viral messenger RNA, which is required for viral replication.

● Spectrum

Baloxavir exhibits potent antiviral activity in vitro against both influenza A and B viruses. In a PA endonuclease assay, the 50% inhibitory concentrations (IC$_{50}$) of baloxavir for influenza A viruses was 1.4–3.1 nM and the IC$_{50}$ of the drug for influenza B viruses was 4.5–8.9 nM. When susceptibility of laboratory and clinical isolates of influenza A and B viruses was determined in an MDCK cell-based plaque reduction assay, the 50% effective concentration (EC$_{50}$) of baloxavir was 0.20-1.85 nM for influenza A (H1N1), 0.35–2.63 nM for influenza A (H3N2), and 2.67–14.23 nM for influenza B.

Viral surveillance data indicate that almost all influenza A (H1N1)pdm09, influenza A (H3N2), and influenza B viruses circulating during recent influenza seasons have been susceptible to baloxavir in vitro.

Baloxavir is active against some influenza strains resistant to neuraminidase inhibitors (e.g., oseltamivir, peramivir, zanamivir), including influenza A (H1N1) with the H275Y mutation, influenza A (H3N2) with the E119V or R292K mutation, influenza B with the R152K or D198E mutation, avian influenza A (H5N1) with the H275Y mutation, and avian influenza A (H7N9) with the R292K mutation.

Baloxavir has been active in vitro in cell culture against some avian influenza A viruses, including some strains of avian influenza A (H5N1) and (H7N9). In an MDCK cell-based virus titer reduction assay, the 90% effective concentration (EC$_{90}$) of baloxavir for avian influenza A (H5N1) and (H7N9) ranged from 0.80–3.16 nM.

The relationship between in vitro antiviral activity of baloxavir in cell culture and clinical response to treatment with baloxavir marboxil has not been established.

● Resistance

Resistance to baloxavir has been produced in vitro by serial passage of influenza A viruses in the presence of increasing concentrations of the drug. In addition, influenza A and B viruses with treatment-emergent amino acid substitutions associated with reduced in vitro susceptibility to baloxavir have been reported in some patients treated with baloxavir marboxil.

Reduced in vitro susceptibility to baloxavir has been reported only rarely in influenza A (H1N1)pdm09 and influenza A (H3N2) circulating during recent influenza seasons.

Influenza viruses with reduced susceptibility to baloxavir have amino acid substitutions in the PA protein of the viral RNA polymerase complex. Treatment-emergent amino acid substitutions that have been associated with reduced in vitro susceptibility to baloxavir include E23K/R and I38F/N/S/T (influenza A [H1N1]); E23G/K, A37T, I38M/T, and E199G (influenza A [H3N2]); and I38T (influenza B). Pooled data from 3 clinical trials evaluating a single dose of baloxavir marboxil for the treatment of RT-PCR-confirmed influenza in adults and adolescents 12 years of age or older indicate that the overall frequencies of treatment-emergent amino acid substitutions associated with reduced susceptibility to baloxavir were 4.5% (influenza A [H1N1]), 10.9% (influenza A [H3N2]), and 0.9% (influenza B).

Oseltamivir may be active against influenza viruses with reduced susceptibility to baloxavir, including influenza A (H1N1) with amino acid substitutions E23K or I38F/T; influenza A (H3N2) with substitutions E23G/K, A37T, I38M/T, or E199G; and influenza B with the substitution I38T.

Cross-resistance between baloxavir and neuraminidase inhibitors (oseltamivir, peramivir, zanamivir) or adamantane derivatives (amantadine, rimantadine) is not expected since these drugs have different mechanisms of action against influenza viruses. However, influenza viruses with amino acid substitutions in the PA protein of the viral RNA polymerase complex that confer resistance to baloxavir may also have substitutions that confer resistance to neuraminidase inhibitors or adamantane derivatives. The clinical relevance of phenotypic cross-resistance evaluations has not been established.

ADVICE TO PATIENTS

Importance of reading patient information provided by the manufacturer.

Treatment of influenza: Importance of initiating baloxavir marboxil as soon as possible after the first appearance of influenza symptoms (within 48 hours after symptom onset).

Postexposure prophylaxis of influenza: Importance of initiating baloxavir marboxil as soon as possible after exposure.

Advise patients that baloxavir marboxil may be taken with or without food, but should not be taken with dairy products or calcium-fortified beverages or with antacids, laxatives, multivitamins, or dietary supplements containing polyvalent cations (e.g., calcium, iron, magnesium, selenium, zinc).

Importance of taking baloxavir marboxil as a single dose as prescribed (either as a tablet or oral suspension).

If the oral suspension is used, advise patients and/or caregivers that the total prescribed dose may require 1 or 2 bottles of the oral suspension, depending on patient's weight. Importance of administering the oral suspension as soon as possible, but no later than 10 hours after preparation. Expiration date and time should appear on the bottle(s) of oral suspension.

Advise patients and/or caregivers of the risk of severe allergic reactions (e.g., anaphylaxis, angioedema, urticaria, erythema multiforme) and importance of seeking immediate medical attention if an allergic-like reaction occurs or is suspected.

Advise patients that influenza antivirals such as baloxavir marboxil may decrease effectiveness of LAIV; importance of consulting clinician before receiving the live intranasal influenza vaccine.

Importance of informing clinicians of existing or contemplated concomitant therapy, including prescription and OTC drugs, as well as any concomitant illnesses.

Importance of women informing clinicians if they are or plan to become pregnant or plan to breast-feed.

Importance of informing patients of other important precautionary information. (See Cautions.)

PREPARATIONS

Excipients in commercially available drug preparations may have clinically important effects in some individuals; consult specific product labeling for details.

Baloxavir Marboxil

Oral

Granules, for suspension	40 mg per bottle	**Xofluza®**, Genentech
Tablets, film-coated	40 mg	**Xofluza®**, Genentech
	80 mg	**Xofluza®**, Genentech

† Use is not currently included in the labeling approved by the US Food and Drug Administration.

Selected Revisions June 10, 2024, © Copyright, November 12, 2018, American Society of Health-System Pharmacists, Inc.

Acyclovir
Acyclovir Sodium

8:18.32 · NUCLEOSIDES AND NUCLEOTIDES

■ Acyclovir is a synthetic purine nucleoside analog antiviral agent derived from guanine and is active against Herpesviridae.

USES

IV acyclovir sodium is used for the treatment of initial and recurrent mucocutaneous herpes simplex virus (HSV-1 and HSV-2) infections and the treatment of varicella-zoster infections in immunocompromised adults and children; for the treatment of severe first episodes of genital herpes infections in immunocompetent individuals; and for the treatment of HSV encephalitis and neonatal HSV infections. Acyclovir is used orally for the treatment of initial and recurrent episodes of genital herpes; for the acute treatment of herpes zoster (shingles, zoster) in immunocompetent individuals; and for the treatment of varicella (chickenpox) in immunocompetent individuals.

For topical uses of acyclovir, see 84:04.06.

● Mucocutaneous, Ocular, and Systemic Herpes Simplex Virus (HSV) Infections

Acyclovir is considered the drug of choice for the treatment of mucocutaneous herpes simplex virus (HSV) infections in immunocompromised adults, adolescents, and children and also is considered the drug of choice for the treatment of severe HSV infections such as HSV encephalitis and neonatal HSV infections.

Controlled studies of initial and recurrent mucocutaneous HSV-1 and HSV-2 infections (e.g., orofacial, esophageal, genital, nasal, labial) in immunocompromised adults and children have shown that IV acyclovir therapy decreases the duration of viral shedding (time from onset of therapy until the last positive culture), the duration of pain and itching, the time required for crusting and healing of lesions, and the duration of positive cultures. In one study, the median duration of viral shedding was 3 days in acyclovir-treated patients compared with 17 days in placebo-treated patients; pain ceased within 10 days of initiating therapy in acyclovir-treated patients compared with 16 days in placebo-treated patients. The time required for crusting and healing of lesions was 7 and 14 days, respectively, in acyclovir-treated patients compared with 14 and 28 days, respectively, in placebo-treated patients. IV acyclovir was not effective in reducing the frequency or delaying the onset of subsequent recurrent infection with HSV-1, HSV-2, or other herpesviruses or in eliminating an established latent infection.

Acyclovir has been used for the treatment of orolabial HSV infections, including gingivostomatitis, in adults and children; the drug is not effective or is minimally effective for the prevention of recurrence of herpes labialis† in immunocompetent individuals.

Oral or IV acyclovir has been reported to be effective in the treatment of eczema herpeticum† caused by HSV in several patients with a history of atopic dermatitis; the drug decreased fever and/or the appearance of new lesions, and promoted crusting and healing of lesions.

HIV-Infected Individuals

Acyclovir generally is considered the drug of choice for the treatment of primary or recurrent mucocutaneous HSV infections in individuals with human immunodeficiency virus (HIV) infection. Mucocutaneous HSV infections in HIV-infected individuals can involve severe lesions that persist longer than those in immunocompetent individuals. Infections often progress to visceral disease and CNS or disseminated HSV may occur. HSV oral lesions in HIV-infected individuals generally are erosive, painful ulcerations that persist for several weeks and can extend to the esophagus. While these lesions may heal spontaneously, initiation of oral acyclovir at the onset of symptoms is recommended since severe pain and local tissue destruction may occur; IV acyclovir may be necessary for severe cases.

In patients with advanced HIV infection, reactivation of HSV frequently occurs and can result in chronic, persistent mucocutaneous disease that may be severe. The Prevention of Opportunistic Infections Working Group of the US Public Health Service and the Infectious Diseases Society of America (USPHS/IDSA) has established guidelines for the prevention of opportunistic infections in HIV-infected individuals that include recommendations concerning prevention of exposure to opportunistic pathogens, prevention of first disease episodes, and prevention of disease recurrence. The USPHS/IDSA does not currently recommend primary prophylaxis against initial episodes of HSV infection in HIV-infected adults, adolescents, or children. In addition, the USPHS/IDSA does not recommend routine chronic suppressive or maintenance therapy (secondary prophylaxis) against HSV disease in HIV-infected individuals since acute episodes generally can be treated successfully with acyclovir. However, long-term prophylaxis against recurrence of HSV can be considered for adults, adolescents, and children who have frequent or severe recurrences. If secondary prophylaxis of HSV disease is indicated in HIV-infected adults or adolescents, the USPHS/IDSA and other experts recommend use of oral acyclovir, oral famciclovir, or oral valacyclovir as the regimen of choice. If indicated in infants and children, the USPHS/IDSA and other experts recommend oral acyclovir.

HIV-infected patients receiving acyclovir may develop acyclovir-resistant strains of HSV; these infections have been reported most often in patients with advanced HIV infection or those who have received long-term acyclovir therapy. IV foscarnet or IV cidofovir can be used for the management of HSV infections in HIV-infected patients when the HSV infection is known or suspected of being caused by acyclovir-resistant strains. Additional study is needed to determine whether long-term suppression of HSV reduces or facilitates the emergence of drug-resistant strains of the virus and to determine optimal strategies for suppressive therapy of acyclovir-resistant HSV infections. It has been postulated that alternating the use of antiviral agents (e.g., acyclovir, foscarnet) may prevent emergence and subsequent predominance of drug-resistant isolates.

Ocular HSV Infections

Oral acyclovir (400 mg 5 times daily) has been used for the treatment of HSV keratitis† in HIV-infected patients. Long-term antiviral therapy may be necessary to prevent recurrent ocular HSV disease in these patients. Oral acyclovir (400 mg twice daily for 12 months) has been used for the prevention of recurrent ocular HSV disease† in immunocompetent adults and children 12 years of age or older who had an episode of ocular HSV disease (blepharitis, conjunctivitis, epithelial keratitis, stromal keratitis, iritis) in one or both eyes within the preceding 12 months. Results of one study in adults indicate that long-term oral acyclovir (400 mg twice daily for up to 18 months) is effective in decreasing the number of HSV recurrences. Oral acyclovir (400 mg twice daily for 6 months) has been used to prevent HSV recurrences in patients undergoing penetrating keratoplasty for herpetic eye disease. The optimum duration of prophylaxis remains to be determined.

HSV Encephalitis

Controlled studies in adults and children 6 months of age or older have shown that IV acyclovir is effective for the treatment of HSV encephalitis. Many clinicians consider acyclovir the drug of choice for the treatment of HSV encephalitis, and the American Academy of Pediatrics (AAP) and other experts also consider acyclovir the drug of choice for the treatment of neonatal HSV infections involving the CNS.

HSV encephalitis and neonatal HSV infections of the CNS are associated with substantial morbidity and mortality despite antiviral treatment. In one study in patients 6 months to 79 years of age with brain biopsy-proven HSV encephalitis randomized to receive 10 days of IV acyclovir (10 mg/kg every 8 hours) or IV vidarabine (15 mg/kg daily; no longer commercially available in the US), the overall mortality rate at 12 months was 25% in those who received acyclovir versus 59% in those who received vidarabine. Morbidity assessments at 12 months indicated that 32% of patients who received acyclovir were functioning normally or had only mild neurologic sequelae (e.g., decreased attention span); the remaining survivors had moderate (e.g., hemiparesis, speech impediment, seizures) or severe (continuous supportive care required) sequelae. Patients who were younger than 30 years of age and those with less severe neurologic involvement at the time of treatment had the best outcome. Initiation of acyclovir early in the course of the infection (prior to the development of semicoma or coma) may enhance its efficacy.

Neonatal HSV Infections

The AAP, US Centers for Disease Control and Prevention (CDC), and other experts consider IV acyclovir the drug of choice for the treatment of mucosal, cutaneous, CNS, or disseminated HSV infections in neonates.

Neonatal HSV infection is associated with substantial morbidity and mortality, and approximately 25% of neonates with disseminated HSV disease die despite antiviral therapy. Because the risk of morbidity and mortality increases substantially with systemic (CNS or disseminated) infection compared with mucocutaneous infection, early recognition of neonates with HSV infection confined to the skin, eyes, and mouth and early initiation of antiviral therapy are important. The AAP recommends that IV acyclovir therapy be initiated in all neonates with HSV infection, irrespective of presenting clinical findings. In addition, the AAP states that infants with HSV disease that has ocular involvement should received a topical ophthalmic antiviral agent (e.g., trifluridine, vidarabine) in addition to parenteral therapy.

In one study in infants with neonatal HSV disease who were randomized to receive a 10-day regimen of IV acyclovir (10 mg/kg every 8 hours) or vidarabine (30 mg/kg daily; no longer commercially available in the US), mortality at 1 year in the acyclovir group was 0/54 in those with localized disease (limited to skin, eye, and/or mouth), 5/35 in those with CNS infections, and 11/18 in those with visceral organ involvement such as hepatitis or pneumonitis with or without CNS involvement.

Relapse of neonatal HSV disease involving the skin, eyes, mouth, or CNS can occur after acyclovir therapy is discontinued; however, optimal management of these recurrences has not been established. The safety and efficacy of long-term suppressive or intermittent acyclovir therapy for neonates with HSV disease of the skin, eyes, and mouth are being evaluated.

The care of infants exposed to HSV during delivery depends on the status of the mother's infection and mode of delivery; infants exposed to HSV during birth should be monitored carefully in consultation with a specialist. Most experts recommend that women with recurrent genital herpetic lesions at the onset of labor should deliver by cesarean section to prevent neonatal herpes. However, cesarean section does not completely eliminate the risk for HSV transmission to the infant. Women without symptoms or signs of genital herpes can deliver vaginally. The AAP states that all neonates born to women with active genital HSV lesions, regardless of whether the child was delivered by vaginal or cesarean delivery, should be observed carefully and viral cultures for HSV should be obtained 24–48 hours after birth. Because the infection rate in infants born by vaginal delivery to mothers with recurrent genital herpes infection is low, most experts recommend that these infants not be given empiric acyclovir therapy. These infants should be observed for signs of infection and undergo surveillance cultures. For neonates whose mothers have presumed or proven primary genital herpes infection, some experts recommend empiric acyclovir treatment at birth (despite the fact that data are not available to support the efficacy of such a strategy) because the risk of infection in these neonates may exceed 50%; other experts would only initiate acyclovir therapy if HSV cultures are positive. All infants with neonatal herpes should be evaluated and treated with acyclovir. Symptoms suggestive of neonatal HSV infection include skin or scalp rash (especially vesicular lesions) and unexplained clinical manifestations (such as respiratory distress, seizures, signs of sepsis). The fact that neonatal HSV infection can occur as late as 4–6 weeks after delivery should be considered.

Hematopoietic Stem Cell Transplant Recipients

The CDC, the Infectious Diseases Society of America (IDSA), and the American Society of Blood and Marrow Transplantation (ASBMT) have established guidelines for preventing opportunistic infections in hematopoietic stem cell transplant (HSCT) recipients. These guidelines recommend that candidates for HSCT whose screening tests before HSCT are seropositive for HSV receive acyclovir to prevent HSV recurrence†. Acyclovir prophylaxis is initiated at the beginning of the conditioning regimen and continued until engraftment occurs or mucositis resolves (approximately 30 days after HSCT). Routine prophylaxis for longer than 30 days is not recommended. Prophylaxis is not indicated for HSCT recipients who are seronegative for HSV.

● Genital Herpes
Treatment of First Episode Infections

Acyclovir is used in the treatment of initial episodes of genital herpes. First episode genital herpes infections occur in patients experiencing their first vesicular or ulcerative lesion of the genitalia and can be either a true primary infection or a non-primary infection. Primary infections frequently are asymptomatic, in which case the first symptomatic episode actually represents a reactivated recurrent infection. Individuals with true primary HSV infections lack antibody to HSV-1 and/or HSV-2 in their serum.

The severity of first episodes of genital herpes may vary from asymptomatic to disabling; however, untreated primary infections are generally characterized by severe and prolonged symptoms (average duration of 14 days) and a large number

of lesions (average duration of 24 days). Symptoms of primary genital herpes usually appear 2–20 days (average: 6 days) following sexual contact with an individual who has a symptomatic or asymptomatic genital herpes infection. Untreated non-primary infections are generally less severe, of shorter duration, and involve fewer systemic complications; lesions of non-primary infections are present for an average of 14 days. Viral shedding occurs in both primary and non-primary infections, and usually lasts about 12 days in untreated primary infections and 7 days in untreated non-primary infections.

Because many patients with first episodes of genital herpes present with mild clinical symptoms but later develop severe or prolonged symptoms, the CDC states that most patients with initial genital herpes should receive antiviral therapy. The CDC and some clinicians recommend that first episodes of genital herpes in immunocompetent adults and adolescents should be treated with a regimen of oral acyclovir (400 mg 3 times daily or 200 mg 5 times daily for 7–10 days), oral famciclovir (250 mg 3 times daily for 7–10 days), or oral valacyclovir (1 g twice daily for 7–10 days). Oral acyclovir also can be used for the treatment of first episodes of genital herpes in pediatric patients. Topical antiviral agents are not recommended for the treatment of genital herpes since these agents offer only minimal clinical benefit.

Controlled studies have shown that oral acyclovir is effective for the treatment of first episodes of genital herpes in immunocompetent patients. Several studies have shown that oral acyclovir therapy decreases viral shedding and the time required for crusting and healing of lesions; in some patients, the formation of new lesions and the duration of pain, pruritus, or dysuria were decreased.

IV acyclovir should be used for the initial treatment of genital herpes when the infection is severe or when there are complications that necessitate hospitalization, including disseminated infection, pneumonitis, hepatitis, CNS involvement (e.g., meningitis, encephalitis). Controlled studies of severe first episodes of genital herpes in immunocompetent individuals have shown that IV acyclovir decreases viral shedding (time from onset of therapy until last positive culture) from genital and cervical lesions, the time necessary for crusting and healing of lesions, the duration of positive cultures, the formation of new lesions, the duration of dysuria and abnormal vaginal discharge, and the degree and duration of pain and pruritus. In one study, the duration of viral shedding was 2 days in acyclovir-treated patients compared with 8 days in placebo-treated patients; the time required for healing of lesions was 7 days in acyclovir-treated patients compared with 15 days in placebo-treated patients. No substantial reduction in the duration of pain was noted in acyclovir-treated patients compared with placebo-treated patients.

Oral acyclovir has been used at higher dosages (400 mg 5 times daily) for the treatment of first episodes of herpes proctitis†.

Episodic Treatment of Recurrent Infections

Oral acyclovir is used in the treatment of recurrent episodes of genital herpes in immunocompetent adults and adolescents. Antiviral therapy for recurrent genital herpes can be given episodically to ameliorate or shorten the duration of lesions or can be given continuously as suppressive therapy to reduce the frequency of recurrences. For episodic treatment of recurrent genital herpes in immunocompetent adults and adolescents, the CDC and some clinicians recommend oral acyclovir (400 mg 3 times daily for 5 days, 800 mg twice daily for 5 days, or 800 mg 3 times daily for 2 days), oral famciclovir (125 mg twice daily for 5 days or 1 g twice daily for 1 day), or oral valacyclovir (500 mg twice daily for 3 days or 1 g once daily for 5 days). Episodic antiviral therapy should be initiated within 1 day of lesion onset or during the prodrome that precedes some outbreaks.

Suppressive Therapy of Recurrent Infections

Oral acyclovir is used for chronic suppressive therapy of recurrent genital herpes in immunocompetent adults and adolescents. Data are not available regarding use of acyclovir for suppressive therapy in children. The CDC states that suppressive antiviral therapy can reduce the frequency of genital herpes recurrences by 70–80% in patients who have frequent recurrences (i.e., 6 or more per year) and many patients report no symptomatic outbreaks during such therapy. Quality of life often is improved in patients who receive suppressive therapy rather than episodic treatment for recurrent genital herpes. For chronic suppressive therapy of recurrent genital herpes, the CDC and some clinicians recommend that immunocompetent adults and adolescents receive a regimen of oral acyclovir (400 mg twice daily), oral famciclovir (250 mg twice daily), or oral valacyclovir (500 mg or 1 g once daily). The CDC states that data suggest that famciclovir and valacyclovir are as effective as acyclovir in terms of clinical outcome, although the 500-mg once-daily valacyclovir regimen might be less effective than the acyclovir regimen or other valacyclovir regimens in patients who have very frequent recurrences (i.e., 10 or more episodes per year).

Controlled studies have shown that prophylactic administration of oral acyclovir for suppressive therapy may reduce the frequency and/or severity of subsequent recurrent genital herpes infections or delay the onset of subsequent episodes in immunocompetent patients and can prevent clinical recurrences of genital herpes infections in a substantial proportion of patients. The efficacy of prophylactic administration of oral acyclovir therapy in patients with recurrent herpes proctitis remains to be established. In a study in patients with frequent recurrences of genital herpes infections (6 or more per year) receiving chronic suppressive therapy (400 mg of oral acyclovir twice daily), 45, 52, and 63% of patients were free of recurrences during the first, second, and third years, respectively; serial analyses of 3-month recurrence rates revealed that 71–87% were recurrence free during each quarter, and the annual frequency of recurrences during the third year of therapy relative to the baseline frequency was reduced in 97% of patients. The proportion of these patients (i.e., those receiving chronic suppressive therapy) who remained recurrence free during the first year of the study was substantially higher than that of another group of patients who received intermittent (initiated within 48 hours of onset of a herpes episode) therapy instead; in addition, approximately 25% of patients who received chronic suppressive therapy for 3 years remained recurrence free during the entire period.

Safety and efficacy of oral acyclovir for suppressive therapy of recurrent genital herpes infections have been established in patients receiving daily therapy for up to 5–6 years. Because the frequency of recurrent episodes diminishes over time in many patients, the manufacturer and CDC recommend that suppressive antiviral therapy be discontinued periodically (e.g., once yearly) to assess the need for continued therapy.

HIV-Infected Individuals

Immunocompromised individuals may have prolonged or severe episodes of genital, perianal, or oral herpes; HSV lesions are common in those with human immunodeficiency virus (HIV) infection and may be severe, painful, and atypical. (See Uses: Mucocutaneous Herpes Simplex Virus Infections.)

The CDC states that episodic treatment or suppressive therapy with oral antiviral agents often is beneficial in HIV-infected individuals with genital herpes. While the drugs of choice for episodic treatment or suppressive therapy of genital herpes in HIV-infected individuals are the same as those in immunocompetent individuals, higher dosages and/or more prolonged therapy may be necessary. For episodic treatment of recurrences of genital herpes in HIV-infected individuals, the CDC recommends a 5- to 10-day regimen of oral acyclovir (400 mg 3 times daily), oral famciclovir (500 mg twice daily), or oral valacyclovir (1 g twice daily). If chronic suppressive therapy of recurrent genital herpes is used in HIV-infected individuals, the CDC recommends oral acyclovir (400–800 mg 2–3 times daily), oral famciclovir (500 mg twice daily), or oral valacyclovir (500 mg twice daily).

Although rare, clinically important resistance to acyclovir is more likely to occur with prolonged or repeated therapy in severely immunocompromised patients with active lesions. Acyclovir-resistant HSV are resistant to valacyclovir and most strains also are resistant to famciclovir. The potential clinical benefits of acyclovir therapy in immunocompromised patients must be weighed against the potential for selecting resistant HSV strains. If presence of acyclovir-resistant HSV are suspected, specimens should be obtained for in vitro susceptibility testing. Patients whose therapy for the prevention or treatment of recurrence fails because of resistance should be managed in consultation with an expert. IV foscarnet can be used for the management of severe HSV infections known or suspected of being caused by acyclovir-resistant strains; IV foscarnet (40 mg/kg every 8 hours given until clinical resolution is attained) often is effective for the treatment of acyclovir-resistant genital herpes.

Pregnant Women

Although safe use of acyclovir during pregnancy has not been established, the CDC states that oral acyclovir may be used to treat first episodes of genital herpes or severe recurrent genital herpes in pregnant women and that IV acyclovir may be used to treat severe HSV infection in pregnant women.

The risk for transmission of HSV to the neonate from an infected mother during vaginal delivery is high (30–50%) among women who acquire genital herpes near the time of delivery (primary infections) and low (0–5%) among women with histories of recurrent genital herpes at term or women who acquire genital herpes during the first half of pregnancy. Administration of acyclovir late in pregnancy in women who have recurrent genital herpes decreases the frequency of recurrences at term and reduces the frequency of cesarean sections; many clinicians recommend such treatment. There are no data to support administration of acyclovir to HSV-seropositive women who do not have a history of genital herpes.

Because the risk of herpes is high in infants of women who acquire genital herpes in late pregnancy, such women should be managed in consultation with an HSV expert. Some experts recommend acyclovir therapy and/or routine cesarean section in these women to decrease the risk of transmission of HSV to the neonate. (See Pregnancy under Cautions: Pregnancy, Fertility, and Lactation.)

Patient Counseling and Management of Sexual Partners

Counseling of infected individuals and their sex partners is critical to management of genital herpes. The goals of such counseling are to help patients understand and cope with the infection and to prevent sexual and perinatal transmission of the virus. Antiviral therapy offers clinical benefit to most symptomatic patients and is the mainstay of management; however, genital herpes is a recurrent, life-long viral infection. Although antiviral therapy can be used to control the symptoms and signs of genital herpes episodes, it cannot eradicate latent HSV or affect the risk, frequency, or severity of recurrences of genital herpes following discontinuance of antiviral therapy.

The majority of genital herpes infections are transmitted by individuals unaware that they have the infection or by individuals who are asymptomatic when transmission occurs. Patients should be advised that acyclovir is not a cure for genital herpes, and there are no data evaluating whether acyclovir prevents transmission of HSV to others. Because genital herpes is a sexually transmitted disease, patients should be advised to avoid sexual contact with uninfected partners when lesions and/or prodromal symptoms are present. In addition, patients should be advised that sexual transmission of the virus can occur during asymptomatic periods and that suppressive antiviral therapy reduces, but does not eliminate, subclinical viral shedding.

Sex partners of individuals with genital herpes should be advised that they may be infected even if they have no symptoms. Asymptomatic partners of patients with genital herpes should be questioned regarding a history of genital lesions, educated to recognize symptoms of genital herpes, and offered type-specific serologic testing to determine whether risk for HSV acquisition exists. Antiviral therapy is not recommended for sex partners who do not have clinical manifestations of infection, but symptomatic sex partners of individuals with genital herpes should be evaluated and treated.

The risk for neonatal HSV infection should be discussed with all genital herpes patients, including men. Pregnant women and women of childbearing potential who have genital herpes should inform their providers who care for them during pregnancy as well as those who will care for their neonate.

Information to assist patients and clinicians in counseling regarding genital herpes is available at http://www.ashastd.org and http://www.ihmf.org.

● Varicella-Zoster Infections
Varicella (Chickenpox)

Oral acyclovir is used in the treatment of varicella (chickenpox) in immunocompetent adults and children to reduce the severity and duration of the illness. Use of oral acyclovir therapy (initiated within 24 hours of the onset of rash) in otherwise healthy children, postpubertal adolescents, or adults with varicella can decrease the appearance of new lesions, accelerate vesicle healing (vesicles often progress directly from the maculopapular stage to the crusted or healed stage), reduce new vesicle formation by the second day of treatment, and reduce the frequency, duration, and/or severity of fever, pruritus, and constitutional symptoms (e.g., anorexia, lethargy, coryza). In one study in otherwise healthy children 2–12 years of age, nearly all patients receiving oral acyclovir therapy initiated within 24 hours of the onset of rash developed only mild illness of 3–4 days duration with manifestations characteristic of the infection, whereas untreated children generally developed more severe disease of longer duration and many had progressive cutaneous lesions that persisted for more than 6 days.

Some patients who received oral acyclovir therapy reportedly had decreased numbers of residual hypopigmented lesions 4 weeks after initial appearance of rash, and it has been suggested that this possibly indicates a reduction in cutaneous sequelae. However, the clinical relevance, if any, of this finding remains to be established. There currently is no evidence that acyclovir therapy for acute varicella in immunocompetent patients can affect the frequency and/or severity of early complications associated with the disease, in part because such complications generally are uncommon even in untreated individuals. In addition, there currently is no evidence that such therapy can affect the frequency and/or severity of subsequent herpes zoster (shingles, zoster) later in life. It remains to be established whether acyclovir can affect transmission of varicella within households. Current regimens, in which acyclovir is initiated within 24 hours of the appearance of rash, have not reduced such transmission, possibly because therapy was initiated after the period of greatest infectivity. Many clinicians suggest that amelioration, rather than prevention, of varicella in otherwise healthy household contacts should be the principal goal of therapy since prevention could result in the individual being at ongoing risk of primary infection at an older age when manifestations of the disease generally are more severe.

Oral acyclovir therapy in immunocompetent patients generally does not appear to affect antibody response to varicella-zoster infection when measured 1 month and 1 year following treatment with the drug, although somewhat reduced response occasionally has been observed 1 month following treatment with the drug. However, some theoretical concern persists since use of acyclovir in patients with primary herpes simplex infection may result in decreased humoral and cellular immune responses in some patients.Although these altered responses generally have not been associated with increased rates of recurrence or relapse of herpes simplex, the severity of the first subsequent episode of the disease may be increased. Some clinicians also have raised theoretical concerns that potential pathophysiologic and/or immunologic alterations induced by early treatment of varicella infection may predispose to subsequent development of, or more severe, herpes zoster infection, but such concerns have been questioned and remain to be substantiated. Acyclovir should *not* be used prophylactically in an attempt to prevent infection or illness in otherwise healthy children exposed to varicella.

Because of the usually benign course of varicella, the current lack of evidence of effect of acyclovir therapy on early and delayed complications of the disease, and the lack of established substantial cost-benefit of such therapy, the role of acyclovir in the treatment of varicella in otherwise healthy patients currently is controversial.Therefore, the AAP and other clinicians state that oral acyclovir *should not be used routinely* in otherwise healthy children with uncomplicated varicella since administration within 24 hours of rash results in only a modest decrease in symptoms. However, use of oral acyclovir may be considered in certain individual cases when family or clinical circumstances justify the drug's modest benefit and only when the drug can be initiated within the first 24 hours after the onset of rash. The AAP and other clinicians state that use of acyclovir can be considered for otherwise healthy individuals at increased risk of moderate to severe varicella, including those older than 12 years of age, those who contract the disease from siblings or other household contacts, those with chronic cutaneous or pulmonary disorders, those receiving long-term salicylate therapy, and those receiving short, intermittent, or aerosolized courses of corticosteroids. Although it is not known whether children receiving short, intermittent, or aerosolized courses of corticosteroid therapy are at increased risk of complicated or severe varicella, the AAP states that use of acyclovir to minimize the likelihood of severe disease should be considered for these children since no data currently exist to confirm their immunocompetence. Because these children are unlikely to have clinically important immunosuppression, oral acyclovir may used; however, children immunocompromised because of high-dose corticosteroid therapy should receive IV acyclovir therapy. If possible, corticosteroid therapy should be discontinued after known exposure to varicella.

The fact that it may be difficult to recognize varicella and initiate acyclovir therapy soon enough after onset of rash to be of appreciable benefit in many patients, particularly the index case, should be considered. Oral acyclovir provides maximum benefit when initiated as soon as possible after the first manifestation of varicella appears; little if any benefit is apparent if treatment is delayed (e.g., for 48 hours after onset of rash).

IV acyclovir is used for the treatment of varicella in immunocompromised adults and children and many clinicians currently consider IV acyclovir the drug of choice for the treatment of varicella in immunocompromised patients. In immunocompromised adults and children with varicella, IV acyclovir therapy may produce negative viral cultures, decrease the appearance of new lesions, and promote the crusting of lesions; the drug also appears to prevent disseminated, life-threatening infection in some patients. Although limited data suggest that oral acyclovir also may be beneficial in some immunocompromised children with varicella†, the AAP states that oral therapy generally is not recommended for these patients because of poor oral bioavailability. However, high dosage of oral acyclovir has been used in highly selected immunocompromised patients perceived to be at lower risk of developing severe varicella, such as HIV-infected patients with relatively normal CD4+ T-cell counts and children with leukemia in whom careful follow-up is assured. Acyclovir has been used IV in immunocompetent adults for the treatment of complicated varicella (e.g., pneumonia, encephalitis). IV acyclovir therapy appeared to be effective in the treatment of varicella-zoster

pneumonia in at least one immunocompetent adult; however, it could not be conclusively determined that the drug was responsible for resolution of infection. In addition, efficacy of the drug may be reduced substantially if initiation of acyclovir is delayed until the disease has advanced to pneumonitis, particularly in immunocompromised patients; therefore, early initiation of therapy is recommended.

Herpes Zoster (Shingles, Zoster)

Controlled studies have shown that oral acyclovir is effective for the acute treatment of herpes zoster (shingles, zoster) in immunocompetent adults. Oral acyclovir may prevent the appearance of new lesions, decrease viral shedding, decrease the severity and/or duration of pain, promote healing and crusting of lesions, and reduce the prevalence of localized zoster-associated neurologic manifestations (paresthesia, dysesthesia, or hyperesthesia) in immunocompetent adults with localized herpes zoster, at least when given in high dosages within 2 days of the onset of rash. In these studies, acyclovir was particularly effective in adults 50 years of age or older. In immunocompetent adults, high-dose oral acyclovir therapy also may ameliorate cutaneous manifestations, if initiated within 72 hours of rash onset, and acute pain, and may reduce some anterior inflammatory ocular complications (pseudodendritic keratopathy, stromal keratitis, uveitis), if initiated within 7 days of rash onset, but not early cutaneous and external ocular complications (e.g., lid margin vesiculation, conjunctivitis, corneal hypoesthesia, episcleritis). Longer than usual courses of acyclovir (e.g., 21-day therapy) appear to be associated only with marginal additional benefits with regard to the incidence, duration, and severity of pain during the acute phase of the disease in immunocompetent patients when compared with those receiving a 7-day course of therapy. Therefore, because of cost considerations and insufficient evidence of clinical benefits to support such prolonged use, acyclovir therapies longer than 10 days' duration are not recommended for treatment of acute herpes zoster in immunocompetent individuals.

The effect of oral acyclovir on postherpetic neuralgia remains to be clearly determined. In most studies to date, the drug did not appear to prevent postherpetic neuralgia; however, there is some evidence that high-dose therapy may reduce the occurrence of pain in the second and third months after treatment and the associated local neurologic symptoms 3–6 months after treatment. In a limited number of patients with acute herpes zoster, addition of corticosteroids to acyclovir therapy did not appear to influence incidence or severity of postherpetic neuralgia. In one double-blind, placebo-controlled study in immunocompetent adults older than 50 years of age with localized herpes zoster, patients were randomized to received oral acyclovir (800 mg 5 times daily for 21 days) with oral prednisone (daily dosage of 60 mg for days 1–7, then 30 mg for days 8–14 and 15 mg for days 15–21), oral acyclovir with placebo, oral prednisone with placebo, or 2 placebos. Patients were evaluated for persistence of pain and quality of life (i.e., return to 100% usual activity, return to uninterrupted sleep, cessation of analgesic therapy); acute neuritis was assessed during the first month and chronic pain was assessed for up to 6 months. While patients who received prednisone had a shorter duration of acute pain and improved quality of life during the first month after disease onset compared with those who did not receive the drug, the incidence of pain at 3 or 6 months was similar in all 4 treatment groups.

IV acyclovir is used for the treatment of herpes zoster infections in immunocompromised patients, and some clinicians suggest that IV acyclovir is the preferred antiviral agent for the treatment of primary or disseminated herpes zoster in immunocompromised patients, including HIV-infected patients. IV acyclovir also has been used for the treatment of herpes zoster in immunocompetent patients† who have both localized and disseminated infections. In a placebo-controlled study in immunocompromised patients with herpes zoster, reductions in cutaneous and visceral dissemination were greater in those who received IV acyclovir (500 mg/m² every 8 hours for 7 days) compared with those who received placebo. In a limited number of immunocompetent adults and immunocompromised adults and children with localized and disseminated herpes zoster infections, IV acyclovir therapy appeared to decrease pain and fever, prevent the appearance of new lesions, produce negative cultures, and promote crusting and healing of lesions; however, the principal therapeutic effect of acyclovir in immunocompromised patients appears to be in preventing progression of disease as manifested by cutaneous or visceral dissemination. IV acyclovir therapy has also produced rapid clinical response in a limited number of immunocompetent and immunocompromised patients with herpes zoster-associated encephalitis. There is no evidence that IV acyclovir prevents postherpetic neuralgia.

Oral acyclovir has been used for the treatment of dermatomal herpes zoster in immunocompromised patients†, including transplant recipients and HIV-infected patients.

IV acyclovir (10 mg/kg 3 times daily for 7 days) followed by oral acyclovir (800 mg 3–5 times daily) as maintenance therapy has been used for the treatment of herpes zoster ophthalmicus† in HIV-infected patients.

Several cases of acyclovir-resistant varicella-zoster virus infections have been reported in adults and children with acquired immunodeficiency syndrome (AIDS) following chronic suppressive courses of therapy with the drug; because pretreatment isolates were not obtained, it is not known whether the original virus developed resistance or a resistant strain was selected during chronic therapy. Another case of therapeutic failure secondary to resistant varicella-zoster has been reported in an immunocompromised patient; however, limited data to date suggest that resistance of the virus to acyclovir occurs only rarely, but additional study and experience are necessary.

● Cytomegalovirus Infections

Acyclovir generally is ineffective in the treatment of cytomegalovirus (CMV) infections†. IV acyclovir therapy reportedly reduced fever, improved radiographic findings of pneumonia, and resulted in negative blood cultures in some immunocompromised patients with pneumonia caused by CMV. However, in one randomized study in HIV-infected patients, there was no evidence that oral acyclovir therapy suppressed CMV excretion in these patients. IV acyclovir therapy produced little clinical improvement in several infants with congenital CMV infection.

Oral acyclovir has been used for the prevention of CMV disease in organ transplant recipients† considered at risk for the disease. There are conflicting data concerning the effectiveness of the drug for this use, however, and further study is necessary. There is some evidence that IV acyclovir may be effective for suppression of CMV infections in some immunocompromised patients undergoing bone marrow transplantation. Results of a randomized, double-blind study in bone marrow allograft recipients at risk for developing CMV infection (i.e., CMV-seropositive or -seronegative recipients of bone marrow from a CMV-seropositive donor) indicate that in patients who received acyclovir (IV [given 500 mg/m² 3 times daily beginning 5 days before bone marrow transplantation until 30 days after transplantation] followed by either placebo or oral acyclovir [800 mg 4 times daily for 6 months]) the probability of developing CMV infection and delaying its onset was reduced compared with those receiving oral acyclovir (200-400 mg 4 times daily beginning 5 days before bone marrow transplantation until 30 days after transplantation) followed by placebo. If acute CMV infection developed in patients receiving oral acyclovir followed by placebo, it occurred at a median time of 41 days after transplantation while if the infection developed in patients receiving IV acyclovir followed by placebo or oral acyclovir, it occurred at a median time of 54 or 57 days, respectively. In addition, survival rate appeared to be increased in patients receiving IV acyclovir followed by oral acyclovir therapy, compared with those receiving oral acyclovir followed by placebo. While IV acyclovir also has been used in an attempt to prevent CMV disease in patients undergoing autologous bone marrow transplantation†, the drug does not appear to be effective for this use. In one retrospective study in CMV-seropositive autologous bone marrow recipients, patients who received IV acyclovir (500 mg/m² every 8 hours beginning 5 days before transplantation and continued to day 30) did not have a lower incidence of CMV disease and CMV pneumonia during the first 200 days after transplantation than a control group of CMV-seropositive autograft recipients who did not receive the drug.

There is some evidence that high-dose, oral acyclovir therapy may decrease the incidence of CMV disease in certain renal transplant patients, and results of one study indicate that the drug may decrease the incidence of CMV infection in some liver transplant patients. Although some clinicians recommend use of high-dose, oral acyclovir in renal transplant patients, there is little evidence to date that use of oral acyclovir (with or without concomitant immune globulin IV) is associated with a clinically important effect on CMV infection or disease in patients undergoing heart, lung, liver, or kidney transplantation who are considered at risk. In one randomized study in patients undergoing liver transplantation, acyclovir (10 mg/kg IV every 8 hours from day 1 after transplantation until discharge, then 800 mg orally 4 times daily until day 100) was less effective than ganciclovir (6 mg/kg daily IV from day 1–30 after transplantation, then 6 mg/kg daily 5 days weekly until day 100) in preventing CMV disease in these patients. During the first 120 days after the procedure, CMV infections occurred in 38% of those receiving acyclovir and in only 5% of those receiving ganciclovir.

Acyclovir is not effective in preventing CMV disease in HIV-infected individuals, and the drug is not recommended for this use in such patients.

Acyclovir is not effective in preventing CMV disease in hematopoietic stem cell transplant (HSCT) recipients, and the drug is not recommended for this use in such patients. Ganciclovir is the drug of choice for this indication.

● Epstein-Barr Virus Infections and Disorders

Because acyclovir exhibits in vitro activity against Epstein-Barr virus (EBV), the drug has been used in the treatment of uncomplicated or complicated infectious mononucleosis, chronic infectious mononucleosis, and various disorders (e.g., oral hairy leukoplakia) associated with EBV infections†. While the role of acyclovir in EBV infections remains to be more fully elucidated, current evidence suggests that efficacy of the drug is variable and probably depends on the linear or circular state of EBV DNA, clonality of EBV-infected cells, immune responsiveness of the host, and role of ongoing EBV replication in the pathophysiology of the infection.

Although high-dose oral acyclovir or IV acyclovir has transiently inhibited oropharyngeal shedding of EBV in patients with uncomplicated or complicated infectious mononucleosis, therapy with the drug generally has had little clinical benefit in immunocompetent patients with signs and symptoms of infectious mononucleosis† or in immunocompromised patients with EBV infections†. There are some reports that IV acyclovir may decrease fever and interstitial pneumonitis and improve lymphocyte CD4⁺/CD8⁺ ratio in patients with chronic infectious mononucleosis; however, these effects do not occur in all patients who receive the drug.

In a limited number of HIV-infected patients, oral acyclovir therapy was effective in producing clinical regression of oral hairy leukoplakia† (apparently caused by EBV), which recurred following discontinuance of the drug; leukoplakia in patients with acquired immunodeficiency syndrome (AIDS) appeared to be less responsive than in patients whose HIV infection had not progressed to this stage. Some clinicians suggest that, because oral hairy leukoplakia is benign and usually asymptomatic, it may not require treatment. If treatment is required, topical therapy (e.g., topical trichloracetic acid, glycolic acid, podophyllum resin) may be effective; oral acyclovir can be used in severe cases. However, all of these should be considered palliative since the condition recurs when treatment is discontinued. While there is some evidence that oral acyclovir may suppress oral hairy leukoplakia†, the benefit of prolonged suppressive therapy with acyclovir is questionable because such use could promote emergence of acyclovir-resistant HSV in HIV-infected patients.

Acyclovir appeared to produce a beneficial response in several patients with an atypical EBV-associated syndrome manifested as fever, interstitial pneumonitis, pancytopenia, and extremely high titers of antibody to replicative antigens of EBV. IV acyclovir has been reported to be effective in some renal allograft recipients for the treatment of the early stages of posttransplant EBV-associated polyclonal B-cell lymphoproliferative disorders†; however, the drug does not appear to be effective once the tumor progresses into monoclonal lymphoma.

Because Epstein-Barr virus (EBV) has been suggested as a cause of chronic fatigue syndrome (chronic Epstein-Barr virus syndrome), acyclovir has been used in a limited number of patients for the treatment of this condition. However, in a placebo-controlled study in adults with chronic (average duration of 6.8 years), debilitating fatigue, oral acyclovir therapy (3.2 g daily for 30 days) was no more effective than placebo in ameliorating symptoms of the syndrome and there was no correlation between clinical improvement and reduction in EBV antibody levels.

DOSAGE AND ADMINISTRATION

● Reconstitution and Administration

Acyclovir is administered orally and acyclovir sodium is administered by slow IV infusion at a constant rate over at least 1 hour. Acyclovir sodium should *not* be administered by rapid IV infusion (over less than 10 minutes) or rapid IV injection. (See Cautions: Renal Effects.) Acyclovir sodium also should *not* be administered orally or by IM or subcutaneous injection and should *not* be applied topically or to the eye.

Oral Administration

Food does not appear to affect oral absorption of acyclovir, and the drug may be administered without regard to meals.

For oral administration, acyclovir is commercially available as capsules, tablets, or an oral suspension. The commercially available capsules and oral suspension are bioequivalent; in addition, one commercially available 800-mg tablet of acyclovir is bioequivalent to four 200-mg capsules of the drug.

IV Infusion

Prior to IV infusion, commercially available acyclovir sodium powder for injection must be reconstituted and then diluted with a compatible IV solution or the commercially available acyclovir sodium concentrate for injection containing acyclovir 50 mg/mL must be diluted with a compatible IV solution. Infusion concentrations of 7 mg/mL or lower are recommended.

Acyclovir sodium powder for injection is reconstituted by adding 10 or 20 mL of sterile water for injection to a vial labeled as containing 500 mg or 1 g of acyclovir, respectively, to provide a solution containing 50 mg/mL. For use in most patients, the appropriate dose of reconstituted solution should then be withdrawn from the vial and diluted with 50–125 mL of a compatible IV infusion solution. (See Chemistry and Stability: Stability.) Before withdrawing the dose of acyclovir, the vial containing the reconstituted solution should be shaken well to ensure complete dissolution of the drug. For use in fluid-restricted patients, the appropriate dose of reconstituted solution can be diluted in a ratio of about 1 part reconstituted solution of acyclovir to 9 parts infusion solution; however, because of the risk of adverse effects (e.g., phlebitis), concentrations of the infusion generally should not exceed 7 mg/mL. In addition, higher concentrations (e.g., 10 mg/mL) may produce phlebitis or inflammation at the infusion site if inadvertent extravasation occurs. Reconstituted acyclovir sodium solutions should be used within 12 hours and reconstituted solutions that have been further diluted in a compatible infusion solution should be used within 24 hours. (See Chemistry and Stability: Stability.)

Rate of Administration

Acyclovir sodium solutions generally should be given by IV infusion at a constant rate over a 1-hour period. Because of the risk of adverse renal effects (see Cautions: Renal Effects), diluted solutions of acyclovir *should not be infused over a period less than 1 hour.*

● *Oral Dosage*

Mucocutaneous, Ocular, and Systemic Herpes Simplex Virus Infections

Treatment of Mucocutaneous HSV Infections

When oral acyclovir is used for the *treatment* of mucocutaneous HSV infections in immunocompromised adults†, including those infected with human immunodeficiency virus (HIV), some clinicians recommend a dosage of 400 mg every 4 hours while awake (5 times daily) for 7–14 days. For the treatment of these infections in immunocompromised children†, the American Academy of Pediatrics (AAP) recommends an oral dosage of 1 g daily given in 3–5 divided doses for 7–14 days.

For the treatment of orolabial HSV infections in HIV-infected adults, the US Centers for Disease Control and Prevention (CDC) recommends an oral acyclovir dosage of 400 mg 3 times daily for 7–14 days. For the treatment of mild symptomatic HSV gingivostomatitis† in HIV-infected children, CDC recommends a dosage of 20 mg/kg (up to 400 mg) 3 times daily for 7–14 days. A dosage of 15 mg/kg (up to 200 mg) 5 times daily for 7 days has been used for the treatment of HSV gingivostomatitis† in immunocompetent children 1–6 years of age.

Chronic Suppressive and Maintenance Prophylaxis of HSV

When oral acyclovir is used for chronic suppressive or maintenance *prophylaxis* (secondary prophylaxis) of HSV† in HIV-infected adults or adolescents who have frequent or severe recurrences of HSV disease, a dosage of 200 mg 3 times daily or 400 mg twice daily has been recommended by the Prevention of Opportunistic Infections Working Group of the US Public Health Service and the Infectious Diseases Society of America (USPHS/IDSA).

The USPHS/IDSA recommends that HIV-infected infants and children who have frequent or severe recurrences of HSV receive oral acyclovir in a dosage of 80 mg/kg daily given in 3 or 4 divided doses for suppressive therapy.

Ocular HSV Infections

For the treatment of HSV keratitis† in HIV-infected patients, oral acyclovir has been given in a dosage of 400 mg 5 times daily; long-term antiviral therapy may be necessary to prevent recurrent ocular HSV disease in these patients. For the prevention of recurrent ocular HSV disease† in immunocompetent adults and

children 12 years of age or older, oral acyclovir has been given in a dosage of 400 mg twice daily for 12–18 months. For prevention of recurrent ocular HSV disease† following penetrating keratoplasty for herpetic eye disease, oral acyclovir has been given in a dosage of 400 mg twice daily for 6 months. Optimum duration of prophylaxis remains to be determined.

Hematopoietic Stem Cell Transplant Recipients

When oral acyclovir is used for the prevention of recurrent HSV disease† in HSV-seropositive adults and adolescents undergoing hematopoietic stem cell transplantation (HSCT), some clinicians recommend an acyclovir dosage of 200 mg 3 times daily. For HSV-seropositive children, clinicians recommend an oral acyclovir dosage of 0.6–1 g daily given in 3–5 divided doses.

Acyclovir therapy is initiated at the beginning of the conditioning regimen and continued until engraftment occurs or mucositis resolves (i.e., approximately 30 days after HSCT). Routine prophylaxis for longer than 30 days is not recommended.

Genital Herpes

Treatment of Initial Episodes in Immunocompetent Individuals

For the treatment of initial episodes of genital herpes in immunocompetent individuals, the dosage of oral acyclovir recommended by the manufacturer is 200 mg every 4 hours while awake (5 times daily) for 10 days. The CDC and other clinicians state that the usual dosage of oral acyclovir for the treatment of initial genital herpes in immunocompetent adults or adolescents is 400 mg 3 times daily or 200 mg 5 times daily given for 7–10 days. The CDC states that the duration of therapy may be extended if healing is incomplete after 10 days.

For the treatment of initial episodes of genital herpes in immunocompetent children, the AAP recommends a dosage of 40–80 mg/kg daily (maximum 1 g daily) given in 3 or 4 divided doses for 5–10 days.

If acyclovir is used for the treatment of initial episodes of herpes proctitis† in adults, an oral acyclovir dosage of 400 mg 5 times daily for 10 days or until clinical resolution occurs has been used. Alternatively, some clinicians recommend an oral dosage of 800 mg every 8 hours for 7–10 days for the treatment of initial episodes of herpes proctitis.

Episodic Treatment of Recurrent Episodes

For the episodic treatment of recurrent genital herpes in immunocompetent adults, the manufacturer recommends a dosage of 200 mg every 4 hours while awake (5 times daily) for 5 days. The CDC states that the usual dosage of oral acyclovir for the episodic treatment of recurrent genital herpes in immunocompetent adults and adolescents is 400 mg 3 times daily for 5 days, 800 mg twice daily for 5 days, or 800 mg 3 times daily for 2 days.

In HIV-infected adults and children, the CDC recommends a dosage of 400 mg 3 times daily given for 5–10 days for episodic treatment of recurrent episodes; alternatively, acyclovir can be given for 7–14 days. Acyclovir should be initiated at the earliest prodromal sign or symptom of recurrence or within 1 day of the onset of lesions.

Chronic Suppressive Therapy of Recurrent Episodes

For chronic suppressive therapy of recurrent episodes of genital herpes in immunocompetent adults and adolescents, the usual dosage of oral acyclovir is 400 mg orally twice daily. Alternatively, the manufacturer states that dosages of 200 mg orally 3–5 times daily have been be used.

In HIV-infected adults and adolescents, the CDC recommends a dosage of 400–800 mg 2- or 3-times daily for chronic suppressive therapy of recurrent genital herpes. Oral acyclovir has been used for chronic suppressive therapy for up to 5–6 years; however, the manufacturer and CDC recommend that suppressive antiviral therapy be discontinued periodically (e.g., once yearly) to assess the need for continued therapy.

Varicella-Zoster Infections

Varicella (Chickenpox)

For the treatment of varicella (chickenpox) in immunocompetent adults and children 2 years of age and older, the recommended oral dosage of acyclovir is 20 mg/kg (maximum 800 mg per dose) 4 times daily for 5 days. The manufacturer recommends that adults and children who weigh more than 40 kg receive 800 mg orally 4 times daily for 5 days and that children 2 years of age and older weighing 40 kg or less receive 20 mg/kg 4 times daily (maximum daily dosage 80 mg/kg) for 5 days. While lower dosages of oral acyclovir also have been used in immunocompetent children with varicella, some evidence indicates that such dosages may be less effective than the currently recommended dosage. Although the manufacturer states that safety and efficacy of oral acyclovir have not been adequately studied for children younger than 2 years of age, the AAP states that certain children older than 12 months of age† may receive the currently recommended oral dosage of the drug but that data are insufficient to make a recommendation for children 12 months of age or younger. For HIV-infected children with mild immunosuppression and mild varicella, CDC recommends oral acyclovir 20 mg/kg (maximum 800 mg per dose) 4 times daily for 7 days or until no new lesions appear for 48 hours.

If oral acyclovir is used for the treatment of varicella, the drug must be initiated at the earliest sign or symptom of infection. Oral acyclovir offers maximum benefit when initiated as soon as possible after the first manifestation of chickenpox appears; little if any benefit is apparent if treatment is delayed (e.g., for 48 hours after onset of rash). AAP recommends that oral acyclovir therapy be initiated within the first 24 hours after the onset of rash.

Herpes Zoster (Shingles, Zoster)

For the treatment of acute herpes zoster (shingles, zoster) in immunocompetent adults and children 12 years of age or older, the recommended oral dosage of acyclovir is 800 mg every 4 hours 5 times daily (4 g daily) for 5–10 days, preferably initiated within 48 hours of rash onset. Acyclovir also has been used for longer periods (e.g., for 21 days) in the management of acute herpes zoster in immunocompetent patients.

For HIV-infected children with mild immunosuppression and mild zoster, CDC recommends oral acyclovir 20 mg/kg (maximum 800 mg per dose) 4 times daily for 7–10 days.

For the treatment of acute herpes zoster ophthalmicus† in immunocompetent adults, an acyclovir oral dosage of 600 mg every 4 hours 5 times daily (3 g daily) for 10 days, preferably initiated within 72 hours but no later than 7 days of rash onset, has been used.

For the treatment of dermatomal herpes zoster in immunocompromised patients†, including transplant recipients or HIV-infected adults, acyclovir has been given in a dosage of 800 mg orally 5 times daily for 10 days.

● IV Dosage

Dosage of acyclovir sodium is expressed in terms of acyclovir. The manufacturer states that the maximum dosage of IV acyclovir is 20 mg/kg every 8 hours. The manufacturer recommends that obese patients receive IV acyclovir dosages based on ideal body weight.

Mucocutaneous and Systemic Herpes Simplex Virus Infections
Treatment of Mucocutaneous HSV Infections

For the treatment of mucocutaneous HSV infections in immunocompromised patients, including HIV-infected individuals, the usual IV dosage of acyclovir for adults and children 12 years of age or older with normal renal function (i.e., creatinine clearance greater than 50 mL/minute per 1.73 m²) is 5 mg/kg every 8 hours (15 mg/kg daily) for 7–14 days; in children younger than 12 years of age, the recommended dosage is 10 mg/kg every 8 hours for 7–14 days.

For the treatment of moderate to severe symptomatic HSV gingivostomatitis† in HIV-infected children, CDC recommends an IV acyclovir dosage of 5–10 mg/kg 3 times daily for 7–14 days.

Treatment of HSV Encephalitis

For the treatment of HSV encephalitis, the recommended IV dosage of acyclovir for adults and children 12 years of age or older is 10–15 mg/kg every 8 hours. In children between 3 months and 12 years of age, the recommended IV dosage is 20 mg/kg every 8 hours. The manufacturer recommends 10 days of IV acyclovir therapy for the treatment of HSV encephalitis; however, because relapses have been reported after only 10 days' treatment, some clinicians recommend a longer duration of parenteral treatment (e.g., 14–21 days).

Treatment of Neonatal HSV Infection

For the treatment of neonatal HSV infection in infants from birth to 3 months of age, the manufacturer recommends an IV acyclovir dosage of 10 mg/kg every 8 hours for 10 days. The AAP and other clinicians recommend an IV acyclovir

dosage of 20 mg/kg every 8 hours for 14–21 days; however, the manufacturer states that safety and efficacy of doses greater than 10 mg/kg for the treatment of neonatal HSV infection have not been established. The AAP states that IV acyclovir should be given for 14 days if disease is limited to the skin, eye, and mouth or for 21 days if disease is disseminated or involves the CNS.

Hematopoietic Stem Cell Transplant Recipients

For the prevention of recurrent HSV disease† in HSV-seropositive adults and adolescents undergoing hematopoietic stem cell transplantation (HSCT), some clinicians recommend an IV acyclovir dosage of 250 mg/m² every 12 hours. For HSV-seropositive children, some clinicians recommend an IV acyclovir dosage of 250 mg/m² every 8 hours or 125 mg/m² every 6 hours. Therapy can be switched to oral acyclovir when appropriate. Acyclovir therapy is initiated at the beginning of the conditioning regimen and continued until engraftment occurs or mucositis resolves (i.e., approximately 30 days after HSCT). Routine prophylaxis for longer than 30 days is not recommended.

Genital Herpes

For the treatment of severe first episodes of genital herpes, the usual IV dosage of acyclovir for immunocompetent adults and children 12 years of age and older is 5–10 mg/kg every 8 hours. The manufacturer and some clinicians states that IV acyclovir should be given for 5–7 days; the CDC states that IV acyclovir should be given for 2–7 days or until clinical improvement occurs and then an oral antiviral agent should be substituted to complete at least 10 days of therapy.

Varicella-Zoster Infections

For the treatment of varicella (chickenpox) or herpes zoster (shingles, zoster) in immunocompromised adults and children 12 years of age and older with normal renal function, the manufacturer recommends an IV dosage of acyclovir of 10 mg/kg every 8 hours for 7 days. In children younger than 12 years of age, the manufacturer recommends an IV acyclovir dosage of 20 mg/kg every 8 hours for 7 days.

For the treatment of varicella in HIV-infected adults, CDC recommends an IV dosage of 10 mg/kg every 8 hours for 7–10 days. Therapy can be switched to oral acyclovir (800 mg 4 times daily) after defervescence if there is no evidence of visceral involvement.

For the treatment of varicella in immunocompetent children 2 years of age or older, AAP recommends an IV acyclovir dosage of 30 mg/kg daily in divided doses or 500 mg/m² every 8 hours for 7–10 days. For the treatment of varicella in immunocompromised children younger than 1 year of age, AAP and others recommend an IV acyclovir dosage of 10 mg/kg every 8 hours for 7–10 days. For immunocompromised children 1 year of age and older, AAP recommends 500 mg/m² every 8 hours for 7–10 days; other experts recommend 30 mg/kg daily in divided doses.

For the treatment of herpes zoster in immunocompromised children younger than 12 years of age, AAP recommends an IV acyclovir dosage of 20 mg/kg every 8 hours for 7–10 days. For immunocompromised children 12 years of age or older, AAP recommends an IV acyclovir dosage of 10 mg/kg every 8 hours for 7 days. For the treatment of herpes zoster in immunocompetent children younger than 1 year of age, AAP recommends an IV acyclovir dosage of 10 mg/kg every 8 hours for 7–10 days. For immunocompetent children 1 year of age and older, AAP recommends 500 mg/m² every 8 hours for 7–10 days; other experts recommend 30 mg/kg daily in divided doses.

For the treatment of extensive multidermatomal zoster or zoster with trigeminal nerve involvement in HIV-infected children with severe immunosuppression, CDC recommends an IV acyclovir dosage of 10 mg/kg 3 times daily for 7–10 days.

● Dosage in Renal Impairment

In patients with impaired renal function, doses and/or frequency of administration of acyclovir must be modified in response to the degree of impairment. Generally, the decrease in total body clearance of acyclovir is directly related to the decrease in body-surface-area-corrected creatinine clearance; however, clearance of acyclovir is usually greater than predicted from creatinine clearance, since the drug undergoes some renal tubular secretion.

Oral Dosage

Based on pharmacokinetic studies of IV acyclovir in patients with renal impairment, the manufacturer recommends the following oral dosage of acyclovir based on the usual dosage regimen and the patient's creatinine clearance (see Table 1):

TABLE 1. Oral Dosage Adjustment in Patients with Renal Impairment

Usual Dosage Regimen	Creatinine Clearance (mL/min per 1.73 m²)	Adjusted Dosage Regimen
200 mg every 4 h 5 times daily	>10	No adjustment necessary
	0–10	200 mg every 12 h
400 mg every 12 h	>10	No adjustment necessary
	0–10	200 mg every 12 h
800 mg every 4 h 5 times daily	>25	No adjustment necessary
	10–25	800 mg every 8 h
	0–10	800 mg every 12 h

Because acyclovir is removed by hemodialysis, the manufacturer recommends that patients undergoing hemodialysis receive a supplemental oral dose of the drug immediately after each dialysis period. The manufacturer states that supplemental doses of oral acyclovir do not appear to be necessary following peritoneal dialysis.

For HIV-infected patients with impaired renal function, the following oral dosages of acyclovir have been suggested based on a usual dosage regimen of 200–800 mg every 4–6 hours and the patient's creatinine clearance (see Table 2):

TABLE 2. Oral Dosage Adjustment in HIV-Infected Patients with Impaired Renal Function

Creatinine Clearance (mL/min per 1.73 m²)	Adjusted Dosage Regimen
>80	No adjustment necessary
50–80	200–800 mg every 6–8 h
25–50	200–800 mg every 8–12 h
10–25	200–800 mg every 12–24 h
<10	200–400 mg every 24 h
Hemodialysis	supplement usual dose after each hemodialysis

Parenteral Dosage

The manufacturer recommends the following IV dosage of acyclovir based on the patient's creatinine clearance (see Table 3):

TABLE 3. IV Dosage Adjustment in Patients with Renal Impairment

Creatinine Clearance (mL/min per 1.73 m²)	Percent of Recommended Dose	Dosing Interval (hours)
>50	100%	8
25–50	100%	12
10–25	100%	24
0–10	50%	24

The manufacturer states that patients undergoing hemodialysis may require a supplemental acyclovir dose after each dialysis period. The patient's dosing schedule should be adjusted so that an additional dose is administered after each

dialysis. Alternatively in patients undergoing hemodialysis, some clinicians recommend that 2.5 mg/kg be administered every 24 hours and that an additional 2.5-mg/kg dose be administered after each dialysis period.

Other IV acyclovir dosage regimens have been suggested for patients with end-stage renal disease. In one regimen, an initial loading dose of 93–185 mg/m², a maintenance dosage of 35–70 mg/m² every 8 hours, and a dose of 56–185 mg/m² immediately after dialysis have been used. Alternatively, an initial loading dose of 250–500 mg/m², a maintenance dosage of 250–500 mg/m² every 48 hours, and a dose of 150–500 mg/m² immediately after dialysis have been suggested.

Because acyclovir is removed by continuous ambulatory peritoneal dialysis (CAPD) to a lesser extent than by hemodialysis, the manufacturer states that supplemental doses of acyclovir do not appear to be necessary following CAPD.

For HIV-infected patients with impaired renal function, the following IV dosages of acyclovir have been suggested based on a usual dosage regimen of 5 mg/kg every 8 hours and the patient's creatinine clearance:

TABLE 4. IV Dosage Adjustment in HIV-Infected Patients with Impaired Renal Function

Creatinine Clearance (mL/min per 1.73 m²)	Adjusted Dosage Regimen
greater than 80	No adjustment necessary
50–80	No adjustment necessary
25–50	5 mg/kg every 12–24 hours
10–25	5 mg/kg every 12–24 hours
less than 10	2.5 mg/kg every 24 hours
Hemodialysis	administer usual dose after hemodialysis

CAUTIONS

Adverse reactions generally have been minimal following oral or IV administration of acyclovir. However, potentially serious reactions (e.g., renal failure, thrombotic thrombocytopenic purpura/hemolytic uremic syndrome) can occur and fatalities have been reported.

● Local Effects

The most frequent adverse effects of IV acyclovir are local reactions at the injection site. Inflammation or phlebitis has been reported in approximately 9% of patients. Severe local inflammatory reactions, including tissue necrosis, have occurred following infusion of acyclovir into extravascular tissues.

● Renal Effects

Increased BUN and/or serum creatinine concentrations, anuria, and hematuria have been reported in patients receiving acyclovir. Abnormal urinalysis (characterized by an increase in formed elements in urine sediment) and pain or pressure on urination have been reported rarely with IV acyclovir.

Transient increases in BUN and/or serum creatinine concentrations and decreases in creatinine clearance occur in about 5–10% of patients receiving IV acyclovir, and have been reported most frequently when the drug was administered by rapid (over less than 10 minutes) IV infusion rather than over the recommended period for IV infusion (at least 1 hour).

Renal failure, resulting in death in some patients, has occurred in patients receiving acyclovir. The risk of adverse renal effects during IV acyclovir therapy depends on the patient's degree of hydration, urine output, concomitant therapy (i.e., other nephrotoxic drugs), preexisting renal disease, and the rate of administration of acyclovir. Precipitation of the drug in the renal tubules can occur when the solubility of free acyclovir in the collecting duct is exceeded or following rapid IV administration of the drug; ensuing renal tubular damage may result in acute renal failure. In some cases, alterations in renal function during IV acyclovir therapy progress to acute renal failure; however, in most cases, alterations in renal function are transient and resolve spontaneously or following improved hydration and electrolyte balance, dosage adjustment, or discontinuance of the drug.

● Nervous System Effects

Headache is one of the most common nervous system adverse effects of oral acyclovir, occurring in about 2% of patients receiving the drug as chronic suppressive therapy. Aggressive behavior, agitation, ataxia, coma, confusion, decreased consciousness, delirium, dizziness, encephalopathy, hallucinations, obtundation, paresthesia, psychosis, seizures, somnolence, and tremors have been reported during oral or IV acyclovir therapy and these effects may be marked, particularly in older adults or patients with renal impairment. In patients receiving oral acyclovir for the treatment of herpes zoster (shingles, zoster), malaise was reported in 11.5% of patients receiving the drug and 11.1% of those receiving placebo.

Encephalopathic effects including lethargy, obtundation, tremors, confusion, hallucinations, agitation, seizures, and coma have occurred in approximately 1% of patients receiving IV acyclovir. Agitation, delirium, diaphoresis, dizziness, headache, lightheadedness, somnolence, and psychosis have occurred rarely. Coarse tremor and clonus developed in at least one immunocompromised patient during IV acyclovir therapy. Cerebral edema, coma, and death, probably resulting from cerebral anoxia, occurred during IV acyclovir therapy in an immunocompromised bone marrow transplant patient with pneumonitis.

● GI Effects

Nausea, vomiting, and diarrhea are among the most common adverse effects of oral acyclovir. In a study in patients receiving oral acyclovir for treatment of recurrent genital herpes, nausea occurred in about 5% and diarrhea in about 2% of patients receiving the drug for chronic suppressive therapy and these adverse GI effects occurred in 2.4–2.7% of those receiving episodic treatment of recurrences. In patients receiving oral acyclovir for the treatment of initial episodes of genital herpes, nausea and/or vomiting occurred in 2.7%. Diarrhea was reported in 3.2% of patients receiving the drug for the treatment of varicella (chickenpox). GI distress also has been reported in patients receiving oral acyclovir.

Nausea and/or vomiting have been reported in about 7% of patients receiving IV acyclovir therapy (mainly occurring in nonhospitalized patients receiving acyclovir dosages of 10 mg/kg 3 times daily). Anorexia, diarrhea, and GI distress also have been reported with IV acyclovir.

● Hematologic Effects

Anemia, leukocytoclastic vasculitis, leukopenia, lymphadenopathy, and thrombocytopenia have been reported in patients receiving oral acyclovir.

Anemia, disseminated intravascular coagulation, hemoglobinemia, hemolysis, leukocytoclastic vasculitis, leukocytosis, leukopenia, lymphadenopathy, neutropenia, neutrophilia, thrombocytopenia, and thrombocytosis have been reported rarely in patients receiving IV acyclovir.

● Dermatologic and Sensitivity Reactions

Rash, pruritus, or urticaria occasionally occurs during oral or IV acyclovir therapy. Alopecia and angioedema have been reported. At least one case of erythematous rash and vasculitis has been reported following administration of IV acyclovir to an immunocompromised patient exposed to chickenpox; however, this reaction has not been directly attributed to the drug.

Anaphylaxis has been reported rarely in patients receiving oral or IV acyclovir. Stevens-Johnson syndrome, erythema multiforme, photosensitivity rash, and toxic epidermal necrolysis have occurred rarely in patients receiving acyclovir.

● Other Adverse Effects

Fever and pain have been reported in patients receiving oral or IV acyclovir. Elevated liver function test results, hepatitis, hyperbilirubinemia, jaundice, hypotension, myalgia, peripheral edema, thirst, and visual abnormalities have been reported rarely in patients receiving oral or IV acyclovir.

● Precautions and Contraindications

Oral and IV acyclovir are contraindicated in patients who develop hypersensitivity to acyclovir or valacyclovir.

Patients receiving acyclovir for the treatment of genital herpes should be advised that the drug is not a cure for genital herpes and that, because genital herpes is a sexually transmitted disease, they should avoid sexual contact while visible lesions are present since there is a risk of infecting their sexual partner. (See Patient Counseling and Management of Sexual Partners under Uses: Genital

Herpes.) If acyclovir is used for chronic suppressive therapy of genital herpes, the drug should be discontinued after 1 year of therapy so that the frequency and severity of the patient's genital herpes infection can be reevaluated to determine the need for continuing acyclovir therapy. Oral acyclovir has been used for suppressive therapy of genital herpes in immunocompetent adults for up to 5–6 years without evidence of long-term adverse effects.

All patients receiving oral acyclovir should be instructed to consult their clinician if severe or troublesome adverse effects occur during acyclovir therapy. Female patients receiving the drug should be instructed to consult their physician if they become pregnant or intend to become pregnant or if they intend to breastfeed. (See Cautions: Pregnancy, Fertility, and Lactation.)

The manufacturer states that the recommended dosage and duration of acyclovir therapy should not be exceeded. The manufacturer also cautions that both the dose and dosage interval should be carefully adjusted in patients with renal failure or in patients undergoing hemodialysis to prevent drug accumulation, decrease the risk of toxicity, and maintain adequate plasma concentrations of acyclovir. The manufacturer states that when dosage adjustment is required, they should be based on estimated creatinine clearance. (See Dosage and Administration: Dosage in Renal Impairment.)

Acyclovir should be used with caution in patients receiving other nephrotoxic drugs concurrently since the risk of acyclovir-induced renal impairment and/or reversible CNS symptoms is increased in these patients. Adequate hydration should be maintained in patients receiving acyclovir; however, in patients with encephalitis, the recommended hydration should be balanced by the risk of cerebral edema. Because the risk of acyclovir-induced renal impairment is increased during rapid IV administration of the drug, acyclovir should be given only by slow IV infusion (over at least 1 hour).

Parenteral acyclovir therapy can cause signs and symptoms of encephalopathy. (See Cautions: Nervous System Effects.) The manufacturer states that acyclovir should be used with caution in patients with underlying neurologic abnormalities and in patients with serious renal, hepatic, or electrolyte abnormalities or substantial hypoxia. The drug also should be used with caution in patients who have manifested prior neurologic reactions to cytotoxic drugs or those receiving intrathecal methotrexate or interferon.

● Pediatric Precautions

The manufacturer states that safety and efficacy of *oral* acyclovir in children younger than 2 years of age have not been established.

● Geriatric Precautions

In a clinical study evaluating use of oral acyclovir for the treatment of herpes zoster (shingles, zoster) in immunocompetent adults 50 years of age or older, approximately 65% of patients were 65 years of age or older and more than 30% were 75 years of age or older. There was no overall difference in effectiveness for time to cessation of new lesion formation or time to healing between geriatric patients and younger adults. However, the duration of pain after healing was longer in those 65 years of age and older and nausea, vomiting, and dizziness were reported more frequently in geriatric patients. Clinical studies evaluating IV acyclovir have not included sufficient numbers of patients 65 years of age or older to determine whether they respond differently than younger patients.

Geriatric patients are more likely than younger adults to have adverse CNS effects (e.g., coma, confusion, hallucinations, somnolence) during acyclovir therapy. Geriatric patients also are more likely to have adverse renal effects during acyclovir therapy and to have reduced renal function requiring dosage adjustment. Acyclovir dosage should be carefully selected for this age group and it may be useful to monitor renal function.

● Mutagenicity and Carcinogenicity

Mutagenic changes and chromosomal damage have occurred in vitro in human lymphocytes and mouse lymphoma cells at acyclovir concentrations at least 25 times greater than plasma drug concentrations achievable with usual dosage in humans. In other in vitro microbial and mammalian cell assays, no evidence of mutagenicity or inconclusive results were observed. The manufacturer states that acyclovir was tested in 16 in vitro and in vivo genetic toxicity assays and was positive in 5 of these assays.

In lifetime bioassays in rats and mice receiving single daily dosages of up to 450 mg/kg administered by gastric lavage, there was no statistically significant difference in the incidence of tumors between treated and control animals and no evidence that acyclovir shortened the latency of tumors. Maximum plasma concentrations in the mouse or rat bioassay were 3–6 or 1–2 times, respectively, the usual human concentrations (based on steady-state plasma concentrations observed in humans receiving 200 or 800 mg of acyclovir orally 5 times daily).

Evidence of mutagenicity or carcinogenicity in humans has not been reported to date.

● Pregnancy, Fertility, and Lactation

Pregnancy

There are no adequate and controlled studies to date using acyclovir in pregnant women, and the drug should be used during pregnancy only when the potential benefits justify the possible risks to the fetus.

Acyclovir administered during organogenesis was not teratogenic in the mouse (450 mg/kg daily orally), rabbit (50 mg/kg daily subcutaneously or IV), or rat (50 mg/kg daily subcutaneously). These dosages resulted in plasma concentrations that were 106, 11, and 22 times, respectively, the steady-state plasma concentrations observed in humans receiving 200 or 800 mg of acyclovir orally 5 times daily. However, in nonstandard tests in rats, fetal abnormalities (e.g., head and tail anomalies) and maternal toxicity were observed with subcutaneous acyclovir. Acyclovir crosses the placenta in humans and the clinical relevance of these animal findings currently is not known.

IV acyclovir has been used during the second or third trimester of pregnancy without apparent adverse effects to the fetus. The US Centers for Disease Control and Prevention (CDC) state that first clinical episodes of genital herpes occurring during pregnancy may be treated with oral acyclovir and that use of IV acyclovir therapy may be indicated for the treatment of severe maternal HSV infections. Preliminary data suggest that acyclovir treatment late in pregnancy might reduce the frequency of cesarean sections among women who have recurrent genital herpes by diminishing the frequency of recurrences at term. The risk for HSV is high in infants born to women who acquired genital herpes in late pregnancy, and such women should be managed in consultation with an HSV specialist. Some experts recommend acyclovir therapy in this circumstance, some recommend routine cesarean section to reduce the risk for neonatal HSV, and others recommend both. (See Pregnant Women under Uses: Genital Herpes.)

Many clinicians do not recommend use of oral acyclovir in pregnant adolescents or women with uncomplicated varicella because the risk or benefit to the fetus currently is not known. However, other clinicians recommend use of oral acyclovir for the treatment of varicella in pregnant women, especially during the second and third trimesters. In addition, use of IV acyclovir is recommended in pregnant women with serious complications of varicella such as extensive cutaneous disease, high fever, or systemic symptoms. It is not known whether acyclovir administered to the mother prevents congenital varicella syndrome (i.e., low birthweight, hypotrophic limbs, ocular abnormalities, brain damage, mental retardation) in the neonate.

To monitor fetal outcomes of pregnant women exposed either inadvertently or intentionally to systemic acyclovir, the manufacturer established a prospective registry of acyclovir use during pregnancy and collected data from 1984 to April 1999. A total of 749 pregnancies were followed over this time period involving 756 outcomes, and comparison of registry data with birth defect surveillance data revealed no evidence of an increased risk for birth defects in infants of mothers treated with acyclovir during the first trimester of pregnancy. However, the sample size of the registry is insufficient to evaluate the risk for less common defects or to permit reliable or definitive conclusions regarding the safety of acyclovir in pregnant women and their developing fetuses.

Fertility

Reproduction studies using oral acyclovir dosages of 450 mg/kg daily in mice and subcutaneous dosages of 25 mg/kg daily in rats have not revealed evidence of impaired fertility. Following subcutaneous dosages of 50 mg/kg daily in rats and rabbits, a decrease in implantation efficiency was observed; decreases in the numbers of corpora lutea, implantation sites, and live fetuses were observed in rats. No effect on implantation efficiency was observed in rabbits following IV dosages of 50 mg/kg daily. Although no drug-related reproductive effects were observed in rabbits following IV dosages of 50 mg/kg daily, increases in fetal resorptions and corresponding decreases in litter size were observed following IV dosages of 100 mg/kg daily. Following intraperitoneal acyclovir dosages of 320 or 80 mg/kg daily in male rats for 1 or 6 months, respectively, testicular atrophy was observed; some evidence of recovery of sperm production was apparent 30 days after discontinuance of the drug. Aspermatogenesis was observed in dogs following IV dosages of

100 and 200 mg/kg daily for 31 days. No adverse testicular effects were observed in dogs given IV dosages of 50 mg/kg daily for one month or given 60 mg/kg daily for one year. In a controlled study in men receiving chronic oral acyclovir (400 mg or 1 g daily) therapy, there was no evidence of clinically important effects on sperm count, motility, or morphology during 6 months of therapy and 3 months of posttreatment follow-up.

Lactation

Limited data indicate that acyclovir is distributed into milk, generally in concentrations greater than concurrent maternal plasma concentrations, and can be absorbed by nursing infants. Acyclovir should be administered to nursing women with caution and only when indicated.

DRUG INTERACTIONS

● Antifungal Agents

Amphotericin B has been shown to potentiate the antiviral effect of acyclovir against pseudorabies virus in vitro when both drugs are added to the culture medium. Ketoconazole and acyclovir have shown dose-dependent, synergistic, antiviral activity against herpes simplex virus types 1 and 2 (HSV-1 and -2) in in vitro replication studies. The clinical importance of these interactions has not been established, and additional study is necessary to determine potential antiviral synergy between these antifungal agents and acyclovir.

● Probenecid

Concomitant administration of probenecid and acyclovir has reportedly increased the mean plasma half-life and area under the plasma concentration-time curve (AUC) and decreased urinary excretion and renal clearance of acyclovir. In one study following oral administration of a 1-g dose of probenecid 1 hour prior to a 1-hour IV infusion of acyclovir 5 mg/kg, the half-life and AUC for acyclovir increased by 18% and 40%, respectively, and urinary excretion and renal clearance of acyclovir decreased by 13% and 32%, respectively. This interaction may result from competitive inhibition of the renal secretion of acyclovir by probenecid.

● Interferon

The manufacturer states that IV acyclovir should be used with caution in patients receiving interferon. In vitro, when acyclovir and interferon are both added to cultures of herpes simplex virus type 1 (HSV-1), the drugs have an additive or synergistic antiviral effect; however, the clinical importance of this interaction is not known.

● Methotrexate

The manufacturer states that IV acyclovir should be used with caution in patients receiving intrathecal methotrexate.

● Zidovudine

Acyclovir has been used concomitantly with zidovudine in some patients with human immunodeficiency virus (HIV) infections without evidence of increased toxicity; however, neurotoxicity (profound drowsiness and lethargy), which recurred on rechallenge, has been reported in at least one patient with acquired immunodeficiency syndrome (AIDS) during concomitant therapy with the drugs. Neurotoxicity was evident within 30–60 days after initiation of IV acyclovir therapy, persisted with some improvement when acyclovir was administered orally, and resolved following discontinuance of acyclovir in this patient. Because use of acyclovir for the treatment and prevention of opportunistic infections may be necessary in patients receiving zidovudine, such patients should be monitored closely during combined therapy.

ACUTE TOXICITY

Acyclovir overdosage involving ingestion of up to 20 g of the drug have been reported. Overdosage of IV acyclovir has been reported following administration of rapid IV injections or inappropriately high doses and in patients with fluid and electrolyte imbalance, resulting in elevations in BUN and serum creatinine concentration and subsequent renal failure. Other adverse effects reported with acyclovir overdosage include agitation, coma, lethargy, and seizures. At renal concentrations exceeding 2.5 mg/mL, acyclovir crystals may precipitate in the renal tubules, possibly causing renal dysfunction and eventual renal failure and anuria. (See Cautions: Renal Effects.)

If acute renal failure and anuria occur, use of hemodialysis should be considered until renal function is restored. A 6-hour period of hemodialysis may result in a 60% decrease in plasma acyclovir concentrations. Data are limited regarding peritoneal dialysis but this method does not appear to appreciably remove the drug.

MECHANISM OF ACTION

Acyclovir exerts its antiviral effect against herpes simplex viruses (HSV) and varicella-zoster virus by interfering with DNA synthesis and inhibiting viral replication. The exact mechanisms of action against other susceptible viruses have not been fully elucidated.

In cells infected with herpesvirus in vitro, the antiviral activity of acyclovir appears to depend principally on the intracellular conversion of the drug to acyclovir triphosphate. Acyclovir is converted to acyclovir monophosphate principally via virus-coded thymidine kinase (TK); the monophosphate is phosphorylated to the diphosphate via cellular guanylate kinase and then to the triphosphate via other cellular enzymes (e.g., phosphoglycerate kinase, pyruvate kinase, phosphoenolpyruvate carboxykinase). In uninfected cells in vitro, acyclovir is only minimally phosphorylated by cellular (host cell) enzymes. The formation of acyclovir monophosphate appears to be the rate-limiting step in the formation of acyclovir triphosphate. In vitro studies have shown that the extent of formation of acyclovir monophosphate, diphosphate, and triphosphate by both uninfected and virus-infected cells is directly related to the concentration of acyclovir in the culture medium. Acyclovir also is apparently converted to acyclovir triphosphate by other mechanisms since the drug has some activity against several viruses that apparently do not code for viral TK (e.g., Epstein-Barr virus, cytomegalovirus). In vitro studies indicate that acyclovir triphosphate is produced in low concentrations via unidentified cellular phosphorylating enzymes in cells infected with Epstein-Barr virus and cytomegalovirus.

In vitro studies with HSV indicate that acyclovir triphosphate is the pharmacologically active form of the drug; the triphosphate functions as both a substrate for and preferential inhibitor of viral DNA polymerase. In herpesviruses, acyclovir triphosphate inhibits DNA synthesis by competing with deoxyguanosine triphosphate for viral DNA polymerase and incorporation principally into viral DNA. In vitro in herpesviruses, acyclovir can be incorporated into growing chains of DNA via viral DNA polymerase and to a much lesser extent via cellular α-DNA polymerase. Viral DNA polymerase exhibits a 10- to 30-fold or greater affinity in vitro for acyclovir triphosphate than does cellular α-DNA polymerase. Following incorporation of acyclovir triphosphate into the DNA chain, DNA synthesis is terminated. In vitro studies have shown that acyclovir triphosphate also partially inhibits the synthesis of γ-polypeptides within cells that are infected with herpesvirus. Acyclovir has minimal pharmacologic effects in vitro in uninfected cells since uptake of the drug into these cells is poor, phosphorylation of acyclovir and intracellular formation of acyclovir triphosphate are minimal, and cellular α-DNA polymerase has a low affinity for acyclovir triphosphate.

Non-phosphorylated acyclovir, acyclovir monophosphate, and acyclovir diphosphate are thought to have minimal or no effect on viral or cellular α-DNA polymerase and therefore have no antiviral activity.

The antiviral activity of acyclovir against Epstein-Barr virus and cytomegalovirus (CMV) appears to differ from that against HSV. The antiviral activity against Epstein-Barr virus may result from increased sensitivity of its viral DNA polymerase to inhibition by low concentrations of acyclovir triphosphate (formed via cellular phosphorylating enzymes). The antiviral activity against human CMV may result from inhibition of virus-specific polypeptide synthesis; such inhibition requires high concentrations of acyclovir or its triphosphate in vitro. In vitro studies indicate that DNA polymerase of murine CMV is substantially more sensitive to inhibition by acyclovir triphosphate than that of human CMV; this difference in sensitivity appears to correlate with the difference in in vitro susceptibility of murine and human CMV to the drug. Further studies are needed to evaluate the antiviral activity of acyclovir against Epstein-Barr virus and CMV.

SPECTRUM

Following intracellular conversion to a pharmacologically active triphosphate metabolite, acyclovir is active in vitro against various Herpesviridae

including herpes simplex virus types 1 and 2 (HSV-1 and HSV-2), varicella-zoster virus, Epstein-Barr virus, herpesvirus simiae (B virus), and cytomegalovirus (CMV).

● In Vitro Susceptibility Testing

Various methods (e.g., cytopathic effect inhibition, plaque inhibition, dye-uptake, disk-agar diffusion) have been used to test the in vitro susceptibility of viruses to acyclovir. The results and interpretations of these tests are method dependent. Although IDs (inhibitory doses) and EDs (effective doses) of acyclovir for various viruses have been reported, a standardized method for determining these values does not currently exist. In addition, the relationship between in vitro susceptibility of viruses to acyclovir and clinical response has not been determined. In viral susceptibility testing, 1 mcg of acyclovir per mL is approximately equivalent to 4.4 µmol/L.

● Herpesviridae

In several studies using a cytopathic effect inhibition assay (CPE-inhibition assay), the ID_{50} (concentration of drug required to produce 50% inhibition of viral cytopathic effect or plaque formation) of acyclovir reported for susceptible strains of HSV-1 ranged from 0.02–0.7 mcg/mL; in studies using a plaque inhibition assay, the ID_{50} of the drug reported for susceptible HSV-1 was 0.018–0.043 mcg/mL. In several studies using a CPE-inhibition assay, the ID_{50} of acyclovir reported for susceptible strains of HSV-2 ranged from 0.01–3.2 mcg/mL; in studies using a plaque inhibition assay, the ID_{50} of the drug reported for susceptible HSV-2 was 0.027–0.36 mcg/mL. In several studies using a plaque inhibition assay, the ID_{50} of acyclovir for susceptible strains of varicella-zoster ranged from 0.34–1.43 mcg/mL.

In several studies using a cytohybridization assay, the ID_{50} of acyclovir for susceptible strains of Epstein-Barr virus ranged from 1.4–1.6 mcg/mL. In several studies using a plaque inhibition assay, the ID_{50} of acyclovir for susceptible strains of herpes simiae ranged from 5–10 mcg/mL.

Acyclovir is much less active against CMV than against many other Herpesviridae. This may occur because CMV does not produce thymidine kinase (TK) and therefore is less able than other viruses to phosphorylate acyclovir to its pharmacologically active triphosphate derivative. In several studies using a plaque inhibition assay, the ID_{50} of acyclovir for susceptible strains of CMV ranged from 2 to greater than 50 mcg/mL.

Acyclovir is inactive against vaccinia virus, adenovirus type 5, and several RNA viruses. Preliminary data indicate that acyclovir may inhibit replication of hepatitis B virus; however, additional study of the susceptibility of this virus to acyclovir is needed.

RESISTANCE

Resistance to acyclovir in Herpesviridae can result from qualitative and quantitative changes in viral thymidine kinase (TK) and/or DNA polymerase. Since the antiviral activity of acyclovir generally appears to depend on phosphorylation of the drug to acyclovir triphosphate (see Mechanism of Action), resistance to the drug may result from low concentrations or absence of virus-coded TK in infected cells or from alterations in substrate specificity of virus-coded TK. Other mechanisms of resistance to acyclovir may also exist.

Acyclovir resistance in HSV-1 and HSV-2 may result from production of a virus-coded TK with altered substrate specificity or from an impaired ability to produce active virus-coded TK; either of these mechanisms may result in minimal amounts or absence of phosphorylated drug. Resistance to acyclovir in varicella-zoster may result from production of a virus-coded TK or DNA polymerase with altered substrate specificity or from an impaired ability to produce active virus-coded TK or DNA polymerase. The relative resistance of Epstein-Barr virus and cytomegalovirus (CMV) compared with HSV-1 and HSV-2 is thought to result from the inability of Epstein-Barr virus and CMV to code for virus-specific TK. In addition, although cellular TK may be present, its low affinity for acyclovir may result in concentrations of acyclovir triphosphate that are insufficient to effectively inhibit the DNA polymerase of Epstein-Barr virus or CMV. Presence of virus-coded TK is not the only determinant of susceptibility to acyclovir. Cells infected with vaccinia virus produce virus-coded TK, but the enzyme does not phosphorylate acyclovir and the drug does not inhibit replication of the virus. In addition to qualitative or quantitative alterations in virus-coded TK, resistance of herpesviruses to acyclovir may result from production of an altered DNA polymerase capable of synthesizing DNA in the presence of acyclovir triphosphate.

Clinical isolates of HSV or varicella-zoster with reduced susceptibility to acyclovir have been obtained from immunocompromised individuals, especially those with advanced human immunodeficiency virus (HIV) infection. It has been suggested that repeated treatment of recurrent viral infections with acyclovir may favor the selection of preexisting, or development of drug-resistant strains. While most of the acyclovir-resistant mutants isolated from immunocompromised individuals have been found to be TK-deficient, other mutants involving the viral TK gene (TK partial and TK altered) and DNA polymerase have been isolated. TK-negative mutants may cause severe disease in infants and immunocompromised adults, and the possibility of acyclovir resistance should be considered in patients who show poor clinical response to the drug.

Although lack of virus-coded TK is apparently responsible for resistance in some strains of viruses, this lack has also been associated with a loss of or decrease in virulence in some strains. In addition, in one study, inoculation of mice with acyclovir-resistant HSV-1 mutants afforded protection against infection with virulent acyclovir-susceptible HSV-1 strains.

During the course of an acute or asymptomatic herpesvirus infection, the virus usually leaves the initial site of infection and invades other cells and tissues where it establishes a site of latent infection. HSV-1, HSV-2, and varicella-zoster are thought to establish latent infections principally within the ganglia. Animal studies indicate that colonization of sensory neurons by HSV-1 may occur as soon as 24–48 hours after initial infection and latency may develop within 2–3 weeks. Epstein-Barr virus and CMV are thought to establish latent infections within B cells and leukocytes, respectively. The exact nature of the virus during the latent state is not well understood; however, current evidence suggests that the virus is not actively replicating and, therefore, would not be susceptible to the antiviral action of drugs such as acyclovir. Despite the host's immunity, latency usually persists for life and the virus can be periodically reactivated by various stimuli (e.g., fever, stress, trauma, exposure to sunlight, menstruation, sexual intercourse, immunosuppression). Once reactivated, the virus usually reinfects the site(s) of initial infection. Acyclovir is apparently unable to eliminate an established latent infection. Acyclovir-resistant HSV mutants appear to be less capable of establishing latent infections than susceptible strains.

PHARMACOKINETICS

In the studies described in the Pharmacokinetics section involving IV administration of the drug, acyclovir was administered as the sodium salt; dosages and concentrations of the drug are expressed in terms of acyclovir. A concentration of 1 mcg of acyclovir per mL is approximately equivalent to 4.4 µmol/L.

The pharmacokinetics of acyclovir in children generally are similar to that reported in adults.

Acyclovir plasma concentrations are higher in geriatric patients than in younger adults, in part due to age-related changes in renal function.

● Absorption

Oral Administration

Absorption of acyclovir from the GI tract is variable and incomplete. It is estimated that 10–30% of an oral dose of the drug is absorbed. Some data suggest that GI absorption of acyclovir may be saturable; in a crossover study in which acyclovir was administered orally to healthy adults as 200-mg capsules, 400-mg tablets, or 800-mg tablets 6 times daily, the extent of absorption decreased with increasing dose, resulting in bioavailabilities of 20, 15, or 10%, respectively. The manufacturer states that this decrease in bioavailability appears to be a function of increasing dose, not differences in dosage forms. In addition, steady-state peak and trough plasma acyclovir concentrations were not dose proportional over the oral dosing range of 200–800 mg 6 times daily, averaging 0.83 and 0.46, 1.21 and 0.63, or 1.61 and 0.83 mcg/mL for the 200-, 400-, or 800-mg dosing regimens, respectively.

Peak plasma concentrations of acyclovir usually occur within 1.5–2.5 hours after oral administration.

In immunocompromised individuals, steady-state peak and trough plasma acyclovir concentrations averaged 0.49–0.56 and 0.29–0.31 mcg/mL, respectively, following oral administration of 200 mg every 4 hours, 1.2 and 0.62 mcg/mL, respectively, following oral administration of 400 mg every 4 hours, and 2.8 and 1.8 mcg/mL, respectively, following oral administration of 800 mg (as capsules) every 4 hours. In another study in immunocompromised individuals, steady-state

peak and trough plasma acyclovir concentrations averaged 1.4 and 0.55 mcg/mL, respectively, following oral administration of 800 mg (as capsules) every 6 hours.

Food does not appear to affect absorption of acyclovir.

The commercially available capsules and oral suspension are bioequivalent; in addition, one commercially available 800-mg tablet of acyclovir is bioequivalent to four 200-mg capsules of the drug.

IV Infusion

Results of studies in adults with normal renal function receiving single acyclovir doses ranging from 0.5- to 15-mg/kg or multiple doses ranging from 2.5- to 15-mg/kg every 8 hours indicate that plasma concentrations of the drug are dose proportional.

In adults with normal renal function receiving 5 or 10 mg/kg of acyclovir IV over 1 hour every 8 hours, mean steady-state peak plasma concentrations were 9.8 or 22.9 mcg/mL, respectively, and trough plasma concentrations were 0.7 or 1.9 mcg/mL. In a multiple-dose study in adults with malignancies and normal renal and liver function, 1-hour IV infusions of 2.5, 5, 10, or 15 mg/kg of acyclovir every 8 hours resulted in mean steady-state peak serum concentrations of 5.1, 9.8, 20.7, and 23.6 mcg/mL, respectively, and mean steady-state trough serum concentrations of 0.5, 0.7, 2.3, and 2 mcg/mL, respectively.

In several studies in adults with malignancies and normal renal and hepatic function, IV infusion over 1 hour of a single acyclovir dose of 0.5, 1, 2.5, or 5 mg/kg resulted in serum concentrations of the drug that averaged 0.7–1.4, 1.4–2.5, 3.4–4.9, or 7.7 mcg/mL, respectively, at the end of the infusion and 0.14, 0.27, 0.34, or 0.93 mcg/mL, respectively, 6 hours after the end of the infusion.

Serum concentrations in children 3 months to 16 years of age receiving IV acyclovir 10 mg/kg or 20 mg/kg every 8 hours are similar to those achieved in adults receiving IV acyclovir 5 mg/kg or 10 mg/kg every 8 hours. In a multiple-dose study in neonates up to 3 months of age, IV infusion over 1 hour of 5, 10, or 15 mg/kg of acyclovir every 8 hours resulted in mean steady-state peak serum concentrations of 6.8, 13.9, or 19.6 mcg/mL, respectively, and mean steady-state trough serum concentrations of 1.2, 2.3, or 3.1 mcg/mL, respectively. In another multiple-dose study in pediatric patients, IV infusion over 1 hour of 250 or 500 mg/m² of acyclovir every 8 hours resulted in mean steady-state peak serum concentrations of 10.3 or 20.7 mcg/mL, respectively.

In a single-dose study in adults with end-stage renal disease, a 1-hour IV infusion of 2.5 mg/kg of acyclovir resulted in serum concentrations of the drug that averaged 8.5, 4, 2.3, 2, and 1.5 mcg/mL at 1, 2, 8, 12, and 24 hours after the start of infusion, respectively. When these patients underwent hemodialysis, predialysis (48 hours after the start of drug infusion) and postdialysis (54.5 hours after the start of drug infusion) plasma acyclovir concentrations were 0.6 and 0.3 mcg/mL, respectively.

● Distribution

Acyclovir is widely distributed into body tissues and fluids including the brain, kidney, saliva, lung, liver, muscle, spleen, uterus, vaginal mucosa and secretions, CSF, and herpetic vesicular fluid. The drug also is distributed into semen, achieving concentrations about 1.4 and 4 times those in plasma during chronic oral therapy at dosages of 400 mg and 1 g daily, respectively.

The apparent volume of distribution of acyclovir is reported to be 32.4–61.8 L/1.73 m² in adults and 28.8, 31.6, 42, or 51.2–53.6 L/1.73 m² in neonates up to 3 months of age, children 1–2 years, 2–7 years, or 7–12 years of age, respectively.

In vitro, acyclovir is approximately 9–33% bound to plasma proteins at plasma concentrations of 0.41–5.2 mcg/mL.

Following IV infusion, acyclovir generally diffuses well into CSF. In patients with uninflamed meninges, CSF concentrations of acyclovir are reported to be approximately 50% of concurrent serum acyclovir concentrations.

Acyclovir crosses the placenta. Limited data indicate that the drug is distributed into milk, generally in concentrations greater than concurrent maternal plasma concentrations, possibly via an active transport mechanism.

● Elimination

Plasma concentrations of acyclovir appear to decline in a biphasic manner. In adults with normal renal function, the half-life of acyclovir in the initial phase ($t_{½α}$) averages 0.34 hours and the half-life in the terminal phase ($t_{½β}$) averages 2.1–3.5 hours. In adults with renal impairment, both $t_{½α}$ and $t_{½β}$ may be prolonged, depending on the degree of renal impairment. In a study in adults with anuria, the

$t_{\frac{1}{2}\alpha}$ of acyclovir averaged 0.71 hours. In several studies, the $t_{\frac{1}{2}\beta}$ of acyclovir averaged 3, 3.5, or 19.5 hours in adults with creatinine clearances of 50–80 or 15–50 mL/minute per 1.73 m² or with anuria, respectively. In patients undergoing hemodialysis, the $t_{\frac{1}{2}\beta}$ of acyclovir during hemodialysis averaged 5.4–5.7 hours.

In neonates, the half-life of acyclovir depends principally on the maturity of renal mechanisms for excretion as determined by gestational age, chronologic age, and weight. In children older than 1 year of age, the half-life of the drug appears to be similar to that of adults. The $t_{\frac{1}{2}\beta}$ averages 3.8–4.1, 1.9, 2.2–2.8, or 3.6 hours in neonates up to 3 months of age, children 1–2 years, 2–12 years, or 12–17 years of age, respectively.

Acyclovir is metabolized partially to 9-carboxymethoxymethylguanine (CMMG) and minimally to 8-hydroxy-9-(2-hydroxyethoxymethyl)guanine. In vitro, acyclovir also is metabolized to acyclovir monophosphate, diphosphate, and triphosphate in cells infected with herpesviruses, principally by intracellular phosphorylation of the drug by virus-coded thymidine kinase (TK) and several cellular enzymes. (See Mechanism of Action.)

Acyclovir is excreted principally in urine via glomerular filtration and tubular secretion. Most of a single IV dose of acyclovir is excreted in urine as unchanged drug within 24 hours after administration. In adults with normal renal function, approximately 30–90% of a single IV dose is excreted unchanged in urine within 72 hours; approximately 8–14% and less than 0.2% are excreted in urine as CMMG and 8-hydroxy-9-(2-hydroxyethoxymethyl) guanine, respectively, within 72 hours. In a study in neonates up to 2 months of age, 62–72% of a single dose was excreted in urine unchanged. Less than 2% of a single IV dose of acyclovir is recovered in feces and only trace amounts in expired CO_2; the drug apparently does not accumulate in tissues.

Total body clearance of acyclovir is reported to be 327, 248, 190, or 29 mL/minute per 1.73 m² in patients with creatinine clearances of greater than 80, 50–80, 15–50, or 0 mL/minute per 1.73 m², respectively.

Oral administration of 1 g of probenecid 1 hour before a single 1-hour IV infusion of 5 mg/kg of acyclovir increased the plasma half-life and the area under the plasma concentration-time curve, produced higher and more prolonged plasma concentrations, and decreases the renal clearance of acyclovir. The volume of distribution of acyclovir does not appear to be affected by concomitant administration of oral probenecid. (See Drug Interactions: Probenecid.)

Acyclovir is removed by hemodialysis. The amount of acyclovir removed during hemodialysis depends on several factors (e.g., type of coil used, dialysis flow-rate); a 6-hour period of hemodialysis in one study removed into the dialysate approximately 60% of a single 2.5-mg/kg dose of acyclovir when the dose was given by a 60-minute IV infusion 48 hours prior to dialysis. Data are limited, but peritoneal dialysis and blood exchange transfusions do not appear to appreciably remove the drug.

CHEMISTRY AND STABILITY

● Chemistry

Acyclovir is a synthetic purine nucleoside analog derived from guanine. The drug differs structurally from guanine by the presence of an acyclic side chain. Acyclovir is commercially available for parenteral use as the sodium salt and for oral use as the base. Potency of commercially available acyclovir sodium powder or concentrate for injection is expressed in terms of acyclovir.

Acyclovir occurs as a white, crystalline powder and has a maximum solubility of 2.5 mg/mL in water at 25°C. The drug has pK$_a$s of 2.27 and 9.25. Commercially available acyclovir sodium powder for injection occurs as a white, crystalline, lyophilized powder. Acyclovir sodium has a maximum solubility of greater than 100 mg/mL in water at 25°C, but at physiologic pH and 37°C the drug is almost completely un-ionized and has a maximum solubility of 2.5 mg/mL. The sodium salt of acyclovir contains 4.2 mEq of sodium per gram of acyclovir. Following reconstitution with sterile water for injection, acyclovir sodium solutions containing 50 mg of acyclovir per mL have a pH of approximately 11 and are clear and colorless.

● Stability

Acyclovir capsules and tablets should be stored in tight, light-resistant containers at 15–25°C. Acyclovir suspension should be stored at 15–25°C.

Commercially available acyclovir sodium powder for injection should be stored at 15–25°C. Following reconstitution with sterile water for injection, acyclovir sodium solutions containing 50 mg of acyclovir per mL are stable for 12 hours. Refrigeration of the reconstituted solution may result in formation of a precipitate which will redissolve at room temperature; potency of the drug does not appear to be affected by precipitation and subsequent redissolution. Acyclovir sodium also is compatible with bacteriostatic water for injection containing *benzyl alcohol*, exhibiting the stability noted above for sterile water for injection; however, use of this diluent is not recommended because of the potential risk of benzyl alcohol exposure if such reconstituted drug were administered to a neonate. Bacteriostatic water for injection containing *parabens* should *not* be used to reconstitute acyclovir sodium powder for injection since this diluent is incompatible with the drug and may cause precipitation.

The manufacturer states that acyclovir sodium is physically and chemically compatible for 24 hours at 25°C when diluted with 50–100 mL of a standard, commercially available electrolyte and/or dextrose solution. Although yellowish discoloration may occur when acyclovir sodium is diluted with greater than 10% dextrose, potency of the drug is not affected. The manufacturer states that acyclovir sodium is incompatible with biologic and/or colloidal fluids (e.g., blood products, protein-containing solutions).

PREPARATIONS

Excipients in commercially available drug preparations may have clinically important effects in some individuals; consult specific product labeling for details.

Acyclovir

Oral

Capsules	200 mg*	**Acyclovir Capsules®**
		Zovirax®, GlaxoSmithKline
Suspension	200 mg/5 mL*	**Acyclovir Suspension**
		Zovirax®, GlaxoSmithKline
Tablets	400 mg*	**Acyclovir Tablets®**
		Zovirax®, GlaxoSmithKline
	800 mg*	**Acyclovir Tablets®**
		Zovirax®, GlaxoSmithKline

* available from one or more manufacturer, distributor, and/or repackager by generic (nonproprietary) name

Acyclovir Sodium

Parenteral

For injection, concentrate, for IV infusion only	50 mg (of acyclovir) per mL (500 mg, 1 g)*	**Acyclovir Sodium Injection**
For injection, for IV infusion only	500 mg (of acyclovir)*	**Acyclovir Sodium for Injection**
		Zovirax®, GlaxoSmithKline
	1 g (of acyclovir)*	**Acyclovir Sodium for Injection**
		Zovirax®, GlaxoSmithKline

* available from one or more manufacturer, distributor, and/or repackager by generic (nonproprietary) name

† Use is not currently included in the labeling approved by the US Food and Drug Administration.

Selected Revisions January 1, 2007, © Copyright, October 1, 1983, American Society of Health-System Pharmacists, Inc.

Adefovir Dipivoxil

8:18.32 • NUCLEOSIDES AND NUCLEOTIDES

■ Adefovir dipivoxil is a prodrug of adefovir, an acyclic nucleotide analog antiviral agent that is active against human hepatitis B virus (HBV) and certain other viruses.

USES

• Chronic Hepatitis B Virus Infection

Adefovir dipivoxil is used for the treatment of chronic hepatitis B virus (HBV) infection in adults and adolescents 12 years of age and older with evidence of active HBV replication and either persistent elevations in serum aminotransferase (ALT or AST) concentrations or histologic evidence of active liver disease. This indication is based on histologic, virologic, biochemical, and serologic responses in adults with hepatitis B e antigen (HBeAg)-positive or HBeAg-negative chronic HBV infection with compensated liver function and with clinical evidence of lamivudine-resistant HBV with either compensated or decompensated liver function. For adolescents 12 years of age or older, this indication is based on virologic and biochemical responses in patients in this age group with HBeAg-positive chronic HBV infection with compensated liver function.

The goal of antiviral therapy in patients with chronic HBV infection is to decrease the morbidity and mortality related to the infection (e.g., cirrhosis, hepatic failure, hepatocellular carcinoma). Sustained suppression of HBV replication has been associated with normalization of serum ALT concentrations, loss of HBeAg with or without detection of antibody to HBeAg (anti-HBe), and improvement in liver histology. Currently available therapies for chronic HBV infection (e.g., adefovir, entecavir, lamivudine, telbivudine, tenofovir alafenamide, tenofovir disoproxil fumarate [tenofovir DF], interferon alfa, peginterferon alfa) are used in an attempt to provide an immunologic cure (HBsAg loss and sustained HBV DNA suppression), but cannot provide a virologic cure (eradication of HBV).

Treatment of chronic HBV infection is complex and evolving, and specialized references and experts should be consulted. Information from the American Association for the Study of Liver Diseases (AASLD) regarding management of HBV infection, including recommendations for initial treatment, is available at https://www.aasld.org.

HBeAg-Positive Adults

Efficacy of adefovir dipivoxil for the management of HBeAg-positive chronic HBV infection was evaluated in a phase III, randomized, double-blind, placebo-controlled study (study 437) in adults with active HBV replication (median baseline serum HBV DNA levels of 8.36 $\log_{10}$ copies/mL), persistent elevations in serum ALT concentrations (median elevations 2.3 times the upper limit of normal), and histologic evidence of active liver disease (median baseline total Knodell Histology Activity Index [HAI] scores of 10). Seventy-four percent of patients in the study were male, 59% were Asian, 36% were Caucasian, and 24 or 2% had prior treatment with interferon alfa or lamivudine, respectively.

Data analysis at 48 weeks indicated that 53% of patients receiving adefovir dipivoxil in a dosage of 10 mg daily had histologic improvement (defined as a reduction of at least 2 points in the Knodell necroinflammatory score with no concurrent worsening of the Knodell fibrosis score) compared with 25% of those receiving placebo. Forty-eight percent of patients receiving adefovir dipivoxil (10 mg daily) had normal serum ALT concentrations (i.e., biochemical response) at week 48 compared with 16% of those receiving placebo. In addition, the mean decrease in serum HBV DNA levels from baseline was 3.57 $\log_{10}$ copies/mL at week 48 in those receiving adefovir dipivoxil compared with a decrease of 0.98 $\log_{10}$ copies/mL in those receiving placebo. Twenty-one percent of patients who received adefovir dipivoxil (10 mg daily) had undetectable levels of serum HBV DNA (defined as less than 400 copies/mL by a polymerase chain reaction [PCR] assay) at week 48 compared with 0% of those who received placebo. Loss of HBeAg and seroconversion to anti-HBe also occurred in 24 and 12% of patients, respectively, who received adefovir dipivoxil (10 mg daily) compared with 11 and 6%, respectively, of those who received placebo. Although this study initially included a treatment arm that involved administering adefovir dipivoxil in a dosage of 30 mg daily, this arm of the study was discontinued at 48 weeks based on data from

a phase II study indicating that the higher dosage might be associated with mild, reversible nephrotoxicity. At 48 weeks, patients who were receiving adefovir dipivoxil in a dosage of 10 mg daily were re-randomized to receive either continued treatment with 10 mg daily or placebo and those who were receiving placebo were all given adefovir dipivoxil 10 mg daily for an additional 48 weeks. There was evidence that treatment with adefovir dipivoxil 10 mg daily for up to 72 weeks resulted in continued maintenance of mean reductions in serum HBV DNA levels observed at week 48 and an increase in the proportion of patients with ALT normalization and/or HBeAg seroconversion. In one study in patients who received adefovir dipivoxil for up to 240 weeks (4.6 years), the median change from baseline serum HBV DNA at study week 144, 192, and 240 was –3.69, –3.55, and –4.05 $\log_{10}$ copies/mL, respectively, and 48% of patients had confirmed HBeAg seroconversion at week 240. The effect of continued adefovir dipivoxil therapy on seroconversion is unknown.

HBeAg-Negative Adults

Efficacy of adefovir dipivoxil for the management of HBeAg-negative, anti-HBe- and HBV-DNA-positive chronic HBV infection was evaluated in a phase III, randomized, double-blind, placebo-controlled study (study 438) in 184 adults with active HBV replication (median baseline serum HBV DNA levels of 7.08 $\log_{10}$ copies/mL by a PCR-based assay), persistent elevations in serum ALT concentrations (median elevations 2.3 times the upper limit of normal), and histologic evidence of active liver disease (median baseline total HAI scores of 10). Eighty-three percent of patients in the study were male, 66% were Caucasian, 30% were Asian, and 41 or 8% had prior treatment with interferon alfa or lamivudine, respectively.

Data analysis at 48 weeks indicated that 64% of patients who received adefovir dipivoxil (10 mg daily) had histologic improvement (defined as a reduction of at least 2 points in the Knodell necroinflammatory score with no concurrent worsening of the Knodell fibrosis score) compared with 33–35% of those who received placebo. Serum ALT concentrations also normalized at week 48 in 72% of patients who received adefovir dipivoxil compared with 29% of those who received placebo. In addition, the mean decrease in serum HBV DNA levels from baseline was 3.65 $\log_{10}$ copies/mL at week 48 in patients receiving adefovir dipivoxil 10 mg daily compared with a mean decrease of 1.32 $\log_{10}$ copies/mL in those receiving placebo. Fifty-one percent of patients who received adefovir dipivoxil had undetectable levels of serum HBV DNA (defined as less than 400 copies/mL by a PCR-based assay) at week 48 compared with 0% of those who received placebo. After 48 weeks, patients receiving adefovir dipivoxil were re-randomized to continue the drug or to receive placebo and those receiving placebo were all given adefovir dipivoxil for an additional 48 weeks. Data analysis of patients who received continuous adefovir dipivoxil therapy for 96 weeks indicates that 71% had serum HBV DNA levels less than 1000 copies/mL, 73% had normalization of serum ALT concentrations, and 74 or 89% of patients with available liver biopsy results at year 2 had improvements in necroinflammation or fibrosis, respectively. After 96 weeks, patients who were receiving adefovir dipivoxil were able to enroll in an open-label study that involved using the drug for an additional 144 weeks. Data analysis of patients who received continuous adefovir dipivoxil therapy for 192 weeks (placebo-adefovir group) indicates that 71–73% had serum HBV DNA levels less than 1000 copies/mL, 73–74% had normalization of serum ALT concentrations, and 86 or 73% of patients with available liver biopsy results had improvements in necroinflammation or fibrosis, respectively. Data analysis of patients who received continuous adefovir dipivoxil therapy for 240 weeks (adefovir-adefovir group) indicates that 67% had serum HBV DNA levels less than 1000 copies/mL, 66–69% had normalization of serum ALT concentrations, and 83 or 75% of patients with available liver biopsy results had improvement in necroinflammation or fibrosis, respectively.

Because patients with HBeAg-negative chronic HBV infections rarely have hepatitis B surface antigen (HBsAg) seroconversion, these patients are likely to require long-term antiviral therapy. While there is evidence that adefovir dipivoxil monotherapy continued for at least 96 weeks may provide some benefits, further study is needed to determine the effect of such therapy on clearance of HBsAg and the frequency of virologic and biochemical relapse after discontinuance of the drug. In addition, further study is needed to investigate the possibility of emergence of adefovir-resistant strains of HBV with long-term therapy with the drug. Although there was no evidence of emergence of HBV resistant to adefovir dipivoxil during 48-week clinical studies evaluating adefovir dipivoxil monotherapy in HBV-infected patients, there are concerns about the potential for such resistance with single-agent use of the drug for long-term treatment of chronic HBV infection. This concern is based in part on experience with use of monotherapy with lamivudine (a nucleoside antiviral agent) for the treatment of chronic HBV infection. (See Patients with Lamivudine-Resistant HBV under Uses: Chronic Hepatitis B Virus Infection.) Although the clinical importance is unclear, there is evidence that reduced susceptibility to adefovir dipivoxil develops in some patients during long-term use. (See Resistance in HBV under Description: Resistance.)

HBeAg-Positive Pediatric Patients

Efficacy of adefovir dipivoxil for the management of HBeAg-positive chronic HBV infection in adolescents was evaluated in a phase III, randomized, double-blind, placebo-controlled study (study 518) that included adolescents 12–17 years of age with active HBV replication (median baseline serum HBV DNA levels of 8.69–8.85 $\log_{10}$ copies/mL) and elevated serum ALT concentrations at baseline (median elevations 2.3 times the upper limit of normal). Seventy-five percent of adolescents 12–17 years of age in the study were male, 22% were Asian, and 75% were Caucasian. Data analysis at 48 weeks indicated that 23% of adolescents receiving adefovir dipivoxil (10 mg daily) had HBV DNA levels less than 1000 copies/mL with normalization of serum ALT concentrations compared with none of those receiving placebo.

Although study 518 also evaluated efficacy and safety of adefovir dipivoxil for the treatment of chronic HBV infection in pediatric patients 2–11 years of age†, the drug was no more effective than placebo in patients younger than 12 years of age. Adefovir dipivoxil is not recommended for and should not be used in children younger than 12 years of age.

Pre- and Post-Liver Transplantation Patients

Adefovir dipivoxil has been shown to be well tolerated and to achieve significant reduction in serum HBV DNA levels and improvement in biochemical indices (e.g., ALT, bilirubin, albumin, prothrombin time [PT]) and Child-Pugh scores in a clinical trial involving HBeAg-positive and HBeAg-negative, compensated and decompensated, pre- and post-liver transplant patients with clinical evidence of lamivudine resistance. In one open-label, uncontrolled study (study 435) in adults, a 48-week regimen of adefovir dipivoxil monotherapy resulted in a mean decrease from baseline serum HBV DNA levels of 3.5–3.7 or 4 $\log_{10}$ copies/mL in pre- or post-liver transplant patients, respectively; these reductions occurred regardless of baseline patterns of lamivudine-resistant HBV DNA polymerase mutations. In addition, normalization of serum ALT, bilirubin, or albumin concentrations occurred in 74–77 or 51%, 58–60 or 76%, and 76–80 or 81% of pre- or post-liver transplant patients, respectively, at 48 weeks. Normalization of PT occurred in 84–85 or 56% of pre- or post-liver transplant patients, respectively. Child-Pugh scores remained stable or improved in 96 or 93% of pre- or post-liver transplant patients, respectively. The clinical importance of these findings as they relate to clinical outcomes is as yet unknown.

Patients with Lamivudine-Resistant HBV

Adefovir dipivoxil has been evaluated for the treatment of chronic HBV infection in patients with clinical evidence of lamivudine-resistant YMDD mutant strains of HBV. Lamivudine-resistant strains of HBV have been reported in up to 24–32% of patients after 1 year of lamivudine monotherapy and in up to 70% of patients after 4–5 years of such treatment; however, there is in vitro evidence that adefovir usually is active against these lamivudine-resistant HBV. Data from a randomized, double-blind, active-controlled study (study 461) in patients 16–65 years of age suggest that adefovir dipivoxil monotherapy is as effective as a regimen of adefovir dipivoxil and lamivudine and more effective than lamivudine monotherapy in decreasing serum HBV DNA in patients with clinical and virologic evidence of lamivudine-resistant HBV. Data analysis at 48 weeks indicates that time-weighted average serum HBV DNA levels decreased approximately 3–4 $\log_{10}$ copies/mL in patients who received adefovir dipivoxil alone or in conjunction with lamivudine compared with a time-weighted average decrease of 0 $\log_{10}$ copies/mL in those who received lamivudine monotherapy. An increase in the proportion of patients with ALT normalization, HBeAg loss, and/or HBeAg seroconversion also was observed at week 48 in patients receiving adefovir dipivoxil alone or in conjunction with lamivudine. The clinical importance of these findings as they relate to clinical outcomes are unknown.

DOSAGE AND ADMINISTRATION

● Administration

Adefovir dipivoxil is administered orally without regard to food.

● Dosage

Adult Dosage
Chronic Hepatitis B Virus Infection

For the treatment of chronic hepatitis B virus (HBV) infection in adults, the usual dosage of adefovir dipivoxil is 10 mg once daily.

The optimal duration of adefovir dipivoxil therapy in patients with chronic HBV infection is not known. The drug has been continued for up to 5 years in controlled clinical studies in adults.

Pediatric Dosage
Chronic Hepatitis B Virus Infection

For the treatment of chronic HBV infection in adolescents 12 years of age or older, the usual dosage of adefovir dipivoxil is 10 mg once daily.

The optimal duration of adefovir dipivoxil therapy in patients with chronic HBV infection is not known. The drug has been continued for up to 5 years in controlled clinical studies in adults.

● Special Populations
Hepatic Impairment

Dosage adjustments are not necessary in patients with hepatic impairment.

Renal Impairment

The dosing interval of adefovir dipivoxil should be adjusted in adults with preexisting renal impairment (i.e., baseline creatinine clearances less than 50 mL/minute). (See Table 1.)

TABLE 1. Dosage of Adefovir Dipivoxil for Treatment of HBV Infection in Adults with Renal Impairment

Creatinine Clearance (mL/min)	Dosage
30–49	10 mg once every 48 hours
10–29	10 mg once every 72 hours
Less than 10 (not undergoing hemodialysis)	Dosage recommendations not available
Hemodialysis patients	10 mg once every 7 days following dialysis

The safety and efficacy of these dosage guidelines for adults with renal impairment have not been clinically evaluated. The manufacturers state these dosage guidelines were derived from data for patients with preexisting renal impairment and may not be appropriate for patients in whom renal impairment evolves during therapy with the drug. Therefore, clinical response and renal function should be monitored closely.

The safety and efficacy of adefovir dipivoxil have not been studied in adolescents 12 years of age or older with renal impairment. Data are insufficient to make dosage recommendations for adolescents 12 years of age or older with underlying renal impairment; the drug should be used with caution and renal function monitored closely in such adolescents.

Geriatric Patients

Dosage of adefovir dipivoxil should be selected with caution in geriatric patients because of possible age-related decreases in renal function, and patients should be monitored closely. (See Geriatric Use under Warnings/Precautions: Specific Populations, in Cautions.)

CAUTIONS

● Contraindications

Adefovir dipivoxil is contraindicated in patients with known hypersensitivity to the drug or any ingredient in the formulation.

● Warnings/Precautions

Warnings

Exacerbation of Hepatitis

Severe acute exacerbations of hepatitis have been reported following discontinuance of hepatitis B virus (HBV) therapy, including adefovir dipivoxil therapy.

In clinical studies, exacerbations of hepatitis (ALT elevations at least 10 times the upper limit of normal) occurred in up to 25% of patients following discontinuance of adefovir dipivoxil, usually within 12 weeks after discontinuance. These exacerbations generally occurred in the absence of hepatitis B e antigen (HBeAg) seroconversion and presented as elevations in ALT and reemergence of viral replication.

Although these exacerbations appeared to be self-limited or resolved with reinitiation of therapy, severe exacerbations (including fatalities) have been reported.

In patients with compensated liver function, exacerbations of hepatitis generally have not been accompanied by hepatic decompensation. However, patients with advanced liver disease or cirrhosis may be at higher risk for hepatic decompensation than those with compensated liver function.

Hepatic function should be closely monitored with both clinical and laboratory follow-up for at least several months after adefovir dipivoxil is discontinued. If appropriate, resumption of HBV therapy may be warranted.

Nephrotoxicity

Nephrotoxicity, characterized by a delayed onset, is the principal dose-limiting toxicity of adefovir dipivoxil and also may occur in patients receiving chronic (long-term) therapy with the recommended dosage of the drug.

Delayed onset of gradual increases in serum creatinine and decreases in serum phosphorus were the treatment-limiting toxicities of adefovir dipivoxil therapy in clinical studies evaluating use of high dosages of the drug for the treatment of human immunodeficiency virus (HIV) infection† (60 or 120 mg daily) or use of high dosages for the treatment of chronic HBV infection (30 mg daily).

Long-term administration of adefovir dipivoxil in dosages recommended for the treatment of HBV infection (10 mg daily) also may result in delayed nephrotoxicity. By week 96 or week 240, 2 or 3% of patients who received adefovir dipivoxil had serum creatinine increases of 0.5 mg/dL or greater from baseline (by Kaplan Meier estimates), respectively.

In pre- or postliver transplant patients receiving the usually recommended dosage of the drug (10 mg daily), most of whom had some degree of baseline renal insufficiency, 37 or 32% had increases in serum creatinine concentrations of 0.3 mg/dL or greater from baseline by week 48, respectively, and 53 or 51% had serum creatinine increases of 0.3 mg/dL or greater from baseline by week 96, respectively.

Although the overall risk of nephrotoxicity is low in patients with adequate renal function, the possibility of nephrotoxicity should be considered in patients at risk of or having underlying renal dysfunction and in those receiving concomitant therapy with nephrotoxic agents. (See Drug Interactions: Nephrotoxic Drugs or Drugs Eliminated by Renal Excretion.)

Renal function should be monitored closely in all patients receiving adefovir dipivoxil, especially those with preexisting renal impairment or other risks for renal impairment. Dosage adjustments may be necessary. (See Renal Impairment under Dosage and Administration: Special Populations.)

HBV-infected Individuals Coinfected with HIV

Use of adefovir dipivoxil for the treatment of chronic HBV infection in patients with unrecognized or untreated HIV infection may result in emergence of HIV resistance. Although adefovir has some in vitro activity against HIV, dosage of the drug used for the treatment of HBV infection (10 mg daily) has not been shown to suppress HIV RNA levels in HIV-infected patients.

Some experts state that adefovir dipivoxil alone or in conjunction with other antivirals should not be used for the treatment of HBV infection in HIV-infected patients.

HIV antibody testing should be offered to all patients prior to initiating adefovir dipivoxil therapy.

Lactic Acidosis and Severe Hepatomegaly with Steatosis

Lactic acidosis and severe hepatomegaly with steatosis, including some fatalities, have been reported in patients receiving nucleoside analogs alone or in conjunction with antiretrovirals. Most reported cases have involved women; obesity and long-term therapy with nucleoside reverse transcriptase inhibitors also may be risk factors.

Nucleoside analogs should be used with particular caution in patients with known risk factors for liver disease; however, lactic acidosis and severe hepatomegaly with steatosis have been reported in patients with no known risk factors.

Adefovir dipivoxil therapy should be discontinued in any patient with clinical or laboratory findings suggestive of lactic acidosis or pronounced hepatotoxicity (which may include hepatomegaly and steatosis even in the absence of marked aminotransferase elevations).

HBV Resistance

Resistance to adefovir dipivoxil may result in hepatitis B viral load rebound, which may lead to exacerbation of HBV infection; if the patient has impaired hepatic function, this may lead to liver decompensation and death.

To reduce risk of clinical resistance in patients with lamivudine-resistant HBV, adefovir dipivoxil should be used in conjunction with lamivudine; adefovir dipivoxil should not be used as monotherapy.

Patients with serum HBV DNA levels greater than 1000 copies/mL after 48 weeks of adefovir dipivoxil treatment are at greater risk of developing clinical resistance. To reduce risk of clinical resistance in patients receiving monotherapy with adefovir dipivoxil, treatment modification should be considered if serum HBV DNA levels remain greater than 1000 copies/mL with continued treatment.

Concomitant Use with Other Drugs

Adefovir dipivoxil should not be used concomitantly with tenofovir disoproxil fumarate (tenofovir DF) or fixed-combination preparations containing tenofovir DF.

Specific Populations

Pregnancy

Category C. (See Users Guide.)

To monitor maternal-fetal outcomes of pregnant women exposed to adefovir dipivoxil, clinicians are encouraged to contact the pregnancy registry at 800-258-4263 to enroll such women.

There are no adequate, well-controlled studies of adefovir dipivoxil in pregnant women. The drug should be used during pregnancy only if potential benefits justify potential risks to the fetus.

There was no evidence of embryotoxicity or teratogenicity in rats or rabbits at systemic exposures 23 or 40 times, respectively, exposures in humans at the therapeutic dosage. However, embryotoxicity and increased incidence of fetal malformations (anasarca, depressed eye bulge, umbilical hernia, kinked tail) occurred in rats at adefovir dipivoxil exposures 38 times human exposures at the therapeutic dosage.

The American Association for the Study of Liver Diseases (AASLD) and other experts state that recommendations regarding antiviral therapy for the management of HBV infection in pregnant women generally are the same as those for other adults. AASLD also suggests that hepatitis B surface antigen (HBsAg)-positive pregnant women with HBV DNA levels exceeding 200,000 IU/mL receive antiviral therapy since this may reduce the risk of perinatal transmission of HBV; however, preferred antiviral agents, exact viral load threshold, and optimal gestational week during the third trimester to initiate such therapy have not been clearly identified.

Data are not available regarding the effect of adefovir dipivoxil therapy during pregnancy on transmission of HBV to the infant. Routine screening for HBV infection is recommended for all pregnant women. For prevention of perinatal transmission of HBV, US Public Health Service Advisory Committee on Immunization Practices (ACIP), American Academy of Pediatrics (AAP), and other experts state that infants born to HBsAg-positive women should receive their first dose of hepatitis B vaccine and a dose of hepatitis B immune globulin (HBIG) within 12 hours of birth.

Lactation

It is not known whether adefovir dipivoxil is distributed into milk.

A decision should be made to discontinue nursing or adefovir dipivoxil, taking into account the importance of the drug to the woman.

Pediatric Use

Safety and efficacy of adefovir dipivoxil have not been established in children younger than 12 years of age. (See HBeAg-Positive Pediatric Patients under Uses: Chronic Hepatitis B Virus Infection.)

Geriatric Use

Experience in those 65 years of age or older is insufficient to determine whether geriatric adults respond differently than younger adults.

Adefovir dipivoxil should be used with caution in geriatric patients because of age-related decreases in hepatic, renal, and/or cardiac function and concomitant disease and drug therapy.

Renal Impairment

Dosage adjustments are recommended for adults with creatinine clearance less than 50 mL/minute. (See Renal Impairment under Dosage and Administration: Special Populations.)

Adefovir dipivoxil has not been evaluated in adolescents 12 years of age or older with renal impairment. The drug should be used with caution in such adolescents and renal function should be monitored closely.

• Common Adverse Effects

Adverse effects reported in 3% or more of patients with adequate renal function who received adefovir dipivoxil for 48 weeks in clinical studies include asthenia (13%), headache (9%), abdominal pain (9%), nausea (5%), flatulence (4%), diarrhea (3%) and dyspepsia (3%); these frequencies were similar to those observed in patients receiving placebo (2–14%).

Adverse effects reported in 2% or greater of pre- and post-liver transplantation patients who received adefovir dipivoxil in clinical studies include asthenia, abdominal pain, headache, nausea, vomiting, diarrhea, increases in ALT and AST, pruritus, rash, increases in creatinine, renal failure, and renal insufficiency. In addition, transient serum phosphorus concentrations less than 2 mg/dL were observed in approximately 2% of these patients; adefovir dipivoxil therapy was continued and the patients did not require phosphorus supplementation. Four percent (19 of 467) of pre- and post-liver transplantation patients discontinued adefovir dipivoxil therapy because of adverse renal effects. However, a causal relationship to changes in serum creatinine and serum phosphorus is difficult to assess because of the presence of multiple concomitant risk factors for renal dysfunction in these patients.

DRUG INTERACTIONS

• Drugs Affecting or Metabolized by Hepatic Microsomal Enzymes

Adefovir dipivoxil is not an inhibitor or a substrate for any of the major cytochrome P-450 (CYP) isoenzymes, including CYP1A2, CYP2C9, CYP2C19, CYP2D6, or CYP3A4; pharmacokinetic interactions unlikely. However, the potential for adefovir dipivoxil to induce CYP isoenzymes is unknown.

• Nephrotoxic Drugs or Drugs Affecting Eliminated by Renal Excretion

Potential increased risk of nephrotoxicity in patients receiving other nephrotoxic drugs (e.g., aminoglycosides, cyclosporine, tacrolimus, vancomycin, certain nonsteroidal anti-inflammatory agents [NSAIAs]); patients should be monitored closely.

Potential pharmacokinetic interactions with drugs that compete for active tubular secretion (increased plasma concentration of adefovir dipivoxil and/or the other drug); patients should be monitored closely.

• Acetaminophen

No pharmacokinetic interactions with acetaminophen.

• Antiretroviral Agents

HIV Nucleoside and Nucleotide Reverse Transcriptase Inhibitors (NRTIs)

Didanosine

No pharmacokinetic interactions with didanosine delayed-release capsules containing enteric-coated pellets.

Lamivudine

No pharmacokinetic interactions with lamivudine.

Additive antiviral effects against hepatitis B virus (HBV).

Tenofovir Disoproxil Fumarate

Tenofovir disoproxil fumarate (tenofovir DF) and adefovir dipivoxil should not be used concomitantly.

• Co-trimoxazole

No pharmacokinetic interactions with co-trimoxazole.

• Entecavir

No clinically important pharmacokinetic interactions with entecavir.

• Ibuprofen

Pharmacokinetic interaction (33% increase in peak plasma concentration and 23% increase in area under the plasma concentration-time curve [AUC] of adefovir dipivoxil; no effect on pharmacokinetics of ibuprofen). Clinical importance unknown. This pharmacokinetic interaction may occur because of increased oral bioavailability of adefovir.

• Immunosuppressive Agents

No pharmacokinetic interactions with tacrolimus.

Effect of adefovir dipivoxil on cyclosporine concentrations not known.

Concomitant use of adefovir dipivoxil and cyclosporine or tacrolimus may increase the risk of nephrotoxicity.

• Telbivudine

No pharmacokinetic interactions with telbivudine.

In vitro studies indicate additive antiviral effects between telbivudine and adefovir against HBV.

DESCRIPTION

Adefovir dipivoxil is a prodrug of adefovir, an acyclic nucleotide analog antiviral agent active against human hepatitis B virus (HBV). Following initial diester hydrolysis in vivo to form adefovir, the drug undergoes subsequent phosphorylation by cellular enzymes to form its active metabolite, adefovir diphosphate. Adefovir diphosphate inhibits HBV DNA polymerase (reverse transcriptase) by competing with the natural substrate deoxyadenosine triphosphate and by causing DNA chain termination after its incorporation into viral DNA. Adefovir diphosphate is a weak inhibitor of human DNA polymerases, including α- and γ-polymerases.

• Spectrum

Adefovir is active in vitro and in vivo against human HBV. The drug also has some in vitro activity against certain other human viruses, including herpes simplex virus types 1 and 2 (HSV-1 and HSV-2), human immunodeficiency virus types 1 and 2 (HIV-1 and HIV-2), human papillomavirus (HPV), Epstein-Barr virus, and varicella zoster virus, but has not been shown to be effective in clinical infections caused by these viruses.

Adefovir is active in vivo against some lamivudine-resistant HBV isolates and has demonstrated anti-HBV activity (median reduction in serum HBV DNA levels of 4.1 $\log_{10}$ copies/mL) against clinical isolates of HBV containing lamivudine-associated mutations. In vitro studies indicate that adefovir is active against HBV variants containing substitutions that confer resistance to lamivudine (rtL180M, rtM204I, rtM204V, rtL180M + rtM204V, rtV173L + rtL180M + rtM204V) or entecavir (rtT184G, rtS202I, rtM250V). (See Patients with Lamivudine-Resistant HBV under Uses: Chronic Hepatitis B Virus Infection.)

• Resistance

Resistance in HBV

Although the clinical importance is unclear, there is evidence that HBV with reduced susceptibility to adefovir dipivoxil develop in some patients during long-term use of the drug.

There was no evidence of emergence of HBV resistant to adefovir dipivoxil during 48-week clinical studies evaluating adefovir dipivoxil monotherapy in HBV-infected patients; however, resistance or diminished virologic response was reported in some patients with HBV infection following at least 56 weeks of adefovir dipivoxil monotherapy.

Genotypic analysis of isolates obtained from patients who showed renewed evidence of HBV replication while receiving adefovir dipivoxil indicates that mutations at rtN236T and rtA181T/V are associated with resistance to adefovir. After 96 weeks of adefovir dipivoxil monotherapy, the N236T mutation was detected in 2 patients (1.6% of patients) and this mutation was associated with reduced in vitro susceptibility to the drug. In studies of patients who received adefovir dipivoxil for up to 5 years, mutations associated with adefovir resistance developed in 20–42% of patients.

Cross-resistance can occur among the nucleoside and nucleotide antivirals used for treatment of HBV. Some strains of HBV may be cross-resistant to both adefovir and lamivudine. Preliminary data suggest that the N236T mutation alone does not confer cross-resistance to lamivudine since isolates with the mutation remained susceptible to lamivudine in vitro and in vivo, but cross-resistance to adefovir and lamivudine can occur in isolates with the rtA181V mutation. In vitro studies indicate that some HBV with mutations associated with adefovir resistance may have decreased susceptibility to entecavir. Some adefovir-resistant HBV (e.g., those with adefovir resistance-associated substitution rtA181V, rtA181S, rt181T) have reduced susceptibility to telbivudine; other strains (e.g., those with rtN236T substitution) remain susceptible to telbivudine. HBV isolates with rtA181T, rtA181V, or rtN236T single adefovir resistance-associated substitutions also have less than twofold reduced susceptibility to tenofovir alafenamide. Isolates with double adefovir resistance-associated substitutions of rtA181V *and* rtN236T have 3.7-fold reduced susceptibility to tenofovir alafenamide.

ADVICE TO PATIENTS

Advise patient of the risks and benefits of adefovir dipivoxil and other alternatives for treatment of hepatitis B virus (HBV) infection and importance of reading the patient package insert for the drug before starting treatment.

Importance of remaining under the care of a clinician while taking adefovir dipivoxil and not discontinuing the drug without first informing a clinician.

Importance of following a regular dosage schedule and avoiding missed doses.

Risk of exacerbations of hepatitis when adefovir dipivoxil is discontinued and importance of close monitoring of liver function and HBV levels for several months or longer after the drug is stopped.

Risk of nephrotoxicity and importance of monitoring renal function during treatment, especially in those with preexisting renal impairment or other risks for renal impairment.

Importance of immediately reporting any signs or symptoms of lactic acidosis (e.g., weakness/fatigue, unusual muscle pain, trouble breathing, stomach pain with nausea and vomiting, cold intolerance especially in the arms and legs, dizziness or feeling light-headed, fast or irregular heart beat) or any signs or symptoms of hepatotoxicity (e.g., jaundice, dark urine, bowel movements light in color, anorexia, nausea, stomach pain). Importance of reporting any other unusual symptoms or any known symptom persists or worsens.

Risk of rapid emergence of human immunodeficiency virus (HIV) resistance in HBV-infected patients with unrecognized or untreated HIV infection; importance of HIV antibody testing prior to initiation of adefovir dipivoxil therapy and any time during therapy if possible exposure to HIV occurs.

Advise patients with lamivudine-resistant HBV that they should receive adefovir dipivoxil in conjunction with lamivudine and should not receive adefovir dipivoxil monotherapy.

Advise patients that the optimal duration of treatment and the relationship between treatment response and long-term outcomes of HBV infection (hepatocellular carcinoma, decompensated cirrhosis) are not known.

Importance of informing clinician of existing or contemplated concomitant therapy, including prescription and OTC drugs, and any concomitant illnesses.

Importance of women immediately informing clinician if they are or plan to become pregnant or plan to breast-feed.

Importance of advising patients of other important precautionary information. (See Cautions.)

PREPARATIONS

Excipients in commercially available drug preparations may have clinically important effects in some individuals; consult specific product labeling for details.

Adefovir Dipivoxil

Oral

| Tablets | 10 mg* | **Adefovir Dipivoxil Tablets** |
| | | Hepsera®, Gilead |

* available from one or more manufacturer, distributor, and/or repackager by generic (nonproprietary) name

† Use is not currently included in the labeling approved by the US Food and Drug Administration.

Selected Revisions October 23, 2017, © Copyright, July 1, 2003, American Society of Health-System Pharmacists, Inc.

Cidofovir

8:18.32 • NUCLEOSIDES AND NUCLEOTIDES

- Cidofovir, an acyclic nucleotide analog (acyclic nucleoside phosphonate), is an antiviral agent active against herpesviruses and certain other viruses.

USES

● Treatment of Cytomegalovirus Infection and Disease

Cytomegalovirus Retinitis

Cidofovir is used for initial treatment (induction therapy) and maintenance therapy (secondary prophylaxis) of cytomegalovirus (CMV) retinitis in adults with human immunodeficiency virus (HIV) infection, including those with acquired immunodeficiency syndrome (AIDS). The drug also is used for the management of CMV retinitis in HIV-infected adolescents and children†. Safety and efficacy of cidofovir have not been established for the treatment of other CMV infections (e.g., pneumonitis, gastroenteritis), congenital or neonatal CMV disease, or CMV disease in individuals not infected with HIV.

Like other antivirals, cidofovir is not a cure for CMV retinitis. Although cidofovir can induce stabilization or improvement of ocular manifestations of CMV retinitis, the retinitis may relapse and/or progress during or after discontinuance of the drug.

Retinitis is the most common clinical manifestation of CMV end-organ disease in HIV-infected patients and ideally should be managed in consultation with an ophthalmologist familiar with the diagnosis and treatment of retinal diseases. Antiviral regimens for initial treatment of CMV retinitis in HIV-infected individuals should be selected based on the location and severity of CMV retinal lesions, severity of underlying immunosuppression, concomitant drug therapy, and the patient's ability to adhere to the treatment regimen. The antiviral regimen used for maintenance therapy of CMV retinitis in HIV-infected individuals should be selected with consideration for the location of the CMV retinal lesions, vision in the contralateral eye, the patient's immunologic and virologic status, and the patient's response to antiretroviral therapy.

For the management of immediate sight-threatening CMV retinal lesions (i.e., within 1.5 mm of the fovea) in HIV-infected adults and adolescents, the US Centers for Disease Control and Prevention (CDC), National Institutes of Health (NIH), and HIV Medicine Association of the Infectious Diseases Society of America (IDSA) state that the preferred regimen is initial treatment (induction therapy) with intravitreal ganciclovir or intravitreal foscarnet (1–4 doses given over a period of 7–10 days) in conjunction with oral valganciclovir (twice daily for 14–21 days) followed by maintenance therapy (secondary prophylaxis) with oral valganciclovir (once daily). One alternative regimen recommended by these experts for management of sight-threatening CMV retinitis in HIV-infected adults and adolescents is intravitreal ganciclovir or intravitreal foscarnet (1–4 doses given over a period of 7–10 days) in conjunction with IV cidofovir (once weekly for 2 weeks) followed by maintenance therapy (secondary prophylaxis) with IV cidofovir (once every other week). Use of systemic antivirals (without an intravitreal antiviral) usually is adequate for the management of CMV retinitis in patients who have only small peripheral lesions.

For the management of CMV retinitis in HIV-infected pediatric patients, CDC, NIH, IDSA, and others state that IV ganciclovir is the drug of choice for initial treatment (induction therapy) and is one of several options for maintenance therapy (secondary prophylaxis). These experts state that IV cidofovir has not been studied in children with CMV disease, but is a possible alternative for the management of CMV retinitis in HIV-infected children† when other options cannot be used.

Because of the risk of relapse, HIV-infected patients who have received adequate initial treatment of CMV retinitis should receive chronic maintenance therapy (secondary prophylaxis) until immune reconstitution occurs as a result of effective antiretroviral therapy. CDC, NIH, and IDSA state that consideration can be given to discontinuing maintenance therapy of CMV retinitis in HIV-infected adults and adolescents if CMV lesions have been treated for at least 3–6 months

and are inactive and there has been a sustained (i.e., 3–6 months) increase in CD4+ T-cell count to greater than 100/mm³ in response to antiretroviral therapy. The safety of discontinuing maintenance therapy of CMV retinitis in HIV-infected pediatric patients has not been well studied; however, CDC, NIH, IDSA, and others state that consideration can be given to discontinuing such maintenance therapy in HIV-infected children who are receiving antiretroviral therapy and have a sustained (i.e., greater than 6 months) increase in CD4+ T-cell percentage to greater than 15% (children younger than 6 years of age) or an increase in CD4+ T-cell count to greater than 100/mm³ (children 6 years of age or older). These experts state that a decision to discontinue maintenance therapy of CMV retinitis should be made in consultation with an ophthalmologist and, if maintenance therapy is discontinued, the patient should continue to receive regular ophthalmologic monitoring (optimally every 3–6 months) for early detection of CMV relapse or immune reconstitution uveitis. If CD4+ T-cell count decreases to less than 100/mm³ (adults, adolescents, children 6 years of age or older) or if CD4+ T-cell percentage decreases to less than 15% (children younger than 6 years of age), maintenance therapy of CMV retinitis should be reinitiated.

For additional information on the management of CMV retinitis and other CMV infections in HIV-infected individuals, the current clinical practice guidelines from CDC, NIH, and IDSA on the prevention and treatment of opportunistic infections in HIV-infected individuals available at http://www.aidsinfo.nih.gov should be consulted.

Clinical Experience

Efficacy of cidofovir for the treatment of previously untreated CMV retinitis and the treatment of CMV retinitis that relapsed (progressed) despite prior therapy with other antivirals has been established in several phase 2/3 controlled trials in HIV-infected patients.

In one trial (study 106) in which previously untreated patients with peripheral CMV retinitis received either immediate or delayed (until progression) cidofovir therapy (induction with 5 mg/kg IV once weekly for 2 weeks, then maintenance therapy with 5 mg/kg IV once every other week), the median time to progression of CMV retinitis as evidenced by changes in retinal photographs was 120 or 22 days for the immediate or delayed groups, respectively. However, because of the limited number of patients in the immediate-treatment group who continued to receive cidofovir therapy over time (only 3 of 25 patients received the drug for 120 days or longer), estimates of the median time to progression are imprecise. For alternative indicators of retinal progression or drug discontinuance, the median times for the immediate- and delayed-treatment groups were 52 and 22 days, respectively. Estimates of clinical efficacy from this trial may not be directly comparable to estimates reported for other therapies.

In an open-label, dose-response trial (study 107) in which HIV-infected patients with relapsing CMV retinitis received cidofovir 5 mg/kg IV once weekly for 2 weeks (induction) followed by either 5 or 3 mg/kg IV once every other week (maintenance therapy), the median time to CMV retinitis progression as evidenced by changes in retinal photographs was 115 or 49 days, respectively. For alternative indicators of retinal progression or drug discontinuance, the median times for the 5- and 3-mg/kg maintenance therapy groups were 49 and 35 days, respectively. In this trial, patients had been diagnosed with CMV retinitis approximately 1 year prior to randomization and had undergone a median of 4 prior courses of systemic antiviral therapy (ganciclovir and/or foscarnet) and 20% had received intraocular antiviral therapy active against CMV.

● Mucocutaneous Herpes Simplex Virus Infections

IV cidofovir has been used for the management of mucocutaneous infections caused by acyclovir-resistant herpes simplex virus types 1 and 2† (HSV-1 and HSV-2) in immunocompromised patients, including HIV-infected individuals.

The drugs of choice for the management of orolabial lesions or initial or recurrent genital lesions caused by HSV are valacyclovir, famciclovir, and acyclovir. For the management of mucocutaneous lesions caused by acyclovir-resistant HSV in HIV-infected adults and adolescents†, CDC, NIH, and IDSA recommend IV foscarnet as the drug of choice and state that IV cidofovir is a potential alternative. These experts also recommend IV foscarnet as the drug of choice for the management of acyclovir-resistant HSV infections in HIV-infected children† and state that IV cidofovir is recommended for infections caused by HSV resistant to acyclovir and foscarnet.

Although a topical preparation of cidofovir is not commercially available in the US, the drug has been used topically† for the management of mucocutaneous HSV infections†, including genital herpes†, caused by acyclovir-resistant strains. CDC, NIH, and IDSA suggest that topical cidofovir (extemporaneously prepared) can be considered another option for the treatment of acyclovir-resistant genital herpes†.

● Adenovirus Infections

Although safety and efficacy have not been established and data are limited, cidofovir has been used with some success for the treatment of adenovirus infections† in some immunocompromised patients (e.g., allogeneic hematopoietic stem cell transplant recipients, solid organ transplant recipients).

● Varicella-Zoster Virus Infections

Cidofovir has been recommended as a possible alternative for the management of varicella-zoster virus (VZV) infections†.

The preferred antivirals for the management of acute, localized herpes zoster (shingles) in HIV-infected adults and adolescents are acyclovir, famciclovir, and valacyclovir. For the management of proven or suspected acyclovir-resistant VZV infections† in HIV-infected adults or adolescents, CDC, NIH, and IDSA recommend IV foscarnet and state that IV cidofovir is a possible alternative.

Although optimal regimens for the management of progressive outer retinal necrosis caused by VZV† in HIV-infected individuals have not been identified, CDC, NIH, and IDSA recommend treatment with at least one IV antiviral (acyclovir, ganciclovir, foscarnet, cidofovir) used in conjunction with at least one intravitreal antiviral (ganciclovir or foscarnet). The prognosis for visual preservation in patients with progressive outer retinal necrosis caused by VZV is poor and such infections should be managed in consultation with an ophthalmologist.

● Smallpox

Smallpox Vaccination Complications

Cidofovir is recommended as an alternative for the treatment of certain serious complications of smallpox vaccination†, including eczema vaccinatum, progressive vaccinia, severe generalized vaccinia, and aberrant vaccinia infection caused by inadvertent autoinoculation (if severe because of large numbers of lesions, toxicity, or pain). While cidofovir has antiviral activity against vaccinia virus in vitro and in animal models, safety and efficacy of the drug for the treatment of complications of smallpox vaccination have not been determined and the possible benefits for this use are not known.

Vaccinia immune globulin IV (VIGIV) is considered first-line treatment for serious complications of smallpox vaccination.

If VIGIV alone is inadequate or if VIGIV is not readily available, certain antivirals (e.g., cidofovir, tecovirimat, brincidofovir) may be considered for the treatment of complications of smallpox vaccination after consultation with CDC.

For assistance with diagnosis and management of suspected complications of smallpox vaccination, clinicians should contact their state or local health department or the CDC Emergency Operations Center at 770-488-7100.

Treatment of Smallpox

The role, if any, of cidofovir in the treatment of smallpox† remains to be determined. Cidofovir is active in vitro against poxviruses, including variola virus (the causative agent of smallpox), and has in vivo activity in mice against cowpox and vaccinia virus. Although limited in vitro and in vivo data suggest that cidofovir might prove useful in preventing smallpox infection if administered within 1–2 days after exposure, there is no evidence that the antiviral would be more effective than smallpox vaccination in this early period. Data are not available to date regarding the safety and efficacy of cidofovir for the treatment or prevention of smallpox in humans and it has been suggested that the potential usefulness of the drug for the treatment of smallpox may be limited because of the need for IV administration and potential renal toxicity. The US Working Group on Civilian Biodefense and US Army Medical Research Institute of Infectious Diseases, while acknowledging the potential activity of cidofovir against the virus, state that clinical efficacy in the treatment of smallpox has not been established for any antiviral agent to date.

● Monkeypox

Although no specific treatments are available for monkeypox infection, CDC states that human monkeypox outbreaks can be controlled through use of smallpox vaccine, VIGIV, and certain antivirals (e.g., cidofovir, tecovirimat, brincidofovir). Monkeypox virus is an orthopoxvirus closely related to the causative agent of smallpox.

Efficacy of cidofovir for the treatment of human monkeypox† remains to be established; however, the drug is active in vitro against monkeypox and has in vivo activity against the virus in animal models. While it is not known whether an individual with severe monkeypox infection would benefit from treatment with an antiviral (e.g., cidofovir, brincidofovir), CDC states that use of an antiviral may be considered in such patients.

If an outbreak of human monkeypox occurs in the US, CDC will establish updated guidelines regarding use of smallpox vaccine, VIGIV, or antivirals for treatment of monkeypox infection and/or postexposure prophylaxis of exposed individuals.

DOSAGE AND ADMINISTRATION

● General

Renal function *must* be assessed prior to initiation of cidofovir and monitored during therapy with the drug.

Cidofovir *must* not be initiated in patients with serum creatinine concentration exceeding 1.5 mg/dL, calculated creatinine clearance of 55 mL/minute or less, or urine protein concentration of 100 mg/dL or greater (equivalent to 2+ or greater). (See Renal Impairment under Dosage and Administration: Special Populations.)

Patients *must* receive adequate hydration prior to each dose of cidofovir.

A regimen of oral probenecid *must* be administered concomitantly with each dose of cidofovir.

The recommended dosage of cidofovir and recommended frequency and rate of administration of the drug *must* not be exceeded.

Hydration

To reduce the risk of cidofovir-induced nephrotoxicity, patients should receive at least 1 L of 0.9% sodium chloride infused IV over 1–2 hours immediately before each IV infusion of cidofovir.

For patients who can tolerate additional fluid, an additional 1 L of 0.9% sodium chloride should be administered; this second IV infusion of 0.9% sodium chloride should be initiated either concomitantly with or immediately after the cidofovir IV infusion and should be administered over 1–3 hours.

Volume repletion and maintenance are particularly important in patients with potential volume depletion secondary to conditions such as chronic diarrhea, poor fluid intake, or wasting related to human immunodeficiency virus (HIV) infection.

Concomitant Probenecid

To reduce the risk of cidofovir-induced nephrotoxicity, a regimen of oral probenecid must be administered concomitantly with each dose of cidofovir. Cidofovir undergoes renal tubular secretion, suggesting that use of probenecid may reduce the risk of cidofovir renal toxicity by decreasing concentrations of the drug within proximal tubular cells.

For each dose of cidofovir, the recommended regimen of *oral probenecid* is 2 g given 3 hours prior to initiation of the cidofovir IV infusion, followed by 1-g doses given 2 and 8 hours after completion of the cidofovir IV infusion, for a total *probenecid* dose of 4 g.

To reduce the risk of nausea and/or vomiting associated with oral probenecid, food can be ingested prior to each probenecid dose and concomitant administration of an effective antiemetic can be considered. For patients who develop allergic or other hypersensitivity manifestations with probenecid, appropriate prophylactic or therapeutic use of antihistamines and/or acetaminophen can be considered. Because concomitant probenecid is required, cidofovir is contraindicated in patients with a history of severe hypersensitivity to probenecid or other sulfa-containing drugs since probenecid is contraindicated in such patients.

Because probenecid can affect the pharmacokinetics of many drugs, a careful assessment should be made of other drugs that the patient may be receiving. (See Drug Interactions: Probenecid.)

● Administration

Cidofovir is administered by slow IV infusion using a controlled-infusion device (e.g., pump).

Although cidofovir has been administered by intravitreal injection†, a preparation specifically for intravitreal administration is not commercially available in the US and the manufacturer states that *direct intraocular injection of the currently available IV preparation of cidofovir (even if diluted) is contraindicated since such administration has been associated with iritis, ocular hypotony, and permanent visual impairment.*

Cidofovir has been administered topically† as a gel or cream for the management of certain mucocutaneous viral infections (e.g., acyclovir-resistant herpes simplex virus [HSV] infections). Although topical preparations of cidofovir are not commercially available in the US, a topical gel containing 1% cidofovir has been prepared extemporaneously using the IV preparation of cidofovir.

IV Infusion

Cidofovir *must* be administered using a controlled-infusion device (e.g., pump).

Cidofovir is commercially available as a concentrate for injection containing 75 mg of cidofovir per mL and *must* be diluted prior to IV infusion.

Cidofovir concentrate should appear clear and colorless and should not be used if it appears discolored or contains particles.

Caution should be exercised when preparing, administering, and discarding solutions of cidofovir according to guidelines for handling mutagenic substances. If cidofovir concentrate for injection or a diluted solution of the drug comes in contact with the skin or mucosa, the affected area should be washed immediately and thoroughly with soap and water. Partially used vials of cidofovir and diluted solutions of the drug should be discarded by high temperature incineration.

Dilution

For IV infusion, the appropriate dose of cidofovir concentrate for injection containing 75 mg/mL should be withdrawn from the vial and diluted in 100 mL of 0.9% sodium chloride injection in a compatible infusion container (e.g., PVC, glass, ethylene/propylene copolymer). The entire volume of diluted solution should then be administered by IV infusion.

Diluted solutions of cidofovir should be administered within 24 hours of preparation and should *not* be refrigerated or frozen to extend the storage period beyond this 24-hour limit. However, if a diluted solution will not be used immediately, it may be prepared in advance and refrigerated at 2–8°C for up to 24 hours; the refrigerated diluted solution should be allowed to reach room temperature before administration and should be administered within 24 hours of initial preparation.

Compatibility of cidofovir with Ringer's, lactated Ringer's, or bacteriostatic infusion fluids has not been evaluated.

Rate of Administration

IV infusions of cidofovir should be given at a constant rate over 1 hour using a controlled-infusion device (e.g., pump).

To minimize the risk of nephrotoxicity, the IV dose must *not* be infused over a shorter time period.

● Dosage

Cidofovir is commercially available as the dihydrate; dosage is expressed in terms of anhydrous drug.

Adult Dosage
Cytomegalovirus Retinitis

For the treatment of cytomegalovirus (CMV) retinitis in HIV-infected adults with serum creatinine concentration of 1.5 mg/dL or less, a calculated creatinine clearance exceeding 55 mL/minute, and urine protein concentration less than 100 mg/dL (equivalent to less than 2+), the recommended dosage of IV cidofovir for initial treatment (induction therapy) is 5 mg/kg once weekly for 2 consecutive weeks. In patients with immediate sight-threatening CMV retinal lesions (i.e., within 1.5 mm of the fovea), the US Centers for Disease Control and Prevention (CDC), National Institutes of Health (NIH), and HIV Medicine Association of the Infectious Diseases Society of America (IDSA) recommend that initial treatment also

include an appropriate intravitreal antiviral. (See Cytomegalovirus Retinitis under Uses: Treatment of Cytomegalovirus Infection and Disease.)

After completion of initial treatment, the recommended dosage of IV cidofovir for maintenance therapy (secondary prophylaxis) of CMV retinitis in HIV-infected adults is 5 mg/kg once every 2 weeks (i.e., every other week). If renal function declines during cidofovir therapy, maintenance dosage must be reduced or the drug discontinued depending on the degree of impairment. (See Renal Impairment under Dosage and Administration: Special Populations.)

Decisions regarding discontinuance of maintenance therapy of CMV retinitis in HIV-infected individuals who have been treated for at least 3–6 months, have inactive CMV retinal lesions, and have achieved immune reconstitution as the result of antiretroviral therapy should be made in consultation with an ophthalmologist. (See Cytomegalovirus Retinitis under Uses: Treatment of Cytomegalovirus Infection and Disease.)

Mucocutaneous Herpes Simplex Virus Infections

For the management of mucocutaneous herpes simplex virus type 1 and 2 (HSV-1 and HSV-2) infections† known or suspected to be caused by acyclovir-resistant strains in immunocompromised individuals, including HIV-infected adults, the recommended dosage of IV cidofovir is 5 mg/kg once weekly for a treatment duration of 2–4 weeks or longer until a response is obtained. CDC states that a cidofovir dosage of 5 mg/kg IV once weekly may be effective for the management of acyclovir-resistant genital herpes.

For the topical treatment of mucocutaneous HSV infections†, including genital herpes†, caused by acyclovir-resistant HSV, an extemporaneously prepared gel† containing cidofovir 1% has been applied topically once daily for 5 days. If an extemporaneously prepared gel containing cidofovir 1% is used for the topical treatment of acyclovir-resistant HSV lesions in HIV-infected individuals, a treatment duration of 3–4 weeks or longer is recommended depending on clinical response.

Pediatric Dosage
Cytomegalovirus Retinitis

If cidofovir is used as an alternative for the management of CMV retinitis in HIV-infected adolescents†, CDC, NIH, IDSA, and others recommend initial treatment (induction therapy) with a dosage of 5 mg/kg IV once weekly for 2 consecutive weeks.

After completion of initial treatment, the recommended dosage of cidofovir for maintenance therapy (secondary prophylaxis) in HIV-infected adolescents† is 5 mg/kg IV once every 2 weeks (i.e., every other week). If renal function declines during cidofovir therapy, dosage must be reduced or the drug discontinued depending on the degree of impairment. (See Renal Impairment under Dosage and Administration: Special Populations.)

Decisions regarding discontinuance of maintenance therapy of CMV retinitis in HIV-infected individuals who have been treated for at least 3–6 months, have inactive CMV retinal lesions, and have achieved immune reconstitution as the result of antiretroviral therapy should be made in consultation with an ophthalmologist. (See Cytomegalovirus Retinitis under Uses: Treatment of Cytomegalovirus Infection and Disease.)

Mucocutaneous Herpes Simplex Virus Infections

For the management of mucocutaneous HSV-1 or HSV-2 infections† known or suspected to be caused by acyclovir-resistant strains in HIV-infected adolescents†, the recommended dosage of cidofovir is 5 mg/kg IV once weekly for a treatment duration of 2–4 weeks or longer until a response is obtained.

For the topical treatment of mucocutaneous HSV infections†, including genital herpes†, caused by acyclovir-resistant HSV, an extemporaneously prepared gel† containing cidofovir 1% has been applied topically once daily for 5 days. If an extemporaneously prepared gel containing cidofovir 1% is used for the topical treatment of acyclovir-resistant HSV lesions in HIV-infected individuals, a treatment duration of 3–4 weeks or longer is recommended depending on clinical response.

● Special Populations
Hepatic Impairment

The manufacturer makes no specific dosage recommendation for use of cidofovir in patients with hepatic impairment; the effect of hepatic impairment on the pharmacokinetics of the drug has not been evaluated to date.

Renal Impairment

Initiation of cidofovir is contraindicated in patients with serum creatinine concentration exceeding 1.5 mg/dL, calculated creatinine clearance of 55 mL/minute or less, or urine protein concentration of 100 mg/dL or greater (equivalent to proteinuria of 2+ or greater).

If serum creatinine concentration increases by 0.3–0.4 mg/dL above baseline during cidofovir therapy, the dose must be reduced to 3 mg/kg. If this occurs in HIV-infected adults or adolescents† receiving cidofovir for maintenance therapy (secondary prophylaxis) of CMV retinitis, dosage of the drug should be reduced to 3 mg/kg once every 2 weeks (i.e., every other week).

If serum creatinine concentration increases by 0.5 mg/dL or more above baseline or if proteinuria of 3+ or greater develops, cidofovir *must* be discontinued.

Patients who develop 2+ proteinuria in the face of a stable serum creatinine during cidofovir therapy should be observed carefully (including close monitoring of serum creatinine and urinary protein) to detect potential deterioration that would warrant dose reduction or discontinuance of the drug.

Geriatric Patients

Dosage of cidofovir for geriatric patients should be selected with caution because of age-related decreases in renal function. (See Geriatric Use under Warnings/Precautions: Specific Populations, in Cautions.)

CAUTIONS

● *Contraindications*

Initiation of cidofovir is contraindicated in patients with serum creatinine concentration exceeding 1.5 mg/dL, calculated creatinine clearance of 55 mL/minute or less, or urine protein concentration of 100 mg/dL or greater (equivalent to proteinuria of 2+ or greater).

Cidofovir is contraindicated in patients receiving other drugs with nephrotoxic potential. (See Drug Interactions: Nephrotoxic Drugs.)

Cidofovir is contraindicated in patients hypersensitive to the drug. Cidofovir also is contraindicated in patients with a history of clinically severe hypersensitivity to probenecid or other sulfa-containing drugs since an oral probenecid regimen *must* be given in conjunction with each cidofovir dose.

Direct intraocular injection of cidofovir is contraindicated; intraocular injection of the drug has been associated with iritis, ocular hypotony, and permanent vision impairment.

● *Warnings/Precautions*

Warnings

Renal Effects

Dose-dependent nephrotoxicity is the major dose-limiting toxicity associated with cidofovir. In clinical trials in patients with cytomegalovirus (CMV) retinitis, renal toxicity (manifested by an increase in serum creatinine concentration of 0.4 mg/dL or greater, decrease in creatinine clearance to 55 mL/minute or less, or proteinuria of 2+ or greater) occurred in 59% of patients receiving cidofovir at the recommended maintenance dosage of 5 mg/kg IV every other week.

There have been reports of severe renal impairment in patients receiving the drug, including acute renal failure resulting in dialysis and/or contributing to death, in patients who received as few as 1 or 2 doses of cidofovir. In some patients, there were associated risk factors for nephrotoxicity, such as preexisting mild renal insufficiency or cidofovir administration proximal to completion of aminoglycoside therapy in a patient with preexisting normal serum creatinine concentrations. In some patients, renal function failed to return to baseline following discontinuance of cidofovir therapy.

Proteinuria may be an early sign of cidofovir-induced nephrotoxicity. In patients who develop proteinuria during cidofovir therapy, the manufacturer recommends that IV hydration be administered and the test repeated. If renal function deteriorates during cidofovir therapy, dosage reduction or discontinuance of the drug may be required. (See Renal Impairment under Dosage and Administration: Special Populations.) Continued administration of cidofovir may lead to additional proximal tubular cell injury, which may result in glycosuria; decreases

in serum phosphate, uric acid, and bicarbonate concentrations; increases in serum creatinine concentrations; and/or acute renal failure which may require dialysis.

A diagnosis of Fanconi syndrome, manifested as multiple abnormalities of proximal renal tubular function, has been reported in 1% of patients receiving cidofovir. (See Metabolic Acidosis under Warnings/Precautions: Other Warnings and Precautions, in Cautions.)

To reduce the risk of nephrotoxicity, IV hydration with 0.9% sodium chloride injection is required prior to administration of each cidofovir dose and a regimen of oral probenecid is required with each cidofovir dose. (See Dosage and Administration: General.) In addition, concomitant use of cidofovir and potentially nephrotoxic drugs is contraindicated and at least 7 days should elapse between discontinuance of such drugs and administration of cidofovir. (See Drug Interactions: Nephrotoxic Drugs.)

Prior to initiation of cidofovir therapy, renal function *must* be assessed. The drug is contraindicated and should *not* be initiated in patients with serum creatinine concentration exceeding 1.5 mg/dL, calculated creatinine clearance of 55 mL/minute or less, or urine protein concentration of 100 mg/dL or greater (equivalent to proteinuria of 2+ or greater). Because serum creatinine concentrations may not provide an accurate assessment of renal function in patients with severe acquired immunodeficiency deficiency syndrome (AIDS) and CMV retinitis, Cockcroft-Gault calculations should be used *initially* to estimate creatinine clearance more precisely when determining the eligibility of such patients to receive cidofovir; for subsequent assessments, serum creatinine and *not* Cockcroft-Gault calculations of creatinine clearance should be used.

During cidofovir therapy, renal function (i.e., serum creatinine concentration and urine protein) *must* be determined within 48 hours prior to *each* dose of cidofovir, and the cidofovir dose should be adjusted or withheld as appropriate based on any changes in renal function. (See Renal Impairment under Dosage and Administration: Special Populations.)

Hematologic Effects

Neutropenia may occur during cidofovir therapy. In clinical trials in patients with CMV retinitis, neutropenia (500/mm³ or less) occurred in 24% of patients receiving recommended maintenance dosages of cidofovir; 39% of these patients received treatment with filgrastim (G-CSF).

Neutrophil counts should be monitored during cidofovir therapy.

Carcinogenic and Mutagenic Potential

Cidofovir should be considered a potential carcinogen in humans. In animal studies, the drug was carcinogenic and mutagenic.

In rats receiving cidofovir by subscapular subcutaneous injection, mammary adenocarcinomas were observed in the females at dosages as low as 0.6 mg/kg once weekly (equivalent to 0.04 times the human systemic exposure achieved at recommended IV dosages); the first mass was detected after 6 doses of cidofovir. In another study in rats receiving IV cidofovir, mammary adenocarcinomas were observed in females and Zymbal gland carcinomas were observed in males and females at a dosage of 15 mg/kg once weekly (equivalent to 1.1 times the human systemic exposure achieved at recommended IV dosages).

In mutagenicity studies in mice, an increase in micronucleated polychromatic erythrocytes was seen at cidofovir dosages of 2 g/kg or greater (equivalent to approximately 65 times the maximum recommended human IV dose). Cidofovir has induced chromosomal aberrations in human peripheral blood lymphocytes in vitro without metabolic activation, but there was no evidence of mutagenicity in microbial mutagenicity assays involving *Salmonella typhimurium* (Ames) and *Escherichia coli* in the presence and absence of metabolic activation.

Effects on Fertility

Cidofovir has caused reduced testes weight and hypospermia in animals and it is possible that such effects could occur in humans and cause infertility.

Although cidofovir caused inhibition of spermatogenesis in rats and monkeys, no adverse effects on fertility or reproduction were observed in male rats receiving IV cidofovir at dosages up to 15 mg/kg once weekly (equivalent to 1.1 times the recommended human dosage) for 13 consecutive weeks.

In female rats receiving IV cidofovir at a dosage of 1.2 mg/kg once weekly (equivalent to 0.09 times the recommended human dosages) for up to 6 weeks prior to mating and for 2 weeks after mating, decreased litter size, decreased live births per litter, and increased early resorptions per litter were observed. In peri- and postnatal development studies in female rats receiving subcutaneous injections of cidofovir at dosages up to 1 mg/kg daily from day 7 of gestation through day 21 postpartum (approximately 5 weeks), there were no observed adverse effects on viability, growth, behavior, sexual maturation, or reproductive capacity in the offspring.

Women of childbearing potential and men should be advised to use an effective method of contraception during cidofovir therapy and for certain periods of time after the drug is discontinued. (See Pregnancy under Warnings/Precautions: Specific Populations, in Cautions.)

Selection and Use of Antivirals

Cidofovir is labeled by the FDA *only* for the treatment of CMV retinitis in patients with human immunodeficiency virus (HIV) infection, including those with AIDS.

Safety and efficacy of the drug have not been established for the treatment of other CMV infections or for the treatment of CMV disease in individuals not infected with HIV.

Other Warnings and Precautions
Administration Precautions

Cidofovir should be administered *only* by IV infusion. The commercially available IV preparation of the drug must *not* be administered by intraocular injection because iritis, ocular hypotony, and permanent visual impairment have been reported when this route was used.

Patients *must* receive IV hydration prior to each cidofovir dose and *must* receive a regimen of oral probenecid concomitantly with each cidofovir dose. (See Dosage and Administration: General.)

Because of the potential for nephrotoxicity, the recommended cidofovir dosage, frequency, and rate of administration *must* not be exceeded. (See Dosage and Administration.)

Ophthalmologic Effects

Decreased intraocular pressure (IOP) may occur during cidofovir therapy. In some cases, decreased IOP has been associated with decreased visual acuity. Among patients in clinical trials who received IV cidofovir doses of 5 mg/kg for maintenance therapy of CMV retinitis and whose IOP was monitored, 24% experienced at least a 50% decrease in IOP from baseline and severe hypotony (i.e., IOP of 0–1 mm Hg) was reported in 3 patients. The risk of ocular hypotony may be increased in patients with preexisting diabetes mellitus.

Uveitis or iritis has been reported in patients in clinical trials receiving IV cidofovir for the treatment of CMV retinitis. Among those receiving IV cidofovir maintenance therapy of CMV retinitis, uveitis or iritis was reported in 11%.

Patients receiving cidofovir should receive periodic ophthalmic examinations to monitor IOP and visual acuity and to monitor for symptoms of uveitis or iritis.

If anterior uveitis or iritis develops, appropriate therapy (e.g., topical corticosteroids with or without cycloplegic therapy) should be considered as indicated.

Metabolic Acidosis

Decreased serum bicarbonate associated with proximal tubule injury and renal wasting syndrome (including Fanconi syndrome) has been reported in patients receiving cidofovir. Decreased serum bicarbonate concentration (16 mEq/L or less) has been reported in 16% of cidofovir-treated patients.

Fatal cases of metabolic acidosis in association with liver dysfunction and pancreatitis have been reported in patients receiving cidofovir.

Specific Populations
Pregnancy

There are no adequate and well-controlled studies to date using cidofovir in pregnant women. Cidofovir should be used during pregnancy only if potential benefits justify potential risks to the fetus.

In animal studies, embryotoxicity (reduced fetal body weights) and maternal toxicity were observed in rats and rabbits receiving IV cidofovir at dosages of 1.5 and 1 mg/kg daily, respectively, during organogenesis. In rabbits receiving IV cidofovir in a dosage of 1 mg/kg daily, maternal toxicity and an increased

incidence of fetal external, soft tissue, and skeletal anomalies (meningocele, short snout, and short maxillary bones) were observed.

Women of childbearing potential should be informed that cidofovir is embryotoxic in animals and should be advised to use an effective method of contraception during and for at least 1 month after cidofovir therapy.

Men should be advised to use a reliable method of barrier contraception during and for at least 3 months after cidofovir therapy.

Lactation

It is not known whether cidofovir is distributed into human milk.

Since there is a potential for adverse effects in nursing infants and because carcinogenicity has been shown in animal studies, cidofovir should not be used in breast-feeding women.

Because of the risk of adverse effects in the infant and the risk of HIV transmission, HIV-infected women should not breast-feed infants.

Pediatric Use

Safety and efficacy of cidofovir have not been established in pediatric patients younger than 18 years of age.

Because of the risks of potential long-term carcinogenic and reproductive toxicity, cidofovir should be used with extreme caution in children† with AIDS. The manufacturer states that the drug should be used in children *only* after careful evaluation and *only* when potential benefits outweigh risks.

Some experts state that cidofovir has not been studied in children with CMV disease, but can be considered for the management of CMV retinitis in HIV-infected children† if other options cannot be used.

Geriatric Use

Safety and efficacy of cidofovir have not been evaluated in geriatric patients older than 60 years of age.

Because geriatric patients frequently have reduced glomerular filtration, particular attention should be paid to monitoring renal function prior to and during cidofovir therapy in this age group, and dosage should be modified in response to changes in renal function. (See Renal Impairment under Dosage and Administration: Special Populations.)

Renal Impairment

Initiation of cidofovir is contraindicated in patients with serum creatinine concentration exceeding 1.5 mg/dL, calculated creatinine clearance of 55 mL/minute or less, or urine protein concentration of 100 mg/dL or greater (equivalent to proteinuria of 2+ or greater).

Pharmacokinetic data in individuals with renal impairment (creatinine clearance as low as 11 mL/minute) indicate that cidofovir clearance decreases proportionally with creatinine clearance.

High-flux hemodialysis reduces serum cidofovir concentrations by approximately 75%.

● Common Adverse Effects

Adverse effects reported in 15% or more of patients receiving cidofovir (with concomitant probenecid regimen) include nephrotoxicity (proteinuria, elevated serum creatinine), nausea and/or vomiting, fever, neutropenia, asthenia, headache, rash, infection, alopecia, diarrhea, pain, anemia, decreased IOP, anorexia, dyspnea, chills, increased cough, oral moniliasis, and decreased serum bicarbonate.

DRUG INTERACTIONS

● Nephrotoxic Drugs

Concomitant use of cidofovir and nephrotoxic drugs (e.g., aminoglycosides [amikacin, gentamicin, tobramycin], amphotericin B, foscarnet, nonsteroidal anti-inflammatory agents, IV pentamidine, vancomycin) may increase the risk of nephrotoxicity and is contraindicated. Such drugs *must* be discontinued at least 7 days prior to initiating cidofovir therapy.

● *Foscarnet*

Concomitant use of foscarnet and cidofovir is contraindicated. Foscarnet must be discontinued at least 7 days prior to initiating cidofovir therapy. In addition, because the risk of cidofovir-associated nephrotoxicity is increased in patients who previously received foscarnet, such patients must be monitored closely after cidofovir is initiated.

● *Probenecid*

Concomitant use of probenecid and cidofovir decreases renal clearance of cidofovir to a level consistent with creatinine clearance, suggesting that probenecid blocks active renal tubular secretion of cidofovir. This pharmacokinetic interaction is used to therapeutic advantage to reduce the risk of cidofovir-associated nephrotoxicity.

Because a regimen of oral probenecid *must* be administered with each dose of cidofovir (see Concomitant Probenecid under Dosage and Administration: General), drug interactions reported for probenecid must also be considered in patients receiving cidofovir. Probenecid interacts with the metabolism or renal tubular excretion of many drugs (e.g., acetaminophen, acyclovir, angiotensin-converting enzyme inhibitors, aminosalicylic acid, barbiturates, benzodiazepines, bumetanide, famotidine, furosemide, methotrexate, nonsteroidal anti-inflammatory agents, theophylline, zidovudine).

● *Zidovudine*

Although concomitant use of cidofovir (without probenecid) and zidovudine does not affect zidovudine pharmacokinetics, probenecid reduces metabolic clearance of zidovudine.

Patients receiving zidovudine may continue taking the antiretroviral agent while receiving cidofovir therapy. However, on the days that the patient receives a dose of cidofovir, zidovudine should be temporarily discontinued or, alternatively, the zidovudine dosage should be reduced by 50% because the probenecid regimen used concomitantly with the cidofovir dose can increase zidovudine concentrations.

DESCRIPTION

Cidofovir, an acyclic nucleotide analog of cytosine (acyclic nucleoside phosphonate), is an antiviral agent.

Cidofovir is a prodrug and exhibits no antiviral activity until converted intracellularly to the active metabolite, cidofovir diphosphate. Unlike other nucleoside and nucleotide antivirals that require conversion within viral cells to an active metabolite (e.g., acyclovir, ganciclovir), the presence of the phosphonate group in cidofovir is believed to account for the drug's ability to become phosphorylated by cellular (host cell) enzymes to its active intracellular metabolite without initial virus-dependent phosphorylation by viral nucleoside kinases.

Cidofovir is converted intracellularly by pyrimidine nucleoside monophosphate kinase to cidofovir monophosphate, which is further converted to the diphosphate and cidofovir phosphate-choline via other cellular enzymes. Cidofovir diphosphate is a viral DNA polymerase inhibitor and exerts its antiviral effects by interfering with DNA synthesis and inhibiting viral replication. Cidofovir diphosphate stops replication of viral DNA by competitive inhibition of viral DNA polymerase (an enzyme encoded by CMV UL54 gene), incorporation and termination of the growing viral DNA chain, and inactivation of the viral DNA polymerase. The inhibitory activity of cidofovir diphosphate is highly selective because of its greater affinity for viral DNA polymerases than for human DNA polymerases.

The pharmacokinetics of IV cidofovir have been evaluated in patients with human immunodeficiency virus (HIV) infection when the drug was given with or without a regimen of oral probenecid. In patients with normal renal function, approximately 80–100% of a dose of IV cidofovir (without oral probenecid) was recovered unchanged in urine within 24 hours. Renal clearance of cidofovir (without oral probenecid) is greater than creatinine clearance, indicating that renal tubular secretion contributes to cidofovir elimination. Following IV administration of cidofovir (with oral probenecid regimen), approximately 70–85% of the dose was excreted unchanged in urine within 24 hours. Renal clearance of cidofovir (with oral probenecid regimen) is consistent with creatinine clearance, indicating that probenecid blocks renal tubular secretion of cidofovir. This effect of probenecid on the pharmacokinetics of cidofovir is used to therapeutic advantage, and a regimen of oral probenecid must be given with each dose of cidofovir. (See Concomitant Probenecid under Dosage and Administration: General.) In vitro studies indicate that cidofovir is less than 6% bound to plasma or serum proteins. In one patient who received a single cidofovir dose of 5 mg/kg by IV infusion over 1 hour (with IV prehydration and concomitant oral probenecid regimen), cidofovir serum concentrations were 8.7 mcg/mL at 15 minutes after completion of the infusion and the drug was undetectable in CSF.

● *Spectrum*

Following intracellular conversion of cidofovir to the pharmacologically active diphosphate metabolite, the drug has in vitro and in vivo inhibitory activity against human herpesviruses, including cytomegalovirus (CMV), herpes simplex virus types 1 and 2 (HSV-1 and HSV-2), varicella-zoster virus (VZV), and Epstein-Barr virus (EBV). The drug also has in vitro activity against adenovirus, human papillomavirus (HPV), and human polyomavirus.

Cidofovir has in vitro activity against poxviruses, including vaccinia virus (cowpox), monkeypox, and variola virus (the causative agent of smallpox). Studies in mice indicate that cidofovir has in vivo activity against vaccinia virus. In vivo activity against monkeypox has been demonstrated in animal models.

Because of the drug's ability to become phosphorylated to its active metabolite without dependence on virally encoded kinases, cidofovir has been shown to exert its antiviral effect on acyclovir-resistant strains of HSV and ganciclovir-resistant strains of CMV. Cidofovir has been shown to exhibit greater in vitro activity against CMV than ganciclovir. In vitro and in vivo studies indicate that cidofovir diphosphate has an extended intracellular half-life, which may result in the drug's ability to exert a prolonged antiviral effect, and activation to the diphosphate by cellular rather than virally encoded enzymes as well as the extended intracellular half-life offer protection against subsequent viral infection in uninfected cells.

● *Resistance*

CMV isolates with reduced susceptibility to cidofovir have been selected in vitro in the presence of high concentrations of the drug, and the possibility of cidofovir-resistant CMV should be considered in patients with CMV retinitis who fail to respond to cidofovir or experience recurrent CMV retinitis progression during therapy with the drug.

Some cidofovir-resistant CMV isolates selected in vitro following exposure to increasing concentrations of cidofovir have been cross-resistant to ganciclovir, but remained susceptible to foscarnet. Ganciclovir-resistant or ganciclovir- and foscarnet-resistant isolates that were cross-resistant to cidofovir have been obtained from drug-naive patients and patients who were treated with ganciclovir with or without foscarnet. Although CMV strains with ganciclovir-resistance caused by mutations in DNA polymerase (UL54) are likely to be cross-resistant to cidofovir, strains with ganciclovir resistance secondary only to mutations in CMV UL97 may remain susceptible to cidofovir. Clinical isolates exhibiting high-level resistance to ganciclovir due to mutations in both CMV UL54 and UL97 have been cross-resistant to cidofovir. Cidofovir is active in vitro against some, but not all, CMV isolates resistant to foscarnet.

ADVICE TO PATIENTS

Advise patients that cidofovir is not a cure for cytomegalovirus (CMV) retinitis; progression of retinitis may continue during or following treatment. Advise patients that regular ophthalmologic examinations are necessary. Other manifestations of CMV disease may also occur.

Advise patients with human immunodeficiency virus (HIV) infection who are receiving zidovudine to temporarily discontinue zidovudine or decrease the zidovudine dose by 50% on days cidofovir is administered because the probenecid regimen used with each cidofovir dose reduces metabolic clearance of zidovudine.

Inform patients that the major toxicity of cidofovir is renal impairment; dosage modifications, including reduction, interruption, and, possibly, discontinuance of the drug may be required. Importance of close monitoring of renal function (routine urinalysis, serum creatinine) during cidofovir therapy.

Importance of receiving IV hydration prior to each cidofovir dose and importance of taking the recommended regimen of oral probenecid with each cidofovir dose to minimize the risk of cidofovir-associated nephrotoxicity.

Inform patients of possible adverse effects associated with the probenecid regimen, including headache, nausea, vomiting, and hypersensitivity reactions (e.g., rash, fever, chills, anaphylaxis). Advise patients that taking probenecid after a meal or concomitant use of an antiemetic may decrease nausea; antihistamines and/or acetaminophen can be used to ameliorate hypersensitivity reactions.

Inform patients that cidofovir has caused tumors (principally mammary adenocarcinomas) in rats and that the drug should be considered a potential carcinogen in humans.

Inform patients that cidofovir has caused reduced testes weight and hypospermia in animals and such effects may occur in humans and cause infertility.

Importance of informing clinician of existing or contemplated concomitant therapy, including prescription and OTC drugs, as well as any concomitant illnesses.

Importance of women informing clinicians if they are or plan to become pregnant or plan to breast-feed. Inform women of childbearing potential that cidofovir is embryotoxic in animals and should not be used during pregnancy.

Advise women of childbearing potential to use effective contraception during and for 1 month after cidofovir therapy. Advise men to practice barrier contraceptive methods during and for 3 months after cidofovir treatment.

Importance of advising patients of other important precautionary information. (See Cautions.)

PREPARATIONS

For the treatment of serious complications of smallpox vaccination† or the treatment of human monkeypox†, cidofovir is stored in the US Strategic National Stockpile (SNS). The SNS ensures that certain drugs and medical supplies are readily available to prevent or treat specific diseases, including during public health emergencies, and is managed by the US Department of Health and Human Services (HHS) Office of the Assistant Secretary for Preparedness and Response (ASPR). To request a drug from the SNS, state health departments can contact the US Centers for Disease Control and Prevention (CDC) Emergency Operations Center at 770-488-7100 or the HHS Secretary's Operations Center at 202-619-7800.

Excipients in commercially available drug preparations may have clinically important effects in some individuals; consult specific product labeling for details.

Cidofovir

Parenteral

Concentrate, for injection, for IV infusion only	75 mg (of anhydrous cidofovir) per mL*	Cidofovir Injection

* available from one or more manufacturer, distributor, and/or repackager by generic (nonproprietary) name

† Use is not currently included in the labeling approved by the US Food and Drug Administration.

Selected Revisions August 19, 2019, © Copyright, January 1, 1997, American Society of Health-System Pharmacists, Inc.

Entecavir

8:18.32 • NUCLEOSIDES AND NUCLEOTIDES

■ Entecavir, a synthetic purine nucleoside analog derived from guanine, is an antiviral agent that is active against human hepatitis B virus (HBV).

USES

● Chronic Hepatitis B Virus Infection

Entecavir is used for the treatment of chronic hepatitis B virus (HBV) infection in adult and pediatric patients 2 years of age and older with evidence of active HBV replication and either persistent elevations in serum aminotransferase (ALT or AST) concentrations or histologic evidence of active disease.

Clinical Experience

The indication for use of entecavir in adults is based on clinical trial data in adults and adolescents 16 years of age or older with hepatitis B e antigen (HBeAg)-positive or HBeAg-negative chronic HBV infection with compensated liver disease who were nucleoside-inhibitor-naïve (had not previously received treatment with nucleoside antivirals) or had lamivudine-refractory HBV; although most study patients had compensated liver disease, a limited number had decompensated liver disease. The indication for use of the drug in pediatric patients is based on clinical trial data in nucleoside-naïve pediatric patients 2 years of age and older and in a limited number of lamivudine-experienced patients with HBeAg-positive chronic HBV infection and compensated liver disease.

Entecavir has not been evaluated for the treatment of chronic HBV infection in patients with human immunodeficiency virus (HIV) coinfection who were not receiving antiretroviral therapy; the drug should *not* be used for the treatment of HBV infection in such patients.

Only limited data are available regarding the efficacy and safety of entecavir for the treatment of HBV infection in liver transplant recipients.

HBeAg-positive Adults

Efficacy of entecavir for the management of HBeAg-positive chronic HBV infection was evaluated in a phase III, randomized, double-blind, active-controlled study (AI463022) in nucleoside-inhibitor-naïve adults with active HBV replication (median baseline serum HBV DNA levels 9.66 $\log_{10}$ copies/mL), persistent elevations in serum ALT concentrations (mean serum ALT of 143 IU/L), and histologic evidence of active liver disease (mean Knodell necroinflammatory score of 7.8). Seventy-five percent of patients in the study were male, 57% were Asian, 40% were white, and 13% had prior treatment with interferon alfa.

Data analysis at 48 weeks indicated that 72% of patients who received entecavir in a dosage of 0.5 mg daily had histologic improvement (defined as a reduction of at least 2 points in the Knodell necroinflammatory score with no concurrent worsening of the Knodell fibrosis score) compared with 62% of those who received lamivudine in a dosage of 100 mg daily. Sixty-eight percent of patients receiving entecavir (0.5 mg daily) had normal serum ALT concentrations (i.e., biochemical response) at week 48 compared with 60% of those receiving lamivudine (100 mg daily). In addition, the mean decrease in serum HBV DNA levels from baseline was 6.86 $\log_{10}$ copies/mL at week 48 in those receiving entecavir compared with a decrease of 5.39 $\log_{10}$ copies/mL in those receiving lamivudine. Sixty-seven percent of patients who received entecavir had undetectable levels of serum HBV DNA (defined as <300 copies/mL by a polymerase chain reaction [PCR] assay) at week 48 compared with 36% of those who received lamivudine. Seroconversion to anti-HBe also occurred in 21 or 18% of patients who received entecavir or lamivudine, respectively. The optimal duration of therapy with entecavir is not known. According to the study protocol, patients who met the response criteria (determined at 48 weeks based on HBV virologic suppression [less than 0.7 MEq/mL by bDNA assay] and loss of HBeAg [in HBeAg-positive patients] or ALT normalization [less than 1.25 times the upper limit of normal in HBeAg-negative patients]) discontinued therapy at week 52 while patients who did not meet the response criteria

continued treatment through week 96 or until they met the response criteria. Twenty-one percent of patients treated with entecavir who met the response criteria discontinued entecavir at 52 weeks per protocol; 82% of these patients maintained such a response during an additional 24 weeks of post-treatment follow-up. Approximately 69% of patients treated with entecavir continued treatment for up to 96 weeks; 74% of these patients had undetectable levels of serum HBV DNA after the last dose of the drug and 79% had normal ALT concentrations. Seroconversion to anti-HBe occurred in 11% of patients receiving entecavir.

HBeAg-negative Adults

Efficacy of entecavir for the management of HBeAg-negative, anti-HBe- and HBV-DNA-positive chronic HBV infection was evaluated in a phase III, randomized, double-blind, active-controlled study (AI463027) in nucleoside-inhibitor-naïve adults with active HBV replication (median baseline serum HBV DNA levels 7.58 $\log_{10}$ copies/mL by a PCR-based assay), persistent elevations in serum ALT concentrations (mean serum ALT of 142 IU/L), and histologic evidence of active liver disease (mean Knodell necroinflammatory score of 7.8). Seventy-six percent of patients in the study were male, 58% were white, 39% were Asian, and 13% had prior treatment with interferon alfa.

Data analysis at 48 weeks indicated that 70% of patients who received entecavir (0.5 mg daily) had histologic improvement (defined as a reduction of at least 2 points in the Knodell necroinflammatory score with no concurrent worsening of the Knodell fibrosis score) compared with 61% of those who received lamivudine (100 mg daily). Serum ALT concentrations also normalized at week 48 in 78% of patients who received entecavir compared with 71% of those who received lamivudine. In addition, the mean decrease in serum HBV DNA levels from baseline was 5.04 $\log_{10}$ copies/mL at week 48 in patients receiving entecavir compared with a mean decrease of 4.53 $\log_{10}$ copies/mL in those receiving lamivudine. Ninety percent of patients who received entecavir had undetectable levels of serum HBV DNA (defined as <300 copies/mL by PCR assay) at week 48 compared with 72% of those who received lamivudine. Eighty-five percent of patients treated with entecavir met the response criteria (determined at 48 weeks based on HBV virologic suppression [less than 0.7 MEq/mL by bDNA assay] and loss of HBeAg) and discontinued entecavir at 52 weeks per protocol; very few of these patients had undetectable levels of serum HBV DNA and 46% of patients maintained normal ALT concentrations during an additional 24 weeks of follow-up.

Adults with Lamivudine-refractory HBV

Entecavir was evaluated for the treatment of lamivudine-refractory chronic HBV infection in a phase III, randomized, double-blind, active-controlled study (AI463026) in adults with active HBV replication (median baseline serum HBV DNA levels 9.36 $\log_{10}$ copies/mL), persistent elevations in serum ALT concentrations (mean serum ALT of 128 IU/L), and histologic evidence of compensated liver disease (mean Knodell necroinflammatory score of 6.5). Seventy-six percent of patients in the study were male, 37% were Asian, 62% were white, and 52% had prior treatment with interferon alfa.

Patients in the study had previously received lamivudine therapy for a mean duration of 2.7 years and lamivudine-resistant mutations were identified at baseline in 85% of patients. Patients were randomized to switch (without a washout or an overlap period) from lamivudine to entecavir (1 mg daily) or to continue lamivudine (100 mg daily) for 52 weeks. Data analysis at 48 weeks indicated that 55% of patients switched to entecavir had histologic improvement (defined as a reduction of at least 2 points in the Knodell necroinflammatory score with no concurrent worsening of the Knodell fibrosis score) compared with 28% of those who continued to receive lamivudine. Sixty-one percent of patients receiving entecavir had normal serum ALT concentrations (i.e., biochemical response) at week 48 compared with 15% of those receiving lamivudine. In addition, the mean decrease in serum HBV DNA levels from baseline was 5.11 $\log_{10}$ copies/mL at week 48 in those receiving entecavir compared with a decrease of 0.48 $\log_{10}$ copies/mL in those receiving lamivudine. Nineteen percent of patients who received entecavir had undetectable levels of serum HBV DNA (defined as <300 copies/mL by PCR assay) at week 48 compared with 1% of those who received lamivudine. Seroconversion to anti-HBe occurred in 8 or 3% of patients who received entecavir or lamivudine, respectively. Approximately 55% of patients treated with entecavir continued treatment for up to 96 weeks; 40% of these patients had undetectable levels of serum HBV DNA, 81% had normal ALT concentrations, and 10% achieved seroconversion.

Adults with Decompensated Liver Disease

Entecavir was evaluated for the treatment of chronic HBV infection in patients with decompensated liver disease in a randomized, open-label study (AI463048). The study included 191 adults with HBeAg-positive or HBeAg-negative chronic HBV infection and evidence of hepatic decompensation (Child-Turcotte-Pugh score of 7 or higher); mean age 52 years, 74% male, 54% Asian, 33% white, 5% Black, baseline HBV DNA levels 7.83 $\log_{10}$ copies/mL, mean ALT concentration 100 U/L, 54% HBeAg-positive, 35% with evidence of lamivudine resistance, baseline mean Child-Turcotte-Pugh score 8.6. Patients were randomized to receive entecavir 1 mg once daily or adefovir dipivoxil 10 mg once daily. At 48 weeks, 57 or 20% of patients receiving entecavir or adefovir dipivoxil, respectively, achieved undetectable levels of HBV DNA (<300 copies/mL [the lower limit of quantification]) and 61 or 67% of patients, respectively, had stable or improved Child-Turcotte-Pugh scores.

HBeAg-positive Pediatric Patients

Efficacy, safety, and pharmacokinetics of entecavir in pediatric patients were initially evaluated in 43 pediatric patients 2 years to less than 18 years of age with chronic HBV infection (HBeAg-positive) with compensated liver disease and elevated ALT concentration (Study AI463028); 24 patients were treatment-naïve and 19 patients were previously treated with lamivudine (lamivudine-experienced). Nucleoside-naïve (had not previously received treatment with nucleoside antivirals) patients received entecavir in a dosage of 0.015 mg/kg (up to 0.5 mg) once daily and lamivudine-experienced patients received 0.03 mg/kg (up to 1 mg) once daily. At 48 weeks, 58 or 47% of treatment-naïve or lamivudine-experienced patients, respectively, achieved HBV DNA levels <50 IU/mL; ALT concentrations normalized in 83 or 95% of patients, respectively.

Efficacy of entecavir in pediatric patients was confirmed in a randomized, placebo-controlled, double-blind study (AI463189) in 180 pediatric patients 2 years to less than 18 years of age who were nucleoside-naïve with HBeAg-positive chronic HBV infection, compensated liver disease, and elevated ALT concentrations (mean HBV DNA levels 8.1 $\log_{10}$ IU/mL, mean ALT concentrations 103 U/L). Patients were randomized in a 2:1 ratio to receive entecavir in a dosage of 0.015 mg/kg (up to 0.5 mg) once daily or placebo. At 48 weeks, 24% of patients receiving entecavir met the composite primary efficacy end point of HBeAg seroconversion *and* serum HBV DNA levels <50 IU/mL. An HBV DNA level <50 IU/mL was achieved in 46 or 2% of patients receiving entecavir or placebo, respectively; ALT normalization and HBeAg seroconversion were attained in 67 or 24%, respectively, of patients receiving entecavir compared with 22 or 12%, respectively, of patients receiving placebo.

HBV-infected Individuals Coinfected with HIV

Efficacy of entecavir for the treatment of chronic HBV infection in HIV-infected patients was evaluated in a phase III, randomized, double-blind, active-controlled study (AI463038) in patients receiving highly active antiretroviral therapy (HAART) that included lamivudine. These HIV-infected patients had recurrent HBV viremia (99% were HBeAg-positive), active HBV replication (median baseline serum HBV DNA levels 9.13 $\log_{10}$ copies/mL), and persistent elevations in serum ALT concentrations (mean serum ALT of 71.5 IU/L). Patients continued HAART (including lamivudine 300 mg daily) and were randomized to receive concurrent therapy with entecavir (1 mg daily) or placebo for 24 weeks followed by an additional 24-week open-label period during which all patients received entecavir (1 mg daily).

Analysis of limited data at 24 weeks indicated that 6% of patients who received entecavir in conjunction with lamivudine-containing HAART had undetectable levels of serum HBV DNA (defined as <300 copies/mL by PCR assay) compared with 0% of those who received placebo and lamivudine-containing HAART. Thirty-four percent of patients receiving the regimen that included entecavir had normal serum ALT concentrations (i.e., biochemical response) at week 24 compared with 8% of those who did not receive entecavir. In addition, the mean decrease in serum HBV DNA levels from baseline was 3.65 $\log_{10}$ copies/mL at week 24 in those receiving the regimen that included entecavir compared with an increase of 0.11 $\log_{10}$ copies/mL in those receiving a lamivudine-containing HAART regimen alone. Median serum HIV-1 RNA levels remained stable at approximately 2 $\log_{10}$/mL during the 24-week blinded study period.

Entecavir should *not* be used for the treatment of HBV infection in HIV-infected patients who are not receiving antiretroviral therapy. Although the drug has not been systematically evaluated in HIV-infected patients with HBV who were not receiving concomitant antiretroviral therapy, limited clinical experience suggests there is a potential for development of HIV resistance in such patients.

Liver Transplant Recipients

Efficacy of entecavir in liver transplant recipients was evaluated in a single-arm, open-label trial that included 65 patients who received a liver transplant for complications of chronic HBV infection. Patients had HBV DNA levels <172 IU/mL and 89% had HBeAg-negative disease at the time of transplant; mean age was 49 years, 82% were male, 39% were white, and 37% were Asian. All patients received entecavir 1 mg once daily in addition to usual posttransplant management, including hepatitis B immune globulin (HBIG). Of the 53 patients who completed the trial and had HBV DNA levels tested at or after 72 weeks of posttransplant treatment, all achieved HBV DNA levels <50 IU/mL. Of the 61 evaluable patients, all lost HBsAg posttransplant and 2 patients experienced recurrence of measurable HBsAg without recurrence of HBV viremia.

Clinical Perspective

The American Association for the Study of Liver Diseases (AASLD) recommends antiviral therapy for adults with immune-active chronic HBV to decrease the risk of liver-related complications. Immune-active chronic HBV is characterized by an elevation of ALT ≥2 times the upper limit of normal or evidence of significant histologic disease plus elevated HBV DNA (>2000 IU/mL if HBeAg negative or >20,000 IU/mL if HBeAg positive). Recommended initial antiviral options for adults with immune-active chronic HBV include peginterferon alfa-2a, entecavir, tenofovir disoproxil fumarate (TDF), or tenofovir alafenamide (TAF). Selection of a specific antiviral medication should be individualized based on patient characteristics and comorbidities, treatment tolerability, and cost; consult the AASLD guideline for more details. Antiviral therapy is also recommended for HBeAg-positive children 2 years of age and older with both elevated ALT and measurable HBV DNA levels; the goal of therapy is to achieve sustained HBeAg seroconversion. Preferred initial treatment options for pediatric patients include interferon alfa-2b, entecavir, or TDF.

DOSAGE AND ADMINISTRATION

● General

Pretreatment Screening

- Offer human immunodeficiency virus (HIV) antibody testing to all patients prior to initiating entecavir therapy.

- Carefully monitor renal function before initiating entecavir therapy in liver transplant recipients who have received or are receiving an immunosuppressant that may affect renal function (e.g., cyclosporine, tacrolimus).

Patient Monitoring

- Carefully monitor renal function during treatment with entecavir in elderly patients and in liver transplant recipients who have received or are receiving an immunosuppressant that may affect renal function (e.g., cyclosporine, tacrolimus).

- Closely monitor hepatic function with both clinical and laboratory follow-up for at least several months after discontinuing treatment with entecavir.

- Monitor hepatic function periodically during treatment.

- Monitor for adverse events if entecavir is coadministered with other drugs that are renally eliminated or are known to affect renal function.

Dispensing and Administration Precautions

- **Handling and Disposal:** Entecavir meets the National Institute for Occupational Safety and Health (NIOSH) definition of a hazardous drug, but does not have manufacturer's safe handling instructions or is not classified as a known or probable carcinogen by the National Toxicology Program or International Agency for Research on Cancer. Use appropriate precautions for receiving, handling, administration, and disposal.

• Administration

Entecavir is administered orally; it is available as tablets and oral solution.

Because the presence of food in the GI tract may decrease the rate and extent of absorption, entecavir should be administered on an empty stomach at least 2 hours before or 2 hours after meals.

Administer the oral solution using the supplied oral dosing spoon according to the patient instructions provided by the manufacturer. The oral solution contains 0.05 mg of entecavir per mL; do not dilute or mix the solution with water or any other liquid. Refer to the full prescribing information for specific instructions for administration of the oral solution.

Store entecavir tablets and oral solution at 25°C (excursions permitted between 15–30°C); the tablets should be stored in a tightly-closed container. Store both the tablets and the oral solution in the outer carton to protect from light. After opening, the oral solution can be used up to the expiration date on the bottle.

• Dosage

Adult Dosage

Chronic Hepatitis B Virus Infection

For the treatment of chronic hepatitis B virus (HBV) infection in adults with compensated liver disease who are nucleoside-naïve (not previously treated with nucleoside antivirals), the recommended dosage of entecavir is 0.5 mg once daily.

For the treatment of chronic HBV infection in adults with compensated liver disease and a history of HBV viremia while receiving lamivudine or with HBV known to have lamivudine- or telbivudine-associated resistance mutations (rtM204I/V ± rtL180M, rtL80I/V, or rtV173L), the recommended dosage of entecavir is 1 mg once daily.

For the treatment of HBV infection in adults with decompensated liver disease, the recommended dosage of entecavir is 1 mg once daily.

The optimal duration of entecavir therapy and the relationship between treatment and long-term outcomes (e.g., cirrhosis, hepatocellular carcinoma) are unknown.

Pediatric Dosage

Chronic Hepatitis B Virus Infection

For the treatment of chronic HBV infection in pediatric patients 2 years of age and older weighing at least 10 kg, dosage of entecavir is based on weight. (See Table 1.) Use entecavir oral solution for patients weighing 30 kg or less.

TABLE 1: Dosage of Entecavir for Treatment of HBV Infection in Pediatric Patients ≥2 Years of Age Weighing ≥10 kg

Body Weight	Dosage of Oral Solution Containing 0.05 mg/mL in Treatment-naïve Patients	Dosage of Oral Solution Containing 0.05 mg/mL in Lamivudine-experienced Patients
10–11 kg	0.15 mg (3 mL) once daily	0.3 mg (6 mL) once daily
>11 to 14 kg	0.2 mg (4 mL) once daily	0.4 mg (8 mL) once daily
>14 to 17 kg	0.25 mg (5 mL) once daily	0.5 mg (10 mL) once daily
>17 to 20 kg	0.3 mg (6 mL) once daily	0.6 mg (12 mL) once daily
>20 to 23 kg	0.35 mg (7 mL) once daily	0.7 mg (14 mL) once daily
>23 to 26 kg	0.4 mg (8 mL) once daily	0.8 mg (16 mL) once daily
>26 to 30 kg	0.45 mg (9 mL) once daily	0.9 mg (18 mL) once daily
>30 kg	0.5 mg (10 mL) once daily[a]	1 mg (20 mL) once daily[b]

[a] Treatment-naive pediatric patients weighing more than 30 kg should receive 0.5 mg (10 mL) of entecavir oral solution once daily or one 0.5-mg tablet of entecavir once daily.

[b] Lamivudine-experienced pediatric patients weighing more than 30 kg should receive 1 mg (20 mL) of entecavir oral solution once daily or one 1-mg tablet of entecavir once daily.

For the treatment of chronic hepatitis B virus (HBV) infection in adolescents ≥16 years of age with compensated liver disease who are nucleoside-naïve (not previously treated with nucleoside antivirals), the recommended dosage of entecavir is 0.5 mg once daily.

For the treatment of chronic HBV infection in adolescents ≥16 years of age with compensated liver disease and a history of HBV viremia while receiving lamivudine or with HBV known to have lamivudine- or telbivudine-associated resistance mutations (rtM204I/V ± rtL180M, rtL80I/V, or rtV173L), the recommended dosage of entecavir is 1 mg once daily.

The optimal duration of entecavir and the relationship between treatment and long-term outcomes (e.g., cirrhosis, hepatocellular carcinoma) are unknown.

• Special Populations

Hepatic Impairment

Dosage adjustments are not necessary in patients with hepatic impairment.

Renal Impairment

Adjust the dosage of entecavir in adults with creatinine clearance <50 mL/minute, including patients on hemodialysis or continuous ambulatory peritoneal dialysis (CAPD). (See Table 2.) The manufacturer states that the once-daily regimens are preferred.

TABLE 2. Dosage of Entecavir for Treatment of HBV Infection in Adults with Renal Impairment

Creatinine Clearance (mL/min)	Nucleoside-naive Individuals (Usual Dose: 0.5 mg)	Lamivudine-refractory HBV or Decompensated Liver Disease (Usual Dose: 1 mg)
30 to <50	0.25 mg once daily[a] or 0.5 mg once every 48 hours	0.5 mg once daily or 1 mg once every 48 hours
10 to <30	0.15 mg once daily[a] or 0.5 mg once every 72 hours	0.3 mg once daily[a] or 1 mg once every 72 hours
<10, or on hemodialysis[b] or CAPD	0.05 mg once daily[a] or 0.5 mg once every 7 days	0.1 mg once daily[a] or 1 mg once every 7 days

[a] For doses <0.5 mg, use entecavir oral solution.

[b] When a dose is indicated on a hemodialysis day, give the dose after the hemodialysis session.

There are insufficient data to recommend specific dose adjustments for pediatric patients with renal impairment; however, consider a dose reduction or an increase in the dosing interval similar to adjustments for adults.

Geriatric Use

Select dosage of entecavir for geriatric patients with caution due to possible age-related decreases in renal function; monitoring renal function also may be helpful.

CAUTIONS

• Contraindications

None.

• Warnings/Precautions

Warnings

Severe Acute Exacerbations of Hepatitis B Virus (HBV) Infection

Severe acute exacerbations of HBV have been reported following discontinuance of anti-HBV therapy, including entecavir, and a boxed warning about this risk has been included in the prescribing information for the drug.

In studies that evaluated safety of entecavir, exacerbations of hepatitis or ALT flare was defined as ALT elevations >10 times the upper limit of normal

(ULN) and >2 times baseline serum concentrations. In clinical studies, ALT flare occurred in 2, 8, or 12% of nucleoside-naïve HBeAg-positive, nucleoside-naïve HBeAg-negative, or lamivudine-refractory patients, respectively, following discontinuance of entecavir. The median time to exacerbations of hepatitis was 23 week. Rates of post-treatment ALT flare may be higher if entecavir therapy is discontinued without regard to previous response to therapy.

Exacerbations of hepatitis also have been reported during entecavir treatment of HBV, but generally resolved with continued therapy. In clinical studies, exacerbations of hepatitis (e.g., ALT elevations >10 times the ULN and >2 times baseline serum concentrations) occurring during therapy were generally associated with a reduction in viral load of ≥2 $\log_{10}$ copies/mL that preceded or coincided with the ALT elevations.

Closely monitor hepatic function with both clinical and laboratory follow-up for at least several months after entecavir is discontinued. If appropriate, resumption of anti-HBV therapy may be warranted.

Coinfection with Human Immunodeficiency Virus (HIV)

A boxed warning about the risk of development of resistance to HIV nucleoside reverse transcriptase inhibitors is included in the prescribing information for entecavir. Entecavir has not been systematically evaluated in HBV-infected patients coinfected with HIV who were not receiving concomitant antiretroviral therapy. Use of entecavir is not recommended for the treatment of patients with HBV/HIV coinfection in patients who are not receiving highly active antiretroviral therapy, since limited clinical evidence suggests there is potential for development of resistance to HIV nucleoside reverse transcriptase inhibitors if entecavir is used to treat chronic HBV infection in patients with untreated HIV infection. Prior to initiation of entecavir therapy, offer HIV testing to all patients. Entecavir has not been systematically evaluated for the treatment of HIV infection and such use is not recommended.

Lactic Acidosis and Severe Hepatomegaly with Steatosis

A boxed warning about the risk of lactic acidosis and severe hepatomegaly with steatosis is included in the prescribing information for entecavir. Lactic acidosis and severe hepatomegaly with steatosis, including some fatalities, have been reported in patients receiving nucleoside analogs alone or in conjunction with antiretrovirals. Most reported cases have involved women; obesity and long-term therapy with nucleoside reverse transcriptase inhibitors also may be risk factos Use nucleoside analogs with particular caution in patients with known risk factors for liver disease; however, lactic acidosis and severe hepatomegaly with steatosis have also been reported in patients with no known risk factors.

Lactic acidosis in patients receiving entecavir often is reported in association with hepatic decompensation, other serious medical conditions, or drug exposures. Patients with decompensated liver disease may be at higher risk of lactic acidosis.

Discontinue entecavir therapy in any patient with clinical or laboratory findings suggestive of lactic acidosis or pronounced hepatotoxicity (which may include hepatomegaly and steatosis even in the absence of marked aminotransferase elevations).

Specific Populations

Pregnancy

A pregnancy exposure registry (the Antiretroviral Pregnancy Registry [APR]) monitors maternal-fetal outcomes of pregnant women exposed to entecavir; clinicians are encouraged to enroll patients in the registry by calling 800-258-4263.

Prospective data from the APR are insufficient to adequately evaluate the risk of birth defects, miscarriage, or adverse maternal or fetal outcomes. The limited number of entecavir exposures reported to the APR is not sufficient to inform a risk assessment in comparison to a reference population. The rate of miscarriage is not reported in the APR.

In animal reproduction studies, there was no evidence of developmental toxicities in rats or rabbits at systemic entecavir exposures approximately 28 or 212 times, respectively, human exposures achieved at the maximum recommended human dose (MRHD) of 1 mg daily. In a pre/postnatal development study, no adverse effects on the offspring were observed when entecavir (≤30 mg/kg per day) was administered orally to pregnant rats from gestation day 6 to lactation/post-partum day 20, resulting in exposures >94 times those in humans at the MRHD.

Lactation

It is not known whether entecavir is distributed into human milk, affects human milk production, or has effects on the breastfed infant. Entecavir was present in milk when administered to lactating rats.

Consider the benefits of breastfeeding and the importance of entecavir to the mother along with the potential adverse effects on the breastfed infant from the drug or from the underlying maternal condition.

Pediatric Use

Safety and efficacy of entecavir were evaluated in clinical trials of pediatric patients ≥2 years of age with HBeAg-positive chronic HBV infection and compensated liver disease.

Steady-state pharmacokinetics of entecavir were evaluated in pediatric patients 2 to <18 years of age with compensated liver disease. Entecavir exposures in nucleoside inhibitor-naïve children receiving the oral solution in a dosage of 0.015 mg/kg (≤0.5 mg) once daily were similar to exposures observed in adults receiving a 0.5-mg tablet once daily. Exposures in lamivudine-experienced children receiving the oral solution in a dosage of 0.03 mg/kg (≤1 mg) once daily were similar to exposures observed in adults receiving a 1-mg tablet once daily.

There are limited data available on the use of entecavir in lamivudine-experienced pediatric patients; use entecavir in these patients only if potential benefits justify potential risks. Since some pediatric patients may require long-term or lifetime management of chronic active HBV infection, consider the impact of entecavir use on future treatment options.

Safety and efficacy of entecavir have not been established in pediatric patients <2 years of age; entecavir has not been evaluated in these patients since treatment of HBV is rarely required in this age group.

Geriatric Use

Clinical studies did not include sufficient numbers of patients ≥65 years of age to determine whether they respond differently to entecavir than younger adults.

Entecavir is substantially excreted by the kidneys, and the risk of entecavir-induced toxicity may be increased in patients with impaired renal function. The area under the plasma concentration-time curve (AUC) of entecavir is increased compared with younger adults, possibly as the result of age-related changes in renal function. Since geriatric patients may be more likely to have decreased renal function, select dosage with caution; it also may be useful to monitor renal function in geriatric patients.

Hepatic Impairment

Pharmacokinetics of entecavir are similar between adults (without HBV infection) with moderate or severe hepatic impairment (Child-Pugh class B or C) and adults without hepatic impairment. No dosage adjustments are recommended for patients with hepatic impairment.

Pharmacokinetics of entecavir have not been studied in pediatric patients with hepatic impairment.

Renal Impairment

Entecavir plasma concentrations and AUC are increased and clearance of the drug is decreased in adults with impaired renal function (without HBV infection) compared with adults without renal impairment. Dosage adjustments are recommended for adults with creatinine clearance <50 mL/minute, including patients on hemodialysis or continuous ambulatory peritoneal dialysis. See Table 2 for dosing strategies.

Hispanic Patients

Safety and efficacy of entecavir have not been established in the US Hispanic population because of low enrollment of such patients in clinical trials.

Liver Transplant Recipients

Limited data are available regarding safety and efficacy of entecavir in liver transplant recipients. In an open-label, post-liver transplant trial, the frequency and nature of adverse events were consistent with those expected in patients who have received a liver transplant and the known safety profile of entecavir.

If entecavir is necessary in liver transplant recipients who have received or are receiving an immunosuppressive agent that may affect renal function (e.g., cyclosporine, tacrolimus), monitor renal function carefully prior to and during entecavir treatment.

● **Common Adverse Effects**

The most common adverse effects (≥3%, all severity grades) in adults were headache, fatigue, dizziness, and nausea. Adverse effects observed in pediatric patients were consistent with those observed in adults.

DRUG INTERACTIONS

● **Drugs Affecting or Metabolized by Hepatic Microsomal Enzymes**

Pharmacokinetics of entecavir are unlikely to be affected by coadministration of drugs that are metabolized by, inhibit, or induce the cytochrome P-450 (CYP) isoenzymes, including 1A2, 2C9, 2C19, 2D6, 3A4, 2B6, 2E1, or 3A5. Pharmacokinetics of known CYP substrates are unlikely to be affected by coadministration of entecavir.

● **Nephrotoxic Drugs or Drugs Eliminated by Renal Excretion**

Coadministration of entecavir with drugs that reduce renal function or compete for active renal tubular secretion may increase serum concentrations of either entecavir or the concomitantly used drug. Although the effect of concomitant use of such drugs with entecavir has not been specifically studied, closely monitor patients for adverse effects if entecavir is coadministered with such drugs.

● **Adefovir Dipivoxil**

No clinically important pharmacokinetic interactions were observed with adefovir dipivoxil.

● **HIV Nucleoside and Nucleotide Reverse Transcriptase Inhibitors**

No clinically important pharmacokinetic interactions were observed between entecavir and lamivudine or tenofovir disoproxil fumarate (TDF).

In vitro evidence indicates that concurrent use of human immunodeficiency virus (HIV) nucleoside reverse transcriptase inhibitors (NRTIs) and entecavir is unlikely to reduce the antiretroviral activity of entecavir against hepatitis B virus (HBV) or of the HIV NRTIs (abacavir, didanosine, lamivudine, tenofovir, or zidovudine) against HIV. Concurrent use of these HIV NRTIs or emtricitabine did not antagonize the antiviral activity of entecavir against HBV in vitro.

● **Immunosuppressive Agents**

In a small pilot study, entecavir exposures in HBV-infected liver transplant recipients receiving a stable dose of cyclosporine or tacrolimus were approximately 2-fold higher than those observed in healthy individuals with normal renal function. Altered renal function contributed to the increase in entecavir exposure in these patients. The potential for pharmacokinetic interactions between entecavir and cyclosporine or tacrolimus was not formally evaluated.

Monitor renal function prior to and during entecavir treatment in patients (e.g., transplant patients) receiving cyclosporine, tacrolimus, or other immunosuppressive agents that may affect renal function.

DESCRIPTION

Entecavir, a synthetic purine nucleoside analog derived from guanine, is an antiviral agent that is selectively active against human hepatitis B virus (HBV). The drug undergoes phosphorylation by cellular enzymes to form its active metabolite, entecavir triphosphate, which has an intracellular half-life of 15 hours. By competing with the natural substrate deoxyguanosine triphosphate, entecavir triphosphate inhibits all 3 activities of HBV DNA polymerase (reverse transcriptase): base priming, reverse transcription of the negative strand from the pregenomic messenger RNA, and synthesis of the positive strand of HBV DNA.

Following oral administration, peak plasma concentrations of entecavir are attained within 0.5–1.5 hours. Steady-state concentrations are achieved after 6–10 days of once-daily administration with approximately 2-fold accumulation. Commercially available entecavir tablets and oral solution are bioequivalent and may be used interchangeably. Food delays absorption, decreases peak plasma concentrations, and decreases the area under the plasma concentration-time curve (AUC) of entecavir.

Entecavir is extensively distributed into tissues, and is approximately 13% bound to serum proteins in vitro. Following oral administration, entecavir undergoes phosphorylation by cellular enzymes to form the active metabolite, entecavir triphosphate. Entecavir is partially metabolized to glucuronide and sulfate conjugates. Entecavir is not a substrate for and does not inhibit or induce cytochrome P-450 (CYP) isoenzymes.

Entecavir is excreted principally in urine via by both glomerular filtration and tubular secretion. Approximately 62–73% of an oral dose is eliminated unchanged in urine. Hemodialysis removes approximately 13% of a dose in 4 hours; continuous ambulatory peritoneal dialysis removes approximately 0.3% of a dose over 7 days. The terminal elimination half-life of entecavir is approximately 128–149 hours. There are no significant gender or racial differences in the pharmacokinetics of entecavir.

● **Spectrum**

Entecavir is active in vitro and in vivo against human HBV, including some strains of lamivudine-resistant HBV. The drug also has limited in vitro activity against certain other human viruses, including herpes simplex virus types 1 and 2 (HSV-1 and HSV-2), varicella zoster virus, and cytomegalovirus, but has not been shown to be effective in clinical infections caused by these viruses.

● **Resistance**

Resistance in HBV

There is some evidence that HBV with reduced susceptibility to entecavir can develop slowly in some patients during long-term therapy. In nucleoside-naïve patients receiving entecavir for up to 96 weeks, viral rebound due to resistance occurred in <1% of patients.. In lamivudine-refractory patients, viral rebound due to entecavir resistance occurred in 1% of patients after the first year of therapy and in 9% of patients during the second year of therapy.

Resistance to entecavir occurs in a 2-step process, with initial selection of M204V/I mutation followed by amino acid substitutions at rtI169, rtT184, stS202, or rtM250.

Cross-resistance can occur among the nucleoside and nucleotide antivirals used for treatment of HBV. Lamivudine- and telbivudine-resistant HBV with reduced in vitro susceptibility to entecavir have been reported. Adefovir-resistant HBV may have reduced susceptibility to entecavir in vitro. HBV isolates from lamivudine-refractory patients who failed entecavir therapy have retained in vitro susceptibility to adefovir.

ADVICE TO PATIENTS

- Inform patients to take entecavir on a regular dosing schedule on an empty stomach at least 2 hours before or 2 hours after meals, and to avoid missing doses in order to prevent development of resistance. Advise patients of the importance of regular medical follow-up during treatment with entecavir.

- Inform patients that if they miss a dose of their medicine, take the dose as soon as they remember. If it is almost time for the next dose, skip the missed dose and take the dose that is due. Patients should not take two doses at a time.

- Inform patients that severe acute exacerbations of hepatitis B virus (HBV) infection have been reported following discontinuance of HBV treatment, including entecavir. Advise patients to not discontinue entecavir without first informing a clinician.

- Advise patients that lactic acidosis and severe hepatomegaly with steatosis, including fatalities, have occurred in patients receiving drugs similar to entecavir. Inform patients to contact their clinician immediately if they experience any signs or symptoms of lactic acidosis (e.g., weakness/fatigue, unusual muscle pain, trouble breathing, stomach pain with nausea and vomiting, feeling cold especially in arms and legs, dizziness or feeling light-headed, fast or irregular heart beat) or hepatotoxicity (e.g., jaundice, dark urine, bowel movements light in color, anorexia, nausea, stomach pain). Inform patients that the clinician may discontinue entecavir therapy if such signs and symptoms occur.

- Inform patients that it is important to test for HIV prior to initiation of entecavir therapy. Advise patients that, if they have HIV infection and are not receiving effective HIV treatment, entecavir may increase the risk of resistance to HIV treatment.

- Inform patients using entecavir oral solution to measure the prescribed dose using the calibrated dosing spoon provided by the manufacturer, and to refer to the patient information for specific instructions for use.

- Advise patients that the optimal duration of entecavir therapy for the treatment of chronic hepatitis B and the relationship between response to treatment and long-term prevention of outcomes such as hepatocellular carcinoma are unknown.

- Inform patients that entecavir is not a cure for HBV infection, and that HBV transmission via sexual contact, sharing needles, or blood contamination is not prevented by entecavir therapy. Inform patients of available measures to prevent spread of HBV infection to close contacts.

- Advise patients to inform their clinician if they are or plan to become pregnant or plan to breastfeed. Inform patients that there is a registry to monitor fetal outcomes of pregnant women exposed to entecavir.

- Advise patients to inform their clinician of existing or contemplated concomitant therapy, including prescription and OTC drugs and dietary or herbal supplements, and any concomitant illnesses (e.g., renal disease).

- Advise patients of other important precautionary information.

PREPARATIONS

Excipients in commercially available drug preparations may have clinically important effects in some individuals; consult specific product labeling for details.

Entecavir

Oral Solution	0.05 mg/mL	Baraclude®, Bristol-Myers Squibb
Oral Tablets, film-coated	0.5 mg*	Baraclude®, Bristol-Myers Squibb Entecavir Tablets
	1 mg*	Baraclude®, Bristol-Myers Squibb Entecavir Tablets

* available from one or more manufacturer, distributor, and/or repackager by generic (nonproprietary) name

† Use is not currently included in the labeling approved by the US Food and Drug Administration.

Selected Revisions December 16, 2023, © Copyright, November 1, 2005, American Society of Health-System Pharmacists, Inc.

Famciclovir

8:18.32 • NUCLEOSIDES AND NUCLEOTIDES

■ Famciclovir (FCV), a synthetic, acyclic purine nucleoside analog antiviral, is a prodrug of the antiviral penciclovir and is active against herpesviruses and hepatitis B virus.

USES

Oral famciclovir is used for the treatment of acute, localized herpes zoster (shingles, zoster). Oral famciclovir also is used for the treatment of genital herpes infections and for the suppression of recurrent episodes of genital herpes in immunocompetent adults. The drug also is used for the treatment of recurrent mucocutaneous herpes simplex virus (HSV) infections in adults with human immunodeficiency virus (HIV) infection. In addition, oral famciclovir is used for the episodic treatment of herpes labialis (perioral herpes, cold sores, fever blisters) in immunocompetent adults.

● Genital Herpes
Treatment of First Episodes

Although the manufacturer states that efficacy of famciclovir for the treatment of initial episodes of genital herpes simplex virus (HSV) infection† has not been established, famciclovir is considered a drug of choice for the treatment of initial episodes of genital herpes. Because many patients with first episodes of genital herpes present with mild clinical symptoms but later develop severe or prolonged symptoms, the US Centers for Disease Control and Prevention (CDC) states that most patients with initial genital herpes should receive antiviral therapy. The CDC and some clinicians recommend that first episodes of genital herpes be treated with a regimen of oral acyclovir (400 mg 3 times daily or 200 mg 5 times daily for 7–10 days), oral famciclovir (250 mg 3 times daily given for 7–10 days), or oral valacyclovir (1 g twice daily given for 7–10 days).

Studies have been initiated to compare the relative efficacy of oral famciclovir and oral acyclovir for the treatment of initial episodes of genital herpes in immunocompetent adults, and preliminary results indicate that oral famciclovir (125, 250, 500, or 750 mg 3 times daily) is as effective as oral acyclovir (200 mg 5 times daily) in terms of time to complete healing of lesions, resolution of symptoms, and time to cessation of viral shedding.

Episodic Treatment of Recurrent Episodes

Oral famciclovir is used in the treatment of recurrent episodes of genital herpes in immunocompetent adults. Antiviral therapy for recurrent genital herpes can be given episodically to ameliorate or shorten the duration of lesions or can be given continuously as suppressive therapy to reduce the frequency of recurrences. For episodic treatment of recurrent genital herpes, the CDC and some clinicians recommend oral acyclovir (400 mg 3 times daily for 5 days, 800 mg twice daily for 5 days, or 800 mg 3 times daily for 2 days), oral famciclovir (125 mg twice daily for 5 days or 1 g twice daily for 1 day), or oral valacyclovir (500 mg twice daily for 3 days or 1 g once daily for 5 days). Episodic antiviral therapy should be initiated within 1 day of lesion onset or during the prodrome that precedes some outbreaks. The manufacturer states that patients should be advised to initiate oral famciclovir at the first sign or symptom of an episode and that there are no data on the effectiveness of the drug initiated more than 6 hours after the onset of signs and symptoms of a recurrent episode.

Efficacy of oral famciclovir for the episodic treatment of recurrent genital herpes has been evaluated in randomized double-blind, placebo-controlled studies. In one study involving 329 immunocompetent adults who self-initiated treatment within 6 hours of appearance of lesions or onset of symptoms of recurrence, the median time to lesion healing of nonaborted lesions and resolution of all symptoms was 4.3 and 3.3 days, respectively, in patients who received oral famciclovir (1 g twice daily for 1 day) compared with 6.1 and 5.4 days, respectively, in those who received placebo. The proportion of patients with aborted lesions (no development beyond erythema) was larger in the famciclovir group than in the placebo group (23 versus 13%).

Combined data from 2 studies involving 626 otherwise healthy adults who self-initiated treatment within 6 hours of appearance of lesions or onset of symptoms of recurrence indicate that the median time to lesion healing and cessation of viral shedding was 4 and 1.8 days, respectively, in patients who received oral famciclovir (125 mg twice daily for 5 days) compared with 5 and 3.4 days, respectively, in those who received placebo. The median time to resolution of all symptoms was 3.2 days in those who received famciclovir versus 3.8 days in placebo-treated patients. There is no evidence that higher dosages of famciclovir (i.e., 250 or 500 mg twice daily) provide additional benefit in terms of time to lesion healing or relief of symptoms in immunocompetent adults.

Suppressive Therapy of Recurrent Episodes

Famciclovir is used for chronic suppressive therapy of recurrent genital herpes in immunocompetent adults. The CDC states that suppressive antiviral therapy can reduce the frequency of genital herpes recurrences by 70–80% in patients who have frequent recurrences (i.e., 6 or more per year) and many patients report no symptomatic outbreaks during such therapy. For chronic suppressive therapy of recurrent genital herpes, the CDC and some clinicians recommend a regimen of oral acyclovir (400 mg twice daily), oral famciclovir (250 mg twice daily), or oral valacyclovir (500 mg or 1 g once daily). The CDC states that data suggest that therapy with famciclovir or valacyclovir is as effective as acyclovir in terms of clinical outcome, although the 500 mg once-daily valacyclovir regimen might be less effective than acyclovir or other valacyclovir regimens in patients who have very frequent recurrences (i.e., 10 or more episodes per year).

In a study of patients with frequent recurrences of genital herpes infections (6 or more per year), 39 or 29% of those receiving famciclovir suppressive therapy (250 mg twice daily) were free of recurrences at 6 or 12 months, respectively, and 10 or 6% of those receiving placebo were free of recurrences at these time points. Safety and efficacy of oral famciclovir for suppressive therapy of recurrent genital herpes infections have been established in patients receiving daily therapy for up to 1 year.

HIV-Infected Individuals

Immunocompromised individuals may have prolonged or severe episodes of genital, perianal, or oral herpes; HSV lesions are common in those with human immunodeficiency virus (HIV) infection and may be severe, painful, and atypical. (See Uses: Mucocutaneous Herpes Simplex Virus Infections.)

The CDC states that episodic treatment or suppressive therapy with oral antiviral agents often is beneficial in HIV-infected individuals with genital herpes. While the drugs of choice for episodic treatment or suppressive therapy of genital herpes in HIV-infected individuals are the same as those in immunocompetent adults, higher dosages and/or more prolonged therapy may be necessary. For episodic treatment of recurrences of genital herpes in HIV-infected individuals, the CDC recommends a 5- to 10-day regimen of oral acyclovir (400 mg 3 times daily), oral famciclovir (500 mg twice daily), or oral valacyclovir (1 g twice daily). For daily suppressive therapy of recurrent genital herpes in HIV-infected individuals, the CDC recommends oral acyclovir (400–800 mg 2–3 times daily), oral famciclovir (500 mg twice daily), or oral valacyclovir (500 mg twice daily).

Patient Counseling and Management of Sexual Partners

Counseling of infected individuals and their sex partners is critical to management of genital herpes. The goals of such counseling are to help patients understand and cope with the infection and to prevent sexual and perinatal transmission of the virus. Antiviral therapy offers clinical benefit to most symptomatic patients and is the mainstay of management; however, genital herpes is a recurrent, life-long viral infection. Although antiviral therapy can be used to control the symptoms and signs of genital herpes episodes, it cannot eradicate latent HSV or affect the risk, frequency, or severity of recurrences of genital herpes when antiviral therapy is discontinued.

The majority of genital herpes infections are transmitted by individuals unaware that they have the infection or by individuals who are asymptomatic when transmission occurs. Patients should be advised that famciclovir is not a cure for genital herpes, and there are no data evaluating whether famciclovir prevents transmission of HSV to others. Because genital herpes is a sexually transmitted disease, patients should be advised to avoid sexual contact with uninfected partners when lesions and/or prodromal symptoms are present. In addition, patients should be advised that sexual transmission of the virus can occur during asymptomatic periods and that suppressive antiviral therapy reduces, but does not eliminate, subclinical viral shedding.

Sex partners of individuals with genital herpes should be advised that they may be infected even if they have no symptoms. Asymptomatic partners of patients with genital herpes should be questioned regarding a history of genital lesions, educated to recognize symptoms of genital herpes, and offered type-specific serologic testing to determine whether risk for HSV acquisition exists. Antiviral therapy is not recommended for sexual partners who do not have clinical manifestations of infection, but symptomatic sex partners of individuals with genital herpes should be evaluated and treated.

The risk for neonatal HSV infection should be discussed with all genital herpes patients, including men. Pregnant women and women of childbearing age who have genital herpes should inform their providers who care for them during pregnancy as well as those who will care for their neonates.

Information to assist patients and clinicians in counseling regarding genital herpes is available at http://www.ashastd.org and http://www.ihmf.org. For further information on treatment of initial or recurrent episodes of genital herpes or suppression of recurrent infections, see Uses: Genital Herpes in Acyclovir 8:18.32.

● *Herpes Labialis*

Famciclovir is used for the episodic treatment of herpes labialis (perioral herpes, cold sores, fever blisters) in immunocompetent adults.

Efficacy of a 1-day regimen of famciclovir was evaluated in healthy adults with a history of recurrent cold sores. Patients were randomized to famciclovir 1.5 g as a single dose, famciclovir 750 mg twice daily for 1 day, or placebo; patients self-initiated therapy within 1 hour of symptom onset. The median time to lesion healing of nonaborted lesions and resolution of symptoms (pain and tenderness) was 4.4 and 1.7 days, respectively, in patients who received the single-dose oral famciclovir regimen compared with 6.2 and 2.9 days, respectively, in those who received placebo. There was no difference between the famciclovir-treated and placebo-treated patients in aborted lesions (no development beyond the papular stage).

● *Mucocutaneous Herpes Simplex Virus Infections*

Oral famciclovir is used for the treatment of recurrent mucocutaneous HSV infections (HSV-1 and HSV-2) in HIV-infected adults. The CDC, National Institutes of Health (NIH), Infectious Diseases Society of America (IDSA), and other experts state that orolabial HSV infections in HIV-infected individuals may be treated with oral acyclovir, oral famciclovir, or oral valacyclovir. IV acyclovir usually is indicated for *initial* treatment of moderate to severe mucocutaneous HSV infections in HIV-infected individuals but may be switched to oral antiviral therapy (acyclovir, famciclovir, valacyclovir) after lesions begin to regress. If acyclovir-resistant HSV is suspected, IV foscarnet or IV cidofovir is recommended for treatment.

In a comparative study in HIV-infected patients (40% had CD4+ T-cell counts below 200/mm³) with recurrent mucocutaneous HSV infections (54% with anogenital lesions, 35% with orolabial lesions) who initiated therapy within 48 hours of the onset of lesions, oral famciclovir (500 mg twice daily for 7 days) was as effective as oral acyclovir (400 mg 5 times daily for 7 days) in reducing formation of new lesions and time to complete healing. (See HIV-infected Individuals under Uses: Genital Herpes.)

Famciclovir also has been recommended for chronic suppressive or maintenance therapy (secondary prophylaxis) against HSV disease† in HIV-infected adults or adolescents with frequent or severe recurrences. In patients with advanced HIV infection, reactivation of HSV frequently occurs and can result in chronic, persistent mucocutaneous disease that may be severe. The Prevention of Opportunistic Infections Working Group of the US Public Health Service and the Infectious Diseases Society of America (USPHS/IDSA) has established guidelines for the prevention of opportunistic infections in HIV-infected individuals that include recommendations concerning prevention of exposure to opportunistic pathogens, prevention of first disease episodes, and prevention of disease recurrence. The USPHS/IDSA does *not* recommend primary prophylaxis against initial episodes of HSV infection in HIV-infected adults, adolescents, or children. In addition, the USPHS/IDSA does not recommend routine chronic suppressive or maintenance therapy (secondary prophylaxis) against HSV disease in HIV-infected individuals since acute episodes of mucocutaneous disease generally can be treated successfully with acyclovir. However, these and other experts state that long-term prophylaxis against recurrence of HSV disease can be considered for HIV-infected adults, adolescents, and children who have frequent or severe recurrences. If secondary prophylaxis is indicated in HIV-infected adults or adolescents, the USPHS/IDSA, CDC, NIH, IDSA, and other experts recommend use of oral acyclovir, oral famciclovir, or oral valacyclovir. If indicated in infants and children, the USPHS/IDSA and other experts recommend use of oral acyclovir.

● *Herpes Zoster (Shingles, Zoster)*

Oral famciclovir is used for the treatment of acute, localized herpes zoster (shingles, zoster) in immunocompetent adults. Some clinicians suggest that the drugs of choice for the treatment of herpes zoster in immunocompetent adults are oral acyclovir, oral famciclovir, or oral valacyclovir.

Efficacy of famciclovir in the treatment of acute, localized herpes zoster has been evaluated in a randomized, double-blind, placebo-controlled trial in immunocompetent adults and in a dose-ranging, double-blind trial in immunocompetent adults who were randomized to receive oral famciclovir (250, 500, or 750 mg 3 times daily for 7 days) or oral acyclovir (800 mg every 4 hours 5 times daily for 7 days). Results of these studies indicate that famciclovir may prevent the appearance of new lesions, decrease the duration of viral shedding, decrease the duration of pain, and promote healing and crusting of lesions in immunocompetent adults with localized herpes zoster when given within 72 hours of the onset of rash, particularly if initiated within 48 hours of rash onset. Like acyclovir, famciclovir does not appear to *prevent* the development of postherpetic neuralgia; the drug significantly *decreases the median duration* of neuralgia, particularly in patients older than 50 years of age. In comparative studies, 7 days of oral therapy with famciclovir (250–750 mg 3 times daily) was comparably effective to 7 days of oral therapy with acyclovir (800 mg 5 times daily). There were no statistically significant differences in the duration of postherpetic neuralgia between famciclovir- and acyclovir-treated patients.

Oral famciclovir has been used in a limited number of patients for the treatment of ophthalmic herpes zoster† or disseminated herpes zoster† or for the treatment of herpes zoster in immunocompromised patients; however, the manufacturer states that efficacy of famciclovir for the treatment of these infections has not been established. The CDC and other experts state that oral famciclovir or oral valacyclovir is the treatment of choice for localized dermatomal herpes zoster in HIV-infected adults or adolescents.

● *Hepatitis B Virus Infection*

Famciclovir has been used for the management of chronic hepatitis B virus (HBV) infection† in a limited number of patients. The drug also has been evaluated for the control of HBV recurrence in organ or bone marrow transplant recipients†. While there is some evidence suggesting that famciclovir (250–500 mg 3 times daily) is effective for the management of HBV infection, further study is needed to establish safety and efficacy.

The CDC, NIH, IDSA, and other experts state that famciclovir is *not* recommended for the treatment of HBV infection in HIV-infected individuals since the drug is less active than lamivudine against HBV and is not active against lamivudine-resistant HBV.

DOSAGE AND ADMINISTRATION

● *Administration*

Famciclovir is administered orally without regard to meals. Food does not affect the systemic bioavailability or elimination of famciclovir.

● *Dosage*
Genital Herpes
Treatment of First Episodes

If oral famciclovir is used for the treatment of initial episodes of genital herpes simplex virus (HSV) infection† in immunocompetent adults or adolescents, the US Centers for Disease Control and Prevention (CDC) and other clinicians recommend that adults receive 250 mg 3 times daily for 7–10 days. The CDC states that the duration of treatment may be extended if healing is incomplete after 10 days of therapy.

In HIV-infected individuals, the CDC and other clinicians recommend a dosage of 500 mg twice daily for 7–14 days for the treatment of initial episodes of genital HSV infection.

Episodic Treatment of Recurrent Episodes

For the episodic treatment of recurrent genital herpes in immunocompetent adults, the dosage of oral famciclovir recommended by the manufacturer is 1 g twice daily for 1 day. The CDC and other clinicians recommend a dosage of 1 g twice daily for 1 day or 125 mg twice daily for 5 days.

In HIV-infected individuals, the CDC and other clinicians recommend a dosage of 500 mg twice daily for 5–10 days for the episodic treatment of recurrent genital herpes; alternatively, this dosage can be given for 7–14 days.

Patients should be advised to initiate famciclovir therapy at the first sign or symptom of an episode. Data are not available concerning efficacy of oral famciclovir initiated more than 6 hours after the onset of signs or symptoms of a recurrent episode of genital herpes.

Suppressive Therapy of Recurrent Episodes

For chronic suppressive therapy of recurrent episodes of genital herpes in immunocompetent adults, the recommended dosage of oral famciclovir is 250 mg every 12 hours.

In HIV-infected individuals, the CDC recommends a dosage of 500 mg twice daily for suppressive therapy of recurrent episodes of genital herpes. The manufacturer states that chronic suppressive therapy with oral famciclovir may be given for up to 1 year. Because the frequency of recurrent episodes diminishes over time in many patients, the CDC recommends that suppressive antiviral therapy be discontinued periodically (e.g., once yearly) to assess the need for continued therapy.

Herpes Labialis

For the treatment of herpes labialis (perioral herpes, cold sores, fever blisters) in immunocompetent adults, the recommended dosage of oral famciclovir is 1.5 g given as a single dose.

Treatment should be initiated at the first prodromal symptom of a cold sore (e.g., tingling, itching, burning).

Mucocutaneous Herpes Simplex Virus Infections

For the treatment of recurrent mucocutaneous HSV infections (i.e., orolabial or anogenital lesions) in adults with human immunodeficiency virus (HIV) infection, the usual dosage of oral famciclovir is 500 mg every 12 hours for 7 days. Some experts recommend a duration of 7–14 days.

If oral famciclovir is used for chronic suppressive or maintenance prophylaxis (secondary prophylaxis) of HSV† in HIV-infected adults and adolescents who have frequent or severe recurrences of HSV disease, a dosage of 250 mg twice daily has been recommended by the Prevention of Opportunistic Infections Working Group of the US Public Health Service and the Infectious Diseases Society of America (USPHS/IDSA).

Herpes Zoster

For the treatment of acute, localized herpes zoster (shingles, zoster) in immunocompetent adults, the recommended dosage of oral famciclovir is 500 mg every 8 hours for 7 days.

For the treatment of local dermatomal herpes zoster in HIV-infected adults†, the CDC and other experts recommend 500 mg of famciclovir three times daily for 7–10 days.

Therapy should be initiated promptly after herpes zoster is diagnosed. Efficacy of famciclovir initiated more than 72 hours after rash onset has not been established.

● Dosage in Renal and Hepatic Impairment
Dosage in Renal Impairment

Famciclovir is eliminated mainly by the kidneys via tubular secretion and glomerular filtration. In patients with moderately or severely impaired renal function, the frequency of administration of famciclovir should be decreased in response to the degree of impairment as indicated by creatinine clearance.

Because penciclovir (the active metabolite) is readily removed from plasma during hemodialysis, famciclovir should be administered after each hemodialysis session when the drug is used for the treatment of herpes zoster, treatment of recurrent mucocutaneous HSV infections in HIV-infected patients, or suppression of recurrent genital herpes. Famciclovir is administered once as a single dose after a hemodialysis session when the drug is used for the treatment of recurrent genital herpes or treatment of recurrent herpes labialis. The manufacturer recommends that a famciclovir dose (250 mg for patients with herpes zoster, 250 mg for HIV-infected patients with recurrent mucosal or cutaneous HSV infection, or 125 mg for patients receiving the drug for suppression of recurrent genital herpes) be administered following each hemodialysis session. The manufacturer recommends that a famciclovir dose (250 mg for patients with recurrent genital herpes, 250 mg for patients with recurrent herpes labialis) be administered once as a single dose after a hemodialysis session.

Genital Herpes

For episodic treatment of recurrent genital herpes in immunocompetent adults, the manufacturer states that patients with creatinine clearances of 60 mL/minute

or greater may receive the usual oral famciclovir dosage of 1 g every 12 hours for 1 day. However, those with creatinine clearances of 40–59 mL/minute should receive 500 mg every 12 hours for 1 day, those with clearances of 20–39 mL/minute should receive 500 mg given as a single dose, and those with creatinine clearances less than 20 mL/minute should receive 250 mg given as a single dose.

For chronic suppressive therapy of recurrent genital herpes in immunocompetent adults with impaired renal function, the manufacturer states that patients with a creatinine clearance of 40 mL/minute or greater may receive the usual oral famciclovir dosage of 250 mg every 12 hours; those with creatinine clearances of 20–39 mL/minute or less than 20 mL/minute should receive 125 mg every 12 or 24 hours, respectively.

Herpes Labialis

For episodic treatment of recurrent herpes labialis in immunocompetent adults, the manufacturer states that patients with creatinine clearances of 60 mL/minute or greater may receive the usual oral famciclovir dosage of 1.5 g given as a single dose. However, those with creatinine clearances of 40–59 mL/minute should receive a single 750-mg dose, those with clearances of 20–39 mL/minute should receive a single 500-mg dose, and those with creatinine clearances less than 20 mL/minute should receive a single 250-mg dose.

Mucocutaneous Herpes Simplex Virus Infections

For the treatment of recurrent mucocutaneous HSV infections in HIV-infected adults with impaired renal function, the manufacturer states that patients with creatinine clearances of 40 mL/minute or greater may receive the usual oral famciclovir dosage of 500 mg every 12 hours; however those with creatinine clearances of 20–39 mL/minute should receive 500 mg once every 24 hours, and those with creatinine clearances less than 20 mL/minute should receive 250 mg once every 24 hours.

Herpes Zoster

For the treatment of localized herpes zoster in immunocompetent adults, the manufacturer states that patients with creatinine clearances of 60 mL/minute or greater may receive the usual oral famciclovir dosage of 500 mg every 8 hours. However, those with creatinine clearances of 40–59 mL/minute should receive 500 mg every 12 hours, those with creatinine clearances of 20–39 mL/minute should receive 500 mg once every 24 hours, and those with creatinine clearances less than 20 mL/minute should receive 250 mg once every 24 hours.

Dosage in Hepatic Impairment

Famciclovir is metabolized mainly in the liver to the active drug penciclovir. In patients with well-compensated chronic liver disease such as chronic hepatitis, chronic alcohol abuse, or primary biliary cirrhosis, bioavailability of penciclovir was not affected. Therefore, modification of famciclovir dosage is not necessary in patients with well-compensated liver disease. The manufacturer does not make specific recommendations for patients with uncompensated hepatic impairment, since the pharmacokinetics of famciclovir has not been evaluated in these patients.

CAUTIONS

Famciclovir is well tolerated in immunocompetent patients with herpes zoster, genital herpes, or herpes labialis with an adverse effect profile similar to that of placebo. The most common adverse effects of the drug in both types of patients are headache, nausea, and diarrhea, and adverse effects usually are mild or moderate in severity. In controlled clinical trials in immunocompetent patients with herpes zoster, less than 1% of patients discontinued famciclovir as a result of severe adverse effects.

Similar adverse effects have been reported when famciclovir was used in patients with human immunodeficiency virus (HIV) infection, and the most frequent adverse effects in these patients are headache, nausea, and diarrhea.

● Nervous System Effects

The most common adverse effect of famciclovir is headache, which occurred in approximately 23% of patients receiving the drug (versus in 18% of placebo recipients) in a large, controlled clinical trial for herpes zoster. Headache resulted in discontinuance of famciclovir in less than 1% of patients in clinical trials for herpes zoster or genital herpes. Fatigue was reported in 4.4% of patients receiving the drug (versus in 3.4% of placebo recipients) in a large, controlled clinical trial for herpes zoster. Dizziness, fever, paresthesia, and somnolence have occurred in patients receiving famciclovir in this clinical trial for herpes zoster.

Headache or fatigue occurred in 16 or 4%, respectively, of HIV-infected patients receiving famciclovir in clinical studies.

● **GI Effects**

The most frequent adverse GI effect of famciclovir is nausea which occurred in approximately 13% of patients receiving the drug (versus in 11.6% in placebo recipients) in a large, controlled clinical trial for herpes zoster. Nausea resulted in discontinuance of famciclovir in less than 1% of patients in clinical trials for herpes zoster or genital herpes. Diarrhea was reported in approximately 8% of patients (5% of placebo recipients) and vomiting in approximately 5% of patients (3.4% of placebo recipients) in a large, controlled clinical trial for herpes zoster. Vomiting only rarely resulted in discontinuance of famciclovir in clinical trials for herpes zoster or genital herpes. Constipation, anorexia, abdominal pain, flatulence, and dyspepsia have occurred in patients receiving famciclovir in clinical trials for herpes zoster. Acute necroticohemorrhagic pancreatitis resulting in death has been reported following famciclovir administration for severe hepatitis B virus infection in a kidney graft recipient who was receiving cyclosporine concomitantly; a causal relationship to famciclovir was not established.

Nausea, diarrhea, vomiting, or abdominal pain has been reported in 11, 7, 5, or 3%, respectively, of HIV-infected patients receiving famciclovir in clinical studies.

● **Hepatic Effects**

Increased serum concentrations of ALT (SGPT) occurred in 1.4–2.4% of patients receiving famciclovir in clinical trials for herpes zoster or genital herpes. Increased serum concentrations of alkaline phosphatase, total bilirubin, and albumin each occurred rarely in patients receiving the drug in clinical trials for herpes zoster or genital herpes.

● **Other Adverse Effects**

Pruritus occurred in approximately 4% of patients (versus in about 3% of placebo recipients) receiving famciclovir in a large, controlled clinical trial for herpes zoster. Worsening of herpes zoster manifestations or complications has been reported in patients receiving the drug. Pharyngitis, sinusitis, injury, generalized pain, rigors, back pain, and arthralgia have occurred in patients receiving famciclovir in this clinical trial for herpes zoster. Increased serum phosphate concentrations occurred in 1.6% of patients receiving famciclovir in a large, placebo-controlled clinical trial for herpes zoster, and increased serum sodium or potassium concentrations and abnormal leukocyte counts each occurred rarely in patients receiving the drug in clinical trials for herpes zoster or genital herpes. Purpura has been reported rarely.

Acute renal failure has been reported in patients with renal disease who received doses of famciclovir that were inappropriately high for their level of renal function.

● **Precautions and Contraindications**

Famciclovir is contraindicated in patients with known hypersensitivity to the drug.

The manufacturer recommends that the dosage interval of famciclovir be adjusted carefully in patients with impaired renal function to prevent drug accumulation while maintaining adequate plasma concentrations of penciclovir, the active metabolite of famciclovir. (See Dosage and Administration: Dosage in Renal and Hepatic Impairment.)

Concomitant administration of famciclovir and probenecid or other drugs that are excreted extensively by active renal tubular secretion may result in increased plasma concentrations of penciclovir.

Each 125-, 250-, or 500-mg tablet of famciclovir contains 26.9, 53.7, or 107.4 mg of lactose, respectively. Patients with a history of galactose intolerance, severe lactase deficiency, or glucose-galactose malabsorption should not be given famciclovir tablets.

● **Pediatric Precautions**

Safety and efficacy of famciclovir in children younger than 18 years of age have not been established.

● **Geriatric Precautions**

Safety and efficacy of famciclovir in geriatric patients have not been specifically studied to date; however, in clinical studies of famciclovir for the treatment of herpes zoster involving over 800 patients, approximately 56% of the patients were 50 years of age or older, 30% were 65 years of age or older, and 13% were 75 years of age and older. As in the overall population of patients, headache and nausea were the most frequently reported adverse effects among geriatric patients. Although no overall differences were observed between geriatric and younger patients in the type or frequency of adverse effects in clinical studies, the possibility that some older patients may exhibit increased sensitivity to the drug cannot be ruled out. Based on comparisons from different studies of the oral administration of famciclovir, the mean renal clearance of penciclovir (the active metabolite of famciclovir) was 22% lower and the area under the plasma concentration-time curve (AUC) for penciclovir was 40% higher in healthy geriatric individuals 65–79 years of age than in healthy younger individuals.

Clinical studies of famciclovir for the treatment of recurrent herpes simplex did not include a sufficient number of patients 65 years of age or older to determine whether geriatric patients respond differently than younger adults

Caution is advised when famciclovir is used in geriatric patients. The greater frequency of decreased hepatic, renal, and/or cardiac function and of concomitant disease and drug therapy observed in the elderly should be considered.

● *Mutagenicity and Carcinogenicity*

Famciclovir and penciclovir (the active metabolite of famciclovir) did not show evidence of genotoxicity in in vitro tests for gene mutations in bacteria (*Salmonella typhimurium* and *Escherichia coli*) or unscheduled DNA synthesis in mammalian HeLa 83 cells at doses up to 10,000 and 5000 mcg/plate, respectively. Famciclovir was not mutagenic in the L5178Y mouse lymphoma assay at a concentration of 5000 mcg/mL, in the in vivo mouse micronucleus test at a dose of 4.8 g/kg, or in the rat dominant lethal study at a dose of 5 g/kg. Famciclovir caused increases in polyploidy in human lymphocytes in vitro in the absence of chromosomal damage at a concentration of 1200 mcg/mL. Penciclovir was mutagenic in the L5178Y mouse lymphoma assay for gene mutation/chromosomal aberrations, with and without metabolic activation at a concentration of 1000 mcg/mL. In human lymphocytes, penciclovir caused chromosomal aberrations in the absence of metabolic activation at a concentration of 250 mcg/mL. Penciclovir caused an increased incidence of micronuclei in mouse bone marrow in vivo when administered IV at a dose highly toxic to bone marrow (500 mg/kg) but not when administered orally.

Two-year dietary carcinogenicity studies of famciclovir were performed in rats and mice. After 7–8 months of drug administration, dosage was decreased from 750 to 600 mg/kg daily in female rats and in male and female mice and from 300 to 240 mg/kg daily in male rats to ensure long-term survival. An increase in the incidence of mammary adenocarcinoma was seen in female rats receiving 600 mg/kg daily (1.5–9 times the human systemic exposure at the recommended oral dosage of 500 mg 3 times daily or 125 mg twice daily based on the 24-hour AUC for penciclovir). Marginal increases in the incidence of subcutaneous tissue fibrosarcomas or squamous cell carcinomas of the skin were seen in female rats and male mice, respectively, at a dosage of 600 mg/kg daily (0.4–2.4 times the human systemic exposure based on the 24-hour AUC for penciclovir). No increases in tumor incidence occurred in male rats receiving dosages up to 240 mg/kg daily (0.9–5.4 times the human systemic exposure) or in female mice receiving dosages up to 600 mg/kg daily (0.4–2.4 times the human systemic exposure).

There currently is no evidence of mutagenicity or carcinogenicity in humans.

● *Pregnancy, Fertility, and Lactation*
Pregnancy

Reproduction studies using oral famciclovir dosages up to 1 g/kg daily in rats and rabbits (approximately 3.6–21.6 and 1.8–10.8 times the human systemic exposure to penciclovir, respectively, based on AUC comparisons) and IV dosages of 360 mg/kg daily in rats (2–12 times the human dose based on body surface area comparisons) or 120 mg/kg daily in rabbits (1.5–9 times the human dose based on body surface area comparisons) have not revealed evidence of adverse effects on embryofetal development. Similar studies using IV penciclovir dosages up to 80 mg/kg daily in rats (0.4–2.6 times the human dose based on body surface area comparisons) or 60 mg/kg daily in rabbits (0.7–4.2 times the human dose based on body surface area comparisons) also did not reveal evidence of adverse effects on embryofetal development. There are no adequate and well-controlled studies to date using famciclovir in pregnant women, and the drug should be used during pregnancy only when clearly needed.

To monitor maternal-fetal outcome of pregnant women exposed to famciclovir, the manufacturer maintains a Famciclovir Pregnancy Registry. The registry may be contacted by calling 888-669-6682.

Reproduction studies using famciclovir or penciclovir in rats, mice, and dogs revealed evidence of testicular toxicity following repeated oral administration of high dosages. Testicular changes, including atrophy of the seminiferous tubules, reduction in sperm count, and/or increased incidence of sperm with abnormal morphology or reduced motility, were observed. The degree of toxicity was related to dose and duration of exposure. In male rats, decreased fertility was observed following 10 weeks of dosing at 500 mg/kg daily (1.9–11.4 times the human AUC). Administration of famciclovir to male rats in dosages of 50 mg/kg daily (0.2–1.2 times the human systemic exposure based on AUC comparisons) for 26 weeks did not reveal evidence of sperm or testicular toxicity. Testicular toxicity was observed following administration of dosages of 600 mg/kg daily (0.4–2.4 times the human systemic exposure based on AUC comparisons) for 104 weeks in male mice and dosages of 150 mg/kg daily (1.7–10.2 times the human system exposure based on AUC comparisons) for 26 weeks in male dogs. No effect on spermatogenesis was observed in human males with genital herpes following oral famciclovir dosages of 250 mg twice daily for 18 weeks.

Fertility

Reproduction studies using oral famciclovir dosages up to 1 g/kg daily (3.6–21.6 times the human systemic exposure based on AUC comparisons) in female rats have not revealed evidence of impaired fertility or reproductive performance.

Lactation

It is not known whether famciclovir or penciclovir is distributed into milk in humans. Following oral administration of famciclovir to lactating rats, penciclovir was distributed into breast milk at concentrations higher than those observed in plasma. Data on safety of famciclovir in infants currently is not available.

DRUG INTERACTIONS

Famciclovir not metabolized by CYP isoenzymes.

● Drugs Eliminated by Renal Excretion

Potential increased plasma penciclovir concentrations when used concomitantly with other drugs eliminated by active renal tubular secretion (e.g., probenecid).

● Drugs Metabolized by Aldehyde Oxidase

Potential pharmacokinetic interaction with other drugs metabolized by aldehyde oxidase.

PHARMACOKINETICS

● Absorption

Bioavailability

Famciclovir, a prodrug of penciclovir, is rapidly and well absorbed following oral administration and metabolized to penciclovir. Little or no prodrug is present in plasma or urine.

Absolute bioavailability of penciclovir is 77% following oral administration of famciclovir; peak penciclovir plasma concentrations attained within 0.5–0.9 hours.

Pharmacokinetics in HIV-infected patients similar to healthy individuals.

Food

Administration of famciclovir with food decreases peak penciclovir plasma concentrations and delays time to peak concentrations but does not affect penciclovir AUC.

● Distribution

Extent

Not known whether penciclovir crosses the placenta or is distributed into human milk.

Plasma Protein Binding

Penciclovir <20% bound to plasma proteins.

● Elimination

Metabolism

Famciclovir is deacetylated and oxidized to penciclovir. Penciclovir is phosphorylated to penciclovir triphosphate (the active metabolite) in cells infected with HSV-1, HSV-2, or VZV. The inactive metabolite 6-deoxy penciclovir is converted to penciclovir by aldehyde oxidase.

Famciclovir not metabolized by CYP enzymes.

Elimination Route

Famciclovir eliminated principally by the kidneys as penciclovir and other metabolites. 73% of an oral famciclovir dose eliminated in urine and 27% eliminated in feces within 72 hours.

Half-life

Elimination half-life of penciclovir after oral administration of famciclovir 1.6–3 hours.

Intracellular half-life of penciclovir triphosphate in cells infected with HSV-1 or HSV-2 is 10 and 20 hours, respectively; intracellular half-life in VZV-infected cells is 7–14 hours.

Special Populations

AUC of penciclovir not affected when oral famciclovir used in patients with well-compensated chronic liver disease (chronic hepatitis, chronic ethanol abuse, primary biliary cirrhosis). Pharmacokinetics not evaluated in severe uncompensated hepatic impairment.

Renal clearance decreased and terminal elimination half-life increased in patients with renal impairment; half-life 6.2 hours if Cl_{cr} 20–39 mL/minute and 13.4 hours if Cl_{cr} <20 mL/minute.

AUC may be greater and renal clearance decreased in geriatric patients ≥65 years of age, presumably because of decreased renal function.

DESCRIPTION

Famciclovir (FCV) is a synthetic, acyclic purine nucleoside analog derived from guanine. The drug is the diacetyl 6-deoxy ester of penciclovir (PCV); penciclovir is structurally related to ganciclovir but pharmacologically and microbiologically related to acyclovir. Famciclovir is a prodrug of penciclovir and exhibits no antiviral activity until hydrolyzed in vivo to penciclovir and its active metabolites (e.g., penciclovir triphosphate).

Following metabolism of famciclovir in the intestinal wall and liver to penciclovir and intracellular conversion to the active triphosphate, the drug is active against various Herpesviridae including herpes simplex virus types 1 and 2 (HSV-1 and HSV-2), varicella-zoster virus, and Epstein-Barr virus (EBV). The drug also is active against hepatitis B virus (HBV). The drug exhibits only limited activity in vitro against cytomegalovirus (CMV).

PREPARATIONS

Excipients in commercially available drug preparations may have clinically important effects in some individuals; consult specific product labeling for details.

Famciclovir

Oral		
Tablets, film-coated	125 mg	**Famvir®**, Novartis
	250 mg	**Famvir®**, Novartis
	500 mg	**Famvir®**, Novartis

† Use is not currently included in the labeling approved by the US Food and Drug Administration.

Selected Revisions November 1, 2007, © Copyright, October 1, 1994, American Society of Health-System Pharmacists, Inc.

Ganciclovir Sodium

8:18.32 • NUCLEOSIDES AND NUCLEOTIDES

■ Ganciclovir, a synthetic nucleoside analog of guanine, is an antiviral agent active against herpesviruses.

USES

● Treatment of Cytomegalovirus Infection and Disease

Ganciclovir is used for the management of cytomegalovirus (CMV) retinitis in immunocompromised patients, including individuals with human immunodeficiency virus (HIV) infection. Ganciclovir also has been used for the management of other CMV infections (e.g., GI infections†, pneumonitis†, CNS infections†) in immunocompromised patients, but experience with the drug in these extraocular infections is less extensive.

Like other herpesviruses, CMV usually establishes a site(s) of latent infection following primary infection with the virus. Latency usually persists for life and the virus can be reactivated by various stimuli (e.g., immunosuppression), especially during periods of impaired cell-mediated immunity. Reactivation of the virus may result in subclinical infections or active end-organ CMV disease (e.g., retinitis, GI infections, pneumonitis, encephalitis), including serious, potentially life-threatening CMV disease.

Cytomegalovirus Retinitis

Ganciclovir is used for initial treatment (induction therapy) and maintenance therapy (secondary prophylaxis) of CMV retinitis in immunocompromised adults, including those with HIV infection and acquired immunodeficiency syndrome (AIDS), those with iatrogenic (e.g., chemotherapy-induced) immunosuppression, and transplant recipients. The drug also is used for the management of CMV retinitis in HIV-infected pediatric patients†.

Like other antivirals, ganciclovir is not a cure for CMV retinitis. Although ganciclovir can induce stabilization or improvement of ocular manifestations, the retinitis may relapse and/or progress during or after discontinuance of the drug.

Retinitis is the most common clinical manifestation of CMV end-organ disease in HIV-infected patients and ideally should be managed in consultation with an ophthalmologist familiar with the diagnosis and treatment of retinal diseases. Antiviral regimens for initial treatment of CMV retinitis in HIV-infected individuals should be selected based on the location and severity of CMV retinal lesions, severity of underlying immunosuppression, concomitant drug therapy, and the patient's ability to adhere to the treatment regimen. The antiviral regimen used for maintenance therapy of CMV retinitis in HIV-infected individuals should be selected with consideration for the location of the CMV retinal lesions, vision in the contralateral eye, the patient's immunologic and virologic status, and the patient's response to antiretroviral therapy.

For the management of immediate sight-threatening CMV retinal lesions (i.e., within 1.5 mm of the fovea) in HIV-infected adults and adolescents, the US Centers for Disease Control and Prevention (CDC), National Institutes of Health (NIH), and the HIV Medicine Association of the Infectious Diseases Society of America (IDSA) state that the preferred regimen is initial treatment (induction therapy) with intravitreal ganciclovir† or intravitreal foscarnet (1–4 doses given over a period of 7–10 days) in conjunction with oral valganciclovir (twice daily for 14–21 days) followed by maintenance therapy (secondary prophylaxis) with oral valganciclovir (once daily). One alternative regimen recommended by these experts for management of sight-threatening CMV retinitis in HIV-infected adults and adolescents is intravitreal ganciclovir† or intravitreal foscarnet (1–4 doses given over a period of 7–10 days) in conjunction with IV ganciclovir (twice daily for 14–21 days) followed by maintenance therapy (secondary prophylaxis) with oral valganciclovir (once daily). Use of systemic antivirals (without an intravitreal antiviral) usually is adequate for the management of CMV retinitis in patients who have only small peripheral lesions.

For the management of CMV retinitis in HIV-infected pediatric patients†, CDC, NIH, IDSA, and others state that IV ganciclovir is the drug of choice for initial treatment (induction therapy) and is one of several options for maintenance therapy (secondary prophylaxis). These experts state that oral valganciclovir is an option for the management of CMV retinitis in HIV-infected pediatric patients and can be considered for induction and/or maintenance therapy in adolescents and older children who can receive the recommended adult dosage of the drug and can also be considered in children who are able to transition from initial IV ganciclovir therapy to an oral regimen to complete treatment and/or for maintenance therapy. Data are limited regarding use of intravitreal antivirals in children, and intravitreal injections are impractical in most children.

Because of the risk of relapse, HIV-infected patients who have received adequate initial treatment of CMV retinitis should receive chronic maintenance therapy (secondary prophylaxis) until immune reconstitution occurs as a result of effective antiretroviral therapy. CDC, NIH, and IDSA state that consideration can be given to discontinuing maintenance therapy of CMV retinitis in HIV-infected adults and adolescents if CMV lesions have been treated for at least 3–6 months and are inactive and there has been a sustained (i.e., 3–6 months) increase in CD4+ T-cell count to greater than 100/mm³ in response to antiretroviral therapy. The safety of discontinuing maintenance therapy of CMV retinitis in HIV-infected pediatric patients has not been well studied; however, CDC, NIH, IDSA, and others state that consideration can be given to discontinuing such maintenance therapy in HIV-infected children who are receiving antiretroviral therapy and have a sustained (i.e., greater than 6 months) increase in CD4+ T-cell percentage to greater than 15% (children younger than 6 years of age) or an increase in CD4+ T-cell count to greater than 100/mm³ (children 6 years of age or older). These experts state that a decision to discontinue maintenance therapy of CMV retinitis should be made in consultation with an ophthalmologist and, if maintenance therapy is discontinued, the patient should continue to receive regular ophthalmologic monitoring (optimally every 3–6 months) for early detection of CMV relapse or immune reconstitution uveitis. If CD4+ T-cell count decreases to less than 100/mm³ (adults, adolescents, children 6 years of age or older) or if CD4+ T-cell percentage decreases to less than 15% (children younger than 6 years of age), maintenance therapy of CMV retinitis should be reinitiated.

For additional information on management of CMV retinitis and other CMV infections in HIV-infected individuals, the current clinical practice guidelines from CDC, NIH, and IDSA on the prevention and treatment of opportunistic infections in HIV-infected individuals available at http://www.aidsinfo.nih.gov should be consulted.

Clinical Experience

Efficacy of IV ganciclovir for the management of CMV retinitis has been established in uncontrolled and randomized controlled studies.

Initial ocular response (improvement or stabilization of vision and/or other ophthalmologic findings) reportedly occurs in 70–80% or more of immunocompromised patients receiving IV ganciclovir induction therapy. Stabilization of retinal lesions usually is apparent within 2 weeks of initiating ganciclovir therapy, although optimum clinical response to induction therapy may be delayed for several weeks to a month after initiating the drug. Ophthalmologic evidence of response to ganciclovir therapy may include decreased retinal opacification and inflammation, improvement in ocular hemorrhage and vasculitis (vascular sheathing) and in visual acuity, and development of atrophic changes in previously inflamed retinal areas, although reversal of resultant visual abnormalities may not occur. Stabilization or improvement in visual acuity reportedly occurs in 50% or more of patients receiving induction therapy with the drug and depends in part on the extent of macular (more specifically, foveal) and optic nerve involvement; however, such visual improvement rarely is dramatic, and rhegmatogenous retinal detachment can develop as a consequence of ganciclovir-induced resolution of retinitis, especially in patients with AIDS. (See Cautions: Ocular Effects.) In one study, visual acuity stabilized in 73%, improved (by more than 2 lines on the Snellen chart) in 15%, and deteriorated in 12% of ganciclovir-treated AIDS patients; there was no foveal involvement in those patients whose acuity improved. Extraocular (e.g., blood, urine) virologic response (negative cultures and/or decreased viral shedding) reportedly occurs in almost all ganciclovir-treated patients with CMV retinitis and usually is apparent within several days to 2 weeks after initiating therapy; however, a direct relationship between extraocular virologic response and clinical improvement of the retinitis has not been demonstrated.

In a retrospective, nonrandomized analysis of data from a study in 41 patients with AIDS and CMV retinitis who received IV ganciclovir induction therapy (5 mg/kg every 12 hours) for 14–21 days followed by IV ganciclovir maintenance therapy (5 mg/kg once daily every day or 6 mg/kg once daily 5 days each week), treatment with ganciclovir resulted in a delay in median time from diagnosis to initial retinitis progression compared with untreated patients (71 days versus 29 days).

In a randomized, prospective study in a limited number of patients with AIDS and peripheral CMV retinitis who received IV ganciclovir that was either initiated immediately or deferred, the median time to retinitis progression was 50 versus 13.5 days for those receiving immediate versus deferred ganciclovir treatment. This study indicates that all patients with HIV-related CMV retinitis, regardless of whether the lesions are peripheral or central, should be offered CMV treatment.

Extraocular Cytomegalovirus Infections

Although safety and efficacy of ganciclovir have not been established for the treatment of extraocular CMV infections, the drug has been used in immunocompromised patients for the management of CMV GI disease† and/or pneumonitis†, and, less frequently, for the management of CMV encephalitis†, hepatic†, cardiac†, and/or other CMV infections†.

GI Infections

Ganciclovir has been used for the management of CMV GI infections†, including colitis†, esophagitis†, gastritis†, and rectal disease†.

There is evidence that the clinical response rate of CMV GI infections† to ganciclovir is similar to or less than that of CMV retinitis. Approximately 70% or more of immunocompromised patients with CMV GI infections exhibit stabilization or improvement of the infection with ganciclovir induction therapy. Similarly, there is clearing of viremia and/or viruria and decreased viral shedding, with the frequency of virologic response usually exceeding clinical response. Response generally is apparent within 1–2 weeks of initiating therapy with the drug. In patients with colitis, response to ganciclovir therapy usually manifests as a reduction in stool frequency and diarrhea and in abdominal pain. In patients with esophagitis, response to the drug usually manifests as a reduction in dysphagia and odynophagia and in esophageal and epigastric pain. Improvement in rectal ulcers usually is observed in those with rectal disease, and weight gain also may be observed in response to ganciclovir therapy in patients with CMV GI infections.

Relapse, usually based on symptomatic recurrence or worsening but occasionally confirmed histologically, has occurred following ganciclovir induction therapy and discontinuance of the drug in immunosuppressed patients with CMV GI infections†. In some patients, particularly those with AIDS, long-term maintenance and/or intermittent induction therapy with the drug may be required.

CDC, NIH, and IDSA state that IV ganciclovir usually is the preferred antiviral for initial management of CMV GI disease† in HIV-infected adults and that a transition to oral valganciclovir may be considered when the patient can tolerate and absorb oral drugs. These experts state that IV foscarnet is a possible alternative to IV ganciclovir for the management of CMV esophagitis or colitis in those who cannot receive ganciclovir or have infections caused by ganciclovir-resistant CMV.

Pneumonitis

Ganciclovir has been used for the treatment of CMV pneumonitis† with variable results; in part, this variability in response appears to depend on the patient's underlying immunologic disorder. Clinical outcome in bone marrow transplant (BMT) recipients treated with ganciclovir alone has been particularly disappointing. Although CMV can be isolated from the respiratory tract of many AIDS patients, the virus rarely is the only pulmonary pathogen recovered, and its role as the principal pathogen in these patients has not been fully defined; in one study in AIDS patients with serious pulmonary disorders, CMV was isolated in 17% of patients but was the sole pathogen isolated in only 4%. Coexistent infections also may be present in organ (e.g., kidney) and BMT recipients, but presence of the virus as the principal pulmonary pathogen in these patients is better defined, especially in BMT recipients. Response to ganciclovir therapy appears to be better if the infection is treated early in its course; therefore, prompt recognition and diagnosis of the infection and initiation of ganciclovir therapy appear important.

There is some evidence that the clinical response rate of CMV pneumonitis† to ganciclovir therapy alone generally is less than that of CMV retinitis, especially in BMT recipients. In some studies, approximately 50–60% of immunocompromised patients with CMV pneumonitis exhibited clinical improvement with ganciclovir induction therapy alone. Up to about 80% of patients whose immunodeficiency resulted from AIDS or organ transplantation exhibited a clinical response to therapy with the drug alone, whereas response rates reportedly have ranged from 10–45% in BMT recipients receiving the drug alone. Response to

ganciclovir therapy usually manifests as improvement in respiratory symptoms and function; radiographic evidence of response usually is somewhat delayed. Evidence of virologic response occurs in almost all ganciclovir-treated patients with CMV pneumonitis, even in those who do not respond clinically. CMV pneumonitis may be less likely to require maintenance therapy after initial treatment than CMV retinitis.

The reasons for the poor response to ganciclovir monotherapy in BMT recipients with CMV pneumonitis† have not been fully elucidated, but in part the poor response may depend on differences in immunologic responses to the infection. Untreated CMV pneumonitis may be fatal in 85% or more of BMT recipients. These patients are more prone than AIDS or organ transplant recipients to develop respiratory failure and die despite pulmonary and extrapulmonary (e.g., blood, urine) clearing of the virus during ganciclovir therapy. There is animal and human evidence to suggest that CMV pneumonitis in BMT recipients is a complex immunopathologic disease. While it is possible that poor response in these patients may result from progressive infection, it has been suggested that a pulmonary immunologic reaction to the infection (e.g., secondary to a T-cell-mediated cytotoxic effect against viral and/or HLA antigens expressed on infected pulmonary cells) and/or exacerbation of the infection by some underlying factor not related to CMV (e.g., graft-versus-host disease, radiation/chemotherapy-induced inflammation, pulmonary toxicity from high oxygen concentrations used during ventilatory support) may be responsible. An association between graft-versus-host disease and development of CMV pneumonitis has been observed in humans and animals. In addition, an association between presence of functional T cells and development of CMV pneumonitis has been observed in animals and is further supported by the more favorable clinical response of the pneumonitis observed in AIDS patients in whom cytotoxic cellular immune responses generally are poorer.

For the management of well-documented CMV pneumonitis† in HIV-infected adults, CDC, NIH, and IDSA state that either IV ganciclovir or IV foscarnet is a reasonable choice.

Neurologic Disease

Ganciclovir has been used with variable results in immunosuppressed patients with CMV encephalitis†. Neurologic and magnetic resonance imaging findings improved with induction and/or maintenance therapy with the drug in some of these patients, while other patients failed to respond. Many patients with CMV encephalitis also have other active CMV infections.

A combination regimen of IV ganciclovir and IV foscarnet has been used for the management of CMV neurologic disease† (e.g., CMV encephalitis or myelitis), and is recommended by CDC, NIH, IDSA, and others for such infections in HIV-infected individuals.

Congenital Cytomegalovirus Disease

Although safety and efficacy of ganciclovir have not been established in neonates or infants with congenital CMV infection, the drug has been used for the management of symptomatic congenital CMV disease† when an antiviral was indicated.

Transmission of CMV from infected mothers to their fetuses occurs as a result of maternal viremia and transplacental infection. Perinatal infection also can occur from exposure of the neonate to CMV shedding in the mother's genital tract. Approximately 10% of neonates with congenital CMV infection are symptomatic at birth; mortality in symptomatic infants is about 10% and approximately 50–90% of symptomatic surviving neonates experience substantial morbidity (e.g., mental retardation, sensorineural hearing loss, microcephaly, seizures). The risk of congenital CMV infection resulting from primary maternal CMV infection may be higher and the disease may be more severe than that resulting from reactivation of maternal CMV infection.

Because there is some evidence that antivirals (i.e., ganciclovir, valganciclovir) may help prevent hearing deterioration and/or improve developmental delay in neonates and infants with moderate to severe symptomatic congenital CMV disease, the American Academy of Pediatrics (AAP) and other clinicians state that use of an antiviral regimen should be considered in such neonates if it can be initiated within the first month of life. Antivirals are not usually recommended for neonates with asymptomatic congenital CMV infection or only mildly symptomatic infection without evidence of CNS involvement.

AAP and others recommend that a 6-month regimen of oral valganciclovir be considered in neonates with moderate to severe symptomatic congenital CMV disease (with or without CNS involvement). A 6-week regimen of IV ganciclovir either alone or followed by a regimen of oral valganciclovir (continued until up to 12 months of age) also has been used in neonates with symptomatic congenital CMV disease.

CDC, NIH, IDSA, and others state that IV ganciclovir can be considered for initial treatment of symptomatic congenital CMV disease with CNS involvement in HIV-exposed or HIV-infected infants†.

Decisions regarding antiviral treatment in neonates with congenital CMV disease should be made in consultation with a pediatric infectious diseases specialist. Because of the risk of serious sequelae (e.g., late-onset hearing loss), long-term ophthalmologic and audiologic monitoring is necessary in patients with congenital CMV infection, regardless of antiviral treatment.

● Prevention of Cytomegalovirus Infection and Disease

IV ganciclovir is used for prophylaxis to prevent CMV infection and disease in solid organ transplant recipients, BMT recipients, and hematopoietic stem cell transplant (HSCT) recipients considered at high risk for the disease. The drug also has been used for preemptive treatment of CMV infection and disease† in transplant recipients.

CMV infection in transplant recipients can occur either as a primary infection in CMV-seronegative recipients of organs and cells from CMV-positive donors or as reactivation of latent CMV infection in CMV-seropositive recipients. CMV infection in transplant recipients is associated with substantial morbidity and mortality. The risk for CMV infection or reactivation is greatest during the first 3 months after transplantation and depends on several factors, including the serologic status of the recipient and donor, CMV-specific T-cell immunity in the recipient, and immunosuppressive regimens used in the recipient. Certain antiviral strategies have been used to prevent severe, life-threatening CMV disease in transplant recipients, including antiviral prophylaxis (initiated posttransplantation and continued for at least 3 months) and/or preemptive antiviral treatment (i.e., initiated when CMV infection is detected, but before clinical progression to symptomatic CMV disease). These antiviral strategies each have certain advantages and disadvantages.

Specialized references should be consulted for specific information regarding prevention and management of CMV infections in BMT, HSCT, or solid organ transplant recipients.

Clinical Experience

In a randomized, double-blind, placebo-controlled study in 149 cardiac allograft recipients at risk for developing CMV disease (i.e., CMV-seropositive or CMV-seronegative recipients of an organ from a CMV-seropositive donor), patients who received IV ganciclovir (5 mg/kg twice daily for 14 days beginning 1 day after cardiac allotransplantation, followed by 6 mg/kg once daily for 5 days per week for an additional 2 weeks) had a substantial decrease in the overall incidence of CMV disease compared with those receiving placebo. During the 120-day period following transplantation, 16% of patients who received ganciclovir developed acute CMV disease (GI infection, pneumonitis, myocarditis, CMV syndrome) compared with 43% of patients who received placebo. However, a clinically important decrease in the incidence of CMV disease was evident only in those cardiac allograft recipients who were CMV-seropositive before transplantation; patients who were at highest risk for serious disease (CMV-seronegative recipients of hearts from CMV-seropositive donors) did not have a clinically important decrease in the incidence of CMV disease. In patients who were CMV-seropositive prior to transplantation, 9% of those who received ganciclovir developed CMV disease compared with 46% who received placebo. In patients who were CMV-seronegative prior to transplantation and received hearts from CMV-positive donors, 35% of those who received ganciclovir developed CMV disease compared with 29% who received placebo. If acute CMV disease developed in patients receiving placebo, it occurred at an average of 45 or 56 days after transplantation in CMV-seropositive patients or CMV-seronegative recipients of CMV-seropositive hearts, respectively. If it developed in patients receiving ganciclovir, it occurred at an average of 71 days after transplantation.

In a randomized study in patients undergoing liver transplantation, IV ganciclovir (6 mg/kg daily from day 1–30 after transplantation, then 6 mg/kg daily 5 days weekly until day 100) was more effective than acyclovir (10 mg/kg IV every 8 hours from day 1 after transplantation until discharge, then 800 mg orally 4 times daily until day 100) in preventing CMV disease in these patients. During the first 120 days after the procedure, CMV infection occurred in only 5% of patients receiving ganciclovir but occurred in 38% of those receiving acyclovir. Symptomatic CMV disease developed in less than 1% of patients receiving ganciclovir and in 10% of those receiving acyclovir. Ganciclovir reduced the incidence of CMV disease in both CMV-seropositive and -seronegative individuals.

In several randomized, double-blind, placebo-controlled studies in bone marrow allograft recipients with asymptomatic CMV infection (CMV-positive culture of urine, throat, or blood) who were at risk for developing CMV disease, patients who received IV ganciclovir (5 mg/kg twice daily for 5–7 days, followed by 5 mg/kg once daily until 100 days after transplantation) had a substantial decrease in the incidence of CMV disease compared with those receiving placebo. During the 100-day period following transplantation, 0–3% of patients receiving ganciclovir and 29–43% of patients receiving placebo developed CMV disease. During the first 6-month period following transplantation, 9–16% of patients who had received ganciclovir and 32–43% of patients who had received placebo developed CMV disease. In one study, the overall survival rate 100 and 180 days after transplantation was higher in patients who had received ganciclovir. In another study, mortality at 100 and 180 days after transplantation was similar in both groups; it was suggested that this lack of difference in survival may have occurred because of a reduction in excess deaths in the placebo group since any patient who began to excrete the virus was removed from the study and given ganciclovir. The incidence of neutropenia was higher in patients receiving ganciclovir compared with those receiving placebo. In another study in bone marrow allograft recipients, patients were evaluated for presence of pulmonary CMV by bronchoscopy with bronchoalveolar lavage at days 35 and 49 after transplantation. Those patients with histologic, immunologic, or virologic evidence of asymptomatic pulmonary CMV infection were identified as at risk for developing interstitial pneumonia and randomly assigned to receive IV ganciclovir (5 mg/kg twice daily for 14 days followed by 5 mg/kg once daily 5 days per week until 120 days after transplantation) or no ganciclovir treatment. The incidence of subsequent interstitial pneumonia was lower in patients who received ganciclovir; interstitial pneumonia developed in 20% of those who received ganciclovir and 70% of those who received no antiviral therapy.

● Varicella-Zoster Virus Infections

Although optimal regimens for the management of progressive outer retinal necrosis caused by varicella-zoster virus† (VZV) in HIV-infected individuals have not been identified, CDC, NIH, and IDSA recommend treatment with at least one IV antiviral (acyclovir, ganciclovir, foscarnet, cidofovir) used in conjunction with at least one intravitreal antiviral (ganciclovir or foscarnet). Some experts recommend a regimen of IV ganciclovir and/or IV foscarnet used in conjunction with intravitreal† ganciclovir and/or intravitreal foscarnet. The prognosis for visual preservation in patients with progressive outer retinal necrosis caused by VZV is poor and such infections should be managed in consultation with an ophthalmologist.

DOSAGE AND ADMINISTRATION

● Reconstitution and Administration

Ganciclovir is administered by IV infusion.

Ganciclovir should not be administered by rapid IV infusion or direct IV injection since potentially toxic plasma concentrations of the drug may result.

Ganciclovir should *not* be administered by IM or subcutaneous injection because reconstituted and diluted solutions of the drug are alkaline (pH of 11) and may cause severe tissue irritation.

Ganciclovir has been administered by intravitreal injection†; however, a preparation of the drug specifically for intravitreal administration is not commercially available in the US.

Ganciclovir has been administered orally, but oral preparations of the drug are no longer commercially available in the US.

Females of childbearing potential should be tested for pregnancy prior to initiation of ganciclovir. (See Cautions: Pregnancy, Fertility, and Lactation.)

Renal function should be assessed prior to initiation of ganciclovir and monitored during therapy with the drug; dosage should be adjusted as necessary.

Complete blood counts with differential and platelet counts should be performed frequently during ganciclovir therapy, especially in those who developed cytopenias during previous therapy with ganciclovir or other nucleoside analogs and in those with neutrophil counts less than 1000/mm³ prior to initiation of ganciclovir. (See Cautions: Hematologic Effects.)

Patients receiving ganciclovir should be adequately hydrated.

The recommended dosage of ganciclovir and the recommended frequency and rate of administration of the drug should not be exceeded.

IV Infusion

IV infusions of ganciclovir should be given via a large peripheral or central vein. To avoid phlebitis and pain at the IV infusion site, the drug preferably should be administered using a plastic cannula and infused into a vein that will provide adequate blood flow for rapid dilution and distribution of the drug.

For IV infusion, single-dose vials of lyophilized ganciclovir sodium labeled as containing 500 mg of ganciclovir are reconstituted by adding 10 mL of preservative-free sterile water for injection to provide a solution containing 50 mg/mL. The vial should be gently swirled until the drug is completely wetted and a clear reconstituted solution is obtained. Bacteriostatic water for injection containing parabens should *not* be used to reconstitute ganciclovir sodium. (See Chemistry and Stability: Stability.) The appropriate dose of reconstituted solution should then be withdrawn from the vial and diluted in a compatible IV infusion solution (usually 100 mL). Solutions containing ganciclovir concentrations exceeding 10 mg/mL are not recommended for IV infusion.

Alternatively, if the commercially available ganciclovir sodium concentrate for injection for IV use containing 500 mg of ganciclovir (50 mg/mL) is used, the single-dose vial of solution should be shaken and the appropriate dose withdrawn from the vial and diluted in a compatible IV infusion solution (usually 100 mL). Solutions containing ganciclovir concentrations exceeding 10 mg/mL are not recommended for IV infusion.

Alternatively, commercially available single-dose IV bags containing 500 mg of ganciclovir in 250 mL of 0.8% sodium chloride (2 mg/mL) can be used for IV infusion without further dilution. The premixed solution in the bag should appear clear. If any crystals have formed in the solution, the bag should be gently shaken to redissolve the crystals prior to use. Any unused portions of the premixed solution should be discarded.

Ganciclovir solutions should be inspected visually for discoloration and particulate matter prior to administration; if either is present, the solution should be discarded.

Ganciclovir lyophilized powder and solutions of the drug should be handled cautiously because of the high pH of some preparations and because of the mutagenic and/or carcinogenic potential of the drug (see Cautions: Mutagenicity and Carcinogenicity). The use of disposable gloves is recommended. If ganciclovir powder or solutions of the drug contact the skin or mucous membranes, the affected area should be washed immediately and thoroughly with soap and water. If the drug comes in contact with the eyes, the eyes should flushed thoroughly with water.

Since ganciclovir shares some of the properties of cytotoxic drugs (i.e., mutagenicity, carcinogenicity), the manufacturers state that consideration should be given to handling and disposing the drug according to guidelines issued for cytotoxic drugs. For further information on the handling of cytotoxic drugs, see the ASHP Guidelines on Handling Hazardous Drugs at http://ahfsdruginformation.com.

Rate of Administration

Ganciclovir solutions should be administered by IV infusion at a constant rate over 1 hour.

• *Dosage*

Ganciclovir is commercially available as the base and as ganciclovir sodium; dosage is expressed in terms of ganciclovir.

Adult Dosage

Cytomegalovirus Retinitis

For the treatment of cytomegalovirus (CMV) retinitis in adults with normal renal function (creatinine clearance of 70 mL/minute or greater), including those with human immunodeficiency virus (HIV) infection, the recommended dosage of IV ganciclovir for initial treatment (induction therapy) is 5 mg/kg every 12 hours for 14–21 days. In patients with immediate sight-threatening CMV retinal lesions (i.e., within 1.5 mm of the fovea), the US Centers for Disease Control and Prevention (CDC), National Institutes of Health (NIH), and HIV Medicine Association of the Infectious Diseases Society of America (IDSA) recommend that initial treatment also include an appropriate intravitreal antiviral. (See Cytomegalovirus Retinitis under Uses: Treatment of Cytomegalovirus Infection and Disease.)

After completion of initial treatment, the usual dosage of IV ganciclovir for maintenance therapy (secondary prophylaxis) of CMV retinitis in adults with normal renal function is 5 mg/kg once daily. Alternatively, IV ganciclovir can be given in a dosage of 6 mg/kg once daily 5 days each week for maintenance therapy.

Decisions regarding discontinuance of maintenance therapy of CMV retinitis in HIV-infected individuals who have received CMV treatment for at least 3–6 months, have inactive CMV retinal lesions, and have achieved immune reconstitution as the result of antiretroviral therapy should be made in consultation with an ophthalmologist. (See Cytomegalovirus Retinitis under Uses: Treatment of Cytomegalovirus Infection and Disease.)

Cytomegalovirus Esophagitis or Colitis

For the treatment of CMV GI infections† in adults with normal renal function, a ganciclovir dosage of 5 mg/kg IV every 12 hours for 14–21 days has been used for initial treatment (induction); alternatively, a dosage of 2.5 mg/kg IV every 8 hours also has been used. If maintenance therapy is required, dosages comparable to those used for maintenance therapy of CMV retinitis have been used.

For the management of CMV esophagitis† or colitis† in HIV-infected adults, CDC, NIH, and IDSA recommend that IV ganciclovir be given in a dosage of 5 mg/kg every 12 hours and state that a switch to oral valganciclovir can be made after the patient can absorb and tolerate oral therapy. These experts recommend that antiviral therapy be continued for 21–42 days or until signs and symptoms of the infection have resolved. Maintenance therapy (secondary prophylaxis) usually is not necessary, but should be considered if relapse occurs.

Cytomegalovirus Pneumonitis

For the treatment of CMV pneumonitis† in adults with normal renal function, a ganciclovir dosage of 5 mg/kg IV every 12 hours for 14–21 days has been used for initial treatment (induction); alternatively, a dosage of 2.5 mg/kg IV every 8 hours also has been used. If maintenance therapy is required, dosages comparable to those used for maintenance therapy of CMV retinitis have been used.

If IV ganciclovir is used for the management of well-documented CMV pneumonitis† in HIV-infected adults, CDC, NIH, and IDSA state that the same dosage recommended for the management of CMV retinitis in HIV-infected adults should be used. The optimal duration of treatment in such patients has not been established.

Cytomegalovirus Neurologic Disease

If IV ganciclovir is used for the management of CMV neurologic disease† in HIV-infected adults, CDC, NIH, and IDSA state that the same dosage recommended for the management of CMV retinitis in HIV-infected adults should be used in conjunction with IV foscarnet. The optimal duration of treatment in such patients has not been established.

Prevention of Cytomegalovirus Infection and Disease in Transplant Recipients

For prophylaxis to prevent CMV infection and disease in transplant recipients with normal renal function, the manufacturers recommend that IV ganciclovir be given in a dosage of 5 mg/kg every 12 hours for 7–14 days followed by a maintenance dosage of 5 mg/kg once daily 7 days each week or 6 mg/kg once daily 5 days each week. Prophylaxis should be continued until 100–120 days posttransplantation.

Some experts recommend that IV ganciclovir be given in a dosage of 5 mg/kg once daily for prophylaxis of CMV infection and disease in transplant recipients with normal renal function. These experts recommend that antiviral prophylaxis be continued for 3 months in CMV-seropositive recipients of solid organs (kidney, pancreas, kidney/pancreas, liver, heart) and for 3–6 months in CMV-seronegative recipients of solid organs (kidney, pancreas, kidney/pancreas, liver, heart) from CMV-seropositive donors.

If IV ganciclovir is used for preemptive treatment of CMV infection in solid organ transplant recipients†, a dosage of 5 mg/kg twice daily is recommended in those with normal renal function.

Varicella-Zoster Virus Infections

For the management of progressive outer retinal necrosis caused by varicella-zoster virus† (VZV) in HIV-infected adults, CDC, NIH, and IDSA state that a regimen that includes IV ganciclovir in a dosage of 5 mg/kg every 12 hours (used with or without IV foscarnet) in conjunction with intravitreal ganciclovir† (used with or without intravitreal foscarnet) can be considered.

Pediatric Dosage
Cytomegalovirus Retinitis

For initial treatment (induction therapy) of CMV retinitis in pediatric patients†, including HIV-infected children†, CDC, NIH, IDSA, and others recommend that IV ganciclovir be given in a dosage of 5 mg/kg IV every 12 hours for 14–21 days (may be increased to 7.5 mg/kg every 12 hours if needed). After completion of initial treatment, these experts recommend that pediatric patients receive IV ganciclovir in a dosage of 5 mg/kg once daily for 5–7 days each week for maintenance therapy (secondary prophylaxis).

Decisions regarding discontinuance of maintenance therapy of CMV retinitis in HIV-infected individuals who have inactive CMV retinal lesions and have achieved immune reconstitution as the result of antiretroviral therapy should be made in consultation with an ophthalmologist. (See Cytomegalovirus Retinitis under Uses: Treatment of Cytomegalovirus Infection and Disease.)

CNS or Disseminated Cytomegalovirus Infections

For initial treatment (induction therapy) of CNS infections caused by CMV in HIV-infected children†, CDC, NIH, IDSA, and others recommend that IV ganciclovir be given in a dosage of 5 mg/kg every 12 hours in conjunction with IV foscarnet. Initial treatment should be continued until symptomatic improvement.

For initial treatment (induction therapy) of disseminated CMV infections in HIV-infected children†, CDC, NIH, IDSA, and others state that IV ganciclovir be given in a dosage of 5 mg/kg IV every 12 hours (may be increased to 7.5 mg/kg every 12 hours if needed). Initial treatment should be continued for 14–21 days.

After completion of initial treatment, the recommended dosage of IV ganciclovir for maintenance therapy (secondary prophylaxis) of CNS or disseminated CMV infections in HIV-infected children† is 5 mg/kg once daily for 5–7 days each week.

Congenital Cytomegalovirus Disease

If IV ganciclovir is used for the management of symptomatic congenital CMV disease† when an antiviral is indicated (see Congenital Cytomegalovirus Disease under Uses: Treatment of Cytomegalovirus Infection and Disease), the American Academy of Pediatrics (AAP) and other clinicians recommend a dosage of 6 mg/kg twice daily.

AAP and other clinicians recommend that, if an antiviral is indicated, it should be initiated within the first month of life and continued for a total of 6 months. If IV ganciclovir is used initially, treatment should be transitioned to oral valganciclovir when the infant is able to tolerate and absorb oral drugs.

Prevention of Cytomegalovirus Infection and Disease in Transplant Recipients

For prophylaxis to prevent CMV infection and disease in pediatric transplant recipients†, some clinicians recommend that IV ganciclovir be given in a dosage of 5 mg/kg every 12 hours for 5–7 days (or 7–14 days) followed by a maintenance regimen of 5 mg/kg once daily 7 days each week or 6 mg/kg once daily 5 days each week. Prophylaxis should be continued for 100–120 days posttransplantation.

Other clinicians recommend that IV ganciclovir be given in a dosage of 5 mg/kg once daily for prophylaxis in pediatric transplant recipients† and that antiviral prophylaxis be continued for 3 months or longer depending on the immune status of the recipient and type of transplant.

If IV ganciclovir is used for preemptive treatment of CMV infection in pediatric patients†, a dosage of 5 mg/kg twice daily for 7–14 days followed by 5 mg/kg once daily has been recommended.

Varicella-Zoster Virus Infections

For the management of progressive outer retinal necrosis caused by VZV in HIV-infected children†, CDC, NIH, IDSA, and others state that a regimen that includes IV ganciclovir given in a dosage of 5 mg/kg every 12 hours (used with IV foscarnet) in conjunction with intravitreal ganciclovir† (used with or without intravitreal foscarnet) can be considered.

● Dosage in Renal Impairment

In patients with impaired renal function, doses and/or frequency of administration of ganciclovir must be modified in response to the degree of impairment.

Dosage should be based on the patient's measured or estimated creatinine clearance. The patient's creatinine clearance (Ccr) can be estimated by using the following formulas:

$$Ccr\ male = \frac{(140 - age) \times weight}{72 \times serum\ creatinine}$$

$$Ccr\ female = 0.85 \times Ccr\ male$$

where age is in years, weight is in kg,
and serum creatinine is in mg/dL.

When IV ganciclovir is used for the management of CMV retinitis in adults with renal impairment, the manufacturers recommend the following dosage for initial treatment (induction therapy) and maintenance therapy (secondary prophylaxis) based on creatinine clearance. (See Table 1.)

TABLE 1. Dosage of IV Ganciclovir for Management of CMV Retinitis in Adults with Renal Impairment

Creatinine Clearance (mL/minute)	Initial Treatment (Induction) Dosage	Maintenance Dosage
50–69	2.5 mg/kg every 12 hours	2.5 mg/kg every 24 hours
25–49	2.5 mg/kg every 24 hours	1.25 mg/kg every 24 hours
10–24	1.25 mg/kg every 24 hours	0.625 mg/kg every 24 hours
Less than 10	1.25 mg/kg 3 times weekly	0.625 mg/kg 3 times weekly

In adults undergoing hemodialysis, dosage of IV ganciclovir for initial treatment (induction therapy) of CMV retinitis should not exceed 1.25 mg/kg 3 times weekly and dosage for maintenance therapy should not exceed 0.625 mg/kg 3 times weekly. Because hemodialysis may reduce ganciclovir plasma concentrations by approximately 50% (see Pharmacokinetics: Elimination), dosing of the drug should be timed so that doses administered on the days of dialysis are given shortly after completion of dialysis.

CAUTIONS

Adverse reactions to ganciclovir occur frequently, but usually are reversible following discontinuance of therapy with the drug. Because most patients receiving ganciclovir have serious underlying disease with multiple baseline symptomatology and clinical abnormalities and are receiving multiple drugs concomitantly and because clinical studies generally did not include a placebo control, it is difficult to establish whether a causal relationship to ganciclovir exists for many reported adverse effects.

Adverse effects reported in 20% of more of patients receiving ganciclovir in clinical trials include hematologic effects (leukopenia, neutropenia, thrombocytopenia, anemia), pyrexia, GI effects (diarrhea, nausea, decreased appetite, abdominal pain), catheter-associated effects (sepsis), hyperhidrosis, asthenia, headache, cough, dyspnea, and increased creatinine concentrations. In clinical trials evaluating ganciclovir in patients with cytomegalovirus (CMV) retinitis, adverse reactions necessitated discontinuance of the drug in 9% of patients.

● Hematologic Effects

Hematologic toxicity, including granulocytopenia (neutropenia), anemia, thrombocytopenia, and pancytopenia, have been reported in patients receiving ganciclovir. Hematologic effects, which may be severe, are one of the most common adverse reactions to the drug.

Neutropenia (absolute neutrophil count less than 1000/mm³), which is potentially fatal, has been reported in up to 25–60% of patients receiving ganciclovir and is the most common dose-limiting adverse effect of the drug. Absolute neutrophil count declines to less than 500/mm³ in approximately 15–25% of patients receiving the drug for the treatment of CMV infection. Granulocytopenia (neutropenia) usually develops early in treatment (e.g., during the first or second week of induction therapy), but can occur at any time. In most cases, interruption of ganciclovir therapy or a decrease in dosage will result in increased neutrophil counts, which usually is evident within 3–7 days; however, prolonged or irreversible neutropenia has occurred, and bacterial or fungal sepsis and subsequent death have been reported occasionally in patients with ganciclovir-induced neutropenia. Neutropenia has recurred following reinitiation of ganciclovir therapy, occasionally even at reduced dosage. If severe neutropenia (absolute neutrophil count less than 500/mm³) occurs, ganciclovir therapy is not recommended.

Patients with human immunodeficiency virus (HIV) infection and acquired immunodeficiency syndrome (AIDS) may be at greater risk of developing neutropenia compared with other immunosuppressed patients receiving the drug. There also is limited evidence to suggest that bone marrow transplant (BMT) recipients may be at greater risk than organ transplant recipients for developing ganciclovir-induced neutropenia, but the possibility exists that other factors (e.g., concurrently administered drugs) may have contributed to the observed differences. In controlled studies in patients who received IV ganciclovir for prevention of CMV disease following transplantation, the absolute neutrophil count decreased to 1000/mm³ or less in 7% of cardiac allograft recipients (mean duration of IV ganciclovir 28 days) and in 41% of bone marrow allograft recipients (mean duration of IV ganciclovir 45 days); 11% of cardiac allograft recipients who received placebo and 23% of bone marrow allograft recipients who did not receive ganciclovir therapy also had neutrophil counts this low.

Thrombocytopenia occurs frequently in patients receiving ganciclovir, developing in approximately 20% of patients who receive the drug. Interruption of ganciclovir therapy or a decrease in dosage usually results in increased platelet counts. Patients with low baseline platelet counts (less than 100,000/mm³) appear to be more prone to develop this reaction. In addition, patients who are iatrogenically immunosuppressed appear to be at greater risk than AIDS patients of developing thrombocytopenia, which occurred in 46 and 14% of such patients, respectively, in one study. In controlled studies in patients who received IV ganciclovir for prevention of CMV disease following transplantation, platelet counts decreased to less than 25,000/mm³ in 3% of cardiac allograft recipients (mean duration of IV ganciclovir 28 days) and in 32% of bone marrow allograft recipients (mean duration of IV ganciclovir 45 days); 1% of cardiac allograft recipients who received placebo and 28% of bone marrow allograft recipients who did not receive ganciclovir therapy in these studies also had platelet counts this low. If the platelet count declines to less than 25,000/mm³, ganciclovir therapy is not recommended.

Leukopenia has been reported in 41% and anemia has been reported in 25% of patients receiving ganciclovir for maintenance therapy of CMV retinitis. Anemia with hemoglobin concentrations less than 6.5 g/dL occurred in 5% of patients. If hemoglobin concentrations decline to less than 8 g/dL, ganciclovir therapy is not recommended.

Pancytopenia and bone marrow failure have been reported in clinical studies in patients receiving ganciclovir for the treatment of CMV retinitis or in transplant recipients receiving the drug for prophylaxis of CMV. Hemolytic anemia, agranulocytosis, and granulocytopenia have been reported during postmarketing experience in patients receiving ganciclovir.

Although experience is limited, intravitreal injection† of ganciclovir does not appear to be associated with appreciable systemic toxicity and this route has been suggested as an alternative to IV ganciclovir in patients with CMV retinitis in whom hematologic toxicity is not tolerated.

Ganciclovir-induced neutropenia and thrombocytopenia appear to result from a direct, dose-dependent myelotoxic effect of the drug. This effect probably results from nonspecific activation of the drug by cellular (host cell) enzymes and subsequent inhibition of cellular DNA synthesis, particularly in rapidly dividing cells (e.g., in bone marrow). In vitro, ganciclovir has been shown to exhibit dose-dependent inhibitory effects on both myeloid and erythroid human progenitor cells, with erythroid precursors being slightly less sensitive than myeloid precursors to the cytotoxic effects. In one in vitro study, ganciclovir exhibited substantial and acyclovir minimal cytotoxic effects as determined by inhibition of colony formation of human granulocyte-macrophage precursors, which could in part explain the apparent differences in in vivo hematologic toxicity of these drugs.

Careful monitoring for potential hematologic toxicity is necessary during ganciclovir therapy. (See Cautions: Precautions and Contraindications.)

● **Ocular Effects**

Rhegmatogenous retinal detachment has been reported in patients with CMV retinitis, both before and after initiation of ganciclovir therapy; however, the relationship between ganciclovir and retinal detachment is not known. Such detachment

is thought to result from the hastening of the involutional stage of the disease in which the retina thins as necrotic tissue is mobilized and edema fluid resorbs; these changes predispose the retina to tears and detachment. Retinal detachment has been reported in 11–30% of ganciclovir-treated patients with CMV retinitis. This complication appears to occur more frequently in AIDS patients than in other immunosuppressed patients and may be related to the inability of AIDS patients to form firm scar tissue, secondary to impaired inflammatory responses, as the retina heals.

Intravitreal injection† of ganciclovir (0.05–0.1 mL of a solution containing 2–8 mg/mL) did not produce any apparent oculotoxic effects in animal studies or in a limited number of patients being treated for CMV retinitis. In one study in several patients with CMV retinitis, there was no evidence during 77–244 days of observation of oculotoxic effects (e.g., lens changes, anterior segment or vitreal inflammation, retinal detachment) associated with intravitreal injection of 9–30 (mean: 16.6) doses of the drug per eye. In a study in rabbits, intravitreal injection of single ganciclovir doses ranging from 10–400 mcg at concentrations of 1–20 mcg/mL produced no discernible ophthalmologic or histologic changes in the eye or in electroretinographic B waves.

Although intravitreal injection† of ganciclovir has been well tolerated, local reactions, such as foreign body sensation, small conjunctival or vitreal hemorrhage, and mattering, have been associated with such administration. In addition, conjunctival scarring and scleral induration have been observed occasionally in patients receiving multiple intravitreal injections of the drug. Staphylococcal endophthalmitis, which responded to intravitreal antibacterial therapy alone or combined with systemic therapy, has been reported in several patients receiving intravitreal ganciclovir. In addition, rhegmatogenous retinal detachment occurred in several patients during intravitreal injection; while this complication also has been associated with IV ganciclovir therapy, the possibility exists that local trauma associated with intravitreal injection may have contributed to its occurrence in these patients.

● **Nervous System Effects**

Adverse nervous system effects, including headache, insomnia, dizziness, paresthesia, hypoesthesia, seizures, somnolence, and tremor, have been reported in clinical studies in patients receiving ganciclovir for the treatment of CMV retinitis or in transplant recipients receiving the drug for prophylaxis of CMV. Peripheral neuropathy has been reported in 9% of patients receiving IV ganciclovir for maintenance therapy of CMV retinitis. Dysesthesia, dysphasia, extrapyramidal disorder, facial paralysis, amnesia, anosmia, myelopathy, cerebrovascular accident, third cranial nerve paralysis, aphasia, encephalopathy, and intracranial hypertension have been reported during postmarketing experience in patients receiving ganciclovir. In some cases, observed nervous system effects may have resulted from causes other than the drug itself, such as opportunistic infections (e.g., toxoplasmosis, cryptococcosis) or HIV encephalopathy, and this possibility should be considered in any ganciclovir-treated patient who develops such effects.

Psychiatric disorders, including depression, confused state, anxiety, agitation, psychotic disorder, abnormal thinking, and abnormal dreams, have been reported in clinical studies in patients receiving ganciclovir for the treatment of CMV retinitis or in transplant recipients receiving the drug for prophylaxis of CMV. Irritability and hallucinations have been reported during postmarketing experience in patients receiving ganciclovir.

● **GI Effects**

Diarrhea, decreased appetite, and vomiting have been reported in 44, 14, and 13% of patients, respectively, receiving IV ganciclovir for maintenance treatment of CMV retinitis. Other adverse GI effects that have been reported in clinical studies in patients receiving ganciclovir for the treatment of CMV retinitis or in transplant recipients receiving the drug for prophylaxis of CMV include nausea, GI perforation, abdominal pain, dyspepsia, flatulence, constipation, mouth ulceration, dysphagia, abdominal distention, pancreatitis, eructation, dysgeusia, and dry mouth. Intestinal ulcer has been reported during postmarketing experience in patients receiving ganciclovir.

● **Renal and Genitourinary Effects**

Increased serum creatinine concentrations have been reported when IV ganciclovir was used in geriatric patients or in transplant patients, including transplant patients receiving concomitant therapy with nephrotoxic drugs (e.g., cyclosporine, amphotericin B). In a placebo-controlled study in cardiac allograft recipients, increased serum creatinine concentrations (2.5 mg/dL or greater) occurred in 18% of those receiving IV ganciclovir and 4% of those receiving placebo. In a study in bone marrow allograft recipients, 20% of patients receiving ganciclovir had serum creatinine concentrations of 2.5 mg/dL or greater whereas no patients receiving placebo had these increased concentrations. In a study in bone marrow allograft recipients, increased serum creatinine concentrations were not reported in patients receiving ganciclovir.

Kidney failure, abnormal renal function, urinary frequency, and hematuria have been reported in clinical studies in patients receiving ganciclovir for the treatment of CMV retinitis or in transplant recipients receiving the drug for prophylaxis of CMV. Renal tubular disorder and hemolytic uremic syndrome have been reported during postmarketing experience in patients receiving ganciclovir.

● Local Effects

Inflammation, edema, phlebitis, and/or pain at the site of IV infusion have been reported in patients receiving ganciclovir and probably are related to the high pH of the infusion solution. (See Dosage and Administration: Reconstitution and Administration.) To minimize the risk of phlebitis, the use of a vein with adequate blood flow is recommended to allow for rapid dilution and distribution of the drug.

Infection at the IV catheter site and other catheter-associated events (e.g., sepsis) have been reported in patients receiving IV ganciclovir.

Intravitreal injection† of ganciclovir in a limited number of animals and humans did not appear to produce oculotoxic effects, although other local ocular effects occasionally were observed. (See Cautions: Ocular Effects.)

● Other Adverse Effects

Pyrexia has been reported in 48% of patients receiving IV ganciclovir for maintenance therapy of CMV retinitis. Other adverse effects reported in 5–13% of patients receiving IV ganciclovir include sepsis, infection, hyperhidrosis, chills, and pruritus.

Hypersensitivity, including anaphylactic or allergic reactions, have been reported in patients receiving ganciclovir.

● Precautions and Contraindications

Ganciclovir is contraindicated in patients who have had a clinically important hypersensitivity reaction (e.g., anaphylaxis) to ganciclovir, valganciclovir, or any component of the formulation.

Because ganciclovir therapy is associated with hematologic toxicity (e.g., neutropenia, anemia, and/or thrombocytopenia), complete blood counts with differential and platelet counts should be monitored frequently in all patients, especially in those with renal impairment, baseline neutrophil counts less than 1000/mm³, or a history of leukopenia during treatment with ganciclovir or other nucleoside analogs and in those receiving myelosuppressive drugs or radiation therapy. Ganciclovir is not recommended in patients with absolute neutrophil counts less than 500/mm³, platelet counts less than 25,000/mm³, or hemoglobin concentrations less than 8 g/dL. Patients should be informed about the potential hematologic toxicities of the drug and the importance of close monitoring of blood cell counts.

Because plasma concentrations and half-life of ganciclovir are increased in patients with renal impairment, the drug should be used with caution in such patients and dosage should be adjusted based on the degree of renal impairment. (See Dosage and Administration: Dosage in Renal Impairment.) Renal function monitoring is essential in all patients receiving ganciclovir therapy, especially in geriatric patients and in transplant recipients receiving concomitant nephrotoxic drugs (e.g., cyclosporine, amphotericin B). (See Drug Interactions.) Patients receiving ganciclovir should be adequately hydrated since the drug is almost entirely excreted renally and normal clearance depends on adequate renal function. Patients should be informed that ganciclovir has been associated with decreased renal function and that serum creatinine concentrations or creatinine clearance should be monitored during treatment with the drug and that dosage adjustments are necessary in patients with renal impairment.

Safety and efficacy of ganciclovir have not been evaluated in patients with hepatic impairment.

Frequent ophthalmologic examinations are necessary in patients being treated for CMV retinitis to monitor status of the CMV retinitis and assess for other retinal abnormalities. Patients should be informed that ganciclovir is not a cure for CMV retinitis and that they may continue to experience progression and/or recurrence of the retinitis during or following treatment with the drug. Patients also should be advised about the necessity of frequent ophthalmologic

examinations and that some patients may require more frequent ophthalmologic follow-up.

Patients should be advised that ganciclovir may cause seizures, dizziness, and/or confusion, which may affect cognitive abilities (e.g., ability to drive or operate machinery).

Patients should be advised that animal data suggest that ganciclovir is a potential carcinogen. (See Cautions: Mutagenicity and Carcinogenicity.)

Patients should be advised that ganciclovir may cause temporary or permanent inhibition of spermatogenesis in males and suppression of fertility in females. (See Cautions: Pregnancy, Fertility, and Lactation.)

Because of the mutagenic potential of ganciclovir and the potential for fetal harm, women of reproductive potential should undergo pregnancy testing before initiation of ganciclovir. In addition, females of childbearing potential should use effective contraception during and for at least 30 days after ganciclovir therapy and male patients should use barrier contraceptive methods during and for at least 90 days after ganciclovir therapy. (See Cautions: Pregnancy, Fertility, and Lactation.)

● Pediatric Precautions

Safety and efficacy of ganciclovir have not been established in pediatric patients.

Granulocytopenia and thrombocytopenia were the most common adverse effects reported in pediatric patients† who received ganciclovir in clinical trials.

Although the pharmacokinetics of IV ganciclovir reported in pediatric patients are similar to those reported in adults (see Pharmacokinetics), safety and efficacy of such ganciclovir exposures in pediatric patients have not been established.

● Geriatric Precautions

Clinical studies of ganciclovir did not include sufficient numbers of patients 65 years of age or older to determine whether geriatric patients respond differently than younger adults. Dosage in geriatric patients generally should be selected carefully, taking into account the greater frequency of decreased hepatic, renal, and/or cardiac function and of concomitant disease and drug therapy in the elderly.

Because geriatric patients may have decreased renal function and because patients with renal impairment may be at increased risk of ganciclovir-induced toxicity, particular attention should be paid to evaluating renal function prior to and during ganciclovir therapy in this age group. If evidence of renal impairment exists or develops, appropriate dosage adjustments should be made. (See Dosage and Administration: Dosage in Renal Impairment.)

● Mutagenicity and Carcinogenicity

Based on animal data, ganciclovir should be considered a potential carcinogen in humans.

Ganciclovir increased mutations in mouse lymphoma cells and DNA damage in human lymphocytes in vitro at concentrations between 50–500 and 250–2000 mcg/mL, respectively. In the mouse micronucleus assay, ganciclovir was clastogenic at doses of 150 and 500 mg/kg (2.8–10 times exposures attained in humans with the recommended human dose), but such effects were not observed at doses comparable to the recommended human dose. Ganciclovir was not mutagenic in the Ames *Salmonella* assay at concentrations of 500–5000 mcg/mL.

Ganciclovir was carcinogenic in mice at mean drug exposures equal to those attained in humans with the recommended dose of 5 mg/kg. At exposures 1.4 times the human exposure at the recommended human dose, there was a significant increase in the incidence of tumors of the preputial gland in males, forestomach (nonglandular mucosa) in males and females, and reproductive tissues (ovaries, uterus, mammary gland, clitoral gland, vagina) and liver in females. At exposures 0.1 times the human exposure at the recommended human dose, there was a slightly increased incidence of tumors in the preputial and harderian glands in males, forestomach in males and females, and liver in females. Carcinogenic effects were not observed in mice at exposures estimated to be 0.01 times those attained in humans with the recommended human dose.

● Pregnancy, Fertility, and Lactation
Pregnancy

Animal data indicate that ganciclovir has the potential to cause fetal toxicity, including birth defects, in humans. Data regarding use of ganciclovir in pregnant women are inadequate to establish whether the drug poses a risk to pregnancy outcomes. Ganciclovir appears to cross the placenta based on ex vivo experiments with human placenta and at least one case report in a pregnant woman.

In animal studies, ganciclovir caused maternal and fetal toxicity and embryofetal mortality in pregnant mice and rabbits and teratogenic effects in rabbits at systemic exposures that were approximately 2 times those attained in humans at the recommended human dose. IV ganciclovir administered to pregnant mice (108 mg/kg daily) and rabbits (60 mg/kg daily) and administered to female mice (90 mg/kg) prior to mating, during gestation, and during lactation resulted in fetal resorptions in at least 85% of the mice and rabbits. Fetal growth retardation, embryolethality, and teratogenic effects (cleft palate, anophthalmia/microphthalmia, hydrocephaly, brachygnathia, aplastic organs [kidney, pancreas]) were reported in the rabbits. In pre/postnatal development studies in mice, maternal/fetal toxicity and embryolethality were observed and included hypoplasia of the testes and seminal vesicles in male offspring, as well as pathologic changes in the nonglandular region of the stomach.

Although most maternal CMV infections are asymptomatic or may be associated with a self-limited mononucleosis-like syndrome, CMV infections in pregnant immunocompromised patients (e.g., HIV-infected patients with AIDS, transplant recipients) may be symptomatic and result in substantial maternal morbidity and mortality. Perinatal transmission of CMV from an infected mother to her fetus can occur resulting in congenital CMV infection and disease. (See Congenital Cytomegalovirus Disease under Uses: Treatment of Cytomegalovirus Infection and Disease.)

Females of childbearing potential should undergo pregnancy testing before initiation of ganciclovir.

Females of childbearing potential should use effective contraception during and for at least 30 days after ganciclovir therapy and male patients should use effective barrier contraceptive methods during and for at least 90 days after ganciclovir therapy.

Fertility

Based on animal data and limited human data, ganciclovir at the usually recommended dosages may cause temporary or permanent inhibition of spermatogenesis in men and may cause suppression of fertility in women.

In female mice, ganciclovir caused decreased mating behavior, decreased fertility, and increased incidence of embryolethality at exposures approximately 1.7 times those attained in humans at the recommended human dose. Ganciclovir caused decreased fertility in male mice and hypospermatogenesis in male mice and dogs following oral or IV doses ranging from 0.2–10 mg/kg. Systemic exposures at the lowest dose associated with toxicity in each species ranged from 0.03–0.1 times the human exposures attained with the recommended human dose.

In a small, open-label, nonrandomized clinical study, adult male renal transplant patients receiving CMV prophylaxis with valganciclovir (prodrug of ganciclovir) for up to 200 days posttransplantation were followed for 6 months after the drug was discontinued and data compared with an untreated control group. Among 24 evaluable patients in the valganciclovir group, the mean sperm density at the end-of-treatment visit was *decreased* by 11 million/mL from baseline; whereas, among 14 evaluable patients in the control group, the mean sperm density at the end-of-treatment visit had *increased* by 33 million/mL. However, at the final follow-up visit, the mean sperm density among 20 evaluable patients in the valganciclovir group was comparable to that observed among 10 evaluable patients in the untreated control group (mean sperm density increased by 41 or 43 million/mL from baseline, respectively).

Patients receiving ganciclovir should be advised that the drug may be associated with infertility.

Lactation

It is not known whether ganciclovir is distributed into human milk, affects the breast-fed infant, or affects milk production. The drug is distributed into milk in lactating rats; the milk-to-serum ratio at steady state is approximately 1.6 in rats.

Because of the potential for serious adverse reactions to ganciclovir in breast-fed infants, nursing women should be instructed not to breast-feed while they are receiving the drug. HIV-infected mothers should be instructed not to breast-feed their infants because of the risk of transmission of HIV.

DRUG INTERACTIONS

Drug interaction studies with ganciclovir were performed in patients with normal renal function. In patients with renal impairment, concomitant use of ganciclovir

and other drugs eliminated by renal excretion may result in increased concentrations of ganciclovir and the concomitant drug and such patients should be closely monitored for toxicity associated with ganciclovir and the concomitant drug.

• Antibacterial Agents

Imipenem and Cilastatin Sodium

Generalized seizures have occurred in several patients who received concomitant therapy with the fixed combination of imipenem and cilastatin sodium (imipenem/cilastatin) and ganciclovir. While the mechanism of this potential interaction is not known, the seizures resolved in all but one patient when both imipenem/cilastatin and ganciclovir or just imipenem/cilastatin was discontinued. In the patient whose seizures failed to resolve following discontinuance of imipenem/cilastatin, continued seizures were attributed to encephalitis rather than the drugs.

Because of the risk of seizures, concomitant use of imipenem/cilastatin and ganciclovir is not recommended.

Trimethoprim

Concomitant use of trimethoprim and oral ganciclovir (no longer commercially available in the US) did not affect the pharmacokinetics of either drug.

Because of possible increased toxicity, concomitant use of trimethoprim and ganciclovir should be considered only if potential benefits outweigh risks.

Other Antibacterials

Because of possible increased toxicity if ganciclovir is used with certain anti-infectives (e.g., co-trimoxazole, dapsone, pentamidine, sulfamethoxazole), concomitant use of ganciclovir and such anti-infectives should be considered only if potential benefits outweigh risks.

• Antifungal Agents

Amphotericin B

Concomitant use of amphotericin B and ganciclovir may result in increased serum creatinine concentrations.

Renal function should be monitored if amphotericin B and ganciclovir are used concomitantly.

Flucytosine

Because of possible increased toxicity, concomitant use of flucytosine and ganciclovir should be considered only if potential benefits outweigh risks.

• Antiretroviral Agents

Didanosine

Although the clinical importance is unclear, there is some in vitro evidence that ganciclovir may antagonize the antiretroviral activity of didanosine against human immunodeficiency virus (HIV).

Concomitant use of didanosine (200 mg every 12 hours) with IV ganciclovir (5 mg/kg twice daily) has resulted in a 70% increase in the area under the plasma concentration-time curve (AUC_{0-12}) and 49% increase in peak plasma concentrations of didanosine, but did not affect the pharmacokinetics of ganciclovir.

Patients receiving didanosine and ganciclovir concomitantly should be monitored closely for didanosine toxicity (e.g., pancreatitis).

Tenofovir

Concomitant use of ganciclovir and tenofovir alafenamide or tenofovir disoproxil fumarate may result in increased serum concentrations of ganciclovir and/or tenofovir and patients should be monitored for dose-related tenofovir toxicities.

Zidovudine

Although the clinical importance is unclear, there is some in vitro evidence that ganciclovir may antagonize the antiretroviral activity of zidovudine against HIV.

Concomitant use of zidovudine with ganciclovir can increase the risk of hematologic toxicity. Both zidovudine and ganciclovir alone produce direct, dose-dependent inhibitory effects on myeloid and erythroid progenitor cells, and combined use of the drugs may result in additive or synergistic myelotoxic effects.

In several studies in patients with acquired immunodeficiency syndrome (AIDS) and cytomegalovirus (CMV) infection, profound, intolerable myelosuppression, evidenced principally as severe neutropenia, occurred in all patients receiving oral zidovudine (200 mg every 4 hours) concomitantly with IV ganciclovir (5 mg/kg 1–4 times daily); anemia also occurred in many of these patients. Severe hematologic toxicity, which required a reduction in zidovudine dosage, also occurred in more than 80% of patients receiving oral zidovudine (100 mg every 4 hours) concomitantly with IV ganciclovir (5 mg/kg 1–2 times daily). Several other patients with initially stable hematologic findings on ganciclovir alone, developed prolonged pancytopenia during concomitant therapy with oral zidovudine and IV ganciclovir. The increased risk of hematologic toxicity does not appear to be related to a pharmacokinetic interaction between ganciclovir and zidovudine.

Because of the risk of hematologic toxicity, concomitant use of zidovudine and ganciclovir should be considered only if potential benefits outweigh risks. If combined therapy is considered necessary, the drugs should be used with extreme caution and careful monitoring of hematologic function.

● Antiviral Agents

Foscarnet

Concomitant use of ganciclovir and foscarnet does not affect the pharmacokinetics of either drug. However, ganciclovir and foscarnet are physically incompatible and must not be admixed.

Foscarnet has exhibited additive or synergistic antiviral activity with ganciclovir in vitro against CMV and herpes simplex virus type 2 (HSV-2). There was no in vitro evidence of antagonistic antiviral effects between ganciclovir and foscarnet.

In addition, combined therapy with the drugs may be effective in the treatment of CMV infection resistant to either drug alone. In several AIDS patients with CMV retinitis and/or GI infections that progressed during therapy with either ganciclovir or foscarnet alone, concomitant use of the drugs appeared to effectively reduce the symptoms and halt progression of the disease. Concomitant therapy was effective in some patients who previously had received monotherapy with both drugs. Although the incidence of anemia during concomitant therapy was higher than that reported during use of ganciclovir alone, adverse effects were not severe enough to require discontinuance of concomitant therapy.

Letermovir

In vitro, there was no evidence of antagonistic anti-CMV effects between letermovir and ganciclovir.

● Immunosuppressive Agents

Patients receiving immunosuppressive agents (e.g., azathioprine, cyclosporine, corticosteroids) may require decreased dosages or temporary withdrawal of these drugs during ganciclovir therapy to prevent excessive suppression of bone marrow or the immune system.

Cyclosporine

When oral cyclosporine at therapeutic doses was used concomitantly with IV ganciclovir (5 mg/kg every 12 hours) in liver allograft recipients, there was no evidence of any change in cyclosporine whole blood concentrations. However, concomitant use of these drugs may increase serum creatinine concentrations.

If ganciclovir is used concomitantly with cyclosporine, renal function should be monitored.

Mycophenolate Mofetil

Concomitant use of mycophenolate mofetil and ganciclovir in patients with normal renal function does not affect the pharmacokinetics of either drug.

Because of possible increased risk, the patient should be monitored for hematologic and renal toxicity if mycophenolate mofetil and ganciclovir are used concomitantly.

Tacrolimus

Because of possible increased toxicity, concomitant use of tacrolimus and ganciclovir should be considered only if potential benefits outweigh risks.

● Myelosuppressive Drugs

Concomitant use of ganciclovir and myelosuppressive drugs may have additive toxicity. Such drugs include dapsone, pentamidine, pyrimethamine, flucytosine, cytotoxic antineoplastic agents (e.g., vincristine, vinblastine, doxorubicin, hydroxyurea), amphotericin B, co-trimoxazole, or other nucleoside analogs. These drugs should be used concomitantly with ganciclovir only when the potential benefits of such therapy are thought to outweigh the possible risks. In addition, the possibility that AIDS patients may be at particular risk for potential toxicity during combined therapy should be considered, since such patients appear to be at increased risk of hematologic toxicity with some of these drugs alone (e.g., co-trimoxazole).

● Probenecid

Concomitant use of probenecid (500 mg every 6 hours) with oral ganciclovir (no longer commercially available in the US) has resulted in a 53% increase in the AUC of ganciclovir and a 22% decrease in renal clearance of ganciclovir.

If probenecid and ganciclovir are used concomitantly, reduced ganciclovir dosage may be required and the patient should be monitored for ganciclovir toxicity.

ACUTE TOXICITY

The acute lethal dose of ganciclovir in humans is not known.

Overdosages of IV ganciclovir, including some fatalities, have been reported during clinical trials and postmarketing experience. In general, overdosage may be expected to produce toxicities that are extensions of the drug's pharmacologic and adverse effects. Ganciclovir overdosage has resulted in hematologic toxicity (pancytopenia, leukopenia, neutropenia, granulocytopenia, thrombocytopenia, bone marrow failure), hepatotoxicity (hepatitis, liver function disorder), renal toxicity (worsening of hematuria, acute kidney injury, elevated creatinine concentration), GI toxicity (abdominal pain, diarrhea, vomiting), and neurotoxicity (seizure).

Management of ganciclovir overdosage generally involves symptomatic and supportive care. Because the drug is removed by dialysis (see Pharmacokinetics: Elimination), hemodialysis or peritoneal dialysis might be useful in the management of overdosage. Adequate hydration should be maintained. Protective measures for neutropenia may be necessary until bone marrow function returns; use of hematopoietic growth factors should be considered in patients with cytopenias.

MECHANISM OF ACTION

Ganciclovir exerts its antiviral effect on human cytomegalovirus (CMV) and other human herpesviruses by interfering with DNA synthesis via competition with deoxyguanosine for incorporation into viral DNA and thereby inhibiting viral DNA polymerase as well as being incorporated into growing viral DNA chains.

Ganciclovir is a prodrug and exhibits no antiviral activity until converted intracellularly to the active metabolite, ganciclovir triphosphate. In CMV-infected cells, ganciclovir is initially phosphorylated to ganciclovir monophosphate by the viral protein kinase pUL97. Further phosphorylation occurs by cellular kinases to produce the pharmacologically active ganciclovir triphosphate. Ganciclovir triphosphate is a viral DNA polymerase inhibitor that competitively inhibits viral DNA polymerase pUL54. The drug also is incorporated into growing DNA chains as a false nucleotide, thus interfering with chain elongation (prematurely terminating DNA synthesis) and/or resulting in formation of a mutant DNA chain and thereby inhibiting viral replication.

Because conversion of ganciclovir to the pharmacologically active triphosphate is largely dependent on viral kinase, phosphorylation of the drug occurs preferentially in virus-infected cells. The formation of ganciclovir monophosphate appears to be the rate-limiting step in the formation of ganciclovir triphosphate. In vitro in herpesviruses, ganciclovir triphosphate functions both as substrate for, and a preferential inhibitor of, viral DNA polymerase and as a false nucleotide base. In cells infected with herpes simplex virus type 1 or 2 (HSV-1 or HSV-2) or varicella-zoster virus (VZV), ganciclovir is converted to ganciclovir monophosphate via virus-coded thymidine kinase. The pathway for conversion to the monophosphate in cells infected with CMV or Epstein-Barr virus (EBV) differs since these viruses do not code for thymidine kinase. A cellular deoxyguanosine kinase, found in the cytosol and in mitochondria, may be involved. In CMV-infected cells, increased concentrations of deoxyguanosine kinase (mitochondrial origin) have been detected, suggesting that the virus may induce production of the enzyme.

Ganciclovir is virustatic in action. Following removal of the drug from the culture medium in vitro, viral DNA synthesis (which previously was inhibited) resumes, resulting in restored viral replication. In addition, clinical evidence of reactivated disease suggests that ganciclovir acts principally to suppress virus activity and that eradication of the virus does not occur.

During the course of an acute or asymptomatic herpesvirus infection, the virus usually leaves the initial site of infection and invades other cells and tissues where it establishes a latent infection. HSV-1, HSV-2, and VZV are thought to establish latent infections principally within the ganglia. CMV and Epstein-Barr virus are thought to establish latent infections within leukocytes and B cells, respectively. CMV also may establish a site of latent infection in solid organ tissue (e.g., lung, kidney). The exact nature of the virus in the latent state is not well understood; however, evidence suggests that the virus is not actively replicating and, therefore, would not be susceptible to the action of antiviral agents such as ganciclovir. Despite the host's immunity, herpesvirus latency usually persists for life and the viruses can be reactivated periodically by various stimuli, including immunosuppression. Reactivation of latent CMV has been specifically linked to pregnancy and to decreases in host immunocompetence, either iatrogenic or via disease process (i.e., acquired immunodeficiency syndrome). Once reactivated, the virus usually reinfects the site of initial infection. Ganciclovir, like other antivirals, is unable to eliminate an established latent infection, as demonstrated in animal tests.

SPECTRUM

Following intracellular conversion of ganciclovir to the pharmacologically active ganciclovir triphosphate, the drug is active against human herpesviruses, including cytomegalovirus (CMV), herpes simplex virus types 1 and 2 (HSV-1 and HSV-2), and varicella-zoster virus (VZV). Although the clinical importance is unclear, ganciclovir has some in vitro activity against Epstein-Barr virus (EBV) and human herpesvirus type 6 and type 8. Ganciclovir is not active against human immunodeficiency virus (HIV).

RESISTANCE

Cytomegalovirus (CMV) isolates resistant to ganciclovir have been selected in vitro in the presence of increasing concentrations of the drug. Ganciclovir-resistant CMV have been reported in ganciclovir-naive patients and may emerge in patients receiving prolonged treatment or prophylaxis with the drug. The possibility of ganciclovir-resistant CMV should be considered in patients who show poor clinical response or relapse or experience persistent viral shedding during ganciclovir therapy.

Several mechanisms of resistance to ganciclovir apparently exist. Since the antiviral activity of ganciclovir depends on phosphorylation of the drug to ganciclovir triphosphate (see Mechanism of Action), resistance to the drug may result from decreased phosphorylation. In some viruses, such as herpes simplex virus (HSV) and varicella-zoster virus (VZV), resistance to ganciclovir might result from low or absent concentrations of virus-coded thymidine kinase or from alterations in substrate specificity of the enzyme. However, other mechanisms also appear to be involved since some thymidine-kinase deficient or mutant strains of acyclovir-resistant HSV are susceptible to ganciclovir.

Ganciclovir resistance usually is the result of amino acid substitutions in the viral protein kinase pUL97 and/or the viral DNA polymerase pUL54. Certain pUL97 ganciclovir resistance-associated substitutions (e.g., M460V/I, H520Q, C529G, A594V, L595S, C603W) have been reported most frequently in clinical isolates. Numerous other pUL97 and pUL54 ganciclovir resistance-associated mutations also have been reported.

Cross-resistance can occur between ganciclovir and some other antivirals (e.g., acyclovir, cidofovir, foscarnet). Certain amino acid substitutions selected in vitro in cell culture following exposure of CMV to ganciclovir, cidofovir, or foscarnet have resulted in cross-resistance. Amino acid substitutions in pUL54 that confer cross-resistance between ganciclovir and cidofovir generally have involved the exonuclease domains and region V of the viral DNA polymerase. A variety of amino acid substitutions have conferred cross-resistance between ganciclovir and foscarnet, but concentrate at and between regions II and III of viral DNA polymerase.

PHARMACOKINETICS

Dosages and concentrations of ganciclovir sodium are expressed in terms of ganciclovir. A concentration of 1 mcg of ganciclovir per mL is approximately equivalent to 3.92 μmol/L.

● Absorption

Following IV administration of ganciclovir given in a dosage of 5 mg/kg every 12 hours by IV infusion over 1 hour, peak plasma concentrations of the drug ranged from 8.3–9 mcg/mL. In immunocompromised patients with cytomegalovirus (CMV) infection and normal renal function who received 2.5 mg/kg of ganciclovir every 8 hours by IV infusion over 1 hour, peak and trough plasma concentrations of the drug averaged 4.09–5.36 (range: 1.66–7.78 mcg/mL) and 0.33–1.07 mcg/mL (range: 0.2–1.66 mcg/mL), respectively. In a limited number of such patients receiving 5 mg/kg every 8 hours by IV infusion over 1 hour, peak and trough plasma concentrations averaged 6.53–11.41 and 1.13–2.23 mcg/mL, respectively. Following IV administration, ganciclovir exhibits linear pharmacokinetics over the dosage range of 1.6–5 mg/kg. Accumulation of the drug does not appear to occur in patients with normal renal function receiving IV dosages of 3–15 mg/kg daily in divided doses.

Studies have not been performed to specifically evaluate the pharmacokinetics of IV ganciclovir in geriatric adults 65 years of age and older.

In a limited number of neonates 2–49 days of age†, IV administration of a ganciclovir dose of 4 or 6 mg/kg resulted in peak plasma concentrations of 5.5 or 7 mcg/mL, respectively. In pediatric patients 9 months to 12 years of age† who received IV ganciclovir (single or multiple doses of 5 mg/kg every 12 hours), peak plasma concentrations of the drug were 7.9 mcg/mL.

Limited data regarding intravitreal injection† of ganciclovir suggest that minimal systemic absorption of the drug occurs, although adequate intravitreal ganciclovir concentrations appear to be achievable with this route. In a patient with CMV retinitis receiving five 200-mcg intravitreal doses of ganciclovir over 15 days, plasma concentrations of the drug were less than 0.1 mcg/mL. A vitreous humor concentration of 1.17 mcg/mL and an aqueous humor concentration of 0.66 mcg/mL were achieved 51.4 hours after the initial dose in this patient, and a vitreous humor concentration of 0.1 mcg/mL was achieved 97.3 hours after the fourth dose. Data from rabbits also indicate that antiviral intravitreal concentrations of the drug are achievable with small intravitreal but *not* subconjunctival doses of ganciclovir. Following intravitreal injection of a single 400-mcg dose in rabbits, vitreous humor ganciclovir concentrations averaged 543, 423, 57.7, 16, 2.02, and 1.2 mcg/mL at 2, 5, 12, 24, 48, and 60 hours after injection. Following subconjunctival injection of a single 1.25-mg dose in rabbits, ganciclovir concentrations at 1, 2, 3, and 8 hours after injection averaged 0.09, 0.31, 0.16, and 0.02 mcg/mL, respectively, in vitreous humor and 2.18, 3.27, 2.22, and 0.07 mcg/mL, respectively, in aqueous humor.

● Distribution

Following IV administration, ganciclovir is widely distributed. Autopsy findings in several patients who had been receiving IV ganciclovir suggest that the drug concentrates in the kidneys, with substantially lower concentrations occurring in lung, liver, brain, and testes. While efficacy of ganciclovir in CMV pneumonitis has been reported to be substantially less than in some other CMV infections (e.g., retinitis), lung ganciclovir concentrations that exceed the ID_{50} for CMV appear to be achievable with usual IV dosages of the drug. Concentrations attained in lung and liver were 99 and 92%, respectively, of those attained concurrently in heart/blood in several adults receiving the drug IV. Following IV administration in mice, ganciclovir was distributed widely, achieving highest concentrations in the kidney and lowest concentrations in the brain. Substantial distribution of ganciclovir into lung, liver, heart, spleen, stomach, intestines, muscle, and testes also occur, exceeding concurrent blood concentrations in these tissues; concentrations achieved in brain, eyes, and fat were lower than concurrent blood concentrations. Accumulation of the drug did not appear to occur, although measurable concentrations persisted for at least 30 hours in stomach, liver, and intestines in these animals. In addition, there was no evidence of testicular ganciclovir accumulation in several men receiving 15 mg/kg IV daily for 8–13 days.

The volume of distribution of ganciclovir at steady state following IV administration is 0.74 L/kg. The volume of distribution appears to be reduced in patients with renal impairment.

Data on intraocular concentrations of ganciclovir following IV administration are limited, but it appears that the drug has good ocular distribution following administration by this route. In one adult patient, subretinal ganciclovir concentrations were 0.87 and 2 times concurrent plasma concentrations at 5.5 and 8 hours after IV administration, respectively. In another adult patient, aqueous and vitreous humor ganciclovir concentrations were 0.4 and 0.6 times simultaneous plasma concentrations, respectively, at 2.5 hours after IV infusion of the drug; at 21 hours after IV infusion, plasma concentrations were undetectable, while the vitreous humor concentration was still 0.2 mcg/mL. Following intravitreal injection† of ganciclovir in an adult with CMV retinitis, the apparent volume of distribution in vitreous humor was 11.7 mL, suggesting that the drug may distribute into the retina.

Ganciclovir crosses the blood-brain barrier. Following IV administration in several adult patients, ganciclovir concentrations in CSF at 0.25–5.7 hours after a dose ranged from 0.31–0.68 mcg/mL and averaged 41% (range: 24–70%) of corresponding plasma concentration of the drug. Autopsy findings revealed similar evidence of CNS distribution of the drug in several other patients, with brain tissue concentrations of ganciclovir averaging 38% of corresponding blood concentrations.

Ganciclovir appears to cross the placenta based on ex vivo experiments with human placenta and at least one case report in a pregnant woman.

It is not known whether ganciclovir is distributed into milk in humans, but the drug is distributed into milk following IV administration in rats.

Ganciclovir is 1–2% bound to plasma proteins at drug concentrations of 0.5–51 mcg/mL.

● Elimination

Following IV administration in adults with normal renal function, the half-life of ganciclovir is 3.5 hours. Plasma concentrations of the drug may be higher and the elimination half-life prolonged in patients with impaired renal function. In a limited number of immunocompromised patients with renal impairment who received IV ganciclovir doses ranging from 1.25–5 mg/kg, mean plasma half-life of the drug was 4.4 hours in those with creatinine clearances of 25–59 mL/minute and 10.7 hours in those with creatinine clearances less than 25 mL/minute. In adults with moderate to severe renal impairment (creatinine clearances less than 50 mL/minute per 1.73 m^2), the terminal half-life ($t_{\frac{1}{2}\beta}$) of IV ganciclovir ranged from 4.4–30 hours, depending on the degree of impairment.

Although the pharmacokinetics of ganciclovir have not been specifically evaluated in geriatric patients, renal clearance decreases with age and decreased ganciclovir total body clearance and prolonged half-life of the drug are expected in adults 65 years of age and older.

In a limited number of neonates 2–49 days of age† who received IV ganciclovir, the plasma half-life of the drug was 2.4 hours. In pediatric patients 9 months to 12 years of age† who received IV ganciclovir, the plasma half-life of the drug also was approximately 2.4 hours.

Following intravitreal injection† of ganciclovir in a patient with CMV retinitis, the elimination half-life of the drug from the vitreous humor was estimated to be 13.3 hours. In this patient, intravitreal ganciclovir concentrations were estimated to exceed the ID$_{50}$ (0.66 mcg/mL) of the virus for about 62 hours after a single 200-mcg intravitreal dose. In rabbits, the elimination half-life from vitreous humor after intravitreal injection of a single 400-mcg dose was 8.6 hours, and intravitreal ganciclovir concentrations exceeded the ID$_{50}$ (range: 0.24–1.5 mcg/mL) of many strains of CMV for at least 60 hours.

With the exception of intracellular phosphorylation of the drug (see Mechanism of Action), ganciclovir does not appear to be metabolized appreciably in humans. The drug appears to undergo little, if any, extrarenal elimination, and approximately 90–99% of an IV dose is excreted unchanged in urine. Renal excretion of ganciclovir appears to occur principally via glomerular filtration and active tubular secretion.

Total body clearance of ganciclovir from plasma reportedly averages 170–203 mL/minute per 1.73 m^2 in adults with normal renal function. Total body clearance of the drug is decreased in adults with renal impairment and appears to correlate positively with creatinine clearance. In a limited number of patients, total body clearance from plasma averaged 128, 57, or 30 mL/minute in adults with creatinine clearances of 50–79, 25–49, or less than 25 mL/minute, respectively.

Ganciclovir is removed by hemodialysis. The amount of ganciclovir removed during hemodialysis depends on several factors (e.g., type of coil used, dialysis flow rate); however, in several patients, a 4-hour period of hemodialysis removed into the dialysate approximately 40–50% of a dose.

CHEMISTRY AND STABILITY

● Chemistry

Ganciclovir, a synthetic nucleoside analog of guanine, is an antiviral agent. Ganciclovir is structurally and pharmacologically related to acyclovir, differing from acyclovir only by the addition of a second terminal hydroxymethyl group at C-2 of the acyclic side chain on the ribose ring. Compared with acyclovir, this structural difference results in substantially increased antiviral activity against cytomegalovirus (CMV) and less selectivity for viral DNA.

Ganciclovir occurs as a white to off-white powder and has an aqueous solubility of 2.6 mg/mL at 25°C. Aqueous solubility of the drug is relatively constant over a pH range of 3.5–8.5, but increases substantially in strongly acidic or basic solutions. The drug has pK$_a$s of 2.2 and 9.4.

Ganciclovir is commercially available for IV use as the monosodium salt, which is formed in situ by the addition of sodium hydroxide during the manufacturing process. At physiologic pH, ganciclovir sodium exists as the unionized form with a solubility of approximately 6 mg/mL at 37°C. Potency of ganciclovir sodium is expressed in terms of ganciclovir.

Commercially available ganciclovir sodium sterile powder for IV use provided in single-use vials containing 500 mg of ganciclovir occurs as a white to off-white lyophilized powder. The lyophilized powder has an aqueous solubility that is greater than 50 mg/mL at 25°C. Following reconstitution of the powder with preservative-free sterile water for injection, ganciclovir sodium solutions containing 50 mg of ganciclovir per mL are alkaline with a pH of 11 and are colorless.

Commercially available sterile ganciclovir sodium concentrate for IV use provided in single-use vials containing 500 mg of ganciclovir (50 mg/mL) should appear as a clear solution.

Commercially available premixed injection for IV use containing 500 mg of ganciclovir in 250 mL of 0.8% sodium chloride (2 mg/mL) is provided in single-use polymeric IV bags. The premixed solution has a pH of 7.5 and does not contain any preservatives.

● Stability

Ganciclovir sodium lyophilized powder for IV use provided in single-use vials should be stored at 25°C, but may be exposed to temperatures ranging from 15–30°C. Following reconstitution with sterile water for injection, ganciclovir sodium solutions containing 50 mg of ganciclovir per mL are stable for 12 hours at 25°C and should not be refrigerated or frozen. Bacteriostatic water for injection containing parabens should *not* be used for reconstitution of ganciclovir sodium since a precipitate may form. The manufacturer states that reconstituted ganciclovir sodium that has been further diluted in 0.9% sodium chloride or other compatible IV infusion solution should be stored under refrigeration at 2–8°C and used within 24 hours. The solution should not be frozen.

Ganciclovir sodium concentrate for IV use containing 500 mg of ganciclovir (50 mg/mL) provided in single-use vials should be stored at 25°C, but may be exposed to temperatures ranging from 15–30°C. Following dilution in 0.9% sodium chloride or other compatible IV infusion solution, the manufacturer states that the solution should be stored under refrigeration at 2–8°C and used within 24 hours. The solution should not be frozen.

The premixed injection for IV use containing 500 mg of ganciclovir in 250 mL of 0.8% sodium chloride (2 mg/mL) provided in single-use IV bags should be stored at 20–25°C, but may be exposed to temperatures ranging from 15–30°C. Crystals may form in the premixed solution if it is exposed during transportation or storage to temperatures lower than recommended; the crystals should redissolve if the bag is gently shaken.

At a concentration of 10 mg or less of ganciclovir per mL, ganciclovir sodium is physically and chemically stable in the following IV solutions: 0.9% sodium chloride, 5% dextrose, Ringer's, or lactated Ringer's. Solutions containing approximately 2.5 mg of ganciclovir per mL reportedly are physically and chemically stable for at least 5 days at 4–25°C in 0.9% sodium chloride injection or 5% dextrose injection. Although sterility of the solutions was not assessed, results of one study indicate that ganciclovir is stable for up to 35 days when diluted in 0.9% sodium chloride or 5% dextrose to a concentration of 1 or 5 mg/mL and stored in polyvinyl chloride (PVC) containers at 5°C or 25°C. In another study, ganciclovir was stable for up to 28 days when diluted in 0.9% sodium chloride or 5% dextrose to a concentration of 5 or 10 mg/mL and stored in PVC containers at 4°C or -20°C or stored in ADFuse syringes (Healthtek) at 4°C. Protection of diluted ganciclovir sodium solutions from usual room light is not necessary. The drug does not appear to adsorb appreciably to PVC containers.

PREPARATIONS

Excipients in commercially available drug preparations may have clinically important effects in some individuals; consult specific product labeling for details.

Ganciclovir

Parenteral

Injection, for IV infusion only	2 mg/mL (500 mg) in 0.8% Sodium Chloride*	Ganciclovir Injection

* available from one or more manufacturer, distributor, and/or repackager by generic (nonproprietary) name

Ganciclovir Sodium

Parenteral

Concentrate, for injection, for IV infusion only	50 mg (of ganciclovir) per mL (500 mg)*	Ganciclovir Injection
For injection, for IV infusion only	500 mg (of ganciclovir)*	Cytovene®-IV, Roche Ganciclovir Sodium for Injection

* available from one or more manufacturer, distributor, and/or repackager by generic (nonproprietary) name

† Use is not currently included in the labeling approved by the US Food and Drug Administration.

Selected Revisions August 12, 2019, © Copyright, December 1, 1989, American Society of Health-System Pharmacists, Inc.

Tenofovir Alafenamide Fumarate

8:18.32 • NUCLEOSIDES AND NUCLEOTIDES

■ Tenofovir alafenamide fumarate, an antiviral agent, is a nucleotide reverse transcriptase inhibitor that is active against hepatitis B virus (HBV) and human immunodeficiency virus (HIV).

USES

Tenofovir alafenamide fumarate is commercially available as a single entity for the treatment of chronic hepatitis B virus (HBV) infection in adults and pediatric patients ≥12 years of age with compensated liver disease.

Tenofovir alafenamide fumarate is also available in various fixed-combination preparations that contain additional antiretroviral agents; these products are used for the treatment of human immunodeficiency virus (HIV) infection and/or for HIV pre-exposure prophylaxis (PrEP). Refer to separate combination product monographs for information related to the specific uses of these products and the role of tenofovir alafenamide fumarate-containing regimens in the treatment and prevention of HIV infection.

● Chronic Hepatitis B Virus Infection

Tenofovir alafenamide fumarate is used for the treatment of chronic HBV infection in adults and pediatric patients ≥12 years of age with compensated liver disease. Safety and efficacy of tenofovir alafenamide fumarate have not been established in patients with decompensated cirrhosis (Child-Pugh class B or C), and the drug is not recommended for treatment of HBV infection in such patients. Tenofovir alafenamide is a preferred initial treatment option in adults when chronic HBV treatment is indicated; choice of antiviral medication should be individualized based on patient characteristics and comorbidities, treatment tolerability, and cost.

Clinical Experience

Adults

Efficacy and safety of tenofovir alafenamide fumarate for the treatment of HBV infection in adults were primarily evaluated in 2 randomized, double-blind, active-controlled studies enrolling treatment-naïve (have not previously received nucleoside or nucleotide antivirals) and previously treated adults with compensated liver disease (study 108 and study 110). The primary efficacy end point in both studies was the proportion of patients with plasma HBV DNA levels <29 IU/mL at week 48.

In study 108, 425 adults with chronic HBV infection who were negative for serum hepatitis B e antigen (HBeAg; mean age 46 years, 61% male; 72% Asian, 25% white, 2% Black; 24% HBV genotype B infection, 38% HBV genotype C infection, 31% HBV genotype D infection; 21% previously treated; mean baseline plasma HBV DNA level 5.8 $\log_{10}$ IU/mL; mean serum ALT concentration 94 units/L, 9% with history of cirrhosis) were randomized in a 2:1 ratio to receive tenofovir alafenamide fumarate (25 mg of tenofovir alafenamide once daily) or tenofovir disoproxil fumarate (tenofovir DF; 300 mg once daily) for 96 weeks. Concomitant use of other nucleoside or nucleotide antivirals or interferons was not permitted. At 48 weeks, 94 or 93% of patients receiving tenofovir alafenamide or tenofovir DF, respectively, had plasma HBV DNA levels <29 IU/mL, meeting preestablished criteria for noninferiority. In patients with baseline serum ALT concentrations above the upper limit of normal (based on American Association for the Study of Liver Diseases [AASLD] criteria), normalized ALT concentrations were achieved in 50% of those treated with tenofovir alafenamide and 32% of those treated with tenofovir DF.. At week 96, 90 or 91% of patients receiving tenofovir alafenamide or tenofovir DF, respectively, had plasma HBV DNA levels <29 IU/mL, and 50 or 40%, respectively, achieved normalized ALT according to AASLD criteria.

In study 110, 873 adults with chronic HBV infection who were positive for serum HBeAg (mean age 38 years, 64% male; 82% Asian, 17% white, 1% Black

or other races; 17% HBV genotype B infection, 52% HBV genotype C infection, 23% HBV genotype D infection; 26% previously treated; mean baseline plasma HBV DNA level 7.6 $\log_{10}$ IU/mL; mean serum ALT concentration 120 units/L, 7% with history of cirrhosis) were randomized in a 2:1 ratio to receive tenofovir alafenamide fumarate (25 mg of tenofovir alafenamide once daily) or tenofovir DF (300 mg once daily) for 96 weeks. Concomitant use of other nucleoside or nucleotide antivirals or interferons was not permitted. At 48 weeks, 64 or 67% of patients receiving tenofovir alafenamide or tenofovir DF, respectively, had plasma HBV DNA levels <29 IU/mL, meeting prespecified criteria for noninferiority. In patients with baseline serum ALT concentrations above the upper limit of normal (based on AASLD criteria), normalized ALT concentrations were achieved by 45% of those treated with tenofovir alafenamide and 36% of those treated with tenofovir DF. At week 96, 73 or 75% of patients receiving tenofovir alafenamide or tenofovir DF, respectively, had plasma HBV DNA levels <29 IU/mL, and 52 or 42%, respectively, achieved normalized ALT according to AASLD criteria.

An additional randomized, double-blind, active-controlled study (study 4018) examined the safety and efficacy of switching from tenofovir DF to tenofovir alafenamide in 488 virologically-suppressed adults with chronic HBV infection. Patients had to have taken tenofovir DF 300 mg once daily for ≥12 months prior to enrollment, and have HBV DNA less than the lower limit of quantitation by local laboratory assessment for ≥12 weeks prior to screening and HBV DNA <20 IU/mL at screening. Patients were randomized in a 1:1 ratio (stratified by HBeAg status and age ≥50 or <50 years) to either switch to tenofovir alafenamide 25 mg once daily or to stay on tenofovir DF 300 mg once daily. The primary efficacy endpoint was the proportion of patients with plasma HBV DNA levels ≥20 IU/mL at week 48. The mean age of patients in the trial was 51 years; 71% were male, 82% were Asian, 14% were white, and 68% were HBeAg-negative. Mean serum ALT at baseline was 27 U/L, and 16% of patients had a history of cirrhosis. At week 48, <1% of patients in each treatment group had HBV DNA ≥20 IU/mL, meeting prespecified criteria for noninferiority. In patients with baseline serum ALT concentrations above the upper limit of normal (based on AASLD criteria), normalized ALT concentrations were achieved in 50% of patients who switched to tenofovir alafenamide and 26% of patients who continued to receive tenofovir DF.

An open-label study (study 4035) evaluated the efficacy and safety of switching from tenofovir DF and/or other antivirals to tenofovir alafenamide in virologically-suppressed, chronically HBV-infected adults with moderate to severe renal impairment (estimated creatinine clearance 15–59 mL/minute; 78 patients) or end-stage renal disease (estimated creatinine clearance <15 mL/minute) on hemodialysis (15 patients). The median age of patients in the trial was 65 years; 74% were male, 77% were Asian, 16% were white, 83% were HBeAg-negative, 98% had baseline HBV DNA <20 IU/mL, and 95% had baseline ALT less than or equal to the upper limit of normal based on AASLD criteria. The median estimated creatinine clearance at baseline was 43 mL/minute, and 34% of patients had a history of cirrhosis. At week 24, 98% of patients achieved HBV DNA <20 IU/mL. The mean change from baseline in ALT was +1 U/L at week 24.

Pediatric Patients

The safety and efficacy of tenofovir alafenamide fumarate were evaluated in a randomized, double-blind, placebo-controlled trial of 70 treatment-naïve and treatment-experienced patients with chronic HBV infection who were 12 to <18 years of age and weighed at least ≥35 kg (study 1092). Among patients who were randomized to receive tenofovir alafenamide once daily, 57% were male, 70% were Asian, 19% were white, and 9, 23, 26, and 40% had HBV genotype A, B, C, or D, respectively. At baseline, median HBV DNA was 8.1 $\log_{10}$ IU/mL, mean ALT was 112 U/L, and 98% of patients were HBeAg-positive. At week 24, 21% of patients receiving tenofovir alafenamide fumarate achieved HBV DNA <20 IU/mL, compared with 0% of patients receiving placebo. Normalization of ALT (based on AASLD criteria) was achieved in 44% of patients receiving tenofovir alafenamide and 0% of patients receiving placebo.

Clinical Perspective

The American Association for the Study of Liver Diseases (AASLD) recommends antiviral therapy for adults with immune-active chronic HBV to decrease the risk of liver-related complications. Immune-active chronic HBV is characterized by an elevation of ALT ≥2 times the upper limit of normal or evidence of significant histologic disease plus elevated HBV DNA (>2000 IU/mL if HBeAg-negative or >20,000 IU/mL if HBeAg-positive). Recommended initial antiviral options for adults with immune-active chronic HBV include peginterferon alfa-2a; entecavir, tenofovir DF, and tenofovir alafenamide. Selection of a specific antiviral medication should be individualized based on patient characteristics and comorbidities, treatment tolerability, and cost; consult the AASLD guideline for more details. Antiviral therapy is also recommended for HBeAg-positive children 2 years of age and older with both elevated ALT and measurable HBV DNA levels; the goal of therapy is to achieve sustained HBeAg seroconversion. Preferred initial treatment options for pediatric patients include interferon alfa-2b, entecavir, and tenofovir DF. At the time of publication of this 2018 AASLD guideline, tenofovir alafenamide had not yet been studied in children 12 years of age and older.

DOSAGE AND ADMINISTRATION

● General

Pretreatment Screening

● Perform testing for human immunodeficiency virus type 1 (HIV-1) infection prior to initiating tenofovir alafenamide. Do not use tenofovir alafenamide alone to treat HIV-1 infection.

● Assess serum creatinine, estimated creatinine clearance, urine glucose, and urine protein prior to initiating tenofovir alafenamide in all patients. In patients with chronic kidney disease, also assess serum phosphorus.

Patient Monitoring

● Assess serum creatinine, estimated creatinine clearance, urine glucose, and urine protein on a clinically appropriate schedule during treatment with tenofovir alafenamide in all patients. In patients with chronic kidney disease, also monitor serum phosphorus.

● After discontinuing treatment with tenofovir alafenamide, closely monitor hepatic function with both clinical and laboratory follow-up for at least several months.

Dispensing and Administration Precautions

● Tenofovir alafenamide is commercially available as a single entity and in various fixed-combination preparations containing additional antiretroviral agents. Refer to the full prescribing information for specific, distinct uses of the combination products. Since the antiretroviral agents contained in the fixed-combination preparations also may be available in single-entity or other fixed-combination preparations, exercise care to ensure that therapy is not duplicated if a fixed combination is used in conjunction with other antiretrovirals.

● Administration

Tenofovir alafenamide fumarate is administered orally once daily with food.

Store at <30°C in the original container; keep container tightly closed.

Fixed Combinations Containing Tenofovir Alafenamide

Tenofovir alafenamide is also commercially available in the following fixed-combination tablets for oral use: elvitegravir, cobicistat, emtricitabine, and tenofovir alafenamide (Genvoya®); emtricitabine, rilpivirine, and tenofovir alafenamide (Odefsey®); emtricitabine and tenofovir alafenamide (Descovy®); bictegravir, emtricitabine, and tenofovir alafenamide (Biktarvy®); and darunavir, cobicistat, emtricitabine, and tenofovir alafenamide (Symtuza®). See the full prescribing information for administration of each of these combination products.

● Dosage

Dosage of tenofovir alafenamide fumarate is expressed in terms of tenofovir alafenamide.

Pediatric Dosage

Chronic Hepatitis B Virus Infection

For the treatment of chronic HBV infection in pediatric patients ≥12 years of age, the recommended dosage of tenofovir alafenamide is 25 mg once daily.

Adult Dosage

Chronic Hepatitis B Virus Infection

For the treatment of chronic HBV infection in adults, the recommended dosage of tenofovir alafenamide is 25 mg once daily.

● Special Populations

Hepatic Impairment

Dosage adjustments are not necessary if tenofovir alafenamide is used in patients with mild hepatic impairment (Child-Pugh class A).

Tenofovir alafenamide is *not* recommended in patients with decompensated hepatic impairment (Child-Pugh class B or C).

Renal Impairment

Dosage adjustments are not necessary if tenofovir alafenamide is used in patients with creatinine clearance ≥15 mL/minute, or in patients with end-stage renal disease (ESRD; creatinine clearance <15 mL/minute) who are receiving chronic hemodialysis. On days of hemodialysis, administer tenofovir alafenamide after completion of hemodialysis treatment.

Tenofovir alafenamide is not recommended in patients with ESRD who are not receiving chronic hemodialysis.

No data are available to make specific dosage recommendations for pediatric patients with renal impairment.

Geriatric Patients

The manufacturer makes no specific dosage recommendations for geriatric patients.

CAUTIONS

● Contraindications

None.

● Warnings/Precautions

Warnings

Severe Acute Exacerbation of Hepatitis B Virus Infection after Discontinuance of Treatment

A boxed warning regarding the risk of severe acute exacerbation of hepatitis B virus (HBV) infection is included in the prescribing information for tenofovir alafenamide. Severe acute exacerbations of HBV infection may occur following discontinuance of HBV treatment, including tenofovir alafenamide.

Closely monitor hepatic function with clinical and laboratory follow-up for at least several months after tenofovir alafenamide is discontinued. If appropriate, resumption of HBV treatment may be warranted.

Other Warnings/Precautions

Individuals with HBV and Human Immunodeficiency Virus Type 1 Coinfection

Safety and efficacy of tenofovir alafenamide have not been established in patients with HBV and human immunodeficiency virus type 1 (HIV-1) coinfection.

Do not use tenofovir alafenamide alone for the treatment of HIV-1 infection due to the risk of development of HIV-1 resistance.

Prior to initiation of tenofovir alafenamide, offer HIV antibody testing to all patients with HBV infection and, if positive, use an appropriate antiretroviral regimen recommended for patients with HBV and HIV-1 coinfection.

New Onset or Worsening Renal Impairment

Postmarketing cases of renal impairment, including acute renal failure, proximal renal tubulopathy, and Fanconi syndrome, have been reported in patients receiving tenofovir alafenamide fumarate-containing products. While potential confounders may have contributed to the reported renal events, these factors may have also predisposed patients to tenofovir-related adverse events.

Patients receiving a tenofovir prodrug who have impaired renal function or are receiving nephrotoxic agents (e.g., nonsteroidal anti-inflammatory agents [NSAIAs]) are at increased risk of developing adverse renal effects.

Assess serum creatinine, estimated creatinine clearance, urine glucose, and urine protein on a clinically appropriate schedule in all patients prior to or when initiating tenofovir alafenamide, and during treatment with the drug. In patients with chronic kidney disease, also assess serum phosphorus.

Discontinue tenofovir alafenamide in patients who develop clinically important decreases in renal function or evidence of Fanconi syndrome.

Lactic Acidosis and Severe Hepatomegaly with Steatosis

Lactic acidosis and severe hepatomegaly with steatosis, including fatal cases, have been reported in patients receiving nucleoside analogs (e.g., tenofovir disoproxil fumarate [tenofovir DF], another tenofovir prodrug) alone or in conjunction with other antiretroviral agents.

Discontinue tenofovir alafenamide therapy in any patient who develops clinical or laboratory findings suggestive of lactic acidosis or pronounced hepatotoxicity (which may include hepatomegaly and steatosis even in the absence of marked increases in serum aminotransferase concentrations).

Bone Mineral Density Effects

In clinical trials, tenofovir prodrugs (tenofovir alafenamide, tenofovir DF) have been associated with changes in bone mineral density (BMD). The long-term clinical importance of these BMD changes is not known.

In a pooled analysis of 2 clinical studies in adults with chronic HBV infection (study 108 and study 110), the mean percentage change in BMD from baseline to week 96 was assessed by dual-energy X-ray absorptiometry (DXA). At the lumbar spine, the mean percentage change in BMD was -0.7% in patients treated with tenofovir alafenamide compared with -2.6% in those treated with tenofovir DF; 11% of those treated with tenofovir alafenamide and 25% of those treated with tenofovir DF had lumbar spine BMD declines that were ≥5%. At the total hip, the mean percentage change in BMD was -0.3% in patients treated with tenofovir alafenamide compared with -2.5% in those treated with tenofovir DF. At the femoral neck, 5% of patients treated with tenofovir alafenamide and 13% of those treated with tenofovir DF had BMD declines that were ≥7%.

In patients who remained on blinded treatment past week 96, the mean percentage change in BMD in each group at week 120 was similar to that at week 96. In the open-label phase, the mean percentage change in BMD from week 96 to week 120 in patients who remained on tenofovir alafenamide was 0.6% and 0% at the lumbar spine and at the total hip, respectively, compared to 1.7% and 0.6% at the lumbar spine and at the total hip, respectively, in those who switched from tenofovir DF to tenofovir alafenamide.

Specific Populations

Pregnancy

The Antiretroviral Pregnancy Registry (APR) monitors pregnancy outcomes in women exposed to tenofovir alafenamide during pregnancy. Clinicians are encouraged to register patients in the APR by calling 800-258-4263.

Data from the APR of >800 exposures to tenofovir alafenamide-containing regimens showed that the prevalence of birth defects in live births was 3.5% and 3.3% following first and second/third trimester exposure, respectively. The rate of miscarriage is not reported in the APR. The overall risk of birth defects for tenofovir alafenamide was not markedly different compared to the background rate for major birth defects of 2.7% in the United States reference population of the Metropolitan Atlanta Congenital Defects Program (MACDP). Use of the MACDP population as the comparator group has several limitations; the MACDP is not disease-specific, assesses populations from a limited geographic area, and does not include outcomes for births that occurred at <20 weeks' gestation.

In animal studies, there was no evidence of impaired fertility or harm to the fetus. Adverse developmental effects were not observed when tenofovir alafenamide was administered during organogenesis to rats or rabbits in dosages that resulted in exposures equal to or 51 times higher, respectively, than human exposures reported with the recommended daily dosage of tenofovir alafenamide.

Lactation

It is not known whether tenofovir alafenamide and its metabolites are distributed into human milk, affect human milk production, or have effects on the breast-fed infant. Tenofovir is distributed into milk of lactating rats and rhesus monkeys receiving tenofovir DF.

Consider the benefits of breast-feeding and the importance of tenofovir alafenamide to the mother along with the potential adverse effects on the breast-fed infant from the drug or from the underlying maternal condition.

Pediatric Use

The steady-state pharmacokinetics, safety, and efficacy of tenofovir alafenamide for the treatment of chronic HBV infection have been established in pediatric patients 12 to <18 years of age. No clinically meaningful differences in pharmacokinetics or safety were observed in comparison to adults.

Safety and efficacy of tenofovir alafenamide have not been established in pediatric patients with chronic HBV infection <12 years of age.

Geriatric Use

In clinical trials of tenofovir alafenamide, no clinically significant differences in safety or efficacy were observed between patients ≥65 years of age and patients 18 to <65 years of age.

Hepatic Impairment

Safety and efficacy of tenofovir alafenamide have not been established in patients with decompensated cirrhosis (Child-Pugh class B or C), and the drug is not recommended in such patients.

Dosage adjustments are not necessary in patients with mild hepatic impairment (Child-Pugh class A). Pharmacokinetics of tenofovir alafenamide and its metabolite tenofovir are similar in patients with mild hepatic impairment (Child-Pugh class A) and in individuals with normal hepatic function.

Renal Impairment

Dosage adjustments are not necessary in patients with mild, moderate, or severe renal impairment, or in patients with end-stage renal disease (ESRD; creatinine clearance <15 mL/minute) receiving chronic hemodialysis. On days of hemodialysis, administer tenofovir alafenamide after completion of hemodialysis treatment. In clinical studies, the pharmacokinetics of tenofovir alafenamide were similar among patients with normal renal function, with severe renal impairment, and with ESRD receiving chronic hemodialysis.

In the clinical study evaluating the safety and efficacy of tenofovir alafenamide in adults infected with HBV with moderate to severe renal impairment (creatinine clearance 15–59 mL/minute) and with ESRD (creatinine clearance <15 mL/minute) receiving chronic hemodialysis, 98% of patients achieved HBV DNA <20 IU/mL at week 24. The safety of tenofovir alafenamide was similar to that observed in clinical trials of tenofovir alafenamide in patients with compensated liver disease but without renal impairment. In the study of virologically-suppressed, HIV-1-infected patients with ESRD receiving chronic hemodialysis and treated with elvitegravir/cobicistat/emtricitabine/tenofovir alafenamide, tenofovir alafenamide exposures were similar when comparing tenofovir alafenamide 25 mg and tenofovir alafenamide 10 mg as part of the combination.

Patients with severe renal impairment or ESRD receiving chronic hemodialysis had increased tenofovir exposures relative to those with normal renal function. In patients receiving chronic hemodialysis, those with HBV had increased tenofovir exposures relative to those with HIV; the clinical importance of these higher exposures is not established.

Safety of tenofovir alafenamide has not been established in patients with ESRD who are not receiving chronic hemodialysis, and the drug is not recommended in such patients.

● Common Adverse Effects

The most common adverse effect (incidence ≥10%, all grades) is headache.

DRUG INTERACTIONS

Tenofovir alafenamide is a substrate of the efflux transporters, P-glycoprotein (P-gp) transport system and breast cancer resistance protein (BCRP), as well as the uptake transporters organic anion transport protein (OATP) 1B1 and OATP1B3; tenofovir alafenamide does not inhibit any transporters.

The following drug interactions are based on studies that used tenofovir alafenamide fumarate, or are predicted to occur with use of tenofovir alafenamide; refer to the prescribing information for specific details. Additional drug interactions may exist for fixed-dose combinations containing elvitegravir, cobicistat, emtricitabine, and tenofovir alafenamide (Genvoya®); emtricitabine, rilpivirine, and tenofovir alafenamide (Odefsey®); emtricitabine and tenofovir alafenamide (Descovy®); bictegravir, emtricitabine, and tenofovir alafenamide (Biktarvy®); and darunavir, cobicistat, emtricitabine, and tenofovir alafenamide (Symtuza®). See the full prescribing information for drug interactions of each of these combination products.

● *Drugs Affecting or Metabolized by Hepatic Microsomal Enzymes*

Tenofovir alafenamide is a weak inhibitor of CYP3A in vitro; tenofovir alafenamide does not induce or inhibit other CYP isoenzymes.

● *Drugs Affecting or Affected by P-glycoprotein Transport System and Breast Cancer Resistance Protein*

Drugs that strongly affect P-gp transport or BCRP activity may lead to changes in tenofovir alafenamide absorption.

Concomitant use of tenofovir alafenamide and P-gp inducers is expected to decrease absorption of tenofovir alafenamide and may result in decreased plasma concentrations and loss of therapeutic effect of tenofovir alafenamide.

Concomitant use of tenofovir alafenamide and inhibitors of P-gp or BCRP may increase absorption of tenofovir alafenamide resulting in increased plasma concentrations of the drug.

● *Nephrotoxic Drugs or Drugs Eliminated by Renal Excretion*

Tenofovir is principally excreted by a combination of glomerular filtration and active tubular secretion. Concomitant use of tenofovir alafenamide with drugs that reduce renal function or compete for active tubular secretion (e.g., acyclovir, cidofovir, ganciclovir, valacyclovir, valganciclovir, gentamicin, high-dose or multiple nonsteroidal anti-inflammatory agents [NSAIAs]) may increase concentrations of tenofovir and other drugs that are renally eliminated, which may increase the risk of adverse effects.

● *Anticonvulsants*

Carbamazepine

Concomitant use of carbamazepine (300 mg twice daily) and the fixed combination of emtricitabine and tenofovir alafenamide (emtricitabine/tenofovir alafenamide) substantially decreases tenofovir alafenamide plasma concentrations and AUC.

If tenofovir alafenamide and carbamazepine are used concomitantly, increase dosage of tenofovir alafenamide to 50 mg once daily.

Oxcarbazepine, Phenobarbital, and Phenytoin

Concomitant use of tenofovir alafenamide and oxcarbazepine, phenobarbital, or phenytoin is expected to decrease tenofovir alafenamide plasma concentrations.

Avoid concomitant use of tenofovir alafenamide and oxcarbazepine, phenobarbital, or phenytoin.

● *Antimycobacterial Agents*

Concomitant use of tenofovir alafenamide and rifabutin, rifampin, or rifapentine is expected to decrease plasma concentrations of tenofovir alafenamide.

Avoid concomitant use of tenofovir alafenamide and rifabutin, rifampin, or rifapentine.

● *Cobicistat*

Concomitant use of cobicistat (150 mg once daily) and tenofovir alafenamide (8 mg once daily) results in increased peak plasma concentrations and AUC of tenofovir alafenamide.

● *Estrogens and Progestins*

No clinically important pharmacokinetic interactions were reported when tenofovir alafenamide was used concomitantly with ethinyl estradiol or norgestimate.

● *HBV Antivirals*

There is no in vitro evidence of antagonistic anti-HBV effects between tenofovir and other HBV nucleoside or nucleotide reverse transcriptase inhibitor antivirals (e.g., entecavir, lamivudine).

● *HCV Antivirals*

Sofosbuvir

No clinically important pharmacokinetic interactions were reported when tenofovir alafenamide was used concomitantly with sofosbuvir.

Ledipasvir and Sofosbuvir

No clinically important pharmacokinetic interactions were reported when tenofovir alafenamide was used concomitantly with the fixed combination of ledipasvir and sofosbuvir (ledipasvir/sofosbuvir).

Sofosbuvir and Velpatasvir

No clinically important pharmacokinetic interactions were reported when tenofovir alafenamide was used concomitantly with the fixed combination of sofosbuvir and velpatasvir (sofosbuvir/velpatasvir).

Sofosbuvir, Velpatasvir, and Voxilaprevir

No clinically important pharmacokinetic interactions were reported when tenofovir alafenamide was used concomitantly with the fixed combination of sofosbuvir, velpatasvir, and voxilaprevir (sofosbuvir/velpatasvir/voxilaprevir).

● *Midazolam*

No clinically important pharmacokinetic interactions were reported when tenofovir alafenamide was used concomitantly with midazolam.

● *Sertraline*

No clinically important pharmacokinetic interactions were reported when tenofovir alafenamide was used concomitantly with sertraline.

● *St. John's Wort*

Concomitant use of St. John's wort (*Hypericum perforatum*) and tenofovir alafenamide is expected to decrease plasma concentrations of tenofovir alafenamide.

Avoid concomitant use of tenofovir alafenamide and St. John's wort.

DESCRIPTION

Tenofovir alafenamide fumarate is a nucleotide reverse transcriptase inhibitor antiviral agent.

Tenofovir alafenamide fumarate is a phosphonamidate prodrug of tenofovir (2'-deoxyadenosine monophosphate analog) and is inactive until converted intracellularly to the active metabolite (tenofovir diphosphate). Tenofovir alafenamide enters primary hepatocytes by passive diffusion and by the hepatic uptake transporters organic anion transport protein (OATP) 1B1 and 1B3. The prodrug is converted to tenofovir within hepatocytes by hydrolysis, principally by carboxylesterase 1 (CES1); tenofovir alafenamide also is hydrolyzed to tenofovir intracellularly within peripheral blood mononuclear cells (PBMCs) and macrophages by cathepsin A. Tenofovir is subsequently phosphorylated by cellular kinases to tenofovir diphosphate. Tenofovir diphosphate is active against hepatitis B virus (HBV) and human immunodeficiency virus type-1 (HIV-1) and has some in vitro activity against HIV-2.

Tenofovir diphosphate inhibits HBV replication through incorporation into viral DNA by HBV reverse transcriptase, which results in DNA chain termination. Tenofovir diphosphate is a weak inhibitor of mammalian DNA polymerases, including mitochondrial DNA polymerase γ, and there is no evidence of toxicity to mitochondria in cell culture.

The antiviral activity of tenofovir alafenamide was assessed in a transient transfection assay (HepG2 cells) against a panel of HBV clinical isolates representing genotypes A–H. The EC_{50} (50% effective concentration) for tenofovir alafenamide ranged from 34.7–134.4 nM, with an overall mean EC_{50} of 86.6 nM. The CC_{50} (50% cytotoxicity concentration) for the drug in HepG2 cells was greater than 44,400 nM.

Genotypic resistance analysis was performed on paired baseline and on-treatment HBV isolates from those who either experienced virologic breakthrough (2 consecutive visits with plasma HBV DNA levels ≥69 IU/mL [400 copies/mL] after having been less than 69 IU/mL, or a 1-log_{10} or greater increase in HBV DNA from nadir) through week 48 or had plasma HBV DNA levels ≥69 IU/mL at early discontinuation at or after week 24. In a pooled analysis of clinical studies evaluating tenofovir alafenamide for treatment of HBV infection in treatment-naive and previously treated patients, treatment-emergent amino acid substitutions in the HBV reverse transcriptase domain, all occurring at polymorphic positions, were observed in 25% (5/20) of HBV isolates evaluated; however, no specific substitutions occurred at a sufficient frequency to be associated with resistance to tenofovir alafenamide. In a study of virologically-suppressed patients receiving tenofovir alafenamide, no patients qualified for resistance analysis through 48 weeks of treatment. In the pediatric trial (N=47), 30 patients 12 to <18 years of age receiving tenofovir alafenamide qualified for resistance analysis at week 24, and results were obtained for 27 out of these 30 patients. No HBV amino acid substitutions known to be associated with resistance to tenofovir alafenamide were detected through 24 weeks of treatment.

HBV isolates resistant to some other nucleoside or nucleotide antivirals used for the treatment of HBV infection (e.g., adefovir, entecavir, lamivudine) may also have reduced susceptibility to tenofovir. HBV isolates with lamivudine resistance-associated substitutions rtM204V/I and entecavir resistance-associated substitutions rtT184G, rtS202G, or rtM250V in the presence of rtL180M and rtM204V result in less than twofold reduced susceptibility to tenofovir alafenamide. HBV isolates with rtA181T, rtA181V, or rtN236T single adefovir resistance-associated substitutions also have less than twofold reduced susceptibility to tenofovir alafenamide. Isolates with double adefovir resistance-associated substitutions of rtA181V *and* rtN236T have 3.7-fold reduced susceptibility to tenofovir alafenamide. The clinical importance of these substitutions is not known.

Tenofovir alafenamide at the recommended dosage or 5 times the recommended dosage does not affect the QT or QT interval corrected for rate (QT_c), and does not prolong the PR interval. Following oral administration of tenofovir alafenamide, peak plasma concentrations occur at approximately 0.5 hours after the dose. After administration of tenofovir alafenamide with a high-fat meal, the AUC increases by 1.65-fold relative to administration in the fasting state. Tenofovir alafenamide is 80% bound to plasma proteins. In vivo, tenofovir alafenamide is hydrolyzed within cells to tenofovir (the major metabolite), which is phosphorylated to tenofovir diphosphate (the pharmacologically active metabolite). Tenofovir alafenamide is metabolized within hepatocytes by CES1 and within PBMCs and macrophages by cathepsin A. Tenofovir alafenamide is also metabolized by cytochrome P-450 (CYP) isoenzyme 3A to a minor extent. The major route of elimination is metabolism (>80% of the oral dose). Following a single oral dose of tenofovir alafenamide fumarate (25 mg of tenofovir alafenamide), approximately 32% of the dose is excreted in feces and <1% is eliminated in urine. The median terminal plasma half-life of tenofovir alafenamide is approximately 0.5 hours.

Limited data suggest that there are no clinically important differences in the pharmacokinetics of tenofovir alafenamide or its metabolite tenofovir in geriatric patients (≥65 years of age) compared with younger adults. No clinically important differences in the pharmacokinetics of tenofovir alafenamide or tenofovir due to race or gender have been identified. The pharmacokinetics of tenofovir alafenamide have not been fully evaluated in patients with HCV and HIV coinfection.

ADVICE TO PATIENTS

- Advise patients to read the patient information provided by the manufacturer.

- Inform patients to take tenofovir alafenamide fumarate on a regular dosing schedule with food and to avoid missed doses in order to prevent the development of resistance.

- Inform patients that severe acute exacerbations of hepatitis B virus (HBV) infection have been reported following discontinuance of HBV treatment, including tenofovir alafenamide. Advise patients not to discontinue tenofovir alafenamide without first informing a clinician.

- Inform patients that if they have or develop human immunodeficiency virus (HIV) infection and are not receiving effective HIV treatment, use of tenofovir alafenamide alone may increase the risk of development of resistance to HIV treatment.

- Advise patients that postmarketing cases of renal impairment, including cases of acute renal failure, have been reported in patients receiving tenofovir alafenamide fumarate-containing formulations.

- Advise patients that lactic acidosis and severe hepatomegaly with steatosis, including fatalities, have occurred in patients receiving drugs similar to tenofovir alafenamide. Inform patients to contact their clinician immediately and discontinue tenofovir alafenamide if they develop clinical symptoms suggestive of lactic acidosis or pronounced hepatotoxicity.

- Advise women to inform their clinician if they are or plan to become pregnant or plan to breast-feed. Inform patients that there is a pregnancy registry to monitor fetal outcomes of pregnant women exposed to tenofovir alafenamide.

- Advise patients to inform their clinician of existing or contemplated concomitant therapy, including prescription and OTC drugs and dietary or herbal products (e.g., St. John's wort), as well as any concomitant illnesses.

- Advise patients of other important precautionary information.

PREPARATIONS

Excipients in commercially available drug preparations may have clinically important effects in some individuals; consult specific product labeling for details.

Tenofovir Alafenamide Fumarate

Oral

Tablets, film-coated	25 mg (of tenofovir alafenamide)	Vemlidy®, Gilead

† Use is not currently included in the labeling approved by the US Food and Drug Administration.

Selected Revisions April 10, 2024, © Copyright, May 29, 2017, American Society of Health-System Pharmacists, Inc.

valACYclovir Hydrochloride

8:18.32 • NUCLEOSIDES AND NUCLEOTIDES

■ Valacyclovir, the L-valine ester of acyclovir, is an antiviral agent that is a prodrug of acyclovir and is active against herpes viruses.

USES

Oral valacyclovir is used for the treatment of initial and recurrent episodes of genital herpes infections in immunocompetent adults and adolescents and for the suppression of recurrent episodes of genital herpes in immunocompetent adults and adolescents and individuals infected with human immunodeficiency virus (HIV). Valacyclovir also is used for the episodic treatment of herpes labialis (perioral herpes, cold sores, fever blisters) in adults and adolescents and for the treatment of acute, localized herpes zoster (shingles, zoster) in adults and adolescents.

The manufacturer states that safety and efficacy of valacyclovir in immunocompromised patients have not been established for any use other than suppression of genital herpes and safety and efficacy of the drug have not been established for any use in prepubertal pediatric patients.

● Genital Herpes

Treatment of First Episodes

Oral valacyclovir is used in the treatment of initial episodes of genital herpes simplex virus (HSV-2) infection in immunocompetent adults and adolescents. Because many patients with first episodes of genital herpes present with mild clinical symptoms but later develop severe or prolonged symptoms, the US Centers for Disease Control and Prevention (CDC) states that most patients with initial genital herpes should receive antiviral therapy. The CDC and some clinicians recommend that first episodes of genital herpes be treated with a regimen of oral acyclovir (400 mg 3 times daily or 200 mg 5 times daily for 7–10 days), oral famciclovir (250 mg 3 times daily for 7–10 days), or oral valacyclovir (1 g twice daily for 7–10 days).

Oral valacyclovir appears to be as effective as oral acyclovir in the treatment of first episodes of genital herpes. Efficacy of oral valacyclovir (1 g twice daily for 10 days) was compared with that of oral acyclovir (200 mg 5 times daily for 10 days) in a randomized, double-blind trial in immunocompetent adults who presented for treatment within 72 hours of the onset of symptoms. Results of this study indicate that, for both drugs, the median time to lesion healing was 9 days, the median time to cessation of pain was 5 days, and the median time to cessation of viral shedding was 3 days.

Episodic Treatment of Recurrent Episodes

Oral valacyclovir is used in the treatment of recurrent episodes of genital herpes in immunocompetent adults and adolescents. Antiviral therapy for recurrent genital herpes can be given episodically to ameliorate or shorten the duration of lesions or can be given continuously as suppressive therapy to reduce the frequency of recurrences. For episodic treatment of recurrent genital herpes, the CDC and some clinicians recommend oral acyclovir (400 mg 3 times daily for 5 days, 800 mg twice daily for 5 days, or 800 mg 3 times daily for 2 days), oral famciclovir (125 mg twice daily for 5 days or 1 g twice daily for 1 day), or oral valacyclovir (500 mg twice daily for 3 days or 1 g once daily for 5 days). Episodic antiviral therapy should be initiated within 1 day of lesion onset or during the prodrome that precedes some outbreaks. The manufacturer states that patients should be advised to initiate oral valacyclovir at the first sign or symptoms of an episode and that there are no data on the effectiveness of the drug initiated more than 24 hours after the onset of signs and symptoms of a recurrent episode.

Efficacy of oral valacyclovir in the treatment of recurrent episodes of genital herpes has been evaluated in 3 double-blind (2 of them placebo-controlled) studies in which immunocompetent adults self-initiated therapy within 24 hours of the first sign or symptom of a recurrent genital herpes episode. In one study, the median time to lesion healing and cessation of pain was 4 and 3 days, respectively, in those randomized to receive oral valacyclovir (500 mg twice daily for 5 days) compared with 6 and 4 days, respectively, in those randomized to receive placebo.

The median time to cessation of viral shedding was 2 days in those who received valacyclovir versus 4 days in those who received placebo. Results of this study were duplicated in a second study.

There is evidence that a 3-day regimen of oral valacyclovir is as effective as a 5-day regimen of the drug for the episodic treatment of recurrent genital herpes. In a double-blind study, patients were randomized to receive valacyclovir 500 mg twice daily for 3 or 5 days (patients receiving the 3-day regimen received placebo on days 4 and 5). The median time to lesion healing was about 4.5 days and the median time to cessation of pain was about 3 days in both treatment groups.

Suppressive Therapy of Recurrent Episodes

Valacyclovir is used for chronic suppressive therapy of recurrent genital herpes in immunocompetent and HIV-infected adults and adolescents. The CDC states that suppressive antiviral therapy can reduce the frequency of genital herpes recurrences by 70–80% in patients who have frequent recurrences (i.e., 6 or more per year) and many patients report no symptomatic outbreaks during such therapy. For chronic suppressive therapy of recurrent genital herpes, the CDC and some clinicians recommend a regimen of oral acyclovir (400 mg twice daily), oral famciclovir (250 mg twice daily), or oral valacyclovir (500 mg or 1 g once daily). The CDC states that data suggest that famciclovir and valacyclovir are as effective as acyclovir in terms of clinical outcome, although the 500 mg once-daily valacyclovir regimen might be less effective than the acyclovir regimen or other valacyclovir regimens in patients who have very frequent recurrences (i.e., 10 or more episodes per year).

Efficacy of oral valacyclovir for chronic suppressive therapy of recurrent genital herpes infections has been evaluated in a double-blind, placebo-controlled study in immunocompetent adults with a history of frequent recurrences (6 or more per year). Patients were randomized to receive oral valacyclovir (1 g once daily), oral acyclovir (400 mg twice daily), or placebo. At 6 months, 55% of those receiving valacyclovir and 54% of those receiving acyclovir were free of recurrences compared with only 7% of those receiving placebo; at 12 months, 34% of patients in both groups receiving antiviral therapy were still free of recurrences. When valacyclovir is used for suppressive therapy in immunocompetent individuals, the risk of heterosexual transmission to susceptible partners is reduced. (See Reduction of Transmission under Uses: Genital Herpes.)

Efficacy of oral valacyclovir for suppressive therapy of recurrent genital herpes has been evaluated in HIV-infected adults 18 years of age or older (median HIV-1 RNA level 2.6 $\log_{10}$ copies/mL and median CD4+ T-cell count 336/mm³ at study entry) with a history of frequent recurrences (4 or more per year). At 6 months, 65% of those receiving valacyclovir were free of recurrences compared with 26% of those receiving placebo. Safety and efficacy of valacyclovir for suppression of recurrent genital herpes in patients with advanced HIV disease (CD4+ T-cell counts less than 100/mm³) have not been established.

Safety and efficacy of oral valacyclovir for suppressive therapy of recurrent genital herpes infections have been established in immunocompetent patients receiving daily therapy for up to 1 year; safety and efficacy for this indication have been established in HIV-infected patients receiving daily therapy for up to 6 months.

Reduction of Transmission

When valacyclovir is used for suppressive therapy of genital herpes in immunocompetent individuals, the risk of heterosexual transmission to susceptible partners is reduced. Transmission of genital herpes was assessed in a double-blind, placebo-controlled study in monogamous, heterosexual, immunocompetent couples discordant for HSV-2 infection; the infected partner received valacyclovir (500 mg once daily) or placebo for 8 months. Clinically symptomatic HSV-2 infection developed in 0.5% of susceptible individuals whose partner received valacyclovir and in 2.2% of those whose partner received placebo. Acquisition of HSV-2 was observed in 1.9% of susceptible individuals whose partner received valacyclovir and in 3.6% of those whose partner received placebo. Efficacy for reducing transmission of HSV-2 has not been established in individuals with multiple partners or in non-heterosexual couples.

HIV-infected Individuals

Immunocompromised individuals may have prolonged or severe episodes of genital, perianal, or oral herpes; HSV-2 lesions are common in those with human immunodeficiency virus (HIV) infection and may be severe, painful, and atypical. (See Uses: Mucocutaneous Herpes Simplex Virus Infections.)

The CDC states that episodic treatment or suppressive therapy with oral antiviral agents often is beneficial in HIV-infected individuals with genital herpes. While the drugs of choice for episodic treatment or suppressive therapy of genital herpes in HIV-infected individuals are the same as those in immunocompetent individuals, higher dosages and/or more prolonged therapy may be necessary. Although safety and efficacy of valacyclovir for treatment of genital herpes have not been established in immunocompromised patients, CDC recommends valacyclovir for the treatment of genital herpes in HIV-infected individuals†. For episodic treatment of recurrences of genital herpes in HIV-infected individuals, the CDC recommends a 5- to 10-day regimen of oral acyclovir (400 mg 3 times daily), oral famciclovir (500 mg twice daily), or oral valacyclovir (1 g twice daily). Valacyclovir is used for suppression of recurrent genital herpes in HIV-infected individuals. For chronic suppressive therapy of recurrent genital herpes, CDC recommends oral acyclovir (400–800 mg 2–3 times daily), oral famciclovir (500 mg twice daily), or oral valacyclovir (500 mg twice daily).

Patient Counseling and Management of Sexual Partners

Counseling of infected individuals and their sex partners is critical to management of genital herpes. The goals of such counseling are to help patients understand and cope with the infection and to prevent sexual and perinatal transmission of the virus. Antiviral therapy offers clinical benefit to most symptomatic patients and is the mainstay of management; however, genital herpes is a recurrent, lifelong viral infection. Use of valacyclovir for suppressive therapy in immunocompetent individuals is associated with reduced risk of heterosexual transmission to susceptible partners. However, antiviral therapy does not eradicate latent HSV-2 or affect the risk, frequency, or severity of recurrences of genital herpes following discontinuance of therapy.

The majority of genital herpes infections are transmitted by individuals unaware that they have the infection or by individuals who are asymptomatic when transmission occurs. Patients should be advised that valacyclovir is not a cure for genital herpes. While use of valacyclovir for suppressive therapy is associated with a reduced risk of heterosexual transmission, safer sex practices should be used even in patients receiving suppressive therapy. Because genital herpes is a sexually transmitted disease, patients should be advised to avoid sexual contact with uninfected partners when lesions and/or prodromal symptoms are present. In addition, patients should be advised that sexual transmission of the virus can occur during asymptomatic periods and that suppressive antiviral therapy reduces, but does not eliminate, subclinical viral shedding.

Sex partners of individuals with genital herpes should be advised that they may be infected even if they have no symptoms. Asymptomatic partners of patients with genital herpes should be questioned regarding a history of genital lesions, educated to recognize symptoms of genital herpes, and offered type-specific serologic testing to determine whether risk for HSV-2 acquisition exists. Antiviral therapy is not recommended for sex partners who do not have clinical manifestations of infection, but symptomatic sex partners of individuals with genital herpes should be evaluated and treated.

The risk for neonatal HSV-2 infection should be discussed with all genital herpes patients, including men. Pregnant women and women of childbearing age who have genital herpes should inform their providers who care for them during pregnancy as well as those who will care for their neonate.

Information to assist patients and clinicians in counseling regarding genital herpes is available at http://www.ashastd.org and http://www.ihmf.org. For further information on treatment of initial or recurrent episodes of genital herpes or suppression of recurrent infections, see Uses: Genital Herpes in Acyclovir 8:18.32.

● Herpes Labialis

Valacyclovir is used for the episodic treatment of herpes labialis (perioral herpes, cold sores, fever blisters) in adults and adolescents.

Efficacy of a short-duration regimen of valacyclovir was evaluated in healthy adults and adolescents 12 years of age or older with a history of recurrent cold sores (at least 3 episodes in the past year). Patients were randomized to 1-day treatment (valacyclovir 2 g twice daily), 2-day treatment (valacyclovir 2 g twice daily on day 1 then valacyclovir 1 g twice daily on day 2), or placebo; patients self-initiated therapy at the earliest prodromal symptom and before clinical signs of a cold sore (most initiated treatment within 2 hours of symptom onset). The

mean duration of the cold sore episode was reduced by about 1 day in patients receiving valacyclovir compared with those given placebo; the 2-day regimen was not more effective than the 1-day regimen. The proportion of valacyclovir-treated patients with prevented and/or blocked cold sore lesions (44–46%) was essentially the same as the proportion of patients given placebo (38%).

The manufacturer states that safety and efficacy of valacyclovir for the treatment of cold sores in immunocompromised patients have not been established.

● Mucocutaneous Herpes Simplex Virus Infections

Oral valacyclovir has been used for the treatment of recurrent mucocutaneous HSV-1 infections in HIV-infected adults† and for chronic suppressive or maintenance therapy (secondary prophylaxis) against HSV-1 disease in HIV-infected individuals†.

In patients with advanced HIV infection, reactivation of HSV-1 frequently occurs and can result in chronic, persistent mucocutaneous disease that may be severe. The Prevention of Opportunistic Infections Working Group of the US Public Health Service and the Infectious Diseases Society of America (USPHS/ IDSA) has established guidelines for the prevention of opportunistic infections in HIV-infected individuals that include recommendations concerning prevention of exposure to opportunistic pathogens, prevention of first disease episodes, and prevention of disease recurrence. The USPHS/IDSA does not currently recommend primary prophylaxis against initial episodes of HSV-1 infection in HIV-infected adults, adolescents, or children. In addition, the USPHS/IDSA does not recommend routine chronic suppressive or maintenance therapy (secondary prophylaxis) against HSV-1 disease in HIV-infected individuals since acute episodes generally can be treated successfully with acyclovir. However, long-term prophylaxis against recurrence of HSV-1 can be considered for adults, adolescents, and children who have frequent or severe recurrences. If secondary prophylaxis of HSV-1 disease is indicated in HIV-infected adults or adolescents, the USPHS/ IDSA recommends oral acyclovir or oral famciclovir as the drugs of choice and oral valacyclovir as an alternative. If indicated in infants and children, the USPHS/ IDSA recommends oral acyclovir. If acyclovir-resistant HSV-1 is suspected, IV foscarnet or IV cidofovir can be used to treat the infection.

● Herpes Zoster

Oral valacyclovir is used for the treatment of acute, localized herpes zoster (shingles, zoster) in immunocompetent adults. Some clinicians suggest that the drugs of choice for the treatment of herpes zoster in immunocompetent adults are oral acyclovir, oral famciclovir, or oral valacyclovir.

Efficacy of oral valacyclovir in the treatment of acute, localized herpes zoster has been evaluated in a randomized, double-blind, placebo-controlled trial in immunocompetent adults younger than 50 years of age and in a double-blind trial in immunocompetent adults 50 years of age or older who were randomized to receive oral valacyclovir (1 g every 8 hours for 7 or 14 days) or oral acyclovir (800 mg 5 times daily for 7 days). Results of these studies indicate that valacyclovir may prevent the appearance of new lesions, decrease viral shedding, decrease the duration of pain, and promote healing and crusting of lesions in immunocompetent adults with localized herpes zoster, at least when given within 72 hours of onset of rash. In one study, there was no evidence of additional benefit on pain duration when valacyclovir was initiated within 48 hours versus between 48–72 hours of rash onset; however, the effect of time on other clinical endpoints (e.g., appearance of new lesions, viral shedding) was not determined, and antiviral therapy for herpes zoster generally is most effective when initiated within 48 hours of rash onset. Like acyclovir, valacyclovir does not appear to *prevent* the development of postherpetic neuralgia; the drug may *decrease the median duration* of neuralgia, particularly in patients older than 50 years of age. In comparative studies, 7 or 14 days of oral valacyclovir (1 g 3 times daily) was as effective as 7 days of oral acyclovir (800 mg 5 times daily) in reducing the duration of virus shedding and accelerating the resolution of herpes zoster-associated pain and cutaneous healing in patients 50 years of age or older, and the drugs exhibited comparable safety profiles. Although there was a trend toward a shorter median duration of postherpetic pain with the valacyclovir regimens compared with the acyclovir regimen in patients 50 years of age or older, the difference was not statistically significant. The principal potential benefits relative to acyclovir are valacyclovir's improved oral bioavailability and resultant more convenient dosing regimen. In these studies, there were no gender-related differences in safety or efficacy.

Valacyclovir has been used for the treatment of localized dermatomal herpes zoster in HIV-infected adults or adolescents†. If cutaneous lesions are extensive or there is clinical evidence of visceral involvement, IV acyclovir should be used for initial treatment.

The manufacturer states that the efficacy of valacyclovir in the treatment of disseminated herpes zoster or for the treatment of herpes zoster in immunocompromised patients has not been established.

● Prevention of Cytomegalovirus Disease

HIV-infected Individuals

Although some evidence indicates that use of valacyclovir for prophylaxis of cytomegalovirus (CMV) disease in HIV-infected individuals† reduces the incidence of CMV disease in these patients, the USPHS/IDSA states that valacyclovir should not be used for primary prophylaxis against CMV in HIV-infected individuals because an unexplained trend toward increased mortality has been observed in HIV-infected patients receiving the drug for such prophylaxis.

Transplant Recipients

Valacyclovir has been evaluated for the prevention of CMV disease in renal transplant recipients† considered at risk for the disease. Results of a randomized placebo-controlled study in renal transplant recipients at risk of developing CMV infection (i.e., CMV-seropositive or -seronegative recipients of a kidney from a CMV-seropositive donor) indicate that in patients who received valacyclovir (2 g four times daily, dosage reduced for those with a creatinine clearance less than 75 mL/minute) the probability of CMV disease was reduced compared with those receiving placebo.

Although valacyclovir is being investigated for prophylaxis of CMV disease in hematopoietic stem cell transplant (HSCT) recipients†, the CDC, IDSA, and American Society of Blood and Marrow Transplantation (ASBMT) state the valacyclovir currently is not recommended for this use since it is presumed to be less effective against CMV than ganciclovir.

DOSAGE AND ADMINISTRATION

● Administration

Valacyclovir hydrochloride is administered orally without regard to meals. Food does not affect systemic bioavailability of the drug.

Patients should maintain adequate hydration during valacyclovir treatment.

Extemporaneously Compounded Oral Liquid

Extemporaneously compounded oral liquid formulations of valacyclovir containing 50 mg/mL have been prepared using the commercially available caplets and commonly used syrups.

Standardize 4 Safety

Standardized concentrations for an extemporaneously prepared oral liquid formulation of valacyclovir have been established through Standardize 4 Safety (S4S), a national patient safety initiative to reduce medication errors, especially during transitions of care. Multidisciplinary expert panels were convened to determine recommended standard concentrations. Because recommendations from the S4S panels may differ from the manufacturer's prescribing information, caution is advised when using concentrations that differ from labeling, particularly when using rate information from the label. For additional information on S4S (including updates that may be available), see https://www.ashp.org/pharmacy-practice/standardize-4-safety-initiative.

TABLE 1. Standardize 4 Safety Compounded Oral Liquid Standards for Valacyclovir

Concentration Standards
50 mg/mL

● Dosage

Dosage of valacyclovir hydrochloride is expressed in terms of valacyclovir.

Valacyclovir dosage modification according to renal function may be necessary in geriatric patients, depending on the underlying renal status of the patient. (See Dosage and Administration: Dosage in Renal and Hepatic Impairment.)

Genital Herpes

Treatment of First Episodes

For the treatment of initial episodes of genital herpes simplex virus (HSV-2) infection in immunocompetent adults and adolescents, the dosage of oral valacyclovir recommended by the manufacturer, the US Centers for Disease Control and Prevention (CDC), and other clinicians is 1 g twice daily for 7–10 days. The manufacturer recommends a duration of 10 days; the CDC states that the usual duration of treatment is 7–10 days but that this may be extended if healing is incomplete after 10 days.

In HIV-infected adults and adolescents†, the CDC and other experts recommend 1 g twice daily for 7–14 days for the treatment of initial episodes of genital herpes.

Valacyclovir has been most effective when administered within 48 hours of the onset of signs and symptoms of genital herpes; efficacy of the drug initiated more than 72 hours after the onset of signs and symptoms has not been established.

Episodic Treatment of Recurrent Episodes

For the episodic treatment of recurrent genital herpes in immunocompetent adults and adolescents, the manufacturer and some clinicians recommend that oral valacyclovir be given in a dosage of 500 mg twice daily for 3 days. The CDC states that oral valacyclovir can be given in a dosage of 500 mg twice daily for 3 days or 1 g once daily for 5 days for the episodic treatment of recurrent genital herpes in immunocompetent adults and adolescents.

In HIV-infected adults and adolescents†, the CDC recommends a dosage of 1 g twice daily for 5–10 days for the episodic treatment of recurrent genital herpes. Alternatively, treatment may be continued for 7–14 days in these patients.

Patients should be advised to initiate valacyclovir therapy at the first sign or symptom of an episode. Data are not available concerning efficacy of oral valacyclovir initiated more than 24 hours after the onset of signs or symptoms of a recurrent episode of genital herpes.

Suppressive Therapy of Recurrent Episodes

For chronic suppression of recurrent episodes of genital herpes in immunocompetent adults and adolescents, the usual dosage of oral valacyclovir is 1 g once daily; however, a dosage of 500 mg once daily may be used in patients with infrequent recurrences. The manufacturer states that those with a history of 9 or fewer recurrences per year may receive 500 mg once daily for chronic suppressive therapy; the CDC cautions that the 500 mg once daily regimen might be less effective in those who have very frequent recurrences (i.e., 10 or more per year).

In HIV-infected adults and adolescents, the usual dose of oral valacyclovir for chronic suppression of recurrent episodes of genital herpes is 500 mg twice daily.

Data are not available to date concerning efficacy and safety of oral valacyclovir administered for more than 1 year in immunocompetent patients or for more than 6 months in HIV-infected patients for chronic suppressive therapy of recurrent genital herpes infections.

Because the frequency of recurrent episodes diminishes over time in many patients, the CDC recommends that suppressive antiviral therapy be discontinued periodically (e.g., once yearly) to assess the need for continued therapy.

Reduction of Transmission

For reduction of transmission of genital herpes in patients with a history of 9 or fewer recurrences per year, the recommended dosage of oral valacyclovir for the infected partner is 500 mg once daily. Valacyclovir is used in conjunction with safer sex practices.

Efficacy for reducing transmission in discordant couples has not been established beyond 8 months.

Herpes Labialis

For the treatment of herpes labialis (perioral herpes, cold sores, fever blisters) in immunocompetent adults and adolescents, the recommended dosage of oral valacyclovir is 2 g every 12 hours for 1 day; initiate at the first prodromal symptom of a cold sore (e.g., tingling, itching, burning). Efficacy has not been established if initiated after development of clinical signs of a cold sore (e.g., papule, vesicle, ulcer).

Mucocutaneous Herpes Simplex Virus Infections

If oral valacyclovir is used for chronic suppressive or maintenance prophylaxis (secondary prophylaxis) of HSV† in HIV-infected adults and adolescents who have frequent or severe recurrences of HSV disease, a dosage of 500 mg twice daily has been recommended by the Prevention of Opportunistic Infections Working Group of the US Public Health Service and the Infectious Diseases Society of America (USPHS/IDSA).

Herpes Zoster (Shingles, Zoster)

For the treatment of acute, localized herpes zoster (shingles, zoster) in immunocompetent adults and adolescents, the recommended dosage of oral valacyclovir is 1 g 3 times daily at 8-hour intervals for 7 days.

Therapy should be initiated at the earliest sign or symptom of herpes zoster, preferably within 48 hours of rash onset. Efficacy of oral valacyclovir initiated longer than 72 hours after rash onset has not been established. Limited evidence indicates that extending the valacyclovir regimen to 14 days in immunocompetent adults with acute, localized herpes zoster does not provide additional clinical benefit.

For the treatment of local dermatomal herpes zoster in HIV-infected adults or adolescents†, the CDC and others recommend 1 g of valacyclovir 3 times daily for 7–10 days.

Dosage in Renal and Hepatic Impairment

The manufacturer states that valacyclovir should be used with caution in patients receiving potentially nephrotoxic agents because this may increase the risk of renal dysfunction and/or reversible CNS manifestations. In patients with impaired renal function, doses and/or frequency of administration of valacyclovir must be modified in response to the degree of impairment.

For the treatment of first episodes of genital herpes in immunocompetent adults with impaired renal function, the manufacturer states that patients with creatinine clearances of 30 mL/minute per 1.73 m^2 or greater may receive the usual oral valacyclovir dosage of 1 g every 12 hours; however, those with creatinine clearances of 10–29 or less than 10 mL/minute per 1.73 m^2 should receive 1 g or 500 mg, respectively, once every 24 hours. For the episodic treatment of recurrent genital herpes in immunocompetent adults with impaired renal function, patients with creatinine clearances of 30 mL/minute per 1.73 m^2 may receive the usual dosage of 500 mg every 12 hours, but those with clearances of 29 mL/minute per 1.73 m^2 or less should receive 500 mg once every 24 hours.

For chronic suppression of recurrent episodes of genital herpes in immunocompetent adults with renal impairment, those with creatinine clearances of 30 mL/minute per 1.73 m^2 or greater may receive the usually recommended dosage of oral valacyclovir. Patients with creatinine clearances less than 30 mL/minute per 1.73 m^2 should receive 500 mg once every 24 hours; alternatively, those with a history of 9 or fewer recurrences per year may receive 500 mg once every 48 hours.

For chronic suppression of recurrent episodes of genital herpes in HIV-infected adults with renal impairment, those with creatinine clearances of 30 mL/minute per 1.73 m^2 or greater may receive the usually recommended dosage of oral valacyclovir and those with creatinine clearances less than 30 mL/minute per 1.73 m^2 should receive 500 mg once every 24 hours.

For the treatment of herpes labialis (cold sores) in patients with renal impairment, patients with creatinine clearances of 50 mL/minute or greater per 1.73 m^2 may receive the usual oral valacyclovir dosage of 2 g every 12 hours for 1 day. Those with creatinine clearances of 30–49 mL/minute per 1.73 m^2 should receive 1 g every 12 hours for 1 day, those with creatinine clearances of 10–29mL/minute per 1.73 m^2 should receive 500 mg every 12 hours for 1 day, and those with creatinine clearances less than 10 mL/minute per 1.73 m^2 should receive a single 500-mg dose.

For the treatment of acute, localized herpes zoster in adults, the manufacturer states that patients with creatinine clearances of 50 mL/minute or greater per 1.73 m^2 may receive the usual oral valacyclovir dosage of 1 g every 8 hours. Those with creatinine clearances of 30–49 mL/minute per 1.73 m^2 should receive 1 g every 12 hours, and those with creatinine clearances of 10–29 or less than 10 mL/minute per 1.73 m^2 should receive 1 g or 500 mg, respectively, once every 24 hours.

Because acyclovir is removed by hemodialysis, the manufacturer states that patients undergoing hemodialysis may require a supplemental dose of valacyclovir after each dialysis period. However, if usual dosing coincides with a valacyclovir dose being administered soon after hemodialysis and subsequent dialysis takes place toward the end of the dosing interval, a supplemental dose would not be necessary.

Information regarding use of valacyclovir in patients undergoing peritoneal dialysis is not available. Based on experience with acyclovir, the manufacturer states that supplemental doses of valacyclovir do not appear to be necessary following peritoneal dialysis, either continuous ambulatory peritoneal dialysis (CAPD) or continuous arteriovenous hemofiltration/dialysis (CAVHD).

The rate but not the extent of conversion of valacyclovir to acyclovir may be reduced in patients with moderate (biopsy-proven cirrhosis) or severe (with and without ascites and biopsy-proven cirrhosis) hepatic impairment. Therefore, the manufacturer states that dosage modification is not necessary for patients with cirrhosis.

CAUTIONS

● Contraindications

Known hypersensitivity or intolerance to valacyclovir, acyclovir, or any component of the formulation.

● Warnings/Precautions

Warnings

Hematologic Effects

Thrombotic thrombocytopenic purpura/hemolytic uremic syndrome (sometimes fatal) reported in patients with advanced HIV infection and in allogeneic bone marrow or renal transplant recipients receiving high dosages (8 g daily).

General Precautions

Renal Effects

Use of inappropriately high dosage for the level of renal function has resulted in acute renal failure in patients with underlying renal disease. Acyclovir may precipitate in renal tubules if solubility exceeds 2.5 mg/mL in intratubular fluid.

Adequate hydration should be maintained during therapy.

If acute renal failure and anuria occur, hemodialysis recommended until normal renal function returns.

CNS Effects

Use of inappropriately high dosage for the level of renal function has resulted in CNS symptoms in patients with underlying renal disease.

Genital Herpes

Valacyclovir is not a cure for genital herpes. Patients should avoid sexual contact while lesions and/or symptoms are present due to risk of infecting sexual partners. Infection can be transmitted in the absence of symptoms through asymptomatic viral shedding. Although use of valacyclovir for suppressive therapy in immunocompetent individuals with genital herpes decreases the risk for heterosexual transmission, safer sex practices also should be used. Efficacy for reducing transmission not established in individuals with multiple partners or in non-heterosexual couples. Type-specific serologic testing of asymptomatic partners of individuals with genital herpes can determine whether risk for HSV-2 acquisition exists. Valacyclovir has not been shown to reduce transmission of sexually transmitted infections other than HSV-2.

Although recommended by CDC and others for episodic treatment of genital herpes or chronic suppressive therapy of recurrent episodes in HIV-infected adults and adolescents, manufacturer says efficacy not established for treatment of genital herpes in HIV-infected individuals and safety and efficacy not established for chronic suppressive therapy in those with advanced HIV disease (CD4+ T-cell count <100/mm³).

Herpes Labialis

Valacyclovir is not a cure for cold sores. Treatment should not exceed a single day; therapy beyond 1 day does not provide additional clinical benefits. Because of high dosage, use caution when prescribing valacyclovir for treatment of cold sores in geriatric individuals or those with renal impairment.

Herpes Zoster

Safety and efficacy not established for treatment of disseminated herpes zoster or for treatment of herpes zoster in immunocompromised individuals.

Specific Populations
Pregnancy

Category B.

Lactation

Acyclovir distributed into human milk following oral administration of valacyclovir. Use valacyclovir with caution.

Pediatric Use

Safety and efficacy not established in prepubertal children.

Geriatric Use

Increased risk of adverse renal or CNS effects. CNS effects reported more frequently in geriatric adults than in younger adults include agitation, hallucinations, confusion, delirium, and encephalopathy. In herpes zoster, longer duration of pain after healing (post-herpetic neuralgia) than in younger adults. Consider age-related decreases in renal function when selecting dosage and adjust dosage if necessary. (See Renal Impairment under Dosage and Administration.)

Renal Impairment

Decreased clearance; increased risk of adverse renal and CNS effects in patients with underlying renal disease receiving high dosages. Adjust dosage as necessary. (See Renal Impairment under Dosage and Administration.)

● Common Adverse Effects

Headache, nausea, vomiting.

DRUG INTERACTIONS

● Antacids

Concomitant use of valacyclovir and aluminum- or magnesium-containing antacids does not affect the pharmacokinetics of acyclovir; no dosage adjustments are necessary.

● Cimetidine

Concomitant use of valacyclovir and cimetidine may increase peak plasma concentrations and AUC of acyclovir. This pharmacokinetic interaction is not considered clinically important in patients with normal renal function; no dosage adjustments are necessary in these patients.

● Digoxin

Concomitant use of valacyclovir and digoxin does not affect the pharmacokinetics of acyclovir or digoxin; no dosage adjustments are necessary.

● Probenecid

Concomitant use of valacyclovir and probenecid may increase peak plasma concentrations and AUC of acyclovir. This pharmacokinetic interaction is not

considered clinically important in patients with normal renal function and no dosage adjustments are necessary in these patients.

● Thiazide Diuretics

Concomitant use of valacyclovir and thiazide diuretics does not affect the pharmacokinetics of acyclovir; no dosage adjustments are necessary.

PHARMACOKINETICS

● Absorption
Bioavailability

Valacyclovir hydrochloride, a prodrug of acyclovir, is rapidly absorbed following oral administration and almost completely converted to acyclovir and L-valine by first-pass intestinal and/or hepatic metabolism.

Absolute bioavailability of acyclovir approximately 54% following oral administration of valacyclovir hydrochloride; peak acyclovir plasma concentrations attained within 1.7 hours.

Food

Administration of valacyclovir with food does not alter acyclovir bioavailability.

● Distribution
Extent

Although there are no adequate studies using valacyclovir in pregnant women, acyclovir crosses the placenta.

Following oral administration of valacyclovir to the mother, peak plasma concentrations of acyclovir in breast milk generally are similar to corresponding maternal plasma concentrations.

Plasma Protein Binding

13.5–17.9% bound to plasma proteins.

● Elimination
Metabolism

Valacyclovir hydrochloride rapidly converted to acyclovir and L-valine by first-pass intestinal and/or hepatic metabolism. Acyclovir converted to acyclovir monophosphate, diphosphate, and triphosphate in cells infected with herpesviruses.

Neither valacyclovir nor acyclovir metabolized by CYP enzymes.

Elimination Route

Valacyclovir principally eliminated as acyclovir; 46 and 47% of an oral dose eliminated in urine and feces, respectively.

Half-life

Plasma elimination half-life of acyclovir after oral administration of valacyclovir averages 2.5–3.3 hours.

Special Populations

Renal clearance and elimination half-life decreased in patients with renal impairment; half-life averages 14 hours in end-stage renal disease.

Pharmacokinetics in geriatric patients vary depending on renal function.

DESCRIPTION

Valacyclovir, the L-valine ester of acyclovir, is an antiviral agent. Valacyclovir is a prodrug and exhibits no antiviral activity until hydrolyzed in the intestinal wall and/or liver to acyclovir and subsequently to its active metabolite (acyclovir triphosphate). Valacyclovir is commercially available as the hydrochloride salt and differs structurally from acyclovir by the presence of the l-amino acid, valine, attached to the 5′-hydroxyl group of the nucleoside and by the presence of the monohydrochloride salt. These structural modifications result in substantially increased GI absorption of valacyclovir and resultant plasma acyclovir concentrations compared with those achieved orally with the parent drug acyclovir, which is poorly absorbed from the GI tract.

Valacyclovir is rapidly converted to acyclovir in vivo and subsequently to the pharmacologically active triphosphate metabolite, which has in vitro and in vivo inhibitory activity against herpes simplex virus types 1 (HSV-1) and 2 (HSV-2), varicella-zoster virus (VZV), and cytomegalovirus (CMV). Acyclovir triphosphate exerts its antiviral effect on HSV and VZV by interfering with DNA synthesis and inhibiting viral replication. The inhibitory activity of acyclovir triphosphate is highly selective because of its affinity for the enzyme thymidine kinase encoded by HSV and VZV; however, other mechanisms may be involved since the drug exhibits activity against viruses that apparently do not code for this enzyme. Virus-coded thymidine kinase converts acyclovir into acyclovir monophosphate, a nucleotide analog. The monophosphate is further converted to the diphosphate via cellular guanylate kinase and then to the triphosphate via other cellular enzymes. In vitro, acyclovir triphosphate stops replication of herpes viral DNA by competitive inhibition of viral DNA polymerase, incorporation and termination of the growing viral DNA chain, and inactivation of the viral DNA polymerase.For additional information, see Mechanism of Action in Acyclovir 8:18.32.

PREPARATIONS

Excipients in commercially available drug preparations may have clinically important effects in some individuals; consult specific product labeling for details.

valACYclovir Hydrochloride

Oral

Tablets, film-coated	500 mg (of valacyclovir)	**Valtrex® Caplets**, GlaxoSmithKline
	1 g (of valacyclovir)	**Valtrex® Caplets**, GlaxoSmithKline

† Use is not currently included in the labeling approved by the US Food and Drug Administration.

valGANciclovir Hydrochloride

8:18.32 • NUCLEOSIDES AND NUCLEOTIDES

■ Valganciclovir, a prodrug of ganciclovir, is an antiviral agent; after in vivo conversion to an active metabolite, the drug is active against herpes viruses.

USES

● Treatment of Cytomegalovirus Infection and Disease

Cytomegalovirus Retinitis

Valganciclovir hydrochloride is used for initial treatment (induction therapy) and maintenance therapy (secondary prophylaxis) of cytomegalovirus (CMV) retinitis in adults with human immunodeficiency virus (HIV) infection, including those with acquired immunodeficiency syndrome (AIDS). The drug also is used for the management of CMV retinitis in certain HIV-infected pediatric patients†.

Like others antivirals, valganciclovir is not a cure for CMV retinitis; the retinitis may relapse and/or progress during or after discontinuance of the drug.

Retinitis is the most common clinical manifestation of CMV end-organ disease in HIV-infected patients and ideally should be managed in consultation with an ophthalmologist familiar with the diagnosis and treatment of retinal diseases. Antiviral regimens for initial treatment of CMV retinitis in HIV-infected individuals should be selected based on the location and severity of the CMV retinal lesions, severity of underlying immunosuppression, concomitant drug therapy, and the patient's ability to adhere to the treatment regimen. The antiviral regimen used for maintenance therapy of CMV retinitis in HIV-infected individuals should be selected with consideration for the location of the CMV retinal lesions, vision in the contralateral eye, the patient's immunologic and virologic status, and the patient's response to antiretroviral therapy.

For the management of immediate sight-threatening CMV retinal lesions (i.e., within 1.5 mm of the fovea) in HIV-infected adults and adolescents, the US Centers for Disease Control and Prevention (CDC), National Institutes of Health (NIH), and HIV Medicine Association of the Infectious Diseases Society of America (IDSA) state that the preferred regimen is initial treatment (induction therapy) with intravitreal ganciclovir or intravitreal foscarnet (1–4 doses given over a period of 7–10 days) in conjunction with oral valganciclovir (twice daily for 14–21 days) followed by maintenance therapy (secondary prophylaxis) with oral valganciclovir (once daily). One alternative regimen recommended by these experts for management of sight-threatening CMV retinitis in HIV-infected adults and adolescents is intravitreal ganciclovir or intravitreal foscarnet (1–4 doses given over a period of 7–10 days) in conjunction with IV ganciclovir (twice daily for 14–21 days) followed by maintenance therapy (secondary prophylaxis) with oral valganciclovir (once daily). Use of systemic antivirals (without an intravitreal antiviral) usually is adequate for the management of CMV retinitis in patients who have only small peripheral lesions.

For the management of CMV retinitis in HIV-infected pediatric patients, CDC, NIH, IDSA, and others state that IV ganciclovir is the drug of choice for initial treatment (induction therapy) and is one of several options for maintenance therapy (secondary prophylaxis). These experts state that oral valganciclovir is an option for the management of CMV retinitis in HIV-infected pediatric patients† and can be considered for induction and/or maintenance therapy in adolescents and older children who can receive the recommended adult dosage of the drug and can also be considered in children who are able to transition from initial IV ganciclovir therapy to an oral regimen to complete treatment and/or for maintenance therapy.

Because of the risk of relapse, HIV-infected patients who have received adequate initial treatment of CMV retinitis should receive chronic maintenance therapy (secondary prophylaxis) until immune reconstitution occurs as a result of effective antiretroviral therapy. CDC, NIH, and IDSA state that consideration can be given to discontinuing maintenance therapy of CMV retinitis in HIV-infected adults and adolescents if CMV lesions have been treated for at least 3–6 months

and are inactive and there has been a sustained (i.e., 3–6 months) increase in CD4⁺ T-cell count to greater than 100/mm³ in response to antiretroviral therapy. The safety of discontinuing maintenance therapy of CMV retinitis in HIV-infected pediatric patients has not been well studied; however, CDC, NIH, IDSA, and others state that consideration can be given to discontinuing such maintenance therapy in HIV-infected children who are receiving antiretroviral therapy and have a sustained (i.e., greater than 6 months) increase in CD4⁺ T-cell percentage to greater than 15% (children younger than 6 years of age) or increase in CD4⁺ T-cell count to greater than 100/mm³ (children 6 years of age or older). These experts state that a decision to discontinue maintenance therapy of CMV retinitis should be made in consultation with an ophthalmologist and, if maintenance therapy is discontinued, the patient should continue to receive regular ophthalmologic monitoring (optimally every 3–6 months) for early detection of CMV relapse or immune reconstitution uveitis. If CD4⁺ T-cell count decreases to less than 100/mm³ (adults, adolescents, children 6 years of age or older) or if CD4⁺ T-cell percentage decreases to less than 15% (children younger than 6 years of age), maintenance therapy of CMV retinitis should be reinitiated.

For additional information on the management of CMV retinitis and other CMV infections in HIV-infected individuals, the current clinical practice guidelines from CDC, NIH, and IDSA on the prevention and treatment of opportunistic infections in HIV-infected individuals available at http://www.aidsinfo.nih.gov should be consulted.

Clinical Experience

In a randomized, open-label, comparative study (study WV15376) in HIV-infected adults with AIDS (median age 39 years, baseline plasma HIV-1 RNA levels of 4.9 log₁₀, median CD4⁺ T-cell count of 23/mm³, 91% male, 53% white, 31% Hispanic, 11% black) with previously untreated CMV retinitis, oral valganciclovir (900 mg twice daily for 21 days followed by 900 mg once daily for 7 days) was as effective as IV ganciclovir (5 mg/kg twice daily for 21 days followed by 5 mg/kg once daily for 7 days) in delaying CMV retinitis progression based on a masked evaluation of retinal photographs at week 4 of the study (the primary outcome measure).

All patients enrolled in study WV15376 received maintenance therapy with open-label valganciclovir after week 4; the median time to photographically determined first CMV retinitis progression in patients who had received initial treatment (induction therapy) with oral valganciclovir or IV ganciclovir was 180 days (mean: 226) or 126 days (mean: 219), respectively.

Extraocular Cytomegalovirus Infections

Safety and efficacy of valganciclovir have not been established for the management of extraocular CMV infections.

CDC, NIH, and IDSA state that IV ganciclovir usually is the preferred antiviral for initial management of CMV GI disease (e.g., colitis, esophagitis) in HIV-infected adults and that a transition to oral valganciclovir may be considered when the patient can tolerate and absorb oral drugs. These experts also state that oral valganciclovir can be considered for initial management of CMV esophagitis† or colitis† in patients with GI symptoms that do not interfere with oral absorption.

Congenital Cytomegalovirus Disease

Although safety and efficacy of valganciclovir have not been established in neonates or infants with congenital CMV infection, the drug has been used for the management of symptomatic congenital CMV disease† when an antiviral was indicated.

Transmission of CMV from infected mothers to their fetuses occurs as a result of maternal viremia and transplacental infection. Perinatal infection also can occur from exposure of the neonate to CMV shedding in the mother's genital tract. Approximately 10% of children with congenital CMV infection are symptomatic at birth; mortality in symptomatic infants is about 10% and approximately 50–90% of symptomatic surviving neonates experience substantial morbidity (e.g., mental retardation, sensorineural hearing loss, microcephaly, seizures). The risk of congenital CMV infection resulting from primary maternal CMV infection may be higher and the disease may be more severe than that resulting from reactivation of maternal CMV infection.

Because there is some evidence that antivirals (i.e., ganciclovir, valganciclovir) may help prevent hearing deterioration and/or improve developmental delay in neonates and infants with moderate to severe symptomatic congenital CMV disease, the American Academy of Pediatrics (AAP) and other clinicians state that use of an antiviral regimen should be considered in such neonates if it can be initiated within the first month of life. Antivirals are not usually recommended for neonates with asymptomatic congenital CMV infection or only mildly symptomatic infection without evidence of CNS involvement.

A 6-month regimen of oral valganciclovir has been used in neonates with symptomatic congenital CMV disease (with or without CNS involvement), and there is some evidence that this regimen is associated with some improvement in audiologic and neurodevelopmental outcomes at 12 and 24 months compared with a 6-week regimen of oral valganciclovir. A 6-week regimen of IV ganciclovir either alone or followed by a regimen of oral valganciclovir (continued until up to 12 months of age) also has been used in neonates with symptomatic congenital CMV disease. CDC, NIH, IDSA, and others state that IV ganciclovir can be considered for initial treatment in HIV-exposed or HIV-infected infants with symptomatic congenital CMV disease with CNS involvement.

Decisions regarding antiviral treatment in neonates with congenital CMV disease should be made in consultation with a pediatric infectious diseases specialist. Because of the risk of serious sequelae (e.g., late-onset hearing loss), long-term ophthalmologic and audiologic monitoring is necessary in patients with congenital CMV infection, regardless of antiviral treatment.

● Prevention of Cytomegalovirus Infection and Disease

Valganciclovir hydrochloride is used for prophylaxis to prevent CMV infection and disease in certain adult and pediatric solid organ transplant recipients at high risk for the disease. The drug also has been used for prophylaxis or preemptive treatment of CMV infection and disease in hematopoietic stem cell transplant (HSCT) recipients† at risk for the disease.

CMV infection in transplant recipients can occur either as a primary infection in CMV-seronegative recipients of organs and cells from CMV-positive donors or as reactivation of latent CMV infection in CMV-seropositive recipients. CMV infection in transplant recipients is associated with substantial morbidity and mortality. The risk for CMV infection or reactivation is greatest during the first 3 months after transplantation and depends on several factors, including the serologic status of the recipient and donor, CMV-specific T-cell immunity in the recipient, and immunosuppressive regimens used in the recipient. Certain antiviral strategies have been used to prevent severe, life-threatening CMV disease in transplant recipients, including antiviral prophylaxis (initiated posttransplantation and continued for at least 3 months) and/or preemptive antiviral treatment (i.e., initiated when CMV infection is detected, but before clinical progression to symptomatic CMV disease). These antiviral strategies each have certain advantages and disadvantages.

Specialized references should be consulted for specific information regarding prevention and management of CMV infections in HSCT or solid organ transplant recipients.

Solid Organ Transplant Recipients

Valganciclovir hydrochloride is used for prophylaxis to prevent CMV infection and disease in adult kidney, heart, and kidney-pancreas transplant recipients considered at high risk (CMV-seronegative recipient of an organ from a CMV-seropositive donor). The drug also is used for prophylaxis to prevent CMV infection and disease in pediatric kidney transplant recipients 4 months to 16 years of age and pediatric heart transplant recipients 1 month to 16 years of age considered at high risk (CMV-seronegative recipient of an organ from a CMV-seropositive donor).

Valganciclovir also has been used for preemptive treatment of CMV infection in solid organ transplant recipients† (e.g., kidney, heart, pancreas); however, safety and efficacy of the drug have not been established for preemptive treatment of CMV infections in transplant recipients.

Although safety and efficacy of valganciclovir have not been established in adult or pediatric liver transplant recipients and low efficacy was reported in one study in adult patients (see Clinical Experience under Prevention of Cytomegalovirus Infection and Disease: Solid Organ Transplant Recipients, in Uses), the drug has been used and is recommended by some clinicians for prophylaxis or preemptive treatment of CMV infection in liver transplant recipients†.

Clinical Experience

Safety and efficacy of valganciclovir for prevention of CMV disease in 372 solid organ transplant recipients were evaluated in a double-blind, double-dummy, active comparator study (study PV16000) in heart, liver, kidney, and kidney-pancreas transplant patients at high risk (CMV-seronegative recipient of an organ from a CMV-seropositive donor). Patients were randomized to receive oral valganciclovir (900 mg once daily) or oral ganciclovir (1 g 3 times daily; not commercially

available in the US) initiated within 10 days of transplantation and continued until 100 days after transplantation. During the first 6 months following transplantation, 12% of those receiving valganciclovir and 15% of those receiving ganciclovir developed CMV disease (CMV syndrome and/or tissue-invasive disease). However, in liver transplant recipients, the incidence of CMV disease was greater in those receiving valganciclovir (19%) than in those receiving ganciclovir (12%); tissue-invasive CMV disease was reported most frequently. Mortality at 6 months was 3.7% in the oral valganciclovir group and 1.6% in the oral ganciclovir group.

Safety and efficacy of a longer duration (200 days) of valganciclovir prophylaxis against CMV disease in kidney transplant recipients were established in a double-blind, placebo-controlled trial that included 326 adult kidney transplant patients at high risk (CMV-seronegative recipient of an organ from a CMV-seropositive donor). Patients were randomized to receive valganciclovir prophylaxis (900 mg once daily) starting within 10 days of transplantation and continued for either 200 days posttransplantation or for 100 days posttransplantation followed by placebo for 100 days. At 1 year posttransplantation, the incidence of CMV disease was about 17% in those who received 200 days of valganciclovir prophylaxis compared with 37% in those who received only 100 days of such prophylaxis. There was no overall difference in the safety profile between the 2 groups.

Safety and pharmacokinetics of oral valganciclovir for prevention of CMV disease in pediatric patients were established in an open-label study of 63 solid organ transplant (i.e., kidney, liver, heart, kidney-liver) recipients 4 months to 16 years of age. These pediatric patients received once-daily valganciclovir (tablets or oral solution) given in a dose calculated based on body surface area (BSA) and estimated creatinine clearance (modified Schwartz formula) and limited to a maximum dosage of 900 mg daily. Valganciclovir treatment was initiated within 10 days posttransplantation and continued for a maximum of 100 days (median duration was approximately 92 days). Systemic ganciclovir exposures in these pediatric solid organ transplant patients were somewhat higher compared with exposures reported in adult solid organ transplant patients receiving the drug at a dosage of 900 mg once daily. Although CMV viremia was reported in 11% of patients in this study, CMV disease was not reported in any pediatric patient up to 26 weeks posttransplantation. Use of valganciclovir for the prevention of CMV disease in pediatric kidney or heart transplant recipients 4 months to 16 years of age at high risk for the disease is based on pharmacokinetic, safety, and efficacy data from this open-label study and efficacy extrapolated from a study in adults.

Valganciclovir in pediatric patients also was evaluated in an open-label tolerability study that included 57 renal transplant recipients 1 month to 16 years of age who were at risk for developing CMV disease. All patients received once-daily valganciclovir (tablets or oral solution) given in a dose calculated based on BSA and modified creatinine clearance. Valganciclovir treatment was initiated within 10 days posttransplantation and continued for a maximum of 200 days. No cases of CMV syndrome or tissue-invasive CMV disease were reported within the first 12 months posttransplantation.

Hematopoietic Stem Cell Transplant Recipients

Valganciclovir has been used for prophylaxis or preemptive treatment of CMV infection and disease in HSCT recipients†.

DOSAGE AND ADMINISTRATION

● Administration

Valganciclovir hydrochloride is administered orally as tablets or an oral solution and should be given with food.

Adults should receive valganciclovir tablets (not the oral solution). Valganciclovir tablets should not be broken or crushed.

Valganciclovir oral solution is the preferred dosage form for pediatric patients. Valganciclovir tablets should be used in pediatric patients *only* if the calculated dose is within 10% of the tablet strength (i.e., a single 450-mg tablet may be used if the calculated dose is 405–495 mg). (See Pediatric Dosage under Dosage and Administration: Dosage.)

Patients receiving valganciclovir should be adequately hydrated.

Females of childbearing potential should be tested for pregnancy prior to initiation of valganciclovir. (See Pregnancy under Warnings/Precautions: Specific Populations, in Cautions.)

Because of the mutagenic and/or carcinogenic potential of valganciclovir, the tablets, powder for oral solution, and reconstituted oral solutions of the drug should be handled carefully according to guidelines issued for cytotoxic drugs. (See Handling and Disposal under Warnings/Precautions: Other Warnings/Precautions, in Cautions.)

Oral Solution

Valganciclovir hydrochloride powder for oral solution should be reconstituted at the time of dispensing by adding 91 mL of purified water to provide a solution containing 250 mg of valganciclovir per 5 mL. After tapping the bottle to loosen the powder, the water should be added in 2 approximately equal portions and the bottle should be shaken for about 1 minute after each addition. Following reconstitution, the solution is colorless to brownish yellow.

The reconstituted oral solution should be stored at 2–8°C for up to 49 days and should not be frozen.

Just prior to each dose, the oral solution should be shaken for about 5 seconds.

The appropriate dose of the reconstituted oral solution should be administered using the bottle adapter and dosing dispenser provided by the manufacturer.

• Dosage

Dosage of valganciclovir hydrochloride is expressed in terms of valganciclovir.

Adult Dosage
Cytomegalovirus Retinitis

For initial treatment (induction therapy) of cytomegalovirus (CMV) retinitis in adults with normal renal function (creatinine clearance 60 mL/minute or greater), the recommended dosage of valganciclovir tablets is 900 mg orally twice daily for 21 days. The US Centers for Disease Control and Prevention (CDC), National Institutes of Health (NIH), and HIV Medicine Association of the Infectious Diseases Society of America (IDSA) recommend that initial treatment (induction therapy) be continued for 14–21 days in adults with human immunodeficiency virus (HIV) infection. In patients with immediate sight-threatening CMV retinal lesions (i.e., within 1.5 mm of the fovea), these experts recommend that initial treatment also include an appropriate intravitreal antiviral. (See Cytomegalovirus Retinitis under Uses: Treatment of Cytomegalovirus Infection and Disease.)

After completion of initial treatment or in patients with inactive CMV retinitis, the recommended dosage of valganciclovir tablets for maintenance therapy (secondary prophylaxis) in adults with normal renal function is 900 mg orally once daily.

Decisions regarding discontinuance of maintenance therapy of CMV retinitis in HIV-infected individuals who have received CMV treatment for at least 3–6 months, have inactive CMV retinal lesions, and have achieved immune reconstitution as the result of antiretroviral therapy should be made in consultation with an ophthalmologist. (See Cytomegalovirus Retinitis under Uses: Treatment of Cytomegalovirus Infection and Disease.)

Cytomegalovirus Esophagitis or Colitis

If oral valganciclovir is used for the management of CMV esophagitis† or colitis† in HIV-infected adults, CDC, NIH, and IDSA recommend a dosage of 900 mg every 12 hours for 21–42 days or until signs and symptoms of the infection have resolved. Maintenance therapy (secondary prophylaxis) usually is not necessary, but should be considered if relapse occurs.

Prevention of Cytomegalovirus Infection and Disease in Transplant Recipients

For prophylaxis to prevent CMV infection and disease in adult *heart* or *kidney-pancreas* transplant recipients, the usual dosage of valganciclovir tablets is 900 mg once daily initiated within 10 days of transplantation and continued until 100 days posttransplantation. Some experts recommend that antiviral prophylaxis be continued for 3–6 months in CMV-seronegative recipients of heart, liver†, or pancreas transplants from CMV-seropositive donors.

For prophylaxis to prevent CMV infection and disease in adult *kidney* transplant recipients, the usual dosage of valganciclovir tablets is 900 mg once daily initiated within 10 days of transplantation and continued until 200 days posttransplantation. Some experts recommend that antiviral prophylaxis be continued for 6 months in CMV-seronegative recipients of kidney transplants from CMV-seropositive donors.

If oral valganciclovir is used for preemptive treatment of CMV infection in solid organ transplant recipients†, a dosage of 900 mg twice daily is recommended in those with normal renal function.

Pediatric Dosage
Cytomegalovirus Retinitis

If oral valganciclovir is used for initial treatment (induction therapy) of CMV retinitis in HIV-infected older children† and adolescents† who can receive adult dosage, CDC, NIH, IDSA, and others recommend a dosage of 900 mg twice daily for 14–21 days.

If oral valganciclovir is used for maintenance therapy (secondary prophylaxis) of CMV retinitis in HIV-infected older children† and adolescents† who can receive adult dosage, CDC, NIH, IDSA, and others recommend a dosage of 900 mg once daily.

Decisions regarding discontinuance of maintenance therapy of CMV retinitis in HIV-infected individuals who have been treated at least 3–6 months, have inactive CMV retinal lesions, and have achieved immune reconstitution as the result of antiretroviral therapy should be made in consultation with an ophthalmologist. (See Cytomegalovirus Retinitis under Uses: Treatment of Cytomegalovirus Infection and Disease.)

Congenital Cytomegalovirus Disease

If oral valganciclovir is used for the management of symptomatic congenital CMV disease† when an antiviral is indicated (see Congenital Cytomegalovirus Disease under Uses: Treatment of Cytomegalovirus Infection and Disease), the American Academy of Pediatrics (AAP) and other clinicians recommend a dosage of 16 mg/kg twice daily.

AAP and other clinicians recommend that, if an antiviral is indicated, it should be initiated within the first month of life and continued for a total of 6 months. If IV ganciclovir is used initially, treatment should be transitioned to oral valganciclovir when the infant is able to tolerate and absorb oral drugs.

Prevention of Cytomegalovirus Infection and Disease in Transplant Recipients

For prophylaxis to prevent CMV infection and disease in pediatric *heart* transplant patients 1 month to 16 years of age, oral valganciclovir should be given once daily initiated within 10 days of transplantation and continued until 100 days posttransplantation.

For prophylaxis to prevent CMV infection and disease in pediatric *kidney* transplant patients 4 months to 16 years of age, oral valganciclovir should be given once daily initiated within 10 days of transplantation and continued until 200 days posttransplantation.

The pediatric dose of oral valganciclovir for prevention of CMV infection and disease should be individualized based on body surface area (BSA) and estimated creatinine clearance (Cl_{cr}, modified Schwartz formula), and is calculated using the following pediatric dosage equation:

$$\text{Pediatric dose (in mg)} = 7 \times \text{BSA (in m}^2\text{)} \times Cl_{cr} \text{ (modified Schwartz formula)}$$

Modified Schwartz formula for Cl_{cr} (in mL/minute per 1.73 m^2) =

$$\frac{k \times \text{height (in cm)}}{\text{serum creatinine (in mg/dL)}}$$

Where k =
0.33 for infants less than 1 year of age with low birth weight for gestational age
0.45 for infants less than 1 year of age with birth weight appropriate for gestational age
0.45 for children 1 to less than 2 years of age
0.55 for girls 2 to less than 16 years of age
0.55 for boys 2 to less than 13 years of age
0.7 for boys 13–16 years of age

To prevent overdosage in pediatric patients, the estimated creatinine clearance used to calculate the pediatric dose should not exceed 150 mL/minute per 1.73 m^2, regardless of the value calculated using the modified Schwartz formula. If the estimated creatinine clearance exceeds 150 mL/minute per 1.73 m^2, the value of 150 mL/minute per 1.73 m^2 should be used to calculate the dose for that patient. The calculated dose should be rounded to the nearest 10-mg increment. The *maximum* dose in pediatric patients is 900 mg.

● Special Populations

Renal Impairment

In patients with impaired renal function, dosage and/or frequency of administration of valganciclovir must be modified in response to the degree of impairment.

Dosage for adults with renal impairment should be based on the patient's creatinine clearance, which can be estimated using the following formula:

$$Ccr\ male = \frac{(140 - age) \times weight}{72 \times serum\ creatinine}$$

$$Ccr\ female = 0.85 \times Ccr\ male$$

where age is in years, weight is in kg,
and serum creatinine is in mg/dL.

Dosage for pediatric patients with renal impairment can be calculated using the usually recommended pediatric dosage equation since this is based on both BSA and estimated creatinine clearance. (See Pediatric Dosage under Dosage and Administration: Dosage.)

Valganciclovir should not be used in adults undergoing hemodialysis (creatinine clearance less than 10 mL/minute). (See Renal Impairment under Warnings/Precautions: Specific Populations, in Cautions.)

Cytomegalovirus Retinitis

When valganciclovir is used for initial treatment (induction therapy) and maintenance therapy (secondary prophylaxis) of CMV retinitis in adults with renal impairment, dosage should be based on the patient's creatinine clearance. (See Table 1.)

TABLE 1. Dosage of Valganciclovir for Management of CMV Retinitis in Adults with Renal Impairment

Creatinine Clearance (mL/minute)	Initial Treatment (Induction) Dosage	Maintenance Dosage
40–59	450 mg twice daily	450 mg once daily
25–39	450 mg once daily	450 mg once every 2 days
10–24	450 mg once every 2 days	450 mg twice weekly
Less than 10 (hemodialysis patients)	Not recommended	Not recommended

Geriatric Patients

Dosage of valganciclovir for geriatric patients should be selected with caution, usually starting at the low end of the dosage range, because of age-related decreases in hepatic, renal, and/or cardiac function. Renal function should be assessed before and during valganciclovir therapy and appropriate dosage adjustments made as necessary. (See Geriatric Use under Warnings/Precautions: Specific Populations, in Cautions.)

CAUTIONS

● Contraindications

Valganciclovir is contraindicated in patients who have had a clinically important hypersensitivity reaction (e.g., anaphylaxis) to valganciclovir, ganciclovir, or any ingredient in the formulation.

● Warnings/Precautions

Warnings

Hematologic Effects

Severe leukopenia, neutropenia, anemia, thrombocytopenia, pancytopenia, and bone marrow failure (including aplastic anemia) have been reported in patients receiving valganciclovir or ganciclovir. Cytopenia may occur at any time during valganciclovir therapy and the degree of cytopenia may increase with continued therapy with the drug. Cell counts usually begin to return to baseline within 3–7 days after valganciclovir is discontinued.

Complete blood cell counts (CBCs) with differential and platelet counts should be performed frequently, especially in infants and in patients with baseline neutrophil counts less than 1000/mm³, in those who previously experienced leukopenia while receiving ganciclovir or other nucleoside analogs, and in those with renal impairment. Because oral valganciclovir results in comparatively increased plasma ganciclovir concentrations compared with oral ganciclovir (not commercially available in the US), more frequent monitoring for cytopenias may be warranted if therapy is changed from oral ganciclovir to valganciclovir.

Valganciclovir should be avoided in patients with absolute neutrophil counts less than 500/mm³, platelet counts less than 25,000/mm³, or hemoglobin concentrations less than 8 g/dL.

Valganciclovir should be used with caution in patients with preexisting cytopenias and in those who have received or are receiving concomitant myelosuppressive drugs or irradiation.

In patients experiencing severe leukopenia, neutropenia, anemia, and/or thrombocytopenia, treatment with hematopoietic growth factors may be considered.

Impairment of Fertility

Animal data from studies using ganciclovir and limited data from patients receiving valganciclovir indicate that valganciclovir may cause temporary or permanent inhibition of spermatogenesis in males and may cause suppression of fertility in females.

In a small, open-label, nonrandomized clinical study, adult male renal transplant patients receiving cytomegalovirus (CMV) prophylaxis with oral valganciclovir for up to 200 days posttransplantation were followed for 6 months after the drug was discontinued and data compared with an untreated control group. Among 24 evaluable patients in the valganciclovir group, the mean sperm density at the end-of-treatment visit was *decreased* by 11 million/mL from baseline; whereas, among 14 evaluable patients in the control group, the mean sperm density at the end-of-treatment visit had *increased* by 33 million/mL. However, at the final follow-up visit, the mean sperm density among 20 evaluable patients in the valganciclovir group was comparable to that observed among 10 evaluable patients in the untreated control group (mean sperm density increased by 41 or 43 million/mL from baseline, respectively).

Patients receiving valganciclovir should be advised that the drug may be associated with infertility.

Teratogenesis

Animal data from studies using ganciclovir indicate that valganciclovir may cause fetal toxicity and has the potential to cause birth defects if administered to pregnant women.

In studies in pregnant mice and rabbits receiving ganciclovir at dosages resulting in 2 times the human exposure, maternal toxicity and embryofetal toxicity (e.g., fetal resorptions, embryofetal mortality) was observed. In addition, teratogenic effects (cleft palate, anophthalmia/microphthalmia, hydrocephalus, brachygnathia, aplastic organs [kidney, pancreas]) were reported in rabbits.

Females of childbearing potential should undergo pregnancy testing before valganciclovir is initiated.

Females of childbearing potential should be advised to use an effective method of contraception during and for at least 30 days after valganciclovir is discontinued. Male patients should be advised to use a reliable method of barrier contraception during and for at least 90 days after valganciclovir is discontinued.

Mutagenicity and Carcinogenicity

Animal studies using ganciclovir indicate the drug is mutagenic and carcinogenic.

Valganciclovir should be considered a potential carcinogen in humans.

Other Warnings/Precautions

Renal Effects

Acute renal failure may occur in geriatric patients (with or without renal impairment), patients receiving potentially nephrotoxic drugs, and inadequately hydrated patients.

Adequate hydration should be maintained in all patients.

Valganciclovir should be used with caution in geriatric patients and in patients receiving concomitant therapy with potentially nephrotoxic drugs.

Dosage adjustment of valganciclovir is recommended in patients with renal impairment. (See Renal Impairment under Dosage and Administration: Special Populations.)

Handling and Disposal

Because valganciclovir is considered a potential teratogen and carcinogen, caution should be exercised when handling the drug. Valganciclovir tablets should not be broken or crushed. Direct contact of broken or crushed tablets, powder for oral solution, or reconstituted oral solution with skin or mucous membranes should be avoided. If such contact occurs, skin should be washed thoroughly with soap and water; eyes should be rinsed thoroughly with water. For further information on handling of cytotoxic drugs, see the ASHP Guidelines on Handling Hazardous Drugs at http://ahfsdruginformation.com.

Specific Populations

Pregnancy

In animal studies, ganciclovir caused maternal and fetal toxicity, embryofetal mortality, and teratogenicity. Valganciclovir is expected to have reproductive toxicity similar to ganciclovir. (See Teratogenesis under Warnings/Precautions: Warnings, in Cautions.)

Data are not available regarding use of valganciclovir in pregnant women to establish the presence or absence of drug-associated risk. An ex vivo placental model indicates that ganciclovir crosses the human placenta by passive diffusion and is not saturable over a concentration range of 1–10 mg/mL.

Although most maternal CMV infections are asymptomatic or may be associated with a self-limited mononucleosis-like syndrome, CMV infections in pregnant immunocompromised patients (e.g., those with human immunodeficiency virus [HIV] infection and acquired immunodeficiency syndrome [AIDS], transplant recipients) may be symptomatic and result in substantial maternal morbidity and mortality. Perinatal transmission of CMV from infected mothers to their neonates can occur resulting in congenital CMV infection and disease. (See Congenital Cytomegalovirus Disease under Uses: Treatment of Cytomegalovirus Infection and Disease.)

Females of childbearing potential should undergo pregnancy testing before initiation of valganciclovir. In addition, pregnancy should be avoided in female patients receiving valganciclovir and in females with male partners receiving valganciclovir.

Females of childbearing potential should be advised to use an effective method of contraception during and for at least 30 days after valganciclovir therapy and male patients should be advised to use a reliable method of barrier contraception during and for at least 90 days after valganciclovir therapy.

Lactation

It is not known whether valganciclovir or ganciclovir is distributed into human milk, affects the breast-fed infant, or affects milk production. Animal data from studies using ganciclovir indicate that the drug is distributed into milk of lactating rats.

Because of the potential for serious adverse effects in nursing infants, valganciclovir is not recommended in breast-feeding women. HIV-infected mothers should be instructed not to breast-feed their infants because of the risk of transmission of HIV.

Pediatric Use

Safety and efficacy of valganciclovir have not been established in pediatric patients younger than 1 month of age.

Use of valganciclovir for the prevention of CMV disease in pediatric *heart* transplant recipients 1 month to 16 years of age is based on safety and pharmacokinetic data from 2 studies in pediatric solid organ transplant recipients and is supported by efficacy data from studies in adult solid organ transplant recipients.

Use of valganciclovir for the prevention of CMV disease in pediatric *kidney* transplant recipients 4 months to 16 years of age is based on safety, tolerability, and pharmacokinetic data from 2 open-label studies in solid organ transplant recipients in this age group and is supported by efficacy data from studies in adult solid organ transplant recipients.

Safety and efficacy of valganciclovir have not been established for prevention of CMV disease in pediatric heart transplant recipients younger than 1 month of age, pediatric kidney transplant recipients younger than 4 months of age, or pediatric liver transplant recipients of any age.

The safety profile of valganciclovir in pediatric patients generally is similar to that observed in adults. However, upper respiratory tract infection, pyrexia, nasopharyngitis, anemia, abdominal pain, and neutropenia have been reported more frequently in pediatric patients than in adults.

Geriatric Use

Safety and efficacy of valganciclovir have not been specifically evaluated in geriatric patients 65 years of age or older and there were insufficient numbers of individuals in this age group in clinical studies to determine whether they respond differently than younger adults. Pharmacokinetics of the drug have been not studied in geriatric patients.

Because geriatric individuals frequently have decreased renal function and because valganciclovir is substantially excreted by the kidneys, particular attention should be paid to assessing renal function before and during valganciclovir therapy in this age group. If evidence of renal impairment exists or develops, appropriate dosage adjustments should be made. In general, dosage should be selected carefully, usually starting at the low end of the dosage range, taking into account the greater frequency of decreased hepatic, renal, and/or cardiac function and of concomitant disease and drug therapy observed in the elderly.

Hepatic Impairment

Safety and efficacy of valganciclovir have not been evaluated in patients with hepatic impairment.

Renal Impairment

The major route of elimination of valganciclovir is renal excretion as ganciclovir. If renal function is impaired, dosage of valganciclovir must be adjusted based on measured or estimated creatinine clearance. (See Renal Impairment under Dosage and Administration: Special Populations.)

Hemodialysis reduces plasma concentrations of ganciclovir by approximately 50%. Valganciclovir should not be used in adults undergoing hemodialysis (creatinine clearance less than 10 mL/minute) because the appropriate daily dose for such patients is lower than 450 mg (i.e., would require breaking a tablet); such patients should receive ganciclovir instead.

● Common Adverse Effects

Adverse effects occurring in 20% or more of adults receiving valganciclovir include diarrhea, pyrexia, fatigue, nausea, tremor, neutropenia, anemia, leukopenia, thrombocytopenia, headache, insomnia, urinary tract infection, and vomiting.

Adverse effects occurring in 20% or more of pediatric patients receiving valganciclovir include diarrhea, pyrexia, upper respiratory tract infection, urinary tract infection, vomiting, neutropenia, leukopenia, and headache.

DRUG INTERACTIONS

No formal drug interaction studies have been performed using valganciclovir. However, valganciclovir is rapidly and extensively converted to ganciclovir and interactions reported with ganciclovir are expected to occur in patients receiving valganciclovir.

Drug interaction studies with ganciclovir were performed in patients with normal renal function. In patients with renal impairment, concomitant use of valganciclovir and other drugs eliminated by renal excretion may result in increased concentrations of ganciclovir and the concomitant drug and such patients should be closely monitored for toxicity associated with ganciclovir and the concomitant drug.

● Antibacterial Agents

Imipenem and Cilastatin Sodium

Generalized seizures have been reported in patients who received ganciclovir concomitantly with the fixed combination of imipenem and cilastatin sodium (imipenem/cilastatin).

Concomitant use of valganciclovir and imipenem/cilastatin is not recommended.

Trimethoprim

Concomitant use of ganciclovir and trimethoprim does not affect the pharmacokinetics of either drug.

Because of the potential for increased toxicity (e.g., nephrotoxicity), concomitant use of valganciclovir and trimethoprim should be considered only if potential benefits outweigh potential risks.

Other Antibacterials

Because of the potential for increased toxicity (e.g., myelosuppression, nephrotoxicity) if valganciclovir is used with certain anti-infectives (e.g., co-trimoxazole, dapsone, pentamidine), concomitant use of valganciclovir and such anti-infectives should be considered only if potential benefits outweigh potential risks.

● Antifungal Agents

Amphotericin B

If valganciclovir and amphotericin B are used concomitantly, renal function should be monitored since there is a potential for increased serum creatinine concentrations.

Flucytosine

Because of the potential for increased toxicity (e.g., myelosuppression, nephrotoxicity), concomitant use of valganciclovir and flucytosine should be considered only if potential benefits outweigh potential risks.

● Antineoplastic Agents

Because of the potential for increased toxicity (e.g., myelosuppression, nephrotoxicity), concomitant use of valganciclovir and certain antineoplastic agents (e.g., doxorubicin, hydroxyurea, vinblastine, vincristine) should be considered only if potential benefits outweigh potential risks.

● Antiretroviral Agents

Didanosine

Concomitant use of ganciclovir and didanosine increases peak plasma concentrations and area under the plasma concentration-time curve (AUC) of didanosine, but does not affect the pharmacokinetics of ganciclovir.

If valganciclovir and didanosine are used concomitantly, the patient should be closely monitored for didanosine toxicity (e.g., pancreatitis).

Tenofovir

Concomitant use of valganciclovir and tenofovir alafenamide or tenofovir disoproxil fumarate may result in increased serum concentrations of ganciclovir and/or tenofovir; patients receiving such concomitant therapy should be monitored for dose-related toxicities.

Zidovudine

Concomitant use of ganciclovir and zidovudine has resulted in additive or synergistic bone marrow toxicity.

If valganciclovir and zidovudine are used concomitantly, there is an increased risk of hematologic toxicity. Concomitant use of valganciclovir and zidovudine should be considered only if potential benefits outweigh potential risks.

● Immunosuppressive Agents

Cyclosporine

Concomitant use of ganciclovir and cyclosporine does not appear to affect cyclosporine whole blood concentrations.

If valganciclovir and cyclosporine are used concomitantly, renal function should be monitored since there is potential for increased serum creatinine concentrations.

Mycophenolate Mofetil

Concomitant use of ganciclovir and mycophenolate mofetil in patients with normal renal function does not affect the pharmacokinetics of either drug.

If valganciclovir and mycophenolate mofetil are used concomitantly, the patient should be monitored for hematologic and renal toxicity because of increased risk.

Tacrolimus

Because of the potential for increased toxicity (e.g., nephrotoxicity) if valganciclovir is used with tacrolimus, concomitant use should be considered only if potential benefits outweigh potential risks.

● Probenecid

Concomitant use of ganciclovir and probenecid decreases renal clearance and increases the AUC of ganciclovir.

If valganciclovir and probenecid are used concomitantly, dosage of valganciclovir may need to be reduced and the patient should be monitored for evidence of ganciclovir toxicity.

PHARMACOKINETICS

● Absorption

Bioavailability

Valganciclovir, a prodrug of ganciclovir, is well absorbed from the GI tract and rapidly metabolized by intestinal and hepatic esterases to ganciclovir. Systemic exposure to the prodrug is transient and low.

Following an oral dose of valganciclovir given with food, absolute bioavailability of ganciclovir is approximately 60% and the median time to peak ganciclovir concentrations is 2.2 hours. The area under the plasma concentration-time curve (AUC) of ganciclovir is proportional to the valganciclovir dose when given under fed conditions.

Food

Administration of valganciclovir with a high-fat meal (approximately 600 calories, 31 g fat) increases the AUC and peak plasma concentrations of ganciclovir at steady state by 30 and 14%, respectively.

Plasma Concentrations

Results from pharmacokinetic studies in adults indicate that oral valganciclovir (900 mg once daily with food) results in a ganciclovir AUC similar to that reported following IV ganciclovir (5 mg/kg once daily).

● Distribution

Extent

It is not known whether valganciclovir is distributed into CSF; ganciclovir is distributed into CSF.

Ganciclovir crosses the placenta (based on an ex vivo human placental model).

It is not known whether valganciclovir or ganciclovir is distributed into human milk; animal data indicate that ganciclovir is distributed into milk of lactating rats.

Plasma Protein Binding

Ganciclovir is 1–2% bound to plasma proteins; protein binding of valganciclovir has not been determined because of rapid conversion to ganciclovir.

● Elimination

Metabolism

Valganciclovir is rapidly hydrolyzed to ganciclovir. Ganciclovir is then phosphorylated by viral protein kinase (pUL97) to ganciclovir monophosphate within cytomegalovirus (CMV)-infected cells. Ganciclovir monophosphate is further phosphorylated by cellular kinases to ganciclovir triphosphate, which is slowly metabolized intracellularly.

Elimination Route

The major route of elimination of valganciclovir is renal excretion as ganciclovir by glomerular filtration and active tubular secretion.

Half-life

The mean half-life of ganciclovir after administration of oral valganciclovir (900 mg once daily with food) is approximately 4 hours in healthy adults, adults with human immunodeficiency virus (HIV) infection, or HIV-positive/CMV-positive adults (with or without retinitis).

The mean half-life of ganciclovir after administration of oral valganciclovir (900 mg once daily with food) in adult heart, kidney, and kidney-pancreas transplant recipients is 6.6–6.8 hours.

In pediatric solid organ transplant recipients, the mean half-life of ganciclovir after administration of oral valganciclovir is 2.8–4.8 hours in those 4 months to less than 12 years of age and 4.4–6 hours in those 12 years of age or older. Clearance is influenced by body surface area (BSA) and renal function.

The intracellular half-life of ganciclovir in CMV-infected cells is 18 hours.

Special Populations

In patients with renal impairment, the half-life of ganciclovir after administration of oral valganciclovir is increased and renal clearance is decreased. Data from otherwise healthy adults with renal impairment indicate that the mean half-life of ganciclovir following a single 900-mg dose of oral valganciclovir is about 10, 22, or 68 hours in those with creatinine clearances of 21–50, 11–20, or up to 10 mL/minute, respectively.

Following administration of oral valganciclovir, hemodialysis reduces plasma concentrations of ganciclovir by approximately 50%.

DESCRIPTION

Valganciclovir, the L-valyl ester of ganciclovir, is an antiviral agent. Valganciclovir is a prodrug and exhibits no antiviral activity until converted by intestinal and hepatic esterases to ganciclovir and subsequently to the active form ganciclovir triphosphate.

Valganciclovir is commercially available as the hydrochloride salt and differs structurally from ganciclovir by the presence of the L-amino acid, valine, attached to the 2-hydroxyl group of the nucleoside and by the presence of the monohydrochloride salt. These structural modifications result in substantially increased GI absorption of valganciclovir relative to oral ganciclovir (no longer commercially available in the US), resulting in plasma ganciclovir concentrations comparable to those achieved with IV ganciclovir.

Valganciclovir is rapidly converted to ganciclovir in vivo and subsequently phosphorylated within cytomegalovirus (CMV)-infected cells to ganciclovir triphosphate. Since initial phosphorylation of ganciclovir depends largely on the presence of a viral kinase (pUL97), phosphorylation occurs preferentially in virus-infected cells. Ganciclovir triphosphate is a viral DNA polymerase inhibitor and exerts its antiviral activity on CMV by inhibiting the viral DNA polymerase. Other mechanisms also are involved. For additional information, see Mechanism of Action in Ganciclovir 8:18.32.

The absolute bioavailability of ganciclovir following oral administration of valganciclovir is about 60%. Results from pharmacokinetic studies in adults indicate that oral administration of valganciclovir 900 mg once daily with food provides a mean area under the plasma concentration-time curve$_{0-24\ hour}$ (AUC$_{0-24\ hour}$) for ganciclovir comparable to that following IV ganciclovir 5 mg/kg once daily. However, at these dosages, oral valganciclovir produces lower peak plasma ganciclovir concentrations than IV ganciclovir.

• Spectrum

Following conversion of valganciclovir to the pharmacologically active ganciclovir triphosphate, the drug is active against human herpes viruses, including CMV, herpes simplex virus types 1 and 2 (HSV-1 and HSV-2), and varicella-zoster virus (VZV). Although the clinical importance is unclear, ganciclovir has some in vitro activity against Epstein-Barr virus (EBV) and human herpes viruses types 6 and 8 (HHV-6 and HHV-8). Ganciclovir is not active against human immunodeficiency virus type 1 (HIV-1).

• Resistance

CMV isolates with reduced susceptibility or resistance to ganciclovir have been selected in vitro in the presence of the drug. CMV resistant to ganciclovir may emerge after prolonged treatment or prophylaxis with the drug, and the possibility of ganciclovir-resistant CMV should be considered in patients who show poor clinical response or relapse or experience persistent viral shedding during valganciclovir therapy.

Resistance can occur as the result of amino acid substitutions in the viral protein kinase pUL97 and/or the viral DNA polymerase pUL54. Certain pUL97 ganciclovir resistance-associated substitutions (e.g., M460V/I, H520Q, C529G, A594V, L595S, C603W) have been reported most frequently in clinical isolates. Numerous other pUL97 and pUL54 ganciclovir resistance-associated mutations also have been reported.

Cross-resistance can occur between ganciclovir and some other antivirals (e.g., acyclovir, cidofovir, foscarnet). Certain amino acid substitutions selected in vitro in cell culture following exposure of CMV to ganciclovir, cidofovir, or foscarnet have resulted in cross-resistance. Amino acid substitutions in pUL54 that confer cross-resistance between ganciclovir and cidofovir generally have involved the exonuclease domains and region V of the viral DNA polymerase. A variety of amino acid substitutions have conferred cross-resistance between ganciclovir and foscarnet, but concentrate at and between regions II and III of viral DNA polymerase.

ADVICE TO PATIENTS

Importance of reading the patient information and instructions for use provided by the manufacturer.

Importance of taking valganciclovir with food. Inform adults that they should receive valganciclovir tablets, not valganciclovir oral solution.

Inform patients that valganciclovir may cause granulocytopenia (neutropenia), anemia, thrombocytopenia, and elevated creatinine concentrations and that dosage modification or discontinuance of the drug may be required. Necessity of frequent monitoring of blood cell counts, platelet counts, and serum creatinine concentrations.

Advise patients that valganciclovir may cause seizures, dizziness, and/or confusion, which may affect tasks requiring alertness (e.g., ability to drive or operate machinery).

When valganciclovir is used for the management of cytomegalovirus (CMV) retinitis, advise patients that the drug is not a cure for CMV retinitis; progression of retinitis may occur during or after treatment with valganciclovir. Advise patients that regular ophthalmologic examinations during valganciclovir therapy (at least every 4–6 weeks) are necessary and some patients require more frequent follow-up.

Importance of informing clinicians of existing or contemplated concomitant therapy, including prescription and OTC drugs, as well as any concomitant illnesses.

Advise patients that valganciclovir is a potential carcinogen.

Advise patients that valganciclovir may cause temporary or permanent female and male infertility.

Advise females of reproductive potential that the drug causes birth defects in animals.

Importance of women informing clinicians if they are or plan to become pregnant or plan to breast-feed. Advise women to avoid pregnancy and to not breast-feed infants.

Importance of both women and men using effective contraception during valganciclovir therapy. Advise females of reproductive potential to use effective contraception during and for at least 30 days after valganciclovir therapy. Advise male patients to use effective barrier contraception during and for at least 90 days after valganciclovir therapy.

Importance of advising patients of other important precautionary information. (See Cautions.)

PREPARATIONS

Excipients in commercially available drug preparations may have clinically important effects in some individuals; consult specific product labeling for details.

valGANciclovir Hydrochloride

Oral			
For solution	250 mg (of valganciclovir) per 5 mL*	Valcyte®, Roche	
		Valganciclovir for Oral Solution	
Tablets, film-coated	450 mg (of valganciclovir)*	Valcyte®, Roche	
		Valganciclovir Tablets	

* available from one or more manufacturer, distributor, and/or repackager by generic (nonproprietary) name

† Use is not currently included in the labeling approved by the US Food and Drug Administration.

Selected Revisions August 12, 2019, © Copyright, July 1, 2001, American Society of Health-System Pharmacists, Inc.

Sofosbuvir, Velpatasvir, and Voxilaprevir

8:18.40.16 • HCV POLYMERASE INHIBITORS

■ Sofosbuvir, velpatasvir, and voxilaprevir (sofosbuvir/velpatasvir/voxilaprevir) is a fixed combination containing 3 hepatitis C virus (HCV) antivirals; sofosbuvir is a nucleotide analog HCV nonstructural 5B (NS5B) polymerase inhibitor, velpatasvir is an HCV nonstructural 5A (NS5A) replication complex inhibitor (NS5A inhibitor), and voxilaprevir is an HCV nonstructural 3/4A (NS3/4A) protease inhibitor.

USES

● Chronic Hepatitis C Virus Infection

The fixed combination of sofosbuvir, velpatasvir, and voxilaprevir (sofosbuvir/velpatasvir/voxilaprevir) is used for the treatment of chronic hepatitis C virus (HCV) genotype 1, 2, 3, 4, 5, or 6 infection in adults previously treated with an HCV regimen containing an HCV nonstructural 5A (NS5A) replication complex inhibitor (NS5A inhibitor), including those without cirrhosis or with compensated cirrhosis (Child-Pugh class A).

Sofosbuvir/velpatasvir/voxilaprevir also is used for the treatment of HCV genotype 1a or 3 infection in adults previously treated with an HCV regimen containing sofosbuvir *without* an HCV NS5A inhibitor, including those without cirrhosis or with compensated cirrhosis (Child-Pugh class A). Clinical trial data to date indicate that sofosbuvir/velpatasvir/voxilaprevir does not provide any additional benefit over the fixed combination of sofosbuvir and velpatasvir (sofosbuvir/velpatasvir) for the treatment of HCV genotype 1b, 2, 4, 5, or 6 infection in adults previously treated with sofosbuvir *without* an HCV NS5A inhibitor.

Although sofosbuvir/velpatasvir/voxilaprevir has been used for treatment of chronic HCV infection caused by HCV genotypes 1, 2, 3, 4, 5, or 6 in some treatment-naive† (previously untreated) adults, the drug is not labeled by FDA for use in such patients.

Because the treatment of chronic HCV infection is complex and rapidly evolving, it is recommended that treatment be directed by clinicians who are familiar with the disease and that a specialist be consulted to obtain the most up-to-date information. Information from the American Association for the Study of Liver Diseases (AASLD) and Infectious Diseases Society of America (IDSA) regarding diagnosis and management of HCV infection, including recommendations for initial treatment, is available at http://www.hcvguidelines.org.

HCV Genotype 1 Infection

Efficacy and safety of sofosbuvir/velpatasvir/voxilaprevir for the treatment of chronic HCV genotype 1 infection in adults have been evaluated in 3 randomized, phase 3 trials (POLARIS-1, POLARIS-2, and POLARIS-4). The primary end point in each study was sustained virologic response at 12 weeks after the end of treatment (SVR12; defined as plasma HCV RNA level less than 15 IU/mL [the lower limit of quantification] at 12 weeks after end of treatment).

POLARIS-1, a double-blind, placebo-controlled trial, included 415 adults with chronic HCV genotype 1, 2, 3, 4, 5, or 6 infection who were noncirrhotic or had compensated cirrhosis and had previously failed treatment with an HCV regimen containing an HCV NS5A inhibitor (median age 59 years, 77% male, 74% with baseline HCV RNA levels 800,000 IU/mL or greater, 41% with compensated cirrhosis). Patients were previously treated with HCV treatment regimens containing ledipasvir (51%), daclatasvir (27%), ombitasvir (11%), velpatasvir (7%), or elbasvir (3%). Those with HCV genotype 1 infection were randomized in a 1:1 ratio to receive a 12-week regimen of sofosbuvir/velpatasvir/voxilaprevir (a fixed-combination tablet containing 400 mg of sofosbuvir, 100 mg of velpatasvir, and 100 mg of voxilaprevir) or placebo once daily. Of the 101 patients with HCV genotype 1a infection treated with sofosbuvir/velpatasvir/voxilaprevir, 96% achieved SVR12; of the 45 patients with HCV genotype 1b infection treated with sofosbuvir/velpatasvir/voxilaprevir, 100% achieved SVR12. No patients treated with placebo achieved SVR12.

POLARIS-4, a randomized, open-label trial, included 333 previously treated adults with chronic HCV genotype 1, 2, 3, or 4 infection who were noncirrhotic or had compensated cirrhosis and had previously failed treatment with an HCV regimen that included a direct acting antiviral (DAA), but did *not* include an HCV NS5A inhibitor (median age 58 years, 77% male, 75% with baseline HCV RNA levels 800,000 IU/mL or greater, 81% with non-CC IL28B alleles [CT or TT], 46% with compensated cirrhosis). Patients whose only DAA exposure was an HCV NS3/4A protease inhibitor were excluded. Those with HCV genotype 1 infection were randomized in a 1:1 ratio to receive sofosbuvir/velpatasvir/voxilaprevir (a fixed-combination tablet containing 400 mg of sofosbuvir, 100 mg of velpatasvir, and 100 mg of voxilaprevir) or sofosbuvir/velpatasvir (a fixed-combination tablet containing 400 mg of sofosbuvir and 100 mg of velpatasvir) once daily for 12 weeks. Of the 54 patients with HCV genotype 1 infection treated with a regimen of sofosbuvir/velpatasvir/voxilaprevir, 96% achieved SVR12 (97 or 94% of those with HCV genotype 1a or 1b, respectively). Of the 40 patients with HCV genotype 1 infection treated with a regimen of sofosbuvir/velpatasvir, 85% achieved SVR12 (82 or 92% of those with HCV genotype 1a or 1b, respectively).

POLARIS-2, a randomized, open-label trial, evaluated sofosbuvir/velpatasvir/voxilaprevir in adults with any genotype of HCV infection who were treatment naive or previously failed treatment with an HCV regimen that did not include a DAA. Enrolled patients were noncirrhotic or had compensated cirrhosis, although those with HCV genotype 3 infection were excluded if they had cirrhosis. Patients were randomized in a 1:1 ratio to receive sofosbuvir/velpatasvir/voxilaprevir (a fixed-combination tablet containing 400 mg of sofosbuvir, 100 mg of velpatasvir, and 100 mg of voxilaprevir) once daily for 8 weeks or sofosbuvir/velpatasvir (a fixed-combination tablet containing 400 mg of sofosbuvir and 100 mg of velpatasvir) once daily for 12 weeks. Results showed that the 8-week regimen of sofosbuvir/velpatasvir/voxilaprevir in these patients did *not* meet noninferiority criteria when compared with the 12-week regimen of sofosbuvir/velpatasvir (overall SVR12 achieved by 95 or 98% of patients, respectively).

HCV Genotype 2 Infection

Efficacy and safety of sofosbuvir/velpatasvir/voxilaprevir for the treatment of chronic HCV genotype 2 infection in adults have been evaluated in 3 randomized, phase 3 trials (POLARIS-1, POLARIS-2, and POLARIS-4). The primary end point in each study was sustained virologic response at 12 weeks after the end of treatment (SVR12; defined as plasma HCV RNA level less than 15 IU/mL [the lower limit of quantification] at 12 weeks after end of treatment).

POLARIS-1, a double-blind, placebo-controlled trial, included 415 adults with chronic HCV genotype 1, 2, 3, 4, 5, or 6 infection who were noncirrhotic or had compensated cirrhosis and had previously failed treatment with an HCV regimen containing an HCV NS5A inhibitor (median age 59 years, 77% male, 74% with baseline HCV RNA levels 800,000 IU/mL or greater, 41% with compensated cirrhosis). Patients were previously treated with HCV treatment regimens containing ledipasvir (51%), daclatasvir (27%), ombitasvir (11%), velpatasvir (7%), or elbasvir (3%). All enrolled patients with HCV genotype 2 infection received a 12-week regimen of sofosbuvir/velpatasvir/voxilaprevir (a fixed-combination tablet containing 400 mg of sofosbuvir, 100 mg of velpatasvir, and 100 mg of voxilaprevir) once daily. Of the 5 patients with HCV genotype 2 infection treated with sofosbuvir/velpatasvir/voxilaprevir, 100% achieved SVR12.

POLARIS-4, a randomized, open-label trial, included 333 previously treated adults with chronic HCV genotype 1, 2, 3, or 4 infection who were noncirrhotic or had compensated cirrhosis and had previously failed treatment with an HCV regimen that included a DAA, but did *not* include an HCV NS5A inhibitor (median age 58 years, 77% male, 75% with baseline HCV RNA levels 800,000 IU/mL or greater, 81% with non-CC IL28B alleles [CT or TT], 46% with compensated cirrhosis). Patients whose only DAA exposure was an HCV NS3/4A protease inhibitor were excluded. Those with HCV genotype 2 infection were randomized in a 1:1 ratio to receive sofosbuvir/velpatasvir/voxilaprevir (a fixed-combination tablet containing 400 mg of sofosbuvir, 100 mg of velpatasvir, and 100 mg of voxilaprevir) or sofosbuvir/velpatasvir (a fixed-combination tablet containing 400 mg of sofosbuvir and 100 mg of velpatasvir) once daily for 12 weeks. Of the 31 patients with HCV genotype 2 infection treated with a regimen of sofosbuvir/velpatasvir/voxilaprevir, 100% achieved SVR12. Of the 33 patients with HCV genotype 2 infection treated with a regimen of sofosbuvir/velpatasvir, 97% achieved SVR12.

POLARIS-2, a randomized, open-label trial, evaluated sofosbuvir/velpatasvir/voxilaprevir in adults with any genotype of HCV infection who were treatment naive or previously failed treatment with an HCV regimen that did not include a DAA. Enrolled patients were noncirrhotic or had compensated cirrhosis, although those with HCV genotype 3 infection were excluded if they had cirrhosis. Patients were randomized in a 1:1 ratio to receive sofosbuvir/velpatasvir/voxilaprevir (a fixed-combination tablet containing 400 mg of sofosbuvir, 100 mg of velpatasvir, and 100 mg of voxilaprevir) once daily for 8 weeks or sofosbuvir/velpatasvir (a fixed-combination tablet containing 400 mg of sofosbuvir and 100 mg of velpatasvir) once daily for 12 weeks. Results showed that the 8-week regimen of sofosbuvir/velpatasvir/voxilaprevir did *not* meet noninferiority criteria in these patients when compared with the 12-week regimen of sofosbuvir/velpatasvir (overall SVR12 achieved by 95 or 98% of patients, respectively).

HCV Genotype 3 Infection

Efficacy and safety of sofosbuvir/velpatasvir/voxilaprevir for the treatment of chronic HCV genotype 3 infection in adults have been evaluated in 4 randomized, phase 3 trials (POLARIS-1, POLARIS-2, POLARIS-3, and POLARIS-4). The primary end point in each study was sustained virologic response at 12 weeks after the end of treatment (SVR12; defined as plasma HCV RNA level less than 15 IU/mL [the lower limit of quantification] at 12 weeks after end of treatment).

POLARIS-1, a double-blind, placebo-controlled trial, included 415 adults with chronic HCV genotype 1, 2, 3, 4, 5, or 6 infection who were noncirrhotic or had compensated cirrhosis and had previously failed treatment with an HCV regimen containing an HCV NS5A inhibitor (median age 59 years, 77% male, 74% with baseline HCV RNA levels 800,000 IU/mL or greater, 41% with compensated cirrhosis). Patients were previously treated with HCV treatment regimens containing ledipasvir (51%), daclatasvir (27%), ombitasvir (11%), velpatasvir (7%), or elbasvir (3%). All patients with HCV genotype 3 infection received a 12-week regimen of sofosbuvir/velpatasvir/voxilaprevir (a fixed-combination tablet containing 400 mg of sofosbuvir, 100 mg of velpatasvir, and 100 mg of voxilaprevir) once daily. Of the 78 patients with HCV genotype 3 infection treated with sofosbuvir/velpatasvir/voxilaprevir, 95% achieved SVR12.

POLARIS-4, a randomized, open-label trial, included 333 previously treated adults with chronic HCV genotype 1, 2, 3, or 4 infection who were noncirrhotic or had compensated cirrhosis and had previously failed treatment with an HCV regimen that included a DAA, but did *not* include an HCV NS5A inhibitor (median age 58 years, 77% male, 75% with baseline HCV RNA levels 800,000 IU/mL or greater, 81% with non-CC IL28B alleles [CT or TT], 46% with compensated cirrhosis). Patients whose only DAA exposure was an HCV NS3/4A protease inhibitor were excluded. Those with HCV genotype 3 infection were randomized in a 1:1 ratio to receive sofosbuvir/velpatasvir/voxilaprevir (a fixed-combination tablet containing 400 mg of sofosbuvir, 100 mg of velpatasvir, and 100 mg of voxilaprevir) or sofosbuvir/velpatasvir (a fixed-combination tablet containing 400 mg of sofosbuvir and 100 mg of velpatasvir) once daily for 12 weeks. Of the 54 patients with HCV genotype 3 infection treated with a regimen of sofosbuvir/velpatasvir/voxilaprevir, 96% achieved SVR12. Of the 52 patients with HCV genotype 3 infection treated with a regimen of sofosbuvir/velpatasvir, 85% achieved SVR12.

POLARIS-2, a randomized, open-label trial, evaluated sofosbuvir/velpatasvir/voxilaprevir in adults with any genotype of HCV infection who were treatment naive or previously failed treatment with an HCV regimen that did not include a DAA. Enrolled patients were noncirrhotic or had compensated cirrhosis, although those with HCV genotype 3 infection were excluded if they had cirrhosis. Patients were randomized in a 1:1 ratio to receive sofosbuvir/velpatasvir/voxilaprevir (a fixed-combination tablet containing 400 mg of sofosbuvir, 100 mg of velpatasvir, and 100 mg of voxilaprevir) once daily for 8 weeks or sofosbuvir/velpatasvir (a fixed-combination tablet containing 400 mg of sofosbuvir and 100 mg of velpatasvir) once daily for 12 weeks. Results showed that the 8-week regimen of sofosbuvir/velpatasvir/voxilaprevir did *not* meet noninferiority criteria in these patients when compared with the 12-week regimen of sofosbuvir/velpatasvir (overall SVR12 achieved by 95 or 98% of patients, respectively).

POLARIS-3, a randomized, open-label trial, evaluated sofosbuvir/velpatasvir/voxilaprevir in treatment-naive patients with HCV genotype 3 infection who also had compensated cirrhosis. Patients were randomized in a 1:1 ratio to receive sofosbuvir/velpatasvir/voxilaprevir (a fixed-combination tablet containing 400 mg of sofosbuvir, 100 mg of velpatasvir, and 100 mg of voxilaprevir) once daily for 8 weeks or a fixed combination of sofosbuvir and velpatasvir (a fixed-combination tablet containing 400 mg of sofosbuvir and 100 mg of velpatasvir) once daily for 12 weeks. SVR12 was achieved by 96% of patients in each group. Both groups exceeded the performance goal of 83%, but the two groups were not statistically compared with each other.

HCV Genotype 4 Infection

Efficacy and safety of sofosbuvir/velpatasvir/voxilaprevir for the treatment of chronic HCV genotype 4 infection in adults have been evaluated in 3 randomized, phase 3 trials (POLARIS-1, POLARIS-2, and POLARIS-4). The primary end point in each study was sustained virologic response at 12 weeks after the end of treatment (SVR12; defined as plasma HCV RNA level less than 15 IU/mL [the lower limit of quantification] at 12 weeks after end of treatment).

POLARIS-1, a double-blind, placebo-controlled trial, included 415 adults with chronic HCV genotype 1, 2, 3, 4, 5, or 6 infection who were noncirrhotic or had compensated cirrhosis and had previously failed treatment with an HCV regimen containing an HCV NS5A inhibitor (median age 59 years, 77% male, 74% with baseline HCV RNA levels 800,000 IU/mL or greater, 41% with compensated cirrhosis). Patients were previously treated with HCV treatment regimens containing ledipasvir (51%), daclatasvir (27%), ombitasvir (11%), velpatasvir (7%), or elbasvir (3%). All patients with HCV genotype 4 infection received a 12-week regimen of sofosbuvir/velpatasvir/voxilaprevir (a fixed-combination tablet containing 400 mg of sofosbuvir, 100 mg of velpatasvir, and 100 mg of voxilaprevir) once daily. Of the 22 patients with HCV genotype 4 infection treated with sofosbuvir/velpatasvir/voxilaprevir, 91% achieved SVR12.

POLARIS-4, a randomized, open-label trial, included 333 previously treated adults with chronic HCV genotype 1, 2, 3, or 4 infection who were noncirrhotic or had compensated cirrhosis and had previously failed treatment with an HCV regimen that included a DAA, but did *not* include an HCV NS5A inhibitor (median age 58 years, 77% male, 75% with baseline HCV RNA levels 800,000 IU/mL or greater, 81% with non-CC IL28B alleles [CT or TT], 46% with compensated cirrhosis). Patients whose only DAA exposure was an HCV NS3/4A protease inhibitor were excluded. All patients with HCV genotype 4 infection received sofosbuvir/velpatasvir/voxilaprevir (a fixed-combination tablet containing 400 mg of sofosbuvir, 100 mg of velpatasvir, and 100 mg of voxilaprevir) once daily for 12 weeks. Of the 18 patients with HCV genotype 4 infection treated with a regimen of sofosbuvir/velpatasvir/voxilaprevir, 100% achieved SVR12.

POLARIS-2, a randomized, open-label trial, evaluated sofosbuvir/velpatasvir/voxilaprevir in adults with any genotype of HCV infection who were treatment naive or previously failed treatment with an HCV regimen that did not include a DAA. Enrolled patients were noncirrhotic or had compensated cirrhosis, although those with HCV genotype 3 infection were excluded if they had cirrhosis. Patients were randomized in a 1:1 ratio to receive sofosbuvir/velpatasvir/voxilaprevir (a fixed-combination tablet containing 400 mg of sofosbuvir, 100 mg of velpatasvir, and 100 mg of voxilaprevir) once daily for 8 weeks or sofosbuvir/velpatasvir (a fixed-combination tablet containing 400 mg of sofosbuvir and 100 mg of velpatasvir) once daily for 12 weeks. Results showed that the 8-week regimen of sofosbuvir/velpatasvir/voxilaprevir did *not* meet noninferiority criteria in these patients when compared with the 12-week regimen of sofosbuvir/velpatasvir (overall SVR12 achieved by 95 or 98% of patients, respectively).

HCV Genotype 5 Infection

Efficacy and safety of sofosbuvir/velpatasvir/voxilaprevir for the treatment of chronic HCV genotype 5 infection in adults have been evaluated in 2 randomized, phase 3 trials (POLARIS-1 and POLARIS-2). The primary end point in both studies was sustained virologic response at 12 weeks after the end of treatment (SVR12; defined as plasma HCV RNA level less than 15 IU/mL [the lower limit of quantification] at 12 weeks after end of treatment).

POLARIS-1, a double-blind, placebo-controlled trial, included 415 adults with chronic HCV genotype 1, 2, 3, 4, 5, or 6 infection who were noncirrhotic or had compensated cirrhosis and had previously failed treatment with an HCV regimen containing an HCV NS5A inhibitor (median age 59 years, 77% male, 74% with baseline HCV RNA levels 800,000 IU/mL or greater, 41% with compensated cirrhosis). Patients were previously treated with HCV treatment regimens containing ledipasvir (51%), daclatasvir (27%), ombitasvir (11%), velpatasvir (7%), or elbasvir (3%). The single patient with HCV genotype 5 infection enrolled in the study received a 12-week regimen of sofosbuvir/velpatasvir/voxilaprevir (a fixed-combination tablet containing 400 mg of sofosbuvir, 100 mg of velpatasvir, and 100 mg of voxilaprevir) once daily and achieved SVR12.

POLARIS-2, a randomized, open-label trial, evaluated sofosbuvir/velpatasvir/voxilaprevir in adults with any genotype of HCV infection who were treatment naive or previously failed treatment with an HCV regimen that did not include a DAA. Enrolled patients were noncirrhotic or had compensated cirrhosis, although those with HCV genotype 3 infection were excluded if they had cirrhosis. Patients were randomized in a 1:1 ratio to receive sofosbuvir/velpatasvir/voxilaprevir (a fixed-combination tablet containing 400 mg of sofosbuvir, 100 mg of velpatasvir, and 100 mg of voxilaprevir) once daily for 8 weeks or sofosbuvir/velpatasvir (a fixed-combination tablet containing 400 mg of sofosbuvir and 100 mg of velpatasvir) once daily for 12 weeks. Results showed that the 8-week regimen of sofosbuvir/velpatasvir/voxilaprevir did *not* meet noninferiority criteria in these patients when compared with the 12-week regimen of sofosbuvir/velpatasvir (overall SVR12 achieved by 95 or 98% of patients, respectively).

HCV Genotype 6 Infection

Efficacy and safety of sofosbuvir/velpatasvir/voxilaprevir for the treatment of chronic HCV genotype 6 infection in adults have been evaluated in 2 randomized, phase 3 trials (POLARIS-1 and POLARIS-2). The primary end point in both studies was sustained virologic response at 12 weeks after the end of treatment (SVR12; defined as plasma HCV RNA level less than 15 IU/mL [the lower limit of quantification] at 12 weeks after end of treatment).

POLARIS-1, a double-blind, placebo-controlled trial, included 415 adults with chronic HCV genotype 1, 2, 3, 4, 5, or 6 infection who were noncirrhotic or had compensated cirrhosis and had previously failed treatment with an HCV regimen containing an HCV NS5A inhibitor (median age 59 years, 77% male, 74% with baseline HCV RNA levels 800,000 IU/mL or greater, 41% with compensated cirrhosis). Patients were previously treated with HCV treatment regimens containing ledipasvir (51%), daclatasvir (27%), ombitasvir (11%), velpatasvir (7%), or elbasvir (3%). All patients with HCV genotype 6 infection received a 12-week regimen of sofosbuvir/velpatasvir/voxilaprevir (a fixed-combination tablet containing 400 mg of sofosbuvir, 100 mg of velpatasvir, and 100 mg of voxilaprevir) once daily. Of the 6 patients with HCV genotype 6 infection treated with sofosbuvir/velpatasvir/voxilaprevir, 100% achieved SVR12.

POLARIS-2, a randomized, open-label trial, evaluated sofosbuvir/velpatasvir/voxilaprevir in adults with any genotype of HCV infection who were treatment naive or previously failed treatment with an HCV regimen that did not include a DAA. Enrolled patients were noncirrhotic or had compensated cirrhosis, although those with HCV genotype 3 infection were excluded if they had cirrhosis. Patients were randomized in a 1:1 ratio to receive sofosbuvir/velpatasvir/voxilaprevir (a fixed-combination tablet containing 400 mg of sofosbuvir, 100 mg of velpatasvir, and 100 mg of voxilaprevir) once daily for 8 weeks or sofosbuvir/velpatasvir (a fixed-combination tablet containing 400 mg of sofosbuvir and 100 mg of velpatasvir) once daily for 12 weeks. Results showed that the 8-week regimen of sofosbuvir/velpatasvir/voxilaprevir did *not* meet noninferiority criteria in these patients when compared with the 12-week regimen of sofosbuvir/velpatasvir (overall SVR12 achieved by 95 or 98% of patients, respectively).

DOSAGE AND ADMINISTRATION

● General

Pretreatment Screening

- Prior to initiating HCV treatment, test all patients for evidence of current or prior HBV infection by measuring hepatitis B surface antigen (HBsAg), hepatitis B surface antibody (anti-HBs), and hepatitis B core antibody (anti-HBc).
- In patients with serologic evidence of HBV infection, measure baseline HBV DNA level.
- Perform appropriate laboratory tests to evaluate liver function.

Patient Monitoring

- Perform appropriate laboratory tests to evaluate liver function during therapy.
- *In all patients with evidence of current or prior HBV infection*: Monitor for clinical and laboratory signs (i.e., HBsAg, HBV DNA levels, serum aminotransferase and bilirubin concentrations) of hepatitis flare or HBV reactivation during and after treatment with HCV DAAs.

Other General Considerations

- If amiodarone is used concomitantly with sofosbuvir/velpatasvir/voxilaprevir, perform cardiac monitoring in an inpatient setting during the first 48 hours of concomitant use; perform heart rate monitoring daily

(outpatient or self-monitoring) through at least the first 2 weeks of concomitant use. Similar cardiac monitoring is recommended in patients who discontinue amiodarone just prior to initiation of sofosbuvir/velpatasvir/voxilaprevir.

● Administration

Sofosbuvir/velpatasvir/voxilaprevir is administered orally once daily with food.

● Dosage

Sofosbuvir/velpatasvir/voxilaprevir is commercially available as fixed-combination tablets containing 400 mg of sofosbuvir, 100 mg of velpatasvir, and 100 mg of voxilaprevir.

Chronic Hepatitis C Virus Infection

HCV Genotype 1, 2, 3, 4, 5, or 6 Infection

For the treatment of chronic HCV genotype 1, 2, 3, 4, 5, or 6 infection in adults who previously failed treatment with an HCV regimen containing an HCV NS5A replication complex inhibitor (NS5A inhibitor) and who are noncirrhotic or have compensated cirrhosis (Child-Pugh class A), the recommended dosage of sofosbuvir/velpatasvir/voxilaprevir is 1 tablet (400 mg of sofosbuvir, 100 mg of velpatasvir, and 100 mg of voxilaprevir) once daily. A treatment duration of 12 weeks is recommended.

HCV Genotype 1a or 3 Infection

For the treatment of chronic HCV genotype 1a or 3 infection in adults who previously failed treatment with an HCV regimen containing sofosbuvir *without* an HCV NS5A inhibitor and who are noncirrhotic or have compensated cirrhosis (Child-Pugh class A), the recommended dosage of sofosbuvir/velpatasvir/voxilaprevir is 1 tablet (400 mg of sofosbuvir, 100 mg of velpatasvir, and 100 mg of voxilaprevir) once daily. A treatment duration of 12 weeks is recommended.

● Special Populations

Hepatic Impairment

Dosage adjustments are not necessary if sofosbuvir/velpatasvir/voxilaprevir is used in adults with mild hepatic impairment or compensated cirrhosis (Child-Pugh class A). However, such patients should be monitored for signs and symptoms of hepatic decompensation. (See Hepatic Impairment under Warnings/Precautions: Specific Populations, in Cautions.)

Sofosbuvir/velpatasvir/voxilaprevir is not recommended in adults with moderate or severe hepatic impairment (Child-Pugh class B or C) or in those with any history of hepatic decompensation. (See Hepatic Impairment under Warnings/Precautions: Specific Populations, in Cautions.)

Renal Impairment

Dosage adjustments are not necessary if sofosbuvir/velpatasvir/voxilaprevir is used in adults with mild, moderate, or severe renal impairment, including those with end-stage renal disease undergoing dialysis.

Geriatric Patients

Dosage adjustments are not necessary if sofosbuvir/velpatasvir/voxilaprevir is used in geriatric patients. (See Geriatric Use under Warnings/Precautions: Specific Populations, in Cautions.)

CAUTIONS

● Contraindications

Concomitant use of the fixed combination of sofosbuvir, velpatasvir, and voxilaprevir (sofosbuvir/velpatasvir/voxilaprevir) and rifampin is contraindicated.

● Warnings/Precautions

Warnings

Risk of HBV Reactivation in Patients Coinfected with HCV and HBV

Reactivation of hepatitis B virus (HBV) infection has been reported during postmarketing experience when direct-acting antivirals (DAAs) were used for the treatment of chronic hepatitis C virus (HCV) infection in patients with HBV coinfection. In some cases, HBV reactivation resulted in fulminant hepatitis, hepatic failure, and death.

HBV reactivation (defined as an abrupt increase in HBV replication manifested as a rapid increase in serum HBV DNA levels or detection of hepatitis B surface antigen [HBsAg] in an individual who was previously HBsAg negative and hepatitis B core antibody [anti-HBc] positive) has been reported in patients with HCV and HBV coinfection who were receiving HCV treatment with a regimen that included HCV DAAs without interferon alfa. Reactivation also may be accompanied by hepatitis (i.e., increased aminotransferase concentrations) and, in severe cases, may lead to increased bilirubin concentrations, liver failure, or death.

Data to date indicate that HBV reactivation usually occurs within 4–8 weeks after initiation of HCV treatment. Patients with HBV reactivation have been heterogeneous in terms of HCV genotype and in terms of baseline HBV disease. While some patients with HBV reactivation were HBsAg positive, others had serologic evidence of resolved HBV infection (i.e., HBsAg negative and anti-HBc positive). HBV reactivation also has been reported in patients receiving certain immunosuppressant or chemotherapeutic drugs; the risk of reactivation associated with HCV DAAs may be increased in such patients.

The mechanism for HBV reactivation in patients with HCV and HBV coinfection receiving HCV DAAs is unknown. Although HCV DAAs are not known to cause immunosuppression, HBV reactivation in coinfected patients may result from a complex interplay of host immunologic responses in the setting of infection with 2 hepatitis viruses.

Prior to initiating treatment with an HCV DAA, including sofosbuvir/velpatasvir/voxilaprevir, all patients should be screened for evidence of current or prior HBV infection by measuring HBsAg, hepatitis B surface antibody (anti-HBs), and anti-HBc. If there is serologic evidence of HBV infection, baseline HBV DNA levels should be measured.

Patients with evidence of current or prior HBV infection should be monitored for clinical and laboratory signs (i.e., HBsAg, HBV DNA levels, serum aminotransferase concentrations, bilirubin concentrations) of hepatitis flare or HBV reactivation during and after treatment with HCV DAAs, including sofosbuvir/velpatasvir/voxilaprevir. Appropriate management for HBV infection should be initiated as clinically indicated.

Patients with HCV and HBV coinfection receiving sofosbuvir/velpatasvir/voxilaprevir should be advised to immediately contact a clinician if they develop any signs or symptoms of serious liver injury. (See Advice to Patients.)

When making decisions regarding HBV monitoring or HBV treatment in coinfected patients, consultation with a clinician who has expertise in managing HBV infection is recommended.

Other Warnings and Precautions

Risk of Hepatic Decompensation or Failure in Patients with Evidence of Advanced Liver Disease

Hepatic decompensation or failure, including some fatalities, have been reported during postmarketing experience in patients receiving HCV treatment regimens containing an HCV nonstructural 3/4A (NS3/4A) protease inhibitor, including sofosbuvir/velpatasvir/voxilaprevir. Data are insufficient to estimate the frequency of such events and a causal relationship has not been established. Hepatic decompensation or failure usually occurred within the first 4 weeks of HCV treatment.

Many of the reported cases of hepatic decompensation or failure occurred in patients with evidence of advanced liver disease with moderate or severe hepatic impairment (Child-Pugh class B or C) prior to initiation of HCV treatment. Some cases occurred in patients who were reported as noncirrhotic or as having compensated cirrhosis with mild liver impairment (Child-Pugh class A) at baseline, but had a history of a decompensation event or had evidence of portal hypertension or decreased platelet counts at baseline. Some cases also were reported in patients who had confounding factors (e.g., serious liver-related comorbidities).

If sofosbuvir/velpatasvir/voxilaprevir is used in patients with compensated cirrhosis (Child-Pugh class A) or evidence of advanced liver disease (e.g., portal hypertension), hepatic function tests should be performed as clinically indicated and patients should be monitored for signs and symptoms of hepatic decompensation (e.g., jaundice, ascites, hepatic encephalopathy, variceal hemorrhage).

Sofosbuvir/velpatasvir/voxilaprevir is not recommended in patients with moderate or severe hepatic impairment (Child-Pugh class B or C) or any history

of hepatic decompensation. (See Hepatic Impairment under Warnings/Precautions: Specific Populations, in Cautions.)

The drug should be discontinued in patients who develop evidence of hepatic decompensation or failure.

Patients should be advised to contact a clinician if they develop any signs or symptoms of worsening liver disease. (See Advice to Patients.)

● Cardiovascular Effects

Symptomatic bradycardia, sometimes requiring pacemaker intervention, has been reported during postmarketing experience in patients receiving amiodarone concomitantly with an HCV treatment regimen containing sofosbuvir in conjunction with daclatasvir or simeprevir (drugs no longer commercially available). Symptomatic bradycardia, including a fatal cardiac arrest, has been reported in patients receiving amiodarone concomitantly with the fixed combination containing ledipasvir and sofosbuvir (ledipasvir/sofosbuvir).

In most reported cases, bradycardia occurred within hours to days after HCV treatment was initiated in patients receiving amiodarone, but has been observed up to 2 weeks after initiation of HCV treatment. Bradycardia generally resolved after HCV treatment was discontinued. The mechanism for this adverse cardiovascular effect is unknown.

Patients who may be at increased risk for symptomatic bradycardia if amiodarone is used concomitantly with an HCV treatment regimen containing sofosbuvir and another HCV DAA include those also receiving a β-adrenergic blocking agent, those with underlying cardiac comorbidities, and/or those with advanced liver disease.

Concomitant use of amiodarone with sofosbuvir/velpatasvir/voxilaprevir is *not* recommended. If there are no alternative HCV treatment options and sofosbuvir/velpatasvir/voxilaprevir must be used in a patient receiving amiodarone, the patient should be advised about the risk of serious symptomatic bradycardia before sofosbuvir/velpatasvir/voxilaprevir is initiated. Cardiac monitoring should be performed in an inpatient setting during the first 48 hours of concomitant use of amiodarone and sofosbuvir/velpatasvir/voxilaprevir; heart rate monitoring should then be performed daily (outpatient or self-monitoring) through at least the first 2 weeks of concomitant use. Similar cardiac monitoring is recommended in patients who discontinued amiodarone just prior to initiation of sofosbuvir/velpatasvir/voxilaprevir or if there are no other treatment options and amiodarone must be initiated in a patient already receiving sofosbuvir/velpatasvir/voxilaprevir.

Patients receiving amiodarone concomitantly with sofosbuvir/velpatasvir/voxilaprevir should be advised to immediately contact a clinician if they develop signs or symptoms of bradycardia (e.g., near-fainting or fainting, dizziness, lightheadedness, malaise, weakness, excessive tiredness, shortness of breath, chest pain, confusion, memory problems).

● Interactions

Concomitant use of sofosbuvir/velpatasvir/voxilaprevir and inducers of the P-glycoprotein (P-gp) transport system and/or moderate or potent inducers of cytochrome P-450 (CYP) isoenzyme 2B6, 2C8, or 3A4 (e.g., carbamazepine and other anticonvulsants, St. John's wort [*Hypericum perforatum*]) may result in clinically important decreases in plasma concentrations of sofosbuvir, velpatasvir, and/or voxilaprevir and may lead to reduced therapeutic effect of sofosbuvir/velpatasvir/voxilaprevir. Concomitant use of such drugs with sofosbuvir/velpatasvir/voxilaprevir is not recommended. (See Drug Interactions.)

● Precautions Related to Fixed Combinations

When sofosbuvir/velpatasvir/voxilaprevir is used, the cautions, precautions, contraindications, and drug interactions associated with each drug in the fixed combination must be considered. Cautionary information applicable to specific populations (e.g., pregnant or nursing women, individuals with hepatic or renal impairment, geriatric patients) should be considered for each drug.

Specific Populations

Pregnancy

Adequate data are not available regarding use of sofosbuvir/velpatasvir/voxilaprevir in pregnant women. In animal studies, there was no evidence that sofosbuvir, velpatasvir, or voxilaprevir affected fetal development at exposures greater than those in humans receiving the recommended human dosage.

Lactation

It is not known whether sofosbuvir/velpatasvir/voxilaprevir or their metabolites are distributed into human milk, affect milk production, or have effects on the breast-fed infant.

The predominant metabolite of sofosbuvir (GS-331007) is distributed into milk in rats; velpatasvir is distributed into milk in rats and has been detected in plasma of suckling rat pups; and voxilaprevir has been detected in plasma of suckling rat pups. GS-331007, velpatasvir, and voxilaprevir had no apparent effects on nursing pups.

The benefits of breast-feeding and the importance of sofosbuvir/velpatasvir/voxilaprevir to the woman should be considered along with the potential adverse effects on the breast-fed child from the drug or from the underlying maternal condition.

Pediatric Use

Safety and efficacy of sofosbuvir/velpatasvir/voxilaprevir have not been established in pediatric patients younger than 18 years of age.

Geriatric Use

No overall differences in safety and efficacy of sofosbuvir/velpatasvir/voxilaprevir have been observed between patients 65 years of age and older and younger adults. However, greater sensitivity in some older individuals cannot be ruled out.

Population pharmacokinetic analysis in HCV-infected adults up to 85 years of age indicates that age does not have a clinically important effect on sofosbuvir, GS-331007, velpatasvir, or voxilaprevir exposures.

Hepatic Impairment

Patients with mild hepatic impairment or compensated cirrhosis (Child-Pugh class A) should be monitored for signs and symptoms of hepatic decompensation (e.g., jaundice, ascites, hepatic encephalopathy, variceal hemorrhage) during sofosbuvir/velpatasvir/voxilaprevir treatment.

Sofosbuvir/velpatasvir/voxilaprevir is not recommended in HCV-infected patients with moderate or severe hepatic impairment (Child-Pugh class B or C) or with any history of hepatic decompensation. There have been postmarketing reports of hepatic decompensation or failure in such patients. (See Risk of Hepatic Decompensation or Failure in Patients with Evidence of Advanced Liver Disease under Warnings/Precautions: Other Warnings and Precautions, in Cautions.)

In HCV-infected individuals with moderate or severe hepatic impairment (Child-Pugh class B or C), sofosbuvir (400 mg daily for 7 days) results in sofosbuvir and GS-331007 plasma exposures higher than those reported in individuals with normal hepatic function.

In individuals with moderate or severe hepatic impairment (Child-Pugh class B or C) without HCV infection, a single 100-mg dose of velpatasvir results in plasma exposures similar to those reported when the same dose is given to individuals with normal hepatic function.

In individuals with moderate or severe hepatic impairment (Child-Pugh class B or C) without HCV infection, a single 100-mg dose of voxilaprevir results in plasma exposures substantially higher than those reported in individuals with normal hepatic function (area under the plasma concentration-time curve [AUC] 299 or 500% higher, respectively).

Renal Impairment

Dosage adjustments are not necessary if sofosbuvir/velpatasvir/voxilaprevir is used in adults with any degree of renal impairment, including those with end-stage renal disease (ESRD) undergoing dialysis.

In individuals with mild, moderate, or severe renal impairment without HCV infection, sofosbuvir and GS-331007 plasma exposures are higher than those reported in individuals with normal renal function. In those with ESRD, sofosbuvir and GS-331007 exposures were higher when the drug was administered 1 hour before or 1 hour after hemodialysis compared with exposures in those with normal renal function; a 4-hour hemodialysis session removed approximately 18% of the dose.

In individuals with severe renal impairment (estimated glomerular filtration rate [eGFR] less than 30 mL/minute per 1.73 m²) without HCV infection, velpatasvir pharmacokinetics following a single 100-mg dose of the drug are similar to pharmacokinetics reported in healthy individuals. Velpatasvir is not expected to be removed to any clinically important extent by hemodialysis.

In individuals with severe renal impairment without HCV infection, voxilaprevir pharmacokinetics following a single 100-mg dose of the drug are similar to pharmacokinetics reported in healthy individuals. Voxilaprevir is not expected to be removed to any clinically important extent by hemodialysis.

In HCV-infected individuals with ESRD requiring dialysis who were receiving the fixed combination of sofosbuvir and velpatasvir (sofosbuvir/velpatasvir), the pharmacokinetics of sofosbuvir, GS-331007, and velpatasvir were similar to the pharmacokinetics reported in those without HCV infection who had ESRD requiring dialysis. The pharmacokinetics of voxilaprevir have not been studied in individuals with ESRD; however, voxilaprevir exposures in HCV-infected individuals with ESRD requiring dialysis who are receiving sofosbuvir/velpatasvir/voxilaprevir are not expected to be affected to any clinically important extent compared with exposures in those with normal renal function.

● Common Adverse Effects

Adverse effects reported in 5% or more of patients receiving sofosbuvir/velpatasvir/voxilaprevir include headache, fatigue, diarrhea, nausea, asthenia, and insomnia.

DRUG INTERACTIONS

The following drug interactions are based on studies using the fixed combination containing sofosbuvir, velpatasvir, voxilaprevir (sofosbuvir/velpatasvir/voxilaprevir), the fixed combination of sofosbuvir and velpatasvir (sofosbuvir/velpatasvir), sofosbuvir alone, velpatasvir alone, or voxilaprevir alone, or are predicted to occur. When sofosbuvir/velpatasvir/voxilaprevir is used, interactions associated with each drug in the fixed combination should be considered.

● Drugs Affecting or Metabolized by Hepatic Microsomal Enzymes

In vitro studies indicate slow metabolic turnover of velpatasvir by cytochrome P-450 (CYP) isoenzymes 2B6, 2C8, and 3A4 and slow metabolic turnover of voxilaprevir by CYP3A4 and, to a lesser extent, 1A2 and 2C8. Sofosbuvir and the predominant metabolite of sofosbuvir (GS-331007) do not inhibit or induce CYP isoenzymes; velpatasvir and voxilaprevir do not inhibit CYP isoenzymes at clinically important concentrations.

Pharmacokinetic interactions are possible with moderate or potent inducers of CYP2B6, 2C8, or 3A4, which may decrease sofosbuvir, velpatasvir, and/or voxilaprevir plasma concentrations potentially leading to reduced therapeutic effect of sofosbuvir/velpatasvir/voxilaprevir. Concomitant use of sofosbuvir/velpatasvir/voxilaprevir with moderate or potent inducers of CYP2B6, 2C8, or 3A4 is not recommended.

Although inhibitors of CYP2B6, 2C8, or 3A4 may increase velpatasvir and/or voxilaprevir plasma concentrations, sofosbuvir/velpatasvir/voxilaprevir may be used concomitantly with inhibitors of CYP2B6, 2C8, or 3A4.

● Drugs Affecting or Affected by P-glycoprotein Transport System

Velpatasvir and voxilaprevir are inhibitors of the P-glycoprotein (P-gp) transport system; sofosbuvir and GS-331007 are not inhibitors of P-gp. Concomitant use of sofosbuvir/velpatasvir/voxilaprevir and P-gp substrates may alter the exposure of such drugs.

Sofosbuvir, velpatasvir, and voxilaprevir are substrates of P-gp; GS-331007 is not a P-gp substrate. Pharmacokinetic interactions are possible with P-gp inducers, which may decrease sofosbuvir, velpatasvir, and/or voxilaprevir plasma concentrations potentially leading to reduced therapeutic effect of sofosbuvir/velpatasvir/voxilaprevir. Concomitant use of sofosbuvir/velpatasvir/voxilaprevir with P-gp inducers is not recommended.

Inhibitors of P-gp may increase plasma concentrations of sofosbuvir, velpatasvir, and/or voxilaprevir without increasing plasma concentrations of GS-331007. Sofosbuvir/velpatasvir/voxilaprevir may be used concomitantly with P-gp inhibitors.

• Drugs Affecting or Affected by Breast Cancer Resistance Protein

Velpatasvir and voxilaprevir are inhibitors of breast cancer resistance protein (BCRP); sofosbuvir and GS-331007 are not BCRP inhibitors. Pharmacokinetic interactions are possible if sofosbuvir/velpatasvir/voxilaprevir and BCRP substrates are used concomitantly; altered exposure of such drugs may occur. Concomitant use of sofosbuvir/velpatasvir/voxilaprevir and BCRP substrates is not recommended.

Sofosbuvir, velpatasvir, and voxilaprevir are substrates of BCRP; GS-331007 is not a BCRP substrate. Inhibitors of BCRP may increase plasma concentrations of sofosbuvir, velpatasvir, and/or voxilaprevir without increasing plasma concentrations of GS-331007. Sofosbuvir/velpatasvir/voxilaprevir may be used concomitantly with BCRP inhibitors.

• Drugs Affecting or Affected by Organic Anion Transporting Polypeptides

Velpatasvir and voxilaprevir inhibit organic anion transporting polypeptide (OATP) 1B1 and 1B3; velpatasvir also inhibits OATP2B1, but does not inhibit OATP1A2 at clinically relevant concentrations. Sofosbuvir and GS-331007 do not inhibit OATP1B1 or 1B3. Concomitant use of sofosbuvir/velpatasvir/voxilaprevir and OATP1B1, 1B3, or 2B1 substrates may alter exposures of such drugs.

Voxilaprevir and, to a lesser extent, velpatasvir are substrates of OATP1B1 and 1B3. Inhibitors of OATP may substantially increase plasma concentrations of voxilaprevir. Therefore, concomitant use of sofosbuvir/velpatasvir/voxilaprevir and OATP inhibitors is not recommended.

• Drugs Affecting or Affected by Other Membrane Transporters

Sofosbuvir and GS-331007 do not inhibit organic cation transporter (OCT) 1; GS-331007 does not inhibit organic anion transporter (OAT) 1, OAT3, OCT2, or multidrug and toxin extrusion protein (MATE) 1. Sofosbuvir and GS-331007 do not inhibit or induce uridine diphosphate-glucuronosyl transferase (UGT) 1A1.

Velpatasvir and voxilaprevir do not inhibit OAT1, OAT3, OCT1, OCT2, MATE1, or UGT1A1 at clinically relevant concentrations.

• Drugs Affecting Gastric pH

The solubility of velpatasvir decreases as pH increases. Therefore, drugs that increase gastric pH are expected to decrease velpatasvir plasma concentrations.

Antacids

Administration of sofosbuvir/velpatasvir/voxilaprevir and antacids (e.g., aluminum and magnesium hydroxide) should be separated by 4 hours.

Histamine H$_2$-Receptor Antagonists

H$_2$-receptor antagonists may be administered concurrently with or staggered from sofosbuvir/velpatasvir/voxilaprevir; dosage of the H$_2$-receptor antagonist should not exceed dosages comparable to famotidine 40 mg twice daily.

Proton-pump Inhibitors

Administration of omeprazole 20 mg 2 hours before or 4 hours after sofosbuvir/velpatasvir/voxilaprevir results in decreased velpatasvir plasma concentrations and area under the plasma concentration-time curve (AUC).

Sofosbuvir/velpatasvir/voxilaprevir may be administered with omeprazole 20 mg. Use of sofosbuvir/velpatasvir/voxilaprevir with other proton-pump inhibitors has not been studied.

• Antiarrhythmic Agents

Amiodarone

Concomitant use of amiodarone and sofosbuvir/velpatasvir/voxilaprevir may result in serious symptomatic bradycardia and is not recommended. If there are no alternative hepatitis C virus (HCV) treatment options and a regimen of sofosbuvir/velpatasvir/voxilaprevir must be used in a patient receiving amiodarone, the patient should be advised about the risk of serious symptomatic bradycardia and cardiac monitoring should be performed in an inpatient setting during the first 48 hours of concomitant use and then heart rate monitoring (outpatient or self-monitoring) should be performed daily through at least the first 2 weeks of concomitant use. Similar cardiac monitoring is recommended in patients who discontinued amiodarone just prior to initiation of sofosbuvir/velpatasvir/voxilaprevir or if there are no other treatment options and amiodarone must be initiated in a patient already receiving sofosbuvir/velpatasvir/voxilaprevir. (See Cardiovascular Effects under Warnings/Precautions: Other Warnings and Precautions, in Cautions.)

The effect of concomitant use of amiodarone and sofosbuvir/velpatasvir/voxilaprevir on plasma concentrations of amiodarone, sofosbuvir, velpatasvir, and voxilaprevir is unknown.

• Anticoagulants

Dabigatran

Concomitant use of sofosbuvir/velpatasvir/voxilaprevir once daily and a single 75-mg dose of dabigatran etexilate results in 2.9- and 2.6-fold increased dabigatran peak plasma concentrations and AUC, respectively.

If sofosbuvir/velpatasvir/voxilaprevir and dabigatran are used concomitantly, clinical effects of the anticoagulant should be monitored; recommendations from the manufacturer of dabigatran etexilate should be consulted regarding dosage modifications.

Warfarin

In patients receiving warfarin, subtherapeutic international normalized ratios (INRs) have been reported after initiation of sofosbuvir-containing HCV treatment regimens. INR fluctuations have been reported in patients receiving warfarin and sofosbuvir/velpatasvir/voxilaprevir concomitantly.

If a sofosbuvir-containing regimen (e.g., sofosbuvir/velpatasvir/voxilaprevir) is used in patients receiving warfarin, INR should be frequently monitored at the time of initiation, during treatment, and after discontinuance of the sofosbuvir-containing regimen. Adjustment of warfarin dosage may be needed.

• Anticonvulsants

Concomitant use of sofosbuvir/velpatasvir/voxilaprevir and certain anticonvulsants (i.e., carbamazepine, oxcarbazepine, phenobarbital, phenytoin) is expected to decrease sofosbuvir, velpatasvir, and voxilaprevir plasma concentrations.

Concomitant use of sofosbuvir/velpatasvir/voxilaprevir and carbamazepine, oxcarbazepine, phenobarbital, or phenytoin is not recommended.

• Antifungal Agents

Ketoconazole

No clinically important pharmacokinetic interactions were observed when sofosbuvir/velpatasvir was used concomitantly with ketoconazole.

No clinically important pharmacokinetic interactions were observed when a single 100-mg dose of velpatasvir was used concomitantly with ketoconazole (200 mg twice daily).

Voriconazole

No clinically important pharmacokinetic interactions were observed when sofosbuvir/velpatasvir/voxilaprevir was used concomitantly with voriconazole.

No clinically important pharmacokinetic interactions were observed when a single 100-mg dose of voxilaprevir was used concomitantly with voriconazole (200 mg twice daily).

• Antimycobacterial Agents

Rifabutin

Rifabutin is expected to decrease plasma concentrations of sofosbuvir, velpatasvir, and voxilaprevir.

Concomitant use of rifabutin and sofosbuvir/velpatasvir/voxilaprevir is not recommended.

Rifampin

Concomitant use of rifampin (600 mg once daily) and sofosbuvir (single 400-mg dose), velpatasvir (single 100-mg dose), or voxilaprevir (single 100-mg dose) results in decreased plasma concentrations and AUCs of sofosbuvir, velpatasvir, and voxilaprevir. Concomitant use of rifampin (single 600-mg dose) and velpatasvir (single 100-mg dose) or voxilaprevir (single 100-mg dose) results in increased velpatasvir or voxilaprevir plasma concentrations and AUC.

Concomitant use of rifampin and sofosbuvir/velpatasvir/voxilaprevir is contraindicated.

Rifapentine

Rifapentine is expected to decrease plasma concentrations of sofosbuvir, velpatasvir, and voxilaprevir.

Concomitant use of rifapentine and sofosbuvir/velpatasvir/voxilaprevir is not recommended.

● Antineoplastic Agents

Concomitant use of sofosbuvir/velpatasvir/voxilaprevir and imatinib, irinotecan, lapatinib, methotrexate, mitoxantrone, or topotecan is not recommended.

● Antiretroviral Agents

HIV Entry and Fusion Inhibitors

Maraviroc

Concomitant use of maraviroc and sofosbuvir/velpatasvir/voxilaprevir is not expected to affect maraviroc pharmacokinetics.

Dosage adjustments are not necessary if maraviroc is used concomitantly with sofosbuvir/velpatasvir/voxilaprevir.

HIV Integrase Inhibitors (INSTIs)

Bictegravir

Pharmacokinetic interactions are not expected if bictegravir is used concomitantly with sofosbuvir/velpatasvir/voxilaprevir.

Dosage adjustments are not necessary if bictegravir is used concomitantly with sofosbuvir/velpatasvir/voxilaprevir.

Dolutegravir

No clinically important pharmacokinetic interactions were observed when dolutegravir was used concomitantly with sofosbuvir/velpatasvir.

Dosage adjustments are not necessary if dolutegravir is used concomitantly with sofosbuvir/velpatasvir/voxilaprevir.

Elvitegravir

Concomitant use of *cobicistat-boosted* elvitegravir results in increased AUCs of sofosbuvir and voxilaprevir, but does not affect velpatasvir concentrations. Dosage adjustments are not necessary if *cobicistat-boosted* elvitegravir is used concomitantly with sofosbuvir/velpatasvir/voxilaprevir.

No clinically important pharmacokinetic interactions were observed when the fixed combination of elvitegravir, cobicistat, emtricitabine, and tenofovir alafenamide fumarate (EVG/c/FTC/TAF) was used concomitantly with sofosbuvir/velpatasvir/voxilaprevir.

If sofosbuvir/velpatasvir/voxilaprevir is used concomitantly with the fixed combination of elvitegravir, cobicistat, emtricitabine, and tenofovir disoproxil fumarate (EVG/c/FTC/TDF), increased tenofovir concentrations may occur. Patients should be monitored for tenofovir-associated adverse effects if sofosbuvir/velpatasvir/voxilaprevir is used concomitantly with EVG/c/FTC/TDF. (See Tenofovir under Antiretroviral Agents: HIV Nucleoside and Nucleotide Reverse Transcriptase Inhibitors [NRTIs], in Drug Interactions.)

Raltegravir

No clinically important pharmacokinetic interactions were observed when raltegravir was used concomitantly with sofosbuvir/velpatasvir.

Concomitant use of sofosbuvir/velpatasvir and an HIV antiretroviral regimen of raltegravir in conjunction with the fixed combination of emtricitabine and TDF (emtricitabine/TDF) did not have a clinically important effect on the pharmacokinetics of raltegravir or emtricitabine, but tenofovir plasma concentrations and AUC were increased.

Dosage adjustments are not necessary if raltegravir is used concomitantly with sofosbuvir/velpatasvir/voxilaprevir.

If sofosbuvir/velpatasvir/voxilaprevir is used concomitantly with an HIV antiretroviral regimen that includes raltegravir and TDF, patients should be monitored for tenofovir-associated adverse effects. (See Tenofovir under Antiretroviral Agents: HIV Nucleoside and Nucleotide Reverse Transcriptase Inhibitors [NRTIs], in Drug Interactions.)

HIV Nonnucleoside Reverse Transcriptase Inhibitors (NNRTIs)

Doravirine

Clinically important pharmacokinetic interactions are not expected if doravirine is used concomitantly with sofosbuvir/velpatasvir/voxilaprevir.

Dosage adjustments are not necessary if doravirine is used concomitantly with sofosbuvir/velpatasvir/voxilaprevir.

Efavirenz

Decreased velpatasvir and voxilaprevir concentrations are expected if efavirenz is used concomitantly with sofosbuvir/velpatasvir/voxilaprevir.

Concomitant use of the fixed combination of efavirenz, emtricitabine, and TDF (efavirenz/emtricitabine/TDF) and sofosbuvir/velpatasvir did not have a clinically important effect on the pharmacokinetics of sofosbuvir, but velpatasvir plasma concentrations and AUC were decreased and tenofovir plasma concentrations and AUC were increased.

Concomitant use of efavirenz and sofosbuvir/velpatasvir/voxilaprevir is not recommended.

Etravirine

Concomitant use of the etravirine and sofosbuvir/velpatasvir/voxilaprevir is expected to result in decreased velpatasvir and voxilaprevir plasma concentrations.

Concomitant use of etravirine and sofosbuvir/velpatasvir/voxilaprevir is not recommended.

Nevirapine

Concomitant use of nevirapine and sofosbuvir/velpatasvir/voxilaprevir is expected to result in decreased velpatasvir and voxilaprevir plasma concentrations.

Concomitant use of nevirapine and sofosbuvir/velpatasvir/voxilaprevir is not recommended.

Rilpivirine

No clinically important pharmacokinetic interactions when rilpivirine is used concomitantly with sofosbuvir/velpatasvir/voxilaprevir.

Concomitant use of the fixed combination of emtricitabine, rilpivirine, and TAF and sofosbuvir/velpatasvir/voxilaprevir did not have a clinically important effect on the pharmacokinetics of sofosbuvir, velpatasvir, or voxilaprevir.

Concomitant use of the fixed combination of emtricitabine, rilpivirine, and TDF (emtricitabine/rilpivirine/TDF) and sofosbuvir/velpatasvir/voxilaprevir did not have a clinically important effect on the pharmacokinetics of emtricitabine or rilpivirine, but tenofovir plasma concentrations and AUC were increased.

Dosage adjustments are not necessary if rilpivirine is used concomitantly with sofosbuvir/velpatasvir/voxilaprevir.

If sofosbuvir/velpatasvir/voxilaprevir is used concomitantly with an HIV antiretroviral regimen that contains rilpivirine and TDF, patients should be monitored for tenofovir-associated adverse effects. (See Tenofovir under Antiretroviral Agents: HIV Nucleoside and Nucleotide Reverse Transcriptase Inhibitors [NRTIs], in Drug Interactions.)

HIV Nucleoside and Nucleotide Reverse Transcriptase Inhibitors (NRTIs)

Emtricitabine

No clinically important pharmacokinetic interactions were observed when sofosbuvir/velpatasvir/voxilaprevir was used concomitantly with emtricitabine.

Tenofovir

No clinically important pharmacokinetic interactions were observed when tenofovir alafenamide fumarate (TAF) was used concomitantly with sofosbuvir/

velpatasvir/voxilaprevir. Dosage adjustments are not necessary if TAF is used concomitantly with sofosbuvir/velpatasvir/voxilaprevir.

Concomitant use of tenofovir disoproxil fumarate (TDF; tenofovir DF) or HIV antiretroviral regimens that include TDF and certain other antiretroviral agents (e.g., EVG/c/FTC/TDF, emtricitabine/rilpivirine/TDF, raltegravir in conjunction with emtricitabine/TDF, *ritonavir-boosted* darunavir in conjunction with emtricitabine/TDF) may result in increased tenofovir peak plasma concentrations and AUC. Patients should be monitored for tenofovir-associated adverse effects if sofosbuvir/velpatasvir/voxilaprevir is used concomitantly with any HIV antiretroviral regimen containing TDF. Some experts recommend that TAF should be considered instead of TDF in patients who are receiving sofosbuvir/velpatasvir/voxilaprevir and are at risk of TDF-associated adverse effects.

HIV Protease Inhibitors (PIs)

Atazanavir

Concomitant use of *ritonavir-boosted* atazanavir and sofosbuvir/velpatasvir/voxilaprevir results in substantially increased voxilaprevir peak plasma concentrations and AUC.

Concomitant use of sofosbuvir/velpatasvir/voxilaprevir and *ritonavir-boosted*, *cobicistat-boosted*, or unboosted atazanavir is not recommended.

Darunavir

No clinically important pharmacokinetic interactions were observed when sofosbuvir/velpatasvir/voxilaprevir was used concomitantly with *ritonavir-boosted* darunavir in conjunction with emtricitabine/TDF, but tenofovir plasma concentrations and AUC were increased.

Dosage adjustments are not necessary if *ritonavir-boosted* or *cobicistat-boosted* darunavir is used concomitantly with sofosbuvir/velpatasvir/voxilaprevir.

Lopinavir

Pharmacokinetic interactions are expected if the fixed combination of lopinavir and ritonavir (lopinavir/ritonavir) is used concomitantly with sofosbuvir/velpatasvir/voxilaprevir (increased voxilaprevir concentrations).

Concomitant use of lopinavir/ritonavir and sofosbuvir/velpatasvir/voxilaprevir is not recommended.

Tipranavir

Pharmacokinetic interactions are expected if *ritonavir-boosted* tipranavir is used concomitantly with sofosbuvir/velpatasvir/voxilaprevir (decreased sofosbuvir and velpatasvir plasma concentrations); the effect of *ritonavir-boosted* tipranavir on voxilaprevir concentrations is not known.

Concomitant use of *ritonavir-boosted* tipranavir and sofosbuvir/velpatasvir/voxilaprevir is not recommended.

● Digoxin

Concomitant use of velpatasvir 100 mg once daily and a single 0.25-mg dose of digoxin results in increased digoxin concentrations and AUC.

If sofosbuvir/velpatasvir/voxilaprevir and digoxin are used concomitantly, therapeutic concentration monitoring of digoxin is recommended.

● Estrogens and Progestins

Concomitant use of sofosbuvir/velpatasvir/voxilaprevir and an oral contraceptive containing ethinyl estradiol and norgestimate does not have a clinically important effect on the pharmacokinetics of ethinyl estradiol or norgestimate.

● Gemfibrozil

Concomitant use of sofosbuvir/velpatasvir/voxilaprevir and gemfibrozil does not result in clinically important pharmacokinetic interactions.

● HCV Antivirals

In vitro in replicon studies, there was no evidence of antagonistic anti-HCV effects between sofosbuvir and velpatasvir or voxilaprevir.

In vitro in replicon studies, there was no evidence of antagonistic anti-HCV effects between velpatasvir and voxilaprevir.

● HMG-CoA Reductase Inhibitors

Atorvastatin

Concomitant use of sofosbuvir/velpatasvir once daily and a single 40-mg dose of atorvastatin results in increased atorvastatin peak plasma concentrations and AUC, which is associated with increased risk of myopathy and rhabdomyolysis.

If sofosbuvir/velpatasvir/voxilaprevir and atorvastatin are used concomitantly, the lowest atorvastatin dosage should be used. If higher atorvastatin dosages are required, the lowest necessary dosage should be used taking into account the risks and benefits.

Fluvastatin, Lovastatin, and Simvastatin

Concomitant use of sofosbuvir/velpatasvir/voxilaprevir with fluvastatin, lovastatin, or simvastatin may increase concentrations of the statin, which is associated with increased risk of myopathy and rhabdomyolysis.

If sofosbuvir/velpatasvir/voxilaprevir is used concomitantly with fluvastatin, lovastatin, or simvastatin, the lowest statin dosage should be used. If higher statin dosages are required, the lowest necessary dosage should be used taking into account the risks and benefits.

Pitavastatin

Concomitant use of sofosbuvir/velpatasvir/voxilaprevir and pitavastatin may increase pitavastatin concentrations, which is associated with increased risk of myopathy and rhabdomyolysis.

Concomitant use of sofosbuvir/velpatasvir/voxilaprevir and pitavastatin is not recommended.

Pravastatin

Concomitant use of sofosbuvir/velpatasvir/voxilaprevir once daily and a single 40-mg dose of pravastatin results in increased pravastatin peak plasma concentrations and AUC, which is associated with increased risk of myopathy and rhabdomyolysis.

If sofosbuvir/velpatasvir/voxilaprevir and pravastatin are used concomitantly, the pravastatin dose should not exceed 40 mg.

Rosuvastatin

Concomitant use of sofosbuvir/velpatasvir/voxilaprevir and rosuvastatin (single 10-mg dose) results in substantially increased rosuvastatin plasma concentrations and AUC, which is associated with increased risk of myopathy and rhabdomyolysis.

Concomitant use of sofosbuvir/velpatasvir/voxilaprevir and rosuvastatin is not recommended.

● Immunosuppressive Agents

Cyclosporine

Concomitant use of cyclosporine (single 600-mg dose) and voxilaprevir (single 100-mg dose) results in substantially increased voxilaprevir peak plasma concentrations and AUC. Increased sofosbuvir or velpatasvir exposures are observed when cyclosporine (single 600-mg dose) is used concomitantly with sofosbuvir (single 400-mg dose) or velpatasvir (single 100-mg dose).

Concomitant use of sofosbuvir/velpatasvir/voxilaprevir and cyclosporine is not recommended.

Tacrolimus

No clinically important pharmacokinetic interactions were observed when tacrolimus (single 5-mg dose) was used concomitantly with sofosbuvir (single 400-mg dose).

● Methadone

No clinically important pharmacokinetic interactions were observed when sofosbuvir (400 mg once daily) was used concomitantly with methadone hydrochloride (30–130 mg daily).

● St. John's Wort

Concomitant use of St. John's wort (*Hypericum perforatum*) and sofosbuvir/velpatasvir/voxilaprevir may result in clinically important decreases in sofosbuvir, velpatasvir, and voxilaprevir plasma concentrations.

Concomitant use of sofosbuvir/velpatasvir/voxilaprevir and St. John's wort is not recommended.

● *Sulfasalazine*

Concomitant use of sulfasalazine and sofosbuvir/velpatasvir/voxilaprevir is not recommended.

DESCRIPTION

Sofosbuvir, velpatasvir, and voxilaprevir (sofosbuvir/velpatasvir/voxilaprevir) is a fixed combination containing 3 hepatitis C virus (HCV) antivirals. Sofosbuvir is a nucleotide analog HCV nonstructural 5B (NS5B) polymerase inhibitor. Velpatasvir is an HCV nonstructural 5A (NS5A) replication complex inhibitor (NS5A inhibitor). Voxilaprevir is an HCV nonstructural 3/4A (NS3/4A) protease inhibitor. All three drugs are direct-acting antivirals (DAAs) with activity against HCV. There is no in vitro evidence of antagonistic anti-HCV effects between sofosbuvir and velpatasvir or voxilaprevir and no in vitro evidence of antagonistic anti-HCV effects between velpatasvir and voxilaprevir.

Sofosbuvir is a prodrug that is converted in the liver to a pharmacologically active uridine analog triphosphate (GS-461203), which can be incorporated into HCV RNA by NS5B polymerase and acts as an RNA chain terminator. In vitro studies using biochemical assays indicate that GS-461203 has activity against HCV genotypes 1b, 2a, 3a, and 4a. Sofosbuvir has shown in vitro activity against full-length or chimeric replicons of HCV genotypes 1a, 1b, 2a, 2b, 3a, 4a, 4d, 5a, and 6a (median concentration of the drug required to inhibit viral replication by 50% [EC_{50}] has ranged from 15–110 nM).

Velpatasvir inhibits the HCV NS5A protein, which is required for viral replication. Velpatasvir has shown in vitro activity against full-length or chimeric replicons of HCV genotypes 1a, 1b, 2a, 2b, 3a, 4a, 4d, 4r, 5a, 6a, and 6e (median EC_{50} has ranged from 0.002–0.13 nM).

Voxilaprevir reversibly binds to the active site of HCV NS3/4A protease, thereby blocking enzyme activity essential for viral replication (i.e., blocking cleavage of the HCV-encoded polyproteins into mature forms of NS3, NS4A, NS4B, NS5A, and NS5B). In vitro studies using biochemical assays indicate that voxilaprevir has activity against HCV genotypes 1b and 3a. Voxilaprevir has shown in vitro activity against full-length or chimeric replicons of HCV genotypes 1a, 1b, 2a, 2b, 3a, 4a, 4d, 4r, 5a, 6a, 6e, and 6n (median EC_{50} has ranged from 0.2–6.6 nM).

Certain amino acid substitutions in NS5B polymerase of HCV genotypes 1b, 2a, 2b, 3a, 4a, 5a, and 6a have been selected in cell culture and have been associated with reduced susceptibility to sofosbuvir in vitro in replicon studies. In all replicon genotypes tested, the S282T substitution was associated with reduced susceptibility to sofosbuvir; in genotypes 2a, 5, and 6 replicons, an M289L substitution developed along with the S282T substitution. Treatment-emergent NS5B resistance-associated substitutions were not detected in patients who experienced virologic failure or relapsed with sofosbuvir/velpatasvir/voxilaprevir in phase 3 clinical trials (POLARIS-1, POLARIS-4).

Certain amino acid substitutions in NS5A of HCV genotype 1a (e.g., L31V, Y93H/N), genotype 1b (e.g., L31V, Y93H), genotype 2a (e.g., F28S, Y93H), genotype 3a (e.g., Y93H/S), genotype 4a (e.g., Y93H), and genotype 6 (e.g., L31V, P32A/L/Q/R) have been selected in cell culture and have been associated with reduced susceptibility to velpatasvir in vitro in replicon studies. Combinations of these NS5A substitutions often resulted in greater reductions in susceptibility to velpatasvir compared with a single NS5A substitution. Treatment-emergent NS5A resistance-associated substitutions were detected in phase 3 clinical trials evaluating sofosbuvir/velpatasvir/voxilaprevir in patients with HCV genotype 1a (e.g., L31M, Y93H, K24R), genotype 3a (e.g., E92K), or genotype 4 (e.g., Y93H) infection who relapsed or experienced virologic failure. Some of these patients also had baseline NS5A polymorphisms at resistance-associated amino acid positions.

Certain amino acid substitutions in NS3/4A protease inhibitor resistance-associated positions of HCV genotypes 1a (e.g., A156 L/T), 1b (e.g., A156T/V), 2a (e.g., A156L/V), 3a (e.g., A156T/V), 4a (e.g., A156L/T/V), 5a, and 6a have been selected in cell culture and have been associated with reduced susceptibility to voxilaprevir in vitro in replicon studies. Combinations of these NS3 substitutions often resulted in greater reductions in susceptibility to voxilaprevir compared

with a single NS3 substitution. Treatment-emergent NS3 resistance-associated substitutions were detected in phase 3 clinical trials evaluating sofosbuvir/velpatasvir/voxilaprevir in patients with HCV genotype 1a (e.g., V36A) or genotype 3a (e.g., Q41K, V55A, R155M) infection who relapsed.

Sofosbuvir, velpatasvir, and voxilaprevir are each active against HCV with substitutions associated with resistance to other HCV DAAs that have different mechanisms of action. Cross-resistance is possible among the HCV NS5A inhibitors and among the HCV NS3/4A protease inhibitors.

Following oral administration of sofosbuvir/velpatasvir/voxilaprevir, peak plasma concentrations of sofosbuvir occur 2 hours after the dose and peak plasma concentrations of velpatasvir and voxilaprevir both occur 4 hours after the dose. Administration of sofosbuvir/velpatasvir/voxilaprevir with food increases sofosbuvir exposures by 64–144%, increases velpatasvir exposures by 40–166%, and increases voxilaprevir exposures by 112–435%.

Sofosbuvir is a prodrug that undergoes intracellular metabolic activation in the liver (hydrolysis by human cathepsin A [CatA] or carboxylesterase 1 [CES1], phosphoramidate cleavage by histidine triad nucleotide-binding protein 1 [HINT1], and phosphorylation by pyrimidine nucleotide biosynthesis pathway). This results in formation of the pharmacologically active metabolite, GS-461203; desphosphorylation subsequently occurs leading to formation of GS-331007 (the predominant circulating metabolite), which has no anti-HCV activity. Sofosbuvir is approximately 61–65% bound to plasma proteins. The major route of elimination is renal clearance (glomerular filtration and active tubular secretion). Following a single oral dose of sofosbuvir, 80% is eliminated in urine (mainly as GS-331007) and 14% is excreted in feces. The median terminal plasma half-lives of sofosbuvir and GS-331007 are 0.5 and 29 hours, respectively.

Velpatasvir is metabolized by cytochrome P-450 (CYP) isoenzymes 2B6, 2C8, and 3A4. The drug is greater than 99% bound to plasma proteins. The major route of elimination of velpatasvir is biliary excretion (approximately 77% excreted as the parent drug). Following a single oral dose of velpatasvir, 94% is excreted in feces and 0.4% is eliminated in urine. The median terminal plasma half-life of velpatasvir is 17 hours.

Voxilaprevir is metabolized by CYP3A4. The drug is greater than 99% bound to plasma proteins. The major route of elimination of velpatasvir is biliary excretion (approximately 40% excreted as the parent drug). Following a single oral dose of voxilaprevir, 94% is excreted in feces and no drug is eliminated in urine. The median terminal plasma half-life of velpatasvir is 33 hours.

ADVICE TO PATIENTS

Importance of reading patient information provided by the manufacturer.

Advise patients that the fixed-combination preparation of sofosbuvir, velpatasvir, and voxilaprevir (sofosbuvir/velpatasvir/voxilaprevir) should be taken once daily with food on a regular dosing schedule.

Importance of taking the recommended dosage of sofosbuvir/velpatasvir/voxilaprevir for the recommended duration of treatment; importance of not missing doses.

Inform patients that reactivation of hepatitis B virus (HBV) infection has occurred in patients being treated for hepatitis C virus (HCV) infection who were coinfected with HBV. Importance of informing clinician of any history of HBV infection or other liver problems (e.g., cirrhosis). Importance of immediately contacting a clinician if any signs or symptoms of serious liver injury (e.g., fatigue, weakness, loss of appetite, nausea and vomiting, yellowing of the eyes or skin, light-colored bowel movements) occur. (See Risk of HBV Reactivation in Patients Coinfected with HCV and HBV under Warnings/Precautions: Warnings, in Cautions.)

Advise patients to immediately contact a clinician if they have symptoms of worsening liver problems (e.g., nausea, tiredness, yellowing of skin or white part of the eyes, bleeding or bruising more easily than normal, confusion, loss of appetite, diarrhea, dark or brown urine, dark or bloody stool, abdominal swelling, pain in upper right side of stomach area, sleepiness, vomiting of blood). (See Risk of Hepatic Decompensation or Failure in Patients with Evidence of Advanced Liver Disease under Warnings/Precautions: Other Warnings and Precautions, in Cautions.)

If sofosbuvir/velpatasvir/voxilaprevir is used in a patient receiving amiodarone, advise the patient about the risk of serious symptomatic bradycardia and the importance of immediately contacting a clinician if signs or symptoms of bradycardia (e.g., near-fainting or fainting, dizziness, lightheadedness, malaise, weakness, excessive tiredness, shortness of breath, chest pain, confusion, memory problems) occur. (See Cardiovascular Effects under Warnings/Precautions: Other Warnings and Precautions, in Cautions.)

Importance of informing clinicians of existing or contemplated concomitant therapy, including prescription and OTC drugs and dietary or herbal supplements, as well as any concomitant illnesses.

Importance of women informing clinicians if they are or plan to become pregnant or plan to breast-feed.

Importance of informing patients of other important precautionary information. (See Cautions.)

PREPARATIONS

Excipients in commercially available drug preparations may have clinically important effects in some individuals; consult specific product labeling for details.

Sofosbuvir, Velpatasvir, and Voxilaprevir

Oral

Tablets, film-coated	Sofosbuvir 400 mg, Velpatasvir 100 mg, and Voxilaprevir 100 mg	**Vosevi®**, Gilead

† Use is not currently included in the labeling approved by the US Food and Drug Administration.

Selected Revisions February 23, 2022, © Copyright, July 1, 2000, American Society of Health-System Pharmacists, Inc.

Glecaprevir and Pibrentasvir

8:18.40.20 • HCV PROTEASE INHIBITORS

■ Glecaprevir and pibrentasvir (glecaprevir/pibrentasvir) is a fixed combination containing 2 hepatitis C virus (HCV) antivirals; glecaprevir is an HCV nonstructural 3/4A (NS3/4A) protease inhibitor and pibrentasvir is an HCV nonstructural 5A (NS5A) replication complex inhibitor (NS5A inhibitor).

USES

● Chronic Hepatitis C Virus Infection

The fixed combination of glecaprevir and pibrentasvir (glecaprevir/pibrentasvir) is used for the treatment of chronic hepatitis C virus (HCV) genotype 1, 2, 3, 4, 5, or 6 infection in adults and pediatric patients ≥3 years of age without cirrhosis or with compensated cirrhosis (Child-Pugh class A), including liver or kidney transplant recipients and those with human immunodeficiency virus (HIV) coinfection. In patients with HCV genotype 1 infection, glecaprevir/pibrentasvir is indicated in those who previously have been treated with a regimen containing an HCV NS5A inhibitor or an NS3/4A protease inhibitor (PI), but not both.

HCV Genotype 1 Infection

Efficacy and safety of glecaprevir/pibrentasvir for the treatment of chronic HCV genotype 1 infection in adults have been evaluated in at least 5 clinical trials that included more than 1000 patients with HCV genotype 1 infection (ENDURANCE-1, EXPEDITION-1, EXPEDITION-4, EXPEDITION-8, MAGELLAN-1). The primary end point in each study was sustained virologic response at 12 weeks after the end of treatment (SVR12; defined as plasma HCV RNA level less than the lower limit of quantification at 12 weeks after end of treatment).

ENDURANCE-1 (NCT02604017) was an open-label, randomized, phase 3 trial, in 703 treatment-naive or previously treated adults with chronic HCV genotype 1 infection who were noncirrhotic, including patients with HIV type 1 (HIV-1) coinfection (median age 52–53 years, 49% male, 84% white, 4% Black, 13% with baseline HCV RNA levels ≥6 million IU/mL, 38% previously treated). Previously treated patients had treatment experience with regimens containing interferon, peginterferon, ribavirin, and/or sofosbuvir, but no prior treatment experience with an HCV NS3/4A protease inhibitor (PI) or HCV NS5A inhibitor. Patients were randomized in a 1:1 ratio to receive glecaprevir/pibrentasvir (300 mg of glecaprevir and 120 mg of pibrentasvir) once daily for 8 or 12 weeks. SVR12 was achieved in 99.1% of patients treated with the 8-week regimen and 99.7% of those treated with the 12-week regimen.

EXPEDITION-1 (NCT02642432), an open-label, single-arm, phase 3 trial, included 146 treatment-naive or previously treated adults with chronic HCV genotype 1, 2, 4, 5, or 6 infection with compensated cirrhosis (median age 60 years, 62% male, 82% white, 10% Black, 12% with baseline HCV RNA levels 6 million IU/mL or greater, 25% previously treated). Previously treated patients had prior treatment experience with regimens containing interferon, peginterferon, ribavirin, and/or sofosbuvir, but no prior treatment experience with an HCV NS3/4A PI or HCV NS5A inhibitor. All patients received glecaprevir/pibrentasvir (300 mg of glecaprevir and 120 mg of pibrentasvir) once daily for 12 weeks. Of the 90 patients with HCV genotype 1 infection, 99% achieved SVR12.

EXPEDITION-4 (NCT02651194), an open-label, single-arm, phase 3 trial, included 104 treatment-naive or previously treated adults with chronic HCV genotype 1, 2, 3, 4, 5, or 6 infection who were noncirrhotic or had compensated cirrhosis; all patients also had severe renal impairment (chronic kidney disease stages 4 and 5). The median age of patients was 57 years, 76% were male, 62% were white, 24% were Black, 82% were receiving hemodialysis, 19% had compensated cirrhosis, and 42% were previously treated; 53% had HCV genotype 1 infection. Previously treated patients had treatment experience with regimens containing interferon, peginterferon, ribavirin, and/or sofosbuvir, but no prior treatment

experience with an HCV NS3/4A PI or HCV NS5A inhibitor. All patients received glecaprevir/pibrentasvir (300 mg of glecaprevir and 120 mg of pibrentasvir) once daily for 12 weeks. Overall, 98% of patients achieved SVR12. The presence of renal impairment did not affect efficacy of glecaprevir/pibrentasvir; dosage adjustments were not required.

EXPEDITION-8 (NCT03089944), an open-label, single-arm, phase 3 trial, included 343 treatment-naive adults with chronic HCV genotype 1, 2, 3, 4, 5, or 6 infection who had compensated cirrhosis (median age of 58 years, 63% male, 83% white, 8% Black). All patients received glecaprevir/pibrentasvir (300 mg of glecaprevir and 120 mg of pibrentasvir) once daily for 8 weeks. SVR12 was achieved in 98% of the 231 patients with HCV genotype 1 infection.

MAGELLAN-1 (NCT02446717), a multi-part, randomized, open-label, phase 2 trial, included adults with HCV genotype 1 or 4 infection who previously failed a treatment regimen containing an HCV NS5A inhibitor and/or HCV NS3/4A PI. In part 1 of the trial, 50 patients with HCV genotype 1 infection were randomized to receive a 12-week regimen of glecaprevir/pibrentasvir (200 mg of glecaprevir and 80 mg of pibrentasvir) once daily (arm A), glecaprevir/pibrentasvir (300 mg of glecaprevir and 120 mg of pibrentasvir) once daily in conjunction with ribavirin (arm B), or glecaprevir/pibrentasvir (300 mg of glecaprevir and 120 mg of pibrentasvir) once daily (arm C). The protocol was later amended to halt enrollment for arm A (lower dosage) so that glecaprevir/pibrentasvir dosage was optimized. In part 2 of the trial, 91 patients with HCV genotype 1 or 4 infection who were noncirrhotic or had compensated cirrhosis were randomized in a 1:1 ratio to receive glecaprevir/pibrentasvir (300 mg of glecaprevir and 120 mg of pibrentasvir) once daily for 12 or 16 weeks (arms D and E, respectively). The median age of patients was 56 years, 75% were male, 72% were white, 26% were Black, 97% had HCV genotype 1 infection, 33% were previously treated with an HCV NS5A inhibitor *and* an HCV NS3/4A PI, 30% were previously treated with an HCV NS5A inhibitor (HCV NS3/4A inhibitor-naive), 37% were previously treated with an HCV NS3/4A PI (HCV NS5A inhibitor-naive), and 19% had compensated cirrhosis. In HCV NS5A inhibitor-experienced (HCV NS3/4A PI-naive) patients, SVR12 was achieved in 90 or 94% of those who received the 12- or 16-week treatment regimen, respectively. In HCV NS3/4A PI-experienced (HCV NS5A inhibitor-naive) patients, SVR12 was achieved in 92 or 100% of those who received the 12- or 16-week treatment regimen, respectively. Those who were previously treated with an HCV NS5A inhibitor *and* an HCV NS3/4A PI and received either 12 or 16 weeks of treatment had SVR12 rates of 80% and these patients had higher rates of virologic failure and treatment-emergent drug resistance compared with the other patient groups. Because of higher rates of virologic failure and treatment-emergent drug resistance, data do not support use of glecaprevir/pibrentasvir for treatment of HCV genotype 1 infection in patients who failed previous treatment with a regimen containing both an HCV NS5A inhibitor *and* an HCV NS3/4A PI.

HCV Genotype 2 Infection

Efficacy and safety of glecaprevir/pibrentasvir for the treatment of chronic HCV genotype 2 infection in adults have been evaluated in at least 4 clinical trials that included approximately 270 patients with HCV genotype 2 infection (SURVEYOR-2, EXPEDITION-1, EXPEDITION-4, EXPEDITION-8). The primary end point in each study was sustained virologic response at 12 weeks after the end of treatment (SVR12; defined as plasma HCV RNA level less than the lower limit of quantification at 12 weeks after end of treatment).

SURVEYOR-2 (NCT02243293), a multi-arm, multi-part, open-label, phase 2 trial, evaluated glecaprevir/pibrentasvir with or without ribavirin in adults with HCV genotype 2, 3, 4, 5, or 6 infection who were treatment naive or previously treated, including those with compensated cirrhosis. Previously treated patients had treatment experience with regimens containing interferon, peginterferon, ribavirin, and/or sofosbuvir, but no prior treatment experience with an HCV NS3/4A PI or HCV NS5A inhibitor. Part 2 of the study included 54 noncirrhotic patients with HCV genotype 2 infection and part 4 of the study included 143 noncirrhotic patients with genotype 2 infection (a total of 197 patients in part 2 and part 4 combined). All 197 of these patients received glecaprevir/pibrentasvir (300 mg of glecaprevir and 120 mg of pibrentasvir) for 8 weeks. SVR12 was achieved in 98% of patients with HCV genotype 2 infection (part 2 and part 4 combined).

EXPEDITION-1 (NCT02642432), an open-label, single-arm, phase 3 trial, included 146 treatment-naive or previously treated adults with chronic HCV genotype 1, 2, 4, 5, or 6 infection with compensated cirrhosis (median age 60 years, 62% male, 82% white, 10% Black, 12% with baseline HCV RNA levels ≥6 million IU/m, 25% previously treated). Previously treated patients had received prior regimens containing interferon, peginterferon, ribavirin, and/or sofosbuvir, but had no prior treatment experience with an HCV NS3/4A PI or HCV NS5A inhibitor. All patients received glecaprevir/pibrentasvir (300 mg of glecaprevir and 120 mg of pibrentasvir) once daily for 12 weeks. Of the 31 patients with HCV genotype 2 infection, 100% achieved SVR12.

EXPEDITION-4 (NCT02651194), an open-label, single-arm, phase 3 trial, included 104 treatment-naive or previously treated adults with chronic HCV genotype 1, 2, 3, 4, 5, or 6 infection who were noncirrhotic or had compensated cirrhosis; all patients also had severe renal impairment (chronic kidney disease stages 4 and 5). The median age of patients was 57 years; 76% were male, 62% were white, 24% were Black, 82% were receiving hemodialysis, 19% had compensated cirrhosis, and 42% were previously treated; 15% had HCV genotype 2 infection. Previously treated patients had received regimens containing interferon, peginterferon, ribavirin, and/or sofosbuvir, but had no prior treatment experience with an HCV NS3/4A PI or HCV NS5A inhibitor. All patients received glecaprevir/pibrentasvir (300 mg of glecaprevir and 120 mg of pibrentasvir) once daily for 12 weeks. Overall, 98% of patients achieved SVR12 and no subjects experienced virologic failure. The presence of renal impairment did not affect the efficacy of glecaprevir/pibrentasvir and dosage adjustments were not required.

EXPEDITION-8 (NCT03089944), an open-label, single-arm, phase 3 trial, included 343 treatment-naive adults with chronic HCV genotype 1, 2, 3, 4, 5, or 6 infection who had compensated cirrhosis. The median age of patients was 58 years; 63% of patients were male, 83% were white, and 8% were Black. All patients received glecaprevir/pibrentasvir (300 mg of glecaprevir and 120 mg of pibrentasvir) once daily for 8 weeks. SVR12 was achieved in 100% of the 26 patients with HCV genotype 2 infection.

HCV Genotype 3 Infection

Efficacy and safety of glecaprevir/pibrentasvir for the treatment of chronic HCV genotype 3 infection in adults have been evaluated in at least 4 clinical trials that included approximately 375 patients with HCV genotype 3 infection (ENDURANCE-3, SURVEYOR-2, EXPEDITION-4, EXPEDITION-8). The primary end point in each study was sustained virologic response at 12 weeks after the end of treatment (SVR12; defined as plasma HCV RNA level less than the lower limit of quantification at 12 weeks after end of treatment).

ENDURANCE-3 (NCT02640157), a partially randomized, open-label, active-controlled, phase 3 trial, evaluated the efficacy of glecaprevir/pibrentasvir in treatment-naive, noncirrhotic patients with HCV genotype 3 infection (median age 47–49 years, 52% male, 88% white, 2% Black, 22% with baseline HCV RNA levels 6 million IU/mL or greater). Patients were randomized in a 2:1 ratio to receive glecaprevir/pibrentasvir (300 mg of glecaprevir and 120 mg of pibrentasvir) once daily for 12 weeks or a regimen of sofosbuvir in conjunction with daclatasvir for 12 weeks. The study subsequently included an additional nonrandomized study arm evaluating an 8-week regimen of glecaprevir/pibrentasvir (300 mg of glecaprevir and 120 mg of pibrentasvir) once daily. SVR12 was achieved in 95 or 97% of patients with HCV genotype 3 infection treated with glecaprevir/pibrentasvir or a regimen of sofosbuvir in conjunction with daclatasvir, respectively. SVR12 was achieved in 95% of those in the nonrandomized arm treated with an 8-week regimen of glecaprevir/pibrentasvir. These data indicated that 8- and 12-week regimens of glecaprevir/pibrentasvir have similar efficacy in noncirrhotic patients with HCV genotype 3 infection.

SURVEYOR-2 (NCT02243293), a multi-arm, multi-part, open-label, phase 2 trial, evaluated glecaprevir/pibrentasvir with or without ribavirin in adults with HCV genotype 2, 3, 4, 5, or 6 infection who were treatment-naive or previously treated, including those with compensated cirrhosis. Previously treated patients had received regimens containing interferon, peginterferon, ribavirin, and/or sofosbuvir, but had no prior treatment experience with an HCV NS3/4A protease inhibitor or HCV NS5A inhibitor. In part 3 of the study, previously treated, noncirrhotic patients with HCV genotype 3 infection were randomized to receive glecaprevir/pibrentasvir (300 mg of glecaprevir and 120 mg of pibrentasvir) once daily for 12 or 16 weeks. In addition, a 12- or 16- week regimen of glecaprevir/pibrentasvir (300 mg of glecaprevir and 120 mg of pibrentasvir) once daily was evaluated in patients with HCV genotype 3 infection who had compensated cirrhosis and were treatment naive or previously treated, respectively. In a pooled

analysis of all previously treated patients with HCV genotype 3 infection (with or without compensated cirrhosis), SVR12 was achieved in 96% of patients.

EXPEDITION-4 (NCT02651194), an open-label, single-arm, phase 3 trial, included 104 treatment-naive or previously treated adults with chronic HCV genotype 1, 2, 3, 4, 5, or 6 infection who were noncirrhotic or had compensated cirrhosis; all patients also had severe renal impairment (chronic kidney disease stages 4 and 5). The median age of patients was 57 years, 76% were male, 62% were white, 24% were Black, 82% were receiving hemodialysis, 19% had compensated cirrhosis, and 42% were previously treated; 11% had HCV genotype 3 infection. Previously treated patients had received regimens containing interferon, peginterferon, ribavirin, and/or sofosbuvir, but had no prior treatment experience with an HCV NS3/4A PI or HCV NS5A inhibitor. All patients received glecaprevir/pibrentasvir (300 mg of glecaprevir and 120 mg of pibrentasvir) once daily for 12 weeks. Overall, 98% of patients achieved SVR12 and no subjects experienced virologic failure. The presence of renal impairment did not affect the efficacy of glecaprevir/pibrentasvir and dosage adjustments were not required.

EXPEDITION-8 (NCT03089944), an open-label, single-arm, phase 3 trial, included 343 treatment-naive adults with chronic HCV genotype 1, 2, 3, 4, 5, or 6 infection who had compensated cirrhosis (median age 58 years, 63% male, 83% white, 8% Black). All patients received glecaprevir/pibrentasvir (300 mg of glecaprevir and 120 mg of pibrentasvir) once daily for 8 weeks. SVR12 was achieved in 95% of the 63 patients with HCV genotype 3 infection.

Patients (treatment naive or previously treated) with genotype 3 HCV infection were also included in 2 Asian regional studies (VOYAGE-1 and VOYAGE-2). VOYAGE-1 was a randomized, double-blind, placebo-controlled study enrolling patients without cirrhosis from China, South Korea, and Singapore. VOYAGE-2 was a single-arm, open-label study enrolling patients with compensated cirrhosis from China and South Korea. Patients in both trials received 300 mg of glecaprevir and 120 mg of pibrentasvir once daily; treatment duration was 8 weeks in patients without cirrhosis, 12 weeks in patients with cirrhosis, and 16 weeks in treatment-experienced patients with HCV genotype 3. The primary end point of SVR12 was achieved in 97.2% of patients in VOYAGE-1 and 99.4% of patients in VOYAGE-2. In a pooled analysis of both trials, 70% of 20 patients with HCV genotype 3b achieved SVR12; SVR12 was achieved in 58% of patients without cirrhosis and in 88% of patients with compensated cirrhosis. All 6 patients with genotype 3b who did not achieve SVR12 experienced virologic failure.

HCV Genotype 4 Infection

Efficacy and safety of glecaprevir/pibrentasvir for the treatment of chronic HCV genotype 4 infection in adults have been evaluated in at least 5 clinical trials that included approximately 170 patients with HCV genotype 4 infection (SURVEYOR-2, ENDURANCE-4, EXPEDITION-1, EXPEDITION-4, EXPEDITION-8). The primary end point in each study was sustained virologic response at 12 weeks after the end of treatment (SVR12; defined as plasma HCV RNA level less than the lower limit of quantification at 12 weeks after end of treatment).

SURVEYOR-2 (NCT02243293), a multi-arm, multi-part, open-label, phase 2 trial, evaluated glecaprevir/pibrentasvir with or without ribavirin in adults with HCV genotype 2, 3, 4, 5, or 6 infection who were treatment naive or previously treated, including those with compensated cirrhosis. Previously treated patients had treatment experience with regimens containing interferon, peginterferon, ribavirin, and/or sofosbuvir, but no prior treatment experience with an HCV NS3/4A protease inhibitor or HCV NS5A inhibitor. In one arm of the study, there were 46 patients with HCV genotype 4 infection; 39 were treatment naive and 7 were previously treated. All 46 patients received glecaprevir/pibrentasvir (300 mg of glecaprevir and 120 mg of pibrentasvir) once daily for 8 weeks. SVR12 was achieved in 93% of patients with HCV genotype 4 infection.

ENDURANCE-4 (NCT02636595), a single-arm, open-label, phase 3 trial, evaluated the efficacy and safety of glecaprevir/pibrentasvir in noncirrhotic treatment-naive and previously treated patients with HCV genotype 4, 5, or 6 infection. Previously treated patients had prior treatment experience with regimens containing interferon, peginterferon, ribavirin, and/or sofosbuvir, but no prior treatment experience with an HCV NS3/4A protease inhibitor or HCV NS5A inhibitor. There were 76 patients with HCV genotype 4 infection; 45 were treatment naive and 31 were previously treated. All 76 patients received glecaprevir/pibrentasvir (300 mg of glecaprevir and 120 mg of pibrentasvir) once daily for 12 weeks. SVR12 was achieved in 99% of patients with HCV genotype 4 infection.

EXPEDITION-1 (NCT02642432), an open-label, single-arm, phase 3 trial, included 146 treatment-naive or previously treated adults with chronic HCV genotype 1, 2, 4, 5, or 6 infection with compensated cirrhosis (median age 60 years, 62% male, 82% white, 10% Black, 12% with baseline HCV RNA levels 6 million IU/mL or greater, 25% previously treated). Previously treated patients had prior treatment experience with regimens containing interferon, peginterferon, ribavirin, and/or sofosbuvir, but no prior treatment experience with an HCV NS3/4A protease inhibitor or HCV NS5A inhibitor. All patients received glecaprevir/pibrentasvir (300 mg of glecaprevir and 120 mg of pibrentasvir) once daily for 12 weeks. Of the 16 patients with HCV genotype 4 infection, 100% achieved SVR12.

EXPEDITION-4 (NCT02651194), an open-label, single-arm, phase 3 trial, included 104 treatment-naive or previously treated adults with chronic HCV genotype 1, 2, 3, 4, 5, or 6 infection who were noncirrhotic or had compensated cirrhosis; all patients also had severe renal impairment (chronic kidney disease stages 4 and 5). Patients had a median age of 57 years, 76% were male, 62% were white, 24% were Black, 82% were receiving hemodialysis, 19% had compensated cirrhosis, and 42% were previously treated; 19% had HCV genotype 4 infection. Previously treated patients had treatment experience with regimens containing interferon, peginterferon, ribavirin, and/or sofosbuvir, but no prior treatment experience with an HCV NS3/4A protease inhibitor or HCV NS5A inhibitor. All patients received glecaprevir/pibrentasvir (300 mg of glecaprevir and 120 mg of pibrentasvir) once daily for 12 weeks. Overall, 98% of patients achieved SVR12 and no subjects experienced virologic failure. The presence of renal impairment did not affect the efficacy of glecaprevir/pibrentasvir and dosage adjustments were not required.

EXPEDITION-8 (NCT03089944), an open-label, single-arm, phase 3 trial, included 343 treatment-naive adults with chronic HCV genotype 1, 2, 3, 4, 5, or 6 infection who had compensated cirrhosis. Patients had a median age of 58 years, 63% were male, 83% were white, and 8% were Black. All patients received glecaprevir/pibrentasvir (300 mg of glecaprevir and 120 mg of pibrentasvir) once daily for 8 weeks. SVR12 was achieved in 100% of the 13 patients with HCV genotype 4 infection.

HCV Genotype 5 Infection

Efficacy and safety of glecaprevir/pibrentasvir for the treatment of chronic HCV genotype 5 infection in adults have been evaluated in at least 6 clinical trials that included approximately 54 patients with HCV genotype 5 infection (SURVEYOR-2, ENDURANCE-4, ENDURANCE-5,6, EXPEDITION-1, EXPEDITION-4, EXPEDITION-8). The primary end point in each study was sustained virologic response at 12 weeks after the end of treatment (SVR12; defined as plasma HCV RNA level less than the lower limit of quantification at 12 weeks after end of treatment).

SURVEYOR-2 (NCT02243293), a multi-arm, multi-part, open-label, phase 2 trial, evaluated glecaprevir/pibrentasvir with or without ribavirin in adults with HCV genotype 2, 3, 4, 5, or 6 infection who were treatment naive or previously treated, including those with compensated cirrhosis. Previously treated patients had received regimens containing interferon, peginterferon, ribavirin, and/or sofosbuvir, but had no prior treatment experience with an HCV NS3/4A protease inhibitor or HCV NS5A inhibitor. There were 2 patients with HCV genotype 5 infection who received glecaprevir/pibrentasvir (300 mg of glecaprevir and 120 mg of pibrentasvir) once daily for 8 weeks. SVR12 was achieved in both patient.

ENDURANCE-4 (NCT02636595), a single-arm, open-label, phase 3 trial, evaluated the efficacy and safety of glecaprevir/pibrentasvir in noncirrhotic treatment-naive and previously treated patients with HCV genotype 4, 5, or 6 infection. Previously treated patients had received regimens containing interferon, peginterferon, ribavirin, and/or sofosbuvir, but had no prior treatment experience with an HCV NS3/4A protease inhibitor or HCV NS5A inhibitor. There were 26 patients with HCV genotype 5 infection; 20 were treatment naive and 6 were previously treated. All 26 patients received glecaprevir/pibrentasvir (300 mg of glecaprevir and 120 mg of pibrentasvir) once daily for 12 weeks. SVR12 was achieved in 100% of patients with HCV genotype 5 infection.

EXPEDITION-1 (NCT02642432), an open-label, single-arm, phase 3 trial, included 146 treatment-naive or previously treated adults with chronic HCV genotype 1, 2, 4, 5, or 6 infection with compensated cirrhosis (median age 60 years, 62% male, 82% white, 10% Black, 12% with baseline HCV RNA levels ≥6 million IU/mL, 25% previously treated). Previously treated patients had received regimens containing interferon, peginterferon, ribavirin, and/or sofosbuvir, but had

no prior treatment experience with an HCV NS3/4A protease inhibitor or HCV NS5A inhibitor. All patients received glecaprevir/pibrentasvir (300 mg of glecaprevir and 120 mg of pibrentasvir) once daily for 12 weeks. Of the 2 patients with HCV genotype 5 infection, both achieved SVR12.

EXPEDITION-4 (NCT02651194), an open-label, single-arm, phase 3 trial, included 104 treatment-naive or previously treated adults with chronic HCV genotype 1, 2, 3, 4, 5, or 6 infection who were noncirrhotic or had compensated cirrhosis; all patients also had severe renal impairment (chronic kidney disease stages 4 and 5). The median age of patients was 57 years, 76% were male, 62% were white, 24% were Black, 82% were receiving hemodialysis, 19% had compensated cirrhosis, and 42% were previously treated; 1% had HCV genotype 5 infection. All patients received glecaprevir/pibrentasvir (300 mg of glecaprevir and 120 mg of pibrentasvir) once daily for 12 weeks. Overall, 98% of patients achieved SVR12 and no subjects experienced virologic failure. The presence of renal impairment did not affect the efficacy of glecaprevir/pibrentasvir and dosage adjustments were not required.

ENDURANCE-5,6 (NCT02966795), an open-label, single-arm, phase 3b trial, included 84 treatment-naive or previously treated adults with chronic HCV genotype 5 or 6 infection who were noncirrhotic or had compensated cirrhosis. Of the 23 patients with HCV genotype 5 infection, median age was 68 years, 43% were male, 91% were white, 13% had compensated cirrhosis, and 17% were previously treated. Noncirrhotic patients received glecaprevir/pibrentasvir (300 mg of glecaprevir and 120 mg of pibrentasvir) once daily for 8 weeks and those with compensated cirrhosis received the same glecaprevir/pibrentasvir dosage for 12 weeks. Of the patients with HCV genotype 5 infection, 95.7% achieved SVR12.

EXPEDITION-8 (NCT03089944), an open-label, single-arm, phase 3 trial, included 343 treatment-naive adults with chronic HCV genotype 1, 2, 3, 4, 5, or 6 infection who had compensated cirrhosis. Patients had a median age of 58 years, 63% were male, 83% were white, and 8% were Black. All patients received glecaprevir/pibrentasvir (300 mg of glecaprevir and 120 mg of pibrentasvir) once daily for 8 weeks. SVR12 was achieved in the single patient with HCV genotype 5 infection.

HCV Genotype 6 Infection

Efficacy and safety of glecaprevir/pibrentasvir for the treatment of chronic HCV genotype 6 infection in adults have been evaluated in at least 6 clinical trials that included approximately 107 patients with HCV genotype 6 infection (SURVEYOR-2, ENDURANCE-4, ENDURANCE-5,6, EXPEDITION-1, EXPEDITION-4, EXPEDITION-8). The primary end point in each study was sustained virologic response at 12 weeks after the end of treatment (SVR12; defined as plasma HCV RNA level less than the lower limit of quantification at 12 weeks after end of treatment).

SURVEYOR-2 (NCT02243293), a multi-arm, multi-part, open-label, phase 2 trial, evaluated glecaprevir/pibrentasvir with or without ribavirin in adults with HCV genotype 2, 3, 4, 5, or 6 infection who were treatment naive or previously treated, including those with compensated cirrhosis. Previously treated patients had treatment experience with regimens containing interferon, peginterferon, ribavirin, and/or sofosbuvir, but no prior treatment experience with an HCV NS3/4A protease inhibitor or HCV NS5A inhibitor. There were 10 patients with HCV genotype 6 infection; 8 were treatment naive and 2 were previously treated. All 10 patients received glecaprevir/pibrentasvir (300 mg of glecaprevir and 120 mg of pibrentasvir) once daily for 8 weeks. SVR12 was achieved in 88% of patients with HCV genotype 6 infection.

ENDURANCE-4 (NCT02636595), a single-arm, open-label, phase 3 trial, evaluated the efficacy and safety of glecaprevir/pibrentasvir in noncirrhotic treatment-naive and previously treated patients with HCV genotype 4, 5, or 6 infection. Previously treated patients had treatment experience with regimens containing interferon, peginterferon, ribavirin, and/or sofosbuvir, but no prior treatment experience with an HCV NS3/4A protease inhibitor or HCV NS5A inhibitor. There were 19 patients with HCV genotype 6 infection; 17 were treatment naive and 2 were previously treated. All 19 patients received glecaprevir/pibrentasvir (300 mg of glecaprevir and 120 mg of pibrentasvir) once daily for 12 weeks. SVR12 was achieved in 100% of patients with HCV genotype 6 infection.

EXPEDITION-1 (NCT02642432), an open-label, single-arm, phase 3 trial, included 146 treatment-naive or previously treated adults with chronic HCV genotype 1, 2, 4, 5, or 6 infection with compensated cirrhosis (median age 60 years, 62% male, 82% white, 10% Black, 12% with baseline HCV RNA levels ≥6 million

IU/mL, 25% previously treated). Previously treated patients had received regimens containing interferon, peginterferon, ribavirin, and/or sofosbuvir, but had no prior treatment experience with an HCV NS3/4A protease inhibitor or HCV NS5A inhibitor. All patients received glecaprevir/pibrentasvir (300 mg of glecaprevir and 120 mg of pibrentasvir) once daily for 12 weeks. Of the 7 patients with HCV genotype 6 infection, 100% achieved SVR12.

EXPEDITION-4 (NCT02651194), an open-label, single-arm, phase 3 trial, included 104 treatment-naive or previously treated adults with chronic HCV genotype 1, 2, 3, 4, 5, or 6 infection who were noncirrhotic or had compensated cirrhosis; all patients also had severe renal impairment (chronic kidney disease stages 4 and 5). The median age of patients was 57 years, 76% were male, 62% were white, 24% were Black, 82% were receiving hemodialysis, 19% had compensated cirrhosis, and 42% were previously treated; 1% had HCV genotype 6 infection. All patients received glecaprevir/pibrentasvir (300 mg of glecaprevir and 120 mg of pibrentasvir) once daily for 12 weeks. Overall, 98% of patients achieved SVR12 and no subjects experienced virologic failure. The presence of renal impairment did not affect the efficacy of glecaprevir/pibrentasvir and dosage adjustments were not required.

ENDURANCE-5,6 (NCT02966795), an open-label, single-arm, phase 3b trial, included 84 treatment-naive or previously treated adults with chronic HCV genotype 5 or 6 infection who were noncirrhotic or had compensated cirrhosis. Of the 61 patients with HCV genotype 6 infection, median age was 54 years, 48% were male, 7% were white, 92% were Asian, 10% had compensated cirrhosis, and 7% were previously treated. Noncirrhotic patients received glecaprevir/pibrentasvir (300 mg of glecaprevir and 120 mg of pibrentasvir) once daily for 8 weeks and those with compensated cirrhosis received the same glecaprevir/pibrentasvir dosage for 12 weeks. Of the patients with HCV genotype 6 infection, 98.4% achieved SVR12.

EXPEDITION-8 (NCT03089944), an open-label, single-arm, phase 3 trial, included 343 treatment-naive adults with chronic HCV genotype 1, 2, 3, 4, 5, or 6 infection who had compensated cirrhosis. The median age of patients was 58 years, 63% were male, 83% were white, and 8% were Black. All patients received glecaprevir/pibrentasvir (300 mg of glecaprevir and 120 mg of pibrentasvir) once daily for 8 weeks. SVR12 was achieved in 100% of the 9 patients with HCV genotype 6 infection.

Transplant Recipients

Efficacy and safety of glecaprevir/pibrentasvir for the treatment of chronic HCV genotype 1, 2, 3, 4, or 6 infection in treatment-naive or previously treated adults who were noncirrhotic and had received a kidney or liver transplant were evaluated in a single-arm, open-label, phase 3 clinical trial (MAGELLAN-2; NCT02692703). Of the 100 patients included in the study, 66% were treatment-naive and 34% were previously treated with interferon, peginterferon, ribavirin, and/ or sofosbuvir; all patients with HCV genotype 3 infection were treatment-naive. The median age of patients was 60 years, 75% were male, 8% were Black, 80% had received liver transplants, 20% had received kidney transplants, and 11% had normal renal function at baseline; 57, 13, 24, 4, or 2% had HCV genotype 1, 2, 3, 4, or 6 infection, respectively. All patients received glecaprevir/pibrentasvir (300 mg of glecaprevir and 120 mg of pibrentasvir) once daily for 12 weeks. Concomitant use of immunosuppressive agents was allowed (e.g., cyclosporine [dosage <100 mg daily], tacrolimus, sirolimus, everolimus, azathioprine, mycophenolic acid, low-dose corticosteroids [prednisone or prednisolone dosage ≤10 mg daily at baseline]). The primary end point was sustained virologic response at 12 weeks after end of treatment (SVR12; defined as plasma HCV RNA level less than the lower limit of quantification at 12 weeks after end of treatment). SVR12 was achieved in 98% of patients; one patient experienced relapse and no patients experienced on-treatment virologic failure.

In another open-label, prospective study (MYTHIC) evaluating the efficacy and safety of glecaprevir/pibrentasvir for the treatment of HCV-negative patients 21–65 years of age, 30 of the 63 patients who underwent kidney transplantation were recipients of transplanted kidneys from donors with HCV infection. The median age of these patients was 57 years, 70% were male, 30% were Black, and the most common cause of end-stage renal disease was diabetes and/or hypertension (66.7%). Patients received glecaprevir/pibrentasvir (300 mg of glecaprevir and 120 mg of pibrentasvir) once daily for 8 weeks, starting 2 to 5 days after transplant. At baseline, 23 of 29 patients had detectable plasma HCV RNA viral loads. All 30 patients (100%) achieved the primary end point of SVR12; no patients had a detectable viral load by week 4 of treatment.

HCV-infected Individuals Coinfected with HIV

Efficacy and safety of glecaprevir/pibrentasvir for the treatment of chronic HCV infection in adults with HIV coinfection have been evaluated in 2 clinical trials (ENDURANCE-1, EXPEDITION-2). The primary end point in each study was sustained virologic response at 12 weeks after end of treatment (SVR12; defined as plasma HCV RNA level less than the lower limit of quantification at 12 weeks after end of treatment).

ENDURANCE-1 (NCT02604017), an open-label, randomized, phase 3 trial, included 703 treatment-naive or previously treated adults with chronic HCV genotype 1 infection who were noncirrhotic, including 33 patients with HIV-1 coinfection. Previously treated patients had treatment experience with regimens containing interferon, peginterferon, ribavirin, and/or sofosbuvir, but no prior treatment experience with an HCV NS3/4A protease inhibitor or HCV NS5A inhibitor. Patients were randomized in a 1:1 ratio to receive glecaprevir/pibrentasvir (300 mg of glecaprevir and 120 mg of pibrentasvir) once daily for 8 or 12 weeks. Overall, SVR12 was achieved in 99.1% of patients treated with the 8-week regimen and 99.7% of those treated with the 12-week regimen. In the subset of patients with HIV-1 coinfection, 100% achieved SVR12.

EXPEDITION-2 (NCT02738138), a nonrandomized, open-label, phase 3 trial, included 153 treatment-naive or previously treated adults with chronic HCV infection and HIV-1 coinfection. Previously treated patients had treatment experience with regimens containing interferon, peginterferon, ribavirin, and/or sofosbuvir. The median age of patients was 45 years, 84% were male, 16% were Black, and 11% had compensated cirrhosis; 63, 7, 17, 11, or 2% had HCV genotype 1, 2, 3, 4, or 6 infection, respectively. All patients with HCV genotype 3 infection were treatment-naive. Noncirrhotic patients or those with compensated cirrhosis received glecaprevir/pibrentasvir (300 mg of glecaprevir and 120 mg of pibrentasvir) once daily for 8 or 12 weeks, respectively. SVR12 was achieved in 98% of patients with HCV and HIV-1 coinfection (100% of noncirrhotic patients and 93% of patients with compensated cirrhosis).

Persons Who Inject Drugs (PWID) or Receive Medication-Assisted Treatment (MAT) for Opioid Use Disorder

Of 4655 adolescents and adults with chronic HCV genotype 1, 2, 3, 4, 5, or 6 infection who received glecaprevir/pibrentasvir in phase 2 and 3 trials, 1373 patients self-reported use of injection drugs (62 and 959 patients reported current/recent and former use of injection drugs, respectively, and 352 patients who did not specify the timing of injection drug use were excluded from the analysis) and 3282 patients did not report injection drug use (non-PWID). The overall SVR12 rate was 98% in former PWID/non-PWID patients compared to 89% in current/recent PWID patients; the difference between the two groups was primarily due to missing data at the time of the SVR12 measurement window in the current/recent PWID group. Virologic failure rates, however, were similar in both groups: 2% in current/recent users and 1% in former PWIDs/non-PWIDs.

In this study, 225 patients reported concomitant use of MAT for opioid use disorder and 4098 patients reported no use of MAT. Among the patients receiving concomitant MAT, 74% were non-cirrhotic, and 7% were co-infected with HIV, similar to those not on MAT. The SVR12 rates were similar between subjects on MAT (96%) and those not on MAT (98%), with low rates of virologic failure in both groups (<1% and 1%, respectively).

Pediatric Patients

Efficacy and safety of glecaprevir/pibrentasvir for the treatment of chronic HCV infection in treatment-naive or previously treated noncirrhotic pediatric patients 12 to <18 years of age were evaluated in a nonrandomized, open-label, phase 2/3 trial (DORA [Part 1]; NCT03067129). Patients received glecaprevir/pibrentasvir (300 mg of glecaprevir and 120 mg of pibrentasvir) once daily for 8 or 16 weeks; treatment duration was chosen to match adult durations based on HCV genotype and prior treatment experience. Of the 47 patients included in the study, median age was 14 years (range: 12–17 years), mean weight was 59 kg (range: 32–109 kg), 55% were female, 9% were Black, 77% were treatment-naive, 23% were previously treated with interferon, and 4% had HIV-1 coinfection; 79, 6, 9, or 6% had HCV genotype 1, 2, 3, or 4 infection, respectively. The primary end point was sustained virologic response at 12 weeks after end of treatment (SVR12; defined as plasma HCV RNA level less than the lower limit of quantification at 12 weeks after end of treatment). The overall SVR12 rate in these pediatric patients was 100%.

Part 2 of the DORA trial evaluated efficacy and safety of glecaprevir/pibrentasvir oral pellets in 80 children 3 to <12 years of age with chronic HCV with genotype 1, 2, 3, 4, 5, or 6. Patients were divided into 3 cohorts based on age: 9 to <12 years of age, 6 to <9 years of age, and 3 to <6 years of age. Patients received glecaprevir/pibrentasvir oral film-coated pellets mixed with 1 to 2 teaspoonfuls of a soft food, such as hazelnut spread, Greek yogurt, or peanut butter. Dosing of glecaprevir/pibrentasvir was based on weight. The median age of the 80 patients included in the study was 7 years (range: 3–11 years), mean weight was 26 kg (range: 13–44 kg), 55% were female, 4% were Black, 97.5% were treatment-naive, 2.5% were previously treated with interferon, 1% had HIV-1 coinfection, and none had cirrhosis; 73, 3, 23, or 3% had HCV genotype 1, 2, 3, or 4 infection, respectively. Overall, 98.4% of patients who received the recommended weight-based dosage achieved SVR12.

Clinical Perspective

Because the treatment of chronic HCV infection is complex and rapidly evolving, it is recommended that treatment be directed by clinicians who are familiar with the disease and that a specialist be consulted to obtain the most up-to-date information. Information from the American Association for the Study of Liver Diseases (AASLD) and Infectious Diseases Society of America (IDSA) regarding diagnosis and management of HCV infection, including recommendations for initial treatment, is available at https://www.hcvguidelines.org.

DOSAGE AND ADMINISTRATION

● General

Pretreatment Screening

● Prior to initiating glecaprevir/pibrentasvir, test all patients for evidence of current or prior HBV infection by measuring hepatitis B surface antigen (HBsAg) and hepatitis B core antibody (anti-HBc).

Patient Monitoring

● In patients with serologic evidence of HBV infection, monitor for clinical and laboratory signs of hepatitis flare or HBV reaction both during and after treatment with glecaprevir/pibrentasvir.

● Monitor patients with compensated cirrhosis (Child-Pugh A) or evidence of advanced liver disease (e.g., portal hypertension) for signs and symptoms of hepatic decompensation (e.g., jaundice, ascites, hepatic encephalopathy, variceal hemorrhage) during treatment with glecaprevir/pibrentasvir.

● Administration

Glecaprevir/pibrentasvir is administered orally once daily with food. The fixed-combination drug is commercially available as film-coated tablets and oral pellets.The pellets must be swallowed whole, and should not be crushed or chewed.

Preparation and Administration of Glecaprevir/Pibrentasvir Oral Pellets

Administer glecaprevir/pibrentasvir pellets with a small amount of soft food that has low water content and will stick to a spoon (e.g., peanut butter, chocolate hazelnut spread, cream cheese, thick jam, Greek yogurt). The pellets should not be mixed with liquids or foods that can drip or slide off a spoon as the drug may dissolve more readily and become less effective when mixed with foods with higher water content. Sprinkle the entire contents of the appropriate number of packets containing glecaprevir/pibrentasvir pellets onto the food. Do not crush or chew the pellets. The entire mixture should be swallowed within 15 minutes after preparation. No pellets should remain in the packet(s). Discard any unused portion of the mixture.

● Dosage

Glecaprevir/pibrentasvir is commercially available as fixed-combination tablets containing 100 mg of glecaprevir and 40 mg of pibrentasvir in each tablet, and fixed-combination pellets containing 50 mg of glecaprevir and 20 mg of pibrentasvir in each packet.

Adult Dosage

HCV Genotype 1, 2, 3, 4, 5, or 6 Infection

For the treatment of chronic HCV genotype 1, 2, 3, 4, 5, or 6 infection in treatment-naive (previously untreated) or previously treated adults without cirrhosis or with compensated cirrhosis (Child-Pugh class A), the recommended dosage of glecaprevir/pibrentasvir is 3 tablets (total of 300 mg of glecaprevir and 120 mg of pibrentasvir) once daily. The treatment duration depends on the HCV genotype, the patient's previous HCV treatment experience, and presence of cirrhosis. (See Tables 1 and 2.)

TABLE 1. Recommended Treatment Duration of Glecaprevir/Pibrentasvir in Treatment-naive Adults with HCV Genotype 1, 2, 3, 4, 5, or 6 Infection.

HCV Genotype	Hepatic Impairment	Duration of Glecaprevir/Pibrentasvir
HCV genotype 1, 2, 3, 4, 5, or 6 infection	Noncirrhotic	8 weeks
	Compensated cirrhosis (Child-Pugh class A)	8 weeks

TABLE 2. Recommended Treatment Duration of Glecaprevir/Pibrentasvir in Previously Treated Adults with HCV Genotype 1, 2, 3, 4, 5, or 6 Infection.

HCV Genotype	Treatment Experience	Hepatic Impairment	Duration of Glecaprevir/Pibrentasvir
HCV genotype 1 infection	Previously treated without HCV NS3/4A protease inhibitors or HCV NS5A inhibitors[a]	Noncirrhotic	8 weeks
		Compensated cirrhosis (Child-Pugh class A)	12 weeks
	Previously treated with an HCV NS5A inhibitor; no prior treatment with HCV NS3/4A protease inhibitors[b]	Noncirrhotic	16 weeks
		Compensated cirrhosis	16 weeks
	Previously treated with an HCV NS3/4A protease inhibitor; no prior treatment with HCV NS5A inhibitors[c]	Noncirrhotic	12 weeks
		Compensated cirrhosis	12 weeks
HCV genotype 2, 4, 5, or 6 infection	Previously treated without HCV NS3/4A protease inhibitors or HCV NS5A inhibitors[a]	Noncirrhotic	8 weeks
		Compensated cirrhosis	12 weeks
HCV genotype 3 infection	Previously treated without HCV NS3/4A protease inhibitors or HCV NS5A inhibitors[a]	Noncirrhotic	16 weeks
		Compensated cirrhosis	16 weeks

[a] Previously received HCV regimen containing interferon, peginterferon, ribavirin, and/or sofosbuvir; no previous treatment with HCV NS3/4A protease inhibitors or HCV NS5A inhibitors.

[b] In clinical trials, patients previously received HCV regimens containing the fixed combination of ledipasvir and sofosbuvir (ledipasvir/sofosbuvir) or daclatasvir (no longer commercially available) in conjunction with peginterferon and ribavirin.

[c] In clinical trials, patients previously received HCV regimens containing simeprevir (no longer commercially available) in conjunction with sofosbuvir or simeprevir, boceprevir, or telaprevir (drugs no longer commercially available) in conjunction with peginterferon and ribavirin.

HCV-infected Individuals with HIV Coinfection

Glecaprevir/pibrentasvir dosage and duration of therapy recommended for the treatment of chronic HCV genotype 1, 2, 3, 4, 5, or 6 infection in adults without cirrhosis or with compensated cirrhosis (Child-Pugh class A) who are coinfected with human immunodeficiency virus type 1 (HIV-1) generally are the same as those recommended for adults without HIV coinfection.

Liver or Kidney Transplant Recipients

For the treatment of chronic HCV genotype 1, 2, 3, 4, 5, or 6 infection in treatment-naive or previously treated adults without cirrhosis or with compensated cirrhosis (Child-Pugh class A) who are liver or kidney transplant recipients, the recommended dosage of glecaprevir/pibrentasvir is 3 tablets (total of 300 mg of glecaprevir and 120 mg of pibrentasvir) once daily for 12 weeks.

A treatment duration of 16 weeks is recommended in those with HCV genotype 1 infection who were previously treated with an HCV NS5A inhibitor, but have not received an HCV NS3/4A protease inhibitor, and in those with HCV genotype 3 infection who were previously treated with regimens containing interferon, peginterferon, ribavirin, and/or sofosbuvir, but have not received an HCV NS3/4A protease inhibitor or HCV NS5A inhibitor.

Pediatric Dosage

HCV Genotype 1, 2, 3, 4, 5, or 6 Infection

For the treatment of chronic HCV genotype 1, 2, 3, 4, 5, or 6 infection in treatment-naive or previously treated pediatric patients ≥3 years of age, the recommended dosage of glecaprevir/pibrentasvir is based on weight. (See Table 3.)

TABLE 3. Recommended Glecaprevir/Pibrentasvir Dosage for Treatment of HCV Genotype 1, 2, 3, 4, 5, or 6 Infection in Pediatric Patients ≥3 Years of Age.

Weight (kg) or Age (years of age)	Dosage of Glecaprevir/ Pibrentasvir Tablets or Pellets	Total Daily Glecaprevir/ Pibrentasvir Dosage
<20 kg	*Pellets:* Three packets containing glecaprevir 50 mg/pibrentasvir 20 mg pellets once daily	Glecaprevir 150 mg/ pibrentasvir 60 mg daily
20 to <30 kg	*Pellets:* Four packets containing glecaprevir 50 mg/pibrentasvir 20 mg pellets once daily	Glecaprevir 200 mg/ pibrentasvir 80 mg daily
30 to <45 kg	*Pellets:* Five packets containing glecaprevir 50 mg/pibrentasvir 20 mg pellets once daily	Glecaprevir 250 mg/ pibrentasvir 100 mg daily
≥45 kg or ≥12 years of age	*Tablets:* Three tablets containing glecaprevir 100 mg/pibrentasvir 40 mg once daily or *Pellets:* Six packets containing glecaprevir 50 mg/pibrentasvir 20 mg pellets once daily[a]	Glecaprevir 300 mg/ pibrentasvir 120 mg daily Glecaprevir 300 mg/ pibrentasvir 120 mg daily

[a] Dosing with oral pellets has not been studied in pediatric patients weighing >45 kg.

The treatment duration depends on the HCV genotype, the patient's previous HCV treatment experience, and presence of cirrhosis. (See Tables 4 and 5.)

TABLE 4. Recommended Treatment Duration of Glecaprevir/ Pibrentasvir in Treatment-naive Pediatric Patients ≥3 Years of Age with HCV Genotype 1, 2, 3, 4, 5, or 6 Infection.

HCV Genotype	Hepatic Impairment	Duration of Glecaprevir/ Pibrentasvir
HCV genotype 1, 2, 3, 4, 5, or 6 infection	Noncirrhotic	8 weeks
	Compensated cirrhosis (Child-Pugh class A)	8 weeks

TABLE 5. Recommended Treatment Duration of Glecaprevir/ Pibrentasvir in Previously Treated Pediatric Patients ≥3 Years of Age with HCV Genotype 1, 2, 3, 4, 5, or 6 Infection.

HCV Genotype	Treatment Experience	Hepatic Impairment	Duration of Glecaprevir/ Pibrentasvir
HCV genotype 1 infection	Previously treated *without* HCV NS3/4A protease inhibitors or HCV NS5A inhibitors[a]	Noncirrhotic	8 weeks
		Compensated cirrhosis (Child-Pugh class A)	12 weeks
	Previously treated with an HCV NS5A inhibitor; no prior treatment with HCV NS3/4A protease inhibitors[b]	Noncirrhotic	16 weeks
		Compensated cirrhosis	16 weeks
	Previously treated with an HCV NS3/4A protease inhibitor; no prior treatment with HCV NS5A inhibitors[c]	Noncirrhotic	12 weeks
		Compensated cirrhosis	12 weeks
HCV genotype 2, 4, 5, or 6 infection	Previously treated *without* HCV NS3/4A protease inhibitors or HCV NS5A inhibitors[a]	Noncirrhotic	8 weeks
		Compensated cirrhosis	12 weeks
HCV genotype 3 infection	Previously treated *without* HCV NS3/4A protease inhibitors or HCV NS5A inhibitors[a]	Noncirrhotic	16 weeks
		Compensated cirrhosis	16 weeks

[a] Previously received HCV regimen containing interferon, peginterferon, ribavirin, and/or sofosbuvir; no previous treatment with HCV NS3/4A protease inhibitors or HCV NS5A inhibitors.

[b] In clinical trials, patients previously received HCV regimens containing the fixed combination of ledipasvir and sofosbuvir (ledipasvir/sofosbuvir) or daclatasvir (no longer commercially available) in conjunction with peginterferon *and* ribavirin.

[c] In clinical trials, patients previously received HCV regimens containing simeprevir (no longer commercially available) in conjunction with sofosbuvir or simeprevir, boceprevir, or telaprevir (drugs no longer commercially available) in conjunction with peginterferon *and* ribavirin.

HCV-infected Individuals with HIV Coinfection

Glecaprevir/pibrentasvir dosage and duration of therapy recommended for the treatment of chronic HCV genotype 1, 2, 3, 4, 5, or 6 infection in pediatric patients ≥12 years of age weighing at least 45 kg without cirrhosis or with compensated cirrhosis (Child-Pugh class A) who are coinfected with HIV-1 generally are the same as those recommended for pediatric patients without HIV coinfection.

Transplant Recipients

For the treatment of chronic HCV genotype 1, 2, 3, 4, 5, or 6 infection in treatment-naive or previously treated pediatric patients ≥12 years of age weighing at least 45 kg without cirrhosis or with compensated cirrhosis (Child-Pugh class A) who are liver or kidney transplant recipients, the recommended dosage of glecaprevir/pibrentasvir is 3 tablets (total of 300 mg of glecaprevir and 120 mg of pibrentasvir) once daily for 12 weeks.

A treatment duration of 16 weeks is recommended in those with HCV genotype 1 infection who were previously treated with an HCV NS5A inhibitor, but have not received an HCV NS3/4A protease inhibitor, and in those with HCV genotype 3 infection who were previously treated with regimens containing interferon, peginterferon, ribavirin, and/or sofosbuvir, but have not received an HCV NS3/4A protease inhibitor or HCV NS5A inhibitor.

● *Special Populations*

Hepatic Impairment

Dosage adjustments are not necessary if glecaprevir/pibrentasvir is used in patients with mild hepatic impairment (Child-Pugh class A). However, such patients should be monitored for signs and symptoms of hepatic decompensation.

Glecaprevir/pibrentasvir is contraindicated in patients with moderate or severe hepatic impairment (Child-Pugh class B or C) and in those with any history of hepatic decompensation.

Renal Impairment

Dosage adjustments are not necessary if glecaprevir/pibrentasvir is used in patients with mild, moderate, or severe renal impairment, including those receiving hemodialysis. Glecaprevir and pibrentasvir are not removed by hemodialysis to any clinically important extent.

Geriatric Patients

Dosage adjustments of glecaprevir/pibrentasvir are not necessary in geriatric patients.

Persons Who Inject Drugs (PWID) or Receive Medication-Assisted Treatment (MAT) for Opioid Use Disorder

Dosage adjustments of glecaprevir/pibrentasvir are not necessary in PWID or patients who are receiving MAT for opioid use disorder.

CAUTIONS

● *Contraindications*

- Patients with moderate or severe hepatic impairment (Child-Pugh class B or C) and those with any history of hepatic decompensation.
- Concomitant use with atazanavir or rifampin.

● *Warnings/Precautions*

Warnings

Risk of HBV Reactivation in Patients Coinfected with HCV and HBV

A boxed warning about the risk of reactivation of hepatitis B virus (HBV) infection is included in the prescribing information for glecaprevir/pibrentasvir. Reactivation of HBV infection has been reported during postmarketing experience when direct-acting antivirals (DAAs) were used for the treatment of chronic hepatitis C virus (HCV) infection in patients with HBV coinfection. In some cases, HBV reactivation resulted in fulminant hepatitis, hepatic failure, and death.

HBV reactivation (defined as an abrupt increase in HBV replication manifested as a rapid increase in serum HBV DNA levels or detection of hepatitis B surface antigen [HBsAg] in an individual who was previously HBsAg negative and hepatitis B core antibody [anti-HBc] positive) has been reported in patients with HCV and HBV coinfection who were receiving HCV treatment with a regimen that included HCV DAAs without HBV antiviral therapy. Reactivation also may be accompanied by hepatitis (i.e., increased aminotransferase concentrations) and, in severe cases, may lead to increased bilirubin concentrations, liver failure, or death.

Data to date indicate that HBV reactivation usually occurs within 4–8 weeks after initiation of HCV treatment. Patients with HBV reactivation have been heterogeneous in terms of HCV genotype and in terms of baseline HBV disease. While some patients with HBV reactivation were HBsAg positive, others had serologic evidence of resolved HBV infection (i.e., HBsAg negative and anti-HBc positive). HBV reactivation also has been reported in patients receiving certain immunosuppressant or chemotherapeutic drugs; the risk of reactivation associated with HCV DAAs may be increased in such patients.

The mechanism for HBV reactivation in patients with HCV and HBV coinfection receiving HCV DAAs is unknown. Although HCV DAAs are not known to cause immunosuppression, HBV reactivation in coinfected patients may result from a complex interplay of host immunologic responses in the setting of infection with 2 hepatitis viruses.

Prior to initiating treatment with an HCV DAA, including glecaprevir/pibrentasvir, all patients should be screened for evidence of current or prior HBV infection by measuring HBsAg and anti-HBc. If there is serologic evidence of HBV infection, baseline HBV DNA levels should be measured.

Patients with evidence of current or prior HBV infection should be monitored for clinical and laboratory signs (i.e., HBsAg, HBV DNA levels, serum aminotransferase concentrations, bilirubin concentrations) of hepatitis flare or HBV reactivation during and after treatment with HCV DAAs, including glecaprevir/pibrentasvir. Appropriate management for HBV infection should be initiated as clinically indicated.

Patients with HCV and HBV coinfection receiving glecaprevir/pibrentasvir should be advised to immediately contact a clinician if they develop any signs or symptoms of serious liver injury.

When making decisions regarding HBV monitoring or HBV treatment in coinfected patients, consultation with a clinician who has expertise in managing HBV infection is recommended.

Other Warnings and Precautions

Risk of Hepatic Decompensation or Failure in Patients with Evidence of Advanced Liver Disease

Hepatic decompensation or failure, including some fatalities, have been reported during postmarketing experience in patients receiving HCV treatment regimens containing an HCV nonstructural 3/4A (NS3/4A) protease inhibitor, including glecaprevir/pibrentasvir. Data are insufficient to estimate the frequency of such events and a causal relationship has not been established. Hepatic decompensation or failure usually occurred within the first 4 weeks of HCV treatment.

The majority of reported cases of hepatic decompensation or failure with severe outcomes in patients receiving glecaprevir/pibrentasvir occurred in those with evidence of advanced liver disease with moderate or severe hepatic impairment (Child-Pugh class B or C) prior to initiation of the drug. Some cases occurred in patients who had compensated cirrhosis with mild liver impairment (Child-Pugh class A) at baseline, but had a history of a decompensation event (i.e., history of ascites, variceal bleeding, encephalopathy). Rare cases of hepatic decompensation or failure were reported in patients without cirrhosis or with compensated cirrhosis (Child-Pugh A); many of these patients had evidence of portal hypertension. Some cases have also been reported in patients receiving concomitant therapy with drugs not recommended for concomitant use with the HCV treatment regimen and in those with confounding factors (e.g., serious liver-related medical or surgical comorbidities).

If glecaprevir/pibrentasvir is used in patients who have compensated cirrhosis (Child-Pugh class A) or evidence of advanced liver disease (e.g., portal hypertension), hepatic function tests should be performed as clinically indicated and patients should be monitored for signs and symptoms of hepatic decompensation (e.g., jaundice, ascites, hepatic encephalopathy, variceal hemorrhage).

Glecaprevir/pibrentasvir should be discontinued in patients who develop evidence of hepatic decompensation or failure.

Patients should be advised to contact a clinician if they develop any signs or symptoms of worsening liver disease.

Interactions

Concomitant use of glecaprevir/pibrentasvir with certain drugs (i.e., carbamazepine, efavirenz, St. John's wort) may result in clinically important decreases in glecaprevir and pibrentasvir plasma concentrations and may lead to reduced therapeutic effect of glecaprevir/pibrentasvir. Concomitant use with such drugs is not recommended.

Precautions Related to Fixed Combinations

When glecaprevir/pibrentasvir is used, the cautions, precautions, contraindications, and drug interactions associated with each drug in the fixed combination must be considered. Cautionary information applicable to specific populations (e.g., pregnant or nursing women, individuals with hepatic or renal impairment, geriatric patients) should be considered for each drug.

Specific Populations

Pregnancy

Adequate data are not available regarding use of glecaprevir/pibrentasvir in pregnant women. In animal studies, there was no evidence of adverse effects on fetal development at glecaprevir or pibrentasvir exposures 53 or 51 times greater, respectively, than human exposures at the recommended human dosage.

Lactation

It is not known whether glecaprevir and pibrentasvir are distributed into human milk, affect human milk production, or have effects on the breast-fed infant.

Glecaprevir and pibrentasvir are distributed into milk in rodents, but no apparent effects on growth and postnatal development were observed in nursing pups.

The benefits of breast-feeding and the importance of glecaprevir/pibrentasvir to the woman should be considered along with potential adverse effects on the breast-fed child from the drug or from the underlying maternal condition.

Pediatric Use

Safety, efficacy, and pharmacokinetics of glecaprevir/pibrentasvir have not been established in pediatric patients <3 years of age.

Safety and efficacy of glecaprevir/pibrentasvir for the treatment of HCV genotype 1, 2, 3, or 4 infection in pediatric patients ≥3 years of age are based on safety, efficacy, and pharmacokinetic data from an open-label phase 2/3 trial in treatment-naive or previously treated noncirrhotic pediatric patients (DORA [Part 1 and Part 2]). Trial data indicated that safety and efficacy of glecaprevir/pibrentasvir in these pediatric patients are consistent with those observed in HCV-infected adults receiving the drug in clinical trials, except for vomiting, rash, and abdominal pain, which occurred more frequently in patients <12 years of age compared to adults.

Safety and efficacy of glecaprevir/pibrentasvir for the treatment of HCV genotype 5 or 6 infection in pediatric patients with cirrhosis or those who have received a kidney and/or liver transplant are supported by data indicating that glecaprevir and pibrentasvir systemic exposures in pediatric patients are comparable to those reported in adults.

Geriatric Use

No overall differences in safety and efficacy of glecaprevir/pibrentasvir have been observed between patients ≥65 years of age and younger adults. Pooled analysis of data from 9 clinical trials (phase 2 or 3) that evaluated safety and efficacy of glecaprevir/pibrentasvir for the treatment of chronic HCV infection in adults indicated that, in the subset of patients with severe renal impairment, those ≥65 years of age had a higher incidence of adverse effects (79 or 68%, respectively) and treatment-related adverse effects (57 or 46%, respectively) compared with younger adults.

Hepatic Impairment

Patients with mild hepatic impairment or compensated cirrhosis (Child-Pugh class A) should be monitored for signs and symptoms of hepatic decompensation (e.g., jaundice, ascites, hepatic encephalopathy, variceal hemorrhage) during glecaprevir/pibrentasvir treatment.

Glecaprevir/pibrentasvir is contraindicated in patients with moderate or severe hepatic impairment (Child-Pugh class B or C) and in those with any history of hepatic decompensation. There have been postmarketing reports of hepatic decompensation or failure in such patients.

Increased glecaprevir and pibrentasvir exposures have been reported in patients with moderate or severe hepatic impairment.

In HCV-infected individuals with compensated cirrhosis (Child-Pugh class A), administration of glecaprevir/pibrentasvir results in glecaprevir exposures approximately twofold higher than those reported in HCV-infected individuals without cirrhosis; pibrentasvir exposures are similar to those observed in HCV-infected individuals without cirrhosis.

In individuals with moderate or severe hepatic impairment (Child-Pugh class B or C), administration of glecaprevir/pibrentasvir results in glecaprevir plasma exposures twofold and 11-fold higher, respectively, than those reported in individuals with normal hepatic function; pibrentasvir plasma exposures are 26 and 114% higher, respectively, than those reported in individuals with normal hepatic function.

Renal Impairment

In individuals with mild, moderate, severe, or end-stage renal impairment without HCV infection, glecaprevir and pibrentasvir exposures were up to 56 and 46% higher, respectively, than exposures reported in individuals with normal renal function. In dialysis-dependent individuals without HCV infection, pibrentasvir and glecaprevir exposures were similar with or without dialysis (up to 18% difference).

In HCV-infected individuals with end-stage renal disease (with or without dialysis), glecaprevir and pibrentasvir exposures were 86 and 54% higher, respectively, than exposures reported in individuals with normal renal function.

Persons Who Inject Drugs (PWID) or Receive Medication-Assisted Treatment (MAT) for Opioid Use Disorder

No overall differences in safety and efficacy of glecaprevir/pibrentasvir have been observed between patients who self-identify as recent or current injection drug users and patients who self-identify as former or noninjection drug users. Safety and efficacy have also been found to be similar between patients who report concomitant use of MAT for opioid use disorder compared to those who do not report such concomitant therapy.

● Common Adverse Effects

Adverse effects reported in ≥10% of patients receiving glecaprevir/pibrentasvir include headache and fatigue.

DRUG INTERACTIONS

● Drugs Affecting or Metabolized by Hepatic Microsomal Enzymes

Glecaprevir and pibrentasvir are weak inhibitors of cytochrome P-450 (CYP) isoenzymes 3A and 1A2. Clinically important pharmacokinetic interactions are not expected if the fixed combination of glecaprevir and pibrentasvir (glecaprevir/pibrentasvir) is used concomitantly with substrates of CYP3A, 1A2, 2C9, 2C19, or 2D6.

Pharmacokinetic interactions are possible with inducers of CYP3A4, which may decrease glecaprevir and pibrentasvir plasma concentrations.

● Drugs Affecting or Affected by P-glycoprotein Transport System

Glecaprevir and pibrentasvir are inhibitors of the P-glycoprotein (P-gp) transport system. Concomitant use of glecaprevir/pibrentasvir and P-gp substrates may increase exposure of such drugs.

Glecaprevir and pibrentasvir are substrates of P-gp. Pharmacokinetic interactions are possible with P-gp inducers, which may decrease glecaprevir and pibrentasvir plasma concentrations. Pharmacokinetic interactions are possible with P-gp inhibitors, which may increase glecaprevir and pibrentasvir plasma concentrations.

● Drugs Affecting or Affected by Breast Cancer Resistance Protein

Glecaprevir and pibrentasvir are inhibitors of breast cancer resistance protein (BCRP). Concomitant use of glecaprevir/pibrentasvir and BCRP substrates may increase exposure of such drugs.

Glecaprevir and pibrentasvir are substrates of BCRP. Pharmacokinetic interactions are possible with BCRP inducers, which may decrease glecaprevir and pibrentasvir plasma concentrations. Pharmacokinetic interactions are possible with BCRP inhibitors, which may increase glecaprevir and pibrentasvir plasma concentrations.

● Drugs Affecting or Affected by Organic Anion Transporting Polypeptides

Glecaprevir and pibrentasvir are inhibitors of organic anion transporting polypeptide (OATP) 1B1 and 1B3. Concomitant use of glecaprevir/pibrentasvir and OATP1B1 or 1B3 substrates may increase exposure of such drugs.

Glecaprevir is a substrate of OATP1B1 and 1B3. Pharmacokinetic interactions are possible with OATP1B1 and 1B3 inducers, which may decrease glecaprevir plasma concentrations. Pharmacokinetic interactions are possible with OATP1B1 and 1B3 inhibitors, which may increase glecaprevir plasma concentrations.

● *Drugs Affecting or Affected by Other Membrane Transporters*

Glecaprevir and pibrentasvir are weak inhibitors of uridine diphosphate-glucuronosyl transferase (UGT) 1A1. Clinically important pharmacokinetic interactions are not expected if glecaprevir/pibrentasvir is used concomitantly with substrates of UGT1A1 or 1A4.

● *Angiotensin II Receptor Antagonists*

No clinically important pharmacokinetic interactions were observed when losartan or valsartan was used concomitantly with glecaprevir/pibrentasvir.

Dosage adjustments are not necessary if losartan or valsartan is used concomitantly with glecaprevir/pibrentasvir.

● *Anticoagulants*

Dabigatran

Concomitant use of dabigatran etexilate (single 150-mg dose) and glecaprevir/pibrentasvir (300 mg of glecaprevir and 120 mg of pibrentasvir once daily) results in increased dabigatran peak plasma concentrations and area under the concentration-time curve (AUC).

If dabigatran etexilate and glecaprevir/pibrentasvir are used concomitantly in patients with renal impairment, the recommendations from the manufacturer of dabigatran etexilate regarding dosage modifications for concomitant use with P-gp inhibitors should be followed.

Warfarin

If warfarin is used in patients receiving treatment for hepatitis C virus (HCV) infection, including treatment with glecaprevir/pibrentasvir, fluctuations in the international normalized ratio (INR) may occur. INR should be closely monitored during glecaprevir/pibrentasvir treatment; adjustment of warfarin dosage may be needed.

● *Anticonvulsants*

Carbamazepine

Concomitant use of carbamazepine (200 mg twice daily) and glecaprevir/pibrentasvir (300 mg of glecaprevir and 120 mg of pibrentasvir as a single dose) results in clinically important decreases in glecaprevir and pibrentasvir plasma concentrations and AUCs, which may lead to reduced therapeutic effect of glecaprevir/pibrentasvir.

Concomitant use of carbamazepine and glecaprevir/pibrentasvir is not recommended.

Lamotrigine

No clinically important pharmacokinetic interactions were observed when lamotrigine was used concomitantly with glecaprevir/pibrentasvir.

Dosage adjustments are not necessary if lamotrigine is used concomitantly with glecaprevir/pibrentasvir.

Phenytoin

Concomitant use of phenytoin and glecaprevir/pibrentasvir may result in decreased glecaprevir and pibrentasvir plasma concentrations and may lead to reduced therapeutic effect of glecaprevir/pibrentasvir.

Concomitant use of phenytoin and glecaprevir/pibrentasvir is not recommended.

● *Antimycobacterial Agents*

Rifampin

Concomitant use of rifampin (600 mg once daily) and a single dose of glecaprevir/pibrentasvir (300 mg of glecaprevir and 120 mg of pibrentasvir) results in clinically important decreases in plasma concentrations and AUCs of glecaprevir and pibrentasvir and may lead to reduced therapeutic effect of glecaprevir/pibrentasvir. Concomitant use of rifampin (single 600-mg dose) and glecaprevir/pibrentasvir results in increased glecaprevir plasma concentrations and AUC.

Concomitant use of rifampin and glecaprevir/pibrentasvir is contraindicated.

● *Antiretroviral Agents*

HIV Integrase Inhibitors (INSTIs)

Dolutegravir

No clinically important pharmacokinetic interactions were observed when the fixed combination of abacavir, dolutegravir, and lamivudine (abacavir/dolutegravir/lamivudine) was used concomitantly with glecaprevir/pibrentasvir.

Dosage adjustments are not necessary if dolutegravir is used concomitantly with glecaprevir/pibrentasvir.

Elvitegravir

Dosage adjustments are not necessary if *cobicistat-boosted* elvitegravir is used concomitantly with glecaprevir/pibrentasvir.

Raltegravir

Concomitant use of raltegravir and glecaprevir/pibrentasvir results in increased plasma concentrations and AUC of raltegravir.

Dosage adjustments are not necessary if raltegravir is used concomitantly with glecaprevir/pibrentasvir.

HIV Nonnucleoside Reverse Transcriptase Inhibitors (NNRTIs)

Efavirenz

Concomitant use of efavirenz and glecaprevir/pibrentasvir may result in decreased glecaprevir and pibrentasvir plasma concentrations and may lead to reduced therapeutic effect of glecaprevir/pibrentasvir.

Concomitant use of efavirenz and glecaprevir/pibrentasvir is not recommended.

Rilpivirine

Concomitant use of rilpivirine and glecaprevir/pibrentasvir results in increased plasma concentrations and AUC of rilpivirine; this is not considered clinically important.

Dosage adjustments are not necessary if rilpivirine is used concomitantly with glecaprevir/pibrentasvir.

HIV Nucleoside and Nucleotide Reverse Transcriptase Inhibitors (NRTIs)

Abacavir

No clinically important pharmacokinetic interactions were observed when abacavir/dolutegravir/lamivudine was used concomitantly with glecaprevir/pibrentasvir.

Dosage adjustments are not necessary if abacavir is used concomitantly with glecaprevir/pibrentasvir.

Emtricitabine

Concomitant use of the fixed combination of elvitegravir, cobicistat, emtricitabine, and tenofovir alafenamide fumarate (TAF) and glecaprevir/pibrentasvir results in increased plasma concentrations and AUCs of glecaprevir and pibrentasvir.

Dosage adjustments are not necessary if emtricitabine is used concomitantly with glecaprevir/pibrentasvir.

Lamivudine

No clinically important pharmacokinetic interactions were observed when abacavir/dolutegravir/lamivudine was used concomitantly with glecaprevir/pibrentasvir.

Dosage adjustments are not necessary if lamivudine is used concomitantly with glecaprevir/pibrentasvir.

Tenofovir

Concomitant use of EVG/c/FTC/TAF and glecaprevir/pibrentasvir results in increased plasma concentrations and AUCs of glecaprevir and pibrentasvir, but does not affect tenofovir concentrations or AUC. Concomitant use of the fixed combination of efavirenz, emtricitabine, and TDF (efavirenz/emtricitabine/TDF) and glecaprevir/pibrentasvir results in increased plasma concentrations and AUC of tenofovir.

Dosage adjustments are not necessary if TAF or TDF is used concomitantly with glecaprevir/pibrentasvir.

HIV Protease Inhibitors (PIs)

Atazanavir

Concomitant use of *ritonavir-boosted* atazanavir (300 mg of atazanavir and 100 mg of ritonavir once daily) and glecaprevir/pibrentasvir (300 mg of glecaprevir and 120 mg of pibrentasvir once daily) results in 4-, 14.3-, and 6.5-fold increases in glecaprevir peak plasma concentrations, trough plasma concentrations, and AUC, respectively, and 1.3-, 2.3-, and 1.6-fold increases in pibrentasvir peak plasma concentrations, trough plasma concentrations, and AUC, respectively. Concomitant use may result in increased ALT concentrations.

Concomitant use of glecaprevir/pibrentasvir and *ritonavir-boosted, cobicistat-boosted*, or unboosted atazanavir is contraindicated.

Darunavir

Concomitant use of *ritonavir-boosted* darunavir (800 mg of darunavir and 100 mg of ritonavir once daily) and glecaprevir/pibrentasvir (300 mg of glecaprevir and 120 mg of pibrentasvir once daily) results in 3.1-, 8.2-, and 5-fold increases in glecaprevir peak plasma concentrations, trough plasma concentrations, and AUC, respectively, and 1.7-fold increases in pibrentasvir trough plasma concentrations.

Concomitant use of glecaprevir/pibrentasvir and *ritonavir-boosted* or *cobicistat-boosted* darunavir is not recommended.

Lopinavir

Concomitant use of the fixed combination of lopinavir 400 mg and ritonavir 100 mg (lopinavir/ritonavir once daily) and glecaprevir/pibrentasvir (300 mg of glecaprevir and 120 mg of pibrentasvir once daily) results in 2.6-, 18.6-, and 4.4-fold increases in glecaprevir peak plasma concentrations, trough plasma concentrations, and AUC, respectively, and 1.4-, 5.2-, and 2.5-fold increases in pibrentasvir peak plasma concentrations, trough plasma concentrations, and AUC, respectively.

Concomitant use of lopinavir/ritonavir and glecaprevir/pibrentasvir is not recommended.

Ritonavir

Concomitant use of ritonavir and glecaprevir/pibrentasvir is expected to increase plasma concentrations of glecaprevir and pibrentasvir.

Concomitant use of ritonavir and glecaprevir/pibrentasvir is not recommended.

● Benzodiazepines

No clinically important pharmacokinetic interactions were observed when midazolam was used concomitantly with glecaprevir/pibrentasvir.

Dosage adjustments are not necessary if midazolam is used concomitantly with glecaprevir/pibrentasvir.

● Caffeine

No clinically important pharmacokinetic interactions were observed when caffeine was used concomitantly with glecaprevir/pibrentasvir.

Dosage adjustments are not necessary if caffeine is used concomitantly with glecaprevir/pibrentasvir.

● Calcium-channel Blocking Agents

Amlodipine and Felodipine

No clinically important pharmacokinetic interactions were observed when amlodipine or felodipine was used concomitantly with glecaprevir/pibrentasvir.

Dosage adjustments are not necessary if amlodipine or felodipine is used concomitantly with glecaprevir/pibrentasvir.

● Dextromethorphan

No clinically important pharmacokinetic interactions were observed when dextromethorphan was used concomitantly with glecaprevir/pibrentasvir.

Dosage adjustments are not necessary if dextromethorphan is used concomitantly with glecaprevir/pibrentasvir.

● Digoxin

Concomitant use of digoxin and glecaprevir/pibrentasvir increases digoxin exposures.

Serum digoxin concentrations should be measured prior to and monitored during concomitant glecaprevir/pibrentasvir therapy. Digoxin serum concentrations should be reduced by decreasing the digoxin dosage by 50% or modifying the frequency of administration of the drug.

● Estrogens

Concomitant use of glecaprevir/pibrentasvir and an ethinyl estradiol-containing product (e.g., oral contraceptives) does not affect glecaprevir or pibrentasvir concentrations. Coadministration of glecaprevir/pibrentasvir with products containing more than 20 mcg of ethinyl estradiol may increase the risk of ALT elevations and is not recommended.

No dose adjustment is required when glecaprevir/pibrentasvir is coadministered with products containing ≤20 mcg of ethinyl estradiol.

● HCV Antivirals

HCV Polymerase Inhibitors

Sofosbuvir

No clinically important pharmacokinetic interactions were observed when sofosbuvir was used concomitantly with glecaprevir/pibrentasvir.

Dosage adjustments are not necessary if sofosbuvir is used concomitantly with glecaprevir/pibrentasvir.

● HMG-CoA Reductase Inhibitors

Atorvastatin

Concomitant use of atorvastatin (10 mg once daily) and glecaprevir/pibrentasvir (400 mg of glecaprevir and 120 mg of pibrentasvir once daily) results in 22- and 8.3-fold increases in atorvastatin peak plasma concentrations and AUC, respectively, which may increase the risk of myopathy and rhabdomyolysis.

Concomitant use of atorvastatin and glecaprevir/pibrentasvir is not recommended.

Fluvastatin

Concomitant use of fluvastatin and glecaprevir/pibrentasvir may increase plasma concentrations of fluvastatin, which may increase the risk of myopathy and rhabdomyolysis.

If fluvastatin and glecaprevir/pibrentasvir are used concomitantly, the lowest dosage of fluvastatin should be used. If higher fluvastatin dosages are required, the lowest necessary dosage should be used taking into account the risks and benefits.

Lovastatin

Concomitant use of lovastatin (10 mg once daily) and glecaprevir/pibrentasvir (300 mg of glecaprevir and 120 mg of pibrentasvir once daily) results in 5.7- and 4.1-fold increases in lovastatin peak plasma concentrations and AUC, respectively, which may increase the risk of myopathy and rhabdomyolysis.

Concomitant use of lovastatin and glecaprevir/pibrentasvir is not recommended.

Pitavastatin

Concomitant use of pitavastatin and glecaprevir/pibrentasvir may increase plasma concentrations of pitavastatin, which may increase the risk of myopathy and rhabdomyolysis.

If pitavastatin and glecaprevir/pibrentasvir are used concomitantly, the lowest dosage of pitavastatin should be used. If higher pitavastatin dosages are required, use the lowest necessary dosage taking into account the risks and benefits.

Pravastatin

Concomitant use of pravastatin (10 mg once daily) and glecaprevir/pibrentasvir (400 mg of glecaprevir and 120 mg of pibrentasvir once daily) results in 2.2- and

2.3-fold increases in pravastatin peak plasma concentrations and AUC, respectively, which may increase the risk of myopathy and rhabdomyolysis.

If pravastatin is used concomitantly with glecaprevir/pibrentasvir, the pravastatin dosage should be reduced by 50%.

Rosuvastatin

Concomitant use of rosuvastatin (5 mg once daily) and glecaprevir/pibrentasvir (400 mg of glecaprevir and 120 mg of pibrentasvir once daily) results in 5.6- and 2.2-fold increases in rosuvastatin peak plasma concentrations and AUC, respectively, which may increase the risk of myopathy and rhabdomyolysis.

If rosuvastatin is used concomitantly with glecaprevir/pibrentasvir, the rosuvastatin dosage should not exceed 10 mg.

Simvastatin

Concomitant use of simvastatin (5 mg once daily) and glecaprevir/pibrentasvir (300 mg of glecaprevir and 120 mg of pibrentasvir once daily) results in 10.7- and 4.5-fold increases in simvastatin peak plasma concentrations and AUC, respectively, which may increase the risk of myopathy and rhabdomyolysis.

Concomitant use of simvastatin and glecaprevir/pibrentasvir is not recommended.

● Immunosuppressive Agents

Cyclosporine

Concomitant use of low-dose cyclosporine (single 100-mg dose) and glecaprevir/pibrentasvir (300 mg of glecaprevir and 120 mg of pibrentasvir once daily) results in 1.3-, 1.3-, and 1.4-fold increases in glecaprevir peak plasma concentrations, trough plasma concentrations, and AUC, respectively, and 1.3-fold increases in pibrentasvir trough plasma concentrations. Concomitant use of high-dose cyclosporine (single 400-mg dose) and glecaprevir/pibrentasvir (300 mg of glecaprevir and 120 mg of pibrentasvir once daily) results in 4.5- and 5-fold increases in glecaprevir peak plasma concentrations and AUC, respectively, and 1.9-fold increases in pibrentasvir AUC. Cyclosporine exposures following single 100- or 400-mg doses are not substantially affected by concomitant glecaprevir/pibrentasvir.

Concomitant use of cyclosporine and glecaprevir/pibrentasvir is not recommended in patients receiving stable cyclosporine dosages exceeding 100 mg daily.

Tacrolimus

No clinically important pharmacokinetic interactions were observed when tacrolimus was used concomitantly with glecaprevir/pibrentasvir.

Dosage adjustments are not necessary if tacrolimus is used concomitantly with glecaprevir/pibrentasvir.

● Medication-Assisted Treatment (MAT) for Opioid Use Disorder

No clinically important pharmacokinetic interactions were observed when methadone, buprenorphine, naloxone, or the fixed combination of buprenorphine and naloxone (buprenorphine/naloxone) was used concomitantly with glecaprevir/pibrentasvir. Dosage adjustments are not necessary if methadone, buprenorphine, naloxone, or buprenorphine/naloxone is used concomitantly with glecaprevir/pibrentasvir.

Data are insufficient regarding concomitant use of naltrexone and glecaprevir/pibrentasvir.

● Proton-pump Inhibitors

No clinically important pharmacokinetic interactions were observed when omeprazole (20 mg once daily) was used concomitantly with glecaprevir/pibrentasvir (single dose of 300 mg of glecaprevir and 120 mg of pibrentasvir). Concomitant use of omeprazole (40 mg once daily) given 1 hour before glecaprevir/pibrentasvir (single dose of 300 mg of glecaprevir and 120 mg of pibrentasvir) decreased peak plasma concentrations and AUC of glecaprevir, but did not affect plasma concentrations or AUC of pibrentasvir. Concomitant use of glecaprevir/pibrentasvir and omeprazole 40 mg has been reported to decrease glecaprevir exposures by 51%.

In a clinical study evaluating glecaprevir/pibrentasvir for the treatment of chronic HCV genotype 1, 2, 4, 5, or 6 infection (EXPEDITION-1), 21% of patients reported concomitant use of a proton-pump inhibitor (PPI); PPI use did not appear to affect rates of sustained virologic response at 12 weeks after end of treatment (SVR12). In a pooled analysis of data from 9 clinical trials (phase 2 or 3) that evaluated efficacy and safety of glecaprevir/pibrentasvir for the treatment of chronic HCV infection in adults, 263 patients were identified who received a PPI during the trial; 59% received low PPI doses (omeprazole 20 mg daily [or equivalent]) and 41% received high PPI doses (at least 1 dose greater than omeprazole 20 mg daily [or equivalent]). SVR12 rates were 97.4% in those receiving low PPI doses and 96.3% in those receiving high PPI doses.

The manufacturer states that dosage adjustments are not necessary if omeprazole is used concomitantly with glecaprevir/pibrentasvir. Some clinicians recommend that long-term concomitant use of glecaprevir/pibrentasvir and omeprazole 40 mg once daily should be avoided.

● St. John's Wort

Concomitant use of St. John's wort (Hypericum perforatum) and glecaprevir/pibrentasvir may result in clinically important decreases in glecaprevir and pibrentasvir plasma concentrations and may lead to reduced therapeutic effect of glecaprevir/pibrentasvir.

Concomitant use of St. John's wort and glecaprevir/pibrentasvir is not recommended.

DESCRIPTION

Glecaprevir and pibrentasvir (glecaprevir/pibrentasvir) is a fixed combination containing 2 hepatitis C virus (HCV) antivirals. Glecaprevir is an HCV nonstructural 3/4A (NS3/4A) protease inhibitor. Pibrentasvir is an HCV nonstructural 5A (NS5A) replication complex inhibitor (NS5A inhibitor). Both drugs are direct-acting antivirals (DAAs) with activity against HCV. There was no in vitro evidence of antagonistic anti-HCV effects between glecaprevir and pibrentasvir when the combination was evaluated in HCV genotype 1 replicon cell culture assays.

Glecaprevir binds to the active site of HCV NS3/4A protease, thereby blocking enzyme activity essential for viral replication (i.e., blocking cleavage of the HCV-encoded polyproteins into mature forms of NS3, NS4A, NS4B, NS5A, and NS5B). In vitro studies using biochemical assays indicate that glecaprevir has activity against clinical isolates of HCV genotypes 1a, 1b, 2a, 2b, 3a, 4a, 5a, and 6a. In HCV replicon assays, glecaprevir has shown in vitro activity against laboratory and clinical isolates of HCV genotypes 1a, 1b, 2a, 2b, 3a, 4a, 4d, 5a, and 6a (median EC_{50} ranging from 0.08–4.6 nM).

Pibrentasvir inhibits the HCV NS5A protein, which is required for viral replication and virion assembly. In HCV replicon assays, pibrentasvir has shown in vitro activity against laboratory and clinical isolates of HCV genotypes 1a, 1b, 2a, 2b, 3a, 4a, 4b, 4d, 5a, 6a, 6e, and 6p (median EC_{50} ranging from 0.5–4.3 nM).

Certain amino acid substitutions in NS3/4A protease inhibitor resistance-associated positions of HCV genotypes 1a (e.g., D168F/Y), 1b, 2a, 3a (e.g., Q168R), 4a, and 6a (e.g., D168A/G/H/V/Y) have been selected in cell culture and have been associated with reduced susceptibility to glecaprevir in vitro in replicon studies. Emergence of amino acid substitutions occurred most commonly at NS3 positions A156 or D/Q168. The combination of NS3 resistance-associated substitutions Y56H and D/Q168 resulted in greater reductions in glecaprevir susceptibility. Treatment-emergent NS3 resistance-associated substitutions were detected in clinical trials evaluating glecaprevir/pibrentasvir in patients with HCV genotype 1 (e.g., A156V, V36A/M, Y56H, R155K/T, A156G/T/V, D168A/T) or genotype 3 (e.g., Y56H/N, Q80K/R, A156G, Q168L/R) infection who experienced virologic failure.

Certain amino acid substitutions in NS5A of HCV genotype 1a (e.g., Q30D/deletion, Y93D/H/N, H58D and Y93H, M28G), genotype 1b (e.g., P32-deletion), genotype 2a (e.g., F28S and M31I, P29S and K30G), and genotype 3a (e.g., K30, M31,Y93H) have been selected in cell culture and have been associated with reduced susceptibility to pibrentasvir in vitro in replicon studies. Combinations of these NS5A substitutions often resulted in greater reductions in susceptibility to pibrentasvir compared with a single NS5A substitution. Treatment-emergent NS5A resistance-associated substitutions were detected in clinical trials evaluating glecaprevir/pibrentasvir in patients with HCV genotype 1 (e.g., Q30R, L31M, M28A/G, L28M, P29Q/R, Q30K/R, H58D, Y93H/N) or genotype 3a (e.g., S24F, M28G/K, A30G/K, L31F, P58T, Y93H) infection who experienced virologic failure. Some of these patients also had baseline NS5A polymorphisms at resistance-associated amino acid positions.

Cross-resistance is possible between glecaprevir and other HCV NS3/4A protease inhibitors and between pibrentasvir and other HCV NS5A inhibitors. Cross-resistance is not expected between glecaprevir/pibrentasvir and sofosbuvir, peginterferon, or ribavirin.

Following oral administration of glecaprevir/pibrentasvir tablets in healthy individuals, peak plasma concentrations of glecaprevir and pibrentasvir occur 5 hours after the dose. Following oral administration of glecaprevir/pibrentasvir pellets in healthy individuals, peak plasma concentrations of glecaprevir and pibrentasvir occur 3 and 5 hours, respectively, after the dose. Administration of glecaprevir/pibrentasvir tablets with a low/moderate- to high-fat meal increased glecaprevir exposures by 83–163% and increased pibrentasvir exposures by 40–53% relative to administration in the fasting state. Administration of glecaprevir/pibrentasvir oral pellets with a low/moderate- to high-fat meal increased systemic exposure of glecaprevir and pibrentasvir by 131–167% and 56–114%, respectively, compared with the fasting state.

Following oral administration of glecaprevir/pibrentasvir in patients with HCV without cirrhosis, peak plasma concentrations of glecaprevir were lower, AUC over 24 hours at steady state was similar, and trough levels at steady state were higher, compared to healthy individuals. In the same patient population, peak plasma concentrations of pibrentasvir were lower, AUC over 24 hours at steady state was lower, and trough levels were lower compared to healthy individuals. Following daily administration of glecaprevir/pibrentasvir to pediatric patients 3 years of age and older infected with HCV, all pharmacokinetic parameters fell within the range observed in adult patients.

Glecaprevir is metabolized to some extent by cytochrome P-450 (CYP) isoenzyme 3A. The drug is 97.5% bound to plasma proteins. The major route of elimination is biliary and fecal excretion. Following a single oral dose of glecaprevir, 92.1% of the dose is excreted in feces and 0.7% is eliminated in urine. The plasma half-life of glecaprevir is 6 hours.

Pibrentasvir is only minimally metabolized. The drug is more than 99.9% bound to plasma proteins. The major route of elimination is biliary and fecal excretion. Following a single oral dose of pibrentasvir, 96.6% of the dose is excreted in feces; no drug is eliminated in urine. The plasma half-life of pibrentasvir is 13 hours.

ADVICE TO PATIENTS

- Advise patients to read the patient information provided by the manufacturer.
- Advise patients that glecaprevir/pibrentasvir should be taken once daily with food on a regular dosing schedule.
- Advise patients or their caregivers to read and follow the manufacturer's instructions to prepare the correct dose of glecaprevir/pibrentasvir oral pellets.

- Importance of taking the recommended dosage of glecaprevir/pibrentasvir for the recommended duration of treatment; importance of not missing doses.
- If a dose is missed and remembered <18 hours after scheduled administration time, take glecaprevir/pibrentasvir as soon as possible and then take the next dose at the usual time. If a dose is missed and remembered >18 hours after schedule administration time, skip the missed dose and take the next dose at the usual time.
- Inform patients that reactivation of HBV infection has occurred in patients being treated for HCV infection who were coinfected with HBV. Importance of informing clinician of any history of HBV infection or other liver problems (e.g., cirrhosis). Importance of immediately contacting a clinician if any signs or symptoms of serious liver injury (e.g., fatigue, weakness, loss of appetite, nausea and vomiting, yellowing of the eyes or skin, light-colored bowel movements) occur.
- Advise patients to immediately contact a clinician if they have symptoms of worsening liver problems (e.g., nausea, tiredness, yellowing of skin or white part of the eyes, bleeding or bruising more easily than normal, confusion, loss of appetite, diarrhea, dark or brown urine, dark or bloody stool, abdominal swelling, pain in upper right side of stomach area, sleepiness, vomiting of blood).
- Advise patients that glecaprevir/pibrentasvir may interact with some drugs. Importance of informing clinicians of existing or contemplated concomitant therapy, including prescription and OTC drugs and dietary or herbal supplements, as well as any concomitant illnesses.
- Importance of women informing clinicians if they are or plan to become pregnant or plan to breast-feed.
- Inform patients of other important precautionary information.

PREPARATIONS

Excipients in commercially available drug preparations may have clinically important effects in some individuals; consult specific product labeling for details.

Glecaprevir and Pibrentasvir

Oral

Pellets	Glecaprevir 50 mg and Pibrentasvir 20 mg	**Mavyret®**, AbbVie
Tablets, film-coated	Glecaprevir 100 mg and Pibrentasvir 40 mg	**Mavyret®**, AbbVie

† Use is not currently included in the labeling approved by the US Food and Drug Administration.

Elbasvir and Grazoprevir

8:18.40.24 • HCV REPLICATION COMPLEX INHIBITORS

■ Elbasvir and grazoprevir (elbasvir/grazoprevir) is a fixed combination containing 2 hepatitis C virus (HCV) antivirals; elbasvir is an HCV nonstructural 5A (NS5A) replication complex inhibitor (NS5A inhibitor) and grazoprevir is an HCV nonstructural 3/4A (NS3/4A) protease inhibitor.

USES

● Chronic Hepatitis C Virus Infection

The fixed combination of elbasvir and grazoprevir (elbasvir/grazoprevir) is used for the treatment of chronic hepatitis C virus (HCV) genotype 1 or genotype 4 infection in adults and pediatric patients 12 years of age and older or weighing at least 30 kg, without cirrhosis or with compensated cirrhosis (Child-Pugh class A), who are treatment-naive (have not previously received HCV treatment) or in whom prior treatment with peginterferon alfa and ribavirin (with or without an HCV protease inhibitor) failed, including those with human immunodeficiency virus (HIV) coinfection.

Elbasvir/grazoprevir is used alone or in conjunction with ribavirin, depending on HCV genotype and certain patient factors (e.g., previous treatment experience, presence of baseline polymorphisms).

Because efficacy of a 12-week regimen of elbasvir/grazoprevir for the treatment of HCV genotype 1a infection is reduced when 1 or more NS5A resistance-associated polymorphisms at certain amino acid positions (28, 30, 31, 93) are present at baseline, screening for NS5A resistance-associated polymorphisms is recommended prior to initiation of treatment in patients with HCV genotype 1a infection.

Because the treatment of chronic HCV infection is complex and rapidly evolving, it is recommended that treatment be directed by clinicians who are familiar with the disease and that a specialist be consulted to obtain the most up-to-date information. Information from the American Association for the Study of Liver Diseases (AASLD), Infectious Diseases Society of America (IDSA), and International Antiviral Society–USA (IAS–USA) regarding diagnosis and management of HCV infection, including recommendations for initial treatment, is available at https://www.hcvguidelines.org.

Clinical Experience

HCV Genotype 1 Infection in Treatment-naive Adults

Efficacy and safety of elbasvir/grazoprevir for the treatment of chronic HCV genotype 1 infection in treatment-naive adults have been evaluated in a randomized, double-blind, placebo-controlled, phase 3 trial (C-EDGE TN; NCT02105467). A total of 421 treatment-naive adults with chronic HCV genotype 1, 4, or 6 infection (noncirrhotic or with compensated cirrhosis) were randomized in a 3:1 ratio to receive elbasvir/grazoprevir (a fixed-combination tablet containing 50 mg of elbasvir and 100 mg of grazoprevir once daily) or placebo for 12 weeks. Those with decompensated liver disease and those with HIV coinfection were excluded. Patients who initially received placebo then received open-label elbasvir/grazoprevir for 12 weeks (deferred-treatment group). The primary end point was sustained virologic response at 12 weeks after the end of treatment (SVR12; defined as plasma HCV RNA level less than 15 IU/mL [the lower limit of quantification] at 12 weeks after end of treatment). The study included 382 patients with HCV genotype 1 infection (288 in the immediate-treatment group, 94 in the deferred-treatment group); among those in the immediate-treatment group, the median age was 55 years, 56% were male, 72% had baseline HCV RNA levels exceeding 800,000 IU/mL, 55% had HCV genotype 1a infection, 67% had non-CC IL28B alleles, and 24% had cirrhosis. SVR12 was achieved in 95% of patients with HCV genotype 1 infection in the immediate-treatment group (92 or 98% of those with HCV genotype 1a or 1b infection, respectively).

HCV Genotype 1 Infection in Previously Treated Adults

Efficacy and safety of elbasvir/grazoprevir for the treatment of chronic HCV genotype 1 infection in previously treated adults have been evaluated in a randomized,

open-label, phase 3 trial (C-EDGE TE) and a single-arm, open-label, phase 2 trial (C-SALVAGE). The primary end point in both studies was SVR12 (defined as plasma HCV RNA level less than 15 IU/mL [the lower limit of quantification] at 12 weeks after end of treatment).

C-EDGE TE (NCT02105701) included 414 noncirrhotic or cirrhotic adults with chronic HCV genotype 1, 4, or 6 infection (with or without HIV coinfection) who previously failed a treatment regimen of peginterferon alfa and ribavirin. Patients were randomized in a 1:1:1:1 ratio to receive elbasvir/grazoprevir (a fixed-combination tablet containing 50 mg of elbasvir and 100 mg of grazoprevir once daily) for 12 or 16 weeks or elbasvir/grazoprevir once daily in conjunction with ribavirin for 12 or 16 weeks. C-EDGE TE included 377 previously treated patients with HCV genotype 1 infection (median age 57 years [range 19–77 years], 64% male, 78% with baseline HCV RNA levels exceeding 800,000 IU/mL, 60% with HCV genotype 1a infection, 79% with non-CC IL28B alleles, 34% with cirrhosis). In those with HCV genotype 1 infection, SVR12 was achieved in 94% of patients treated with elbasvir/grazoprevir alone for 12 weeks and in 97% of those treated with elbasvir/grazoprevir with ribavirin for 16 weeks.

C-SALVAGE (NCT02105454) included 79 noncirrhotic or cirrhotic adults with HCV genotype 1 infection who previously failed a treatment regimen of peginterferon alfa, ribavirin, and an HCV protease inhibitor (e.g., boceprevir, simeprevir, telaprevir; drugs no longer commercially available) (median age 55 years, 58% male, 63% with baseline HCV RNA levels exceeding 800,000 IU/mL, 38% with HCV genotype 1a infection, 97% with non-CC IL28B alleles, 43% with cirrhosis, 46% with baseline NS3 resistance-associated substitutions). All patients received elbasvir/grazoprevir (a fixed-combination tablet containing 50 mg of elbasvir and 100 mg of grazoprevir once daily) in conjunction with ribavirin for 12 weeks. SVR12 was achieved in 96% of patients overall; 4% of patients did not achieve SVR12 and experienced relapse after the end of treatment. The SVR12 rates were similar in those with HCV genotype 1a or 1b infection, cirrhotic or noncirrhotic patients, and those with varying response to previous HCV treatments. All patients who achieved SVR12 also achieved SVR24 (defined as plasma HCV RNA level less than 15 IU/mL [the lower limit of quantification] at 24 weeks after end of treatment).

HCV Genotype 4 Infection in Treatment-naive Adults

Efficacy and safety of elbasvir/grazoprevir for the treatment of chronic HCV genotype 4 infection in treatment-naive adults have been evaluated in a randomized, open-label, phase 2 trial (C-SCAPE), a randomized, double-blind, placebo-controlled, phase 3 trial (C-EDGE TN), and an open-label, single-arm, phase 3 trial (C-EDGE COINFECTION).

In C-SCAPE (NCT01932762), 20 treatment-naive, noncirrhotic adults with HCV genotype 4 infection were randomized to receive elbasvir/grazoprevir (a ixed-combination tablet containing 50 mg of elbasvir and 100 mg of grazoprevir once daily) alone or in conjunction with ribavirin for 12 weeks. The primary end point was sustained virologic response at 12 weeks after the end of treatment (SVR12; defined as plasma HCV RNA level less than 25 IU/mL [the lower limit of quantification] at 12 weeks after end of treatment).

In C-EDGE TN (NCT02105467), treatment-naive adults with chronic HCV genotype 1, 4, or 6 infection (without cirrhosis or with compensated cirrhosis) were randomized in a 3:1 ratio to receive elbasvir/grazoprevir (a fixed-combination tablet containing 50 mg of elbasvir and 100 mg of grazoprevir once daily) or placebo for 12 weeks followed by open-label elbasvir/grazoprevir for 12 weeks (deferred treatment group). The primary end point was sustained virologic response at 12 weeks after the end of treatment (SVR12; defined as plasma HCV RNA level less than 15 IU/mL [the lower limit of quantification] at 12 weeks after end of treatment). The immediate-treatment group in C-EDGE TN included 18 treatment-naive patients with HCV genotype 4 infection.

In C-EDGE COINFECTION (NCT02105662), treatment-naive adults with HCV genotype 1, 4, or 6 infection coinfected with HIV received elbasvir/grazoprevir (a fixed-combination tablet containing 50 mg of elbasvir and 100 mg of grazoprevir once daily) for 12 weeks. The primary end point was sustained virologic response at 12 weeks after the end of treatment (SVR12; defined as plasma HCV RNA level less than 15 IU/mL [the lower limit of quantification] at 12 weeks after end of treatment). C-EDGE COINFECTION included 28 treatment-naive patients with HCV genotype 4 infection.

When data from these 3 studies were combined, a total of 66 treatment-naive adults with HCV genotype 4 infection received 12 weeks of treatment with elbasvir/grazoprevir and SVR12 was achieved in 97% of these patients.

HCV Genotype 4 Infection in Previously Treated Adults

Efficacy and safety of elbasvir/grazoprevir for the treatment of chronic HCV genotype 4 infection in previously treated adults have been evaluated in a randomized, open-label, phase 3 trial, C-EDGE TE (NCT02105701). This trial included cirrhotic or noncirrhotic adults with chronic HCV genotype 1, 4, or 6 (with or without HIV coinfection) who previously failed a treatment regimen of peginterferon alfa and ribavirin. Patients were randomized (stratified by presence or absence of cirrhosis and by type of prior treatment failure [relapse, partial response, or null response] to peginterferon/ribavirin) in a 1:1:1:1 ratio to receive elbasvir/grazoprevir (a fixed-combination tablet containing 50 mg of elbasvir and 100 mg of grazoprevir once daily) for 12 or 16 weeks or elbasvir/grazoprevir (once daily) in conjunction *with* ribavirin (twice daily) for 12 or 16 weeks. The primary end point was SVR12 (defined as plasma HCV RNA level less than 15 IU/mL [the lower limit of quantification] at 12 weeks after end of treatment). In C-EDGE TE, a total of 37 previously treated patients with HCV genotype 4 infection received a 12- or 16-week regimen of elbasvir/grazoprevir with or without ribavirin. Among the 8 patients who received a 16-week regimen of elbasvir/grazoprevir *with* ribavirin, the SVR12 rate was 100%.

HCV-infected Individuals Coinfected with HIV

Efficacy and safety of elbasvir/grazoprevir for the treatment of HCV genotype 1, 4, or 6 infection in treatment-naive adults coinfected with HIV have been evaluated in an open-label, single-arm, phase 3 study (C-EDGE COINFECTION; NCT02105662). A total of 218 HCV-infected patients who were coinfected with HIV (mean age 49 years, 84% male, 58% with baseline HCV RNA levels exceeding 800,000 IU/mL, 66% with HCV genotype 1a infection, 20% with HCV genotype 1b infection, 13% with HCV genotype 4 infection, 1% with HCV genotype 6 infection, 65% with non-CC IL28B alleles, 16% with METAVIR F4 [cirrhosis], 97% receiving HIV antiretroviral therapy and with undetectable HIV RNA levels) received elbasvir/grazoprevir (a fixed-combination tablet containing 50 mg of elbasvir and 100 mg of grazoprevir once daily) for 12 weeks. The primary end point was SVR12 (defined as plasma HCV RNA level less than 15 IU/mL [the lower limit of quantification] at 12 weeks after end of treatment). SVR12 was achieved in 96% of patients overall (97, 96, or 96% of those with HCV genotype 1a, 1b, or 4 infection, respectively).

HCV-infected Individuals with Severe Renal Impairment

Efficacy and safety of elbasvir/grazoprevir for the treatment of HCV genotype 1 infection in treatment-naive or previously treated adults with severe renal impairment were evaluated in a randomized, double-blind, placebo-controlled phase 3 study (C-SURFER; NCT02092350). A total of 235 patients with compensated liver disease (with or without cirrhosis) and with stage 4 or 5 chronic kidney disease (estimated glomerular filtration rate [eGFR] 15–29 mL/minute per 1.73 m² or less than 15 mL/minute per 1.73 m², respectively, including those undergoing hemodialysis) were randomized in a 1:1 ratio to receive elbasvir/grazoprevir (a fixed-combination tablet containing 50 mg of elbasvir and 100 mg of grazoprevir once daily) or placebo for 12 weeks followed by open-label elbasvir/grazoprevir for 12 weeks (deferred treatment group). In addition, 11 patients in an intensive pharmacokinetic group received open-label treatment with elbasvir/grazoprevir once daily for 12 weeks. The primary end point was sustained virologic response at 12 weeks after the end of treatment (SVR12; defined as plasma HCV RNA level less than 15 IU/mL [the lower limit of quantification] at 12 weeks after end of treatment). A total of 122 patients were included in the immediate-treatment group and intensive pharmacokinetic group (median age 58 years, 75% male, 57% with baseline HCV RNA levels exceeding 800,000 IU/mL, 72% with non-CC IL28B alleles, 52% with HCV genotype 1a infection, 6% with cirrhosis). SVR12 was achieved in 94% of patients in the pooled immediate-treatment group and intensive pharmacokinetic group (97 or 92% of those with HCV genotype 1a or 1b infection, respectively). SVR12 was achieved in 95% of those without cirrhosis compared with 86% of those with cirrhosis and in 100% of those with stage 4 renal impairment compared with 93% of those with stage 5 renal impairment.

Pediatric Patients

Efficacy and safety of elbasvir/grazoprevir for the treatment of HCV genotype 1 or 4 chronic HCV infection in 22 treatment-naive or previously treated noncirrhotic pediatric patients 12 to less than 18 years of age were evaluated in an open-label trial. Patients with HCV genotype 1a and at least one NS5A RAS mutation at baseline were excluded from participating. Patients received treatment with elbasvir/grazoprevir (a fixed-combination tablet containing 50 mg of elbasvir and 100 mg of grazoprevir once daily) for 12 weeks. Of the 22 patients included in the study, 95.5% had HCV genotype 1 and 4.5% had genotype 4; the median age was 13.5 years (range: 12–17 years), weight ranged from 28.1 to 96.5 kg, 50% were female, 95% were white, and 64% were treatment-naive. After 12 weeks of treatment, 100% of patients in this trial achieved SVR12.

Clinical Perspective

Because the treatment of chronic HCV infection is complex and rapidly evolving, it is recommended that treatment be directed by clinicians who are familiar with the disease and that a specialist be consulted to obtain the most up-to-date information. Information from the American Association for the Study of Liver Diseases (AASLD), Infectious Diseases Society of America (IDSA), and International Antiviral Society–USA (IAS–USA) regarding diagnosis and management of HCV infection, including recommendations for initial treatment, is available at https://www.hcvguidelines.org/.

DOSAGE AND ADMINISTRATION

● General

Pretreatment Screening

- Test for evidence of current or prior HBV infection by measuring hepatitis B surface antigen (HBsAg) and hepatitis B core antibody (anti-HBc).
- Screen for the presence of HCV nonstructural 5A (NS5A) resistance-associated polymorphisms in patients with HCV genotype 1a infection to determine the appropriate treatment regimen and treatment duration.
- Perform appropriate laboratory tests to evaluate liver function.

Patient Monitoring

- Perform appropriate laboratory tests to evaluate liver function at treatment week 8 and as clinically indicated. For patients receiving 16 weeks of therapy, perform additional hepatic laboratory testing at treatment week 12.
- *In patients with compensated cirrhosis (Child-Pugh class A) or evidence of advanced liver disease (e.g., portal hypertension), more frequent hepatic laboratory testing may be warranted.*
- *In all patients with evidence of current or prior HBV infection:* Monitor for clinical and laboratory signs (i.e., HBsAg, HBV DNA levels, serum aminotransferase and bilirubin concentrations) of hepatitis flare or HBV reactivation during and after treatment.
- Monitor for signs and symptoms of hepatic decompensation (e.g., jaundice, ascites, hepatic encephalopathy, variceal hemorrhage).

Other General Considerations

- For the treatment of chronic HCV infection, elbasvir and grazoprevir (elbasvir/grazoprevir) is used alone or in conjunction with ribavirin.
- Specific regimen and duration of treatment depend on HCV genotype and certain patient factors (e.g., presence of compensated or decompensated cirrhosis, liver transplantation). Consider that relapse rates following treatment are affected by baseline host and viral factors and differ between treatment durations for certain subgroups.

● Administration

Elbasvir/grazoprevir is administered orally once daily without regard to food.

Store elbasvir/grazoprevir at 20–25°C (excursions permitted between 15–30°C). Protect from moisture by storing in the original blister package until used.

● Dosage

Elbasvir/grazoprevir is commercially available as fixed-combination tablets containing 50 mg of elbasvir and 100 mg of grazoprevir.

Adult Dosage

HCV Genotype 1a Infection

For the treatment of HCV genotype 1a infection in adults without cirrhosis or with compensated cirrhosis (Child-Pugh class A), the recommended dosage of elbasvir/grazoprevir is 1 tablet (50 mg of elbasvir and 100 mg of grazoprevir) once daily. Elbasvir/grazoprevir is used alone in patients *without* baseline NS5A polymorphisms who are treatment-naive or were previously treated with peginterferon alfa and ribavirin, but is used in conjunction with ribavirin in those *with* baseline NS5A polymorphisms or in those previously treated with peginterferon alfa, ribavirin, and an HCV protease inhibitor. (See Table 1.)

A treatment duration of 12 weeks is recommended for most patients, but a treatment duration of 16 weeks is recommended in those *with* baseline NS5A polymorphisms. (See Table 1.)

TABLE 1. Recommended Treatment Regimen and Duration of Elbasvir/Grazoprevir for HCV Genotype 1a Infection in Adults without Cirrhosis or with Compensated Cirrhosis.

Patient Type	Multiple-drug Regimen	Duration of Treatment
Treatment-naive or previously treated[a] *without* baseline NS5A polymorphisms[b]	Elbasvir/grazoprevir	12 weeks
Treatment-naive or previously treated[a] *with* baseline NS5A polymorphisms[b]	Elbasvir/grazoprevir *with* ribavirin	16 weeks
Previously treated with an HCV protease inhibitor[d, e]	Elbasvir/grazoprevir *with* ribavirin[c]	12 weeks

[a] Previously treated defined as patients who failed treatment with peginterferon alfa and ribavirin.

[b] NS5A resistance-associated polymorphisms at amino acid positions 28, 30, 31, or 93.

[c] Use weight-based ribavirin dosage in patients with creatinine clearance >50 mL/minute (800 mg daily in those <66 kg, 1 g daily in those 66–80 kg, 1.2 g daily in those 81–105 kg, 1.4 g daily in those >105 kg); give ribavirin daily dosage in 2 divided doses with food.

[d] Previously treated with an HCV protease inhibitor defined as patients who failed treatment with a regimen of peginterferon alfa, ribavirin, and an HCV NS3/4A protease inhibitor (e.g., boceprevir, simeprevir, telaprevir; drugs no longer commercially available).

[e] The optimal elbasvir/grazoprevir-based regimen and duration of treatment not established for patients with HCV genotype 1a infection who previously failed treatment with peginterferon alfa, ribavirin, and an HCV protease inhibitor and have 1 or more baseline NS5A resistance-associated polymorphisms at positions 28, 30, 31, and 93.

HCV Genotype 1b Infection

For the treatment of HCV genotype 1b infection in adults without cirrhosis or with compensated cirrhosis (Child-Pugh class A), the recommended dosage of elbasvir/grazoprevir is 1 tablet (50 mg of elbasvir and 100 mg of grazoprevir) once daily. Elbasvir/grazoprevir is used alone in patients who are treatment-naive or were previously treated with peginterferon alfa and ribavirin, but is used in conjunction with ribavirin in those previously treated with peginterferon alfa, ribavirin, and an HCV protease inhibitor. (See Table 2.)

A treatment duration of 12 weeks is recommended. (See Table 2.)

TABLE 2. Recommended Treatment Regimen and Duration of Elbasvir/Grazoprevir for HCV Genotype 1b Infection in Adults without Cirrhosis or with Compensated Cirrhosis.

Patient Type	Multiple-drug Regimen	Duration of Treatment
Treatment-naive or previously treated[a]	Elbasvir/grazoprevir	12 weeks
Previously treated with an HCV protease inhibitor[b]	Elbasvir/grazoprevir *with* ribavirin[c]	12 weeks

[a] Previously treated defined as patients who failed treatment with peginterferon alfa and ribavirin.

[b] Previously treated with an HCV protease inhibitor defined as patients who failed treatment with a regimen of peginterferon alfa, ribavirin, and an HCV NS3/4A protease inhibitor (e.g., boceprevir, simeprevir, telaprevir; drugs no longer commercially available).

[c] Use weight-based ribavirin dosage in patients with creatinine clearance >50 mL/minute (800 mg daily in those <66 kg, 1 g daily in those 66–80 kg, 1.2 g daily in those 81–105 kg, 1.4 g daily in those >105 kg); give ribavirin daily dosage in 2 divided doses with food.

HCV Genotype 4 Infection

For the treatment of HCV genotype 4 infection in adults without cirrhosis or with compensated cirrhosis (Child-Pugh class A), the recommended dosage of elbasvir/grazoprevir is 1 tablet (50 mg of elbasvir and 100 mg of grazoprevir) once daily. Elbasvir/grazoprevir is used alone in patients who are treatment-naive, but is used in conjunction with ribavirin in those previously treated with peginterferon alfa and ribavirin. (See Table 3.)

A treatment duration of 12 weeks is recommended for treatment-naive patients, but a treatment duration of 16 weeks is recommended in patients previously treated with peginterferon alfa and ribavirin. (See Table 3.)

TABLE 3. Recommended Treatment Regimen and Duration of Elbasvir/Grazoprevir for HCV Genotype 4 Infection in Adults without Cirrhosis or with Compensated Cirrhosis.

Patient Type	Multiple-drug Regimen	Duration of Treatment
Treatment-naive	Elbasvir/grazoprevir	12 weeks
Previously treated[a]	Elbasvir/grazoprevir *with* ribavirin[a]	16 weeks

[a] Previously treated defined as patients who failed treatment with peginterferon alfa and ribavirin.

[b] Use weight-based ribavirin dosage in patients with creatinine clearance >50 mL/minute (800 mg daily in those <66 kg, 1 g daily in those 66–80 kg, 1.2 g daily in those 81–105 kg, 1.4 g daily in those >105 kg); give ribavirin daily dosage in 2 divided doses with food.

HCV-infected Individuals Coinfected with HIV

For the treatment of chronic HCV genotype 1 or genotype 4 infection in adults with human immunodeficiency virus (HIV) coinfection without cirrhosis or with compensated cirrhosis (Child-Pugh class A), the same elbasvir/grazoprevir dosage and same HCV genotype-specific multiple-drug regimen and treatment duration recommended for HCV-infected patients without HIV coinfection should be used. (See Table 1, Table 2, and Table 3.)

Pediatric Dosage

HCV Genotype 1a Infection

For the treatment of HCV genotype 1a infection in pediatric patients 12 years of age and older or weighing at least 30 kg without cirrhosis or with compensated cirrhosis (Child-Pugh class A), the recommended dosage of elbasvir/grazoprevir is 1 tablet (50 mg of elbasvir and 100 mg of grazoprevir) once daily. Elbasvir/grazoprevir is used alone in patients without baseline NS5A polymorphisms who are treatment-naive or were previously treated with peginterferon alfa and ribavirin. In patients with baseline NS5A polymorphisms or those previously treated with peginterferon alfa, ribavirin, and an HCV protease inhibitor, elbasvir/grazoprevir is used in conjunction with ribavirin. (See Table 4.)

A treatment duration of 12 weeks is recommended for most patients, but a treatment duration of 16 weeks is recommended in those with baseline NS5A polymorphisms. (See Table 4.)

TABLE 4. HCV Genotype 1a Infection: Recommended Treatment Regimen and Duration of Elbasvir/Grazoprevir in Pediatric Patients ≥12 Years of Age or Weighing ≥30 kg without Cirrhosis or with Compensated Cirrhosis.

Patient Type	Multiple-drug Regimen	Duration of Treatment
Treatment-naive or previously treated[a] *without* baseline NS5A polymorphisms[b]	Elbasvir/grazoprevir	12 weeks
Treatment-naive or previously treated[a] *with* baseline NS5A polymorphisms[b]	Elbasvir/grazoprevir *with* ribavirin[c]	16 weeks
Previously treated with an HCV protease inhibitor[d, e]	Elbasvir/grazoprevir *with* ribavirin[c]	12 weeks

[a] Previously treated defined as patients who failed treatment with peginterferon alfa and ribavirin.

[b] NS5A resistance-associated polymorphisms at amino acid positions 28, 30, 31, or 93.

TABLE 4. Continued

c Use weight-based ribavirin dosage in patients with creatinine clearance >50 mL/minute (800 mg daily in those <66 kg, 1 g daily in those 66–80 kg, 1.2 g daily in those 81–105 kg, 1.4 g daily in those >105 kg); give ribavirin daily dosage in 2 divided doses with food.

d Previously treated with an HCV protease inhibitor defined as patients who failed treatment with a regimen of peginterferon alfa, ribavirin, and an HCV NS3/4A protease inhibitor (e.g., boceprevir, simeprevir, telaprevir; drugs no longer commercially available).

e The optimal elbasvir/grazoprevir-based regimen and duration of treatment not established for patients with HCV genotype 1a infection who previously failed treatment with peginterferon alfa, ribavirin, and an HCV protease inhibitor and have 1 or more baseline NS5A resistance-associated polymorphisms at positions 28, 30, 31, and 93.

HCV Genotype 1b Infection

For the treatment of HCV genotype 1b infection in pediatric patients 12 years of age and older or weighing at least 30 kg without cirrhosis or with compensated cirrhosis (Child-Pugh class A), the recommended dosage of elbasvir/grazoprevir is 1 tablet (50 mg of elbasvir and 100 mg of grazoprevir) once daily. Elbasvir/grazoprevir is used alone in patients who are treatment-naive or were previously treated with peginterferon alfa and ribavirin. In patients previously treated with peginterferon alfa, ribavirin, and an HCV protease inhibitor, elbasvir/grazoprevir is used in conjunction with ribavirin. (See Table 5.)

A treatment duration of 12 weeks is recommended. (See Table 5.)

TABLE 5. HCV Genotype 1b Infection: Recommended Treatment Regimen and Duration of Elbasvir/Grazoprevir in Pediatric Patients ≥12 Years of Age or Weighing ≥30 kg without Cirrhosis or with Compensated Cirrhosis.

Patient Type	Multiple-drug Regimen	Duration of Treatment
Treatment-naive or previously treated[a]	Elbasvir/grazoprevir	12 weeks
Previously treated with an HCV protease inhibitor[b]	Elbasvir/grazoprevir with ribavirin[c]	12 weeks

a Previously treated defined as patients who failed treatment with peginterferon alfa and ribavirin.

b Previously treated with an HCV protease inhibitor defined as patients who failed treatment with a regimen of peginterferon alfa, ribavirin, and an HCV NS3/4A protease inhibitor (e.g., boceprevir, simeprevir, telaprevir; drugs no longer commercially available).

c Use weight-based ribavirin dosage in patients with creatinine clearance >50 mL/minute (800 mg daily in those <66 kg, 1 g daily in those 66–80 kg, 1.2 g daily in those 81–105 kg, 1.4 g daily in those >105 kg); give ribavirin daily dosage in 2 divided doses with food.

HCV Genotype 4 Infection

For the treatment of HCV genotype 4 infection in pediatric patients 12 years of age and older or weighing at least 30 kg without cirrhosis or with compensated cirrhosis (Child-Pugh class A), the recommended dosage of elbasvir/grazoprevir is 1 tablet (50 mg of elbasvir and 100 mg of grazoprevir) once daily. Elbasvir/grazoprevir is used alone in patients who are treatment-naive. In patients previously treated with peginterferon alfa and ribavirin, elbasvir/grazoprevir is used in conjunction with ribavirin. (See Table 6.)

A treatment duration of 12 weeks is recommended for treatment-naive patients, but a treatment duration of 16 weeks is recommended in patients previously treated with peginterferon alfa and ribavirin. (See Table 6.)

TABLE 6. HCV Genotype 4 Infection: Recommended Treatment Regimen and Duration of Elbasvir/Grazoprevir in Pediatric Patients ≥12 Years of Age or Weighing ≥30 kg without Cirrhosis or with Compensated Cirrhosis.

Patient Type	Multiple-drug Regimen	Duration of Treatment
Treatment-naive	Elbasvir/grazoprevir	12 weeks
Previously treated[a]	Elbasvir/grazoprevir with ribavirin[b]	16 weeks

TABLE 6. Continued

a Previously treated defined as patients who failed treatment with peginterferon alfa and ribavirin.

b Use weight-based ribavirin dosage in patients with creatinine clearance >50 mL/minute (800 mg daily in those <66 kg, 1 g daily in those 66–80 kg, 1.2 g daily in those 81–105 kg, 1.4 g daily in those >105 kg); give ribavirin daily dosage in 2 divided doses with food.

HCV-infected Individuals Coinfected with HIV

For the treatment of chronic HCV genotype 1 or genotype 4 infection in pediatric patients 12 years of age and older or weighing at least 30 kg, with human immunodeficiency virus (HIV) coinfection without cirrhosis or with compensated cirrhosis (Child-Pugh class A), the same elbasvir/grazoprevir dosage and same HCV genotype-specific multiple-drug regimen and treatment duration recommended for HCV-infected patients without HIV coinfection should be used. (See Table 4, Table 5, and Table 6.)

● Special Populations

Hepatic Impairment

Dosage adjustments of elbasvir/grazoprevir are not needed in patients with mild hepatic impairment or compensated cirrhosis (Child-Pugh class A). However, monitor such patients for signs and symptoms of hepatic decompensation.

Elbasvir/grazoprevir is contraindicated in patients with moderate or severe hepatic impairment (Child-Pugh class B or C) and in those with any history of hepatic decompensation.

Renal Impairment

Dosage adjustments of elbasvir/grazoprevir are not needed in patients with mild, moderate, or severe renal impairment, including those requiring hemodialysis.

Geriatric Patients

Dosage adjustments of elbasvir/grazoprevir are not necessary in geriatric patients.

CAUTIONS

● Contraindications

The fixed combination of elbasvir and grazoprevir (elbasvir/grazoprevir) is contraindicated in patients with moderate or severe hepatic impairment (Child-Pugh class B or C) and in those with any history of hepatic decompensation.

Concomitant use of elbasvir/grazoprevir with certain drugs (e.g., inhibitors of organic anion transporting polypeptides [OATP] 1B1 and 1B3, potent inducers of cytochrome P-450 [CYP] 3A, efavirenz) is contraindicated.

When elbasvir/grazoprevir is used in conjunction with ribavirin, the contraindications for ribavirin apply.

● Warnings/Precautions

Warnings

Risk of HBV Reactivation in Patients Coinfected with HCV and HBV

A boxed warning about the risk of hepatitis B virus (HBV) reactivation is included in the prescribing information for elbasvir/grazoprevir. Reactivation of hepatitis B virus (HBV) infection has been reported during postmarketing experience when direct-acting antivirals (DAAs) were used for the treatment of chronic hepatitis C virus (HCV) infection in patients with HBV coinfection. In some cases, HBV reactivation resulted in fulminant hepatitis, hepatic failure, and death.

HBV reactivation (defined as an abrupt increase in HBV replication manifested as a rapid increase in serum HBV DNA levels or detection of hepatitis B surface antigen [HBsAg] in an individual who was previously HBsAg negative and hepatitis B core antibody [anti-HBc] positive) has been reported in patients with HCV and HBV coinfection who were receiving HCV treatment with a regimen that included HCV DAAs without interferon alfa. Reactivation also may be accompanied by hepatitis (i.e., increased aminotransferase concentrations) and, in severe cases, may lead to increased bilirubin concentrations, liver failure, or death. Data to date indicate that HBV reactivation usually occurs within 4–8 weeks after initiation of HCV treatment. Patients with HBV reactivation have been heterogeneous in terms of HCV genotype and in terms of baseline HBV disease. While some patients with HBV reactivation were HBsAg positive, others had serologic evidence of resolved HBV infection (i.e., HBsAg negative and anti-HBc positive). HBV reactivation also has been reported in patients receiving certain immunosuppressant or chemotherapeutic drugs; the risk of reactivation associated with HCV DAAs may be increased in such patients.

The mechanism for HBV reactivation in patients with HCV and HBV coinfection receiving HCV DAAs is unknown. Although HCV DAAs are not known to cause immunosuppression, HBV reactivation in coinfected patients may result from a complex interplay of host immunologic responses in the setting of infection with 2 hepatitis viruses.

Prior to initiating treatment with an HCV DAA, including elbasvir/grazoprevir, screen all patients for evidence of current or prior HBV infection by measuring HBsAg, anti-HBs, and anti-HBc. If there is serologic evidence of HBV infection, measure baseline HBV DNA levels.

Patients with evidence of current or prior HBV infection should be monitored for clinical and laboratory signs (i.e., HBsAg, HBV DNA levels, serum aminotransferase concentrations, bilirubin concentrations) of hepatitis flare or HBV reactivation during and after treatment with HCV DAAs, including elbasvir/grazoprevir. Initiate appropriate management for HBV infection as clinically indicated.

Advise patients with HCV and HBV coinfection receiving elbasvir/grazoprevir to immediately contact a clinician if they develop any signs or symptoms of serious liver injury.

When making decisions regarding HBV monitoring or HBV treatment in coinfected patients, consult with a clinician who has expertise in managing HBV infection.

Other Warnings/Precautions

Risk of Hepatic Decompensation or Failure in Patients with Evidence of Advanced Liver Disease

Hepatic decompensation or failure, including some fatalities, have been reported during postmarketing experience in patients receiving HCV treatment regimens containing an HCV nonstructural 3/4A (NS3/4A) protease inhibitor, including elbasvir/grazoprevir. Data are insufficient to estimate the frequency of such events and a causal relationship has not been established. Hepatic decompensation or failure usually occurred within the first 4 weeks of HCV treatment.

Many of the reported cases of hepatic decompensation or failure occurred in patients with evidence of advanced liver disease with moderate or severe hepatic impairment (Child-Pugh class B or C) prior to initiation of HCV treatment. Some cases occurred in patients who were reported as noncirrhotic or as having compensated cirrhosis with mild liver impairment (Child-Pugh class A) at baseline, but had a history of a decompensation event or had evidence of portal hypertension or decreased platelet counts at baseline. Some cases also were reported in patients who had confounding factors (e.g., serious liver-related comorbidities).

If elbasvir/grazoprevir is used in patients who have compensated cirrhosis (Child-Pugh class A) or evidence of advanced liver disease (e.g., portal hypertension), perform hepatic function tests as clinically indicated and monitor patients for signs and symptoms of hepatic decompensation (e.g., jaundice, ascites, hepatic encephalopathy, variceal hemorrhage).

Discontinue elbasvir/grazoprevir in patients who develop evidence of hepatic decompensation or failure. (See Cautions: Contraindications.)

Patients should be advised to contact a clinician if they develop any signs or symptoms of worsening liver disease.

● Hepatic Effects

In clinical trials evaluating elbasvir/grazoprevir with or without ribavirin, increased ALT concentrations (exceeding 5 times the upper limit of normal [ULN]) were reported in 1% of patients, usually at 8 weeks or longer after initiation of treatment (mean onset 10 weeks; range 6–12 weeks). ALT elevations usually were asymptomatic and resolved with ongoing treatment or completion of treatment. Increased rates of late-onset ALT elevations were reported in patients with increased grazoprevir plasma concentrations and in certain patient groups (e.g., 65 years of age or older, Asian descent, females). The incidence of late-onset ALT elevations did not appear to be affected by presence of cirrhosis or treatment duration.

In clinical trials, increased bilirubin concentrations (exceeding 2.5 times the ULN) were reported in 6% of patients receiving elbasvir/grazoprevir in conjunction *with* ribavirin compared with less than 1% of patients receiving elbasvir/grazoprevir alone. These bilirubin increases were predominately indirect bilirubin and typically were not associated with increased ALT concentrations.

Perform hepatic laboratory testing prior to initiation of elbasvir/grazoprevir, at treatment week 8, and as clinically indicated. For patients receiving 16 weeks of elbasvir/grazoprevir treatment, perform additional hepatic laboratory testing at treatment week 12.

If ALT concentrations remain persistently greater than 10 times the ULN, consider discontinuation of elbasvir/grazoprevir. If ALT elevations are accompanied by signs or symptoms of liver inflammation or increasing conjugated bilirubin, alkaline phosphatase, or international normalized ratio (INR), discontinue the drug. Advise patients to immediately contact a clinician if they have onset of fatigue, weakness, lack of appetite, nausea and vomiting, jaundice, or discolored feces.

● Interactions

Concomitant use of elbasvir/grazoprevir and certain drugs is contraindicated or not recommended. Concomitant use with some drugs may result in drug interactions leading to loss of therapeutic effect and possible development of resistance to elbasvir/grazoprevir. Certain other drug interactions may result in clinically important adverse reactions due to increased exposures of the concomitant drugs or components of elbasvir/grazoprevir.

Consider potential drug interactions prior to and during elbasvir/grazoprevir treatment. Review drugs used concomitantly with elbasvir/grazoprevir during the course of treatment and monitor the patient for adverse reactions associated with these drugs.

● Precautions Related to Fixed Combinations and Multiple-drug Treatment Regimens

When elbasvir/grazoprevir is used, consider the cautions, precautions, contraindications, and drug interactions associated with both drugs in the fixed combination. Consider cautionary information applicable to specific populations (e.g., pregnant or nursing women, individuals with hepatic or renal impairment, geriatric patients) for each drug.

When elbasvir/grazoprevir is used in conjunction *with* ribavirin, consider the cautions, precautions, and contraindications associated with ribavirin. (See Cautions in Ribavirin 8:18.32.)

Specific Populations

Pregnancy

Adequate data are not available regarding use of elbasvir/grazoprevir in pregnant women. Animal reproduction studies using elbasvir or grazoprevir have not revealed evidence of fetal harm at exposures greater than those attained with recommended human dosage.

When elbasvir/grazoprevir is used in conjunction *with* ribavirin, consider the cautions, precautions, and contraindications associated with ribavirin. (See Cautions in Ribavirin 8:18.32.)

Lactation

It is not known whether elbasvir/grazoprevir is distributed into human milk, affects human milk production, or affects the breast-fed infant. Both elbasvir and grazoprevir are distributed into milk in rats.

Consider the benefits of breast-feeding and the importance of elbasvir/grazoprevir to the woman along with the potential adverse effects on the breast-fed child from the drug or from the underlying maternal condition.

When elbasvir/grazoprevir is used in conjunction *with* ribavirin, consider the potential for adverse reactions to ribavirin in nursing infants. A decision should be made whether to discontinue nursing or the ribavirin-containing regimen, taking into account the importance of the treatment regimen to the woman.

Pediatric Use

Safety and efficacy of elbasvir/grazoprevir have not been established in pediatric patients younger than 12 years of age or who weigh less than 30 kg.

Safety and efficacy of elbasvir/grazoprevir for the treatment of HCV genotype 1 or 4 infection in pediatric patients 12 years of age and older or weighing greater than 30 kg are based on safety, efficacy, and pharmacokinetic data from an open-label trial that included 22 treatment-naive or previously treated non-cirrhotic pediatric patients. Trial data indicated that safety, efficacy, and pharmacokinetics of elbasvir/grazoprevir in these pediatric patients were consistent with those observed in HCV-infected adults receiving the drug in clinical trials.

In a pharmacokinetic study of 22 pediatric patients 12 years of age and older with HCV genotype 1 or 4, administration of elbasvir 50 mg/grazoprevir 100 mg once daily led to similar drug exposures to those observed in adult patients.

Geriatric Use

In clinical trials, a higher rate of late-onset ALT elevations was reported in individuals 65 years of age and older.

In population pharmacokinetic analyses, the areas under the plasma concentration-time curves (AUCs) of elbasvir and grazoprevir are estimated to be increased by 16 and 45%, respectively, in individuals 65 years of age and older compared with AUCs in younger adults.

Hepatic Impairment

Patients with mild hepatic impairment or compensated cirrhosis (Child-Pugh class A) should be monitored for signs and symptoms of hepatic decompensation (e.g., jaundice, ascites, hepatic encephalopathy, variceal hemorrhage) during elbasvir/grazoprevir treatment.

Elbasvir/grazoprevir is contraindicated in patients with moderate or severe hepatic impairment (Child-Pugh class B or C) and in those with any history of hepatic decompensation. There have been postmarketing reports of hepatic decompensation or failure in such patients.

Efficacy and safety of elbasvir/grazoprevir have not been established in liver transplant recipients or pretransplant patients.

In population pharmacokinetic analyses of elbasvir and grazoprevir in adults with mild, moderate, or severe hepatic impairment (Child-Pugh class A, B, or C) without HCV infection, the AUC of grazoprevir is increased by 1.7-, 5-, and 12-fold, respectively, compared with AUCs reported in adults with normal hepatic function. There are no clinically important differences in the AUCs of elbasvir in adults with mild, moderate, or severe hepatic impairment compared with AUCs reported in adults with normal hepatic function.

Although elbasvir AUCs in HCV-infected adults with compensated cirrhosis are similar to those reported in HCV-infected adults without cirrhosis, grazoprevir AUCs in HCV-infected adults with compensated cirrhosis are 1.65-fold higher than those reported in HCV-infected adults without cirrhosis.

Renal Impairment

In population pharmacokinetic analyses of elbasvir and grazoprevir in adults with severe renal impairment (not dependent on dialysis) and adults requiring hemodialysis, the AUC of elbasvir was increased by 46 and 25%, respectively, and the AUC of grazoprevir was increased by 40 and 10%, respectively, compared with adults without severe renal impairment. These changes in elbasvir and grazoprevir exposures in HCV-infected adults with renal impairment (with or without hemodialysis) are not considered clinically important.

Elbasvir and grazoprevir are not removed by hemodialysis; the drugs are unlikely to be removed by peritoneal dialysis since they are highly bound to plasma proteins.

Race

In clinical trials, a higher rate of late-onset ALT elevations was observed in Asian individuals. In population pharmacokinetic analyses, elbasvir and grazoprevir AUCs were estimated to be increased by 15 and 50%, respectively, in Asian patients compared with AUCs reported in white patients; dosage adjustments are not needed based on race.

Estimated elbasvir and grazoprevir exposures in Black or African American individuals are comparable to those reported in white individuals.

Gender

In clinical trials, a higher rate of late-onset ALT elevations was observed in females.

In population pharmacokinetic analyses, elbasvir and grazoprevir AUCs were estimated to be increased by 50 and 30%, respectively, in females compared with AUCs reported in males; dosage adjustments are not needed based on gender.

● *Common Adverse Effects*

Elbasvir/grazoprevir (≥5%): Fatigue, headache, and nausea.

Elbasvir/grazoprevir in conjunction *with* ribavirin (≥5%): Anemia and headache.

DRUG INTERACTIONS

The following drug interactions are based on studies that used the fixed combination of elbasvir and grazoprevir (elbasvir/grazoprevir), elbasvir alone, or grazoprevir alone, or are predicted drug interactions that may occur with elbasvir/grazoprevir. When elbasvir/grazoprevir is used, consider interactions associated with both drugs in the fixed combination.

● *Drugs Affecting or Metabolized by Hepatic Microsomal Enzymes*

Elbasvir and grazoprevir are both substrates of cytochrome P-450 (CYP) isoenzyme 3A. Elbasvir does not inhibit CYP3A in vitro; grazoprevir is a weak inhibitor of CYP3A in vivo.

Pharmacokinetic interactions are possible if elbasvir/grazoprevir is used concomitantly with moderate or potent inducers of CYP3A (decreased elbasvir and grazoprevir concentrations and possible loss of therapeutic effect) or potent inhibitors of CYP3A (increased elbasvir and grazoprevir concentrations).

Concomitant use of elbasvir/grazoprevir and potent CYP3A inducers is contraindicated and concomitant use with moderate CYP3A inducers is not recommended. Concomitant use of elbasvir/grazoprevir and certain potent CYP3A inhibitors is not recommended.

In vitro, elbasvir and grazoprevir both inhibit CYP1A2, 2B6, 2C8, 2C9, 2C19, and 2D6. However, clinically important pharmacokinetic interactions are not expected if elbasvir/grazoprevir is used concomitantly with substrates of these CYP isoenzymes. Based on in vitro data, it is unlikely that administration of multiple doses of elbasvir or grazoprevir would induce metabolism of drugs metabolized by CYP1A2, 2B6, or 3A.

● *Drugs Affecting or Affected by P-glycoprotein Transport*

Elbasvir and grazoprevir are both substrates of P-glycoprotein (P-gp) transport; the role of intestinal P-gp in absorption of elbasvir and grazoprevir appears to be minimal.

In vitro, elbasvir inhibits P-gp; grazoprevir is not an inhibitor of P-gp.

● *Drugs Affecting or Affected by Breast Cancer Resistance Protein*

Elbasvir and grazoprevir are both inhibitors of intestinal breast cancer resistance protein (BCRP). Concomitant use of elbasvir/grazoprevir and drugs that are BCRP substrates may result in increased concentrations of such substrate drugs.

● *Drugs Affecting or Affected by Organic Anion Transport Polypeptides*

Grazoprevir is a substrate and inhibitor of organic anion transporting polypeptide (OATP) 1B1 and 1B3. Elbasvir is not a substrate of OATP1B.

Pharmacokinetic interactions are possible if elbasvir/grazoprevir is used concomitantly with OATP1B1 or 1B3 inhibitors (increased grazoprevir concentrations). Concomitant use of elbasvir/grazoprevir and OATP1B1 or 1B3 inhibitors that are known or expected to substantially increase grazoprevir plasma concentrations is contraindicated.

● *Drugs Affecting or Affected by Other Enzymes*

In vitro, elbasvir and grazoprevir do not inhibit carboxylesterase (CES) 1, CES2, cathepsin A (CatA), or uridine diphosphate-glucuronosyl transferase (UGT) 1A1. Clinically important pharmacokinetic interactions are not expected if elbasvir/grazoprevir is used concomitantly with CES1, CES2, CatA, or UGT1A1 substrates.

● Drugs Affecting Gastric pH

Antacids

Dosage adjustments are not needed if antacids are used concomitantly with elbasvir/grazoprevir.

Histamine H₂-receptor Antagonists

Concomitant use of famotidine and elbasvir/grazoprevir does not result in clinically important changes in the pharmacokinetics of elbasvir or grazoprevir.

Dosage adjustments are not needed if a histamine H₂-receptor antagonist is used concomitantly with elbasvir/grazoprevir.

Proton-pump Inhibitors

Concomitant use of pantoprazole and elbasvir/grazoprevir does not result in clinically important changes in the pharmacokinetics of elbasvir or grazoprevir.

Dosage adjustments are not needed if a proton-pump inhibitor is used concomitantly with elbasvir/grazoprevir.

● Antibacterial Agents

Penicillins

Nafcillin

Concomitant use of nafcillin and elbasvir/grazoprevir may result in decreased elbasvir and grazoprevir concentrations due to moderate CYP3A induction by nafcillin, which may lead to reduced therapeutic effect of the HCV antiviral.

Concomitant use of nafcillin and elbasvir/grazoprevir is not recommended.

● Anticonvulsants

Carbamazepine

Concomitant use of carbamazepine and elbasvir/grazoprevir may result in substantially decreased elbasvir and grazoprevir concentrations due to potent CYP3A induction by carbamazepine, which may lead to loss of virologic response to the HCV antiviral.

Concomitant use of carbamazepine and elbasvir/grazoprevir is contraindicated.

Phenytoin

Concomitant use of phenytoin and elbasvir/grazoprevir may result in substantially decreased elbasvir and grazoprevir concentrations due to potent CYP3A induction by phenytoin, which may lead to loss of virologic response to the HCV antiviral.

Concomitant use of phenytoin and elbasvir/grazoprevir is contraindicated.

● Antidiabetic Agents

Altered blood glucose control resulting in serious symptomatic hypoglycemia has been reported during postmarketing experience when direct-acting antivirals (DAAs) were used in diabetic patients receiving antidiabetic agents. Management of hypoglycemia in these cases required either discontinuance or dosage modification of the antidiabetic agent. Frequently monitor blood glucose concentrations; adjustment of antidiabetic agent dosage may be necessary.

● Antifungal Agents

Ketoconazole

In healthy adults, concomitant use of ketoconazole (400 mg once daily) and elbasvir (single 50-mg dose) or grazoprevir (single 100-mg dose) results in increased plasma concentrations and areas under the plasma concentration-time curves (AUCs) of elbasvir and grazoprevir, which may increase the overall risk of hepatotoxicity.

Concomitant use of ketoconazole and elbasvir/grazoprevir is not recommended.

● Antimycobacterial Agents

Rifampin

Concomitant use of rifampin (single 600-mg oral or IV dose) and elbasvir (single 50-mg dose) results in slightly increased elbasvir plasma concentrations and AUC. Although specific studies are not available, concomitant use of multiple doses of

rifampin and elbasvir is expected to result in clinically important decreases in elbasvir plasma concentrations because of potent CYP3A induction and may lead to loss of virologic response to the HCV antiviral.

Concomitant use of rifampin (single 600-mg oral or IV dose) and grazoprevir (single 200-mg dose) results in substantially increased grazoprevir plasma concentrations and AUC, presumably due to OATP1B1 inhibition by rifampin. However, concomitant use of multiple doses of rifampin and grazoprevir results in clinically important decreases in grazoprevir concentrations, most likely because of the mixed effects of rifampin on OATP1B (inhibition) and CYP3A4 (induction) and may lead to loss of virologic response to the HCV antiviral.

Concomitant use of rifampin and elbasvir/grazoprevir is contraindicated.

● Antiretroviral Agents

HIV Entry and Fusion Inhibitors

Maraviroc

Concomitant use of maraviroc and elbasvir/grazoprevir is not expected to affect maraviroc pharmacokinetics. Dosage adjustments are not needed.

HIV Integrase Inhibitors (INSTIs)

Bictegravir

Concomitant use of bictegravir and elbasvir/grazoprevir is not expected to affect bictegravir pharmacokinetics. Dosage adjustments are not needed.

Dolutegravir

Concomitant use of dolutegravir and elbasvir/grazoprevir does not result in clinically important changes in the pharmacokinetics of elbasvir, grazoprevir, or dolutegravir. Dosage adjustments are not needed.

Elvitegravir

Concomitant use of cobicistat-boosted elvitegravir and elbasvir/grazoprevir is expected to result in increased elbasvir and grazoprevir concentrations.

Concomitant use of the fixed combination of elvitegravir, cobicistat, emtricitabine, and tenofovir disoproxil fumarate (EVG/c/FTC/TDF) and elbasvir/grazoprevir results in increased elbasvir and grazoprevir concentrations. Concomitant use of the fixed combination of elvitegravir, cobicistat, emtricitabine, and tenofovir alafenamide fumarate (EVG/c/FTC/TAF) and elbasvir/grazoprevir is expected to result in increased elbasvir and grazoprevir concentrations.

Concomitant use of elbasvir/grazoprevir and cobicistat-boosted elvitegravir, including EVG/c/FTC/TAF or EVG/c/FTC/TDF, is not recommended.

Raltegravir

Concomitant use of raltegravir and elbasvir/grazoprevir does not result in clinically important changes in the pharmacokinetics of elbasvir, grazoprevir, or raltegravir. Dosage adjustments are not needed.

HIV Nonnucleoside Reverse Transcriptase Inhibitors (NNRTIs)

Doravirine

Concomitant use of doravirine and elbasvir/grazoprevir does not result in clinically important changes in the pharmacokinetics of elbasvir or grazoprevir, but may increase the AUC of doravirine.

Some experts state that dosage adjustments are not needed if doravirine is used concomitantly with elbasvir/grazoprevir.

Efavirenz

Concomitant use of efavirenz (600 mg once daily) and elbasvir (50 mg once daily) or grazoprevir (200 mg once daily) results in substantially decreased elbasvir or grazoprevir concentrations due to potent CYP3A induction by efavirenz, which may lead to loss of virologic response to the HCV antiviral.

Concomitant use of efavirenz and elbasvir/grazoprevir is contraindicated.

Etravirine

Concomitant use of etravirine and elbasvir/grazoprevir may result in decreased elbasvir and grazoprevir concentrations due to moderate CYP3A induction by etravirine, which may lead to reduced therapeutic effect of the HCV antiviral.

Concomitant use of etravirine and elbasvir/grazoprevir is not recommended.

Nevirapine

Concomitant use of nevirapine and elbasvir/grazoprevir is expected to result in decreased elbasvir and grazoprevir concentrations.

Concomitant use of nevirapine and elbasvir/grazoprevir is not recommended.

Rilpivirine

Concomitant use of rilpivirine and elbasvir/grazoprevir does not result in clinically important changes in the pharmacokinetics of elbasvir, grazoprevir, or rilpivirine. Dosage adjustments are not needed.

HIV Nucleoside and Nucleotide Reverse Transcriptase Inhibitors (NRTIs)

Abacavir

Clinically important pharmacokinetic interactions are not expected if abacavir is used concomitantly with elbasvir/grazoprevir.

Emtricitabine

Clinically important pharmacokinetic interactions are not expected if emtricitabine is used concomitantly with elbasvir/grazoprevir.

Lamivudine

Clinically important pharmacokinetic interactions are not expected if lamivudine is used concomitantly with elbasvir/grazoprevir.

Tenofovir

Concomitant use of tenofovir disoproxil fumarate (TDF; tenofovir DF) and elbasvir or grazoprevir does not result in clinically important changes in the pharmacokinetics of elbasvir, grazoprevir, or tenofovir. Dosage adjustments are not needed.

HIV Protease Inhibitors (PIs)

Atazanavir

Concomitant use of ritonavir-boosted atazanavir (300 mg of atazanavir and 100 mg of ritonavir once daily) and elbasvir (50 mg once daily) results in increased elbasvir concentrations. Concomitant use of ritonavir-boosted atazanavir (300 mg of atazanavir and 100 mg of ritonavir once daily) and grazoprevir (200 mg once daily) results in substantially increased grazoprevir concentrations due to OATP1B1 and 1B3 inhibition by ritonavir-boosted atazanavir. Increased grazoprevir concentrations may increase the risk of ALT elevations.

Concomitant use of elbasvir/grazoprevir and ritonavir-boosted, cobicistat-boosted, or unboosted atazanavir is contraindicated.

Darunavir

Concomitant use of ritonavir-boosted darunavir (600 mg of darunavir and 100 mg of ritonavir twice daily) and elbasvir (50 mg once daily) results in increased elbasvir concentrations. Concomitant use of ritonavir-boosted darunavir (600 mg of darunavir and 100 mg of ritonavir twice daily) and grazoprevir (200 mg once daily) results in substantially increased grazoprevir concentrations due to OATP1B1 and 1B3 inhibition by ritonavir-boosted darunavir. Increased grazoprevir concentrations may increase the risk of ALT elevations.

Concomitant use of elbasvir/grazoprevir and ritonavir-boosted or cobicistat-boosted darunavir is contraindicated.

Lopinavir

Concomitant use of the fixed combination of lopinavir and ritonavir (lopinavir/ritonavir) and elbasvir (50 mg once daily) results in increased elbasvir concentrations. Concomitant use of lopinavir/ritonavir and grazoprevir (200 mg once daily) results in substantially increased grazoprevir concentrations due to OATP1B1 and 1B3 inhibition by lopinavir/ritonavir. Increased grazoprevir concentrations may increase the risk of ALT elevations.

Concomitant use of lopinavir and elbasvir/grazoprevir is contraindicated.

Ritonavir

Concomitant use of ritonavir (100 mg twice daily) and grazoprevir (single 200-mg dose) results in increased grazoprevir concentrations.

Saquinavir

Pharmacokinetic interactions are expected if saquinavir and elbasvir/grazoprevir are used concomitantly (substantially increased grazoprevir concentrations due to potent OATP1B1 and 1B3 inhibition by saquinavir). Increased grazoprevir concentrations may increase the risk of ALT elevations.

Concomitant use of elbasvir/grazoprevir and saquinavir or ritonavir-boosted saquinavir is contraindicated.

Tipranavir

Pharmacokinetic interactions are expected if tipranavir and elbasvir/grazoprevir are used concomitantly (substantially increased grazoprevir concentrations due to potent OATP1B1 and 1B3 inhibition by tipranavir). Increased grazoprevir concentrations may increase the risk of ALT elevations.

Concomitant use of elbasvir/grazoprevir and ritonavir-boosted tipranavir is contraindicated.

● Benzodiazepines

Midazolam

Concomitant use of midazolam (single 2-mg dose) and grazoprevir (200 mg once daily) results in a 34% increase in midazolam exposures due to weak CYP3A inhibition by grazoprevir.

● Bosentan

Possible pharmacokinetic interactions if bosentan and elbasvir/grazoprevir are used concomitantly (decreased elbasvir and grazoprevir concentrations due to moderate CYP3A induction by bosentan, which may lead to reduced therapeutic effect of the HCV antiviral).

Concomitant use of bosentan and elbasvir/grazoprevir is not recommended.

● Cardiac Agents

Digoxin

Concomitant use of digoxin (single 0.25-mg dose) and elbasvir (50 mg once daily) does not result in clinically important changes in digoxin plasma concentrations or AUC.

Dosage adjustments are not needed if digoxin is used concomitantly with elbasvir/grazoprevir.

● Corticosteroids

Prednisone

Concomitant use of prednisone and elbasvir/grazoprevir does not result in clinically important changes in the pharmacokinetics of elbasvir, grazoprevir, or prednisone. Dosage adjustments are not needed.

● Entecavir

Clinically important pharmacokinetic interactions are not expected if entecavir is used concomitantly with elbasvir/grazoprevir.

● Estrogens and Progestins

Concomitant use of elbasvir or grazoprevir with an oral contraceptive containing ethinyl estradiol and levonorgestrel does not result in clinically important changes in the pharmacokinetics of ethinyl estradiol or levonorgestrel. Dosage adjustments are not needed.

● HCV Antivirals

HCV Polymerase Inhibitors

Sofosbuvir

Concomitant use of sofosbuvir and elbasvir/grazoprevir does not result in clinically important pharmacokinetic interactions. Dosage adjustments are not needed.

● HMG-CoA Reductase Inhibitors

Atorvastatin

Concomitant use of atorvastatin (single 10-mg dose) and elbasvir (50 mg once daily) in conjunction with grazoprevir (200 mg once daily) results in increased atorvastatin plasma concentrations and AUC.

If atorvastatin is used concomitantly with elbasvir/grazoprevir, atorvastatin dosage should not exceed 20 mg once daily.

Fluvastatin

Possible pharmacokinetic interaction if fluvastatin and elbasvir/grazoprevir are used concomitantly (increased fluvastatin concentrations).

If fluvastatin and elbasvir/grazoprevir are used concomitantly, use the lowest necessary dosage of fluvastatin and monitor the patient closely for statin-associated adverse effects (e.g., myopathy).

Lovastatin

Possible pharmacokinetic interaction if lovastatin and elbasvir/grazoprevir are used concomitantly (increased lovastatin concentrations).

If lovastatin and elbasvir/grazoprevir are used concomitantly, use the lowest necessary dosage of lovastatin and monitor the patient closely for statin-associated adverse effects (e.g., myopathy).

Pitavastatin

Concomitant use of pitavastatin (single 1-mg dose) and grazoprevir (200 mg once daily) does not have a clinically important effect on the pharmacokinetics of pitavastatin. Dosage adjustments are not needed.

Pravastatin

Concomitant use of pravastatin (single 40-mg dose) and elbasvir (50 mg once daily) in conjunction with grazoprevir (200 mg once daily) does not have a clinically important effect on the pharmacokinetics of pravastatin. Dosage adjustments are not needed.

Rosuvastatin

Concomitant use of rosuvastatin (single 10-mg dose) and elbasvir (50 mg once daily) in conjunction with grazoprevir (200 mg once daily) results in increased rosuvastatin plasma concentrations and AUC.

If rosuvastatin is used concomitantly with elbasvir/grazoprevir, do not exceed a rosuvastatin dosage of 10 mg once daily.

Simvastatin

Possible pharmacokinetic interaction if simvastatin and elbasvir/grazoprevir are used concomitantly (increased simvastatin concentrations).

If simvastatin and elbasvir/grazoprevir are used concomitantly, use the lowest necessary dosage of simvastatin and monitor the patient closely for statin-associated adverse effects (e.g., myopathy).

● Immunosuppressive Agents

Cyclosporine

Concomitant use of cyclosporine (single 400-mg dose) and elbasvir (50 mg once daily) in conjunction with grazoprevir (200 mg once daily) results in increased elbasvir plasma concentrations and AUC and substantially increased grazoprevir plasma concentrations and AUC. Substantially increased grazoprevir concentrations are caused by OATP1B1 and 1B3 inhibition by cyclosporine and may increase the risk of ALT elevations.

Concomitant use of cyclosporine and elbasvir/grazoprevir is contraindicated.

Tacrolimus

Concomitant use of tacrolimus (single 2-mg dose) and elbasvir (50 mg once daily) in conjunction with grazoprevir (200 mg once daily) results in a 43% increase in tacrolimus exposures due to weak CYP3A inhibition by grazoprevir; elbasvir and grazoprevir concentrations are not affected.

If tacrolimus and elbasvir/grazoprevir are used concomitantly, monitor tacrolimus whole blood concentrations, renal function, and for tacrolimus-associated adverse effects frequently.

● Modafinil

Possible pharmacokinetic interactions if modafinil and elbasvir/grazoprevir are used concomitantly (decreased elbasvir and grazoprevir concentrations due to moderate CYP3A induction by modafinil, which may lead to reduced therapeutic effect of the HCV antiviral).

Concomitant use of modafinil and elbasvir/grazoprevir is not recommended.

● Montelukast

Concomitant use of montelukast and grazoprevir does not result in clinically important changes in the pharmacokinetics of montelukast.

● Mycophenolate

Concomitant use of mycophenolate mofetil and elbasvir in conjunction with grazoprevir does not result in clinically important changes in elbasvir, grazoprevir, or mycophenolic acid plasma concentrations or AUC. Dosage adjustments are not needed.

● Opiate Agonists and Opiate Partial Agonists

Buprenorphine

Concomitant use of the fixed combination of buprenorphine and naloxone (buprenorphine/naloxone) and elbasvir does not result in clinically important effects on plasma concentrations or AUCs of elbasvir or buprenorphine. Concomitant use of buprenorphine/naloxone and grazoprevir does not result in clinically important effects on plasma concentrations or AUC of buprenorphine. Dosage adjustments are not needed.

Methadone

Concomitant use of methadone does not result in clinically important effects on plasma concentrations or AUCs of elbasvir or grazoprevir. Dosage adjustments are not needed.

● Phosphate Binders

Concomitant use of sevelamer carbonate or calcium acetate and elbasvir/grazoprevir does not result in clinically important changes in the pharmacokinetics of elbasvir or grazoprevir.

Dosage adjustments are not needed if elbasvir/grazoprevir is used concomitantly with phosphate binders.

● Ribavirin

Concomitant use of ribavirin and elbasvir/grazoprevir does not have clinically important effects on peak plasma concentrations or AUCs of elbasvir or grazoprevir compared with administration of elbasvir/grazoprevir alone. Dosage adjustments are not needed if elbasvir/grazoprevir is used in conjunction with ribavirin.

There was no in vitro evidence of antagonistic anti-HCV effects between ribavirin and elbasvir or ribavirin and grazoprevir when the combinations were evaluated in HCV replicon studies.

● St. John's Wort

Concomitant use of St. John's wort (*Hypericum perforatum*) and elbasvir/grazoprevir may result in substantially decreased elbasvir and grazoprevir concentrations due to potent CYP3A induction by St. John's wort, which may lead to loss of virologic response to the HCV antiviral.

Concomitant use of St. John's wort and elbasvir/grazoprevir is contraindicated.

● Warfarin

Fluctuations in international normalized ratios (INRs) have been reported in patients receiving elbasvir/grazoprevir. Monitor INR frequently; adjust warfarin dosage if necessary.

DESCRIPTION

Elbasvir and grazoprevir (elbasvir/grazoprevir) is a fixed combination containing 2 hepatitis C virus (HCV) antivirals. Elbasvir is an HCV nonstructural 5A (NS5A) replication complex inhibitor (NS5A inhibitor). Grazoprevir is an HCV nonstructural 3/4A (NS3/4A) protease inhibitor. Both drugs are direct-acting antivirals (DAAs) with activity against HCV. There was no in vitro evidence of antagonistic anti-HCV effects between elbasvir and grazoprevir when the combination was evaluated in HCV replicon studies.

Elbasvir targets HCV NS5A protein, which is required for viral replication and virion assembly. In vitro studies using cell-based replicon assays indicate that elbasvir has activity against HCV genotypes 1a, 1b, and 4.

Grazoprevir inhibits HCV NS3/4A protease, which is required for viral replication. Inhibition of NS3/4A protease prevents proteolytic cleavage of the HCV-encoded polyprotein to form mature forms of NS3, NS4A, NS4B, NS5A, and NS5B. In vitro studies using cell-based replicon assays indicate that grazoprevir has activity against HCV genotypes 1a, 1b, and 4.

Certain amino acid substitutions in NS5A of HCV genotypes 1a, 1b, and 4 have been selected in cell culture and have been associated with reduced susceptibility to elbasvir in vitro in replicon studies. In HCV genotype 1a replicons, single M28A/G/T, Q30D/E/H/K/R, L31M/V, H28D, and Y93C/H/N substitutions in NS5A are associated with reduced susceptibility to elbasvir (up to 2000-fold lower); in HCV genotype 1b replicons, single L28M, L31F, and Y93H substitutions in NS5A are associated with reduced susceptibility to elbasvir (up to 17-fold lower). In HCV genotype 4 replicons, single L30S, M31V, and Y93H substitutions in NS5A are associated with reduced susceptibility to elbasvir (up to 23-fold lower). In general, combinations of elbasvir resistance-associated substitutions further reduce elbasvir antiviral activity in HCV genotypes 1a, 1b, and 4 replicons. In phase 2 and 3 clinical trials, treatment-emergent amino acid substitutions in NS5A were detected in patients with HCV genotype 1a infection (M28A/G/T, Q30H/K/R/Y, L31F/M/V, H58D, Y93H/N/S), HCV genotype 1b infection (L28M, L31F/V, Y93H), or HCV genotype 4 infection (L28S/T, M31I/V, P58D, Y93H) experiencing virologic failure.

Certain amino acid substitutions in NS3 of HCV genotypes 1a, 1b, and 4 have been selected in cell culture and have been associated with reduced susceptibility to grazoprevir in vitro in replicon studies. In HCV genotype 1a replicons, single Y56H, R155K, A156G/T/V, and D168A/E/G/N/S/V/Y substitutions in NS3 are associated with reduced susceptibility to grazoprevir (up to 81-fold lower); in HCV genotype 1b replicons, single F43S, Y56F, V107I, A156S/T/V, and D168A/G/V substitutions in NS3 are associated with reduced susceptibility to grazoprevir (up to 375-fold lower). In HCV genotype 4 replicons, single D168A/V substitutions in NS3 are associated with reduced susceptibility to grazoprevir (up to 320-fold lower). In general, combinations of grazoprevir resistance-associated substitutions further reduce grazoprevir antiviral activity in HCV genotypes 1a, 1b, and 4 replicons. In phase 2 and 3 clinical trials, treatment-emergent amino acid substitutions in NS3 were detected in patients with HCV genotype 1a infection (V36L/M, Y56H, V107I, R155I/K, A156G/T/V, V158A, D168A/G/N/V/Y), HCV genotype 1b infection (Y56F, V107I, A156T), or HCV genotype 4 infection (A156M/T/V, D168A/G, V170I) experiencing virologic failure.

Cross-resistance among HCV NS5A inhibitors and among HCV NS3/4A protease inhibitors is possible. Efficacy of elbasvir/grazoprevir has not been established in patients in whom previous treatment with a regimen that included an HCV NS5A inhibitor failed. Only limited data are available regarding efficacy of elbasvir/grazoprevir in patients who previously failed treatment with a regimen of peginterferon alfa, ribavirin, and an HCV NS3/4A protease inhibitor (e.g., boceprevir, simeprevir, telaprevir; drugs no longer commercially available) and have HCV NS3 resistance-associated substitutions at baseline prior to administration of elbasvir/grazoprevir. Elbasvir and grazoprevir are active against HCV with amino acid substitutions associated with resistance to HCV NS5B polymerase inhibitors.

Following oral administration of elbasvir/grazoprevir in HCV-infected adults, peak plasma concentrations of elbasvir and grazoprevir occur approximately 3 and 2 hours, respectively, after the dose. Although not considered clinically important, administration of elbasvir/grazoprevir with a high-fat meal (approximately 900 kcal, 500 kcal from fat) in healthy adults decreases the area under the plasma concentration-time curve (AUC) and peak plasma concentrations of elbasvir by approximately 11 and 15%, respectively, and increases the AUC and peak plasma concentrations of grazoprevir by approximately 1.5- and 2.8-fold, respectively, relative to administration in the fasting state. When a once-daily regimen of elbasvir/grazoprevir is used, steady-state concentrations of elbasvir and grazoprevir are attained within approximately 6 days. Concomitant use of elbasvir and grazoprevir does not have a clinically important effect on the pharmacokinetics of either drug compared with administration alone.

Elbasvir pharmacokinetics are similar in healthy and HCV-infected adults; elbasvir exposures increase in a dose-proportional manner over the dosage range of 5–200 mg once daily. Grazoprevir exposures are approximately two-fold higher in HCV-infected adults compared with healthy adults; studies using grazoprevir dosages of 10–800 mg once daily in HCV-infected adults indicate that peak plasma concentrations and AUC increase in a more-than-dose-proportional manner. Preclinical studies indicate that elbasvir is distributed into most tissues (including the liver) and grazoprevir is distributed principally into the liver, which is likely facilitated by active transport of the drug through organic anion transporting polypeptide (OATP) 1B1 and 1B3 liver uptake transporters. Elbasvir and grazoprevir are both partially eliminated by oxidative metabolism, principally by cytochrome P-450 (CYP) 3A; both drugs are extensively (99.9 and 98.8%, respectively) bound to plasma proteins (e.g., serum albumin, α_1-acid glycoprotein). Both elbasvir and grazoprevir are eliminated principally in feces. Over 90% of each dose is excreted in feces and less than 1% is excreted in urine. In HCV-infected adults, the geometric mean apparent terminal half-lives of elbasvir and grazoprevir are approximately 24 and 31 hours, respectively.

In a pharmacokinetic study of 22 pediatric patients 12 years of age and older with HCV genotype 1 or 4, administration of elbasvir 50 mg/grazoprevir 100 mg once daily led to similar drug exposures to those observed in adult patients.

ADVICE TO PATIENTS

- Inform patients of the importance of reading patient information provided by the manufacturer.
- Advise patients that the fixed-combination preparation of elbasvir and grazoprevir (elbasvir/grazoprevir) should be taken once daily (with or without food) on a regular dosing schedule.
- Inform patients of the importance of taking the recommended dosage of elbasvir/grazoprevir for the recommended duration of treatment; importance of not missing or skipping doses.
- Inform patients that reactivation of hepatitis B virus (HBV) infection has occurred in coinfected patients being treated for hepatitis C virus (HCV) infection. Inform patients of the importance of informing clinician of any history of HBV infection or other liver problems (e.g., cirrhosis). Inform patients of the importance of immediately contacting a clinician if any signs or symptoms of serious liver injury (e.g., fatigue, weakness, loss of appetite, nausea and vomiting, yellowing of the eyes or skin, light-colored bowel movements) occur.
- Advise patients to immediately contact a clinician if they have symptoms of worsening liver problems (e.g., nausea, vomiting, yellowing of skin or white part of the eyes, bleeding or bruising more easily than normal, confusion, loss of appetite, diarrhea, dark or brown urine, dark or bloody stools, abdominal swelling, pain in upper right side of stomach area, sleepiness, vomiting of blood).
- Advise patients to inform their clinicians of existing or contemplated concomitant therapy, including prescription and OTC drugs and dietary or herbal supplements, as well as any concomitant illnesses.
- Advise women to inform clinicians if they are or plan to become pregnant or plan to breast-feed. If used in conjunction with ribavirin, advise men and women of importance of using 2 forms of effective contraception during and for 6 months after ribavirin therapy.
- Advise patients of other important precautionary information.

PREPARATIONS

Excipients in commercially available drug preparations may have clinically important effects in some individuals; consult specific product labeling for details.

Elbasvir and Grazoprevir

Oral			
Tablets, film-coated		Elbasvir 50 mg and Grazoprevir 100 mg	Zepatier®, Merck

†Use is not currently included in the labeling approved by the US Food and Drug Administration.

Ledipasvir and Sofosbuvir

8:18.40.24 • HCV REPLICATION COMPLEX INHIBITORS

■ Ledipasvir and sofosbuvir (ledipasvir/sofosbuvir) is a fixed combination containing 2 hepatitis C virus (HCV) antivirals; ledipasvir is an HCV non-structural 5A (NS5A) replication complex inhibitor (NS5A inhibitor) and sofosbuvir is a nucleotide analog HCV nonstructural 5B (NS5B) polymerase inhibitor.

USES

● Chronic Hepatitis C Virus Infection

The fixed combination of ledipasvir and sofosbuvir (ledipasvir/sofosbuvir) is used for the treatment of chronic hepatitis C virus (HCV) genotype 1 infection in treatment-naive (have not previously received HCV treatment) or previously treated adults and pediatric patients 3 years of age or older without cirrhosis or with compensated or decompensated cirrhosis (Child-Pugh class A, B, or C), including those with human immunodeficiency virus (HIV) coinfection and liver transplant recipients without cirrhosis or with compensated cirrhosis (Child-Pugh class A).

Ledipasvir/sofosbuvir is used for the treatment of chronic HCV genotype 4 infection in treatment-naive or previously treated adults and pediatric patients 3 years of age or older without cirrhosis or with compensated cirrhosis (Child-Pugh class A), including those with HIV coinfection and liver transplant recipients.

Ledipasvir/sofosbuvir also is used for the treatment of chronic HCV genotype 5 or 6 infection in treatment-naive or previously treated adults and pediatric patients 3 years of age or older without cirrhosis or with compensated cirrhosis (Child-Pugh class A), including those with HIV coinfection.

Ledipasvir/sofosbuvir is used alone for the treatment of chronic HCV infection in patients without cirrhosis or with compensated cirrhosis (Child-Pugh class A) and is used in conjunction with ribavirin for the treatment of chronic HCV infection in patients with decompensated cirrhosis (Child-Pugh class B or C) and in liver transplant recipients.

Because the treatment of chronic HCV infection is complex and rapidly evolving, it is recommended that treatment be directed by clinicians who are familiar with the disease and that a specialist be consulted to obtain the most up-to-date information. Information from the American Association for the Study of Liver Diseases (AASLD) and Infectious Diseases Society of America (IDSA) regarding diagnosis and management of HCV infection, including recommendations for initial treatment, is available at http://www.hcvguidelines.org.

HCV Genotype 1 Infection

Treatment-naive Adults

Efficacy and safety of ledipasvir/sofosbuvir for the treatment of chronic HCV genotype 1 infection in treatment-naive adults have been evaluated in 2 randomized, open-label, phase 3 trials (ION-1 [NCT01701401] and ION-3 [NCT01851330]). The primary end point for both studies was sustained virologic response at 12 weeks after the end of treatment (SVR12; defined as plasma HCV RNA level less than 25 IU/mL [the lower limit of quantification] at 12 weeks after end of treatment).

In ION-1, 865 treatment-naive cirrhotic or noncirrhotic adults with chronic HCV genotype 1 infection (median age 54 years, 59% male, 79% with baseline HCV RNA levels 800,000 IU/mL or greater, 67% with HCV genotype 1a infection, 70% with non-CC IL28B alleles [CT or TT], 16% with cirrhosis) were randomized to receive ledipasvir/sofosbuvir (a fixed-combination tablet containing 90 mg of ledipasvir and 400 mg of sofosbuvir once daily) with or without ribavirin for 12 or 24 weeks. Of the 213 patients treated with ledipasvir/sofosbuvir *without* ribavirin for 12 weeks, 99% achieved SVR12. No additional benefit was observed with the addition of ribavirin or with the extended 24-week treatment duration. In patients who received the 12-week regimen of ledipasvir/sofosbuvir *without* ribavirin, the SVR12 rate was 98% in those with HCV genotype 1a infection and 100% in those with HCV genotype 1b infection. In a subgroup analysis of patients with or without cirrhosis who received the 12-week regimen of ledipasvir/sofosbuvir

without ribavirin, 94% of those with cirrhosis and 99% of those without cirrhosis achieved SVR12.

ION-3 evaluated ledipasvir/sofosbuvir in 647 treatment-naive, noncirrhotic patients with chronic HCV genotype 1 infection. Patients were randomized to receive ledipasvir/sofosbuvir (a fixed-combination tablet containing 90 mg of ledipasvir and 400 mg of sofosbuvir once daily) with or without ribavirin for 8 weeks or ledipasvir/sofosbuvir (a fixed-combination tablet containing 90 mg of ledipasvir and 400 mg of sofosbuvir once daily) alone for 12 weeks. Baseline characteristics were balanced among treatment groups (median age 55 years, 58% male, 81% with baseline HCV RNA levels 800,000 IU/mL or greater, 80% with HCV genotype 1a infection, 73% with non-CC IL28B alleles [CT or TT]). SVR12 was achieved in 94 or 96% of patients treated with ledipasvir/sofosbuvir *without* ribavirin for 8 or 12 weeks, respectively. No additional benefit was observed with the addition of ribavirin to the 8-week treatment regimen. Among patients with baseline HCV RNA levels less than 6 million IU/mL, the SVR12 rate was 97 or 96% in patients treated with ledipasvir/sofosbuvir *without* ribavirin for 8 or 12 weeks, respectively; 2% of patients in both treatment groups experienced relapse. In patients who received the 12-week regimen of ledipasvir/sofosbuvir *without* ribavirin, the SVR12 rate was 96% in those with HCV genotype 1a infection and 98% in those with HCV genotype 1b infection.

Previously Treated Adults

Efficacy and safety of ledipasvir/sofosbuvir for the treatment of chronic HCV genotype 1 infection in previously treated adults have been evaluated in a randomized, open-label, phase 3 trial (ION-2; NCT01768286) and a randomized, double-blind, placebo-controlled, phase 2 trial (SIRIUS; NCT01965535). The primary end point for both studies was SVR12 (defined as plasma HCV RNA level less than 25 IU/mL [the lower limit of quantification] at 12 weeks after end of treatment).

ION-2 included 440 cirrhotic or noncirrhotic adults with chronic HCV genotype 1 infection who previously failed therapy with an interferon-based regimen, including regimens containing an HCV protease inhibitor. Patients were randomized to receive ledipasvir/sofosbuvir (a fixed-combination tablet containing 90 mg of ledipasvir and 400 mg of sofosbuvir once daily) with or without ribavirin for 12 or 24 weeks. Baseline characteristics were balanced among treatment groups (median age 57 years, 65% male, 89% with baseline HCV RNA levels 800,000 IU/mL or greater, 79% with HCV genotype 1a infection, 88% with non-CC IL28B alleles, 20% with cirrhosis, 47% failed prior therapy with peginterferon alfa and ribavirin, 53% failed prior therapy with peginterferon alfa, ribavirin, and an HCV protease inhibitor). SVR12 was achieved in 94 or 99% of patients treated with ledipasvir/sofosbuvir *without* ribavirin for 12 or 24 weeks, respectively. Use of ribavirin in conjunction with ledipasvir/sofosbuvir did not affect response rates, regardless of treatment duration. In patients who received a 12- or 24-week regimen of ledipasvir/sofosbuvir *without* ribavirin, the SVR rate was 95 or 99%, respectively, in those with HCV genotype 1a infection and 87 or 100%, respectively, in those with HCV genotype 1b infection. In a subgroup analysis of patients with or without cirrhosis, the SVR12 rate in those treated with ledipasvir/sofosbuvir *without* ribavirin was 86 or 100% with the 12- or 24-week regimen, respectively, in those with cirrhosis and 95 or 99% with the 12- or 24-week regimen, respectively, in those without cirrhosis.

SIRIUS included 155 adults with chronic HCV genotype 1 infection who had compensated cirrhosis and previously failed therapy with peginterferon alfa and ribavirin *and* failed subsequent therapy with peginterferon alfa, ribavirin, and an HCV protease inhibitor. Patients were randomized in a 1:1 ratio to receive ledipasvir/sofosbuvir (a fixed-combination tablet containing 90 mg of ledipasvir and 400 mg of sofosbuvir once daily) in conjunction with ribavirin for a duration of 12 weeks or ledipasvir/sofosbuvir *without* ribavirin for a duration of 24 weeks. Demographics and baseline characteristics were balanced among treatment groups (median age 56 years, 74% male, 97% white, 63% with HCV genotype 1a infection, 94% with non-CC IL28B alleles [CT or TT]). The SVR12 rate was 96% in patients treated with a 12-week regimen of ledipasvir/sofosbuvir *with* ribavirin and 97% in those treated with a 24-week regimen of ledipasvir/sofosbuvir alone.

HCV Genotype 4 Infection

Treatment-naive or Previously Treated Adults

Efficacy and safety of ledipasvir/sofosbuvir for the treatment of chronic HCV genotype 4 infection in treatment-naive or previously treated adults with or without cirrhosis have been evaluated in an open-label, phase 2 trial (Study 1119; NCT02081079). The primary end point was sustained virologic response at

12 weeks after the end of treatment (SVR12; defined as plasma HCV RNA level less than 15 IU/mL [the lower limit of quantification] at 12 weeks after end of treatment). Study 1119 included 22 treatment-naive patients (mean age 52 years, 50% male, 5% with cirrhosis) and 22 previously treated patients (mean age 50 years, 77% male, 41% with cirrhosis) who received ledipasvir/sofosbuvir (a fixed-combination tablet containing 90 mg of ledipasvir and 400 mg of sofosbuvir once daily) for 12 weeks. The overall SVR12 rate was 93%; SVR12 rates were similar based on prior HCV treatment history and cirrhosis status.

HCV Genotype 5 Infection

Treatment-naive or Previously Treated Adults

Efficacy and safety of ledipasvir/sofosbuvir for the treatment of chronic HCV genotype 5 infection in treatment-naive or previously treated adults with or without cirrhosis have been evaluated in an open-label, phase 2 trial (Study 1119; NCT02081079). The primary end point was sustained virologic response at 12 weeks after the end of treatment (SVR12; defined as plasma HCV RNA level less than 15 IU/mL [the lower limit of quantification] at 12 weeks after end of treatment). Study 1119 included 21 treatment-naive patients (mean age 61 years, 50% male, 100% white, 14% with cirrhosis) and 20 previously treated patients (mean age 64 years, 50% male, 100% white, 30% with cirrhosis) who received ledipasvir/sofosbuvir (a fixed-combination tablet containing 90 mg of ledipasvir and 400 mg of sofosbuvir once daily) for 12 weeks. The overall SVR12 rate was 93%; SVR12 rates were similar based on prior HCV treatment history and cirrhosis status.

HCV Genotype 6 Infection

Treatment-naive or Previously Treated Adults

Efficacy and safety of ledipasvir/sofosbuvir for the treatment of chronic HCV genotype 6 infection in treatment-naive or previously treated adults have been evaluated in an open-label trial (ELECTRON-2). The primary end point was sustained virologic response at 12 weeks after the end of treatment (SVR12; defined as plasma HCV RNA level less than 15 IU/mL [the lower limit of quantification] at 12 weeks after end of treatment). A total of 25 patients with or without cirrhosis received ledipasvir/sofosbuvir (a fixed-combination tablet containing 90 mg of ledipasvir and 400 mg of sofosbuvir once daily) for 12 weeks. The overall SVR12 was 96%; SVR12 rates were similar based on prior HCV treatment history and cirrhosis status.

Pediatric Patients

HCV Genotype 1 or 4 Infection

Efficacy and safety of ledipasvir/sofosbuvir for the treatment of chronic HCV genotype 1 or 4 infection in pediatric patients were evaluated in a phase 2 open-label study that included 224 treatment-naive or previously treated pediatric patients 3 years of age or older without cirrhosis or with compensated cirrhosis (study 1116; NCT02249182). The majority of these pediatric patients were treatment naive and had been infected through vertical transmission. Patients 3 to less than 6 years of age received a ledipasvir/sofosbuvir dosage based on weight (ledipasvir 33.75 mg/sofosbuvir 150 mg once daily in those weighing less than 17 kg or ledipasvir 45 mg/sofosbuvir 200 mg once daily in those weighing 17 kg or greater), patients 6 to less than 12 years of age received a dosage of ledipasvir 22.5 mg/sofosbuvir 100 mg once daily, and those 12 to less than 18 years of age received a dosage of ledipasvir 90 mg/sofosbuvir 400 mg once daily. The duration of ledipasvir/sofosbuvir treatment was 12 weeks. The primary efficacy end point was SVR12. Results were stratified based on age.

Study 1116 included 34 treatment-naive patients 3 to less than 6 years of age with HCV genotype 1 or 4 infection (median age 5 years, 71% female, 79% white, 18% Hispanic/Latino, 6% Asian, 3% black, mean weight 19 kg, 56% with baseline HCV RNA levels 800,000 IU/mL or greater, 82% with HCV genotype 1a infection, no patients with known cirrhosis). The SVR12 rate was 97% in the 33 patients with HCV genotype 1 infection; the single patient with HCV genotype 4 infection also achieved SVR12. No patient had virologic nonresponse or relapse after treatment. One patient discontinued ledipasvir/sofosbuvir treatment after 5 days because of an adverse event (abnormal taste).

Study 1116 included 90 patients 6 to less than 12 years of age with HCV genotype 1 or 4 infection (median age 9 years, 59% male, 79% white, 10% Hispanic/Latino, 8% black, 6% Asian, 80% treatment-naive, 59% with baseline HCV RNA levels 800,000 IU/mL or greater, 86% with HCV genotype 1a infection, 2 patients

with known compensated cirrhosis). The SVR12 rate was 99% in the 87 patients with HCV genotype 1 infection and 100% in the 2 patients with HCV genotype 4 infection. One patient with HCV genotype 1 infection who received ledipasvir/sofosbuvir for 24 weeks also achieved SVR12. The one patient with HCV genotype 1 infection who did not achieve SVR12 and relapsed had been treated with ledipasvir/sofosbuvir for 12 weeks.

Study 1116 included 100 pediatric patients 12 to less than 18 years of age with HCV genotype 1 infection (median age 15 years, 63% female, 91% white, 13% Hispanic/Latino, 7% black, 2% Asian, 20% previously treated, 55% with baseline HCV RNA levels 800,000 IU/mL or greater, 81% with HCV genotype 1a infection, 76% with non-CC IL28B alleles, 1% with known compensated cirrhosis). The SVR12 rate was 98% in the 80 patients who were treatment-naive and 100% in the 20 patients who were previously treated. No patient experienced on-treatment virologic failure or relapse.

HCV Genotype 5 or 6 Infection

Efficacy and safety of ledipasvir/sofosbuvir for the treatment of HCV genotype 5 or 6 infection in treatment-naive or previously treated pediatric patients 3 years of age or older without cirrhosis or with compensated cirrhosis are supported by data indicating that ledipasvir, sofosbuvir, and G-331007 (predominant metabolite of sofosbuvir) exposures in pediatric patients 3 years of age or older with HCV genotype 1, 3, or 4 infection are similar to exposures in adults.

Transplant Recipients

HCV Genotype 1 or 4 Infection

Efficacy and safety of ledipasvir/sofosbuvir in conjunction with ribavirin for the treatment of HCV genotype 1 or 4 infection in 670 treatment-naive or previously treated adults who were liver transplant recipients and/or had decompensated liver disease were evaluated in 2 identical, open-label, phase 2 trials (SOLAR-1 and SOLAR-2). Study patients were enrolled in 1 of 7 groups based on liver transplantation status and severity of hepatic impairment; those with Child-Pugh scores greater than 12 were excluded. Within each group, patients were randomized in a 1:1 ratio to receive either a 12- or 24-week regimen of ledipasvir/sofosbuvir with ribavirin; patients with decompensated cirrhosis received an initial ribavirin dosage of 600 mg daily regardless of transplantation status and ribavirin dosage adjustments were performed according to ribavirin prescribing information. Demographics and baseline characteristics were balanced across the treatment groups (median age 59 years, 77% male, 91% white, 94% with HCV genotype 1 infection, 6% with HCV genotype 4 infection, 78% failed previous HCV therapy). The primary end point was SVR12 (defined as plasma HCV RNA level less than 15 IU/mL [the lower limit of quantification] at 12 weeks after end of treatment).

In patients with HCV genotype 1 infection enrolled in SOLAR-1 and SOLAR-2, the SVR12 rates observed with the 12- and 24-week regimens of ledipasvir/sofosbuvir in conjunction with ribavirin were similar. Pooled SVR12 rates for patients with HCV genotype 1 infection who were liver transplant recipients and received the 12-week regimen were 95% in those with METAVIR score F0–F3 and 98, 89, or 57% in those with Child-Pugh class A, B, or C, respectively. Pooled SVR12 rates in pretransplant patients with HCV genotype 1 infection were 87 or 88% in those with Child-Pugh class B or C, respectively. The relapse rate was 7% in those with HCV genotype 1 infection *with* baseline NS5A polymorphisms at baseline and 5% in those with HCV genotype 1 infection *without* NS5A polymorphisms at baseline. In patients with HCV genotype 4 infection who received the 12-week regimen of ledipasvir/sofosbuvir with ribavirin, SVR12 rates in transplant recipients without cirrhosis or with compensated cirrhosis were similar to SVR12 rates reported in those with HCV genotype 1 infection. Data were insufficient to determine the SVR rates in transplant recipients or pretransplant patients who had HCV genotype 4 infection and decompensated cirrhosis.

HCV-infected Individuals Coinfected with HIV

HCV Genotype 1 or 4 Infection

Efficacy and safety of ledipasvir/sofosbuvir for the treatment of chronic HCV genotype 1 or 4 infection in adults coinfected with HIV-1 have been evaluated in an open-label, phase 3 trial (ION-4; NCT02073656). Patients were HCV treatment-naive or had failed previous HCV treatment with a regimen of peginterferon alfa and ribavirin (with or without an HCV protease inhibitor) or a regimen of sofosbuvir and ribavirin. The primary end point was sustained virologic response at 12 weeks after the end of treatment (SVR12; defined as plasma HCV RNA level less than 25 IU/mL [the lower limit of quantification] at 12 weeks after end of treatment). A total of 335 adults (median age 52 years, 82% male, 61% white, 34% black, 75% with HCV genotype 1a infection, 23% with HCV genotype 1b infection, 2% with HCV genotype 4 infection, 76% with non-CC IL28B alleles [CT or TT], 20% with compensated cirrhosis, 55% previously treated) received ledipasvir/sofosbuvir (a fixed-combination tablet containing 90 mg of ledipasvir and 400 mg of sofosbuvir once daily) for 12 weeks. All patients also were receiving a stable HIV antiretroviral regimen (emtricitabine and tenofovir disoproxil fumarate [TDF; tenofovir DF] in conjunction with efavirenz, rilpivirine or raltegravir). The overall SVR12 rate was 96%; SVR12 rates were similar based on prior HCV treatment history and cirrhosis status. However, black patients had lower SVR12 rates compared with patients of other races (90 versus 99%, respectively) and the relapse rate was 9% in black patients (all patients who relapsed had non-CC IL28B alleles). HCV treatment did not appear to interfere with maintenance of HIV virologic suppression; the percentage of CD4+ T-cells remained stable and there was no evidence of HIV-1 virologic rebound in any patient during the study.

HCV-infected Individuals with Severe Renal Impairment

Efficacy and safety of ledipasvir/sofosbuvir for the treatment of chronic HCV infection in adults with severe renal impairment were evaluated in 2 open-label studies.

One open-label study evaluated a 12-week regimen of ledipasvir/sofosbuvir in 18 treatment-naive or previously treated adults with HCV genotype 1 infection who had severe renal impairment not requiring dialysis (study 0154; NCT01958281). At baseline, the mean estimated glomerular filtration rate (eGFR) was 24.9 mL/minute and 2 patients had cirrhosis. SVR-12 was achieved in all 18 of these patients with severe renal impairment.

In the second open-label study, adults with chronic HCV genotype 1, 5, or 6 infection with end-stage renal disease (ESRD) requiring dialysis received ledipasvir/sofosbuvir given for 8, 12, or 24 weeks (study 4063; NCT03036839). This study included 63 adults (24% previously treated, 10% with cirrhosis, 95% on hemodialysis, 5% on peritoneal dialysis, mean duration on dialysis was 12 years). The SVR12 rate was 93% in the 45 noncirrhotic treatment-naive patients with HCV genotype 1 infection who received an 8-week regimen of ledipasvir/sofosbuvir and 100% in the 12 noncirrhotic treatment-naive or previously treated patients with HCV genotype 1, 5, or 6 infection who received a 12-week regimen of ledipasvir/sofosbuvir. The SVR12 rate was 83% in the 6 previously treated patients with HCV genotype 1 infection who had compensated cirrhosis and received a 24-week regimen of ledipasvir/sofosbuvir.

DOSAGE AND ADMINISTRATION

● General

Pretreatment Screening

- Prior to initiating HCV treatment, test all patients for evidence of current or prior HBV infection by measuring hepatitis B surface antigen (HBsAg), hepatitis B surface antibody (anti-HBs), and hepatitis B core antibody (anti-HBc).
- In patients with serologic evidence of HBV infection, measure baseline HBV DNA level.
- Perform appropriate laboratory tests to evaluate liver function, especially in patients with decompensated cirrhosis receiving a regimen of ledipasvir/sofosbuvir in conjunction with ribavirin.
- When used in conjunction with ribavirin, women of childbearing potential should have a negative pregnancy test immediately prior to initiating ribavirin therapy; perform pregnancy tests periodically during and for 6 months after completion of ribavirin therapy.

Patient Monitoring

- Perform appropriate laboratory tests to evaluate liver function during therapy, especially in patients with decompensated cirrhosis receiving a regimen of ledipasvir/sofosbuvir in conjunction with ribavirin.
- *In all patients with evidence of current or prior HBV infection*: Monitor for clinical and laboratory signs (i.e., HBsAg, HBV DNA levels, serum

aminotransferase and bilirubin concentrations) of hepatitis flare or HBV reactivation during and after treatment with HCV DAAs.

Other General Considerations

- For treatment of chronic HCV infection, ledipasvir/sofosbuvir is used alone or in conjunction with ribavirin.
- Specific regimen and duration of treatment depend on HCV genotype and certain patient factors (e.g., presence of compensated or decompensated cirrhosis, liver transplantation). Consider that relapse rates following treatment are affected by baseline host and viral factors and differ between treatment durations for certain subgroups.
- If amiodarone is used concomitantly with ledipasvir/sofosbuvir, perform cardiac monitoring in an inpatient setting during the first 48 hours of concomitant use; perform heart rate monitoring daily (outpatient or self-monitoring) through at least the first 2 weeks of concomitant use. Similar cardiac monitoring is recommended in patients who discontinue amiodarone just prior to initiation of ledipasvir/sofosbuvir.

● Administration

Ledipasvir/sofosbuvir is administered orally once daily with or without food.

Ledipasvir/sofosbuvir is commercially available for oral administration as film-coated tablets and as pellets that should be swallowed whole or mixed with soft food and swallowed whole. The pellets can be used in pediatric patients who cannot swallow tablets.

Ledipasvir/sofosbuvir pellets taken with food: One or more spoonfuls of nonacidic soft food at or below room temperature (e.g., pudding, chocolate syrup, mashed potato, ice cream) should be added to a bowl. The entire contents of the appropriate number of single-dose packets of pellets (see Table 4) should be sprinkled onto the food and gently mixed with a spoon. No pellets should remain in the packet(s). The entire mixture containing the pellets should be ingested within 30 minutes after preparation; the pellets in the mixture should be swallowed whole without chewing to avoid a bitter aftertaste. Any unused portion of the mixture should be discarded and should not be stored or used later.

Ledipasvir/sofosbuvir pellets taken without food: The entire contents of a single-dose packet of pellets should be poured directly into the mouth and the pellets swallowed whole without chewing to avoid a bitter aftertaste. Water may be swallowed after the pellets, if needed. If 2 packets of pellets are indicated (see Table 4), the process should be repeated. No pellets should remain in the packet(s).

● Dosage

Ledipasvir/sofosbuvir is commercially available as fixed-combination pellets containing 33.75 mg of ledipasvir and 150 mg of sofosbuvir, fixed-combination pellets containing 45 mg of ledipasvir and 200 mg of sofosbuvir, fixed-combination tablets containing 45 mg of ledipasvir and 200 mg of sofosbuvir, and fixed-combination tablets containing 90 mg of ledipasvir and 400 mg of sofosbuvir.

Adult Dosage

HCV Genotype 1 Infection

For the treatment of chronic HCV genotype 1 infection in treatment-naive or previously treated adults, the recommended dosage of ledipasvir/sofosbuvir is ledipasvir 90 mg/sofosbuvir 400 mg (given as 1 tablet containing 90 mg of ledipasvir and 400 mg of sofosbuvir) once daily.

Ledipasvir/sofosbuvir is used alone for the treatment of HCV genotype 1 infection in patients without cirrhosis or with compensated cirrhosis (Child-Pugh class A), but is used in conjunction with ribavirin for the treatment of HCV genotype 1 infection in those with decompensated cirrhosis (Child-Pugh class B or C) and in liver transplant recipients without cirrhosis or with compensated cirrhosis (Child-Pugh class A). A treatment duration of 12 weeks is recommended for most patients with HCV genotype 1 infection, but a treatment duration of 24 weeks is recommended for previously treated patients with compensated cirrhosis (Child-Pugh class A). (See Table 1.)

If ledipasvir/sofosbuvir (without ribavirin) is used for the treatment of HCV genotype 1 infection in adults with decompensated cirrhosis who cannot receive ribavirin, some experts recommend a treatment duration of 24 weeks. HCV-infected patients with decompensated cirrhosis should be referred to an expert for treatment (ideally at a liver transplant center).

TABLE 1. Recommended Treatment Regimen and Duration of Ledipasvir/Sofosbuvir for HCV Genotype 1 Infection in Adults.

Patient Type	Treatment Regimen	Duration of Treatment
Treatment-naive *without* cirrhosis	Ledipasvir/sofosbuvir	12 weeks[a]
Treatment-naive *with* compensated cirrhosis (Child-Pugh class A)	Ledipasvir/sofosbuvir	12 weeks
Previously treated[b] *without* cirrhosis	Ledipasvir/sofosbuvir	12 weeks
Previously treated[b] *with* compensated cirrhosis (Child-Pugh class A)	Ledipasvir/sofosbuvir	24 weeks[c]
Treatment-naive or previously treated[b] *with* decompensated cirrhosis (Child-Pugh class B or C)	Ledipasvir/sofosbuvir and ribavirin[d]	12 weeks
Treatment-naive or previously treated[b] liver transplant recipients *without* cirrhosis or *with* compensated cirrhosis (Child-Pugh class A)	Ledipasvir/sofosbuvir and ribavirin[d]	12 weeks

[a] Manufacturer states treatment duration of 8 weeks can be considered in treatment-naive patients *without* cirrhosis who have pretreatment HCV RNA levels less than 6 million IU/mL.

[b] Previously treated defined as patients who failed treatment with peginterferon alfa (with or without ribavirin) with or without an HCV protease inhibitor.

[c] Alternatively, a regimen of ledipasvir/sofosbuvir *and* ribavirin for a duration of 12 weeks can be considered in previously treated patients with compensated cirrhosis who are eligible to receive ribavirin.

[d] Use weight-based ribavirin dosage in adults without cirrhosis or with compensated cirrhosis (1 g daily for patients weighing <75 kg or 1.2 g daily for those weighing ≥75 kg). In adults with decompensated cirrhosis, the starting ribavirin dosage is 600 mg daily and can be titrated up to weight-based ribavirin dosage (up to 1 g daily for patients weighing <75 kg or up to 1.2 g daily for those weighing ≥75 kg). Give ribavirin daily dosage in 2 divided doses with food. If ribavirin starting dosage not well tolerated, reduce dosage as clinically indicated based on hemoglobin concentrations.

HCV Genotype 4 Infection

For the treatment of chronic HCV genotype 4 infection in treatment-naive or previously treated adults, the recommended dosage of ledipasvir/sofosbuvir is ledipasvir 90 mg/sofosbuvir 400 mg (given as 1 tablet containing 90 mg of ledipasvir and 400 mg of sofosbuvir) once daily.

Ledipasvir/sofosbuvir is used alone for the treatment of HCV genotype 4 infection in patients without cirrhosis or with compensated cirrhosis (Child-Pugh class A), but is used in conjunction with ribavirin for the treatment of HCV genotype 4 infection in liver transplant recipients without cirrhosis or with compensated cirrhosis. The usual treatment duration is 12 weeks. (See Table 2.)

For the treatment of HCV genotype 4 infection in adults with decompensated cirrhosis† (Child-Pugh class B or C), some experts recommend a 12-week regimen of ledipasvir/sofosbuvir given in a dosage of 1 tablet (90 mg of ledipasvir and 400 mg of sofosbuvir) once daily in conjunction *with* ribavirin. If ledipasvir/sofosbuvir (without ribavirin) is used for the treatment of HCV genotype 4 infection in patients with decompensated cirrhosis who cannot receive ribavirin, these experts recommend a treatment duration of 24 weeks. HCV-infected patients with decompensated cirrhosis should be referred to an expert for treatment (ideally at a liver transplant center).

TABLE 2. Recommended Treatment Regimen and Duration of Ledipasvir/Sofosbuvir for HCV Genotype 4 Infection in Adults.

Patient Type	Treatment Regimen	Duration of Treatment
Treatment-naive *without* cirrhosis or *with* compensated cirrhosis (Child-Pugh class A)	Ledipasvir/ sofosbuvir	12 weeks
Previously treated[a] *without* cirrhosis or *with* compensated cirrhosis (Child-Pugh class A)	Ledipasvir/ sofosbuvir	12 weeks

TABLE 2. Continued

Patient Type	Treatment Regimen	Duration of Treatment
Treatment-naive or previously treated[a] liver transplant recipients *without* cirrhosis or *with* compensated cirrhosis (Child-Pugh class A)	Ledipasvir/ sofosbuvir *and* ribavirin[b]	12 weeks

[a] Previously treated defined as patients who failed treatment with peginterferon alfa (with or without ribavirin) with or without an HCV protease inhibitor.

[b] Use weight-based ribavirin dosage in adults without cirrhosis or with compensated cirrhosis (1 g daily for patients weighing <75 kg or 1.2 g daily for those weighing ≥75 kg). In adults with decompensated cirrhosis, the starting ribavirin dosage is 600 mg daily and can be titrated up to weight-based ribavirin dosage (up to 1 g daily for patients weighing <75 kg or up to 1.2 g daily for those weighing ≥75 kg). Give ribavirin daily dosage in 2 divided doses with food. If ribavirin starting dosage not well tolerated, reduce dosage as clinically indicated based on hemoglobin concentrations.

HCV Genotype 5 or 6 Infection

For the treatment of chronic HCV genotype 5 or 6 infection in treatment-naive or previously treated adults without cirrhosis or with compensated cirrhosis (Child-Pugh class A), the recommended dosage of ledipasvir/sofosbuvir is ledipasvir 90 mg/sofosbuvir 400 mg (given as 1 tablet containing 90 mg of ledipasvir and 400 mg of sofosbuvir) once daily.

Ledipasvir/sofosbuvir is used alone for the treatment of HCV genotype 5 or 6 infection in patients without cirrhosis or with compensated cirrhosis (Child-Pugh class A). The usual treatment duration is 12 weeks. (See Table 3.)

For the treatment of HCV genotype 5 or 6 infection in adults with decompensated cirrhosis† (Child-Pugh class B or C), some experts recommend a 12-week regimen of ledipasvir/sofosbuvir given in a dosage of 1 tablet (90 mg of ledipasvir and 400 mg of sofosbuvir) once daily in conjunction *with* ribavirin. If ledipasvir/sofosbuvir (without ribavirin) is used for the treatment of HCV genotype 5 or 6 infection in patients with decompensated cirrhosis who cannot receive ribavirin, these experts recommend a treatment duration of 24 weeks. HCV-infected patients with decompensated cirrhosis should be referred to an expert for treatment (ideally at a liver transplant center).

TABLE 3. Recommended Treatment Regimen and Duration of Ledipasvir/Sofosbuvir for HCV Genotype 5 or 6 Infection in Adults.

Patient Type	Treatment Regimen	Duration of Treatment
Treatment-naive *without* cirrhosis or *with* compensated cirrhosis (Child-Pugh class A)	Ledipasvir/ sofosbuvir	12 weeks
Previously treated[a] *without* cirrhosis or *with* compensated cirrhosis (Child-Pugh class A)	Ledipasvir/ sofosbuvir	12 weeks

[a] Previously treated defined as patients who failed treatment with peginterferon alfa (with or without ribavirin) with or without an HCV protease inhibitor.

HCV-infected Adults Coinfected with HIV

For the treatment of chronic HCV genotype 1, 4, 5, or 6 infection in adults with human immunodeficiency virus (HIV) coinfection, the same ledipasvir/sofosbuvir dosage and same HCV genotype-specific multiple-drug regimen and treatment duration recommended for HCV-infected patients without HIV coinfection should be used.

Pediatric Dosage

HCV Genotype 1 Infection

For the treatment of chronic HCV genotype 1 infection in treatment-naive or previously treated pediatric patients 3 years of age or older, the recommended dosage of ledipasvir/sofosbuvir is based on weight. (See Table 4.)

Ledipasvir/sofosbuvir is used alone for the treatment of HCV genotype 1 infection in patients without cirrhosis or with compensated cirrhosis (Child-Pugh class A), but is used in conjunction with ribavirin for the treatment of HCV genotype 1 infection in those with decompensated cirrhosis (Child-Pugh class B or C) and in liver transplant recipients without cirrhosis or with compensated cirrhosis (Child-Pugh class A). A treatment duration of 12 weeks is recommended for most patients with HCV genotype 1 infection, but a treatment duration of 24 weeks is recommended for previously treated patients with compensated cirrhosis (Child-Pugh class A). (See Table 5.)

TABLE 4. Recommended Ledipasvir/Sofosbuvir Dosage for Treatment of HCV Genotype 1, 4, 5, or 6 Infection in Pediatric Patients 3 Years of Age or Older.

Weight (kg)	Dosage of Ledipasvir/Sofosbuvir Tablets or Oral Pellets	Total Daily Ledipasvir/ Sofosbuvir Dosage
<17 kg	One packet of pellets containing ledipasvir 33.75 mg/sofosbuvir 150 mg once daily	Ledipasvir 33.75 mg/ sofosbuvir 150 mg daily
17 to <35 kg	One tablet containing ledipasvir 45 mg/sofosbuvir 200 mg once daily	Ledipasvir 45 mg/ sofosbuvir 200 mg daily
	or	
	One packet of pellets containing ledipasvir 45 mg/sofosbuvir 200 mg once daily	
≥35 kg	One tablet containing ledipasvir 90 mg/sofosbuvir 400 mg once daily	Ledipasvir 90 mg/ sofosbuvir 400 mg daily
	or	
	Two tablets containing ledipasvir 45 mg/sofosbuvir 200 mg once daily	
	or	
	Two packets of pellets containing ledipasvir 45 mg/sofosbuvir 200 mg once daily	

TABLE 5. Recommended Treatment Regimen and Duration of Ledipasvir/Sofosbuvir for HCV Genotype 1 Infection in Pediatric Patients 3 Years of Age or Older.

Patient Type	Treatment Regimen	Duration of Treatment
Treatment-naive *without* cirrhosis	Ledipasvir/sofosbuvir	12 weeks
Treatment-naive *with* compensated cirrhosis (Child-Pugh class A)	Ledipasvir/sofosbuvir	12 weeks[a]
Previously treated[b] *without* cirrhosis	Ledipasvir/sofosbuvir	12 weeks
Previously treated[b] *with* compensated cirrhosis (Child-Pugh class A)	Ledipasvir/sofosbuvir	24 weeks[c]
Treatment-naive or previously treated[b] *with* decompensated cirrhosis (Child-Pugh class B or C)	Ledipasvir/sofosbuvir *and* ribavirin[d]	12 weeks
Treatment-naive or previously treated[b] liver transplant recipients *without* cirrhosis or *with* compensated cirrhosis (Child-Pugh class A)	Ledipasvir/sofosbuvir *and* ribavirin[d]	12 weeks

[a] Manufacturer states treatment duration of 8 weeks can be considered in treatment-naive patients *without* cirrhosis who have pretreatment HCV RNA levels less than 6 million IU/mL.

[b] Previously treated defined as patients who failed treatment with peginterferon alfa (with or without ribavirin) with or without an HCV protease inhibitor

[c] Alternatively, a regimen of ledipasvir/sofosbuvir *and* ribavirin for a duration of 12 weeks can be considered in previously treated patients with compensated cirrhosis who are eligible to receive ribavirin.

[d] Use weight-based ribavirin dosage in pediatric patients 3 years of age or older (7.5 mg twice daily in those weighing <47 kg; 200 mg in a.m. and 400 mg in p.m. in those 47–49 kg; 400 mg twice daily in those 50–65 kg; 400 mg in a.m. and 600 mg in p.m. in those 66–80 kg; 600 mg twice daily in those >80 kg). Give each ribavirin dose with food.

HCV Genotype 4 Infection

For the treatment of chronic HCV genotype 4 infection in treatment-naive or previously treated pediatric patients 3 years of age or older, the recommended dosage of ledipasvir/sofosbuvir is based on weight. (See Table 4.)

Ledipasvir/sofosbuvir is used alone for the treatment of HCV genotype 4 infection in patients without cirrhosis or with compensated cirrhosis (Child-Pugh class A), but is used in conjunction with ribavirin for the treatment of HCV genotype 4 infection in liver transplant recipients without cirrhosis or with compensated cirrhosis. The treatment duration is 12 weeks. (See Table 6.)

TABLE 6. Recommended Treatment Regimen and Duration of Ledipasvir/Sofosbuvir for HCV Genotype 4 Infection in Pediatric Patients 3 Years of Age or Older.

Patient Type	Treatment Regimen	Duration of Treatment
Treatment-naive *without* cirrhosis or *with* compensated cirrhosis (Child-Pugh class A)	Ledipasvir/ sofosbuvir	12 weeks
Previously treated[a] *without* cirrhosis or *with* compensated cirrhosis (Child-Pugh class A)	Ledipasvir/ sofosbuvir	12 weeks
Treatment-naive or previously treated[a] liver transplant recipients *without* cirrhosis or *with* compensated cirrhosis (Child-Pugh class A)	Ledipasvir/ sofosbuvir *and* ribavirin[b]	12 weeks

[a] Previously treated defined as patients who failed treatment with peginterferon alfa (with or without ribavirin) with or without an HCV protease inhibitor.

[b] Use weight-based ribavirin dosage in pediatric patients 3 years of age or older (7.5 mg twice daily in those weighing <47 kg; 200 mg in a.m. and 400 mg in p.m. in those 47–49 kg; 400 mg twice daily in those 50–65 kg; 400 mg in a.m. and 600 mg in p.m. in those 66–80 kg; 600 mg twice daily in those >80 kg). Give each ribavirin dose with food.

HCV Genotype 5 or 6 Infection

For the treatment of chronic HCV genotype 5 or 6 infection in treatment-naive or previously treated pediatric patients 3 years of age or older, the recommended dosage of ledipasvir/sofosbuvir is based on weight. (See Table 4.)

Ledipasvir/sofosbuvir is used alone for the treatment of HCV genotype 5 or 6 infection in patients without cirrhosis or with compensated cirrhosis (Child-Pugh class A). The treatment duration is 12 weeks. (See Table 7.)

TABLE 7. Recommended Treatment Regimen and Duration of Ledipasvir/Sofosbuvir for HCV Genotype 5 or 6 Infection in Pediatric Patients 3 Years of Age or Older.

Patient Type	Treatment Regimen	Duration of Treatment
Treatment-naive *without* cirrhosis or *with* compensated cirrhosis (Child-Pugh class A)	Ledipasvir/ sofosbuvir	12 weeks
Previously treated[a] *without* cirrhosis or *with* compensated cirrhosis (Child-Pugh class A)	Ledipasvir/ sofosbuvir	12 weeks

[a] Previously treated defined as patients who failed treatment with peginterferon alfa (with or without ribavirin) with or without an HCV protease inhibitor.

HCV-infected Pediatric Patients Coinfected with HIV

For the treatment of chronic HCV genotype 1, 4, 5, or 6 infection in pediatric patients 3 years of age or older with HIV coinfection, the same ledipasvir/sofosbuvir dosage and same HCV genotype-specific multiple-drug regimen and treatment duration recommended for HCV-infected patients without HIV coinfection should be used.

● Special Populations

Hepatic Impairment

Ledipasvir/sofosbuvir dosage adjustments are not necessary in patients with mild, moderate, or severe hepatic impairment (Child-Pugh class A, B, or C). (See Hepatic Impairment under Warnings/Precautions: Specific Populations, in Cautions.)

Renal Impairment

Ledipasvir/sofosbuvir dosage adjustments are not necessary in patients with mild, moderate, or severe renal impairment, including those with end-stage renal disease (ESRD) requiring dialysis. (See Renal Impairment under Warnings/Precautions: Specific Populations, in Cautions.)

Geriatric Patients

Ledipasvir/sofosbuvir dosage adjustments are not necessary in geriatric patients.

CAUTIONS

● Contraindications

If the fixed combination of ledipasvir and sofosbuvir (ledipasvir/sofosbuvir) is used in conjunction with ribavirin, the contraindications to ribavirin also apply. (See Precautions Related to Fixed Combinations and Multiple-drug Treatment Regimens under Warnings/Precautions: Other Warnings/Precautions, in Cautions.)

● Warnings/Precautions

Warnings

Risk of HBV Reactivation in Patients Coinfected with HCV and HBV

Reactivation of hepatitis B virus (HBV) infection has been reported during postmarketing experience when direct-acting antivirals (DAAs) were used for the treatment of chronic hepatitis C virus (HCV) infection in patients with HBV coinfection. In some cases, HBV reactivation resulted in fulminant hepatitis, hepatic failure, and death.

HBV reactivation (defined as an abrupt increase in HBV replication manifested as a rapid increase in serum HBV DNA levels or detection of hepatitis B surface antigen [HBsAg] in an individual who was previously HBsAg negative and hepatitis B core antibody [anti-HBc] positive) has been reported in patients with HCV and HBV coinfection who were receiving HCV treatment with a regimen that included HCV DAAs without interferon alfa. Reactivation also may be accompanied by hepatitis (i.e., increased aminotransferase concentrations) and, in severe cases, may lead to increased bilirubin concentrations, liver failure, or death. Data to date indicate that HBV reactivation usually occurs within 4–8 weeks after initiation of HCV treatment. Patients with HBV reactivation have been heterogeneous in terms of HCV genotype and in terms of baseline HBV disease. While some patients with HBV reactivation were HBsAg positive, others had serologic evidence of resolved HBV infection (i.e., HBsAg negative and anti-HBc positive). HBV reactivation also has been reported in patients receiving certain immunosuppressant or chemotherapeutic drugs; the risk of reactivation associated with HCV DAAs may be increased in such patients.

The mechanism for HBV reactivation in patients with HCV and HBV coinfection receiving HCV DAAs is unknown. Although HCV DAAs are not known to cause immunosuppression, HBV reactivation in coinfected patients may result from a complex interplay of host immunologic responses in the setting of infection with 2 hepatitis viruses.

Prior to initiating treatment with an HCV DAA, including ledipasvir/sofosbuvir, all patients should be screened for evidence of current or prior HBV infection by measuring HBsAg, anti-HBs, and anti-HBc. If there is serologic evidence of HBV infection, baseline HBV DNA levels should be measured.

Patients with evidence of current or prior HBV infection should be monitored for clinical and laboratory signs (i.e., HBsAg, HBV DNA levels, serum aminotransferase concentrations, bilirubin concentrations) of hepatitis flare or HBV reactivation during and after treatment with HCV DAAs, including ledipasvir/sofosbuvir. Appropriate management for HBV infection should be initiated as clinically indicated.

Patients with HCV and HBV coinfection receiving ledipasvir/sofosbuvir should be advised to immediately contact a clinician if they develop any signs or symptoms of serious liver injury (e.g., fatigue, weakness, loss of appetite, nausea and vomiting, yellowing of the eyes or skin, light-colored bowel movements).

When making decisions regarding HBV monitoring or HBV treatment in coinfected patients, consultation with a clinician who has expertise in managing HBV infection is recommended.

Sensitivity Reactions

Angioedema and rash, sometimes with blisters or angioedema-like swelling, have been reported during postmarketing experience.

Other Warnings/Precautions

Cardiovascular Effects

Symptomatic bradycardia, sometimes requiring pacemaker intervention, has been reported during postmarketing experience in patients receiving amiodarone concomitantly with an HCV treatment regimen containing sofosbuvir in conjunction with another HCV DAA. Symptomatic bradycardia, including a fatal cardiac arrest, has been reported in patients receiving amiodarone concomitantly with the fixed combination containing ledipasvir and sofosbuvir (ledipasvir/sofosbuvir). In most reported cases, bradycardia occurred within hours to days after HCV treatment was initiated in patients receiving amiodarone, but has been observed up to 2 weeks after initiation of HCV treatment. Bradycardia generally resolved after HCV treatment was discontinued. The mechanism for this adverse cardiovascular effect is unknown.

Patients who may be at increased risk for symptomatic bradycardia if amiodarone is used concomitantly with an HCV treatment regimen containing sofosbuvir and another HCV DAA include those also receiving a β-adrenergic blocking agent, those with underlying cardiac comorbidities, and/or those with advanced liver disease.

Concomitant use of amiodarone with ledipasvir/sofosbuvir is *not* recommended. If there are no alternative HCV treatment options and ledipasvir/sofosbuvir must be used in a patient receiving amiodarone, the patient should be advised about the risk of serious symptomatic bradycardia before ledipasvir/sofosbuvir is initiated. Cardiac monitoring should be performed in an inpatient setting during the first 48 hours of concomitant use of amiodarone and ledipasvir/sofosbuvir; heart rate monitoring should then be performed daily (outpatient or self-monitoring) through at least the first 2 weeks of concomitant use. Similar cardiac monitoring is recommended in patients who discontinued amiodarone just prior to initiation of ledipasvir/sofosbuvir or if there are no other treatment options and amiodarone must be initiated in a patient already receiving ledipasvir/sofosbuvir.

Patients receiving amiodarone concomitantly with ledipasvir/sofosbuvir should be advised to immediately contact a clinician if they develop signs or symptoms of bradycardia (e.g., near-fainting or fainting, dizziness, lightheadedness, malaise, weakness, excessive tiredness, shortness of breath, chest pain, confusion, memory problems).

Interactions

Concomitant use of ledipasvir/sofosbuvir and inducers of the P-glycoprotein (P-gp) transport system (e.g., rifampin, St. John's wort [*Hypericum perforatum*]) may decrease ledipasvir and sofosbuvir plasma concentrations and may lead to reduced therapeutic effect of ledipasvir/sofosbuvir. Concomitant use of ledipasvir/sofosbuvir and P-gp inducers is not recommended. (See Drug Interactions.)

Precautions Related to Fixed Combinations and Multiple-drug Treatment Regimens

When ledipasvir/sofosbuvir is used, the cautions, precautions, contraindications, and drug interactions associated with both drugs in the fixed combination (i.e., ledipasvir, sofosbuvir) must be considered. Cautionary information applicable to specific populations (e.g., pregnant or nursing women, individuals with hepatic or renal impairment, geriatric patients) should be considered for both drugs. (For cautionary information specific for sofosbuvir, see Cautions in Sofosbuvir 8:18.40.16.)

When ledipasvir/sofosbuvir is used in conjunction with ribavirin, the cautions, precautions, and contraindications associated with ribavirin also should be considered. (See Cautions in Ribavirin 8:18.32.) Ribavirin may cause fetal toxicity and/or death and extreme care *must* be taken to avoid pregnancy in female patients and in female partners of male patients receiving ribavirin-containing regimens. Women of childbearing potential should have a negative pregnancy test immediately prior to initiating ribavirin and pregnancy tests should be performed periodically during and for 6 months after ribavirin treatment is completed. Women of childbearing potential (and their male partners) and male patients (and their female partners) *must* use effective contraception during and for 6 months after ribavirin treatment is completed. (See Cautions: Pregnancy, Fertility, and Lactation, in Ribavirin 8:18.32.)

Specific Populations

Pregnancy

Adequate data are not available regarding use of ledipasvir/sofosbuvir in pregnant women. In animal studies, neither ledipasvir nor sofosbuvir affected fetal development at the dosages tested.

When ledipasvir/sofosbuvir is used in conjunction *with* ribavirin, clinicians should consider that ribavirin may cause fetal toxicity and/or death and extreme care must be taken to avoid pregnancy in female patients and in female partners of male patients receiving the ribavirin-containing regimen. (See Cautions: Pregnancy, Fertility, and Lactation, in Ribavirin 8:18.32.)

Lactation

It is not known whether ledipasvir, sofosbuvir, or their metabolites are distributed into human milk, affect milk production, or have effects on a breast-fed child.

The predominant metabolite of sofosbuvir (GS-331007) is distributed into milk in rats, and ledipasvir has been detected in plasma of suckling rat pups. Ledipasvir and GS-331007 had no apparent effects on the nursing pups.

The benefits of breast-feeding and the importance of ledipasvir/sofosbuvir to the woman should be considered along with the potential adverse effects on the breast-fed child from the drug or from the underlying maternal condition.

When ledipasvir/sofosbuvir is used in conjunction *with* ribavirin, the potential for adverse reactions to ribavirin in nursing infants should be considered. (See Precautions Related to Fixed Combinations and Multiple-drug Treatment Regimens under Warnings/Precautions: Other Warnings/Precautions, in Cautions.)

Pediatric Use

Safety and efficacy of ledipasvir/sofosbuvir have not been established in pediatric patients younger than 3 years of age.

Safety and efficacy of ledipasvir/sofosbuvir for the treatment of HCV genotype 1 or 4 infection in treatment-naive and previously treated pediatric patients 3 years of age or older without cirrhosis or with compensated cirrhosis (Child-Pugh class A) have been established in an open-label clinical study.

Safety and efficacy of ledipasvir/sofosbuvir for the treatment of HCV genotype 1 infection in pediatric patients 3 years of age or older with decompensated cirrhosis (Child-Pugh class B or C) and for the treatment of HCV genotype 1 or 4 infection in pediatric patients 3 years of age or older who are liver transplant recipients without cirrhosis or with compensated cirrhosis (Child-Pugh class A) are supported by pharmacokinetic data indicating that ledipasvir, sofosbuvir, and GS-331007 exposures in pediatric patients 3 years of age or older with HCV genotype 1, 3, or 4 infection are similar to exposures in adults.

Safety and efficacy of ledipasvir/sofosbuvir for the treatment of HCV genotype 5 or 6 infection in pediatric patients 3 years of age or older are supported by pharmacokinetic data indicating that ledipasvir, sofosbuvir, and GS-331007 exposures in pediatric patients 3 years of age or older with HCV genotype 1, 3, or 4 infection are similar to exposures in adults.

Adverse effects of ledipasvir/sofosbuvir reported in pediatric patients 3 years of age and older are similar to those observed in adults.

Data are not available regarding the safety and pharmacokinetics of ledipasvir/sofosbuvir in pediatric patients with renal impairment.

Geriatric Use

No overall differences in safety and efficacy of ledipasvir/sofosbuvir have been observed between patients 65 years of age and older and younger adults. However, greater sensitivity in some older individuals cannot be ruled out.

Hepatic Impairment

In individuals with severe hepatic impairment (Child-Pugh class C) without HCV infection, a single 90-mg dose of ledipasvir results in plasma exposures similar to those reported when the same dose is given to individuals with normal hepatic function. In HCV-infected individuals with moderate or severe hepatic impairment (Child-Pugh class B or C), sofosbuvir (400 mg daily for 7 days) results in

sofosbuvir and GS-331007 plasma exposures higher than those reported in individuals with normal hepatic function.

When ledipasvir/sofosbuvir is used in conjunction with ribavirin in patients with decompensated cirrhosis (Child-Pugh class B or C), clinical and hepatic laboratory monitoring is recommended as clinically indicated.

Data are not available regarding the safety of ledipasvir/sofosbuvir in patients with decompensated cirrhosis *and* severe renal impairment, including those requiring dialysis.

Renal Impairment

In individuals with severe renal impairment without HCV infection, ledipasvir pharmacokinetics following a single 90-mg dose of the drug are similar to pharmacokinetics reported in healthy individuals. In individuals with severe renal impairment or end-stage renal disease (ESRD) requiring hemodialysis without HCV infection, a single 400-mg dose of sofosbuvir results in sofosbuvir and GS-331007 plasma exposures that are substantially higher than those reported in individuals with normal renal function.

Data are not available regarding the safety of ledipasvir/sofosbuvir in patients with severe renal impairment, including those requiring dialysis, who also have decompensated cirrhosis.

Although hemodialysis removes the predominant metabolite of sofosbuvir (GS-331007), it is unlikely that ledipasvir will be substantially removed by dialysis since it is highly bound to plasma proteins.

HCV-infected Individuals Coinfected with HIV

The safety profile of ledipasvir/sofosbuvir in individuals with HCV genotype 1 or 4 infection and HIV-1 coinfection generally has been comparable to that reported in HCV-infected individuals without HIV-1 coinfection.

● Common Adverse Effects

Ledipasvir/sofosbuvir: Adverse effects reported in 5% or more of patients receiving ledipasvir/sofosbuvir include fatigue, headache, nausea, diarrhea, abdominal pain, insomnia or sleep disorder, irritability, rash, pruritus, dry skin, arthralgia, myalgia, back pain, asthenia, cough, upper respiratory tract infection, and dizziness.

Ledipasvir/sofosbuvir in conjunction with ribavirin: Adverse effects reported in 5% or more of patients receiving ledipasvir/sofosbuvir in conjunction with ribavirin include fatigue, headache, nausea, diarrhea, insomnia, asthenia, cough, bronchitis, dyspnea, irritability, pruritus, dry skin, myalgia, and decreased hemoglobin.

DRUG INTERACTIONS

The following drug interactions are based on studies using the fixed combination of ledipasvir and sofosbuvir (ledipasvir/sofosbuvir), ledipasvir alone, or sofosbuvir alone. When ledipasvir/sofosbuvir is used, interactions associated with both drugs in the fixed combination should be considered.

● Drugs Affecting or Affected by P-glycoprotein Transport System

Ledipasvir is an inhibitor of the P-glycoprotein (P-gp) transport system; sofosbuvir and the predominant sofosbuvir metabolite (GS-331007) are not inhibitors of P-gp. Concomitant use of ledipasvir and P-gp substrates may increase intestinal absorption of such drugs.

Ledipasvir and sofosbuvir are substrates of P-gp; GS-331007 is not a P-gp substrate. Pharmacokinetic interactions are possible with P-gp inducers (e.g., rifampin, St. John's wort), which may decrease ledipasvir and sofosbuvir plasma concentrations leading to reduced therapeutic effect of ledipasvir/sofosbuvir. Concomitant use of ledipasvir/sofosbuvir with P-gp inducers is not recommended.

● Drugs Affecting or Affected by Breast Cancer Resistance Protein

Ledipasvir is an inhibitor of breast cancer resistance protein (BCRP); sofosbuvir and GS-331007 are not BCRP inhibitors. Concomitant use of ledipasvir and BCRP substrates may increase intestinal absorption of such drugs.

Ledipasvir and sofosbuvir are substrates of BCRP; GS-331007 is not a BCRP substrate. Inhibitors of BCRP may increase plasma concentrations of ledipasvir and sofosbuvir without increasing plasma concentrations of GS-331007.

● Drugs Affecting or Affected by Other Membrane Transporters

At concentrations exceeding those achieved in the clinical setting, ledipasvir inhibits organic anion transporting polypeptide (OATP) 1B1, OATP1B3, and the bile salt export pump (BSEP).

Ledipasvir does not inhibit organic anion transporter (OAT) 1, OAT3, organic cation transporter (OCT) 1, OCT2, multidrug and toxin extrusion protein (MATE) 1, multidrug resistance-associated protein (MRP) 2, or MRP4.

● Drugs Affecting Gastric pH

The solubility of ledipasvir decreases as pH increases. Therefore, drugs that increase gastric pH are expected to decrease ledipasvir plasma concentrations.

Antacids

Administration of ledipasvir/sofosbuvir and antacids (e.g., aluminum and magnesium hydroxides) should be separated by 4 hours.

Histamine H$_2$-Receptor Antagonists

H$_2$-receptor antagonists may be administered concomitantly with or 12 hours apart from ledipasvir/sofosbuvir; dosage of the H$_2$-receptor antagonist should not exceed dosages comparable to famotidine 40 mg twice daily.

Proton-pump Inhibitors

Proton-pump inhibitors in dosages comparable to omeprazole 20 mg once daily or lower may be administered concomitantly with ledipasvir/sofosbuvir under fasting conditions.

● Antiarrhythmic Agents

Amiodarone

Concomitant use of amiodarone and ledipasvir/sofosbuvir may result in serious symptomatic bradycardia and is not recommended. If there are no alternative hepatitis C virus (HCV) treatment options and a regimen of ledipasvir/sofosbuvir must be used in a patient receiving amiodarone, the patient should be advised about the risk of serious symptomatic bradycardia and cardiac monitoring should be performed in an inpatient setting during the first 48 hours of concomitant use and then heart rate monitoring (outpatient or self-monitoring) should be performed daily through at least the first 2 weeks of concomitant use. Similar cardiac monitoring is recommended in patients who discontinued amiodarone just prior to initiation of ledipasvir/sofosbuvir or if there are no other treatment options and amiodarone must be initiated in a patient already receiving ledipasvir/sofosbuvir. (See Cardiovascular Effects under Warnings/Precautions: Other Warnings/Precautions, in Cautions.)

The effect of concomitant use of amiodarone and ledipasvir/sofosbuvir on plasma concentrations of amiodarone, ledipasvir, and sofosbuvir is unknown.

● Anticonvulsants

Concomitant use of carbamazepine (300 mg twice daily) and sofosbuvir (single 400-mg dose) results in decreased peak plasma concentrations and area under the plasma concentration-time curve (AUC) of sofosbuvir. Concomitant use of ledipasvir/sofosbuvir and certain other anticonvulsants (i.e., phenobarbital, phenytoin) is expected to decrease ledipasvir and sofosbuvir plasma concentrations, leading to reduced therapeutic effect of ledipasvir/sofosbuvir.

Concomitant use of ledipasvir/sofosbuvir and carbamazepine, phenytoin, or phenobarbital is not recommended.

● Antidiabetic Agents

Altered blood glucose control resulting in serious symptomatic hypoglycemia has been reported during postmarketing experience when HCV direct-acting antivirals (DAAs) were used in diabetic patients receiving antidiabetic agents. Management of hypoglycemia in these patients required either discontinuance or dosage modification of the antidiabetic agents. Blood glucose concentrations should be frequently monitored; adjustment of antidiabetic agent dosage may be necessary.

● Antimycobacterial Agents

Rifabutin

Concomitant use of rifabutin (300 mg once daily) and sofosbuvir (single 400-mg dose) results in decreased peak plasma concentrations and AUC of sofosbuvir. Rifabutin is expected to decrease plasma concentrations of ledipasvir.

Concomitant use of rifabutin and ledipasvir/sofosbuvir is not recommended.

Rifampin

Concomitant use of rifampin (a P-gp inducer) and ledipasvir/sofosbuvir may result in a clinically important decrease in plasma concentrations of ledipasvir and sofosbuvir and may lead to decreased therapeutic effect of ledipasvir/sofosbuvir.

Concomitant use of rifampin and ledipasvir/sofosbuvir is not recommended.

Rifapentine

Rifapentine is expected to decrease plasma concentrations of ledipasvir and sofosbuvir, which may lead to decreased therapeutic effect of ledipasvir/sofosbuvir.

Concomitant use of rifapentine and ledipasvir/sofosbuvir is not recommended.

● Antiretroviral Agents

HIV Entry and Fusion Inhibitors

Maraviroc

Concomitant use of ledipasvir/sofosbuvir and maraviroc is not expected to affect the pharmacokinetics of maraviroc.

Dosage adjustments are not necessary if maraviroc is used concomitantly with ledipasvir/sofosbuvir.

HIV Integrase Inhibitors (INSTIs)

Bictegravir

Concomitant use of the fixed combination of bictegravir, emtricitabine, and tenofovir alafenamide fumarate (bictegravir/emtricitabine/TAF) and ledipasvir/sofosbuvir does not result in clinically important pharmacokinetic interactions.

Dolutegravir

Concomitant use of dolutegravir and ledipasvir/sofosbuvir is not expected to result in clinically important pharmacokinetic interactions. Dosage adjustments are not necessary if dolutegravir is used concomitantly with ledipasvir/sofosbuvir.

If ledipasvir/sofosbuvir is used concomitantly with an HIV antiretroviral regimen that contains dolutegravir *and* tenofovir disoproxil fumarate (TDF), patients should be monitored for tenofovir-associated adverse effects.

Elvitegravir

Concomitant use of *cobicistat-boosted* elvitegravir and ledipasvir/sofosbuvir increases peak plasma concentrations and AUC of ledipasvir and cobicistat, but does not have clinically important effects on the pharmacokinetics of sofosbuvir or elvitegravir.

Concomitant use of the fixed combination of elvitegravir, cobicistat, emtricitabine, and TAF (EVG/c/FTC/TAF) and ledipasvir/sofosbuvir does not result in clinically important effects on the pharmacokinetics of any of the drugs. Dosage adjustments are not necessary if EVG/c/FTC/TAF is used concomitantly with ledipasvir/sofosbuvir.

Concomitant use of the fixed combination of elvitegravir, cobicistat, emtricitabine, and TDF (EVG/c/FTC/TDF) and ledipasvir/sofosbuvir is expected to result in increased tenofovir and ledipasvir concentrations. Concomitant use of ledipasvir/sofosbuvir and EVG/c/FTC/TDF is not recommended.

Raltegravir

Concomitant use of raltegravir (400 mg twice daily) and either ledipasvir (90 mg once daily) or sofosbuvir (single 400-mg dose) did not have a clinically important effect on the pharmacokinetics of raltegravir, ledipasvir, or sofosbuvir. Dosage adjustments are not necessary if raltegravir is used concomitantly with ledipasvir/sofosbuvir.

If ledipasvir/sofosbuvir is used concomitantly with an HIV antiretroviral regimen that contains raltegravir *and* TDF, the patient should be monitored for tenofovir-associated adverse effects.

HIV Nonnucleoside Reverse Transcriptase Inhibitors (NNRTIs)

Doravirine

Concomitant use of doravirine and ledipasvir/sofosbuvir does not result in clinically important pharmacokinetic interactions. Dosage adjustments are not necessary if doravirine is used concomitantly with ledipasvir/sofosbuvir.

Concomitant use of the fixed combination of doravirine, lamivudine, and TDF (doravirine/lamivudine/TDF) and ledipasvir/sofosbuvir results in increased tenofovir concentrations. If doravirine/lamivudine/TDF is used concomitantly with ledipasvir/sofosbuvir, the patient should be monitored for tenofovir-associated adverse effects.

Efavirenz

Concomitant use of efavirenz and ledipasvir/sofosbuvir may decrease ledipasvir plasma concentrations and AUC, but has no clinically important effect on sofosbuvir or efavirenz pharmacokinetics. Dosage adjustments are not necessary if efavirenz and ledipasvir/sofosbuvir are used concomitantly.

Concomitant use of the fixed combination of efavirenz, emtricitabine, and TDF (efavirenz/emtricitabine/TDF) and ledipasvir/sofosbuvir does not have a clinically important effect on the pharmacokinetics of efavirenz or sofosbuvir, but results in decreased ledipasvir plasma concentrations and AUC and increased tenofovir plasma concentrations and AUC.

If ledipasvir/sofosbuvir is used concomitantly with an HIV antiretroviral regimen that includes efavirenz *and* TDF, the patient should be monitored for tenofovir-associated adverse effects.

Etravirine

Concomitant use of etravirine and ledipasvir/sofosbuvir is not expected to result in clinically important drug interactions. Dosage adjustments are not necessary if etravirine and ledipasvir/sofosbuvir are used concomitantly.

If ledipasvir/sofosbuvir is used concomitantly with an HIV antiretroviral regimen that includes etravirine *and* TDF, the patient should be monitored for tenofovir-associated adverse effects.

Nevirapine

Concomitant use of nevirapine and ledipasvir/sofosbuvir is not expected to result in clinically important drug interactions. Dosage adjustments are not necessary if nevirapine and ledipasvir/sofosbuvir are used concomitantly.

If ledipasvir/sofosbuvir is used concomitantly with an HIV antiretroviral regimen that includes nevirapine *and* TDF, the patient should be monitored for tenofovir-associated adverse effects.

Rilpivirine

Concomitant use of rilpivirine and ledipasvir/sofosbuvir does not have clinically important effects on the pharmacokinetics of rilpivirine, ledipasvir, or sofosbuvir. Dosage adjustments are not necessary if rilpivirine and ledipasvir/sofosbuvir are used concomitantly.

If ledipasvir/sofosbuvir is used concomitantly with an HIV antiretroviral regimen that includes rilpivirine *and* TDF, the patient should be monitored for tenofovir-associated adverse effects.

HIV Nucleoside and Nucleotide Reverse Transcriptase Inhibitors (NRTIs)

No clinically important pharmacokinetic interactions are expected if ledipasvir/sofosbuvir is used concomitantly with abacavir, emtricitabine, or lamivudine.

Abacavir and Lamivudine

Concomitant use of the fixed combination of abacavir and lamivudine (abacavir/lamivudine) and ledipasvir/sofosbuvir does not have a clinically important effect on the pharmacokinetics of abacavir, lamivudine, ledipasvir, or sofosbuvir.

Tenofovir Alafenamide Fumarate

Concomitant use of tenofovir alafenamide fumarate (TAF) and ledipasvir/sofosbuvir may result in a 27% increase in the AUC of tenofovir; this increase is not considered clinically important. Dosage adjustments are not needed if TAF is used concomitantly with ledipasvir/sofosbuvir.

Tenofovir Disoproxil Fumarate

Concomitant use of tenofovir disoproxil fumarate (TDF; tenofovir DF) and ledipasvir/sofosbuvir results in increased tenofovir concentrations and AUC. If ledipasvir/sofosbuvir is used concomitantly with TDF, the patient should be monitored for tenofovir-associated adverse effects

Concomitant use of ledipasvir/sofosbuvir and HIV antiretroviral regimens that include TDF and a *ritonavir-boosted* or *cobicistat-boosted* HIV protease inhibitor (PI) is expected to result in increased tenofovir concentrations; the safety of increased tenofovir concentrations in this setting has not been established. An alternative HCV regimen or alternative antiretroviral regimen should be considered. If concomitant use of ledipasvir/sofosbuvir and an HIV antiretroviral regimen that includes TDF and a *ritonavir-boosted* or *cobicistat-boosted* HIV PI is necessary, the patient should be monitored for tenofovir-associated adverse effects.

Concomitant use of ledipasvir/sofosbuvir and HIV antiretroviral regimens that include TDF and an HIV INSTI may result in increased tenofovir concentrations. Concomitant use of ledipasvir/sofosbuvir and EVG/c/FTC/TDF is not recommended. If ledipasvir/sofosbuvir is used concomitantly with an HIV antiretroviral regimen that includes TDF and other HIV INSTIs (e.g., dolutegravir, raltegravir), the patient should be monitored for tenofovir-associated adverse effects.

Concomitant use of ledipasvir/sofosbuvir and HIV antiretroviral regimens that include TDF and an HIV NNRTI may result in increased tenofovir concentrations. If ledipasvir/sofosbuvir is used concomitantly with an HIV antiretroviral regimen that includes TDF and an HIV NNRTI (e.g., doravirine, efavirenz, etravirine, nevirapine, rilpivirine), the patient should be monitored for tenofovir-associated adverse effects.

HIV Protease Inhibitors (PIs)

Concomitant use of ledipasvir/sofosbuvir and any HIV antiretroviral regimen that includes TDF *and* a *ritonavir-boosted* PI (e.g., *ritonavir-boosted* atazanavir, *ritonavir-boosted* darunavir, fixed combination of lopinavir and ritonavir [lopinavir/ritonavir], *ritonavir-boosted* saquinavir) or TDF *and cobicistat-boosted* atazanavir or *cobicistat-boosted* darunavir may result in increased tenofovir concentrations. Safety of increased tenofovir concentrations in patients receiving ledipasvir/sofosbuvir and these HIV treatment regimens has not been established. Alternative HCV treatment or an alternative antiretroviral regimen should be considered to avoid increased tenofovir exposure. If concomitant use of ledipasvir/sofosbuvir and any of these HIV PI regimens is necessary, the patient should be monitored for tenofovir-associated adverse effects.

Atazanavir

Concomitant use of *ritonavir-boosted* atazanavir (atazanavir 300 mg and ritonavir 100 mg) and ledipasvir/sofosbuvir increases the AUCs of atazanavir and ledipasvir by 33 and 113%, respectively, but does not have a clinically important effect on the pharmacokinetics of sofosbuvir.

Concomitant use of *cobicistat-boosted* atazanavir or unboosted atazanavir and ledipasvir/sofosbuvir is not expected to result in clinically important pharmacokinetic interactions.

Dosage adjustments are not necessary if ledipasvir/sofosbuvir is used concomitantly with *ritonavir-boosted* atazanavir, *cobicistat-boosted* atazanavir, or unboosted atazanavir.

Darunavir

Concomitant use of *ritonavir-boosted* darunavir once daily (darunavir 800 mg and ritonavir 100 mg) and either ledipasvir (90 mg once daily) or sofosbuvir (single 400-mg dose) does not have a clinically important effect on the pharmacokinetics of darunavir, ritonavir, ledipasvir, or sofosbuvir.

Concomitant use of *cobicistat-boosted* darunavir and ledipasvir/sofosbuvir is not expected to result in clinically important pharmacokinetic interactions.

Dosage adjustments are not necessary if *ritonavir-boosted* or *cobicistat-boosted* darunavir is used concomitantly with ledipasvir/sofosbuvir.

Tipranavir

Concomitant use of *ritonavir-boosted* tipranavir and ledipasvir/sofosbuvir is expected to decrease ledipasvir and sofosbuvir concentrations, leading to reduced therapeutic effect of ledipasvir/sofosbuvir.

Concomitant use of *ritonavir-boosted* tipranavir and ledipasvir/sofosbuvir is not recommended.

● Calcium-channel Blockers

Concomitant use of ledipasvir/sofosbuvir and verapamil is not expected to result in any clinically important drug interactions.

● Digoxin

Concomitant use of ledipasvir/sofosbuvir and digoxin may increase digoxin concentrations. Therapeutic concentration monitoring of digoxin is recommended if used concomitantly with ledipasvir/sofosbuvir.

● Estrogens and Progestins

When studied in healthy women, concomitant use of ledipasvir or sofosbuvir and an oral contraceptive containing ethinyl estradiol and norgestimate did not have a clinically important effect on the pharmacokinetics of ethinyl estradiol or norgestimate and its active metabolites (norelgestromin, norgestrel). Concomitant use of ledipasvir/sofosbuvir is not expected to affect efficacy of oral contraceptives containing ethinyl estradiol and norgestimate.

● Benzodiazepines

Concomitant use of midazolam (single 2.5-mg dose) and ledipasvir (single 90-mg dose) did not affect the pharmacokinetic of midazolam.

● HMG-CoA Reductase Inhibitors

Atorvastatin

Concomitant use of atorvastatin and ledipasvir/sofosbuvir may increase atorvastatin concentrations and increase the risk of myopathy and rhabdomyolysis.

If atorvastatin is used concomitantly with ledipasvir/sofosbuvir, patients should be monitored closely for adverse reactions associated with hydroxymethylglutaryl-CoA (HMG-CoA) reductase inhibitors (statins), including myopathy and rhabdomyolysis.

Pravastatin

Concomitant use of pravastatin and ledipasvir/sofosbuvir is not expected to result in any clinically important drug interactions.

Rosuvastatin

Concomitant use of rosuvastatin and ledipasvir/sofosbuvir may result in increased rosuvastatin concentrations, which is associated with increased risk of myopathy and rhabdomyolysis.

Concomitant use of rosuvastatin and ledipasvir/sofosbuvir is not recommended.

● Immunosuppressive Agents

Cyclosporine

Cyclosporine pharmacokinetics are not affected by ledipasvir or sofosbuvir. Concomitant use of ledipasvir/sofosbuvir and cyclosporine is not expected to result in any clinically important drug interactions.

Tacrolimus

Concomitant use of ledipasvir/sofosbuvir and tacrolimus is not expected to result in any clinically important drug interactions.

● Methadone

Methadone pharmacokinetics are not affected by ledipasvir or sofosbuvir. Concomitant use of ledipasvir/sofosbuvir and methadone is not expected to result in any clinically important drug interactions.

● St. John's Wort

Concomitant use of St. John's wort (*Hypericum perforatum*) and ledipasvir/sofosbuvir may result in a clinically important decrease in ledipasvir and sofosbuvir plasma concentrations because of P-gp induction by St. John's wort and may result in loss of therapeutic effect of ledipasvir/sofosbuvir. Concomitant use of ledipasvir/sofosbuvir and St. John's wort is not recommended.

● Warfarin

In patients receiving warfarin, subtherapeutic international normalized ratios (INRs) have been reported after initiation of sofosbuvir-containing regimens, including ledipasvir/sofosbuvir.

INR should be closely monitored, especially when initiating or discontinuing ledipasvir/sofosbuvir in patients receiving warfarin. Adjustment of warfarin dosage may be necessary.

DESCRIPTION

Ledipasvir and sofosbuvir is a fixed combination containing 2 hepatitis C virus (HCV) antivirals. Ledipasvir is an HCV nonstructural 5A (NS5A) replication complex inhibitor (NS5A inhibitor). Sofosbuvir is a nucleotide analog HCV nonstructural 5B (NS5B) polymerase inhibitor. Both drugs are direct-acting antivirals (DAAs) with activity against HCV. There was no in vitro evidence of antagonistic anti-HCV effects between ledipasvir and sofosbuvir when the combination was evaluated in HCV replicon studies.

Ledipasvir targets HCV NS5A protein, which is required for viral replication. In vitro studies using cell-based replicon assays indicate that ledipasvir has activity against HCV genotypes 1a and 1b. Ledipasvir also has some antiviral activity against HCV genotypes 4a, 5a, and 6a, but substantially lower activity against HCV genotype 6e.

Sofosbuvir is a prodrug that is converted in the liver to a pharmacologically active uridine analog triphosphate (GS-461203), which can be incorporated into HCV RNA by NS5B polymerase and acts as an RNA chain terminator. In vitro studies using biochemical and cell-based replicon assays indicate that GS-461203 has activity against HCV genotypes 1a, 1b, 4a, 5a, and 6a.

Certain amino acid substitutions in NS5A of HCV genotype 1a (e.g., Y93H, Q30E) and genotype 1b (e.g., Y93H) have been selected in cell culture and have been associated with reduced susceptibility to ledipasvir in vitro in replicon studies. In phase 2 and 3 clinical trials evaluating ledipasvir/sofosbuvir in patients with HCV genotype 1 infection, treatment-emergent NS5A resistance-associated substitutions (e.g., K24R, M28T/V, Q30R/H/K/L, L31M/V, H58D/P, and/or Y93H/N/C) were detected in patients with HCV genotype 1a infection who experienced virologic failure, and treatment-emergent resistance-associated substitutions (e.g., L31V/M/I, R30Q, and/or Y93H/N) were detected in patients with HCV genotype 1b infection who experienced virologic failure. Some of these patients also had baseline NS5A polymorphisms at resistance-associated amino acid positions. In clinical trials evaluating ledipasvir/sofosbuvir in patients with HCV genotype 4, 5, or 6 infection, patients with relapse who had NS5A sequencing data available had pretreatment NS5A resistance-associated polymorphisms (single polymorphism or combinations at positions 24, 28, 30, 31 and 58); NS5A resistance-associated substitutions Y93C or L28V emerged posttreatment in a few of the patients with HCV genotype 4 relapse who also had NS5A polymorphisms pretreatment.

Certain amino acid substitutions in NS5B polymerase of HCV genotypes 1b, 4a, 5a, and 6a have been selected in cell culture and have been associated with reduced susceptibility to sofosbuvir in vitro in replicon studies. In all replicon genotypes tested, the S282T substitution was associated with reduced susceptibility to sofosbuvir; in genotypes 5 and 6 replicons, an M289L substitution developed along with the S282T substitution. Although the clinical importance is unknown, treatment-emergent NS5B resistance-associated substitutions (e.g., L159, V321, D61G, A112T, E237G, S473T, S282T, L320V/I, V321I) were detected in phase 3 clinical trials evaluating ledipasvir/sofosbuvir in patients with HCV genotype 1 infection. Treatment-emergent sofosbuvir resistance-associated NS5B substitution S282T has been reported at the time of relapse in patients with HCV genotype 4, 5, or 6 infection who received ledipasvir/sofosbuvir in clinical trials; treatment-emergent nucleotide inhibitor substitution M289I also was reported in a patient with HCV genotype 5 relapse.

Cross-resistance between ledipasvir and other NS5A inhibitors is expected; efficacy of ledipasvir/sofosbuvir has not been established in patients in whom previous treatment with other regimens that included an NS5A inhibitor failed.

Ledipasvir and sofosbuvir are both active against HCV with amino acid substitutions associated with resistance to other classes of HCV DAAs that have different mechanisms of action (e.g., HCV NS5B nonnucleoside inhibitors, HCV NS3 protease inhibitors).

Following oral administration of ledipasvir/sofosbuvir, peak plasma concentrations of ledipasvir occur approximately 4–4.5 hours after the dose and peak plasma concentrations of sofosbuvir and the predominant sofosbuvir metabolite (GS-331007; accounts for more than 90% of total systemic exposure) occur approximately 0.8–1 and 3.5–4 hours, respectively, after the dose. Administration with a moderate-fat (approximately 600 kcal, 25–30% fat) or high-fat (approximately 1000 kcal, 50% fat) meal does not substantially affect ledipasvir or GS-331007 exposures relative to administration in the fasting state; sofosbuvir peak plasma concentrations are not affected, but the AUC of the drug is increased approximately twofold.

Ledipasvir appears to undergo slow oxidative metabolism by an unknown mechanism; however, systemic exposure is almost exclusively the parent drug. The drug is greater than 99.8% bound to plasma proteins. The major route of elimination of ledipasvir is biliary excretion. Following a single 90-mg oral dose of ledipasvir, 86% is excreted in feces (70% as unchanged ledipasvir, 2.2% as the oxidative metabolite) and 1% is excreted in urine. Following oral administration of ledipasvir/sofosbuvir, the median terminal half-life of ledipasvir is 47 hours.

Sofosbuvir is a prodrug that undergoes intracellular metabolic activation in the liver (hydrolysis by human cathepsin A [CatA] or carboxylesterase 1 [CES1], phosphoramidate cleavage by histidine triad nucleotide-binding protein 1 [HINT1], and phosphorylation by pyrimidine nucleotide biosynthesis pathway). This results in formation of the pharmacologically active metabolite, GS-461203; desphosphorylation subsequently occurs leading to formation of GS-331007 (the predominant circulating metabolite), which has no anti-HCV activity. Sofosbuvir is approximately 61–65% bound and GS-331007 is minimally bound to plasma proteins. The major route of elimination is renal clearance. Following a single 400-mg oral dose of sofosbuvir, 80% is eliminated in urine (mainly as GS-331007), 14% is excreted in feces, and 2.5% is eliminated in expired air. Following oral administration of ledipasvir/sofosbuvir, the median terminal half-lives of sofosbuvir and GS-331007 are 0.5 and 27 hours, respectively.

In individuals with severe hepatic impairment (Child-Pugh class C) without HCV infection, AUC of ledipasvir after a single 90-mg dose is similar to that observed in individuals with normal hepatic function. In HCV-infected individuals with moderate or severe hepatic impairment (Child-Pugh class B or C), sofosbuvir AUC is 126 or 143% higher, respectively, compared with HCV-infected individuals with normal hepatic function; GS-331007 AUC is 18 or 9% higher, respectively. Population pharmacokinetic analysis in HCV-infected patients indicates that cirrhosis has no clinically important effect on ledipasvir, sofosbuvir, or GS-331007 exposure. Following a single 90-mg dose, there were no clinically important differences in ledipasvir pharmacokinetics between individuals with severe renal impairment without HCV infection and healthy individuals. In individuals with mild, moderate, or severe renal impairment without HCV infection, sofosbuvir AUC is 61, 107, or 171% higher, respectively, compared with individuals with normal renal function; GS-331007 AUC is 55, 88, or 451% higher, respectively. Pharmacokinetics of ledipasvir, sofosbuvir, and GS-331007 in pediatric patients 3 years of age or older with HCV genotype 1, 3, or 4 infection are similar to the pharmacokinetics of the drugs in adults; pharmacokinetics of ledipasvir, sofosbuvir, and GS-331007 have not been established in pediatric patients younger than 3 years of age. Although not considered clinically important, population pharmacokinetic analysis in HCV-infected individuals indicates that peak plasma concentrations and AUC of ledipasvir are 58 and 77% higher, respectively, in females than in males; gender does not affect sofosbuvir or GS-331007 exposure. Population pharmacokinetic analysis indicates that age (range 18–80 years)

and race do not have clinically important effects on ledipasvir, sofosbuvir, or GS-331007 exposures.

ADVICE TO PATIENTS

Advise patients that the fixed-combination preparation of ledipasvir and sofosbuvir (ledipasvir/sofosbuvir) should be taken once daily (with or without food) on a regular dosing schedule.

Inform patients that reactivation of hepatitis B virus (HBV) infection has occurred in coinfected patients being treated for hepatitis C virus (HCV) infection. Importance of informing clinician of any history of HBV infection or other liver problems (e.g., cirrhosis). Importance of immediately contacting a clinician if any signs or symptoms of serious liver injury (e.g., fatigue, weakness, loss of appetite, nausea and vomiting, yellowing of the eyes or skin, light-colored bowel movements) occur. (See Risk of HBV Reactivation in Patients Coinfected with HCV and HBV under Warnings/Precautions: Warnings, in Cautions.)

Importance of taking the recommended dosage of ledipasvir/sofosbuvir for the recommended duration of treatment; importance of not missing or skipping doses.

If ledipasvir/sofosbuvir is used in a patient receiving amiodarone, advise the patient about the risk of serious symptomatic bradycardia and the importance of immediately contacting a clinician if signs or symptoms of bradycardia (e.g., near-fainting or fainting, dizziness, lightheadedness, malaise, weakness, excessive tiredness, shortness of breath, chest pain, confusion, memory problems) occur. (See Cardiovascular Effects under Warnings/Precautions: Other Warnings/Precautions, in Cautions.)

Importance of informing clinicians of existing or contemplated concomitant therapy, including prescription and OTC drugs and dietary or herbal supplements, as well as any concomitant illnesses.

Importance of women informing clinicians if they are or plan to become pregnant or plan to breast-feed. If used in conjunction with ribavirin, advise men and women of importance of using effective contraception during and for 6 months after ribavirin therapy. (See Precautions Related to Fixed Combinations and Multiple-drug Treatment Regimens under Warnings/Precautions: Other Warnings/Precautions, in Cautions.)

Importance of informing patients of other important precautionary information. (See Cautions.)

PREPARATIONS

Excipients in commercially available drug preparations may have clinically important effects in some individuals; consult specific product labeling for details.

Ledipasvir and Sofosbuvir

Oral		
Pellets	Ledipasvir 33.75 mg and Sofosbuvir 150 mg	Harvoni®, Gilead
	Ledipasvir 45 mg and Sofosbuvir 200 mg	Harvoni®, Gilead
Tablets, film-coated	Ledipasvir 45 mg and Sofosbuvir 200 mg	Harvoni®, Gilead
	Ledipasvir 90 mg and Sofosbuvir 400 mg	Harvoni®, Gilead

† Use is not currently included in the labeling approved by the US Food and Drug Administration.

Foscarnet Sodium

8:18.92 • MISCELLANEOUS ANTIVIRALS

■ Foscarnet sodium (phosphonoformic acid), an organic analog of inorganic pyrophosphate, is an antiviral agent active against herpesviruses.

USES

● Treatment of Cytomegalovirus Infection and Disease

Cytomegalovirus Retinitis

Foscarnet sodium is used for initial treatment (induction therapy) and maintenance therapy (secondary prophylaxis) of cytomegalovirus (CMV) retinitis in adults with human immunodeficiency virus (HIV) infection, including those with acquired immunodeficiency syndrome (AIDS). The drug also is used for the management of CMV retinitis in HIV-infected adolescents and children†. Foscarnet can be used in conjunction with ganciclovir for the management of CMV retinitis that relapsed after monotherapy with either drug. Safety and efficacy of foscarnet have not been established for the treatment of CMV retinitis in immunocompetent individuals.

Like other antivirals, foscarnet, is not a cure for CMV retinitis. Although foscarnet can induce stabilization or improvement of ocular manifestations of CMV retinitis, the retinitis may relapse and/or progress during or after discontinuance of the drug. The possibility of foscarnet-resistant CMV should be considered in patients who fail to respond to foscarnet or who experience persistent CMV shedding while receiving maintenance therapy with the drug; some strains resistant to foscarnet may be susceptible to ganciclovir. In some patients whose retinitis progressed with foscarnet or ganciclovir monotherapy, combined therapy with the drugs stabilized progression of the disease.

Retinitis is the most common clinical manifestation of CMV end-organ disease in HIV-infected patients and ideally should be managed in consultation with an ophthalmologist familiar with the diagnosis and treatment of retinal diseases. Antiviral regimens for initial treatment of CMV retinitis in HIV-infected individuals should be selected based on the location and severity of CMV retinal lesions, severity of underlying immunosuppression, concomitant drug therapy, and the patient's ability to adhere to the treatment regimen. The antiviral regimen used for maintenance therapy of CMV retinitis in HIV-infected individuals should be selected with consideration for the location of the CMV retinal lesions, vision in the contralateral eye, the patient's immunologic and virologic status, and the patient's response to antiretroviral therapy.

For the management of immediate sight-threatening CMV retinal lesions (i.e., within 1.5 mm of the fovea) in HIV-infected adults and adolescents, the US Centers for Disease Control and Prevention (CDC), National Institutes of Health (NIH), and HIV Medicine Association of the Infectious Diseases Society of America (IDSA) state that the preferred regimen is initial treatment (induction therapy) with intravitreal ganciclovir or intravitreal foscarnet† (1–4 doses given over a period of 7–10 days) in conjunction with oral valganciclovir (twice daily for 14–21 days) followed by maintenance therapy (secondary prophylaxis) with oral valganciclovir (once daily). One alternative regimen recommended by these experts for management of sight-threatening CMV retinitis in HIV-infected adults and adolescents is intravitreal ganciclovir or intravitreal foscarnet† (1–4 doses given over a period of 7–10 days) in conjunction with IV foscarnet (2 or 3 times daily for 2–3 weeks) followed by maintenance therapy (secondary prophylaxis) with IV foscarnet (once daily). Use of systemic antivirals (without an intravitreal antiviral) usually is adequate for the management of CMV retinitis in patients who have only small peripheral lesions.

For the management of CMV retinitis in HIV-infected pediatric patients, CDC, NIH, IDSA, and others state that IV ganciclovir is the drug of choice for initial treatment (induction therapy) and is one of several options for maintenance therapy (secondary prophylaxis). These experts state that IV foscarnet is a preferred alternative for the management of CMV retinitis in HIV-infected children† and is recommended for infections known or suspected to be caused by ganciclovir-resistant CMV. These experts state that a regimen of IV ganciclovir and IV foscarnet can be considered for initial treatment (induction therapy) in HIV-

infected children with sight-threatening CMV retinitis or when the infection failed to respond to or relapsed after monotherapy. Data are limited regarding use of intravitreal antivirals in children, and intravitreal injections are impractical in most children.

Because of the risk of relapse, HIV-infected patients who have received adequate initial treatment of CMV retinitis should receive chronic maintenance therapy (secondary prophylaxis) until immune reconstitution occurs as a result of effective antiretroviral therapy. CDC, NIH, and IDSA state that consideration can be given to discontinuing maintenance therapy of CMV retinitis in HIV-infected adults and adolescents if CMV lesions have been treated for at least 3–6 months and are inactive and there has been a sustained (i.e., 3–6 months) increase in $CD4^+$ T-cell count to greater than $100/mm^3$ in response to antiretroviral therapy. The safety of discontinuing maintenance therapy of CMV retinitis in HIV-infected pediatric patients has not been well studied; however, CDC, NIH, IDSA, and others state that consideration can be given to discontinuing such maintenance therapy of CMV retinitis in HIV-infected children who are receiving antiretroviral therapy and have a sustained (i.e., greater than 6 months) increase in $CD4^+$ T-cell percentage to greater than 15% (children younger than 6 years of age) or increase in $CD4^+$ T-cell count to greater than $100/mm^3$ (children 6 years of age and older). These experts state that a decision to discontinue maintenance therapy of CMV retinitis should be made in consultation with an ophthalmologist and, if maintenance therapy is discontinued, the patient should continue to receive regular ophthalmologic monitoring (optimally every 3–6 months) for early detection of CMV relapse or immune reconstitution uveitis. If $CD4^+$ T-cell count decreases to less than $100/mm^3$ (adults, adolescents, children 6 years of age or older) or if $CD4^+$ T-cell percentage decreases to less than 15% (children younger than 6 years of age), maintenance therapy of CMV retinitis should be reinitiated.

For additional information on the management of CMV retinitis and other CMV infections in HIV-infected individuals, the current clinical practice guidelines from CDC, NIH, and IDSA on the prevention and treatment of opportunistic infections in HIV-infected individuals available at http://www.aidsinfo.nih.gov should be consulted.

Clinical Experience

Efficacy of IV foscarnet sodium for the treatment of CMV retinitis was evaluated in a prospective, randomized, controlled trial in 24 patients with AIDS. Patients received induction treatment with foscarnet sodium (60 mg/kg IV every 8 hours for 3 weeks), followed by maintenance treatment with the drug (90 mg/kg IV once daily until retinitis progression [appearance of a new lesion or advancement of the border of a posterior lesion greater than 750 μm in diameter]). All diagnoses and determinations of retinitis progression were made from masked reading of retinal photographs. The 13 patients randomized to receive IV foscarnet had a delay in progression of CMV retinitis compared with untreated controls. The median time to retinitis progression from study entry was 93 days (range: 21 to greater than 364 days) in those treated with IV foscarnet compared with 22 days (range: 7–42 days) in untreated controls.

In another prospective trial in AIDS patients with CMV retinitis, 33 patients received induction treatment with IV foscarnet sodium (60 mg/kg IV 3 times daily for 2–3 weeks) and were randomized to receive maintenance therapy with the drug in a dosage of 90 or 120 mg/kg IV once daily. The median time from study entry to retinitis progression was not significantly different between the treatment groups; 96 days (range: 14 to greater than 176 days) in those receiving the lower maintenance dosage and 140 days (range: 16 to greater than 233 days) in those receiving the higher maintenance dosage.

The comparative efficacy of IV foscarnet and IV ganciclovir for the treatment of newly diagnosed CMV retinitis was evaluated in a study that included 107 patients randomized to receive foscarnet sodium (induction treatment with 60 mg/kg IV 3 times daily for 2 weeks followed by maintenance therapy with 90 mg/kg IV once daily) and 127 patients randomized to receive ganciclovir (induction treatment with 5 mg/kg IV twice daily followed by maintenance therapy with 5 mg/kg IV once daily). The median time to retinitis progression was similar with both drugs (59 days in those receiving foscarnet and 56 days in those receiving ganciclovir).

In a study evaluating efficacy of combination therapy with IV foscarnet and IV ganciclovir versus monotherapy with either drug alone for the treatment of persistently active or relapsed CMV retinitis in patients with AIDS, patients who were randomized to combination therapy while receiving IV foscarnet alone continued to receive the usual maintenance dosage of foscarnet sodium (i.e., 90 mg/kg IV once daily) while IV ganciclovir therapy was initiated using usual ganciclovir induction and maintenance dosages (i.e., 5 mg/kg IV every 12 hours for 14 days followed by 5 mg/kg IV once daily). Patients who were randomized to combination therapy while receiving IV ganciclovir alone continued to receive the usual maintenance dosage of ganciclovir (i.e., 5 mg/kg IV once daily) while IV foscarnet therapy was initiated using usual foscarnet sodium induction and maintenance dosages (i.e., 90 mg/kg IV every 12 hours for 14 days followed by 90 mg/kg IV once daily). Therapy was then continued using maintenance dosages of both drugs. Patients who relapsed while receiving combination therapy were reinduced with both drugs using usual induction dosages (i.e., ganciclovir 5 mg/kg IV every 12 hours and foscarnet sodium 90 mg IV every 12 hours for 14 days) followed by usual maintenance dosages (i.e., ganciclovir 5 mg/kg IV once daily and foscarnet sodium 90 mg/kg IV once daily). The median time to retinitis progression in the foscarnet group, ganciclovir group, or combination group was 1.3, 2, or 4.3 months, respectively.

Extraocular Cytomegalovirus Infections

Although safety and efficacy of foscarnet sodium have not been established for the treatment of extraocular CMV infections (e.g., pneumonitis, gastroenteritis), the drug has been used for the management of extraocular CMV infections†.

CDC, NIH, and IDSA state that IV ganciclovir usually is the preferred antiviral for initial management of CMV GI disease (e.g., colitis, esophagitis) in HIV-infected adults; however, IV foscarnet is a possible alternative for the management of CMV esophagitis† or colitis† in those who cannot receive ganciclovir or have infections caused by ganciclovir-resistant CMV.

For the management of well-documented CMV pneumonitis† in HIV-infected adults, CDC, NIH, and IDSA state that either IV ganciclovir or IV foscarnet is a reasonable choice.

A combination regimen of IV ganciclovir and IV foscarnet has been used for the management of CMV neurologic disease† (e.g., CMV encephalitis or myelitis) and is recommended by CDC, NIH, IDSA, and others for such infections in HIV-infected individuals.

● Prevention of Cytomegalovirus Infection and Disease

Foscarnet sodium has been used for prophylaxis or preemptive treatment of CMV infection and disease in hematopoietic stem cell transplant (HSCT) recipients†. Although safety and efficacy have not been established, IV foscarnet sodium is considered a second-line or alternative antiviral for prophylaxis or preemptive treatment of CMV infection in HSCT recipients and usually is reserved for resistant and refractory CMV infections or when first-line antivirals cannot be used because of intolerance. Foscarnet also has been recommended as a second-line or alternative antiviral for treatment of CMV infection in solid organ transplant recipients† when first-line antivirals cannot be used because of resistance or intolerance.

CMV infection in transplant recipients can occur either as a primary infection in CMV-seronegative recipients of organs and cells from CMV-positive donors or as reactivation of latent CMV infection in CMV-seropositive recipients. CMV reactivation commonly occurs in CMV-seropositive transplant recipients and can result in severe CMV disease with substantial morbidity and mortality. The risk for CMV infection or reactivation is greatest during the first 3 months after transplantation and depends on several factors, including the serologic status of the recipient and donor and CMV-specific T-cell immunity and immunosuppressive regimens used in the recipient. Certain antiviral strategies have been used to prevent severe, life-threatening CMV disease in HSCT or solid organ transplant patients, including antiviral prophylaxis (initiated posttransplant and continued for at least 3 months) and/or preemptive antiviral treatment (i.e., initiated when CMV infection is detected, but before clinical progression to symptomatic CMV disease). These strategies each have certain advantages and disadvantages.

Specialized references should be consulted for specific information regarding management of CMV infections in HSCT or solid organ transplant recipients.

● Mucocutaneous Herpes Simplex Virus Infections

Foscarnet sodium is used for the management of mucocutaneous infections (e.g., orofacial, genital, digital) caused by acyclovir-resistant herpes simplex virus types 1 and 2 (HSV-1 and HSV-2) in immunocompromised patients, including HIV-infected individuals with AIDS. Safety and efficacy of foscarnet have not been established for the treatment of other HSV infections (e.g., retinitis, encephalitis), congenital or neonatal HSV disease, or HSV infections in immunocompetent individuals.

The drugs of choice for the management of orolabial lesions or initial or recurrent genital lesions caused by HSV are valacyclovir, famciclovir, and acyclovir. For the management of mucocutaneous lesions caused by acyclovir-resistant HSV in HIV-infected adults and adolescents†, CDC, NIH, and IDSA recommend IV foscarnet as the drug of choice. These experts also recommend IV foscarnet as the drug of choice for the management of acyclovir-resistant HSV infections in HIV-infected children†.

Like other antivirals, foscarnet is not a cure for mucocutaneous HSV infections. While complete healing is possible, relapse occurs in most patients. Repeated foscarnet treatment of HSV infections has led to development of resistance that was associated with poor response. If there is a poor therapeutic response to foscarnet therapy, in vitro susceptibility testing of the HSV isolate is advised.

Clinical Experience

Efficacy of IV foscarnet sodium for the treatment of mucocutaneous acyclovir-resistant HSV infections was evaluated in a study in AIDS patients that included 8 patients randomized to receive IV foscarnet sodium (40 mg/kg IV 3 times daily), 6 patients randomized to receive vidarabine (15 mg/kg daily; not commercially available in the US), and 11 patients nonrandomly assigned to receive treatment with IV foscarnet sodium because of prior intolerance to vidarabine. HSV lesions in the 8 patients randomized to foscarnet healed after 11–25 days and HSV lesions in 7 of the 11 patients nonrandomly treated with foscarnet healed in 10–30 days. In a second trial, 40 patients with AIDS and 3 bone marrow transplant recipients with mucocutaneous acyclovir-resistant HSV infections were randomized to receive IV foscarnet sodium (40 mg/kg 2 or 3 times daily). HSV lesions in 15 of the 43 patients healed in 11–72 days with no difference in response between the 2 groups.

Foscarnet sodium (40 mg/kg IV every 8 hours until clinical resolution is attained) often is effective in the treatment of acyclovir-resistant genital herpes. Limited data have shown that foscarnet may decrease duration of viral shedding and time required for crusting and healing of lesions, and the duration of positive cultures in AIDS patients with HSV infections that did not respond to oral or parenteral acyclovir therapy. However, eventual recurrence of HSV has been reported in virtually all such patients following discontinuance of foscarnet therapy; median time to recurrence reportedly was 42.5 days (range: 14–191 days) following discontinuance of the drug. Such recurrences may or may not be associated with acyclovir-resistant strains of the virus. In some patients who had received foscarnet (repeated or chronic therapy) for management of acyclovir-resistant HSV infection, foscarnet-resistant strains of the virus were reported. Patients who developed foscarnet-resistant HSV infections subsequently received oral or parenteral acyclovir or, alternatively, concomitant therapy with acyclovir and foscarnet.

● Varicella-Zoster Virus Infections

Foscarnet sodium is used in the management of acyclovir-resistant varicella-zoster virus (VZV) infections† in immunocompromised patients, including those with AIDS.

The preferred antivirals for the management of acute, localized herpes zoster (shingles) in HIV-infected adults and adolescents are acyclovir, famciclovir, and valacyclovir. For the management of proven or suspected acyclovir-resistant VZV infections† in HIV-infected adults or adolescents, CDC, NIH, and IDSA recommend IV foscarnet.

In HIV-infected children, acyclovir is the drug of choice for VZV infections and foscarnet is the preferred alternative for the management of acyclovir-resistant VZV infections†.

Although optimal regimens for the management of progressive outer retinal necrosis caused by VZV† in HIV-infected individuals have not been identified, CDC, NIH, and IDSA recommend treatment with at least one IV antiviral (acyclovir, ganciclovir, foscarnet, cidofovir) used in conjunction with at least one intravitreal antiviral (ganciclovir or foscarnet). Some experts recommend a regimen of IV ganciclovir and/or IV foscarnet used in conjunction with intravitreal ganciclovir and/or intravitreal foscarnet†. The prognosis for visual preservation in patients with progressive outer retinal necrosis caused by VZV is poor and such infections should be managed in consultation with an ophthalmologist.

DOSAGE AND ADMINISTRATION

● General

Renal function *must* be assessed prior to initiation of foscarnet sodium and monitored during therapy with the drug. (See Renal Impairment under Dosage and Administration: Special Populations.)

To reduce the risk of foscarnet-associated nephrotoxicity, patients *must* receive adequate hydration prior to and during foscarnet sodium therapy.

The recommended dosage of foscarnet sodium and recommended frequency and rate of administration of the drug *must* not be exceeded.

Hydration

Patients *must* be adequately hydrated before and during administration of foscarnet sodium.

Patients who are clinically dehydrated should have their hydration status corrected before the drug is initiated.

Prior to the first dose of foscarnet, patients should receive IV hydration with 750–1000 mL of 0.9% sodium chloride or 5% dextrose injection to establish diuresis. With each subsequent dose of foscarnet, 750–1000 mL of IV hydration fluid should be administered concurrently with each foscarnet sodium dose of 90–120 mg/kg or 500 mL of IV hydration fluid should be administered concurrently with each foscarnet sodium dose of 40–60 mg/kg. The volume of IV hydration fluid may be decreased if clinically appropriate.

Oral rehydration using similar regimens may be considered in some patients.

● Administration

Foscarnet sodium is administered by slow IV infusion using a controlled-infusion device (e.g., pump). The drug should *not* be administered by rapid IV infusion or direct IV injection since potentially toxic plasma foscarnet concentrations may result.

Foscarnet has been administered by intravitreal injection†; however, a preparation of the drug specifically for intravitreal administration is not commercially available in the US.

IV Infusion

IV infusions of foscarnet sodium *must* be administered using a controlled-infusion device (e.g., pump) and the rate of administration carefully controlled to avoid adverse effects and unintentional overdosage.

Foscarnet sodium is commercially available as a solution for IV infusion containing 24 mg/mL.

If a central venous line is used for IV infusion, the commercially available solution of foscarnet sodium can be administered either undiluted or diluted.

If a peripheral vein is used for IV infusion, the commercially available solution of the drug *must* be diluted prior to administration with a compatible infusion solution to a concentration of 12 mg/mL. In addition, care should be taken to select a vein that will provide adequate blood flow for rapid dilution and distribution of the drug.

Foscarnet sodium solution should appear clear and colorless and should not be used if it appears discolored or contains particles.

Commercially available foscarnet sodium solution should be stored at 20–25°C. Precipitates may form if the solution is refrigerated or exposed to freezing temperatures, but may be brought into solution again if kept at room temperature with repeated shaking.

IV solutions of foscarnet sodium should *not* be admixed or administered through the same catheter with other drugs. Foscarnet sodium injection is physically and/or chemically incompatible with certain infusion solutions (e.g., calcium-containing solutions such as Ringer's or lactated Ringer's) and certain drugs (e.g., ganciclovir). Specialized references should be consulted for specific information.

Caution should be exercised when preparing and administering solutions of foscarnet sodium. Accidental skin and eye contact with solutions of the drug may cause local irritation and burning sensation. If accidental contact occurs, the exposed area should be flushed with water.

Dilution

When a diluted solution of foscarnet sodium is indicated for IV infusion (e.g., for infusion via a peripheral vein), the commercially available solution of the drug containing 24 mg/mL *must* be diluted with a compatible infusion solution (i.e., 0.9% sodium chloride injection or 5% dextrose injection) to a concentration of 12 mg/mL.

Diluted solutions of foscarnet sodium should be used within 24 hours after first entry into the sealed bottle.

Rate of Administration

IV infusions of foscarnet sodium should be administered at a constant rate using a controlled-infusion device (e.g., pump) and usually are given over 1–2 hours depending on dosage.

The IV infusion rate *must* not exceed 1 mg/kg per minute.

● Dosage

Foscarnet is commercially available as the hydrated trisodium salt (i.e., foscarnet sodium); dosage is expressed in terms of foscarnet sodium.

Adult Dosage
Cytomegalovirus Retinitis

For the treatment of cytomegalovirus (CMV) retinitis in adults with human immunodeficiency virus (HIV) infection and normal renal function, the recommended dosage of IV foscarnet sodium for initial treatment (induction therapy) is 60 mg/kg (by IV infusion over at least 1 hour) every 8 hours for 14–21 days or 90 mg/kg (by IV infusion over 1.5–2 hours) every 12 hours for 14–21 days. In patients with immediate sight-threatening CMV retinal lesions (i.e., within 1.5 mm of the fovea), the US Centers for Disease Control and Prevention (CDC), National Institutes of Health (NIH), and HIV Medicine Association of the Infectious Diseases Society of America (IDSA) recommend that initial treatment also include an appropriate intravitreal antiviral. (See Cytomegalovirus Retinitis under Uses: Treatment of Cytomegalovirus Infection and Disease.)

After completion of initial treatment, the recommended dosage of IV foscarnet sodium for maintenance therapy (secondary prophylaxis) of CMV retinitis in adults with normal renal function is 90–120 mg/kg (by IV infusion over 2 hours) once daily. Because superiority of the 120-mg/kg daily dosage has not been established in controlled studies and because such dosage is likely to be associated with an increased risk of toxicity, the manufacturer recommends that most patients initially receive a maintenance dosage of 90 mg/kg IV once daily. However, dosage may be increased up to 120 mg/kg daily in patients in whom early reinduction therapy is required because of progression of CMV retinitis. In addition, some patients exhibiting excellent tolerance to the drug may benefit from early initiation of a maintenance dosage of 120 mg/kg daily.

Patients who experience relapse or progression of CMV retinitis while receiving foscarnet maintenance therapy may be retreated with foscarnet using the usual dosages for initial treatment (induction therapy) and maintenance therapy (secondary prophylaxis) or, alternatively, these patients may receive combination therapy with foscarnet and ganciclovir.

Decisions regarding discontinuance of maintenance therapy of CMV retinitis in HIV-infected individuals who have been treated for at least 3–6 months, have inactive CMV retinal lesions, and have achieved immune reconstitution as the result of antiretroviral therapy should be made in consultation with an ophthalmologist. (See Cytomegalovirus Retinitis under Uses: Treatment of Cytomegalovirus Infection and Disease.)

Cytomegalovirus Esophagitis or Colitis

If IV foscarnet sodium is used as an alternative for the management of CMV esophagitis† or colitis† in HIV-infected adults, CDC, NIH, and IDSA recommend a dosage of 60 mg/kg every 8 hours or 90 mg/kg every 12 hours given for 21–42 days or until signs and symptoms of the infection have resolved. Maintenance therapy (secondary prophylaxis) usually is not necessary, but should be considered if relapse occurs.

Cytomegalovirus Pneumonitis

If IV foscarnet sodium is used as an alternative for the management of well-documented CMV pneumonitis† in HIV-infected adults, CDC, NIH, and IDSA state that the same dosage recommended for the management of CMV retinitis in HIV-infected adults should be used. The optimal duration of treatment in such patients has not been established.

Cytomegalovirus Neurologic Disease

If IV foscarnet sodium is used in conjunction with IV ganciclovir for the management of CMV neurologic disease† in HIV-infected adults, CDC, NIH, and IDSA state that the same dosage recommended for the management of CMV retinitis in HIV-infected adults should be used. The optimal duration of treatment in such patients has not been established.

Mucocutaneous Herpes Simplex Virus Infections

For the management of mucocutaneous herpes simplex virus (HSV) infections known or suspected to be caused by acyclovir-resistant strains in immunocompromised patients, the manufacturer and some clinicians recommend that IV foscarnet sodium be given in a dosage of 40 mg/kg (by IV infusion over at least 1 hour) every 8 or 12 hours for 2–3 weeks or until clinical resolution. For the management of acyclovir-resistant genital herpes, CDC states that foscarnet sodium has been effective when given in a dosage of 40–80 mg/kg IV every 8 hours until clinical resolution.

For the management of acyclovir-resistant mucocutaneous HSV infections in HIV-infected adults, CDC, NIH, and IDSA recommend that IV foscarnet sodium be given in a dosage of 80–120 mg/kg daily in 2 or 3 divided doses until a clinical response is obtained.

Varicella-Zoster Virus Infections

For the management of mucocutaneous varicella-zoster virus (VZV) infections† known or suspected to be caused by acyclovir-resistant strains in immunocompromised patients, some clinicians recommend that IV foscarnet sodium be given in a dosage of 40–60 mg/kg IV every 8 hours for 10–21 days.

For the management of progressive outer retinal necrosis caused by VZV† in HIV-infected adults, CDC, NIH, and IDSA state that a regimen that includes IV foscarnet sodium in a dosage of 90 mg/kg IV every 12 hours (used with or without IV ganciclovir) in conjunction with intravitreal foscarnet† (used with or without intravitreal ganciclovir) can be considered.

Pediatric Dosage
Cytomegalovirus Retinitis

If IV foscarnet sodium is used with or without IV ganciclovir for initial treatment (induction therapy) of CMV retinitis in HIV-infected children†, CDC, NIH, IDSA, and others recommend a dosage of 60 mg/kg IV every 8 hours or 90 mg/kg IV every 12 hours for 14–21 days or until symptomatic improvement.

After completion of initial treatment, the recommended dosage of IV foscarnet sodium for maintenance therapy (secondary prophylaxis) of CMV retinitis in HIV-infected children† is 90–120 mg/kg IV once daily.

Decisions regarding discontinuance of maintenance therapy of CMV retinitis in HIV-infected individuals who have been treated at least 3–6 months, have inactive CMV retinal lesions, and have achieved immune reconstitution as the result of antiretroviral therapy should be made in consultation with an ophthalmologist. (See Cytomegalovirus Retinitis under Uses: Treatment of Cytomegalovirus Infection and Disease.)

Disseminated Cytomegalovirus Infections

If IV foscarnet sodium is used with or without IV ganciclovir for initial treatment (induction therapy) of disseminated CMV infections in HIV-infected children†, CDC, NIH, IDSA, and others recommend a dosage of 60 mg/kg IV every 8 hours or 90 mg/kg IV every 12 hours until symptomatic improvement.

After completion of initial treatment, the recommended dosage of IV foscarnet sodium for maintenance therapy (secondary prophylaxis) of disseminated CMV infection in HIV-infected children† is 90–120 mg/kg IV once daily.

Mucocutaneous Herpes Simplex Virus Infections

If IV foscarnet sodium is used for the management of mucocutaneous acyclovir-resistant HSV infections in HIV-infected children†, CDC, NIH, IDSA, and others recommend a dosage of 40 mg/kg every 8 hours or 60 mg/kg every 12 hours (by IV infusion over 2 hours).

Varicella-Zoster Virus Infections

If IV foscarnet sodium is used for the management of VZV infections caused by acyclovir-resistant strains in HIV-infected children†, CDC, NIH, IDSA, and others recommend a dosage of 40–60 mg/kg (by IV infusion over 2 hours) given 3 times daily for 7–10 days or until no new lesions have appeared for at least 48 hours.

For the management of progressive outer retinal necrosis caused by VZV† in HIV-infected children, CDC, NIH, IDSA, and others state that a regimen that includes IV foscarnet given in a dosage of 90 mg/kg IV every 12 hours (used with or without IV ganciclovir) in conjunction with intravitreal foscarnet† given in a dosage of 1.2 mg/0.05 mL by intravitreal injection twice weekly (with or without intravitreal ganciclovir) can be considered.

● Special Populations
Hepatic Impairment

The manufacturer makes no specific dosage recommendations for use of foscarnet sodium in patients with hepatic impairment; some clinicians state that dosage of the drug does not need to be adjusted in such patients.

Renal Impairment

In patients with impaired renal function, dosage of foscarnet sodium *must* be modified based on the degree of impairment. Dosage adjustment may be required in patients with initially normal renal function since most patients will experience a decrease in renal function during foscarnet therapy.

Renal function (i.e., measured and estimated creatinine clearance) should be assessed prior to initiating foscarnet sodium, 2 or 3 times weekly during induction therapy, and at least once every 1 or 2 weeks during maintenance therapy with the drug and dosage should be adjusted accordingly. (See Table 1 and Table 2.)

Dosage of foscarnet sodium should be based on the patient's measured or estimated creatinine clearance. Creatinine clearance (mL/minute per kg) should be calculated even if serum creatinine is within the normal range.

If creatinine clearance declines to less than 0.4 mL/minute per kg during foscarnet therapy, the drug should be discontinued and the patient should be hydrated and monitored daily until resolution of renal impairment is ensured.

To determine dosage of foscarnet sodium in patients with renal impairment, the patient's weight-adjusted 24-hour creatinine clearance (Ccr divided by body weight in kg) is used or Ccr (per kg) can be calculated using the following formulas:

$$Ccr\ male = \frac{(140 - age) \times weight}{72 \times serum\ creatinine}$$
$$Ccr\ female = 0.85 \times Ccr\ male$$

where age is in years, weight is in kg, and serum creatinine is in mg/dL.

TABLE 1. Recommended Foscarnet Sodium Dosage for Initial Treatment (Induction Therapy) of CMV Retinitis or HSV Infections in Adults Based on Patient's Creatinine Clearance.

Creatinine Clearance (mL/minute per kg)	Induction Dosage for CMV (in mg/kg) Equivalent to 60 mg/kg Every 8 Hours	Induction Dosage for CMV (in mg/kg) Equivalent to 90 mg/kg Every 12 Hours	Induction Dosage for HSV (in mg/kg) Equivalent to 40 mg/kg Every 12 Hours	Induction Dosage for HSV (in mg/kg) Equivalent to 40 mg/kg Every 8 Hours
>1.4	60 every 8 hours	90 every 12 hours	40 every 12 hours	40 every 8 hours
>1–1.4	45 every 8 hours	70 every 12 hours	30 every 12 hours	30 every 8 hours
>0.8–1	50 every 12 hours	50 every 12 hours	20 every 12 hours	35 every 12 hours
>0.6–0.8	40 every 12 hours	80 every 24 hours	35 every 24 hours	25 every 12 hours
>0.5–0.6	60 every 24 hours	60 every 24 hours	25 every 24 hours	40 every 24 hours
≥0.4–0.5	50 every 24 hours	50 every 24 hours	20 every 24 hours	35 every 24 hours
<0.4	Not recommended	Not recommended	Not recommended	Not recommended

TABLE 2. Recommended Foscarnet Sodium Dosage for Maintenance Therapy of CMV Retinitis in Adults Based on Patient's Creatinine Clearance.

Creatinine Clearance (mL/minute per kg)	Maintenance Dosage for CMV (in mg/kg) Equivalent to 90 mg/kg Once Daily	Maintenance Dosage for CMV (in mg/kg) Equivalent to 120 mg/kg Once Daily
>1.4	90 every 24 hours	120 every 24 hours
>1–1.4	70 every 24 hours	90 every 24 hours
>0.8–1	50 every 24 hours	65 every 24 hours
>0.6–0.8	80 every 48 hours	105 every 48 hours
>0.5–0.6	60 every 48 hours	80 every 48 hours
≥0.4–0.5	50 every 48 hours	65 every 48 hours
<0.4	Not recommended	Not recommended

Dosage recommendations are not available for use of foscarnet sodium in patients undergoing hemodialysis. Use of the drug is not recommended in patients undergoing hemodialysis or peritoneal dialysis.

● **Geriatric Patients**

Dosage of foscarnet sodium for geriatric patients should be selected with caution because of age-related decreases in renal function. (See Geriatric Use under Warnings/Precautions: Specific Populations, in Cautions.)

CAUTIONS

● **Contraindications**

Foscarnet sodium is contraindicated in patients with clinically important hypersensitivity to the drug.

● **Warnings/Precautions**

Warnings

Renal Effects

Foscarnet appears to be nephrotoxic. Renal impairment and/or failure, manifested mainly as an increase in serum creatinine concentration and/or a decrease in creatinine clearance, is the major toxicity of foscarnet and occurs to some degree in most patients receiving the drug. Renal impairment may be accompanied by polyuria and associated polydipsia and, less frequently, by oliguria. In at least one patient, polyuria and polydipsia were attributed to nephrogenic diabetes insipidus temporally related to foscarnet therapy.

In initial clinical trials in patients with human immunodeficiency virus (HIV) infection and acquired immunodeficiency syndrome (AIDS) who received foscarnet sodium for the treatment of cytomegalovirus (CMV) retinitis, 27% of patients developed abnormal renal function. Approximately 33% of patients who received a dosage of 60 mg/kg 3 times daily *without* adequate hydration developed renal impairment (serum creatinine concentration of 2 mg/dL or greater). In subsequent clinical trials in patients who received 1 L of 0.9% sodium chloride or 5% dextrose injection with each dose of foscarnet, only 12% developed renal impairment.

Based on measurement of serum creatinine, renal impairment is most likely to become clinically evident during the second week of induction therapy in patients receiving foscarnet sodium in a dosage of 180 mg/kg daily; however, renal impairment may occur at any time during therapy with the drug. Foscarnet-induced increases in serum creatinine concentration are usually, but not uniformly, reversible following dosage adjustment or discontinuance of the drug, although maximum deterioration in renal function may not be apparent until several weeks after discontinuance of the drug. Foscarnet is removed by hemodialysis, and some clinicians have suggested that hemodialysis may be useful in the management of foscarnet-induced nephrotoxicity when elevated plasma concentrations of the drug are present and the degree of renal failure is severe.

The risk of foscarnet-induced renal impairment may be decreased by adequate hydration before and during administration of the drug. It is imperative that patients receive adequate hydration to establish diuresis prior to the first dose of foscarnet and also receive a recommended hydration regimen with each subsequent dose of the drug. (See Hydration under Dosage and Administration: General.)

The mechanism of foscarnet-induced nephrotoxicity has not been fully determined. While underlying disease and concomitant therapy may contribute to the development and degree of acute renal impairment in some patients, foscarnet alone appears to be nephrotoxic. Autopsy findings of extensive tubular necrosis have been reported in at least one patient, and clinical and laboratory findings in other patients, as well as evidence of a potential beneficial prophylactic effect of adequate hydration, have been consistent with acute tubulopathy. Biopsy or autopsy findings of tubular interstitial nephritis also have been reported, as well as the presence of crystals within glomerular capillary lumen; while positive identification was not made, the physicochemical characteristics of the crystals were suggestive of foscarnet crystals.

Because renal impairment is the principal toxicity of foscarnet and occurs to some degree in most patients receiving the drug, foscarnet must be used with caution, particularly in patients with a history of renal impairment, and it is imperative that renal function be assessed prior to initiation of foscarnet and continually during therapy with the drug and that dosage be modified as needed based on renal function. In patients with impaired renal function, reduced plasma clearance of foscarnet will result in elevated plasma concentrations of the drug; in addition, foscarnet potentially may further impair renal function in these patients. Therefore, dosage modification based on renal function (i.e., creatinine clearance) is essential.

The manufacturer recommends that creatinine clearance (measured or estimated based on serum creatinine) be determined at baseline prior to initiating foscarnet therapy, 2 or 3 times weekly during induction therapy, and at least once every 1 or 2 weeks during maintenance therapy, and dosage should be adjusted accordingly. More frequent monitoring may be necessary for some patients. It is also recommended that a 24-hour creatinine clearance be determined at baseline and periodically thereafter to ensure appropriate dosing (assuming verification of an adequate urine collection using the creatinine index). If creatinine clearance declines to less than 0.4 mL/minute per kg during foscarnet therapy, the drug should be discontinued and the patient should be hydrated and monitored daily until resolution of renal impairment is ensured. (See Renal Impairment under Dosage and Administration: Special Populations.)

Electrolyte and Metabolic Effects

Foscarnet therapy has been associated with changes in serum electrolyte concentrations, which potentially may contribute to the risk of cardiac disturbances and seizures. Hypocalcemia has occurred in 15–30%, hypophosphatemia in 8–26%, hyperphosphatemia in 6%, hypomagnesemia in 15–30%, and hypokalemia in 16–48% of patients receiving the drug. Hyponatremia, hypercalcemia, decreased body weight, acidosis, cachexia, and thirst (including polydipsia) have been reported in 1–5% of patients receiving foscarnet. The higher incidences of these electrolyte changes were derived from patients receiving hydration. Increased serum creatine kinase (CK; creatine phosphokinase, CPK) concentration, hematuria, and hypoproteinemia have been reported in less than 1% of patients. Rarely, nephrogenic diabetes mellitus has been associated with foscarnet therapy.

Foscarnet has been shown to produce a dose-related decrease in ionized serum calcium concentration that may not be reflected in total serum calcium concentration. Decreased serum concentrations of ionized calcium may result in symptoms such as perioral tingling, numbness in the extremities, or paresthesias. Foscarnet-induced changes in serum concentrations of calcium or other electrolytes most likely result from the drug's ability to chelate divalent metal ions, such as calcium and magnesium, and form stable coordination compounds.

Because foscarnet has a propensity to chelate divalent metal ions and alter serum concentrations of calcium and other electrolytes (including magnesium, potassium, or phosphate), which may contribute to the risk of cardiac disturbances and seizures, patients receiving the drug must be monitored carefully and frequently for such changes and their potential sequelae. The manufacturer recommends that serum calcium (particularly ionized calcium), magnesium, potassium, and phosphorous concentrations be determined on a schedule similar to that recommended for creatinine clearance. Foscarnet should be used with particular caution in patients with altered serum concentrations of calcium or other electrolytes at baseline and especially in those who have neurologic or cardiac abnormalities or are receiving other drugs known to influence electrolytes (especially calcium).

Patients should be advised about the symptoms of low ionized serum calcium concentration (e.g., perioral tingling, numbness in the extremities, paresthesias) and the importance of reporting such symptoms to a clinician. In patients who experience mild (e.g., perioral tingling) or severe (e.g., seizures) symptoms of electrolyte abnormalities, serum electrolyte concentrations should be determined as soon as possible in temporal relation to the symptoms. If adverse nervous system manifestations (e.g., perioral tingling) occur during IV infusion of foscarnet, the infusion should be discontinued, appropriate laboratory samples obtained for assessment of serum electrolyte concentrations, and a clinician consulted before resuming treatment; if the infusion is restarted, the rate of IV infusion should not exceed 1 mg/kg per minute. Clinicians should be prepared to treat manifestations resulting from electrolyte abnormalities, including severe manifestations such as tetany, seizures, or cardiac disturbances. Careful monitoring and appropriate management of serum electrolyte (including calcium and magnesium) concentrations are particularly important in patients with conditions that may predispose to seizures. (See Nervous System Effects under Warning/Precautions: Warnings, in Cautions.) Since the rate of infusion of foscarnet may affect the transient decrease in ionized serum calcium concentrations, a controlled-infusion device (e.g., pump) must be used for administration of foscarnet; in addition, slowing the rate of infusion may decrease or prevent symptoms.

Since foscarnet may decrease serum concentrations of ionized calcium, other drugs known to influence serum calcium concentrations should be administered concomitantly with caution. In addition, elimination of foscarnet may be impaired by drugs that inhibit renal tubular secretion, although no studies have been performed to determine whether this occurs. Because foscarnet may cause renal impairment, concomitant administration with other potentially nephrotoxic drugs (e.g., aminoglycosides, amphotericin B, IV pentamidine) should be avoided unless potential benefits outweigh possible risks. (See Drug Interactions.)

Nervous System Effects

Seizures related to mineral and electrolyte abnormalities have been associated with foscarnet therapy. Several cases of seizures were associated with death. Cases of status epilepticus have been reported. There have been at least 3 reports of seizures associated with overdosage of the drug. In initial clinical studies evaluating foscarnet in patients with AIDS, seizures occurred in 10% of patients; the rate of seizures did not increase with the duration of treatment.

Risk factors associated with seizures during foscarnet therapy have included impaired baseline renal function, low total serum calcium concentration, and underlying CNS conditions. Close monitoring of plasma electrolytes and minerals and appropriate electrolyte and/or mineral supplementation is particularly important in patients predisposed to seizures. (See Electrolyte and Metabolic Effects under Warnings/Precautions: Warnings, in Cautions.)

Cardiovascular Effects

Foscarnet therapy has been associated with prolongation of the QT interval, which may increase the risk of torsades de pointes. There have been postmarketing reports of torsades de pointes in patients receiving foscarnet. Some of these patients had confounding risk factors (e.g., underlying cardiac disease, electrolyte abnormalities, concomitant drug therapy). Foscarnet-associated transient changes in serum concentrations of calcium or other electrolytes may contribute to the risk of cardiac disturbances. (See Electrolyte and Metabolic Effects under Warnings/Precautions: Warnings, in Cautions.)

Foscarnet should be used with caution in patients with a history of QT-interval prolongation and in those receiving other drugs known to prolong the QT interval, those with electrolyte abnormalities, and those with other risk factors for QT-interval prolongation. Electrocardiograms (ECGs) and electrolyte concentrations should be assessed prior to and periodically during foscarnet therapy.

If any cardiovascular adverse effects occur, the foscarnet IV infusion should be stopped, electrolyte concentrations determined, and a clinician consulted before treatment with the drug is resumed.

Selection and Use of Antivirals

Foscarnet is labeled by the FDA *only* for the treatment of CMV retinitis in HIV-infected patients and the treatment of acyclovir-resistant mucocutaneous herpes simplex virus (HSV) infections in immunocompromised patients.

Safety and efficacy of foscarnet have not been established for the treatment of extraocular CMV infections (e.g., pneumonitis, gastroenteritis), congenital or neonatal CMV disease, or CMV disease in individuals not infected with HIV.

Safety and efficacy of foscarnet have not been established for the treatment of systemic HSV infections (e.g., retinitis, encephalitis), congenital or neonatal HSV disease, or HSV infections in immunocompetent individuals.

When used for the management of mucocutaneous HSV infections, repeated treatment with foscarnet has led to the development of resistance associated with poor response. If there is a poor therapeutic response to foscarnet therapy, in vitro susceptibility testing of the HSV isolate is advised.

Sensitivity Reactions
Hypersensitivity Reactions

Serious acute hypersensitivity reactions (e.g., anaphylactic shock, urticaria, angioedema) have been reported in patients receiving foscarnet.

If an acute hypersensitivity reaction occurs, foscarnet therapy should be discontinued and appropriate medical therapy should be immediately initiated.

Other Warnings and Precautions
Administration Precautions

To avoid local irritation, the commercially available preparation of foscarnet sodium containing 24 mg/mL *must* be diluted before IV administration via a peripheral vein. In addition, particular care must be taken to select a vein with adequate blood flow to permit rapid dilution and distribution of the drug. (See Dosage and Administration: Administration.)

Because of the potential for nephrotoxicity, patients *must* receive adequate hydration prior to the initial dose of foscarnet and also receive a recommended hydration regimen with each subsequent dose of the drug. (See Hydration under Dosage and Administration: General.)

To avoid unintentional overdosage, foscarnet *must* be administered by slow IV infusion using a controlled-infusion device (e.g., pump) to carefully control the infusion rate. (See Rate of Administration under Administration: IV Infusion, in Dosage and Administration.)

Genitourinary Effects

Local irritation and ulceration of the penile epithelium (resembling fixed drug eruption grossly but not histologically) have been reported in male patients and vulvovaginal ulceration has been reported in at least one female patient receiving foscarnet. The genital lesions are often painful, erythematous, and erosive and may require discontinuance of the drug. The lesions usually resolve spontaneously within several weeks after discontinuing foscarnet, but may recur when the drug is reinstituted. Occasionally, the lesions may resolve despite continued foscarnet therapy.

The local irritation and ulceration effects may be related to exposure to high concentrations of unchanged foscarnet in the urine; it also has been suggested that precipitation of the drug in arterioles and capillaries may contribute to ulceration. Adequate hydration and close attention to personal hygiene may minimize the risk of genital irritation and lesions associated with foscarnet therapy.

Hematologic Effects

Anemia, manifested as decreased hemoglobin concentration and hematocrit, is the most common adverse hematologic effect of foscarnet and has been reported in 33% of AIDS patients in controlled clinical trials receiving the drug for the treatment of CMV retinitis. The risk of anemia may be increased in patients receiving foscarnet and ganciclovir concomitantly for progressive retinitis.

Granulocytopenia was reported in 17% of AIDS patients with CMV retinitis receiving foscarnet in controlled clinical trials, but resulted in discontinuance of the drug in only 1% of patients. Leukopenia was reported in 5% or more of AIDS patients with CMV retinitis receiving foscarnet, while thrombocytopenia, platelet abnormalities, thrombosis, leukocyte abnormalities, and lymphadenopathy were reported in 1–5% and pancytopenia was reported in less than 1% of patients.

Foscarnet generally is not myelosuppressive. Only 1% of patients did not complete clinical studies because of neutropenia.

Sodium Content

Commercially available foscarnet sodium solution containing 24 mg of the drug per mL contains 5.5 mg (0.24 mEq) of sodium per mL.

Foscarnet should be avoided in patients who may not tolerate large amounts of sodium or water (e.g., patients with cardiomyopathy) and in patients on a sodium-controlled diet.

Carcinogenic and Mutagenic Potential

Foscarnet caused genotoxic effects in the BALB/3T3 in vitro transformation assay at concentrations exceeding 0.5 mcg/mL and an increased frequency of chromosomal aberrations in the sister chromatid exchange assay at a concentration of 1 mg/mL. A high dose of foscarnet (350 mg/kg) produced an increase in micronucleated polychromatic erythrocytes in vivo in mice at doses that produced exposures (as measured by the area under the plasma concentration-time curve [AUC]) comparable to that anticipated clinically.

There was no evidence of oncogenicity in studies in rats and mice receiving oral foscarnet dosages of 500 and 250 mg/kg daily, respectively, which resulted in plasma foscarnet concentrations equal to 33 and 20%, respectively, of those in humans (at the maximum recommended human daily dose) as measured by the AUC.

Effects on Fertility

Foscarnet did not adversely affect fertility and general reproductive performance in rats. The results of perinatal and postnatal studies in rats were also negative; however, these studies used exposures that were inadequate to define the potential for impairment of fertility at human foscarnet exposure levels.

Specific Populations
Pregnancy

There are no adequate and well-controlled studies to date using foscarnet sodium in pregnant women. The drug should be used during pregnancy only when clearly needed.

Reproduction studies in female rats given subcutaneous foscarnet sodium in doses up to 75 mg/kg daily prior to and during mating, during gestation, and through 21 days postpartum caused a slight increase (less than 5%) in the number of skeletal anomalies compared with the control group. Daily subcutaneous doses up to 75 mg/kg administered to rabbits and 150 mg/kg administered to rats during gestation also caused an increased frequency of skeletal anomalies and variations. On the basis of estimated drug exposure (as measured by AUC), the 150- and 75-mg/kg doses were approximately one-eighth (rats) and one-third (rabbits) the estimated maximal daily human exposure. These data were inadequate to define the potential teratogenicity of foscarnet at dosages used in humans.

Lactation

It is not known whether foscarnet is distributed into human milk. In lactating rats that received a dose of 75 mg/kg, the drug was distributed in maternal milk at concentrations 3 times higher than peak maternal blood concentrations.

Since there is potential for serious adverse reactions to foscarnet in nursing infants, a decision should be made to discontinue nursing or the drug, taking into consideration the importance of the drug to the woman.

Because of the risk of adverse effects in the infant and the risk of HIV transmission, HIV-infected women should not breast-feed infants.

Pediatric Use

Safety and efficacy of foscarnet sodium have not been established in pediatric patients younger than 18 years of age.

The manufacturer states that the drug should be used in children† *only* after careful evaluation and *only* when potential benefits of the drug outweigh possible risks.

Some experts recommend foscarnet as the preferred alternative for the management of CMV retinitis, acyclovir-resistant mucocutaneous HSV infections, and acyclovir-resistant varicella-zoster virus (VZV) infections in HIV-infected children†.

In animals, foscarnet is deposited in teeth and bone and such deposition is greater in those that are young and growing. Foscarnet adversely affects tooth enamel development in mice and rats; the effects of drug deposition on skeletal development have not been studied. There is evidence that foscarnet accumulates in bone in humans, but the extent to which this occurs has not been studied. Since foscarnet is deposited in human bone, it is likely that it does so to a greater degree in developing bone in children.

Geriatric Use

Safety and efficacy of foscarnet have not been specifically studied in geriatric patients 65 years of age or older.

Adverse effects reported in patients 65 years of age or older have been similar to those reported in younger adults.

Because geriatric patients frequently have decreased renal function and because foscarnet is substantially excreted by the kidneys, particular attention should be paid to evaluating renal function prior to and during foscarnet therapy in this age group. If evidence of renal impairment exists or develops, appropriate dosage adjustments should be made. (See Renal Impairment under Dosage and Administration: Special Populations.)

Renal Impairment

Foscarnet sodium should be used with particular caution in patients with impaired renal function since reduced clearance of the drug will result in increased plasma concentrations and increase the risk of toxicity. In addition, foscarnet has the potential to further impair renal function in patients with preexisting renal impairment. (See Renal Effects under Warnings/Precautions: Warnings, in Cautions.)

Due to the risk of nephrotoxicity, renal function should be assessed at baseline and monitored carefully during foscarnet therapy. Dosage of the drug must be individualized and adjusted as needed based on renal function. (See Renal Impairment under Dosage and Administration: Special Populations.)

If creatinine clearance declines to less than 0.4 mL/minute per kg during foscarnet therapy, the drug should be discontinued and the patient should be hydrated and monitored daily until resolution of renal impairment is ensured.

Only limited safety and efficacy data are available regarding use of foscarnet in patients with baseline serum creatinine concentrations greater than 2.8 mg/dL or measured 24-hour creatinine clearances less than 50 mL/minute.

Foscarnet is not recommended in patients undergoing hemodialysis or peritoneal dialysis. Foscarnet is removed by hemodialysis.

● Common Adverse Effects

Adverse effects reported in 10% or more of patients receiving foscarnet include fever, nausea, anemia, diarrhea, abnormal renal function, vomiting, headache, seizures, and marrow suppression.

DRUG INTERACTIONS

● Drugs Affecting Calcium

Because foscarnet sodium can decrease serum concentrations of ionized calcium, possibly because the drug chelates divalent metal ions such as calcium, extreme caution and close monitoring of serum electrolytes is advised if foscarnet is used concomitantly with other drugs known to influence serum calcium concentrations (e.g., IV pentamidine).

● Drugs That Prolong QT Interval

Because foscarnet sodium may increase the risk of QT-interval prolongation and the potential for torsades de pointes, concomitant use of foscarnet with drugs known to prolong the QT interval (e.g., class IA antiarrhythmics [procainamide, quinidine], class III antiarrhythmics [amiodarone, dofetilide, sotalol], other antiarrhythmic agents, phenothiazines, tricyclic antidepressants, certain macrolide antibiotics, certain fluoroquinolones) should be avoided. (See Cardiovascular Effects under Warnings/Precautions: Warnings, in Cautions.)

● Nephrotoxic Drugs

Concomitant use of foscarnet sodium with potentially nephrotoxic drugs (e.g., acyclovir, aminoglycosides, amphotericin B, cyclosporine, methotrexate, tacrolimus) may increase the risk of nephrotoxicity and should be avoided unless potential benefits outweigh potential risks. If foscarnet is used with another drug known to be nephrotoxic, renal function must be monitored closely.

• *Antiretroviral Agents*

Didanosine and Zidovudine

There are no clinically important pharmacokinetic interactions between foscarnet and didanosine or zidovudine.

Ritonavir

Abnormal renal function has been observed when foscarnet was used concomitantly with ritonavir (with or without saquinavir).

• *Antivirals*

Acyclovir

Because acyclovir and foscarnet have both been associated with renal impairment, concomitant use of the drugs should be avoided unless potential benefits outweigh potential risks.

There was no in vitro evidence of antagonistic antiviral effects between acyclovir and foscarnet.

Cidofovir

The manufacturer of cidofovir states that concomitant use of cidofovir and foscarnet is contraindicated and foscarnet must be discontinued at least 7 days prior to initiating cidofovir therapy.

Ganciclovir

Concomitant use of ganciclovir and foscarnet does not affect the pharmacokinetics of either drug. However, ganciclovir and foscarnet are physically incompatible and *must* not be admixed. (See IV Infusion under Dosage and Administration: Administration.)

There was no in vitro evidence of antagonistic antiviral effects between ganciclovir and foscarnet. Although the clinical importance is unclear, some in vitro studies indicate that the combination of ganciclovir and foscarnet results in synergistic or additive antiviral effects against cytomegalovirus (CMV).

Letermovir

In vitro, there was no evidence of antagonistic anti-CMV effects between letermovir and foscarnet.

• *Diuretics*

Concomitant use of foscarnet and loop diuretics may impair elimination of foscarnet due to inhibition of renal tubular excretion, which may lead to toxicity. If concomitant use of foscarnet and a diuretic is required, the manufacturer of foscarnet states that thiazide diuretics are preferred over loop diuretics.

• *Pentamidine*

Concomitant use of IV pentamidine and foscarnet may cause hypocalcemia; severe hypocalcemia resulting in death occurred in at least one patient receiving the drugs concomitantly. Renal impairment also has been observed when IV pentamidine and foscarnet were used concomitantly. Toxicity associated with concomitant use of foscarnet and pentamidine administered by oral inhalation via nebulization (aerosolized pentamidine) has not been reported.

Concomitant use of IV pentamidine and foscarnet should be avoided unless potential benefits outweigh potential risks. If the drugs are used concomitantly, extreme caution is advised and renal function should be monitored closely (e.g., daily assessment of renal function).

• *Probenecid*

There are no clinically important pharmacokinetic interactions between probenecid and foscarnet.

DESCRIPTION

Foscarnet (phosphonoformic acid), an organic analog of inorganic pyrophosphate, is an antiviral agent. The drug is commercially available as the trisodium salt. Foscarnet is structurally unrelated to other currently available antiviral agents. Unlike nucleoside and nucleotide antivirals (e.g., acyclovir, cidofovir, ganciclovir, valganciclovir), foscarnet does not require intracellular enzyme conversion to an active metabolite.

Foscarnet acts as a viral DNA polymerase inhibitor. The mechanism of action of foscarnet against herpesviruses involves selective inhibition of the pyrophosphate binding site on virus-specific DNA polymerases at concentrations that do not affect cellular DNA polymerases.

The pharmacokinetics of foscarnet sodium have been evaluated in patients with human immunodeficiency virus (HIV) infection and acquired immunodeficiency syndrome (AIDS) receiving intermittent IV infusions of the drug for the management of cytomegalovirus (CMV) retinitis. Considerable interindividual variation in plasma concentrations of the drug has been reported. Following a single 90-mg/kg dose of IV foscarnet sodium in one study, plasma concentrations of the drug ranged from 297–1775 mcg/mL. Foscarnet is distributed into CSF; the CSF-to-plasma ratio has been reported to be 0.2–0.7. Postmortem data indicate that foscarnet accumulates in human bones, but the extent to which this occurs has not been determined. In vitro studies indicate that foscarnet is 14–17% bound to plasma proteins. Foscarnet is not substantially metabolized and is principally excreted unchanged in urine by glomerular filtration. Following a single IV infusion of 60 mg/kg of foscarnet sodium, the plasma half-life of the drug was 1.9 hours in adults with normal renal function (creatinine clearance greater than 80 mL/minute) and approximately 3, 13, and 25 hours in those with creatinine clearances of 50–80, 25–49, and 10–24 mL/minute, respectively. However, the terminal half-life of foscarnet determined by urinary excretion has been reported to be 87.5 hours, most likely because of slow release of the drug from bone.

SPECTRUM

Foscarnet is active in vitro against human herpesviruses, including CMV, herpes simplex virus types 1 and 2 (HSV-1 and HSV-2), and varicella-zoster virus (VZV). Although the clinical importance is unclear, foscarnet has some in vitro activity against Epstein-Barr virus (EBV) and human herpes viruses types 6 and 8 (HHV-6 and HHV-8). Foscarnet also has some in vitro activity against human hepatitis B virus (HBV) and human immunodeficiency virus types 1 and 2 (HIV-1 and HIV-2), but is not used for the treatment of infections caused by these viruses.

RESISTANCE

CMV and HSV isolates with reduced susceptibility to foscarnet have been selected in vitro in cell culture. In CMV strains, foscarnet resistance-associated substitutions are located in the viral DNA polymerase pUL54; in HSV strains, foscarnet resistance-associated substitutions are located in the viral DNA polymerase pUL30. Limited data are available on clinical resistance to foscarnet and several pathways to resistance likely exist.

Certain foscarnet resistance-associated substitutions also result in reduced susceptibility to some other antivirals (e.g., acyclovir, cidofovir, ganciclovir). In CMV strains, foscarnet resistance-associated substitutions associated with cross-resistance to ganciclovir and/or cidofovir have been identified. In HSV-1 and HSV-2 strains, foscarnet resistance-associated substitutions with cross-resistance to acyclovir have been identified; strains marginally cross-resistant to cidofovir also have been identified.

ADVICE TO PATIENTS

Advise patients that foscarnet is not a cure for cytomegalovirus (CMV) retinitis; progression and/or recurrence can occur, particularly during periods of continued immunosuppression. Regular ophthalmologic examinations are necessary.

Advise patients that foscarnet is not a cure for herpes simplex virus (HSV) infections. Although complete healing of HSV lesions is possible, relapse occurs in most patients. Repeated treatment with foscarnet may lead to development of resistance and poor response; in vitro susceptibility testing may be necessary if there is a poor therapeutic response or if relapse occurs.

Inform patients about the major toxicities of foscarnet (e.g., renal impairment, electrolyte disturbances, seizures) and that dosage modifications and possibly discontinuance of the drug may be necessary. The importance of close monitoring during foscarnet therapy must be emphasized.

Advise patients of the importance of adequate hydration to establish and maintain diuresis and minimize the risk of renal impairment during foscarnet therapy.

Advise patients of the importance of promptly informing clinicians if symptoms of electrolyte imbalance (e.g., perioral tingling, numbness in the extremities, paresthesias) or any cardiac symptoms occur during or after IV infusion of foscarnet. If such symptoms occur, the IV infusion should be stopped, electrolyte concentrations determined, and a clinician consulted before treatment with the drug is resumed.

Advise patients that dizziness and convulsions may occur during foscarnet therapy. Patients who experience seizures, dizziness, somnolence, or other adverse reactions that could result in cognitive impairment should avoid driving or operating machinery.

Importance of informing clinicians of existing or contemplated concomitant therapy, including prescription and OTC drugs, as well as any concomitant illnesses.

Importance of women informing clinicians if they are or plan to become pregnant or plan to breast-feed.

Importance of advising patients of other important precautionary information. (See Cautions.)

PREPARATIONS

Excipients in commercially available drug preparations may have clinically important effects in some individuals; consult specific product labeling for details.

Foscarnet Sodium

Parenteral		
Injection, for IV infusion only	24 mg/mL	Foscavir®, Hospira

† Use is not currently included in the labeling approved by the US Food and Drug Administration.

Selected Revisions August 19, 2019, © Copyright, May 1, 1992, American Society of Health-System Pharmacists, Inc.

Pentamidine Isethionate

8:30.12 • ANTIPROTOZOALS, *PNEUMOCYSTIS JIROVECII* PNEUMONIA

- Pentamidine isethionate, an aromatic diamidine derivative, is an antiprotozoal and antifungal agent.

USES

● *Pneumocystis jirovecii Pneumonia*

Pentamidine isethionate is used as an alternative for treatment of *Pneumocystis jirovecii* (formerly *Pneumocystis carinii*) pneumonia (PCP) and prevention of *P. jirovecii* infections. Pentamidine is designated an orphan drug by the US Food and Drug Administration (FDA) for treatment and prevention of PCP in patients at high risk for the disease.

Treatment of Pneumocystis jirovecii Pneumonia

Parenteral pentamidine is used alone as an alternative for treatment of PCP in patients who cannot tolerate or do not respond to co-trimoxazole, including adults, adolescents, and children with human immunodeficiency virus (HIV) infection. Pentamidine administered by oral inhalation via nebulization (aerosolized pentamidine) should *not* be used for treatment of PCP.

Co-trimoxazole is the drug of choice for treatment of mild, moderate, or severe PCP, including PCP in HIV-infected adults, adolescents, and children.

The US Centers for Disease Control and Prevention (CDC), National Institutes of Health (NIH), and Infectious Diseases Society of America (IDSA) state that alternatives for treatment of moderate to severe PCP in HIV-infected adults and adolescents who cannot tolerate or have not responded to co-trimoxazole are IV pentamidine or a regimen of primaquine in conjunction with clindamycin. Some clinicians prefer the primaquine and clindamycin regimen in such patients since it may be more effective and may be associated with lower toxicity compared with IV pentamidine. For treatment of PCP in HIV-infected children who cannot tolerate co-trimoxazole or have not responded after 5–7 days of co-trimoxazole, CDC, NIH, IDSA, and the American Academy of Pediatrics (AAP) recommend IV pentamidine; these experts state that treatment in such children can be switched to an appropriate oral regimen (e.g., atovaquone) after an initial response is obtained with IV pentamidine.

Parenteral pentamidine is associated with a cure rate of approximately 50–70% in patients with PCP, and has been effective in some patients whose infection did not respond to initial co-trimoxazole treatment. In patients with PCP who respond to pentamidine, a therapeutic clinical response manifested by defervescence and improved respiratory function may be apparent within 24–48 hours, but is generally evident within 2–8 days after initiation of the drug. While improvement in pulmonary radiographic signs generally occurs within several days to a week after the clinical response, complete clearing of radiographic signs may not occur for up to 20–30 days or longer.

Prior to the commercial availability of co-trimoxazole, pentamidine was considered the drug of choice for treatment of PCP; however, because co-trimoxazole has excellent tissue penetration and is associated with rapid clinical response (e.g., 3–5 days in patients with mild to moderate PCP), co-trimoxazole became the drug of choice for treatment of PCP in most patients. Results of limited comparative studies suggest that pentamidine is about as effective as or slightly less effective than co-trimoxazole for treatment of PCP in patients with AIDS and the drugs produce a similar incidence of adverse reactions, including those severe enough to require discontinuance of treatment.

Prevention of Pneumocystis jirovecii Infections

Pentamidine administered by oral inhalation via nebulization (aerosolized pentamidine) is used for prevention of initial episodes of PCP (primary prophylaxis) in patients at high risk (e.g., HIV-infected patients with CD4$^+$ T-cell counts of 200/mm^3 or less) and for prevention of recurrence (secondary prophylaxis) in those with a history of PCP.

Prevention of Initial Episode (Primary Prophylaxis)

CDC, NIH, and IDSA recommend that primary prophylaxis to prevent initial episodes of PCP be initiated in HIV-infected adults and adolescents with CD4$^+$ T-cell counts less than 200/mm^3 or a history of oropharyngeal candidiasis. These experts state that primary PCP prophylaxis should be considered in HIV-infected adults and adolescents with CD4$^+$ T-cell percentages less than 14% or a history of an AIDS-defining illness who would not otherwise qualify for prophylaxis and also should be considered in those with CD4$^+$ T-cell counts greater than 200/mm^3 but less than 250/mm^3 if frequent monitoring of CD4$^+$ T-cell counts (e.g., every 3 months) is not possible.

CDC, NIH, and IDSA state that primary PCP prophylaxis should be discontinued in HIV-infected adults and adolescents who have responded to antiretroviral therapy and have CD4$^+$ T-cell counts that have remained greater than 200/mm^3 for longer than 3 months. Discontinuance of primary PCP prophylaxis is recommended in these individuals since it appears to add little benefit in terms of disease prevention (PCP, toxoplasmosis, bacterial infections) and discontinuance reduces the medication burden, cost, and potential for drug toxicity, drug interactions, and selection of drug-resistant pathogens. Primary PCP prophylaxis should be reinitiated if CD4$^+$ T-cell counts decrease to less than 200/mm^3.

Co-trimoxazole is the drug of choice for primary PCP prophylaxis in HIV-infected adults and adolescents. CDC, NIH, and IDSA recommend that co-trimoxazole prophylaxis be continued, if clinically feasible, in individuals who experience adverse reactions to the drug that are not life-threatening; however, co-trimoxazole prophylaxis should be permanently discontinued and an alternative used in those with life-threatening adverse reactions to the drug.

Alternative regimens recommended by CDC, NIH, and IDSA for primary PCP prophylaxis in HIV-infected adults and adolescents who cannot tolerate co-trimoxazole are dapsone alone, dapsone in conjunction with pyrimethamine (and leucovorin), aerosolized pentamidine, atovaquone alone, or atovaquone in conjunction with pyrimethamine (and leucovorin). In HIV-infected adults or adolescents who cannot tolerate co-trimoxazole and are seropositive for *Toxoplasma gondii*, dapsone with pyrimethamine (and leucovorin), atovaquone alone, or atovaquone with pyrimethamine (and leucovorin) would provide prophylaxis against both PCP and toxoplasmosis.

In an 18-month, randomized, dose-response study in which 408 HIV-infected patients with or without a history of previous PCP received orally inhaled pentamidine isethionate 30 mg every 2 weeks, 150 mg every 2 weeks, or 300 mg every 4 weeks via a Respirgard® II nebulizer, the risk of developing PCP (either as an initial episode or as recurrence) was reduced by 50–70% in patients receiving the 300-mg dosage regimen compared with patients receiving the 30-mg regimen. Although not statistically significant, a dose-response effect also was apparent in patients receiving the 300-mg regimen versus the 150-mg regimen, and the benefit of the 300-mg dosage was evident even after considering the effect of zidovudine in patients receiving the antiretroviral concurrently. Although the pentamidine dosage had no effect on reduction of overall mortality in this study, mortality was low in all 3 dosage groups. In a study in which oral inhalation therapy with pentamidine isethionate (300 mg every 4 weeks via a Respirgard® II nebulizer) was limited to HIV-infected adults at high risk of PCP (e.g., those with AIDS, advanced AIDS-related complex [ARC], CD4$^+$ T-cell count less than 200/mm^3) but with no history of previous PCP (primary prevention), the 1-year estimated risk of developing PCP was reduced by about 70% relative to placebo.

Prevention of Recurrence (Secondary Prophylaxis)

CDC, NIH, and IDSA recommend that HIV-infected adults and adolescents who have a history of PCP receive long-term suppressive or chronic maintenance therapy (secondary prophylaxis) to prevent recurrence.

Secondary PCP prophylaxis generally is administered for life, unless immune recovery occurs as a result of antiretroviral therapy. CDC, NIH, and IDSA state that secondary PCP prophylaxis generally can be discontinued in HIV-infected adults and adolescents who have responded to antiretroviral therapy and have CD4$^+$ T-cell counts that have remained greater than 200/mm^3 for longer than 3 months, but should be reinitiated if CD4$^+$ T-cell counts decrease to less than 200/mm^3. In addition, these experts state that it may be prudent to continue secondary PCP prophylaxis for life (regardless of CD4$^+$ T-cell count) if PCP occurred or recurred when CD4$^+$ T-cell counts were greater than 200/mm^3.

Co-trimoxazole is the drug of choice for secondary PCP prophylaxis in HIV-infected adults and adolescents. CDC, NIH, and IDSA recommend that co-trimoxazole prophylaxis be continued, if clinically feasible, in individuals who experience adverse reactions to the drug that are not life-threatening; however, co-trimoxazole prophylaxis should be permanently discontinued and an alternative used in those with life-threatening adverse reactions to the drug.

Alternative regimens recommended by CDC, NIH, and IDSA for secondary PCP prophylaxis in HIV-infected adults and adolescents who cannot tolerate co-trimoxazole are the same as those recommended for primary prophylaxis and include dapsone alone, dapsone in conjunction with pyrimethamine (and leucovorin), aerosolized pentamidine, atovaquone alone, or atovaquone in conjunction with pyrimethamine (and leucovorin). In HIV-infected adults or adolescents who cannot tolerate co-trimoxazole and are seropositive for *T. gondii*, dapsone with pyrimethamine (and leucovorin), atovaquone alone, or atovaquone with pyrimethamine (and leucovorin) would provide prophylaxis against both PCP and toxoplasmosis.

Primary and Secondary Prophylaxis in Children

CDC, NIH, IDSA, and AAP recommend that primary prophylaxis to prevent initial episodes of PCP be initiated in HIV-infected children 1 to less than 6 years of age with CD4+ T-cell counts less than 500/mm³ or CD4+ T-cell percentages less than 15% and in HIV-infected children 6–12 years of age with CD4+ T-cell counts less than 200/mm³ or CD4+ T-cell percentages less than 15%. These experts recommend that all HIV-infected infants younger than 1 year of age (regardless of CD4+ T-cell count or percentage) receive primary PCP prophylaxis. In addition, infants born to HIV-infected mothers should be considered for primary PCP prophylaxis beginning at 4–6 weeks of age and those with indeterminate HIV status should continue to receive prophylaxis until they are determined to be non-HIV-infected or presumptively non-HIV-infected. Those found to be HIV-infected should receive primary PCP prophylaxis throughout the first year of life; at 1 year of age, the need for continued PCP prophylaxis should be reassessed based on age-specific CD4+ T-cell thresholds.

HIV-infected children who have a history of PCP should receive long-term suppressive or chronic maintenance therapy (secondary prophylaxis) to prevent recurrence.

CDC, NIH, IDSA, and AAP state that, in HIV-infected children who have received at least 6 months of antiretroviral therapy, discontinuance of primary or secondary PCP prophylaxis should be considered in those 1 to less than 6 years of age if CD4+ T-cell counts have remained at 500/mm³ or greater or CD4+ T-cell percentages have remained at 15% or greater for more than 3 consecutive months and in those 6–12 years of age if CD4+ T-cell counts have remained at 200/mm³ or greater or CD4+ T-cell percentages have remained at 15% or greater for more than 3 consecutive months. If primary or secondary PCP prophylaxis is discontinued in HIV-infected children, CD4+ T-cell counts and CD4+ T-cell percentages should be assessed every 3 months and PCP prophylaxis reinitiated if indicated based on age-specific CD4+ T-cell thresholds.

Co-trimoxazole is the drug of choice for primary and secondary PCP prophylaxis in HIV-infected infants and children. CDC, NIH, IDSA, and AAP recommend that co-trimoxazole be continued, if clinically feasible, in individuals who experience adverse reactions to the drug that are not life-threatening; however, co-trimoxazole should be permanently discontinued and an alternative used in those with life-threatening adverse reactions to the drug.

Alternative regimens recommended by CDC, NIH, IDSA, and AAP for primary and secondary PCP prophylaxis in HIV-infected infants and children who cannot tolerate co-trimoxazole are dapsone (1 month of age or older), atovaquone (1 month of age or older), or aerosolized pentamidine (5 years of age or older†).

• African Trypanosomiasis

Pentamidine is used for treatment of early or first-stage (hemolymphatic) trypanosomiasis caused by *Trypanosoma brucei gambiense†* (West African trypanosomiasis, gambiense sleeping sickness) and has been used as an alternative for treatment of early or first-stage (hemolymphatic) trypanosomiasis caused by *Trypanosoma brucei rhodesiense†* (East African trypanosomiasis, rhodesiense sleeping sickness).

Pentamidine penetrates the CNS poorly and is *not* effective for and should *not* be used for treatment of second-stage (meningoencephalitic) *T. b. gambiense* or *T. b. gambiense* infections when trypanosomes have invaded the CNS.

T. b. gambiense and *T. b. rhodesiense* are transmitted to humans by the bite of infected tsetse flies; transmission via blood or perinatal transmission from mother to infant is rare.

Trypanosoma brucei gambiense Infections

T. b. gambiense is endemic in West and Central Africa, and more than 95% of reported trypanosomiasis cases involve *T. b. gambiense*. *T. b. gambiense* infection occurs only rarely in short-term travelers to endemic areas, but has been reported in immigrants and expatriates from such areas.

Pentamidine usually is the drug of choice for treatment of first-stage (hemolymphatic) trypanosomiasis caused by *T. b. gambiense*. Suramin (not commercially available in the US, but may be available from CDC) also is effective for these first-stage infections, but is considered an alternative since pentamidine is better tolerated.

For treatment of *T. b. gambiense* infection with CNS involvement, eflornithine (with or without nitfurtimox) or melarsoprol (drugs not commercially available in the US, but may be available from CDC) usually is recommended. In untreated patients, CNS invasion and symptoms may not occur for months or years after infection with *T. b. gambiense*.

For assistance with diagnosis or treatment of *T. b. gambiense* trypanosomiasis in the US, clinicians can contact CDC Parasitic Diseases Hotline at 404-718-4745 from 8:00 a.m. to 4:00 p.m. Eastern Standard Time or CDC Emergency Operation Center at 770-488-7100 after business hours and on weekends and holidays. CDC Drug Service should be contacted at 404-639-3670 for information on how to obtain antiparasitic drugs not commercially available in the US.

Trypanosoma brucei rhodesiense Infections

T. b. rhodesiense is endemic in Eastern and Southern Africa. The disease has been reported occasionally in short-term travelers to endemic areas, especially tourists visiting wildlife reserves in such areas. *T. b. rhodesiense* infections are reported much less frequently than *T. b. gambiense* infections, but usually are associated with more rapidly progressive disease.

For treatment of first-stage (hemolymphatic) trypanosomiasis caused by *T. b. rhodesiense*, suramin (not commercially available in the US, but may be available from CDC) usually is the drug of choice. Pentamidine has been recommended as an alternative to suramin for treatment of first-stage *T. b. rhodesiense* infection because it is better tolerated, but pentamidine may be less active against this infection than against *T. b. gambiense* infection.

Melarsoprol (not commercially available in the US, but may be available from CDC) usually is the drug of choice for treatment of *T. b. rhodesiense* infection with CNS involvement. Clinicians should consider that CNS invasion may occur as soon as 3 weeks to 2 months after infection with *T. b. rhodesiense*.

For assistance with diagnosis or treatment of *T. b. rhodesiense* trypanosomiasis in the US, clinicians can contact CDC Parasitic Diseases Hotline at 404-718-4745 from 8:00 a.m. to 4:00 p.m. Eastern Standard Time or CDC Emergency Operation Center at 770-488-7100 after business hours and on weekends and holidays. CDC Drug Service should be contacted at 404-639-3670 for information on how to obtain antiparasitic drugs not commercially available in the US.

• Leishmaniasis

Pentamidine has been used for treatment of cutaneous and mucocutaneous leishmaniasis† caused by various *Leishmania* species and also has been used for treatment of visceral leishmaniasis† (also known as kala-azar).

Leishmaniasis is caused by more than 15 different species of *Leishmania* that are transmitted to humans by the bite of infected sand flies. *Leishmania* also can be transmitted via blood (e.g., blood transfusions, needles shared by IV drug abusers) and transmitted perinatally from mother to infant. In the Eastern Hemisphere, leishmaniasis is found most frequently in parts of Asia, the Middle East, Africa, and southern Europe; in the Western Hemisphere, the disease is found most frequently in Mexico and Central and South America and has been reported occasionally in Texas and Oklahoma. Leishmaniasis has been reported in short-term travelers to endemic areas and in immigrants and expatriates from such areas, and also has been reported in US military personnel and contract workers serving or working in endemic areas (e.g., Iraq, Afghanistan).

Leishmania infection in humans may cause uncomplicated cutaneous leishmaniasis, diffuse cutaneous leishmaniasis, mucosal leishmaniasis, visceral leishmaniasis, or post-kala-azar leishmaniasis and may be termed Old World (Eastern Hemisphere) or New World (Western Hemisphere). The specific form of leishmaniasis and disease severity depend on the *Leishmania* species involved, geographic area of origin, location of sand fly bite, and patient factors (e.g., nutritional and immune status). Treatment of leishmaniasis (e.g., drug, dosage, duration of treatment) must be individualized based on the region where the disease was acquired, likely infecting species, drug susceptibilities reported in the area of origin, form of the disease, and patient factors (e.g., age, pregnancy, immune status). No single treatment approach is appropriate for all possible clinical presentations. Consultation with clinicians experienced in management of leishmaniasis is recommended.

For assistance with diagnosis or treatment of leishmaniasis in the US, clinicians can contact CDC Parasitic Diseases Hotline at 404-718-4745 from 8:00 a.m. to 4:00 p.m. Eastern Standard Time or CDC Emergency Operation Center at 770-488-7100 after business hours and on weekends and holidays. CDC Drug Service should be contacted at 404-639-3670 for information on how to obtain antiparasitic drugs not commercially available in the US.

Cutaneous and Mucocutaneous Leishmaniasis

Although some cases of cutaneous leishmaniasis (usually Old World) may subside or resolve spontaneously over months or years, treatment of cutaneous leishmaniasis is recommended if there are multiple or large lesions, lesions are disabling or disfiguring or fail to heal within 6 months, the patient is immunocompromised, or dissemination to mucosal leishmaniasis is likely (e.g., New World disease caused by *L. braziliensis* or *L. panamensis*). Local treatment (e.g., topical paromomycin [not commercially available in the US], thermotherapy, intralesional pentavalent antimonials [not commercially available in the US], cryotherapy) may be appropriate in selected cases. For systemic treatment of cutaneous leishmaniasis, pentavalent antimonials (i.e., sodium stibogluconate or meglumine antimonate [drugs not commercially available in the US, but may be available from CDC]) usually are used. Other treatment options for cutaneous leishmaniasis include amphotericin B, miltefosine, pentamidine, and ketoconazole, especially when antimonials cannot be used because of tolerance or resistance. Pentamidine may be particularly useful for and has been recommended for treatment of New World cutaneous leishmaniasis† caused by *L. guyanensis* or *L. panamensis*. Variable efficacy and potential adverse effects limit usefulness of pentamidine for other types of cutaneous leishmaniasis.

For treatment of mucosal leishmaniasis, pentavalent antimonials (i.e., sodium stibogluconate or meglumine antimonate [drugs not commercially available in the US, but may be available from CDC]), amphotericin B, or miltefosine usually are used. Although data are limited, pentamidine also has been used as an alternative for these infections.

Visceral Leishmaniasis

Pentavalent antimonials (i.e., sodium stibogluconate or meglumine antimonate [drugs not commercially available in the US, but may available from CDC]) have historically been considered the drugs of first choice for initial treatment of visceral leishmaniasis; however, drug resistance and treatment failures have become a major concern in some areas (e.g., India, Nepal). Relapse of visceral leishmaniasis is common in immunocompromised patients (e.g., HIV-infected patients), regardless of treatment regimen.

Other treatment options for visceral leishmaniasis include amphotericin B, miltefosine, or paromomycin. Pentamidine has been used for treatment of visceral leishmaniasis, especially when antimonials may be not be effective because of resistance, but pentamidine is not usually recommended for treatment of visceral leishmaniasis, including in HIV-infected individuals, because of variable or suboptimal efficacy and potential adverse effects.

● Babesiosis

Because of its activity against *Babesia* infections in animals, pentamidine has been used in a small number of patients for treatment of babesiosis† caused by *B. microti*; however, efficacy has not been established and use of the drug alone has not been shown to be effective. Although parenteral pentamidine used in conjunction with co-trimoxazole has been beneficial for treatment of infection caused by *B. divergens* in at least one patient, potential adverse effects associated with pentamidine limit use of this regimen.

When anti-infective treatment of babesiosis is indicated, IDSA and other clinicians recommend either a regimen of clindamycin and quinine or a regimen of atovaquone and azithromycin.

DOSAGE AND ADMINISTRATION

● Reconstitution and Administration

Pentamidine isethionate is administered by deep IM injection or slow IV infusion. The drug should *not* be administered by rapid IV injection or infusion. (See Cautions: Cardiovascular Effects.)

Pentamidine isethionate also is administered by oral inhalation via nebulization (aerosolized pentamidine) using a Respirgard® II jet nebulizer.

IV infusion (not IM injection) is usually recommended for treatment of *Pneumocystis jirovecii* (formerly *Pneumocystis carinii*) pneumonia (PCP); oral inhalation via nebulization is used *only* for prevention of PCP.

Parenteral Administration

Because sudden, severe hypotensive reactions can occur following IM or IV administration of pentamidine, the patient should be in a supine position and blood pressure should be monitored closely during administration of the drug and several times thereafter until blood pressure is stable. Equipment and supportive therapy to treat a hypotensive reaction should be readily available. (See Precautions Related to Parenteral Pentamidine under Cautions: Precautions and Contraindications.)

Reconstituted and diluted solutions of pentamidine should be inspected visually for particulate matter and discoloration prior to administration whenever solution and container permit.

IM Injection

For IM injection, a vial of pentamidine isethionate lyophilized powder labeled as containing 300 mg of the drug for IM or IV use should be reconstituted by adding 3 mL of sterile water for injection at 22–30°C to provide a solution containing approximately 100 mg/mL. The powder for IM or IV use should be reconstituted using *only* sterile water for injection; sodium chloride injection should *not* be used since precipitation of the drug will occur.

The desired dose of reconstituted solution should then be withdrawn and administered by deep IM injection. Unused portions of reconstituted solution should be discarded.

Some clinicians suggest that local adverse effects (e.g., sterile abscess, pain) associated with IM administration of pentamidine may be minimized by using the Z-track technique of injection, in which the subcutaneous tissue over the site of injection is firmly pushed aside before inserting the needle at a 90-degree angle, preferably into the upper outer quadrant of the buttock. (See Cautions: Local Effects.)

IV Infusion

For IV infusion, a vial of pentamidine isethionate lyophilized powder labeled as containing 300 mg of the drug for IM or IV use should be reconstituted by adding 3–5 mL of sterile water for injection or 5% dextrose injection at 22–30°C (e.g., using 3, 4, or 5 mL of diluent will provide solutions containing approximately 100, 75, or 60 mg/mL, respectively). The powder for IM or IV use should be reconstituted using *only* sterile water for injection; sodium chloride injection should *not* be used since precipitation of the drug will occur.

The desired dose of reconstituted solution should then be withdrawn and diluted in 50–250 mL of 5% dextrose injection.

The reconstituted and diluted solution of pentamidine should be administered by slow IV infusion over 60–120 minutes. Rapid IV infusion should be avoided. (See Cautions: Cardiovascular Effects.)

The IV needle or catheter should be positioned carefully and closely observed throughout the period of administration. Extravasation should be avoided; if extravasation occurs, the infusion should be immediately discontinued and restarted at another site. (See Cautions: Local Effects.)

Oral Inhalation via Nebulization

For oral inhalation via nebulization (aerosolized pentamidine), a vial of pentamidine isethionate lyophilized powder labeled as containing 300 mg of the drug for oral inhalation solution should be reconstituted by adding 6 mL of sterile water for injection. The powder for oral inhalation solution should be reconstituted using *only* sterile water for injection; sodium chloride injection should *not* be used since precipitation of the drug will occur.

Prior to administration of pentamidine oral inhalation solution, the manufacturer's information on administering pentamidine via the Respirgard® II jet nebulizer should be reviewed to assure thorough familiarity with the use and operation of the nebulizer.

The entire contents of the reconstituted vial of pentamidine should be placed into the reservoir of the Respirgard® II jet nebulizer and delivered until the nebulizer chamber is empty (approximately 30–45 minutes) using a flow rate of 5–7 L/minute and an air or oxygen source at 40–50 PSI. Alternatively, an air compressor delivering 40–50 PSI may be used by setting the flowmeter at 5–7 L/minute or the pressure at 22–25 PSI; low-pressure (i.e., less than 20 PSI) air compressors should not be used.

Pentamidine for oral inhalation solution should not be admixed with any other drugs, and the Respirgard® II jet nebulizer should not be used to administer a bronchodilator.

• Dosage

Pneumocystis jirovecii Pneumonia

Treatment of Pneumocystis jirovecii Pneumonia

When parenteral pentamidine isethionate is used for treatment of PCP in adults and adolescents, including those with human immunodeficiency virus (HIV) infection, the usual dosage is 4 mg/kg once daily given IV or IM. The US Centers for Disease Control and Prevention (CDC), National Institutes of Health (NIH), and Infectious Diseases Society of America (IDSA) recommend that the drug be given IV for treatment of moderate to severe PCP in HIV-infected adults and adolescents and also state that dosage in these patients can be reduced to 3 mg/kg IV once daily if necessary because of toxicity.

When parenteral pentamidine isethionate is used for treatment of PCP in children and infants 4 months of age or older, including those with HIV infection, the usual dosage is 4 mg/kg once daily given IV or IM. CDC, NIH, IDSA, and American Academy of Pediatrics (AAP) recommend that the drug be given IV for treatment of PCP in HIV-infected children and also state that patients who have clinical improvement after 7–10 days of IV pentamidine can be switched to an appropriate oral regimen (e.g., atovaquone) to complete 21 days of treatment.

CDC, NIH, IDSA, and AAP recommend a total treatment duration of 21 days. The manufacturer recommends a treatment duration of 14–21 days and states that parenteral pentamidine has been continued for longer than 21 days, but such treatment may be associated with increased toxicity.

Prevention of Pneumocystis jirovecii Infections

When pentamidine isethionate is administered by oral inhalation via nebulization (aerosolized pentamidine) for prevention of initial episodes (primary prophylaxis) of PCP in adults, adolescents, and children 5 years of age or older†, including HIV-infected individuals, the usual dosage is 300 mg once every 4 weeks (once monthly). CDC, NIH, and IDSA state that primary PCP prophylaxis should be discontinued in HIV-infected adults and adolescents if CD4+ T-cell counts have remained greater than 200/mm³ for longer than 3 months in response to antiretroviral therapy, but should be reinitiated if CD4+ T-cell counts decrease to less than 200/mm³. In HIV-infected children who have received at least 6 months of antiretroviral therapy, CDC, NIH, IDSA, and AAP state that discontinuance of primary PCP prophylaxis should be considered based on age-related CD4+ T-cell counts or CD4+ T-cell percentages, but should be reinitiated if these parameters decrease below the age-related thresholds. (See Prevention of Pneumocystis jirovecii Infections under Uses: Pneumocystis jirovecii Pneumonia.)

When pentamidine isethionate is administered by oral inhalation via nebulization (aerosolized pentamidine) for prevention of recurrence (secondary prophylaxis) of PCP in adults, adolescents, and children 5 years of age or older†, including HIV-infected individuals, the usual dosage is 300 mg once every 4 weeks (once monthly). CDC, NIH, and IDSA state that secondary PCP prophylaxis generally can be discontinued in HIV-infected adults and adolescents if CD4+ T-cell counts have remained greater than 200/mm³ for longer than 3 months in response to antiretroviral therapy, but should be reinitiated if CD4+ T-cell counts decrease to less than 200/mm³. However, secondary PCP prophylaxis probably should be continued for life (regardless of CD4+ T-cell count) if PCP occurred or recurred when CD4+ T-cell counts were greater than 200/mm³. In HIV-infected children who have received at least 6 months of antiretroviral therapy, CDC, NIH, IDSA, and AAP state that discontinuance of secondary PCP prophylaxis should be considered based on age-related CD4+ T-cell counts or CD4+ T-cell percentages, but should be reinitiated if these parameters decrease below the age-related thresholds. (See Prevention of Pneumocystis jirovecii Infections under Uses: Pneumocystis jirovecii Pneumonia.)

African Trypanosomiasis

For treatment of first-stage (hemolymphatic) trypanosomiasis caused by *Trypanosoma brucei gambiense*† (West African trypanosomiasis, gambiense sleeping sickness), the World Health Organization (WHO) and others recommend that adults and children receive pentamidine isethionate in a dosage of 4 mg/kg once daily for 7–10 days given IM or, alternatively, by IV infusion over 2 hours.

If pentamidine isethionate is used as an alternative for treatment of first-stage (hemolymphatic) trypanosomiasis caused by *T. b. rhodesiense*† (East African trypanosomiasis, rhodesiense sleeping sickness), WHO recommends that adults and children receive 4 mg/kg once daily for 7 days given IM or, alternatively, by IV infusion over 2 hours.

Leishmaniasis

For treatment of cutaneous leishmaniasis† caused by various *Leishmania* species, some clinicians recommend that adults and children receive pentamidine isethionate in a dosage of 2–3 mg/kg IM or IV once daily or every other day for 4–7 doses. Others recommend 3–4 mg/kg IM or IV once every other day for 4–10 doses. For treatment of New World cutaneous leishmaniasis caused by *L. guyanensis* or *L. panamensis*, WHO recommends that pentamidine isethionate be given in a dosage of 4 mg/kg IM or IV once every other day for 3 doses.

If pentamidine isethionate is used as an alternative for treatment of visceral leishmaniasis†, some clinicians recommend a dosage of 4 mg/kg IM or IV once every other day or 3 times weekly for 15–20 doses.

• Dosage in Renal and Hepatic Impairment

The manufacturer of parenteral pentamidine isethionate states that efficacy and safety of alternative dosage regimens have not been established in patients with impaired renal or hepatic function, and the drug should be used with caution in such patients. (See Precautions Related to Parenteral Pentamidine under Cautions: Precautions and Contraindications.)

When IV pentamidine isethionate is used for treatment of PCP in HIV-infected adults and adolescents with renal impairment, some experts recommend that those with creatinine clearances of 10–50 mL/minute receive a dosage of 3 mg/kg once every 24 hours and that those with creatinine clearances less than 10 mL/minute receive 4 mg/kg once every 48 hours.

CAUTIONS

The most common adverse effects reported with parenteral pentamidine isethionate are nephrotoxic effects; the most common adverse effects reported with pentamidine isethionate administered by oral inhalation via nebulization (aerosolized pentamidine) are cough and bronchospasm.

• Renal Effects

Nephrotoxicity is common in patients receiving parenteral pentamidine for treatment of *Pneumocystis jirovecii* (formerly *Pneumocystis carinii*) pneumonia (PCP). Pentamidine-induced nephrotoxicity is manifested by impaired renal function, increased serum creatinine concentration and/or BUN concentrations, and azotemia. Renal impairment usually is mild to moderate in severity and reversible following discontinuance of pentamidine; however, acute renal failure or severe renal insufficiency requiring discontinuance of the drug may occur. Nephrotoxicity and hyperkalemia both may occur more frequently in patients with acquired immunodeficiency syndrome (AIDS) than in other patients treated with parenteral pentamidine; hyperkalemia has been severe in some patients. (See Precautions Related to Parenteral Pentamidine under Cautions: Precautions and Contraindications.) Rarely, pentamidine-induced acute renal failure has been associated with myoglobinuria or gross hematuria. The risk and degree of pentamidine-induced renal impairment may be increased in the presence of dehydration or by concomitant use of other nephrotoxic drugs. (See Drug Interactions: Nephrotoxic Drugs.)

Flank pain, incontinence, increased BUN and serum creatinine concentrations, nephritis, renal failure, renal pain, and syndrome of inappropriate antidiuretic hormone secretion (SIADH) have been reported rarely in patients receiving pentamidine administered by oral inhalation via nebulization.

● Cardiovascular Effects

Hypotension, which may develop suddenly and may be moderate to severe (e.g., less than 60 mm Hg systolic), can occur following a single IM or IV dose of pentamidine. Deaths resulting from severe hypotension and cardiac arrhythmias have been reported in patients receiving the drug IM or IV. The risk of hypotensive reactions following IM or IV administration of pentamidine has not been directly compared, but some data suggest that there is no difference in the frequency of these reactions following either route of administration when IV infusions of the drug are administered over a period of at least 60 minutes. Hypotensive reactions may be particularly likely to occur following rapid IV injection or infusion. To minimize the risk of this adverse effect when pentamidine is administered IV, infusions of the drug should be given over a period of 60–120 minutes. In some patients, hypotension was not ameliorated by adjustment of the infusion rate, persisted beyond completion of the infusion, and required volume expansion for correction.

Cardiorespiratory arrest (following rapid IV injection), ventricular tachycardia, atypical ventricular tachycardia (torsades de pointes), ECG abnormalities (abnormal ST segment), facial flushing, cerebrovascular accident, hypertension, palpitations, syncope, vasodilation, and vasculitis have also been reported in patients receiving parenteral pentamidine.

Cerebrovascular accident, hypotension, hypertension, palpitations, poor circulation, syncope, tachycardia, torsades de pointes, vasodilatation, and vasculitis have been reported rarely in patients receiving pentamidine administered by oral inhalation via nebulization.

● Hypersensitivity and Dermatologic Effects

There have been rare reports of anaphylaxis and anaphylactoid reactions with shock with parenteral pentamidine. Stevens-Johnson syndrome and toxic epidermal necrolysis have been reported.

Anaphylaxis, allergic reaction, and nonspecific allergy have been reported in patients receiving pentamidine administered by oral inhalation via nebulization.

Pruritus and local or generalized urticaria or rash (e.g., maculopapular, pruritic) occur infrequently in patients receiving parenteral pentamidine.

Rash, including severely pruritic, maculopapular eruption on the upper chest and back, also has occurred when the drug was administered by oral inhalation via nebulization.

Erythema, dry skin, dry and breaking hair, dermatitis, and desquamation have been reported occasionally in patients receiving pentamidine.

● Local Effects

Following IM injection of pentamidine, adverse effects at the site of injection, including sterile abscess and/or necrosis, pain, erythema, tenderness, and induration, have been reported in 10–20% of patients. To minimize some of these local adverse effects associated with IM administration of the drug, some clinicians recommend that the Z-track technique of injection be used. (See Parenteral Administration under Dosage and Administration: Reconstitution and Administration.)

Phlebitis may occur following IV administration of pentamidine. Extravasation, sometimes resulting in ulceration, tissue necrosis, and/or sloughing at the injection site, has been reported in patients receiving pentamidine. Surgical debridement and skin grafting have been necessary in a few patients; long-term sequelae have occurred. Because prevention is the most effective means of limiting the severity of pentamidine extravasation, the IV needle or catheter should be properly positioned and closely observed throughout the infusion. If extravasation occurs, the infusion should be discontinued immediately and restarted in another vein; management of the extravasation site is symptomatic.

● Hypoglycemia and Diabetogenic Effects

Hypoglycemia, which may be severe (e.g., blood glucose concentration less than 25 mg/dL) and/or prolonged, appears to occur in at least 5–10% of patients

receiving parenteral pentamidine. Hyperglycemia insulin-dependent diabetes mellitus (which appears to be permanent in some cases), with or without preceding hypoglycemia, and ketoacidosis, have also occurred in patients receiving parenteral pentamidine; these adverse effects sometimes occurred several months after discontinuance of parenteral pentamidine. The exact mechanism(s) is not clearly established, but pentamidine-induced hypoglycemia has been associated with pancreatic islet cell necrosis and inappropriately high plasma insulin concentrations and the drug may produce insulin-dependent diabetes mellitus via direct toxic effects on beta cells of the pancreas.

Hypoglycemia, hyperglycemia, and diabetes also have occurred when pentamidine was administered by oral inhalation via nebulization.

Although pentamidine-induced hypoglycemia may occur after initial doses of the drug, it generally occurs after at least 5–7 days of treatment and can even occur up to several days after the drug is discontinued. The duration of hypoglycemia appears to be quite variable, persisting for one or more days up to several weeks. While often asymptomatic, pentamidine-induced hypoglycemia is occasionally severe and has resulted in death. Some data suggest that the occurrence of hypoglycemia caused by the drug in patients with AIDS may be associated with the development of nephrotoxicity. Other apparent risk factors associated with the occurrence of hypoglycemia reportedly include duration of treatment (or total cumulative dosage) and previous treatment with the drug (particularly within the prior 3 months).

Management of pentamidine-induced hypoglycemia depends on the severity and duration of the reaction. Hypoglycemia is usually, but not always, readily controlled by administration of IV dextrose; in some cases, large dosages of IV dextrose and/or supplemental IV dextrose therapy for several days or longer may be required. In a few cases of recurring, severe hypoglycemia, short-term therapy with oral diazoxide was useful.

● Hematologic Effects

Leukopenia (e.g., neutropenia) and thrombocytopenia, which can be severe (e.g., leukocyte count less than 1000/mm³, platelet count less than 20,000/mm³), occur occasionally in patients receiving parenteral pentamidine. Leukopenia occurs more frequently than thrombocytopenia. Anemia, defibrination, eosinophilia, pancytopenia, and prolonged clotting time have been reported rarely in patients receiving parenteral pentamidine. Severe thrombocytopenic purpura also has been reported rarely. Although decreased serum folate concentrations (associated with megaloblastic changes in bone marrow in at least one case) have been observed rarely in patients receiving parenteral pentamidine, it is not clear whether the drug can cause folic acid deficiency.

Anemia has been reported occasionally in patients receiving pentamidine by oral inhalation via nebulization; eosinophilia, neutropenia, nonspecific cytopenia, pancytopenia, and thrombocytopenia also have been reported.

● GI Effects

Adverse GI effects reported with parenteral pentamidine or oral inhalation of the drug via nebulization include abdominal cramping or pain, anorexia or decreased appetite, diarrhea, dry mouth, dyspepsia, hematochezia, increased sputum production (hypersalivation), loss of taste, melena, nausea, splenomegaly, and vomiting. An unpleasant (e.g., metallic) taste (dysgeusia) sensation in the mouth or unpleasant feeling on the tongue also have been reported. Dysgeusia may be more severe and persistent with IV than oral inhalation therapy.

Gingivitis, oral ulcer or abscess, gastritis, gastric ulcer, hiatal hernia, esophagitis, constipation, colitis, and numb lips also have been reported in patients receiving pentamidine by oral inhalation via nebulization.

Acute pancreatitis (sometimes fatal) has occurred with parenteral pentamidine; acute pancreatitis also has been reported rarely with pentamidine oral inhalation therapy. (See Cautions: Precautions and Contraindications.)

● Hepatic Effects

Elevated liver function test results, including increased serum AST and ALT concentrations, occur occasionally in patients receiving parenteral pentamidine. Hepatitis, hepatomegaly, and hepatic dysfunction have been reported in patients receiving pentamidine parenterally or by oral inhalation via nebulization.

Respiratory Effects

Cough and bronchospasm are frequent effects attributed to pentamidine oral inhalation therapy. Cough and bronchospasm also have been reported with parenteral pentamidine.

Cough has occurred in up to 63% of patients receiving pentamidine by oral inhalation via nebulization (38% of patients in initial clinical trials). Cough is most likely in and may be most severe in patients who smoke, and occasionally may be severe enough to require discontinuance of oral inhalation therapy. Bronchospasm has occurred in patients receiving pentamidine oral inhalation via nebulization (15% of patients in initial clinical trials), and is most likely in those with a history of smoking or asthma. Although the exact cause of this bronchospasm has not been elucidated, it has been suggested that it may result, at least in part, from local histamine release and/or anticholinesterase activity induced by the drug.

Cough or bronchospasm occurring during pentamidine oral inhalation therapy can be controlled in most patients by interruption of oral inhalation therapy and administration of a bronchodilator. Coughing also may be controlled by slowing the delivery or intensity of the aerosol stream. In patients who experience cough or bronchospasm with pentamidine oral inhalation, use of an orally inhaled bronchodilator prior to each dose may minimize recurrence of these symptoms. Limited evidence suggests that pretreatment with orally inhaled cromolyn sodium is less effective than bronchodilators in preventing such bronchoconstriction.

Other adverse respiratory effects reported in patients receiving parenteral pentamidine or pentamidine administered by oral inhalation via nebulization include asthma, bronchitis, chest congestion or tightness, coryza, cyanosis, dyspnea, eosinophilic or interstitial pneumonitis, gagging, hemoptysis, hyperventilation, laryngitis (sometimes severe), laryngospasm, nonspecific lung disorder, nasal congestion, pleuritis, pneumothorax, rales, rhinitis, shortness of breath, tachypnea, and wheezing. Bronchial bleeding during bronchoscopy or severe pulmonary hemorrhage following bronchoscopic biopsy also have occurred in association with pentamidine oral inhalation therapy.

Nervous System Effects

Anxiety, confusion, depression, dizziness, drowsiness, emotional lability, hallucinations, hypesthesia, insomnia, memory loss, nervousness, neuralgia, neuropathy (peripheral or nonspecific), paranoia, paresthesia, seizure, tremors, unsteady gait, and vertigo have been reported in patients receiving parenteral pentamidine and pentamidine oral inhalation therapy.

Fatigue was reported in about 66% of patients receiving pentamidine by oral inhalation via nebulization in initial clinical trials.

Other Adverse Effects

Other adverse effects reported in patients receiving parenteral pentamidine or pentamidine by oral inhalation via nebulization include arthralgia, body odor, chills, edema (facial or leg), fever, gout, headache, hypocalcemia (sometimes severe), hypomagnesemia, lethargy, low or abnormal body temperature, myalgia, miscarriage, night sweats, nonspecific odor, and extrapulmonary pneumocystosis (sometimes fatal). (See Precautions Related to Pentamidine Oral Inhalation via Nebulization under Cautions: Precautions and Contraindications.)

Blepharitis, blurred vision, conjunctivitis, contact lens discomfort, eye pain or discomfort, hemianopsia, loss of hearing, bad taste, and loss of taste or smell also have been reported in patients receiving pentamidine.

Environmental Exposure of Health-care Personnel and Visitors

When pentamidine is administered by oral inhalation via nebulization, health-care personnel and visitors or other individuals present during administration of the drug may be at risk of environmental exposure to aerosolized pentamidine and may also be at risk of exposure to pathogens (e.g., *Mycobacterium tuberculosis*) that can be transmitted by patients who cough during the oral inhalation procedure.

There is evidence from several studies that measurable levels of pentamidine can be present in room air when pentamidine is administered by oral inhalation via nebulization. This level may depend on several factors, including room ventilation, proper use of the nebulizer, and variations in treatment practices (e.g., turning off the nebulizer 2–5 minutes before the mouthpiece is removed from the patient). In one study, area air samples were collected using an ambient air sampler over a 4-hour period in an unventilated treatment room where patients received a median dose of 150 mg of aerosolized pentamidine isethionate over 35–40 minutes via a nebulizer (Respirgard® II, which included an expiratory filter); pentamidine concentrations in area air samples averaged about 45 ng/m³ during this period. Theoretical estimates based on exposure data from this study indicate that the amount of aerosolized pentamidine isethionate that potentially could be deposited in the lungs of health-care personnel would be 22 ng per 8-hour workday or 4.9 mcg per 225-day workyear, assuming continuous exposure during each 8-hour period. Although it was postulated that the relatively low estimated amounts of drug deposited in the lungs following environmental exposure and the low systemic absorption of pentamidine from the lungs might minimize risk, the potential risk for extrapulmonary toxicity that this or other exposure would represent remains to be established. In another study in a limited number of health-care personnel and other individuals with varying levels of potential exposure to patients receiving the drug via a jet nebulizer (Respirgard® II or AeroTech® II, with expiratory filters), the likelihood of a positive urinary sample for pentamidine appeared to be increased by increasing degrees of potential exposure, with treatment providers being at greatest risk for measurable exposure and personnel simply working in the vicinity of the treatment area or in other areas of the institution being at minimal risk. In this study, approximately 90% of positive samples occurred in treatment providers; urinary concentrations in positive samples ranged from 0.15–8.19 ng/mL, and the number of treatment exposures in providers ranged from 1 monthly in various areas of the institution to 80 monthly in designated rooms with 6 or 35 exchanges of nonrecirculated air per hour.

Adverse effects that have been reported in health-care personnel and others exposed to aerosolized pentamidine in the environment include eye irritation (e.g., conjunctivitis); perioral and perinasal paresthesia; numbness of the mouth and nose; bitter metallic taste; burning sensation of the eyes, nose, and throat; sinus irritation; increased mucous discharge; nasal stuffiness; sneezing; shortness of breath; cough; tightness of the chest; acute bronchospasm; wheezing; hoarseness; fatigue; headache; and light-headedness. Asymptomatic reduction in carbon monoxide diffusion capacity was reported in a nonsmoking, apparently otherwise healthy, respiratory therapist following occupational exposure over a 14-month period to aerosolized pentamidine that was being administered to patients via a Respirgard® II jet nebulizer; this individual's diffusion capacity improved upon removal from exposure and remained stable despite reexposure when ventilation fans were installed in the area used for administration of orally inhaled pentamidine. Reduction in diffusion capacity also has been reported in other health-care personnel.

Because of concerns about the potential risks of environmental exposure to aerosolized pentamidine by health-care personnel and visitors while in contact with patients undergoing oral inhalation therapy with the drug and because of the lack of data on potential effects of pentamidine on the fetus or pregnancy, environmental exposure to aerosolized pentamidine by pregnant women and possibly those planning to become pregnant (e.g., within 8 weeks of potential exposure) should be avoided. (See Pregnancy under Cautions: Pregnancy, Fertility, and Lactation.)

Exposure to tuberculosis is possible in settings where cough-inducing procedures, including administration of aerosolized pentamidine, are performed on patients with undiagnosed *M. tuberculosis* infection. Therefore, it has been suggested that appropriate diagnostic procedures be performed to rule out potentially infectious tuberculosis (e.g., sputum smear, tuberculin skin test, chest radiographs) or other active pulmonary infections prior to initiation of pentamidine oral inhalation therapy. Antituberculosis therapy should be initiated before pentamidine oral inhalation therapy is started in patients with suspected or confirmed potentially infectious tuberculosis. While the risk of tuberculosis transmission to individuals in contact with HIV-infected patients undergoing pentamidine prophylaxis has not been elucidated and some evidence suggests that it may be low overall in some areas (but variable depending on demographics and other factors), epidemiologic studies in one health clinic in which a substantial number of employees developed significant (positive) reactions to a tuberculin skin test (Mantoux) within a 6-month period suggest that occupational exposure to patients with positive *M. tuberculosis* sputum cultures who were receiving pentamidine oral inhalation therapy may have contributed to transmission of the infection. Inadequate fresh air ventilation in this clinic probably contributed substantially to transmission of tuberculosis; several months after installation of adequate ventilation in the facility, no additional significant reactions to a tuberculin skin test were observed. Therefore, adequate air exchange and exhaust to the outside and away from intake vents should be ensured in rooms and booths used for administering aerosolized pentamidine. However, it should be recognized that such ensurance cannot completely eliminate the risk of transmission. Other appropriate preventive measures (e.g., minimizing contact of coughing patients with health-care personnel and others, appropriate use of ultraviolet air disinfection, use of properly constructed and vented and/or filtered [using high-efficiency particulate air filters] administration booths) aimed at reducing the risk of tuberculosis transmission in this setting also should be considered.

The potential risks, particularly long-term and cumulative effects, associated with environmental exposure to aerosolized pentamidine have not been elucidated, and health-care facilities should have procedures to minimize environmental exposure to aerosolized pentamidine. Whenever possible, patients receiving pentamidine oral inhalation via nebulization should be located in rooms where potential exposure to personnel and other patients is minimized (e.g., using separate treatment rooms with closed doors, using properly constructed and vented and/or filtered [with an exhaust HEPA filter] booths or hoods, using nebulizers that have an expiratory filter [e.g., Respirgard® II], instructing the patient to turn off the nebulizer when the mouthpiece is removed). Proper room ventilation can reduce ambient concentrations of the drug. Some clinicians suggest that use of gowns, gloves, goggles, and masks by health-care personnel be considered, although the level of protection provided is not known and some experts state that measures aimed at isolating and engineering out potential exposure generally should be emphasized over *personal* protective apparel and equipment. Use of surgical masks by health-care personnel caring for pentamidine-treated patients probably is unlikely to provide an effective means for reducing environmental exposure to the drug; therefore, if a face mask is used, alternative, appropriately designed (e.g., for adequate particle-size filtration) and well-fitted face masks (e.g., 3M Company model 9970 or 9920) should be employed since they are more likely to substantially reduce respiratory exposure levels. In addition, health-care personnel administering aerosolized pentamidine should be familiar with the manufacturer's instructions for use of the nebulizer delivery system, since improper use of the nebulizer potentially could result in release of substantial amounts of pentamidine into the environment and exposure of health-care personnel to the same risks of adverse effects as patients receiving orally inhaled pentamidine prophylaxis.

● *Precautions and Contraindications*

Parenteral pentamidine isethionate is contraindicated in patients with a history of hypersensitivity to the drug.

Pentamidine isethionate administered by oral inhalation via nebulization is contraindicated in patients with a history of anaphylactic reaction following parenteral or oral inhalation of the drug.

Precautions Related to Parenteral Pentamidine

Parenteral pentamidine isethionate should be used with caution in patients with hypertension, hypotension, ventricular tachycardia, pancreatitis, Stevens-Johnson syndrome, hyperglycemia, hypoglycemia, hypocalcemia, leukopenia, thrombocytopenia, anemia, or hepatic or renal dysfunction.

Parenteral pentamidine causes adverse effects in a high percentage of patients, and deaths resulting from severe hypotension, hypoglycemia, acute pancreatitis, or cardiac arrhythmias have occurred in patients receiving the drug IM or IV. Therefore, parenteral pentamidine should be used for treatment of PCP only after presence of the organism has been demonstrated. In addition, patients receiving the drug should be closely monitored for the development of severe adverse reactions (e.g., leukopenia, hypoglycemia, nephrotoxicity).

Because sudden, severe hypotension can occur following a single IM or IV dose of pentamidine, patients receiving the drug should be in a supine position and blood pressure should be monitored closely during administration of the drug and several times thereafter until blood pressure is stable. Appropriate equipment for maintenance of an adequate airway and other supportive measures and agents (e.g., IV fluids, vasopressor agents) for the management of hypotensive reactions should be readily available whenever pentamidine is administered parenterally. Since cardiac arrhythmias have been reported in patients receiving pentamidine, the manufacturers recommend that ECGs be performed before, during, and after parenteral therapy with the drug.

Because parenteral pentamidine often causes nephrotoxicity, renal function should be frequently and carefully monitored in patients receiving the drug. Limited evidence suggests that nephrotoxicity associated with parenteral pentamidine

may occur more frequently in patients with AIDS than in other patients treated with the drug and may be accompanied by severe, sometimes life-threatening, hyperkalemia despite modest elevations in BUN and/or serum creatinine concentration. Therefore, some clinicians suggest that, in addition to routine monitoring of renal function, serum potassium concentrations should be monitored and patients well hydrated during pentamidine therapy, particularly in AIDS patients. The manufacturers recommend that BUN and serum creatinine concentrations be determined prior to initiation of parenteral pentamidine therapy, daily during therapy with the drug, and after the drug is discontinued.; some clinicians suggest that renal function may be monitored less frequently during therapy (e.g., every other day), unless substantial increases in serum creatinine concentration become evident during treatment and/or other nephrotoxic drugs are administered concomitantly. In addition, to minimize the risk and degree of pentamidine-induced nephrotoxicity, fluid status should be carefully monitored in patients with PCP, particularly patients with AIDS who may be at high risk of dehydration as a result of diarrhea, fever, and poor oral intake. Concurrent administration of IV sodium chloride injection with each dose of parenteral pentamidine has been reported to decrease the incidence and/or severity of adverse effects (e.g., GI symptoms) associated with pentamidine administration.

Since pentamidine commonly causes hypoglycemia (which can occur up to several days after the drug is discontinued) and has diabetogenic effects (which may not be preceded by hypoglycemia and which can sometimes occur several months after therapy with the drug), blood glucose concentration should be frequently and carefully monitored in patients receiving the drug parenterally. The manufacturers recommend that blood glucose concentration be determined before, daily during, and after parenteral pentamidine therapy. Some clinicians suggest that blood glucose concentration may be monitored less frequently during therapy (e.g., every other day), but should be determined daily in patients with a history of diabetes mellitus or hypoglycemia or in those with poor oral intake and should be determined whenever signs and/or symptoms suggestive of hypoglycemia occur.

The manufacturers and some clinicians also recommend that complete blood counts, platelet counts, liver function tests (including serum bilirubin, alkaline phosphatase, AST, and ALT concentrations), and serum calcium concentrations be determined before and at periodic intervals during and after pentamidine therapy.

Because acute pancreatitis has been reported rarely in patients receiving parenteral pentamidine, some clinicians suggest that periodic monitoring of serum amylase concentrations may be warranted in patients receiving the drug. Pentamidine should be discontinued if signs or symptoms of acute pancreatitis develop.

Precautions Related to Pentamidine Oral Inhalation via Nebulization

Although pentamidine isethionate administered by oral inhalation via nebulization is generally considered not to be associated with substantial risk of serious adverse effects, the extent and consequences of accumulation of pentamidine following chronic oral inhalation therapy are not known. Therefore, patients receiving pentamidine oral inhalation therapy should be closely monitored for development of serious adverse effects that have been reported with parenteral pentamidine (e.g., hypotension, hypoglycemia, hyperglycemia, hypocalcemia, anemia, thrombocytopenia, leukopenia, hepatic or renal dysfunction, ventricular tachycardia, pancreatitis, Stevens-Johnson syndrome, hyperkalemia, ECG abnormalities [abnormal ST segment]).

Prior to initiating prophylaxis with pentamidine oral inhalation via nebulization, symptomatic patients should be evaluated appropriately to exclude the presence of PCP. Dosage of pentamidine isethionate oral inhalation therapy recommended for prevention of PCP is insufficient for treatment of PCP.

Patients receiving pentamidine oral inhalation via nebulization for prevention of PCP may still develop acute PCP. Relapse of PCP with atypical clinical or radiographic features (e.g., mild disease, granulomatous pulmonary lesions, focal infection confined to the upper lobes of the lung) may occur; such relapses have been treated successfully with parenteral pentamidine, suggesting that inadequate dosage or drug distribution rather than drug resistance is responsible for failure of prophylaxis.

Extrapulmonary and/or disseminated infection caused by *P. jirovecii*, which can be fatal, has been reported occasionally in patients receiving pentamidine oral inhalation therapy for prevention of PCP; most cases have occurred in patients with a history of PCP. The presence of extrapulmonary pneumocystosis should be considered when evaluating patients with unexplained signs and symptoms.

Patients receiving pentamidine by oral inhalation via nebulization for prevention of PCP should be monitored closely for signs and symptoms of pulmonary infection (e.g., fever, cough, dyspnea); those who exhibit such signs or symptoms should have thorough medical evaluations and appropriate diagnostic tests to rule out infection caused by *P. jirovecii* or other opportunistic or nonopportunistic pathogens. If PCP develops in a patient receiving prophylaxis with pentamidine oral inhalation therapy, prophylaxis should be discontinued and treatment with co-trimoxazole, parenteral pentamidine, or other effective treatment regimen should be initiated. Upon completion of treatment, PCP prophylaxis can be reinstituted.

Because acute pancreatitis has been reported rarely in patients receiving orally inhaled pentamidine, some clinicians suggest that periodic monitoring of serum amylase concentrations may be warranted in patients receiving the drug. Pentamidine should be discontinued if signs or symptoms of acute pancreatitis develop.

● Pediatric Precautions

Safety and efficacy of parenteral pentamidine isethionate has been established for treatment of PCP in children and infants older than 4 months of age, and there appear to be no unusual risks associated with use of the drug in this age group. Parenteral pentamidine isethionate also has been used effectively and apparently without unusual risks in children for treatment of first-stage (hemolymphatic) African trypanosomiasis† and treatment of leishmaniasis†.

The manufacturer states that safety and efficacy of orally inhaled pentamidine isethionate have not been established in children 16 years of age or younger. The US Centers for Disease Control and Prevention (CDC), National Institutes of Health (NIH), Infectious Diseases Society of America (IDSA), and American Academy of Pediatrics (AAP) recommend pentamidine administered by oral inhalation via nebulization as an alternative for prevention of PCP in children 5 years of age or older† who are capable of effectively using a nebulizer. (See Primary and Secondary Prophylaxis in Children under Pneumocystis jirovecii Pneumonia: Prevention of Pneumocystis jirovecii Infections, in Uses.)

● Mutagenicity and Carcinogenicity

Pentamidine was not mutagenic in the Ames bacteria (*Salmonella typhimurium*) test and did not induce an increase in chromosomal aberrations in Chinese hamster ovary (CHO) cells or human lymphocytes in vitro.

Studies have not been performed to date to evaluate the carcinogenic potential of pentamidine isethionate.

● Pregnancy, Fertility, and Lactation

Pregnancy

In a study in pregnant rats, IV pentamidine 4 mg/kg daily was embryolethal; teratogenicity was not observed in this study. It is not known whether pentamidine isethionate can cause fetal harm when administered to pregnant women, and parenteral pentamidine or pentamidine administered by oral inhalation via nebulization should be used during pregnancy only when clearly needed.

For treatment of first-stage (hemolymphatic) trypanosomiasis† or treatment of leishmaniasis† in pregnant women, the World Health Organization (WHO) states that parenteral pentamidine should not be used during the first trimester of pregnancy, but may be used after the first trimester.

Although fetal exposure would theoretically not be substantial, some clinicians recommend that pregnant women and possibly those planning to become pregnant (e.g., within 8 weeks of potential exposure) avoid environmental exposure to aerosolized pentamidine. (See Cautions: Environmental Exposure of Health-Care Personnel and Visitors.)

Fertility

It is not known whether pentamidine isethionate affects fertility in humans.

Lactation

It is not known whether pentamidine isethionate is distributed into milk. Because of the potential for serious adverse reactions to pentamidine isethionate in nursing infants, a decision should be made whether to discontinue nursing or the

drug, taking into account the importance of the drug to the woman. The manufacturers state that pentamidine isethionate should not be administered parenterally or by oral inhalation via nebulization in nursing mothers unless potential benefits outweigh potential risks.

DRUG INTERACTIONS

● Nephrotoxic Drugs

Concurrent or sequential use of pentamidine isethionate and other nephrotoxic drugs (e.g., aminoglycosides, amphotericin B, capreomycin, colistin [commercially available in the US as colistimethate sodium], cisplatin, foscarnet, polymyxin B, vancomycin) should be closely monitored or avoided, if possible, since nephrotoxic effects may be additive.

LABORATORY TEST INTERFERENCES

Pentamidine appears to affect the results of bronchoalveolar lavage and induced sputum diagnostic tests for *Pneumocystis jirovecii* (formerly *Pneumocystis carinii*) in patients receiving prophylaxis with the drug administered by oral inhalation via nebulization. The diagnostic yield of bronchoalveolar lavage in patients receiving the drug via oral inhalation was 62% compared with 100% in patients not receiving oral inhalation therapy; similar decreases in diagnostic yield have been observed for induced sputum tests. It is suggested that in the case of bronchoalveolar lavage, both bronchoalveolar and transbronchial biopsy specimens be obtained to optimize the diagnosis of *P. jirovecii* pneumonia (PCP); however, the yield from these tests is still considered high enough to maintain their diagnostic utility in these patients.

ACUTE TOXICITY

Renal and hepatic impairment, hypotension, and cardiopulmonary arrest occurred following inadvertent administration of a 1.6-g dose of IV pentamidine isethionate in a 17-month-old infant. Treatment included cardiopulmonary resuscitation, intubation, epinephrine, atropine, intubation, and 4 hours of charcoal hemoperfusion (resulting in a reduction in serum pentamidine concentrations). The patient recovered from this event, but later died from an unknown cause. One patient with *Pneumocystis jirovecii* (formerly *Pneumocystis carinii*) pneumonia (PCP) inadvertently received a 2-g IM dose of the drug, reportedly without ill effect. In general, overdosage of pentamidine isethionate would be expected to produce effects that are extensions of common adverse reactions.

Overdosage of pentamidine isethionate administered by oral inhalation via nebulization has not been reported to date and the signs and symptoms of such an overdose are not known. Currently available pharmacokinetic data suggest that a dose up to 40 times the recommended dose of orally inhaled pentamidine isethionate would be required to produce plasma concentrations similar to those of a single IV dose of 4 mg/kg; such an overdosage would have the potential of producing adverse effects similar to those seen after parenteral administration of the drug.

In mice, the LD_{50} of pentamidine isethionate has been reported to be 15, 63, or 120 mg/kg following IV, intraperitoneal, or subcutaneous administration, respectively.

MECHANISM OF ACTION

● Antiprotozoal Effects

The exact mechanism(s) of antiprotozoal action of pentamidine has not been fully elucidated. Several mechanisms of action may be involved, and the role of the mechanism(s) may vary among the different types of protozoa. The effects of pentamidine on various organisms (e.g., bacteria, protozoa) and cells (e.g., murine ascites tumor cells) have been studied to elucidate the mechanism(s) of action, and most information on the antiprotozoal activity of aromatic diamidines such as pentamidine has been derived from studies involving Trypanosomatidae (e.g., *Crithidia*, *Leishmania*, *Trypanosoma*).

In vitro studies indicate that pentamidine interferes with protozoal nuclear metabolism by inhibition of DNA, RNA, phospholipid, and protein synthesis. Mechanisms that may play a role include binding to nucleic acids, disruption of kinetoplast DNA, inhibition of RNA editing in trypanosomes, and inhibition of mRNA trans-splicing. In vitro, pentamidine has been shown to inhibit protein and nucleic acid synthesis in cell-free extracts of *Crithidia oncopelti*. The drug has also been shown to bind to and aggregate ribosomes in cell-free extracts of *C. oncopelti* in vitro, but pentamidine-induced inhibition of protein and nucleic acid synthesis is not associated with marked ribosomal aggregation in intact organisms. In vitro, pentamidine has also been shown to inhibit polyamine synthesis in *Leishmania* spp. and DNA, RNA, protein, and phospholipid synthesis and thymidylate synthetase activity in *C. fasciculata*; in addition, the drug partially inhibits respiration in *C. fasciculata* and in mitochondria-kinetoplast fractions obtained from the organism. The exact mechanism(s) by which pentamidine may impair energy-yielding reactions in trypanosomes is not known, but it has been suggested that the drug may inhibit oxidative phosphorylation. It has also been suggested that the susceptibility of different species of trypanosomes to pentamidine may be related to the relative importance of aerobic and anaerobic glycolysis in their metabolic processes, with the drug being more active against those species that rely more on aerobic glycolysis. There is also some evidence suggesting that susceptibility of different species and subspecies of trypanosomes to pentamidine may be correlated with the rate and/or extent of drug uptake by the organisms. The trypanosomicidal activity of pentamidine and related aromatic diamidine derivatives (e.g., diaminazene, hydroxystilbamidine) may be related in a large part to the ability of the drugs to bind to nucleic acids and DNA, particularly that of mitochondrial kinetoplasts, and thereby produce disruptive effects including inhibition of DNA and RNA synthesis. Ultrastructural studies in various trypanosomes indicate that pentamidine rapidly causes mitochondrial enlargement and fragmentation and condensation of kinetoplast DNA.

● Antifungal Effects

In vitro, pentamidine appears to be directly lethal to *Pneumocystis jirovecii* (formerly *Pneumocystis carinii*), although the drug only moderately inhibits glucose metabolism, protein and RNA synthesis, and intracellular amino acid transport in the organism at concentrations attainable in vivo.

● Hypotensive Effect

Pentamidine can cause hypotension, which can be severe. (See Cautions: Cardiovascular Effects.) The exact mechanism(s) of pentamidine-induced hypotension is not known, but studies in animals suggest that the drug has a direct vasodilatory action on peripheral small arteries and arterioles. It has also been suggested that histamine release may contribute to the hypotensive effect, since other aromatic diamidine derivatives have been shown to have histamine-releasing activity.

● Hypoglycemic and Diabetogenic Effects

Pentamidine can produce hypoglycemia, which may be severe and/or prolonged; in addition, the drug may produce hyperglycemia and insulin-dependent diabetes mellitus, with or without preceding hypoglycemia. (See Cautions: Hypoglycemic and Diabetogenic Effects.) The effect of pentamidine on blood glucose concentration can be multiphasic; an initial increase in blood glucose concentration may occur immediately following administration of the drug (possibly attributed to an adrenergic reaction), followed by a period of hypoglycemia lasting several hours and then hyperglycemia. Although the exact mechanism is not clearly established, pentamidine-induced hypoglycemia has been associated with pancreatic islet cell necrosis and inappropriately elevated plasma insulin concentrations. In vitro studies using pancreatic islet cells and malignant insulinoma cells suggest that pentamidine causes an acute release of insulin from beta cells of the pancreas, possibly via a cytolytic effect, followed by inhibition of insulin release and by cytolysis of the cells. The results of these in vitro studies and in vivo metabolic studies in patients receiving the drug indicate that pentamidine-induced diabetes mellitus probably results from a direct, selective cytotoxic effect of the drug on beta cells of the pancreas.

● Other Effects

At concentrations greater than 1 mcg/mL in vitro, pentamidine inhibits platelet aggregation induced by thrombin, epinephrine, adenosine diphosphate (ADP), collagen, and ristocetin in a concentration-dependent manner, with complete inhibition occurring at a concentration of 10 mcg/mL. In vitro, the drug also prolongs thrombin time by a few seconds at a concentration of 5 mcg/mL and slightly prolongs prothrombin and partial thromboplastin times, but only at substantially higher concentrations. At concentrations attained in vivo, pentamidine probably does not affect platelet function or coagulation. Pentamidine also has inhibited cholinesterases in vitro.

SPECTRUM

● Protozoa

Pentamidine is active in vitro and/or in vivo against a variety of protozoa, including Trypanosomatidae that are pathogenic to humans—*Trypanosoma* and *Leishmania*.

Pentamidine is active in vivo against the causative agents of African trypanosomiasis, including most strains of *Trypanosoma brucei gambiense* and some strains of *T. b. rhodesiense*, but is not active against *T. cruzi* (causative agent of American trypanosomiasis [Chagas disease]).

Pentamidine is active in vitro and in vivo against *Leishmania donovani*, including antimony-resistant strains of the organism. In vitro, pentamidine concentrations of 0.05–0.5 mcg/mL result in elimination of 85–90% of *L. donovani* amastigotes in human monocyte-derived macrophages and 20–40% of *L. donovani* promastigotes in cell-free media. The drug is also active in vivo against *L. aethiopica* and has some activity in vitro and possibly in vivo against *L. tropica*. In vitro, pentamidine concentrations of 0.1–0.5 mcg/mL result in elimination of about 85% of *L. tropica* amastigotes in human monocyte-derived macrophages and 10–20% of *L. tropica* promastigotes in cell-free media. Pentamidine also has some activity in vivo against *L. braziliensis* (including *L. b. guyanensis*) and in vitro against *L. mexicana* (including *L. m. amazonensis*) and possibly in vivo against *L. mexicana*.

Pentamidine also is active in vitro against *Crithidia fasciculata* and *C. oncopelti*, which are not pathogenic to humans.

Pentamidine has been shown to have some activity against pathogenic strains of *Acanthamoeba* in vitro, against *Babesia canis* in dogs, and against *B. microti* in rodents. The drug also has some antiplasmodial activity in animals. Pentamidine was inactive in vitro against pathogenic strains of *Naegleria* in one study.

● Fungi

Pentamidine is active in vitro and in vivo against *Pneumocystis jirovecii* (formerly *Pneumocystis carinii*). In vitro, the drug appears to be directly lethal to the organism at concentrations attainable in vivo.

Pentamidine is active in vitro and in vivo against some strains of *Candida albicans*. The drug also has some activity in vitro against various *Trichophyton*, *Microsporum*, *Cryptococcus*, *Blastomyces*, and *Histoplasma*, but usually only at very high concentrations.

● Other Organisms

In vitro, pentamidine has some antibacterial activity against *Escherichia coli* and *Staphylococcus aureus* and some antiviral activity.

RESISTANCE

Little information is available on natural or acquired resistance of protozoa to pentamidine. Pentamidine resistance can be induced in vitro. Evidence from in vitro studies using *Trypanosoma brucei brucei* and *Crithidia oncopelti* with induced pentamidine resistance and *T. b. brucei* with a degree of natural resistance to the drug suggests that resistance to pentamidine results primarily because of reduced uptake of the drug by the organisms. Studies using trypanosomes indicate that the P2 aminopurine transporter is important for uptake of pentamidine and loss of this transporter results in emergence of resistance. In addition, there is evidence that loss of the P2 transporter and the high-affinity pentamidine transporter appears to be associated with high-level resistance to both pentamidine and melarsoprol (not commercially available in the US, but may be available from the CDC). Trypanosomes resistant to pentamidine are generally cross-resistant to other aromatic diamidine derivatives (e.g., stilbamidine).

PHARMACOKINETICS

● *Absorption*

Following daily IM administration of single 4-mg/kg doses of pentamidine isethionate (2.3 mg/kg of pentamidine) in an early study in patients with *Pneumocystis jirovecii* (formerly *Pneumocystis carinii*) pneumonia (PCP), plasma pentamidine concentrations (determined using a fluorometric assay) after 1–10 days of therapy averaged 0.3–0.5 mcg/mL (range: 0.3–1.4 mcg/mL). In these patients, plasma drug concentrations did not vary appreciably throughout the day and did not increase with successive doses of the drug. Although plasma pentamidine concentrations generally did not increase immediately after administration of a dose, if an increase did occur, it was usually within 1 hour after administration. Highest plasma drug concentrations occurred in patients with varying degrees of renal impairment.

Following a single 4-mg/kg IM or IV (given as a 2-hour infusion) dose of pentamidine isethionate in patients with acquired immunodeficiency syndrome (AIDS) and PCP, peak plasma pentamidine concentrations (determined using an HPLC assay) averaged 209 ng/mL approximately 40 minutes after the IM dose and 612 ng/mL after completion of the IV infusion. Following IV administration of pentamidine isethionate 3.7–4 mg/kg daily (given as a 4-hour infusion) in HIV-infected patients with PCP, mean peak plasma concentrations were 175.3, 210.9, or 256.7 ng/mL on day 1, 4, or 7, respectively. Data from this study suggest that steady state was not achieved by day 7.

Following oral inhalation of pentamidine isethionate via nebulization (aerosolized pentamidine), bronchoalveolar lavage fluid concentrations of the drug are substantially higher (at least 5–10 times higher) than those attained following IV administration; however, plasma concentrations following oral inhalation are substantially lower than those attained with a comparable IV dose. In a small number of patients with AIDS and suspected PCP, concentrations of pentamidine determined 18–24 hours after oral inhalation of pentamidine isethionate 300 mg via a Respirgard® II jet nebulizer or IV administration of pentamidine isethionate 4 mg/kg averaged 23.2 ng/mL (range: 5.1–43 ng/mL) or 2.6 ng/mL (range: 1.5–4 ng/mL), respectively, in bronchoalveolar lavage fluid and 705 ng/mL (range: 140–1336 ng/mL) or 9.3 ng/mL (range: 6.9–12.8 ng/mL), respectively, in bronchoalveolar lavage sediment; plasma pentamidine concentrations in all but one patient receiving pentamidine by oral inhalation were at or below the level of detection of the HPLC assay (2–3 ng/mL). In other studies in patients receiving orally inhaled pentamidine isethionate 600 mg daily via the Respirgard® II jet nebulizer, mean plasma concentrations after the dose on day 21 reportedly averaged 11.8–13.8 ng/mL. Pentamidine appears to undergo limited absorption from the respiratory tract into systemic circulation; peak plasma concentrations appear to occur at or near completion of oral inhalation administration and appear to be 5% or less of those attained following IV administration. The extent of pentamidine accumulation following chronic oral inhalation therapy is not known.

● *Distribution*

Distribution of pentamidine into human body tissues and fluids has not been well characterized, but the drug appears to be rapidly and extensively distributed and/or bound to tissues. Data from patients with AIDS indicate that following parenteral administration of pentamidine, highest concentrations of the drug (determined using a bioassay) are found in the liver, followed by the kidneys, adrenals, spleen, lungs, and pancreas. Further studies are needed, but these data also suggest that continued parenteral administration beyond the first week of therapy may not substantially increase accumulation of the drug in lung tissue. Since pentamidine is not effective for the treatment of trypanosomiasis involving the CNS, the drug has been believed to poorly penetrate the CNS; this is supported by limited data from patients with AIDS which indicate that pentamidine may distribute into the CNS in some patients, but only in very low concentrations and after prolonged therapy (a month or longer). Following intraperitoneal or IM administration of pentamidine isethionate in mice or rats, respectively, highest concentrations of the drug are found in the kidneys, followed by the liver and lungs. Following IV administration in dogs, highest concentrations of pentamidine are found in the liver, followed by the kidneys, lungs, and spleen; the drug is also distributed into bile and the CNS. IV administration of pentamidine isethionate 5 mg/kg in rats reportedly produced concentrations

in the liver and kidney that were 87.5 and 62.3 times higher, respectively, than those produced by an identical dose of pentamidine isethionate administered by oral inhalation.

Deposition of orally inhaled pentamidine shows considerable interindividual variation and appears to depend on several factors, including delivery device, particle size of aerosolized drug, dose, patient position, and nebulization efficiency. Limited data from patients with HIV infections indicate that distribution of the drug in the lungs following oral inhalation via nebulization is more uniform when the patient is in the supine rather than the sitting position. In one study, differences in pulmonary deposition of pentamidine appeared to relate principally to aerosol delivery from the nebulizer system rather than from lung parameters (e.g., breathing pattern, pulmonary function tests, regional ventilation). In this study, the fraction of a dose deposited (amount deposited versus amount inhaled, *not* the amount deposited versus the amount of drug added to the nebulizer) averaged 62% in patients with HIV infection and did not differ substantially as a fraction of that inhaled for the Respirgard® II or AeroTech® II jet nebulizers, although the latter nebulizer was substantially more efficient in delivering the drug to the patient (i.e., the amount inhaled per minute was higher). In an in vitro study simulating clinical conditions, the amount of drug that would be delivered for oral inhalation versus that originally added to the nebulizer (nebulizer efficiency) averaged 4.6, 21, and 16% for the Respirgard® II, AeroTech® II, and FISONeb® nebulizers, respectively, at a simulated tidal volume of 750 cm³ and a frequency of 20 breaths/minute.

In vitro, pentamidine is reportedly 69% bound to serum proteins. Pentamidine apparently crosses the placenta. In a child delivered by cesarean section from an HIV-infected woman receiving IV pentamidine (3.4 mg/kg daily), concentrations of the drug in cord blood were 13.2 ng/mL; the sample was obtained 16.5 hours after the mother's last dose and blood concentrations of the drug in the mother that day were 81.3 ng/mL. It is not known whether pentamidine isethionate is distributed into milk.

● *Elimination*

Following a single pentamidine isethionate dose of 4 mg/kg given by IM injection or IV infusion over 2 hours in patients with AIDS and PCP who had normal renal function, plasma concentrations of the drug declined in a biphasic manner with a mean half-life of 54 or 18 minutes in the initial phase, respectively, and 9.4 or 6.4 hours in the elimination phase, respectively. Pentamidine appears to be eliminated very slowly from tissues in which the drug principally accumulates (e.g., liver, lungs), and terminal half-lives of 2.8–12 days have been reported with IV dosages of 2–4 mg/kg daily. Following a single pentamidine isethionate dose of 3–4.8 mg/kg given by IV infusion in patients with *Trypanosoma brucei gambiense* infection, the mean terminal elimination half-life was 11 days (range 4–19 days). Limited data suggest that the elimination half-life of pentamidine is not substantially altered in patients with mild to moderate renal impairment but may be prolonged up to 2 days or longer in patients with severe renal impairment.

In mice, pentamidine is excreted in urine and feces in a ratio of about 4:1, respectively; the ratio remains constant for at least 90 hours after administration. In humans, pentamidine is excreted in urine, apparently as unchanged drug; it is not known if the drug is excreted in feces. Following daily IM administration of pentamidine isethionate in a study in patients with PCP who had varying degrees of renal function, 24-hour urinary drug excretion (determined using a fluorometric assay) after 1–10 days of therapy was generally 15–20% (range: 11–29%) of the daily dose; most urinary excretion occurred within the first 6 hours after administration of a dose. In several patients, decreasing amounts of pentamidine were excreted in urine for up to 6–8 weeks after discontinuance of the drug. Following a single 4-mg/kg IM or IV dose of pentamidine isethionate in patients with AIDS and PCP who had normal renal function, about 2.5–5% of the dose (determined using an HPLC assay) was excreted in urine as unchanged drug in 24 hours, mainly within the first 8 hours after administration of the drug; similar amounts (about 1–4% of the dose) were also excreted in urine as unchanged drug in 24 hours in patients with mild to moderate renal impairment. Studies in dogs and humans suggest that renal clearance accounts for about 5% or less of the total body clearance of the drug.

Limited data suggest that pentamidine is not appreciably removed by hemodialysis or peritoneal dialysis.

Data are not available regarding the pharmacokinetics of pentamidine isethionate after oral inhalation via nebulization in patients with hepatic or renal dysfunction.

CHEMISTRY AND STABILITY

● *Chemistry*

Pentamidine isethionate is an aromatic diamidine-derivative antiprotozoal and antifungal agent. The presence of the benzenecarboximidamide (aromatic amidine, benzamidine) group is associated with pentamidine's trypanosomicidal activity, and the presence of both benzenecarboximidamide groups is necessary for this activity.

Pentamidine isethionate is commercially available as a sterile, lyophilized powder for preparation of solutions for IM or IV use and as a sterile, lyophilized powder for preparation of solutions for oral inhalation via nebulization (aerosolized pentamidine). Pentamidine isethionate occurs as white or almost white crystals or powder; the drug is hygroscopic and may be odorless or have a slight butyric odor. The drug is soluble in water, having an aqueous solubility of approximately 100 mg/mL at 25°C, and is slightly soluble in alcohol. Each 1.74 mg of pentamidine isethionate is equivalent to 1 mg of pentamidine. Pentamidine reportedly has a pK_{a1} and pK_{a2} of 11.4.

Following reconstitution with sterile water for injection or 5% dextrose injection, pentamidine isethionate solutions for parenteral use are clear and colorless. After reconstitution with sterile water for injection, solutions of the drug for parenteral use containing 60–100 mg/mL have a pH of approximately 5.4. Following reconstitution with 5% dextrose injection, pentamidine isethionate solutions for parenteral use containing 60 or 100 mg/mL have a pH of 4.09 or 4.38, respectively. Pentamidine isethionate solutions for parenteral use containing 100 mg/mL in sterile water for injection or 5% dextrose injection have osmolalities of 160 or 455 mOsm/kg, respectively.

When pentamidine isethionate lyophilized powder for oral inhalation solution is reconstituted and administered using the Respirgard® II jet nebulizer, the resultant mist contains nebulized particles of the drug with a median mass aerodynamic diameter of 0.8–1.4 μm.

● *Stability*

Prior to reconstitution, pentamidine isethionate lyophilized powders should be stored at 20–25°C and protected from light.

Following reconstitution with sterile water for injection, pentamidine isethionate solutions for parenteral use containing 60–100 mg/mL are stable in the original vial for 48 hours at room temperature if protected from light; to avoid crystallization, reconstituted solutions should be stored at 22–30°C. Unused portions of the reconstituted solutions should be discarded. Reconstituted solutions of the drug for parenteral use that have been further diluted in 5% dextrose injection to a concentration of 1 or 2.5 mg/mL for IV infusion are stable for up to 24 hours at room temperature. Reconstituted solutions that have been diluted to a concentration of 1 or 2 mg/mL in 5% dextrose or 0.9% sodium chloride injection in PVC bags are reportedly stable for 48 hours exposed to normal fluorescent light at 22–26°C; some data suggest that small amounts of the drug may be adsorbed onto PVC infusion sets.

Following reconstitution with sterile water for injection, pentamidine isethionate solutions for oral inhalation are stable in the original vial for 48 hours at room temperature if protected from light.

PREPARATIONS

Excipients in commercially available drug preparations may have clinically important effects in some individuals; consult specific product labeling for details.

Pentamidine Isethionate

Oral-inhalation		
For solution, for nebulization	300 mg	NebuPent®, APP

Parenteral		
For injection	300 mg*	Pentam® 300, APP
		Pentamidine Isethionate for Injection

* available from one or more manufacturer, distributor, and/or repackager by generic (nonproprietary) name

† Use is not currently included in the labeling approved by the US Food and Drug Administration.

Selected Revisions April 10, 2024, © Copyright, May 1, 1985, American Society of Health-System Pharmacists, Inc.

Secnidazole

8:30.16 • ANTIPROTOZOALS, NITROIMIDAZOLE-DERIVATIVE

■ Secnidazole, a nitroimidazole derivative, is an antiprotozoal and antibacterial agent.

USES

● Bacterial Vaginosis

Secnidazole is used for the treatment of bacterial vaginosis.

Bacterial vaginosis is a polymicrobial syndrome that can occur when normal hydrogen peroxide-producing *Lactobacillus* in the vagina are replaced by overgrowth of various anaerobic bacteria (e.g., *Atopobium vaginae, Bacteroides, Mobiluncus, Prevotella*), *Gardnerella vaginalis, Ureaplasma urealyticum, Mycoplasma hominis*, or other bacteria. Treatment of bacterial vaginosis is usually recommended in symptomatic women to relieve the signs and symptoms of infection; routine treatment of male sexual partner(s) is not usually recommended. Relapse or recurrence of bacterial vaginosis is common, regardless of the treatment regimen used.

Clinical Experience

Efficacy and safety of secnidazole for the treatment of bacterial vaginosis in nonpregnant women were evaluated in 2 similarly designed randomized, placebo-controlled studies (Trial 1 and Trial 2). In both studies, bacterial vaginosis was diagnosed by presence of an off-white (milky or gray), thin, homogeneous vaginal discharge, vaginal pH 4.7 or greater, presence of clue cells as 20% or greater of total epithelial cells on a microscopic examination of vaginal saline wet mount, detection of amine odor on addition of 10% potassium hydroxide (KOH) solution to a sample of vaginal discharge (positive "whiff" test), and a Nugent score 4 or greater. The 144 women enrolled in Trial 1 (19–54 years of age) and 189 women enrolled in Trial 2 (18–54 years of age) were randomized to receive a single 2-g dose of secnidazole oral granules or placebo. The primary end point was clinical response (defined as normal vaginal discharge, negative detection of amine odor on addition of 10% KOH solution, and clue cells less than 20% of total epithelial cells) at the test-of-cure visit (21–30 days after the dose).

In the modified intent-to-treat (MITT) population in Trial 1, clinical response was achieved in 67.7 or 17.7% of patients treated with secnidazole or placebo, respectively; in Trial 2, clinical response was achieved in 53.3 or 19.3% of patients in the MITT population treated with secnidazole or placebo, respectively. In Trial 1, Nugent score cure (i.e., Nugent score 0–3) was achieved in 40.3 or 6.5% of patients treated with secnidazole or placebo, respectively; in Trial 2, Nugent score cure was achieved in 43.9 or 5.3% of patients treated with secnidazole or placebo, respectively.

DOSAGE AND ADMINISTRATION

● Administration

Secnidazole is administered orally without regard to meals.

Secnidazole is commercially available as single-dose packets containing oral granules that are taken by sprinkling onto applesauce, yogurt, or pudding. The granules will not dissolve and are not intended to be administered in any liquid.

The entire contents of a single-dose packet of secnidazole granules (2 g of secnidazole) should be sprinkled onto applesauce, yogurt, or pudding and the entire mixture should be consumed within 30 minutes without chewing or crunching the granules. A glass of water may be taken after administration of secnidazole granules to aid in swallowing.

● Dosage

Bacterial Vaginosis

For the treatment of bacterial vaginosis in adult women, secnidazole is administered as a single 2-g dose.

● Special Populations

The manufacturer makes no specific dosage recommendations for patients with hepatic or renal impairment or for geriatric patients.

CAUTIONS

● Contraindications

Secnidazole is contraindicated in patients with known hypersensitivity to secnidazole, other ingredients in the formulation, or other nitroimidazole derivatives.

● Warnings/Precautions

Vulvovaginal Candidiasis

The use of secnidazole may result in vulvovaginal candidiasis. In clinical trials in nonpregnant women with bacterial vaginosis, vulvovaginal candidiasis developed in 9.6% of patients who received secnidazole and 2.9% of patients who received placebo. Symptomatic vulvovaginal candidiasis may require treatment with an antifungal.

Carcinogenicity

Carcinogenicity has been observed in mice and rats treated chronically with nitroimidazole derivatives structurally related to secnidazole (e.g., metronidazole). In some rodent studies, lifetime exposure to nitroimidazoles was associated with tumors affecting liver, lung, mammary, and lymphatic tissues.

It is not known if positive tumor findings in rodent studies using other nitroimidazoles indicate a risk to patients receiving a single dose of secnidazole to treat bacterial vaginosis. The manufacturer states that chronic use of secnidazole should be avoided.

Selection and Use of Anti-infectives

To reduce development of drug-resistant bacteria and maintain effectiveness of secnidazole and other anti-infectives, the drug should be used only for treatment of infections proven or strongly suspected to be caused by susceptible bacteria.

Prescribing secnidazole in the absence of proven or strongly suspected bacterial infection or for prophylaxis is unlikely to provide benefit to the patient and increases the risk of development of drug-resistant bacteria.

When selecting or modifying anti-infective therapy, results of culture and in vitro susceptibility testing should be used. In the absence of such data, local epidemiology and susceptibility patterns should be considered when selecting anti-infectives for empiric therapy.

Specific Populations

Pregnancy

There are insufficient data on use of secnidazole in pregnant women. In animal reproduction studies, there was no evidence of adverse developmental outcomes when oral secnidazole was administered to pregnant rats and rabbits during organogenesis at doses up to fourfold greater than the recommended human dose.

Lactation

It is not known whether secnidazole is distributed into human milk, affects the breast-fed infant, or affects milk production. Other nitroimidazole derivatives are distributed into human milk.

Due to the potential for serious adverse effects, including tumorigenicity, breast-feeding is not recommended during secnidazole treatment and for 96 hours after administration of the drug. In this situation, a nursing mother may choose to pump and discard her breast milk during and for 96 hours after secnidazole treatment and feed her infant stored human milk or formula during this period.

Pediatric Use

Safety and efficacy of secnidazole have not been established in pediatric patients younger than 18 years of age.

Geriatric Use

Clinical studies of secnidazole did not include a sufficient number of patients 65 years of age and older to determine if geriatric adults respond differently than younger adults.

Hepatic Impairment

Secnidazole has not been studied in patients with hepatic impairment.

Renal Impairment

Secnidazole has not been studied in patients with renal impairment.

● Common Adverse Effects

Adverse effects reported in 2% or more of patients receiving secnidazole in clinical trials include vulvovaginal candidiasis, headache, GI effects (nausea, vomiting, diarrhea, dysgeusia, abdominal pain), and vulvovaginal pruritus.

DRUG INTERACTIONS

● Drugs Affecting or Metabolized by Hepatic Microsomal Enzymes

Secnidazole is minimally metabolized by cytochrome P-450 (CYP) isoenzymes and the drug is unlikely to be affected by CYP inducers or inhibitors.

● Estrogens and Progestins

Concomitant administration of secnidazole (single 2-g oral dose) and an oral contraceptive containing ethinyl estradiol and norethindrone (single dose) in healthy adult females resulted in a 29% decrease in the mean peak plasma concentration of ethinyl estradiol, but did not affect the area under the plasma concentration-time curve (AUC) of ethinyl estradiol; the mean peak plasma concentration and AUC of norethindrone were increased by 13 and 16%, respectively. However, none of these effects on the oral contraceptive were considered clinically important. Administration of secnidazole (single 2-g dose) 1 day prior to the oral contraceptive did not have a clinically important effect on mean peak plasma concentrations or AUCs of ethinyl estradiol or norethindrone.

Secnidazole may be used concomitantly with oral estrogen-progestin combination contraceptives (e.g., containing ethinyl estradiol and norethindrone).

● Ethanol

In vitro studies indicate secnidazole has no effect on aldehyde dehydrogenase activity at clinically important doses.

DESCRIPTION

Secnidazole is a 5-nitroimidazole antiprotozoal and antibacterial agent.

The exact mechanism of action of secnidazole has not been fully elucidated. Secnidazole is a prodrug that is activated after entry into bacterial cells where the nitro group is reduced by bacterial enzymes to form short-lived radical anions. It is believed that these radical anions interfere with DNA synthesis of susceptible bacteria.

Secnidazole is active in vitro against some anaerobic bacteria, including *Bacteroides*, *Gardnerella vaginalis*, *Prevotella*, *Mobiluncus*, and *Megasphaera*-like type I/II. *G. vaginalis* and *Mobiluncus* with reduced in vitro susceptibility or resistance to secnidazole have been reported. Some bacteria with reduced in vitro susceptibility to metronidazole also have reduced susceptibility to secnidazole; the clinical importance of this possible cross-resistance is not known.

Secnidazole is active against some protozoa, including *Giardia duodenalis* (also known as *G. lamblia* or *G. intestinalis*), *Trichomonas vaginalis*, and *Entamoeba histolytica*.

Following oral administration of a single 2-g dose of secnidazole (as granules admixed with applesauce) in healthy, fasting adult females, mean peak plasma concentrations of the drug were 45.4 mcg/mL and the median time to peak plasma concentrations was 4 hours; mean plasma concentrations were 22.1, 9.2, 3.8, and 1.4 mcg/mL at 24, 48, 72, and 96 hours, respectively, after the dose. Peak plasma concentrations and area under the plasma concentration-time curve (AUC) following administration of secnidazole granules admixed in applesauce are similar to those observed when secnidazole granules are admixed in pudding or yogurt. Administration of a single 2-g dose of secnidazole admixed with applesauce followed by a high-fat meal does not affect peak plasma concentrations or AUC of the drug compared with administration in the fasting state. Secnidazole is less than 5% bound to plasma proteins. In vitro studies indicate that no more than 1% of secnidazole is metabolized by cytochrome P-450 (CYP) isoenzymes. Following a single 2-g dose of oral secnidazole, approximately 15% is excreted unchanged in urine. The plasma elimination half-life of secnidazole is approximately 17 hours.

ADVICE TO PATIENTS

Advise patients to read the patient information provided by the manufacturer.

Advise patients that antibacterials (including secnidazole) should only be used to treat bacterial infections and not used to treat viral infections (e.g., the common cold).

Instruct patients that the entire contents of the single-dose packet of secnidazole granules should be sprinkled on applesauce, yogurt, or pudding and the entire mixture should be consumed within 30 minutes (without chewing or crunching the granules). Inform patients that the granules are not intended to be dissolved in any liquid.

Advise patients that secnidazole may be taken without regard to meals.

Advise patients that use of secnidazole may result in vulvovaginal candidiasis that may require treatment with an antifungal.

Importance of informing clinicians of existing or contemplated concomitant therapy, including prescription and OTC drugs and herbal supplements, as well as any concomitant illnesses.

Importance of women informing clinicians if they are or plan to become pregnant or plan to breast-feed. Advise women not to breast-feed during and for 96 hours following administration of secnidazole.

Importance of informing patients of other important precautionary information. (See Cautions.)

PREPARATIONS

Excipients in commercially available drug preparations may have clinically important effects in some individuals; consult specific product labeling for details.

Secnidazole

Oral		
Granules	2 g	Solosec®, Lupin

† Use is not currently included in the labeling approved by the US Food and Drug Administration.

Selected Revisions April 10, 2024, © Copyright, October 9, 2017, American Society of Health-System Pharmacists, Inc.

Nitazoxanide

8:30.20 • ANTIPROTOZOALS, CRYPTOSPORIDIOSIS

- Nitazoxanide, a synthetic nitrothiazolyl-salicylamide derivative, is an antiprotozoal agent.

USES

• Cryptosporidiosis

Nitazoxanide is used for the treatment of diarrhea caused by *Cryptosporidium parvum* in immunocompetent adults, adolescents, and children 1 year of age or older. The drug is designated an orphan drug by FDA for the treatment of cryptosporidiosis.

Cryptosporidium is an important cause of infectious diarrhea in children and adults in developed and developing countries. Cryptosporidiosis can occur as the result of ingestion of contaminated water, vegetables, fruits, or unpasteurized milk; exposure to infected livestock (e.g., cattle, sheep); or person-to-person transmission via the fecal-oral route. Outbreaks in the US have occurred in childcare centers and have occurred as a result of contaminated municipal water supplies or swimming pools (including chlorinated pools) or infected animals in petting zoos. The duration and severity of clinical symptoms of cryptosporidiosis vary depending on the immune status of the patient. Immunocompetent individuals usually have disease that is asymptomatic or self-limited (i.e., acute, watery diarrhea that persists for up to 2–3 weeks and may be accompanied by nausea, vomiting, abdominal pain, fever); however, immunocompromised individuals can have disease that manifests either as asymptomatic shedding of cryptosporidial oocysts or as transient infection with diarrhea lasting less than 2 months, chronic diarrhea lasting 2 months or longer with persistence of parasites in stool or biopsy specimens, or fulminant cholera-like illness.

Nitazoxanide is considered the drug of choice for the treatment of cryptosporidiosis.

Adults and Adolescents 12 Years of Age or Older

Efficacy of nitazoxanide for the treatment of diarrhea caused by *C. parvum* in adults and adolescents 12 years of age or older has been evaluated in several double-blind, controlled studies in Egypt. In one study, patients were randomized to receive nitazoxanide (500 mg as tablets twice daily) or placebo for 3 days; a third group of patients received open label nitazoxanide oral suspension in a dosage of 500 mg twice daily for 3 days. At 4–7 days following the end of treatment, an intent-to-treat analysis in those with *C. parvum* as the sole pathogen indicated that a clinical response (defined as well with no symptoms, no watery stools, and no more than 2 soft stools within the past 24 hours or well with no symptoms and no unformed stools within the past 48 hours) was attained in 96% of those who received nitazoxanide tablets, 87% of those who received nitazoxanide oral suspension, and 41% of those who received placebo.

In another study in Egypt in adults and adolescents with diarrhea caused by *C. parvum* (the sole pathogen), clinical response evaluated 2–6 days following the end of treatment was 71% in those who received nitazoxanide and 43% in those who received placebo.

Although the relevance is unknown, some patients in the above studies categorized as having a clinical response defined as well had *C. parvum* oocysts in their stool at 4–7 days following the end of treatment. Patients should be managed based on clinical response to treatment.

Children 1–11 Years of Age

Efficacy of nitazoxanide for the treatment of diarrhea caused by *C. parvum* in children 1–11 years of age has been evaluated in several double-blind, controlled studies. In these studies, clinical response was evaluated 3–7 days following completion of therapy and was defined as well with no symptoms, no watery stools, no more than 2 soft stools, and no hematochezia within the previous 24 hours or well with no symptoms and no unformed stools within the previous 48 hours. In a study in Egypt that included children 1–11 years of age with diarrhea caused by *C. parvum*, clinical response was observed in 88% of those receiving a 3-day regimen

of oral nitazoxanide (100 mg twice daily in those 12–47 months of age or 200 mg twice daily in those 4–11 years of age) compared with 38% of those receiving placebo (intent-to-treat analysis).

In a study in malnourished (60% severely underweight, 19% moderately underweight, 17% mildly underweight) hospitalized Zambian children 12–35 months of age with diarrhea caused by *C. parvum*, clinical response was achieved in 56 or 23% of children receiving a 3-day regimen of oral nitazoxanide (100 mg twice daily for 3 days) or placebo, respectively.

HIV-infected Individuals

Nitazoxanide has not been shown to be more effective than placebo for the treatment of diarrhea caused by *C. parvum* in immunocompromised patients, including those with human immunodeficiency virus (HIV) infection. Although nitazoxanide has been used for the treatment of cryptosporidiosis in immunocompromised patients, including HIV-infected individuals, no anti-infective has been found to reliably eradicate *Cryptosporidium* in such patients.

In a study in malnourished hospitalized Zambian children with diarrhea caused by *C. parvum*, the clinical response to a 3-day regimen of oral nitazoxanide (100 mg twice daily in those 12–47 months of age or 200 mg twice daily in those 4–11 years of age) in the subgroup of HIV-seropositive patients was no better than that reported for children receiving placebo.

The US Centers for Disease Control and Prevention (CDC), National Institutes of Health (NIH), HIV Medicine Association of the Infectious Diseases Society of America (IDSA), and other clinicians state that the most appropriate treatment for cryptosporidiosis in HIV-infected individuals is the use of potent antiretroviral therapy and supportive care (e.g., aggressive oral and/or IV hydration, correction of electrolyte abnormalities, symptomatic treatment of diarrhea). A highly potent antiretroviral regimen that results in immune restoration (CD4+ T-cell counts exceeding 100/mm^3) may lead to microbiologic and clinical resolution of *Cryptosporidium* infection. These experts state that adjunctive use of nitazoxanide can be considered for the treatment of cryptosporidiosis in HIV-infected adults, adolescents, or children† receiving effective antiretroviral therapy; however, nitazoxanide should not be used in HIV-infected patients who are not receiving antiretroviral therapy.

• Giardiasis

Nitazoxanide is used for the treatment of diarrhea caused by *Giardia intestinalis* (also known as *G. lamblia* or *G. duodenalis*) in immunocompetent adults, adolescents, and children 1 year of age or older. Nitazoxanide is designated an orphan drug by FDA for the treatment of intestinal giardiasis.

Drugs of choice for the treatment of giardiasis are metronidazole, tinidazole, and nitazoxanide; alternative agents include paromomycin (especially in pregnant women), furazolidone (no longer commercially available in the US), or quinacrine (not commercially available in the US).

Adults and Adolescents 12 Years of Age or Older

In double-blind controlled studies in Peru and Egypt in adults and adolescents with diarrhea caused by *Giardia*, clinical response was observed in 85–100% of those receiving nitazoxanide tablets (500 mg twice daily for 3 days), 83% of those receiving nitazoxanide oral suspension (500 mg twice daily for 3 days), and in 30–44% of those receiving placebo. Clinical response was evaluated 4–7 days following completion of therapy and was defined as no symptoms, no watery stools, no more than 2 soft stools, and no hematochezia within the previous 24 hours or no symptoms and no unformed stools within the previous 48 hours.

Children 1–11 Years of Age

In a controlled study in Peru in children with diarrhea caused by *Giardia*, clinical response rates in children receiving a 3-day regimen of oral nitazoxanide (100 mg twice daily in those 12–47 months of age or 200 mg twice daily in those 4–11 years of age) were similar (80–85%) to response rates achieved in children receiving a 5-day regimen of oral metronidazole (125 mg twice daily in those 2–5 years of age or 250 mg twice daily in those 6–11 years of age). In this study, clinical response was evaluated 7–10 days following initiation of therapy and was defined as no symptoms, no watery stools, no more than 2 soft stools, and no hematochezia within the previous 24 hours or no symptoms and no unformed stools within the previous 48 hours.

HIV-infected Individuals

Safety and efficacy of nitazoxanide have not been established for the treatment of diarrhea caused by *Giardia* in HIV-infected patients or other individuals with immunodeficiency. However, CDC, NIH, and IDSA state that tinidazole and nitazoxanide are the drugs of choice for the treatment of giardiasis in HIV-infected infants and children† and metronidazole is the preferred alternative.

● *Amebiasis*

Nitazoxanide has been used for the treatment of amebiasis caused by *Entamoeba*†. The drug is designated an orphan drug by FDA for the treatment of intestinal amebiasis.

The regimen of choice for symptomatic intestinal amebiasis or extraintestinal disease is treatment with a nitroimidazole derivative (tinidazole or metronidazole) followed by treatment with a luminal amebicide (iodoquinol or paromomycin).

Although nitazoxanide has been effective in some patients for the treatment of mild to moderate intestinal amebiasis, data are limited and some clinicians state that additional study is needed to evaluate efficacy of the drug for the treatment of amebiasis.

● *Isosporiasis (Cystoisosporiasis)*

Nitazoxanide has been used in some patients for the treatment of isosporiasis† (also known as cystoisosporiasis) caused by *Isospora belli* (*Cystoisospora belli*).

Co-trimoxazole is the drug of choice for the treatment of infections caused by *I. belli* (*C. belli*); pyrimethamine and ciprofloxacin are recommended as alternatives. Although data are limited, some experts state that nitazoxanide is a potential alternative for the treatment of isosporiasis (cystoisosporiasis) in HIV-infected infants and children† who cannot tolerate co-trimoxazole.

● *Cestode (Tapeworm) Infections*

Nitazoxanide has been used for the treatment of hymenolepiasis caused by *Hymenolepis nana*† (dwarf tapeworm). Praziquantel is considered the drug of choice for the treatment of *H. nana* infections and niclosamide (not commercially available in the US) and nitazoxanide are recommended as alternatives.

In a randomized study comparing efficacy of nitazoxanide and praziquantel for the treatment of hymenolepiasis in children in Peru, nitazoxanide was effective in 82% and praziquantel was effective in 96% of patients.

● *Nematode (Roundworm) Infections*

Nitazoxanide has been used for the treatment of ascariasis† caused by *Ascaris lumbricoides*. Albendazole, mebendazole, and ivermectin are considered the drugs of choice for the treatment of ascariasis. In a randomized study comparing efficacy of nitazoxanide and albendazole for the treatment of ascariasis in children in Peru, nitazoxanide was effective in 89% and albendazole was effective in 91% of patients.

Nitazoxanide has been used for the treatment of trichuriasis† caused by *Trichuris trichiura* (whipworm). Albendazole is considered the drug of choice for treatment of trichuriasis and mebendazole and ivermectin are recommended as alternatives. In a randomized study comparing efficacy of nitazoxanide and albendazole for the treatment of trichuriasis in children in Peru, nitazoxanide was effective in 89% and albendazole was effective in 58% of patients.

● *Trematode (Fluke) Infections*

Nitazoxanide has been used in some patients for the treatment of fascioliasis caused by *Fasciola hepatica*† (sheep liver fluke).

Triclabendazole is considered the drug of choice for the treatment of infections caused by *F. hepatica* and bithionol (not commercially available in the US) and nitazoxanide are recommended as alternatives.

DOSAGE AND ADMINISTRATION

● *Reconstitution and Administration*

Nitazoxanide is administered orally twice daily with food.

Nitazoxanide tablets containing 500 mg of the drug should not be used in pediatric patients 11 years of age or younger since the amount of the drug contained in the tablets exceeds the recommended dosage in this age group.

Nitazoxanide powder for oral suspension should be reconstituted at the time of dispensing by adding 48 mL of water to provide a suspension containing 100 mg/5 mL. After tapping the bottle gently to loosen the powder, the water should be added in 2 portions, and the suspension shaken vigorously after each addition.

Reconstituted nitazoxanide oral suspension may be stored for up to 7 days at room temperature; any unused portion should be discarded after that time.

Prior to administration of each dose, the oral suspension should be shaken well.

● *Dosage*

Nitazoxanide tablets and oral suspension are not bioequivalent. Bioavailability of the oral suspension is 70% relative to that of the tablet.

Adult Dosage

Cryptosporidiosis

For the treatment of diarrhea caused by *Cryptosporidium parvum* in immunocompetent adults, the usual dosage of nitazoxanide (as tablets or oral suspension) is 500 mg every 12 hours for 3 days.

If nitazoxanide is used for the treatment of cryptosporidiosis in adults with human immunodeficiency virus (HIV) infection† who are receiving an optimized antiretroviral regimen, the US Centers for Disease Control and Prevention (CDC), National Institutes of Health (NIH), and HIV Medicine Association of the Infectious Diseases Society of America (IDSA) recommend a dosage of 0.5–1 g twice daily for 14 days.

Giardiasis

For the treatment of diarrhea caused by *Giardia intestinalis* (also known as *G. lamblia* or *G. duodenalis*) in immunocompetent adults, the recommended dosage of nitazoxanide (as tablets or oral suspension) is 500 mg every 12 hours for 3 days.

Cestode (Tapeworm) Infections

For the treatment of hymenolepiasis caused by *Hymenolepis. nana*† (dwarf tapeworm) in adults, some clinicians recommend a nitazoxanide dosage of 500 mg twice daily for 3 days.

Trematode (Fluke) Infections

If nitazoxanide is used as an alternative for the treatment of fascioliasis caused by *Fasciola hepatica*† (sheep liver fluke) in adults, some clinicians recommend a dosage of 500 mg twice daily for 7 days.

Pediatric Dosage

Cryptosporidiosis

For the treatment of diarrhea caused by *C. parvum* in immunocompetent children, the recommended dosage of nitazoxanide (as oral suspension) is 100 mg every 12 hours for 3 days for those 1–3 years of age or 200 mg every 12 hours for 3 days for those 4–11 years of age.

For the treatment of diarrhea caused by *C. parvum* in immunocompetent adolescents 12 years of age or older, the usual dosage of nitazoxanide (as tablets or oral suspension) is 500 mg every 12 hours for 3 days.

If nitazoxanide is used for the treatment of cryptosporidiosis in HIV-infected pediatric patients† who are receiving an optimized antiretroviral regimen, CDC, NIH, and IDSA recommend a dosage of 100 mg twice daily in those 1–3 years of age, 200 mg twice daily in those 4–11 years of age, and 500 mg twice daily in those 12 years of age or older. The recommended duration of nitazoxanide treatment in these HIV-infected patients is 3–14 days.

Giardiasis

For the treatment of diarrhea caused by *Giardia* in immunocompetent children, the recommended dosage of nitazoxanide (as oral suspension) is 100 mg every 12 hours for 3 days for those 1–3 years of age or 200 mg every 12 hours for 3 days for those 4–11 years of age.

For the treatment of diarrhea caused by *Giardia* in immunocompetent adolescents 12 years of age or older, the recommended dosage of nitazoxanide (as tablets or oral suspension) is 500 mg every 12 hours for 3 days.

If nitazoxanide is used for the treatment of giardiasis in HIV-infected pediatric patients†, CDC, NIH, and IDSA recommend a dosage of 100 mg every 12 hours in those 1–3 years of age, 200 mg every 12 hours in those 4–11 years of age, and 500 mg every 12 hours in those 12 years of age or older. The recommended duration of nitazoxanide treatment is 3 days.

Isosporiasis (Cystoisosporiasis)

If nitazoxanide is used for the treatment of infections caused by *Isospora belli* (*Cystoisospora belli*) in HIV-infected pediatric patients†, CDC, NIH, and IDSA recommend a dosage of 100 mg every 12 hours in those 1–3 years of age, 200 mg every 12 hours in those 4–11 years of age, and 500 mg every 12 hours in those 12 years of age or older. The recommended duration of nitazoxanide treatment in HIV-infected patients is 3 days.

Cestode (Tapeworm) Infections

For the treatment of hymenolepiasis caused by *H. nana*† (dwarf tapeworm) in pediatric patients, some clinicians recommend a nitazoxanide dosage of 100 mg twice daily in those 1–3 years of age, 200 mg twice daily in those 4–11 years of age, and 500 mg twice daily in those 12 years of age or older. The recommended duration of treatment is 3 days.

Nematode (Roundworm) Infections

For the treatment of ascariasis† caused by *Ascaris lumbricoides* in pediatric patients, some clinicians recommend a nitazoxanide dosage of 100 mg twice daily in those 1–3 years of age, 200 mg twice daily in those 4–11 years of age, and 500 mg twice daily in those 12 years of age or older. The recommended duration of treatment is 3 days.

For the treatment of trichuriasis† caused by *Trichuris trichiura* (whipworm) in pediatric patients, some clinicians recommend a nitazoxanide dosage of 100 mg twice daily for 3 days in those 1–3 years of age and 200 mg twice daily for 3 days in those 4–11 years of age.

Trematode (Fluke) Infections

If nitazoxanide is used as an alternative for the treatment of fascioliasis caused by *F. hepatica*† (sheep liver fluke) in pediatric patients, some clinicians recommend a dosage of 100 mg twice daily in those 1–3 years of age, 200 mg twice daily in those 4–11 years of age, and 500 mg twice daily in those 12 years of age or older. The recommended duration of treatment is 7 days.

CAUTIONS

● Contraindications

Nitazoxanide is contraindicated in patients hypersensitive to the drug or any ingredient in the formulation.

● Warnings/Precautions

General Precautions

Immunodeficiency

Nitazoxanide has not been shown to be more effective than placebo for the treatment of diarrhea caused by *Cryptosporidium parvum* in immunodeficient individuals, including those with human immunodeficiency virus (HIV) infection.

Nitazoxanide has not been evaluated for the treatment of diarrhea caused by *Giardia* in HIV-infected or other immunodeficient individuals.

Specific Populations

Pregnancy

Data are not available on use of nitazoxanide in pregnant women to inform a drug-associated risk.

In animal reproduction studies, there was no evidence of teratogenicity or fetotoxicity in rats or rabbits when nitazoxanide was given during organogenesis at exposures 30 or 2 times, respectively, the human exposure at the recommended human dosage of 500 mg twice daily based on body surface area.

Lactation

It is not known whether nitazoxanide is distributed into human milk, affects milk production, or affects a breast-fed child.

The developmental and health benefits of breast-feeding should be considered along with the mother's clinical need for nitazoxanide and potential adverse effects on the breast-fed infant from the drug or from the underlying maternal condition.

Pediatric Use

Safety and efficacy of nitazoxanide have not been established in pediatric patients younger than 1 year of age.

Nitazoxanide oral suspension: Safety and efficacy for the treatment of diarrhea caused by *C. parvum* or *G. intestinalis* (also known as *G. lamblia* or *G. duodenalis*) in pediatric patients 1–11 years of age have been established based on results of 3 randomized, controlled studies. Safety and efficacy of the oral suspension for the treatment of diarrhea caused by *C. parvum* or *G. intestinalis* in pediatric patients 12–17 years of age have been established based on results of 2 randomized, controlled studies.

Nitazoxanide tablets: Safety and efficacy for the treatment of diarrhea caused by *C. parvum* or *G. intestinalis* have been established in pediatric patients 12–17 years of age based on results of 3 randomized, controlled studies. The commercially available 500-mg tablets of nitazoxanide should not be used in pediatric patients 11 years of age or younger since the tablets contain a greater amount of the drug than is recommended in this age group.

Geriatric Use

Clinical studies of nitazoxanide did not include a sufficient number of individuals 65 years of age and older to determine whether geriatric adults respond differently than younger individuals. The greater frequency of decreased hepatic, renal, and/or cardiac function and of concomitant disease or drug therapy in this age group should be considered.

Hepatic Impairment

Some clinicians suggest that nitazoxanide should be used with caution in patients with hepatic impairment. Pharmacokinetics of the drug have not been evaluated in patients with hepatic impairment.

Renal Impairment

Some clinicians suggest that nitazoxanide should be used with caution in patients with renal impairment. Pharmacokinetics of the drug have not been evaluated in patients with renal impairment.

● Common Adverse Effects

Adverse effects reported in 2% or more of patients receiving nitazoxanide include abdominal pain, headache, chromaturia, and nausea.

DRUG INTERACTIONS

● Protein-bound Drugs

The active metabolite of nitazoxanide (tizoxanide) is highly bound to plasma proteins and pharmacokinetic interactions with other highly protein-bound drugs are possible. Patients should be closely monitored for adverse effects if nitazoxanide is used concomitantly with highly protein-bound drugs that have a narrow therapeutic index (e.g., warfarin).

● Drugs Metabolized by Hepatic Microsomal Enzymes

In vitro studies indicate that tizoxanide does not inhibit cytochrome P-450 (CYP) isoenzymes.

● Warfarin

Concomitant use of warfarin and nitazoxanide should be avoided. If the drugs are used concomitantly, the patient should be closely monitored for adverse effects.

DESCRIPTION

Nitazoxanide is a synthetic nitrothiazolyl-salicylamide-derivative antiprotozoal agent. Nitazoxanide is rapidly hydrolyzed in vivo to tizoxanide, an active metabolite. Both nitazoxanide and tizoxanide have antiprotozoal activity against the sporozoites and oocysts of *Cryptosporidium parvum* and the trophozoites of *Giardia intestinalis* (also known as *G. lamblia* or *G. duodenalis*). The antiprotozoal activity of nitazoxanide may be related principally to its ability to interfere with the pyruvate:ferredoxin 2-oxidoreductase enzyme-dependent electron transfer reaction essential to anaerobic energy metabolism in susceptible organisms such as *C. parvum* and *Giardia*. Nitazoxanide and tizoxanide also are active against some other protozoa, including *Entamoeba histolytica*, *Trichomonas vaginalis*, *Cyclospora cayetanensis*, and *Isospora belli* (*Cystoisospora belli*).

Nitazoxanide is active against certain helminths, including some cestodes (tapeworms). Although the clinical importance is unclear, nitazoxanide is active in vitro against some anaerobic and microaerophilic gram-positive and gram-negative bacteria, including *Clostridioides difficile* (formerly known as *Clostridium difficile*) and *Helicobacter pylori*, and also is active against some viruses.

Following oral administration, nitazoxanide is rapidly hydrolyzed to tizoxanide (desacetyl-nitazoxanide) and tizoxanide then undergoes conjugation, primarily by glucuronidation. Peak plasma concentrations of tizoxanide and tizoxanide glucuronide usually are attained within 1–5 and 2–8 hours, respectively; nitazoxanide is undetectable in plasma. When nitazoxanide tablets or oral suspension is administered with food, the areas under the plasma concentration-time curves for tizoxanide and tizoxanide glucuronide are increased. Nitazoxanide tablets and oral suspension are not bioequivalent; the relative bioavailability of the oral suspension compared to that of the tablet is 70%. Tizoxanide is more than 99% bound to plasma proteins. The plasma half-life of nitazoxanide is reported to be 6 minutes. The median plasma half-lives of tizoxanide and tizoxanide glucuronide are reported to be 1.2–1.5 and 1.9–2.9 hours, respectively, following a single nitazoxanide dose of 0.5–1 g taken with food and 1.8–6.4 and 3.5–5.6 hours, respectively, following repeated nitazoxanide doses of 0.5–1 g taken with food. Tizoxanide is eliminated in urine, bile, and feces; tizoxanide glucuronide is eliminated in urine and bile. Approximately two-thirds of an oral dose of nitazoxanide is excreted in feces and approximately one-third of the dose is excreted in urine.

ADVICE TO PATIENTS

Advise patients that nitazoxanide tablets or oral suspension should be taken with food.

Advise patients using the oral suspension to keep the container tightly closed and to shake the suspension well prior to each dose. Inform patients that the oral suspension may be stored at room temperature for up to 7 days and any unused portion must be discarded after that time.

Importance of informing clinicians of existing or contemplated concomitant therapy, including prescription and OTC drugs, and any concomitant illnesses. Importance of avoiding concomitant use of warfarin.

Importance of women informing clinicians if they are or plan to become pregnant or to breast-feed.

Importance of informing patients of other important precautionary information. (See Cautions.)

PREPARATIONS

Excipients in commercially available drug preparations may have clinically important effects in some individuals; consult specific product labeling for details.

Nitazoxanide

Oral		
For suspension	100 mg/5 mL	Alinia®, Romark
Tablets	500 mg	Alinia®, Romark

† Use is not currently included in the labeling approved by the US Food and Drug Administration.

Table of Contents

10:00 ANTINEOPLASTIC AGENTS

§ Omitted from the print version of *AHFS Drug Information* because of space limitations. This monograph is available on the *AHFS Drug Information* web site, http://www.ahfsdruginformation.com. See the Preface for details on accessing this site.

Abemaciclib

10:00 • ANTINEOPLASTIC AGENTS

- Abemaciclib, a selective inhibitor of cyclin-dependent kinases 4 (CDK4) and 6 (CDK6), is an antineoplastic agent.

USES

● Breast Cancer

Adjuvant Therapy for Early-stage Breast Cancer

Abemaciclib is used in combination with an aromatase inhibitor or tamoxifen for the adjuvant treatment of hormone receptor-positive, human epidermal growth factor receptor type 2 (HER2)-negative, node-positive, early-stage breast cancer in adults who are at high risk for recurrence. Guidelines generally recommend abemaciclib as a treatment option (in combination with endocrine therapy) for hormone receptor-positive, HER2-negative, early-stage breast cancer in patients with a Ki-67 score of ≥20%, ≥4 positive axillary lymph nodes, or 1–3 positive axillary lymph nodes with additional high-risk features (e.g., grade 3 histology, tumor size ≥5 cm).

This indication for abemaciclib is based principally on the results of a randomized, open-label, two cohort, multicenter, phase 3 study (monarchE) in a cohort of female (any menopausal status) and male patients with hormone receptor-positive, HER2-negative, node-positive, resected early-stage breast cancer with clinical and pathological features consistent with a high risk of recurrence. In cohort 1, patients were required to have ≥4 positive axillary lymph nodes or 1–3 positive axillary lymph nodes and at least one of the following: grade 3 histology or tumor size ≥5 cm. Patients enrolled in cohort 2 could not meet the eligibility requirements for cohort 1 and were required to have 1–3 positive axillary lymph nodes and a Ki-67 score ≥20%. Patients with available untreated breast tumor samples were tested retrospectively at central sites using the Ki-67 immunohistochemistry (IHC) MIB-1 pharmDx assay to establish if the Ki-67 score was ≥20%. Eligible patients were randomized within 16 months of surgical resection to receive abemaciclib 150 mg twice daily in combination with the investigator's choice of standard endocrine therapy for 2 years. The primary measure of efficacy was invasive disease-free survival as defined by the Standardized Definitions for Efficacy End Points in Adjuvant Breast Cancer Trials (STEEP) criteria; an additional outcome was overall survival. In cohort 1, the median age of patients was 51 years (range: 22–89); 99% were women, 70% were white, 24% were Asian, 43% were premenopausal, 37% received prior neoadjuvant chemotherapy, 59% received prior adjuvant chemotherapy, and 96% received prior radiotherapy. Initial endocrine therapy included letrozole (39%), tamoxifen (31%), anastrozole (22%), or exemestane (8%).

At the time of the final analysis, patients in cohort 1 who received abemaciclib in combination with endocrine therapy had fewer invasive disease events compared with those receiving standard endocrine therapy alone (12.4 versus 18.5%; hazard ratio: 0.653). At the time of data analysis, a significant difference was noted for invasive disease-free survival in the intent to treat population, which was primarily attributed to patients treated in cohort 1. Invasive disease-free survival at 48 months was 85.5% in patients receiving abemaciclib in combination with endocrine therapy and 78.6% in those receiving standard endocrine therapy in cohort 1. The overall survival (OS) analysis for cohort 2 remains immature, but more deaths were observed in patients receiving abemaciclib in combination with endocrine therapy (10/253) compared to those receiving standard endocrine therapy alone (5/264).

Initial Therapy for Advanced Breast Cancer

Abemaciclib is used in combination with an aromatase inhibitor for the initial treatment of hormone receptor-positive, HER2-negative advanced or metastatic breast cancer in adults. Guidelines generally recommend CDK 4/6 inhibitors, including abemaciclib, in combination with an aromatase inhibitor for the first-line treatment of hormone receptor-positive metastatic breast cancer in men and postmenopausal women.

This indication for abemaciclib is based principally on the results of a randomized, double-blind, placebo-controlled phase 3 study (MONARCH-3) in postmenopausal women with previously untreated hormone receptor-positive, HER2-negative advanced or metastatic breast cancer. In this study, 493 patients were randomized (stratified by site of metastases and prior neoadjuvant or adjuvant endocrine therapy) in a 2:1 ratio to receive either abemaciclib (150 mg orally twice daily) in combination with an aromatase inhibitor (letrozole 2.5 mg or anastrozole 1 mg orally once daily) or placebo in combination with an aromatase inhibitor. Treatment was continued until disease progression, death, or unacceptable toxicity occurred or treatment was discontinued for other reasons. Cross over to the opposite treatment arm was not permitted. The primary measure of efficacy was progression-free survival as assessed by the investigator according to Response Evaluation Criteria in Solid Tumors (RECIST). In this study, the median age of patients was 63 years; 58% were white, 30% were Asian, 40% had de novo metastatic disease, 53% had visceral involvement, 22% had bone-only disease, 51% had received prior systemic therapy, and 39% had received prior chemotherapy. All patients enrolled in the study had a baseline Eastern Cooperative Oncology Group (ECOG) performance status of 0 or 1. Patients who had received prior therapy with a cyclin-dependent kinase (CDK) 4/6 inhibitor or everolimus were excluded from the study.

At the time of the interim analysis, patients receiving abemaciclib in combination with an aromatase inhibitor had a longer median progression-free survival than those receiving placebo in combination with an aromatase inhibitor (28.2 versus 14.8 months; hazard ratio: 0.54). Final analyses for progression-free survival at a median follow-up of 26.7 months showed that progression-free survival benefit was maintained in patients receiving abemaciclib in combination with an aromatase inhibitor compared with those receiving placebo in combination with an aromatase inhibitor (28.2 versus 14.8 months, respectively; hazard ratio: 0.54). The results of the final progression-free survival analysis based on an independent, blinded, central radiologic assessment were consistent with the investigator assessment. Among patients with measurable disease, patients receiving abemaciclib in combination with an aromatase inhibitor also had higher overall response rates compared with those receiving placebo in combination with an aromatase inhibitor (55.4 versus 40.2%). Overall response rate for abemaciclib- and placebo-treated patients at the time of the final analysis remained similar to the interim results. A subset analysis of progression-free survival based on site of metastases and prior endocrine therapy consistently showed progression-free survival benefit in patients receiving abemaciclib in combination with an aromatase inhibitor compared with those receiving placebo in combination with an aromatase inhibitor. Median overall survival had not been reached at the time of the interim analysis.

Previously Treated Advanced Breast Cancer

Abemaciclib is used alone or in combination with fulvestrant for the treatment of adults with hormone receptor-positive, HER2-negative advanced or metastatic breast cancer with disease progression following previous therapy. Guidelines state that abemaciclib must be used in combination with either an aromatase inhibitor or fulvestrant in men and postmenopausal women with hormone receptor-positive, HER2-negative advanced or metastatic breast cancer depending on previous exposure to endocrine therapy.

Combination Therapy

Abemaciclib is used in combination with fulvestrant for the treatment of hormone receptor-positive, HER2-negative advanced or metastatic breast cancer in adults with disease progression following endocrine therapy. A statistically significant progression-free survival benefit has been observed in women with previously treated, hormone receptor-positive, HER2-negative advanced or metastatic breast cancer receiving combined therapy with abemaciclib and fulvestrant compared with patients receiving placebo in combination with fulvestrant.

This indication for abemaciclib is based principally on the results of a randomized, double-blind, placebo-controlled phase 3 study (MONARCH-2) in women with hormone receptor-positive, HER2-negative metastatic breast cancer. Patients enrolled in this study had disease progression following prior endocrine therapy. In this study, 669 patients were randomized (stratified according to sensitivity to endocrine therapy and site of metastases) in a 2:1 ratio to receive either abemaciclib in combination with fulvestrant or placebo in combination with fulvestrant. Patients randomized to abemaciclib received 200 mg orally twice daily upon initiation of the study, but the protocol was amended to reduce the abemaciclib dosage to 150 mg twice daily following review of safety data and dosage reduction rates. All patients enrolled in the study received fulvestrant 500 mg IM on days 1 and 15 during cycle 1 followed by day 1 of each 28-day cycle thereafter.

Patients were treated until disease progression, unacceptable toxicity, or death occurred. Premenopausal or perimenopausal patients received goserelin acetate for at least 4 weeks prior to and during the study. The primary measure of efficacy was progression-free survival as assessed by the investigator according to RECIST. In this study, the median age of patients was 60 years; 56% were Caucasian, 20% had de novo metastatic disease, 56% had visceral disease, 27% had bone-only disease, 25% had primary resistance to endocrine therapy (defined as disease that relapsed during the initial 2 years of adjuvant endocrine therapy or disease progression within the initial 6 months of first-line endocrine therapy for metastatic disease), and 17% were premenopausal or perimenopausal. The majority of patients (99%) had an ECOG performance status of 0 or 1. Patients who had received chemotherapy for metastatic disease or prior therapy with a CDK4/6 inhibitor, fulvestrant, or everolimus were excluded from the study.

At a median follow-up of 19.5 months, patients receiving abemaciclib in combination with fulvestrant had a longer median progression-free survival compared with patients receiving placebo in combination with fulvestrant (16.4 versus 9.3 months; hazard ratio: 0.55). The results of the progression-free survival analysis based on an independent, blinded, central radiologic assessment were consistent with the investigator assessment. Among patients with measurable disease, patients receiving abemaciclib in combination with fulvestrant also had higher overall response rates compared with those receiving placebo in combination with fulvestrant (48.1 versus 21.3%). At a median follow-up of 47.7 months, patients receiving abemaciclib in combination with fulvestrant had a longer median overall survival compared with patients receiving placebo in combination with fulvestrant (46.7 versus 37.3 months; hazard ratio: 0.76). A subset analysis of progression-free survival and overall survival based on site of metastases and sensitivity to endocrine therapy consistently showed treatment benefit with abemaciclib and fulvestrant combination therapy compared with placebo and fulvestrant therapy. An additional analysis suggests that the clinical outcomes in a subgroup of 114 premenopausal women were consistent with the overall study population.

Monotherapy

Abemaciclib monotherapy is used for the treatment of hormone receptor-positive, HER2-negative advanced or metastatic breast cancer in adults with disease progression following endocrine therapy and prior chemotherapy for metastatic disease.

This indication for abemaciclib is based principally on the results of an open-label, noncomparative phase 2 study (MONARCH-1) in women with hormone receptor-positive, HER2-negative metastatic breast cancer. Patients enrolled in this study had received a taxane in any setting and 1–2 prior chemotherapy regimens for metastatic disease and had disease progression during or following prior endocrine therapy. In this study, 132 patients received abemaciclib 200 mg orally twice daily until disease progression or unacceptable toxicity occurred. The primary measure of efficacy was overall response rate as assessed by the investigator according to RECIST. The median age of patients was 58 years and 85% of patients were Caucasian. All patients enrolled in the study had an ECOG performance status of 0 or 1. The median duration of metastatic disease was 27.6 months; 90% had visceral disease and 51% had at least 3 sites of metastases. Approximately one-half (51%) of patients received one prior line of chemotherapy in the metastatic setting; 69% of patients received a taxane-based regimen and 55% received capecitabine. Patients who had received prior therapy with a CDK4/6 inhibitor were excluded from the study.

In this study, the investigator-assessed overall response rate was 19.7%; none of the patients achieved a complete response. At the time of data analysis, the median duration of response was 8.6 months. Effects of abemaciclib on overall response rate as assessed by an independent review facility and investigator-assessed overall response rate were comparable. At the time of the final analysis at a follow-up of 18 months, the median overall survival was 22.3 months.

DOSAGE AND ADMINISTRATION

● General

Pretreatment Screening

- Obtain baseline complete blood cell (CBC) counts and liver function tests.
- Verify pregnancy status in females of reproductive potential prior to initiation of therapy.

Patient Monitoring

- Monitor CBC counts and liver function tests every 2 weeks for the initial 2 months of therapy, monthly for the next 2 months, and then as clinically indicated.
- Monitor for signs or symptoms of interstitial lung disease or pneumonitis.
- Monitor for signs or symptoms of venous thromboembolism (e.g., deep-vein thrombosis, pulmonary embolism).

Dispensing and Administration Precautions

- Based on the Institute for Safe Medication Practices (ISMP), abemaciclib is a high-alert medication that has a heightened risk of causing significant patient harm when used in error.

Other General Considerations

- Premenopausal or perimenopausal women receiving abemaciclib in combination with fulvestrant or an aromatase inhibitor should be treated with a gonadotropin-releasing hormone (GnRH, luteinizing hormone-releasing hormone) agonist (e.g., goserelin) according to current standards of care.
- Men receiving combination therapy with abemaciclib and an aromatase inhibitor should be treated with a GnRH agonist according to current standards of care.
- Consult the respective manufacturers' labelings on the dosage, method of administration, and administration sequence of other antineoplastic agents used in combination regimens.

● Administration

Abemaciclib is administered orally without regard to food at approximately the same time each day. The tablets should be swallowed intact and should *not* be broken, chewed, crushed, or split.

If a dose of abemaciclib is missed or vomited, patients should not take an extra dose. The next dose should be taken at the regularly scheduled time.

Store abemaciclib at 20–25°C (excursions permitted to 15–30°C).

● Dosage

Breast Cancer

Adjuvant Therapy for Early-stage Breast Cancer

For the adjuvant treatment of patients with hormone receptor-positive, human epidermal growth factor receptor type 2 (HER2)-negative, node-positive, early-stage breast cancer with high risk of recurrence, the recommended adult dosage of abemaciclib is 150 mg twice daily in combination with an aromatase inhibitor (e.g., anastrozole, letrozole) or tamoxifen. Therapy should be continued for 2 years or until disease progression or unacceptable toxicity occurs.

Premenopausal or perimenopausal women receiving abemaciclib in combination with fulvestrant or an aromatase inhibitor should be treated with a gonadotropin-releasing hormone (GnRH, luteinizing hormone-releasing hormone) agonist (e.g., goserelin) according to current standards of care.

Men receiving combination therapy with abemaciclib and an aromatase inhibitor should be treated with a GnRH agonist according to current standards of care.

Initial Therapy for Advanced Breast Cancer

For the initial treatment of hormone receptor-positive, HER2-negative advanced or metastatic breast cancer in men or postmenopausal women, the recommended adult dosage of abemaciclib is 150 mg twice daily in combination with an aromatase inhibitor (e.g., anastrozole, letrozole). Therapy should be continued until disease progression or unacceptable toxicity occurs.

Premenopausal or perimenopausal patients receiving combination therapy with abemaciclib and aromatase inhibitor should be treated with a GnRH agonist (e.g., goserelin) according to current standards of care.

Men receiving combination therapy with abemaciclib and an aromatase inhibitor should be treated with a GnRH agonist according to current standards of care.

Previously Treated Advanced Breast Cancer

For use in combination with fulvestrant in the treatment of hormone receptor-positive, HER2-negative advanced or metastatic breast cancer in patients with disease progression following endocrine therapy, the recommended adult dosage of abemaciclib is 150 mg twice daily. Fulvestrant 500 mg is administered IM on days 1, 15, and 29, and then once monthly thereafter. Premenopausal or perimenopausal patients receiving combination therapy with abemaciclib and fulvestrant should be treated with a GnRH agonist (e.g., goserelin) according to current standards of care.

For use as a single-agent in the treatment of hormone receptor-positive, HER2-negative advanced or metastatic breast cancer in patients with disease progression following endocrine therapy and chemotherapy in the metastatic setting, the recommended adult dosage of abemaciclib is 200 mg twice daily.

Therapy should be continued until disease progression or unacceptable toxicity occurs.

Dosage Modification for Toxicity

Dosage interruption and/or reduction or discontinuance of abemaciclib therapy may be necessary based on severity of adverse reactions. The following table on Dosage Modifications for Abemaciclib Toxicity indicates the recommended dosage modifications for abemaciclib during monotherapy or combination therapy with fulvestrant or an aromatase inhibitor.

TABLE 1. Dosage Modifications for Abemaciclib Toxicity

| Toxicity Occurrence | Dosage Modification after Recovery from Toxicity | |
	Single-agent Abemaciclib (Starting Dosage = 200 mg twice daily)	Abemaciclib in Combination with Fulvestrant, Tamoxifen, or an Aromatase Inhibitor (Starting Dosage = 150 mg twice daily)
First	Restart at 150 mg twice daily	Restart at 100 mg twice daily
Second	Restart at 100 mg twice daily	Restart at 50 mg twice daily
Third	Restart at 50 mg twice daily	Discontinue abemaciclib
Fourth	Discontinue abemaciclib	

Hematologic Toxicity

For grade 4 hematologic toxicity, abemaciclib therapy should be interrupted until the toxicity improves to grade 2 or less. Upon resumption of therapy, the dosage of abemaciclib should be reduced. Hematopoietic growth factors (e.g., granulocyte colony-stimulating factor [G-CSF]) may be administered if clinically indicated; however, abemaciclib therapy should be withheld for at least 48 hours after the last dose of a hematopoietic growth factor and until the toxicity improves to grade 2 or less.

For the first occurrence of grade 3 hematologic toxicity, abemaciclib therapy should be interrupted; therapy may be resumed at the same dosage when the toxicity improves to grade 2 or less. If grade 3 hematologic toxicity recurs, abemaciclib therapy should be withheld again; therapy may then be resumed at a reduced dosage when the toxicity improves to grade 2 or less.

For grade 1 or 2 hematologic toxicity, no dosage adjustment is necessary.

Diarrhea

For grade 3 or 4 diarrhea or diarrhea requiring hospitalization, abemaciclib therapy should be interrupted until the toxicity improves to grade 1 or less. Upon resumption of therapy, the dosage of abemaciclib should be reduced.

For persistent grade 2 diarrhea lasting 24 hours or longer, abemaciclib therapy should be interrupted; therapy may be resumed at the same dosage when the toxicity resolves. If grade 2 diarrhea persists or recurs despite optimal supportive measures, abemaciclib therapy should be withheld again; therapy may then be resumed at a reduced dosage when the toxicity improves to grade 1 or less.

For grade 1 diarrhea, no dosage adjustment is necessary.

Hepatic Toxicity

For grade 4 serum aminotransferase (ALT and/or AST) elevations (i.e., exceeding 20 times the upper limit of normal [ULN]) or serum ALT and/or AST

elevations exceeding 3 times the ULN with total bilirubin concentrations exceeding 2 times the ULN in the absence of cholestasis, abemaciclib therapy should be discontinued.

For grade 3 serum ALT and/or AST elevations (i.e., exceeding 5 times the ULN, but no more than 20 times the ULN) with total bilirubin concentrations no more than 2 times the ULN, abemaciclib therapy should be interrupted until the toxicity improves to grade 1 or baseline. Upon resumption of therapy, the dosage of abemaciclib should be reduced.

For grade 2 serum ALT and/or AST elevations (i.e., exceeding 3 times the ULN, but no more than 5 times the ULN) with total bilirubin concentrations no more than 2 times the ULN, no dosage adjustment is necessary. If grade 2 serum ALT and/or AST elevations with total bilirubin concentrations no more than 2 times the ULN persist or recur, abemaciclib therapy should be interrupted until the toxicity improves to grade 1 or baseline. Upon resumption of therapy, the dosage of abemaciclib should be reduced.

For grade 1 serum ALT and/or AST elevations (i.e., exceeding the ULN, but no more than 3 times the ULN) with total bilirubin concentrations no more than 2 times the ULN, no dosage adjustment is necessary.

Interstitial Lung Disease/Pneumonitis

For grade 3 or 4 interstitial lung disease (ILD)/pneumonitis, abemaciclib therapy should be permanently discontinued.

For grade 2 ILD/pneumonitis, abemaciclib therapy may be continued at the same dosage. If grade 2 ILD/pneumonitis persists or recurs despite optimal supportive measures for up to 7 days, abemaciclib therapy should be interrupted until the toxicity improves to grade 1 or baseline. Upon resumption of therapy, the dosage of abemaciclib should be reduced.

For grade 1 ILD/pneumonitis, no dosage adjustment is necessary.

Venous Thromboembolic Event

For venous thromboembolic events of any grade in patients with early-stage breast cancer, interrupt abemaciclib therapy and treat as clinically indicated. When the patient is clinically stable, resume abemaciclib therapy.

For grade 1 or 2 venous thromboembolic events in patients with advanced or metastatic breast cancer, no dosage adjustment is necessary.

For grade 3 or 4 venous thromboembolic events in patients with advanced or metastatic breast cancer, interrupt abemaciclib therapy and treat as clinically indicated. When the patient is clinically stable, resume abemaciclib therapy.

Other Toxicity

For grade 3 or 4 adverse reactions, abemaciclib therapy should be interrupted until the toxicity improves to grade 1 or baseline. Upon resumption of therapy, the dosage of abemaciclib should be reduced.

For grade 2 adverse reactions, abemaciclib therapy may be continued at the same dosage. If grade 2 adverse reactions persist or recur despite optimal supportive measures for up to 7 days, abemaciclib therapy should be interrupted until the toxicity improves to grade 1 or baseline. Upon resumption of therapy, the dosage of abemaciclib should be reduced.

For grade 1 adverse reactions, no dosage adjustment is necessary.

Dosage Modification with Concomitant Drugs or Foods Affecting Hepatic Microsomal Enzymes

Concomitant use of abemaciclib with ketoconazole, a potent inhibitor of cytochrome P-450 (CYP) isoenzyme 3A (CYP3A), must be avoided; however, when abemaciclib is used concomitantly with *other* potent CYP3A inhibitors, the manufacturer recommends reducing the initial dosage of abemaciclib (200 or 150 mg twice daily depending on indication) to 100 mg twice daily or, in those already receiving a reduced dosage of abemaciclib (100 mg twice daily), further reducing the dosage of abemaciclib to 50 mg twice daily. When concomitant use of the potent CYP3A inhibitor is discontinued, the abemaciclib dosage should be returned (after at least 3–5 elimination half-lives of the CYP3A inhibitor) to the dosage used prior to initiation of the potent CYP3A inhibitor.

Patients receiving abemaciclib concomitantly with moderate CYP3A inhibitors should be monitored for signs of abemaciclib toxicity and dosage modifications for adverse reactions (see Table 1) should be considered.

• Special Populations

For patients with severe preexisting hepatic impairment (Child-Pugh class C), the manufacturer recommends reducing the dosage frequency from twice daily to once daily. No dosage adjustment is necessary in patients with mild or moderate preexisting hepatic impairment (Child-Pugh class A or B).

Dosage adjustment is not necessary in patients with mild or moderate renal impairment (creatinine clearance 30–89 mL/minute). The effects of severe renal impairment (creatinine clearance less than 30 mL/minute), end-stage renal disease, or dialysis on the pharmacokinetics of abemaciclib have not been established, and the manufacturer makes no specific dosage recommendations for such patients.

The manufacturer makes no specific dosage recommendations for geriatric patients.

CAUTIONS

• Contraindications

The manufacturer states there are no known contraindications to the use of abemaciclib.

• Warnings/Precautions

Diarrhea

Severe diarrhea, sometimes resulting in dehydration or infection, has occurred in patients receiving abemaciclib, generally during the initial month of therapy. Across 4 clinical studies, diarrhea was reported in 81–90% of abemaciclib-treated patients; grade 3 diarrhea occurred in 8–20% of patients. The median time to first occurrence of diarrhea was 6–8 days in patients receiving abemaciclib and the median duration of grade 2 or 3 diarrhea was 6–11 or 5–8 days, respectively. Temporary interruption or dosage reduction of abemaciclib was necessary in 19–26 or 13–23% of patients, respectively.

Patients receiving abemaciclib should be monitored for development of diarrhea and immediately treated as necessary with appropriate therapy (e.g., antidiarrheal agents, fluid replacement) at the first sign of loose stools. Temporary interruption, dosage reduction, or discontinuance of abemaciclib may be necessary depending on the severity of the diarrhea.

Neutropenia

Neutropenia, including febrile neutropenia and fatal neutropenic sepsis, has occurred in patients receiving abemaciclib. Across 4 clinical studies, neutropenia was reported in 37–46% of abemaciclib-treated patients; grade 3 or greater neutropenia occurred in 19–32% of patients. The median time to first occurrence of grade 3 or greater neutropenia was 29–33 days and the median duration was 11–16 days. Febrile neutropenia was reported in less than 1% of abemaciclib-treated patients. In the MONARCH-2 study, fatal neutropenic sepsis occurred in 2 patients receiving abemaciclib in combination with fulvestrant.

Complete blood cell (CBC) counts should be monitored at baseline, every 2 weeks during the initial 2 months of therapy, monthly during the next 2 months, and then as clinically indicated. Temporary interruption, dosage reduction, or discontinuance of abemaciclib may be necessary if neutropenia occurs during therapy with the drug.

Interstitial Lung Disease/Pneumonitis

Severe, life-threatening, or fatal interstitial lung disease (ILD)/pneumonitis has occurred in patients receiving cyclin-dependent kinases 4 (CDK4) and 6 (CDK6) inhibitors, including abemaciclib. In the monarchE trial evaluating abemaciclib in patients with early-stage breast cancer, ILD or pneumonitis occurred in 3% of patients receiving abemaciclib in combination with an aromatase inhibitor, grade 3 or 4 ILD or pneumonitis occurred in 0.4% of patients and 1 patient died. In the MONARCH-1, MONARCH-2, and MONARCH-3 studies evaluating abemaciclib in patients with advanced or metastatic breast cancer, ILD or pneumonitis occurred in 3.3% of abemaciclib-treated patients, and grade 3 or 4 ILD or pneumonitis occurred in 0.6% of abemaciclib-treated patients. ILD or pneumonitis resulting in death occurred in 0.4% of abemaciclib-treated patients. Cases of ILD or pneumonitis, including fatal cases, also have been reported during postmarketing experience in patients receiving abemaciclib.

Patients receiving abemaciclib should be monitored clinically and by radiographic imaging for manifestations of ILD or pneumonitis. If manifestations suggestive of ILD or pneumonitis (e.g., hypoxia, cough, dyspnea, interstitial infiltrates) occur, the possibility of other etiologies (e.g., infection, neoplastic) should be excluded. Temporary interruption, dosage reduction, or discontinuance of abemaciclib may be necessary if ILD or pneumonitis occurs during therapy with the drug.

Hepatic Toxicity

Hepatotoxicity has occurred in patients receiving abemaciclib. In the monarchE, MONARCH-2, and MONARCH-3 studies, grade 3 or greater elevations in serum ALT or AST concentrations were reported in 2–6 or 2–3%, respectively, of abemaciclib-treated patients. The median time to onset of grade 3 or greater elevations in AST concentrations was 71–185 days in abemaciclib-treated patients and the median time to resolution to less than grade 3 severity was 11–15 days.

Liver function tests (i.e., serum ALT, AST, and bilirubin concentrations) should be monitored at baseline, every 2 weeks during the initial 2 months of therapy, monthly during the next 2 months, and then as clinically indicated. Temporary interruption, dosage reduction, or discontinuance of abemaciclib may be necessary if hepatotoxicity occurs during therapy with the drug.

Thromboembolic Events

Venous thromboembolic events (i.e., deep-vein thrombosis, pulmonary embolism, pelvic venous thrombosis, cerebral venous sinus thrombosis, subclavian and axillary vein thrombosis, inferior vena cava thrombosis) have occurred in patients receiving abemaciclib. Venous thromboembolic events occurred in 2–5% of abemaciclib-treated patients across 3 clinical trials (monarchE, MONARCH-2, MONARCH-3). Fatal venous thromboembolic events have occurred in clinical trials. Abemaciclib has not been studied in patients with early-stage breast cancer with a history of venous thromboembolism.

Patients should be monitored for signs or symptoms of venous thromboembolic events, including pulmonary embolism. If a venous thromboembolic event occurs, patients should receive appropriate medical intervention. Interrupt treatment with abemaciclib in patients with early-stage breast cancer who develop a venous thromboembolic event of any grade and in patients with advanced or metastatic breast cancer who develop a grade 3 or 4 venous thromboembolic event.

Fetal/Neonatal Morbidity and Mortality

There are no adequate and well-controlled studies of abemaciclib in pregnant females; however, based on its mechanism of action and animal findings, abemaciclib may cause fetal harm. Embryofetal toxicity (e.g., decreased fetal weight) and teratogenicity (e.g., cardiovascular and skeletal abnormalities) have been demonstrated in rats receiving abemaciclib at exposure levels similar to the human exposure at the maximum recommended dosage.

Pregnancy should be avoided during abemaciclib therapy. The manufacturer recommends confirmation of pregnancy status prior to initiation of abemaciclib, and females of reproductive potential should be advised to use effective contraceptive methods during and for at least 3 weeks after discontinuance of the drug. Patients should be apprised of the potential hazard to the fetus if abemaciclib is used during pregnancy.

Specific Populations

Pregnancy

Abemaciclib may cause fetal harm if administered to pregnant females based on its mechanism of action and animal findings.

Verify pregnancy status prior to initiation of abemaciclib therapy.

Lactation

It is not known whether abemaciclib is distributed into human milk. Because of the potential for serious adverse reactions to abemaciclib in nursing infants, women should be advised to discontinue nursing during and for at least 3 weeks after discontinuance of abemaciclib therapy. The effects of the drug on nursing infants or on milk production are unknown.

Females and Males of Reproductive Potential

Results of animal studies suggest that abemaciclib may impair male fertility.

In a general toxicology study, degeneration of reproductive tissues, decreased reproductive organ weights, intratubular cellular debris, hypospermia, and tubular dilation were observed in male animals receiving abemaciclib at exposure levels as low as 0.02 times the human exposure at the maximum recommended dosage for up to 3 months. Additional animal studies did not find any adverse effects on mating or fertility among male animals receiving abemaciclib at exposure levels 2–3 times the human exposure at the maximum recommended dosage.

Pediatric Use

Safety and efficacy of abemaciclib have not been established in pediatric patients.

Geriatric Use

In the monarchE study, 15% of patients were 65 years of age or older and 2.7% were 75 years of age or older.

In the MONARCH-1, MONARCH-2, and MONARCH-3 studies, 38% of patients were 65 years of age or older and 10% were 75 years of age or older. No overall differences in safety and efficacy were observed between geriatric patients and younger adults. Grade 3 or 4 adverse reactions occurring in at least 5% of geriatric patients in MONARCH-1, MONARCH-2, and MONARCH-3 were neutropenia, diarrhea, fatigue, nausea, dehydration, leukopenia, anemia, infection, and elevated serum ALT concentrations.

Among patients 24–91 years of age, age did not appear to substantially affect systemic exposure to abemaciclib.

Hepatic Impairment

Following administration of a single 200-mg dose of abemaciclib, potency-adjusted total exposure to unbound drug and active metabolites in individuals with mild, moderate, or severe hepatic impairment (Child-Pugh class A, B, or C) increased by 1.2-, 1.1-, or 2.4-fold, respectively, compared with individuals with normal hepatic function; however, the mean elimination half-life of abemaciclib was prolonged by more than twofold in patients with severe hepatic impairment (55 hours) compared with individuals with normal hepatic function (24 hours). Dosage adjustment is required in patients with severe hepatic impairment.

Renal Impairment

Population pharmacokinetic analysis indicated that mild or moderate renal impairment (creatinine clearance 30 to less than 90 mL/minute) did not appear to substantially affect systemic exposure to abemaciclib.

Pharmacokinetics of abemaciclib have not been established in patients with severe renal impairment (creatinine clearance less than 30 mL/minute).

Abemaciclib has been shown to increase serum creatinine concentrations; however, it does not cause a clinically important change in glomerular filtration rate (GFR). Abemaciclib inhibits tubular secretion of creatinine by inhibiting renal organic cation transporter (OCT) 2, multidrug and toxin extrusion transporter (MATE) 1, and MATE2K. In clinical studies, the mean increase in serum creatinine concentrations was 0.2–0.3 mg/dL. Elevated concentrations of serum creatinine generally occurred during the initial month of therapy and were reversible after discontinuance of abemaciclib. The manufacturer states that parameters not based on serum creatinine concentrations (e.g., BUN or cystatin C concentrations, estimated GFR) may be considered to evaluate renal function.

● Common Adverse Effects

Adverse effects reported in 20% or more of patients treated with abemaciclib include diarrhea, neutropenia, nausea, abdominal pain, infections, fatigue, anemia, leukopenia, decreased appetite, vomiting, headache, alopecia, and thrombocytopenia.

DRUG INTERACTIONS

Metabolism of abemaciclib to the active N-desethyl (M-2), hydroxy-N-desethyl (M-18), and hydroxy (M-20) metabolites is mediated principally by cytochrome P-450 (CYP) isoenzyme 3A4.

Autoinhibition of abemaciclib metabolism via CYP3A4 has not been observed.

In vitro studies indicate that abemaciclib inhibits P-glycoprotein (P-gp) and breast cancer resistance protein (BCRP). Abemaciclib and its major active metabolites also inhibit organic cation transporter (OCT) 2, multidrug and toxic compound extrusion protein (MATE) 1, and MATE2K, but do not inhibit OCT1, organic anion transport protein (OATP) 1B1, OATP1B3, organic anion transporter (OAT) 1, and OAT3 at clinically relevant concentrations. In vitro, the drug is a substrate for P-gp and BCRP, but the drug and its major active metabolites are not substrates for OCT1, OATP1B1, or OATP1B3.

● Drugs and Foods Affecting Hepatic Microsomal Enzymes
Inhibitors of CYP3A

Concomitant use of abemaciclib with potent or moderate inhibitors of CYP3A may result in increased systemic exposure (area under the concentration-time curve [AUC]) of abemaciclib and its active metabolites and an increased incidence of adverse effects. When the potent CYP3A inhibitor clarithromycin (500 mg twice daily) was administered concomitantly with abemaciclib (single 50-mg dose) in healthy individuals, the potency-adjusted total AUC of unbound abemaciclib and its active metabolites was increased 2.5-fold compared with cancer patients receiving the drug alone. Simulations using physiologically based pharmacokinetic models suggest that the potent CYP3A inhibitor itraconazole may increase the potency-adjusted total AUC of unbound abemaciclib and its active metabolites by 2.2-fold; however, ketoconazole may increase the AUC of abemaciclib by up to 16-fold. Simulations using physiologically based pharmacokinetic models suggest that the moderate CYP3A inhibitors diltiazem and verapamil may increase the potency-adjusted total AUC of unbound abemaciclib and its active metabolites approximately 2.4- and 1.6-fold, respectively.

Concomitant use of abemaciclib with the potent CYP3A inhibitor ketoconazole *must* be avoided; however, when abemaciclib is used concomitantly with *other* potent CYP3A inhibitors (e.g., clarithromycin, itraconazole), the manufacturer of abemaciclib recommends reducing the initial dosage of abemaciclib (200 or 150 mg twice daily depending on indication) to 100 mg twice daily or, in those already receiving a reduced dosage of abemaciclib (100 mg twice daily), further reducing the dosage of abemaciclib to 50 mg twice daily. When concomitant use of the potent CYP3A inhibitor is discontinued, the abemaciclib dosage should be returned (after at least 3–5 elimination half-lives of the CYP3A inhibitor) to the dosage used prior to initiation of the potent CYP3A inhibitor.

If abemaciclib is used concomitantly with moderate CYP3A inhibitors, patients should be monitored for signs of abemaciclib toxicity and dosage modifications for adverse reactions should be considered.

Grapefruit products are CYP3A inhibitors and should be avoided because of the potential for increased systemic exposure of abemaciclib during concurrent use.

Inducers of CYP3A

Concomitant use of abemaciclib with potent or moderate inducers of CYP3A may result in decreased peak plasma concentrations and AUC of abemaciclib and its active metabolites and reduced abemaciclib efficacy. When the potent CYP3A inducer rifampin (600 mg daily) was administered concomitantly with abemaciclib (single 200-mg dose) in healthy individuals, the potency-adjusted total AUC of unbound abemaciclib and its active metabolites was decreased by approximately 70%. Moderate CYP3A inducers efavirenz, bosentan, and modafinil are predicted to decrease the potency-adjusted total AUC of unbound abemaciclib and its active metabolites by 53, 41, and 29%, respectively.

Concomitant use of abemaciclib with potent or moderate inducers of CYP3A should be avoided, and selection of an alternative drug with less CYP3A induction potential should be considered.

● Drugs Affected by Hepatic Microsomal Enzymes

A drug interaction study indicated that administration of abemaciclib 200 mg twice daily for 7 days in patients with cancer does not result in clinically significant alterations to the pharmacokinetics of CYP isoenzymes 1A2, 2C9, 2D6, and 3A4 substrates.

● Drugs Affected by Transport Systems

Abemaciclib and its active metabolites inhibit OCT2, MATE1, and MATE2K at clinically relevant concentrations. When a single 1-g dose of metformin (a substrate of OCT2, MATE1, and MATE2K) was administered with a single

400-mg dose of abemaciclib, peak plasma concentrations and AUC of metformin increased by 22 and 37%, respectively. Abemaciclib reduced the renal clearance and renal secretion of metformin by 45 and 62%, respectively.

● Anastrozole

Concomitant administration of abemaciclib and anastrozole did not affect the pharmacokinetics of either drug.

● Exemestane

Concomitant administration of abemaciclib and exemestane did not affect the pharmacokinetics of either drug.

● Fulvestrant

Concomitant administration of abemaciclib and fulvestrant did not affect the pharmacokinetics of either drug.

● Letrozole

Concomitant administration of abemaciclib and letrozole did not affect the pharmacokinetics of either drug.

● Loperamide

Concomitant administration of loperamide (single 8-mg dose) in healthy individuals receiving abemaciclib (single 400-mg dose) did not have a clinically relevant effect on the pharmacokinetics of abemaciclib and its active metabolites or loperamide.

● Tamoxifen

Concomitant administration of abemaciclib and tamoxifen did not affect the pharmacokinetics of either drug.

DESCRIPTION

Abemaciclib, a selective inhibitor of cyclin-dependent kinases 4 (CDK4) and 6 (CDK6), is an antineoplastic agent. Several mechanisms contribute to the dysregulation of the cell cycle during the G1 into S phase, including amplification or overexpression of the cyclin D oncogene or the loss of intrinsic CDK inhibitors (i.e., p16, p15, p18, p19, p21, p27, p57) in breast cancer. Abemaciclib specifically inhibits CDK4 and CDK6 and blocks the interaction of CDK4 and CDK6 with cyclin D, resulting in inhibition of phosphorylation of the tumor suppressor protein retinoblastoma and inhibition of progression of the cell cycle from the G1 into S phase. In vitro, abemaciclib has demonstrated decreased phosphorylation of retinoblastoma protein and reduced cellular proliferation of breast cancer cell lines by inhibiting the G1 into S phase of the cell cycle. The combination of abemaciclib with an antiestrogen agent or as a single-agent demonstrated reduced tumor volume in xenograft models of breast cancer.

Area under the serum concentration-time curve (AUC) and peak plasma concentrations of abemaciclib are dose proportional over a dosage range of 50–200 mg. Peak plasma concentrations of abemaciclib are achieved in a median of 8 hours following oral administration of the drug. Following repeated doses of abemaciclib twice daily, steady-state concentrations of the drug are achieved in 5 days and the mean accumulation ratio for the drug based on AUC or peak plasma concentration is 3.2 or 2.3, respectively. Oral administration of abemaciclib with a high-fat, high-calorie meal (approximately 800–1000 calories with fat accounting for over 50% of the caloric content) increases systemic exposure and peak plasma concentrations of abemaciclib and its active metabolites by 9 and 26%, respectively. Abemaciclib and its active metabolites are highly bound (more than 93%) to plasma proteins, albumin, and α_1-acid glycoprotein. Abemaciclib is metabolized principally by cytochrome P-450 (CYP) isoenzyme 3A4. The main circulating metabolites, M-2 (an N-desethyl metabolite), M-18 (a hydroxy-N-desethyl metabolite), and M-20 (a hydroxy metabolite) have been shown to be equipotent to abemaciclib, and these metabolites account for 25, 13, and 26%, respectively, of total plasma concentrations of the drug. In patients with advanced cancer, including breast cancer, CSF concentrations of abemaciclib and its active metabolites M-2 and M-20 are similar to unbound plasma concentrations. Following oral administration of a single radiolabeled dose of abemaciclib, approximately 81% of the radioactivity was recovered in feces (mainly as metabolites) and

approximately 3% was recovered in urine. The mean plasma elimination half-life of the drug is 18.3 hours.

Population pharmacokinetic analysis indicated that age (24–91 years), gender, and body weight (36–175 kg) do not have clinically important effects on the exposure of abemaciclib.

ADVICE TO PATIENTS

- Advise patients to swallow abemaciclib tablets whole and *not* to break, chew, crush, or split the tablets.
- If a dose is missed or vomited, importance of administering the next dose at the regularly scheduled time; an additional dose should not be administered to make up for a missed dose.
- Risk of diarrhea. Importance of informing patients that early identification and intervention is critical for the optimal management of diarrhea. Importance of informing patients how to manage diarrhea (e.g., oral hydration, antidiarrheal agents) at the first sign of loose stools. Importance of informing clinician if diarrhea occurs.
- Risk of neutropenia. Importance of promptly informing clinician if signs or symptoms of neutropenia or infection (e.g., fever) occur.
- Risk of severe, life-threatening, or fatal ILD/pneumonitis. Importance of informing clinician immediately if new or worsening cough, chest pain, or shortness of breath occurs.
- Risk of hepatotoxicity. Importance of promptly informing clinician if symptoms of hepatotoxicity (e.g., fatigue, anorexia, right upper quadrant pain, bleeding diathesis) occur.
- Risk of venous thromboembolic events. Importance of promptly informing clinician if any symptoms suggestive of a thromboembolic event occur (e.g., extremity pain or swelling, chest pain, shortness of breath, tachypnea, tachycardia).
- Risk of fetal harm. Necessity of advising females of reproductive potential to use an effective method of contraception during treatment and for ≥3 weeks after discontinuance of therapy. Importance of females informing clinicians if they are or plan to become pregnant. Apprise patient of potential fetal hazard if used during pregnancy.
- Importance of advising females to discontinue nursing during therapy and for >3 weeks after discontinuance of the drug.
- Importance of informing clinicians of existing or contemplated concomitant therapy, including prescription and OTC drugs (e.g., ketoconazole) and dietary (e.g,. ketoconazole, grapefruit products) or herbal supplements, as well as any concomitant illnesses.
- Inform males of reproductive potential that abemaciclib may impair fertility.
- Importance of informing patients of other important precautionary information.

PREPARATIONS

Obtain abemaciclib through designated specialty pharmacies and authorized distributors.

Excipients in commercially available drug preparations may have clinically important effects in some individuals; consult specific product labeling for details.

Abemaciclib

Oral		
Tablets	50 mg	Verzenio®, Lilly
	100 mg	Verzenio®, Lilly
	150 mg	Verzenio®, Lilly
	200 mg	Verzenio®, Lilly

† Use is not currently included in the labeling approved by the US Food and Drug Administration.

Selected Revisions August 24, 2023, © Copyright, October 16, 2017, American Society of Health-System Pharmacists, Inc.

Afatinib Dimaleate

10:00 • ANTINEOPLASTIC AGENTS

■ Afatinib dimaleate, a second-generation inhibitor of receptor tyrosine kinases, is an antineoplastic agent.

USES

● *Non-small Cell Lung Cancer*

First-line Therapy for Metastatic Non-small Cell Lung Cancer

Afatinib is used for the first-line treatment of metastatic non-small cell lung cancer (NSCLC) in patients whose tumors harbor nonresistant epidermal growth factor receptor (EGFR) mutations (e.g., exon 19 deletions [del19], exon 21 substitution [L858R]) mutations as detected by an FDA-approved diagnostic test. Nonresistant EGFR mutations are those where efficacy of afatinib may be predicted by a clinically meaningful reduction in tumor size at the recommended dosage of the drug and/or inhibition of cellular proliferation or EGFR tyrosine kinase phosphorylation is expected at the recommended dosage.

EGFR-activating mutations are present in approximately 15–22% of NSCLC cases in North America and Europe and are present in up to 30–50% of cases in patients of East Asian descent. The majority of EGFR mutations are exon 19 deletions and an L858R substitution in exon 21, which together account for about 90% of EGFR mutations in patients with NSCLC; less frequently occurring EGFR mutations are a heterogeneous group of molecular alterations within exons 18–21 (i.e., uncommon EGFR mutations), which exhibit variable responses to EGFR tyrosine kinase inhibitor therapy.

The current indication for afatinib in the first-line treatment of metastatic NSCLC is based principally on the results of a randomized, multinational, open-label phase 3 study (LUX-Lung 3) in adults with previously untreated EGFR mutation-positive locally advanced or metastatic (stage IIIB with pleural and/or pericardial effusion or stage IV) NSCLC. In this study, 345 patients were randomized (stratified by type of EGFR mutation and race) in a 2:1 ratio to receive either afatinib (40 mg orally once daily) alone or cisplatin (75 mg/m² by IV infusion) in combination with pemetrexed (500 mg/m² by IV infusion) once every 3 weeks (for a maximum of 6 cycles) until disease progression. The primary measure of efficacy was progression-free survival as assessed by an independent review committee (IRC); secondary end points included objective response rate (complete plus partial responses) and overall survival. The median age of patients was 61 years. The majority (72%) of patients were of East Asian ancestry. Patients enrolled in the study were required to have evidence of an EGFR mutation as determined by a standardized polymerase chain reaction (PCR) assay; the majority of patients had exon 19 deletions (49%) or exon 21 (L858R) substitution mutations (40%), while the remaining (11%) had other mutations.

At a median follow-up of 16.4 months, patients receiving afatinib had a longer median IRC-assessed progression-free survival compared with patients receiving combined therapy with cisplatin and pemetrexed (11.1 versus 6.9 months). Effects of afatinib on investigator-assessed progression-free survival and IRC-assessed progression-free survival were comparable. Patients receiving afatinib also had a higher objective response rate (50.4 versus 19.1%) and a longer median duration of response (12.5 versus 6.7 months) compared with those receiving combined therapy with cisplatin and pemetrexed. A planned subgroup analysis indicated that the magnitude of progression-free survival benefit from afatinib was greater in patients with common EGFR mutations (del19 and L858R) compared with those in the general study population; among patients with common EGFR mutations, the median IRC-assessed progression-free survival reportedly was 13.6 months in those receiving afatinib and 6.9 months in those receiving combined therapy with cisplatin and pemetrexed. No significant difference in overall survival was observed between patients receiving afatinib and those receiving combined therapy with cisplatin and pemetrexed at the time of final analysis. Another planned subgroup analysis indicated that the magnitude of progression-free survival and overall survival benefit in Japanese patients with common EGFR mutations was greater in those receiving afatinib compared with those receiving combined therapy with cisplatin and pemetrexed; however, no significant difference in overall survival was observed between treatment groups in Japanese patients with L858R mutations. In a pooled analysis of 3 clinical studies involving 32 patients with

uncommon EGFR mutations (i.e., S768I; S768I and G719X; S768I and L858R; G719X; G719X and L861Q; L861Q; L861Q and del19 mutations) receiving afatinib (40 or 50 mg orally once daily), responses were observed in 66% of patients. At the time of analysis, 52% of responders maintained a response for 12 months or longer and 33% had ongoing responses. In the LUX-Lung 3 study, approximately 10% of patients were long-term responders who received afatinib therapy for at least 3 years; baseline characteristics of these patients were similar to the overall study population except a higher proportion of long-term responders were female or had NSCLC harboring an *EGFR* del19 mutation. The median duration of treatment in long-term responders was 50 months, and median progression-free survival was 49.5 months.

In a randomized, open-label phase 3 study (LUX-Lung 6) evaluating afatinib or combined therapy with gemcitabine and cisplatin in 364 patients with previously untreated EGFR mutation-positive locally advanced or metastatic (stage IIIB with pleural effusion or stage IV) NSCLC in East Asia (i.e., China, Thailand, South Korea), patients receiving afatinib had longer IRC-assessed progression-free survival (11 versus 5.6 months), higher objective response rates (66.9 versus 23%) and disease control rates (92.6 versus 76.2%), and a longer median duration of response (9.7 versus 4.3 months) compared with those receiving combined therapy with gemcitabine and cisplatin. In a planned subgroup analysis of 86 patients 65 years of age or older, the median progression-free survival was substantially longer in patients receiving afatinib compared with combined therapy with gemcitabine and cisplatin (13.7 versus 4.1 months; HR of 0.16; 95% CI of 0.07–0.39); however, no substantial difference in overall survival was observed between patients receiving afatinib and those receiving combined gemcitabine and cisplatin. In the LUX-Lung 6 study, approximately 10% of patients were long-term responders who received afatinib therapy for at least 3 years; baseline characteristics of these patients were similar to the overall study population except a higher proportion of long-term responders were female or had NSCLC harboring an *EGFR* del19 mutation. The median duration of treatment was 56 months, and median progression-free survival was 55.5 months.

In a planned subgroup analysis of 134 patients 65 years of age or older, median PFS was prolonged in patients receiving afatinib compared with those receiving combined therapy with cisplatin and pemetrexed (11.3 versus 8.2 months; hazard ratio [HR] of 0.64; 95% confidence interval [CI] of 0.39–1.03). Although a trend toward overall survival was observed in older adults in the LUX-Lung 6 study and in those with tumors harboring common *EGFR* mutations in the LUX-Lung 3 study, overall survival was substantially prolonged in older afatinib-treated adults with NSCLC harboring an *EGFR* del19 mutation compared with those who received combined therapy with cisplatin and pemetrexed (41.5 versus 14.3 months; HR of 0.39; 95% CI of 0.19–0.80).

The safety and efficacy of afatinib compared with gefitinib was evaluated in a multinational, randomized, open-label, phase 2b trial (LUX-Lung 7) in 319 patients with previously untreated *EGFR* mutation-positive stage IIIB (ineligible for curative surgery or local radiotherapy) or recurrent or metastatic stage IV NSCLC. Median progression-free survival (11 versus 10.9 months) and time to treatment failure (13.7 versus 11.5 months) were prolonged in patients receiving afatinib compared with those receiving gefitinib. At a median duration of follow-up of 42.6 months, median overall survival was not significantly different between patients receiving afatinib and those receiving gefitinib (27.9 versus 24.5 months). In the LUX-Lung 7 study, approximately 12% of patients were long-term responders who received afatinib for at least 3 years. The median duration of treatment was 42 months, and median progression-free survival was 42.2 months.

A prospective, observational, phase II study evaluated a lower initial dosage of afatinib (30 mg daily) in 40 treatment-naive patients 70 years of age or older with *EGFR* mutation-positive stage IIIB or IV NSCLC. In this study, 19 patients required a dosage reduction to 20 mg daily. After a median follow-up duration of 17.6 months, the objective overall response was 72.5% and progression-free survival was 12.9 months. Median overall survival had not been reached at the time of analysis.

In a pooled analysis of 3 clinical studies involving 32 patients with nonresistant *EGFR* mutations (i.e., S768I; S768I and G719X; S768I and L858R; G719X; G719X and L861Q; L861Q; L861Q and del19 mutations) receiving afatinib (40 or 50 mg orally once daily), responses were confirmed in 66% of patients. At the time of analysis, responses were ongoing in 33% of these patients, and 52% of responders had a durable response of at least 12 months. Safety and efficacy of afatinib have not been established in patients whose tumors harbor resistant EGFR mutations.

Previously Treated Metastatic Non-small Cell Lung Cancer

Afatinib is used for the treatment of metastatic squamous NSCLC that has progressed following therapy with platinum-based chemotherapy.

The current indication for afatinib in the treatment of previously treated metastatic squamous NSCLC is based principally on the results of a randomized, multicenter, open-label, active-controlled study (LUX-Lung 8) in 795 adults with stage IIIb or IV squamous NSCLC whose disease progressed following a platinum-based doublet chemotherapy regimen for at least 4 cycles. Patients were randomized (stratified by geographic region) in a 1:1 ratio to receive afatinib (40 mg orally once daily) or erlotinib (150 mg orally once daily). Treatment was continued until disease progression, unacceptable toxicity, or study withdrawal occurred. The primary efficacy end point of the study was progression-free survival as assessed by an independent review committee according to Response Evaluation Criteria in Solid Tumors (RECIST 1.1); secondary end points included objective response rate and overall survival. The median age of patients was 64 years; the majority of patients were male (84%), 73% were Caucasian, 24% were of Asian ancestry, 95% were current or former smokers, 96% had squamous cell histology, and 3.5% had mixed cell histology. All patients enrolled in the study had an Eastern Cooperative Oncology Group (ECOG) performance status of 0 or 1.

At a median follow-up of 6.7 months, patients receiving afatinib had a longer median progression-free survival compared with patients receiving erlotinib (2.4 versus 1.9 months). At a median follow-up of 18.4 months, median overall survival also was prolonged in patients receiving afatinib compared with those receiving erlotinib (7.9 versus 6.8 months). The objective response rate was 3 or 2% in afatinib-treated or erlotinib-treated patients, respectively. Results of subgroup analyses (based on age, gender, ethnicity, response to first-line chemotherapy, interval between first- and second-line therapies, histology, smoking status, ECOG performance status, use of maintenance therapy) suggested that the effect of afatinib on progression-free survival and overall survival was consistent across all subgroups. Improved global health status and quality of life scores have been observed in a larger proportion of patients receiving afatinib compared with those receiving erlotinib (36 versus 28%). Afatinib substantially delayed the time to deterioration of dyspnea compared with erlotinib. No differences were observed between the treatment groups in time to deterioration of cough or pain.

Clinical Perspective

First-line Therapy for Metastatic Non-small Cell Lung Cancer

The American Society of Clinical Oncology (ASCO) and Ontario Health (OH; formerly known as Cancer Care Ontario) 2021 joint guideline specifically addresses treatment of stage IV NSCLC harboring driver alterations such as *EGFR* mutations. For patients with previously untreated stage IV NSCLC harboring sensitizing *EGFR* mutations (L858R/exon 19 deletion) and a performance status of 0 to 2, ASCO/OH states that afatinib monotherapy or the combination of erlotinib with a VEGF inhibitor (e.g., bevacizumab, ramucirumab) may be used when first-line treatment with osimertinib, dacomitinib, or gefitinib in combination with carboplatin and pemetrexed are not treatment options. Although progression-free survival benefit has been demonstrated with afatinib monotherapy or combination erlotinib therapy, overall survival benefit has not been demonstrated compared with first-generation EGFR tyrosine kinase inhibitors alone. For patients with previously untreated stage IV NSCLC harboring sensitizing *EGFR* mutations (L858R/exon 19 deletion) and a performance status of 3, monotherapy with an EGFR tyrosine kinase inhibitor may be offered based on access and toxicity. For patients with an activating *EGFR* mutation other than exon 20 insertion mutations, T790M, L858R, or exon 19 deletion (e.g., G719X, L861Q, and S768I), and a performance status of 0 to 2, who have not received systemic therapy, ASCO/OH states that clinicians may offer afatinib monotherapy, osimertinib, or standard treatment based on the ASCO/OH nondriver mutation guideline.

A 2021 Cochrane review on first-line treatment options for patients with *EGFR* mutation-positive NSCLC concluded that erlotinib, gefitinib, afatinib, and icotinib (not commercially available in the US market) demonstrate increased tumor response, prolonged progression-free survival, less toxicity, and greater quality of life compared to cytotoxic chemotherapy. The analysis also states that single agent tyrosine kinase inhibitor therapy remains the standard of care and the benefit of combining a tyrosine kinase inhibitor with chemotherapy remains uncertain. Cytotoxic chemotherapy is less effective for the treatment of NSCLC harboring *EGFR* mutations compared with erlotinib, gefitinib, afatinib or icotinib, and is associated with greater toxicity.

Previously Treated Metastatic Squamous Non-small Cell Lung Cancer

The ASCO guideline on systemic therapy for patients with stage IV NSCLC states that a recommendation for or against use of afatinib in patients with squamous cell carcinoma who are not eligible for further therapy cannot be made due to the minor survival gain compared with erlotinib and the potential benefit of therapy with immune checkpoint inhibitors.

● Other Uses

Afatinib also has been used for the treatment of malignant brain and central nervous system tumors† and pancreatic cancer†.

DOSAGE AND ADMINISTRATION

● General

Pretreatment Screening

- Confirm nonresistant *EGFR* mutation-positive (e.g., del19, L858R) NSCLC by an FDA-approved diagnostic test prior to initiating therapy.
- Verify pregnancy status in females of reproductive potential prior to initiating therapy.

Patient Monitoring

- Periodically monitor liver function.
- Monitor for diarrhea.

● Administration

Administer orally once daily. Administer on an empty stomach, at least 1 hour before or 2 hours after a meal.

If a dose of afatinib is missed, the prescribed dose should be taken as soon as possible unless the next dose is within 12 hours; an additional dose should not be administered to replace the missed dose.

Store at 25°C (excursions permitted between 15–30°C). Store in original container and protect from excessive humidity and light.

● Dosage

Dosage of afatinib dimaleate is expressed in terms of afatinib.

Non-small Cell Lung Cancer

For the first-line treatment of metastatic NSCLC in patients whose tumors harbor nonresistant EGFR mutations (e.g., exon 19 deletions or exon 21 substitution [L858R] mutations), the recommended dosage of afatinib in adults is 40 mg once daily. Therapy should be continued until disease progression or unacceptable toxicity occurs. In the LUX-Lung 3 study, afatinib therapy was continued for a median of 11 months. Approximately one-half (53.3%) of patients required dosage reductions within the initial 6 months of therapy; however, median progression-free survival was similar among patients who received a dosage reduction and those who received the recommended dosage.

For the treatment of metastatic squamous NSCLC that has progressed following therapy with platinum-based chemotherapy, the recommended dosage of afatinib in adults is 40 mg once daily. Therapy should be continued until disease progression or unacceptable toxicity occurs. In the LUX-Lung 8 study, afatinib therapy was continued for a median of 2.1 months.

Dosage Modification

If adverse effects occur during afatinib therapy, temporary interruption of therapy, dosage reduction, and/or permanent discontinuance of the drug may be necessary.

Permanently discontinue afatinib in patients who develop life-threatening bullous, blistering, or exfoliative skin lesions; interstitial lung disease; severe drug-induced hepatic impairment; GI perforation; persistent ulcerative keratitis; or symptomatic left ventricular dysfunction. The drug also should be permanently discontinued in patients who experience severe or intolerable adverse reactions to an afatinib dosage of 20 mg daily.

Grade 3 or 4 Toxicity

If grade 3 or 4 toxicity occurs, interrupt afatinib therapy. When the toxicity resolves completely or improves to grade 1, resume afatinib at a reduced dosage (i.e., 10 mg less than the daily dosage used prior to the event).

Diarrhea

If grade 2 diarrhea persists for 2 or more consecutive days despite anti-diarrheal therapy or grade 3 or greater diarrhea occurs, interrupt afatinib therapy. When diarrhea improves to grade 1 or less, resume afatinib at a reduced dosage (i.e., 10 mg less than the daily dosage used prior to the event).

Dermatologic Toxicity

If intolerable or prolonged (lasting more than 7 days) grade 2 cutaneous reactions or grade 3 cutaneous reactions occur, interrupt afatinib therapy. When the cutaneous reaction improves to grade 1 or less, resume afatinib at a reduced dosage (i.e., 10 mg less than the daily dosage used prior to the event).

If life-threatening bullous, blistering, or exfoliating lesions occur, permanently discontinue afatinib.

Concomitant Use with Drugs Affecting the P-glycoprotein Transport System

If afatinib is used concomitantly with an inhibitor of P-glycoprotein (P-gp), reduce daily dosage of afatinib by 10 mg daily if not tolerated. If concomitant use of the P-gp inhibitor is discontinued, the afatinib dosage should be returned to the dosage used prior to initiation of the P-gp inhibitor as tolerated.

If afatinib is used concomitantly with an inducer of P-gp, increase daily dosage of afatinib by 10 mg daily as tolerated. If concomitant use of the P-gp inducer is discontinued, return the afatinib dosage (2–3 days following discontinuance of the P-gp inducer) to the dosage used prior to initiation of the P-gp inducer.

● Special Populations

Hepatic Impairment

No initial dosage adjustment is necessary in patients with mild or moderate hepatic impairment (Child-Pugh class A or B). Closely monitor patients with severe hepatic impairment (Child-Pugh class C), and adjust dosage of afatinib if not tolerated. Afatinib has not been studied in patients with severe hepatic impairment.

Renal Impairment

For patients with severe renal impairment (estimated glomerular filtration rate [eGFR] 15–29 mL/minute per 1.73 m²), the manufacturer recommends a reduced afatinib dosage of 30 mg once daily. Dosage adjustment is not necessary in patients with mild or moderate renal impairment (eGFR 30–89 mL/minute per 1.73 m²). Afatinib has not been studied in patients with eGFR less than 15 mL/minute per 1.73 m² or in those receiving dialysis.

Geriatric Patients

The manufacturer makes no specific dosage recommendations for geriatric patients.

CAUTIONS

● Contraindications

The manufacturer states there are no known contraindications to the use of afatinib.

● Warnings/Precautions

Diarrhea

Diarrhea, resulting in dehydration with or without renal impairment, has been reported in patients receiving afatinib; some of these cases were fatal. In clinical studies, grade 3 or 4 diarrhea was reported in 16% of patients receiving afatinib. In the LUX-Lung 3 study in patients with previously untreated metastatic non-small cell lung cancer (NSCLC), diarrhea was reported in 96% of patients receiving afatinib and was grade 3 in 15% of patients; diarrhea occurred within the first 6 weeks of therapy. In the LUX-Lung 8 study in patients with previously treated

metastatic squamous NSCLC, diarrhea was reported in 75% of patients receiving afatinib and was grade 3 or 4 in 10 or 0.8%, respectively, of patients. In the LUX-Lung 3 and LUX-Lung 8 studies, renal impairment secondary to diarrhea was reported in 6 and 7% of patients receiving afatinib, respectively, and was grade 3 in 1.3 and 2%, respectively, of patients.

Although the mechanism for development of diarrhea has not been fully determined, an increased incidence and greater severity of diarrhea have been observed with second-generation pan-human epidermal growth factor receptor (pan-HER) inhibitors (e.g., afatinib, dacomitinib) compared with single-target tyrosine kinase inhibitors selective for epidermal growth factor receptor (EGFR) (e.g., erlotinib, gefitinib); therefore, it has been suggested that other members of the HER tyrosine kinase family may have an essential role in the development of diarrhea.

If persistent or severe diarrhea occurs, temporary interruption of therapy followed by dosage reduction may be required. Antidiarrheal therapy (e.g., loperamide) should be provided for subsequent home use by the patient as needed. Patients should be advised to take an antidiarrheal agent at the onset of diarrhea and to continue antidiarrheal therapy until loose bowel movements have ceased for 12 hours.

Dermatologic Effects

Cutaneous reactions have been reported frequently in patients receiving afatinib. Grade 3 cutaneous reactions (characterized by bullous, blistering, and exfoliating lesions) occurred in 0.2% of 4257 patients receiving afatinib across clinical trials. In the LUX-Lung 3 study in patients with previously untreated metastatic NSCLC, cutaneous reactions (i.e., rash, erythema, acneiform rash) were reported in 90% of patients receiving afatinib, and grade 3 cutaneous reactions were reported in 16% of patients. In the LUX-Lung 8 study in patients with previously treated metastatic squamous NSCLC, cutaneous reactions were reported in 70% of patients receiving afatinib, and grade 3 cutaneous reactions were reported in 7% of patients. In the LUX-Lung 3 and LUX-Lung 8 studies, grade 1–3 palmar-plantar erythrodysesthesia (hand-foot syndrome) was reported in 7 and 1.5%, respectively, of patients receiving afatinib.

Management of afatinib-associated rash may include use of topical or systemic corticosteroids, anti-infectives, or antihistamines. If persistent or severe cutaneous reactions occur, temporary interruption of therapy followed by dosage reduction may be required. Afatinib should be permanently discontinued in patients who develop life-threatening bullous, blistering, or exfoliating lesions.

Toxic epidermal necrolysis and Stevens-Johnson syndrome have been reported during postmarketing experience in patients receiving afatinib. Toxic epidermal necrolysis and Stevens-Johnson syndrome bullous cutaneous reactions have occurred from a distinct and separate mechanism of toxicity than bullous lesions secondary to inhibition of EGFR. If toxic epidermal necrolysis or Stevens-Johnson syndrome is suspected, afatinib should be discontinued.

Pulmonary Effects

Interstitial lung disease or interstitial lung disease-like events (e.g., lung infiltration, pneumonitis, acute respiratory distress syndrome [ARDS], allergic alveolitis) occurred in 1.6% of 4257 patients receiving afatinib across clinical trials; fatal interstitial lung disease occurred in 0.4% of patients receiving the drug. In the LUX-Lung 3 study in patients with previously untreated metastatic NSCLC, grade 3 or greater interstitial lung disease was reported in 1.3% of patients receiving afatinib and was fatal in 1% of patients. In the LUX-Lung 8 study in patients with previously treated metastatic squamous NSCLC, grade 3 or greater interstitial lung disease was reported in 0.9% of patients receiving afatinib and was fatal in 0.8% of patients. The incidence of interstitial lung disease appears to be higher in Asian patients (2.3%) compared with Caucasian patients (1%).

If interstitial lung disease is suspected, afatinib therapy should be interrupted. If a diagnosis of interstitial lung disease is confirmed, afatinib should be permanently discontinued.

Hepatic Toxicity

Abnormal liver function tests were reported in 9.7% of 4257 patients receiving afatinib across clinical trials; fatal hepatic toxicity occurred in 0.2% of patients receiving the drug. In the LUX-Lung 3 study in patients with previously untreated metastatic NSCLC, liver function test abnormalities of any grade were reported in 17.5% of patients receiving afatinib, and were grade 3 or 4 in 3.5% of patients. In the LUX-Lung 8 study in patients with previously treated metastatic squamous

NSCLC, liver function test abnormalities of any grade were reported in 6% of patients receiving afatinib, and were grade 3 or 4 in 0.2% of patients.

Liver function tests should be performed periodically during afatinib therapy. Afatinib therapy should be temporarily interrupted in patients who develop worsening of liver function. Afatinib should be permanently discontinued in patients who develop severe hepatic impairment.

GI Perforation

GI perforation were reported in 0.2% of 3213 patients receiving afatinib across clinical trials. Factors that may increase the risk of GI perforation include increased age, history of GI ulceration, underlying diverticular disease or bowel metastases, or concomitant use of corticosteroids, nonsteroidal anti-inflammatory agents (NSAIAs) or anti-angiogenic agents.

Ocular Effects

Keratitis (characterized as acute or worsening eye inflammation, lacrimation, light sensitivity, blurred vision, eye pain, and/or red eye) occurred in 0.7% of 4257 patients receiving afatinib across clinical trials; grade 3 keratitis occurred in 0.05% of patients receiving the drug. In the LUX-Lung 3 study in patients with previously untreated metastatic NSCLC, keratitis was reported in 2.2% of patients receiving afatinib; grade 3 keratitis was reported in 0.4% of patients. In the LUX-Lung 8 study in patients with previously treated metastatic squamous NSCLC, keratitis was reported in 0.3% of patients receiving afatinib; grade 3 or greater keratitis was reported in none of the patients.

If keratitis is suspected, afatinib therapy should be interrupted; if a diagnosis of keratitis is confirmed, the potential benefit of the drug to the patient must be carefully weighed against the risks of continued therapy. Afatinib therapy should be temporarily interrupted or discontinued in patients with confirmed ulcerative keratitis; therapy should be permanently discontinued in patients with persistent ulcerative keratitis.

Afatinib should be used with caution in patients with a history of keratitis, ulcerative keratitis, or severe dry eye. Contact lens use is a risk factor for development of keratitis and ulceration.

Fetal/Neonatal Morbidity and Mortality

Afatinib may cause fetal harm if administered to pregnant women based on its mechanism of action and animal findings. Embryofetal toxicity (e.g., decreased fetal weight, abortion) and teratogenicity (e.g., skeletal alterations) have been demonstrated in animals. Females of reproductive potential should use effective contraception while receiving afatinib and for at least 2 weeks after the drug is discontinued. Patients should be apprised of the potential fetal hazard if afatinib is used during pregnancy.

Cardiovascular Effects

Left ventricular dysfunction has been reported in patients receiving afatinib. In the principal efficacy study in patients with previously untreated NSCLC, left ventricular dysfunction was reported in 2.2% of patients receiving afatinib compared with 0.9% of patients receiving combined therapy with cisplatin and pemetrexed. Afatinib therapy should be permanently discontinued if symptomatic left ventricular dysfunction occurs.

Afatinib does not appear to have substantial effects on the corrected QT (QT$_c$) interval. In an open-label, single-arm study evaluating potential effects of afatinib on the QT$_c$ interval, substantial (i.e., by more 20 msec) increases in the mean QT$_c$ interval were not observed in patients with relapsed or refractory solid tumors who received multiple doses of the drug (50 mg once daily).

Impairment of Fertility

Results of animal studies suggest that afatinib may impair female and male fertility; it is not known whether these effects are reversible.

In female rats, administration of afatinib at exposure levels approximately 0.63 times the human exposure at the recommended dosage resulted in decreased corpora lutea and increased postimplantation loss. In a general toxicology study, the effects of afatinib on reduced ovarian weights were not reversible at 2 weeks.

In male rats, administration of afatinib at exposure levels approximately equal to the human exposure at the recommended dosage resulted in reduced or absent sperm count; however overall fertility was not affected. In a general toxicology study, increased apoptosis in the testes and atrophy in seminal vesicles were observed.

Specific Populations

Pregnancy

Afatinib may cause fetal harm if administered to pregnant women based on its mechanism of action and animal findings.

Lactation

Afatinib is distributed into milk in rats; it is not known whether the drug is distributed into milk in humans or if the drug has any effect on milk production or the nursing infant. Because of the potential for serious adverse reactions to afatinib in nursing infants, women should be advised to discontinue nursing while receiving the drug and for 2 weeks after the drug is discontinued.

Pediatric Use

Safety and efficacy of afatinib have not been established in pediatric patients.

Geriatric Use

The LUX-Lung 3 study evaluating afatinib in patients with previously untreated metastatic NSCLC did not include sufficient numbers of patients 65 years of age and older to determine whether geriatric patients respond differently than younger adults. In subgroup analyses of 3 clinical studies, including LUX-Lung 3, evaluating afatinib as first-line therapy in patients with EGFR mutation-positive NSCLC, efficacy of afatinib in patients 65 years of age and older was consistent with that observed in the overall study population.

In the LUX-Lung 8 study evaluating afatinib in patients with previously treated metastatic squamous NSCLC, 53% of patients were 65 years of age or older and 11% were 75 years of age or older. In an exploratory subgroup analysis, afatinib reduced the risk of death by 5% in patients 65 years of age and older and 32% in those younger than 65 years of age. No overall differences in safety were observed between geriatric patients and younger adults.

Hepatic Impairment

Following administration of a single dose of afatinib, systemic exposure to the drug was not affected by mild or moderate hepatic impairment (Child-Pugh class A or B). Afatinib has not been studied in patients with severe hepatic impairment (Child-Pugh class C); therefore, such patients should be monitored closely.

Renal Impairment

Following administration of a single 40-mg dose of afatinib, peak plasma concentrations and systemic exposure of afatinib in individuals with severe renal impairment (estimated glomerular filtration rate [eGFR] 15–29 mL/minute per 1.73 m^2) were increased by 22 and 50%, respectively, compared with individuals with normal renal function; however, peak plasma concentrations of afatinib in individuals with moderate renal impairment (eGFR 30–59 mL/minute per 1.73 m^2) were similar to those in individuals with normal renal function but systemic exposure was increased by 22%. Dosage adjustment is required in patients with severe renal impairment. Afatinib has not been studied in patients with eGFR less than 15 mL/minute per 1.73 m^2 or in those receiving dialysis.

● Common Adverse Effects

The most common adverse reactions (≥20%) in patients receiving afatinib include diarrhea, rash/acneiform dermatitis, stomatitis, paronychia, dry skin, decreased appetite, nausea, vomiting, and pruritus.

DRUG INTERACTIONS

In vitro studies in human hepatocytes indicate that afatinib does not inhibit or induce cytochrome P-450 (CYP) isoenzyme 1A2, 2B6, 2C8, 2C9, 2C19, or 3A4. CYP-mediated mechanisms play a minor role in the drug's overall metabolism.

In vitro data indicate that afatinib is a substrate and inhibitor of the efflux transporters P-glycoprotein (P-gp) and breast cancer resistance protein (BCRP).

● *Drugs Affecting Hepatic Microsomal Enzymes*

Clinically important pharmacokinetic interactions with CYP inhibitors and inducers are unlikely.

● *Drugs Metabolized by Hepatic Microsomal Enzymes*

Clinically important pharmacokinetic interactions with drugs metabolized by CYP isoenzymes are unlikely.

● *Drugs Affecting the P-glycoprotein Transport System*

Inhibitors of P-gp

Concomitant use of afatinib with inhibitors of P-gp may result in increased systemic exposure to afatinib. When the P-gp inhibitor ritonavir (200 mg twice daily for 3 days) was administered 1 hour prior to afatinib (single 20-mg dose) in healthy individuals, area under the plasma concentration-time curve (AUC) and peak plasma concentrations of afatinib were increased by 48 and 39%, respectively. However, AUC of afatinib was not substantially affected when ritonavir (200 mg twice daily for 3 days) was administered concomitantly with or 6 hours following administration of afatinib (single 40-mg dose) in healthy individuals. If afatinib is used concomitantly with a P-gp inhibitor (e.g., amiodarone, cyclosporine, erythromycin, itraconazole, ketoconazole, nelfinavir, quinidine, ritonavir, saquinavir, tacrolimus, verapamil), dosage of afatinib should be reduced by 10 mg daily if not tolerated. If concomitant use of the P-gp inhibitor is discontinued, the afatinib dosage should be returned to the dosage used prior to initiation of the P-gp inhibitor as tolerated.

Inducers of P-gp

Concomitant use of afatinib with inducers of P-gp may result in decreased systemic exposure to afatinib. When the potent P-gp inducer rifampin (600 mg once daily for 7 days) was administered concomitantly with afatinib, AUC and peak plasma concentrations of afatinib were decreased by 34 and 22%, respectively. If afatinib is used concomitantly with a P-gp inducer (e.g., carbamazepine, phenobarbital, phenytoin, rifampin, St. John's wort [*Hypericum perforatum*]), dosage of afatinib should be increased by 10 mg daily as tolerated. If concomitant use of the P-gp inducer is discontinued, the afatinib dosage should be returned (2–3 days following discontinuance of the P-gp inducer) to the dosage used prior to initiation of the P-gp inducer.

● *Antiangiogenic Agents*

Concomitant use of afatinib with antiangiogenic agents may increase the risk of GI perforation.

● *Antineoplastic Agents*

Cisplatin

In patients receiving a cisplatin-containing regimen concomitantly with afatinib, the pharmacokinetics of cisplatin were not substantially altered when cisplatin (50–100 mg/m² as a 1-hour IV infusion) was given 3 or 5 days prior to administration of afatinib (20–50 mg orally once daily).

Paclitaxel

In patients receiving a paclitaxel-containing regimen concomitantly with afatinib, the pharmacokinetics of paclitaxel were not substantially altered when paclitaxel (175 mg/m² as a 3-hour IV infusion) was given 3 days prior to administration of afatinib (20–50 mg orally once daily).

Fluorouracil

In patients receiving a fluorouracil-containing regimen concomitantly with afatinib, the pharmacokinetics of fluorouracil were not substantially altered when afatinib (20–40 mg orally once daily) was given 1 day after completion of fluorouracil IV infusion (750 or 1000 mg/m² infused over 96 hours).

● *Corticosteroids*

Concomitant use of afatinib with corticosteroids may increase the risk of GI perforation.

● *Nonsteroidal Anti-Inflammatory Agents*

Concomitant use of afatinib with nonsteroidal anti-inflammatory agents (NSAIAs) may increase the risk of GI perforation.

DESCRIPTION

Afatinib dimaleate, a second-generation inhibitor of receptor tyrosine kinases, is an antineoplastic agent. The drug covalently binds to the kinase domains of epidermal growth factor receptor (EGFR/human epidermal growth factor receptor type 1 [HER1]/ErbB1), HER2/ErbB2, and HER4/ErbB4, and irreversibly inhibits tyrosine kinase phosphorylation, resulting in downregulation of ErbB signaling. Some EGFR-activating mutations, including nonresistant mutations, increase autophosphorylation and activation, sometimes independent of ligand binding, of the tyrosine kinase receptor resulting in increased cell proliferation in non-small cell lung cancer (NSCLC) cells harboring these mutations. Nonresistant EGFR mutations are defined as kinase domain mutations in EGFR that lead to activation of tyrosine kinase activity and where efficacy of afatinib is predicted by a clinically meaningful reduction in tumor size at the recommended dosage of the drug and/ or inhibition of cellular proliferation or EGFR tyrosine kinase phosphorylation is expected at afatinib concentrations sustainable at the recommended dosage.

Although first-generation (reversible) EGFR tyrosine kinase inhibitors (e.g., erlotinib, gefitinib) have demonstrated improved outcomes in patients with NSCLC harboring EGFR mutations (e.g., EGFR exon 19 deletion [del19], exon 21 substitution [L858R]), secondary resistance to these agents eventually develops following 9–13 months of treatment. Clinical resistance to first-generation EGFR tyrosine kinase inhibitors has been attributed to several mechanisms, but development of the secondary T790M mutation in exon 20 appears to be the most common, occurring in 50–60% of patients who develop this resistance; this mutation results in production of a bulky methionine side chain in the receptor kinase domain of EGFR that is thought to sterically hinder the binding of first-generation EGFR tyrosine kinase inhibitors to EGFR. It has been suggested that second-generation EGFR tyrosine kinase inhibitors (e.g., afatinib, dacomitinib) may theoretically delay or prevent the emergence of secondary resistance through their irreversible inhibition of EGFR, more complete blockade of the EGFR signaling pathway (i.e., inhibition of EGFR as well as HER2/ErbB2 and HER4/ErbB4), and inhibitory effects against tumors harboring the T790M mutation. Afatinib has been shown to inhibit phosphorylation and in vitro proliferation of cell lines expressing wild-type EGFR and cell lines expressing del19 or L858R mutations, including other less common EGFR-activating (nonresistant) mutations. The drug also has been shown to inhibit in vitro proliferation of cell lines that overexpress HER2. Treatment with afatinib has resulted in inhibition of tumor growth in mice implanted with tumors overexpressing wild-type EGFR, HER2/ErbB2, or the EGFR L858R/T790M mutation. In vitro, afatinib appears to be approximately 100 times more potent than gefitinib against EGFR L858R/T790M EGFR mutations and as potent as lapatinib against HER2.

Following oral administration, peak plasma concentrations of afatinib are achieved within 2–5 hours. The area under the plasma concentration-time curve (AUC) and peak plasma concentration of afatinib increase in a slightly more than dose-proportional manner over a dosage range of 20–50 mg. The geometric mean bioavailability of 20 mg afatinib tablets is 92% compared to an oral solution. Steady-state concentrations are achieved within 8 days of repeated afatinib dosing. Administration of afatinib with a high-fat meal decreased the peak plasma concentration and AUC of afatinib by 50 and 39%, respectively, compared with administration in the fasted state. Cytochrome P-450 (CYP)-mediated mechanisms play a minor role in the drug's overall metabolism; however, in vitro data indicate that afatinib is a substrate for P-glycoprotein (P-gp) and breast cancer resistance protein (BCRP). In vitro, afatinib is approximately 95% bound to plasma proteins. Biliary and fecal excretion are the principal routes of elimination of the drug. Following oral administration of a single radiolabeled dose of afatinib as an oral solution (not commercially available in the US), 85% of the dose was recovered in feces and 4% was recovered in urine, mostly (88%) as unchanged drug. Following repeated administration of afatinib in cancer patients, the elimination half-life of afatinib was 37 hours.

ADVICE TO PATIENTS

● Importance of advising patients to take afatinib on an empty stomach, at least 1 hour before or 2 hours after a meal. If a dose is missed, instruct patients to take the missed dose as soon as it is remembered unless it is within 12 hours of the next scheduled dose, in which case they should not take the missed dose. Advise patients to not take 2 doses at the same time to make up for a missed dose.

- Risk of diarrhea; importance of advising patient about appropriate countermeasures to manage diarrhea. Importance of informing clinician if diarrhea develops and promptly seeking medical attention if severe or persistent diarrhea occurs.
- Risk of cutaneous reactions. Importance of limiting exposure to sunlight by wearing protective clothing and using sunscreen (minimum SPF of 15).
- Risk of interstitial lung disease. Importance of immediately informing clinician if new or worsening respiratory symptoms occur or if any combination of the following symptoms occur: difficulty breathing, shortness of breath, cough, and/or fever.
- Risk of hepatotoxicity and importance of periodic liver function test monitoring. Importance of immediately reporting any manifestations of hepatotoxicity (e.g., jaundice, unusually dark or "tea-colored" urine, right upper quadrant pain, fatigue, bleeding or bruising more easily than normal).
- Instruct patients to seek medical attention if severe abdominal pain occurs.
- Risk of ocular effects. Importance of immediately informing clinician if ocular problems (e.g., eye pain, swelling, redness, blurred vision, other vision changes) occur.
- Risk of left ventricular dysfunction; importance of immediately informing clinicians if new-onset or worsening shortness of breath, exercise intolerance, cough, fatigue, peripheral edema, palpitations, or sudden weight gain occurs.
- Risk of fetal harm. Necessity of advising females of reproductive potential to use adequate methods of contraception while receiving afatinib and for at least 2 weeks after the drug is discontinued. Importance of patients informing their clinicians if they are pregnant or think they may be pregnant.
- Risk of impaired female and male fertility.
- Importance of advising females to avoid breast-feeding while receiving afatinib therapy and for 2 weeks after discontinuance of therapy.

- Importance of informing clinicians of existing or contemplated concomitant therapy, including prescription and OTC drugs and dietary or herbal supplements, as well as any concomitant illnesses.
- Importance of informing patients of other important precautionary information. (See Cautions.)

For further information on the handling of antineoplastic agents, see the ASHP Guidelines on Handling Hazardous Drugs at http://www.ahfsdrug information.com.

PREPARATIONS

Afatinib is available only be obtained through specialty distributors. Consult the manufacturer's website for specific availability information.

Excipients in commercially available drug preparations may have clinically important effects in some individuals; consult specific product labeling for details.

Afatinib Dimaleate

Oral

Tablets, film-coated	20 mg (of afatinib)	**Gilotrif®**, Boehringer Ingelheim
	30 mg (of afatinib)	**Gilotrif®**, Boehringer Ingelheim
	40 mg (of afatinib)	**Gilotrif®**, Boehringer Ingelheim

† Use is not currently included in the labeling approved by the US Food and Drug Administration.

Selected Revisions April 15, 2022, © Copyright, June 30, 2014, American Society of Health-System Pharmacists, Inc.

Alectinib Hydrochloride

10:00 • ANTINEOPLASTIC AGENTS

■ Alectinib hydrochloride, an inhibitor of several receptor tyrosine kinases including anaplastic lymphoma kinase (ALK), is an antineoplastic agent.

USES

● Non-small Cell Lung Cancer

Alectinib is used for the treatment of metastatic non-small cell lung cancer (NSCLC) in adult patients whose cancer is anaplastic lymphoma kinase (*ALK*)-positive as detected by an FDA-approved diagnostic test. The drug has been designated an orphan drug by FDA for use in this condition. Alectinib is also used as adjuvant treatment in adults following tumor resection of *ALK*-positive NSCLC (tumors ≥4 cm or node positive), as detected by an FDA-approved test.

Clinical Experience
Treatment of Metastatic ALK-Positive NSCLC

The indication for alectinib in the treatment of *ALK*-positive metastatic NSCLC is based principally on the results of a multicenter, open-label, randomized phase 3 study (ALEX) in patients with previously untreated metastatic disease and 2 non-comparative phase 2 studies (NP28761 and NP28673) in patients whose cancer had progressed during crizotinib therapy.

In the ALEX study, 303 adults with previously untreated *ALK*-positive metastatic NSCLC were randomized (stratified by Eastern Cooperative Oncology Group [ECOG] performance status, race, and presence of brain metastases) in a 1:1 ratio to receive either alectinib (600 mg orally twice daily) or crizotinib (250 mg orally twice daily) until disease progression or unacceptable toxicity. The primary measure of efficacy was progression-free survival as assessed by the investigator according to Response Evaluation Criteria in Solid Tumors (RECIST 1.1); additional outcome measures included time to progression of brain metastases as assessed by an independent review committee (IRC), overall response rate, duration of response, overall survival, and IRC-assessed progression-free survival. Presence of *ALK* rearrangement was determined using an FDA-approved diagnostic test (e.g., Ventana ALK [D5F3] CDx assay). The median age of patients enrolled in the study was 56 years; 50% of patients were white, 46% were Asian, 56% were female, 63% had never smoked, and 92% had adenocarcinoma histology. Approximately one-half (40%) of patients had brain metastases at baseline and 35% of these patients had measurable brain metastases at baseline.

In the ALEX study, median IRC-assessed progression-free survival was prolonged in patients receiving alectinib compared with those receiving crizotinib (25.7 versus 10.4 months; hazard ratio: 0.53). Overall response rate (as assessed by the IRC) in patients receiving alectinib or crizotinib was 79 or 72%, respectively; complete response was achieved in 13 or 6% of patients receiving these respective treatments. At the time of analysis, 82, 64, or 37% of patients who responded to alectinib had durable responses of 6, 12, or 18 months or more, respectively, and 57, 36, or 14% of patients who responded to crizotinib had durable responses of 6, 12, or 18 months or more, respectively. Median overall survival had not been reached at the time of analysis. In the subgroup of 43 patients with measurable brain metastases at baseline, CNS overall response rate was 81 or 50% in patients receiving alectinib or crizotinib, respectively; complete response was achieved in 38 or 5% of patients receiving these respective treatments. At the time of analysis, durable responses of 12 months or more were observed in 59 or 36% of alectinib- or crizotinib-treated patients, respectively, with measurable brain metastases at baseline.

In the NP28761 and NP28673 studies, 225 adults (87 patients in the NP28761 study and 138 in the NP28673 study) with locally advanced or metastatic ALK-positive NSCLC (as detected by an FDA-approved diagnostic test) who had experienced disease progression during crizotinib therapy received alectinib (600 mg orally twice daily). Treatment was continued until disease progression, death, or unacceptable toxicity occurred or treatment was discontinued for other reasons. Most patients enrolled in both studies had received systemic chemotherapy prior to crizotinib therapy for NSCLC, and, among those with CNS metastases, most had received CNS radiation therapy. The primary efficacy end point in both

studies was the objective response rate according to Response Evaluation Criteria in Solid Tumors (RECIST 1.1) as assessed by an IRC. The objective response rate and duration of response in the CNS in patients with CNS metastases were key secondary end points. IRC-assessed objective response rates with alectinib therapy were 38 and 44% in the NP28761 and NP28673 studies, respectively, and investigator-assessed objective response rates were 46 and 48%, respectively; all responses were partial responses. The median IRC-assessed duration of response was 7.5 and 11.2 months in the NP28761 and NP28673 studies, respectively.

In the subgroup of 51 patients in both studies with baseline measurable CNS metastases according to RECIST 1.1 criteria, the CNS objective response rate with alectinib therapy was 61% (18% complete responses and 43% partial responses) and the median duration of CNS response was 9.1 months. CNS responses were observed irrespective of prior CNS irradiation.

Alectinib also was compared with chemotherapy in a randomized, multicenter, open-label, phase 3 (ALUR) study. In the ALUR study, 107 patients with advanced or metastatic *ALK*-positive NSCLC previously treated with 2 prior lines of systemic therapy (including a platinum-based doublet chemotherapy and crizotinib therapy) were randomized in a 2:1 ratio to receive either alectinib 600 mg orally twice daily or chemotherapy (pemetrexed 500 mg/m^2 IV every 3 weeks or docetaxel 75 mg/m^2 IV every 3 weeks). Treatment was continued until disease progression, death, or withdrawal. The median age of patients was approximately 56 years in the alectinib-treated group and 59 years in the chemotherapy-treated group; approximately 82% of patients were white, 47% were females, and 100% had adenocarcinoma histology. In the alectinib-treated group, 6.9% of patients were Asian and 48.6% had never smoked. In the chemotherapy-treated group, 20% of patients were Asian and 45.7% had never smoked. At baseline, CNS metastases were present in 65.3 or 74.3% of patients randomized to alectinib or chemotherapy, respectively; 59.6 or 57.7% of these patients, respectively, had received treatment for CNS metastases.

The primary end point in the ALUR study (investigator-assessed progression-free survival) was substantially greater in patients receiving alectinib compared with those receiving chemotherapy (9.6 versus 1.4 months; hazard ratio, 0.15; 95% confidence interval, 0.08–0.29). CNS objective response rate in patients with measurable baseline CNS disease also was substantially improved in patients receiving alectinib (54.2%) compared with those receiving chemotherapy (0%).

Adjuvant Treatment of Resected ALK-Positive NSCLC

The indication for alectinib in the adjuvant treatment of resected *ALK*-positive NSCLC is based principally on the results of an open-label, randomized, phase 3 study (ALINA) in patients who had completely resected, histologically confirmed stage IB (tumors ≥4 cm), II, or IIIA NSCLC with documented *ALK*-positive disease. Additionally, enrolled patients had to be eligible for platinum-based chemotherapy, an ECOG performance status of 0 or 1, and no prior systemic anticancer therapy. In ALINA, 257 patients were randomly assigned to alectinib 600 mg orally twice daily or IV platinum-based chemotherapy for 4 cycles, with each cycle lasting 21 days. Treatment with alectinib continued for 24 months or until disease recurrence, unacceptable toxicity, or withdrawal of consent, whichever first. The primary end point was disease-free survival, defined as time from randomization to the first documented disease recurrence, new primary NSCLC, or death from any cause. Overall survival was a secondary end point.

The median age of patients enrolled in the study was 56 years (range, 26-87 years); 42% of patients were white, 56% were Asian, 0.4% were Black or African American, 0.4% were Hispanic or Latino, 52% were female, 60% had never smoked, and 53% had an ECOG performance status of 0. In the ALINA study, alectinib therapy was associated with a significant improvement in disease-free survival as compared to chemotherapy The percentage of patients alive and disease-free at 2 years was 93.8% in the alectinib group and 63% in the chemotherapy group among patients with stage II or IIIA NSCLC. Overall survival data were not mature at the time of study publication.

Clinical Perspective

Approximately 60% of patients with lung cancer have driver alterations (e.g., mutations in *EGFR*, *ALK*, or *BRAF*; *ROS-1* fusions, *RET* fusions, *MET* exon 14 skipping mutations, and *NTRK* fusions). A relatively small subset of patients with NSCLC (approximately 3–7%) have *ALK*-positive disease, which indicates potential responsiveness to ALK inhibitor therapy (e.g., alectinib, brigatinib, ceritinib, crizotinib, lorlatinib). Patients with this form of lung cancer typically are nonsmokers or have a history of light smoking, are female, and are younger in age and often have adenocarcinoma histology.

First-line Therapy for Metastatic Non-small Cell Lung Cancer

The American Society of Clinical Oncology (ASCO) and Ontario Health (OH; formerly known as Cancer Care Ontario) 2021 joint guideline specifically addresses treatment of stage IV NSCLC harboring driver alterations such as *ALK* mutations. In a recent update, ASCO states that alectinib, brigatinib, or lorlatinib should be offered in the first-line setting in patients with stage IV NSCLC and driver alterations in *ALK*. ASCO also states that if alectinib, brigatinib, or lorlatinib are not available, ceritinib or crizotinib should be offered in the first-line setting.

Previously Treated Metastatic Non-small Cell Lung Cancer

In the second-line setting, ASCO states that alectinib, brigatinib, or ceritinib should be offered in patients who received initial therapy with crizotinib. ASCO also states that for patients who previously received other *ALK* inhibitors including alectinib or brigatinib, clinicians may offer lorlatinib.

Adjuvant Treatment for Early Stage Resectable Non-small Cell Lung Cancer

The International Association for the Study of Lung Cancer recommends that, at a minimum, determination of *EGFR* and *ALK* alteration status is required for patients under consideration for neoadjuvant or adjuvant systemic therapy. The Association recommends adjuvant alectinib for patients with stage IB (tumors ≥4 cm) to IIIA disease with *ALK* alterations. Adjuvant chemotherapy prior to alectinib may be considered at provider discretion.

DOSAGE AND ADMINISTRATION

● General

Pretreatment Screening

- Select patients for treatment of metastatic non-small cell lung cancer (NSCLC) with alectinib based on presence of anaplastic lymphoma kinase (*ALK*) rearrangement in tumor tissue or plasma specimens. If undetected in plasma specimen, test tumor tissue for *ALK* rearrangement, if feasible.

- Select patients with resectable tumors for adjuvant treatment of NSCLC with alectinib based on presence of *ALK* rearrangement in tumor tissue.

- Verify pregnancy status in females of reproductive potential.

Patient Monitoring

- Monitor liver function tests (e.g., ALT, AST, and total bilirubin) every 2 weeks during the first 3 months of therapy, then once monthly and as clinically indicated. More frequent monitoring may be necessary in patients who experience elevated serum aminotransferase and bilirubin concentrations.

- Monitor heart rate and blood pressure regularly. More frequent monitoring may be necessary as clinically indicated.

- Monitor serum creatine kinase (CK, creatine phosphokinase, CPK) every 2 weeks during the first month of treatment and as clinically indicated in symptomatic patients.

● Administration

Alectinib hydrochloride is administered orally twice daily with food. The capsules should be swallowed whole and should *not* be dissolved or opened.

If a dose of alectinib is missed or vomiting occurs after administration of a dose, take the next dose at the regularly scheduled time.

Do *not* store the capsules at temperatures above 30°C. Store in the original container to protect the drug from light and moisture.

● Dosage

Dosage of alectinib hydrochloride is expressed in terms of alectinib.

Non-small Cell Lung Cancer

The recommended adult dosage of alectinib for the treatment of *ALK*-positive metastatic non-small cell lung cancer (NSCLC) is 600 mg orally twice daily.

Alectinib therapy should be continued until disease progression or unacceptable toxicity occurs.

The recommended adult dosage of alectinib for the adjuvant treatment of *ALK*-positive resected NSCLC is 600 mg orally twice daily. Alectinib therapy should be continued for a total of 2 years or until disease progression or unacceptable toxicity occurs.

Dosage Modification for Toxicity

When dosage reduction is necessary, an initial dosage reduction to 450 mg twice daily is recommended. If further dosage reduction is necessary, the dosage should be reduced to 300 mg twice daily. If a dosage of 300 mg twice daily is not tolerated, alectinib should be discontinued.

Hepatic Toxicity

If an elevation in serum ALT or AST concentrations exceeding 5 times the upper limit of normal (ULN) occurs with a total bilirubin concentration of no more than 2 times the ULN, alectinib therapy should be withheld until liver function test results return to baseline values or decrease to no more than 3 times the ULN. Alectinib therapy may then be resumed at a reduced dosage.

If an elevation in ALT or AST concentrations exceeding 3 times the ULN occurs with an elevation in total bilirubin concentrations exceeding 2 times the ULN in the absence of cholestasis or hemolysis, therapy with alectinib should be permanently discontinued.

If an elevation in total bilirubin concentrations exceeding 3 times the ULN occurs, alectinib therapy should be withheld until total bilirubin concentrations return to baseline values or decrease to no more than 1.5 times the ULN. Alectinib therapy may then be resumed at a reduced dosage.

Interstitial Lung Disease/Pneumonitis

If treatment-related interstitial lung disease/pneumonitis of any grade occurs, alectinib therapy should be permanently discontinued.

Renal Toxicity

If grade 3 renal impairment occurs, alectinib therapy should be withheld until serum creatinine improves to 1.5 times the ULN or less. Alectinib therapy may then be resumed at a reduced dosage.

If grade 4 renal impairment occurs, alectinib therapy should be permanently discontinued.

Bradycardia

If symptomatic, but non-life-threatening, bradycardia occurs, therapy with alectinib should be withheld until recovery to asymptomatic bradycardia or to a heart rate of at least 60 beats/minute. If concomitant drugs known to cause bradycardia or hypotension are identified and the dosage of the concomitant drug can be adjusted or the drug can be discontinued, alectinib therapy can be resumed at the previous dosage upon recovery to asymptomatic bradycardia or to a heart rate of at least 60 beats/minute. If dosage adjustment or discontinuance of such concomitant drugs is not possible, or if no concomitant contributory drugs are identified, alectinib should be resumed at a reduced dosage upon recovery to asymptomatic bradycardia or to a heart rate of at least 60 beats/minute.

If life-threatening bradycardia or bradycardia requiring urgent intervention occurs in patients receiving concomitant drugs known to cause bradycardia or hypotension, therapy with alectinib should be withheld until recovery to asymptomatic bradycardia or to a heart rate of at least 60 beats/minute. If the dosage of the concomitant drug can be adjusted or the drug can be discontinued, alectinib therapy may then be resumed at a reduced dosage with frequent monitoring; alectinib therapy should be permanently discontinued in case of recurrence.

If life-threatening bradycardia or bradycardia requiring urgent intervention occurs in patients not receiving concomitant therapy with drugs known to cause bradycardia or hypotension, alectinib therapy should be permanently discontinued.

Creatine Kinase Elevation

If an elevation in serum CK concentrations exceeding 5 times the ULN occurs, alectinib therapy should be withheld until serum CK concentrations return to baseline values or decrease to no more than 2.5 times the ULN. Alectinib therapy may then be resumed at the previous dosage. If an elevation in serum CK concentrations exceeding 5 times the ULN *recurs*, alectinib therapy should be withheld until serum CK concentrations return to baseline values or decrease to no more than 2.5 times the ULN; alectinib therapy may then be resumed at a reduced dosage.

If an elevation in serum CK concentrations exceeding 10 times the ULN occurs, alectinib therapy should be withheld until serum CK concentrations return to baseline values or decrease to no more than 2.5 times the ULN. Alectinib therapy may then be resumed at a reduced dosage.

Hemolytic Anemia

Withhold alectinib if hemolytic anemia is suspected and initiate appropriate testing. If hemolytic anemia is confirmed, consider resuming alectinib at a reduced dosage upon resolution or permanently discontinue the drug.

● Special Populations

Hepatic Impairment

No initial dosage adjustment is necessary in patients with mild (Child-Pugh class A) or moderate (Child-Pugh class B) hepatic impairment. For patients with severe hepatic impairment (Child-Pugh class C), the manufacturer recommends an alectinib dosage of 450 mg twice daily.

Renal Impairment

No initial dosage adjustment is necessary in patients with mild or moderate renal impairment (creatinine clearance of 30–89 mL/minute). Pharmacokinetics and safety of alectinib have not been established in patients with severe renal impairment (creatinine clearance less than 30 mL/minute) or end-stage renal disease.

Geriatric Patients

The manufacturer makes no specific dosage recommendations for geriatric patients.

CAUTIONS

● Contraindications

● None.

● Warnings/Precautions

Hepatic Toxicity

Severe hepatotoxicity, including drug-induced liver injury, has been reported in patients receiving alectinib. In a pooled safety analysis, hepatotoxicity occurred in 41% of patients, with grade ≥3 hepatotoxicity reported in 8%. In the adjuvant therapy clinical trial (ALINA), hepatotoxicity was seen in 61% of patients administered alectinib, with grade ≥3 hepatotoxicity occurring in 4.7%. Most patients experienced elevated transaminases during the initial 3 months of treatment. Discontinuation of alectinib due to hepatotoxicity occurred in 3.6% of patients in the pooled analysis and 1.6% of patients in the ALINA study.

In the pooled safety analysis, elevations in ALT or AST concentrations of 3 or more times the ULN with total bilirubin concentrations of 2 or more times the ULN and alkaline phosphatase concentrations within normal limits were reported in less than 1% of alectinib-treated patients. Drug-induced liver injury with grade 3-4 AST/ALT elevations was reported in 3 patients.

The manufacturer states that liver function tests, including ALT, AST, and total bilirubin concentrations, should be monitored every 2 weeks for the first 3 months of alectinib therapy, then once every month, and as clinically indicated, with more frequent testing in patients who develop aminotransferase or bilirubin elevations during therapy. Temporary interruption followed by dosage reduction or permanent discontinuance of alectinib may be necessary depending on the severity of the hepatic toxicity.

Interstitial Lung Disease/Pneumonitis

Interstitial lung disease (ILD)/pneumonitis may occur in patients receiving alectinib. In a pooled safety analysis, ILD/pneumonitis occurred in 1.3% of alectinib-treated patients; grade 3 ILD/pneumonitis occurred in 0.4% of patients. Discontinuation of therapy due to ILD/pneumonitis occurred in 5 patients. The median time to onset of grade ≥3 ILD/pneumonitis was 2.1 months (range, 0.6-3.6 months).

Patients receiving alectinib should be monitored for pulmonary symptoms indicative of ILD or pneumonitis, and other potential causes of ILD or pneumonitis should be excluded. Alectinib should be permanently discontinued in patients who are diagnosed with treatment-related ILD or pneumonitis of any grade.

Renal Toxicity

Renal impairment, sometimes with fatal outcome, has occurred in patients receiving alectinib. In a pooled safety analysis, renal impairment was reported in 12% of alectinib-treated patients; 1.7% of patients receiving the drug experienced grade 3 or greater renal impairment (0.4% of these events resulted in death). The median time to grade 3 or 4 renal impairment was 3.7 months (range, 0.5-31.8 months). Dosage modification of alectinib was necessary because of renal impairment in 2.4% of patients.

Temporary interruption followed by dosage reduction or permanent discontinuance of alectinib may be necessary depending on the severity of renal impairment.

Bradycardia

Alectinib may cause symptomatic bradycardia. In a pooled safety population, bradycardia (defined as a heart rate of less than 60 beats/minute) was reported in 11% of alectinib-treated patients; a heart rate of less than 50 beats/minute was reported in 20% of patients in whom serial ECGs were obtained.

Heart rate and blood pressure should be monitored regularly in all patients receiving alectinib. For asymptomatic bradycardia, dose modification is not required. If symptomatic bradycardia occurs, temporary interruption of alectinib therapy, subsequent dosage reduction, or permanent discontinuance of the drug may be necessary depending on the severity of the bradycardia, the concomitant use of drugs known to cause bradycardia or hypotension, and the feasibility of modifying such concomitant therapy. Any concomitantly used drugs that may cause bradycardia or hypotension should be identified and the dosage should be adjusted or the drug should be discontinued if possible.

Severe Myalgia and Creatine Kinase Elevation

Severe myalgia and creatine kinase (CK) elevation have been reported with alectinib therapy. In a pooled safety analysis, myalgia events were reported in 31% of alectinib-treated patients; 0.8% of patients receiving the drug experienced grade 3 or greater myalgia events. Elevated serum CK (creatine phosphokinase, CPK) concentrations were reported in 56% of patients receiving alectinib; 6% of patients receiving the drug had grade 3 or greater elevations in CK concentrations. Median time to grade 3 or greater CK elevations was 15 days (interquartile range, 15-337 days). Dosage modification because of myalgia events or elevated serum CK concentrations was required in 2.1 or 5%, respectively, of patients. In ALINA, elevated CK levels were reported in 77% of patients, with grade 3 or greater elevations occurring in 6%.

The manufacturer states that serum CK concentrations should be monitored every 2 weeks for the first month of alectinib therapy and as clinically indicated in patients reporting muscle symptoms (e.g., unexplained or persistent muscle pain, tenderness, or weakness). Temporary interruption followed by dosage reduction or permanent discontinuance of alectinib may be necessary depending on the severity of the CK elevation.

Hemolytic Anemia

Hemolytic anemia, including cases associated with a negative direct antiglobulin test result, have been reported in patients receiving alectinib. In the ALINA study, hemolytic anemia was reported in 3.1% of patients administered alectinib.

Withhold alectinib if hemolytic anemia is suspected and initiate appropriate testing. If hemolytic anemia is confirmed, consider resuming alectinib at a reduced dosage upon resolution or permanently discontinue the drug.

Fetal/Neonatal Morbidity and Mortality

Based on its mechanism of action, alectinib may cause fetal harm. There are no adequate and well-controlled studies in humans; developmental toxicity, abortion, and embryolethality were observed when alectinib was administered to pregnant animals at maternally toxic dosages. Pregnancy should be avoided during therapy. If alectinib is used during pregnancy or if the patient becomes pregnant while receiving the drug, the patient should be apprised of the potential fetal hazard.

Specific Populations

Pregnancy

Based on findings from animal studies and its mechanism of action, alectinib may cause fetal harm if administered to pregnant females.

Lactation

It is not known whether alectinib or its metabolites are distributed into human milk. Because of the potential for serious adverse reactions to alectinib in nursing infants, women should be advised not to breast-feed while receiving the drug and for 1 week after the last dose.

Females and Males of Reproductive Potential

Verify pregnancy status in females of reproductive potential prior to initiation of alectinib therapy. Females of reproductive potential should use effective methods of contraception while receiving the drug and for 5 weeks after the last dose.

Males with female partners of reproductive potential should use effective methods of contraception while receiving the drug and for 3 months after the last dose.

Pediatric Use

Safety and efficacy of alectinib have not been established in pediatric patients. In animal toxicology studies, alectinib has been associated with changes in growing teeth (discoloration, changes in tooth size, histopathologic disarrangement of ameloblast and odontoblast layers) and bones (decreases in trabecular bone, increased osteoclast activity).

Geriatric Use

In clinical studies, 19% of 533 patients were 65 years of age and older and 3.2% were 75 years of age and older. No overall differences in effectiveness based on age were observed. Exploratory analysis suggests that patients 65 years of age or older experience an increased incidence of serious adverse events (38% versus 25%), more adverse events leading to treatment discontinuation (18% versus 6%), and more adverse events leading to dose modifications (48% versus 35%) as compared to patients younger than 65 years of age.

Hepatic Impairment

Mild hepatic impairment (Child-Pugh class A) did not have clinically important effects on systemic exposure to alectinib and its M4 metabolite. Following administration of a single 300-mg dose of alectinib, moderate (Child-Pugh class B) or severe (Child-Pugh class C) hepatic impairment increased the area under the concentration-time curve (AUC) of the total active forms of alectinib (i.e., alectinib plus M4) by 36 or 76%, respectively, compared with individuals with normal hepatic function; peak plasma concentration of the total active forms of alectinib was similar to that reported in individuals with normal hepatic function. Dosage adjustment is required in patients with severe hepatic impairment.

Renal Impairment

Mild to moderate renal impairment (creatinine clearance of 30–89 mL/minute) did not have clinically important effects on systemic exposure to alectinib and its M4 metabolite. Pharmacokinetics and safety of alectinib have not been established in patients with severe renal impairment (creatinine clearance less than 30 mL/minute) or end-stage renal disease.

Hemodialysis is not expected to enhance clearance of alectinib because the drug and its M4 metabolite are extensively bound to plasma proteins.

● Common Adverse Effects

Adverse effects reported in 20% or more of patients receiving alectinib in clinical trials include hepatotoxicity, constipation, fatigue, myalgia, edema, rash, and cough.

DRUG INTERACTIONS

Clinically important drug interactions with alectinib have not been identified to date.

Alectinib is metabolized by cytochrome P-450 (CYP) isoenzyme 3A4 to its major active metabolite, M4. In vitro studies suggest that M4, but not alectinib,

is a substrate of P-glycoprotein (P-gp); neither alectinib nor M4 is a substrate of breast cancer resistance protein (BCRP), organic anion transport protein (OATP) 1B1, or OATP1B3.

In vitro studies indicate that alectinib and M4 do not inhibit CYP isoenzymes 1A2, 2B6, 2C9, 2C19, or 2D6. Alectinib also does not inhibit OATP1B1 or OATP1B3, organic anion transporter (OAT) 1 and OAT3, or organic cation transporter (OCT) 2 in vitro.

In vitro studies suggest that alectinib and M4 inhibit P-gp and BCRP.

● Drugs Affecting or Metabolized by Hepatic Microsomal Enzymes

Clinically important drug interactions with alectinib have not been identified to date. Concomitant administration of alectinib and posaconazole (a potent CYP3A inhibitor) or rifampin (a potent CYP3A inducer) did not have a clinically important effect on the combined systemic exposure to alectinib and its M4 metabolite. Clinically important pharmacokinetic interactions between alectinib and midazolam (a CYP3A substrate) or repaglinide (a CYP2C8 substrate) are unlikely.

● Drugs Associated with Bradycardia

Alectinib has been associated with bradycardia. If clinically important bradycardia occurs with concomitant use of alectinib and other drugs known to cause bradycardia (including hypotensive agents), the dosage of the concomitant drug should be adjusted or the concomitant drug should be discontinued, if possible.

● Drugs Affecting Gastric Acidity

Concomitant administration of alectinib and esomeprazole did not have a clinically important effect on the combined systemic exposure to alectinib and its M4 metabolite.

DESCRIPTION

Alectinib hydrochloride, an inhibitor of receptor tyrosine kinases, including anaplastic lymphoma kinase (ALK) and ret proto-oncogene (RET), is an antineoplastic agent. The drug inhibits ALK phosphorylation and ALK-mediated activation of the downstream signaling proteins signal transducer and activator of transcription 3 (STAT3) and AKT serine/threonine kinase. The drug also inhibits leukocyte tyrosine kinase receptor (LTK) and cyclin-G-associated kinase (GAK).

Activating mutations or translocations of the ALK gene have been identified in several malignancies and can result in the expression of oncogenic fusion proteins (e.g., echinoderm microtubule-associated protein-like 4 [EML4]-ALK). Such ALK gene rearrangements have been identified in approximately 3–7% of patients with non-small cell lung cancer (NSCLC). Formation of ALK fusion proteins such as EML4-ALK results in activation and dysregulation of the gene's expression and signaling, which can contribute to increased cell proliferation and survival in tumors expressing these proteins.

Although the ALK inhibitor crizotinib has demonstrated improved outcomes in patients with NSCLC harboring ALK mutations, secondary resistance to crizotinib eventually develops, generally within the first 1–2 years of treatment. Clinical resistance to crizotinib has been attributed to several possible mechanisms, including acquired resistance mutations of ALK, amplification of gene expression, and activation of alternate signaling pathways. Secondary mutations of ALK are responsible for about 30% of cases of acquired crizotinib resistance and gene amplification is implicated in 9% of these cases.

In vitro, alectinib is approximately fivefold more potent than crizotinib in activity against ALK. Alectinib demonstrated dose-dependent antitumor activity and increased survival in mice bearing NSCLC tumor xenografts that expressed EML4-ALK, including several cell lines with demonstrated resistance to crizotinib. In preclinical studies in vitro and in vivo, alectinib was active against several crizotinib-resistant ALK mutations (e.g., L1196M, C1156Y, F1174L, G1269A).

The CNS is a common site of disease progression in crizotinib-treated patients because of poor distribution of crizotinib into CSF; development and/or progression of brain metastases occurs in approximately one-half of patients during crizotinib treatment. Alectinib crosses the blood-brain barrier, distributing into CSF at concentrations similar to estimated alectinib free plasma concentrations; the drug demonstrated antitumor activity and increased survival in mice bearing intracranial *ALK*-positive NSCLC tumor xenografts. In clinical studies, alectinib demonstrated antitumor activity in patients with crizotinib-resistant disease and baseline CNS metastases.

Exposure to alectinib is dose proportional over the oral dose range of 460–900 mg in the fed state. Following oral administration under fed conditions, peak plasma concentrations of alectinib are achieved within 4 hours. Steady-state concentrations of alectinib and its major active metabolite (M4) are achieved within 7 days. The absolute oral bioavailability of alectinib under fed conditions is 37%. Oral administration of a single 600-mg dose of the drug with a high-calorie, high-fat meal increases total systemic exposure to alectinib and M4 by 3.1-fold compared with administration in the fasting state. Alectinib and M4 are more than 99% bound to plasma proteins; the drug distributes into CSF at concentrations similar to estimated alectinib free plasma concentrations. Alectinib is metabolized by cytochrome P-450 (CYP) isoenzyme 3A4 to its major active metabolite, M4, which also is metabolized by CYP3A4. M4 exhibits in vitro potency and activity similar to those of alectinib. Following oral administration of radiolabeled alectinib, 98% of the dose is eliminated in feces, mainly as unchanged drug (84%) and, to a lesser extent, as M4 (6%); less than 0.5% of the dose is eliminated in urine. The mean elimination half-lives of alectinib and M4 in patients with *ALK*-positive NSCLC are 33 and 31 hours, respectively.

ADVICE TO PATIENTS

- Advise patients to read the manufacturer's patient information.

- Stress importance of taking alectinib exactly as prescribed and of not altering the dosage or discontinuing therapy unless advised to do so by a clinician. Advise patients to swallow alectinib capsules whole with food and not dissolve or open the capsules.

- If a dose is missed or if vomiting occurs after taking a dose, advise patients to take the next dose at the regularly scheduled time; do not take the missed dose or take an extra dose to replace the vomited dose.

- Risk of hepatotoxicity; stress importance of liver function test monitoring. Immediately inform clinician if manifestations suggestive of hepatotoxicity (e.g., fatigue, anorexia, nausea, vomiting, right upper quadrant pain, jaundice, dark urine, generalized pruritus, unusual bleeding or bruising) occur.

- Risk of renal toxicity. Stress importance of informing clinician if manifestations of renal toxicity (e.g., decreased urine output, hematuria, peripheral edema) occur.

- Risk of severe or fatal ILD/pneumonitis. Symptoms may be similar to those of lung cancer. Immediately inform clinician if any new or worsening pulmonary symptoms (e.g., dyspnea, shortness of breath, cough, fever) occur.

- Risk of bradycardia. Immediately inform clinician if dizziness, lightheadedness, or faintness occurs.

- Risk of muscle problems or myalgia; importance of CK monitoring. Stress importance of promptly informing clinician if any unexplained or persistent muscle pain, tenderness, or weakness occurs.

- Risk of photosensitivity. Advise patients to avoid prolonged sun exposure during therapy and for ≥7 days after drug discontinuance and of using a broad-spectrum sunscreen and lip balm (minimum SPF of 50).

- Risk of fetal harm. Advise women of reproductive potential to use effective methods of contraception during therapy and for 5 weeks after the last dose. Advise men who are partners of such women to use adequate methods of contraception during therapy and for 3 months after the last dose.

- Advise women to avoid breast-feeding during therapy and for 1 week after the last dose.

- Stress importance of informing clinicians of existing or contemplated concomitant therapy, including prescription and OTC drugs (e.g., cardiac or hypotensive agents) and dietary or herbal supplements, as well as any concomitant illnesses (e.g., hepatic impairment).

- Advise patients to inform their clinician of other important precautionary information.

For further information on the handling of antineoplastic agents, see the ASHP Guidelines on Handling Hazardous Drugs at https://www.ahfsdruginformation.com.

PREPARATIONS

Excipients in commercially available drug preparations may have clinically important effects in some individuals; consult specific product labeling for details.

Alectinib is available only from designated specialty distributors and pharmacies. The manufacturer should be contacted for additional information.

Alectinib Hydrochloride

Oral

Capsules	150 mg (of alectinib)	**Alecensa®**, Genentech

† Use is not currently included in the labeling approved by the US Food and Drug Administration.

Selected Revisions November 10, 2024, © Copyright, October 17, 2016, American Society of Health-System Pharmacists, Inc.

Alpelisib

10:00 • ANTINEOPLASTIC AGENTS

■ Alpelisib, a selective inhibitor of the α isoform of phosphoinositide 3-kinase (PI3Kα), is an antineoplastic agent.

USES

● Breast Cancer

Alpelisib is used in combination with fulvestrant for the treatment of adults with hormone receptor-positive, human epidermal growth factor receptor type 2 (HER2)-negative, phosphatidylinositol-3-kinase catalytic subunit α (*PIK3CA*)-mutated, advanced or metastatic breast cancer as detected by an FDA-approved diagnostic test (e.g., *therascreen*® PIK3CA RGQ PCR Kit) following progression on or after an endocrine-based regimen. The alpelisib preparation labeled as Piqray® is specifically indicated for this use. In patients with hormone receptor-positive, HER2-negative, advanced or metastatic breast cancer that has progressed during or following endocrine-based therapy, combined therapy with alpelisib and fulvestrant has been shown to prolong progression-free survival compared with fulvestrant alone. Guidelines generally recommend alpelisib in combination with fulvestrant in postmenopausal women and men with hormone receptor-positive, HER-2 negative, *PIK3CA*-mutated advanced or metastatic breast cancer previously treated with endocrine therapy (e.g., aromatase inhibitor with or without a cyclin-dependent kinase [CDK] 4/6 inhibitor).

Clinical Experience

This indication for alpelisib is based principally on the results of a randomized, double-blind, placebo-controlled, phase 3 study (SOLAR-1; NCT02437318) in patients with hormone receptor-positive, HER2-negative, advanced or metastatic breast cancer that had progressed during or following endocrine-based therapy. In this study, a cohort of 341 patients with tumors harboring at least one *PIK3CA* mutation were randomized (stratified by presence of lung or liver metastases and prior therapy with a cyclin-dependent kinase [CDK] 4 and 6 inhibitor) in a 1:1 ratio to receive either alpelisib (300 mg orally once daily) or placebo, each given in combination with fulvestrant (500 mg by IM injection on days 1 and 15 during cycle 1 and then on day 1 of each 4-week cycle thereafter). Treatment was continued until disease progression, death, or unacceptable toxicity occurred or treatment was discontinued for other reasons. The primary measure of efficacy was progression-free survival as assessed by the investigator according to Response Evaluation Criteria in Solid Tumors (RECIST); secondary end points included overall response rate and overall survival.

In the SOLAR-1 study, the median age of patients with PIK3CA-mutated tumors was 63 years (range: 25–92 years); 99.8% were female, 66% were Caucasian, 22% were Asian, 50% had lung or liver metastases, 23% had metastasis to bone only, 6% had received prior therapy with a CDK 4 and 6 inhibitor, and 98% had received hormonal therapy as their most recent treatment (52% in the adjuvant setting and 48% in the setting of metastatic disease). In this study, 13% of patients with *PIK3CA*-mutated tumors had primary resistance and 72% had secondary resistance to endocrine therapy. Primary resistance was defined as relapse within 24 months while the patient was receiving adjuvant endocrine therapy or progression within 6 months while the patient was receiving endocrine therapy for advanced or metastatic disease; secondary resistance was defined as relapse after at least 24 months while the patient was receiving adjuvant endocrine therapy, relapse within 12 months following discontinuance of adjuvant endocrine therapy, or progression after at least 6 months while the patient was receiving endocrine therapy for advanced or metastatic disease. All patients enrolled in the study had a baseline ECOG performance status of 0 or 1.

The median duration of combined therapy with alpelisib and fulvestrant was 8.2 months; treatment was continued for at least 6 months in 59% of patients. At a median follow-up of 20 months, patients with *PIK3CA*-mutated tumors receiving alpelisib in combination with fulvestrant had longer median progression-free survival (11 versus 5.7 months) and a higher overall response rate (35.7 versus 16.2%) compared with those receiving fulvestrant and placebo. Median overall survival had not been reached at the time of the analysis. Subgroup analysis based on stratification criteria and important demographic and prognostic factors suggested that the progression-free survival benefit of alpelisib given in combination with fulvestrant was consistent across these subgroups. In a final survival analysis of patients with PIK3CA-mutated tumors from the SOLAR-1 study, median overall survival was 39.3 months among patients receiving alpelisib in combination with fulvestrant and 31.4 months among patients treated with fulvestrant plus placebo; this difference was not statistically significant.

Clinical Perspective

Guidelines from the American Society of Clinical Oncology (ASCO) provide recommendations for treatment of postmenopausal women and men with hormone receptor-positive, HER2-negative advanced or metastatic breast cancer.

ASCO recommends CDK4/6 inhibitor therapy with endocrine therapy as first-line treatment. Second and third-line treatment options include targeted therapies (e.g., capivasertib, alpelisib) based on tumor genomics and prior endocrine therapy. Alpelisib combined with endocrine therapy is an option for tumors harboring PIK3CA mutations, but not AKT1 mutations or PTEN inactivation. No comparative efficacy data are available to guide selection between capivasertib or alpelisib when targeting PIK3CA mutations. In this situation, ASCO recommends choosing the targeted agent based on perceived risk-benefit considerations (e.g., hyperglycemia, diarrhea, or treatment discontinuation for adverse events).

● Phosphatidylinositol-3-kinase Catalytic Subunit α (PIK3CA)-Related Overgrowth Spectrum

Alpelisib is used to treat adults and pediatric patients 2 years of age or older who require systemic therapy for severe manifestations of PIK3CA-related overgrowth spectrum (PROS). The alpelisib preparation labeled as Vijoice® is specifically indicated for this use.The accelerated approval of alpelisib for this indication is based on radiological response rate and duration of response. Continued approval for this indication may be contingent on verification and description of clinical benefit of alpelisib in confirmatory studies. Alpelisib has been designated an orphan drug by FDA for the treatment of PROS.

Clinical Experience

This indication for alpelisib is based principally on the results of a single-arm clinical study (EPIK-P1) that enrolled patients 2 years of age or older with severe or life-threatening clinical manifestations of PROS requiring systemic therapy. Patients were required to have a confirmed *PIK3CA* mutation. In this study, 37 patients with PROS and at least 1 target lesion (identified on imaging performed within 24 weeks prior to receipt of the first dose of alpelisib) were treated with alpelisib at dosages ranging from 50–250 mg orally once daily. The primary measure of efficacy was the proportion of patients with radiological response at week 24, defined as a reduction of 20% or greater from baseline in the sum of measurable target lesion volume (1–3 lesions). An additional efficacy outcome was duration of response, which was measured from the time of the first documented response to the time of disease progression or death.

In EPIK-P1 study, the median age of patients was 14 years (range: 2–38 years); 22%, 22%, and 27% of patients were 2–5 years, 6–11 years, and 12 to <18 years of age, respectively. Fifty-seven percent of the patients were female and 92% had congenital overgrowth; manifestations of PROS varied and included Congenital Lipomatous Overgrowth, Vascular Malformations, Epidermal Nevi, Scoliosis/Skeletal and Spinal Syndrome (CLOVES; 81%), Megalencephaly-Capillary Malformation Polymicrogyria (MCAP; 8%), Klippel-Trenaunay Syndrome (KTS; 2.7%), Facial Infiltrating Lipomatosis (FIL; 8%), and other (5%).

After 24 weeks of treatment with alpelisib, 10 patients (27%) had a radiological response, confirmed by blinded independent central review. Seventy percent and 60% of patients had a duration of response of at least 6 or 12 months, respectively.

Clinical Perspective

Phosphatidylinositol-3-kinase catalytic subunit α-related overgrowth spectrum (PROS) is an umbrella term that comprises a heterogeneous group of disorders characterized by vascular malformations and abnormal tissue growth. Examples of disorders classified as PROS include CLOVES, Klippel-Trenaunay syndrome, and megalencephaly capillary malformation. All disorders classified as PROS originate from a mutation in *PIK3CA* that causes hyperactivation of the gene, which results in abnormal growth of epithelial and other tissues. Patients affected by these disorders have a wide array of potential complications, including pain, vascular and neurologic complications (e.g., thromboembolism, seizures), functional impairment, and risk of malignancy.

Currently, various procedures (e.g., sclerotherapy, laser therapy, debulking surgery) are used to treat the disorder; however, these procedures are often not curative. Traditional management of overgrowth syndromes has been conservative and limited to addressing complications as they arise; however, targeted therapies (e.g., alpelisib, sirolimus) have emerged as therapeutic options for various syndromes across the spectrum of PROS.

DOSAGE AND ADMINISTRATION

● General

Pretreatment Screening

* *Breast cancer*: Confirmation of at least one phosphatidylinositol-3-kinase catalytic subunit α (*PIK3CA*) mutation in tumor or plasma specimens by an FDA-approved diagnostic test is necessary prior to initiating therapy with alpelisib (Piqray®). Reevaluate patients with a negative plasma *PIK3CA* mutation result for the feasibility of a tumor biopsy.

* Assess fasting plasma glucose and hemoglobin A_{1c} (HbA_{1c}); serum glucose levels should be normalized prior to initiation of the drug.

* Verify pregnancy status in females of reproductive potential.

Patient Monitoring

* Monitor fasting plasma glucose at least once per week for the first 2 weeks of therapy with alpelisib, then at least once every 4 weeks, and as clinically indicated. More frequent monitoring during the first few weeks may be necessary in patients with risk factors for hyperglycemia (e.g., obesity [body mass index ≥30 kg/m²], elevated fasting glucose, HbA_{1c} at or above the upper limit of normal, concomitant use of corticosteroids, ≥75 years of age).

* Monitor HbA_{1c} every 3 months and as clinically indicated.

* Monitor for signs or symptoms of hyperglycemia. Closely monitor patients with diabetes.

* If hyperglycemia following initiation of alpelisib therapy occurs, monitor fasting glucose as clinically indicated, and at least twice weekly until fasting glucose decreases to normal levels. During treatment with antihyperglycemic medication, continue monitoring fasting glucose at least once a week for 8 weeks, followed by once every 2 weeks, and as clinically indicated.

* Monitor for signs or symptoms of hypersensitivity reactions.

* Monitor for signs or symptoms of severe cutaneous adverse reactions (SCARs).

* Monitor for clinical symptoms or radiological changes of pneumonitis.

* Monitor for diarrhea and other symptoms of colitis, including abdominal pain and mucus or blood in stool.

Premedication and Prophylaxis

* Prophylactic administration of an oral antihistamine may decrease incidence and severity of rash.

* Consider metformin therapy prior to initiation of alpelisib in combination with fulvestrant based on patient risk factors for hyperglycemia, GI tolerability, and clinical situation.

Other General Considerations

* *Breast cancer*: Consult manufacturer's labeling for information on dosage adjustments, adverse effects, and contraindications of other antineoplastic agents used in combination regimens.

● Administration

Alpelisib is commercially available as oral tablets (Piqray®, Vijoice®) or oral granules (Vijoice®). The Vijoice® tablets may also be administered as an oral suspension for patients who have difficulty swallowing the whole tablets.

The most appropriate dosage form of Vijoice® (tablets or granules) should be prescribed based on patient needs and dosage requirements.

The oral granules are single use and *only* for patients prescribed a 50 mg daily dose. Clinicians should *not* use multiple packets to achieve a prescribed dose of 125 mg or 250 mg, and should not use partial quantities of the oral granule packets to prepare a dose. The oral granules should not be used if the packet seal is broken.

The tablets should be swallowed whole; do *not* chew, crush, or split. Do not use tablets that are cracked, broken, or otherwise not intact.

Administer orally with food. Take at approximately the same time each day.

If a dose of alpelisib is missed and cannot be taken within 9 hours of the regularly scheduled time, skip the missed dose and take the next dose at the regularly scheduled time.

If a dose of alpelisib is vomited, do not take an extra dose; take the next dose at the regularly scheduled time.

Store alpelisib at 20–25°C (excursions permitted between 15–30°C).

Preparation of Oral Suspension from Vijoice® Tablets

In individuals who are unable to swallow the intact tablets, the appropriate dose of alpelisib (Vijoice®) tablets may be placed in a cup containing 2–4 ounces of water and allowed to sit for approximately 5 minutes. The manufacturer states that *no* other liquid should be used. After allowing the tablets to sit for 5 minutes, a spoon should be used to crush the tablets in the water and to stir the suspension; the resultant suspension should be administered immediately and should not be stored for later use. If immediate administration is not possible, the suspension should be discarded within 60 minutes of preparation. Following administration of the dose, add 1-2 ounces of water to the cup, stir the water with the same spoon to resuspend any remaining drug and administer the resultant suspension; repeat these steps as necessary.

Preparation of Vijoice® Oral Granules

For the administration of a 50 mg daily dose, oral granules can be administered via 1 of 2 methods:

* The contents of 1 granule packet may be poured directly onto the tongue and swallowed with approximately 2-4 ounces of water. The mouth may be rinsed with additional water with subsequent swallowing to ensure that no particles remain, if necessary.

* The contents of 1 granule packet may be poured into a cup with 1-3 teaspoons (about 0.5 ounces) of a beverage (e.g., water, milk, or apple juice) or soft food (e.g., applesauce or yogurt) and administered immediately. The cup may be rinsed with up to 2 additional ounces of a beverage (e.g., water, milk, or apple juice) and administered immediately to ensure delivery of the entire dose. This procedure may be repeated if particles remain until the full dose is administered. If not used within 2 hours after preparation, the mixed oral granules should be discarded.

● Dosage

Pediatric Patients

PIK3CA-related Overgrowth Spectrum (PROS)

For the treatment of PROS in pediatric patients 2–18 years of age, the recommended dosage of alpelisib is 50 mg orally once daily.

After 24 weeks of therapy at a dosage of 50 mg once daily, consider increasing the dosage to 125 mg once daily in patients ≥6 years of age. An increase in dosage has not been established in pediatric patients <6 years of age.

When a patient turns 18 years of age, consider gradually increasing the dosage to the recommended adult dosage of 250 mg once daily.

Continue treatment until disease progression or unacceptable toxicity occurs.

Adults

Breast Cancer

For use in combination with fulvestrant in the treatment of hormone receptor-positive, HER2-negative, *PIK3CA*-mutated, advanced or metastatic breast cancer in men and postmenopausal women with disease progression following endocrine therapy, the recommended adult dosage of alpelisib is 300 mg (two 150-mg tablets) once daily. The recommended adult dosage of fulvestrant is 500 mg administered by IM injection on days 1, 15, and 29 and then once monthly thereafter.

Continue treatment until disease progression or unacceptable toxicity occurs.

PIK3CA-related Overgrowth Spectrum (PROS)

For the treatment of PROS, the recommended adult dosage of alpelisib is 250 mg orally once daily. Continue treatment until disease progression or unacceptable toxicity occurs.

Dosage Modification for Toxicity

Temporary interruption of therapy, dosage reduction, and/or permanent discontinuance of alpelisib may be necessary in patients experiencing certain adverse effects.

The following tables on dosage modifications for alpelisib toxicity indicate the recommended dosage modifications in adults and pediatric patients receiving alpelisib (see Table 1 and Table 2).

TABLE 1. Adults: Recommended Dosage Reduction for Alpelisib Toxicity.

	Dosage Reduction after Recovery from Toxicity	Dosage Reduction after Recovery from Toxicity
Dose Reduction Level	Breast Cancer (Dosage = 300 mg once daily)	PROS (Dosage = 250 mg once daily)
First	Reduce dosage to 250 mg (one 200 mg and one 50 mg tablet) once daily	Reduce dosage to 125 mg once daily
Second	Reduce dosage to 200 mg once daily	Reduce dosage to 50 mg once daily
Third	Permanently discontinue drug	Permanently discontinue drug

TABLE 2. Pediatric Patients: Recommended Dosage Reduction for Alpelisib Toxicity in Patients with PROS.

	Dosage Reduction after Recovery from Toxicity	Dosage Reduction after Recovery from Toxicity
Dose Reduction Level	Dosage = 50 mg once daily	Dosage = 125 mg once daily
First	Permanently discontinue drug	Reduce dosage to 50 mg once daily
Second		Permanently discontinue drug

Hyperglycemia

If grade 1 hyperglycemia (fasting plasma glucose concentration exceeding the upper limit of normal [ULN] but not more than 160 mg/dL) occurs in *adults or pediatric patients*, continue alpelisib therapy at the same dosage. Oral antihyperglycemic therapy (e.g., metformin in adults and pediatric patients ≥10 year of age; a sodium-glucose cotransporter 2 [SGLT2] inhibitor, a thiazolidinedione, a dipeptidyl peptidase-4 [DPP-4] inhibitor in adults) should be initiated or intensified.

If grade 2 hyperglycemia (fasting plasma glucose concentration exceeding 160 mg/dL but not more than 250 mg/dL) occurs in *adults*, may continue alpelisib therapy at the same dosage. Oral antihyperglycemic therapy should be initiated or intensified. If grade 2 hyperglycemia persists for longer than 21 days despite oral antihyperglycemic therapy, reduce the dosage of alpelisib by one dose level.

If grade 2 hyperglycemia (fasting plasma glucose concentration exceeding 160 mg/dL but not more than 250 mg/dL) occurs in *pediatric patients*, may continue alpelisib therapy at the same dosage. Oral antihyperglycemic therapy should be initiated or intensified. If grade 2 hyperglycemia persists for longer than 21 days despite oral antihyperglycemic therapy, interrupt alpelisib therapy; when hyperglycemia improves to grade 1 or less, resume alpelisib at a dosage of 50 mg once daily.

If grade 3 hyperglycemia (fasting plasma glucose concentration exceeding 250 mg/dL but not more than 500 mg/dL) occurs in *adults*, interrupt alpelisib therapy. Oral antihyperglycemic therapy should be initiated or intensified and additional antihyperglycemic therapy with insulin may be considered for 1–2 days until hyperglycemia improves. The manufacturer states that most patients experiencing alpelisib-induced hyperglycemia may not require insulin therapy because of the short half-life of alpelisib. Administer IV fluids and appropriate treatment for electrolyte disorders, ketoacidosis, and/or hyperosmolar disturbances, if required. If hyperglycemia improves to 160 mg/dL or less within 3–5 days with appropriate antihyperglycemic therapy, resume alpelisib therapy at a dosage reduced by one dose level. If grade 3 hyperglycemia does not improve to 160 mg/dL or less within 3–5 days despite antihyperglycemic therapy, consultation with a clinician with expertise in the management of hyperglycemia is recommended. If improvement to 160 mg/dL or less does not occur within 21 days despite oral antihyperglycemic therapy, permanently discontinue alpelisib.

cIf grade 3 hyperglycemia (fasting plasma glucose concentration exceeding 250 mg/dL but not more than 500 mg/dL) occurs in *pediatric patients*, interrupt alpelisib therapy. Oral antihyperglycemic therapy should be initiated or intensified and additional antihyperglycemic therapy with insulin may be considered for 1–2 days until hyperglycemia improves. The manufacturer states that most patients experiencing alpelisib-induced hyperglycemia may not require insulin therapy because of the short half-life of alpelisib. Administer IV fluids and appropriate treatment for electrolyte disorders, ketoacidosis, and/or hyperosmolar disturbances, if required. If hyperglycemia improves to 160 mg/dL or less within 3–5 days with appropriate antihyperglycemic therapy, resume alpelisib therapy at 50 mg once daily. If grade 3 hyperglycemia does not improve to 160 mg/dL or less within 3–5 days despite antihyperglycemic therapy, consultation with a clinician with expertise in the management of hyperglycemia is recommended to determine if alpelisib may be resumed or permanently discontinued. If improvement to 160 mg/dL or less does not occur within 21 days despite oral antihyperglycemic therapy, permanently discontinue alpelisib. If grade 3 or greater hyperglycemia recurs, consider permanently discontinuing the drug.

If grade 4 hyperglycemia (fasting plasma glucose concentration exceeding 500 mg/dL) occurs in *adults or pediatric patients*, interrupt alpelisib therapy. Appropriate antihyperglycemic therapy should be initiated or intensified, IV fluids should be administered, and appropriate treatment for electrolyte disorders, ketoacidosis, and/or hyperosmolar disturbances should be considered, if required. Reassess fasting plasma glucose concentration within 24 hours and as clinically indicated. If hyperglycemia improves to grade 3 or less, follow recommendations for management of grade 3 hyperglycemia. If grade 4 hyperglycemia persists, permanently discontinue alpelisib.

Dermatologic Toxicity

If grade 1 dermatologic toxicity (active skin toxicity affecting less than 10% of the body surface area [BSA]) occurs in *adults or pediatric patients*, may continue alpelisib therapy at the same dosage. Topical corticosteroid therapy should be administered and an oral antihistamine also should be considered for symptomatic management. If an active rash does not improve within 28 days of appropriate treatment, add a low dose systemic corticosteroid.

If grade 2 dermatologic toxicity (active skin toxicity affecting 10–30% of BSA) occurs in *adults or pediatric patients*, may continue alpelisib therapy at the same dosage. Topical corticosteroid and oral antihistamine therapy should be initiated or intensified, and low-dose systemic corticosteroid therapy also considered. If rash improves to grade 1 or less within 10 days, may discontinue systemic corticosteroid therapy.

If grade 3 dermatologic toxicity (e.g., severe rash not responsive to therapy; active skin toxicity affecting more than 30% of BSA) occurs in *adults or pediatric patients*, interrupt alpelisib therapy. Topical/systemic corticosteroid and oral antihistamine therapy should be initiated or intensified. If the etiology is not a severe cutaneous adverse reaction (SCAR) in *adults*, may resume alpelisib therapy at a dosage reduced by one dose level when the toxicity improves to grade 1 or less. If the etiology is not a SCAR in *pediatric patients*, may resume alpelisib therapy at 50 mg once daily while continuing oral antihistamine therapy when the toxicity improves to grade 1 or less or permanently discontinue alpelisib. Permanently discontinue alpelisib in *pediatric patients* if a grade 3 or greater rash recurs or if the patient was already receiving antihistamines at the time of rash onset and the antihistamine dosage cannot be increased further.

If the etiology of any dermatologic reaction is confirmed to be a SCAR in *adults or pediatric patients*, permanently discontinue alpelisib. Do *not* reinitiate therapy with alpelisib in patients who have previously experienced SCAR during alpelisib therapy.

If grade 4 dermatologic toxicity (e.g., severe bullous, blistering, or exfoliating skin conditions; involvement of any percentage of BSA accompanied by extensive superinfection requiring IV anti-infective therapy; life-threatening consequences) occurs in *adults or pediatric patients*, permanently discontinue alpelisib.

Diarrhea or Colitis

If grade 1 diarrhea or colitis occurs in *adults or pediatric patients*, may continue alpelisib therapy at the same dosage; however, initiate appropriate therapy for diarrhea and additional monitoring as clinically indicated.

If grade 2 diarrhea or colitis occurs in *adults*, interrupt alpelisib therapy; may resume alpelisib at the same dosage when the toxicity improves to grade 1 or less. Appropriate therapy for diarrhea should be initiated or intensified, and patients should receive additional monitoring as clinically indicated. If grade 2 diarrhea recurs, interrupt alpelisib therapy. Resume alpelisib at a dosage reduced by one level when the toxicity improves to grade 1 or less.

If grade 2 diarrhea or colitis occurs in *pediatric patients*, interrupt alpelisib therapy; may resume alpelisib at the same dosage when the toxicity improves to grade 1 or less. Appropriate therapy for diarrhea should be initiated or intensified, and patients should receive additional monitoring as clinically indicated. If grade 2 diarrhea recurs, interrupt alpelisib therapy. Resume alpelisib at 50 mg once daily when the toxicity improves to grade 1 or less.

If grade 3 diarrhea or colitis occurs in *adults*, interrupt alpelisib therapy; resume alpelisib at a dosage reduced by one level when the toxicity improves to grade 1 or less. Appropriate therapy for diarrhea should be initiated or intensified, and patients should receive additional monitoring as clinically indicated.

If grade 3 diarrhea or colitis occurs in *pediatric patients*, interrupt alpelisib therapy; when the toxicity improves to grade 1 or less, alpelisib may be resumed at 50 mg once daily or permanently discontinued. Appropriate therapy for diarrhea should be initiated or intensified, and patients should receive additional monitoring as clinically indicated. If grade 3 or greater diarrhea recurs, consider permanently discontinuing alpelisib therapy.

If grade 4 diarrhea or colitis occurs in *adults or pediatric patients*, permanently discontinue alpelisib.

Pancreatitis

If grade 2 or 3 pancreatitis occurs in *adults*, interrupt alpelisib therapy; may resume alpelisib at a reduced dosage when the toxicity improves to less than grade 2. The manufacturer states that only one dosage reduction for pancreatitis is permitted; if pancreatitis recurs, permanently discontinue alpelisib.

If grade 2 pancreatitis occurs in *pediatric patients*, interrupt alpelisib; may resume alpelisib at a dosage of 50 mg once daily when the toxicity improves to less than grade 2. If pancreatitis recurs or grade 3 pancreatitis occurs, permanently discontinue alpelisib.

If grade 4 pancreatitis occurs in *adults or pediatric patients*, permanently discontinue alpelisib.

Pneumonitis

If pneumonitis is suspected in *adults or pediatric patients*, interrupt alpelisib therapy. If pneumonitis of any grade is confirmed, permanently discontinue alpelisib.

Hepatic Toxicity

For grade 2 elevations in total bilirubin concentrations in *adults*, interrupt alpelisib therapy; may resume alpelisib at the same dosage if the toxicity resolves or improves to grade 1 or less within 14 days. If toxicity improves to grade 1 or less in more than 14 days, resume alpelisib at a dosage reduced by one level.

For grade 2 elevations in total bilirubin concentrations in *pediatric patients*, interrupt alpelisib therapy; may resume alpelisib at the same dosage if the toxicity resolves or improves to grade 1 or less within 14 days. If toxicity improves to grade 1 or less in more than 14 days, resume alpelisib at a dosage of 50 mg once daily.

Other Toxicity

If other grade 1 or 2 adverse reactions occur in *adults or pediatric patients*, may continue alpelisib therapy at the same dosage; however, patients should receive appropriate therapy and additional monitoring as clinically indicated.

If other grade 3 adverse reactions occur in *adults*, interrupt alpelisib therapy; may resume alpelisib at a dosage reduced by one level when the toxicity improves

to grade 1 or less. Appropriate therapy for the toxicity should be initiated or intensified, and patients should receive additional monitoring as clinically indicated.

If other grade 3 adverse reactions occur in *pediatric patients*, interrupt alpelisib therapy; when the toxicity improves to grade 1 or less, alpelisib may be resumed at 50 mg once daily or permanently discontinued. Appropriate therapy for the toxicity should be initiated or intensified, and patients should receive additional monitoring as clinically indicated. If the adverse reaction recurs at grade 3 or greater severity, consider permanent discontinuance of the drug. Consultation with a clinician with expertise in a field related to the adverse reaction should be considered in pediatric patients experiencing other grade 3 adverse reactions.

If other grade 4 adverse reactions occur in *adults or pediatric patients*, permanently discontinue alpelisib.

● Special Populations

Hepatic Impairment

The manufacturer makes no specific dosage recommendations for patients with hepatic impairment.

Renal Impairment

No dosage adjustment is necessary in patients with mild to moderate renal impairment (creatinine clearance 30–89 mL/minute). Insufficient data are available to provide dosage recommendations for patients with severe renal impairment (creatinine clearance less than 30 mL/minute).

Geriatric Patients

The manufacturer makes no specific dosage recommendations for geriatric patients.

CAUTIONS

● Contraindications

- History of serious hypersensitivity reactions to alpelisib or any ingredient in the formulation.

● Warnings/Precautions

Severe Hypersensitivity

Serious hypersensitivity reactions, including anaphylaxis, anaphylactic shock, and angioedema have been reported in patients receiving alpelisib in the oncology setting. Manifestations may include dyspnea, flushing, rash, fever, and tachycardia. In the SOLAR-1 study, grade 3 or 4 hypersensitivity reactions were reported in 0.7% of patients receiving the drug. Alpelisib should be permanently discontinued and supportive treatment instituted in patients who experience a severe hypersensitivity reaction.

Dermatologic Effects

Severe cutaneous adverse reactions (SCARs), including erythema multiforme and Stevens-Johnson syndrome, toxic epidermal necrolysis, and drug reaction with eosinophilia and systemic symptoms may occur in patients receiving alpelisib in the oncology setting. In the SOLAR-1 study, erythema multiforme and Stevens-Johnson syndrome were reported in 1.1 and 0.4%, respectively, of patients receiving the drug. Drug reaction with eosinophilia and systemic symptoms has been reported in the postmarketing surveillance in alpelisib-treated patients.

If rash (any grade) occurs, consultation with a dermatologist should be considered. If signs and symptoms of SCARs (e.g., progressive rash, mucosal lesions, fever, lymphadenopathy, flu-like symptoms) occur, alpelisib therapy should be interrupted and the etiology should be evaluated; consultation with a dermatologist is recommended. Permanently discontinue alpelisib if SCARs are confirmed; do not reinitiate in patients who previously experienced SCARs during treatment with alpelisib. If SCARs are not confirmed, dosage modification, administration of corticosteroids and/or oral antihistamines, or treatment discontinuance may be necessary.

Rash (i.e., generalized, macular, maculopapular, papular, or pruritic rash) was reported in 52% of patients receiving alpelisib in the oncology setting; grade 3 rash was reported in 20% of patients. Prophylactic administration of an oral antihistamine prior to onset of rash may decrease the incidence and severity of alpelisib-induced rash.

Hyperglycemia

Severe hyperglycemia (including cases of hyperglycemic hyperosmolar nonketotic syndrome or ketoacidosis) has been reported in patients receiving alpelisib in the oncology setting; some cases reported in the postmarketing setting have been fatal. In the SOLAR-1 study, hyperglycemia occurred in 65% of patients receiving alpelisib; grade 3 or 4 hyperglycemia (based on fasting plasma glucose concentrations) occurred in 33 or 3.9%, respectively, of patients receiving the drug. Ketoacidosis occurred in 0.7% of patients receiving the drug. In the SOLAR-1 study, 87% of patients receiving alpelisib who experienced hyperglycemia received antihyperglycemic agents; 76% of patients with hyperglycemia received metformin alone or in combination with other antihyperglycemic agents (e.g., insulin, dipeptidyl peptidase-4 [DPP-4] inhibitors, sulfonylureas). The median time to occurrence of hyperglycemia (grade 2 or higher) was 15 days (range: 5–517 days), and the median time to at least 1 grade improvement of hyperglycemia was 8 days (range: 2–65 days). Hyperglycemia resolved and fasting plasma glucose concentrations returned to baseline in 96% of patients who discontinued alpelisib but continued fulvestrant therapy. In the EPIK-P1 study, grade 1 or 2 hyperglycemia occurred in 12% of patients receiving alpelisib for phosphatidylinositol-3-kinase catalytic subunit α-related overgrowth spectrum (PROS).

Fasting plasma glucose concentrations and glycosylated hemoglobin [hemoglobin A_{1c}; HbA_{1c}] should be assessed and blood glucose concentrations optimized prior to initiation of alpelisib therapy. Blood glucose concentrations and/or fasting plasma glucose concentrations should be monitored at least once weekly for the first 2 weeks of alpelisib therapy, at least once monthly thereafter, and as clinically indicated. More frequent monitoring may be necessary for the first few weeks in patients with risk factors for hyperglycemia (e.g., obesity [body mass index ≥30 kg/m²], elevated fasting glucose, HbA_{1c} at or above the upper limit of normal, concomitant use of corticosteroids, or ≥75 years of age). Monitor HbA_{1c} once every 3 months and as clinically indicated.

If hyperglycemia occurs, fasting plasma glucose concentrations should be assessed as clinically indicated and at least twice weekly until hyperglycemia resolves. antihyperglycemic agents should be initiated or optimized as necessary; fasting plasma glucose concentrations and/or blood glucose concentrations should be monitored at least once weekly for 8 weeks after initiating antihyperglycemic therapy and then at least once every 2 weeks and as clinically indicated. Consultation with a clinician with expertise in the management of hyperglycemia should be considered. Temporary interruption of therapy, dosage reduction, or permanent discontinuance of alpelisib may be necessary depending on the severity of hyperglycemia.

Patients with a history of type 2 diabetes mellitus should be monitored closely during alpelisib therapy; such patients may require intensified antihyperglycemic therapy. Safety of alpelisib has not been established in patients with type 1 diabetes mellitus or uncontrolled type 2 diabetes mellitus.

Consider premedication with metformin prior to initiation of alpelisib in combination with fulvestrant based on patient risk factors for hyperglycemia, GI tolerability, and clinical situation. In a clinical study, metformin administration starting 7 days prior to alpelisib therapy reduced the incidence and severity of hyperglycemia events, but increased the incidence and severity of nausea, vomiting, and diarrhea.

Pneumonitis

Severe pneumonitis (e.g, acute interstitial pneumonitis and interstitial lung disease [ILD]) has occurred in patients receiving alpelisib in the oncology setting. In the SOLAR-1 study, pneumonitis was reported in 1.8% of patients receiving the drug.

If new or progressive respiratory manifestations (e.g., cough, dyspnea, hypoxia, interstitial infiltrates) occur, alpelisib therapy should be interrupted and patients should be evaluated for ILD/pneumonitis or other causes of respiratory symptoms (e.g., tumor progression, pneumonia). If pneumonitis is confirmed, alpelisib should be permanently discontinued.

Diarrhea or Colitis

Diarrhea, sometimes severe and resulting in dehydration or in some cases acute kidney injury or colitis, has occurred in patients receiving alpelisib in the oncology setting. In the SOLAR-1 study, diarrhea was reported in 58% of patients receiving alpelisib; grade 3 diarrhea occurred in 7% of patients. The median time to first occurrence of diarrhea (grade 2 or 3) was 46 days (range: 1–442 days). Diarrhea

requiring dosage reduction or discontinuance of therapy was reported in 6 or 2.8%, respectively, of patients receiving the drug; 63% of patients who experienced diarrhea required antidiarrhea medications (e.g., loperamide). In the EPIK-P1 study, grade 1 diarrhea was reported in 16% of patients receiving alpelisib.

Monitor patients for diarrhea and additional symptoms of colitis, such as abdominal pain and mucus or blood in stool. If diarrhea occurs, appropriate therapy (e.g., antidiarrhea agents, fluid replacement) should be initiated. Patients with colitis may require additional treatment, such as enteric-acting and/or systemic steroids. Temporary interruption, dosage reduction, or permanent discontinuance of alpelisib may be necessary depending on the severity of the diarrhea or colitis.

Fetal/Neonatal Morbidity and Mortality

Based on its mechanism of action and animal findings, alpelisib may cause fetal harm if administered to pregnant females. Maternal toxicity and postimplantation loss were observed in rats receiving alpelisib at exposure levels of approximately 3 times the human exposure at the recommended dosage, and reduced fetal weight and teratogenicity (i.e., skeletal malformations, fetal variations) were observed at exposure levels of approximately equivalent to the recommended pediatric and adult dosage. In rabbits, postimplantation loss was observed at exposure levels of approximately 10 times the human exposure at the recommended dosage, and embryofetal deaths, reduced fetal weight, and malformations were observed at exposure levels of approximately 5 times human exposure.

Pregnancy should be avoided during alpelisib therapy. The manufacturer states that a pregnancy test should be performed prior to initiation of alpelisib therapy in females of reproductive potential and that such females should be advised to use effective contraceptive methods while receiving the drug and for at least one week after discontinuance of therapy. Males who are partners of such females should be advised to use condoms and effective contraception during treatment and for at least one week after discontinuance of therapy. If alpelisib is used during pregnancy or if the patient becomes pregnant while receiving the drug, the patient should be apprised of the potential fetal hazard.

Specific Populations

Pregnancy

Alpelisib may cause fetal harm if administered to pregnant females based on its mechanism of action and animal findings.

Lactation

It is not known whether alpelisib is distributed into milk. Because of the potential for serious adverse reactions to alpelisib in breast-fed infants, females should be advised to discontinue breast-feeding during alpelisib therapy and for one week after discontinuance of the drug. The effects of the drug on breast-fed infants or on milk production are unknown.

Females and Males of Reproductive Potential

Females should be advised to use effective contraceptive methods while receiving the drug and for at least one week after discontinuance of therapy.

Males who are partners of such females should be advised to use condoms and effective contraception during treatment and for at least one week after discontinuance of therapy.

Results of animal studies suggest that alpelisib may impair male and female fertility.

Pediatric Use

Safety and efficacy of alpelisib for the treatment of breast cancer have not been established in pediatric patients.

Safety and efficacy of alpelisib for the treatment of PROS have not been established in pediatric patients <2 years of age.

Geriatric Use

No adults ≥65 years of age were enrolled in the EPIK-P1 study evaluating alpelisib in patients with PROS.

In the SOLAR-1 study evaluating alpelisib in patients with breast cancer, 41% of patients receiving alpelisib were 65 years of age or older, while 12% were 75 years of age or older. No overall differences in efficacy were observed between geriatric patients 65 years of age or older and younger adults; however, grade 3 or 4 hyperglycemia occurred more frequently in geriatric patients (44 versus 32%). Experience with alpelisib in patients 75 years of age or older is insufficient to determine whether efficacy and safety of the drug in this age group are similar to those in younger adults. However, in the SOLAR-1 study, hyperglycemia (74 versus 66%) and grade 3–4 hyperglycemia (56 versus 36%) occurred more frequently in patients 75 years of age or older compared to patients younger than 75 years of age, respectively.

Hepatic Impairment

Population pharmacokinetic analysis suggests that the pharmacokinetics of alpelisib are not substantially altered in patients with mild to severe hepatic impairment (Child-Pugh class A, B, or C).

Renal Impairment

Population pharmacokinetic analysis suggests that the pharmacokinetics of alpelisib are not substantially altered in patients with mild to moderate renal impairment (creatinine clearance of 30–89 mL/minute). The effect of severe renal impairment (creatinine clearance less than 30 mL/minute) on the pharmacokinetics of alpelisib has not been established.

● Common Adverse Effects

Adverse effects reported in 20% or more of patients receiving alpelisib for the treatment of breast cancer include increased serum glucose, increased serum creatinine, diarrhea, rash, decreased lymphocyte count, increased gamma glutamyl transferase, nausea, increased alanine aminotransferase, fatigue, decreased hemoglobin, increased lipase, decreased appetite, stomatitis, vomiting, decreased weight, decreased calcium, decreased glucose, prolonged activated partial thromboplastin time, and alopecia.

Adverse effects reported in 10% or more of patients receiving alpelisib for the treatment of PROS include diarrhea, stomatitis, and hyperglycemia.

DRUG INTERACTIONS

Alpelisib is metabolized principally by chemical and enzymatic hydrolysis and to a lesser extent by cytochrome P-450 (CYP) isoenzyme 3A4.

In vitro studies indicate that alpelisib inhibits CYP isoenzyme 3A4 in a time-dependent manner and also induces CYP isoenzymes 2B6, 2C9, and 3A4.

In vitro studies also indicate that alpelisib inhibits the efflux transporter P-glycoprotein (P-gp), but has a low potential to inhibit breast cancer resistance protein (BCRP), multidrug resistance protein 2 (MRP2), bile salt export pump (BSEP), organic anion transport protein (OATP) 1B1, OATP1B3, organic anion transporter (OAT) 1, OAT3, organic cation transporter (OCT) 1, OCT2, multidrug and toxin extrusion (MATE) transporter 1, and MATE2-K at clinically relevant concentrations. In vitro, alpelisib is a substrate of BCRP.

● Drugs Affecting Hepatic Microsomal Enzymes
Inducers of CYP3A4

Concomitant use of alpelisib and potent inducers of CYP3A4 may result in decreased systemic exposure to, and decreased therapeutic efficacy of, alpelisib. Avoid concomitant use of alpelisib with potent CYP3A4 inducers and consider an alternative concomitant drug with no or minimal potential to induce CYP3A4.

Drugs Metabolized by Hepatic Microsomal Enzymes

Coadministration of repeated doses of alpelisib 300 mg with a single dose of sensitive substrates of CYP3A4 (midazolam), CYP2C8 (repaglinide), CYP2C9 (warfarin), CYP2C19 (omeprazole), and CYP2B6 (bupropion) did not reveal clinically significant pharmacokinetic interactions. No clinically significant differences in the pharmacokinetics of everolimus (CYP3A4 and P-gp substrate) were seen when given concomitantly with alpelisib.

● Inhibitors of Breast Cancer Resistance Protein

Alpelisib is a substrate of BCRP in vitro. Concomitant use of alpelisib and BCRP inhibitors may result in increased alpelisib plasma concentrations and a possible increased risk of alpelisib toxicity. Avoid concomitant use of alpelisib and BCRP inhibitors. If concomitant use cannot be avoided, closely monitor for adverse effects.

● Drugs Affecting Gastric Acidity

Concomitant administration of alpelisib with drugs that increase the pH of the upper GI tract (e.g., histamine H_2-receptor antagonists) may decrease the solubility of alpelisib, which may result in decreased plasma alpelisib concentrations. Concomitant administration of ranitidine and alpelisib with a low-fat, low-calorie meal or in a fasted state decreased the area under the concentration-time curve (AUC) of alpelisib by 21 or 30%, respectively, and decreased peak plasma concentrations of alpelisib by 36 or 51%, respectively. Because alpelisib is administered with food and food has a more pronounced effect on solubility of the drug than does gastric pH, the manufacturer states that alpelisib may be administered concomitantly with drugs that increase the pH of the upper GI tract.

● Bone Resorption Inhibitors

Use of alpelisib with bone resorption inhibitors (a bisphosphonate [e.g., alendronate, ibandronate, risedronate, zoledronic acid] or human receptor activator of nuclear factor kappa-B ligand [RANKL] inhibitor [e.g., denosumab]) may increase the risk of osteonecrosis of the jaw. In the SOLAR-1 study, osteonecrosis of the jaw was reported in 4.2 or 1.4% of patients receiving alpelisib or placebo, respectively, in combination with fulvestrant; all patients who experienced osteonecrosis of the jaw were receiving or had previously received therapy with a bisphosphonate or RANKL inhibitor.

DESCRIPTION

Alpelisib, a selective inhibitor of the α isoform of phosphatidylinositol-3-kinase (PI3Kα), is an antineoplastic agent. Phosphatidylinositol-3-kinases are lipid kinases consisting of a catalytic subunit that exists in 4 different isoforms (α, β, γ, δ). Alpelisib is predominantly active against the PI3K-α isoform. Mutations in the gene that encodes the PI3Kα isoform (PIK3CA) are expressed in approximately 40% of hormone receptor-positive, human epidermal growth factor receptor type 2 (HER2)-negative breast cancers and result in PI3Kα/Akt signaling, cellular transformation, and generation of tumors. In breast cancer cell lines, alpelisib inhibited phosphorylation of PI3K/Akt downstream targets and exhibited activity in cell lines harboring a PIK3CA mutation. In xenograft models of PI3Kα-dependent tumors in mice, alpelisib blocked PI3K/Akt signaling and decreased tumor growth. PI3K inhibition by alpelisib has been shown to induce estrogen receptor transcription in breast cancer cells. The combination of alpelisib and the estrogen antagonist fulvestrant demonstrated increased antitumor activity compared with either drug alone in xenograft models of PIK3CA-mutated, estrogen receptor-positive breast cancer.

Activating mutations in PIK3CA also induce various overgrowth and malformations that ultimately cause PIK3CA-related overgrowth spectrum (PROS) disorders. In an animal model of Congenital Lipomatous Overgrowth, Vascular Malformations, Epiderman Nevi, Scoliosis/Skeletal and Spinal syndrome (CLOVES), a phenotype of PROS, alpelisib therapy was associated with improvements in organ dysfunction via inhibition of the PIK3 pathway.

Systemic exposure to alpelisib increases in a dose-proportional manner over a dose range of 30–450 mg in a fed state. Bioavailability of alpelisib in the fasted state is limited by low solubility. Following oral administration of a single dose of alpelisib with a high-fat, high-calorie or low-fat, low-calorie meal, systemic exposure to the drug was increased by 73 or 77%, respectively, and peak plasma concentrations were increased by 84 or 145%, respectively, compared with administration in the fasted state. Peak plasma concentrations of the drug are attained 2–4 hours following oral administration. With once-daily dosing, the accumulation ratio is 1.3–1.5 and steady-state concentrations are reached within 3 days. Alpelisib is 89% bound to plasma proteins. Alpelisib is metabolized to its major metabolite, BZG791, principally by chemical and enzymatic hydrolysis; the drug is metabolized to a lesser extent by cytochrome P-450 (CYP) isoenzyme 3A4. Following oral administration of a single 400-mg dose of radiolabeled alpelisib in the fasted state, 81% of the dose was recovered in feces (36% as unchanged drug) and 14% was recovered in urine (2% as unchanged drug); approximately 12% of the dose was recovered as metabolites formed by CYP3A4-mediated metabolism. The terminal half-life of alpelisib is 8–9 hours.

Population pharmacokinetic analysis indicated that age (21–87 years), sex, race (Japanese, Caucasian), and body weight (37–181 kg) do not have clinically important effects on the pharmacokinetics of alpelisib.

ADVICE TO PATIENTS

- Instruct patients to read the manufacturer's patient information.

- Advise patients to take alpelisib exactly as prescribed and to not alter the dosage or discontinue therapy unless advised to do so by their clinician. Advise patients to take the drug with food.

- Advise patients that a missed dose should be taken as soon as it is remembered, up to 9 hours after the scheduled administration time; if a dose is missed by more than 9 hours, the missed dose should be omitted and the next dose taken at the regularly scheduled time. If a dose is vomited, administer the next dose at the regularly scheduled time; an additional dose should not be administered to make up for a vomited dose.

- Risk of serious hypersensitivity reactions, including anaphylaxis. Immediately contact a clinician if signs or symptoms of a hypersensitivity reaction (e.g., dyspnea, flushing, rash, fever, tachycardia) occur.

- Risk of serious cutaneous adverse reactions (SCARs). Immediately contact a clinician if signs or symptoms of SCARs (e.g., severe or progressive rash; redness; flu-like symptoms; blistering or peeling skin; swollen lymph nodes; blistering of the lips, eyes, or mouth) occur.

- Risk of hyperglycemia. Stress importance of periodic fasting blood glucose monitoring and of immediately reporting signs or symptoms of hyperglycemia (e.g., excessive thirst, dry mouth, frequent urination, increased appetite with weight loss).

- Risk of interstitial lung disease or pneumonitis. Immediately contact a clinician if any new or worsening respiratory symptoms (e.g., cough, shortness of breath, difficulty breathing, chest pain) occur.

- Risk of diarrhea and colitis with potential for dehydration and acute kidney injury if diarrhea is severe. Advise patients on how to manage diarrhea (e.g., oral hydration, antidiarrhea agents) at the first sign of loose stools. Inform clinician if diarrhea occurs and notify healthcare provider immediately of any symptoms of colitis, such as abdominal pain and mucus or blood in stool.

- Advise patients and caregivers that alpelisib may cause alopecia.

- Risk of fetal harm. Advise females of reproductive potential to use effective contraceptive methods while receiving alpelisib and for ≥1 week after

discontinuance of therapy. Advise males who are partners of such females to use condoms and effective contraception during treatment and for ≥1 week after discontinuance of therapy. Stress importance of females informing clinicians if they are or plan to become pregnant. Apprise patient of potential fetal hazard if used during pregnancy.

- Advise females to discontinue breast-feeding during therapy and for ≥1 week after discontinuance of the drug.

- Advise patients with reproductive potential that alpelisib may impair male and female fertility.

- Stress importance of informing clinicians of existing or contemplated concomitant therapy, including prescription and OTC drugs and dietary or herbal supplements, as well as any concomitant illnesses (e.g., diabetes mellitus). Stress importance of close monitoring if certain interacting drugs must be used concomitantly.

- Inform patients of other important precautionary information.

For further information on the handling of antineoplastic agents, see the ASHP Guidelines on Handling Hazardous Drugs at https://www.ahfsdrug information.com.

PREPARATIONS

Excipients in commercially available drug preparations may have clinically important effects in some individuals; consult specific product labeling for details.

Alpelisib

Oral		
Granules	50 mg	Vijoice® (Single-use packet), Novartis
Tablets, film-coated	50 mg	Piqray®, Novartis
		Vijoice®, Novartis
	125 mg	Vijoice®, Novartis
	150 mg	Piqray®, Novartis
	200 mg	Piqray®, Novartis
		Vijoice®, Novartis

† Use is not currently included in the labeling approved by the US Food and Drug Administration.

Selected Revisions April 10, 2024, © Copyright, June 10, 2019, American Society of Health-System Pharmacists, Inc.

Apalutamide

10:00 · ANTINEOPLASTIC AGENTS

■ Apalutamide, a nonsteroidal antiandrogen, is an antineoplastic agent.

USES

● Prostate Cancer

Metastatic Castration-Sensitive Prostate Cancer

Apalutamide is used for the treatment of metastatic castration-sensitive prostate cancer in patients who are either receiving concomitant treatment with a gonadotropin-releasing hormone (GnRH) analog or who have had a bilateral orchiectomy. Guidelines recommend androgen deprivation therapy combined with abiraterone, apalutamide, enzalutamide, or docetaxel for the treatment of metastatic castration-sensitive prostate cancer.

Clinical Experience

The indication for apalutamide in metastatic castration-sensitive prostate cancer is based principally on the results of a randomized, double-blind, placebo-controlled phase 3 study (TITAN) in 1052 patients. Patients were randomized in a 1:1 ratio to receive either apalutamide (240 mg once daily) or placebo; androgen deprivation therapy was continued in all patients. Patients were stratified by Gleason score at diagnosis, prior docetaxel use, and region of the world. The primary measures of efficacy were radiographic progression-free survival and overall survival. The median age of patients enrolled in the study was 68 years; 23% of patients were 75 years of age or older. The majority of patients (63%) had high-volume disease; 67% had a Gleason score of 8 or higher, 68% had received prior treatment with an antiandrogen (bicalutamide, flutamide, or nilutamide), 16% had prior surgery, radiotherapy, or both for prostate cancer, and all patients except 1 had an Eastern Cooperative Oncology Group (ECOG) performance status of 0 or 1 at baseline.

At a median follow-up of 44 months, the median radiographic progression-free survival was not reached in the apalutamide group and was 22.1 months in the placebo group. Median overall survival was not reached in the apalutamide group and was 52 months in the placebo group. Improvements in radiographic progression-free survival and overall survival were consistent across subgroups based on disease volume and Gleason score at diagnosis. Patients receiving apalutamide also had a longer time to initiation of cytotoxic chemotherapy. Time to pain worsening was prolonged with apalutamide, and health-related quality of life did not worsen with the addition of apalutamide to androgen deprivation therapy.

Clinical Perspective

According to a joint guideline from the American Urological Association (AUA), American Society for Radiation Oncology (ASTRO), and the Society of Urologic Oncology (SUO), clinicians should offer androgen deprivation therapy in combination with androgen pathway directed therapy (abiraterone plus prednisone, apalutamide, or enzalutamide) or docetaxel for the treatment of metastatic castration-sensitive prostate cancer. Oral androgen pathway directed therapy should not be offered without concomitant androgen deprivation therapy. A guideline from the American Society of Clinical Oncology (ASCO) similarly states that standard of care therapy for noncastration-sensitive metastatic prostate cancer is androgen deprivation therapy combined with docetaxel, abiraterone, enzalutamide, or apalutamide. No specific agent is recommended over another. Apalutamide plus androgen deprivation therapy should be offered to men with metastatic noncastration-sensitive prostate cancer, including those with de novo metastatic disease and those who have received prior therapy (e.g., radical prostatectomy or radiotherapy for localized disease).

Nonmetastatic Castration-Resistant Prostate Cancer

Apalutamide is used for the treatment of nonmetastatic castration-resistant prostate cancer in patients who are either receiving concomitant treatment with a GnRH analog or who have had a bilateral orchiectomy. The use of an androgen receptor antagonist (i.e., darolutamide, apalutamide, enzalutamide) is recommended for patients with nonmetastatic castration-resistant prostate cancer who are at high risk of metastases.

Clinical Experience

The indication for apalutamide in nonmetastatic castration-resistant prostate cancer is based principally on the results of a randomized, double-blind, placebo-controlled phase 3 study (SPARTAN) in 1207 patients who were at high risk for metastasis (i.e., prostate specific antigen [PSA] doubling time of 10 months or less despite continuous androgen deprivation therapy). Patients were randomized in a 2:1 ratio to receive either apalutamide (240 mg once daily) or placebo; androgen deprivation therapy was continued in all patients. Patients were stratified by PSA doubling time, use of bone resorption inhibitors, and presence of locoregional nodal disease. Treatment was continued until disease progression or unacceptable toxicity occurred, new treatment was initiated, or the patient withdrew from the study. The primary measure of efficacy was metastasis-free survival; secondary end points included time to metastasis, progression-free (including locoregional or distant metastatic progression) survival, time to symptomatic progression, overall survival, and time to initiation of cytotoxic chemotherapy. The median age of patients enrolled in the study was 74 years; 26% of patients were 80 years of age or older. Most patients (77%) had undergone prior surgery or radiation therapy of the prostate; 78% had a Gleason score of 7 or higher, 73% had received prior treatment with a nonsteroidal antiandrogen (69% had received bicalutamide and 10% had received flutamide), and all had an ECOG performance status of 0 or 1.

At a median follow-up of 20.3 months, metastasis-free survival was substantially longer in apalutamide-treated patients compared with those who received placebo (40.5 and 16.2 months, respectively). Results of a subgroup analysis (based on PSA doubling time, baseline PSA concentration, number of prior hormonal therapies, use of bone resorption inhibitors, locoregional nodal disease, age, race, ECOG performance status, and geographic region) suggested that the drug's effect on metastasis-free survival was consistent across all subgroups. Patients receiving apalutamide also had longer time to metastasis, progression-free survival, time to symptomatic progression, and time to initiation of cytotoxicity chemotherapy compared with those receiving placebo. In the final overall survival analysis (conducted 32 months after the primary endpoint analysis), median overall survival was significantly prolonged in patients receiving apalutamide compared with those receiving placebo (73.9 months versus 59.9 months).

Clinical Perspective

According to a joint guideline from AUA, ASTRO, and SUO, the decision to add an androgen receptor antagonist to androgen deprivation therapy in patients with nonmetastatic castration-resistant prostate cancer is dependent on metastatic risk. The risk of metastasis is determined by the time to doubling of PSA levels. If the PSA doubling time is 10 months or less, metastatic risk is high and the guideline recommends use of either apalutamide, darolutamide, or enzalutamide in addition to androgen deprivation therapy. Continuation of androgen deprivation therapy with observation is recommended for patients who have a PSA doubling time greater than 10 months as risk of metastasis is considered to be lower.

DOSAGE AND ADMINISTRATION

● General

Pretreatment Screening

● Evaluate patients for fracture and fall risk.

Patient Monitoring

● Monitor for signs and symptoms of ischemic heart disease and cerebrovascular disorders. Optimize management of cardiovascular risk factors (e.g., hypertension, diabetes, dyslipidemia).

● In patients at risk for fracture, monitor and manage fracture risk.

● Monitor patients for the development of severe cutaneous adverse reactions.

Other General Considerations

- Patients receiving apalutamide should receive concurrent therapy with a gonadotropin-releasing hormone (GnRH) analog unless they have undergone bilateral orchiectomy.

● Administration

Apalutamide is administered orally once daily without regard to food. The tablets should be swallowed whole; do not crush or split tablets. Store tablets in the original package at 20–25°C (excursions permitted between 15–30°C); protect from light and moisture, and do not discard the desiccant. If a dose is missed, the dose should be taken as soon as possible on the same day, with a return to the normal dosing schedule on the following day. Patients should not take extra tablets to make up for the missed dose.

For patients who have difficulty swallowing, apalutamide 240 mg tablet may be dispersed in non-carbonated water and then administered with either orange juice, applesauce, or additional water. Place the whole apalutamide 240 mg tablet in a cup; do not crush or split the tablet. Add approximately 2 teaspoons (10 mL) of non-carbonated water to fully immerse the tablet in water. Wait 2 minutes until the tablet is broken up, then stir the mixture. Add 2 tablespoons (30 mL) of either orange juice, applesauce, or additional water and stir the mixture. Swallow the mixture immediately. Rinse the cup with enough water to ensure the whole dose is administered and drink immediately. Do not store apalutamide mixed with non-carbonated water, orange juice, or applesauce for later use.

For patients who have difficulty swallowing, apalutamide 60 mg tablets may be mixed in applesauce. Mix whole apalutamide 60 mg tablets in 4 ounces (120 mL) of applesauce by stirring; do not crush or split the tablets. After stirring, wait 15 minutes, then stir the mixture again. Wait another 15 minutes and stir the mixture until the tablets are dispersed with no chunks remaining. Use a spoon to administer the mixture, and swallow it right away. After administration of the mixture, rinse the container with 2 ounces (60 mL) of water and immediately drink the contents. Repeat this rinse with 2 ounces (60 mL) of water a second time to ensure that the entire dose is administered. Administer the entire mixture within 1 hour of preparation. Do not store apalutamide that is mixed with applesauce.

The apalutamide 240 mg tablet can be administered through a feeding tube (8 French or greater). Place one 240 mg tablet in the barrel of at least a 20 mL syringe and draw up 10 mL of non-carbonated water into the syringe. Wait 10 minutes and then shake the syringe vigorously to disperse contents completely. Administer immediately through the feeding tube. Refill the syringe with non-carbonated water and administer. Repeat this process until no tablet residue is left in the syringe or feeding tube.

● Dosage

Prostate Cancer

Metastatic Castration-Sensitive Prostate Cancer

For the treatment of metastatic castration-sensitive prostate cancer, the recommended dosage of apalutamide in adults is 240 mg once daily.

Nonmetastatic Castration-Resistant Prostate Cancer

For the treatment of nonmetastatic castration-resistant prostate cancer, the recommended dosage of apalutamide in adults is 240 mg once daily.

Dosage Modification for Toxicity

General Toxicity

If an intolerable adverse effect or grade 3 or greater toxicity occurs, apalutamide therapy should be interrupted until symptoms improve to grade 1 or less or return to baseline. Apalutamide therapy may then be resumed with or without a dosage reduction. If a dosage reduction is warranted, the dosage of apalutamide may be reduced to 180 or 120 mg once daily.

Consider permanent discontinuation of apalutamide for grade 3 or 4 cerebrovascular and ischemic cardiovascular events. Permanently discontinue apalutamide for confirmed severe cutaneous adverse reactions or for other grade 4 skin reactions.

● Special Populations

Hepatic Impairment

Initial dosage adjustment is not necessary in patients with mild or moderate hepatic impairment (Child-Pugh class A or B).

Apalutamide has not been studied in patients with severe hepatic impairment (Child-Pugh class C).

Renal Impairment

Initial dosage adjustment is not necessary in patients with mild or moderate renal impairment (estimated glomerular filtration rate [eGFR] of 30–89 mL/minute per 1.73 m²).

Apalutamide has not been studied in patients with severe renal impairment (eGFR ≤29 mL/minute per 1.73 m²).

Geriatric Patients

The manufacturer makes no special dosage recommendations for geriatric patients; most patients (81%) in the principal efficacy studies were ≥65 years of age.

CAUTIONS

● Contraindications

None.

● Warnings/Precautions

Cerebrovascular and Ischemic Cardiovascular Events

Cerebrovascular and ischemic cardiovascular events, including events leading to death, occurred in patients receiving apalutamide. In a study of patients with non-metastatic castration-resistant prostate cancer (SPARTAN), 3.7% of apalutamide-treated patients experienced ischemic cardiovascular events compared to 2% of patients receiving placebo. In a study of patients with metastatic castration-sensitive prostate cancer (TITAN), 4.4% of apalutamide-treated patients experienced ischemic cardiovascular events compared to 1.5% of patients receiving placebo. Across both studies, 4 patients (0.3%) receiving apalutamide died from an ischemic cardiovascular event, compared to 2 patients (0.2%) receiving placebo.

In the SPARTAN study, cerebrovascular events occurred in 2.5% of apalutamide-treated patients and 1% of patients receiving placebo; in the TITAN study, cerebrovascular events occurred in 1.9% of apalutamide-treated patients and 2.1% of patients receiving placebo. Across both studies, death due to a cerebrovascular event occurred in 3 apalutamide-treated patients (0.2%) and 2 patients receiving placebo (0.2%).

Patients with a history of unstable angina, myocardial infarction, congestive heart failure, stroke, or transient ischemic attack within 6 months of randomization were excluded from the SPARTAN and TITAN studies.

Monitor for signs and symptoms of ischemic heart disease and cerebrovascular disorders during apalutamide therapy. Optimize management of cardiovascular risk factors (e.g., hypertension, diabetes, dyslipidemia), and consider discontinuation of apalutamide for grade 3 and 4 events.

Fractures

Fractures have occurred in patients receiving apalutamide. In a study of patients with nonmetastatic castration-resistant prostate cancer (SPARTAN), fractures were reported in 12% of apalutamide-treated patients compared with 7% of those receiving placebo; grade 3 or 4 fractures occurred in 2.7% of patients receiving the drug compared with 0.8% of those receiving placebo. The median time to onset of fracture was 314 days (range: 20–953 days) in patients receiving apalutamide. In a study of patients with metastatic castration-sensitive prostate cancer (TITAN), fractures were reported in 9% of apalutamide-treated patients and 6% of patients receiving placebo; grade 3 or 4 fractures occurred in 1.5% of patients in both study arms. The median time to onset of fracture was 56 days (range: 2–111 days) in patients receiving apalutamide. Routine bone density assessment and treatment of osteoporosis with bone-targeted agents were not performed during either study.

Evaluate patients for fracture risk. Monitor and manage patients at risk for fractures according to established treatment guidelines; consider therapy with bone-targeted agents.

Falls

Falls have occurred in patients receiving apalutamide, with increased frequency observed in geriatric patients. In a study of patients with nonmetastatic castration-resistant prostate cancer (SPARTAN), falls occurred in 16% of apalutamide-treated patients and 9% of patients receiving placebo. In clinical studies, falls occurred in 8% of patients <65 years of age, 10% of patients 65–74 years of age, and 19% of patients ≥75 years of age receiving the drug. Falls were not associated with loss of consciousness or seizure.

Evaluate patients for fall risk.

Seizures

Seizures have occurred in patients receiving apalutamide. In 2 randomized studies in patients with prostate cancer, seizures were reported in 0.4% of patients receiving apalutamide compared with 0.1% of those receiving placebo. Patients with a history of seizures, predisposing factors for seizures, or concomitant use of drugs that can lower the seizure threshold or induce seizures were excluded from these studies. Time to onset of seizures ranged from 159–650 days following initiation of the drug.

It is not known whether anticonvulsants will prevent seizures in patients receiving apalutamide. The safety of resuming apalutamide therapy in patients who experienced a seizure while receiving the drug has not been established. Permanently discontinue apalutamide in patients who develop a seizure during treatment.

Severe Cutaneous Adverse Reactions

Fatal and life-threatening severe cutaneous adverse reactions (e.g., Stevens-Johnson syndrome/toxic epidermal necrolysis and drug reaction with eosinophilia and systemic symptoms [DRESS]) have been reported in patients receiving apalutamide. Inform patients of the signs and symptoms of these reactions (e.g., a prodrome of fever, flu-like symptoms, mucosal lesions, progressive skin rash, or lymphadenopathy) and monitor for development.

If a severe cutaneous adverse reaction is suspected, interrupt apalutamide therapy until the cause of the reaction is determined. Consulting a dermatologist is recommended. If a severe cutaneous adverse reaction (or other grade 4 skin reaction) is confirmed, permanently discontinue apalutamide.

Fetal/Neonatal Morbidity and Mortality

Safety and efficacy of apalutamide have not been established in females. Based on its mechanism of action and findings from animal studies, apalutamide may cause fetal harm and loss of pregnancy. Fetal abnormalities and embryofetal lethality were observed in pregnant rats when oral apalutamide was administered during and after organogenesis at maternal exposures ≥2 times the human clinical exposure at the recommended dose.

Advise males with female partners of reproductive potential to use effective methods of contraception during apalutamide therapy and for 3 months after the last dose of the drug; in addition, males should not donate sperm while receiving the drug and for 3 months after the drug is discontinued. Male patients receiving the drug should use a condom during sexual encounters with pregnant females.

Specific Populations

Pregnancy

Safety and efficacy of apalutamide have not been established in females. Based on its mechanism of action and findings from animal studies, apalutamide may cause fetal harm and loss of pregnancy. Fetal abnormalities and embryofetal lethality were observed in pregnant rats when oral apalutamide was administered during and after organogenesis at maternal exposures ≥2 times the human clinical exposure at the recommended dose.

Lactation

Safety and efficacy of apalutamide have not been established in females. It is not known whether apalutamide or its metabolites are distributed into human milk. The effects of apalutamide on nursing infants or on milk production also are not known.

Females and Males of Reproductive Potential

Advise males with female partners of reproductive potential to use effective methods of contraception during apalutamide therapy and for 3 months after the last dose of the drug; in addition, males should not donate sperm while receiving the drug and for 3 months after the drug is discontinued. Male patients receiving the drug should use a condom during sexual encounters with pregnant females.

Based on animal studies, apalutamide may impair male fertility. In male rats, apalutamide was associated with decreased sperm concentration and motility, increased abnormal sperm morphology, reduced epididymis and secondary sex gland weights, lower copulation and fertility rates upon pairing with untreated females, and a reduced number of live fetuses secondary to increased pre- and/or post-implantation loss; effects on male rats were reversible following discontinuance of the drug.

Pediatric Use

Safety and efficacy of apalutamide have not been established in pediatric patients.

Geriatric Use

In the principal efficacy studies evaluating apalutamide, 81% of patients were ≥65 years of age and 40% were ≥75 years of age. No overall differences in efficacy were observed between geriatric patients and younger adults. Grade 3 or 4 adverse reactions occurred in 39% of patients <65 years of age, 41% of patients 65–74 years of age, and 49% of patients ≥75 years of age. Falls occurred more frequently in geriatric patients, with falls reported in 8% of patients <65 years of age, 10% of patients 65–74 years of age, and 19% of patients ≥75 years of age.

Hepatic Impairment

No clinically important differences in systemic exposure of apalutamide or N-desmethylapalutamide were observed in patients with mild or moderate hepatic impairment (Child-Pugh class A or B) compared with individuals with normal hepatic function. The unbound fraction of apalutamide or N-desmethylapalutamide was not affected by hepatic impairment.

Pharmacokinetics of apalutamide have not been established in patients with severe hepatic impairment (Child-Pugh class C).

Renal Impairment

Renal impairment is not expected to affect the elimination of apalutamide or N-desmethylapalutamide. No clinically important differences in systemic exposure of apalutamide or N-desmethylapalutamide were observed in patients with mild or moderate renal impairment (estimated glomerular filtration rate [eGFR] of 30–89 mL/minute per 1.73 m²) compared with individuals with normal renal function.

Pharmacokinetics of apalutamide have not been established in patients with severe renal impairment (eGFR ≤29 mL/minute per 1.73 m²).

● Common Adverse Effects

Adverse effects reported in ≥10% of patients receiving apalutamide include fatigue, arthralgia, rash, decreased appetite, falls, decreased weight, hypertension, hot flush, diarrhea, and fracture.

DRUG INTERACTIONS

Apalutamide is metabolized principally by cytochrome P-450 (CYP) isoenzymes 2C8 and 3A4 to form its major active metabolite, N-desmethylapalutamide.

Apalutamide is a potent inducer of CYP3A4 and 2C19 and a weak inducer of CYP2C9 in humans. In addition, in vitro studies indicate that apalutamide and N-desmethylapalutamide are moderate to potent inducers of CYP3A4 and 2B6, moderate inhibitors of CYP2B6 and 2C8, and weak inhibitors of CYP2C9, 2C19, and 3A4. Apalutamide and N-desmethylapalutamide neither inhibit nor induce CYP1A2 or 2D6 at clinically relevant concentrations.

Apalutamide and N-desmethylapalutamide are substrates of P-glycoprotein (P-gp) in vitro; however, apalutamide absorption is not limited by P-gp.

Apalutamide and *N*-desmethylapalutamide are not substrates of breast cancer resistance protein (BCRP), organic anion transport protein (OATP) 1B1, or OATP1B3.

Apalutamide is a weak inducer of P-gp, BCRP, and OATP1B1 in humans. In vitro, apalutamide and *N*-desmethylapalutamide inhibit organic cation transporter 2 (OCT2), organic anion transporter 3 (OAT3), and multidrug and toxin extrusion (MATE) transporters. Apalutamide may induce uridine diphosphate-glucuronosyltransferase (UGT). Apalutamide and *N*-desmethylapalutamide do not inhibit organic anion transporter 1 (OAT1).

● *Drugs Affecting Hepatic Microsomal Enzymes*

Concomitant use of apalutamide with potent inhibitors of CYP2C8 or 3A4 may result in increased steady-state exposure of the total active forms of apalutamide (i.e., unbound apalutamide plus potency-adjusted unbound *N*-desmethylapalutamide). No initial dosage adjustment is necessary; however, reduction of apalutamide dosage may be necessary based on tolerability.

Mild or moderate inhibitors of CYP2C8 or 3A4 are not expected to affect the exposure of apalutamide.

● *Drugs Metabolized by Hepatic Microsomal Enzymes*

Concomitant use of apalutamide with drugs that are principally metabolized by CYP3A4, 2C9, or 2C19 may result in decreased exposure of the CYP substrate. The manufacturer of apalutamide recommends that concomitant use be avoided when possible (e.g., by switching to an alternative drug that is not metabolized by these isoenzymes); if concomitant use cannot be avoided, patients should be monitored for decreased therapeutic effect of the CYP substrate.

Concomitant administration of apalutamide with a CYP2C8 substrate did not result in clinically important changes in exposure of the CYP2C8 substrate.

● *Drugs Affecting or Affected by P-glycoprotein Transport*

Inhibition or induction of P-gp is not expected to affect the bioavailability of apalutamide.

Concomitant use of apalutamide and P-gp substrates may result in decreased exposure of the P-gp substrate. If concomitant use is necessary, caution should be exercised and patients should be monitored for decreased therapeutic effect of the P-gp substrate.

● *Drugs Affected by Breast Cancer Resistance Protein and/or Organic Anion Transport Polypeptide 1B1*

Concomitant use of apalutamide with drugs that are substrates of BCRP or OATP1B1 may result in decreased exposure of the BCRP or OATP1B1 substrate. If concomitant use is necessary, caution should be exercised and patients should be monitored for decreased therapeutic effect of the BCRP or OATP1B1 substrate.

● *Drugs Metabolized by Uridine Diphosphate-glucuronosyltransferase*

Concomitant use of apalutamide with drugs that are substrates of UGT may result in decreased exposure of the UGT substrate. If concomitant use is necessary, caution should be exercised and patients should be monitored for decreased therapeutic effect of the UGT substrate.

● *Drugs Affected by Other Transporters*

In vitro, apalutamide and *N*-desmethylapalutamide inhibit OCT2, OAT3, and MATE transporters, but do not inhibit OAT1. Apalutamide is not expected to cause clinically important changes in exposure of OAT3 substrates (e.g., penicillin G).

● *Drugs Affecting Gastric Acidity*

Because apalutamide remains un-ionized at physiologic pH, concomitant administration of apalutamide and drugs that increase gastric pH (e.g., proton-pump inhibitors, histamine H_2-receptor antagonists, antacids) are not expected to have a clinically important effect on the solubility and bioavailability of apalutamide.

● *Antifungal Agents*

Itraconazole

Concomitant administration of the potent CYP3A4 inhibitor itraconazole and apalutamide (single 240-mg dose) decreased peak plasma concentrations of apalutamide and *N*-desmethylapalutamide by 22 and 15%, respectively; areas under the concentration-time curve (AUCs) were not affected.

No initial dosage adjustment is necessary; however, reduction of apalutamide dosage may be necessary based on tolerability in patients receiving concomitant itraconazole therapy.

Ketoconazole

Based on pharmacokinetic modeling, concomitant use of ketoconazole (a potent CYP3A4 inhibitor) and apalutamide is expected to increase AUC of single-dose apalutamide by 24% with no change in apalutamide peak plasma concentration, and to increase steady-state AUC and peak plasma concentration of apalutamide by 51 and 38%, respectively. At steady state, AUC and peak plasma concentration of the total active forms of apalutamide (i.e., unbound apalutamide plus potency-adjusted unbound *N*-desmethylapalutamide) are expected to increase by 28 and 23%, respectively.

No initial dosage adjustment is necessary; however, reduction of apalutamide dosage may be necessary based on tolerability in patients receiving concomitant ketoconazole therapy.

● *Fexofenadine*

Concomitant administration of the P-gp substrate fexofenadine (single dose) and apalutamide (240 mg daily at steady state) decreased fexofenadine AUC by 30%. If concomitant use of fexofenadine and apalutamide is necessary, caution should be exercised and patients should be monitored for decreased therapeutic effect of fexofenadine.

● *Gemfibrozil*

Concomitant administration of the potent CYP2C8 inhibitor gemfibrozil and apalutamide decreased peak plasma concentration of apalutamide by 21% and increased AUC of apalutamide by 68%. Based on pharmacokinetic modeling, gemfibrozil is expected to increase steady-state AUC and peak plasma concentrations of apalutamide by 44 and 32%, respectively, and to increase steady-state AUC and peak plasma concentrations of the total active forms of apalutamide (i.e., unbound apalutamide plus potency-adjusted unbound *N*-desmethylapalutamide) by 23 and 19%, respectively.

No initial dosage adjustment is necessary; however, reduction of apalutamide dosage may be necessary based on tolerability in patients receiving concomitant gemfibrozil therapy.

● *Leuprolide*

Pharmacokinetic data indicate that apalutamide has no apparent effect on steady-state exposure to leuprolide when co-administered.

● *Midazolam*

Concomitant administration of the CYP3A4 substrate midazolam (single oral dose) and apalutamide (240 mg daily) decreased midazolam AUC by 92%. Concomitant use of apalutamide and midazolam should be avoided when possible (e.g., by switching to an alternative drug that is not metabolized by CYP3A4); if concomitant use cannot be avoided, patients should be monitored for decreased therapeutic effect of midazolam.

● *Omeprazole*

Concomitant administration of the CYP2C19 substrate omeprazole (single dose) and apalutamide (240 mg daily) decreased omeprazole AUC by 85%. Concomitant use of apalutamide and omeprazole should be avoided when possible (e.g., by switching to an alternative drug that is not metabolized by CYP2C19); if concomitant use cannot be avoided, patients should be monitored for decreased therapeutic effect of omeprazole.

● *Pioglitazone*

Concomitant administration of the CYP2C8 substrate pioglitazone (single dose) and apalutamide (240 mg daily) decreased pioglitazone AUC by 18%.

● *Rifampin*

Based on pharmacokinetic modeling, concomitant use of the potent CYP3A4 and moderate CYP2C8 inducer rifampin (600 mg daily) and apalutamide is expected to decrease steady-state AUC and peak plasma concentrations of apalutamide by 34 and 25%, respectively, and to decrease steady-state AUC and peak plasma concentrations of the total active forms of apalutamide (i.e., unbound apalutamide plus potency-adjusted unbound N-desmethylapalutamide) by 19 and 15%, respectively. However, no pharmacokinetic interactions were observed between apalutamide and CYP3A4 inducers in a population pharmacokinetic analysis based on limited data.

● *Rosuvastatin*

Concomitant administration of the BCRP and OATP1B1 substrate rosuvastatin (single dose) and apalutamide (240 mg daily) decreased rosuvastatin AUC by 41% with no change in rosuvastatin peak plasma concentration. If concomitant use of rosuvastatin and apalutamide is necessary, caution should be exercised and patients should be monitored for decreased therapeutic effect of rosuvastatin.

● *Warfarin*

Concomitant administration of the CYP2C9 substrate warfarin (single dose) and apalutamide (240 mg daily) decreased AUC of S-warfarin by 46%. If apalutamide is used concomitantly with warfarin, international normalized ratio (INR) should be monitored at initiation of concomitant therapy and upon discontinuance of apalutamide.

DESCRIPTION

Apalutamide, a nonsteroidal antiandrogen, is an antineoplastic agent. The drug competitively inhibits androgen binding to androgen receptors; its mechanisms of action are similar to those of enzalutamide. Apalutamide binds directly to the ligand-binding domain of the androgen receptor and inhibits nuclear translocation of the activated androgen receptor, androgen-dependent binding of the androgen receptor complex to DNA, and androgen receptor-mediated gene transcription in cells that overexpress the androgen receptor. Apalutamide reduced tumor growth and induced apoptosis of tumor cells, leading to decreased tumor volume, in xenograft models of castration-resistant prostate cancer in mice.

In castration-resistant prostate cancer, alterations in androgen receptor signaling (e.g., androgen receptor gene mutation or amplification, androgen receptor overexpression) have been shown to result in persistence of androgen receptor signaling and to contribute to disease progression despite castrate levels of androgens. Resistance to conventional antiandrogens (e.g., bicalutamide, flutamide, nilutamide) in castration-resistant prostate cancer has been associated with paradoxical agonistic effects of these drugs and continued androgen receptor signaling. Unlike these conventional antiandrogens but similar to enzalutamide, apalutamide does not exhibit agonistic activity in cells that overexpress the androgen receptor.

The binding affinity of apalutamide at the androgen receptor is 7–10 times greater than that of bicalutamide. Although apalutamide and enzalutamide exhibit similar antiandrogenic activity in vitro, apalutamide demonstrated greater activity than enzalutamide in xenograft models of castration-resistant prostate cancer. At equivalent dosages, steady-state concentrations of apalutamide and enzalutamide in xenograft tumors in mice were similar, but steady-state plasma and CNS concentrations of apalutamide were twofold to fourfold lower and fourfold lower, respectively, compared with concentrations of enzalutamide. Whether these higher murine tumor-to-plasma and tumor-to-CNS ratios for apalutamide translate into a lower risk of adverse effects, including seizures and other CNS toxicity, remains to be established.

Apalutamide exhibits dose-proportional pharmacokinetics over a dosage range of 30–480 mg once daily. Following oral administration, the median time to peak plasma concentrations is 2 hours; the mean absolute bioavailability of apalutamide is approximately 100%. Steady-state concentrations of apalutamide are achieved after 4 weeks of once-daily dosing and the mean accumulation ratio is approximately fivefold. Oral administration of apalutamide tablets dispersed in applesauce did not result in any clinically relevant changes in time to peak plasma concentration or area under the concentration-time curve (AUC) when compared with administration of intact tablets under fasting conditions. Administration of apalutamide with a high-fat meal delays time to peak plasma concentration by approximately 2 hours but has no clinically important effects on AUC. Apalutamide is metabolized principally by cytochrome P-450 (CYP) isoenzymes 2C8 and 3A4 to form its major active metabolite, N-desmethylapalutamide, which exhibits antiandrogenic activity at one-third the potency of the parent drug in vitro. The contributions of CYP2C8 and 3A4 to the metabolism of apalutamide are approximately 58 and 13%, respectively, following a single dose and 40 and 37%, respectively, at steady state. Apalutamide and N-desmethylapalutamide account for 45 and 44%, respectively, of the total drug exposure following a single 240-mg dose of apalutamide.

Apalutamide and N-desmethylapalutamide are 96 and 95% bound, respectively, to plasma proteins; the extent of binding is independent of plasma concentration. Clearance of apalutamide is increased at steady state, suggesting that the drug may induce its own metabolism by CYP3A4. The mean steady-state half-life of apalutamide is approximately 3 days. Following oral administration of a single radiolabeled dose of apalutamide, 65% of the dose was recovered in urine (1.2% as unchanged drug and 2.7% as N-desmethylapalutamide) and 24% of the dose was recovered in feces (1.5% as unchanged drug and 2% as N-desmethylapalutamide).

ADVICE TO PATIENTS

- Importance of reading the manufacturer's patient information.

- For patients concurrently receiving GnRH analog therapy, importance of continuing this therapy during apalutamide therapy.

- Importance of taking apalutamide at the same time each day without regard to food and of swallowing tablets whole. Instruct patients who cannot swallow tablets whole to follow the instructions for the prescribed strength of apalutamide tablets for alternate methods of administration. If a dose is missed, importance of taking the missed dose as soon as possible on the same day and taking the next dose at the regularly scheduled time on the following day. Advise patients that they should not take extra tablets to make up for a missed dose.

- Risk of cerebrovascular and ischemic cardiovascular events. Importance of advising patients to seek immediate medical attention if any symptoms of a cardiovascular or cerebrovascular event develop.

- Risk of falls and fractures.

- Risk of seizures; discuss conditions that may predispose to seizures and drugs that may lower the seizure threshold. Advise patients of the risk of engaging in activities where sudden loss of consciousness could cause serious harm to self or others. Importance of immediately informing clinician if a seizure occurs.

- Risk of severe cutaneous adverse reactions. Inform patients of the signs and symptoms of severe cutaneous adverse reactions (e.g., a prodrome of fever, flu-like symptoms, mucosal lesions, progressive skin rash, or lymphadenopathy).

- Risk of fetal harm. Necessity of advising male patients with female partners of reproductive potential to use effective methods of contraception during apalutamide therapy and for 3 months after the last dose of the drug; also advise male patients receiving the drug to use a condom during sexual encounters with pregnant females.

- Potential for apalutamide to impair male fertility. Advise patients that they should not donate sperm during apalutamide therapy and for 3 months after the last dose of the drug.

- Importance of informing clinicians of existing or contemplated concomitant therapy, including prescription and OTC drugs and dietary or herbal supplements, as well as any concomitant illnesses (e.g., seizures).

- Importance of informing patients of other important precautionary information.

PREPARATIONS

Apalutamide can only be obtained through designated specialty pharmacies and specialty distributors. Contact Janssen CarePath at 877-227-3728 or consult the Janssen CarePath website for specific availability information (https://www.janssencarepath.com/hcp/erleada).

Excipients in commercially available drug preparations may have clinically important effects in some individuals; consult specific product labeling for details.

Apalutamide

Oral

Tablets, film-coated	60 mg	Erleada®, Janssen
	240 mg	Erleada®

† Use is not currently included in the labeling approved by the US Food and Drug Administration.

Selected Revisions May 10, 2024, © Copyright, February 26, 2018, American Society of Health-System Pharmacists, Inc.

Atezolizumab

10:00 • ANTINEOPLASTIC AGENTS

■ Atezolizumab, a humanized anti-programmed-death ligand-1 (anti-PD-L1) monoclonal antibody, is an antineoplastic agent.

USES

● Urothelial Carcinoma

Atezolizumab is used as a single agent for the treatment of locally advanced or metastatic urothelial carcinoma in adult patients with high programmed-death ligand-1 (PD-L1) expression (defined as PD-L1 staining in tumor-infiltrating immune cells covering at least 5% of the tumor area) who are not candidates for cisplatin-containing therapy; an FDA-approved diagnostic test is required to confirm the presence of PD-L1 expression prior to initiation of therapy in patients who are not candidates for cisplatin-containing therapy.

Atezolizumab also is used as a single agent for the treatment of locally advanced or metastatic urothelial carcinoma in adult patients who are not candidates for platinum-containing chemotherapy regardless of PD-L1 expression.

The accelerated approval of atezolizumab for these indications is based on objective response rate and duration of response. Continued approval for these indications may be contingent on verification and description of clinical benefit of atezolizumab in confirmatory studies.

The current indications for atezolizumab in the treatment of locally advanced or metastatic urothelial carcinoma are based principally on the results of a single cohort (cohort 1) from an open-label, multicenter, noncomparative, 2-cohort, phase 2 study (IMvigor210). Cohort 1 consisted of 119 patients with locally advanced or metastatic urothelial carcinoma who were ineligible for cisplatin-containing chemotherapy and were either previously untreated or had disease progression at least 12 months after neoadjuvant or adjuvant chemotherapy. The primary measure of efficacy was objective response rate as assessed by an independent review facility according to Response Evaluation Criteria in Solid Tumors (RECIST). Patients received atezolizumab 1200 mg administered as an IV infusion every 3 weeks until disease progression or unacceptable toxicity occurred. Patients with a history of autoimmune disease; those with active or corticosteroid-dependent brain metastases; those who had received a live, attenuated vaccine within 28 days prior to enrollment; and those who had received systemic immunostimulatory agents within 6 weeks or immunosuppressive agents within 2 weeks prior to enrollment were excluded from the study.

In the cisplatin-ineligible cohort (cohort 1), the median age of patients was 73 years; 91% were Caucasian, 81% were male, 80% had a baseline Eastern Cooperative Oncology Group (ECOG) performance status of 0 or 1, 66% had visceral metastases, 35% had non-bladder urothelial carcinoma, and 20% had disease progression following platinum-containing therapy in the neoadjuvant or adjuvant setting. Most patients (73%) had low expression of PD-L1 (defined as PD-L1 staining in tumor-infiltrating immune cells covering less than 5% of the tumor area) as detected by an immunohistochemistry assay (Ventana PD-L1 [SP142]). Approximately 27% of patients had high expression of PD-L1 (defined as PD-L1 staining in tumor-infiltrating immune cells covering 5% or more of the tumor area). The median age of patients with high expression of PD-L1 was 67 years; 88% were Caucasian, 81% were male, 72% had a baseline ECOG performance status of 0 or 1, 56% had visceral metastases, 28% had non-bladder urothelial carcinoma, and 31% had disease progression following platinum-containing therapy in the neoadjuvant or adjuvant setting. Reasons for cisplatin ineligibility included baseline renal impairment (creatinine clearance 30–59 mL/minute), poor performance status (ECOG performance status of 2), hearing loss (25-decibel or more loss at 2 contiguous frequencies), or baseline grade 2–4 peripheral neuropathy in 70, 20, 14, or 6%, respectively, of patients in the entire cohort and in 66, 28, 16, or 9%, respectively, of those in the subset with high PD-L1 expression. The objective response rate for patients in the cisplatin-ineligible cohort of this study was 23.5%; complete response was achieved in 6.7% of patients in this cohort. Among patients who had disease progression following therapy in the neoadjuvant or adjuvant setting, the objective response rate was 33%. Objective response rates in patients with high or low levels of PD-L1 expression were 28.1 or 21.8%,

respectively; complete response was achieved in 6.3 or 6.9% of patients, respectively. At a median follow-up of 14.4 months, the median duration of response had not been reached.

Decreased survival with atezolizumab monotherapy compared with platinum-based therapy has been reported in an ongoing clinical trial (IMvigor130) in patients with previously untreated metastatic urothelial carcinoma with low PD-L1 expression; atezolizumab monotherapy is *not* currently FDA-labeled for use in such patients. In this trial, patients with previously untreated metastatic urothelial carcinoma who were eligible for platinum-containing therapy were randomized to receive atezolizumab monotherapy, atezolizumab in combination with platinum-based therapy (cisplatin or carboplatin in combination with gemcitabine), or platinum-based therapy alone. A preliminary data analysis showed decreased survival of patients with low PD-L1 expression who were receiving atezolizumab monotherapy compared with those receiving platinum-based therapy. Therefore, at the request of the independent data monitoring committee, enrollment in the atezolizumab monotherapy group was halted for patients with low expression of PD-L1 (defined as PD-L1 staining in tumor-infiltrating immune cells covering less than 5% of the tumor area) as detected by an immunohistochemistry assay (Ventana PD-L1 [SP142]). At a median follow-up of 11.8 months, median progression-free or overall survival in the intent-to-treat population was 8.2 or 16 months, respectively, in patients receiving atezolizumab plus platinum-based chemotherapy, and 6.3 or 13.4 months, respectively, in patients receiving placebo plus platinum-based chemotherapy. No difference in median overall survival was observed in patients receiving single-agent atezolizumab compared with those receiving placebo plus platinum-based chemotherapy.

Regulatory History

Atezolizumab received FDA approval for use in patients with locally advanced or metastatic urothelial carcinoma who progressed during or following platinum-containing chemotherapy or within 12 months of neoadjuvant or adjuvant treatment with platinum-containing chemotherapy in 2016 under the principles and procedures of FDA's accelerated review process that allows approval based on analysis of surrogate markers of response rather than clinical end points (e.g., prolongation of overall survival). Approval for this indication was based principally on the results of a cohort of patients previously treated with platinum-containing therapy in the IMvigor210 study. As a condition of the accelerated approval process, the manufacturer of atezolizumab was required to submit data from a phase 3 study (IMvigor211) to confirm overall survival benefit of the drug in patients with platinum-refractory locally advanced or metastatic urothelial carcinoma. In the IMvigor211 study, patients were randomized (stratified by PD-L1 expression, chemotherapy, presence of liver metastases, and prognostic factors) to receive atezolizumab 1200 mg or investigator's choice of chemotherapy IV every 3 weeks. The primary end point of overall survival in the IMvigor211 study was not met in patients with platinum-refractory metastatic urothelial carcinoma with high expression of PD-L1; therefore, the manufacturer voluntarily withdrew use of atezolizumab for the treatment of platinum-refractory locally advanced or metastatic urothelial carcinoma from labeling in recognition of the principles of the accelerated approval program. The manufacturer states that patients currently receiving atezolizumab for the treatment of metastatic urothelial carcinoma previously treated with platinum-containing chemotherapy should consult their clinician about whether to continue atezolizumab therapy or consider other treatment options.

● Non-small Cell Lung Cancer

Monotherapy for Previously Untreated Metastatic Non-small Cell Lung Cancer

Atezolizumab is used as monotherapy for the initial treatment of metastatic non-small cell lung cancer (NSCLC) with high PD-L1 expression and without epidermal growth factor receptor (*EGFR*) or anaplastic lymphoma kinase (*ALK*) genomic aberrations. High PD-L1 expression is defined as PD-L1 staining of at least 50% of tumor cells or PD-L1 stained tumor-infiltrating immune cells covering at least 10% of the tumor area; an FDA-approved diagnostic test is required to confirm the presence of PD-L1 expression prior to initiation of therapy.

The current indication for atezolizumab for previously untreated metastatic NSCLC in adult patients with high PD-L1 expression and without *EGFR* or *ALK* genomic aberrations is based principally on the results of a randomized, open-label, phase 3 study (IMpower110). In this study, 572 adults with metastatic NSCLC with squamous or nonsquamous histology who had previously untreated metastatic disease were randomized (stratified by sex, ECOG status, histology, and PD-L1 expression) in a 1:1 ratio to receive atezolizumab 1200 mg every 3 weeks or investigator's choice of platinum-based chemotherapy. Patients with non-squamous NSCLC were randomized to an investigator's choice of platinum-based chemotherapy received either cisplatin (75 mg/m²) in combination with pemetrexed (500 mg/m²) or carboplatin (dose required to obtain an AUC of 6 mg/mL per minute) in combination with pemetrexed (500 mg/m²); chemotherapy was administered on day 1 of each 21-day cycle for up to 4 or 6 cycles, followed by pemetrexed (500 mg/m²) as a single agent until disease progression or unacceptable toxicity occurred. Patients with squamous NSCLC randomized to an investigator's choice of platinum-based therapy received cisplatin (75 mg/m²) on day 1 in combination with gemcitabine (1250 mg/m²) on days 1 and 8 of each 21-day cycle or carboplatin (dose required to obtain an AUC of 5 mg/mL per minute) on day 1 in combination with gemcitabine (1000 mg/m²) on days 1 and 8 of each 21-day cycle for up to 4 or 6 cycles. Treatment was continued for the specified duration or until disease progression or unacceptable toxicity occurred; however, clinically stable patients with disease progression could continue treatment if they were considered to be deriving clinical benefit. In this study, the primary measure of efficacy was overall survival in a cohort of patients with wild-type EGFR and ALK expression.

In the cohort of 205 patients with wild-type *EGFR* and *ALK* and high PD-L1 expression, the median age was 65 years; 70% were male, 82% were White, and 17% were Asian. All patients had a baseline ECOG performance status of 0 or 1, 88% were current or former smokers, and 76% had non-squamous disease histology. The study excluded patients with a history of autoimmune disease; those with active or untreated CNS metastases; those who had received a live, attenuated vaccine within 28 days prior to randomization; and those who had received systemic immunostimulatory agents within 4 weeks or systemic immunosuppressive agents within 2 weeks prior to randomization.

In the cohort of patients with wild-type *EGFR* and *ALK* and high PD-L1 expression, median overall survival was prolonged in those receiving atezolizumab compared with those receiving platinum-based chemotherapy (20.2 versus 13.1 months; hazard ratio: 0.59). Median investigator-assessed progression-free survival in this cohort of patients was also prolonged in those receiving atezolizumab compared with those receiving platinum-based chemotherapy (8.1 versus 5 months; hazard ratio: 0.63). Investigator-assessed overall response rates were 38 or 29% in patients receiving atezolizumab or platinum-based chemotherapy, respectively.

At the time of the interim analysis, no difference in median overall survival was observed in patients with high or intermediate PD-L1 expression (PD-L1 staining of at least 1%, but less than 50%, of tumor cells or PD-L1 stained tumor-infiltrating immune cells covering at least 1%, but less than 10%, of the tumor area) receiving atezolizumab or platinum-based chemotherapy (18.2 versus 14.9 months).

Combination Therapy for Previously Untreated Metastatic Nonsquamous Non-small Cell Lung Cancer

Combination with Bevacizumab, Paclitaxel, and Carboplatin

Atezolizumab is used in combination with bevacizumab, carboplatin, and paclitaxel for the initial treatment of metastatic nonsquamous NSCLC without *EGFR* or *ALK* genomic aberrations.

The current indication for atezolizumab in combination with bevacizumab, carboplatin, and paclitaxel for the initial treatment of metastatic nonsquamous NSCLC is based principally on the results of a randomized, open-label, phase 3 study (IMpower150). In this study, 1202 adults with metastatic NSCLC with non-squamous histology who had not received prior chemotherapy for metastatic disease were randomized (stratified by sex, presence of liver metastases, and PD-L1 expression) in a 1:1:1 ratio to receive 4 or 6 cycles of therapy with atezolizumab in combination with carboplatin and paclitaxel (atezolizumab-carboplatin-paclitaxel); atezolizumab in combination with bevacizumab, carboplatin, and paclitaxel (atezolizumab-bevacizumab-carboplatin-paclitaxel); or bevacizumab, carboplatin, and paclitaxel alone (bevacizumab-carboplatin-paclitaxel). Following the initial 4 or 6 cycles of therapy, carboplatin and paclitaxel were discontinued and patients continued receiving atezolizumab and/or bevacizumab as initially assigned until disease progression or unacceptable toxicity occurred; however, atezolizumab-treated patients with disease progression could continue receiving treatment if they were considered to be deriving clinical benefit. The treatment regimens were administered in 3-week cycles at the following dosages:

atezolizumab 1200 mg every 3 weeks, bevacizumab 15 mg/kg every 3 weeks, carboplatin at the dose required to obtain an area under the concentration-time curve (AUC) of 6 mg/mL per minute every 3 weeks, and paclitaxel 200 mg/m² (175 mg/m² in patients of Asian ancestry) every 3 weeks. The primary measures of efficacy were overall survival in patients with wild-type EGFR and ALK expression (wild-type population) and progression-free survival as assessed by investigators according to RECIST in the wild-type population and in the subset of the wild-type population with high expression of an effector T-cell (Teff) gene signature.

The median age of patients receiving atezolizumab-bevacizumab-carboplatin-paclitaxel or bevacizumab-carboplatin-paclitaxel in the IMpower150 study was 63 years; within these 2 treatment groups, 82% of patients were Caucasian, 80% were current or prior smokers, 60% were male, 49% had negative PD-L1 expression (defined as PD-L1 expression on less than 1% of tumor cells and tumor-infiltrating immune cells, as detected by the Ventana PD-L1 [SP142] immunohistochemistry assay), 39% had high Teff gene-signature expression (defined as a score of −1.91 or greater based on PD-L1, CXCL9, and interferon gamma mRNA expression in tumor tissue, as detected by a clinical trial assay), 14% had liver metastases at baseline, 13% were of Asian ancestry, and 10% were Hispanic. All patients had a baseline ECOG performance status of 0 or 1. The study excluded patients with a history of autoimmune disease; those with active or untreated CNS metastases; those who had received a live, attenuated vaccine within 28 days prior to randomization; those who had received systemic immunostimulatory agents within 4 weeks or systemic immunosuppressive agents within 2 weeks prior to randomization; and those with tumor infiltration into the thoracic great vessels or cavitation of pulmonary lesions. Neoadjuvant or adjuvant chemotherapy must have been completed at least 6 months before randomization into the IMpower150 study.

In the subset of patients with wild-type EGFR and ALK expression, median progression-free survival was prolonged in those receiving atezolizumab-bevacizumab-carboplatin-paclitaxel compared with those receiving bevacizumab-carboplatin-paclitaxel (8.5 versus 7 months; hazard ratio: 0.71). At a median follow-up of approximately 20 months, median overall survival also was prolonged in those receiving atezolizumab-bevacizumab-carboplatin-paclitaxel compared with those receiving bevacizumab-carboplatin-paclitaxel (19.2 versus 14.7 months; hazard ratio: 0.78). However, neither progression-free survival (6.7 or 7 months, respectively; hazard ratio: 0.94) nor overall survival (19.4 or 14.7 months, respectively; hazard ratio: 0.84) was prolonged in those receiving atezolizumab-carboplatin-paclitaxel compared with those receiving bevacizumab-carboplatin-paclitaxel. In patients with wild-type EGFR and ALK expression, the objective response rate was 55% in those receiving atezolizumab-bevacizumab-carboplatin-paclitaxel, 43% in those receiving atezolizumab-carboplatin-paclitaxel, and 42% in those receiving bevacizumab-carboplatin-paclitaxel; complete responses were achieved in 4, 3, or 1% of patients receiving these respective treatments. The median duration of response was 10.8 months in patients receiving atezolizumab-bevacizumab-carboplatin-paclitaxel, 9.5 months in those receiving atezolizumab-carboplatin-paclitaxel, and 6.5 months in those receiving bevacizumab-carboplatin-paclitaxel. In patients with wild-type EGFR and ALK expression, subset analyses indicated a progression-free survival benefit for atezolizumab-bevacizumab-carboplatin-paclitaxel compared with bevacizumab-carboplatin-paclitaxel regardless of level of PD-L1 or Teff gene-signature expression and across subgroups based on sex, age, ECOG performance status, smoking status, presence of liver metastases, and KRAS mutation status.

In the subset of patients with wild-type EGFR and ALK expression and high Teff gene-signature expression, median progression-free survival was prolonged in patients receiving atezolizumab-bevacizumab-carboplatin-paclitaxel compared with those receiving bevacizumab-carboplatin-paclitaxel; however, progression-free survival was not prolonged in patients receiving atezolizumab-carboplatin-paclitaxel compared with those receiving bevacizumab-carboplatin-paclitaxel.

In an exploratory analysis, efficacy in patients receiving atezolizumab-bevacizumab-carboplatin-paclitaxel appeared to be similar in those who tested positive for anti-atezolizumab antibodies by week 4 compared with those who did not develop anti-atezolizumab antibodies by week 4. (See Immunogenicity under Cautions.)

Combination with Albumin-bound Paclitaxel and Carboplatin

Atezolizumab is used in combination with albumin-bound paclitaxel and carboplatin for the initial treatment of metastatic nonsquamous NSCLC without *EGFR* or *ALK* genomic aberrations.

The current indication for atezolizumab in combination with albumin-bound paclitaxel and carboplatin for the initial treatment of metastatic nonsquamous NSCLC is based principally on the results of a randomized, open-label, phase 3 study (IMpower130). In this study, 724 adults with stage IV metastatic NSCLC with nonsquamous histology who had not received prior chemotherapy for metastatic disease were randomized (stratified by sex, presence of liver metastases, and PD-L1 expression as detected by Ventana PD-L1 [SP142] immunochemistry assay) in a 2:1 ratio to receive atezolizumab (1200 mg) and carboplatin (dose required to obtain an AUC of 6 mg/mL per minute) on day 1 and albumin-bound paclitaxel 100 mg/m^2 on days 1, 8, and 15 of each 21-day cycle for up to 4 or 6 cycles, followed by atezolizumab (1200 mg) once every 3 weeks until disease progression or unacceptable toxicity occurred or carboplatin in combination with albumin-bound paclitaxel at the same dosage, followed by best supportive care or pemetrexed. Patients who received prior therapy with an EGFR or ALK kinase inhibitor, if appropriate, were eligible for enrollment. The primary measures of efficacy were overall survival and investigator-assessed progression-free survival according to RECIST in the subgroup of patients with wild-type EGFR and ALK.

In the subgroup of 681 patients with wild-type EGFR and ALK, the median age of patients was 64 years; 90% were current or prior smokers, 52% had negative PD-L1 expression (defined as PD-L1 expression on less than 1% of tumor cells and tumor-infiltrating immune cells), 59% were male, 90% were White, 5% were Hispanic, 4% were Black, and 2% were of Asian ancestry. Baseline ECOG performance status was 0 or 1 in 99% of patients. The study excluded patients with a history of autoimmune disease; those with active or untreated CNS metastases; those who had received a live, attenuated vaccine within 28 days prior to randomization; and those who had received systemic immunostimulatory agents within 4 weeks or systemic immunosuppressive agents within 2 weeks prior to randomization. In this subgroup of patients, median progression-free survival was prolonged in those receiving atezolizumab with carboplatin and albumin-bound paclitaxel compared with those receiving carboplatin and albumin-bound paclitaxel (7.2 versus 6.5 months; hazard ratio: 0.75). Median overall survival also was prolonged in those receiving atezolizumab combined with carboplatin and albumin-bound paclitaxel compared with those receiving carboplatin and albumin-bound paclitaxel (18.6 versus 13.9 months; hazard ratio: 0.80). In patients with wild-type EGFR and ALK, the objective response rate was 46% in those receiving atezolizumab combined with carboplatin and albumin-bound paclitaxel and 32% in those receiving carboplatin and albumin-bound paclitaxel; complete responses were achieved in 5 or 1% of patients receiving these respective treatments. The median duration of response was 10.8 months in patients receiving atezolizumab combined with carboplatin and albumin-bound paclitaxel and 7.8 months in patients receiving carboplatin and albumin-bound paclitaxel. In a subgroup analysis based on age, sex, ECOG performance status, smoking status, presence of liver metastases, and PD-L1 expression, clinical benefit (i.e., progression-free and overall survival) associated with atezolizumab plus chemotherapy compared with chemotherapy alone was consistent across subgroups in IMpower130; however, atezolizumab was not associated with an overall survival benefit in patients with liver metastases or those with EGFR or ALK genomic aberrations.

Monotherapy for Previously Treated Metastatic Non-small Cell Lung Cancer

Atezolizumab is used as a single agent for the treatment of metastatic NSCLC that has progressed during or following platinum-based chemotherapy. Patients with EGFR- or ALK-positive tumors also should have documented disease progression during or following an FDA-labeled anti-EGFR or anti-ALK therapy prior to initiating therapy with atezolizumab.

The current indication for atezolizumab in the treatment of previously treated NSCLC is based principally on the results of a randomized, open-label phase 3 study (OAK), with supporting data from a similarly designed phase 2 study (POPLAR), in patients with locally advanced or metastatic NSCLC that had progressed during or following platinum-based chemotherapy. Patients in these studies were randomized (stratified by level of PD-L1 expression in tumor-infiltrating immune cells, number of prior chemotherapy regimens, and histology) in a 1:1 ratio to receive either atezolizumab (1200 mg IV every 3 weeks) or docetaxel (75 mg/m^2 IV every 3 weeks). Treatment was continued until disease progression or unacceptable toxicity occurred; however, atezolizumab-treated patients with disease progression could continue receiving treatment if they were considered to be deriving clinical benefit. The studies excluded patients with a history of

autoimmune disease; those with symptomatic or corticosteroid-dependent brain metastases; and those who received systemic immunosuppressive agents within 2 weeks prior to enrollment. In both studies, the primary measure of efficacy was overall survival.

In the OAK study, the primary efficacy population consisted of the initial 850 patients randomized in the study. In the primary efficacy population, the median age of patients was 64 years; 94% had metastatic disease, 74% had nonsquamous histology, 70% were Caucasian, 67% were former smokers, 61% were male, 55% had positive PD-L1 expression, 47% were 65 years of age or older, 21% were of Asian ancestry, 15% were current smokers, 10% had EGFR mutation-positive disease, 7% had KRAS mutation-positive disease, and less than 1% had ALK-positive disease. All patients had a baseline ECOG performance status of 0 or 1. Most patients (75%) had received one prior platinum-based chemotherapy regimen. In the primary efficacy population, patients receiving atezolizumab had longer median overall survival (13.8 versus 9.6 months; hazard ratio: 0.74) compared with patients receiving docetaxel; however, progression-free survival appeared to be shorter in patients receiving atezolizumab compared with those receiving docetaxel (2.8 versus 4 months). At the time of analysis, no difference in objective response rates was observed between patients receiving atezolizumab and those receiving docetaxel (14 and 13%, respectively); however, median response duration was prolonged in patients receiving atezolizumab compared with those receiving docetaxel (16.3 versus 6.2 months). Effects of atezolizumab on overall survival in the total patient population were comparable to those observed in the primary efficacy population. In the primary efficacy population, a planned subgroup analysis indicated that the risk of death was decreased with atezolizumab compared with docetaxel regardless of PD-L1 expression; however, survival benefit for atezolizumab compared with docetaxel was more pronounced in patients with high levels of PD-L1 expression (defined as PD-L1 expression on 50% or more of tumor cells or 10% or more of tumor-infiltrating immune cells) as detected by an immunohistochemistry assay (Ventana PD-L1 [SP142]) (hazard ratio: 0.41) compared with those with lower levels of PD-L1 expression (hazard ratio: 0.82). In an exploratory analysis, efficacy appeared to be reduced in patients who tested positive for anti-atezolizumab antibodies by week 4 compared with those who did not develop anti-atezolizumab antibodies by week 4. (See Immunogenicity under Cautions.)

In the POPLAR study, the median age of patients was 62 years. All patients enrolled in the study had a baseline ECOG performance status of 0 or 1, 66% had nonsquamous histology, 7% had EGFR mutation-positive disease, and 1% had ALK-positive disease. Approximately 67% had received one prior platinum-based chemotherapy regimen. After a median follow-up of 22 months, patients receiving atezolizumab had longer median overall survival (12.6 versus 9.7 months) compared with patients receiving docetaxel. Although objective response rates were similar between both treatment groups, patients receiving atezolizumab had a longer median duration of response (18.6 versus 7.2 months) compared with those receiving docetaxel. A subgroup analysis also indicated that increasing levels of PD-L1 expression were associated with an overall survival benefit for atezolizumab compared with docetaxel. Overall survival benefit for atezolizumab compared with docetaxel also was apparent regardless of histology and prior tobacco use.

● Breast Cancer

Atezolizumab is used in combination with albumin-bound paclitaxel for the treatment of unresectable locally advanced or metastatic triple-negative breast cancer in adult patients with PD-L1 expression (defined as PD-L1 staining in tumor-infiltrating immune cells of any intensity covering at least 1% of the tumor area); an FDA-approved diagnostic test is required to confirm the presence of PD-L1 expression prior to initiation of therapy. Atezolizumab is not indicated for use in combination with conventional paclitaxel for treating triple-negative breast cancer. (See Treatment-related Mortality under Cautions.)

The accelerated approval of atezolizumab for this indication is based on progression-free survival. Continued approval for this indication may be contingent on verification and description of clinical benefit of atezolizumab in confirmatory studies.

The current indication for use of atezolizumab in combination with albumin-bound paclitaxel in the treatment of unresectable locally advanced or metastatic triple-negative breast cancer in adults with PD-L1 expression is based principally on the results of a phase 3, double-blind, placebo-controlled study (IMpassion130). In this study, 902 patients with locally advanced or metastatic triple-negative breast cancer who had not received prior chemotherapy for metastatic disease were randomized (stratified by presence of liver metastases, prior taxane treatment, and PD-L1 expression) in a 1:1 ratio to receive atezolizumab 840 mg IV or placebo on days 1 and 15 in combination with albumin-bound paclitaxel 100 mg/m^2 IV on days 1, 8, and 15 of each 28-day cycle. Treatment was continued until radiographic disease progression per RECIST v1.1 or until unacceptable toxicity occurred. The primary measures of efficacy were investigator-assessed progression-free survival per RECIST v1.1 and overall survival in the intent-to-treat population and the subset of patients with PD-L1 expression on at least 1% of tumor-infiltrating immune cells, as detected by the Ventana PD-L1 (SP142) immunohistochemistry assay.

The median age of patients in the IMpassion130 study was 55 years and 99.6% of patients were women; 68% of patients were White, 18% were of Asian ancestry, 7% were Black or African American, 4% were American Indian or Alaskan Native, baseline ECOG performance status was 0 or 1 in 99% of patients, 41% of patients had PD-L1 expression on at least 1% of tumor-infiltrating immune cells, and liver and brain metastases were present in 27 and 7% of patients, respectively. The study excluded patients with a history of autoimmune disease; those with untreated or corticosteroid-dependent CNS metastases; those who had received a live, attenuated vaccine within 28 days prior to randomization; and those who had received systemic immunostimulatory agents within 4 weeks or systemic immunosuppressive agents within 2 weeks prior to randomization.

In the subset of patients with PD-L1 expression on at least 1% of tumor-infiltrating immune cells, median progression-free survival was prolonged in those receiving atezolizumab combined with albumin-bound paclitaxel compared with those receiving placebo and albumin-bound paclitaxel (7.4 versus 4.8 months; hazard ratio: 0.60). Median overall survival also was prolonged in those receiving atezolizumab combined with albumin-bound paclitaxel compared with those receiving placebo and albumin-bound paclitaxel (25.4 versus 17.9 months; hazard ratio: 0.67). The objective response rate was 53% in those receiving atezolizumab combined with albumin-bound paclitaxel and 33% in those receiving placebo and albumin-bound paclitaxel; complete responses were achieved in 9 and <1% of patients receiving these respective treatments. The median duration of response was 9.2 months in atezolizumab-treated patients and 6.2 months in those randomized to the placebo arm.

In the subset of patients in the IMpassion130 study with *negative* PD-L1 expression, no difference in median overall survival was observed between patients receiving atezolizumab in combination with albumin-bound paclitaxel compared with those receiving placebo in combination with albumin-bound paclitaxel (19.7 and 19.6 months, respectively; hazard ratio: 0.97).

Atezolizumab did not confer a survival benefit when used in combination with conventional paclitaxel in a clinical trial (IMpassion131) in patients with unresectable locally advanced or metastatic triple-negative breast cancer who had not received prior chemotherapy for metastatic disease. Atezolizumab is not indicated for use in combination with conventional paclitaxel in such patients. In this randomized, double-blind, placebo-controlled trial, patients with previously untreated, unresectable locally advanced or metastatic triple-negative breast cancer were randomized (stratified by presence of liver metastases, prior taxane treatment, and PD-L1 expression) to receive either atezolizumab 840 mg or placebo on days 1 and 15 in combination with conventional paclitaxel 90 mg/m^2 on days 1, 8, and 15 of each 28-day cycle. Treatment was continued until radiographic disease progression or unacceptable toxicity occurred. The primary measure of efficacy was investigator-assessed progression-free survival according to RECIST v1.1 in patients with PD-L1 expression (defined as PD-L1 expression on at least 1% of tumor-infiltrating immune cells, as detected by the Ventana PD-L1 [SP142] immunohistochemistry assay). In the subset of patients with PD-L1 expression, no difference in median progression-free survival was observed between patients receiving atezolizumab in combination with conventional paclitaxel and those receiving placebo in combination with conventional paclitaxel (6 versus 5.7 months; hazard ratio: 0.82 with a 95% confidence interval of 0.6–1.12). Median overall survival in the subset of patients with PD-L1 expression was 22.1 months in patients receiving atezolizumab and conventional paclitaxel and 28.3 months in patients receiving placebo and conventional paclitaxel.

● **Small Cell Lung Cancer**

Atezolizumab is used in combination with carboplatin and etoposide for the initial treatment of extensive-stage small cell lung cancer (SCLC). Atezolizumab has been designated an orphan drug by FDA for the treatment of this cancer.

The current indication for use of atezolizumab in combination with carboplatin and etoposide for the initial treatment of extensive-stage SCLC is based principally on the results of a phase 3, double-blind, placebo-controlled study (IMpower133). In this study, 403 patients with extensive-stage SCLC were randomized (stratified by sex, ECOG status, and presence of brain metastases) in a 1:1 ratio to receive atezolizumab 1200 mg on day 1 in combination with carboplatin (dose required to obtain an AUC of 5 mg/mL per minute) on day 1 and etoposide 100 mg/m^2 on days 1, 2, and 3 of each 21-day cycle for up to 4 cycles, followed by atezolizumab 1200 mg once every 3 weeks until disease progression or unacceptable toxicity occurred, or placebo in combination with carboplatin and etoposide at the same dosages for up to 4 cycles, followed by placebo once every 3 weeks until disease progression or unacceptable toxicity occurred. The primary measures of efficacy were overall and progression-free survival as assessed by investigators according to RECIST v1.1.

The median age of patients in IMpower133 was 64 years; 97% were current or previous smokers, 65% were male, 80% were White, 17% were of Asian ancestry, 4% were Hispanic, and 1% were Black. All patients had a baseline ECOG performance status of 0 or 1 and 9% of patients had a history of brain metastases. The study excluded patients with a history of autoimmune disease; those with active or untreated CNS metastases; those who had received a live, attenuated vaccine within 4 weeks prior to randomization; and those who had received systemic immunosuppressive agents within 1 week prior to randomization.

At a median follow-up of 13.9 months, median overall survival was prolonged in patients receiving atezolizumab combined with carboplatin and etoposide compared with those receiving placebo, carboplatin, and etoposide (12.3 versus 10.3 months; hazard ratio: 0.70). Median progression-free survival also was longer in patients receiving atezolizumab combined with carboplatin and etoposide compared with those receiving placebo, carboplatin, and etoposide (5.2 versus 4.3 months; hazard ratio: 0.77). Clinical benefit (e.g., overall and progression-free survival) associated with the addition of atezolizumab to chemotherapy was consistent across relevant subgroups. The objective response rate was 60% in those receiving atezolizumab combined with carboplatin and etoposide and 64% in those receiving placebo, carboplatin, and etoposide; complete responses were achieved in 2 and 1% of patients receiving these respective treatments. The median duration of response was 4.2 months in patients receiving atezolizumab combined with carboplatin and etoposide and 3.9 months in those receiving placebo, carboplatin, and etoposide.

● **Hepatocellular Carcinoma**

Atezolizumab is used in combination with bevacizumab for the treatment of patients with unresectable or metastatic hepatocellular carcinoma (HCC) who have not received prior systemic therapy. Atezolizumab has been designated an orphan drug by FDA for the treatment of this cancer.

The current indication for use of atezolizumab in combination with bevacizumab for the treatment of patients with previously untreated unresectable or metastatic HCC is primarily based on the results of a phase 3, open-label study (IMbrave150). In this study, 501 patients with unresectable locally advanced or metastatic HCC who had not received prior systemic therapy were randomized in a 2:1 ratio to receive atezolizumab 1200 mg in combination with bevacizumab 15 mg/kg, administered on the same day, once every 3 weeks, or sorafenib 400 mg orally twice daily; therapy was continued until disease progression or unacceptable toxicity occurred. The primary measures of efficacy were overall survival and progression-free survival as assessed by an independent review facility (IRF) according to RECIST v1.1; IRF-assessed overall response rate was also assessed using RECIST v1.1 and hepatocellular carcinoma-specific modified RECIST (mRECIST) criteria.

The median age of patients in the IMbrave150 study was 65 years; 83% of patients were male, 57% of patients were of Asian ancestry, 40% were from Asia (excluding Japan), and 35% were White. At baseline, macrovascular invasion and/or extrahepatic spread were present in approximately 75% of patients and AFP serum glycoprotein concentrations were at least 400 ng/mL in 37% of patients. All patients enrolled in the study had an ECOG performance status of 0 or 1 at baseline. The majority (82%) of patients had BCLC stage C disease at baseline, while 16 or 3% had stage B or A disease, respectively. Hepatitis B, hepatitis C, or nonviral liver disease were risk factors for HCC in 48, 22, or 31% of patients, respectively. The study excluded patients with a history of variceal bleeding within 6 months before treatment, and those with untreated or incompletely treated bleeding varices, high risk of bleeding, history of hepatic encephalopathy, Child-Pugh class B or C cirrhosis, or moderate or severe ascites. Patients with a history of autoimmune disease; those with untreated or corticosteroid-dependent CNS metastases; those who had received a live, attenuated vaccine within 4 weeks prior to randomization; and those who had received systemic immunostimulatory agents within 4 weeks or systemic immunosuppressive agents within 2 weeks prior to randomization also were excluded from the study.

At a median follow-up of 8.6 months, median overall survival was prolonged in patients receiving atezolizumab in combination with bevacizumab compared with those receiving sorafenib (71 versus 61%; hazard ratio: 0.58). Median progression-free survival also was prolonged in patients receiving atezolizumab-bevacizumab compared with those receiving sorafenib (6.8 versus 4.3 months; hazard ratio: 0.59). The overall response rate (according to RECIST v1.1) was 28% in patients receiving atezolizumab-bevacizumab and 12% in patients receiving sorafenib; complete responses were achieved in 7% of those treated with atezolizumab-bevacizumab and in none of the patients receiving sorafenib. The overall response rate (according to mRECIST) was 33% in patients receiving atezolizumab-bevacizumab and 13% in patients receiving sorafenib; complete responses were achieved in 11 and 1.8% of patients receiving these respective treatments. Median duration of response was not reached at the time of analysis in patients receiving atezolizumab-bevacizumab, but was 6.3 months in patients treated with sorafenib.

An exploratory analysis indicated reduced efficacy (e.g., overall survival) in patients receiving atezolizumab-bevacizumab who developed anti-atezolizumab antibodies by week 6 of therapy compared with those who did not develop anti-atezolizumab antibodies by week 6; no difference in overall survival was observed in patients who developed anti-atezolizumab antibodies and those treated with sorafenib. (See Immunogenicity under Cautions.)

● **Melanoma**

Atezolizumab is used in combination with cobimetinib and vemurafenib for the treatment of unresectable or metastatic melanoma harboring *BRAF* V600 mutation. Atezolizumab has been designated an orphan drug by FDA for the treatment of this cancer.

The current indication for use of atezolizumab in combination with cobimetinib and vemurafenib for the treatment of patients with unresectable or metastatic melanoma harboring *BRAF* V600 mutation is based principally on the results of a phase 3, double-blind, placebo-controlled study (IMspire150). In this study, 514 patients with previously untreated *BRAF* mutation-positive unresectable or metastatic melanoma were randomized (stratified by geographical location and baseline lactate dehydrogenase) in a 1:1 ratio to receive atezolizumab or placebo combined with cobimetinib and vemurafenib. Atezolizumab was initiated after patients received one 28-day cycle of cobimetinib 60 mg orally once daily on days 1–21 and vemurafenib 960 mg orally twice daily on days 1–21, followed by vemurafenib 720 mg orally twice daily on days 22–28; for subsequent cycles, patients received atezolizumab 840 mg administered by IV infusion over 60 minutes on days 1 and 15, cobimetinib 60 mg orally once daily on days 1–21, and vemurafenib 720 mg orally twice daily on days 1–28 of a 28-day cycle. Patients randomized to placebo received cobimetinib 60 mg orally once daily on days 1–21 and vemurafenib 960 mg twice daily on days 1–28 of each 28-day cycle. The primary measure of efficacy was investigator-assessed progression-free survival according to RECIST v1.1.

The median age of patients in the IMspire150 study was 54 years; 58% were male, 95% were White, 33% had elevated lactate dehydrogenase, 94% had metastatic disease, 60% had stage IV disease, 14% had received prior adjuvant systemic therapy, and 3% had received prior treatment for brain metastases. At baseline, 56% of patients had fewer than 3 metastatic sites and 30% had liver metastases. Most (74%) patients had *BRAF* V600E mutation, 11% had *BRAF* V600K mutation, and 1% had *BRAF* V600D or V600R mutation. All patients had an ECOG performance status of 0 or 1 (77 or 23%, respectively). The study excluded patients with a history of autoimmune disease; those with active or untreated CNS metastases; those who had received a live, attenuated vaccine within 28 days prior to randomization; and those who had received systemic immunostimulatory agents within 4 weeks or immunosuppressive agents within 2 weeks prior to randomization.

At a median follow-up of 18.9 months, median progression-free survival was prolonged in patients receiving atezolizumab-cobimetinib-vemurafenib compared with those receiving placebo-cobimetinib-vemurafenib (15.1 versus 10.6 months; hazard ratio: 0.78). The overall response rate was 66% in patients

receiving atezolizumab-cobimetinib-vemurafenib and 65% in those receiving placebo-cobimetinib-vemurafenib; complete responses were achieved in 16 and 18% of patients receiving these respective treatments. The median duration of response was 20.4 months in patients treated with atezolizumab-cobimetinib-vemurafenib and 12.5 months in patients treated with placebo-cobimetinib-vemurafenib. Overall survival data were not mature at the time of analysis; however, median overall survival was 28.8 months in patients receiving atezolizumab-cobimetinib-vemurafenib and 25.1 months in patients receiving placebo-cobimetinib-vemurafenib at the time of the interim analysis.

DOSAGE AND ADMINISTRATION

● **General**

Pretreatment Screening
● Verify pregnancy status in females of reproductive potential.
● Liver function tests.
● Thyroid function.

Biomarker Testing
● Select patients for treatment with atezolizumab based on the presence of biomarkers. (See Table 1.)

TABLE 1. Biomarker Testing for Patient Selection

Indication	Biomarker
Locally advanced or metastatic urothelial carcinoma in patients who are not candidates for cisplatin-containing chemotherapy	PD-L1 expression on tumor-infiltrating immune cells
Monotherapy for the treatment of metastatic NSCLC	PD-L1 expression on tumor cells or tumor-infiltrating immune cells
Locally advanced or metastatic triple-negative breast cancer (in combination with albumin-bound paclitaxel)	PD-L1 expression on tumor-infiltrating immune cells
Unresectable or metastatic melanoma (in combination with cobimetinib and vemurafenib)	BRAF V600 mutation

Patient Monitoring
● Immune-mediated effects during and following therapy.
● Manifestations of pneumonitis.
● Signs and symptoms of hepatitis (e.g., liver function tests) during therapy.
● Signs and symptoms of colitis (e.g., diarrhea, abdominal pain, lower GI bleeding).
● Thyroid function periodically during therapy. Monitor for thyroiditis.
● Signs and symptoms of adrenal insufficiency.
● Signs and symptoms of diabetes mellitus (e.g., hyperglycemia).
● Signs and symptoms of hypophysitis (e.g., headache, photophobia, visual field changes, hypopituitarism).
● Signs and symptoms of dermatologic effects.
● Signs and symptoms of infusion-related reactions.

Other General Considerations
● Consider potential benefits and risks of anti-PD-1 monoclonal antibody therapy administered either before or after allogeneic stem cell transplantation. Closely monitor for early manifestations of stem cell transplantation-related complications and manage promptly if they occur.

● **Administration**

Atezolizumab is administered by IV infusion. The initial dose of atezolizumab should be administered as an IV infusion over 60 minutes; if the first infusion is tolerated, subsequent doses may be administered by IV infusion over 30 minutes. *The drug should not be administered by rapid IV injection, such as IV push or bolus.*

Unopened vials of atezolizumab injection concentrate should be protected from light, stored at 2–8°C, and should *not* be frozen or shaken.

Atezolizumab injection concentrate must be diluted prior to administration. The appropriate vial size should be selected based on the dose required. Prior to dilution and administration, atezolizumab injection concentrate should be inspected visually for particulate matter and discoloration. The undiluted solution should be colorless to slightly yellow; the solution should *not* be used if it is cloudy or discolored or if particulate matter is present. Atezolizumab is diluted by adding the required volume of atezolizumab injection concentrate (containing 60 mg/mL) to a polyvinyl chloride (PVC), polyethylene, or polyolefin infusion bag containing 0.9% sodium chloride injection. No other diluent should be used. The final concentration of the diluted atezolizumab solution should be 3.2–16.8 mg/mL. The diluted solution should be mixed by gentle inversion and should *not* be shaken. The manufacturer recommends immediate administration of diluted solutions of the drug. If immediate administration is not possible, the diluted solution of the drug should be stored at room temperature for up to 6 hours from the time of preparation (including infusion time) or 2–8°C for up to 24 hours from time of preparation; diluted solutions of the drug should *not* be frozen.

Atezolizumab should *not* be administered simultaneously through the same IV line with any other drug. Use of a low-protein-binding 0.2- to 0.22-μm inline filter is optional. Atezolizumab injection concentrate contains no preservatives and is intended for single use only; any partially used vials should be discarded.

● Dosage

Urothelial Carcinoma

For the treatment of locally advanced or metastatic urothelial carcinoma in patients with high programmed-death ligand-1 (PD-L1) expression (defined as PD-L1 staining in tumor-infiltrating immune cells covering at least 5% of the tumor area) who are not candidates for cisplatin-containing therapy, and in those who are not candidates for platinum-containing chemotherapy regardless of PD-L1 expression, the manufacturer recommends one of the following dosages for atezolizumab in adults: 840 mg as an IV infusion every 2 weeks, 1200 mg as an IV infusion every 3 weeks, or 1680 mg as an IV infusion every 4 weeks. Therapy should be continued until disease progression or unacceptable toxicity occurs.

Non-small Cell Lung Cancer

For the initial treatment of metastatic NSCLC with high PD-L1 expression and without *EGFR* or *ALK* genomic aberrations, the manufacturer recommends one of the following dosages for atezolizumab in adults: 840 mg as an IV infusion every 2 weeks, 1200 mg as an IV infusion every 3 weeks, or 1680 mg as an IV infusion every 4 weeks. Continue therapy until disease progression or unacceptable toxicity occurs.

For the initial treatment of metastatic nonsquamous NSCLC without *EGFR* or *ALK* genomic aberrations, atezolizumab is used in combination with bevacizumab, carboplatin, and paclitaxel, or in combination with albumin-bound paclitaxel and carboplatin. The manufacturer recommends one of the following dosages for atezolizumab in adults: 840 mg as an IV infusion every 2 weeks, 1200 mg as an IV infusion every 3 weeks, or 1680 mg as an IV infusion every 4 weeks. Administer atezolizumab prior to concomitant chemotherapy or bevacizumab when scheduled on the same day.

In the IMpower150 study, carboplatin and paclitaxel were administered for a maximum of 4–6 cycles; therapy with atezolizumab and bevacizumab was continued until disease progression or unacceptable toxicity occurred.

In the IMpower130 study, albumin-bound paclitaxel and carboplatin were administered for a maximum of 4–6 cycles; therapy with atezolizumab was continued until disease progression or unacceptable toxicity occurred.

For the treatment of metastatic NSCLC that has progressed during or following platinum-based chemotherapy, the manufacturer recommends one of the following dosages for atezolizumab in adults: 840 mg as an IV infusion every 2 weeks, 1200 mg as an IV infusion every 3 weeks, or 1680 mg as an IV infusion every 4 weeks. Therapy should be continued until disease progression or unacceptable toxicity occurs.

Breast Cancer

For the treatment of locally advanced or metastatic triple-negative breast cancer (in combination with albumin-bound paclitaxel) in patients with PD-L1 expression (defined as PD-L1 staining in tumor-infiltrating immune cells of any intensity covering at least 1% of the tumor area), the manufacturer recommends one of the following dosages for atezolizumab in adults: 840 mg as an IV infusion every 2 weeks, 1200 mg as an IV infusion every 3 weeks, or 1680 mg as an IV infusion every 4 weeks.

Albumin-bound paclitaxel 100 mg/m² is administered on days 1, 8, and 15 of each 28-day cycle; conventional paclitaxel should not be substituted for albumin-bound paclitaxel. Administer atezolizumab prior to albumin-bound paclitaxel when scheduled on the same day. Continue therapy until disease progression or unacceptable toxicity occurs.

If toxicity occurs, atezolizumab and albumin-bound paclitaxel may be discontinued independently of each other.

Atezolizumab is not indicated for use in combination with conventional paclitaxel for the treatment of triple-negative breast cancer. (See Treatment-related Mortality under Cautions.)

Small Cell Lung Cancer

For the treatment of adult patients with previously untreated, extensive-stage small cell lung cancer (in combination with carboplatin and etoposide), the manufacturer recommends one of the following dosages for atezolizumab in adults: 840 mg as an IV infusion every 2 weeks, 1200 mg as an IV infusion every 3 weeks, or 1680 mg as an IV infusion every 4 weeks. Administer atezolizumab prior to carboplatin and etoposide when scheduled on the same day.

In the principal efficacy study, carboplatin and etoposide were administered for up to 4 cycles, and atezolizumab therapy was continued until disease progression or unacceptable toxicity occurred.

Hepatocellular Carcinoma

For the treatment of unresectable or metastatic hepatocellular carcinoma (in combination with bevacizumab) in patients who have not received prior systemic therapy, the manufacturer recommends one of the following dosages for atezolizumab in adults: 840 mg as an IV infusion every 2 weeks, 1200 mg as an IV infusion every 3 weeks, or 1680 mg as an IV infusion every 4 weeks.

Administer atezolizumab prior to bevacizumab when scheduled on the same day. Therapy should be continued until disease progression or unacceptable toxicity occurs.

Melanoma

For the treatment of *BRAF* V600 mutation-positive unresectable or metastatic melanoma (in combination cobimetinib and vemurafenib), the manufacturer recommends one of the following dosages for atezolizumab in adults: 840 mg as an IV infusion every 2 weeks, 1200 mg as an IV infusion every 3 weeks, or 1680 mg as an IV infusion every 4 weeks.

Atezolizumab should be initiated *after* patients receive one 28-day cycle of cobimetinib 60 mg orally once daily on days 1–21 and vemurafenib 960 mg orally twice daily on days 1–21, followed by vemurafenib 720 mg orally twice daily on days 22–28; for subsequent cycles, patients should receive atezolizumab in combination with cobimetinib 60 mg orally once daily on days 1–21 and vemurafenib 720 mg orally twice daily on days 1–28 of a 28-day cycle. Continue therapy until disease progression or unacceptable toxicity occurs.

Therapy Interruption for Toxicity

If adverse effects occur, temporary or permanent discontinuance of atezolizumab may be required based on the toxicity and severity of the reaction; the manufacturer does not recommend dosage reductions for managing toxicity.

In general, temporarily interrupt atezolizumab therapy if severe (grade 3) immune-mediated adverse effects occur.

Permanently discontinue atezolizumab therapy in patients experiencing grade 4 immune-mediated adverse effects, recurrent grade 3 immune-mediated adverse effects requiring systemic immunosuppressive therapy, and in patients unable to reduce corticosteroid dosage to 10 mg or less of prednisone daily (or equivalent) within 12 weeks of initiating corticosteroids.

Immune-mediated Pulmonary Effects

If grade 2 immune-mediated pneumonitis occurs, atezolizumab therapy should be interrupted until the toxicity resolves to grade 0 or 1 *and* the corticosteroid dosage has been tapered. Atezolizumab should be permanently discontinued if immune-mediated pneumonitis does not resolve to grade 0 or 1 within 12 weeks of starting corticosteroids or if the patient is unable to reduce corticosteroid dosage to 10 mg or less of prednisone daily (or equivalent) within 12 weeks of initiating corticosteroids. (See Immune-mediated Pulmonary Effects under Cautions.)

If grade 3 or 4 immune-mediated pneumonitis occurs, atezolizumab therapy should be permanently discontinued.

Immune-mediated Hepatic Effects

For patients without tumor involvement of the liver experiencing immune-mediated hepatitis characterized by serum ALT or AST elevations exceeding 3 times but not more than 8 times the upper limit of normal (ULN), or total bilirubin concentrations exceeding 1.5 times but not more than 3 times the ULN, atezolizumab therapy should be interrupted until the toxicity resolves to grade 0 or 1 *and* the corticosteroid dosage has been tapered. Atezolizumab should be permanently discontinued if immune-mediated hepatitis does not resolve to grade 0 or 1 within 12 weeks of starting corticosteroids or if the patient is unable to reduce corticosteroid dosage to 10 mg or less of prednisone daily (or equivalent) within 12 weeks of initiating corticosteroids. (See Immune-mediated Hepatic Effects under Cautions.)

For patients without tumor involvement of the liver experiencing immune-mediated hepatitis characterized by ALT or AST elevations exceeding 8 times the ULN, or total bilirubin concentrations exceeding 3 times the ULN, atezolizumab therapy should be permanently discontinued.

For patients with liver involvement and baseline ALT or AST concentrations exceeding the ULN but not more than 3 times the ULN who develop immune-mediated hepatitis characterized by ALT or AST elevations exceeding 5 times but not more than 10 times the ULN, or in those with baseline ALT or AST concentrations exceeding 3 times the ULN but not more than 5 times the ULN who develop immune-mediated hepatitis characterized by ALT or AST elevations exceeding 8 times the ULN but not more than 10 times the ULN, atezolizumab therapy should be interrupted until immune-mediated hepatitis resolves to grade 0 or 1 and the corticosteroid dosage has been tapered. Atezolizumab should be permanently discontinued if immune-mediated hepatitis does not resolve to grade 0 or 1 within 12 weeks of starting corticosteroids or if the patient is unable to reduce corticosteroid dosage to 10 mg or less of prednisone daily (or equivalent) within 12 weeks of initiating corticosteroids. (See Immune-mediated Hepatic Effects under Cautions.)

For patients with liver involvement who develop immune-mediated hepatitis characterized by ALT or AST elevations exceeding 10 times the ULN or total bilirubin increases exceeding 3 times the ULN, atezolizumab therapy should be permanently discontinued.

For patients with liver involvement and baseline AST and ALT less than or equal to the ULN who develop immune-mediated hepatitis characterized by serum ALT or AST elevations exceeding 3 times but not more than 8 times the upper limit of normal ULN, or total bilirubin concentrations exceeding 1.5 times but not more than 3 times the ULN, atezolizumab therapy should be interrupted until the toxicity resolves to grade 0 or 1 and the corticosteroid dosage has been tapered. Atezolizumab should be permanently discontinued if immune-mediated hepatitis does not resolve to grade 0 or 1 within 12 weeks of starting corticosteroids or if the patient is unable to reduce corticosteroid dosage to 10 mg or less of prednisone daily (or equivalent) within 12 weeks of initiating corticosteroids.

For patients with liver involvement and baseline AST and ALT less than or equal to the ULN who develop immune-mediated hepatitis characterized by ALT or AST elevations exceeding 8 times the ULN, or total bilirubin concentrations exceeding 3 times the ULN, atezolizumab therapy should be permanently discontinued.

Immune-mediated GI Effects

If grade 2 or 3 immune-mediated colitis occurs, atezolizumab therapy should be interrupted until the toxicity resolves to grade 0 or 1 *and* the corticosteroid dosage has been tapered. Atezolizumab should be permanently discontinued if immune-mediated colitis does not resolve to grade 0 or 1 within 12 weeks of starting corticosteroids or if the patient is unable to reduce corticosteroid dosage to 10 mg or less of prednisone daily (or equivalent) within 12 weeks of initiating corticosteroids. (See Immune-mediated GI Effects under Cautions.)

If grade 4 immune-mediated colitis occurs, atezolizumab therapy should be permanently discontinued.

Immune-mediated Endocrine Effects

If grade 3 or 4 immune-mediated endocrinopathies (e.g., hypophysitis, adrenal insufficiency, thyroid disorders, type 1 diabetes mellitus) occur, atezolizumab therapy should either be interrupted until the patient is clinically stable or permanently discontinued according to the severity of the adverse effect. (See Immune-mediated Endocrine Effects under Cautions.)

Immune-mediated Renal Effects

If immune-mediated nephritis characterized by grade 2 or 3 elevations in serum creatinine concentration occur, atezolizumab therapy should be interrupted until the toxicity resolves to grade 0 or 1 and the corticosteroid dosage is tapered. Atezolizumab should be permanently discontinued if immune-mediated nephritis does not resolve to grade 0 or 1 within 12 weeks of starting corticosteroids or if the patient is unable to reduce corticosteroid dosage to 10 mg or less of prednisone daily (or equivalent) within 12 weeks of initiating corticosteroids. (See Immune-mediated Renal Effects under Cautions.)

If immune-mediated nephritis characterized by grade 4 elevations in serum creatinine concentration occurs, atezolizumab therapy should be permanently discontinued.

Immune-mediated Dermatologic Effects

If exfoliative dermatitis (i.e., Stevens Johnson syndrome [SJS], toxic epidermal necrolysis [TEN], drug rash with eosinophilia and systemic symptoms [DRESS]) is suspected, therapy with atezolizumab should be temporarily interrupted; if the diagnosis is confirmed, atezolizumab therapy should be permanently discontinued. (See Immune-mediated Dermatologic Effects under Cautions.)

Immune-mediated Cardiac Effects

If grade 2-4 immune-mediated myocarditis occurs, atezolizumab therapy should be permanently discontinued.

Immune-mediated Neurologic Effects

If grade 2 immune-mediated neurologic toxicity (e.g., meningitis, encephalitis, myasthenia gravis, Guillain-Barré syndrome, autoimmune neuropathy) occurs, atezolizumab therapy should be interrupted until the toxicity resolves to grade 0 or 1 and the corticosteroid dosage is tapered. Atezolizumab should be permanently discontinued if toxicity does not resolve to grade 0 or 1 within 12 weeks of starting corticosteroids or if the patient is unable to reduce corticosteroid dosage to 10 mg or less of prednisone daily (or equivalent) within 12 weeks of initiating corticosteroids. (See Other Immune-mediated Effects under Cautions.)

If grade 3 or 4 immune-mediated neurologic toxicity occurs, atezolizumab therapy should be permanently discontinued.

Infusion-related Reactions

If grade 1 or 2 infusion-related reactions occur, the infusion should be interrupted or the infusion rate should be reduced. (See Infusion-related Effects under Cautions.)

If grade 3 or 4 infusion-related reactions occur, atezolizumab therapy should be permanently discontinued.

• Special Populations

The manufacturer makes no special dosage recommendations for patients with hepatic or renal impairment or for geriatric patients. (See Specific Populations under Cautions: Warnings/Precautions.)

CAUTIONS

• Contraindications

The manufacturer states there are no known contraindications to the use of atezolizumab.

• Warnings/Precautions

Severe and Fatal Immune-mediated Effects

As an anti-PD-L1 monoclonal antibody, atezolizumab interferes with immune response inhibition, potentially eliciting immune-mediated adverse effects, which can be severe or even fatal. Atezolizumab-related immune-mediated adverse effects can occur in any tissue or organ system; immune-mediated adverse effects usually appear during treatment, but can also occur after discontinuance of therapy.

Patients should be closely monitored during and following therapy with atezolizumab; it is important to promptly identify and manage immune-mediated adverse effects if they occur. If an immune-mediated adverse effect is suspected, the patient should be assessed for potential alternative causes, and treatment should begin promptly; consultation with a specialist should be considered if appropriate.

Temporary interruption or discontinuance of atezolizumab therapy may be necessary to manage immune-mediated adverse effects. (See Therapy Interruption for Toxicity under Dosage and Administration.) In general, if interruption or discontinuance of atezolizumab is necessary, systemic corticosteroids should be initiated (1–2 mg/kg of prednisone daily [or equivalent]) followed by a taper over at least 1 month when the immune-mediated adverse effect improves to grade 1 or less. If immune-mediated adverse effects are not controlled with corticosteroid therapy, other systemic immunosuppressants may be considered. Some immune-mediated effects may not require treatment with systemic corticosteroids (e.g., mild or moderate non-exfoliative dermatologic rash, certain immune-mediated endocrine effects).

Immune-mediated Pulmonary Effects

Immune-mediated pneumonitis, sometimes fatal, has occurred in patients receiving atezolizumab therapy. Patients who have received thoracic radiation may be at increased risk.

In clinical studies, immune-mediated pneumonitis occurred in 3% of patients receiving atezolizumab as a single agent; the reaction was fatal in less than 0.1% of patients. Grade 2, 3, or 4 immune-mediated pneumonitis occurred in 1.1, 0.8, or 0.2% of atezolizumab-treated patients, respectively. Temporary interruption of atezolizumab was necessary due to pneumonitis in 1.5% of patients, and therapy was permanently discontinued in 0.5% of patients. Treatment with systemic corticosteroids was needed in 55% of patients who developed immune-mediated pneumonitis, and pneumonitis resolved in 69% of patients who received corticosteroid therapy. Of the patients in whom atezolizumab was temporarily interrupted, 64% were able to restart atezolizumab therapy; however, pneumonitis recurred in 4% of these patients.

In clinical studies evaluating atezolizumab in combination with cobimetinib and vemurafenib, immune-mediated pneumonitis occurred in 13% of patients; immune-mediated pneumonitis was grade 2 or 3 in 7 or 1.3% of patients, respectively. Temporary interruption of atezolizumab was necessary due to pneumonitis in 7.4% of patients, and therapy was permanently discontinued in 2.6% of patients. Treatment with systemic corticosteroids was needed in 55% of patients who developed immune-mediated pneumonitis, and pneumonitis resolved in 97% of patients who received corticosteroid therapy. Of the patients in whom atezolizumab was temporarily interrupted, 59% were able to restart atezolizumab therapy; however, pneumonitis recurred in 50% of these patients.

Patients receiving atezolizumab should be monitored for manifestations of pneumonitis. Temporary interruption or discontinuance of atezolizumab may be necessary if immune-mediated pneumonitis occurs during therapy with the drug. (See Immune-mediated Pulmonary Effects under Dosage and Administration and also see Severe and Fatal Immune-mediated Effects under Cautions.)

Immune-mediated Hepatic Effects

Immune-mediated hepatitis, sometimes fatal, has occurred in patients receiving atezolizumab therapy.

In clinical studies, immune-mediated hepatitis occurred in 1.8% of patients receiving atezolizumab as a single agent; the reaction was fatal in less than 0.1% of patients; immune-mediated hepatitis was grade 2, 3, or 4 in 0.5, 0.5, or 0.2% of patients, respectively. Temporary interruption or permanent discontinuance of atezolizumab therapy were each necessary in 0.2% of patients. Treatment with systemic corticosteroids was needed in 25% of patients who developed immune-mediated hepatitis, and resolved in 50% of patients who received corticosteroid therapy. Among 6 patients in whom atezolizumab was temporarily interrupted, 4 patients were able to restart atezolizumab therapy; hepatitis recurred in none of these patients.

In clinical studies evaluating atezolizumab in combination with cobimetinib and vemurafenib, immune-mediated hepatitis occurred in 6.1% of patients;

immune-mediated hepatitis was grade 2, 3, or 4 in 1.3, 1.7 or, 1.3% of patients, respectively. Temporary interruption of atezolizumab was necessary due to hepatitis in 1.7% of patients, and therapy was permanently discontinued in 2.2% of patients. Treatment with systemic corticosteroids was needed in 50% of patients who developed immune-mediated hepatitis, and hepatitis resolved in 93% of patients who received corticosteroid therapy. Among 4 patients in whom atezolizumab was temporarily interrupted, 3 were able to restart atezolizumab therapy; hepatitis recurred in one of these patients.

Patients receiving atezolizumab should be monitored for signs and symptoms of hepatitis (including liver function tests) at baseline and during atezolizumab therapy. Temporary interruption or discontinuance of atezolizumab may be necessary if immune-mediated hepatitis or liver function test abnormalities occur during therapy with the drug. (See Immune-mediated Hepatic Effects under Dosage and Administration and also see Severe and Fatal Immune-mediated Effects under Cautions.)

Immune-mediated GI Effects

Immune-mediated colitis has occurred in patients receiving atezolizumab therapy. Manifestations of colitis include diarrhea, abdominal pain, and lower GI bleeding.

In clinical studies, immune-mediated colitis occurred in 1% of patients receiving atezolizumab as a single agent; immune-mediated colitis was grade 2 or 3 in 0.3 or 0.5% of patients, respectively. Temporary interruption of atezolizumab was necessary due to colitis in 0.5% of patients, and therapy was permanently discontinued in 0.2% of patients. Treatment with systemic corticosteroids was needed in 50% of patients who developed immune-mediated colitis, and colitis resolved in 73% of patients who received corticosteroids. Of the patients in whom atezolizumab was temporarily interrupted, 67% were able to restart atezolizumab therapy; however, colitis recurred in 25% of these patients.

Patients receiving atezolizumab should be monitored for signs and symptoms of colitis. Temporary interruption or discontinuance of atezolizumab may be necessary if immune-mediated colitis or diarrhea occurs during therapy with the drug. (See Immune-mediated GI Effects under Dosage and Administration and also see Severe and Fatal Immune-mediated Effects under Cautions.) Cytomegalovirus (CMV) infection or reactivation has occurred in patients with immune-mediated colitis that is refractory to corticosteroid therapy. If corticosteroid-refractory colitis occurs, consider assessing the patient for alternative etiologies.

Immune-mediated Endocrine Effects

Immune-mediated endocrinopathies, such as thyroid dysfunction (i.e., thyroiditis, hypothyroidism, hyperthyroidism), adrenal insufficiency (primary or secondary), hypophysitis/hypopituitarism, and diabetes mellitus (including ketoacidosis), have occurred in patients receiving atezolizumab therapy. Immune-mediated hyperthyroidism may be followed by hypothyroidism.

Thyroid Dysfunction

Atezolizumab can cause immune-mediated thyroiditis that presents with or without endocrinopathy. In clinical studies, thyroiditis occurred in 0.2% of patients receiving atezolizumab as a single agent; immune-mediated thyroiditis was grade 2 in less than 0.1% of patients. Temporary interruption or discontinuance of atezolizumab was necessary due to thyroiditis in 1 or 0 patients, respectively. Thyroid hormone replacement therapy was required in 3 of 4 patients who developed immune-mediated thyroiditis and systemic corticosteroid therapy was required in 1 of 4 patients who developed immune-mediated thyroiditis. Thyroiditis resolved in 50% of patients. One patient resumed atezolizumab therapy following temporary interruption, and did not experience recurrence of thyroiditis.

In clinical studies, immune-mediated hypothyroidism occurred in 4.9% of patients receiving atezolizumab as a single agent; immune-mediated hypothyroidism was grade 2 or 3 in 3.4 or 0.2% of patients, respectively. Thyroid hormone replacement was required in 81% of patients receiving atezolizumab who experienced hypothyroidism, with the majority of patients remaining on thyroid replacement. Temporary interruption of atezolizumab was necessary due to hypothyroidism in 0.6% of patients, but no patients required permanent discontinuance of atezolizumab. Of the patients in whom therapy was temporarily interrupted, 47% were able to restart atezolizumab following improvement of symptoms. In clinical studies evaluating atezolizumab in combination with platinum-based chemotherapy in patients with NSCLC or SCLC, immune-mediated hypothyroidism occurred in 11% of atezolizumab-treated patients; immune-mediated hypothyroidism was grade 2, 3, or 4 in 5.7, 0.3, or less than 0.1% of patients, respectively. Thyroid hormone replacement was required in 71% of patients receiving atezolizumab in combination with platinum-based therapy who experienced hypothyroidism, with the majority of patients remaining on thyroid replacement. Temporary interruption of atezolizumab was necessary due to hypothyroidism in 1.6% of patients, and permanent discontinuance of atezolizumab was needed in 0.1% of patients. Of the patients in whom therapy was temporarily interrupted, 23% were able to restart atezolizumab following improvement of symptoms.

In a clinical study evaluating atezolizumab in combination with cobimetinib and vemurafenib in patients with melanoma, immune-mediated hypothyroidism occurred in 26% of patients; severity was grade 2 in 9.1% of patients. Thyroid hormone replacement was required in 52% of patients receiving atezolizumab in combination with cobimetinib and vemurafenib who experienced hypothyroidism, with the majority of patients remaining on thyroid replacement. Temporary interruption of atezolizumab was necessary due to hypothyroidism in 2.6% of patients, but no patients required permanent discontinuance of atezolizumab. Of 6 patients in whom therapy was temporarily interrupted for hypothyroidism, 4 patients were able to restart atezolizumab following improvement of symptoms.

In clinical studies, immune-mediated hyperthyroidism occurred in 0.8% of patients receiving atezolizumab as a single agent; severity was grade 2 in 0.4% of patients. Treatment with an antithyroid agent was required in 29% of patients receiving atezolizumab who experienced hyperthyroidism, with the majority of patients remaining on antithyroid therapy. Temporary interruption of atezolizumab was necessary due to hyperthyroidism in 0.1% of patients, but no patients required permanent discontinuance of atezolizumab. Of 3 patients in whom therapy was temporarily interrupted for hyperthyroidism, one patient was able to restart atezolizumab without recurrence of hyperthyroidism.

In a clinical study evaluating atezolizumab in combination with cobimetinib and vemurafenib in patients with melanoma, immune-mediated hyperthyroidism occurred in 19% of patients; immune-mediated hyperthyroidism was grade 2 or 3 in 7.8 or 0.9% of patients, respectively. Treatment with an antithyroid agent was required in 53% of patients receiving atezolizumab who experienced hyperthyroidism, with the majority of patients remaining on antithyroid therapy. Temporary interruption of atezolizumab was necessary due to hyperthyroidism in 10% of patients, and permanent discontinuance was necessary in 0.4% of patients. Of the patients in whom therapy was temporarily interrupted for hyperthyroidism, 78% were able to restart atezolizumab; hyperthyroidism recurred in 28% of these patients.

Thyroid function should be evaluated prior to initiation of atezolizumab therapy and periodically during therapy. In patients who develop immune-mediated hypothyroidism, thyroid hormone replacement therapy should be initiated as clinically indicated. If immune-mediated hyperthyroidism occurs, medical therapy should be initiated as clinically indicated. Temporary interruption or permanent discontinuance of atezolizumab may be necessary for immune-mediated thyroid disorders. (See Immune-mediated Endocrine Effects under Dosage and Administration and also see Severe and Fatal Immune-mediated Effects under Cautions.)

Adrenal Insufficiency

In clinical studies, immune-mediated adrenal insufficiency occurred in 0.4% of patients receiving atezolizumab as a single agent and was grade 2 or 3 in 0.2 or less than 0.1%, respectively, of patients receiving the drug. Adrenal insufficiency led to permanent discontinuation of atezolizumab in one patient and temporary interruption of therapy in one patient; however, atezolizumab was not restarted in the patient who temporarily interrupted therapy. Treatment with systemic corticosteroids was needed in 81% of patients experiencing immune-mediated adrenal insufficiency; 33% of these patients remained on systemic corticosteroids.

Patients receiving atezolizumab should be monitored for signs and symptoms of adrenal insufficiency. Temporary interruption or discontinuance of atezolizumab may be necessary if immune-mediated adrenal insufficiency occurs during therapy with the drug. (See Immune-mediated Endocrine Effects under Dosage and Administration and also see Severe and Fatal Immune-mediated Effects under Cautions.) If grade 2 or greater immune-mediated adrenal insufficiency occurs, symptomatic treatment (e.g., hormone replacement therapy) should be initiated as clinically indicated.

Hypophysitis

In clinical studies, immune-mediated hypophysitis occurred in 2 patients (less than 0.1%) receiving atezolizumab as a single agent; severity was grade 2 in one patient. Atezolizumab therapy was permanently discontinued in one patient and the other patient received systemic corticosteroid therapy; hypophysitis did not resolve in either patient.

Patients receiving atezolizumab should be monitored for signs and symptoms of hypophysitis. Hypophysitis can present with acute symptoms associated with mass effect such as headache, photophobia, or visual field changes; hypopituitarism can be caused by hypophysitis. If immune-mediated hypophysitis occurs, temporary interruption or discontinuance of atezolizumab may be necessary. (See Immune-mediated Endocrine Effects under Dosage and Administration and also see Severe and Fatal Immune-mediated Effects under Cautions.) Hormone replacement therapy should be initiated as clinically indicated.

Diabetes Mellitus

In clinical studies, immune-mediated type 1 diabetes mellitus occurred in 0.3% of patients receiving atezolizumab as a single agent; immune-mediated type 1 diabetes mellitus was grade 2 or 3 in less than 0.1 or 0.2% of patients, respectively. Temporary interruption of treatment was necessary in 2 patients and permanent discontinuance of therapy was necessary in 1 patient. Of the patients in whom therapy was temporarily interrupted for type 1 diabetes mellitus, both patients restarted atezolizumab therapy. Long-term insulin therapy was required in all patients with confirmed type 1 diabetes mellitus.

Patients receiving atezolizumab should be monitored for signs and symptoms of diabetes mellitus (e.g., hyperglycemia). If immune-mediated type 1 diabetes mellitus occurs, temporary interruption or discontinuance of atezolizumab may be necessary and insulin therapy should be initiated as clinically indicated. (See Immune-mediated Endocrine Effects under Dosage and Administration and also see Severe and Fatal Immune-mediated Effects under Cautions.)

Immune-mediated Renal Effects

Immune-mediated nephritis has occurred in patients receiving atezolizumab therapy.

In clinical studies evaluating single-agent atezolizumab, 1 of 2616 patients developed immune-mediated nephritis with renal dysfunction; this adverse reaction was grade 3 in severity. Atezolizumab was permanently discontinued in this patient.

In clinical studies evaluating atezolizumab in combination with cobimetinib and vemurafenib, 3 patients (1.3%) developed immune-mediated nephritis with renal dysfunction; atezolizumab therapy was temporarily interrupted in 2 patients and permanently discontinued in 1 patient. Treatment with systemic corticosteroids was required in 2 patients. Nephritis resolved in all 3 patients. Both patients in whom atezolizumab was temporarily interrupted were able to restart atezolizumab therapy without recurrence of nephritis.

Patients receiving atezolizumab should be monitored for signs and symptoms of nephritis and renal impairment (including serum creatinine concentration) at baseline and periodically during atezolizumab therapy. Temporary interruption or discontinuance of atezolizumab may be necessary if immune-mediated nephritis or renal dysfunction occurs during therapy with the drug. (See Immune-mediated Renal Effects under Dosage and Administration and also see Severe and Fatal Immune-mediated Effects under Cautions.)

Immune-mediated Dermatologic Effects

Immune-mediated rash and dermatitis have occurred in patients receiving atezolizumab therapy. Severe exfoliative dermatitis, including SJS, TEN, or DRESS, has been reported in patients receiving anti-PD-L1 and anti-PD-1 monoclonal antibodies.

In clinical studies evaluating single-agent atezolizumab, immune-mediated dermatologic effects occurred in 0.6% of patients; grade 2 or 3 immune-mediated dermatologic effects occurred in 0.2 or less than 0.1% of patients, respectively. Interruption of atezolizumab was necessary due to dermatologic effects in 0.2% of patients, and therapy was permanently discontinued in 0.1% of patients. Treatment with systemic corticosteroids was required in 20% of patients experiencing immune-mediated dermatologic effects, and symptoms resolved in 87% of these patients. Among the patients in whom atezolizumab therapy was interrupted, none restarted the drug.

Topical corticosteroids and/or topical emollients may be adequate to treat mild to moderate non-exfoliative rashes. Temporary interruption or discontinuance of atezolizumab may be necessary for more severe immune-mediated dermatologic conditions. (See Immune-mediated Dermatologic Effects under Dosage and Administration and also see Severe and Fatal Immune-mediated Effects under Cautions.)

Other Immune-mediated Effects

Other immune-mediated adverse effects, including myocarditis, pericarditis, vasculitis, meningitis, encephalitis, myelitis and demyelination, myasthenic syndrome/myasthenia gravis, Guillain-Barré syndrome, nerve paresis, autoimmune neuropathy, ocular inflammatory conditions (e.g., uveitis, iritis), retinal detachment, visual impairment, blindness, pancreatitis (including elevation of serum amylase and lipase concentrations), gastritis, duodenitis, myositis/polymyositis, rhabdomyolysis (including renal failure), arthritis, polymyalgia rheumatic, hypoparathyroidism, hemolytic anemia, aplastic anemia, hemophagocytic lymphohistiocytosis, systemic inflammatory response syndrome, histiocytic necrotizing lymphadenitis (Kikuchi lymphadenitis), sarcoidosis, immune thrombocytopenic purpura, and solid organ transplant rejection, have occurred rarely in patients receiving atezolizumab or other anti-programmed-death ligand-1 (anti-PD-L1) or anti-programmed-death receptor-1 (anti-PD-1) antibodies. Some cases have resulted in death.

Temporary interruption or discontinuance of atezolizumab may be necessary if immune-mediated adverse effects occur during therapy with the drug. (See Therapy Interruption for Toxicity under Dosage and Administration and also see Severe and Fatal Immune-mediated Effects under Cautions.)

If uveitis occurs in conjunction with other immune-mediated adverse effects, a Vogt-Koyanagi-Harada-like syndrome should be considered. Systemic corticosteroid therapy may be required to reduce the risk of permanent vision loss.

Allogeneic Stem Cell Transplantation-related Complications

Patients who undergo allogeneic stem cell transplantation either before or after receiving therapy with an anti-PD-1 or anti-PD-L1 monoclonal antibody, including atezolizumab, may experience serious or fatal transplant-related complications, including hyperacute, acute, or chronic graft-versus-host disease (GVHD); hepatic veno-occlusive disease following allogeneic stem cell transplantation with a reduced-intensity conditioning regimen; and corticosteroid-requiring febrile syndrome with no identified infectious cause. These complications may occur despite other intervening therapy between administration of the anti-PD-1 or anti-PD-L1 monoclonal antibody and transplantation.

Potential benefits and risks of anti-PD-1 or anti-PD-L1 monoclonal antibody therapy administered before or after allogeneic stem cell transplantation should be considered. Patients who receive atezolizumab should be monitored closely for early manifestations of stem cell transplantation-related complications, and such conditions should be promptly managed if they occur.

Treatment-related Mortality

In a clinical trial, a higher rate of mortality was reported in PD-L1-positive patients with metastatic triple-negative breast cancer receiving atezolizumab in combination with conventional paclitaxel compared with patients receiving placebo and conventional paclitaxel. Efficacy of atezolizumab in combination with conventional paclitaxel in patients with unresectable locally advanced or metastatic triple-negative breast cancer has not been demonstrated. Albumin-bound paclitaxel should not be substituted with conventional paclitaxel in patients with metastatic triple-negative breast cancer outside of a controlled clinical trial.

Infusion-related Effects

Severe or life-threatening infusion-related reactions may occur in patients receiving atezolizumab therapy. In clinical studies, infusion-related reactions occurred in 1.3% of patients receiving atezolizumab as a single agent and were grade 3 in 0.2% of patients receiving the drug. The frequency and severity of infusion-related reactions were similar regardless of whether atezolizumab was administered as a single agent in patients with various cancers, in combination with other antineoplastic drugs in patients with NSCLC or SCLC, or the dosage administered (i.e. 840 mg every 2 weeks to 1680 mg every 4 weeks).

Patients receiving atezolizumab should be monitored for signs and symptoms of infusion-related reactions. In patients experiencing infusion-related reactions, interruption of the infusion, reduction in the infusion rate, or discontinuance

of atezolizumab may be necessary. (See Infusion-related Reactions under Dosage and Administration.) For patients experiencing grade 1 or 2 infusion-related reactions, premedication may be considered prior to subsequent atezolizumab infusions.

Fetal/Neonatal Morbidity and Mortality

Atezolizumab may cause fetal harm if administered to pregnant women. Blockade of signaling of the PD-1 and PD-L1 pathway in animals has been shown to disrupt maternal immune tolerance to the fetus and has been associated with increased fetal loss (e.g., abortion, stillbirth) and immune-mediated disorders; however, teratogenicity has not been observed.

Pregnancy should be avoided during atezolizumab therapy. The manufacturer states that pregnancy status should be verified prior to initiation of atezolizumab. Females of reproductive potential should be advised to use an effective method of contraception while receiving atezolizumab and for at least 5 months after discontinuance of therapy. Females of reproductive potential should be apprised of the potential fetal hazard if atezolizumab is used during pregnancy.

Immunogenicity

There is a potential for immunogenicity with atezolizumab therapy. Anti-atezolizumab antibodies were detected at one or more post-dose time points in the OAK, IMvigor210 (cohort 1), IMpower150, IMpassion130, IMbrave150, and IMspire150 studies. The neutralizing capacity of anti-atezolizumab antibodies has not been established. Median clearance of atezolizumab increased by 22% in the presence of anti-atezolizumab antibodies. In general, presence of anti-atezolizumab antibodies did not have a clinically substantial effect on the incidence or severity of adverse effects. Exploratory analysis of the OAK study (in patients with NSCLC) and the IMbrave150 study (in patients with hepatocellular carcinoma) suggests reduced efficacy in patients who develop anti-atezolizumab antibodies by week 4 and 6, respectively.

In the OAK study in patients with NSCLC, anti-atezolizumab antibodies were detected in 30% of 565 patients, with a median time to antibody formation of 3 weeks. Systemic exposure was reduced in patients who developed anti-atezolizumab antibodies. Exploratory analysis also suggests that efficacy (i.e., overall survival) is reduced in patients who are positive for anti-atezolizumab antibodies by week 4. The incidence and severity of adverse effects were not substantially impacted by the presence of anti-atezolizumab antibodies.

In cohort 1 of the IMvigor210 study in patients with urothelial carcinoma, anti-atezolizumab antibodies were detected in 48% of 111 patients at one or more post-dose time points. Systemic exposure was reduced in patients who developed anti-atezolizumab antibodies, but the incidence and severity of adverse effects were not substantially impacted by the presence of anti-atezolizumab antibodies.

In the IMpower150 study in patients with NSCLC who received atezolizumab in combination with bevacizumab, paclitaxel, and carboplatin, anti-atezolizumab antibodies were detected in 36% of 364 patients at one or more post-dose time points, and 83% of patients had detectable anti-atezolizumab antibodies prior to receiving the second dose of atezolizumab. Systemic exposure was reduced in patients who developed anti-atezolizumab antibodies; however, the incidence and severity of adverse effects were not substantially impacted by the presence of anti-atezolizumab antibodies. Exploratory analysis suggests that efficacy (i.e., overall survival) is similar in patients who develop anti-atezolizumab antibodies by week 4 and those without antibodies.

In the IMpassion130 study in patients with triple-negative breast cancer who received atezolizumab in combination with albumin-bound paclitaxel, anti-atezolizumab antibodies were detected in 13% of 434 patients at one or more post-dose time points; the rate of detection was 12% among patients whose tumors expressed PD-L1. Systemic exposure was reduced in patients who developed anti-atezolizumab antibodies; however, the number of PD-L1-positive patients who developed anti-drug antibodies was insufficient to determine whether patients who develop anti-drug antibodies respond differently than those who do not develop anti-drug antibodies. The incidence and severity of adverse effects were not substantially impacted by the presence of anti-atezolizumab antibodies.

In the IMbrave150 study in patients with hepatocellular carcinoma who received atezolizumab in combination with bevacizumab, anti-atezolizumab antibodies were detected in 28% of 315 patients at one or more post-dose time points; 66% of these patients had detectable anti-drug antibodies prior to receiving the third dose of atezolizumab. Systemic exposure was reduced in patients who developed anti-atezolizumab antibodies. Exploratory analysis suggests that efficacy (i.e., overall survival) is reduced in patients who develop anti-atezolizumab antibodies by week 6 compared with those who do not develop anti-drug antibodies at week 6. The incidence and severity of adverse effects were not substantially impacted by the presence of anti-atezolizumab antibodies.

In the IMspire150 study in patients with melanoma who received atezolizumab in combination with cobimetinib and vemurafenib, anti-atezolizumab antibodies were detected in 13% of 218 patients. Systemic exposure was reduced in patients who developed anti-atezolizumab antibodies; however, the number of patients who developed anti-drug antibodies was insufficient to determine whether patients who develop anti-drug antibodies respond differently than those who do not develop anti-drug antibodies.

Impairment of Fertility

Results of animal studies suggest that atezolizumab may impair female fertility. In a 26-week general toxicology study, irregular menstrual cycle patterns and absence of corpora lutea were observed in female animals receiving atezolizumab at exposure levels approximately 6 times the human exposure at the recommended dosage; however, these adverse effects were reversible. Adverse reproductive effects in male animals were not observed.

Specific Populations

Pregnancy

Atezolizumab may cause fetal harm if administered to pregnant women based on its mechanism of action and animal findings. (See Fetal/Neonatal Morbidity and Mortality under Cautions.)

Pregnancy status should be verified prior to initiation of atezolizumab.

Lactation

It is not known whether atezolizumab is distributed into human milk. Because human immunoglobulin G (IgG) is distributed into milk and because of the potential for serious adverse reactions to atezolizumab in nursing infants, women should be advised to discontinue nursing during atezolizumab therapy and for at least 5 months after discontinuance of therapy. The effects of the drug on nursing infants or on milk production are unknown.

Pediatric Use

Safety and efficacy of atezolizumab have not been established in pediatric patients.

Safety and antitumor activity of atezolizumab were assessed, but not established, in 60 pediatric patients 7 months to less than 17 years of age with relapsed or progressive solid tumors or lymphomas in a phase ½ study (iMATRIX). No new safety signals were observed in this study. The median duration of atezolizumab therapy was 0.8 months.

The iMATRIX study also compared the pharmacokinetic parameters of atezolizumab in pediatric patients and adults 18-29 years of age. Pediatric patients received a weight-based dose of 15 mg/kg (up to a maximum of 1200 mg per dose) every 3 weeks and adults received a fixed dose of 1200 mg every 3 weeks. Overall, steady-state area under the concentration-time curve (AUC) was similar between patients 12 to less than 18 years of age and adults, but systemic exposure trended lower in pediatric patients younger than 12 years of age. Peak plasma concentrations increased from children to adolescents to young adults. Terminal elimination half-lives of atezolizumab in pediatric patients and young adults were consistent with those estimated in adults.

Geriatric Use

In clinical studies evaluating single-agent atezolizumab for the treatment of metastatic urothelial carcinoma, metastatic NSCLC, or other tumor types, 49% of patients were 65 years of age or older and 15% were 75 years of age or older. In clinical studies of atezolizumab in combination with other antineoplastic agents for the treatment of SCLC and NSCLC, 48% of patients were 65 years of age or older, and 10% were 75 years of age or older. No overall differences in safety or efficacy were observed between geriatric patients and younger adults.

Hepatic Impairment

The effects of hepatic impairment on the pharmacokinetics of atezolizumab have not been formally studied. Analysis of population pharmacokinetic data indicates that clearance and systemic exposure of atezolizumab are similar between patients with mild (total bilirubin concentration not exceeding the ULN with AST concentration exceeding the ULN, or total bilirubin concentration more than 1 time but no more than 1.5 times the ULN with any AST concentration) or moderate (total bilirubin concentration more than 1.5 times but no more than 3 times the ULN with any AST concentration) hepatic impairment and those with normal hepatic function. Pharmacokinetic data in patients with severe hepatic impairment are lacking.

Renal Impairment

The effects of renal impairment on the pharmacokinetics of atezolizumab have not been formally studied. Analysis of population pharmacokinetic data indicates that atezolizumab clearance is not substantially affected by mild or moderate renal impairment (estimated glomerular filtration rate [GFR] 30–89 mL/minute per 1.73 m²). Pharmacokinetic data in patients with severe renal impairment are limited.

● Common Adverse Effects

Adverse effects reported in 20% or more of patients receiving atezolizumab as a single agent include fatigue or asthenia, nausea, cough, dyspnea, and decreased appetite.

Adverse effects reported in 20% or more of patients with NSCLC or SCLC receiving atezolizumab in combination with other antineoplastic agents include fatigue or asthenia, nausea, alopecia, constipation, diarrhea, and decreased appetite.

Adverse effects reported in 20% or more of patients with triple-negative breast cancer receiving atezolizumab in combination with albumin-bound paclitaxel include alopecia, peripheral neuropathy, fatigue, nausea, diarrhea, constipation, cough, headache, vomiting, and decreased appetite; laboratory abnormalities occurring in 50% or more of patients include decreased concentrations of hemoglobin, leukocytes, neutrophils, and lymphocytes.

Adverse effects reported in 20% or more of patients with hepatocellular carcinoma receiving atezolizumab in combination with bevacizumab include hypertension, fatigue, and proteinuria.

Adverse effects reported in 20% or more of patients with melanoma receiving atezolizumab in combination with cobimetinib and vemurafenib include rash, musculoskeletal pain, fatigue, hepatotoxicity, pyrexia, nausea, pruritus, edema, stomatitis, hypothyroidism, and photosensitivity.

DRUG INTERACTIONS

No formal drug interaction studies have been performed to date.

DESCRIPTION

Atezolizumab, a humanized anti-programmed-death ligand-1 (anti-PD-L1) monoclonal antibody, is an antineoplastic agent. The drug is an IgG_1 kappa immunoglobulin.

The immune-checkpoint receptor PD-1 is expressed on activated T-cells, monocytes, B-cells, natural killer (NK) T-cells, and dendritic cells. Overexpression of PD-1 ligands on the surface of tumor cells results in activation of PD-1 and B7.1 and suppression of cytotoxic T-cell activity, T-cell proliferation, and cytokine production. Atezolizumab blocks the interaction between PD-L1 and the receptors PD-1 and B7.1, resulting in activation of the antitumor immune response without inducing antibody-dependent cell-mediated cytotoxicity (ADCC). The drug also has been shown to reduce tumor growth in syngeneic mouse tumor models. In mouse models of cancer, dual inhibition of the PD-1/PD-L1 and MAPK pathways suppresses tumor growth and improves tumor immunogenicity through increased antigen presentation and T-cell infiltration and activation compared to targeted therapy alone.

Systemic exposure to atezolizumab is proportional to dose over the dose range of 1–20 mg/kg, including the fixed dosage of 1.2 g every 3 weeks. Following repeated doses of atezolizumab 1200 mg every 3 weeks, steady-state concentrations are reached by 6–9 weeks; systemic accumulation of the drug is 3.3- or 1.9-fold when administered every 2 or 3 weeks, respectively. Atezolizumab clearance decreases over time by approximately 17% from baseline values; however, this difference is not considered clinically important. The terminal half-life of atezolizumab is 27 days.

Systemic exposure to atezolizumab does not appear to be affected by age (range of 21–89 years), body weight, sex, serum albumin concentration, tumor burden, geographic region, race, PD-L1 expression, or performance status.

ADVICE TO PATIENTS

Importance of advising patients to read the manufacturer's medication guide.

Risk of immune-mediated pneumonitis. Importance of informing clinician immediately if new or worsening cough, chest pain, or shortness of breath occurs.

Risk of immune-mediated colitis. Importance of informing clinician immediately if diarrhea or severe abdominal pain occurs or if mucus or blood is present in stool.

Risk of immune-mediated hepatitis. Importance of informing clinician immediately if signs and symptoms of liver damage (e.g., jaundice, severe nausea or vomiting, abdominal pain [particularly in the right upper quadrant], lethargy, easy bruising or bleeding, lack of appetite, dark urine, drowsiness) occur.

Risk of immune-mediated endocrine effects. Importance of informing clinician immediately if manifestations of hypophysitis, hyperthyroidism, hypothyroidism, adrenal insufficiency, or diabetes mellitus (including ketoacidosis) occur.

Risk of immune-mediated nephritis. Importance of informing clinician immediately if signs or symptoms of nephritis (e.g., pelvic pain, frequent urination, unusual swelling) occur.

Risk of immune-mediated dermatologic adverse effects. Importance of informing clinician immediately if skin eruption, generalized rash, or painful lesions on the skin or mucous membranes develop.

Risk of other immune-mediated adverse effects. Importance of informing clinician immediately if manifestations of other potential immune-mediated adverse effects occur.

Risk of infusion-related reactions. Importance of informing clinician if signs and symptoms of such reactions, including dizziness, chills, fever, breathing difficulty (i.e., shortness of breath, wheezing), pruritus, flushing, feeling of faintness, back or neck pain, and angioedema, occur.

Risk of allogeneic stem cell transplantation-related complications.

Risk of fetal harm. Necessity of advising women of childbearing potential that they should use an effective method of contraception while receiving atezolizumab and for at least 5 months after discontinuance of therapy. Importance of women informing clinicians if they are or plan to become pregnant. If pregnancy occurs, advise pregnant women of potential risk to the fetus.

Importance of advising women to avoid breast-feeding while receiving atezolizumab and for at least 5 months after discontinuance of therapy.

Importance of informing clinicians of existing or contemplated concomitant therapy, including prescription and OTC drugs and dietary or herbal supplements, as well as any concomitant illnesses.

Importance of informing patients of other important precautionary information. (See Cautions.)

For further information on the handling of antineoplastic agents, see the ASHP Guidelines on Handling Hazardous Drugs at http://www.ahfsdrug information.com.

PREPARATIONS

Obtain atezolizumab through a limited network of specialty distributors. Contact manufacturer for additional information.

Excipients in commercially available drug preparations may have clinically important effects in some individuals; consult specific product labeling for details.

Atezolizumab

Parenteral

Concentrate, for injection, for IV infusion	60 mg/mL (840 mg and 1200 mg)	Tecentriq®, Genentech

Selected Revisions October 18, 2021, © Copyright, September 8, 2016, American Society of Health-System Pharmacists, Inc.

Bevacizumab

10:00 • ANTINEOPLASTIC AGENTS

- Bevacizumab, a recombinant humanized monoclonal antibody, is an antineoplastic agent.

USES

• Colorectal Cancer

First-line Treatment of Metastatic Cancer of the Colon or Rectum

Bevacizumab is used in combination with IV fluorouracil-based chemotherapy for the first-line treatment of metastatic cancer of the colon or rectum.

The indication for use of bevacizumab in combination with IV fluorouracil-based chemotherapy for the first-line treatment of metastatic cancer of the colon or rectum is based mainly on the results of 2 randomized, controlled clinical studies (one phase 2 and one phase 3).

In the phase 3, randomized, double-blind, active-controlled study, 813 patients received either a placebo (administered every 2 weeks) or bevacizumab (5 mg/kg administered by IV infusion every 2 weeks until disease progression occurred) in conjunction with a combination irinotecan/fluorouracil/leucovorin regimen. The combination regimen consisted of irinotecan 125 mg/m², fluorouracil 500 mg/m², and leucovorin 20 mg/m², administered as an IV bolus injection once weekly for 4 out of every 6 weeks. Patients who received bevacizumab in combination with the irinotecan/fluorouracil/leucovorin regimen had a higher median overall response rate (45 versus 35%, respectively) and prolonged median overall survival (20.3 versus 15.6 months, respectively), median progression-free survival (10.6 versus 6.2 months, respectively), and median duration of response (10.4 versus 7.1 months, respectively) than patients receiving placebo in conjunction with the same combination regimen. Grade 3–4 adverse effects, including leukopenia (37 versus 31%), diarrhea (34 versus 25%), neutropenia (21 versus 14%), hypertension (12 versus 2%), asthenia (10 versus 7%), deep-vein thrombosis (9 versus 5%), pain (8 versus 5%), abdominal pain (8 versus 5%), constipation (4 versus 2%), intra-abdominal thrombosis (3 versus 1%), and syncope (3 versus 1%), occurred more frequently in patients receiving bevacizumab rather than placebo in conjunction with the irinotecan/fluorouracil/leucovorin regimen.

This phase 3 study also included initial enrollment of patients by random assignment into a third group receiving fluorouracil/leucovorin and bevacizumab to establish a comparison group for determining the toxicity of bevacizumab combined with irinotecan. When the toxicity of bevacizumab with the irinotecan/fluorouracil/leucovorin regimen was deemed acceptable, enrollment of patients into this treatment group was discontinued. Among 110 patients receiving bevacizumab (5 mg/kg administered by IV infusion every 2 weeks) with fluorouracil and leucovorin (each 500 mg/m² IV once weekly for 6 out of every 8 weeks), the objective response rate was 39%, median overall survival was 18.3 months, median progression-free survival was 8.8 months, and median duration of response was 8.5 months.

In the phase 2, open-label, dose-ranging study, 104 patients with previously untreated metastatic colorectal cancer were randomized to receive a combination regimen of fluorouracil and leucovorin (leucovorin 500 mg/m² administered by IV infusion over 2 hours, followed by fluorouracil 500 mg/m² administered by slow IV injection [1 hour after initiation of leucovorin] given once weekly for the first 6 weeks out of every 8-week cycle) alone or in conjunction with either low-dose bevacizumab (5 mg/kg every 2 weeks) or high-dose bevacizumab (10 mg/kg every 2 weeks); bevacizumab was given for a total of 6 cycles (i.e., 48 weeks) or until disease progression occurred. Results of this study suggest that patients receiving combination therapy with bevacizumab and the fluorouracil-containing regimen may have a higher overall response rate and prolonged median overall survival and median progression-free survival than those receiving the fluorouracil-containing regimen alone. Although progression-free survival was longer in patients receiving low-dose bevacizumab in conjunction with the fluorouracil-containing regimen than in those receiving the fluorouracil-containing regimen alone, overall survival and overall response rate were similar between the 2 groups. In addition, overall outcomes for patients receiving high-dose bevacizumab in conjunction with the fluorouracil-containing regimen were similar to outcomes in those receiving the fluorouracil-containing regimen alone. In this

study, median overall survival was 13.6, 17.7, or 15.2 months in patients receiving the fluorouracil-containing combination alone, with the 5 mg/kg-bevacizumab regimen, or with the 10 mg/kg-bevacizumab regimen, respectively. Median survival was 13.8, 21.5, or 16.1 months in patients receiving the fluorouracil-containing combination alone, in conjunction with the 5-mg/kg bevacizumab regimen, or in conjunction with the 10-mg/kg bevacizumab regimen, respectively. Median progression-free survival was 5.2, 9, or 7.2 months in patients receiving the fluorouracil-containing combination alone, in conjunction with the 5-mg/kg bevacizumab regimen, or in conjunction with the 10-mg/kg bevacizumab regimen, respectively. In addition, the overall response rate was 17, 40, or 24% among patients receiving the fluorouracil-containing combination alone, in conjunction with the 5-mg/kg bevacizumab regimen, or in conjunction with the 10-mg/kg bevacizumab regimen, respectively.

The combination of bevacizumab with fluorouracil/leucovorin for previously untreated metastatic colorectal cancer also has been studied in patients who were not optimal candidates for first-line irinotecan-containing therapy (i.e., 65 years of age or older, ECOG performance status of 1 or 2, serum albumin concentration of 3.5 g/dL or less, or prior pelvic or abdominal radiation therapy). In a phase 2 randomized trial involving 209 patients with previously untreated metastatic colorectal cancer who were not considered optimal candidates for irinotecan-containing therapy, median progression-free survival was prolonged (9.2 versus 5.5 months) but median overall survival was similar (16.6 versus 12.9 months) in patients receiving bevacizumab/fluorouracil/leucovorin compared with those receiving fluorouracil/leucovorin. Grade 3 or 4 toxicity occurred more frequently in patients receiving bevacizumab versus placebo (87 versus 71%) in combination with fluorouracil/leucovorin, including grade 3 hypertension (16 versus 3%). Proteinuria (38 versus 19%) and arterial thrombotic events (10 versus 5%) also occurred more often in patients receiving bevacizumab. Combined analysis of pooled individual data from this trial as well as the 2 primary efficacy studies suggests that survival is prolonged when bevacizumab is added to the fluorouracil/leucovorin regimen for the first-line treatment of metastatic colorectal cancer.

Bevacizumab also has been used in combination with oxaliplatin-containing regimens† as first-line therapy for metastatic colorectal cancer. In a randomized phase 3 trial, the addition of bevacizumab to oxaliplatin-containing chemotherapy (either capecitabine and oxaliplatin [XELOX] or fluorouracil/leucovorin and oxaliplatin [FOLFOX4]) in first-line therapy for metastatic colorectal cancer prolonged median progression-free survival, but no difference in overall survival was observed.

Second-line Treatment of Metastatic Cancer of the Colon or Rectum

Bevacizumab is used in combination with IV fluorouracil-based chemotherapy for the second-line treatment of metastatic cancer of the colon or rectum.

The indication for use of bevacizumab in combination with IV fluorouracil-based chemotherapy for the second-line treatment of metastatic cancer of the colon or rectum is based mainly on the results of a randomized, controlled clinical study and an open-access single-arm study.

In an open-label, randomized, 3-arm, active-controlled, multicenter clinical study, 829 patients received bevacizumab in combination with FOLFOX4 (i.e., fluorouracil/leucovorin and oxaliplatin), FOLFOX4 alone, or bevacizumab alone, for the second-line treatment of metastatic carcinoma of the colon or rectum. Patients had received prior treatment with irinotecan, with or without fluorouracil, as initial therapy for metastatic disease (99%) or irinotecan and fluorouracil as adjuvant therapy (1%). The FOLFOX4 regimen consisted of oxaliplatin 85 mg/m² and leucovorin 200 mg/m² concurrently IV, then fluorouracil 400 mg/m² by IV bolus, followed by fluorouracil 600 mg/m² by continuous IV infusion on day 1; and leucovorin 200 mg/m² IV, then fluorouracil 400 mg/m² by IV bolus, followed by fluorouracil 600 mg/m² by continuous IV infusion on day 2; with treatment cycles repeated every 2 weeks. Bevacizumab was administered at a dose of 10 mg/kg every 2 weeks. For patients receiving the combination of the 2 regimens, bevacizumab was administered prior to the FOLFOX4 regimen on day 1 of the treatment cycle. The median age of patients was 61 years, 40% were female, 87% were Caucasian, and 49% had an ECOG performance status of 0. Most patients (80%) had received adjuvant chemotherapy, and 26% had received prior radiation therapy.

Following an interim analysis that showed decreased survival in patients receiving bevacizumab alone compared with those receiving FOLFOX4 alone, the bevacizumab monotherapy arm was closed to accrual after enrollment of 244 of the planned 290 patients. In patients receiving bevacizumab in combination with

FOLFOX4, median overall survival was prolonged (13 versus 10.8 months), and progression-free survival and overall response rate based on investigator assessment were higher than in patients receiving FOLFOX4 alone. Grade 3–5 nonhematologic and grade 3–4 hematologic adverse effects, including fatigue (19 versus 13%), diarrhea (18 versus 13%), sensory neuropathy (17 versus 9%), nausea (12 versus 5%), vomiting (11 versus 4%), dehydration (10 versus 5%), hypertension (9 versus 2%), abdominal pain (8 versus 5%), hemorrhage (5 versus 1%), other neurologic adverse effects (5 versus 3%), ileus (4 versus 1%), and headache (3 versus 0%), occurred more frequently in patients receiving bevacizumab with FOLFOX4 compared with those receiving FOLFOX4 alone. Because of the reporting mechanisms used in this study, the manufacturer states that the true incidence of adverse effects associated with bevacizumab therapy may have been underestimated.

In a multicenter, single-arm, open-access protocol, 339 patients received bevacizumab in combination with fluorouracil/leucovorin (administered by either IV infusion or rapid IV injection) for metastatic colorectal cancer with disease progression following both irinotecan-containing and oxaliplatin-containing regimens. Most patients (73%) received concurrent fluorouracil and leucovorin according to a rapid IV injection ("bolus") regimen. Among the first 100 evaluable patients, there was one objective partial response for an overall response rate of 1%. The median progression-free survival of the first 100 evaluable patients was 3.5 months, and the median overall survival was 9 months. Among 322 patients evaluated for toxicity, 47% had at least one grade 3 or higher adverse event, and 14% discontinued treatment because of adverse effects.

Adjuvant Therapy for Early-stage Colon Cancer

Bevacizumab has been investigated for use in combination with fluorouracil, leucovorin, and oxaliplatin (modified FOLFOX6)† as adjuvant therapy following surgery for early-stage (i.e., stage II or III)† colon cancer. Results of a phase 3, randomized, open-label study (National Surgical Adjuvant Breast and Bowel Project [NSABP] C-08) demonstrated no improvement in disease-free survival following use of bevacizumab (5 mg/kg administered by IV infusion every 2 weeks for 1 year) in combination with modified FOLFOX6 (leucovorin 400 mg/m² IV on day 1, fluorouracil 400 mg/m² by IV injection on day 1 followed by fluorouracil 2400 mg/m² by continuous IV infusion over 46 hours, and oxaliplatin 85 mg/m² IV on day 1; regimen administered every 2 weeks for 6 months). The 3-year disease-survival rate was 77.4% in patients with stage II or III colon adenocarcinoma who received bevacizumab in combination with modified FOLFOX6 compared with 75.5% in those who received modified FOLFOX6 alone. Because of the lack of improvement in disease-free survival, investigators of this study recommended that bevacizumab *not* be used in combination with modified FOLFOX6 as adjuvant therapy for stage II or III colon cancer.

● Non-small Cell Lung Cancer

Bevacizumab is used in combination with carboplatin and paclitaxel for the first-line treatment of unresectable, locally advanced, recurrent or metastatic nonsquamous non-small cell lung cancer.

This indication is based on the results of a randomized, active-controlled, open-label, multicenter study (supported by a randomized, dose-ranging, active-controlled phase 2 study) in which 878 chemotherapy-naive patients with locally advanced, metastatic, or recurrent nonsquamous non-small cell lung cancer were randomized to receive paclitaxel and carboplatin either with or without bevacizumab. Patients received paclitaxel 200 mg/m² and carboplatin (dose required to obtain an area under the plasma concentration-time curve [AUC] of 6 mg/mL per minute) both by IV infusion on day 1 with bevacizumab 15 mg/kg by IV infusion on day 1 or the same regimen of paclitaxel/carboplatin alone (without bevacizumab); each regimen was administered every 21 days for up to 6 cycles. Upon completion or discontinuance of chemotherapy, patients receiving bevacizumab continued to receive bevacizumab alone until disease progression or intolerable toxicity occurred. Most of the patients (89%) had newly diagnosed disease (stage IV in 76%), 46% were female, 43% were 65 years of age or older (median age: 63 years), and 28% of the patients had at least a 5% weight loss at the time of entry to the study. Excluded from the study were patients with disease of predominantly squamous histology, CNS metastasis, gross hemoptysis (0.5 teaspoon of red blood or more), unstable angina, and those receiving anticoagulant therapy.

The median overall survival was prolonged (12.3 versus 10.3 months) in patients receiving chemotherapy (paclitaxel and carboplatin) and bevacizumab compared with those receiving chemotherapy alone for advanced nonsquamous non-small cell lung cancer. Subgroup analysis suggested that the benefit of the addition of bevacizumab to this chemotherapy regimen was less certain in

women, patients 65 years of age or older, and patients with at least a 5% weight loss at study entry. Grade 3–5 nonhematologic and grade 4–5 hematologic adverse effects, including neutropenia (27 versus 17%), fatigue (16 versus 13%), hypertension (8 versus 0.7%), infection without neutropenia (7 versus 3%), venous thrombosis or embolism (5 versus 3%), febrile neutropenia (5 versus 2%), pneumonitis or pulmonary infiltrates (5 versus 3%), infection with grade 3 or 4 neutropenia (4 versus 2%), hyponatremia (4 versus 1%), headache (3 versus 1%), and proteinuria (3 versus 0%), occurred more frequently in patients receiving bevacizumab and chemotherapy than in those receiving chemotherapy alone.

Bevacizumab has been investigated for use in combination with cisplatin and gemcitabine† for the first-line treatment of locally advanced, metastatic, or recurrent nonsquamous non-small cell lung cancer. In a randomized, double-blind, active-controlled study, 1043 patients with locally advanced, metastatic, or recurrent nonsquamous non-small cell lung cancer were randomized to receive bevacizumab 7.5 mg/kg in combination with cisplatin and gemcitabine, bevacizumab 15 mg/kg in combination with cisplatin and gemcitabine, or cisplatin and gemcitabine with placebo. Most of the patients (77%) had stage IV disease, 8% had recurrent disease, 36% were female, and 29% were 65 years of age or older. Patients receiving bevacizumab 7.5 or 15 mg/kg in combination with cisplatin and gemcitabine had longer progression-free survival, but not a significantly longer overall survival, compared with patients receiving cisplatin and gemcitabine alone.

● Glioblastoma

Bevacizumab is used as a single agent for the treatment of glioblastoma (also known as glioblastoma multiforme) in patients whose disease has progressed following radiation therapy and chemotherapy (i.e., temozolomide). Labeling for use of bevacizumab for the management of previously treated glioblastoma was approved under the principles and procedures of the US Food and Drug Administration's (FDA's) accelerated review process that allows approval based on analysis of surrogate markers of response. As a result of the accelerated review, labeling of bevacizumab for management of previously treated glioblastoma was based on improvement in objective response rate; currently, there are no data demonstrating amelioration of disease-related symptoms or prolonged survival with use of the drug for this condition.

The current indication for use of bevacizumab in the management of previously treated glioblastoma is based principally on the results of 2 studies (one open-label, multicenter, randomized, noncomparative study and one single-arm, single-institution study).

In the phase 2, open-label, multicenter, randomized, noncomparative study (AVF3708g, BRAIN), 167 patients with previously treated glioblastoma were randomized to receive either bevacizumab (10 mg/kg administered by IV infusion every 2 weeks) alone or bevacizumab in combination with irinotecan (340 mg/m² in patients receiving enzyme-inducing antiepileptic drugs or 125 mg/m² in those not receiving enzyme-inducing antiepileptic drugs, administered by IV infusion over 90 minutes every 2 weeks); treatment was continued until disease progression or unacceptable toxicity occurred, up to a maximum of 104 weeks. Because this study design did not permit isolation of the contribution of each drug to the efficacy of the bevacizumab plus irinotecan regimen, efficacy data for the combination regimen could not be used to support drug approval and were not analyzed by FDA; only efficacy data for bevacizumab monotherapy were evaluated. Patients enrolled in this study had received prior radiation therapy (completed at least 8 weeks prior to receiving bevacizumab) and chemotherapy (i.e., temozolomide); patients with active brain hemorrhage were excluded. Of the 85 patients randomized to receive bevacizumab monotherapy, the median age was 54 years (range: 23–78 years), 32% were female, 81% were in first relapse, and 45 or 55% had a Karnofsky performance status of 90–100 or 70–80, respectively; the mean treatment duration was 4.8 months (range: 0–12.9 months). Response to bevacizumab was determined by magnetic resonance imagery (MRI) (using WHO radiographic criteria) and by evaluation of corticosteroid usage (i.e., stabilization or reduction of corticosteroid dosage). Analysis of efficacy data differed between FDA and the manufacturer; only FDA's analysis is discussed. Treatment with bevacizumab monotherapy resulted in an objective response rate of 25.9% (partial responses only), a median duration of response of 4.2 months, a 6-month progression-free survival rate of 36%, and a median overall survival of 9.3 months. In addition, corticosteroid dosage decreased by a median of 37.5% at the time of response compared with baseline. The most common adverse effects reported with bevacizumab monotherapy included infection (55%), fatigue (45%), headache (37%), hypertension (30%), epistaxis (19%), and diarrhea (21%). Serious (grade 3 or greater) adverse effects included infection (10%), fatigue (4%), headache (4%), hypertension (8%), and diarrhea (1%). Two deaths (one from retroperitoneal hemorrhage and one from neutropenic infection), possibly associated with bevacizumab, also have been reported in patients receiving bevacizumab monotherapy. Other serious (grade 3–5) adverse effects reported in patients receiving bevacizumab alone or in combination with irinotecan included bleeding or hemorrhage (2%), CNS hemorrhage (1%), venous thromboembolic events (7%), arterial thromboembolic events (3%), wound healing complications (3%), proteinuria (1%), and GI perforation (2%); because some of these adverse effects (i.e., CNS hemorrhage, wound healing complications, venous thromboembolic events) are inherent in patients with glioblastoma and associated with prior surgery and radiation therapy, a causal relationship of such adverse effects to bevacizumab has not been established.

In the single-arm, single-institution study (study NCI 06-C-0064E), 56 patients with previously treated glioblastoma received bevacizumab (10 mg/kg administered by IV infusion every 2 weeks) until disease progression or unacceptable toxicity occurred. All patients had documented disease progression after receiving temozolomide and radiation therapy. The median age was 54 years, 54% were male, 68% had a Karnofsky performance status of 90–100, and 54% were receiving corticosteroids. Treatment with bevacizumab resulted in an objective response rate of 19.6% (partial responses only) and a median duration of response of 3.9 months. Although evaluation of corticosteroid usage was not a required efficacy end point, it was noted that 58% of patients were able to reduce their corticosteroid dosage during treatment with bevacizumab; the average reduction in corticosteroid dosage was 59%. Grade 3 or greater adverse effects associated with bevacizumab included thromboembolic events (12.7%), hypertension (3.6%), arterial thromboembolic events (1.8%), GI perforation (1.8%), and wound healing complications (1.8%).

● **Renal Cell Carcinoma**

Bevacizumab is used in combination with interferon alfa for the first-line treatment of metastatic renal cell carcinoma and is designated an orphan drug by FDA for use in this condition.

The current indication for use of bevacizumab in combination with interferon alfa in patients with metastatic renal cell carcinoma is based principally on the results of a multicenter, randomized, double-blind, placebo-controlled study (AVOREN).

In the AVOREN study, 649 patients with previously untreated metastatic renal cell carcinoma (predominantly [more than 50%] clear-cell histology) who had undergone nephrectomy (or partial nephrectomy) were randomized to receive bevacizumab (10 mg/kg administered by IV infusion every 2 weeks) in combination with interferon alfa-2a (9 million units by subcutaneous injection 3 times weekly) or interferon alfa-2a in combination with placebo; treatment was continued until disease progression or unacceptable toxicity occurred (up to a maximum of 52 weeks for interferon alfa-2a). The median age of the patients was 60 years (range: 18–82 years), and 70% were male; 28, 56, or 8% of patients had Motzer scores of 0 (favorable risk), 1–2 (intermediate risk), or 3–5 (poor risk), respectively. In this study, patients receiving bevacizumab in combination with interferon alfa-2a had prolonged median progression-free survival (10.2 versus 5.4 months) and a higher overall response rate (30 versus 12%), but similar median overall survival (23 versus 21 months), compared with those receiving interferon alfa-2a alone. Grade 3–5 adverse effects occurring at a higher incidence (2% or greater) in patients receiving bevacizumab in combination with interferon alfa-2a than in those receiving interferon alfa-2a monotherapy included fatigue (13 versus 8%), asthenia (10 versus 7%), proteinuria (7 versus 0%), hypertension (6 versus 1%), and hemorrhage (3 versus 0.3%).

● **Breast Cancer**

First-line Treatment of Metastatic Breast Cancer

Although bevacizumab in combination with paclitaxel previously was labeled for use as first-line treatment of metastatic HER2-negative breast cancer†, FDA concluded that such use has not been shown in postmarketing studies to prolong overall survival or provide sufficient clinical benefit (e.g., prolongation of progression-free survival, amelioration of disease-related symptoms, improvement in quality of life) to outweigh the risk of severe, potentially fatal, adverse effects (e.g., myocardial infarction [MI], heart failure, severe hypertension, bleeding or hemorrhage, perforation and fistula/abscess formation, wound healing complications). On November 18, 2011, the agency rescinded approval of bevacizumab for use (in combination with paclitaxel) as first-line treatment of metastatic HER2-negative breast cancer; as a result, this indication no longer appears in bevacizumab's current approved labeling. (See FDA Decisions Regarding Breast Cancer Indication under Breast Cancer:

First-line Treatment of Metastatic Breast Cancer, in Uses.) Following FDA's decision, Health Canada, but not the European Medicines Agency (EMA), took similar action. The United Kingdom's National Institute for Health and Clinical Excellence (NICE) reached similar conclusions about the lack of evidence of clinical benefit and has not supported this use. The AHFS Oncology Expert Committee concluded that use of bevacizumab in combination with paclitaxel for the first-line treatment of metastatic breast cancer currently is not fully established because of equivocal evidence; additional studies are needed to identify subgroups of patients who might derive clinical benefit from bevacizumab treatment. (See AHFS Oncology Expert Committee Decision Regarding Use as First-line Therapy under Breast Cancer: First-line Treatment of Metastatic Breast Cancer, in Uses.)

Patients currently receiving bevacizumab for breast cancer should consult their clinician about whether to continue bevacizumab therapy or consider other treatment options. Clinicians should use clinical judgment in deciding whether patients should continue receiving bevacizumab in combination with paclitaxel, receive paclitaxel monotherapy, or consider other treatment options.

FDA Decisions Regarding Breast Cancer Indication

Bevacizumab (in combination with paclitaxel) received approval for use as first-line treatment of metastatic HER2-negative breast cancer in February 2008 under the principles and procedures of FDA's accelerated review process that allows approval based on analysis of surrogate markers of response (i.e., prolongation of progression-free survival) rather than clinical endpoints (e.g., prolongation of overall survival, amelioration of disease-related symptoms). Approval for this indication was based principally on the results of a single multicenter, open-label, randomized study (E2100) in which 722 patients received bevacizumab and paclitaxel or paclitaxel alone as first-line therapy for locally recurrent or metastatic breast cancer. Patients with HER2-overexpressing breast cancer were not eligible for the study unless they had received previous therapy with trastuzumab. Patients who had received hormonal therapy for metastatic disease or adjuvant therapy (chemotherapy or hormonal therapy) for breast cancer were eligible for the study. Patients who had received adjuvant taxane therapy were eligible for the study if they had completed treatment at least 12 months prior to entry to the study. Patients with CNS metastasis were excluded from the study. The median age of patients was 55 years (range: 27–85 years), 76% were white, about 55% were postmenopausal, and 64% had estrogen receptor-positive and/or progesterone receptor-positive disease; 36% had received hormonal therapy for advanced disease and 66% had received adjuvant therapy for breast cancer, including 20% with previous taxane use and 50% with previous anthracycline use. Treatment consisted of paclitaxel 90 mg/m² IV once weekly for 3 out of 4 weeks, with or without bevacizumab 10 mg/kg by IV infusion every 2 weeks, until disease progression or unacceptable toxicity occurred. Among patients randomized to receive the combination regimen in whom paclitaxel was withheld or discontinued, bevacizumab monotherapy was allowed to continue until disease progression or unacceptable toxicity occurred.

Because study E2100 was open-label and included patients without measurable disease, efficacy data from a planned interim analysis were subjected to independent, retrospective, blinded review. Although some data points were missing, this analysis of interim data confirmed a higher response rate (48.9 versus 22.2%, partial responses only) and a progression-free survival benefit (11.3 versus 5.8 months) for combined therapy with bevacizumab and paclitaxel compared with paclitaxel alone, and achieved 76–80% concordance with investigator assessments of individual patient results. Final analyses performed by the investigators indicated that patients receiving bevacizumab and paclitaxel had longer progression-free survival (11.8 versus 5.9 months), similar overall survival (26.7 versus 25.2 months), and a higher response rate (36.9 versus 21.2%) compared with those receiving paclitaxel alone as first-line therapy for metastatic breast cancer. Grade 3–4 adverse effects, including sensory neuropathy (24 versus 18%), hypertension (15 versus 0%), fatigue (9 versus 5%), infection (9 versus 3%), proteinuria (4 versus 0%), nausea (3 versus 1%), arthralgia (3 versus 1%), headache (2 versus 0%), and cerebrovascular ischemia (2 versus 0%) occurred more frequently in patients receiving bevacizumab and paclitaxel than in those receiving paclitaxel alone.

As a condition of the accelerated approval process, the manufacturer of bevacizumab was required to submit data from 2 controlled clinical studies (AVADO and RIBBON1) to confirm the progression-free survival benefit that was observed with use of bevacizumab in study E2100 and to provide additional information regarding effects of the drug on overall survival of patients with metastatic HER2-negative breast cancer. In the AVADO study, 736 patients were randomized to receive bevacizumab (7.5 or 15 mg/kg) plus docetaxel (100 mg/m²) or docetaxel (100 mg/m²) plus placebo every 3 weeks as first-line therapy for metastatic or locally recurrent HER2-negative breast cancer; bevacizumab or placebo was continued until disease progression or unacceptable toxicity occurred, while docetaxel was administered for up to 9 cycles. In the RIBBON1 study, 1237 patients were randomized to receive either bevacizumab (15 mg/kg every 3 weeks) or placebo in conjunction with a taxane- or anthracycline-based regimen or in conjunction with capecitabine as first-line therapy for metastatic or locally recurrent HER2-negative breast cancer; treatment was continued until disease progression or unacceptable toxicity occurred.

In the AVADO study, objective response rates were higher for patients receiving bevacizumab 7.5 or 15 mg/kg plus docetaxel (55.2 or 64.1%, respectively) compared with those receiving docetaxel alone (46.4%). Inclusion of bevacizumab in the treatment regimen prolonged median progression-free survival by 0.8–1.9 months but did not prolong overall survival. Among patients receiving bevacizumab 7.5 mg/kg plus docetaxel, bevacizumab 15 mg/kg plus docetaxel, or docetaxel alone, median progression-free survival was 9, 10.1, or 8.2 months, respectively, and median overall survival was 30.8, 30.2, or 31.9 months, respectively.

In the RIBBON1 study, patients receiving bevacizumab in conjunction with capecitabine or in conjunction with a taxane- or anthracycline-based regimen had higher objective response rates and longer progression-free survival than did those receiving either capecitabine or a taxane- or anthracycline-based regimen alone; inclusion of bevacizumab in the treatment regimen did not significantly prolong overall survival. Patients receiving bevacizumab and capecitabine had a higher objective response rate (35.4 versus 23.6%) and longer median progression-free survival (8.6 versus 5.7 months), but not a significantly longer median overall survival (25.7 versus 22.8 months), compared with patients receiving capecitabine alone. Similarly, patients receiving bevacizumab in conjunction with a taxane- or anthracycline-based regimen had a higher objective response rate (51.3 versus 37.9%) and longer median progression-free survival (9.2 versus 8 months) compared with patients receiving a taxane- or anthracycline-based regimen alone; inclusion of bevacizumab in these regimens did not provide an overall survival benefit (hazard ratio of 1.11 favoring the use of a taxane- or anthracycline-based regimen).

In both the AVADO and RIBBON1 studies, adverse effects described as grade 3–5 in severity and serious adverse effects (i.e., those requiring medical intervention or hospitalization or resulting in death) were more common in patients receiving bevacizumab-containing regimens compared with those receiving comparator regimens. In the AVADO study, patients were more likely to experience adverse effects requiring docetaxel modification (discontinuance, interruption, dosage reduction) if they received concomitant therapy with bevacizumab.

The FDA Oncologic Drugs Advisory Committee (ODAC) reviewed data from the AVADO and RIBBON1 studies in July 2010 and concluded that these studies did not provide evidence of an overall survival benefit for bevacizumab in patients with metastatic HER2-negative breast cancer; the committee also concluded that the increases in progression-free survival observed in the confirmatory studies were marginal compared with that observed in study E2100 and not clinically meaningful. The committee recommended that the current indication for use of bevacizumab in combination with paclitaxel in the first-line treatment of metastatic HER2-negative breast cancer be removed from the drug's approved labeling.

In December 2010, after reviewing the committee's recommendation and data from 4 clinical studies (i.e., E2100, AVADO, RIBBON1, AVF2119g), FDA's Center for Drug Evaluation and Research (CDER) concurred with the committee, stating that bevacizumab does not prolong overall survival in patients with metastatic HER2-negative breast cancer or provide a sufficient benefit in slowing disease progression to outweigh the substantial risk of serious adverse effects (e.g., hypertension, bleeding or hemorrhage, wound healing complications or wound dehiscence, perforation and fistula/abscess formation, MI, heart failure). Because bevacizumab (in combination with paclitaxel) has not been shown to be safe and effective for first-line treatment of metastatic HER2-negative breast cancer, CDER recommended that this indication be removed from the drug's approved labeling. A public hearing on this recommendation was held on June 28–29, 2011.

On November 18, 2011, after reviewing submissions from the manufacturer and CDER, recommendations from ODAC, and public comments, the FDA Commissioner issued a final decision to rescind approval of bevacizumab for use in combination with paclitaxel as first-line treatment of metastatic HER2-negative breast cancer, citing 3 main reasons for the decision: lack of clinical benefit, unfavorable benefit-to-risk ratio, and lack of other compelling reasons (i.e., special circumstances) to support continued accelerated approval. In evaluating clinical benefit, the commissioner noted that confirmatory studies (AVADO and RIBBON1) failed to verify the magnitude of effect on progression-free survival observed in study E2100, and that none of the 5 studies submitted by the

manufacturer (E2100, AVADO, RIBBON1, AVF2119g, RIBBON2) demonstrated an overall survival benefit or an improvement in quality of life. In evaluating the regimen's safety profile, it was noted that the addition of bevacizumab to chemotherapy resulted in an increased risk of severe (grade 3 or greater) adverse effects (e.g., neutropenia, sensory neuropathy, hypertension, febrile neutropenia, proteinuria, arterial thromboembolic events, left ventricular systolic dysfunction, hemorrhage, wound healing complications, fistula formation, GI perforation) that was considered unacceptable for a regimen that has not demonstrated clinical benefit. In evaluating special circumstances that may justify continuing accelerated approval (e.g., until clinical benefit is fully established or until a subset of patients likely to benefit from therapy is identified), the commissioner concluded that continuing an approval that is no longer supported by current data and allowing a substantial length of time for additional studies to be completed would be inconsistent with the protection of public health. The commissioner noted that because FDA does not regulate the practice of medicine, clinicians may continue to prescribe bevacizumab for the treatment of metastatic breast cancer (i.e., unlabeled [off-label] use) despite withdrawal of approval for this use.

AHFS Oncology Expert Committee Decision Regarding Use as First-line Therapy

The AHFS Oncology Expert Committee was concerned that the E2100 study failed to demonstrate an overall survival benefit despite showing prolonged disease-free survival in patients receiving combined therapy with bevacizumab and paclitaxel, and also was concerned by the failure of the confirmatory studies (AVADO and RIBBON1) to verify the same magnitude of effect on progression-free survival as observed in the E2100 study. These studies provide a basis for assessing tolerability of bevacizumab in patients with previously untreated metastatic breast cancer, but the results provide equivocal evidence of the drug's efficacy for this use. In the absence of additional data, attempts to identify subgroups of patients in whom bevacizumab might provide clinical benefit (e.g., prolonged progression-free survival, prolonged overall survival, improved quality of life) and achieve a favorable benefit-to-risk ratio are speculative; additional studies are needed to identify subgroups of patients with previously untreated metastatic breast cancer who might derive clinical benefit from bevacizumab treatment. Therefore, the committee concluded that use of bevacizumab in combination with paclitaxel for the first-line treatment of metastatic breast cancer currently is not fully established because of equivocal evidence.

Previously Treated Metastatic Breast Cancer

The efficacy and safety of bevacizumab for the treatment of metastatic breast cancer† previously treated with cytotoxic chemotherapy has been studied in several randomized studies.

The first study (AVF2119g) was an open-label, randomized study in which 462 patients received either bevacizumab and capecitabine or capecitabine alone. Patients with metastatic breast cancer who had received prior therapy with both an anthracycline (or anthracenedione) and a taxane and had received 1 or 2 prior chemotherapy regimens for metastatic disease were eligible to enroll in the study; patients who relapsed within 12 months of completing adjuvant anthracycline (or anthracenedione) and taxane therapy also were eligible to enroll in the study without having received additional chemotherapy. Patients with HER2-overexpressing breast cancer were not eligible for the study unless their disease had progressed following treatment with trastuzumab. Patients with CNS disease and those who had received prior therapy with bevacizumab or capecitabine were excluded from the study. The mean age of patients was about 51 years (range: 29–78 years), about 81% were white, 47% had estrogen receptor-positive disease, and 37% had progesterone receptor-positive disease. Treatment consisted of capecitabine (1.25 g/m^2 orally twice daily on days 1–14 of each 3-week cycle) given alone or in combination with bevacizumab (15 mg/kg by IV infusion on day 1 of each 3-week cycle) for a maximum of 35 cycles or until disease progression or unacceptable toxicity occurred. Patients without disease progression following 35 cycles of therapy could continue to receive their assigned treatment in an extension study. Patients randomized to receive bevacizumab and capecitabine could continue to receive bevacizumab either alone or in combination with other therapies following initial disease progression.

Patients receiving bevacizumab and capecitabine had higher response rates (19.8 versus 9.1%) but similar median progression-free survival (4.9 versus 4.2 months) and overall survival (15.1 months versus 14.5 months) compared with those receiving capecitabine alone. Hypertension (23.6 versus 2.3%, frequently grade 3), proteinuria (22.3 versus 7.4%, mostly grade 1 or 2), and hemorrhage

(28.8 versus 11.2%, mostly grade 1) occurred more frequently in patients receiving bevacizumab and capecitabine than in those receiving capecitabine alone.

The second study (AVF3693g, RIBBON2) was a double-blind, placebo-controlled trial evaluating safety and efficacy of bevacizumab in combination with taxanes (paclitaxel, albumin-bound paclitaxel, or docetaxel), capecitabine, gemcitabine, or vinorelbine as second-line therapy for locally recurrent or metastatic breast cancer in 684 patients who had received one prior cytotoxic chemotherapy regimen for metastatic disease. Patients with HER2-overexpressing breast cancer, those with untreated CNS metastases, and those who had received prior therapy with bevacizumab or other vascular endothelial growth factor (VEGF) inhibitors were not eligible to enroll in the study. The median age of patients was 55 years (range: 23–90 years) and about 72% had hormone receptor-positive disease. Patients were randomized in a 2:1 ratio to receive either bevacizumab (15 mg/kg every 3 weeks or 10 mg/kg every 2 weeks depending on the chemotherapy regimen) or placebo in combination with the investigator-selected chemotherapy regimen. Most patients received a taxane (44.4%), gemcitabine (23.4%), or capecitabine (21.1%). Bevacizumab could be continued until disease progression or unacceptable toxicity occurred, up to a maximum of 36 months of therapy; the chemotherapy regimen could be continued until disease progression or unacceptable toxicity occurred. If chemotherapy was discontinued before disease progression occurred, patients could continue receiving bevacizumab (or placebo, as assigned) as monotherapy.

At a median follow-up of 15 months, combined therapy with bevacizumab and chemotherapy prolonged median progression-free survival (7.2 versus 5.1 months) but was not associated with an overall survival benefit compared with chemotherapy alone; in patients receiving bevacizumab and chemotherapy, median overall survival was 18 months and the one-year survival rate was 69.5%, compared with 16.4 months and 66.2%, respectively, for those receiving chemotherapy alone. No significant difference in objective response rate was observed between patients receiving bevacizumab in combination with chemotherapy and those receiving chemotherapy alone (39.5 and 29.6%, respectively). Subgroup analysis showed that the progression-free survival benefit observed when bevacizumab and chemotherapy were given in combination was not uniform across all 4 chemotherapy regimens. When bevacizumab was used in combination with capecitabine, gemcitabine, or a taxane, median progression-free survival was prolonged by 0.5–2.8 months (depending on the regimen) compared with the chemotherapy regimen alone; however, when bevacizumab was used in combination with vinorelbine, median progression-free survival was 1.3 months shorter than when vinorelbine was used alone. Grade 3 or greater hypertension (9 versus 0.5%), neutropenia (17.7 versus 14.5%), proteinuria (3.1 versus 0.5%), and hemorrhage (1.7 versus 0%) occurred more frequently in patients receiving bevacizumab in combination with chemotherapy than in those receiving chemotherapy alone. In each chemotherapy subgroup, the incidence of adverse effects requiring study drug discontinuance was higher when the chemotherapy regimen was given in combination with bevacizumab.

Although combined therapy with bevacizumab and chemotherapy prolonged progression-free survival in the RIBBON2 study, the same benefit was not observed in the AVF2119g study; in addition, combined therapy did not prolong overall survival in either study. Therefore, usefulness of the drug in combination with chemotherapy for the treatment of metastatic breast cancer previously treated with cytotoxic chemotherapy is unclear. Use of bevacizumab in combination with chemotherapy for the treatment of metastatic breast cancer previously treated with cytotoxic chemotherapy currently is not fully established because of equivocal evidence.

Other Uses

Bevacizumab has been investigated for use in the treatment of ovarian cancer†. Results of two phase 3 randomized trials indicate that addition of bevacizumab to chemotherapy (carboplatin and paclitaxel) prolonged progression-free survival by approximately 1.5–4 months in patients with advanced ovarian epithelial cancer, primary peritoneal cancer, or fallopian-tube cancer. Effects on overall survival have not been fully elucidated (i.e., no difference in overall survival reported in one study, final overall survival data not yet available for the second study). Bevacizumab in combination with chemotherapy was associated with an increased risk of hypertension and GI perforation compared with chemotherapy alone. Further study is needed to determine the optimal timing and duration of bevacizumab therapy and to identify patient populations most likely to benefit from this drug.

Intravitreal injection† of bevacizumab has been used for the treatment of neovascular age-related macular degeneration†. Results of several randomized controlled studies suggest that intravitreal bevacizumab has similar efficacy as ranibizumab in improving visual acuity. In one study, the incidence of serious systemic adverse effects (primarily hospitalizations) appeared to be higher with bevacizumab

compared with ranibizumab; however, other studies, including a systematic review of 9 randomized controlled studies, directly comparing intravitreal injections of bevacizumab and ranibizumab in patients with neovascular age-related macular degeneration have found no such difference. Patient-specific factors, which may vary the level of risk associated with these VEGF antagonists, should be considered prior to the use of intravitreal bevacizumab. (See Ocular Effects under Warnings/Precautions: Other Warnings and Precautions, in Cautions.)

Intravitreal injection† of bevacizumab also has been used for the treatment of diabetic macular edema†. Results of a study comparing intravitreal ranibizumab, aflibercept, and bevacizumab for the treatment of diabetic macular edema suggest that the relative treatment effect of these drugs may be dependent upon a patient's baseline visual acuity. (See Uses: Diabetic Macular Edema, in Aflibercept 52:92.) Further study is needed to establish the role of bevacizumab in the treatment of diabetic macular edema.

DOSAGE AND ADMINISTRATION

Administration

Bevacizumab is administered by IV infusion. The drug should *not* be administered by rapid IV injection, such as IV push or bolus. The initial dose of bevacizumab should be infused over 90 minutes (following other antineoplastic agents); if the infusion is well tolerated, the second dose may be infused over 60 minutes. If this second infusion also is well tolerated, subsequent doses may be infused over 30 minutes. One institution has reported use of shorter infusion times for bevacizumab at an infusion rate of 0.5 mg/kg per minute.

For IV infusion, the appropriate dose of bevacizumab should be withdrawn into a syringe and diluted in a total volume of 100 mL of 0.9% sodium chloride using aseptic technique. Bevacizumab infusions should not be administered or mixed with dextrose solutions. Bevacizumab injection should be inspected visually for particulate matter and discoloration prior to administration. Any unused portion left in the vial should be discarded since the injection contains no preservative. The diluted drug may be stored at 2–8°C for up to 8 hours.

The manufacturer states that no incompatibilities between bevacizumab and polyvinylchloride or polyolefin bags have been observed.

Bevacizumab injection should be protected from light and stored in the original carton at 2–8°C until use; freezing should be avoided. The injection should not be shaken prior to use.

General Dosage

Bevacizumab therapy should *not* be initiated for at least 28 days following major surgery, and the surgical incision should be fully healed prior to initiation of the drug. (See Surgery and Wound Healing Complications under Warnings/Precautions: Warnings, in Cautions.)

Clinicians should consult the respective manufacturers or published protocols for information on the dosage, method of administration, and administration sequence of other antineoplastic agents used in combination regimens.

First-line Treatment for Metastatic Colorectal Cancer

For the first-line treatment of metastatic cancer of the colon or rectum in adults, a bevacizumab dosage of 5 mg/kg, administered by IV infusion every 2 weeks, is used in combination with IV irinotecan/fluorouracil/leucovorin. Bevacizumab therapy should be continued until disease progression or unacceptable toxicity occurs.

Second-line Treatment for Metastatic Colorectal Cancer

For the second-line treatment of metastatic cancer of the colon or rectum in adults, a bevacizumab dosage of 10 mg/kg, administered by IV infusion every 2 weeks, is used in combination with FOLFOX4 (IV fluorouracil/leucovorin and oxaliplatin). Bevacizumab therapy should be continued until disease progression or unacceptable toxicity occurs.

First-line Treatment for Advanced Nonsquamous Non-small Cell Lung Cancer

For the first-line treatment of unresectable, locally advanced, recurrent or metastatic nonsquamous non-small cell lung cancer, the recommended dosage of bevacizumab is 15 mg/kg by IV infusion on day 1 every 3 weeks. In the pivotal study, bevacizumab was administered in combination with paclitaxel and carboplatin. Bevacizumab therapy should be continued until disease progression or unacceptable toxicity occurs.

Second-line Treatment for Glioblastoma

For the second-line treatment of glioblastoma in adults whose disease has progressed following radiation therapy and chemotherapy, the recommended dosage of bevacizumab is 10 mg/kg by IV infusion every 2 weeks. Bevacizumab therapy should be continued until disease progression or unacceptable toxicity occurs.

First-line Treatment for Renal Cell Carcinoma

For the first-line treatment of metastatic renal cell carcinoma in adults, a bevacizumab dosage of 10 mg/kg, administered by IV infusion every 2 weeks, is used in combination with interferon alfa. Bevacizumab therapy should be continued until disease progression or unacceptable toxicity occurs.

First-line Treatment for Metastatic Breast Cancer

For the first-line treatment of metastatic breast cancer†, a bevacizumab dosage of 10 mg/kg, administered by IV infusion every 2 weeks, has been used in combination with IV paclitaxel. However, this combination regimen has not been shown to prolong overall survival or provide sufficient clinical benefit to outweigh the risk of severe, potentially fatal, adverse effects. (See Uses: Breast Cancer.)

Dosage Modification for Toxicity

Bevacizumab dosage reductions are not recommended in any patient; instead, the drug should either be temporarily suspended or permanently discontinued, according to causality.

Bevacizumab should be *permanently discontinued* in patients who develop GI perforation (GI perforation, fistula formation in the GI tract, and/or intra-abdominal abscess), non-GI fistula formation involving an internal organ, wound dehiscence and wound healing complications requiring medical intervention, severe hemorrhage requiring medical intervention, severe arterial thromboembolic events, hypertensive crisis, hypertensive encephalopathy, or nephrotic syndrome.

Bevacizumab therapy also should be *permanently discontinued* in patients who develop reversible posterior leukoencephalopathy syndrome (RPLS). Treatment of hypertension should be initiated as clinically indicated. The risk of reinitiating bevacizumab therapy in patients previously experiencing RPLS is not known.

Temporary suspension is recommended in patients who develop moderate to severe proteinuria (pending further evaluation) and in those with severe hypertension (not controlled by medical management). The risk of continuing bevacizumab therapy in patients with moderate to severe proteinuria is not known. Bevacizumab infusion should be interrupted in patients with severe infusion reactions, and appropriate medical therapy should be initiated. Adequate information regarding rechallenge with bevacizumab is unavailable; whether therapy with the drug may be safely resumed following resolution of a severe bevacizumab-induced infusion reaction has not been determined. Bevacizumab therapy should be suspended at least 28 days prior to elective surgery and should not be resumed until at least 28 days following major surgery and after the surgical incision has fully healed.

● Special Populations

No special populations dosage recommendations at this time.

CAUTIONS

● Contraindications

The manufacturer states that there are no contraindications to the use of bevacizumab.

● Warnings/Precautions

Warnings

Because the bevacizumab therapeutic regimen may include the use of other antineoplastic agents, the usual cautions, precautions, and contraindications of these drugs also should be considered.

● GI Perforation

Severe GI perforation, sometimes fatal, occurs more frequently in patients receiving bevacizumab than in those receiving placebo or active controls. GI perforation has been reported in 0.3–2.4% of patients receiving bevacizumab in clinical studies. Manifestations may include abdominal pain, nausea, emesis, constipation, and fever. GI perforation can be complicated by intra-abdominal abscess and fistula formation. The majority of cases occurred within the first 50 days of initiation of bevacizumab.

Bevacizumab should be *permanently discontinued* in patients with GI perforation (GI perforation, fistula formation in the GI tract, and/or intra-abdominal abscess).

● Surgery and Wound Healing Complications

Wound healing and bleeding complications (including wound dehiscence) have occurred in patients who underwent surgery during bevacizumab therapy. In a randomized trial involving patients with metastatic colorectal cancer, wound healing and/or bleeding complications, including serious and fatal complications, occurred in 15% (6/39) of patients undergoing surgery during or within 60 days following therapy with bevacizumab and chemotherapy compared with 4% (1/25) of patients undergoing surgery within the same time period following chemotherapy alone; the incidence of wound dehiscence was also higher in the patients receiving bevacizumab (1 versus 0.5%). In one patient, dehiscence occurred 56 days after the last dose of bevacizumab.

Bevacizumab therapy should not be initiated until at least 28 days following major surgery and after the surgical incision has fully healed.

The appropriate interval between discontinuance of bevacizumab and subsequent elective surgery has not been established, but the long half-life of the drug (approximately 20 days) should be considered. The manufacturer recommends that bevacizumab be suspended at least 28 days prior to elective surgery and not resumed until the surgical incision has fully healed.

Bevacizumab should be *permanently discontinued* if wound dehiscence and wound healing complications requiring medical intervention occur.

● Hemorrhage

Severe or fatal hemorrhages, including hemoptysis, GI bleeding, hematemesis, CNS hemorrhage, epistaxis, and vaginal bleeding, occurred up to fivefold more frequently in patients receiving bevacizumab and chemotherapy than in those receiving chemotherapy alone.

Grade 3 or greater hemorrhagic events have been reported in 1.2–4.6% of patients receiving bevacizumab in clinical studies. Serious or fatal pulmonary hemorrhage occurred in 31% (4/13) of patients with squamous cell carcinoma of the lung and 4% (2/53) of patients with nonsquamous non-small cell lung cancer receiving bevacizumab with chemotherapy compared with 0% (0/32) of patients receiving chemotherapy alone. Symptomatic grade 2 CNS hemorrhage occurred in 1.2% (1/83) of patients with non-small cell lung cancer with CNS metastases receiving bevacizumab in clinical studies. Intracranial hemorrhage (including grade 3–4 hemorrhage) has been reported in 4.9% (8/163) of patients with previously treated glioblastoma receiving bevacizumab.

Mild to moderate hemorrhagic events also have been reported more frequently in patients receiving bevacizumab. Grade 1 epistaxis was common in clinical studies and occurred in up to 35% of patients receiving bevacizumab in conjunction with other antineoplastic agents for metastatic colorectal cancer. Epistaxis generally was mild and resolved without medical intervention. Other grade 1–2 hemorrhagic events reported more frequently in patients receiving bevacizumab in conjunction with other antineoplastic agents for metastatic colorectal cancer when compared with those not receiving bevacizumab included GI hemorrhage (24 versus 6%, respectively), minor gum bleeding (2 versus 0%, respectively), and vaginal hemorrhage (4 versus 2%, respectively).

Patients with a history of recent hemoptysis (0.5 teaspoon of red blood or more) should not receive bevacizumab. Bevacizumab should be *permanently discontinued* in patients with severe hemorrhage requiring medical intervention.

Sensitivity Reactions

Infusion Reactions

In clinical studies, infusion reactions with the first bevacizumab dose were uncommon (less than 3%). Severe infusion reactions occurred in 0.2% of patients receiving bevacizumab. Infusion reactions include hypertension, hypertensive crises associated with neurologic manifestations, wheezing, oxygen desaturation, grade 3 hypersensitivity, chest pain, headaches, rigors, and diaphoresis.

Initial doses of bevacizumab should be infused slowly; if well tolerated, the rate of IV infusion may be increased during administration of subsequent doses. (See Dosage and Administration: Administration.)

Bevacizumab infusion should be interrupted if severe infusion reaction occurs, and appropriate medical therapy should be initiated.

Other Warnings and Precautions

Non-GI Fistula Formation

Severe, sometimes fatal, non-GI fistula formation involving tracheo-esophageal, bronchopleural, biliary, vaginal, renal, and bladder sites has been reported more frequently in patients receiving bevacizumab compared with those receiving controls. Non-GI fistula formation was reported in 0.3% or less of patients in controlled clinical studies and typically occurred within the first 6 months of bevacizumab therapy.

Bevacizumab should be *permanently discontinued* in patients with non-GI fistula formation involving an internal organ.

Thromboembolism

Severe, sometimes fatal, arterial thromboembolic events (e.g., cerebral infarction, transient ischemic attacks [TIAs], myocardial infarction [MI], angina) occurred at a higher incidence in patients receiving bevacizumab in combination with chemotherapy compared with those receiving chemotherapy alone. In clinical studies, grade 3 or greater arterial thromboembolic events have been reported in 2.6% of patients receiving bevacizumab in combination with chemotherapy compared with 0.8% of those receiving chemotherapy alone. The relative risk of arterial thromboembolic events in patients receiving bevacizumab in combination with chemotherapy was increased in patients with a history of arterial thromboembolism and in patients older than 65 years of age.

Whether bevacizumab therapy can be safely resumed following resolution of an arterial thromboembolic event has not been studied. Bevacizumab should be *permanently discontinued* in patients who experience severe arterial thromboembolic events.

Grade 3 or 4 venous thromboembolic events, such as deep-vein thrombosis and intra-abdominal venous thrombosis, occurred more often in patients receiving bevacizumab with chemotherapy than in those receiving chemotherapy alone for metastatic colorectal cancer or advanced non-small cell lung cancer. In addition, the risk of developing a second thromboembolic event was increased in patients receiving bevacizumab with chemotherapy compared with those receiving chemotherapy alone for metastatic colorectal cancer despite the use of full-dose warfarin therapy following an initial venous thromboembolic event.

Hypertension

The incidence of severe hypertension was increased in patients receiving bevacizumab in combination with chemotherapy compared with those receiving chemotherapy alone. Grade 3 or 4 hypertension occurred in 5–18% of patients receiving bevacizumab in clinical studies. Hypertension was more common in patients with previous history of hypertension and may respond to antihypertensive therapy. Hypertension also occurred more frequently in patients who received higher dosages of bevacizumab (e.g., 10 mg/kg).

Blood pressure should be monitored every 2–3 weeks during bevacizumab therapy. If hypertension occurs, patients should be treated with appropriate antihypertensive therapy, and blood pressure should be monitored regularly.

Temporary suspension of bevacizumab therapy is recommended in patients with severe hypertension that is not controlled with medical management. Bevacizumab should be *permanently discontinued* in patients who develop hypertensive crisis or hypertensive encephalopathy. If bevacizumab is discontinued because of hypertension, blood pressure should be monitored at regular intervals thereafter.

Reversible Posterior Leukoencephalopathy Syndrome

Reversible posterior leukoencephalopathy syndrome (RPLS) has occurred in patients receiving bevacizumab. This complication occurred in less than 0.1% of patients receiving bevacizumab in clinical studies.

RPLS, a brain-capillary leak syndrome associated with hypertension, fluid retention, and the cytotoxic effects of immunosuppressive drugs on the vascular endothelium, is a neurological disorder that may manifest with headache, seizure, lethargy, confusion, blindness, and other visual and neurologic disturbances. Mild to severe hypertension may occur, but it is not necessary for the diagnosis of RPLS. Magnetic resonance imaging is necessary to confirm the diagnosis of RPLS. The onset of symptoms has occurred from 16 hours to 1 year after initiation of bevacizumab therapy.

Blood pressure should be closely monitored and strictly controlled during and following bevacizumab infusion. If RPLS develops, bevacizumab should be *permanently discontinued*, and treatment of hypertension should be initiated as clinically indicated. Symptoms of RPLS usually lessen or resolve within days of discontinuance of bevacizumab, but some patients have experienced ongoing neurologic sequelae. The risk of reinitiating bevacizumab therapy in patients previously experiencing RPLS is not known.

Proteinuria

Increased incidence and severity of proteinuria have been reported in patients receiving bevacizumab. In clinical trials, proteinuria ranged in severity from clinically silent to nephrotic syndrome. Grade 3 or 4 proteinuria (defined as greater than 3.5 g of protein in the urine collected over 24 hours) occurred in 0.7–7.4% of patients receiving bevacizumab for colorectal cancer, non-small cell lung cancer, or renal cell carcinoma. In the randomized clinical study in patients with metastatic renal cell carcinoma, proteinuria (all grades) was reported in 20% of those receiving bevacizumab. In this study, the median onset of proteinuria was 5.6 months (range: 15 days to 37 months) after initiation of bevacizumab; median time to resolution was 6.1 months. Proteinuria did not resolve in 40% of patients after a median follow-up of 11.2 months, and 30% of patients required permanent discontinuance of bevacizumab. Proteinuria with findings of thrombotic microangiopathy on renal biopsy has been reported in patients receiving bevacizumab alone or in combination with other antineoplastic agents for various cancers. Nephrotic syndrome, sometimes fatal, occurred in less than 1% of patients receiving bevacizumab in clinical studies.

Patients receiving bevacizumab should be monitored for the development or worsening of proteinuria. Patients with a 2+ or greater urine dipstick reading should undergo further assessment with a 24-hour urine collection.

Bevacizumab therapy should be interrupted for proteinuria of or exceeding 2 g per 24 hours and resumed when proteinuria declines below this level. The safety of continued treatment in patients with moderate to severe proteinuria has not been evaluated.

Bevacizumab should be *permanently discontinued* in patients with nephrotic syndrome.

Ovarian Failure

Ovarian failure has been reported more frequently in premenopausal women receiving bevacizumab in combination with chemotherapy (i.e., fluorouracil, leucovorin, and oxaliplatin [modified FOLFOX6]†) (34%) compared with those receiving chemotherapy alone (2%) for adjuvant treatment of colorectal cancer. Following discontinuance of bevacizumab, recovery of ovarian function occurred in 22% of patients. The long-term effects of bevacizumab exposure on fertility are unknown.

Women of childbearing potential should be informed of the risk of ovarian failure prior to initiating bevacizumab therapy.

Neutropenia and Infection

Increased rates of severe (grade 3 or 4) neutropenia, febrile neutropenia, infection with severe neutropenia (sometimes fatal), and serious infections (e.g., pneumonia, catheter infections, wound infections) have been observed in patients receiving bevacizumab and chemotherapy compared with those receiving chemotherapy alone.

Congestive Heart Failure

Congestive heart failure has been reported in patients receiving bevacizumab. Grade 3 or greater left ventricular dysfunction was reported in 1% of patients receiving bevacizumab in clinical studies. Among patients receiving bevacizumab and paclitaxel for metastatic breast cancer† in a randomized trial, grade 3 or 4 congestive heart failure occurred in 2.2%; of these patients, those who had received previous anthracycline therapy had a higher rate of congestive heart failure (3.8%). The safety of continuation or resumption of bevacizumab in patients who develop cardiac dysfunction has not been studied.

Microangiopathic Hemolytic Anemia

Cases of microangiopathic hemolytic anemia have been reported in patients with solid tumors receiving bevacizumab and sunitinib†. In a phase 1 study involving 25 patients receiving bevacizumab at a fixed dose and sunitinib at escalating dose levels, 5 of 12 patients receiving bevacizumab with the highest dose level of sunitinib had laboratory findings consistent with microangiopathic hemolytic anemia. Of these 5 patients, 2 patients had evidence of severe microangiopathic hemolytic anemia, including thrombocytopenia, anemia, reticulocytosis, reduced serum haptoglobin concentrations, schistocytes on peripheral smear, modest increases in serum creatinine concentrations, severe hypertension, RPLS, and proteinuria. These findings were reversed within 3 weeks following discontinuance of both drugs without other interventions. Use of bevacizumab in combination with sunitinib is *not* recommended. Clinicians should report cases of microangiopathic hemolytic anemia associated with bevacizumab therapy to the manufacturer or the US Food and Drug Administration (FDA).

Immunogenicity

As with all therapeutic proteins, there is a potential for immunogenicity. The incidence of antibody formation to bevacizumab has not been established.

Ocular Effects

Permanent loss of vision, endophthalmitis (infectious and sterile), intraocular inflammation, retinal detachment, increased intraocular pressure, hemorrhage (including conjunctival, vitreous, or retinal hemorrhage), vitreous floaters, ocular hyperemia, and ocular pain or discomfort have been reported during postmarketing experience in patients receiving intravitreal injection† of bevacizumab for treatment of various ocular disorders†.

Specific Populations

Pregnancy

Category C. (See Users Guide.)

Lactation

It is not known whether bevacizumab is distributed into milk. Human immunoglobulin G_1 (IgG_1) is distributed into milk; however, published data suggest that antibodies in breast milk do not enter the neonatal and infant circulations in substantial amounts. Because many drugs are distributed into milk and because of the potential for serious adverse reactions in nursing infants from bevacizumab, a decision should be made whether to discontinue nursing or the drug, taking into account the long half-life (approximately 20 days [range: 11–50 days]) and the importance of the drug to the woman.

Pediatric Use

Safety and efficacy of bevacizumab have not been established in children younger than 18 years of age.

Geriatric Use

No difference in overall survival relative to younger adults was observed in patients receiving bevacizumab and chemotherapy (irinotecan, fluorouracil, and leucovorin) for metastatic colorectal cancer; experience in those 65 years of age and older is insufficient to determine whether overall adverse effect profile differs compared with younger adults. Severe adverse effects reported more frequently among patients 65 years of age and older than among younger adults receiving bevacizumab and chemotherapy for metastatic colorectal cancer included asthenia, sepsis, deep thrombophlebitis, hypertension, hypotension, myocardial infarction, congestive heart failure, diarrhea, constipation, anorexia, leukopenia, anemia, dehydration, hypokalemia, and hyponatremia. Geriatric patients receiving bevacizumab and chemotherapy (fluorouracil, leucovorin, and oxaliplatin) for metastatic colorectal cancer also may be at greater risk for nausea, vomiting (emesis), ileus, or fatigue. Geriatric patients receiving bevacizumab and chemotherapy (carboplatin and paclitaxel) for advanced non-small cell lung cancer may be at greater risk for proteinuria than younger patients. Other adverse effects reported more frequently among patients 65 years of age and older included dyspepsia, GI hemorrhage, edema, epistaxis, increased cough, and voice alteration.

Analysis of pooled data from 5 randomized controlled trials involving 1745 patients (35% aged 65 years or older) showed that arterial thromboembolic events occurred more frequently in all patients receiving bevacizumab with chemotherapy compared with those receiving chemotherapy alone, regardless of age. However, the increase in the incidence of arterial thromboembolic events associated with concomitant bevacizumab therapy was greater in patients 65 years of age or older (8.5 versus 2.9%) compared with those younger than 65 years of age (2.1 versus 1.4%). (See Thromboembolism under Warnings/Precautions: Other Warnings and Precautions, in Cautions.)

● Common Adverse Effects

Adverse effects reported in more than 10% of patients receiving bevacizumab and at a frequency at least twice that reported among patients receiving controls include epistaxis, headache, hypertension, rhinitis, proteinuria, taste alteration, dry skin, rectal hemorrhage, lacrimation disorder, back pain, and exfoliative dermatitis.

DRUG INTERACTIONS

● Carboplatin

Pharmacokinetic interaction is unlikely (no effect on mean carboplatin exposure). (See Drug Interactions: Paclitaxel.)

● Interferon Alfa

Pharmacokinetic interaction is unlikely (no effect on mean interferon alfa exposure).

● Irinotecan

Pharmacokinetic interaction is unlikely (no effect on pharmacokinetics of irinotecan or the active metabolite of irinotecan [SN38]).

● Paclitaxel

Limited data indicate that although mean paclitaxel exposure was not altered following concomitant use of bevacizumab with carboplatin and paclitaxel, paclitaxel exposure after 4 treatment cycles decreased in patients receiving concomitant therapy (lower paclitaxel exposure observed on day 63 than on day 0) compared with that in patients receiving carboplatin and paclitaxel alone (higher paclitaxel exposure observed on day 63 than on day 0).

● Sunitinib

Cases of microangiopathic hemolytic anemia have been reported. (See Microangiopathic Hemolytic Anemia under Warnings/Precautions: Other Warnings and Precautions, in Cautions.) Use of bevacizumab in combination with sunitinib is *not* recommended.

DESCRIPTION

Bevacizumab, a recombinant humanized monoclonal antibody, is an antineoplastic agent. The drug is an IgG_1 antibody that contains human framework regions and murine complementarity-determining regions.

Bevacizumab binds to human vascular endothelial growth factor (VEGF) and prevents interaction of VEGF with its receptors (Flt-1, KDR) on the surface of endothelial cells. In vitro models of angiogenesis have shown that interaction of VEGF with its receptors may lead to endothelial cell proliferation and new blood vessel formation. Evidence from animal models has suggested that administration of an anti-VEGF monoclonal antibody (e.g., bevacizumab) may inhibit angiogenesis and thus may reduce microvascular growth of tumors and inhibit metastatic disease progression. Bevacizumab is metabolized and eliminated via the reticuloendothelial system.

ADVICE TO PATIENTS

Importance of understanding potential risks associated with therapy, including severe hypertension, wound healing complications, arterial thromboembolic events, and ovarian failure.

Importance of routine monitoring of blood pressure and informing clinician if blood pressure is elevated.

Importance of immediately informing clinician if unusual bleeding, high fever, rigors, sudden worsening of neurologic function, persistent or severe abdominal pain, severe constipation, or vomiting occurs.

Risk of fetal toxicity. Necessity of advising women to use an effective method of contraception during and for at least 6 months after the last dose of bevacizumab.

Importance of informing clinicians of existing or contemplated concomitant therapy, including prescription and OTC drugs, as well as any concomitant illnesses.

Importance of informing patients of other important precautionary information. (See Cautions.)

PREPARATIONS

Excipients in commercially available drug preparations may have clinically important effects in some individuals; consult specific product labeling for details.

Bevacizumab (Recombinant)

Parenteral

For injection, concentrate, for IV infusion	25 mg/mL (100 and 400 mg)		Avastin®, Genentech

† Use is not currently included in the labeling approved by the US Food and Drug Administration.

Bicalutamide

10:00 • ANTINEOPLASTIC AGENTS

■ Bicalutamide, a nonsteroidal antiandrogen, is an antineoplastic agent.

USES

● Prostate Cancer

Bicalutamide 50 mg daily is used in combination with a luteinizing hormone-releasing hormone (LHRH) analog (e.g., goserelin or leuprolide acetate) for the treatment of metastatic (stage D2) prostate cancer.

Guidelines state that clinicians should not offer first-generation antiandrogens, including bicalutamide, in combination with LHRH agonists in patients with metastatic hormone-sensitive prostate cancer, except to block testosterone flare.

Bicalutamide 150 mg daily should not be used alone or in combination with other treatments; this dosage regimen was associated with a potentially increased risk of mortality compared to castration in studies enrolling patients with locally advanced (T3–4, NX, M0) or metastatic (M1) prostate cancer†.

Clinical Experience

Safety and efficacy of bicalutamide for this use are based principally on the results of a double-blind, multicenter, randomized study in 813 patients with previously untreated advanced prostate cancer. Patients were randomized to receive bicalutamide 50 mg once daily or flutamide 250 mg 3 times daily, each in combination with an LHRH analog (goserelin acetate implant or leuprolide acetate depot). The mean age of patients in the trial was 70 years, and approximately 71% of patients were white. Approximately 39% of patients had 6 or more metastases. The final analysis of this trial was conducted after a median follow-up time of 160 weeks. At the time of final analysis, 52.7% of bicalutamide-treated patients had died, and 57.5% of flutamide-treated patients had died. There was no difference in survival between treatment groups (hazard ratio, 0.87; 95% confidence interval, 0.72–1.05). Quality of life measurements were also found to be similar among treatment groups.

A phase 2, double-blind, randomized controlled trial (TERRAIN) compared bicalutamide 50 mg daily to enzalutamide 160 mg daily (each in combination with LHRH agonist or antagonist therapy) in patients with metastatic castration-resistant prostate cancer. The primary endpoint was progression-free survival. The mean age of patients in this trial was 71 years, and approximately 93% were white. The median follow-up time was 20 months in the enzalutamide group and 16.7 months in the bicalutamide group. Median progression-free survival was substantially prolonged among patients who received enzalutamide compared with bicalutamide (15.7 versus 5.8 months, respectively).

Clinical Perspective

According to a joint guideline from the American Urological Association (AUA), American Society for Radiation Oncology (ASTRO), and Society of Urologic Oncology (SUO), clinicians should not offer first-generation antiandrogens (i.e., bicalutamide, flutamide, nilutamide) in combination with LHRH agonists in patients with metastatic hormone-sensitive prostate cancer, except to block testosterone flare. In light of the compelling evidence to support the use of other therapies (i.e., docetaxel, abiraterone acetate plus prednisone, apalutamide, or enzalutamide) in combination with androgen deprivation therapy in men with newly diagnosed metastatic hormone-sensitive prostate cancer, long-term use of first-generation antiandrogens in lieu of these agents cannot be supported. Androgen pathway-directed therapy (e.g., abiraterone plus prednisone, apalutamide, bicalutamide, darolutamide, enzalutamide, flutamide, nilutamide) should not be offered without concomitant androgen deprivation therapy in metastatic hormone-sensitive prostate cancer.

DOSAGE AND ADMINISTRATION

● General

Pretreatment Screening

● Measure serum transaminase levels prior to treatment with bicalutamide.

Patient Monitoring

● Monitor serum transaminase levels at regular intervals during the first 4 months of treatment, and periodically thereafter. If signs or symptoms of liver dysfunction occur (e.g., nausea, vomiting, abdominal pain, fatigue, anorexia, "flu-like" symptoms, dark urine, jaundice, or right upper quadrant tenderness), assess serum transaminase levels. If jaundice occurs, or alanine aminotransferase (ALT) increases above 2 times the upper limit of normal (ULN), discontinue bicalutamide and closely monitor liver function.

● Consider monitoring prostate specific antigen (PSA) concentrations periodically to assess response to therapy; if PSA levels rise while on bicalutamide, evaluate for clinical disease progression.

● Closely monitor the prothrombin time (PT) and international normalized ratio (INR) in patients on concomitant warfarin therapy, and adjust the anticoagulant dosage as necessary.

● Consider monitoring blood glucose in patients treated with bicalutamide in combination with LHRH agonists.

Other General Considerations

● Initiate bicalutamide and LHRH analog therapy concomitantly.

● Administration

Bicalutamide is administered orally once daily at the same time each day (morning or evening) without regard to meals.

If a dose of bicalutamide is missed, the prescribed dose should be taken at the next scheduled time; an additional dose should not be administered to replace the missed dose.

Store bicalutamide tablets between 20–25°C.

● Dosage

Prostate Cancer

For use in combination with a luteinizing hormone-releasing hormone (LHRH) analog in the treatment of metastatic (stage D2) prostate cancer, the usual adult dosage of bicalutamide is 50 mg once daily in the morning or evening. Treatment with bicalutamide and the LHRH analog should be initiated concomitantly.

Hepatic Impairment

No adjustment of bicalutamide dosage is necessary in patients with mild to moderate hepatic impairment. Although data indicate that delayed excretion and accumulation of bicalutamide can occur in severe hepatic impairment, no dosage adjustment is necessary.

Renal Impairment

No adjustment of bicalutamide dosage is necessary in patients with renal impairment.

Geriatric Use

The manufacturer provides no recommendations regarding modification of bicalutamide dosage in geriatric patients.

CAUTIONS

● Contraindications

● Pregnancy.

● Not indicated for use in females.

- History of hypersensitivity to bicalutamide or any component of the preparation. Hypersensitivity reactions such as angioneurotic edema and urticaria have occurred.

• Warnings/Precautions

Hepatitis

Severe liver injury, in some cases leading to hospitalization and/or death, has been reported rarely in association with bicalutamide therapy. Hepatotoxicity generally occurred within the first 3–4 months of bicalutamide therapy. Hepatitis or marked increases in serum concentrations of hepatic transaminases leading to discontinuance of bicalutamide therapy were reported in 1% of patients receiving the drug in controlled clinical trials.

Serum transaminase concentrations should be measured prior to initiation of bicalutamide therapy, at regular intervals during the first 4 months of treatment, and periodically thereafter. If clinical signs or symptoms suggestive of liver dysfunction (e.g., nausea, vomiting, abdominal pain, fatigue, anorexia, "flu-like" symptoms, dark urine, jaundice, or right upper quadrant tenderness) occur, serum transaminase (especially ALT) concentrations should be measured immediately. Bicalutamide should be discontinued immediately in any patient who develops jaundice or an increase in serum ALT concentration to greater than 2 x ULN, and liver function should be monitored closely.

Hemorrhage with Concomitant Use of Coumarin Anticoagulant

Post-marking reports of excessive prolongation of the prothrombin time (PT) and international normalized ratio (INR) occurring days to weeks after introduction of bicalutamide have been reported in patients who were previously stable on anticoagulation with coumarin anticoagulants. Some cases resulted in serious intracranial, retroperitoneal, or GI bleeding that required blood transfusion and/or vitamin K administration. When patients on warfarin are started on bicalutamide, closely monitor the PT/INR and adjust the dosage of warfarin as necessary.

Gynecomastia and Breast Pain

In clinical trials, gynecomastia and breast pain were reported in 38 and 39% of patients, respectively, who were receiving bicalutamide 150 mg as monotherapy for prostate cancer.

Glucose Tolerance

A reduction of glucose tolerance, presenting as diabetes or loss of glycemic control has occurred in patients receiving luteinizing hormone-releasing hormone (LHRH) agonists. Consider monitoring blood glucose in patients on bicalutamide and LHRH analog combination therapy.

Laboratory Tests

Regular monitoring of prostate specific antigen (PSA) concentrations can be helpful when assessing response to therapy. If PSA levels rise while on bicalutamide, the patient should undergo evaluation for clinical disease progression.

For patients who have objective progression of disease together with an elevated PSA, a treatment-free period of antiandrogen, while continuing the LHRH analog, may be considered.

Specific Populations

Pregnancy

Bicalutamide is contraindicated for use in pregnancy due to the risk of fetal harm and is not indicated for use in females. No human data are available evaluating bicalutamide in pregnancy; in animal studies, abnormal development of male reproductive organs occurred when bicalutamide was administered during organogenesis.

Lactation

Bicalutamide is not indicated for use in females. It is not known whether bicalutamide or its metabolites are distributed into human milk. The effects of the drug on the breast-fed infant or on the production of milk are unknown. The presence of bicalutamide has been detected in rat milk.

Females and Males of Reproductive Potential

Morphological changes of spermatozoa may occur with antiandrogen therapy. Advise male patients with female partners of reproductive potential to use effective contraception during treatment with bicalutamide and for 130 days after the final dose. Bicalutamide can inhibit spermatogenesis and impair fertility in males of reproductive potential; the long-term effects of bicalutamide on male fertility have not been evaluated.

Pediatric Use

The safety and efficacy of bicalutamide have not been established in pediatric patients.

Geriatric Use

No significant relationship has been shown between age and steady state levels of bicalutamide or the active R-enantiomer of bicalutamide.

Hepatic Impairment

Use bicalutamide with caution in patients with moderate to severe hepatic impairment. Bicalutamide is extensively metabolized in the liver; however, the pharmacokinetics of the drug do not appear to be altered in patients with mild to moderate hepatic impairment. Limited pharmacokinetic data in severe hepatic impairment indicate that the half-life of the bicalutamide R-enantiomer is increased by approximately 76%. Consider periodic liver function tests in patients with hepatic impairment receiving long-term therapy.

Renal Impairment

Renal impairment has no significant impact on the elimination of bicalutamide or its active R-enantiomer.

• Common Adverse Effects

Adverse effects reported in ≥10% of patients in clinical trials receiving bicalutamide plus a LHRH analog include hot flashes, pain (including general, back, pelvic, and abdominal), asthenia, constipation, infection, nausea, peripheral edema, dyspnea, diarrhea, hematuria, nocturia, and anemia.

DRUG INTERACTIONS

Bicalutamide does not induce cytochrome P-450 (CYP) isoenzymes. In vitro, the R-enantiomer of bicalutamide has been shown to inhibit CYP3A4 to a greater extent than CYP2C9, CYP2C19, and CYP2D6. Clinical data have not demonstrated an interaction between LHRH analogs (eg, leuprolide, goserelin) and bicalutamide.

• Drugs Metabolized by Hepatic Microsomal Enzymes

CYP3A4 substrates

Use caution with coadministration of bicalutamide and CYP3A4 substrates. Studies have shown that concomitant use of bicalutamide with midazolam, a sensitive CYP3A4 substrate, can increase the maximum serum concentration (Cmax) and AUC of midazolam by 1.5- and 1.9-fold, respectively.

Protein-bound Drugs

Bicalutamide is highly protein bound (96%); in vitro, studies have shown bicalutamide to displace coumarin anticoagulants from protein binding sites. Monitor the PT/INR closely and adjust the warfarin dosage as necessary in patients receiving concomitant bicalutamide and warfarin.

DESCRIPTION

Bicalutamide is a nonsteroidal antiandrogen that is structurally and pharmacologically related to flutamide and nilutamide.

Bicalutamide inhibits the action of androgens by competitively blocking nuclear androgen receptors in target tissues such as the prostate, seminal vesicles, and adrenal cortex; blockade of androgen receptors in the hormone-sensitive tumor cells may result in growth arrest or transient tumor regression through inhibition of androgen-dependent DNA and protein synthesis. Bicalutamide is a selective antiandrogen with no androgenic or progestational activity in various animal models. The relative binding affinity of bicalutamide at the androgen receptor is more than that of nilutamide and approximately 4 times that of hydroxyflutamide, the active metabolite of flutamide.

Common pharmacologic therapies for prostate cancer (i.e., gonadotropin-releasing hormone [GnRH] analogs, nonsteroidal antiandrogens) when used as monotherapy initially result in increased serum testosterone concentrations, which may limit the effects of the drugs. Androgen receptors in the hypothalamus are blocked by bicalutamide, which disrupts the inhibitory feedback of testosterone on luteinizing hormone (LH) release, resulting in a temporary increase in secretion of LH; the increase in LH stimulates an increase in the production of testosterone. As GnRH analogs have potent GnRH agonist properties, testicular steroidogenesis continues during the first few weeks after initiating therapy. However, the combination of orchiectomy or GnRH analog therapy to suppress testicular androgen production and an antiandrogen to block response of remaining adrenal androgens provides maximal androgen blockade. Concomitant administration of antiandrogens such as bicalutamide in patients initiating therapy with a GnRH analog can inhibit initial androgenic stimulation and potential exacerbation of symptoms (e.g., bone pain, urinary obstruction, liver pain, impending spinal cord compression) that may occur during the first month of GnRH analog therapy.

Although the absolute bioavailability is not known, bicalutamide is well absorbed following oral administration. Administration of bicalutamide with food does not affect the rate or extent of drug absorption. Bicalutamide exhibits high protein-binding (96%). The S (inactive) enantiomer of bicalutamide is metabolized primarily by glucuronidation. The R (active) enantiomer also undergoes glucuronidation but is predominantly oxidized to an inactive metabolite followed by glucuronidation. Metabolites are eliminated in the urine or feces. The S-enantiomer undergoes rapid clearance in comparison to the R-enantiomer; the R-enantiomer accounts for the majority of steady-state plasma levels (99%). In healthy males, the half-life of the R-enantiomer of bicalutamide is approximately 5.8 days.

ADVICE TO PATIENTS

- Risk of potential liver toxicity. Importance of notifying clinicians if nausea, vomiting, abdominal pain, or jaundice occurs.

- Importance of initiating bicalutamide concomitantly with luteinizing hormone-releasing hormone (LHRH) analog and of not interrupting or discontinuing therapy without consulting a clinician.

- Advise male patients with female partners of reproductive potential to use effective contraception during treatment with bicalutamide and for 130 days after the final dose.

- Importance of closely monitoring the prothrombin time (PT) and international normalized ratio (INR) in patients on concomitant warfarin therapy. Advise patients to notify their clinician of any bleeding or spontaneous bruising while on bicalutamide and anticoagulants.

- Inform patients that diabetes or loss of glycemic control can occur with use of a luteinizing hormone-releasing hormone (LHRH) analog. Consider advising patients to monitor blood glucose levels.

- Inform patients of risk of photosensitivity with bicalutamide therapy. Patients should avoid excessive direct exposure to sunlight or ultraviolet light and wear sunscreen.

- Advise patients that bicalutamide may increase somnolence; patients who experience somnolence should exercise caution when driving or operating machinery.

- Importance of informing clinicians of existing or contemplated concomitant therapy, including prescription and OTC drugs and dietary or herbal supplements, as well as any concomitant illnesses.

- Importance of informing patients of other important precautionary information.

For further information on the handling of antineoplastic agents, see the ASHP Guidelines on Handling Hazardous Drugs at https://www.ahfsdrug information.com.

PREPARATIONS

Excipients in commercially available drug preparations may have clinically important effects in some individuals; consult specific product labeling for details.

Bicalutamide

Oral

Tablets, film-coated	50 mg	Casodex®, ANI Pharmaceuticals

† Use is not currently included in the labeling approved by the US Food and Drug Administration.

Selected Revisions July 25, 2023, © Copyright, June 1, 1996, American Society of Health-System Pharmacists, Inc.

Binimetinib

10:00 • ANTINEOPLASTIC AGENTS

■ Binimetinib, a reversible inhibitor of mitogen-activated extracellular signal-regulated kinase (MEK) 1 and MEK2, is an antineoplastic agent.

USES

● *Melanoma*

Binimetinib is used in combination with encorafenib for the treatment of unresectable or metastatic melanoma with b-Raf serine-threonine kinase (BRAF) V600E or V600K mutation. Binimetinib has been designated an orphan drug by FDA for the treatment of this cancer. An FDA-approved diagnostic test is required to confirm the presence of the BRAF V600E or V600K mutation in tumor specimens prior to initiation of therapy. In patients with unresectable or metastatic melanoma with BRAF V600E or V600K mutation, combined therapy with binimetinib and encorafenib has been shown to prolong progression-free survival and overall survival, and increase response rate compared with vemurafenib alone.

Clinical Experience

This indication for binimetinib use is based principally on the results of a randomized, open-label, phase 3 study (COLUMBUS) in patients with unresectable locally advanced or metastatic melanoma positive for V600E or V600K BRAF mutation as detected by the bioMerieux THxID® BRAF V600 mutation test. In this study, 577 patients were randomized (stratified by disease stage, Eastern Cooperative Oncology Group [ECOG] performance status, and prior immunotherapy use) in a 1:1:1 ratio to receive binimetinib 45 mg twice daily with encorafenib 450 mg once daily (binimetinib-encorafenib), encorafenib 300 mg once daily alone, or vemurafenib 960 mg twice daily. Treatment was continued until disease progression or unacceptable toxicity occurred or the patient withdrew from the study. The primary measure of efficacy was progression-free survival (as evaluated by a blinded independent central review committee). The median age of patients randomized to the binimetinib-encorafenib or vemurafenib treatment groups was 56 years; 91% of patients were white, 59% were male, 95% had metastatic disease, 65% had stage M1c disease, 72% had a baseline ECOG performance status of 0, 28% had elevated LDH concentrations, 45% had tumor involvement in at least 3 organs, and 3% of patients had brain metastases. Approximately 4% of patients enrolled in the binimetinib-encorafenib or vemurafenib treatment groups received prior therapy with an anti-programmed-death 1 (anti-PD-1), anti-programmed-death ligand-1 (anti-PD-L1), or anti-cytotoxic T-lymphocyte-associated antigen 4 (anti-CTLA-4) antibody. Most patients (88%) randomized to receive binimetinib-encorafenib or vemurafenib had BRAF V600E mutation; 11% had V600K mutation and <1% had both BRAF V600E and V600K mutations. Patients who had received immunotherapy in the adjuvant setting or one prior immunotherapy regimen for unresectable locally advanced or metastatic melanoma were eligible for this study; however, patients with prior exposure to BRAF or mitogen-activated extracellular signal-regulated kinase (MEK) inhibitors were not eligible to enroll in the study.

At a median follow-up of 16.7 or 14.4 months in patients receiving binimetinib-encorafenib or vemurafenib alone, respectively, median progression-free survival was 14.9 months in patients receiving binimetinib-encorafenib compared with 7.3 months in those receiving vemurafenib. The overall response rate was 63% for patients receiving binimetinib-encorafenib and 40% for those receiving vemurafenib; complete response was achieved in 8% of patients receiving binimetinib-encorafenib and 6% of those receiving vemurafenib. The median duration of response in patients receiving binimetinib-encorafenib or vemurafenib alone was 16.6 or 12.3 months, respectively. After a median follow-up of 48.8 months for the overall study population, the median overall survival was 33.6 or 16.9 months in patients receiving binimetinib-encorafenib or vemurafenib alone, respectively. The risk for death was reduced by 39% with binimetinib-encorafenib as compared to vemurafenib alone. In general, the overall survival benefit for combination therapy with binimetinib and encorafenib versus vemurafenib was consistent in most subgroup analyses (e.g., age, gender, race, ECOG performance status, geographic region, baseline serum LDH concentration, BRAF mutation status,

disease stage, organ involvement, presence of brain metastases, prior use of first-line immunotherapy or adjuvant therapy).

Clinical Perspective

The American Society of Clinical Oncology (ASCO) guidelines on systemic therapy for melanoma recommends that in the setting of unresectable or metastatic melanoma, patients with confirmed BRAF wild type cutaneous melanoma should be offered (in no particular order) ipilimumab plus nivolumab, nivolumab alone, or pembrolizumab alone. In patients with confirmed BRAF-mutant (V600) disease, ASCO recommends offering treatment (in no particular order) with the 3 previous regimens or combination BRAF/MEK inhibitor therapy with dabrafenib plus trametinib, encorafenib plus binimetinib, or vemurafenib plus cobimetinib. For patients who progress after first-line therapy with programmed-death receptor-1 (PD-1) inhibitors, combination BRAF/MEK inhibitors may be offered; PD-1 inhibitors may be offered after progression on first-line combination BRAF/MEK inhibitors. Patients with mucosal melanoma may be offered the same treatment options as those with cutaneous melanoma; enrollment in clinical trials should be offered where possible.

● *Non-small Cell Lung Cancer*

Binimetinib is used in combination with encorafenib for the treatment of adults with metastatic non-small cell lung cancer (NSCLC) with a BRAF V600E mutation. An FDA-approved diagnostic test is required to confirm the presence of the BRAF V600E mutation in tumor or plasma specimens prior to initiation of therapy. If no mutation is detected in a plasma specimen, test tumor tissue.

Clinical Experience

This indication for binimetinib use is based principally on the results of an open-label, single-arm, multicenter, phase 2 study (PHAROS) in patients with metastatic NSCLC positive for a BRAF V600E mutation. In this study, 98 patients received binimetinib 45 mg orally twice daily in combination with encorafenib 450 mg orally once daily in 28-day cycles; 59 patients were treatment-naïve and 39 were previously treated. Treatment was continued until disease progression or unacceptable toxicity occurred. The primary end point was confirmed objective response rate per RECIST version 1.1 criteria.

The median age of enrolled patients was 70 years (range: 47 to 86 years); 88% of patients were white, 7% Asian, 3% Black or African American, and 1% American Indian or Alaska Native; 53% were female; 57% were former smokers; 73% had an ECOG performance status of 1; and 97% had adenocarcinoma. Results revealed an objective response rate of 75% in treatment-naïve patients and 46% in previously treated patients. A complete response was observed in 9 (15%) and 4 (10%) patients in the treatment-naïve and previously treated groups, respectively, with a partial response documented in 35 (59%) and 14 (36%) patients, respectively. At the time of this analysis, the median duration of response was not estimable in the treatment naïve group and was 16.7 months in the previously treated group. Durable responses lasting ≥12 months were seen in 59% of treatment naïve and 33% of previously treated patients. The disease control rate after 24 weeks was 64% among treatment naïve patients and 41% in previously treated patients. Median progression-free survival was not estimable in the treatment naïve group and was 9.3 months in the previously treated group.

Clinical Perspective

Approximately 60% of patients with lung cancer have driver alterations (e.g., mutations in EGFR, ALK, or BRAF; ROS-1 fusions, RET fusions, MET exon 14 skipping mutations, and NTRK fusions). The ASCO and Ontario Health (OH; previously known as Cancer Care Ontario) 2021 guideline specifically addresses treatment of stage IV NSCLC with driver alterations, including BRAF gene alterations. The 2023 update to this guideline recommends that, for patients with stage IV NSCLC with a BRAF V600E mutation, clinicians may offer dabrafenib and trametinib or encorafenib and binimetinib as first-line treatment. If these treatment options are unavailable, clinicians may offer standard first-line therapy following the nondriver alteration guideline.

In the second-line setting, standard first-line treatment based on the ASCO/OH nondriver mutation guideline should be offered in patients with stage IV NSCLC harboring BRAF V600E driver alterations who were previously treated with BRAF/MEK inhibitor combination therapy. In patients who did not receive BRAF-targeted therapy in the first-line setting, dabrafenib and trametinib or encorafenib and binimetinib may be offered. For patients with stage IV NSCLC with BRAF mutations other than V600E, standard treatment based on the ASCO/OH nondriver mutation guideline should be offered.

DOSAGE AND ADMINISTRATION

• General

Pretreatment Screening

- Confirm presence of BRAF V600E or V600K mutation, dependent upon indication, using an FDA-approved diagnostic test prior to initiation of therapy.

- Assess left ventricular ejection fraction (LVEF) using echocardiogram or multigated radionuclide angiography (MUGA) prior to the initiation of binimetinib.

- Monitor liver function tests, creatine phosphokinase (CPK), and creatinine levels prior to initiation of therapy.

- Verify the pregnancy status of females of reproductive potential prior to initiating binimetinib.

- Monitor patients for the development of new malignancies prior to treatment initiation.

Patient Monitoring

- Assess LVEF using echocardiogram or MUGA one month after initiation of binimetinib and then every 2 to 3 months during therapy.

- Assess for visual symptoms at each visit. Perform an ophthalmologic examination at regular intervals, for new or worsening visual disturbances, and to follow new or persistent ophthalmologic findings.

- Assess new or progressive unexplained pulmonary symptoms or findings for possible interstitial lung disease (ILD).

- Monitor liver function tests monthly during treatment, and as clinically indicated.

- Monitor CPK and creatinine levels periodically during treatment, and as clinically indicated.

- Monitor for signs of bleeding, as well as blood clots, during therapy.

- Monitor patients for the development of new malignancies during therapy and after treatment discontinuation.

• Administration

Binimetinib is administered orally twice daily, with doses given approximately 12 hours apart; the drug can be taken without regard to meals.

If a dose of binimetinib is missed by more than 6 hours, the missed dose should be skipped and the next dose should be taken at the regularly scheduled time. Patients should *not* take extra tablets of the drug to make up for the missed dose.

If vomiting occurs following administration of binimetinib, a replacement dose should *not* be administered, and the next dose should be taken at the regularly scheduled time.

Store at 20-25°C (excursions permitted between 15-30°C).

• Dosage

Melanoma

For use in combination with encorafenib in the treatment of unresectable or metastatic melanoma with BRAF V600E or V600K mutation, the recommended adult dosage of binimetinib is 45 mg twice daily. Therapy should be continued until disease progression or unacceptable toxicity occurs.

If encorafenib therapy is permanently discontinued, binimetinib also should be discontinued. Clinicians should consult the manufacturer's labeling for information on recommended dosage modifications for encorafenib.

Non-small Cell Lung Cancer (NSCLC)

For use in combination with encorafenib in the treatment of adults with metastatic NSCLC with a BRAF V600E mutation, the recommended adult dosage of binimetinib is 45 mg twice daily. Therapy should be continued until disease progression or unacceptable toxicity occurs.

If encorafenib therapy is permanently discontinued, binimetinib also should be discontinued. Clinicians should consult the manufacturer's labeling for information on recommended dosage modifications for encorafenib.

Dosage Modification for Toxicity

If adverse reactions occur, interruption of therapy, dosage reduction, and/or permanent discontinuance of binimetinib may be required based on severity of the reaction. If dosage modification of binimetinib for adverse reactions is necessary, a dosage reduction to 30 mg twice daily is initially recommended. If a dosage of 30 mg twice daily is not tolerated, binimetinib should be permanently discontinued.

Cardiovascular Toxicity

If an asymptomatic absolute decrease in left ventricular ejection fraction (LVEF) from baseline of >10% and to a level below the lower limit of normal (LLN) occurs, binimetinib therapy should be withheld for up to 4 weeks and left ventricular function should be reassessed every 2 weeks; therapy may be resumed at a reduced dosage if the following are present: LVEF is at or above the LLN and the absolute decrease from baseline is 10% or less and the patient is asymptomatic. If the toxicity does not improve within 4 weeks of withholding binimetinib, the drug should be permanently discontinued.

If symptomatic congestive heart failure or an absolute decrease in LVEF from baseline of >20% and to a level below the LLN occurs, binimetinib therapy should be permanently discontinued.

If prolongation of QT interval occurs during combination therapy with binimetinib and encorafenib, no dosage modification of binimetinib is necessary.

Venous Thromboembolism

If uncomplicated deep-vein thrombosis (DVT) or pulmonary embolism (PE) occurs, binimetinib therapy should be withheld; therapy may be resumed at a reduced dosage when the toxicity improves to grade 1 or less. If the toxicity does not improve, the drug should be permanently discontinued.

If life-threatening PE occurs, binimetinib therapy should be permanently discontinued.

Ocular Effects

If symptomatic serous retinopathy or retinal pigment epithelial detachment occurs, binimetinib therapy should be withheld for up to 10 days; therapy may be resumed at the same dosage when the toxicity improves and the patient becomes asymptomatic. If the toxicity does not improve within 10 days of withholding therapy, therapy may be resumed at a reduced dosage or permanently discontinued.

If grade 1 or 2 uveitis unresponsive to ocular therapy occurs, binimetinib therapy should be withheld for up to 6 weeks. If the toxicity improves within 6 weeks of withholding therapy, therapy may be resumed at the same or reduced dosage. If the toxicity does not improve within 6 weeks of withholding therapy, binimetinib therapy should be permanently discontinued.

If grade 3 uveitis occurs, binimetinib therapy should be withheld for up to 6 weeks. If grade 3 uveitis improves within 6 weeks of withholding therapy, therapy may be resumed at the same or reduced dosage. If grade 3 uveitis does not improve within 6 weeks of withholding therapy, binimetinib therapy should be permanently discontinued.

If retinal vein occlusion or grade 4 uveitis occurs, binimetinib therapy should be permanently discontinued.

Pulmonary Effects

If grade 2 interstitial lung disease occurs, binimetinib therapy should be withheld for up to 4 weeks; therapy may be resumed at a reduced dosage when the toxicity improves to grade 1 or less. If grade 2 interstitial lung disease does not improve within 4 weeks of withholding therapy, the drug should be permanently discontinued.

If grade 3 or 4 interstitial lung disease occurs, binimetinib therapy should be permanently discontinued.

Hepatotoxicity

In patients who develop grade 2 elevations of serum aminotransferases (ALT or AST), binimetinib therapy may be continued at the same dosage for up to 2 weeks. If the toxicity persists, binimetinib therapy should be withheld; therapy may be resumed at the same dosage when the toxicity improves to grade 1 or less or to baseline.

For the first occurrence of grade 3 elevations of serum ALT or AST, binimetinib therapy should be withheld for up to 4 weeks; therapy may be resumed at a reduced dosage when the toxicity improves to grade 1 or less or to baseline. If the toxicity does not improve to grade 1 or less or to baseline within 4 weeks of withholding therapy, the drug should be permanently discontinued. If grade 3 elevations of serum ALT or AST recur, permanent discontinuance of binimetinib should be considered.

For the first occurrence of grade 4 elevations of serum ALT or AST, binimetinib therapy may be permanently discontinued or temporarily interrupted. If binimetinib therapy is temporarily interrupted, the drug should be withheld for up to 4 weeks; therapy may be resumed at a reduced dosage when the toxicity improves to grade 1 or less or to baseline. If the toxicity does not improve to grade 1 or less or to baseline within 4 weeks of withholding therapy, the drug should be permanently discontinued. For recurrent grade 4 serum ALT or AST elevations, binimetinib therapy should be permanently discontinued.

Musculoskeletal Effects

In patients who exhibit asymptomatic grade 4 creatine kinase (CK, creatine phosphokinase, CPK) elevations or any grade of CK elevation with symptoms or concomitant renal impairment, binimetinib therapy should be withheld for up to 4 weeks; therapy may be resumed at a reduced dosage when the toxicity improves to grade 1 or less. If the toxicity does not improve within 4 weeks of withholding therapy, the drug should be permanently discontinued.

Dermatologic Effects

For the first occurrence of grade 2 dermatologic reactions, binimetinib therapy should be continued at the same dosage. If the toxicity does not improve within 2 weeks, binimetinib therapy should be withheld; therapy may be resumed at the same dosage when the toxicity improves to grade 1 or less. If grade 2 dermatologic reactions recur and do not improve within 2 weeks, binimetinib therapy should be withheld; therapy may be resumed at a reduced dosage when the toxicity improves to grade 1 or less.

For the first occurrence of grade 3 dermatologic reactions, binimetinib therapy should be withheld; therapy may be resumed at the same dosage when the toxicity improves to grade 1 or less. If grade 3 dermatologic reactions recur, binimetinib therapy should be withheld; therapy may be resumed at a reduced dosage when the toxicity improves to grade 1 or less.

If grade 4 dermatologic reactions occur, binimetinib therapy should be permanently discontinued.

If palmar-plantar erythrodysesthesia syndrome (hand-foot syndrome) develops during combination therapy with binimetinib and encorafenib, no dosage modification of binimetinib is necessary.

Development of New Primary Malignancies

No dosage adjustment of binimetinib is necessary in patients who develop new primary RAS mutation-positive, noncutaneous malignancies during combination therapy with binimetinib and encorafenib.

Other Toxicity

If grade 2 adverse reaction recurs, binimetinib therapy should be withheld for up to 4 weeks; therapy may be resumed at a reduced dosage when the toxicity improves to grade 0 or 1 or to pretreatment baseline levels. If the toxicity does not improve to grade 0 or 1 or to pretreatment baseline levels within 4 weeks of withholding therapy, the drug should be permanently discontinued.

For the first occurrence of grade 3 adverse reaction, binimetinib therapy should be withheld for up to 4 weeks; therapy may be resumed at a reduced dosage when the toxicity improves to grade 0 or 1 or to pretreatment baseline levels. If the toxicity does not improve to grade 0 or 1 or to pretreatment baseline levels within 4 weeks of withholding therapy, the drug should be permanently discontinued. If grade 3 adverse reaction recurs, permanent discontinuance of binimetinib should be considered.

For the first occurrence of grade 4 adverse reaction, binimetinib therapy may be permanently discontinued or temporarily interrupted. If binimetinib therapy is temporarily interrupted, the drug should be withheld for up to 4 weeks; therapy may be resumed at a reduced dosage when the toxicity improves to grade 0 or 1 or to pretreatment baseline levels. If the grade 4 adverse reaction does not improve to grade 0 or 1 or to pretreatment baseline levels within 4 weeks of withholding therapy, the drug should be permanently discontinued. For recurrent grade 4 adverse reactions, binimetinib therapy should be permanently discontinued.

● Special Populations

Hepatic Impairment

In patients with moderate (total bilirubin concentration exceeding 1.5 times the upper limit of normal [ULN], but no more than 3 times the ULN, with any AST concentration) or severe (total bilirubin concentration exceeding 3 times the ULN, with any AST concentration) hepatic impairment, the manufacturer recommends a reduced binimetinib dosage of 30 mg twice daily. No dosage adjustment is necessary in patients with mild hepatic impairment (total bilirubin concentration not exceeding the ULN with AST concentration exceeding the ULN or total bilirubin concentration exceeding the ULN, but no more than 1.5 times the ULN, with any AST concentration).

Renal Impairment

The manufacturer makes no specific dosage recommendations for patients with renal impairment.

Geriatric Patients

The manufacturer makes no specific dosage recommendations for geriatric patients.

CAUTIONS

● Contraindications

- None.

● Warnings/Precautions

Combination Therapy

When binimetinib is used in combination with encorafenib, the usual cautions, precautions, and contraindications associated with encorafenib must be considered in addition to those associated with binimetinib.

New Primary Malignancies

New primary malignancies, both cutaneous and non-cutaneous, can occur with use of binimetinib. In the PHAROS study, cutaneous squamous cell carcinoma and skin papilloma each occurred in 2% of patients receiving binimetinib in combination with encorafenib. Monitor patients for the development of new malignancies prior to treatment initiation, during therapy, and after discontinuation.

Cardiomyopathy

Cardiomyopathy, which may manifest as a symptomatic or asymptomatic decrease in left ventricular ejection fraction (LVEF), has been reported in patients receiving binimetinib in combination with encorafenib. In the COLUMBUS study, cardiomyopathy (defined as an absolute decrease in LVEF from baseline of ≥10% and to a level below the lower limit of normal [LLN]) occurred in 7% of patients receiving binimetinib in combination with encorafenib; grade 3 left ventricular dysfunction occurred in 1.6% of patients receiving combination therapy. The median time to first onset of left ventricular dysfunction was 3.6 months (range: 0–21 months). Cardiomyopathy resolved in 87% of patients receiving combination therapy with binimetinib and encorafenib.

Evidence of cardiomyopathy was observed in 11% of patients administered binimetinib in combination with encorafenib in the PHAROS study, with grade 3 left ventricular dysfunction occurring in 1% of patients. Cardiomyopathy resolved in 82% of patients.

Safety of combination therapy with binimetinib and encorafenib has not been established in patients with a baseline LVEF below the LLN or <50%.

LVEF should be assessed using echocardiogram or multigated radionuclide angiography (MUGA) prior to and 1 month after initiation of binimetinib and then every 2–3 months during therapy. Close monitoring during therapy is indicated in patients with preexisting cardiovascular risk factors. If left ventricular dysfunction occurs, temporary interruption followed by dosage reduction or discontinuance of binimetinib may be necessary.

Venous Thromboembolism

Venous thromboembolism (VTE) has been reported in patients receiving binimetinib in combination with encorafenib. In the COLUMBUS study, VTE occurred in 6% of patients receiving binimetinib in combination with encorafenib; 3.1% of patients receiving combination therapy developed pulmonary embolism (PE). In the PHAROS study, VTE was reported in 7% of patients receiving binimetinib in combination with encorafenib; 1% of patients administered this combination therapy developed PE.

If deep-vein thrombosis (DVT) or PE occurs, temporary interruption followed by dosage reduction or discontinuance of binimetinib may be necessary.

Ocular Effects

Serous retinopathy, retinal vein occlusion, retinal pigment epithelial detachment, and macular edema have been reported in patients receiving binimetinib in combination with encorafenib. Uveitis, including iritis and iridocyclitis, also has occurred in patients receiving binimetinib in combination with encorafenib.

In the COLUMBUS study, serous retinopathy occurred in 20% of patients receiving combination therapy with binimetinib and encorafenib; macular edema and retinal detachment were reported in 6 and 8%, respectively, of patients receiving combination therapy. Symptomatic serous retinopathy occurred in 8% of patients receiving combination therapy with binimetinib and encorafenib; blindness was not reported in these patients. The median time to initial onset of serous retinopathy was 1.2 months (range: 0–17.5 months). Discontinuance of binimetinib therapy was not necessary in patients experiencing serous retinopathy; however, dosage modification or interruption of binimetinib therapy was necessary in 6% of patients.

In the PHAROS study, serous retinopathy (retinal detachment) occurred in 2% of patients receiving binimetinib in combination with encorafenib, with no cases of blindness reported with the combination therapy. No patient permanently discontinued binimetinib due to serous retinopathy; 1% of patients required dose interruptions.

Retinal vein occlusion is a known risk of mitogen-activated extracellular signal-regulated kinase (MEK) inhibitors. In clinical trials evaluating combination therapy with binimetinib and encorafenib, retinal vein occlusion occurred in 1 of 690 patients (0.1%) with b-Raf serine-threonine kinase (BRAF) mutation-positive melanoma. In the COLUMBUS study, uveitis was reported in 4% of patients receiving binimetinib in combination with encorafenib. In the PHAROS study, uveitis was reported in 1% of patients receiving binimetinib in combination with encorafenib.

Safety of binimetinib has not been established in patients with a history of or predisposition to retinal vein occlusion, including those with uncontrolled glaucoma or a history of hyperviscosity or hypercoagulability syndromes.

Ophthalmologic examinations should be performed regularly and as clinically indicated (i.e., if new or worsening visual disturbances occur; to follow new or persistent ophthalmologic findings) during binimetinib therapy. Patients should be monitored for visual symptoms at each visit. If visual disturbances are reported, ophthalmologic evaluations should be performed urgently (within 24 hours). Temporary interruption, dosage reduction, or discontinuance of binimetinib may be necessary if ocular toxicities occur during therapy with the drug.

Pulmonary Effects

Interstitial lung disease or pneumonitis has been reported in patients receiving combination therapy with binimetinib and encorafenib. In clinical trials evaluating combination therapy with binimetinib and encorafenib, interstitial lung disease and pneumonitis occurred in 2 of 690 patients (0.3%) with BRAF mutation-positive melanoma. One patient receiving binimetinib in combination with encorafenib developed pneumonitis in the PHAROS study.

Patients presenting with manifestations of interstitial lung disease (e.g., new or progressive pulmonary symptoms) should be evaluated. If a diagnosis of interstitial lung disease is confirmed, temporary interruption followed by dosage reduction or discontinuance of binimetinib may be necessary.

Hepatotoxicity

Liver function test abnormalities have been reported in patients receiving combination therapy with binimetinib and encorafenib. In the COLUMBUS study, grade 3 or 4 elevations in ALT, AST, or alkaline phosphatase concentrations occurred in 6, 2.6, or 0.5%, respectively, of patients receiving combination therapy with binimetinib and encorafenib; grade 3 or 4 elevations in serum bilirubin were not reported. In the PHAROS study, grade 3 or 4 elevations in ALT, AST, or alkaline phosphatase concentrations occurred in 9%, 10%, and 3.2%, respectively, of patients receiving binimetinib in combination with encorafenib.

Liver function tests should be performed prior to initiation of binimetinib therapy and then monthly, or more frequently as clinically indicated, during therapy with the drug. Temporary interruption, dosage reduction, or discontinuance of binimetinib may be necessary if liver function test abnormalities occur during therapy with the drug.

Musculoskeletal Effects

Rhabdomyolysis has been reported in patients receiving combination therapy with binimetinib and encorafenib. In clinical trials evaluating combination therapy with binimetinib and encorafenib, rhabdomyolysis occurred in 1 of 690 patients (0.1%) with BRAF mutation-positive melanoma. In the COLUMBUS study, elevations of serum creatine kinase (CK, creatine phosphokinase, CPK) occurred in 58% of patients receiving combination therapy with binimetinib and encorafenib. In the PHAROS study, 41% of patients experienced CK elevations with combination therapy; however, no patient experienced rhabdomyolysis.

Serum CK and creatinine concentrations should be evaluated at baseline, periodically during binimetinib therapy, and as clinically indicated. If elevated CK concentrations occur, therapy interruption followed by dosage reduction or discontinuance of binimetinib may be necessary.

Hemorrhage

Hemorrhage has been reported in patients receiving combination therapy with binimetinib and encorafenib. In the COLUMBUS study, hemorrhage occurred in 19% of patients and was grade 3 or greater in 3.2% of patients receiving binimetinib in combination with encorafenib. The most common hemorrhagic events in patients receiving binimetinib in combination with encorafenib were GI hemorrhage, including rectal hemorrhage (4.2%), hematochezia (3.1%), and hemorrhoidal hemorrhage (1%). Intracranial hemorrhage was fatal in 1.6% of patients with new or progressive brain metastases receiving combination therapy with binimetinib and encorafenib.

In the PHAROS study, hemorrhage occurred in 12% of patients receiving binimetinib in combination with encorafenib, including fatal intracranial hemorrhage in 1% of patients. Grade 3 or 4 hemorrhage was reported in 4.1% of patients. The most frequent hemorrhagic events were anal hemorrhage and hemothorax (2% each).

If hemorrhagic events occur, therapy interruption followed by dosage reduction or discontinuance of binimetinib may be necessary.

Fetal/Neonatal Morbidity and Mortality

Binimetinib may cause fetal harm in humans based on its mechanism of action and animal findings; the drug has been shown to be embryotoxic, fetotoxic, and teratogenic in animals. There are no available data regarding the risk of binimetinib use in pregnant women to date. In animal reproduction studies, embryofetal toxicity (i.e., decreases in fetal body weight, postimplantation loss, abortion) and teratogenic effects were observed in rabbits receiving binimetinib at exposure levels of approximately 5 times the human exposure at the recommended dosage; fetal ventricular septal defects and pulmonary trunk alterations were increased at exposure levels less than 8 times the human exposure. Skeletal anomalies also were observed in rats receiving binimetinib at exposure levels of approximately 37 times the human exposure at the recommended dosage.

Pregnancy should be avoided during binimetinib therapy. The manufacturer states that pregnancy status should be verified prior to initiation of binimetinib therapy in women of childbearing potential and that such women should be advised to use effective contraception while receiving binimetinib and for at least 30 days after the last dose. Patients should be apprised of the potential hazard to the fetus if the drug is used during pregnancy.

Specific Populations

Pregnancy

Binimetinib may cause fetal harm if administered to pregnant women based on its mechanism of action and animal findings.

Lactation

It is not known whether binimetinib or its metabolites are distributed into human milk. Because of the potential for serious adverse reactions to binimetinib in nursing infants, women should be advised not to breast-feed while receiving the drug and for 3 days after the last dose. The effects of the drug on nursing infants or on the production of milk are unknown.

Females and Males of Reproductive Potential

Pregnancy status should be verified in women of childbearing potential prior to initiation of binimetinib therapy. Advise females of reproductive potential to use effective contraception during treatment and for ≥30 days after the final dose of binimetinib.

Pediatric Use

Safety and efficacy of binimetinib have not been established in pediatric patients.

Geriatric Use

In clinical trials evaluating binimetinib (45 mg twice daily) in combination with encorafenib (300–600 mg once daily) in patients with BRAF mutation-positive melanoma, 20% of patients were 65–74 years of age and 8% were ≥75 years of age. In a clinical trial of patients with BRAF V600E mutation-positive metastatic NSCLC administered binimetinib in combination with encorafenib, 63.2% of patients were ≥65 years of age and 20.4% were ≥75 years of age. No overall differences in safety or efficacy were observed between geriatric patients and younger adults.

Hepatic Impairment

Systemic exposure of binimetinib is increased by 80 or 110% in individuals with moderate (total bilirubin concentration exceeding 1.5 times the ULN, but not more than 3 times the ULN, with any AST concentration) or severe (total bilirubin concentration exceeding 3 times the ULN, with any AST concentration) hepatic impairment, respectively, compared with individuals with normal hepatic function; therefore, dosage adjustment is recommended in patients with moderate or severe hepatic impairment.

No clinically important differences in systemic exposure of binimetinib were observed between individuals with mild hepatic impairment (total bilirubin concentration not exceeding the ULN with AST concentration exceeding the ULN or total bilirubin concentration exceeding the ULN, but no more than 1.5 times the ULN, with any AST concentration) and those with normal hepatic function; no dosage adjustment is necessary in patients with mild hepatic impairment.

Renal Impairment

No clinically important differences in systemic exposure of binimetinib were observed between individuals with severe renal impairment (estimated glomerular filtration rate ≤29 mL/minute per 1.73 m^2) and those with normal renal function.

● Common Adverse Effects

The most common adverse effects (≥25%) for binimetinib, in combination with encorafenib, for the treatment of melanoma include fatigue, nausea, diarrhea, vomiting, and abdominal pain.

The most common adverse effects (≥25%) for binimetinib, in combination with encorafenib, for the treatment of NSCLC include fatigue, nausea, diarrhea, musculoskeletal pain, vomiting, abdominal pain, visual impairment, constipation, dyspnea, rash, and cough.

DRUG INTERACTIONS

Binimetinib is metabolized principally by uridine diphosphate-glucuronosyltransferase (UGT) 1A1 and, to a lesser extent, by cytochrome P-450 (CYP) isoenzymes 1A2 and 2C19 to form a minor active metabolite (M3). Binimetinib is a weak inhibitor of UGT1A. The drug does not demonstrate time-dependent inhibition of CYP isoenzymes 1A2, 2C9, 2D6, and 3A, and shows little to no induction of CYP2C9.

In vitro studies indicate that binimetinib is a substrate of P-glycoprotein (P-gp) and breast cancer resistance protein (BCRP); the drug is not a substrate of organic cation transporter (OCT) 1 or organic anion transport protein (OATP) 1B1, OATP1B3, and OATP2B1. In vitro, binimetinib is a weak inhibitor of OCT2, but does not inhibit OCT1.

● Drugs Affected by Hepatic Microsomal Enzymes

Concomitant administration of binimetinib (30 mg orally twice daily for 7 or 15 days) with the CYP3A4 substrate midazolam (single oral dose of 4 mg) did not substantially alter systemic exposure of midazolam.

● Drugs Affected by Other Enzymes

Uridine Diphosphate glucuronosyltransferase

Binimetinib is a substrate of UGT1A1; however, in vitro studies indicate that binimetinib is unlikely to interact with drugs affecting UGT1A1.

Concomitant administration of binimetinib with the UGT1A1 inhibitor encorafenib did not substantially alter systemic exposure of binimetinib. Pharmacokinetic simulations also suggest that concomitant administration of atazanavir (single 400-mg dose), a UGT1A1 inhibitor, and binimetinib (single 45-mg dose) does not substantially alter peak plasma concentrations of binimetinib.

Cigarette smoking has been shown to induce UGT1A1; however, cigarette smoking did not have a clinically important effect on systemic exposure of binimetinib.

Organic Cation Transporters

Clinically important pharmacokinetic interactions between drugs that are substrates of OCT1 or OCT2 and binimetinib are not expected during concurrent use.

● Drugs Affecting Gastric Acidity

Concomitant administration of the proton-pump inhibitor rabeprazole (20 mg once daily for 4 days) with binimetinib (single 45-mg dose) did not result in clinically important changes in peak plasma concentrations and systemic exposure of binimetinib and M3.

DESCRIPTION

Binimetinib, a reversible inhibitor of mitogen-activated extracellular signal-regulated kinase (MEK) 1 and MEK2, is an antineoplastic agent. MEK proteins are upstream regulators of the extracellular signal-related kinase (ERK) pathway, which promotes cellular proliferation. Approximately 40–60% of cutaneous melanomas carry a b-Raf serine-threonine kinase (BRAF) mutation. The most common BRAF mutation is the substitution of glutamic acid for valine at codon 600 in exon 15 (BRAF V600E); a less frequently occurring BRAF mutation is the substitution of lysine for valine at codon 600 in exon 15 (BRAF V600K). BRAF V600 mutations result in activation of the BRAF pathway that includes MEK 1 and 2. The mutation of BRAF V600E activates the mitogen-activated protein kinase (MAPK) and ERK signal transduction pathway, which enhances cell proliferation and tumor progression (e.g., metastasis). In vitro studies have demonstrated that binimetinib inhibits phosphorylation of ERK in cell-free assays and MEK-dependent phosphorylation of melanoma cells harboring BRAF mutation. The drug also has demonstrated inhibition of ERK phosphorylation and tumor growth in xenograft models of melanoma harboring BRAF mutation in mice.

Clinical resistance to monotherapy with a BRAF inhibitor, generally occurring 6–7 months following initiation of therapy, has been attributed to several possible resistance mechanisms mostly relying on reactivation of the MAPK/ERK pathway. Complete inhibition of the MAPK/ERK pathway resulting in durable responses may be achieved with the use of combination therapy with a BRAF inhibitor (i.e., dabrafenib, encorafenib, vemurafenib) and an MEK inhibitor (i.e., binimetinib, cobimetinib, trametinib). In vitro, use of binimetinib in combination with encorafenib resulted in increased antiproliferative activity compared with either drug alone in BRAF mutation-positive cell lines. The combination of binimetinib and encorafenib also has demonstrated increased inhibition of tumor growth and delayed emergence of resistance compared with either drug alone in xenograft models of melanoma harboring BRAF V600E mutation in mice.

Following oral administration of binimetinib 45 mg twice daily, at least 50% of the dose is rapidly absorbed with peak plasma concentrations occurring in 1.6 hours. Peak plasma concentrations and systemic exposure of binimetinib and its active metabolite (M3) are proportional to dose following single or repeated administration of the drug over the dosage range of 5–80 mg or 5–60 mg once daily, respectively. Repeated administration of binimetinib 45 mg twice daily resulted in a 1.5-fold binimetinib accumulation ratio. Administration of a single 45-mg dose of binimetinib with a high-fat, high-calorie meal (approximately 150 calories from protein, 350 calories from carbohydrates, 500 calories from fat) did not affect systemic exposure of the drug in healthy individuals. Binimetinib is highly bound (97%) to plasma proteins. The mean terminal half-life of binimetinib is 3.5 hours. Binimetinib is metabolized principally by uridine diphosphate-glucuronosyltransferase (UGT) 1A1 and, to a lesser extent, by N-dealkylation and amide hydrolysis by cytochrome P-450 (CYP) isoenzymes 1A2 and 2C19 to form its minor active metabolite (M3). Following oral administration of a single radiolabeled dose of binimetinib, 62% of the radioactivity was recovered in feces (32% of the dose as unchanged drug) and 31% was recovered in urine (6.5% of the dose as unchanged drug). Single agent MEK inhibitor treatment is no longer recommended by experts as combination BRAF/MEK inhibition has demonstrated superior outcomes with a similar safety profile.

The pharmacokinetics of binimetinib do not appear to be affected substantially by age (20–94 years), gender, body weight, or UGT1A1 genotype.

ADVICE TO PATIENTS

- Advise patients to read the manufacturer's patient information.

- If a dose of binimetinib is missed by >6 hours or vomited, instruct patients to administer the next dose at the regularly scheduled time. A replacement dose should not be administered.

- Risk of hemorrhage. Advise patients to contact a clinician promptly and seek immediate medical attention if signs and/or symptoms of unusual bleeding (e.g., headache, dizziness, weakness, blood in stool, coughing up blood, vomiting blood) occur.

- Risk of venous thromboembolism (VTE). Advise patients to contact a clinician promptly and seek immediate medical attention if sudden onset of breathing difficulty, chest pain, leg pain, or swelling occurs.

- Risk of cardiomyopathy. Advise patients to contact a clinician promptly if manifestations of heart failure (e.g., tachycardia, shortness of breath, peripheral edema, feeling lightheaded) occur.

- Risk of serous retinopathy or retinal vein occlusion. Advise patients to contact a clinician promptly if ocular pain, swelling, redness, changes in vision, or blurred vision occurs.

- Risk of interstitial lung disease. Advise patients to contact a clinician if new or progressive pulmonary symptoms (e.g., cough, dyspnea) occur.

- Risk of hepatotoxicity. Advise patients of the importance of liver function test monitoring before and during binimetinib therapy. Instruct patients to report any possible manifestations of hepatotoxicity (e.g., jaundice, dark or tea-colored urine, nausea, vomiting, fatigue, loss of appetite, bruising, bleeding).

- Risk of rhabdomyolysis. Advise patients of the importance of monitoring CK concentrations before and during binimetinib therapy. Instruct patients to immediately report any possible manifestations of rhabdomyolysis (e.g., dark or red urine, muscle pain, unusual or new-onset weakness).

- Risk of new primary malignancy. Advise patients to contact their clinician immediately for any new skin lesions, changes to existing skin lesions, or other signs and symptoms of malignancies.

- Risk of fetal harm. Advise women of childbearing potential that they should use an effective method of contraception while receiving the drug and for ≥30 days after the last dose. Advise women to inform their clinicians if they are or plan to become pregnant. Apprise patient of potential fetal hazard if used during pregnancy.

- Advise women to avoid breast-feeding while receiving binimetinib and for 3 days after the last dose.

- Advise patients to inform their clinicians of existing or contemplated concomitant therapy, including prescription and OTC drugs and herbal supplements, as well as any concomitant illnesses.

- Advise patients of other important precautionary information.

PREPARATIONS

Binimetinib can only be obtained through select specialty pharmacies. Contact the manufacturer or consult the Braftovi® and Mektovi® website for specific availability information (https://braftovimektovi.pfizerpro.com/)

Excipients in commercially available drug preparations may have clinically important effects in some individuals; consult specific product labeling for details.

Binimetinib

Oral		
Tablets, film-coated	15 mg	**Mektovi®**, Array BioPharma

† Use is not currently included in the labeling approved by the US Food and Drug Administration.

Selected Revisions May 10, 2024, © Copyright, July 16, 2018, American Society of Health-System Pharmacists, Inc.

Bortezomib

10:00 • ANTINEOPLASTIC AGENTS

■ Bortezomib, an inhibitor of the 26S proteasome, is an antineoplastic agent.

USES

● Multiple Myeloma

Previously Untreated Multiple Myeloma

Bortezomib is used in combination with melphalan and prednisone for the treatment of previously untreated multiple myeloma.

The current indication for bortezomib in patients with previously untreated multiple myeloma is based principally on the results of a phase 3, open-label, randomized study (Velcade as Initial Standard Therapy in Multiple Myeloma: Assessment with Melphalan and Prednisone [VISTA]) involving 682 patients with newly diagnosed multiple myeloma who were considered ineligible (e.g., because of a coexisting medical condition, an age of 65 years or older) for high-dose chemotherapy followed by stem cell transplantation. Patients were assigned to receive either melphalan plus prednisone (MP) or bortezomib plus melphalan and prednisone (VMP). Patients were stratified according to their baseline β_2-microglobulin concentration (less than 2.5, 2.5–5.5, or above 5.5 mg/L), baseline serum albumin concentration (below 3.5 g/dL, equal to or above 3.5 g/dL), and the geographic region where they received treatment. The planned course of therapy for both regimens was 9 six-week courses for a total treatment duration of 54 weeks. Patients in the control group received melphalan 9 mg/m² orally plus prednisone 60 mg/m² orally (both administered once daily on days 1–4). Patients in the study group received the same regimen of melphalan plus prednisone with the addition of bortezomib (1.3 mg/m² by IV injection) on days 1, 4, 8, 11, 22, 25, 29, and 32 during cycles 1–4; during cycles 5–9, bortezomib was administered on days 1, 8, 22, and 29.

At the time of the initial interim analysis (median follow-up of 16.3 months), the complete response rates, defined by immunofixation negativity and using the European Group for Blood and Marrow Transplantation (EBMT) response criteria, were 30 and 4% for VMP and MP, respectively; rates for partial response or better (i.e., partial plus complete) were 69 and 34%, respectively. Using the International Uniform Response criteria, rates for partial response or better (i.e., partial response plus very good partial response plus complete response) were 74 and 39%, respectively, for VMP and MP. The median time to disease progression (20.7 months versus 15 months) and median progression-free survival (18.3 versus 14 months) were prolonged with VMP compared with MP. This study was terminated prematurely at the request of the independent data monitoring committee because of improved time to disease progression, tumor response rate, and progression-free and overall survival observed during the initial prespecified interim analysis in patients receiving VMP. Updated analysis of overall survival after a median follow-up of 36.7 months indicated a survival benefit (hazard ratio of 0.65) in patients receiving VMP despite subsequent therapies, including bortezomib-based regimens. After a median follow-up of 60.1 months, analysis of data also indicated that median overall survival was prolonged in patients receiving VMP compared with those receiving MP (56.4 versus 43.1 months, respectively; hazard ratio of 0.7). No important differences in the complete response rates, time to progression, or overall survival were reported for patients with impaired renal function (i.e., creatinine clearance less than 60 mL/minute) compared with patients with normal renal function in the VMP group. Similar complete response rates (28%), time to progression, and overall survival rates were reported for patients with high-risk cytogenetic features (e.g., t(4;14), t(14;16) translocation; a 17p or 13q deletion) receiving VMP compared with standard-risk patients.

Results from this study demonstrated superiority of the VMP regimen compared with the MP regimen for previously untreated patients ineligible for peripheral blood stem cell transplantation and for patients older than 65 years of age.

Relapsed Multiple Myeloma

Bortezomib is used alone for the treatment of relapsed multiple myeloma in patients who have received at least one prior therapy, including those who previously responded to bortezomib-containing therapy and relapsed at least 6 months following completion of therapy.

The current indication for bortezomib in patients with relapsed multiple myeloma is based principally on the results of a phase 3, randomized, open-label study involving 669 patients and several open-label studies in more than 250 patients with multiple myeloma.

In the prospective phase 3 open-label study, random assignment of patients with progressive multiple myeloma was stratified according to number of lines of prior therapy (1 versus greater than 1 line), time of progression relative to prior treatment (during or within 6 months of stopping most recent therapy versus greater than 6 months following completion of most recent therapy), and screening β_2-microglobulin concentration (2.5 mg/L or less versus greater than 2.5 mg/L). Exclusion criteria included disease refractory to prior therapy with high-dose dexamethasone, grade 2 or higher peripheral neuropathy at baseline, or platelet count less than 50,000/mm³. Treatment regimens consisted of either bortezomib or high-dose dexamethasone according to the following schedules: bortezomib (1.3 mg/m² by IV bolus injection) administered in a 3-week standard treatment cycle (twice weekly for 2 weeks on days 1, 4, 8, and 11 followed by a 10-day rest period) for 8 cycles followed by 5-week maintenance treatment cycles (once weekly for 4 weeks on days 1, 8, 15, and 22 followed by a 13-day rest period) for 3 cycles; or dexamethasone (40 mg orally) administered in a 5-week standard treatment cycle (once daily on days 1–4, 9–12, and 17–20, followed by a 15-day rest period) for 4 cycles followed by 4-week maintenance treatment cycles (once daily on days 1–4 followed by a 24-day rest period) for 5 cycles. Patients experiencing progression of disease during dexamethasone therapy were offered enrollment in a companion study allowing crossover to bortezomib therapy. Bortezomib was administered for a maximum of 11 cycles (9 months). Responses and disease progression were assessed according to EBMT response criteria. A complete response was defined as less than 5% plasma cells in the bone marrow, 100% reduction in serum myeloma (M) protein, and a negative immunofixation test; a partial response was defined as reductions in myeloma protein concentrations of at least 50% in serum and at least 90% in urine on at least 2 occasions for a minimum of 6 weeks, and stable bone disease and normal serum calcium concentrations.

At a planned interim analysis, the study was terminated early and patients receiving dexamethasone were offered therapy with bortezomib. At the time of early termination of the study, at a median follow-up of 8.3 months, prolonged median time to progression of disease (6.2 versus 3.5 months), prolonged survival (hazard ratio of 0.57), and higher response rates (complete plus partial responses) (38 versus 18%) were observed in patients receiving bortezomib compared with those receiving dexamethasone. Overall survival was prolonged in patients receiving bortezomib, both for those who had received one prior treatment (hazard ratio of 0.39) and for those who had received more than one prior treatment (hazard ratio of 0.65). The median duration of response was 8 months in patients receiving bortezomib and 5.6 months in patients receiving dexamethasone. A higher response rate was observed in patients receiving bortezomib regardless of baseline β_2-microglobulin concentration. Limitations of the study that may have affected the outcome include previous corticosteroid therapy in most patients, higher dose intensity for bortezomib than dexamethasone, and the short period of follow-up. Patients receiving bortezomib experienced a greater frequency of grade 3 toxicity (61 versus 44%) than patients receiving dexamethasone.

The primary phase 2 efficacy study enrolled 202 patients with multiple myeloma who had received at least 2 prior chemotherapy regimens and had experienced disease progression following the most recent regimen; patients in this study had received a median of 6 prior chemotherapy regimens, and 64% of patients had received prior stem cell transplantation or other high-dose therapy. Ninety-eight percent of enrolled patients received the standard 21-day regimen of bortezomib (1.3 mg/m² by IV injection twice weekly for 2 weeks on days 1, 4, 8, and 11, followed by a 10-day rest period) with subsequent doses adjusted as needed if serious adverse effects occurred; patients exhibiting progressive disease after 2 cycles or stable disease after 4 cycles were eligible to receive oral dexamethasone (20 mg) on the day of and the day after each dose of bortezomib. A mean of 6 treatment cycles was administered.

Using the EBMT response criteria, complete responses or partial responses were observed in 3 or 25%, respectively, of 188 evaluable patients receiving bortezomib. Clinical remission, as determined by the Southwest Oncology Group (SWOG) criteria (defined as reductions in serum M protein concentrations of at least 75% in serum and/or 90% in urine on at least 2 occasions for a minimum of at least 6 weeks, and stable bone disease and normal serum calcium concentrations), was observed in 18% of these patients. Among the 202 enrolled patients, the median time to first response was 38 days, and median survival was 17 months. In this study, response to bortezomib was not influenced by gender, type of myeloma, serum concentrations of β_2-microglobulin, or number or types of prior chemotherapy treatments. However, the likelihood of attaining a response was reduced in patients with more than 50% plasma cells or abnormal cytogenetics in the bone marrow. Responses were observed in patients with or without chromosome 13 abnormalities.

In a small dose-response phase 2 study in 54 patients with relapsed multiple myeloma, the overall response rate (complete plus partial responses) was approximately 30 or 38% in patients receiving bortezomib 1 or 1.3 mg/m², respectively, by IV injection twice weekly for 2 weeks on days 1, 4, 8, and 11, followed by a 10-day rest period. A mean of 7 or 6 treatment cycles was administered in patients receiving the 1- or 1.3-mg/m² dose, respectively.

Patients from the two phase 2 studies who were expected to benefit from extended therapy were able to continue receiving bortezomib therapy beyond 8 cycles in an extension study. A total of 63 patients from the phase 2 multiple myeloma studies were enrolled and received a median of 7 additional cycles of bortezomib therapy for a total median of 14 cycles (range: 7–32 cycles). The overall median dosing intensity in this study was similar to that in the phase 2 studies. In this study, 67% of patients initiated bortezomib at the same or higher dose intensity compared with that used at the end of the phase 2 studies, and 89% of patients maintained the standard 3-week dosing schedule during the study. No new cumulative or long-term toxicities were observed with prolonged bortezomib treatment.

Efficacy and safety of retreatment with bortezomib (with or without dexamethasone) is based principally on the results of a phase 2 open-label study involving 130 adults with multiple myeloma who had previously achieved at least a partial response to bortezomib-based therapy but had relapsed 6 or more months following completion of therapy. In this study, patients received the last tolerated dose of bortezomib (up to 1.3 mg/m² by IV injection) on days 1, 4, 8, and 11 of each 21-day cycle for up to 8 cycles; however, lower doses of bortezomib could be increased to 1.3 mg/m². Patients who had received treatment for multiple myeloma (except for maintenance therapy with an immunomodulatory agent or corticosteroid) following the prior course of bortezomib therapy and those with baseline grade 2 or greater peripheral neuropathy or neuropathic pain were excluded from the study. The primary measure of efficacy was best confirmed response according to EBMT response criteria. The overall best confirmed response rate was 38.5%; complete response was achieved in 1 patient. At the time of analysis, the median duration of response for all responders was 6.5 months (range: 0.6–19.3 months). Results of a subgroup analysis suggested that the drug's effect on overall response rate decreased with increasing number of prior therapies. The overall response rate with bortezomib retreatment appeared to be higher in patients who had achieved a complete response rather than a partial response to prior bortezomib-based therapy.

Subcutaneous Versus IV Administration

Efficacy and safety of bortezomib administered by subcutaneous injection are based principally on the results of an open-label, randomized, phase 3 study (MMY-3021) in patients with relapsed multiple myeloma who had not previously received bortezomib. Patients with baseline grade 2 or greater peripheral neuropathy or neuropathic pain or platelet count less than 50,000/mm³ were excluded from the study. In this study, 222 patients were randomized in a 2:1 ratio to receive bortezomib 1.3 mg/m² by either subcutaneous or IV injection on days 1, 4, 8, and 11 of each 21-day cycle for up to 8 cycles. The median number of cycles of bortezomib administered by either route was 8. Patients with a suboptimal response (less than a complete response, without disease progression) after 4 cycles could receive oral dexamethasone (20 mg on the day of and the day after bortezomib administration); approximately one-half of patients in both treatment groups received oral dexamethasone. The primary objective of the study was to show that single-agent bortezomib administered by subcutaneous injection retains at least 60% of the overall response rate attained after 4 cycles with single-agent IV bortezomib.

At a median follow-up of 11.8 months, no significant difference in median time to progression (10.4 versus 9.4 months, respectively), median progression-free survival (10.2 versus 8 months, respectively), and 1-year overall survival (72.6 versus 76.7%, respectively) were observed in patients receiving bortezomib by subcutaneous injection compared with those receiving the drug by IV injection. The overall response rates with subcutaneous and IV injection were 43 and 42%, respectively, following 4 cycles of bortezomib and 53 and 51%, respectively, following 8 cycles; complete response rates following 8 cycles of bortezomib were 11 and 12%, respectively. Overall response rates, median time to progression, median progression-free survival, and overall survival remained similar in

both groups at the time of the final analysis after a median follow-up of 17.3 or 17.8 months for patients receiving subcutaneous or IV bortezomib, respectively. Adverse effects generally were similar in both treatment groups, although grade 3 or 4 neuralgia (3 versus 9%), peripheral neuropathy (6 versus 15%), neutropenia (13 versus 18%), and thrombocytopenia (8 versus 16%) occurred less frequently in patients receiving bortezomib by subcutaneous injection compared with those receiving the drug by IV injection.

Induction Therapy Prior to Stem Cell Transplantation in Newly Diagnosed Multiple Myeloma

Bortezomib has been studied as a component of various induction regimens for newly diagnosed multiple myeloma in transplant-eligible patients†.

Bortezomib and Dexamethasone

Efficacy and safety of bortezomib in combination with dexamethasone† as induction therapy for newly diagnosed multiple myeloma in transplant-eligible patients† have been studied in an open-label, randomized phase 3 study (IFM 2005-01).

In the IFM 2005-01 study, 482 patients with previously untreated multiple myeloma were randomized to receive bortezomib in combination with dexamethasone (bortezomib-dexamethasone) or the combination of vincristine, doxorubicin, and dexamethasone (vincristine-doxorubicin-dexamethasone) as an induction regimen; both regimens were administered with or without dexamethasone, cyclophosphamide, etoposide, and cisplatin (DCEP) consolidation therapy. Patients receiving the bortezomib-dexamethasone induction regimen received bortezomib 1.3 mg/m² as an IV injection on days 1, 4, 8, and 11 of each 3-week cycle for 4 cycles along with dexamethasone 40 mg orally on days 1–4 and 9–12 during cycles 1 and 2 and then on days 1–4 of cycles 3 and 4. Those receiving the vincristine-doxorubicin-dexamethasone induction regimen received vincristine sulfate 0.4 mg and doxorubicin hydrochloride 9 mg/m² per day by continuous IV infusion on days 1–4 of each 4-week cycle for 4 cycles along with dexamethasone 40 mg orally on days 1–4, 9–12, and 17–20 during cycles 1 and 2 and then on days 1–4 of cycles 3 and 4. The median age of patients enrolled in the study was 57.1 years; 22% had International Staging System (ISS) stage III disease, 57.5% had a baseline β_2-microglobulin concentration exceeding 3 mg/L, 42.3% had chromosome 13 deletion (del(13)), and 14.3% had t(4;14) translocation with or without chromosome 17p deletion (del(17p)).

The primary measure of efficacy was complete plus near-complete response rate following induction therapy. Tumor responses were assessed using EBMT response criteria. The postinduction complete plus near-complete response rate (14.8 versus 6.4%) and the postinduction overall response rate (78.5 versus 62.8%) were higher in patients receiving bortezomib-dexamethasone compared with those receiving vincristine-doxorubicin-dexamethasone. The complete plus near-complete response rate also was higher following initial transplantation (35 versus 18.4%) and overall (39.5 versus 22.5%), including responses following second transplants when required, in patients receiving bortezomib-dexamethasone compared with those receiving vincristine-doxorubicin-dexamethasone. Postinduction response rates were higher in patients receiving bortezomib-dexamethasone compared with those receiving vincristine-doxorubicin-dexamethasone regardless of disease stage or presence of high-risk cytogenetic features (i.e., del(13), t(4;14) translocation and/or del(17p) chromosomal abnormality). Among patients who received bortezomib-dexamethasone induction therapy, rates of attaining a very good partial response or better were similar regardless of disease stage, use of consolidation therapy, or presence of the t(4;14) translocation with or without del(17p), but were slightly higher in patients with del(13) compared with those without this chromosomal abnormality. Following initial autologous stem cell transplantation, 38.6% of patients who had received bortezomib-dexamethasone induction therapy required a second stem cell transplant compared with 56% of those who had received vincristine-doxorubicin-dexamethasone. Although median overall survival had not been reached at a median follow-up of 32.2 months, median progression-free survival at a median follow-up of 31.2 months was numerically, but not significantly, longer in patients who received induction therapy with bortezomib-dexamethasone compared with those who received vincristine-doxorubicin-dexamethasone (36 versus 29.7 months).

Infection (48.1 versus 38.1%), peripheral neuropathy (45.6 versus 28%), thrombocytopenia (10.9 versus 4.6%), and herpes zoster infection (9.2 versus 2.1%) occurred more frequently in patients receiving bortezomib-dexamethasone, while neutropenia (13.8 versus 8%) and thrombosis (12.1 versus 4.6%) occurred more frequently in patients receiving vincristine-doxorubicin-dexamethasone.

Based on current evidence, use of bortezomib in combination with dexamethasone may be considered a reasonable choice (accepted, with possible conditions) as induction therapy for newly diagnosed multiple myeloma in transplant-eligible patients; factors that should be considered when selecting a combination chemotherapy regimen for use as induction therapy include performance status and pre-existing conditions (e.g., peripheral neuropathy).

Bortezomib, Dexamethasone, and Thalidomide

Efficacy and safety of bortezomib in combination with thalidomide and dexamethasone† (bortezomib-thalidomide-dexamethasone) as induction therapy for newly diagnosed multiple myeloma in transplant-eligible patients† have been studied in several phase 3, open-label, randomized studies.

The GIMEMA and PETHEMA/GEM studies compared bortezomib-thalidomide-dexamethasone with the combination of thalidomide and dexamethasone (thalidomide-dexamethasone). In the GIMEMA study, 480 patients were randomized to receive bortezomib-thalidomide-dexamethasone or thalidomide-dexamethasone; both induction regimens were followed by tandem autologous stem cell transplantation and consolidation therapy with the same drug combination used for induction therapy. Patients receiving bortezomib-thalidomide-dexamethasone induction therapy received bortezomib 1.3 mg/m^2 as an IV injection on days 1, 4, 8, and 11 along with thalidomide 200 mg orally daily (after initial dose escalation during cycle 1) and dexamethasone 40 mg orally on days 1, 2, 4, 5, 8, 9, 11, and 12 of each 21-day cycle. Those receiving thalidomide-dexamethasone induction therapy received the same dosage of thalidomide; however, dexamethasone 40 mg was administered orally on days 1–4 and 9–12 of each 21-day cycle. Both regimens were continued for a total of 3 cycles. In the PETHEMA/GEM study, 386 patients were randomized to receive bortezomib-thalidomide-dexamethasone, thalidomide-dexamethasone, or alternating cycles of vincristine, carmustine, melphalan, cyclophosphamide, and prednisone (VBMCP) and vincristine, carmustine, doxorubicin, and dexamethasone (VBAD) followed by bortezomib as induction therapy. Patients receiving bortezomib-thalidomide-dexamethasone received bortezomib 1.3 mg/m^2 as an IV injection on days 1, 4, 8, and 11 along with thalidomide 200 mg orally daily (after initial dose escalation during cycle 1) and dexamethasone 40 mg orally on days 1–4 and 9–12 of each 4-week cycle for 6 cycles. Patients receiving thalidomide-dexamethasone received the same dosages of thalidomide and dexamethasone. Those receiving VBMCP/VBAD received each regimen in alternating cycles for 4 cycles followed by two 3-week cycles of bortezomib 1.3 mg/m^2 administered as an IV injection on days 1, 4, 8, and 11. In the GIMEMA study, the primary measure of efficacy was postinduction complete plus near-complete response rate. In the PETHEMA/GEM study, the primary measures of efficacy were postinduction and posttransplant complete response rates. In both studies, responses were assessed according to EBMT response criteria. In both studies, a higher postinduction response rate and prolonged progression-free survival were observed in patients who received bortezomib-thalidomide-dexamethasone compared with those who received the comparator regimens; however, addition of bortezomib to thalidomide and dexamethasone induction therapy did not provide an overall survival benefit in either study.

In the GIMEMA study, postinduction complete plus near-complete response rate was 31% in patients receiving bortezomib-thalidomide-dexamethasone compared with 11% in those receiving thalidomide-dexamethasone; improved responses also were observed with bortezomib-thalidomide-dexamethasone following first (52 versus 31%) and second (55 versus 41%) autologous stem cell transplants and subsequent consolidation therapy (62 versus 45%). The median time to best complete or near-complete response was shorter in patients receiving bortezomib-thalidomide-dexamethasone compared with those receiving thalidomide-dexamethasone (9 versus 14 months). At a median follow-up of 36 months, progression-free survival was prolonged in patients who received bortezomib-thalidomide-dexamethasone compared with those who received thalidomide-dexamethasone (hazard ratio 0.63); however, no difference in estimated 3-year overall survival (86 versus 84%, respectively) was observed between the groups. Subgroup analysis based on poor prognostic factors (i.e., older than 60 years of age, advanced disease stage, elevated serum LDH concentration, high infiltration of bone marrow plasma cells, del(13q), t(4;14) translocation with or without del(17p) chromosomal abnormality) suggested that the progression-free survival benefit of bortezomib-thalidomide-dexamethasone was consistent across these subgroups; however, because the proportion of patients with the del(17p) chromosomal abnormality was substantially smaller than the proportion of patients with other high-risk cytogenetic abnormalities, the effect of bortezomib-thalidomide-dexamethasone on progression-free survival in patients with the del(17p) chromosomal abnormality was not evaluated.

In the PETHEMA/GEM study, the complete response rate (35 versus 14%) was higher following induction therapy with bortezomib-thalidomide-dexamethasone compared with thalidomide-dexamethasone; improved complete response rates also were maintained following autologous stem cell transplantation (46 versus 24%). Among patients evaluated for high-risk cytogenetic features, 21% had high-risk features (i.e., t(4;14), t(14;16), and/or del(17p) chromosomal abnormalities); 64 or 31% of these patients had t(4;14) or del(17p) chromosomal abnormalities, respectively. Among the patients with high-risk cytogenetic features, complete response rate was substantially higher in patients who received bortezomib-thalidomide-dexamethasone compared with those who received thalidomide-dexamethasone (35 versus 0%); complete responses were achieved in 38 or 58% of patients receiving bortezomib-thalidomide-dexamethasone who had t(4;14) or del(17p) chromosomal abnormalities, respectively, compared with 0% of patients receiving thalidomide-dexamethasone who had either chromosomal abnormality. At a median follow-up of 35.2 months, median progression-free survival was prolonged in patients who received bortezomib-thalidomide-dexamethasone compared with those who received thalidomide-dexamethasone (56.2 versus 28.2 months); however, no difference in estimated 4-year overall survival (74 versus 65%, respectively) was observed between the treatment groups.

In both the GIMEMA and PETHEMA/GEM studies, grade 3 or 4 peripheral neuropathy occurred more frequently in patients receiving bortezomib-thalidomide-dexamethasone (10 and 14%, respectively) compared with those receiving thalidomide-dexamethasone (2 and 5%, respectively).

In the third study (IFM2013-04), 340 patients were randomized to receive bortezomib by subcutaneous injection in combination with thalidomide and dexamethasone or in combination with cyclophosphamide and dexamethasone. Patients receiving bortezomib-thalidomide-dexamethasone received bortezomib 1.3 mg/m^2 by subcutaneous injection on days 1, 4, 8, and 11 along with thalidomide 100 mg orally daily and dexamethasone 40 mg orally on days 1–4 and 9–12 of each 3-week cycle. Those receiving bortezomib-cyclophosphamide-dexamethasone received the same dosages of bortezomib and dexamethasone along with cyclophosphamide 500 mg/m^2 orally on days 1, 8, and 15 of each 3-week cycle. Both induction regimens were continued for a total of 4 cycles. The median age of patients enrolled in the study was approximately 60 years; 22% had ISS stage III disease, and 18% had t(4;14) translocation and/or del(17p) chromosomal abnormalities. The primary measure of efficacy was the rate of very good partial response or better, as assessed according to the International Myeloma Working Group Uniform Response criteria, following induction therapy. Overall response rate (92.3 versus 83.4%) and the rate of very good partial response or better (66.3 versus 56.2%) based on intent-to-treat analysis were higher following induction therapy with bortezomib-thalidomide-dexamethasone compared with bortezomib-cyclophosphamide-dexamethasone; however, no significant difference in complete response rate was observed between the treatment groups. Grade 2 or greater peripheral neuropathy (21.9 versus 12.9%) occurred more frequently in patients receiving bortezomib-thalidomide-dexamethasone, while grade 3 or 4 neutropenia (33.1 versus 18.9%), thrombocytopenia (10.6 versus 4.7%), and anemia (9.5 versus 4.1%) occurred more frequently in patients receiving bortezomib-cyclophosphamide-dexamethasone.

Because peripheral neuropathy occurs frequently with bortezomib- and thalidomide-based induction regimens, a modified bortezomib-thalidomide-dexamethasone induction regimen was compared with bortezomib-dexamethasone in another phase 3 study in 199 patients. Patients receiving bortezomib-dexamethasone received bortezomib 1.3 mg/m^2 as an IV injection on days 1, 4, 8, and 11 of each 3-week cycle for 4 cycles along with dexamethasone 40 mg orally on days 1–4 and 9–12 during cycles 1 and 2 and then on days 1–4 during cycles 3 and 4. Patients receiving the modified bortezomib-thalidomide-dexamethasone regimen received the same dosage of dexamethasone along with bortezomib 1 mg/m^2 as an IV injection on days 1, 4, 8, and 11 and thalidomide 100 mg orally daily during each 3-week cycle for 4 cycles. In patients with an inadequate (less than partial) response after 2 cycles of the modified bortezomib-thalidomide-dexamethasone regimen (7% of patients receiving the regimen), the dose of bortezomib was increased to 1.3 mg/m^2 and the dosage of thalidomide was increased to 200 mg daily during subsequent cycles. The median age of patients enrolled in the study was approximately 58 years; 22% had ISS stage III disease and, among those with cytogenetic test results, 20% had t(4;14) translocation or del(17p) chromosomal abnormalities. The primary measure of efficacy was complete response rate, as assessed according to the International Myeloma Working Group Uniform Response criteria, following induction therapy. The rate of very good partial response or better following induction therapy was higher with bortezomib-thalidomide-dexamethasone compared with bortezomib-dexamethasone (49 versus

36%); however, postinduction complete response (13 and 12%, respectively) and overall response (88 and 81%, respectively) rates were similar for both treatment groups. At a median follow-up of 32 months, median progression-free survival was similar in patients who received bortezomib-thalidomide-dexamethasone compared with those who received bortezomib-dexamethasone (26 versus 30 months, respectively). Peripheral neuropathy occurred more frequently in patients receiving bortezomib-dexamethasone compared with those receiving bortezomib-thalidomide-dexamethasone (70 versus 53%).

Use of bortezomib in combination with thalidomide and dexamethasone also was investigated in an open-label, noncomparative phase 2 study in 98 patients randomized to receive bortezomib-thalidomide-dexamethasone with or without cyclophosphamide. Patients receiving bortezomib-thalidomide-dexamethasone received bortezomib 1.3 mg/m^2 as an IV injection on days 1, 4, 8, and 11 along with thalidomide 100 mg orally daily and dexamethasone 40 mg orally on days 1–4 and 9–12 of each 21-day cycle. Patients receiving bortezomib-thalidomide-dexamethasone-cyclophosphamide received the same dosages of bortezomib, thalidomide, and dexamethasone along with cyclophosphamide 400 mg/m^2 IV on days 1 and 8 of each 21-day cycle. Both induction regimens were continued for a total of 4 cycles. Postinduction rates of overall response and complete plus near-complete response were 100 and 51%, respectively, in patients receiving bortezomib-thalidomide-dexamethasone and 94 and 43%, respectively, in those receiving bortezomib-thalidomide-dexamethasone-cyclophosphamide. At a median follow-up of 64.8 months, median progression-free survival was 56.3 months with bortezomib-thalidomide-dexamethasone and 36.3 months with bortezomib-thalidomide-dexamethasone-cyclophosphamide; the difference was not statistically significant and was largely related to an imbalance between treatment groups in the number of patients receiving subsequent therapy for relapsed disease prior to meeting the specified criteria for disease progression. A trend toward improved quality of life (assessed using the European Organisation for Research and Treatment of Cancer Quality of Life Questionnaire C30 [EORTC QLQ-C30] and EuroQoL EQ-5D health status questionnaire) was observed following the first posttransplantation follow-up visit in patients who received bortezomib-thalidomide-dexamethasone compared with those who received bortezomib-thalidomide-dexamethasone-cyclophosphamide.

Use of bortezomib-thalidomide-dexamethasone as induction therapy for newly diagnosed multiple myeloma in transplant-eligible patients has improved postinduction response rates and prolonged progression-free survival in several randomized controlled studies; however, the same benefits were not observed in a study evaluating a modified bortezomib-thalidomide-dexamethasone regimen (i.e., reduced bortezomib and thalidomide dosages). Therefore, the role of a modified bortezomib-thalidomide-dexamethasone regimen using reduced dosages of bortezomib and thalidomide is unclear. In addition, in the absence of studies including adequate numbers of patients with the del(17p) chromosomal abnormality, attempts to identify whether these patients might derive clinical benefit (e.g., prolonged progression-free survival) from bortezomib-thalidomide-dexamethasone induction therapy are speculative; additional studies are needed to identify subgroups of patients with high-risk cytogenetic features who might benefit from such therapy. The AHFS Oncology Expert Committee concluded that use of bortezomib in combination with thalidomide and dexamethasone as induction therapy for newly diagnosed multiple myeloma in transplant-eligible patients may be considered a reasonable choice (accepted; with possible conditions); however, use of a modified bortezomib-thalidomide-dexamethasone regimen using reduced dosages of bortezomib and thalidomide is not fully established because of unclear risk/benefit and/or inadequate experience. Factors that should be considered when selecting a combination chemotherapy regimen for use as induction therapy for newly diagnosed multiple myeloma in transplant-eligible patients include performance status and preexisting conditions (e.g., peripheral neuropathy).

Bortezomib, Dexamethasone, and Doxorubicin (or Pegylated Liposomal Doxorubicin)

Efficacy and safety of bortezomib in combination with dexamethasone and conventional doxorubicin† (bortezomib-doxorubicin-dexamethasone) as induction therapy for newly diagnosed multiple myeloma in transplant-eligible patients† have been studied in an open-label, randomized phase 3 study (HOVON-65/GMMG-HD4).

In the HOVON-65/GMMG-HD4 study, 827 patients with newly diagnosed multiple myeloma were randomized to receive conventional doxorubicin and dexamethasone in combination with either bortezomib or vincristine as an induction regimen. Patients receiving the bortezomib-doxorubicin-dexamethasone induction regimen received bortezomib 1.3 mg/m^2 as an IV injection on days 1, 4, 8, and 11 along with doxorubicin hydrochloride 9 mg/m^2 IV per day on days 1–4 and dexamethasone 40 mg orally on days 1–4, 9–12, and 17–20 during each 28-day cycle for 3 cycles. Those receiving the vincristine-doxorubicin-dexamethasone induction regimen received vincristine sulfate 0.4 mg and doxorubicin hydrochloride 9 mg/m^2 IV per day on days 1–4 and dexamethasone 40 mg orally on days 1–4, 9–12, and 17–20 during each 28-day cycle for 3 cycles. Patients who received bortezomib-doxorubicin-dexamethasone induction therapy received 2 years of maintenance therapy with bortezomib (1.3 mg/m^2 every 2 weeks) following stem cell transplantation, while those who received vincristine-doxorubicin-dexamethasone induction therapy received thalidomide (50 mg daily) as maintenance therapy. The median age of patients enrolled in the study was 57 years; 87% had World Health Organization (WHO) performance status of 0 or 1, and 23% had ISS stage III disease. Among patients for whom cytogenetic tests were performed, 43, 14, or 11% had del(13q), t(4;14) translocation, or del(17p13) chromosomal abnormalities, respectively.

The primary measure of efficacy in the HOVON-65/GMMG-HD4 study was progression-free survival. Tumor responses were assessed using EBMT response criteria. At a median follow-up of 41 months, patients who received bortezomib-doxorubicin-dexamethasone had prolonged progression-free survival (35 versus 28 months; hazard ratio: 0.75) and higher postinduction (11 versus 5%) and posttransplant (31 versus 15%) complete plus near-complete response rates compared with those who received vincristine-doxorubicin-dexamethasone. Median overall survival had not been reached at a median follow-up of 66 months; however, no significant difference in 5-year overall survival was observed between the groups. Subgroup analyses based on presence of renal insufficiency or high-risk cytogenetic features (i.e., del(13q14), t(4;14), del(17p13) chromosomal abnormalities) suggested prolonged progression-free and overall survival with bortezomib-doxorubicin-dexamethasone compared with vincristine-doxorubicin-dexamethasone induction therapy in patients with serum creatinine concentrations exceeding 2 mg/dL and in those with del(17p13) chromosomal abnormality, as well as an overall survival benefit for bortezomib-doxorubicin-dexamethasone compared with vincristine-doxorubicin-dexamethasone in patients with del(13q14) chromosomal abnormality. Herpes zoster (2 versus 0%) and grade 3 or 4 thrombocytopenia (10 versus 5%), GI toxicity (11 versus 7%), and peripheral neuropathy (24 versus 10%) occurred more frequently in patients receiving bortezomib-doxorubicin-dexamethasone compared with those receiving vincristine-doxorubicin-dexamethasone.

Use of bortezomib and dexamethasone also has been studied in combination with pegylated liposomal doxorubicin† (bortezomib-pegylated liposomal doxorubicin-dexamethasone) as induction therapy for previously untreated multiple myeloma† in 2 open-label, noncomparative phase 2 studies.

In the first study, 40 patients with newly diagnosed multiple myeloma received bortezomib 1.3 mg/m^2 as an IV injection on days 1, 4, 8, and 11 along with pegylated liposomal doxorubicin hydrochloride 30 mg/m^2 IV on day 4 and dexamethasone 40 mg orally on days 1, 2, 4, 5, 8, 9, 11, and 12 during cycle 1. During cycles 2–6, the same dosages of bortezomib and pegylated liposomal doxorubicin were administered, but the dexamethasone dosage was 20 mg orally daily. Treatment cycles were repeated every 3 weeks for a total of 6 cycles. Overall response rate and complete plus near-complete response rate were 85 and 38%, respectively, following 6 cycles of induction therapy with bortezomib-pegylated liposomal doxorubicin-dexamethasone. Among patients who underwent stem cell transplantation, the complete plus near-complete response rate increased to 57% following transplantation, but the overall response rate did not improve substantially. At a median follow-up of 45.1 months, median progression-free survival had not been reached; however, among patients who underwent stem cell transplantation, actuarial 2- and 4-year progression-free survival rates were 93 and 65%, respectively, and actuarial 2- and 4-year overall survival rates were 97 and 67%, respectively. Grade 1 or 2 peripheral neuropathy, fatigue, palmar-plantar erythrodysesthesia (hand-foot syndrome), and constipation occurred in 90, 88, 75, and 70% of patients, respectively.

Because bortezomib and pegylated liposomal doxorubicin frequently cause adverse effects, another phase 2 study evaluated a modified bortezomib-pegylated liposomal doxorubicin-dexamethasone regimen in 35 patients with previously untreated multiple myeloma. Patients received bortezomib 1 mg/m^2 as an IV injection, pegylated liposomal doxorubicin hydrochloride 5 mg/m^2 IV, and dexamethasone phosphate 40 mg IV on days 1, 4, 8, and 11 of each 28-day cycle for a maximum of 8 cycles. Overall response rate was 86%; complete response was achieved in 20% of patients. At a median follow-up of 17.7 months, median time to progression, duration of response, and overall survival had not been reached. Constipation, fatigue, peripheral neuropathy, insomnia, and nausea occurred in 51, 46, 34, 29, and 26%, respectively, of patients.

Based on current evidence, use of bortezomib in combination with doxorubicin (or pegylated liposomal doxorubicin) and dexamethasone as induction therapy for newly diagnosed multiple myeloma in transplant-eligible patients may be considered a reasonable choice (accepted; with possible conditions); however, in the absence of longer follow-up data, use of a modified bortezomib-pegylated liposomal doxorubicin-dexamethasone regimen (i.e., reduced dosages of bortezomib and pegylated liposomal doxorubicin) is not fully established because of unclear risk/benefit and/or inadequate experience. Factors that should be considered when selecting a combination chemotherapy regimen for use as induction therapy include performance status and preexisting conditions (e.g., peripheral neuropathy).

Bortezomib, Dexamethasone, and Cyclophosphamide

Efficacy and safety of bortezomib in combination with cyclophosphamide and dexamethasone† (bortezomib-cyclophosphamide-dexamethasone) as induction therapy for newly diagnosed multiple myeloma in transplant-eligible patients† have been studied in 2 noncomparative phase 2 studies and an open-label, randomized phase 3 study (GMMG-MM5).

In the first phase 2 study, patients with newly diagnosed multiple myeloma receiving bortezomib in combination with cyclophosphamide and dexamethasone were compared with a historical control group (34 patients who received lenalidomide 25 mg orally on days 1–21 and dexamethasone 40 mg orally on days 1–4, 9–12, and 17–20 during each 28-day cycle for 4 cycles). In this study, 33 patients received bortezomib 1.3 mg/m² as an IV injection twice weekly (days 1, 4, 8, and 11) along with cyclophosphamide 300 mg/m² orally on days 1, 8, 15, and 22 and dexamethasone 40 mg orally on days 1–4, 9–12, and 17–20 during each 28-day cycle for 4 cycles. The mean age of patients enrolled in the study was 60 years; 48% were female and 30% had ISS stage III disease. Among patients for whom cytogenetic tests were performed, 50, 18, or 13% had del(13q), t(4;14) translocation, or del(17) chromosomal abnormalities, respectively. The overall response rate and rate of very good partial response or better after 4 cycles of therapy were 88 and 61%, respectively, in patients who received bortezomib-cyclophosphamide-dexamethasone compared with 91 and 44%, respectively, in the historical control group based on intent-to-treat analysis. Among patients who underwent stem cell transplantation following bortezomib-cyclophosphamide-dexamethasone induction therapy, the posttransplant complete or near-complete response rate was 70%.

Patients from this study (twice-weekly bortezomib; cohort 1) also were compared with a subsequent cohort of 30 patients who received bortezomib 1.5 mg/m² as an IV injection once weekly (days 1, 8, 15, and 22) along with cyclophosphamide (same dosage as in cohort 1) and dexamethasone (same dosage as in cohort 1 during cycles 1 and 2, followed by 40 mg once weekly during cycles 3 and 4). Comparison of the 2 cohorts suggested that overall response rates and rates of very good partial response or better for the regimens containing once-weekly (93 and 60%, respectively) or twice-weekly (88 and 61%, respectively) bortezomib were similar; however, the incidences of grade 3 or 4 thrombocytopenia (0 versus 25%), neutropenia (7 versus 13%), anemia (0 versus 12%), and peripheral neuropathy (0 versus 7%) were lower in patients receiving the regimen containing once-weekly bortezomib compared with those receiving the regimen containing twice-weekly bortezomib. Analysis of pooled data for the 2 cohorts indicated a median progression-free survival of 40 months; in addition, 5-year progression-free and overall survival rates for the 2 cohorts combined were 42 and 70%, respectively. Although the overall response rate was similar in patients with high-risk cytogenetic features and those with standard-risk cytogenetic features, median progression-free survival was shorter and 5-year progression-free and overall survival rates were lower in patients with high-risk cytogenetic features (27.6 months, 33%, and 54%, respectively) compared with those with standard-risk cytogenetic features (55.7 months, 48%, and 81%, respectively).

In another phase 2 study, patients with newly diagnosed multiple myeloma received the combination of bortezomib-cyclophosphamide-dexamethasone followed by bortezomib-thalidomide-dexamethasone to determine if sequential combination therapy could improve response rates and tolerability. In this study, 44 patients received bortezomib 1.3 mg/m² as an IV injection on days 1, 4, 8, and 11 along with cyclophosphamide 300 mg/m² IV on days 1 and 8 and dexamethasone 40 mg orally on days 1, 2, 4, 5, 8, 9, 11, and 12 during each 21-day cycle for 3 cycles (cycles 1–3) followed by bortezomib 1 mg/m² as an IV injection on days 1, 4, 8, and

11 along with thalidomide 100 mg orally daily and dexamethasone 40 mg orally on days 1, 2, 4, 5, 8, 9, 11, and 12 during each 21-day cycle for 3 cycles (cycles 4–6). The median age of patients enrolled in the study was 58 years, and the median Karnofsky performance status was 90%; 60% of patients had ISS stage II or III disease, 49% had a baseline β₂-microglobulin concentration of 3.5 mg/L or greater, and 7 patients had cytogenetic abnormalities, including t(4;14) translocation, del(17p), and/or del(13) chromosomal abnormalities. Very good partial response or better was observed in 31 or 57% of 42 evaluable patients following 3 cycles of bortezomib-cyclophosphamide-dexamethasone or 6 cycles of sequential combination therapy, respectively; near-complete response or better was observed following 3 or 6 cycles of therapy in 2 or 36% of patients, respectively. At a median follow-up of 20.9 months, median event-free and overall survival had not been reached; however, estimated 1-year event-free and overall survival rates were 81 and 91%, respectively.

In the GMMG-MM5 study, 502 patients with newly diagnosed multiple myeloma were randomized to receive bortezomib in combination with either cyclophosphamide and dexamethasone or doxorubicin and dexamethasone. Patients receiving bortezomib-cyclophosphamide-dexamethasone received bortezomib 1.3 mg/m² as an IV injection on days 1, 4, 8, and 11 along with cyclophosphamide 900 mg/m² IV on day 1 and dexamethasone 40 mg orally on days 1, 2, 4, 5, 8, 9, 11, and 12 during each 21-day cycle. Those receiving bortezomib-doxorubicin-dexamethasone received the same dosage of bortezomib along with doxorubicin hydrochloride 9 mg/m² IV per day on days 1–4 and dexamethasone 20 mg orally on days 1–4, 9–12, and 17–20 of each 28-day cycle. Both regimens were continued for a total of 3 cycles. The route of administration for bortezomib was changed from IV to subcutaneous injection when data from a prior study in patients with relapsed multiple myeloma demonstrated no apparent loss in efficacy or increase in toxicity with subcutaneous administration. The median age of patients enrolled in the GMMG-MM5 study was 59 years, and 29% had ISS stage III disease. Among patients for whom cytogenetic tests were performed, 11, 11, or 40% had del(17p), t(4;14) translocation, or chromosome 1q21 duplication (i.e., 1q21 gain) abnormalities, respectively. The primary measure of efficacy was the rate of very good partial response or better, as assessed according to the International Myeloma Working Group Uniform Response criteria, following induction therapy.

Rates of overall response (78.1 versus 72.1%, respectively) and very good partial response or better (37 versus 34.3%, respectively) in the GMMG-MM5 study did not differ significantly between patients receiving bortezomib-cyclophosphamide-dexamethasone and those receiving bortezomib-doxorubicin-dexamethasone. In subgroups of patients with poor prognostic factors (i.e., t(4;14) translocation, del(17p), and/or 1q21 gain; renal impairment [serum creatinine concentration of 2 mg/dL or higher]), response rates attained with bortezomib-cyclophosphamide-dexamethasone appeared to be at least as high as those attained with bortezomib-doxorubicin-dexamethasone; the rate of progressive disease in patients with high-risk cytogenetic features, ISS stage III disease, or renal impairment appeared to be higher in those receiving bortezomib-doxorubicin-dexamethasone compared with those receiving bortezomib-cyclophosphamide-dexamethasone. In an exploratory analysis, overall response rates were similar with IV or subcutaneous injection of bortezomib, including in patients with poor prognostic factors. Grade 3 or greater leukopenia and/or neutropenia (35.2 versus 11.3%) occurred more frequently in patients receiving bortezomib-cyclophosphamide-dexamethasone, while grade 2 or greater neuropathy (14.9 versus 8.4%) occurred more frequently in patients receiving bortezomib-doxorubicin-dexamethasone.

Based on current evidence, use of bortezomib in combination with cyclophosphamide and dexamethasone may be considered a reasonable choice (accepted, with possible conditions) as induction therapy for newly diagnosed multiple myeloma in transplant-eligible patients; factors that should be considered when selecting a combination chemotherapy regimen for use as induction therapy include cytogenetic features, performance status, preexisting conditions (e.g., peripheral neuropathy), and tolerability.

● Non-Hodgkin's Lymphoma
Previously Untreated Mantle Cell Lymphoma

Bortezomib is used in combination with rituximab, cyclophosphamide, doxorubicin, and prednisone for the treatment of previously untreated mantle cell lymphoma.

The current indication for bortezomib in patients with previously untreated mantle cell lymphoma is based principally on the results of a phase 3, open-label, randomized study (LYM-3002) in patients with newly diagnosed stage II–IV mantle cell lymphoma who were considered ineligible for or were not considered for stem cell transplantation. In this study, 487 patients were randomized (stratified by International Prognostic Index [IPI] score and disease stage) in a 1:1 ratio to receive either rituximab plus cyclophosphamide, doxorubicin, vincristine, and prednisone (R-CHOP) or bortezomib plus rituximab, cyclophosphamide, doxorubicin, and prednisone (VR-CAP). The planned course of therapy for both regimens was six 21-day cycles; patients were permitted to receive up to 2 additional cycles if a response was first observed at cycle 6. Patients in the control group received rituximab 375 mg/m² IV, cyclophosphamide 750 mg/m² IV, doxorubicin hydrochloride 50 mg/m² IV, and vincristine sulfate 1.4 mg/m² (maximum dose of 2 mg) IV on day 1 plus prednisone 100 mg/m² orally on days 1–5 of each 21-day cycle. Patients in the study group received the same dosages of rituximab, cyclophosphamide, doxorubicin hydrochloride, and prednisone with the addition of bortezomib 1.3 mg/m² by IV injection on days 1, 4, 8, and 11 of each 21-day cycle. The median number of cycles for patients receiving R-CHOP or VR-CAP was 6; 17 or 14% of patients receiving R-CHOP or VR-CAP, respectively, received up to 2 additional cycles of their respective chemotherapy regimen. The primary end point of this study was progression-free survival as assessed by an independent review committee. The median age of patients enrolled in the study was 66 years; 74% of patients were male, 66% were white, 54% had an IPI score of 3 or greater, 76% had stage IV disease, and 69% had a positive bone marrow aspirate and/or bone marrow biopsy for mantle cell lymphoma.

At a median follow-up of 40 months, median progression-free survival was prolonged in patients who received VR-CAP compared with those who received R-CHOP (25 versus 14 months; hazard ratio of 0.63). The overall response rates with VR-CAP and R-CHOP were 88 and 85%, respectively, with 44% of patients receiving VR-CAP and 34% of those receiving R-CHOP achieving complete responses. Median overall survival had not been reached at the time of the analysis.

Relapsed Mantle Cell Lymphoma

Bortezomib is used for treatment of mantle cell lymphoma in patients who have received at least one prior therapy. The current indication for bortezomib in patients with relapsed mantle cell lymphoma is based principally on the results of a phase 2, open-label, single-arm, clinical study involving 155 patients (median age: 65 years; range: 42–89 years). Patients received bortezomib 1.3 mg/m² by IV injection administered in 21-day treatment cycles (on days 1, 4, 8, and 11 followed by a 10-day rest period on days 12–21) for a maximum of 17 cycles; patients achieving a complete response or an unconfirmed complete response were treated for 4 cycles beyond the first evidence of complete response or unconfirmed complete response. Therapy was discontinued if progressive disease or unacceptable toxicity occurred or based on a decision by the patient and clinician. The median number of cycles administered in all patients was 4; in responding patients, the median number of cycles was 8.

Responses were assessed according to International Workshop Response Criteria (IWRC) based on independent review of CT scans. The median time to response was 40 days (range: 31–204 days). The overall response rate (complete responses, unconfirmed complete responses, and partial responses) was 31%, and the median duration of response was 9.3 months. A complete response or an unconfirmed complete response was reported in 8%.

Other Non-Hodgkin's Lymphomas

Bortezomib is being investigated for use in the treatment of other non-Hodgkin's lymphomas†. In small phase 2 uncontrolled studies, bortezomib has shown activity in the treatment of relapsed or refractory B-cell lymphomas.

DOSAGE AND ADMINISTRATION

● General

Clinicians should consult the respective manufacturers' labelings for information on the dosage and method of administration of other antineoplastic agents used in combination regimens.

Because reactivation of latent varicella zoster virus infection has been reported in bortezomib-treated patients, the manufacturer recommends that antiviral prophylaxis be considered in patients receiving the drug.

● Reconstitution and Administration

Bortezomib is administered by IV injection (over 3–5 seconds) or by subcutaneous injection; the drug should *not* be administered by any other route. (See Cautions: Contraindications.) A sticker indicating the route of administration is provided by the manufacturer and should be affixed directly to the syringe following

reconstitution. Subcutaneous administration of bortezomib may be considered in patients with preexisting peripheral neuropathy and those at high risk for developing peripheral neuropathy. (See Relapsed Multiple Myeloma under Uses: Multiple Myeloma.) Recommended sites for subcutaneous injection of bortezomib include the thigh and abdominal region. Injection sites should be rotated, with new injections administered at least one inch from the previous injection site; any area that is tender, erythematous, bruised, or indurated should be avoided.

The manufacturer recommends that procedures for proper handling (e.g., use of gloves or protective clothing) and disposal of bortezomib be used.

Prior to administration, bortezomib powder for injection must be reconstituted using proper aseptic technique. The manufacturer states that only 0.9% sodium chloride injection should be used to reconstitute the lyophilized powder. The reconstituted bortezomib solution should be inspected visually for particulate matter and/or discoloration prior to administration and should be discarded if either is present.

For IV injection, bortezomib sterile powder for injection is reconstituted by adding 3.5 mL of 0.9% sodium chloride injection to a vial labeled as containing 3.5 mg of the drug to yield a final concentration of 1 mg/mL.

For subcutaneous injection, bortezomib sterile powder for injection is reconstituted by adding 1.4 mL of 0.9% sodium chloride injection to a vial labeled as containing 3.5 mg of the drug to yield a final concentration of 2.5 mg/mL. If local injection site reactions occur following subcutaneous administration of the drug at a reconstituted concentration of 2.5 mg/mL, the manufacturer states that the solution may be reconstituted to a lower concentration of 1 mg/mL; however, administration of subsequent doses of the drug by IV injection also should be considered.

Unreconstituted bortezomib powder for injection should be stored in unopened vials at a controlled room temperature of 25°C but may be exposed to temperatures ranging from 15–30°C. Unopened vials should be retained in the original package to protect from light. The reconstituted drug may be stored at 25°C in the original vial and/or syringe but should be administered within 8 hours after reconstitution.

● Dosage

The amount of bortezomib contained in one 3.5-mg vial may exceed the usual single dose required. Because the final concentration of reconstituted bortezomib solutions varies depending on the route of administration, caution should be exercised in calculating the dose and respective volume of bortezomib to be administered to prevent overdosage.

Previously Untreated Multiple Myeloma

For the treatment of previously untreated multiple myeloma, bortezomib is administered in combination with melphalan and prednisone as part of the VMP regimen. The recommended adult dosage of bortezomib during cycles 1–4 (of the recommended nine 6-week cycles) is 1.3 mg/m² by IV injection over 3–5 seconds or by subcutaneous injection twice weekly during weeks 1, 2, 4, and 5 (days 1, 4, 8, 11, 22, 25, 29, and 32 of the 6-week cycle) followed by a 10-day rest period (days 33–42). For cycles 5–9, the same dosage of bortezomib is administered once weekly during weeks 1, 2, 4, and 5 (days 1, 8, 22, and 29) followed by a 13-day rest period. In all 9 cycles, melphalan 9 mg/m² and prednisone 60 mg/m² are administered orally once daily on days 1–4. The manufacturer states that at least 72 hours should elapse between consecutive doses of bortezomib.

Previously Untreated Mantle Cell Lymphoma

For the treatment of previously untreated mantle cell lymphoma, bortezomib is administered in combination with rituximab, cyclophosphamide, doxorubicin, and prednisone as part of the VR-CAP regimen in 3-week cycles for 6 cycles. The recommended adult dosage of bortezomib is 1.3 mg/m² by IV injection over 3–5 seconds twice weekly for 2 weeks (days 1, 4, 8, and 11), followed by a 10-day rest period (days 12–21). Rituximab 375 mg/m², cyclophosphamide 750 mg/m², and doxorubicin hydrochloride 50 mg/m² are administered IV on day 1 and prednisone 100 mg/m² is administered orally on days 1–5 of each 3-week cycle. For patients in whom a response is first observed at cycle 6, the manufacturer recommends 2 additional cycles of the VR-CAP regimen. The manufacturer states that at least 72 hours should elapse between consecutive doses of bortezomib.

Relapsed Multiple Myeloma and Mantle Cell Lymphoma

For the treatment of relapsed multiple myeloma and mantle cell lymphoma, the recommended adult dosage of bortezomib for the standard schedule is 1.3 mg/m² by IV injection over 3–5 seconds or by subcutaneous injection twice weekly for 2 weeks (days 1, 4, 8, and 11), followed by a 10-day rest period (days 12–21). For extended therapy of more than 8 treatment cycles, bortezomib may be administered on the standard schedule or, for patients with relapsed multiple myeloma, on a maintenance schedule consisting of bortezomib 1.3 mg/m^2 by IV injection or by subcutaneous injection once weekly for 4 weeks (days 1, 8, 15, and 22), followed by a 13-day rest period (days 23–35). The manufacturer states that at least 72 hours should elapse between consecutive doses of bortezomib.

For the retreatment of multiple myeloma in patients who previously responded to bortezomib-based therapy and relapsed at least 6 months following therapy, the last tolerated dose of bortezomib is administered twice weekly for 2 weeks (days 1, 4, 8, and 11), followed by a 10-day rest period (days 12–21) for up to 8 cycles. Bortezomib may be reinitiated with or without dexamethasone. The manufacturer states that at least 72 hours should elapse between consecutive doses of bortezomib.

Induction Therapy Prior to Stem-Cell Transplantation in Newly Diagnosed Multiple Myeloma
Bortezomib and Dexamethasone

When bortezomib has been used in combination with dexamethasone† as induction therapy for newly diagnosed multiple myeloma in transplant-eligible patients†, bortezomib 1.3 mg/m^2 has been administered by IV injection twice weekly for 2 weeks (days 1, 4, 8, and 11) followed by a 10-day rest period (days 12–21) of each 21-day cycle for 4 cycles. In cycles 1 and 2, dexamethasone 40 mg was administered orally on days 1–4 and 9–12; in cycles 3 and 4, dexamethasone 40 mg was administered orally on days 1–4.

Bortezomib, Dexamethasone, and Thalidomide

Bortezomib has been used in several regimens in combination with thalidomide and dexamethasone† as induction therapy for newly diagnosed multiple myeloma in transplant-eligible patients†.

When bortezomib has been used in combination with thalidomide and dexamethasone as induction therapy for newly diagnosed multiple myeloma in transplant-eligible patients, bortezomib 1.3 mg/m^2 has been administered by IV injection twice weekly for 2 weeks (days 1, 4, 8, and 11) along with dexamethasone 40 mg orally on days 1, 2, 4, 5, 8, 9, 11, and 12 and thalidomide 200 mg orally daily (after initial dosage escalation during cycle 1 with 100 mg orally on days 1–14 followed by 200 mg orally daily thereafter). Treatment cycles were repeated every 21 days for 3 cycles.

Bortezomib 1.3 mg/m^2 also has been administered by IV injection twice weekly for 2 weeks (days 1, 4, 8, and 11) along with dexamethasone 40 mg orally on days 1–4 and 9–12 and thalidomide 200 mg orally daily (after initial dosage escalation during cycle 1 with 50 mg orally on days 1–14 followed by 100 mg orally on days 15–28). Treatment cycles were repeated every 4 weeks for 6 cycles.

Bortezomib 1.3 mg/m^2 also has been administered by subcutaneous or IV injection twice weekly for 2 weeks (days 1, 4, 8, and 11) along with dexamethasone 40 mg orally on days 1–4 and 9–12 and thalidomide 100 mg orally daily. Treatment cycles were repeated every 3 weeks for 4 cycles.

A modified regimen using reduced dosages of bortezomib and thalidomide is not fully established.

Bortezomib, Dexamethasone, and Doxorubicin (or Pegylated Liposomal Doxorubicin)

Bortezomib has been used in several regimens in combination with doxorubicin (or pegylated liposomal doxorubicin) and dexamethasone† as induction therapy for newly diagnosed multiple myeloma in transplant-eligible patients†.

When bortezomib has been used in combination with doxorubicin and dexamethasone as induction therapy for newly diagnosed multiple myeloma in transplant-eligible patients, bortezomib 1.3 mg/m^2 has been administered by IV injection twice weekly for 2 weeks (days 1, 4, 8, and 11) along with doxorubicin hydrochloride 9 mg/m^2 IV per day on days 1–4 and dexamethasone 40 mg orally on days 1–4, 9–12, and 17–20 of each 28-day cycle for 3 cycles.

Bortezomib 1.3 mg/m^2 also has been administered by IV injection twice weekly for 2 weeks (days 1, 4, 8, and 11) along with pegylated liposomal doxorubicin hydrochloride 30 mg/m^2 IV on day 4 and dexamethasone 40 mg orally on days 1, 2, 4, 5, 8, 9, 11, and 12 during cycle 1. During cycles 2–6, the same dosages of bortezomib and pegylated liposomal doxorubicin were administered along with

dexamethasone 20 mg orally daily. Treatment cycles were repeated every 3 weeks for a total of 6 cycles.

A modified regimen using reduced dosages of bortezomib and pegylated liposomal doxorubicin is not fully established.

Bortezomib, Dexamethasone, and Cyclophosphamide

Bortezomib has been used in several regimens in combination with cyclophosphamide and dexamethasone† as induction therapy for newly diagnosed multiple myeloma in transplant-eligible patients†.

When bortezomib has been used in combination with cyclophosphamide and dexamethasone as induction therapy for newly diagnosed multiple myeloma in transplant-eligible patients, bortezomib 1.3 mg/m^2 has been administered by IV injection twice weekly for 2 weeks (days 1, 4, 8, and 11) along with cyclophosphamide 300 mg/m^2 orally on days 1, 8, 15, and 22 and dexamethasone 40 mg orally on days 1–4, 9–12, and 17–20 of each 28-day cycle for 4 cycles.

Bortezomib 1.5 mg/m^2 also has been administered by IV injection once weekly (days 1, 8, 15, and 22) along with cyclophosphamide 300 mg/m^2 orally on days 1, 8, 15, and 22 of each 28-day cycle for 4 cycles, with dexamethasone 40 mg administered orally on days 1–4, 9–12, and 17–20 during cycles 1 and 2 and then once weekly during cycles 3 and 4.

Bortezomib 1.3 mg/m^2 also has been administered by IV injection twice weekly for 2 weeks (days 1, 4, 8, and 11) along with cyclophosphamide 300 mg/m^2 IV on days 1 and 8 and dexamethasone 40 mg orally on days 1, 2, 4, 5, 8, 9, 11, and 12 of each 21-day cycle for 3 cycles (cycles 1–3) followed by bortezomib 1 mg/m^2 by IV injection twice weekly for 2 weeks (days 1, 4, 8, and 11) along with thalidomide 100 mg orally daily and dexamethasone 40 mg orally on days 1, 2, 4, 5, 8, 9, 11, and 12 of each 21-day cycle for 3 cycles (cycles 4–6).

Bortezomib 1.3 mg/m^2 also has been administered by subcutaneous or IV injection twice weekly for 2 weeks (days 1, 4, 8, and 11) along with cyclophosphamide 900 mg/m^2 IV on day 1 and dexamethasone 40 mg orally on days 1, 2, 4, 5, 8, 9, 11, and 12 of each 21-day cycle for 3 cycles.

● Dosage Modification for Toxicity
Dosage Modification in Patients with Newly Diagnosed Multiple Myeloma Receiving Bortezomib with Melphalan and Prednisone (VMP)

The manufacturer of bortezomib states that before administration of any cycle of VMP, platelet counts should be 70,000/mm^3 or higher and the absolute neutrophil count (ANC) should be 1000/mm^3 or above. In addition, any nonhematologic toxicities should have resolved to grade 1 or baseline before any VMP cycle is administered.

Hematologic Toxicity

If prolonged grade 4 neutropenia or thrombocytopenia, or thrombocytopenia with bleeding, was observed in the previous VMP cycle, reduction of the melphalan dose by 25% in the next cycle should be considered.

If the platelet count is 30,000/mm^3 or less or if the ANC is 750/mm^3 or less on a day when bortezomib is to be administered (other than on day 1), the dose of bortezomib should be withheld. If several doses of bortezomib were withheld because of toxicity in consecutive cycles, it is recommended that the dose of bortezomib be reduced by one dose level (i.e., a dose of 1.3 mg/m^2 reduced to 1 mg/m^2; a dose of 1 mg/m^2 reduced to 0.7 mg/m^2).

Nonhematologic Effects

If nonhematologic toxicities (other than neuropathy) of grade 3 or more in severity occur during VMP therapy, bortezomib therapy should be withheld until symptoms of the toxicity have resolved to grade 1 or baseline. Bortezomib may then be reinitiated with a reduction of one dose level (i.e., a dose of 1.3 mg/m^2 reduced to 1 mg/m^2; a dose of 1 mg/m^2 reduced to 0.7 mg/m^2).

If neuropathic pain and/or peripheral neuropathy occurs during VMP therapy, bortezomib should be withheld or the dose reduced as recommended in patients with relapsed multiple myeloma or mantle cell lymphoma who develop such manifestations. (See Peripheral Neuropathy under Dosage Modification for Toxicity: Dosage Modification in Patients with Relapsed Multiple Myeloma or Mantle Cell Lymphoma, in Dosage and Administration.)

Dosage Modification in Patients with Newly Diagnosed Mantle Cell Lymphoma Receiving Bortezomib with Rituximab, Cyclophosphamide, Doxorubicin, and Prednisone (VR-CAP)

The manufacturer of bortezomib states that before administration of cycles 2–6 of VR-CAP therapy, platelet counts should be at least 100,000/mm³, ANC should be at least 1500/mm³, hemoglobin concentration should be at least 8 g/dL, and any nonhematologic toxicities should have resolved to grade 1 or baseline.

Hematologic Toxicity

If neutropenia of grade 3 or more in severity or platelet count less than 25,000/mm³ occurs on a day when bortezomib is to be administered (other than on day 1 of the cycle), the dose of bortezomib should be withheld for up to 2 weeks until ANC reaches or exceeds 750/mm³ and platelet count reaches or exceeds 25,000/mm³; bortezomib may then be resumed at one dose level lower than the previous dosage (i.e., a dose of 1.3 mg/m² reduced to 1 mg/m²; a dose of 1 mg/m² reduced to 0.7 mg/m²). If hematologic toxicity has not resolved after withholding bortezomib for 2 weeks, bortezomib therapy should be discontinued.

Nonhematologic Effects

If nonhematologic toxicities (other than neuropathy) of grade 3 or more in severity occur during VR-CAP therapy on a day when bortezomib is to be administered (other than on day 1 of the cycle), bortezomib therapy should be withheld until symptoms of the toxicity have resolved to grade 2 or less. Bortezomib may then be reinitiated with a reduction of one dose level (i.e., a dose of 1.3 mg/m² reduced to 1 mg/m²; a dose of 1 mg/m² reduced to 0.7 mg/m²).

If neuropathic pain and/or peripheral neuropathy occurs during VR-CAP therapy, bortezomib should be withheld or the dose reduced as recommended in patients with relapsed multiple myeloma or mantle cell lymphoma who develop such manifestations. (See Peripheral Neuropathy under Dosage Modification for Toxicity: Dosage Modification in Patients with Relapsed Multiple Myeloma or Mantle Cell Lymphoma, in Dosage and Administration.)

Dosage Modification in Patients with Relapsed Multiple Myeloma or Mantle Cell Lymphoma

Peripheral Neuropathy

Adjustment of the dose and/or frequency of administration of bortezomib may be required in patients who develop new or worsening peripheral neuropathy. In patients who develop grade 1 peripheral neuropathy (asymptomatic, loss of deep tendon reflexes or paresthesia) *without* pain or loss of function, no dosage modification is necessary. However, in patients who develop grade 1 peripheral neuropathy *with* pain or grade 2 peripheral neuropathy (moderate symptoms resulting in interference with instrumental activities of daily living), the dose of bortezomib should be reduced to 1 mg/m². In patients who develop grade 2 peripheral neuropathy with pain or grade 3 peripheral neuropathy (severe symptoms resulting in interference with self-care activities of daily living), bortezomib therapy should be temporarily discontinued; once manifestations of toxicity have resolved, the drug may be reinitiated at a dosage of 0.7 mg/m² once weekly. Bortezomib therapy should be discontinued in patients who develop grade 4 peripheral neuropathy (sensory neuropathy that is disabling or motor neuropathy that is life threatening or leads to paralysis). The manufacturer states that bortezomib should be used in patients with preexisting severe neuropathy only after careful assessment of the risks and benefits for the individual patient.

Other Nonhematologic or Hematologic Effects

Bortezomib therapy should be temporarily discontinued in patients who develop any grade 3 nonhematologic or grade 4 hematologic toxicities (e.g., grade 4 thrombocytopenia [platelet count less than 25,000/mm³]). Once manifestations of toxicity have resolved, bortezomib may be reinitiated but dosage of the drug should be reduced by 25% (i.e., a dose of 1.3 mg/m² reduced to 1 mg/m²; a dose of 1 mg/m² reduced to 0.7 mg/m²).

● Special Populations

Bortezomib is metabolized by hepatic enzymes, and exposure to the drug is increased in patients with moderate hepatic impairment (defined as bilirubin concentrations ranging from more than 1.5 to 3 times the upper limit of normal with any AST concentrations) or severe hepatic impairment (defined as bilirubin concentrations exceeding 3 times the upper limit of normal with any AST concentrations). The manufacturer recommends that doses of bortezomib during the first cycle of treatment be reduced to 0.7 mg/m² in patients with moderate or severe hepatic impairment. Based on patient tolerance, dosage in subsequent cycles may be increased to 1 mg/m² or further reduced to 0.5 mg/m². The manufacturer states that no adjustment in the initial dose is needed in patients with mild hepatic impairment (defined as bilirubin concentrations at or below the upper limit of normal with AST concentrations exceeding the upper limit of normal *or* bilirubin concentrations ranging from more than 1 to 1.5 times the upper limit of normal with any AST concentrations); such patients should be treated with the usual recommended initial dosage.

The pharmacokinetics of bortezomib are not influenced by the degree of renal impairment; therefore, dosage adjustment is not necessary in such patients. Because dialysis may decrease bortezomib concentrations, the drug should be administered after a dialysis procedure. (See Renal Impairment under Warnings/Precautions: Specific Populations, in Cautions.)

CAUTIONS

● Contraindications

Bortezomib is contraindicated in patients with known hypersensitivity (except for local reactions) to bortezomib, boron, or mannitol. Anaphylactic reactions have been reported in patients receiving bortezomib.

Intrathecal administration of bortezomib is contraindicated. Intrathecal administration of bortezomib has resulted in death.

● Warnings/Precautions

Peripheral Neuropathy

Bortezomib mainly causes sensory peripheral neuropathy, but severe motor peripheral neuropathy also has been reported. Patients with preexisting manifestations of peripheral neuropathy (e.g., numbness, pain, or burning sensation in feet or hands) may experience worsening peripheral neuropathy (including grade 3 or higher) during therapy with bortezomib.

In clinical studies in patients with relapsed multiple myeloma or mantle cell lymphoma, peripheral neuropathy occurred in 38% of patients receiving IV bortezomib and was grade 3 or higher in approximately 11% of patients receiving the drug. In the phase 3 randomized study in patients with relapsed multiple myeloma, dosage adjustments resulted in amelioration or resolution of peripheral neuropathy in 48% of patients with grade 2 or higher peripheral neuropathy within a median of 3.8 months from onset. In the phase 2 trials in patients with relapsed multiple myeloma, amelioration or resolution of peripheral neuropathy occurred in 73% of patients who discontinued bortezomib therapy because of grade 2 peripheral neuropathy or who had grade 3 or 4 peripheral neuropathy; the median time to improvement of one grade or more from the last dose of bortezomib was 47 days. The long-term outcome of peripheral neuropathy has not been elucidated in patients with mantle cell lymphoma. About 8% of patients with multiple myeloma or mantle cell lymphoma discontinued IV bortezomib therapy because of peripheral neuropathy.

In the phase 3 study evaluating subcutaneous administration of bortezomib in patients with relapsed multiple myeloma, grade 2 or higher peripheral neuropathy occurred in 39% of patients receiving bortezomib by IV injection compared with 24% of those receiving subcutaneous bortezomib. Grade 3 or higher peripheral neuropathy occurred more frequently in patients receiving bortezomib by IV injection compared with those receiving subcutaneous bortezomib (15 versus 6%). (See Dosage and Administration: Reconstitution and Administration.)

Patients receiving bortezomib should be monitored for manifestations of neuropathy (e.g., burning sensation, hyperesthesia, hypoesthesia, paresthesia, discomfort, neuropathic pain or weakness). Adjustment of the dose and/or frequency of administration of bortezomib may be required in patients who experience new onset or exacerbation of peripheral neuropathy. (See Dosage and Administration: Dosage Modification for Toxicity.)

Hypotension

In clinical studies in patients with relapsed multiple myeloma or mantle cell lymphoma, hypotension, including orthostatic hypotension, was reported in 8% of patients receiving IV bortezomib; grade 3 or higher hypotension occurred in approximately 2% of patients receiving the drug. Hypotension was reported as a serious adverse event in 2% of patients receiving bortezomib, and 1% of patients discontinued bortezomib therapy because of hypotension. In addition, less than 1% of patients who developed hypotension also experienced a concurrent syncopal event.

The manufacturer states that bortezomib should be used with caution in patients with a history of syncope, in patients receiving drugs known to be associated with hypotension, and in patients who are dehydrated. Orthostatic hypotension may be managed with adjustment of antihypertensive therapy, hydration, and administration of mineralocorticoids and/or sympathomimetic agents.

Cardiovascular Effects

Death from cardiogenic shock, congestive heart failure, or cardiac arrest has occurred in patients receiving bortezomib. Acute development or exacerbation of congestive heart failure and new onset of decreased left ventricular ejection fraction have been reported in association with bortezomib therapy, including in patients who had no risk factors for decreased left ventricular ejection fraction. Patients with existing heart disease and patients with increased risk for heart disease should be monitored closely during bortezomib therapy. In the phase 3 study in patients with relapsed multiple myeloma, the incidence of any treatment-emergent cardiac disorder was 8 or 5% in patients receiving bortezomib or dexamethasone, respectively. The incidence of cardiac failure and congestive cardiac failure was similar in patients receiving bortezomib versus dexamethasone (less than 1%); however, acute pulmonary edema, cardiogenic shock, and pulmonary edema each occurred in less than 1% of patients receiving bortezomib compared with none of those receiving dexamethasone. Isolated cases of prolonged QT interval have been reported; a causal relationship to bortezomib has not been established.

Pulmonary Effects

Death from respiratory insufficiency has occurred in patients receiving bortezomib. Acute diffuse infiltrative pulmonary disease of unknown etiology (e.g., pneumonitis, interstitial pneumonia, lung infiltration) and acute respiratory distress syndrome, sometimes fatal, have been reported in patients receiving bortezomib. Pulmonary hypertension in the absence of left heart failure or substantial pulmonary disease also has been reported. If new or worsening cardiopulmonary symptoms occur, a prompt comprehensive diagnostic evaluation should be conducted; temporary interruption of therapy should be considered pending evaluation of symptoms.

Reversible Posterior Leukoencephalopathy Syndrome

Reversible posterior leukoencephalopathy syndrome (RPLS) has occurred in patients receiving bortezomib. RPLS may manifest with seizures, hypertension, headache, lethargy, confusion, blindness, and other visual and neurologic disturbances. Brain imaging, preferably magnetic resonance imaging, is used to confirm the diagnosis. Bortezomib should be discontinued in patients who develop RPLS. The safety of reinitiating bortezomib in patients previously experiencing RPLS has not been established.

GI Effects

Nausea, diarrhea, constipation, vomiting, loss of appetite, dyspepsia, and dysgeusia can occur in patients receiving bortezomib therapy; ileus also may occur. In clinical studies in patients with relapsed multiple myeloma or mantle cell lymphoma, 75% of patients receiving IV bortezomib experienced at least one GI disorder; grade 3 or higher adverse GI effects occurred in approximately 14% of patients receiving the drug, and serious adverse GI effects occurred in 7% of patients. About 4% of patients receiving bortezomib discontinued therapy because of adverse GI effects.

Because adverse GI effects may be severe and sometimes may require use of antiemetics and antidiarrheals, the manufacturer states that fluid and electrolyte replacement should be used in patients receiving bortezomib therapy to prevent dehydration. If severe adverse GI effects occur, temporary interruption of therapy is recommended.

Hematologic Effects

In clinical studies in patients with relapsed multiple myeloma or mantle cell lymphoma, thrombocytopenia was reported in 32% of patients receiving IV bortezomib and was grade 3 or higher in 26% of patients receiving the drug. Neutropenia was reported in 15% of patients receiving bortezomib and was grade 3 or higher in approximately 10% of patients receiving the drug. Thrombocytopenia or neutropenia was reported as a serious adverse event in 2 or less than 1%, respectively, of patients receiving bortezomib. In these studies, thrombocytopenia or neutropenia occurred during days 1–11 of each cycle and platelet and neutrophil counts returned toward baseline during the 10-day rest period.

Dose-related decreases in absolute neutrophil count (ANC) and platelet count followed a cyclical pattern with nadirs occurring following the last dose of each cycle and typically recovering prior to initiation of the subsequent cycle. The pattern of ANC and platelet count decreases and recovery remained consistent with no evidence of cumulative neutropenia or thrombocytopenia in the regimens evaluated for the treatment of multiple myeloma or mantle cell lymphoma.

In the phase 3 randomized study in patients with relapsed multiple myeloma, the platelet count nadir in patients receiving bortezomib averaged approximately 40% of the baseline platelet count. The severity of thrombocytopenia associated with bortezomib was related to pretreatment platelet count. In this study, platelet count less than 10,000/mm³ occurred in 1 (14%) of 7 patients with a baseline platelet count of 10,000–49,999/mm³, in 2 (14%) of 14 patients with a baseline platelet count of 50,000–74,999/mm³, and in 8 (3%) of 309 patients with a baseline platelet count of at least 75,000/mm³; platelet count of 10,000–25,000/mm³ occurred in 5 (71%) of 7 patients with a baseline platelet count of 10,000–49,999/mm³, in 11 (79%) of 14 patients with a baseline platelet count of 50,000–74,999/mm³, and in 36 (12%) of 309 patients with a baseline platelet count of at least 75,000/mm³. Grade 3 or higher bleeding events occurred in 2% of patients receiving bortezomib compared with less than 1% of patients receiving dexamethasone. GI and intracerebral hemorrhage associated with thrombocytopenia have been reported in patients receiving bortezomib.

In the phase 3 clinical study evaluating bortezomib in combination with rituximab, cyclophosphamide, doxorubicin, and prednisone (VR-CAP) in patients with previously untreated mantle cell lymphoma, grade 4 or higher thrombocytopenia or neutropenia was reported in 32 or 70%, respectively, of patients receiving VR-CAP compared with 1 or 52%, respectively, of those receiving rituximab plus cyclophosphamide, doxorubicin, vincristine, and prednisone (R-CHOP). Grade 3 or higher bleeding events or grade 4 or higher febrile neutropenia occurred in 1 or 5%, respectively, of patients receiving VR-CAP compared with less than 1 or 6%, respectively, of those receiving R-CHOP. Platelet transfusions were administered in 23 or 3% of patients receiving VR-CAP or R-CHOP, respectively. Granulocyte colony-stimulating factor or granulocyte-macrophage colony-stimulating factor support was administered in 78 or 61% of patients receiving VR-CAP or R-CHOP, respectively.

The manufacturer states that complete blood cell counts should be performed frequently in patients receiving bortezomib therapy. Platelet counts should be monitored prior to the administration of each dose of bortezomib. Depending on the severity of thrombocytopenia or neutropenia, temporary interruption of bortezomib followed by dosage reduction may be required. (See Dosage and Administration: Dosage Modification for Toxicity.) Supportive care (e.g., transfusions) should be administered according to published guidelines.

Tumor Lysis Syndrome

Tumor lysis syndrome has been reported in patients receiving bortezomib. The risk of tumor lysis syndrome is increased in patients with a large tumor burden; such patients should be monitored closely and appropriate precautions should be taken.

Hepatic Effects

Acute liver failure has been reported in patients with serious underlying medical conditions who were receiving bortezomib with multiple concomitant drugs. Increases in hepatic enzyme concentrations, hyperbilirubinemia, and hepatitis also have been reported. If such effects occur, the manufacturer recommends interrupting therapy with the drug to assess reversibility of adverse hepatic effects. Information on the results of rechallenge with the drug in these patients is limited.

Fetal/Neonatal Morbidity and Mortality

There are no adequate and well-controlled studies of bortezomib in pregnant women; however, based on animal findings, bortezomib may cause fetal harm. Embryofetal toxicity (i.e., decreased fetal weight) and lethality were observed in pregnant animals receiving bortezomib at a dosage approximately 0.5 times the recommended human dosage; no evidence of teratogenicity was observed.

Pregnancy should be avoided during therapy. (See Advice to Patients.) If bortezomib is used during pregnancy or if the patient becomes pregnant while receiving the drug, the patient should be apprised of the potential hazard to the fetus.

Herpes Virus Infections

In randomized studies in patients with previously untreated or relapsed multiple myeloma, reactivation of varicella zoster virus infection was more common in patients receiving bortezomib (6–11%) compared with those receiving other therapies (3–4%). The frequency of herpes simplex virus infection was similar in patients receiving bortezomib and those receiving other therapies (1–3%). In the phase 3 study in patients with previously untreated multiple myeloma, reactivation of latent varicella zoster virus infection occurred less frequently in patients receiving bortezomib plus melphalan and prednisone (VMP) with prophylactic antiviral therapy (3%) compared with patients receiving VMP without antiviral prophylaxis (17%).

Specific Populations

Pregnancy

Category D. (See Fetal/Neonatal Morbidity and Mortality under Cautions: Warnings/Precautions.)

Lactation

It is not known whether bortezomib is distributed into milk. Because of the potential for serious adverse reactions to bortezomib in nursing infants, a decision should be made whether to discontinue nursing or the drug, taking into account the importance of the drug to the woman.

Pediatric Use

Efficacy of bortezomib has not been established in pediatric patients with relapsed pre-B acute lymphoblastic leukemia (ALL). In a study evaluating the activity and safety of bortezomib (1.3 mg/m² IV) in combination with intensive reinduction chemotherapy in pediatric patients and young adults with lymphoid malignancies, bortezomib did not alter complete remission rates at day 36 in the subset of patients with pre-B ALL compared with a historical control. No new safety concerns were identified in this study.

In pediatric patients, clearance of bortezomib normalized to body surface area (BSA) was comparable to that observed in adults.

Geriatric Use

Although no overall differences in efficacy or safety were observed between geriatric and younger patients receiving bortezomib, the possibility that some older patients may exhibit increased sensitivity to the drug cannot be ruled out. Exposure to bortezomib may be increased in geriatric patients compared with younger adults.

Of the 669 patients with relapsed multiple myeloma enrolled in the phase 3 randomized trial, 245 (37%) were 65 years of age or older. Among geriatric patients, longer median time to progression (5.5 versus 4.3 months), longer median duration of response (8 versus 4.9 months), and higher rates of overall response (40 versus 18%) were observed for those receiving bortezomib versus dexamethasone. Among patients receiving bortezomib, grade 3 or 4 adverse effects were reported in 64% of patients 50 years of age or younger, 78% of patients 51–64 years of age, and 75% of patients 65 years of age or older.

In patients with multiple myeloma, exposure to bortezomib (based on dose-normalized area under the concentration-time curve [AUC] and peak plasma concentrations) following the first 1- or 1.3-mg/m² IV dose of the drug was 25% lower in patients younger than 65 years of age compared with older adults.

Renal Impairment

In a pharmacokinetic study in patients with normal renal function or with varying degrees of renal impairment, exposure to bortezomib (based on dose-normalized AUC and peak plasma concentrations) was comparable among all the groups. However, because dialysis may decrease bortezomib concentrations, the drug should be administered after a dialysis procedure. (See Dosage and Administration: Special Populations.)

Hepatic Impairment

Bortezomib is metabolized by hepatic enzymes (e.g., cytochrome P-450 [CYP] microsomal enzymes), and exposure to the drug is increased in patients with moderate or severe hepatic impairment. In a pharmacokinetic study in cancer patients, exposure to bortezomib (based on dose-normalized AUC) was increased by approximately 60% in patients with moderate or severe hepatic impairment compared with patients with normal hepatic function; mild hepatic impairment did not alter the dose-normalized AUC of bortezomib. Patients with moderate or severe hepatic impairment should receive reduced initial dosages of bortezomib and be closely monitored for adverse effects. (See Dosage and Administration: Special Populations.)

● Common Adverse Effects

Adverse effects reported in 10% or more of patients with previously untreated multiple myeloma receiving IV bortezomib plus melphalan and prednisone (VMP) include thrombocytopenia, neutropenia, peripheral neuropathy, nausea, diarrhea, neuralgia, anemia, leukopenia, vomiting, fatigue, constipation, lymphopenia, anorexia, asthenia, pyrexia, paresthesia, herpes zoster, rash, abdominal pain (upper quadrant), and insomnia. Serious (grade 3 or higher) adverse effects reported in 5% or more of patients receiving VMP include neutropenia, leukopenia, thrombocytopenia, lymphopenia, anemia, peripheral neuropathy, neuralgia, diarrhea, fatigue, asthenia, hypokalemia, and pneumonia.

Adverse effects reported in 10% or more of patients with relapsed multiple myeloma receiving IV bortezomib include nausea, diarrhea, fatigue, peripheral neuropathy, thrombocytopenia, constipation, vomiting, anorexia, pyrexia, paresthesia, anemia, headache, neutropenia, rash, decreased appetite, dyspnea, abdominal pain, dizziness (excluding vertigo), and weakness. Serious (grade 3 or higher) adverse effects reported in 5% or more of patients receiving bortezomib include thrombocytopenia, neutropenia, diarrhea, peripheral neuropathy, anemia, and fatigue.

Adverse effects reported in 10% or more of patients with relapsed multiple myeloma receiving bortezomib by subcutaneous injection include peripheral neuropathy, thrombocytopenia, neuralgia, neutropenia, anemia, diarrhea, leukopenia, nausea, pyrexia, vomiting, asthenia, weight loss, constipation, and fatigue. Serious (grade 3 or higher) adverse effects reported in 5% or more of patients receiving bortezomib by subcutaneous injection include neutropenia, anemia, leukopenia, peripheral neuropathy, thrombocytopenia, and pneumonia.

Adverse effects reported in 10% or more of patients with previously untreated mantle cell lymphoma receiving IV bortezomib plus rituximab, cyclophosphamide, doxorubicin, and prednisone (VR-CAP) include neutropenia, thrombocytopenia, leukopenia, anemia, peripheral neuropathy, lymphopenia, diarrhea, nausea, pyrexia, cough, constipation, fatigue, febrile neutropenia, loss of appetite, peripheral edema, alopecia, asthenia, pneumonia, neuralgia, and vomiting. Serious (grade 3 or higher) adverse effects reported in 5% or more of patients receiving VR-CAP include thrombocytopenia, leukopenia, neutropenia, anemia, febrile neutropenia, lymphopenia, peripheral neuropathy, pneumonia, diarrhea, and fatigue.

Adverse effects reported in 10% or more of patients with relapsed mantle cell lymphoma receiving IV bortezomib include peripheral neuropathy, fatigue, diarrhea, nausea, constipation, rash, vomiting, dizziness (excluding vertigo), thrombocytopenia, anorexia, anemia, weakness, headache, and pyrexia. Serious (grade 3 or higher) adverse effects reported in 5% or more of patients receiving bortezomib include peripheral neuropathy, fatigue, thrombocytopenia, and diarrhea.

DRUG INTERACTIONS

Bortezomib is metabolized principally by cytochrome P-450 (CYP) isoenzymes 1A2, 2C19, and 3A4 and, to a lesser extent, by CYP2C9 and 2D6. In vitro, bortezomib may inhibit CYP2C19. However, bortezomib is a poor inhibitor of CYP1A2, 2C9, 2D6, and 3A4 and does not induce CYP1A2 or CYP3A4 in vitro.

● Drugs Affecting Hepatic Microsomal Enzymes

Inhibitors of CYP3A4

Concomitant use of bortezomib with potent inhibitors of CYP3A4 may result in increased systemic exposure of bortezomib. Concomitant administration of the potent CYP3A4 inhibitor ketoconazole with bortezomib increased systemic exposure of bortezomib by 35%.

If bortezomib is used concomitantly with a potent CYP3A4 inhibitor, patients should be monitored for bortezomib-associated toxicity and a reduced dosage of bortezomib should be considered.

Inducers of CYP3A4

Concomitant use of bortezomib with potent inducers of CYP3A4 may result in decreased systemic exposure and reduced efficacy of bortezomib. Concomitant administration of the potent CYP3A4 inducer rifampin with bortezomib is expected to decrease bortezomib exposure by at least 45%, although larger reductions in exposure may occur. Concomitant use with St. John's wort (Hypericum perforatum) may result in unpredictable decreases in bortezomib exposure. Concomitant use of bortezomib with potent inducers of CYP3A4 (e.g., rifampin, St. John's wort) should be avoided.

Concomitant administration of the weak CYP3A4 inducer dexamethasone with bortezomib did not alter systemic exposure of bortezomib.

Inhibitors of CYP2C19

Concomitant administration of the potent CYP2C19 inhibitor omeprazole with bortezomib did not alter systemic exposure of bortezomib.

● *Melphalan and Prednisone*

Concomitant administration of melphalan and prednisone with bortezomib resulted in a 17% increase in systemic exposure of bortezomib. However, the manufacturer states that this increase is unlikely to be clinically relevant.

● *Oral Antidiabetic Agents*

In clinical studies, hypoglycemia and hyperglycemia have been reported in patients with diabetes mellitus who received bortezomib concomitantly with oral antidiabetic agents. If bortezomib is used concomitantly with oral antidiabetic agents, blood glucose concentrations should be monitored carefully and dosage of the antidiabetic agent adjusted as necessary.

● *Hypotensive Agents*

Concomitant use of bortezomib with drugs that can cause hypotension may result in an increased risk of hypotension. Dosage adjustment of hypotensive agents may be necessary.

DESCRIPTION

Bortezomib, a modified dipeptidyl boronic acid, is an antineoplastic agent. The drug reversibly inhibits the 26S proteasome, a large protein complex that degrades ubiquitinated proteins. The ubiquitin-proteasome pathway plays an essential role in regulating the intracellular concentration of specific proteins, thereby maintaining homeostasis within cells. Inhibition of the 26S proteasome by bortezomib prevents targeted proteolysis and causes disruption of normal homeostatic mechanisms, which can lead to cell death. In vitro studies indicate that bortezomib is cytotoxic to a variety of cancer cell types. Bortezomib has been shown to cause a delay in tumor growth in vivo in tumor models, including multiple myeloma.

Systemic exposure to bortezomib was similar following IV or subcutaneous administration in patients with multiple myeloma receiving repeated 1.3-mg/m² doses of the drug. Bortezomib is approximately 83% bound to plasma proteins. In vitro studies indicate that bortezomib is metabolized by the cytochrome P-450 (CYP) enzyme system, principally by isoenzymes 1A2, 2C19, and 3A4, to inactive metabolites; metabolism by isoenzymes 2C9 and 2D6 is minor. Following repeated IV administration of bortezomib 1 or 1.3 mg/m² in patients with multiple myeloma, the mean terminal half-life of the drug was 40–193 or 76–108 hours, respectively. Exposure to bortezomib is increased in patients with moderate or severe hepatic impairment and in patients 65 years of age or older; pharmacokinetics of bortezomib are not influenced by renal impairment or gender. (See Dosage and Administration: Special Populations and see Specific Populations under Cautions: Warnings/Precautions.)

ADVICE TO PATIENTS

Risk of fatigue, dizziness, syncope, or orthostatic hypotension; do not drive a motor vehicle or operate machinery if any of these symptoms are experienced.

Risk of dehydration secondary to vomiting and/or diarrhea. Importance of advising patients regarding appropriate measures (e.g., adequate fluid intake) to avoid dehydration. Importance of advising patients to inform a clinician if dizziness, lightheadedness, fainting spells, or muscle cramps develop.

Necessity of advising women to use an effective method of contraception and to avoid breast-feeding while receiving bortezomib therapy. Importance of women informing a clinician immediately if they are or plan to become pregnant or plan to breast-feed. Advise pregnant women of risk to the fetus.

If used concomitantly with oral antidiabetic agents, importance of frequent monitoring of blood glucose concentrations and informing a clinician of any unusual change.

Risk of peripheral neuropathy. Importance of informing a clinician of new-onset or worsening symptoms of peripheral neuropathy (e.g., tingling, numbness, pain, burning sensation in hands or feet, weakness in arms or legs).

Risk of reversible posterior leukoencephalopathy syndrome (RPLS). Importance of reporting any possible manifestations of RPLS (e.g., seizure, persistent headache, reduced eyesight, blurred vision, confusion, lethargy, inability to think, difficulty walking).

Risk of cardiac effects. Importance of informing clinician if swelling (of the feet, ankles, or legs) or other cardiac-related problems occur.

Risk of pulmonary effects. Importance of informing clinician if shortness of breath, cough, or other pulmonary problems occur.

Risk of hepatotoxicity. Importance of reporting any possible manifestations of hepatotoxicity (e.g., jaundice, abdominal pain [particularly in the right upper quadrant]).

Importance of informing clinician if rash, severe injection site reactions, or dermatologic pain occurs.

Risk of reactivation of latent varicella zoster virus infection. Importance of discussing with clinician whether antiviral prophylaxis should be initiated.

Importance of informing clinician if increase in blood pressure, bleeding, fever, constipation, or loss of appetite occurs.

Importance of informing clinicians of existing or contemplated concomitant therapy, including prescription and OTC drugs and dietary or herbal supplements (e.g., St. John's wort), as well as any concomitant illnesses.

Importance of informing patients of other important precautionary information. (See Cautions.)

For further information on the handling of antineoplastic agents, see the ASHP Guidelines on Handling Hazardous Drugs at http://www.ahfsdruginformation.com.

PREPARATIONS

Excipients in commercially available drug preparations may have clinically important effects in some individuals; consult specific product labeling for details.

Bortezomib

Parenteral		
For injection, for IV or subcutaneous use	3.5 mg	Velcade®, Millennium

† Use is not currently included in the labeling approved by the US Food and Drug Administration.

Selected Revisions August 6, 2018, © Copyright, October 1, 2003, American Society of Health-System Pharmacists, Inc.

Bosutinib

10:00 • ANTINEOPLASTIC AGENTS

■ Bosutinib, an inhibitor of multiple tyrosine kinases, is an antineoplastic agent.

USES

● Philadelphia Chromosome-Positive Chronic Myelogenous Leukemia

Bosutinib is used for the treatment of chronic phase Philadelphia chromosome-positive (Ph+) chronic myelogenous leukemia (CML) in adults and pediatric patients 1 year of age and older who are newly diagnosed or resistant or intolerant to prior therapy. Bosutinib is also used for the treatment of chronic, accelerated, or blast phase Ph+ CML in adults after failure (secondary to resistance or intolerance) of prior therapy. Bosutinib is designated an orphan drug by FDA for use in the treatment of CML.

Treatment of Newly Diagnosed Chronic Phase CML in Adults

Bosutinib is used for the treatment of newly diagnosed Ph+ CML in adults who are in the chronic phase of the disease. This indication is based principally on the results of an open-label, randomized, multicenter trial (BFORE trial). In this study, 487 patients with Ph+ CML harboring b2a2 and/or b3a2 transcripts at baseline with Bcr-Abl gene copies >0 were randomized (stratified by Sokal score and geographical region) in a 1:1 ratio to receive bosutinib 400 mg once daily or imatinib 400 mg once daily. The median treatment duration was 55.1 months in the bosutinib group and 55 months in the imatinib group. The median age of patients was 53 years, and distribution of Sokal scores in the bosutinib and imatinib groups was similar (35 and 39% were low risk, 44 and 38% were intermediate risk, and 22 and 22% were high risk in the bosutinib and imatinib groups, respectively).

The primary efficacy end point was major molecular response at 12 months (48 weeks), defined as ≤0.1% Bcr-Abl ratio on international scale (corresponding to ≥3 log reduction from standardized baseline) with a minimum of 3000 Abl transcripts as assessed by the central laboratory. Complete cytogenetic response was also assessed at 12 months; complete cytogenetic response was defined as the absence of Ph+ metaphases in chromosome banding analysis of ≥20 metaphases derived from bone marrow aspirate, or major molecular response if adequate cytogenetic assessment was unavailable. At 12 months, 78 and 72% of patients receiving bosutinib and imatinib, respectively, were still receiving the assigned treatment. The major molecular response rate at 12 months was 47 and 37% in patients receiving bosutinib and those receiving imatinib, respectively. The complete cytogenetic response rate at 12 months was 77 and 66% in bosutinib- and imatinib-treated patients, respectively. By month 60 (week 240), the rates of major molecular response were 74 and 66% in the bosutinib and imatinib groups, respectively. Median time to major molecular response was 9 months in patients receiving bosutinib and 11.9 months in patients receiving imatinib. Transformation to acute phase or blast phase occurred in 2 and 3% of bosutinib- and imatinib-treated patients, respectively, after 60 months of follow-up.

Treatment of Chronic, Accelerated, or Blast Phase CML Following Prior Treatment Failure in Adults

Bosutinib is used for the treatment of chronic, accelerated, or blast phase Ph+ CML in adults after failure (secondary to resistance or intolerance) of prior therapy.

This indication is based principally on the results of an open-label, single-arm, multicenter, phase 1/phase 2 study in adults with chronic, accelerated, or blast phase CML following therapy with either imatinib alone or imatinib followed by dasatinib and/or nilotinib; patients were intolerant of or had disease that was resistant to imatinib. In this study, 546 patients received bosutinib 500 mg once daily (increased to 600 mg daily if complete hematologic or cytogenetic response was not achieved by week 8 or 12, respectively). The median duration of therapy with bosutinib was 26 months in patients with chronic phase CML previously treated with only imatinib; patients previously treated with imatinib followed by dasatinib and/or nilotinib received therapy with bosutinib for a median duration

of 9 months. The median duration of therapy with bosutinib in patients previously treated with at least imatinib who were in the accelerated or blast phase of the disease was 10 or 3 months, respectively.

The primary efficacy end point of this study was major cytogenetic response (defined as elimination or substantial reduction [by at least 65%] of Ph+ hematopoietic cells) at 24 weeks. In this study, resistance to imatinib was defined as failure to achieve or maintain any hematologic improvement within 4 weeks of therapy; or failure to achieve a complete hematologic response by 3 months, a cytogenetic response by 6 months, or a major cytogenetic response by 12 months; or disease progression after a previous cytogenetic or hematologic response; or evidence of the genetic mutation in the Bcr-Abl gene associated with imatinib resistance. Imatinib intolerance was defined as inability to tolerate imatinib because of toxicity, or disease progression with imatinib and inability to receive a higher dosage because of toxicity. Definitions of resistance and intolerance to both dasatinib and nilotinib were similar to those for imatinib. Major cytogenetic response was achieved at 24 weeks in 40.1% of patients in chronic phase CML who were previously treated with imatinib alone and in 25.9% of those previously treated with imatinib followed by dasatinib or nilotinib. Major cytogenetic response was achieved at any time during the study in 59.5% of patients in chronic phase CML who were previously treated with imatinib alone and 40.2% of those previously treated with imatinib followed by dasatinib or nilotinib. In an exploratory analysis, treatment with bosutinib resulted in confirmed complete hematologic responses at 48 weeks in 30.6 or 16.7% of patients in accelerated or blast phase CML, respectively. Overall hematologic response at 48 weeks was observed in 56.9 or 28.3% of patients in accelerated or blast phase CML, respectively. Long-term follow-up data was based on a minimum of 60 months for patients with chronic phase CML previously treated with imatinib alone, and a minimum of 48 months for patients with chronic phase CML previously treated with imatinib and at least one other tyrosine kinase inhibitor, patients with accelerated phase CML, and patients with blast phase CML. Median duration of major cytogenetic response was not reached in patients with chronic phase CML previously treated with imatinib alone or in those with chronic phase CML previously treated with imatinib and at least one other tyrosine kinase inhibitor. Among patients with chronic phase CML previously treated with imatinib alone, 65.4 and 42.9% had a major cytogenetic response lasting at least 18 and 54 months, respectively. Among patients with chronic phase CML previously treated with imatinib and at least one other tyrosine kinase inhibitor, 64.4 and 35.6% had a major cytogenetic response lasting at least 9 and 42 months, respectively. Twenty of the 403 patients with chronic phase CML at baseline had disease transformation to accelerated or blast phase during bosutinib therapy, and 3 of 79 patients with accelerated phase CML at baseline had disease transformation to blast phase CML during bosutinib therapy.

A single-arm, open-label, phase 4 study (BYOND) confirmed the results of the initial approval trial in patients with chronic or advanced Ph+ CML who had failed previous tyrosine kinase inhibitor therapy. In this trial, the cumulative confirmed major cytogenetic response rate at 1 year was 75.8% among patients with chronic phase CML who had received 1 or 2 prior tyrosine kinase inhibitors and 62.2% in those with chronic phase CML who had received 3 prior tyrosine kinase inhibitors.

Pediatric Use

Bosutinib is used for the treatment of chronic phase Ph+ CML in pediatric patients 1 year of age and older who are newly diagnosed or resistant or intolerant to prior therapy. This indication is based primarily on the results of a multicenter, nonrandomized, open-label study (BCHILD).

The BCHILD study enrolled 28 patients with chronic phase Ph+ CML with resistance or intolerance to prior therapy and 21 patients with newly diagnosed chronic phase Ph+ CML. Patients in the prior treatment failure group received bosutinib at doses of 300 to 400 mg/m² orally once daily and those in the newly diagnosed group were administered bosutinib 300 mg/m² orally once daily. Efficacy outcomes included complete cytogenetic response, major cytogenetic response, and major molecular response.

Patients with newly diagnosed chronic phase Ph+ CML had a median age of 14 years (range, 5 to 17 years); 68% were male; 81% were white and 14% were Black/African American. In the chronic phase Ph+ CML with resistance or intolerance to prior therapy group, the median age was 11.5 years (range, 1 to 17 years); 57% were male; 43% were white, 7% were Black/African American, and 14% were Asian.

The major and complete cytogenetic responses among newly diagnosed patients were 76.2% and 71.4%, respectively. The major molecular response was 28.6%. The median duration of follow-up was 14.2 months (range, 1.1 to 26.3 months) in this group. For patients in the prior treatment failure group, the major and complete cytogenetic responses were 82.1% and 78.6%, respectively. The major molecular response was 50.0%. Among 14 patients who achieved major molecular response, 2 lost this response after 13.6 months and 24.7 months on treatment, respectively . The median duration of follow-up for overall survival was 23.2 months (range, 1.0 to 61.5 months) in this patient group.

Clinical Perspective

Most adult patients with chronic phase CML can expect a normal life expectancy. With the exception of newly diagnosed cases during pregnancy, first-line treatment of CML is a tyrosine kinase inhibitor (TKI). The choice of TKI in the first-line setting is individualized based on efficacy, tolerability, toxicity, and cost, particularly since adherence to therapy is life-long.

If treatment failure or resistance develops with first-line TKI therapy, second-line treatment requires changing to another TKI with investigation of potential BCR-ABL1 KD-mutations. If intolerance or treatment-related complications related to the initial TKI occurs, the decision to change to another TKI is partly subjective and dependent upon the patient, clinician, supportive care options, and level of response.

If BCR-ABL1 resistance mutations occur with imatinib (the first generation TKI), second generation TKIs (dasatinib, nilotinib, bosutinib) are an option dependent upon the specific mutation. If there are no BCR-ABL1 KD-mutations present, there is no clear recommendation for any particular second generation TKI as all are effective. Choice of TKI is almost entirely patient-related and depends on age, comorbidities, toxicity of the initial TKI, and other factors.

DOSAGE AND ADMINISTRATION

● General

Pretreatment Screening

- Assess renal function at baseline.

- Verify pregnancy status in females of reproductive potential prior to initiation of therapy.

Patient Monitoring

- Monitor complete blood cell counts (CBC) weekly for the first month of therapy and monthly (or as clinically indicated) thereafter.

- Monitor liver function tests monthly for the first 3 months of therapy and then as clinically indicated; more frequent monitoring is recommended if increased aminotransferase concentrations occur.

- Monitor renal function during therapy, particularly in patients with preexisting renal impairment or risk factors for renal impairment.

- Monitor for signs and symptoms of cardiac failure or ischemia, fluid retention, or GI toxicity (e.g., diarrhea, nausea, vomiting, abdominal pain) and treat as clinically indicated.

Dispensing and Administration Precautions

Handling and Disposal

- Follow procedures for proper handling and disposal of antineoplastic drugs when preparing and administering bosutinib.

● Administration

Bosutinib is administered orally once daily with food; tolerability of the drug may be increased when taken with food. Bosutinib is available as tablets and capsules.

Swallow tablets whole. Tablets should *not* be crushed, broken, chewed, or cut. Touching or handling of crushed or broken tablets should be avoided.

Capsules may be swallowed whole. If a patient is unable to swallow a whole capsule, the required number of capsules for the dose can be opened and contents mixed with room temperature applesauce or yogurt in a clean container (see Table 1). Patients should immediately consume the full mixture without chewing;

do not store for later use. If the entire mixture is not swallowed, do not administer an additional dose. Resume dosing on the next day.

TABLE 1. Bosutinib Dose Using Capsules and Soft Food Volume

Dose (mg)	Volume of Applesauce or Yogurt
100	10 mL (2 teaspoons)
150	15 mL (3 teaspoons)
200	20 mL (4 teaspoons)
250	25 mL (5 teaspoons)
300	30 mL (6 teaspoons)
350	30 mL (6 teaspoons)
400	35 mL (7 teaspoons)
450	40 mL (8 teaspoons)
500	45 mL (9 teaspoons)
550	45 mL (9 teaspoons)
600	50 mL (10 teaspoons)

If a dose of bosutinib is missed by more than 12 hours, the dose should be omitted, and the next dose should be taken at the regularly scheduled time. Do *not* double the dose to make up for the missed dose.

Store bosutinib tablets and capsules at 20–25°C (excursions permitted between 15–30°C).

● Dosage

Bosutinib is commercially available as the monohydrate; dosage is expressed in terms of anhydrous bosutinib.

Adults

Treatment of Newly Diagnosed Chronic Phase Chronic Myelogenous Leukemia

The recommended initial adult dosage of bosutinib for the treatment of newly-diagnosed chronic phase Philadelphia chromosome-positive (Ph⁺) chronic myelogenous leukemia (CML) is 400 mg once daily. In clinical studies, patients who did not achieve or maintain a hematologic, cytogenetic, or molecular response could increase the dosage in increments of 100 mg once daily up to a maximum dosage of 600 mg once daily if they did not experience grade 3 or higher adverse effects while receiving the original starting dosage (400 mg daily). Therapy should be continued until disease progression or intolerance to therapy occurs.

Treatment of Chronic, Accelerated, or Blast Phase CML Following Prior Treatment Failure

The recommended initial adult dosage of bosutinib for the treatment of Ph⁺ chronic, accelerated, or blast phase CML following prior treatment failure is 500 mg once daily. In clinical studies, patients who did not achieve or maintain a hematologic, cytogenetic, or molecular response could increase the dosage in increments of 100 mg once daily up to a maximum dosage of 600 mg once daily if they did not experience grade 3 or higher adverse effects while receiving the original starting dosage (500 mg daily). Therapy should be continued until disease progression or intolerance to therapy occurs.

Pediatric Patients

Treatment of Newly Diagnosed Chronic Phase CML

The recommended initial pediatric (≥1 year of age) dosage of bosutinib for the treatment of newly-diagnosed chronic phase Ph⁺ CML is 300 mg/m² once daily. In pediatric patients with a body surface area (BSA) <1.1 m² and an insufficient response after 3 months of therapy, consider increasing the dosage in increments of 50 mg up to a maximum of 100 mg above the starting dose. Dose increases for insufficient response in pediatric patients with BSA ≥1.1 m² can be performed similarly to adult 100 mg increment recommendations. The maximum dose in pediatric patients is 600 mg once daily. Therapy should be continued until disease progression or intolerance to therapy occurs.

Treatment of Chronic Phase CML Following Prior Treatment Failure

The recommended initial pediatric (≥1 year of age) dosage of bosutinib for the treatment of chronic phase Ph⁺ CML following prior treatment failure is 400 mg/ m² once daily. In pediatric patients with BSA <1.1 m² and an insufficient response after 3 months of therapy, consider increasing the dosage in increments of 50 mg up to a maximum of 100 mg above the starting dose. Dose increases for insufficient response in pediatric patients with BSA ≥1.1 m² can be performed similarly to adult 100 mg increment recommendations. The maximum dose in pediatric patients is 600 mg once daily. Therapy should be continued until disease progression or intolerance to therapy occurs.

Dose Recommendations

Dose recommendations for pediatric patients with newly diagnosed chronic phase Ph⁺ CML or with chronic phase Ph⁺ CML with resistance or intolerance to prior therapy are presented in Table 2.

TABLE 2. Dose Recommendations for Bosutinib in Pediatric Patients.

Body Surface Area (m²)	Newly Diagnosed Recommended Dose (Once Daily)	Resistant or Intolerant Recommended Dose (Once Daily)
<0.55	150 mg	200 mg
0.55 to <0.63	200 mg	250 mg
0.63 to <0.75	200 mg	300 mg
0.75 to <0.9	250 mg	350 mg
0.9 to <1.1	300 mg	400 mg
≥1.1	400 mg[a]	500 mg[a]

[a] Maximum starting dose (corresponds to maximum starting dose for adult indication).

Dosage Modification for Toxicity

Myelosuppression

In patients who experience neutropenia (i.e., absolute neutrophil counts [ANC] less than 1000/mm³) or thrombocytopenia (i.e., platelet counts less than 50,000/ mm³) unrelated to the underlying CML, therapy with bosutinib should be withheld until ANC reaches or exceeds 1000/mm³ and platelet counts reach or exceed 50,000/mm³. Bosutinib therapy may then be resumed at the original starting dosage if recovery occurs within 2 weeks; if recovery is delayed (exceeding 2 weeks), the dose of bosutinib should be reduced by 100 mg (e.g., a dose of 500 mg reduced to 400 mg), or by 50 mg in pediatric patients with BSA <1.1 m², upon resumption of therapy. If neutropenia or thrombocytopenia recurs, withhold bosutinib therapy until recovery, then reduce the dose by an additional 100 mg or by an additional 50 mg in pediatric patients with BSA <1.1 m² upon resumption of therapy. Dosages less than 300 mg daily have been used, but efficacy has not been established.

Hepatotoxicity

In patients who exhibit increases in serum aminotransferase concentrations (ALT or AST exceeding 5 times the upper limit of normal [ULN]), therapy with bosutinib should be withheld until serum aminotransferase concentrations decrease to no more than 2.5 times the ULN. Bosutinib therapy may then be resumed at a dosage of 400 mg once daily. If recovery is delayed (exceeding 4 weeks), discontinue treatment with bosutinib.

In patients who exhibit increases in aminotransferase concentrations (ALT or AST 3 or more times the ULN) concurrently with total bilirubin concentrations exceeding 2 times the ULN and alkaline phosphatase concentrations less than 2 times the ULN, discontinue treatment with bosutinib.

Diarrhea

In patients with grade 3 or 4 diarrhea (7 or more stools per day over baseline), withhold therapy with bosutinib until diarrhea resolves to no more than grade 1. Bosutinib therapy may then be resumed at a dosage of 400 mg once daily.

Other Nonhematologic Effects

In patients who exhibit other clinically important, moderate or severe nonhematologic toxicity, therapy with bosutinib should be withheld until the toxicity has resolved. Bosutinib therapy may then be resumed at a dosage reduced by 100 mg once daily. If clinically appropriate, bosutinib may be re-escalated to the original starting dosage.

In pediatric patients, dose adjustments for non-hematologic toxicities can be conducted similarly to adults, however dose reduction increments may differ. For pediatric patients with BSA <1.1 m², reduce dose by 50 mg initially followed by additional 50 mg increment if the adverse reactions persist. For pediatric patients with BSA ≥1.1 m², reduce dose similarly to adults.

● Special Populations

Hepatic Impairment

For adult patients with mild to severe preexisting hepatic impairment (Child-Pugh class A, B, or C), the manufacturer recommends a bosutinib dosage of 200 mg daily.

For pediatric patients with mild to severe preexisting hepatic impairment (Child-Pugh class A, B, or C), the manufacturer recommends the following initial doses based on indication for use and BSA group:

Newly Diagnosed Ph⁺ Chronic Phase CML

- BSA <0.55 m²; 0.55 to <0.9 m²: 100 mg once daily
- BSA 0.9 to <1.1 m²: 150 mg once daily
- BSA ≥1.1 m²: 200 mg once daily

Chronic Phase CML Following Prior Treatment Failure

- BSA <0.55 m²; 0.55 to <0.63 m²: 100 mg once daily
- BSA 0.63 to <0.9 m²: 150 mg once daily
- BSA 0.9 to <1.1 m²; ≥1.1 m²: 200 mg once daily

Renal Impairment

Newly Diagnosed Ph⁺ Chronic Phase CML

For adult patients with creatinine clearance 30–50 mL/minute, the recommended dosage of bosutinib is 300 mg daily.

For adult patients with creatinine clearance <30 mL/minute, the recommended dosage of bosutinib is 200 mg daily.

For pediatric patients with newly diagnosed chronic phase Ph⁺ CML and renal impairment, dosage adjustments are presented in Table 3.

TABLE 3. Recommended Initial Doses for Pediatric Patients with Renal Impairment and Newly Diagnosed Chronic Phase Ph⁺ CML

BSA Band (m²)	Creatinine Clearance: 30-50 mL/min	Creatinine Clearance: <30 mL/min
<0.55	100 mg once daily	100 mg once daily
0.55 to <0.63	150 mg once daily	100 mg once daily
0.63 to <0.75	150 mg once daily	100 mg once daily
0.75 to <0.9	200 mg once daily	150 mg once daily
0.9 to <1.1	200 mg once daily	200 mg once daily
≥1.1	300 mg once daily	200 mg once daily

Chronic, Accelerated, or Blast Phase Ph⁺ CML Following Prior Treatment Failure

For adult patients with creatinine clearance 30–50 mL/minute, the recommended dosage of bosutinib is 400 mg daily.

For adult patients with creatinine clearance <30 mL/minute, the recommended dosage of bosutinib is 300 mg daily.

For pediatric patients with chronic phase Ph⁺ CML following prior treatment failure and renal impairment, dosage adjustments are presented in Table 4.

TABLE 4. Recommended Initial Doses for Pediatric Patients with Renal Impairment and Chronic Phase Ph⁺ CML Following Prior Treatment Failure

BSA Band (m²)	Creatinine Clearance: 30-50 mL/min	Creatinine Clearance: <30 mL/min
<0.55	150 mg once daily	100 mg once daily
0.55 to <0.63	200 mg once daily	150 mg once daily
0.63 to <0.75	200 mg once daily	200 mg once daily
0.75 to <0.9	250 mg once daily	200 mg once daily
0.9 to <1.1	300 mg once daily	250 mg once daily
≥1.1	400 mg once daily	300 mg once daily

Bosutinib has not been studied in adult or pediatric patients receiving hemodialysis.

Geriatric Use

The manufacturer makes no specific dosage recommendations for geriatric patients.

CAUTIONS

● *Contraindications*

● Known hypersensitivity to bosutinib.

● *Warnings/Precautions*

GI Toxicity

Nausea, vomiting, abdominal pain, and diarrhea occur frequently in patients receiving bosutinib. In a randomized clinical trial in adult patients with newly diagnosed Philadelphia chromosome-positive (Ph⁺) chronic myelogenous leukemia (CML), the median time to onset of diarrhea was 4 days and the median duration of each episode of diarrhea was 3 days. In a single-arm study of adult patients with CML who were resistant or intolerant to prior therapy, the median time to onset of diarrhea was 2 days and the median duration of each episode of diarrhea was 2 days. Among patients who experienced diarrhea, the median number of episodes of diarrhea per patient during therapy with bosutinib was 3 (range: 1–268 episodes).

Among pediatric patients with newly-diagnosed chronic phase Ph⁺ CML or who had chronic phase Ph⁺ CML with prior treatment failure, the median time to onset for diarrhea (all grades) was 2 days and the duration was 2 days. For those who experienced diarrhea, the median number of episodes per patient during treatment with bosutinib was 2 (range, 1 to 198).

Monitor patients for GI adverse effects and treat as clinically indicated with appropriate therapy (e.g., antidiarrheal, antiemetic, fluid replacement). Temporary interruption, dosage reduction, or discontinuance of bosutinib may be necessary if GI toxicity occurs during therapy with the drug.

Myelosuppression

Cytopenias, including thrombocytopenia, anemia, and neutropenia, have been reported in patients receiving bosutinib. Complete blood cell (CBC) counts should be monitored weekly for the first month of therapy and monthly thereafter, or as clinically indicated.

Temporary interruption, dosage reduction, or discontinuance of bosutinib may be necessary if myelosuppression occurs during therapy with the drug.

Hepatic Toxicity

Elevations in aminotransferase (ALT or AST) concentrations have occurred in patients receiving bosutinib.

In clinical trials, 2 of 1711 bosutinib-treated adult patients developed drug-induced hepatic injury without other etiology. In a randomized clinical trial evaluating adult patients with newly diagnosed CML, increased serum ALT and AST concentrations occurred in 68.3 and 56% of patients, respectively; increased aminotransferase concentrations occurred within the first 3 months of bosutinib therapy in 73% of these patients. The median time to onset of increased ALT and AST concentrations was 29 and 56 days, respectively, and the median duration was 19 and 15 days, respectively. In a single-arm study evaluating bosutinib in adult patients with CML who were resistant or intolerant to prior therapy, ALT and AST elevations occurred in 53.3 and 46.7% of patients, respectively; increased aminotransferase concentrations occurred within the first 3 months of bosutinib therapy in 81% of these patients. The median time to onset of increased ALT and AST concentrations was 22 and 29 days, respectively, and the median duration was 21 days for both ALT and AST elevations.

Among pediatric patients with newly diagnosed chronic phase Ph⁺ CML or who had chronic phase Ph⁺ CML with prior treatment failure, the incidence of increased ALT and AST from baseline was 59% and 51%, respectively. Most cases of increased transaminases occurred early in treatment; 84% of patients experienced initial increases within the first 3 months of treatment. The median time to onset for increased ALT and AST was 22 and 15 days, respectively. The median duration for grade 3 or 4 increased ALT or AST was 26 and 12 days, respectively.

Liver function tests should be monitored monthly for the first 3 months of therapy and then as clinically indicated. More frequent monitoring is recommended if elevations in aminotransferase concentrations occur. Temporary interruption, dosage reduction, or discontinuance of bosutinib may be necessary if hepatic toxicity occurs during therapy with the drug.

Cardiovascular Toxicity

Cardiovascular toxicity, including cardiac failure, left ventricular dysfunction, and cardiac ischemic events, has been reported with bosutinib. In a randomized study of adult patients with newly diagnosed CML, cardiac failure occurred in 1.9% of patients receiving bosutinib and 0.8% of patients receiving imatinib. Cardiac ischemic events occurred in 4.9 and 0.8% of bosutinib- and imatinib-treated patients, respectively. In a single-arm study of patients with CML who were resistant or intolerant to prior therapy, rates of cardiac failure and cardiac ischemic events were 5.3 and 4.9%, respectively.

Cardiac failure occurred more frequently in adult patients with previously treated CML and in those with advanced age or risk factors for cardiac failure (e.g., previous history of cardiac failure). Cardiac ischemic events were more common in patients with risk factors for coronary artery disease (e.g., history of diabetes mellitus, body mass index >30 kg/m², hypertension, vascular disorders).

Among pediatric patients with newly diagnosed chronic phase Ph⁺ CML or who had chronic phase Ph⁺ CML with prior treatment failure, 4 (8%) patients had grade 1-2 cardiac events, including tachycardia (n=2), angina pectoris, right bundle branch block, and sinus tachycardia (n=1 each).

Monitor patients for signs and symptoms of cardiac failure and cardiac ischemia and treat as clinically indicated. Temporary interruption of therapy, dosage reduction, or discontinuance of bosutinib may be necessary if cardiovascular toxicity occurs during therapy.

Fluid Retention

Fluid retention has occurred in patients receiving bosutinib and may manifest as pericardial effusion, pleural effusion, pulmonary edema, and/or peripheral edema. In a randomized trial evaluating bosutinib in 268 adult patients with newly diagnosed CML, 1.1% of patients experienced grade 3 fluid retention, 1 patient experienced grade 3 pericardial effusion, and 2 patients experienced grade 3 pleural effusion. In a single-arm study of 546 adult patients with CML who were resistant or intolerant to prior therapy, grade 3 or 4 fluid retention was reported in 6% of patients. Some patients experienced more than 1 fluid retention event; 24 patients had grade 3 or 4 pleural effusions, 9 patients had grade 3 or 4 pericardial effusions, and 6 patients had grade 3 edema.

Among pediatric patients with newly diagnosed chronic phase Ph⁺ CML or who had chronic phase Ph⁺ CML with prior treatment failure, grade 1-2 pericardial effusion, peripheral edema, and face edema were seen in 1 patient each.

If fluid retention occurs, patients should be monitored and managed according to current standards of care. Temporary interruption, dosage reduction, or discontinuance of bosutinib therapy may be necessary.

Renal Toxicity

Renal impairment has been reported during bosutinib therapy. In patients with normal baseline renal function who received bosutinib therapy for a median duration of 24 months, mild, mild to moderate, moderate to severe, or severe renal impairment occurred in 62.6, 9.5, 4.4, or 0.6% of patients, respectively; kidney failure was reported in 0.9% of bosutinib-treated patients. In patients with mild renal impairment at baseline who received bosutinib therapy for a median duration of 24 months, mild to moderate, moderate to severe, or severe renal impairment occurred in 40.3, 14.3, or 3.9% of patients, respectively; kidney failure was reported in 0.9% of bosutinib-treated patients. In patients with mild to moderate renal impairment at baseline who received bosutinib therapy for a median duration of 24 months, moderate to severe or severe renal impairment occurred in 48.2 or 17.5% of patients, respectively; kidney failure was reported in 0.7% of bosutinib-treated patients. In patients with moderate to severe renal dysfunction at baseline who received bosutinib therapy for a median duration of 24 months, severe renal dysfunction occurred in 57.6% of patients and kidney failure occurred in 12.1% of patients.

Among pediatric patients with a normal estimated glomerular filtration rate (eGFR) at baseline and newly diagnosed chronic phase Ph⁺ CML or chronic phase Ph⁺ CML with prior treatment failure, 45% shifted to a maximum of mild renal impairment, and 40% of patients who had mild eGFR at baseline shifted to a maximum of moderate renal impairment during treatment.

Monitor renal function at baseline and during therapy with bosutinib; patients with preexisting renal impairment or risk factors for renal impairment should be monitored more closely. Consider dosage adjustment in patients with baseline and/or drug-induced renal impairment.

Fetal/Neonatal Morbidity and Mortality

Bosutinib may cause fetal harm when administered to pregnant patients; there are no available data in pregnant patients to inform the drug-associated risk, but bosutinib was associated with structural abnormalities, embryofetal mortality, and alterations in growth when administered to pregnant rats and rabbits during the period of organogenesis. Pregnancy should be avoided during therapy. If used during pregnancy or if the patient becomes pregnant while receiving the drug, the patient should be apprised of the potential fetal hazard.

Specific Populations

Pregnancy

Based on findings from animal studies and its mechanism of action, bosutinib may cause fetal harm when administered to a pregnant patient. If used during pregnancy or if the patient becomes pregnant while receiving the drug, inform the patient of the potential fetal hazard.

Lactation

No data are available regarding the presence of bosutinib or its metabolites in human milk, its effects on a breast-fed child, or its effects on milk production. However, bosutinib is present in the milk of lactating rats. Breast-feeding during bosutinib treatment is not recommended due to the potential for serious adverse reactions; breast-feeding should be avoided during bosutinib therapy and for 2 weeks following the last bosutinib dose.

Females and Males of Reproductive Potential

Verify pregnancy status in females of reproductive potential prior to starting bosutinib therapy. Advise females of reproductive potential to use effective contraception during bosutinib therapy and for 2 weeks following the last dose of the drug.

Pediatric Use

Safety and efficacy of bosutinib in pediatric patients ≥1 year of age with newly diagnosed chronic phase Ph⁺ CML or who had chronic phase Ph⁺ CML with prior treatment failure has been established.. Use of bosutinib for these indications is based on data from a clinical study that included pediatric patients with newly diagnosed chronic phase Ph⁺ CML in the following age groups: 1 to <6 years of age (2 patients), 6 to <12 years of age (3 patients), and 12 to <17 years of age (10 patients). The study also included pediatric patients with chronic phase Ph⁺ CML with prior treatment failure in the following age groups: 1 to <6 years of age (4 patients), 6 to <12 years of age (10 patients), and 12 to <17 years of age (10 patients).

Geriatric Use

In clinical trials evaluating bosutinib in patients with Ph⁺ CML who were resistant or intolerant to prior therapy, 20% of patients were ≥65 years of age and 4% were ≥75 years of age. In clinical trials evaluating bosutinib for newly diagnosed CML, 20% of patients were ≥65 years of age and 5% were ≥75 years of age. No overall differences in safety or efficacy were observed between geriatric and younger adults. However, the possibility of increased sensitivity to the drug in some geriatric patients cannot be ruled out.

Hepatic Impairment

Following oral administration of a single 200-mg dose of bosutinib with food, peak plasma concentrations of bosutinib were increased by 2.4-, 2-, or 1.5-fold in patients with preexisting mild (Child-Pugh class A), moderate (Child-Pugh class B), or severe (Child-Pugh class C) hepatic impairment, respectively, compared with healthy individuals with normal hepatic function. In the same study, systemic exposure of bosutinib was increased by 2.3-, 2-, and 1.9-fold, respectively. Systemic exposure following administration of bosutinib 200 mg daily in patients with hepatic impairment is expected to be similar to that observed in those with normal hepatic function receiving bosutinib 500 mg once daily; however, efficacy of bosutinib 200 mg once daily in patients with hepatic impairment and CML is unknown. In addition, the elimination half-life of bosutinib was prolonged in patients with preexisting mild to severe hepatic impairment compared with healthy individuals with normal hepatic function. The incidence of QT interval prolongation (i.e., QT interval corrected for rate [QT$_c$] exceeding 450 msec or increased by more than 30 msec compared with baseline) increased with declining hepatic function; QT$_c$ interval prolongation was observed in all patients with severe (Child-Pugh class C) hepatic impairment enrolled in the study. Dosage adjustment is required in patients with preexisting mild, moderate, or severe hepatic impairment.

Renal Impairment

Following oral administration of a single 200-mg dose of bosutinib with food, systemic exposure of bosutinib was increased by 1.4- or 1.6-fold in patients with preexisting moderate (creatinine clearance 30–50 mL/minute) or severe (creatinine clearance less than 30 mL/minute) renal impairment, respectively, compared with healthy individuals with normal renal function. Systemic exposure of bosutinib was not affected by mild (creatinine clearance 51–80 mL/minute) renal impairment. Bosutinib has not been studied in patients receiving hemodialysis. Dosage adjustment is required in patients with preexisting moderate or severe renal impairment.

● Common Adverse Effects

Adverse effects reported in 20% or more of adult and pediatric patients receiving bosutinib include diarrhea, abdominal pain, vomiting, nausea, rash, fatigue, hepatic dysfunction, headache, pyrexia, decreased appetite, respiratory tract infection, and constipation.

Laboratory abnormalities reported in 20% or more of adult and pediatric patients receiving bosutinib include increased serum creatinine concentrations, decreased hemoglobin concentrations, decreased lymphocyte count, decreased white blood cell count, decreased absolute neutrophil count, decreased platelet count, increased aminotransferase concentrations (ALT, AST), increased alkaline phosphatase concentrations, decreased calcium concentrations, decreased phosphorus concentrations, increased glucose concentrations, increased urate concentrations, increased lipase concentrations, increased creatine kinase (CK, creatine phosphokinase, CPK) concentrations, and increased amylase concentrations.

DRUG INTERACTIONS

Bosutinib is principally metabolized by cytochrome P-450 (CYP) isoenzyme 3A4.

Bosutinib may inhibit breast cancer resistance protein (BRCP) in the GI tract but has a low potential to inhibit BRCP systemically. Bosutinib is also unlikely to inhibit organic anion transporting polypeptide (OATP) 1B1, OATP1B3, organic anion transporter (OAT) 1, OAT3, organic cation transporter (OCT) 1, or OCT2 at clinically relevant concentrations.

● Drugs and Foods Affecting Hepatic Microsomal Enzymes

Inhibitors of CYP3A

Concomitant use of bosutinib with moderate or potent inhibitors of CYP3A may result in increased systemic exposure of bosutinib and possible bosutinib toxicity. When the potent CYP3A inhibitor ketoconazole (400 mg once daily for 5 days) was administered concomitantly with bosutinib (single 100-mg dose) under fasting conditions, peak plasma concentrations and systemic exposure of bosutinib were increased 5.2- and 8.6-fold, respectively; however, in another study, adverse effects generally were mild in severity when a single bosutinib dose ranging from 100–600 mg was administered with ketoconazole (400 mg once daily for 5 days). When bosutinib (single 500-mg dose) was administered concomitantly with the moderate CYP3A inhibitor aprepitant (125 mg with food), aprepitant increased peak plasma concentrations and systemic exposure of bosutinib by 1.5- and 2-fold, respectively.

Concomitant use of bosutinib with moderate or potent inhibitors of CYP3A should be avoided.

Inducers of CYP3A

Concomitant use of bosutinib with potent inducers of CYP3A may decrease bosutinib exposure. When the potent CYP3A inducer rifampin (600 mg once daily) was administered concomitantly with bosutinib (single 500-mg dose) with meals, peak plasma concentrations and systemic exposure of bosutinib were decreased by 86 and 94%, respectively.

Concomitant use of bosutinib with potent inducers of CYP3A should be avoided.

● Substrates of P-glycoprotein Transport Systems

When a single 500-mg dose of bosutinib was administered concomitantly with the P-glycoprotein (P-gp) substrate dabigatran etexilate mesylate (150-mg dose), no clinically significant difference in dabigatran pharmacokinetics was observed.

● Drugs that Prolong the QT Interval

When bosutinib (single 500-mg dose) was administered concomitantly with ketoconazole, clinically important changes in the QT$_c$ interval were not observed.

● Proton-pump Inhibitors

When bosutinib (single 400-mg dose) was administered in combination with lansoprazole (multiple 60-mg doses) under fasting conditions, peak plasma concentrations and AUC of bosutinib were reduced by 46 and 26%, respectively. Concomitant use of bosutinib and proton-pump inhibitors is not recommended. Instead, use of histamine H$_2$-receptor antagonists or short-acting antacids, administered at least 2 hours before or after a dose of bosutinib, should be considered.

DESCRIPTION

Bosutinib, an inhibitor of multiple tyrosine kinases (including Bcr-Abl and the Src family [Src, Lyn, Hck]), is an antineoplastic agent; the drug has minimal inhibitory activity against c-Kit or platelet-derived growth factor (PDGF)-β.

The Philadelphia chromosome, characteristic of chronic myelogenous leukemia (CML), is created by a reciprocal translocation between chromosomes 9 and 22. Translocation between these chromosomes results in production of an abnormal protein (Bcr-Abl tyrosine kinase) that exhibits enhanced tyrosine kinase activity (i.e., increased phosphorylation of tyrosine residues); phosphorylation of tyrosine residues on growth factor receptors is thought to be important in stimulating cell proliferation and inhibiting cell death (apoptosis). Bosutinib competitively and selectively inhibits Bcr-Abl tyrosine kinase, thereby inhibiting tyrosine phosphorylation of proteins involved in Bcr-Abl signal transduction. In vitro studies show the drug inhibits the growth of leukemic cell lines expressing Bcr-Abl.

Clinical resistance to imatinib in CML has been attributed to several mechanisms, but point mutations in the Bcr-Abl kinase domain appear to be the most common, occurring in 30–90% of patients who develop resistance. In preclinical studies in cell-line models, bosutinib inhibited most (16 of 18) imatinib-resistant Bcr-Abl kinase domain mutant forms except for T315I and V299L mutant cells. Data from preclinical and clinical studies also implicate signaling pathways involving the Src family kinases (Lyn, Hck) in imatinib resistance.

Bosutinib is 94–96% bound to plasma proteins in vitro. In a dose escalation study, bosutinib exhibited linear and dose proportional pharmacokinetics under fed conditions; AUC and peak plasma concentrations of the drug are dose proportional over the bosutinib dosage range of 200–800 mg. The median time to peak plasma concentrations of bosutinib is 6 hours, and the absolute bioavailability of the drug is 34%. Administration of bosutinib tablets with a high-fat meal resulted in increases in systemic exposure and peak plasma concentrations of 1.7- and 1.8-fold, respectively. No clinically significant differences in the pharmacokinetics of bosutinib were observed following administration of either the tablet or capsule dosage forms at the same dose, under fed conditions. Bosutinib is extensively metabolized by the cytochrome P-450 (CYP) microsomal enzyme system, principally by the isoenzyme 3A4 to inactive metabolites. Following administration of a single radiolabeled dose of bosutinib, 91.3% of the dose was recovered in feces and 3.3% was recovered in urine. Following administration of single 500-mg doses of bosutinib with food, the elimination half-life of bosutinib was 22.5 hours. No clinically significant differences in the pharmacokinetics of bosutinib were observed following administration of bosutinib capsule that was opened and the contents mixed with applesauce or yogurt immediately before use.

ADVICE TO PATIENTS

- Advise patients not to alter the dosage or discontinue therapy without first consulting a clinician.

- If a dose is missed by >12 hours, take the next dose at the regularly scheduled time. Do *not* double the dose.

- Advise patients to take bosutinib with food. Advise patients to swallow bosutinib tablets whole and not to crush, break, chew, or cut the tablets. Importance of not touching or handling crushed or broken tablets.

- Advise patients that bosutinib capsules may be swallowed whole. For patients that cannot swallow the whole capsule, the capsule can be opened and the contents mixed with applesauce or yogurt.

- Risk of diarrhea, nausea, vomiting, abdominal pain, or bloody stools. Advise patients to promptly seek medical attention if any of these symptoms occur.

- Risk of cytopenias. Inform a clinician if fever, easy bruising, or other signs and symptoms of infection or bleeding occur.

- Risk of liver function abnormalities. Contact a clinician promptly if jaundice occurs.

- Risk of cardiac problems. Inform patients to seek immediate medical attention if symptoms of cardiac failure or cardiac ischemia (e.g., shortness of breath, weight gain, fluid retention) occur.

- Risk of fluid retention. Contact a clinician promptly if swelling, weight gain, or shortness of breath occurs.

- Risk of renal impairment. Immediately report symptoms of frequent urination, polyuria, or oliguria to a clinician.

- Importance of females informing clinicians if they become pregnant. Advise pregnant females of risk to fetus. Advise females of reproductive potential to use an effective method of contraception while receiving bosutinib and for 2 weeks after discontinuance of therapy.

- Advise females to avoid breast-feeding during therapy and for 2 weeks after discontinuance of therapy.

- Inform clinicians of existing or contemplated concomitant therapy, including prescription and OTC drugs and herbal supplements (e.g., St. John's wort), as well as any concomitant illnesses.

- Inform patients of other important precautionary information.

For further information on the handling of antineoplastic agents, see the ASHP Guidelines on Handling Hazardous Drugs at https://www.ahfsdrug information.com.

PREPARATIONS

Excipients in commercially available drug preparations may have clinically important effects in some individuals; consult specific product labeling for details.

Bosutinib

Oral		
Tablets, film-coated	100 mg	Bosulif®, Pfizer
	400 mg	Bosulif®, Pfizer
	500 mg	Bosulif®, Pfizer
Capsules	50 mg	Bosulif®
	100 mg	Bosulif®

† Use is not currently included in the labeling approved by the US Food and Drug Administration.

Selected Revisions June 10, 2024, © Copyright, October 21, 2013, American Society of Health-System Pharmacists, Inc.

Brentuximab Vedotin

10:00 • ANTINEOPLASTIC AGENTS

■ Brentuximab vedotin, a chimeric human-murine anti-CD30 antibody conjugated with the microtubule inhibitor monomethyl auristatin E (MMAE), is an antineoplastic agent.

USES

● Hodgkin Lymphoma

Newly Diagnosed Classical Hodgkin Lymphoma

Brentuximab vedotin is used in combination with doxorubicin, vinblastine, and dacarbazine (AVD) for the treatment of previously untreated stage III or IV classical Hodgkin lymphoma (cHL). Brentuximab vedotin is designated an orphan drug by FDA for the treatment of this cancer. In adults with previously untreated stage III or IV cHL, combination therapy with brentuximab vedotin and AVD substantially reduced the risk of progression, death, or, in those who did not achieve a complete response, receipt of subsequent anticancer therapy compared with combination therapy with doxorubicin, bleomycin, vinblastine, and dacarbazine (ABVD).

Efficacy of brentuximab vedotin in combination with AVD for previously untreated stage III or IV cHL is based principally on the results of an open-label, randomized phase 3 study (ECHELON-1) in 1334 patients with previously untreated advanced cHL. The primary measure of efficacy was progression-free survival (based on time to disease progression, death, or receipt of subsequent anticancer therapy following failure to achieve complete response) as assessed by an independent review facility. The median age of patients was 36 years; 84% of patients were white, 64% had stage IV disease, and 62% had extranodal involvement at diagnosis.

In this study, patients were randomized in a 1:1 ratio to receive therapy with brentuximab vedotin in combination with AVD (brentuximab vedotin-AVD) or ABVD alone. Patients in the brentuximab vedotin-AVD group received brentuximab vedotin 1.2 mg/kg by IV infusion over 30 minutes in combination with IV doxorubicin hydrochloride 25 mg/m^2, IV vinblastine sulfate 6 mg/m^2, and IV dacarbazine 375 mg/m^2 on days 1 and 15 of each 28-day cycle for a maximum of 6 cycles. Patients in the ABVD group received the same dosages of doxorubicin hydrochloride, vinblastine sulfate, and dacarbazine with the addition of IV bleomycin 10 units/m^2 on days 1 and 15 of each 28-day cycle for a maximum of 6 cycles.

At a median follow-up of 24.6 months, median progression-free survival had not been reached in either group; however, the risk of disease progression, death, or receipt of subsequent anticancer therapy following failure to achieve complete response was reduced by 23% in patients receiving brentuximab vedotin-AVD compared with those receiving ABVD alone. Disease progression, death, or receipt of subsequent anticancer therapy following failure to achieve complete response occurred in 14, 3, or 1%, respectively, of patients receiving brentuximab vedotin-AVD and 15, 3, or 3%, respectively, of those receiving ABVD alone. Subsequent anticancer therapy consisted of salvage chemotherapy (71%) and radiation therapy (29%). At the time of analysis, overall survival was not substantially different between the treatment groups. Complete response was achieved in 73% of patients receiving brentuximab vedotin-AVD and 70% of those receiving ABVD alone. Results of a subgroup analysis based on relevant baseline patient and disease characteristics suggested lack of a progression-free survival benefit for brentuximab vedotin-AVD compared with ABVD alone in patients 60 years of age or older and in those without extranodal involvement.

Consolidation Therapy

Brentuximab vedotin is used as single-agent consolidation therapy for cHL in patients at high risk of relapse or progression following autologous stem cell transplantation. Brentuximab vedotin is designated an orphan drug by FDA for the treatment of this cancer. In adults with cHL at high risk of relapse or progression following autologous stem cell transplantation, consolidation therapy with brentuximab vedotin substantially prolonged median progression-free survival compared with placebo.

Efficacy of brentuximab vedotin as consolidation therapy for cHL in patients at high risk of relapse or progression following autologous stem cell transplantation is based principally on the results of a randomized, double-blind, placebo-controlled phase 3 study (AETHERA) in 329 patients with relapsed or refractory cHL

(i.e., disease progression within 12 months or, in those with extranodal involvement, at 12 or more months following first-line therapy). Patients were enrolled in the study if they achieved a complete or partial response or had stable disease following their most recent pre-stem cell transplantation salvage therapy. The primary measure of efficacy was progression-free survival as assessed by an independent review facility. The median age of patients was 32 years; the patients had received a median of 2 prior systemic therapies for their disease. In this study, patients were randomized in a 1:1 ratio to receive brentuximab vedotin (1.8 mg/kg by IV infusion over 30 minutes) or placebo every 3 weeks for a maximum of 16 cycles; treatment was initiated 30–45 days after autologous stem cell transplantation. At a median follow-up of 22 months, median progression-free survival was prolonged in brentuximab vedotin-treated patients compared with placebo recipients (at least 42.9 versus 24.1 months; hazard ratio: 0.57). At the time of analysis, overall survival was not substantially different between the treatment groups. At a follow-up of 5 years, median progression-free survival for brentuximab vedotin-treated patients had not been reached and was 15.8 months in those receiving placebo; however, 5-year progression-free survival rate was 59% in patients receiving brentuximab vedotin and 41% in those receiving placebo.

Relapsed Classical Hodgkin Lymphoma

Brentuximab vedotin is used as a single agent for the treatment of cHL following failure of autologous stem cell transplantation or following failure of 2 or more multiple-agent chemotherapy regimens in patients who are not candidates for autologous stem cell transplantation. Brentuximab vedotin is designated an orphan drug by FDA for the treatment of this cancer. This indication is based on objective response rate in a noncomparative, open-label study in patients with relapsed cHL.

Efficacy of brentuximab vedotin for cHL following failure of autologous stem cell transplantation or following failure of 2 or more multiple-agent chemotherapy regimens in patients who are not candidates for autologous stem cell transplantation is based principally on the results of an open-label, noncomparative, phase 2 study in 102 patients with Hodgkin lymphoma who relapsed following autologous stem cell transplantation. The primary measure of efficacy was objective response rate (complete plus partial responses). The median age of patients was 31 years; the patients had received a median of 5 prior therapies for their disease. In this study, all patients received brentuximab vedotin (1.8 mg/kg IV every 3 weeks) for a maximum of 16 cycles or until disease progression or unacceptable toxicity occurred. At the time of interim analysis, objective response rate was 73%; 32% of patients receiving the drug achieved a complete response. At the time of analysis, the median duration of response for all responders was 6.7 months (range: 1.3–21.9 months); the median duration of response was 20.5 months for patients achieving a complete response but only 3.5 months for those achieving a partial response. Complete response rates at the time of final analysis (at a median follow-up of 35.1 months) remained similar to the interim results. At the time of final analysis, median overall survival and progression-free survival were 40.5 and 9.3 months, respectively; estimated 5-year overall survival and progression-free survival rates were 41 and 22%, respectively.

● Peripheral T-cell Lymphoma

Previously Untreated Systemic Anaplastic Large Cell Lymphoma or other Peripheral T-cell Lymphomas

Brentuximab vedotin is used in combination with cyclophosphamide, doxorubicin, and prednisone (CHP) for the treatment of previously untreated systemic anaplastic large cell lymphoma (sALCL) or other CD30-positive peripheral T-cell lymphomas (PTCLs), including angioimmunoblastic T-cell lymphoma (AITL) and PTCL not otherwise specified (PTCL-NOS). Brentuximab vedotin is designated an orphan drug by FDA for the treatment of these cancers. In adults with previously untreated sALCL or other CD30-positive PTCLs, brentuximab vedotin in combination with CHP prolonged progression-free survival and overall survival compared with cyclophosphamide, doxorubicin, vincristine, and prednisone (CHOP).

Efficacy of brentuximab vedotin in combination with CHP for previously untreated sALCL or other CD30-positive PTCLs is based principally on the results of a double-blind, double-dummy, active-controlled, randomized phase 3 study (ECHELON-2) in 452 patients with previously untreated CD30-positive (defined as CD30 expression of at least 10% per immunohistochemistry) PTCL. The primary measure of efficacy was progression-free survival (based on time to disease progression, death, or receipt of subsequent systemic chemotherapy for the treatment of residual or progressive disease) as assessed by a blinded independent review facility.

In this study, patients were randomized in a 1:1 ratio to receive therapy with brentuximab vedotin in combination with CHP (brentuximab vedotin-CHP) or CHOP alone. Patients in the brentuximab vedotin-CHP group received brentuximab vedotin 1.8 mg/kg by IV infusion over 30 minutes on day 1 in combination with IV cyclophosphamide 750 mg/m² on day 1, IV doxorubicin hydrochloride 50 mg/m² on day 1, and oral prednisone 100 mg on days 1–5 of each 21-day cycle for up to 6–8 cycles. Patients in the CHOP group received the same dosages of cyclophosphamide, doxorubicin hydrochloride, and prednisone with the addition of IV vincristine sulfate 1.4 mg/m² on day 1 of each 21-day cycle for up to 6–8 cycles.

The median age of patients enrolled in this study was 58 years; 78% of the patients had an Eastern Cooperative Oncology Group (ECOG) performance status of 0 or 1, 81% had stage III or IV disease, and 63% had a baseline International Prognostic Index score of 2 or 3. Most patients (70%) enrolled in the study had sALCL; 16% had PTCL-NOS, 12% had AITL, 2% had adult T-cell leukemia/lymphoma, and less than 1% had enteropathy-associated T-cell lymphoma. Approximately one-half (48%) of patients with sALCL had anaplastic lymphoma kinase (ALK)-negative disease. This study excluded patients with primary cutaneous CD30-positive T-cell lymphoproliferative disorders and lymphomas.

Overall, patients receiving brentuximab vedotin-CHP had longer median progression-free survival (48.2 versus 20.8 months; hazard ratio: 0.71), higher objective response rates (83 versus 72%), and higher complete response rates (68 versus 56%) compared with those receiving CHOP alone. In the subset of patients with sALCL, those receiving brentuximab vedotin-CHP also had longer median progression-free survival compared with those receiving CHOP alone (55.7 versus 54.2 months; hazard ratio: 0.59). In the overall study population at a median follow-up of 41.9 months for those receiving brentuximab vedotin-CHP and 42.2 months for those receiving CHOP, median overall survival had not been reached in either group; however, overall survival appeared to be prolonged in patients receiving brentuximab vedotin-CHP compared with those receiving CHOP alone. Results of a subgroup analysis (based on age, sex, ECOG performance status, International Prognostic Index score, disease stage, histologic subtype) suggested lack of progression-free survival and overall survival benefits for brentuximab vedotin-CHP compared with CHOP alone in patients with an International Prognostic Index score of 4 or 5 or ECOG performance status score of 2; a progression-free survival benefit for brentuximab vedotin-CHP compared with CHOP alone also was not apparent in the subgroup of patients with AITL or stage I or II disease.

Relapsed Systemic Anaplastic Large Cell Lymphoma

Brentuximab vedotin is used as a single agent for the treatment of sALCL following failure of 1 or more multiple-agent chemotherapy regimens; brentuximab vedotin is designated an orphan drug by FDA for the treatment of this cancer. This indication is based on objective response rate in a noncomparative, open-label, phase 2 study in patients with relapsed sALCL.

This noncomparative, open-label study included 58 patients with sALCL who relapsed following prior therapy. The primary measure of efficacy was objective response rate (complete plus partial responses). The median age of patients was 52 years; the patients had received a median of 2 prior therapies, 26% of the patients had received prior autologous stem cell transplantation for their disease, and 72% of the patients had ALK-negative disease, which is associated with a worse prognosis. In this study, all patients received brentuximab vedotin (1.8 mg/kg IV every 3 weeks) for a maximum of 16 cycles or until disease progression or unacceptable toxicity occurred.

At the time of interim analysis, the objective response rate was 86%; 57% of patients receiving the drug achieved a complete response. At the time of analysis, the median duration of response for all responders was 12.6 months (range: 0.1–15.9 months); the median duration of response was 13.2 months for patients achieving a complete response but only 2.1 months for those achieving a partial response. Objective response rates at the time of final analysis (at a median follow-up of 58.4 months) remained similar to the interim results; 66% of patients receiving the drug achieved a complete response. At the time of final analysis, the median duration of response for all responders was 25.6 months. Although median overall survival had not been reached at the time of final analysis, median progression-free survival was 20 months and estimated 5-year overall survival and progression-free survival rates were 60 and 39%, respectively. Subgroup analysis suggested that objective response rates were similar in patients with ALK-negative or ALK-positive disease (88 or 81%, respectively).

Relapsed Primary Cutaneous T-cell Lymphoma or Mycosis Fungoides

Brentuximab vedotin is used as a single agent for the treatment of primary cutaneous anaplastic large cell lymphoma (pcALCL) or CD30-positive mycosis fungoides previously treated with systemic therapy. Brentuximab vedotin is designated an orphan drug by FDA for the treatment of these conditions. In patients with previously treated CD30-positive pcALCL or mycosis fungoides, durable response rates were higher in patients receiving brentuximab vedotin compared with those receiving standard chemotherapy.

Efficacy of brentuximab vedotin for the treatment of pcALCL or CD30-positive mycosis fungoides previously treated with systemic therapy is based principally on the results of an open-label, multicenter, randomized phase 3 study (ALCANZA) in 131 patients with previously treated CD30-positive (defined as CD30 expression of at least 10% on at least one skin biopsy specimen) pcALCL or mycosis fungoides. Patients were eligible for this study if they had pcALCL previously treated with systemic therapy or radiation therapy or mycosis fungoides previously treated with systemic therapy. The primary measure of efficacy was durable response rate (complete plus partial responses lasting at least 4 months) as assessed by an independent review facility according to global response scoring.

In this study, patients were randomized in a 1:1 ratio to receive therapy with brentuximab vedotin 1.8 mg/kg by IV infusion over 30 minutes on day 1 of each 21-day cycle for a maximum of 16 cycles or investigator's choice of standard chemotherapy (methotrexate 5–50 mg orally once weekly or bexarotene 300 mg/m² orally once daily) for a maximum of 48 weeks. The median age of patients was 60 years; 85% of patients were white, 63% had stage I or II disease, and 13% had stage IV disease. Patients enrolled in the study had received a median of 4 prior therapies, including a median of 1 skin-directed therapy and 2 systemic therapies.

At a median follow-up of 22.9 months, the durable response rate was 56.3% in patients receiving brentuximab vedotin compared with 12.5% in those receiving standard chemotherapy. The objective response rate was 67.2% in patients receiving brentuximab vedotin and 20.3% in those receiving standard chemotherapy; complete responses were achieved in 15.6 and 1.6% of patients receiving these respective treatments. Patients receiving brentuximab vedotin also had longer median progression-free survival (16.7 versus 3.5 months) and event-free survival (9.4 versus 2.3 months) compared with those receiving standard chemotherapy. Results of a subgroup analysis based on relevant baseline patient and disease characteristics suggested that the effect of brentuximab vedotin on durable response rate and progression-free survival was consistent across all subgroups.

DOSAGE AND ADMINISTRATION

● General

Because brentuximab vedotin may cause neutropenia, the manufacturer states that complete blood cell (CBC) counts should be obtained prior to each dose; more frequent monitoring should be considered in patients with evidence of grade 3 or 4 neutropenia.

Primary prophylaxis with a granulocyte colony-stimulating factor (G-CSF) is recommended for patients receiving brentuximab vedotin in combination with doxorubicin, vinblastine, and dacarbazine (AVD) or cyclophosphamide, doxorubicin, and prednisone (CHP) beginning with cycle 1.

Patients who experience an infusion-related reaction to brentuximab vedotin should receive a premedication regimen (e.g., a corticosteroid, an antihistamine, and acetaminophen) prior to each subsequent dose of the drug. (See Sensitivity Reactions under Warnings/Precautions: Other Warnings and Precautions, in Cautions.)

Clinicians should consult the respective manufacturers' labelings or published protocols for information on the dosage, method of administration, and administration sequence of other antineoplastic agents used in combination regimens.

● Administration

Procedures for proper handling (e.g., use of gloves or protective clothing) and disposal of antineoplastic agents should be followed.

Brentuximab vedotin is administered by IV infusion over 30 minutes.

Unreconstituted brentuximab vedotin powder for injection should be stored in unopened vials at 2–8°C. Unopened vials should be retained in the original package for protection from light.

Prior to administration, commercially available brentuximab vedotin powder for injection must be reconstituted and diluted using proper aseptic technique. The powder is reconstituted by adding 10.5 mL of sterile water for injection to a vial labeled as containing 50 mg of the drug to provide a solution containing 5 mg/mL. The diluent should be directed toward the wall of the vial and not directly at the brentuximab vedotin cake or powder. The vial should be gently swirled and inspected visually for particulate matter and discoloration prior to dilution and administration. The resulting solution should *not* be shaken. The solution should be clear to slightly opalescent, colorless, and free of visible particulates. The reconstituted brentuximab vedotin solution may be diluted immediately or stored at 2–8°C for use within 24 hours, and should be protected from direct sunlight until time of use. The reconstituted solution should not be frozen.

For preparation of the final diluted brentuximab vedotin solution for infusion, the required amount of reconstituted brentuximab vedotin solution should be injected into an infusion bag containing a minimum volume of 100 mL of 0.9% sodium chloride injection, 5% dextrose injection, or lactated Ringer's injection to produce a final solution with brentuximab vedotin concentration of 0.4–1.8 mg/mL. The final diluted brentuximab vedotin solution for infusion should be mixed by gentle inversion. The solution may be infused immediately or stored at 2–8°C and used within 24 hours following reconstitution; the solution for infusion should not be frozen and should be protected from direct sunlight until use. Any partially used vials should be discarded. Brentuximab vedotin should not be admixed with any other drug, nor should any other drug be administered simultaneously in the same IV line with brentuximab vedotin infusion.

● **Dosage**

In patients who weigh 100 kg or less, dosage of brentuximab vedotin should be based on actual body weight; however, in patients who weigh more than 100 kg, dosage should be calculated based on a weight of 100 kg.

Hodgkin Lymphoma

Combination Therapy for Previously Untreated Classical Hodgkin Lymphoma

When used in combination with doxorubicin, vinblastine, and dacarbazine (AVD) for the treatment of previously untreated stage III or IV classical Hodgkin lymphoma (cHL), the recommended adult dosage of brentuximab vedotin is 1.2 mg/kg (up to a maximum dose of 120 mg) administered as a 30-minute IV infusion on days 1 and 15 of each 28-day cycle. Therapy should be continued for up to 6 cycles or until disease progression or unacceptable toxicity occurs. In the ECHELON-1 study, brentuximab vedotin was administered approximately 1 hour after administration of the AVD regimen.

Consolidation Therapy for Classical Hodgkin Lymphoma

For consolidation therapy as a single agent in patients with cHL at high risk of relapse or progression following autologous stem cell transplantation, the recommended adult dosage of brentuximab vedotin is 1.8 mg/kg (up to a maximum dose of 180 mg) administered as a 30-minute IV infusion every 3 weeks. Therapy should be continued for up to 16 cycles or until disease progression or unacceptable toxicity occurs. Brentuximab vedotin should be initiated upon recovery from or within 4–6 weeks following autologous stem cell transplantation.

Monotherapy for Relapsed Classical Hodgkin Lymphoma

For the treatment of cHL following failure of autologous stem cell transplantation or following failure of 2 or more multiple-agent chemotherapy regimens in patients who are not autologous stem cell transplantation candidates, the recommended adult dosage of brentuximab vedotin is 1.8 mg/kg (up to a maximum dose of 180 mg) administered as a 30-minute IV infusion every 3 weeks. Therapy should be continued until disease progression or unacceptable toxicity occurs.

Peripheral T-cell Lymphoma

Combination Therapy for Previously Untreated Peripheral T-cell Lymphoma

When used in combination with cyclophosphamide, doxorubicin, and prednisone (CHP) for the treatment of previously untreated systemic anaplastic large cell lymphoma (sALCL) or other CD30-positive peripheral T-cell lymphomas (PTCLs), including angioimmunoblastic T-cell lymphoma (AITL) and PTCL not otherwise specified (PTCL-NOS), the recommended adult dosage of brentuximab vedotin is

1.8 mg/kg (up to a maximum dose of 180 mg) administered as a 30-minute IV infusion on day 1 of each 21-day cycle. Therapy should be continued for 6–8 cycles.

In the ECHELON-2 study, 70 or 18% of patients received 6 or 8 cycles, respectively, of brentuximab vedotin in combination with CHP.

Monotherapy for Relapsed Peripheral T-cell Lymphoma

For the treatment of sALCL following failure of 1 or more multiple-agent chemotherapy regimens, the recommended adult dosage of brentuximab vedotin is 1.8 mg/kg (up to a maximum dose of 180 mg) administered as a 30-minute IV infusion every 3 weeks. Therapy should be continued until disease progression or unacceptable toxicity occurs.

For the treatment of primary cutaneous anaplastic large cell lymphoma (pcALCL) or CD30-positive mycosis fungoides previously treated with systemic therapy, the recommended adult dosage of brentuximab vedotin is 1.8 mg/kg (up to a maximum dose of 180 mg) administered as a 30-minute IV infusion every 3 weeks. Therapy should be continued for up to 16 cycles or until disease progression or unacceptable toxicity occurs.

Dosage Modification for Toxicity

Dosing interruption and/or dosage reduction or discontinuance of brentuximab vedotin therapy may be necessary based on severity of an adverse effect as described in Tables 1, 2, and 3.

TABLE 1. Dosage Modifications for Toxicity of Single-agent Brentuximab Vedotin

Toxicity	Dosage Modification
	Relapsed cHL, Consolidation Therapy for cHL, Relapsed sALCL, or Relapsed pcALCL or Mycosis Fungoides (Initial Dosage = 1.8 mg/kg every 3 weeks)
Peripheral neuropathy	New or worsening grade 2 or 3: Interrupt brentuximab vedotin; when toxicity resolves to grade 1 or baseline, resume at reduced dosage of 1.2 mg/kg (maximum 120 mg) every 3 weeks
	Grade 4: Discontinue brentuximab vedotin
Neutropenia	Grade 3 or 4: Interrupt brentuximab vedotin; when toxicity improves to grade 2 or less or to baseline, resume at same dosage; consider G-CSF use during subsequent cycles
	Recurrent grade 4 (despite G-CSF use): Consider drug discontinuance or dosage reduction (i.e., reduced brentuximab vedotin dosage of 1.2 mg/kg [maximum 120 mg] every 3 weeks)

TABLE 2. Dosage Modifications for Brentuximab Vedotin During Combination Therapy with Doxorubicin, Vinblastine, and Dacarbazine (AVD)

Toxicity	Dosage Modification
	Previously Untreated cHL (Initial Dosage = 1.2 mg/kg every 2 weeks)
Peripheral neuropathy	Grade 2: Reduce brentuximab vedotin dosage to 0.9 mg/kg (maximum 90 mg) every 2 weeks
	Grade 3: Consider dosage modification of concomitant neurotoxic drugs and interrupt brentuximab vedotin; when toxicity improves to grade 2 or less, resume brentuximab vedotin at reduced dosage of 0.9 mg/kg (maximum 90 mg) every 2 weeks
	Grade 4: Discontinue brentuximab vedotin
Neutropenia	Grade 3 or 4 (patient not receiving primary G-CSF prophylaxis): Administer G-CSF during subsequent cycles

TABLE 3. Dosage Modifications for Brentuximab Vedotin During Combination Therapy with Cyclophosphamide, Doxorubicin, and Prednisone (CHP)

Toxicity	Dosage Modification
	Previously Untreated sALCL or Other PTCL (Initial Dosage = 1.8 mg/kg every 3 weeks)
Peripheral sensory neuropathy	Grade 2: Continue same dosage
	Grade 3: Reduce brentuximab vedotin dosage to 1.2 mg/kg (maximum 120 mg) every 3 weeks
	Grade 4: Discontinue brentuximab vedotin
Peripheral motor neuropathy	Grade 2: Reduce brentuximab vedotin dosage to 1.2 mg/kg (maximum 120 mg) every 3 weeks
	Grade 3 or 4: Discontinue brentuximab vedotin
Neutropenia	Grade 3 or 4 (patient not receiving primary G-CSF prophylaxis): Administer G-CSF during subsequent cycles

● Special Populations

For patients with mild hepatic impairment (Child-Pugh class A), the manufacturer recommends a reduced dosage of brentuximab vedotin. When the usual recommended dosage is 1.2 mg/kg every 2 weeks, the manufacturer recommends that patients with mild hepatic impairment (Child-Pugh class A) receive an initial brentuximab vedotin dosage of 0.9 mg/kg (up to a maximum dose of 90 mg) every 2 weeks. When the usual recommended dosage is 1.8 mg/kg every 3 weeks, the manufacturer recommends that patients with mild hepatic impairment (Child-Pugh class A) receive an initial brentuximab vedotin dosage of 1.2 mg/kg (up to a maximum dose of 120 mg) every 3 weeks. Use of brentuximab vedotin in patients with moderate or severe hepatic impairment (Child-Pugh class B or C) should be avoided. (See Hepatic Impairment under Warnings/Precautions: Specific Populations, in Cautions.)

No dosage adjustment is necessary in patients with mild or moderate renal impairment (creatinine clearance of 30–80 mL/minute). Use of brentuximab vedotin in patients with severe renal impairment (creatinine clearance less than 30 mL/minute) should be avoided. (See Renal Impairment under Warnings/Precautions: Specific Populations, in Cautions.)

The manufacturer makes no specific dosage recommendations for geriatric patients. (See Geriatric Use under Warnings/Precautions: Specific Populations, in Cautions.)

CAUTIONS

● Contraindications

Concomitant use with bleomycin. (See Respiratory Effects under Warnings/Precautions: Other Warnings and Precautions, in Cautions.)

● Warnings/Precautions

Warnings

Progressive Multifocal Leukoencephalopathy

JC virus infection causing progressive multifocal leukoencephalopathy (PML), sometimes fatal, has been reported in patients receiving brentuximab vedotin. Other factors that might increase the risk for PML include prior therapies and underlying disease that may cause immunosuppression. Signs and symptoms of PML may develop over several weeks or months; some cases have occurred within 3 months of initiation of brentuximab vedotin.

The possible diagnosis of PML should be considered in any patient receiving brentuximab vedotin who experiences new neurologic manifestations suggestive of PML (e.g., changes in mood or behavior, confusion, changes in thinking, memory loss, vision changes, changes in speech or walking, decreased strength or weakness on one side of the body). If PML is suspected, the drug should be withheld. If PML is confirmed, brentuximab vedotin should be permanently discontinued.

Other Warnings and Precautions

Peripheral Neuropathy

Peripheral neuropathy has been reported in patients receiving brentuximab vedotin. Brentuximab vedotin mainly causes sensory neuropathy, but motor neuropathy also has been reported.

In clinical studies evaluating single-agent brentuximab vedotin, peripheral neuropathy occurred in 62% of patients receiving the drug. The median time to onset of peripheral neuropathy was 3 months (range: 0–12 months), and the median time to resolution or improvement of any grade was 5 months. Peripheral neuropathy was managed with treatment delays, drug discontinuance, and/or dosage reductions; 62% of patients had complete resolution, 24% had partial improvement, and 14% had no improvement.

In the ECHELON-1 study evaluating brentuximab vedotin in combination with doxorubicin, vinblastine, and dacarbazine (AVD), peripheral neuropathy occurred in 67% of patients receiving brentuximab vedotin in combination with AVD. The median time to onset of peripheral neuropathy was 2 months (range: 0–7 months). The median time to resolution or improvement of any grade was 2 months; however, the median time to resolution or improvement increased with severity. Among patients who experienced peripheral neuropathy, 43% of patients had complete resolution, 24% had partial improvement, and 33% had no improvement.

In the ECHELON-2 study evaluating brentuximab vedotin in combination with cyclophosphamide, doxorubicin, and prednisone (CHP), new or worsening peripheral neuropathy occurred in 52% of patients receiving brentuximab vedotin in combination with CHP; sensory or motor neuropathy occurred in 94 or 16%, respectively, of these patients. The median time to onset of peripheral neuropathy was 2 months (range: less than 1 month to 5 months), and the median time to resolution or improvement of any grade was 4 months. Among patients who experienced peripheral neuropathy, 50% of patients had complete resolution, 12% had partial improvement, and 38% had no improvement.

Patients receiving brentuximab vedotin should be monitored for manifestations of neuropathy (e.g., hypoesthesia, hyperesthesia, paresthesia, discomfort, burning sensation, neuropathic pain, weakness). Dosage reduction, treatment delay, or drug discontinuance may be required in patients who experience new or worsening neuropathic symptoms. (See Dosage Modification for Toxicity under Dosage and Administration: Dosage.)

Sensitivity Reactions

Infusion-related reactions, including anaphylaxis, have been reported in patients receiving brentuximab vedotin. In clinical studies evaluating single-agent brentuximab vedotin, infusion-related reactions, including chills, nausea, dyspnea, pruritus, pyrexia, and/or cough, occurred in 13% of patients receiving the drug; grade 3 infusion-related reactions were reported in 5 of these patients. In the ECHELON-1 study evaluating brentuximab vedotin in combination with AVD, infusion-related reactions occurred in 57 of 662 patients (9%) receiving brentuximab vedotin in combination with AVD; grade 3 infusion-related reactions were reported in 3 of these patients. In the ECHELON-2 study evaluating brentuximab vedotin in combination with CHP, infusion-related reactions occurred in 10 of 223 patients (4%) receiving brentuximab vedotin in combination with CHP; grade 3 or greater infusion-related reactions were reported in 2 of these patients. Patients should be monitored during infusions of the drug for manifestations of infusion-related reactions.

In patients experiencing infusion-related reactions, the brentuximab vedotin infusion should be interrupted and appropriate therapy should be instituted. The drug should be immediately and permanently discontinued in patients who experience anaphylaxis. The manufacturer states that patients who experience an infusion-related reaction to brentuximab vedotin should be premedicated (e.g., with a corticosteroid, an antihistamine, and acetaminophen) prior to each subsequent dose of the drug.

Hematologic Effects

Severe and prolonged (lasting 1 week or longer) neutropenia and grade 3 or 4 anemia or thrombocytopenia may occur. Febrile neutropenia, sometimes fatal, also has been reported in patients receiving brentuximab vedotin. Complete blood cell (CBC) counts should be monitored prior to each dose of brentuximab vedotin; if grade 3 or 4 neutropenia occurs, more frequent monitoring should be considered. Patients should be monitored for fever. The manufacturer recommends primary prophylaxis with a granulocyte colony-stimulating factor (G-CSF) for patients receiving brentuximab vedotin in combination with chemotherapy for classical Hodgkin lymphoma (cHL) or previously untreated peripheral T-cell lymphomas (PTCL). In patients who develop grade 3 or 4 neutropenia, temporary interruption of therapy, dosage reduction, drug discontinuance or, in those who did not receive primary G-CSF prophylaxis, use of a G-CSF may be required. (See Dosage Modification for Toxicity under in Dosage and Administration: Dosage.)

Infectious Complications

Serious infections and opportunistic infections, such as pneumonia, bacteremia, and sepsis/septic shock, sometimes fatal, have been reported in patients receiving brentuximab vedotin.

Patients receiving brentuximab vedotin should be monitored closely for signs and symptoms of bacterial, fungal, or viral infections.

Tumor Lysis Syndrome

Tumor lysis syndrome may occur following rapid lysis of malignant cells. The risk of tumor lysis syndrome is increased in patients with a large tumor burden; such patients should be monitored closely and appropriate precautions should be taken.

Hepatic Toxicity

Hepatotoxicity (i.e., findings suggestive of hepatocellular injury, including elevations in aminotransferases [ALT or AST] or bilirubin concentrations), sometimes serious or fatal, has been reported following initiation of or rechallenge with brentuximab vedotin. Patients with preexisting hepatic disease or elevations in liver enzymes at baseline and those receiving other potentially hepatotoxic drugs may be at greater risk for developing treatment-related hepatotoxicity. (See Hepatic Impairment under Warnings/Precautions: Specific Populations, in Cautions.)

Liver function tests should be monitored during therapy. In patients presenting with new, worsening, or recurrent hepatotoxicity, temporary interruption of therapy, dosage reduction, or drug discontinuance may be required.

Respiratory Effects

Concomitant use of brentuximab vedotin and bleomycin may increase the risk of pulmonary toxicity; such concomitant use is contraindicated. In a clinical trial, the incidence of noninfectious pulmonary reactions (e.g., cough, dyspnea, interstitial infiltration, inflammation) in patients receiving brentuximab vedotin in combination with chemotherapy containing bleomycin (40%) was higher than the historical incidence of pulmonary reactions in patients receiving bleomycin-based regimens (e.g., doxorubicin, bleomycin, vinblastine, and dacarbazine [ABVD]) (10–25%). Most patients responded to corticosteroid therapy. In the ECHELON-1 study evaluating brentuximab vedotin in combination with AVD, noninfectious pulmonary reactions (i.e., pulmonary infiltration, pneumonitis, interstitial lung disease) occurred in 12 of 662 patients (2%) receiving brentuximab vedotin in combination with AVD. In the ECHELON-2 study evaluating brentuximab vedotin in combination with CHP, noninfectious pneumonitis occurred in 5 of 223 patients (2%) receiving brentuximab vedotin in combination with CHP. In the AETHERA study evaluating single-agent brentuximab vedotin, pulmonary toxicity occurred in 5% of patients receiving the drug compared with 3% of placebo recipients.

Patients receiving brentuximab vedotin should be monitored for signs or symptoms of pulmonary toxicity (e.g., cough, dyspnea). In patients presenting with new or progressive pulmonary symptoms, brentuximab vedotin should be withheld pending results of clinical investigation and until symptoms resolve.

Dermatologic Effects

Serious or fatal cases of Stevens-Johnson syndrome and toxic epidermal necrolysis have been reported in patients receiving brentuximab vedotin. If Stevens-Johnson syndrome or toxic epidermal necrolysis occurs, brentuximab vedotin should be discontinued and appropriate treatment should be provided.

GI Complications

GI complications (i.e., acute pancreatitis; GI perforation, hemorrhage, erosion, or ulcer; intestinal obstruction; enterocolitis; neutropenic colitis; ileus), sometimes fatal or serious, have been reported in patients receiving brentuximab vedotin. Patients with preexisting lymphoma-related GI involvement may be at greater risk for developing treatment-related GI perforation.

In patients presenting with new or progressive GI symptoms (e.g., severe abdominal pain), prompt diagnostic evaluation should be performed and appropriate therapy should be instituted.

Hyperglycemia

Serious or fatal episodes of hyperglycemia, including new-onset hyperglycemia, exacerbation of preexisting diabetes mellitus, and ketoacidosis, have been reported in patients receiving brentuximab vedotin. In clinical studies evaluating single-agent brentuximab vedotin, hyperglycemia occurred in 8% of patients receiving the drug and was grade 3 or 4 in 6% of those receiving the drug. The median time to onset of hyperglycemia was 1 month (range: 0–10 months). Hyperglycemia occurred more frequently in patients with high body mass index or preexisting diabetes mellitus. Serum glucose concentrations should be monitored in patients receiving brentuximab vedotin; if hyperglycemia occurs, antidiabetic agents should be administered as clinically indicated.

Fetal/Neonatal Morbidity and Mortality

Brentuximab vedotin may cause fetal harm in humans based on its mechanism of action and animal findings; the drug has been shown to be embryotoxic, fetotoxic, and teratogenic in animals. Available data on use of brentuximab vedotin in pregnant women are insufficient to inform a drug-associated risk of adverse developmental outcomes. Reproduction studies in rats revealed post-implantation loss, early resorption, decreased number of live fetuses, umbilical hernia, and malrotated hindlimbs at exposure levels similar to those achieved with the maximum recommended human dosage of brentuximab vedotin (1.8 mg/kg every 3 weeks).

Pregnancy should be avoided during brentuximab vedotin therapy. The manufacturer recommends confirmation of pregnancy status prior to initiation of brentuximab vedotin, and women of reproductive potential and men who are partners of such women should use effective methods of contraception while receiving the drug and for at least 6 months after the drug is discontinued. If brentuximab vedotin is used during pregnancy or if the patient or the patient's partner becomes pregnant during therapy, the patient should be apprised of the potential fetal hazard.

Immunogenicity

Antibodies to brentuximab vedotin have been detected in patients receiving the drug; the clinical relevance of such antibodies is not known. In phase 2 clinical trials evaluating brentuximab vedotin in patients with cHL or sALCL, testing for anti-brentuximab vedotin antibodies was performed every 3 weeks using a sensitive electrochemiluminescent immunoassay; test results were persistently (at more than 2 time points) or transiently (at 1 or 2 postbaseline time points) positive in approximately 7 or 30%, respectively, of patients. A higher incidence of infusion-related reactions was observed in patients who persistently tested positive for anti-brentuximab vedotin antibodies. Neutralizing antibodies were detected in 62% of patients who tested positive (either transiently or persistently) for anti-brentuximab vedotin antibodies.

Impairment of Fertility

Results of animal studies suggest that brentuximab vedotin may impair male fertility.

Specific Populations

Pregnancy

Brentuximab vedotin may cause fetal harm if administered to pregnant women based on animal findings. (See Fetal/Neonatal Morbidity and Mortality under Warnings/Precautions: Other Warnings and Precautions, in Cautions.)

Lactation

It is not known whether brentuximab vedotin is distributed into milk in humans; because of the potential for serious adverse reactions to brentuximab vedotin in nursing infants, women should be advised to discontinue nursing during brentuximab vedotin therapy. The effects of the drug on nursing infants or on the production of milk are unknown.

Pediatric Use

Safety and efficacy of brentuximab vedotin have not been established in pediatric patients.

Geriatric Use

The ECHELON-1 study did not include sufficient numbers of patients 65 years of age and older to determine whether geriatric patients with previously untreated stage III or IV cHL receiving brentuximab vedotin in combination with AVD respond differently than younger adults; however, febrile neutropenia occurred more frequently in geriatric patients (39 versus 17%).

In the ECHELON-2 study, 31% of patients with previously untreated CD30-positive PTCL receiving brentuximab vedotin in combination with CHP were 65 years of age or older. Grade 3 or greater adverse effects (74 versus 62%) and serious adverse effects (49 versus 33%) occurred more frequently in geriatric patients compared with younger adults. In this study, geriatric patients were at greater risk for developing febrile neutropenia compared with younger adults (29 versus 14%).

Clinical studies evaluating single-agent brentuximab vedotin for relapsed cHL, cHL following autologous stem cell transplantation, and relapsed systemic anaplastic large cell lymphoma (sALCL) did not include sufficient numbers of patients 65 years of age and older to determine whether geriatric patients respond differently than younger adults.

In the ALCANZA study, 42% of patients with relapsed primary cutaneous ALCL (pcALCL) or CD30-positive mycosis fungoides receiving single-agent brentuximab vedotin were 65 years of age or older. No overall differences in safety and efficacy were observed between these geriatric patients and younger adults.

Hepatic Impairment

Following administration of brentuximab vedotin (1.2 mg/kg), systemic exposure of the microtubule disrupting component (monomethyl auristatin E [MMAE]) of the drug was increased by approximately 2.3-fold in individuals with mild, moderate, or severe hepatic impairment (Child-Pugh class A, B, or C, respectively) compared with individuals with normal hepatic function. Dosage adjustment is required in patients with mild hepatic impairment. (See Dosage and Administration: Special Populations.) Brentuximab vedotin should be avoided in patients with moderate or severe hepatic impairment since an increased incidence of grade 3 or greater adverse effects, including fatalities, has been observed in such patients compared with those with normal hepatic function. (See Hepatic Toxicity under Warnings/Precautions: Other Warnings and Precautions, in Cautions.)

Renal Impairment

Following administration of brentuximab vedotin (1.2 mg/kg), systemic exposure of the microtubule disrupting component (MMAE) of the drug in individuals with mild to moderate renal impairment (creatinine clearance 30–80 mL/minute) was similar to that in individuals with normal renal function; systemic exposure of MMAE was approximately twofold higher in those with severe renal impairment (creatinine clearance less than 30 mL/minute). No dosage adjustment is required in patients with mild or moderate renal impairment. Brentuximab vedotin should be avoided in patients with severe renal impairment since an increased incidence of grade 3 or greater adverse effects, including fatalities, has been observed in such patients compared with those with normal renal function. (See Dosage and Administration: Special Populations.)

● Common Adverse Effects

Adverse effects reported in 10% or more of patients with previously untreated stage III or IV cHL receiving brentuximab vedotin in combination with AVD in the ECHELON-1 study include anemia, neutropenia, peripheral sensory neuropathy, constipation, vomiting, fatigue, diarrhea, pyrexia, abdominal pain, decreased weight, stomatitis, febrile neutropenia, bone pain, insomnia, decreased appetite, back pain, rash, dyspnea, peripheral motor neuropathy, and elevated concentrations of alanine aminotransferase (ALT).

Adverse effects reported in 10% or more of patients with cHL at high risk for relapse or progression following autologous stem cell transplantation receiving brentuximab vedotin consolidation therapy in the AETHERA study include neutropenia, peripheral sensory neuropathy, thrombocytopenia, anemia, upper respiratory tract infection, fatigue, peripheral motor neuropathy, nausea, cough, diarrhea, decreased weight, pyrexia, arthralgia, vomiting, abdominal pain, constipation, dyspnea, decreased appetite, pruritus, headache, muscle spasms, myalgia, and chills.

Adverse effects reported in 10% or more of patients with relapsed cHL receiving brentuximab vedotin as a single agent include neutropenia, peripheral sensory neuropathy, fatigue, upper respiratory tract infection, nausea, diarrhea, anemia, pyrexia, thrombocytopenia, rash, abdominal pain, vomiting, arthralgia/myalgia,

headache, pruritus, constipation, cough, peripheral motor neuropathy, back pain, insomnia, alopecia, chills, dyspnea, night sweats, anxiety, decreased appetite, dizziness, lymphadenopathy, oropharyngeal pain, and extremity pain.

Adverse effects reported in 10% or more of patients with previously untreated CD30-positive PTCL receiving brentuximab vedotin in combination with CHP in the ECHELON-2 study include anemia, neutropenia, peripheral neuropathy, lymphopenia, nausea, diarrhea, fatigue/asthenia, mucositis, constipation, alopecia, pyrexia, vomiting, febrile neutropenia, abdominal pain, decreased appetite, thrombocytopenia, rash, edema, dyspnea, headache, upper respiratory tract infection, cough, dizziness, hypokalemia, decreased weight, insomnia, and myalgia.

Adverse effects reported in 10% or more of patients with relapsed sALCL receiving brentuximab vedotin as a single agent include neutropenia, peripheral sensory neuropathy, anemia, fatigue, nausea, pyrexia, rash, diarrhea, pain, constipation, dyspnea, pruritus, cough, vomiting, decreased appetite, dizziness, headache, insomnia, myalgia, peripheral edema, thrombocytopenia, alopecia, decreased weight, chills, upper respiratory tract infection, back pain, dry skin, extremity pain, lymphadenopathy, and muscle spasms.

Adverse effects reported in 10% or more of patients with relapsed pcALCL or CD30-positive mycosis fungoides receiving brentuximab vedotin as a single agent in the ALCANZA study include anemia, peripheral sensory neuropathy, nausea, diarrhea, fatigue/asthenia, neutropenia, pruritus, pyrexia, vomiting, alopecia, decreased appetite, thrombocytopenia, arthralgia, myalgia, dyspnea, peripheral edema, and rash.

DRUG INTERACTIONS

In vitro studies indicate that monomethyl auristatin E (MMAE), the microtubule-disrupting component of brentuximab vedotin, is a substrate and an inhibitor of cytochrome P-450 (CYP) isoenzymes 3A4/5. (See Description.) In vitro studies also indicate that MMAE does not inhibit other CYP isoenzymes and does not induce major CYP isoenzymes. MMAE is a substrate of P-glycoprotein (P-gp) and is not an inhibitor of P-gp.

● Drugs Affecting Hepatic Microsomal Enzymes

Concomitant use of brentuximab vedotin with potent inhibitors of CYP3A4 may result in increased systemic exposure of MMAE and possible adverse effects. When the potent CYP3A4 inhibitor ketoconazole (400 mg once daily from day 19 of cycle 1 to day 21 of cycle 2) was administered concomitantly with brentuximab vedotin (1.2 mg/kg on day 1 of each cycle), the systemic exposure of MMAE was increased by approximately 34%. The manufacturer states that patients receiving brentuximab vedotin concomitantly with potent CYP3A4 inhibitors should be closely monitored for adverse effects.

When the potent CYP3A4 inducer rifampin (600 mg once daily from day 14 of cycle 1 to day 21 of cycle 2) was administered concomitantly with brentuximab vedotin (1.8 mg/kg on day 1 of each cycle), the systemic exposure of MMAE was decreased by approximately 46%. However, dosage adjustment is not necessary. Clinically important effects on MMAE concentrations are not expected when other inducers of CYP3A4 (i.e., carbamazepine, dexamethasone, phenobarbital, phenytoin) are used concomitantly with brentuximab vedotin.

● Drugs Metabolized by Hepatic Microsomal Enzymes

Brentuximab vedotin is not expected to alter the systemic exposure of drugs that are metabolized by CYP3A4. When the CYP3A4 substrate midazolam was administered 2 days after brentuximab vedotin (at approximately peak MMAE concentrations), systemic exposure of midazolam was unchanged.

● Protein-bound Drugs

MMAE is not likely to displace or be displaced by other highly protein-bound drugs.

● Bleomycin

The incidence of noninfectious pulmonary reactions (e.g., cough, dyspnea, interstitial infiltration, inflammation) in patients receiving brentuximab vedotin in combination with chemotherapy containing bleomycin was higher than the historical incidence of pulmonary reactions in patients receiving bleomycin-based regimens. Concomitant use of brentuximab vedotin and bleomycin is contraindicated. (See Respiratory Effects under Warnings/Precautions: Other Warnings and Precautions, in Cautions.)

DESCRIPTION

Brentuximab vedotin, an anti-CD30 antibody-drug conjugate, is an antineoplastic agent. The anti-CD30 antibody, a chimeric human-murine IgG₁ immunoglobulin, is conjugated with the microtubule inhibitor monomethyl auristatin E (MMAE), a synthetic analog of dolastatin 10, a naturally occurring product isolated from the sea hare *Dolabella auricularia*. A dipeptide bond covalently links MMAE to the antibody component; on average, 4 molecules of MMAE are attached to each antibody molecule. The antibody portion of brentuximab vedotin binds specifically to antigen CD30, a membrane glycoprotein and member of the tumor necrosis factor (TNF) family that is expressed on malignant cells in approximately 98% of Hodgkin lymphoma cases. The CD30 antigen also is expressed in other hematologic malignancies, including anaplastic large cell lymphoma and T-cell lymphoma, but has limited expression in normal tissue. Following binding of the antibody portion of brentuximab vedotin to antigen CD30, the resultant complex is internalized by the cell. MMAE is released via proteolytic cleavage of the dipeptide bond and binds to tubulin, resulting in cell cycle arrest, apoptosis, and antibody-dependent cellular phagocytosis (ADCP).

The pharmacokinetic profile of brentuximab vedotin in combination with chemotherapy is similar to that of single-agent brentuximab vedotin. Areas under the serum concentration-time curve (AUCs) of the antibody-drug conjugate and free MMAE are approximately dose proportional over the brentuximab vedotin single-dose range of 1.2–2.7 mg/kg. Peak MMAE concentrations are achieved about 1–3 days following an IV dose of brentuximab vedotin. When brentuximab vedotin 1.8 mg/kg is administered IV every 3 weeks, steady-state concentrations of the antibody-drug conjugate and MMAE are reached within 21 days; minimal systemic accumulation of the antibody-drug conjugate occurs. When brentuximab vedotin 1.2 mg/kg is administered IV every 2 weeks, steady-state concentrations of the antibody-drug conjugate and MMAE are reached within 56 days; the accumulation ratio of the antibody-drug conjugate is 1.27-fold. Following multiple doses of brentuximab vedotin, systemic exposure of MMAE is decreased to about 50–80% of the exposure achieved following the initial dose. In vitro, MMAE is 68–82% bound to plasma proteins. A small fraction of free MMAE is metabolized, mainly via oxidation by the cytochrome P-450 (CYP) 3A4/5 isoenzyme. Elimination of MMAE appears to be limited by the rate of release from the antibody-drug conjugate. Following administration of a single 1.8-mg/kg dose of brentuximab vedotin, approximately 24% of the total administered dose of MMAE is excreted over a 1-week period in feces (72%) and to a lesser extent in urine, mainly as unchanged drug. The terminal half-lives of the antibody-drug conjugate and MMAE are 4–6 and 3–4 days, respectively.

ADVICE TO PATIENTS

Risk of progressive multifocal leukoencephalopathy (PML). Importance of patients, family, and caregivers being alert to and immediately reporting emergence of signs and symptoms suggestive of PML (e.g., changes in mood, unusual changes in behavior, confusion, changes in thinking, memory loss, vision changes, changes in speech or walking, decreased strength or weakness on one side of the body).

Risk of infusion-related reactions. Importance of reporting signs and symptoms of such reactions, including fever, chills, rash, or breathing difficulty, that occur within 24 hours of an infusion of the drug.

Risk of peripheral neuropathy. Importance of informing clinician of new or worsening symptoms of peripheral neuropathy (e.g., tingling or numbness of the hands or feet, any muscle weakness).

Risk of neutropenia. Importance of informing clinician of fever or other signs and symptoms of infection (e.g., chills, cough, painful urination).

Risk of hepatotoxicity. Importance of informing clinician if signs and symptoms of liver damage (e.g., jaundice, fatigue, dark urine, abdominal pain [particularly in the right upper quadrant], lack of appetite) occur.

Risk of pulmonary reactions. Importance of informing clinician if signs and symptoms of pulmonary reactions (e.g., cough, dyspnea) occur.

Risk of acute pancreatitis. Importance of informing clinician of severe abdominal pain.

Risk of adverse GI effects. Importance of informing clinician if severe abdominal pain, chills, fever, nausea, vomiting, or diarrhea occurs.

Risk of hyperglycemia. Importance of learning how to recognize symptoms of hyperglycemia.

Risk of fetal harm. Necessity of advising women of reproductive potential and men who are partners of such women that they should use an effective method of contraception while receiving the antibody-drug conjugate and for at least 6 months after the last dose. Importance of women informing clinicians if they are or plan to become pregnant. If pregnancy occurs, advise pregnant women of potential risk to the fetus.

Importance of advising women to avoid breast-feeding while receiving brentuximab vedotin therapy.

Importance of informing clinicians of existing or contemplated concomitant therapy, including prescription and OTC drugs, as well as any concomitant illnesses.

Importance of informing patients of other important precautionary information. (See Cautions.)

For further information on the handling of antineoplastic agents, see the ASHP Guidelines on Handling Hazardous Drugs at http://www.ahfsdrug information.com.

PREPARATIONS

Excipients in commercially available drug preparations may have clinically important effects in some individuals; consult specific product labeling for details.

Brentuximab Vedotin

Parenteral
For injection, for IV infusion only   50 mg   **Adcetris®**, Seattle Genetics

Selected Revisions June 1, 2020, © Copyright, September 1, 2012, American Society of Health-System Pharmacists, Inc.

Brigatinib

10:00 · ANTINEOPLASTIC AGENTS

■ Brigatinib, an inhibitor of multiple tyrosine kinases, including anaplastic lymphoma kinase (ALK), is an antineoplastic agent.

USES

● Non-small Cell Lung Cancer

Brigatinib is used for the treatment of anaplastic lymphoma kinase (*ALK*)-positive metastatic non-small cell lung cancer (NSCLC) as detected by an FDA-approved test. Information on FDA-approved tests for the detection of *ALK* rearrangements in NSCLC may be found at https://www.fda.gov/CompanionDiagnostics. Brigatinib has been designated an orphan drug by the FDA for the treatment of *ALK*-positive, c-ros oncogene-1 (*ROS-1*)-positive, or epidermal growth factor receptor (*EGFR*) mutation-positive NSCLC. Guidelines for the treatment of stage IV NSCLC in patients with *ALK* driver alterations generally support the use of brigatinib as an option in the first-line setting and in the second-line setting following therapy with crizotinib.

A relatively small subset of patients with NSCLC (approximately 3–7%) have *ALK*-positive disease, which indicates potential responsiveness to ALK inhibitor therapy (e.g., alectinib, brigatinib, ceritinib, crizotinib). Patients with this form of lung cancer typically are nonsmokers or have a history of light smoking, are female, and are younger in age and often have adenocarcinoma histology. Although crizotinib is highly active in patients with *ALK*-positive NSCLC, most patients treated with the drug eventually experience disease progression, limiting the drug's long-term therapeutic potential. Disease progression in patients receiving crizotinib can result from acquired resistance mutations in *ALK*, amplification of gene expression, activation of alternate signaling pathways, and/or progression of brain metastases (because of poor distribution of crizotinib into the CSF).

ALK Inhibitor-naive NSCLC

Efficacy and safety of brigatinib for the treatment of advanced *ALK*-positive NSCLC in patients naive to ALK inhibitor therapy were demonstrated in a randomized, open-label, multicenter trial (ALTA 1L). Patients enrolled in the study had received up to 1 prior chemotherapy regimen in the locally advanced or metastatic setting. Neurologically stable patients with treated or untreated CNS metastases, including leptomeningeal metastases, were eligible. Patients with a history of interstitial lung disease, drug-related pneumonitis, or radiation pneumonitis were excluded from the study. The primary efficacy end point was progression-free survival as assessed by a blinded independent review committee.

In this study, 275 patients were randomized to receive brigatinib 180 mg once daily (following an initial dosage of 90 mg once daily for 7 days) or crizotinib 250 mg orally twice daily. The median age of patients enrolled in this study was 59 years (range: 27–89); 59% of patients were white, 39% were Asian, 55% were female, 58% were never smokers, 39% had an ECOG performance status of 0, and 56% had an ECOG performance status of 1. Most (93%) of the patients had stage IV disease, 27% had received prior chemotherapy for locally advanced or metastatic disease, 14% had received prior CNS radiation, 31% had bone metastases, and 20% had liver metastases. The median duration of therapy was 9.2 months (range: 0.1–18.4) in the brigatinib treatment group and 7.4 months (range: 0.1–19.2 months) in the crizotinib treatment group.

At the time of the interim analysis (median follow-up of 11 months), median progression-free survival was substantially prolonged in brigatinib-treated patients compared with crizotinib-treated patients (24 versus 11 months). Overall response rate, intracranial overall response rate, and intracranial confirmed response were also substantially improved in patients receiving brigatinib compared with those receiving crizotinib. Progression-free survival at the time of final analysis (at a median follow-up of 40.4 months) remained similar to the interim results.

Previously-treated NSCLC

Efficacy and safety of brigatinib for the treatment of NSCLC previously treated with crizotinib are based principally on the results of a multicenter, two-arm, open-label, phase 2 study (ALTA) that enrolled a total of 222 adults with locally advanced or metastatic *ALK*-positive NSCLC who had experienced disease progression while receiving crizotinib therapy. *ALK* rearrangement was required for study entry and was confirmed by an FDA-approved diagnostic test or a different test with adequate archival tissue to confirm *ALK* rearrangement by the Vysis® ALK Break Apart fluorescence in situ hybridization (FISH) Probe Kit test. Patients were randomized in a 1:1 ratio to initially receive brigatinib in a dosage of 90 mg once daily (arm A) or 180 mg once daily (following an initial dosage of 90 mg once daily for 7 days) (arm B) until disease progression, unacceptable toxicity, or consent withdrawal occurred. Patients in arm A could receive brigatinib 180 mg once daily after objective progression occurred on a dosage of 90 mg once daily. The primary efficacy end point was confirmed overall response rate according to the Response Evaluation Criteria in Solid Tumors (RECIST 1.1) as evaluated by a central independent review committee (IRC); additional outcome measures included investigator-assessed overall response rate, duration of response, overall response rate in patients with CNS metastases, and duration of response in patients with CNS metastases. The median age of patients enrolled in the study was 54 years (range: 18–82 years); 67% of enrolled patients were white and 31% were Asian; and 57% were female. Stage IV disease was present in 98% of the patients and 97% had adenocarcinoma histology, 74% of the patients had received prior systemic chemotherapy, and 64% of patients had an objective response to prior crizotinib treatment. CNS metastases were present in 69% of patients and 61% had previously received radiation to the brain.

The median duration of follow-up in the ALTA study was 8 months (range: 0.1–20.2 months). The IRC-assessed overall response rate in patients receiving brigatinib 180 mg daily was 53%; partial responses were achieved in 48% of patients and 4.5% had a complete response. The investigator-assessed overall response rate in patients receiving brigatinib 180 mg daily was 54%; partial responses were achieved in 50% of patients and 3.6% had a complete response. Patients receiving brigatinib 90 mg daily had IRC- or investigator-assessed overall response rates of 48 or 45%, respectively; IRC- or investigator-assessed partial responses were achieved in 45 or 44% of patients, respectively, and complete responses were achieved in 3.6 or 0.9% of patients, respectively. The median IRC-assessed duration of response was 13.8 months in both dosage groups and the median investigator-assessed duration of response was 13.8 months in the 90-mg dosage group and 11.1 months in the 180-mg dosage group.

In the subgroup of 44 patients with measurable brain metastases at baseline in the ALTA study, the IRC-assessed intracranial overall response rate was 67% (all partial responses) in patients receiving brigatinib 180 mg daily and 42% (7.7% complete responses and 35% partial responses) in patients receiving brigatinib 90 mg daily. The median duration of intracranial response was 5.6 months in the 180-mg dosage group and could not be estimated at the time of analysis in the 90-mg dosage group. Among the 23 patients who demonstrated an intracranial response to brigatinib therapy, 78% of the patients receiving 90 mg once daily and 68% of the patients receiving 180 mg once daily maintained a response for at least 4 months.

Clinical Perspective

First-line Therapy for Metastatic Non-small Cell Lung Cancer

The American Society of Clinical Oncology (ASCO) and Ontario Health (OH; formerly known as Cancer Care Ontario) 2021 joint guideline specifically addresses treatment of stage IV NSCLC harboring driver alterations such as *ALK* mutations. ASCO/OH state that alectinib or brigatinib should be offered in the first-line setting in patients with stage IV NSCLC and driver alterations in *ALK*. ASCO/OH also state that if alectinib or brigatinib are not available, ceritinib or crizotinib should be offered in the first-line setting.

Previously Treated Metastatic Non-small Cell Lung Cancer

In the second-line setting, ASCO/OH state that alectinib, brigatinib, or ceritinib should be offered in patients who received initial therapy with crizotinib.

DOSAGE AND ADMINISTRATION

● General

Pretreatment Screening

● Control blood pressure before initiating therapy.

● Measure fasting serum glucose concentrations prior to initiating therapy, and initiate or optimize antihyperglycemic therapy as clinically indicated.

Patient Monitoring

- Monitor blood pressure 2 weeks after starting therapy and at least monthly thereafter.

- Monitor heart rate during therapy. More frequent monitoring may be necessary in patients receiving concomitant therapy with drugs known to cause bradycardia.

- Monitor serum creatine kinase (CK, creatine phosphokinase, CPK) and pancreatic enzyme (e.g., amylase, lipase) concentrations during therapy.

- Measure fasting serum glucose concentrations periodically during therapy.

- Monitor for new or worsening respiratory symptoms, particularly during the initial week of therapy.

- Monitor for visual disturbances.

- Monitor AST, ALT, and total bilirubin during treatment, especially during the first 3 months.

Other General Considerations

- Advise patients to limit sun exposure (e.g., wear protective clothing and sunscreen) during therapy and for at least 5 days after discontinuing the drug.

● Administration

Brigatinib is administered orally once daily without regard to food. Swallow brigatinib tablets whole and do *not* crush or chew.

If a dose of brigatinib is missed or vomiting occurs after taking a dose, the prescribed dose should be taken at the next scheduled time; an additional dose should not be administered to replace the missed dose.

Store brigatinib tablets at 20–25°C (excursions permitted between 15–30°C).

● Dosage

Non-small Cell Lung Cancer

The recommended adult dosage of brigatinib for the treatment of anaplastic lymphoma kinase (*ALK*)-positive metastatic non-small cell lung cancer (NSCLC) is 90 mg once daily for the first 7 days, followed by an increase to 180 mg once daily. Continue therapy until disease progression or unacceptable toxicity occurs.

Following treatment interruptions of 14 or more days for reasons other than adverse reactions, resume brigatinib at a dosage of 90 mg once daily for 7 days, then increase to the previously tolerated dosage.

Dosage Modification for Toxicity

Dosing interruption and/or dosage reduction of brigatinib may be necessary based on individual safety and tolerability.

In the ALTA study, dosage reduction because of adverse effects was necessary in 7.3 or 20% of patients receiving brigatinib 90 mg daily or 180 mg daily, respectively (most commonly because of elevated serum CK concentrations). In the ALTA 1L trial, dosage reduction because of any adverse event occurred in 29% of patients treated with brigatinib 180 mg once daily.

If dosage reduction is necessary in a patient receiving 90 mg of brigatinib once daily, the dosage should be reduced to 60 mg once daily. If further dosage reduction is necessary, the drug should be permanently discontinued.

If dosage reduction is necessary in a patient receiving 180 mg of brigatinib once daily, an initial dosage reduction to 120 mg once daily is recommended. If further dosage reduction is necessary, the dosage should be reduced to 90 mg once daily. If dosage reduction from 90 mg once daily is necessary, a dosage of 60 mg once daily is recommended. If a dosage of 60 mg once daily is not tolerated, brigatinib should be permanently discontinued.

Once the dosage of brigatinib has been reduced because of adverse reactions, the dosage should not be subsequently increased.

Interstitial Lung Disease/Pneumonitis

If new grade 1 pulmonary symptoms occur *during* the first 7 days of treatment, withhold brigatinib therapy until recovery to baseline. Therapy may then be resumed at the same dosage; dosage should *not* be increased to 180 mg once daily if interstitial lung disease (ILD)/pneumonitis is suspected.

If new grade 1 pulmonary symptoms occur *after* the first 7 days of treatment, withhold brigatinib therapy until recovery to baseline. Therapy may then be resumed at the same dosage.

If new grade 2 pulmonary symptoms occur *during* the first 7 days of treatment, withhold brigatinib therapy until recovery to baseline. Therapy may then be resumed at the next lower dosage; dosage should *not* be increased if ILD/pneumonitis is suspected.

If new grade 2 pulmonary symptoms occur *after* the first 7 days of treatment, withhold brigatinib therapy until recovery to baseline. If ILD/pneumonitis is suspected, therapy may be resumed at the next lower dosage; otherwise, therapy may be resumed at the same dosage.

If grade 1 or 2 ILD/pneumonitis *recurs*, permanently discontinue brigatinib therapy.

If grade 3 or 4 ILD/pneumonitis occurs, permanently discontinue brigatinib therapy.

Hypertension

If grade 3 hypertension (i.e., systolic blood pressure of 160 mm Hg or greater or diastolic blood pressure of 100 mm Hg or greater requiring medical intervention and more than one antihypertensive agent or more intensive therapy than previously used) occurs, withhold brigatinib therapy until recovery to grade 1 or less hypertension (i.e., systolic blood pressure less than 140 mm Hg and diastolic blood pressure less than 90 mm Hg). Therapy may then be resumed at the next lower dosage.

If grade 3 hypertension *recurs*, withhold brigatinib therapy until recovery to grade 1 or less; resume therapy at the next lower dosage *or* permanently discontinue brigatinib.

If grade 4 hypertension (i.e., life-threatening consequences, requiring urgent intervention) occurs, withhold brigatinib therapy until recovery to grade 1 or less; therapy may then be resumed at the next lower dosage or permanently discontinue brigatinib.

If grade 4 hypertension *recurs*, permanently discontinue brigatinib.

Bradycardia

If symptomatic, but non-life-threatening, bradycardia occurs, withhold brigatinib therapy until recovery to asymptomatic bradycardia or to a resting heart rate of at least 60 beats/minute. If concomitant drugs known to cause bradycardia are identified and discontinued or their dosage is adjusted, brigatinib therapy may be resumed at the same dosage upon recovery to asymptomatic bradycardia or to a resting heart rate of at least 60 beats/minute. If no concomitant drugs known to cause bradycardia are identified or if discontinuance or dosage adjustment of such concomitant drugs is not possible, resume brigatinib at the next lower dosage upon recovery to asymptomatic bradycardia or to a resting heart rate of at least 60 beats/minute.

If life-threatening bradycardia requiring urgent intervention occurs in patients receiving concomitant contributory drugs, withhold brigatinib therapy until recovery to asymptomatic bradycardia or to a resting heart rate of at least 60 beats/minute. If such concomitant drugs are discontinued or the dosage adjusted, brigatinib therapy may be resumed at the next lower dosage with frequent monitoring as clinically indicated. Brigatinib should be permanently discontinued in case of recurrence.

If life-threatening bradycardia requiring urgent intervention occurs in patients not receiving concomitant contributory drugs, permanently discontinue brigatinib.

Visual Disturbances

If grade 2 or 3 visual disturbance occurs, withhold brigatinib therapy until recovery to grade 1 or baseline. Therapy may then be resumed at the next lower dosage.

If grade 4 visual disturbance occurs, permanently discontinue brigatinib.

Creatine Kinase Elevation

If an elevation in serum CK concentrations exceeding 5 times the upper limit of normal (ULN; i.e., grade 3 or 4) occurs concomitantly with grade 2 or higher muscle pain or weakness, withhold brigatinib therapy until CK concentrations return to baseline values or decrease to no more than 2.5 times the ULN (i.e., grade 1 or less). Brigatinib may then be resumed at the same dosage. If an elevation in serum CK concentrations exceeding 5 times the ULN *recurs*, withhold brigatinib until CK concentrations return to baseline values or decrease to grade 1 or less; brigatinib therapy may then be resumed at the next lower dosage.

Pancreatic Enzyme Elevation

If an elevation in serum amylase or lipase concentrations exceeding 2 times the ULN (i.e., grade 3) occurs, withhold brigatinib therapy until amylase or lipase concentrations return to baseline values or decrease to no more than 1.5 times the ULN (i.e., grade 1 or less). Brigatinib may then be resumed at the same dosage. If grade 3 elevation in serum amylase or lipase concentrations *recurs*, withhold brigatinib until amylase or lipase concentrations return to baseline values or decrease to grade 1 or less; brigatinib therapy may then be resumed at the next lower dosage.

If an elevation in serum amylase or lipase concentrations exceeding 5 times the ULN (i.e., grade 4) occurs, withhold brigatinib therapy until amylase or lipase concentrations return to baseline values or decrease to grade 1 or less. Brigatinib therapy may then be resumed at the next lower dosage.

Hepatotoxicity

If a grade 3 or 4 elevation (>5 times the ULN) of either AST or ALT with bilirubin ≤2 times the ULN occurs, withhold brigatinib therapy until recovery to grade 1 or less (≤3 times the ULN) or to baseline. Brigatinib may then be resumed at the next lower dose.

If grade 2 to 4 elevation (>3 times the ULN) of ALT or AST with concurrent total bilirubin elevation >2 times the ULN in the absence of cholestasis or hemolysis occurs, brigatinib therapy should be permanently discontinued.

Hyperglycemia

If hyperglycemia with serum glucose concentrations exceeding 250 mg/dL (i.e., grade 3) occurs and adequate hyperglycemic control cannot be achieved despite optimal antidiabetic agent therapy, withhold brigatinib until adequate control of hyperglycemia is achieved; brigatinib may then be resumed at the next lower dosage or discontinued permanently.

Other Toxicity

If any other grade 3 adverse reaction occurs, withhold brigatinib therapy until recovery to baseline. Brigatinib therapy may then be resumed at the same dosage. If the grade 3 adverse reaction *recurs*, brigatinib therapy should be withheld until recovery to baseline; brigatinib may then be resumed at the next lower dosage or the drug discontinued.

If any other grade 4 adverse reaction occurs, withhold brigatinib therapy until recovery to baseline. Brigatinib therapy may then be resumed at the next lower dosage or permanently discontinued. If the grade 4 adverse reaction *recurs*, brigatinib therapy should be permanently discontinued.

Concomitant Use of Drugs Affecting Hepatic Microsomal Enzymes

Inhibitors of CYP3A

Avoid concomitant use of brigatinib with drugs that are potent or moderate inhibitors of cytochrome P-450 (CYP) isoenzyme 3A.

If concomitant use of brigatinib with a *potent* CYP3A inhibitor cannot be avoided, reduce the once daily dosage of brigatinib by approximately 50% (e.g., from 180 mg to 90 mg once daily; from 90 mg to 60 mg once daily).

If concomitant use of brigatinib with a *moderate* CYP3A inhibitor cannot be avoided, reduce the dosage of brigatinib by approximately 40% (e.g., from 180 mg to 120 mg once daily; from 120 mg to 90 mg once daily; from 90 mg to 60 mg once daily).

If concomitant use of the potent or moderate CYP3A inhibitor is discontinued, resume brigatinib dosage that was tolerated prior to initiation of the CYP3A inhibitor.

Inducers of CYP3A

Avoid concomitant use of brigatinib with drugs that are potent or moderate inducers of CYP3A.

If concomitant use of brigatinib with a *moderate* CYP3A inducer cannot be avoided, increase the dosage of brigatinib in 30-mg increments (as tolerated) after 7 days of therapy, up to a maximum of twice the brigatinib dose that was tolerated prior to initiation of the moderate CYP3A inducer. If concomitant use of the moderate CYP3A inducer is discontinued, resume the brigatinib dose that was tolerated prior to initiation of the moderate CYP3A inducer.

● Special Populations

Hepatic Impairment

In patients with severe hepatic impairment (Child-Pugh class C), reduce the dosage of brigatinib by approximately 40% (e.g., from 180 mg to 120 mg once daily; from 120 mg to 90 mg once daily; from 90 mg to 60 mg once daily).

No dosage adjustment is necessary in patients with mild or moderate hepatic impairment (Child-Pugh class A or B).

Renal Impairment

In patients with severe renal impairment (creatinine clearance 15–29 mL/minute), reduce the dosage of brigatinib by approximately 50% (e.g., from 180 mg to 90 mg once daily; from 90 mg to 60 mg once daily).

No dosage adjustment is necessary in patients with mild or moderate renal impairment (creatinine clearance of 30–89 mL/minute).

Geriatric Patients

The manufacturer makes no specific dosage recommendations for geriatric patients.

CAUTIONS

● Contraindications

- None.

● Warnings/Precautions

Interstitial Lung Disease/Pneumonitis

Severe, life-threatening, or fatal adverse pulmonary reactions consistent with interstitial lung disease (ILD)/pneumonitis may occur in patients receiving brigatinib. In the ALTA study, ILD or pneumonitis occurred in 3.7% of patients receiving brigatinib 90 mg once daily and in 9.1% of patients receiving the recommended dosage regimen (180 mg once daily with a 7-day lead-in at 90 mg once daily), and grade 3 or 4 adverse reactions consistent with possible ILD or pneumonitis occurred in 2.7% of patients receiving the drug. Adverse pulmonary symptoms consistent with possible ILD/pneumonitis occurred early (i.e., within 9 days of initiation of therapy; median onset was 2 days) in 6.4% of patients in this study, and all patients were receiving brigatinib 90 mg once daily at the time of symptom onset. In the ALTA 1L trial, ILD or pneumonitis occurred in 5.1% of patients receiving brigatinib 180 mg once daily (with a 7-day lead-in at 90 mg once daily). These events occurred within 8 days of initiation of brigatinib therapy in 2.9% of patients and grade 3 or 4 adverse reactions occurred in 2.2% of patients.

Monitor patients receiving brigatinib for new or worsening respiratory symptoms (e.g., dyspnea, cough), particularly during the first week of initiating therapy. If such respiratory manifestations occur, interrupt brigatinib therapy and promptly evaluate for ILD/pneumonitis or other causes of respiratory symptoms (e.g., pulmonary embolism, tumor progression, pneumonia). If ILD/pneumonitis is confirmed or ILD/pneumonitis recurs, dosage reduction or discontinuance of therapy may be necessary depending on the severity.

Hypertension

Brigatinib may cause hypertension. In the ALTA study, hypertension occurred in 21% of patients; grade 3 or 4 hypertension occurred in 5.9% of patients receiving the recommended dosage regimen of brigatinib (180 mg once daily with a 7-day lead-in at 90 mg once daily). Among patients receiving brigatinib 90 mg once daily in the ALTA study, hypertension occurred in 11% of patients. In the ALTA 1L trial, hypertension occurred in 32% of patients receiving brigatinib 180 mg once daily (with a 7-day lead-in at 90 mg once daily); grade 3 hypertension occurred in 13% of patients.

Blood pressure should be controlled prior to initiating therapy with brigatinib. Blood pressure should be monitored 2 weeks after treatment initiation and at least monthly during therapy with the drug. If severe hypertension (i.e., grade 3) occurs despite optimal antihypertensive therapy, interrupt brigatinib therapy until blood pressure is controlled. Upon resolution or improvement of hypertension to grade 1, resume brigatinib at the same dosage. Consider permanent discontinuance of brigatinib therapy if grade 4 hypertension occurs or if grade 3 hypertension recurs.

Bradycardia

Brigatinib may cause bradycardia. In the ALTA study, bradycardia with a heart rate of less than 50 beats/minute was reported in 7.6 or 5.7% of patients receiving brigatinib 180 mg once daily (with a 7-day lead-in at 90 mg once daily) or 90 mg once daily, respectively. Grade 2 bradycardia occurred in one patient (0.9%) receiving the 90-mg daily dosage. In the ALTA 1L trial, bradycardia occurred in 8.1% of patients treated with brigatinib 180 mg once daily (with a 7-day lead-in at 90 mg once daily); grade 3 bradycardia occurred in 1 patient (0.7%).

Monitor heart rate and blood pressure periodically during brigatinib therapy. Monitor patients more frequently if concomitant use with a drug known to cause bradycardia cannot be avoided. If symptomatic or life-threatening bradycardia occurs, withhold brigatinib therapy. Evaluate concomitant therapy to identify any drugs that may cause bradycardia; adjust dosage or discontinue such drugs, and then resume brigatinib at the same dosage following resolution of symptomatic bradycardia. If no concomitant therapy with a drug known to cause bradycardia is identified, reduce the dosage of brigatinib following resolution of symptomatic bradycardia. Discontinue brigatinib if life-threatening bradycardia occurs in the absence of contributing concomitant medications.

Visual Disturbances

In the ALTA study, adverse reactions leading to visual disturbances, including blurred vision, diplopia, and reduced visual acuity, were reported in 10 or 7.3% of patients receiving brigatinib 180 mg once daily (with a 7-day lead-in at 90 mg once daily) or 90 mg once daily, respectively. Grade 3 macular edema and cataract each occurred in one patient receiving brigatinib 180 mg once daily (with a 7-day lead-in at 90 mg once daily). In the ALTA 1L trial, grade 1 or 2 adverse reactions resulting in visual disturbance were reported in 7.4% of patients receiving brigatinib.

In patients who report new or worsening visual symptoms of grade 2 or higher severity, interrupt brigatinib therapy and perform an ophthalmologic evaluation. Dosage reduction or drug discontinuance may be required depending on the severity.

Creatine Kinase Elevation

In the ALTA study, elevated serum creatine kinase (CK, creatine phosphokinase, CPK) concentrations were reported in 48% and were grade 3 or 4 in 12% of patients receiving brigatinib 180 mg once daily (with a 7-day lead-in at 90 mg once daily). Among patients receiving brigatinib 90 mg once daily, elevated serum CK concentrations were reported in 27% of patients; 2.8% of these patients had grade 3 or 4 elevations in CK concentrations. Dosage modification because of elevated serum CK concentrations was required in 4.5 or 1.8% of patients receiving brigatinib 180 or 90 mg daily, respectively. In the ALTA 1L trial, elevated serum CK concentrations were reported in 81% of patients treated with brigatinib 180 mg once daily (with a 7-day lead-in at 90 mg once daily); grade 3 or 4 elevations occurred in 24% of patients. In the ALTA 1L trial, dosage modification because of elevated serum CK concentrations was required in 15% of patients.

Monitor serum CK concentrations periodically during brigatinib therapy. Temporary interruption followed by resumption of therapy at the same or at a reduced dosage of brigatinib may be necessary, depending on the severity of the CK elevation.

Pancreatic Enzyme Elevation

In the ALTA study, elevated serum amylase concentrations and grade 3 or 4 elevated serum amylase concentrations were reported in 39 and 2.7% of patients receiving brigatinib 180 mg once daily (with a 7-day lead-in at 90 mg once daily), respectively. Elevated serum lipase concentrations and grade 3 or 4 elevated serum lipase concentrations were reported in 45 and 5.5% of patients receiving the 180-mg daily dosage, respectively. Among patients receiving brigatinib 90 mg once daily, elevated serum amylase concentrations and grade 3 or 4 elevated serum amylase concentrations were reported in 27 and 3.7% of patients, respectively. Elevated serum lipase concentrations and grade 3 or 4 elevated serum lipase concentrations were reported in 21 and 4.6% of patients receiving the 90-mg daily dosage of brigatinib, respectively. In the ALTA 1L trial, elevated serum amylase or lipase concentrations were reported in 52 or 59%, respectively, of patients treated with brigatinib 180 mg once daily (with a 7-day lead-in at 90 mg once daily); grade 3 or 4 elevations of serum amylase or lipase concentrations occurred in 6.8 or 17% of patients, respectively.

Serum amylase and lipase concentrations should be monitored periodically during brigatinib therapy. Temporary interruption followed by resumption of therapy at the same or a reduced dosage of brigatinib may be necessary, depending on the severity of the amylase and/or lipase elevation.

Hepatotoxicity

Hepatotoxicity may occur in patients receiving brigatinib. In the ALTA study, elevated AST concentrations and grade 3 or 4 AST elevations were reported in 38% and 0.9% of patients in the brigatinib 90 mg once daily group. Elevations in ALT concentrations and grade 3 or 4 ALT elevations occurred in 34% and 0 patients in the brigatinib 90 mg once daily group. In the brigatinib 180 mg once daily (with a 7-day lead-in at 90 mg once daily) group, AST elevations occurred in 65% of patients, ALT elevations in 40%, grade 3 or 4 AST elevations in 0 patients, and grade 3 or 4 ALT elevations in 2.7% of patients.

In the ALTA 1L trial, AST elevations and grade 3 or 4 AST elevations occurred in 72% and 4.5% of patients, respectively. ALT elevations were reported in 52% of patients and grade 3 or 4 ALT elevations in 5.2% of patients. One patient (0.7%) experienced serious hepatocellular injury.

Monitor AST, ALT, and total bilirubin during treatment with brigatinib, especially during the initial 3 months. Withhold brigatinib for grade 3 or 4 hepatic enzyme elevation with bilirubin ≤2 times the ULN. Upon resolution or recovery to grade 1 or less (≤3 times the ULN) or to baseline, resume brigatinib at a next lower dose. Permanently discontinue brigatinib for grade 2 or 4 hepatic enzyme elevation with concurrent total bilirubin elevations >2 times the ULN in the absence of cholestasis or hemolysis.

Hyperglycemia

Hyperglycemia may occur in patients receiving brigatinib. In the ALTA study, new or worsening hyperglycemia occurred in 43% of brigatinib-treated patients; grade 3 hyperglycemia (based on fasting serum glucose concentrations) occurred in 3.7% of patients receiving the drug. Among patients with diabetes mellitus or glucose intolerance at baseline, 10% required initiation of insulin during brigatinib therapy. In the ALTA 1L trial, new or worsening hyperglycemia occurred in 56% of patients receiving brigatinib 180 mg once daily (with a 7-day lead-in at 90 mg once daily); grade 3 hyperglycemia occurred in 7.5% of patients.

Assess fasting serum glucose concentrations prior to initiation of brigatinib and monitor periodically during treatment. Antidiabetic agents should be initiated or optimized as necessary. If adequate glycemic control cannot be achieved despite optimal medical management, interrupt brigatinib therapy until hyperglycemia is adequately controlled. Dosage reduction or discontinuance of therapy may be necessary depending on the severity of hyperglycemia.

Photosensitivity

Photosensitivity may occur in patients receiving brigatinib. In the ALTA study, photosensitivity occurred in 0.9% of patients receiving brigatinib 90 mg daily; however, grade 3 to 4 photosensitivity was not reported in patients receiving brigatinib 90 mg daily or 180 mg once daily (with a 7-day lead-in at 90 mg once daily). In the ALTA 1L trial, photosensitivity occurred in 3.7% of patients receiving brigatinib 180 mg once daily (with a 7-day lead-in at 90 mg once daily); grade 3 or 4 photosensitivity occurred in 0.7% of patients.

Advise patients to limit sun exposure during brigatinib therapy, and for at least 5 days after discontinuation of treatment. Counsel patients to wear a hat and protective clothing when outdoors, and to use a broad-spectrum sunscreen and lip balm (SPF ≥30) for protection against sunburn.

Fetal/Neonatal Morbidity and Mortality

Brigatinib may cause fetal harm if administered to pregnant women based on its mechanism of action and animal findings. There are no clinical data on the use of brigatinib in pregnant women. Dose-related skeletal abnormalities were observed when the drug was administered to pregnant animals during the period of organogenesis at dosages equivalent to approximately 0.7 times the human exposure achieved with the recommended dosage. In addition, increased post-implantation loss, malformations, and decreased fetal body weight were observed in animals at dosages equivalent to approximately 1.26 times the human exposure achieved at the recommended dosage.

Avoid pregnancy during brigatinib therapy. Females of reproductive potential should use effective nonhormonal contraception during brigatinib therapy and for at least 4 months after the drug is discontinued. In addition, men with female partners of reproductive potential should use effective methods of contraception while receiving brigatinib therapy and for at least 3 months after the drug is discontinued. If brigatinib is used during pregnancy or if the patient becomes pregnant while receiving the drug, the patient should be apprised of the potential fetal hazard.

Specific Populations
Pregnancy

Although there are no clinical data in pregnant women to date, animal studies and its mechanism of action suggest that brigatinib may cause fetal harm.

Females and Males of Reproductive Potential

Verify pregnancy status in females of reproductive potential prior to initiating brigatinib therapy. Advise females of reproductive potential to use effective contraception during therapy and for at least 4 months after the final dose. Advise males with female partners of reproductive potential to use effective contraception during brigatinib therapy and for at least 3 months after the final dose.

Based on findings from animal studies, brigatinib may reduce fertility in males.

Lactation

It is not known whether brigatinib is distributed into human milk or if the drug has any effect on milk production or the breast-fed infant. Because of the potential for adverse reactions to brigatinib in breast-fed infants, advise females not to breast-feed while receiving the drug and for at least 1 week after the drug is discontinued.

Pediatric Use

Safety and efficacy of brigatinib have not been established in pediatric patients.

Geriatric Use

Clinical studies of brigatinib did not include sufficient numbers of patients 65 years of age and older to determine whether geriatric patients respond differently than younger adults. In the principal efficacy studies evaluating brigatinib in patients with NSCLC, 26.7% were ≥65 years of age and 7.5% were ≥75 years of age. No clinically important differences in safety or efficacy were observed between geriatric patients and younger adults in this study.

Age does not have a clinically important effect on the pharmacokinetics of brigatinib.

Hepatic Impairment

In a population pharmacokinetic analysis, mild hepatic impairment (total bilirubin concentrations not exceeding the upper limit of normal [ULN] with AST concentrations exceeding the ULN, or total bilirubin concentrations exceeding 1 but not exceeding 1.5 times the ULN with any AST concentration) did not affect systemic exposure to brigatinib.

Following a single dose of brigatinib 90 mg, unbound systemic exposure of brigatinib was 37% higher in subjects with severe hepatic impairment (Child-Pugh class C) compared to subjects with normal hepatic function. In patients with mild to moderate hepatic impairment (Child-Pugh class A or B), systemic exposure of the drug was similar to that in patients with normal hepatic function.

Renal Impairment

In a population pharmacokinetic analysis, mild or moderate renal impairment (creatinine clearance of 30–89 mL/minute) did not affect systemic exposure to brigatinib.

Following administration of a single 90-mg dose of brigatinib, AUC of brigatinib was 86% higher in individuals with severe renal impairment (creatinine clearance 15–29 mL/minute) compared with individuals with normal renal function.

● Common Adverse Effects

The most common adverse reactions (reported in at least 25% of patients) include diarrhea, fatigue, nausea, rash, cough, myalgia, headache, hypertension, vomiting, and dyspnea.

DRUG INTERACTIONS

Brigatinib is metabolized principally by cytochrome P-450 (CYP) isoenzymes 2C8 and 3A4. In vitro studies indicate that brigatinib is a substrate of P-glycoprotein (P-gp) and breast cancer resistance protein (BCRP), but not a substrate of organic anion transport protein (OATP) 1B1, OATP1B3, organic anion transporter (OAT) 1, OAT3, organic cation transporter (OCT) 1, OCT2, multidrug and toxin extrusion transporter (MATE) 1, MATE2K, or bile salt export pump (BSEP).

In vitro studies indicate that brigatinib inhibits P-gp, BCRP, OCT1, MATE1, and MATE2K. Brigatinib does not inhibit OATP1B1, OATP1B3, OAT1, OAT3, OCT2, or BSEP.

Brigatinib induces CYP3A and also may induce CYP2C isoenzymes via activation of the pregnane X receptor (PXR). Brigatinib and its principal metabolite do not inhibit CYP isoenzymes 1A2, 2B6, 2C8, 2C9, 2C19, 2D6, or 3A4/5 at clinically relevant concentrations.

● Drugs and Foods Affecting Hepatic Microsomal Enzymes
Inhibitors of CYP3A

Concomitant use of brigatinib with potent or moderate inhibitors of CYP3A may increase plasma concentrations of brigatinib, which may result in increased adverse effects. Concurrent administration of the potent CYP3A inhibitor itraconazole (200 mg twice daily) and brigatinib (single 90-mg dose) increased peak plasma concentrations and AUC of brigatinib by 21 and 101%, respectively, compared with administration of brigatinib alone. Concomitant use of brigatinib with a moderate CYP3A inhibitor is expected to increase the AUC of brigatinib by approximately 40%.

The manufacturer states that concomitant use of potent or moderate CYP3A inhibitors, including grapefruit products, should be avoided during brigatinib therapy. If concomitant use of a *potent* CYP3A inhibitor cannot be avoided, reduce the once daily dosage of brigatinib by approximately 50% (e.g., from 180 mg to 90 mg once daily; from 90 mg to 60 mg once daily). If concomitant use of brigatinib with a *moderate* CYP3A inhibitor cannot be avoided, reduce the dosage of brigatinib by approximately 40% (e.g., from 180 mg to 120 mg once daily; from 120 mg to 90 mg once daily; from 90 mg to 60 mg once daily). If concomitant use of the potent or moderate CYP3A inhibitor is discontinued, the brigatinib dosage should be returned to the dosage that was tolerated prior to initiation of the potent CYP3A inhibitor.

Inhibitors of CYP2C8

Concomitant administration of the potent CYP2C8 inhibitor gemfibrozil (600 mg twice daily) and brigatinib (single 90-mg dose) decreased peak plasma concentrations and the AUC of brigatinib by 41 and 12%, respectively. The manufacturer states that the effect of gemfibrozil on the pharmacokinetics of brigatinib is not considered clinically important and that the underlying mechanism for the decreased exposure of brigatinib is not known.

Inducers of CYP3A

Concomitant use of brigatinib with potent or moderate inducers of CYP3A (e.g., carbamazepine, phenytoin, rifampin) may decrease plasma concentrations and reduce efficacy of brigatinib and should be avoided. When the potent CYP3A inducer rifampin (600 mg daily) was administered concomitantly with brigatinib (single 180-mg dose), peak plasma concentrations and AUC of brigatinib decreased by 60 and 80%, respectively.

Avoid concomitant use of brigatinib with potent or moderate CYP3A inducers. If concomitant use of brigatinib with a *moderate* CYP3A inducer cannot be avoided, increase the dosage of brigatinib in 30-mg increments (as tolerated) after 7 days of therapy, up to a maximum of twice the brigatinib dose that was tolerated prior to initiation of the moderate CYP3A inducer. If concomitant use of the moderate CYP3A inducer is discontinued, resume the brigatinib dose that was tolerated prior to initiation of the moderate CYP3A inducer.

● *Drugs Metabolized by Hepatic Microsomal Enzymes*

Brigatinib induces CYP3A in vitro; therefore, concomitant use of brigatinib and drugs metabolized by CYP3A may result in decreased concentrations and loss of efficacy of the CYP3A substrate.

● *Substrates of Drug Transport Systems*

Brigatinib inhibits P-gp, BCRP, OCT1, MATE1, and MATE2K in vitro and potentially may increase concentrations of drugs that are substrates of these transport systems.

● *Drugs Associated with Bradycardia*

Because brigatinib has been associated with bradycardia, caution is advised when brigatinib is used concurrently with other drugs known to cause bradycardia. Heart rate should be monitored more frequently if such concomitant use cannot be avoided. If clinically important bradycardia occurs with concomitant use of brigatinib and drugs known to cause bradycardia (including antihypertensive agents), the dosage of the concomitant drug should be adjusted or the concomitant drug should be discontinued, if possible.

● *Hormonal Contraceptives*

Concomitant use of brigatinib and hormonal contraceptives, which are CYP3A substrates, may result in decreased plasma concentrations and reduced efficacy of the hormonal contraceptive. Women of childbearing potential should therefore use effective nonhormonal contraception during brigatinib therapy and for at least 4 months after the drug is discontinued.

● *Grapefruit*

Grapefruit products are CYP3A inhibitors and should be avoided because of the potential for increased plasma brigatinib concentrations during concurrent use.

DESCRIPTION

Brigatinib, an inhibitor of multiple tyrosine kinases, including anaplastic lymphoma kinase (ALK), c-ros oncogene-1 (ROS-1), insulin-like growth factor receptor-1 (IGFR-1), and fms-like tyrosine kinase 3 (FLT-3) as well as epidermal growth factor receptor (EGFR) deletion and point mutations, is an antineoplastic agent. The drug inhibits autophosphorylation of ALK and ALK-mediated phosphorylation of the downstream signaling proteins signal transducer and activator of transcription 3 (STAT3), AKT serine/threonine kinase, extracellular signal-regulated kinase (ERK) 1/2, and ribosomal protein S6 in vitro and in vivo.

Activating mutations or translocations of the ALK gene have been identified in several malignancies and can result in the expression of oncogenic fusion proteins (e.g., echinoderm microtubule-associated protein-like 4 [EML4]-ALK). Such ALK gene rearrangements have been identified in approximately 3–7% of patients with non-small cell lung cancer (NSCLC). Formation of ALK fusion proteins such as EML4-ALK results in activation and dysregulation of the gene's expression and signaling, which can contribute to increased cell proliferation and survival in tumors expressing these proteins.

Although the ALK inhibitor crizotinib has demonstrated improved outcomes in patients with NSCLC harboring ALK mutations, secondary resistance to crizotinib eventually develops, generally within the first 1–2 years of treatment. Clinical resistance to crizotinib has been attributed to several possible mechanisms, including acquired resistance mutations of ALK, amplification of gene expression, and activation of alternate signaling pathways. Secondary mutations of ALK are responsible for about 30% of cases of acquired crizotinib resistance and gene amplification is implicated in 9% of these cases. The CNS is a common site of disease progression in crizotinib-treated patients because of poor distribution of the drug into CSF; development and/or progression of brain metastases occurs in approximately one-half of patients during crizotinib treatment.

In vitro, brigatinib is approximately 12-fold more potent than crizotinib in its activity against native ALK-positive cell lines and is active against cell lines expressing EML4-ALK and nucleophosmin (NPM)-ALK fusion proteins and many mutant forms associated with resistance to alectinib, ceritinib, and/or crizotinib, as well as EGFR-Del (E746-A750), ROS1-L2026M, FLT3-F691L, and FLT3-D835Y. Brigatinib also demonstrated dose-dependent antitumor activity in mice bearing NSCLC tumor xenografts that expressed EML4-ALK, including those with the crizotinib resistance-conferring L1196M mutation and the G1202R mutation that also confers resistance to ceritinib and alectinib. In addition, brigatinib reduced tumor burden and prolonged survival in mice bearing intracranial ALK-positive NSCLC tumor xenografts. Brigatinib also has demonstrated antitumor activity in patients with crizotinib-resistant disease and baseline CNS metastases.

Systemic exposure to brigatinib is dose proportional over the oral dosage range of 60–240 mg following single or multiple doses. Following oral administration, peak plasma concentrations of brigatinib are achieved in 1–4 hours. Administration of brigatinib with a high-fat meal decreases peak plasma concentrations of brigatinib by 13% but has no effect on systemic exposure compared with administration in the fasting state. Brigatinib is 66% bound to plasma proteins and binding is independent of drug concentration. Brigatinib is primarily metabolized by cytochrome P-450 (CYP) isoenzymes 2C8 and 3A4; its major active metabolite, AP26123, inhibits ALK with approximately threefold lower potency than the parent drug. Steady-state systemic exposure of AP26123 is less than 10% of the parent drug. Following oral administration of radiolabeled brigatinib, 65% of the dose is eliminated in feces (41% as unchanged drug) and 25% of the dose is eliminated in urine (86% as unchanged drug). The mean elimination half-life of brigatinib is 25 hours. Age, gender, race, body weight, and serum albumin concentration do not have clinically important effects on the pharmacokinetics of brigatinib.

ADVICE TO PATIENTS

- Instruct patients to read the manufacturer's patient information.

- Advise patients to take brigatinib exactly as prescribed and to not alter the dosage or discontinue therapy unless advised to do so by their clinician. Advise patients to swallow brigatinib tablets whole without regard to food and not to crush or chew the tablets. If a dose is missed or if vomiting occurs after a dose is administered, the next dose should be taken at the regularly scheduled time; the missed dose should not be taken, and an additional dose should not be administered to replace the vomited dose.

- Inform patients of the symptoms and risks of serious adverse pulmonary reactions such as ILD/pneumonitis, which occur particularly during the first week of brigatinib therapy. Advise patients to immediately report any new or worsening pulmonary symptoms (e.g., dyspnea or shortness of breath, cough with or without mucus, chest pain, fever) to their clinician and inform them that such symptoms may be similar to those of lung cancer.

- Risk of hypertension. Advise patients to promptly report signs or symptoms of hypertension (e.g., headache, dizziness, blurred vision, chest pain, shortness of breath).

- Risk of bradycardia. Advise patients to immediately contact their clinician if they experience dizziness, lightheadedness, or faintness.

- Risk of visual disturbances. Advise patients to inform clinician of any new or worsening visual symptoms (e.g., diplopia, blurred vision, flashes of light, photophobia, new or increased floaters).

- Risk of muscle problems or myalgia; importance of CK monitoring. Inform patients to promptly report any new or worsening signs or symptoms of muscle problems (e.g., unexplained or persistent muscle pain, tenderness, weakness).

- Risk of elevated concentrations of pancreatic enzymes and importance of monitoring amylase and lipase concentrations. Inform patients to immediately contact their clinician if they experience manifestations of pancreatitis (e.g., upper abdominal pain that may spread to the back and get worse with eating, weight loss, nausea).

- Risk of new or worsening hyperglycemia and importance of periodically monitoring blood glucose concentrations. Immediately inform clinician if manifestations of hyperglycemia occur (e.g., increased thirst, increased urination, increased appetite, nausea, weakness, fatigue, confusion). Patients with diabetes mellitus or glucose intolerance may require dosage adjustment of antidiabetic therapy during brigatinib treatment.

- Risk of hepatotoxicity. Inform patients of the signs and symptoms of hepatotoxicity (e.g., yellowing of the skin or whites of the eyes, dark urine, nausea or vomiting, feeling tired, decreased appetite) and the need to monitor for liver function during treatment. Advise patients to inform their clinician of any new or worsening symptoms.

- Risk of photosensitivity. Advise patients to limit sun exposure while taking brigatinib and for at least 5 days after discontinuance of the drug.

- Risk of fetal harm. Advise females of reproductive potential that they should use effective, nonhormonal methods of contraception while receiving brigatinib and for ≥4 months after discontinuance of therapy and advise such females that oral contraceptives and other hormonal forms of contraception may not be effective during brigatinib therapy. Advise males with female partners of reproductive potential to use effective methods of contraception while receiving the drug and for ≥3 months after the drug is discontinued. Also advise males that brigatinib may cause fertility problems and to discuss any concerns about fertility with their clinician.

- Importance of females informing their clinicians if they are or plan to become pregnant. If pregnancy occurs, advise of potential fetal risk.

- Advise females to avoid breast-feeding while receiving brigatinib and for ≥1 week after discontinuance of therapy.

- Importance of informing clinicians of existing or contemplated concomitant therapy, including prescription and OTC drugs (e.g., cardiac or antihypertensive agents, antidiabetic agents) and dietary or herbal supplements

(e.g., St. John's wort, grapefruit-containing products), as well as any concomitant illnesses (e.g., cardiovascular disease, diabetes mellitus, pancreatitis).

- Advise patients to avoid grapefruit and grapefruit juice while taking brigatinib.
- Inform patients of other important precautionary information.

PREPARATIONS

Brigatinib can only be obtained through a limited network of specialty pharmacies. Consult manufacturer's website for specific information regarding distribution of the drug.

Excipients in commercially available drug preparations may have clinically important effects in some individuals; consult specific product labeling for details.

Brigatinib

Oral			
Tablets, film-coated		30 mg	Alunbrig®, Ariad
		90 mg	Alunbrig®, Ariad
		180 mg	Alunbrig®, Ariad

† Use is not currently included in the labeling approved by the US Food and Drug Administration.

Selected Revisions April 10, 2024, © Copyright, May 15, 2017, American Society of Health-System Pharmacists, Inc.

Cabazitaxel

10:00 · ANTINEOPLASTIC AGENTS

■ Cabazitaxel, a semisynthetic taxoid derived from the major natural taxoid (10-deacetyl baccatin III) extracted from the needles of various species of yew trees (*Taxus* species), is an antineoplastic agent.

USES

● Prostate Cancer

Cabazitaxel is used in combination with prednisone for the treatment of hormone-refractory metastatic prostate cancer in patients with disease that has progressed following prior treatment with docetaxel-based therapy.

The current indication for cabazitaxel is based principally on the results of a randomized, multicenter, phase 3 study (TROPIC) in 755 men with hormone-refractory metastatic prostate cancer who had experienced disease progression during or after completion of a docetaxel-containing regimen. Approximately 92% of patients had received a cumulative docetaxel dose of at least 225 mg/m^2 at time of study entry. Patients with measurable disease who were enrolled in the study had disease progression documented by Response Evaluation Criteria in Solid Tumors (RECIST) with at least one visceral or soft-tissue metastatic lesion, while those with nonmeasurable disease were required to have either rising serum prostate specific antigen (PSA) concentrations or the presence of at least one new radiographic lesion. Patients were randomized to receive either cabazitaxel and prednisone or mitoxantrone and prednisone. Treatment consisted of cabazitaxel 25 mg/m^2 administered IV over 1 hour or mitoxantrone 12 mg/m^2 administered IV over 15–30 minutes on day 1 of each 21-day treatment cycle; prednisone 10 mg daily (or an equivalent dosage of prednisolone) was administered orally throughout both treatment courses. Patients receiving cabazitaxel were premedicated with an antihistamine, a histamine H$_2$-receptor antagonist (excluding cimetidine), and a corticosteroid at least 30 minutes prior to cabazitaxel administration. Treatment duration in both groups was limited to 10 cycles to minimize the risk of mitoxantrone-induced cardiotoxicity. Prophylactic use of granulocyte colony-stimulating factors was not permitted during the first cycle of treatment, but use of these agents was allowed after the first occurrence of prolonged neutropenia (i.e., lasting 7 days or longer) or neutropenia associated with fever or infection.

At a median follow-up of 12.8 months, patients receiving cabazitaxel and prednisone had longer median overall survival (15.1 versus 12.7 months) and progression-free survival (2.8 versus 1.4 months) compared with those receiving mitoxantrone and prednisone. A subset analysis of overall survival based on prognostic features at baseline consistently favored the cabazitaxel regimen over the mitoxantrone regimen. Patients receiving cabazitaxel and prednisone also had higher objective tumor response rates (14.4 versus 4.4%) and PSA response rates (39.2 versus 17.8%) and longer median times to tumor progression (8.8 versus 5.4 months) and PSA progression (6.4 versus 3.1 months), but had similar times to pain progression, compared with those receiving mitoxantrone and prednisone. In both treatment groups, the most common reason for drug discontinuance was disease progression; discontinuance because of disease progression was more common (71 versus 48%) in patients receiving mitoxantrone and prednisone, whereas discontinuance because of adverse effects was more common (18 versus 8%) in patients receiving cabazitaxel and prednisone.

Higher frequencies of severe (grade 3 or greater) neutropenia (82 versus 58%), severe febrile neutropenia (7 versus 1%), diarrhea (47 versus 11%, severe in 6 versus less than 1%), and peripheral neuropathy (13 versus 3%) were observed in patients receiving cabazitaxel and prednisone compared with those receiving mitoxantrone and prednisone. The frequency of peripheral edema was similar in both treatment groups (9%). About 5% of cabazitaxel-treated patients compared with 2% of mitoxantrone-treated patients died within 30 days of the last dose of the drug; disease progression was the most common cause of early death among patients receiving mitoxantrone, whereas adverse reactions, including neutropenic complications and renal failure, were the most frequent causes of early death among patients receiving cabazitaxel.

DOSAGE AND ADMINISTRATION

● General

Cabazitaxel should administered under the supervision of a qualified clinician experienced in therapy with cytotoxic agents; appropriate diagnostic and treatment facilities should be readily available for the management of treatment-related complications.

To minimize the risk and/or severity of hypersensitivity reactions, patients should be premedicated with an IV antihistamine (diphenhydramine hydrochloride 25 mg or equivalent), IV histamine H$_2$-receptor antagonist (ranitidine 50 mg or equivalent [except cimetidine]), and IV corticosteroid (dexamethasone 8 mg or equivalent) at least 30 minutes prior to each cabazitaxel infusion.

Antiemetic prophylaxis, administered orally or IV as needed, also is recommended in patients receiving cabazitaxel.

● Reconstitution and Administration

Cabazitaxel is administered by IV infusion over 1 hour.

Caution should be exercised when preparing and handling cabazitaxel solutions, and the use of protective equipment (e.g., gloves) is recommended. If the drug (as a concentrate or diluted solution) comes into contact with mucous membranes, the affected area should be flushed immediately and thoroughly with water. Skin accidentally exposed to the drug should be washed immediately and thoroughly with soap and water.

Cabazitaxel injection concentrate must be diluted prior to IV infusion. First, the cabazitaxel injection concentrate is diluted to prepare the initial diluted cabazitaxel solution and then the initial diluted cabazitaxel solution is further diluted to prepare the final dilution of cabazitaxel solution for infusion. Both the cabazitaxel injection concentrate and diluent vials contain an overfill to compensate for the loss of liquid during preparation.

For preparation of the *initial* diluted solution, the entire contents of the diluent vial supplied by the manufacturer (approximately 5.7 mL of 13% [w/w] ethanol in water for injection) is withdrawn and transferred to a vial labeled as containing cabazitaxel 60 mg in 1.5 mL; the resultant solution contains cabazitaxel 10 mg/mL. The diluent should be directed toward the wall of the vial and injected slowly to minimize foaming. The vial should be inverted repeatedly for at least 45 seconds to fully mix the injection concentrate and diluent; the vial should not be shaken. The solution should be allowed to stand for a few minutes to let any foam dissipate; then preparation may continue even if some foam remains. The initial diluted cabazitaxel solution should be further diluted within 30 minutes of preparation.

For preparation of the *final* diluted cabazitaxel solution, the required amount of the initial diluted cabazitaxel solution (cabazitaxel 10 mg/mL) should be injected into a 250-mL non-PVC infusion bag or bottle containing 0.9% sodium chloride injection or 5% dextrose injection to produce a final solution with a cabazitaxel concentration of 0.1–0.26 mg/mL. If the required dose exceeds 65 mg, the volume of IV solution should be increased accordingly so that a cabazitaxel concentration of 0.26 mg/mL is not exceeded. The final diluted cabazitaxel solution for infusion should be mixed thoroughly by gently inverting the bag or bottle. Infusion of the final diluted cabazitaxel solution should be completed within 8 hours if stored at room temperature or within 24 hours if stored under refrigeration. The infusion solution should be at room temperature for administration. Any unused portion should be discarded. Cabazitaxel should not be admixed with other drugs.

Because both the initial and final diluted cabazitaxel solutions are supersaturated, crystallization may occur over time. Diluted solutions of the drug should be inspected visually for particulate matter, including crystals, and discoloration; the drug should be discarded if either the initial or final diluted solution is cloudy or contains a precipitate. Cabazitaxel should be administered through a 0.22-μm in-line filter.

Cabazitaxel injection concentrate contains polysorbate 80, which can cause leaching of diethylhexyl phthalate (DEHP) from PVC containers. PVC infusion containers and polyurethane administration sets should not be used during preparation or administration of the drug.

● Dosage
Prostate Cancer

The recommended adult dosage of cabazitaxel for the treatment of hormone-refractory metastatic prostate cancer in patients previously treated with a docetaxel-containing regimen is 25 mg/m^2 administered as a 1-hour IV infusion every 3 weeks. Prednisone (10 mg orally once daily) is administered continuously throughout cabazitaxel treatment. In the phase 3 clinical trial supporting use of cabazitaxel for this indication, treatment duration was limited to 10 cycles because of the potential for cumulative cardiotoxicity with the comparator regimen (mitoxantrone). Although no cumulative dose-limiting toxicities have been described with cabazitaxel use, the manufacturer states there are no data to support use of the drug beyond 10 cycles.

Dosage Modification for Toxicity

Dosage Modification for Hematologic Toxicity

Complete blood cell counts should be monitored weekly during the first cycle of cabazitaxel therapy and prior to *each* treatment cycle thereafter. In patients who experience severe prolonged neutropenia (i.e., grade 3 or greater neutropenia lasting longer than one week) despite appropriate use of a granulocyte colony-stimulating factor (e.g., filgrastim, pegfilgrastim), cabazitaxel therapy should be interrupted until the neutrophil count exceeds 1500/mm³; upon resumption of therapy, the cabazitaxel dosage should be reduced to 20 mg/m² every 3 weeks. In patients who experience an episode of febrile neutropenia, therapy should be interrupted until improvement or resolution occurs and the neutrophil count exceeds 1500/mm³; upon resumption of therapy, the cabazitaxel dosage should be reduced to 20 mg/m² every 3 weeks. The manufacturer recommends use of a granulocyte colony-stimulating factor for secondary prophylaxis in patients who have experienced severe prolonged neutropenia or an episode of febrile neutropenia. Cabazitaxel therapy should be discontinued if severe prolonged neutropenia or febrile neutropenia recurs following reduction of the cabazitaxel dosage to 20 mg/m² every 3 weeks.

Dosage Modification for GI Toxicity

In patients who experience severe diarrhea (grade 3 or greater) or persistent diarrhea despite use of appropriate medical therapy (e.g., antidiarrheals, fluid and electrolyte replacement), cabazitaxel therapy should be interrupted until the diarrhea improves or resolves; upon resumption of therapy, the cabazitaxel dosage should be reduced to 20 mg/m² every 3 weeks. Cabazitaxel therapy should be discontinued if severe or persistent diarrhea recurs following reduction of the cabazitaxel dosage to 20 mg/m² every 3 weeks.

● Special Populations

The manufacturer makes no special population dosage recommendations at this time. The manufacturer states that cabazitaxel should *not* be used in patients with hepatic impairment (serum AST and/or ALT concentrations of 1.5 or more times the upper limit of normal [ULN] or total serum bilirubin concentrations at or above the ULN). (See Specific Populations under Cautions: Warnings/Precautions.)

CAUTIONS

● Contraindications

Known severe hypersensitivity reaction to cabazitaxel or other formulations containing polysorbate 80.

Baseline neutrophil count of 1500/mm³ or less.

● Warnings/Precautions

Warnings

Neutropenia

Neutropenia, including fatal neutropenic episodes, have been reported in patients receiving cabazitaxel. In the TROPIC study in patients with prostate cancer, grade 3 or 4 neutropenia was reported in 82% and febrile neutropenia was reported in 7% of patients receiving cabazitaxel and prednisone. Five deaths due to sepsis or septic shock were reported with this regimen in the TROPIC study; all 5 patients had severe (grade 4) neutropenia, and one patient had febrile neutropenia. One additional death was attributed to neutropenia without documented infection.

Granulocyte colony-stimulating factors (G-CSF) (e.g., filgrastim, pegfilgrastim) may be used to reduce the risk of neutropenic complications associated with cabazitaxel. The manufacturer recommends that primary prophylaxis with G-CSF be considered in patients with high-risk clinical features that could potentially increase the risk of complications associated with prolonged neutropenia, including patients older than 65 years of age and those with poor performance status, prior episodes of febrile neutropenia, extensive prior radiation, poor nutritional status, or other serious comorbidities. The manufacturer recommends that therapeutic use of G-CSF and secondary prophylaxis be considered in all patients at increased risk for neutropenic complications.

Complete blood cell counts should be monitored weekly during the first treatment cycle and prior to *each* treatment cycle thereafter. After administration of the recommended dosage for the initial cycle, dosage for each subsequent cycle should be adjusted as needed based on hematologic recovery. Cabazitaxel should *not* be administered until neutrophil counts exceed 1500/mm³. In patients who experience severe prolonged neutropenia despite appropriate treatment (e.g.,

G-CSF) or febrile neutropenia, temporary interruption of cabazitaxel therapy followed by dosage reduction or discontinuance of cabazitaxel therapy may be required. (See Dosage Modification for Hematologic Toxicity under Dosage: Dosage Modification for Toxicity, in Dosage and Administration.)

Sensitivity Reactions

Cabazitaxel can cause severe hypersensitivity reactions (e.g., generalized rash/erythema, hypotension, bronchospasm), and all patients receiving the drug should be premedicated to minimize the risk and/or severity of these reactions. (See Dosage and Administration: General.) Patients should be observed closely for hypersensitivity reactions, especially during the first and second infusions of the drug. Appropriate facilities and equipment for the treatment of hypotension and bronchospasm should be readily available, since hypersensitivity reactions may occur within minutes following initiation of a cabazitaxel infusion. If a severe hypersensitivity reaction develops, the infusion should be discontinued immediately and appropriate supportive treatment instituted. Cabazitaxel injection concentrate contains polysorbate 80 and should *not* be used in patients with a history of severe hypersensitivity to cabazitaxel or to other formulations containing polysorbate 80.

Other Warnings and Precautions

GI Effects

Cabazitaxel can cause nausea, vomiting, and severe diarrhea. Death related to diarrhea and associated dehydration and electrolyte imbalance has been reported in a patient who received the drug. Antiemetic prophylaxis, administered orally or IV as needed, is recommended in patients receiving cabazitaxel. Rehydration therapy and antidiarrheal and antiemetic agents should be used as needed; intensive measures may be required for the management of severe diarrhea and electrolyte imbalance. In patients with severe or persistent diarrhea, temporary interruption of therapy followed by dosage reduction, or discontinuance of cabazitaxel therapy, may be required. (See Dosage Modification for GI Toxicity under Dosage: Dosage Modification for Toxicity, in Dosage and Administration.)

Renal Effects

Renal failure, sometimes fatal, has been reported in patients receiving cabazitaxel, generally in association with sepsis, dehydration, or obstructive uropathy; some deaths due to renal failure did not have a clear etiology. If renal failure develops during cabazitaxel therapy, appropriate measures should be taken to identify the cause and the renal failure should be treated aggressively.

Fetal/Neonatal Morbidity and Mortality

Cabazitaxel may cause fetal harm if administered to pregnant women; the drug has been shown to be embryotoxic, fetotoxic, and abortifacient in animals. Pregnancy should be avoided during therapy. If cabazitaxel is used during pregnancy or if the patient becomes pregnant while receiving the drug, the patient should be apprised of the potential fetal hazard.

Specific Populations

Pregnancy

Category D. (See Fetal/Neonatal Morbidity and Mortality under Warnings/Precautions: Other Warnings and Precautions, in Cautions.) (See Users Guide.)

Lactation

Cabazitaxel or its metabolites are distributed into milk in lactating rats. It is not known whether cabazitaxel or its metabolites are distributed into human milk. Because of the potential for serious adverse reactions to cabazitaxel in nursing infants, a decision should be made whether to discontinue nursing or the drug, taking into account the importance of the drug to the woman.

Pediatric Use

Safety and efficacy of cabazitaxel have not been established in pediatric patients.

Geriatric Use

In the TROPIC study in patients with prostate cancer, 65% of patients receiving cabazitaxel and prednisone were 65 years of age or older, while 19% were 75 years of age or older. Although no substantial differences in efficacy or pharmacokinetics of cabazitaxel were observed between individuals 65 years of age or older and younger adults, reported frequencies of neutropenia, fatigue, asthenia, pyrexia, dizziness, urinary tract infection, and dehydration were at least 5 percentage points higher in patients 65 years of age or older compared with younger adults. In addition, 6% of patients 65 years of age or older, compared with 2% of patients younger than 65 years of age, died within 30 days of the last cabazitaxel dose from a cause other than disease progression.

Hepatic Impairment

Safety and efficacy of cabazitaxel have not been established in patients with hepatic impairment. Patients with serum transaminase (AST, ALT) concentrations of 1.5 or more times the upper limit of normal (ULN) or serum bilirubin concentrations at or above the ULN were excluded from the TROPIC study.

Because cabazitaxel is extensively metabolized in the liver, hepatic impairment is expected to result in increased serum concentrations of the drug. Hepatic impairment increases the risk of severe or life-threatening complications of other taxanes (e.g., docetaxel). The manufacturer states that cabazitaxel should *not* be used in patients with hepatic impairment (i.e., AST and/or ALT concentrations of 1.5 or more times the ULN or total serum bilirubin concentrations at or above the ULN).

Renal Impairment

Safety and efficacy of cabazitaxel in patients with renal impairment have not been studied specifically to date. Only minimal amounts of cabazitaxel (3.7%) are excreted as unchanged drug or metabolites in urine. A population pharmacokinetic analysis indicated that mild to moderate renal impairment (creatinine clearance of 30 to less than 80 mL/minute) did not substantially alter cabazitaxel clearance. However, no data are available for patients with severe renal impairment (creatinine clearance less than 30 mL/minute) or end-stage renal disease, and the manufacturer states that cabazitaxel should be used with caution in patients with severe renal impairment or end-stage renal disease.

● Common Adverse Effects

Adverse effects reported in 10% or more of patients receiving cabazitaxel in combination with prednisone include neutropenia, leukopenia, anemia, thrombocytopenia, diarrhea, fatigue, nausea, vomiting, constipation, asthenia, abdominal pain, anorexia, back pain, hematuria, peripheral neuropathy, pyrexia, dyspnea, cough, dysgeusia, arthralgia, and alopecia. Serious (grade 3 or 4) adverse effects reported in 5% or more of patients receiving cabazitaxel in combination with prednisone include neutropenia, leukopenia, anemia, febrile neutropenia, diarrhea, fatigue, and asthenia.

DRUG INTERACTIONS

No formal drug interaction studies have been performed to date.

The manufacturer states that cabazitaxel is unlikely to inhibit multidrug resistance proteins MRP1 and MRP2, the efflux transporter P-glycoprotein (P-gp, ABCB1), or breast cancer resistance protein (BCRP) in vivo following administration of the drug at a dose of 25 mg/m². In vitro data indicate that cabazitaxel does not inhibit MRP1 or MRP2; although in vitro inhibition of P-gp transport and BCRP has been observed, inhibition occurred at concentrations at least 38 times those achieved clinically.

In vitro data indicate that cabazitaxel is a substrate of P-gp, but not a substrate of MRP1, MRP2, or BCRP.

● Drugs Affecting or Metabolized by Hepatic Microsomal Enzymes

Because cabazitaxel is extensively metabolized by cytochrome P-450 (CYP) isoenzyme 3A (CYP3A), potent inhibitors or inducers of this isoenzyme are expected to alter the drug's pharmacokinetics. Cabazitaxel does not induce CYP isoenzymes in vitro. In vitro data also indicate that cabazitaxel is unlikely to inhibit metabolism of drugs that are substrates of CYP isoenzymes 1A2, 2B6, 2C8, 2C9, 2C19, 2D6, 2E1, or 3A4/5.

Concomitant use of cabazitaxel with potent inhibitors of CYP3A (e.g., atazanavir, clarithromycin, indinavir, itraconazole, ketoconazole, nefazodone, nelfinavir, ritonavir, saquinavir, telithromycin, voriconazole) is expected to result in increased plasma cabazitaxel concentrations and should be avoided. Moderate CYP3A inhibitors should be used concomitantly with caution.

Concomitant use of cabazitaxel with potent inducers of CYP3A (e.g., carbamazepine, phenobarbital, phenytoin, rifampin, rifabutin, rifapentine) is expected to result in decreased plasma cabazitaxel concentrations and should be avoided. Concomitant use of St. John's wort (*Hypericum perforatum*) also should be avoided.

● Corticosteroids

Administration of prednisone or prednisolone at a dosage of 10 mg daily did not affect the pharmacokinetics of cabazitaxel.

DESCRIPTION

Cabazitaxel, a semisynthetic taxoid derived from the major natural taxoid (10-deacetyl baccatin III) extracted from the needles of various species of yew trees (*Taxus* species), is an antimicrotubule antineoplastic agent. Cabazitaxel is the 7,10-dimethoxy analog of docetaxel. Like other taxanes (e.g., docetaxel, paclitaxel), cabazitaxel binds to β-tubulin subunits on microtubules and stabilizes and suppresses microtubule activity, thereby resulting in mitotic arrest and cell death.

In preclinical studies, cabazitaxel was active against some cell lines that are resistant to other antineoplastic agents, including anthracyclines, vinca alkaloids, and other taxanes (i.e., docetaxel, paclitaxel). Cabazitaxel, a weak substrate for the efflux transporter P-glycoprotein (P-gp), has demonstrated activity in cell lines with acquired resistance to docetaxel resulting from P-gp overexpression and in cell lines with primary resistance to taxanes resulting from increased expression of the multidrug resistance (MDR) gene and its product P-gp. Cabazitaxel has demonstrated activity against some taxane-resistant tumors in vivo, including activity against docetaxel-resistant prostate cancer.

Evidence from animal studies suggests that cabazitaxel may cross the blood-brain barrier to a greater extent than docetaxel or paclitaxel, possibly because of cabazitaxel's lower affinity for P-gp, which is expressed in the blood-brain barrier. Animal data suggest that P-gp-mediated transport across the blood-brain barrier can be saturated, resulting in nonlinear accumulation of the drug in the brain. The clinical relevance of these findings to neurotoxicity or antitumor effects of the drug in humans is unknown.

Cabazitaxel is extensively metabolized in the liver, primarily by cytochrome P-450 (CYP) isoenzyme 3A4/5 and to a lesser extent by CYP isoenzyme 2C8. About 76% of a dose of cabazitaxel is eliminated in feces as metabolites, and about 3.7% is eliminated in urine as unchanged drug or metabolites; about 20 metabolites of the drug have been identified in urine or feces. The terminal elimination half-life of cabazitaxel is 95 hours.

ADVICE TO PATIENTS

Risk of hypersensitivity reactions. Importance of informing clinician immediately if manifestations of severe hypersensitivity (e.g., rash, itching, dizziness or faintness, difficulty breathing, chest or throat tightness, facial swelling) occur. Importance of informing clinician of any history of hypersensitivity to cabazitaxel or other formulations containing polysorbate 80.

Risk of infection, including severe or potentially fatal infection. Importance of routine monitoring of blood cell counts. Importance of patients monitoring their temperature frequently and immediately notifying their clinician if fever or other manifestations of infection (e.g., cough, burning on urination, myalgia) occur.

Risk of dehydration and renal failure. Importance of informing clinician if substantial vomiting or diarrhea occurs, decreased urine output occurs, or edema develops.

Importance of informing geriatric patients that certain adverse effects may be more frequent or severe in older patients. (See Geriatric Use under Warnings/Precautions: Specific Populations, in Cautions.)

Importance of taking the oral prednisone component of the cabazitaxel/prednisone regimen for prostate cancer as directed. Importance of informing clinician if not adherent to the oral prednisone regimen.

Importance of women informing clinicians if they are or plan to become pregnant or plan to breast-feed. Apprise patient of potential hazard to the fetus if used during pregnancy; women of childbearing potential should avoid becoming pregnant.

Importance of informing clinician of existing or contemplated concomitant therapy, including prescription and OTC drugs and herbal supplements, as well as any concomitant illnesses.

Importance of informing patients of other important precautionary information. (See Cautions.)

For further information on the handling of antineoplastic agents, see the ASHP Guidelines on Handling Hazardous Drugs at http://www.ahfsdrug information.com.

PREPARATIONS

Excipients in commercially available drug preparations may have clinically important effects in some individuals; consult specific product labeling for details.

Cabazitaxel

Parenteral

Injection concentrate, for IV infusion only	40 mg/mL (60 mg)	Jevtana® (with water for injection containing alcohol 13% w/w diluent), Sanofi-Aventis

Cabozantinib *S*-malate

10:00 • ANTINEOPLASTIC AGENTS

■ Cabozantinib *S*-malate, an inhibitor of multiple receptor tyrosine kinases, is an antineoplastic agent.

USES

● Medullary Thyroid Cancer

Cabozantinib *S*-malate capsules (Cometriq®) are used for the treatment of progressive, metastatic medullary thyroid cancer. Cabozantinib (Cometriq®) has been designated an orphan drug by the US Food and Drug Administration (FDA) for the treatment of this cancer. Guidelines generally support the use of tyrosine kinase inhibitors, including cabozantinib, in the first-line treatment of progressive and metastatic medullary thyroid cancer.

Clinical Experience

The current indication for cabozantinib (Cometriq®) is based principally on the results of a randomized, multicenter, double-blind, placebo-controlled, phase 3 study (EXAM) in patients with unresectable, locally advanced or metastatic medullary thyroid cancer who had evidence of actively progressive disease within 14 months prior to study entry according to Response Evaluation Criteria in Solid Tumors (RECIST). In the EXAM study, 330 patients were randomized in a 2:1 ratio to receive either cabozantinib (140 mg) or placebo orally once daily, without food, until disease progression or intolerable toxicity occurred. The primary efficacy end point of this study was progression-free survival according to RECIST; secondary endpoints included overall survival, objective response rate, and duration of response. The median age of patients enrolled in the study was 55 years; 25% of the patients had received 2 or more prior systemic therapies and 21% had previously received a tyrosine kinase inhibitor. Rearranged during transfection (RET) mutation status was positive, negative, or unknown in 48, 12, or 39% of the enrolled patients, respectively.

Patients receiving cabozantinib in the EXAM study demonstrated a longer median progression-free survival than those receiving placebo (11.2 versus 4 months, respectively). The favorable treatment effect of cabozantinib on progression-free survival was consistent across patient subgroups, including RET mutation status and previous therapy with a tyrosine kinase inhibitor. Patients receiving cabozantinib also had higher overall response rates (all were partial responses) compared with those receiving placebo (27 versus 0%), and their median duration of response was 14.7 months. Overall survival was not substantially different between the cabozantinib and placebo groups in a planned interim analysis, an unplanned analysis requested by the FDA, and the final analysis.

Clinical Perspective

The American Thyroid Association (ATA) published a guideline on management of medullary thyroid cancer in 2015. Single agent or combination cytotoxic chemotherapy regimens in patients with medullary thyroid cancer is characterized by low response rates and short durations of response; therefore, single agent or combination cytotoxic chemotherapy regimens are not recommended as first-line therapy in patients with persistent or recurrent medullary thyroid cancer. Systemic therapy with tyrosine kinase inhibitors targeting both rearranged during transfection (RET) proto-oncogene and vascular endothelial growth factor receptor (VEGFR) should be considered in patients with significant tumor burden and symptomatic or progressive metastatic disease. The ATA states that cabozantinib or vandetanib can be used as single-agent first-line therapy in patients with advanced progressive disease. Other experts also recommend cabozantinib and vandetanib (both strong recommendations based on high-quality evidence) as first-line systemic therapy in patients with progressive metastatic medullary thyroid cancer.

● Differentiated Thyroid Cancer

Cabozantinib *S*-malate tablets (Cabometyx®) is used for the treatment of locally advanced or metastatic differentiated thyroid cancer (DTC) that has progressed following VEGFR-targeted therapy in adult and pediatric patients ≥12 years of age who are refractory to or ineligible for radioactive iodine (iodine-131). Safety and efficacy of cabozantinib tablets (Cabometyx®) for the treatment of previously treated, locally advanced or metastatic DTC in pediatric patients ≥12 years of age is supported by extrapolation of data from clinical studies evaluating cabozantinib tablets in adults and population pharmacokinetic data indicating that exposure to the drug in pediatric patients ≥12 years of age is similar to that in adults. Guidelines state that tyrosine kinase inhibitors should be considered in patients with metastatic radioactive iodine-refractory DTC that is rapidly progressive, symptomatic, and/or imminently threatening and not amenable to control with other approaches.

Clinical Experience

Efficacy of cabozantinib tablets (Cabometyx®) has been evaluated in a randomized, double-blind, placebo-controlled trial (COSMIC-311) in patients with locally advanced or metastatic DTC. Patients were enrolled in the study if they had DTC that progressed following VEGFR-targeted therapy and were refractory to or ineligible for radioactive iodine. Patients were randomized to receive cabozantinib tablets 60 mg orally once daily or placebo with supportive care until disease progression or unacceptable toxicity occurred. Patients randomized to placebo were permitted to cross-over to cabozantinib tablets following confirmed disease progression. The primary efficacy end points were progression-free survival in the intent-to-treat population (187 patients) and objective response rate in the initial 100 randomized patients. In this study, the median age of patients was 65 years (range: 31–85 years); 53% were female, 70% were white, 19% were Asian, 2% were Black, 2% were American Indian or Alaska Native, 63% previously received lenvatinib, and 93% had metastatic disease. Baseline Eastern Cooperative Oncology Group (ECOG) performance status was 0 or 1 in 46 or 54% of patients, respectively.

At a median follow-up of 6.2 months in the intent-to-treat population, median progression-free survival had not been reached in patients receiving cabozantinib tablets and was 1.9 months in those receiving placebo (hazard ratio: 0.22 with a 95% confidence interval of 0.14–0.35). At the time of an updated progression-free survival analysis in 258 patients, median progression-free survival was 11 months in patients receiving cabozantinib tablets and was 1.9 months in those receiving placebo (hazard ratio: 0.22 with a 95% confidence interval of 0.15–0.31). At a median follow-up duration of 8.9 months in the initial 100 randomized patients, objective response was achieved in 15% of patients receiving cabozantinib tablets compared with none of those receiving placebo; these results did not meet the prespecified significance level.

Clinical Perspective

The American Thyroid Association (ATA) published a guideline on the management of patients with thyroid nodules and DTC in 2015. The basic goals of initial therapy for patients with DTC are to improve overall and disease-specific survival, reduce the risk of persistent/recurrent disease and associated morbidity, and permit accurate disease staging and risk stratification, while minimizing treatment-related morbidity and unnecessary therapy. In patients with metastatic disease, ATA states that the preferred hierarchy of treatment is surgical excision of locoregional disease in potentially curable patients, iodine-131 therapy for radioactive iodine-responsive disease, directed treatment modalities (e.g., external beam radiation therapy, thermal ablation), TSH-suppressive thyroid hormone therapy for patients with stable or slowly progressive asymptomatic disease, and systemic therapy with kinase inhibitors, especially for patients with significantly progressive macroscopic refractory disease.

At the time of publication of the ATA guideline, limited evidence of efficacy was available for certain kinase inhibitors (e.g., sorafenib, lenvatinib, vandetanib); however, a 2019 guideline published by international experts states that lenvatinib and sorafenib should be considered the standard first-line systemic therapy in patients with radioactive iodine-refractory DTC.

● Renal Cell Carcinoma

Cabozantinib *S*-malate tablets (Cabometyx®) are used as a single agent for the treatment of patients with advanced renal cell carcinoma (RCC); the drug also is used in combination with nivolumab as first-line treatment in patients with advanced RCC. Guidelines generally support the use of tyrosine kinase inhibitors, including cabozantinib, in patients with treatment-naïve and treatment-experienced advanced RCC.

Monotherapy

METEOR Study

Efficacy of cabozantinib tablets (Cabometyx®) has been compared with everolimus in one open-label, randomized controlled trial (METEOR) in 658 patients with advanced RCC who had previously received at least 1 anti-angiogenic therapy. Patients were randomized to receive cabozantinib tablets 60 mg orally once daily or everolimus 10 mg orally once daily until disease progression or unacceptable toxicity occurred. The primary efficacy end point was progression-free survival in the initial 375 randomized patients; other efficacy end points were objective response rate and overall survival. The median age of enrolled patients was 62 years; 75% were male, 69% received only one prior anti-angiogenic therapy, 46% were Memorial Sloan Kettering Cancer Center (MSKCC) favorable risk (0 risk factors), 42% were MSKCC intermediate risk (1 risk factor), and 13% were MSKCC poor risk (2 or 3 risk factors). Metastatic disease was present in 3 or more organs in 54% of patients and included the lung (63%), lymph nodes (62%), liver (29%), and bone (22%). Analysis of progression-free survival and overall survival occurred after a minimum duration of follow-up of 11 and 6 months, respectively. In this study, a substantial improvement in progression-free survival (7.4 versus 3.8 months; hazard ratio [HR] of 0.58 with a 95% confidence interval [CI] of 0.45–0.74), overall survival (21.4 versus 16.5 months; HR of 0.66 with a 95% CI of 0.53–0.83), and objective response rate (17% versus 3%) was observed in patients receiving cabozantinib compared with those receiving everolimus. Overall survival, progression-free survival, and objective response rates for cabozantinib- and everolimus-treated patients at the time of final analysis (at a median follow-up of 18.7 months) remained similar to the initial results.

CABOSUN Study

Cabozantinib tablets (Cabometyx®) are used for the first-line treatment of patients with advanced RCC. Efficacy of cabozantinib tablets (Cabometyx®) has been compared with sunitinib in an open-label randomized trial (CABOSUN) in 157 patients with previously untreated advanced RCC. Patients were randomized to receive cabozantinib tablets 60 mg orally once daily or sunitinib 50 mg orally once daily (4 weeks on treatment followed by 2 weeks off) until disease progression or unacceptable toxicity occurred. All patients were required to have intermediate- or poor-risk disease as defined by the International Metastatic RCC Database Consortium (IMDC). The primary efficacy end point was progression-free survival; secondary end points included overall survival and objective response rate. The median age of enrolled patients was 63 years; 78% were male, 81% were categorized as IMDC intermediate risk, and 19% had IMDC poor-risk disease. Bone metastases were present in 36% of patients. ECOG performance status scores were 0, 1, or 2 in 46, 41%, or 13% of patients, respectively. At a median follow-up duration of 34.5 months, a substantial improvement in progression-free survival in patients receiving cabozantinib compared with those receiving sunitinib (8.6 versus 5.3 months; HR of 0.48 with a 95% CI of 0.31–0.74) was observed. Median overall survival was 26.6 months with cabozantinib and 21.2 months with sunitinib (HR of 0.80 with a 95% CI of 0.53–1.21). Objective response rate (partial responses only) was 20% in patients receiving cabozantinib and 9% in those receiving sunitinib.

Combination Therapy with Nivolumab

The CHECKMATE-9ER study was an open-label, randomized controlled trial comparing the combination of cabozantinib tablets (Cabometyx®) and nivolumab with sunitinib in 651 patients with previously untreated advanced RCC. Patients were randomized to receive cabozantinib tablets 40 mg orally daily in combination with nivolumab 240 mg IV every 2 weeks, or sunitinib 50 mg orally daily for the first 4 weeks of each 6-week cycle (4 weeks on treatment followed by 2 weeks off). The primary efficacy end point was progression-free survival; secondary end points were overall survival and objective response rate.

The median age of patients in the CHECKMATE-9ER study was 61 years; 74% were male, 82% were white, and 23% and 77% of patients had a baseline Karnofsky Performance Score (KPS) of 70–80% and 90–100%, respectively. Risk status by IMDC was favorable in 22% of patients, intermediate in 58%, and poor in 20%. At a median follow-up duration of 18.1 months, a substantial improvement in progression-free survival (16.6 versus 8.3 months; HR of 0.51 with a 95% CI, 0.41–0.64), overall survival (HR of 0.60; 95% CI, 0.40–0.89), and objective response rate (55.7% versus 27.1%; p<0.0001) was observed in patients receiving cabozantinib plus nivolumab compared with those receiving sunitinib. Consistent

results for progression-free survival were observed across prespecified subgroups of IMDC risk categories and PD-L1 tumor expression status.

Clinical Perspective

Prognosis is generally poor in patients with metastatic RCC, including those who have undergone complete tumor resection. First-line therapy with vascular endothelial growth factor receptor (VEGFR) inhibitors has been shown to provide benefits in patients with advanced RCC; however, relapsed or refractory RCC eventually develops in most patients. Combination regimens (e.g., immune checkpoint inhibitor in combination with a tyrosine kinase inhibitor) have generally become a standard for the treatment of advanced RCC. A limited number of randomized controlled trials have compared sunitinib with other treatment options for advanced renal cell carcinoma (e.g., pembrolizumab plus axitinib, avelumab plus axitinib, atezolizumab plus bevacizumab, nivolumab plus ipilimumab, nivolumab plus cabozantinib, or lenvatinib plus pembrolizumab). In clinical trials, combination chemotherapy resulted in longer progression-free survival compared with sunitinib alone in patients with previously untreated advanced renal cell carcinoma.

In addition, some experts state that subsequent monotherapy with a tyrosine kinase inhibitor (e.g., sunitinib, pazopanib) may be offered as an alternative to programmed death 1 (PD-1) inhibitor-based combinations in the first-line setting when immune checkpoint therapy is contraindicated or not available or as a second-line option following disease progression during immune checkpoint inhibitor-based therapy.

● Hepatocellular Carcinoma

Cabozantinib S-malate tablets (Cabometyx®) are used for the treatment of patients with hepatocellular carcinoma (HCC) previously treated with sorafenib. Cabozantinib (Cabometyx®) has been designated an orphan drug by the US FDA for the treatment of patients with HCC. Safety and efficacy of cabozantinib tablets (Cabometyx®) for this use is based principally on the results of a randomized controlled trial (CELESTIAL) in patients with HCC previously treated with sorafenib. Guidelines generally support second-line use of another tyrosine kinase inhibitor (e.g., cabozantinib), in patients with HCC treated with sorafenib or lenvatinib in the first-line setting.

Clinical Experience

Efficacy of cabozantinib tablets (Cabometyx®) has been evaluated in a randomized, double-blind, placebo-controlled trial (CELESTIAL) in 704 patients with HCC previously treated with sorafenib. In this study, patients were required to have Child-Pugh class A hepatic impairment. Patients were randomized in a 2:1 ratio to receive cabozantinib tablets 60 mg orally once daily or placebo until disease progression or unacceptable toxicity occurred. The primary efficacy end point was overall survival; secondary end points were progression-free survival and objective response rate.

The median age of patients in the CELESTIAL study was 64 years; 81% were male, 56% were white, and 34% were Asian. At baseline, 53% of patients had an ECOG performance status of 0 and 47% had performance status of 1. The etiology of HCC was attributed to hepatitis B virus, hepatitis C virus, or other etiology in 38, 21, or 40% of patients, respectively. Macroscopic vascular invasion or extrahepatic tumor spread was present in 78% of patients and 41% had serum alpha-fetoprotein (AFP) concentrations ≥0.4 mg/L. All patients had received prior sorafenib and 27% had received 2 prior systemic therapy regimens.

In the CELESTIAL study, substantial improvements in overall survival (10.2 versus 8.0 months; hazard ratio of 0.76, 95% CI of 0.63–0.92), progression-free survival (5.2 versus 1.9 months; hazard ratio of 0.44, 95% CI of 0.36–0.52), and objective response rate (4% versus 0.4%) was observed in patients receiving cabozantinib compared with those receiving placebo.

Clinical Perspective

Management of early stage hepatocellular carcinoma generally includes liver transplantation, surgical resection, and ablation. Survival is usually less than 6 months in patients with untreated advanced stage hepatocellular carcinoma. Treatment of hepatocellular carcinoma is complicated by the presence of underlying liver disease, the extent and location of tumor, comorbidities, and performance status. The American Society of Clinical Oncology (ASCO) states that the risk of potential toxicities and benefits of therapy should be considered when selecting therapy.

The 2024 ASCO guideline update on systemic therapy for advanced hepatocellular carcinoma states that lenvatinib, sorafenib, or durvalumab may be offered as first-line therapy for patients with advanced hepatocellular carcinoma, Child-Pugh class A, and an ECOG performance status of 0 or 1 when therapy with atezolizumab plus bevacizumab or durvalamab plus tremelimumab is contraindicated. ASCO also states that tyrosine kinase inhibitors (i.e., cabozantinib, lenvatinib, sorafenib) may be used as second-line therapy† following therapy with various first-line treatment options.

The decision to pursue second-line therapy and choice of treatment should be based on patient and clinician preferences and other factors (i.e., comorbidities, liver function, performance status, and potential for benefit and risk of harm).

DOSAGE AND ADMINISTRATION

• *General*

Pretreatment Screening

- Assess for recent history of hemorrhage, including hemoptysis, hematemesis, or melena; do not use in patients with a history of these events.
- Blood pressure should be adequately controlled prior to initiating therapy. Do not initiate in patients with uncontrolled hypertension.
- Perform oral examination prior to initiating therapy.
- Verify pregnancy status of females of reproductive potential prior to initiation of therapy.
- The manufacturer of Cabometyx® also recommends assessing for signs of thyroid dysfunction prior to the initiation of Cabometyx®.

Patient Monitoring

- Monitor for signs and symptoms of GI perforation/fistula, including abscess and sepsis.
- Monitor blood pressure regularly during therapy.
- Perform oral examination periodically during therapy.
- Assess urine protein regularly during therapy.
- Monitor for hemorrhage.
- Monitor for arterial or venous thromboembolic events.
- The manufacturer of Cabometyx® also recommends monitoring for signs and symptoms of thyroid dysfunction during Cabometyx® therapy. Perform thyroid function testing and manage thyroid dysfunction as clinically indicated.
- The manufacturer of Cabometyx® recommends physeal and longitudinal growth monitoring in children with open growth plates during therapy.
- Monitor and correct serum calcium levels as clinically indicated during therapy.

Other General Considerations

- Withhold cabozantinib ≥3 weeks prior to elective surgery, and for ≥2 weeks following major surgery and until adequate wound healing has occurred.
- Withhold cabozantinib ≥3 weeks prior to scheduled dental surgery or invasive dental procedures, if possible.
- Maintain good oral hygiene during therapy.
- Clinicians should consult published protocols for information on the dosage, method of administration, and administration sequence of other antineoplastic agents used in combination regimens with cabozantinib tablets. When used in combination with nivolumab, the usual cautions, precautions, and contraindications associated with nivolumab must be considered in addition to those associated with cabozantinib tablets.

• *Administration*

Cabozantinib S-malate is administered orally as capsules (Cometriq®) or tablets (Cabometyx®).

Cometriq® capsules: Cabozantinib S-malate is administered orally once daily. The drug should *not* be administered with food; patients should not eat for at least 2 hours before and at least 1 hour after taking cabozantinib capsules. Cabozantinib capsules should be swallowed whole with a full glass (at least 240 mL) of water; the capsules should *not* be opened or crushed.

Cabometyx® tablets: Cabozantinib S-malate is administered orally once daily. The drug should *not* be administered with food; patients should take cabozantinib tablets at least 1 hour before or at least 2 hours after eating. Cabozantinib tablets should be swallowed whole; the tablets should *not* be crushed.

If a dose of cabozantinib is missed, the missed dose should not be taken within 12 hours of the next dose.

Store cabozantinib capsules (Cometriq®) or tablets (Cabometyx®) at 20–25°C; excursions are permitted from 15–30°C.

• *Dosage*

Dosage of cabozantinib, which is commercially available as cabozantinib S-malate, is expressed in terms of cabozantinib.

Cometriq® capsules and Cabometyx® tablets are *not* interchangeable.

Medullary Thyroid Cancer

The recommended adult dosage of cabozantinib (Cometriq®) as a single agent for the treatment of progressive, metastatic medullary thyroid cancer is 140 mg (one 80-mg and three 20-mg capsules) once daily. Therapy should be continued until disease progression or unacceptable toxicity occurs.

Differentiated Thyroid Cancer

The recommended *adult* dosage of cabozantinib (Cabometyx®) as a single agent for the treatment of locally advanced or metastatic differentiated thyroid cancer in adults with a body surface area (BSA) ≥1.2 m² is 60 mg once daily. Continue therapy until disease progression or unacceptable toxicity occurs.

The recommended *pediatric* dosage of cabozantinib (Cabometyx®) as a single agent for the treatment of locally advanced or metastatic differentiated thyroid cancer in pediatric patients ≥12 years of age and with a BSA ≥1.2 m² is 60 mg once daily. The recommended pediatric dosage in patients ≥12 years of age and a BSA <1.2 m² is 40 mg once daily. Continue therapy until disease progression or unacceptable toxicity occurs.

Renal Cell Carcinoma
Monotherapy

The recommended adult dosage of cabozantinib (Cabometyx®) as a single agent for advanced renal cell carcinoma is 60 mg once daily. Continue therapy until disease progression or unacceptable toxicity occurs.

Combination Therapy with Nivolumab

The recommended adult dosage of cabozantinib (Cabometyx®) for the first-line treatment of advanced renal cell carcinoma is 40 mg once daily in combination with nivolumab (240 mg every 2 weeks by IV infusion over 30 minutes or 480 mg every 4 weeks by IV infusion over 30 minutes). Continue therapy for up to 2 years or until disease progression or unacceptable toxicity occurs.

Hepatocellular Carcinoma

The recommended adult dosage of cabozantinib (Cabometyx®) as a single agent for the treatment of previously treated hepatocellular carcinoma is 60 mg once daily. Continue therapy until disease progression or unacceptable toxicity occurs.

Dosage Modification for Toxicity
Cabometyx® Tablets

Cabozantinib tablets should be *withheld* if intolerable grade 2 adverse reactions, grade 3 or 4 adverse reactions, or osteonecrosis of the jaw (ONJ) occurs.

Upon resolution or improvement of the adverse effect (i.e., return to baseline or resolution to grade 1), the dosage should be reduced; however, in some cases, the drug should be permanently discontinued. (See Tables 1, 2, 3, and 4.) If dosage reduction is required, the adult and pediatric dosage of cabozantinib should be reduced as described in Tables and 1 and 2, respectively.)

TABLE 1. Adults: Recommended Dosage Reduction for Cabometyx® (Cabozantinib Tablets) Toxicity.

Dosage Reduction Level	Cabozantinib Monotherapy in Adults with BSA ≥1.2 m² (Starting Dosage = 60 mg daily)	Cabozantinib in Combination with Nivolumab (Starting Dosage = 40 mg daily in combination with nivolumab)
First	Restart at 40 mg once daily	Restart at 20 mg once daily
Second	Restart at 20 mg once daily[a]	Restart at 20 mg every other day[a]

[a] If previously receiving lowest dosage, resume therapy at same dosage. If lowest dosage not tolerated, discontinue cabozantinib tablets.

TABLE 2. Pediatric Patients: Recommended Dosage Reduction for Cabometyx® (Cabozantinib Tablets) Toxicity.

Dosage Reduction Level	Cabozantinib Monotherapy in Pediatric Patients ≥12 years of age with BSA ≥1.2 m² (Starting Dosage = 60 mg daily)	Cabozantinib Monotherapy in Pediatric Patients ≥12 years of age with BSA <1.2 m² (Starting Dosage = 40 mg daily)
First	Restart at 40 mg once daily	Restart at 20 mg once daily
Second	Restart at 20 mg once daily[a]	Restart at 20 mg every other day[a]

[a] If previously receiving lowest dosage, resume therapy at same dosage. If lowest dosage not tolerated, discontinue cabozantinib tablets.

If an adverse reaction occurs during therapy with cabozantinib tablets, modify dosage accordingly (see Table 3).

TABLE 3. Recommended Dosage Modification for Cabometyx® (Cabozantinib Tablets) Toxicity.

Adverse Reaction and Severity	Modification
Hemorrhage	
Grade 3 or 4	Permanently discontinue therapy
GI Perforation	
Any grade	Permanently discontinue therapy
Fistula Formation	
Grade 4	Permanently discontinue therapy
Thromboembolic Events	
Any grade acute myocardial infarction (MI)	Permanently discontinue therapy
Grade 2 or higher cerebral infarction	Permanently discontinue therapy
Grade 3 or 4 arterial thromboembolic events	Permanently discontinue therapy
Grade 4 venous thromboembolic events	Permanently discontinue therapy
Hypertension	
Grade 3 hypertension or hypertensive crisis	Withhold therapy; when blood pressure is adequately controlled to grade 2 or less, resume at reduced dosage (see Tables 1 and 2); permanently discontinue therapy for uncontrolled hypertension
Grade 4 hypertension or hypertensive crisis	Permanently discontinue therapy

TABLE 3. Continued

Adverse Reaction and Severity	Modification
Diarrhea	
Grade 2–4	Withhold therapy; when diarrhea improves to grade 1 or less, resume at reduced dosage (see Tables 1 and 2)
Palmar-plantar Erythrodysesthesia	
Grade 2 (intolerable) or grade 3	Withhold therapy; when palmar-plantar erythrodysesthesia improves to grade 1 or less, resume at reduced dosage (see Tables 1 and 2)
Proteinuria	
Grade 2 or 3	Withhold therapy; when proteinuria improves to grade 1 or less, resume at reduced dosage (see Tables 1 and 2)
Nephrotic syndrome	Permanently discontinue therapy
Osteonecrosis of the Jaw (ONJ)	
Any grade	Withhold therapy; when ONJ completely resolves, resume at reduced dosage (see Tables 1 and 2)
Reversible Posterior Leukoencephalopathy Syndrome (RPLS)	
Any grade	Permanently discontinue therapy
Other Adverse Effects	
Grade 2 (intolerable) or grade 3–4	Withhold therapy; when adverse effect resolves or improves to grade 1 or less, resume at reduced dosage (see Tables 1 and 2)

If hepatotoxicity occurs when cabozantinib tablets (Cabometyx®) are used in combination with nivolumab, the dosage of cabozantinib tablets should be reduced as described in Table 4. When used in combination with nivolumab, the recommended dosage modifications, usual cautions, precautions, and contraindications associated with nivolumab must be considered in addition to those associated with cabozantinib tablets.

TABLE 4. Combination Therapy with Nivolumab: Recommended Dosage Reduction for Cabometyx® (Cabozantinib Tablets) for Hepatotoxicity.

Liver Function Test Abnormalities	Dosage Modification (Starting Dosage = 40 mg daily)
ALT or AST >3 times ULN but ≤10 times ULN with concurrent total bilirubin <2 times ULN	Withhold both cabozantinib tablets and nivolumab and consider corticosteroid therapy; when hepatotoxicity resolves or improves to grade 1 or less, may resume one or both of the drugs
ALT or AST >10 times ULN or >3 times ULN with concurrent total bilirubin ≥2 times ULN	Permanently discontinue cabozantinib and nivolumab

Cometriq® Capsules

Cabozantinib capsules should be *withheld* if grade 4 hematologic adverse effects, grade 3 or greater nonhematologic adverse effects, intolerable grade 2 adverse effects (as defined by the National Cancer Institute [NCI] Common Terminology Criteria for Adverse Events [CTCAE]), or osteonecrosis of the jaw (ONJ) occurs. Upon resolution or improvement of the adverse effect (i.e., return to baseline or resolution to grade 1), the dosage of cabozantinib should be reduced as follows: in patients previously receiving 140 mg daily, cabozantinib therapy should be resumed at a dosage of 100 mg daily; in patients previously receiving 100 mg daily, cabozantinib therapy should be resumed at a dosage of 60 mg daily; and in patients previously receiving 60 mg daily, cabozantinib therapy should be resumed at a dosage of 60 mg daily, if tolerated. Otherwise, cabozantinib therapy should be discontinued.

Cabozantinib capsules should be *permanently discontinued* in patients who develop GI perforation or grade 4 fistula formation, severe hemorrhage, acute myocardial infarction or arterial or venous thromboembolic events requiring medical intervention, nephrotic syndrome, hypertensive crisis, persistent uncontrolled hypertension despite optimal medical management, or reversible posterior leukoencephalopathy syndrome.

Dosage Modification for Concomitant Use with Drugs Affecting Hepatic Microsomal Enzymes

Cabometyx® Tablets

Concomitant use of cabozantinib tablets with drugs that are potent inhibitors of cytochrome P-450 (CYP) isoenzyme 3A4 should be *avoided*. If concomitant use of a potent CYP3A4 inhibitor cannot be avoided, reduce the daily dosage of cabozantinib tablets by 20 mg (e.g., from 60 mg to 40 mg daily, or from 40 mg to 20 mg daily, or from 20 mg daily to 20 mg every other day in pediatric patients with BSA <1.2 m²). If concomitant use of the potent CYP3A4 inhibitor is discontinued, the dosage of cabozantinib tablets should be returned to the dosage used prior to initiation of the potent CYP3A4 inhibitor 2–3 days following discontinuance of the potent CYP3A4 inhibitor.

Concomitant use of cabozantinib tablets with drugs that are potent inducers of CYP3A4 should be *avoided*. Foods or dietary supplements (e.g., St. John's wort [*Hypericum perforatum*]) that are known to induce CYP450 activity should be avoided during therapy. If concomitant use of a potent CYP3A4 inducer cannot be avoided, increase the daily dosage of cabozantinib tablets by 20 mg (e.g., from 60 mg to 80 mg daily, or from 40 mg to 60 mg daily) as tolerated. If concomitant use of the potent CYP3A4 inducer is discontinued, the dosage of cabozantinib tablets should be returned to the dosage used prior to initiation of the potent CYP3A4 inducer 2–3 days following discontinuance of the potent CYP3A4 inducer. The daily dosage of cabozantinib tablets should not exceed 80 mg.

Cometriq® Capsules

Concomitant use of cabozantinib capsules with drugs that are potent inhibitors of cytochrome P-450 (CYP) isoenzyme 3A4 should be *avoided*. If concomitant use of a potent CYP3A4 inhibitor cannot be avoided, reduce the daily dosage of cabozantinib capsules by 40 mg (e.g., from 140 mg daily to 100 mg daily or from 100 mg daily to 60 mg daily). If concomitant use of the potent CYP3A4 inhibitor is discontinued, the dosage of cabozantinib capsules should be returned to the dosage used prior to initiation of the potent CYP3A4 inhibitor 2–3 days following discontinuance of the potent CYP3A4 inhibitor.

Chronic concomitant use of potent CYP3A4 inducers should be *avoided* in patients receiving cabozantinib tablets if alternative therapy is available. Foods or dietary supplements (e.g., St. John's wort [*Hypericum perforatum*]) that are known to induce CYP3A4 should be avoided during therapy with the drug. If concomitant use of a potent CYP3A4 inducer cannot be avoided, increase the daily dosage of cabozantinib capsules by 40 mg (e.g., from 140 mg daily to 180 mg daily or from 100 mg daily to 140 mg daily) as tolerated. If concomitant use of the potent CYP3A4 inducer is discontinued, the dosage of cabozantinib capsules should be returned to the dosage used prior to initiation of the potent CYP3A4 inducer 2–3 days following discontinuance of the potent CYP3A4 inducer. The daily dosage of cabozantinib capsules should not exceed 180 mg.

● Special Populations

Hepatic Impairment

Cabometyx®: In patients with moderate hepatic impairment (Child-Pugh class B), the initial dosage of cabozantinib tablets should be reduced from 60 mg daily to 40 mg daily or, in pediatric patients with a BSA <1.2 m², the initial dosage should be reduced from 40 mg daily to 20 mg daily.

Cometriq®: In patients with mild to moderate hepatic impairment, the recommended initial dosage of cabozantinib capsules is 80 mg.

Renal Impairment

Dosage adjustment is not necessary in patients with mild or moderate renal impairment. The manufacturer states that there is no experience with cabozantinib capsules or tablets in patients with severe renal impairment and does not make specific dosage recommendations for such patients.

Geriatric Use

The manufacturer makes no specific dosage recommendations for geriatric patients.

CAUTIONS

● Contraindications

None.

● Warnings/Precautions

Perforations and Fistulas

GI perforations and fistulas, including serious and fatal cases, were reported in 1–3 and 1%, respectively, of cabozantinib-treated patients. Non-GI fistulas, including tracheal/esophageal fistulas, were reported in 4% of patients receiving cabozantinib capsules (Cometriq®), and were fatal in two (1%) of these cases.

Patients receiving cabozantinib should be monitored for symptoms of perforations and fistulas. Cabozantinib should be permanently discontinued in patients who develop a GI perforation or grade 4 fistula.

Hemorrhage

Serious, sometimes fatal, hemorrhage, including hemoptysis and GI hemorrhage, has been reported with cabozantinib. The incidence of grade 3 or greater adverse hemorrhagic events was higher in patients receiving cabozantinib capsules (Cometriq®) compared with those receiving placebo (3 versus 1%, respectively). In clinical trials, grade 3 to 5 hemorrhagic events occurred in 5% of patients receiving cabozantinib tablets (Cabometyx®) for the treatment of renal cell carcinoma (RCC), hepatocellular carcinoma (HCC), or differentiated thyroid cancer (DTC).

Patients receiving cabozantinib should be monitored for signs and symptoms of bleeding. The drug should not be used in patients with severe hemorrhage or a recent history of hemorrhage, hemoptysis, hematemesis, or melena. Cabozantinib should be discontinued prior to surgery or if grade 3 or 4 hemorrhage occurs.

Thromboembolic Events

Cabozantinib therapy is associated with an increased incidence of thromboembolic events. Venous thromboembolism was reported in 6 or 3% of patients receiving cabozantinib capsules (Cometriq®) or placebo, respectively, and arterial thromboembolism was reported in 2 or 0% of patients receiving cabozantinib capsules (Cometriq®) or placebo, respectively. Venous or arterial thromboembolism, including fatal cases, was reported in 7 or 2%, respectively, of patients receiving cabozantinib tablets (Cabometyx®).

Cabozantinib should be permanently discontinued in patients who develop an acute myocardial infarction or arterial or venous thromboembolic event that requires medical intervention.

Impaired Wound Healing

Inhibitors of vascular endothelial growth factor receptor (VEGFR) may impair wound healing, and wound-healing complications have been reported in patients receiving cabozantinib.

The manufacturer recommends that cabozantinib be discontinued at least 3 weeks prior to elective surgery, including invasive dental procedures. Therapy with the drug may be resumed at least 2 weeks following major surgery based on clinical judgment of adequate wound healing. The safety of resuming cabozantinib after resolution of wound healing complications has not been established.

Hypertension

Cabozantinib is associated with an increased incidence of treatment-induced hypertension. Nearly all patients receiving cabozantinib capsules (Cometriq®)

experienced elevated blood pressure; stage 1 or 2 hypertension occurred in 61% of patients receiving cabozantinib compared with 30% of those receiving placebo in the phase 3 clinical study. Hypertension was reported in 37% of patients receiving cabozantinib tablets (Cabometyx®); grade 3 or 4 hypertension occurred in 16% and <1% of patients, respectively.

Do not initiate cabozantinib in patients with uncontrolled hypertension. Blood pressure should be monitored prior to initiation of cabozantinib and periodically during therapy. Cabozantinib should be temporarily withheld for hypertension that is not adequately controlled with medical management; when controlled, cabozantinib therapy should be resumed at a reduced dosage. Cabozantinib should be permanently discontinued for hypertensive crisis, or persistent uncontrolled hypertension despite optimal medical management (i.e., antihypertensive therapy).

Osteonecrosis of the Jaw

Osteonecrosis of the jaw (ONJ) has been reported in <1% of cabozantinib-treated patients. The condition may manifest as jaw pain, osteomyelitis, osteitis, bone erosion, tooth or periodontal infection, toothache, gingival ulceration or erosion, persistent jaw pain, or delayed healing of the mouth or jaw following dental surgery.

An oral examination should be performed prior to initiation of cabozantinib and periodically during therapy. Patients should be advised to maintain good oral hygiene during treatment. For patients requiring invasive dental procedures, cabozantinib therapy should be withheld for at least 3 weeks prior to scheduled surgery, if possible. In patients who develop ONJ, cabozantinib should be withheld until complete resolution of ONJ.

The manufacturer of cabozantinib tablets (Cabometyx®) states that therapy may be resumed at a reduced dosage following resolution of ONJ.

Diarrhea

Diarrhea has been reported in 62–63% of patients receiving cabozantinib therapy; grade 3–4 diarrhea has been reported in 10–16% of patients.

Withhold cabozantinib until diarrhea improves to grade 1, and then resume the drug at a reduced dosage. When resuming cabozantinib capsules (Cometriq®), the dosage should be reduced only for intolerable grade 2 diarrhea, grade 3 diarrhea unresponsive to standard antidiarrheal therapy, or grade 4 diarrhea.

Palmar-plantar Erythrodysesthesia Syndrome

Palmar-plantar erythrodysesthesia syndrome (hand-foot syndrome) occurred in 45–50% of cabozantinib-treated patients, and was severe (grade 3 or greater) in 13% of patients. In addition, a hand-foot skin reaction with subungual splinter hemorrhages and hypertension has been reported in at least one patient receiving the drug.

If palmar-plantar erythrodysesthesia syndrome occurs, temporary interruption of cabozantinib and dosage reduction may be necessary.

Proteinuria

Proteinuria was observed in 2–8% of patients receiving cabozantinib, including one patient with nephrotic syndrome, compared with none of those receiving placebo. Urine protein should be monitored regularly during cabozantinib therapy. Cabozantinib should be permanently discontinued in patients who develop nephrotic syndrome. If proteinuria occurs, temporary interruption of cabozantinib and dosage reduction may be necessary.

Reversible Posterior Leukoencephalopathy Syndrome

Reversible posterior leukoencephalopathy syndrome (RPLS) has occurred in one (less than 1%) patient receiving cabozantinib. RPLS is a syndrome of subcortical vasogenic edema that may manifest with seizures, headache, visual disturbances, confusion, or altered mental function. Magnetic resonance imaging (MRI) is necessary to confirm the diagnosis of RPLS.

The possible diagnosis of RPLS should be considered in any patient receiving cabozantinib who presents with neurologic manifestations suggestive of RPLS. Cabozantinib should be permanently discontinued in patients who develop RPLS.

Hepatotoxicity

Grade 3 or 4 hepatotoxicity and elevated ALT/AST concentrations occurred in patients receiving cabozantinib tablets (Cabometyx®) in combination with nivolumab at a higher frequency compared with cabozantinib alone. Grade 3 and 4 elevations in serum ALT or AST concentrations were observed in 11% of patients receiving cabozantinib tablets in combination with nivolumab. Grade 2 elevations in ALT/AST concentrations (ALT or AST >3 times ULN) were reported in 83 patients, 23 of whom received systemic corticosteroids; elevated ALT/AST concentrations resolved to grade 0 or 1 in 89% of patients who experienced grade 2 elevations. Among 44 patients with grade 2 or greater elevations in ALT or AST concentrations who were rechallenged with either cabozantinib tablets or nivolumab as a single agent or with both drugs, recurrence of grade 2 or greater elevations in ALT or AST concentrations was observed in 2 patients receiving cabozantinib, 2 patients receiving nivolumab, and 7 patients receiving both cabozantinib and nivolumab.

Withhold cabozantinib tablets (Cabometyx®) and resume at a reduced dosage based on severity. Monitor liver enzymes prior to and periodically during therapy; more frequent monitoring should be considered when cabozantinib is used in combination with nivolumab. For elevated liver enzymes, temporarily interrupt therapy with cabozantinib tablets (Cabometyx®) and nivolumab and consider administration of systemic corticosteroids.

Adrenal Insufficiency

Primary or secondary adrenal insufficiency has been reported in patients receiving cabozantinib tablets (Cabometyx®) in combination with nivolumab. Adrenal insufficiency occurred in 4.7% (grade 3 in 2.2% and grade 2 in 1.9%) of patients with RCC who received cabozantinib tablets (Cabometyx®) in combination with nivolumab. Approximately 80% of 15 patients who developed adrenal insufficiency received hormone replacement therapy, including systemic corticosteroids; adrenal insufficiency resolved in 4 of 15 patients. Combination therapy with cabozantinib and nivolumab was withheld because of development of adrenal insufficiency in 9 patients and 6 of these patients were rechallenged with therapy following improvement of symptoms; all 6 patients received hormone replacement therapy and adrenal insufficiency recurred in 2 patients.

For grade 2 or higher adrenal insufficiency, initiate symptomatic treatment, including hormone replacement therapy, as clinically indicated. Withhold cabozantinib (Cabometyx®) and/or nivolumab therapy and resume cabozantinib (Cabometyx®) at a reduced dosage depending on severity.

Thyroid Dysfunction

Thyroid dysfunction, primarily hypothyroidism, occurred in 19% of patients receiving cabozantinib tablets (Cabometyx®), including grade 3 in 0.4% of patients. Assess patients for signs of thyroid dysfunction prior to initiation of cabozantinib (Cabometyx®); monitor for signs and symptoms of thyroid dysfunction during treatment and manage as clinically indicated.

Hypocalcemia

Hypocalcemia has been reported in 13% of patients receiving cabozantinib tablets (Cabometyx®), including grade 3 in 2% and grade 4 in 1% of patients. In the COSMIC-311 trial of patients with differentiated thyroid cancer, hypocalcemia occurred in 36% of patients receiving cabozantinib tablets (Cabometyx®), including grade 3 in 6% and grade 4 in 3% of patients. Hypocalcemia occurred in 52% of patients treated with cabozantinib capsules (Cometriq®), including Grade 3 or 4 in 12% of patients.

Monitor serum calcium levels and replace calcium as necessary. Withhold cabozantinib and resume at reduced dosage following recovery of hypocalcemia or permanently discontinue therapy depending on severity.

Fetal/Neonatal Morbidity and Mortality

Cabozantinib may cause fetal harm if administered to pregnant women; the drug has been shown to be embryotoxic, fetotoxic, and teratogenic in animals (e.g., fetal loss, skeletal variations, visceral variations, malformations).

Females of reproductive potential should be advised to use an effective method of contraception while receiving cabozantinib and for 4 months after discontinuance of therapy. If cabozantinib is used during pregnancy or if the patient becomes pregnant while receiving the drug, the patient should be apprised of the potential fetal hazard.

Specific Populations

Pregnancy

May cause fetal harm.

A pregnancy test should be performed prior to initiation of the drug in females of reproductive potential and such females should be advised to use effective contraceptive methods while receiving the drug and for 4 months after the last dose. Patients should be apprised of the potential hazard to the fetus if the drug is used during pregnancy.

Lactation

It is not known whether cabozantinib or its metabolites are distributed into human milk. The effects of the drug on breast-fed infants or on the production of milk are unknown. Because of the potential for serious adverse reactions to cabozantinib in breast-fed infants, advise women not to breast-feed during treatment with cabozantinib and for 4 months after the last dose.

Females and Males of Reproductive Potential

Females of reproductive potential should be advised to use an effective method of contraception while receiving cabozantinib and for 4 months after the last dose.

There are no data on the effect of cabozantinib on human fertility. However, cabozantinib impaired male and female fertility in animal studies.

Pediatric Use

Safety and effectiveness of cabozantinib tablets (Cabometyx®) for the treatment of differentiated thyroid cancer (DTC) have been established in pediatric patients ≥12 years of age; safety and effectiveness in patients <12 years of age have not been established.

Safety and efficacy of cabozantinib tablets (Cabometyx®) for the treatment of previously treated, locally advanced or metastatic DTC in pediatric patients ≥12 years of age is supported by extrapolation of data from clinical studies evaluating cabozantinib tablets in adults and population pharmacokinetic data indicating that exposure to the drug in pediatric patients ≥12 years of age is similar to that in adults.

Physeal widening has been observed in children with open growth plates when treated with cabozantinib tablets (Cabometyx®). Physeal and longitudinal growth monitoring is recommended in children with open growth plates.

Safety, efficacy, and pharmacokinetics of cabozantinib capsules (Cometriq®) have not been established in pediatric patients. Systemic exposure of cabozantinib (Cabometyx®) in pediatric patients ≥12 years of age at the recommended dosages is expected to be comparable to the exposure in adults at a dosage of 60 mg once daily.

Geriatric Use

Clinical studies of cabozantinib capsules (Cometriq®) did not include sufficient numbers of patients ≥65 years of age to determine whether geriatric patients respond differently than younger adults. The pharmacokinetics of cabozantinib capsules (Cometriq®) do not appear to be affected by age in adults (20–86 years of age).

Clinical studies of cabozantinib (Cabometyx®) included patients ≥65 years of age at frequencies of 41–50% for patients ≥65 years of age and of 8–15% for patients ≥75 years of age. No overall differences in safety or effectiveness were observed between these patients and younger patients.

Hepatic Impairment

Results of a population pharmacokinetic analysis showed no clinically important differences in cabozantinib exposure between patients with normal liver function and those with mild hepatic impairment. In a pharmacokinetic study, cabozantinib exposure increased by 63% in patients with moderate hepatic impairment. The pharmacokinetics of cabozantinib have not been studied in patients with severe (Child-Pugh class C) hepatic impairment.

Cometriq®: In patients with mild to moderate hepatic impairment, the recommended initial dosage of cabozantinib capsules (Cometriq®) is 80 mg daily. Use of cabozantinib (Cometriq®) is not recommended in patients with severe hepatic impairment.

Cabometyx®: In patients with moderate hepatic impairment (Child-Pugh class B), the initial dosage of cabozantinib tablets (Cabometyx®) should be reduced from 60 mg daily to 40 mg daily or, in pediatric patients with a BSA <1.2 m², the initial dosage should be reduced from 40 mg daily to 20 mg daily. Use of cabozantinib (Cabometyx®) should be avoided in patients with severe hepatic impairment.

Renal Impairment

The pharmacokinetics of cabozantinib capsules (Cometriq®) have not been studied in patients with severe renal impairment (estimated glomerular filtration rate <29 mL/minute per 1.73 m² as estimated by Modification of Diet in Renal Disease equation) or renal impairment requiring dialysis.

Dosage adjustment of cabozantinib is not recommended in patients with mild or moderate renal impairment.

● Common Adverse Effects

Adverse effects reported in ≥25% of patients receiving cabozantinib capsules (Cometriq®) include diarrhea, stomatitis, palmar-plantar erythrodysesthesia syndrome (hand-foot syndrome), weight loss, decreased appetite, nausea, fatigue, oral pain, hair color changes, dysgeusia, hypertension, abdominal pain, and constipation.

Laboratory abnormalities reported in ≥25% of patients receiving cabozantinib capsules (Cometriq®) include increased AST concentrations, increased ALT concentrations, lymphopenia, increased alkaline phosphatase concentrations, hypocalcemia, neutropenia, thrombocytopenia, hypophosphatemia, and hyperbilirubinemia.

Adverse effects reported in ≥20% of patients receiving cabozantinib tablets (Cabometyx®) as a single-agent: Diarrhea, fatigue, palmar-plantar erythrodysesthesia syndrome (hand-foot syndrome), decreased appetite, hypertension, nausea, vomiting, weight decreased, and constipation.

Adverse effects reported in ≥20% of patients receiving cabozantinib tablets (Cabometyx®) in combination with nivolumab: Diarrhea, fatigue, hepatotoxicity, palmar-plantar erythrodysesthesia syndrome (hand-foot syndrome), stomatitis, rash, hypertension, hypothyroidism, musculoskeletal pain, decreased appetite, nausea, dysgeusia, abdominal pain, cough, and upper respiratory tract infection.

DRUG INTERACTIONS

Cabozantinib is metabolized in the liver by cytochrome P-450 (CYP) isoenzyme 3A4. Inhibition of CYP3A4 reduced the formation of the drug's *N*-oxide metabolite by more than 80%. Inhibition of CYP2C9 had minimal effects on cabozantinib metabolite formation (i.e., less than a 20% reduction). Inhibition of CYP isoenzymes 1A2, 2A6, 2B6, 2C8, 2C19, 2D6, and 2E1 had no effect on cabozantinib metabolite formation.

In vitro, cabozantinib is an inhibitor of CYP2C8. Cabozantinib is not an inhibitor of CYP isoenzymes 1A2 or 2D6.

Cabozantinib is an inducer of CYP1A1 messenger RNA (mRNA) in human hepatocyte incubations, but does not induce CYP1A2, CYP2B6, CYP2C8, CYP2C9, CYP2C19, or CYP3A4 mRNA or isoenzyme-associated enzyme activities.

Cabozantinib is an inhibitor, but not a substrate, of P-glycoprotein (P-gp) transport activities in a bi-directional assay system. Cabozantinib is a substrate of MRP2 in vitro.

● Drugs and Foods Affecting Hepatic Microsomal Enzymes

Inhibitors of CYP3A4 and Other CYP-450 Isoenzymes

Concomitant use of cabozantinib with potent inhibitors of CYP3A4 may increase systemic exposure of cabozantinib. When the potent CYP3A4 inhibitor ketoconazole (400 mg daily for 27 days) was administered concomitantly with cabozantinib capsules (as a single 140-mg dose) in healthy individuals, plasma cabozantinib exposure increased by 38%.

Concomitant use of cabozantinib with potent CYP3A4 inhibitors (e.g., atazanavir, clarithromycin, indinavir, itraconazole, ketoconazole, nefazodone, nelfinavir, ritonavir, saquinavir, telithromycin, voriconazole) should be *avoided* if alternative therapy is available. If concomitant use of a potent CYP3A4 inhibitor cannot be avoided, reduce the daily dosage of cabozantinib capsules (Cometriq®) by 40 mg (e.g., from 140 mg daily to 100 mg daily or from 100 mg daily to 60 mg daily) and the daily dosage of cabozantinib tablets (Cabometyx®) by 20 mg (e.g., from 60 mg to 40 mg daily, or from 40 mg to 20 mg daily, or from 20 mg daily to 20 mg every other day in pediatric patients with BSA <1.2 m²). If concomitant use of the potent CYP3A4 inhibitor is discontinued, the cabozantinib dosage should be returned (2–3 days following discontinuance of the potent CYP3A4 inhibitor) to the dosage used prior to initiation of the potent CYP3A4 inhibitor.

The manufacturer states that foods (e.g., grapefruit, grapefruit juice) or nutritional supplements that are known to inhibit CYP isoenzymes, including CYP3A4, should *not* be ingested during cabozantinib therapy.

Inducers of CYP3A4 and Other CYP-450 Isoenzymes

Chronic concomitant use of potent inducers of CYP3A4 with cabozantinib may reduce systemic exposure of cabozantinib. When the potent CYP3A4 inducer rifampin (600 mg daily for 31 days) was administered concomitantly with cabozantinib capsules (as a single 140-mg dose) in healthy individuals, plasma cabozantinib exposure decreased by 77%.

Chronic concomitant use of potent CYP3A4 inducers (e.g., carbamazepine, dexamethasone, rifabutin, rifampin, rifapentine, phenobarbital, phenytoin, St. John's wort [*Hypericum perforatum*]) with cabozantinib should be *avoided* if alternative therapy is available. If concomitant use with a potent CYP3A4 inducer cannot be avoided, increase the daily dosage of cabozantinib capsules (Cometriq®) by 40 mg (e.g., from 140 mg daily to 180 mg daily or from 100 mg daily to 140 mg daily) as tolerated and the daily dosage of cabozantinib tablets (Cabometyx®) by 20 mg (e.g., from 60 mg to 80 mg daily or from 40 mg to 60 mg daily) as tolerated. If concomitant use of the potent CYP3A4 inducer is discontinued, the cabozantinib dosage should be returned (2–3 days following the discontinuance of the potent CYP3A4 inducer) to the dosage used prior to initiation of the potent CYP3A4 inducer. The daily dosage of cabozantinib capsules (Cometriq®) should not exceed 180 mg. The daily dosage of cabozantinib tablets (Cabometyx®) should not exceed 80 mg.

The manufacturer states that foods or dietary supplements (e.g., St. John's wort [*Hypericum perforatum*]) that are known to induce CYP activity, including CYP3A4, should be avoided during cabozantinib therapy.

● *Drugs Affected by Hepatic Microsomal Enzymes*

Cabozantinib is an inhibitor of CYP2C8 in vitro; however, a clinical study suggests that clinically relevant effects on exposure to CYP2C8 substrate drugs is unlikely.

● *Drugs Affecting Multidrug Resistance Protein*

Cabozantinib is a substrate of multidrug resistance protein (MRP) 2 in vitro. Therefore, MRP2 inhibitors (e.g., abacavir, cidofovir, furosemide, lamivudine, nevirapine, ritonavir, probenecid, saquinavir, tenofovir) may have the potential to increase plasma concentrations of cabozantinib; monitor for increased cabozantinib toxicity.

● *Drugs Affected by the P-glycoprotein Transport System*

Cabozantinib is an inhibitor, but not a substrate, of P-gp transport activities in a bidirectional assay system. Therefore, cabozantinib may have the potential to increase plasma concentrations of concomitantly administered substrates of P-gp.

● *Grapefruit*

Grapefruit products are CYP3A4 inhibitors and should be avoided during cabozantinib therapy because of the potential for increased cabozantinib concentrations.

● *Rosiglitazone*

Cabozantinib at steady-state plasma concentrations (100 mg or more daily of the capsule formulation for a minimum of 21 days) did not affect single-dose rosiglitazone (a CYP2C8 substrate) plasma exposure (peak concentration and area under the concentration-time curve [AUC]) in patients with solid tumors. A clinically important pharmacokinetic interaction with these drugs therefore appears unlikely.

DESCRIPTION

Cabozantinib *S*-malate, an inhibitor of multiple receptor tyrosine kinases, is an antineoplastic agent. Receptor tyrosine kinases (RTKs) are involved in the initiation of various cascades of intracellular signaling events that lead to cell proliferation and/or influence processes critical to cell survival and tumor progression (e.g., angiogenesis, metastasis, inhibition of apoptosis), based on the respective kinase. Various tyrosine kinases and pathways are abnormally activated in medullary thyroid carcinoma cells (e.g., rearranged during transfection [RET] proto-oncogene mutations are associated with the development of hereditary medullary thyroid cancer). In vitro biochemical and/or cellular assays have shown that cabozantinib inhibits the activity of multiple receptor tyrosine kinases, including RET; met proto-oncogene encoding hepatocyte growth factor (c-MET); vascular endothelial growth factor receptors (VEGFR)-1, VEGFR-2, and VEGFR-3; stem cell factor receptor (c-Kit); tropomyosin receptor kinase B (trkB); fms-like tyrosine kinase 3 (Flt-3); AXL; and TIE-2. These receptor tyrosine kinases are involved in both normal cellular function and pathologic processes (e.g., oncogenesis, metastasis, tumor angiogenesis, and maintenance of the tumor microenvironment).

The absolute oral bioavailability of cabozantinib has not been established. Following oral administration of cabozantinib capsules or tablets, median time to peak plasma concentrations of cabozantinib ranged from 2–5 or 3–4 hours, respectively. Repeated daily administration of cabozantinib capsules (Cometriq®) for 19 days resulted in fourfold to fivefold mean cabozantinib accumulation (based on area under the concentration-time curve [AUC]) compared with single-dose administration; steady-state concentrations of the drug were achieved in 15 days. Following a single 140-mg dose of cabozantinib capsules or tablets, peak plasma concentration of cabozantinib tablets was 19% higher compared with cabozantinib capsules; however, a less than 10% difference in AUC was observed between the tablet and capsule formulations. A high-fat meal increased the peak plasma concentration and AUC of cabozantinib by 41 and 57%, respectively, relative to fasted conditions following administration of a single 140-mg oral dose of cabozantinib capsules (Cometriq®) in healthy individuals. Cabozantinib is highly bound (99.7% or more) to plasma proteins. Cabozantinib is metabolized in the liver by cytochrome P-450 (CYP) isoenzyme 3A4, and is a substrate of CYP3A4 in vitro. Inhibition of CYP3A4 reduced the formation of the cabozantinib *N*-oxide metabolite by greater than 80%; inhibition of CYP2C9 had minimal effects on cabozantinib metabolite formation (i.e., less than a 20% reduction). Inhibition of CYP isoenzymes 1A2, 2A6, 2B6, 2C8, 2C19, 2D6, and 2E1 had no effect on cabozantinib metabolite formation. Following administration of a single dose of radiolabeled cabozantinib in healthy individuals, approximately 81% of the total administered radioactivity was recovered with 54% in feces and 27% in urine within 48 days. The elimination half-life of cabozantinib capsules or tablets is approximately 55 or 99 hours, respectively.

ADVICE TO PATIENTS

- Inform patients that cabozantinib should *not* be taken with food. Importance of swallowing cabozantinib capsules whole with a full glass (at least 240 mL) of water and not to open or crush the capsules. Importance of swallowing cabozantinib tablets whole and not to crush the tablets. Importance of avoiding grapefruit or grapefruit juice while taking the drug.

- If a dose of cabozantinib is missed and it is ≥12 hours before the next scheduled dose, importance of taking the dose as soon as it is remembered, and taking the next dose at the regularly scheduled time. If a dose is missed and there are <12 hours before the next scheduled dose, importance of taking the next dose at the regularly scheduled time; the missed dose should not be replaced.

- Inform patients that diarrhea often occurs and may be severe in some cases. Importance of contacting clinician if severe diarrhea occurs during therapy.

- Risk of palmar-plantar erythrodysesthesia syndrome. Importance of contacting clinician if progressive or intolerable rash occurs. Advise patients to protect their skin to avoid subclinical vascular damage and subsequent adverse cutaneous effects that may interrupt ongoing therapy.

- Risk of mouth sores, oral pain, taste changes, nausea, or vomiting. Importance of contacting clinician if any of these symptoms are severe or prevent eating or drinking.

- Risk of weight loss, which may be substantial in some cases. Inform clinician if substantial weight loss occurs.

- Risk of osteonecrosis of the jaw; symptoms may include jaw pain, toothache, or sores on the gums. Advise patients that their clinician should examine their mouth before and during cabozantinib therapy. Importance of informing dentist about therapy with the drug. Importance of maintaining good oral hygiene during treatment.

- Risk of hypertension. Importance of informing clinician of signs or symptoms of elevated blood pressure and of regular monitoring.

- Risk of hemorrhage. Importance of informing clinician of any signs or symptoms of bleeding.

- Risk of thromboembolic events. Advise patients to seek emergency medical care for signs or symptoms of blood clots, stroke, heart attack, or chest pain.

- Risk of GI perforation and development of fistulas. Importance of informing clinician of any abdominal tenderness or pain.

- Risk of adrenal insufficiency. Importance of informing clinician of extreme fatigue, dizziness, fainting, weakness, nausea, or vomiting.

- Risk of hypocalcemia. Importance of informing clinician of muscle stiffness, numbness, seizures, weight gain, and swelling of extremities.

- Risk of wound healing complications. Importance of contacting clinician before any planned surgeries, including dental procedures, or if any recent surgery has occurred.

- Risk of fetal harm. Advise females of reproductive potential that they must use an effective method of contraception while receiving cabozantinib and for 4 months after discontinuance of therapy. Importance of patients informing their clinicians if they become pregnant. If pregnancy occurs, apprise patient of potential hazard to the fetus.

- Importance of discontinuing breast-feeding while receiving cabozantinib therapy and for 4 months after discontinuance of therapy.

- Importance of informing clinician of existing or contemplated concomitant therapy, including prescription and OTC drugs and dietary and herbal supplements (e.g., St. John's wort), as well as any concomitant illnesses (e.g., hypertension, bleeding or wound disorders, hepatic impairment).

- Inform patients of other important precautionary information.

For further information on the handling of antineoplastic agents, see the ASHP Guidelines on Handling Hazardous Drugs at https://www.ahfsdruginformation.com.

PREPARATIONS

Cabozantinib S-malate can only be obtained through a specialty pharmacy. Specific information regarding distribution of the drug is available by telephone at 855-253-3273 or at https://www.cometriq.com/hcp).

Excipients in commercially available drug preparations may have clinically important effects in some individuals; consult specific product labeling for details.

Cabozantinib S-malate

Oral		
Capsules	20 mg (of cabozantinib)	**Cometriq®**, Exelixis
	80 mg (of cabozantinib)	**Cometriq®**, Exelixis
Tablets	20 mg (of cabozantinib)	**Cabometyx®**, Exelixis
	40 mg (of cabozantinib)	**Cabometyx®**, Exelixis
	60 mg (of cabozantinib)	**Cabometyx®**, Exelixis
Kit	84 Capsules, Cabozantinib S-malate 20 mg (of cabozantinib) (Cometriq®)	**Cometriq® 60 mg Daily Dose Blister Cards** (available in a package containing 4 blister cards), Exelixis
	28 Capsules, Cabozantinib S-malate 20 mg (of cabozantinib) (Cometriq®)	**Cometriq® 100 mg Daily Dose Blister Cards** (available in a package containing 4 blister cards), Exelixis
	28 Capsules, Cabozantinib S-malate 80 mg (of cabozantinib) (Cometriq®)	
	84 Capsules, Cabozantinib S-malate 20 mg (of cabozantinib) (Cometriq®)	**Cometriq® 140 mg Daily Dose Blister Cards** (available in a package containing 4 blister cards), Exelixis
	28 Capsules, Cabozantinib S-malate 80 mg (of cabozantinib) (Cometriq®)	

† Use is not currently included in the labeling approved by the US Food and Drug Administration.

Capecitabine

10:00 • ANTINEOPLASTIC AGENTS

- Capecitabine, a prodrug that has little pharmacologic activity until it is converted to fluorouracil (an antimetabolite) in tumor tissue, is an antineoplastic agent.

USES

• Breast Cancer

Capecitabine is used in combination with docetaxel for the treatment of advanced or metastatic breast cancer after disease progression on prior anthracycline-containing chemotherapy. Capecitabine is also used for the treatment of advanced or metastatic breast cancer as a single agent if an anthracycline- or taxane-containing chemotherapy is not indicated.

Combination Therapy

The efficacy of capecitabine as a component of combination chemotherapy in patients with metastatic breast cancer is based principally on the results of an open-label, multicenter, randomized trial (Study SO14999). The study included 511 patients with metastatic breast cancer resistant to or recurring during or following anthracycline-containing therapy, or relapsing during or recurring within 2 years of completion of anthracycline-containing adjuvant therapy.

Patients received either combination therapy with capecitabine 1250 mg/m^2 twice daily for 14 days followed by 1 week without treatment and docetaxel 75 mg/m^2 as a 1-hour IV infusion administered on the first day of each 3-week cycle or monotherapy with docetaxel 100 mg/m^2 as a 1-hour IV infusion administered on the first day of each 3-week cycle. The median patient age was 52 and 51 years in the capecitabine/docetaxel combination group and docetaxel monotherapy group, respectively; the median Karnofsky performance status score was 90 in both treatment groups. The median time to disease progression was 6.1 and 4.2 months, median overall survival was 14.5 and 11.6 months, and response rate was 32 and 22% for the capecitabine/docetaxel and docetaxel groups, respectively.

Monotherapy

The efficacy of capecitabine monotherapy in the treatment of metastatic breast cancer is based principally on the results of a multicenter, open-label, single-arm, phase 2 trial (SO14697) in 162 patients (135 patients with measurable disease) with previously treated stage IV breast cancer resistant to both paclitaxel and an anthracycline or resistant to paclitaxel and where further anthracycline therapy was not indicated. Patients received capecitabine 1255 mg/m^2 twice daily for 2 weeks followed by a 1-week rest period in each 3-week treatment cycle. The median patient age was 55—56 years, and the Karnofsky Performance Status score was 90 in all patients.

For the subgroup of 43 patients whose disease was resistant to both paclitaxel and an anthracycline, response rate was 25.6%, with a median duration of response of 5.1 months, median time to progression of 3.4 months, and median survival of 8.4 months. For the 135 patients with measurable disease, the objective response rate was 18.5%, median time to progression was 3 months, and median survival was 10.1 months.

Clinical Perspective

According to the National Cancer Institute, treatment options for locally advanced breast cancer include surgery, chemotherapy, radiation therapy, and hormone therapy, with targeted therapies (e.g., trastuzumab) added for locoregional recurrent disease. For metastatic disease, treatment options include surgery for metastases, hormone therapy, targeted therapies, chemotherapy, immunotherapy, and radiation. Various chemotherapy agents have been used for metastatic disease, including anthracyclines, taxanes, capecitabine or fluorouracil, vinca alkaloids, and platinum agents.

• Colorectal Cancer

Capecitabine is used as adjuvant treatment of patients with stage III colon cancer alone or as part of a combination chemotherapy regimen. The drug is also used as perioperative treatment for adults with locally advanced rectal cancer as part of a combination chemoradiotherapy regimen. Capecitabine is also is used for treatment of patients with unresectable or metastatic colorectal cancer as a single agent or as part of a combination chemotherapy regimen.

Adjuvant Treatment of Colon Cancer

Monotherapy

The efficacy of capecitabine as a single-agent adjuvant therapy in patients with stage III colon cancer is based principally on the results of a multicenter, randomized, controlled, phase 3 clinical study (X-ACT).

In this study, 1987 patients were randomized to receive either capecitabine 1250 mg/m^2 orally twice daily for the first 14 days of a 21-day cycle for a total of 8 cycles or fluorouracil 425 mg/m^2 and leucovorin 20 mg/m^2 IV on days 1—5 of each 28-day cycle for a total of 6 cycles. The primary outcome was disease-free survival; secondary outcomes included relapse-free survival and overall survival.

The median age of patients was 62 and 63 years for the capecitabine and fluorouracil/leucovorin groups, respectively; 54% of patients were male, 85% had an Eastern Cooperative Oncology Group (ECOG) performance status score of 0, and 76% had a primary tumor staging of 3. Median follow-up was 6.9 years. The 5-year disease-free survival rate was 60.8% for patients receiving capecitabine and 56.7% for patients receiving fluorouracil/leucovorin, demonstrating noninferiority of capecitabine to fluorouracil/leucovorin. The 5-year overall survival was 71.4 and 68.4% for the capecitabine and fluorouracil/leucovorin groups, respectively. The 5-year relapse-free survival rate was 63.2 and 59.8% for the capecitabine and fluorouracil/leucovorin groups, respectively.

Combination Therapy

The efficacy of capecitabine as a component of an adjuvant combination chemotherapy regimen for stage III colon cancer is based on several published studies, including a randomized, open-label, phase 3 clinical study (NO16968). In this study, patients were randomly assigned to treatment with either oxaliplatin 130 mg/m^2 on day 1 plus capecitabine 1000 mg/m^2 twice daily on days 1—14 of a 3-week cycle for a total of 8 cycles or a fluorouracil/leucovorin regimen. A total of 1886 patients were enrolled. At a median follow-up of 74 months, 33.9% of patients who received capecitabine experienced a relapse, developed a new colon cancer, or died versus 40.2% of patients who received fluorouracil/leucovorin. Overall survival was also higher with the capecitabine regimen versus fluorouracil/leucovorin; at a median follow-up of 83 months, deaths occurred in 25.6% and 30.4% of patients in the respective treatment groups.

Perioperative Treatment of Rectal Cancer

The efficacy of capecitabine as perioperative treatment of adults with locally advanced rectal cancer is based on several published studies, including an open-label, phase 3 trial comparing fluorouracil with capecitabine (Rektum-III). In Rektum-III, patients were randomized (1:1 ratio) to preoperative treatment with either capecitabine- or fluorouracil-based chemoradiotherapy. The 5-year overall survival was 76 and 67% with capecitabine and fluorouracil, respectively, with capecitabine found to be noninferior to fluorouracil.

Metastatic or Unresectable Colorectal Cancer

Monotherapy

The efficacy of capecitabine monotherapy in patients with metastatic colorectal cancer is based principally on the results of 2 open-label, randomized trials (SO14695 and SO14796). Enrolled patients were randomized to treatment with either capecitabine 1250 mg/m^2 twice daily for 14 days of a 21-day cycle or leucovorin 20 mg/m^2 IV followed by fluorouracil 425 mg/m^2 as an IV bolus on days 1–5 of each 28-day cycle. Outcomes assessed were overall survival, time to progression, and response rate (complete plus partial response).

A total of 1207 patients were enrolled in the 2 trials; the median age of patients was 63 or 64 years; 57—65% were male, the median Karnofsky performance status score was 90, 65—77% of patients had disease in the colon, and 23–35% had disease in the rectum. In Study SO14695, the overall response rate was 24.8 and 15.5%, median time to progression was 4.3 and 4.7 months, and overall median survival was 12.5 and 13.3 months for the capecitabine and fluorouracil/leucovorin groups, respectively. In Study SO14796, the overall response rate was 18.9 and 15%, median time to progression was 5.2 and 4.7 months, and overall median survival was 13.2 or 12.1 months for the capecitabine and fluorouracil/leucovorin groups, respectively.

Combination Therapy

The efficacy of capecitabine in the treatment of unresectable or metastatic colorectal cancer as part of a combination chemotherapy regimen is based on several published trials, including Study NO16966, a randomized, noninferiority, 2-arm study evaluating capecitabine in combination with oxaliplatin versus FOLFOX-4 (fluorouracil/folinic acid/oxaliplatin). The protocol was later revised to include 4 treatment arms (capecitabine/oxaliplatin/placebo; capecitabine/oxaliplatin/bevacizumab; FOLFOX-4/placebo; or FOLFOX-4/bevacizumab). Treatment was continued until disease progression or for 48 weeks, whichever came first. A total of 2034 patients were enrolled. Median progression-free survival was 8 and 8.5 months for the capecitabine-containing and FOLFOX-4 based regimens, respectively. Results for secondary outcomes (overall response rate, median overall survival, and median duration of response) were similar between treatment groups.

Clinical Perspective

According to the National Cancer Institute, surgery is the first-line treatment for patients with any stage of colon or rectal cancer. The use of chemotherapy or other systemic therapy after surgery is recommended for recurrent, late-stage, or metastatic disease. Various chemotherapy regimens have been used, including folic acid/fluorouracil/irinotecan, capecitabine/oxaliplatin, and fluorouracil/oxaliplatin. For stage IV or recurrent colon or rectal cancer, surgical resection (based on site of metastasis) and/or systemic therapy (e.g., targeted therapies, palliative chemotherapy) is recommended.

The American Society of Clinical Oncology (ASCO) guideline on metastatic colorectal cancer recommends the use of a chemotherapy (doublet or triplet) backbone as first-line therapy for previously untreated, unresectable microsatellite stable (MSS) or proficient mismatch repair (pMMR) metastatic colorectal cancer, in combination with anti-vascular endothelial growth factor (VEGF) antibodies (e.g., bevacizumab). Doublet chemotherapy regimens include folinic acid/fluorouracil/oxaliplatin and folinic acid/fluorouracil/irinotecan. Capecitabine plus oxaliplatin may be used as a substitute for folinic acid/fluorouracil/oxaliplatin. Triplet chemotherapy includes folinic acid/fluorouracil/oxaliplatin/irinotecan.

● Gastric, Esophageal, or Gastroesophageal Junction Cancer

Capecitabine is used for the treatment of adults with unresectable or metastatic gastric, esophageal, or gastroesophageal junction cancer as part of a combination chemotherapy regimen. Capecitabine is also used for treatment of adults with human epidermal growth factor receptor (HER)2-overexpressing metastatic gastric or gastroesophageal junction adenocarcinoma who have not been previously treated for metastatic disease as part of a combination regimen.

Unresectable or Metastatic Gastric, Esophageal, or Gastroesophageal Junction Cancer

The efficacy of capecitabine in the treatment of unresectable or metastatic gastric, esophageal, or gastroesophageal cancer was derived from several published studies, including REAL-2, a randomized noninferiority trial. A total of 1002 patients were randomized to treatment with 1 of 4 combination regimens (epirubicin/cisplatin/fluorouracil [ECF]; epirubicin/cisplatin/capecitabine [ECX]; epirubicin/oxaliplatin/fluorouracil [EOF]; or epirubicin/oxaliplatin/capecitabine [EOX]). The primary endpoint was overall survival. At a median follow-up of 17.1 months, median overall survival was 9.9, 9.9, 9.3, and 11.2 months for ECF, ECX, EOF, and EOX, respectively, demonstrating noninferiority of capecitabine to oxaliplatin.

HER2-overexpressing Metastatic Gastric or Gastroesophageal Junction Adenocarcinoma

The efficacy of capecitabine in the treatment of HER2-overexpressing metastatic gastric or gastroesophageal junction adenocarcinoma was derived from several published studies, including ToGA, a phase 3, open-label, randomized trial. A total of 594 patients with HER2-overexpressing metastatic cancer were randomized (1:1 ratio) to treatment with trastuzumab plus chemotherapy (capecitabine plus cisplatin or fluorouracil plus cisplatin) or chemotherapy alone. Median overall survival was 13.8 or 11.1 months for trastuzumab plus chemotherapy and chemotherapy alone, respectively.

Clinical Perspective

According to the National Cancer Institute, therapies for the treatment of stage IV or recurrent gastric cancers include a combination of chemotherapy, targeted therapies, immunotherapies, and palliative treatment. First-line palliative systemic therapies for HER2-negative tumors include chemotherapy with or without immunotherapy (e.g., fluorouracil or capecitabine with oxaliplatin and nivolumab), triplet chemotherapy regimens (e.g., fluorouracil and either epirubicin and cisplatin, etoposide and leucovorin, or doxorubicin and methotrexate), doublet regimens (e.g., a taxane and either cisplatin or carboplatin, or capecitabine plus oxaliplatin), or single agents (e.g., fluorouracil or capecitabine). For HER-2 positive tumors, first-line palliative systemic therapy includes immunotherapy with chemotherapy (nivolumab or trastuzumab with chemotherapy, including cisplatin plus fluorouracil, or capecitabine plus oxaliplatin).

The National Cancer Institute guidelines for esophageal cancer include surgery, endoscopic resection, chemotherapy (including capecitabine and fluorouracil), chemoradiation, and immunotherapies as treatment options, based on stage and extent of disease.

● Pancreatic Cancer

Capecitabine is used as adjuvant treatment of adults with pancreatic adenocarcinoma as part of a combination chemotherapy regimen.

Clinical Experience

The efficacy of capecitabine in the treatment of pancreatic adenocarcinoma was derived from ESPAC-4, an open-label, randomized trial. A total of 732 patients were randomized to treatment (1:1 ratio) with either capecitabine plus gemcitabine or gemcitabine alone, with a primary outcome of overall survival. At a median follow-up of 43.2 months, median overall survival with capecitabine plus gemcitabine was 28 months versus 25.5 months with gemcitabine alone, with results favoring the combination regimen.

Clinical Perspective

According to the National Cancer Institute, treatment options for pancreatic cancer are based on clinical stage of the disease and include surgery, chemotherapy, radiation, and chemotherapy with targeted therapy. For patients with resectable or borderline resectable pancreatic cancer, postoperative chemotherapy includes adjuvant FOLFIRINOX (leucovorin, fluorouracil, irinotecan, and oxaliplatin) or gemcitabine plus capecitabine. For both locally advanced and metastatic or recurrent pancreatic cancer, chemotherapy with or without targeted therapy is a primary treatment option. Evidence for several chemotherapy regimens is discussed, including FOLFIRINOX, gemcitabine-based regimens, fluorouracil/leucovorin/oxaliplatin, and capecitabine-based regimens.

DOSAGE AND ADMINISTRATION

● General

Pretreatment Screening

- Consider testing for genetic variants of dihydropyrimidine dehydrogenase (DPYD), the gene encoding dihydropyrimidine dehydrogenase (DPD), prior to initiating treatment with capecitabine.

- Obtain complete blood count (CBC) at baseline. Do not initiate capecitabine therapy if baseline neutrophil count <1500/mm³ and/ or baseline platelet count <100,000/mm³.

- Assess renal function and hydration status prior to initiating treatment with capecitabine. Optimize hydration prior to initiating treatment.

- Verify pregnancy status in females of reproductive potential prior to initiating treatment with capecitabine.

Patient Monitoring

- Obtain CBC prior to each treatment cycle.

- Monitor renal function and hydration status as clinically indicated during treatment with capecitabine. Promptly correct dehydration, which can develop rapidly in patients with anorexia, asthenia, nausea, vomiting, or diarrhea, and can result in acute renal failure; patients with preexisting renal impairment and those receiving concomitant therapy with nephrotoxic agents are at increased risk.

- Monitor for new or worsening serious skin reactions during treatment with capecitabine.

- If capecitabine is used in patients receiving a coumarin-derivative anticoagulant, prothrombin time (PT) or international normalized ratio (INR) should be monitored frequently, and the anticoagulant dosage should be adjusted accordingly.

- Liver function should be monitored carefully during capecitabine therapy in patients with mild to moderate hepatic impairment.

Premedication and Prophylaxis

- If used concomitantly with docetaxel, administer premedication prior to docetaxel administration. Consult docetaxel manufacturer's labeling for specific information.

Dispensing and Administration Precautions

- Based on the Institute for Safe Medication Practices (ISMP), capecitabine is a high-alert medication that has a heightened risk of causing significant patient harm when used in error.

Handling and Disposal

- Procedures for proper handling and disposal of antineoplastic drugs should be followed when preparing or administering capecitabine.

- Capecitabine should be used under the supervision of a qualified clinician experienced in therapy with cytotoxic agents.

● Administration

Capecitabine is administered orally. Capecitabine tablets should be swallowed whole with water within 30 minutes after the end of a meal. The recommended dose should be rounded to the nearest 150-mg dose so that whole tablets are administered. Capecitabine tablets should not be chewed, cut, or crushed. If a dose is missed or vomited, skip the missed/vomited dose and continue with the next scheduled dose.

Capecitabine tablets should be stored in tightly closed containers at 20–25°C; excursions are permitted to 15–30°C.

Pharmacogenomic Considerations in Dosing

Patients who are intermediate or poor metabolizers of dihydropyrimidine dehydrogenase (DPYD) may be at an increased risk for severe and sometimes fatal adverse effects with fluoropyrimidines (5-fluorouracil and capecitabine). Genetic DPYD variants associated with reduced DPD enzyme activity (particularly DPYD c.1905+1G>A and c.1679T>G) have been linked to decreased 5-fluorouracil clearance and increased risk for 5-fluorouracil toxicity. The Clinical Pharmacogenetics Implementation Consortium (CPIC) provides recommendations for fluoropyrimidine dosing guided by DPYD phenotype. For patients who are DPYD intermediate metabolizers (i.e., DPYD activity score of 1 or 1.5), the starting dose should be reduced based on the enzyme activity score; when the activity score is 1, the dose should be reduced by 50% and when the score is 1.5, the dose should be reduced by 25—50%. Further dose titration should be guided by toxicity or therapeutic drug monitoring (if available). For patients who are DPYD poor metabolizers (i.e., DPYD activity score of 0 or 0.5), it is strongly recommended to avoid use of fluoropyrimidines. In patients with an activity score of 0.5 who do not have suitable alternative therapeutic options, fluoropyrimidines should be administered at a markedly reduced dose (i.e., estimated via phenotyping test or <25% of the normal starting dose), with therapeutic drug monitoring completed as early as possible. Consult the CPIC guideline for additional details.

● Dosage

Breast Cancer

Combination Therapy

When used in combination with docetaxel for the treatment of advanced or metastatic breast cancer in patients with disease that failed to respond to or recurred following anthracycline-containing chemotherapy, the recommended dosage of capecitabine is 1000 or 1250 mg/m² twice daily (morning and evening), for the first 14 days of a 21-day cycle until disease progression or unacceptable toxicity

occurs, in combination with docetaxel. Docetaxel 75 mg/m² is administered as an IV infusion on the first day of each 21-day cycle.

Monotherapy

For the treatment of advanced or metastatic breast cancer in patients who are not candidates for anthracycline- or taxane-containing chemotherapy, the recommended initial dosage of capecitabine is 1000 or 1250 mg/m² twice daily (morning and evening), for the first 14 days of a 21-day cycle until disease progression or unacceptable toxicity occurs. Individualize the dosing schedule based on patient-specific factors (i.e., risk factors, adverse reactions).

Colorectal Cancer

Adjuvant Therapy for Colon Cancer

For adjuvant therapy following the complete resection of the primary tumor in patients with stage III colon cancer when treatment with fluoropyrimidine therapy alone is preferred, the recommended dosage of capecitabine is 1250 mg/m² twice daily (morning and evening) for the first 14 days of each 21-day cycle for a maximum of 8 cycles.

When used in combination with oxaliplatin-containing regimens as adjuvant therapy following the complete resection of the primary tumor in patients with stage III colon cancer, the dosage of capecitabine is 1000 mg/m² given twice daily (morning and evening) for the first 14 days of each 21-day cycle for a maximum of 8 cycles in combination with oxaliplatin 130 mg/m² administered IV on day 1 of each cycle.

Perioperative Treatment of Rectal Cancer

When used as a component of chemoradiotherapy for the perioperative treatment of locally advanced rectal cancer, the recommended dosage of capecitabine is 825 mg/m² twice daily (morning and evening) when administered with concomitant radiation therapy or 1250 mg/m² twice daily when administered as part of a perioperative combination regimen that does not include radiation therapy.

Unresectable or Metastatic Colorectal Cancer

When used as monotherapy for the treatment of unresectable or metastatic colorectal cancer, the recommended dosage of capecitabine is 1250 mg/m² twice daily (morning and evening) for the first 14 days of a 21-day cycle until disease progression or unacceptable toxicity occurs.

When used in combination with oxaliplatin for the treatment of unresectable or metastatic colorectal cancer, the recommended dosage of capecitabine is 1000 mg/m² twice daily for the first 14 days of each 21-day cycle. Continue treatment until disease progression or unacceptable toxicity occurs. Oxaliplatin 130 mg/m² is administered as an IV infusion on day 1 of each cycle.

Gastric, Esophageal, or Gastroesophageal Junction Cancer

Unresectable or Metastatic Gastric, Esophageal, or Gastroesophageal Junction Cancer

When used in combination with platinum-containing chemotherapy for the treatment of unresectable or metastatic gastric, esophageal, or gastroesophageal junction cancer, the recommended dosage of capecitabine is 625 mg/m² twice daily (morning and evening) on days 1—21 of each 21-day cycle for a maximum of 8 cycles. Alternately, a capecitabine dosage of 850 or 1000 mg/m² twice daily (morning and evening) for the first 14 days of each 21-day cycle can be administered in combination with oxaliplatin 130 mg/m² IV given on day 1 of each cycle. Continue treatment until disease progression or unacceptable toxicity occurs.

Human Epidermal Growth Factor Receptor (HER)2-overexpressing Metastatic Gastric or Gastroesophageal Junction Adenocarcinoma

For treatment of HER2-overexpressing metastatic gastric or gastroesophageal junction adenocarcinoma, the recommended dosage of capecitabine is 1000 mg/m² twice daily (morning and evening), for the first 14 days of each 21-day cycle until disease progression or unacceptable toxicity occurs. Capecitabine is given in combination with cisplatin and trastuzumab for this indication. Refer to the prescribing information for dosing recommendations for combination agents.

Pancreatic Adenocarcinoma

For adjuvant therapy patients with pancreatic adenocarcinoma (as a component of a combination chemotherapy regimen), the recommended dosage of capecitabine is 830 mg/m² twice daily (morning and evening) for the first 21 days of each 28-day cycle until disease progression or unacceptable toxicity occurs. If used in combination with gemcitabine 1000 mg/m² IV, given on days 1, 8, and 15 of each cycle, administer capecitabine for a maximum of 6 cycles.

Dosage Modification for Toxicity

Monitor patients for adverse reactions during treatment with capecitabine and modify dosages as indicated in Table 1 below. When capecitabine is administered in combination with docetaxel, withhold both capecitabine and docetaxel until the requirements for resuming both agents are met. Refer to the prescribing information for docetaxel for additional dosing information.

TABLE 1. Recommended Capecitabine Dosage Modifications for Adverse Reactions

Severity	Dosage Modification	Resume at Same or Reduce Dose (Percent of Current Dose)
Grade 2 toxicity		
First appearance	Withhold therapy until resolved to grade 0 or 1	100%
Second appearance	Withhold therapy until resolved to grade 0 or 1	75%
Third appearance	Withhold therapy until resolved to grade 0 or 1	50%
Fourth appearance	Permanently discontinue capecitabine	
Grade 3 toxicity		
First appearance	Withhold therapy until resolved to grade 0 or 1	75%
Second appearance	Withhold therapy until resolved to grade 0 or 1	50%
Third appearance	Permanently discontinue capecitabine	
Grade 4 toxicity		
First appearance	Permanently discontinue capecitabine OR withhold until resolved to grade 0 or 1	50%

If patients develop grade 3 or 4 hyperbilirubinemia during treatment with capecitabine, withhold treatment and resume once the event is grade 2 or less (i.e., bilirubin level below 3 times the upper limit of normal); use the percent of current dose column of Table 1 to determine the appropriate dose of capecitabine to resume therapy.

● Special Populations

Hepatic Impairment

The manufacturer makes no specific dosage recommendations for patients with hepatic impairment; however, more frequent monitoring of such patients is recommended.

Renal Impairment

In patients with mild to moderate renal impairment (i.e., creatinine clearance of 30—50 mL/min as determined by the Cockroft-Gault equation), reduce the dose of capecitabine by 25%. The manufacturer states that a dosage has not been established for patients with severe renal impairment (creatinine clearance <30 mL/min). If no alternative treatment exists for such patients, capecitabine can be administered on an individual basis using a reduced starting dose, close monitoring, and dosage modifications guided by adverse events.

Geriatric Patients

The manufacturer makes no specific dosage recommendations for geriatric patients.

CAUTIONS

● Contraindications

- History of severe hypersensitivity reactions to fluorouracil or capecitabine.

● Warnings/Precautions

Warnings

Increased Risk of Bleeding with Concomitant Use of Vitamin K Antagonists

A boxed warning about an increased risk of bleeding with concomitant use of vitamin K antagonists is included in the prescribing information for capecitabine. Altered coagulation and/or bleeding parameters, including fatal cases of bleeding, have been reported in patients taking capecitabine concomitantly with vitamin K antagonists such as warfarin. There have been reports of clinically significant increases in the prothrombin time and international normalized ratio (INR) following initiation of capecitabine in patients on stable therapy with oral vitamin K antagonists. These events have occurred anywhere from several days to several months after initiation of capecitabine, with a few cases occurring within 1 month following discontinuation of capecitabine. Such bleeding events have occurred in patients with and without liver metastases. In patients receiving capecitabine with concomitant vitamin K antagonist therapy, monitor INR more frequently and adjust the dose of the vitamin K antagonist as appropriate.

Other Warnings and Precautions

Cardiotoxicity

Cardiotoxicity can occur with capecitabine. Myocardial infarction or ischemia, angina, dysrhythmias, cardiac arrest, cardiac failure, sudden death, electrocardiographic changes, and cardiomyopathy have been reported in patients taking capecitabine. Patients with a past history of coronary artery disease may be more likely to experience these adverse reactions. If cardiotoxicity occurs, withhold capecitabine as appropriate. The safety of resuming capecitabine therapy in patients with resolution of symptoms after development of cardiotoxicity has not been established.

Diarrhea

Diarrhea, sometimes severe, can occur with capecitabine. In clinical trials including 875 patients with metastatic breast or colorectal cancer who received treatment with capecitabine monotherapy, grade 2 to 4 diarrhea first occurred after a median of 34 days (range, 1 day to 1 year). Grade 3 to 4 diarrhea lasted for a median of 5 days. If diarrhea occurs, withhold treatment; dosage modification or permanent discontinuation of capecitabine may be necessary upon resumption depending on the frequency and severity of symptoms.

Dehydration

Dehydration can occur with capecitabine. Patients with anorexia, asthenia, nausea, vomiting, or diarrhea may be more likely to develop dehydration during treatment with capecitabine. Prior to treatment with capecitabine, optimize hydration. Monitor hydration status and kidney function at baseline and during treatment as clinically indicated. If dehydration occurs, withhold treatment; dosage modification or permanent discontinuation of capecitabine may be necessary upon resumption depending on the frequency and severity of symptoms.

Renal Toxicity

Serious and sometimes fatal renal failure can occur with capecitabine. Patients with renal impairment or who are receiving concomitant therapy with capecitabine and other drugs that are known to cause renal toxicity may increase this risk. Prior to treatment with capecitabine, optimize hydration. Monitor renal function at baseline and during treatment as clinically indicated. If renal toxicity occurs, withhold treatment; dosage modification or permanent discontinuation of capecitabine may be necessary upon resumption depending on the frequency and severity of symptoms.

Serious Skin Toxicities

Serious, sometimes fatal severe cutaneous adverse reactions, including Stevens-Johnson Syndrome and toxic epidermal necrolysis, can occur with capecitabine. Monitor for new or worsening skin reactions during treatment with capecitabine and permanently discontinue treatment if such reactions occur.

Palmar-Plantar Erythrodysesthesia Syndrome

Palmar-plantar erythrodysesthesia syndrome can occur with capecitabine. Among patients who developed grade 1 to 3 palmar-plantar erythrodysesthesia syndrome in clinical trials of capecitabine monotherapy for treatment of metastatic breast or colorectal cancer, the median time to onset was 2.6 months (range, 11 days to 1 year). If palmar-plantar erythrodysesthesia syndrome occurs, withhold treatment; dosage modification or permanent discontinuation of capecitabine may be necessary upon resumption depending on the frequency and severity of symptoms.

Myelosuppression

Myelosuppression can occur with capecitabine. In clinical trials including 875 patients with metastatic breast or colorectal cancer who received treatment with capecitabine monotherapy, grade 3 or 4 neutropenia, thrombocytopenia, and anemia occurred in 3.2, 1.7, and 2.4% of patients, respectively. In 251 patients with metastatic breast cancer who received combination therapy with capecitabine and docetaxel, grade 3 or 4 neutropenia, thrombocytopenia, and anemia occurred in 68, 2.8, and 10% of patients, respectively. Necrotizing enterocolitis (typhlitis) has also been reported with capecitabine. Consider a diagnosis of typhlitis in patients taking capecitabine who experience fever, neutropenia, and abdominal pain.

Monitor CBC at baseline and prior to each capecitabine treatment cycle. Treatment with capecitabine is not recommended if the neutrophil count is below 1500/mm^3 or the platelet count is below 100,000/mm^3 at baseline. If grade 3 or 4 myelosuppression occurs during treatment with capecitabine, withhold treatment; dosage modification or permanent discontinuation of capecitabine may be necessary upon resumption depending on the frequency of symptoms.

Hyperbilirubinemia

Hyperbilirubinemia can occur with capecitabine. In clinical trials including 875 patients with metastatic breast or colorectal cancer who received treatment with capecitabine monotherapy, grade 3 and 4 hyperbilirubinemia occurred in 15 and 3.9% of patients, respectively. Grade 3 or 4 hyperbilirubinemia occurred more frequently in the 566 patients with hepatic metastases at baseline (23%) compared to 309 without hepatic metastases at baseline (12%). Among the 167 patients who developed grade 3 or 4 hyperbilirubinemia, post-baseline increases in alkaline phosphatase and transaminases at any time (not necessarily concurrent) occurred in 19 and 28% of patients, respectively; most patients who experienced these increases had liver metastases at baseline. Of the patients who developed grade 3 or 4 hyperbilirubinemia, pre- and post-baseline values of alkaline phosphatase and transaminases were elevated in 58 and 35% of patients, respectively. Grade 3 or 4 elevations of alkaline phosphatase and transaminases occurred in 8 and 3% of patients, respectively.

Among 596 patients with metastatic colorectal cancer who were treated with capecitabine, grade 3 or 4 hyperbilirubinemia occurred at a similar rate as seen for the pooled population described above. The median time to onset of grade 3 or 4 hyperbilirubinemia was 64 days; median total bilirubin levels increased from a median of 8 μm/L at baseline to 13 μm/L during treatment with capecitabine.

Of the 251 patients with metastatic breast cancer who received combination therapy with capecitabine and docetaxel, grade 3 and 4 hyperbilirubinemia occurred in 7 and 2% of patients, respectively.

If hyperbilirubinemia develops, withhold treatment; dosage modification or permanent discontinuation of capecitabine may be necessary upon resumption depending on the frequency of symptoms. If grade 3 or 4 hyperbilirubinemia occurs, capecitabine may be resumed once the event is classified as grade 2 or less than 3 times the upper limit of normal.

Eye Irritation, Skin Rash, and Other Adverse Reactions from Exposure to Crushed Tablets

Eye irritation and swelling, skin rash, diarrhea, paresthesia, headache, gastric irritation, nausea, and vomiting have occurred following exposure to crushed capecitabine tablets. Advise patients not to cut or crush capecitabine tablets. If the tablets must be cut or crushed, this should be done by a professional who is trained in the safe handling of cytotoxic drugs using appropriate equipment and safety procedures. Safety and effectiveness of administering crushed capecitabine tablets have not been established.

Pharmacogenomics of Capecitabine-Induced Serious Adverse Reactions Due to Dihydropyrimidine Dehydrogenase (DPD) Deficiency

Dihydropyrimidine dehydrogenase, encoded by the DPYD gene, is responsible for catabolism of >80% of fluorouracil. Capecitabine is metabolized to fluorouracil in vivo. Capecitabine should be withheld or permanently discontinued in patients experiencing acute early-onset or unusually severe toxicity, which may indicate near complete or total absence of dihydropyrimidine dehydrogenase (DPD) activity. Patients with certain homozygous or certain compound heterozygous mutations in the DPYD gene resulting in complete or near complete absence of DPD activity (i.e., DPYD poor metabolizers) are at increased risk for acute early-onset toxicity and severe, life-threatening, or fatal toxicity (e.g., mucositis, diarrhea, neutropenia, neurotoxicity) caused by capecitabine; patients with partial DPD activity (i.e., DPYD intermediate metabolizers) also may be at increased risk for severe, life-threatening, or fatal toxicity. No dosage of capecitabine has been proven safe for patients with complete absence of DPD activity, and there are insufficient data to support dosage recommendations for those with partial DPD activity. Consider testing patients for genetic variants of DPYD prior to initiating treatment with capecitabine. However, serious adverse reactions can still occur even if no variants are identified.

Genetic DPYD variants associated with reduced DPD enzyme activity (particularly DPYD c.1905+1G>A and c.1679T>G) have been linked to decreased 5-fluorouracil clearance and increased risk for 5-fluorouracil toxicity. The Clinical Pharmacogenetics Implementation Consortium (CPIC) provides recommendations for fluoropyrimidine dosing guided by DPYD phenotype. Dosage adjustments are recommended for patients who are DPYD intermediate metabolizers, and fluoropyrimidines should be avoided in patients who are DPYD poor metabolizers. (See Pharmacogenomic Considerations in Dosing under Dosage and Administration.) Consult the CPIC guideline for more details and definitions of DPYD phenotypes based on genotype.

Fetal/Neonatal Morbidity and Mortality

Based on its mechanism of action and animal findings, capecitabine can cause fetal harm when administered to a pregnant patient. Human data are not sufficient to inform the drug-associated risk of capecitabine use in pregnancy. In animal studies, administration of capecitabine during the period of organogenesis at 0.2 times the human exposure in patients receiving the recommended dose of 1250 mg/m^2 twice daily in pregnant mice and 0.6 times the human exposure in pregnant monkeys led to embryolethality and teratogenicity in mice and embryolethality in monkeys. Additionally, animal studies have shown that capecitabine may impair fertility in females and males of reproductive potential.

Verify pregnancy status in female patients of reproductive potential prior to initiating treatment with capecitabine and advise pregnant patients of the potential risk to a fetus. Advise females of reproductive potential to use effective contraception during treatment with capecitabine and for 6 months following discontinuation. Advise male partners of such females to use effective contraception during treatment with capecitabine and for 3 months following discontinuation.

Specific Populations

Pregnancy

Based on its mechanism of action and animal findings, capecitabine can cause fetal harm when administered to a pregnant patient. (See Fetal/Neonatal Morbidity and Mortality under Cautions.) Advise pregnant patients of the potential risk to a fetus.

Lactation

In lactating mice receiving a single dose of capecitabine, significant amounts of capecitabine metabolites were distributed into milk. It is not known whether capecitabine or its metabolites are distributed into human milk. The effects of the drug on nursing infants or on milk production are unknown. Because of the potential for serious adverse reactions to capecitabine in nursing infants, women should be advised to discontinue nursing during capecitabine therapy and for 1 week after discontinuance of therapy.

Females and Males of Reproductive Potential

Based on animal studies, capecitabine may impair fertility in females and males of reproductive potential. Verify pregnancy status in female patients of reproductive potential prior to initiating treatment with capecitabine. Advise females of reproductive potential to use effective contraception during treatment with capecitabine and for 6 months following discontinuation. Advise male partners of such females to use effective contraception during treatment with capecitabine and for 3 months following discontinuation.

Pediatric Use

The manufacturer states that safety and efficacy of capecitabine in children younger than 18 years of age have not been established.

Geriatric Use

In clinical trials of patients with colorectal cancer (N=7938), metastatic breast cancer (N=4536), gastric, esophageal, or gastrointestinal junction cancer (N=1951), or pancreatic cancer (N=364) who were treated with capecitabine, 33, 18, 26, and 47% of patients, respectively, were ≥65 years of age. No differences in efficacy were noted in geriatric patients compared to younger patients in these trials. However, geriatric patients experienced increased GI toxicity from capecitabine. Deaths have been reported from severe enterocolitis, diarrhea, and dehydration in geriatric patients treated with weekly leucovorin and fluorouracil.

Hepatic Impairment

In pharmacokinetic studies, systemic exposure and maximum serum concentrations of fluorouracil (the active principle of capecitabine) were not affected in patients with mild or moderate hepatic impairment compared to patients with normal hepatic function. The maximum serum concentration and systemic exposure of capecitabine increased by 60%. The effect of severe hepatic impairment on the pharmacokinetics of capecitabine and its metabolites are not known.

Renal Impairment

The effect of renal impairment on the elimination of capecitabine has been evaluated in cancer patients. Renal impairment causes increased systemic exposure to capecitabine and its metabolites. Following oral administration of capecitabine 1250 mg/m^2 twice daily, systemic exposure to the FBAL metabolite on day 1 was 85% higher in patients with moderate renal impairment (creatinine clearance of 30–50 mL/min) and 258% higher in patients with severe renal impairment (creatinine clearance <30 mL/min) than in patients with normal renal function (creatinine clearance >80 mL/min). Systemic exposure to the 5′-DFUR metabolite was 42 or 71% greater in patients with moderate or severe renal impairment, respectively, than in those with normal renal function. Systemic exposure to 5-fluorouracil did not increase in patients with moderate renal impairment, but increased by 24% in patients with severe renal impairment, compared to those with normal renal function. Systemic exposure to capecitabine was about 25% greater in patients with moderate or severe renal impairment than in those with normal renal function.

The effect of dialysis on the elimination of capecitabine has not been determined; however, the manufacturer reports that dialysis may reduce circulating concentrations of 5′-DFUR, a low molecular weight metabolite of the drug.

● Common Adverse Effects

Adverse effects reported in ≥30% of patients receiving capecitabine monotherapy for adjuvant treatment of colon cancer include palmar-plantar erythrodysesthesia syndrome, diarrhea, and nausea.

Adverse effects reported in ≥30% of patients receiving capecitabine monotherapy for metastatic colorectal cancer include anemia, diarrhea, palmar-plantar erythrodysesthesia syndrome, hyperbilirubinemia, nausea, fatigue, and abdominal pain.

Adverse effects reported in ≥30% of patients receiving capecitabine monotherapy for metastatic breast cancer include lymphopenia, anemia, diarrhea, hand-and-foot syndrome, nausea, fatigue, vomiting, and dermatitis.

Adverse effects reported in ≥30% of patients receiving capecitabine in combination with docetaxel for metastatic breast cancer include lymphocytopenia, leukopenia, neutropenia, anemia, diarrhea, stomatitis, palmar-plantar erythrodysesthesia syndrome, nausea, alopecia, thrombocytopenia, vomiting, edema, and abdominal pain.

DRUG INTERACTIONS

Capecitabine is not metabolized by cytochrome P-450 (CYP) isoenzymes. In vitro studies indicate that capecitabine and its metabolites do not inhibit CYP isoenzymes 1A2, CYP2A6, CYP3A4, CYP2C19, CYP2D6, or CYP2E1.

● Drugs Affecting Hepatic Microsomal Enzymes

Capecitabine increases exposure of CYP2C9 substrates, which may increase the likelihood for development of adverse events from such substrates. Concomitant administration of celecoxib (a sensitive CYP2C9 substrate) with capecitabine 1000 mg/m^2 twice daily for 14 days increased systemic exposure to celecoxib and its maximum serum concentration by 28 and 24%, respectively.

In patients receiving concomitant therapy with capecitabine and CYP2C9 substrates where minimal concentration changes may lead to serious adverse reactions (e.g., anticoagulants, antidiabetic drugs), closely monitor for adverse events.

● Nephrotoxic Drugs

Due to the additive pharmacologic effect, concomitant use of capecitabine with other drugs that are known to cause renal toxicity may increase the risk of renal toxicity. When capecitabine is used concomitantly with nephrotoxic drugs (e.g., platinum salts, irinotecan, methotrexate, IV bisphosphonates), closely monitor for signs of renal toxicity.

● Allopurinol

Concomitant use of allopurinol and capecitabine may decrease conversion of capecitabine to the active metabolites, 5-fluoro-2′-deoxyuridine 5′-monophosphate (FdUMP) and 5-fluorouridine triphosphate (FUTP), and result in reduced capecitabine efficacy. Concomitant use of capecitabine with allopurinol should be avoided.

● Antacids

In a small number of patients, administration of an antacid containing aluminum hydroxide and magnesium hydroxide immediately following capecitabine (1250 mg/m^2) resulted in an increased rate and extent of absorption of capecitabine; AUC and peak plasma concentration increased by 16 and 35%, respectively, for capecitabine and by 18 and 22%, respectively, for the 5′-DFCR metabolite. Antacid administration had no effect on the other 3 major metabolites of capecitabine (i.e., 5′-DFUR, fluorouracil, and FBAL).

● Anticoagulants

Capecitabine increases exposure of vitamin K antagonists (i.e., warfarin), which may alter coagulation parameters and/or bleeding and could result in death. Such events may occur within days after initiation of treatment with capecitabine, and up to 1 month following its discontinuation. In 4 patients receiving chronic administration of capecitabine 1250 mg/m^2 twice daily with a single dose of warfarin 20 mg, the mean AUC of S-warfarin was increased by 57% and clearance was decreased by 37%. The baseline corrected AUC of INR in these patients increased by 2.8-fold, and the maximum observed mean international normalized ratio (INR) increased by 91%.

In patients receiving concomitant treatment with capecitabine and a vitamin K antagonist, monitor the INR more frequently; reduction in the dosage of the vitamin K antagonist may be necessary.

● Docetaxel

When used in combination, capecitabine had no impact on the pharmacokinetics of docetaxel and docetaxel did not affect the pharmacokinetics of capecitabine or its metabolite 5'-DFUR.

● Leucovorin

Leucovorin potentiates the antineoplastic activity of fluorouracil (the active drug of capecitabine) and also may increase its toxicity. Deaths from severe enterocolitis, diarrhea, and dehydration have been reported in geriatric patients receiving a weekly regimen of combination therapy with leucovorin and fluorouracil. Instruct patients to avoid taking products that contain folic acid or folate analog products unless directed to do so by their healthcare provider.

● *Phenytoin*

Concomitant use of phenytoin and capecitabine may result in toxicity from increased serum phenytoin concentrations. In patients receiving capecitabine, serum concentrations of phenytoin must be monitored carefully, and reduction in the phenytoin dosage may be necessary.

DESCRIPTION

Capecitabine, a fluoropyrimidine carbamate, is an antineoplastic agent. Capecitabine is a prodrug of 5′-deoxy-5-fluorouridine (doxifuridine, 5′-DFUR) and has little pharmacologic activity until it is converted to fluorouracil, a fluorinated pyrimidine antagonist, in tumor tissue. Because capecitabine is converted to fluorouracil by enzymes that are expressed at higher concentrations in many tumors than in adjacent normal tissues or plasma, it is thought that high tumor concentrations of the active drug may be achieved with less systemic toxicity. Fluorouracil is metabolized in both normal and tumor cells to 5-fluoro-2′-deoxyuridine 5′-monophosphate (FdUMP) and 5-fluorouridine triphosphate (FUTP). The main mechanism of fluorouracil is via the binding of the deoxyribonucleotide of the drug (FdUMP) and the folate cofactor (N5–10-methylenetetrahydrofolate) to thymidylate synthase (TS) to form a covalently bound ternary complex, which inhibits the formation of thymidylate from 2′-deoxyuridylate, thereby interfering with DNA synthesis. In addition, FUTP can be incorporated into RNA in place of uridine triphosphate (UTP), producing a fraudulent RNA and interfering with RNA processing and protein synthesis. Capecitabine has been shown to be active in xenograft tumors that are resistant to fluorouracil indicating incomplete cross-resistance between the drugs.

Over a dosage range of 500–3500 mg/m^2 daily, the pharmacokinetics of capecitabine and its metabolite, 5′-deoxy-5-fluorocytidine (5′-DFCR), were dose proportional and did not change over time. However, the manufacturer reports that increases in area under the concentration-time curves (AUCs) of metabolites 5′-DFUR and fluorouracil were greater than proportional to the increase in dose. Considerable interindividual variations (i.e., exceeding 85%) in peak plasma concentrations and AUCs have been reported following oral administration of capecitabine. According to the manufacturer, peak plasma concentrations of capecitabine occur in about 1.5 hours, and peak plasma concentrations of fluorouracil, its active metabolite, occur at 2 hours.

Administration of capecitabine after a breakfast that is medium-rich in fat and carbohydrates resulted in decreases in the peak plasma concentration and AUC of capecitabine by 60 and 34%, respectively. The peak plasma concentration and AUC of fluorouracil were also decreased by 37 and 12%, respectively. The time to maximum concentration of both capecitabine and fluorouracil were delayed by 1.5 hours. Plasma protein binding (mainly to albumin) of capecitabine and its metabolites is less than 60% and is not concentration dependent. Capecitabine is extensively metabolized in the liver and tumors. The plasma elimination half-life of capecitabine and fluorouracil is about 45 minutes.

In the liver, capecitabine is largely hydrolyzed to 5′-DFCR by carboxylesterase. 5′-DFCR subsequently is converted to another noncytotoxic intermediate, 5′-deoxy-5-fluorouridine (5′-DFUR), by cytidine deaminase. Hydrolysis of 5′-DFUR to the active drug fluorouracil is catalyzed by thymidine phosphorylase. Once capecitabine is converted to the active drug fluorouracil, mainly in tumor tissue, fluorouracil is anabolized to 5-fluoro-2′-deoxyuridine-5′-monophosphate (FdUMP) and 5-fluorouridine triphosphate (FUTP), the active metabolites of the drug. Fluorouracil is catabolized to dihydrofluorouracil (FUH$_2$), by dihydropyrimidine dehydrogenase. Dihydropyrimidinase cleaves the pyrimidine ring of FUH$_2$, yielding 5-fluoro-ureido-propionic acid (FUPA), which is then cleaved by β-ureido-propionase to form α-fluoro-β-alanine (FBAL). Capecitabine and its metabolites are excreted predominantly in urine (96%); fecal excretion is minimal (2.6%). Most of the capecitabine dose is excreted in urine as metabolites, principally FBAL, a catabolite of fluorouracil (57% of an administered dose); about 3% of an administered dose is excreted in urine as unchanged drug.

Following therapeutic doses of capecitabine, no clinically meaningful differences in the pharmacokinetics of 5′-DFUR, fluorouracil, or FBAL were observed based on sex and race; additionally, no clinically meaningful differences of 5′-DFUR and fluorouracil were observed based on age (range, 27—86 years). The exposure to FBAL increased by 15% following a 20% increase in age. Data from a study in Japanese and white patients receiving capecitabine 825 mg/m^2 twice daily for 14 days showed differences in the pharmacokinetic disposition of capecitabine and its catabolite, FBAL. Peak plasma concentration and the AUC of capecitabine were reduced by about 36 and 24%, respectively, and peak plasma concentration and AUC of FBAL were about 25 and 34% lower, respectively, in the Japanese patients than in the white patients. The clinical importance of these differences is not known. No clinically significant differences in the pharmacokinetics of 5′-DFCR, 5′-DFUR, or fluorouracil were observed.

ADVICE TO PATIENTS

- Stress importance of reading the manufacturer's patient information.

- Advise patients on vitamin K antagonists, such as warfarin, that they are at an increased risk of severe bleeding while taking capecitabine. Advise these patients that the international normalized ratio (INR) should be monitored more frequently, and dosage modifications of the vitamin K antagonist may be required, while taking and after discontinuation of capecitabine. Advise these patients to immediately contact their healthcare provider if signs or symptoms of bleeding occur.

- Inform patients of the potential for serious and life-threatening adverse reactions due to dihydropyrimidine dehydrogenase (DPD) deficiency and discuss whether they should be tested for genetic variants that are associated with an increased risk of serious adverse reactions from the use of capecitabine. Advise patients to immediately contact their healthcare provider if symptoms of severe mucositis, diarrhea, neutropenia, and neurotoxicity occur.

- Advise patients of the risk of cardiotoxicity and to immediately contact their healthcare provider for new onset of chest pain, shortness of breath, dizziness, or lightheadedness.

- Inform patients experiencing grade 2 diarrhea (an increase of 4 to 6 stools/day or nocturnal stools) or greater or experiencing severe bloody diarrhea with severe abdominal pain and fever to stop taking capecitabine. Advise patients on the use of antidiarrheal treatments (e.g., loperamide) to manage diarrhea.

- Instruct patients experiencing grade 2 or greater dehydration to stop taking capecitabine immediately and to contact their healthcare provider. Advise patients to not restart capecitabine until rehydrated and any precipitating causes have been corrected or controlled.

- Instruct patients experiencing decreased urinary output or other signs and symptoms of renal toxicity to immediately contact their healthcare provider.

- Instruct patients with skin rash, blistering, or peeling to immediately contact their healthcare provider.

- Instruct patients experiencing grade 2 or greater palmar-plantar erythrodysesthesia syndrome to stop taking capecitabine immediately and to contact their healthcare provider. Inform patients that initiation of symptomatic treatment is recommended and hand-and-foot syndrome can lead to loss of fingerprints, which could impact personal identification.

- Inform patients who develop a fever of 100.5°F or greater or other evidence of potential infection to immediately contact their healthcare provider.

- Inform patients who develop jaundice or icterus to immediately contact their healthcare provider.

- Advise women to inform their clinician if they are or plan to become pregnant or plan to breast-feed. Advise pregnant women and females of reproductive potential of the potential risk to a fetus. Advise females of reproductive potential to inform their healthcare provider of a known or suspected pregnancy. Advise females not to breast-feed during treatment with capecitabine and for 1 week after the last dose.

- Advise males and females of reproductive potential that capecitabine may impair fertility. Advise females of reproductive potential to use effective contraception during treatment with capecitabine and for 6 months after the last dose. Advise males with female partners of reproductive potential to use effective contraception during treatment with capecitabine and for 3 months after the last dose.

- Advise patients that capecitabine may cause severe hypersensitivity reactions and angioedema. Advise patients who have known hypersensitivity to capecitabine or 5-fluorouracil to inform their healthcare provider. Instruct patients who develop hypersensitivity reactions or mucocutaneous symptoms (e.g., urticaria, rash, erythema, pruritus, or swelling of the face, lips, tongue, or throat which make it difficult to swallow or breathe) to stop taking capecitabine and immediately contact their healthcare provider or go to an emergency room.

- Instruct patients experiencing grade 2 nausea (food intake significantly decreased but able to eat intermittently) or greater to stop taking capecitabine and to immediately contact their healthcare provider for management of nausea. Instruct patients experiencing grade 2 vomiting (2 to 5 episodes in a 24-hour period) or greater to stop taking capecitabine immediately and to contact their healthcare provider for management of vomiting.

- Inform patients experiencing grade 2 stomatitis (painful erythema, edema, or ulcers of the mouth or tongue, but able to eat) or greater to stop taking capecitabine immediately and to contact their healthcare provider.

- Advise patients to swallow capecitabine tablets whole with water within 30 minutes after a meal. Advise patients and caregivers not to chew, crush, or cut capecitabine tablets. Advise patients if they cannot swallow capecitabine tablets whole to inform their healthcare provider.

- Instruct patients not to take products containing folic acid or folate analog products (e.g., leucovorin, levoleucovorin) unless directed to do so by their healthcare provider. Advise patients to inform their clinician of existing or contemplated concomitant therapy, including prescription and OTC drugs and dietary and herbal supplements, as well as any concomitant illnesses.

- Inform patients of other important precautionary information.

For further information on the handling of antineoplastic agents, see the ASHP Guidelines on Handling Hazardous Drugs at https://www.ahfsdruginformation.com.

PREPARATIONS

Excipients in commercially available drug preparations may have clinically important effects in some individuals; consult specific product labeling for details.

Capecitabine

Oral		
Tablets	150 mg*	**Capecitabine Tablets**
		Xeloda®, H2 Pharma
	500 mg*	**Capecitabine Tablets**
		Xeloda®, H2 Pharma

* available from one or more manufacturer, distributor, and/or repackager by generic (nonproprietary) name

† Use is not currently included in the labeling approved by the US Food and Drug Administration.

Selected Revisions October 10, 2024, © Copyright, June 1, 1999, American Society of Health-System Pharmacists, Inc.

CARBOplatin

10:00 · ANTINEOPLASTIC AGENTS

■ Carboplatin is a platinum-containing antineoplastic agent.

USES

While the relative efficacy of carboplatin and cisplatin in the treatment of specific malignancies remains to be more fully elucidated, the drugs appear to have similar efficacy in platinum-responsive ovarian tumors, lung cancers, and certain head and neck cancers, but carboplatin is less effective than cisplatin in certain testicular cancers. Carboplatin and cisplatin are associated with different toxicity profiles and carboplatin may be effective in patients with platinum-responsive tumors who are unable to tolerate cisplatin because of renal impairment, refractory nausea, hearing impairment, or neuropathy. It has been suggested that while carboplatin may be preferred in patients with renal failure or patients at high risk for ototoxicity or neurotoxicity, cisplatin may be preferred in patients who have decreased bone marrow reserve or a high risk of sepsis, or who require anticoagulation therapy.

● Ovarian Cancer

Carboplatin is used alone or in combination therapy for the treatment of ovarian cancer.

First-line Therapy for Advanced Ovarian Epithelial Cancer
Combination Chemotherapy

Carboplatin in combination with paclitaxel† is a preferred regimen for the initial treatment of advanced ovarian epithelial cancer. The best combination or sequential therapy with multiple agents in the treatment of advanced ovarian tumors has not been established, and comparative efficacy is continually being evaluated.

Carboplatin versus Cisplatin: Randomized trials have demonstrated that carboplatin is as effective as but less toxic than cisplatin when used in combination with either paclitaxel or cyclophosphamide for the initial treatment of advanced ovarian cancer. Further study is needed to determine optimal dosing for carboplatin.

Carboplatin has been substituted for cisplatin in combination therapy with paclitaxel. In randomized trials in advanced ovarian cancer, carboplatin was as effective as cisplatin when combined with paclitaxel but was better tolerated.

In a randomized trial designed to establish noninferiority of the studied carboplatin-containing regimen, 792 women with small-volume stage III ovarian cancer (i.e., no tumor nodule greater than 1 cm in diameter following the initial surgery) received either carboplatin/paclitaxel or cisplatin/paclitaxel. The treatment regimens consisted of carboplatin at the dose required to obtain an area under the plasma concentration-time curve (AUC) of 7.5 mg/mL per minute (using the Calvert formula in which creatinine clearance, calculated using the Jellife formula, was substituted for GFR) and paclitaxel 175 mg/m² as a 3-hour IV infusion; or cisplatin 75 mg/m² IV administered at 1 mg per minute and paclitaxel 135 mg/m² as a 24-hour continuous IV infusion every 3 weeks for a total of six courses. Based on median overall survival and median progression-free survival, carboplatin with paclitaxel was as effective as cisplatin with paclitaxel for small-volume stage III ovarian epithelial cancer. Grade 2 to 4 thrombocytopenia and grade 1 to 2 pain occurred more frequently in patients receiving the carboplatin regimen, whereas leukopenia and GI, renal (genitourinary), and metabolic toxicities (e.g., hypomagnesemia or abnormal electrolytes) occurred more frequently in patients receiving the cisplatin regimen. Grade 2 to 4 neurologic toxicity, mainly peripheral neuropathy, occurred with similar frequency (about 30%) in both groups.

In another randomized trial designed to establish noninferiority of carboplatin, 798 women with FIGO stage IIb–IV ovarian cancer received either carboplatin/paclitaxel or cisplatin/paclitaxel. The treatment regimens consisted of paclitaxel 185 mg/m² administered IV over 3 hours followed by carboplatin at the dose required to obtain an AUC of 6 mg/mL per minute (using the Calvert formula in which GFR was estimated using the Jellife formula) administered IV over 30–60 minutes; or paclitaxel 185 mg/m² administered IV over 3 hours followed by cisplatin 75 mg/m² administered IV over 30 minutes. Regardless of calculated doses, the maximal absolute doses administered for each drug were paclitaxel 400 mg, carboplatin 880 mg, and cisplatin 165 mg. Based on the proportion of patients without disease progression at 2 years, median overall survival, and

median progression-free survival, carboplatin with paclitaxel was as effective as cisplatin with paclitaxel for FIGO stage IIa–IV ovarian epithelial cancer. Grade 3 or 4 hematologic toxicity and grade 3 or 4 non-neutropenic infections occurred more frequently in patients receiving the carboplatin regimen, whereas certain grade 3 or 4 nonhematologic toxicities, including nausea, vomiting, and peripheral sensory neuropathy, occurred more frequently in patients receiving the cisplatin regimen.

Carboplatin also has been substituted for cisplatin in combination therapy with cyclophosphamide. In randomized trials comparing the use of carboplatin versus cisplatin in combination with cyclophosphamide for advanced ovarian cancer, similar efficacy was observed but carboplatin appeared to have a more favorable therapeutic index than cisplatin.

Because carboplatin is as effective as cisplatin in combination regimens for advanced ovarian cancer, it is preferred except in patients who are unable to tolerate carboplatin (e.g., those who have decreased bone marrow reserve, a high risk of sepsis, or imperative need for anticoagulation therapy).

Platinum-containing Agent with Paclitaxel Versus Platinum-containing Agent with Cyclophosphamide: Evidence from randomized trials indicates that combined therapy with a platinum-containing agent and paclitaxel is superior to therapy with cyclophosphamide and a platinum-containing agent for the initial treatment of advanced epithelial ovarian carcinoma and therefore is the preferred regimen. In a comparative study of patients with suboptimally debulked (greater than 1 cm residual tumor mass) stage III or IV ovarian cancer who had no prior chemotherapy, combined therapy with cisplatin and paclitaxel produced higher rates of overall objective response (73 versus 60%), increased disease-free survival (median: 18 versus 13 months), and increased overall survival (median: 38 versus 24 months) compared with a combined regimen of cisplatin and cyclophosphamide. A higher frequency of neutropenia, fever, alopecia, and allergic reactions was observed in patients receiving cisplatin and paclitaxel compared with those receiving cisplatin and cyclophosphamide. In another randomized trial, a higher rate of complete response and prolonged overall survival was observed in patients receiving paclitaxel and cisplatin versus cyclophosphamide and cisplatin for advanced epithelial ovarian cancer. At a follow-up of 6.5 years, the survival benefit associated with the cisplatin and paclitaxel regimen in both randomized trials has been maintained.

Carboplatin and Docetaxel: Carboplatin in combination with docetaxel† has been used for the first-line treatment of ovarian cancer. In a phase III randomized trial, response rates, progression-free survival, and 2-year survival rates were similar in patients receiving docetaxel and carboplatin versus paclitaxel and carboplatin for stage Ic–IV epithelial ovarian cancer or primary peritoneal cancer. Severe or life-threatening neutropenia and neutropenic complications occurred more frequently in patients receiving docetaxel and carboplatin, whereas neurotoxicity was more common in patients receiving paclitaxel and carboplatin.

Monotherapy

Carboplatin also has been used as a single agent in the first-line treatment of advanced ovarian cancer†. However, the specific role of carboplatin monotherapy for this advanced cancer remains to be established.

In a large randomized trial known as the ICON3 (International Collaborative Ovarian Neoplasm 3) trial, 2074 patients with invasive ovarian cancer were randomly assigned to receive carboplatin alone, carboplatin and paclitaxel, or cyclophosphamide/doxorubicin/cisplatin (also known as CAP). About 95% of the patients were randomly assigned to a control group (carboplatin alone or CAP) or the standard regimen (carboplatin and paclitaxel) on a 2:1 basis favoring the control group. Patients enrolled in the study had invasive ovarian cancer that was FIGO stage I (9%), FIGO stage II (11%), FIGO stage III (64%), or FIGO stage IV (16%). Treatment regimens consisted of carboplatin at the dose required to obtain an AUC of 5–6 mg/mL per minute; paclitaxel 175 mg/m² IV over 3 hours followed by carboplatin (at the same dose used for carboplatin monotherapy); or cyclophosphamide 500 mg/m², doxorubicin 50 mg/m², and cisplatin 50 mg/m². At least 80% of the patients received 6 cycles of chemotherapy, and approximately one-third of patients receiving a control regimen (carboplatin alone or CAP) received taxane-based therapy as second-line treatment upon progression of disease.

At a median follow-up of 4.25 years, median overall survival and median progression-free survival were similar among the treatment groups. Alopecia, fever, and sensory neuropathy occurred more frequently in patients receiving carboplatin combined with paclitaxel than in those receiving carboplatin alone. Sensory neuropathy also occurred more frequently in patients receiving carboplatin and paclitaxel than in those receiving CAP. Fever occurred more frequently in patients receiving CAP than in those receiving carboplatin and paclitaxel.

The combination regimen of carboplatin plus paclitaxel generally remains preferred for the initial treatment of advanced ovarian cancer. However, because of the comparable efficacy and lesser toxicity demonstrated in this randomized trial, some clinicians consider single-agent carboplatin a reasonable option for the first-line treatment of advanced ovarian cancer.

Second-line Therapy for Advanced Ovarian Epithelial Cancer
Combination Chemotherapy

Carboplatin is being studied for use in combination regimens for the second-line treatment of advanced ovarian epithelial cancer†. Most experience to date has been with platinum-based regimens that included paclitaxel.

Combined analysis of data from 2 randomized trials in which a total of 802 patients with platinum-responsive ovarian cancer received either paclitaxel with platinum-based chemotherapy or conventional platinum-based chemotherapy for relapsed disease suggested a survival benefit associated with combination therapy. The median age of the patients was 59–60 years, and 75% of the patients did not experience relapse of ovarian cancer until at least 12 months following prior therapy. About 92% of patients had received only 1 prior line of treatment, and prior therapy included a taxane in only 43% of patients. Inclusion criteria and treatment regimens differed among the 3 protocols used in the 2 randomized trials.

In all 3 protocols, courses of treatment were administered every 3 weeks. Treatment regimens included carboplatin alone in 71% of patients receiving a platinum-based regimen alone and paclitaxel combined with carboplatin in 80% of patients receiving combination therapy. Dosages for the agents were paclitaxel 175 mg/m² or 185 mg/m² administered as a 3-hour IV infusion; cisplatin 75 mg/m² as monotherapy or 50 mg/m² in combination; carboplatin at the dose required to obtain a minimum AUC of 5–6 mg/mL per minute.

At a median follow-up of 3.5 years, median overall survival and median progression-free survival were prolonged in patients receiving paclitaxel and platinum-based chemotherapy versus platinum-based chemotherapy alone. Grade 2–4 neurologic toxicity (20 versus 1%) and alopecia (86 versus 25%) occurred more frequently in patients receiving combination therapy with paclitaxel and a platinum agent than in those receiving a platinum agent alone.

Carboplatin also is being studied in combination with other agents for the treatment of relapsed ovarian cancer. In a phase III randomized trial, patients with platinum-responsive recurrent ovarian cancer receiving combination therapy with carboplatin and gemcitabine appear to have prolonged progression-free survival compared with those receiving carboplatin alone; combination therapy was associated with a higher frequency of grade 3 or 4 hematologic toxicity.

Monotherapy

Carboplatin is used alone as second-line (salvage) therapy for the palliative treatment of patients with advanced ovarian carcinoma who have recurrence following an initial chemotherapy regimen, including ones that had cisplatin as a component. Either cisplatin or carboplatin can be used when retreatment is indicated in patients with platinum-responsive disease who relapse; however, some clinicians suggest that carboplatin may be preferred because it is associated with a more favorable toxicity profile than cisplatin.

Although some patients who failed to respond to cisplatin or had a response of only short duration have responded to carboplatin, nonplatinum-based regimens generally are preferred for retreatment of patients with platinum-refractory disease.

Adjuvant Therapy for Early-stage Ovarian Epithelial Cancer

Carboplatin also has been used alone or in combination therapy for the adjuvant treatment of early-stage ovarian cancer†. In 2 large randomized trials, patients receiving adjuvant therapy with single-agent or combination platinum-based therapy experienced prolonged overall survival and/or prolonged recurrence-free survival compared with patients undergoing observation (i.e., no adjuvant chemotherapy until chemotherapy was clinically indicated). However, evidence from one study (EORTC–ACTION trial) suggests that survival benefit may be limited to patients whose early-stage disease is associated with a poorer prognosis.

In a large randomized trial known as the EORTC–ACTION trial (i.e., European Organisation for Research and Treatment of Cancer–Adjuvant ChemoTherapy in Ovarian Neoplasm trial), 448 patients who underwent appropriate surgery and had disease identified with surgical staging as any of the qualifying FIGO stages (i.e., stages Ia–Ib, grade II–III; all stages Ic and IIa; and all stages I–IIa with

clear-cell epithelial cancer of the ovary) were randomly assigned to either adjuvant chemotherapy or observation. The median age of patients in the study was 54–55 years.

Adjuvant chemotherapy consisted of at least 4 courses (but preferably 6 courses) of a platinum-based regimen following surgery. Platinum-based therapy included single-agent therapy or combination therapy with either carboplatin (at a required dose of 350 mg/m²) or cisplatin (at a required dose of 75 mg/m²). Most patients in the chemotherapy arm received cisplatin combined with cyclophosphamide (about half of the patients) or single-agent carboplatin (about one third of the patients).

At a median follow-up of 5.5 years, patients receiving adjuvant chemotherapy had similar 5-year overall survival (85 versus 78%) and prolonged recurrence-free survival (76 versus 68%) compared with patients under observation. About 66% of the patients in the trial had undergone nonoptimal surgical staging, and completeness of surgical staging was identified as an independent prognostic factor. Optimal surgical staging of ovarian cancer minimizes the likelihood of undetected residual disease. Subgroup analysis showed that overall survival and recurrence-free survival were prolonged in patients with nonoptimally staged disease who received adjuvant chemotherapy, but not in patients with optimally staged disease who received adjuvant chemotherapy. The results of this analysis suggest that the observed benefit of adjuvant therapy may be limited to patients with inadequately staged epithelial ovarian cancer who are likely to have appreciable residual disease.

In another large randomized trial known as the ICON1 (International Collaborative Ovarian Neoplasm 1) trial, 477 patients with early-stage ovarian cancer were randomly assigned to either adjuvant chemotherapy or observation. The adequacy of surgical staging was not monitored; 93% of the patients had FIGO stage I disease, and most patients had well differentiated (32%) or moderately differentiated (41%) tumors. The median age of patients in the study was 55 years.

Recommended adjuvant chemotherapy following surgery consisted of 6 courses of a platinum-based regimen administered at 3-week intervals. Platinum-based therapy included either carboplatin or cisplatin, as single-agent therapy or in combination therapy (e.g., cyclophosphamide, doxorubicin, and cisplatin, also known as CAP). Using the Calvert formula, the recommended dose of carboplatin when used as a single agent was based on the dose required to obtain an area under the plasma concentration-time curve (AUC) of 5 mg/mL per minute; the recommended dose of carboplatin when used in combination was based on the dose required to obtain an AUC of 4 mg/mL per minute. The recommended dose of cisplatin when used as a single agent was 70 mg/m². The recommended doses for the CAP regimen were cyclophosphamide 500 mg/m², doxorubicin 50 mg/m², and cisplatin 50 mg/m².

Of the 241 patients assigned to adjuvant chemotherapy, 197 patients received chemotherapy that was documented; among these patients, 171 (87%) received single-agent carboplatin, 21 (11%) received cisplatin-based combination therapy, 3 (2%) received carboplatin-based combination therapy, 1 (less than 1%) received single-agent cisplatin, and 1 (less than 1%) received an unspecified regimen. Among the patients receiving adjuvant chemotherapy, a total of 168 patients (85%) received all 6 cycles of chemotherapy but 65 patients required delayed doses or reduced dosage typically because of treatment toxicity.

At a median follow-up of 4.25 years, patients receiving adjuvant chemotherapy had prolonged 5-year overall survival (79 versus 70%; hazard ratio: 0.66) and prolonged 5-year recurrence-free survival (73 versus 62%; hazard ratio: 0.65) compared with patients under observation.

Interpretation of the results of each of the 2 randomized trials is limited by the small sample size; enrollment in both studies was stopped before the planned number of patients (i.e., at least 1000 patients in the ACTION trial and 2000 patients in the ICON1 trial) was accrued. Although the outcomes of the 2 randomized trials were similar, some important differences between the studies include the broader inclusion criteria and lack of strict surgical staging in the ICON1 trial. Combined analysis of the data from the ACTION and the ICON1 trials showed that at a median follow-up of at least 4 years, patients receiving adjuvant chemotherapy had prolonged 5-year overall survival (82 versus 74%; hazard ratio: 0.67) and prolonged 5-year recurrence-free survival (76 versus 65%; hazard ratio: 0.64) compared with patients under observation. Subgroup analyses of the combined data from the 2 trials according to age, tumor stage, histologic cell type, and cell differentiation did not identify any prognostic factor for the effect of adjuvant chemotherapy; subgroup analysis according to the completeness of surgical staging was not done because information about surgical staging was not collected in the ICON1 trial.

In patients with FIGO stage Ia or Ib ovarian epithelial cancer, surgery alone generally is adequate. However, some prognostic factors, including grade III tumor, densely adherent tumor, or FIGO stage Ic disease, are associated with higher risk of recurrence of the disease, and additional treatment options may be considered. The results of these 2 randomized trials, individually or combined, suggest that adjuvant chemotherapy may benefit some patients with early-stage (FIGO stage I or II) ovarian epithelial cancer. However, further study is needed to differentiate patients with good-prognosis early-stage ovarian epithelial cancer who can be treated with surgery alone from patients with poor-prognosis early-stage disease who may benefit from surgery with immediate adjuvant chemotherapy. Various regimens were used for adjuvant chemotherapy in the 2 trials, and further study also is needed to compare the efficacy and toxicity of different regimens.

● Lung Cancer

Small Cell Lung Cancer

Carboplatin is used as a component of combination regimens for the treatment of small cell lung cancer†. Combination chemotherapy regimens are superior to single-agent therapy for the treatment of small cell lung cancer and moderately intensive drug doses are superior to doses that produce minimal toxicity. Various regimens have been used in combination therapy and many 2- to 4-drug combination regimens, including carboplatin-containing regimens, have produced objective response rates of 65–90 or 70–85% and complete response rates of 45–75 or 20–30% in patients with limited-stage or extensive-stage disease, respectively.

Carboplatin-containing regimens are used in chemotherapy for extensive-stage small cell lung cancer and in combined modality treatment (i.e., combination chemotherapy with concurrent thoracic irradiation administered early in the course of treatment) for limited-stage disease. In the treatment of small cell lung cancer, carboplatin has been used in conjunction with etoposide with or without ifosfamide. In a randomized study, patients with small cell lung cancer receiving carboplatin and etoposide had similar response rates and median survival but less toxicity than those receiving cisplatin and etoposide.

Although optimum duration of chemotherapy has not been clearly defined, additional improvement in survival has not been observed when the duration of drug administration exceeds 3–6 or 6 months in patients with limited-stage or extensive-stage small cell lung cancer, respectively. While efficacy of the various available regimens is continually being evaluated, combination chemotherapy regimens containing carboplatin and etoposide (with or without ifosfamide) currently are considered preferred or alternative regimens for the treatment of small cell lung carcinoma.

Because the current prognosis for small cell lung carcinoma is unsatisfactory regardless of stage and despite considerable diagnostic and therapeutic advances, all patients with this cancer are candidates for inclusion in clinical trials at the time of diagnosis.

Non-small Cell Lung Cancer

Carboplatin is an active agent in non-small cell lung carcinoma†. A small survival benefit has been demonstrated for the use of platinum-based (cisplatin) chemotherapy alone or combined with radiation therapy in selected patients with metastatic or unresectable, locally advanced non-small cell lung cancer who have a good performance status.

Carboplatin in combination with paclitaxel is used as an alternative to cisplatin-containing regimens in the treatment of advanced non-small cell lung cancer. Similar response rates and median survival were observed in a randomized trial in which patients received carboplatin and paclitaxel versus regimens of cisplatin in combination with paclitaxel, gemcitabine, or docetaxel for advanced non-small cell lung cancer. However, in another randomized trial, response rates were similar but median survival was shorter for patients receiving carboplatin and paclitaxel than for those receiving cisplatin and paclitaxel for advanced non-small cell lung cancer. In other randomized trials, response rates and median survival were similar in patients receiving either carboplatin and paclitaxel or cisplatin and vinorelbine for advanced non-small cell lung cancer; grade 3 peripheral neurotoxicity occurred more frequently in patients receiving paclitaxel and carboplatin whereas leukopenia/neutropenia and nausea and vomiting were more frequent in patients receiving vinorelbine and cisplatin.

Carboplatin also is used as an alternative to cisplatin in combination with docetaxel for the treatment of advanced non-small cell lung cancer. In a randomized phase III trial comparing a platinum agent and docetaxel with cisplatin and vinorelbine for the treatment of locally advanced, recurrent, or metastatic non-small cell lung cancer, patients receiving carboplatin and docetaxel had similar response rates and median survival as those receiving cisplatin and vinorelbine; higher response rates and a trend toward prolonged median survival were observed in patients receiving cisplatin and docetaxel compared with those receiving cisplatin and vinorelbine.

Various chemotherapy regimens used alone or in combination with other treatment modalities, such as radiation therapy, are continually being evaluated for the treatment of advanced non-small cell lung cancer. Because current treatment is not satisfactory for almost all patients with non-small cell lung cancer except selected patients with early-stage, resectable disease, all patients may be considered for enrollment in clinical trials at the time of diagnosis.

● Cervical Cancer

The role of carboplatin in the treatment of cervical cancer† remains to be established. (See Uses: Cervical Cancer in Cisplatin 10:00 for an overview of treatment for cervical cancer.)

Concurrent Chemotherapy and Radiation Therapy for Invasive Cervical Cancer

Concurrent platinum (i.e., cisplatin)-containing chemotherapy and radiation therapy is recommended in women with invasive cervical cancer (FIGO stage IB2 through IVA disease or FIGO stage IA2, IB, or IIA disease with poor prognostic factors). Although carboplatin often is used as a less toxic substitute for cisplatin, current evidence supports the use of cisplatin in chemotherapy regimens given concurrently with radiation therapy in patients with locally advanced cervical cancer, and similar benefit with the use of carboplatin-containing chemotherapy cannot be assumed.

Metastatic or Recurrent Cervical Cancer

Carboplatin is an active agent in the treatment of metastatic or recurrent cervical cancer†. Objective response rates of 15% have been reported with the use of carboplatin as a single agent for the treatment of metastatic or recurrent squamous cervical cancer. Because of its lesser toxicity, carboplatin may be considered as an alternative to cisplatin, particularly in patients with nephrotoxicity or neurotoxicity caused by advanced cervical tumor who are not suitable candidates for cisplatin therapy. However, randomized controlled trials comparing carboplatin and cisplatin have not been performed to date, and because of superior response rates and lesser hematologic toxicity, most experts consider cisplatin the current drug of choice in the treatment of advanced cervical cancer, particularly in patients who have received radiation therapy. Some experts suggest that study of higher dosages and various dosage schedules is needed to fully establish the activity of carboplatin in advanced cervical cancer.

Various single agents and combination regimens for the treatment of advanced cervical cancer have been evaluated mostly in phase II studies, and optimal treatment has not been established. Combination regimens have not been consistently shown to be superior to the use of single agents, such as cisplatin, one of the most active drugs in the treatment of metastatic or recurrent cervical cancer. In addition, the benefit of chemotherapy versus best supportive care has not been studied in patients with metastatic or recurrent cervical cancer. Because the prognosis of patients with advanced cervical cancer remains poor and optimal therapy has not been established, all such patients may be considered for enrollment in clinical trials investigating new agents or combination regimens.

● Head and Neck Cancer

Carboplatin may be useful in the treatment of recurrent or metastatic squamous cell carcinoma of the head and neck†. Therapy that includes carboplatin has been suggested as one of several alternatives to various cisplatin-containing regimens for recurrent or metastatic squamous cell carcinoma of the head and neck, but experience with carboplatin is less extensive than with cisplatin. In a randomized study, patients with recurrent or metastatic squamous cell carcinoma of the head and neck who received cisplatin and fluorouracil, carboplatin and fluorouracil, or methotrexate alone had objective response rates of 32, 21, and 10%, respectively. Median survival was similar among the groups. Combination chemotherapy was associated with increased toxicity (particularly hematologic toxicity for cisplatin and carboplatin and renal toxicity for cisplatin).

In males younger than 50 years of age with metastatic squamous neck cancer who have a poorly differentiated tumor, an occult primary, and elevated β-human chorionic gonadotropin (β-hCG) and α-fetoprotein (AFP), chemotherapy with a platinum-containing regimen should be considered because these tumors may respond to such therapy in a manner similar to extragonadal germ cell malignancies. Although surgical resection, radiation therapy, or both are preferred therapy for the initial management of cancer of the head and neck, chemotherapy before or after surgery or radiation therapy can be considered for such tumors.

● **Wilms' Tumor**

Carboplatin has shown activity in the management of Wilms' tumor†. Second-line (salvage) therapy with ifosfamide, carboplatin, and etoposide may be considered for patients with recurrent tumors of unfavorable histology, abdominal recurrence after radiation therapy, or recurrence within 6 months of nephrectomy or after initial 3-drug combination chemotherapy (e.g., vincristine, dactinomycin, and doxorubicin); however, this regimen is associated with substantial hematologic toxicity. Cyclophosphamide and etoposide alternating with carboplatin and etoposide has been used as an induction regimen preceding surgery and then as maintenance chemotherapy for patients with high-risk, relapsed Wilms' tumor. Patients with recurrent disease failing to respond to such attempts with salvage therapy should be offered treatment under protocol conditions in ongoing clinical trials.

● **Brain Tumors**

Carboplatin has been used for the palliative treatment of various primary brain tumors†. Regimens that include carboplatin have been used principally in the treatment of germ cell tumors. Most primary brain tumors are treated with surgery and/or radiation therapy, but adjuvant chemotherapy may prolong survival in some tumor types and has increased disease-free survival in patients with medulloblastoma, certain germ cell tumors, and gliomas.

Malignant Gliomas

Astrocytic Tumors

Carboplatin has shown activity in the treatment of progressive or recurrent low-grade gliomas in children†. Use of carboplatin in combination with vincristine for the treatment of progressive low-grade gliomas in children is being investigated.

Responses to IV carboplatin have been observed in adults with recurrent gliomas, including those who had received previous chemotherapy with nitrosoureas.

Medulloblastoma

Carboplatin has shown activity in the treatment of recurrent medulloblastoma†. The use of carboplatin in myeloablative chemotherapy regimens (e.g., carboplatin, thiotepa, and etoposide) with autologous bone marrow or stem cell rescue has been studied in a limited number of children with recurrent medulloblastoma. In children with newly diagnosed medulloblastoma, combination regimens containing carboplatin are being investigated for use as neoadjuvant therapy preceding radiation therapy or as a component of intensive chemotherapy accompanied by autologous bone marrow rescue to avoid the need for radiotherapy in young children. Further study is needed to compare the efficacy and toxicity of carboplatin versus cisplatin in the treatment of medulloblastoma. (For further discussion of the treatment of medulloblastoma, see Uses: Brain Tumors in Cisplatin 10:00.)

Intracranial Germ Cell Tumors

Combination therapy with a platinum-containing agent (i.e., cisplatin or carboplatin) and etoposide is used in the treatment of intracranial germ cell tumors†.

● **Neuroblastoma**

Carboplatin is used as a component of combination therapy for neuroblastoma†. Combination chemotherapy with moderate doses of carboplatin, cyclophosphamide, doxorubicin, and etoposide is used in conjunction with surgery (with or without radiation therapy) for the treatment of neuroblastoma in patients with intermediate-risk tumors or, in some cases, low-risk tumors. Although surgery alone typically is adequate for the treatment of low-risk tumors, combination chemotherapy is administered if surgical resection is incomplete (less than 50% of the primary tumor is resected) or if life-threatening or organ-threatening symptomatic disease is present (e.g., spinal cord compression). In patients with high-risk tumors, aggressive chemotherapy using higher doses of these drugs and additional drugs (e.g., ifosfamide, high-dose cisplatin, vincristine) is used. If high-risk disease responds to the initial regimen of chemotherapy, further therapy consists of surgical resection of the primary tumor, myeloablative therapy and autologous stem cell transplantation (bone marrow transplantation or peripheral blood stem

cell transplantation), and radiation therapy (radiation to the primary tumor site and sometimes total-body irradiation); following recovery, 6 months of therapy with oral 13-*cis*-retinoic acid (isotretinoin) is administered.

● **Testicular Cancer**

Randomized trials indicate that a cisplatin-based regimen (i.e., cisplatin/etoposide or cisplatin/etoposide/bleomycin) is more effective than a carboplatin-based regimen (i.e., carboplatin/etoposide or carboplatin/etoposide/bleomycin) in the initial treatment of good-prognosis metastatic nonseminomatous germ cell tumors, and treatment with a carboplatin regimen generally is reserved for patients who do not tolerate or who refuse cisplatin. Limited data suggest that high-dose carboplatin and etoposide may be effective in the treatment of relapsed or refractory germ cell tumors† in some patients. High-dose carboplatin and etoposide with autologous bone marrow transplant has been associated with complete remission in 10–20% of patients with cisplatin-resistant germ cell tumors. Even higher rates of durable complete response (exceeding 50%) have been observed when high-dose carboplatin and etoposide, followed by peripheral blood stem cell transplantation or autologous bone marrow transplantation, is used as initial salvage therapy in patients with relapsed testicular cancer.

● **Bladder Cancer**

Carboplatin has been substituted as a less toxic alternative to cisplatin in some patients receiving combination chemotherapy for advanced bladder cancer†. Inadequate dosing of carboplatin may have contributed to its lesser efficacy compared with cisplatin in earlier studies of platinum-based regimens for the treatment of advanced or metastatic bladder cancer.

Combination therapy with paclitaxel followed by carboplatin is being investigated as a tolerable and active regimen in patients with advanced bladder cancer, including patients with abnormal renal function. In a phase III randomized trial, 80 patients received paclitaxel 225 mg/m² IV over 3 hours, followed by carboplatin (at the dose required to obtain an AUC of 6 mg/mL per minute) IV over 30 minutes, every 21 days, or the standard MVAC regimen (i.e., cisplatin, methotrexate, vinblastine, and doxorubicin) every 28 days, for a maximum of 6 treatment cycles. The response rates were similar; at a median follow-up of 2.7 years, patients receiving paclitaxel and carboplatin had similar median overall survival as patients receiving MVAC. Severe neutropenia occurred more frequently in patients receiving MVAC than in those receiving paclitaxel and carboplatin. Interpretation of the results is limited by the failure to meet the planned accrual of 330 patients in the trial.

● **Retinoblastoma**

Carboplatin has been used in combination with etoposide in a limited number of children† with recurrent or progressive retinoblastoma†. While regimens including doxorubicin, cyclophosphamide, and/or vincristine have been used, some clinicians consider carboplatin one of several alternative agents that can be used in children with extraocular retinoblastoma. Therapy with carboplatin in combination with etoposide has been associated with partial or complete responses in up to 85% of children with recurrent disease; the role of carboplatin-containing regimens as adjuvant therapy after enucleation or as neoadjuvant therapy of ocular tumors remains to be determined.

● **Other Uses**

Carboplatin has been used for the treatment of breast cancer†. In a phase III randomized trial, higher response rates and prolonged median progression-free survival were observed with the addition of carboplatin to trastuzumab and paclitaxel for the treatment of HER2-overexpressing metastatic breast cancer; grade 4 neutropenia occurred more frequently in patients receiving carboplatin with trastuzumab and paclitaxel.

Carboplatin is being studied for use in the treatment of endometrial cancer†. A phase III randomized trial comparing carboplatin and paclitaxel versus doxorubicin, cisplatin, paclitaxel and filgrastim (G-CSF) for advanced or recurrent endometrial cancer is under way.

DOSAGE AND ADMINISTRATION

● **Reconstitution and Administration**

Carboplatin is administered by IV infusion. Infusions of the drug usually are administered IV over a period of 15 minutes or longer; carboplatin has been administered by continuous IV infusion over 24 hours. Unlike precautions required during cisplatin administration, pretreatment and posttreatment hydration and/or diuresis are *not* necessary when carboplatin is administered. Carboplatin also has been administered intraperitoneally†. Needles, syringes, catheters, and IV administration sets that contain aluminum parts which may come in contact with carboplatin should *not* be used for preparation or administration of the drug. (See Chemistry and Stability: Stability.) The usual precautions for handling and preparing cytotoxic drugs should be observed when preparing or administering carboplatin.

Commercially available carboplatin injection is a premixed aqueous solution containing 10 mg of carboplatin per mL. The manufacturer states that carboplatin aqueous solution may be further diluted with 0.9% sodium chloride injection or 5% dextrose injection to a concentration as low as 0.5 mg/mL. Prior to administration, carboplatin solutions should be inspected visually for particulate matter and discoloration.

● Dosage

Dosage of carboplatin must be based on the clinical, renal, and hematologic response and tolerance of the patient in order to obtain optimum therapeutic response with minimum adverse effects. While initial carboplatin dosage can be based on body surface area, dosage may be more accurately calculated using formula dosing methods based on the patient's renal function. Because renal function often is reduced in geriatric patients, the manufacturer recommends that dosing formulas incorporating estimates of glomerular filtration rate be used in geriatric patients to help minimize the risk of toxicity. (See Dosage: Individualization of Dosage.) The manufacturer recommends that carboplatin generally be given no more frequently than once every 4 weeks at usual dosage. *A repeat course of carboplatin should not be administered until the patient's hematologic functions are within acceptable limits, and precautions must always be taken to treat a hypersensitivity reaction if it occurs.* (See Cautions: Precautions and Contraindications.) When carboplatin is used as a component of a multiple-drug regimen, clinicians should consult published protocols for the dosage of each chemotherapeutic agent and the method and sequence of administration.

Because carboplatin is an antineoplastic agent of moderate emetic risk, antiemetic therapy is recommended. (See Cautions: GI Effects.)

Ovarian Cancer

For the treatment of advanced ovarian carcinoma (stage III and IV) in combination chemotherapy regimens (i.e., with cyclophosphamide), an initial IV carboplatin dose of 300 mg/m² can be used in adults. Subsequent dosage of the drug should be adjusted according to the patient's hematologic tolerance of the previous dose (e.g., as described below); doses should not be administered until the patient's hematologic function is within acceptable limits. Alternatively, carboplatin dosage can be calculated using formula dosing methods based on renal function. (See Dosage: Individualization of Dosage.) A course of carboplatin consists of single doses administered once every 4 weeks (or longer if delayed for hematologic toxicity) for a total of 6 cycles.

When carboplatin is used alone in the treatment of recurrent ovarian carcinoma, an initial dose of 360 mg/m² can be used, administering the drug once every 4 weeks (or longer if delayed for hematologic toxicity). Doses of carboplatin generally should not be repeated until the patient's hematologic function is within acceptable limits, adjusting dosage according to the patient's hematologic tolerance of the most recent dose (e.g., as described in the following paragraph).

For patients who experience no hematologic toxicity (i.e., platelet counts greater than 100,000/mm³ and neutrophil counts greater than 2000/mm³) with the previous dose, dosage of carboplatin in single or combination therapy may be increased by 25%. In studies used to establish efficacy of carboplatin in combination with cyclophosphamide, dosage escalation above 25% of the initial dose was not evaluated. For patients who experience only mild to moderate hematologic toxicity (i.e., platelet counts of 50,000–100,000 mm³ or neutrophil counts of 500–2000/mm³, respectively) with the previous dose, dosage adjustment is not necessary in single agent or combination regimens. For patients who experience moderate to severe hematologic toxicity (e.g., platelet counts lower than 50,000 mm³ or neutrophil counts lower than 500/mm³, respectively) with the previous dose, the dosage of carboplatin in single agent or combination regimens should be reduced by 25%. In studies used to establish efficacy of carboplatin in stage III and IV ovarian carcinoma, carboplatin therapy was continued only at the investigator's discretion in patients who experienced hematologic toxicity following 2 dosage

reductions (i.e., while receiving a carboplatin dosage equivalent to 50% of the initial dosage). Some authorities suggest that, rather than compromise carboplatin's efficacy by dosage reduction in patients who experience substantial hematologic toxicity, carboplatin therapy should be replaced with cisplatin (which is less myelosuppressive) therapy if possible. Whether concomitant hematopoietic agents (colony-stimulating factor) can obviate carboplatin dosage reduction in patients who experience substantial hematologic toxicity remains to be established.

Other Neoplasms

Dosage of carboplatin used in the treatment of other malignant neoplasms† generally has been similar to that used in the treatment of ovarian carcinoma; however, various dosage schedules and regimens of carboplatin alone or in conjunction with other antineoplastic agents have been used. Clinicians should consult published protocols for dosages and the method and sequence of administration. In general, escalation of carboplatin dosages above 400 mg/m² results in substantial hematologic toxicity, but high-dose carboplatin (900–2000 mg/m²) has been used with colony-stimulating factors, autologous bone marrow rescue, and/or peripheral stem cell rescue.

Individualization of Dosage

Several alternative methods for calculating initial carboplatin dosage have been suggested based on the patient's pretreatment renal function or pretreatment renal function and desired platelet nadir. These methods, compared with empiric dosage calculations based only on body surface area, compensate for patient variations in pretreatment renal function that may otherwise result in carboplatin underdosing (e.g., in patients with above average renal function) or overdosing (e.g., in patients with impaired renal function). The methods incorporate considerations about the direct relationship between renal clearance of carboplatin and glomerular filtration rate (GFR) over widely ranging renal function and about the predictive relationship between the area under the plasma concentration-time curve (AUC) of ultrafilterable platinum and the degree of subsequent thrombocytopenia and neutropenia.

One commonly employed method for carboplatin dosage calculation in adults is the Calvert formula based on the patient's GFR (in mL/minute) and the target AUC (in mg/mL per minute). *Using the Calvert formula, carboplatin dosage is calculated in mg, not mg/m².* Because the predictability of this calculation has been established using chromic edetate Cr 51 (^{51}Cr-EDTA) clearance to establish GFR, some clinicians have recommended that other methods for estimating creatinine clearance (e.g., Cockcroft-Gault equation, Jelliffe equation) not be substituted for this determination since carboplatin dosing based on such estimates may not be predictive. However, other clinicians have successfully employed such methods for estimating creatinine clearance because of their simplicity and/or unavailability of ^{51}Cr-EDTA clearance, although they may not be as precisely predictive.

Calvert Formula for Carboplatin Dosing:

total dose (mg) =

target AUC (in mg/mL per min) x [GFR (in mL/min) + 25]

In studies used to derive the Calvert formula, the GFR was measured by ^{51}Cr-EDTA, which correlates well with creatinine clearance. A target AUC of 5 (range: 4–6) mg/mL per minute appears to provide the most appropriate dosage range for use of carboplatin alone in patients previously treated with chemotherapeutic agents. Analysis of toxicity in previously treated patients receiving carboplatin alone indicates that substantial thrombocytopenia (grade 3 or 4 [platelet counts less than 50,000/ mm³]) occurs in 16% and leukopenia (grade 3 or 4 [leukocyte counts less than 200,000/ mm³]) occurs in 13% of patients with target AUCs of 4–5 mg/mL per minute. A higher incidence of myelotoxicity was reported in patients with target AUCs of 6–7 mg/mL per minute with thrombocytopenia (grade 3 or 4) occurring in 33% and leukopenia (grade 3 or 4) occurring in 34% of patients. For patients who previously did not receive chemotherapy, a target AUC of 7 (range: 6–8) mg/mL per minute has been recommended when carboplatin is used alone. Higher target AUCs (e.g., 7.5 mg/mL) also have been used (e.g., when carboplatin was used as a component of high-intensity dosing with paclitaxel and a hematopoietic agent for non-small cell lung carcinoma). Subsequent carboplatin dosage has been adjusted according to hematologic tolerance to the previous dose (e.g., reducing the dose by 25% for moderate to severe hematologic toxicity).

The Calvert formula is not sufficiently accurate to determine carboplatin dosage for children or for adults with severe renal impairment (i.e., GFR less than 20 mL/minute); therefore, this formula should *not* be used in such patients.

An alternative pediatric formula has been suggested, but specialized references should be consulted.

Another method (the Chatelut or French formula) for carboplatin dosage calculation in adults that is simplified by not requiring determination of GFR has been suggested. While this method is more recent and therefore has not been employed as extensively as the Calvert method, it offers a means of estimating carboplatin clearance that relies only on patient age, gender, and serum creatinine concentration. *Using the Chatelut formula, carboplatin dosage is calculated in mg, not mg/m^2.*

Chatelut (French) Formula for Carboplatin Dosing:

total dose (mg) = target AUC (in mg/mL/min) × carboplatin clearance (in mL/min)

When carboplatin clearance is calculated as follows:

Carboplatin clearance (mL/min) =

$$[0.134 \times wt] + \frac{[218 \times wt \times (1 - \{0.00457 \times age\})] \times [1 - \{0.314 \times gender\}]}{serum\ creatinine\ (\mu mol/L)}$$

*where weight is in kg, age is in years,
and gender is 0 for males and 1 for females*

This formula should *not* be used for calculating carboplatin dosage in pediatric patients or those undergoing hemodialysis.

● Dosage in Renal Impairment

Dosage of carboplatin should be reduced in patients with impaired renal function. Because patients with creatinine clearances less than 60 mL/minute are at increased risk of myelosuppression during carboplatin therapy, dosage in such patients should be adjusted according to the degree of renal impairment. When carboplatin is used alone in the treatment of recurrent ovarian carcinoma in patients with renal impairment, the manufacturer recommends that those with creatinine clearances of 41–59 mL/minute receive an initial dose of 250 mg/m^2 and those with creatinine clearances of 16–40 mL/minute receive an initial dose of 200 mg/m^2. The incidence of severe leukopenia, neutropenia, or thrombocytopenia in these patients at these dosages is about 25%. Subsequent carboplatin dosage should be adjusted according to the patient's hematologic tolerance to the previous dose. Although carboplatin has been used in a limited number of patients with creatinine clearances less than 15 mL/minute, the manufacturer states that experience in these patients is too limited to make dosage recommendations.

CAUTIONS

Although carboplatin and cisplatin are both platinum-coordination compounds and have similar mechanism(s) of action, they have different toxicologic profiles, with carboplatin being better tolerated overall. While the major dose-limiting adverse effects associated with cisplatin therapy include nonhematologic toxicities such as nephrotoxicity, ototoxicity, neurotoxicity, and emesis, the major dose-limiting adverse effects associated with carboplatin therapy are hematologic toxicities such as thrombocytopenia and leukopenia. The improved overall toxicity profile of carboplatin relative to cisplatin appears to result at least partly from the presence of a cyclobutane dicarboxylate ligand on carboplatin which results in a more stable compound; decreased reactivity with macromolecules and differences in renal handling appear to be important factors in this improvement. Differences in the toxicity and pharmacokinetic profiles of the drugs may be important determinants in the selection of carboplatin versus cisplatin for specific patients. In addition, differences in toxicity profile may make it possible to escalate carboplatin dosages beyond those usually recommended particularly when autologous bone marrow transplantation (ABMT), peripheral stem cell transplantation, and/or hematopoietic agents (colony-stimulating factors) are used concomitantly.

Information on safety and efficacy of carboplatin has been obtained from clinical studies in patients with malignancy who received the drug alone or in conjunction with other antineoplastic agents (i.e., cyclophosphamide).

● Hematologic Effects

The major and dose-limiting adverse effect of carboplatin is bone marrow suppression, which is manifested as thrombocytopenia, leukopenia, neutropenia, and/or anemia and is more pronounced than that with cisplatin. Carboplatin-induced myelosuppression is dose related and appears to be most common and more severe in patients who have received prior antineoplastic therapy (especially cisplatin-containing regimens), those who are receiving concurrently or have received recently other myelosuppressive drugs or radiation therapy, and those who have renal impairment. The correlation between renal function and degree of thrombocytopenia and neutropenia is related to the pharmacokinetic characteristics of carboplatin and has resulted in the development of individualized dosing schedules based on glomerular filtration rate. (See Dosage: Individualization of Dosage, in Dosage and Administration.) Patients with poor performance status also appear to be at increased risk for severe leukopenia and thrombocytopenia during carboplatin therapy.

At usual dosages, carboplatin-induced thrombocytopenia is more common and pronounced than leukopenia. Thrombocytopenia (platelet counts less than 100,000/mm^3) occurred in about 60–70% of patients receiving usual dosages of carboplatin alone or in conjunction with cyclophosphamide in clinical trials; more severe thrombocytopenia (platelet counts less than 50,000/mm^3) occurred in 22–41% of patients. Thrombocytopenia may be cumulative and occasionally require platelet transfusions. Leukopenia (leukocyte count less than 4000/mm^3) was reported in up to 85–98% of patients receiving usual dosages of the drug alone or in conjunction with cyclophosphamide in clinical trials. Leukopenia was pronounced (leukocyte count less than 2000/mm^3) in 15–26% of patients receiving usual dosages of carboplatin alone and in 68–76% of patients receiving the drug in conjunction with cyclophosphamide. In patients who received carboplatin alone, neutrophil counts less than 2000/mm^3 occurred in 67% and neutrophil counts less than 1000/mm^3 occurred in 16–21% of patients. When the drug was used in conjunction with cyclophosphamide, neutrophil counts less than 2000/mm^3 occurred in 95–97% and counts less than 1000/mm^3 occurred in up to 84% of patients. At high doses (i.e., 1.2 g/m^2 or greater), more than 90% of patients reportedly experience grade IV thrombocytopenia and neutropenia (platelet counts less than 25,000/mm^3 and neutrophil counts less than 500/mm^3, respectively), and decreases in hemoglobin concentrations of 3–3.5 g/dL.

When carboplatin is administered alone, leukocyte and platelet nadirs generally occur 21 days (range: 14–28 days) following administration of the drug, and recovery of platelet counts (exceeding 100,000/mm^3), leukocyte counts (exceeding 4000/mm^3, and neutrophil counts (exceeding 2000/mm^3) occurs within 28 days in 90, 67, and 74% of patients, respectively. In most patients, recovery generally is adequate to permit a repeat carboplatin dose 4 weeks after a previous dose. In clinical studies, at least one episode of infection occurred in 5% of patients receiving carboplatin alone and in 14–18% of patients receiving the drug in conjunction with cyclophosphamide.

Anemia (hemoglobin less than 11 g/dL), which may be symptomatic (e.g., accompanied by asthenia), occurred in 71–91% of patients receiving usual dosages of carboplatin alone or in conjunction with cyclophosphamide in clinical trials, and anemia was severe (hemoglobin less than 8 g/dL) in 8–21% of such patients. The incidence of anemia appears to increase with increased exposure to carboplatin. Since anemia may be cumulative, transfusions may be needed during carboplatin therapy, particularly in patients receiving prolonged (e.g., more than 6 cycles) therapy. In clinical studies, bleeding was reported in 5–10% and transfusions were administered to 25–44% of patients.

While hematologic toxicity associated with the standard dosages of carboplatin usually is not of sufficient magnitude to warrant routine administration of hematopoietic agents, autologous bone marrow transplant (ABMT), peripheral stem cell transplantation, and/or colony-stimulating factors (e.g., granulocyte colony-stimulating factor) have been used in patients receiving high-dose carboplatin or carboplatin in conjunction with other myelosuppressive therapy.

● GI Effects

Nausea and/or vomiting, which generally are mild to moderate in severity, have occurred in 65–94% of patients receiving carboplatin alone or in conjunction with cyclophosphamide. Carboplatin is classified as an antineoplastic agent of *moderate emetic risk* (i.e., incidence of emesis without antiemetics exceeds 30% but does not exceed 90%). Although nausea and/or vomiting occur in most patients receiving carboplatin, the drug is substantially less emetogenic and better tolerated than cisplatin. When carboplatin is used alone, nausea occurs in 10–15% and vomiting occurs in 65–81% of patients. Nausea and vomiting usually begin within 6–12 hours after administration of carboplatin and may persist up to 24 hours or longer; in some patients, vomiting may persist for up to 3 days. Delayed vomiting beginning 24 hours or longer after chemotherapy also has occurred in some patients. The incidence and severity of emesis may be reduced by pretreatment with antiemetics, although nausea and vomiting rarely may be refractory to antiemetic therapy. Carboplatin-induced acute vomiting episodes appear to be mediated by local GI and central mechanisms involving serotonin, and are most common in patients who have received prior emetogenic antineoplastic regimens (especially cisplatin-containing regimens) and in those who are receiving other emetogenic agents concurrently.

There is some evidence that the incidence of nausea and vomiting is reduced when carboplatin is given as a 24-hour continuous IV infusion or administered IV in divided doses over 5 consecutive days rather than as a single IV infusion; however, efficacy of these administration schedules in the treatment of ovarian carcinoma has not been established. For the prevention of *acute* emesis, the American Society of Clinical Oncology (ASCO) currently recommends a 2-drug antiemetic regimen consisting of a 5-HT₃ serotonin receptor antagonist and dexamethasone given before the administration of carboplatin or other chemotherapy with moderate emetic risk. Delayed or anticipatory vomiting is more difficult to manage. For the prevention of *delayed* emesis, ASCO currently recommends single-agent therapy with dexamethasone or a 5-HT₃ serotonin receptor antagonist following the administration of carboplatin or other chemotherapy regimens with moderate emetic risk. Because anticipatory vomiting is a learned response conditioned by the severity and duration of previous emetic reactions to chemotherapy, optimal use of antiemetics for prevention of acute and delayed emesis during early courses of therapy is the most important means for preventing this effect; behavioral modification, hypnosis, and drug therapy (e.g., a benzodiazepine such as alprazolam or lorazepam [for anxiolytic, sedative, amnesic, and possibly antiemetic effects] with or without conventional antiemetics) also may be useful. For additional information on the mechanisms and management of nausea and vomiting induced by platinum compounds, see Cautions: GI Effects in Cisplatin 10:00.

Adverse GI effects other than nausea and vomiting have been reported in 21% of patients receiving carboplatin alone and in 40–50% of patients receiving carboplatin in conjunction with cyclophosphamide. When carboplatin is used alone, GI pain, diarrhea, and constipation have been reported in 6–17% of patients. Anorexia also has been reported in patients receiving carboplatin.

Mucositis (i.e., oral ulceration) has been reported in 1% of patients receiving carboplatin alone and in 6–10% of patients receiving the drug in conjunction with cyclophosphamide.

● **Nervous System Effects**

Carboplatin-containing regimens are associated with a lower incidence of, and less severe, neurotoxicity than cisplatin-containing regimens. Neurotoxicity associated with carboplatin usually is characterized by peripheral neuropathies, which generally are sensory in nature (e.g., paresthesia). Peripheral neuropathies have occurred in 4–6% of patients receiving carboplatin alone and in 13–16% of patients receiving the drug in conjunction with cyclophosphamide. Carboplatin-induced peripheral neuropathy appears to be more common in patients older than 65 years of age than in younger adults. In addition, carboplatin-induced peripheral neuropathies appear to be cumulative occurring most commonly in patients receiving prolonged therapy and/or those who have received prior cisplatin therapy; in some cases, the neurotoxicity may be a delayed effect of cisplatin rather than secondary to carboplatin. Patients with preexisting cisplatin-induced peripheral neurotoxicity generally do not experience additional neurologic deterioration during carboplatin therapy.

Adverse sensory effects, including otic and ocular effects (see Cautions: Otic and Ocular Effects) and taste abnormalities, have been reported in up to 13% of patients receiving usual dosages of carboplatin. Central neurotoxicity has been reported in 5% of patients receiving carboplatin alone and in 23–28% of patients receiving carboplatin in conjunction with cyclophosphamide. It has been suggested that central neurotoxicity in many of these patients may have been related to concomitant antiemetic therapy. Fatigue was one of the most common nonhematologic effects reported in patients receiving carboplatin concomitantly with paclitaxel.

● **Otic and Ocular Effects**

Ototoxicity has been reported in 12–13% of patients receiving usual dosages of carboplatin in conjunction with cyclophosphamide. When carboplatin has been used alone, ototoxicity and adverse sensory effects have been reported in only 1% of patients. While carboplatin is associated with a low incidence of hearing loss at usual dosages, ototoxicity may be dose-limiting at carboplatin doses of 2 g/m² or greater. The risk of ototoxicity also may be increased by concomitantly administered ototoxic drugs (e.g., aminoglycosides, furosemide, ifosfamide). (See Drug Interactions: Other Drugs.) Clinically important hearing loss has occurred in pediatric patients receiving carboplatin at higher than recommended doses in combination with other ototoxic agents.

Other adverse sensory effects, including visual abnormalities, have been reported in 4–6% of patients receiving usual dosages of carboplatin in conjunction with cyclophosphamide. Loss of vision (which can be complete for light and colors) has been reported rarely in patients receiving carboplatin doses higher than those usually recommended; improvement and/or total recovery of vision occurred within weeks after the drug was discontinued.

● **Renal and Electrolyte Effects**

Mild and transient elevations of serum creatinine and BUN concentrations have occurred in 6–22% of patients receiving carboplatin alone or in conjunction with cyclophosphamide. Acute renal failure has been reported rarely. Nephrotoxicity is less common and severe than that associated with cisplatin, and concomitant IV hydration and diuresis generally are not necessary with carboplatin. As a result, administration regimens and monitoring requirements with carboplatin generally are less complex, and outpatient therapy is easier to accomplish. However, the risk of carboplatin-induced nephrotoxicity (e.g., impaired creatinine clearance) becomes more prominent at relatively high dosages. Animal studies indicate that carboplatin's reduced nephrotoxic potential relative to cisplatin may relate to differences in renal handling of the drugs and reactivity with macroglobulins; differences in risk do not appear to correlate with renal platinum concentrations.

Carboplatin may cause electrolyte abnormalities, principally hyponatremia, hypokalemia, hypocalcemia, and/or hypomagnesemia. Such electrolyte changes, unlike those reported with cisplatin, usually are not symptomatic and do not require administration of supplemental electrolytes. Hyponatremia, hypocalcemia, and hypokalemia have been reported in 10–47% and hypomagnesemia has been reported in 29–62% of patients receiving carboplatin alone or in conjunction with cyclophosphamide.

● **Hepatic Effects**

Mild and usually transient elevations of serum alkaline phosphatase, aspartate aminotransferase (AST, SGOT), or bilirubin concentrations have been reported in 24–37, 15–23, or 5% of patients, respectively, receiving carboplatin alone or in conjunction with cyclophosphamide. Substantial abnormalities in liver function test results have been reported in a few patients receiving high doses of carboplatin (more than 4 times higher than the usually recommended dosage) and autologous bone marrow transplantation.

● **Sensitivity Reactions**

Allergic reactions have been reported in 2% of patients receiving carboplatin alone and in 10–12% of patients receiving carboplatin in conjunction with other antineoplastic agents. Allergic reactions associated with carboplatin are similar in nature and severity to those associated with other platinum-containing antineoplastic agents (e.g., cisplatin) and have included anaphylaxis and anaphylactoid reactions. Although allergic reactions usually have occurred following multiple courses of platinum-containing therapy, such reactions can occur with the initial dose. The risk of allergic reactions, including anaphylaxis, is increased in patients who previously have received treatment with platinum-containing agents. Rash, perioral tingling, urticaria, erythema, pruritus, bronchospasm, hypotension, and hypoxia have occurred within a few minutes after IV administration of carboplatin in patients who previously received a platinum-containing antineoplastic agent. Exfoliative dermatitis has been reported rarely.

In many cases, allergic reactions appear to be immediate type I IgE-mediated hypersensitivity reactions, although some reactions may result from direct, nonimmunologic histamine release. In addition, some reactions may have been secondary to mannitol (which was present in the previous formulation) hypersensitivity rather than to carboplatin. Hypersensitivity reactions may be alleviated by IV epinephrine, corticosteroids, and/or antihistamines; in some cases, continued therapy with carboplatin may be possible with prophylactic corticosteroid and antihistamine therapy. While the manufacturer states that carboplatin is contraindicated in patients with a history of sensitivity reactions to other platinum-containing compounds, switching to cisplatin may be tolerated by some, but not all, patients who have experienced hypersensitivity reactions to carboplatin and vice versa.

Other Adverse Effects

Although alopecia is uncommon in patients receiving carboplatin alone, occurring in about 2–3% of such patients, it occurs in 43–50% of patients receiving carboplatin in conjunction with cyclophosphamide. In patients receiving concurrent cyclophosphamide, the frequency and severity of alopecia was attributed to the cyclophosphamide dosage.

Pain, most likely related to tumor size, has been reported in 36–54% of patients receiving carboplatin in conjunction with cyclophosphamide. In addition, asthenia, presumably secondary to carboplatin-induced anemia, has occurred in 40–43% of patients receiving carboplatin in conjunction with cyclophosphamide. Malaise also has been reported in patients receiving the drug. Adverse respiratory and genitourinary effects have occurred in 2–6% of patients receiving carboplatin alone and in 8–12% of patients receiving the drug in conjunction with cyclophosphamide. Hemolytic uremic syndrome has occurred rarely. Myalgias/arthralgias were one of the most common nonhematologic adverse effects reported in patients receiving carboplatin concomitantly with paclitaxel; these effects were cumulative with repeated cycles.

Although not attributed to antineoplastic therapy, adverse cardiovascular effects, including cardiac failure, embolism, and cerebrovascular accident, have been reported in up to 23% of patients receiving carboplatin. Fatalities associated with cardiovascular events occurred in less than 1% of patients receiving the drug. Hypertension also has been reported in patients receiving carboplatin.

Precautions and Contraindications

Carboplatin is a highly toxic drug with a low therapeutic index, and a therapeutic response is not likely to occur without some evidence of toxicity. The drug should be used under the supervision of physicians experienced in therapy with cytotoxic agents. In addition, the manufacturer states that carboplatin should be used only when adequate treatment facilities for appropriate management of therapy and complications are readily available.

Patients receiving carboplatin should be observed closely for possible hypersensitivity reactions, and appropriate equipment for maintenance of an adequate airway and other supportive measures and agents for the treatment of such reactions (e.g., antihistamines, epinephrine, oxygen, corticosteroids) should be readily available whenever carboplatin is administered. Patients with prior exposure to other platinum-containing agents are at increased risk for carboplatin-induced allergic reactions, including anaphylaxis. The manufacturer states that carboplatin is contraindicated in patients with a history of sensitivity reactions to the drug or other platinum-containing compounds (e.g., cisplatin); however, cross-sensitivity is not absolute, and occasionally with appropriate precautions patients sensitive to one platinum-containing compound have tolerated another. Exposure (e.g., industrial) to platinum-containing compounds can cause asthma and immediate and delayed hypersensitivity reactions, and the possibility that patients with a history of such exposure may be cross-sensitive to carboplatin should be considered.

The emetogenic potential of carboplatin should be considered. (See Cautions: GI Effects.) The neurotoxic potential of the drug also should be considered, particularly in geriatric patients older than 65 years of age and patients previously treated with cisplatin. (See Cautions: Nervous System Effects.) Vision loss is possible in patients receiving carboplatin, particularly at high doses. (See Cautions: Otic and Ocular Effects.)

Because patients who receive myelosuppressive drugs experience an increased frequency of infection and/or bleeding, hematologic status must be carefully monitored. While the hematologic toxicity of carboplatin usually is moderate and reversible, severe myelosuppression may occur in patients who received prior antineoplastic therapy (especially cisplatin-containing regimens), those who are receiving concurrently or have received recently other myelosuppressive drugs or radiation therapy, and those with renal impairment. To monitor for the occurrence of carboplatin-induced bone marrow suppression, the manufacturer recommends that peripheral blood counts be performed at frequent intervals in all patients receiving the drug. In studies used to establish efficacy of carboplatin, peripheral blood counts were determined weekly. Carboplatin usually should not be administered to patients with severe bone marrow depression or substantial bleeding. Pretreatment platelet counts and performance status are important prognostic factors for severity of myelosuppression in previously treated patients. In patients who experience myelosuppression following a dose of carboplatin, the manufacturer recommends that subsequent cycles of the drug be withheld until neutrophil counts exceed 2000/mm^3 and platelet counts exceed 100,000/mm^3. Treatment of severe hematologic toxicity may consist of supportive care,

anti-infective agents for complicating infections, blood product transfusions, autologous bone marrow rescue, peripheral stem cell transplantation, and hematopoietic agents (colony-stimulating factors).

Because patients with renal impairment are at risk for severe bone marrow depression, renal function must be monitored carefully in patients receiving carboplatin. Creatinine clearance appears to most accurately reflect kidney function in patients receiving the drug. Although carboplatin has a low nephrotoxic potential, concomitant administration of an aminoglycoside has been associated with an increased risk of nephrotoxicity and/or ototoxicity. The possibility that carboplatin's nephrotoxicity may be potentiated by other nephrotoxic drugs also should be considered. (See Drug Interactions: Other Drugs.)

Pediatric Precautions

The manufacturer states that safety and efficacy of carboplatin in children have not been established. Although experience is limited, carboplatin has been used in the treatment of germ cell tumors in adolescents 16 year of age or older, in the treatment of various brain tumors or neuroblastoma in children and adolescents 6 months to 19 years of age, and in the treatment of Wilms' tumor in children 2–15 years of age. Adverse effects reported to date in children are similar to those reported in adults and include hematologic toxicity (principally thrombocytopenia), adverse GI effects such as nausea and vomiting, and hypersensitivity reactions such as urticaria, facial swelling, abdominal pain, coryza, and cough. Hearing loss also has been reported in children receiving carboplatin. (See Cautions: Otic and Ocular Effects.)

Geriatric Precautions

While the safety and efficacy of carboplatin in geriatric patients have not been established specifically, a substantial number of patients who received the drug in clinical trials as part of combination therapy for ovarian cancer were elderly (i.e., 36% were 65 years of age or older and 6% were 75 years of age or older). Age was not found to be a prognostic factor for survival in these studies.

Severe thrombocytopenia associated with carboplatin therapy occurred more frequently in geriatric patients than in younger patients. In addition, carboplatin-induced peripheral neuropathy appears to be more common in adults older than 65 years of age than in younger patients. Among a total of 1942 patients (21% of whom were 65 years of age or older) receiving carboplatin monotherapy for different tumor types, a similar incidence of adverse effects was observed in older and younger patients; other clinical experience has not revealed age-related differences among patients receiving the drug. However, the possibility of greater sensitivity of some older patients and increased risk for other effects of carboplatin related to age cannot be ruled out.

Because dosage of carboplatin generally is based on the clinical and hematologic response, renal function, and tolerance of the patient, the fact that geriatric patients may have decreased renal function as well as decreased hematopoietic function should be considered. The manufacturer recommends that dosing formulas based on estimates of glomerular filtration rate be used to determine the appropriate dosage of carboplatin in geriatric patients.

Mutagenicity and Carcinogenicity

Carboplatin is mutagenic in both in vitro and in vivo experimental models.

Although the carcinogenic potential of carboplatin has not been fully studied, the manufacturer states that drugs with similar mechanisms of action and evidence of mutagenic effects have been reported to be carcinogenic. Secondary malignancies have been reported in patients receiving carboplatin in combination with other agents.

Pregnancy, Fertility, and Lactation
Pregnancy

Carboplatin can cause fetal toxicity when administered to pregnant women, but potential benefits from use of the drug may be acceptable in certain conditions despite possible risks to the fetus. Carboplatin has been shown to be embryotoxic and teratogenic in rats. Reproductive studies in rats receiving carboplatin during organogenesis revealed evidence of embryotoxicity and teratogenicity. There are no adequate or controlled studies to date using carboplatin in pregnant women. Carboplatin should be used during pregnancy only in life-threatening situations or for disease for which safer drugs cannot be used or are ineffective. If the drug is administered during pregnancy or if the patient becomes pregnant while receiving carboplatin, the patient should be informed of the potential hazard to the fetus. Women of childbearing potential should be advised to avoid becoming pregnant during carboplatin therapy.

Fertility

The effects of carboplatin on the gonads and fertility have not been fully determined.

Lactation

It is not known whether carboplatin or its platinum-containing products are distributed into human milk. Because of the potential for serious adverse reactions to carboplatin in nursing infants if the drug were distributed into milk, nursing should be discontinued during carboplatin therapy.

DRUG INTERACTIONS

● Myelosuppressive Therapy

Concomitant use of carboplatin and other myelosuppressive agents or radiation therapy may potentiate the hematologic toxicity of the other agents and vice versa. Patients receiving concurrently or who have received recently such therapy should be monitored carefully, and dosage of the drugs and time of administration should be managed to minimize additive toxic effects. In addition, the fact that use of carboplatin in individuals who have received prior antineoplastic therapy is associated with an increased risk of bone marrow suppression should be considered.

● Other Drugs

Concomitant administration of carboplatin and aminoglycosides results in an increased risk of nephrotoxicity and/or ototoxicity, and the drugs should be used concurrently with caution. Clinically important hearing loss has been reported in children receiving carboplatin at higher than recommended doses in combination with other ototoxic medications. The manufacturer states that the renal effects of other nephrotoxic drugs may be potentiated by carboplatin.

Concomitant use of carboplatin and other emetogenic drugs or use of carboplatin in individuals who previously received emetogenic therapy is associated with an increased incidence of emesis.

ACUTE TOXICITY

● Manifestations

Limited information is available on the acute toxicity of carboplatin. Overdosage of the drug would be expected to produce complications secondary to bone marrow suppression and/or hepatotoxicity. In addition, typical nonhematologic toxicity associated with platinum-containing antineoplastic agents (e.g., nephrotoxicity, neurotoxicity, ototoxicity) would be expected to become prominent with carboplatin overdosage. Carboplatin is substantially less toxic on a mg-for-mg basis than cisplatin, and inadvertent substitution of *cisplatin* (which usually is administered at substantially lower dosages) for carboplatin has resulted in massive cisplatin overdosage, including fatalities. (See Acute Toxicity in Cisplatin 10:00.)

● Treatment

There currently is no established specific antidote for carboplatin overdosage. Management of overdosage currently consists principally in discontinuance of the drug and initiation of supportive measures appropriate for the type of toxicity observed. The use of colony-stimulating factors (CSFs), platelet transfusions, and/or red blood cell transfusions should be considered in patients experiencing substantial myelosuppression. Whether measures suggested for the management of cisplatin overdosage, including the possible merits of chemoprotectants,would be of benefit in the event of massive carboplatin overdosage remains to be established. (For additional information on acute toxicity associated with platinum compounds, see Acute Toxicity in Cisplatin 10:00.)

Although carboplatin is removed by hemodialysis, it is not known whether this procedure would enhance elimination of the drug following overdosage. Plasmapheresis has been used effectively in the management of cisplatin overdosage, and the possibility that it may be useful in the management of massive carboplatin overdosage should be considered.

PHARMACOLOGY

The exact mechanism(s) of action of carboplatin has not been conclusively determined. Platinum-containing antineoplastic agents such as carboplatin and cisplatin appear to exert their effects by binding to DNA, thereby inhibiting DNA synthesis. The drugs are cycle-phase nonspecific. Carboplatin and cisplatin appear to act on tumor cells by the same general molecular mechanisms and, once bound to DNA, have virtually the same action. Although the principal mechanism of action of the drugs appears to be inhibition of DNA synthesis, other mechanisms also are involved in their antineoplastic activity.

Carboplatin, like cisplatin, must undergo activation before antineoplastic activity occurs. The bidentate dicarboxylate ligands of carboplatin presumably are displaced by water (aquation), forming positively charged platinum complexes that react with nucleophilic sites on DNA. Although both carboplatin and cisplatin are activated by an initial aquation reaction, carboplatin is a more stable compound and is activated more slowly than cisplatin.

Carboplatin produces predominantly DNA intrastrand interstrand cross-links rather than DNA-protein cross-links. The relative importance of intrastrand or interstrand DNA cross-linking in the antineoplastic activity of carboplatin remains to be clearly determined; however, interstrand cross-linking appears to correlate well with the cytotoxicity of the drug. Intrastrand cross-links result from the formation of adducts between the activated platinum complexes of the drug and (but not exclusively) the N-7 atom on guanine to produce 1,2-intrastrand links between adjacent guanosine molecules, between neighboring guanosine and adenosine molecules, or between neighboring guanosine molecules. Interstrand cross-linking within the DNA helix also occurs. The resultant interstrand intrastrand cross-links are stable bonds that do not dissociate easily. While the mechanism through which DNA adducts exert their cytotoxic effects has not been determined, limited evidence indicates that platinum adducts may inhibit DNA replication, transcription, and ultimately cell division.

Higher concentrations of carboplatin than cisplatin are required to produce equivalent levels of DNA binding. In one in vitro study comparing the relative potency of the drugs in L1210 cells, carboplatin was 45 times less cytotoxic than cisplatin on a molar basis and peak levels of cross-linking occurred 6-12 hours later with carboplatin than with cisplatin. These differences are believed to result from the difference in rates of aquation or activation of the drugs. When the drugs are compared at concentrations that produce equivalent levels of DNA binding, however, both drugs induce equal numbers of drug-DNA cross-links, resulting in equivalent lesions and biologic activity. In various studies in mice, the antitumor activity of carboplatin was comparable to or slightly less than that of cisplatin.

Further study is needed to elucidate more fully the extent of cross-resistance between cisplatin and carboplatin. Although some cisplatin-refractory tumors may respond to carboplatin, a high degree of cross-resistance appears to occur between the drugs. The mechanisms of cellular resistance to platinum-containing antineoplastic agents have not been fully elucidated, but studies using cisplatin indicate that resistance can be related to decreased cellular uptake of the drug or enhanced DNA repair and may be related to elevated cellular levels of sulfhydryl (thiol) compounds including glutathione or metallothionein. Glutathione appears to play an essential role in protecting cells from the effects of certain toxins including certain antineoplastic agents, and increased levels of this sulfhydryl compound have been demonstrated in certain cell lines resistant to cisplatin and other analogs. Increased repair of platinum complex-induced DNA adducts also has been demonstrated in certain resistant cell lines. The relative roles of these mechanisms of resistance and their relationship to treatment failure in patients who do not respond to platinum-containing antineoplastic agents has not been fully determined.

PHARMACOKINETICS

The pharmacokinetics of carboplatin are complex and involve the parent compound as well as total platinum and ultrafilterable platinum. Total platinum consists of both protein-bound and nonprotein-bound platinum, while ultrafilterable platinum consists of carboplatin and nonprotein-bound carboplatin metabolites. Measurement of ultrafilterable platinum is commonly used in pharmacokinetic studies of carboplatin since only nonprotein-bound platinum or its platinum-containing products are cytotoxic.

The pharmacokinetics of carboplatin have been studied principally in adults with various malignancies who received the drug IV either alone or in conjunction with other antineoplastic agents. The pharmacokinetics of the drug are similar to those of cisplatin; however, a smaller percentage of carboplatin's total platinum is protein-bound, carboplatin has a longer initial distribution half-life ($t_{1/2\alpha}$), and carboplatin undergoes more extensive renal excretion.

● Absorption

Following IV infusion of a single dose of carboplatin in adults with malignancies, peak plasma concentrations of carboplatin, total platinum, and ultrafilterable platinum occur immediately. When a single carboplatin dose of 290–370 mg/m² is administered IV over 30–40 minutes in cancer patients with normal renal function, peak plasma concentrations of carboplatin, total platinum, and ultrafilterable platinum range from 84–140, 84–134, and 90–130 µmol/L, respectively; these plasma concentrations are essentially the same over the first 6 hours. Over a dosage range of 20–500 mg/m², peak plasma concentrations of carboplatin and free platinum and area under the plasma concentration-time curve (AUC) of the drug increase linearly with dose.

Carboplatin is absorbed following intraperitoneal administration†, and peak concentrations of total platinum, free platinum, and carboplatin are attained within 2–4 hours following instillation. In a limited number of patients receiving intraperitoneal carboplatin dosages of 200–300 mg/m², approximately 65% of the dose was absorbed over a 4-hour dwell period. Although peak concentrations of ultrafilterable platinum in peritoneal fluid substantially exceed those achieved in plasma, penetration of platinum from the peritoneal cavity into tumor tissue is limited. While the clinical importance is unclear, data from studies in rats indicate that cisplatin is able to penetrate tumor tissue more effectively than carboplatin following intraperitoneal administration.

● Distribution

Following IV administration of carboplatin, platinum is widely distributed into body tissues and fluids, with highest concentrations in the kidney, liver, skin, and tumor tissue. Lower concentrations are found in fat and brain. Platinum also is distributed into erythrocytes, with maximum platinum concentrations of 2.5 µmol/L obtained 6 hours after IV infusion of a carboplatin dose of 290–370 mg/m². Following IV administration, the initial distribution half-lives of carboplatin, total platinum, and ultrafilterable platinum are essentially the same; the $t_{1/2}\alpha$ of carboplatin has been reported to be 1–2 hours. The volumes of distribution at steady-state of carboplatin, total platinum, and ultrafilterable platinum average 9–25, 23–117, and 10–20 L/m² respectively.

In vitro studies indicate that carboplatin is not bound to plasma proteins, but degrades to platinum-containing products which rapidly bind to protein. In vivo, protein binding increases over time as the platinum-containing products of carboplatin become bound to tissue and plasma proteins. During the first 4 hours following IV administration of carboplatin, less than 24% of platinum is bound to plasma proteins; however, within 24 hours, 87% of platinum is protein-bound.

It is not known whether carboplatin or its platinum-containing products cross the placenta or are distributed into milk.

● Elimination

Following IV administration of carboplatin, plasma concentrations of carboplatin and ultrafilterable platinum has been reported to decline in a biphasic manner, while plasma concentrations of total platinum reportedly decline in a triphasic manner. In adults with malignancy and normal renal function, plasma elimination half-lives ($t_{1/2}\beta$) of 2–3 hours have been reported for carboplatin and ultrafilterable platinum. A terminal elimination half-life ($t_{1/2}\gamma$) of 4–6 days has been reported for total platinum. Small amounts of total platinum can be detected in plasma 4 weeks after administration of carboplatin, indicating that the rate of elimination of total platinum may decrease with time.

The mean elimination half-life of total platinum from erythrocytes reportedly is about 12 days following IV administration of the drug. Following intraperitoneal administration of carboplatin, the peritoneal elimination half-life of ultrafilterable platinum is about 4.2 hours.

Renal clearance and total body clearance of platinum are reduced in patients with impaired renal function. In patients undergoing hemodialysis, the $t_{1/2}\beta$ of total and ultrafilterable platinum is increased compared with values reported in individuals with normal renal function.

The metabolic fate of carboplatin has not been completely elucidated. There is no evidence to date that the drug undergoes enzymatic biotransformation; the bidentate dicarboxylate ligands of carboplatin are believed to be displaced by water, forming positively charged platinum complexes that react with nucleophilic sites on DNA.

Carboplatin and its platinum-containing product(s) are excreted principally in urine; there are insufficient data to date to determine whether intestinal secretion or fecal elimination occurs. Renal excretion predominantly occurs via glomerular filtration. The clearance of carboplatin is directly affected by the glomerular filtration rate (GFR), and this parameter of renal function often is decreased in geriatric patients. Dosing formulas that incorporate estimates of GFR to provide predictable areas under the plasma concentration-time curve (AUCs) for carboplatin should be used in geriatric patients to minimize the risk of toxicity. The relationship between GFR and AUC of ultrafilterable platinum has been used to develop several formulas for calculating carboplatin dosage. (See Dosage: Individualization of Dosage, in Dosage and Administration.) In patients with malignancy and normal renal function, about 65% of an IV dose of carboplatin is eliminated in urine within 12 hours and 71% is eliminated within 24 hours; a substantial portion of the amount excreted is unchanged carboplatin. Carboplatin (as ultrafilterable carboplatin) is removed extensively by hemodialysis.

CHEMISTRY AND STABILITY

● Chemistry

Carboplatin is a platinum-containing antineoplastic agent. Carboplatin, like cisplatin, is a platinum coordination compound composed of a platinum atom surrounded in a plane by 2 ammonia groups and 2 other ligands in the *cis* position; presence of the ammonia groups, the *cis* configuration, and neutrality in plasma are necessary for the activity of both drugs. However, the other 2 ligands in carboplatin are present in a bidentate dicarboxylate chelate ring structure rather than as 2 chloride atoms present in cisplatin. The cyclobutane dicarboxylate moiety has greater chemical stability than the chlorides contained in cisplatin and this difference results in a less reactive compound that is associated with reduced toxicity (e.g., nephrotoxicity) but with antineoplastic activity that may be comparable to or slightly less than that of cisplatin.

Carboplatin occurs as a white to off-white crystalline powder. The drug has a solubility of 14 mg/mL in water and is insoluble in alcohol. A 1% solution of carboplatin has a pH of 5–7. Carboplatin is commercially available as a sterile, pyrogen-free, aqueous solution containing 10 mg of carboplatin per mL.

● Stability

Commercially available carboplatin aqueous solution in unopened vials is stable until the date indicated on the package when protected from light and stored as directed; the solution should be stored at 25°C, but may be exposed to temperatures ranging from 15–30°C. Carboplatin injection in multidose vials is stable for up to 14 days at 25°C.

Carboplatin aqueous solution may be further diluted in 5% dextrose injection or 0.9% sodium chloride injection to concentrations as low as 0.5 mg/mL, and these dilutions are stable for 8 hours at 25°C; because there is no preservative in the formulation, the manufacturer states that unused portions of diluted carboplatin solution for infusion should be discarded 8 hours after preparation.

Because some platinum coordination compounds (e.g., cisplatin) are unstable in certain sodium chloride solutions and because there is evidence that carboplatin dissolved in sodium chloride solutions is converted partially in vitro to cisplatin, it previously was suggested that these solutions not be used to dilute carboplatin. However, while the rate of carboplatin decomposition in 0.9% sodium chloride or 5% dextrose and 0.9% sodium chloride is greater than that in sterile water for injection (i.e., 4% loss in 7 days at 27°C), it still does not exceed 10% per day at room temperature (i.e., 4-5% loss in 24 hours at 25°C). In addition, while the process responsible for the loss of carboplatin potency in these solutions has not been fully characterized, a study using carboplatin solutions containing 1 mg/mL in 0.9% sodium chloride indicates that only a minimal amount of carboplatin (less than 0.7%) is converted to cisplatin within 24 hours at 25°C. Therefore, previous recommendations not to use sodium chloride solutions to dilute carboplatin no longer appear to be justified.

Aluminum displaces platinum from the carboplatin molecule, resulting in the formation of a black precipitate and loss of potency. Carboplatin solutions should not be prepared or administered with needles, syringes, catheters, or IV administration sets containing aluminum parts that might come in contact with the drug.

For further information on the handling of antineoplastic agents, see the ASHP Guidelines on Handling Hazardous Drugs at http://www.ahfsdruginformation.com.

PREPARATIONS

Excipients in commercially available drug preparations may have clinically important effects in some individuals; consult specific product labeling for details.

CARBOplatin

Parenteral		
For injection, concentrate, for IV infusion	10 mg/mL (50, 150, 450, or 600 mg)*	CARBOplatin for Injection Paraplatin®, Bristol-Myers Squibb
For injection, for IV infusion	50 mg*	CARBOplatin for Injection Paraplatin®, Bristol-Myers Squibb
	150 mg*	CARBOplatin for Injection Paraplatin®, Bristol-Myers Squibb
	450 mg*	CARBOplatin for Injection Paraplatin®, Bristol-Myers Squibb

* available from one or more manufacturer, distributor, and/or repackager by generic (nonproprietary) name

† Use is not currently included in the labeling approved by the US Food and Drug Administration.

Selected Revisions January 1, 2009, © Copyright, January 1, 1996, American Society of Health-System Pharmacists, Inc.

Cemiplimab-rwlc

10:00 · ANTINEOPLASTIC AGENTS

■ Cemiplimab, a fully human anti-programmed-death receptor-1 (anti-PD-1) monoclonal antibody, is an antineoplastic agent.

USES

● Cutaneous Squamous Cell Carcinoma

Cemiplimab-rwlc is used for the treatment of metastatic or locally advanced cutaneous squamous cell carcinoma in patients who are not candidates for curative surgery or radiation therapy.

The current indication for cemiplimab-rwlc is based principally on the combined results of an open-label, multicenter, nonrandomized, phase 1 study (Study 1423) and an open-label, multicenter, nonrandomized, multicohort phase 2 study (Study 1540) in 108 adults with metastatic or locally advanced cutaneous squamous cell carcinoma who were not candidates for curative surgery or radiation therapy. In these studies, patients received cemiplimab-rwlc 3 mg/kg administered as an IV infusion every 2 weeks for up to 48 or 96 weeks. Treatment was continued for the specified duration or until the occurrence of unacceptable toxicity or disease progression. The primary measures of efficacy were objective response rate and duration of response as evaluated by an independent central review committee. Response was evaluated according to Response Evaluation Criteria in Solid Tumors (RECIST) in patients without externally visible target lesions or by a composite end point that included radiographic assessment according to RECIST and digital medical images according to World Health Organization (WHO) criteria in patients with externally visible target lesions.

The median age of patients in the combined analysis of Study 1423 and Study 1540 was 71 years (range: 38–96 years); 97% were white, 85% were male, 50% had received at least one prior systemic therapy, 96% had previously undergone surgery, and 79% had received prior radiation therapy. All patients enrolled in the studies had an Eastern Cooperative Oncology Group (ECOG) performance status of 0 or 1. Most patients (69%) had metastatic cutaneous squamous cell carcinoma and 31% had locally advanced disease. Among patients with metastatic cutaneous squamous cell carcinoma, 69% had distant metastases and 31% had nodal metastases only. These studies excluded patients with active autoimmune disease that required systemic therapy in the past 5 years; those who had received a solid organ transplant; those who had received prior therapy with other anti-programmed-death 1 (anti-PD-1) or anti-PD ligand 1 (anti-PD-L1) antibodies or other immune-checkpoint inhibitors; those with an ECOG performance status of 2 or greater; and those with human immunodeficiency virus (HIV), hepatitis B virus (HBV), or hepatitis C virus (HCV) infection.

At a median follow-up of 8.9 months, the objective response rate was 47.2%; complete responses were achieved in 3.7% of patients. In the cohort of patients with metastatic cutaneous squamous cell carcinoma at a median follow-up of 8.1 months, the objective response rate was 46.7%; complete responses were achieved in 5.3% of patients. In the cohort of patients with locally advanced cutaneous squamous cell carcinoma at a median follow-up 10.2 months, the objective response rate was 48.5%; there were no complete responses. At the time of analysis, the overall median duration of response had not been reached; however, 60 or 63% of patients with metastatic or locally advanced cutaneous squamous cell carcinoma, respectively, had durable responses of 6 months or more.

DOSAGE AND ADMINISTRATION

● General

Because immune-mediated adverse effects may occur in any organ system or tissue, the manufacturer states that blood chemistries and liver and thyroid function tests should be assessed prior to initiation of cemiplimab therapy and periodically during therapy.

Restricted Distribution

Cemiplimab-rwlc can only be obtained through a limited network of speciality distributors or pharmacies. Clinicians may contact the manufacturer (Regeneron)

at 877-542-8296 or consult the Libtayo® website (https://www.libtayohcp.com) for specific ordering and availability information.

● Administration

Cemiplimab-rwlc is administered by IV infusion over 30 minutes.

Unopened vials of cemiplimab-rwlc injection concentrate should be stored at 2–8°C in the original carton to protect the drug from light, and should *not* be frozen or shaken.

Cemiplimab-rwlc injection concentrate must be diluted prior to administration. Prior to administration, cemiplimab-rwlc injection concentrate should be inspected visually for particulate matter and discoloration. The undiluted solution should be clear to slightly opalescent and colorless to pale yellow; the solution should *not* be used if it is cloudy or discolored or if foreign particles other than translucent to white particles are present. Cemiplimab-rwlc is diluted by adding 7 mL of cemiplimab-rwlc injection concentrate (containing 50 mg/mL) to an appropriate volume of 0.9% sodium chloride or 5% dextrose injection to a final concentration of 1–20 mg/mL. The diluted solution should be mixed by gentle inversion and should *not* be shaken. Cemiplimab-rwlc should be administered through a sterile, 0.2- to 5-µm inline or add-on filter.

Diluted solutions of the drug are stable for up to 8 hours after dilution (including infusion time) when stored at room temperature (up to 25°C) or up to 24 hours after dilution (including infusion time) when stored under refrigeration (2–8°C); diluted solutions of the drug should be brought to room temperature prior to administration. Diluted solutions of the drug should *not* be frozen.

Cemiplimab-rwlc injection concentrate is intended for single use only; any unused portion in the vial should be discarded.

● Dosage

Cutaneous Squamous Cell Carcinoma

For the treatment of metastatic or locally advanced cutaneous squamous cell carcinoma, the recommended adult dosage of cemiplimab-rwlc is 350 mg administered every 3 weeks. Therapy should be continued until disease progression or unacceptable toxicity occurs.

Therapy Interruption for Toxicity

If immune-mediated adverse effects occur, temporary or permanent discontinuance of cemiplimab may be required based on the severity of the reaction.

Cemiplimab should be *permanently discontinued* in patients experiencing recurrent grade 3 or 4 immune-mediated adverse effects or persistent grade 2 or 3 immune-mediated adverse effects lasting 12 weeks or longer, and in those requiring a corticosteroid dosage of 10 mg or more of prednisone daily (or equivalent) for 12 weeks or longer.

Immune-mediated Pneumonitis

If grade 2 immune-mediated pneumonitis occurs, cemiplimab therapy should be interrupted. Once the toxicity has resolved to grade 0 or 1, cemiplimab therapy may be resumed following completion of the corticosteroid taper. (See Immune-mediated Pneumonitis under Cautions: Warnings/Precautions.)

If grade 3 or 4 immune-mediated pneumonitis occurs, cemiplimab therapy should be permanently discontinued.

Immune-mediated GI Effects

If grade 2 or 3 immune-mediated colitis occurs, cemiplimab therapy should be interrupted. Once the toxicity has resolved to grade 0 or 1, cemiplimab therapy may be resumed following completion of the corticosteroid taper. (See Immune-mediated GI Effects under Cautions: Warnings/Precautions.)

If grade 4 immune-mediated colitis occurs, cemiplimab therapy should be permanently discontinued.

Immune-mediated Hepatic Effects

For serum aminotransferase (ALT or AST) elevations exceeding 3 times but not more than 10 times the upper limit of normal (ULN) or total bilirubin concentrations exceeding the ULN but not more than 3 times the ULN, cemiplimab therapy should be interrupted. Once the toxicity has resolved to grade 0 or 1, cemiplimab therapy may be resumed following completion of the corticosteroid taper. (See Immune-mediated Hepatic Effects under Cautions: Warnings/Precautions.)

For ALT or AST elevations exceeding 10 times the ULN or total bilirubin concentrations exceeding 3 times the ULN, cemiplimab therapy should be permanently discontinued.

Immune-mediated Endocrine Effects

If grade 2–4 endocrinopathies (e.g., adrenal insufficiency, hypophysitis, hypothyroidism, hyperthyroidism, diabetes mellitus) occur, cemiplimab therapy should be interrupted if clinically necessary. (See Immune-mediated Endocrine Effects under Cautions: Warnings/Precautions.)

Other Immune-mediated Adverse Effects

If any other grade 3 immune-mediated adverse effects involving a major organ occur, cemiplimab therapy should be interrupted. Once the toxicity has resolved to grade 0 or 1, cemiplimab therapy may be resumed following completion of the corticosteroid taper. (See Other Immune-mediated Effects under Cautions: Warnings/Precautions.)

If any other grade 4 immune-mediated adverse effects involving a major organ occur, cemiplimab therapy should be permanently discontinued.

Infusion-related Reactions

If grade 1 or 2 infusion-related reactions occur, the infusion should be interrupted or the infusion rate should be reduced. (See Infusion-related Effects under Cautions: Warnings/Precautions.)

If grade 3 or 4 infusion-related reactions occur, cemiplimab therapy should be permanently discontinued.

● Special Populations

The manufacturer makes no special population dosage recommendations at this time. (See Specific Populations under Cautions: Warnings/Precautions.)

CAUTIONS

● Contraindications

The manufacturer states there are no known contraindications to the use of cemiplimab.

● Warnings/Precautions

Immune-mediated Pneumonitis

Immune-mediated pneumonitis, sometimes fatal, has occurred in patients receiving cemiplimab therapy. Immune-mediated adverse effects generally occur during therapy with anti-programmed-death 1 (anti-PD-1) and anti-PD ligand 1 (anti-PD-L1) antibodies, but also may occur following discontinuance of the drug.

In clinical trials, immune-mediated pneumonitis occurred in 2.4% of 534 patients receiving cemiplimab-rwlc and was fatal in 0.2% of patients. Grade 2 or 3 immune-mediated pneumonitis was reported in 2% of patients. Cemiplimab-rwlc was permanently discontinued because of immune-mediated pneumonitis in 1.3% of patients receiving the drug. All patients experiencing immune-mediated pneumonitis received systemic corticosteroid therapy and 85% received high-dose corticosteroid therapy (40 mg or more of prednisone daily [or equivalent]). Immune-mediated pneumonitis resolved in 62% of patients.

Patients receiving cemiplimab should be monitored for manifestations of pneumonitis. Temporary interruption or discontinuance of cemiplimab may be necessary if immune-mediated pneumonitis occurs during therapy with the drug. (See Immune-mediated Pneumonitis under Dosage: Therapy Interruption for Toxicity, in Dosage and Administration.) In patients who develop grade 2 or greater pneumonitis, systemic corticosteroid therapy should be initiated (1–2 mg/kg of prednisone daily [or equivalent]) followed by tapering of the corticosteroid dosage over 1 month once symptoms improve to grade 0 or 1. Systemic immunosuppressive therapy may be considered in patients experiencing immune-mediated pneumonitis inadequately controlled with systemic corticosteroid therapy.

Immune-mediated GI Effects

Immune-mediated colitis has occurred in patients receiving cemiplimab therapy. Immune-mediated adverse effects generally occur during therapy with anti-PD-1 and anti-PD-L1 antibodies, but also may occur following discontinuance of the drug.

In clinical trials, grade 2 or 3 immune-mediated colitis occurred in 0.9% of 534 patients receiving cemiplimab-rwlc. Cemiplimab-rwlc was permanently discontinued because of immune-mediated colitis in 0.2% of patients. All patients experiencing immune-mediated colitis received systemic corticosteroid therapy and 60% received high-dose corticosteroid therapy (40 mg or more of prednisone daily [or equivalent]). Immune-mediated colitis resolved in 80% of patients.

Patients receiving cemiplimab should be monitored for manifestations of colitis. Temporary interruption or discontinuance of cemiplimab may be necessary if immune-mediated colitis occurs during therapy with the drug. (See Immune-mediated GI Effects under Dosage: Therapy Interruption for Toxicity, in Dosage and Administration.) In patients who develop grade 2 or greater colitis, systemic corticosteroid therapy should be initiated (1–2 mg/kg of prednisone daily [or equivalent]) followed by tapering of the corticosteroid dosage over 1 month once symptoms improve to grade 0 or 1. Systemic immunosuppressive therapy may be considered in patients experiencing immune-mediated colitis inadequately controlled with systemic corticosteroid therapy.

Immune-mediated Hepatic Effects

Immune-mediated hepatitis, sometimes fatal, has occurred in patients receiving cemiplimab therapy. Immune-mediated adverse effects generally occur during therapy with anti-PD-1 and anti-PD-L1 antibodies, but also may occur following discontinuance of the drug.

In clinical trials, immune-mediated hepatitis occurred in 2.1% of 534 patients receiving cemiplimab-rwlc and was fatal in 0.2% of patients. Grade 3 or 4 immune-mediated hepatitis was reported in 1.9% of patients. Cemiplimab-rwlc was permanently discontinued because of immune-mediated hepatitis in 0.9% of patients receiving the drug. All patients experiencing immune-mediated hepatitis received systemic corticosteroid therapy and 91% received high-dose corticosteroid therapy (40 mg or more of prednisone daily [or equivalent]). Immune-mediated hepatitis resolved in 64% of patients.

Patients receiving cemiplimab should be monitored for manifestations of hepatitis. Liver function tests should be assessed prior to initiation of cemiplimab therapy and periodically during therapy. Temporary interruption or discontinuance of cemiplimab may be necessary if immune-mediated hepatitis occurs during therapy with the drug. (See Immune-mediated Hepatic Effects under Dosage: Therapy Interruption for Toxicity, in Dosage and Administration.) If serum aminotransferase (ALT or AST) elevations exceeding 3 times the upper limit of normal (ULN) (i.e., grade 2 or greater) or total bilirubin concentrations exceeding the ULN occur, systemic corticosteroid therapy should be initiated (1–2 mg/kg of prednisone daily [or equivalent]) followed by tapering of the corticosteroid dosage over 1 month once the toxicity improves to grade 0 or 1. Systemic immunosuppressive therapy may be considered in patients experiencing immune-mediated hepatitis inadequately controlled with systemic corticosteroid therapy.

Immune-mediated Endocrine Effects

Immune-mediated endocrinopathies, such as adrenal insufficiency, hypophysitis (including hypopituitarism), thyroid dysfunction (i.e., hypothyroidism, hyperthyroidism), and diabetes mellitus (including ketoacidosis), have occurred in patients receiving cemiplimab therapy. Immune-mediated adverse effects generally occur during therapy with anti-PD-1 and anti-PD-L1 antibodies, but also may occur following discontinuance of the drug.

Temporary interruption or discontinuance of cemiplimab may be necessary if immune-mediated endocrinopathies occur during therapy with the drug. (See Immune-mediated Endocrine Effects under Dosage: Therapy Interruption for Toxicity, in Dosage and Administration.) Certain grade 2 or greater endocrinopathies may require initiation of systemic corticosteroid therapy (1–2 mg/kg of prednisone daily [or equivalent]) followed by tapering of the corticosteroid dosage over 1 month once the toxicity improves to grade 0 or 1. Systemic immunosuppressive therapy may be considered in patients experiencing certain immune-mediated endocrinopathies inadequately controlled with systemic corticosteroid therapy. Hormone replacement therapy, including antidiabetic therapy (e.g., insulin), also should be administered as clinically indicated.

Adrenal Insufficiency

In clinical trials, grade 2 or 3 immune-mediated adrenal insufficiency occurred in 0.4% of 534 patients receiving cemiplimab-rwlc.

Patients receiving cemiplimab should be monitored for signs and symptoms of adrenal insufficiency.

Hypophysitis

In clinical trials, grade 3 immune-mediated hypophysitis occurred in 1 of 534 patients (0.2%) receiving cemiplimab-rwlc.

Patients receiving cemiplimab should be monitored for manifestations of hypophysitis.

Thyroid Dysfunction

In clinical trials, immune-mediated hypothyroidism occurred in 6% of 534 patients receiving cemiplimab-rwlc therapy and was grade 3 in 0.2% of patients. None of the patients experiencing immune-mediated hypothyroidism were able to discontinue thyroid hormone replacement therapy.

In clinical trials, immune-mediated hyperthyroidism occurred in 1.5% of 534 patients receiving cemiplimab-rwlc and was grade 2 or 3 in 0.6% of patients. Immune-mediated hyperthyroidism resolved in 38% of patients.

Patients receiving cemiplimab should be monitored for manifestations of thyroid dysfunction. Thyroid function should be evaluated prior to initiation of cemiplimab therapy and periodically during therapy.

Diabetes Mellitus

In clinical trials, grade 3 or 4 immune-mediated type 1 diabetes mellitus and ketoacidosis occurred in 0.7% of 534 patients receiving cemiplimab-rwlc. Cemiplimab-rwlc was permanently discontinued because of immune-mediated type 1 diabetes mellitus in 0.2% of patients receiving the drug.

Patients should be monitored for manifestations of diabetes mellitus. Blood glucose concentrations should be assessed prior to initiation of cemiplimab therapy and periodically during therapy.

Immune-mediated Renal Effects

Immune-mediated nephritis has occurred in patients receiving cemiplimab therapy. Immune-mediated adverse effects generally occur during therapy with anti-PD-1 and anti-PD-L1 antibodies, but also may occur following discontinuance of the drug.

In clinical trials, grade 2 or 3 immune-mediated nephritis occurred in 0.6% of 534 patients receiving cemiplimab-rwlc. Cemiplimab-rwlc was permanently discontinued because of immune-mediated nephritis in 0.2% of patients receiving the drug. All patients experiencing immune-mediated nephritis received systemic corticosteroid therapy and 67% received high-dose corticosteroid therapy (40 mg or more of prednisone daily [or equivalent]). Complete resolution of immune-mediated nephritis occurred in all patients.

Patients receiving cemiplimab should be monitored for changes in renal function. Serum creatinine should be assessed prior to initiation of cemiplimab therapy and periodically during therapy. Temporary interruption or discontinuance of cemiplimab may be necessary if immune-mediated nephritis occurs. (See Other Immune-mediated Adverse Effects under Dosage: Therapy Interruption for Toxicity, in Dosage and Administration.) If grade 2 or greater nephritis occurs, systemic corticosteroid therapy should be initiated (1–2 mg/kg of prednisone daily [or equivalent]) followed by tapering of the corticosteroid dosage over 1 month once the toxicity improves to grade 0 or 1. Systemic immunosuppressive therapy may be considered in patients experiencing immune-mediated nephritis inadequately controlled with systemic corticosteroid therapy.

Immune-mediated Dermatologic Effects

Immune-mediated dermatologic reactions, including Stevens-Johnson syndrome, toxic epidermal necrolysis, erythema multiforme, and pemphigoid, have occurred in patients receiving cemiplimab therapy. Immune-mediated adverse effects generally occur during therapy with anti-PD-1 and anti-PD-L1 antibodies, but also may occur following discontinuance of the drug.

In clinical trials, grade 2 or 3 immune-mediated dermatologic reactions, including erythema multiforme and pemphigoid, occurred in 1.7% of 534 patients receiving cemiplimab-rwlc. Stevens-Johnson syndrome and toxic epidermal necrolysis also have occurred in patients receiving anti-PD-1 and anti-PD-L1 antibodies, including cemiplimab-rwlc. All patients experiencing immune-mediated dermatologic reactions received systemic corticosteroid therapy and 89% received high-dose corticosteroid therapy (40 mg or more of prednisone daily [or equivalent]). Immune-mediated dermatologic reactions resolved in 33% of patients. Following reinitiation of cemiplimab-rwlc, immune-mediated dermatologic reactions recurred in approximately 22% of patients.

Patients receiving cemiplimab should be monitored for dermatologic reactions. Temporary interruption or discontinuance of cemiplimab may be necessary if immune-mediated dermatologic reactions occur. (See Other Immune-mediated Adverse Effects under Dosage: Therapy Interruption for Toxicity, in Dosage and Administration.) If grade 2 or greater dermatologic reactions occur, systemic corticosteroid therapy should be initiated (1–2 mg/kg of prednisone daily [or equivalent]) followed by tapering of the corticosteroid dosage over 1 month once the toxicity improves to grade 0 or 1. Systemic immunosuppressive therapy may be considered in patients experiencing immune-mediated dermatologic reactions inadequately controlled with systemic corticosteroid therapy.

Other Immune-mediated Effects

Other immune-mediated adverse effects, sometimes severe or fatal, including meningitis, encephalitis, myelitis and demyelination, myasthenic syndrome/myasthenia gravis, Guillain-Barré syndrome, nerve paresis, autoimmune neuropathy, myocarditis, pericarditis, vasculitides, pancreatitis (including elevations in serum amylase and lipase concentrations), gastritis, duodenitis, myositis, rhabdomyolysis and associated sequelae (e.g., renal failure), arthritis, polymyalgia rheumatica, hemolytic anemia, aplastic anemia, hemophagocytic lymphohistiocytosis, systemic inflammatory response syndrome, histiocytic necrotizing lymphadenitis, sarcoidosis, and immune thrombocytopenic purpura, were observed in less than 1% of 534 patients receiving cemiplimab-rwlc in clinical trials or have been reported in patients receiving other anti-PD-1 or anti-PD-L1 antibodies. Immune-mediated rejection of solid organ transplants also was reported in patients who received cemiplimab. Immune-mediated adverse effects generally occur during therapy with anti-PD-1 and anti-PD-L1 antibodies, but also may occur following discontinuance of the drug.

Ocular inflammatory toxicity (e.g., uveitis, iritis), sometimes associated with retinal detachment, visual impairment, or blindness, also has been reported rarely in patients receiving cemiplimab-rwlc in clinical trials. If uveitis occurs in conjunction with other immune-mediated adverse effects, a Vogt-Koyanagi-Harada-like syndrome should be considered. Systemic corticosteroid therapy may be required to reduce the risk of permanent vision loss.

Patients receiving cemiplimab should be monitored for immune-mediated adverse effects. Temporary interruption or discontinuance of cemiplimab may be necessary if immune-mediated adverse effects occur. (See Other Immune-mediated Adverse Effects under Dosage: Therapy Interruption for Toxicity, in Dosage and Administration.) If grade 2 or greater adverse effects occur, systemic corticosteroid therapy should be initiated (1–2 mg/kg of prednisone daily [or equivalent]) followed by tapering of the corticosteroid dosage over 1 month once the toxicity improves to grade 0 or 1. Systemic immunosuppressive therapy may be considered in patients experiencing immune-mediated adverse effects inadequately controlled with systemic corticosteroid therapy.

Infusion-related Effects

Severe infusion-related reactions have occurred in 0.2% of patients receiving cemiplimab-rwlc.

Patients receiving cemiplimab should be monitored for manifestations of infusion-related reactions. In patients experiencing infusion-related reactions, interruption of the infusion, reduction in the infusion rate, or permanent discontinuance of the drug may be necessary. (See Infusion-related Reactions under Dosage: Therapy Interruption for Toxicity, in Dosage and Administration.)

Fetal/Neonatal Morbidity and Mortality

Cemiplimab may cause fetal harm if administered to pregnant women. Blockade of signaling of the PD-1 and PD-L1 pathway in animals has been shown to disrupt maternal immune tolerance to the fetus and has been associated with increased fetal loss and immune-mediated disorders. Therefore, inhibition of this pathway by cemiplimab may increase the risk of fetal loss (e.g., abortion, stillbirth). Human immunoglobulin G_4 (IgG_4) has been shown to cross the placenta; therefore, fetal exposure to cemiplimab may occur and increase the risk of immune-mediated disorders or alter normal immune response of the developing fetus.

Pregnancy should be avoided during cemiplimab therapy. The manufacturer recommends confirmation of pregnancy status prior to initiation of cemiplimab. Women of childbearing potential should be advised to use an effective method of contraception while receiving cemiplimab and for at least 4 months after the last dose. If cemiplimab is used during pregnancy or if the patient becomes pregnant while receiving the drug, the patient should be apprised of the potential fetal hazard.

Immunogenicity

There is a potential for immunogenicity with cemiplimab therapy. Development of anti-cemiplimab antibodies was detected by electrochemiluminescence (ECL) in 5 of 398 patients (1.3%) receiving cemiplimab-rwlc. Among the 5 patients who tested positive for antibody formation during treatment, one patient had persistently positive test results and none of the patients had evidence of neutralizing antibodies to the drug. Data are insufficient to determine the clinical importance of such anti-drug antibodies; however, no effects of antibody formation on pharmacokinetics or safety (i.e., infusion-related reactions) of the drug were observed.

Specific Populations

Pregnancy

Cemiplimab may cause fetal harm if administered to pregnant women based on its mechanism of action and animal findings. (See Fetal/Neonatal Morbidity and Mortality under Cautions: Warnings/Precautions.)

Lactation

It is not known whether cemiplimab is distributed into human milk. Because many drugs are distributed into human milk and because of the potential for serious adverse reactions to cemiplimab in nursing infants, women should be advised to discontinue nursing during cemiplimab therapy and for at least 4 months after the last dose. The effects of the drug on nursing infants or on milk production are unknown.

Pediatric Use

Safety and efficacy of cemiplimab have not been established in pediatric patients.

Geriatric Use

In clinical trials evaluating cemiplimab-rwlc for metastatic or locally advanced cutaneous squamous cell carcinoma, 72% of patients were 65 years of age or older and 37% were 75 years of age or older. No overall differences in safety or efficacy were observed between geriatric patients and younger adults.

Hepatic Impairment

Systemic exposure of cemiplimab-rwlc was unaffected following administration of the drug in individuals with total bilirubin concentrations of 0.02–2.63 mg/dL. Cemiplimab has not been studied in patients with moderate or severe hepatic impairment.

Renal Impairment

Systemic exposure of cemiplimab-rwlc was unaffected following administration of the drug in individuals with creatinine clearance of 25 mL/minute or greater.

● Common Adverse Effects

Adverse effects reported in 10% or more of patients receiving cemiplimab-rwlc for the treatment of metastatic or locally advanced cutaneous squamous cell carcinoma include fatigue, rash, diarrhea, nausea, musculoskeletal pain, pruritus, cough, headache, constipation, dry skin, vomiting, and decreased appetite. Grade 3 or 4 laboratory abnormalities reported in 1% or more of patients receiving cemiplimab-rwlc for the treatment of metastatic or locally advanced cutaneous squamous cell carcinoma include lymphopenia, hypophosphatemia, elevated concentrations of aspartate aminotransferase (AST), hyponatremia, increased international normalized ratio (INR), anemia, hypoalbuminemia, and hypercalcemia.

DRUG INTERACTIONS

No formal drug interaction studies have been performed to date.

DESCRIPTION

Cemiplimab, a fully human anti-programmed-death receptor-1 (anti-PD-1) monoclonal antibody, is an antineoplastic agent. The drug is an IgG_4 immunoglobulin.

Cemiplimab is highly selective for PD-1, an immune-checkpoint receptor expressed on activated T cells, monocytes, B cells, natural killer (NK) T cells, and dendritic cells. Overexpression of PD-1 ligands on the surface of tumor cells results in activation of PD-1 and suppression of cytotoxic T-cell activity. Cemiplimab blocks the interaction between PD-1 and its ligands, resulting in enhanced immune response, including enhanced antitumor immune response. The drug also has been shown to reduce tumor growth in syngeneic mouse tumor models.

Cemiplimab-rwlc exhibits linear and dose-proportional pharmacokinetics over the dosage range of 1–10 mg/kg IV every 2 weeks and at a dosage of 350 mg IV every 3 weeks. Following repeated doses of cemiplimab-rwlc 350 mg IV every 3 weeks, steady-state concentrations are reached by approximately 4 months. Clearance of cemiplimab-rwlc is approximately 34% lower at steady state than following the initial dose. The elimination half-life of cemiplimab-rwlc is 19 days.

Systemic exposure to cemiplimab-rwlc does not appear to be affected by age (range: 27–96 years), gender, body weight (range: 31–156 kg), race, cancer type, or serum albumin concentration (2.2–4.8 g/dL).

ADVICE TO PATIENTS

Importance of advising patients to read the manufacturer's medication guide.

Risk of immune-mediated pneumonitis. Importance of informing clinician immediately if new or worsening cough, chest pain, or shortness of breath occurs.

Risk of immune-mediated colitis. Importance of informing clinician immediately if diarrhea, severe abdominal pain, or changes in stool occur.

Risk of immune-mediated hepatitis. Importance of informing clinician immediately if signs and symptoms of liver damage (e.g., jaundice, severe nausea or vomiting, abdominal pain [particularly in the right upper quadrant], drowsiness, dark urine, easy bruising or bleeding, lack of appetite) occur.

Risk of immune-mediated endocrine effects. Importance of informing clinician immediately if signs and symptoms of hypothyroidism, hyperthyroidism, adrenal insufficiency, hypophysitis, or diabetes mellitus occur.

Risk of immune-mediated nephritis or renal dysfunction. Importance of informing clinician immediately if signs and symptoms of nephritis (e.g., decreased urine output, hematuria, peripheral edema, lack of appetite) occur.

Risk of immune-mediated rash. Importance of informing clinician immediately if a new rash develops.

Risk of infusion-related reactions. Importance of informing clinician immediately if signs and symptoms of such reactions (e.g., chills, pruritus, flushing, difficulty breathing, dizziness, fever, feeling of faintness, back or neck pain, angioedema) occur.

Risk of fetal harm. Necessity of advising women of childbearing potential that they should use an effective method of contraception while receiving the drug and for at least 4 months after the last dose. Importance of women informing clinicians if they are or plan to become pregnant. If pregnancy occurs, advise pregnant women of potential risk to the fetus.

Importance of advising women to avoid breast-feeding while receiving cemiplimab therapy and for at least 4 months after the last dose.

Importance of informing clinicians of existing or contemplated concomitant therapy, including prescription and OTC drugs, as well as any concomitant illnesses (e.g., autoimmune disorders, history of solid organ transplantation, hepatic or renal dysfunction, pulmonary disorders, diabetes mellitus).

Importance of informing patients of other important precautionary information. (See Cautions.)

For further information on the handling of antineoplastic agents, see the ASHP Guidelines on Handling Hazardous Drugs at http://www.ahfsdrug information.com.

PREPARATIONS

Cemiplimab-rwlc can only be obtained through a limited network of speciality distributors or specialty pharmacies. (See Restricted Distribution under Dosage and Administration: General.)

Excipients in commercially available drug preparations may have clinically important effects in some individuals; consult specific product labeling for details.

Cemiplimab-rwlc

Parenteral

Concentrate, for injection, for IV infusion	50 mg/mL (350 mg)	Libtayo®, Regeneron (comarketed by Sanofi-Aventis)

Selected Revisions August 26, 2019, © Copyright, October 22, 2018, American Society of Health-System Pharmacists, Inc.

Ceritinib

10:00 • ANTINEOPLASTIC AGENTS

■ Ceritinib, an inhibitor of several receptor tyrosine kinases including anaplastic lymphoma kinase (ALK), is an antineoplastic agent.

USES

● Non-small Cell Lung Cancer

Ceritinib is used for the treatment of metastatic non-small cell lung cancer (NSCLC) in patients whose cancer is anaplastic lymphoma kinase (*ALK*)-positive as detected by an FDA-approved diagnostic test. Information on FDA-approved tests for the detection of ALK rearrangements in NSCLC is available at https://www.fda.gov/CompanionDiagnostics. Ceritinib has been designated an orphan drug by the FDA for this use. Guidelines for the treatment of patients with stage IV NSCLC with driver alterations in ALK generally support the use of ceritinib as an option in the first-line setting if alectinib and brigatinib are not available; ceritinib also may be offered in the second-line setting if crizotinib was given in the first-line setting.

Clinical Experience

Efficacy and safety of ceritinib for the treatment of *ALK*-positive metastatic NSCLC are based principally on the results of a multicenter, open-label, randomized phase 3 study (ASCEND-4) in patients with previously untreated advanced disease and a multicenter, single-arm, open-label study (ASCEND-1) in patients whose cancer had progressed during crizotinib therapy or who were intolerant to crizotinib.

In the ASCEND-4 study, 376 adults with previously untreated *ALK*-positive metastatic NSCLC were randomized (stratified by World Health Organization [WHO] performance status, prior chemotherapy, and presence of brain metastases) in a 1:1 ratio to receive either ceritinib (750 mg orally once daily in a fasted state) alone or standard chemotherapy (pemetrexed 500 mg/m² IV and either cisplatin 75 mg/m² IV or carboplatin at the dose required to obtain an AUC of 5–6 mg/mL per minute IV every 3 weeks for up to 4 cycles followed by maintenance therapy with pemetrexed 500 mg/m² IV every 3 weeks). Treatment was continued until disease progression, death, or unacceptable toxicity occurred or treatment was discontinued for other reasons. The primary measure of efficacy was progression-free survival as assessed by a blinded independent review committee according to Response Evaluation Criteria in Solid Tumors (RECIST 1.1); additional outcome measures included overall survival, overall response rate, duration of response, intracranial overall response rate, and duration of intracranial response. Presence of *ALK* rearrangement was determined using an FDA-approved diagnostic test (Ventana ALK [D5F3] CDx assay). The median age of patients enrolled in the study was 54 years; 54% of patients were white, 42% were Asian, 57% were female, 61% had never smoked, and 97% had adenocarcinoma histology. At the time of analysis, 43% of patients previously randomized to receive standard chemotherapy had subsequently received ceritinib therapy.

In the ASCEND-4 study, median progression-free survival was prolonged in patients receiving ceritinib compared with those receiving standard chemotherapy (16.6 versus 8.1 months; hazard ratio: 0.55). Overall response rate in patients receiving ceritinib or standard chemotherapy was 73 or 27%, respectively; complete response was achieved in 1 or 0% of patients, respectively. At the time of analysis, the median duration of response in patients receiving ceritinib or standard chemotherapy was 23.9 or 11.1 months, respectively. No substantial difference in overall survival was observed between patients receiving ceritinib and those receiving standard chemotherapy at the time of an interim analysis. In the subgroup of 55 patients with measurable brain metastases at baseline, intracranial overall response rate was 57 or 22% in patients receiving ceritinib or standard chemotherapy, respectively; complete responses were achieved in 7% of patients in both treatment groups. The median duration of intracranial response had not been reached in patients receiving standard chemotherapy, but was 16.6 months in ceritinib-treated patients. Results of an exploratory analysis (based on patient-reported symptoms) suggested that ceritinib therapy delayed the time to new onset or worsening of shortness of breath compared with standard chemotherapy;

however, because patients were not blinded to treatment assignment, differences in patient-related symptoms cannot be assessed reliably.

In the ASCEND-1 study, 163 adults with metastatic *ALK*-positive NSCLC whose cancer had progressed with or who were intolerant of crizotinib received ceritinib 750 mg once daily in a fasted state. The primary efficacy end point was overall response rate as assessed by a blinded independent review committee (IRC) according to RECIST 1.1; an additional outcome measure was duration of response. The median age of patients enrolled in the study was 52 years; 91% of patients had experienced disease progression during crizotinib therapy and 93% had adenocarcinoma histology. At the time of analysis, overall response rate in patients receiving ceritinib was 44%; complete responses were achieved in 2.5% of patients. Median duration of response was 7.1 months. Effects of ceritinib on investigator-assessed progression-free survival and IRC-assessed progression-free survival were comparable.

Use of ceritinib also was investigated in ASCEND-7, a 5-arm, multicenter, open-label phase 2 study in 156 patients with ALK-positive NSCLC with active brain and/or leptomeningeal metastases. The study arms were defined as follows: arm 1 (patients previously treated with radiation to the brain and with prior exposure to an ALK inhibitor [ALKi]), arm 2 (patients previously not treated with radiation to the brain but with prior exposure to an ALKi), arm 3 (patients previously treated with radiation to the brain but no prior ALKi exposure), arm 4 (patients previously not treated with radiation to the brain and no prior ALKi exposure), and arm 5 (patients with leptomeningeal carcinomatosis). Patients in each arm were treated with ceritinib 750 mg orally once daily, in a fasted state; treatment was continued until disease progression, discontinuation, or withdrawal of study consent.

The median age of patients ranged from 46 to 53.5 years and the majority of patients in arms 1, 2, and 5 had received crizotinib previously. The primary efficacy endpoint was investigator-assessed overall response rate according to RECIST 1.1. A key secondary outcome was investigator-assessed whole-body disease control rate.

At the time of analysis, overall response rate was higher in arm 4 (59.1%) compared to other arms: arm 1 (35.7%), arm 2 (30%), arm 3 (50%), and arm 5 (16.7%). Investigator-assessed whole-body disease control rate was highest in arm 2 (82.5%) compared to other arms.

Clinical Perspective

Approximately 60% of patients with lung cancer have driver alterations (e.g., in the epidermal growth factor receptor and ALK and BRAF genes). A relatively small subset of patients with NSCLC (approximately 3–7%) have ALK-positive disease, which indicates potential responsiveness to ALK inhibitor therapy (e.g., alectinib, brigatinib, ceritinib, crizotinib). Patients with this form of lung cancer typically are nonsmokers or have a history of light smoking, are female, and are younger in age and often have adenocarcinoma histology. Although crizotinib is highly active in patients with ALK-positive NSCLC, most patients treated with the drug eventually experience disease progression, limiting the drug's long-term therapeutic potential. Disease progression in patients receiving crizotinib can result from acquired resistance mutations in ALK, amplification of gene expression, activation of alternate signaling pathways, and/or progression of brain metastases (because of poor distribution of crizotinib into the CSF).

The American Society of Clinical Oncology (ASCO)/Cancer Care Ontario (CCO) March 2021 guideline addresses treatment of stage IV NSCLC with driver alterations, including ALK-positive disease. For patients with stage IV NSCLC and driver alterations in ALK, alectinib or brigatinib should be offered in the first-line setting. If alectinib and brigatinib are not available, ceritinib or crizotinib should be offered. In the second-line setting, alectinib, brigatinib, or ceritinib should be offered if crizotinib was given in the first-line setting.

DOSAGE AND ADMINISTRATION

● General

Pretreatment Screening

- Confirmation of the presence of anaplastic lymphoma kinase (*ALK*) rearrangement in tumor specimens of patients with metastatic non-small cell lung cancer (NSCLC) is necessary prior to initiating therapy with ceritinib.
- Perform pregnancy testing in females of reproductive potential.

Patient Monitoring

- Monitor lipase and amylase levels prior to initiating ceritinib treatment and periodically as clinically indicated.
- Monitor liver function tests (ALT and AST) and total bilirubin monthly and as clinically indicated. More frequent monitoring is warranted in patients who develop elevations of aminotransferase levels.
- Monitor fasting serum glucose prior to initiating ceritinib treatment and periodically as clinically indicated.
- Monitor blood pressure and heart rate regularly. Monitor ECGs and electrolytes periodically in patients with congestive heart failure, electrolyte abnormalities, bradyarrhythmia, or patients taking QT_c-prolonging medications.
- Monitor for pulmonary symptoms suggestive of pneumonitis or interstitial lung disease.
- Monitor for severe GI adverse reactions. Manage patients with the standard of care which may include antidiarrhea agents, fluid replacement, or antiemetics.

● Administration

Ceritinib is administered orally once daily with food.

If a dose of ceritinib is missed, the missed dose should be taken as soon as it is remembered unless the next dose is due within 12 hours.

If a dose of ceritinib is vomited after administration, an additional dose should not be administered to replace the vomited dose. The next dose should be administered at the next scheduled time.

Store ceritinib tablets and capsules at 20–25°C (excursions permitted between 15–30°C).

● Dosage

Non-small Cell Lung Cancer

The recommended adult dosage of ceritinib for the treatment of *ALK*-positive metastatic NSCLC is 450 mg once daily with food. Therapy should be continued until disease progression or unacceptable toxicity occurs.

Dosage Modification for Toxicity

If adverse reactions occur during ceritinib therapy, temporary interruption of therapy, dosage reduction, and/or discontinuance of the drug may be necessary. If dosage reduction is required, the dosage of ceritinib should be reduced as described in Table 1. Ceritinib should be discontinued if patients are unable to tolerate 150 mg once daily.

TABLE 1: Recommended Dosage Reduction for Ceritinib Toxicity

Dose Reduction Level	Dosage Reduction after Recovery from Toxicity (Initial Dosage = 450 mg once daily)
First	Resume at 300 mg once daily
Second	Resume at 150 mg once daily

GI Toxicity

In patients experiencing severe or intolerable nausea, vomiting, or diarrhea despite optimal antiemetic or antidiarrheal therapy, ceritinib therapy should be withheld until improvement of GI symptoms. Ceritinib may then be resumed at the next lower dosage as described in Table 1.

Hepatic Toxicity

If an elevation in serum ALT or AST concentrations exceeding 5 times the upper limit of normal (ULN) occurs with an elevation in total bilirubin concentrations no more than 2 times the ULN, ceritinib therapy should be withheld until the liver function test results return to baseline values or decrease to no more than 3 times the ULN. Ceritinib therapy may then be resumed at the next lower dosage as described in Table 1.

If an elevation in ALT or AST concentrations exceeding 3 times the ULN occurs with an elevation in total bilirubin concentrations exceeding 2 times the ULN in the absence of cholestasis or hemolysis, therapy with ceritinib should be permanently discontinued.

Interstitial Lung Disease/Pneumonitis

If treatment-related interstitial lung disease/pneumonitis of any grade occurs, ceritinib therapy should be permanently discontinued.

Prolongation of QT Interval

If corrected QT (QT_c) interval exceeds 500 msec on at least 2 separate ECGs, ceritinib therapy should be withheld until the QT_c interval is less than 481 msec or returns to baseline (if baseline QT_c interval is 481 msec or more). Ceritinib therapy may then be resumed at the next lower dosage as described in Table 1.

If QT_c-interval prolongation occurs concurrently with torsades de pointes, polymorphic ventricular tachycardia, or signs and/or symptoms of serious arrhythmia, ceritinib therapy should be permanently discontinued.

Bradycardia

If symptomatic, but non-life-threatening, bradycardia (heart rate less than 60 beats/minute) occurs, therapy with ceritinib should be withheld until recovery to asymptomatic bradycardia or to a heart rate of at least 60 beats/minute. If no concomitant drugs known to cause bradycardia are identified, ceritinib therapy may be resumed at the next lower dosage as described in Table 1.

If clinically important bradycardia requiring intervention or life-threatening bradycardia occurs in patients receiving concomitant drugs known to cause bradycardia or hypotension, ceritinib should be withheld until recovery to asymptomatic bradycardia or to a heart rate of at least 60 beats/minute. If such concomitant drugs are discontinued or the dosage adjusted, ceritinib therapy may be resumed at the next lower dosage as described in Table 1 with frequent monitoring.

If life-threatening bradycardia occurs in patients not receiving concomitant drugs known to cause bradycardia or hypotension, ceritinib therapy should be permanently discontinued.

Hyperglycemia

If persistent hyperglycemia with serum glucose concentrations exceeding 250 mg/dL occurs despite optimal antidiabetic agent therapy, ceritinib therapy should be withheld until adequate control of the hyperglycemia is achieved. Ceritinib therapy may then be resumed at the next lower dosage as described in Table 1. If hyperglycemia persists despite optimal medical management, ceritinib therapy should be discontinued.

Pancreatitis

If elevation in serum lipase or amylase concentration exceeding 2 times the ULN occurs, ceritinib therapy should be withheld until serum lipase or amylase concentrations improve to less than 1.5 times the ULN. Ceritinib therapy may then be resumed at the next lower dosage as described in Table 1.

Concomitant Use of Drugs Affecting Hepatic Microsomal Enzymes

Concomitant use of ceritinib with drugs that are potent inhibitors of cytochrome P-450 (CYP) isoenzyme 3A should be avoided. If concomitant use of a potent CYP3A inhibitor cannot be avoided, the manufacturer recommends reducing the daily dosage of ceritinib by approximately 33% and rounding dosage to the nearest 150-mg strength of ceritinib capsules or tablets (e.g., from 450 mg daily to 300 mg daily). If concomitant use of the potent CYP3A inhibitor is discontinued, the ceritinib dosage should be returned to the dosage used prior to initiation of the potent CYP3A inhibitor.

● Special Populations

Hepatic Impairment

Patients with hepatic impairment may have an increased exposure to ceritinib. The manufacturer recommends reducing the daily dosage of ceritinib by approximately 33% and rounding dosage to the nearest 150-mg strength of ceritinib capsules or tablets (e.g., from 450 mg daily to 300 mg daily) in patients with severe hepatic impairment (Child-Pugh class C). No dosage adjustment is necessary in patients with mild or moderate hepatic impairment (Child-Pugh class A or B).

Renal Impairment

The manufacturer makes no specific dosage recommendations for patients with renal impairment.

Geriatric Patients

The manufacturer makes no specific dosage recommendations for geriatric patients.

CAUTIONS

● Contraindications

● None.

● Warnings/Precautions

GI Toxicity

Severe adverse GI effects may occur in patients receiving ceritinib. In clinical trials evaluating ceritinib 750 mg once daily, diarrhea, nausea, vomiting, or abdominal pain occurred in 95% of patients receiving the drug in a fasting state, including severe cases in 14% of these patients; permanent discontinuance of ceritinib therapy or dosage modification (i.e., temporary interruption of therapy, dosage reduction) was necessary in 1.6 or 36%, respectively, of patients receiving the drug. In a dose-optimization study (ASCEND-8), the incidence and severity of adverse GI effects were reduced in patients receiving ceritinib 450 mg daily with food. In the ASCEND-8 study, diarrhea, nausea, vomiting, or abdominal pain occurred in 79% of 108 patients receiving ceritinib 450 mg daily with food; 53% of these cases were grade 1 in severity. Grade 3 diarrhea and grade 3 vomiting each occurred in one patient. Diarrhea or nausea resulted in temporary interruption of ceritinib therapy in 10% of patients receiving the drug; no dosage reduction was necessary in patients experiencing these adverse GI effects.

Patients receiving ceritinib should be monitored for development of GI toxicity and treated as necessary with appropriate therapy (e.g., antidiarrhea agents, antiemetics, fluid replacement). Temporary interruption followed by dosage reduction or discontinuance of ceritinib may be necessary depending on the severity of the GI toxicity.

Hepatic Toxicity

Drug-induced hepatotoxicity has occurred in patients receiving ceritinib. In clinical trials evaluating ceritinib 750 mg once daily, elevations in ALT or AST concentrations exceeding 5 times the upper limit of normal (ULN) were reported in 28 or 16%, respectively, of patients receiving the drug in a fasting state. Concurrent elevations in ALT concentrations exceeding 3 times the ULN and total bilirubin concentrations exceeding 2 times the ULN with alkaline phosphatase concentrations less than 2 times the ULN have been reported in 0.3% of ceritinib-treated patients. Permanent discontinuance of the drug due to hepatotoxicity was necessary in approximately 1% of patients.

The manufacturer states that liver function tests (i.e., ALT, AST, total bilirubin) should be monitored once monthly and as clinically indicated during ceritinib therapy, with more frequent testing in patients who develop aminotransferase elevations during therapy. Temporary interruption followed by dosage reduction or permanent discontinuance of ceritinib may be necessary depending on the severity of the hepatic toxicity.

Interstitial Lung Disease/Pneumonitis

Severe, life-threatening, or fatal interstitial lung disease (ILD) or pneumonitis may occur in patients receiving ceritinib. In clinical trials evaluating ceritinib 750 mg once daily, ILD or pneumonitis occurred in 2.4% of patients receiving the drug in a fasting state; grade 3 or 4 ILD or pneumonitis occurred in 1.3% of patients and fatal ILD or pneumonitis was reported in 0.2% of patients. Discontinuance of ceritinib due to ILD or pneumonitis occurred in 10 (1.1%) patients in these clinical trials.

Patients receiving ceritinib should be monitored for pulmonary symptoms indicative of ILD or pneumonitis, and other potential causes of ILD or pneumonitis should be excluded. Ceritinib should be permanently discontinued in patients who are diagnosed with treatment-related ILD or pneumonitis.

Prolongation of QT Interval

Prolongation of the corrected QT (QT$_c$) interval, which may increase the risk for ventricular arrhythmias (e.g., torsades de pointes) or sudden death, has been reported in patients receiving ceritinib. The prolongation appears to occur in a plasma concentration-dependent manner. In clinical trials, an increase in the QT$_c$ interval exceeding 60 msec from baseline occurred in 6% of patients receiving ceritinib. QT$_c$ interval exceeding 500 msec has been reported in approximately 1.3% of patients receiving ceritinib 750 mg once daily in a fasting state. Discontinuance of ceritinib due to prolongation of the QT$_c$ interval was necessary in 0.2% of patients in clinical trials.

Ceritinib should be avoided in patients with congenital long QT syndrome, if possible. The manufacturer recommends periodic monitoring of ECGs and serum electrolytes during ceritinib therapy in patients with congestive heart failure, bradyarrhythmias, or electrolyte abnormalities and in those who are receiving drugs known to prolong the QT interval.

Temporary interruption followed by dosage reduction or discontinuance of ceritinib may be necessary depending on the severity of the prolongation of QT$_c$ interval.

Hyperglycemia

Hyperglycemia has been reported in patients receiving ceritinib. In clinical trials evaluating ceritinib 750 mg once daily, grade 3 or 4 hyperglycemia occurred in 13% of patients receiving the drug in a fasting state. The risk of hyperglycemia may be increased in patients with diabetes mellitus or glucose intolerance and in those concurrently receiving corticosteroids.

Fasting serum glucose concentrations should be monitored prior to initiation of ceritinib, during therapy, and as clinically indicated. Antidiabetic agents should be initiated or optimized as necessary. Temporary interruption followed by dosage reduction or discontinuance of ceritinib may be necessary depending on the severity of the hyperglycemia.

Bradycardia

Ceritinib may cause bradycardia. In clinical trials evaluating ceritinib 750 mg once daily, sinus bradycardia (defined as a heart rate of less than 50 beats/minute) was reported as a new finding in 1.1% of patients receiving the drug in a fasting state; bradycardia was reported as an adverse drug reaction in 1% of patients. In patients experiencing bradycardia, temporary interruption of ceritinib therapy followed by dosage reduction was necessary in 0.1% of patients receiving the drug; discontinuance of ceritinib therapy was not required in any patients experiencing bradycardia.

Ceritinib should be avoided in patients who are receiving other drugs known to cause bradycardia when possible.

Heart rate and blood pressure should be monitored regularly in all patients receiving ceritinib. Temporary interruption followed by dosage reduction or discontinuance of ceritinib may be necessary depending on the severity of bradycardia.

Pancreatitis

Pancreatitis, sometimes fatal, has been reported in patients receiving ceritinib. In clinical trials, pancreatitis occurred in less than 1% of ceritinib-treated patients; grade 3 or 4 elevations of serum amylase or lipase concentrations were reported in 7 or 14% of patients, respectively.

Serum lipase and amylase concentrations should be monitored prior to initiation of ceritinib, periodically during therapy, and as clinically indicated. Temporary interruption followed by dosage reduction or discontinuance of ceritinib may be necessary depending on the severity of the toxicity.

Fetal/Neonatal Morbidity and Mortality

Based on its mechanism of action, ceritinib may cause fetal harm if administered to pregnant women. Ceritinib produced developmental toxicity, including dose-related skeletal abnormalities (e.g., delayed or incomplete ossification, skeletal variations) and a low incidence of visceral abnormalities, when administered to pregnant animals in dosages associated with exposure levels lower than those associated with the recommended human dosage; maternal toxicity, abortion, and embryolethality also were observed.

Pregnancy should be avoided during therapy. (See Females and Males of Reproductive Potential under Cautions.)

Specific Populations

Pregnancy

Ceritinib may cause fetal harm if administered to pregnant women based on its mechanism of action and animal findings. (See Fetal/Neonatal Morbidity and Mortality under Cautions.) If ceritinib is used during pregnancy or if the patient becomes pregnant while receiving the drug, the patient should be apprised of the potential fetal hazard.

Lactation

It is not known whether ceritinib or its metabolites are distributed into human milk or if the drug has any effect on milk production or the nursing infant. Because of the potential for serious adverse reactions to ceritinib in nursing infants, women should be advised not to breast-feed while receiving the drug and for 2 weeks after the drug is discontinued.

Females and Males of Reproductive Potential

Prior to initiation of ceritinib therapy, verify pregnancy status of females of reproductive potential. Females of reproductive potential should be advised to use effective methods of contraception while receiving the drug and for 6 months after the drug is discontinued. Men who are partners of such women should use effective contraceptive methods during and for 3 months after discontinuance of the drug.

Pediatric Use

Safety and efficacy of ceritinib have not been established in pediatric patients.

Geriatric Use

In clinical trials evaluating ceritinib 750 mg once daily in patients with *ALK*-positive non-small cell lung cancer (NSCLC), 18% of patients were ≥65 years of age and 5% were ≥75 years of age. No substantial differences in safety or efficacy of ceritinib were observed between geriatric patients and younger adults.

In pharmacokinetic population analyses, age did not have a clinically important effect on the systemic exposure of ceritinib in adults.

Hepatic Impairment

Following administration of a single 750-mg dose of ceritinib in a fasting state in individuals with severe hepatic impairment (Child-Pugh class C), mean systemic exposure to total and unbound ceritinib was increased by 66 and 108%, respectively, compared with exposure in individuals with normal hepatic function. Systemic exposure to total and unbound ceritinib in individuals with mild or moderate hepatic impairment (Child-Pugh class A or B) was similar to that observed in individuals with normal hepatic function.

The manufacturer recommends dosage adjustment in patients with severe hepatic impairment.

Renal Impairment

Population pharmacokinetic analysis suggests that systemic exposure to ceritinib is not substantially altered in patients with mild to moderate renal impairment (creatinine clearance of 30–89 mL/minute). Patients with severe renal impairment (creatinine clearance less than 30 mL/minute) were not included in the clinical trials.

● Common Adverse Effects

Adverse effects reported in ≥25% of patients receiving ceritinib 450 mg with food include nausea, diarrhea, vomiting, abdominal pain, and fatigue.

DRUG INTERACTIONS

Ceritinib is metabolized principally by cytochrome P-450 (CYP) isoenzyme 3A. In vitro, ceritinib is a substrate of P-glycoprotein (P-gp). In vitro studies also indicate that ceritinib may inhibit CYP isoenzymes 3A and 2C9 at clinically relevant concentrations. In vitro, ceritinib induces CYP3A4, but does not induce CYP isoenzymes 1A2, 2B6, or 2C9.

In vitro, ceritinib is not a substrate of breast cancer resistance protein (BCRP), multidrug resistance protein (MRP) 2, organic cation transporter (OCT) 1, organic anion transporter (OAT) 2, or organic anion transport protein (OATP) 1B1. Ceritinib is unlikely to inhibit P-gp, BCRP, MRP2, OATP1B1, OATP1B3, OAT1, OAT3, OCT1, or OCT2 in vitro at clinically relevant concentrations.

● Drugs or Foods Affecting Hepatic Microsomal Enzymes

Inhibitors of CYP3A

Concomitant use of ceritinib with potent inhibitors of CYP3A may result in increased systemic exposure of ceritinib and possible toxicity. When the potent CYP3A and P-gp inhibitor ketoconazole (200 mg twice daily for 14 days) was administered concomitantly with ceritinib (as a single 450-mg dose in a fasted state) in healthy individuals, AUC and peak plasma concentrations of ceritinib increased by 2.9-fold and 22%, respectively. The steady-state AUC of ceritinib following concomitant administration of the drug at a dosage of 450 mg once daily in a fasted state and ketoconazole for 14 days is expected to be similar to the steady-state AUC of ceritinib alone at a dosage of 750 mg once daily in a fasted state.

Concomitant use of potent CYP3A inhibitors should be avoided during ceritinib therapy. If concomitant use of a potent CYP3A inhibitor cannot be avoided, the manufacturer recommends reducing the daily dosage of ceritinib by approximately 33% and rounding to the nearest 150-mg strength of ceritinib capsules or tablets (e.g., from 450 mg daily to 300 mg daily). If concomitant use of the potent CYP3A inhibitor is discontinued, the ceritinib dosage should be returned to the dosage used prior to initiation of the potent CYP3A inhibitor.

Grapefruit products are CYP3A inhibitors and should be avoided because of the potential for increased plasma ceritinib concentrations during concomitant use.

Inducers of CYP3A

Concomitant use of ceritinib with potent inducers of CYP3A may result in decreased systemic exposure to ceritinib and reduced ceritinib efficacy. When the potent CYP3A4 and P-gp inducer rifampin (600 mg daily for 14 days) was administered concomitantly with ceritinib (as a single 750-mg dose) in healthy individuals, AUC and peak plasma concentrations of ceritinib decreased by 70 and 44%, respectively.

Concomitant use of ceritinib with potent CYP3A inducers should be avoided.

● Drugs Metabolized by Hepatic Microsomal Enzymes

Substrates of CYP3A

Ceritinib may inhibit CYP3A at clinically relevant concentrations and potentially can increase plasma concentrations of other drugs metabolized by CYP3A. When a single dose of the sensitive CYP3A substrate midazolam was administered concomitantly with ceritinib (750 mg once daily in a fasted state for 3 weeks), AUC and peak plasma concentration of midazolam increased 5.4- and 1.8-fold, respectively, compared with midazolam alone.

Concomitant use of ceritinib with CYP3A substrates with a narrow therapeutic index (e.g., midazolam) should be avoided. If concomitant use of CYP3A substrates with a narrow therapeutic index cannot be avoided, a dosage reduction of the CYP3A substrate should be considered.

Substrates of CYP2C9

Ceritinib may inhibit CYP2C9 at clinically relevant concentrations and potentially can increase plasma concentrations of other drugs metabolized by CYP2C9. When a single dose of the CYP2C9 substrate warfarin was administered concomitantly with ceritinib (750 mg once daily in a fasted state for 3 weeks), AUC of *S*-warfarin increased by 54% and peak plasma concentrations remained unchanged compared with warfarin alone. Concomitant use of ceritinib with CYP2C9 substrates that have a narrow therapeutic index (e.g., warfarin) should be avoided. If concomitant use of warfarin cannot be avoided, the manufacturer recommends more frequent INR monitoring for increased anticoagulant effects. If concomitant use of CYP2C9 substrates with a narrow therapeutic index cannot be avoided, a dosage reduction of the CYP2C9 substrate should be considered.

● Drugs Affecting Efflux Transport Systems

Ceritinib is a substrate of the efflux transporter P-glycoprotein (P-gp). If ceritinib is administered with drugs that inhibit P-gp (e.g., ketoconazole), increased concentrations of ceritinib may occur.

● Drugs Associated with QT Prolongation

Because ceritinib has been associated with QT-interval prolongation, the manufacturer recommends that concomitant use of ceritinib with other drugs known to prolong the QT interval be avoided, if possible. If concomitant use of other drugs known to prolong the QT interval cannot be avoided, the manufacturer recommends periodic monitoring of electrocardiograms (ECGs) and serum electrolytes.

● Drugs Associated with Bradycardia

Because ceritinib has been associated with bradycardia, the manufacturer recommends that concurrent use with other drugs known to cause bradycardia (e.g., β-adrenergic blocking agents, nondihydropyridine calcium-channel blocking agents [e.g., diltiazem, verapamil], clonidine, digoxin) be avoided, if possible.

● Drugs Affecting Gastric Acidity

Concomitant use of ceritinib with drugs that increase gastric pH (e.g., antacids, histamine H_2-receptor antagonists, proton-pump inhibitors) may decrease the solubility of ceritinib and subsequently reduce its bioavailability. When ceritinib (single 750-mg dose in fasted state) was administered concomitantly with the proton-pump inhibitor esomeprazole for 6 days in healthy individuals, AUC and peak plasma concentration of ceritinib decreased by 76 and 79%, respectively. However, in the ASCEND-1 study, decreases in ceritinib AUC and peak plasma concentration were only 30 and 25%, respectively, in a subgroup of patients who received ceritinib (single 750-mg dose in a fasted state) with a proton-pump inhibitor (for a duration of 6 days); no clinically meaningful effect on the pharmacokinetics of ceritinib were observed in these patients at steady state.

DESCRIPTION

Ceritinib, an inhibitor of receptor tyrosine kinases, including anaplastic lymphoma kinase (ALK), insulin-like growth factor 1 receptor (IGF-1R), insulin receptor, and c-ros oncogene-1 (ROS-1), is an antineoplastic agent. Among these tyrosine kinases, ceritinib is most active against ALK.

Activating mutations or translocations of the *ALK* gene have been identified in several malignancies and can result in the expression of oncogenic fusion proteins (e.g., echinoderm microtubule-associated protein-like 4 [EML4]-ALK). Such *ALK* gene rearrangements have been identified in approximately 3–7% of patients with NSCLC. Formation of ALK fusion proteins such as EML4-ALK results in activation and dysregulation of the gene's expression and signaling, which can contribute to increased cell proliferation and survival in tumors expressing these proteins. In vitro and in vivo, ceritinib has demonstrated inhibition of ALK phosphorylation, ALK-mediated phosphorylation of the downstream signaling protein signal transducer and activator of transcription-3 (STAT-3), and proliferation of ALK-dependent cancer cells. In vitro, ceritinib inhibited proliferation of cell lines that expressed EML4-ALK and nucleophosmin (NPM)-ALK fusion proteins. The drug also has demonstrated dose-dependent inhibition of EML4-ALK in mice and rats bearing NSCLC tumor xenografts that expressed EML4-ALK. In vitro, ceritinib is approximately 20-fold more potent than crizotinib in its activity against ALK.

At clinically relevant concentrations, ceritinib has demonstrated dose-dependent antitumor activity in mice bearing NSCLC tumor xenografts that expressed EML4-ALK with demonstrated resistance to crizotinib. Clinical resistance to crizotinib has been attributed to several possible mechanisms, including acquired resistance mutations of *ALK*, amplification of gene expression, and activation of alternate signaling pathways. Limited data to date suggest that secondary mutations of *ALK* (e.g., L1196M, G1269A) are responsible for only about 30% of cases of acquired crizotinib resistance. The CNS is a common site of disease progression in crizotinib-treated patients because of poor distribution of the drug into CSF; development and/or progression of brain metastases occurs in approximately one-half of patients during crizotinib treatment. In preclinical studies in cell-line models, ceritinib inhibited several crizotinib-resistant ALK kinase domain mutant forms.

Peak plasma concentrations of ceritinib are achieved about 4–6 hours following single-dose, oral administration of the drug. Following repeated administration of ceritinib 50–750 mg once daily, systemic exposure increases in a greater than dose-proportional manner. Following multiple-dose administration of ceritinib 750 mg daily, steady-state concentrations of the drug were achieved in approximately 15 days. Systemic exposure to ceritinib is increased when the drug is administered with food. Oral administration of a single 500-mg dose of ceritinib with a low-fat (approximately 330 calories and 9 g of fat) or high-fat meal (approximately 1000 calories and 58 g of fat) resulted in increases in systemic exposure of 58 or 73%, respectively, and increases in peak plasma concentrations by 43 or 41%, respectively, compared with the fasted state. Oral administration of a single 750-mg dose of ceritinib with a low- or high-fat meal resulted in increases in systemic exposure of 39 or 64%, respectively, and increases in peak plasma concentrations of 42 or 58%, respectively, compared with the fasted state. Systemic exposure to ceritinib was not substantially altered following oral administration of ceritinib 450 mg daily with food compared with administration of ceritinib 750 mg daily in a fasted state. Ceritinib is predominantly metabolized by the cytochrome P-450 (CYP) isoenzyme 3A. The drug is 97% bound to plasma proteins. Following oral administration of a single 750-mg radiolabeled dose of ceritinib, 92% of the dose was recovered in feces and 1.3% was recovered in urine; unchanged drug accounted for 68% of the dose recovered in feces. The mean terminal half-life of ceritinib is 41 hours.

ADVICE TO PATIENTS

- Advise patients to read the FDA-approved patient labeling.
- If a dose is missed, importance of advising patients to take it as soon as they remember unless it is less than 12 hours before the next dose, in which case they should not take the missed dose.
- If a dose is vomited, advise patients to not take an additional dose to replace the vomited dose. The next dose should be administered at the next scheduled time.
- Importance of informing patients that ceritinib should be taken with food. Importance of also advising patients to avoid grapefruit and grapefruit juice while taking ceritinib.
- Importance of informing patients that nausea, vomiting, diarrhea, and abdominal pain are the most common adverse effects associated with ceritinib therapy, as well as supportive treatment options (e.g., antiemetic and/or antidiarrhea agents). Importance of contacting clinician if severe or persistent adverse GI effects occur.
- Risk of hepatotoxicity; importance of liver function test monitoring. Importance of informing patients of the signs and symptoms of hepatotoxicity (e.g., fatigue, anorexia, nausea, vomiting, abdominal pain [especially right upper quadrant pain], jaundice, dark or "tea-colored" urine, generalized pruritus, unusual bleeding or bruising) and advising them to immediately report possible symptoms of hepatotoxicity to their clinician.
- Risk of severe or fatal interstitial lung disease/pneumonitis. Importance of advising patients that pneumonitis symptoms may be similar to those of lung cancer and to contact their clinician immediately if they experience any new or worsening pulmonary symptoms (e.g., dyspnea, shortness of breath, cough with or without mucus, chest pain, fever).
- Risk of QT_c-interval prolongation and bradycardia. Importance of informing clinicians immediately if new chest pain or discomfort, changes in heartbeat, palpitations, dizziness, lightheadedness, faintness, or changes in or new use of cardiovascular or antihypertensive therapy occurs.
- Risk of hyperglycemia, particularly in patients with diabetes or glucose intolerance and in those receiving corticosteroid medications. Importance of informing patients of the signs and symptoms of hyperglycemia (e.g., increased thirst, increased urination, increased appetite, fatigue, blurred vision, headache, difficulty thinking or concentrating, breath that smells like fruit) and advising patients to immediately contact their clinician if they experience such signs and symptoms.
- Risk of pancreatitis. Importance of informing clinicians immediately if signs or symptoms of pancreatitis (e.g., upper abdominal pain that may spread to the back) occur.
- Risk of fetal harm. Importance of patients informing their clinicians if they are pregnant or plan to become pregnant. If pregnancy occurs, advise patient of potential risk to the fetus.

- Advise women of reproductive potential that they should use effective methods of contraception while receiving ceritinib and for 6 months after discontinuance of therapy. Advise men who are partners with women of reproductive potential to use effective methods of contraception while receiving the drug and for 3 months after the drug is discontinued.
- Advise women to avoid breast-feeding while receiving ceritinib and for 2 weeks after discontinuance of therapy.
- Advise patients to inform their clinician of existing or contemplated concomitant therapy, including prescription and OTC drugs and dietary or herbal supplements (e.g., St. John's wort), as well as any concomitant illnesses (e.g., hepatic impairment, cardiovascular disease [including congenital long QT syndrome], diabetes mellitus or hyperglycemia).
- Advise patients of other important precautionary information. (See Cautions.)

For further information on the handling of antineoplastic agents, see the ASHP Guidelines on Handling Hazardous Drugs at http://www.ahfsdrug information.com.

PREPARATIONS

Ceritinib is available only from designated specialty distributors and pharmacies. The manufacturer should be contacted for additional information.

Excipients in commercially available drug preparations may have clinically important effects in some individuals; consult specific product labeling for details.

Ceritinib

Oral		
Capsules	150 mg	Zykadia®, Novartis
Tablets, film-coated	150 mg	Zykadia®, Novartis

Cetuximab

10:00 · ANTINEOPLASTIC AGENTS

■ Cetuximab, a recombinant chimeric (human-murine) monoclonal antibody that binds to epidermal growth factor receptors (EGFR), is an antineoplastic agent.

USES

● Colorectal Cancer

Patients enrolled in clinical studies for the use of cetuximab for colorectal cancer were required to have immunohistochemical (IHC) evidence of epidermal growth factor receptor (EGFR) expression; however, response rates in these clinical studies did not correlate with either the percentage of positive cells or the intensity of EGFR expression. In addition, responses to cetuximab therapy have been observed in patients with EGFR-negative colorectal cancer. Some authorities state that routine EGFR expression testing is not recommended in patients with colorectal cancer and that patients should not be included or excluded from cetuximab therapy based solely on EGFR test results.

Because retrospective stratified analyses of metastatic colorectal cancer trials have not shown a treatment benefit for cetuximab in patients whose tumors had *KRAS* mutations in codon 12 or 13, use of the drug is *not* recommended for the treatment of colorectal cancer with such mutations. (See *KRAS* Testing in Patients Receiving Cetuximab for Colorectal Cancer under Uses: Colorectal Cancer.)

Cetuximab Monotherapy for Advanced Colorectal Cancer

Cetuximab is used as a single agent for the treatment of EGFR-expressing metastatic colorectal cancer in patients with disease that has failed treatment with both irinotecan-based and oxaliplatin-based regimens. Cetuximab also is used as a single agent for the treatment of EGFR-expressing, metastatic colorectal cancer in patients who are intolerant of irinotecan-based chemotherapy.

The current indication for cetuximab monotherapy for recurrent EGFR-expressing metastatic colorectal cancer is based mainly on the results of a multicenter, open-label, randomized trial in 572 patients receiving either cetuximab and best supportive care or best supportive care alone for EGFR-expressing metastatic colorectal cancer. All patients had progression of disease following previous treatment with an irinotecan-containing regimen and an oxaliplatin-containing regimen or had contraindications to treatment with these agents. The treatment regimen consisted of an initial dose of cetuximab 400 mg/m² as a 2-hour IV infusion followed by cetuximab 250 mg/m² as a 1-hour IV infusion weekly until disease progression or unacceptable toxicity occurred. The median age of the patients was 63 years, 64% were male, and most of the patients (89%) were Caucasian; 77% had a baseline ECOG performance status of 0–1.

Median overall survival was prolonged in patients receiving cetuximab and best supportive care compared with those receiving best supportive care alone (6.1 versus 4.6 months; hazard ratio for death 0.77 with a 95% confidence interval of 0.64–0.92). Adverse effects were more frequent in patients receiving cetuximab therapy and best supportive care than in those receiving best supportive care alone, particularly rash/desquamation (89 versus 16%, grade 3 or 4 in 12 versus less than 1%).

Cetuximab and Irinotecan for Advanced Colorectal Cancer

Cetuximab is used in combination with irinotecan for the treatment of EGFR-expressing metastatic colorectal cancer that is refractory to irinotecan-based chemotherapy. The indication for cetuximab in combination with irinotecan for EGFR-expressing, metastatic colorectal cancer is based on objective response rates; there currently are no data demonstrating a clinical benefit (e.g., improvement in disease-related symptoms, increased survival).

The current indication for cetuximab in combination with irinotecan is based principally on the results of a phase 2, multicenter, randomized, controlled study that compared safety and efficacy of cetuximab monotherapy with the combination regimen of cetuximab and irinotecan.

This phase 2 study enrolled 329 patients with EGFR-expressing, metastatic colorectal cancer refractory to irinotecan-based chemotherapy; approximately two thirds of enrolled patients had previously failed oxaliplatin therapy. In this study, 111 patients were randomized to receive cetuximab monotherapy (400 mg/m²

initially, followed by 250 mg/m² weekly until disease progression or unacceptable toxicity occurred), and 218 patients were randomized to receive cetuximab (at the same dosage) in combination with irinotecan (350 mg/m² every 3 weeks, 180 mg/m² every 2 weeks, *or* 125 mg/m² weekly for 4 doses every 6 weeks).

The overall response rate (complete plus partial responses) was higher in patients receiving the combination regimen (about 23%) than in those receiving cetuximab monotherapy (about 11%). In addition, median time to radiographic disease progression and median duration of response were longer in patients receiving the combination regimen (4.1 and 5.7 months, respectively) than in those receiving cetuximab alone (1.5 and 4.2 months, respectively). Median survival was not substantially different between the 2 groups (8.6 months for the combination regimen versus 6.9 months for cetuximab monotherapy).

Cetuximab and Combination Chemotherapy as First-line Therapy for Metastatic Colorectal Cancer

Cetuximab has been used with combination chemotherapy regimens for the first-line treatment of metastatic colorectal cancer.

In a phase 3 randomized trial that enrolled 238 patients with previously untreated metastatic colorectal cancer before closing early because of slow accrual, the addition of cetuximab to either FOLFIRI (irinotecan/fluorouracil/leucovorin) or FOLFOX (oxaliplatin/fluorouracil/leucovorin) appeared to increase response rates; at a median follow-up of about 1 year, analysis of the data did not show any effect of the addition of cetuximab on progression-free survival or duration of response. A phase 3 randomized trial comparing the addition of cetuximab, bevacizumab, or both to combination chemotherapy (FOLFOX or FOLFIRI) for the first-line treatment of metastatic colorectal cancer is under way.

KRAS Testing in Patients Receiving Cetuximab for Colorectal Cancer

The presence of mutations in the *KRAS* (also called *K-ras*) gene in codon 12 or 13 in colorectal cancer tumor tissue has been associated with a lack of benefit from therapy with anti-EGFR monoclonal antibodies (e.g., cetuximab, panitumumab); such mutations appear to be present in approximately 30–50% of primary colorectal tumors. Retrospective subset analyses from 7 randomized clinical studies evaluating cetuximab or panitumumab either as monotherapy or in combination with chemotherapy in metastatic colorectal cancer suggest that these anti-EGFR monoclonal antibodies are not effective for the treatment of patients with colorectal cancer containing *KRAS* mutations in codon 12 or 13. The American Society of Clinical Oncology (ASCO) and some clinicians recommend that all patients with metastatic colorectal cancer who are potential candidates for EGFR inhibitor therapy (e.g., cetuximab, panitumumab) have their tumor tested for *KRAS* mutations in a Clinical Laboratory Improvement Amendments (CLIA)-accredited laboratory. If *KRAS* mutation in codon 12 or 13 is detected, the use of cetuximab is *not* recommended.

● Head and Neck Cancer

Because expression of EGFR has been detected in nearly all head and neck cancers, patients enrolled in the studies on which the labeled indications for cetuximab for this neoplasm were based were not required to have immunohistochemical evidence of EGFR expression.

Cetuximab and Radiation Therapy for Locally or Regionally Advanced Disease

Cetuximab is used in combination with radiation therapy for the initial treatment of locally or regionally advanced squamous cell carcinoma of the head and neck, particularly for patients who cannot tolerate platinum-based chemotherapy with radiation therapy.

In a multicenter randomized controlled trial, 424 patients with stage III or IV squamous cell carcinoma of the oropharynx (60%), larynx (25%), or hypopharynx (15%) received initial treatment with either cetuximab and radiation therapy or radiation therapy alone. Stratification factors were Karnofsky performance status (60–80 versus 90–100), nodal stage (N0 versus N+), tumor stage (T1–3 versus T4 according to AJCC 1998 staging criteria), and radiation therapy fractionation (concomitant boost, once daily, or twice daily).

Patients receiving cetuximab were given premedication with IV diphenhydramine hydrochloride 50 mg or an equivalent histamine H_1-receptor antagonist to reduce the risk of infusion-related reactions. Patients receiving cetuximab were given a 20-mg test dose of the drug on day 1; an initial dose of cetuximab 400 mg/m² was administered by 2-hour IV infusion 1 week before the initiation of radiation therapy followed by cetuximab 250 mg/m² by 1-hour IV infusion 1 hour prior to radiation therapy once weekly for 6–7 weeks. Radiation therapy was administered for 6–7 weeks as concomitant boost (56%), once daily fractionation (26%), or twice daily fractionation (18%). For patients with stage N1 or higher neck disease, neck dissection at 4–8 weeks following completion of radiation therapy was recommended. The patients enrolled in the trial were mostly Caucasian men with a baseline Karnofsky performance status of at least 80; the median age of the patients was 57 years.

Patients with locally or regionally advanced squamous cell carcinoma of the head and neck receiving cetuximab and radiation therapy had prolonged median duration of locoregional control (24 versus 15 months, hazard ratio for locoregional progression or death: 0.68) and prolonged median overall survival (49 versus 29 months, hazard ratio for death: 0.74) compared with those receiving radiation therapy alone. Subgroup analysis according to tumor type suggested efficacy of cetuximab and radiation therapy for oropharyngeal tumors, but not for hypopharyngeal or laryngeal tumors. Acneiform rash (all grades: 87 versus 10%, grade 3 or 4: 17 versus 1%) and infusion reactions (all grades: 15 versus 2%, grade 3 or 4: 3 versus 0%) occurred more frequently in patients receiving cetuximab and radiation therapy than in those receiving radiation therapy alone.

The use of platinum-based chemotherapy with radiation therapy is the current standard of care for the treatment of advanced head and neck cancer. Further study is needed to compare the efficacy and toxicity for cetuximab and radiation therapy versus platinum-based chemotherapy and radiation therapy.

Monotherapy for Advanced Disease

Cetuximab is used alone for the treatment of recurrent or metastatic squamous cell carcinoma of the head and neck in patients with disease that has failed platinum-based therapy.

The current indication for use of cetuximab as a single agent for the treatment of recurrent or metastatic squamous cell carcinoma of the head and neck is based principally on the results of a single-arm, multicenter clinical trial involving 103 patients with disease that progressed within 30 days following 2–6 cycles of platinum-based chemotherapy. Patients received a 20-mg test dose of cetuximab on day 1, an initial dose of cetuximab 400 mg/m², and then cetuximab 250 mg/m² once weekly until disease progression or unacceptable toxicity. The patients enrolled in the trial were mostly Caucasian men, and 62% of the patients had a baseline Karnofsky performance status of at least 80; the median age of the patients was 57 years.

The objective response rate was 13% and the median duration of response was 5.8 months for patients receiving cetuximab monotherapy for recurrent or metastatic head and neck cancer.

Cetuximab and Chemotherapy With or Without Radiation Therapy for Advanced Disease

Cetuximab has been used in combination with chemotherapy, with or without radiation therapy†, for the treatment of recurrent or metastatic squamous cell carcinoma of the head and neck.

In two phase 2 studies, cetuximab with platinum-based chemotherapy demonstrated activity in the treatment of recurrent or metastatic platinum-refractory squamous cell carcinoma of the head and neck. In a phase 3 randomized trial, the addition of cetuximab to cisplatin improved response rates but did not affect progression-free survival or overall survival in patients receiving first-line treatment for recurrent or metastatic squamous cell carcinoma of the head and neck. In another phase 3 randomized trial, the addition of cetuximab to a platinum agent (cisplatin or carboplatin) and fluorouracil prolonged median overall survival (10.1 versus 7.4 months) and median progression-free survival (5.6 versus 3.3 months) and increased the response rate (36 versus 20%) in the first-line treatment of recurrent and/or metastatic squamous cell cancer of the head and neck. Grade 3 or 4 adverse effects that occurred more frequently in patients receiving cetuximab with a platinum agent and fluorouracil than in those receiving a platinum agent and fluorouracil included skin reactions (grade 3 only, in 9 versus less than 1%), hypomagnesemia and anorexia (each in 5 versus 1%), and sepsis, including septic shock (in 4 versus less than 1%).

In a pilot study, cetuximab and cisplatin were administered with delayed, accelerated (concomitant boost) fractionation radiation therapy for the treatment of locoregionally advanced squamous cell head and neck cancer. The study was closed early because of safety concerns regarding fatalities and serious adverse

events. Of the 21 patients enrolled in the study, one patient died from and one patient died of an unknown cause. Four patients disconti because of adverse events; adverse cardiac events were the re uation of treatment in two of these patients with myoca patient and arrhythmia, diminished cardiac output, and hypote patient. Although use of this regimen is not recommended outside of a clinical trial because of safety concerns, high rates of response and high 3-year survival rates suggest that further study of cetuximab in combined modality treatment for advanced head and neck cancer is warranted.

A phase 3 randomized trial studying the effect of the addition of cetuximab to a regimen of concurrent accelerated fractionated radiation therapy and cisplatin for stage III or IV squamous cell carcinoma of the oropharynx, hypopharynx, or larynx is under way.

● Non-small Cell Lung Cancer

Efficacy and safety of cetuximab in combination with various chemotherapy regimens as first-line therapy for advanced (stage IIIB [with malignant pleural effusion] or IV [metastatic]) non-small cell lung cancer (NSCLC)† has been studied in several randomized studies.

Use of cetuximab either concurrently with or following carboplatin and paclitaxel therapy was investigated in a randomized phase 2 study (S0342) in 242 patients with previously untreated stage IIIB or IV NSCLC. Patients in both treatment groups received carboplatin (at the dose required to obtain an area under the plasma concentration-time curve [AUC] of 6 mg/mL per minute) and paclitaxel (225 mg/m² by IV infusion) in 21-day cycles for 4 cycles; cetuximab (initial dose of 400 mg/m² by IV infusion followed by 250 mg/m² by IV infusion once weekly) was initiated either concurrently with or following completion of carboplatin and paclitaxel therapy and was continued until disease progression, unacceptable toxicity, or withdrawal of patient consent. At a median follow-up of 32 months, overall survival (10.9 versus 10.7 months), progression-free survival (4.3 versus 4.4 months), and response rates (32 versus 30%) were similar in both treatment groups; however, the incidence of grade 3/4 sensory neuropathy was higher in patients receiving concurrent therapy compared with those receiving sequential therapy (15 versus 5%, respectively). About one-third of patients underwent EGFR testing (using fluorescent in situ hybridization [FISH] methodology); those with EGFR-positive tumors had longer median progression-free survival (6 versus 3 months) and overall survival (15 versus 7 months) compared with those with EGFR-negative tumors. Overall survival favored EGFR-positive patients receiving cetuximab concurrently with chemotherapy.

Efficacy and safety of cetuximab administered concurrently with up to 6 cycles of chemotherapy and then continued alone as maintenance therapy have been evaluated in two phase 3, open-label, randomized studies (First-line Erbitux in Lung Cancer [FLEX] and BMS-099) in patients with previously untreated stage IIIB or IV NSCLC. Patients in these studies received either cetuximab and chemotherapy (either cisplatin and vinorelbine or carboplatin and a taxane) or chemotherapy alone. The studies included patients with any histologic cell type but excluded those with metastatic CNS disease and those who had received prior anti-EGFR therapy. Patient enrollment in the BMS-099 study was independent of EGFR expression status, while enrollment in the FLEX study required immunohistochemical (IHC) evidence of EGFR expression (using the Dako EGFR pharmDx® test kit). In the BMS-099 study, patients were stratified according to their baseline ECOG performance status (0 or 1), intended taxane (paclitaxel or docetaxel), and study site.

In the FLEX study, 1125 patients were randomized to receive vinorelbine (25 mg/m² by IV infusion on days 1 and 8) and cisplatin (80 mg/m² by IV infusion on day 1) in 21-day cycles either alone or in combination with cetuximab (initial dose of 400 mg/m² as a 2-hour IV infusion on day 1 followed by 250 mg/m² by IV infusion over 1 hour once weekly); cetuximab was continued until disease progression or unacceptable toxicity occurred, while vinorelbine and cisplatin were administered for up to 6 cycles. In the BMS-099 study, 676 patients were randomized to receive carboplatin (administered on day 1 at the dose required to obtain an AUC of 6 mg/mL per minute) and a taxane (paclitaxel 225 mg/m² as a 3-hour IV infusion or docetaxel 75 mg/m² as a 1-hour IV infusion on day 1) in 21-day cycles either alone or in combination with cetuximab (initial dose of 400 mg/m² as a 2-hour IV infusion followed by 250 mg/m² by IV infusion over 1 hour once weekly); cetuximab was continued until disease progression or unacceptable toxicity occurred, while carboplatin and a taxane were administered for up to 6 cycles.

In the FLEX study, the primary measure of efficacy was overall survival. At a median follow-up of 23.8 months, median overall survival was 1.2 months longer

10.1 months; hazard ratio of 0.87) and the rate of survival at 1 year _____ versus 42%) for patients receiving cetuximab in combination with _____ elbine compared with those receiving cisplatin and vinorelbine alone. Median progression-free survival was 4.8 months in both treatment groups. The overall response rate was 36% for patients receiving cetuximab in combination with chemotherapy and 29% for those receiving chemotherapy alone. Subset analysis suggested that ECOG performance status, smoking status, histologic type, gender, and age did not influence the treatment effect on overall survival.

Subset analysis of the FLEX study results based on ethnicity indicated that characteristics associated with a more favorable prognosis (i.e., adenocarcinoma histology, female gender, never smoked) were more common in Asian patients than in Caucasian patients and that the median survival of Asian patients was 10 months longer than that of Caucasian patients. However, a higher proportion of Asian patients received oral tyrosine kinase inhibitors following their assigned study treatment, and the possibility that additional EGFR-targeted therapy might have contributed to an improved survival rate for these patients cannot be ruled out. The addition of cetuximab to chemotherapy did not significantly improve survival of Asian patients or other non-Caucasian patients. In contrast, median overall survival of Caucasian patients (84% of patients in the study) was longer for those receiving cetuximab in combination with chemotherapy compared with those receiving chemotherapy alone (10.5 versus 9.1 months). Subset analysis based on tumor histology indicated that median survival times for patients receiving cetuximab in combination with chemotherapy compared with those receiving chemotherapy alone were 12 versus 10.3 months, respectively, for patients with adenocarcinoma and 10.2 versus 8.9 months, respectively, for those with squamous cell carcinoma.

In the FLEX study, grade 3 or 4 febrile neutropenia (22 versus 15%), acneiform rash (10 versus less than 1%), infusion-related reactions (4 versus 1%), and diarrhea (5 versus 2%) occurred more frequently in patients receiving cetuximab in combination with cisplatin and vinorelbine than in those receiving cisplatin and vinorelbine alone.

In the BMS-099 study, the primary measure of efficacy was progression-free survival assessed by an independent radiologic review committee. The addition of cetuximab to carboplatin and taxane therapy improved the overall response rate (25.7 versus 17.2%) but did not substantially improve median progression-free survival (4.4 versus 4.2 months) or median overall survival (9.7 versus 8.4 months). Subgroup analyses suggested that the addition of cetuximab to chemotherapy had a greater effect on progression-free survival in certain subgroups of patients (those with an ECOG performance status of 0, those receiving docetaxel, and those with squamous cell histology) than in the overall study population; however, similar trends were not observed for overall survival. Grade 3 or 4 acneiform rash (10.5 versus 0%), infusion-related reactions (4.6 versus 0.9%), hypomagnesemia (8.8 versus 0.7%), diarrhea (5.2 versus 2.5%), dehydration (8.6 versus 4.7%), and neutropenia (62.5 versus 56%) occurred more frequently in patients receiving cetuximab in combination with carboplatin and a taxane than in those receiving carboplatin and a taxane alone.

Post-hoc analyses of the FLEX and BMS-099 studies were performed in an attempt to identify tumor markers that would predict which patients might benefit from the addition of cetuximab to chemotherapy as first-line treatment for advanced NSCLC. Comparisons of outcomes between treatment groups according to tumor marker status revealed no significant associations between efficacy (i.e., overall survival, progression-free survival, tumor response) and *KRAS* mutation status, EGFR mutation status, EGFR gene copy number (assessed by FISH methodology), or phosphatase and tensin homolog (PTEN) gene expression (assessed by IHC methodology) that would identify patients who might benefit from receiving cetuximab in addition to chemotherapy. In the BMS-099 study, EGFR expression (assessed by IHC methodology and described as either positive or negative) was not associated with improved efficacy for cetuximab and chemotherapy compared with chemotherapy alone. However, in the FLEX study, addition of cetuximab to chemotherapy was associated with a survival benefit in patients with high EGFR expression (IHC score of 200 or greater on a scale of 0–300); among patients with high EGFR expression, overall survival was 12 months for those receiving cetuximab and chemotherapy compared with 9.6 months for those receiving chemotherapy alone.

Although combined therapy with cetuximab and chemotherapy prolonged overall survival in the FLEX study, the magnitude of the benefit was modest and the same benefit was not observed in the BMS-099 study; in addition, combined therapy did not prolong progression-free survival in either study. Therefore, the role of the drug in combination with chemotherapy for the treatment of previously untreated advanced NSCLC is unclear. In addition, although exploratory analyses in the FLEX and BMS-099 studies suggested that overall survival results were generally consistent across most patient subgroups, exploratory analyses of progression-free survival in the BMS-099 study suggested some differences in treatment effect in certain patient subgroups (as compared with the overall population). Additional studies are needed to validate predictive tumor biomarkers and identify subgroups of patients with previously untreated advanced NSCLC who might derive clinical benefit (e.g., prolonged progression-free survival, prolonged overall survival, improved quality of life) from the addition of cetuximab to chemotherapy. The AHFS Oncology Expert Committee concluded that use of cetuximab in combination with various chemotherapy regimens as first-line therapy for advanced (stage IIIB [with malignant pleural effusion] or IV [metastatic]) NSCLC currently is not fully established because of equivocal evidence.

DOSAGE AND ADMINISTRATION

● Administration

Cetuximab is administered by IV infusion. *The drug should not be administered by rapid IV injection, such as IV push or bolus.* The initial dose of cetuximab is administered over 2 hours, and the subsequent weekly dose is administered over 1 hour. The maximum infusion rate should not exceed 10 mg/minute.

Cetuximab injection should be inspected visually for particulate matter and discoloration whenever solution and container permit. Cetuximab injection for IV infusion should be clear and colorless and may contain a small amount of easily visible, white, amorphous cetuximab particulates. Cetuximab injection for IV infusion should not be diluted, and vials should not be shaken.

Cetuximab may be administered using either an infusion pump or a syringe pump. The drug must be administered through a low-protein-binding 0.22-μm inline filter. Patients should be monitored for signs of infusion reactions during and for 1 hour following cetuximab infusion. For patients experiencing infusion reactions requiring treatment, monitoring should be continued until the event is resolved. (See Infusion-related Effects under Warnings/Precautions: Warnings, in Cautions.)

Cetuximab solution should be stored in unopened vials under refrigeration at 2–8°C and protected from freezing. Preparations of cetuximab solution in infusion containers are chemically and physically stable for up to 12 hours at 2–8°C and up to 8 hours at controlled room temperature (20–25°C); any solution remaining in the infusion container after 8 hours (if stored at room temperature) or after 12 hours (if refrigerated) should be discarded. Cetuximab contains no preservatives; any unused portion of the vial should be discarded.

● General Dosage
Premedication

To minimize the risk of infusion-related reactions associated with cetuximab, premedication with an antihistamine (e.g., 50 mg of IV diphenhydramine hydrochloride 30–60 minutes prior to the first dose of cetuximab) is recommended. Based on the occurrence and severity of previous infusion reactions, premedication with an antihistamine may be administered for subsequent cetuximab doses as clinically indicated.

Colorectal Cancer

For the management of previously treated EGFR-expressing metastatic colorectal cancer, either as monotherapy or in combination therapy with irinotecan, an initial dose of cetuximab 400 mg/m² is administered by IV infusion over 2 hours, followed by cetuximab 250 mg/m² as a 1-hour IV infusion once weekly until disease progression or unacceptable toxicity occurs; the maximum infusion rate should not exceed 10 mg/minute.

Head and Neck Cancer

For use in combination with radiation therapy for the treatment of locally or regionally advanced squamous cell cancer of the head and neck, an initial dose of cetuximab 400 mg/m² is administered by IV infusion over 2 hours at 1 week prior to the initiation of a course of radiation therapy. For the duration of radiation therapy (6–7 weeks), cetuximab 250 mg/m² is administered by 1-hour IV infusion once weekly. Administration of cetuximab should be completed 1 hour prior to radiation therapy. The maximum infusion rate for cetuximab should not exceed 10 mg/minute. In a randomized trial for locally or regionally advanced head and neck cancer, a median of 8 doses of cetuximab was administered in patients receiving cetuximab and radiation therapy.

For use as monotherapy for the treatment of recurrent or metastatic squamous cell cancer of the head and neck, an initial dose of cetuximab 400 mg/m^2 is administered as a 2-hour IV infusion followed by cetuximab 250 mg/m^2 as a 1-hour IV infusion once weekly (maximum infusion rate of 10 mg/min for initial and subsequent doses) until disease progression or unacceptable toxicity occurs.

Dosage Modification for Toxicity and Contraindications for Continued Therapy

Infusion-related Reactions

In patients who develop grade 1 or 2 or nonserious grade 3 or 4 infusion-related reactions, the infusion rate should be reduced by 50%. In patients who develop serious infusion-related reactions, requiring medical intervention and/or hospitalization, cetuximab therapy should be immediately and permanently discontinued. (See Infusion-related Effects under Warning/Precautions: Warnings, in Cautions.)

Dermatologic Toxicity

In patients who experience severe acneiform rash, cetuximab therapy should be temporarily delayed, and subsequent doses should be reduced or therapy discontinued depending on the patient's response (see Table 1).

TABLE 1. Cetuximab Dosage Modification for Severe Acneiform Rash

Occurrence of Severe Acneiform Rash	Intervention	Outcome	Cetuximab Dosage
First occurrence	Delay cetuximab infusion for 1–2 weeks	Improvement	Continue subsequent weekly dose of 250 mg/m^2
		No improvement	Discontinue cetuximab therapy
Second occurrence	Delay cetuximab infusion for 1–2 weeks	Improvement	Reduce subsequent weekly dose to 200 mg/m^2
		No improvement	Discontinue cetuximab therapy
Third occurrence	Delay cetuximab infusion for 1–2 weeks	Improvement	Reduce subsequent weekly dose to 150 mg/m^2
		No improvement	Discontinue cetuximab therapy
Fourth occurrence	Discontinue cetuximab therapy		

Pulmonary Toxicity

If acute onset or worsening of pulmonary symptoms occurs, cetuximab therapy should be interrupted. If interstitial lung disease is confirmed, cetuximab therapy should be permanently discontinued.

Special Populations

No special population dosage recommendations at this time.

CAUTIONS

Contraindications

The manufacturer states that there are no contraindications to the use of cetuximab.

Warnings/Precautions

Warnings

Infusion-related Effects

Infusion-related effects (e.g., chills, fever, rigors, dyspnea, bronchospasm, angioedema, urticaria, hypertension, hypotension) have been reported in 15–21% of patients receiving cetuximab in clinical trials. Serious infusion-related effects, requiring medical intervention and immediate, permanent discontinuance of cetuximab, have included rapid airway obstruction (bronchospasm, stridor, hoarseness), hypotension, shock, loss of consciousness, myocardial infarction, and cardiac arrest. Severe (grade 3 or 4) infusion reactions occurred in 2–5% of 1373 patients in clinical trials; one patient died. Approximately 90% of severe infusion reactions occurred in association with the initial infusion of cetuximab despite premedication with antihistamines.

Patients should be monitored for signs of infusion reactions during and for 1 hour following cetuximab infusion in a setting where resuscitation equipment and agents necessary to treat anaphylaxis are readily available. For patients experiencing infusion reactions requiring treatment, monitoring should be continued until the event is resolved.

If grade 1 or 2 or nonserious grade 3 or 4 infusion-related reactions occur, the infusion rate for cetuximab should be reduced by 50%. If serious infusion-related effects occur, cetuximab therapy should be immediately and permanently discontinued, and appropriate therapy (e.g., epinephrine, corticosteroids, IV antihistamines, bronchodilators, oxygen) initiated. Patients should be monitored until all infusion-related manifestations have completely resolved.

Cardiac Effects

Cardiopulmonary arrest and/or sudden death occurred in 4 (2%) of 208 patients receiving cetuximab and radiation therapy compared with none of 212 patients receiving radiation therapy alone for squamous cell carcinoma of the head and neck in a randomized, controlled trial. One patient with no history of coronary artery disease died 1 day following the last dose of cetuximab. Three patients with histories of coronary artery disease died at home at 27, 32, and 43 days following the last dose of cetuximab; myocardial infarction was the presumed cause of death. One of these patients had arrhythmia and one patient had congestive heart failure.

Cetuximab and radiation therapy for the treatment of head and neck cancer should be used with caution in patients with a history of coronary artery disease, congestive heart failure, or arrhythmias. Serum concentrations of electrolytes, including magnesium, potassium, and calcium, should be monitored closely during and following cetuximab therapy.

Adverse cardiac events—myocardial infarction in one patient and arrhythmia, diminished cardiac output, and hypotension in another patient—caused discontinuation of treatment in patients with head and neck cancer receiving cetuximab with cisplatin and radiation therapy in a clinical trial. The safety of cetuximab in combination with cisplatin and radiation therapy has not been established.

Pulmonary Effects

Interstitial lung disease, interstitial pneumonitis (fatal in one case), and exacerbation of preexisting fibrotic lung disease have been reported in patients receiving cetuximab alone or in combination with other antineoplastic agents (e.g., cisplatin, irinotecan). Interruption or discontinuance of cetuximab therapy may be required in patients with pulmonary symptoms. (See Pulmonary Toxicity under Dosage Modification for Toxicity and Contraindications for Continued Therapy, in Dosage and Administration.)

Electrolyte Effects

Electrolyte abnormalities, sometimes severe, including hypomagnesemia, hypocalcemia, and hypokalemia, have occurred in patients receiving cetuximab. Hypomagnesemia occurred in 199 (55%) of 365 patients receiving cetuximab in clinical trials and was severe (grade 3 or 4) in 6–17% of patients. The onset of hypomagnesemia and accompanying electrolyte abnormalities may occur from days to months following initiation of cetuximab therapy. Manifestations of hypomagnesemia may include fatigue and hypocalcemia. Patients should be monitored for hypomagnesemia, hypocalcemia, and hypokalemia during and for at least 8 weeks following completion of cetuximab therapy. Electrolyte repletion therapy should be administered as necessary and, in severe cases, intravenous replacement therapy is required.

Sensitivity Reactions

Dermatologic Effects

Acneiform rash occurred in 76–88% of 1373 patients receiving cetuximab in clinical trials and was severe in 1–17% of patients. Acneiform rash generally appears within the first 2 weeks of cetuximab therapy and may resolve following discontinuance of cetuximab; however, manifestations have persisted beyond 28 days in nearly 50% of cases.

Other adverse dermatologic effects, including skin drying/fissuring, paronychial inflammation, infectious sequelae (e.g., abscess formation, blepharitis, conjunctivitis, keratitis, cheilitis, cellulitis, *Staphylococcus aureus* sepsis), and hypertrichosis also have been reported. Fatal toxic epidermal necrolysis has been reported in a patient receiving cetuximab for colorectal cancer. Abnormal hair growth has been reported in a patient receiving cetuximab for head and neck cancer.

Reduction of dosage or discontinuance of therapy is required in patients who develop severe acneiform rash. (See Dermatologic Toxicity under Dosage Modification for Toxicity and Contraindications for Continued Therapy, in Dosage and Administration.)

Major Toxicities

Serious Adverse Effects

Other serious adverse effects associated with cetuximab include radiation dermatitis, sepsis, renal failure, and pulmonary embolus. Sepsis occurred in 1–4% of patients receiving cetuximab. Renal failure was reported in 1% of patients receiving cetuximab for colorectal cancer. Across all studies, cetuximab therapy was discontinued in 3–10% of patients because of adverse effects. (See Warnings under Cautions: Warnings/Precautions.)

General Precautions

EGFR Testing

In clinical trials for colorectal cancer, testing for evidence of EGFR expression was required. However, some authorities state that routine EGFR expression testing is not recommended in patients with colorectal cancer and that patients should not be included or excluded from cetuximab therapy based solely on EGFR test results.

Because expression of EGFR has been detected in nearly all head and neck cancers, EGFR testing was not required in these clinical trials.

Therapy Monitoring

Patients receiving cetuximab should be monitored for dermatologic toxicity and infectious sequelae.

Patients should be monitored periodically for hypomagnesemia, and accompanying hypocalcemia and hypokalemia, during and following the completion of cetuximab therapy. Monitoring should be continued for at least 8 weeks following completion of therapy.

Immunologic Effects

Non-neutralizing anticetuximab antibodies were detected in about 5% of patients (49/1001) receiving cetuximab; although the incidence of antibody development to cetuximab has not been fully established, there appears to be no effect on the safety and efficacy of the drug.

Specific Populations

Pregnancy

Category C. (See Users Guide.)

Lactation

It is not known whether cetuximab is distributed into milk; however, human immunoglobulin G_1 (IgG_1) is distributed into milk. Because of the potential for distribution of IgG antibodies such as cetuximab into milk and the risks for serious adverse reactions from cetuximab in nursing infants, a decision should be made whether to discontinue nursing or the drug, taking into account the importance of the drug to the woman. Based on the long half-life of cetuximab, women should be advised to discontinue nursing while receiving cetuximab therapy and for at least 60 days following the last dose of the drug (see Description).

Pediatric Use

Safety and efficacy of cetuximab have not been established in pediatric patients.

Geriatric Use

Approximately 34% of the 1062 patients receiving cetuximab (alone or in combination with irinotecan) in clinical studies for advanced colorectal cancer were 65 years of age or older. No overall differences in safety and efficacy relative to younger adults were observed.

Clinical studies of cetuximab for head and neck cancer did not include sufficient numbers of patients 65 years of age and older to determine whether geriatric patients respond differently than younger patients. Of 208 patients with advanced head and neck cancer receiving cetuximab and radiation therapy in a clinical trial, 45 patients (22%) were 65 years of age or older.

● Common Adverse Effects

The most common adverse effects, observed in at least 25% of patients receiving cetuximab, are adverse dermatologic effects (including rash, pruritus, and nail changes), headache, diarrhea, and infection. Across studies, infection occurred in 13–35% of patients receiving cetuximab.

The most common adverse effects in patients receiving cetuximab in combination with irinotecan for advanced colorectal cancer include acneiform rash (88%), asthenia/malaise (73%), diarrhea (72%), and nausea (55%); the most common grade 3 or 4 adverse effects include diarrhea (22%), leukopenia (17%), asthenia/malaise (16%), and acneiform rash (14%).

The most common adverse effects in patients receiving cetuximab and best supportive care for advanced colorectal cancer include rash/desquamation (89%), fatigue (89%), abdominal pain (59%), pain (51%), dry skin (49%), dyspnea (48%), and constipation (46%).

The most common adverse effects in patients receiving cetuximab in combination with radiation therapy for advanced head and neck cancer include acneiform rash (87%); radiation dermatitis (86%); weight loss (84%); asthenia (56%); nausea (49%); and elevated serum ALT (43%), AST (38%), and alkaline phosphatase concentrations (33%).

DRUG INTERACTIONS

● Antineoplastic Agents

Pharmacokinetic interaction with irinotecan unlikely.

● Radiation Therapy

Potential pharmacologic interaction (death, cardiotoxicity, increased risk of adverse dermatologic effects). Death and serious cardiotoxicity occurred in patients with locally advanced squamous cell head and neck cancer receiving cetuximab, cisplatin, and radiation therapy. Rash was reported in 87% of patients with locally advanced squamous cell head and neck cancer who received cetuximab concomitantly with radiation therapy. The incidence of late radiation toxicities was higher in patients receiving cetuximab and radiation therapy than in those receiving radiation therapy alone.

DESCRIPTION

Cetuximab, a recombinant chimeric (human-murine) monoclonal antibody, is an antineoplastic agent. The drug is an immunoglobulin containing human framework (i.e., IgG_1 heavy and kappa light constant regions) and murine Fv regions.

Cetuximab binds specifically to the extracellular domain of the human epidermal growth factor receptor (EGFR, HER1, c-erbB-1) on both normal and tumor cells and competitively blocks the cellular action of EGF and other ligands (e.g., transforming growth factor [TGF]-α). EGFR is a transmembrane glycoprotein that belongs to the subfamily of type I receptor tyrosine kinases, which includes EGFR (HER1), HER2, HER3, and HER4. While EGFR is expressed in many normal epithelial tissues (e.g., skin, hair follicle), overexpression of the glycoprotein is detected in human carcinomas (e.g., colon, rectum, head and neck). In vitro assays and in vivo animal studies have shown that binding of cetuximab to EGFR blocks phosphorylation and activation of receptor-associated kinases; this results in inhibition of cell growth, induction of apoptosis (programmed cell death), and decreased matrix metalloproteinase and vascular endothelial growth factor production. Signal transduction through EGFR leads to activation of the wild-type (nonmutated) KRAS gene. However, the presence of an activating somatic mutation of the KRAS gene (mutated KRAS) in a cancer cell can lead to dysregulation of signaling pathways and resistance to EGFR inhibitor therapy (e.g., cetuximab, panitumumab). In vitro, cetuximab can mediate antibody-dependent cellular cytotoxicity against certain types of human tumors.

In vitro tests and in vivo animal studies have suggested that cetuximab inhibits growth and survival of tumor cells that express EGFR, while such antitumor effects were not observed in human cancer xenografts that lacked EGFR expression. In xenograft models for human tumors in mice, addition of cetuximab to radiation therapy or irinotecan resulted in an increased antitumor effect when compared with radiation therapy or chemotherapy alone.

The pharmacokinetic disposition of cetuximab was similar in patients receiving the drug for head and neck cancer or colorectal cancer. Following administration of the recommended regimen of cetuximab (initial dose, followed by subsequent weekly doses), steady-state cetuximab concentrations are achieved by the third weekly infusion; the mean half-life of cetuximab following multiple dosing is approximately 112 hours. The major route of clearance from the circulation is believed to be through internalization of the cetuximab EGFR complex on hepatocytes and skin.

ADVICE TO PATIENTS

Risk of infusion-related effects and adverse pulmonary and dermatologic effects. Advise patients to report signs or symptoms of infusion reactions, such as fever, chills, or breathing problems.

Importance of advising patients to use sunscreen and hats and limit sun exposure during and for 2 months following discontinuance of cetuximab therapy to avoid exacerbation of adverse dermatologic effects.

Necessity of advising men and women to use an effective method of contraception during and for 6 months following the last dose of cetuximab therapy. Advise pregnant women of risk to the fetus. Advise women to avoid breast-feeding during and for 2 months following the last dose of cetuximab.

Importance of informing clinicians of existing or contemplated concomitant therapy, including prescription and OTC drugs, as well as any concomitant illnesses.

PREPARATIONS

Excipients in commercially available drug preparations may have clinically important effects in some individuals; consult specific product labeling for details.

Cetuximab (Recombinant)

Parenteral		
Injection, for IV infusion only	2 mg/mL (100 and 200 mg)	Erbitux®, Bristol-Myers Squibb

† Use is not currently included in the labeling approved by the US Food and Drug Administration.

Selected Revisions April 28, 2015, © Copyright, November 1, 2004, American Society of Health-System Pharmacists, Inc.

CISplatin

10:00 · ANTINEOPLASTIC AGENTS

■ Cisplatin is a platinum-containing antineoplastic agent.

USES

Cisplatin is often used as a component of combination chemotherapeutic regimens because of its relative lack of hematologic toxicity.

● Testicular Cancer

Cisplatin is used as a component of various chemotherapeutic regimens for the treatment of metastatic testicular tumors, including nonseminomatous testicular carcinoma, seminoma testis, and extragonadal germ-cell tumors, in patients who have already received appropriate surgery and/or radiation therapy.

Nonseminomatous Testicular Carcinoma

In the treatment of disseminated nonseminomatous testicular carcinoma (stage III), cisplatin is one of the most active single agents; however, combination chemotherapy for induction of remissions is superior to single-agent therapy. Various regimens have been used in combination therapy, and comparative efficacy is continually being evaluated. Most clinicians use cisplatin in combination with other antineoplastic agents as initial therapy in patients with stage III or unresectable stage II nonseminomatous testicular carcinoma; if the patient has persistent, localized tumor following chemotherapy, the residual tumor is removed surgically, and if the residual disease contains malignant elements, additional chemotherapy is administered.

Cisplatin has been used in combination with bleomycin and vinblastine, with or without other antineoplastic agents, for the induction of remissions. Cisplatin also has been used in combination with bleomycin and etoposide for the treatment of disseminated disease. These chemotherapy regimens usually produce a complete remission in 60–70% of patients with disseminated disease;response rates generally are higher in patients with minimal stage III disease and less advanced disease and lower in patients with advanced stage III disease. An additional 10–20% of patients can attain a complete remission following surgical removal of localized residual disease after chemotherapy-induced partial remissions. Most patients who attain a complete remission remain disease free, and those patients who have continuous disease-free remission for longer than 2 years generally are considered cured. Maintenance chemotherapy does not appear to be necessary following the attainment of a complete remission. Although not clearly established, patients with embryonal carcinoma may have a better response to chemotherapy than do patients with choriocarcinoma or teratocarcinoma.

For the initial treatment of advanced nonseminomatous testicular carcinoma, most clinicians recommend regimens containing cisplatin and bleomycin, in combination with etoposide rather than vinblastine, particularly because of the reduced neuromuscular toxicity and evidence suggesting greater efficacy in poor-risk patients. In addition, while a regimen of etoposide, cisplatin, and bleomycin appears to be as effective overall as a regimen of vinblastine, cisplatin, and bleomycin, the etoposide-containing regimen may be more effective than the vinblastine-containing regimen in a subgroup of patients with advanced disease (i.e., high tumor load). However, the best combination or sequential therapy in the treatment of advanced nonseminomatous testicular tumors has not been established, and comparative efficacy is continually being evaluated.

A regimen of cisplatin, ifosfamide with mesna, and either vinblastine or etoposide has induced complete responses in 20–45% of patients who previously received other cisplatin-based chemotherapy regimens, and is considered by most clinicians to be the standard initial salvage (i.e., second-line) regimen in patients with recurrent testicular cancer. Patients with minimal or moderate disease have a more favorable outcome with this salvage regimen than those with extensive disease. In a clinical study in patients with recurrent germ cell tumors (who had previously received at least 2 cisplatin-based chemotherapy regimens and were considered to have cisplatin-responsive disease), a regimen of cisplatin, ifosfamide, and either vinblastine or etoposide resulted in disease-free status in 36% of patients (with or without surgery) and median duration of disease

control ranged from 3 to more than 42 weeks, median survival was 53 weeks, and 20% of patients had survival of 2 years or longer. In patients with refractory disease, high-dose chemotherapy with autologous bone marrow transplant (ABMT) or peripheral stem cell rescue may produce durable complete remissions in some patients. Patients with progressive tumors during initial or salvage therapy and those with refractory mediastinal germ cell tumors generally appear to benefit less from high-dose chemotherapy and ABMT or peripheral stem cell rescue than those whose disease relapses after a response. Salvage surgery also may be considered for certain highly selected patients (e.g., those with chemorefractory disease confined to a single site).

The role of chemotherapy in the treatment of stage I and resectable stage II nonseminomatous testicular carcinoma has not been clearly established. Although most patients with stage I disease are cured by surgery alone, cisplatin-containing combination chemotherapy regimens have been used successfully to induce complete remissions in a limited number of these patients whose disease relapsed following surgical treatment. Cisplatin-containing combination chemotherapy regimens have also been used successfully as an adjuvant to surgery (orchiectomy and retroperitoneal lymphadenectomy) to induce complete remissions in patients with resectable stage II disease. Although the precise role of chemotherapy as an adjuvant to surgery in the treatment of stage II disease remains to be clearly established, such therapy with cisplatin-containing combination regimens is effective in preventing tumor recurrence in patients with such disease. When surgery, follow-up, and chemotherapy are optimal in patients with stage II disease who have no postoperative evidence of residual or recurrent disease, including absence of elevated tumor markers, cure rates appear to be similar whether cisplatin-containing chemotherapy is administered as an adjuvant to surgery (i.e., beginning postoperatively) or is withheld and used to treat relapse in closely monitored patients. In patients with residual gross disease or residual elevated tumor markers following retroperitoneal lymphadenopathy, some clinicians recommend that all such patients receive cisplatin-containing combination chemotherapy.

Seminoma Testis

Cisplatin-containing combination chemotherapy regimens have been used successfully in the treatment of disseminated seminoma testis, with complete remission rates comparable to those in patients with disseminated nonseminomatous disease. Further evaluation is needed to determine the optimum therapy.

Extragonadal Germ-Cell Tumors

Although data are limited and some reports indicate a low response rate, cisplatin-containing combination chemotherapy regimens (followed by surgery when feasible) have reportedly been successful in the treatment of advanced extragonadal germ-cell tumors, with complete remission rates comparable to those in patients with nonseminomatous tumors of similar advanced stages. Cisplatin-containing combination chemotherapy regimens have also been reported to be successful in a few cases for the treatment of extragonadal endodermal sinus tumor (yolk-sac carcinoma) in males, although this tumor is generally considered poorly responsive to chemotherapy.

● Ovarian Cancer

Cisplatin is used alone or in combination therapy for the treatment of ovarian cancer.

Adjuvant Therapy for Early-stage Ovarian Epithelial Cancer

Platinum-based therapy has been used for adjuvant treatment following surgery in early-stage ovarian epithelial cancer†. (See Uses: Ovarian Cancer: Adjuvant Therapy for Early-stage Ovarian Epithelial Cancer in Carboplatin 10:00.)

First-line Therapy for Advanced Ovarian Epithelial Cancer

A platinum-containing agent in combination with paclitaxel is a preferred regimen for the treatment of advanced ovarian epithelial cancer. The best combination or sequential therapy with multiple agents in the treatment of advanced ovarian tumors has not been established, and comparative efficacy is continually being evaluated.

Combination chemotherapy regimens containing platinum are associated with higher response rates and improved survival compared with non-platinum-containing regimens as first-line treatment for advanced ovarian cancer. The benefit of cisplatin used in combination therapy rather than as monotherapy has not been fully established. In a large randomized trial, cisplatin combined with paclitaxel produced higher response rates than paclitaxel alone and similar response rates but less toxicity than cisplatin alone; median survival did not differ among the groups.

Carboplatin versus Cisplatin

Randomized trials have demonstrated that carboplatin is as effective as but less toxic than cisplatin when used in combination with either paclitaxel or cyclophosphamide for the initial treatment of advanced ovarian cancer. Carboplatin in combination with paclitaxel currently is a preferred regimen for the initial treatment of advanced ovarian epithelial cancer. (See Uses: Ovarian Cancer: First-line Therapy for Advanced Ovarian Epithelial Cancer in Carboplatin 10:00.)

Platinum-Containing Agent with Paclitaxel Versus Platinum-containing Agent with Cyclophosphamide

The combination of IV cisplatin and IV paclitaxel has been used for the initial treatment of advanced epithelial ovarian carcinoma, and evidence from randomized trials indicates that this combination is superior to combined cisplatin and cyclophosphamide for initial treatment. In a comparative study of patients with suboptimally debulked (greater than 1 cm residual tumor mass) stage III or IV ovarian cancer who had no prior chemotherapy, combined therapy with paclitaxel and cisplatin produced higher rates of overall objective response (73 versus 60%), increased disease-free survival (median: 18 versus 13 months), and increased overall survival (median: 38 versus 24 months) compared with a combined regimen of cisplatin and cyclophosphamide. A higher frequency of neutropenia, fever, alopecia, and allergic reactions was observed in patients receiving cisplatin and paclitaxel compared with those receiving cisplatin and cyclophosphamide. In another randomized trial, higher rates of overall and complete response (59 versus 45% and 41 versus 27%, respectively) and prolonged median overall survival (36 versus 26 months) were observed in patients receiving paclitaxel and cisplatin versus cyclophosphamide and cisplatin for advanced epithelial ovarian cancer. At a follow-up of 6.5 years, the survival benefit associated with the cisplatin and paclitaxel regimen in both randomized trials has been maintained.

Intraperitoneal Cisplatin and Paclitaxel

Combined IV and intraperitoneal therapy with IV paclitaxel, intraperitoneal cisplatin, and intraperitoneal paclitaxel† has been used for the treatment of optimally debulked stage III epithelial ovarian cancer.

The National Cancer Institute (NCI) recommends use of a combined IV and intraperitoneal regimen for eligible patients with advanced epithelial ovarian cancer because of a substantial survival benefit. Based on clinical trials, NCI recommends that use of a regimen containing intraperitoneal cisplatin (100 mg/m²) and a taxane (either IV only or IV plus intraperitoneal) should be strongly considered following primary surgery in patients with optimally debulked stage III epithelial ovarian cancer. Although an optimal intraperitoneal chemotherapy regimen has not been established, favorable results were observed following sequential administration of IV paclitaxel, intraperitoneal cisplatin, and intraperitoneal paclitaxel in the Gynecologic Oncology Group (GOG)-172 study.

In this randomized phase 3 trial (GOG-172), 429 patients with previously untreated stage III epithelial ovarian cancer or primary peritoneal cancer, with no residual mass exceeding 1 cm in diameter following surgery, received either combined IV and intraperitoneal therapy or IV therapy. All patients enrolled in this study had good baseline GOG performance status (0–2) and adequate bone marrow, renal, and hepatic function. Most patients (88%) had ovarian cancer, and serous adenocarcinoma was the most common histologic type (79% of patients). The primary end points of the study were progression-free survival and overall survival. Combined IV and intraperitoneal therapy consisted of IV paclitaxel 135 mg/m² by 24-hour infusion on day 1, followed by intraperitoneal cisplatin 100 mg/m² on day 2 and intraperitoneal paclitaxel 60 mg/m² on day 8. IV therapy consisted of IV paclitaxel 135 mg/m² by 24-hour infusion on day 1 followed by IV cisplatin 75 mg/m² on day 2. Both regimens were repeated every 21 days for up to 6 cycles. Patients who received combined IV and intraperitoneal therapy had longer median progression-free (23.8 versus 18.3 months) and overall (65.6 versus 49.7 months) survival compared with patients who received IV therapy.

Most (83%) of the patients receiving IV therapy completed 6 cycles of their assigned chemotherapy regimen; however, only 42% of patients receiving combined IV and intraperitoneal therapy completed 6 cycles of assigned chemotherapy; patients who could not complete the intraperitoneal regimen received IV

therapy for the remaining treatment cycles. The most common reason for discontinuance of intraperitoneal therapy was catheter-related complications. Grade 3 or 4 leukopenia (76 versus 64%), GI effects (46 versus 24%), metabolic effects (27 versus 7%), fatigue (18 versus 4%), neurologic effects (19 versus 9%), infection (16 versus 6%), thrombocytopenia (12 versus 4%), and pain (11 versus 1%) occurred more frequently in patients receiving combined IV and intraperitoneal therapy than in those receiving IV therapy. Although patients receiving combined IV and intraperitoneal therapy reported less improvement in abdominal discomfort before cycle 4, improvement in abdominal discomfort was similar in both treatment groups 1 year after completion of therapy. Among patients who received combined IV and intraperitoneal therapy, quality of life was worse during and shortly after completion of therapy (before cycle 4 and at 3–6 weeks following therapy) compared with those who received IV therapy. Quality-of-life scores were similar for the groups at 1 year after completion of treatment, except for greater persistence of moderate paresthesias in patients receiving combined IV and intraperitoneal therapy.

Retrospective review of baseline data (patient and disease characteristics) from two phase 3 clinical trials (including GOG-172) for patients receiving intraperitoneal therapy for optimally debulked stage III epithelial ovarian cancer suggested that extent of residual tumor mass, histology, and age were important predictors of survival in such patients. Patients with clear cell histology appeared to derive less benefit from intraperitoneal therapy compared with those with serous histology (hazard ratio for progression-free and overall survival of 2.66 and 3.88, respectively). In addition, each additional year of age was associated with a 1% increase in the risk of death. Although patients enrolled in the studies had optimally debulked (1 cm or less residual tumor mass) disease, survival was greater in patients with only microscopic residual disease.

Retrospective analysis of data from patients receiving a modified IV and intraperitoneal regimen suggests that a reduced dosage of intraperitoneal cisplatin administered in conjunction with a shortened IV paclitaxel infusion time may result in less toxicity and produce a survival benefit similar to that reported in the GOG-172 study (67 months versus 65.6 months reported in GOG-172). The modified IV and intraperitoneal regimen consisted of IV paclitaxel 135 mg/m² by 3-hour infusion on day 1, followed by intraperitoneal cisplatin 75 mg/m² on day 2 and intraperitoneal paclitaxel 60 mg/m² on day 8 of each 21-day cycle. Most patients (80%) completed 4 or more cycles of therapy and 55% completed 6 cycles. The frequency of grade 3 or 4 neutropenia (12%), GI effects (8%), metabolic effects (5%), neurologic effects (6%), infection (2%), fatigue (2%), and thrombocytopenia (0%) in this series of patients receiving the modified IV and intraperitoneal regimen appeared to be lower than toxicity rates reported in the GOG-172 study. By shortening the infusion time for IV paclitaxel to 3 hours, the modified regimen also may provide an outpatient alternative to inpatient administration over 24 hours. However, randomized controlled trials are needed to establish comparative safety and efficacy of this modified regimen. The modified IV and intraperitoneal schedule containing the lower intraperitoneal cisplatin dosage and the 3-hour IV paclitaxel infusion also has been studied in conjunction with a third cytotoxic drug, but with evidence of excessive toxicity.

Based on current evidence, combined IV and intraperitoneal therapy with IV paclitaxel, intraperitoneal cisplatin, and intraperitoneal paclitaxel is recommended (accepted) for use as initial adjuvant treatment of optimally debulked stage III epithelial ovarian cancer in patients with good performance status (GOG performance status of 0–2).

Second-line Therapy for Advanced Ovarian Epithelial Cancer

Either cisplatin or carboplatin can be used when retreatment is indicated in patients with platinum-sensitive disease who relapse; however, some clinicians suggest that carboplatin may be preferred because it is associated with a more favorable toxicity profile than cisplatin. Although some patients who failed to respond to cisplatin or had a response of only short duration have responded to carboplatin, nonplatinum-based regimens (e.g., paclitaxel) generally are preferred for retreatment of patients with platinum-resistant disease. Responses to cisplatin also have been observed in patients with disease resistant to initial treatment with paclitaxel monotherapy.

Dosage and Other Therapeutic Considerations

While some evidence indicates that dose intensity (i.e., amount of platinum per unit time) is an important factor in achieving optimum results in patients with stage III or IV ovarian carcinoma, other evidence suggests that total platinum dose or duration of exposure is a more important factor in improving progression-free survival in responding patients. However, no improvement in response appears to occur with increased dose intensity or increased total dose once a certain threshold is reached. Although optimum duration of chemotherapy has not been clearly defined, there currently is no evidence of improved response and/or survival when the duration of drug administration exceeds 6 cycles. Despite the fact that platinum-containing combination chemotherapy regimens are associated with high response rates, no regimen has been found that is sufficiently active to prevent disease progression and/or recurrence in most women with stage III or IV ovarian carcinoma.

Other therapeutic techniques, such as interval debulking surgery, may improve survival in patients with advanced ovarian carcinoma. In a randomized study involving patients with residual lesions (greater than 1 cm) following primary surgery for advanced ovarian cancer (stages IIB through IV) who responded to cisplatin-based induction chemotherapy, those who received interval debulking surgery accompanied by subsequent chemotherapy had improved survival compared with those who received chemotherapy alone.

Ovarian Germ Cell Tumors

Cisplatin-containing chemotherapy regimens are used in the treatment of ovarian germ-cell tumors, including endodermal sinus tumors. Combination chemotherapy with cisplatin, bleomycin, and etoposide currently is a regimen of choice for the adjuvant therapy of ovarian germ-cell tumors.

● Bladder Cancer

Cisplatin is used widely in the treatment of muscle-invasive and advanced bladder cancer. Approximately 20–25% of patients with bladder cancer are initially diagnosed with invasive tumors. Radical cystectomy is the standard therapy for muscle-invasive bladder cancer; however, because of the high rate of metastasis following local therapy, combined modality treatment including chemotherapy (neoadjuvant or adjuvant), radiation therapy, and surgery is being evaluated for the management of invasive disease and also has been used to allow bladder preservation in selected patients. Combination chemotherapy alone or as an adjunct to local therapy with surgery and/or radiation therapy is used for the palliative and occasionally curative treatment of locally advanced (unresectable) or metastatic bladder cancer.

Over 90% of bladder tumors are transitional cell carcinomas originating from the uroepithelium. Other histologic types of bladder cancer, such as squamous cell carcinoma (6–8%) and adenocarcinoma (2%), are associated with greater resistance to treatment and a more aggressive pattern of local spread than transitional cell carcinoma. Bladder carcinoma is clinically staged according to the TNM classification. Major prognostic factors in patients with carcinoma of the bladder include the depth of tumor invasion into the bladder wall and the degree of differentiation or grade of the tumor.

Muscle-invasive Bladder Carcinoma
Overview

Choice of therapy in muscle-invasive cancer must be individualized according to prognostic factors, the patient's medical condition, expected benefits and risks of therapy, and patient preference. Important prognostic factors used to guide selection of therapy for invasive bladder cancer include stage of tumor, particularly whether the tumor is organ-confined (stage 2 or T3a) or not organ-confined (stage T3b, 4, 4a, or 4b); presence of lymph node involvement, and lymphatic or vascular invasion of the tumor.

There is a 30–50% risk of nodal or distant metastases in patients with muscle-invasive bladder carcinoma. Radical cystectomy (i.e., removal of the bladder, prostate, and seminal vesicles in men or removal of the bladder, uterus, fallopian tubes, ovaries, and upper vagina in women) with pelvic lymphadenectomy is considered standard therapy in the US; depending on the location of the tumor, partial cystectomy rarely may be adequate in some patients. A retrospective analysis demonstrated that radical cystectomy with urinary diversion is well tolerated and effective for the definitive treatment of muscle-invasive bladder cancer in geriatric patients (70 years of age or older) in good health (i.e., good cardiac performance and absence of cardiovascular or pulmonary problems) in comparison with younger patients (younger than 70 years).

Rarely, transurethral resection (TUR) alone has been effective in selected patients with a small (less than 2 cm), solitary papillary tumor that is minimally invasive into muscle and is not associated with carcinoma in situ, a palpable mass, or hydronephrosis; however, in the treatment of muscle-invasive bladder carcinoma, TUR more often is used to debulk tumors prior to the administration of

systemic therapy with chemotherapy and/or radiation therapy in selected patients receiving combined modality treatment with bladder preservation. Some clinicians perform a second TUR in selected patients to further reduce tumor burden or to pursue findings (e.g., progression of disease, absence of residual tumor) that may influence treatment strategy.

The addition of preoperative radiation has not been shown to affect overall survival in patients undergoing radical cystectomy for muscle-invasive bladder cancer and is not standard care in the US; however, limited evidence from a matched analysis suggests that preoperative radiation therapy may reduce the rate of local recurrence in patients with T3b tumors. Although overall survival in patients receiving sole treatment with radiation for invasive disease is inferior to that obtained with radical cystectomy, treatment with radiation therapy alone with external beam radiation may be considered in patients who refuse or are unable to tolerate surgery. Treatment with radiation therapy followed by salvage cystectomy does not appear to adversely affect survival or rate of metastasis compared with immediate cystectomy in patients with muscle-invasive bladder cancer.

Despite treatment with radical cystectomy, 50% of patients with muscle-invasive bladder cancer will develop metastases within 18 months. Because of the high rates of metastasis following local therapy with cystectomy and/or radiation therapy, the addition of chemotherapy to the treatment regimen for muscle-invasive bladder cancer is being investigated. Randomized trials are being conducted to determine the benefit of chemotherapy (adjuvant or neoadjuvant) added to cystectomy or used in conjunction with radiation therapy for muscle-invasive bladder carcinoma; studies to date have shown no effect on overall survival. Combined modality therapy with combination chemotherapy, radiation therapy, and conservative surgery (aggressive transurethral resection or partial cystectomy) has been used to allow organ preservation in selected patients with muscle-invasive bladder cancer; however, the effect on survival with use of organ-sparing treatment versus standard therapy with radical cystectomy is not known.

Neoadjuvant or Adjuvant Chemotherapy

In patients with muscle-invasive bladder cancer, chemotherapy has been given prior to (i.e., as neoadjuvant therapy) or following (i.e., as adjuvant therapy) local treatment with surgery and/or radiation therapy. The benefit of adjuvant or neoadjuvant chemotherapy has not been established, and use of chemotherapy as a component of therapy currently is considered investigational in the treatment of muscle-invasive bladder cancer.

Although no survival benefit has been conclusively demonstrated with the use of adjuvant chemotherapy, some experts recommend systemic therapy following either cystectomy or aggressive transurethral resection in patients with adverse prognostic factors (e.g., stage T3b or greater, node-positive disease, lymphatic or vascular invasion of the tumor). Use of adjuvant chemotherapy may be unnecessary or excessive treatment, particularly in patients with muscle-invasive bladder cancer that is organ-confined (e.g., stage T2 or T3a) and node-negative.

Trials evaluating the use of single chemotherapeutic agents as adjuvant therapy have not shown any benefit, and combination regimens consisting of cisplatin, methotrexate, and vinblastine with or without doxorubicin (abbreviated as M-VAC or CMV, respectively) currently are used for the adjuvant treatment of muscle-invasive bladder cancer. Combination chemotherapy used as adjuvant treatment has been demonstrated to delay progression of disease and decrease local recurrence of tumor in patients with muscle-invasive bladder cancer. When chemotherapy is administered in the adjuvant setting, it is recommended that a minimum of 4 cycles (at full doses) be given; however, the optimal dose, schedule, and number of courses for adjuvant chemotherapy in the treatment of muscle-invasive bladder carcinoma has not been determined. Additional study in randomized trials is needed to determine the benefit of adjuvant chemotherapy for invasive bladder cancer.

Single-agent cisplatin or cisplatin-containing combination chemotherapy has been used as neoadjuvant therapy preceding cystectomy and/or radiation therapy or as concurrent therapy with definitive or preoperative radiation therapy in patients with muscle-invasive bladder cancer. The addition of neoadjuvant chemotherapy to local treatment appears to cause regression of existing tumor, decrease local recurrence of tumor, and increase time to relapse of disease in patients with muscle-invasive bladder cancer; however, no effect on overall survival has been conclusively demonstrated. Results of a pooled analysis that mostly included randomized trials of single-agent cisplatin did not demonstrate a difference in survival with the addition of chemotherapy (neoadjuvant or concurrent) in patients undergoing cystectomy and/or radiation therapy for muscle-invasive bladder cancer; however, based on experience with treatment of advanced bladder cancer, single-agent cisplatin is considered less effective than combination cisplatin-based chemotherapy.

Results from large randomized trials of neoadjuvant therapy with cisplatin-based combination regimens (e.g., cisplatin, methotrexate, and vinblastine; cisplatin and doxorubicin) have not shown a survival benefit in patients with muscle-invasive bladder cancer. Subgroup analysis suggests a possible effect of neoadjuvant chemotherapy on overall survival in patients with cancers of histologic grade G3 or stage T3 or T4a disease, and further randomized trials may identify prognostic factors that allow selection of a subgroup of patients with locally advanced bladder cancer who are likely to benefit from neoadjuvant chemotherapy. Because a conclusive survival benefit has not been shown, routine use of neoadjuvant therapy with combination chemotherapy regimens (e.g., cisplatin, methotrexate, and vinblastine with or without doxorubicin) for muscle-invasive bladder cancer is *not* recommended, and such therapy is considered investigational. Longer periods of follow-up in ongoing randomized trials are needed to establish the benefit (if any) of neoadjuvant chemotherapy in patients undergoing cystectomy and/or radiation therapy for muscle-invasive bladder cancer.

The effect of sequence of therapy when chemotherapy is used in conjunction with local treatment (i.e., cystectomy and/or radiation therapy) for invasive bladder cancer is not known. Interim analysis of a randomized trial of patients with stage T3b or T4a tumors receiving either adjuvant or neoadjuvant chemotherapy did not detect any difference in survival. Further study is needed to establish the benefit of adding chemotherapy (adjuvant or neoadjuvant) to cystectomy and/or radiation therapy for the treatment of muscle-invasive bladder cancer.

Neoadjuvant chemotherapy for muscle-invasive bladder cancer typically is administered IV. In a limited number of patients with muscle-invasive bladder cancer, neoadjuvant chemotherapy has been administered intra-arterially; however, this method of administration is associated with substantial toxicity, and the comparative efficacy of intra-arterial chemotherapy versus IV chemotherapy for the neoadjuvant treatment of muscle-invasive bladder cancer is not known.

Combined Modality Therapy with Bladder Preservation

Single-agent cisplatin or cisplatin-containing combination chemotherapy (e.g., cisplatin with methotrexate and vinblastine [CMV]) has been used in conjunction with radiation therapy and conservative surgery as a bladder-sparing approach for the treatment of selected patients with muscle-invasive bladder cancer. Clinical trials are under way to investigate whether bladder preservation is a reasonable goal in patients with small-volume, organ-confined (stage T2 or T3a) disease when total eradication of the tumor can be achieved; patients with bulky tumors, tumors with overexpression of p53 nuclear protein, nontransitional or mixed histology carcinoma, hydronephrosis, and/or ureteral obstruction are at high risk for relapse of invasive bladder tumor and generally are not good candidates for clinical trials of organ-preserving therapy.

Following aggressive transurethral resection (TUR), use of chemotherapy with radiation therapy appears to produce survival rates comparable to those reported for radical cystectomy in patients with muscle-invasive bladder cancer. In one case series, patients with muscle-invasive bladder cancer (stages T2 through T4, node-negative disease) underwent TUR followed by combination chemotherapy with cisplatin, methotrexate, and vinblastine (CMV) and then radiation therapy with concurrent cisplatin therapy. At 5 years, the overall survival rate was 52%, and 43% of all patients who entered the study had survived with a functioning bladder. However, in a randomized trial of patients with muscle-invasive bladder cancer (stages T2 through T4, node-negative disease) undergoing aggressive TUR followed by radiation therapy with concurrent cisplatin therapy, with or without the addition of neoadjuvant combination chemotherapy with cisplatin, methotrexate, and vinblastine (CMV) preceding concurrent chemoradiation therapy, neoadjuvant chemotherapy caused substantial toxicity (particularly severe neutropenia and sepsis) and did not provide additional benefit in rate of overall survival (48 versus 49%), rate of survival with a functioning bladder (36 versus 40%), or rate of distant metastases (33 versus 39%). Combination chemotherapy with cisplatin, methotrexate, vinblastine, and doxorubicin (M-VAC) followed by partial cystectomy also has been used as an organ-preserving approach to the treatment of muscle-invasive bladder cancer. Response to induction chemotherapy and/or radiation therapy confirmed by cystoscopy and/or bladder biopsy is an important predictor of survival in patients with muscle-invasive bladder cancer.

Bladder preservation is attempted only in patients with disease that responds to induction chemotherapy and/or radiation therapy. Patients with disease that does not demonstrate a complete response to chemotherapy and/or radiation

therapy are immediately referred for radical cystectomy; further study is needed to determine whether delay of cystectomy adversely affects outcome in such patients. All patients who receive organ-sparing therapy must be carefully monitored for tumor recurrence and/or occurrence of new tumors; local therapy (e.g., intravesical instillation) and/or cystectomy eventually is required in some patients. Combined modality treatment with conservative surgery and radiation therapy with concurrent cisplatin-containing chemotherapy may be a reasonable alternative in patients with muscle-invasive bladder cancer who refuse or are unable to tolerate radical cystectomy, and clinical trials are under way to investigate this approach; however, unless randomized trials demonstrate that survival is comparable to that achieved with radical cystectomy, organ-preserving treatment cannot be routinely recommended in patients with muscle-invasive bladder cancer.

Advanced Bladder Carcinoma

Combination chemotherapy is used alone or as an adjunct to local therapy with surgery and/or radiation therapy for the palliative treatment of advanced (unresectable) or metastatic bladder carcinoma. The prognosis for patients with advanced or metastatic bladder cancer generally is poor, particularly in patients with bony or hepatic metastases. Although complete response to combination chemotherapy has been observed in some patients with metastatic bladder cancer, median survival with current treatment is only 12 months.

Combination Cisplatin-based Chemotherapy

Cisplatin-based combination chemotherapy regimens (e.g., cisplatin, methotrexate, and vinblastine with or without doxorubicin, abbreviated as M-VAC or CMV, respectively; cisplatin and gemcitabine) currently are used for the palliative treatment of advanced or metastatic bladder cancer. In patients with metastatic bladder cancer, the potential benefit must be weighed against the substantial toxicity associated with aggressive chemotherapy. The activity of new agents and optimal regimens for the treatment of advanced or metastatic bladder cancer are continually being evaluated.

Combination cisplatin-based therapy is superior to single-agent cisplatin, and combination chemotherapy regimens consisting of 3 or 4 drugs are considered standard therapy for patients with metastatic bladder cancer. Overall response rates with cisplatin-based combination regimens range from 40–70%, with complete responses rates of 10–20%.

In randomized trials, patients with advanced or metastatic bladder cancer receiving combination chemotherapy with cisplatin, methotrexate, vinblastine, and doxorubicin (M-VAC) had higher response rates and more prolonged survival compared with single-agent cisplatin or combination therapy with cisplatin, doxorubicin, and cyclophosphamide. The use of M-VAC also is associated with greater toxicity than single-agent cisplatin, particularly leukopenia, mucositis, granulocytopenia, and drug-related mortality. At 6 years of follow-up, patients receiving M-VAC have more prolonged survival than those receiving cisplatin, but despite the superior efficacy of this regimen, only 3.7% of patients receiving M-VAC are alive and continuously disease-free.

Combination therapy with cisplatin and gemcitabine is an alternative to M-VAC for the treatment of advanced or metastatic bladder cancer. In a large randomized trial of patients receiving either M-VAC or cisplatin and gemcitabine for the treatment of advanced or metastatic bladder cancer, overall median survival (14.8 versus 13.8 months, respectively), median time to progressive disease (7.4 months for each regimen), and response rates (38 versus 44%, respectively, using intent-to-treat analysis) were similar. Prophylactic hematopoietic agents (growth factors) were not administered to either group; grade 3 or 4 neutropenia, neutropenic sepsis, grade 3 or 4 mucositis, and alopecia occurred more frequently in patients receiving M-VAC whereas grade 3 or 4 anemia or grade 3 or 4 thrombocytopenia were observed more often in patients receiving cisplatin and gemcitabine.

Patients receiving combination chemotherapy with cisplatin, methotrexate, and vinblastine (CMV) had a higher rate of survival at 1 year (29 versus 16%) but experienced more toxicity than those receiving methotrexate and vinblastine for advanced or metastatic bladder cancer. The comparative efficacy of M-VAC and CMV has not been investigated in randomized trials; some clinicians favor M-VAC as the established regimen of choice for the treatment of advanced or metastatic bladder cancer whereas others prefer CMV because of decreased toxicity associated with this regimen. Because of the cardiac toxicity associated with doxorubicin, CMV generally is preferable to M-VAC in patients with cardiac dysfunction. Non-transitional cell bladder cancers are less sensitive to standard cisplatin-based chemotherapy regimens than is transitional cell bladder carcinoma, and most clinicians recommend that standard regimens such as M-VAC or CMV not be used in patients with metastatic adenocarcinoma or squamous cell carcinoma of the bladder.

Because of the substantial toxicity and poor survival associated with current regimens, optimal therapy for advanced bladder cancer continually is being evaluated and all eligible candidates should be considered for entry into clinical trials; randomized trials are under way to compare the efficacy and toxicity of M-VAC with other regimens (e.g., paclitaxel and carboplatin) for the treatment of advanced or metastatic bladder cancer.

Dosage Considerations

The usual dosage schedule for the M-VAC regimen is a monthly cycle consisting of IV cisplatin 70 mg/m^2 (administered on day 2), IV methotrexate 30 mg/m^2 (administered on days 1, 15, and 22), IV vinblastine 3 mg/m^2 (administered on days 2, 15, and 22), and IV doxorubicin 30 mg/m^2 (administered on day 2).

Higher doses of cisplatin are administered in the CMV regimen. The usual dosage schedule for the CMV regimen is a 21-day cycle consisting of IV cisplatin 100 mg/m^2 (administered on day 2), IV methotrexate 30 mg/m^2 (administered on days 1 and 8), and IV vinblastine 4 mg/m^2 (administered on days 1 and 8).

Escalated doses in the M-VAC regimen with concomitant administration of hematopoietic therapy (GM-CSF or G-CSF) have been used in patients with advanced urothelial carcinoma. In a randomized, phase III trial, a higher rate of complete response but no difference in overall survival was observed in patients receiving high-dose M-VAC with G-CSF versus classic M-VAC alone (without G-CSF) for advanced bladder cancer.

Treatment with cisplatin-based regimens should be discontinued if objective response is not observed following 2 or 3 cycles of therapy. Although the optimal duration of therapy has not been fully determined, some experts recommend 4–6 cycles of therapy as tolerated for patients showing clinical response; additional cycles of therapy do not appear to improve outcome. Surgical resection, when indicated, generally is considered after 4 cycles of therapy; additional cycles of chemotherapy following surgery have not been shown to provide benefit.

Administration of cisplatin in divided doses may be necessary in patients with renal impairment receiving cisplatin-based regimens for the treatment of advanced bladder cancer.

Adverse Effects and Other Considerations

Substantial toxicity, including myelosuppression and mucositis, is associated with use of the M-VAC regimen in patients with advanced or metastatic bladder cancer. The administration of hematopoietic agents (e.g., G-CSF, GM-CSF) has been used to reduce the incidence and severity of myelosuppression in patients receiving M-VAC for advanced bladder cancer. Prophylactic use of G-CSF should be strongly considered in patients receiving M-VAC.

Carboplatin has been substituted as a less toxic alternative to cisplatin in some patients receiving combination chemotherapy for advanced bladder cancer. Inadequate dosing of carboplatin may have contributed to its lesser efficacy compared with cisplatin in earlier studies of platinum-based regimens for the treatment of advanced or metastatic bladder cancer. Combination therapy with paclitaxel followed by carboplatin is being investigated as an active regimen in patients with advanced bladder cancer, including patients with abnormal renal function.

● Head and Neck Cancer

Cisplatin is commonly used in combination with fluorouracil for the palliative treatment of recurrent or metastatic head and neck cancer†. Combination therapy with cisplatin, methotrexate, bleomycin, and vincristine also has been used for the treatment of recurrent or metastatic squamous cell carcinoma of the head and neck. Methotrexate alone also may be used for the treatment of recurrent or metastatic head and neck cancer, particularly in patients who cannot tolerate aggressive chemotherapy.

Cisplatin-containing combination therapy is superior to single-agent therapy in producing higher response rates; however, no effect on overall survival has been demonstrated. In a randomized study, patients with recurrent or metastatic squamous cell carcinoma of the head and neck who received cisplatin and fluorouracil, carboplatin and fluorouracil, or methotrexate alone had objective response rates of 32, 21, and 10%, respectively. Although the objective response rate achieved with cisplatin and fluorouracil was greater than that observed with methotrexate alone, combination chemotherapy was associated with increased toxicity (particularly hematologic and renal toxicity), and no difference in survival was observed. Patients receiving cisplatin and fluorouracil for advanced head and neck cancer had a higher response rate and delayed progression of disease but no difference in survival compared with those receiving either cisplatin or fluorouracil alone. In another randomized trial, patients receiving cisplatin, methotrexate, bleomycin, and vincristine for recurrent or metastatic head and neck cancer had higher rates of complete response than those receiving cisplatin and fluorouracil; although both combination regimens produced a higher rate of objective response than cisplatin alone, no difference in survival was detected among the treatment groups.

Cisplatin has been administered concurrently with radiation therapy for the palliative treatment of head and neck cancer in patients with locally advanced disease that is unresectable. The use of cisplatin-containing chemotherapy administered concurrently with radiation therapy is being investigated as an approach to resectable disease in cases where surgical resection would lead to functional deficit. Cisplatin also has been used in combination with docetaxel and fluorouracil as induction therapy prior to radiotherapy or chemoradiotherapy in the treatment of locally advanced squamous cell carcinoma of the head and neck. (See Uses: Head and Neck Cancer, in Docetaxel 10:00.)

In males younger than 50 years of age with metastatic squamous neck cancer who have a poorly differentiated tumor, an occult primary tumor, and elevated β-human chorionic gonadotropin (β-hCG) and α-fetoprotein (AFP), chemotherapy with a platinum-containing regimen should be considered because these tumors may respond to such therapy in a manner similar to extragonadal germ cell malignancies.

● Cervical Cancer

Cisplatin is used, alone or in combination therapy, concurrently with radiation therapy for the treatment of invasive cervical cancer† (FIGO stages IB2 through IVA cervical cancer or FIGO stage IA2, IB, or IIA cervical cancer with poor prognostic factors, such as metastatic disease in pelvic lymph nodes, parametrial disease, or positive surgical margins, identified at the time of primary surgery). Cisplatin also is used in the treatment of metastatic or recurrent cervical cancer†.

Overview

About 13,000–16,000 new cases of invasive cervical cancer and 5,000 deaths from this disease occur in the US each year. The most common histologic types of cervical cancer are squamous cell carcinoma (approximately 80–90%) and adenocarcinoma (approximately 10–20%); adenosquamous carcinoma and small cell carcinoma of the cervix occur less frequently, and other types of cancers of the cervix are relatively rare. The principal risk factor for the development of preinvasive cervical lesions or invasive cervical cancer is infection with certain subtypes of human papilloma virus (HPV).

Procedures routinely used to determine the clinical stage of cervical cancer include physical examination, radiologic studies, and cervical biopsy; although they are not included in the process of clinical staging, imaging procedures, such as computed tomography (CT) or magnetic resonance imaging (MRI), and/or lymphangiography with fine-needle aspiration may be used to establish the extent of invasive disease. HIV testing should be considered, particularly in younger (less than 50 years of age), at-risk patients diagnosed with invasive cervical cancer, because of the higher prevalence of HIV infection, often asymptomatic, in these women compared with women in the general population. Prognostic factors for cervical cancer include the stage of disease, the volume and grade of tumor, histologic type, spread of disease to pelvic or para-aortic lymph nodes, and vascular invasion. Controversy exists regarding whether adenocarcinoma of the cervix carries a worse prognosis than squamous cell carcinoma of the cervix, and most treatment recommendations for cervical cancer are based on experience in patients with squamous cell carcinoma. The clinical staging system established by the Federation Internationale de Gynecologie et d'Obstetrique (FIGO) is commonly used to classify cervical cancer.

The earliest stage of invasive cervical cancer (FIGO stage IA1) may be treated surgically. Other early-stage, small-volume cervical cancer (FIGO stage IA2, IB1, or IIA) may be treated initially with surgery or radiation therapy. According to the findings from randomized trials, strong consideration should be given to the concurrent administration of cisplatin-based chemotherapy to prolong overall survival and progression-free survival in women who require postoperative radiation therapy for the treatment of stage IA2, IB1, or IIA cervical cancer with poor prognostic factors identified at the time of primary surgery or in women who require primary radiation therapy for the treatment of stage IB1 or IIA cervical cancer with poor prognostic factors.

For the initial treatment of early stages of cervical cancer, surgery is preferred for younger women who have concerns about preservation of the ovaries and avoidance of vaginal atrophy and stenosis; radiation therapy is advisable in women who have bulky disease, women who have disease with poor prognostic factors (e.g., metastasis to pelvic lymph nodes), or women who are not suitable candidates for surgery. Although randomized controlled studies are needed, some evidence suggests that survival may be prolonged in patients receiving primary treatment with surgery rather than radiation therapy for early stages of adenocarcinoma of the cervix. Patients initially treated with surgery may require postoperative radiation therapy to reduce the risk of local recurrence if tumor is present in the margins of the surgical specimen or has metastasized to pelvic or para-aortic lymph nodes. Because the combination of radical surgery and adjuvant radiation therapy increases both morbidity and the cost of treatment, careful staging and identification of prognostic factors are important in the selection of the optimal mode of initial treatment.

Although controversy exists regarding the optimal treatment of stage IB2 cervical cancer, many experts prefer the use of primary radiation therapy. Initial treatment with radiation therapy generally is recommended in women with stages IIB through IVA cervical cancer. According to the findings from randomized trials, strong consideration should be given to the concurrent administration of cisplatin-based chemotherapy to prolong overall survival and progression-free survival in women receiving primary radiation therapy for the treatment of stage IB2 or stages IIB through IVA cervical cancer. Results of randomized trials and pooled data from randomized trials did *not* demonstrate prolonged survival or improved local control of disease with use of neoadjuvant chemotherapy followed by radiation therapy in locally advanced cervical cancer; evidence from at least 2 randomized trials suggests that use of neoadjuvant chemotherapy may adversely affect survival in patients receiving radiation therapy for locally advanced cervical cancer.

Palliative treatment with radiation and/or chemotherapy has been used in patients with metastatic or recurrent cervical cancer. The benefit of chemotherapy and/or radiation therapy versus best supportive care has not been established in patients with advanced cervical cancer.

FIGO Stage IA1 Cervical Cancer

Chemotherapy currently is not usually recommended for FIGO stage IA1 cervical cancer. Instead, simple hysterectomy or cone biopsy are initial treatments of choice. The use of conservative surgical management of adenocarcinoma in situ of the uterine cervix with conization has not been established. Radiation therapy alone (intracavitary insertion only) may be used to treat stage IA1 disease in women who are not suitable candidates for surgery.

FIGO Stage IA2 Cervical Cancer

In patients with FIGO stage IA2 cervical cancer, surgery or pelvic radiation therapy is the initial treatment of choice. Concurrent cisplatin-based chemotherapy may be strongly considered for certain women with this stage of the cancer.

Primary surgical treatment for FIGO stage IA2 cervical cancer generally consists of radical hysterectomy with pelvic lymph node dissection. The use of conservative surgical management with cone biopsy alone is not established as an appropriate treatment option for stage IA2 cervical cancer. Postoperative radiation therapy is required in women with stage IA2 cervical cancer with poor prognostic factors (i.e., metastatic disease in pelvic lymph nodes, parametrial disease, positive surgical margins) identified at the time of primary surgery. According to the findings from randomized trials, strong consideration should be given to the concurrent administration of cisplatin-based chemotherapy in women who require postoperative radiation therapy for the treatment of stage IA2 cervical cancer with poor prognostic factors.

Primary radiation therapy for FIGO stage IA2 cervical cancer consists of intracavitary brachytherapy with or without external-beam radiation therapy.

FIGO Stage IB1 or IIA Cervical Cancer

In patients with FIGO stage IB1 or IIA cervical cancer, the use of surgery or pelvic radiation therapy as initial treatment appears to produce equivalent results. Concurrent cisplatin-based chemotherapy may be strongly considered for certain women with this stage of the cancer.

Primary surgical treatment for FIGO stage IB1 or IIA cervical cancer generally consists of radical hysterectomy with pelvic lymph node dissection (with or without para-aortic lymph node dissection); depending on the extent of vaginal involvement in patients with stage IIA disease, a more extensive upper vaginectomy also is performed. Postoperative radiation therapy is required in women with stage IB1 or IIA cervical cancer with poor prognostic factors (i.e., metastatic disease in pelvic or para-aortic lymph nodes, parametrial disease, or positive surgical margins) identified at the time of primary surgery. According to the findings from randomized trials, strong consideration should be given to the concurrent administration of cisplatin-based chemotherapy in women who require postoperative radiation therapy for the treatment of stage IB1 or IIA cervical cancer with poor prognostic factors.

Primary radiation therapy for stage IB1 or IIA cervical cancer consists of a combination of external-beam radiation and intracavitary implants. Some evidence suggests that the use of prophylactic radiation of the para-aortic nodes may prolong overall survival in patients receiving pelvic radiation therapy for bulky stage IIA cervical cancer. According to the findings from randomized trials, strong consideration should be given to the concurrent administration of cisplatin-based chemotherapy in women who require primary radiation therapy for the treatment of stage IB1 or IIA cervical cancer with poor prognostic factors.

FIGO Stage IB2 Cervical Cancer

The treatment of stage IB2 cervical cancer is controversial, and numerous methods have been used including surgery alone, radiation therapy alone, surgery with adjuvant radiation therapy, radiation therapy with adjuvant surgery, and neoadjuvant chemotherapy and surgery.

Many experts currently prefer initial treatment with pelvic radiation therapy consisting of a combination of external-beam radiation and intracavitary implants for bulky stage IB cervical tumors. According to the findings from randomized trials, strong consideration should be given to the concurrent administration of cisplatin-based chemotherapy in women receiving primary radiation therapy for the treatment of stage IB2 cervical cancer. Some evidence suggests that the use of prophylactic radiation of the para-aortic nodes may prolong overall survival in patients receiving pelvic radiation therapy for stage IB2 cervical cancer. Although it does not improve survival and many experts discourage its routine practice, extrafascial hysterectomy has been performed following primary radiation therapy for stage IB2 cervical tumors to reduce the risk of recurrence of central pelvic disease. In a randomized controlled trial, the addition of neoadjuvant chemotherapy did not improve control of local disease or prolong disease-free survival in patients receiving radiation therapy for invasive cervical cancer, including those with bulky stage IB tumors.

Primary surgery for bulky stage IB cervical cancer consists of radical hysterectomy with pelvic node and para-aortic lymph node dissection. The addition of adjuvant radiation therapy to primary surgery increases morbidity in patients with stage IB cervical cancer, including those with bulky tumors, and routine use of this combination is not advised in such patients. Long-term follow-up from a randomized controlled trial involving patients with stage IB squamous carcinoma of the cervix suggests that the addition of neoadjuvant cisplatin-containing chemotherapy reduces tumor volume, improves tumor operability, and consequently prolongs survival and disease-free survival in patients receiving surgery and adjuvant pelvic radiation therapy for bulky tumors.

FIGO Stages IIB–IVA Cervical Cancer

Because of high rates of local relapse, extensive locoregional disease (FIGO stages IIB through IVA) generally is treated with pelvic radiation therapy consisting of external-beam radiation therapy and brachytherapy. According to the findings from randomized trials, strong consideration should be given to the concurrent administration of cisplatin-based chemotherapy in women receiving radiation therapy for the treatment of stages IIB through IVA cervical cancer. Some evidence suggests that the use of prophylactic radiation of the para-aortic nodes may prolong overall survival in patients receiving pelvic radiation therapy for stage IIB cervical cancer.

FIGO Stage IVB Cervical Cancer

Patients with distant metastases (FIGO stage IVB) may receive chemotherapy for control of systemic disease; such patients also may benefit from palliative treatment with radiation therapy for symptoms from pelvic disease and/or distant metastases. The benefit of chemotherapy and/or radiation therapy versus best supportive care has not been established in patients with metastatic cervical cancer.

Recurrent Cervical Cancer

Depending on the initial treatment of cervical cancer, local recurrence of disease is treated with the treatment modality the patient did not previously receive. Radiation therapy can prolong survival and improve local control of disease in patients with locally recurrent cervical cancer following hysterectomy. In patients with local recurrence of disease following primary radiation therapy for cervical cancer, the overall survival rate following pelvic exenteration is 30–60%.

Most patients with recurrent cervical cancer have disease at local and distant sites. Palliative treatment with chemotherapy may be considered in patients with recurrent cervical cancer, but responses to treatment typically are short-lived. Radiation therapy may be useful in the palliation of symptoms in such patients, although many patients are symptomatic from recurrence of disease in a previously irradiated field where additional radiation may be contraindicated. The benefit of palliative chemotherapy versus best supportive care has not been established in patients with recurrent cervical cancer.

Treatment of Cervical Cancer during Pregnancy

Treatment for preinvasive cervical lesions (i.e., CIN 2, CIN 3, cervical carcinoma in situ) in pregnant women may be delayed and followed up with reevaluation in the postpartum period, but expert colposcopy and cervical biopsy should be performed promptly to confirm the absence of invasive disease. Diagnostic cone biopsy should be performed when microinvasive or invasive cervical carcinoma is suspected; cone biopsy is associated with substantial morbidity, such as excessive blood loss and increased risk of miscarriage, in pregnant women.

Most patients with cervical cancer during pregnancy are diagnosed with early-stage disease. The prognosis of early-stage cervical cancer appears to be similar in pregnant and nonpregnant women receiving standard treatment. Although surgery and radiation therapy are equally effective for the treatment of early-stage cervical cancer, surgical treatment is preferred in pregnant women because it allows preservation of ovarian and sexual function in this younger patient population.

The choice and timing of treatment of invasive cervical cancer during pregnancy depend on the stage of disease, duration of the pregnancy (i.e., gestational age of the fetus) at the time of diagnosis, risk to the mother and the fetus, and the wishes of the patient. The treatment of invasive cervical cancer diagnosed before fetal maturity (less than 20 weeks' gestation) is controversial; although many experts traditionally have recommended immediate treatment (according to stage of disease) with loss of the pregnancy, some clinicians support longer delays in treatment for patients with early-stage, nonbulky cervical tumors who desire completion of the pregnancy. If invasive cervical cancer is detected later in pregnancy when the fetus is viable (generally at greater than 20 weeks' gestation), planned delay of treatment is offered to appropriate candidates (according to stage and extent of disease, histology, and lesion size) who are placed under close surveillance for progression of disease, and delivery of the fetus by cesarean section is followed by surgery or radiation therapy for invasive cervical cancer according to the stage of disease. Most experts agree that planned delay of treatment to improve fetal viability is a reasonable option in women with early-stage cervical cancer (FIGO stage IA or IB1) detected in the third trimester or late second trimester of pregnancy.

Treatment of Cervical Cancer in HIV-infected Women

The prevalence of cervical squamous intraepithelial lesions and HPV infection with oncogenic genotypes is high among women with human immunodeficiency virus (HIV) infection, and the US Centers for Disease Control and Prevention (CDC) has designated invasive cervical cancer in HIV-positive women as an acquired immunodeficiency syndrome (AIDS)-defining illness. Some evidence suggests that antiretroviral therapy (triple-drug therapy including an HIV protease inhibitor) may reduce the prevalence and/or lower the grade of cervical lesions in HIV-infected women despite the persistence of HPV infection. Women with HIV infection who are diagnosed with invasive cervical cancer often have more aggressive and advanced disease with a poorer prognosis. The same standard treatment for preinvasive cervical lesions or invasive cervical cancer used in non-HIV-infected women generally is recommended in HIV-infected women, but response to treatment may be poor; close surveillance is required, and repetitive treatment of cervical intraepithelial neoplasia (CIN) may be necessary in

HIV-infected women to prevent progression of disease. Evidence from a phase III, nonblinded, randomized trial indicates that the recurrence rate of CIN is reduced and time to recurrence is prolonged in women with HIV infection receiving adjunctive therapy with vaginal fluorouracil† versus observation only following excisional or ablative treatment of high-grade cervical dysplasia (i.e., CIN 2 or 3).

Concurrent Chemotherapy and Radiation Therapy for Invasive Cervical Cancer

Results from 3 large randomized, controlled, phase III trials at 3 years or more of follow-up show that the addition of cisplatin-based chemotherapy given concurrently with radiation therapy decreases the risk of death by 40–50% in women receiving primary radiation therapy for FIGO stages IB2 through IVA cervical cancer and in women receiving postoperative radiation therapy for FIGO stage IA2, IB, or IIA cervical cancer with poor prognostic factors (i.e., metastatic disease in pelvic lymph nodes, parametrial disease, positive surgical margins) identified at the time of primary surgery. Results from 2 other large randomized trials show that in patients receiving concomitant chemotherapy and radiation therapy for FIGO stages IIB through IVA cervical cancer, risk of death is decreased by about 30–40% among those receiving cisplatin-containing versus non-cisplatin-containing chemotherapeutic regimens.

Because of the findings from these randomized trials, NCI recommends that strong consideration be given to the concurrent administration of cisplatin-based chemotherapy in women who require radiation therapy for the treatment of cervical cancer. Substitution of carboplatin for cisplatin is not recommended because of the lack of evidence supporting comparable efficacy of this agent for cervical cancer. Further study is needed to establish the magnitude of benefit when chemotherapy is given concurrently with optimal-dose radiation therapy in patients with locally advanced cervical cancer.

Clinical Trials

In addition to its cytotoxic effects, chemotherapy is believed to have a synergistic antineoplastic effect with radiation therapy by mechanisms that include increased sensitivity of tumor to radiation and inhibition of the repair of sublethal damage to tumor induced by radiation. The current recommendation for concurrent cisplatin-containing chemotherapy and radiation therapy in women with invasive cervical cancer (FIGO stage IB2 through IVA disease or FIGO stage IA2, IB, or IIA disease with poor prognostic factors) is based principally on the findings from 5 large, randomized trials (3 randomized trials showing prolonged survival with the concurrent use of chemotherapy and radiation therapy versus radiation therapy alone and 2 randomized trials showing the superiority of cisplatin-containing regimens versus non-cisplatin-containing regimens for concurrent use with radiation therapy).

In a randomized trial of 403 patients (386 evaluable patients) with advanced squamous cell carcinoma, adenocarcinoma, or adenosquamous carcinoma of the cervix confined to the pelvis (FIGO stages IIB through IVA or FIGO stage IB or IIA with a tumor diameter of at least 5 cm or involvement of the pelvic lymph nodes), the estimated overall rate of survival at 5 years (calculated at a median follow-up of 43 months) was higher (73 versus 58%) among those receiving concurrent chemotherapy (with cisplatin and fluorouracil) and pelvic radiation therapy than among those receiving radiation therapy alone (consisting of pelvic radiation therapy and irradiation of the para-aortic lymph nodes). The estimated rate of disease-free survival at 5 years was 67% among patients who received combined therapy with chemotherapy and radiation and 40% among those who received radiation therapy alone. According to stage of disease, overall survival was prolonged with the addition of chemotherapy to radiation therapy in patients with FIGO stage IB, IIA, or IIB cervical cancer but not in patients with stage III or IVA disease; however, the study was not designed to test for differences in survival within these subgroups. The rates of distant or locoregional metastases were lower among patients receiving combined modality treatment (14 versus 33% and 19 versus 35%, respectively); a higher rate of reversible adverse hematologic effects was observed in patients receiving combined chemotherapy and radiation therapy, but the severity of late adverse effects was similar between the groups.

In a randomized trial of 374 patients (369 evaluable patients) with bulky or barrel-shaped stage IB (i.e., FIGO stage IB2) squamous cell carcinoma, adenocarcinoma, or adenosquamous carcinoma of the cervix, higher rates of overall survival (83 versus 74% at 3 years) and progression-free survival were observed at 4 years in those receiving concurrent chemotherapy (with cisplatin) and radiation therapy with adjuvant hysterectomy than in those receiving radiation therapy with adjuvant hysterectomy. The relative risks of progression of disease and death among women receiving combined chemotherapy and radiation therapy were 0.51 and 0.54, respectively, compared with those receiving radiation therapy alone. Higher frequencies of adverse hematologic effects (21 versus 2%) and adverse GI effects (14 versus 5%) were observed in patients receiving combined chemotherapy and radiation therapy than in those receiving radiation therapy alone.

At a median follow-up of 42 months in a randomized trial of 268 patients (243 evaluable patients) with clinical stage IA2, IB, or IIA cervical cancer initially treated with radical hysterectomy and pelvic node dissection, higher rates of overall survival (estimated 4-year survival of 81 versus 71%) and progression-free survival (estimated 4-year progression-free survival of 80 versus 63%) were observed in those receiving concurrent chemotherapy (with cisplatin and fluorouracil) and pelvic radiation therapy versus pelvic radiation therapy alone for high risk factors, such as positive pelvic lymph nodes, positive surgical margins, and/or microscopic involvement of the parametrium, identified at the time of primary surgery.

Optimal chemotherapy regimens for the treatment of invasive cervical cancer have not been established. Current evidence from large, randomized, phase III trials indicates that cisplatin is a drug of choice for chemotherapy to be used concomitantly with radiation therapy for locally advanced cervical cancer. Cisplatin may be used alone or in combination therapy (e.g., cisplatin and fluorouracil) as an adjunct to radiation therapy in patients with locally advanced cervical cancer; however, results from at least one randomized trial suggest that cisplatin alone is as effective but less toxic than cisplatin-containing combination regimens for concomitant use with radiation therapy. Improvement in survival with the combination of chemotherapy and radiation therapy in patients with locally advanced cervical cancer has been observed only with *concurrent* administration of chemotherapy. Analysis of pooled data from several randomized trials did *not* demonstrate prolonged survival or improved local control of disease with use of neoadjuvant chemotherapy followed by radiation therapy in locally advanced cervical cancer.

In a randomized trial of 575 patients (526 evaluable patients) receiving concurrent chemotherapy and radiation therapy for stage IIB, III, or IVA squamous cell carcinoma, adenocarcinoma, or adenosquamous carcinoma of the cervix without involvement of the para-aortic lymph nodes, follow-up at a median duration of 35 months showed higher rates of survival and progression-free survival among those receiving cisplatin alone or a combination regimen of cisplatin, fluorouracil, and hydroxyurea than among those receiving hydroxyurea alone. The rates of progression-free survival at 24 months were 67, 64, and 47% in patients receiving radiation therapy and concomitant chemotherapy with cisplatin alone; cisplatin, fluorouracil, and hydroxyurea; and hydroxyurea alone, respectively. Relative risk of death was 0.61 or 0.58 in those receiving cisplatin alone or combination therapy with cisplatin, fluorouracil, and hydroxyurea, respectively, compared with those receiving hydroxyurea alone. The rate of local recurrences was lower in patients receiving radiation therapy with cisplatin or cisplatin-containing combination therapy (19 and 20%, respectively) than in those receiving radiation therapy with hydroxyurea alone (30%); the rate of distant metastases (i.e., lung metastases) also was lower in patients receiving radiation therapy with cisplatin alone or radiation therapy with cisplatin in combination chemotherapy (3 and 4%, respectively) than in those receiving radiation therapy with hydroxyurea alone (10%). Compared with patients receiving either cisplatin or hydroxyurea alone, the frequency of moderate or severe leukopenia was more than double and the frequency of moderate or severe granulocytopenia was approximately double in patients receiving the 3-drug regimen (cisplatin, fluorouracil, and hydroxyurea).

In a randomized trial of 388 patients (368 evaluable patients) receiving concomitant chemotherapy and radiation therapy for FIGO stage IIB, III, or IVA squamous cell carcinoma, adenocarcinoma, or adenosquamous carcinoma of the cervix without involvement of the para-aortic lymph nodes, follow-up at a median duration of 8.7 years showed higher rates of survival (55 versus 43%) and progression-free survival in those receiving cisplatin and fluorouracil than in those receiving hydroxyurea alone. Relative risk of progression of disease or death was 0.79 and relative risk of death was 0.74 in those receiving cisplatin and fluorouracil compared with those receiving hydroxyurea. Severe (grade 3) or life-threatening (grade 4) leukopenia occurred less frequently in patients receiving combination therapy with cisplatin and fluorouracil (4%) than in those receiving hydroxyurea alone (24%).

The results of these randomized trials suggest that agents other than hydroxyurea, particularly cisplatin (alone or in combination with other agents), are preferred for concurrent use with radiation therapy in the treatment of locally advanced cervical cancer. Fluorouracil is used in combination with cisplatin for

concurrent chemotherapy and radiation therapy in patients with locally advanced cervical cancer, but randomized controlled studies are needed to determine if this combination regimen is superior to cisplatin alone. Although carboplatin often is used as a less toxic substitute for cisplatin, current evidence supports the use of cisplatin-containing chemotherapy given concurrently with radiation therapy in patients with locally advanced cervical cancer, and similar benefit with carboplatin-containing chemotherapy cannot be assumed. Additional comparative studies are needed to determine the optimal chemotherapy regimens and schedules to be used concurrently with radiation therapy for the treatment of locally advanced cervical cancer.

Chemotherapy for Metastatic or Recurrent Cervical Cancer

Cisplatin is used in the palliative treatment of metastatic or recurrent squamous cell carcinoma of the cervix†. The drug is considered one of the most active agents in the treatment of cervical neoplasms. Response rates of 18–31% have been reported with use of cisplatin as a single agent in advanced cervical cancer.

Cisplatin also has been used as a component of various combination chemotherapeutic regimens (e.g., bleomycin, cisplatin and ifosfamide [BIP]; bleomycin, cisplatin, mitomycin, and vincristine [BOMP]) for the treatment of metastatic or recurrent cervical cancer. Limited evidence from a small randomized trial of patients with advanced cervical cancer suggests that cisplatin-based chemotherapy is superior to hydroxyurea, which has minimal activity as a single agent in the treatment of metastatic or recurrent cervical cancer. Combination regimens have not been consistently shown to be superior to the use of single agents, such as cisplatin, one of the most active drugs in the treatment of metastatic or recurrent cervical cancer. Although relatively high response rates have been reported with cisplatin-containing combination chemotherapy regimens, these regimens generally are more toxic and do not appear to be superior to cisplatin alone in the treatment of metastatic or recurrent cervical cancer. For example, high objective response rates have been observed with the combination regimen of bleomycin, ifosfamide, and cisplatin in women with metastatic or recurrent cervical cancer, but toxicity is greater and survival is not improved in women receiving the combination regimen rather than cisplatin alone. Similarly, higher response rates and prolonged progression-free survival but greater toxicity and no difference in overall survival has been observed with use of the combination of cisplatin and ifosfamide (with mesna) compared with cisplatin alone in patients with metastatic or recurrent squamous cell carcinoma of the cervix.

Because of its lesser toxicity, carboplatin may be considered as an alternative to the parent compound cisplatin, particularly in patients with nephrotoxicity or neurotoxicity caused by advanced cervical tumor who are not suitable candidates for cisplatin therapy; however, randomized controlled trials comparing carboplatin and cisplatin have not been performed to date, and because of superior response rates and lesser hematologic toxicity, most experts consider cisplatin the current drug of choice in the treatment of advanced cervical cancer, particularly in patients who have received radiation therapy.

Various single agents and combination regimens for the treatment of advanced cervical cancer have been evaluated mostly in phase II studies, and optimal treatment has not been established. In addition, the benefit of chemotherapy versus best supportive care has not been studied in patients with metastatic or recurrent cervical cancer. Because the prognosis of patients with advanced cervical cancer remains poor and optimal therapy has not been established, all such patients may be considered for enrollment in clinical trials investigating new agents or combination regimens. The use of cisplatin with other agents (e.g., paclitaxel, gemcitabine, fluorouracil, vinorelbine) or in other combination regimens (e.g., cisplatin, methotrexate, vinblastine, and doxorubicin [MVAC]) is being evaluated in patients with metastatic or recurrent cervical cancer.

● *Non-small Cell Lung Cancer*
Overview

Cisplatin is used as a component of various chemotherapeutic regimens for advanced non-small cell lung cancer†. Non-small cell lung cancer, which includes squamous cell carcinoma, adenocarcinoma, and large cell carcinoma, accounts for approximately 80% of all lung cancers; the prognosis for this neoplasm is poor with a 5-year survival of less than 10% in patients with advanced disease.

Cisplatin-containing chemotherapy is used for the treatment of advanced non-small cell lung cancer. A small survival benefit has been demonstrated for the use of platinum-based (cisplatin) chemotherapy alone or combined with radiation therapy in selected patients with unresectable, locally advanced or metastatic non-small cell lung cancer who have a good performance status. Analysis of pooled data from individual patients enrolled in published and unpublished randomized trials or from published randomized trials indicates a 13% reduction in risk of death and an absolute increase in survival rate of 4% at 2 years for cisplatin-based chemotherapy combined with radiation therapy compared with radiation therapy alone in the treatment of unresectable, locally advanced non-small cell lung cancer. The optimal timing of chemotherapy used in conjunction with radiation therapy (sequential, concurrent, or alternating) has not been established. Analysis of pooled data from individual patients enrolled in published and unpublished randomized trials indicates that the addition of cisplatin-containing chemotherapy to supportive care in patients with advanced non-small cell lung cancer provides a small survival advantage (i.e., absolute increase in survival rate of approximately 10% at 1 year or increased median survival of about 1.5 months). Results from two small randomized trials suggest that the administration of cisplatin-containing chemotherapy preceding surgery prolongs survival in patients with resectable, locally advanced non-small cell lung cancer although further study is needed to confirm these findings.

Because many patients with earlier stages of disease treatable with surgical resection subsequently develop metastases, the use of adjuvant chemotherapy and/or radiotherapy is being investigated. Current evidence does not show improvement in survival with radiation therapy and/or chemotherapy administered following surgery in patients with resectable non-small cell lung cancer. Although limited by the inclusion of mostly studies involving now-obsolete equipment, analysis of pooled data from individual patients enrolled in published and unpublished randomized trials indicates that postoperative treatment with conventional radiation therapy reduces local recurrence of disease but adversely affects survival in patients with completely resected stage I and II non-small cell lung cancer. The effect of postoperative radiation therapy in patients with later stages of non-small cell lung cancer (e.g., stage IIIA with N2) has not been established. Differing regimens of radiation therapy (e.g., accelerated versus conventional radiation therapy) also are being investigated.

Combination Chemotherapy for Advanced Non-small Cell Lung Cancer

Platinum-based chemotherapy regimens currently are preferred for the treatment of non-small cell lung cancer. A detrimental effect on survival has been observed for patients with non-small cell lung cancer receiving treatment based on alkylating agents, such as busulfan and cyclophosphamide, and such regimens are *not* recommended. Currently preferred regimens for the treatment of advanced non-small cell lung cancer include the combination of cisplatin with another agent, such as paclitaxel, vinorelbine, gemcitabine, or docetaxel.

In randomized trials, patients with advanced non-small cell lung cancer receiving cisplatin combined with paclitaxel or gemcitabine had higher response rates and similar median survival compared with those receiving combination therapy with cisplatin and etoposide; consequently, paclitaxel-containing regimens or other platinum-based regimens currently are preferred in the treatment of patients with advanced non-small cell lung cancer. (See Uses: Non-small Cell Lung Carcinoma in Paclitaxel 10:00 or Gemcitabine 10:00.) Cisplatin combined with gemcitabine is associated with improved survival (estimated median survival of 9.1 versus 7.6 months) and higher response rates (30 versus 11%) compared with cisplatin alone in patients with advanced non-small cell lung cancer. Patients with stage IIIB or IV non-small cell lung carcinoma receiving cisplatin and vinorelbine had a longer median survival, higher survival rate at 1 year, a longer median progression-free survival, and higher response rate than those receiving cisplatin alone. (See Uses: Non-small Cell Lung Carcinoma in Vinorelbine 10:00.)

Use of chemotherapy for the treatment of advanced non-small cell lung cancer generally is advised only in patients with good performance status (ECOG performance status of 0 or 1, and 2 in selected patients) and evaluable lesions so that treatment can be discontinued if the disease does not respond. The decision to use chemotherapy must be individualized according to several factors, including patient preference, toxicity, survival benefit, quality of life, and cost of treatment. Once the decision is made to use chemotherapy, treatment should begin promptly to allow for optimal response in patients receiving chemotherapy combined with radiation therapy for unresectable stage III disease and to allow treatment before deterioration of performance status in patients with stage IV disease. Although the optimal duration of chemotherapy has not been fully established, treatment with 2–8 cycles generally is advised in patients with stage IV or unresectable stage III non-small cell lung cancer; periodic imaging studies are used to monitor response and determine whether to continue treatment.

Cisplatin, an active agent in the treatment of non-small cell lung carcinoma, produces an objective response in about 10–20% of patients, No single chemotherapy regimen currently can be recommended as superior in the treatment of non-small cell lung cancer. Analysis of pooled data from published randomized trials involving patients with advanced non-small cell lung cancer indicates higher response rates and a small increase in survival rates at 6 months and 1 year but greater toxicity in patients receiving combination chemotherapy versus single-agent chemotherapy. A large randomized trial showed a higher response rate but no difference in median survival in patients receiving combination therapy with cisplatin and paclitaxel for advanced non-small cell lung cancer compared with those receiving high-dose cisplatin alone.

Various chemotherapy regimens used alone or in combination with other treatment modalities, such as radiation therapy, are continually being evaluated for the treatment of advanced non-small cell lung cancer. Because current treatment is not satisfactory for almost all patients with non-small cell lung cancer except selected patients with early-stage, resectable disease, all patients may be considered for enrollment in clinical trials at the time of diagnosis.

● Small Cell Lung Cancer

Cisplatin is used in combination chemotherapy for the treatment of small cell lung cancer†. Combination chemotherapy regimens are superior to single-agent therapy for the treatment of small cell lung cancer and moderately intensive drug doses are superior to doses that produce minimal toxicity. Various regimens have been used in combination therapy, and many 2- to 4-drug combination regimens, including cisplatin-containing regimens, have produced response rates of 65–90 or 70–85% and complete response rates of 45–75 or 20–30% in patients with limited-stage or extensive-stage disease, respectively; however, comparative efficacy is continually being evaluated. While efficacy of the various available regimens is continually being evaluated, combination chemotherapy containing cisplatin and etoposide currently is considered a preferred regimen for the treatment of small cell lung carcinoma. Combination therapy with cisplatin and etoposide used in combined modality treatment with concurrent thoracic irradiation that is administered early in the course of treatment is a preferred regimen for limited-stage small cell lung cancer. Cisplatin in conjunction with etoposide also is used in the treatment of extensive-stage small cell lung cancer.

In a randomized study, patients with previously untreated extensive-stage small cell lung cancer receiving combination therapy with cisplatin and etoposide (PE); cyclophosphamide, doxorubicin, and vincristine (CAV); or an alternation of these regimens (PE/CAV) had similar objective response rates, complete response rates, and median survival; because of a higher frequency of severe thrombocytopenia associated with the alternation of regimens, therapy with PE/CAV generally is not recommended. Cisplatin in combination with etoposide and ifosfamide with mesna is used as an alternative regimen for the treatment of small cell lung cancer. Second-line therapy with combination regimens (e.g., cisplatin and etoposide) or single agents (e.g., paclitaxel, topotecan) may be of some value for the treatment of small cell lung cancer refractory to other chemotherapy regimens (particularly when relapse occurs more than 6 months following completion of initial treatment).

Although optimum duration of chemotherapy has not been clearly defined, additional improvement in survival has not been observed when the duration of drug administration exceeds 3–6 or 6 months in patients with limited-stage or extensive-stage small cell lung cancer, respectively. Because the current prognosis for small cell lung carcinoma is unsatisfactory regardless of stage and despite considerable diagnostic and therapeutic advances, all patients with this cancer are candidates for inclusion in clinical trials at the time of diagnosis.

● Malignant Pleural Mesothelioma

Cisplatin is used in combination with pemetrexed for the treatment of malignant pleural mesothelioma in patients who are not eligible for surgery. (See Uses: Malignant Pleural Mesothelioma in Pemetrexed 10:00.)

Cisplatin alone or in combination with other agents (e.g., doxorubicin, mitomycin) is used in the palliative treatment of advanced malignant pleural mesothelioma†. Combination chemotherapy regimens are associated with greater toxicity and do not appear to prolong survival or improve control of symptoms in patients with unresectable malignant pleural mesothelioma.

● Esophageal Cancer

Cisplatin has been used alone and in combination therapy for the treatment of localized or advanced esophageal cancer†. Optimum therapy for esophageal cancer has not been established, and new therapies are continually being evaluated. Because the prognosis for most patients with esophageal cancer remains poor, all newly diagnosed patients should be considered for enrollment in clinical trials comparing various treatment modalities.

Localized Esophageal Cancer

For the treatment of patients with localized esophageal cancer, combined modality treatment consisting of combination chemotherapy with cisplatin and fluorouracil and concurrent radiation therapy may be used prior to surgery (as neoadjuvant therapy) or as an alternative to surgery (i.e., in patients who are not considered suitable surgical candidates or in an attempt to avoid perioperative mortality [less than 10%] and to relieve dysphagia).

Combined modality therapy consisting of combination chemotherapy with cisplatin and fluorouracil and concurrent radiation therapy is more effective than radiation therapy alone in patients with localized esophageal carcinoma. Patients with locally advanced esophageal cancer (most patients had squamous cell carcinoma) who received combined modality therapy with cisplatin and fluorouracil and concurrent radiation therapy had longer survival (12.5 versus 8.9 months) and higher survival rates (38 versus 10% at 24 months) than patients who received radiation therapy alone. Cisplatin 75 mg/m^2 (up to a maximum dose of 150 mg) was administered IV on day 1 and fluorouracil 1 g/m^2 (up to a maximum dose of 8 g) was administered by 96-hour continuous IV infusion on days 1–4 every 4 weeks during concurrent radiation therapy and every 3 weeks following the completion of radiation therapy. At 5 years, 26% of patients who received combined modality therapy were alive compared with none of the patients who received radiation therapy alone. In patients with localized esophageal cancer, particularly squamous cell carcinoma, who are not considered suitable candidates for surgery, combined modality treatment with cisplatin and fluorouracil and concurrent radiation therapy may be used as an alternative therapy. Although the comparative benefit of combined chemotherapy and radiation versus surgery has not been established, some experts recommend combined modality treatment with combination chemotherapy (e.g., cisplatin and fluorouracil) and concurrent radiation therapy with or without surgery as primary treatment for localized, resectable esophageal cancer.

Because of high rates of distant metastasis or locoregional recurrence of disease in patients undergoing surgery for localized esophageal cancer, the addition of systemic therapy was proposed to provide early treatment of disseminated but undetected disease and to reduce the risk of recurrent locoregional disease. Neoadjuvant therapy may reduce tumor size and increase the chances of complete resection in patients with locally advanced esophageal cancer. Variable results have been observed in studies of induction therapy with cisplatin-based chemotherapy and concurrent radiation therapy followed by surgery in patients with squamous cancer or adenocarcinoma of the esophagus. In a large, randomized trial, surgery combined with preoperative and postoperative chemotherapy with cisplatin and fluorouracil did not improve survival compared with surgery alone in patients with localized, operable esophageal carcinoma. Combined modality treatment of esophageal cancer may be associated with substantial toxicity, and choice of therapy must be individualized. Histologic type also influences choice of therapy for esophageal carcinoma. Clinical trials for esophageal cancer have included mostly patients with squamous cell carcinomas, and surgical resection remains standard therapy for esophageal adenocarcinoma. Further study is needed to determine the role of neoadjuvant or adjuvant therapy in combination with surgery in the treatment of localized esophageal cancer.

Advanced Esophageal Cancer

Combination therapy with cisplatin and fluorouracil is used for the palliative treatment of metastatic (local or distant) disease or recurrent or locally advanced disease that is not amenable to surgery or radiation therapy, and such combined therapy currently is considered a regimen of choice. Cisplatin also has been used alone in the palliative treatment of advanced esophageal cancer. Although higher response rates are achieved with cisplatin and fluorouracil than with cisplatin alone in patients with metastatic disease, no overall difference in survival has been observed. Combination therapy with cisplatin and other active agents for advanced esophageal cancer (e.g., paclitaxel) is being investigated.

● *Biliary Tract Cancer*

Cisplatin has been used in combination with gemcitabine for the treatment of unresectable locally advanced or metastatic biliary tract cancer† (intrahepatic or extrahepatic cholangiocarcinoma, gallbladder cancer, or ampullary cancer), including unresectable recurrent disease following surgical resection.

Experts state that, in patients with biliary tract adenocarcinoma (the most common type of biliary tract cancer), chemotherapy can be recommended in individuals with unresectable locally advanced or metastatic disease and in those with recurrent disease following surgical resection. Chemotherapy is recommended in such individuals with good performance status (ECOG performance status of 0 or 1). However, in patients with poor performance status (ECOG performance status of 2 or 3) or insufficient biliary decompression, the benefits of chemotherapy are limited and use of alternative therapy for palliation of associated symptoms (e.g., pain) and improvement in quality of life is recommended.

In a phase 3 trial in 410 patients with unresectable locally advanced or metastatic biliary tract carcinoma, including unresectable recurrent disease following surgical resection, patients who received cisplatin in combination with gemcitabine had longer median overall (11.7 versus 8.1 months) and progression-free (8 versus 5 months) survival, a higher 6-month progression-free survival rate (59.3 versus 42.5%), and higher rates of tumor control (complete or partial responses or stable disease) (81.4 versus 71.8%) compared with those who received gemcitabine alone. Only one patient in each treatment group achieved a complete response. Patients enrolled in the study generally had good baseline performance status (ECOG performance status of 0 or 1 in 88% of patients). Based on current evidence, combination therapy with cisplatin and gemcitabine is recommended (accepted) for use in the treatment of unresectable locally advanced or metastatic biliary tract cancer (intrahepatic or extrahepatic cholangiocarcinoma, gallbladder cancer, or ampullary cancer), including unresectable recurrent disease following surgical resection, in patients with good performance status (ECOG performance status of 0 or 1).

For further information on the treatment of unresectable locally advanced or metastatic biliary tract cancer, including use of combination therapy with cisplatin and gemcitabine, see Uses: Biliary Tract Cancer, in Gemcitabine 10:00.

● *Melanoma*

Cisplatin and other platinum analogs, such as carboplatin, have minimal activity but substantial toxicity in metastatic melanoma†. Although cisplatin has been used in combination therapy (e.g., carmustine, cisplatin, dacarbazine, and tamoxifen) for the palliative treatment of metastatic melanoma, evidence suggests that the addition of cisplatin to dacarbazine-containing regimens increases toxicity but does not improve survival. Evidence from large, randomized trials has not established the superiority of combination regimens compared with dacarbazine alone, and dacarbazine monotherapy currently is a systemic treatment of choice for metastatic melanoma (see Uses: Melanoma in Dacarbazine 10:00 for an overview of therapy for melanoma). The use of cisplatin-containing chemotherapy in combination with biologic therapy using aldesleukin and interferon alfa is being investigated for the treatment of metastatic melanoma.

Intra-arterial† infusions of cisplatin have been used in the treatment of regionally confined metastases from malignant melanoma. Cisplatin also has been used for hyperthermic isolated limb perfusion for recurrent melanoma of the extremity.

● *Brain Tumors*

Cisplatin has been used for the palliative treatment of various primary brain tumors†. Regimens that include cisplatin have been used principally in the treatment of medulloblastoma and germ cell tumors. Most primary brain tumors are treated with surgery and/or radiation therapy, but adjuvant chemotherapy may prolong survival in some tumor types and has increased disease-free survival in patients with medulloblastoma, certain germ cell tumors, and gliomas.

Malignant Gliomas

Astrocytic Tumors

Cisplatin has been used as an adjunct for the treatment of astrocytic tumors†, such as anaplastic astrocytoma and glioblastoma multiforme. Although brief in duration, responses to high-dose IV cisplatin have been observed in patients with malignant glioma that recurred following previous chemotherapy with nitrosoureas. (For further discussion of the treatment of astrocytic tumors, see Uses: Brain Tumors in Carmustine 10:00.)

The use of cisplatin and carmustine as adjuvant and/or neoadjuvant therapy in conjunction with radiation therapy for the treatment of high-grade gliomas† is being investigated. In a large randomized trial, cisplatin and carmustine administered by continuous IV infusion prior to postoperative radiation therapy in patients with newly diagnosed glioblastoma multiforme did not increase survival and was associated with greater toxicity than standard adjuvant therapy consisting of IV carmustine administered concurrently with radiation therapy.

Medulloblastoma

Cisplatin is used in combination with lomustine and vincristine as adjuvant therapy following surgical resection and radiation therapy for the treatment of medulloblastoma†, the most common malignant childhood brain tumor. Such adjuvant chemotherapy is associated with improved progression-free survival in patients with poor prognostic factors (i.e., younger than 3 years of age, metastatic disease and/or subtotal resection with >1.5 cm³ of residual disease and/or nonposterior fossa location), but the role of adjuvant chemotherapy in children with average-risk medulloblastoma has not been established.

The use of adjuvant chemotherapy coupled with reduced-dose radiation therapy in children with average-risk medulloblastoma (i.e., older than 3 years of age, total or near-total resection with <1.5 cm³ of residual disease, no dissemination) is being investigated. Because of the debilitating effects of radiation on growth and neurologic development, the use of postoperative chemotherapy (e.g., induction therapy with cyclophosphamide and vincristine followed by cisplatin and etoposide, with or without bone marrow rescue) to delay, modify, or possibly avoid the need for radiation therapy in children younger than 3–6 years of age is being studied.

Cisplatin is an active agent in the treatment of recurrent medulloblastoma in children; response to chemotherapy is observed in more than 50% of patients with disease that recurs following treatment with surgery and radiation therapy, but long-term control of the disease is rare.

Oligodendroglioma

Cisplatin also has been used, alone or in combination with other agents (e.g., cisplatin and etoposide) as salvage therapy for recurrent oligodendroglioma†, a uniquely chemosensitive form of glioma.

Intracranial Germ Cell Tumors

Combination therapy with a platinum-containing agent (i.e., cisplatin or carboplatin) and etoposide is used in the treatment of intracranial germ cell tumors†. Other combination chemotherapy regimens (e.g., cisplatin, vinblastine, bleomycin) also have been used. The role of adjuvant chemotherapy in addition to radiation therapy for the treatment of such tumors remains to be established.

Intra-arterial Therapy

Intra-arterial† administration of cisplatin, alone or in combination with other agents, has been investigated in the treatment of newly diagnosed or recurrent gliomas; severe adverse effects, including renal, otologic, neurologic, and retinal toxicity, have been reported in patients receiving such therapy, and the role of intra-arterial cisplatin in the treatment of primary brain tumors has not been established.

• Neuroblastoma

Cisplatin is used as a component of combination therapy for high-risk neuroblastoma†. Combination chemotherapy with moderate doses of carboplatin, cyclophosphamide, doxorubicin, and etoposide is used in conjunction with surgery (with or without radiation therapy) for the treatment of neuroblastoma in patients with intermediate-risk tumors or, in some cases, low-risk tumors. Although surgery alone typically is adequate for the treatment of low-risk tumors, combination chemotherapy is administered if surgical resection is incomplete (less than 50% of the primary tumor is resected) or if life-threatening or organ-threatening symptomatic disease is present (e.g., spinal cord compression). In patients with high-risk tumors, aggressive chemotherapy using higher doses of these drugs and additional drugs (e.g., ifosfamide, high-dose cisplatin, vincristine) is used. If high-risk disease responds to the initial regimen of chemotherapy, further therapy consists of surgical resection of the primary tumor, myeloablative therapy and autologous stem cell transplantation (bone marrow transplantation or peripheral blood stem cell transplantation), and radiation therapy (radiation to the primary tumor site and sometimes total-body irradiation); following recovery, 6 months of therapy with oral 13-cis-retinoic acid (isotretinoin) is administered.

• Other Uses

Cisplatin is used in the treatment of adrenocortical cancer†, anal cancer†, GI carcinoid tumors†, choriocarcinoma†, endometrial cancer†, gastric cancer†, hepatoblastoma†, liver cancer†, certain types of non-Hodgkin's lymphoma†,

osteosarcoma†, and soft-tissue sarcomas in adults†. Cisplatin also is used in the treatment of penile cancer†, malignant thymoma†, and anaplastic thyroid cancer†. Cisplatin has been used in the treatment of rhabdoid tumor of the kidney†, a highly malignant form of childhood kidney cancer. The drug also has shown some activity in the palliative treatment of advanced medullary thyroid cancer†.

Intra-arterial† infusions of cisplatin have been used with some success in the treatment of regionally confined malignancies, including osteogenic sarcomas. Cisplatin has also been administered intraperitoneally† alone or in conjunction with IV sodium thiosulfate in patients with various tumors (e.g., adenocarcinoma of the breast, carcinoid, mesothelioma) that were associated with malignant ascites and/or were confined to the peritoneal cavity. (See also Intraperitoneal Cisplatin and Paclitaxel under Ovarian Cancer: First-line Therapy for Advanced Ovarian Epithelial Cancer, in Uses.)

DOSAGE AND ADMINISTRATION

• Reconstitution and Administration

Cisplatin is administered by IV infusion. The drug has also been administered intra-arterially† and intraperitoneally†. Needles, syringes, catheters, or IV administration sets that contain aluminum parts which may come in contact with cisplatin should *not* be used for preparation or administration of the drug. (See Chemistry and Stability: Stability.)

The manufacturer recommends that protective gloves be used during handling of commercially available cisplatin injection and during preparation of cisplatin solutions, since skin reactions associated with accidental exposure to the drug may occur. If cisplatin solution comes in contact with the skin or mucosa, the affected area should be washed with soap and water (skin) or flushed with water (mucosa) immediately and thoroughly. Rarely, adverse local effects have occurred following extravasation of cisplatin during administration. (See Cautions: Local Effects.)

Patients should be adequately hydrated before and for 24 hours after administration of cisplatin to ensure good urinary output and minimize nephrotoxicity. (See Cautions: Renal and Electrolyte Effects.) Various regimens of IV hydration, with or without mannitol and/or furosemide diuresis, and various rates of administration of cisplatin have been employed. The clinician should consult published protocols for information related to specific regimens. The manufacturer and many clinicians recommend IV infusion of 1–2 L of fluid over 8–12 hours prior to administration of the drug. In adults, unless contraindicated, IV fluids are usually administered alone or with mannitol and/or furosemide at an initial rate sufficient to maintain hydration and a diuresis of 150–400 mL/hour during and for at least 4–6 hours after administration of cisplatin, and then a diuresis of 100–200 mL or more per hour for the next 18–24 hours or until vomiting stops and oral fluids are tolerated. Patients must be closely monitored for fluid and serum electrolyte disturbances. (See Cautions: Renal and Electrolyte Effects.) Potassium chloride is often added (e.g., 10–20 mEq/L) to IV fluids infused during and/or following administration of cisplatin to replace losses and prevent deficiencies.

IV Infusion

For IV infusion, the manufacturer recommends that the required dose of cisplatin (as the commercially available injection) be diluted in 2 L of 5% dextrose and 0.33 or 0.45% sodium chloride injection containing 18.75 g of mannitol per liter (i.e., 37.5 g in 2 L), and infused IV over 6–8 hours. Various other methods of dilution and/or rates of administration are used, and the clinician should consult published protocols for information related to specific regimens. IV infusions over 15 minutes to 2 hours are commonly employed and have been used with minimal adverse renal effects. Continuous 24-hour or 5-day IV infusions of the drug have also been used. While cisplatin has been administered by rapid IV injection (e.g., over 1–5 minutes), such rapid administration may be associated with increased nephrotoxicity or ototoxicity compared with slower IV infusion of the drug.

Intra-arterial Infusion

For intra-arterial† infusion, cisplatin has been administered via an appropriately placed catheter using a controlled-infusion device. The cisplatin dose has generally been diluted in 0.9% sodium chloride injection (300 mL for doses less than 300 mg and 450 mL for doses greater than 300 mg) containing small amounts of heparin sodium (e.g., 3000 units) and infused over 2–4 hours (range 1–24 hours).

Intraperitoneal Instillation

For intraperitoneal† administration in the Gynecologic Oncology Group (GOG)-172 study in patients with advanced epithelial ovarian cancer, the cisplatin dose was diluted in 2 L of 0.9% sodium chloride solution that was warmed to 37°C and administered as rapidly as possible through a surgically implanted peritoneal catheter. Following peritoneal infusion, patients were asked to roll into a different position every 15 minutes for the next 2 hours to disperse the drug throughout the peritoneal cavity. In this study, the paclitaxel dose was diluted in a liter of saline solution that was warmed to 37°C and infused through the intraperitoneal catheter, followed by intraperitoneal infusion of an additional liter of warmed saline solution. Some clinicians have recommended that intraperitoneal chemotherapeutic agents be mixed in 1 L of 0.9% sodium chloride solution warmed to 37°C and administered by gravity flow as rapidly as possible; after infusion and in the absence of pain, an additional 1 L of 0.9% sodium chloride solution may be administered to ensure adequate distribution within the peritoneal cavity.

Cisplatin also has been diluted in 2 L of lactated Ringer's injection and administered by gravity flow over 10–12 minutes; after a 15- to 20-minute dwell, the peritoneal cavity was drained as completely as possible. Alternatively, the cisplatin dose has been diluted in 500 mL of 0.9% sodium chloride solution and administered by gravity flow over 15–20 minutes; after 24 hours, paracentesis was begun. There is some evidence that the risk of systemic anaphylactoid reactions may be increased when doses of 100 mg/m² are administered relatively rapidly into the peritoneal cavity; therefore, some clinicians have recommended that intraperitoneal administration of such doses be over 45 minutes or longer.

Various implanted access ports and connecting catheters have been used for intraperitoneal administration of chemotherapeutic agents. The intraperitoneal catheter may be placed at the time of primary (cytoreductive) surgery as long as contamination of the peritoneal cavity has not occurred. Timing of placement of the intraperitoneal catheter (at the time of primary surgery versus delayed insertion) does not appear to affect tolerance of intraperitoneal therapy or treatment completion rates. The intraperitoneal catheter should be removed as soon as intraperitoneal therapy is completed to avoid catheter-related complications. Further study is needed to optimize techniques for intraperitoneal therapy to minimize the risk of complications (e.g., infection, catheter obstruction, catheter retraction, bowel perforation, pain, leakage, port access problems). Specialized sources should be consulted for guidance on how to administer intraperitoneal therapy.

Supportive therapy should include hydration and antiemetic therapy for the intraperitoneal infusion of cisplatin.

● **Dosage**

Dosage of cisplatin must be based on the clinical, renal, hematologic, and otic response and tolerance of the patient in order to obtain optimum therapeutic results with minimum adverse effects. The clinician should consult published protocols for the dosage of cisplatin and other chemotherapeutic agents and the method and sequence of administration. At the usual dosage, courses of cisplatin therapy should not be given more frequently than once every 3–4 weeks. *A repeat course of cisplatin should not be administered until the patient's renal, hematologic, and otic functions are within acceptable limits, and precautions must always be taken to treat an anaphylactoid reaction if it occurs.* (See Cautions: Precautions and Contraindications.)

Inadvertent substitution of cisplatin for carboplatin can result in potentially fatal overdosage. Therefore, care should be taken to ensure that such mix-ups do not occur. In addition, care should be taken to avoid prescribing practices by clinicians that fail to differentiate between daily doses of cisplatin and a total cisplatin dosage used in one course of therapy. To minimize the risk of overdosage, the manufacturer recommends that an alerting mechanism be instituted to verify any prescription or order for cisplatin doses exceeding 100 mg/m² per course. IV dosages exceeding 100 mg/m² per course once every 3–4 weeks are rarely used. Other safeguard procedures to minimize the risk of accidental overdosage of cisplatin (e.g., overdosage resulting from inadvertent administration of the drug when carboplatin was intended) also should be considered.

Because cisplatin is considered an antineoplastic agent of high emetic risk, antiemetic therapy for the prevention of acute and delayed emesis is recommended. (See Emetogenic Effects in Cautions: GI Effects.)

Testicular Cancer

For remission induction in the treatment of metastatic testicular neoplasms, the usual dosage of cisplatin in combination chemotherapy regimens (e.g., with bleomycin and etoposide) is 20 mg/m² IV daily for 5 consecutive days every 3 weeks for 3 or 4 courses of therapy. Randomized trials indicate that 3 cycles of therapy

are sufficient for favorable-prognosis germ cell tumors since similar results are achieved with either 3 or 4 cycles of therapy in such patients. Use of high-dose cisplatin in combination chemotherapy for poor-risk germ cell tumors results in increased toxicity without additional clinical benefit.

Ovarian Cancer

For the treatment of advanced ovarian carcinoma, a cisplatin dosage of 75 mg/m² IV once every 3 weeks has been used in combination therapy with paclitaxel. The usual dosage of cisplatin when used in combination with cyclophosphamide is 50–100 mg/m² IV once every 3–4 weeks. In combination therapy, cisplatin and cyclophosphamide are administered sequentially. When cisplatin is used as a single agent, the manufacturer's recommended dosage is 100 mg/m² IV once every 4 weeks, but some experts recommend dosages of 50–100 mg/m² IV once every 3 weeks, and dosages of 30–120 mg/m² IV once every 3–4 weeks have been used.

Bladder Cancer

For the treatment of advanced bladder cancer, the usual dosage of cisplatin is 50–70 mg/m² IV once every 3–4 weeks, depending on the extent of prior radiation therapy and/or chemotherapy. For patients who have been extensively pretreated, the recommended initial dosage is 50 mg/m² IV once every 4 weeks. For additional information, see Advanced Bladder Carcinoma: Dosage Considerations, under Uses: Bladder Cancer.

Head and Neck Cancer

When used alone in the treatment of recurrent or advanced head and neck cancer†, cisplatin has been given in a dosage of 80–120 mg/m² IV once every 3 weeks or 50 mg/m² IV on the first and eighth days of every 4 weeks. In combination chemotherapy regimens, the usual dose of cisplatin has generally been 50–120 mg/m² IV, with the frequency of administration depending on the specific regimen employed. When used as induction chemotherapy in combination with docetaxel and fluorouracil, cisplatin 75–100 mg/m² has been administered IV once every 3 weeks. (See Head and Neck Cancer under Dosage and Administration: Dosage, in Docetaxel 10:00.)

Cervical Cancer

Invasive Cervical Cancer

For the treatment of invasive cervical cancer† (FIGO stages IB2 through IVA or FIGO stages I through IIA with poor prognostic factors), cisplatin doses of 40–75 mg/m² have been given concurrently with radiation therapy. Weekly or daily infusions of cisplatin have been used concomitantly with radiation therapy in patients with invasive cervical cancer. When used alone for the treatment of invasive cervical cancer, cisplatin 40 mg/m² IV once weekly has been administered concurrently with radiation therapy up to a maximum of 6 doses. When used in combination chemotherapy regimens (e.g., cisplatin and fluorouracil) for the treatment of invasive cervical cancer, cisplatin 50–75 mg/m² has been administered IV concurrently with radiation therapy according to various dosage schedules. Various regimens, doses, and dosage schedules have been used for concurrent cisplatin-based chemotherapy and radiation therapy, and the optimal treatment for locally advanced cervical cancer has not been established.

Metastatic or Recurrent Cervical Cancer

For the treatment of metastatic or recurrent cervical carcinoma†, the usual dosage of cisplatin used alone or in combination therapy is 50 mg/m² IV once every 3 weeks up to a maximum of 6 courses. Higher dosages of cisplatin (e.g., 100 mg/m² IV once every 3 weeks) produce higher response rates in patients with advanced cervical cancer, but duration of response, survival, and progression-free survival are similar to those observed with the usual dosage, and toxicity is greater.

Non-small Cell Lung Cancer

When used in combination chemotherapy for the treatment of non-small cell lung carcinoma†, cisplatin typically has been given in a dosage of 75–100 mg/m² IV once every 3–4 weeks depending on the specific regimen used.

Esophageal Cancer

When used alone in the treatment of advanced esophageal cancer†, cisplatin has been given in a dosage of 50–120 mg/m² IV once every 3–4 weeks. In combination chemotherapy regimens for esophageal cancer, the usual dosage of cisplatin is 75–100 mg/m² IV once every 3–4 weeks.

Biliary Tract Cancer

When cisplatin has been used in combination with gemcitabine for the treatment of unresectable locally advanced or metastatic biliary tract cancer† in adults, including treatment of unresectable recurrent disease following surgical resection, cisplatin 25 mg/m² has been administered by 1-hour IV infusion on days 1 and 8 of each 21-day cycle, and gemcitabine 1 g/m² has been administered by 30-minute IV infusion on days 1 and 8 after cisplatin administration. Treatment has been continued for 24 weeks (8 cycles of therapy) in the absence of disease progression or unacceptable toxicity.

Intra-arterial Dosage

When cisplatin has been administered intra-arterially† for the treatment of regionally confined malignancies, including advanced bladder cancer, metastases from malignant melanoma, and osteogenic sarcomas, a dose of 75–150 mg/m² at intervals ranging from 2–5 weeks for at least 1–4 courses of therapy has been used.

Intraperitoneal Dosage

For the management of intraperitoneal tumors (e.g., advanced ovarian carcinoma, carcinoid, mesothelioma) that are confined to the peritoneal cavity and/or are associated with malignant ascites, cisplatin has been administered intraperitoneally† in doses of 60–100 mg/m².

When combined therapy with intraperitoneal cisplatin and IV and intraperitoneal paclitaxel† has been used for the initial adjuvant treatment of optimally debulked stage III epithelial ovarian cancer, IV paclitaxel 135 mg/m² by 24-hour infusion on day 1, followed by intraperitoneal cisplatin 100 mg/m² on day 2 and intraperitoneal paclitaxel 60 mg/m² on day 8, has been administered every 21 days for up to 6 cycles. Modified IV and intraperitoneal regimens are being investigated. (See Uses: Ovarian Cancer.)

Pediatric Dosage

Pediatric dosage of cisplatin has not been fully established. For the treatment of osteogenic sarcoma† or neuroblastoma†, cisplatin has been given in a dosage of 90 mg/m² IV once every 3 weeks or 30 mg/m² IV once weekly. For the treatment of recurrent brain tumors†, cisplatin has been given in a dosage of 60 mg/m² IV once daily for 2 consecutive days every 3–4 weeks.

• Dosage in Renal Impairment

Cisplatin therapy is contraindicated in patients with preexisting renal impairment. Because cisplatin-induced renal toxicity may become more prolonged and severe with repeated doses of the drug, the manufacturer states that cisplatin therapy should be resumed only when the patient has recovered normal renal function. (See Cautions: Precautions and Contraindications.)

CAUTIONS

Cisplatin is a highly toxic drug, and generally is more poorly tolerated overall compared with carboplatin, another platinum-coordination compound. While the major dose-limiting adverse effects associated with cisplatin therapy include nonhematologic toxicities such as nephrotoxicity, ototoxicity, neurotoxicity, and emesis, the major dose-limiting adverse effects associated with carboplatin therapy are hematologic toxicities such as thrombocytopenia and leukopenia. Differences in the toxicity and pharmacokinetic profiles of the drugs may be important determinants in the selection of cisplatin versus carboplatin for specific patients.

• Renal and Electrolyte Effects

Renal Effects

Nephrotoxicity, which is dose related and can be severe, may occur in patients receiving cisplatin and is more common and severe than that associated with carboplatin. Geriatric patients may be at increased risk for nephrotoxicity associated with cisplatin therapy. (See Cautions: Geriatric Precautions.) When cisplatin formerly was administered without concomitant IV hydration and diuresis, nephrotoxicity was clearly cumulative and was the major dose-limiting adverse effect. Renal toxicity has occurred in 28–36% of patients receiving a single dose of cisplatin 50 mg/m². Renal toxicity is manifested by an increase in serum creatinine, BUN, serum uric acid, and/or a decrease in creatinine clearance and glomerular filtration rate.

Cisplatin-induced renal impairment has been associated with renal tubular damage as evidenced by renal pathologic changes and by increased urinary excretion of β₂-microglobulin and enzymes such as N-acetyl-β-glucosaminidase (NAG), leucine aminopeptidase (LAP), and β-glucuronidase. Focal acute tubular necrosis may occur, with tubular degeneration, interstitial edema and fibrosis, dilation of convoluted tubules, and cast formation. Both proximal and distal tubules are affected, but glomeruli appear intact. While the exact mechanism(s) is not known, renal toxicity may be caused by the positively charged products of cisplatin that are formed in vivo.

If renal toxicity occurs in patients receiving cisplatin, it generally appears during the second week after administration of the drug; with high-dose regimens, it may occur within several days. Renal insufficiency is usually mild to moderate and reversible with usual doses of the drug; however, high or repeated doses can increase the severity and duration of renal impairment and may produce irreversible renal insufficiency (sometimes fatal). The risk and degree of renal impairment may be increased by concomitant use of other nephrotoxic drugs. (See Drug Interactions: Nephrotoxic Drugs.) There is some evidence that cisplatin-induced renal impairment is not age dependent and that nephrotoxic effects may actually be less severe in patients with a single functional kidney.

Regimens of IV hydration, diuresis, and 6- to 8-hour infusions of cisplatin are used to decrease the incidence and severity of nephrotoxicity (see Dosage and Administration: Reconstitution and Administration), possibly by decreasing renal and urinary concentrations of the drug or its platinum-containing product(s). While several regimens have been shown to be very effective in reducing and minimizing renal toxicity, the most effective regimen remains to be established. The value of diuretics in minimizing nephrotoxicity is not clearly defined, and hydration alone may be equally effective. There is some evidence that intensive IV hydration with 0.9% sodium chloride injection and administration of cisplatin in 3% sodium chloride injection may substantially reduce the risk of nephrotoxicity, possibly by providing a chloride concentration that minimizes the formation and renal tubular concentration of nephrotoxic product(s) of the drug. Use of prophylactic amifostine (ethiofos), a phosphorylated sulfhydryl compound, reduces the incidence and severity of cisplatin-induced nephrotoxicity in patients with advanced ovarian cancer. (See Amifostine 92:56.) There is also some evidence that concurrent administration of IV sodium thiosulfate with cisplatin may reduce the risk of nephrotoxicity, but further studies are needed to determine whether the therapeutic efficacy of cisplatin is also affected; although the exact mechanism in preventing nephrotoxicity is not known, sodium thiosulfate may be concentrated in renal tubules, where it could react covalently with cisplatin to form an inactive compound and thereby protect the kidneys.

The effect of the rate of administration of cisplatin on the incidence and severity of nephrotoxicity has not been fully elucidated. While there is some evidence that 6- to 8-hour infusions are less nephrotoxic than rapid IV administration, infusions over 15 minutes to 2 hours are commonly employed and have been used with minimal adverse renal effects. Continuous 24-hour or 5-day IV infusions of the drug have generally not been associated with a reduction in renal toxicity compared with shorter periods of drug administration; while there is some evidence that continuous 5-day IV infusions with IV hydration and diuresis may be employed with minimal adverse renal effects, a relative therapeutic advantage has not been established.

The value of plasma platinum concentrations for predicting or monitoring nephrotoxicity has not been defined, but there is some evidence that patients who eventually develop cisplatin-induced renal toxicity may have elevated plasma platinum concentrations early in the course of 24-hour IV infusions of the drug.

Recovery of renal function generally occurs within 2–4 weeks after administration of cisplatin, but may be delayed or rarely not occur. The long-term effects of the drug on renal function are not fully known. In patients who received cisplatin without concomitant hydration and diuresis, decreases in creatinine clearance have been reported to persist for up to 1–2 years after discontinuance of the drug. While subclinical renal impairment (which may be detected only by measurement of creatinine clearance) may develop and persist even when regimens of hydration and diuresis are employed, the evidence to date suggests that clinically important chronic renal failure or cumulative, delayed nephrotoxicity does not occur following discontinuance of therapy with usual doses of the drug (total cumulative doses of about 300–700 mg/m²) and regimens of hydration and diuresis.

Hypomagnesemia and Other Electrolyte Effects

Cisplatin may cause serious electrolyte disturbances, principally hypomagnesemia, hypocalcemia, and hypokalemia; hypophosphatemia may also occur, and hyponatremia has occurred in some patients receiving cisplatin-containing combination chemotherapy. The disturbances in serum electrolytes have been associated principally with cisplatin-induced renal tubular dysfunction. The drug markedly increases urinary excretion of magnesium and calcium; urinary excretion of potassium, zinc, copper, and amino acids is also increased. Although the exact mechanism(s) is not known, the renal tubular dysfunction caused by cisplatin may result from a specific drug-induced membrane or transport-system defect.

Hypomagnesemia and hypocalcemia may develop during cisplatin therapy or following discontinuance of the drug; although these electrolyte disturbances may occur within several days after an initial dose of the drug, hypomagnesemia usually develops within 3–4 weeks after therapy is initiated and appears to increase in severity with progressive courses of treatment. Children may be particularly susceptible to the development of cisplatin-induced hypomagnesemia. Hypomagnesemia and/or hypocalcemia may become symptomatic, with muscle irritability or cramps, clonus, tremor, carpopedal spasm, and/or tetany. Generally, these manifestations are managed and normal serum electrolyte concentrations may be restored by administration (usually parenteral) of appropriate supplemental electrolytes and discontinuance of the drug; however, hypomagnesemia may persist for several months to years after cisplatin therapy is discontinued and, in some patients, has persisted for longer than 3 years. The long-term effects of the drug on renal tubular dysfunction remain to be fully evaluated. The severity of hypomagnesemia has been associated with an increased risk of subsequently developing Raynaud's phenomenon, but a causal relationship has not been clearly established. (See Cautions: Cardiovascular Effects.)

Methods of preventing cisplatin-induced hypomagnesemia and optimum management of persistent hypomagnesemia have not been fully established. In patients with advanced ovarian cancer, use of prophylactic amifostine reduces the incidence and severity of cisplatin-induced hypomagnesemia. (See Amifostine 92:56.) Although not universally recommended, prophylactic administration of magnesium supplements during cisplatin therapy to patients without renal insufficiency has been suggested. Specific dosage recommendations have not been established, but some clinicians have given 3 g of magnesium sulfate IV during a 6-hour IV infusion of cisplatin in each course of therapy with the drug, or 1 g of magnesium sulfate IV daily for 5 days with each 5-day course of cisplatin when the serum magnesium concentration was less than 1.2 mEq/L. However, some data indicate that hypomagnesemia may develop despite replacement therapy. The value of oral magnesium supplements in the management of asymptomatic cisplatin-induced hypomagnesemia has not been established; chronic oral magnesium supplements do not appear to increase serum magnesium concentrations or hasten the resolution of such hypomagnesemia. It is also uncertain whether continuous administration of oral magnesium supplements is of value in preventing the development of symptomatic hypomagnesemia; however, to minimize the risk of recurrent, symptomatic episodes, adequate magnesium intake is generally recommended in patients who become symptomatic.

● GI Effects

Emetogenic Effects

Cisplatin, one of the most emetogenic antineoplastic agents, induces marked nausea and vomiting in virtually all patients. Because of its universal emetogenic potential, cisplatin is classified as an antineoplastic agent of *high emetic risk* (i.e., incidence of emesis exceeds 90% if no antiemetic agents are administered). In the absence of effective antiemetic therapy, patients develop an average of 10–12 vomiting episodes within the first 24 hours after an initial dose. Although cisplatin-induced nausea and vomiting generally are self-limited and seldom life-threatening, they occasionally are severe enough to require discontinuance of the drug. In addition, of all the adverse effects of cisplatin, patients often are most fearful of the emetogenic effects and may develop anticipatory nausea and vomiting and/or refuse further therapy with the drug.

Nausea and vomiting, which appear to be mediated via local GI stimulation of central mechanisms, generally begin within 1–6 (usually 2–3) hours after administration of cisplatin; this early period of emesis after a dose is the most severe and generally persists for about 8 hours with repeating emetic episodes but may persist up to 24 hours or longer. Various degrees of nausea, vomiting, and anorexia may persist for up to 5–10 days. Delayed nausea and vomiting beginning or persisting 24 hours or longer (although occasionally beginning 16–20 hours) following chemotherapy has occurred in patients who had attained complete emetic control on the day of cisplatin therapy. The incidence and severity of cisplatin-induced nausea and vomiting appear to be increased in females, in young patients, and in patients receiving the drug in high doses, by rapid infusion, and/or in combination with other emetogenic drugs such as anthracyclines (e.g., doxorubicin); patients with a history of chronic heavy alcohol use appear to experience less frequent and severe emetogenic effects.

Mechanism

The role of serotonin as a mediator of acute cisplatin-induced emesis has been strongly suggested by the temporal relationship between the emetogenic action of the drug and the release (e.g., from GI enterochromaffin cells) of serotonin (e.g., as reflected by increases in plasma and urine concentrations of the serotonin metabolite 5-hydroxyindoleacetic acid (5-HIAA)) as well as by the clinical efficacy of antiemetic agents that act as inhibitors of the type 3 (5-HT$_3$) serotonin receptor (e.g., dolasetron, granisetron, ondansetron, palonosetron, tropisetron [not commercially available in the US]). In addition, the severity of emetogenic activity and degree of serotonin release appear to be dose related and increased with repeated cisplatin courses. Studies in animals have shown that cisplatin-induced emesis can be prevented completely by ablation of the area postrema (the locus of the chemoreceptor trigger zone [CTZ]) or depletion of serotonin from this area; in addition, high levels of 5-HT$_3$ receptors have been demonstrated in this area, and direct injection of 5-HT$_3$ receptor antagonists into the area postrema also can prevent cisplatin-induced emesis. Therefore, current evidence suggests that the emetogenic action of cisplatin may be initiated by degenerative changes in the GI tract (e.g., small intestine) induced by the drug and associated increases in endogenous serotonin release; serotonin then stimulates vagal and splanchnic nerve receptors that project to the medullary vomiting (emetic) center of the brain and also appears to stimulate 5-HT$_3$ receptors in the area postrema. Thus, 5-HT$_3$ receptor antagonists appear to prevent or ameliorate acute cisplatin-induced emesis by inhibiting visceral (from the GI tract) afferent stimulation of the vomiting center probably indirectly at the level of the area postrema and by directly inhibiting serotonin activity within the area postrema and CTZ.

Alternative mechanisms appear to be principally responsible for delayed nausea and vomiting induced by cisplatin, since similar temporal relationships between serotonin and emesis beyond the first day after a dose have not been established, and inhibitors of 5-HT$_3$ receptors do not appear to be effective alone in preventing or ameliorating delayed effects. Antagonists at substance P/neurokinin 1 (NK$_1$) receptors represent another class of antiemetic agents. The binding of the tachykinin substance P to NK$_1$ receptors in the GI tract and the brainstem emetic center appears to cause emesis. Substance P/NK$_1$ receptor antagonists, such as aprepitant, block the binding of substance P and therefore prevent acute and delayed emesis. (See Aprepitant 56:22.92.) Anticipatory vomiting is a learned response conditioned by the severity and duration of previous emetic reactions to chemotherapy.

Management

There is some evidence that the incidence and/or severity of nausea and vomiting may be reduced with 5-day continuous IV infusions of cisplatin compared with rapid, intermittent IV administration.

For the prevention of *acute* emesis, the American Society of Clinical Oncology (ASCO) currently recommends a 3-drug antiemetic regimen consisting of a type 3 serotonin receptor antagonist, dexamethasone, and aprepitant given before the administration of cisplatin or other chemotherapy regimens with high emetic risk. (See Aprepitant 56:22.92.) Currently available selective 5-HT$_3$ receptor antagonists (e.g., dolasetron, granisetron, ondansetron, palonosetron, or tropisetron [not commercially available in the US], are comparably effective in preventing acute chemotherapy-induced nausea and vomiting. (For additional information, see the individual monographs for 5-HT$_3$ receptor antagonists in 56:22.20.)

For the prevention of *delayed* emesis, ASCO currently recommends a 2-drug regimen of dexamethasone and aprepitant following the administration of cisplatin or other chemotherapy associated with high emetic risk.

Antiemetic agents with a lower therapeutic index (i.e., less efficacious and generally associated with more frequent adverse effects), including cannabinoids (e.g., dronabinol, nabilone), metoclopramide, butyrophenones, and phenothiazines, are *not* considered by ASCO to be appropriate first-line antiemetics for chemotherapy of high emetic risk; these drugs should be reserved for patients with refractory emesis or unacceptable toxicity from first-line agents. Although antihistamines (e.g., diphenhydramine) and benzodiazepines (e.g., alprazolam, lorazepam) may be useful as adjunctive antiemetic agents, they should *not* be used as monotherapy.

Aggressive antiemetic therapy for the prevention of acute and delayed emesis during early courses of emetogenic chemotherapy is the best way to prevent *anticipatory* nausea and vomiting; behavioral modification and hypnosis also may be useful. Although evidence is lacking, many clinicians also find benzodiazepines useful in the management of anticipatory emesis.

Other GI Effects

Diarrhea also has occurred in patients receiving cisplatin.

● *Otic Effects*

Ototoxicity, manifested as tinnitus, with or without clinical hearing loss, and occasional deafness, may occur in patients receiving cisplatin and may be more severe in children than in adults. Rarely, temporary unilateral otalgia and recruitment have also occurred.

Tinnitus has occurred in about 9% of patients receiving cisplatin and is usually reversible; it is not clear whether tinnitus is dose related. The most common cisplatin-induced hearing changes are audiogram abnormalities, which occur in about 24% of patients receiving usual doses of the drug, but high-frequency loss on audiograms has been reported in up to 74–100% of patients receiving cumulative doses of 200 mg/m² or more. Audiogram abnormalities usually appear within 4 days after administration of the drug, consist of at least a 15-dB loss in pure-tone threshold, and are principally bilateral but can be unilateral. Cisplatin-induced audiogram abnormalities are dose related (increasing with higher single doses and total cumulative dosage) and cumulative; there is also some evidence that audiogram abnormalities may occur more frequently when the drug is administered by rapid IV injection compared with infusion over 1–3 hours or 24 hours. The audiogram abnormalities appear to be most severe in older adults and in children, especially young children. Although not clearly established, patients with preexisting hearing impairment may be more susceptible to cisplatin-induced ototoxicity. The long-term effects have not been fully determined, but the audiogram abnormalities generally appear to be irreversible; however, partial or complete recovery has been reported.

Cisplatin-induced audiogram abnormalities are most common and usually most severe in the high frequency range (4000–8000 Hz); however, audiogram abnormalities may occur at frequencies up to 20,000 Hz, and with increasing cumulative dosage, abnormalities may become evident at lower frequencies (1000–4000 Hz) and result in clinical hearing loss. About 6% of patients receiving the drug have developed clinical hearing loss, manifested as decreased hearing acuity. Although audiogram abnormalities and clinical hearing loss usually develop gradually, rapid-onset clinical hearing loss has occurred rarely. Rarely, deafness after the initial dose of cisplatin has been reported. Clinically important hearing loss may occasionally require dosage reduction or discontinuance of cisplatin therapy.

Although the exact mechanism of cisplatin-induced ototoxicity is not known, the drug has been shown to cause loss of hair cells of the organum spirale in animals and there are limited data to suggest that a similar effect occurs in humans. Electrophysiologic studies have shown the site of principal damage to be the apical stereocilia on the hair cell surface. The possibility that concomitant administration of other potentially ototoxic drugs (e.g., aminoglycosides) may increase the risk of ototoxicity in patients receiving cisplatin should be considered. (See Drug Interactions: Ototoxic Drugs.) In addition, ototoxicity may be enhanced in patients with prior or simultaneous cranial irradiation.

Rarely, cisplatin has been reported to cause vestibular ototoxicity, manifested as vertigo or vestibular dysfunction. Although data are limited, cisplatin-induced vestibular ototoxicity may increase with increasing cumulative dosage and may be most likely to occur in patients with preexisting vestibular dysfunction.

● *Nervous System Effects*

Neurotoxicity produced by cisplatin usually is characterized by peripheral neuropathies, which are generally sensory in nature (e.g., paresthesias of the upper and lower extremities)but can also include motor (especially gait) difficulties; reduced or absent deep-tendon reflexes and leg weakness may also occur. A myasthenic-like syndrome characterized by ptosis and proximal muscle weakness also has been associated with cisplatin. Geriatric patients may be at increased risk for peripheral neuropathy associated with cisplatin therapy. (See Cautions: Geriatric Precautions.) Cisplatin-containing regimens are associated with a higher incidence of, and more severe, neurotoxicity than carboplatin-containing regimens, and neurotoxic effects of cisplatin have become the principal dose-limiting toxicity of the drug subsequent to institution of more effective means of controlling renal and GI toxicities.

Cisplatin-induced peripheral neuropathies occur infrequently with usual doses of the drug and usually only with prolonged therapy (4–7 months) or high cumulative doses; however, neurologic manifestations have been reported after a single dose of the drug, and some evidence suggests that both cumulative-dose intensity and single-dose intensity may be risk factors in the development of neurotoxicity.Manifestations of cisplatin-induced neuropathy usually develop during treatment; rarely, neurologic manifestations may occur 3–8 weeks or longer after the last dose of cisplatin.

The incidence of peripheral neuropathy may be increased when cisplatin is administered concurrently with other potentially neurotoxic agents (e.g., altretamine, paclitaxel, vincristine). Peripheral nerve damage caused by cisplatin has been documented by sensory and motor nerve conduction studies. Sural nerve biopsies from patients with cisplatin-induced paresthesias of the upper and lower extremities and gait disturbances have shown microscopic features consistent with a segmented demyelination pattern of peripheral nerve injury; loss of axons may also be present. In one case of cisplatin neurotoxicity, the spinal cord showed loss of myelinated fibers and gliosis of the dorsal columns at autopsy. Muscle cramps, defined as localized, painful, involuntary skeletal muscle contractions of sudden onset and short duration, have been reported and usually occurred in patients with symptomatic peripheral neuropathy who received relatively high cumulative doses of cisplatin.

Lhermitte's sign (a sensation during neck flexion resembling electric shock) often is present with cisplatin-induced neuropathy. The occurrence of Lhermitte's sign may be particularly likely to coincide with the onset of peripheral neuropathy. Lhermitte's sign has persisted for 2–8 months. As the neuropathy progresses, the sense of joint position also becomes impaired, and severely affected patients may become markedly impaired by sensory ataxia. Temperature and pain sensations remain relatively preserved.

Dorsal column myelopathy and autonomic neuropathy have occurred in some patients receiving cisplatin. Transient partial (focal) or tonic-clonic (grand mal) seizures have also occurred in some patients receiving the drug. Other manifestations of focal neurologic deficits induced by the drug have included cortical blindness and aphasia with seizures or with homonymous hemianopia. Other reported adverse nervous system effects include slurred speech, loss of taste, memory loss, and intention tremor. Postmortem findings of leukoencephalopathy also have been reported.

If manifestations of neuropathy occur, cisplatin therapy should immediately be discontinued; however, neuropathy may worsen even after discontinuance of the drug. Peripheral neuropathy may be irreversible in some patients but has been partially or completely reversible in others following discontinuance of cisplatin therapy.

Management

The role, if any, of neurotrophic peptides (e.g., Org 2766, an analog of corticotropin devoid of glucocorticoid activity) or other drugs on neurotoxic effects of cisplatin remains to be more fully elucidated. There is limited evidence from a study in women receiving cisplatin (75 mg/m² every 3 weeks) and cyclophosphamide (750 mg/m² every 3 weeks) for ovarian cancer that Org 2766 (1 mg/m² administered subcutaneously before and after each cycle of chemotherapy) can prevent or attenuate cisplatin-induced neuropathy, as determined by effects on the threshold value for vibration perception, without apparently affecting the cytotoxic effects of the drugs adversely; fewer neurologic manifestations relative to placebo also were observed in patients receiving Org 2766. However, the drug does not appear to prevent delayed neurotoxic effects several months after discontinuance of cisplatin and Org 2766 therapy; therefore, it has been suggested that continued therapy with this drug may be necessary for up to several months after discontinuance of cisplatin. Although the mechanism of possible neuroprotection by Org 2766 is unclear, the drug is a melanocortin and has been postulated to trigger or facilitate peripheral-nerve repair. Amifostine (ethiofos), a phosphorylated sulfhydryl compound, and glutathione, another sulfhydryl compound, also have exhibited neuroprotective effects. In a randomized study of patients with advanced ovarian cancer, the incidence and severity of cisplatin-induced neurotoxicity appeared to be reduced in patients who received prophylactic amifostine. Additional study and experience are needed to determine the usefulness of potential neuroprotectant compounds in patients receiving cisplatin.

● Hematologic Effects

The hematologic toxicity of cisplatin is usually moderate and reversible and affects all 3 blood lineages. Myelosuppression, which is manifested as leukopenia, thrombocytopenia, and anemia (a decrease in hemoglobin of greater than 2 g/dL), occurs in about 25–30% of patients receiving the drug. Geriatric patients may be at increased risk for myelosuppression associated with cisplatin therapy. (See Cautions: Geriatric Precautions.) Bone marrow suppression associated with cisplatin is less pronounced than that associated with carboplatin.

Cisplatin-induced myelosuppression may be cumulative and may be more severe in patients previously treated with other antineoplastic agents or radiation therapy. Leukopenia and thrombocytopenia are dose related and more pronounced at doses exceeding 50 mg/m². Leukocyte and platelet nadirs generally occur 18–23 days (range: 7.2–45 days) following a single dose of cisplatin, with levels returning to pretreatment values in most patients within 39 days (range: 13–62 days). The incidence and severity of cisplatin-induced anemia are not clearly related to dose. The anemia is usually normochromic and normocytic and generally occurs over the same time course as leukopenia and thrombocytopenia; occasionally, the anemia may be severe, and patients may require transfusions.

The etiology of cisplatin-induced anemia appears to be complex and several mechanisms may be involved. It has been suggested that anemia caused by cisplatin may result from a drug-induced decrease in erythropoietin or erythroid stem cells. There is also some evidence that both hemolysis and decreased erythropoiesis may contribute to the anemia. Rarely, cisplatin has reportedly caused hemolytic anemia; in a few of these cases, positive direct antiglobulin (Coombs') test results were observed, but it is not clear if this effect is immunologically mediated. Positive direct antiglobulin test results can apparently occur without evidence of hemolysis in patients receiving cisplatin.

● Sensitivity Reactions

Anaphylactoid reactions consisting principally of facial edema, flushing, bronchoconstriction, wheezing or respiratory difficulty (e.g., dyspnea), tachycardia, and hypotension have occurred within a few minutes after IV administration of cisplatin in patients who previously received the drug; diaphoresis, nasal stuffiness, rhinorrhea, conjunctivitis, generalized erythema, apprehension, and sensation of chest constriction also may occur. Anaphylactoid reactions also have occurred following intravesical† or intraperitoneal† administration of the drug. Cisplatin-induced anaphylactoid reactions usually have occurred only after multiple cycles (e.g., at least 5 doses) of the drug, but also can occur after the initial dose. The exact mechanism(s) is not known, but the reactions may be immune mediated in some patients. The reactions may be controlled by IV epinephrine, corticosteroids, and/or antihistamines as clinically indicated. Occasionally, patients who experienced anaphylactoid reactions reportedly have been safely retreated with cisplatin following pretreatment with corticosteroids and/or antihistamines; however, such prophylaxis is not uniformly effective in preventing recurrence.

Rarely, urticarial or nonspecific maculopapular rashes, recurrent dermatitis, exfoliative dermatitis, and erythema have been reported in patients receiving cisplatin. In at least one patient, severe exfoliative dermatitis (diffuse erythroderma, desquamation, and eosinophilia) occurred after the second cycle of carboplatin and recurred with subsequent administration of cisplatin despite antihistamine and corticosteroid prophylaxis; with cisplatin, the dermatitis was associated with fever, facial edema, hypotension, tachycardia, and edema and cyanosis of the hands (as well as hypoesthesia and pain consistent with local ischemia).

● Ocular Effects

Optic neuritis (principally retrobulbar), papilledema, and cerebral (cortical) blindness have been reported infrequently in patients receiving recommended dosages of cisplatin. Improvement and/or total recovery usually occur after discontinuance of the drug. Corticosteroids, with or without mannitol, have been used in the management of these adverse ocular effects; however, the efficacy of such treatment has not been established.

● Cardiovascular Effects

Rarely, bradycardia, left bundle-branch block, and ST-T-wave changes with congestive heart failure have been associated with cisplatin therapy. Postural hypotension, which has been attributed to cisplatin-induced neurotoxicity, has also occurred. Hypertension, which persisted for up to 6 months and in some cases required treatment, has occurred following intra-arterial† infusion of the drug.

Rarely, vascular toxicities have been associated with the use of cisplatin-containing combination chemotherapy. The adverse vascular effects are clinically heterogeneous and may include thrombotic microangiopathy, renovascular lesions, severe coronary artery disease, myocardial infarction, cerebrovascular accident, or cerebral arteritis. Various mechanisms have been suggested, including endothelial cell damage. Raynaud's phenomenon has also occurred in patients receiving bleomycin and vinblastine, with or without cisplatin. It has been suggested that cisplatin-induced hypomagnesemia may be an additional, although not essential, factor associated with its occurrence. (See Hypomagnesemia and Other Electrolyte Effects in Cautions: Renal and Electrolyte Effects.) The cause of Raynaud's phenomenon in these cases, however, is not clearly established and may involve the underlying disease or vascular compromise, bleomycin, vinblastine, hypomagnesemia, or some combination of these factors.

● Hepatic Effects

Mild and transient elevations of serum AST (SGOT), ALT (SGPT), and bilirubin concentrations may occur in patients receiving cisplatin. There has been one report of acute, reversible liver toxicity, manifested by transient elevations of serum bilirubin and hepatic enzymes, associated with cisplatin therapy.

● Local Effects

Rarely, local phlebitis has been associated with IV administration of cisplatin. There also have been rare reports of severe cellulitis with residual fibrosis and full-thickness skin necrosis following extravasation of the drug. Severity of local tissue toxicity appears to be related to the concentration of the cisplatin solution. Infusion of solutions with a cisplatin concentration exceeding 0.5 mg/mL may result in tissue cellulitis, fibrosis, and necrosis. Intra-arterial† infusion of cisplatin may result in local pain, edema, and erythema.

● Other Adverse Effects

Hyperuricemia may occur in patients receiving cisplatin, principally as a result of drug-induced nephrotoxicity. Hyperuricemia is more pronounced with doses greater than 50 mg/m², and peak serum concentrations of uric acid generally occur 3–5 days after administration of the drug. Allopurinol has been given to reduce serum uric acid concentrations.

Elevated serum amylase concentrations have been reported infrequently in patients receiving cisplatin. Other adverse effects associated with cisplatin include mild alopecia or thinning of the hair, malaise, asthenia, hiccups, myalgia, pyrexia, and gingival platinum line. Although the exact mechanism(s) has not been determined, gynecomastia has occurred in some males with testicular carcinomas treated with cisplatin-containing combination chemotherapy; a direct causal relationship to cisplatin has not been established. Cisplatin has also been associated with the occurrence of syndrome of inappropriate antidiuretic hormone secretion (SIADH).

● Precautions and Contraindications

Cisplatin is a highly toxic drug with a low therapeutic index, and a therapeutic response is not likely to occur without some evidence of toxicity. The drug must be used only under constant supervision by clinicians experienced in therapy with cytotoxic agents.

Patients receiving cisplatin should be observed closely for possible anaphylactoid reactions, and appropriate equipment for maintenance of an adequate airway and other supportive measures and agents for the treatment of anaphylactoid reactions (e.g., antihistamines, epinephrine, oxygen, corticosteroids) should be readily available whenever cisplatin is administered. The manufacturer states that cisplatin is contraindicated in patients with a history of sensitivity reactions to the drug or other platinum-containing compounds; however, cross-sensitivity is not absolute, and occasionally with appropriate precautions patients sensitive to one platinum-containing compound have tolerated another. Exposure (e.g., industrial) to platinum-containing compounds can cause asthma and immediate and delayed hypersensitivity reactions, and the possibility that patients with a history of such exposure may be cross-sensitive to cisplatin should be considered.

Renal, hematologic, otic, and neurologic function must be frequently and carefully monitored in patients receiving cisplatin; hepatic function should also be monitored periodically. Patients receiving the drug should be adequately hydrated, and serum electrolyte concentrations and fluid requirements carefully monitored; if serum electrolyte and/or fluid disturbances occur, appropriate treatment should be instituted.

Cisplatin therapy is contraindicated in patients with preexisting renal impairment. The manufacturer recommends that serum magnesium, sodium, potassium, calcium, and creatinine concentrations and creatinine clearance and BUN be determined prior to beginning cisplatin therapy and prior to each additional course of therapy. While creatinine clearance appears to most accurately reflect the degree of renal insufficiency produced by the drug, some clinicians suggest that it is usually necessary to repeat measurement of creatinine clearance during cisplatin therapy only when the serum creatinine concentration increases by more than 33% over the baseline value. Since renal toxicity may become more prolonged and severe with repeated doses of cisplatin, the manufacturer states that another cisplatin dose should not be given until serum creatinine concentration is less than 1.5 mg/dL and/or BUN is less than 25 mg/dL. Cisplatin has been used successfully, however, in some patients with obstructive uropathy caused by tumors sensitive to the drug; in some of these patients, renal function improved following treatment with the drug. The drug has also been used successfully in some patients with a single functional kidney.

The manufacturer recommends that peripheral blood cell counts be monitored weekly in patients receiving cisplatin; some clinicians suggest that blood counts can be monitored less frequently (e.g., every 2 weeks). While the hematologic toxicity of the drug is usually moderate and reversible, treatment of severe hematologic toxicity may consist of supportive therapy, anti-infectives for complicating infections, and blood product transfusions. The manufacturer states that a repeat dose of cisplatin should not be administered unless circulating blood elements are at an acceptable level (i.e., leukocyte count of at least 4000/mm³ and platelet count of at least 100,000/mm³). Fever and infection have been reported in patients with neutropenia. In the presence of cisplatin-induced hemolytic anemia, a further course of treatment may be accompanied by increased hemolysis, and the risk should be considered. The manufacturer states that cisplatin is contraindicated in patients with myelosuppression.

Since cisplatin-induced ototoxicity is cumulative, the manufacturer recommends that audiometry be performed prior to initiating cisplatin therapy and prior to each additional course of therapy and that additional doses be withheld until audiometric determinations indicate that auditory acuity is within normal limits. Many clinicians believe that repeat audiograms are of limited value in the routine management of most patients receiving the drug and suggest that repeat audiometry be performed only when auditory symptoms occur or clinical hearing changes become apparent. Clinically important hearing changes may require dosage modification or discontinuance of therapy. The manufacturer states that cisplatin is contraindicated in patients with hearing impairment.

Neurologic examinations should be performed regularly in patients receiving cisplatin, and the manufacturer recommends discontinuing therapy when symptoms of neurotoxicity first appear.

● Pediatric Precautions

Safety and efficacy of cisplatin in children have not been established. The drug has been used in the treatment of osteogenic sarcoma†, neuroblastoma†, and brain tumors† in children, but additional evaluation is needed. Some adverse effects (e.g., ototoxicity) appear to be more severe in children.

● Geriatric Precautions

While the safety and efficacy of cisplatin in geriatric patients have not been established specifically, data from 4 clinical trials involving a total of 1484 patients (29% of whom were older than 65 years of age) receiving cisplatin in combination with cyclophosphamide or paclitaxel for advanced ovarian cancer indicate that a higher incidence and greater severity of certain adverse effects may occur in older patients. Although age was not found to be a prognostic factor for survival in these studies, secondary analysis of data from one of these clinical trials demonstrated shorter survival in older patients compared with younger patients. Data from clinical trials involving the use of cisplatin in the treatment of metastatic testicular cancer or advanced bladder cancer are insufficient to determine whether elderly patients respond to the drug differently than younger patients.

In all 4 clinical trials, severe neutropenia associated with cisplatin-containing chemotherapy occurred more frequently in geriatric patients than in younger patients; higher incidences of severe thrombocytopenia and leukopenia were observed in elderly patients receiving some cisplatin-containing regimens. A numerically higher incidence of peripheral neuropathy was observed in geriatric patients in 2 of the clinical trials, which evaluated nonhematologic toxicity according to age. Other clinical experience suggests that geriatric patients are at increased risk for myelosuppression, infectious complications, and nephrotoxicity associated with cisplatin therapy.

Cisplatin is excreted mainly by the kidney and is contraindicated in patients with preexisting renal impairment. Because geriatric patients may have decreased renal function, careful dosage selection and monitoring of renal function are advised.

● Mutagenicity and Carcinogenicity

In vitro, cisplatin has been shown to be mutagenic in bacteria and has produced chromosomal aberrations in animal cells in tissue culture.

Cisplatin has been shown to be carcinogenic in mice and rats. In studies in BD IX rats receiving intraperitoneal cisplatin at a dosage of 1 mg/kg body weight weekly for 3 weeks, 66% of the animals died within 450 days following the first application of the drug; approximately 40% of the deaths were related to malignancies (i.e., predominantly leukemias and 1 renal fibrosarcoma). Cisplatin-containing combination chemotherapy has been associated with the development of bladder cancer in a patient treated for nonseminomatous testicular carcinoma; however, other drugs and radiation therapy were used in this patient, and a direct causal relationship to cisplatin has not been established. Rarely, acute leukemia (e.g., lymphocytic, myeloid) has developed in patients receiving cisplatin therapy; in such patients, cisplatin generally has been given in combination with other leukemogenic agents and/or radiation.

● Pregnancy, Fertility, and Lactation

Pregnancy

Cisplatin and/or its platinum-containing products appear to cross the placenta. Cisplatin may cause fetal harm when administered to a pregnant woman, but potential benefits from use of the drug may be acceptable in certain conditions despite possible risks to the fetus. Cisplatin has been shown to be teratogenic in mice and embryotoxic in mice and rats. Cisplatin should be used during pregnancy only in life-threatening situations or severe disease for which safer drugs cannot be used or are ineffective. When the drug is administered during pregnancy or if the patient becomes pregnant while receiving the drug, the patient should be informed of the potential hazard to the fetus. Patients should be advised to avoid becoming pregnant during the period in which they are receiving cisplatin therapy.

Fertility

The effects of cisplatin on the gonads and fertility have not been fully determined. Since the drug has produced testicular atrophy in animals and platinum is distributed in high concentration into testes, a risk of adverse testicular effects in humans exists. Although impairment of spermatogenesis is present in many males with testicular carcinomas prior to treatment, most males with these tumors become aspermic during and after treatment with cisplatin-containing combination chemotherapy; however, in some of these males, disease- and drug-induced impairment of spermatogenesis are apparently reversible. In one study in males with disseminated nonseminomatous testicular carcinoma treated with cisplatin, bleomycin, and vinblastine, with or without doxorubicin, 77% were initially oligospermic and 96% became aspermic within 2 months after initiation of therapy; however, there appears to be a high degree of reversibility as evidenced by a return of spermatogenesis with normal sperm counts 2–3 years after initiation of therapy. In addition, some of the males with recovery of spermatogenesis successfully impregnated their wives, resulting in 5 normal births, 3 ongoing pregnancies at the time of the study, and 1 spontaneous abortion. While recovery of spermatogenesis may occur, abnormal sperm may be present.

Lactation

Cisplatin is distributed into milk. Because of the potential for serious adverse reactions to cisplatin in nursing infants, nursing should not be undertaken by women receiving the drug.

DRUG INTERACTIONS

● Nephrotoxic Drugs

Cisplatin produces cumulative nephrotoxicity that is potentiated by aminoglycoside antibiotics. Concurrent administration of the drugs or administration of an aminoglycoside within 1–2 weeks after cisplatin therapy has been associated with an increased risk of nephrotoxicity and acute renal failure (sometimes severe). Aminoglycosides should be used with extreme caution, if at all, during or shortly after cisplatin therapy. Some clinicians suggest that the risk of this drug interaction may be reduced if the aminoglycoside is administered at least 2 weeks after cisplatin. Concomitant use of other potentially nephrotoxic drugs (e.g., amphotericin B) should probably also be avoided during cisplatin therapy.

● Ototoxic Drugs

Patients receiving cisplatin and other potentially ototoxic drugs such as aminoglycoside antibiotics or loop diuretics (e.g., ethacrynic acid, furosemide) concomitantly should be carefully monitored for signs of ototoxicity. A study in guinea pigs has shown that cisplatin and ethacrynic acid potentiate the ototoxic effects of each other.

● Antineoplastic Agents

Studies in animals and clinical trials in humans indicate that the antineoplastic activity of cisplatin and etoposide may be synergistic against some tumors. In mice implanted with P388 or L1210 leukemia or B16 melanoma, a combination of cisplatin and etoposide was shown to act synergistically in reducing the body burden of tumor cells and/or increasing survival. Response rates in humans receiving combination chemotherapy with cisplatin and etoposide suggest that the combination has synergistic antineoplastic activity against testicular carcinomas, small cell carcinoma of the lung, or non-small cell carcinoma of the lung. Studies in animals also indicate that the antineoplastic activity of cisplatin and some other antineoplastic agents (e.g., bleomycin, doxorubicin, fluorouracil, methotrexate, vinblastine, vincristine) is potentially synergistic.

Limited data indicate that elimination of etoposide may be impaired in patients previously treated with cisplatin. In a randomized trial in patients with advanced ovarian cancer, response duration was adversely affected when pyroxidine was used in combination with altretamine (hexamethylmelamine) and cisplatin.

● Renally Excreted Drugs

Limited data suggest that cisplatin may alter the renal elimination of bleomycin and methotrexate, possibly as a result of cisplatin-induced nephrotoxicity. Although further documentation is needed, the possibility that cisplatin may affect the elimination of renally excreted drugs should be considered.

● Phenytoin

In patients receiving cisplatin and phenytoin, serum concentrations of phenytoin may be decreased, possibly as a result of decreased absorption and/or increased metabolism of phenytoin. In patients receiving cisplatin therapy, serum concentrations of phenytoin should be monitored and dosage adjustments made as necessary.

ACUTE TOXICITY

● Manifestations

Overdosage of cisplatin may be fatal. In some cases, cisplatin overdosage resulted from inadvertent substitution of the drug for carboplatin; the latter drug is substantially less toxic than cisplatin and generally is administered at much higher dosages. Caution should be exercised to avoid inadvertent overdosage with cisplatin. (See Dosage and Administration: Dosage.)

Acute overdosage with cisplatin may result in acute renal failure, ototoxicity that can progress to irreversible deafness, severe myelosuppression, intractable nausea and vomiting, and neuritis. Less commonly, hepatotoxicity (e.g., hepatic failure manifested as increased serum transaminase concentrations and elevations in clotting times, prothrombin time, and partial thromboplastin time), central neurotoxicity (e.g., manifested as generalized seizures and hallucinations), and ocular toxicity (e.g., manifested as visual changes such as blurring and altered color perception that are attributable to retinal damage, including retinal detachment) can occur. Other manifestations of neurotoxicity have included dysarthria, paresthesias, and impaired taste perception. Myelosuppression, nephrotoxicity, ocular toxicity, and neuropathy may be partially or totally reversible. However, ototoxicity (e.g., bilateral sensorineural hearing loss) often is irreversible and, in patients whose overdosage was not accompanied by IV hydration (e.g., when cisplatin inadvertently was given instead of carboplatin), renal failure also may be irreversible.

● Treatment

Although there currently is no established antidote for cisplatin overdosage, nucleophilic (reducing) sulfhydryl (thiol) compounds (e.g., glutathione, acetylcysteine, mesna) can inactivate cisplatin and act as chemoprotectants (e.g., protecting against nephrotoxicity). However, the potential benefits of such therapy in the management of cisplatin overdosage remain to be established, and many of these compounds

would be of limited, if any, benefit if administration were delayed for several hours after cisplatin administration since most platinum would be protein bound and not in its reactive form. Theoretically offering potentially greater usefulness would be dithiocarbamates (e.g., dithiocarb [diethyldithiocarbamate, DDTC], amifostine [ethiofos]) since the drugs can react with platinum even after protein binding has occurred and can stimulate substantial biliary excretion of the metal. *Since most experience to date with the effects of various chemoprotectants on cisplatin toxicity has been in animal or in vitro studies or in preliminary studies in humans, the role, if any, of these agents in treating cisplatin toxicity remains to be elucidated. The role, if any, of neurotrophic peptides (e.g., Org 2766, an analog of corticotropin devoid of glucocorticoid activity) on neurotoxic effects of cisplatin also remains to be elucidated.*

Management of cisplatin overdosage currently consists principally of discontinuance of the drug and general supportive measures to sustain the patient throughout any period of toxicity that may occur. Hemodialysis, even when initiated within 4 hours following overdosage of cisplatin, appears to have little effect on removing platinum from the body because of cisplatin's rapid and high degree of protein binding. However, limited evidence suggests that aggressive plasmapheresis may be useful in removing protein-bound platinum and thus ameliorating toxicity. Antiemetics that are recommended for the prevention of acute or delayed emesis associated with cisplatin (type 3 serotonin receptor antagonists, dexamethasone and aprepitant) may be useful for managing acute intractable nausea and vomiting. Hematopoietic agents (e.g., sargramostim [GM-CSF]) may be useful in managing myelosuppression, and hemodialysis may be required for the management of renal failure.

PHARMACOLOGY

The exact mechanism(s) of action of cisplatin has not been conclusively determined, but the drug has biochemical properties similar to those of bifunctional alkylating agents. Platinum-containing antineoplastic agents appear to exert their effects by binding to DNA, thereby inhibiting DNA synthesis. Cisplatin is cycle-phase nonspecific. Although the principal mechanism of action of cisplatin appears to be inhibition of DNA synthesis, other mechanisms, possibly including enhancement of tumor immunogenicity, are involved in its antineoplastic activity.

Neutrality of charge and the *cis* configuration are necessary for the cisplatin complex to exert antineoplastic activity. In the relatively high chloride concentration of plasma, the cisplatin complex is believed to be un-ionized, allowing passage of the drug through cell membranes. Intracellularly, in the presence of a low chloride concentration, the chloride ligands of the complex are displaced by water (aquation), resulting in formation of positively charged platinum complexes that are toxic and react with the nucleophilic sites on DNA. Cisplatin binds to DNA and inhibits DNA synthesis; protein and RNA synthesis also are inhibited but less extensively. The drug produces predominately DNA intrastrand and interstrand cross-links, with intrastrand cross-links resulting from the formation of adducts between activated platinum complexes of the drug and areas of specific base sequences; DNA-protein cross-links also are formed. The relative importance of intrastrand or interstrand DNA cross-links in the antineoplastic activity of cisplatin remains to be clearly determined; however, interstrand cross-linking appears to correlate well with the cytotoxicity of the drug. Interstrand cross-linking within the DNA helix also occurs. The resultant interstrand and intrastrand cross-links are stable bonds that do not dissociate easily. While the mechanism through which DNA adducts exert their cytotoxic effects has not been determined, limited evidence indicates that platinum adducts may inhibit DNA replication, transcription, and ultimately cell division.

Cisplatin also has immunosuppressive, radiosensitizing, and antimicrobial properties.

Further study is needed to elucidate more fully the extent of cross-resistance between cisplatin and carboplatin. Although some cisplatin-refractory tumors may respond to carboplatin, a high degree of cross-resistance appears to occur between the drugs. The mechanisms of cellular resistance to platinum-containing antineoplastic agents have not been fully elucidated, but resistance can be related to decreased cellular uptake of the drug or enhanced DNA repair and may be related to elevated cellular levels of sulfhydryl (thiol) compounds including glutathione or metallothionein. Glutathione appears to play an essential role in protecting cells from the effects of certain toxins including certain antineoplastic agents, and increased levels of this sulfhydryl compound have been demonstrated in certain cell lines resistant to cisplatin and other analogs. Increased repair of platinum complex-induced DNA adducts also has been demonstrated in certain resistant cell lines. The relative roles of these mechanisms of resistance and their relationship to treatment failure in patients who do not respond to platinum-containing antineoplastic agents have not been fully determined.

PHARMACOKINETICS

The pharmacokinetics of cisplatin are complex and have been studied principally by using assays for elemental platinum or by using preparations of the drug containing radioactive platinum; only a few studies have used analytical methods capable of measuring intact cisplatin. Published studies on the pharmacokinetics of cisplatin have varied widely in the doses administered, the rate of administration, the use of IV hydration, and the concurrent use of diuretics; the effects of these factors, if any, on the pharmacokinetics of the drug and their clinical importance remain to be fully elucidated. The chemical identities of platinum-containing products of cisplatin that are formed in vivo have not been definitely determined. In addition, relationships between therapeutic activity or toxicity and plasma concentrations of cisplatin or platinum have not been clearly established; however, results of in vitro studies have suggested that only nonprotein-bound cisplatin or its platinum-containing products are cytotoxic.

● Absorption

Following rapid IV injection of cisplatin over 1–5 minutes or rapid IV infusion over 15 minutes or 1 hour, peak plasma drug and platinum concentrations occur immediately. Following rapid IV injection of a 50-mg/m² dose of cisplatin over 3–5 minutes to patients with normal renal function in one study, peak plasma concentrations of intact cisplatin, total platinum, and nonprotein-bound platinum averaged 2.3, 4.7, and 2.7 mcg/mL, respectively; after a 100-mg/m² dose, peak plasma concentrations averaged 3.3, 6.2, and 4.5 mcg/mL, respectively. Following rapid IV infusion of a 100-mg/m² dose of the drug over 15 minutes to patients with normal renal function in another study, peak plasma concentrations of nonprotein-bound platinum averaged 2.73 mcg/mL. Following 1-hour IV infusions of 50 and 70 mg/m² to patients with normal renal function, peak plasma total platinum concentrations of 2.26–2.45 and 4.25–7.02 mcg/mL, respectively, have been reported.

When cisplatin is administered by IV infusion over 6 or 24 hours, plasma concentrations of total platinum increase gradually during the infusion and peak immediately following the end of the infusion. Following 6-hour IV infusions of 100 mg/m² to patients with normal renal function, peak plasma total and nonprotein-bound platinum concentrations ranging from 2.5–5.3 and 0.22–0.73 mcg/mL, respectively, have been reported. Following a 24-hour IV infusion of 80 mg/m² in one study, peak plasma total platinum concentrations ranged from 1.03–1.90 mcg/mL. When equal doses of cisplatin are administered by rapid IV infusion or infusion over 2–3 or 24 hours in patients with normal renal and hepatic function, the areas under the plasma nonprotein-bound platinum concentration-time curves (AUCs) appear to be equivalent.

Concomitant IV administration of cisplatin and mannitol appeared to increase peak plasma concentrations of nonprotein-bound platinum in one study, but in another study mannitol appeared to have no effect on plasma concentrations of intact cisplatin, total platinum, or nonprotein-bound platinum. In one study comparing the effects of IV furosemide or mannitol on the pharmacokinetics of cisplatin, plasma concentrations of total platinum and nonprotein-bound platinum were similar following administration of either diuretic.

Following intra-arterial† infusion of cisplatin, local tumor exposure to the drug is increased compared with IV administration as evidenced by increased plasma platinum concentrations in local veins draining the infused region compared with systemic veins and by increased AUCs calculated for local versus systemic exposure. Following local infusion, systemic plasma platinum concentrations are similar to those attained following IV administration of comparable doses of the drug. Local venous plasma platinum concentrations are reportedly lower following infusion of cisplatin into the hepatic artery compared with other arteries (e.g., brachial, femoral), suggesting that the drug is highly extracted by the liver.

Cisplatin is rapidly and well absorbed systemically following intraperitoneal administration†, resulting in 50–100% of the degree of systemic exposure compared with IV administration when comparable doses are given; however, peak intraperitoneal fluid concentrations of nonprotein-bound platinum are greatly increased, and intraperitoneal exposure to nonprotein-bound platinum is increased by about 15- to 30-fold compared with IV administration.

● Distribution

Following IV administration of cisplatin, platinum is widely distributed into body fluids and tissues, with highest concentrations in the kidneys, liver, and prostate. Lower concentrations are found in the bladder, muscle, testes,pancreas, and spleen; platinum is also distributed into the small and large intestines, adrenals, heart, lungs, lymph nodes, thyroid, gallbladder, thymus, cerebrum, cerebellum, ovaries, and uterus. Platinum appears to accumulate in body tissues following administration of cisplatin and has been detected in many of these tissues for up to 6 months after the last dose of the drug. Platinum is also distributed minimally into leukocytes and erythrocytes.

The volume of distribution of platinum in adults following IV administration of cisplatin has been reported to range from 20–80 L and averaged 41 L/m² in one study. Platinum is rapidly distributed into pleural effusions and ascitic fluid following IV administration of cisplatin. The manufacturer states that small amounts of platinum have been detected in the bile and large intestine following administration of cisplatin, but fecal excretion of platinum appears to be insignificant. Cisplatin is distributed into milk, and limited evidence indicates that the drug and/or its platinum-containing products cross the placenta.

Although there is some evidence to the contrary, cisplatin and/or its platinum-containing products apparently do not readily penetrate the CNS. Following IV administration of cisplatin, platinum is distributed into intracerebral tumor tissue and edematous brain tissue adjacent to tumor; however, only low concentrations of platinum have been detected in healthy brain tissue. In one study in patients with brain tumors, platinum was barely or not detectable in CSF following IV administration of cisplatin, but, in other reports, platinum was detected in the CSF of patients with or without brain tumors following IV administration of the drug. When platinum has been detected in CSF, peak CSF platinum concentrations occurred within 30–60 minutes after IV administration of cisplatin and CSF platinum concentrations ranged from less than 5% to up to 100% of concurrent plasma concentrations.

Cisplatin does not undergo the instantaneous and reversible binding to plasma proteins that is characteristic of typical drug-protein binding. The platinum from cisplatin, but not cisplatin itself, is rapidly and extensively bound to tissue and plasma proteins, including albumin, γ-globulins, and transferrin. Binding to tissue and plasma proteins appears to be essentially irreversible.Protein binding increases with time, and less than 2–10% of platinum in blood remains unbound several hours after IV administration of cisplatin.

● Elimination

Following rapid IV injection or infusion of cisplatin, plasma concentrations of intact cisplatin, total platinum, and nonprotein-bound platinum have generally been reported to decline in a monophasic, biphasic, and biphasic manner, respectively; however, some reports indicate that plasma concentrations of nonprotein-bound platinum decline in a monophasic manner and that plasma concentrations of total platinum may exhibit triphasic or quadraphasic elimination with a prolonged terminal phase. In adults with normal renal function, the following plasma elimination half-lives have been reported after rapid IV injection or infusion of cisplatin: intact cisplatin, about 20–30 minutes; total platinum, 8.1–49 minutes in the initial phase and 30.5–107 hours or possibly longer in the terminal phase; and nonprotein-bound platinum, 2.7–30 minutes in the initial phase and 32–53.5 minutes in the terminal phase. Concomitant administration of IV mannitol does not alter the terminal plasma half-life of nonprotein-bound platinum. Following 6-hour IV infusions of cisplatin in patients with normal renal function, a terminal plasma elimination half-life for total platinum of 73–290 hours has been reported. Some data suggest that the rate of elimination of total plasma platinum in patients with normal renal function may decrease with time. In one patient with acute oliguric renal failure requiring hemodialysis, the terminal plasma half-life of total platinum was approximately 10 days.

In children with normal renal function, the serum elimination half-lives of total platinum reportedly average about 25 minutes in the initial phase and 44 hours in the terminal phase, and the serum elimination half-life of nonprotein-bound platinum averages 1.3 hours.

Following IV administration of cisplatin, the elimination half-lives of total platinum from CSF and pleural effusion fluid are reportedly about 0.75–1.5 hours and 22 days, respectively. Following IV administration of the drug, a mean elimination half-life of total platinum from erythrocytes of about 30 hours has been reported, suggesting that cisplatin may increase the breakdown of erythrocytes. Following intraperitoneal administration of cisplatin, the peritoneal elimination half-lives of total platinum and nonprotein-bound platinum are about 33 hours and 1 hour, respectively.

The metabolic fate of cisplatin has not been completely elucidated. There is no evidence to date that the drug undergoes enzymatic biotransformation; the chloride ligands of the cisplatin complex are believed to be displaced by water, forming positively charged platinum complexes that react with nucleophilic sites. The chemical identities of platinum-containing products of the drug that are formed in vivo have not been definitely determined. Intact cisplatin and its platinum-containing product(s) are excreted principally in urine; fecal elimination of platinum appears to be insignificant. The presence of a secondary peak in plasma platinum concentration during the principal elimination phase of platinum has been reported, suggesting that cisplatin or its platinum-containing products may undergo enterohepatic circulation.

Renal excretion appears to occur predominantly via glomerular filtration, but there is some evidence that secretion and possibly reabsorption of cisplatin or a platinum-containing product(s) also occurs. Following a 6-hour IV infusion of the drug, the renal clearance of total platinum decreases substantially to a relatively low, constant value about 6–12 hours after the end of the infusion; this appears to be consistent with a relatively high, initial renal clearance of intact cisplatin and nonprotein-bound platinum, followed by clearance of nonprotein-bound platinum-containing product(s). The urinary excretion of 2 platinum-containing compounds has been partially characterized. The first, a water-elutable compound believed to be intact cisplatin, represents most of the platinum initially excreted in urine but rapidly decreases to represent a very small fraction of excreted platinum. The second, a hydrochloric acid-elutable compound believed to be a positively charged complex formed by replacement of one of cisplatin's chloride ligands with water, initially represents a small fraction of platinum excreted in urine but rapidly increases to represent a large fraction of urinary platinum. A third, unidentified platinum-containing compound also appears to be excreted in urine.

Following rapid IV injection or infusion of cisplatin in patients with normal renal function, approximately 15–50% of a dose is excreted in urine within 24–48 hours; most urinary excretion occurs within the first 4–6 hours following administration of the drug, apparently principally as intact cisplatin. Following IV infusion of the drug over 6 hours in patients with normal renal function, 24-hour urinary excretion has generally ranged from about 10–35% of a dose; however, in some reports as much as 65–80% of the dose administered was excreted within 24 hours. Concomitant IV administration of mannitol and a 15-minute or 6-hour IV infusion of cisplatin reportedly results in substantially decreased 24-hour urinary excretion of platinum. An average of 14% of the administered dose was excreted in urine within 24 hours in one study when cisplatin was given as a 24-hour IV infusion to patients with normal renal function. There is some evidence that the circadian timing of cisplatin administration has a pronounced effect on urinary platinum excretion, with evening administration of the drug resulting in greater urine output and lower peak urinary platinum concentrations than morning administration.

The effects of renal impairment on the elimination of cisplatin and its platinum-containing products have not been fully evaluated; individuals with decreased renal function may have impaired elimination. There is also some evidence that patients with impaired renal function may have elevated plasma concentrations of nonprotein-bound platinum.

Limited data indicate that cisplatin and/or its platinum-containing products are minimally removed by hemodialysis. In one patient, 4- to 5.5-hour periods of hemodialysis removed into the dialysate about 8% of individual doses of cisplatin given by IV infusion over 0.75–1.5 hours immediately prior to dialysis; about 3% of a dose was removed into the dialysate per period during periods of hemodialysis 24 and 48 hours after the first period.

CHEMISTRY AND STABILITY

● Chemistry

Cisplatin is a platinum-containing antineoplastic agent. The drug is an inorganic complex that contains a platinum atom surrounded in a plane by 2 chloride atoms and 2 ammonia molecules in the *cis* position. Cisplatin occurs as a yellow to orange crystalline powder and has a solubility of 1 mg/mL in water or in 0.9% sodium chloride solution.

Commercially available cisplatin injection is a clear, colorless solution and contains hydrochloric acid and/or sodium hydroxide to adjust pH and sodium chloride. The commercially available injection has a pH of 3.7–6, an osmolality of about 285–286 mOsm/kg, and contains a sodium chloride concentration of 0.9%.

Cisplatin powder for injection (no longer commercially available in the US; see Preparations) occurs as a white, lyophilized powder and contains sodium chloride and mannitol, and hydrochloric acid to adjust pH. Following reconstitution of the powder for injection with sterile water for injection as recommended (see Dosage and Administration: Reconstitution and Administration), solutions containing 1 mg of cisplatin per mL are clear and colorless and have a pH of 3.5–5.5 and sodium chloride and mannitol concentrations of 0.9 and 1%, respectively.

● Stability

Commercially available cisplatin injection should be protected from light. The injection should be stored at 15–25°C and refrigeration avoided (since precipitation of the drug may occur); however, if cisplatin injection is inadvertently refrigerated, the precipitate will dissolve at room temperature, without loss of potency. If freezing occurs, cisplatin injection may be thawed at room temperature until precipitate dissolves; the manufacturer states that the chemical or physical stability of the injection is not affected. When stored under recommended conditions, commercially available cisplatin injection is stable for 17 months following the date of manufacture; cisplatin injection remaining in the amber vial following initial entry is stable for 28 days when protected from light or for 7 days when stored under fluorescent room light. Cisplatin powder for injection should be stored at room temperature. Unopened vials of the powder for injection are stable for 2 years at room temperature (27°C).

The manufacturer states that, when reconstituted as directed from cisplatin powder for injection, cisplatin solutions are stable for 20 hours when stored at 27°C. Following reconstitution of the powder for injection with bacteriostatic water for injection containing benzyl alcohol or parabens, cisplatin solutions containing 1 mg/mL are reportedly stable for at least 72 hours at 25°C. Reconstituted solutions of cisplatin removed from the amber vial should be protected from light if they are not to be used within 6 hours. Reconstituted solutions of cisplatin should be stored at room temperature and should *not* be refrigerated, since precipitation may occur; a precipitate reportedly forms within 1 hour when solutions containing 1 mg of cisplatin per mL of 0.9% sodium chloride injection are refrigerated (2–6°C). Redissolution of the precipitate may occur very slowly when the solution is warmed to room temperature, but such warming to effect redissolution is not recommended and cisplatin solutions containing a precipitate should be discarded.

In aqueous solutions or solutions containing less than 0.2% sodium chloride, cisplatin is decomposed with displacement of chloride ions by water. Increasing the chloride concentration in the solvent up to 0.9% improves the stability of cisplatin in solution. The stability of cisplatin in various IV solutions and admixtures is reported as follows:

IV Solution	Cisplatin Concentration (mg/mL)	Duration of Stability (time and temperature)
5% Dextrose and 0.45 or 0.9% Sodium Chloride	0.05, 0.5	at least 24 h at room temperature
5% Dextrose and 0.33% Sodium Chloride with 1.875% Mannitol (with or without 0.15% Potassium Chloride)	0.05, 0.1, 0.2	at least 72 h at 4 or 25°C
5% Dextrose and 0.45% Sodium Chloride with 1.875% Mannitol	0.05, 0.1, 0.2	at least 72 h at 4 or 25°C
0.2% Sodium Chloride	0.2	at least 24 h at room temperature
0.225% Sodium Chloride	0.05, 0.1, 0.2	at least 72 h at 4 or 25°C
0.3% Sodium Chloride	0.05, 0.1, 0.2	at least 72 h at 4 or 25°C
0.45% Sodium Chloride	0.2	at least 24 h at room temperature
	0.05, 0.5	at least 24 h at 25°C
0.9% Sodium Chloride	0.2	at least 24 h at room temperature
	0.05, 0.5	at least 24 h at 25°C

The stability of cisplatin in solution is reportedly not adversely affected by the presence of up to 5% mannitol; however, cisplatin-mannitol complexes may form after several days, and advanced preparation and storage of such admixtures should be avoided. Cisplatin solutions should generally not be diluted in sodium bicarbonate or other alkaline solutions because of enhanced decomposition of cisplatin; formation of a bright gold precipitate has occurred after admixture of 5% sodium bicarbonate and a cisplatin solution. Cisplatin may react covalently with sodium thiosulfate to form a pharmacologically inactive compound and may also react with sodium bisulfite. Specialized references should be consulted for specific stability and compatibility information.

Aluminum displaces platinum from the cisplatin molecule, causing the formation of a black precipitate and loss of potency. Cisplatin solutions should not be prepared or administered with needles or IV administration sets containing aluminum parts that might come in contact with the drug. Stainless steel needles and plated brass hubs do not react with cisplatin within 24 hours.

For further information on the handling of antineoplastic agents, see the ASHP Guidelines on Handling Hazardous Drugs at http://www.ahfsdrug information.com.

PREPARATIONS

Excipients in commercially available drug preparations may have clinically important effects in some individuals; consult specific product labeling for details.

CISplatin

Parenteral

Injection, for IV infusion	1 mg/mL (50 or 100 mg)*	**Cisplatin Injection**
		Platinol®-AQ, Bristol-Myers Squibb

* available from one or more manufacturer, distributor, and/or repackager by generic (nonproprietary) name

† Use is not currently included in the labeling approved by the US Food and Drug Administration.

Selected Revisions August 10, 2017, © Copyright, April 1, 1984, American Society of Health-System Pharmacists, Inc.

Cobimetinib Fumarate

10:00 · ANTINEOPLASTIC AGENTS

■ Cobimetinib, a potent, selective, and reversible inhibitor of mitogen-activated extracellular signal-regulated kinase (MEK) 1 and MEK2, is an antineoplastic agent.

USES

● Melanoma

Cobimetinib is used in combination with vemurafenib for the treatment of adult patients with unresectable or metastatic melanoma with b-Raf serine-threonine kinase (BRAF) V600E or V600K mutation. Cobimetinib has been designated an orphan drug by FDA for the treatment of this cancer. An FDA-approved diagnostic test (e.g., cobas® 4800 BRAF V600 mutation test) is required to confirm the presence of the BRAF V600E or V600K mutation prior to initiation of therapy.

Clinical Experience

The current indication for cobimetinib is based principally on the results of a randomized, double-blind, placebo-controlled phase 3 study (coBRIM) in patients with previously untreated, unresectable or metastatic melanoma with BRAF V600E or V600K mutation as detected by the cobas® 4800 BRAF V600 mutation test. In this study, 495 patients were randomized (stratified by disease stage and geographic region) in a 1:1 ratio to receive either cobimetinib (60 mg once daily for 21 days followed by a 7-day rest period) in combination with vemurafenib (960 mg twice daily) or placebo in combination with vemurafenib (960 mg twice daily). Treatment was continued until disease progression or unacceptable toxicity occurred or the patient withdrew from the study. Patients randomized to receive placebo were not permitted to cross over to open-label cobimetinib therapy upon disease progression. The primary end point of this study was progression-free survival as assessed by the investigator according to Response Evaluation Criteria in Solid Tumors (RECIST).

The median age of patients enrolled in the study was 55 years; 93% of patients were white, 60% had stage M1c disease, 72% had a baseline ECOG performance status of 0, 45% had elevated LDH concentrations, 10% had previously received adjuvant therapy, and less than 1% of patients had previously received therapy for brain metastases. Most patients (86% of those with known mutation status) had BRAF V600E mutations.

At initial analysis at a median follow-up of 7.3 months, the median duration of progression-free survival was 6.2 or 9.9 months for placebo and vemurafenib or vemurafenib and cobimetinib. Objective response rates (complete or partial) were higher with cobimetinib and vemurafenib compared to placebo and vemurafenib (68 versus 45%). Median overall survival had not been reached at the time of the analysis.

In a long-term extension of coBRIM, patients were followed for a median duration of 21.2 or 16.6 months for cobimetinib and vemurafenib or placebo and vemurafenib, respectively. Median progression-free survival was 12.3 months for patients receiving cobimetinib and vemurafenib compared with 7.2 months for those receiving placebo and vemurafenib. A progression-free survival benefit for cobimetinib and vemurafenib was confirmed by independent blinded review. In addition, patients receiving cobimetinib and vemurafenib had higher objective response rates (70 versus 50%) compared with those receiving placebo and vemurafenib. The median duration of response for patients receiving cobimetinib and vemurafenib or receiving placebo and vemurafenib was 13 or 9.2 months, respectively. Median overall survival was 22.3 or 17.4 months, respectively, for cobimetinib and vemurafenib compared with placebo and vemurafenib.

Use of cobimetinib in combination with vemurafenib also was investigated in a phase 1b, open-label study (BRIM7) in 129 patients with unresectable stage IIIc or IV advanced melanoma with BRAF V600 mutation. Patients enrolled in the study were either BRAF inhibitor therapy naïve (BRAF inhibitor-naïve) or had experienced disease progression during prior vemurafenib monotherapy. Patients received cobimetinib with vemurafenib, both given in a dose-escalating regimen.

Initial analysis reported a median progression-free survival of 2.8 months for patients who had progressed on vemurafenib, compared to 13.7 months for BRAF inhibitor naïve patients. Response rates were also higher among BRAF inhibitor naïve patients, with 88% achieving a complete (10%) or partial (78%) response. For patients who had progressed on prior vemurafenib monotherapy, none achieved a complete response and 15% had a partial response; the remainder had stable (42%) or progressive (36%) disease. At a later analysis, with a median follow-up of 28 or 8.4 months for BRAF inhibitor naïve or vemurafenib-experienced patients, respectively, progression-free survival rates were similar, with a median of 13.8 or 2.8 months. Median overall survival was 31.8 or 8.5 months for BRAF inhibitor naïve patients or vemurafenib-experienced patients, respectively. At 5 years, the overall survival rate was 39.2%, similar to the 3 and 4 year rates (41.5 and 39.2%, respectively), for BRAF inhibitor naïve patients. Among patients who had progressed on prior vemurafenib monotherapy, the 3, 4, and 5 year survival rates were the same for each year, at 14%.

Clinical Perspective

The 2023 American Society for Clinical Oncology (ASCO) guideline on systemic therapy for unresectable and/or metastatic cutaneous melanoma with BRAF mutant (V600) recommends one of the following as first-line therapy: programmed cell death protein (PD-1) inhibitors (nivolumab plus ipilimumab followed by nivolumab; or nivolumab plus relatlimab; or nivolumab); or combination BRAF/MEK inhibitor therapy (dabrafenib plus trametinib; or encorafenib plus binimetinib; or vemurafenib plus cobimetinib). Per the ASCO guidelines, nivolumab plus ipilimumab is preferred as first-line therapy for patients with unresectable and/or metastatic BRAF mutant (V600) disease over BRAF/MEK inhibitor combination therapy.

For patients with BRAF mutation-positive (V600) unresectable/metastatic cutaneous melanoma who progress on first-line PD-1 inhibitor therapy, combination BRAF/MEK inhibitor therapy may be offered. Patients with BRAF mutation-positive (V600) unresectable/metastatic cutaneous melanoma who had disease progression following combination BRAF/MEK inhibitor therapy may be offered PD-1 inhibitor therapy.

● Histiocytic Neoplasms

Cobimetinib is used as a single agent for treatment of adult patients with histiocytic neoplasms. Cobimetinib has been designated an orphan drug by FDA for the treatment of this cancer.

Clinical Experience

The current indication for cobimetinib is based on the results of a single-center, single-arm, phase 2 trial. Twenty-six adult patients with histiocytic neoplasms (multi-system disease, recurrent or refractory disease, or single-system disease unlikely to benefit from conventional therapies), regardless of tumor genotype, were enrolled; patients with documented BRAF V600E mutations could be enrolled if access to a BRAF inhibitor was not available or if BRAF inhibitor therapy was discontinued due to toxicity. Histiocytic neoplasms present in enrolled patients included Langerhans cell histiocytosis (n=4), Rosai-Dorfman disease (n=4), Erdheim-Chester disease (n=13), xanthogranuloma (n=2), and mixed histiocytosis (n=3). The median patient age was 50.5 years, 65% of patients were male, and 85% were white. Cobimetinib was given at a dose of 60 mg once daily for 21 days and then off for 7 days, in a 28-day cycle. The primary outcome was best overall response rate, maintained on 2 occasions at least 4 weeks apart, as assessed by PET response criteria (PRC). PRC-based duration of response and best overall response rate assessed using RECIST, maintained on 2 occasions at least 4 weeks apart, were also assessed.

The median duration of follow-up was 11.4 months; with a median time to a PRC-based response of 2 months. The overall response rate was 76.9%, with a complete response seen in 61.5% and a partial response in 15.4% of patients, based on PRC. The median PRC-based duration of response was 31 months. The overall response rate based on RECIST was 46.2%; complete or partial response was seen in 11.5 or 34.6% of patients, respectively.

DOSAGE AND ADMINISTRATION

● General

Pretreatment Screening

- Confirm presence of b-Raf serine-threonine kinase (BRAF) V600E or V600K mutation in patients with melanoma prior to initiation of combination therapy with cobimetinib and vemurafenib.

- Perform a dermatologic evaluation prior to initiation of cobimetinib.

- Evaluate left ventricular ejection fraction (LVEF) prior to initiation of cobimetinib.

- Monitor liver function tests prior to initiation of cobimetinib.

- Obtain baseline serum creatine phosphokinase (CPK) and serum creatinine (S_{cr}) concentrations prior to initation of cobimetinib.

Patient Monitoring

- Perform dermatologic evaluation every 2 months during monotherapy with cobimetinib or when used in combination with vemurafenib. Continue monitoring for 6 months following discontinuance of cobimetinib when used in combination with vemurafenib.

- Monitor for new noncutaneous malignancies during combination therapy with cobimetinib and vemurafenib.

- Assess LVEF 1 month after initiation of cobimetinib therapy and then every 3 months during therapy. In patients restarting cobimetinib after dose reduction or interruption, assess LVEF at 2 weeks, 4 weeks, 10 weeks, 16 weeks, then as clinically appropriate.

- Perform ophthalmologic examinations regularly and as clinically indicated (i.e., if new or worsening visual disturbances occur) during cobimetinib therapy.

- Perform liver function tests monthly or more frequently as clinically indicated, during therapy.

- Evaluate serum CPK and creatinine concentrations periodically and as clinically indicated, during therapy.

Other General Considerations

- Avoid exposure to sunlight during therapy.

- When used in combination with vemurafenib, the usual cautions, precautions, and contraindications associated with vemurafenib must be considered in addition to those associated with cobimetinib.

● Administration

Cobimetinib fumarate is administered orally without regard to meals.

Store below 30°C.

● Dosage

Dosage of cobimetinib fumarate is expressed in terms of cobimetinib.

Melanoma

For use in combination with vemurafenib for the treatment of unresectable or metastatic melanoma with BRAF V600E or V600K mutation, the recommended adult dosage of cobimetinib is 60 mg once daily for 21 days followed by a 7-day rest period; courses of therapy are given in 28-day cycles. Continue therapy until disease progression or unacceptable toxicity occurs.

Histiocytic Neoplasms

For use as a single agent for the treatment of histiocytic neoplasms, the recommended adult dosage of cobimetinib is 60 mg once daily for 21 days followed by a 7-day rest period; courses of therapy are given in 28-day cycles. Continue therapy until disease progression or unacceptable toxicity occurs.

Dosage Modifications

If adverse reactions occur, consider interruption of therapy, dosage reduction, and/or permanent discontinuation of cobimetinib. If dosage modification of cobimetinib is necessary, an initial dosage reduction to 40 mg once daily is recommended. If further dosage reduction is necessary, reduce the dosage to 20 mg once daily. Dosages less than 20 mg once daily are not recommended; permanently discontinue the drug if the 20-mg daily dosage is not tolerated.

Hemorrhage

If grade 3 hemorrhage occurs, withhold cobimetinib therapy for up to 4 weeks; resume therapy at a reduced dosage when the toxicity improves to grade 1 or less. If the toxicity does not improve within 4 weeks of withholding cobimetinib, permanently discontinue the drug.

If grade 4 hemorrhage occurs, permanently discontinue cobimetinib therapy.

Cardiomyopathy

If an asymptomatic absolute decrease in left ventricular ejection fraction (LVEF) from baseline of more than 10% and to a level below the lower limit of normal (LLN) occurs, withhold cobimetinib therapy for 2 weeks and reassess left ventricular function; resume therapy at a reduced dosage when LVEF recovers to at least the LLN *and* the absolute decrease in LVEF from baseline is 10% or less.

If a symptomatic decrease in LVEF from baseline occurs, withhold cobimetinib therapy for up to 4 weeks and reassess left ventricular function; resume therapy at a reduced dosage when symptoms resolve, LVEF recovers to at least the LLN, *and* the absolute decrease from baseline is 10% or less.

If LVEF remains below the LLN, the absolute decrease from baseline remains above 10%, or symptoms persist, permanently discontinue cobimetinib therapy.

If QT-interval prolongation occurs during combination therapy with cobimetinib and vemurafenib, dosage modifications for vemurafenib may be required.

Dermatologic Reactions

If intolerable grade 2 dermatologic reactions or grade 3 or 4 dermatologic reactions occur, withhold cobimetinib therapy or reduce the dose.

Serous Retinopathy or Retinal Vein Occlusion

If serous retinopathy occurs, withhold cobimetinib therapy for up to 4 weeks; resume therapy at a reduced dosage when visual manifestations improve. If the toxicity does not improve or if symptoms recur within 4 weeks of resuming therapy at a reduced dosage, permanently discontinue the drug.

If retinal vein occlusion occurs, permanently discontinue cobimetinib therapy.

Liver Laboratory Abnormalities and Hepatotoxicity

For the first occurrence of grade 4 liver function test abnormalities, withhold cobimetinib therapy for up to 4 weeks; resume therapy at a reduced dosage when the toxicity improves to grade 1 or less. If liver function test abnormalities do not improve to grade 1 or less within 4 weeks of withholding therapy, permanently discontinue the drug.

If grade 4 liver function test abnormalities recur, permanently discontinue cobimetinib therapy.

Rhabdomyolysis and CPK Elevations

In patients who exhibit grade 4 CPK elevations or any grade of CPK elevation with concomitant myalgia, withhold cobimetinib therapy for up to 4 weeks; resume therapy at a reduced dosage when the toxicity improves to grade 3 or less. If the toxicity does not improve within 4 weeks of withholding therapy, permanently discontinue the drug.

Photosensitivity

If intolerable grade 2 photosensitivity or grade 3 or 4 photosensitivity occurs, withhold cobimetinib therapy for up to 4 weeks; resume therapy at a reduced dosage when the toxicity improves to grade 1 or less. If the toxicity does not improve within 4 weeks of withholding therapy, permanently discontinue the drug.

Development of New Primary Malignancies

No dosage adjustment is necessary in patients who develop new primary cutaneous or noncutaneous malignancies.

Other Toxicity

If an intolerable grade 2 or any grade 3 adverse reaction occurs, withhold cobimetinib therapy for up to 4 weeks; resume therapy at a reduced dosage when the toxicity improves to grade 1 or less. If the toxicity does not improve within 4 weeks of withholding therapy, permanently discontinue the drug.

For the first occurrence of any grade 4 adverse reaction, withhold *or* permanently discontinue cobimetinib therapy; if withheld, resume therapy at a reduced dosage when the toxicity improves to grade 1 or less. If the grade 4 adverse reaction recurs, permanently discontinue cobimetinib therapy.

Concomitant Use with Drugs and Foods Affecting Hepatic Microsomal Enzymes

Avoid concomitant use of cobimetinib with drugs that are moderate or potent inhibitors of cytochrome P-450 (CYP) isoenzyme 3A. If concomitant short-term (14 days or less) therapy with a moderate CYP3A inhibitor cannot be avoided, the manufacturer recommends reducing the dosage of cobimetinib from 60 mg once daily to 20 mg once daily. When concomitant use of the moderate CYP3A inhibitor is discontinued, resume the prior cobimetinib dosage of 60 mg once daily.

In patients receiving a reduced dosage of cobimetinib (40 or 20 mg once daily), select an alternative drug with no or only mild CYP3A inhibitory activity.

● Special Populations

Hepatic Impairment

No dosage adjustment is necessary in patients with mild, moderate, or severe pre-existing hepatic impairment (Child-Pugh class A, B, or C).

Renal Impairment

No dosage adjustment is necessary in patients with mild or moderate renal impairment (creatinine clearance of 30–89 mL/minute). The manufacturer states that an appropriate dosage for patients with severe renal impairment has not been established.

Geriatric Patients

The manufacturer makes no specific dosage recommendations for geriatric patients.

CAUTIONS

● Contraindications

- None.

● Warnings/Precautions

Severe Photosensitivity

Photosensitivity reactions, sometimes severe, have been reported in patients receiving cobimetinib. In the coBRIM study in patients with unresectable or metastatic melanoma, photosensitivity reactions occurred in 47% of patients receiving combination therapy with cobimetinib and vemurafenib; grade 3 reactions occurred in 4% of patients receiving combined therapy. The median time to first onset of photosensitivity reactions in patients receiving combined therapy was 2 months (range: 1 day to 14 months). The median duration of photosensitivity reactions was 3 months (range: 2 days to 14 months). Most patients (63%) had resolution of photosensitivity reactions.

The manufacturer recommends that patients avoid exposure to sunlight during cobimetinib therapy. Temporary interruption, dosage reduction, or discontinuance of cobimetinib may be necessary if photosensitivity reactions occur during therapy with the drug.

Combination Therapy

When cobimetinib is used in combination with vemurafenib, the usual cautions, precautions, and contraindications associated with vemurafenib must be considered in addition to those associated with cobimetinib.

New Primary Malignancies

New primary cutaneous or noncutaneous malignancies have been reported in patients receiving cobimetinib.

In the coBRIM study in patients with unresectable or metastatic melanoma, cutaneous squamous cell carcinoma or keratoacanthoma, basal cell carcinoma, or new primary melanoma occurred in 6, 4.5, or 0.8%, respectively, of patients receiving cobimetinib in combination with vemurafenib compared with 20, 2.4, or 2.4%, respectively, of those receiving vemurafenib alone. In this study, the median time to detection of cutaneous squamous cell carcinoma, including keratoacanthoma, or basal cell carcinoma was 4 months in patients receiving combination therapy with cobimetinib and vemurafenib. Development of new primary melanoma occurred 9 and 12 months after initiation of combination therapy with cobimetinib and vemurafenib in 2 patients.

In the coBRIM study, noncutaneous malignancies were reported in 0.8% of patients receiving cobimetinib in combination with vemurafenib compared with 1.2% of those receiving vemurafenib alone.

Perform a dermatologic evaluation at baseline and every 2 months during monotherapy with cobimetinib or when cobimetinib is used in combination with vemurafenib. Continue monitoring for 6 months following discontinuance of cobimetinib, when administered in combination with vemurafenib. Treat suspicious cutaneous lesions and excise for pathologic evaluation as appropriate. Monitor for new noncutaneous malignancies when cobimetinib is used in combination with vemurafenib.

Hemorrhage

Hemorrhage, including major hemorrhagic events (defined as symptomatic bleeding in a critical area or organ), has been reported in patients receiving cobimetinib. In the coBRIM study in patients with unresectable or metastatic melanoma, hemorrhage occurred in 13% of patients receiving cobimetinib in combination with vemurafenib compared with 7% of those receiving vemurafenib alone. Grade 3 or 4 hemorrhage was reported in 1.2% of patients receiving combination therapy compared with 0.8% of those receiving vemurafenib alone. An increased incidence of GI hemorrhage, reproductive system hemorrhage, or hematuria was observed in patients receiving combination therapy with cobimetinib and vemurafenib (3.6, 2, or 2.4%, respectively) compared with those receiving vemurafenib alone (1.2, 0.4, or 0.8%, respectively). Cerebral hemorrhage occurred in 0.8% of patients receiving combination therapy compared with none of those receiving vemurafenib alone. Hemorrhagic events (all grade 1 severity) occurred in 19% of patients with histiocytic neoplasms receiving cobimetinib monotherapy.

Temporary interruption, dosage reduction, or discontinuance of cobimetinib may be necessary if hemorrhagic events occur during therapy with the drug.

Cardiomyopathy

Cardiomyopathy (defined as a symptomatic or asymptomatic decrease in left ventricular ejection fraction [LVEF]) has been reported in patients receiving cobimetinib. Safety of cobimetinib has not been established in patients with a baseline LVEF below the lower limit of normal (LLN) or less than 50%.

In the coBRIM study in patients with unresectable or metastatic melanoma, grade 2 or 3 decreases in LVEF occurred in 26% of patients receiving combination therapy with cobimetinib and vemurafenib and in 19% of those receiving vemurafenib alone; temporary interruption and/or dosage modification or permanent discontinuance of therapy was necessary in 22 or 14%, respectively, of those with left ventricular dysfunction. The median time to first onset of left ventricular dysfunction was 4 months (range: 23 days to 13 months). Left ventricular dysfunction resolved (i.e., LVEF improved to above the LLN or to within 10% of baseline) in 62% of patients receiving combination therapy with cobimetinib and vemurafenib; the median time to resolution was 3 months (range: 4 days to 12 months).

In patients with histiocytic neoplasms receiving monotherapy with cobimetinib, grade 2 or grade 3—4 decreases in LVEF occurred in 8 or 12% of patients, respectively. The median time to first onset of left ventricular dysfunction was 29 days (range: 22—114 days). Patients who experienced left ventricular dysfunction had dosage reductions or interruptions in therapy with cobimetinib, and none required permanent discontinuation. Left ventricular dysfunction resolved (i.e., LVEF improved to above the LLN or within 10% of baseline) in 60% of patients, with a median time to resolution of 31 days (range: 13—126 days).

Assess LVEF prior to and 1 month after initiation of cobimetinib therapy and then every 3 months during therapy. If left ventricular dysfunction occurs, temporary interruption, dosage reduction, or discontinuance of cobimetinib may be necessary; reassess LVEF at approximately 2, 4, 10, and 16 weeks following reinitiation of the drug and then as clinically indicated.

Severe Dermatologic Reactions

Severe dermatologic reactions, sometimes requiring hospitalization, have been reported in patients receiving cobimetinib. In the coBRIM study in patients with unresectable or metastatic melanoma, grade 3 or 4 rash occurred in 16% (grade 4 in 1.6%) of patients receiving combination therapy with cobimetinib and vemurafenib and in 17% (grade 4 in 0.8%) of those receiving vemurafenib alone; hospitalization was required in 3.2 or 2% of patients receiving combination therapy with cobimetinib and vemurafenib or vemurafenib alone, respectively. The median time to onset of grade 3 or 4 rash in patients receiving combination therapy with cobimetinib and vemurafenib was 11 days (range: 3 days to 2.8 months). Complete resolution occurred in 95% of patients with grade 3 or 4 rash; the median time to resolution was 21 days (range: 4 days to 17 months). In patients with histiocytic neoplasms receiving monotherapy with cobimetinib, rash events were reported in 81% of patients; all were grade 1—2 in severity.

Temporary interruption, dosage reduction, or discontinuance of cobimetinib may be necessary if dermatologic reactions occur during therapy with the drug.

Serous Retinopathy and Retinal Vein Occlusion

Ocular toxicities, such as serous retinopathy, have been reported in patients receiving cobimetinib. In the coBRIM study in patients with unresectable or metastatic melanoma, symptomatic or asymptomatic serous retinopathy occurred in 26% of patients receiving combination therapy with cobimetinib and vemurafenib; the most common events were chorioretinopathy and retinal detachment. The time to initial onset of serous retinopathy ranged from 2 days to 9 months and the duration ranged from 1 day to 15 months. Retinal vein occlusion occurred in one patient in each treatment group. In patients with histiocytic neoplasms receiving monotherapy with cobimetinib, grade 2 retinopathy and grade 3 retinal vascular disorders each occurred in 4% of patients.

Perform ophthalmologic examinations regularly and as clinically indicated (i.e., if new or worsening visual disturbances occur) during cobimetinib therapy. Temporary interruption, dosage reduction, or discontinuance of cobimetinib may be necessary if ocular toxicities occur during therapy with the drug.

Hepatotoxicity

Liver function test abnormalities have been reported in patients receiving cobimetinib. In the coBRIM study in patients with unresectable or metastatic melanoma, grade 3 or 4 elevations in ALT, AST, total bilirubin, or alkaline phosphatase concentrations occurred in 11, 8, 1.6, or 7%, respectively, of patients receiving combination therapy with cobimetinib and vemurafenib and in 5, 2.1, 1.2, or 3.3%, respectively, of patients receiving vemurafenib alone. Concurrent elevations in ALT (exceeding 3 times the upper limit of normal [ULN]) and total bilirubin concentrations (exceeding 2 times the ULN) with normal alkaline phosphatase concentrations (not exceeding 2 times the ULN) occurred in 1 of 247 patients (0.4%) receiving combination therapy with cobimetinib and vemurafenib and in none of those receiving vemurafenib alone. In patients with histiocytic neoplasms receiving cobimetinib monotherapy, grade 3 or 4 elevations in AST and ALT occurred in 9 and 5% of patients, respectively.

Perform liver function tests prior to initiation of cobimetinib therapy and then monthly, or more frequently as clinically indicated, during therapy with the drug. Temporary interruption, dosage reduction, or discontinuance of cobimetinib may be necessary if liver function test abnormalities occur during therapy with the drug.

Rhabdomyolysis

Rhabdomyolysis has been reported in patients receiving cobimetinib. In the coBRIM study in patients with unresectable or metastatic melanoma, grade 3 or 4 elevations of serum CPK, including asymptomatic elevations over baseline, occurred in 14% of patients receiving combination therapy with cobimetinib and vemurafenib and in 0.5% of patients receiving vemurafenib alone. The median time to first occurrence of grade 3 or 4 elevations in CPK concentrations was 16 days (range: 12 days to 11 months) in patients receiving combination therapy with cobimetinib and vemurafenib. The median time to complete resolution of elevated CPK concentrations was 15 days (range: 9 days to 11 months). Concurrent elevations in CPK concentrations (exceeding 10 times the baseline value) and serum creatinine concentrations (1.5 or more times the baseline value) occurred in 3.6% of patients receiving combination therapy with cobimetinib and vemurafenib and in 0.4% of patients receiving vemurafenib alone. In patients with histiocytic

neoplasms receiving cobimetinib monotherapy, grade 2 CPK elevations occurred in 27% of patients and grade 3—4 CPK elevations occurred in 27% of patients.

Evaluate serum CPK and creatinine concentrations at baseline, periodically during cobimetinib therapy, and as clinically indicated. Patients with elevated CPK concentrations should be evaluated for manifestations of rhabdomyolysis and for other potential causes. Temporary interruption, dosage reduction, or discontinuance of cobimetinib may be necessary if increased CPK concentrations occur during therapy with the drug.

Fetal/Neonatal Morbidity and Mortality

There are no adequate and well-controlled studies of cobimetinib in pregnant women; however, based on its mechanism of action and animal findings, cobimetinib may cause fetal harm. Embryotoxicity (i.e., post-implantation loss) and teratogenicity (i.e., great vessel and eye socket abnormalities) were observed in pregnant animals receiving cobimetinib at exposure levels equivalent to 0.9–1.4 times the human exposure at the recommended dosage.

Avoid pregnancy during cobimetinib therapy. Advise women of childbearing potential to use an effective method of contraception while receiving cobimetinib and for at least 2 weeks after discontinuance of therapy. Apprise patients of the potential hazard to the fetus if the drug is used during pregnancy.

Specific Populations

Pregnancy

Cobimetinib may cause fetal harm if administered to pregnant women based on its mechanism of action and animal findings.

Lactation

It is not known whether cobimetinib is distributed into human milk. The effects of the drug on nursing infants or on the production of milk are unknown. Because of the potential for serious adverse reactions to cobimetinib in nursing infants, advise women not to breast-feed during cobimetinib therapy and for 2 weeks following the final dose.

Females and Males of Reproductive Potential

Results of animal studies suggest that cobimetinib may impair female and male fertility. In a general toxicology study, degeneration of reproductive tissues was observed in female (apoptosis and necrosis of corpora lutea and vaginal epithelial cells) and male (testicular degeneration) animals receiving cobimetinib at exposure levels approximately 2 and 0.1 times, respectively, the human exposure at the recommended dosage.

Avoid pregnancy during cobimetinib therapy and for at least 2 weeks after drug discontinuance. Advise women of childbearing potential to use an effective method of contraception while receiving cobimetinib and for at least 2 weeks after discontinuance of therapy.

Pediatric Use

Safety and efficacy of cobimetinib have not been established in pediatric patients.

Safety and efficacy were assessed, but were not established, in a clinical study of 55 pediatric patients 2—17 years of age with solid tumors; no new safety events were observed. Cobimetinib exposure at the maximally tolerated dosage in pediatric patients was lower than that observed in adult patients receiving the recommended dosage.

Mortality from unknown cause has been observed in immature rats receiving cobimetinib (exposure level on postnatal days 10–17 of approximately 0.13–0.5 times the AUC at the recommended human adult dosage).

Geriatric Use

Clinical studies of cobimetinib did not include sufficient numbers of patients 65 years of age and older to determine whether geriatric patients respond differently than younger adults.

Hepatic Impairment

Following administration of a single 10-mg dose of cobimetinib, systemic exposure to cobimetinib was similar in individuals with mild or moderate hepatic impairment and those with normal hepatic function, but systemic exposure to cobimetinib was decreased by 31% in individuals with severe hepatic impairment. Cobimetinib dosage adjustment is not necessary in patients with hepatic impairment.

Renal Impairment

Formal pharmacokinetic studies of cobimetinib have not been conducted in patients with renal impairment; however, cobimetinib undergoes minimal renal elimination.

In a population pharmacokinetic analysis, systemic exposure to cobimetinib was similar in patients with mild (creatinine clearance of 60–89 mL/minute) or moderate (creatinine clearance of 30–59 mL/minute) renal impairment compared with patients with normal renal function. Cobimetinib dosage adjustment is not necessary in patients with mild to moderate renal impairment. Cobimetinib has not been studied in patients with severe renal impairment; therefore, the manufacturer states that an appropriate dosage for these patients has not been established.

● Common Adverse Effects

Adverse effects reported in 20% or more of patients receiving cobimetinib in combination with vemurafenib for the treatment of unresectable or metastatic melanoma with BRAF V600E or V600K mutation include diarrhea, photosensitivity reaction, nausea, pyrexia, and vomiting. Laboratory abnormalities of grade 3 or 4 severity reported in 5% or more of patients receiving cobimetinib in combination with vemurafenib include elevated concentrations of CPK, elevated concentrations of aminotransferases (i.e., AST, ALT), lymphopenia, elevated concentrations of alkaline phosphatase, hypophosphatemia, elevated concentrations of γ-glutamyltransferase (γ-glutamyltranspeptidase, GGT, GGTP), and hyponatremia.

Adverse effects reported in 20% or more of patients receiving cobimetinib monotherapy for histiocytic neoplasms include acneiform dermatitis, diarrhea, infection, fatigue, nausea, edema, dry skin, maculopapular rash, pruritis, dyspepsia, vomiting, dyspnea, and urinary tract infections. Laboratory abnormalities of grade 3 or 4 severity reported in 5% or more of patients receiving cobimetinib monotherapy for histiocytic neoplasms include hyponatremia, elevated concentrations of CPK, hypokalemia, increased serum creatinine, elevated concentrations of AST, hypocalcemia, lymphopenia, leukopenia, and anemia.

DRUG INTERACTIONS

Cobimetinib is metabolized principally by cytochrome P-450 (CYP) isoenzyme 3A and uridine diphosphate-glucuronosyltransferase (UGT) 2B7. In vitro, cobimetinib is a substrate of CYP3A and P-glycoprotein (P-gp). In vitro studies also indicate that cobimetinib may inhibit CYP isoenzymes 3A and 2D6. In vitro, cobimetinib does not inhibit CYP isoenzymes 1A2, 2B6, 2C8, 2C9, and 2C19 or induce CYP isoenzymes 1A2, 2B6, and 3A4 at clinically relevant concentrations. Cobimetinib also does not inhibit P-gp in vitro at clinically relevant concentrations.

In vitro studies indicate that cobimetinib is not a substrate or inhibitor of breast cancer resistance protein (BCRP), organic cation transporter (OCT) 1, OCT2, organic anion transport protein (OATP) 1B1, OATP1B3, organic anion transporter (OAT) 1, and OAT3 at clinically relevant concentrations.

● Drugs and Foods Affecting Hepatic Microsomal Enzymes

Inhibitors of CYP3A

Concomitant use of cobimetinib with potent or moderate inhibitors of CYP3A may result in increased systemic exposure (AUC) of cobimetinib. Concomitant administration of the potent CYP3A inhibitor itraconazole (200 mg daily for 14 days) with cobimetinib (single 10-mg dose) in healthy individuals increased the peak plasma concentration and AUC of cobimetinib by 3.2- and 6.7-fold, respectively. Simulations suggest that steady-state concentrations of cobimetinib following concomitant administration of a reduced dosage of cobimetinib (20 mg once daily) with a moderate CYP3A inhibitor for less than 14 days are similar to steady-state concentrations attained with cobimetinib alone at a dosage of 60 mg once daily.

Avoid concomitant use of cobimetinib with potent or moderate inhibitors of CYP3A. If concomitant short-term (14 days or less) therapy with a moderate CYP3A inhibitor (e.g., an anti-infective agent [e.g., erythromycin, ciprofloxacin])

cannot be avoided, the manufacturer recommends reducing the dosage of cobimetinib from 60 mg once daily to 20 mg once daily. When concomitant use of the moderate CYP3A inhibitor is discontinued, resume the prior cobimetinib dosage of 60 mg once daily. In patients receiving a reduced dosage of cobimetinib (40 or 20 mg once daily), select an alternative drug with no or only mild CYP3A inhibitory activity.

Inducers of CYP3A

Concomitant use of cobimetinib with potent or moderate inducers of CYP3A may result in decreased systemic exposure and reduced efficacy of cobimetinib. Simulations suggest that concomitant administration of a potent or moderate CYP3A inducer and cobimetinib may decrease systemic exposure of cobimetinib by 83 or 73%, respectively.

Avoid concomitant use of cobimetinib with potent or moderate inducers of CYP3A (e.g., carbamazepine, efavirenz, phenytoin, rifampin, St. John's wort [*Hypericum perforatum*]).

● Drugs Metabolized by Hepatic Microsomal Enzymes

Concomitant administration of cobimetinib (60 mg once daily for 15 days) with the CYP2D6 substrate dextromethorphan (single 30-mg dose) or the CYP3A substrate midazolam (single 2-mg dose) in patients with solid tumors did not substantially alter systemic exposure to dextromethorphan or midazolam.

● Drugs Affecting Efflux Transport Systems

Cobimetinib is a substrate of the efflux transporter P-gp. Concomitant use of cobimetinib with drugs that inhibit P-gp may result in increased concentrations of cobimetinib.

● Drugs Affecting Gastric Acidity

Concomitant administration of the proton-pump inhibitor rabeprazole (20 mg once daily for 5 days) with cobimetinib (single 20-mg dose) under fed and fasted conditions did not result in clinically important changes in systemic exposure of cobimetinib.

● Vemurafenib

Concomitant use of cobimetinib (60 mg once daily) with vemurafenib (960 mg twice daily) did not result in clinically important pharmacokinetic interactions.

DESCRIPTION

Cobimetinib, a potent, selective, and reversible inhibitor of mitogen-activated extracellular signal-regulated kinase (MEK) 1 and MEK2, is an antineoplastic agent. MEK proteins are upstream regulators of the extracellular signal-related kinase (ERK) pathway, which promotes cellular proliferation. Approximately 40–60% of cutaneous melanomas carry a BRAF mutation. The most common BRAF mutation is the substitution of glutamic acid for valine at codon 600 in exon 15 (BRAF V600E); a less frequently occurring BRAF mutation is the substitution of lysine for valine at codon 600 in exon 15 (BRAF V600K). BRAF V600 mutations result in activation of the BRAF pathway that includes MEK 1 and 2. The mutation of BRAF V600E activates the mitogen-activated protein kinase (MAPK) and ERK signal transduction pathway, which enhances cell proliferation and tumor progression (e.g., metastasis). Cobimetinib has demonstrated antitumor activity in mice bearing tumor xenografts that expressed BRAF V600E.

Clinical resistance to monotherapy with a BRAF inhibitor, generally occurring 6–7 months following initiation of therapy, has been attributed to several possible resistance mechanisms mostly relying on reactivation of the MAPK/ERK pathway. Complete inhibition of the MAPK/ERK pathway resulting in durable responses may be achieved with the use of combination therapy with a BRAF inhibitor (i.e., dabrafenib, encorafenib, vemurafenib) and an MEK inhibitor (i.e., binimetinib, cobimetinib, trametinib). In vitro, use of cobimetinib in combination with vemurafenib resulted in increased apoptosis and reduced tumor growth of melanoma cell lines testing positive for BRAF V600E compared with either drug alone. In addition, cobimetinib prevented vemurafenib-mediated growth enhancement of a wild-type BRAF tumor cell line in mice bearing tumor xenografts.

Following oral administration of cobimetinib in healthy individuals, the absolute bioavailability of the drug is 46%. Cobimetinib exhibits linear pharmacokinetics over a dose range of 3.5–100 mg. Following oral administration in cancer patients, median time to peak plasma concentrations of cobimetinib is 2.4 hours. Repeated administration of cobimetinib 60 mg daily resulted in a 2.4-fold mean cobimetinib accumulation ratio. Steady-state concentrations are reached within 9 days. Administration of a single 20-mg dose of cobimetinib with a high-fat meal did not affect systemic exposure (AUC) and peak plasma concentration of the drug in healthy individuals. Cobimetinib is highly bound (95%) to plasma proteins. Following oral administration of cobimetinib 60 mg once daily in cancer patients, the mean terminal half-life of cobimetinib was 44 hours. Cobimetinib is metabolized mainly by cytochrome P-450 (CYP) isoenzyme 3A and uridine diphosphate-glucuronosyltransferase (UGT) 2B7. Following oral administration of a single radiolabeled dose of cobimetinib, 76% of the radioactivity was recovered in feces (6.6% of the dose as unchanged drug) and 17.8% was recovered in urine (1.6% of the dose as unchanged drug).

The pharmacokinetics of cobimetinib do not appear to be affected substantially by age (19–88 years), gender, or ethnicity.

ADVICE TO PATIENTS

- If a dose is missed or vomited, administer the next dose at the regularly scheduled time; do not take an additional dose to replace the missed or vomited dose.

- Risk of new primary cutaneous malignancies. Contact a clinician promptly if dermatologic changes (e.g., new wart, skin sore or reddish bump that bleeds or does not heal, mole that changes in size or color) occur.

- Risk of hemorrhage. Contact a clinician promptly and seek immediate medical attention if signs and/or symptoms of unusual bleeding (e.g., blood in stool or urine, unusual vaginal bleeding) occur.

- Risk of cardiomyopathy. Importance of cardiac monitoring before and during cobimetinib therapy. Contact a clinician promptly if manifestations of left ventricular dysfunction (e.g., shortness of breath, persistent coughing or wheezing, fatigue, peripheral edema, tachycardia) occur.

- Risk of serious adverse dermatologic effects. Contact a clinician promptly if a serious reaction (e.g., rash affecting a large area, blistering or peeling of the skin) occurs.

- Risk of serous retinopathy or retinal vein occlusion. Contact a clinician promptly if visual disturbances (i.e., blurred, distorted, partial, or halo vision) occur.

- Risk of hepatotoxicity. Importance of liver function test monitoring before and during cobimetinib therapy. Immediately report any possible manifestations of hepatotoxicity (e.g., jaundice, dark or tea-colored urine, nausea, vomiting, fatigue, loss of appetite).

- Risk of rhabdomyolysis. Importance of monitoring creatine kinase (CK, creatine phosphokinase, CPK) concentrations before and during cobimetinib therapy. Immediately report any possible manifestations of rhabdomyolysis (e.g., dark or red urine; muscle pain, spasms, or weakness).

- Risk of photosensitivity reactions. Use a broad-spectrum sunscreen and lip balm (minimum SPF of 30), wear protective clothing, and avoid exposure to sunlight during therapy. Contact a clinician if skin becomes red, painful, itchy, warm to touch, irritated, or thick, dry, or wrinkled; if bumps or small papules develop; or if a rash from sunlight exposure occurs.

- Risk of fetal harm. Advise women of childbearing potential that they should use an effective method of contraception while receiving the drug and for at least 2 weeks after discontinuance of therapy. Importance of women informing clinicians if they are or plan to become pregnant. If pregnancy occurs, advise pregnant women of potential risk to the fetus.

- Advise women to avoid breast-feeding while receiving cobimetinib and for 2 weeks after discontinuance of therapy.

- Importance of informing clinicians of existing or contemplated concomitant therapy, including prescription and OTC drugs and dietary or herbal supplements (e.g., St. John's wort), as well as any concomitant illnesses.

- Inform patients of other important precautionary information.

For further information on the handling of antineoplastic agents, see the ASHP Guidelines on Handling Hazardous Drugs at https://www.ahfsdruginformation.com.

PREPARATIONS

Cobimetinib is obtained through specialty pharmacies. Contact manufacturer or consult the Cotellic® product website https://www.cotellic.com/hcp/support-resources/helpful-resources-for-your-practice.html#distribution for specific availability information.

Excipients in commercially available drug preparations may have clinically important effects in some individuals; consult specific product labeling for details.

Cobimetinib Fumarate

Oral

Tablets, film-coated	20 mg (of cobimetinib)	Cotellic®, Genentech

† Use is not currently included in the labeling approved by the US Food and Drug Administration.

Selected Revisions March 10, 2024, © Copyright, August 2, 2016, American Society of Health-System Pharmacists, Inc.

Crizotinib

10:00 • ANTINEOPLASTIC AGENTS

■ Crizotinib, an inhibitor of multiple receptor tyrosine kinases including anaplastic lymphoma kinase (*ALK*) and c-ros oncogene-1 (*ROS-1*), is an antineoplastic agent.

USES

● Non-small Cell Lung Cancer

Crizotinib is used for the treatment of metastatic non-small cell lung cancer (NSCLC) in patients whose cancer is anaplastic lymphoma kinase (*ALK*)- or c-ros oncogene-1 (*ROS-1*)-positive as detected by an FDA-approved diagnostic test. The drug has been designated an orphan drug by the FDA for use in this condition. Use of crizotinib for the treatment of metastatic NSCLC is supported by several randomized controlled trials. Guidelines generally support use of crizotinib for the treatment of stage IV NSCLC when other ALK inhibitors are unavailable or were previously used in the first-line setting.

The current indication for crizotinib in the treatment of *ALK*- or *ROS-1*-positive metastatic NSCLC is based principally on the results of 2 multicenter, open-label, randomized, phase 3 studies (PROFILE 1014 and PROFILE 1007) and a multicenter, open-label, noncomparative study (PROFILE 1001).

In the PROFILE 1014 study, 343 adults with previously untreated *ALK*-positive metastatic NSCLC were randomized (stratified by Eastern Cooperative Oncology Group [ECOG] performance status, race, and presence of brain metastases) in a 1:1 ratio to receive either crizotinib (250 mg orally twice daily) alone or standard chemotherapy (pemetrexed 500 mg/m² IV and either cisplatin 75 mg/m² IV or carboplatin at the dose required to obtain an AUC of 5–6 mg/mL per minute IV every 3 weeks for up to 6 cycles). Treatment was continued until disease progression, death, or unacceptable toxicity occurred or treatment was discontinued for other reasons. At the time of documented disease progression, patients randomized to chemotherapy were offered crizotinib. The primary measure of efficacy was progression-free survival as assessed by an independent review committee according to Response Evaluation Criteria in Solid Tumors (RECIST 1.1); additional outcome measures included objective response rate, duration of response, and overall survival. Presence of *ALK* rearrangement was determined using an FDA-approved diagnostic test (i.e., Vysis ALK Break-Apart fluorescence in situ hybridization [FISH] probe kit).

The median age of patients enrolled in the PROFILE 1014 study was 53 years; 51% of patients were white, 46% were Asian, 62% were female, 95% had an ECOG performance status of 0 or 1, 64% had never smoked, 92% had adenocarcinoma histology, 27% had brain metastases, and 7% had received adjuvant or neoadjuvant chemotherapy. At the time of final analysis for overall survival, 84% of patients previously randomized to receive standard chemotherapy subsequently received crizotinib therapy. At a median follow-up of 17.4 months for those receiving crizotinib and 16.7 months for those receiving chemotherapy, median progression-free survival was prolonged in patients receiving crizotinib compared with those receiving standard chemotherapy (10.9 versus 7 months; hazard ratio: 0.45). Objective response rate in patients receiving crizotinib or standard chemotherapy was 74 or 45%, respectively; complete response was achieved in 2 or 1% of patients, respectively. At the time of analysis, the median duration of response in patients receiving crizotinib or standard chemotherapy was 11.3 or 5.3 months, respectively. No substantial difference in overall survival was observed between patients receiving crizotinib and those receiving standard chemotherapy. In a final overall survival analysis (median duration of follow-up of 46 months), no substantial difference in overall survival was observed; however, analysis adjusted for crossover demonstrated an overall survival benefit with crizotinib therapy. Results of an exploratory analysis (based on patient-reported symptoms) suggested that crizotinib therapy delayed the time to new onset or worsening of dyspnea compared with chemotherapy; however, because patients were not blinded to treatment assignment, differences in patient-related symptoms cannot be assessed reliably.

In the PROFILE 1007 study, 347 adults with *ALK*-positive metastatic NSCLC previously treated with one platinum-containing regimen were randomized (stratified by ECOG performance status, presence of brain metastases, and prior epidermal growth factor receptor [EGFR] tyrosine kinase inhibitor therapy) in a 1:1 ratio to receive either crizotinib (250 mg orally twice daily) or standard chemotherapy (pemetrexed 500 mg/m² IV or docetaxel 75 mg/m² IV every 21 days). Treatment was continued until unacceptable toxicity or disease progression occurred or the patient was no longer experiencing clinical benefit. The primary measure of efficacy was progression-free survival as assessed by an independent review committee according to RECIST 1.1; additional outcome measures included objective response rate, duration of response, and overall survival. Presence of *ALK* rearrangement was determined using an FDA-approved diagnostic test (i.e., Vysis ALK Break-Apart FISH probe kit).

The median age of patients enrolled in the PROFILE 1007 study was 50 years; 52% of patients were white, 45% were Asian, 56% were female, 90% had an ECOG performance status of 0 or 1, and 63% had never smoked. Most patients (approximately 95%) had metastatic disease and at least 93% had adenocarcinoma histology. At the time of final analysis for overall survival, 89% of patients previously randomized to receive standard chemotherapy subsequently received crizotinib therapy. At a median follow-up of 12.2 months for those receiving crizotinib and 12.1 months for those receiving standard chemotherapy, median progression-free survival was prolonged in patients receiving crizotinib compared with those receiving standard chemotherapy (7.7 versus 3 months; hazard ratio: 0.49). Objective response rate in patients receiving crizotinib or standard chemotherapy was 65 or 20%, respectively; complete response was achieved in one crizotinib-treated patient and none of those receiving standard chemotherapy. At the time of analysis, the median duration of response in patients receiving crizotinib or standard chemotherapy was 7.4 or 5.6 months, respectively. No substantial difference in overall survival was observed between patients receiving crizotinib and those receiving chemotherapy.

In the PROFILE 1001 study, 50 patients with *ROS-1*-positive metastatic NSCLC received crizotinib (250 mg orally twice daily) until disease progression, death, or unacceptable toxicity occurred or treatment was discontinued for other reasons. The primary measures of efficacy were objective response rate according to RECIST 1.1 and duration of response. Presence of *ROS-1* rearrangement was determined by reverse transcription-polymerase chain reaction (RT-PCR) or FISH (defined as *ROS-1* rearrangement on at least 15% of at least 50 tumor cells). The median age of patients enrolled in the study was 53 years; 54% of patients were white, 42% were Asian, 56% were female, 98% had an ECOG performance status of 0 or 1, and 78% had never smoked. Most patients (92%) had metastatic disease and 96% had adenocarcinoma histology. The majority (80%) of patients had previously received platinum-based chemotherapy for metastatic disease. At the time of analysis, objective response rate as assessed by an independent review committee (IRC) or the investigator was 66 or 72%, respectively; complete response was achieved in 1 or 5 patients, respectively. The median duration of IRC-assessed response was 18.3 months; median duration of investigator-assessed response had not been reached at the time of analysis.

Crizotinib also has been compared with alectinib, brigatinib, and lorlatinib in clinical trials enrolling ALK inhibitor-naïve NSCLC patients.

Clinical Perspective

A relatively small subset of patients with NSCLC have *ALK*- or *ROS-1*-positive disease (approximately 3–7% or 1–2%, respectively), which indicates potential responsiveness to ALK or ROS-1 inhibitor therapy. Patients with these forms of lung cancer typically are nonsmokers or have a history of light smoking, are female, and are younger in age and often have adenocarcinoma histology. Although crizotinib is highly active in patients with *ALK*-positive NSCLC, most patients treated with the drug eventually experience disease progression, limiting the drug's long-term therapeutic potential. Disease progression in patients receiving crizotinib can result from acquired resistance mutations in *ALK*, amplification of gene expression, activation of alternate signaling pathways, and/or progression of brain metastases (because of poor distribution of crizotinib into the CSF).

ALK-positive Non-small Cell Lung Cancer

The American Society of Clinical Oncology (ASCO) and Ontario Health (OH; formerly known as Cancer Care Ontario) 2021 joint guideline specifically addresses treatment of stage IV NSCLC harboring driver alterations such as *ALK* mutations. ASCO/OH state that alectinib or brigatinib should be offered in the first-line setting in patients with stage IV NSCLC and driver alterations in *ALK*. If alectinib or brigatinib are not available, ceritinib or crizotinib should be offered in the first-line setting.

In the second-line setting, ASCO/OH state that alectinib, brigatinib, or ceritinib should be offered in patients who received initial therapy with crizotinib.

ROS-1-*positive Non-small Cell Lung Cancer*

The American Society of Clinical Oncology (ASCO) and Ontario Health (OH; formerly known as Cancer Care Ontario) 2021 joint guideline specifically addresses treatment of stage IV NSCLC harboring driver alterations such as *ROS-1* mutations. ASCO/OH state that crizotinib or entrectinib may be offered in patients with driver alterations in *ROS-1*. ASCO/OH also state that if nontargeted therapy was given in the first-line setting in patients with *ROS-1*-positive NSCLC, ceritinib, crizotinib, or entrectinib may be offered in the second-line setting.

● *Anaplastic Large Cell Lymphoma*

Crizotinib is used for the treatment of pediatric patients ≥1 year of age and young adults with relapsed or refractory *ALK*-positive systemic anaplastic large cell lymphoma (ALCL). The drug has been designated an orphan drug by the FDA for use in this condition. The principal efficacy study did not include any patients >21 years of age; the manufacturer states that safety and efficacy of crizotinib have not been established in older adults with relapsed or refractory systemic *ALK*-positive ALCL.

Safety and efficacy of crizotinib for the treatment of relapsed or refractory systemic *ALK*-positive ALCL are based principally on the results of a multi-center, single-arm, open-label study in 26 patients 1–21 years of age with systemic *ALK*-positive ALCL that relapsed or was refractory to at least 1 systemic treatment. Patients with primary cutaneous ALCL or CNS involvement by lymphoma were excluded. In this study, patients received crizotinib 280 mg/m² (20 patients) or 165 mg/m² (6 patients) orally twice daily until disease progression or unacceptable toxicity occurred. Discontinuance of crizotinib therapy was permitted to undergo hematopoietic stem cell transplantation (HSCT). The median age of patients enrolled in the study was 11 years (range, 3 to 20); 69% were male, 54% were white, 19% were Black, and 8% were Asian. All patients had received systemic combination therapy, 8% had previously undergone HSCT, and 15% had received at least 3 prior therapies. The objective response rate was 88% (95% confidence interval, 71–96%); complete response occurred in 81% of patients and partial response occurred in 8% of patients. Of those with an objective response, 57% maintained a response at 3 months, 39% maintained a response at 6 months, and 22% maintained a response at 12 months.

Clinical Perspective

Anaplastic large cell lymphoma occurs in approximately 2 and 15% of adult and pediatric patients with non-Hodgkin lymphoma, respectively. The prevalence of *ALK*-positive ALCL is unknown, but the disease typically affects children and young adults. Anthracycline-based therapy is generally considered first-line treatment for ALCL. Hematopoietic stem cell transplantation (HSCT) may be considered in specific patients and may improve survival; however, the clinical role of HSCT in patients with relapsed or refractory ALCL remains unclear. Targeted therapy and immunotherapy, including ALK inhibitors such as crizotinib, histone deacetylase inhibitors, and brentuximab vedotin, are generally considered emerging therapies for ALCL and have demonstrated high rates of response and survival in patients with *ALK*-positive or CD30-positive relapsed or refractory ALCL.

● *Inflammatory Myofibroblastic Tumor*

Crizotinib is used for the treatment of adult and pediatric patients ≥1 year of age with unresectable, recurrent, or refractory inflammatory myofibroblastic tumor (IMT) that is ALK-positive. The drug has been designated an orphan drug by the FDA for use in this condition. Efficacy of crizotinib for treatment of *ALK*-positive IMT was established in 2 separate clincial studies; one study was conducted in patients 1 to ≤21 years of age and the other study was conducted in adults.

The efficacy of crizotinib for treatment of *ALK*-positive IMT for pediatric patients 1 to ≤21 years of age was evaluated in a multicenter, single-arm, open-label study that included 14 pediatric patients with unresectable, recurrent, or refractory ALK-positive IMT. Twelve patients received crizotinib 280 mg/m² twice daily until disease progression or unacceptable toxicity; 2 patients received

a lower dose. The median age of patients in this study was 6.5 years (range: 2 to 13); 64% were female, 71% were white, 7% were Black, and 71% had a Lansky/Karnofsky Score of 100. A total of 12 (86%) patients received prior therapy; the most common prior therapy was surgery (57%). The primary efficacy outcome was objective response rate with 86% of patients having a complete (36%) or partial (50%) response rate. The duration of response was ≥6 and 12 months in 58% of the patients.

The efficacy of crizotinib for treatment of *ALK*-positive IMT for adult patients was evaluated in a multicenter, single-arm, open-label study that included 7 adult patients with unresectable, recurrent, or refractory ALK-positive IMT. Patients received crizotinib 250 mg twice daily. The median age of patients was 38 years (range: 23 to 73); 57% were male, 57% were white, 43% were Asian, and 86% had an ECOG performance status of 0 or 1. Two (29%) patients had at least one prior systemic treatment. The primary efficacy outcome was objective response rate with 5 patients experiencing a response, including 1 complete response. The duration of response was ≥6 months for all 5 patients and ≥12 months for 2 patients.

Clinical Perspective

Inflammatory myofibroblastic tumors (IMTs) occur throughout the body, with the lungs as the most commonly involved organ. If possible, surgical resection is the treatment of choice as patients with completely resected tumors have an excellent prognosis. Molecular rearrangement of the ALK locus on chromosome 2p23 is seen in approximately 50% of IMT cases; therefore, patients with unresectable or recurrent tumors may respond to crizotinib if the ALK mutation is present and crizotinib administration is followed by complete or incomplete resection.

DOSAGE AND ADMINISTRATION

● *General*

Pretreatment Screening

- *In patients with metastatic non-small cell lung cancer (NSCLC)*: Confirm presence of anaplastic lymphoma kinase (*ALK*)- or c-ros oncogene-1 (*ROS-1*) rearrangement in tumor specimens prior to initiating therapy with crizotinib.

- Verify pregnancy status in females of reproductive potential.

- *In pediatric and young adult patients with anaplastic large cell lymphoma (ALCL) or pediatric patients with IMT*: Perform ophthalmologic examination prior to initiating therapy.

Patient Monitoring

- Monitor complete blood cell counts (CBCs) including differential counts weekly for the first month of therapy and then at least monthly. More frequent testing is recommended in patients with grade 3 or 4 hematologic toxicity, or if fever or infection occurs.

- Monitor liver function tests every 2 weeks during the initial 2 months of therapy, monthly thereafter, and as clinically indicated. More frequent testing is recommended if elevated aminotransferase concentrations occur.

- Monitor for pulmonary symptoms indicative of interstitial lung disease or pneumonitis.

- Monitor ECGs and serum electrolytes in patients with congestive heart failure, bradyarrhythmias, or electrolyte abnormalities and in those who are receiving drugs known to prolong the QT interval.

- Monitor heart rate and blood pressure regularly during therapy.

- *In pediatric and young adult patients with ALCL or pediatric patients with IMT*: Ophthalmologic examination including retinal examination is recommended within 1 month of initiating crizotinib therapy, every 3 months thereafter.

- Assess visual symptoms monthly during treatment in all patients receiving crizotinib. Patients with new symptoms should be referred to an eye specialist.

Premedication and Prophylaxis

- *In pediatric and young adult patients with ALCL or pediatric patients with IMT*: Administer standard antiemetic and antidiarrheal agents for GI adverse effects; antiemetics are recommended prior to and during treatment with crizotinib.

- Consider IV or oral hydration for patients at risk of dehydration; serum electrolytes also should be corrected as clinically indicated.

Dispensing and Administration Precautions

- Based on the Institute for Safe Medication Practices (ISMP), crizotinib is a high-alert mediation that has a heightened risk of causing significant patient harm when used in error.

● Administration

Crizotinib is administered orally twice daily without regard to meals. The capsules should be swallowed whole; do not crush, chew, or split.

The pellets are supplied encapsulated in shells. Do not chew or crush the pellets and do not swallow pellets encapsulated in the shell.

Crizotinib pellets may be administered by opening the shells containing the pellets and emptying the contents directly into the patient's mouth or by emptying the contents into an oral dosing aid (e.g., spoon, medicine cup) and administering the pellets via the dosing aid directly into the patient's mouth. Give the patient a sufficient amount of water immediately after administration to ensure that all medication is swallowed.

If a dose of crizotinib is missed, take it as soon as it is remembered unless the next dose is due within 6 hours.

If a dose of crizotinib is vomited after administration, an additional dose should not be administered to replace the vomited dose. The next dose should be administered at the next scheduled time.

Store capsules and pellets at room temperature (20°-25°C); excursions permitted between 15°-30°C.

● Dosage

Non-small Cell Lung Cancer

The recommended adult dosage of crizotinib for the treatment of *ALK*- or *ROS-1*-positive metastatic NSCLC is 250 mg twice daily. Therapy should be continued until disease progression or unacceptable toxicity occurs.

Anaplastic Large Cell Lymphoma

The recommended dosage of crizotinib in pediatric patients ≥1 year of age and young adults with anaplastic large cell lymphoma (ALCL) is 280 mg/m² orally twice daily until disease progression or unacceptable toxicity occurs. The recommended dosage of crizotinib is based on body surface area (BSA). See Table 1.

TABLE 1. Recommended Crizotinib Dosage Based on BSA in Pediatric Patients ≥1 Year of Age and Young Adults with ALK-positive ALCL or Pediatric Patients ≥1 Year of Age with ALK-positive IMT

Body Surface Area (m²)	Recommended Dosage (280 mg/m² twice daily)
0.38–0.46	120 mg twice daily
0.47–0.51	140 mg twice daily
0.52–0.61	150 mg twice daily
0.62–0.80	200 mg twice daily
0.81-0.97	250 mg twice daily
0.98-1.16	300 mg twice daily
1.17-1.33	350 mg twice daily
1.34-1.51	400 mg twice daily
1.52-1.69	450 mg twice daily
≥1.7	500 mg twice daily

Inflammatory Myofibroblastic Tumor

The recommended dosage of crizotinib in pediatric patients ≥1 year of age with IMT is 280 mg/m² orally twice daily until disease progression or unacceptable toxicity occurs. The recommended dosage of crizotinib is based on BSA. See Table 1.

The recommended adult dosage of crizotinib in patients with IMT is 250 mg orally twice daily until disease progression or unacceptable toxicity occurs.

Dosage Modification for Toxicity

If adverse reactions occur during crizotinib therapy, temporary interruption of therapy, dosage reduction, and/or discontinuance of the drug may be necessary. If dosage reduction is required, the dosage of crizotinib should be reduced as described in Table 2 in adult patients with NSCLC or IMT or in Table 3 for pediatric patients with ALCL or IMT and young adults with ALCL; the recommended dosage modifications for pediatric patients with ALCL or IMT and young adults with ALCL are based on BSA.

TABLE 2. Recommended Dosage Reduction for Crizotinib Toxicity in Adults with NSCLC or IMT.

Dose Reduction Level	Dosage Reduction after Recovery from Toxicity (Initial Adult Dosage = 250 mg twice daily)
First	Resume at 200 mg twice daily
Second	Resume at 250 mg once daily
Third	Permanently discontinue drug

TABLE 3. Recommended Dosage Reductions for Crizotinib Toxicity in Pediatric Patients with ALCL or IMT and Young Adults with ALCL

Body Surface Area (m²)	First Dose Reduction	Second Dose Reduction[a]
0.38-0.46	90 mg twice daily	70 mg twice daily
0.47-0.51	100 mg twice daily	80 mg twice daily
0.52-0.61	120 mg twice daily	90 mg twice daily
0.62-0.80	150 mg twice daily	120 mg twice daily
0.81-0.97	200 mg twice daily	150 mg twice daily
0.98-1.16	220 mg twice daily	170 mg twice daily
1.17-1.33	250 mg twice daily	200 mg twice daily
1.34-1.69	250 mg twice daily	200 mg twice daily
≥1.7	400 mg twice daily	250 mg twice daily

[a] Permanently discontinue in patients who are unable to tolerate crizotinib therapy after 2 dose reductions.

Hematologic Toxicity

In adult patients receiving crizotinib for the treatment of NSCLC or IMT:

If grade 3 hematologic toxicity occurs, withhold crizotinib therapy until the hematologic toxicity resolves to ≤grade 2, then resume therapy at the same dosage.

If grade 4 hematologic toxicity occurs, withhold crizotinib therapy until the hematologic toxicity resolves to ≤grade 2, then resume therapy at the next lower dosage.

Dosage modification is not recommended for lymphopenia unless it is associated with clinical events (e.g., opportunistic infections).

In pediatric and young adult patients receiving crizotinib for the treatment of ALCL or pediatric patients with IMT:

If absolute neutrophil count (ANC) <500/mm³ occurs, withhold crizotinib until ANC recovers to >1000/mm³, then resume crizotinib at the next lower dosage. If ANC <500/mm³ recurs, permanently discontinue crizotinib if recurrence is complicated by febrile neutropenia or infection. If uncomplicated grade 4 neutropenia occurs, withhold therapy until ANC recovers to >1000/mm³ and then resume at the next lower dosage or permanently discontinue therapy. Permanently discontinue crizotinib in patients who are unable to tolerate the drug after 2 dosage reductions, unless indicated otherwise.

If platelet count of 25,000–50,000/mm³ occurs with concurrent bleeding, withhold crizotinib until platelet count recovers to >50,000/mm³ and bleeding resolves, then resume at the same dosage. If platelet count <25,000/mm³ occurs, withhold crizotinib until platelet count recovers to >50,000/mm³, then resume at the next lower dosage; permanently discontinue for recurrence.

If hemoglobin concentration <8 g/dL occurs, withhold crizotinib until hemoglobin concentration recovers to ≥8 g/dL, then resume at the same dosage. If life-threatening anemia occurs and urgent intervention is needed, withhold crizotinib until hemoglobin recovers to ≥8 g/dL, then resume at the next lower dosage. If life-threatening anemia recurs, permanently discontinue crizotinib therapy.

Hepatic Toxicity

If elevations in serum alanine aminotransferase (ALT) or aspartate aminotransferase (AST) concentrations exceeding 5 times the upper limit of normal (ULN) with total bilirubin concentrations ≤1.5 times the ULN occur, withhold crizotinib therapy until liver function test results return to baseline values or improve to ≤3 times the ULN. Crizotinib therapy may then be resumed at the next lower dosage.

If elevations in ALT or AST concentrations exceeding 3 times the ULN with total bilirubin concentrations exceeding 1.5 times the ULN (in the absence of cholestasis or hemolysis) occur, permanently discontinue crizotinib therapy.

Pulmonary Effects

If treatment-related interstitial lung disease/pneumonitis of any grade occurs, permanently discontinue crizotinib therapy.

Prolongation of QT Interval

If corrected QT (QT_c) interval exceeds 500 msec on at least 2 separate electrocardiograms (ECGs), withhold crizotinib therapy until the QT_c-interval returns to baseline values or improves to <481 msec. Crizotinib therapy may then be resumed at the next lower dosage.

If QT_c interval exceeds 500 msec or a change from baseline of ≥60 msec occurs with torsades de pointes, polymorphic ventricular tachycardia, or signs and/or symptoms of serious arrhythmia, permanently discontinue crizotinib therapy.

Bradycardia

If *symptomatic, but non-life-threatening*, bradycardia requiring medical intervention occurs, withhold therapy with crizotinib until recovery to a resting heart rate according to the patient's age (based on the 2.5th percentile per age-specific norms) as seen in Table 4. If concomitant drugs known to cause bradycardia are identified and discontinued or their dosage is adjusted, crizotinib therapy may be resumed at the same dosage upon recovery to asymptomatic bradycardia or to the age-specific heart rate. If no concomitant drugs known to cause bradycardia are identified or if discontinuance or dosage adjustment of such concomitant drugs is not possible, resume crizotinib at the next lower dosage upon recovery to asymptomatic bradycardia or to the age-specific heart rate.

If *life-threatening* bradycardia requiring urgent intervention occurs in patients not receiving concomitant contributory drugs, permanently discontinue crizotinib therapy. If concomitant drugs known to cause bradycardia are identified and discontinued or their dosage is adjusted, crizotinib therapy may be resumed at the second dose reduction level in Table 2 or 3 upon recovery to asymptomatic bradycardia or to the heart rate criteria listed for management of symptomatic, but non-life-threatening bradycardia, with frequent monitoring. Permanently discontinue crizotinib therapy for recurrence.

TABLE 4. Resting Heart Rate Based on the 2.5th Percentile Per Age-specific Norms.

Age (years)	Resting Heart Rate
1 to <2	≥91 beats/minute
2–3	≥82 beats/minute
4–5	≥72 beats/minute
6–8	≥64 beats/minute
>8	≥60 beats/minute

Visual Disturbances

If visual loss (grade 3 or 4 ocular disorder, marked decrease in vision) occurs, discontinue crizotinib therapy and perform an ophthalmologic evaluation. Permanently discontinue crizotinib for grade 3 or 4 ocular disorders or severe visual loss if no other etiology is discovered during the ophthalmologic evaluation.

If visual symptoms (grade 1 or 2 ocular toxicity) occur, monitor symptoms and consult an eye specialist; consider dosage reduction of crizotinib for grade 2 visual disorders. I

GI Toxicity

In pediatric and young adult patients receiving crizotinib for the treatment of ALCL or pediatric patients with IMT:

If grade 3 nausea occurs, withhold crizotinib until symptoms resolve and then resume at the next lower dosage level.

If grade 3 or 4 vomiting occurs, withhold crizotinib until symptoms resolve and then resume at the next lower dosage level.

If grade 3 or 4 diarrhea occurs, withhold crizotinib until symptoms resolve and then resume at the next lower dosage level.

In patients experiencing GI toxicity who are unable to tolerate crizotinib after 2 dosage reductions, permanently discontinue crizotinib unless otherwise indicated.

Concomitant Use of Drugs or Foods Affecting Hepatic Microsomal Enzymes

Concomitant use of crizotinib with potent cytochrome P-450 (CYP) isoenzyme 3A inhibitors should be avoided. If concomitant use of a potent CYP3A inhibitor cannot be avoided, the manufacturer recommends reducing the dose of crizotinib to the second dose reduction (see Table 2 for adults with NSCLC or IMT and Table 3 for pediatric patients with ALCL or IMT and young adults with ALCL). When concomitant use of the potent CYP3A inhibitor is discontinued, resume the crizotinib dosage used prior to initiation of the potent CYP3A inhibitor.

● Special Populations

Hepatic Impairment

For adult patients with severe preexisting hepatic impairment (total bilirubin concentration exceeding 3 times the upper limit of normal [ULN] with any AST concentration), the manufacturer recommends a crizotinib dosage of 250 mg *once daily in patients with NSCLC or IMT* and reducing the dosage according to the second dosage reduction level *in pediatric and young adult patients with ALCL or pediatric patients with IMT* (see Table 3).

For adult patients with moderate preexisting hepatic impairment (total bilirubin concentration exceeding 1.5 times ULN, but no more than 3 times ULN, with any AST concentration), the manufacturer recommends a crizotinib dosage of 200 mg twice daily *in patients with NSCLC or IMT* and reducing the dosage according to the first dosage reduction level *in pediatric and young adult patients with ALCL or pediatric patients with IMT* (see Table 3).

No dosage adjustment is necessary in patients with mild preexisting hepatic impairment (AST concentration exceeding the ULN with total bilirubin concentration no more than the ULN, or total bilirubin concentration exceeding the ULN, but no more than 1.5 times the ULN, with any AST concentration).

Renal Impairment

For adult patients with severe renal impairment (creatinine clearance <30 mL/minute, calculated using the modified Cockroft-Gault equation) who do not require dialysis, the manufacturer recommends a crizotinib dosage of 250 mg *once daily* in *patients with NSCLC or IMT*.

For patients with severe renal impairment (creatinine clearance <30 mL/minute, calculated using the modified Cockroft-Gault equation for adults and the Schwartz equation for pediatric patients) who do not require dialysis, the manufacturer recommends a crizotinib dosage according to the second dosage reduction level in *pediatric and young adult patients with ALCL or pediatric patients with IMT* (see Table 3).

No dosage adjustment is necessary in patients with mild or moderate renal impairment (creatinine clearance 30–89 mL/minute).

Geriatric Patients

The manufacturer makes no specific dosage recommendations for geriatric patients.

CAUTIONS

● *Contraindications*

- None.

● *Warnings/Precautions*

Hepatic Toxicity

Drug-induced hepatotoxicity with fatal outcome has occurred; such cases were reported in 0.1% of patients receiving crizotinib in clinical trials. Concurrent alanine aminotransferase (ALT) or aspartate aminotransferase (AST) elevations of ≥3 times the upper limit of normal (ULN) and total bilirubin elevations of ≥2 times the ULN with normal alkaline phosphatase concentrations occurred in less than 1% of crizotinib-treated patients in clinical trials. ALT or AST elevations occurred in 11 or 6% of patients, respectively, in clinical trials in patients with NSCLC. ALT or AST elevations exceeding 5 times the ULN occurred in 4 or 4% of patients, respectively, in clinical trials in patients with ALCL. In clinical trials in patients with IMT treated with crizotinib, AST or ALT elevations occurred in 71% and 71% of pediatric patients, respectively and 57% and 43% of adult patients, respectively. Permanent discontinuance of crizotinib was required in 1% of patients with elevated ALT or AST concentrations in clinical trials in patients with NSCLC. Elevations in aminotransferase concentrations usually occurred within the first 2 months of treatment.

The manufacturer states that liver function tests, including ALT, AST, and total bilirubin, should be monitored every 2 weeks during the first 2 months of therapy, monthly thereafter, and as clinically indicated. More frequent repeat testing for increased aminotransferases, alkaline phosphatase, or total bilirubin is necessary in patients who develop aminotransferase elevations during therapy. If hepatotoxicity occurs, temporary interruption, dosage reduction, or discontinuance of crizotinib may be necessary.

Pulmonary Effects

Severe, life-threatening, or fatal interstitial lung disease or pneumonitis can occur in patients treated with crizotinib. In patients with NSCLC receiving crizotinib in clinical studies, grade 3 or 4 interstitial lung disease occurred in 1% of patients and fatal interstitial lung disease occurred in 0.5% of patients. Interstitial lung disease generally occurred within the first 3 months of therapy. In clinical studies of patients 1 to ≤21 years of age with relapsed or refractory tumors, including ALCL and IMT, interstitial lung disease occurred in 0.8% of patients.

Patients receiving the drug should be monitored for pulmonary symptoms indicative of interstitial lung disease or pneumonitis, and other causes of interstitial lung disease or pneumonitis should be excluded. Crizotinib should be permanently discontinued in patients who are diagnosed with treatment-related interstitial lung disease or pneumonitis.

Prolongation of QT Interval

Prolongation of the corrected QT (QT$_c$) interval has been observed in crizotinib-treated patients. The prolongation appears to occur in a plasma concentration-dependent manner. An increase in the QT$_c$ interval (corrected for heart rate using Fridericia's formula [QT$_c$F]) of ≥60 msec from baseline occurred in 5% of patients receiving crizotinib 250 mg twice daily, and QT$_c$F intervals of ≥500 msec occurred in 2.1% of crizotinib-treated patients. Prolongation of the QT$_c$ interval occurred in 8% of patients with ALCL and 7% of pediatric patients with IMT in clinical studies.

Crizotinib should be avoided in patients with congenital long QT syndrome. Electrocardiograms (ECGs) and serum electrolytes should be monitored in patients with congestive heart failure, bradyarrhythmias, or electrolyte abnormalities and in those who are receiving drugs known to prolong the QT interval.

If QT$_c$-interval prolongation occurs, temporary interruption, dosage reduction, or discontinuance of crizotinib may be necessary.

Bradycardia

Symptomatic bradycardia has been observed in crizotinib-treated patients. In clinical studies, bradycardia occurred in 13% of crizotinib-treated patients with NSCLC. Grade 3 syncope was reported in 2.4 or 0.6% of patients receiving crizotinib or standard chemotherapy, respectively. Bradycardia (all grade 1 severity) occurred in 19% of crizotinib-treated patients with ALCL in clinical studies. In pediatric patients with IMT treated with crixotinib, bradycardia occured in 14% of patients, including grade 3 bradycardia in 0.8% of patients.

Crizotinib should be avoided in patients who are receiving other drugs known to cause bradycardia (e.g., β-adrenergic blockers, nondihydropyridine calcium-channel blockers, clonidine, digoxin) when possible.

Heart rate and blood pressure should be monitored regularly during crizotinib therapy. If symptomatic or life-threatening bradycardia occurs, temporary interruption, dosage reduction, or discontinuance of crizotinib may be necessary depending on concomitant use of other drugs known to cause bradycardia.

Visual Disturbances

Visual disturbances, which may result in partial or complete loss of vision in one or both eyes, have been observed in crizotinib-treated patients; visual disturbances generally occur within 1 week of initiating therapy. In clinical studies, grade 4 visual field defects leading to vision loss occurred in 0.2% of crizotinib-treated patients with NSCLC. Visual disorders occurred in 65% of crizotinib-treated patients with ALCL and 50% of patients with IMT in clinical studies. Optic atrophy and optic nerve disorder also may cause vision loss.

In pediatric and young adult patients with ALCL or pediatric patients with IMT, perform ophthalmologic examination prior to starting crizotinib. Follow-up ophthalmologic examination including retinal examination is recommended within 1 month of treatment initiation, every 3 months thereafter. Assess visual symptoms monthly for all patients during treatment. If visual disturbances occur, consult an eye specialist. Permanently discontinue crizotinib for any grade 3 or 4 ocular disorders or for severe vision loss (best corrected vision less than 20/200 in one or both eyes) unless other etiology is identified. The manufacturer states that insufficient data are available to determine the risks of resuming crizotinib in patients who develop severe vision loss; the potential benefit of the drug to the patient must be carefully weighed against the potential risks of continued therapy.

GI Toxicity

Severe GI toxicities have been observed in pediatric and young adult patients with ALCL or in pediatric patients with IMT receiving crizotinib. GI toxicity has been reported in all patients receiving crizotinib for the treatment of ALCL; grade 3 toxicity (i.e., diarrhea, nausea, vomiting, stomatitis) has been reported in 27% of patients. In pediatric patients with IMT, vomiting occurred in 93%, nausea occurred in 86%, and diarrhea occurred in 64% of patients. Provide standard antiemetic and antidiarrheal agents for GI toxicities in pediatric and young adult patients with ALCL and pediatric patients with IMT.

Antiemetics are recommended prior to and during treatment with crizotinib to prevent nausea and vomiting. In patients who develop grade 3 nausea lasting 3 days or grade 3 or 4 diarrhea or vomiting despite maximum medical therapy, withhold crizotinib until symptoms resolve, and then resume at the next lower dosage level. When clinically indicated, consider supportive care such as hydration, electrolyte supplementation, and nutritional support.

Fetal/Neonatal Morbidity and Mortality

Crizotinib may cause fetal harm if administered to pregnant women; the drug has been shown to be embryotoxic and fetotoxic in animals. There are no adequate and well-controlled studies in humans.

Pregnancy should be avoided during therapy. Advise females of reproductive potential to use effective contraception during treatment with crizotinib and for 45 days following the last dose. Advise male patients with female partners of reproductive potential to use condoms during treatment with crizotinib and for 90 days after the last dose. If crizotinib is used during pregnancy or if the patient or their partner becomes pregnant during therapy, the patient should be apprised of the potential fetal hazard.

Specific Populations

Pregnancy

Crizotinib may cause fetal harm if administered to pregnant females based on its mechanism of action and animal findings.

Lactation

It is not known whether crizotinib is distributed into human milk. Because of the potential for serious adverse reactions to crizotinib in nursing infants, females should be advised not to breast-feed while receiving the drug and for 45 days after the drug is discontinued.

Females and Males of Reproductive Potential

The manufacturer states that a pregnancy test should be performed prior to initiation of crizotinib in females of reproductive potential and that such females should use effective contraceptive methods while receiving the drug and for at least 45 days after the drug is discontinued. Males with female partners should use condoms during and for at least 90 days after discontinuance of the drug.

Based on findings from animal studies, crizotinib may impair male and female fertility.

In repeat-dose toxicity studies, testicular pachytene spermatocyte degeneration and single-cell necrosis of ovarian follicles were observed in male and female rats, respectively, receiving crizotinib at exposure levels exceeding human exposure at the recommended dosage; whether these effects on fertility are reversible has not been established.

Pediatric Use

Safety and efficacy of crizotinib have been established in pediatric patients ≥12 months of age with relapsed or refractory systemic anaplastic lymphoma kinase (ALK)-positive ALCL or with unresectable, recurrent, or refractory (ALK)-positive IMT. Safety and efficacy have not been established in pediatric patients <12 months of age with ALCL or IMT or in any pediatric patients with NSCLC.

In a study of crizotinib in combination with chemotherapy in pediatric patients with newly diagnosed ALCL, 20% of patients experienced a grade 2 or higher thromboembolic event, including pulmonary embolism in 6% of the patients. The safety and efficacy of crizotinib in combination with chemotherapy have not been established in patients with newly diagnosed ALCL.

Decreased bone formation in growing long bones has been observed in immature rats receiving crizotinib for 28 days (at a dosage of 150 mg/kg daily, approximately 5.4 times the recommended human dosage based on AUC); other toxicities of potential concern in pediatric patients have not been evaluated to date in juvenile animal studies.

Geriatric Use

In clinical studies, 16% of patients with anaplastic lymphoma kinase (ALK)-positive metastatic NSCLC receiving crizotinib were ≥65 years of age and 3.8% were ≥75 years of age. No overall differences in safety or efficacy were observed between these geriatric patients and younger adults.

Clinical studies evaluating crizotinib in patients with c-ros oncogene-1 (ROS-1)-positive metastatic NSCLC did not include sufficient numbers of patients ≥65 years of age to determine whether geriatric patients respond differently than younger adults.

Hepatic Impairment

Dosage of crizotinib should be reduced in patients with preexisting moderate or severe hepatic impairment. Systemic exposure to crizotinib was increased in patients with moderate (total bilirubin concentration exceeding 1.5 times the upper limit of normal [ULN], but not exceeding 3 times ULN, with any AST concentration) or severe (total bilirubin concentration exceeding 3 times the ULN with any AST concentration) hepatic impairment; dosage adjustment is necessary in patients with preexisting moderate or severe hepatic impairment. Following administration of a reduced crizotinib dosage of 200 mg twice daily in patients with moderate hepatic impairment, mean AUC and peak plasma concentrations at steady state were increased by 14 and 9%, respectively, compared with patients with normal hepatic function receiving the recommended dosage of crizotinib (250 mg twice daily). Following administration of a reduced crizotinib dosage of 250 mg once daily in patients with severe hepatic impairment, mean AUC and peak plasma concentrations were decreased by 35 and 27%, respectively, compared with patients with normal hepatic function receiving the recommended dosage of crizotinib (250 mg twice daily).

Mean AUC and peak plasma concentrations of crizotinib at steady state were decreased by 9% in patients with mild hepatic impairment (AST concentration exceeding the ULN with total bilirubin concentration no more than the ULN, or total bilirubin concentration exceeding the ULN, but no more than 1.5 times the ULN, with any AST concentration) compared with patients with normal hepatic function following the recommended dosage of crizotinib (250 mg twice daily); no dosage adjustment is necessary in patients with preexisting mild hepatic impairment.

Renal Impairment

Following administration of a single 250-mg dose of crizotinib in patients with severe renal impairment (creatinine clearance <30 mL/minute) who did not require dialysis, mean peak plasma concentrations and AUC of crizotinib were increased by 34 and 79%, respectively, compared with patients with normal renal function; similar effects on the AUC and peak plasma concentrations of the active metabolite of crizotinib were observed in patients with severe renal impairment. The manufacturer recommends dosage adjustment in patients with severe renal impairment.

Systemic exposure of crizotinib was unaffected following administration of the drug in patients with mild (creatinine clearance 60–89 mL/minute) or moderate (creatinine clearance 30–59 mL/minute) renal impairment.

● Common Adverse Effects

Adverse effects reported in ≥25% of patients receiving crizotinib for the treatment of ALK-positive metastatic NSCLC include vision disorders, nausea, diarrhea, vomiting, edema, constipation, elevated aminotransferase concentrations, fatigue, decreased appetite, upper respiratory infection, dizziness, and neuropathy.

Adverse effects reported in ≥35% of pediatric patients receiving crizotinib for the treatment of IMT include vomiting, nausea, diarrhea, abdominal pain, rash, vision disorder, upper respiratory tract infection, cough, pyrexia, musculoskeletal pain, fatigue, edema, constipation, and headache. Adverse effects reported in ≥20% of adult patients receiving crizotinib for the treatment of IMT include vision disorders, nausea, and edema.

Adverse effects reported in ≥35% of patients receiving crizotinib for the treatment of ALCL include diarrhea, vomiting, nausea, vision disorder, headache, musculoskeletal pain, stomatitis, fatigue, decreased appetite, pyrexia, abdominal pain, cough, and pruritus.

Grade 3 or 4 laboratory abnormalities reported in ≥15% of patients receiving crizotinib for the treatment of ALCL include include neutropenia, lymphopenia, and thrombocytopenia.

DRUG INTERACTIONS

Crizotinib is metabolized principally by cytochrome P-450 (CYP) isoenzyme 3A. In vitro studies indicate that crizotinib is an inhibitor of CYP isoenzyme 2B6.

Crizotinib does not inhibit CYP isoenzymes 1A2, 2C8, 2C9, 2C19, or 2D6, or uridine diphosphate-glucuronosyl transferases (UGT) 1A1, 1A4, 1A6, 1A9, or 2B7. The drug also does not induce CYP isoenzymes 1A2, 2B6, 2C8, 2C9, 2C19, or 3A.

In vitro, crizotinib is an inhibitor and substrate of P-glycoprotein (P-gp). Crizotinib inhibits organic cation transporter (OCT) 1 and OCT2, but does not inhibit organic anion transport protein (OATP) B1, OATP1B3, organic anion transporter (OAT) 1, OAT3, or bile salt export pump (BSEP).

● Drugs and Foods Affecting Hepatic Microsomal Enzymes

Inhibitors of CYP3A

Concomitant use of crizotinib with potent inhibitors of CYP3A may result in increased systemic exposure to crizotinib and possible toxicity. When the potent CYP3A inhibitor ketoconazole was administered concomitantly with crizotinib (single 150-mg dose), peak plasma concentration and area under the concentration-time curve (AUC) of crizotinib were increased by 44 and 216%, respectively, compared with crizotinib administration alone. When the potent CYP3A inhibitor itraconazole was administered concomitantly with crizotinib (250 mg once daily), peak plasma concentration and AUC of crizotinib were increased by 33 and 57%, respectively, compared with crizotinib administration alone.

Concomitant use of crizotinib with potent CYP3A inhibitors (e.g., ketoconazole, itraconazole) should be avoided. If concomitant use of a potent CYP3A inhibitor cannot be avoided, the manufacturer recommends reducing the dosage of crizotinib to 250 mg *once daily* in adult patients with NSCLC or IMT and reducing the dosage according to the second dosage reduction level in pediatric and young adult patients with ALCL or pediatric patients with IMT (see Table 3). When concomitant use of the potent CYP3A inhibitor is discontinued, the crizotinib dosage should be returned to the dosage used prior to initiation of the potent CYP3A inhibitor.

Caution should be exercised with concomitant use of crizotinib and moderate CYP3A inhibitors.

Grapefruit products are CYP3A inhibitors and should be avoided because of the potential for increased plasma crizotinib concentrations during concurrent use.

Inducers of CYP3A

Concomitant use of crizotinib with potent inducers of CYP3A may result in decreased plasma concentrations of crizotinib and reduced crizotinib efficacy. When the potent CYP3A inducer rifampin was administered concomitantly with crizotinib (250 mg twice daily), AUC and peak plasma concentration of crizotinib were decreased by 84 and 79%, respectively, compared with crizotinib administration alone.

Concomitant use of crizotinib with potent CYP3A4 inducers should be avoided.

● Drugs Metabolized by Hepatic Microsomal Enzymes

Substrates of CYP3A

Concomitant use of crizotinib and substrates of CYP3A may result in increased plasma concentrations of the CYP3A substrate and possible toxicity. When the CYP3A substrate midazolam was administered concomitantly with crizotinib (250 mg twice daily for 28 days), AUC of midazolam increased 3.7-fold compared with midazolam administration alone.

Concomitant use of crizotinib with CYP3A substrates that have a narrow therapeutic index should be avoided. If concomitant use of CYP3A substrates that have a narrow therapeutic index cannot be avoided, the manufacturer recommends reducing the dosage of the substrate drug.

● Drugs that Prolong the QT Interval

Because crizotinib has been associated with QT-interval prolongation, the manufacturer recommends that concomitant use of crizotinib with other drugs known to prolong the QT interval be avoided. If concomitant use of other drugs known to prolong the QT interval cannot be avoided, the manufacturer recommends monitoring electrocardiograms (ECGs) and serum electrolytes.

● Drugs Associated with Bradycardia

Because crizotinib has been associated with bradycardia, concomitant use of crizotinib with other drugs known to cause bradycardia (e.g., β-adrenergic blocking agents, nondihydropyridine calcium-channel blocking agents, clonidine, digoxin) should be avoided, when possible.

● Drugs Affecting Gastric Acidity

Concomitant administration of crizotinib and the proton-pump inhibitor esomeprazole did not substantially affect the pharmacokinetics of crizotinib.

DESCRIPTION

Crizotinib, an inhibitor of receptor tyrosine kinases, including anaplastic lymphoma kinase (ALK), hepatocyte growth factor receptor (HGFR, c-Met), c-ros oncogene-1 (ROS-1), and recepteur d'origine nantais (RON), is an antineoplastic agent. Activating mutations or translocations of the *ALK* gene have been identified in several malignancies and can result in the expression of oncogenic fusion proteins (e.g., echinoderm microtubule-associated protein-like 4 [EML4]-ALK). Such *ALK* gene rearrangements have been identified in approximately 3–7% of patients with non-small cell lung cancer (NSCLC). Approximately 1–2% of patients with NSCLC have *ROS-1*-positive disease. Formation of ALK fusion proteins such as EML4-ALK results in activation and dysregulation of the gene's expression and signaling, which can contribute to increased cell proliferation and survival in tumors expressing these proteins. In vitro, crizotinib has demonstrated concentration-dependent inhibition of ALK, ROS-1, and c-Met phosphorylation. The drug has also demonstrated antitumor activity in mice bearing tumor xenografts that expressed EML4-ALK or nucleophosmin (NPM)-ALK fusion proteins or c-Met. In vitro, crizotinib induced apoptosis and inhibited proliferation and ALK-mediated signaling in anaplastic large cell lymphoma (ALCL)-derived cell lines at clinically achievable exposures.

Although crizotinib has demonstrated improved outcomes in patients with NSCLC harboring *ALK* mutations, secondary resistance to crizotinib eventually develops, generally within the first 1–2 years of treatment. Clinical resistance to crizotinib has been attributed to several possible mechanisms, including acquired resistance mutations of *ALK*, amplification of gene expression, and activation of alternate signaling pathways. Secondary mutations of *ALK* are responsible for about 30% of cases of acquired crizotinib resistance and gene amplification is implicated in 9% of these cases. The CNS is a common site of disease progression in crizotinib-treated patients because of poor distribution of the drug into CSF; development and/or progression of brain metastases occurs in approximately one-half of patients during crizotinib treatment.

Crizotinib is predominantly metabolized by the cytochrome P-450 (CYP) isoenzyme 3A. Following oral administration of a single 250-mg radiolabeled dose of crizotinib, approximately 63% of the radioactivity was recovered in feces and 22% was recovered in urine; unchanged drug accounted for 53% of the dose recovered in feces and 2.3% of the dose recovered in urine. The mean terminal half-life of crizotinib is 42 hours. The mean absolute bioavailability of crizotinib following oral administration as capsules is approximately 43%. Bioavailability of the oral pellets is comparable to that of the oral capsules. Following administration of a single capsule dose of crizotinib, peak plasma concentrations of the drug are achieved in a median of 4–6 hours. In vitro, crizotinib is 91% bound to plasma proteins, and binding is independent of crizotinib concentration. Following administration of crizotinib over the dose range of 200 to 300 mg twice daily, trough plasma concentrations and AUC increase in a greater than dose-proportional manner; steady-state concentrations of the drug are achieved in 15 days, with a median accumulation ratio of 4.8. AUC and peak plasma concentrations were reduced by approximately 14% when crizotinib in the capsule formulation was administered with a high-fat meal; for the pellet formulation, AUC and peak plasma concentrations were reduced by 15% and 23%, respectively. The pharmacokinetics of crizotinib are not affected by age, sex, or ethnicity (Asian or non-Asian). In patients ≤18 years of age, crizotinib exposure is lower in patients with higher body weight.

ADVICE TO PATIENTS

- Importance of taking crizotinib exactly as prescribed and of not altering the dosage or discontinuing therapy unless advised to do so by clinician. Importance of swallowing crizotinib capsules whole. Administer crizotinib pellets by opening the shells containing the pellets and emptying the contents directly into the patient's mouth or via use of a dosing aid (e.g., spoon, medicine cup).

- If a dose is missed, importance of taking the missed dose as soon as it is remembered, unless it is less than 6 hours before the next dose, in which case the missed dose should be omitted. Do not take a double dose to make up for a missed dose. If a dose is vomited after administration, an additional dose should not be administered to replace the vomited dose. The next dose should be administered at the next scheduled time.

- Importance of avoiding grapefruit products while taking crizotinib.

- Risk of fetal harm. Necessity of advising females of reproductive potential that they should use effective contraceptive methods while receiving the drug and for ≥45 days after the drug is discontinued. Importance of advising males who are partners with females of reproductive potential to use a condom while receiving the drug and for ≥90 days after the drug is discontinued. Importance of patients informing their clinicians if they or their partners are pregnant or think they may be pregnant. If pregnancy occurs, advise of potential risk to fetus.

- Importance of advising females to avoid breast-feeding while receiving crizotinib therapy and for 45 days after discontinuance of therapy.

- Risk of impaired female and male fertility.

- Risk of hepatotoxicity; importance of regular liver function test monitoring. Importance of immediately reporting possible symptoms of hepatotoxicity (e.g., weakness, fatigue, anorexia, nausea, vomiting, abdominal pain [especially right upper quadrant pain], jaundice, dark urine, generalized pruritus, bleeding diathesis), particularly in combination with fever and rash.

- Risk of GI toxicity in pediatric and young adult patients with anaplastic large cell lymphoma (ALCL) and in pediatric patients with IMT. Inform patients of the risk of severe nausea, vomiting, diarrhea, and stomatitis, and to immediately inform their clinician if problems with swallowing, vomiting, or diarrhea occur.

- Risk of photosensitivity. Advise patients to avoid prolonged sun exposure and to use sunscreen or protective clothing.

- Risk of interstitial lung disease/pneumonitis. Importance of immediately reporting any new or worsening pulmonary symptoms (e.g., dyspnea, shortness of breath, cough with or without mucus, fever); interstitial lung disease/pneumonitis symptoms may be similar to those from lung cancer.

- Risk of QT-interval prolongation or bradycardia. Importance of informing clinicians immediately if changes in heartbeat or feelings of dizziness or faintness occur.

- Risk of visual disturbances, sometimes severe, that may result in vision loss; such changes occur commonly, usually during the first week of therapy. Importance of immediately reporting loss of vision or other visual disturbances (e.g., double vision, blurred vision, flashes of light, photosensitivity, floaters) to clinicians.

- Importance of exercising caution when driving or operating machinery in the event that visual changes, dizziness, or fatigue occurs.

- Importance of informing clinician of existing or contemplated concomitant therapy, including prescription (e.g., cardiac or antihypertensive agents) and OTC drugs and herbal supplements (e.g., grapefruit-containing products), as well as any concomitant illnesses (e.g., hepatic or renal impairment, cardiovascular disease [including congenital long QT syndrome]).

- Importance of informing patients of other important precautionary information.

For further information on the handling of antineoplastic agents, see the ASHP Guidelines on Handling Hazardous Drugs at https://www.ahfsdrug information.com.

PREPARATIONS

Crizotinib is available only from designated specialty pharmacies. Consult the manufacturer's website for additional information.

Excipients in commercially available drug preparations may have clinically important effects in some individuals; consult specific product labeling for details.

Crizotinib

Oral		
Capsules	200 mg	**Xalkori®**, Pfizer
	250 mg	**Xalkori®**, Pfizer
Pellets	20 mg	**Xalkori®**
	50 mg	**Xalkori®**
	150 mg	**Xalkori®**

† Use is not currently included in the labeling approved by the US Food and Drug Administration.

Selected Revisions February 10, 2024, © Copyright, October 31, 2012, American Society of Health-System Pharmacists, Inc.

Cyclophosphamide

10:00 · ANTINEOPLASTIC AGENTS

■ Cyclophosphamide, a nitrogen mustard-derivative, polyfunctional alkylating agent, is an antineoplastic agent and immunosuppressant.

USES

● Hodgkin's Disease

Cyclophosphamide is used in combination regimens (e.g., bleomycin, etoposide, doxorubicin, cyclophosphamide, vincristine, procarbazine, and prednisone [BEACOPP]) for the treatment of Hodgkin's disease.

● Non-Hodgkin's Lymphoma

Cyclophosphamide is used in combination therapy for the treatment of non-Hodgkin's lymphoma, including high-grade lymphomas, such as Burkitt's lymphoma and lymphoblastic lymphoma, as well as intermediate- and low-grade lymphomas. For example, cyclophosphamide is commonly used with doxorubicin, vincristine, and prednisone (known as the CHOP regimen), with or without other agents, in the treatment of various types of intermediate-grade non-Hodgkin's lymphoma. Cyclophosphamide also has been used as a single agent in the treatment of low-grade lymphomas.

● Multiple Myeloma

Cyclophosphamide is used in combination with prednisone, or as a component of combination chemotherapy (i.e., vincristine, carmustine, melphalan, cyclophosphamide, and prednisone [VBMCP]) for the treatment of multiple myeloma. Comparative studies have shown the effectiveness of cyclophosphamide in the treatment of multiple myeloma to be equivalent to that of melphalan, and the combination of either agent with prednisone is considered a treatment of choice. Some authorities prefer melphalan to cyclophosphamide because of the lesser severity of adverse effects; in the presence of severe thrombocytopenia, others prefer cyclophosphamide because of its relative platelet-sparing effect.

Use of cyclophosphamide in combination with bortezomib and dexamethasone (bortezomib-cyclophosphamide-dexamethasone) as induction therapy for newly diagnosed multiple myeloma in transplant-eligible patients may be considered a reasonable choice (accepted, with possible conditions) based on current evidence from 2 noncomparative phase 2 studies and an open-label, randomized phase 3 study (GMMG-MM5); factors that should be considered when selecting a combination chemotherapy regimen for use as induction therapy include cytogenetic features, performance status, preexisting conditions (e.g., peripheral neuropathy), and tolerability.

In the first phase 2 study, the overall response rate and rate of very good partial response or better after 4 cycles of therapy were 88 and 61%, respectively, in the study group (cohort of 33 patients with newly diagnosed multiple myeloma who received cyclophosphamide in combination with bortezomib [twice weekly] and dexamethasone) compared with 91 and 44%, respectively, in a historical control group (34 patients who received lenalidomide and dexamethasone). Among patients who underwent stem cell transplantation following bortezomib-cyclophosphamide-dexamethasone induction therapy, the posttransplant complete or near-complete response rate was 70%. A subsequent cohort of 30 patients who received cyclophosphamide with bortezomib (once weekly) and dexamethasone achieved similar overall response rates and rates of very good partial response or better (93 and 60%, respectively). Median progression-free survival for the 2 cohorts combined was 40 months, and 5-year progression-free and overall survival rates for the 2 cohorts were 42 and 70%, respectively. Although the overall response rate was similar in patients with high-risk cytogenetic features and those with standard-risk cytogenetic features, median progression-free survival was shorter and 5-year progression-free and overall survival rates were lower in patients with high-risk cytogenetic features (27.6 months, 33%, and 54%, respectively) compared with those with standard-risk cytogenetic features (55.7 months, 48%, and 81%, respectively).

In another phase 2 study in 44 patients with newly diagnosed multiple myeloma who received 3 cycles of bortezomib-cyclophosphamide-dexamethasone followed by 3 cycles of bortezomib-thalidomide-dexamethasone, very good partial response or better was observed in 31 or 57% of 42 evaluable patients following 3 or 6 treatment cycles, respectively; near-complete response or better was observed following 3 or 6 cycles in 2 or 36% of patients, respectively. At a median follow-up of 20.9 months, estimated 1-year event-free and overall survival rates were 81 and 91%, respectively.

In the GMMG-MM5 study in 502 patients with newly diagnosed multiple myeloma, rates of overall response (78.1 versus 72.1%, respectively) and very good partial response or better (37 versus 34.3%, respectively) did not differ significantly between patients receiving bortezomib-cyclophosphamide-dexamethasone and those receiving bortezomib-doxorubicin-dexamethasone. In subgroups of patients with poor prognostic factors (i.e., t(4;14) translocation, chromosome 17p deletion [del(17p)], and/or chromosome 1q21 duplication [1q21 gain]; renal impairment), response rates attained with bortezomib-cyclophosphamide-dexamethasone appeared to be at least as high as those attained with bortezomib-doxorubicin-dexamethasone; the rate of progressive disease in patients with high-risk cytogenetic features, International Staging System (ISS) stage III disease, or renal impairment appeared to be higher in those receiving bortezomib-doxorubicin-dexamethasone compared with those receiving bortezomib-cyclophosphamide-dexamethasone.

For further information on the use of combination therapy with cyclophosphamide, bortezomib, and dexamethasone as induction therapy for newly diagnosed multiple myeloma in transplant-eligible patients, see Induction Therapy Prior to Stem Cell Transplantation in Newly Diagnosed Multiple Myeloma under Uses: Multiple Myeloma, in Bortezomib 10:00.

● Leukemias

In the treatment of chronic lymphocytic (lymphoblastic) leukemia, cyclophosphamide is considered one of the drugs of choice. Cyclophosphamide is used in combination with busulfan as a conditioning regimen prior to allogeneic hematopoietic progenitor cell transplantation in patients with chronic myelogenous leukemia.

Cyclophosphamide is used in the treatment of acute lymphoblastic leukemia, especially in children.

In the treatment of acute myeloid (myelogenous, nonlymphocytic) leukemia (AML, ANLL), cyclophosphamide has been used as an additional drug for induction or post induction therapy.

Although cyclophosphamide and its metabolites appear in the brain and CSF, concentrations are probably insufficient to treat meningeal leukemia.

● Cutaneous T-cell Lymphoma

Cyclophosphamide is used alone or in combination regimens for the treatment of advanced mycosis fungoides, a form of cutaneous T-cell lymphoma.

● Neuroblastoma

In the treatment of disseminated neuroblastoma, cyclophosphamide used alone has been reported to produce objective responses in up to 65% of patients; used in combinations, the response rate and duration of survival may increase. Combination chemotherapy that includes cyclophosphamide is a treatment of choice for this neoplasm.

● Ovarian Cancer

Cyclophosphamide is used in combination chemotherapy (vincristine, dactinomycin, and cyclophosphamide [VAC]) as an alternative regimen for the treatment of ovarian germ cell tumors†.

Although cyclophosphamide has been used in combination with a platinum-containing agent for the treatment of advanced (stage III or IV) epithelial ovarian cancer, evidence from randomized trials indicates that combined therapy with paclitaxel and a platinum-containing agent is superior (higher response rates, prolonged overall survival) and therefore is the preferred regimen. (See Uses: Ovarian Cancer, in Carboplatin 10:00 and Cisplatin 10:00.)

● Retinoblastoma

Cyclophosphamide is used in combination therapy for the treatment of retinoblastoma.

● Breast Cancer

In the treatment of breast cancer, cyclophosphamide used alone has been reported to produce objective responses in about 35% of patients. Used in combination regimens, objective responses have been reported in up to 90% of patients, and cyclophosphamide-containing combinations are believed by some experts to be the treatment of choice.

Combination chemotherapy used as an adjunct to surgery has been shown to increase both disease-free (i.e., decreased recurrence) and overall survival in premenopausal and postmenopausal women with node-negative or -positive early (TNM stage I or II) breast cancer. Adjuvant combination chemotherapy has produced overall reductions in the annual rates of recurrence and death of 28 and 16%, respectively, with overall 5-year disease-free survival rates of 58.8 versus 49.6% for patients receiving combination chemotherapy versus those who did not. Adjuvant combination chemotherapy that includes cyclophosphamide, methotrexate, and fluorouracil has been used extensively and is considered a regimen of choice. Although adjuvant hormonal therapy with tamoxifen (with or without combination chemotherapy) generally is used for node-positive, estrogen-receptor-positive postmenopausal women, adjuvant combination chemotherapy (with or without tamoxifen) also can be used in such patients, but differences in toxicity profiles may influence the choice of regimen. For node-positive premenopausal women, adjuvant combination chemotherapy (with or without tamoxifen) generally is used. Adjuvant therapy with combination chemotherapy and/or tamoxifen has been used in women with node-negative disease.

Controversy currently exists regarding which patients with node-negative and estrogen-receptor-negative breast cancer are most likely to benefit from such adjuvant therapy following surgery (see Uses: Breast Cancer, in Fluorouracil 10:00), but such patients with poor prognosis are reasonable candidates for adjuvant chemotherapy with an effective regimen (e.g., 6–12 months of cyclophosphamide, methotrexate, and fluorouracil initiated within 6 weeks of surgery); other node-negative patients also may be suitable candidates, but toxicities, costs, and other quality-of-life considerations should be weighed in assessing potential benefit. All patients with node-negative breast cancer are at some risk of recurrence, and effective adjuvant combination chemotherapy can increase both disease-free and overall survival, albeit less markedly than in patients with node-positive disease.

In patients with node-positive early breast cancer (i.e., stage II), an effective regimen of adjuvant combination chemotherapy (e.g., cyclophosphamide, methotrexate, and fluorouracil; cyclophosphamide, doxorubicin, and fluorouracil; cyclophosphamide and doxorubicin with or without tamoxifen) is used to reduce the rate of recurrence and improve survival in both premenopausal and postmenopausal patients once treatment to control local disease (surgery, with or without radiation therapy) has been undertaken. These combinations have been tested and established as providing therapeutic benefit, and are superior to single-agent therapy with conventional agents; numerous other combination regimens providing apparently similar outcomes also have been used but are less common or have been studied less extensively. Although long-term (e.g., 6 months or longer) chemotherapy with adjuvant regimens is clinically superior to short-term (e.g., preoperative and perioperative) adjuvant regimens, clinical superiority between 6- versus 12-month regimens has not been demonstrated. There is some evidence that the addition of doxorubicin to a regimen of cyclophosphamide, methotrexate, and fluorouracil can improve outcome further in patients with more than 3 positive axillary lymph nodes, and that sequential (i.e., administering several courses of doxorubicin first) regimens are more effective than alternating regimens in such patients; in patients with fewer positive nodes, no additional benefit from doxorubicin has been demonstrated. The dose intensity of adjuvant combination chemotherapy also appears to be an important factor influencing clinical outcome in patients with early node-positive breast cancer, with response increasing with increasing dose intensity; therefore, arbitrary reductions in dose intensity should be avoided.

In stage III (locally advanced) breast cancer, combination chemotherapy (with or without hormonal therapy) is used sequentially following surgery and radiation therapy for operable disease and following biopsy and radiation therapy for inoperable disease; commonly employed effective regimens include cyclophosphamide, methotrexate, and fluorouracil; cyclophosphamide, doxorubicin, and fluorouracil; and cyclophosphamide, methotrexate, fluorouracil, and prednisone. These and other regimens also have been used in the treatment or more advanced (stage IV) and recurrent disease.

• Small Cell Lung Cancer

Cyclophosphamide is used in combination chemotherapy regimens (e.g., cyclophosphamide, doxorubicin, and vincristine [CAV]; cyclophosphamide, doxorubicin, and etoposide [CAE]) for the treatment of extensive-stage small cell lung

cancer†. Survival outcomes are similar in patients with extensive-stage small cell lung cancer receiving CAV or cisplatin/etoposide. Combination chemotherapy regimens have produced response rates of 70–85% and complete response rates of 20–30% in patients with extensive-stage disease; however, comparative efficacy is continually being evaluated. Because the current prognosis for small cell lung cancer is unsatisfactory regardless of stage and despite considerable diagnostic and therapeutic advances, all patients with this cancer are candidates for inclusion in clinical trials at the time of diagnosis.

• Sarcomas

Cyclophosphamide has been used in combination regimens (usually with dactinomycin and vincristine) and as an adjunct to surgery and radiation therapy in the treatment of rhabdomyosarcoma†. In children in groups I and II, 2-year relapse-free survival rates of 80–90% have been reported. Intensive regimens of dactinomycin, cyclophosphamide, and vincristine (with or without doxorubicin) followed by radiation therapy have produced an objective response in 80% of patients having residual tumor following surgery (group III) or with metastatic tumor (group IV). Cyclophosphamide used in combination regimens as an adjunct to surgery and radiation therapy is considered one of the treatments of choice for Ewing's sarcoma†.

• Other Uses

Cyclophosphamide is used in selected cases of biopsy-proven minimal change nephrotic syndrome in children; the drug should not be used as initial therapy in such patients. Cyclophosphamide has induced remission in patients whose disease has not responded to appropriate corticosteroid therapy or in whom such therapy produces intolerable adverse effects (e.g., growth failure).

Cyclophosphamide is used in combination with vincristine and dacarbazine for the treatment of pheochromocytoma†. Cyclophosphamide also is used in the treatment of brain tumors†, choriocarcinoma†, and Wilms' tumor†.

As an immunosuppressant, cyclophosphamide has been used to control rejection following kidney, heart, liver, and bone marrow transplants†. Some experts consider cyclophosphamide as effective as azathioprine for the maintenance of renal allografts and superior to azathioprine for the maintenance of hepatic allografts. Cyclophosphamide has also been used with some success in the treatment of severe, active and progressive rheumatoid disorders†. In the treatment of glomerulonephritis,† especially in children, cyclophosphamide alone or in conjunction with corticosteroids has been useful. Other disorders of altered immune reactivity in which cyclophosphamide has been used with some success include Wegener's granulomatosis†, idiopathic pulmonary hemosiderosis†, myasthenia gravis†, multiple sclerosis†, polymyositis†, pyoderma gangrenosum†, bullous pemphigoid†, pemphigus vulgaris†, autoallergic ocular disease†, uveitis†, orbital pseudotumor†, scleromalacia perforans†, thyroid exophthalmopathy†, corneal transplant rejection†, systemic lupus erythematosus†, lupus nephritis†, autoimmune hemolytic anemia†, idiopathic thrombocytic purpura†, macroglobulinemia†, cryoglobulinemia†, and antibody-induced pure red cell aplasia†. The drug has also been used for the treatment of bleeding syndromes in patients with acquired antibodies to clotting factors†. Because of the potential for serious adverse effects, cyclophosphamide must be used as an immunosuppressant† with caution, and some experts advocate reserving use of cyclophosphamide for patients who become refractory to corticosteroids or other less toxic agents, or limiting it to short-term use whenever feasible.

DOSAGE AND ADMINISTRATION

• Reconstitution and Administration

Cyclophosphamide is administered orally or by IV injection or infusion. Less frequently, the drug has been administered IM and by intracavitary (e.g., intrapleural, intraperitoneal) injection and direct perfusion, but some experts believe the drug should not be administered via routes which bypass activation in the liver.

The choice of diluent for reconstituting cyclophosphamide powder for injection containing cyclophosphamide monohydrate depends on the route of administration to be used. If the solution is to be used for direct injection, cyclophosphamide powder for injection (containing cyclophosphamide monohydrate) is reconstituted by adding 0.9% sterile sodium chloride solution. If the solution is to be used for IV infusion, cyclophosphamide powder for injection (containing cyclophosphamide monohydrate) is reconstituted by adding sterile water for injection. Cyclophosphamide powder for injection (containing cyclophosphamide monohydrate) reconstituted in water is *hypotonic* and should *not* be injected directly. Cyclophosphamide powder for injection (containing cyclophosphamide monohydrate) is reconstituted by adding 25 mL of diluent to the vial labeled as containing 500 mg, 50 mL to the vial labeled as containing 1 g, or 100 mL to the vial labeled as containing 2 g. After adding the diluent to the vial, the vial should be shaken vigorously to dissolve the drug. If the powder fails to dissolve immediately and completely, the vial should be allowed to stand for a few minutes.

Reconstituted solutions of cyclophosphamide to be used for IV infusion may be diluted in one of the following compatible solutions: 5% dextrose injection, 5% dextrose and 0.9% sodium chloride injection, 5% dextrose and Ringer's injection, lactated Ringer's injection, 0.45% sodium chloride injection, or (1/6) *M* sodium lactate injection.

Cyclophosphamide solutions should be inspected visually for particulate matter and discoloration prior to administration whenever solution and container permit.

Extemporaneous liquid preparations of the drug for oral administration may be prepared by dissolving cyclophosphamide powder for injection in aromatic elixir. The manufacturer states that such solutions should be stored under refrigeration in glass containers and used within 14 days.

• Dosage

Because of the risk of certain toxicities (e.g., cardiotoxicity) and overdosage with high doses of cyclophosphamide, particular care should be taken to ensure that correct dosages and administration schedules have been prescribed and appropriate monitoring instituted when higher than usual dosages (e.g., those employed under protocol conditions) are encountered.

Clinicians should consult published protocols for the dosage of cyclophosphamide and other chemotherapeutic agents in combination regimens and the method and sequence of administration.

General Dosage

The manufacturers state that, in patients with no hematologic deficiencies receiving cyclophosphamide monotherapy, induction therapy in adults and children is usually initiated with an IV cyclophosphamide loading dose of 40–50 mg/kg administered in divided doses over 2–5 days. Other regimens for IV administration include 10–15 mg/kg every 7–10 days or 3–5 mg/kg twice weekly.

If cyclophosphamide is administered orally, the usual dose for induction or maintenance therapy is 1–5 mg/kg daily, depending on the tolerance of the patient.

Various other regimens for IV or oral cyclophosphamide have been reported. Dosage of cyclophosphamide must be adjusted according to tumor response and/or leukopenia. The total leukocyte count is used as a guide for regulating cyclophosphamide dosage. Transient decreases in the total leukocyte count to 2000/mm³ (following short courses of therapy) or more persistent reduction to 3000/mm³ (with continuing therapy) may be tolerated without serious risk of infection if there is no marked granulocytopenia.

When cyclophosphamide is included in combination regimens with other cytotoxic agents, dosage reduction for cyclophosphamide as well as for the other agents may be necessary.

Breast Cancer

Various cyclophosphamide-containing combination chemotherapy regimens have been used in the treatment of breast cancer, and published protocols should be consulted for dosages and the method and sequence of administration. The dose intensity of adjuvant combination chemotherapy appears to be an important factor influencing clinical outcome in patients with early node-positive breast cancer, with response increasing with increasing dose intensity; therefore, *arbitrary* reductions in dose intensity should be avoided.

One commonly employed regimen for the treatment of early breast cancer includes a cyclophosphamide dosage of 100 mg/m² orally on days 1 through 14 of each cycle combined with methotrexate 40 mg/m² IV on days 1 and 8 of each cycle and fluorouracil 600 mg/m² IV on days 1 and 8 of each cycle. In patients older than 60 years of age, the initial methotrexate dosage was reduced to 30 mg/m² IV and the initial fluorouracil dosage was reduced to 400 mg/m² IV. Dosage also was reduced if myelosuppression developed. Cycles generally were repeated monthly (i.e., allowing a 2-week rest period between cycles) for a total of 6–12 cycles (i.e., 6–12 months of therapy). Clinical superiority between 6- versus 12-month regimens has not been demonstrated.

There is some evidence that the addition of doxorubicin to a regimen of cyclophosphamide, methotrexate, and fluorouracil can improve outcome further in patients with early breast cancer and more than 3 positive axillary lymph nodes, and that sequential (i.e., administering several courses of doxorubicin first) regimens are more effective than alternating regimens in such patients; in patients with fewer positive nodes, no additional benefit from doxorubicin has been demonstrated. In the sequential regimen, 4 doses of doxorubicin hydrochloride 75 mg/m² IV were administered initially at 3-week intervals followed by 8 cycles of cyclophosphamide 600 mg/m² IV, methotrexate 40 mg/m² IV, and fluorouracil 600 mg/m² IV at 3-week intervals for a total of approximately 9 months of therapy. If myelosuppression developed with this sequential regimen, the subsequent cycle generally was delayed rather than reducing dosage.

Nephrotic Syndrome

In the treatment of minimal change nephrotic syndrome in children, an oral dosage of 2.5–3 mg/kg daily for 60–90 days has been recommended. In males, treatment for longer than 60 days increases the incidence of oligospermia and azoospermia; treatment for longer than 90 days increases the risk of sterility. Corticosteroid therapy may be tapered and discontinued during the course of cyclophosphamide therapy.

Multiple Myeloma

Cyclophosphamide has been used in several regimens in combination with bortezomib and dexamethasone as induction therapy for newly diagnosed multiple myeloma in transplant-eligible patients.

When cyclophosphamide has been used in combination with bortezomib and dexamethasone as induction therapy for newly diagnosed multiple myeloma in transplant-eligible patients, cyclophosphamide 300 mg/m² has been administered orally on days 1, 8, 15, and 22 along with bortezomib 1.3 mg/m² by IV injection twice weekly for 2 weeks (days 1, 4, 8, and 11) and dexamethasone 40 mg orally on days 1–4, 9–12, and 17–20 of each 28-day cycle for 4 cycles.

Cyclophosphamide 300 mg/m² also has been administered orally on days 1, 8, 15, and 22 along with bortezomib 1.5 mg/m² by IV injection once weekly (days 1, 8, 15, and 22) during each 28-day cycle for 4 cycles. In this regimen, dexamethasone 40 mg has been administered orally on days 1–4, 9–12, and 17–20 during cycles 1 and 2 and then once weekly during cycles 3 and 4.

Cyclophosphamide 300 mg/m² also has been administered IV on days 1 and 8 along with bortezomib 1.3 mg/m² by IV injection twice weekly for 2 weeks (days 1, 4, 8, and 11) and dexamethasone 40 mg orally on days 1, 2, 4, 5, 8, 9, 11, and 12 of each 21-day cycle for 3 cycles (cycles 1–3) followed by bortezomib 1 mg/m² by IV injection twice weekly for 2 weeks (days 1, 4, 8, and 11) along with thalidomide 100 mg orally daily and dexamethasone 40 mg orally on days 1, 2, 4, 5, 8, 9, 11, and 12 of each 21-day cycle for 3 cycles (cycles 4–6).

Cyclophosphamide 900 mg/m² also has been administered IV on day 1 along with bortezomib 1.3 mg/m² by subcutaneous or IV injection twice weekly for 2 weeks (days 1, 4, 8, and 11) and dexamethasone 40 mg orally on days 1, 2, 4, 5, 8, 9, 11, and 12 of each 21-day cycle for 3 cycles.

• Dosage in Renal and Hepatic Impairment

The effects of renal or hepatic impairment on the elimination of cyclophosphamide have not been elucidated. The manufacturers recommend caution and careful monitoring for toxicity in patients with renal and/or hepatic impairment, but makes no specific recommendations for adjustment of cyclophosphamide dosage. Measurable changes in pharmacokinetic parameters for cyclophosphamide may be observed in patients with renal impairment, but there is no consistent evidence demonstrating the need for dosage adjustment.

CAUTIONS

• Hematologic Effects

One of the major and dose-limiting adverse effects of cyclophosphamide is hematologic toxicity, which is usually reversible after discontinuance of the drug. Hematopoietic adverse effects include leukopenia, thrombocytopenia, hypothrombinemia, and anemia. Leukopenia is considered to be an expected effect of cyclophosphamide therapy and may be severe. Leukopenia nadirs generally occur at 8–15 days following a single dose of cyclophosphamide and recovery usually occurs within 17–28 days. Fever in the absence of documented infection has been reported in some patients with neutropenia. Thrombocytopenia reportedly is less common, with nadirs occurring 10–15 days after administration of the drug. Anemia, particularly after large doses or prolonged therapy, and rarely, hypoprothrombinemia have been reported. Rarely, cyclophosphamide has been reported to produce positive direct antiglobulin (Coombs') test results and hemolytic anemia.

GI and Hepatic Effects

Anorexia, nausea, and vomiting occur commonly with cyclophosphamide, especially at high doses; some clinicians reported that these effects respond to treatment with antiemetics. Occasionally, diarrhea, hemorrhagic colitis, mucosal irritation, and oral ulceration have been reported. Rarely, aphthous stomatitis, enterocolitis, and hepatotoxicity as evidenced by jaundice and hepatic dysfunction have occurred.

Genitourinary Effects

Sterile hemorrhagic cystitis has been reported to occur in up to 20% of patients (especially children) on long-term cyclophosphamide therapy. This effect, which rarely can be severe and even fatal, is attributed to chemical irritation by active metabolites of cyclophosphamide that accumulate in concentrated urine. Hematuria usually resolves spontaneously within a few days after discontinuance of cyclophosphamide therapy but may persist for several months. Fibrosis of the bladder (sometimes extensive), with or without cystitis, also has occurred, but less frequently. Atypical epithelial cells may be found in the urinary sediment. These adverse effects appear to be related to the dosage and duration of cyclophosphamide therapy. Nephrotoxicity, including hemorrhagic ureteritis and renal tubular necrosis, has been reported; such lesions reportedly resolve in most instances following discontinuance of cyclophosphamide therapy.

Although the incidence of hemorrhagic cystitis associated with cyclophosphamide therapy appears to be lower than that associated with ifosfamide therapy, mesna (sodium 2-mercaptoethanesulfonate) has been used prophylactically as a uroprotective agent in some patients receiving cyclophosphamide. (See Drug Interactions: Mesna.) Evidence from animal and clinical studies suggests that prophylactic mesna therapy, when used concomitantly with cyclophosphamide, can substantially decrease the incidence and severity of, or prevent, cyclophosphamide-induced urothelial toxicity (e.g., hemorrhagic cystitis). Mesna also has uroprotective activity in preventing or ameliorating recurrent or worsening bladder toxicity during subsequent cyclophosphamide therapy in patients with a history of such toxicity induced by the drug or other oxazaphosphorine derivatives (e.g., ifosfamide). Clinical studies indicate that mesna generally is more effective than, but at least as effective as, standard prophylactic measures (e.g., forced diuresis, hydration) in preventing bladder toxicity (e.g., hematuria, hemorrhagic cystitis) commonly associated with cyclophosphamide therapy, although prophylactic mesna therapy is not effective in all patients.

Dermatologic Effects

Alopecia occurs frequently in patients who receive cyclophosphamide, and patients should be forewarned of this possibility. In usual doses, about 33% of patients who receive the drug experience alopecia, generally beginning about 3 weeks after initiation of therapy; the condition is usually reversible, but new hair may be a different color or texture. Transverse ridging, retarded growth, and/or pigmentation of fingernails may occur, as well as skin pigmentation. Nonspecific dermatitis has also been reported.

Stevens-Johnson syndrome and toxic epidermal necrolysis have been reported rarely in patients receiving cyclophosphamide; a causal relationship to the drug has not been established.

Respiratory Effects

Patients who receive high doses of cyclophosphamide over prolonged periods may develop interstitial pulmonary fibrosis, which can be fatal. In some cases, discontinuance of the drug and administration of corticosteroids has failed to reverse this syndrome. Interstitial pneumonitis also has been reported in patients receiving cyclophosphamide.

Metabolic Effects

As a result of extensive purine catabolism accompanying rapid cellular destruction, hyperuricemia may occur in some patients receiving cyclophosphamide, especially those with non-Hodgkin's lymphomas or leukemias. Hyperuricemia

may be minimized by adequate hydration, alkalinization of the urine, and/or administration of allopurinol. If allopurinol is administered, the patient should be watched carefully for cyclophosphamide toxicity. (See Drug Interactions: Drugs Affecting Hepatic Microsomal Enzymes.) Hyperkalemia has been reported in patients receiving cyclophosphamide. Hyperkalemia probably is related to rapid lysis of tumor cells which occurs especially in connection with lymphomas or leukemias.

A syndrome of inappropriate antidiuretic hormone secretion has occurred during cyclophosphamide therapy. Hyponatremia resulting from impaired excretion of water associated with progressive weight gain without edema occurs. The tendency toward water retention in these patients is aggravated by the common practice of encouraging fluid intake to prevent formation of uric acid calculi and the occurrence of chemical cystitis.

Cardiac Effects

Cardiotoxicity, which is uncommon at usual dosages, has been reported in patients receiving high doses of cyclophosphamide (120 [i.e., 60 mg/kg daily] to 270 mg/kg over a period of a few days), generally as part of an intensive, multiple-drug antineoplastic regimen or in conjunction with transplantation procedures. Potentially fatal cardiotoxicity also has occurred when cyclophosphamide (given concomitantly with mesna and followed with autologous bone marrow transplant) was administered inadvertently in a dosage of 4 g/m^2 daily for 4 doses rather than in a total dosage of 4 g/m^2 administered over 4 days in equally divided doses of 1 g/m^2 daily as part of a phase I protocol. Deaths have occurred from diffuse hemorrhagic myocardial necrosis and from a syndrome of acute myopericarditis when cyclophosphamide was used in high doses alone or in combination regimens; severe, sometimes fatal congestive heart failure has occurred rarely within a few days after the first dose of cyclophosphamide in such cases. Hemopericardium secondary to hemorrhagic myocarditis and myocardial necrosis, and pericarditis without evidence of hemopericardium, also have been reported. Acute myocardial infarction occurred in a patient with no history of cardiac conditions who received conventional doses of cyclophosphamide in conjunction with vincristine.

The precise mechanism of cyclophosphamide-induced cardiotoxicity is not known, but it has been postulated that the drug and/or its metabolites may affect the endothelium directly with secondary extravasation of blood containing high concentrations of cyclophosphamide. The antidiuretic effect of cyclophosphamide observed with high doses also may contribute to cardiopulmonary manifestations. Although clear risk factors have not been established, patients who have received or are receiving concomitantly radiation therapy and/or other potentially cardiotoxic drugs (e.g., anthracyclines) appear to be at increased risk. Some indicators of cyclophosphamide-induced cardiotoxicity include sudden weight gain, ECG abnormalities, dyspnea, and/or other signs of congestive heart failure, and patients receiving higher than usual dosages of the drug should be monitored for such effects. In addition to death, possible consequences of the cardiotoxicity include debilitating heart failure, arrhythmias, and potentially irreversible cardiomyopathy and/or pericarditis.

Other Adverse Effects

Malaise and asthenia have been reported in patients receiving cyclophosphamide. Other reported adverse effects of cyclophosphamide include headache, dizziness, and myxedema. Faintness, facial flushing, diaphoresis, and oropharyngeal sensation have occurred following IV administration. Rarely, decreased serum cholinesterase concentrations, especially following IV administration of cyclophosphamide, have been reported. The drug may interfere with normal wound healing.

Anaphylactic reaction, including fatality, has been reported with cyclophosphamide therapy. Possible cross-sensitivity with other alkylating agents also has been reported. Positive reactions to skin test antigens (e.g., tuberculin purified protein derivative, mumps, trichophyton, candida) are reported to be frequently suppressed in patients receiving cyclophosphamide.

Precautions and Contraindications

Cyclophosphamide is a highly toxic drug with a low therapeutic index, and a therapeutic response is not likely to occur without some evidence of toxicity. The drug must be used only under constant supervision by clinicians experienced in therapy with cytotoxic agents.

Patients who receive myelosuppressive drugs experience an increased frequency of infections, as well as possible hemorrhagic complications. Because these complications are potentially fatal, the patient should be instructed to notify the clinician if fever, sore throat, or unusual bleeding or bruising occurs. The patient's hematologic status must be carefully monitored, at least weekly for the first few months of therapy or until the maintenance dosage is determined, and then at intervals of 2–3 weeks. Leukopenia is dose-related and can be used as a guide to adjusting dosage of cyclophosphamide. A reduction in leukocyte count to less than 2000/mm³ occurs commonly with initial loading doses of the drug, and less frequently in patients maintained on smaller doses. Transient decreases in leukocyte count to 2000/mm³ (during short courses of treatment) or more persistent reductions to 3000/mm³ (with continuing therapy) reportedly are tolerated without serious risk of infection if marked granulocytopenia is not present.

To prevent the occurrence of hemorrhagic cystitis in patients receiving cyclophosphamide, many experts recommend adequate hydration and frequent voiding. Patients should be instructed to increase their fluid intake for 24 hours before, during, and for at least 24 hours after receiving cyclophosphamide and to void frequently for 24 hours after receiving the drug. Urine also should be examined regularly for the presence of red cells, which may precede hemorrhagic cystitis. Since hemorrhagic cystitis can be severe and even fatal, the drug should be discontinued and not resumed if possible in patients who develop this complication. In severe cases, replacement of blood may be needed. Protracted cases have been treated with 1–10% formaldehyde irrigations, electrocautery to the telangiectatic areas of the bladder, diversion of urine flow, and cryosurgery.

Because of the immunosuppressive activity of cyclophosphamide, interruption or reduction of dosage should be considered for patients who develop bacterial, fungal, protozoan, helminthic, or viral infections, especially those patients who are receiving or perhaps in those who have recently received corticosteroid therapy. Infections in some of these patients have been fatal; varicella-zoster infections appear to be particularly dangerous. Cyclophosphamide has been reported to be more toxic in adrenalectomized dogs, and adjustment of both replacement corticosteroids and cyclophosphamide may be necessary in adrenalectomized patients.

Cyclophosphamide should be administered with caution to patients with severe leukopenia, thrombocytopenia, tumor cell infiltration of bone marrow, previous therapy with radiation or other cytotoxic agents, impaired hepatic function, or impaired renal function. The drug is contraindicated in patients with severely depressed bone marrow function and in those who have demonstrated hypersensitivity to cyclophosphamide.

Patients should be informed that exposure to large doses of cyclophosphamide causes gonadal toxicity (see Cautions: Pregnancy, Fertility, and Lactation); counseling on fertility options, prior to such therapy whenever possible for young patients, and long-term follow-up for evaluation of gonadal function is advised.

● **Pediatric Precautions**

According to the manufacturers, the safety profile of cyclophosphamide in children is similar to that observed in adult patients. Children receiving large doses of cyclophosphamide are at high risk for long-term gonadal damage and infertility. (See Cautions: Pregnancy, Fertility, and Lactation.)

● **Geriatric Precautions**

Safety and efficacy of cyclophosphamide in geriatric patients have not been studied specifically to date. Clinical studies of cyclophosphamide for malignant lymphoma, multiple myeloma, leukemia, mycosis fungoides, neuroblastoma, retinoblastoma, and breast cancer did not include sufficient numbers of patients 65 years of age and older to determine whether geriatric patients respond differently than younger patients. In 2 clinical trials in which cyclophosphamide and cisplatin were compared with paclitaxel and cisplatin for the treatment of advanced ovarian cancer, 154 (28%) of 552 patients receiving cyclophosphamide and cisplatin were 65 years or older. Subset analyses according to age (younger than 65 years versus 65 years or older) from these trials, published reports of clinical trials of cyclophosphamide-containing regimens in breast cancer and non-Hodgkin's lymphoma, and postmarketing experience suggest that geriatric patients may be more susceptible to cyclophosphamide-induced toxicity. In general, dosage should be titrated carefully in geriatric patients, usually initiating therapy at the low end of the dosage range.

● **Mutagenicity and Carcinogenicity**

Some patients who have received cyclophosphamide alone, as part of a combination regimen, or as adjunctive therapy have developed secondary malignancies, most frequently urinary bladder, myeloproliferative, and lymphoproliferative malignancies. Although a causal relationship has not been definitely established, the possibility of development of a secondary malignancy should be considered in weighing the possible benefit from the drug against the potential risk. Secondary malignancies have occurred most frequently in patients who have been treated with cyclophosphamide for primary myeloproliferative and lymphoproliferative malignancies and primary nonmalignant diseases in which immune processes are believed to be involved. Secondary urinary bladder malignancies generally have occurred in patients who previously developed hemorrhagic cystitis. In some cases, the secondary malignancy was not detected until several years after discontinuance of cyclophosphamide therapy. In one study in patients with breast cancer who received 2–4 times the standard dose of cyclophosphamide in conjunction with doxorubicin, cases of secondary acute myeloid leukemia were reported within 2 years of treatment initiation. Long-term follow-up of women who received cyclophosphamide-containing adjuvant chemotherapy regimens for the treatment of early breast cancer indicates that the incidence of other solid tumors and secondary leukemia in these women is not substantially greater than that in the general population.

● **Pregnancy, Fertility, and Lactation**

Pregnancy

Cyclophosphamide can cause fetal toxicity when administered to pregnant women, but potential benefits from use of the drug may be acceptable in certain conditions despite the possible risks to the fetus. Abnormalities, including ectrodactylia, have occurred in infants born to women treated with the drug during pregnancy. Normal infants also have been born to women who received cyclophosphamide, including during the first trimester. Cyclophosphamide should be used during pregnancy only in life-threatening situations or severe disease for which safer drugs cannot be used or are ineffective. When the drug is administered during pregnancy or if the patient becomes pregnant while receiving cyclophosphamide, the patient should be informed of the potential hazard to the fetus. Women of childbearing potential should be advised to avoid becoming pregnant.

Fertility

Gonadal suppression, which appears to be related to dose and duration of therapy, has been reported in patients who received cyclophosphamide. The drug interferes with oogenesis and spermatogenesis. Amenorrhea, azoospermia, oligospermia, and ovarian fibrosis have been reported in patients who receive cyclophosphamide. Sterility may occur in both men and women and may be permanent. Although the full effect of cyclophosphamide on prepubertal gonads has not been established, ovarian failure and testicular atrophy have occurred. Male patients who receive high-dose cyclophosphamide for childhood cancer, including treatment prior to the onset of puberty, are at high risk for long-term, irreversible gonadal damage, such as infertility and subclinical Leydig cell insufficiency.

Lactation

Cyclophosphamide is distributed into milk. Because of the potential for serious adverse reactions to cyclophosphamide in nursing infants, a decision should be made whether to discontinue nursing or the drug, taking into account the importance of the drug to the woman.

DRUG INTERACTIONS

● **Mesna**

Mesna (sodium 2-mercaptoethanesulphonate) is a synthetic sulfhydryl compound that can chemically interact with urotoxic metabolites (and/or their precursors) of cyclophosphamide (e.g., acrolein, 4-hydroxycyclophosphamide) and other oxazaphosphorine derivatives (e.g., ifosfamide) to decrease the incidence and severity of, or prevent, bladder toxicity (e.g., hemorrhagic cystitis) induced by these drugs. (See Mesna 92:56.)

Mesna is rapidly oxidized in systemic circulation to dimesna (mesna disulfide), which is substantially less chemically reactive than mesna; following glomerular filtration, dimesna is reduced to mesna by the glutathione system in the renal tubular epithelium and is excreted by the kidneys. In urine, mesna reacts chemically (e.g., binding with 4-hydroxycyclophosphamide to form 4-sulfoethylthiocyclophosphamide and/or binding with double-bonds of acrolein) with the urotoxic metabolites (and/or their precursors) of cyclophosphamide thought to be principally responsible for drug-induced hematuria and hemorrhagic cystitis and thus detoxifies these metabolites. In addition, mesna enhances urinary excretion of cysteine, which also can react chemically with acrolein, and this effect may contribute to the uroprotective activity of mesna. While limited evidence in animals suggests that mesna also may enhance systemic deactivation of cyclophosphamide to some extent, pharmacokinetic characteristics of mesna may differ in mice compared with humans, and the poor lipophilicity of mesna and dimesna (resulting in poor distribution into tumor cells in humans), evidence from in vitro and in vivo tumor models, and clinical evidence in humans indicate that mesna does not substantially deactivate active cyclophosphamide metabolites in tumor cells or interfere with the systemic antineoplastic activity of the drug.

● Cardiotoxic Drugs

Because potentiation of cardiotoxic effects may result, caution should be exercised in the concomitant administration of cyclophosphamide and other cardiotoxic drugs such as doxorubicin.

● Drugs Affecting Hepatic Microsomal Enzymes

Barbiturates and other drugs which induce liver microsomal enzymes may result in an increased pharmacologic effect and increased toxicity of cyclophosphamide because of increased conversion of the drug to active metabolites. Although the full clinical importance of this interaction has not been assessed, it is advisable to monitor patients who receive both drugs closely for cyclophosphamide toxicity.

Although it has been proposed that corticosteroids and sex hormones may inhibit liver microsomal enzymes and that discontinuance or reduction in steroid dosage can cause an increase in the toxicity of previously well-tolerated doses of cyclophosphamide, the clinical importance of this effect has not been established. Other drugs which may inhibit microsomal enzyme activity in the liver and therefore interfere with the metabolism of cyclophosphamide include allopurinol, chloramphenicol, chloroquine, imipramine, phenothiazines, potassium iodide, and vitamin A. In one controlled study, concomitant administration of cyclophosphamide and allopurinol increased the incidence of bone marrow depression as compared to cyclophosphamide alone, but the mechanism or clinical importance of the interaction has not been established.

● Succinylcholine

Cyclophosphamide reportedly reduces serum pseudocholinesterase concentrations and may prolong the neuromuscular blocking activity of succinylcholine, especially in very ill patients who are receiving large IV doses of cyclophosphamide. Although the clinical importance has not been established, it has been suggested that succinylcholine be administered with caution in patients receiving cyclophosphamide and that succinylcholine or cyclophosphamide be avoided in patients with substantially depressed pseudocholinesterase concentrations. The anesthesiologist should be informed before general anesthesia is administered if a patient has received cyclophosphamide within the previous 10 days.

ACUTE TOXICITY

Limited information is available on acute overdosage of cyclophosphamide.

● Manifestations

Overdosage with cyclophosphamide would be expected to produce effects that are mainly extensions of common adverse reactions, particularly severe leukopenia and thrombocytopenia; cardiotoxicity also may be prominent. In patients who received 4- to 10-day courses of cyclophosphamide with total dosage of the drug per course exceeding 140 mg/kg (5.2 g/m²), cardiac damage manifested by heart failure occurred within 15 days of the initial dose. Impairment of water excretion with hyponatremia, weight gain, and inappropriately concentrated urine has been reported after cyclophosphamide doses exceeding 50 mg/kg (2 g/m²).

Overdosage, which was fatal in at least one case, also has occurred in several patients who were enrolled in high-dose protocols in which cyclophosphamide (given concomitantly with mesna and followed with autologous bone marrow transplant) was administered inadvertently in a dosage of 4 g/m² daily for 4 doses rather than in a total dosage of 4 g/m²administered over 4 days in equally divided doses of 1 g/m² daily; potentially irreversible or fatal cardiotoxicity was the most serious consequence of overdosage in these patients. Potentially fatal cardiotoxicity, manifested as congestive heart failure, ECG abnormalities, cardiomyopathy, and/or pericarditis, also has been reported in other patients receiving high doses of cyclophosphamide (120 mg/kg [60 mg/kg daily] or more over several days), and the risk of such toxicity appears to be increased in patients who have received

or are receiving concomitantly radiation therapy or other potentially cardiotoxic drugs (e.g., anthracyclines). (See Cautions: Cardiac Effects.)

● Treatment

If overdosage of cyclophosphamide is known or suspected, the patient should be hospitalized for general supportive therapy. There is no known specific antidote. Although cyclophosphamide theoretically is dialyzable, no studies have been performed to date to evaluate efficacy of dialysis in the treatment of acute overdosage of the drug.

PHARMACOLOGY

Following conversion to active metabolites in the liver, cyclophosphamide functions as an alkylating agent, interfering with DNA replication and transcription of RNA, and ultimately resulting in the disruption of nucleic acid function. The drug exhibits phosphorylating properties that also enhance its cytotoxicity. Cyclophosphamide also possesses potent immunosuppressive activity.

PHARMACOKINETICS

● Absorption

Cyclophosphamide appears to be well absorbed following oral administration, with a reported bioavailability greater than 75%. Maximum plasma concentrations of cyclophosphamide occur at about 1 hour. Concentrations of cyclophosphamide metabolites reportedly reach maximum levels 2–3 hours after an IV dose of the drug.

● Distribution

Cyclophosphamide and its metabolites appear to be distributed throughout the body, including the brain and CSF, but probably not in concentrations sufficient to treat meningeal leukemia. It is assumed that cyclophosphamide crosses the placenta. The drug is distributed into milk.

Although in vitro binding of cyclophosphamide to plasma proteins has not been demonstrated, in vivo binding generally has been reported to range from 0–10% and protein binding for some alkylating metabolites has been reported to exceed 60%.

● Elimination

The serum half-life after IV administration of cyclophosphamide has been reported to range from 3–12 hours; however, the drug and/or its metabolites can be detected in the serum up to 72 hours after administration.

Cyclophosphamide is metabolized in the liver by the enzymatic mixed-function oxidase system of liver microsomes to 4-hydroxycyclophosphamide, which is in equilibrium with aldophosphamide, the acyclic tautomer. 4-Hydroxycyclophosphamide may be enzymatically metabolized to 4-ketocyclophosphamide, and aldophosphamide may be enzymatically metabolized to carboxyphosphamide, phosphoramide mustard, and acrolein. Some authorities believe that phosphoramide mustard and acrolein account for the cytotoxic properties of the drug, and that 4-ketocyclophosphamide and carboxyphosphamide do not possess substantial biologic activity. However, there is controversy regarding the toxicity of 4-ketocyclophosphamide.

Cyclophosphamide and its metabolites are excreted principally in urine, with about 36–99% of a dose being eliminated within 48 hours; of the amount excreted, about 5–30% is unchanged drug.

CHEMISTRY AND STABILITY

● Chemistry

Cyclophosphamide is a nitrogen mustard-derivative, polyfunctional alkylating agent. The drug occurs as a monohydrate, white, crystalline powder and is soluble in water and in alcohol. Potency of cyclophosphamide is calculated on the anhydrous basis.

Cyclophosphamide is commercially available as cyclophosphamide tablets containing anhydrous cyclophosphamide. Cyclophosphamide for injection is commercially available as a sterile white powder containing cyclophosphamide monohydrate.

When reconstituted as directed with sterile 0.9% sodium chloride solution (for direct injection), solutions of cyclophosphamide monohydrate (Cytoxan®)

have an osmolarity of 374 mOsm/L. When reconstituted as directed with sterile water for injection (for IV infusion), solutions of cyclophosphamide monohydrate (Cytoxan®) have an osmolarity of 74 mOsm/L and are hypotonic.

● *Stability*

Commercially available cyclophosphamide tablets should be stored at a temperature not exceeding 25°C; the tablets will withstand brief exposure to temperatures up to 30°C, but should be protected from temperatures exceeding 30°C.

Commercially available cyclophosphamide powder for injection containing cyclophosphamide monohydrate should be stored at a temperature not exceeding 25°C. During storage or transport, exposure of the vials to temperature fluctuations may result in melting of the contents; vials should be visually inspected, and any vials with signs of melting of the cyclophosphamide monohydrate into a clear or yellowish viscous liquid, in droplets or as a connected phase, should be discarded.

Following reconstitution as directed with sterile 0.9% sodium chloride solution or sterile water for injection, solutions of cyclophosphamide powder for injection containing cyclophosphamide monohydrate are stable for 24 hours at room temperature or 6 days when refrigerated. Reconstituted solutions of the drug to be used for IV infusion are compatible with 5% dextrose, 5% dextrose and 0.9% sodium chloride, 5% dextrose and Ringer's, lactated Ringer's, 0.45% sodium chloride, or (1/6) *M* sodium lactate injection.

Extemporaneous oral liquid preparations of cyclophosphamide, prepared by dissolving the powder for injection in aromatic elixir, are stable for 14 days in glass containers when refrigerated.

For further information on the handling of antineoplastic agents, see the ASHP Guidelines on Handling Hazardous Drugs at http://www.ahfsdrug information.com.

PREPARATIONS

Excipients in commercially available drug preparations may have clinically important effects in some individuals; consult specific product labeling for details.

Cyclophosphamide

Oral

Tablets	25 mg (of anhydrous cyclophosphamide)*	**Cyclophosphamide Tablets**
		Cytoxan®, Bristol-Myers Squibb
	50 mg (of anhydrous cyclophosphamide)*	**Cyclophosphamide Tablets**
		Cytoxan®, Bristol-Myers Squibb

Parenteral

For injection	500 mg (of anhydrous cyclophosphamide)*	**Cyclophosphamide for Injection**
		Cytoxan®, Bristol-Myers Squibb
	1 g (of anhydrous cyclophosphamide)*	**Cyclophosphamide for Injection**
		Cytoxan®, Bristol-Myers Squibb
	2 g (of anhydrous cyclophosphamide)*	**Cyclophosphamide for Injection**
		Cytoxan®, Bristol-Myers Squibb

* available from one or more manufacturer, distributor, and/or repackager by generic (nonproprietary) name

† Use is not currently included in the labeling approved by the US Food and Drug Administration.

Selected Revisions August 6, 2018, © Copyright, March 1, 1978, American Society of Health-System Pharmacists, Inc.

Dabrafenib Mesylate

10:00 • ANTINEOPLASTIC AGENTS

■ Dabrafenib, an inhibitor of b-Raf serine-threonine kinase (BRAF) with V600E or V600K mutation, is an antineoplastic agent.

USES

● Melanoma

Dabrafenib is used as combination therapy for the adjuvant treatment of melanoma in patients with b-Raf serine-threonine kinase (BRAF) V600E or V600K mutations and involvement of lymph node(s), following complete resection. Dabrafenib is also used for the treatment of unresectable or metastatic melanoma in patients with a BRAF V600E mutation (as monotherapy) or BRAF V600E or V600K mutations (as combination therapy).

Dabrafenib is not indicated for treatment of patients with wild-type BRAF solid tumors.

Adjuvant Therapy for Melanoma

Dabrafenib is used in combination with trametinib as adjuvant therapy following complete resection of melanoma with a BRAF V600E or V600K mutation and nodal involvement. An FDA-approved diagnostic test (e.g., THxID® BRAF kit) is required to confirm the presence of the BRAF V600E or V600K mutation prior to initiation of therapy.

This indication for dabrafenib is based principally on the results of a randomized, double-blind, placebo-controlled, phase 3 study (COMBI-AD) in patients who had undergone complete resection of stage III melanoma with BRAF V600E or V600K mutation (as detected by the bioMerieux THxID® BRAF V600 mutation test) and involvement of regional lymph nodes. In this study, 870 patients were randomized (stratified by disease stage and BRAF mutation status) in a 1:1 ratio to receive dabrafenib 150 mg twice daily with trametinib 2 mg once daily or placebo for up to 12 months. Enrolled patients were required to have undergone complete resection of melanoma with complete lymphadenectomy within 12 weeks of randomization. The primary measure of efficacy was relapse-free survival. The median age of patients was 51 years; 99% of patients were Caucasian, 55% were male, 91% had a baseline Eastern Cooperative Oncology Group (ECOG) performance status of 0, 65% had macroscopic lymph node involvement, 41% had tumor ulceration, 41% had stage IIIb disease, and 40% had stage IIIc disease. The majority (91%) of patients had BRAF V600E mutation and 9% had a V600K mutation. Patients who had mucosal or ocular melanoma, unresectable in-transit metastases, or distant metastatic disease and those who had previously received systemic therapy (including radiation therapy) were not eligible to enroll in the study.

After a median follow-up of 2.8 years, median relapse-free survival had not been reached in patients receiving dabrafenib in combination with trametinib and was 16.6 months in those receiving placebo; however, dabrafenib in combination with trametinib reduced the risk of relapse by 53% compared with placebo. In an updated analysis at a median follow-up of 44 or 42 months for patients receiving dabrafenib in combination with trametinib or those receiving placebo, respectively, relapse-free survival remained similar to the primary results. Dabrafenib in combination with trametinib was associated with a numerically, but not significantly, higher estimated 3-year overall survival rate as compared with placebo. Results of a subgroup analysis (based on disease stage, lymph node involvement, presence of tumor ulceration) suggested that the effect of dabrafenib in combination with trametinib was consistent across all subgroups.

Unresectable or Metastatic Melanoma

Dabrafenib, alone or in combination therapy, is used for the treatment of unresectable or metastatic melanoma in selected patients.

Monotherapy

Dabrafenib is used as monotherapy for the treatment of unresectable or metastatic melanoma with BRAF V600E mutation. Dabrafenib has been designated

an orphan drug by the FDA for this use. An FDA-approved diagnostic test (e.g., THxID® BRAF kit) is required to confirm the presence of the BRAF V600E mutation prior to initiation of monotherapy.

This indication is based principally on the results of an open-label, randomized, phase 3 study (BREAK-3) in patients with previously untreated stage IV or unresectable stage III melanoma positive for BRAF V600E mutation. Patients receiving dabrafenib experienced longer progression-free survival when compared with those receiving dacarbazine. In the BREAK-3 study, 250 adults (median age of 52 years, 60% male, 99% white, 67% with ECOG performance status of 0, 66% with stage M1c disease, 62% with normal lactate dehydrogenase [LDH]) were randomized in a 3:1 ratio to receive oral dabrafenib 150 mg twice daily or IV dacarbazine 1 g/m² every 3 weeks; treatment was continued until disease progression, death, or study withdrawal occurred. Patients who experienced disease progression while receiving dacarbazine were allowed to cross over to dabrafenib treatment. The median duration of follow-up was 5.1 months in patients receiving dabrafenib and 3.5 months in those receiving dacarbazine. The median progression-free survival assessed radiographically or photographically by the investigator was 5.1 or 2.7 months for those receiving dabrafenib or dacarbazine, respectively. Progression-free survival as assessed by an independent review committee was 6.7 or 2.9 months for patients receiving dabrafenib or dacarbazine, respectively. The independent review committee reported a confirmed objective response in 50% of patients receiving dabrafenib compared with 6% of those receiving dacarbazine. The estimated median duration of response was 5.5 months for those receiving dabrafenib and was not yet reached for those receiving dacarbazine.

Dabrafenib treatment has been shown to be effective in patients with melanoma with brain metastasis. Dabrafenib was evaluated in a single-arm, open-label, phase 2 study (BREAK-MB) of 139 adults with melanoma positive for BRAF mutation (V600E) and at least one asymptomatic brain metastasis. Patients received oral dabrafenib 150 mg twice daily until disease progression, death, or unacceptable toxicity occurred. Up to 2 previous treatment regimens for extracranial metastatic melanoma were allowed, but patients could not have received prior treatment with a BRAF inhibitor or a mitogen-activated extracellular signal regulated kinase (MEK) inhibitor. The BREAK-MB study consisted of 2 cohorts: patients with no prior treatment for brain metastasis (median 50 years of age, 72% male, 59% with ECOG performance status of 0, 57% with elevated LDH) and those with prior local treatment for brain metastasis (median 51 years of age, 63% male, 66% with ECOG performance status of 0, 54% with elevated LDH). Among 139 patients with melanoma positive for BRAF V600E mutation, 18% in each cohort achieved an overall intracranial response (i.e., best intracranial response was a complete or partial response) as assessed by an independent review committee. The median duration of overall intracranial response was 4.6 months in both cohorts.

Combination Therapy

Dabrafenib is used in combination with trametinib for the treatment of unresectable or metastatic melanoma with BRAF V600E or V600K mutation. Dabrafenib has been designated an orphan drug by the FDA for this use. When dabrafenib is used in combination with trametinib, the presence of BRAF V600E or V600K mutation should be confirmed using an FDA-approved diagnostic test (e.g., THxID® BRAF kit) prior to initiation of therapy.

This indication is based principally on the results of 2 randomized phase 3 studies (COMBI-d and COMBI-v) in patients with previously untreated stage IIIc or IV cutaneous melanoma with BRAF V600E or V600K mutation and a non-randomized open-label phase 2 study in previously treated or untreated patients with metastatic disease (COMBI-MB). In the COMBI-d and COMBI-v studies, the primary measures of efficacy were progression-free survival and overall survival, respectively. In the COMBI-MB study, the primary outcome measure was intracranial response rate in patients with BRAF V600E mutation and asymptomatic melanoma brain metastases who had not received prior local brain-directed therapy.

In the COMBI-d study, 423 patients were randomized in a 1:1 ratio to receive either dabrafenib (150 mg twice daily) in combination with trametinib (2 mg once daily) or dabrafenib in combination with placebo. Treatment was continued until disease progression or unacceptable toxicity occurred or the patient withdrew from the study; however, patients with disease progression could continue receiving treatment if they met prespecified criteria for continuation. The median age of patients was 56 years; almost all patients (>99%) were white, 72% had an ECOG performance status of 0, 66% had stage M1c disease, 65% had normal LDH concentrations, and 2 patients had a history of brain metastases. Most patients (85%) had *BRAF* V600E mutation and 15% had a V600K mutation. At a median follow-up of 9 months, median progression-free survival or overall survival was 9.3 or 25.1 months, respectively, in patients receiving dabrafenib in combination with trametinib compared with 8.8 or 18.7 months, respectively, in those receiving dabrafenib and placebo. An updated analysis confirmed prolonged median progression-free survival in patients receiving dabrafenib in combination with trametinib compared with those receiving placebo and dabrafenib (11 versus 8.8 months). A final analysis for overall survival estimated a prolonged median overall survival in the dabrafenib and trametinib group versus the dabrafenib only group (25.1 versus 18.7 months). In addition, patients receiving dabrafenib and trametinib had a higher overall response rate (66 versus 51%) compared with those receiving dabrafenib and placebo; complete responses were achieved in 10% of patients receiving dabrafenib in combination with trametinib and 8% of those receiving dabrafenib and placebo. The median duration of response in patients receiving dabrafenib and trametinib or those dabrafenib and placebo was 9.2 or 10.2 months, respectively. Results of a subgroup analysis (based on age, gender, disease stage, baseline ECOG performance status, baseline serum LDH concentration, visceral involvement, number of disease sites, and *BRAF* V600 mutation status) suggested that the effects of combination therapy with dabrafenib and trametinib on progression-free survival and overall survival were consistent across all subgroups.

In the COMBI-v study, 704 patients were randomized in a 1:1 ratio to receive either dabrafenib (150 mg twice daily) in combination with trametinib (2 mg once daily) or vemurafenib (960 mg twice daily). The median age of patients was 55 years; 96% were Caucasian, 70% had an ECOG performance status of 0, 67% had normal LDH concentrations, 61% had stage M1c disease, 6% had stage IIIc disease, and one patient had a history of brain metastases. Most patients (89%) had *BRAF* V600E mutation and 10% had a V600K mutation. The median follow-up period at the time of the interim analysis was 11 months for those receiving dabrafenib in combination with trametinib and 10 months for those receiving vemurafenib alone. Median overall survival had not been reached in patients receiving dabrafenib in combination with trametinib and was 17.2 months in those receiving vemurafenib alone; however, dabrafenib in combination with trametinib reduced the risk of death by 31% compared with vemurafenib alone. Patients receiving dabrafenib in combination with trametinib also had longer median progression-free survival (11.4 versus 7.3 months) and higher overall response rates (64 versus 51%) compared with patients receiving vemurafenib alone. Because of the survival benefit observed at the interim analysis, study investigators permitted patients previously randomized to receive vemurafenib alone to cross over to combination therapy with dabrafenib and trametinib. Results of a subgroup analysis (based on age, gender, *BRAF* mutation status, ECOG performance status, and baseline LDH concentration) suggested that the effect of dabrafenib in combination with trametinib was consistent across most subgroups; an overall survival benefit for combination therapy with dabrafenib and trametinib versus vemurafenib was not apparent in the subgroup of patients with an ECOG performance status of 1 (hazard ratio: 1.03).

Dabrafenib in combination with trametinib also has been evaluated in adults with melanoma with brain metastases in an open-label, multicohort, phase 2 study (COMBI-MB). In this study, 121 patients with previously treated metastatic melanoma received dabrafenib 150 mg twice daily in combination with trametinib 2 mg daily. Treatment was continued until disease progression or unacceptable toxicity occurred. Most patients (85%) had *BRAF* V600E and 15% had a V600K mutation. Eligible patients were required to have at least one measurable intracranial lesion, but no leptomeningeal disease, parenchymal brain metastases greater than 4 cm in diameter, ocular melanoma, or primary mucosal melanoma. Prior to study entry, patients could have received up to two previous systemic treatments, except BRAF or MEK inhibitors, for the treatment of metastatic melanoma. The primary efficacy outcome was confirmed intracranial response rate as assessed by an independent review committee using a modified Response Evaluation Criteria in Solid Tumors (RECIST) v1.1 to allow up to 5 intracranial target lesions ≥5 mm in diameter. The median age of patients in this study was 54 years; 58% were male, 100% were white, 65% had a normal LDH level at baseline, and 97% had an ECOG performance status of 0 or 1. Intracranial metastases were asymptomatic in 87% of patients and were symptomatic in 13% of patients; 87% had extracranial metastases and 22% had received prior local therapy for brain metastases. Confirmed intracranial response rate was 50%; complete or partial response was achieved in 4.1 or 46% of patients, respectively.

The median duration of response was 6.4 months (range 1–31 months). Stable or progressive disease was the best overall response in 9% of patients with an intracranial response.

Trametinib in combination with dabrafenib has also been compared to immunotherapy in patients with unresectable stage III or IV melanoma in the 2-arm, 2-step, open-label, randomized phase 3, DREAMseq trial. The aim of DREAMseq was to determine whether immunotherapy or the combination of BRAF and MEK inhibition should be preferred as initial therapy in patients with *BRAF*-mutant melanoma. Patients were required to have an ECOG performance status of 0 or 1 and be untreated in the metastatic setting, but were eligible if they had received adjuvant therapy that did not include a programmed death 1 (PD-1), programmed death-ligand 1, cytotoxic T-cell lymphocyte-4, BRAF, or MEK inhibitor. In step 1 of this study, 265 patients were randomized in a 1:1 ratio to receive either trametinib (2 mg once daily) in combination with dabrafenib (150 mg twice daily) until disease progression or unacceptable toxicity occurred or nivolumab in combination with ipilimumab (1 mg/kg and 3 mg/kg, respectively, once every 3 weeks for 4 doses) followed by nivolumab alone (240 mg once every 2 weeks for up to 72 weeks); patients who experienced disease progression by RECIST criteria proceeded to step 2, in which they crossed over to the alternate therapy. The primary endpoint of DREAMseq was 2-year overall survival among patients followed for at least 2 years.

The median age of patients enrolled in DREAMseq was 61 years; 63% were male, 95% were white, and 60% had baseline LDH within normal limits. Most patients had *BRAF* V600E mutations; a higher proportion of patients randomized in step 1 to receive trametinib in combination with dabrafenib had BRAF V600K mutations (25%) compared to those randomized to immunotherapy (12%).

Study accrual was halted by an independent data safety monitoring committee after an interim analysis; at the time, 265 patients were randomized in step 1 and 73 patients had crossed over in step 2 (63% of whom were initially randomized to trametinib in combination with dabrafenib). The median follow-up was 27.7 months. The 2-year overall survival rate was substantially lower in patients initially randomized to trametinib in combination with dabrafenib compared to those initially randomized to immunotherapy (51.5% versus 71.8%, respectively). The data safety monitoring committee determined that this difference was clinically meaningful and recommended closing the study to accrual, with patients initially randomized to trametinib in combination with dabrafenib given the option to cross over to immunotherapy without prerequisite disease progression. Overall response rates to step 1 treatment were similar between groups; patients who received trametinib in combination with dabrafenib in step 1 appeared to have similar response rates to those who received this combination in step 2 (43% versus 48%, respectively), whereas response rates appeared to be higher in patients who received immunotherapy in step 1 compared to those who received immunotherapy in step 2 (46% versus 30%, respectively). Duration of response among responders to step 1 therapy was significantly prolonged with immunotherapy compared to trametinib in combination with dabrafenib (median not reached versus 12.7 months, respectively).

Clinical Perspective

Adjuvant Therapy for Melanoma

The 2020 American Society of Clinical Oncology (ASCO) guideline on systemic therapy for melanoma recommends offering nivolumab or pembrolizumab for a duration of 52 weeks to patients with completely resected stage IIIA/B/C/D *BRAF* wild-type cutaneous melanoma and, in those with *BRAF* mutation-positive (V600E/K) cutaneous melanoma, nivolumab alone, pembrolizumab alone, or combination therapy with dabrafenib and trametinib for a duration of 52 weeks. ASCO makes no recommendation for or against dabrafenib in combination with trametinib in patients with completely resected stage III/IV melanoma with *BRAF* mutations other than V600E/K. Ipilimumab and high-dose interferon are not recommended for routine use in adjuvant therapy. Because patients with stage III disease (regardless of *BRAF* mutation status) with microscopic sentinel node metastasis <1 mm in diameter generally have a relatively better prognosis and lower risk of relapse, ASCO states that treatment should be individualized after discussing the potential risks and benefits of therapy in these patients. ASCO states that pembrolizumab, nivolumab, or the combination of dabrafenib and trametinib in the adjuvant setting should not be offered to patients with completely resected stage II melanoma outside of a clinical trial.

For the treatment of melanoma, monotherapy with a BRAF inhibitor is no longer recommended by experts since combination BRAF/MEK inhibition has demonstrated superior outcomes with a similar safety profile.

Unresectable or Metastatic Melanoma

The 2020 ASCO guideline on systemic therapy for melanoma recommends offering ipilimumab plus nivolumab followed by nivolumab, nivolumab alone, or pembrolizumab alone in patients with unresectable or metastatic *BRAF* wild-type cutaneous melanoma and, in those with *BRAF* mutation-positive (V600E/K) cutaneous melanoma, ipilimumab plus nivolumab followed by nivolumab, nivolumab alone, pembrolizumab alone, or combination BRAF/MEK inhibitor therapy (i.e., dabrafenib and trametinib; encorafenib and binimetinib; vemurafenib and cobimetinib) may be offered. For patients with *BRAF* mutation-positive (V600) unresectable/metastatic cutaneous melanoma who progress on first-line PD-1 inhibitor therapy, combination BRAF/MEK inhibitor therapy may be offered. Similarly, patients with *BRAF* mutation-positive (V600) unresectable/metastatic cutaneous melanoma who had disease progression following combination BRAF/MEK inhibitor therapy may be offered PD-1 inhibitor therapy. Patients with mucosal melanoma may be offered the same treatment regimens as those recommended for cutaneous melanoma; however, in the absence of additional data, the ASCO Expert Panel states that patients with unresectable/metastatic mucosal melanoma should be offered or referred for enrollment in clinical trials whenever possible.

ASCO states that switching between BRAF/MEK inhibitor combination regimens may be reasonable if patients experience toxicity since toxicity profiles may differ for each combination; however, no data exist regarding the efficacy of switching to a different BRAF/MEK combination.

● Non-small Cell Lung Cancer

Dabrafenib is used in combination with trametinib for the treatment of metastatic non-small cell lung cancer (NSCLC) with *BRAF* V600E mutation. Dabrafenib has been designated an orphan drug by the FDA when used in combination with trametinib for the treatment of this cancer. An FDA-approved diagnostic test (e.g., THxID® BRAF kit) is required to confirm the presence of the *BRAF* V600E mutation prior to initiation of therapy.

Dabrafenib is not indicated for treatment of patients with wild-type *BRAF* solid tumors.

Clinical Experience

This indication for dabrafenib in combination with trametinib in the treatment of metastatic NSCLC with *BRAF* V600E mutation is based principally on the results of an open-label, multicenter, nonrandomized, 3-cohort, phase 2 study (BRF113928). Patients in the BRF113928 study were enrolled into 2 cohorts: those previously treated with 1–3 systemic therapies with disease progression following at least one platinum-containing regimen and those with treatment-naive metastatic NSCLC. The cohort of patients with previously treated disease consisted of 2 cohorts who received either single-agent dabrafenib (150 mg twice daily) or dabrafenib (150 mg twice daily) in combination with trametinib (2 mg once daily). The cohort of patients with previously untreated disease received dabrafenib (150 mg twice daily) in combination with trametinib (2 mg once daily). Treatment was continued until disease progression or unacceptable toxicity occurred or the patient withdrew from the study. Patients with prior exposure to BRAF or MEK inhibitors were not eligible to enroll in the study; however, prior exposure to epidermal growth factor receptor (EGFR) or anaplastic lymphoma kinase (ALK) inhibitors was permitted in patients with EGFR- or ALK-positive tumors. The primary measure of efficacy was objective response rate as assessed by an independent review committee according to RECIST and duration of response. The median age of patients was 66 years; 98% had squamous cell histology, 90% had an ECOG performance status of 0 or 1, 81% were Caucasian, 60% had a history of smoking, 48% were male, 32% were nonsmokers, 14% were Asian, 11% had received adjuvant chemotherapy, 8% were current smokers, 3% were black, and 2% were Hispanic. The majority (99%) of patients had metastatic disease; brain or liver metastases were present in 6 or 14% of these patients, respectively. Among the cohort of patients with previously treated disease, 58% had received only one prior systemic therapy for metastatic disease.

In the cohort of patients with previously treated disease, the objective response rate was 27 or 63% in patients receiving single-agent dabrafenib or combination therapy with dabrafenib and trametinib, respectively, and the median duration of

response was 9.9 or 12.6 months, respectively. In the cohort of patients receiving dabrafenib in combination with trametinib for treatment-naive disease, the objective response rate was 61%. In the overall study population, 52 or 59–64% of the patients who responded to single-agent dabrafenib or dabrafenib and trametinib combination therapy, respectively, had durable responses of 6 months or more.

Clinical Perspective

Approximately 60% of patients with lung cancer have driver alterations (e.g., mutations in *EGFR*, *ALK*, or *BRAF*; *ROS-1* fusions, *RET* fusions, *MET* exon 14 skipping mutations, and *NTRK* fusions). The ASCO and Ontario Health (OH; previously known as Cancer Care Ontario) 2021 guideline specifically addresses treatment of stage IV NSCLC with driver alterations, including *BRAF* gene alterations.

For patients with stage IV NSCLC with a *BRAF* V600E mutation, dabrafenib and trametinib combination therapy should be offered as first line treatment; however, standard first-line therapy based on the ASCO/OH nondriver mutation guideline may also be offered. The 2022 update to this guideline leaves these recommendations unchanged.

In the second-line setting, standard treatment based on the ASCO/OH nondriver mutation guideline should be offered in patients with stage IV NSCLC harboring *BRAF* V600E driver alterations who were previously treated with BRAF/MEK inhibitor combination therapy. In patients who did not receive BRAF-targeted therapy in the first-line setting, dabrafenib in combination with trametinib, dabrafenib alone, or vemurafenib alone may be offered. For patients with stage IV NSCLC with *BRAF* mutations other than V600E, second-line treatment based on the ASCO/OH nondriver mutation guideline should be offered.

● Anaplastic Thyroid Cancer

Dabrafenib is used in combination with trametinib for the treatment of locally advanced or metastatic anaplastic thyroid cancer with *BRAF* V600E mutation when no satisfactory locoregional treatment options are available. Dabrafenib has been designated an orphan drug by the FDA for this use. The presence of the *BRAF* V600E mutation should be confirmed prior to initiation of therapy. There is currently no FDA-approved diagnostic test for the detection of *BRAF* V600E mutation in anaplastic thyroid cancer.

Dabrafenib is not indicated for treatment of patients with wild-type *BRAF* solid tumors.

Clinical Experience

This indication for dabrafenib in combination with trametinib in the treatment of anaplastic thyroid cancer with *BRAF* V600E mutation is based principally on the results of an open-label, multicenter, nonrandomized, multi-cohort, phase 2, basket trial (BRF117019; ROAR) in patients with rare *BRAF* V600E mutation-positive malignancies. In this trial, a cohort of 36 patients with locally advanced, unresectable, or metastatic anaplastic thyroid cancer received dabrafenib (150 mg twice daily) in combination with trametinib (2 mg once daily). Treatment was continued until disease progression or unacceptable toxicity occurred or the patient withdrew from the study. Patients with prior exposure to BRAF or MEK inhibitors, symptomatic or untreated CNS metastases, airway obstruction, or inability to swallow or retain oral drugs were not eligible to enroll in the study. The primary measure of efficacy was objective response rate as assessed by an independent review committee according to RECIST and duration of response. The median age of patients enrolled in the anaplastic thyroid cancer cohort was 71 years; 44% were male, 50% were Caucasian, 44% were Asian, and 94% had an ECOG performance status of 0 or 1. The majority of patients had received prior surgery and external beam radiation therapy (83% each) and 67% had previously received systemic therapy. The objective response rate in 36 evaluable patients in the anaplastic thyroid cancer cohort was 53%; complete response was achieved in 6% of the evaluable patients. The median duration of response was 13.6 months.

Clinical Perspective

Approximately 40–70% of patients with anaplastic thyroid cancer have *BRAF* V600E driver alterations. Mainstays of therapy in addition to surgery involve locoregional approaches (commonly radiotherapy with or without concurrent chemotherapy) or systemic therapy (cytotoxic therapy or targeted therapy).

The 2021 American Thyroid Association (ATA) guidelines for the management of anaplastic thyroid cancer recommend BRAF/MEK inhibitor combination therapy (dabrafenib in combination with trametinib) over other systemic therapies in patients with stage 4C or unresectable stage 4B anaplastic thyroid cancer harboring *BRAF* V600E mutation who decline radiation therapy. If radiotherapy is feasible in patients with *BRAF* V600E mutation-positive unresectable stage 4B anaplastic thyroid cancer, ATA recommends chemoradiotherapy or neoadjuvant dabrafenib-trametinib combination therapy as alternatives to initial treatment.

● Solid Tumors

Dabrafenib is used in combination with trametinib for the treatment of adults and pediatric patients 1 year of age and older with unresectable or metastatic solid tumors (excluding colorectal cancer) harboring the *BRAF* V600E mutation who have progressed following prior treatment and have no satisfactory alternative treatment. This indication is approved under accelerated approval based on overall response rate and duration of response. Continued approval for this indication may be contingent upon verification and description of clinical benefit in a confirmatory trial(s). Confirmation of the presence of the *BRAF* V600E mutation is necessary prior to initiation of therapy; no FDA-approved diagnostic test for the detection of the *BRAF* V600E mutation in solid tumors other than melanoma and NSCLC is currently available. Dabrafenib is designated an orphan drug by FDA for the treatment of malignant glioma.

Dabrafenib is not indicated for use in patients with *BRAF*-mutant colorectal cancer because of intrinsic resistance to BRAF inhibition. Dabrafenib is not indicated for the treatment of patients with wild-type *BRAF* solid tumors.

Clinical Experience

The indication for dabrafenib in combination with trametinib for the treatment of unresectable or metastatic *BRAF* V600E-mutant solid tumors is based on the results of the phase 2 ROAR trial in adults (including patients with anaplastic thyroid cancer), additional phase 2 trials in adults (protocol EAY131-H of the NCI-MATCH study) and pediatric patients (CTMT212X2101), and previously-described data from the COMBI-d and COMBI-v trials in patients with melanoma and the BRF113928 study in patients with NSCLC. In addition to adults with anaplastic thyroid cancer, the ROAR trial enrolled adults with high-grade glioma, low-grade glioma, GI stromal tumor, biliary tract cancer, and adenocarcinoma of the small intestine. EAY131-H was a multicenter, single-arm, open-label, phase 2, basket trial in patients with solid tumors, lymphoma, or multiple myeloma with *BRAF* V600 mutations who had received at least 1 prior line of standard therapy. Patients in the study received trametinib (2 mg once daily) and dabrafenib (150 mg twice daily) until disease progression or unacceptable toxicity occurred. Patients with melanoma, thyroid cancer, colorectal cancer, or NSCLC (following a protocol amendment), prior exposure to BRAF or MEK inhibitors, history of any RAS-mutant cancer, left ventricular ejection fraction below the lower limit of normal, or no measurable disease were excluded. The primary endpoint of both the ROAR and EAY131-H studies was objective response rate.

A pooled analysis of ROAR and EAY131-H included a total of 131 patients with *BRAF* V600E-mutant solid tumors (excluding patients with NSCLC and anaplastic thyroid cancer). Among patients in the pooled analysis, 37% had biliary tract cancers, 37% had high-grade gliomas, 11% had low-grade gliomas, and 15% had other GI, lung, gynecologic, or peritoneal tumors. In this pooled cohort, the median age was 51 years; 56% were female, 85% were white, 9% were Asian, and 93% had an ECOG performance status of 0 or 1. Most patients (90%) had received prior systemic therapy.

Among disease groups composed of more than 5 patients, RECIST objective response rate was 33% in those with high-grade gliomas, 46% in those with biliary tract cancers, and 50% in those with low-grade gliomas. Median duration of response was 13.6 months and 9.8 months in patients with high-grade gliomas and biliary tract cancers, respectively.

CTMT212X2101 was a multicenter, multi-cohort, open-label, phase 2 trial investigating trametinib monotherapy and trametinib in combination with dabrafenib in pediatric patients with recurrent or refractory solid tumors. Part C of this study was a dose escalation of trametinib and dabrafenib in pediatric patients with *BRAF* V600-mutant tumors; part D was an expansion cohort in pediatric patients with *BRAF* V600-mutant low-grade glioma or Langerhans cell histiocytosis. Patients received trametinib and dabrafenib at recommended dosage levels according to weight and age.

A pooled analysis of parts C and D of the CTMT212X2101 trial included a total of 48 pediatric patients with *BRAF* V600E-mutant tumors, including 34 patients

with low-grade gliomas and 2 patients with high-grade gliomas. Among the patients with gliomas, the median age was 10 years (range: 1 to 17 years); 50% were male, 75% were white, 8% were Asian, 3% were Black, and 58% had a Karnofsky/Lansky performance status of 100. Most patients had undergone prior surgical (83%) and/or systemic treatment (92%). Objective response rate by independent review according to Response Assessment in Neuro-Oncology (RANO) criteria for gliomas, the major efficacy outcome in the pooled glioma analysis, was 25%. Among responders, duration of response was 6 months or longer in 78% and 24 months or longer in 44% of patients.

● Low-grade Glioma

Dabrafenib is used in combination with trametinib for the treatment of pediatric patients 1 year of age and older with low-grade glioma with a *BRAF* V600E mutation who require systemic therapy. Confirmation of the presence of the *BRAF* V600E mutation is necessary prior to initiation of therapy; no FDA-approved diagnostic test for the detection of the *BRAF* V600E mutation in low-grade glioma is currently available. Safety and efficacy of dabrafenib in this use are principally supported by results of an open-label, multicenter, randomized, phase 2 trial in pediatric patients with *BRAF* V600E mutation-positive low-grade glioma. Guidelines on management of certain CNS tumors support consideration of BRAF and/or MEK inhibitors in patients with *BRAF*-altered pilocytic astrocytoma, pleomorphic xanthoastrocytoma, or ganglioglioma.

Dabrafenib is not indicated for treatment of patients with wild-type *BRAF* solid tumors.

Clinical Experience

This indication for dabrafenib in combination with trametinib for the treatment of *BRAF* V600E mutation-positive low-grade glioma in pediatric patients ≥1 year of age is based on the results from a phase 2 study (Study CDRB436G2201; NCT 02684058) involving 110 patients. In this study, patients with low-grade glioma who required systemic therapy were randomly assigned to dabrafenib plus trametinib or carboplatin plus vincristine (standard care) in a 2:1 ratio. The dosing of dabrafenib plus trametinib was age- and weight-based, with administration until disease progression or unacceptable toxicity occurred. The dosing of carboplatin and vincristine was body surface area-based at doses of 175 mg/m² and 1.5 mg/m² (0.05 mg/kg for patients <12 kg), respectively, with a single 10-week induction course followed by eight 6-week maintenance cycles.

The median age of enrolled patients was 9.5 years (range: 1 to 17) and 60% were female. The primary outcome was overall response rate; additional efficacy outcomes were progression-free survival and overall survival. The primary efficacy analysis was conducted after all patients had completed at least 32 weeks of therapy. Results revealed a substantial improvement in overall response rate and progression-free survival with dabrafenib plus trametinib in comparison to carboplatin plus vincristine. The overall response rate was 47% with dabrafenib plus trametinib and 11% with carboplatin plus vincristine; median progression-free survival was 20.1 months for the combination of dabrafenib plus trametinib versus 7.4 months with carboplatin plus vincristine. At the time of the interim analysis of overall survival, there was one death in the carboplatin plus vincristine arm with no deaths reported in the dabrafenib plus trametinib arm. The overall survival results at interim analysis did not reach statistical significance.

Clinical Perspective

Recurrent somatic alterations in *BRAF*, particularly V600E mutations and gene fusions, are encountered in certain CNS tumors in adults and children. These include select low- and high-grade gliomas in adults, such as pilocytic astrocytoma, pleomorphic xanthoastrocytoma (up to 70% with *BRAF* V600E), and ganglioglioma (20 to 60% with *BRAF* V600E), and pediatric low-grade gliomas. Surgery and/or radiation are the cornerstones of management of adult gliomas, with cytotoxic chemotherapy typically reserved for cases refractory to these interventions. In children, surgery is frequently utilized for diagnosis and symptomatic management, while cytotoxic chemotherapy is a typical mainstay of therapy for disease control due to long-term sequalae associated with radiotherapy.

The 2022 European Association of Neuro-Oncology, European Network for Rare Cancers, and Society for Neuro-Oncology joint guidelines for management of circumscribed astrocytic gliomas, glioneuronal, and neuronal tumors make general recommendations for treatment of these conditions in adults and children. In patients with *BRAF*-altered pilocytic astrocytoma, pleomorphic xanthoastrocytoma, or ganglioglioma, these guidelines recommend that use of BRAF and/or MEK inhibitors be considered.

DOSAGE AND ADMINISTRATION

• *General*

Pretreatment Screening

- *Melanoma*: Confirm presence of the *BRAF* V600E mutation in tumor specimens prior to initiation of dabrafenib as a single agent, and presence of *BRAF* V600E or V600K mutation in tumor specimens prior to initiation of combination therapy with dabrafenib and trametinib.

- *Non-small cell lung cancer (NSCLC)*: Confirm presence of the *BRAF* V600E mutation in tumor specimens prior to initiation of combination therapy with dabrafenib and trametinib for the treatment of metastatic NSCLC.

- *Anaplastic thyroid cancer*: Confirm presence of the *BRAF* V600E mutation in tumor specimens prior to initiation of combination therapy with dabrafenib and trametinib for the treatment of locally advanced or metastatic anaplastic thyroid cancer.

- *Solid tumors*: Confirm presence of the *BRAF* V600E mutation in tumor specimens prior to initiation of combination therapy with dabrafenib and trametinib for the treatment of unresectable or metastatic solid tumors.

- *Low-grade glioma*: Confirm presence of the *BRAF* V600E mutation in tumor specimens prior to initiation of combination therapy with dabrafenib and trametinib for the treatment of low-grade glioma.

- Perform a dermatologic evaluation prior to initiation of therapy.

- Assess left ventricular ejection fraction (LVEF) by echocardiogram or multigated radionuclide angiography (MUGA) scan prior to the initiation of dabrafenib in combination with trametinib.

- Monitor serum glucose concentrations prior to initiation of therapy in patients with preexisting diabetes mellitus or hyperglycemia.

- Verify pregnancy status in females of reproductive potential prior to initiation of therapy.

Patient Monitoring

- Perform dermatologic evaluations every 2 months during therapy and for up to 6 months following discontinuance of dabrafenib.

- Monitor for signs and symptoms of new noncutaneous malignancies.

- In patients receiving combination therapy with dabrafenib and trametinib, assess LVEF by echocardiogram or MUGA scan 1 month after initiation of therapy, and then every 2–3 months during combination therapy.

- Monitor serum glucose concentrations as clinically appropriate in patients with preexisting diabetes mellitus or hyperglycemia.

- Monitor for signs and symptoms of uveitis (e.g., vision change, photophobia, eye pain).

- Monitor patients with glucose-6-phosphate dehydrogenase (G-6-PD) deficiency for manifestations of hemolytic anemia.

- Monitor for signs and symptoms of bleeding due to the risk of hemorrhage.

- Monitor for new or worsening serious skin reactions during therapy, including Stevens-Johnson syndrome (SJS) and drug reaction with eosinophilia and systemic symptoms (DRESS).

Premedication and Prophylaxis

- Administer antipyretics as secondary prophylaxis when resuming dabrafenib therapy following resolution of a severe febrile reaction or fever associated with complications.

Dispensing and Administration Precautions

- Based on the Institute for Safe Medication Practices (ISMP), dabrafenib is a high-alert medication that has a heightened risk of causing significant patient harm when used in error.

Other General Considerations

- Clinicians should consult published protocols for information on the dosage, method of administration, and administration sequence of other antineoplastic agents used in combination regimens with dabrafenib. When used in combination with trametinib, the usual cautions, precautions, and contraindications associated with trametinib must be considered in addition to those associated with dabrafenib.

• *Administration*

Administer dabrafenib orally twice daily (as capsules or tablets for oral suspension), approximately every 12 hours, at least 1 hour before or 2 hours after a meal.

Dabrafenib capsules: Do not open, crush, or break the capsules.

Dabrafenib tablets for oral suspension: Do not chew or crush tablets and do not swallow whole. Prepare the suspension by dissolving the tablets with approximately 5 mL (1 to 4 tablets) or 10 mL (5 to 15 tablets) of water in the provided cup. Gently stir the mixture with the handle of a teaspoon; full dissolution may take at least 3 minutes. The resulting suspension should be cloudy white in appearance. Administer the suspension immediately after preparation from the cup, oral dosing syringe, or feeding tube. Discard the suspension if not administered within 30 minutes after preparation.

If a dose of dabrafenib is missed, take the dose as soon as it is remembered, but only if it can be taken at least 6 hours prior to the next scheduled dose.

If vomiting occurs after administration, do not take an additional dose. Take the next dose at its scheduled time.

Store dabrafenib capsules and tablets for oral suspension in the original bottle with the dessicant at 20–25°C (excursions permitted between 15–30°C).

• *Dosage*

Dosage of dabrafenib mesylate is expressed in terms of dabrafenib. Refer to the trametinib prescribing information for recommended trametinib dosage regimens.

Adults

Adjuvant Therapy for Melanoma

For use in combination with trametinib as adjuvant treatment following complete resection of melanoma with *BRAF* V600E or V600K mutation and nodal involvement, the recommended adult dosage of dabrafenib is 150 mg (two 75 mg capsules) twice daily. Continue therapy for up to 1 year or until disease progression or unacceptable toxicity occurs.

Monotherapy for Unresectable or Metastatic Melanoma

For use as a single-agent for the treatment of unresectable or metastatic melanoma with *BRAF* V600E mutation, the recommended adult dosage of dabrafenib is 150 mg (two 75 mg capsules) twice daily. Continue therapy until disease progression or unacceptable toxicity occurs.

Combination Therapy for Unresectable or Metastatic Melanoma

For use in combination with trametinib for the treatment of unresectable or metastatic melanoma with *BRAF* V600E or V600K mutation, the recommended adult dosage of dabrafenib is 150 mg (two 75 mg capsules) twice daily. Continue therapy until disease progression or unacceptable toxicity occurs.

Non-small Cell Lung Cancer

For use in combination with trametinib for the treatment of metastatic NSCLC with *BRAF* V600E mutation, the recommended adult dosage of dabrafenib is 150 mg (two 75 mg capsules) twice daily. Continue therapy until disease progression or unacceptable toxicity occurs.

Anaplastic Thyroid Cancer

For use in combination with trametinib for the treatment of locally advanced or metastatic anaplastic thyroid cancer with *BRAF* V600E mutation when no satisfactory locoregional treatment options are available, the recommended adult dosage of dabrafenib is 150 mg (two 75 mg capsules) twice daily. Continue therapy until disease progression or unacceptable toxicity occurs.

Solid Tumors

For use in combination with trametinib for the treatment of unresectable or metastatic solid tumors with *BRAF* V600E mutation in patients who have progressed following prior treatment and have no satisfactory alternative treatment options, the recommended adult dosage of dabrafenib is 150 mg (two 75 mg capsules) twice daily. Continue therapy until disease progression or unacceptable toxicity occurs.

Pediatric Patients

Solid Tumors

Dabrafenib capsules: For use in combination with trametinib for the treatment of unresectable or metastatic solid tumors in pediatric patients 1 year of age or older with *BRAF* V600E mutation, the recommended pediatric dosage of dabrafenib *capsules* is 150 mg (two 75 mg capsules) twice daily for patients who weigh ≥51 kg, 100 mg (two 50 mg capsules) twice daily for those who weigh 38–50 kg, and 75 mg twice daily for those who weigh 26–37 kg. Continue therapy until disease progression or unacceptable toxicity occurs. A recommended dosage of dabrafenib *capsules* has not been established for patients weighing <26 kg.

Dabrafenib tablets for oral suspension: The recommended dosage of the tablets for oral suspension is based on body weight (see Table 1).

TABLE 1. Recommended Dosage for Dabrafenib Tablets for Oral Suspension

Body Weight (kg)	Recommended Dosage
8 to 9	20 mg twice daily
10 to 13	30 mg twice daily
14 to 17	40 mg twice daily
18 to 21	50 mg twice daily
22 to 25	60 mg twice daily
26 to 29	70 mg twice daily
30 to 33	80 mg twice daily
34 to 37	90 mg twice daily
38 to 41	100 mg twice daily
42 to 45	110 mg twice daily
46 to 50	130 mg twice daily
≥51	150 mg twice daily

Low-grade Glioma

Dabrafenib capsules: For use in combination with trametinib for the treatment of low-grade glioma in pediatric patients 1 year of age or older with a *BRAF* V600E mutation, the recommended pediatric dosage of dabrafenib *capsules* is 150 mg (two 75 mg capsules) twice daily for patients who weigh ≥51 kg, 100 mg (two 50 mg capsules) twice daily for those who weigh 38–50 kg, and 75 mg twice daily for those who weigh 26–37 kg. Continue therapy until disease progression or unacceptable toxicity occurs. A recommended dosage of dabrafenib *capsules* has not been established for patients weighing <26 kg.

Dabrafenib tablets for oral suspension: The recommended dosage is based on body weight (see Table 1).

Dosage Modification for Toxicity

Dosage of dabrafenib may be reduced or therapy temporarily interrupted or discontinued in patients who develop adverse effects. Dosage reductions for dabrafenib *capsules* and dabrafenib *tablets for oral suspension* for adverse reactions are presented in Tables 2 and 3. Permanently discontinue dabrafenib *capsules* if a patient is unable to tolerate the 50 mg twice daily dosage regimen.

TABLE 2. Recommended Dosage Reductions for Dabrafenib Capsules for Adverse Reactions

Recommended Dosage	75 mg orally twice daily	100 mg orally twice daily	150 mg orally twice daily
First Dose Reduction	50 mg orally twice daily	75 mg orally twice daily	100 mg orally twice daily
Second Dose Reduction	Not applicable	50 mg orally twice daily	75 mg orally twice daily
Third Dose Reduction	Not applicable	Not applicable	50 mg orally twice daily

TABLE 3. Recommended Dosage Reductions for Dabrafenib Tablets for Oral Suspension for Adverse Reactions

Body Weight (Recommended Dosage)	First Dose Reduction	Second Dose Reduction	Third Dose Reduction
8 to 9 kg (20 mg twice daily)	10 mg twice daily	Not applicable	Not applicable
10 to 13 kg (30 mg twice daily)	20 mg twice daily	10 mg twice daily	Not applicable
14 to 17 kg (40 mg twice daily)	30 mg twice daily	20 mg twice daily	10 mg twice daily
18 to 21 kg (50 mg twice daily)	30 mg twice daily	20 mg twice daily	10 mg twice daily
22 to 25 kg (60 mg twice daily)	40 mg twice daily	30 mg twice daily	20 mg twice daily
26 to 29 kg (70 mg twice daily)	50 mg twice daily	40 mg twice daily	20 mg twice daily
30 to 33 kg (80 mg twice daily)	50 mg twice daily	40 mg twice daily	30 mg twice daily
34 to 37 kg (90 mg twice daily)	60 mg twice daily	50 mg twice daily	30 mg twice daily
38 to 41 kg (100 mg twice daily)	70 mg twice daily	50 mg twice daily	30 mg twice daily
42 to 45 kg (110 mg twice daily)	70 mg twice daily	60 mg twice daily	40 mg twice daily
46 to 50 kg (130 mg twice daily)	90 mg twice daily	70 mg twice daily	40 mg twice daily
≥51 kg (150 mg twice daily)	100 mg twice daily	80 mg twice daily	50 mg twice daily

New Primary Cutaneous Malignancies

If new primary cutaneous malignancies occur, no dosage modification of dabrafenib is recommended.

New Primary Noncutaneous Malignancies

If new RAS mutation-positive, noncutaneous malignancies occur, permanently discontinue dabrafenib.

Febrile Drug Reactions

If fever (temperature of 38–40°C) or any initial symptom of fever recurrence occurs, interrupt dabrafenib treatment until the adverse reaction resolves. Once fever resolves, resume dabrafenib at the same or a reduced dosage.

If a higher fever (temperature >40°C) or fever complicated by rigors, hypotension, dehydration, or renal failure occurs, permanently discontinue dabrafenib treatment or interrupt dabrafenib treatment until such adverse reactions resolve for at least 24 hours. Once fever resolves, resume dabrafenib at a reduced dosage.

Dermatologic Effects

If grade 2 skin toxicity develops and is intolerable, withhold dabrafenib for up to 3 weeks. If grade 2 toxicity improves within 3 weeks of withholding dabrafenib, resume the drug at a reduced dosage. If grade 2 skin toxicity does not improve within 3 weeks of withholding dabrafenib, permanently discontinue the drug.

If grade 3 or 4 skin toxicity occurs, withhold dabrafenib for up to 3 weeks. If grade 3 or 4 skin toxicity improves within 3 weeks of withholding dabrafenib, resume the drug at a reduced dosage. If grade 3 or 4 skin toxicity does not improve within 3 weeks of withholding dabrafenib, permanently discontinue the drug.

If severe cutaneous adverse reactions (SCARs) such as Stevens-Johnson syndrome (SJS) and drug reaction with eosinophilia and systemic symptoms (DRESS) occur, permanently discontinue dabrafenib.

Cardiac Effects

If symptomatic congestive heart failure (CHF) occurs or LVEF decreases by >20% from baseline and to a level below the lower limit of normal (LLN), withhold dabrafenib therapy; resume therapy at the same dosage when LVEF improves to at least the institutional LLN and absolute decrease to ≤10% compared to baseline.

Hemorrhage

If an intolerable grade 2 or any grade 3 hemorrhagic events occur, withhold dabrafenib therapy. If improvement to grade 0 or 1 is observed, resume dabrafenib at a reduced dosage. If no improvement, permanently discontinue dabrafenib.

Permanently discontinue dabrafenib for all grade 4 hemorrhagic events.

Venous Thromboembolism

If uncomplicated venous thromboembolism (VTE) occurs in patients receiving dabrafenib in combination with trametinib, no dosage modification of dabrafenib is recommended.

Ocular Effects

If retinal pigment epithelial detachment or retinal vein occlusion occurs in patients receiving combination therapy with trametinib, no dosage modification of dabrafenib is needed.

If iritis occurs, continue dabrafenib therapy at the same dosage and initiate ocular therapy.

If mild or moderate uveitis occurs and is unresponsive to ocular therapy, interrupt dabrafenib treatment for up to 6 weeks. If improvement to grade 0 or 1 is observed within 6 weeks, resume dabrafenib therapy at the same or a reduced dosage. If no improvement is observed within 6 weeks, permanently discontinue dabrafenib therapy.

If severe uveitis occurs, interrupt dabrafenib treatment for up to 6 weeks and initiate ocular therapy as clinically indicated. If improvement to grade 0 or 1 is observed within 6 weeks, resume dabrafenib therapy at the same or a reduced dosage. If no improvement is observed within 6 weeks or for persistent uveitis of grade 2 or greater, permanently discontinue dabrafenib therapy.

Pulmonary Effects

If interstitial lung disease or pneumonitis occurs during combination therapy with dabrafenib and trametinib, no dosage modification of dabrafenib is needed.

Other Toxicity

If an intolerable grade 2 adverse reaction or any grade 3 adverse reaction occurs, interrupt dabrafenib treatment until the adverse reaction resolves to grade 1 or less. Once the adverse reaction has resolved, resume dabrafenib at a reduced dosage. If no improvement is observed, permanently discontinue dabrafenib.

For a first occurrence of any grade 4 adverse reaction, permanently discontinue dabrafenib treatment or interrupt until the adverse reaction resolves to grade 1 or less. Once the adverse reaction has resolved, resume dabrafenib at a reduced dosage. If a grade 4 adverse reaction recurs, permanently discontinue dabrafenib therapy.

• Special Populations

Hepatic Impairment

In patients with mild hepatic impairment (bilirubin ≤ the upper limit of normal [ULN] and AST >ULN or bilirubin >1–1.5 times the ULN and any AST level), dosage adjustments are not necessary.

Patients with moderate hepatic impairment (bilirubin >1.5–3 times the ULN and any AST) or severe hepatic impairment (bilirubin >3–10 times the ULN and any AST) may have increased exposure to dabrafenib; however, an appropriate dosage has not been established for these patients.

Renal Impairment

The manufacturer makes no specific dosage recommendations for patients with renal impairment.

Geriatric Use

The manufacturer makes no specific dosage recommendations for geriatric patients.

CAUTIONS

• Contraindications

• None.

• Warnings/Precautions

Combination Therapy

When combination therapy with dabrafenib includes the use of trametinib, the manufacturer's prescribing information for trametinib should be consulted for detailed information on the usual cautions, precautions, and contraindications of this drug.

New Primary Malignancies

New primary cutaneous or noncutaneous malignancies have been reported in patients receiving b-Raf serine-threonine kinase (BRAF) inhibitors, including dabrafenib.

Cutaneous Malignancies

In clinical trials, cutaneous squamous cell carcinomas and keratoacanthomas occurred in 11% and 4%, respectively, of adult patients receiving dabrafenib monotherapy. Basal cell carcinoma and new primary melanoma occurred in 4% and 1% of patients, respectively.

Among adults receiving dabrafenib in combination with trametinib, cutaneous squamous cell carcinomas including keratoacanthomas occurred in 2% of patients in clinical studies. Basal cell carcinoma and new primary melanoma occurred in approximately 3% and <1% of patients, respectively.

Among pediatric patients receiving dabrafenib in combination with trametinib, new primary melanoma occurred in <1% of patients.

Although the mechanism for development of cutaneous squamous cell carcinoma has not been fully determined, it has been suggested that paradoxical activation of mitogen-activated protein kinase (MAPK) signaling may lead to accelerated growth of such skin lesions as well as development of other primary malignancies. MAPK-mediated events in wild-type *BRAF* cells have been observed in a study evaluating the pathology and immunohistochemistry of normal and proliferating skin lesions in patients receiving the weak b-Raf kinase inhibitor sorafenib. Another study performed a molecular analysis of DNA extracted from tumor specimens of patients receiving the BRAF inhibitor vemurafenib; results indicated that these patients have a secondary mutation (in addition to the *BRAF* V600E mutation) that appears to be activated by vemurafenib treatment. Some clinicians suggest that advanced age (i.e., 65 years of age or older), history of skin cancer, and chronic sun exposure may be risk factors for developing cutaneous squamous cell carcinoma. Some data suggest that mitogen-activated extracellular signal-regulated kinase (MEK) inhibitors (i.e., binimetinib, cobimetinib, trametinib) block the paradoxical activation of the MAPK pathway induced by BRAF inhibitors (i.e., dabrafenib, encorafenib, vemurafenib); therefore, combination therapy with a BRAF inhibitor and an MEK inhibitor may reduce the risk of developing cutaneous squamous cell carcinoma. Findings from a meta-analysis of randomized controlled studies that assessed the relative risk of development of cutaneous squamous cell carcinoma in cancer patients receiving a BRAF inhibitor indicate that the risk of cutaneous squamous cell carcinoma is higher in patients receiving a BRAF inhibitor than in patients receiving combination therapy with a BRAF inhibitor and an MEK inhibitor.

Perform dermatologic evaluations prior to initiation of therapy, every 2 months during therapy, and for up to 6 months following discontinuance of dabrafenib monotherapy or combination therapy with trametinib. In patients who develop new primary cutaneous malignancies during combination therapy with dabrafenib and trametinib, the manufacturer states that no dosage adjustment of dabrafenib is necessary.

Noncutaneous Malignancies

In clinical trials, noncutaneous malignancies occurred in 1% of patients receiving dabrafenib monotherapy or dabrafenib in combination with trametinib.

Monitor for signs and symptoms of new noncutaneous malignancies. If new primary RAS mutation-positive, noncutaneous malignancies occur, permanently discontinue dabrafenib therapy.

Tumor Promotion in Wild-Type BRAF Tumors

In vitro evidence of increased MAPK signaling and cell proliferation in wild-type BRAF cells exposed to BRAF inhibitors has been observed.

Confirm presence of BRAF V600E or V600K mutation prior to initiating dabrafenib monotherapy or combination therapy with trametinib. Use of dabrafenib is not recommended in patients with wild-type BRAF solid tumors.

Hemorrhage

Hemorrhage, including major hemorrhagic events (i.e., symptomatic bleeding in a critical area or organ), has occurred when dabrafenib is used in combination with trametinib; some cases have been fatal. In clinical trials in adults, hemorrhagic events occurred in 17% of patients receiving dabrafenib in combination with trametinib. Gastrointestinal hemorrhage and intracranial hemorrhage occurred in 3% and 0.6%, respectively, of adult patients receiving dabrafenib in combination with trametinib. Fatal hemorrhagic events (e.g., cerebral hemorrhage, brainstem hemorrhage) occurred in 0.5% of adults receiving the combination therapy. In clinical trials in pediatric patients, hemorrhagic events occurred in 25% of patients, with epistaxis the most common type of bleeding. Serious bleeding events, including GI hemorrhage, cerebral hemorrhage, uterine hemorrhage, postprocedural hemorrhage, and epistaxis, were observed in 3.6% of pediatric patients.

If hemorrhagic events occur, dosage modification and/or treatment discontinuance may be necessary.

Cardiomyopathy

Cardiomyopathy has been reported in patients receiving dabrafenib in combination with trametinib.

In clinical trials in adults, cardiomyopathy (defined as an absolute decrease in left ventricular ejection fraction [LVEF] from baseline of ≥10% and to a level below institution-specific lower limit of normal) occurred in 6% of adults receiving dabrafenib in combination with trametinib. Dosage interruption or discontinuance of dabrafenib was necessary in 3% or <1%, respectively, of patients receiving dabrafenib in combination with trametinib. Cardiomyopathy resolved in 45 of 50 patients receiving the combination therapy.

In clinical trials in pediatric patients, cardiomyopathy occurred in 9% of patients receiving dabrafenib in combination with trametinib.

Assess LVEF using echocardiogram or multigated radionuclide angiography (MUGA) prior to and 1 month after initiation of dabrafenib in combination with trametinib and then every 2–3 months during therapy. If left ventricular dysfunction occurs, temporary interruption of dabrafenib may be necessary.

Uveitis

Uveitis has occurred in patients receiving dabrafenib monotherapy or combination therapy with trametinib. In clinical trials, uveitis has been reported in 1% of adults receiving dabrafenib and in 2% and 1.2% of adult and pediatric patients, respectively, receiving dabrafenib in combination with trametinib. Symptomatic treatment (e.g., ophthalmic corticosteroid or mydriatic preparations) was used during clinical trials for management of this condition.

Monitor patients receiving dabrafenib for signs and symptoms of uveitis (e.g., vision change, photophobia, eye pain). Temporary interruption, dosage reduction, or discontinuance of dabrafenib and/or initiation of ocular therapy may be necessary if uveitis occurs during therapy with the drug.

Serious Febrile Reactions

Serious febrile drug reactions (including fever accompanied by hypotension, rigors/chills, dehydration, or renal failure) have occurred in patients receiving dabrafenib as monotherapy or as combination therapy with trametinib. In clinical trials in adults, fever occurred in 30% of adults receiving dabrafenib monotherapy. Serious febrile reactions and fever of any severity complicated by hypotension, rigors, or chills, dehydration or renal failure occurred in 6% of adult patients receiving dabrafenib monotherapy. Increased incidence and severity of pyrexia have been observed during combination therapy with dabrafenib and trametinib compared with dabrafenib alone. In clinical trials, fever occurred in 58% of adults receiving dabrafenib in combination with trametinib. Serious febrile reactions and fever of any severity complicated by hypotension, rigors, chills, dehydration, or renal failure occurred in 5% of adult patients. In pooled safety data in pediatric patients, pyrexia was reported in 66% of patients during combination therapy with dabrafenib and trametinib in clinical trials.

Interrupt dabrafenib monotherapy and combination treatment with trametinib and evaluate the patient for manifestations of infection if the patient's temperature is ≥38°C. If severe pyrexia occurs, monitor renal function (e.g., serum creatinine) during and following severe pyrexia. Administer prophylactic antipyretics in patients resuming dabrafenib following a serious febrile reaction or fever associated with complications. For second or subsequent occurrences of prolonged fever (lasting longer than 3 days) or fever associated with complications (e.g., dehydration, hypotension, renal failure, severe chills/rigors) without evidence of an active infection, administer corticosteroids (e.g., prednisone 10 mg daily) for at least 5 days.

Serious Skin Toxicities

Severe cutaneous adverse reactions (SCARs), including Stevens-Johnson syndrome and drug reaction with eosinophilia and systemic symptoms (DRESS), have been reported in postmarketing surveillance during therapy with dabrafenib in combination with trametinib. Across clinical trials, other serious dermatologic toxicity occurred in <1% of adults receiving dabrafenib in combination with trametinib; serious adverse events of skin and subcutaneous tissue disorders occurred in 1.8% of pediatric patients receiving dabrafenib in combination with trametinib.

Monitor for new or worsening serious skin toxicities. If dermatologic toxicity occurs, dosage modification or treatment discontinuance may be necessary. Permanently discontinue dabrafenib if SCARs occur. For other skin toxicities, withhold dabrafenib for intolerable or severe skin toxicity. Resume treatment at a lower dose in patients with improvement or recovery from skin toxicity within 3 weeks; permanently discontinue dabrafenib if skin toxicity has not improved within 3 weeks.

Hyperglycemia

Hyperglycemia requiring increased dosage of insulin or oral hypoglycemic agents or requiring initiation of these agents has occurred in patients receiving dabrafenib as monotherapy or as combination therapy with trametinib. Across clinical trials of dabrafenib monotherapy, 14% of adults with a history of diabetes mellitus required intensification of hypoglycemic therapy; grade 3 and 4 hyperglycemia occurred in 3% of patients. Across clinical trials of adults receiving dabrafenib in combination with trametinib, grade 3 or 4 hyperglycemia occurred in 2% of patients; grade 3 or 4 hyperglycemia occurred in <1% of pediatric patients receiving the combination therapy.

Monitor serum glucose concentrations prior to initiation of therapy and as clinically appropriate in patients with preexisting diabetes mellitus or hyperglycemia. Initiate or optimize antihyperglycemic therapy as clinically indicated.

Glucose-6-Phosphate Dehydrogenase Deficiency

Dabrafenib contains a sulfonamide moiety and has the potential to induce hemolytic anemia in patients with glucose-6-phosphate dehydrogenase (G-6-PD) deficiency.

Monitor patients with G-6-PD deficiency for manifestations of hemolytic anemia during dabrafenib therapy.

Hemophagocytic Lymphohistiocytosis

Dabrafenib in combination with trametinib may result in hemophagocytic lymphohistiocytosis (HLH). Interrupt therapy if HLH is suspected. If a diagnosis is confirmed, discontinue therapy and initiate appropriate management of HLH.

Fetal/Neonatal Morbidity and Mortality

Dabrafenib may cause fetal harm based on its mechanism of action and animal findings; the drug has been shown to be teratogenic and embryotoxic in rats administered dabrafenib dosages equivalent to 3 times the human exposure achieved with recommended dosages.

Verify pregnancy status in females of reproductive potential prior to initiation of therapy. Advise females of reproductive potential to use effective nonhormonal contraception during treatment and for 2 weeks after the last dabrafenib dose.

Advise females to contact their clinician if pregnancy is suspected or confirmed.

Specific Populations

Pregnancy

Dabrafenib may cause fetal harm if administered to pregnant females based on its mechanism of action and animal findings. If dabrafenib is used during pregnancy, the patient should be informed of the potential hazard to the fetus.

Lactation

It is not known whether dabrafenib is distributed into human milk. Because of the potential for serious adverse reactions to dabrafenib in breast-fed infants, females should be advised not to breast-feed while receiving the drug and for 2 weeks after the last dose. The effects of the drug on breast-fed infants or on the production of milk are unknown.

Females and Males of Reproductive Potential

Verify pregnancy status in females of reproductive potential prior to initiation of therapy.

Since hormonal contraceptives may be ineffective when used concomitantly with dabrafenib, female patients of reproductive potential should use an effective nonhormonal method of contraception during dabrafenib therapy and for 2 weeks after the last dose.

To avoid potential drug exposure to pregnant partners and female partners of reproductive potential, advise male patients (including those who have had vasectomies) with female partners of reproductive potential to use condoms during treatment with dabrafenib and for at least 2 weeks after the last dose.

Results of animal studies suggest that dabrafenib may reduce male and female fertility. In fertility studies, impairment of fertility (reduced corpora lutea in females and impaired spermatogenesis in males) was observed in animals receiving dabrafenib at exposure levels approximately or up to 3 times the human exposure at the recommended dosage.

Pediatric Use

The safety and efficacy of dabrafenib in combination with trametinib have been established in pediatric patients 1 year of age and older with unresectable or metastatic solid tumors with *BRAF* V600E mutation who have progressed following prior treatment and have no satisfactory alternative treatment options, or with low-grade glioma with *BRAF* V600E mutation who require systemic therapy. Dabrafenib in combination with trametinib for these indications is supported by evidence from 2 studies that enrolled 171 patients (between the ages of 1 to <18 years) with *BRAF* V600 mutation-positive advanced solid tumors. Safety and efficacy of dabrafenib in combination with trametinib have not been established in pediatric patients younger than 1 year of age.

Safety and efficacy of dabrafenib as monotherapy have not been established in pediatric patients.

Geriatric Use

No substantial differences in safety and efficacy of dabrafenib monotherapy have been observed in patients ≥65 years of age relative to younger adults.

In clinical trials evaluating dabrafenib in combination with trametinib in patients with melanoma, 21% of patients were ≥65 years of age and 5% were ≥75 years of age. No overall differences in efficacy were observed between geriatric patients and younger adults, but some adverse effects (i.e., peripheral edema, anorexia) occurred more frequently in geriatric patients with metastatic melanoma.

Clinical experience with dabrafenib and trametinib combination therapy in patients ≥65 years of age with non-small cell lung cancer (NSCLC) is insufficient to determine whether geriatric patients respond differently than younger adults.

In clinical trials evaluating dabrafenib and trametinib combination therapy in patients with anaplastic thyroid cancer, 77% of patients were ≥65 years of age. An insufficient number of younger adults were included in the study to determine whether geriatric patients respond differently than younger adults.

Hepatic Impairment

Patients with moderate hepatic impairment (bilirubin >1.5–3 times the ULN and any AST) or severe hepatic impairment (bilirubin >3–10 times the ULN and any AST) may have increased exposure to dabrafenib; however, an appropriate dosage has not been established for these patients.

Renal Impairment

Clinically relevant pharmacokinetic differences have not been observed in patients with renal impairment (estimated glomerular filtration rate [eGFR] of 15–89 mL/minute per 1.73 m^2).

● Common Adverse Effects

Adverse effects reported in ≥20% of adult patients receiving dabrafenib monotherapy include hyperkeratosis, headache, pyrexia, arthralgia, papilloma, alopecia, and palmar-plantar erythrodysesthesia syndrome (hand-foot syndrome).

Adverse effects reported in ≥20% of adult patients receiving dabrafenib in combination with trametinib for the treatment of previously untreated unresectable or metastatic melanoma include pyrexia, rash, chills, headache, arthralgia, and cough.

Adverse effects reported in ≥20% of adult patients receiving dabrafenib in combination with trametinib for the adjuvant treatment of melanoma include pyrexia, fatigue, nausea, headache, rash, chills, diarrhea, vomiting, arthralgia, and myalgia.

Adverse effects reported in ≥20% of adult patients receiving dabrafenib in combination with trametinib for the treatment of metastatic NSCLC include pyrexia, fatigue, nausea, vomiting, diarrhea, dry skin, decreased appetite, edema, rash, chills, hemorrhage, cough, and dyspnea.

Adverse effects reported in ≥20% of adult patients receiving dabrafenib in combination with trametinib for the treatment of solid tumors include: pyrexia, fatigue, nausea, rash, chills, headache, hemorrhage, cough, vomiting, constipation, diarrhea, myalgia, arthralgia, and edema.

Adverse effects reported in ≥20% of pediatric patients receiving dabrafenib in combination with trametinib for the treatment of solid tumors include: pyrexia, rash, vomiting, fatigue, dry skin, cough, diarrhea, dermatitis acneiform, headache, abdominal pain, nausea, hemorrhage, constipation, and paronychia.

Adverse effects reported in ≥20% of pediatric patients receiving dabrafenib in combination with trametinib for the treatment of low-grade glioma incude pyrexia, rash, headache, vomiting, musculokeletal pain, fatigue, diarrhea, dry skin, nausea, hemorrhage, abdominal pain, and dermatitis acneiform.

DRUG INTERACTIONS

Dabrafenib is metabolized primarily by cytochrome P-450 (CYP) isoenzymes 3A4 and 2C8.

Dabrafenib is an inducer of CYP isoenzymes 3A4, 1A2, and 2C9. In vitro studies show that dabrafenib induces CYP3A4 and CYP2B6 via activation of the pregnane X receptor and constitutive androstane receptor. Dabrafenib also may induce CYP2C isoenzymes via this same mechanism of action.

Dabrafenib and its metabolites, hydroxyl-dabrafenib and desmethyldabrafenib, are substrates of human P-glycoprotein (P-gp) and breast cancer resistance protein (BCRP). Dabrafenib and its hydroxy, carboxy, and desmethyl metabolites are inhibitors of organic anion-transporting polypeptide (OATP) 1B1 and 1B3 as well as organic anion transporters (OAT) 1 and 3 in vitro.

● Drugs Affecting Hepatic Microsomal Enzymes

Inhibitors of CYP3A4 and CYP2C8

Potential pharmacokinetic interactions may occur when dabrafenib is used concomitantly with potent inhibitors of CYP isoenzymes 3A4 or 2C8 (e.g., gemfibrozil, ketoconazole) resulting in increased dabrafenib concentrations. In a pharmacokinetic study, concomitant administration of dabrafenib 75 mg twice daily and ketoconazole 400 mg once daily (a potent CYP3A4 inhibitor) for 4 days resulted in a 71% increase in AUC of dabrafenib, an 82% increase in the AUC of hydroxy-dabrafenib, and a 68% increase in the AUC of desmethyl-dabrafenib. In another study, concomitant administration of dabrafenib 75 mg twice daily and gemfibrozil 600 mg twice daily (a potent CYP2C8 inhibitor) for 4 days resulted in a 47% increase in the AUC of dabrafenib with no change in the AUC of dabrafenib's metabolites. Alternative therapy to potent inhibitors of CYP3A4 or 2C8 is recommended during dabrafenib therapy. If concomitant use is unavoidable, monitor the patient closely for dabrafenib-associated adverse reactions.

Inducers of CYP3A4 and CYP2C8

Potential pharmacokinetic interactions may occur when dabrafenib is used concomitantly with potent inducers of CYP3A4 or moderate inducers of CYP2C8 (e.g., rifampin) resulting in decreased dabrafenib concentrations. In a pharmacokinetic study, concomitant administration of dabrafenib 150 mg twice daily and rifampin 600 mg once daily (a potent CYP3A4 and moderate CYP2C8 inducer) for 10 days resulted in a 34% decrease in AUC of dabrafenib, a 30% decrease in the AUC of desmethyl-dabrafenib, and no change in the AUC of hydroxy-dabrafenib.

● Drugs Metabolized by Hepatic Microsomal Enzymes

In a pharmacokinetic study, concomitant use of dabrafenib 150 mg twice daily for 15 days and a single dose of midazolam 3 mg (a CYP3A4 substrate) resulted in a 65% decrease in midazolam AUC. In another study, concomitant administration of dabrafenib 150 mg twice daily for 15 days and a single dose of warfarin sodium 15 mg resulted in a 37% decrease in the AUC of S-warfarin (a CYP2C9 substrate) and a 33% reduction in the AUC of R-warfarin (a CYP3A4/CYP1A2 substrate). Monitor the international normalized ratio (INR) frequently in patients receiving warfarin during initiation or discontinuance of dabrafenib.

Potential pharmacokinetic interactions may occur when dabrafenib is used concomitantly with substrates of CYP isoenzymes 3A4, 1A2, 2B6, 2C8, 2C9, or 2C19 (e.g., dexamethasone, hormonal contraceptives, midazolam, warfarin sodium) possibly resulting in decreased concentrations and reduced efficacy of the substrate drug. Alternative therapy to the substrate drug is recommended. If concomitant use is unavoidable, monitor the patient closely for reduced efficacy of the substrate drug.

● Drugs Affected by Transport Proteins

Potential pharmacokinetic interactions may occur when dabrafenib is used concomitantly with drugs transported by OATP1B1, OATP1B3, OAT1, or OAT3. Concomitant administration of a single dose of the sensitive OATP1B1 and OATP1B3 substrate rosuvastatin with dabrafenib (150 mg twice daily) resulted in a 2.6-fold increase in peak plasma concentrations of rosuvastatin and no change in AUC of rosuvastatin.

● Drugs Affecting Gastric Acidity

Concomitant use of dabrafenib (150 mg twice daily) with the proton-pump inhibitor rabeprazole (40 mg once daily for 4 days) resulted in no clinically important changes in peak plasma concentration or systemic exposure of dabrafenib or its metabolites.

● Hormonal Contraceptives

Concomitant use of dabrafenib with hormonal contraceptives that are metabolized by CYP3A4, 1A2, or 2C9 may result in decreased systemic exposure and reduced efficacy of the contraceptive. Alternative nonhormonal contraception is recommended. If concomitant use is unavoidable, monitor the patient closely for reduced efficacy of the hormonal contraceptive.

● Trametinib

Concomitant administration of dabrafenib 150 mg twice daily with trametinib 2 mg once daily resulted in a 23% increase in AUC of dabrafenib, a 33% increase in AUC of desmethyl-dabrafenib, and no change in AUC of hydroxy-dabrafenib compared with administration of dabrafenib alone.

● Warfarin

Dabrafenib is an inducer of CYP isoenzymes 3A4, 1A2, and 2C9. Concomitant use of dabrafenib with warfarin may result in decreased systemic exposure to S-warfarin (a CYP2C9 substrate) and R-warfarin (a CYP3A4/CYP1A2 substrate). Monitor INR frequently in patients receiving warfarin during initiation or discontinuance of dabrafenib.

DESCRIPTION

Dabrafenib, a potent inhibitor of b-Raf serine-threonine kinase (BRAF) with V600E or V600K mutation, is an antineoplastic agent. Approximately 50% of cutaneous melanomas carry a BRAF mutation. The most common BRAF mutation is the substitution of glutamic acid for valine at codon 600 in exon 15 (BRAF V600E); a less frequently occurring BRAF mutation is the substitution of lysine for valine at codon 600 in exon 15 (BRAF V600K). The mutation of BRAF V600E activates the mitogen-activated protein kinase (MAPK) and extracellular signal-regulated kinase (ERK) signal transduction pathway, which enhances cell proliferation and tumor progression (e.g., metastasis). In vitro studies indicate that dabrafenib also inhibits BRAF with V600D mutation. Paradoxical activation of MAPK and increased cell proliferation have been observed in BRAF wild-type cells exposed to BRAF inhibitors.

Clinical resistance to monotherapy with a BRAF inhibitor, generally occurring 6–7 months following initiation of therapy, has been attributed to several possible resistance mechanisms mostly relying on reactivation of the MAPK/ERK pathway. Complete inhibition of the MAPK/ERK pathway resulting in durable responses may be achieved with the use of combination therapy with a BRAF inhibitor (i.e., dabrafenib, encorafenib, vemurafenib) and an MEK inhibitor (i.e., binimetinib, cobimetinib, trametinib). Use of dabrafenib and trametinib in combination resulted in greater growth inhibition of melanoma cell lines testing positive for BRAF V600 mutations in vitro. In addition, combination therapy was associated with prolonged inhibition of tumor growth in melanoma xenografts testing positive for BRAF V600 mutations compared with either drug alone.

Following oral administration, the absolute bioavailability of dabrafenib is 95%. Peak plasma concentrations of dabrafenib occur within 2 hours after oral administration. Following administration of a single dabrafenib dose within the dosage range of 12–300 mg, the drug exhibits dose-proportional increases in peak plasma concentrations and AUC; however, these increases are less than dose proportional after repeated twice-daily dosing. Administration of a single dose of dabrafenib with a high-fat meal (approximately 1000 calories) decreased peak plasma concentrations and AUC of the drug by 51 and 31%, respectively, and delayed the rate of absorption (time to reach peak concentrations delayed by 3.6 hours). Dabrafenib is more than 99% bound to plasma proteins; in vitro studies suggest that dabrafenib is a substrate of P-glycoprotein (P-gp) and breast cancer resistance protein (BCRP). Dabrafenib is principally metabolized by cytochrome P-450 (CYP) isoenzymes 3A4 and 2C8. Dabrafenib is an inducer of CYP3A4 and 2C19 and may induce other CYP isoenzymes. The metabolites hydroxy- and desmethyl-dabrafenib are likely to contribute to the clinical activity of dabrafenib. The mean terminal half-life of dabrafenib is 8 hours. Following oral administration of a radiolabeled dose of dabrafenib, about 71% of the dose is recovered in feces and 23% is recovered in urine.

The pharmacokinetics of dabrafenib in pediatric patients (1 to 18 years of age) with glioma and other solid tumors following single or multiple doses are with range of values observed in adults given the same dose based on weight. Weight (6 to 156 kg) had a statistically significant effect of dabrafenib oral clearance in this population.

ADVICE TO PATIENTS

- Take dabrafenib exactly as prescribed and do not alter the dosage or discontinue therapy unless advised to do so by a clinician.

- Advise patient or caregiver to read instructions for use for dabrafenib tablets for oral suspension for directions on preparing and administering the drug.

- Advise patients to take dabrafenib at least 1 hour before or 2 hours after a meal.

- Advise patients to take a missed dose as soon as remembered, but only if it can be taken at least 6 hours prior to the next scheduled dose.

- Inform patients of the risk of new primary cutaneous and noncutaneous malignancies. Advise patients to inform their clinician promptly if dermatologic changes (i.e., new lesions, changes to existing lesions) or signs and/or symptoms of other malignancies occur.

- Inform patients of the risk of intracranial and GI hemorrhage. Advise patients to inform their clinician promptly if signs and/or symptoms of unusual bleeding or hemorrhage occur.

- Inform patients of the risk of cardiomyopathy. Advise patients to inform their clinician promptly if signs and/or symptoms of heart failure occur.

- Inform patients of the risk of serious febrile drug reactions and the increased incidence and severity of pyrexia with dabrafenib/trametinib combination therapy. Advise patients to inform their clinician if fever occurs.

- Inform patients of the risk of serious skin toxicities. Advise patients to inform their clinician if progressive or intolerable rash occurs.

- Inform patients of the risk of impaired glucose control in patients with diabetes mellitus resulting in need for more intensive antidiabetic treatment. Advise patients to inform their clinician if symptoms of severe hyperglycemia occur.

- Inform patients of the risk of hemolytic anemia in patients with G-6-PD deficiency. Advise patients with known G-6-PD deficiency to contact their clinician if manifestations of anemia or hemolysis occur.

- Inform females of the risk of fetal harm if taken during pregnancy. Advise females of reproductive potential to use effective nonhormonal contraception during treatment and for 2 weeks after the last dose. Advise males (including those who have had vasectomies) with female partners of reproductive potential to use condoms during treatment and for at least 2 weeks after the last dose. Advise patients to contact their clinician if pregnancy is suspected or confirmed during treatment.

- Advise females to avoid breast-feeding while receiving dabrafenib and for 2 weeks after the last dose.

- Advise males and females of reproductive potential that dabrafenib may reduce male and female fertility.

- Inform patients of the risk of uveitis, iritis, and iridocyclitis. Advise patients to contact their clinician promptly if any vision changes or other ocular effects (e.g., ocular pain, swelling, redness, blurred vision) occur.

- Advise patients to inform their clinician of existing or contemplated concomitant therapy, including prescription and OTC drugs and dietary or herbal supplements, as well as any concomitant illnesses (e.g., diabetes).

- Inform patients of other important precautionary information.

For further information on the handling of antineoplastic agents, see the ASHP Guidelines on Handling Hazardous Drugs at https://www.ahfsdrug information.com.

PREPARATIONS

Excipients in commercially available drug preparations may have clinically important effects in some individuals; consult specific product labeling for details.

Dabrafenib Mesylate

Oral

Capsules	50 mg (of dabrafenib)	Tafinlar®, Novartis
	75 mg (of dabrafenib)	Tafinlar®, Novartis
Tablets, for oral suspension	10 mg (of dabrafenib)	Tafinlar®

† Use is not currently included in the labeling approved by the US Food and Drug Administration.

Selected Revisions November 16, 2023, © Copyright, January 30, 2014, American Society of Health-System Pharmacists, Inc.

Darolutamide

10:00 • ANTINEOPLASTIC AGENTS

■ Darolutamide, a nonsteroidal antiandrogen, is an antineoplastic agent.

USES

● Nonmetastatic Castration-resistant Prostate Cancer

Darolutamide is used for the treatment of nonmetastatic castration-resistant prostate cancer (nmCRPC) in adults; patients treated with darolutamide should also receive a gonadotropin-releasing hormone (GnRH) analog concurrently or have had a bilateral orchiectomy. In a clinical trial, metastasis-free survival was substantially longer in darolutamide-treated patients compared with those receiving placebo. The use of an androgen receptor antagonist (i.e., darolutamide, apalutamide, enzalutamide) is recommended for patients with nmCRPC who are at high risk of metastases.

Clinical Experience

Darolutamide has been shown to prolong metastasis-free survival in patients with nmCRPC. The drug was evaluated in a randomized, double-blind, placebo-controlled phase 3 study (ARAMIS) in 1509 patients with nmCRPC at high risk for metastasis (i.e., prostate-specific antigen [PSA] doubling time of 10 months or less despite continuous androgen deprivation therapy). Patients were randomized to receive either darolutamide (600 mg twice daily) or placebo; androgen deprivation therapy was continued in all patients. Patients were stratified by PSA doubling time and use of bone resorption inhibitors. Treatment was continued until disease progression or unacceptable toxicity occurred or the patient withdrew from the study. The primary measure of efficacy was metastasis-free survival. The median age of patients enrolled in the study was 74 years; 9% of patients were 85 years of age or older. Nearly half of patients (42%) had undergone prior surgery or radiation therapy of the prostate; 73% had a Gleason score of 7 or higher, 73% had received prior treatment with a nonsteroidal antiandrogen (66% had received bicalutamide and 13% had received flutamide), and all had an Eastern Cooperative Oncology Group (ECOG) performance status of 0 or 1. Patients with a history of seizures or with conditions predisposing to seizures were not excluded. At a median follow-up of 17.9 months, median metastasis-free survival was substantially longer in darolutamide-treated patients compared with those receiving placebo (40.4 and 18.4 months, respectively). Results of a subgroup analysis (based on PSA doubling time, baseline PSA concentration, number of prior hormonal therapies, use of bone resorption inhibitors, regional nodal disease, Gleason score, age, race, ECOG performance status, and geographic region) suggested that the drug's effect on metastasis-free survival was consistent across subgroups. Time to pain progression and time to initiation of cytotoxic chemotherapy were delayed in patients receiving darolutamide compared with those receiving placebo. Deterioration of health-related quality of life measures was significantly delayed with use of darolutamide compared to placebo. At the end of the initial study, patients continued open-label treatment. After a median follow-up time of 29 months, overall survival at 3 years was 83% with darolutamide and 77% with placebo. The risk of death was reduced by 31% with darolutamide treatment compared to placebo.

Clinical Perspective

According to a joint guideline from the American Urological Association (AUA) and the Society of Urologic Oncology (SUO), the decision to add an androgen receptor antagonist to androgen deprivation therapy (ADT) in patients with nonmetastatic castration-resistant prostate cancer is dependent on metastatic risk. The risk of metastasis is determined by the time to doubling of PSA levels. If the PSA doubling time is 10 months or less, metastatic risk is high and the guideline recommends use of either apalutamide, darolutamide, or enzalutamide in addition to ADT. Continuation of ADT with observation is recommended for patients who have a PSA doubling time greater than 10 months as risk of metastasis is considered to be lower in such patients.

● Metastatic Hormone-sensitive Prostate Cancer

Darolutamide is used for the treatment of metastatic hormone-sensitive prostate cancer (mHSPC) in combination with docetaxel in adults; patients treated with darolutamide should also receive a gonadotropin-releasing hormone (GnRH) analog concurrently or have had a bilateral orchiectomy In a clinical trial, overall survival was substantially longer in darolutamide-treated patients compared with those receiving placebo. The use of either abiraterone acetate plus prednisone or darolutamide in combination with ADT is recommended in selected patients with de novo mHSPC who are free of major comorbidities.

Clinical Experience

Darolutamide has been shown to prolong overall survival in patients with mHSPC. The drug was evaluated in a multicenter, double-blind, placebo-controlled clinical trial in 1306 patients with mHSPC. Patients were randomized 1:1 to receive 600 mg darolutamide orally twice daily or matching placebo, concomitantly with 75 mg/m² of docetaxel for 6 cycles. All patients received a GnRH analog concurrently or had a bilateral orchiectomy. Treatment with darolutamide or placebo continued until symptomatic progressive disease, change of antineoplastic therapy, or unacceptable toxicity. Patients with regional lymph node involvement only (M0) were excluded from the study; patients were stratified by extent of disease (non–regional lymph nodes metastases only (M1a), bone metastases with or without lymph node metastases (M1b) or visceral metastases with or without lymph node metastases or with or without bone metastases (M1c) and by alkaline phosphatase level (< or ≥ upper limit of normal) at study entry. The median age of patients was 67 years (range 41–89) and 17% of patients were 75 years of age or older. In this study, 78% of patients had a Gleason score of ≥8 at diagnosis, 71% of patients had an ECOG performance status score of 0, and 29% of patients had an ECOG performance status score of 1. The study population included 86% with de novo disease and 13% with recurrent disease.

The major efficacy outcome measure was overall survival (OS). Treatment with darolutamide with docetaxel resulted in OS of 65%, a substantial improvement compared to 54% in patients receiving placebo with docetaxel.

Clinical Perspective

The American Urological Association (AUA) and the Society of Urologic Oncology (SUO) published updated guidelines in 2023 for the management of advanced prostate cancer. The guidelines state that in selected patients with de novo mHSPC, clinicians should offer ADT in combination with docetaxel and either abiraterone acetate plus prednisone or darolutamide.

DOSAGE AND ADMINISTRATION

● General

Patient Monitoring

• Monitor for signs and symptoms of ischemic heart disease.

Other General Considerations

• Ensure patient is receiving concomitant treatment with a gonadotropin-releasing hormone (GnRH) analog or has had a bilateral orchiectomy.

● Administration

Darolutamide is administered orally twice daily with food. Tablets should be swallowed whole.

If a dose of darolutamide is missed, the missed dose should be taken as soon as it is remembered prior to the next scheduled dose. The dose should not be doubled to make up for a missed dose.

Store darolutamide tablets at 20–25°C (excursions permitted between 15–30°C).

● Dosage

Nonmetastatic Castration-resistant Prostate Cancer

For the treatment of nonmetastatic castration-resistant prostate cancer, the recommended adult dosage of darolutamide is 600 mg twice daily. Continue until disease progression or unacceptable toxicity occurs.

Metastatic Hormone-sensitive Prostate Cancer

For the treatment of metastatic hormone-sensitive prostate cancer in combination with docetaxel, the recommended adult dosage of darolutamide is 600 mg twice daily.

Administer the first of 6 cycles of docetaxel within 6 weeks after the start of darolutamide treatment. Refer to docetaxel prescribing information for additional dosing information, including dosage modifications.

Continue treatment until disease progression or unacceptable toxicity occurs, even if a cycle of docetaxel is delayed, interrupted, or discontinued.

Dosage Modification for Toxicity

General Toxicity

If an intolerable or grade 3 or greater adverse effect occurs, interrupt darolutamide therapy or reduce dosage to 300 mg twice daily until symptoms improve. Resume dosage of 600 mg twice daily when the adverse reaction returns to baseline. Dosage reduction below 300 mg twice daily is not recommended.

● Special Populations

Hepatic Impairment

The recommended dosage of darolutamide in patients with moderate hepatic impairment (Child-Pugh class B) is 300 mg twice daily. No initial dosage adjustment is necessary in patients with mild hepatic impairment (Child-Pugh class A). Pharmacokinetics of darolutamide have not been established in patients with severe hepatic impairment (Child-Pugh class C).

Renal Impairment

The recommended dosage of darolutamide in patients with severe renal impairment (estimated glomerular filtration rate [eGFR] of 15–29 mL/minute per 1.73 m²) not receiving hemodialysis is 300 mg twice daily. No initial dosage adjustment is necessary in patients with mild or moderate renal impairment (eGFR of 30–89 mL/minute per 1.73 m²). Pharmacokinetics of darolutamide have not been established in patients with end-stage renal disease (eGFR of less than 15 mL/minute per 1.73 m²).

Geriatric Use

The manufacturer makes no special dosage recommendations for geriatric patients; most patients (88%) in the principal efficacy study were 65 years of age or older.

CAUTIONS

● Contraindications

● None.

● Warnings/Precautions

Ischemic Heart Disease

Ischemic heart disease, including fatalities, have been reported in patients receiving darolutamide. In a randomized study of patients with nonmetastatic castration-resistant prostate cancer (nmCRPC), ischemic heart disease occurred in 3.2% of patients receiving darolutamide and 2.5% of patients receiving placebo, including Grade 3-4 events in 1.7% and 0.4% of the respective groups. Ischemic events led to death in 0.3% of patients receiving darolutamide and 0.2% of patients receiving placebo. In a randomized study of patients with metastatic hormone-sensitive prostate cancer (mHSPC), ischemic heart disease occurred in 3.2% of patients receiving darolutamide with docetaxel and 2% of patients receiving placebo with docetaxel, including grade 3-4 events in 1.3% and 1.1% of the respective treatment groups. Ischemic events led to death in 0.3% of patients receiving darolutamide with docetaxel and 0% of patients receiving placebo with docetaxel.

Monitor for signs and symptoms of ischemic heart disease. Optimize management of cardiovascular risk factors, such as hypertension, diabetes, or dyslipidemia. Discontinue darolutamide for Grade 3 or 4 ischemic heart disease.

Seizures

Seizures have been reported in patients receiving darolutamide.

In a clinical study in patients with nmCRPC, grade 1 or 2 seizures occurred in 0.2% of patients receiving darolutamide and 0.2% of those receiving placebo. Seizures occurred 261 and 456 days after initiation of darolutamide.

In a study in patients with mHSPC, seizures occurred in 0.6% of patients receiving darolutamide with docetaxel, including one Grade 3 event, and 0.2% of those receiving placebo with docetaxel. Seizures occurred 38 to 340 days after initiation of darolutamide.

It is unknown whether anti-epileptic medications will prevent seizures with darolutamide. Advise patients of the risk of developing a seizure while receiving darolutamide and of engaging in any activity where sudden loss of consciousness could cause harm to themselves or others. Consider discontinuation of darolutamide in patients who develop a seizure during treatment.

Fetal/Neonatal Morbidity and Mortality

Darolutamide may cause fetal harm and potential loss of pregnancy in humans based on its mechanisms of action. Safety and efficacy of darolutamide have not been established in females.

Males with female partners of reproductive potential should use effective methods of contraception during darolutamide therapy and for 1 week after the last dose of the drug.

Specific Populations

Pregnancy

Based on its mechanism of action, darolutamide can cause fetal harm and potential loss of pregnancy if administered to pregnant women.

Lactation

It is not known whether darolutamide or its metabolites are distributed into milk. The effects of darolutamide on nursing infants or on milk production also are not known.

Female and Males of Reproductive Potential

Males with female partners of reproductive potential should use effective methods of contraception during darolutamide therapy and for 1 week after the last dose of the drug.

Based on animal studies, darolutamide may impair fertility in males of reproductive potential. Darolutamide was associated with tubular dilation of the testes, hypospermia, and atrophy of the seminal vesicles, testes, prostate gland, and epididymides in rats and dogs at exposure levels approximately 0.6 and 1 times the human exposure, respectively.

Pediatric Use

Safety and efficacy of darolutamide have not been established in pediatric patients.

Geriatric Use

In the principal efficacy study evaluating darolutamide in men with nmCRPC, 88% of patients were 65 years of age or older, and 49% were 75 years of age or older. In the principal efficacy study evaluating darolutamide in men with mHSPC, 63% of patients were 65 years and over, and 16% were 75 years and over. No overall differences in safety or efficacy were observed between geriatric patients and younger adults in both studies.

Hepatic Impairment

Exposure to darolutamide in individuals with moderate hepatic impairment (Child-Pugh class B) is increased about 1.9-fold compared with individuals with normal hepatic function.

Pharmacokinetics of darolutamide have not been established in patients with severe hepatic impairment (Child-Pugh class C).

Renal Impairment

Exposure to darolutamide in individuals without cancer with severe renal impairment (estimated glomerular filtration rate [eGFR] of 15–29 mL/minute per 1.73 m²) not receiving dialysis is increased about 2.5-fold compared with those with normal renal function.

Pharmacokinetics of darolutamide have not been established in patients with end-stage renal disease (eGFR of less than 15 mL/minute per 1.73 m²).

● Common Adverse Effects

Adverse effects reported in ≥2% of patients receiving darolutamide in the principal efficacy study of patients with nmCRPC include fatigue, pain in extremity, and rash. Laboratory test abnormalities reported in ≥2% of patients receiving darolutamide in the study include increased AST, decreased neutrophil count, and increased bilirubin.

Adverse effects reported in ≥10% of patients receiving darolutamide in the principal efficacy study of patients with mHSPC include constipation, decreased appetite, rash, hemorrhage, increased weight, and hypertension. The most common laboratory test abnormalities (≥30%) in this group include anemia, hyperglycemia, decreased lymphocyte count, decreased neutrophil count, increased AST and ALT, and hypocalcemia.

DRUG INTERACTIONS

Darolutamide is metabolized principally by cytochrome P-450 (CYP) isoenzyme 3A4; the drug also is metabolized by uridine diphosphate-glucuronosyltransferase (UGT) 1A9 and UGT1A1.

In vitro, darolutamide is an inducer of CYP3A4 and an inhibitor of P-glycoprotein (P-gp) and breast cancer resistance protein (BCRP); darolutamide also inhibits organic anion transport protein (OATP) 1B1 and OATP1B3 in vitro.

Darolutamide did not inhibit the major CYP enzymes 1A2, 2A6, 2B6, 2C8, 2C9, 2C19, 2D6, 2E1, and 3A4 or transporters, including multidrug resistance protein 2 (MRP2), bile salt export pump (BSEP), organic anion transporters (OATs), organic cation transporters (OCTs), multidrug and toxin extrusion transporters (MATEs), OATP2B1, and sodium taurocholate co-transporting polypeptide (NTCP), at clinically relevant concentrations.

● *Drugs Affecting Hepatic Microsomal Enzymes and Efflux Transport Systems*

Inhibitors of CYP3A4 and Efflux Transport Systems

Concomitant use of darolutamide with drugs that are combined P-gp and potent CYP3A4 inhibitors increases exposure of darolutamide and may increase the risk of darolutamide adverse effects. Concomitant use of the combined P-gp and potent CYP3A4 inhibitor itraconazole (200 mg twice daily) with darolutamide (single 600-mg dose) increased the mean area under the concentration-time curve (AUC) and peak plasma concentration of darolutamide by 1.7- and 1.4-fold, respectively.

Patients receiving darolutamide with a drug that is a combined P-gp and potent CYP3A4 inhibitor should be monitored more frequently for darolutamide toxicity, and the dosage of darolutamide should be modified as needed.

Inducers of CYP3A4 and Efflux Transport Systems

Concomitant use of darolutamide with drugs that are combined P-gp and moderate or potent CYP3A4 inducers decreases exposure of darolutamide and may decrease darolutamide activity. Concomitant use of the P-gp and potent CYP3A4 inducer rifampin (600 mg once daily) with darolutamide (single 600-mg dose) decreased the mean AUC and peak plasma concentration of darolutamide by 72 and 52%, respectively. Concomitant use of moderate CYP3A4 inducers with darolutamide is expected to decrease darolutamide exposure by 36–58%.

Concomitant use of darolutamide with combined P-gp and moderate or potent CYP3A4 inducers should be avoided.

● *Drugs Metabolized by Hepatic Microsomal Enzymes*

Concomitant use of darolutamide (600 mg twice daily) and the sensitive CYP3A4 substrate midazolam (single 1-mg dose) decreased the mean AUC and peak plasma concentration of midazolam by 29 and 32%, respectively. These effects were not considered clinically important.

● *Drugs Affected by Breast Cancer Resistance Protein and Organic Anion Transport Protein*

Concomitant use of darolutamide with drugs that are BCRP, OATP1B1, and/or OATP1B3 substrates increases exposure of the substrate and may increase the risk of substrate-related toxicity.

Concomitant use of darolutamide (600 mg twice daily) and the BCRP, OATP1B1, and OATP1B3 substrate rosuvastatin (single 5-mg dose) increased the mean AUC and peak plasma concentration of rosuvastatin by approximately

fivefold. No clinically important effects on the pharmacokinetics of darolutamide were observed. In the principal efficacy study evaluating darolutamide (ARAMIS), approximately 30% of patients received concomitant antilipemic therapy with a statin that was a BCRP substrate. In this subset of patients, elevations in serum creatinine, aminotransferase, and bilirubin concentrations were observed more frequently in those receiving darolutamide compared with those receiving placebo.

Concomitant use of darolutamide with BCRP substrates should be avoided when possible. If concomitant use cannot be avoided, patients should be monitored more frequently for adverse effects; the manufacturer's prescribing information for the BCRP substrate should be consulted and dosage reduction of the BCRP substrate should be considered.

Concomitant use of darolutamide with OATP1B1 or OATP1B3 substrates requires close monitoring for adverse reactions of these drugs and may require dosage reduction while taking darolutamide. The manufacturer's prescribing information for the OATP1B1 or OATP1B3 substrate should be consulted.

Docetaxel

Concomitant use of darolutamide and docetaxel resulted in no clinically important effects on the pharmacokinetics of docetaxel in metastatic hormone-sensitive prostate cancer (mHSPC) patients. There were no clinically important effects on the pharmacokinetics of darolutamide, when used in combination with docetaxel.

● *Drugs Affected by P-glycoprotein Transport*

Concomitant use of darolutamide (600 mg twice daily) with the P-gp substrate dabigatran etexilate (single 75-mg dose) did not result in clinically important effects on the pharmacokinetics of dabigatran.

DESCRIPTION

Darolutamide, a nonsteroidal antiandrogen, is an antineoplastic agent. The drug competitively inhibits androgen binding to androgen receptors; its mechanisms of action are similar to those of enzalutamide and apalutamide (nonsteroidal antiandrogens structurally unrelated to darolutamide). Darolutamide inhibits nuclear translocation of the androgen receptor, interaction of the androgen receptor with DNA, and androgen receptor-mediated gene transcription. Compared with enzalutamide and apalutamide, darolutamide appears to cross the blood-brain barrier to a negligible or lesser extent and to have less affinity for γ-aminobutyric acid type A (GABA$_A$) receptors in preclinical models, which has theoretical implications for a potentially improved CNS adverse effect profile (e.g., decreased risk of seizures). Darolutamide inhibited tumor growth in vitro and decreased tumor volume in xenograft models of castration-resistant prostate cancer in mice.

In castration-resistant prostate cancer, alterations in androgen receptor signaling (e.g., androgen receptor gene mutation or amplification, androgen receptor overexpression) have been shown to result in persistence of androgen receptor signaling and to contribute to disease progression despite castrate levels of androgens. Resistance to conventional antiandrogens (e.g., bicalutamide, flutamide, nilutamide) in castration-resistant prostate cancer has been associated with paradoxical agonistic effects of these drugs and continued androgen receptor signaling. Unlike these conventional antiandrogens but similar to other second generation antiandrogens (e.g., enzalutamide, apalutamide), darolutamide does not exhibit agonistic activity in cells that overexpress the androgen receptor. In addition to inhibition of wild-type androgen receptors, darolutamide also has demonstrated inhibition of mutant androgen receptors known to trigger bicalutamide, enzalutamide, and apalutamide antagonist-to-agonist switch.

Darolutamide exhibits nearly dose-proportional exposure over a dose range of 100–700 mg. Following oral administration of a single 600-mg dose, peak plasma concentration is attained in approximately 4 hours. Absolute bioavailability of a 300-mg dose of darolutamide administered orally under fasted conditions is approximately 30%; bioavailability increases 2 to 2.5-fold when administered with food. Steady-state concentrations of darolutamide are achieved after 2–5 days of repeated dosing with food, and the accumulation ratio is approximately twofold. Darolutamide is metabolized principally by cytochrome P-450 (CYP) isoenzyme 3A4 to form its major active metabolite, keto-darolutamide. Keto-darolutamide has been shown to have activity similar to that of the parent drug in vitro; however, its contribution to the overall pharmacologic effect of the drug in vivo is expected to be minor, owing to its small unbound fraction (0.2%). Uridine diphosphate-glucuronosyltransferase (UGT) enzymes 1A9 and 1A1 also contribute to the metabolism of darolutamide. Darolutamide and keto-darolutamide are 92 and 99.8% bound, respectively, to plasma proteins, mainly albumin. The half-life of both darolutamide and keto-darolutamide is approximately 20 hours. Following oral administration of a single radiolabeled dose of darolutamide, 63.4% of the dose was recovered in urine (7% as unchanged drug) and 32.4% was recovered in feces (30% as unchanged drug).

ADVICE TO PATIENTS

- Inform patients that darolutamide has been associated with an increased risk of ischemic heart disease. Advise patients to seek immediate medical attention if any symptoms suggestive of an ischemic heart disease event occur.

- Inform patients that darolutamide has been associated with an increased risk of seizures and discuss conditions that may predispose to seizures and medications that may lower the seizure threshold. Advise patients of the risk of engaging in any activity where sudden loss of consciousness could cause serious harm to themselves or others. Inform patients to contact their healthcare provider right away if they experience loss of consciousness or a seizure.

- Advise patients currently receiving gonadotropin-releasing hormone (GnRH) analog therapy to continue this therapy during darolutamide therapy.

- Advise patients to take darolutamide as instructed with food and to swallow tablets whole. If a dose is missed, the missed dose should be taken as soon as it is remembered prior to the next scheduled dose. The dose should not be doubled to make up for a missed dose.

- Risk of fetal harm and loss of pregnancy. Advise patients with female partners of reproductive potential to use effective methods of contraception during darolutamide therapy and for 1 week after the last dose of the drug.

- Advise patients that darolutamide may impair male fertility.

- Advise patients to inform clinicians of existing or contemplated concomitant therapy, including prescription and OTC drugs and dietary or herbal supplements, as well as any concomitant illnesses.

- Inform patients of other important precautionary information.

For further information on the handling of antineoplastic agents, see the ASHP Guidelines on Handling Hazardous Drugs at https://www.ahfsdrug information.com.

PREPARATIONS

Darolutamide can only be obtained through designated specialty pharmacies. Contact the manufacturer or consult the Nubeqa specialty pharmacy network (https://www.nubeqahcp.com/nubeqa_specialty_pharmacy_network.pdf) for specific information.

Excipients in commercially available drug preparations may have clinically important effects in some individuals; consult specific product labeling for details.

Darolutamide

Oral		
Tablets, film-coated	300 mg	**Nubeqa®**, Bayer

† Use is not currently included in the labeling approved by the US Food and Drug Administration.

Selected Revisions May 10, 2024, © Copyright, August 12, 2019, American Society of Health-System Pharmacists, Inc.

DOCEtaxel

10:00 · ANTINEOPLASTIC AGENTS

- Docetaxel, a semisynthetic taxoid produced from the needles of the European yew (*Taxus baccata*) tree, is an antineoplastic agent.

USES

● Breast Cancer

Adjuvant Therapy for Early-stage Breast Cancer

Docetaxel is used in combination with doxorubicin and cyclophosphamide for the adjuvant treatment of operable node-positive breast cancer.

The current indication is based on a multicenter, open-label, randomized trial (the BCIRG 001 trial) in which 1491 patients with axillary node-positive breast cancer and no evidence of metastatic disease received either doxorubicin and cyclophosphamide followed by docetaxel (TAC) or doxorubicin followed by fluorouracil and cyclophosphamide (FAC). The median age of women participating in this study was 49 years. Treatment regimens consisted of doxorubicin 50 mg/m² as a 15-minute IV infusion and cyclophosphamide 500 mg/m² IV administered over 1–5 minutes followed by a 1-hour interval and then docetaxel 75 mg/m² as a 1-hour IV infusion on day 1 (TAC regimen), or doxorubicin 50 mg/m² followed by fluorouracil 500 mg/m² each administered as a 15-minute IV infusion and then cyclophosphamide 500 mg/m² as a 1- to 5-minute IV infusion on day 1 (FAC regimen); each regimen was administered once every 3 weeks for up to 6 cycles. Stratification was performed according to the number of positive lymph nodes (1–3, 4+). Following the completion of chemotherapy, patients with hormone receptor-positive disease received tamoxifen 20 mg daily for up to 5 years. About 70% of patients in each group received adjuvant radiation therapy.

Results of a second interim analysis of the data at a median follow-up of 55 months indicate that disease-free survival was prolonged in patients receiving the docetaxel-containing regimen. The estimated rate of disease-free survival at 5 years was 75% in patients receiving the TAC regimen compared with 68% in those receiving the FAC regimen. An overall reduction of about 26% in risk of relapse, including local or distant recurrence, contralateral breast cancer, and death from any cause, was observed in patients receiving the TAC regimen. At the time of this interim analysis, overall survival also was prolonged in patients receiving the docetaxel-containing regimen. Subgroup analysis suggests that those most likely to benefit from docetaxel-containing adjuvant treatment are patients with 1–3 positive nodes. Because this trial was restricted to women who were 70 years of age or younger, the benefit and risk associated with use of the TAC regimen as adjuvant therapy for breast cancer in older patients is not known.

Patients receiving TAC generally experienced increased toxicity compared with those receiving FAC. A higher rate of severe nonhematologic treatment-emergent adverse events occurred in patients receiving TAC (36%) than in those receiving FAC (27%). Treatment was discontinued because of adverse effects in 6% of patients receiving TAC compared with about 1% of those receiving FAC. Fever in the absence of infection and allergy were the most common reasons for withdrawal from the study among patients receiving TAC. Anemia (92 versus 72%), stomatitis (69 versus 53%), grade 3 or 4 neutropenia (66 versus 49%), fever in the absence of infection (46 versus 17%), fluid retention (35 versus 15%) including peripheral edema (27 versus 7%), myalgia (27 versus 10%), sensory neuropathy (26 versus 10%), and febrile neutropenia (25 versus 2%) occurred more frequently in patients receiving TAC. Neutropenia of any grade (82 versus 71%) and vomiting (59 versus 44%) occurred more frequently in those receiving FAC. The most frequent adverse effects in patients receiving TAC included alopecia (98%), hematologic toxicity (anemia [92%], neutropenia [71%], grade 3 or 4 neutropenia [66%]), asthenia (81%), GI toxicity (nausea [80%], stomatitis [69%], vomiting [44%]), amenorrhea (62%), and fever in the absence of infection (46%).

In this trial (BCIRG 001), patients receiving TAC experienced a higher rate of febrile neutropenia than those receiving FAC (25 versus 2.5%). Primary prophylaxis with granulocyte colony-stimulating factor (G-CSF) was not allowed, but use of G-CSF was mandatory in subsequent cycles for any patient experiencing febrile neutropenia or infection. Another randomized trial (RAPP-01), which compared doxorubicin and docetaxel versus doxorubicin and cyclophosphamide as adjuvant therapy for intermediate-risk breast cancer, was prematurely terminated because of serious adverse events, including 2 deaths, associated with febrile neutropenia in patients receiving the docetaxel-containing regimen. Some clinicians, including the investigators in these trials (BCIRG 001 and RAPP-01), currently recommend primary prophylaxis with G-CSF in patients receiving docetaxel with an anthracycline agent as adjuvant therapy for early-stage breast cancer.

Other docetaxel-containing regimens are being investigated as adjuvant therapy for early-stage breast cancer, including nonanthracycline-containing regimens†. In a randomized trial involving 1016 patients, patients receiving docetaxel and cyclophosphamide as adjuvant therapy for operable breast cancer had prolonged disease-free survival and similar overall survival compared with those receiving doxorubicin and cyclophosphamide. Grade 1 or 2 edema, myalgia, and arthralgia occurred more frequently in patients receiving docetaxel and cyclophosphamide whereas grade 1 to 4 nausea and vomiting were more frequent in patients receiving doxorubicin and cyclophosphamide.

Docetaxel and Doxorubicin as First-line Therapy for Advanced Breast Cancer

Docetaxel is used in combination with doxorubicin for the first-line treatment of metastatic breast cancer†.

In a multicenter, randomized, phase 3 trial, 429 patients received either doxorubicin and docetaxel or doxorubicin and cyclophosphamide for the initial treatment of metastatic breast cancer. Treatment consisted of doxorubicin 50 mg/m² as a 15-minute IV infusion followed 1 hour later by docetaxel 75 mg/m² as a 1-hour IV infusion, or doxorubicin 60 mg/m² as a 15-minute IV infusion followed by cyclophosphamide 600 mg/m² as a 15-minute IV infusion, on day 1 once every 3 weeks for up to 8 cycles. Among patients receiving doxorubicin and docetaxel, median time to progression was prolonged (37 versus 32 weeks), overall response rate was higher (59 versus 47%), and overall survival was similar compared with those receiving doxorubicin and cyclophosphamide as initial treatment for metastatic breast cancer. Diarrhea, febrile neutropenia, edema, neurosensory toxicity, nail changes, rashes, and grade 3 or 4 infections occurred more frequently in patients receiving doxorubicin and docetaxel whereas nausea and vomiting were more frequent in patients receiving doxorubicin and cyclophosphamide.

Other dosage schedules have been investigated for the use of doxorubicin and docetaxel as first-line therapy for metastatic breast cancer. In a multicenter, randomized, phase 3 trial involving 144 patients, sequential administration of doxorubicin and docetaxel was shown to be as effective but less toxic than concomitant administration of these drugs for the first-line treatment of metastatic breast cancer. Patients who had not received previous treatment with anthracycline agents received either 3 cycles of doxorubicin 75 mg/m² every 21 days followed by 3 cycles of docetaxel 100 mg/m² every 21 days (sequential treatment) or 6 cycles of doxorubicin 50 mg/m² and docetaxel 75 mg/m² every 21 days (concomitant treatment). Dosage adjustments were made for patients who had received previous treatment with anthracycline agents, so these patients received either 2 cycles of doxorubicin 75 mg/m² every 21 days followed by 4 cycles of docetaxel 100 mg/m² every 21 days (sequential treatment) or 3 cycles of doxorubicin 50 mg/m² and docetaxel 75 mg/m² every 21 days followed by 3 cycles of docetaxel 100 mg/m² every 21 days (concomitant treatment). Patients received premedication with a corticosteroid regimen and prophylactic antiemetic therapy. The use of granulocyte colony-stimulating factor (G-CSF) was not allowed as primary prophylaxis but was allowed following a first episode of febrile neutropenia. Patients receiving sequential treatment with doxorubicin and docetaxel had a higher rate of completion of 6 cycles of therapy (81 versus 67%) and a lower rate of withdrawal from the study because of adverse events (1 versus 14.5%) compared with those receiving concomitant treatment with doxorubicin and docetaxel. Efficacy was similar between the groups, but febrile neutropenia was less frequent (29 versus 48%) in patients receiving sequential administration of doxorubicin and docetaxel than in those receiving concomitant administration of these agents.

Because of the higher rate of febrile neutropenia and increased risk of life-threatening sepsis associated with the use of doxorubicin in combination with docetaxel as adjuvant or neoadjuvant therapy for early-stage breast cancer, some clinicians recommend use of G-CSF and/or antibiotics as primary prophylaxis in patients receiving these agents for metastatic breast cancer.

Second-line Therapy for Advanced Breast Cancer
Docetaxel and Capecitabine

Docetaxel is used in combination with capecitabine for the treatment of metastatic breast cancer in patients with disease that has failed anthracycline-containing chemotherapy. In a randomized trial, patients receiving combination therapy with docetaxel and capecitabine for metastatic breast cancer had longer time to disease progression, prolonged survival, and higher objective response rate than those receiving docetaxel alone. (See Uses: Breast Cancer: Combination Therapy in Capecitabine 10:00.)

Docetaxel Monotherapy

Docetaxel is used as monotherapy for the second-line treatment of locally advanced or metastatic breast cancer after failure of prior chemotherapy. As with paclitaxel, clinical cross-resistance with anthracyclines is incomplete with docetaxel, and patients with metastatic breast cancer refractory to treatment with anthracycline antineoplastic agents (e.g., doxorubicin) may respond to docetaxel therapy.

The current indication for docetaxel is based principally on the results of 2 large randomized trials in patients with locally advanced or metastatic breast cancer that failed to respond to prior chemotherapy regimens.

Docetaxel (100 mg/m^2 IV over 1 hour every 3 weeks) was compared with a combination of mitomycin (12 mg/m^2 IV every 6 weeks) and vinblastine (6 mg/m^2 IV every 3 weeks) in an open-label, multicenter, randomized phase 3 study in 392 patients with a history of treatment failure with an anthracycline regimen. Most patients in the study had received prior anthracycline-based chemotherapy for the treatment of metastatic disease (rather than as adjuvant therapy) and 75% had measurable, visceral metastases; only 15% of patients at study entry were those whose disease had relapsed after adjuvant therapy. Patients receiving docetaxel experienced a longer median survival duration (11.4 versus 8.7 months), longer median time to progression (4.3 versus 2.5 months), and higher overall and complete response rates (28.1 versus 9.5% overall and 3.4 versus 1.6% complete) compared with patients receiving mitomycin and vinblastine. Grade 3 or 4 neutropenia, asthenia, stomatitis, neurosensory toxicity, nail disorder, diarrhea, skin toxicity, grade 3 or 4 infections, and febrile neutropenia occurred more frequently in patients receiving docetaxel whereas thrombocytopenia and constipation occurred more frequently in those receiving mitomycin and vinblastine.

In a second open-label, multicenter phase 3 trial, 326 patients with metastatic breast cancer and a history of treatment failure with an alkylating agent-containing chemotherapy regimen were randomized to receive either docetaxel (100 mg/m^2 IV over 1 hour every 3 weeks) or doxorubicin (75 mg/m^2 IV over 15–20 minutes every 3 weeks). Prior chemotherapy was administered for metastatic disease in about half of the patients studied and as adjuvant therapy in the other half of the patients, and 75% of patients had measurable, visceral metastases. Higher overall and complete response rates (45.3 versus 29.7% overall and 6.8 versus 4.2% complete) were observed in patients receiving docetaxel, and a similar median survival (14.7 and 14.3 months) and median time to progression (6.5 and 5.3 months) were reported with docetaxel and doxorubicin, respectively. Fluid retention, diarrhea, nail disorder, neurosensory toxicity, skin toxicity, allergy, and neuromotor toxicity occurred more frequently in patients receiving docetaxel whereas nausea, vomiting, stomatitis, thrombocytopenia, cardiac toxicity, grade 3 or 4 anemia, red blood cell transfusions, febrile neutropenia, and grade 3 or 4 infections were more frequent in patients receiving doxorubicin.

In another randomized trial, 527 patients with advanced breast cancer that had progressed or relapsed after 1 prior chemotherapy regimen received docetaxel at dose levels of 60, 75, or 100 mg/m^2. Most patients (94%) had metastatic disease and 79% had received prior anthracycline-containing therapy. Response rate and toxicity increased with increase in dose. Patients receiving docetaxel 100 mg/m^2 had a higher response rate (30 versus 20%) than those receiving docetaxel 60 mg/m^2. Grade 3 or 4 adverse events occurred in 49% of patients receiving docetaxel 60 mg/m^2, 55% of those receiving docetaxel 75 mg/m^2, and 66% of those receiving docetaxel 100 mg/m^2. Discontinuance of therapy because of toxicity was reported in 5% of patients receiving docetaxel 60 mg/m^2 compared with 16.5% of patients receiving docetaxel 100 mg/m^2. Adverse effects that occurred at higher frequency in respective order with increasing docetaxel dose (60, 75, and 100 mg/m^2) included neutropenia (92, 94, and 97%), anemia (87, 94, and 97%), fluid retention (26, 38, and 46%), thrombocytopenia (7, 11, and 12%), febrile neutropenia (5, 7, and 14%), and treatment-related grade 3 or 4 infection (2, 3, and 7%).

In phase 2 studies, docetaxel has been evaluated in patients with locally advanced or metastatic breast cancer, including those with disease resistant to treatment with anthracycline antineoplastic agents. Anthracycline resistance was defined as progression of disease while undergoing anthracycline-containing therapy for advanced disease or disease relapse while undergoing anthracycline-containing adjuvant therapy. Among 309 patients receiving a docetaxel dose of 100 mg/m^2 as second-line therapy for metastatic breast cancer in 6 single-arm

studies, 190 patients had anthracycline-resistant disease. Among patients with anthracycline-resistant disease, the overall response rate was about 38% with a complete response rate of 2%. A similar rate of overall response (about 35%) was observed in 26 patients with anthracycline-resistant disease among a total of 174 patients receiving a docetaxel dose of 60 mg/m^2 as second-line therapy for locally advanced or metastatic breast cancer in 3 single-arm studies conducted in Japan.

● Non-small Cell Lung Cancer

Docetaxel and Cisplatin as First-line Therapy for Advanced Disease

Docetaxel is used in combination with cisplatin as first-line therapy for unresectable, locally advanced or metastatic non-small cell lung cancer.

The current indication is based on a randomized trial in which 1218 patients with unresectable stage IIIB or stage IV non-small cell lung cancer received initial treatment with docetaxel and cisplatin, vinorelbine and cisplatin, or docetaxel and carboplatin. Treatment regimens consisted of docetaxel 75 mg/m^2 as a 1-hour IV infusion immediately followed by cisplatin 75 mg/m^2 IV over 30–60 minutes on day 1 once every 3 weeks; vinorelbine 25 mg/m^2 IV over 6–10 minutes on days 1, 8, 15, and 22 followed by cisplatin 100 mg/m^2 IV on day 1 in 4-week cycles; or docetaxel 75 mg/m^2 IV as a 1-hour IV infusion and carboplatin IV at the dose required to obtain an area under the concentration-time curve (AUC) of 6 mg/mL per minute on day 1 once every 3 weeks.

Median survival was similar in patients receiving docetaxel and cisplatin compared with those receiving vinorelbine and cisplatin. Among patients receiving docetaxel and cisplatin, at least 62% of the known survival effect of adding vinorelbine to cisplatin was maintained. The use of the docetaxel/carboplatin regimen did not prolong survival compared with the vinorelbine/cisplatin regimen, and less than 50% of the known survival effect of adding vinorelbine to cisplatin was maintained.

Hematologic toxicity was frequent for all 3 regimens. Alopecia (75 versus 42%), fluid retention (54 versus 42%) including peripheral edema (34 versus 18%), diarrhea (47 versus 25%), and nail disorders (14 versus less than 1%) occurred more frequently in patients receiving docetaxel and cisplatin. Grade 3 or 4 anemia (25 versus 7%), grade 3 or 4 nausea (17 versus 10%), and grade 3 or 4 vomiting (16 versus 8%) were more common in patients receiving vinorelbine and cisplatin.

Docetaxel as Second-line Therapy for Locally Advanced or Metastatic Disease

Docetaxel is used alone as second-line therapy for locally advanced or metastatic non-small cell lung cancer in patients with disease that has recurred or progressed following prior treatment with platinum-based chemotherapy.

A small survival benefit has been demonstrated for the use of platinum-based (cisplatin) chemotherapy in selected patients with unresectable, locally advanced or metastatic non-small cell lung cancer who have a good performance status. Platinum-based chemotherapy regimens currently are preferred for the treatment of non-small cell lung cancer. (See Uses: Non-small Cell Lung Cancer in Cisplatin 10:00 for comprehensive discussion.) Use of chemotherapy for the treatment of advanced non-small cell lung cancer generally is advised only in patients with good performance status (ECOG performance status of 0 or 1, and 2 in selected patients) and evaluable lesions so that treatment can be discontinued if the disease does not respond. The decision to use chemotherapy must be individualized according to several factors, including patient preference, toxicity, survival benefit, quality of life, and cost of treatment.

The current indication is based on the results of 2 randomized trials that established the use of docetaxel 75 mg/m^2 as a tolerable dose level for patients who had previously received platinum-based chemotherapy for advanced non-small cell lung cancer. In a randomized trial, median survival was prolonged and the 1-year survival rate was higher in patients receiving docetaxel (75 mg/m^2) versus best supportive care for the treatment of unresectable locally advanced or metastatic (stage IIIB or IV) non-small cell lung cancer that had previously been treated with platinum-containing chemotherapy. In another randomized trial, patients receiving docetaxel (75 mg/m^2) experienced higher response rates (all partial responses) and a higher 1-year survival rate but similar median survival compared with those receiving a control regimen of vinorelbine or ifosfamide for advanced non-small cell lung cancer previously treated with platinum-containing chemotherapy. In both randomized trials, the optimum dosage of docetaxel was 75 mg/m^2 by 1-hour IV infusion once every 3 weeks; higher doses of docetaxel (100 mg/m^2) were associated with excessive toxicity. Docetaxel at a dose of 100 mg/m^2 caused unacceptable hematologic toxicity, infections, and treatment-related mortality, and the use of this higher dose in this patient population is not recommended. Of the 5 patients who died from treatment-related toxicity while receiving docetaxel 75 mg/m² in the 2 randomized trials, 3 had a performance status of 2 upon entry to the study.

● Prostate Cancer

Docetaxel is used in combination with prednisone for the treatment of androgen-independent (hormone-refractory) metastatic prostate cancer.

The current indication is based on the results of a multicenter, randomized, active-control trial involving 1006 patients with androgen-independent metastatic prostate cancer receiving prednisone with either docetaxel or the active control, mitoxantrone. Treatment consisted of docetaxel 75 mg/m² as a 1-hour IV infusion once every 3 weeks for up to 10 cycles or docetaxel 30 mg/m² as a 30-minute IV infusion once weekly for the first 5 weeks in a 6-week cycle for up to 5 cycles. The active control regimen was mitoxantrone 12 mg/m² as a 30-minute IV infusion once every 3 weeks for 10 cycles. Each patient also received prednisone 5 mg orally twice daily continually.

Median survival was prolonged (18.9 versus 16.5 months) in patients receiving the docetaxel once-every-3-weeks regimen and prednisone compared with those receiving mitoxantrone and prednisone. No difference in survival was observed for patients receiving the docetaxel once-weekly regimen and prednisone compared with those receiving mitoxantrone and prednisone.

Anemia (66 versus 58%), alopecia (65 versus 13%), fatigue (53 versus 35%), grade 3 or 4 neutropenia (32 versus 22%), infection (32 versus 20%), diarrhea (32 versus 10%), nail changes (30 versus 8%), sensory neuropathy (30 versus 7%), fluid retention (24 versus 4%) including peripheral edema (18 versus 2%), stomatitis (20 versus 8%), and taste disturbance (18 versus 7%) occurred more frequently in patients receiving docetaxel and prednisone. Left ventricular cardiac dysfunction (22 versus 10%) was more frequent in patients receiving mitoxantrone and prednisone. The most frequent adverse effects in patients receiving docetaxel and prednisone included anemia (66%), alopecia (65%), fatigue (53%), neutropenia (41%), and nausea (41%).

● Gastric Cancer

Docetaxel is used in combination with cisplatin and fluorouracil for the initial treatment of advanced gastric adenocarcinoma, including adenocarcinoma of the gastroesophageal junction.

The current indication is based on the results of a multicenter, open-label, randomized trial in which 445 patients received either docetaxel/cisplatin/fluorouracil or cisplatin/fluorouracil for the initial treatment of advanced gastric adenocarcinoma, including gastric adenocarcinoma of the gastroesophageal junction. Treatment regimens consisted of docetaxel 75 mg/m² as a 1-hour IV infusion on day 1 in combination with cisplatin 75 mg/m² as a 1-hour to 3-hour IV infusion on day 1 and fluorouracil 750 mg/m² as a continuous IV infusion daily for 5 days (on days 1–5) in 3-week cycles; or cisplatin 100 mg/m² on day 1 and fluorouracil 1000 mg/m² daily for 5 days (on days 1–5) in 4-week cycles. Most (71%) of the patients were Caucasian males, and the median age was 55 years; 19% of the patients had undergone prior curative surgery and 12% of patients had undergone palliative surgery. The median number of cycles of therapy administered per patient was 6 cycles (range: 1–16 cycles) for those receiving docetaxel/cisplatin/fluorouracil and 4 cycles (range: 1–12 cycles) for those receiving cisplatin/fluorouracil.

Patients receiving docetaxel, cisplatin, and fluorouracil had longer median time to progression (5.6 versus 3.7 months) and prolonged survival (9.2 versus 8.6 months) compared with those receiving cisplatin and fluorouracil as first-line therapy for advanced gastric cancer.

Neutropenia (96 versus 83%) including severe neutropenia (82 versus 57%), diarrhea (78 versus 50%) including severe diarrhea (20 versus 8%), alopecia (66 versus 41%), neurosensory toxicity (38 versus 25%), fever in the absence of infection (36 versus 23%), febrile neutropenia (16 versus 4%), and fluid retention (15 versus 4%) occurred more frequently in patients receiving docetaxel with cisplatin and fluorouracil. Thrombocytopenia (39 versus 26%) occurred more frequently in patients receiving cisplatin and fluorouracil. The most frequent adverse effects in patients receiving docetaxel with cisplatin and fluorouracil for advanced gastric cancer were anemia (97%), neutropenia (96%) including severe neutropenia (82%), diarrhea (78%), nausea (73%), vomiting (66%), alopecia (66%), lethargy (63%), stomatitis (59%), and anorexia (51%).

● Head and Neck Cancer

Docetaxel is used in combination with cisplatin and fluorouracil as induction chemotherapy for locally advanced squamous cell carcinoma of the head and neck.

The current indication is based on the results of 2 randomized trials in which patients received induction chemotherapy with cisplatin and fluorouracil, with or without docetaxel, followed by radiotherapy or chemoradiotherapy for locally advanced squamous cell carcinoma of the head and neck.

In the first randomized trial (TAX323), a multicenter, open-label study, 358 patients with inoperable locally advanced squamous cell carcinoma of the head and neck received induction chemotherapy with either docetaxel/cisplatin/fluorouracil or cisplatin/fluorouracil. All patients had a WHO performance status of 0 or 1. The median age of patients in the study was 53 years.

Treatment regimens consisted of docetaxel 75 mg/m² as a 1-hour IV infusion on day 1, followed by cisplatin 75 mg/m² as a 1-hour IV infusion on day 1, followed by fluorouracil 750 mg/m² daily as a continuous IV infusion on days 1–5 (the TPF regimen); or cisplatin 100 mg/m² as a 1-hour IV infusion on day 1, followed by fluorouracil 1000 mg/m² daily as a continuous IV infusion on days 1–5 (the PF regimen). Each regimen was administered every 3 weeks for up to 4 cycles. At an interval of 4–7 weeks following completion of chemotherapy, patients with disease that did not progress also received locoregional radiation therapy with either a conventional fraction regimen (1.8–2 Gy once daily for 5 days per week for a total dose of 66–70 Gy) or an accelerated or hyperfractionated regimen (twice daily with a minimum interfraction interval of 6 hours for 5 days per week for a total dose of 70 Gy or 74 Gy, respectively). Surgical resection was allowed following completion of chemotherapy, preceding or following radiation therapy.

At a median follow-up of 34 months, patients receiving docetaxel in combination with cisplatin and fluorouracil for inoperable locally advanced squamous cell carcinoma of the head and neck had prolonged median progression-free survival (11 versus 8 months) compared with those receiving cisplatin and fluorouracil. At a median follow-up of 51 months, patients receiving the docetaxel-containing regimen also had prolonged median overall survival (19 versus 14 months).

Alopecia (81 versus 43%), grade 3 or 4 neutropenia (76 versus 53%), and grade 3 or 4 leukopenia (42 versus 23%) occurred more frequently in patients receiving docetaxel/cisplatin/fluorouracil. Thrombocytopenia (47 versus 24%) including grade 3 or 4 thrombocytopenia (18 versus 5%), vomiting (39 versus 26%), toxic death (6 versus 2%), and hearing loss (3 versus 0%) occurred more frequently in patients receiving cisplatin/fluorouracil. The most frequent adverse effects in patients receiving docetaxel with cisplatin and fluorouracil as induction chemotherapy for locally advanced head and neck cancer followed by radiotherapy were neutropenia (93%) including grade 3 or 4 neutropenia (76%), anemia (89%), alopecia (81%), nausea (47%), stomatitis (42%), and lethargy (41%).

In the second randomized trial (TAX324), a multicenter, open-label study, 501 patients with locally advanced squamous cell carcinoma of the head and neck who had unresectable disease or disease with low chance of surgical cure, or who were candidates for organ preservation received induction chemotherapy with either docetaxel/cisplatin/fluorouracil or cisplatin/fluorouracil. All patients had a WHO performance status of 0 or 1. The median age of patients in the study was 55–56 years.

Treatment regimens consisted of docetaxel 75 mg/m² as a 1-hour IV infusion on day 1, followed by cisplatin 100 mg/m² as a 30-minute to 3-hour IV infusion on day 1, followed by fluorouracil 1000 mg/m² daily as a continuous IV infusion on days 1–4 (the TPF regimen); or cisplatin 100 mg/m² as a 30-minute to 3-hour IV infusion on day 1, followed by fluorouracil 1000 mg/m² daily as a continuous IV infusion on days 1–5 (the PF regimen). Each regimen was administered every 3 weeks for up to 3 cycles. At 3–8 weeks following the start of the last cycle of induction chemotherapy, patients with disease that did not progress received 7 weeks of chemoradiotherapy. Radiotherapy was administered with megavoltage equipment as once daily fractionation (2 Gy daily for 5 days per week for 7 weeks for a total dose of 70–72 Gy). During radiotherapy, carboplatin (at the dose required to obtain an AUC of 1.5 mg/mL per minute) was administered once weekly as a 1-hour IV infusion for up to 7 doses. Surgical resection was allowed at any time following the completion of chemoradiotherapy.

Patients receiving docetaxel/cisplatin/fluorouracil had prolonged overall survival (71 versus 30 months, hazard ratio for death: 0.70) compared with those receiving cisplatin/fluorouracil as induction chemotherapy for locally advanced squamous cell carcinoma of the head and neck.

Neutropenia of grade 3 or 4 in severity (84 versus 56%) and alopecia (68 versus 44%) occurred more frequently in patients receiving docetaxel/cisplatin/fluorouracil. Constipation (38 versus 27%) was more frequent in patients receiving cisplatin/fluorouracil. The most frequent adverse effects in patients receiving docetaxel with cisplatin and fluorouracil as induction chemotherapy for locally advanced head and neck cancer followed by chemoradiotherapy were neutropenia (95%) including grade 3 or 4 neutropenia (84%), anemia (90%), nausea (76%), alopecia (68%), stomatitis (66%), lethargy (61%), vomiting (56%), diarrhea (48%), and anorexia (40%).

● Ovarian Cancer

Docetaxel in combination with carboplatin is used an as alternative regimen for the first-line treatment of ovarian epithelial cancer†.

In a randomized trial involving 1077 patients with stage Ic–IV ovarian epithelial cancer, patients received either docetaxel/carboplatin or paclitaxel/carboplatin. Treatment regimens consisted of docetaxel 75 mg/m² as a 1-hour IV infusion followed by carboplatin (at the dose required to obtain an AUC of 5 mg/mL per minute) as a 1-hour IV infusion; or paclitaxel 175 mg/m² as a 3-hour IV infusion followed by carboplatin (at the dose required to obtain an AUC of 5 mg/mL per minute) as a 1-hour IV infusion. The treatment regimens were repeated every 3 weeks for 6 cycles of therapy; patients who responded to combination therapy then could receive an additional 3 cycles of carboplatin alone. Median progression-free survival was similar (about 15 months) between the groups. Grade 3 or 4 neutropenia (94 versus 84%) and complicated neutropenia (25 versus 5%) occurred more frequently in patients receiving docetaxel and carboplatin. GI toxicity, peripheral edema, allergic reactions, and nail changes also were more frequent in patients receiving docetaxel and carboplatin. Neurotoxicity, including neurosensory toxicity (78 versus 45%) and neuromotor toxicity (16 versus 9%), occurred more frequently in patients receiving paclitaxel and carboplatin. Arthralgia, myalgia, alopecia, and abdominal pain also were more frequent in patients receiving paclitaxel and carboplatin.

Docetaxel also is used for the treatment of recurrent or persistent ovarian epithelial cancer that is platinum-resistant or platinum-refractory†.

DOSAGE AND ADMINISTRATION

● Reconstitution and Administration

Docetaxel is administered by IV infusion over a 1-hour period under ambient room temperature and lighting conditions. Infusion of the drug over longer periods (e.g., 6 or 24 hours) or the use of frequently repeated infusions (e.g., over 5 days) was associated with clinically important and dose-limiting mucositis in phase 1 studies.

Caution should be exercised when preparing and handling docetaxel solutions, and the use of protective gloves is recommended. Skin accidentally exposed to the drug should be immediately and thoroughly washed with soap and water. If the drug comes into contact with mucous membranes, the affected area should be flushed immediately and thoroughly with water.

Docetaxel is commercially available as an injection concentrate and as a lyophilized powder. The lyophilized powder must be reconstituted and then diluted to prepare a final docetaxel infusion solution. *Docetaxel injection concentrate must be diluted prior to IV administration.* The proper procedure for preparing a final docetaxel infusion solution from an injection concentrate may vary by manufacturer (i.e., some manufacturers' preparations may require one dilution step, whereas other manufacturers' preparations may require 2 dilution steps). Taxotere® injection concentrate has been reformulated to require one dilution step rather than 2 dilution steps. In addition, injection concentrates available from various manufacturers may contain different concentrations of the drug. *The manufacturer's instructions for the specific formulation should be consulted to ensure that the correct preparation procedure is followed.* Formulations requiring 2 dilution steps should not be used with formulations requiring one dilution step.

Because reconstituted and diluted docetaxel solutions are supersaturated, crystallization may occur over time. Docetaxel injection concentrate and reconstituted and diluted solutions of the drug should be inspected visually for particulate matter and discoloration whenever solution and container permit. If the solution is not clear or appears to have precipitation, the solution should be discarded.

Contact of docetaxel injection concentrate or reconstituted docetaxel solution with plasticized polyvinyl chloride (PVC) equipment or devices used to prepare solutions for infusion is *not* recommended. Polysorbate 80 can cause leaching of diethylhexyl phthalate (DEHP) from PVC containers and, following dilution of docetaxel injection concentrate in PVC containers, substantial leaching of DEHP occurs in a time-dependent and concentration-dependent manner. To minimize exposure of the patient to leached DEHP, final diluted docetaxel solutions for infusion preferably should be stored in glass or polypropylene containers or in plastic (polypropylene or polyolefin) bags and administered through polyethylene-lined administration sets.

Dilution of Docetaxel Injection Concentrate Requiring One Dilution Step

If the vial containing docetaxel injection concentrate has been stored in the refrigerator, it should be allowed to stand at room temperature for approximately 5 minutes prior to dilution. When the docetaxel injection concentrate is a formulation that requires one dilution step, the required amount of docetaxel injection concentrate should be withdrawn from the vial using a syringe with a 21-gauge needle and injected into a 250-mL infusion bag or bottle containing either 0.9% sodium chloride injection or 5% dextrose injection to produce a final solution with a docetaxel concentration of 0.3–0.74 mg/mL. If doses larger than 200 mg of docetaxel are required, the volume of IV solution should be increased accordingly so that the docetaxel concentration does not exceed 0.74 mg/mL. The final diluted docetaxel solution for infusion should be mixed thoroughly by gentle manual rotation.

Dilution of Docetaxel Injection Concentrate Requiring Two Dilution Steps

When the docetaxel injection concentrate is a formulation that requires 2 dilution steps, the docetaxel injection concentrate is first diluted with the diluent supplied by the manufacturer (13% w/v polyethylene glycol 400 in water for injection) to prepare the initial diluted docetaxel solution, and then the initial diluted docetaxel solution is further diluted to make the final dilution of docetaxel solution for infusion.

For preparation of the initial diluted docetaxel solution, the entire contents of the vial of diluent supplied by the manufacturer (approximately 1.95 mL of diluent for docetaxel 20 mg and approximately 7.2 mL of diluent for docetaxel 80 mg) should be added to the appropriate vial of docetaxel injection concentrate to create an initial diluted solution of docetaxel 10 mg/mL. The vial should be inverted repeatedly for at least 45 seconds to fully mix the concentrate and the diluent; the vial should not be shaken. The initial diluted docetaxel solution should be clear but there may be some foam on top because of the presence of polysorbate 80. The solution should be allowed to stand for a few minutes to let the foam dissipate, and then preparation may continue even if some foam remains. The initial diluted docetaxel solution may be used immediately to prepare the final diluted docetaxel solution for infusion or it may be stored either in the refrigerator or at room temperature for up to 8 hours.

For preparation of the final diluted docetaxel solution for infusion, the required amount of the initial diluted docetaxel solution (docetaxel 10 mg/mL) should be injected into a 250-mL infusion bag or bottle containing either 0.9% sodium chloride injection or 5% dextrose injection to produce a final solution with a docetaxel concentration of 0.3–0.74 mg/mL. If doses larger than 200 mg of docetaxel are required, the volume of IV solution should be increased accordingly so that the docetaxel concentration does not exceed 0.74 mg/mL. The final diluted docetaxel solution for infusion should be mixed thoroughly by manual rotation.

Reconstitution and Dilution of Docetaxel Lyophilized Powder

Commercially available docetaxel powder for injection must be reconstituted and diluted prior to IV infusion. The drug should be reconstituted with the diluent supplied by the manufacturer (ethanol 35.4% w/w and polysorbate 80). The appropriate number of diluent vials and vials containing docetaxel lyophilized powder should be removed from the refrigerator and allowed to stand at room temperature for approximately 5 minutes prior to reconstitution. The powder is reconstituted by withdrawing 1 mL of diluent using a 1-mL syringe with an 18- or 21-gauge needle and adding the diluent to a vial labeled as containing docetaxel 20 mg to provide a solution containing 20 mg in 0.8 mL or by withdrawing 4 mL of diluent using a 4-mL syringe with an 18- or 21-gauge needle and adding the diluent to a vial labeled as containing docetaxel 80 mg to provide a solution containing 24 mg/mL of the drug. The vial should be shaken well to ensure complete dissolution of the drug. The resulting solution should be clear but may contain some air bubbles because of the presence of polysorbate 80. The solution should be allowed to stand for a few minutes to let the bubbles dissipate. The reconstituted docetaxel solution may be used immediately to prepare the final diluted docetaxel solution for infusion or it may be stored either in a refrigerator or at room temperature for up to 8 hours.

For preparation of the final diluted docetaxel solution for infusion, the required amount of reconstituted docetaxel solution should be injected into a 250-mL infusion bag or bottle containing 0.9% sodium chloride injection or 5% dextrose injection to produce a final solution with a docetaxel concentration of 0.3–0.74 mg/mL. If doses larger than 200 mg of docetaxel are required, the volume of IV solution should be increased accordingly so that the docetaxel concentration does not exceed 0.74 mg/mL. The final diluted docetaxel solution for infusion should be mixed thoroughly by manual rotation.

Dispensing and Administration Precautions

The manufacturer states that formation of particulate matter in docetaxel solutions has not been observed when the drug has been administered at recommended doses; therefore, the use of inline filters with docetaxel infusion solutions is neither required nor recommended. Medication errors have occurred that involved confusion between docetaxel (Taxotere®) and paclitaxel (Taxol®). Two pharmacists should provide independent confirmation that the correct drug is being ordered before chemotherapy is dispensed, and two nurses should confirm that the correct drug has been dispensed for the correct patient before administering the medication. (See Cautions: Precautions and Contraindications.)

● Dosage

The incidence of mortality associated with docetaxel therapy is higher in patients with hepatic impairment (see Dosage and Administration: Dosage in Renal and Hepatic Impairment) and in patients receiving higher doses of the drug.

Concomitant use of potent inhibitors of cytochrome P-450 (CYP) isoenzyme 3A4 (CYP3A4) (e.g., atazanavir, clarithromycin, indinavir, itraconazole, ketoconazole, nefazodone, nelfinavir, ritonavir, saquinavir, telithromycin, voriconazole) may increase docetaxel exposure and should be avoided. If such concomitant use cannot be avoided, a reduction in docetaxel dosage with careful monitoring for toxicity should be considered. Based on limited pharmacokinetic data, the manufacturers state that a 50% reduction in docetaxel dosage may be considered in patients requiring concomitant therapy with a potent CYP3A4 inhibitor; however, there are no clinical data with use of this adjusted docetaxel dosage. (See Drug Interactions: Drugs Affecting or Metabolized by Hepatic Microsomal Enzymes.)

Premedication Regimen

All patients should be premedicated with oral corticosteroids before docetaxel administration to reduce the severity of hypersensitivity reactions and to reduce the incidence and severity of fluid retention. For patients receiving docetaxel for hormone-refractory metastatic prostate cancer, the manufacturers recommend a regimen of oral dexamethasone 8 mg at 12 hours, 3 hours, and 1 hour prior to the infusion of docetaxel. For patients receiving docetaxel for other cancers, the manufacturer recommends a regimen of oral dexamethasone 8 mg twice daily for 3 days, starting 1 day prior to docetaxel administration.

Breast Cancer

The manufacturers state that prophylaxis with granulocyte colony-stimulating factor (G-CSF) may be used to reduce the risk of hematologic toxicity associated with docetaxel therapy. Some clinicians recommend primary prophylaxis with G-CSF in patients receiving docetaxel with an anthracycline agent for breast cancer.

Adjuvant Therapy for Breast Cancer

For the adjuvant treatment of operable node-positive breast cancer, the recommended dosage is docetaxel 75 mg/m^2 as a 1-hour IV infusion administered 1 hour following doxorubicin 50 mg/m^2 IV and cyclophosphamide 500 mg/m^2 IV; this regimen is administered once every 3 weeks for up to 6 courses of therapy.

Advanced Breast Cancer

Optimum dosage of docetaxel for the treatment of advanced or metastatic breast cancer has not been established. The manufacturers currently recommend a docetaxel regimen of 60–100 mg/m^2 infused IV over 1 hour and repeated every

3 weeks as tolerated in patients with locally advanced or metastatic breast cancer after failure of prior chemotherapy.

Among patients who are dosed initially at docetaxel 60 mg/m^2 and who do not experience severe adverse effects (e.g., febrile neutropenia, severe neutropenia for more than 1 week, severe or cumulative cutaneous reactions, or severe peripheral neuropathy), higher doses of docetaxel may be tolerated.

In phase 2 studies, patients received a median of 4 or 5 cycles of docetaxel therapy; however, the usual course of therapy remains to be established.

Non-small Cell Lung Cancer

First-line Therapy for Advanced Disease

For the first-line treatment of unresectable, locally advanced or metastatic non-small cell lung cancer, the recommended dosage is docetaxel 75 mg/m^2 administered as a 1-hour IV infusion followed by cisplatin 75 mg/m^2 IV administered over 30–60 minutes; this regimen is administered once every 3 weeks.

Second-line Therapy for Advanced Disease

When used as monotherapy for the second-line treatment of non-small cell lung cancer, docetaxel 75 mg/m^2 IV is administered as a 1-hour infusion once every 3 weeks; higher doses of docetaxel are associated with excessive toxicity in this patient population, including increased rates of hematologic toxicity, infection, and treatment-related mortality, and are *not* recommended.

Prostate Cancer

For the treatment of hormone-refractory metastatic prostate cancer, the recommended dosage is docetaxel 75 mg/m^2 administered as a 1-hour IV infusion once every 3 weeks. Prednisone 5 mg orally twice daily is administered continually.

Gastric Cancer

Premedication with antiemetic agents and adequate hydration for cisplatin administration are required. Primary prophylaxis with G-CSF should be considered.

For the first-line treatment of gastric adenocarcinoma, the recommended dosage is docetaxel 75 mg/m^2 as a 1-hour IV infusion on day 1 followed by cisplatin 75 mg/m^2 as a 1-hour to 3-hour IV infusion on day 1 followed by fluorouracil 750 mg/m^2 as a 24-hour continuous IV infusion daily for 5 days (days 1–5) initiated upon completion of the cisplatin infusion; this regimen is repeated every 3 weeks.

Head and Neck Cancer

Premedication with antiemetic agents and adequate hydration preceding and following cisplatin administration are required. Prophylaxis for neutropenic infections also should be administered. In the randomized trials, all patients receiving the docetaxel-containing regimen were given prophylactic antibiotic therapy.

Induction Chemotherapy Followed by Radiotherapy

For induction chemotherapy of inoperable locally advanced squamous cell carcinoma of the head and neck, the recommended dosage is docetaxel 75 mg/m^2 as a 1-hour IV infusion (day 1) followed by cisplatin 75 mg/m^2 as a 1-hour IV infusion (day 1) followed by fluorouracil 750 mg/m^2 as a 24-hour continuous IV infusion daily for 5 days (days 1–5) initiated upon completion of the cisplatin infusion; this regimen is administered once every 3 weeks for up to 4 cycles. Following the completion of chemotherapy, patients should receive radiotherapy.

Induction Chemotherapy Followed by Chemoradiotherapy

For induction chemotherapy of locally advanced squamous cell carcinoma of the head and neck in patients who have unresectable disease or disease with low chance of surgical cure, or who are candidates for organ preservation, the recommended dosage is docetaxel 75 mg/m^2 as a 1-hour IV infusion (day 1) followed by cisplatin 100 mg/m^2 as a 30-minute to 3-hour IV infusion (day 1) followed by fluorouracil 1000 mg/m^2 as a 24-hour continuous IV infusion daily for 4 days (days 1–4); this regimen is administered once every 3 weeks for up to 3 cycles. Following the completion of chemotherapy, patients should receive chemoradiotherapy.

Dosage Modification for Toxicity and Contraindications for Continued Therapy

Adjustment of docetaxel dosage may be required according to toxicity. When docetaxel is used in combination regimens, adjustment of dosage for the other drugs may be necessary. In addition to the dosage adjustments for cisplatin and fluorouracil described here, also see the manufacturers' labelings.

Hematologic Toxicity

For patients who experience neutropenia and/or thrombocytopenia, docetaxel doses should be withheld until neutrophil counts are at least 1500/mm^3 and platelet counts exceed 100,000/mm^3.

For patients who have experienced severe neutropenia (neutrophil count less than 500/mm^3) for at least 7 days, febrile neutropenia, or a grade 4 infection during a cycle of therapy, a 25% reduction in the dose of docetaxel is recommended for subsequent cycles.

Among patients receiving docetaxel monotherapy for breast cancer who are dosed initially at 100 mg/m^2 and who experience either febrile neutropenia or severe neutropenia (neutrophil count less than 500/mm^3) for more than 1 week, the manufacturer recommends a 25% reduction in the dose (from 100 to 75 mg/m^2) for subsequent courses of therapy. If the patient continues to experience these reactions, either the dose of docetaxel should be reduced further to 55 mg/m^2 or the drug should be discontinued.

Among patients receiving docetaxel with doxorubicin and cyclophosphamide for the adjuvant treatment of breast cancer who are dosed initially at 75 mg/m^2, those who experience febrile neutropenia should receive G-CSF for all subsequent cycles of therapy. If febrile neutropenia persists, G-CSF should be continued and the docetaxel dose should be reduced to 60 mg/m^2.

Among patients receiving docetaxel monotherapy for advanced non-small cell lung cancer who are dosed initially at 75 mg/m^2 and who experience severe neutropenia (neutrophil count less than 500/mm^3) for more than 1 week or febrile neutropenia, treatment with the drug should be interrupted. Upon resolution of the toxicity, therapy may be resumed at a reduced dose of docetaxel 55 mg/m^2.

Among patients receiving docetaxel in combination with cisplatin for advanced non-small cell lung cancer who are dosed initially at 75 mg/m^2 and who experience a nadir platelet count of less than 25,000/mm^3 during the previous course of therapy or febrile neutropenia, the docetaxel dose should be reduced to 65 mg/m^2 for subsequent cycles. If toxicity persists, further reduction to a docetaxel dose of 50 mg/m^2 is recommended. For recommendations for cisplatin dosage reduction, consult the manufacturer's labeling.

Among patients receiving docetaxel with prednisone for advanced prostate cancer who have experienced severe neutropenia (less than 500/mm^3) for at least 7 days or febrile neutropenia, the docetaxel dose should be reduced from 75 mg/m^2 to 60 mg/m^2. If these reactions persist at a docetaxel dose of 60 mg/m^2, treatment should be discontinued.

Among patients receiving docetaxel in combination with cisplatin and fluorouracil for either advanced gastric cancer or locally advanced head and neck cancer who experience neutropenia lasting more than 7 days, febrile neutropenia, or documented infection with neutropenia, the use of G-CSF during the second or subsequent cycles of therapy is recommended. If the patient experiences an episode of prolonged neutropenia, febrile neutropenia, or neutropenic infection despite use of G-CSF, the docetaxel dose should be reduced from 75 mg/m^2 to 60 mg/m^2. If the patient experiences subsequent episodes of complicated neutropenia, the docetaxel dose should be reduced from 60 mg/m^2 to 45 mg/m^2. If toxicity persists, treatment should be discontinued.

Among patients receiving docetaxel in combination with cisplatin and fluorouracil for either advanced gastric cancer or locally advanced head and neck cancer who experience grade 4 thrombocytopenia, the docetaxel dose should be reduced from 75 mg/m^2 to 60 mg/m^2. If toxicity persists, treatment should be discontinued.

Hypersensitivity

If signs or symptoms of a severe reaction (e.g., hypotension requiring treatment, bronchospasm/dyspnea requiring bronchodilators, generalized rash/erythema, anaphylaxis) occur during administration of the drug, the infusion should be discontinued immediately and aggressive symptomatic therapy instituted as necessary. Docetaxel therapy should *not* be reinitiated in patients experiencing severe hypersensitivity reactions.

Mild manifestations, such as pruritus, flushing, or localized skin reactions, do not require interruption of therapy; however, decreasing the infusion rate until recovery from symptoms may be considered.

Dermatologic Toxicity

Among patients receiving docetaxel monotherapy for breast cancer who are dosed initially at 100 mg/m^2 and who experience severe or cumulative cutaneous reactions, the manufacturer recommends a 25% reduction in the dose (from 100 mg/m^2 to 75 mg/m^2) for subsequent courses of therapy. If the patient continues to experience these reactions, either the docetaxel dose should be reduced further to 55 mg/m^2 or the drug should be discontinued.

Among patients receiving docetaxel with doxorubicin and cyclophosphamide for the adjuvant treatment of breast cancer who experience severe or cumulative cutaneous reactions, the docetaxel dose should be reduced from 75 to 60 mg/m^2. If these reactions persist at docetaxel dose 60 mg/m^2, treatment should be discontinued.

Among patients receiving docetaxel monotherapy for advanced non-small cell lung cancer who are dosed initially at 75 mg/m^2 and who experience severe or cumulative cutaneous reactions, treatment with the drug should be interrupted. Upon resolution of the toxicity, therapy may be resumed at a reduced dose of docetaxel 55 mg/m^2.

Among patients receiving docetaxel with prednisone for advanced prostate cancer who experience severe or cumulative cutaneous reactions, the docetaxel dose should be reduced from 75 mg/m^2 to 60 mg/m^2. If these reactions persist at a docetaxel dose of 60 mg/m^2, treatment should be discontinued.

Among patients receiving docetaxel in combination with cisplatin and fluorouracil who experience palmar-plantar toxicity (hand-foot syndrome) that is grade 2 or higher in severity, fluorouracil should be stopped until recovery and then the fluorouracil dose should be reduced by 20%. This dose modification is based on the adjustment used for the advanced gastric cancer study.

Neurologic Toxicity

Among patients receiving docetaxel monotherapy for advanced breast cancer or advanced non-small cell lung cancer who develop grade 3 or higher peripheral neuropathy, docetaxel therapy should be discontinued.

Among patients receiving docetaxel with doxorubicin and cyclophosphamide for the adjuvant treatment of breast cancer or docetaxel with prednisone for advanced prostate cancer who experience moderate neurosensory manifestations, the docetaxel dose should be reduced from 75 mg/m^2 to 60 mg/m^2. If these reactions persist at a docetaxel dose of 60 mg/m^2, treatment should be discontinued.

Among patients receiving docetaxel in combination with cisplatin and fluorouracil who experience grade 2 peripheral neuropathy, the cisplatin dose should be reduced by 20%. For patients who experience grade 3 peripheral neuropathy, treatment should be discontinued. These dose modifications are based on the adjustments used for the advanced gastric cancer study.

GI Toxicity

Among patients receiving docetaxel with doxorubicin and cyclophosphamide for the adjuvant treatment of breast cancer who experience grade 3 or 4 stomatitis, the docetaxel dose should be reduced from 75 mg/m^2 to 60 mg/m^2.

Among patients receiving docetaxel in combination with cisplatin and fluorouracil for either advanced gastric cancer or locally advanced head and neck cancer who experience grade 3 diarrhea, the guidelines for dosage reduction are as follows: after the first episode, the fluorouracil dose should be reduced by 20%; after the second episode, the docetaxel dose should be reduced by 20%. For patients who experience grade 4 diarrhea, the guidelines for dosage reduction are as follows: after the first episode, both the docetaxel dose and the fluorouracil dose should be reduced by 20%; after the second episode, treatment should be discontinued.

Among patients receiving docetaxel in combination with cisplatin and fluorouracil for either advanced gastric cancer or locally advanced head and neck cancer who experience grade 3 stomatitis/mucositis, the guidelines for dosage reduction are as follows: after the first episode, the fluorouracil dose should be reduced by 20%; after the second episode, fluorouracil should be discontinued for all subsequent cycles; after the third episode, the docetaxel dose should be reduced by 20%. For patients who experience grade 4 stomatitis/mucositis, the guidelines for dosage reduction are as follows: after the first episode, fluorouracil should be discontinued for all subsequent cycles; after the second episode, the docetaxel dose should be reduced by 20%.

Hepatic Toxicity

Among patients receiving docetaxel in combination with cisplatin and fluorouracil for advanced gastric cancer who exhibit increases in serum AST and/or ALT exceeding 2.5 times the upper limit of normal (up to 5 times the upper limit of normal) and alkaline phosphatase up to 2.5 times the upper limit of normal, the docetaxel dose should be reduced by 20%. For patients with serum AST and/or ALT exceeding 1.5 times the upper limit of normal (up to 5 times the upper limit of normal) and alkaline phosphatase exceeding 2.5 times the upper limit of normal (up to 5 times the upper limit of normal), the docetaxel dose should be reduced by 20%. For patients with serum AST and/or ALT exceeding 5 times the upper limit of normal and/or alkaline phosphatase exceeding 5 times the upper limit of normal, docetaxel should be discontinued.

Nephrotoxicity

Among patients receiving docetaxel in combination with cisplatin and fluorouracil who experience a rise in serum creatinine concentration that is grade 2 or higher in severity (greater than 1.5 times the normal value) despite adequate hydration, the creatinine clearance should be determined before each subsequent cycle of therapy and the following dose reductions should be considered. These dose modifications are based on the adjustments used for the advanced gastric cancer study.

For patients with a creatinine clearance of 60 mL/minute or higher, the full dose of cisplatin may be given for the subsequent cycle, and the creatinine clearance should be measured prior to each treatment cycle.

For patients with a creatinine clearance of 40–59 mL/minute, the cisplatin dose should be reduced by 50% for the subsequent cycle. If the creatinine clearance exceeds 60 mL/minute at the end of the cycle using the 50% cisplatin dose, the full cisplatin dose may be given for the next cycle. If recovery does not occur at the end of the cycle using the 50% cisplatin dose, cisplatin should be omitted from the next treatment cycle.

For patients with a creatinine clearance less than 40 mL/minute, the cisplatin dose should be omitted for that treatment cycle only. If the creatinine clearance remains low (less than 40 mL/minute) at the end of the treatment cycle omitting the cisplatin dose, cisplatin should be discontinued. If the creatinine clearance exceeds 40 mL/minute but is less than 60 mL/minute at the end of the treatment cycle omitting the cisplatin dose, a 50% cisplatin dose may be given for the next cycle. If the creatinine clearance exceeds 60 mL/minute at the end of the treatment cycle using the 50% cisplatin dose, the full cisplatin dose may be given for the next cycle.

Ototoxicity

Among patients receiving docetaxel in combination with cisplatin and fluorouracil who experience grade 3 ototoxicity, treatment should be discontinued. This dose modification is based on the adjustment used for the advanced gastric cancer study.

Ocular Toxicity

If cystoid macular edema is diagnosed, docetaxel therapy should be discontinued and appropriate treatment initiated. Alternative therapy with a nontaxane antineoplastic agent should be considered.

Other Toxicity

For patients receiving docetaxel alone or in combination with cisplatin for advanced non-small cell lung cancer who experience grade 3 or 4 nonhematologic toxicities, the same recommendations for reduction of the docetaxel dose should be followed as for patients experiencing hematologic toxicities. (See Hematologic Toxicity under Dosage: Dosage Modification for Toxicity and Contraindications for Continued Therapy, in Dosage and Administration.)

Among patients receiving docetaxel in combination with cisplatin and fluorouracil who experience toxicity (except alopecia and anemia) that is higher than grade 3 in severity, chemotherapy should be delayed for up to 2 weeks from the planned date of infusion until resolution of the toxicity to grade 1 or less in severity occurs and then resumption of chemotherapy may be considered. These dose modifications are based on the adjustments used for the advanced gastric cancer study.

● Dosage in Renal and Hepatic Impairment

Urinary excretion of docetaxel has been reported to be low (less than 10%), and reduction of dosage in patients with impaired renal function does not appear to be necessary.

Docetaxel clearance appears to be reduced in patients with abnormal liver function, and an increased incidence of adverse effects (including treatment-related mortality) has been reported in patients with moderate to severe hepatic impairment. Therefore, patients with serum total bilirubin exceeding the upper limit of normal, and patients with serum AST and/or ALT exceeding 1.5 times the upper limit of normal concomitant with alkaline phosphatase exceeding 2.5 times the upper limit of normal, generally should not receive docetaxel.

For further information on the handling of antineoplastic agents, see the guidelines at the end of Antineoplastic Agents 10:00.

CAUTIONS

The principal, dose-limiting adverse effect of docetaxel is bone marrow suppression, manifested by neutropenia, leukopenia, thrombocytopenia, and anemia.

The incidence of treatment-related adverse effects associated with docetaxel therapy is increased in patients with abnormal liver function and in those receiving higher doses. (See Cautions: Precautions and Contraindications.) The incidence of adverse effects reported here is based principally upon data from 2045 patients with normal liver function receiving docetaxel 100 mg/m^2 for various solid tumors, including a subset of 965 patients with locally advanced or metastatic breast cancer and a subset of 61 patients with various tumor types and hepatic dysfunction manifested by elevated results of liver function tests. The incidence of selected adverse effects is reported for differing dose levels (e.g., 60 mg/m^2 in 174 patients with metastatic breast cancer), combination regimens, and/or patient populations receiving docetaxel for specific cancers when the rates or types of adverse effects differed substantially from the patterns of toxicity reported for the 2045 patients with various solid tumors. This information may include selected adverse effects for patients receiving docetaxel every 3 weeks as follows: at doses of 60, 75, and 100 mg/m^2 for advanced breast cancer; or at a dose of 75 mg/m^2 as adjuvant therapy for breast cancer (with doxorubicin and cyclophosphamide), as second-line therapy for advanced non-small cell lung cancer, as first-line therapy for advanced non-small cell lung cancer (with cisplatin), for androgen-independent (hormone-refractory) metastatic prostate cancer (with prednisone), as first-line therapy for advanced gastric cancer (with cisplatin and fluorouracil), and as induction chemotherapy for advanced head and neck cancer (with cisplatin and fluorouracil). Additional incidence data for adverse effects and information on the comparative toxicity of chemotherapy regimens evaluated in clinical trials is discussed in the corresponding Uses section for each cancer. In general, the safety profile of docetaxel in patients being treated for breast cancer or other types of solid tumors is similar. The most common adverse effects of docetaxel across all labeled indications for the drug are infection, neutropenia, anemia, febrile neutropenia, hypersensitivity, thrombocytopenia, neuropathy, dysgeusia, dyspnea, constipation, anorexia, nail disorders, fluid retention, asthenia, pain, nausea, diarrhea, vomiting, mucositis, alopecia, skin reactions, and myalgia.

Death possibly or probably related to treatment occurred in 2% of patients with normal hepatic function receiving docetaxel 100 mg/m^2 for metastatic breast cancer and in 11.5% of patients receiving docetaxel 100 mg/m^2 for various tumor types who had hepatic dysfunction. Among patients receiving docetaxel 60 mg/m^2 for breast cancer, treatment-related mortality occurred in about 1% of patients with normal liver function and in 3 of 7 patients with hepatic dysfunction. Approximately half of these deaths occurred during the first treatment cycle, and sepsis accounted for a majority of the deaths.

● Hematologic Effects and Infectious Complications

The frequency and severity of docetaxel-induced hematologic toxicity, febrile reactions and infections, and rates of death caused by sepsis increase with dose and in the presence of hepatic dysfunction. As with paclitaxel, docetaxel-induced myelosuppression may be more severe in patients who have received prior radiation therapy.

Docetaxel-induced neutropenia generally is reversible. Neutropenia secondary to docetaxel, in contrast to that caused by paclitaxel, is not schedule-dependent. Neutropenia (neutrophil count less than 2000/mm^3) occurred in almost all patients (96%) receiving docetaxel for solid tumors. Severe (grade 4) neutropenia (less than 500/mm^3) occurred in 75% of patients with solid tumors and lasted more than 7 days in about 3% of treatment cycles. Severe neutropenia occurred at a higher rate among the subsets of patients receiving docetaxel for locally advanced or metastatic breast cancer (86%) or patients with hepatic dysfunction (88%). Similarly high rates of neutropenia were reported in patients receiving docetaxel in combination therapy for other cancers except for advanced prostate cancer (41%, grade 3 or 4 in 32%).

The onset of neutropenia is rapid, with neutrophil nadirs generally occurring 7–8 days following docetaxel administration; the median duration of severe (grade 4) neutropenia is about 7 days. Subsequent courses of docetaxel therapy generally do not result in lower neutrophil nadirs than in the initial course, suggesting that the drug may not be irreversibly toxic to stem cells.

Leukopenia (leukocyte count less than 4000/mm³) occurred in almost all patients (96%) receiving docetaxel for solid tumors. Severe leukopenia (less than 1000/mm³) occurred in 32% of patients with solid tumors and at a higher rate among the subsets of patients receiving docetaxel for locally advanced or metastatic breast cancer (44%) or patients with hepatic dysfunction (47%).

Anemia (hemoglobin less than 11 g/dL) occurred in 90% of patients receiving docetaxel for solid tumors. Severe anemia (hemoglobin less than 8 g/dL) occurred in 9% of patients with solid tumors and in 31% of the subset of patients with hepatic dysfunction. Similarly high rates of anemia were reported in patients receiving docetaxel in combination therapy for other cancers except advanced prostate cancer (66%). A lower rate of anemia was reported in patients receiving docetaxel 60 mg/m² for advanced breast cancer (65%). Packed red blood cell transfusions may be required in some patients.

Fever in the absence of infection occurred in 31% of patients receiving docetaxel for solid tumors and in 41% (severe in 8%) of the subset of patients with hepatic dysfunction. Fever in the absence of infection was reported in 46% of patients receiving docetaxel with doxorubicin and cyclophosphamide as adjuvant therapy for breast cancer.

Febrile neutropenia (neutrophil count less than 500/mm³ with fever greater than 38°C and IV anti-infectives and/or hospitalization required) occurred in 11% of patients receiving docetaxel for solid tumors and in 26% of the subset of patients with hepatic dysfunction. Patients with isolated elevations of serum aminotransferase concentrations (more than 1.5 times the upper limit of normal) had a higher rate of grade 4 febrile neutropenia but the incidence of toxic death was not increased in these patients. Febrile neutropenia (grade 3 or 4 neutropenia with fever greater than 38.1°C) occurred in none of 174 patients receiving docetaxel 60 mg/m² for advanced breast cancer. Febrile neutropenia was reported in 25% of patients receiving docetaxel with doxorubicin and cyclophosphamide as adjuvant therapy for breast cancer. Among patients receiving docetaxel with cisplatin and fluorouracil for gastric cancer, febrile neutropenia and/or neutropenic infection occurred in 28% of patients who did not receive granulocyte colony-stimulating factor (G-CSF) versus 12% of patients who did receive G-CSF.

Infection occurred in 22% of patients receiving docetaxel for solid tumors and was severe in 6%. The rate of infection (33%) and severe infection (16%) was higher in the subset of patients with hepatic dysfunction. Fatal sepsis occurred in about 2% of patients receiving docetaxel for solid tumors and in 5% of the subset of patients with hepatic dysfunction. Higher rates of infection were reported in patients receiving docetaxel in combination therapy for the adjuvant treatment of breast cancer (39%), for advanced non-small cell lung cancer (35%), for advanced prostate cancer (32%), and for advanced gastric cancer (29%, grade 3 or 4 in 16%). Neutropenic infection was reported in patients receiving docetaxel in combination regimens for gastric cancer (16%), head and neck cancer (14 or 12%), and adjuvant treatment of breast cancer (12%). Infection occurred in 1% of patients receiving docetaxel 60 mg/m² for advanced breast cancer.

Thrombocytopenia (platelet count less than 100,000/mm³) occurred in 8% of patients receiving docetaxel for solid tumors and in 25% of the subset of patients with hepatic dysfunction. A higher rate of thrombocytopenia (44%), including grade 4 thrombocytopenia (17%), was reported in 18 patients with hepatic dysfunction receiving docetaxel 100 mg/m² for metastatic breast cancer. Higher rates of thrombocytopenia also were reported in patients receiving docetaxel in combination therapy for the adjuvant treatment of breast cancer (39%), for advanced gastric cancer (26%), for locally advanced head and neck cancer (24 or 28%), and for advanced non-small cell lung cancer (15%).

Bleeding episodes have occurred in patients receiving docetaxel in clinical trials, including 3 breast cancer patients with severe liver impairment (serum total bilirubin value exceeding 1.7 times the upper limit of normal) who developed fatal GI hemorrhage associated with severe docetaxel-induced thrombocytopenia. GI bleeding also was reported in patients receiving docetaxel with cisplatin and fluorouracil as induction chemotherapy for locally advanced head and neck cancer (approximately 5%). Epistaxis occurred in 6% of patients receiving docetaxel and prednisone for advanced prostate cancer. Disseminated intravascular coagulation, often associated with sepsis or multiorgan failure, has occurred in patients receiving docetaxel.

• Sensitivity Reactions

Docetaxel frequently causes hypersensitivity reactions, which can be severe, and all patients receiving the drug should be premedicated to reduce the severity of these reactions. (See Dosage and Administration: Dosage.) Severe hypersensitivity reactions, characterized by generalized rash/erythema, hypotension and/or bronchospasm, or rarely, fatal anaphylaxis, have occurred in patients receiving docetaxel who received the recommended premedication regimen. Discontinuance of therapy and aggressive management is required in patients experiencing severe hypersensitivity reactions associated with docetaxel. (See Hypersensitivity under Dosage: Dosage Modification for Toxicity and Contraindications for Continued Therapy, in Dosage and Administration.)

Hypersensitivity reactions occurred in 21% of patients receiving docetaxel for solid tumors and were severe in 4%; in the subset of 92 patients receiving the 3-day premedication regimen, hypersensitivity reactions occurred in 15% and were severe in 2%. In the subset of patients with hepatic dysfunction, severe hypersensitivity reactions occurred in 10%. Hypersensitivity reactions or allergic reactions were reported in patients receiving docetaxel in combination therapy for adjuvant treatment of breast cancer (13%), for advanced non-small cell lung cancer (12%), for advanced gastric cancer (10%), and for advanced prostate cancer (8%) and in patients receiving docetaxel alone for non-small cell lung cancer (6%). Allergy (6 or 2%) was reported in patients receiving docetaxel with cisplatin and fluorouracil as induction chemotherapy for locally advanced head and neck cancer. A lower rate of hypersensitivity reactions (about 1%, none severe) was reported in patients receiving docetaxel 60 mg/m² for advanced breast cancer.

Docetaxel-induced hypersensitivity reactions almost always occur with the first or second cycle of therapy, usually within a few minutes following initiation of docetaxel infusion. In clinical trials, mild reactions (e.g., flushing, localized skin reactions) generally did not require interruption of docetaxel administration or prevent completion of treatment with the drug. Some mild adverse effects, such as flushing, rash with or without pruritus, chest tightness, back pain, dyspnea, drug fever, or chills, resolved after completion of the infusion and appropriate therapy.

The exact cause of hypersensitivity reactions associated with docetaxel therapy is not known, but they may result from the polysorbate 80 in commercially available docetaxel injection concentrate and/or from docetaxel itself. Both docetaxel and paclitaxel can cause hypersensitivity reactions, despite the fact that the vehicles used for formulation are different; the Cremophor® EL in paclitaxel concentrate for injection has been suggested as a possible cause of hypersensitivity reactions with paclitaxel therapy.

• Nervous System Effects

Because of the alcohol content of parenteral formulations of docetaxel, alcohol intoxication has been reported during postmarketing experience in patients receiving the drug. After a review of the Adverse Event Reporting System (AERS) database and case reports, the US Food and Drug Administration (FDA) identified 3 cases of alcohol intoxication following administration of docetaxel. In these cases, onset of alcohol intoxication occurred during administration or within 24 hours of administration of the drug. Symptoms of alcohol intoxication were transient in one patient. In another patient, symptoms subsided and the infusion was completed at a slower infusion rate.

Adverse neurosensory effects occurred in 49% of patients receiving docetaxel for solid tumors and were severe in 4%. The rate of adverse neurosensory effects was 58% in the subset of patients receiving docetaxel for locally advanced or metastatic breast cancer and 20% in patients receiving docetaxel 60 mg/m² for advanced breast cancer. Severe neurosensory effects (i.e., paresthesia, dysesthesia, pain) were reported in 5.5% of patients receiving docetaxel for metastatic breast cancer in clinical trials and required treatment discontinuance in 6.1% of these patients. Adverse neurosensory effects were reported in patients receiving docetaxel in combination therapy for advanced non-small cell lung cancer (47%), advanced gastric cancer (38%), and locally advanced head and neck cancer (18 or 14%) and in patients receiving docetaxel alone for advanced non-small cell lung cancer (23%). Sensory neuropathy was reported in patients receiving docetaxel in combination therapy for advanced prostate cancer (30%) and the adjuvant treatment of breast cancer (26%).

Docetaxel can cause a predominantly sensory neuropathy similar to that reported with paclitaxel administration. The neuropathy usually is characterized by paresthesia or dysesthesia with numbness and tingling in a stocking-and-glove distribution. Some patients also have experienced pain (including burning sensation) in the hands and/or feet.

The frequency and severity of docetaxel-induced neurotoxicity increase with cumulative dose, especially at cumulative doses exceeding 400–600 mg/m². Sensory manifestations usually improve or resolve following discontinuance of docetaxel, with most patients experiencing improvement within 9 weeks from onset (range: 0–106 weeks); however, neuropathy may continue to worsen after stopping docetaxel in some patients.

Neuromotor toxicity also has been reported with docetaxel. Motor involvement is less frequent than sensory involvement and is usually only seen in patients who experience relatively severe neuropathy secondary to docetaxel therapy. Neuromotor toxicity has been manifested principally as both proximal and distal muscle weakness in the extremities, predominantly in the legs. Neuromotor toxicity was reported in patients receiving docetaxel in combination therapy for advanced non-small cell lung cancer (19%), advanced gastric cancer (9%), advanced prostate cancer (7%), and locally advanced head and neck cancer (2 or 9%) and in patients receiving docetaxel alone for advanced non-small cell lung cancer (16%). Severe peripheral neuromotor toxicity, consisting principally of distal extremity weakness, was reported in about 4% of patients receiving docetaxel for breast cancer in clinical trials. Although docetaxel-induced neuropathy has been reported in some patients with prior cisplatin therapy, no apparent relationship between docetaxel-induced neuropathy and prior treatment with cisplatin has been observed, and prior neurotoxic therapy may not necessarily predispose patients to docetaxel neuropathy. Neurocortical (5%), neuromotor (4%), and neurocerebellar (2%) toxicity were reported in patients receiving docetaxel with doxorubicin and cyclophosphamide for the adjuvant treatment of breast cancer.

Asthenia occurred in 62% of patients receiving docetaxel for solid tumors and was severe in 13%. Severe asthenia occurred in 25% of the subset of patients with hepatic dysfunction. Severe asthenia was reported in about 15% of patients with metastatic breast cancer treated with docetaxel in clinical trials and required discontinuance of the drug in approximately 2% of patients. Higher rates of asthenia were reported in patients receiving docetaxel in combination therapy for the adjuvant treatment of breast cancer (81%) and for advanced non-small cell lung cancer (74%). Symptoms of fatigue and weakness may persist for a few days to several weeks and may be associated with a deterioration in performance status in patients with progressive disease. Among patients receiving docetaxel in combination therapy, lethargy was reported in patients with advanced gastric cancer (63%, grade 3 or 4 in 21%) and in patients with locally advanced head and neck cancer (41% in TAX323 and 61% in TAX324), and fatigue was reported in patients with advanced prostate cancer (53%).

Dizziness occurred in patients receiving docetaxel in combination therapy for advanced gastric cancer (16%) and locally advanced head and neck cancer (2% in TAX323 and 16% in TAX324). Confusion has been reported in patients receiving docetaxel. Seizures or transient loss of consciousness has been reported rarely in patients receiving docetaxel, sometimes occurring during infusion of the drug.

● **Cardiovascular Effects**

Hypotension associated with severe hypersensitivity reactions has occurred in patients receiving docetaxel. (See Cautions: Sensitivity Reactions.)

Hypotension was reported in about 3% of patients receiving docetaxel for solid tumors in clinical trials, with approximately 1% of such patients requiring treatment. In selected phase 1 studies of docetaxel therapy in which continuous Holter monitoring was used, no clinically relevant bradycardia or cardiac rhythm disturbances were observed. However, adverse cardiovascular events such as heart failure, sinus tachycardia, atrial flutter, dysrhythmia, unstable angina, pulmonary edema, and hypertension have been reported rarely in patients receiving the drug. A deterioration in left-ventricular ejection fraction (LVEF) by 10% or more associated with a decline to below the institutional lower limit of normal occurred in 8% of patients with metastatic breast cancer receiving docetaxel 100 mg/m².

Fluid retention, sometimes severe, has occurred in patients receiving docetaxel despite premedication with dexamethasone. Fluid retention generally is manifested by peripheral edema and weight gain; less frequently, pleural or pericardial effusion and/or ascites may occur. During docetaxel therapy, pleural effusion has been reported in patients with non-small cell lung cancer and lymphedema has been reported in patients with breast cancer.

The exact mechanism by which docetaxel causes fluid retention is unknown; renal, hepatic, cardiac, or endocrinologic abnormalities have not been documented. However, limited data based on capillary filtration tests with technetium-99m albumin and capillaroscopy suggest that an abnormality in capillary permeability may be the cause of the fluid retention. Docetaxel-induced fluid retention usually starts in the lower extremities but may become generalized and

appears to be completely (although sometimes slowly) reversible; a median weight gain of 2 kg has been reported with resolution of fluid retention after a median of 16 weeks (range: 0–42+ weeks) from the last infusion of docetaxel. Peripheral edema can be treated with standard measures (e.g., sodium restriction, diuretics).

Fluid retention occurred in 47% of patients receiving docetaxel for solid tumors and was severe in 7%; in the subset of 92 patients receiving the 3-day premedication regimen, fluid retention occurred in 64% and was severe in 6.5%. In the subset of patients receiving docetaxel for locally advanced or metastatic breast cancer, fluid retention occurred in 60% and was severe in 9%. Among patients receiving docetaxel in combination therapy, rates reported for fluid retention were 54% for advanced non-small cell lung cancer, 35% for adjuvant treatment of breast cancer (including peripheral edema in 27% and weight gain in 13%), 15% for advanced gastric cancer (plus edema in 13%), 24% for advanced prostate cancer (including peripheral edema in 18% and weight gain in 7.5%), and 20% (TAX323) or 13% (TAX324) for locally advanced head and neck cancer. Fluid retention was reported in 13% of patients receiving docetaxel 60 mg/m² for advanced breast cancer.

The incidence and severity of fluid retention appear to be related to the cumulative dose of docetaxel, increasing in incidence with cumulative doses of 400 mg/m² or greater. Premedication with oral corticosteroids has been reported to delay the onset and decrease the severity of fluid retention. In a phase 2 clinical trial of docetaxel as first-line therapy in patients with breast cancer in whom no routine premedication was used, 76% of responding patients discontinued treatment because of fluid retention after a median cumulative dose of 574 mg/m². In 92 patients with metastatic breast cancer receiving docetaxel in clinical trials with the recommended 3-day corticosteroid premedication regimen, moderate or severe fluid retention occurred in 27 or 6.5%, respectively; the median cumulative dose associated with the onset of moderate or severe fluid retention was 819 mg/m². Severe fluid retention, characterized by poorly tolerated peripheral edema, generalized edema, pleural effusion requiring urgent drainage, dyspnea at rest, cardiac tamponade, and/or pronounced abdominal distention (caused by ascites), may lead to discontinuance of docetaxel therapy. Discontinuance of docetaxel therapy secondary to fluid retention was required in about 10% of these patients; median cumulative dose to treatment discontinuance was 1021 mg/m².

Vasodilatation was reported in 27% of patients receiving docetaxel with doxorubicin and cyclophosphamide for the adjuvant treatment of breast cancer. Left ventricular cardiac dysfunction was reported in 10% of patients receiving docetaxel and prednisone for advanced prostate cancer. Cardiac dysrhythmias were reported in patients receiving docetaxel in combination therapy for the adjuvant treatment of breast cancer (8%), for advanced gastric cancer (4%), and for locally advanced head and neck cancer (2% in TAX323 and 6% in TAX324). Congestive heart failure (CHF) was reported in 2% of patients receiving docetaxel with doxorubicin and cyclophosphamide for the adjuvant treatment of breast cancer in the randomized trial, including fatal CHF in 1 patient.

Venous thromboembolic events, including superficial and deep-vein thrombosis and pulmonary embolism, were reported in patients receiving docetaxel with cisplatin and fluorouracil as induction chemotherapy for locally advanced head and neck cancer (3 or 4%). Other adverse cardiovascular effects that have been reported in patients receiving docetaxel include ECG abnormalities, atrial fibrillation, tachycardia, thrombophlebitis, acute pulmonary edema, myocardial ischemia, myocardial infarction, and syncope.

● **GI Effects**

Fatal GI hemorrhage associated with thrombocytopenia has been reported in patients receiving docetaxel for locally advanced or metastatic breast cancer. GI bleeding was reported in 4 or 5% of patients receiving docetaxel in combination therapy for locally advanced head and neck cancer. Colitis/enteritis/large intestine perforation was reported in 7 patients receiving docetaxel with doxorubicin and cyclophosphamide for the adjuvant treatment of breast cancer; discontinuance of therapy was required in 5 of these patients.

Pronounced abdominal distention caused by ascites may be a manifestation of severe fluid retention in patients receiving docetaxel. (See Cautions: Cardiovascular Effects.)

Nausea occurred in 39%, diarrhea in 39%, and vomiting in 22% of patients receiving docetaxel for solid tumors; these adverse GI effects generally are mild to moderate in severity in most patients but were severe in 3–5% of patients. Higher rates of nausea, typically ranging from 70–80%, were reported in patients receiving docetaxel in combination therapy for other cancers in some randomized trials, such as advanced non-small cell lung cancer, gastric cancer (grade 3 or 4 in 16%), locally advanced head and neck cancer (grade 3 or 4 in 14% in TAX324), and breast cancer (adjuvant treatment). Higher rates of vomiting and diarrhea also have been reported in patients receiving docetaxel in combination therapy, particularly when docetaxel is used in combination with cisplatin. Among patients receiving docetaxel with cisplatin and fluorouracil, vomiting occurred in 66% (grade 3 or 4 in 15%) of patients with advanced gastric cancer and 56% of patients with locally advanced head and neck cancer in TAX324. Among patients receiving docetaxel with cisplatin and fluorouracil, diarrhea occurred in 78% (grade 3 or 4 in 20%) of patients with advanced gastric cancer and 48% of patients with locally advanced head and neck cancer in TAX324. Among patients receiving docetaxel and cisplatin for advanced non-small cell lung cancer, vomiting was reported in 55% and diarrhea in 47% of patients. Among patients receiving docetaxel in combination therapy for the adjuvant treatment of breast cancer, vomiting occurred in 44% and diarrhea in 35% of patients.

Stomatitis occurred in 42% of patients receiving docetaxel for solid tumors and was severe in 5.5%. Stomatitis occurred in 52% of the subset of patients receiving docetaxel for locally advanced or metastatic breast cancer, and severe stomatitis was more frequent (13%) in the subset of patients with hepatic dysfunction. Stomatitis was reported at various rates in patients receiving docetaxel in combination therapy for the adjuvant treatment of breast cancer (69%), for locally advanced head and neck cancer (42% in TAX323; 66% in TAX324, grade 3 or 4 in 21%), and for advanced gastric cancer (59%, grade 3 or 4 in 21%). Similar rates of stomatitis were reported in patients receiving docetaxel for advanced non-small cell lung cancer as monotherapy (26%) or in combination therapy (24%). Stomatitis/pharyngitis was reported in 20% of patients receiving docetaxel and prednisone for advanced prostate cancer. Lower rates of stomatitis (19%) and severe stomatitis (about 1%) were reported in patients receiving docetaxel 60 mg/m^2 for advanced breast cancer.

Docetaxel-induced stomatitis (mucositis), is characterized by diffuse ulceration of the lips, tongue, and oral cavity. Mucositis reportedly is schedule-dependent and was observed more commonly in patients receiving longer infusions of docetaxel; radiation-recall mucositis also has been reported with docetaxel therapy.

Anorexia was reported in patients receiving docetaxel in combination therapy for gastric cancer (51%, grade 3 or 4 in 13%), advanced non-small cell lung cancer (42%), adjuvant treatment of breast cancer (22%), advanced prostate cancer (17%), and locally advanced head and neck cancer (16% in TAX323 and 40% in TAX324). Constipation was reported in patients receiving docetaxel in combination therapy for the adjuvant treatment of breast cancer (34%), for advanced gastric cancer (25%), and for locally advanced head and neck cancer (17% in TAX323 and 27% in TAX324). Taste perversion/disturbance was reported in patients receiving docetaxel in combination therapy for the adjuvant treatment of breast cancer (28%) and advanced prostate cancer (18%) and in patients receiving docetaxel alone for non-small cell lung cancer (6%). Altered taste or sense of smell was reported in patients receiving docetaxel with cisplatin and fluorouracil as induction chemotherapy for locally advanced head and neck cancer (10% in TAX323 and 20% in TAX324). Esophagitis/dysphagia/odynophagia was reported in patients receiving docetaxel in combination therapy for advanced gastric cancer (16%) and locally advanced head and neck cancer (13% in TAX323 and 25% in TAX324). Also reported in patients receiving docetaxel in combination therapy were abdominal pain (11% of patients receiving adjuvant treatment for breast cancer), GI pain/cramping (11% of patients with advanced gastric cancer; 8% of patients in TAX323 and 15% of patients in TAX324 for locally advanced head and neck cancer), and heartburn (6% of patients in TAX323 and 13% of patients in TAX324 for locally advanced head and neck cancer).

Other adverse GI effects reported in patients receiving docetaxel include duodenal ulcer, ischemic colitis, intestinal obstruction, ileus, and dehydration caused by adverse GI events. In addition, at least one case of typhlitis (neutropenic enterocolitis) and fatal sepsis secondary to *Clostridium septicum* has been reported with docetaxel.

● *Dermatologic Effects*

Alopecia occurred in 76% of patients receiving docetaxel for solid tumors and at similar rates in patients receiving the drug in combination regimens for other cancers. Alopecia occurred in almost all patients (98%) receiving docetaxel with doxorubicin and cyclophosphamide as adjuvant therapy for breast cancer. A lower rate of alopecia was reported in patients receiving docetaxel alone for advanced non-small cell lung cancer (56%).

Alopecia has a sudden onset and occurs 14–21 days after administration of docetaxel. Patients often experience loss of all body hair, including axillary and pubic hair and that on the extremities, eyelashes, and eyebrows. Alopecia is dose-related and generally occurs at docetaxel doses exceeding 55 mg/m^2. Docetaxel-induced alopecia is fully reversible after treatment discontinuance. Limited data suggest that the use of a cold cap during docetaxel infusion may lessen the incidence and severity of alopecia.

Adverse cutaneous reactions occurred in 48% of patients receiving docetaxel for solid tumors and were severe in 5%. In the subset of patients receiving docetaxel for locally advanced or metastatic breast cancer, 1.6% of patients discontinued therapy because of skin toxicity. A lower rate of cutaneous toxicity (30.5%) was reported in patients receiving docetaxel 60 mg/m^2 for advanced breast cancer. Skin toxicity was reported in patients receiving docetaxel in combination therapy for the adjuvant treatment of breast cancer (26%) and for advanced non-small cell lung cancer (16%) and in patients receiving docetaxel alone for advanced non-small cell lung cancer (20%). Also reported in patients receiving docetaxel in combination therapy were rash/itch (12% of patients with advanced gastric cancer; 12% of patients in TAX323 and 20% of patients in TAX324 for locally advanced head and neck cancer), rash/desquamation (6% of patients with advanced prostate cancer), dry skin (6 or 5% of patients with locally advanced head and neck cancer), and desquamation (4 or 2% of patients with locally advanced head and neck cancer; 2% of patients with advanced gastric cancer).

Generalized rash/erythema associated with severe hypersensitivity reactions have occurred in patients receiving docetaxel. (See Cautions: Sensitivity Reactions.) As with paclitaxel, transient skin changes have been observed in patients experiencing hypersensitivity reactions to docetaxel. In addition, cutaneous reactions, which occasionally are severe, appear to occur more frequently with docetaxel than with paclitaxel therapy. Reversible cutaneous reactions, characterized by rash, including localized eruptions (usually on the feet and/or hands, and less commonly on the arms, face, or trunk) usually associated with pruritus, occur frequently in patients receiving docetaxel. Such eruptions generally occurred within 1 week after docetaxel administration, resolved before the next infusion, and were not disabling. Severe cutaneous toxicity, such as localized erythema and edema of the extremities followed by desquamation, has been observed in patients receiving docetaxel.

Other skin reactions such as macular erythema have been observed at sites of previous tissue injury in patients receiving docetaxel. Cutaneous reactions are dose-dependent and cumulative and rarely have been seen at doses less than 85 mg/m^2. A syndrome of erythrodysesthesia, characterized by a painful, tender, erythematous eruption, frequently followed by tingling and decreased sensation, has been reported with docetaxel therapy. In addition, there have been reports of scleroderma-like changes, usually preceded by peripheral lymphedema and affecting the lower extremities, associated with docetaxel therapy.

In cases of severe skin toxicity, the dosage of docetaxel should be reduced or therapy with the drug should be discontinued. (See Dermatologic Toxicity under Dosage: Dosage Modification for Toxicity and Contraindications for Continued Therapy, in Dosage and Administration.)

Treatment of docetaxel-induced cutaneous reactions, when necessary, generally has been symptomatic. Cutaneous reactions in some patients have been successfully treated with an ointment consisting of glycerin and chlorhexidine. Topical corticosteroids and cool compresses also have been used, especially in patients with erythrodysesthesia. A decreased incidence and severity of cutaneous reactions to docetaxel with recommended corticosteroid premedication has been reported by some clinicians, while others have found no benefit. A severe case of erythrodysesthesia that occurred despite pretreatment with corticosteroids and failed to respond to oral pyridoxine treatment reportedly was treated successfully with localized hypothermia during docetaxel infusion.

Nail changes occurred in 31% of patients receiving docetaxel for solid tumors and were severe in 2.5%. Severe nail disorders were characterized by hypopigmentation or hyperpigmentation and, occasionally, onycholysis and pain; onycholysis occurred in about 1% of patients receiving docetaxel for solid tumors. Nail disorders were reported in patients receiving docetaxel in combination therapy for advanced prostate cancer (30%), adjuvant treatment of breast cancer (18%), advanced non-small cell lung cancer (14%), and advanced gastric cancer (8%) and in patients receiving docetaxel alone for advanced non-small cell lung cancer (11%). Thinning and ridging of the nail plates as well as subungual erythema and subungual hemorrhage also have been reported in patients receiving docetaxel. Nail toxicity appears to be related to the cumulative dose of docetaxel.

Cutaneous lupus erythematosus and bullous eruptions, such as erythema multiforme, Stevens-Johnson syndrome, and toxic epidermal necrolysis, have occurred rarely in patients receiving docetaxel.

● *Musculoskeletal Effects*

Musculoskeletal effects, including arthralgia and/or myalgia, have been reported with docetaxel therapy but appear to be less common than with paclitaxel. Myalgia occurred in 19% of patients receiving docetaxel for solid tumors and was severe in 1.5%; arthralgia occurred in 9%. A similar rate of myalgia was reported in patients receiving docetaxel in combination therapy for advanced non-small cell lung cancer. Myalgia was reported in 27% and arthralgia in 19% of patients receiving docetaxel with doxorubicin and cyclophosphamide for the adjuvant treatment of breast cancer. Lower rates of adverse musculoskeletal effects were reported in patients receiving docetaxel in combination therapy for locally advanced head and neck cancer (myalgia in 10 or 7%), patients receiving docetaxel alone for advanced non-small cell lung cancer (myalgia in 6%, arthralgia in 3%), and patients receiving docetaxel 60 mg/m² for advanced breast cancer (myalgia in 3%). Musculoskeletal manifestations usually are mild and transient, occurring within a few days after docetaxel administration and lasting about 4 days, and have been reported to respond to mild analgesics (e.g., acetaminophen) when needed.

● *Hepatic Effects*

Hepatitis, sometimes fatal, has been reported rarely in patients receiving docetaxel. Fatal hepatitis occurred mainly in patients with pre-existing liver disorders. Abnormalities in liver function test results have occurred in patients receiving docetaxel. In clinical trials in the US and Europe in patients with normal liver function test results at baseline, serum total bilirubin values exceeding the upper limit of normal occurred in 8.9% of patients. Increases in serum AST (SGOT) or ALT (SGPT) values to greater than 1.5 times the upper limit of normal were observed in 18.9% of patients, and serum alkaline phosphatase concentrations exceeding 2.5 times normal were observed in 7.3% of patients. In clinical trials, increases in AST or ALT to greater than 1.5 times the upper limit of normal concomitant with increases in serum alkaline phosphatase to greater than 2.5 times the normal value were reported in 4.3% of patients with normal liver function test results at baseline.

● *Respiratory Effects*

Bronchospasm associated with severe hypersensitivity reactions has occurred in patients receiving docetaxel. (See Cautions: Sensitivity Reactions.) Pleural effusion requiring urgent drainage or dyspnea at rest may be manifestations of severe fluid retention in patients receiving docetaxel. (See Cautions: Cardiovascular Effects.)

Adverse pulmonary effects occurred in patients receiving docetaxel (41%), best supportive care (49%), or either vinorelbine or ifosfamide (45%) for advanced non-small cell lung cancer in randomized trials. Dyspnea was reported in 15% of patients receiving docetaxel and prednisone for advanced prostate cancer.

Other adverse pulmonary effects reported in patients receiving docetaxel include acute pulmonary edema, acute respiratory distress syndrome/pneumonitis, interstitial lung disease, and interstitial pneumonia. Pulmonary fibrosis has been reported rarely. Radiation pneumonitis has been reported rarely in patients receiving concomitant radiation therapy.

● *Local Effects*

Local reactions at the injection site occurred in about 4% of patients receiving docetaxel for solid tumors and generally were mild and consisted of hyperpigmentation, inflammation, erythema or dryness of the skin, phlebitis, extravasation, or venous swelling. Extravasation of docetaxel has led to localized pain, discoloration, and erythema, and desquamation has continued for up to 6 weeks in some cases. Specific treatment for docetaxel-induced extravasation reactions currently has not been fully determined. However, the manufacturer recommends using general conservative measures and avoiding the application of warm compresses (which may result in skin discoloration, blistering, and peeling) in the treatment of docetaxel extravasation. Reversible peripheral vein inflammation has been reported rarely with docetaxel administration.

● *Ocular Effects*

Cystoid macular edema has been reported in patients receiving docetaxel.

Lacrimation disorder occurred in 11% and conjunctivitis in 5% of patients receiving docetaxel in combination therapy as adjuvant treatment for breast cancer. Conjunctivitis was reported in 1% of patients receiving docetaxel in combination therapy for locally advanced head and neck cancer. Tearing was reported in patients receiving docetaxel in combination therapy for advanced prostate cancer (10%), advanced gastric cancer (8%), and locally advanced head and neck cancer (2%). Excessive tearing may be caused by lacrimal duct obstruction. Transient visual disturbances, such as flashes, flashing lights, and scotomata, have been reported rarely in patients receiving docetaxel; these visual disturbances typically occurred during the infusion in association with hypersensitivity reactions and were reversible upon discontinuance of the drug.

● *Otic Effects*

Adverse otic effects, including ototoxicity, hearing disorders, and/or hearing loss, have been reported in patients receiving docetaxel, including some cases associated with other ototoxic agents. Altered hearing was reported in patients receiving docetaxel with cisplatin and fluorouracil for advanced gastric cancer (6%) or locally advanced head and neck cancer (6% in TAX323 and 13% in TAX324).

● *Other Adverse Effects*

Amenorrhea was reported in patients receiving either docetaxel (62%) or fluorouracil (52%) (each in combination with doxorubicin and cyclophosphamide) for the adjuvant treatment of breast cancer. Weight loss (21 or 14%) and cancer pain (21 or 17%) were reported in patients receiving docetaxel with cisplatin and fluorouracil as induction chemotherapy for locally advanced head and neck cancer. Cough was reported in patients receiving docetaxel in combination therapy for the adjuvant treatment of breast cancer (14%) and for advanced prostate cancer (12%).

Other adverse effects reported in patients receiving docetaxel include diffuse pain, chest pain, radiation recall phenomenon, and hyponatremia. Renal insufficiency and renal failure also have been reported, generally in patients receiving docetaxel concomitantly with nephrotoxic drugs.

● *Precautions and Contraindications*

Docetaxel is a toxic drug with a low therapeutic index at the maximum recommended dose of 100 mg/m². Appropriate diagnostic and treatment facilities must be readily available in case the patient develops any severe adverse effects, such as severe hypersensitivity reactions to docetaxel (e.g., hypotension requiring treatment, bronchospasm/dyspnea requiring bronchodilators, generalized rash/erythema, anaphylaxis). Patients who respond to docetaxel may not experience an improvement and/or may experience worsening in performance status while receiving the drug. The relationship between changes in performance status, response to therapy, and treatment-related adverse effects has not been established.

Docetaxel should *not* be given to patients with baseline neutrophil counts less than 1500/mm³. Bone marrow suppression with docetaxel is dose-dependent and is the dose-limiting toxicity. To monitor for the occurrence of docetaxel-induced bone marrow suppression, mainly neutropenia, which may be severe and result in infection, it is recommended that frequent peripheral blood cell counts be performed in all patients receiving the drug. Patients receiving docetaxel with cisplatin and fluorouracil should be monitored closely for the occurrence of febrile neutropenia and neutropenic infection.

Because of the alcohol content of parenteral formulations of docetaxel, patients should be advised that alcohol-induced CNS effects (e.g., intoxication) can occur during or following infusions of the drug. Patients should be advised to avoid driving, operating machinery, or performing other dangerous activities for 1–2 hours following administration of the drug. Patients also should be instructed to inform a clinician of symptoms of alcohol intoxication (e.g., confusion, stumbling, drowsiness) during or after docetaxel administration. Clinicians should consider the alcohol content of docetaxel formulations available from various manufacturers, especially when administering the drug to patients with hepatic impairment, patients in whom alcohol intake should be avoided or minimized, patients who experienced alcohol intoxication with a previous infusion of docetaxel, and those receiving concomitant therapy with drugs with CNS depressant effects (see Drug Interactions: CNS Depressants). Patients should be monitored for symptoms of alcohol intoxication during and following infusions of the drug. If such symptoms occur, reduction of the infusion rate may resolve symptoms. For patients who experience alcohol intoxication, use of a formulation of docetaxel containing the least amount of alcohol should be considered. The manufacturer's labeling should be consulted for the alcohol content of the specific formulation, as formulations of docetaxel available from various manufacturers may contain different amounts of alcohol.

Patients experiencing impaired vision during docetaxel therapy should promptly receive a comprehensive ophthalmologic examination. If cystoid macular edema is diagnosed, docetaxel therapy should be discontinued and appropriate treatment initiated. Alternative therapy with a nontaxane antineoplastic agent should be considered.

Fluid retention, generally manifested by peripheral edema and weight gain, occurs frequently in patients receiving docetaxel. Patients with preexisting effusions should be monitored closely beginning with the first dose of docetaxel to detect possible exacerbation of effusions.

Among patients receiving docetaxel with doxorubicin and cyclophosphamide as adjuvant therapy for breast cancer, continued hematologic monitoring is required because of the risk of delayed myelodysplasia or treatment-related acute myeloid leukemia. (See Cautions: Mutagenicity and Carcinogenicity.)

Among patients receiving docetaxel in combination with cisplatin and fluorouracil for advanced gastric cancer in the randomized trial, neurologic examination was performed before entry into the study, periodically during the study (at least after every 2 cycles of therapy), and at the completion of treatment. In patients experiencing peripheral neuropathy or other neurologic manifestations, examinations should be performed more frequently and dosage reduction and/or discontinuance of the drug may be required. (See Neurologic Toxicity under Dosage: Dosage Modification for Toxicity and Contraindications for Continued Therapy, in Dosage and Administration.)

Docetaxel injection concentrate contains polysorbate 80 and should *not* be used in patients with known severe hypersensitivity to polysorbate 80 or to the drug. To reduce the severity of hypersensitivity reactions and to reduce the incidence and severity of fluid retention, the manufacturers recommend that all patients be pretreated with oral corticosteroids. (See Premedication Regimen under Dosage and Administration: Dosage.) Patients should be observed closely for hypersensitivity reactions, particularly during the first and second infusions of docetaxel. Docetaxel therapy should not be undertaken in any patient who experienced a severe hypersensitivity reaction during a previous course of therapy with the drug.

Medication errors have occurred that involved confusion between docetaxel (Taxotere®) and paclitaxel (Taxol®). To avoid medication errors, the prescriber should print both the brand and generic names for docetaxel on the prescription order form. If a handwritten prescription is difficult to read, the pharmacist should confirm the drug name with the prescriber. If the prescription is confirmed verbally, the drug names should be spelled out. Pharmacy labels and preprinted order forms should list both the generic and brand names using upper-case and lower-case fonts (i.e., DOCEtaxel and TaxoTERE). Two pharmacists should provide independent confirmation that the correct drug is being ordered before chemotherapy is dispensed, and two nurses should confirm that the correct drug has been dispensed for the correct patient before administering the medication.

Docetaxel generally should not be given to patients with serum total bilirubin concentrations exceeding the upper limit of normal, or to patients with serum AST (SGOT) and/or ALT (SGPT) concentrations exceeding 1.5 times the upper limit of normal concomitant with serum alkaline phosphatase concentrations exceeding 2.5 times the upper limit of normal. Patients with elevations of serum bilirubin or abnormalities of serum transaminases concurrent with serum alkaline phosphatase are at increased risk for the development of severe or life-threatening complications, including severe neutropenia, febrile neutropenia, infections, severe thrombocytopenia, severe stomatitis, severe skin toxicity, and toxic death. Determinations of serum bilirubin, AST and/or ALT, and alkaline phosphatase concentrations should be obtained prior to each cycle of docetaxel therapy and reviewed by the clinician.

The incidence of mortality was higher in patients with non-small cell lung cancer previously treated with platinum-based chemotherapy who received docetaxel as a single agent at a dose of 100 mg/m². Because of excessive toxicity with higher doses, such patients should receive the recommended dosage of (i.e., docetaxel 75 mg/m² once every 3 weeks). (See Non-small Cell Lung Cancer under Dosage and Administration: Dosage.)

The patient should be instructed to notify a clinician immediately about difficulty breathing or swallowing, facial swelling, or rash during or shortly after the infusion of docetaxel because this may indicate an allergic reaction to the drug. The patient should be informed of the importance of routine monitoring of blood cell counts and should be advised to notify a clinician immediately if he or she develops a fever, because this may be an early sign of infection. The patient should be instructed to monitor for signs of fluid retention (e.g., edema in the lower extremities, weight gain, dyspnea) and should be advised of the importance of taking the corticosteroid premedication as directed to lessen fluid retention and to reduce the severity of hypersensitivity reactions. Patients also should be instructed to inform a clinician of excessive or persistent fatigue, muscle pain, rash, or sensations (numbness, tingling, or burning) in the hands and/or feet after treatment with docetaxel.

● **Pediatric Precautions**

Clinicians should consider the alcohol content of docetaxel formulations available from various manufacturers when administering the drug to pediatric patients. (See Cautions: Nervous System Effects and Cautions: Precautions and Contraindications.)

Efficacy of docetaxel administered as monotherapy or in combination chemotherapy regimens has not been established in pediatric patients. In clinical trials to date, the safety profile of docetaxel in pediatric patients has been similar to that in adults. Clearance of the drug (adjusted for body surface area) also has been similar in pediatric patients and adults.

In a dose-finding study in 61 patients 1–22 years of age (median age: 12.5 years) with various refractory solid tumors, the primary dose-limiting toxicity of docetaxel was neutropenia. The dosage identified in this study (125 mg/m² IV every 21 days) subsequently was evaluated in a phase 2 noncomparative trial in 178 patients 1–26 years of age (median age: 12 years) with various recurrent or refractory solid tumors. This phase 2 trial failed to establish efficacy of docetaxel monotherapy in pediatric patients; tumor responses in this trial included one complete response in a patient with undifferentiated sarcoma and 4 partial responses, one each in patients with Ewing's sarcoma, neuroblastoma, osteosarcoma, and squamous cell carcinoma.

In a study in 75 patients 9–21 years of age (median age: 16 years) with nasopharyngeal carcinoma, 1 of 50 patients receiving an induction regimen of docetaxel, cisplatin, and fluorouracil prior to chemoradiation consolidation achieved a complete response following the induction regimen compared with none out of 25 patients receiving an induction regimen of cisplatin and fluorouracil.

● **Geriatric Precautions**

Certain toxicities associated with docetaxel therapy may occur more frequently and with greater severity in geriatric patients. Because of the greater frequency of decreased hepatic, renal, and/or cardiac function and of concomitant disease and drug therapy observed in the elderly, caution is advised in dose selection for geriatric patients.

Among patients receiving docetaxel and cisplatin as first-line treatment of advanced non-small cell lung cancer in the randomized trial, 36% were 65 years of age or older. Geriatric patients experienced similar survival but greater toxicity than younger patients. Among patients receiving docetaxel and cisplatin, median survival was 12 months in geriatric patients compared with about 10 months in younger patients. Adverse effects that occurred more frequently in geriatric patients than in younger patients receiving docetaxel and cisplatin include diarrhea (55 versus 43%), infections (42 versus 31%), peripheral edema (39 versus 31%), and stomatitis (28 versus 21%). Among geriatric patients, diarrhea (55 versus 24%), peripheral edema (39 versus 20%), and stomatitis (28 versus 20%) occurred more frequently in those receiving docetaxel and cisplatin than in those receiving vinorelbine and cisplatin. Among patients receiving docetaxel and carboplatin as first-line treatment of advanced non-small cell lung cancer in the same randomized trial, 28% were 65 years of age or older. Among geriatric patients, those receiving docetaxel and carboplatin had a higher frequency of infection than those receiving docetaxel and cisplatin and a higher frequency of diarrhea, infection, and peripheral edema than those receiving vinorelbine and cisplatin.

Among patients receiving docetaxel and prednisone for the treatment of androgen-independent (hormone-refractory) advanced prostate cancer in the randomized trial, 63% were 65 years of age or older and 20% were older than 75 years of age. Treatment-emergent adverse effects that occurred more frequently in geriatric patients than in younger patients receiving docetaxel and prednisone included anemia (71 versus 59%), infection (37 versus 24%), nail changes (34 versus 23%), anorexia (21 versus 10%), and weight loss (15 versus 5%).

Among patients receiving docetaxel with cisplatin and fluorouracil for advanced gastric cancer in the randomized trial, 24% were 65 years of age or older. Although this trial did not include sufficient numbers of elderly patients to determine whether geriatric patients respond differently than younger patients, the incidence of serious adverse effects was higher. The incidence rates of lethargy, stomatitis, diarrhea, dizziness, edema, and febrile neutropenia/neutropenic infection were at least 10% higher in geriatric patients than in younger patients, and close monitoring is advised for elderly patients.

Among patients receiving docetaxel with cisplatin and fluorouracil as induction therapy for advanced head and neck cancer in randomized trials, the number of patients 65 years of age or older (10% in TAX323 and 13% in TAX324) was not sufficient to determine whether geriatric patients respond differently than younger patients. Other clinical experience has not revealed age-related differences in response for patients receiving this regimen.

Among patients receiving docetaxel with doxorubicin and cyclophosphamide as adjuvant therapy for breast cancer in the randomized trial, the number of patients 65 years of age or older (6%) was not sufficient to determine age-related differences in response or tolerance.

● **Mutagenicity and Carcinogenicity**

Docetaxel has been shown to be clastogenic in the in vitro chromosome aberration test in CHO-K1 cells and in the in vivo micronucleus test in mice; however, the drug was not mutagenic in the Ames test or the CHO/HGPRT gene mutation assay.

Studies to determine the carcinogenic potential of docetaxel have not been performed to date.

Acute myeloid leukemia and myelodysplastic syndrome have been reported in patients receiving docetaxel in combination therapy with other antineoplastic agents with or without radiation therapy. Acute myeloid leukemia (AML) or myelodysplasia related to treatment has occurred in patients receiving anthracycline agents and/or cyclophosphamide, including those receiving these drugs as adjuvant therapy for breast cancer. In the randomized trial, AML occurred in 3 of 744 patients receiving docetaxel, doxorubicin, and cyclophosphamide and in 1 of 736 patients receiving fluorouracil, doxorubicin, and cyclophosphamide as adjuvant therapy for breast cancer.

● **Pregnancy, Fertility, and Lactation**

Pregnancy

Docetaxel may cause fetal harm when administered to pregnant women, but potential benefits may be acceptable in certain conditions despite possible risks to the fetus. Reproduction studies in rats and rabbits given docetaxel doses greater than or equal to 0.3 and 0.03 mg/kg (about 1/50 and 1/300 the maximum daily recommended human dose on a mg/m^2 basis), respectively, during organogenesis revealed evidence of maternal toxicity, embryotoxicity, and fetotoxicity; fetotoxicity was characterized by intrauterine mortality, increased resorption, reduced fetal weight, and fetal ossification delay. There are no adequate and well-controlled studies to date using docetaxel in pregnant women. Docetaxel should be used during pregnancy only in life-threatening situations or in diseases for which safer drugs cannot be used or are ineffective. Women of childbearing potential should be advised to avoid becoming pregnant during therapy with docetaxel. When docetaxel is used during pregnancy or if the patient becomes pregnant while receiving the drug, the patient should be apprised of the potential hazard to the fetus.

Fertility

When administered in multiple IV doses of up to 0.3 mg/kg (about 1/50 of the recommended human dose on a mg/m^2 basis), docetaxel produced no impairment of fertility in rats, but decreased testicular weights were reported. These findings correlate with those of a 10-cycle toxicity study (dosing once every 21 days for 6 months) in rats and dogs in which testicular atrophy or degeneration was observed at IV doses of 5 mg/kg in rats and 0.375 mg/kg in dogs (about 1/3 and 1/15 the recommended human dose on a mg/m^2 basis, respectively). An increased frequency of dosing in rats produced similar effects at lower dose levels.

Lactation

It is not known whether docetaxel is distributed into milk. Because of the potential for serious adverse reactions to docetaxel in nursing infants, a decision should be made whether to discontinue nursing or the drug, taking into account the importance of the drug to the woman.

DRUG INTERACTIONS

Formal drug interaction studies of docetaxel have not been conducted.

● **Drugs Affecting or Metabolized by Hepatic Microsomal Enzymes**

Results of in vitro studies show that the metabolism of docetaxel may be altered by the concomitant administration of drugs that induce, inhibit, or are metabolized by cytochrome P-450 isoenzyme 3A4 (CYP3A4). In a limited number of patients, administration of ketoconazole (200 mg orally once daily for 3 days) concomitantly with docetaxel (10 mg/m^2 IV) resulted in a 2.2-fold increase in exposure and a 49% reduction in clearance of docetaxel. Concomitant use of potent CYP3A4 inhibitors (e.g., atazanavir, clarithromycin, indinavir, itraconazole, ketoconazole, nefazodone, nelfinavir, ritonavir, saquinavir, telithromycin, voriconazole) with docetaxel should be avoided. If such concomitant use cannot be avoided, a reduction in docetaxel dosage with careful monitoring for toxicity should be considered. Based on extrapolation of limited pharmacokinetic data for ketoconazole, the manufacturers state that a 50% reduction in docetaxel dosage may be considered in patients requiring concomitant therapy with a potent CYP3A4 inhibitor; however, there are no clinical data with use of this adjusted docetaxel dosage in patients receiving potent CYP3A4 inhibitors.

● **CNS Depressants**

Because of the alcohol content of parenteral formulations of docetaxel, concomitant use of drugs with CNS depressant effects (e.g., opiate analgesics, sedatives) may worsen the effects of alcohol. (See Cautions: Nervous System Effects.)

ACUTE TOXICITY

Limited information is available on the acute toxicity of docetaxel. In male and female rats, lethality occurred at a dose of 20 mg/kg (comparable to a human dose of 100 mg/m^2 on a mg/m^2 basis) and was associated with abnormal mitosis and necrosis of multiple organs. In mice, lethality was observed following single IV doses of 154 mg/kg (about 4.5 times a human dose of 100 mg/m^2 on a mg/m^2 basis) or greater. In mice, at a dose of 48 mg/kg (about 1.5 times a human dose of 100 mg/m^2 on a mg/m^2 basis), neurotoxicity associated with paralysis, nonextension of hind limbs, and myelin degeneration was observed.

Overdosage of docetaxel produces symptoms that are mainly extensions of common adverse reactions, including bone marrow suppression, peripheral neurotoxicity, and mucositis. In 2 reports of overdosage, one in a patient receiving docetaxel 150 mg/m^2 and another in a patient receiving docetaxel 200 mg/m^2 (both as 1-hour IV infusions), both patients experienced severe neutropenia, mild asthenia, cutaneous reactions, and mild paresthesias. These patients recovered without incident.

There is no known antidote for docetaxel overdosage. In case of overdosage, the patient should be moved to a specialized unit that allows close monitoring of vital functions. As soon as possible after the discovery of docetaxel overdosage, therapeutic G-CSF should be administered. Other supportive and symptomatic treatment should be initiated as clinically indicated.

PHARMACOLOGY

Like paclitaxel, docetaxel is an antimicrotubule antineoplastic agent. Unlike some other common antimicrotubule agents (e.g., vinca alkaloids, colchicine, podophyllotoxin), however, docetaxel and paclitaxel *promote* rather than inhibit microtubule assembly while simultaneously preventing microtubule disassembly. Microtubules are organelles that exist in a state of dynamic equilibrium with their components, tubulin dimers. They are an essential part of the mitotic spindle and also are involved in maintenance of cell shape and motility, and transport between organelles within the cell.

Docetaxel enhances the polymerization of tubulin, the protein subunit of the spindle microtubules, even in the absence of factors that are normally required for microtubule assembly (e.g., guanosine triphosphate [GTP]); as a result, the drug induces the formation of stable, nonfunctional microtubules. While the precise mechanism of action of the drug is not understood fully, docetaxel disrupts the dynamic equilibrium within the microtubule system and arrests the cell cycle in the late G$_2$ and M phases, inhibiting cell replication.

Docetaxel results in the formation of tubulin polymers that differ structurally from those generated by paclitaxel and, unlike paclitaxel, does not alter the number of protofilaments in the microtubules. As an inhibitor of microtubule depolymerization, docetaxel is approximately twice as potent as paclitaxel; the increased potency of docetaxel may be related to its higher affinity for microtubules, its higher achievable intracellular concentration, and its slower cellular efflux. In addition, higher radiosensitivity effects have been observed with docetaxel as compared with paclitaxel (at equimolar concentrations). Preclinical evidence suggests that cross-resistance between docetaxel and paclitaxel is incomplete; a lack of cross-resistance between docetaxel and fluorouracil or cisplatin also has been noted.

Docetaxel is a schedule-independent antineoplastic agent. Preclinical studies using different dosage schedules revealed no alteration in antitumor activity with splitting of the total dose of docetaxel.

PHARMACOKINETICS

● Absorption

Docetaxel exhibits linear, dose-dependent pharmacokinetics. The area under the concentration-time curve (AUC) was dose-proportional following docetaxel doses of 70–115 mg/m² IV administered over 1–2 hours.

● Distribution

The pharmacokinetic disposition of docetaxel is consistent with a 3-compartment model with initial rapid decline indicating distribution to peripheral compartments and a late (terminal) phase with a half-life of about 11 hours suggesting relatively slow efflux of docetaxel from the peripheral compartment. Following docetaxel doses of 70–115 mg/m² IV administered over 1–2 hours, the steady-state volume of distribution averaged 113 L.

About 94% of docetaxel is bound to plasma proteins (97% in patients with cancer). It is not known whether docetaxel is distributed into milk.

● Elimination

Following docetaxel doses of 70–115 mg/m² IV administered over 1–2 hours, total body clearance averaged 21 L/hour per m².

Docetaxel is metabolized in the liver and undergoes oxidative metabolism of the *tert*-butyl ester group. (See Drug interactions: Drugs Affecting or Metabolized by Hepatic Microsomal Enzymes.) Docetaxel is excreted mainly in the feces (75% of the dose) with minimal excretion (about 6% of the dose) in the urine. Following the administration of a radioactive dose, about 80% of the dose is excreted in the feces during the first 48 hours as a major metabolite and 3 minor metabolites with small amounts (less than 8% of the dose) excreted as unchanged drug.

In patients with mild to moderate hepatic impairment (serum AST and/or ALT concentration exceeding 1.5 times the upper limit of normal and serum alkaline phosphatase concentration exceeding 2.5 times the upper limit of normal), total body clearance was lowered by an average of 27% and resulted in a 38% increase in systemic exposure (AUC) for docetaxel. Docetaxel has not been studied in patients with severe hepatic impairment.

The pharmacokinetics of docetaxel do not appear to be influenced by age or gender.

CHEMISTRY AND STABILITY

● Chemistry

Docetaxel, a semisynthetic taxoid produced from the needles of the European yew (*Taxus baccata*) tree, is an antineoplastic agent. The drug is derived from a noncytotoxic precursor (10-deacetyl baccatin III) and is structurally and pharmacologically similar to paclitaxel.

Docetaxel is a complex diterpene with a taxane ring system linked at positions 4 and 5 to a four-membered oxetane ring and at position 13 to an ester side chain. The taxane nucleus is important for binding of docetaxel to microtubules, and this binding is stabilized by the ester side chain at position 13 of the taxane ring, which is required for the drug's cytotoxic activity. Docetaxel differs structurally from paclitaxel by the presence of a hydroxyl group rather than an acetyl group on position 10 of the baccatin III ring and by a trimethylmethoxy moiety instead of a benzamide phenyl group on the 3′ position of the side chain at position 13 of the taxane ring.

Docetaxel occurs as a white to almost-white powder. Docetaxel is highly lipophilic and practically insoluble in water; however, docetaxel is more water soluble than paclitaxel, permitting its formulation in polysorbate (Tween®) 80 rather than Cremophor® EL (polyoxyl 35 castor oil).

Commercially available docetaxel injection concentrate (Taxotere®) is a sterile solution of the drug in a 50/50 v/v mixture of polysorbate 80 and dehydrated alcohol. The injection concentrate is a pale yellow to brownish-yellow solution. The injection concentrate must be diluted with an appropriate infusion solution prior to administration (one dilution step).

Commercially available docetaxel injection concentrate (Hospira) is a sterile solution of the drug in a vehicle containing polysorbate 80, citric acid, polyethylene glycol 300, and dehydrated alcohol 23% v/v. The injection concentrate is a clear, colorless to pale yellow solution. The injection concentrate must be diluted with an appropriate infusion solution prior to administration (one dilution step).

Commercially available docetaxel injection concentrate requiring one dilution step (one-vial formulation, Accord) is a sterile solution of the drug in a vehicle containing polysorbate 80, citric acid, and dehydrated alcohol. The injection concentrate is a pale yellow to brownish-yellow solution. The injection concentrate must be diluted with an appropriate infusion solution prior to administration (one dilution step).

Commercially available docetaxel injection concentrate requiring 2 dilution steps (2-vial formulation, Accord) is a sterile solution of the drug in polysorbate 80 and dehydrated alcohol with an accompanying diluent of 13% w/v polyethylene glycol 400 in water for injection; citric acid may be added to adjust the pH. The injection concentrate is a clear yellow to brownish-yellow viscous solution. The injection concentrate must be diluted with the diluent supplied by the manufacturer, followed by dilution with an appropriate infusion solution prior to administration (2 dilution steps).

Docetaxel also is commercially available as a lyophilized powder (Docefrez®) with an accompanying diluent of ethanol 35.4% w/w and polysorbate 80. The lyophilized powder must be reconstituted with the diluent supplied by the manufacturer, followed by dilution with an appropriate infusion solution.

● Stability

Commercially available docetaxel injection concentrate (Taxotere®) should be stored in unopened vials at 2–25°C and retained in the original package for protection from light. Freezing does not adversely affect docetaxel for injection concentrate. The final diluted docetaxel solution for infusion (prepared by mixing the required amount of the injection concentrate with either 0.9% sodium chloride injection or 5% dextrose injection) is stable for up to 6 hours at 2–25°C. The infusion solution should be used within 6 hours, so it may be stored for up to 5 hours at 2–25°C before initiating the 1-hour IV infusion. When prepared as directed and stored in non-PVC bags at 2–8°C, the final diluted docetaxel infusion solution is stable for up to 48 hours.

Commercially available docetaxel injection concentrate (Hospira) should be stored in unopened vials at 20–25°C and retained in the original package for protection from light. Between uses, multiple-dose vials of the injection concentrate are stable for up to 28 days when stored at 2–8°C and protected from light. Freezing does not adversely affect docetaxel for injection concentrate. The final diluted docetaxel solution for infusion (prepared by mixing the required amount of the injection concentrate with either 0.9% sodium chloride injection or 5% dextrose injection) is stable for up to 4 hours at 2–25°C. The infusion solution should be used within 4 hours, so it may be stored for up to 3 hours at 2–25°C before initiating the 1-hour IV infusion.

Commercially available docetaxel injection concentrate requiring one dilution step (one-vial formulation, Accord) should be stored in unopened vials at 15–25°C and protected from light. Between uses, multiple-dose vials of the injection concentrate are stable for up to 28 days when stored at room temperature and protected from light. Freezing does not adversely affect this formulation. The final diluted docetaxel solution for infusion (prepared by mixing the required amount of the injection concentrate with either 0.9% sodium chloride injection or 5% dextrose injection) is stable for up to 4 hours at 2–25°C. The infusion solution should be used within 4 hours, so it may be stored for up to 3 hours at 2–25°C before initiating the 1-hour IV infusion.

Commercially available docetaxel injection concentrate requiring 2 dilution steps (2-vial formulation, Accord) should be stored in unopened vials at 25°C (but may be exposed to temperatures ranging from 15–30°C) and protected from light. The initial diluted docetaxel solution (prepared by mixing the contents of the diluent vial with the docetaxel injection concentrate) may be used immediately to prepare the final diluted docetaxel solution for infusion or it may be stored either in the refrigerator or at room temperature for up to 8 hours. The final diluted docetaxel solution for infusion (prepared by mixing the required amount of the initial diluted docetaxel solution with either 0.9% sodium chloride injection or

5% dextrose injection) is stable for up to 4 hours at 2–25°C. The final diluted docetaxel solution for infusion should be used within 4 hours, so it may be stored for up to 3 hours at 2–25°C before initiating the 1-hour IV infusion.

Commercially available docetaxel lyophilized powder (Docefrez®) should be stored at 2–8°C and retained in the original package for protection from bright light. The reconstituted docetaxel solution may be used immediately to prepare the final diluted docetaxel solution for infusion or it may be stored either in the refrigerator or at room temperature for up to 8 hours. The final diluted docetaxel solution for infusion (prepared by mixing the required amount of the reconstituted docetaxel solution with either 0.9% sodium chloride injection or 5% dextrose injection) is stable for up to 6 hours at 2–25°C. The final diluted docetaxel solution for infusion should be used within 6 hours, so it may be stored for up to 5 hours at 2–25°C before initiating the 1-hour IV infusion. When prepared as directed and stored in non-PVC bags at 2–8°C, the final diluted docetaxel infusion solution is stable for up to 48 hours.

For further information on the handling of antineoplastic agents, see the ASHP Guidelines on Handling Hazardous Drugs at http://www.ahfsdruginformation.com.

PREPARATIONS

Excipients in commercially available drug preparations may have clinically important effects in some individuals; consult specific product labeling for details.

DOCEtaxel

Parenteral		
For injection, for IV infusion	20 mg	**Docefrez®** (with ethanol 35.4% w/w in polysorbate 80 diluent), Sun
	80 mg	**Docefrez®** (with ethanol 35.4% w/w in polysorbate 80 diluent), Sun
Injection concentrate, for IV infusion	10 mg (of anhydrous docetaxel) per mL (20, 80, or 160 mg)	**Docetaxel Injection**
	20 mg (of anhydrous docetaxel) per mL (20, 80, or 160 mg)*	**Taxotere®**, Sanofi-Aventis
	40 mg (of anhydrous docetaxel) per mL (20 or 80 mg)	**Docetaxel Injection** (with 13% w/v polyethylene glycol 400 in water for injection diluent)

* available from one or more manufacturer, distributor, and/or repackager by generic (nonproprietary) name

† Use is not currently included in the labeling approved by the US Food and Drug Administration.

Selected Revisions June 24, 2015, © Copyright, November 1, 1996, American Society of Health-System Pharmacists, Inc.

DOXOrubicin Hydrochloride

10:00 · ANTINEOPLASTIC AGENTS

■ Doxorubicin is an anthracycline glycoside antineoplastic antibiotic produced by *Streptomyces peucetius* var. *caesius*.

USES

Since doxorubicin does not cross the blood-brain barrier or achieve a measurable concentration in CSF, there is a possibility of metastases to the brain and meninges from potentially metastatic tumors.

● Breast Cancer

Doxorubicin hydrochloride is used in the treatment of breast cancer. Use of the drug in combination with other chemotherapeutic agents and/or surgery in the early stage of breast cancer has produced clinically important responses in both quantity and duration. Combination chemotherapy used as an adjunct to surgery has been shown to increase both disease-free (i.e., decreased recurrence) and overall survival in premenopausal and postmenopausal women with node-negative or node-positive early (TNM stage I or II) breast cancer. Although adjuvant combination chemotherapy that includes cyclophosphamide, methotrexate, and fluorouracil has been used most extensively and is considered a regimen of choice for early breast cancer, doxorubicin-containing regimens (e.g., combined cyclophosphamide and doxorubicin with or without fluorouracil; combined cyclophosphamide and doxorubicin with or without tamoxifen) appear to be comparably effective and also are considered regimens of choice, but differences in toxicity profiles may influence the choice of regimen. There is some evidence that the addition of doxorubicin to a regimen of cyclophosphamide, methotrexate, and fluorouracil can improve outcome further in patients with early breast cancer and more than 3 positive axillary lymph nodes, and that sequential (i.e., administering several courses of doxorubicin first) regimens are more effective than alternating regimens in such patients; in patients with fewer positive nodes, no additional benefit from doxorubicin has been demonstrated. The dose intensity of adjuvant combination chemotherapy also appears to be an important factor influencing clinical outcome in patients with early node-positive breast cancer, with response increasing with increasing dose intensity; therefore, arbitrary reductions in dose intensity should be avoided. In stage III (locally advanced) breast cancer, combination chemotherapy (with or without hormonal therapy) is used sequentially following surgery and radiation therapy for operable disease and following biopsy and radiation therapy for inoperable disease; commonly employed effective regimens include cyclophosphamide, methotrexate, and fluorouracil; cyclophosphamide, doxorubicin, and fluorouracil; and cyclophosphamide and doxorubicin.

Patients refractory to cyclophosphamide, vincristine sulfate, dactinomycin, or daunorubicin have responded to doxorubicin hydrochloride; however, apparent cross-resistance between doxorubicin and daunorubicin has been noted in some patients with neuroblastoma. Cross-resistance between doxorubicin and vincristine sulfate or dactinomycin in animals or cell cultures has been reported, but clinical evidence of these cross-resistances in humans is lacking.

● AIDS-related Kaposi's Sarcoma

Overview

Doxorubicin hydrochloride as conventional (nonencapsulated) injections has been used alone or in combination chemotherapy for the palliative treatment of AIDS-related Kaposi's sarcoma†, and combination chemotherapy that includes the drug (e.g., doxorubicin, bleomycin, and vincristine) has been a preferred regimen; but many clinicians currently consider a liposomal anthracycline (doxorubicin or daunorubicin) the first-line therapy of choice for advanced AIDS-related Kaposi's sarcoma (see also Uses: AIDS-related Kaposi's Sarcoma in Daunorubicin 10:00).

Although single-agent therapy with conventional (i.e., nonencapsulated) cytotoxic agents generally has been used in the early stage of disease, Kaposi's sarcoma in patients with human immunodeficiency virus (HIV) infection often is rapidly progressive. AIDS-related Kaposi's sarcoma often progresses to multifocal, widespread lesions that may involve the skin, oral mucosa, and lymph nodes as well as visceral organs such as the GI tract, lung, liver, and spleen; such lesions often are numerous and may be cosmetically unattractive or disfiguring and accompanied by lymphedema. Appropriate evaluation of the effects of drug therapies on survival in patients with Kaposi's sarcoma must include assessment of the effects of such therapies on the development of infection as well as on tumor regression. Although treatment may result in disappearance or reduction in the size of Kaposi's sarcoma skin lesions and thereby alleviate the discomfort associated with chronic edema and ulcerations that often accompany multiple skin lesions on the lower extremities and in symptomatic control of mucosal and visceral lesions, there currently are no data demonstrating unequivocal evidence of improved survival with any therapy. Small localized Kaposi's sarcoma lesions may be treated with electrodesiccation and curettage cryotherapy or by surgical excision; the lesions also generally are responsive to local radiation, and excellent palliation often can be achieved. Localized palatal lesions have been treated effectively with intralesional injections of vinblastine or bleomycin.

Alitretinoin gel (Panretin®, Ligand Pharmaceuticals), a topical retinoid, is used for the treatment of localized cutaneous lesions in patients with AIDS-related Kaposi's sarcoma; responses of cutaneous lesions to topical therapy with alitretinoin have been reported in patients who have received prior systemic and/or topical therapy for Kaposi's sarcoma as well as in those with previously untreated disease.

Liposomal Agents

Pegylated liposomal doxorubicin is labeled for use in the palliative treatment of AIDS-related Kaposi's sarcoma in adults intolerant to combination chemotherapy or whose disease has progressed while receiving such therapy. Liposomal daunorubicin citrate is labeled for use as first-line therapy for advanced AIDS-related Kaposi's sarcoma. (See Daunorubicin 10:00.) The results of several randomized, multicenter trials indicate that patients receiving a liposomal anthracycline for the treatment of advanced AIDS-related Kaposi's sarcoma experience similar or higher response rates with a more favorable toxic effects profile than those receiving combination therapy with conventional chemotherapeutic agents.

Administration of doxorubicin hydrochloride encapsulated in PEG-stabilized liposomes (see Chemistry and Stability: Chemistry) allows the drug-containing liposomes to remain circulating in plasma for prolonged periods and reduces extravascular circulation of the drug while substantially increasing concentrations of the drug in the lesions of Kaposi's sarcoma compared with administration of equivalent doses of conventional (nonencapsulated) doxorubicin hydrochloride injections (see Pharmacokinetics: Distribution).

In an open-label, single-arm, multicenter study in patients with moderate to severe AIDS-related Kaposi's sarcoma whose disease had progressed on prior combination chemotherapy (consisting of at least 2 cycles of a regimen containing bleomycin, a vinca alkaloid [vincristine or vinblastine], and/or doxorubicin) or who were intolerant of such therapy, response rates were analyzed according to the investigator assessment of changes in lesions over the entire body or according to changes in indicator lesions; in this study, liposomal doxorubicin was administered IV in doses of 20-mg/m^2 once every 3 weeks, generally until disease progression or intolerance to doxorubicin therapy occurred. According to investigator assessment of changes, partial response, stable disease, or progressive disease was observed in 27, 29, or 44% of patients, respectively, while duration of partial response or time to partial response was 73 (range: 42–210) days or 43 (range: 15–133) days, respectively. According to indicator lesion assessment, partial response, stable disease, or progressive disease was observed in 48, 26, or 26%, respectively, while duration of partial response or time to partial response was 71 (range: 22–210) days or 22 (range: 15–109) days, respectively.

In a large, randomized trial, patients with AIDS-related Kaposi's sarcoma receiving liposomal doxorubicin (20 mg/m^2 by IV infusion over 30 minutes) had a higher objective response rate (58.7 versus 23.3%) than those receiving a combination regimen of bleomycin (15 mg/m^2 by IV infusion over 30 minutes) and vincristine (1.4 mg/m^2 or a maximum of 2 mg by IV bolus); each regimen was administered every 3 weeks for a maximum of 6 cycles. Treatment with liposomal doxorubicin was associated with greater improvement in signs and symptoms of pulmonary Kaposi's sarcoma (e.g., dyspnea, cough, chest pain, effusions) and GI Kaposi's sarcoma (e.g., GI bleeding, early satiety, dysphagia). Early termination from the study, withdrawal because of adverse effects, and withdrawal because of progressive disease occurred less frequently in patients receiving liposomal doxorubicin than in those receiving combination chemotherapy with bleomycin and vincristine. The incidence of paresthesia, peripheral neuropathy, and constipation was higher in patients receiving bleomycin and vincristine, whereas leukopenia and opportunistic infections (particularly oral candidiasis) occurred more frequently in those receiving liposomal doxorubicin. In another large, randomized trial involving 258 patients with advanced AIDS-related Kaposi's sarcoma, a higher rate of objective response (45.9 versus 24.8%) and less toxicity were reported in those receiving liposomal doxorubicin (20 mg/m^2 IV over 30 minutes) versus the ABV regimen, consisting of conventional doxorubicin (20 mg/m^2), bleomycin (10 mg/m^2), and vincristine (1 mg); each regimen was administered every 14 days for a maximum of 6 cycles. Treatment was discontinued because of adverse effects more frequently among those receiving the ABV regimen (37%) than among those receiving liposomal doxorubicin (11%). A higher incidence of nausea and vomiting, alopecia, and peripheral neuropathy was reported in patients receiving the ABV regimen, whereas stomatitis and rash were reported more frequently in patients receiving liposomal doxorubicin.

Preliminary evidence suggests that the mean survival period in patients with pulmonary AIDS-related Kaposi's sarcoma receiving liposomal doxorubicin may be increased compared with those receiving conventional chemotherapy (bleomycin and/or vincristine). Similar response rates, time to treatment failure, and overall survival, with less toxicity, were observed in patients receiving liposomal daunorubicin versus combination chemotherapy with bleomycin, conventional doxorubicin, and vincristine for advanced AIDS-related Kaposi's sarcoma. The comparative efficacy of liposomal doxorubicin relative to liposomal daunorubicin has not been established.

Although treatment may result in the reduction in size or disappearance of specific skin lesions and alleviation of the associated symptoms, no treatment has been shown conclusively to alter the natural history of AIDS-related Kaposi's sarcoma and additional study and experience are needed to establish the optimal regimen.

Conventional Chemotherapy

Response rates observed with single-agent chemotherapy (e.g., doxorubicin, etoposide, vinblastine, vincristine) appear to be similar to those observed with interferon alfa; however, studies directly comparing the efficacy of doxorubicin alone with that of interferon alfa have not been performed. The wide variation in response rates reported in clinical studies generally appear to reflect differences in patient selection and in the heterogeneity of criteria used to evaluate response rather than in drug activity. Combined treatment with chemotherapy (e.g., vinblastine or etoposide) and interferon alfa generally appears to result in enhanced systemic toxicity without added therapeutic benefits.

Combination chemotherapy with conventional antineoplastic agents (e.g., conventional doxorubicin, etoposide, vinblastine, vincristine) has been used for advanced disease (e.g., extensive mucocutaneous disease, lymphedema, symptomatic visceral disease). Evidence from a study in patients with advanced Kaposi's sarcoma indicates that combined therapy with low-dose conventional (nonencapsulated) doxorubicin, bleomycin, and vincristine is more effective than low-dose doxorubicin alone in inducing response and prolonging disease-free survival, although overall survival with either regimen was comparable. In this study, complete and partial tumor remissions as well as disease-free survival were higher in patients receiving combination therapy with low-dose conventional doxorubicin (20 mg/m^2), bleomycin (10 units/m^2), and vincristine (1.4 mg/m^2; up to 2 mg) every 2 weeks than in those receiving low-dose doxorubicin (20 mg/m^2) alone every 2 weeks; complete and partial remissions occurred in 88 or 48% of patients receiving combination or single-agent chemotherapy, respectively, while a median survival of 9 months was observed with both therapies.

● Ovarian Cancer

Liposomal Doxorubicin

Pegylated liposomal doxorubicin is used for the treatment of ovarian cancer that has progressed or recurred following platinum-based chemotherapy.

The current indication for use of liposomal doxorubicin in platinum-refractory ovarian cancer is based principally on data from a subset of patients involved in 3 uncontrolled studies and a randomized trial. In these clinical trials, liposomal doxorubicin was administered at an initial dosage of 50 mg/m^2 IV over 1 hour every 3–4 weeks for 3–6 cycles or more. Among 145 patients with metastatic ovarian carcinoma refractory to paclitaxel- and platinum-based chemotherapy regimens who received liposomal doxorubicin in 3 open-label, phase II studies, the objective response rate was 13.8% (range: 0–22%), the median time to response was 17.6 weeks, the median duration of response was 39.4 weeks, and the median time to progression was 15.9 weeks. In a randomized, open-label trial

involving 474 patients with epithelial ovarian cancer (mostly stage III–IV disease) who had received platinum-based chemotherapy, similar median time to progression (4 months), median overall survival (14 months) and response rates (20 versus 17%) were observed in those receiving liposomal doxorubicin or topotecan. Hand-foot syndrome (51 versus 1%), stomatitis (41 versus 15%), and rash (28 versus 12%) occurred more frequently in patients receiving liposomal doxorubicin, whereas nausea (63 versus 46%), alopecia (52 versus 19%), and constipation (46 versus 30%) occurred more frequently in those receiving topotecan. Severe hematologic toxicity, including neutropenia, anemia, and thrombocytopenia, occurred more frequently in patients receiving topotecan than in those receiving liposomal doxorubicin. Severe neutropenia (less than 500/mm^3) was reported in 4% of patients receiving liposomal doxorubicin compared with 62% of patients receiving topotecan.

Conventional Doxorubicin

Although conventional doxorubicin is labeled for use in the treatment of ovarian carcinoma and has been used in combination regimens for the treatment of this cancer, other agents currently are preferred.

● Bladder Cancer

Doxorubicin has been used intravesically† for the treatment of residual tumor and/or as adjuvant therapy for prophylaxis of superficial bladder carcinoma†.

Complete response rates of about 40–50% have been observed in patients receiving intravesical doxorubicin for the treatment of papillary tumors; complete responses to intravesical doxorubicin also have been reported in a small number of patients with carcinoma in situ. No additional benefit has been shown for the use of maintenance therapy with intravesical doxorubicin. Treatment with intravesical doxorubicin generally is well tolerated; the most common adverse effect observed is chemical cystitis, usually reversible, in approximately 20–30% of patients. Systemic toxicity, including hypersensitivity reactions and cardiovascular events, have been reported in patients receiving intravesical doxorubicin for the prophylaxis or treatment of superficial bladder cancer.

Although evidence from comparative studies is limited, other agents (e.g. mitomycin, epirubicin) that appear to be similar in efficacy but less toxic than doxorubicin generally are preferred for the prophylaxis or treatment of superficial bladder cancer. (See Uses: Bladder Cancer in Mitomycin 10:00 for further discussion of intravesical chemotherapy for superficial bladder cancer.)

Doxorubicin is used in combination regimens with cisplatin, methotrexate, and vinblastine for the treatment of invasive and advanced bladder carcinoma. (See Uses: Bladder Cancer in Cisplatin 10:00.)

● Small Cell Lung Cancer

Doxorubicin is used in combination chemotherapy regimens (e.g., cyclophosphamide, doxorubicin, and vincristine [CAV]; cyclophosphamide, doxorubicin, and etoposide [CAE]) for the treatment of extensive-stage small cell lung cancer†. Survival outcomes are similar in patients with extensive-stage small cell lung cancer receiving CAV or cisplatin/etoposide. Combination chemotherapy regimens have produced response rates of 70–85% and complete response rates of 20–30% in patients with extensive-stage disease; however, comparative efficacy is continually being evaluated. Because the current prognosis for small cell lung carcinoma is unsatisfactory regardless of stage and despite considerable diagnostic and therapeutic advances, all patients with this cancer are candidates for inclusion in clinical trials at the time of diagnosis.

● Multiple Myeloma

Induction Therapy Prior to Stem Cell Transplantation

Conventional Doxorubicin

Use of conventional doxorubicin in combination with bortezomib and dexamethasone† (bortezomib-doxorubicin-dexamethasone) as induction therapy for newly diagnosed multiple myeloma in transplant-eligible patients† may be considered a reasonable choice (accepted; with possible conditions) based on current evidence from an open-label, randomized phase 3 study (HOVON-65/GMMG-HD4). Factors that should be considered when selecting a combination chemotherapy regimen for use as induction therapy include performance status and preexisting conditions (e.g., peripheral neuropathy).

In the HOVON-65/GMMG-HD4 study in 827 patients with newly diagnosed multiple myeloma, patients who received bortezomib-doxorubicin-dexamethasone had prolonged progression-free survival (35 versus 28 months; hazard ratio: 0.75) and higher postinduction (11 versus 5%) and posttransplant (31 versus 15%)

complete plus near-complete response rates compared with those who received vincristine-doxorubicin-dexamethasone at a median follow-up of 41 months. Median overall survival had not been reached at a median follow-up of 66 months; however, no significant difference in 5-year overall survival was observed between the groups. Subgroup analyses based on presence of renal insufficiency or high-risk cytogenetic features (i.e., chromosome 13q14 deletion [del(13q14)], t(4;14) translocation, chromosome 17p13 deletion [del(17p13)]) suggested prolonged progression-free and overall survival with bortezomib-doxorubicin-dexamethasone compared with vincristine-doxorubicin-dexamethasone induction therapy in patients with serum creatinine concentrations exceeding 2 mg/dL and in those with del(17p13) chromosomal abnormality, as well as an overall survival benefit for bortezomib-doxorubicin-dexamethasone compared with vincristine-doxorubicin-dexamethasone in patients with del(13q14) chromosomal abnormality.

For further information on the use of combination therapy with conventional doxorubicin, bortezomib, and dexamethasone as induction therapy for newly diagnosed multiple myeloma in transplant-eligible patients, see Induction Therapy Prior to Stem Cell Transplantation in Newly Diagnosed Multiple Myeloma under Uses: Multiple Myeloma, in Bortezomib 10:00.

Liposomal Doxorubicin

Use of pegylated liposomal doxorubicin also has been studied in combination with bortezomib and dexamethasone† (bortezomib-liposomal doxorubicin-dexamethasone) as induction therapy for previously untreated multiple myeloma† in 2 open-label, noncomparative phase 2 studies. Based on current evidence, use of liposomal doxorubicin in combination with bortezomib and dexamethasone as induction therapy for newly diagnosed multiple myeloma in transplant-eligible patients may be considered a reasonable choice (accepted; with possible conditions); however, in the absence of longer follow-up data, use of a modified bortezomib-liposomal doxorubicin-dexamethasone regimen (i.e., reduced dosages of liposomal doxorubicin and bortezomib) is not fully established because of unclear risk/benefit and/or inadequate experience (see Liposomal Doxorubicin Hydrochloride under Dosage and Administration: Dosage). Factors that should be considered when selecting a combination chemotherapy regimen for induction therapy include performance status and preexisting conditions (e.g., peripheral neuropathy).

In the first study in 40 patients with newly diagnosed multiple myeloma, overall response rate and complete plus near-complete response rate were 85 and 38%, respectively, following 6 cycles of induction therapy with bortezomib-liposomal doxorubicin-dexamethasone. Among patients who underwent stem cell transplantation, the complete plus near-complete response rate increased to 57% following transplantation, but the overall response rate did not improve substantially. At a median follow-up of 45.1 months, median progression-free survival had not been reached; however, among patients who underwent stem cell transplantation, actuarial 2- and 4-year progression-free survival rates were 93 and 65%, respectively, and actuarial 2- and 4-year overall survival rates were 97 and 67%, respectively.

Because liposomal doxorubicin and bortezomib frequently cause adverse effects, another phase 2 study evaluated a modified bortezomib-liposomal doxorubicin-dexamethasone regimen (i.e., reduced dosages of liposomal doxorubicin and bortezomib) in 35 patients with previously untreated multiple myeloma. Overall and complete response rates were 86 and 20%, respectively. At a median follow-up of 17.7 months, median time to progression, duration of response, and overall survival had not been reached.

For further information on the use of combination therapy with liposomal doxorubicin, bortezomib, and dexamethasone as induction therapy for newly diagnosed multiple myeloma in transplant-eligible patients, see Induction Therapy Prior to Stem Cell Transplantation in Newly Diagnosed Multiple Myeloma under Uses: Multiple Myeloma, in Bortezomib 10:00.

Refractory Multiple Myeloma

Doxorubicin is used in combination therapy for refractory multiple myeloma†. A regimen employing continuous IV infusions of doxorubicin and vincristine and high-dose dexamethasone is used in patients with advanced multiple myeloma refractory to alkylating agents and in patients with relapsing disease.

● Other Uses

Doxorubicin hydrochloride is used in the treatment of solid tumors including thyroid cancer, gastric cancer, soft-tissue and osteogenic sarcomas, neuroblastoma, and Wilms' tumor; malignant lymphomas of both Hodgkin and non-Hodgkin type; and acute lymphocytic leukemia.

Doxorubicin is used in the treatment of Ewing's sarcoma†, squamous cell carcinomas of the cervix† and prostate†, and uterine cancer†.

Doxorubicin also is used in the treatment of adrenocortical cancer†, carcinoid tumors†, endometrial cancer†, islet cell carcinoma†, chronic lymphocytic leukemia†, liver cancer†, and mesothelioma†.

Although doxorubicin is labeled for use in the treatment of acute myeloid leukemia, other agents are preferred.

DOSAGE AND ADMINISTRATION

● Reconstitution and Administration

Doxorubicin hydrochloride conventional and PEG-stabilized liposomal for injection concentrate are administered IV. The drug is extremely irritating to tissues and, therefore, must not be given IM or subcutaneously. (See Cautions: Local Effects.) *Care should be taken to avoid extravasation of the drug.*

Because doxorubicin may cause adverse local dermatologic reactions, commercially available conventional and liposomal doxorubicin hydrochloride for injection concentrate, the powder for injection, and solutions of the drug must be prepared and handled cautiously and the use of latex gloves is recommended. If the powder or solutions of the drug contact the skin or mucous membranes, the affected area should be immediately and thoroughly washed with soap and water. Parenteral doxorubicin hydrochloride solutions should be inspected visually for particulate matter and discoloration prior to administration whenever solution and container permit. However, because PEG-stabilized liposomal doxorubicin hydrochloride occurs as a liposomal dispersion, the for injection concentrate is not clear but rather is translucent and red.

Conventional Doxorubicin Hydrochloride

The lyophilized drug is reconstituted by adding 5, 10, 25, 50, or 75 mL of 0.9% sodium chloride injection to a vial labeled as containing 10, 20, 50, 100, or 150 mg of doxorubicin hydrochloride, respectively. The vial should then be shaken and the contents allowed to dissolve. When reconstituted as directed above, the resultant solution contains 2 mg of doxorubicin hydrochloride per mL. Diluents containing preservatives should not be used to reconstitute the powder for injection. Alternatively, to avoid the potential risks associated with reconstitution of the powder, the commercially available injection can be used; however, handling of the solution is *not* without risk.

Solutions of the conventional doxorubicin hydrochloride injection should be administered slowly into the tubing of a freely running IV infusion of 0.9% sodium chloride or 5% dextrose injection, preferably via a Butterfly® needle inserted into a large vein. When possible, veins over joints or in extremities with compromised venous or lymphatic drainage should *not* be used. The rate of the conventional doxorubicin hydrochloride injection depends on the size of the vein and the dose, but the dose should be administered over at least 3–5 minutes. Local erythematous streaking along the vein and/or facial flushing may be indicative of too rapid an administration rate.

Although a stinging or burning sensation may be a symptom of extravasation during IV administration of conventional doxorubicin hydrochloride, extravasation may occur without these symptoms and even when blood returns well during initial aspiration of the infusion needle. If any signs or symptoms of extravasation occur, the injection or infusion of conventional doxorubicin hydrochloride should be immediately stopped and restarted at another site. When extravasation of the conventional injection occurs or is suspected, intermittent application of ice packs to the site for 15 minutes four times daily for 3 days may be helpful in reducing the local reaction. The benefit of local administration of drugs to the extravasation site has not been established. Because of the progressive nature of extravasation reactions, the affected area should be examined frequently and consultation with a specialist in plastic surgery should be obtained. If blistering, ulceration, and/or persistent pain occurs, wide excision of the affected area followed by split-thickness skin grafting should be considered.

Liposomal Doxorubicin Hydrochloride

PEG-stabilized liposomal doxorubicin hydrochloride for injection concentrate must be diluted prior to IV infusion. The concentrate should be diluted in 5% dextrose injection *only*, and no other diluent should be used. Doses of PEG-stabilized liposomal doxorubicin hydrochloride for injection concentrate up to 90 mg should be diluted in 250 mL of 5% dextrose injection. Doses of PEG-stabilized liposomal doxorubicin hydrochloride for injection concentrate exceeding 90 mg should be diluted in 500 mL of 5% dextrose injection. Strict aseptic technique must be observed because the liposomal doxorubicin for injection concentrate does not contain any preservative or bacteriostatic agent. Diluents containing preservatives (e.g., benzyl alcohol) should *not* be used to dilute the liposomal for injection concentrate, and other drugs should *not* be mixed with the solution. Because PEG-stabilized liposomal doxorubicin hydrochloride occurs as a liposomal dispersion of the drug, inline filters should *not* be used. Rapid flushing of the infusion line should be avoided.

The diluted solution of liposomal doxorubicin hydrochloride should be infused at an initial rate of 1 mg/minute in patients receiving the drug for ovarian cancer or AIDS-related Kaposi's sarcoma to reduce the risk of infusion-related reactions; if no infusion-related reactions occur, the rate of infusion may be increased to complete administration of the infusion over a 1-hour period. If infusion reactions manifested as flushing, shortness of breath, facial edema, headache, chills, chest pain, back pain, tightness of the chest or throat, fever, tachycardia, pruritus, rash, cyanosis, syncope, bronchospasm, asthma, apnea, and/or hypotension occur, the rate of infusion should be slowed or the infusion stopped. Because rapid infusion may increase the risk of such reactions, the liposomal injection should *not* be administered by rapid direct injection nor as an undiluted solution.

Although a stinging or burning sensation may be a symptom of extravasation during IV administration of liposomal doxorubicin hydrochloride, extravasation may occur without these symptoms and even when blood returns well during initial aspiration of the infusion needle. If any signs or symptoms of extravasation occur, the injection or infusion of liposomal doxorubicin hydrochloride should be immediately stopped and restarted at another site. When extravasation of liposomal doxorubicin hydrochloride occurs, applying ice packs over the site of extravasation for about 30 minutes may help alleviate the local reaction.

● **Dosage**

To obtain optimum therapeutic results with minimum adverse effects, dosage of doxorubicin hydrochloride must be based on the clinical, cardiac, hepatic, renal, and hematologic response and tolerance of the patient and on other chemotherapy or irradiation being used. Dosage reduction may be necessary in patients who have received extensive prior radiation therapy or in those whose bone marrow has been infiltrated with malignant cells, since severe myelosuppression is likely to occur. Clinicians should consult published protocols for the dosage of doxorubicin hydrochloride and other chemotherapeutic agents and the method and sequence of administration. Dosage of doxorubicin hydrochloride is based indirectly on body weight; if the patient has abnormal fluid retention, the patient's ideal weight is used to calculate body surface area.

Accidental substitution of liposomal doxorubicin for conventional doxorubicin hydrochloride injection has resulted in severe adverse effects. Liposomal doxorubicin hydrochloride should *not* be substituted for conventional doxorubicin hydrochloride, and the drugs are not equivalent on a mg per mg basis.

The total cumulative dose of doxorubicin hydrochloride should not exceed 550 mg/m² because of the risk of potentially irreversible cardiotoxicity, but higher cumulative doses may be tolerated when dexrazoxane (Zinecard®) is used concomitantly as a cardioprotectant. (See Cautions: Cardiac Effects.) If previous or concomitant therapy includes the use of other potentially cardiotoxic agents, such as cyclophosphamide, or irradiation of the cardiac region, total doxorubicin hydrochloride dosage should not exceed 400 mg/m². The total dosage of doxorubicin hydrochloride should include any previous or concomitant therapy with other anthracycline agents or related compounds.

Conventional Doxorubicin Hydrochloride

The usual adult dosage of conventional (nonencapsulated) doxorubicin hydrochloride is 60–75 mg/m², administered as a single dose at 21-day intervals; the lower dose should be considered for patients with poor performance status, inadequate bone marrow reserves secondary to old age, prior therapy, or marrow infiltration with malignant cells. Alternatively, a dosage of 20 mg/m² once weekly may be used; this dosage schedule has been reported to produce a lower incidence of congestive heart failure. A dosage of 30 mg/m² daily on 3 successive days every 4 weeks has also been used; this dosage schedule is usually associated with a higher incidence of stomatitis. When used in combination with other chemotherapy, doxorubicin hydrochloride commonly has been used in a dosage of 40–60 mg/m² given as a single IV dose and repeated at 21- to 28-day intervals.

When doxorubicin hydrochloride has been used in combination with bortezomib and dexamethasone† as induction therapy for newly diagnosed multiple myeloma in transplant-eligible patients†, doxorubicin hydrochloride 9 mg/m² per day has been administered IV on days 1–4 along with bortezomib 1.3 mg/m² by IV injection twice weekly for 2 weeks (days 1, 4, 8, and 11) and dexamethasone 40 mg orally on days 1–4, 9–12, and 17–20 of each 28-day cycle for 3 cycles.

Liposomal Doxorubicin Hydrochloride

For the treatment of AIDS-related Kaposi's sarcoma, the usual adult dosage of pegylated liposomal doxorubicin hydrochloride is 20 mg/m² once every 3 weeks, administered at an initial rate of 1 mg/minute. If no infusion-related adverse effects occur, the rate of infusion may be increased to complete administration of the infusion over a 1-hour period. The duration of therapy depends on response and tolerance of the patient.

When used for the treatment of ovarian cancer that has progressed or recurred following platinum-based chemotherapy, the manufacturer recommends a pegylated liposomal doxorubicin hydrochloride dosage of 50 mg/m² IV once every 4 weeks, administered at an initial rate of 1 mg/minute. If no infusion-related adverse effects occur, the rate of infusion may be increased to complete administration of the infusion over a 1-hour period. In patients without disease progression or intolerable toxicity, the manufacturer recommends a minimum of 4 courses of therapy because the median time to response with liposomal doxorubicin therapy in clinical trials for metastatic ovarian cancer was approximately 4 months.

When pegylated liposomal doxorubicin hydrochloride has been used in combination with bortezomib and dexamethasone† as induction therapy for newly diagnosed multiple myeloma in transplant-eligible patients†, pegylated liposomal doxorubicin hydrochloride 30 mg/m² has been administered IV on day 4 along with bortezomib 1.3 mg/m² by IV injection twice weekly for 2 weeks (days 1, 4, 8, and 11) and dexamethasone 40 mg orally on days 1, 2, 4, 5, 8, 9, 11, and 12 during cycle 1. During cycles 2–6, the same dosages of pegylated liposomal doxorubicin hydrochloride and bortezomib were administered along with dexamethasone 20 mg orally daily. Treatment cycles were repeated every 3 weeks for a total of 6 cycles.

Although a modified regimen using reduced dosages of both pegylated liposomal doxorubicin hydrochloride and bortezomib given in combination with dexamethasone† also has been used as induction therapy for newly diagnosed multiple myeloma in transplant-eligible patients†, use of this regimen is not fully established.

The management of certain adverse effects (e.g., hand-foot syndrome, hematologic toxicity, stomatitis) in patients receiving liposomal doxorubicin hydrochloride may require reduction in dosage and/or delay of doses. The manufacturer recommends the following dosage modifications for liposomal doxorubicin hydrochloride based on drug-induced adverse effects (see Dosage Modification tables). Once the dose of liposomal doxorubicin hydrochloride has been reduced because of drug-related toxicity, such as hand-foot syndrome or stomatitis, the dose should not be increased. For the management of nausea and vomiting associated with liposomal doxorubicin therapy, pretreatment with or concomitant use of antiemetic therapy should be considered.

TABLE 1. Dosage Modification for Hand-Foot Syndrome

Toxicity Grade	Symptoms	Dose Modification
0	No symptoms	None
1	Mild erythema, swelling, or desquamation not interfering with daily activities	Redose unless patient has experienced previous grade 3 or 4 skin toxicity in which case delay dose up to 2 weeks and decrease dose by 25%; then return to original dose interval
2	Erythema, desquamation, or swelling interfering with, but not precluding, normal physical activities; small blisters or ulcerations <2 cm in diameter	Delay dosing up to 2 weeks or until toxicity resolved to grade 0–1; if no resolution after 2 weeks, discontinue liposomal doxorubicin; if resolved to grade 0–1 within 2 weeks and no previous grade 3–4 toxicity, continue treatment at previous dose and return to original dose interval; if patient experienced previous grade 3–4 toxicity, decrease dose by 25% and return to original dose interval

TABLE 1. Continued

Toxicity Grade	Symptoms	Dose Modification
3	Blistering, ulceration, or swelling interfering with walking or normal daily activities; cannot wear regular clothing	Delay dosing up to 2 weeks or until toxicity resolved to grade 0–1, then decrease dose by 25% and return to original dose interval; if no resolution after 2 weeks, discontinue liposomal doxorubicin
4	Diffuse or local process causing infectious complications, or a bedridden state or hospitalization	Delay dosing up to 2 weeks or until toxicity resolved to grade 0–1, then decrease dose by 25% and return to original dose interval; if no resolution after 2 weeks, discontinue liposomal doxorubicin

For further information on reduced dosage of Doxil® (liposomal doxorubicin hydrochloride) based on drug-induced adverse effects, consult the manufacturer at (415) 617-3078.

TABLE 2. Dosage Modification for Hematologic Toxicity

Toxicity Grade	ANC (per mm³)	Platelets (per mm³)	Dose Modification
1	1500–1900	75,000–150,000	None
2	1000–1499	50,000–74,999	Wait until ANC ≥1500 and platelets ≥75,000, then redose with no dose reduction
3	500–999	25,000–49,999	Wait until ANC ≥1500 and platelets ≥75,000, then redose with no dose reduction
4	<500	<25,000	Wait until ANC ≥1500 and platelets ≥75,000, then redose at 25% dose reduction or continue full dose with cytokine support

TABLE 3. Dosage Modification for Stomatitis

Toxicity Grade	Symptoms	Dose Modification
1	Painless ulcers, erythema, or mild soreness	Redose unless patient has experienced previous grade 3 or 4 toxicity, in which case delay up to 2 weeks and decrease dose by 25%, returning to original dose interval
2	Painful erythema, edema, or ulcers, but can eat	Delay dosing up to 2 weeks or until resolved to grade 0–1; if no improvement after 2 weeks, discontinue liposomal doxorubicin; if resolved to grade 0–1 within 2 weeks and no previous grade 3–4 toxicity, continue treatment at previous dose and return to original dose interval; if patient experienced previous grade 3–4 toxicity, decrease dose by 25% and return to original dose interval
3	Painful erythema, edema, or ulcers, and cannot eat	Delay dosing up to 2 weeks or until resolution to grade 0–1, then redose at 25% dose reduction and return to original dose interval; if no improvement after 2 weeks, discontinue liposomal doxorubicin
4	Requires parenteral or enteral support	Delay dosing up to 2 weeks or until resolution to grade 0–1, then redose at 25% dose reduction and return to original dose interval; if no improvement after 2 weeks, discontinue liposomal doxorubicin

● Dosage in Hepatic Impairment

In adults with impairment of hepatic function, conventional or liposomal doxorubicin dosage *must* be reduced. Patients with serum bilirubin concentrations of 1.2–3 mg/dL should receive 50% of the usual dose of doxorubicin hydrochloride and those with serum bilirubin concentrations exceeding 3 mg/dL should receive 25% of the usual dose.

CAUTIONS

● Hematologic Effects

Because of the risk of myelosuppression, hematologic status must be monitored carefully in patients receiving conventional or liposomal doxorubicin.

Conventional Doxorubicin

Leukopenia (principally granulocytopenia) is the predominant manifestation of hematologic toxicity, the severity of which depends on the dose of the drug and on the regenerative capacity of the bone marrow. Leukocyte counts as low as 1000/mm³ should be anticipated during therapy with appropriate doses of doxorubicin, although severe myelosuppression can occur. Thrombocytopenia and anemia may also occur. Deaths from septicemia have been associated with severe leukopenia. Maximum leukopenia, thrombocytopenia, and anemia generally occur during the second week (nadir at 10–14 days) following administration of the drug and generally return to normal by the third week.

Liposomal Doxorubicin

The principal dose-limiting toxicity of pegylated liposomal doxorubicin in patients with AIDS-related Kaposi's sarcoma has been myelosuppression, commonly manifested by leukopenia and neutropenia; anemia and thrombocytopenia also occur frequently. Among 720 patients with AIDS-related Kaposi's sarcoma receiving liposomal doxorubicin in clinical trials, neutropenia less than 2000/mm³ was reported in 85% of patients, neutropenia less than 1000/mm³ was reported in about 49% of patients, and severe or life-threatening neutropenia (less than 500/mm³) occurred in 13% of patients. Leukopenia less than 4000/mm³ was reported in about 91% of patients, and leukopenia less than 1000/mm³ occurred in 11.5% of patients. Anemia was reported in 55.4% of patients and was severe or life-threatening in 18.2% of patients. Hypochromic anemia was reported in about 10% of patients. Thrombocytopenia was reported in 61% of patients and was life-threatening in 4% of patients.

Patients receiving pegylated liposomal doxorubicin for AIDS-related Kaposi's sarcoma often have baseline myelosuppression secondary to their underlying human immunodeficiency virus (HIV) infection and/or numerous concomitant drug therapy. With the recommended dosage schedule, leukopenia associated with liposomal doxorubicin usually is transient, but hematologic toxicity occasionally may be severe enough to require dose reduction or delay or suspension of therapy with the drug. Persistent, severe myelosuppression may result in superinfection or hemorrhage. In patients with AIDS-related Kaposi's sarcoma receiving liposomal doxorubicin, sepsis occurred in 5% of patients and was considered possibly or probably related to the drug in 0.7% of patients. Discontinuance of liposomal doxorubicin because of myelosuppression or neutropenia was required in 1.6% of patients with AIDS-related Kaposi's sarcoma. The development of neutropenic sepsis rarely has resulted in death.

Adverse hematologic effects reported in 1–5% of patients receiving pegylated liposomal doxorubicin for AIDS-related Kaposi's sarcoma include hemolysis and increased prothrombin time.

In patients with relapsed ovarian cancer, myelosuppression associated with pegylated liposomal doxorubicin generally has been moderate and reversible. Anemia was the most common adverse hematologic effect in patients with relapsed ovarian cancer, occurring in about 53% of patients receiving liposomal doxorubicin in 3 single-arm clinical trials. Neutropenia with an absolute neutrophil count less than 2000/mm³ was reported in 52%, and neutropenia with an absolute neutrophil count less than 1000/mm³ was reported in 19%, of patients with relapsed ovarian cancer receiving liposomal doxorubicin. Leukopenia (white blood cell count less than 4000/mm³) was reported in 42%, and thrombocytopenia was reported in 24%, of patients with relapsed ovarian cancer receiving liposomal doxorubicin. In the randomized trial, anemia occurred in 40%, leukopenia in 37%, neutropenia (absolute neutrophil count less than 1000/mm³) in 35%, and thrombocytopenia in 13%, of patients receiving liposomal doxorubicin for ovarian cancer. Granulocyte colony-stimulating factor or granulocyte-macrophage colony-stimulating factor was used in 4.6% of patients receiving liposomal doxorubicin for relapsed ovarian cancer to reduce the severity of myelosuppression associated with therapy.

● *Cardiac Effects*

Types of Cardiotoxicity

Three types of cardiotoxicity may occur in patients receiving an anthracycline (e.g., doxorubicin): an acute transient type; a chronic, subacute type, which is related to cumulative dose and has a later, more indolent onset; and a late-onset type that manifests years after anthracycline therapy and occurs mainly in patients exposed to the drugs as children. The use of conventional or liposomal doxorubicin may cause cardiac toxicity.

Acute anthracycline-induced cardiotoxicity usually is uncommon. It occurs immediately after a single dose or a single course of anthracycline therapy and may involve abnormal ECG findings including ST-T wave changes (e.g., T-wave flattening and ST-segment depression), prolongation of the QT interval, and arrhythmias (e.g., sinus tachycardia; ventricular, supraventricular, and junctional tachycardia). Conduction disturbances (including atrioventricular [AV] and bundle-branch block) have been reported rarely in acute anthracycline-induced cardiotoxicity (they are more usually associated with late-onset anthracycline-induced cardiotoxicity). Although acute cardiotoxicity generally is transient, rarely, pericarditis-myocarditis syndrome (e.g., pericardial effusion and/or decreased myocardial contractility) and possible cardiac failure may occur.

Chronic cardiotoxicity, such as congestive heart failure or cardiomyopathy, usually occurs within 1 year after discontinuance of anthracycline therapy, is more common than acute cardiotoxicity, and is considered clinically the most important anthracycline-associated toxicity. Chronic cardiotoxicity, such as heart failure, may occur as total cumulative dosage of doxorubicin hydrochloride approaches or exceeds 550 mg/m². Heart failure may occur at a lower total cumulative dosage (i.e., 400 mg/m²) in patients who have received radiotherapy to the mediastinal region or in patients receiving concomitant therapy with other potentially cardiotoxic agents, such as cyclophosphamide. Time of onset of chronic cardiotoxicity may vary but usually is manifested within 1 year of anthracycline therapy. In one study, onset of congestive heart failure developed 0–231 days after discontinuance of anthracycline therapy.

Chronic cardiotoxicity reflects a progressive injury and loss of cardiac myocytes, with increasing cumulative anthracycline doses resulting in thinning of ventricular walls and decreased systolic performance. Initially, there is functional compensation by the remaining myocytes allowing overall cardiac function to appear normal despite histologic damage, which can be demonstrated by endomyocardial biopsy. However, as cumulative doses of anthracycline increase, there is a decrease in systolic performance, as measured by a decrease in fractional shortening (FS) and in left-ventricular ejection fraction (LVEF) with eventual progression to symptomatic congestive heart failure, if cardiac reserve is exhausted, and to cardiorespiratory decompensation. Symptoms of the described rapidly progressing syndrome may include tachycardia, tachypnea, dilation of the heart, exercise intolerance, pulmonary and venous congestion, poor perfusion, and pleural effusion; these manifestations may respond to cardiac supportive therapy and may be self-limiting, or, alternatively, may be irreversible and unresponsive to therapy and fatal.

Sensitivity to anthracycline-induced cardiotoxicity exhibits interindividual variation, with some patients occasionally tolerating cumulative doxorubicin hydrochloride doses exceeding 1 g/m² while other patients exhibit histopathologic changes characteristic of doxorubicin-induced cardiotoxicity, decreases in LVEF, and even congestive heart failure at cumulative doses of less than 300 mg/m². Despite such interindividual variation, the risk of developing doxorubicin-induced impairment in myocardial function (based on a combined index of signs, symptoms, and decline in LVEF) increases with increasing cumulative dose, occurring in 1–2% of patients receiving cumulative doses of 300 mg/m² and increasing to 3–5, 5–8, and 6–20% in those receiving cumulative doses of 400, 450, or 500 mg/m² in schedules of rapid IV doses given once every 3 weeks. In one retrospective review, congestive heart failure developed in 3, 7, or 21% of patients at cumulative doses of 430, 575, or 728 mg/m², and the slope of the probability curve for developing congestive heart failure increased at around 550 mg/m². However, in a prospective study in which doxorubicin was administered concomitantly with cyclophosphamide, fluorouracil, and/or vincristine in patients with

breast cancer or small cell lung cancer, the risk of congestive heart failure was 1.5, 4.9, 7.7, or 20.5% at cumulative doses of 300, 400, 450, or 500 mg/m².

Adverse cardiac effects occurred in 9.6% of patients with AIDS-related Kaposi's sarcoma receiving pegylated liposomal doxorubicin in clinical trials and were considered possibly or probably related to the drug in 4.3% of patients. Cardiomyopathy and congestive heart failure have been reported in patients receiving liposomal doxorubicin for AIDS-related Kaposi's sarcoma. Severe adverse cardiac effects, including arrhythmia, cardiomyopathy, heart failure, pericardial effusion, and tachycardia, were reported in 1% of patients receiving liposomal doxorubicin for AIDS-related Kaposi's sarcoma. The manufacturer reports that therapy with liposomal doxorubicin was discontinued because of adverse cardiac events in 3 patients with AIDS-related Kaposi's sarcoma receiving the drug in clinical trials.

In 250 patients with advanced breast cancer receiving pegylated liposomal doxorubicin hydrochloride at a starting dose of 50 mg/m² every 4 weeks, the incidence of cardiac toxicity was 11% at cumulative doses of 450–500 mg/m² and 500–550 mg/m².

Factors reported to increase the risk of anthracycline-induced cardiotoxicity (some of which may cause such toxicity at lower cumulative doxorubicin doses) include irradiation to the mediastinal region, concomitant cyclophosphamide, preexisting heart disease (e.g., occult hypertension, subclinical coronary artery disease), extremes in age, liver disease, whole body hyperthermia, and female gender (mainly in children). In one study in women with early breast cancer receiving cyclophosphamide-based adjuvant chemotherapy following either surgery alone or surgery and mediastinal irradiation, cardiac abnormalities (e.g., ECG changes) developed in about 5% of all (both those who did and did not receive irradiation) patients and about 70% of these cases of cardiac abnormalities occurred in patients receiving irradiation of the left breast; all cases of congestive heart failure (which was fatal in several patients) reported in irradiated patients occurred at cumulative doxorubicin hydrochloride doses that did not exceed 315 mg/m². This and other evidence suggest that irradiation of the left breast may be a more important cardiotoxic cofactor than concomitant alkylating chemotherapy. Anthracycline therapy may potentiate cardiotoxicity caused by high-dose cyclophosphamide therapy used for bone marrow ablation and transplantation. It is unclear if lower doses of cyclophosphamide interact with anthracyclines in the development of cardiotoxicity. Some evidence also suggests that the risk of cardiotoxicity may be increased in patients receiving calcium-channel blocking agents concomitantly. The cardiotoxic risk associated with cumulative doses of doxorubicin also should take into account previous or concomitant therapy with related drugs such as daunorubicin, idarubicin, and mitoxantrone.

Late-onset anthracycline-induced cardiotoxicity, which may include late-onset ventricular dysfunction, heart failure, conduction disturbances, and arrhythmias (e.g., nonsustained ventricular tachycardia) which may be life-threatening, occurs several years or even decades after discontinuance of anthracycline therapy and it may develop after a prolonged asymptomatic interval. In one study in patients with solid tumors or leukemia, those who were followed for 4 to less than 10 or 10–20 years after discontinuance of anthracycline therapy had an 18 or 38% incidence, respectively, of abnormal FS in echocardiograms. In another study in children with acute lymphoblastic leukemia who were followed for up to 15 years after discontinuance of anthracycline therapy, increases in myocardial afterload and/or decreases in myocardial contractility were reported in 65% of patients receiving cumulative doses of at least 228 mg/m²; these cardiac abnormalities appeared to be progressive and were predictive of future cardiac decompensation. It has been suggested that myocyte damage and ventricular dysfunction progress after the initial myocardial insult and may lead to late-onset cardiac decompensation. Some clinicians state that late-onset cardiotoxicity can be clinically manifest in response to stressful situations (e.g., surgery, pregnancy), exercise (e.g., weight lifting), and acute viral infection. In at least one patient, postpartum-associated congestive heart failure occurred 7 years after discontinuance of doxorubicin therapy. Some clinicians suggested that the postpartum effects of anemia, hypertension, and fluid mobilization on subclinical doxorubicin fibrosis resulted in reversible cardiac decompensation. The incidence of late-onset cardiotoxicity may be increased with increasing cumulative doses of anthracyclines, high rates of administration, or irradiation to the mediastinal region; young age at the time of anthracycline therapy and female gender may be contributing factors to such cardiotoxicity, but further study is needed.

Late-onset anthracycline toxicity can be expected to be observed more frequently with the growing census of long-term survivors (e.g., survivors of childhood cancers) who have received anthracyclines. It also is expected that this cardiotoxicity will be associated with increased morbidity and mortality.

Substantial cardiac injury may occur even with low-dose anthracycline therapy. Since the observed incidence of severe anthracycline-induced cardiotoxicity appears to increase (especially after irradiation to the mediastinal region) with duration of long-term monitoring, the full extent of late-onset anthracycline toxicity in asymptomatic patients remains to be elucidated since data currently are inadequate regarding cardiotoxicity occurring 15 years or more after discontinuance of anthracycline therapy. Long-term follow-up shows that overt cardiac failure occurs in about 4.5–7% of patients receiving anthracycline therapy.

Assessment of Cardiotoxicity

Clinical manifestations found on physical examination (e.g., shortness of breath, pulmonary rales) and/or changes detected on electrocardiographic monitoring (e.g., sinus tachycardia) are not specific enough to diagnose anthracycline-induced cardiotoxicity. More sensitive methods are needed to detect early signs of cardiac damage so that the potential benefits from larger than usual dosages of anthracyclines in cancer therapy may be weighed against the possible risks of drug-induced cardiotoxicity. Monitoring of the left-ventricular ejection fraction with serial echocardiographic studies is a sensitive, noninvasive method for the detection and follow-up of anthracycline-induced cardiomyopathy. Radionuclide angiography also has been used to monitor the ejection fraction, but this procedure exposes the patient to ionizing radiation. The combination of exercise stress testing and ejection-fraction studies is a more sensitive indicator for detecting early signs of subclinical cardiomyopathy associated with anthracycline therapy. Endomyocardial biopsy (using a semiquantitative histologic scoring system) currently is considered the most sensitive and specific method for diagnosing and determining the degree of anthracycline-induced cardiotoxicity; however, this invasive procedure is not routinely used. Concerns for safety, especially in children requiring multiple biopsies, and in those with thrombocytopenia, and the lack of experience in obtaining and scoring biopsies have limited the use of endomyocardial biopsy; the correlation between biopsy scores and the long-term effects of anthracycline cardiotoxicity has not been established, and underestimation of cardiac damage may occur. Guidelines for cardiac monitoring of children receiving anthracycline therapy have been published, although their general acceptance remains to be established. Guidelines also have been published for adults using multigated radionuclide angiography (MUGA scans).

Anthracycline-induced cardiomyopathy usually is associated with characteristic histopathologic changes on endomyocardial (EM) biopsy (e.g., fibrosis, myofibrillar dropout, intracellular vacuolar degeneration) and with decreased LVEF, as determined by multi-gated radionuclide angiography (MUGA scans) and/or echocardiogram (ECHO), relative to baseline values. In adults, a 10% decline in LVEF to below the lower limit of normal, a 20% decline in LVEF at any level, or an absolute LVEF of 45% is indicative of a deterioration in cardiac function. Although monitoring the ejection fraction has not been shown to be predictive of impending maximal tolerance of the cumulative doxorubicin dose, the benefits of continued therapy with the drug should be weighed carefully against the risk of irreversible cardiotoxicity whenever test results indicate a deterioration in cardiac function.

Mechanism of Cardiotoxicity

Several anthracycline-induced effects may contribute to the development of cardiotoxicity. In animals, anthracyclines cause a selective inhibition of cardiac muscle gene expression for α-actin, troponin, myosin light-chain 2, and the M isoform of creatine kinase, which may result in myofibrillar loss associated with anthracycline-induced cardiotoxicity. Other potential causes of anthracycline-induced cardiotoxicity include myocyte damage from calcium overload, altered myocardial adrenergic function, release of vasoactive amines, and proinflammatory cytokines. Limited data indicate that calcium-channel blocking agents (e.g., prenylamine) or β-adrenergic blocking agents may prevent calcium overload; however, the cardioprotective effects of β-adrenergic blocking agents have not been studied. It has been suggested that the principal cause of anthracycline-induced cardiotoxicity is associated with free radical damage to DNA.

Anthracyclines intercalate DNA, chelate metal ions to produce drug-metal complexes, and generate oxygen free radicals via oxidation-reduction reactions. Anthracyclines contain a quinone structure that may undergo reduction via NADPH-dependent reactions to produce a semiquinone free radical that initiates a cascade of oxygen-free radical generation. It appears that the metabolite, doxorubicinol, may be the moiety responsible for cardiotoxic effects, and the heart may be particularly susceptible to free-radical injury because of relatively low antioxidant concentrations. Initial attempts at preventing anthracycline-induced cardiotoxicity by administering antioxidants (e.g., vitamin E) to act as free-radical scavengers were not successful. Limited animal data indicate that probucol (no longer commercially available in the US), an antilipemic agent structurally similar to vitamin E, may prevent anthracycline-induced cardiotoxicity without interfering with the antineoplastic effect of doxorubicin. Chelation of metal ions, particularly iron, by the drug results in a doxorubicin-metal complex that catalyzes the generation of reactive oxygen free radicals, and the complex is a powerful oxidant that can initiate lipid peroxidation in the absence of oxygen free radicals. This reaction is not blocked by free-radical scavengers, and probably is the principal mechanism of anthracycline-induced cardiotoxicity. As a result, administration of dexrazoxane (ICRF-187), a cyclic derivative of EDTA that is converted intracellularly to a ring-opened chelating agent, can prevent anthracycline-induced cardiotoxicity, at least in part, by chelating free iron and thus preventing the formation of the anthracycline-iron complex and resultant free radical generation.

Management of Cardiotoxicity

Effective management of anthracycline-induced cardiotoxicity requires early diagnosis and intervention by identifying patients with existing risk factors for cardiotoxicity.

Dexrazoxane has been shown to prevent or reduce the incidence and severity of anthracycline-induced cardiotoxicity, although some, but not all, evidence suggests that the drug also may interfere with the antineoplastic efficacy of certain chemotherapeutic regimens (e.g., when initiated concurrently with cyclophosphamide, doxorubicin, and fluorouracil therapy). This potentially detrimental effect was not observed when dexrazoxane therapy was withheld until several initial courses of chemotherapy could be administered, and results from most clinical studies have failed to demonstrate interference by dexrazoxane with the antineoplastic efficacy of chemotherapeutic regimens. Therefore, the manufacturer of dexrazoxane currently recommends that cardioprotectant therapy with the drug *not* be initiated at the time doxorubicin-containing chemotherapy is initiated but instead be delayed until patients have received a cumulative doxorubicin dose of 300 mg/m². Although patients receiving dexrazoxane generally can tolerate higher cumulative doses of doxorubicin before experiencing cardiotoxicity, the cardioprotectant will not eliminate the risk of cardiotoxicity in patients who have already received cumulative doxorubicin hydrochloride doses of 300 mg/m². Therefore, cardiac function should be monitored carefully even when dexrazoxane is used. Use of dexrazoxane is associated with severe myelosuppression, which is potentiated by doxorubicin, and the long-term effect of the drug on the prevention of doxorubicin-induced cardiotoxicity is not known.

In one study in women receiving doxorubicin with cyclophosphamide and fluorouracil for advanced breast cancer, patients receiving concomitant cardioprotection with dexrazoxane tolerated higher cumulative doxorubicin hydrochloride doses (median: 500 mg/m²) than those who did not receive the cardioprotectant (median: 441 mg/m²), and one-third of cardioprotected patients were able to tolerate cumulative doxorubicin doses of at least 700 mg/m² (about 40% of whom received cumulative doses of 1 g/m² or more) whereas only 4% of unprotected patients could tolerate such doses. There also was some evidence that dexrazoxane may reduce the risk of doxorubicin-induced cardiotoxicity in patients with other contributing risk factors (e.g., mediastinal irradiation).

Doxorubicin-induced cardiotoxicity also has reportedly been reduced by administration of low doses of doxorubicin at weekly intervals or by administration of the drug by prolonged, continuous IV infusion (e.g., over 48–96 hours) via a central venous catheter; the comparative efficacy of these dosage schedules in various cancers and the long-term effects on the development of anthracycline-induced cardiotoxicity have not been established.

Management of doxorubicin-induced congestive heart failure should include cardiac glycosides, inotropic agents (e.g., dobutamine), diuretics, after-load reduction (e.g., with vasodilators), angiotensin-converting enzyme (ACE) inhibitors, restricted sodium intake, and bed rest. β-Blocking agents (β_1-selective adrenergic blocking agents) also have been used in conjunction with other treatment for anthracycline-induced congestive heart failure. Early treatment of subclinical anthracycline-induced systolic dysfunction, possibly with an ACE inhibitor, may reduce mortality rates in these patients. Although such interventions may provide symptomatic relief and improvement in the functional status of the patient, myocardial toxicity can be poorly responsive and irreversible; prognosis for patients with anthracycline-induced cardiomyopathic failure is poor. (See Cautions: Precautions and Contraindications.) Heart transplantation may be a consideration for some patients with cardiac decompensation.

Other Cardiovascular Effects

Adverse cardiovascular effects reported in 1–5% of patients receiving pegylated liposomal doxorubicin for AIDS-related Kaposi's sarcoma include chest pain, hypotension, and tachycardia.

Adverse cardiovascular effects reported in 1–10% of patients receiving pegylated liposomal doxorubicin for ovarian cancer include vasodilation, tachycardia, deep thrombophlebitis, hypotension, pallor, and cardiac arrest.

● GI Effects
Conventional Doxorubicin

Stomatitis and esophagitis (mucositis) may occur in patients receiving doxorubicin, especially when the drug is administered daily on several successive days. Stomatitis usually begins as a burning sensation accompanied by erythema of the oral mucosa, which in 2–3 days may progress to ulceration, particularly in the sublingual and lateral tongue margins and on the palate. Ulceration is sometimes severe enough to result in difficulty in swallowing, but seldom requires cessation of therapy. Stomatitis is maximal during the second week of therapy and lasts an additional 3–7 days. GI toxicity (evidenced frequently by nausea and vomiting and occasionally by anorexia and diarrhea) may occur, usually on the day of drug administration. Nausea and vomiting can be severe but may be alleviated by antiemetic therapy.

Ulceration and necrosis of the colon, particularly the cecum, leading to bleeding or severe and possibly fatal infection, have occurred in patients with acute myelogenous leukemia who received combined doxorubicin and cytarabine therapy.

Liposomal Doxorubicin

Among patients receiving pegylated liposomal doxorubicin for AIDS-related Kaposi's sarcoma in randomized trials, nausea occurred in 17%, vomiting in 8%, diarrhea in 8%, and stomatitis in 7%, of patients. Oral moniliasis was reported in 5.5% of these patients. Adverse GI effects reported in 1–5% of patients receiving liposomal doxorubicin for AIDS-related Kaposi's sarcoma include mouth ulceration, glossitis, constipation, aphthous stomatitis, anorexia, dysphagia, and abdominal pain.

Among patients receiving pegylated liposomal doxorubicin for ovarian cancer in the randomized trial, nausea occurred in 46%, stomatitis in 41%, and vomiting in 33%, of patients. Abdominal pain occurred in 33.5% of these patients. Constipation was reported in 30%, and diarrhea and anorexia each were reported in about 20% of these patients. Dyspepsia occurred in 12%, and intestinal obstruction in 11%, of patients receiving liposomal doxorubicin for ovarian cancer in the randomized trial. Adverse GI effects reported in 1–10% of patients receiving liposomal doxorubicin for ovarian cancer include oral moniliasis, mouth ulceration, dry mouth, gingivitis, esophagitis, dysphagia, flatulence, rectal bleeding, ileus, enlarged abdomen, and ascites.

● Dermatologic Effects
Conventional Doxorubicin

Complete alopecia almost always accompanies doxorubicin therapy, and patients should be advised of this effect. Regrowth of hair usually begins 2–3 months after doxorubicin is discontinued. The degree of doxorubicin-induced alopecia has been reduced by use of scalp hypothermia before and for 30 minutes after administration of the drug. Hyperpigmentation of nailbeds, pigmented banding of fingernails, and phalangeal and other dermal creases may occur in patients receiving doxorubicin. One clinician reported that pigment changes appeared 6 or more weeks following initiation of doxorubicin administration. Onycholysis, plantar callus formation, and epidermolysis also have been reported in patients receiving the drug.

Like dactinomycin, doxorubicin has reactivated latent effects of previous irradiation in some patients, producing erythema with vesiculation, nonpitting edema, severe pain, and moist desquamation in sites which were previously subjected to radiation therapy and which had subsequently returned to normal appearance. The reaction occurred from 4–7 days after each doxorubicin hydrochloride dose was administered and lasted an average of 7 days thereafter.

Liposomal Doxorubicin

Palmar-plantar erythrodysesthesia (PPE), or hand-foot syndrome, characterized by swelling, pain, erythema, and occasionally desquamation of the hands and feet, has been reported in patients receiving pegylated liposomal doxorubicin for ovarian cancer or AIDS-related Kaposi's sarcoma. In patients receiving liposomal doxorubicin for ovarian cancer in the randomized trial, hand-foot syndrome occurred in 51% of patients and was severe (grade 3 or 4) in 24% of patients; 4.2% of patients discontinued therapy with the drug because of hand-foot syndrome

or other dermatologic toxicity. In patients receiving liposomal doxorubicin 20 mg/m^2 every 2 weeks for AIDS-related Kaposi's sarcoma, 3.4% developed palmar-plantar skin eruptions, and 0.9% of patients discontinued therapy with the drug because of such effects.

Hand-foot syndrome generally developed after 2 or 3 cycles (i.e., 6 or more weeks) of therapy but occasionally occurred sooner. Although the reaction generally is mild and resolves within 1–2 weeks so that prolonged delay of therapy usually is not necessary, dose modification may be necessary (see Dosage Modification for Hand-Foot Syndrome table in Dosage section), and discontinuance of liposomal doxorubicin therapy may be required in some patients because of severe and debilitating effects.

Among patients receiving pegylated liposomal doxorubicin for AIDS-related Kaposi's sarcoma in randomized trials, alopecia was reported in about 9% of patients. Adverse dermatologic effects reported in 1–5% of patients receiving liposomal doxorubicin for AIDS-related Kaposi's sarcoma include herpes simplex, rash, and itching.

Among patients receiving pegylated liposomal doxorubicin for ovarian cancer in the randomized trial, rash occurred in 28.5%, and alopecia in 19%, of patients. Adverse dermatologic effects reported in 1–10% of patients receiving liposomal doxorubicin for ovarian cancer include pruritus, skin discoloration, vesiculobullous rash, maculopapular rash, exfoliative dermatitis, herpes zoster, sweating, dry skin, herpes simplex, fungal dermatitis, furunculosis, and acne.

● Infusion-related Effects

Acute infusion-related reactions in patients receiving pegylated liposomal doxorubicin were characterized by one or more of the following manifestations: flushing, shortness of breath, facial edema, headache, chills, chest pain, back pain, tightness of the chest and throat, fever, tachycardia, pruritus, rash, cyanosis, syncope, bronchospasm, asthma, apnea, and hypotension. Allergic or anaphylactoid-like reactions, sometimes life-threatening or fatal, also have been reported.

Acute infusion-related reactions occurred in 7% of patients with ovarian cancer receiving pegylated liposomal doxorubicin in the randomized trial; 2 patients (0.8%) discontinued therapy because of infusion-related reactions. Discontinuance of therapy with liposomal doxorubicin because of infusion-related reactions was required in 1.7% of patients receiving drug for solid tumors and in 0.9% of patients receiving the drug for AIDS-related Kaposi's sarcoma.

Infusion-related reactions typically occur during the first infusion and usually resolve over the course of several hours to a day once the infusion is stopped. Occasionally, the reactions may resolve simply by slowing the rate of infusion. The manufacturer recommends an initial infusion rate of 1 mg/minute to minimize the risk of infusion-related reactions in patients receiving liposomal doxorubicin. Medications and emergency equipment for the treatment of allergic or anaphylactoid-like reactions should be available for immediate use in patients receiving liposomal doxorubicin. Similar reactions have not been reported with conventional doxorubicin and therefore have been attributed to the liposomes or one of their surface components.

● Local Effects
Conventional Doxorubicin

Extravasation of conventional doxorubicin produces severe local tissue necrosis, as well as possible cellulitis, vesication, thrombophlebitis, lymphangitis, or painful induration and may result in limitation of mobility of the adjacent joints. Erythematous streaking along the vein proximal to the site of injection has been reported. Phlebosclerosis may also occur, especially when conventional doxorubicin is administered into small vein or repeatedly into a single vein.

Liposomal Doxorubicin

Although animal evidence suggests that lesions associated with extravasation of pegylated liposomal doxorubicin may be minor and reversible relative to more severe and irreversible lesions associated with conventional doxorubicin, liposomal doxorubicin also should be considered an irritant, and the usual precautions to avoid extravasation of the drug should be followed. For information on the management of extravasation of conventional or liposomal doxorubicin, see Dosage and Administration: Reconstitution and Administration.

● Sensitivity Reactions
Conventional Doxorubicin

Fever, chills, and urticaria have been reported occasionally in patients receiving conventional doxorubicin. Anaphylaxis may occur, and a case of apparent cross-sensitivity to lincomycin has been reported.

Liposomal Doxorubicin

Allergic or anaphylactoid-like reactions, sometimes life-threatening or fatal, have been reported in patients receiving liposomal doxorubicin. Among patients receiving pegylated liposomal doxorubicin for AIDS-related Kaposi's sarcoma, allergic reactions were reported in 1–5% of patients.

• Respiratory Effects

Pulmonary embolism, sometimes fatal, has occurred rarely in patients receiving pegylated liposomal doxorubicin.

Dyspnea and pneumonia were each reported in 1–5% of patients receiving pegylated liposomal doxorubicin for AIDS-related Kaposi's sarcoma.

Pharyngitis occurred in 16%, dyspnea in 15%, and increased cough in about 10%, of patients receiving pegylated liposomal doxorubicin for ovarian cancer in the randomized trial. Adverse respiratory effects reported in 1–10% of patients receiving liposomal doxorubicin for ovarian cancer include rhinitis, pneumonia, pleural effusion, sinusitis, apnea, and epistaxis.

• Nervous System Effects

Conventional Doxorubicin

Peripheral neurotoxicity, manifested as local-regional sensory and/or motor disturbances, has been reported in patients receiving conventional doxorubicin by intra-arterial administration; in most cases, patients also were receiving cisplatin. Seizures and coma have been reported in patients receiving doxorubicin in combination with cisplatin or vincristine. Seizures also have been reported in a patient receiving doxorubicin at 2–3 times the recommended dosage in combination with high-dose cyclophosphamide.

Liposomal Doxorubicin

Adverse neurologic effects reported in 1–5% of patients receiving pegylated liposomal doxorubicin for AIDS-related Kaposi's sarcoma include headache, dizziness, and somnolence.

Among patients receiving pegylated liposomal doxorubicin for ovarian cancer in the randomized trial, paresthesia and headache each occurred in about 10%, and dizziness occurred in 4%, of patients. Adverse neurologic effects reported in 1–10% of patients receiving liposomal doxorubicin for ovarian cancer include somnolence, dizziness, depression, insomnia, anxiety, confusion, neuropathy, hypertonia, agitation, neuralgia, peripheral neuritis, and vertigo.

• Metabolic and Electrolyte Effects

Conventional Doxorubicin

As a result of extensive purine catabolism accompanying rapid cellular destruction, hyperuricemia may occur in patients receiving conventional doxorubicin, and serum uric acid concentrations should be monitored. Hyperuricemia and its potential adverse effects may be minimized or prevented by adequate hydration, alkalinization of the urine, and/or administration of allopurinol.

Liposomal Doxorubicin

Adverse metabolic and electrolyte effects reported in 1–5% of patients receiving pegylated liposomal doxorubicin for AIDS-related Kaposi's sarcoma include weight loss, hypocalcemia, and hyperglycemia.

Adverse metabolic and electrolyte effects reported in 1–10% of patients receiving pegylated liposomal doxorubicin for ovarian cancer include dehydration, weight loss, hypokalemia, hypercalcemia, edema, cachexia, hyperglycemia, and hyponatremia.

• Genitourinary Effects

Albuminuria was reported in 1–5% of patients receiving pegylated liposomal doxorubicin for AIDS-related Kaposi's sarcoma.

Adverse genitourinary effects reported in 1–10% of patients receiving pegylated liposomal doxorubicin for ovarian cancer include urinary tract infection, dysuria, leukorrhea, urinary frequency, cystitis, hematuria, urinary incontinence, urinary urgency, vaginal moniliasis, vaginal bleeding, and pelvic pain.

• Musculoskeletal Effects

Adverse musculoskeletal effects reported in 1–10% of patients receiving pegylated liposomal doxorubicin for ovarian cancer include myalgia, arthralgia, and

pathological fracture. Muscle spasms have been reported rarely in patients receiving liposomal doxorubicin.

• Ocular Effects

Conventional Doxorubicin

Conjunctivitis and lacrimation occur rarely in patients receiving doxorubicin.

Liposomal Doxorubicin

Retinitis was reported in 1–5% of patients receiving pegylated liposomal doxorubicin for AIDS-related Kaposi's sarcoma.

Adverse ocular effects reported in 1–10% of patients receiving pegylated liposomal doxorubicin for ovarian cancer include conjunctivitis and dry eyes.

• Hepatic Effects

Among patients receiving pegylated liposomal doxorubicin for AIDS-related Kaposi's sarcoma in randomized trials, increased serum concentrations of alkaline phosphatase occurred in 8% of patients. Other adverse hepatic effects reported in 1–5% of patients receiving liposomal doxorubicin for AIDS-related Kaposi's sarcoma include increased serum concentrations of ALT (SGPT) and hyperbilirubinemia.

Among patients receiving pegylated liposomal doxorubicin for ovarian cancer, hyperbilirubinemia was reported in 1–10% of patients.

• Other Adverse Effects

Conventional Doxorubicin

Other reported adverse effects of doxorubicin include facial flushes (especially when doxorubicin is injected rapidly) and rarely conjunctivitis and lacrimation.

Acute "recall" pneumonitis, occurring at variable times after local radiation therapy, has been reported in children receiving concomitant doxorubicin and dactinomycin. Prepubertal growth failure and gonadal impairment, usually reversible, have occurred in children receiving doxorubicin-containing regimens.

Liposomal Doxorubicin

Among patients receiving pegylated liposomal doxorubicin for AIDS-related Kaposi's sarcoma in randomized trials, asthenia occurred in 10%, and fever occurred in 9%, of patients. Other adverse effects reported in 1–5% of patients receiving liposomal doxorubicin for AIDS-related Kaposi's sarcoma include back pain, infection, chills, and emotional lability.

Among patients receiving pegylated liposomal doxorubicin for ovarian cancer in the randomized trial, asthenia occurred in 40%, fever in 21%, pain in 21%, mucous membrane disorder in 14%, back pain in 12%, infection in 12%, and peripheral edema in 11%, of patients. Other adverse effects reported in 1–10% of patients receiving liposomal doxorubicin for ovarian cancer include ecchymosis, taste perversion, and ear pain.

• Precautions and Contraindications

The usual precautions and contraindications of doxorubicin apply to both the conventional and liposomal formulations.

Doxorubicin hydrochloride is a toxic drug with a low therapeutic index. A therapeutic response is not likely to occur without some evidence of toxicity. The major toxic effects of the drug are on the normal, rapidly proliferating tissues, particularly those of the bone marrow, GI and oral mucosa, and hair follicles. Patients receiving doxorubicin should be under constant supervision by clinicians experienced in cancer chemotherapy and should be hospitalized during the initial phase of treatment. If feasible, subsequent therapy and patient evaluation may be performed on an outpatient basis. Determinations of hepatic, hematopoietic, and cardiac function should be performed prior to and at regular intervals during doxorubicin therapy. Possible synergism of therapeutic response and toxicity with other antineoplastic agents used in concomitant chemotherapy should be considered.

Medications and emergency equipment for the treatment of allergic or anaphylactoid-like reactions should be available for immediate use in patients receiving liposomal doxorubicin.

Myelosuppression

Leukocyte, erythrocyte, and platelet counts should be performed prior to and at frequent intervals during doxorubicin therapy. Hematopoietic toxicity may require dosage reduction or suspension of the drug until blood cell counts return to normal or may be severe enough to require discontinuance of therapy. If a profound drop in blood cell count occurs, the patient should be closely observed and anti-infective therapy initiated if there are signs of infection; suspension of doxorubicin therapy may be necessary during this period. Platelet and leukocyte transfusions have proved beneficial in patients with severe bone marrow depression; use of hematopoietic agents (colony-stimulating factors) also can be considered. Doxorubicin is contraindicated in patients with preexisting myelosuppression.

Cardiotoxicity

Early recognition of drug-induced cardiac failure appears essential for successful treatment with cardiac glycosides, diuretics, sodium intake restriction, and rest. Cardiac evaluation employing ECGs and determination of left-ventricular ejection fraction with echocardiogram (ECHO) should be performed prior to initiation of doxorubicin therapy and subsequently prior to each dose or course of therapy after a total cumulative dosage of 400 mg/m^2 has been given. Such evaluation is particularly important in patients with preexisting risk factors for cardiotoxicity (e.g., those with heart disease or who received mediastinal irradiation or cyclophosphamide). Although T-wave flattening, ST depression, and arrhythmias may occur and last up to 2 weeks after a dose or course of doxorubicin, these effects currently are not considered indications for suspension of doxorubicin therapy.

Doxorubicin-induced cardiomyopathy has been reported to be associated with persistent reduction in QRS voltage, prolongation of the systolic time interval, and reduction of the ejection fraction (as determined by echocardiography or radionuclide angiography), but none of these tests has been shown to consistently identify those patients who are approaching their maximally tolerated cumulative dose of doxorubicin. If these or other test results indicate changes in cardiac function associated with doxorubicin, the benefit of continued therapy must be carefully weighed against the risk of irreversible cardiac damage. Fatal cardiotoxicity can occur without antecedent ECG alterations.

Administration of low doses of doxorubicin at weekly intervals or administration of the drug by continuous IV infusion (e.g., over 48–96 hours) reportedly has reduced anthracycline-associated cardiotoxicity. Consideration also can be given to cardioprotectant therapy with dexrazoxane, which can reduce substantially but not eliminate fully, the risk of doxorubicin-induced cardiotoxicity. Because anthracycline-induced cardiotoxicity may develop long after discontinuance of therapy with the drug, periodic monitoring of cardiac function with evaluation of ejection fraction should be continued throughout the patient's lifetime.

Patients with a history of cardiovascular disease should receive doxorubicin only when the potential benefit outweighs the risk. Doxorubicin is contraindicated in patients with impaired cardiac function and in patients who have been treated previously with complete cumulative doses of doxorubicin, daunorubicin, and/or epirubicin. In patients who have received anthracyclines previously, addition of further anthracycline therapy can be contemplated *only* after careful assessment of the cardiac status of the patient with noninvasive and/or invasive procedures. However, it also should be considered that functional impairment can be masked by compensatory hypertrophy and patients with previous abnormal test results should still be considered at risk. The potential benefit of additional anthracycline therapy must be weighed carefully against the possible risks of cardiotoxicity associated with such therapy.

Hepatic Impairment

Prolonged and elevated plasma concentrations of doxorubicin and its metabolites in patients with impaired hepatic function have resulted in increased toxicity. Prior to each dose of doxorubicin, it is recommended that liver function tests be performed, including serum AST (SGOT), ALT (SGPT), alkaline phosphatase, and bilirubin concentrations. Dosage of doxorubicin hydrochloride should be reduced in patients with impaired hepatic function.

Advice to Patients

Conventional doxorubicin often imparts a red color to the urine for 1–2 days after administration, and patients should be advised to expect this effect during therapy.

Patients receiving pegylated liposomal doxorubicin should be informed to notify the clinician if they experience signs or symptoms of any of the expected adverse effects of the drug, including hand-foot syndrome (tingling or burning, redness, flaking, bothersome swelling, small blisters, or small sores on the palms of the hands or soles of the feet), stomatitis (painful redness, swelling, or sores in the mouth), fever of 100.5°F or higher, nausea, vomiting, tiredness, weakness,

rash, or mild hair loss. Patients should be informed that urine or other body fluids may appear reddish-orange in color during therapy with liposomal doxorubicin; this is a nontoxic reaction and the color will dissipate as the drug is eliminated from the body.

Other Precautions and Contraindications

Clearance of doxorubicin is reduced in obese women (actual body weight exceeding 130% of ideal body weight).

In addition to the usual precautions and contraindications associated with doxorubicin therapy, use of liposomal doxorubicin hydrochloride is contraindicated in patients who are hypersensitive to conventional doxorubicin preparations or to any component in the liposomal formulation.

● Pediatric Precautions

Cardiotoxicity

Doxorubicin-induced cardiomyopathy impairs myocardial growth as children mature. Therefore, pediatric patients appear to be at particular risk for developing delayed cardiac toxicity with the drug, with possible subsequent development of congestive heart failure during early adulthood.

Results of studies to date are inconclusive concerning the relative risk of children for developing acute or chronic anthracycline-induced cardiotoxicity. Children are at increased risk for developing late-onset anthracycline toxicity since such cardiotoxicity is expected to increase with the growing census of long-term survivors (e.g., survivors of childhood cancers). Children who have received doxorubicin therapy develop subclinical cardiac dysfunction including abnormal fractional shortening (FS) in 23% of patients and abnormal afterload and/or contractility in 65% of patients. Overt congestive heart failure has been reported in about 5% of patients during long-term follow-up with a median length of follow-up of 9 years; 5–10% develop overt congestive heart failure during long-term follow-up. This late cardiotoxicity may be dose related, and the rate of detection increases with increased duration of follow-up. Therefore, periodic long-term follow-up is recommended for children treated with doxorubicin. In children, deterioration in cardiac function during or after therapy with the drug is indicated by a decrease in fractional shortening (FS) that declines by an absolute value of 10 or more percentile units or to less than 29%, and by a decrease in left-ventricular ejection fraction (LVEF) of 10 percentile units or an LVEF less than 55%. Although monitoring the ejection fraction has not been shown to be predictive of impending maximal tolerance of the cumulative doxorubicin dose, the benefits of continued therapy with the drug should be weighed carefully against the risk of irreversible cardiotoxicity whenever test results indicate a deterioration in cardiac function.

Other Precautions

Doxorubicin, when administered as a component of intensive chemotherapy regimens in children, may contribute to prepubertal growth failure. Gonadal impairment, which usually is reversible, also may occur.

The use of doxorubicin or other topoisomerase II inhibitors in children is associated with increased risk of acute myelogenous leukemia and other secondary malignancies.

Caregivers of children receiving doxorubicin should be advised to take precautions (e.g., wearing latex gloves) to prevent contact with the patient's urine and other body fluids for at least 5 days after administration of doxorubicin.

The manufacturer states that safety and efficacy of pegylated liposomal doxorubicin hydrochloride in children have not been established.

● Geriatric Precautions

Safety and efficacy of liposomal doxorubicin in geriatric patients have not been specifically studied to date. In single-arm studies of pegylated liposomal doxorubicin for ovarian cancer, 29% of patients were 60–69 years of age, and 23% were 70 years of age or older. In the randomized trial of pegylated liposomal doxorubicin for ovarian cancer, 35% of patients were 65 years of age or older. No overall differences in efficacy or safety were observed between geriatric and younger patients.

● Mutagenicity and Carcinogenicity

Doxorubicin has been shown to be mutagenic and carcinogenic in experimental models. Secondary acute myeloid (myelogenous) leukemia, sometimes fatal, has been reported in adults and children receiving topoisomerase II inhibitors, including rare cases in patients receiving liposomal doxorubicin. The extent of increased risk of developing secondary malignancies associated with the use of doxorubicin has not been fully established. There was no evidence of mutagenic potential when Stealth® liposomes (see Chemistry and Stability: Chemistry) that were devoid of doxorubicin hydrochloride were tested in vitro in the Ames, mouse lymphoma, and chromosomal aberration assays or in vivo in the mammalian micronucleus assay.

● Pregnancy, Fertility, and Lactation

Pregnancy

Doxorubicin can cause fetal toxicity when administered to pregnant women, but potential benefits from use of the drug may be acceptable in certain conditions despite the possible risks to the fetus. The drug is embryotoxic and teratogenic in rats and embryotoxic and abortifacient in rabbits, and trace amounts of drug have been found in mouse fetuses and in one aborted human fetus following administration of conventional (nonencapsulated) doxorubicin. Liposomal doxorubicin is embryotoxic at doses of 1 mg/kg daily (about one-eighth the 50 mg/m² human dose on a mg/m² basis) in rats and is embryotoxic and abortifacient at doses of 0.5 mg/kg daily (about one-eighth the 50 mg/m² human dose on a mg/m² basis) in rabbits. Embryotoxicity consisted of increased embryo-fetal deaths and reduced live litter sizes.

There are no adequate and well-controlled studies to date using conventional or liposomal doxorubicin in pregnant women. Doxorubicin should be used during pregnancy only in life-threatening situations or for disease for which safer drugs cannot be used or are ineffective. When conventional or liposomal doxorubicin is used during pregnancy, or if the patient becomes pregnant while receiving the drug, the patient should be apprised of the potential hazard to the fetus. If a patient becomes pregnant during the first few months following liposomal doxorubicin therapy, the prolonged elimination half-life of the drug must be taken into account. Women of childbearing potential should be advised to avoid becoming pregnant during doxorubicin therapy.

Fertility

Information on whether conventional or liposomal doxorubicin affects fertility has not been evaluated adequately. Liposomal doxorubicin hydrochloride has been associated with mild to moderate ovarian and testicular atrophy in mice after a single 36-mg/kg dose (about 2 times the 50-mg/m² human dose on a mg/m² basis), decreased testicular weight and hypospermia in rats after repeated dosages of 0.25 mg/kg or more daily (about one-thirtieth of the 50-mg/m² human dosage on a mg/m² basis), and diffuse degeneration of the seminiferous tubules and marked decreases in spermatogenesis in dogs after repeated dosages of 1 mg/kg daily (about one-half the 50-mg/m² human dosage on a mg/m² basis).

Lactation

Conventional (nonencapsulated) doxorubicin is distributed into milk. It is not known whether liposomal doxorubicin is distributed into milk. Because of the potential for serious adverse reactions to doxorubicin in nursing infants, nursing should be discontinued during doxorubicin therapy. Liposomal doxorubicin is contraindicated in nursing women.

DRUG INTERACTIONS

Formal drug interaction studies employing liposomal doxorubicin have not been performed to date; therefore, pending further accumulation of data, drugs known to interact with conventional (nonencapsulated) doxorubicin should be considered to also interact with the liposomal formulation. In addition, although most patients who have received liposomal doxorubicin to date were receiving antiviral therapy concomitantly, the potential for interactions with these drugs has not been evaluated.

● Antineoplastic Agents

Doxorubicin has been used in combination with other antineoplastic agents. Although combination chemotherapy has been shown to be more effective than single-agent therapy in some types of neoplasms, the benefits and risks of such therapy have not been fully elucidated.

Compared with administration of doxorubicin followed by paclitaxel, initial administration of paclitaxel (by IV infusion over 24 hours) followed by

doxorubicin (administered over 48 hours) was shown to result in a decrease in doxorubicin clearance and an increase in the severity of neutropenia and stomatitis.

Doxorubicin may potentiate the toxicity of other antineoplastic therapies and vice versa. Doxorubicin reportedly has exacerbated cyclophosphamide-induced hemorrhagic cystitis and enhanced mercaptopurine-induced hepatotoxicity. Concomitant or previous administration with cyclophosphamide, irradiation of the cardiac region, daunorubicin, idarubicin, or mitoxantrone may potentiate the cardiotoxic effects of doxorubicin, and the maximum cumulative dose of doxorubicin should be reduced. (See Dosage and Administration: Dosage.) Combined therapy with other myelosuppressive agents may increase the severity of hematologic toxicity. Acute "recall" pneumonitis, occurring at variable times after local radiation therapy, has been reported in children receiving concomitant doxorubicin and dactinomycin. Seizures and/or coma have occurred in patients receiving doxorubicin and vincristine concomitantly. Seizures also have been reported in a patient receiving doxorubicin at 2–3 times the recommended dosage in combination with high-dose cyclophosphamide.

● Cyclosporine

The use of cyclosporine in combination with doxorubicin may result in an increase in the area under the plasma concentration-time curve for both doxorubicin and doxorubicinol, possibly due to a decrease in doxorubicin clearance and a decrease in the metabolism of doxorubicinol. Evidence suggests that concomitant use of cyclosporine may result in more severe and prolonged hematologic toxicity associated with doxorubicin. In addition, seizures and/or coma have occurred in patients receiving doxorubicin and cyclosporine concomitantly.

● Other Drugs

Some evidence suggests that doxorubicin-induced cardiotoxicity may be potentiated by concomitant use of calcium-channel blocking agents.

Exacerbation of doxorubicin-induced neutropenia and thrombocytopenia has been reported in patients with advanced malignancies receiving high doses of progesterone (up to 10 g IV over 24 hours) concomitantly with doxorubicin (60 mg/m² by IV bolus).

Phenobarbital has increased the elimination of doxorubicin, doxorubicin has decreased serum phenytoin concentrations, and streptozocin may inhibit hepatic metabolism of doxorubicin.

ACUTE TOXICITY

Overdosage with doxorubicin exacerbates known adverse effects of the drug, including mucositis, leukopenia, and thrombocytopenia.

Management of acute doxorubicin overdosage consists of hospitalization of the severely myelosuppressed patient, anti-infective therapy, platelet and granulocyte transfusions, and symptomatic treatment of mucositis. The use of hematopoietic growth factor (granulocyte colony-stimulating factor or granulocyte-macrophage colony-stimulating factor) to reduce the severity of myelosuppression may be considered.

PHARMACOLOGY

Doxorubicin hydrochloride is an antineoplastic antibiotic with pharmacologic actions similar to those of daunorubicin. Although the drug has anti-infective properties, its cytotoxicity precludes its use as an anti-infective agent. The precise and/or principal mechanism(s) of the antineoplastic action of doxorubicin is not fully understood. It appears that the cytotoxic effect of the drug results from a complex system of multiple modes of action related to free radical formation secondary to metabolic activation of the doxorubicin by electron reduction, intercalation of the drug into DNA, induction of DNA breaks and chromosomal aberrations, and alterations in cell membranes induced by the drug. Evidence from in vitro studies in cells treated with doxorubicin suggests that apoptosis (programmed cell death) also may be involved in the drug's mechanism of action. These and other mechanisms (chelation of metal ions to produce drug-metal complexes) also may contribute to the cardiotoxic effects of the drug. (See Cautions: Cardiac Effects.)

Doxorubicin undergoes enzymatic 1- and 2-electron reduction to the corresponding semiquinone and dihydroquinone. 7-Deoxyaglycones are formed enzymatically by 1-electron reduction, and the resulting semiquinone free radical reacts with oxygen to produce the hydroxyl radical in a cascade of reactions; this radical may lead to cell death by reacting with DNA, RNA, cell membranes, and proteins. The dihydroquinone that results from 2-electron reduction of doxorubicin also can be formed by the reaction of 2 semiquinones. In the presence of oxygen, dihydroquinone reacts to form hydrogen peroxide, and in its absence, loses its sugar and gives rise to the quinone methide, a monofunctional alkylating agent with low affinity for DNA. The contribution of dihydroquinone and the quinone methide to the cytotoxicity of doxorubicin is unclear. Experimental evidence indicates that doxorubicin forms a complex with DNA by intercalation between base pairs, causing inhibition of DNA synthesis and DNA-dependent RNA synthesis by the resulting template disordering and steric obstruction. Doxorubicin also inhibits protein synthesis. Doxorubicin is active throughout the cell cycle including the interphase.

Of the cell types tested in vitro, cardiac cells are the most sensitive to the effects of doxorubicin, followed by sarcoma and melanoma cells, normal muscle fibroblasts, and normal skin fibroblasts. Normal, rapidly proliferating tissues such as those of bone marrow, GI and oral mucosa, and hair follicles are also affected to varying degrees. Doxorubicin hydrochloride also has immunosuppressive activity.

PHARMACOKINETICS

Nonencapsulated (conventional) doxorubicin hydrochloride exhibits linear pharmacokinetics; PEG-stabilized liposomal doxorubicin hydrochloride also exhibits dose-proportional, linear pharmacokinetics over a dosage range of 10–20 mg/m². The pharmacokinetics of liposomally encapsulated doxorubicin at a dose of 50 mg/m² have been reported to be nonlinear. At a dose of 50 mg/m², a longer elimination half-life and lower clearance compared to those observed with a 20 mg/m² dose are expected, with greater-than-proportional increases in area under the plasma concentration-time curve. Encapsulation of doxorubicin hydrochloride in PEG-stabilized (Stealth®) liposomes substantially alters the pharmacokinetics of the drug relative to conventional IV formulations (i.e., nonencapsulated drug), with resultant decreased distribution into the peripheral compartment, increased distribution into Kaposi's lesions, and decreased plasma clearance. The pharmacokinetics of the drug encapsulated in PEG-stabilized liposomes have not been evaluated separately by gender, ethnic group, or hepatic or renal impairment. In the Pharmacokinetics section, liposomal doxorubicin hydrochloride was administered as the drug encapsulated in PEG-stabilized liposomes.

● Absorption

Nonencapsulated doxorubicin hydrochloride is not stable in gastric acid, and animal studies indicate that the drug undergoes little, if any, absorption from the GI tract. The drug is extremely irritating to tissues and, therefore, must be administered IV. Following IV infusion of a single 10- or 20-mg/m² dose of liposomal doxorubicin hydrochloride in patients with AIDS-related Kaposi's sarcoma, average peak plasma doxorubicin (mostly bound to liposomes) concentrations are 4.33 or 10.1 mcg/mL, respectively, following a 15-minute infusion and 4.12 or 8.34 mcg/mL, respectively, following a 30-minute infusion. Following IV infusion over 15 minutes of a 40-mg/m² dose of liposomal doxorubicin hydrochloride in adults with AIDS-related Kaposi's, peak plasma concentrations averaged 20.1 mcg/mL.

● Distribution

Doxorubicin administered as a conventional injection is widely distributed in the plasma and in tissues. As early as 30 seconds after IV administration, doxorubicin is present in the liver, lungs, heart, and kidneys. Doxorubicin is absorbed by cells and binds to cellular components, particularly to nucleic acids. The volume of distribution of doxorubicin hydrochloride administered IV as a conventional injection is about 700–1100 L/m². Nonencapsulated doxorubicin is approximately 50–85% bound to plasma proteins; the protein binding of liposomally encapsulated drug has not been determined.

Encapsulation in PEG-stabilized liposomes substantially slows the rate of distribution of doxorubicin into the extravascular space. As a result, the liposomally encapsulated drug does not distribute into plasma and tissues as widely as doxorubicin hydrochloride administered as the conventional injection; doxorubicin hydrochloride encapsulated in liposomes distributes mainly in intravascular fluid, whereas nonencapsulated drug distributes widely into extravascular fluids and tissues. Animal studies indicate that liposomally encapsulated doxorubicin hydrochloride distributes from blood vessels into tumors, and once distributed into the tissue compartment, the drug is released; the exact mechanism of drug release

from liposomal encapsulation is not known. The steady-state volume of distribution of doxorubicin following IV administration of a single 10–40-mg/m² dose of the drug as a PEG-stabilized liposomal for injection concentrate in patients with AIDS-related Kaposi's sarcoma ranges from 2.2–4.4 L/m².

Doxorubicin hydrochloride administered IV as the liposomally encapsulated drug distributes into Kaposi's sarcoma lesions to a greater extent than into healthy skin. Following IV administration of a single 20-mg/m² dose of liposomal doxorubicin hydrochloride, doxorubicin concentrations in Kaposi's sarcoma lesions were 19 (range: 3–53)-fold higher than those observed in healthy skin; however, blood concentrations in the lesions or in healthy skin were not considered. In addition, distribution of doxorubicin into Kaposi's sarcoma lesions following IV administration of liposomally encapsulated drug was 5.2–11.4 times greater than that following IV administration of comparable doses of a conventional (nonencapsulated) injection. The mechanism by which liposomal encapsulation enhances doxorubicin distribution into Kaposi's sarcoma lesions has not been elucidated fully, but similar PEG-stabilized liposomes containing colloidal gold as a marker have been shown to enter Kaposi's sarcoma-like lesions in animals. Extravasation of the liposomes also may occur by passage of the particles through endothelial cell gaps present in Kaposi's sarcoma. Once within the lesions, the drug presumably is released locally as the liposomes degrade and become permeable in situ.

Doxorubicin does not cross the blood-brain barrier or achieve a measurable concentration in the CSF.

Trace amounts of doxorubicin have been found in fetal mice whose mothers received the drug during pregnancy, and there are limited data to indicate that nonencapsulated doxorubicin crosses the human placenta. Nonencapsulated doxorubicin is distributed into milk, achieving concentrations that often exceed those in plasma; doxorubicinol (the major metabolite) also distributes into milk.

● Elimination

Plasma concentrations of nonencapsulated doxorubicin and its metabolites decline in a biphasic or triphasic manner. In the first phase of the triphasic model, nonencapsulated doxorubicin is rapidly metabolized, presumably by a first-pass effect through the liver. It appears that most of this metabolism is completed before the entire dose is administered. In the triphasic model, nonencapsulated doxorubicin and its metabolites are rapidly distributed into the extravascular compartment with a plasma half-life of approximately 0.2–0.6 hours for doxorubicin and 3.3 hours for its metabolites. This is followed by relatively prolonged plasma concentrations of doxorubicin and its metabolites, probably resulting from tissue binding. During the second phase, the plasma half-life of nonencapsulated doxorubicin is 16.7 hours and that of its metabolites is 31.7 hours. In the biphasic model, the initial distribution $t_{1/2}$ has been reported to average about 5–10 minutes, and the terminal elimination $t_{1/2}$ has been reported to average about 30 hours.

In patients with impaired hepatic function, particularly those who are hyperbilirubinemic, clearance of doxorubicin is reduced and plasma concentrations of both the drug and its metabolites are elevated; doxorubicin dosage must be reduced in patients with hepatic impairment. (See: Dosage and Administration: Dosage in Hepatic Impairment.)

Plasma clearance of nonencapsulated doxorubicin (when administered as a conventional injection) ranges from 8–20 mL/minute per kilogram (or 324–809 mL/minute per m²). Systemic clearance of doxorubicin is reduced in obese women (actual body weight exceeding 130% of ideal body weight). Clearance of doxorubicin was reduced without any change in volume of distribution in obese patients compared with patients with an actual body weight less than 115% of ideal body weight. Limited evidence suggests that the pharmacokinetics of nonencapsulated doxorubicin is influenced by gender. In a clinical study involving 6 men and 21 women with no history of prior anthracycline treatment, doxorubicin clearance was higher in men than in women (1883 versus 750 mL/min, respectively). However, the terminal elimination half-life of the drug was longer in men than in women (54 versus 35 hours, respectively).

The pharmacokinetics of nonencapsulated doxorubicin also appears to be influenced by age. In a pharmacokinetic study in 60 children and adolescents (aged 2 months to 20 years) receiving 10–75 mg/m² nonencapsulated doxorubicin, a mean clearance of 1443 mL/min per m² was reported. Further analysis indicated that doxorubicin clearance in 52 children older than 2 years of age (1540 mL/minute per m²) was increased compared with clearance reported for adults. In contrast, clearance of the drug in children younger than 2 years of age (813 mL/minute per m²) was decreased compared with that in older children and approached the range of clearance values reported for adults.

Plasma concentrations of liposomally encapsulated doxorubicin hydrochloride appear to decline in a biphasic manner. Following IV administration of a single 10- to 40-mg/m² dose of doxorubicin hydrochloride as a liposomal injection in patients with AIDS-related Kaposi's sarcoma, the initial plasma half-life ($t_{\frac{1}{2}\alpha}$) of doxorubicin averaged 3.76–5.2 hours while the terminal elimination half-life ($t_{\frac{1}{2}\beta}$) averaged 39.1–55 hours.

Plasma clearance of doxorubicin encapsulated in PEG-stabilized liposomes appears to be substantially slower than that of nonencapsulated doxorubicin. In adults with AIDS-related Kaposi's sarcoma, plasma clearance of PEG-stabilized liposomal doxorubicin hydrochloride following a single IV dose of 10–40 mg/m² averaged 0.57–1.8 mL/minute per m². This reduction in plasma clearance with liposomal doxorubicin results in a substantial increase in the area under the plasma concentration-time curve (AUC) compared with that of nonencapsulated drug.

Nonencapsulated doxorubicin is metabolized by NADPH-dependent aldoketoreductases to the hydrophilic 13-hydroxyl metabolite doxorubicinol, which exhibits antineoplastic activity and is the major metabolite; these reductases are present in most if not all cells, but particularly in erythrocytes, liver, and kidney. Although not clearly established, doxorubicinol also appears to be the moiety responsible for the cardiotoxic effects of the drug. Undetectable or low plasma concentrations (i.e., 0.8–26.2 ng/mL) of doxorubicinol have been reported following IV administration of a single 10- to 50-mg/m² dose of doxorubicin hydrochloride as a PEG-stabilized liposomal injection; it remains to be established whether such liposomally encapsulated anthracyclines are less cardiotoxic than conventional (nonencapsulated) drug, and the usual precautions for unencapsulated drug currently also should be observed for the liposomal preparation. (See Cautions: Cardiac Effects.) Substantially reduced or absent plasma concentrations of the usual major metabolite of doxorubicin observed with the PEG-stabilized liposomal injection suggests that either the drug is not released appreciably from the liposomes as they circulate or that some doxorubicin may be released but that the rate of doxorubicinol elimination greatly exceeds the release rate; doxorubicin hydrochloride encapsulated in liposomes that have not been PEG-stabilized is metabolized to doxorubicinol.

Other metabolites, which are therapeutically inactive, include the poorly water-soluble aglycones, doxorubicinone (adriamycinone) and 7-deoxydoxorubicinone (17-deoxyadriamycinone), and conjugates. The aglycones are formed in microsomes by NADPH-dependent, cytochrome reductase-mediated cleavage of the amino sugar moiety. The enzymatic reduction of doxorubicin to 7-deoxyaglycones is important to the cytotoxic effect of the drug since it results in hydroxyl radicals that cause extensive cell damage and death. (See Pharmacology.) With nonencapsulated doxorubicin, more than 20% of the total drug in plasma is present as metabolites as soon as 5 minutes after a dose, 70% in 30 minutes, 75% in 4 hours, and 90% in 24 hours.

Nonencapsulated doxorubicin and its metabolites are excreted predominantly in bile; about 10–20% of a single dose is excreted in feces in 24 hours, and 40–50% of a dose is excreted in bile or feces within 7 days. About 50% of the drug in bile is unchanged drug, 23% is doxorubicinol, and the remainder is other metabolites including aglycones and conjugates. About 4–5% (range: 0.7–23%) of the administered dose is excreted in urine after 5 days, principally as unchanged doxorubicin. It appears that very little further urinary excretion of the drug occurs after 5 days. Although only small urinary concentrations of the drug usually are achieved, doxorubicin often imparts a red color to the urine for the first hours to days after administration, and patients should be advised to expect this effect during therapy.

CHEMISTRY AND STABILITY

● Chemistry

Doxorubicin is an anthracycline glycoside antibiotic produced by *Streptomyces peucetius* var. *caesius*. The drug is structurally related to daunorubicin and epirubicin. Doxorubicin differs structurally from daunorubicin in that doxorubicin contains a hydroxyacetyl group instead of an acetyl group in the 8-position. Epirubicin is the 4'-epimer of doxorubicin.

Doxorubicin is commercially available as the hydrochloride salt. Commercially available doxorubicin hydrochloride powder for injection occurs as a sterile, lyophilized, crystalline, red-orange or red powder; the powder for injection also may contain lactose and methylparaben to enhance dissolution. Doxorubicin

hydrochloride is freely soluble in water, slightly soluble in 0.9% sodium chloride solution, and very slightly soluble in alcohol. When doxorubicin hydrochloride powder for injection is reconstituted with 0.9% sodium chloride injection, the pH of the resulting solution is 3.8–6.5.

Doxorubicin hydrochloride also is commercially available as a sterile, isotonic, aqueous solution of the drug. Hydrochloric acid is added during manufacture of the injection to adjust the pH to approximately 3 (range: 2.5–3.5); the injection also contains 0.9% sodium chloride.

As an injection, doxorubicin hydrochloride also is available in a liposomal formulation. In the liposomal doxorubicin hydrochloride for injection concentrate, an aqueous core of doxorubicin hydrochloride is encapsulated in Stealth® liposomes; approximately 90% of the drug present in the commercially available liposomal doxorubicin hydrochloride is encapsulated. Liposomes are microscopic vesicles composed of a phospholipid bilayer that is capable of encapsulating drugs; the lipid bilayer separates the internal aqueous core, which for doxorubicin hydrochloride liposomal for injection concentrate contains the drug, from the external environment. Stealth® liposomes, which contain hydrogenated soy phosphatidylcholine (HSPC) and cholesterol in the phospholipid bilayer, are formulated with methoxypolyethylene glycol (MPEG, a hydrophilic polymer) combined with distearoyl-*sn*-glycerophosphoethanolamine (DSPE) on their surface (combined as MPEG-DSPE). Formulating the liposomes with surface-bound MPEG has been referred to as "pegylation," and the resulting polymer coating protects the liposomes from opsonization by plasma proteins and subsequent detection as a foreign protein by the mononuclear phagocyte system (MPS) and rapid clearance from circulation (e.g., by fixed macrophages in the liver and spleen); as a result, the blood circulation time of the liposomes is prolonged. The Stealth® liposomes also have been referred to as PEG-stabilized; the MPEG groups extend 5 nm from the liposome surface creating a protective wall that inhibits interaction between the lipid bilayer membrane and plasma components. It has been suggested that liposomes can penetrate the altered and often compromised vasculature of tumors because of their small size (about 100 nm) and persistence in the blood circulation. Doxorubicin hydrochloride liposomal for injection concentrate is a sterile, translucent red liposomal dispersion. Hydrochloric acid and/or sodium hydroxide is added during manufacture of the for injection concentrate to adjust the pH to approximately 6.5. Doxorubicin hydrochloride liposomal for injection concentrate also contains sucrose for isotonicity, histidine as a buffer, and ammonium sulfate. During manufacturing, inclusion of sucrose in the external phase and ammonium sulfate in the internal phase creates the chemical gradient needed for promoting diffusion of doxorubicin hydrochloride from the external phase into the aqueous core of the liposomes.

● Stability

Commercially available doxorubicin hydrochloride lyophilized powder for injection should be stored in a dry place protected from sunlight. When stored at 15–30°C, Adriamycin RDF® or Rubex® has an expiration date of 3 or 2 years, respectively, following the date of manufacture. Doxorubicin hydrochloride conventional (nonencapsulated) injection should be protected from light and refrigerated at 2–8°C; when stored under these conditions, the injection is stable for 18 months.

Solutions of doxorubicin hydrochloride should be protected from exposure to sunlight. When reconstituted as directed, solutions prepared from the single-dose or multiple-dose vial of the powder for injection can be stored for up to 7 days at room temperature and under normal room light (100 foot-candles) or for up to 15 days when refrigerated at 2–8°C; unused portions should be discarded after these storage periods. Doxorubicin hydrochloride is unstable in solutions with a pH less than 3 or greater than 7. Acids split the glycosidic bond in doxorubicin, yielding a red-colored, water insoluble aglycone (doxorubicinone, also known as adriamycinone) and a water soluble, reducing amino sugar (daunosamine). Doxorubicin hydrochloride solution is chemically incompatible with heparin sodium injection, and a precipitate may form if the solutions are mixed. Doxorubicin hydrochloride solution also is reportedly incompatible with fluorouracil, and a precipitate may form if the solutions are mixed. The manufacturers recommend that doxorubicin hydrochloride solutions or doxorubicin liposomal dispersion generally *not* be mixed with other drugs; specialized references should be consulted for specific compatibility information.

Commercially available doxorubicin hydrochloride liposomal for injection concentrate should be refrigerated at 2–8°C and protected from freezing. The manufacturer states that prolonged freezing may adversely affect stability of liposomal doxorubicin hydrochloride; however, short-term freezing (less than 1 month) does not appear to affect stability of liposomal doxorubicin hydrochloride. During shipping, vials of doxorubicin hydrochloride for injection concentrate are packaged with a gel refrigerant ("blue ice") to maintain a temperature of 2–8°C. When diluted as directed with 5% dextrose injection, solutions of liposomal doxorubicin hydrochloride are stable for 24 hours when refrigerated at 2–8°C.

For further information on the handling of antineoplastic agents, see the ASHP Guidelines on Handling Hazardous Drugs at http://www.ahfsdruginformation.com.

PREPARATIONS

Excipients in commercially available drug preparations may have clinically important effects in some individuals; consult specific product labeling for details.

DOXOrubicin Hydrochloride

Parenteral

For injection, for IV use only	10 mg*	**Adriamycin®**, Bedford
		Adriamycin RDF®, Pfizer
		Doxorubicin Hydrochloride for Injection
	20 mg*	**Adriamycin®**, Bedford
		Adriamycin RDF®, Pfizer
		Doxorubicin Hydrochloride for Injection
	50 mg*	**Adriamycin®**, Bedford
		Adriamycin RDF®, Pfizer
		Doxorubicin Hydrochloride for Injection
		Rubex®, Bristol-Myers Squibb
	100 mg	**Rubex®**, Bristol-Myers Squibb
	150 mg	**Adriamycin RDF®**, Pfizer
Injection, for IV use only	2 mg/mL (10, 20, 50, 75, 150, and 200 mg)*	**Adriamycin®**, Bedford
		Adriamycin PFS® (available in Cytosafe® and glass vials), Pfizer
		Doxorubicin Hydrochloride Injection (available in polymer vials)

* available from one or more manufacturer, distributor, and/or repackager by generic (nonproprietary) name

DOXOrubicin Hydrochloride Liposomal

Parenteral

For injection concentrate, for IV infusion only	2 mg/mL (20 and 50 mg)	**Doxil®**, Janssen Therapeutics (formerly Tibotec Therapeutics)

† Use is not currently included in the labeling approved by the US Food and Drug Administration.

Selected Revisions August 6, 2018, © Copyright, October 1, 1975, American Society of Health-System Pharmacists, Inc.

Enasidenib Mesylate

10:00 • ANTINEOPLASTIC AGENTS

■ Enasidenib, a potent and selective inhibitor of isocitrate dehydrogenase-2 (IDH2), is an antineoplastic agent.

USES

● Acute Myeloid Leukemia

Enasidenib mesylate is used for the treatment of adults with relapsed or refractory acute myeloid leukemia (AML) with isocitrate dehydrogenase-2 (IDH2) mutation. Enasidenib has been designated an orphan drug by FDA for the treatment of this cancer. An FDA-approved diagnostic test (e.g., Abbott RealTime® IDH2 assay) is required to confirm the presence of IDH2 mutation (peripheral blood or bone marrow) prior to initiation of therapy.

Clinical Experience

Efficacy and safety of enasidenib in the treatment of AML are based principally on the results of an open-label, multicenter, 2-cohort, single-arm study (AG221-C-001) in adults with relapsed or refractory AML with IDH2 mutation as detected by the Abbott RealTime® IDH2 mutation test. The primary measures of efficacy were CR and CRh, duration of response, and loss of transfusion dependence (red blood cells [RBCs] and/or platelets). CR was defined as the presence of less than 5% blasts in bone marrow without evidence of disease and with full recovery of peripheral blood cell counts (platelet count exceeding 100,000/mm³ and absolute neutrophil count [ANC] exceeding 1000/mm³), and CRh was defined as the presence of less than 5% blasts in bone marrow without evidence of disease and with partial recovery of peripheral blood cell counts (platelet count exceeding 50,000/mm³ and ANC exceeding 500/mm³). Overall, the median age of patients was 68 years (range: 19–100 years); 77% were Caucasian, 62% were ≥65 years of age, 52% were male, 62% had an Eastern Cooperative Oncology Group (ECOG) performance status of 1, 52% had refractory AML, 49% had intermediate-risk cytogenetics, 27% had poor-risk cytogenetics, 79% were transfusion dependent at baseline, and 13% had previously undergone stem cell transplantation. Patients enrolled in this study had received a median of 2 prior antineoplastic chemotherapy regimens. IDH2 mutations at codon R140 or R172 were present in 78 or 22% of patients, respectively; mutations detected in peripheral blood were reported if bone marrow and peripheral blood mutations were inconsistent. In this study, 199 adults received an enasidenib dosage of 100 mg orally once daily. Therapy was continued until disease progression or unacceptable toxicity occurred. At a median follow-up of 6.6 months, CR or CRh was achieved in 23% of patients with a median response duration of 8.2 months; 19% of patients achieved CR. The median time to initial CR or CRh was 1.9 months. The median time to best response (CR or CRh) was 3.7 months; the majority (85%) of these patients achieved a best response within 6 months of initiating enasidenib therapy. Approximately one-third (34%) of patients who were transfusion dependent at baseline became transfusion independent during any 56-day period during the study. The majority (76%) of patients who were transfusion independent at baseline remained transfusion independent during any 56-day period during the study.

Clinical Perspective

International experts recommend allogeneic hematopoietic stem cell transplantation in the first-line setting for all patients with primary refractory AML who are candidates for intensive chemotherapy. Patients with relapsed AML who are candidates for intensive chemotherapy should receive salvage chemotherapy followed by allogeneic hematopoietic stem cell transplantation. For patients who are not candidates for intensive chemotherapy, these experts state that such patients may be offered hypomethylating agents or low-dose cytarabine (in combination with venetoclax, if available); gilteritinib (if FLT3-ITD/FLT3-TKD mutation- positive); ivosidenib or enasidenib (if IDH1/2 mutation-positive); melphalan; or best supportive care.

DOSAGE AND ADMINISTRATION

● General

Pretreatment Screening

- Confirm presence of IDH2 mutation (peripheral blood or bone marrow) prior to initiation of therapy.
- Assess complete blood count (CBC) and blood chemistries for leukocytosis and tumor lysis syndrome prior to initiation of therapy.
- Verify pregnancy status in females of reproductive potential prior to initiation of therapy.

Patient Monitoring

- Monitor CBC and blood chemistries at least every 2 weeks for at least the initial 3 months of therapy.
- Monitor for signs and symptoms of differentiation syndrome (e.g., fever, dyspnea, acute respiratory distress, pulmonary infiltrates, pleural or pericardial effusion, rapid weight gain, peripheral edema, lymphadenopathy, bone pain, and hepatic, renal, or multiorgan dysfunction).

● Administration

Enasidenib is administered orally without regard to meals. The drug should be taken at approximately the same time each day. The tablets should be swallowed whole with a glass of water; they should *not* be chewed, crushed, or split.

If a dose is vomited, missed, or not taken at the usual time, administer the dose as soon as possible on the same day, and then return to the normal schedule the following day. Do not take 2 doses to make up for a missed dose.

Store enasidenib tablets in the original container with the desiccant at 20–25°C (excursions permitted between 15–30°C).

● Dosage

Dosage of enasidenib mesylate is expressed in terms of enasidenib.

Acute Myeloid Leukemia

For the treatment of relapsed or refractory acute myeloid leukemia (AML) with IDH2 mutation, the recommended adult dosage of enasidenib is 100 mg once daily. Therapy should be continued until disease progression or unacceptable toxicity occurs. In the principal efficacy study, most patients achieved best response within 6 months of initiating enasidenib; therefore, the manufacturer states that therapy should be continued for at least 6 months to allow time for response.

In patients who present with leukocytosis (leukocyte counts exceeding 30,000/ mm³) in the absence of infection, hydroxyurea therapy should be initiated according to standard practices. If leukocytosis persists, temporary interruption of enasidenib therapy may be necessary.

Dosage Modification for Toxicity

Differentiation Syndrome

If severe pulmonary symptoms requiring respiratory support (i.e., intubation, assisted respiration) occur and/or renal dysfunction persists for more than 48 hours despite systemic corticosteroid therapy, enasidenib should be withheld until the toxicity improves to grade 2 or less.

Noninfectious Leukocytosis

If leukocytosis persists despite hydroxyurea therapy, enasidenib therapy should be withheld until leukocyte counts decrease to less than 30,000/mm³; therapy may then be resumed at the initial dosage (100 mg daily).

Hepatotoxicity

In patients who exhibit increases in serum bilirubin concentrations exceeding 3 times the upper limit of normal (ULN) for 2 weeks or more (in the absence of elevated aminotransferase [ALT/AST] concentrations or other hepatic disorders), enasidenib therapy may be continued at a reduced dosage of 50 mg daily. When serum bilirubin concentrations improve to less than 2 times the ULN, the dosage of enasidenib should be re-escalated to 100 mg daily.

Tumor Lysis Syndrome

In patients who develop grade 3 or greater tumor lysis syndrome, therapy with enasidenib should be withheld. When tumor lysis syndrome improves to grade 2 or less, enasidenib may be resumed at a reduced dosage of 50 mg daily; the dosage of enasidenib may be re-escalated to 100 mg daily when tumor lysis syndrome improves to grade 1 or less.

If grade 3 or greater tumor lysis syndrome recurs, enasidenib therapy should be discontinued.

Other Toxicity

If a grade 3 or greater adverse reaction occurs, therapy with enasidenib should be withheld. When the toxicity improves to grade 2 or less, enasidenib may be resumed at a reduced dosage of 50 mg daily; the dosage of enasidenib may be re-escalated to 100 mg daily when the toxicity improves to grade 1 or less.

If the grade 3 or greater adverse reaction recurs, enasidenib therapy should be discontinued.

● Special Populations

Hepatic Impairment

No dosage adjustment is necessary in patients with mild hepatic impairment (total bilirubin concentration not exceeding the ULN with AST concentration exceeding the ULN *or* total bilirubin concentration 1–1.5 times the ULN with any AST concentration).

Renal Impairment

No dosage adjustment is necessary in patients with renal impairment.

Geriatric Patients

No dosage adjustment is necessary in geriatric patients.

CAUTIONS

● Contraindications

● None.

● Warnings/Precautions

Warnings

Differentiation Syndrome

A boxed warning regarding the risk of differentiation syndrome is included in the prescribing information for enasidenib. Differentiation syndrome, which may be life-threatening or fatal, occurred in 14% of patients receiving enasidenib in the principal efficacy study; approximately one-half of these patients continued therapy without interruption. In a subsequent analysis of the principal efficacy study, the incidence of differentiation syndrome with enasidenib may have been as high as 19%, with 5% of cases resulting in fatality. Differentiation syndrome following therapy with an isocitrate dehydrogenase-2 (IDH2) inhibitor, including enasidenib, is associated with rapid proliferation and differentiation of myeloid cells. Differentiation syndrome has been characterized by acute respiratory distress (dyspnea and/or hypoxia), hypoxia requiring supplemental oxygen, pulmonary infiltrates, renal or hepatic impairment, multiorgan dysfunction, pyrexia, lymphadenopathy, bone pain, peripheral edema, rapid weight gain, rash, and pleural or pericardial effusions in patients receiving enasidenib. Differentiation syndrome has been observed with or without concomitant leukocytosis as early as 1 day or up to 5 months after initiation of enasidenib.

The risk of developing differentiation syndrome associated with IDH2 inhibitor therapy is increased in patients with bone marrow blast counts exceeding 20% and those who have received fewer prior antileukemic therapies. High peripheral blast counts and high serum concentrations of LDH are less predictive of the development of differentiation syndrome associated with IDH2 inhibitor therapy than they are of the development of acute promyelocytic leukemia (APL) differentiation syndrome (also known as retinoic acid-APL [RA-APL] syndrome).

Early recognition and treatment of differentiation syndrome lessens the likelihood of severe illness and death. Manifestations of differentiation syndrome may

be clinically indistinguishable from manifestations of disease progression or other acute comorbidities; therefore, differentiation syndrome should be suspected if there is no clear alternate etiology. If signs or symptoms suggestive of differentiation syndrome occur, IV or oral corticosteroid therapy (e.g., dexamethasone 10 mg every 12 hours) should be initiated and hemodynamic parameters should be monitored until symptoms improve. Because enasidenib has a long half-life, signs or symptoms of differentiation syndrome may recur if systemic corticosteroid therapy is discontinued prematurely; therefore, corticosteroid therapy should be continued until symptoms resolve followed by tapering of the corticosteroid dosage. If severe pulmonary symptoms requiring respiratory support (i.e., intubation, assisted respiration) occur and/or renal dysfunction persists for more than 48 hours despite corticosteroid therapy, enasidenib should be temporarily interrupted until symptoms improve. The manufacturer recommends close monitoring in a hospital setting in patients with pulmonary and/or renal manifestations of differentiation syndrome.

Other Warnings and Precautions

Fetal/Neonatal Morbidity and Mortality

Enasidenib may cause fetal harm in humans based on animal findings; the drug has been shown to be teratogenic, embryotoxic, and fetotoxic in animals. There are no available data regarding the risk of enasidenib use in pregnant patients to date. In animal reproduction studies, postimplantation loss, increased rate of resorption, decreased fetal body weight, and skeletal anomalies were observed in rats receiving enasidenib at a maternally toxic dosage (exposure level equivalent to approximately 1.6 times the human exposure at the recommended human dosage). The drug also was abortifacient in rabbits receiving enasidenib at exposure levels below the human exposure at the recommended dosage.

Pregnancy should be avoided during enasidenib therapy. Females of reproductive potential and males who are partners of such females should use adequate methods of contraception while receiving the drug and for 2 months after the drug is discontinued. Patients using hormonal contraceptives should be advised to use an effective non-hormonal contraceptive method during treatment with enasidenib and for 2 months after the final dose.

Specific Populations

Pregnancy

Enasidenib may cause fetal harm if administered to pregnant patients based on animal findings.

Pregnancy status should be confirmed prior to initiation of enasidenib therapy. If enasidenib is used during pregnancy or if the patient or their partner becomes pregnant during therapy, the patient should be informed of the potential fetal hazard.

Lactation

It is not known whether enasidenib or its metabolites are distributed into human milk. Because of the potential for serious adverse reactions to enasidenib in nursing infants, women should be advised to discontinue nursing during enasidenib therapy. Women may begin nursing 2 months after discontinuance of therapy. The effects of the drug on nursing infants or on the production of milk are unknown.

Females and Males of Reproductive Potential

Pregnancy status should be confirmed prior to initiation of enasidenib therapy. Females of reproductive potential and males who are partners of such females should use adequate methods of contraception while receiving the drug and for 2 months after the drug is discontinued. Patients using hormonal contraceptives should be advised to use an effective non-hormonal contraceptive method during treatment with enasidenib and for 2 months after the final dose.

Results of toxicity studies in animals suggest that enasidenib may impair female and male fertility. In a general toxicology study, decreased corpora lutea, uterine degeneration, and increased ovarian atretic follicles were observed in female animals and seminiferous tubular degeneration, seminal vesicle and prostate atrophy, and hypospermia were observed in male animals receiving enasidenib twice daily for up to 90 days; reversibility of these changes is unknown.

Pediatric Use

Safety and efficacy of enasidenib have not been established in pediatric patients.

Geriatric Use

In the principal efficacy study, 61% of patients receiving enasidenib were ≥65 years of age and 24% were ≥75 years of age. No overall differences in safety and efficacy were observed between these geriatric patients and younger adults.

In a pharmacokinetic population analysis, age (range of 19–100 years) did not have a substantial effect on the pharmacokinetics of enasidenib.

Hepatic Impairment

In a population pharmacokinetic analysis, mild hepatic impairment (total bilirubin concentration not exceeding the upper limit of normal [ULN] with AST concentration exceeding the ULN or total bilirubin concentration 1–1.5 times the ULN with any AST concentration) did not have a substantial effect on the systemic exposure of enasidenib. However, since enasidenib is eliminated principally by hepatic metabolism, hepatic impairment may result in increased exposure to the drug and increased potential for adverse reactions.

Renal Impairment

Enasidenib undergoes minimal renal elimination.

In a population pharmacokinetic analysis, renal impairment (estimated glomerular filtration rate [GFR] of 30 mL/minute or more) did not have a substantial effect on the systemic exposure of enasidenib.

● Common Adverse Effects

Adverse effects reported in ≥20% of patients receiving enasidenib in clinical studies include nausea, vomiting, diarrhea, elevated bilirubin, and decreased appetite.

DRUG INTERACTIONS

Metabolism of enasidenib to the active AGI-16903 metabolite is mediated by cytochrome P-450 (CYP) isoenzymes 1A2, 2B6, 2C8, 2C9, 2C19, 2D6, and 3A4 and by uridine diphosphate-glucuronosyl transferases (UGT) 1A1, 1A3, 1A4, 1A9, 2B7, and 2B15. AGI-16903 is subsequently metabolized by CYP isoenzymes 1A2, 2C19, and 3A4 and by UGT1A1, 1A3, and 1A9.

In vitro, enasidenib inhibits CYP isoenzymes 1A2, 2B6, 2C8, 2C9, 2C19, 2D6, and 3A4; enasidenib also inhibits UGT1A1. In vitro, AGI-16903 inhibits CYP isoenzymes 1A2, 2B6, 2C8, 2C9, 2C19, and 2D6. In vitro studies show that enasidenib induces CYP isoenzymes 2B6 and 3A4.

In vitro studies indicate that enasidenib inhibits P-glycoprotein (P-gp), breast cancer resistance protein (BCRP), organic anion transporter (OAT) 1, organic anion transport protein (OATP) 1B1, OATP1B3, and organic cation transporter (OCT) 2, but does not inhibit multidrug resistance protein 2 (MRP2) or OAT3. In vitro, AGI-16903 inhibits BCRP, OAT1, OAT3, OATP1B1, and OCT2, but does not inhibit P-gp, MRP2, or OATP1B3. In vitro, AGI-16903 is a substrate of efflux transporters P-gp and BCRP; enasidenib is not a substrate of these transporters. Neither enasidenib nor AGI-16903 is a substrate of MRP2, OATP1B1, OATP1B3, OAT1, OAT3, or OCT2.

● Drugs Affecting or Affected by Hepatic Microsomal Enzymes

Substrates of CYP1A2 and CYP2C19

Concomitant use of enasidenib with certain substrates of CYP1A2 and CYP2C19 may increase systemic exposure to the substrate drug and increase the risk of adverse reactions to the drug. When a CYP1A2 substrate (caffeine 100 mg) was administered concomitantly with enasidenib, peak plasma concentrations of caffeine were increased by 18%, and systemic exposure to caffeine was increased by 655%. When a CYP2C19 substrate (omeprazole 40 mg) was administered concomitantly with enasidenib, peak plasma concentrations of omeprazole were increased by 47%, and systemic exposure to omeprazole increased by 86%.

Avoid concomitant use with enasidenib unless otherwise recommended in the prescribing information for CYP1A2 or CYP2C19 substrates where minimal concentration changes may lead to serious adverse reactions. For caffeine, consider reducing the frequency of caffeine intake in a 24 hour period while taking enasidenib as the drug may increase caffeine-related effects in sensitive individuals.

Substrates of CYP3A

Concomitant use of enasidenib with certain substrates of CYP3A may decrease systemic exposure to the substrate drug and reduce the efficacy of the drug. When a CYP3A substrate (midazolam 0.3 mg/kg IV) was administered concomitantly with enasidenib, peak plasma concentrations of midazolam were reduced by 23%, and systemic exposure to midazolam was reduced by 43%. The decrease in midazolam exposure following oral administration is expected to be even larger than that following IV administration.

Avoid concomitant use with enasidenib unless otherwise recommended in the prescribing information for CYP3A substrates where minimal concentration changes may lead to reduced efficacy. Antifungal agents that are CYP3A substrates should *not* be administered with enasidenib. Concomitant administration of enasidenib with hormonal contraceptives may reduce plasma concentrations of the hormonal contraceptive; patients should consider alternative methods of contraception if receiving enasidenib.

● Substrates of Transport Systems

Substrates of OATP1B1, OATP1B3, and BCRP

Concomitant use of enasidenib with substrates of OATP1B1, OATP1B3, and BCRP may increase systemic exposure to the substrate drug and increase the risk of adverse reactions to the drug. When such a substrate drug (rosuvastatin 10 mg) was administered concomitantly with enasidenib, peak plasma concentrations of rosuvastatin were increased by 366%, and systemic exposure to rosuvastatin was increased by 244%. Avoid coadministration of enasidenib with OATP1B1, OATP1B3, and BCRP substrates, for which minimal concentration changes may lead to serious toxicities. If concomitant use of enasidenib with a OATP1B1, OATP1B3, and BCRP substrate is necessary, the dosage of the substrate drug should be reduced in accordance with the respective prescribing information.

Substrates of P-gp

Concomitant use of enasidenib with substrates of P-gp may increase systemic exposure to the substrate drug and increase the risk of adverse reactions of the drug. When a P-gp substrate (digoxin 0.25 mg) was administered concomitantly with enasidenib, peak plasma concentrations of digoxin were increased by 26%, and systemic exposure to digoxin was increased by 20%. If concomitant use of enasidenib with a sensitive P-gp substrate is necessary, follow recommendations within the P-gp substrate prescribing information and monitor more frequently for adverse reactions.

DESCRIPTION

Enasidenib, a potent and selective inhibitor of isocitrate dehydrogenase-2 (IDH2), is an antineoplastic agent. Isocitrate dehydrogenases (IDH) are metabolic enzymes in the citric acid cycle responsible for the oxidative decarboxylation of isocitrate to α-ketoglutarate, which is essential for normal cellular processes. Approximately 15–20% of acute myeloid leukemia (AML) cases carry IDH2 mutations. The most common IDH2 mutation is a point mutation at codon R140Q; a less frequently occurring IDH2 mutation is a point mutation at codon R172K. IDH2 mutations cause a reduction of α-ketoglutarate to the oncometabolite 2-hydroxyglutarate, which competitively inhibits α-ketoglutarate-dependent dioxygenases resulting in epigenetic dysregulation and subsequent histone and DNA hypermethylation and differentiation arrest of hematopoietic stem cells. In vitro studies indicate that enasidenib inhibits IDH2 with R140Q, R172S, or R172K mutation at approximately 40-fold lower concentrations than IDH2 wild-type enzymes. Enasidenib has demonstrated decreased 2-hydroxyglutarate levels and induction of myeloid cell differentiation in vitro and in mice bearing tumor xenografts that expressed IDH2 mutation. Enasidenib also has demonstrated decreased 2-hydroxyglutarate levels, reduced blast cell counts, and increased percentages of mature myeloid cells in patients with AML that expressed IDH2 mutation. In the phase 1/2 study evaluating enasidenib in patients with relapsed or refractory AML, mature granulocytes retained baseline IDH2 mutations and cytogenetic abnormalities in patients who achieved remission, indicating continued differentiation of abnormal myeloblast cells into mature granulocytes.

Following oral administration of enasidenib, the absolute bioavailability of the drug is 57%. Area under the serum concentration-time curve (AUC) of enasidenib is dose proportional over the enasidenib dosage range of 50–450 mg daily.

Following oral administration of a single dose, median time to peak plasma concentrations of enasidenib is 4 hours. Repeated administration of enasidenib resulted in an approximately tenfold mean enasidenib accumulation ratio. Steady-state concentrations are reached within 29 days. Systemic exposure of enasidenib was increased by 50% when enasidenib was administered with a high-fat meal; however, this effect is not considered clinically important. Enasidenib is metabolized to the active AGI-16903 metabolite by cytochrome P-450 (CYP) isoenzymes 1A2, 2B6, 2C8, 2C9, 2C19, 2D6, and 3A4 and by uridine diphosphate-glucuronosyl transferases (UGT) 1A1, 1A3, 1A4, 1A9, 2B7, and 2B15. AGI-16903 is subsequently metabolized by CYP isoenzymes 1A2, 2C19, and 3A4 and by UGT1A1, 1A3, and 1A9. Enasidenib and AGI-16903 are highly bound (98.5 and 96.6%, respectively) to plasma proteins. The terminal half-life of enasidenib is 7.9 days. Following administration of a radiolabeled dose of enasidenib, 89% of the radioactivity was recovered in feces (34% of the dose as unchanged drug) and 11% was recovered in urine (0.4% of the dose as unchanged drug).

The pharmacokinetics of enasidenib do not appear to be affected substantially by age (19–100 years), gender, race, body weight (39–136 kg), or body surface area.

ADVICE TO PATIENTS

- Advise patients to swallow enasidenib tablets whole with a full glass of water and *not* to chew, crush, or split the tablets.

- Advise patients to take enasidenib as directed by their clinician and at approximately the same time each day. If a dose is missed, administer the missed dose on the same day as soon as it is remembered. Advise patients not to take 2 doses on the same day to make up for a missed dose.

- Risk of developing differentiation syndrome. Advise patients to immediately report possible symptoms of differentiation syndrome (e.g., pyrexia, cough, difficulty breathing, bone pain, rapid weight gain, peripheral edema) to their clinician.

- Risk of tumor lysis syndrome. Importance of monitoring blood chemistry and maintaining adequate hydration during enasidenib therapy.

- Risk of diarrhea, nausea, vomiting, decreased appetite, and taste changes. Importance of contacting clinician if any of these adverse reactions occur.

- Risk of elevated serum bilirubin concentrations. Importance of contacting clinician if jaundice occurs.

- Risk of fetal harm. Advise females of reproductive potential and males who are partners of such females that they should use adequate methods of contraception while receiving the drug and for 2 months after the drug is discontinued. Advise females of reproductive potential to use an effective non-hormonal contraceptive method while receiving the drug and for 2 months after the last dose. Importance of patients informing their clinicians if they or their partners are pregnant or think they may be pregnant. If pregnancy occurs, advise patient of potential risk to fetus.

- Advise females to discontinue nursing during therapy and for 2 months after discontinuance of the drug.

- Importance of informing clinicians of existing or contemplated concomitant therapy, including prescription and OTC drugs (e.g,. combination hormonal contraceptives) and dietary or herbal supplements, as well as any concomitant illnesses.

- Inform patients of other important precautionary information.

For further information on the handling of antineoplastic agents, see the ASHP Guidelines on Handling Hazardous Drugs at https://www.ahfsdrug information.com.

PREPARATIONS

Enasidenib mesylate can only be obtained through select specialty pharmacies and distributors. Consult manufacturer's website for specific availability information.

Excipients in commercially available drug preparations may have clinically important effects in some individuals; consult specific product labeling for details.

Enasidenib Mesylate

Oral

Tablets, film-coated	50 mg (of enasidenib)	Idhifa®, Celgene
	100 mg (of enasidenib)	Idhifa®, Celgene

† Use is not currently included in the labeling approved by the US Food and Drug Administration.

Encorafenib

10:00 • ANTINEOPLASTIC AGENTS

■ Encorafenib, an inhibitor of b-Raf serine-threonine kinase (BRAF) V600E or V600K mutation, is an antineoplastic agent.

USES

● Melanoma

Encorafenib is used in combination with binimetinib for the treatment of unresectable or metastatic melanoma with b-Raf serine-threonine kinase (BRAF) V600E or V600K mutation. Encorafenib has been designated an orphan drug by FDA for the treatment of this cancer. An FDA-approved diagnostic test (e.g., bioMerieux THxID® BRAF V600 mutation test) is required to confirm the presence of the BRAF V600E or V600K mutation prior to initiation of therapy. In patients with unresectable or metastatic melanoma with BRAF V600E or V600K mutation, combined therapy with encorafenib and binimetinib has been shown to prolong progression-free and overall survival, and increase response rate compared with vemurafenib alone.

The safety and efficacy of encorafenib in patients with wild-type BRAF melanoma have not been established; encorafenib is not indicated for use in these patients.

Clinical Experience

The melanoma indication for encorafenib is based principally on the results of a randomized, open-label, phase 3 study (COLUMBUS) in patients with unresectable locally advanced or metastatic melanoma positive for BRAF V600E or V600K mutation as detected by the bioMerieux THxID® BRAF V600 mutation test. In this study, 577 patients were randomized (stratified by disease stage, Eastern Cooperative Oncology Group [ECOG] performance status, and prior immunotherapy use) in a 1:1:1 ratio to receive encorafenib 450 mg once daily with binimetinib 45 mg twice daily (encorafenib-binimetinib), encorafenib 300 mg once daily alone, or vemurafenib 960 mg twice daily. Treatment was continued until disease progression or unacceptable toxicity occurred or the patient withdrew from the study. The primary measure of efficacy was progression-free survival (as evaluated by a blinded independent central review committee). The median age of patients randomized to the encorafenib-binimetinib or vemurafenib treatment groups was 56 years; 91% of patients were white, 59% were male, 95% had metastatic disease, 65% had stage M1c disease, 72% had a baseline ECOG performance status of 0, 28% had elevated LDH concentrations, 45% had tumor involvement in at least 3 organs, and 3% of patients had brain metastases. Approximately 4% of patients enrolled in the encorafenib-binimetinib or vemurafenib treatment groups received prior therapy with an anti-programmed-death 1 (anti-PD-1), anti-programmed-death ligand-1 (anti-PD-L1), or anti-cytotoxic T-lymphocyte-associated antigen 4 (anti-CTLA-4) antibody. Most patients (88%) randomized to receive encorafenib-binimetinib or vemurafenib had BRAF V600E mutation; 11% had V600K mutation and <1% had both BRAF V600E and V600K mutations. Patients who had received immunotherapy in the adjuvant setting or one prior immunotherapy regimen for unresectable locally advanced or metastatic melanoma were eligible for this study; however, patients with prior exposure to BRAF or mitogen-activated extracellular signal-regulated kinase (MEK) inhibitors were not eligible to enroll in the study.

At a median follow-up of 16.7 or 14.4 months in patients receiving encorafenib-binimetinib or vemurafenib alone, respectively, median progression-free survival was 14.9 months in patients receiving encorafenib-binimetinib compared with 7.3 months in those receiving vemurafenib. The overall response rate was 63% for patients receiving encorafenib-binimetinib and 40% for those receiving vemurafenib; complete response was achieved in 8% of patients receiving encorafenib-binimetinib and 6% of those receiving vemurafenib. The median duration of response in patients receiving encorafenib-binimetinib or vemurafenib alone was 16.6 or 12.3 months, respectively. After a median follow-up of 48.8 months for the overall study population, the median overall survival was 33.6 or 16.9 months in patients receiving encorafenib-binimetinib or vemurafenib alone, respectively. The risk for death was reduced by 39% with encorafenib-binimetinib as compared

to vemurafenib alone. In general, the overall survival benefit for combination therapy with binimetinib and encorafenib versus vemurafenib was consistent in most subgroup analyses (e.g., age, gender, race, ECOG performance status, geographic region, baseline serum LDH concentration, BRAF mutation status, disease stage, organ involvement, presence of brain metastases, prior use of first-line immunotherapy or adjuvant therapy).

Clinical Perspective

Guidance from the American Society of Clinical Oncology (ASCO) in 2020 on systemic therapy for melanoma recommends that in the setting of unresectable or metastatic melanoma, patients with confirmed BRAF wild-type cutaneous melanoma should be offered (in no particular order) ipilimumab plus nivolumab, nivolumab alone, or pembrolizumab alone. In patients with confirmed BRAF-mutant (V600) disease, ASCO recommends offering treatment (in no particular order) with one of the three previous regimens or combination BRAF/MEK inhibitor therapy with dabrafenib plus trametinib, encorafenib plus binimetinib, or vemurafenib plus cobimetinib. For patients who progress after first-line therapy with programmed-death receptor-1 (PD-1) inhibitors, combination BRAF/MEK inhibitors may be offered; PD-1 inhibitors may be offered after progression on first-line combination BRAF/MEK inhibitors. Patients with mucosal melanoma may be offered the same treatment options as those with cutaneous melanoma; enrollment in clinical trials should be offered where possible.

● Colorectal Cancer

Encorafenib is used in combination with cetuximab for the treatment of metastatic colorectal cancer in adults with a BRAF V600E mutation after prior therapy. An FDA-approved diagnostic test (e.g., Qiagen therascreen BRAF V600E RGQ polymerase chain reaction [PCR] kit) is required to confirm the presence of the BRAF V600E mutation prior to initiation of therapy. In patients with metastatic colorectal cancer with BRAF V600E mutation and disease progression after 1 or 2 prior therapies, combined therapy with encorafenib and cetuximab has been shown to improve overall survival, overall response rate, and progression-free survival compared with combination chemotherapy with cetuximab.

The safety and efficacy of encorafenib in patients with wild-type BRAF colorectal cancer have not been established; encorafenib is not indicated for use in these patients.

Clinical Experience

The colorectal cancer indication for encorafenib is based principally on the results of a randomized, open-label, phase 3 study (BEACON CRC) in patients with metastatic colorectal cancer positive for BRAF V600E mutation with disease progression after 1 or 2 prior therapies. In this study, 665 patients were randomized (stratified by ECOG performance status, history of previous irinotecan use, and cetuximab formulation used [US-licensed versus EU-approved]) in a 1:1:1 ratio to receive encorafenib 300 mg once daily with cetuximab, encorafenib 300 mg once daily with binimetinib 45 mg twice daily and cetuximab, or irinotecan with cetuximab or FOLFIRI (leucovorin, fluorouracil, and irinotecan) with cetuximab (control). In all groups, the cetuximab dosage was 400 mg/m² followed by 250 mg/m² weekly, administered IV. Treatment was administered in 28-day cycles until disease progression or unacceptable toxicity occurred. The primary measure of efficacy for encorafenib-cetuximab doublet therapy was overall survival. In the encorafenib-cetuximab and control groups, the median age of patients randomized was 61 years; 80% of patients were white, 15% were Asian, 53% were female, and 50% had a baseline ECOG performance status of 0. Two-thirds of patients had received 1 prior therapy and the remaining patients previously received 2 therapies; 93% of patients previously had received oxaliplatin. Patients with prior exposure to RAF, MEK, or epidermal growth factor receptor (EGFR) inhibitors were not eligible to enroll in the study.

At a median follow-up of 7.8 months, median overall survival was improved in patients receiving encorafenib-cetuximab (8.4 months) as compared with those in the control group (5.4 months), corresponding to a 40% reduction in the risk for death with encorafenib-cetuximab. Median progression-free survival was 4.2 months and 1.5 months in the encorafenib-cetuximab and control groups, respectively. The overall response rate was 20% for patients receiving encorafenib-cetuximab and 2% for those in the control group; complete response was achieved in 5% of patients receiving encorafenib-cetuximab and in 0 patients in the control group. In an updated survival analysis after a median follow-up of 12.8 months, median overall survival was 9.3 months and 5.9 months in the encorafenib-cetuximab and control groups, respectively; overall survival results were similar between encorafenib-cetuximab and the triplet therapy (encorafenib-binimetinib-cetuximab) groups.

Clinical Perspective

According to the National Cancer Institute, surgery is the first-line treatment for patients with any stage of colon or rectal cancer. The use of chemotherapy or other systemic therapy after surgery is recommended for recurrent, late-stage, or metastatic disease. The use of adjuvant systemic therapy for stages II and III colorectal cancer is less well established.

The American Society of Clinical Oncology (ASCO) guideline on late-stage colorectal cancer states that most patients receive treatment with chemotherapy, where chemotherapy is available. Approximately 12% of patients with metastatic colorectal cancer express mutations in the BRAF gene. Some experts recommend the combination of encorafenib and an EGFR inhibitor (cetuximab) as second- or third-line treatment options for BRAF V600E-mutated metastatic colorectal cancer.

● Non-small Cell Lung Cancer

Encorafenib is used in combination with binimetinib for the treatment of adults with metastatic non-small cell lung cancer (NSCLC) with a BRAF V600E mutation. Encorafenib has been designated an orphan drug by FDA for the treatment of this cancer. An FDA-approved diagnostic test is required to confirm the presence of the BRAF V600E mutation in tumor or plasma specimens prior to initiation of therapy. If no mutation is detected in a plasma specimen, test tumor tissue.

The safety and efficacy of encorafenib in patients with wild-type BRAF NSCLC have not been established; encorafenib is not indicated for use in these patients.

Clinical Experience

This indication for encorafenib use is based principally on the results of an open-label, single-arm, multicenter, phase 2 study (PHAROS) in patients with metastatic NSCLC positive for a BRAF V600E mutation. In this study, 98 patients received binimetinib 45 mg orally twice daily in combination with encorafenib 450 mg orally once daily in 28-day cycles; 59 were treatment-naïve and 39 were previously treated. Treatment was continued until disease progression or unacceptable toxicity occurred. The primary end point was confirmed objective response rate per RECIST version 1.1 criteria.

The median age of enrolled patients was 70 years (range: 47 to 86 years); 88% of patients were white, 7% Asian, 3% Black or African American, and 1% American Indian or Alaska Native; 53% were female; 57% were former smokers; 73% had an ECOG performance status of 1; and 97% had adenocarcinoma. Results revealed an objective response rate of 75% in treatment-naïve patients and 46% in previously treated patients. A complete response was observed in 9 (15%) and 4 (10%) patients in the treatment-naïve and previously treated groups, respectively, with a partial response documented in 35 (59%) and 14 (36%) patients, respectively. At the time of this analysis, the median duration of response was not estimable in the treatment naïve group and was 16.7 months in the previously treated group. Durable responses lasting ≥12 months were seen in 59% of treatment naïve and 33% of previously treated patients. The disease control rate after 24 weeks was 64% among treatment naïve patients and 41% in previously treated patients. Median progression-free survival was not estimable in the treatment naïve group and was 9.3 months in the previously treated group.

Clinical Perspective

Approximately 60% of patients with lung cancer have driver alterations (e.g., mutations in EGFR, ALK, or BRAF; ROS-1 fusions, RET fusions, MET exon 14 skipping mutations, and NTRK fusions). The ASCO and Ontario Health (OH; previously known as Cancer Care Ontario) 2021 guideline specifically addresses treatment of stage IV NSCLC with driver alterations, including BRAF gene alterations. The 2023 update to this guideline recommends that, for patients with stage IV NSCLC with a BRAF V600E mutation, clinicians may offer dabrafenib and trametinib or encorafenib and binimetinib as first-line treatment. If these treatment options are unavailable, clinicians may offer standard first-line therapy following the nondriver alteration guideline.

In the second-line setting, standard first-line treatment based on the ASCO/OH nondriver mutation guideline should be offered in patients with stage IV NSCLC harboring BRAF V600E driver alterations who were previously treated

with BRAF/MEK inhibitor combination therapy. In patients who did not receive BRAF-targeted therapy in the first-line setting, dabrafenib and trametinib or encorafenib and binimetinib may be offered. For patients with stage IV NSCLC with BRAF mutations other than V600E, standard treatment based on the ASCO/OH nondriver mutation guideline should be offered.

DOSAGE AND ADMINISTRATION

● General

Pretreatment Screening

- Confirm presence of the b-Raf serine-threonine kinase (BRAF) V600E or V600K mutation, dependent upon indication, using an FDA-approved diagnostic test prior to initiation of therapy.
- Assess left ventricular ejection fraction (LVEF) using echocardiogram or multigated radionuclide angiography (MUGA).
- Monitor liver function tests.
- Perform dermatologic evaluations.
- Measure and correct any hypokalemia or hypomagnesemia.
- Verify the pregnancy status of females of reproductive potential.

Patient Monitoring

- Assess LVEF using echocardiogram or MUGA one month after initiation of encorafenib and then every 2 to 3 months during therapy.
- Monitor liver function tests monthly during treatment, and as clinically indicated.
- Perform dermatologic evaluations every 2 months during therapy, and for up to 6 months following discontinuance of combination therapy. Monitor for signs and symptoms of new noncutaneous malignancies.
- Perform ophthalmologic examinations at regular intervals and as clinically indicated for visual disturbances.
- Monitor patients who have or are at significant risk for corrected QT (QTc) prolongation; correct any hypokalemia or hypomagnesemia during therapy.

● Administration

Encorafenib is administered orally once daily without regard to meals.

If a dose of encorafenib is missed by more than 12 hours, the missed dose should be skipped and the next dose should be taken at the regularly scheduled time. Patients should *not* take extra capsules of the drug to make up for the missed dose.

If vomiting occurs following administration of encorafenib, a replacement dose should *not* be administered, and the next dose should be taken at the regularly scheduled time.

Store encorafenib capsules at 20–25°C (excursions permitted between 15–30°C). Store in the original container, tightly closed, with desiccant.

● Dosage

Melanoma

For use in combination with binimetinib in the treatment of unresectable or metastatic melanoma with BRAF V600E or V600K mutation, the recommended adult dosage of encorafenib is 450 mg once daily. Therapy should be continued until disease progression or unacceptable toxicity occurs.

Colorectal Cancer

For use in combination with cetuximab in the treatment of metastatic colorectal cancer with BRAF V600E mutation, the recommended adult dosage of encorafenib is 300 mg once daily. Therapy should be continued until disease progression or unacceptable toxicity occurs.

Non-small Cell Lung Cancer (NSCLC)

For use in combination with binimetinib in the treatment of adults with metastatic NSCLC with a BRAF V600E mutation, the recommended dosage of encorafenib is 450 mg (six 75 mg capsules) once daily. Therapy should be continued until disease progression or unacceptable toxicity occurs.

Dosage Modification for Toxicity

If adverse reactions occur, interruption of therapy, dosage reduction, and/or permanent discontinuance of encorafenib may be required based on severity of the reaction.

No dosage adjustment of encorafenib when given in combination with binimetinib or cetuximab is necessary in patients who experience interstitial lung disease, pneumonitis, cardiac dysfunction, increased creatine phosphokinase concentrations, rhabdomyolysis, or venous thromboembolism.

Melanoma or NSCLC Dose Modifications

If dosage modification of encorafenib is necessary, an initial dosage reduction to 300 mg once daily is recommended. If further dosage reduction is necessary, the dosage should be reduced to 225 mg once daily. Dosages less than 225 mg once daily are not recommended; the drug should be permanently discontinued if the 225 mg once daily dosage is not tolerated.

If binimetinib is withheld, reduce encorafenib to a maximum dose of 300 mg once daily until binimetinib is resumed.

Colorectal Cancer Dose Modifications

If dosage modification of encorafenib is necessary, an initial dosage reduction to 225 mg once daily is recommended. If further dosage reduction is necessary, the dosage should be reduced to 150 mg once daily. Dosages less than 150 mg once daily are not recommended; the drug should be permanently discontinued if the 150 mg once daily dosage is not tolerated.

If concomitant therapy with cetuximab is discontinued, discontinue encorafenib.

Development of New Primary Malignancies

If new primary RAS mutation-positive, noncutaneous malignancies occur, encorafenib therapy should be permanently discontinued.

No dosage adjustment of encorafenib is necessary in patients who develop new primary cutaneous malignancies during combination therapy with encorafenib and binimetinib.

Cardiomyopathy

If symptomatic congestive heart failure or an absolute decrease in left ventricular ejection fraction (LVEF) >20% from baseline that is also below the institutional lower limit of normal (LLN) occurs, reduce encorafenib by one dose level. If LVEF improves to at least the institutional LLN and absolute decrease to ≤10% compared to baseline, continue encorafenib at the reduced dose. If no improvement, withhold encorafenib until improvement to at least the institutional LLN and absolute decrease to ≤10% compared to baseline and then resume therapy at the reduced dosage or reduce the encorafenib dosage an additional dosage level.

Uveitis

If grade 1 or 2 uveitis unresponsive to ocular therapy occurs, encorafenib therapy should be withheld for up to 6 weeks. If the toxicity improves within 6 weeks of withholding therapy, therapy may be resumed at the same or reduced dosage. If the toxicity does not improve within 6 weeks of withholding therapy, encorafenib therapy should be permanently discontinued.

If grade 3 uveitis occurs, encorafenib therapy should be withheld for up to 6 weeks. If grade 3 uveitis improves within 6 weeks of withholding therapy, therapy may be resumed at the same or reduced dosage. If the toxicity does not improve within 6 weeks of withholding therapy, encorafenib therapy should be permanently discontinued.

If grade 4 uveitis occurs, encorafenib therapy should be permanently discontinued.

If adverse ocular reactions other than uveitis, iritis, or iridocyclitis occur during combination therapy with encorafenib and binimetinib, no dosage modification of encorafenib is necessary.

Prolongation of QT Interval

If the QT interval (corrected for heart rate using Fridericia's formula [QT$_c$F]) exceeds 500 msec and increases by no more than 60 msec from baseline, encorafenib therapy should be withheld; therapy may be resumed at a reduced dosage when QT$_c$F decreases to 500 msec or less. If there is more than one recurrence, encorafenib therapy should be permanently discontinued.

If QT$_c$F exceeds 500 msec and increases more than 60 msec from baseline, encorafenib therapy should be permanently discontinued.

Hepatotoxicity

In patients who develop grade 2 elevations of serum aminotransferases (ALT or AST), encorafenib therapy may be continued at the same dosage for up to 4 weeks. If the toxicity persists, encorafenib therapy should be withheld; therapy may be resumed at the same dosage when the toxicity improves to grade 1 or less or to baseline.

For the first occurrence of grade 3 elevations of serum ALT or AST, encorafenib therapy should be withheld for up to 4 weeks; therapy may be resumed at a reduced dosage when the toxicity improves to grade 1 or less or to baseline. If the toxicity does not improve to grade 1 or less or to baseline within 4 weeks of withholding therapy, the drug should be permanently discontinued. If recurrent grade 3 hepatic toxicity occurs, permanent discontinuance of encorafenib should be considered.

For the first occurrence of grade 4 elevations of serum ALT or AST, encorafenib therapy may be permanently discontinued or temporarily interrupted. If encorafenib therapy is temporarily interrupted, the drug should be withheld for up to 4 weeks; therapy may be resumed at a reduced dosage when the toxicity improves to grade 1 or less or to baseline. If the toxicity does not improve to grade 1 or less or to baseline within 4 weeks of withholding therapy, the drug should be permanently discontinued. If recurrent grade 4 hepatic toxicity occurs, the drug should be permanently discontinued.

Dermatologic Effects

If grade 2 dermatologic reactions occur (other than hand-foot skin reactions), encorafenib therapy may be continued at the same dosage for up to 2 weeks. If the toxicity persists, encorafenib therapy should be withheld; therapy may be resumed at the same dosage when the toxicity improves to grade 1 or less.

For the first occurrence of grade 3 dermatologic reactions (other than hand-foot skin reactions), encorafenib therapy should be withheld; therapy may be resumed at the same dosage when the toxicity improves to grade 1 or less. If grade 3 dermatologic reactions recur, encorafenib therapy should be withheld; therapy may be resumed at a reduced dosage when the toxicity improves to grade 1 or less.

If grade 4 dermatologic reactions occur (other than hand-foot skin reactions), encorafenib therapy should be permanently discontinued.

Other Toxicities Including Hemorrhage and Hand-Foot Skin Reaction

For recurrent grade 2 adverse reactions, encorafenib therapy should be withheld for up to 4 weeks; therapy may be resumed at a reduced dosage when the toxicity improves to grade 1 or less or to baseline. If the toxicity does not improve to grade 1 or less or to baseline within 4 weeks of withholding therapy, the drug should be permanently discontinued.

For the first occurrence of any grade 3 adverse reaction, encorafenib therapy should be withheld for up to 4 weeks; therapy may be resumed at a reduced dosage when the toxicity improves to grade 1 or less or to baseline. If the toxicity does not improve to grade 1 or less or to baseline within 4 weeks of withholding therapy, the drug should be permanently discontinued. If a grade 3 adverse reaction recurs, permanent discontinuance of encorafenib should be considered.

For the first occurrence of any grade 4 adverse reaction, encorafenib therapy may be permanently discontinued or temporarily interrupted. If encorafenib therapy is temporarily interrupted, the drug should be withheld for up to 4 weeks; therapy may be resumed at a reduced dosage when the toxicity improves to grade 1 or less or to baseline. If the grade 4 adverse reaction does not improve to grade 1 or less or to baseline within 4 weeks of withholding therapy, the drug should be permanently discontinued. For recurrent grade 4 adverse reactions, encorafenib therapy should be permanently discontinued.

Concomitant Use with Drugs and Foods Affecting Hepatic Microsomal Enzymes

Concomitant use of encorafenib with moderate or strong inhibitors of cytochrome P-450 (CYP) isoenzyme 3A4 should be avoided; however, if such concomitant use cannot be avoided, the manufacturer recommends reducing the dosage of encorafenib based on the recommendations in Table 1. If concomitant use of the strong or moderate CYP3A4 inhibitor is discontinued, the encorafenib dosage should be returned (after 3–5 terminal half-lives of the CYP3A4 inhibitor) to the dosage used prior to initiation of the strong or moderate CYP3A4 inhibitor.

TABLE 1. Dosage Reductions for Concomitant Use with Strong or Moderate CYP3A4 Inhibitors.

Current Encorafenib Dosage	Recommended Dosage with *Moderate* CYP3A4 Inhibitor	Recommended Dosage with *Strong* CYP3A4 Inhibitor
450 mg	225 mg	150 mg
300 mg	150 mg	75 mg
225 mg	75 mg	75 mg
150 mg	75 mg	75 mg[a]

[a] When coadministered with a strong CYP3A4 inhibitor, exposure to encorafenib at the 75-mg dosage is expected to be higher than the 150-mg dosage without concomitant CYP3A4 inhibitor and similar to the 225-mg dosage without concomitant CYP3A4 inhibitor. Closely monitor for adverse reactions and use clinical judgement when encorafenib 150 mg is used in combination with a strong CYP3A4 inhibitor.

● Special Populations

Hepatic Impairment

Dosage adjustment is not necessary in patients with mild hepatic impairment (Child-Pugh class A). Use of encorafenib in patients with moderate or severe (Child-Pugh class B or C) hepatic impairment has not been studied, and the manufacturer provides no specific dosage recommendations for such patients.

Renal Impairment

Dosage adjustment is not necessary in patients with mild or moderate renal impairment (creatinine clearance of 30 to <90 mL/minute). Use of encorafenib in patients with severe renal impairment (creatinine clearance <30 mL/minute) has not been studied, and the manufacturer provides no specific dosage recommendations for such patients.

Geriatric Patients

The manufacturer makes no specific dosage recommendations for geriatric patients.

CAUTIONS

● Contraindications

- None.

● Warnings/Precautions

Combination Therapy

When encorafenib is used in combination with binimetinib or cetuximab, the usual cautions, precautions, and contraindications associated with binimetinib or cetuximab, respectively, must be considered in addition to those associated with encorafenib.

Development of New Primary Malignancies

New primary cutaneous or noncutaneous malignancies have been reported in patients receiving b-Raf serine-threonine kinase (BRAF) inhibitors, including encorafenib.

In the COLUMBUS study, cutaneous squamous cell carcinoma (including keratoacanthoma) or basal cell carcinoma occurred in 8 or 1%, respectively, of patients receiving single-agent encorafenib compared with 2.6 or 1.6%, respectively, of those receiving encorafenib in combination with binimetinib. New primary melanoma also was reported in 5% of patients receiving single-agent encorafenib. The median time to first onset of cutaneous squamous cell carcinoma or keratoacanthoma in patients receiving encorafenib in combination with binimetinib was 5.8 months (range: 1–9 months).

In the BEACON CRC study, cutaneous squamous cell carcinoma (including keratoacanthoma) or new primary melanoma occurred in 1.4 or 1.4%, respectively, of patients receiving encorafenib in combination with cetuximab.

In the PHAROS study, cutaneous squamous cell carcinoma and skin papilloma each occurred in 2% of patients receiving encorafenib in combination with binimetinib.

Although the mechanism for development of cutaneous squamous cell carcinoma has not been fully determined, it has been suggested that paradoxical activation of mitogen-activated protein kinase (MAPK) signaling may lead to accelerated growth of such skin lesions as well as development of other primary malignancies. MAPK-mediated events in wild-type BRAF cells have been observed in a study evaluating the pathology and immunohistochemistry of normal and proliferating skin lesions in patients receiving the weak b-Raf kinase inhibitor sorafenib. Another study performed a molecular analysis of DNA extracted from tumor specimens of patients receiving the BRAF inhibitor vemurafenib; results indicated that these patients have a secondary mutation (in addition to the BRAF V600E mutation) that appears to be activated by vemurafenib treatment. Some clinicians suggest that advanced age (i.e., 65 years of age or older), history of skin cancer, and chronic sun exposure may be risk factors for developing cutaneous squamous cell carcinoma. Some data suggest that mitogen-activated extracellular signal-regulated kinase (MEK) inhibitors (i.e., binimetinib, cobimetinib, trametinib) block the paradoxical activation of the MAPK pathway induced by BRAF inhibitors; therefore, combination therapy with a BRAF inhibitor and a MEK inhibitor may reduce the risk of developing cutaneous squamous cell carcinoma. Findings from a meta-analysis of randomized controlled studies that assessed the relative risk of development of cutaneous squamous cell carcinoma in cancer patients receiving a BRAF inhibitor indicate that the risk of cutaneous squamous cell carcinoma is higher in patients receiving a BRAF inhibitor than in patients receiving combination therapy with a BRAF inhibitor and a MEK inhibitor.

A dermatologic evaluation should be performed at baseline, every 2 months during therapy, and for up to 6 months following discontinuance of therapy. Suspicious cutaneous lesions should be treated as appropriate and excised for pathologic evaluation. Patients should be monitored for signs and symptoms of new noncutaneous malignancies. If new primary RAS mutation-positive, noncutaneous malignancies occur, encorafenib therapy should be permanently discontinued. In patients who develop new primary cutaneous malignancies, the manufacturer states that no dosage adjustment of encorafenib is necessary.

Tumor Promotion in Wild-type BRAF Tumors

In vitro, paradoxical activation of MAPK signaling and increased cell proliferation have been observed in wild-type BRAF cells exposed to BRAF inhibitors. Presence of BRAF V600E or V600K mutation must be confirmed prior to initiation of therapy.

Cardiomyopathy

Cardiomyopathy, which may manifest as a symptomatic or asymptomatic decrease in left ventricular ejection fraction (LVEF), has been reported in patients receiving encorafenib in combination with binimetinib. In the COLUMBUS study, cardiomyopathy (defined as an absolute decrease in LVEF from baseline of ≥10% and to a level below the lower limit of normal [LLN]) occurred in 7% of patients receiving encorafenib in combination with binimetinib; grade 3 left ventricular dysfunction occurred in 1.6% of patients receiving combination therapy. The median time to first onset of left ventricular dysfunction was 3.6 months (range: 0–21 months). Cardiomyopathy resolved in 87% of patients receiving combination therapy with encorafenib and binimetinib.

Evidence of cardiomyopathy was observed in 11% of patients administered encorafenib in combination with binimetinb in the PHAROS study, with grade 3 left ventricular dysfunction occurring in 1% of patients. Cardiomyopathy resolved in 82% of patients.

Safety of combination therapy with encorafenib and binimetinib has not been established in patients with a baseline LVEF below the LLN or <50%.

LVEF should be assessed using echocardiogram or multigated radionuclide angiography (MUGA) prior to and 1 month after initiation of encorafenib and then every 2–3 months during therapy. Close monitoring during therapy is indicated in patients with preexisting cardiovascular risk factors. If left ventricular dysfunction occurs, temporary interruption followed by dosage reduction or discontinuance of encorafenib may be necessary.

Hepatotoxicity

Liver function test abnormalities have been reported in patients receiving combination therapy with encorafenib and binimetinib. In the COLUMBUS study, grade 3 or 4 elevations in ALT, AST, and alkaline phosphatase concentrations occurred in 6, 2.6, and 0.5%, respectively, of patients receiving combination therapy with encorafenib and binimetinib. In the PHAROS study, grade 3 or 4 elevations in ALT, AST, and alkaline phosphatase concentrations occurred in 9%, 10%, and 3.2%, respectively, of patients receiving encorafenib in combination with binimetinib.

Liver function tests should be performed prior to initiation of encorafenib therapy and then monthly, or more frequently as clinically indicated, during therapy with the drug. Temporary interruption, dosage reduction, or discontinuance of encorafenib may be necessary if liver function test abnormalities occur during therapy with the drug.

Hemorrhage

Hemorrhage has been reported in patients receiving encorafenib. In the COLUMBUS study, hemorrhage occurred in 19% of patients and was grade 3 or greater in 3.2% of patients receiving encorafenib in combination with binimetinib. The most common hemorrhagic events in patients receiving encorafenib in combination with binimetinib were GI hemorrhage, including rectal hemorrhage (4.2%), hematochezia (3.1%), and hemorrhoidal hemorrhage (1%). Intracranial hemorrhage was fatal in 1.6% of patients with new or progressive brain metastases receiving combination therapy with encorafenib and binimetinib.

In the BEACON CRC study, hemorrhage occurred in 19% of patients and was grade 3 or greater in 1.9% of patients receiving encorafenib in combination with cetuximab. The most common hemorrhagic events in patients receiving encorafenib in combination with cetuximab were epistaxis (6.9%), hematochezia (2.3%), and rectal hemorrhage (2.3%); fatal GI hemorrhage was reported in 0.5% of patients.

In the PHAROS study, hemorrhage occurred in 12% of patients receiving encorafenib in combination with binimetinib, including fatal intracranial hemorrhage in 1% of patients. Grade 3 or 4 hemorrhage was reported in 4.1% of patients. The most frequent hemorrhagic events were anal hemorrhage and hemothorax (2% each).

If hemorrhagic events occur, therapy interruption followed by dosage reduction or discontinuance of encorafenib may be necessary.

Uveitis

Uveitis, including iritis and iridocyclitis, have occurred in patients receiving encorafenib in combination with binimetinib. In the COLUMBUS study, uveitis occurred in 4% of patients receiving encorafenib in combination with binimetinib. In PHAROS, uveitis occurred in 1% of patients administered encorafenib in combination with binimetinib.

Ophthalmologic examinations should be performed regularly and as clinically indicated (i.e., if new or worsening visual disturbances occur; to follow new or persistent ophthalmologic findings) during encorafenib therapy. Patients should be monitored for visual symptoms at each visit. Temporary interruption, dosage reduction, or discontinuance of encorafenib may be necessary if ocular toxicities occur during therapy with the drug.

Prolongation of QT Interval

Encorafenib is associated with dose-dependent prolongation of the QT interval. In the COLUMBUS study, a QT interval (corrected for heart rate using Fridericia's formula [QT_cF]) exceeding 500 msec was observed in 1 of 192 patients (0.5%) receiving encorafenib in combination with binimetinib. In PHAROS, an increase in QT_cF exceeding 500 msec was measured in 2 of 95 patients (2.1%) receiving encorafenib in combination with binimetinib.

Patients at an increased risk for QT_c-interval prolongation, including those with a history of long QT syndromes, clinically important bradyarrhythmias, or severe or uncontrolled heart failure, and those concurrently receiving other drugs known to prolong the QT interval should be monitored. Hypokalemia and hypomagnesemia should be corrected prior to administration of encorafenib and as clinically indicated during therapy. If prolongation of the QT interval occurs, therapy interruption followed by dosage reduction or discontinuance of encorafenib may be necessary.

Fetal/Neonatal Morbidity and Mortality

Encorafenib may cause fetal harm in humans based on its mechanism of action and animal findings; the drug has been shown to be embryotoxic, fetotoxic, and teratogenic in animals. There are no available data regarding the risk of encorafenib use in pregnant women to date. In animal reproduction studies, embryofetal toxicity (i.e., decreases in fetal body weight) and teratogenic effects (i.e., skeletal anomalies) have been demonstrated in pregnant rats receiving encorafenib at exposure levels equivalent to approximately 26 times the human exposure at the recommended human dosage. Postimplantation loss and abortion also were observed in rabbits receiving encorafenib at exposure levels of approximately 178 times the human exposure at the recommended human dosage. Although formal placental transfer studies have not been conducted, encorafenib has been detected in fetal plasma of rats and rabbits at concentrations up to 1.7 and 0.8%, respectively, of maternal plasma concentrations.

Pregnancy should be avoided during encorafenib therapy. The manufacturer states that pregnancy status should be verified prior to initiation of encorafenib therapy in women of childbearing potential and that such women should be advised to use an effective nonhormonal method of contraception while receiving encorafenib and for 2 weeks after the last dose. Patients should be apprised of the potential hazard to the fetus if the drug is used during pregnancy.

Use as a Single Agent

Some adverse effects may occur less frequently during combination therapy with encorafenib and binimetinib compared to single-agent encorafenib. Grade 3 or 4 dermatologic reactions occurred in 21 or 2% of patients receiving single-agent encorafenib or combination therapy with encorafenib and binimetinib, respectively.

Specific Populations

Pregnancy

Encorafenib may cause fetal harm if administered to pregnant women based on its mechanism of action and animal findings.

Pregnancy status should be verified in women of childbearing potential prior to initiation of encorafenib therapy.

Lactation

It is not known whether encorafenib or its metabolites are distributed into human milk. Because of the potential for serious adverse reactions to encorafenib in breast-fed infants, women should be advised not to breast-feed while receiving the drug and for 2 weeks after the last dose. The effects of the drug on breast-fed infants or on the production of milk are unknown.

Females and Males of Reproductive Potential

Results of animal studies suggest that encorafenib may reduce male fertility. The effect of the drug on fertility in humans is not known.

For women of childbearing potential, an effective nonhormonal method of contraception should be used while receiving encorafenib and for 2 weeks after the last dose. Advise patients to use a nonhormonal method as encorafenib can interact with hormonal contraceptives and render them ineffective.

Pediatric Use

Safety and efficacy of encorafenib have not been established in pediatric patients.

Geriatric Use

In the clinical trials evaluating encorafenib (300–600 mg once daily) in combination with binimetinib (45 mg twice daily) in patients with BRAF mutation-positive melanoma, 20% of patients were 65–74 years of age and 8% were 75 years of age or older.

Among 216 patients with metastatic BRAF mutation-positive colorectal cancer who received encorafenib 300 mg once daily in combination with cetuximab in a clinical trial, 29% of patients were 65–74 years of age and 9% were ≥75 years of age.

In a clinical trial of patients with BRAF V600E mutation-positive metastatic NSCLC administered encorafenib in combination with binimetinib, 63% of patients were ≥65 years of age and 20% were ≥75 years of age.

No overall differences in safety or efficacy of encorafenib in combination with binimetinib or cetuximab were observed between geriatric patients and younger adults.

Hepatic Impairment

In population pharmacokinetic analyses, systemic exposure of encorafenib was similar in patients with mild hepatic impairment (Child-Pugh class A) and those with normal hepatic function.

The pharmacokinetic profile of encorafenib has not been established in patients with moderate or severe hepatic impairment (Child-Pugh class B or C).

Renal Impairment

In population pharmacokinetic analyses, systemic exposure of encorafenib was similar in patients with mild or moderate renal impairment (creatinine clearance of 30–89 mL/minute) and those with normal renal function.

The pharmacokinetic profile of encorafenib has not been established in patients with severe renal impairment (creatinine clearance <30 mL/minute).

● Common Adverse Effects

The most common adverse effects (≥25%) in patients with melanoma receiving encorafenib in combination with binimetinib include fatigue, nausea, vomiting, abdominal pain, and arthralgia.

The most common adverse effects (≥25%) in patients with colorectal cancer receiving encorafenib in combination with cetuximab include fatigue, nausea, diarrhea, dermatitis acneiform, abdominal pain, decreased appetite, arthralgia, and rash.

The most common adverse effects (≥25%) in patients with NSCLC receiving encorafenib in combination with binimetinib include fatigue, nausea, diarrhea, musculoskeletal pain, vomiting, abdominal pain, visual impairment, constipation, dyspnea, rash, and cough.

DRUG INTERACTIONS

Encorafenib is metabolized principally by cytochrome P-450 (CYP) isoenzyme 3A4 and, to a lesser extent, by CYP isoenzymes 2C19 and 2D6. In vitro studies also indicate that encorafenib is a reversible inhibitor of uridine diphosphate-glucuronosyltransferase (UGT) 1A1 and CYP isoenzymes 1A2, 2B6, 2C8, 2C9, 2D6, and 3A. The drug has demonstrated time-dependent inhibition of CYP3A4 at clinically relevant concentrations. In vitro, encorafenib induces CYP isoenzymes 2B6, 2C9, and 3A4 at clinically relevant concentrations.

Encorafenib is an inhibitor of P-glycoprotein (P-gp), breast cancer resistance protein (BCRP), organic cation transporter (OCT) 2, organic anion transporter (OAT) 1, OAT3, organic anion transporting polypeptide (OATP) 1B1, and OATP1B3, but does not inhibit OCT1 or multidrug resistance-associated protein (MRP) 2 at clinically relevant concentrations.

In vitro studies indicate that encorafenib is a substrate of P-gp, but is not a substrate for BCRP, MRP2, OATP1B1, OATP1B3, or OCT1 at clinically relevant concentrations.

● Drugs and Foods Affecting Hepatic Microsomal Enzymes

Inhibitors of CYP3A4

Concomitant use of encorafenib with strong or moderate inhibitors of CYP3A4 may result in increased peak plasma concentrations and systemic exposure (AUC) of encorafenib and an increased incidence of adverse effects. When the strong CYP3A4 inhibitor posaconazole was administered concomitantly with encorafenib (single 50-mg dose), the peak plasma concentration and AUC of encorafenib were increased by 68% and 3-fold, respectively. When the moderate

CYP3A4 inhibitor diltiazem hydrochloride was administered concomitantly with encorafenib (single 50-mg dose), the peak plasma concentration and AUC of encorafenib were increased by 45% and 2-fold, respectively.

Concomitant use of encorafenib with strong (e.g., posaconazole) or moderate (e.g., diltiazem) inhibitors of CYP3A4 should be avoided. If such concomitant use cannot be avoided, the manufacturer recommends reducing the dosage of encorafenib based on the recommendations in Table 1. If concomitant use of the strong or moderate CYP3A4 inhibitor is discontinued, the encorafenib dosage should be returned (after 3–5 terminal half-lives of the CYP3A4 inhibitor) to the dosage used prior to initiation of the potent or moderate CYP3A4 inhibitor.

Inducers of CYP3A4

Concomitant use of encorafenib with strong or moderate inducers of CYP3A4 may result in decreased systemic exposure and reduced efficacy of encorafenib. When the moderate CYP3A4 inducer (modafinil) was administered concomitantly with encorafenib 450 mg once daily and binimetinib 45 mg twice daily, the peak plasma concentration and AUC of encorafenib were decreased by 20% and 24%, respectively, compared to encorafenib alone.

Because formal drug interaction studies with strong CYP3A4 inducers have not been performed, the manufacturer states that concomitant use of encorafenib with strong inducers of CYP3A4 should be avoided.

● Drugs Metabolized by Hepatic Microsomal Enzymes

Concomitant administration of encorafenib with sensitive CYP3A4 substrates may decrease plasma concentrations of the CYP3A4 substrate (e.g., midazolam) and result in reduced efficacy of the substrate drug. Avoid concomitant use of encorafenib with CYP3A4 substrates for which a decrease in plasma concentration may lead to reduced substrate efficacy. If concurrent use cannot be avoided, refer to the CYP3A4 substrate prescribing information for recommendations.

● Drugs that Prolong the QT Interval

Because encorafenib has been associated with QT-interval prolongation, concomitant use of encorafenib with drugs known to prolong the QT interval should be avoided.

● Drugs Affecting Gastric Acidity

Concomitant administration of encorafenib (single 100-mg dose) with the proton-pump inhibitor rabeprazole (20 mg once daily for 5 days) resulted in no clinically important changes in peak plasma concentration or systemic exposure of encorafenib.

● Drugs Affecting Efflux Transport Systems

Repeated, concomitant administration of encorafenib (450 mg once daily) and binimetinib (45 mg twice daily) with a single dose of rosuvastatin, a sensitive substrate for OATP1B1, OATP1B3, and BCRP, resulted in an increase in peak plasma concentration and AUC of rosuvastatin by 2.7- and 1.6-fold, respectively.

● Grapefruit

Concomitant use of encorafenib with grapefruit products (CYP3A4 inhibitor) may result in increased peak plasma concentrations and systemic exposure of encorafenib. Patients receiving encorafenib should be advised to avoid consuming grapefruit products.

● Hormonal Contraceptives

Concomitant use of encorafenib with hormonal contraceptives that are metabolized by CYP3A4 may result in decreased systemic exposure to the substrate drug and reduced contraceptive efficacy. Concomitant use of encorafenib with hormonal contraceptives should be avoided.

● Binimetinib

Concomitant administration of encorafenib with binimetinib, a UGT1A1 substrate, did not substantially alter systemic exposure of binimetinib.

● Cetuximab

Concomitant administration of encorafenib with cetuximab did not substantially alter systemic exposure of either drug.

DESCRIPTION

Encorafenib, an inhibitor of b-Raf serine-threonine kinase (BRAF) with V600E or V600K mutation, is an antineoplastic agent. Approximately 40–60% of cutaneous melanomas carry a BRAF mutation. The most common BRAF mutation is the substitution of glutamic acid for valine at codon 600 in exon 15 (BRAF V600E); a less frequently occurring BRAF mutation is the substitution of lysine for valine at codon 600 in exon 15 (BRAF V600K). The mutation of BRAF V600E activates the mitogen-activated protein kinase (MAPK) and extracellular signal-regulated kinase (ERK) signal transduction pathway, which enhances cell proliferation and tumor progression (e.g., metastasis). Encorafenib induced tumor regression associated with inhibition of the MAPK/ERK signal transduction pathway in xenograft models of tumor cells with BRAF V600E mutation in mice. In vitro studies have demonstrated that encorafenib inhibited tumor growth of cell lines testing positive for BRAF with V600E, V600D, or V600K mutation. Encorafenib also inhibits wild-type b-Raf and other kinases such as c-Raf, c-Jun NH(2)-terminal protein kinase (JNK)1, JNK2, JNK3, LIM domain kinase (LIMK)1, LIMK2, mitogen-activated extracellular signal-regulated kinase (MEK)4, and serine/threonine kinase (STK)36 and substantially reduces ligand binding to these kinases at clinically relevant concentrations.

Clinical resistance to monotherapy with a BRAF inhibitor, generally occurring 6–7 months following initiation of therapy, has been attributed to several possible resistance mechanisms mostly relying on reactivation of the MAPK/ERK pathway. Complete inhibition of the MAPK/ERK pathway resulting in durable responses may be achieved with the use of combination therapy with a BRAF inhibitor (i.e., dabrafenib, encorafenib, vemurafenib) and a MEK inhibitor (i.e., binimetinib, cobimetinib, trametinib). In vitro, use of encorafenib in combination with binimetinib resulted in increased antiproliferative activity compared with either drug alone in BRAF mutation-positive cell lines. The combination of encorafenib and binimetinib also has demonstrated increased inhibition of tumor growth and delayed emergence of resistance compared with either drug alone in xenograft models of melanoma harboring BRAF V600E mutations in mice. Single agent BRAF or MEK inhibitor treatment is no longer recommended by experts as combination BRAF/MEK inhibition has demonstrated superior outcomes with a similar safety profile.

In metastatic colorectal cancer, approximately 12% of patients express mutations in the BRAF gene; the BRAF V600E mutation is a poor prognostic factor, associated with a reduced median survival. Single agent BRAF inhibition has demonstrated only modest activity in BRAF mutation-positive colorectal cancer, which may be attributed to resistance mechanisms that reactivate epidermal growth factor receptor (EGFR). Synergistic inhibition of tumor growth and improved activity have been demonstrated with BRAF and EGFR inhibitor combinations in xenograft models and clinical studies.

Following oral administration of encorafenib, at least 86% of the dose is rapidly absorbed with peak plasma concentrations occurring in 2 hours. Systemic exposure of encorafenib is proportional to dose following single administration of the drug over the dosage range of 50–700 mg, but less than proportional to dose following repeated administration of the drug over the dosage range of 50–800 mg once daily. Steady-state concentrations are achieved within 15 days. In a physiologically based pharmacokinetic model, systemic exposure of encorafenib at steady state was 50% lower compared to the systemic exposure following the initial dose, suggesting that encorafenib causes autoinduction of its own metabolism; however, intersubject variability ranged from 12–69%. Administration of a single 100-mg dose of encorafenib with a high-fat, high-calorie meal (approximately 150 calories from protein, 350 calories from carbohydrates, 500 calories from fat) decreased mean peak plasma concentrations of the drug by 36%, but did not affect the extent of absorption (AUC). Encorafenib is 86% bound to plasma proteins. Encorafenib is metabolized principally by cytochrome P-450 (CYP) isoenzyme 3A4 and, to a lesser extent, by CYP2C19 and CYP2D6. The mean terminal half-life of encorafenib is 3.5 hours. Following oral administration of a radiolabeled dose of encorafenib, 47% of the dose is recovered in feces (5% of the dose as unchanged drug) and 47% is recovered in urine (2% of the dose as unchanged drug).

The pharmacokinetics of encorafenib do not appear to be affected substantially by age (19–89 years), gender, or body weight.

ADVICE TO PATIENTS

- Advise patients to read the manufacturer's patient information.

- If a dose of encorafenib is missed by more than 12 hours or vomited, administer the next dose at the regularly scheduled time; an additional dose should not be administered to replace the missed or vomited dose.

- Risk of new primary malignancy. Advise patients to contact their clinician immediately for any new skin lesions, changes to existing skin lesions, or other signs and symptoms of malignancies.

- Risk of hemorrhage. Advise patients to contact a clinician promptly and seek immediate medical attention if signs and/or symptoms of unusual bleeding (e.g., headache, dizziness, weakness, blood in stool, coughing up blood, vomiting blood) occur.

- Risk of cardiomyopathy. Advise patients to contact a clinician promptly if manifestations of heart failure (e.g., tachycardia, shortness of breath, peripheral edema, feeling lightheaded) occur.

- Risk of hepatotoxicity. Advise patients of the importance of liver function test monitoring before and during encorafenib therapy. Instruct patients to report any possible manifestations of hepatotoxicity (e.g., jaundice, dark or tea-colored urine, nausea, vomiting, fatigue, loss of appetite, bruising, bleeding).

- Risk of QT-interval prolongation. Advise patients to contact a clinician promptly if syncope, abnormal heartbeat, or feelings of dizziness or faintness occur.

- Risk of uveitis. Advise patients to contact a clinician promptly if ocular pain, swelling, redness, changes in vision, or blurred vision occurs.

- Risk of fetal harm. Advise women of childbearing potential that they should use an effective nonhormonal method of contraception while receiving the drug and for 2 weeks after the last dose. Importance of women informing clinicians if they are or plan to become pregnant. Apprise patient of potential fetal hazard if used during pregnancy.

- Advise women to avoid breast-feeding while receiving encorafenib and for 2 weeks after the last dose.

- Advise men of reproductive potential that encorafenib may reduce male fertility.

- Importance of informing clinicians of existing or contemplated concomitant therapy, including prescription and OTC drugs and herbal supplements, as well as any concomitant illnesses. Advise patients to avoid grapefruit or grapefruit juice while receiving encorafenib.

- Advise patients of other important precautionary information.

For further information on the handling of antineoplastic agents, see the ASHP Guidelines on Handling Hazardous Drugs at https://www.ahfsdruginformation.com.

PREPARATIONS

Encorafenib can only be obtained through select specialty pharmacies. Contact the manufacturer or consult the Braftovi® and Mektovi® website for specific availability information (https://braftovimektovi.pfizerpro.com/).

Excipients in commercially available drug preparations may have clinically important effects in some individuals; consult specific product labeling for details.

Encorafenib

Oral

Capsules	75 mg	Braftovi®, Array BioPharma

† Use is not currently included in the labeling approved by the US Food and Drug Administration.

Selected Revisions July 10, 2024, © Copyright, July 16, 2018, American Society of Health-System Pharmacists, Inc.

Entrectinib

10:00 • ANTINEOPLASTIC AGENTS

■ Entrectinib, a potent inhibitor of multiple receptor tyrosine kinases including tropomyosin receptor kinases (Trk) A, TrkB, TrkC, c-ros oncogene-1 (*ROS-1*), and anaplastic lymphoma kinase (ALK), is an antineoplastic agent.

USES

• Non-small Cell Lung Cancer

Entrectinib is used for the treatment of c-ros oncogene-1 (*ROS-1*)-positive metastatic non-small cell lung cancer (NSCLC) in adults. The presence of *ROS-1* rearrangement in tumor or plasma specimens should be confirmed by an FDA-approved test prior to initiation of therapy. Testing with plasma specimens is only appropriate for patients for whom tumor tissue is not available. Entrectinib has been designated an orphan drug by FDA for the treatment of tropomyosin receptor kinase (Trk) A-positive, TrkB-positive, TrkC-positive, *ROS-1*-positive, and anaplastic lymphoma kinase (ALK)-positive NSCLC.

Clinical Experience

The indication for entrectinib in the treatment of *ROS-1*-positive metastatic NSCLC is based principally on pooled results for a cohort of 92 adults with metastatic NSCLC harboring a *ROS-1* fusion in 3 multicenter, open-label, noncomparative phase 1 and 2 studies (ALKA-372-001, STARTRK-1, and STARTRK-2). Patients who previously received a *ROS-1* inhibitor were excluded from the primary efficacy analysis. *ROS-1* fusion was determined using fluorescence in situ hybridization (FISH), next-generation sequencing (NGS), or polymerase chain reaction (PCR) and was confirmed by a central laboratory using a validated NGS test in 25% of patients. Patients enrolled in the NSCLC cohort received varying dosages of entrectinib; however, 90% of patients received entrectinib 600 mg orally once daily. The primary efficacy end points were objective response rate (as evaluated by a blinded independent review committee) according to Response Evaluation Criteria in Solid Tumors (RECIST 1.1) and duration of response; an additional outcome measure was intracranial response. The median age of patients included in the NSCLC cohort was 53 years; 96% had adenocarcinoma histology, 88% had an Eastern Cooperative Oncology Group (ECOG) performance status of 0 or 1, 48% were white, 45% were Asian, 65% were female, and 65% had received prior platinum-containing therapy for metastatic or recurrent disease. No patients had disease progression within 6 months of adjuvant or neoadjuvant platinum-based chemotherapy. Most patients (94%) had metastatic disease; CNS metastases were present in 43% of patients.

At the time of data analysis, the objective response rate for patients receiving entrectinib for the treatment of metastatic *ROS-1*-positive NSCLC was 74%; complete response was achieved in 15% of patients. At the time of analysis, 75, 57, or 38% of patients had durable responses of at least 9, 12, or 18 months, respectively. Intracranial response was achieved in 7 of 10 patients with measurable CNS metastases at baseline (as assessed by a blinded independent review committee) who had not received prior radiation therapy to the brain within 2 months of receiving entrectinib. The most common *ROS-1* fusion was *CD74-ROS-1*. The objective response rate in patients with tumors harboring *CD74-ROS-1*, *SLC34A2-ROS-1*, *SDC4-ROS-1*, *EZR-ROS-1*, or *TPM3-ROS-1* was 85, 57, 67, 100, or 50%, respectively. Among patients with tumors harboring an unknown *ROS-1* fusion, the objective response rate was 83%.

• Solid Tumors with Neurotrophic Tyrosine Receptor Kinase Gene Fusion

Entrectinib is used in adults and pediatric patients >1 month of age for the treatment of solid tumors harboring a neurotrophic tyrosine receptor kinase (*NTRK*) gene fusion (without a known acquired mutation for resistance), in patients who have metastatic disease or may experience severe morbidity following surgical resection, and whose disease progressed following prior therapy or those who are not candidates for other treatment options. The presence of *NTRK* fusion should be confirmed in tumor or plasma specimens by an FDA-approved test

prior to initiation of therapy. Testing using plasma specimens is only appropriate for patients for whom tumor tissue is not available. Entrectinib has been designated an orphan drug by FDA for the treatment of these cancers. The accelerated approval of entrectinib for this indication is based on objective response rate and duration of response. Continued approval for this indication may be contingent on verification and description of clinical benefit of entrectinib in confirmatory studies.

The incidence of solid tumors harboring activating *NTRK* fusions has not been fully characterized; however, 1500–5000 cases are estimated per year in the US. Although a relatively small subset (less than 1%) of patients with common solid tumors (e.g., cancers of the lung, colon, or prostate) harbor *NTRK* fusions, such fusions have been frequently reported in certain rare cancers (i.e., 91–100% of mammary analogue secretory carcinomas, secretory breast carcinomas, or infantile fibrosarcomas; 61% of congenital mesoblastic nephromas; 12–15% of papillary thyroid cancers).

Clinical Experience

The indication for entrectinib in the treatment of solid tumors harboring a *NTRK* fusion is based principally on pooled results for a cohort of patients with unresectable or metastatic solid tumors harboring a *NTRK* fusion in 3 multicenter, open-label, noncomparative phase 1 and 2 studies (ALKA-372-001, STARTRK-1, and STARTRK-2). This cohort of patients included the initial 54 adults enrolled in the ALKA-372-001, STARTRK-1, and STARTRK-2 studies with solid tumors harboring a *NTRK* fusion. Patients were included in the *NTRK* fusion-positive solid tumor cohort if they experienced disease progression following prior systemic therapy, if available, or if severe morbidity following surgical resection for locally advanced disease was expected. Patients were also required to have at least 2 years of follow-up from first post-treatment tumor assessment. Patients who previously received a tropomyosin receptor kinase (Trk) inhibitor were excluded from the primary efficacy analysis. *NTRK* fusion was detected using NGS or other nucleic acid-based tests; confirmation of *NTRK* fusion was detected by a validated NGS test in a central laboratory in 83% of patients. Patients enrolled in the *NTRK* fusion-positive solid tumor cohort received varying dosages of entrectinib; however, 94% of patients received entrectinib 600 mg orally once daily. Treatment was continued until disease progression or unacceptable toxicity occurred. The primary efficacy end points were objective response rate according to RECIST 1.1 (as evaluated by a blinded independent review committee) and duration of response; an additional outcome measure was intracranial response. The median age of patients included in the *NTRK* fusion-positive solid tumor cohort was 58 years, 89% had an ECOG performance status of 0 or 1, 80% were white, and 59% were female. Most patients (96%) had metastatic disease and 4% had unresectable locally advanced disease. All patients in the *NTRK* fusion-positive solid tumor cohort had received prior therapy for their disease (i.e., surgery, radiation therapy, systemic therapy); 74 or 17% of patients had received a median of 1 or at least 3 prior systemic therapies for metastatic disease, respectively. CNS metastases were present in 22% of patients. The most common cancers in the *NTRK* fusion-positive solid tumor cohort were sarcoma (24%), lung cancer (19%), salivary gland tumors (13%), breast cancer (11%), thyroid cancer (9%), and colorectal cancer (7%).

At the time of data analysis, the objective response rate in the *NTRK* fusion-positive solid tumor cohort was 59%; complete response was achieved in 13% of patients. At the time of analysis, 72, 66, or 56% of patients had durable responses of at least 6, 9, or 12 months, respectively. Intracranial response was achieved in 3 of 4 patients with measurable CNS metastases at baseline (as assessed by a blinded independent review committee) who had not received prior radiation therapy to the brain within 2 months of receiving entrectinib. Among patients with previously treated metastatic disease, the objective response rate was 53%. The objective response rate in patients with mammary analogue secretory carcinoma, breast cancer, NSCLC, sarcoma, colorectal cancer, or thyroid cancer was 86, 83, 60, 46, 25, or 60%, respectively. All patients with pancreatic cancer, gynecologic cancers, or cholangiocarcinoma achieved partial responses. All patients with neuroendocrine cancers achieved complete responses. The most common documented *NTRK* fusion was *ETV6-NTRK3*. The objective response rate in patients with tumors harboring *TPR-NTRK1*, *ETV6-NTRK3*, or *TPM3-NTRK1* was 100, 72, or 50%, respectively. Although *SQSTM1-NTRK1* fusion was detected in 2 patients and *CD74-NTRK1*, *PLEKHA6-NTRK1*, *CDC42B-PA-NTRK1*, *EPS15L1-NTRK1*, and *RBPMS-NTRK3* fusions were detected in one patient each, most patients with tumors harboring these *NTRK* fusions achieved partial responses.

The efficacy of entrectinib was also evaluated in 33 pediatric patients with unresectable or metastatic solid tumors with a NTRK gene fusion enrolled in 1 of 2 multicenter, open-label clinical trials: STARTRK-NG and TAPISTRY. Patients were administered entrectinib 20 to 600 mg [dosing based on body surface area (BSA)] orally or via enteral feeding tube once daily in 4-week cycles until unacceptable toxicity or disease progression. The primary efficacy outcome measure was overall response rate. The median age of enrolled patients was 4 years (range: 2 months to 15 years). About half (52%) of patients were male; 58% were white, 30% Asian, 9% Hispanic or Latino, and 3% Black or African American. Locally advanced disease was present in 71% of patients and 29% had metastatic disease; a majority (85%) received prior treatment for their cancer including surgery, radiotherapy, and/or systemic therapy.

Results revealed an overall response rate of 70% for the 33 evaluable pediatric patients, with a complete response observed in 42% of patients and a partial response in 27%. A duration of response was assessed in 23 patients with a median duration of 25.4 months. The most common tumor types were primary CNS in 17 patients, infantile fibosarcoma in 8 patients, and spindle cell in 6 patients. The overall response rates for these tumor types were 53%, 88%, and 100%, respectively.

DOSAGE AND ADMINISTRATION

● General

Pretreatment Screening

- Confirm presence of ROS-1 rearrangement with an FDA-approved test in patients with metastatic NSCLC prior to initiation of therapy.
- Confirm presence of NTRK fusion with an FDA-approved test prior to initiation of therapy for the treatment of locally advanced or metastatic solid tumors.
- Evaluate left ventricular ejection fraction (LVEF).
- Assess serum uric acid levels.
- Assess QT interval and serum electrolyte concentrations.
- Verify pregnancy status in females of reproductive potential.

Patient Monitoring

- Monitor for signs and symptoms of heart failure (e.g., dyspnea, edema).
- Monitor liver function tests (e.g., ALT, AST) every 2 weeks during the first month of therapy, monthly thereafter, and as clinically indicated.
- Assess serum uric acid levels periodically during therapy.
- Monitor for signs and symptoms of hyperuricemia.
- Monitor QT interval and serum electrolyte concentrations periodically during therapy. More frequent monitoring may be necessary in patients with preexisting QT_c-interval prolongation or risk factors for developing QT_c-interval prolongation (e.g., long QT syndrome, clinically important bradyarrhythmia, severe or uncontrolled heart failure, electrolyte abnormalities, concomitant use of drugs known to prolong QT interval).

● Administration

Administer entrectinib orally without regard to food.

Entrectinib is commercially available as oral capsules and oral pellets; clinicians should prescribe the most appropriate dosage form based on the dose required and patient needs.

The capsules may be swallowed whole or made into an oral suspension (for oral or enteral tube administration). If swallowed whole, the capsules should not be crushed or chewed.

The oral pellets should be swallowed with soft food. The pellets should not be chewed or crushed in order to avoid a bitter taste.

If a dose of entrectinib is missed, the missed dose should be taken as soon as it is remembered unless the next dose is due within 12 hours. If a dose is vomited immediately after administration, an additional dose should be administered to make up for the vomited dose.

Capsules

Whole capsules are intended for use in patients who can swallow a whole capsule and whose doses are in multiples of 100 mg.

Capsules prepared as an oral suspension are intended for use in patients who have difficulty or inability to swallow whole capsules or patients who require enteral (e.g., gastric or nasogastric tube) administration. Capsules prepared as a suspension should also be used for those patients who require dose increments of 10 mg. The oral suspension is compounded by carefully opening the appropriate number of capsules and pouring the contents into room temperature drinking water or milk. The suspension should sit for 15 minutes after preparation and then be administered immediately. Patients should drink water after taking the oral suspension to ensure the drug has been completely swallowed.

If enteral administration is necessary, the oral suspension should be administered via a gastric or nasogastric tube. For dosing volumes ≥3 mL, an enteral tube that is 8 FR or higher is required for administration. Patients should divide dosing volumes ≥3 mL into at least 2 aliquots and a dosing volume of 30 mL into at least 3 (10 mL aliquots). The tube should be flushed with an equivalent volume of water or milk after administration of each aliquot.

Refer to the entrectinib prescribing information for more specific information on the preparation of entrectinib capsules as a suspension for oral or enteral tube administration.

Store entrectinib capsules at 20-25°C (excursions permitted between 15-30°C) in the original container and keep the bottle tightly closed to protect from moisture. If the capsules are prepared as an oral suspension using drinking water or milk, store at <30°C for no more than 2 hours. Discard any unused suspension if not used within the 2 hours following preparation.

Pellets

The pellet formulation is intended for patients who have difficulty or inability to swallow whole capsules, but can swallow soft foods, and whose doses are in multiples of 50 mg.

The pellets should be sprinkled on 1 or more spoonfuls of soft food (e.g., applesauce, yogurt, pudding) and administered within 20 minutes of preparation, followed by water to ensure the drug has been completely swallowed.

The pellets should not be used to prepare an oral suspension. Partial quantities of pellets from a packet should not be used to prepare a dose. The pellet formulation should not be used for enteral administration as the pellets may clog the tube.

Store entrectinib pellets at 20-25°C (excursions permitted between 15-30°C) in the original container in order to protect from moisture.

● Dosage

Non-small Cell Lung Cancer

For the treatment of ROS-1-positive metastatic NSCLC, the recommended adult dosage of entrectinib is 600 mg orally once daily. Treatment should be continued until disease progression or unacceptable toxicity occurs.

Solid Tumors with Neurotrophic Receptor Tyrosine Kinase Gene Fusion

For the treatment of solid tumors harboring a NTRK fusion (without a known acquired mutation for resistance) in patients who have metastatic disease or may experience severe morbidity following surgical resection and whose disease progressed following prior therapy or those who are not candidates for other treatment options, the recommended dosage of entrectinib in *adults* and *pediatric patients with a body surface area (BSA) ≥1.51 m²* is 600 mg once daily. The recommended dosage in *pediatric patients >1 month to ≤6 months of age* is 250 mg/m² once daily. Table 1 presents the recommended dosage for *pediatric patients >6 months of age*, which is based on BSA. Treatment should be continued until disease progression or unacceptable toxicity occurs.

TABLE 1. Recommended Dosage of Entrectinib in Pediatric Patients >6 Months of Age.

Body Surface Area (BSA)[a]	Recommended Dosage
≤0.50 m²	300 mg/m² once daily
0.51 to 0.80 m²	200 mg once daily
0.81 to 1.10 m²	300 mg once daily
1.11 to 1.50 m²	400 mg once daily

[a] BSA categories and recommended dosage are based on closely matching exposures to a target dose of 300 mg/m².

Dosage Modification for Toxicity

Temporary interruption of therapy, dosage reduction, and/or permanent discontinuance of entrectinib may be necessary in patients experiencing certain adverse effects. When necessary, the dosage of entrectinib should be reduced as described in Table 2. Permanently discontinue entrectinib in patients who are unable to tolerate therapy after 2 dose reductions.

TABLE 2. Dosage Reduction for Entrectinib Toxicity

Starting Dose (once daily)	First Dose Reduction	Second Dose Reduction
250 mg/m² or 300 mg/m²	Reduce dose to two-thirds of the starting dose	Reduce dose to one-third of the starting dose
200 mg	150 mg once daily	100 mg once daily
300 mg	200 mg once daily	100 mg once daily
400 mg	300 mg once daily	200 mg once daily
600 mg	400 mg once daily	200 mg once daily

Table 3 indicates the recommended dosage modification (i.e., temporary interruption of therapy, dosage reduction, discontinuance of therapy) for certain adverse effects according to severity.

TABLE 3. Dosage Modification for Entrectinib Toxicity

Adverse Reaction and Severity	Modification
Heart Failure	
Grade 2 or 3	Withhold therapy; when toxicity resolves to grade 1 or less, resume at reduced dosage
Grade 4	Permanently discontinue therapy
CNS Effects	
Grade 2 (intolerable)	Withhold therapy; when toxicity resolves to baseline or grade 1 or less, resume at same or reduced dosage
Grade 3	Withhold therapy; when toxicity resolves to baseline or grade 1 or less, resume at reduced dosage
Grade 4	Permanently discontinue therapy
Hepatotoxicity	
Grade 3	Withhold therapy. If toxicity resolves to baseline or grade 1 or less within 4 weeks, resume at same dosage; if toxicity does *not* resolve within 4 weeks, permanently discontinue therapy. Resume at a reduced dose for recurrent grade 3 events that resolve within 4 weeks
Grade 4	Withhold therapy. If toxicity resolves to baseline or grade 1 or less within 4 weeks, resume at reduced dosage; if toxicity does *not* resolve within 4 weeks, permanently discontinue therapy. Permanently discontinue therapy for recurrent grade 4 events
Elevated ALT or AST concentrations >3 times the ULN with concomitant total bilirubin concentrations >1.5 times the ULN in absence of cholestasis or hemolysis	Permanently discontinue therapy

TABLE 3. Continued

Adverse Reaction and Severity	Modification
Hyperuricemia	
Symptomatic	Withhold therapy and initiate urate-lowering therapy; when toxicity improves, resume at same or reduced dosage
Grade 4	Withhold therapy and initiate urate-lowering therapy; when toxicity improves, resume at same or reduced dosage
Prolongation of QT Interval	
QT$_c$ interval >500 msec	If other etiology of QT-interval prolongation is present: Withhold therapy and correct other causes of QT-interval prolongation; resume at same dosage when toxicity resolves to baseline If no other etiology of QT-interval prolongation is present: Withhold therapy; resume at reduced dosage when toxicity resolves to baseline
Torsades de pointes, polymorphic ventricular tachycardia, or signs and/or symptoms of serious arrhythmia	Permanently discontinue therapy
Visual Disturbances	
New visual symptoms, including changes that interfere with activities of daily living	Withhold therapy; when toxicity improves or stabilizes, resume at same or reduced dosage
Grade 2 or greater	Withhold therapy; when toxicity improves or stabilizes, resume at same or reduced dosage
Hematologic Toxicity	
Grade 3 or 4 anemia or neutropenia	Withhold therapy; when toxicity improves to grade 2 or less, resume at same or reduced dosage
Other Toxicity	
Grade 3 or 4 (clinically significant)	Withhold therapy. If toxicity resolves to baseline or grade 1 within 4 weeks, resume at same or reduced dosage; if toxicity does *not* resolve within 4 weeks, permanently discontinue therapy Permanently discontinue therapy for recurrent grade 4 events

Concomitant Use with CYP3A Inhibitors

Concomitant use of entrectinib with moderate or strong inhibitors of cytochrome P-450 (CYP) isoenzyme 3A should be avoided. If concomitant use cannot be avoided in adults and pediatric patients 2 years of age or older, the manufacturer recommends reducing the dosage of entrectinib as shown in Table 4 and limiting coadministration to 14 days or less. After discontinuing the strong or moderate CYP3A inhibitor for 3-5 elimination half-lives, resume the entrectinib dose that was taken prior to initiating the CYP3A inhibitor.

TABLE 4. Recommended Dose Modifications of Entrectinib for Concomitant Use with Moderate or Strong CYP3A Inhibitors.

Starting Dose[a]	Moderate CYP3A Inhibitor	Strong CYP3A Inhibitor
200 mg	50 mg once daily	50 mg on alternate days
300 mg	100 mg once daily	50 mg once daily
400 mg	200 mg once daily	50 mg once daily
600 mg	200 mg once daily	100 mg once daily

[a] For pediatric patients with a starting dose <200 mg, avoid coadministration with a strong or moderate CYP3A inhibitor.

● **Special Populations**

Hepatic Impairment

No dosage adjustment is necessary in patients with mild hepatic impairment (total bilirubin concentration 1.5 times or less the ULN).

Renal Impairment

No dosage adjustment is necessary in patients with mild or moderate renal impairment (creatinine clearance of 30 to less than 90 mL/minute).

Geriatric Patients

The manufacturer makes no specific dosage recommendations for geriatric patients.

CAUTIONS

● **Contraindications**

● None.

● **Warnings/Precautions**

Heart Failure

Heart failure has been reported in patients receiving entrectinib. In clinical trials, heart failure occurred in 12 (3.4%) of 355 patients receiving the drug and was grade 3 in 2.3% of patients. The median time to onset of heart failure was 2 months (range: 11 days to 12 months). Entrectinib was interrupted in 6 patients with heart failure (50%) and discontinued in 2 patients (17%). Heart failure resolved in 6 patients (50%) following interruption or discontinuation of entrectinib and initiation of appropriate medical management. Myocarditis in the absence of heart failure also was reported in 0.3% of patients receiving the drug. Routine cardiac function assessment (except electrocardiograms [ECGs]) prior to and during therapy was not performed during these studies.

Patients with symptomatic heart failure, myocardial infarction (MI), unstable angina, or those who underwent coronary artery bypass graft (CABG) within 3 months were excluded from clinical trials.

In patients with symptoms or known risk factors for heart failure, left ventricular ejection fraction (LVEF) should be assessed prior to initiation of entrectinib. Patients should be monitored for signs and symptoms of heart failure (e.g., dyspnea, edema). For patients with myocarditis with or without decreased ejection fraction, magnetic resonance imaging (MRI) or cardiac biopsy may be necessary to confirm the diagnosis of myocarditis. If new onset or worsening heart failure occurs, appropriate therapy for heart failure should be initiated and assessment of left ventricular function should be repeated. Dosage reduction or permanent discontinuance of therapy may be necessary depending on the severity of heart failure or left ventricular dysfunction.

CNS Effects

Entrectinib can cause a wide variety of adverse CNS effects, including cognitive impairment, mood disorder, dizziness, and sleep disturbance. The overall incidence of adverse CNS effects was similar in patients with or without CNS metastases; however, the incidence of dizziness, headache, paresthesia, balance disorder, and confusional state appeared to be higher in patients who received prior radiation therapy to the brain for the treatment of CNS metastases compared with those who had not received prior radiation therapy to the brain.

In clinical trials, 27% of 355 patients receiving entrectinib experienced cognitive impairment, which was grade 3 in 4.5% of patients. Most patients (77%) experienced cognitive impairment within 3 months of initiating the drug. Cognitive impairment included cognitive disorders, confusional state, disturbance in attention, memory impairment, amnesia, aphasia, mental status change, hallucination, and delirium. Dosage interruption, dosage reduction, or drug discontinuance was required in 18, 13, or 1%, respectively, of entrectinib-treated patients experiencing cognitive impairment.

In clinical trials, 10% of 355 patients receiving entrectinib experienced mood disorders, which were grade 3 in 0.6% of patients. The median time to onset of mood disorders was 1 month (range: 1 day to 9 months). Mood disorders included anxiety, depression, and agitation. Suicidality (i.e., completed suicide) was reported in one patient 11 days following discontinuance of entrectinib. Among patients experiencing mood disorders, 6% required dosage reduction and 6% required interruption of therapy. Discontinuance of entrectinib therapy was not required in patients who experienced mood disorders.

In clinical trials, 38% of 355 patients receiving entrectinib experienced dizziness, which was grade 3 in 2.2% of patients. Dosage reduction, dosage interruption, or drug discontinuance was required in 10, 7, or 0.7%, respectively, of entrectinib-treated patients experiencing dizziness.

In clinical trials, 14% of 355 patients receiving entrectinib experienced sleep disturbances and was grade 3 in 0.6% of patients. Sleep disturbances included insomnia, somnolence, hypersomnia, and sleep disorder. Dosage reduction was required in 6% of entrectinib-treated patients experiencing sleep disturbance. Discontinuance of entrectinib therapy was not required in patients who experienced sleep disturbance.

Patients and their caregivers should be informed of the risk of adverse CNS effects associated with entrectinib therapy. Temporary interruption of entrectinib therapy, dosage reduction, or permanent discontinuance of therapy may be necessary in patients experiencing adverse CNS effects during therapy with the drug, and such patients should be advised not to drive or operate machinery.

Fractures

Fractures have been reported in patients receiving entrectinib. In an expanded safety population, fracture occurred in 5% of 338 adults and 25% of 76 pediatric patients receiving the drug; the median time to onset of fracture was 3.8 months (range: 0.3–18.5 months) in adults and 4.3 months (range: 2–28.7 months) in pediatric patients. In both adult and pediatric patients, most fractures were hip or other lower extremity fractures. In 2 pediatric patients, bilateral femoral neck fractures occurred. A total of 41 fracture events were reported in 19 pediatric patients; 13 patients experienced more than one occurrence of fracture. Among the 19 pediatric patients who experienced fractures, 17 patients were <12 years of age. Entrectinib therapy was interrupted in 41% of adults and 16% of pediatric patients who experienced fractures. Five pediatric patients discontinued treatment due to fractures.

Patients experiencing signs or symptoms of fracture (e.g., pain, changes in mobility, deformity) should be promptly evaluated. Effect of entrectinib on healing of known fractures or long-term fracture risk is unknown.

Hepatotoxicity

Hepatotoxicity has been reported in patients receiving entrectinib. In clinical trials, elevations of serum AST or ALT concentrations were reported in 42 or 36%, respectively, of 355 patients receiving entrectinib; grade 3–4 elevations in AST or ALT concentrations occurred in 2.5 or 2.8%, respectively, of patients. Because posttreatment liver function tests were not available for 4.5% of patients, the reported frequency may underestimate the drug's potential to cause elevated aminotransferase concentrations. The median time to onset of elevated ALT or AST concentrations was 2 weeks (range: 1 day to 29.5 months). Dosage interruption, dosage reduction, or drug discontinuance was required in 0.8, 0.8, or 0.8%, respectively, of entrectinib-treated patients who developed elevated ALT or AST concentrations.

Liver function tests (e.g., ALT and AST concentrations) should be monitored every 2 weeks during the first month of therapy, monthly thereafter, and as clinically indicated. Temporary interruption of entrectinib therapy, dosage reduction, or permanent discontinuance of therapy may be necessary in patients experiencing hepatotoxicity.

Hyperuricemia

Hyperuricemia has been reported in patients receiving entrectinib. In clinical trials, 9% of 355 patients receiving entrectinib experienced symptomatic hyperuricemia-associated adverse reactions. Grade 4 hyperuricemia occurred in 1.7% of patients receiving the drug, including one fatal case of tumor lysis syndrome. Urate-lowering therapy, dosage reduction, and interruption of therapy were required in 34, 6, and 6%, respectively, of patients who experienced symptomatic hyperuricemia. Hyperuricemia resolved in 73% of patients following initiation of urate-lowering therapy without interruption of therapy or dosage reduction. Discontinuance of entrectinib therapy was not required in patients experiencing hyperuricemia.

Serum uric acid levels should be assessed prior to initiating entrectinib and periodically during treatment. Patients should be monitored for signs and symptoms of hyperuricemia. In patients who develop signs or symptoms of hyperuricemia, urate-lowering therapy should be initiated as clinically indicated. Temporary interruption of therapy or dosage reduction may be necessary.

Prolongation of QT Interval

Prolongation of the corrected QT (QT_c) interval has been reported in patients receiving entrectinib. In clinical trials, an increase in the QT_c interval (corrected for heart rate using Fridericia's formula [QT_cF]) exceeding 60 msec from baseline occurred in 3.1% of entrectinib-treated patients, and QT_cF intervals exceeding 500 msec occurred in 0.6% of entrectinib-treated patients.

QT interval and electrolyte concentrations should be monitored at baseline and periodically during therapy. More frequent monitoring may be necessary in patients with preexisting QT_c-interval prolongation and those with risk factors for developing QT_c-interval prolongation (e.g., long QT syndromes, clinically important bradyarrhythmia, severe or uncontrolled heart failure, electrolyte abnormalities, concomitant use of drugs known to prolong the QT_c interval). Temporary interruption of entrectinib therapy, dosage reduction, or permanent discontinuance of therapy may be necessary in patients experiencing QT_c-interval prolongation.

Visual Disturbances

Visual disturbances (i.e., blurring, photophobia, diplopia, visual impairment, photopsia, cataract, vitreous floaters), generally mild in severity, have been reported in patients receiving entrectinib. In clinical trials, vision changes occurred in 21% of 355 patients receiving the drug.

In patients who report new visual symptoms, including changes that interfere with activities of daily living, an ophthalmologic evaluation should be performed as clinically appropriate. Temporary interruption of therapy or dosage reduction may be necessary depending on the severity of the visual disturbance.

Embryo-Fetal Toxicity

Entrectinib may cause fetal harm in humans based on its mechanism of action and animal findings; embryofetal toxicity and teratogenicity have been demonstrated in animals. There are no available data regarding use of entrectinib in pregnant women. In animal reproduction studies, body closure defects (omphalocele, gastroschisis) and malformations of vertebrae, ribs, and limbs (micromelia, adactyl) were observed in rats receiving entrectinib at exposure levels up to 2.7 times the human exposure at the recommended dosage; reduced fetal weight and reduced skeletal ossification were observed in rats receiving the drug at exposure levels approximately 0.2 and 0.9 times the human exposure, respectively, at the recommended dosage. Literature reports in individuals with congenital mutations in the tropomyosin receptor kinase (Trk) pathway suggest an association between decreased Trk-mediated signaling and obesity, developmental delays, cognitive impairment, insensitivity to pain, and anhidrosis.

Pregnancy should be avoided during entrectinib therapy. The manufacturer states that a pregnancy test should be performed prior to initiation of entrectinib therapy in women of reproductive potential and states that such women should be advised to use effective contraceptive methods while receiving entrectinib and for at least 5 weeks after the last dose. Men who are partners of such women should use effective methods of contraception while receiving entrectinib and for 3 months after the last dose. Patients should be apprised of the potential hazard to the fetus if entrectinib is used during pregnancy.

Specific Populations

Pregnancy

Entrectinib may cause fetal harm if administered to pregnant women based on its mechanism of action and animal findings.

Lactation

It is not known whether entrectinib or its metabolites are distributed into human milk. The effects of the drug on nursing infants or on the production of milk are unknown. Because of the potential for adverse reactions to entrectinib in nursing infants, women should be advised not to nurse while receiving the drug and for 1 week after the last dose.

Females and Males of Reproductive Potential

Verify the pregnancy status of females of reproductive potential prior to starting entrectinib therapy. Advise female patients of reproductive potential to use effective contraception during treatment and for at least 5 weeks following the last dose. Advise male patients with female partners of reproductive potential to use effective contraception during treatment and for 3 months following the last dose.

Pediatric Use

Safety and efficacy of entrectinib for the treatment of c-ros oncogene-1 (*ROS-1*)-positive non-small cell lung cancer (NSCLC) have not been established in pediatric patients.

Safety and efficacy of entrectinib have been established in pediatric patients older than 1 month of age with solid tumors harboring a neurotrophic receptor tyrosine kinase (*NTRK*) gene fusion. Efficacy of entrectinib in pediatric patients is supported by evidence from adequate and well-controlled studies in adults and pediatric patients with additional population pharmacokinetic data demonstrating that the exposure of drug substance in pediatric patients >1 month of age is expected to be in the adult range, and that the course of disease is sufficiently similar in adult and pediatric patients to allow extrapolation of data in adults to pediatric patients.

Geriatric Use

In clinical trials, 25% of patients receiving entrectinib were 65 years of age or older, while 5% were 75 years of age or older. There is insufficient experience in patients 65 years of age or older to determine whether geriatric patients respond differently than younger adults.

Hepatic Impairment

Population pharmacokinetic analysis suggests that the pharmacokinetics of entrectinib are not substantially altered in patients with mild hepatic impairment (total bilirubin concentration 1.5 times or less the upper limit of normal [ULN]). Following administration of a single oral dose of entrectinib 100 mg (1/6 of the recommended dose), AUC_{INF} was increased by 39%, 39%, and 23% in patients with mild, moderate, and severe hepatic impairment, respectively, compared to individuals with normal hepatic function. The combined AUC_{last} of entrectinib and its M5 metabolite was increased by 16% for the mild, 16% for the moderate, and 4% for the severe hepatic impairment groups compared to the normal hepatic function group. Substantial variability in systemic exposure of entrectinib was observed in these hepatic impairment groups.

The effect of moderate hepatic impairment (total bilirubin > 1.5 – 3 times ULN with any aspartate aminotransferase) or severe hepatic impairment (total bilirubin >3 times ULN with any aspartate aminotransferase) on the safety of entrectinib at the recommended dosage is unknown.

Consider the risk/benefit profile of entrectinib prior to use in patients with moderate to severe hepatic impairment. Monitor for adverse reactions in patients with hepatic impairment more frequently since these patients may be at increased risk for adverse reactions.

Renal Impairment

Population pharmacokinetic analysis suggests that the pharmacokinetics of entrectinib are not substantially altered in patients with mild to moderate renal impairment (creatinine clearance of 30 to less than 90 mL/minute).

The effect of severe renal impairment (creatinine clearance less than 30 mL/minute) on the pharmacokinetics of entrectinib has not been established.

● Common Adverse Effects

Adverse effects reported in at least 20% of patients receiving entrectinib include fatigue, constipation, dysgeusia, edema, dizziness, diarrhea, nausea, dysesthesia, dyspnea, myalgia, cognitive impairment, increased weight, cough, vomiting, pyrexia, arthralgia, and vision disorders.

DRUG INTERACTIONS

Entrectinib is metabolized principally by cytochrome P-450 (CYP) isoenzyme 3A4.

In vitro, entrectinib is not a substrate of P-glycoprotein (P-gp) or breast cancer resistance protein (BCRP), but its major active metabolite M5 is a substrate of both P-gp and BCRP. Neither entrectinib nor M5 is a substrate of organic anion transport protein (OATP) 1B1 or 1B3.

● Drugs and Foods Affecting Hepatic Microsomal Enzymes

Inhibitors of CYP3A

Concomitant use of entrectinib with moderate or strong inhibitors of CYP isoenzyme 3A may increase systemic exposure to entrectinib and possible toxicity. When the strong CYP3A inhibitor itraconazole was administered concomitantly with entrectinib (single 100-mg dose), peak plasma concentration and AUC of entrectinib were increased 1.7- and 6-fold, respectively. Simulations using physiologically based pharmacokinetic models suggest that concomitant use of the moderate CYP3A inhibitor erythromycin (500 mg three times daily) and entrectinib (200 mg once daily) may increase steady-state peak plasma concentration and AUC of entrectinib 2.9- and 3.4-fold, respectively.

In *adults and pediatric patients 2 years of age or older*, concomitant use of entrectinib with moderate or strong CYP3A inhibitors (e.g., itraconazole, grapefruit juice) should be avoided. If concomitant use of a strong CYP3A inhibitor cannot be avoided, the manufacturer recommends reducing the dosage of entrectinib as noted in Table 4 and limiting coadministration to 14 days or less. When concomitant use of the moderate or strong CYP3A inhibitor is discontinued, the entrectinib dosage should be returned (after 3–5 elimination half-lives of the CYP3A inhibitor) to the dosage used prior to initiation of the moderate or strong CYP3A inhibitor.

In *pediatric patients less than 2 years of age*, concomitant use of moderate or strong inhibitors of CYP3A should be avoided.

Inducers of CYP3A

Concomitant use of entrectinib with moderate and strong inducers of CYP3A may decrease systemic exposure to entrectinib and reduce entrectinib efficacy. When the strong CYP3A inducer rifampin (600 mg once daily for 14 days) was administered concomitantly with entrectinib (single 600-mg dose), peak plasma concentration and AUC of entrectinib were decreased by 56 and 77%, respectively. Simulations using physiologically-based pharmacokinetic models suggest that concomitant use of the moderate CYP3A inducer efavirenz (600 mg once daily) and entrectinib (600 mg once daily) may decrease the steady-state peak plasma concentration and AUC of entrectinib by 43 and 56%, respectively.

Concomitant use of entrectinib with moderate or strong CYP3A inducers should be avoided.

● Drugs Metabolized by Hepatic Microsomal Enzymes

Substrates of CYP3A

When the sensitive CYP3A substrate midazolam was administered concomitantly with entrectinib (600 mg once daily), peak plasma concentration of midazolam was decreased by 21% and AUC of midazolam was increased by 50%.

Substrates of P-glycoprotein Transport Systems

When the sensitive P-gp substrate digoxin was administered concomitantly with entrectinib (single 600-mg dose), peak plasma concentration and AUC of digoxin were increased by 28 and 18%, respectively.

● Drugs Affecting Gastric Acidity

When the proton-pump inhibitor lansoprazole was administered concomitantly with entrectinib (single 600-mg capsule dose), peak plasma concentration and AUC of entrectinib were decreased by 23 and 25%, respectively. When lansoprazole was concurrently administered with entrectinib (single 600-mg dose as oral suspension in water), peak plasma concentration and AUC of entrectinib increased by 17 and 25%, respectively.

● Drugs that Prolong the QT Interval

Concomitant use of entrectinib with other drugs known to prolong the QT interval should be avoided.

DESCRIPTION

Entrectinib, a potent inhibitor of multiple receptor tyrosine kinases, including tropomyosin receptor kinases (Trk) A, TrkB, TrkC, c-ros oncogene-1 (*ROS-1*), and anaplastic lymphoma kinase (ALK), is an antineoplastic agent. The Trk family of tyrosine kinases (encoded by the neurotrophic receptor tyrosine kinase genes *NTRK1*, *NTRK2*, and *NTRK3*) is involved in the initiation of various cascades of intracellular signaling events (i.e., Ras/MAPK/ERK, PI3K/Akt, and PLCγ1/Pkc signal transduction pathways), which leads to cell proliferation, differentiation, apoptosis, and regulation of processes critical to neuron survival in the central and peripheral nervous systems. Chromosomal rearrangements of the *NTRK1*, *NTRK2*, and *NTRK3* genes result in fusions with an unrelated gene. These *NTRK* gene fusions encode a constitutively active chimeric Trk oncogenic fusion protein resulting in dysregulation of Trk signaling and subsequent tumorigenesis. Similarly, fusion proteins, including *ROS-1* or ALK kinase domains, activate tumorigenesis through hyperactivation of downstream signaling pathways. In vitro and in vivo, entrectinib has demonstrated inhibition of cancer cell lines derived from multiple tumor types harboring *NTRK*, *ROS-1*, and *ALK* fusion genes. In vitro, entrectinib is 10- to 100-fold more potent than crizotinib in its activity against *ROS-1*, and 7- to 8-fold more potent than crizotinib in its activity against ALK. Entrectinib also has demonstrated inhibition of Janus kinase 2 (JAK2) and tyrosine kinase nonreceptor 2 (TNK2).

Based on limited data, clinical resistance to entrectinib has been attributed to secondary point mutations of the NTRK kinase domain (i.e., G595R and G667C point mutations in the TrkA kinase domain; G623R point mutation in the TrkC kinase domain).

Entrectinib and its active metabolite exhibit linear and time-independent pharmacokinetics over the oral dosage range of 100–400 mg/m² when coadministered with food. Following oral administration of a single 600-mg dose, peak plasma concentration of the drug is achieved in 4–6 hours. Entrectinib exposure following a single oral dose (600 mg) of oral pellets did not differ to a clinically significant extent compared to exposure following capsule administration with a light meal (250 calories; 25% fat) in healthy subjects. Additionally, exposure following a single oral dose (600 mg) of entrectinib capsules as a suspension with water or milk given through a nasogastric or gastric tube did not differ to a clinically significant extent compared to exposure following capsule administration under fasted conditions in healthy subjects. A high-fat, high-calorie meal did not affect the systemic exposure of entrectinib capsules. Steady-state concentrations of entrectinib and its active metabolite are achieved within 1 and 2 weeks, respectively, of daily dosing; systemic accumulation of entrectinib and its active metabolite is approximately 2- and 1.6-fold, respectively. Entrectinib crosses the blood-brain barrier in preclinical models. Entrectinib is metabolized principally by cytochrome P-450 (CYP) isoenzyme 3A4 to form its major active metabolite, M5, which exhibits similar inhibitory activity for TrkA, TrkB, TrkC, *ROS-1*, and ALK to that of the parent drug in vitro. Entrectinib and M5 are more than 99% bound to plasma proteins. Following oral administration of a single radiolabeled dose of entrectinib, 83% of the dose was recovered in feces (36% as unchanged drug and 22% as M5) and 3% of the dose was recovered in urine. The elimination half-lives of entrectinib and M5 are 20 and 40 hours, respectively.

ADVICE TO PATIENTS

- Advise patients to read the FDA-approved patient information.
- Advise patients to swallow entrectinib capsules whole and to not chew or crush the capsules.

- Patients and caregivers should use a provided measuring device (e.g., oral syringe, measuring cup) to prepare and measure the prescribed dose if taking entrectinib capsules as an oral suspension. Instruct patients and/or caregivers on how to use the measuring device and inform patients that they may need to measure out a portion of the prepared oral suspension to receive the prescribed dosage. Instruct patients and/or caregivers that the oral suspension should be taken immediately after preparation or stored at room temperature (<30°C) for no more than 2 hours.

- Instruct patients and caregivers that entrectinib oral pellets should be sprinkled on one or more spoonfuls of a soft food (e.g., applesauce, yogurt, or pudding) and must be taken within 20 minutes of preparation.

- If a dose is missed, advise patients to take the missed dose as soon as it is remembered unless the next dose is due within 12 hours. If a dose is vomited immediately after administration, an additional dose should be administered to make up for the vomited dose.

- Risk of heart failure. Stress importance of informing clinician promptly if new or worsening signs or symptoms of heart failure (e.g., dyspnea, edema) occur.

- Risk of CNS effects. Stress importance of informing clinician if new or worsening CNS effects (i.e., cognitive impairment, mood disorders, dizziness, sleep disturbance) occur. Advise patients to avoid driving or operating hazardous machinery if they experience CNS effects.

- Risk of hepatotoxicity and importance of monitoring liver function. Stress importance of informing clinician promptly if symptoms of hepatotoxicity (e.g., loss of appetite, nausea, vomiting, upper right abdominal pain) occur.

- Risk of fractures. Stress importance of informing clinician if symptoms such as pain, changes in mobility, or deformity occur.

- Risk of hyperuricemia. Stress importance of informing clinician if signs or symptoms associated with hyperuricemia occur.

- Risk of QT-interval prolongation. Stress importance of informing clinician promptly if abnormal heartbeat or feelings of faintness, lightheadedness, or dizziness occur.

- Risk of visual disturbances. Stress importance of informing clinician if visual disturbances (e.g., blurring, photophobia, diplopia, photopsia, light sensitivity, new or increased floaters) occur.

- Risk of fetal harm. Advise females of reproductive potential to use effective methods of contraception while receiving entrectinib and for ≥5 weeks after the last dose. Advise males with female partners of reproductive potential to use effective methods of contraception while receiving the drug and for 3 months after the last dose. Advise females to inform their clinicians if they are or plan to be pregnant. If pregnancy occurs, advise patients of potential risk to the fetus.

- Advise females to avoid breastfeeding while receiving the drug and for 1 week after the last dose.

- Advise patients to inform their clinicians of existing or contemplated concomitant therapy, including prescription and OTC drugs and herbal supplements, as well as any concomitant illnesses.

- Inform patients of other important precautionary information.

For further information on the handling of antineoplastic agents, see the ASHP Guidelines on Handling Hazardous Drugs at https://www.ahfsdruginformation.com

PREPARATIONS

Obtain entrectinib through designated specialty pharmacies and distributors.

Excipients in commercially available drug preparations may have clinically important effects in some individuals; consult specific product labeling for details.

Entrectinib

Oral		
Capsules	100 mg	Rozlytrek®, Genentech
	200 mg	Rozlytrek®, Genentech
Pellets	50 mg	Rozlytrek®

† Use is not currently included in the labeling approved by the US Food and Drug Administration.

Selected Revisions July 10, 2024, © Copyright, September 9, 2019, American Society of Health-System Pharmacists, Inc.

Enzalutamide

10:00 • ANTINEOPLASTIC AGENTS

■ Enzalutamide, a nonsteroidal antiandrogen, is an antineoplastic agent.

USES

● Prostate Cancer

Castration-resistant Prostate Cancer

Enzalutamide is used for the treatment of castration-resistant prostate cancer.

This indication is based principally on the results of 3 randomized, double-blind, placebo-controlled, phase 3 studies (AFFIRM, PREVAIL, and PROSPER) and results of a multicenter, double-blind, randomized, phase 2 study (TERRAIN).

Clinical Experience

In the AFFIRM study, 1199 patients with metastatic, castration-resistant, prostate cancer that had progressed following treatment with 1 or 2 cytotoxic regimens, at least one of which had to contain docetaxel, were randomized in a 2:1 ratio to receive either enzalutamide (160 mg once daily) or placebo; androgen deprivation therapy was continued in all patients. Treatment was continued until disease progression or unacceptable toxicity occurred, new treatment was initiated, or the patient withdrew from the study. Continuation or initiation of glucocorticoid therapy was permitted but not required; 48 or 46% of patients receiving enzalutamide or placebo, respectively, received glucocorticoids. The primary measure of efficacy was overall survival. The median age of patients enrolled in the study was 69 years; 93% were Caucasian, 91% had bone metastases, 59% had disease progression based on radiographic evidence, 41% had prostate specific antigen (PSA)-only progression, 24% had received 2 prior cytotoxic regimens, and 23% had visceral (lung and/or liver) involvement. The majority (92%) of patients had an Eastern Cooperative Oncology Group (ECOG) performance status of 0 or 1, and 28% of patients had a mean Brief Pain Inventory score of 4 or greater.

In the AFFIRM study, a planned interim analysis after a specified number of deaths occurred indicated that patients receiving enzalutamide had a longer median overall survival (18.4 versus 13.6 months) than those receiving placebo. The median follow-up at the time of the interim analysis was 14.4 months, and the median duration of treatment was 8.3 months for patients receiving enzalutamide and 3 months for those receiving placebo. Because of the survival benefit observed at the interim analysis, study investigators permitted patients previously randomized to receive placebo to cross over to open-label enzalutamide therapy. At the interim analysis, patients receiving enzalutamide also had higher PSA response rates (54 versus 2%), higher soft tissue response rates (29 versus 4%), higher quality-of-life response rates (43 versus 18%), longer median time to PSA progression (8.3 versus 3 months), longer median progression-free survival based on radiographic evidence (8.3 versus 2.9 months), and longer median time to the first skeletal-related event (16.7 versus 13.3 months) compared with those receiving placebo.

In the PREVAIL study, 1717 patients with chemotherapy-naïve, metastatic, castration-resistant, prostate cancer were randomized in a 1:1 ratio to receive either enzalutamide (160 mg once daily) or placebo; androgen deprivation therapy was continued in all patients. Treatment was continued until disease progression or unacceptable toxicity occurred, new treatment was initiated, or the patient withdrew from the study. Continuation or initiation of glucocorticoid therapy was permitted but not required; 27 or 30% of patients receiving enzalutamide or placebo, respectively, received glucocorticoids. The primary measures of efficacy were overall survival and progression-free survival based on radiographic evidence (as evaluated by a central review committee according to Prostate Cancer Clinical Trials Working Group [PCCTWG] criteria for bone lesions and/or Response Evaluation Criteria in Solid Tumors [RECIST] for soft tissue lesions). The median age of patients enrolled in the study was 71 years; 77% of patients were Caucasian, 54% had radiographic evidence of disease progression, 43% had PSA-only progression, and 12% had visceral (lung and/or liver) involvement. Baseline pain assessment indicated the presence of mild or no pain in 32 or 67%,

respectively, of patients enrolled in the study. All patients enrolled in the study had an ECOG performance status of 0 or 1.

At a median follow-up of approximately 22 months in the PREVAIL study, patients receiving enzalutamide had longer median overall survival (32.4 versus 30.2 months) and progression-free survival based on radiographic evidence (20 versus 5.4 months) than those receiving placebo. Overall survival for enzalutamide-treated patients at the time of updated analysis (at a median follow-up of 31 months) remained similar to the interim results. At the time of the updated analysis, 52% of enzalutamide-treated patients and 81% of placebo recipients had received subsequent antineoplastic therapy associated with overall survival benefit; 29% of patients randomized to receive placebo crossed over to receive enzalutamide therapy. Results of a subgroup analysis (based on age, geographic region, ECOG performance status, Gleason score, PSA-only progression, disease progression based on radiographic evidence, visceral involvement, baseline PSA concentration, baseline LDH concentration, baseline hemoglobin concentration) suggested that the drug's effect on overall survival was consistent across all subgroups. Patients receiving enzalutamide also had a longer median time to initiation of antineoplastic chemotherapy and first skeletal-related event (i.e., radiation therapy or surgery for prostate cancer-related bone metastases, pathologic bone fracture, spinal cord compression, subsequent antineoplastic therapy for the treatment of prostate cancer-related bone pain) compared with those receiving placebo.

In the TERRAIN study, 375 patients with chemotherapy-naïve, metastatic, castration-resistant, prostate cancer were randomized in a 1:1 ratio to receive either enzalutamide (160 mg once daily) or bicalutamide (50 mg once daily); androgen deprivation therapy was continued in all patients. Treatment was continued until disease progression or unacceptable toxicity occurred, new treatment was initiated, or the patient withdrew from the study. The primary measure of efficacy was progression-free survival based on radiographic evidence (as evaluated by an independent central review committee according to PCCTWG criteria and/or RECIST for soft tissue lesions). The median age of patients enrolled in the study was 71 years; 93% were Caucasian, 98% had radiographic evidence of disease progression, and 46% had received prior therapy with bicalutamide. Baseline pain assessment indicated the presence of mild or no pain in 36 or 58%, respectively, of patients enrolled in the study. All patients enrolled in the study were enzalutamide-naïve and had an ECOG performance status of 0 or 1. Patients were excluded from the study if disease progression occurred during prior treatment with an antiandrogen (e.g., bicalutamide). Patients receiving enzalutamide had longer median progression-free survival based on radiographic evidence than those receiving bicalutamide (19.5 versus 13.4 months).

In the PROSPER study, 1401 patients with nonmetastatic, castration-resistant, prostate cancer were randomized (stratified by PSA doubling time and use of bone resorption inhibitors) in a 2:1 ratio to receive either enzalutamide (160 mg once daily) or placebo; androgen deprivation therapy was continued in all patients. Treatment was continued until disease progression or unacceptable toxicity occurred, new treatment was initiated, or the patient withdrew from the study. The primary measure of efficacy was metastasis-free survival. Patients were enrolled in the study if they had a PSA doubling time of 10 months or less and serum PSA concentration of 2 ng/mL or greater. The median age of patients enrolled in the study was 74 years; 77% had a Gleason score of 7 or higher, 71% were Caucasian, and 54% had undergone prior surgery or radiation therapy of the prostate. The majority (63%) of patients had received therapy with an antiandrogen; 56 or 11% had received bicalutamide or flutamide, respectively. All patients enrolled in the study had an ECOG performance status of 0 or 1.

At a median follow-up of 18.5 or 15.1 months in patients receiving enzalutamide or placebo, respectively, in the PROSPER study, patients receiving enzalutamide had longer median metastasis-free survival than those receiving placebo (36.6 versus 14.7 months). Results of a subgroup analysis (based on PSA doubling time and previous therapy with a bone resorption inhibitor) suggested that the drug's effect on metastasis-free survival was consistent across all subgroups. At 27 months after the metastasis-free survival analysis, patients receiving enzalutamide had longer median overall survival than those receiving placebo (67 versus 56.3 months). The effect of enzalutamide on overall survival was generally consistent across all subgroups, except those who received a bone resorption inhibitor at baseline; however, the sample size of patients who received a bone resorption inhibitor at baseline was small. Patients receiving enzalutamide also had longer median time to initiation of antineoplastic chemotherapy (39.6 versus 17.7 months) and longer median time to PSA progression (37.2 versus 3.9 months) compared with those receiving placebo.

Clinical Perspective

According to a joint guideline from American Urological Association (AUA), American Society for Radiation Oncology (ASTRO), and the Society of Urologic Oncology (SUO), the decision to add an androgen receptor antagonist to androgen deprivation therapy in patients with *non-metastatic*, castration-resistant, prostate cancer is dependent on metastatic risk. The risk of metastasis is determined by the time to doubling of PSA levels. If the PSA doubling time is 10 months or less, metastatic risk is high and the guideline recommends use of either apalutamide, darolutamide, or enzalutamide in addition to androgen deprivation therapy. Continuation of androgen deprivation therapy with observation is recommended for patients who have a PSA doubling time greater than 10 months as risk of metastasis is considered to be lower. In patients with newly diagnosed *metastatic*, castration-resistant, prostate cancer, who have not received prior androgen receptor pathway inhibitors, clinicians should offer continued androgen deprivation therapy with abiraterone acetate plus prednisone, docetaxel, or enzalutamide.

Metastatic Castration-sensitive Prostate Cancer

Enzalutamide is used for the treatment of metastatic, castration-sensitive, prostate cancer.

This indication is based principally on the results of a randomized, double-blind, placebo-controlled, phase 3 study (ARCHES).

Clinical Experience

In the ARCHES study, 1150 patients with metastatic, castration-sensitive, prostate cancer were randomized in a 1:1 ratio to receive either enzalutamide (160 mg once daily) or placebo; concurrent therapy with a gonadotropin-releasing hormone (GnRH) analog was permitted unless the patient had previously undergone bilateral orchiectomy. Patients were stratified by prior docetaxel therapy and volume of disease; concurrent therapy with docetaxel was not permitted during the trial. Enzalutamide therapy was continued until disease progression or unacceptable toxicity occurred, new treatment was initiated, or the patient withdrew from the study. The primary measure of efficacy was progression-free survival based on radiographic evidence (as evaluated by a blinded central review committee according to PCCTWG criteria for bone lesions and/or RECIST for soft tissue lesions). The median age of patients enrolled in the study was 70 years; 81% were Caucasian, 66% had a Gleason score of 8 or greater, and 63% had a high volume of disease. A majority of patients (82%) had not received prior docetaxel therapy. Concomitant bone resorption inhibitors were used in 12% of patients for prostate cancer or other indications. All patients enrolled in the study had an ECOG performance status of 0 or 1.

At a median follow-up of 14.4 months, patients receiving enzalutamide had a lower rate of disease progression (based on radiographic evidence) or death than those receiving placebo (15.5 versus 34.4%). Median progression-free survival based on radiographic evidence and overall survival had not been reached at the time of analysis. Results of a subgroup analysis (based on age, geographic region, ECOG performance status, Gleason score, disease localization, PSA value, disease volume, prior docetaxel therapy, and prior androgen deprivation therapy or orchiectomy) suggested the effect of the drug on progression-free survival was consistent across all subgroups. Patients receiving enzalutamide also had longer median time to PSA progression and median time to initiation of antineoplastic chemotherapy compared with those receiving placebo.

Clinical Perspective

According to a joint guideline from AUA, ASTRO, and SUO, clinicians should offer androgen deprivation therapy in combination with androgen pathway directed therapy (abiraterone plus prednisone, apalutamide, or enzalutamide) or docetaxel for the treatment of metastatic, castration-sensitive, prostate cancer. Oral androgen pathway directed therapy should not be offered without concomitant androgen deprivation therapy. A guideline from the American Society of Clinical Oncology (ASCO) similarly states that standard of care therapy for metastatic, castration-sensitive, prostate cancer is androgen deprivation therapy combined with docetaxel, abiraterone, enzalutamide, apalutamide, or darolutamide. With the exception of the triplet therapies of docetaxel plus abiraterone plus

androgen deprivation therapy and docetaxel plus darolutamide plus androgen deprivation therapy, the use of any of these agents in any other particular combination or in any particular series cannot yet be recommended. Enzalutamide plus androgen deprivation therapy should be offered to men with metastatic, castration-sensitive, prostate cancer, including those with de novo metastatic disease and those who have received prior therapy (e.g., radical prostatectomy or radiotherapy for localized disease).

Non-metastatic Castration-Sensitive Prostate Cancer

Enzalutamide is used for the treatment of non-metastatic, castration-sensitive, prostate cancer with biochemical recurrence at high risk for metastasis. This indication is based principally on the results of a randomized, phase 3 study (EMBARK).

Clinical Experience

In the EMBARK study, 1068 patients with non-metastatic, castration-sensitive, prostate cancer were randomly assigned in a 1:1:1 ratio to either enzalutamide (160 mg once daily) plus leuprolide, enzalutamide (160 mg once daily) as open-label monotherapy, or placebo once daily plus leuprolide. Patients were stratified by screening PSA (≤10 ng/mL versus >10 ng/mL), PSA doubling time (≤3 months versus >3 months to ≤ 9 months), and prior hormonal therapy. For patients with an undetectable PSA level (<0.2 ng/mL) at week 36, treatment was suspended at week 37 and restarted when the PSA level increased to ≥2.0 ng/mL (with prior prostatectomy) or ≥5.0 ng/mL (without prior prostatectomy). Patients continued to receive assigned treatments until confirmed imaging-based disease progression, unacceptable toxicity, study withdrawal, or initiation of a new treatment. The primary endpoint was metastasis-free survival (defined as the time from randomization to the date of earliest evidence of imaging-based disease progression or death from any cause) in patients administered enzalutamide plus leuprolide compared to those receiving placebo plus leuprolide. The median age of patients enrolled in the study was 69 years (range: 49-93 years); 83% of patients were white, 7% Asian, 4% Black, and 5.5% were Hispanic or Latino. The median PSA doubling time was 4.9 months. Seventy-four percent (74%) of patients had prior definitive therapy with radical prostatectomy, 34% had prior primary radiotherapy (including brachytherapy), and 49% had prior therapy with both surgery and radiotherapy (including adjuvant and salvage radiotherapy). A Gleason score of ≥8 was recorded in 32% of patients. All patients enrolled in the study had an ECOG performance status of 0 or 1.

At a median follow-up of 60.7 months, results revealed that patients receiving enzalutamide plus leuprolide had a significant improvement in metastasis-free survival compared to placebo plus leuprolide (12.7% versus 25.7%). A significant improvement in metastasis-free survival was also seen in patients assigned to enzalutamide monotherapy as compared to placebo plus leuprolide (17.7% versus 25.7%). Patients receiving the combination of enzalutamide plus leuprolide also had improvement in time to PSA progression, time to use of new antineoplastic therapy, and overall survival.

DOSAGE AND ADMINISTRATION

● General

Pretreatment Screening

- Assess for fall and fracture risk.

Patient Monitoring

- In patients at risk for fracture, monitor and manage fracture risk.
- Monitor for signs and symptoms of ischemic heart disease.

Other General Considerations

- *Patients with castration-resistant prostate cancer or metastatic castration-sensitive prostate cancer*: Use concurrently with a gonadotropin-releasing hormone (GnRH) analog unless patient has undergone bilateral orchiectomy.

- *Patients with non-metastatic castration-sensitive prostate cancer with high-risk biochemical recurrence*: May receive enzalutamide with or without a GnRH analog.

● Administration

Enzalutamide is administered orally without regard to meals.

Enzalutamide is commercially available in capsule and tablet formulations. The capsules should be swallowed whole and should *not* be chewed, dissolved, or opened. The tablets should be swallowed whole and should *not* be cut, crushed, or chewed.

● Dosage

Enzalutamide is commercially available in capsule and tablet formulations; these formulations are equivalent on a mg-per-mg basis.

Prostate Cancer

Castration-resistant Prostate Cancer

For the treatment of castration-resistant prostate cancer, the recommended dosage of enzalutamide is 160 mg once daily until disease progression or unacceptable toxicity.

Metastatic Castration-sensitive Prostate Cancer

For the treatment of metastatic castration-sensitive prostate cancer, the recommended dosage of enzalutamide is 160 mg once daily until disease progression or unacceptable toxicity.

Non-metastatic Castration-sensitive Prostate Cancer

For the treatment of non-metastatic castration-sensitive prostate cancer with biochemical recurrence at high risk for metastasis, the recommended dosage of enzalutamide is 160 mg once daily until disease progression or unacceptable toxicity.

Treatment can be suspended if prostate specific antigen (PSA) is undetectable (<0.2 ng/mL) after 36 weeks of therapy. Treatment can be reinitiated when PSA has increased to ≥2 ng/mL for patients who have undergone a radical prostatectomy or ≥5 ng/mL for patients who had prior primary radiation therapy.

Dosage Modifications

General Toxicity

If an intolerable adverse effect or grade 3 or greater toxicity occurs, enzalutamide therapy should be interrupted for one week or until symptoms improve to grade 2 or less. Enzalutamide therapy may then be resumed with or without a dosage reduction. If a dosage reduction is necessary, the dosage of enzalutamide should be reduced to 120 or 80 mg daily.

Concomitant Use with Strong CYP2C8 Inhibitors

Concomitant use of enzalutamide with strong CYP2C8 inhibitors should be avoided. If concomitant use cannot be avoided, the enzalutamide dosage should be reduced to 80 mg once daily. Upon discontinuation of the strong CYP2C8 inhibitor, the enzalutamide dosage should be increased to the dosage used prior to initiation of the strong CYP2C8 inhibitor.

Concomitant use with Strong CYP3A4 Inducers

Concomitant use of enzalutamide with strong CYP3A4 inducers should be avoided. If concomitant use cannot be avoided, the enzalutamide dosage should be increased from 160 mg to 240 mg once daily. Upon discontinuation of the strong CYP3A4 inducer, the enzalutamide dosage should be decreased to the dosage used prior to initiation of the strong CYP3A4 inducer.

● Special Populations

Hepatic Impairment

Dosage adjustment is not necessary in patients with mild, moderate, or severe hepatic impairment (Child-Pugh class A, B, or C).

Renal Impairment

Dosage adjustment is not necessary in patients with mild or moderate renal impairment (creatinine clearance 30–89 mL/minute). Enzalutamide has not been evaluated in patients with severe renal impairment (creatinine clearance <30 mL/minute) or end-stage renal disease.

Geriatric Patients

No specific dosage adjustments are recommended in geriatric patients; however, greater sensitivity of some older individuals to therapy cannot be ruled out.

CAUTIONS

● Contraindications

- None.

● Warnings/Precautions

Seizures

Seizures have occurred in patients receiving enzalutamide. In clinical trials, seizure was reported in 0.6% of patients receiving enzalutamide; seizures resolved following permanent discontinuance of the drug. Time to onset of seizures ranged from 13–2250 days following initiation of enzalutamide therapy.

Patients with predisposing factors for seizures generally were excluded from clinical trials. However, in a trial designed to assess the risk of seizures in such patients, seizure was reported in 8 of 366 enzalutamide-treated patients (2.2%) with predisposing factors for seizures (i.e., concomitant use of drugs that lower seizure threshold; history of cerebrovascular accident, transient ischemic attack, head trauma, seizure, cerebral arteriovenous malformation, or CNS infection; Alzheimer's disease; meningioma; prostate cancer with leptomeningeal involvement; unexplained loss of consciousness within the past 12 months; presence of space-occupying brain lesion). Enzalutamide therapy was resumed in all patients experiencing seizure; seizure recurred in 3 patients following resumption of the drug. Approximately 17% of patients had more than one risk factor for developing seizure. It is not known whether anticonvulsants will prevent seizures in patients receiving enzalutamide.

Enzalutamide should be permanently discontinued in patients who develop a seizure during treatment.

Posterior Reversible Encephalopathy Syndrome

Posterior reversible encephalopathy syndrome (PRES) has occurred in patients receiving enzalutamide. PRES is a neurologic disorder that may manifest with seizure, headache, lethargy, confusion, blindness, or other visual and neurologic disturbances. Hypertension may occur, but it is not necessary for the diagnosis of PRES. Brain imaging, preferably magnetic resonance imaging (MRI), is used to confirm the diagnosis. Enzalutamide therapy should be discontinued in patients who develop PRES.

Hypersensitivity

Hypersensitivity reactions, including angioedema, have occurred in patients receiving enzalutamide. In clinical trials, edema of the face, tongue, or lip was reported in 0.5, 0.1, or 0.1%, respectively, of patients receiving enzalutamide. Pharyngeal edema also has been reported during postmarketing experience. Patients who experience symptoms of hypersensitivity should temporarily discontinue enzalutamide and seek immediate medical care.

Enzalutamide should be permanently discontinued in patients who develop a serious hypersensitivity reaction during treatment.

Cardiovascular Effects

Ischemic heart disease, sometimes fatal, has occurred in patients receiving enzalutamide. In clinical studies in patients with prostate cancer, ischemic heart disease was reported in 3.5% of patients receiving enzalutamide compared with 2% of those receiving placebo; grade 3 or 4 ischemic events occurred in 1.8% of patients receiving the drug compared with 1.1% of those receiving placebo. Fatal ischemic events occurred in 0.4% of patients receiving enzalutamide and 0.1% of those receiving placebo.

Patients receiving enzalutamide therapy should be monitored for signs or symptoms of ischemic heart disease, and management of preexisting cardiovascular risk factors (e.g., hypertension, diabetes mellitus, dyslipidemia) should be optimized. Enzalutamide therapy should be discontinued in patients who develop grade 3 or 4 ischemic heart disease.

In a pooled safety analysis of clinical studies, the incidence of hypertension with enzalutamide or placebo was 14 or 7%, respectively. Less than 1% of both enzalutamide- and placebo-treated patients withdrew from the study because of hypertension.

Falls and Fractures

Falls and fractures have occurred in patients receiving enzalutamide. In a pooled safety analysis of clinical studies in patients with prostate cancer, falls were reported in 12% of patients receiving enzalutamide compared with 6% of those receiving placebo and were not associated with loss of consciousness or seizure. Fractures were reported in 13% of patients receiving enzalutamide compared with 6% of those receiving placebo; grade 3 or 4 fractures occurred in 3.4% of patients receiving the drug compared with 1.9% of those receiving placebo. The median time to occurrence of fracture was 420 days (range: 1–2348 days) in patients receiving enzalutamide. Routine bone density assessments were not performed during these studies. In addition, bone-targeting agents for the prevention of bone loss in the setting of osteoporosis were not administered.

Patients receiving enzalutamide should be evaluated for fracture and fall risk. Patients at risk for fractures should be monitored and managed according to established treatment guidelines; therapy with bone-targeting agents should be considered.

Embryo-fetal Toxicity

Enzalutamide may cause fetal harm in humans based on its mechanism of action and animal findings; the drug has been shown to be teratogenic, embryotoxic, and fetotoxic in animals. Safety and efficacy of enzalutamide have not been established in females. Reproduction studies in mice revealed post-implantation loss and resorption, decreased anogenital distance, cleft palate, and absent palatine bone at dosages below the maximum recommended human dosage. However, there was no evidence of developmental toxicity in rabbits at exposure levels approximately 0.4 times the human exposure. If used during pregnancy or if the patient becomes pregnant while receiving enzalutamide, the patient should be apprised of the potential hazard to the fetus and the potential risk for loss of the pregnancy.

Because it is not known whether enzalutamide or its metabolites distribute into semen, males receiving the drug should use a condom during sexual encounters with pregnant females and should use an effective contraceptive method during sexual encounters with females of reproductive potential. These contraceptive measures are required during enzalutamide therapy and for 3 months after the last dose of the drug.

Specific Populations

Pregnancy

Based on its mechanism of action and animal findings, enzalutamide can cause fetal harm and potential loss of pregnancy if administered to pregnant females.

Lactation

Enzalutamide and/or its metabolites are distributed into milk in rats; peak concentrations in milk (achieved 4 hours following oral administration of the drug) are 4 times higher than plasma concentrations. It is not known whether the drug distributes into human milk or if the drug has any effect on milk production or on the nursing infant.

Females and Males of Reproductive Potential

Males with female partners of reproductive potential should use effective contraception during enzalutamide treatment and for 3 months after the last dose of the drug. Males should also use a condom during sexual intercourse with pregnant females.

Results of animal studies suggest that enzalutamide may impair male fertility. In repeat-dose toxicity studies in animals, hypospermatogenesis and atrophy of seminal vesicles, prostate, and epididymis were observed.

Pediatric Use

Safety and efficacy of enzalutamide have not been established in pediatric patients.

Geriatric Use

In clinical trials evaluating enzalutamide in men with prostate cancer, 78% of patients were 65 years of age or older and 33% were 75 years of age or older.

No overall differences in safety and efficacy were observed between geriatric patients and younger adults. However, the possibility of increased sensitivity to the drug in some geriatric patients cannot be ruled out.

Hepatic Impairment

Following a single 160-mg dose of enzalutamide, systemic exposure to the major active forms of the drug (i.e., enzalutamide plus N-desmethylenzalutamide) in individuals with mild, moderate, or severe hepatic impairment (Child-Pugh class A, B, or C) was similar to that in individuals with normal hepatic function.

Renal Impairment

The effect of renal impairment on the pharmacokinetic disposition of enzalutamide has not been specifically studied to date. In a population pharmacokinetic analysis, clearance of enzalutamide in patients with mild to moderate renal impairment (creatinine clearance 30–89 mL/minute) was similar to that in individuals with normal renal function. Enzalutamide has not been evaluated systematically in patients with severe renal impairment (creatinine clearance <30 mL/minute) or end-stage renal disease.

● Common Adverse Effects

Adverse effects reported in 10% or more of patients receiving enzalutamide for the treatment of prostate cancer and at an incidence that is at least 2% higher than that reported with placebo include musculoskeletal pain, fatigue, hot flush, constipation, decreased appetite, diarrhea, hypertension, hemorrhage, fall, fracture, and headache.

DRUG INTERACTIONS

In vivo studies indicate that enzalutamide is a strong inducer of cytochrome P-450 (CYP) isoenzyme 3A4 and a moderate inducer of CYP isoenzymes 2C9 and 2C19; enzalutamide does not induce CYP1A2 at clinically relevant concentrations. Enzalutamide also induces CYP2B6 in vitro. In vitro studies show that enzalutamide and its 2 major metabolites (an active N-desmethyl metabolite and an inactive carboxylic acid metabolite) are inhibitors of CYP isoenzymes 2B6, 2C8, 2C9, 2C19, 2D6, and 3A4/5; enzalutamide also causes time-dependent inhibition of CYP1A2 in vitro. In vitro, N-desmethylenzalutamide is not a substrate of CYP isoenzymes 1A1, 1A2, 2A6, 2B6, 2C8, 2C9, 2C18, 2C19, 2D6, 2E1, or 3A4/5. In vitro studies indicate that neither enzalutamide nor its 2 major metabolites are substrates of P-glycoprotein (P-gp); however, both enzalutamide and N-desmethylenzalutamide are inhibitors of P-gp. Enzalutamide is metabolized by CYP isoenzymes 2C8 and 3A4; formation of the active N-desmethyl metabolite is mediated principally by CYP2C8.

● Drugs Affecting Hepatic Microsomal Enzymes

Strong Inhibitors of CYP2C8

Concomitant use of enzalutamide with strong inhibitors of CYP2C8 may result in increased systemic exposure to enzalutamide and its active N-desmethyl metabolite. When the strong CYP2C8 inhibitor gemfibrozil (600 mg twice daily) was administered concomitantly with enzalutamide (single 160-mg dose) in healthy individuals, systemic exposure to the major active forms of the antiandrogen (i.e., enzalutamide plus N-desmethylenzalutamide) was increased by approximately 2.2-fold; however, peak plasma concentrations of these active forms of the drug were not substantially affected. Concomitant use of enzalutamide with strong CYP2C8 inhibitors should be avoided if possible. If concomitant use cannot be avoided, the dosage of enzalutamide should be reduced to 80 mg once daily. If concomitant use of the strong CYP2C8 inhibitor is discontinued, the enzalutamide dosage should be returned to the dosage used prior to initiation of the strong CYP2C8 inhibitor.

Strong Inhibitors of CYP3A4

When the strong CYP3A4 inhibitor itraconazole (200 mg once daily) was administered concomitantly with enzalutamide (single 160-mg dose) in healthy individuals, systemic exposure to the major active forms of the antiandrogen (i.e., enzalutamide plus N-desmethylenzalutamide) was increased by approximately 1.3-fold; peak plasma concentrations of these active forms of the drug were not affected. Initial dosage adjustment is not necessary.

Inducers of CYP3A4

Concomitant use of enzalutamide with strong inducers of CYP3A4 (e.g., carbamazepine, phenobarbital, phenytoin, rifabutin, rifampin, rifapentine) may result in decreased systemic exposure to enzalutamide. When the combined strong CYP3A4 and moderate CYP2C8 inducer rifampin (600 mg once daily) was administered concomitantly with enzalutamide (single 160-mg dose) in healthy individuals, systemic exposure to the major active forms of the antiandrogen (i.e., enzalutamide plus N-desmethylenzalutamide) was decreased by 37%; however, peak plasma concentrations of these active forms of the drug were not affected.

Concomitant use of enzalutamide with strong CYP3A4 inducers should be avoided if possible. If concomitant use cannot be avoided, the dosage of enzalutamide should be increased from 160 mg to 240 mg once daily. If concomitant use of the strong CYP3A4 inducer is discontinued, the enzalutamide dosage should be returned to the dosage used prior to initiation of the strong CYP3A4 inducer.

St. John's wort (*Hypericum perforatum*) is an inducer of CYP3A4 and can decrease systemic exposure to enzalutamide. Concomitant use of enzalutamide with St. John's wort should be avoided.

● Drugs Metabolized by Hepatic Microsomal Enzymes

Concomitant use of enzalutamide with drugs that are metabolized by CYP isoenzymes 3A4, 2C9, or 2C19 may result in decreased systemic exposure to the substrate drug. When the CYP3A4 substrate midazolam (single 2-mg dose), CYP2C9 substrate warfarin sodium (single 10-mg dose), and CYP2C19 substrate omeprazole (single 20-mg dose) were administered concomitantly with enzalutamide (160 mg daily), systemic exposure and peak plasma concentrations of midazolam were decreased by 86 and 77%, respectively; systemic exposure to S-warfarin was decreased by 56%; and systemic exposure and peak plasma concentrations of omeprazole were decreased by 70%. Concomitant use of enzalutamide with CYP3A4, 2C9, or 2C19 substrates that have a narrow therapeutic index (e.g., alfentanil, clopidogrel, cyclosporine, dihydroergotamine, ergotamine, fentanyl, phenytoin, pimozide, quinidine, sirolimus, tacrolimus, warfarin) should be avoided. If concomitant use with warfarin cannot be avoided, additional monitoring of the international normalized ratio (INR) is recommended.

When the CYP2C8 substrate pioglitazone (single 30-mg dose) was administered concomitantly with enzalutamide (160 mg daily), clinically important changes in systemic exposure to pioglitazone were not observed; therefore, dosage adjustment is not necessary.

When the CYP1A2 substrate caffeine (single 100-mg dose) and CYP2D6 substrate dextromethorphan (single 30-mg dose) were administered concomitantly with enzalutamide (160 mg daily), clinically important changes in systemic exposure to caffeine and dextromethorphan were not observed; therefore, dosage adjustment is not necessary.

● Protein-bound Drugs

Because enzalutamide and N-desmethylenzalutamide are highly protein bound (97–98 and 95%, respectively), the drug could be displaced from binding sites by, or could displace from binding sites, other protein-bound drugs. In vitro data indicate that displacement between enzalutamide and other highly protein-bound drugs (i.e., salicylates, ibuprofen) is unlikely at clinically relevant concentrations.

DESCRIPTION

Enzalutamide, a nonsteroidal antiandrogen, is an antineoplastic agent. Like conventional nonsteroidal antiandrogens (e.g., bicalutamide, flutamide, nilutamide), enzalutamide competitively inhibits androgen binding to androgen receptors; blockade of androgen receptors may result in growth arrest or apoptosis of prostate cancer cells through inhibition of nuclear translocation of the activated androgen receptor and through inhibition of androgen-dependent binding of the androgen receptor complex to DNA. In vitro, enzalutamide has been shown to reduce tumor growth and induce apoptosis of tumor cells; the drug also has been shown to induce tumor regression in mouse models of castration-resistant prostate cancer. The binding affinity of enzalutamide at the androgen receptor is 5–8 times greater than that of bicalutamide. The main circulating metabolite of enzalutamide, an N-desmethyl derivative, has been shown to have activity similar to that of the parent drug in vitro.

In castration-resistant prostate cancer, alterations in androgen receptor signaling (e.g., androgen receptor gene mutation or amplification and androgen receptor overexpression) have been shown to result in persistence of androgen receptor signaling and to contribute to disease progression despite castrate levels of androgens. Androgen receptor overexpression has been associated with resistance to conventional antiandrogens. In cells that overexpress the androgen receptor, conventional antiandrogens (e.g., bicalutamide, flutamide, nilutamide) have been shown to have partial agonist effects on the androgen receptor, which results in continued activation of the androgen receptor signaling axis despite castrate levels of androgens; this paradoxical effect has been attributed to alterations in the androgen signaling cascade (e.g., androgen receptor gene amplification or mutation). Unlike these conventional antiandrogens, enzalutamide appears to lack agonistic effects in cells that overexpress the androgen receptor, which may result in retained antagonism of the androgen receptor despite overexpression of the receptor.

Pharmacokinetics of enzalutamide are dose proportional over a dosage range of 30–360 mg daily. Following oral administration, the median time to peak plasma concentrations is 1 hour. Steady-state concentrations of enzalutamide are achieved after 28 days of once-daily dosing and the accumulation ratio is approximately 8.3-fold. Administration of enzalutamide with a high-fat meal did not affect the extent of absorption. Following a single 160-mg dose of enzalutamide in healthy males, the extent of absorption was comparable between the tablet and capsule formulations; however, mean peak plasma concentration following administration of the tablet formulation was 10–28% lower than that of capsules. Peak plasma concentration and AUC of enzalutamide and N-desmethyl enzalutamide at steady state were comparable between the tablet and capsule formulations. Enzalutamide is metabolized by cytochrome P-450 (CYP) isoenzymes 2C8 and 3A4. Major metabolites of the drug include an active N-desmethyl derivative and an inactive carboxylic acid derivative; formation of N-desmethylenzalutamide is mediated principally by CYP2C8. Enzalutamide and N-desmethylenzalutamide are 97–98 and 95% bound, respectively, to plasma proteins. The terminal half-lives of enzalutamide and N-desmethylenzalutamide following a single oral dose of the drug are 5.8 and approximately 7.8–8.6 days, respectively. Following oral administration of a radiolabeled dose of enzalutamide, about 71% of the dose is recovered in urine (including only trace amounts of unchanged drug and N-desmethylenzalutamide) and 14% of the dose is recovered in feces (0.4% as unchanged drug and 1% as N-desmethylenzalutamide).

In a dose-finding study, the maximum tolerated dosage of enzalutamide was 240 mg daily; decreases in serum prostate specific antigen (PSA) concentrations were dose dependent at dosages of 30–150 mg daily, but reached a plateau at dosages between 150–240 mg daily.

The pharmacokinetics of enzalutamide do not appear to be affected by age, body weight, or race (Asian versus non-Asian).

ADVICE TO PATIENTS

- Advise patients to take enzalutamide as directed by their clinician and at the same time each day. If a dose is missed, administer the missed dose on the same day as soon as it is remembered; do not take 2 doses on the same day to make up for a missed dose.

- Advise patients to swallow enzalutamide capsules whole and not to chew, dissolve, or open the capsules. Advise patients to swallow enzalutamide tablets whole and not to cut, crush, or chew the tablets.

- For patients currently receiving gonadotropin-releasing hormone (GnRH) agonist therapy, stress importance of continuing this therapy during enzalutamide therapy.

- Risk of seizures. Advise patients to avoid activities where sudden loss of consciousness could cause serious harm to themselves or others. Stress importance of informing clinician immediately if loss of consciousness or seizure occurs.

- Risk of posterior reversible encephalopathy syndrome (PRES). Stress importance of informing clinician immediately if rapidly worsening symptoms suggestive of PRES (e.g., seizure, headache, decreased alertness, confusion, visual disturbances) occur.

- Risk of hypersensitivity reactions, including angioedema. Stress importance of seeking immediate medical care if signs or symptoms of hypersensitivity reactions (e.g., edema of the face, lip, tongue, or throat) occur.

- Risk of ischemic heart disease. Stress importance of seeking immediate medical care if signs or symptoms of a cardiovascular event (e.g., angina, shortness of breath) occur.

- Risk of dizziness, vertigo, falls, and fractures. Stress importance of informing clinician if these adverse effects occur.

- Risk of fetal harm. Advise men receiving the drug to use a condom during sexual encounters with pregnant women and to use an effective contraceptive method during sexual encounters with women of childbearing potential; these contraceptive measures are required during enzalutamide therapy and for 3 months after last dose.

- Advise patients to inform their clinicians of existing or contemplated concomitant therapy, including prescription (e.g., drugs that lower seizure threshold) and OTC drugs and herbal supplements, as well as any concomitant illnesses or conditions that might predispose to seizures.

- Inform patients of other important precautionary information.

For further information on the handling of antineoplastic agents, see the ASHP Guidelines on Handling Hazardous Drugs at https://www.ahfsdruginformation.com.

PREPARATIONS

Enzalutamide can only be obtained through designated specialty pharmacies. Contact manufacturer for specific ordering and availability information.

Excipients in commercially available drug preparations may have clinically important effects in some individuals; consult specific product labeling for details.

Enzalutamide

Oral

Capsules, liquid-filled	40 mg	Xtandi®, Astellas
Tablets, film-coated	40 mg	Xtandi®, Astellas
	80 mg	Xtandi®, Astellas

† Use is not currently included in the labeling approved by the US Food and Drug Administration.

Selected Revisions August 10, 2024, © Copyright, September 17, 2013, American Society of Health-System Pharmacists, Inc.

Erdafitinib

10:00 • ANTINEOPLASTIC AGENTS

■ Erdafitinib, a potent inhibitor of fibroblast growth factor receptors (FGFR)-1, FGFR-2, FGFR-3, and FGFR-4, is an antineoplastic agent.

USES

● Urothelial Carcinoma

Erdafitinib is used for the treatment of adults with locally advanced or metastatic urothelial carcinoma with susceptible fibroblast growth factor receptor (*FGFR-3*) genetic alterations that has progressed during or following at least one prior systemic therapy. An FDA-approved companion diagnostic test (e.g., Qiagen *therascreen®* FGFR RGQ RT-PCR Kit) is required to confirm the presence of susceptible *FGFR-3* genetic alterations in tumor specimens prior to initiation of therapy. Erdafitinib is *not* recommended for the treatment of patients who are eligible for and have not received prior programmed cell death (PD)-1 or programmed death-ligand 1 (PD-L1) inhibitor therapy.

Clinical Experience

The current indication for erdafitinib was initially based principally on the results of an open-label, multicenter, noncomparative, phase 2 study (BLC2001) in patients with relapsed or refractory locally advanced or metastatic urothelial carcinoma. In the BLC2001 study, the cohort of patients with relapsed or refractory advanced urothelial carcinoma included 87 adults with locally advanced or metastatic urothelial carcinoma that had progressed during or following at least one prior chemotherapy regimen. Patients enrolled in this cohort also had disease harboring at least one of the following *FGFR* genomic aberrations (as detected by a Clinical Trial Assay [CTA]): *FGFR3* gene mutation (mutations at codon R248C, S249C, G370C, and/or Y373C) and/or gene fusion (*FGFR3-TACC3, FGFR3-BAIAP2L1, FGFR2-BICC1,* and/or *FGFR2-CASP7*). Erdafitinib was administered at an initial dosage of 8 mg orally once daily followed by an increase to 9 mg once daily if serum phosphate concentrations remained below 5.5 mg/dL on days 14–17 during cycle 1; an increase in dosage to 9 mg once daily was achieved in 41% of patients. Erdafitinib therapy was continued until disease progression or unacceptable toxicity occurred. The median age of patients enrolled in the relapsed or refractory cohort of this study was 67 years (range: 36–87 years); 79% were male, 74% were white, 92% had an Eastern Cooperative Oncology Group (ECOG) performance status of 0 or 1, and 66% had visceral metastases. Most (97%) patients enrolled in the cohort had previously received at least one carboplatin- or cisplatin-containing therapy, 10% had received both carboplatin- and cisplatin-containing therapy, and 24% had previously received an anti-PD-1 or anti-PD-L1 monoclonal antibody.

At the time of analysis, the objective response rate for patients in the relapsed or refractory disease cohort of this study was 32.2% with a median duration of response of 5.4 months; complete response was achieved in 2.3% of patients. In an exploratory subgroup analysis, the objective response rate in patients with *FGFR-3* point mutation, *FGFR-3* gene fusion, or *FGFR-2* gene fusion was 40.6, 11.1, or 0%, respectively. These response rates appeared to represent measurable benefits with erdafitinib treatment based on historical objective responses of approximately 10–20% with second-line, single-agent chemotherapy (e.g., taxanes, immune checkpoint inhibitors [e.g., pembrolizumab]) in patients with locally advanced and unresectable or metastatic urothelial carcinoma with *FGFR* aberrations.

In a confirmatory, phase 3, randomized, open-label, multicenter, 2-cohort trial (THOR), the efficacy of erdafitinib was evaluated in patients with previously treated metastatic urothelial carcinoma. In Cohort 1, 266 adult patients with advanced urothelial cancer harboring selected *FGFR-3* alterations were randomly assigned to erdafitinib 8 mg, with titration up to 9 mg, or chemotherapy (docetaxel 75 mg/m^2 once every 3 weeks or vinflunine [not available in the United States] 320 mg/m^2 once every 3 weeks) until unacceptable toxicity or progression. All patients had disease progression after 1 or 2 prior treatments, at least 1 of which included a PD-1 or PD-L1 inhibitor. The primary endpoint was overall survival, defined as the time from randomization to death from any cause. Key secondary efficacy outcome measures included progression-free survival and objective response rate assessed by the investigator using RECIST (Response Evaluation Criteria in Solid Tumors) Version 1.1.

The median age of enrolled patients was 67 years (range, 32-86 years); 71% were male; 54% were white, 29% Asian, and 0.4% Black. Most patients had a baseline ECOG performance status of 0 (43%) or 1 (48%). Eighty-one percent of patients had *FGFR-3* mutations, 17% had fusions, and 2% had both mutations and fusions. The majority (88%) of patients received platinum-containing chemotherapy previously. Results revealed that median overall survival was significantly improved with erdafitinib as compared to chemotherapy (12.1 versus 7.8 months), at a median follow-up of 15.9 months. Median progression-free survival was also significantly longer with erdafitinib (5.6 versus 2.7 months), and investigator-assessed objective response rate was significantly higher with erdafitinib therapy (45.6% vs. 11.5%).

Cohort 2 of the THOR trial involved 351 adults with locally advanced or metastatic urothelial carcinoma with selected *FGFR-3* alterations who received a single prior line of systemic therapy and were PD-1/PDL1 inhibitor naïve. Patients were randomly assigned to erdafitinib 8 mg once daily, with titration up to 9 mg, or pembrolizumab 200 mg every 3 weeks. The primary endpoint was overall survival; however, the study did not meet its major efficacy outcome measure for superiority of overall survival at the pre-specified final analysis. Median overall survival was 10.9 months for erdafitinib as compared to 11.1 months for pembrolizumab.

Clinical Perspective

The European Society of Medical Oncology (ESMO) released updated guidelines on the treatment of advanced urothelial carcinoma in 2024. ESMO recommends administration of enfortumab vedotin in combination with pembrolizumab as first-line therapy for treatment-naïve advanced or metastatic urothelial carcinoma, irrespective of platinum eligibility. If progression occurs on enfortumab vedotin in combination with pembrolizumab, standard platinum-based chemotherapy without maintenance avelumab in unselected patients or erdafitinib in selected *FGFR*-altered tumors can be recommended.

If administration of enfortumab vedotin plus pembrolizumab is not possible, ESMO recommends nivolumab + cisplatin + gemcitabine or platinum-based chemotherapy + maintenance avelumab as alternative regimens. Erdafitinib is also recommended in patients with selected *FGFR* DNA fusions and mutations who have previously been treated with chemotherapy and an immune checkpoint inhibitor.

DOSAGE AND ADMINISTRATION

● General

Pretreatment Screening

● Confirm presence of susceptible fibroblast growth factor receptor (*FGFR-3*) genetic alterations in tumor specimens prior to initiation of erdafitinib therapy.

● Because elevated phosphate concentrations occur frequently in patients receiving erdafitinib, phosphate intake should not exceed 600–800 mg daily during therapy.

● Assess concomitant therapy, including prescription drugs, OTC drugs, and dietary or herbal supplements, for agents that may alter plasma phosphate concentrations.

● Verify pregnancy status in females of reproductive potential prior to initiating therapy.

Patient Monitoring

● Monitor serum phosphate concentrations 14–21 days following initiation of erdafitinib therapy and then monthly thereafter or more frequently as clinically indicated.

● Perform ophthalmologic examination, including visual acuity assessment, slit lamp examination, fundoscopy, and optical coherence tomography, monthly during the first 4 months of erdafitinib therapy; every 3 months thereafter; and as clinically indicated (e.g., if new or worsening visual disturbances occur).

Premedication and Prophylaxis

- To minimize the risk of dry eye, the manufacturer recommends prophylaxis with ophthalmic demulcents (e.g., artificial tears substitutes, hydrating or lubricating ophthalmic gel or ointment). Apply ophthalmic demulcents frequently (i.e., at least every 2 hours) during waking hours.

● Administration

Erdafitinib is administered orally once daily without regard to meals. The tablets should be swallowed whole.

If a dose of erdafitinib is missed, take the dose as soon as possible on the same day and resume the regular dosing schedule the next day. If vomiting occurs at any time following administration of erdafitinib, a replacement dose should not be administered; take the next dose at the regularly scheduled time.

Store between 20–25°C (excursions permitted between 15–30°C).

● Dosage

Urothelial Carcinoma

For the treatment of locally advanced or metastatic urothelial carcinoma with susceptible *FGFR-3* genetic alterations that has progressed during or following at least one prior systemic therapy in adults, the recommended initial dosage of erdafitinib is 8 mg orally once daily; if this initial dosage is tolerated (i.e., serum phosphate concentrations less than 9 mg/dL, absence of ocular disorders or grade 2 or greater adverse effects) for 14–21 days, the dosage of erdafitinib should be increased to a maximum dosage of 9 mg once daily. Therapy should be continued until disease progression or unacceptable toxicity occurs.

Dosage Modification for Toxicity

If adverse reactions occur during erdafitinib therapy, temporary interruption of therapy, dosage reduction, and/or permanent discontinuance of the drug may be necessary. If dosage modification is required, the dosage of erdafitinib should be reduced as described in Table 1.

TABLE 1. Dosage Modification for Erdafitinib Toxicity Following Therapy Interruption

Dose Reduction Level	Current Dosage of 8 mg daily	Current Dosage of 9 mg daily
First	Restart at 6 mg daily	Restart at 8 mg daily
Second	Restart at 5 mg daily	Restart at 6 mg daily
Third	Restart at 4 mg daily	Restart at 5 mg daily
Fourth	Discontinue erdafitinib	Restart at 4 mg daily
Fifth		Discontinue erdafitinib

Hyperphosphatemia

If hyperphosphatemia (≥7 mg/dL) occurs during erdafitinib therapy, temporary interruption, dosage reduction, and/or permanent discontinuance of the drug may be necessary (see Table 2). If serum phosphate with life-threatening consequences occurs and urgent intervention is required (e.g., dialysis), permanently discontinue erdafitinib therapy.

TABLE 2. Dosage Modification for Hyperphosphatemia.

Serum Phosphate Concentration (mg/dL)	Dosage Modification
7–8.99	Continue therapy at the current dosage; start phosphate binder with food until phosphate level <7 mg/dL
	Reduce dose if phosphate level remains ≥7 mg/dL for a period of 2 months or if clinically necessary

TABLE 2. Continued

Serum Phosphate Concentration (mg/dL)	Dosage Modification
9 to 10	Withhold therapy with weekly reassessments until phosphate level <7 mg/dL; then restart at the same dose level
	Start phosphate binder with food until phosphate level <7 mg/dL
	Reduce dose if phosphate level ≥9 mg/dL for a period of 1 month or if clinically necessary
>10	Withhold therapy with weekly reassessments until phosphate level <7 mg/dL; then restart at the first reduced dose level
	If hyperphosphatemia (≥10 mg/dL) for >2 weeks, discontinue therapy permanently
	Utilize medical management of symptoms as clinically relevant

Ocular Effects

If central serous retinopathy occurs, temporary interruption of therapy, dosage reduction, and/or permanent discontinuance of the drug as described in Table 3 may be necessary.

TABLE 3. Dosage Modification for Central Serous Retinopathy.

Severity	Dosage Modification
Any grade	Withhold erdafitinib and perform an ophthalmic evaluation within 2 weeks. If improving within 14 days, restart erdafitinib at the current dose
	If not improving within 14 days, withhold erdafitinib until improving; once improving, may resume at the next lower dose level
	Upon restarting erdafitinib, monitor for recurrence every 1 to 2 weeks for a month
	If recurs or has not improved after 4 weeks of withholding therapy, consider permanent discontinuation

Other Adverse Effects

If other grade 3 adverse reactions occur, erdafitinib therapy should be withheld until the toxicity improves to grade 1 or baseline; therapy may then be resumed at a dosage reduced by 1 dose level.

If grade 4 adverse reactions occur, erdafitinib therapy should be permanently discontinued.

● Special Populations

Hepatic Impairment

No dosage adjustment is necessary in patients with mild to moderate hepatic impairment (Child-Pugh class A or B).

Limited data are available in patients with severe hepatic impairment (Child-Pugh class C).

Renal Impairment

No dosage adjustment is necessary in patients with mild to moderate renal impairment (estimated glomerular filtration rate [eGFR] 30–89 mL/minute per 1.73 m^2).

Limited data are available in patients with severe renal impairment.

Geriatric Patients

The manufacturer makes no specific dosage recommendations for geriatric patients.

CAUTIONS

● *Contraindications*

● None.

● *Warnings/Precautions*

Ocular Disorders

Central serous retinopathy and retinal pigment epithelial detachment resulting in visual field defect have been reported in patients receiving erdafitinib. In the pooled safety population, central serous retinopathy/retinal pigment epithelial detachment occurred in 22% of erdafitinib-treated patients, with a median time to first onset of 46 days. In 104 patients with central serous retinopathy, 40% required dose interruptions and 56% required dose reductions; 2.9% required permanent treatment discontinuation. Of the 24 patients who restarted erdafitinib after dose interruption with or without dose reduction, 67% had recurrence and/or worsening of central serous retinopathy after reinitiation.

Dry eye symptoms also have occurred in 26% of erdafitinib-treated patients. The manufacturer recommends prophylaxis with ocular demulcents as needed.

Ophthalmologic examination, including visual acuity assessment, slit lamp examination, fundoscopy, and optical coherence tomography, should be performed monthly during the first 4 months of erdafitinib therapy; every 3 months thereafter; and as clinically indicated (e.g., if new or worsening visual disturbances occur). If visual symptoms are reported, ophthalmologic evaluations should be performed urgently. Temporary interruption or discontinuance of erdafitinib may be necessary if ocular toxicities occur during therapy with the drug.

Hyperphosphatemia and Soft Tissue Mineralization

Increased serum phosphate concentration is a consequence of inhibition of fibroblast growth factor receptor (FGFR). Erdafitinib can cause hyperphosphatemia leading to soft tissue mineralization, cutaneous calcinosis, nonuremic calciphylaxis, and vascular calcification. In the pooled safety population, hyperphosphatemia was reported in 73% of patients receiving erdafitinib. The median time to onset of increased phosphate was 16 days (range: 8–421 days) following initiation of erdafitinib. Twenty-four percent of patients received phosphate binders during erdafitinib therapy. Vascular calcification was seen in 0.2% of patients treated with erdafitinib.

Because elevated phosphate concentrations occur frequently in patients receiving erdafitinib, phosphate intake should not exceed 600–800 mg daily during therapy and patients should avoid concurrent use of agents that may increase serum phosphate levels. If hyperphosphatemia (serum phosphate concentrations exceeding 7 mg/dL) occurs, an oral phosphate binder should be considered until serum phosphate concentrations improve to less than 7 mg/dL. Treatment interruption, dosage reduction, or permanent discontinuance of therapy may be necessary based on duration and severity of hyperphosphatemia.

Fetal/Neonatal Morbidity and Mortality

Erdafitinib may cause fetal harm in humans based on its mechanism of action and animal findings; embryofetal toxicity and teratogenicity have been demonstrated in animals. There are no data regarding use of erdafitinib in pregnant women. In animal reproduction studies, embryofetal toxicity (i.e., death, decreased fetal body weight) and teratogenic effects (i.e., major blood vessel malformation and other vascular anomalies, limb malformation, skeletal anomalies) were observed in rats receiving erdafitinib at total maternal exposure levels less than 0.1% of total human exposure levels at the maximum recommended human dose.

Pregnancy should be avoided during erdafitinib therapy. The manufacturer recommends confirmation of pregnancy status prior to initiation of erdafitinib in females of reproductive potential and states that such females should be advised to use effective contraceptive methods while receiving erdafitinib and for 1 month after discontinuance of the drug. In addition, males with such female partners should use effective methods of contraception while receiving erdafitinib and for 1 month after discontinuance of the drug. Patients should be apprised of the potential hazard to the fetus if erdafitinib is used during pregnancy.

Specific Populations

Pregnancy

Erdafitinib may cause fetal harm if administered to pregnant females based on its mechanism of action and animal findings.

Lactation

It is not known whether erdafitinib is distributed into human milk. Because of the potential for serious adverse reactions to erdafitinib in breast-fed infants, females should be advised not to breast-feed while receiving the drug and for 1 month after the last dose. The effects of the drug on breast-fed infants or on the production of milk are unknown.

Females and Males of Reproductive Potential

Females of reproductive potential should be advised to use effective contraceptive methods while receiving erdafitinib and for 1 month after discontinuance of the drug. In addition, males with such female partners should use effective methods of contraception while receiving erdafitinib and for 1 month after discontinuance of the drug.

Based on animal studies, erdafitinib may impair female fertility. In a repeat-dose toxicity study, necrosis of ovarian corpora lutea was observed in female rats at exposure levels less than the human exposure at the maximum recommended human dosage.

Pediatric Use

Safety and efficacy of erdafitinib have not been established in pediatric patients.

Chondroid dysplasia or metaplasia in multiple bones and tooth abnormalities (i.e., abnormal or irregular dentin, odontoblast discoloration and degeneration) have been observed in animals receiving erdafitinib for 4 or 13 weeks (at exposure levels less than the AUC in humans at the maximum recommended dosage).

Geriatric Use

In clinical trials, 40% of patients receiving erdafitinib were 65 to 74 years of age, while 20% were 75 years of age or older. Patients 65 years of age and older experienced a higher incidence of adverse reactions requiring treatment discontinuation than younger patients. No overall differences in efficacy were observed between geriatric patients and younger adults.

Hepatic Impairment

Analysis of population pharmacokinetic data indicate that the pharmacokinetics of erdafitinib are not substantially altered in patients with mild or moderate hepatic impairment (Child-Pugh class A or B).

Limited data are available in patients with severe hepatic impairment (Child-Pugh class C).

Renal Impairment

Analysis of population pharmacokinetic data indicate that the pharmacokinetics of erdafitinib are not substantially altered in patients with mild or moderate renal impairment (estimated glomerular filtration rate [eGFR] 30–89 mL/min per 1.73 m^2).

Pharmacokinetics of erdafitinib have not been established in patients with severe renal impairment or renal impairment requiring dialysis.

Pharmacogenomic Considerations

Patients who are known or suspected poor cytochrome P-450 (CYP) isoenzyme 2C9 metabolizers carrying the CYP2C9*3/*3 genotype should be monitored for adverse effects since systemic exposure to the drug may be increased.

● *Common Adverse Effects*

Adverse effects and laboratory abnormalities reported in at least 20% of patients receiving erdafitinib include increased phosphate, nail disorders, stomatitis, diarrhea, increased creatinine, increased alkaline phosphatase, increased ALT, decreased hemoglobin, decreased sodium, increased AST, fatigue, dry mouth, dry skin, decreased phosphate, decreased appetite, dysgeusia, constipation, increased calcium, dry eye, palmar-plantar erythrodysesthesia syndrome, increased potassium, alopecia, and central serous retinopathy.

DRUG INTERACTIONS

Erdafitinib is metabolized principally by cytochrome P-450 (CYP) isoenzymes 2C9 and 3A4. In vitro, erdafitinib demonstrates time-dependent inhibition and induction of CYP3A4. In vitro, the drug is not an inhibitor of other major CYP isoenzymes at clinically relevant concentrations.

In vitro studies indicate that erdafitinib is a substrate of P-glycoprotein (P-gp). In vitro, erdafitinib is an inhibitor of P-gp and organic cation transporter (OCT) 2, but does not inhibit breast cancer resistance protein (BCRP), organic anion transporting polypeptide (OATP) 1B or 1B3, organic anion transporter (OAT) 1 or 3, OCT1, and multidrug and toxin extrusion (MATE) 1 or 2K transporters at clinically important concentrations.

● Drugs Affecting Hepatic Microsomal Enzymes

Inhibitors of CYP2C9 and/or 3A4

Concomitant use of erdafitinib with moderate inhibitors of CYP2C9 or strong inhibitors of 3A4 may result in increased erdafitinib plasma concentrations and increased risk of erdafitinib toxicity. When the strong CYP2C9 and moderate CYP3A4 inhibitor fluconazole (400 mg daily on days 1–11) was administered concomitantly with erdafitinib (single 4-mg dose on day 5) in healthy individuals, peak plasma concentrations and AUC of erdafitinib were increased by 21 and 48%, respectively. When the strong CYP3A4 inhibitor and P-gp inhibitor itraconazole (200 mg daily on days 1–11) was administered concomitantly with erdafitinib (single 4-mg dose on day 5) in healthy individuals, peak plasma concentrations and AUC of erdafitinib were increased by 5 and 34%, respectively.

Concomitant use of erdafitinib with moderate inhibitors of CYP2C9 and strong inhibitors of CYP3A4 (e.g., fluconazole, itraconazole) should be avoided, and selection of an alternative drug with less CYP2C9 or 3A4 inhibition potential should be considered. If concomitant use of a moderate CYP2C9 or strong CYP3A4 inhibitor cannot be avoided, patients should be monitored closely for signs of erdafitinib toxicity and a dose modification considered. When concomitant use of the moderate CYP2C9 or strong CYP3A4 inhibitor is discontinued, resume the erdafitinib dose used before dose modifications in the absence of drug-related toxicity.

Inducers of CYP3A4

Concomitant use of erdafitinib with strong or moderate inducers of CYP3A4 may result in decreased erdafitinib plasma concentrations and reduced erdafitinib efficacy. Simulations suggest that peak plasma concentrations and AUC of erdafitinib are substantially decreased following concomitant administration of the drug with the strong CYP3A4 inducer rifampin.

Concomitant use of erdafitinib with strong (e.g., rifampin) inducers of CYP3A4 should be avoided. If concomitant use of a moderate 3A4 inducer cannot be avoided upon initiation, the manufacturer states that erdafitinib should be initiated at 9 mg once daily. When concomitant use of the moderate CYP3A4 inducer is discontinued, the erdafitinib dosage should be continued at the same dosage, in the absence of drug-related toxicity.

● Drugs Metabolized by Hepatic Microsomal Enzymes

Because erdafitinib is a time-dependent inhibitor and inducer of CYP3A4, concomitant use of erdafitinib with drugs that are substrates of CYP3A4 may result in altered plasma concentrations of the CYP3A4 substrate and either reduced efficacy or increased toxicity of the CYP3A4 substrate; however, the effect of erdafitinib on sensitive CYP3A4 substrates (e.g., midazolam) has not been established.

Concomitant use of erdafitinib with sensitive CYP3A4 substrates that have a narrow therapeutic index should be avoided.

● Drugs Affecting or Affected by P-glycoprotein Transport

Concomitant use of erdafitinib and inhibitors of P-gp are not expected to have a clinically important effect on systemic exposure of erdafitinib.

Concomitant use of erdafitinib with drugs that are substrates of P-gp may result in increased exposure of the P-gp substrate and increased risk of toxicity of the P-gp substrate. If concomitant use is necessary, erdafitinib should be administered at least 6 hours before or after administration of P-gp substrates that have a narrow therapeutic index (e.g., digoxin).

● Drugs Affecting Serum Phosphate Concentrations

Concomitant use of erdafitinib with other drugs that alter serum phosphate concentrations may result in increased or decreased serum phosphate concentrations.

In clinical trials, concomitant use of erdafitinib with other drugs that increase serum phosphate concentrations (e.g., potassium phosphate supplements, vitamin D supplements, antacids, phosphate-containing laxatives, and medications containing phosphate as an excipient) were not permitted. Because the initial dosage titration of erdafitinib is based on serum phosphate concentrations, concomitant use of erdafitinib with other drugs that may alter serum phosphate concentrations should be avoided during the initial dosage titration period (i.e., initial 14–21 days of erdafitinib therapy).

● Drugs Affecting Gastric pH

Concomitant administration of erdafitinib with drugs that reduce gastric acidity such as antacids, histamine H_2-receptor antagonists, and proton-pump inhibitors do not have a clinically meaningful effect on bioavailability of erdafitinib.

DESCRIPTION

Erdafitinib, a potent and reversible inhibitor of fibroblast growth factor receptors (FGFR)-1, FGFR-2, FGFR-3, and FGFR-4, is an antineoplastic agent. Similar to other receptor tyrosine kinases, activation of FGFR tyrosine kinase is involved in the initiation of various cascades of intracellular signaling events leading to cell proliferation and influences processes critical to cell survival and tumor progression (e.g., angiogenesis, metastasis, inhibition of apoptosis). Aberrations in FGFR (e.g., gene amplification, point mutation, chromosomal translocation) resulting in dysregulation of the FGFR signaling cascade have been implicated in various solid tumors; the reversible binding of erdafitinib to and subsequent inhibition of FGFR-1, FGFR-2, FGFR-3, and FGFR-4 reduces cell viability in cell lines expressing aberrant FGFR. The drug also has demonstrated antitumor activity in FGFR-expressing cell lines and xenograft models of tumor types such as bladder cancer. Erdafitinib also has demonstrated binding to ret proto-oncogene (RET), colony stimulating factor receptor type 1 (CSF-1R), platelet-derived growth factor receptors (PDGFR)-α and PDGFR-β, fms-like tyrosine kinase-4 (Flt-4), stem cell factor receptor (c-Kit), and vascular endothelial growth factor receptor (VEGFR)-2.

Serum phosphate concentration is a marker of FGFR inhibition following initiation of erdafitinib therapy. In an exposure-response analysis, a significant relationship between better investigator-assessed clinical outcomes (i.e., objective response rate, disease control rate, progression-free survival) and increased serum phosphate concentrations was observed.

Peak plasma concentrations and AUC of erdafitinib are dose proportional over the erdafitinib dose range of 0.5–12 mg following single or repeated once-daily dosing. The median time to peak plasma concentration of erdafitinib is 2.5 hours. Steady-state concentrations of erdafitinib are reached after 2 weeks of once-daily dosing and the accumulation ratio is approximately 4-fold. Administration of a single 9-mg dose of erdafitinib with a high-fat, high-calorie meal (800–1000 calories with approximately 50% of calories from fat) in healthy individuals did not have a clinically meaningful effect on the pharmacokinetics of erdafitinib.

Erdafitinib is metabolized principally by cytochrome P-450 (CYP) isoenzymes 2C9 and 3A4. Erdafitinib is highly bound (99.8%) to plasma proteins in vivo, primarily to α_1-acid glycoprotein. The mean effective half-life of erdafitinib is 59 hours. Following administration of a single oral radiolabeled dose of erdafitinib, 69% of the recovered dose is excreted in feces (19% as unchanged drug) and 19% is eliminated in urine (13% as unchanged drug). Clearance of erdafitinib does not appear to be affected by age (range: 21–88 years), sex, race, or body weight (range: 36–132 kg).

● Pharmacogenomics

Genetic polymorphism of the CYP2C9 isoenzyme may affect exposure to erdafitinib. Systemic exposure of erdafitinib was similar in patients with CYP2C9*1/*2 and CYP2C9*1/*3 genotypes compared with individuals with the CYP2C9*1/*1 wild-type genotype. Erdafitinib has not been studied in individuals with other CYP2C9 genotypes (e.g., CYP2C9*2/*2, CYP2C9*2/*3, CYP2C9*3/*3); however, pharmacokinetic modeling suggests that no clinically meaningful changes in systemic exposure of erdafitinib are expected in individuals with CYP2C9*2/*2 and CYP2C9*2/*3 genotypes. Pharmacokinetic modeling also suggests that systemic exposure of erdafitinib is expected to increase by 50% in individuals with the CYP2C9*3/*3 genotype compared with individuals with the CYP2C9*1/*1 wild-type genotype.

ADVICE TO PATIENTS

- Instruct patients to read the manufacturer's patient information.

- Advise patients to take erdafitinib tablets once daily without regard to meals. Advise patients to swallow erdafitinib tablets whole. If a dose is vomited, stress the importance of taking the next dose at the regularly scheduled time; an additional dose should not be administered to make up for the vomited dose.

- If a dose is missed, stress the importance of taking the missed dose as soon as possible on the same day and taking the next dose at the regularly scheduled time on the following day. An additional dose should not be taken to make up for a missed dose.

- Risk of ocular disorders. Stress the importance of patients immediately informing their clinician if any visual changes (e.g., blurry or loss of vision) occur. Stress the importance of preventing or treating dry eyes with artificial tears substitutes or hydrating or lubricating eye gels or ointments at least every 2 hours while awake.

- Risk of dermatologic effects. Stress the importance of informing clinician if progressive or intolerable skin, mucous, or nail disorders occur.

- Risk of hyperphosphatemia and soft tissue mineralization. Advise patients that phosphate intake should not exceed 600—800 mg daily during therapy. Advise patients to avoid drugs that may alter serum phosphate concentrations during the first 14–21 days of erdafitinib therapy. Stress the importance of patients immediately informing their clinician if painful skin lesions or any symptoms related to acute change in phosphate levels such as muscle cramps, numbness, or tingling around the mouth occur.

- Risk of fetal harm. Advise females of reproductive potential and males who are partners of such females that they should use effective methods of contraception while receiving the drug and for 1 month after discontinuance of therapy. Stress the importance of females informing clinicians if they are or plan to become pregnant. If pregnancy occurs, advise pregnant females of potential risk to the fetus.

- Advise females to avoid breast-feeding while receiving the drug and for 1 month after discontinuance of therapy.

- Stress the importance of informing clinicians of existing or contemplated concomitant therapy, including prescription and OTC drugs (e.g., potassium phosphate supplements, vitamin D supplements, antacids, phosphate-containing medications), as well as any concomitant illnesses.

- Inform patients of other important precautionary information.

For further information on the handling of antineoplastic agents, see the ASHP Guidelines on Handling Hazardous Drugs at https://www.ahfsdruginformation.com.

PREPARATIONS

Erdafitinib is available only from a designated specialty pharmacy. The manufacturer should be contacted for additional information.

Excipients in commercially available drug preparations may have clinically important effects in some individuals; consult specific product labeling for details.

Erdafitinib

Oral

Tablets, film-coated	3 mg	Balversa®, Janssen
	4 mg	Balversa®, Janssen
	5 mg	Balversa®, Janssen

† Use is not currently included in the labeling approved by the US Food and Drug Administration.

Erlotinib Hydrochloride

10:00 • ANTINEOPLASTIC AGENTS

■ Erlotinib hydrochloride, an epidermal growth factor receptor (EGFR) tyrosine kinase inhibitor, is an antineoplastic agent.

USES

● Non-small Cell Lung Cancer

Erlotinib hydrochloride is used for the first-line or maintenance treatment of metastatic non-small cell lung cancer (NSCLC) in patients whose tumors harbor epidermal growth factor receptor (*EGFR*) exon 19 deletions (del19) or exon 21 (L858R) substitution mutations as detected by an FDA-approved diagnostic test (e.g., cobas® EGFR Mutation Test); the drug also is used for second-line or subsequent treatment in such patients whose disease progressed following at least one chemotherapy regimen. Information on FDA-approved companion diagnostic tests for the detection of *EGFR* mutations in NSCLC is available at https://www.fda.gov/CompanionDiagnostics.

Data from 2 multicenter, randomized, placebo-controlled studies in over 1000 patients did not demonstrate any clinical benefit from concurrent administration of erlotinib with carboplatin and paclitaxel or with gemcitabine and cisplatin in the first-line setting. Therefore, the manufacturer states that use of erlotinib in combination with platinum-based chemotherapy is not recommended.

The manufacturer states that the safety and efficacy of erlotinib have not been established in patients with NSCLC whose tumors harbor *EGFR* mutations other than exon 19 deletions or exon 21 substitution mutations.

First-line Treatment of Metastatic Non-small Cell Lung Cancer

The current indication for erlotinib in the first-line treatment of metastatic NSCLC is based principally on the results of a randomized, multicenter, open-label phase 3 study (EURTAC) in adults with newly diagnosed locally advanced or metastatic NSCLC. In this study, 174 patients were randomized (stratified by type of *EGFR* mutation and Eastern Cooperative Oncology Group [ECOG] performance status) in a 1:1 ratio to receive either erlotinib (150 mg orally once daily until disease progression occurred) or investigator's choice of platinum-based chemotherapy (cisplatin 75 mg/m² and docetaxel 75 mg/m² on day 1 of each 3-week cycle for 4 cycles; gemcitabine 1.25 g/m² on days 1 and 8 and cisplatin 75 mg/m² on day 1 of each 3-week cycle for 4 cycles; carboplatin at the dose required to obtain AUC of 6 mg/mL per minute and docetaxel 75 mg/m² on day 1 of each 3-week cycle for 4 cycles; gemcitabine 1 g/m² on days 1 and 8 and carboplatin at the dose required to obtain an AUC of 5 mg/mL per minute on day 1 of each 3-week cycle for 4 cycles). The primary measure of efficacy was progression-free survival. The median age of patients was 65 years (range: 24–82 years); most patients (99%) were Caucasian, 93% had metastatic disease, 93% had adenocarcinoma histology, 72% were female, 86% had a baseline ECOG performance status of 0 or 1, 69% had never smoked, 20% were former smokers, and 11% were current smokers. The majority (66%) of patients had exon 19 deletions and 34% of patients had L858R substitution mutations as determined by a clinical trial assay. The majority (84%) of patients randomized to investigator's choice of platinum-based chemotherapy received at least one subsequent therapy; 97% of these patients received an EGFR tyrosine kinase inhibitor. Approximately 66% of patients randomized to erlotinib received at least one subsequent therapy.

In the EURTAC study, patients receiving erlotinib had longer median progression-free survival compared with patients receiving platinum-based chemotherapy (10.4 versus 5.2 months; hazard ratio of 0.34). Effects of erlotinib on investigator-assessed progression-free survival and progression-free survival as assessed by an independent review committee were comparable. Patients receiving erlotinib also had a higher objective response rate compared with those receiving platinum-based chemotherapy (65 versus 16%). At the time of analysis, no significant difference in overall survival was observed between patients receiving erlotinib and those receiving platinum-based chemotherapy. An exploratory subgroup analysis based on *EGFR* mutation (del19 or L858R substitution mutations) indicated that the magnitude of progression-free survival benefit from erlotinib was greater in patients with exon 19 deletions than in those with L858R

substitution mutations (hazard ratio: 0.27 and 0.52, respectively); however, an overall survival benefit for the drug in patients with exon 19 deletions or L858R substitution mutations was not apparent. Subgroup analysis suggested that erlotinib had a greater effect on progression-free survival relative to platinum-based chemotherapy in patients who had never smoked than in those who were current smokers (hazard ratio: 0.24 and 0.56, respectively) and in those who had not received prior surgery or radiation therapy than in those who had previously undergone surgery (hazard ratio: 0.32 and 0.61, respectively) or radiation therapy (hazard ratio: 0.31 and 0.79, respectively); a progression-free survival benefit for the drug versus platinum-based chemotherapy was not apparent in patients who were former smokers or those who previously received chemotherapy.

Erlotinib also has been used in combination with ramucirumab† in patients with *EGFR* mutation positive metastatic NSCLC. In a randomized, double-blind, placebo-controlled trial (RELAY), 449 previously untreated patients ≥18 years of age with stage IV NSCLC with an *EGFR* exon 19 deletion or exon 21 substitution mutation were randomized to receive either erlotinib (150 mg once daily orally) with IV ramucirumab (10 mg/kg once every 2 weeks) or erlotinib plus placebo. At a median follow-up of 20.7 months, median progression-free survival was substantially improved in patients receiving erlotinib in combination with ramucirumab compared with those receiving erlotinib alone (19.4 versus 12.4 months, respectively; hazard ratio of 0.59).

Erlotinib also has been used in combination with bevacizumab† in patients with advanced *EGFR* mutation-positive NSCLC. In an open-label, randomized trial (NEJ026) conducted in Japan, 224 patients with stage IIIB or IV *EGFR* mutation-positive NSCLC or recurrent *EGFR* mutation-positive NSCLC were randomized to receive erlotinib 150 mg once daily plus IV bevacizumab 15 mg/kg once every 21 days or erlotinib monotherapy. At a prespecified interim analysis, progression-free survival was 16.9 months in patients receiving erlotinib in combination with bevacizumab versus 13.3 months in those receiving erlotinib monotherapy (hazard ratio: 0.605). At a median follow-up of 39.2 months, median overall survival with combination therapy was 50.7 months compared to 46.2 months with erlotinib alone (hazard ratio: 1.007).

Second-line or Subsequent Treatment of Metastatic Non-small Cell Lung Cancer

Safety and efficacy of erlotinib in the second-line or subsequent treatment of patients with metastatic NSCLC were established in a randomized, double-blind, placebo-controlled study in 731 patients with locally advanced or metastatic non-small cell lung cancer after failure of at least one prior chemotherapy regimen. In this study, patients were randomized on a 2:1 basis to receive either erlotinib (150 mg) or placebo, respectively, orally once daily until disease progression or unacceptable toxicity occurred; therapy was continued for a median of 9.6 weeks. The objective response rate was higher in patients receiving erlotinib (8.9%) than in those receiving placebo (0.9%). In addition, median overall survival and progression-free survival were longer in patients receiving erlotinib (6.7 and 2.3 months, respectively) than in those receiving placebo (4.7 and 1.8 months, respectively).

Maintenance Therapy

The current indication for maintenance therapy with erlotinib is based principally on the results of a randomized, double-blind, placebo-controlled phase 3 study (Sequential Tarceva® in Unresectable NSCLC [SATURN]) in adults with metastatic NSCLC who did not experience disease progression following prior platinum-based chemotherapy. In this study, 889 patients were randomized in a 1:1 ratio to receive either erlotinib (150 mg orally once daily) or placebo until disease progression or unacceptable toxicity occurred. The primary measure of efficacy was progression-free survival. The median age of patients was 60 years (range: 30–83 years); most patients (84%) were Caucasian, 74% were male, 55% were current smokers, 27% were former smokers, 17% had never smoked, and 15% of patients were of Asian ancestry. The majority (75%) of patients had metastatic disease and 25% of patients had stage IIIB disease with pleural effusion; approximately one-half (45%) of patients had adenocarcinoma/bronchoalveolar carcinoma, 40% had squamous histology, and 5% had large cell carcinoma. The majority (70%) of patients had positive EGFR expression as detected by an immunohistochemistry assay; 14% of patients had negative EGFR expression.

In the SATURN study, the risk of disease progression or death was reduced by 29 or 19%, respectively, in patients receiving erlotinib maintenance therapy compared with those receiving placebo. Progression-free survival and overall survival benefits were observed in the overall study population and in patients with positive EGFR expression. Results of a subgroup analysis (based on age, gender, ethnicity, ECOG performance status, disease stage, histology) suggested that the effect of erlotinib on progression-free survival and overall survival was evident across all subgroups.

Efficacy and safety of erlotinib have not been established in patients with NSCLC whose tumors harbor EGFR mutations other than exon 19 deletions or exon 21 substitution mutations. In a multicenter, randomized, placebo-controlled study, clinical benefit was not demonstrated in 643 patients with advanced NSCLC without exon 19 deletions or exon 21 (L858R) substitution mutations who received erlotinib maintenance therapy.

Clinical Perspective

EGFR-activating mutations are present in approximately 15–22% of NSCLC cases in North America and Europe and are present in up to 30–50% of cases in patients of East Asian descent. The majority of EGFR mutations are exon 19 deletions and an L858R substitution in exon 21, which together account for about 90% of EGFR mutations in patients with NSCLC. Patients with this form of lung cancer typically are nonsmokers (49.3%), female (43.7%), and have adenocarcinoma histology (38%).

First-line Therapy for Metastatic Non-small Cell Lung Cancer

The American Society of Clinical Oncology (ASCO) and Ontario Health (OH; formerly known as Cancer Care Ontario) 2021 joint guideline specifically addresses treatment of stage IV NSCLC harboring driver alterations such as EGFR mutations. For patients with previously untreated stage IV NSCLC harboring sensitizing EGFR mutations (L858R/exon 19 deletion) and a performance status of 0 to 2, ASCO/OH states that afatinib monotherapy or the combination of erlotinib with a vascular endothelial growth factor (VEGF) inhibitor† (e.g., bevacizumab, ramucirumab) may be used when first-line treatment with osimertinib, dacomitinib, or gefitinib in combination with carboplatin and pemetrexed are not treatment options. Although progression-free survival benefit has been demonstrated with afatinib monotherapy or combination erlotinib therapy†, overall survival benefit has not been demonstrated compared with first-generation EGFR tyrosine kinase inhibitors alone. For patients with previously untreated stage IV NSCLC harboring sensitizing EGFR mutations (L858R/exon 19 deletion) and a performance status of 3, monotherapy with an EGFR tyrosine kinase inhibitor may be offered based on access and toxicity.

A 2021 Cochrane review on first-line treatment options for patients with EGFR mutation-positive NSCLC concluded that erlotinib, gefitinib, afatinib, and icotinib (not commercially available in the US market) demonstrate increased tumor response, prolonged progression-free survival, less toxicity, and greater quality of life compared to cytotoxic chemotherapy. The analysis also states that single agent tyrosine kinase inhibitor therapy remains the standard of care and the benefit of combining a tyrosine kinase inhibitor with chemotherapy remains uncertain. Cytotoxic chemotherapy is less effective for the treatment of NSCLC harboring EGFR mutations compared with erlotinib, gefitinib, afatinib or icotinib, and is associated with greater toxicity.

● Pancreatic Cancer

Erlotinib is used in combination with gemcitabine for the first-line treatment of locally advanced, unresectable or metastatic pancreatic cancer. Efficacy and safety of this treatment combination is supported by a randomized placebo-controlled trial. Guidelines generally support the use of erlotinib in the treatment of pancreatic cancer for patients unable to receive more intensive therapy.

Efficacy and safety of erlotinib in combination with gemcitabine as first-line therapy for locally advanced, unresectable or metastatic pancreatic cancer have been evaluated in a randomized, double-blind, placebo-controlled trial in 569 patients. Patients received either erlotinib (100 mg or 150 mg) or placebo orally once daily in combination with gemcitabine 1 g/m² IV once weekly (for 7 consecutive weeks of an 8-week cycle and thereafter for 3 consecutive weeks of a 4-week cycle) until disease progression or unacceptable toxicity. Because of the small number of patients receiving erlotinib 150 mg or placebo (24 patients in each group), efficacy and safety results are reported only for the patients receiving erlotinib 100 mg (261 patients) or placebo (260 patients). These groups were comparable except there were more females in the group receiving erlotinib 100 mg (51%) than in the group receiving placebo (44%). Upon entry to the study, most of the patients (about 76%) had metastatic disease as the initial manifestation of pancreatic cancer.

Patients receiving erlotinib plus gemcitabine had longer median overall survival (6.5 versus 6 months) and median progression-free survival (3.8 versus 3.6 months) than those receiving placebo and gemcitabine as first-line therapy for locally advanced, unresectable or metastatic pancreatic cancer. The objective response rate was 8.6 or 7.9% in patients receiving erlotinib plus gemcitabine or placebo plus gemcitabine, respectively. Among the most common adverse effects, rash (70 versus 30%) and diarrhea (48 versus 36%) occurred more frequently in patients receiving erlotinib and gemcitabine than in those receiving gemcitabine alone.

Clinical Perspective

The 2020 American Society of Clinical Oncology (ASCO) guideline specifically addresses treatment of metastatic pancreatic cancer. The guideline states that gemcitabine-based combination therapy such as the combination of gemcitabine and erlotinib may be considered in selected patients with metastatic pancreatic adenocarcinoma, with proactive dose and schedule adjustments to minimize toxicities.

● Other Uses

Erlotinib also has been used as monotherapy and in combination with bevacizumab (with or without imatinib) for the treatment of advanced or metastatic renal cell carcinoma†.

DOSAGE AND ADMINISTRATION

● General

Pretreatment Screening

- Confirm presence of epidermal growth factor receptor (EGFR) exon 19 deletions (del19) or exon 21 (L858R) substitution mutations in tumor or plasma specimens of patients with metastatic non-small cell lung cancer (NSCLC) by an FDA-approved diagnostic test prior to initiating therapy with erlotinib. Patients with a negative plasma del19 or L858R mutation result should be reevaluated for the feasibility of a tumor biopsy.

Patient Monitoring

- Monitor liver function tests periodically during treatment; more frequent monitoring may be necessary in patients with preexisting hepatic impairment or biliary obstruction.
- Monitor for acute onset of new or progressive unexplained pulmonary symptoms such as dyspnea, cough, and fever.
- Monitor renal function and serum electrolytes.
- Monitor for new onset of severe bullous, blistering, or exfoliating skin conditions.
- Monitor for acute or worsening ocular disorders.
- Monitor prothrombin time and international normalized ratio during erlotinib therapy in patients receiving concomitant warfarin or other coumarin derivatives.

● Administration

Administer erlotinib orally once daily. The drug should be administered on an empty stomach (e.g., at least 1 hour before or 2 hours after ingestion of food).

Store erlotinib tablets at 25°C (excursions permitted between 15–30°C).

● Dosage

Dosage of erlotinib hydrochloride is expressed in terms of erlotinib.

Non-small Cell Lung Cancer

For the first-line or subsequent treatment or maintenance treatment of metastatic NSCLC in patients whose tumors harbor EGFR del19 or L858R substitution mutations and progressed following at least one chemotherapy regimen, the usual adult dosage of erlotinib is 150 mg once daily. Treatment should be continued until disease progression or unacceptable toxicity occurs.

Pancreatic Cancer

For the first-line treatment of locally advanced, unresectable or metastatic pancreatic cancer, erlotinib 100 mg once daily, is used in combination with gemcitabine. In the randomized trial, patients received erlotinib in combination with gemcitabine 1 g/m² IV once weekly (for 7 consecutive weeks of an 8-week cycle and thereafter for 3 consecutive weeks of a 4-week cycle). Treatment should be continued until disease progression or unacceptable toxicity occurs.

Dosage Modification

Dosage interruption and/or reduction, or discontinuance of erlotinib therapy, may be necessary based on severity of adverse reactions. When dosage reduction is required, reduce the dose of erlotinib by 50-mg decrements.

Pulmonary Toxicity

In patients who experience acute onset of new or progressive pulmonary manifestations (e.g., dyspnea, cough, fever), interrupt treatment with erlotinib pending diagnostic evaluation. If interstitial lung disease is diagnosed, permanently discontinue erlotinib. If interstitial lung disease is excluded, erlotinib may be resumed at a reduced dosage when pulmonary manifestations resolve completely or improve to ≤grade 1.

Renal Toxicity

If severe (grade 3 or 4) renal toxicity occurs, consider discontinuance of erlotinib therapy. Alternatively, erlotinib therapy may be interrupted; when the toxicity resolves completely or improves to ≤grade 1, erlotinib may be resumed at a reduced dosage.

Hepatotoxicity

If total bilirubin concentrations increase to 2 times baseline values or serum aminotransferase concentrations increase to 3 times baseline values in patients with preexisting hepatic impairment or biliary obstruction, consider discontinuance of erlotinib therapy. Alternatively, erlotinib therapy may be interrupted; when hepatic impairment resolves or improves to ≤grade 1, erlotinib may be resumed at a reduced dosage.

If elevated total bilirubin concentrations greater than 3 times the upper limit of normal (ULN) or serum aminotransferase concentrations greater than 5 times the ULN occur in patients without preexisting hepatic impairment, consider discontinuance of erlotinib therapy. Alternatively, erlotinib therapy may be interrupted; when hepatic impairment resolves or improves to ≤grade 1, erlotinib may be resumed at a reduced dosage.

If severe hepatotoxicity occurs and does not improve substantially or resolve within 3 weeks, discontinue erlotinib therapy.

GI Toxicity

In patients with severe and persistent diarrhea that is unresponsive to medical management (e.g., loperamide), interrupt erlotinib therapy. When the toxicity resolves completely or improves to ≤grade 1, erlotinib may be resumed at a reduced dosage.

If GI perforation occurs, permanently discontinue erlotinib therapy.

Dermatologic Toxicity

If severe rash unresponsive to medical management occurs, interrupt erlotinib therapy. When the rash resolves completely or improves to ≤grade 1, erlotinib may be resumed at a reduced dosage.

In patients with severe skin reactions, such as severe bullous, blistering, or exfoliative conditions, discontinue erlotinib therapy.

Ocular Toxicity

In patients who experience acute or worsening ocular toxicity, such as eye pain, consider discontinuance of erlotinib therapy. Alternatively, erlotinib therapy may be interrupted; when the toxicity resolves completely or improves to ≤grade 1, erlotinib may be resumed at a reduced dosage.

If grade 3 or 4 keratitis or persistent (lasting longer than 2 weeks) grade 2 keratitis occurs, interrupt erlotinib therapy. When toxicity resolves completely or improves to ≤grade 1, erlotinib may be resumed at a reduced dosage.

In patients who experience corneal perforation or severe corneal ulceration, discontinue erlotinib therapy.

Concomitant Use with Drugs and Foods Affecting Hepatic Microsomal Enzymes

Concomitant use with potent inhibitors of cytochrome P-450 (CYP) isoenzyme 3A4 (e.g., atazanavir, clarithromycin, conivaptan, indinavir, itraconazole, ketoconazole, lopinavir/ritonavir, nefazodone, nelfinavir, posaconazole, ritonavir, saquinavir, telithromycin, voriconazole) or combined inhibitors of CYP3A4 and CYP1A2 (e.g., ciprofloxacin) should be avoided. If concomitant use cannot be avoided, the manufacturer recommends reducing the dosage of erlotinib in 50-mg decrements.

Concomitant use with an inducer of CYP3A4 (e.g., carbamazepine, phenobarbital, phenytoin, rifabutin, rifampin, rifapentine, St. John's wort [*Hypericum perforatum*]) should be avoided. If concomitant use cannot be avoided, the manufacturer recommends increasing the dosage of erlotinib in 50-mg increments (not to exceed 450 mg daily) as tolerated at 2-week intervals.

Concomitant use with moderate inducers of CYP1A2 (e.g., phenytoin, rifampin, teriflunomide) should be avoided. If concomitant use cannot be avoided, the manufacturer recommends increasing the dosage of erlotinib.

Cigarette Smoking

Because cigarette smoking reduces systemic exposure to erlotinib, patients should be advised to stop smoking. In patients who continue to smoke, the manufacturer recommends increasing the dosage of erlotinib in 50-mg increments (not to exceed 300 mg daily) at 2-week intervals. Upon cessation of smoking, the erlotinib dose should be reduced immediately to the recommended starting dose.

Drugs Affecting Gastric Acidity

If possible, avoid concomitant use of erlotinib and proton-pump inhibitors.

If use of a histamine H₂-receptor antagonist is necessary, erlotinib must be taken 10 hours after the H₂-receptor antagonist and at least 2 hours before the next dose of the H₂-receptor antagonist.

If use of an antacid is necessary, separate the antacid dose and erlotinib dose by several hours.

Grapefruit

Avoid concomitant use of erlotinib with grapefruit or grapefruit juice, a potent inhibitor of CYP3A4. If concomitant use cannot be avoided, the manufacturer recommends reducing the dosage of erlotinib in 50-mg decrements.

● Special Populations

Hepatic Impairment

Consider dosage interruption or discontinuance of erlotinib therapy if abnormal liver function tests occur in patients with preexisting hepatic impairment.

Renal Impairment

The manufacturer currently makes no special dosage recommendations for patients with renal impairment.

Geriatric Patients

The manufacturer currently makes no special dosage recommendations for geriatric patients.

CAUTIONS

● Contraindications

- The manufacturer states that there are no known contraindications to the use of erlotinib.

● Warnings/Precautions

Pulmonary Toxicity

Serious, sometimes fatal, interstitial lung disease has occurred in patients receiving erlotinib. Interstitial lung disease has been reported in approximately 1.1% of patients receiving erlotinib in controlled and uncontrolled studies. Onset of manifestations occurred from 5 days to more than 9 months (median: 39 days) after initiating erlotinib therapy.

Interruption or discontinuance of erlotinib therapy may be required in patients experiencing pulmonary toxicity.

Renal Failure

Hepatorenal syndrome or acute renal failure, sometimes fatal, and renal insufficiency have been reported in patients receiving erlotinib. Factors contributing to these adverse renal effects included baseline hepatic impairment and severe dehydration. In clinical studies for non-small cell lung cancer (NSCLC), severe renal impairment occurred in 0.5% of patients receiving erlotinib monotherapy compared with 0.8% of those assigned to the control groups. In the principal efficacy study for pancreatic cancer, renal impairment occurred in 1.4% of patients receiving erlotinib and gemcitabine versus 0.4% of those receiving placebo and gemcitabine.

Renal function and serum electrolytes should be monitored periodically.

If severe (grade 3 or 4) renal impairment occurs, interrupt or discontinue erlotinib therapy.

Hepatic Toxicity

Hepatic failure and hepatorenal syndrome, sometimes fatal, have occurred in patients receiving erlotinib, particularly in patients with hepatic impairment prior to treatment. In clinical studies for NSCLC, which excluded patients with baseline moderate to severe hepatic impairment, hepatic failure occurred in 0.4% of patients receiving erlotinib monotherapy compared with none of those assigned to the control groups. In the principal efficacy study for pancreatic cancer, the reported incidence of hepatic failure (0.4%) was similar between patients receiving erlotinib and gemcitabine and those receiving placebo and gemcitabine.

In a small subset of 15 patients with substantial tumor burden in the liver and moderate hepatic impairment (Child-Pugh class B), 10 patients died within 30 days of the last dose of erlotinib; 6 of the 10 patients had baseline total bilirubin concentrations greater than 3 times the upper limit of normal (ULN). Hepatorenal syndrome and rapidly progressing hepatic failure were the cause of death in 2 patients; the remaining 8 patients died from disease progression.

Monitor liver function tests (i.e., serum concentrations of aminotransferases, bilirubin, and alkaline phosphatase) periodically during therapy and more frequently in patients with preexisting hepatic impairment (e.g., total bilirubin concentrations greater than 3 times the ULN) or biliary obstruction. Interrupt or discontinue erlotinib therapy if changes in liver function are severe.

GI Perforation

GI perforation, sometimes fatal, has been reported in patients receiving erlotinib. Patients with a history of peptic ulcer disease or diverticulitis and those who are receiving concomitant therapy with antiangiogenesis drugs, corticosteroids, nonsteroidal anti-inflammatory agents (NSAIAs), and/or taxane-based chemotherapy are at increased risk for perforation while receiving erlotinib therapy. In clinical studies for NSCLC, GI perforation occurred in 0.2% of patients receiving erlotinib monotherapy compared with 0.1% of those assigned to the control groups. In the principal efficacy study for pancreatic cancer, GI perforation occurred in 0.4% of patients receiving erlotinib and gemcitabine compared with none of those receiving placebo and gemcitabine. If GI perforation occurs, permanently discontinue erlotinib therapy.

Bullous and Exfoliative Skin Disorders

Bullous, blistering, and exfoliative skin reactions, including cases suggestive of Stevens-Johnson syndrome or toxic epidermal necrolysis, have been reported in patients receiving erlotinib therapy; some cases have been fatal. In clinical studies for NSCLC, bullous and exfoliative skin reactions occurred in 1.2% of patients receiving erlotinib monotherapy compared with none of those assigned to the control groups. In the principal efficacy study for pancreatic cancer, GI perforation occurred in 0.4% of patients receiving erlotinib and gemcitabine compared with none of those receiving placebo and gemcitabine.

If severe dermatologic reactions occur, interrupt or discontinue erlotinib therapy.

Cerebrovascular Accident

In the principal efficacy study for pancreatic cancer, cerebrovascular accidents occurred in 7 patients (2.5%) receiving erlotinib and gemcitabine compared with none of those receiving placebo and gemcitabine; one of these events was a

hemorrhagic stroke and the patient died. In clinical studies for NSCLC, cerebrovascular accident occurred in 0.6% of patients receiving erlotinib monotherapy.

Microangiopathic Hemolytic Anemia with Thrombocytopenia

In clinical studies for NSCLC, microangiopathic hemolytic anemia with thrombocytopenia occurred in none of the patients receiving erlotinib monotherapy compared with 0.1% of those assigned to the control groups. In the principal efficacy study for pancreatic cancer, microangiopathic hemolytic anemia with thrombocytopenia occurred in 1.4% of patients receiving erlotinib and gemcitabine compared with none of those receiving placebo and gemcitabine.

Corneal Ulceration or Perforation

Abnormal eyelash growth, keratoconjunctivitis sicca (i.e., dry eye), keratitis, and decreased lacrimation may occur in patients receiving erlotinib and are considered risk factors for corneal ulceration or perforation. In clinical studies for NSCLC, ocular disorders occurred in 17.8% of patients receiving erlotinib monotherapy compared with 4% of those assigned to the control groups. In the principal efficacy study for pancreatic cancer, ocular disorders occurred in 12.8% of patients receiving erlotinib and gemcitabine compared with 11.4% of those receiving placebo and gemcitabine.

If patients experience ocular toxicity, interrupt or discontinue erlotinib therapy.

Elevated International Normalized Ratio (INR) and Bleeding

Increased INR and hemorrhagic events, sometimes fatal, have been reported in clinical studies; some of these patients were receiving erlotinib concomitantly with warfarin or a nonsteroidal anti-inflammatory agent (NSAIA). GI bleeding included peptic ulcer bleeding (gastritis, gastroduodenal ulcers), hematemesis, hematochezia, melena, and hemorrhage from possible colitis.

Fetal/Neonatal Morbidity and Mortality

Erlotinib may cause fetal harm in humans based on its mechanism of action and animal findings; the drug has been shown to be embryotoxic and fetotoxic in animals. Limited data are available regarding use of erlotinib in pregnant women; data are insufficient to inform a drug-associated risk of adverse developmental outcomes or miscarriage. Embryofetal toxicity (e.g., embryofetal lethality, abortion) has been demonstrated in animals receiving the drug at exposure levels equivalent to approximately 3 times the human exposure at the recommended erlotinib dosage of 150 mg daily. In a fertility study, increased early resorptions were observed in animals receiving the drug at exposure levels equivalent to 0.3 or 0.7 times the human exposure at the recommended daily dosage.

Pregnancy should be avoided during erlotinib therapy. (See Females and Males of Reproductive Potential under Cautions.) Patients should be apprised of the potential fetal hazard or potential risk for loss of the pregnancy if erlotinib is used during pregnancy.

Specific Populations

Pregnancy

Erlotinib may cause fetal harm if administered to pregnant women based on its mechanism of action and animal findings. (See Fetal/Neonatal Morbidity and Mortality under Cautions.)

Lactation

It is not known whether erlotinib is distributed into human milk or if the drug or its metabolites have any effect on milk production or the nursing infant. Because of the potential for serious adverse reactions to erlotinib in nursing infants, women should be advised not to breast-feed while receiving the drug and for 2 weeks after the last dose of the drug.

Females and Males of Reproductive Potential

Females of childbearing potential should be advised to use effective contraception while receiving erlotinib and for 1 month after the last dose of the drug.

Pediatric Use

Safety and efficacy of erlotinib have not been established in pediatric patients.

In a clinical trial, 25 patients 3–20 years of age with recurrent or refractory ependymoma received erlotinib (85 mg/m² orally daily). No overall difference in safety relative to adults was observed.

Among patients 2–21 years of age, age did not appear to substantially affect erlotinib clearance normalized to body surface area in a population pharmacokinetic analysis.

Geriatric Use

In clinical studies in patients with NSCLC or pancreatic cancer, 40% of patients receiving erlotinib were ≥65 years of age and 10% were ≥75 years of age. No overall differences in safety and efficacy relative to younger adults were observed.

Hepatic Impairment

Although erlotinib is eliminated mainly by the liver, systemic exposure was not substantially altered in patients with Child-Pugh class B hepatic impairment relative to those with adequate hepatic function (including individuals with primary liver cancer or hepatic metastases); however, because hepatic failure and hepatorenal syndrome, sometimes fatal, have been reported in patients with normal hepatic function, the risk of hepatotoxicity is increased in patients with preexisting hepatic impairment. Close monitoring is required during erlotinib therapy in patients with hepatic impairment (total bilirubin concentrations greater than the upper limit of normal [ULN] or Child-Pugh class A, B, or C); patients with biliary obstruction or total bilirubin concentrations greater than 3 times the ULN should be monitored more frequently. If worsening of liver dysfunction occurs, interruption of erlotinib therapy or reduction of erlotinib dosage accompanied by frequent monitoring of liver function tests should be considered before changes in liver function become severe. If severe changes in liver function test results, such as doubling of total bilirubin and/or tripling of serum aminotransferase concentrations, occur in patients with hepatic dysfunction prior to treatment, erlotinib therapy should be interrupted or discontinued.

Renal Impairment

Safety and efficacy of erlotinib have not been established in patients with renal impairment.

● Common Adverse Effects

Adverse effects occurring in ≥20% of patients receiving erlotinib in a pooled analysis of data from patients with NSCLC across all approved lines of therapy, with and without *EGFR* mutations, and in patients with pancreatic cancer were rash, diarrhea, anorexia, fatigue, dyspnea, cough, nausea, and vomiting.

DRUG INTERACTIONS

Erlotinib is metabolized principally by cytochrome P-450 (CYP) isoenzyme 3A4 and, to a lesser extent, CYP1A1 and CYP1A2.

● Drugs and Foods Affecting Hepatic Microsomal Enzymes

Inhibitors of CYP3A4

Concomitant use of erlotinib with potent inhibitors of CYP3A4 may result in increased erlotinib exposure. When the potent CYP3A4 inhibitor ketoconazole was administered concomitantly with erlotinib, the area under the concentration-time curve (AUC) of erlotinib was increased by 67%. Concomitant use of erlotinib with potent CYP3A4 inhibitors (e.g., atazanavir, clarithromycin, conivaptan, indinavir, itraconazole, ketoconazole, lopinavir/ritonavir, nefazodone, nelfinavir, posaconazole, ritonavir, saquinavir, telithromycin, voriconazole, grapefruit or grapefruit juice) should be avoided. If concomitant use cannot be avoided, the manufacturer recommends reducing the dosage of erlotinib in 50-mg decrements.

Combined Inhibitors of CYP3A4 and 1A2

Concomitant use of erlotinib with combined inhibitors of CYP3A4 and 1A2 may result in increased peak plasma concentrations and systemic exposure of erlotinib. When the combined CYP3A4 and CYP1A2 inhibitor ciprofloxacin was administered concomitantly with erlotinib, the peak plasma concentration and AUC of erlotinib was increased by 17 and 39%, respectively. Concomitant use of erlotinib with combined CYP3A4 and CYP1A2 inhibitors (e.g., ciprofloxacin) should be avoided. If concomitant use cannot be avoided, the manufacturer recommends reducing the dosage of erlotinib in 50-mg decrements.

Inducers of CYP3A4

Concomitant use of erlotinib with inducers of CYP3A4 may result in decreased erlotinib exposure. When the CYP3A4 inducer rifampin was administered 7–11 days prior to erlotinib, the AUC of erlotinib was decreased by 58–80%. Concomitant use of erlotinib with CYP3A4 inducers (e.g., carbamazepine, phenobarbital, phenytoin, rifabutin, rifampin, rifapentine, St. John's wort [*Hypericum perforatum*]) should be avoided. If concomitant use with these agents cannot be avoided, the manufacturer recommends increasing the dosage of erlotinib in 50-mg increments (not to exceed 450 mg daily) as tolerated at 2-week intervals.

Inducers of CYP1A2

Concomitant use of erlotinib with moderate inducers of CYP1A2 may result in decreased erlotinib exposure. Concomitant use with moderate CYP1A2 inducers (e.g., phenytoin, rifampin, teriflunomide) should be avoided. If concomitant use with these agents cannot be avoided, the manufacturer recommends increasing the dosage of erlotinib.

● Cigarette Smoking

Because cigarette smoking moderately induces CYP1A2, concomitant cigarette smoking may result in decreased systemic exposure to erlotinib. Patients should be advised to stop smoking. Cigarette smoking decreases the AUC of erlotinib by approximately 64%. In a clinical trial, clearance of erlotinib was increased by 24% resulting in steady-state plasma trough concentrations of erlotinib approximately twofold less in current smokers compared with those who never smoked or were former smokers. In a pharmacokinetic analysis in current smokers, steady-state exposure of erlotinib increased in a dose-proportional manner following an increase in erlotinib dosage from 150 to 300 mg.

If patients continue to smoke, the manufacturer recommends increasing the dosage of erlotinib in 50-mg increments (not to exceed 300 mg daily) at 2-week intervals. Upon cessation of smoking, the erlotinib dose should be reduced immediately to the recommended starting dose.

● Drugs Affecting Gastric Acidity

Drugs that increase the pH of the upper GI tract decrease the solubility of erlotinib and reduce its bioavailability. Concomitant administration of omeprazole, a proton-pump inhibitor, decreased the peak plasma concentration and AUC of erlotinib by 61 and 46%, respectively. In another small study, concomitant administration of pantoprazole and erlotinib decreased AUC and peak plasma concentrations of erlotinib by 50% compared to patients who received erlotinib alone; however, when erlotinib was administered concomitantly with famotidine, a H$_2$-receptor antagonist, no clinically important change in peak plasma concentrations of erlotinib was observed. Increasing the dose level of erlotinib is not likely to compensate for the loss of exposure, and separation of doses may not eliminate the interaction because proton-pump inhibitors have an extended effect on the pH of the upper GI tract. If possible, concomitant use of erlotinib and proton-pump inhibitors should be avoided.

If use of a histamine H$_2$-receptor antagonist (e.g., ranitidine) is necessary, erlotinib must be taken 10 hours after the H$_2$-receptor antagonist and at least 2 hours before the next dose of the H$_2$-receptor antagonist. Concomitant administration of ranitidine (300 mg) administered 2 hours prior to erlotinib decreased the peak plasma concentration and AUC of erlotinib by 54 and 33%, respectively; however, when ranitidine (150 mg twice daily) was administered at least 10 hours before or 2 hours after erlotinib, the peak plasma concentration and AUC of erlotinib decreased by 17 and 15%, respectively.

The effect of antacids on the pharmacokinetics of erlotinib has not been studied. If use of an antacid is necessary, the antacid dose and the erlotinib dose should be separated by several hours.

● Antineoplastic Agents

Concomitant use of erlotinib with gemcitabine did not affect the clearance of erlotinib.

Concomitant use of erlotinib with paclitaxel and carboplatin in patients with cancers other than non-small cell lung cancer (NSCLC) did not substantially alter the pharmacokinetics of these antineoplastic agents.

Concomitant use of erlotinib with gemcitabine and cisplatin in patients with cancers other than NSCLC did not substantially alter the pharmacokinetics of these antineoplastic agents.

Concomitant use of erlotinib with capecitabine and docetaxel in patients with cancers other than NSCLC did not substantially alter the pharmacokinetics of these antineoplastic agents.

Concomitant use of erlotinib with docetaxel in patients with cancers other than NSCLC did not substantially alter the pharmacokinetics of either drug.

Concomitant use of erlotinib with capecitabine in patients with pancreatic cancer did not substantially alter the pharmacokinetics of either drug.

• *Crizotinib*

Concomitant use of erlotinib with crizotinib 150 or 200 mg twice daily in patients with NSCLC increased the AUC of erlotinib by 1.5- or 1.8-fold, respectively.

• *Warfarin*

Increased international normalized ratio (INR) and hemorrhagic events, sometimes fatal, have been reported in patients receiving erlotinib concomitantly with warfarin. Prothrombin time (PT) or INR should be monitored regularly in patients receiving erlotinib concomitantly with warfarin or other coumarin-derivative anticoagulants. Dosage adjustment of erlotinib is not necessary.

DESCRIPTION

Erlotinib, a reversible inhibitor of epidermal growth factor receptor (EGFR/human epidermal growth factor receptor type 1 [HER1]/ErbB1) and mutated *EGFR* (e.g., exon 19 deletion [del19], exon 21 substitution [L858R]) tyrosine kinases, is an antineoplastic agent. EGFR is expressed on the cell surface of many cancer cells, as well as many normal cells; activation of EGFR tyrosine kinase is thought to initiate a cascade of intracellular signaling events leading to cell proliferation and influencing processes critical to cell survival and tumor progression (e.g., angiogenesis, apoptosis, metastasis). Some *EGFR*-activating mutations, such as exon 19 deletion (del19) and exon 21 (L858R) substitution mutation, contribute to increased cell proliferation and survival in non-small cell lung cancer (NSCLC) cells harboring these mutations. The drug binds to the kinase domains of EGFR and reversibly inhibits tyrosine kinase phosphorylation, resulting in downregulation of EGFR signaling. Erlotinib has demonstrated a greater affinity for cell lines expressing del19 or L858R mutations than for wild-type EGFR. Specificity with regard to other tyrosine kinase receptors has not been fully characterized.

Approximately 60% of an oral dose of erlotinib is absorbed from the GI tract; presence of food in the GI tract increases oral bioavailability to approximately 100%. Peak plasma concentrations of erlotinib occur at 4 hours following oral administration. Steady-state concentrations of erlotinib are achieved within 7–8 days. Erlotinib is 93% bound to plasma proteins (mainly to albumin and α_1-acid glycoprotein). Erlotinib is extensively metabolized via the cytochrome P-450 (CYP) enzyme system, mainly by CYP3A4 and, to a lesser extent, by CYP1A1 (principally an extrahepatic enzyme) and CYP1A2. The half-life of erlotinib is approximately 36 hours; the clearance is approximately 24% higher in smokers. Following a 100-mg oral dose, erlotinib is excreted mainly as metabolites in feces (83%) and urine (8%).

Systemic exposure of erlotinib does not appear to be affected substantially by age, body weight, or gender in patients receiving the drug as a single agent for maintenance or second- or third-line therapy in NSCLC or in combination with gemcitabine for the treatment of pancreatic cancer.

ADVICE TO PATIENTS

• Risk of skin rash, bullous and exfoliative skin disorders. Importance of proper skin care (e.g., alcohol-free emollient cream, use of sunscreen or avoidance of sun exposure), to minimize the risk of skin reactions. Advise patients that hyperpigmentation or dry skin, with or without digital skin fissures, have been reported and in the majority of cases were associated with rash. Advise patients to immediately seek medical attention if a severe skin reaction occurs.

• Risk of diarrhea. Diarrhea can usually be managed with loperamide. Importance of informing clinician if severe or persistent diarrhea occurs.

• Risk of interstitial lung disease. Importance of immediately informing clinician if new or worsening respiratory symptoms (e.g., dyspnea, cough) occur.

• Risk of renal failure and importance of periodic monitoring of kidney function and electrolytes.

• Risk of hepatotoxicity and importance of periodic liver function test monitoring. Importance of reporting any manifestations of hepatotoxicity.

• Risk of GI perforation. Importance of advising patients to seek immediate medical attention if they experience symptoms of GI perforation (e.g., severe abdominal pain).

• Risk of cerebrovascular accident. Importance of advising patients to seek immediate medical attention if they experience symptoms of cerebrovascular accident.

• Risk of ocular disorders. Importance of promptly informing clinician if ocular problems (e.g., lacrimation, sensitivity to light, eye pain, redness, blurred vision, other vision changes) occur.

• Risk of hair or nail disorders (e.g., hirsutism, brittle or loose nails).

• Advise smokers to stop smoking; smoking may reduce efficacy of erlotinib.

• Importance of women using an effective method of contraception during and for one month after discontinuance of therapy. If pregnancy occurs, advise patient of risk to the fetus.

• Importance of women informing clinicians if they plan to breast-feed. Importance of advising women to avoid breast-feeding while receiving erlotinib and for 2 weeks after discontinuance of therapy.

• Importance of informing clinicians of existing or contemplated concomitant therapy, including prescription and OTC drugs (e.g., warfarin) and herbal supplements, as well as any concomitant illnesses.

• Importance of informing patients of other important precautionary information. (See Cautions.)

For further information on the handling of antineoplastic agents, see the ASHP Guidelines on Handling Hazardous Drugs at http://www.ahfsdruginformation.com.

PREPARATIONS

Excipients in commercially available drug preparations may have clinically important effects in some individuals; consult specific product labeling for details.

Erlotinib Hydrochloride

Oral		
Tablets	25 mg (of erlotinib)*	**Erlotinib Hydrochloride Tablets**
		Tarceva®, Genentech
	100 mg (of erlotinib)*	**Erlotinib Hydrochloride Tablets**
		Tarceva®, Genentech
	150 mg (of erlotinib)*	**Erlotinib Hydrochloride Tablets**
		Tarceva®, Genentech

† Use is not currently included in the labeling approved by the US Food and Drug Administration.

* available from one or more manufacturer, distributor, and/or repackager by generic (nonproprietary) name

Etoposide

10:00 • ANTINEOPLASTIC AGENTS

■ Etoposide is a semisynthetic podophyllotoxin-derivative antineoplastic agent.

USES

● Testicular Neoplasms

Etoposide or etoposide phosphate may be used IV as a component of various chemotherapeutic regimens for the treatment of refractory testicular tumors in patients who have already received appropriate surgery, chemotherapy, and radiation therapy. Adequate data on the use of oral etoposide for the treatment of testicular tumors are currently not available.

Nonseminomatous Testicular Carcinoma

In the treatment of disseminated nonseminomatous testicular carcinoma (Stage III), etoposide alone produces an objective response in about 35% of patients and is active in some patients whose disease is refractory to cisplatin-containing combination chemotherapy; however, combination chemotherapy for induction of remissions is superior to single-agent therapy. Various regimens have been used in combination therapy, and comparative efficacy is continually being evaluated. Most clinicians use cisplatin-containing combination chemotherapy regimens as initial therapy in patients with Stage III or unresectable Stage II nonseminomatous testicular carcinoma; if the patient has persistent, localized tumor following chemotherapy, the residual tumor is removed surgically, and if the disease contains malignant elements, additional chemotherapy is administered. Combination chemotherapy regimens containing etoposide and cisplatin have been evaluated in the treatment of disseminated nonseminomatous testicular carcinomas. For the initial treatment of advanced nonseminomatous testicular carcinoma, most clinicians recommend regimens containing cisplatin and bleomycin, in combination with etoposide rather than vinblastine, particularly because of the reduced neuromuscular toxicity and evidence suggesting greater efficacy in poor-risk patients. In addition, while a regimen of etoposide, cisplatin, and bleomycin appears to be as effective overall as a regimen of vinblastine, cisplatin, and bleomycin, the etoposide-containing regimen may be more effective than the vinblastine-containing regimen in a subgroup of patients with advanced disease (i.e., high tumor load). However, the best combination or sequential therapy in the treatment of advanced nonseminomatous testicular tumors has not been established, and comparative efficacy is continually being evaluated.

Although studied less extensively than cisplatin-containing regimens, etoposide in combination with carboplatin with or without bleomycin has produced clinical response in the treatment of stage II or stage III nonseminomatous testicular cancer†. However, there is evidence that a regimen of etoposide and cisplatin is more effective than standard dosages of etoposide and carboplatin in the initial treatment of germ cell tumors, and treatment with a carboplatin regimen generally is reserved for patients who do not tolerate or refuse cisplatin. Limited data suggest that high-dose etoposide and carboplatin may be effective in the treatment of relapsed or refractory germ cell tumors in some patients. High-dose etoposide and carboplatin with autologous bone marrow transplant has been associated with complete remission in 10–20% of patients with cisplatin-resistant germ cell tumors.

Etoposide also is used effectively in cisplatin-containing combination chemotherapy regimens for the treatment of those patients whose disease is refractory to chemotherapy, with or without surgery; a complete remission has been produced in about 50% of such patients treated with regimens that include etoposide and cisplatin, followed by surgery when feasible. Some data suggest that combination chemotherapy containing etoposide and cisplatin is effective in the treatment of refractory testicular cancer principally in those patients whose disease relapses after having achieved a complete remission with cisplatin-containing chemotherapy, followed by surgery when necessary. This combination does not appear to be very effective in patients with multiple tumor sites, increasing tumor markers, and refractory disease (as evidenced by incomplete response to conventional chemotherapy). Intensive combination chemotherapy regimens containing etoposide and high-dose cisplatin are currently being evaluated for the initial treatment of patients with disseminated disease associated with a poor prognosis.

Etoposide also is used as a component of various other chemotherapeutic regimens for salvage therapy in patients with recurrent or refractory germ cell testicular cancer. A regimen of ifosfamide, cisplatin, and either etoposide or vinblastine has induced complete responses in 20–45% of patients who previously received other cisplatin-based chemotherapy regimens, and is considered by most clinicians to be the standard initial salvage (i.e., second-line) regimen in patients with recurrent testicular cancer. Patients with minimal or moderate disease have a more favorable outcome with this salvage regimen than those with extensive disease. In a clinical study in patients with recurrent germ cell tumors (who had previously received at least 2 cisplatin-based chemotherapy regimens and were considered to have cisplatin-responsive disease), a regimen of ifosfamide, cisplatin, and either etoposide or vinblastine resulted in disease-free status in 36% of patients (with or without surgery) and median duration of disease control ranged from 3 to more than 42 weeks, median survival was 53 weeks, and 20% of patients had survival of 2 years or longer. In patients with refractory disease, high-dose chemotherapy (e.g., etoposide and carboplatin with or without ifosfamide) with autologous bone marrow transplant (ABMT) or peripheral stem cell rescue may produce durable complete remissions in some patients. Patients with progressive tumors during initial or salvage therapy and those with refractory mediastinal germ cell tumors generally appear to benefit less from high-dose chemotherapy and ABMT or peripheral stem cell rescue than those whose disease relapses after a response. Salvage surgery also may be considered for certain highly selected patients (e.g., those with chemorefractory disease confined to a single site).

The role of chemotherapy in the treatment of Stage I and resectable Stage II nonseminomatous testicular carcinoma has not been clearly established. Although most patients with Stage I disease are cured by surgery alone, combination chemotherapy regimens containing etoposide and cisplatin have been used successfully to induce complete remissions in a limited number of patients whose disease relapsed following surgical treatment.

Seminoma Testis

Etoposide has been used successfully as a component of cisplatin-containing combination chemotherapy regimens in a limited number of patients for the initial treatment of disseminated seminoma testis and for the treatment of disseminated disease refractory to initial chemotherapy regimens, with complete remission rates comparable to those in patients with disseminated nonseminomatous disease. Further evaluation is needed to determine the optimum therapy.

Extragonadal Germ-Cell Tumors

Data are limited, but etoposide-containing combination chemotherapy regimens (usually also containing cisplatin), followed by surgery when feasible, have reportedly been successful in the initial treatment of advanced extragonadal germ-cell tumors, but have generally produced only partial responses in the treatment of advanced extragonadal germ-cell tumors refractory to initial chemotherapy regimens.

● Lung Cancer

Etoposide has been widely used for the treatment of lung cancer, principally as a component of chemotherapeutic regimens in the treatment of small cell lung carcinoma.

Small Cell Lung Cancer

Etoposide is used IV (either as etoposide or etoposide phosphate) in combination chemotherapy regimens for the treatment of small cell lung carcinoma; etoposide also has been used orally, either alone or as a component of combination therapy for this cancer. Combination chemotherapy regimens are superior to single-agent therapy in the treatment of this tumor and moderately intensive drug doses are superior to doses that produce minimal toxicity. Staging the cancer provides useful prognostic information and has implications for the specific course of therapy employed; all patients with small cell lung cancer generally should receive combination chemotherapy initially regardless of the extent of tumor dissemination since this cancer is the most aggressive form of lung cancer and some degree of metastasis is present in most patients regardless of whether it is detected at initial diagnosis.

Various regimens have been used in combination therapy, and many 2- to 4-drug regimens, including etoposide-containing regimens, have produced response rates of 65–90 or 70–85% and complete response rates of 45–75 or 20–30% in patients with limited-stage or extensive-stage disease, respectively; however, comparative efficacy is continually being evaluated. Etoposide-containing regimens are used in chemotherapy for extensive-stage small cell lung cancer and in combined modality treatment (i.e., combination chemotherapy with concurrent thoracic irradiation administered early in the course of treatment) for limited-stage disease.

Etoposide used in combination with cisplatin or carboplatin is a preferred regimen for the treatment of small cell lung cancer; this combination also may be of some value for the treatment of small cell lung carcinoma refractory to other chemotherapy regimens (particularly when relapse occurs more than 6 months following completion of initial treatment). Etoposide also has been employed in conjunction with a platinum agent (i.e., cisplatin or carboplatin) and ifosfamide with mesna. Other etoposide-containing combination chemotherapy regimens (e.g., etoposide, cyclophosphamide, and doxorubicin; etoposide, cyclophosphamide, and vincristine) have been used less commonly for the treatment of extensive-stage small cell lung cancer.

Concomitant administration of granulocyte colony-stimulating factor has been used in some patients with small cell lung carcinoma but is not routinely used to reduce the incidence and severity of myelosuppression associated with therapy.

Monotherapy with oral etoposide is inferior to combination therapy, and even geriatric and/or debilitated patients should be offered standard IV combination chemotherapy regimens for the treatment of advanced small cell lung cancer. In a randomized trial involving patients with poor-prognosis extensive-stage small cell lung cancer and geriatric patients (older than 75 years of age) with any stage of small cell lung cancer, fewer complete responses, reduced survival, and comparable or worse toxicity were observed among patients who received oral etoposide alone compared with those who received IV combination chemotherapy with alternating cycles of cisplatin/etoposide and cyclophosphamide/doxorubicin/vincristine. A randomized trial involving patients with previously untreated extensive-stage small cell lung cancer and poor performance status (WHO grade performance status 2–4) was stopped when interim analysis showed reduced survival and increased hematologic toxicity for those receiving oral etoposide alone compared with those receiving IV combination chemotherapy with etoposide/vincristine or cyclophosphamide/doxorubicin/vincristine.

Etoposide currently is considered one of the most active antineoplastic agents in the treatment of small cell lung carcinoma, producing an objective response in about 35–40% of previously untreated patients when used alone†. Although results of initial studies suggested that etoposide alone had substantial activity in patients whose disease was refractory to initial combination chemotherapy, more extensive studies have shown that monotherapy with the drug generally is of little benefit in these patients.

Although optimum duration of chemotherapy has not been clearly defined, additional improvement in survival has not been observed when the duration of drug administration exceeds 3–6 or 6 months in patients with limited-stage or extensive-stage small cell lung cancer, respectively. Because the current prognosis for small cell lung carcinoma is unsatisfactory regardless of stage and despite considerable diagnostic and therapeutic advances, all patients with this cancer are candidates for inclusion in clinical trials at the time of diagnosis.

Non-small Cell Lung Carcinoma

In the treatment of non-small cell lung carcinoma†, etoposide alone appears to be of little benefit. A small survival benefit has been demonstrated for the use of platinum-based (cisplatin) chemotherapy in selected patients with unresectable, locally advanced or metastatic non-small cell lung cancer who have a good performance status. Etoposide has been used in combination with cisplatin for the treatment of advanced non-small cell lung cancer. However, in randomized trials, patients with stage IIIB or IV non-small cell lung cancer receiving paclitaxel combined with cisplatin or gemcitabine combined with cisplatin had higher response rates and similar median survival compared with those receiving combination therapy with etoposide and cisplatin; consequently, paclitaxel-containing regimens or other platinum-based regimens currently are preferred in the treatment of patients with advanced non-small cell lung cancer. Some clinicians consider etoposide and cisplatin an alternative regimen for the treatment of advanced non-small cell lung cancer.

Various chemotherapy regimens used alone or in combination with other treatment modalities, such as radiation therapy, are continually being evaluated for the treatment of advanced non-small cell lung cancer. A randomized trial is under way to determine the comparative efficacy and toxicity of combination therapy with etoposide and cisplatin versus paclitaxel and carboplatin in patients with advanced non-small cell lung cancer. Because current treatment is not satisfactory for almost all patients with non-small cell lung cancer except selected patients with early-stage, resectable disease, all patients may be considered for enrollment in clinical trials at the time of diagnosis.

● Malignant Lymphomas and Hodgkin's Disease

Etoposide appears to be one of the more active antineoplastic agents in the treatment of advanced non-Hodgkin's lymphomas†. The drug appears to be particularly effective for the treatment of advanced diffuse lymphomas of unfavorable histology such as diffuse histiocytic lymphoma, producing an objective response in about 30–40% of previously treated patients. Etoposide has been used in effective combination chemotherapy regimens (e.g., etoposide, ifosfamide, and methotrexate) for the treatment of refractory advanced diffuse lymphomas of unfavorable histology. Etoposide has also been used in effective alternating combination chemotherapy regimens for the initial treatment of advanced diffuse lymphomas of unfavorable histology.

Data are limited, but etoposide has produced transient responses in a few patients with mycosis fungoides†.

Etoposide has shown some activity in the treatment of advanced Hodgkin's disease†, and combination chemotherapy regimens containing the drug are currently being evaluated in the treatment of refractory disease.

● Leukemias

Although the exact role of etoposide has not been established, the drug has been shown to be active in the treatment of refractory acute myeloid (myelogenous, nonlymphocytic) leukemia (AML, ANLL)† in adults and children. When used alone in patients whose disease is refractory to initial chemotherapy, etoposide induces complete remission in about 10–15% of patients; response rates appear to be higher in patients with acute monocytic and myelomonocytic leukemias. Since etoposide appears to be particularly effective for the treatment of acute monocytic and myelomonocytic leukemias, the drug may be useful when monocytoid cells are not cleared with conventional combination chemotherapy. Because of its antileukemic activity, etoposide also has been employed in various combination chemotherapy regimens for remission induction in adults and children with refractory AML; while some of these regimens are effective (e.g., etoposide and azacitidine), the role of etoposide in these regimens remains to be clearly established. Additional studies are needed to evaluate the role of etoposide as a single agent and in combination chemotherapy for the treatment of AML.

Data are limited, but etoposide has shown activity alone and in combination chemotherapy for remission induction in the treatment of refractory acute lymphocytic (lymphoblastic) leukemia† in children; in adults with acute lymphocytic leukemia, etoposide appears to have little, if any, activity.

● Wilms' Tumor

Etoposide has shown activity in the management of Wilms' tumor and has been used with encouraging results in conjunction with carboplatin in a limited number of children with recurrent (relapsed or refractory) disease. Etoposide also has been used as an alternative to standard preferred regimens (e.g., combined vincristine and dactinomycin with or without doxorubicin) in patients with less severe stages of Wilms' tumor. Second-line (salvage) therapy with etoposide and carboplatin may be considered for patients with recurrent tumors of unfavorable histology, abdominal recurrence after radiation therapy, or recurrence within 6 months of nephrectomy or after initial 3-drug combination chemotherapy (e.g., vincristine, dactinomycin, and doxorubicin). In a study in a limited number of children with recurrent Wilms' tumor, most of whose tumors were of favorable histology, second-line therapy (2 courses separated by 21 days) with etoposide (100 mg/m^2 daily for 5 days) and carboplatin (160 mg/m^2 daily for 5 days) resulted in complete or partial responses in 73% of patients; complete response was maintained for a median follow-up of 40 months (range: 24–56 months) in about 30% of patients. The principal toxicity in these children was high-grade hematologic toxicity, particularly thrombocytopenia. Second-line therapy with high-dose chemotherapy followed by autologous bone marrow transplantation also has been used effectively in patients with recurrent disease, occasionally resulting in long-term survival. Patients with recurrent disease failing to respond to such attempts with salvage therapy should be offered treatment under protocol conditions in ongoing clinical trials.

● Neuroblastoma

Etoposide also has been used in the treatment of disseminated neuroblastoma†, and combination regimens using cyclophosphamide, doxorubicin, cisplatin, and/or etoposide or teniposide generally are preferred in children with this tumor. For localized resectable neuroblastoma, complete gross surgical excision produces disease-free survival that is indistinguishable from that obtained with surgery and adjuvant chemotherapy or adjuvant radiation therapy and therefore is preferred; however, the importance of certain tumor biologic properties (e.g., N-myc amplification and DNA ploidy) and other prognostic factors should be considered in evaluating the possible need for adjuvant therapy. For localized unresectable tumor, subtotal resection followed by chemotherapy is used for initial treatment, and short-term treatment (e.g., 4–6 months) usually is adequate. For regional neuroblastoma in children younger than 1 year of age, chemotherapy generally is limited to relatively resistant tumors since prognosis in less resistant tumors treated with surgery alone is good. In older children with regional neuroblastoma, chemotherapy may be employed for tumor reduction prior to surgery or may be employed aggressively following surgery; the role of aggressive therapy that includes high-dose chemotherapy, radiation therapy, and bone marrow transplant is being evaluated for children older than 1 year of age and/or those with poor prognostic characteristics (e.g., N-myc amplification). For disseminated neuroblastoma, intensive conventional chemotherapy, with or without surgery and radiation therapy (depending on clinical presentation and course), currently is the preferred initial therapy, although the relative efficacy of such therapy compared with myeloablative chemotherapy and autologous bone marrow transplant is being evaluated. For infants with stage IVS (special) neuroblastoma, chemotherapy often is unnecessary, but the management course should be individualized.

● AIDS-related Kaposi's Sarcoma

Etoposide has been used alone or in combination chemotherapy for the palliative treatment of AIDS-related Kaposi's sarcoma†. Single-agent therapy with etoposide is an alternative regimen for treatment of such sarcoma. Combination chemotherapy that includes bleomycin, doxorubicin, and a vinca alkaloid (vinblastine or vincristine) has been considered a regimen of choice for the disease, but many clinicians currently consider a liposomal anthracycline (doxorubicin or daunorubicin) the first-line therapy of choice for advanced AIDS-related Kaposi's sarcoma (see Uses: AIDS-related Kaposi's Sarcoma in Doxorubicin 10:00 or Daunorubicin 10:00).

Although single-agent therapy with conventional (i.e., nonencapsulated) cytotoxic agents generally has been used in the early stage of disease, Kaposi's sarcoma in patients with human immunodeficiency virus (HIV) infection often is rapidly progressive. AIDS-related Kaposi's sarcoma often progresses to multifocal, widespread lesions that may involve the skin, oral mucosa, and lymph nodes as well as visceral organs such as the GI tract, lung, liver, and spleen; such lesions often are numerous and may be cosmetically unattractive or disfiguring and accompanied by lymphedema. Appropriate evaluation of the effects of drug therapies on survival in patients with Kaposi's sarcoma must include assessment of the effects of such therapies on the development of infection as well as on tumor regression. Although treatment may result in disappearance or reduction in the size of Kaposi's sarcoma skin lesions and thereby alleviate the discomfort associated with chronic edema and ulcerations that often accompany multiple skin lesions on the lower extremities and in symptomatic control of mucosal and visceral lesions, there currently are no data demonstrating unequivocal evidence of improved survival with any therapy. Small localized Kaposi's sarcoma lesions may be treated with electrodesiccation and curettage cryotherapy or by surgical excision; the lesions also generally are responsive to local radiation, and excellent palliation often can be achieved. Localized palatal lesions have been treated effectively with intralesional† injections of vinblastine. Alitretinoin gel (Panretin®, Ligand Pharmaceuticals), a topical retinoid, is used for the treatment of localized cutaneous lesions in patients with AIDS-related Kaposi's sarcoma; responses of cutaneous lesions to topical therapy with alitretinoin have been reported in patients who have received prior systemic and/or topical therapy for Kaposi's sarcoma as well as in those with previously untreated disease.

Response rates observed with single-agent chemotherapy (e.g., doxorubicin, etoposide, vinblastine, vincristine) appear to be similar to those observed with interferon alfa; however, studies directly comparing the efficacy of doxorubicin alone with that of interferon alfa have not been performed. Any differences in response rates reported in clinical studies generally appear to reflect differences in patient selection and in the criteria used to evaluate response rather than in drug activity. In one study in patients with AIDS-related Kaposi's sarcoma who received etoposide in an IV dosage of 150 mg/m² daily for 3 consecutive days at the beginning of a 28-day cycle for a median of 6 or 7 cycles (range: 2–26 cycles), complete or partial response was observed in about 30 or 46% of evaluable patients, respectively. Combined treatment with etoposide and interferon alfa generally appears to result in enhanced systemic toxicity without added therapeutic benefit.

Combination chemotherapy with conventional antineoplastic agents (e.g., bleomycin, conventional doxorubicin, etoposide, vinblastine, vincristine) usually

has been used for more advanced disease (e.g., extensive mucocutaneous disease, lymphedema, symptomatic visceral disease). Doxorubicin hydrochloride liposomal injection (Doxil® by Alza Pharmaceuticals) is approved for use in the palliative treatment of AIDS-related Kaposi's sarcoma in adults who are intolerant to combination chemotherapy or whose disease has progressed while receiving such therapy. Liposomal daunorubicin citrate (DaunoXome® by NeXstar) is approved for use as first-line therapy for advanced AIDS-related Kaposi's sarcoma. The results of several randomized, multicenter trials indicate that patients receiving a liposomal anthracycline for the treatment of advanced AIDS-related Kaposi's sarcoma experience similar or higher response rates with a more favorable toxic effects profile than those receiving combination therapy with conventional chemotherapeutic agents. Preliminary evidence suggests that the mean survival period in patients with AIDS-related pulmonary Kaposi's sarcoma receiving liposomal doxorubicin may be increased compared with those receiving conventional chemotherapy (bleomycin and/or vincristine). The comparative efficacy of liposomal daunorubicin relative to liposomal doxorubicin has not been established.

Although treatment may result in the reduction or disappearance of lesions and alleviation of the associated symptoms, no treatment has been shown conclusively to alter the natural history of AIDS-related Kaposi's sarcoma and additional study and experience are needed to establish the optimal regimen.

● Ovarian Neoplasms
Epithelial Ovarian Cancer

Etoposide currently is being investigated as an active agent for use in the treatment of advanced epithelial ovarian cancer†. In phase II studies, objective responses were observed in 6–26% of patients receiving low-dose oral etoposide as salvage therapy for previously treated advanced epithelial ovarian cancer; responses occurred in patients with platinum- and paclitaxel-resistant disease.

Ovarian Germ Cell Tumors

Etoposide is used in combination with cisplatin and bleomycin for the treatment of ovarian germ cell tumors†.

● Other Uses

The use of high-dose† etoposide regimens in conjunction with autogenous (autologous) bone marrow transplantation is currently being evaluated for the treatment of various refractory advanced malignant neoplasms (e.g., nonseminomatous testicular carcinoma). Etoposide has been used with encouraging results in the treatment of gestational trophoblastic tumors† (choriocarcinoma and chorioadenoma destruens) in women. The drug has also shown some activity in the treatment of hepatoma†, Ewing's sarcoma†, rhabdomyosarcoma†, and brain tumors†. The role of etoposide in the treatment of these neoplasms has not been fully elucidated.

DOSAGE AND ADMINISTRATION

● Administration

Etoposide is administered orally and by slow IV infusion. Etoposide phosphate is administered by IV infusion.

Etoposide solutions should not be administered by rapid IV injection. (See Cautions: Cardiovascular Effects.) *Because delayed, severe (sometimes fatal) toxicity has occurred in animals following intraperitoneal and intrapleural administration of etoposide, it is recommended that the drug not be administered by these routes.*

The toxicity of rapidly infused etoposide phosphate in patients with impaired renal or hepatic function has not been adequately evaluated, and the toxicity profile of etoposide phosphate when infused at doses exceeding 175 mg/m² has not been delineated.

To minimize the risk of hypotensive reactions, IV infusions of etoposide should be administered over a period of at least 30–60 minutes. The manufacturer states that a longer duration of administration may be used if the volume of fluid to be infused is a concern. Patients should be observed closely for possible hypotensive or anaphylactoid reactions during administration of the drug. (See Cautions: Precautions and Contraindications.) When a hypotensive reaction occurs and the infusion is discontinued and then restarted after appropriate treatment of the reaction, a slower rate of infusion should be employed. Etoposide has been administered by continuous IV infusion over 5 days, but this method of administration has not been shown to date to have any therapeutic advantage over intermittent IV infusions of the drug.

Etoposide phosphate solutions may be administered over 5–210 minutes.

The manufacturer recommends that protective gloves be used during handling of etoposide concentrate for injection and preparation of etoposide and etoposide phosphate solutions, since skin reactions associated with accidental exposure to the drug may occur. If etoposide concentrate for injection or a solution of the drug comes in contact with the skin, the affected area should be washed immediately and thoroughly with soap and water. If solutions of etoposide phosphate come in contact with the skin or mucosa, the affected skin should be washed immediately and thoroughly with soap and water, and the affected mucosa should be rinsed thoroughly with water.

Etoposide concentrate for injection must be diluted before administration. It is recommended that syringes with Luer-Lok® fittings be used for handling of etoposide concentrate for injection; when under pressure, needles have become displaced from etoposide-containing syringes without Luer-Lok® fittings, an effect which may be related to the drug's vehicle. The manufacturer recommends that the required dose of etoposide concentrate for injection be diluted to a final concentration of 0.2 or 0.4 mg/mL in 0.9% sodium chloride or 5% dextrose injection prior to slow IV infusion. (See Chemistry and Stability: Stability.) Etoposide concentrate for injection and the diluted solution for infusion should be inspected visually for particulate matter and discoloration prior to administration whenever solution and container permit.

Etoposide phosphate powder for injection should be reconstituted with 5 or 10 mL of sterile water for injection, 5% dextrose injection, 0.9% sodium chloride, bacteriostatic water for injection (with benzyl alcohol), or bacteriostatic sodium chloride for injection (with benzyl alcohol), resulting in a concentration equivalent to 20 or 10 mg of etoposide per mL (22.7 or 11.4 mg of etoposide phosphate per mL), respectively. Following reconstitution, the solution may be administered without further dilution, or it may be further diluted to concentrations as low as 0.1 mg of etoposide per mL with either 5% dextrose injection or 0.9% sodium chloride injection.

● Dosage

Dosage of etoposide must be based on the clinical and hematologic response and tolerance of the patient and whether or not other chemotherapy or radiation therapy has been or is also being used in order to obtain optimum therapeutic results with minimum adverse effects. Clinicians should consult published protocols for the dosage of etoposide and other chemotherapeutic agents and the method and sequence of administration. *A repeat course of etoposide should not be administered until the patient's hematologic function is within acceptable limits.* (See Cautions: Precautions and Contraindications.) When etoposide phosphate is used, dosage is expressed in terms of etoposide; 113.6 mg of etoposide phosphate is equivalent to 100 mg of etoposide.

Testicular Neoplasms

For remission induction in the treatment of refractory testicular neoplasms, the usual IV dosage of etoposide in combination chemotherapy regimens is 50–100 mg/m² daily for 5 consecutive days every 3–4 weeks or 100 mg/m² daily on days 1, 3, and 5 every 3–4 weeks, for 3 or 4 courses of therapy. When the consecutive-day dosage regimen is employed, some clinicians administer etoposide for 3–5 days, depending on the patient's hematologic tolerance.

Small Cell Lung Carcinoma

For the treatment of small cell lung carcinoma, the usual IV dosage of etoposide in combination chemotherapy regimens ranges from 35 mg/m² daily for 4 consecutive days to 50 mg/m² daily for 5 consecutive days, every 3–4 weeks. The recommended oral dosage of the drug is twice the IV dosage rounded to the nearest 50 mg.

Other Malignant Neoplasms

For the treatment of other malignant neoplasms†, the optimum dosage of etoposide remains to be clearly established. Various dosage schedules and regimens of etoposide, alone or in combination with other antineoplastic agents, have been used. While the dosage of etoposide employed for the treatment of other malignant neoplasms has generally been similar to that used for the treatment of refractory testicular neoplasms, dosage has varied widely. Some high-dose† IV etoposide regimens (e.g., 400–800 mg/m² daily for 3 consecutive days for 1 or 2 courses of therapy in conjunction with autogenous bone marrow transplantation for the treatment of various advanced malignant neoplasms) have been

investigated. Clinicians should consult published protocols for the dosage of etoposide and other chemotherapeutic agents and the method and sequence of administration.

For the treatment of Kaposi's sarcoma† in patients with AIDS, etoposide has been given in an IV dosage of 150 mg/m² daily for 3 consecutive days every 4 weeks, with cycles of therapy repeated as necessary depending on the patient's response and dosage reduced as necessary depending on the myelosuppressive effect of the drug.

● Dosage in Renal and Hepatic Impairment

The effects of renal or hepatic impairment on the elimination of etoposide have not been fully evaluated. Because a substantial fraction of the drug is excreted unchanged in urine, it is suggested that dosage reductions be considered in patients with impaired renal function. In patients with a measured creatinine clearance of greater than 50 mL/minute, no initial dose modification is required. In patients with a measured creatinine clearance of 15–50 mL/minute, 75% of the initial recommended etoposide dose should be administered. Although specific data are not available in patients with a measured creatinine clearance less than 15 mL/minute, further dose reduction should be considered. Subsequent etoposide dosing should be based on patient tolerance and clinical effect. Since etoposide-induced hematologic toxicity appeared to be more severe in patients with elevated serum bilirubin concentrations in one study and there is some evidence that total plasma clearance and elimination of the drug may be reduced in patients with impaired hepatic function, etoposide should probably be used with caution and the need for dosage reduction considered in patients with hepatic impairment.

CAUTIONS

Because etoposide phosphate is converted rapidly and completely in vivo to etoposide, the adverse effects associated with etoposide can be expected to occur with etoposide phosphate.

● Hematologic Effects

The major and dose-limiting adverse effect of etoposide is hematologic toxicity. Myelosuppression, which is dose related, is manifested mainly by leukopenia (principally granulocytopenia). Myelosuppression resulting in death has been reported in patients receiving etoposide. Thrombocytopenia occurs less frequently, and anemia may also occur; pancytopenia has occurred in some patients. Myelosuppression apparently is not cumulative but may be more severe in patients previously treated with other antineoplastic agents or radiation therapy. Leukopenia has reportedly occurred in 60–91% of patients receiving etoposide and was severe (leukocyte count less than 1000/mm³) in 3–17% of patients. Neutropenia (less than 2000/mm³) occurred in 88% of patients treated with etoposide phosphate; severe neutropenia (less than 500/mm³) occurred in 37% of patients treated. Thrombocytopenia has reportedly occurred in 22–41% of patients receiving the drug and was severe (platelet count less than 50,000/mm³) in 1–20% of patients. Anemia has occurred in up to 33% of patients receiving etoposide. Anemia (hemoglobin less than 11 g/dL) occurred in 72% of patients treated with etoposide phosphate; severe anemia (hemoglobin less than 8 g/dL) occurred in 19% of patients treated. Granulocyte and platelet nadirs usually occur within 7–14 and 9–16 days, respectively, after administration of etoposide, and within 12–19 and 10–15 days, respectively, after administration of etoposide phosphate; leukocyte nadir has been reported to occur within 15–22 days after administration of etoposide, phosphate. Bone marrow recovery is usually complete within 20 days after administration, but may occasionally require longer periods. Fever and infection have been reported in patients with drug-induced neutropenia.

● GI Effects

Nausea and vomiting are the principal adverse GI effects of etoposide, occurring in about 30–40% of patients receiving the drug. Etoposide-induced nausea and vomiting do not appear to be dose related and are usually mild to moderate in severity and readily controlled by conventional antiemetics. Nausea and vomiting have required discontinuance of the drug in about 1% of patients. There is some evidence that the incidence of nausea and vomiting may be reduced with 5-day continuous IV infusions of etoposide compared with intermittent IV administration.

Other adverse GI effects of etoposide include abdominal pain, anorexia, and diarrhea, which have occurred in up to 7%, about 10–16%, and about 1–13%

of patients, respectively. Stomatitis has reportedly occurred in about 1–6% of patients receiving usual dosages of etoposide and may be more likely to occur and/or be more severe in patients previously treated with radiation therapy to the head and neck region; in studies evaluating high-dose† etoposide regimens, stomatitis occurred more frequently and was found to be the dose-limiting adverse effect. Mucositis, constipation, and taste alteration have been reported in 11%, 8%, and 6%, respectively, of patients treated with etoposide phosphate. Aftertaste, dysphagia, and parotitis have also been reported rarely.

Adverse GI effects appear to occur slightly more frequently following oral administration of etoposide than following IV administration.

● Cardiovascular Effects

Transient hypotension has occurred in about 1–2% of patients following rapid IV administration of etoposide, but has not been associated with cardiotoxicity or ECG changes to date. Hypotension also has been reported following administration of etoposide phosphate solution. While delayed hypotension has not been reported with recommended doses and rates of administration, it has occurred following slow IV infusion of higher than recommended doses. Geriatric patients may be particularly susceptible to etoposide-induced hypotension. While etoposide does not consistently induce hypotension following rapid IV administration, to minimize the risk of this adverse effect, etoposide solutions should be infused slowly over a period of at least 30–60 minutes. If hypotension occurs during administration of etoposide or etoposide phosphate solutions, it usually subsides with discontinuance of the infusion and administration of IV fluids or other supportive therapy as necessary. In some patients, etoposide and etoposide phosphate have reportedly caused a transient increase in blood pressure. Blood pressure usually normalizes within a few hours after discontinuance of the infusion.

Etoposide has been associated with myocardial infarction or congestive heart failure in a small number of patients; however, these effects occurred almost exclusively in patients receiving etoposide by continuous IV infusion over 5 days, some of whom had preexisting cardiovascular disease, and were attributed to the large volumes of sodium chloride injection used as the diluent for administration of the drug.

● Sensitivity Reactions

Anaphylactoid reactions consisting principally of chills, rigors, diaphoresis, pruritus, loss of consciousness, nausea, vomiting, fever, bronchospasm, dyspnea, tachycardia, hypertension, and/or hypotension have occurred during or immediately after administration of etoposide or etoposide phosphate in 0.7–3% of patients receiving the drug. Other manifestations have included flushing, rash, substernal chest pain, lacrimation, sneezing, coryza, throat pain, back pain, generalized body pain, abdominal cramps, and auditory impairment. Anaphylactoid reactions have occurred during the initial infusion of etoposide in some patients. Facial/lingual swelling, coughing, diaphoresis, cyanosis, tightness in the throat, laryngospasm, back pain, and/or loss of consciousness have sometimes occurred in association with the above reactions in patients receiving etoposide. Rarely, an apparent hypersensitivity-associated apnea has been reported. Anaphylactoid reactions are usually controlled by discontinuance of the drug infusion and administration of vasopressors, corticosteroids, antihistamines, and/or plasma volume expanders as necessary; however, these reactions can be fatal. In one patient who had experienced several acute anaphylactoid reactions to the drug, prolonging the infusion over 4–6 hours prevented further occurrences of the reactions.

Bronchospasm with severe wheezing, responsive to antihistamine therapy, has been reported, and at least one fatal acute reaction associated with etoposide-induced bronchospasm has occurred. Acute pulmonary dysfunction, with or without hypertension, which may progress to pulmonary edema has also occurred.

● Dermatologic and Local Effects

Reversible alopecia, sometimes progressing to complete baldness, has occurred in 8–66% of patients receiving etoposide. The degree of alopecia may be dose related. Stevens-Johnson syndrome has been reported infrequently in patients receiving etoposide. Rash, pigmentation, urticaria, and severe pruritus have occurred infrequently, and cutaneous radiation-recall reactions associated with etoposide have been reported. At investigational doses, a generalized pruritic erythematous maculopapular rash, consistent with perivasculitis, has been reported. Localized herpes zoster infections have occurred in a few patients with AIDS during therapy with the drug.

Swelling of the forearm and upper arm with erythema was reported in one patient receiving an IV infusion of etoposide via a hand vein. Phlebitis has

occurred following IV administration of undiluted etoposide concentrate for injection, and local pain has occurred following rapid IV injection of the drug diluted with 0.9% sodium chloride injection to a final concentration of 10 mg/mL; these irritant effects may be related to the solubilizing agents in the drug's vehicle. While etoposide and its vehicle have been shown to produce ulceration in mice following intradermal injection, only one case of soft-tissue ulceration following extravasation of an etoposide infusion has been reported to date. In mice, local infiltration of 0.9% sodium chloride injection or hyaluronidase was an effective local antidote, probably by diluting the local tissue concentration of the drug.

● Nervous System Effects

Peripheral neuropathy has occurred in about 1–2% of patients receiving etoposide. Although not clearly established, it has been suggested that the risk and/or severity of peripheral neuropathy may be increased when etoposide is administered concurrently with other potentially neurotoxic agents (e.g., vincristine).

Adverse CNS effects, including somnolence and fatigue, have been reported to occur in up to 3% of patients receiving etoposide. Seizure, occasionally associated with allergic reactions, has been reported infrequently in patients receiving etoposide. Headache, transient cortical blindness, optic neuritis, and transient vertigo have been reported rarely. Transient mental confusion during administration of etoposide has been reported in a few patients receiving high-dose regimens of the drug; this effect appeared to be consistent with alcohol intoxication resulting from the large volume of the drug's vehicle necessary to administer the dose.

● Other Adverse Effects

Hepatotoxicity has been reported in patients receiving etoposide. Hepatic toxicity generally has occurred in those patients receiving doses of the drug higher than recommended. Metabolic acidosis also has been reported in patients receiving such doses of etoposide.

Interstitial pneumonitis or pulmonary fibrosis has been reported infrequently in patients receiving etoposide. Fever and intermittent muscle cramps have been reported rarely in patients receiving etoposide. Although a causal relationship has not been established, etoposide has been associated with increases in serum bilirubin (sometimes resulting in jaundice), AST (SGOT), and alkaline phosphatase concentrations; these effects were transient and resolved without sequelae and occurred almost exclusively in patients in studies evaluating high-dose† regimens of the drug. Transient compensated metabolic acidosis has also occurred in patients receiving high-dose† etoposide regimens and was presumably caused by the agents contained in the drug's vehicle.

● Precautions and Contraindications

Etoposide is a toxic drug with a low therapeutic index, and a therapeutic response is not likely to occur without evidence of toxicity. The drug must be used only under constant supervision by clinicians experienced in therapy with cytotoxic agents and only when the potential benefits of etoposide therapy are thought to outweigh the possible risks. Most adverse effects of etoposide are reversible if detected promptly. When severe adverse effects occur during etoposide therapy, the drug should be discontinued or dosage reduced and appropriate measures instituted as necessary. Etoposide therapy should be reinstituted with caution, with adequate consideration of further need for the drug and awareness of possible recurrence of toxicity.

Patients receiving etoposide should be observed closely for possible hypotensive or anaphylactoid reactions, and appropriate equipment for maintenance of an adequate airway and other supportive measures and agents for the treatment of these reactions should be readily available whenever etoposide is administered. Higher rates of anaphylactoid reactions have been reported in children who received etoposide infusions at concentrations higher than those recommended. The role that the concentration of the infusion (or rate of infusion) plays in the development of anaphylactoid reactions is uncertain. If hypotension occurs during administration of etoposide, it usually subsides with discontinuance of the infusion and administration of IV fluids or other supportive therapy as necessary. If an anaphylactoid reaction occurs during administration of the drug, the infusion should be discontinued and appropriate therapy (e.g., antihistamines, epinephrine, oxygen, corticosteroids) instituted as necessary. Etoposide and etoposide phosphate are contraindicated in patients who are hypersensitive to either etoposide or etoposide phosphate or any ingredient in the formulation.

Hematologic function must be frequently and carefully monitored during and after etoposide therapy. The manufacturer states that complete blood cell counts (leukocyte count with differential, platelet count, hemoglobin) should be performed prior to initiation of etoposide therapy, at appropriate intervals during the course of treatment (e.g., twice weekly), and before each subsequent course of treatment with the drug. The manufacturer also states that therapy should be suspended if the platelet count is less than 50,000/mm³ or the absolute neutrophil count is less than 500/mm³; when blood counts have returned to an acceptable level, therapy may be resumed if indicated. Severe myelosuppression with resulting infection or bleeding may occur in patients receiving the drug. Treatment of severe hematologic toxicity may consist of supportive therapy, antibiotics for complicating infections, and blood product transfusions.

● Pediatric Precautions

Safety and efficacy of etoposide in children have not been established. The drug has been used with encouraging results in children for the treatment of refractory acute myelogenous leukemia†, principally in combination chemotherapy regimens, and has shown some activity in the treatment of refractory acute lymphocytic leukemia† and other pediatric malignancies†, but additional evaluation is needed.

Higher rates of anaphylactoid reactions have been reported in children who received infusions of etoposide at higher-than-recommended concentrations. The role that the concentration or rate of infusion plays in the development of anaphylactoid reactions is uncertain.

Each mL of etoposide concentrate for injection and etoposide for injection pharmacy bulk package contains 30 mg of benzyl alcohol as a preservative. Although a causal relationship has not been established, administration of injections preserved with benzyl alcohol has been associated with toxicity in neonates. Toxicity appears to have resulted from administration of large amounts (i.e., 100–400 mg/kg daily) of benzyl alcohol in these neonates. Although use of drugs preserved with benzyl alcohol should be avoided in neonates whenever possible, the American Academy of Pediatrics states that the presence of small amounts of the preservative in a commercially available injection should not proscribe its use when indicated in neonates.

A complex, potentially fatal syndrome including thrombocytopenia, ascites, and renal, pulmonary, and hepatic failure has occurred in several premature infants who received IV therapy with an injectable vitamin E product containing polysorbate 80; etoposide injection contains polysorbate 80.

● Mutagenicity and Carcinogenicity

Etoposide is mutagenic and potentially carcinogenic; the occurrence of acute leukemia (with or without a preleukemic phase) has been reported rarely in patients receiving etoposide in association with other antineoplastic agents. Etoposide has been shown to induce chromosomal aberrations in embryonic murine cells and in human hematopoietic cell lines in vitro; gene mutations in Chinese hamster ovary cells; and DNA damage via strand breakage and DNA-protein crosslinks in mouse leukemia cells. The drug also caused a dose-related increase in sister chromatid exchanges in Chinese hamster ovary cells. Although etoposide phosphate was nonmutagenic in the in vitro Ames microbial mutagenicity assay and the *E. coli* WP2 uvrA reverse mutation assay, because it is rapidly and completely converted to etoposide in vivo, etoposide phosphate also should be considered as a potential mutagen.

Studies in animals to determine the carcinogenic potential of etoposide have not been performed to date; however, because of its mechanism of action, the drug should be considered a potential carcinogen.

● Pregnancy, Fertility, and Lactation

Pregnancy

Etoposide may cause fetal harm when administered to pregnant women, but potential benefits from use of the drug may be acceptable in certain conditions despite possible risks to the fetus. Etoposide has been shown to be teratogenic and embryocidal in mice and rats at doses of 1–5% of the recommended human dose based on body surface area. In rats, etoposide caused dose-related maternal toxicity, embryotoxicity, and teratogenicity with IV dosages of 0.4–3.6 mg/kg daily. Embryonic resorptions, decreased fetal weights, and fetal abnormalities including major skeletal anomalies, exencephaly, encephalocele, and anophthalmia, were observed; even at an IV dosage of 0.13 mg/kg daily, a substantial increase in retarded ossification occurred. In mice, intraperitoneal etoposide doses of 1–2 mg/kg caused dose-related embryotoxicity, cranial abnormalities, and major skeletal malformations. There are no adequate and controlled studies

to date using etoposide in pregnant women. Women of childbearing potential should be advised to avoid becoming pregnant while receiving the drug. Etoposide should be used during pregnancy only in life-threatening situations or severe disease for which safer drugs cannot be used or are ineffective. When the drug is administered during pregnancy or if the patient becomes pregnant while receiving the drug, the patient should be informed of the potential hazard to the fetus.

Fertility

The effect of etoposide on fertility in humans is not known. In rats, oral doses of etoposide phosphate at 86 mg (of etoposide) per kg daily (approximately 10 times the human dosage based on body surface area) or greater for 5 consecutive days resulted in irreversible testicular atrophy also was observed in rats given IV etoposide phosphate at a dosage of 5.11 mg (of etoposide) per kg daily for 30 days (approximately 50% the human dosage based on body surface area).

Lactation

It is not known whether etoposide is distributed into milk. Because of the potential for serious adverse reactions to etoposide in nursing infants, a decision should be made whether to discontinue nursing or the drug, taking into account the importance of the drug to the woman.

DRUG INTERACTIONS

● Antineoplastic Agents

Studies in animals and clinical trials in humans indicate that the antineoplastic activity of etoposide and cisplatin may be synergistic against some tumors. In mice implanted with P388 or L1210 leukemia or B16 melanoma, a combination of etoposide and cisplatin was shown to act synergistically in reducing the body burden of tumor cells and/or increasing survival. Response rates in humans receiving combination chemotherapy with etoposide and cisplatin suggest that the combination has synergistic antineoplastic activity against testicular carcinomas, small cell carcinoma of the lung, or non-small cell carcinoma of the lung. Studies in animals also indicate that the antineoplastic activity of etoposide and some other antineoplastic agents (e.g., carmustine, cytarabine, cyclophosphamide) is potentially additive or synergistic.

Limited data indicate that patients previously treated with cisplatin may have impaired elimination of etoposide. Although further documentation is needed, the potential effect should be considered when etoposide is administered to patients who received prior cisplatin therapy.

● Other Drugs

Caution should be exercised when administering etoposide phosphate with drugs that are known to inhibit phosphatase activity (e.g., levamisole hydrochloride).

High-dose cyclosporine administration, resulting in blood cyclosporine concentrations greater than 2000 ng/mL, with concomitant oral etoposide administration, resulted in an 80% increase in etoposide exposure with a 38% decrease in total body clearance of etoposide compared with etoposide alone.

PHARMACOLOGY

The exact mechanism(s) of action of etoposide is not known, but the drug appears to produce its cytotoxic effects by damaging DNA and thereby inhibiting or altering DNA synthesis. Although the in vitro cytotoxicity of etoposide phosphate is significantly less than that seen with etoposide, once the drug has undergone dephosphorylation in vivo to the active etoposide moiety, the mechanism of action is believed to be the same as that of etoposide. Etoposide appears to be cell-cycle dependent and cycle-phase specific, inducing G_2-phase arrest and preferentially killing cells in the G_2 and late S phases.

Etoposide has been shown to arrest metaphase in chick fibroblasts, but its principal effect in mammalian cells appears to be in the G_2 phase. At etoposide concentrations of 0.3–10 mcg/mL in vitro, cells are inhibited from entering prophase; at concentrations of 10 mcg/mL or higher, lysis of cells entering mitosis occurs. Unlike podophyllotoxin, etoposide does not inhibit microtubule assembly. Etoposide has been shown to induce single-stranded DNA breaks in HeLa cells and in murine leukemia L1210 cells in vitro; the drug also induces double-stranded DNA breaks and DNA-protein crosslinks in L1210 cells. Etoposide-induced DNA damage appears to correlate well with the cytotoxicity of the drug. While the exact mechanism remains to be determined, etoposide appears to induce single-stranded DNA breaks indirectly, possibly through endonuclease activation, inhibition of intranuclear type II topoisomerase, or formation of a free-radical metabolite via an enzymatic reaction involving the hydroxyl group at the C-4' position of the E ring. Etoposide also reversibly inhibits the facilitated diffusion of nucleosides into HeLa cells in a concentration-dependent manner in vitro; however, the relative importance of this effect to the cytotoxicity of the drug is unclear.

PHARMACOKINETICS

Although some minor differences in etoposide pharmacokinetic parameters between age and gender have been observed, these differences were not considered clinically important.

● Absorption

Etoposide is variably absorbed following oral administration. The extent of absorption of etoposide is not affected by food. Several oral dosage preparations of the drug have been evaluated. Lipophilic capsules containing etoposide were found to be erratically absorbed and produced dose-limiting adverse GI effects. An oral solution of the drug (known as the "drink ampul") was about 50–90% absorbed but was unpalatable. The absolute bioavailability of the currently available hydrophilic liquid-filled soft gelatin capsules containing the drug averages about 50% (range: 25–75%). Following oral administration of the commercially available capsules, peak plasma etoposide concentrations are generally attained within 1–1.5 hours (range: 0.75–4 hours) and peak plasma concentration and area under the plasma concentration-time curve (AUC) exhibit marked intraindividual and interindividual variation. However, peak plasma concentrations and AUCs for a given oral dose consistently fall in the same range as those following an IV dose one half as large. There is some evidence that the extent of absorption of etoposide does not increase proportionately with doses greater than 200 mg and may plateau at doses of 400 mg or more, but further studies are needed to evaluate the dose-bioavailability relationship of the drug. Following oral administration of 160 or 200 mg/m^2 as the commercially available capsules, peak plasma etoposide concentrations of 9 mcg/mL (range: 3–19 mcg/mL) and 9.6 mcg/mL (range: 2.1–15.9 mcg/mL), respectively, were attained. There is no evidence that the drug undergoes first-pass metabolism.

Following IV administration of etoposide phosphate, the drug is rapidly and completely converted to etoposide in plasma. A direct comparison of the pharmacokinetic parameters (area under the plasma concentration-time curve [AUC] and maximum plasma concentration) of etoposide following IV administration of molar equivalent doses of etoposide phosphate and etoposide was made in 2 randomized, crossover studies in patients with a variety of malignancies. Results from both studies demonstrated no statistically significant differences in the AUC and maximum plasma concentration of etoposide when administered as either etoposide phosphate or etoposide. Therefore, the pharmacokinetic data reported for etoposide apply also to etoposide phosphate.

Peak plasma concentrations and AUCs following IV administration of etoposide exhibit marked interindividual variation, but possibly less intraindividual variation than after oral administration. Over the dose range of 100–600 mg/m^2, peak plasma concentration and AUC increase linearly with dose. Following IV infusion of an 80-mg/m^2 dose of etoposide over 1 hour in adults with normal renal and hepatic function, peak plasma drug concentrations occurred at the end of the infusion and averaged 14.9 mcg/mL (range: 7.8–19.3 mcg/mL). Following 500-mg/hour IV infusions of 400, 500, or 600 mg/m^2 in adults with normal renal function in one study, peak plasma etoposide concentrations of 26–53, 27–73, and 42–114 mcg/mL, respectively, were attained. When etoposide was administered as a 72-hour continuous IV infusion in a dosage of 100 mg/m^2 daily in several patients with normal renal and hepatic function, plasma drug concentrations of about 2–5 mcg/mL were attained 2–3 hours after beginning the infusion and were maintained until the end of the infusion. In a limited number of children 3 months to 16 years of age with normal renal and hepatic function who were given IV infusions of 200–250 mg/m^2 over 0.5–2.25 hours, peak serum etoposide concentrations ranged from 17–88 mcg/mL.

● Distribution

Distribution of etoposide into human body tissues and fluids has not been fully characterized. Following IV administration of etoposide in mice and rats, highest concentrations of the drug are attained in the small intestine, kidneys, and liver, with lower concentrations in the lungs, stomach, pancreas, spleen, heart, and skin.

Following IV administration in humans, etoposide undergoes rapid distribution. The apparent steady-state volume of distribution of the drug averages 20–28% of body weight or 18–29 L or 7–17 L/m^2 in adults and 5–10 L/m^2 in children. The major metabolite of etoposide appears to be distributed into a volume approximately equal to total body water. Following IV administration, etoposide is distributed minimally into pleural fluid and has been detected in the saliva, liver, spleen, kidney, myometrium, healthy brain tissue, and brain tumor tissue. Limited data suggest that distribution of the drug into bile is minimal. It is not known if etoposide is distributed into milk. The drug apparently crosses the placenta in animals.

Etoposide and its metabolites apparently do not readily penetrate the CNS. While variable, CSF etoposide concentrations generally range from undetectable to less than 5% of concurrent plasma concentrations during the initial 24 hours after IV administration of the drug, even after administration of very high doses. Limited data suggest that etoposide distributes into brain tumor tissue more readily than into healthy brain tissue. Concentrations of the drug are higher in healthy lung tissue than in lung metastases but those achieved in primary myometrial tumors are similar to those achieved in healthy myometrial tissues.

In vitro, etoposide is approximately 94% bound to serum proteins at a concentration of 10 mcg/mL.

● Elimination

Following IV infusion of etoposide, plasma concentrations of the drug have generally been reported to decline in a biphasic manner; however, some data indicate that the drug may exhibit triphasic elimination with a prolonged terminal phase. In adults with normal renal and hepatic function, the half-life of etoposide averages 0.6–2 hours (range: 0.2–2.5 hours) in the initial phase and 5.3–10.8 hours (range: 2.9–19 hours) in the terminal phase. In one adult with impaired hepatic function, the terminal elimination half-life was reportedly 78 hours. In children with normal renal and hepatic function, the half-life of etoposide averages 0.6–1.4 hours in the initial phase and 3–5.8 hours in the terminal phase.

The metabolic fate of etoposide has not been completely determined. Etoposide appears to be metabolized principally at the D ring to produce the resulting hydroxy acid (probably the trans-hydroxy acid); this metabolite appears to be pharmacologically inactive. The picrolactone isomer of etoposide has been detected in low concentrations in the plasma and urine of some patients but not in others. The aglycone of etoposide and/or its conjugates have not been detected to date in patients receiving the drug. In vitro, the picrolactone isomer and aglycone of etoposide have minimal cytotoxic activity.

Metabolism and excretion of etoposide appear to be similar following oral or IV administration of the drug. Etoposide and its metabolites are excreted principally in urine; fecal excretion of the drug is variable. Following IV infusion of etoposide in patients with normal renal and hepatic function, approximately 40–60% of a dose is excreted in urine as unchanged drug and metabolites within 48–72 hours and from less than 2 to 16% is excreted in feces within 72 hours; about 20–30% of the dose is excreted in urine unchanged within 24 hours and 30–45% within 48 hours. The principal urinary metabolite is the hydroxy acid of the drug. Following oral administration in patients with normal renal and hepatic function, about 5–25% of the dose is excreted in urine within 24–48 hours.

Total plasma clearance of etoposide reportedly averages 19–28 mL/minute per m^2 in adults and 18–39 mL/minute per ^{2} in children with normal renal and hepatic function; renal clearance of the drug is approximately 30–40% of the total plasma clearance. The effects of renal impairment on the elimination of the drug and its metabolites have not been fully evaluated; individuals with decreased renal function may have impaired elimination. Patients with impaired renal function receiving etoposide have exhibited reduced total body clearance, increased AUC, and a lower volume of distribution at steady state. Limited evidence suggests that total plasma clearance and elimination of etoposide may be reduced in patients with impaired hepatic function.

Limited data suggest that etoposide is not appreciably dialyzable.

CHEMISTRY AND STABILITY

● Chemistry

Etoposide is a semisynthetic podophyllotoxin-derivative antineoplastic agent. Etoposide differs structurally from podophyllotoxin by having a glucoside moiety and the epimeric configuration at the C-4 position of the C ring and by the presence of a hydroxyl group, rather than a methoxy group, at the C-4' position of the E ring. The presence of the hydroxyl group at the C-4' position is associated with the drug's ability to induce single-stranded DNA breaks, and the presence of the glucoside moiety is associated with the drug's inability to inhibit microtubule assembly. Etoposide also is commercially available as etoposide phosphate, a water-soluble ester; this chemical modification decreases the potential for precipitation following dilution of the drug in aqueous solution, while maintaining pharmacologic activity in vivo. Etoposide phosphate undergoes dephosphorylation in vivo to etoposide, the active moiety. Each single-dose vial of etoposide phosphate contains 100 mg of etoposide, equivalent to 113.6 mg of etoposide phosphate.

Etoposide occurs as a white to yellow-brown crystalline powder and is sparingly soluble in water (approximately 0.03 mg/mL) and slightly soluble in alcohol (approximately 0.76 mg/mL); the water miscibility of the drug is increased by the presence of organic solvents. Etoposide phosphate occurs as a white to off-white crystalline powder and is freely soluble in water (exceeding 100 mg/mL) and slightly soluble in alcohol. Etoposide concentrate for injection is a sterile, nonaqueous solution of the drug in a vehicle consisting of dehydrated alcohol, benzyl alcohol, citric acid, polyethylene glycol 300, and polysorbate (Tween®) 80. Etoposide phosphate for injection is a sterile, nonpyrogenic, lyophilized powder containing sodium citrate and dextran 40; following reconstitution of etoposide phosphate with water for injection to a concentration of 1 mg/mL, the solution has a pH of 2.9. The concentrate for injection occurs as a clear, yellow solution and has a pH of 3–4. Etoposide is also commercially available as soft gelatin capsules containing the drug in a vehicle consisting of citric acid, glycerin, purified water, and polyethylene glycol 400; the soft gelatin capsules contain gelatin, glycerin, sorbitol, purified water, and parabens.

● **Stability**

Etoposide concentrate for injection should be stored at room temperature. Unopened vials of the drug are stable for 2 years when stored at room temperature (25°C). Etoposide phosphate powder for injection should be stored in unopened vials at 2–8°C and retained in the original package to protect from light; such unopened vials of the drug are stable at least 36 months when refrigerated at 2–8°C. Etoposide liquid-filled capsules should be refrigerated at 2–8°C. The capsules are stable for 2 years when refrigerated at 2–8°C.

Etoposide concentrate for injection must be diluted before administration. The manufacturer states that, following dilution in 0.9% sodium chloride or 5% dextrose injection, etoposide solutions containing 0.2 or 0.4 mg/mL are stable for 96 or 24 hours, respectively, at room temperature (25°C) in glass or plastic (PVC) containers under exposure to normal room fluorescent light; following dilution in lactated Ringer's or 10% mannitol injection, solutions of the drug containing 0.2 or 0.4 mg/mL are stable for 8 hours at 25°C in glass containers under exposure to normal room fluorescent light. Because etoposide is sparingly soluble in water, the drug may crystallize following dilution in the above diluents; if crystallization occurs, the solution should be discarded. Crystallization of etoposide in aqueous solutions appears to be concentration dependent. At a concentration of 1 mg/mL in 0.9% sodium chloride or 5% dextrose injection, crystallization has occurred within 5 minutes upon stirring the solution or within 30 minutes upon allowing the solution to stand; therefore, this concentration is *not* recommended for IV administration. If solutions of etoposide are prepared at concentrations above

0.4 mg/mL, precipitation may occur, and the manufacturer recommends that the concentration not exceed 0.4 mg/mL.

Etoposide solutions containing 0.1–0.4 mg/mL in 0.9% sodium chloride or 5% dextrose injection have been filtered through several commercially available filters (e.g., 0.22-μm Millex®-GS or Millex®-GV) without filter decomposition.

Plastic devices composed of acrylic or ABS (a polymer composed of acrylonitrile, butadiene, and styrene) have been reported to crack and leak when used with undiluted etoposide injection.

When reconstituted and/or diluted as directed, solutions of etoposide phosphate can be stored in glass or plastic containers at controlled room temperature (20–25°C) or under refrigeration (2–8°C) for 24 hours. Refrigerated solutions of etoposide phosphate should be used immediately following return to room temperature.

For further information on the handling of antineoplastic agents, see the ASHP Guidelines on Handling Hazardous Drugs at http://www.ahfsdrug finformation.com.

PREPARATIONS

Excipients in commercially available drug preparations may have clinically important effects in some individuals; consult specific product labeling for details.

Etoposide

Oral		
Capsules, liquid-filled	50 mg	**Etoposide Capsules**
		VePesid®, Bristol-Myers Squibb

Parenteral		
For injection concentrate, for IV infusion only	20 mg/mL (100, 150, 200, 250, and 500 mg)*	**Etoposide for Injection**
		Toposar®, Pfizer
		VePesid®, Bristol-Myers Squibb
	20 mg/mL (1 g) pharmacy bulk package*	**Etoposide for Injection**
		VePesid®, Bristol-Myers Squibb

* available from one or more manufacturer, distributor, and/or repackager by generic (nonproprietary) name

Etoposide Phosphate

Parenteral		
For injection	500 mg (of etoposide) pharmacy bulk package	**Etopophos®**, Bristol-Myers Squibb
	1 g (of etoposide) pharmacy bulk package	**Etopophos®**, Bristol-Myers Squibb
For injection, for IV infusion	100 mg (of etoposide)	**Etopophos®**, Bristol-Myers Squibb

† Use is not currently included in the labeling approved by the US Food and Drug Administration.

Selected Revisions January 1, 2009, © Copyright, July 1, 1984, American Society of Health-System Pharmacists, Inc.

Fluorouracil

10:00 • ANTINEOPLASTIC AGENTS

■ Fluorouracil, a pyrimidine antagonist, is an antimetabolite antineoplastic agent.

USES

Fluorouracil is used for the treatment of adenocarcinoma of the colon, rectum, breast, stomach, and pancreas. The drug also is used as an adjunct to surgery for the treatment of various solid tumors (e.g., adenocarcinoma of the colon, rectal carcinoma, breast cancer).

● GI Cancers

Combination Therapies for Colorectal Cancer

Leucovorin calcium and levoleucovorin calcium are used to potentiate the antineoplastic activity of, and thus improve response to, fluorouracil in the treatment of colorectal carcinoma. Fluorouracil is used in combination with leucovorin or levoleucovorin in an attempt to prolong survival relative to fluorouracil alone in patients with advanced disease. In vitro studies and clinical evidence have shown that the cytotoxicity of fluorouracil may be enhanced by reduced folates (e.g., leucovorin, levoleucovorin); it appears that elevated intracellular concentrations of reduced folates may stabilize the covalent ternary complex formed by fluorodeoxyuridylic acid, 5,10-methylenetetrahydrofolate, and thymidylate synthase, enhancing inhibition of this enzyme and thereby increasing the efficacy of fluorouracil. Leucovorin and levoleucovorin also may potentiate the risk of fluorouracil-induced toxicity (especially GI toxicity, including diarrhea, nausea, stomatitis, and vomiting, and, to a lesser degree, myelosuppression). (See Cautions: GI Effects.)

Combined therapy with fluorouracil and leucovorin or levoleucovorin with or without additional antineoplastic agents (e.g., oxaliplatin, irinotecan hydrochloride) has been evaluated in patients with advanced colorectal cancer in the adjuvant and metastatic settings.

Approximately monthly combination regimens of fluorouracil and leucovorin studied in the North Central Cancer Treatment Group (Mayo/NCCTG) adjuvant study included 5-day courses of IV fluorouracil 370 mg/m² plus IV leucovorin 200 mg/m² daily or fluorouracil 425 mg/m² plus leucovorin 20 mg/m² daily; both regimens were repeated at 4- to 5-week intervals. A commonly used regimen that is administered on a weekly schedule (often referred to as the high-dose leucovorin or Roswell Park regimen), consists of fluorouracil 500 mg/m² and leucovorin 500 mg/m² both given IV once weekly for 6 consecutive weeks. Results from the Intergroup 0089 study have demonstrated equal efficacy between the low-dose (monthly or Mayo Clinic schedule) and the high-dose (weekly or Roswell Park schedule) leucovorin regimens; however, because of ease of use and less toxicity, the high-dose regimen is considered a preferred regimen in the adjuvant setting.

A combination regimen of fluorouracil and leucovorin also has been evaluated as adjuvant treatment of colorectal cancer as a bimonthly continuous IV infusion (i.e., the LV5FU2 or deGramont regimen). The use of this regimen has been shown to be safer compared with the use of a direct IV injection ("bolus") regimen of fluorouracil and leucovorin. A simplified version of the LV5FU2 regimen also has been evaluated.

Although combined therapy with fluorouracil and leucovorin or levoleucovorin has historically been considered the standard of care in the adjuvant or metastatic setting, use of a doublet regimen (i.e., fluorouracil, oxaliplatin, and leucovorin or levoleucovorin [FOLFOX]; fluorouracil, irinotecan, and leucovorin or levoleucovorin [FOLFIRI]; capecitabine and oxaliplatin [CapeOx; CapOx]) is the current standard of care for the adjuvant or palliative treatment of advanced colorectal cancer based on data from randomized controlled trials demonstrating improved response and prolonged survival in such patients.

Use of fluorouracil in combination with oxaliplatin and leucovorin as adjuvant therapy for stage III colon cancer is based principally on evidence of improved disease-free and overall survival from a multicenter, open-label, randomized study (Multicenter International Study of Oxaliplatin/5-Fluorouracil/Leucovorin in the Adjuvant Treatment of Colon Cancer [MOSAIC]) in 2246 patients with stage II or III colon cancer who had undergone complete resection of the primary tumor. Eligible patients were randomized to receive a 2-day combination regimen of oxaliplatin, fluorouracil, and leucovorin (leucovorin 200 mg/m² administered by IV infusion over 2 hours, followed by fluorouracil 400 mg/m² administered by IV injection and fluorouracil 600 mg/m² administered by IV infusion over 22 hours, administered for 2 consecutive days; oxaliplatin 85 mg/m² was administered by IV infusion over 2 hours concurrently with leucovorin on the first day only) or a 2-day combination regimen of fluorouracil and leucovorin (leucovorin 200 mg/m² administered by IV infusion over 2 hours, followed by fluorouracil 400 mg/m² administered by IV injection and fluorouracil 600 mg/m² administered by IV infusion over 22 hours). Treatment with both regimens was repeated at intervals of 2 weeks for a total of 12 cycles. Among patients with stage III colon cancer, treatment with the oxaliplatin/fluorouracil/leucovorin regimen was associated with higher rates of disease-free survival at 5 years and overall survival at 6 years (66 and 73%, respectively) compared with the fluorouracil/leucovorin regimen (59 and 69%, respectively). At a median follow-up of 9.5 years, the disease-free and overall survival benefit of oxaliplatin/fluorouracil/leucovorin in patients with stage III colon cancer was maintained (10-year disease-free and overall survival rates of 62 and 67%, respectively, with oxaliplatin/fluorouracil/leucovorin compared with 54 and 59%, respectively, with fluorouracil/leucovorin). Among patients with stage II disease, the oxaliplatin/fluorouracil/leucovorin regimen was associated with similar 5-year disease-free survival and 6-year overall survival as compared with the fluorouracil/leucovorin regimen. Disease-free and overall survival rates at 10 years also failed to show a benefit for oxaliplatin/fluorouracil/leucovorin compared with fluorouracil/leucovorin in patients with stage II disease. Grade 3 and 4 hematologic toxicity (neutropenia, thrombocytopenia, anemia) occurred more commonly with oxaliplatin/fluorouracil/leucovorin than with fluorouracil/leucovorin, although the incidence of febrile neutropenia was low with both regimens. Grade 3 and 4 GI toxicity (nausea, vomiting, diarrhea) also occurred more commonly with oxaliplatin/fluorouracil/leucovorin. Peripheral sensory neuropathy was reported in 92% of patients receiving oxaliplatin/fluorouracil/leucovorin compared with 16% of those receiving fluorouracil/leucovorin.

Because the duration and severity of peripheral neuropathy appear to increase with increasing cumulative dosage of oxaliplatin, the International Duration Evaluation of Adjuvant Chemotherapy (IDEA) collaboration pooled data from 6 similarly designed prospective, randomized, controlled phase 3 studies (Cancer and Leukemia Group B/Southwest Oncology Group [CALGB/SWOG] study 80702, Short Course Oncology Treatment [SCOT], Adjuvant Chemotherapy for Colon Cancer with High Evidence [ACHIEVE], Three or Six Colon Adjuvant [TOSCA], Hellenic Oncology Research Group [HORG], IDEA France) to evaluate noninferiority of a shortened duration (i.e., 3 months) of adjuvant fluoropyrimidine-oxaliplatin doublet therapy compared to the standard duration of 6 months in patients with stage II or III colon cancer. In this pooled analysis, 12,834 patients with stage III colon cancer received fluoropyrimidine-oxaliplatin doublet therapy with FOLFOX (i.e., FOLFOX4, modified FOLFOX6) or capecitabine in combination with oxaliplatin for 3 or 6 months. At the time of the initial analysis (median follow-up of 41.8 months), 3 months of fluoropyrimidine-oxaliplatin doublet therapy did not meet the noninferiority criterion for 3-year disease-free survival when compared to a duration of 6 months (74.6 versus 75.5%, respectively; hazard ratio of 1.07). In a preplanned subgroup analysis based on treatment regimen, FOLFOX for a duration of 6 months was superior to a treatment duration of 3 months with an absolute difference in 3-year disease-free survival of 2.4% for patients with stage III disease. Subgroup analysis based on risk of recurrence suggested that a duration of 3 months of fluoropyrimidine-oxaliplatin doublet therapy was at least equivalent to a duration of 6 months of therapy in patients with low-risk disease (stage T1–T3 and N1) (hazard ratio of 1.01, which corresponded to an absolute difference in disease-free survival of 0.2% at 3 years); however, a duration of 6 months of therapy was superior to a duration of 3 months in patients with high-risk disease (stage T4 disease and/or N2) (hazard ratio of 1.12, which corresponded to an absolute difference in disease-free survival of 1.7% at 3 years). In patients with low-risk disease receiving FOLFOX, a duration of 3 months did not meet the noninferiority criterion for 3-year disease-free survival when compared to a duration of 6 months; however, in patients with high-risk disease, a duration of 6 months of therapy appeared to be superior to a duration of 3 months (hazard ratio of 1.2). At the time of the final analysis, fluoropyrimidine-oxaliplatin doublet therapy for a duration of 3 months did not meet noninferiority criteria for 5-year disease-free survival (hazard ratio of 1.08) or overall survival (hazard ratio of 1.02) when compared to a duration of 6 months; however, in patients receiving FOLFOX, a duration of 6 months of therapy demonstrated superiority for 5-year disease-free survival (hazard ratio of 1.16), but not for overall survival (hazard ratio of 1.07), compared to a duration of 3 months of therapy. The incidence of grade 3 or 4 neurosensory toxicity was substantially lower in patients receiving 3 months of fluoropyrimidine-oxaliplatin doublet therapy compared with those receiving 6 months of therapy (2.5–2.6 versus 8.9–15.9%, respectively). Although the standard duration of adjuvant fluoropyrimidine-oxaliplatin doublet therapy has been 6 months, a shorter duration of therapy may be considered in certain patients based on these data. Some clinicians state that factors that should be considered when selecting the duration of adjuvant fluoropyrimidine-oxaliplatin doublet therapy include tolerability, patient preference, patient characteristics, preexisting conditions, and other factors.

In a randomized phase 3 study (Gruppo Oncologico Dell'Italia Meridionale) comparing irinotecan, fluorouracil, and leucovorin combination therapy (FOLFIRI) and oxaliplatin, fluorouracil, and leucovorin combination therapy (FOLFOX4) in patients with previously untreated locally advanced or metastatic colorectal cancer, no substantial difference in overall response rate, time to progression, or overall survival was observed between the treatment groups. Efficacy also was similar in another phase 3 study (Groupe Coopérateur Multidisciplinaire en Oncologie [GERCOR]) comparing FOLFIRI followed by FOLFOX6 or the reverse sequence in patients with previously untreated metastatic colorectal cancer. In these studies, mucositis, nausea/vomiting, and alopecia occurred more frequently in patients receiving FOLFIRI, whereas thrombocytopenia and neurosensory toxicity occurred more frequently in patients receiving FOLFOX.

Combined therapy with fluorouracil with leucovorin, oxaliplatin, and irinotecan (FOLFOXIRI) also has been used in patients with metastatic colorectal cancer. In a randomized clinical study (Gastrointestinal Committee of the Hellenic Oncology Research Group [HORG] study) comparing FOLFOXIRI and FOLFIRI, no substantial difference in overall response rate, time to progression, or overall survival was observed between the treatment groups; however, in another randomized clinical study (Gruppo Oncologico Nord Ovest [GONO]), progression-free survival and overall survival were substantially prolonged in patients receiving FOLFOXIRI compared with those receiving FOLFIRI. In these studies, alopecia, diarrhea, neurosensory toxicity, and neutropenia occurred more frequently in patients receiving FOLFOXIRI.

Fluorouracil also has been used in combination with IV levoleucovorin given at one-half the usual dosage of leucovorin. Results from a comparative study demonstrated no substantial differences in response or tolerability between levoleucovorin and leucovorin when used in conjunction with fluorouracil for the palliative treatment of advanced colorectal cancer.

IV fluorouracil also has been used in combination with orally administered leucovorin in a limited number of patients with advanced colorectal cancer.

Monotherapy of Colorectal Cancer

Fluorouracil has been administered as monotherapy of advanced colorectal cancer in various disease regimens. However, these regimens have been replaced by the use of fluorouracil and leucovorin combination regimens in the adjuvant setting for patients with stage III disease.

Hepatic Metastases

Fluorouracil also has been studied as a form of regional adjuvant therapy (e.g., portal vein or hepatic artery infusion) of liver metastases associated with colon cancer†; however, the potential role of this drug in this setting remains to be more fully elucidated.

● Breast Cancer

Outcome may be improved when fluorouracil is used as an adjunct to surgery in certain women with breast cancer. Combination chemotherapy (e.g., cyclophosphamide, methotrexate, and fluorouracil [CMF]) used as an adjunct to surgery has been shown to increase both disease-free (i.e., decreased recurrence) and overall survival in premenopausal and postmenopausal women with node-negative or -positive early (TNM stage I or II) breast cancer. Adjuvant therapy with such combination chemotherapy in both premenopausal and postmenopausal women has been associated with prolongation of disease-free survival and reduction of local, regional, and distant metastases, with tolerable adverse effects.

In patients with hormone receptor-positive early-stage breast cancer, the American Society of Clinical Oncology (ASCO) and other experts state that the decision regarding use of adjuvant endocrine therapy with or without sequential combination chemotherapy may be guided by prognostic tools, such as the recurrence score based on 21-gene assay results, to predict the absolute benefits of

combination chemotherapy in addition to adjuvant endocrine therapy. In patients with node-negative disease, use of adjuvant endocrine therapy with or without sequential combination chemotherapy should be individualized based on consideration of the risk of recurrent disease without such adjuvant therapy, the expected reduction in risk of recurrence and improvement in quality of life with such adjuvant therapy, and the potential adverse effects of such therapy. Some experts state that adjuvant endocrine therapy with sequential chemotherapy may be considered in patients with early-stage, hormone receptor-positive, human epidermal growth factor receptor type 2 (HER2)-negative, node-negative breast cancer whose tumors have recurrence scores greater than 30 based on 21-gene assay results and in those who are 50 years of age or younger with recurrence scores of 16–25. Patients with hormone receptor-positive, HER2-negative, node-negative breast cancer and poor prognosis may be suitable candidates for adjuvant chemotherapy. Although patients with early-stage hormone receptor-positive breast cancer whose tumors have low recurrence scores and limited to no nodal involvement have a favorable prognosis with or without chemotherapy, pooled analysis of a large number of randomized studies and other evidence have shown that effective adjuvant combination chemotherapy can increase both disease-free and overall survival in patients with node-negative disease, albeit less markedly than in those with node-positive disease.

In patients with node-positive early breast cancer, an effective regimen of adjuvant combination chemotherapy (e.g., CMF; cyclophosphamide, doxorubicin, and fluorouracil; cyclophosphamide and doxorubicin with or without tamoxifen) is used to reduce the rate of recurrence and improve survival in both premenopausal and postmenopausal patients once treatment to control local disease (surgery, with or without radiation therapy) has been undertaken. These combinations have demonstrated superiority compared to single-agent therapy with conventional agents. Although long-term (e.g., 6 months or longer) chemotherapy with adjuvant regimens is clinically superior to short-term (e.g., preoperative and perioperative) adjuvant regimens, clinical superiority between 6- versus 12-month regimens has not been demonstrated. The dose intensity of adjuvant combination chemotherapy also appears to be an important factor influencing clinical outcome in patients with early node-positive breast cancer, with response increasing with increasing dose intensity; therefore, arbitrary reductions in dose intensity should be avoided. In a pooled analysis of 14 randomized controlled trials involving 5600 women with early-stage breast cancer and a high risk of recurrence (involvement of multiple local lymph nodes) receiving high-dose chemotherapy followed by autologous transplantation (bone marrow or stem cell) or conventional chemotherapy without autologous transplantation, high-dose chemotherapy followed by autologous transplantation was associated with an increased risk of treatment-related mortality and little or no increase in survival.

Fluorouracil also is used in the treatment of more advanced forms of breast cancer, including inoperable cancer. In stage III (locally advanced) breast cancer, combination chemotherapy (with or without hormonal therapy) is used sequentially following surgery and radiation therapy for operable disease and following biopsy and radiation therapy for inoperable disease; commonly employed effective regimens include cyclophosphamide, methotrexate, and fluorouracil; cyclophosphamide, doxorubicin, and fluorouracil; and cyclophosphamide, methotrexate, fluorouracil, and prednisone. These and other regimens also have been used in the treatment or more advanced (stage IV) and recurrent disease.

Fluorouracil alone has been reported to cause temporary objective remissions in patients with metastatic breast cancer; approximately 10–35% of patients respond. Response is improved in patients with metastatic disease when fluorouracil is used in combination with other antineoplastic agents. While continuous maintenance combination chemotherapy that included fluorouracil has been shown to delay disease progression after initial response or stabilization with induction therapy in women with metastatic disease and may improve quality of life, continuous maintenance therapy has not been shown to prolong overall survival compared with intermittent reinduction therapy that is initiated at the time of progression.

● Esophageal Cancer

Fluorouracil has been used alone and in combination therapy for the treatment of localized or advanced esophageal cancer†.

For the treatment of localized esophageal cancer, combined modality treatment consisting of combination chemotherapy with fluorouracil and cisplatin and concurrent radiation therapy may be used prior to surgery (as neoadjuvant therapy) or as an alternative to surgery (i.e., in patients who are not considered suitable surgical candidates or in an attempt to avoid perioperative mortality [less than 10%] and to relieve dysphagia). Combined modality therapy consisting of combination chemotherapy with fluorouracil and cisplatin and concurrent radiation therapy is more effective than radiation therapy alone in patients with localized esophageal carcinoma. Although the comparative benefit of combined chemotherapy and radiation versus surgery has not been established, some experts recommend combined modality treatment with combination chemotherapy (e.g., fluorouracil and cisplatin) and concurrent radiation therapy with or without surgery as primary treatment for localized, resectable esophageal cancer. (See Uses: Esophageal Cancer, in Cisplatin 10:00.)

For the palliative treatment of metastatic (local or distant) disease or recurrent or locally advanced esophageal disease that is not amenable to surgery or radiation therapy, fluorouracil is used in combination chemotherapy with cisplatin, and such combined therapy is considered a regimen of choice.

● **Head and Neck Cancer**

Fluorouracil has been used in combination chemotherapy for the treatment of metastatic or recurrent squamous cell carcinoma of the head and neck†. Fluorouracil alone produces poor response rates (13–15%) in patients with advanced head or neck cancer; however, fluorouracil has a synergistic antitumor effect when used in combination with cisplatin. Combination chemotherapy with fluorouracil and cisplatin is commonly used for the palliative treatment of recurrent or metastatic head and neck cancer. (See Uses: Head and Neck Cancer in Cisplatin 10:00.)

Chemotherapy also has been administered in combination with radiation therapy for the palliative treatment of head and neck cancer in patients with locally advanced disease that is unresectable. Combination chemotherapy with fluorouracil and cisplatin administered in rapidly alternating sequence with radiation therapy has been shown to prevent local recurrence of tumor and prolong survival compared with radiation therapy alone in patients with unresectable locally advanced head and neck cancer. The use of chemotherapy combined with radiation therapy also is being investigated for larynx preservation; in 2 large randomized trials, patients receiving induction chemotherapy with fluorouracil and cisplatin followed by radiation therapy had similar survival rates as patients receiving laryngectomy and radiation therapy for locally advanced laryngeal or hypopharyngeal cancer. Induction chemotherapy with fluorouracil, cisplatin, and docetaxel also has been used prior to radiotherapy or chemoradiotherapy for the treatment of locally advanced squamous cell carcinoma of the head and neck. (See Uses: Head and Neck Cancer, in Docetaxel 10:00.)

● **Cervical Cancer**

Fluorouracil in combination with cisplatin has been used concurrently with radiation therapy for the treatment of invasive cervical cancer†. Fluorouracil also has been used in the treatment of metastatic or recurrent cervical cancer†. (See Uses: Cervical Cancer in Cisplatin 10:00 for an overview of therapy for cervical cancer.)

Concurrent Chemotherapy and Radiation Therapy for Invasive Cervical Cancer

Fluorouracil is used in combination with cisplatin for concurrent chemotherapy and radiation therapy in patients with invasive cervical cancer (FIGO stages IB2 through IVA cervical cancer or FIGO stage IA2, IB, or IIA cervical cancer with poor prognostic factors, such as metastatic disease in pelvic lymph nodes, parametrial disease, or positive surgical margins, identified at the time of primary surgery), but randomized controlled studies are needed to determine if this combination regimen is superior to cisplatin alone. Results from one randomized trial suggest that cisplatin alone is as effective but less toxic than cisplatin-containing combination regimens for concomitant use with radiation therapy for the treatment of locally advanced cervical cancer.

Chemotherapy for Metastatic or Recurrent Cervical Cancer

Response rates of about 10–20% have been reported with the use of fluorouracil alone or with leucovorin in advanced cervical cancer†. An overall response rate of 14% was observed in a small uncontrolled phase II study of patients receiving fluorouracil and leucovorin for recurrent adenocarcinoma of the cervix. The benefit of combination therapy with fluorouracil and cisplatin compared with cisplatin alone for metastatic or recurrent cervical cancer has not been established. Fluorouracil also has been used concurrently with radiation therapy for the treatment of recurrent pelvic disease following radical surgery for invasive cervical cancer. Further study is needed to define the role of fluorouracil in the treatment of advanced cervical cancer.

● **Renal Cell Carcinoma**

Fluorouracil has been used alone or in combination regimens for the treatment of metastatic renal cell carcinoma†. Fluorouracil alone has minimal activity in the treatment of metastatic renal cell carcinoma with response rates of about 5–7% in phase II studies. Fluorouracil also has been used in combination with aldesleukin and/or interferon alfa for the treatment of metastatic renal cell carcinoma. Because of variable efficacy and/or greater toxicity reported with such regimens, further study is required to establish the role of fluorouracil in combination therapy for the treatment of metastatic renal cell carcinoma. (See discussion of fluorouracil in combination regimens in Uses: Renal Cell Carcinoma in Aldesleukin 10:00 and Interferon Alfa 10:00.)

● **Other Uses**

Fluorouracil has been used as second-line therapy in the treatment of ovarian epithelial cancer†, including platinum-refractory disease. Fluorouracil also is used in the treatment of carcinoid tumors† and cancers of the liver† and biliary tract†. The optimal effectiveness and sequence of combination therapy of fluorouracil with other antineoplastic agents or with irradiation requires further investigation, and it should be kept in mind that any form of therapy that adds to the stress of the patient, interferes with nutrition, or depresses bone marrow function will increase fluorouracil toxicity.

For the use of fluorouracil in the treatment of actinic keratosis, see 84:92.

DOSAGE AND ADMINISTRATION

● **Administration**

Fluorouracil is administered IV. Care should be taken to avoid extravasation of the drug. The usual injection formulation need not be further diluted. The 2.5- or 5-g pharmacy bulk package of fluorouracil is intended for preparation of individual doses of the drug and is *not* for direct IV infusion; after the vial has been entered, any unused portion should be discarded within 4 hours. An established IV line should be used to administer fluorouracil by direct IV injection. For IV infusion regimens, the drug should be administered via a central venous catheter using a controlled-infusion device (e.g., pump). Fluorouracil also has been infused regionally into the venous or arterial blood supply of a tumor† (e.g., portal vein or hepatic artery infusions for liver metastases). For topical administration of fluorouracil, see 84:92.

● **Dosage**

General Dosage

Dosage of fluorouracil is based on the patient's actual weight unless the patient is obese or has fluid retention. In these latter instances, dosage is based on ideal weight. Dosage also can be calculated according to body surface area.

Various dosage schedules for fluorouracil therapy have appeared in literature. Dosage and dosage schedules of fluorouracil should be individualized based on the tumor type, specific regimen, clinical response, and concomitant comorbidities. Clinicians should consult published protocols for the dosage of fluorouracil and other chemotherapeutic agents and the method and sequence of administration.

Colorectal Cancer

If fluorouracil is administered by direct IV injection in combination with leucovorin or levoleucovorin for the treatment of adenocarcinoma of the colon and rectum, the manufacturers of fluorouracil recommend a dosage of 500 mg/m^2 on days 1, 8, 15, 22, 29, and 36 of each 8-week cycle.

If fluorouracil is administered by IV infusion in combination with leucovorin or levoleucovorin (with or without oxaliplatin or irinotecan) for the treatment of adenocarcinoma of the colon and rectum, the manufacturers of fluorouracil recommend a dosage of 400 mg/m^2 by direct IV injection on day 1 followed by 2400–3000 mg/m^2 by continuous IV infusion over 46 hours every 14 days.

Monthly Direct IV Injection ("Bolus") Schedule (Mayo Clinic Regimen)

A monthly regimen administered by direct IV injection is leucovorin 20 mg/m^2 IV *or* an equivalent dose of levoleucovorin (10 mg/m^2 IV) followed by IV fluorouracil 425 mg/m^2; fluorouracil and either leucovorin or levoleucovorin are administered daily for 5 consecutive days. The regimen is repeated at 4-week intervals for 2 additional courses; thereafter, the regimen may be repeated at intervals of 4–5 weeks provided toxicity from the previous course has resolved completely. This regimen is frequently administered for a total of 6 cycles in the adjuvant setting.

Alternatively, leucovorin 200 mg/m^2 *or* an equivalent dose of levoleucovorin (100 mg/m^2) may be administered by slow IV injection (over a minimum of 3 minutes) and followed by IV fluorouracil 370 mg/m^2; fluorouracil and either leucovorin or levoleucovorin are administered daily for 5 consecutive days. The regimen is repeated at 4-week intervals for 2 additional courses; thereafter, the regimen may be repeated at intervals of 4–5 weeks provided toxicity from the previous course has resolved completely.

Weekly IV Infusion Schedule (Roswell Park Regimen)

A weekly regimen administered by IV infusion is leucovorin 500 mg/m^2 as a 2-hour IV infusion followed by fluorouracil 500 mg/m^2 as a slow IV injection administered 1 hour after the start of the leucovorin infusion. Both drugs are administered weekly for 6 consecutive weeks followed by a 2-week rest; cycles are repeated every 8 weeks for a total of 4 courses in the adjuvant setting.

Combination Therapy with Oxaliplatin

Combined therapy with fluorouracil, oxaliplatin, and leucovorin is administered over 2 consecutive days. On day 1, oxaliplatin 85 mg/m^2 and leucovorin 200 mg/m^2 are administered concurrently (in separate containers using a Y-type administration set) by IV infusion over 2 hours. Fluorouracil 400 mg/m^2 then is administered by direct IV injection followed by fluorouracil 600 mg/m^2 administered as an IV infusion over 22 hours. On day 2, leucovorin 200 mg/m^2 is administered by IV infusion over 2 hours, followed by fluorouracil 400 mg/m^2 administered by direct IV injection and then fluorouracil 600 mg/m^2 administered as an IV infusion over 22 hours. This regimen is repeated every 2 weeks.

Combined therapy with fluorouracil, oxaliplatin, and leucovorin also has been administered as oxaliplatin 85–100 mg/m^2 and leucovorin 400 mg/m^2 by IV infusion over 2 hours, followed by fluorouracil 400 mg/m^2 by direct IV injection and then fluorouracil 2400–3000 mg/m^2 by IV infusion over 46 hours of each 2-week cycle.

Combination Therapy with Irinotecan

When fluorouracil is administered in combination with leucovorin and irinotecan for the treatment of colorectal cancer, irinotecan 180 mg/m^2 and leucovorin 400 mg/m^2 are administered concurrently by IV infusion over 2 hours, followed by fluorouracil 400 mg/m^2 by direct IV injection, and then fluorouracil 2400–3000 mg/m^2 by IV infusion over 46 hours of each 2-week cycle.

Combination Therapy with Oxaliplatin and Irinotecan

When fluorouracil is administered in combination with leucovorin, oxaliplatin, and irinotecan (FOLFOXIRI) for the treatment of colorectal cancer, irinotecan 165 mg/m^2 is administered by IV infusion over 1 hour, followed by leucovorin 200 mg/m^2 and oxaliplatin 85 mg/m^2 administered concurrently by IV infusion over 2 hours, and then fluorouracil 3200 mg/m^2 by IV infusion over 48 hours of each 2-week cycle.

Dosage Modification for Mayo Clinic and Roswell Park Regimens

Dosage of fluorouracil in subsequent courses of therapy should be adjusted according to patient tolerance of the prior treatment course; dosage of leucovorin or levoleucovorin in subsequent courses is not adjusted because of toxicity. Daily fluorouracil dosage generally is reduced by 20% in patients who experienced moderate hematologic or GI toxicity in the prior course and by 30% in those patients who experienced severe toxicity. For patients who experienced no toxicity in the prior course of therapy, the dosage of fluorouracil may be increased by 10%. Other combination dosage regimens also have been used. (See Uses: Combination Therapies for GI Cancers.)

Bimonthly Infusion Schedule (Modified deGramont Regimen)

A simplified version of the LV5FU2 regimen (deGramont regimen) consists of leucovorin 400 mg/m^2 as a 2-hour IV infusion on day 1 followed by fluorouracil 400 mg/m^2 as an IV injection on day 1; then fluorouracil 1500 mg/m^2 as a continuous IV infusion over 23 hours on days 1 and 2 (i.e., a total of 3000 mg/m^2 by continuous IV infusion over 46 hours); cycles are repeated every 2 weeks.

Breast Cancer

Various fluorouracil-containing combination chemotherapy regimens have been used in the treatment of breast cancer, and published protocols should be consulted for dosages and the method and sequence of administration. The dose intensity of adjuvant combination chemotherapy appears to be an important factor influencing clinical outcome in patients with early node-positive breast cancer, with response increasing with increasing dose intensity; therefore, *arbitrary* reductions in dose intensity should be avoided.

When fluorouracil is combined with a cyclophosphamide-based regimen for the treatment of breast cancer, the manufacturers of fluorouracil recommend a dosage of 500 or 600 mg/m^2 IV on days 1 and 8 of each 28-day cycle for a total of 6 cycles.

One commonly employed regimen for the treatment of early breast cancer includes a fluorouracil dosage of 600 mg/m^2 IV on days 1 and 8 of each cycle combined with cyclophosphamide 100 mg/m^2 orally on days 1 through 14 of each cycle and methotrexate 40 mg/m^2 IV on days 1 and 8 of each cycle. In patients older than 60 years of age, the initial fluorouracil dosage was reduced to 400 mg/m^2 IV and the initial methotrexate dosage was reduced to 30 mg/m^2 IV. Dosage also was reduced if myelosuppression developed. Cycles generally were repeated monthly (i.e., allowing a 2-week rest period between cycles) for a total of 6–12 cycles (i.e., 6–12 months of therapy). Clinical superiority between 6- versus 12-month regimens has not been demonstrated.

There is some evidence that the addition of doxorubicin to a regimen of cyclophosphamide, methotrexate, and fluorouracil can improve outcome further in patients with early breast cancer and more than 3 positive axillary lymph nodes, and that sequential (i.e., administering several courses of doxorubicin first) regimens are more effective than alternating regimens in such patients; in patients with fewer positive nodes, no additional benefit from doxorubicin has been demonstrated. In the sequential regimen, 4 doses of doxorubicin hydrochloride 75 mg/m^2 IV were administered initially at 3-week intervals followed by 8 cycles of fluorouracil 600 mg/m^2 IV, cyclophosphamide 600 mg/m^2 IV, and methotrexate 40 mg/m^2 IV at 3-week intervals for a total of approximately 9 months of therapy. If myelosuppression developed with this sequential regimen, the subsequent cycle generally was delayed rather than reducing dosage.

Gastric Cancer

When fluorouracil is combined with a platinum-based regimen for the treatment of gastric adenocarcinoma, the manufacturers of fluorouracil recommend a dosage of 200–1000 mg/m^2 as a continuous IV infusion over 24 hours. Clinicians should consult published protocols for the frequency of fluorouracil dosing and duration of each cycle for the specific regimen.

Pancreatic Cancer

When fluorouracil is used in combination with leucovorin or as a component of a multidrug regimen that includes leucovorin for the treatment of pancreatic adenocarcinoma, the manufacturers of fluorouracil recommend a dosage of 400 mg/m^2 by direct IV injection on day 1 followed by 2400 mg/m^2 as a continuous IV infusion over 46 hours every 14 days.

Dosage Modification for Toxicity

If grade 3 or 4 diarrhea or mucositis, grade 4 myelosuppression, or grade 2 or 3 palmar-plantar erythrodysesthesia (hand-foot syndrome) occurs, fluorouracil should be withheld. When the toxicity has resolved or improved to grade 1, fluorouracil may be resumed at a reduced dosage.

Fluorouracil should be temporarily withheld if cardiotoxicity (i.e., angina, myocardial infarction or ischemia, arrhythmia, heart failure) develops in patients with no history of coronary artery disease or cardiac dysfunction. Therapy with the drug also should be withheld if hyperammonemic encephalopathy or neurologic effects (i.e., acute cerebellar syndrome, confusion, disorientation, ataxia, visual disturbance) develop. The manufacturers state that there is no recommended dosage for resumption of fluorouracil therapy following development of cardiotoxicity, hyperammonemic encephalopathy, or neurologic effects.

CAUTIONS

The major toxic effects of fluorouracil are on the normal, rapidly proliferating tissues particularly of the bone marrow and lining of the GI tract.

● GI Effects

Anorexia and nausea are common adverse effects of fluorouracil, and vomiting occurs frequently. These reactions generally occur during the first week of therapy, can often be alleviated by antiemetics, and generally subside within 2 or 3 days following therapy. Mucositis, stomatitis, and esophagopharyngitis and subsequent mucosal sloughing or ulceration also may occur during fluorouracil therapy; these adverse effects have been reported more frequently in patients who received fluorouracil by direct IV injection than in those who received the drug by continuous IV infusion. Stomatitis is one of the most common and often the earliest sign of specific toxicity, appearing as early as the fourth day but more commonly on the fifth to eighth day of therapy. Diarrhea, which occurs frequently and may be severe, usually appears slightly later than stomatitis, but may occur concurrently or even in the absence of stomatitis. Esophagitis, proctitis, and GI ulceration and bleeding have been reported, and paralytic ileus occurred in two patients who received excessive dosage. Patients must be closely monitored for adverse GI effects. (See Cautions: Precautions and Contraindications.)

GI toxicities (particularly stomatitis and diarrhea) occur more frequently and may be more severe or prolonged in patients receiving leucovorin or levoleucovorin concomitantly with fluorouracil. A GI syndrome characterized by progression from mild GI symptoms to potentially fatal enterocolitis has been reported in several studies in patients with advanced colorectal carcinoma receiving combined therapy with the drugs; in these studies, adverse GI effects (e.g., severe diarrhea) were the dose-limiting toxicity. In one comparative study, severe (grade 3 or 4) diarrhea or stomatitis occurred in 18.9 or 8.6%, respectively, of patients receiving IV levoleucovorin (100 mg/m^2), 15.7 and 11.2%, respectively, of those receiving oral leucovorin (500 mg/m^2 in 4 divided doses), and 17.6 and 14.2%, respectively, of those receiving IV leucovorin (200 mg/m^2) concomitantly with fluorouracil. In one study, severe or exacerbated diarrhea occurred in 25 or 13% of patients receiving fluorouracil combined with high- (500-mg/m^2 doses) or low- (25-mg/m^2 doses) dose leucovorin, respectively. In another study, diarrhea required dose reduction in 50% of patients receiving fluorouracil and high-dose leucovorin. Death occurred in several geriatric patients who developed severe diarrhea, with or without nausea and vomiting, and subsequent dehydration during combined therapy. Limited data suggest that once-weekly administration of fluorouracil plus leucovorin may be associated with a higher risk of developing serious adverse GI effects than 5-day regimens administered at approximately monthly intervals. Severe diarrhea appears to be the dose-limiting toxicity associated with once-weekly administration of the combination, while diarrhea and/or mucositis appear to be the dose-limiting toxicities associated with the 5-day regimens. GI bleeding also has been associated with such fatal toxicity in some patients, and neutropenia, fever, sepsis (possibly related to disruption of the GI mucosa), and acute renal failure also were present in some but not all of the patients who died. Autopsy findings in 2 patients revealed evidence of enterocolitis, including hemorrhagic enterocolitis in one, as well as erosions of the gastric mucosa. In a patient who developed hypotension and abdominal pain and tenderness during combined fluorouracil and leucovorin therapy, there was histologic evidence of ileitis, duodenitis, and esophageal ulceration; the patient responded to hydration, parenteral nutrition, transfusions, and anti-infective therapy.

Combined therapy with fluorouracil and a reduced folate (leucovorin or levoleucovorin) should *not* be initiated or continued in patients with symptomatic GI toxicity until such symptoms have completely resolved. Fluorouracil dosage reduction may be necessary in patients who develop adverse GI effects, particularly in geriatric patients. Close monitoring is particularly important in patients who develop diarrhea with such combined therapy since rapid clinical deterioration and death can occur.

● Hematologic Effects

Myelosuppression (e.g., neutropenia, thrombocytopenia, anemia), sometimes severe or fatal, may occur during fluorouracil therapy. Leukopenia, predominantly of the granulocytopenic type, thrombocytopenia, and anemia occur commonly with fluorouracil therapy; leukopenia usually occurs after an adequate course of fluorouracil therapy. Pancytopenia and agranulocytosis also have occurred. (See Cautions: Precautions and Contraindications.) The patient's hematologic status must be carefully monitored. The nadir neutrophil count usually occurs from the ninth to the fourteenth day after therapy is initiated but may occur as late as the 25th day after the first dose of fluorouracil. Maximum thrombocytopenia has been reported to occur from the seventh to seventeenth day of therapy. Hematopoietic recovery is usually rapid and by the thirtieth day, blood cell counts have usually reached the normal range.

● Dermatologic and Sensitivity Reactions

Hair loss occurs frequently with fluorouracil therapy, and cosmetically significant alopecia has occurred in a substantial number of patients. Regrowth of hair has been reported even in patients receiving repeated courses of the drug. Partial loss of nails has occurred rarely, and diffuse melanosis of the nails has been reported. The most common type of dermatologic toxicity is a pruritic maculopapular rash which usually appears on the extremities and less frequently on the trunk. This rash is generally reversible and usually responsive to symptomatic treatment.

Palmar-plantar erythrodysesthesia (commonly referred to as hand-foot syndrome), an erythematous, desquamative rash involving the hands and feet, has been reported in patients receiving fluorouracil. Hand-foot syndrome has been reported more frequently in patients who received fluorouracil by continuous IV infusion than in those who received the drug by direct IV injection. Hand-foot syndrome also has been reported more frequently in patients who have previously received chemotherapy. The rash may be accompanied by a tingling sensation, pain, swelling, desquamation, and erythema with tenderness. Hand-foot syndrome generally occurs within 8–9 weeks of initiation of fluorouracil. Hand-foot syndrome may be treated with oral pyridoxine therapy.

Other dermatologic manifestations of fluorouracil toxicity have included dry skin and fissuring, diffuse erythema, and scaling. Exposure to strong sunlight may intensify skin reactions to the drug. Seborrheic dermatitis has been reported in a few patients, but could not always be definitely attributed to fluorouracil.

Photosensitivity manifested by erythema or increased pigmentation can occur with fluorouracil therapy. Anaphylaxis and generalized allergic reactions have occurred in patients receiving fluorouracil.

● Nervous System Effects

Disorientation, confusion, ataxia, visual disturbances, and acute cerebellar syndrome have occurred in patients receiving fluorouracil. There are insufficient data on the risks of resuming fluorouracil after resolution of neurologic adverse effects.

Hyperammonemic encephalopathy, in the absence of liver disease or other identifiable cause, also has occurred in patients receiving fluorouracil. Manifestations of hyperammonemic encephalopathy, including altered mental status, confusion, disorientation, ataxia, or coma in the presence of elevated serum ammonia concentrations, may begin within 72 hours following initiation of fluorouracil infusion.

● Ocular Effects

Lacrimation, dacryostenosis, visual changes, and photophobia have been reported in patients receiving fluorouracil.

● Cardiovascular Effects

Myocardial ischemia/infarction, heart failure, arrhythmias, and angina (including Prinzmetal variant angina) have occurred in patients receiving fluorouracil. The exact mechanism(s) is not known, but the drug may cause these effects by inducing coronary artery vasospasm. Administration of fluorouracil by continuous IV infusion and presence of coronary artery disease have been reported to increase the risk of cardiotoxicity. Safety of resuming fluorouracil after resolution of cardiotoxicity has not been established.

● Other Adverse Effects

Fever that occurred during the end of the second week following the first dose of fluorouracil, and which usually was not accompanied by demonstrable infection, has been reported. Epistaxis, thrombophlebitis, and vein pigmentation also have been reported.

● Precautions and Contraindications

Fluorouracil is a highly toxic drug with a very low therapeutic index. The drug can produce severe hematologic toxicity, GI hemorrhage, and even death. Fluorouracil should be given only by, or under the supervision of, a clinician who is experienced in cancer chemotherapy and in the use of antimetabolites.

If intractable vomiting occurs, fluorouracil should be immediately discontinued. Patients should be questioned and the mouth examined daily for early evidence of stomatitis. Appearance of stomatitis, as evidenced by either oral mucosal erythema or ulceration at the inner margin of the lips, or of esophagopharyngitis as evidenced by a sore throat or dysphagia, necessitates cessation of therapy.

Diarrhea necessitates immediate discontinuance of the drug. GI ulceration or bleeding, or hemorrhage at any site, also requires prompt cessation of treatment.

If angina, myocardial infarction or ischemia, arrhythmia, or heart failure develops in patients without a history of coronary artery disease or cardiac dysfunction, therapy with fluorouracil should be interrupted. Patients experiencing new-onset angina, shortness of breath, dizziness, or lightheadedness should promptly inform their clinician or seek emergency treatment.

Since leucovorin calcium and levoleucovorin calcium enhance the toxicity of fluorouracil, combined therapy with fluorouracil and either leucovorin or levoleucovorin should be used with extreme caution in geriatric or debilitated patients since such patients are more likely to develop serious toxicity from fluorouracil. If grade 3 or 4 diarrhea or mucositis occurs, therapy with fluorouracil should be interrupted until diarrhea or mucositis resolves or decreases in intensity to grade 1. If diarrhea occurs, fluid and electrolyte replacement or an antidiarrheal agent should be initiated as clinically necessary.

Complete blood cell counts (CBCs) should be performed prior to each treatment cycle, weekly (if administered on a weekly or similar schedule), and as clinically indicated. Leukocyte counts with differential should be made before each dose of fluorouracil is given and if the leukocyte count falls to below 3500/mm^3 or decreases rapidly, or if there is a fall in the platelet count to below 100,000/mm^3, the drug should be discontinued. If the leukocyte count drops to less than 2000/mm^3, the patient should be placed in protective isolation and appropriate measures taken for the prevention of infection. If grade 4 myelosuppression occurs, administration of fluorouracil should be interrupted until the toxicity resolves or decreases in intensity to grade 1.

If grade 2 or 3 hand-foot syndrome occurs, administration of fluorouracil should be interrupted until the toxicity resolves or decreases in intensity to grade 1. Topical emollients (e.g., hand creams, udder balm) or oral pyridoxine therapy may ameliorate the manifestations of hand-foot syndrome in patients receiving fluorouracil.

If hyperammonemic encephalopathy or neurologic effects occur, therapy with fluorouracil should be interrupted. Patients experiencing new-onset confusion, disorientation, visual disturbances, or difficulty with balance or coordination should promptly inform their clinician or seek emergency treatment.

Fluorouracil should be withheld or permanently discontinued in patients experiencing acute early-onset or unusually severe toxicity, which may indicate near-complete or total absence of dihydropyrimidine dehydrogenase (DPD) activity. Patients with certain homozygous or certain compound heterozygous mutations in the DPD gene resulting in complete or near complete absence of DPD activity are at increased risk for acute early-onset toxicity and severe, life-threatening, or fatal toxicity (e.g., mucositis, diarrhea, neutropenia, neurotoxicity); patients with partial DPD activity also may be at increased risk for severe, life-threatening, or fatal toxicity. The manufacturer states that safety of fluorouracil in patients with complete absence of DPD activity has not been established; there are insufficient data to support dosage recommendations for those with partial DPD activity. Patients should be advised to inform their clinician if they are known to have deficient DPD activity.

Results of animal studies suggest that fluorouracil may impair female and male fertility.

● *Pediatric Precautions*

Safety and efficacy of fluorouracil in children have not been established.

● *Mutagenicity and Carcinogenicity*

Fluorouracil has been shown to be mutagenic in vitro in the bacterial reverse mutation (Ames) assay and induced chromosomal aberrations in hamster fibroblasts in vitro and in the micronucleus test on mouse bone marrow cells. Although the risk of mutagenesis in patients receiving fluorouracil has not been evaluated, the possibility must be considered.

Carcinogenicity studies of fluorouracil have not been performed.

● *Pregnancy, Fertility, and Lactation*

Pregnancy

Fluorouracil may cause fetal harm when administered to pregnant women. The drug has been shown to be embryotoxic and teratogenic in animals at dosages lower than a human dose of 12 mg/kg. Fetal malformations included cleft palate,

skeletal defects, and deformed appendages, paws, and tails. In monkeys, doses greater than an approximate human dose of 12 mg/kg resulted in abortion.

There are no adequate and controlled studies using fluorouracil in pregnant women, and the drug should be used during pregnancy only in life-threatening situations or severe disease for which safer drugs cannot be used or are ineffective. Women of childbearing potential and males with female partners of childbearing potential should be advised to use effective contraceptive methods during fluorouracil therapy and for up to 3 months after the last dose of the drug. If the drug is used during pregnancy or if the patient becomes pregnant while receiving the drug, the patient should be informed of the potential hazard to the fetus.

Fertility

Following intraperitoneal administration of fluorouracil at doses greater than or equal to 1.7 times the human dose of 12 mg/kg in male rats, chromosomal aberrations in spermatogonia were induced; spermatogonial differentiation also was inhibited, resulting in transient infertility. Following intraperitoneal administration of fluorouracil at doses greater than or equal to 0.33 times the human dose of 12 mg/kg during the preovulatory phases of oogenesis in female rats, fetotoxicity, decreased fertile matings, and increased preimplantation loss were observed.

Lactation

It is not known whether fluorouracil or its metabolites are distributed into milk. Because many drugs are distributed into human milk and because of the potential for serious adverse reactions to fluorouracil in nursing infants, a decision should be made whether to discontinue nursing or the drug, taking into account the importance of the drug to the mother.

DRUG INTERACTIONS

● *Drugs Metabolized by Hepatic Microsomal Enzymes*
CYP2C9 Substrates

Fluorouracil or its metabolites may inhibit cytochrome P-450 (CYP) isoenzyme 2C9.

● *Anticoagulants*

When fluorouracil was administered concomitantly with warfarin, clinically important elevations in coagulation parameters have been reported. Although concomitant use of fluorouracil with warfarin has not been specifically studied to date, altered coagulation parameters (e.g., increased prothrombin time [PT], increased international normalized ratio [INR]) were accompanied by increased systemic exposure to warfarin in patients receiving the prodrug of fluorouracil (capecitabine) and concomitant warfarin therapy. If fluorouracil is administered with a coumarin anticoagulant, the INR or PT should be closely monitored, and the anticoagulant dosage should be adjusted accordingly.

ACUTE TOXICITY

Overdosage of fluorouracil is often caused by dose calculation errors, confusion between the dose per day and the total dose for infusion over multiple days, ambulatory infusion pump programming errors, lack of pump programming safeguards, use of an incorrect infusion pump in outpatient settings, failure to independently double check dosage calculations, confusing pharmacy labels, and lack of familiarity with the chemotherapy protocol.

● *Manifestations*

Overdosage of fluorouracil would be expected to cause nausea, vomiting, diarrhea, and mucositis approximately 3–8 days following fluorouracil exposure. Myelosuppression generally occurs around 9–14 days following fluorouracil exposure; however, leukopenia has occurred as late as 20 days following fluorouracil exposure.

● *Treatment*

Treatment of toxicity resulting from impaired elimination or overdosage of fluorouracil consists of temporary interruption or permanent discontinuance of the drug, appropriate supportive care for the type of toxicity observed, and administration of the pyrimidine analog antidote uridine triacetate. Uridine triacetate (Vistogard®) is indicated *only* for emergency treatment of adults and pediatric patients following fluorouracil overdosage regardless of the presence of symptoms and for emergency treatment of adults and pediatric patients who exhibit early-onset, severe or life-threatening cardiac or CNS toxicity and/or early-onset, unusually severe adverse reactions (e.g., GI toxicity, neutropenia) within 96 hours following fluorouracil administration; the antidote is *not* recommended for the nonemergency treatment of adverse reactions associated with fluorouracil or capecitabine because it may decrease the clinical efficacy of these drugs. Safety and efficacy of uridine triacetate initiated more than 96 hours following the end of a fluorouracil infusion have not been established. Because delayed adverse effects may occur following fluorouracil overdosage, close monitoring of patients should be continued after discharge from the hospital and throughout the expected neutrophil nadir.

For information on the emergency treatment of fluorouracil toxicity or overdosage with uridine triacetate, see Uridine Triacetate 92:12.

PHARMACOLOGY

Although the precise mechanisms of action of fluorouracil have not been fully elucidated, the main mechanism is thought to be the binding of the deoxyribonucleotide of the drug (FdUMP) and the folate cofactor, N^{5-10}-methylenetetrahydrofolate, to thymidylate synthase (TS) to form a covalently bound ternary complex, which inhibits the formation of thymidylate from uracil, thereby interfering with DNA synthesis. In addition, FUTP can be incorporated into RNA in place of uridine triphosphate (UTP), producing a fraudulent RNA and interfering with RNA processing and protein synthesis.

PHARMACOKINETICS

● Absorption

Following IV administration of fluorouracil, no intact drug is detected in plasma after 3 hours.

● Distribution

Fluorouracil is distributed throughout the body into intestinal mucosa, bone marrow, liver, CSF, and brain tissue. Distribution studies in humans and animals have usually shown a higher concentration of the drug or its metabolites in the tumor than in surrounding tissue or in corresponding normal tissue. It has also been shown that there is a longer persistence of fluorouracil in some tumors than in the normal tissues of the host, perhaps due to impaired uracil catabolism. From these data, it has been suggested that the drug may possibly have some specificity against certain tumors in comparison with normal tissues.

It is not known whether the drug or its metabolites are distributed into human milk.

● Elimination

Following direct IV injection, the plasma elimination half-life ranges from 8–20 minutes and increases with dose.

A small portion of fluorouracil is anabolized in the tissues to 5-fluoro-2'-deoxyuridine and then to 5-fluoro-2'-deoxyuridine-5'-monophosphate, the active metabolite of the drug. The major portion of the drug is degraded in the liver. Following direct IV injection of fluorouracil, 5–20% of the dose is excreted in urine as intact drug within 6 hours. The metabolites (e.g., urea, α-fluoro-β-alanine) are excreted in urine over 3–4 hours.

Dihydropyrimidine dehydrogenase (DPD), a rate-limiting enzyme in the catabolism of fluoropyrimidines, is responsible for the elimination of approximately 80% of the administered dose of fluorouracil. Partial to complete DPD deficiency may result in impaired elimination of fluorouracil.

CHEMISTRY AND STABILITY

● Chemistry

Fluorouracil is a fluorinated pyrimidine antagonist. The drug occurs as a white to practically white, practically odorless, crystalline powder and is sparingly soluble in water and slightly soluble in alcohol. The pH of the commercially available injection has been adjusted to 8.6–9.4 with sodium hydroxide.

● Stability

Fluorouracil injection should be stored at 20–25°C; freezing and exposure to light should be avoided. After the vial has been entered, any unused portion should be discarded within 4 hours. Precipitation of fluorouracil in the injection occurs commonly, particularly following exposure to low temperatures. The frequency of precipitation may increase during cold weather (e.g., winter months), and efforts should be taken to ensure storage in adequately heated areas during these periods to minimize such risk. The ease with which the precipitate will dissolve may depend on the size and location of the precipitated crystals; crystals that become lodged between the stopper and glass container may be more difficult to dissolve. In some cases, attempts to dissolve the precipitate with heat and agitation may be unsuccessful.

Undiluted solutions of fluorouracil may be stored for up to 4 hours at 25°C in a syringe.

Diluted solutions of fluorouracil may be stored for up to 4 hours at 25°C.

For further information on the handling of antineoplastic agents, see the ASHP Guidelines on Handling Hazardous Drugs at http://www.ahfsdrug information.com.

PREPARATIONS

Excipients in commercially available drug preparations may have clinically important effects in some individuals; consult specific product labeling for details.

Fluorouracil

Parenteral		
Injection, for IV use	50 mg/mL*	**Fluorouracil Injection**
	50 mg/mL (2.5 or 5 g) pharmacy bulk package*	**Adrucil®, Teva Fluorouracil Injection**

* available from one or more manufacturer, distributor, and/or repackager by generic (nonproprietary) name

† Use is not currently included in the labeling approved by the US Food and Drug Administration.

Selected Revisions July 26, 2021, © Copyright, November 01, 1970, American Society of Health-System Pharmacists, Inc.

Gemcitabine Hydrochloride

10:00 • ANTINEOPLASTIC AGENTS

■ Gemcitabine hydrochloride, a synthetic pyrimidine nucleoside, is an antimetabolite antineoplastic agent.

USES

● Ovarian Cancer

Gemcitabine is used in combination with carboplatin for the treatment of advanced ovarian epithelial cancer in patients whose disease has relapsed at least 6 months following completion of platinum-based therapy (i.e., platinum-sensitive recurrent ovarian cancer).

The current indication for use of gemcitabine in the treatment of ovarian cancer is based principally on the results of an open-label, randomized, phase 3 study in 356 patients with advanced ovarian cancer whose disease had relapsed at least 6 months following completion of first-line, platinum-based therapy. Patients were randomized to receive either combination therapy with gemcitabine (1 g/m^2 on days 1 and 8) and carboplatin (administered after gemcitabine on day 1 at the dose required to obtain an area under the plasma concentration-time curve [AUC] of 4 mg/mL per minute) or carboplatin alone (administered on day 1 at the dose required to obtain an AUC of 5 mg/mL per minute) on a 21-day cycle; 6 cycles of therapy were administered in the absence of progressive disease or unacceptable toxicity, with up to 10 cycles administered to those who derived benefit from therapy. Patients who received combination therapy with gemcitabine and carboplatin had prolonged median progression-free survival (8.6 versus 5.8 months) and a higher overall response rate (47.2 versus 30.9%) than patients who received carboplatin alone; median overall survival and median duration of response were similar for both groups. Grade 3 or 4 hematologic toxicity occurred more frequently in patients receiving combination therapy with gemcitabine and carboplatin than in those receiving carboplatin alone; neutropenia was the predominant toxicity. A greater proportion of patients receiving the gemcitabine and carboplatin regimen received red blood cell (27 versus 6.7%) and platelet transfusions (8 versus 3%) compared with those who received carboplatin alone. Although use of hematopoietic growth factors was higher in the group receiving gemcitabine and carboplatin (23.6%) than in the group receiving carboplatin alone (10.1%), the incidence of febrile neutropenia was low and similar in both groups.

● Breast Cancer

Gemcitabine is used in combination with paclitaxel for initial treatment of metastatic breast cancer following failure of adjuvant therapy with an anthracycline-containing regimen, unless such therapy was clinically contraindicated.

The current indication for use of gemcitabine in the treatment of breast cancer is based principally on the results of an open-label, randomized, phase 3 study in 529 patients with locally recurrent or metastatic breast cancer following failure of prior adjuvant or neoadjuvant therapy with an anthracycline-containing regimen, unless such therapy was clinically contraindicated. Patients were randomized to receive either combination therapy with gemcitabine (1.25 g/m^2 administered by IV infusion over 30–60 minutes on days 1 and 8) and paclitaxel (175 mg/m^2 administered by IV infusion over 3 hours before gemcitabine on day 1) or paclitaxel alone (175 mg/m^2 administered by IV infusion over 3 hours on day 1) in 21-day cycles; treatment was continued until disease progression, intolerable toxicity, or patient withdrawal occurred. Patients who received combination therapy with gemcitabine and paclitaxel had longer median overall survival (18.6 versus 15.8 months), median time to disease progression (6.14 versus 3.98 months), and median progression-free survival (5.9 versus 3.9 months), and a higher overall response rate (41.4 versus 26.2%) than patients who received paclitaxel alone; median duration of response was similar for both groups. Hematologic toxicity, particularly grade 3/4 neutropenia (47.9 versus 11.5%), was observed more frequently in patients receiving combination therapy with gemcitabine and paclitaxel than in those receiving paclitaxel alone. Febrile neutropenia occurred in 5% of patients who received combination therapy with gemcitabine and paclitaxel and in 1.2% of those who received paclitaxel alone.

● Pancreatic Cancer

Gemcitabine is used for the palliative treatment of locally advanced (nonresectable stage II or III) or metastatic (stage IV) adenocarcinoma of the pancreas. The drug can be used either as first-line therapy or as second-line therapy in patients previously treated with fluorouracil. Pancreatic cancer rarely is curable, and response to conventional chemotherapy, radiation therapy, and/or surgery generally is poor regardless of the stage of the cancer. Therefore, the principal goal of therapy for pancreatic cancer generally has been to provide palliation of associated symptoms (e.g., pain) and improvement in the quality of life.

The current indication for use of gemcitabine in the treatment of pancreatic cancer is based on limited data from a multicenter randomized study comparing the drug with fluorouracil in patients with locally advanced or metastatic pancreatic cancer who had not received previous chemotherapy, and from a multicenter open-label study in patients with advanced pancreatic cancer who previously had received fluorouracil alone or as a component of a chemotherapeutic regimen. In both clinical trials, gemcitabine was administered in an initial cycle of 1 g/m^2 IV over 30 minutes once weekly for up to 7 weeks (as tolerated) followed by a treatment-free week, and in subsequent cycles of once-weekly doses (adjusted according to hematologic tolerance) for 3 consecutive weeks each month. The primary efficacy parameter in these studies involved palliative effects grouped as "clinical benefit response." A clinical benefit response was defined as a reduction in pain intensity or analgesic consumption of at least 50% or an improvement in performance status of at least 20 points (on the Karnofsky scale) for a period of at least 4 consecutive weeks, without sustained worsening in any other parameter, or as a stabilization of these parameters combined with a marked, sustained weight gain (of at least 7% maintained for at least 4 weeks) that was not attributable to fluid accumulation.

In the comparative study, gemcitabine therapy was associated with statistically significant increases in clinical benefit response (occurring in 23.8 versus 4.8% of patients receiving gemcitabine or fluorouracil, respectively), survival (median of 5.65 versus 4.41 months with gemcitabine or fluorouracil therapy, respectively), and time to disease progression (9 versus 4 weeks, respectively) compared with fluorouracil therapy (administered IV over 30 minutes at a weekly dosage of 600 mg/m^2). However, there was no confirmed objective evidence of tumor response nor of weight gain with either therapy in this study. One-year survival probability based on Kaplan-Meier estimates was 18 or 2% for those receiving gemcitabine or fluorouracil, respectively.

In the open-label study, 27% of patients receiving gemcitabine as second-line therapy after previous fluorouracil-containing regimens exhibited a clinical benefit response. The median duration of clinical benefit response was 14 weeks (range: 4–69 weeks), and median survival in this study was 3.9 months.

● Non-small Cell Lung Cancer

Combination Therapy

Gemcitabine is used in combination with cisplatin for the initial treatment of inoperable, locally advanced (stage IIIA or IIIB) or metastatic (stage IV) non-small cell lung cancer.

A small survival benefit has been demonstrated for the use of platinum-based (cisplatin) chemotherapy in selected patients with unresectable, locally advanced or metastatic non-small cell lung cancer who have a good performance status. Platinum-based chemotherapy regimens currently are preferred for the treatment of non-small cell lung cancer. (See Uses: Non-small Cell Lung Cancer in Cisplatin 10:00 for comprehensive discussion.) Use of chemotherapy for the treatment of advanced non-small cell lung cancer generally is advised only in patients with good performance status (ECOG performance status of 0 or 1, and 2 in selected patients) and evaluable lesions so that treatment can be discontinued if the disease does not respond. The decision to use chemotherapy must be individualized according to several factors, including patient preference, toxicity, survival benefit, quality of life, and cost of treatment.

In a large randomized trial comparing 4 chemotherapy regimens for advanced non-small cell lung cancer, median survival (8.1 versus 7.8 months) and response rate (22 versus 21%) were similar for patients receiving gemcitabine and cisplatin versus paclitaxel and cisplatin. Although median time to progression of disease was longer in patients receiving gemcitabine and cisplatin (4.2 months) compared with paclitaxel and cisplatin (3.4 months), patients receiving the gemcitabine-containing regimen were more likely to experience hematologic toxicity (thrombocytopenia or anemia) or renal toxicity. A higher percentage of patients receiving gemcitabine and cisplatin withdrew from the study because of complications of therapy compared with those receiving paclitaxel and cisplatin (27 versus 15%).

The current indication for gemcitabine in combination with cisplatin for the treatment of advanced non-small cell lung cancer is based principally on data from 2 randomized clinical studies involving a total of 657 patients. In a multicenter study, 522 patients with previously untreated, inoperable stage IIIA, IIIB, or IV non-small cell lung cancer were randomized to receive gemcitabine (1 g/m^2 IV on days 1, 8, and 15) and cisplatin (100 mg/m^2 IV on day 1) or cisplatin alone (100 mg/m^2 IV on day 1) on a 28-day cycle. Characteristics of the patients on the 2 study arms were similar except for tumor histology, with more patients receiving cisplatin alone having adenocarcinoma (48 versus 37%). Patients receiving combination therapy with gemcitabine and cisplatin had a longer median survival time (9 versus 7.6 months), a longer median time to disease progression (5.2 versus 3.7 months), and a higher objective response rate (26 versus 10%) than patients receiving cisplatin alone. Duration of response and quality of life (assessed using the FACT-L, a scale incorporating physical, social, emotional, and functional well-being as well as lung cancer symptoms) were similar for the 2 study groups. Combined therapy with gemcitabine and cisplatin was associated with greater toxicity, particularly myelosuppression, compared with cisplatin monotherapy, and dose adjustments were required in 90% of patients receiving gemcitabine and cisplatin compared with 16% of patients receiving cisplatin alone.

In a second multicenter, randomized study in 135 patients with stage IIIB or IV non-small cell lung cancer, patients were treated on 21-day cycles with cisplatin (100 mg/m^2 IV on day 1) and either gemcitabine (1.25 g/m^2 IV on days 1 and 8) or etoposide (100 mg/m^2 IV on days 1, 2, and 3). Median survival (8.7 versus 7 months) and quality of life (using the EORTC QLQ-C30 and LC13, which evaluate physical and psychologic functioning and symptoms related to lung cancer and its treatment) were similar in patients receiving gemcitabine/cisplatin or etoposide/cisplatin, respectively. A longer median time to disease progression (5 versus 4.1 months) and a higher objective response rate (33 versus 14%) were observed in patients receiving gemcitabine and cisplatin compared with those receiving etoposide and cisplatin. Thrombocytopenia (grade 3 or 4) was more frequent in patients receiving the gemcitabine-containing regimen than in those receiving the etoposide-containing regimen; although the incidence of grade 4 neutropenia was lower in patients receiving gemcitabine with cisplatin versus etoposide with cisplatin, the need for dose reductions or omission of scheduled doses for gemcitabine in twice as many patients as needed for etoposide may have contributed to this difference.

The use of gemcitabine in combination with other antineoplastic agents† for the treatment of non-small cell lung cancer is being investigated. In a randomized trial, patients with stage IIIB or IV non-small cell lung cancer receiving gemcitabine and docetaxel had similar response rates, median survival, and 1- or 2-year survival rates compared with those receiving cisplatin and docetaxel. Further study is needed to evaluate the role of platinum- and non-platinum-containing chemotherapy in the treatment of advanced non-small cell lung cancer.

Monotherapy

Gemcitabine is an active agent in non-small cell lung cancer. In nonrandomized phase 2 studies of patients with advanced non-small cell lung cancer who had not received prior chemotherapy, objective response rates of approximately 20% (0–3% complete responses, 17–20% partial responses) have been observed with gemcitabine alone. In these studies, median duration of response ranged from 3.6–12.7 months, and median survival ranged from 7–9 months. Responses to gemcitabine also have been observed in patients with relapsed or refractory advanced non-small cell lung cancer who previously were treated with platinum-containing chemotherapy regimens. Gemcitabine therapy is well tolerated; because of the lower incidence of myelosuppression associated with its use compared with other agents used in the treatment of non-small cell lung cancer, the drug is particularly suited for use in combination chemotherapy regimens. Response rates do not appear to be significantly affected by age; there appears to be similar efficacy and no difference in adverse effects in patients 70 years of age or older versus younger patients receiving gemcitabine alone for advanced non-small cell lung cancer. Noncomparative studies suggest that patients with advanced non-small cell lung cancer receiving gemcitabine experience relief of symptoms (including cough, hemoptysis, chest pain, dyspnea, and anorexia) and improvement in performance status.

In 2 randomized phase 2 studies in patients with inoperable, locally advanced or metastatic non-small cell lung cancer that was previously untreated with

chemotherapy, similar efficacy but less toxicity (leukopenia, nausea and vomiting, alopecia) was observed in those receiving gemcitabine alone versus combination therapy with cisplatin and etoposide.

Dosage and Other Considerations

Although optimum dosage regimens have not been established, gemcitabine dosages of 1 or 1.25 g/m^2 administered by 30-minute IV infusion once weekly for 3 weeks followed by 1 week of rest have been used most commonly in patients receiving gemcitabine as monotherapy for advanced non-small cell lung cancer. Various dosage schedules have been studied for the combination of gemcitabine with cisplatin for the treatment of advanced non-small cell lung cancer; gemcitabine dosages of 1 g/m^2 administered once weekly for 3 weeks on a 4-week cycle or 1.25 g/m^2 administered once weekly for 2 weeks on a 3-week cycle have been used in large randomized trials (see Dosage and Administration: Dosage); gemcitabine doses of 1–1.5 g/m^2 have been used in combination with cisplatin in phase 2 studies. Other dosage schedules for gemcitabine (e.g., higher doses, lower doses administered over longer infusion periods) are being investigated in patients with advanced non-small cell lung cancer.

Further study is needed to define the role of gemcitabine used alone or in combination therapy for the treatment of advanced non-small cell lung cancer. No single chemotherapy regimen currently can be recommended as superior in the treatment of non-small cell lung cancer. Various chemotherapy regimens used alone or in combination with other treatment modalities, such as radiation therapy, are continually being evaluated for the treatment of advanced non-small cell lung cancer. Because current treatment is not satisfactory for almost all patients with non-small cell lung cancer except selected patients with early-stage, resectable disease, all patients may be considered for enrollment in clinical trials at the time of diagnosis.

● Bladder Cancer

Gemcitabine is an active agent that is used alone or in combination therapy for the treatment of advanced or metastatic bladder cancer†. Objective responses to gemcitabine have been observed in patients with metastatic bladder cancer that did not respond to previous treatment with cisplatin-based regimens, including some patients with hepatic metastases.

Gemcitabine is used in combination with cisplatin as an alternative to M-VAC (i.e., cisplatin, methotrexate, and vinblastine with doxorubicin) for the treatment of advanced or metastatic bladder cancer. In a large randomized trial of patients receiving either gemcitabine (1 g/m^2 over 30–60 minutes on days 1, 8, and 15) and cisplatin (70 mg/m^2 on day 2) or M-VAC for the treatment of advanced or metastatic bladder cancer, overall median survival (13.8 versus 14.8 months, respectively), median time to progressive disease (7.4 months for each regimen), and response rates (44 versus 38%, respectively, using intent-to-treat analysis) were similar. Prophylactic hematopoietic agents (growth factors) were not administered to either group; grade 3 or 4 anemia or grade 3 or 4 thrombocytopenia were observed more often in patients receiving gemcitabine and cisplatin whereas grade 3 or 4 neutropenia, neutropenic sepsis, grade 3 or 4 mucositis, and alopecia occurred more frequently in patients receiving M-VAC.

Gemcitabine also is used as a single agent for the treatment of advanced or metastatic bladder cancer. In a phase 2 study, gemcitabine 1.25 g/m^2 was administered IV once weekly for 3 weeks every 4 weeks in patients with advanced bladder cancer that did not respond to previous treatment with cisplatin-based chemotherapy. Among 25 evaluable patients, an overall response rate of 28% (12% complete responses, 16% partial responses) was reported, and symptomatic improvements in hematuria, dysuria, cystitis, and polyuria were observed. In two other phase 2 studies, IV gemcitabine 1.2 g/m^2 was administered once weekly for 3 weeks every 4 weeks in previously untreated patients with advanced or metastatic bladder cancer. Among 76 evaluable patients, overall response rates of 24–29% (8–11% complete responses, 16–18% partial responses) were observed. Gemcitabine appears to be well-tolerated in most patients with only mild toxicity.

Further study is needed to define the precise role of gemcitabine in the treatment of advanced or metastatic bladder cancer, particularly in combination regimens.

● Biliary Tract Cancer

Gemcitabine has been used in combination with cisplatin for the treatment of unresectable locally advanced or metastatic biliary tract cancer† (intrahepatic or extrahepatic cholangiocarcinoma, gallbladder cancer, or ampullary cancer), including unresectable recurrent disease following surgical resection.

Evidence concerning efficacy of chemotherapy regimens in the treatment of advanced biliary tract cancer is derived largely from small, nonrandomized, clinical studies and retrospective analyses; few large, randomized, controlled clinical trials have been conducted. Experts state that, in patients with biliary tract adenocarcinoma (the most common type of biliary tract cancer), chemotherapy can be recommended in individuals with unresectable locally advanced or metastatic disease and in those with recurrent disease following surgical resection, since there is some evidence from a randomized study in patients with unresectable pancreatic or biliary tract cancer indicating that use of chemotherapy for the treatment of unresectable biliary tract cancer is associated with prolonged survival and improved quality of life. Chemotherapy is recommended in such individuals with good performance status (ECOG performance status of 0 or 1). However, in patients with poor performance status (ECOG performance status of 2 or 3) or insufficient biliary decompression, the benefits of chemotherapy are limited and use of alternative therapy for palliation of associated symptoms (e.g., pain) and improvement in quality of life is recommended. In one retrospective analysis comparing chemotherapy with best supportive care in patients with advanced gallbladder cancer, a survival benefit was observed in patients with good performance status but not in those with poor performance status.

In a multicenter, randomized, phase 3 trial (Advanced Biliary Cancer [ABC]-02), 410 patients with unresectable locally advanced or metastatic biliary tract carcinoma, including unresectable recurrent disease following surgical resection, were randomized to receive either combination therapy with gemcitabine (1 g/m² administered by IV infusion over 30 minutes on days 1 and 8) and cisplatin (25 mg/m² administered by IV infusion over 1 hour on days 1 and 8) on a 21-day cycle or gemcitabine alone (1 g/m² administered by IV infusion over 30 minutes on days 1, 8, and 15) on a 28-day cycle. Patients without evidence of disease progression at 12 weeks could continue to receive their assigned regimen for an additional 12 weeks. Patients enrolled in the study generally had good baseline performance status (ECOG score of 0 or 1 in 88% of patients, score of 2 in 12%). Patients who had received prior systemic chemotherapy for locally advanced or metastatic biliary tract carcinoma (other than low-dose radiosensitizing chemotherapy given in conjunction with radiotherapy) were excluded from the study. At a median follow-up of 8.2 months, patients who received combination therapy with gemcitabine and cisplatin had longer median overall (11.7 versus 8.1 months) and progression-free (8 versus 5 months) survival, a higher 6-month progression-free survival rate (59.3 versus 42.5%), and higher rates of tumor control (complete or partial responses or stable disease) (81.4 versus 71.8%) compared with patients who received gemcitabine alone. Only one patient in each treatment group achieved a complete response. Grade 3 or 4 hematologic toxicity (most commonly neutropenia [25.3 versus 16.6%]) occurred more frequently in patients receiving combination therapy with gemcitabine and cisplatin, whereas grade 3 or 4 abnormalities in liver function (27.1 versus 16.7%), including elevations in serum ALT (SGPT) concentrations, occurred more frequently in patients receiving gemcitabine alone. Grade 3 or 4 infection occurred with similar frequency in both groups. Based on current evidence, combination therapy with gemcitabine and cisplatin is recommended (accepted) for use in the treatment of unresectable locally advanced or metastatic biliary tract cancer (intrahepatic or extrahepatic cholangiocarcinoma, gallbladder cancer, or ampullary cancer), including unresectable recurrent disease following surgical resection, in patients with good performance status (ECOG performance status of 0 or 1).

DOSAGE AND ADMINISTRATION

• Reconstitution and Administration

Gemcitabine hydrochloride is administered by IV infusion. The manufacturer states that the drug is for IV use only.

Vials labeled as containing 200 mg or 1 g of gemcitabine should be reconstituted by adding 5 or 25 mL, respectively, of 0.9% sodium chloride injection without preservatives and shaking to dissolve. The resultant solutions have a gemcitabine concentration of 38 mg/mL, which accounts for the displacement volume of lyophilized powder (0.26 or 1.3 mL for vials labeled as containing 200 mg or 1 g, respectively). Smaller volumes should not be used for reconstitution since gemcitabine concentrations greater than 38 mg/mL may exceed the solubility of the drug and result in incomplete dissolution. The total volume upon reconstitution for vials labeled as containing 200 mg or 1 g is about 5.26 or 26.3 mL, respectively, and complete withdrawal of contents of the vials will provide

200 mg or 1 g, respectively. The reconstituted solutions can be infused IV without further dilution or as solutions that have been further diluted in 0.9% sodium chloride injection to gemcitabine concentrations as low as 0.1 mg/mL.

Reconstituted and diluted solutions of gemcitabine hydrochloride generally are infused IV over a period of 30 minutes; any unused portion after preparation of the appropriate dose should be discarded. Increased toxicity, including clinically important myelosuppression, was observed in clinical trials when gemcitabine was infused over periods exceeding 60 minutes. In a phase 1 study designed to assess maximally tolerated infusion rates, the risk of clinically important myelosuppression was particularly great with infusion periods of 4.5 hours (270 minutes) or longer. Because prolonged IV infusion of gemcitabine hydrochloride is associated with a prolonged half-life and increased toxicity, the manufacturer warns that the infusion time for the drug should *not* exceed 60 minutes. (See Description.)

Prior to administration, reconstituted and diluted solutions of gemcitabine hydrochloride should be inspected visually whenever solution and container permit. If discoloration or particulate matter is present, the solution should be discarded. When reconstituted and/or diluted as directed, gemcitabine hydrochloride solutions are stable for 24 hours at controlled room temperatures of 20–25°C. The solutions should *not* be refrigerated since crystallization may occur.

• Dosage

Dosage of gemcitabine hydrochloride is expressed in terms of gemcitabine and must be individualized based on body surface area and patient tolerance and response.

The manufacturer warns that gemcitabine should not be administered more frequently than once weekly since the risk of toxicity is increased with such dosing. In a phase 1 trial designed to assess the maximum tolerated dose on a schedule of 5 consecutive daily doses, patients developed intolerable hypotension and flu-like symptoms at gemcitabine dosages exceeding 10 mg/m² daily; the incidence and severity of these effects were dose related. In other dose-ranging phase 1 trials using twice-weekly schedules, maximum tolerated gemcitabine doses were 65 mg/m² when the drug was infused over 30 minutes and 150 mg/m² when the drug was injected over 5 minutes; in these trials, dose-limiting toxicities included thrombocytopenia and flu-like symptoms, particularly asthenia.

Ovarian Cancer

For the treatment of advanced ovarian cancer in women whose disease has relapsed at least 6 months following completion of platinum-based therapy, the manufacturer recommends a regimen of gemcitabine 1 g/m² administered by 30-minute IV infusion on days 1 and 8 of a 21-day cycle; carboplatin (at a dose required to obtain an area under the plasma concentration-time curve [AUC] of 4 mg/mL per minute) should be administered IV on day 1 after gemcitabine administration.

Patients should have an absolute granulocyte count of at least 1500/mm³ and a platelet count of at least 100,000/mm³ prior to each cycle. If necessary, dosage of gemcitabine should be reduced or withheld according to the degree of hematologic toxicity. (See Hematologic Toxicity under Dosage: Dosage Modification for Toxicity and Contraindications for Continued Therapy, in Dosage and Administration.) For adjustment of carboplatin dosage according to the degree of hematologic toxicity, see Dosage and Administration: Dosage, in Carboplatin 10:00; the manufacturer's prescribing information also should be consulted. In case of severe (i.e., grade 3 or 4) nonhematologic toxicity other than nausea and vomiting, gemcitabine doses should be withheld or reduced. (See Nonhematologic Toxicity under Dosage: Dosage Modification for Toxicity and Contraindications for Continued Therapy, in Dosage and Administration.)

Breast Cancer

For initial treatment of metastatic breast cancer in adults following failure of anthracycline-containing adjuvant chemotherapy or in whom such chemotherapy was contraindicated, the manufacturer recommends a regimen of gemcitabine 1.25 g/m² administered by 30-minute IV infusion on days 1 and 8 of a 21-day cycle; paclitaxel 175 mg/m² should be administered as a 3-hour IV infusion on day 1 before administration of gemcitabine.

Patients should have an absolute granulocyte count of at least 1500/mm³ and a platelet count of at least 100,000/mm³ prior to each cycle. If necessary, dosage of gemcitabine should be reduced or withheld according to the degree of hematologic toxicity. In case of severe (i.e., grade 3 or 4) nonhematologic toxicity other than alopecia or nausea and vomiting, gemcitabine doses should be withheld or reduced. (See Dosage Modification for Toxicity and Contraindications for Continued Therapy under Dosage and Administration: Dosage.) For adjustment of paclitaxel dosage according to the degree of hematologic or nonhematologic toxicity, see Dosage Modification for Toxicity and Contraindications for Continued Therapy under Dosage and Administration: Dosage, in Paclitaxel 10:00; the manufacturer's prescribing information also should be consulted.

Pancreatic Cancer

The usual dosage of gemcitabine currently recommended by the manufacturer for the treatment of locally advanced or metastatic pancreatic carcinoma, either as first-line therapy in chemotherapy-naive patients or as second-line therapy in those previously treated with fluorouracil, is 1 g/m² once weekly. For the initial cycle, this dosage is repeated at weekly intervals as tolerated for up to 7 weeks, followed by a week of rest from treatment. If necessary during the course of the initial cycle, dosage should be reduced or withheld according to the degree of hematologic toxicity. (See Hematologic Toxicity under Dosage: Dosage Modification for Toxicity and Contraindications for Continued Therapy, in Dosage and Administration.) Subsequent cycles consist of once-weekly administration for 3 consecutive weeks of the usual or escalated dosage (see Dosage Escalation under Dosage: Pancreatic Cancer, in Dosage and Administration), if tolerated, or at dosages reduced according to the degree of hematologic toxicity, followed by a week of rest from treatment. In clinical trials, patients with pancreatic cancer reportedly received an average of 3 cycles of gemcitabine therapy. Because clearance of gemcitabine is reduced in women and geriatric patients, dosage reductions, including withholding of doses in some cases, may be more likely in these populations; however, there currently is no evidence that unusual dosage adjustments (i.e., other than those recommended in general for hematologic toxicity) would be required. In clinical trials, women tolerated the drug more poorly than men, were less likely to progress to subsequent cycles, and were more likely to experience hematologic toxicity (i.e., neutropenia and thrombocytopenia).

Dosage Escalation

Dosage escalation can be considered for patients with pancreatic cancer who successfully complete the initial 7-week or subsequent 3-week cycle of gemcitabine therapy at the full weekly dosage of 1 g/m², provided nadirs of the absolute granulocyte and platelet counts exceed 1500 and 100,000/mm³, respectively, and nonhematologic toxicity exceeding a World Health Organization (WHO) grade of 1 is not present. In such patients, the dosage can be increased to 1.25 g/m² weekly. If a complete 3-week course at a dosage of 1.25 g/m² is tolerated (i.e., these hematologic parameters are met and there is no evidence of WHO grade 1 nonhematologic toxicity), dosage can be escalated further to 1.5 g/m² weekly given in 3-week cycles.

Non-small Cell Lung Cancer

The optimum dosage regimen for gemcitabine when used in combination with cisplatin for the treatment of advanced non-small cell lung cancer has not been established. For the initial treatment of patients with inoperable, locally advanced (stage IIIA or IIIB) or metastatic (stage IV) non-small cell lung cancer, gemcitabine used in combination with cisplatin may be administered on either a 4-week schedule or a 3-week schedule with doses specific to the selected dosage schedule. For patients receiving combination therapy with gemcitabine and cisplatin on the *4-week schedule*, the manufacturer recommends a regimen of gemcitabine 1 g/m² administered by 30-minute IV infusion on days 1, 8, and 15 of each 28-day cycle; cisplatin 100 mg/m² should be administered IV on day 1 following completion of the gemcitabine infusion. For patients receiving combination therapy with gemcitabine and cisplatin on the *3-week schedule*, the manufacturer recommends a regimen of gemcitabine 1.25 g/m² administered by 30-minute IV infusion on days 1 and 8 of each 21-day cycle; cisplatin 100 mg/m² should be administered IV on day 1 following completion of the gemcitabine infusion.

If necessary, dosage of gemcitabine should be reduced or withheld according to the degree of hematologic toxicity. (See Hematologic Toxicity under Dosage: Dosage Modification for Toxicity and Contraindications for Continued Therapy, in Dosage and Administration.) For adjustment of cisplatin dosage according to the degree of hematologic toxicity, see Cautions: Precautions and Contraindications, in Cisplatin 10:00; the manufacturer's prescribing information also should be consulted. In case of severe (i.e., grade 3 or 4) nonhematologic toxicity other than alopecia or nausea and vomiting, gemcitabine and cisplatin doses should be withheld or reduced. (See Nonhematologic Toxicity under Dosage: Dosage

Modification for Toxicity and Contraindications for Continued Therapy, in Dosage and Administration.) The manufacturer also recommends careful monitoring of serum concentrations of creatinine, potassium, calcium, and magnesium in patients receiving gemcitabine in combination with cisplatin. Appropriate administration, hydration, and dosage adjustment guidelines for cisplatin should be followed. (See Cisplatin 10:00.)

Biliary Tract Cancer

When gemcitabine has been used in combination with cisplatin for the treatment of unresectable locally advanced or metastatic biliary tract cancer† in adults, including treatment of unresectable recurrent disease following surgical resection, gemcitabine 1 g/m² has been administered by 30-minute IV infusion on days 1 and 8 of each 21-day cycle, and cisplatin 25 mg/m² has been administered by 1-hour IV infusion on days 1 and 8 prior to gemcitabine administration. Treatment has been continued for 24 weeks (8 cycles of therapy) in the absence of disease progression or unacceptable toxicity.

Dosage Modification for Toxicity and Contraindications for Continued Therapy

Hematologic Toxicity

A complete blood cell count (CBC), including differential and platelets, should be performed prior to each dose of gemcitabine. If myelosuppression is detected, therapy should be modified or temporarily withheld according to the degree of hematologic toxicity.

In patients receiving gemcitabine for the treatment of *advanced ovarian cancer*, the dosage of gemcitabine within a cycle of treatment should be adjusted according to the granulocyte and platelet counts obtained on day 8 of therapy. For patients with absolute granulocyte counts of at least 1500/mm³ and platelet counts of at least 100,000/mm³, no adjustment in dosage is necessary. For those with absolute granulocyte counts of 1000–1499/mm³ *and/or* platelet counts of 75,000–99,999/mm³, 50% of the full dose should be given. If the absolute granulocyte count is less than 1000/mm³ *and/or* the platelet count is less than 75,000/mm³, the dose should be withheld. The dosage of gemcitabine in combination with carboplatin for subsequent cycles should be adjusted according to observed toxicity. The dosage of gemcitabine in subsequent cycles should be reduced to 800 mg/m² on days 1 and 8 if any of the following hematologic toxicities occur: absolute granulocyte counts of less than 500/mm³ for more than 5 days or less than 100/mm³ for more than 3 days, febrile neutropenia, platelet counts of less than 25,000/mm³, or cycle delay of more than one week due to toxicity. If any of these toxicities recur after the initial dosage reduction, gemcitabine should be administered on day 1 *only* at a dose of 800 mg/m² for the subsequent cycle.

In patients receiving gemcitabine for the treatment of *metastatic breast cancer*, the dosage of gemcitabine should be adjusted according to the granulocyte and platelet counts obtained on day 8 of therapy. For patients with absolute granulocyte counts of at least 1200/mm³ and platelet counts exceeding 75,000/mm³, no adjustment in dosage is necessary. For those with absolute granulocyte counts of 1000–1199/mm³ *or* platelet counts of 50,000–75,000/mm³, 75% of the full dose should be given. For those with absolute granulocyte counts of 700–999/mm³ *and* platelet counts of at least 50,000/mm³, 50% of the full dose should be given. If the absolute granulocyte count is less than 700/mm³ *or* the platelet count is less than 50,000/mm³, the dose should be withheld.

In patients receiving gemcitabine for the treatment of *locally advanced or metastatic pancreatic carcinoma* or *advanced non-small cell lung cancer* with absolute granulocyte counts of at least 1000/mm³ and platelet counts of at least 100,000/mm³, no adjustment in dosage is necessary. For those with absolute granulocyte counts of 500–999/mm³ *or* platelet counts of 50,000–99,999/mm³, 75% of the full dose should be given weekly. If the absolute granulocyte count is less than 500/mm³ *or* the platelet count is less than 50,000/mm³, the weekly dose should be withheld until the counts exceed these levels.

Nonhematologic Toxicity

The diagnosis of hemolytic-uremic syndrome should be considered and gemcitabine should be discontinued immediately in patients who develop anemia with evidence of microangiopathic hemolysis, elevation of serum bilirubin or LDH, reticulocytosis, and/or severe thrombocytopenia with or without evidence of renal failure (e.g., elevation of serum creatinine or BUN).

Gemcitabine should be discontinued immediately and appropriate supportive care (e.g., diuretics, corticosteroids) provided promptly in patients who develop severe adverse pulmonary effects.

In patients receiving gemcitabine for the treatment of *advanced ovarian cancer* who develop grade 3 or 4 nonhematologic toxicity other than nausea and vomiting, gemcitabine doses should be withheld or reduced by 50%.

In patients receiving gemcitabine for the treatment of *metastatic breast cancer* who develop grade 3 or 4 nonhematologic toxicity other than alopecia or nausea and vomiting, gemcitabine doses should be withheld or reduced by 50%.

In patients receiving gemcitabine in combination with cisplatin for the treatment of *advanced non-small cell lung cancer* who develop grade 3 or 4 nonhematologic toxicity other than alopecia or nausea and vomiting, gemcitabine and cisplatin doses should be withheld or reduced by 50%.

● **Special Populations**

The manufacturer states that there are insufficient data to recommend a dosage of gemcitabine in patients with renal or hepatic impairment. (See Adequate Patient Evaluation and Monitoring under Warnings/Precautions: General Precautions, in Cautions and see Hepatic Impairment and also see Renal Impairment under Warnings/Precautions: Specific Populations, in Cautions.)

CAUTIONS

● **Contraindications**

Known hypersensitivity to gemcitabine or any ingredient in the formulation.

● **Warnings/Precautions**

Warnings

IV Administration

Prolonged IV infusion of gemcitabine (i.e., over periods exceeding 60 minutes) and administration more frequent than once weekly may be associated with increased toxicity (e.g., myelosuppression). (See Dosage and Administration: Reconstitution and Administration.)

Hematologic Effects

The dose-limiting toxicity of gemcitabine is myelosuppression, including leukopenia, anemia, and thrombocytopenia. Patients receiving the drug may require red blood cell transfusions or, less frequently, platelet transfusions. Patients should be monitored for myelosuppression during therapy. A complete blood cell count (CBC), including differential and platelets, should be performed prior to each dose; dosage should be modified accordingly. (See Hematologic Toxicity under Dosage: Dosage Modification for Toxicity and Contraindications for Continued Therapy, in Dosage and Administration.)

Pulmonary Effects

Severe and sometimes fatal adverse pulmonary effects, including pulmonary edema, interstitial pneumonitis, pulmonary fibrosis, and adult respiratory distress syndrome (ARDS), have been reported in patients receiving one or more doses of gemcitabine; the drug should be discontinued immediately and appropriate supportive care (e.g., diuretics, corticosteroids) provided promptly in patients developing such effects. Onset of pulmonary symptoms has occurred up to 2 weeks following administration of the last dose of gemcitabine, and in rare instances, respiratory failure and death have occurred despite discontinuance of gemcitabine therapy. Dyspnea, unrelated to underlying disease and occasionally accompanied by bronchospasm, has been reported in patients receiving gemcitabine. Dose-limiting pulmonary toxicity, including esophagitis, pulmonary fibrosis, and pneumonitis, occurred in patients receiving gemcitabine and concurrent thoracic radiation therapy for non-small cell lung cancer. In addition, fatal pulmonary veno-occlusive disease has been reported in a patient who developed progressive dyspnea during gemcitabine therapy.

Renal Effects

Hemolytic-uremic syndrome and/or renal failure have been reported in patients receiving one or more doses of gemcitabine. In rare cases, renal failure leading to death or requiring dialysis has occurred despite discontinuance of gemcitabine therapy. Cases of renal failure leading to death typically were caused by hemolytic-uremic syndrome. The diagnosis of hemolytic-uremic syndrome should be considered and gemcitabine should be discontinued immediately in patients who develop anemia with evidence of microangiopathic hemolysis, elevation of serum bilirubin or LDH, reticulocytosis, severe thrombocytopenia and/or evidence of renal failure (e.g., elevation of serum creatinine or BUN).

Hepatic Effects

Serious hepatotoxicity, including hepatic failure and death, has been reported rarely in patients receiving gemcitabine alone or in combination with other potentially hepatotoxic drugs. In clinical studies, gemcitabine was associated with transient elevations in serum transaminases; however, there was no evidence of increasing hepatotoxicity with either longer duration of exposure to gemcitabine or with greater total cumulative dose. Elevated liver function test results, including increased concentrations of AST, ALT, γ-glutamyltransferase (GGT, γ-glutamyltranspeptidase, GGTP), alkaline phosphatase, and bilirubin, have been reported rarely during postmarketing surveillance.

Fetal/Neonatal Morbidity and Mortality

Gemcitabine may cause fetal harm; teratogenicity and embryolethality have been demonstrated in animals. There are no studies to date in humans. If gemcitabine is used during pregnancy or the patient becomes pregnant while receiving the drug, the patient should be apprised of the potential fetal hazard.

Sensitivity Reactions

Hypersensitivity Reactions

Anaphylactoid reactions have been reported rarely during postmarketing surveillance in patients receiving gemcitabine.

General Precautions

Adequate Patient Evaluation and Monitoring

Gemcitabine should be used under the supervision of a qualified clinician experienced in therapy with antineoplastic agents. Most adverse effects of the drug are reversible and do not require discontinuance of gemcitabine therapy, although withholding doses or reducing dosage may be necessary. (See Dosage Modification for Toxicity and Contraindications for Continued Therapy under Dosage and Administration: Dosage.)

Renal and hepatic function should be assessed prior to and periodically during gemcitabine therapy. A complete blood cell count, including differential and platelets, should be performed prior to each dose.

Cardiovascular Effects

Cardiovascular toxicity, including congestive heart failure, myocardial infarction, and arrhythmias (mainly supraventricular), has been reported rarely during postmarketing surveillance in patients receiving gemcitabine. Vasculitis and gangrene also have been reported rarely in patients receiving the drug.

Specific Populations

Pregnancy

Category D. (See Fetal/Neonatal Morbidity and Mortality under Warnings/Precautions: Warnings, in Cautions.) (See Users Guide.)

Lactation

It is not known whether gemcitabine is distributed into milk. The manufacturer states that a decision should be made whether to discontinue nursing or the drug, taking into account the importance of the drug to the woman and the potential risk to nursing infants..

Pediatric Use

Efficacy of gemcitabine has not been established in children younger than 18 years of age. In a phase 1 study in pediatric patients with refractory leukemia†, the maximum tolerated dosage of gemcitabine was 10 mg/m² per minute for 6 hours (360 minutes) 3 times weekly, followed by 1 week of rest. When gemcitabine was administered at this dosage in a phase 2 study in patients with relapsed acute lymphoblastic leukemia† or acute myelogenous leukemia†, no clinically important activity was observed. Adverse effects reported in these studies were similar to those reported in adults and included bone marrow suppression, febrile neutropenia, increased serum transaminases, nausea, and rash/desquamation.

Geriatric Use

Because gemcitabine clearance is reduced and half-life is increased in geriatric patients, dosage reductions, including withholding of doses in some cases, may be more likely in this population; however, there currently is no evidence that unusual dosage adjustments (i.e., other than those recommended in general for hematologic and nonhematologic toxicity) would be required. Information derived from the safety database for gemcitabine monotherapy indicates that the frequency of adverse effects in patients older than 65 years of age is similar to that in younger adults; however, severe (grade 3/4) thrombocytopenia has occurred more frequently in geriatric patients. In the clinical study of gemcitabine given in combination with carboplatin for recurrent ovarian cancer, no overall differences in efficacy or safety were observed between geriatric and younger patients; however, grade 3/4 neutropenia occurred more frequently in geriatric patients 65 years of age or older.

Hepatic Impairment

Gemcitabine should be used with caution in patients with hepatic impairment. The effects of substantial hepatic insufficiency on the disposition of the drug have not been established. Use of gemcitabine in patients with current liver metastases or a history of hepatitis, alcoholism, or cirrhosis may lead to exacerbation of the underlying hepatic insufficiency. (See Dosage and Administration: Special Populations and see Adequate Patient Evaluation and Monitoring under Warnings/Precautions: General Precautions, in Cautions.)

Renal Impairment

Gemcitabine should be used with caution in patients with renal impairment. The effects of substantial renal insufficiency on the disposition of the drug have not been established. (See Dosage and Administration: Special Populations and see Adequate Patient Evaluation and Monitoring under Warnings/Precautions: General Precautions, in Cautions.)

Women

Because gemcitabine clearance is reduced and half-life is increased in women, dosage reductions, including withholding of doses in some cases, may be more likely in this population; however, there currently is no evidence that unusual dosage adjustments (i.e., other than those recommended in general for hematologic and nonhematologic toxicity) would be required. In clinical studies with gemcitabine therapy, women, especially older women, were more likely not to proceed to the next cycle and more likely to experience World Health Organization (WHO) grade 3/4 neutropenia and thrombocytopenia.

● Common Adverse Effects

Adverse effects reported in 10% or more of patients receiving gemcitabine monotherapy include myelosuppression (i.e., anemia, leukopenia, neutropenia, thrombocytopenia), proteinuria, hematuria, increased BUN, nausea, vomiting, pain, fever, rash, pruritus, dyspnea, constipation, diarrhea, hemorrhage, peripheral edema, edema, flu-like symptoms, infection, alopecia, stomatitis, somnolence, paresthesias, and increased serum AST, ALT, alkaline phosphatase, and bilirubin concentrations.

DRUG INTERACTIONS

No formal drug interaction studies have been performed to date.

● Antineoplastic Agents

Based on data from patients with metastatic breast cancer, concomitant use of gemcitabine and paclitaxel appears to have minimal or no effect on the pharmacokinetics (i.e., clearance, half-life) of either drug.

Based on data from patients with non-small cell lung cancer, concomitant use of gemcitabine and carboplatin does not appear to alter the pharmacokinetics of either drug compared with use of each drug alone.

● Radiation Therapy

A pattern of tissue injury usually associated with radiation toxicity has been reported in association with concurrent and nonconcurrent use of gemcitabine and radiation therapy. Radiosensitizing activity of gemcitabine was observed in preclinical and clinical studies when the drug was administered with or within 7 days of radiation therapy (i.e., concurrent therapy). Gemcitabine has been associated with radiation recall reactions, but administration more than 7 days before or after radiation therapy (i.e., nonconcurrent therapy) does not otherwise appear to enhance toxicity. Available data suggest that gemcitabine therapy may be initiated

once the acute effects of radiation therapy have resolved, or at least one week following radiation therapy.

Toxicity in patients receiving combined modality treatment is dependent on many factors, including doses of gemcitabine and radiation, frequency of gemcitabine administration, radiotherapy planning technique, and target tissue and volume. In one study in patients with non-small cell lung cancer who received gemcitabine therapy (dose of 1 g/m²) and therapeutic thoracic radiation concurrently for up to 6 consecutive weeks, substantial toxicity (manifested as severe and potentially life-threatening mucositis, especially esophagitis and pneumonitis) was observed, particularly in those receiving large volumes of radiotherapy. Subsequent studies have suggested that toxicity is predictable and less severe when lower doses of gemcitabine are administered concurrently with radiation therapy; however, the optimal regimen for safe administration of gemcitabine with therapeutic dosages of radiation has not been established for all tumor types.

DESCRIPTION

Gemcitabine hydrochloride, a synthetic pyrimidine nucleoside, is an antineoplastic agent. The nucleoside analog consists of the pyrimidine base difluorocytidine, and the sugar moiety deoxyribose.

Like most antimetabolite antineoplastic agents, gemcitabine is cell-cycle specific, acting principally in the S phase of the cell cycle; the drug also may cause cellular arrest at the G_1—S border. The cytotoxic activity of gemcitabine (2'-deoxy-2',2'-difluorocytidine) depends on intracellular conversion to its 5'-diphosphate and -triphosphate metabolites; thus, deoxydifluorocytidine-5'-diphosphate (dFdCDP, gemcitabine diphosphate) and -triphosphate (dFdCTP, gemcitabine triphosphate) and not unchanged gemcitabine are the pharmacologically active forms of the drug. Gemcitabine is phosphorylated by deoxycytidine kinase to gemcitabine monophosphate, which subsequently is phosphorylated to the corresponding diphosphate and triphosphate nucleosides, presumably by deoxycytidylate kinase and nucleoside diphosphate kinase, respectively. The cytotoxic effect of gemcitabine is attributed to the combined actions of its diphosphate and triphosphate nucleosides, which lead to inhibition of DNA synthesis.

Gemcitabine diphosphate inhibits ribonucleotide reductase, which is responsible for catalyzing the formation of deoxynucleoside triphosphates needed in DNA synthesis. By inhibiting this reductase, gemcitabine diphosphate interferes with subsequent de novo nucleotide production. Gemcitabine triphosphate inhibits DNA synthesis by competing with the physiologic substrate, deoxycytidine triphosphate, for DNA polymerase and incorporation into DNA. The reduction in intracellular concentrations of deoxycytidine triphosphate induced by gemcitabine diphosphate actually enhances the incorporation of gemcitabine triphosphate into DNA, a mechanism referred to as "self-potentiation." Following incorporation of gemcitabine triphosphate into the DNA chain, a single additional nucleotide, a normal base pair, is added and DNA synthesis is terminated, resulting in apoptosis (programmed cell death). DNA polymerase ε is unable to recognize the abnormal (gemcitabine) nucleotide and repair the DNA strand as a result of masking by the terminal normal base pair nucleotide (masked chain termination). This inability to recognize and excise the abnormal nucleotide results in a prolonged intracellular half-life of gemcitabine compared with other nucleoside analogs such as cytarabine and is thought to contribute to gemcitabine's expanded spectrum of antineoplastic activity relative to such agents. In CEM T lymphoblastoid cells, gemcitabine induces internucleosomal DNA fragmentation, which is characteristic of programmed cell death.

Following infusion of a single 1-g/m² dose over 30 minutes, gemcitabine is excreted principally in urine as unchanged drug (less than 10%) and as the inactive metabolite, 2'-deoxy-2',2'-difluorouridine (dFdU). The inactive metabolite, dFdU, does not appear to accumulate with weekly dosing; however, it is excreted by the kidneys and may accumulate in patients with decreased renal function. The inactive metabolite also is found in plasma. The active metabolite, deoxy-difluorocytidine-5'-triphosphate (dFdCTP, gemcitabine triphosphate), can be extracted from peripheral blood mononuclear cells. Volume of distribution and half-life of gemcitabine increase with longer infusion times. The half-life of gemcitabine ranges from 42–94 minutes and 4.1–10.6 hours following short and long infusions, respectively, depending on the patient's age and gender. Clearance is reduced and half-life increased in women and geriatric patients. Following a short (less than 70 minutes) infusion, the half-life of gemcitabine is approximately 42, 48, 61, and 79 minutes for men 29, 45, 65, and 79 years of age, respectively, and

49, 57, 73, and 94 minutes for women 29, 45, 65, and 79 years of age, respectively. The terminal phase half-life for the active metabolite, gemcitabine triphosphate, in mononuclear cells ranges from 1.7–19.4 hours.

ADVICE TO PATIENTS

Risk of myelosuppression.

Importance of women informing clinicians if they are or plan to become pregnant or plan to breast-feed; necessity for clinicians to advise women to avoid pregnancy

Importance of informing clinicians of existing or contemplated concomitant therapy, including prescription and OTC drugs, as well as any concomitant illnesses.

Importance of informing patients of other important precautionary information. (See Cautions.)

PREPARATIONS

Excipients in commercially available drug preparations may have clinically important effects in some individuals; consult specific product labeling for details.

Gemcitabine Hydrochloride

Parenteral		
For injection, for IV infusion	200 mg (of gemcitabine)	Gemzar®, Lilly
	1 g (of gemcitabine)	Gemzar®, Lilly

† Use is not currently included in the labeling approved by the US Food and Drug Administration.

Gilteritinib Fumarate

10:00 • ANTINEOPLASTIC AGENTS

- Gilteritinib, an inhibitor of multiple receptor tyrosine kinases, including fms-like tyrosine kinase-3 (Flt-3), is an antineoplastic agent.

USES

• Acute Myeloid Leukemia

Gilteritinib fumarate is used for the treatment of relapsed or refractory acute myeloid leukemia (AML) harboring a fms-like tyrosine kinase-3 (Flt-3) mutation in adults. Gilteritinib has been designated an orphan drug by the Food and Drug Administration (FDA) for the treatment of this cancer. An FDA-approved companion diagnostic test (e.g., LeukoStrat® CDx Flt-3 mutation assay) is required to confirm the presence of the Flt-3 mutation (peripheral blood or bone marrow) prior to initiation of therapy. The current indication is based on complete remission (CR) or complete remission with partial hematologic recovery (CRh) and improvement of hematologic deficits (determined by rate of conversion from transfusion dependence to transfusion independence). Safety and efficacy of gilteritinib in this use is based principally on the results of a phase 3, open-label, controlled trial in adults with relapsed or refractory AML with an internal tandem duplication (ITD) or a point mutation in the tyrosine kinase domain (TKD) of Flt-3 kinase. The National Cancer Institute states there is no standard treatment regimen for relapsed or refractory AML; patients who are unable or unwilling to undergo intensive therapy may be candidates for reduced-intensity therapies, including gilteritinib.

Clinical Experience

The current indication for gilteritinib in the treatment of AML is based principally on the results of a planned interim and final analysis of the open-label, controlled phase 3 study (ADMIRAL) in adults with relapsed or refractory AML with an ITD or a point mutation in the TKD of Flt-3 kinase as detected by the LeukoStrat® CDx Flt-3 mutation assay. The primary measures of efficacy were CR and CRh, duration of response, and loss of transfusion dependence (red blood cells [RBCs] and/or platelets). CR was defined as the presence of <5% blasts in bone marrow without evidence of extramedullary disease or myeloid differentiation, full recovery of peripheral blood cell counts (absolute neutrophil count [ANC] ≥1000/mm^3, platelet count ≥100,000/mm^3), and transfusion independence. Complete remission with partial hematologic recovery was defined as the presence of <5% blasts in bone marrow without evidence of extramedullary disease and with incomplete recovery of peripheral blood cell counts (ANC ≥500/mm^3, platelet count ≥50,000/mm^3).

In this study, 371 adults were randomized in a 2:1 ratio to receive either gilteritinib (initial dosage of 120 mg once daily; dosage escalations up to 200 mg once daily were permitted) or a preselected salvage chemotherapy regimen (cytarabine 20 mg IV or subcutaneously twice daily for 10 days; azacitidine 75 mg/m^2 IV or subcutaneously daily for 7 days; mitoxantrone 8 mg/m^2 IV daily for 5 days in combination with etoposide 100 mg/m^2 IV daily for 5 days and cytarabine 1 g/m^2 IV daily for 5 days [MEC]; fludarabine phosphate 30 mg/m^2 IV daily for 5 days, cytarabine 2 g/m^2 IV daily for 5 days, and idarubicin hydrochloride 10 mg/m^2 IV daily for 3 days with granulocyte colony-stimulating factor [G-CSF] 300 mcg/m^2 IV daily for 5 days [FLAG-IDA]). Gilteritinib therapy was continued until disease progression or unacceptable toxicity occurred. Allogeneic stem cell transplantation was permitted in patients who achieved CR.

The median age of patients randomized to receive gilteritinib was 60 years (range: 20–84 years); 56% were Caucasian, 38% were ≥65 years of age, 46% were male, 82% had an Eastern Cooperative Oncology Group (ECOG) performance status of 0 or 1, 59% had previously untreated relapsed AML, 41% had primary refractory AML, 77% were transfusion dependent at baseline, and 20% had previously undergone stem cell transplantation. Flt-3-ITD mutations were present in 88% of patients and Flt-3-TKD (D835 or I836) mutations were present in 9% of patients.

At a median follow-up of 4.6 months, CR or CRh was achieved in 21% of gilteritinib-treated patients with a median response duration of 4.6 months; 11.6% of patients achieved CR. The median time to initial CR or CRh in gilteritinib-treated patients was 3.6 months. Approximately one-third (31%) of gilteritinib-treated patients who were transfusion dependent at baseline became transfusion independent during any 56-day period during the study. The majority (53%) of gilteritinib-treated patients who were transfusion independent at baseline remained transfusion independent during any 56-day period during the study.

The final analysis of the ADMIRAL trial included 371 patients randomized to gilteritinib (n=247) or chemotherapy (n=124). Patient characteristics were similar to those in the interim analysis. After a median follow-up of 17.8 months, overall survival was substantially longer among patients treated with gilteritinib compared with chemotherapy (median, 9.3 versus 5.6 months, respectively; hazard ratio, 0.64; 95% CI, 0.49–0.83). In the final analysis, the CR/CRh rate in patients treated with gilteritinib was 22.6% and the duration of response was 7.4 months. Among patients treated with gilteritinib who were transfusion-dependent at baseline, 34.5% became transfusion-independent during any 56-day post-baseline period. Among patients who were transfusion-independent at baseline, 59.2% remained transfusion-independent during any 56-day post-baseline period. A follow-up study of the ADMIRAL trial 2 years after the primary analysis found that, after a median survival follow-up of 37.1 months, maintenance treatment with gilteritinib was associated with sustained efficacy and safety.

Clinical Perspective

The National Cancer Institute (NCI) states that there is no standard treatment regimen for patients with refractory or recurrent AML. Treatment options may include chemotherapy (intensive salvage chemotherapy and reduced-intensity therapy, including targeted therapy) and allogeneic hematopoietic cell transplantation (HCT).

Intensive salvage chemotherapy may use a number of regimens, including fludarabine, cytarabine, and filgrastim (FLAG); mitoxantrone, etoposide, and cytarabine (MEC); standard or high-dose cytarabine and mitoxantrone; high-dose etoposide and cyclophosphamide; idarubicin and cytarabine; and other intensive regimens. Patients who are unable or unwilling to undergo intensive therapy may be candidates for reduced-intensity therapies such as gilteritinib, enasidenib, or ivosidenib, depending on the presence of specific mutations; hypomethylating agents, gemtuzumab ozogamicin, and clofarabine with or without cytarabine are also options. Allogeneic HCT may be an option in patients who have not experienced remission with intensive chemotherapy.

DOSAGE AND ADMINISTRATION

• General

Pretreatment Screening

- Confirm presence of the fms-like tyrosine kinase-3 (Flt-3) mutation (peripheral blood or bone marrow) by an FDA-approved companion diagnostic test prior to initiation of therapy with gilteritinib in patients with acute myeloid leukemia (AML).

- Assess complete blood cell (CBC) counts and blood chemistries, including creatine kinase (CK), prior to initiation of therapy.

- Perform electrocardiogram (ECG) prior to initiation of therapy.

- Correct hypokalemia or hypomagnesemia prior to initiation of therapy.

- Confirm pregnancy status in females of reproductive potential within 7 days prior to initiation of gilteritinib therapy.

Patient Monitoring

- Correct hypokalemia or hypomagnesemia during gilteritinib therapy.

- Perform ECG prior to initiation of gilteritinib therapy, on days 8 and 15 of cycle 1, and prior to the start of the next 2 subsequent cycles.

- Monitor for signs and symptoms of pancreatitis.

- Monitor CBC counts and blood chemistries at least weekly for the first month of therapy, every other week for the following month of therapy, and then monthly thereafter.

- If the concomitant use of strong cytochrome P-450 (CYP) 3A inhibitors cannot be avoided, monitor patients more frequently for adverse effects of gilteritinib.

- If the concomitant use of P-glycoprotein (P-gp), breast cancer resistance protein (BCRP), or organic cation transporter 1 (OCT1) substrates cannot be avoided, monitor patients more frequently for adverse effects of these substrates.

Dispensing and Administration Precautions

- **Handling and Disposal:** Intact gilteritinib tablets can be handled without gloves; however, if the tablets are accidentally broken or crushed, chemically resistant protective gloves should be worn.

- Based on the Institute for Safe Medication Practices (ISMP), gilteritinib is a high-alert medication that has a heightened risk of causing significant patient harm.

● Administration

Gilteritinib fumarate is administered orally once daily without regard to meals. The drug should be taken at approximately the same time each day. The tablets should be swallowed whole with a cup of water; they should *not* be chewed, crushed, or broken.

If a dose of gilteritinib is missed by 12 hours or less, administer the missed dose on the same day as soon as it is remembered and take the next dose at the regularly scheduled time on the following day. If a dose of gilteritinib is missed by more than 12 hours, administer the next dose at the regularly scheduled time; do not administer an additional dose to replace the missed dose. Advise patients not to take 2 doses within a 12-hour period.

Intact gilteritinib tablets can be handled without gloves; however, if the tablets are accidentally broken or crushed, chemically resistant protective gloves should be worn.

Store gilteritinib at 20–25°C (excursions permitted between 15–30°C). Store in original container. Protect from light, moisture, and humidity.

● Dosage

Dosage of gilteritinib fumarate is expressed in terms of gilteritinib.

Acute Myeloid Leukemia

For the treatment of relapsed or refractory AML with Flt-3 mutation, the recommended initial adult dosage of gilteritinib is 120 mg once daily. Therapy should be continued for at least 6 months to allow time for response or until disease progression or unacceptable toxicity occurs.

Dosage Modification for Toxicity

Differentiation Syndrome

If differentiation syndrome is suspected, administer systemic corticosteroids and initiate hemodynamic monitoring until symptoms resolve and for a minimum of 3 days.

Interrrupt treatment with gilteritinib if severe signs and/or symptoms continue for more than 48 hours after initiation of corticosteroids.

Resume gilteritinib when signs and symptoms improve to grade 2 (i.e., moderate) or lower.

Posterior Reversible Encephalopathy Syndrome

If posterior reversible encephalopathy syndrome occurs, gilteritinib therapy should be discontinued.

Prolongation of QT Interval

If the corrected QT (QT_c) interval exceeds 500 msec, gilteritinib should be withheld. When the QT_c interval improves to 480 msec or less or no more than 30 msec from baseline, gilteritinib may be resumed at a reduced dosage of 80 mg daily.

If the QT_c interval increases by more than 30 antmsec from baseline on day 8 of cycle 1, confirm with an ECG on day 9. If QT_c interval increase is confirmed on day 9, consider dosage reduction of gilteritinib to 80 mg daily.

Pancreatitis

If pancreatitis occurs, gilteritinib therapy should be withheld. Upon resolution of pancreatitis, gilteritinib may be resumed at a reduced dosage of 80 mg daily.

Other Toxicity

If other grade 3 or 4 adverse reaction occurs, therapy with gilteritinib should be withheld. When the toxicity improves to grade 1 or less, gilteritinib may be resumed at a reduced dosage of 80 mg daily.

● Special Populations

Hepatic Impairment

The manufacturer makes no specific dosage recommendations for patients with hepatic impairment.

Renal Impairment

The manufacturer makes no specific dosage recommendations for patients with renal impairment.

Geriatric Use

The manufacturer makes no specific dosage recommendations for geriatric patients.

CAUTIONS

● Contraindications

Gilteritinib fumarate is contraindicated in patients with hypersensitivity to the drug or any ingredient in the formulation.

● Warnings/Precautions

Warnings

Differentiation Syndrome

The prescribing information of gilteritinib contains a boxed warning regarding the risk of differentiation syndrome, which can be fatal or life-threatening if untreated. Differentiation syndrome is associated with rapid proliferation and differentiation of myeloid cells and may occur as early as day 1 and up to 82 days after gilteritinib initiation. In clinical trials, 3% of patients experienced differentiation syndrome. Of these, 82% recovered after treatment or dose interruption of gilteritinib.

Symptoms of differentiation syndrome and clinical findings may include fever, dyspnea, hypoxia, pulmonary infiltrates, pleural or pericardial effusions, rapid weight gain or peripheral edema, hypotension, rash, or renal dysfunction. If differentiation syndrome is suspected, initiate corticosteroid therapy with dexamethasone 10 mg IV every 12 hours (or an equivalent dose of an alternative oral or IV corticosteroid) and hemodynamic monitoring until symptom resolution. Following symptom resolution, taper corticosteroids and administer corticosteroids for a minimum of 3 days. Symptoms of differentiation syndrome may recur if corticosteroid treatment is prematurely discontinued. If severe signs and/or symptoms continue for more than 48 hours after corticosteroid initiation, interrupt gilteritinib until signs and symptoms are no longer severe.

● Other Warnings/Precautions

Posterior Reversible Encephalopathy Syndrome

Posterior reversible encephalopathy syndrome has been reported rarely in patients receiving gilteritinib. In clinical trials, this syndrome occurred in 1% of patients receiving gilteritinib. Manifestations include seizure and altered mental status, which may resolve upon discontinuance of the drug. Brain imaging, preferably magnetic resonance imaging (MRI), is used to confirm the diagnosis. Gilteritinib therapy should be discontinued in patients who develop posterior reversible encepalopathy syndrome.

Prolongation of QT Interval

Prolongation of the corrected QT (QT_c) interval has been observed in patients receiving gilteritinib. In clinical trials, an increase in the QT_c interval exceeding

60 msec from baseline occurred in 7% of gilteritinib-treated patients, and QT_c intervals exceeding 500 msec occurred in 1% of gilteritinib-treated patients.

Electrocardiograms should be assessed prior to initiation of gilteritinib, on days 8 and 15 of cycle 1, and prior to initiation of cycles 2 and 3. In addition, serum electrolytes (e.g., potassium, magnesium) should be assessed prior to initiation of gilteritinib therapy and monitored at least weekly for the first month of therapy, every other week for the following month of therapy, and then monthly thereafter. Because of the increased risk of QT interval prolongation in patients with hypokalemia and hypomagnesemia, such electrolyte abnormalities should be corrected prior to initiation of and during gilteritinib therapy. Temporary interruption and/or dosage reduction may be necessary in patients who experience prolongation of the QT_c interval during therapy with the drug.

Pancreatitis

Pancreatitis was reported in 4% of patients receiving gilteritinib in clinical trials. Patients presenting with manifestations of pancreatitis (e.g., severe and persistent abdominal pain, which may be accompanied by nausea or vomiting) should be evaluated. Temporary interruption followed by dosage reduction may be necessary in patients who develop pancreatitis.

Fetal/Neonatal Morbidity and Mortality

Gilteritinib may cause fetal harm in humans based on its mechanism of action and animal findings; the drug has been shown to be embryotoxic, fetotoxic, and teratogenic in animals. There are no available data regarding the risk of gilteritinib use in pregnant women to date to inform a drug-associated risk of adverse developmental outcomes. In animal reproduction studies, embryofetal toxicity (i.e., postimplantation loss, decreases in fetal body and placental weight) and teratogenic effects (i.e., gross external, visceral, and skeletal anomalies) were observed in rats receiving gilteritinib at exposure levels approximately 0.4 times the human exposure at the recommended dosage.

Placental transfer of gilteritinib has been observed in rats. Following administration of a radiolabeled dose of gilteritinib on gestation day 14, radioactivity of the drug in the fetus was similar to radioactivity of the drug observed in maternal plasma.

Pregnancy should be avoided during gilteritinib therapy. The manufacturer recommends confirmation of pregnancy status within 7 days prior to initiation of gilteritinib in females of reproductive potential and states that such patients should be advised to use effective contraceptive methods while receiving gilteritinib and for at least 6 months after discontinuance of the drug. In addition, male patients with such female partners should use effective methods of contraception while receiving gilteritinib and for at least 4 months after discontinuance of the drug. Patients should be apprised of the potential hazard to the fetus if gilteritinib is used during pregnancy.

Specific Populations

Pregnancy

Gilteritinib may cause fetal harm if administered to pregnant females based on its mechanism of action and animal findings.

The manufacturer recommends confirmation of pregnancy status in females of reproductive potential within 7 days prior to initiation of gilteritinib therapy.

Lactation

Gilteritinib and/or its metabolite(s) are distributed into milk in rats. It is not known whether the drug or its metabolites distribute into human milk or if the drug has any effect on milk production or the nursing infant. Low amounts of gilteritinib are expected to distribute into human milk since the drug is highly bound to plasma proteins; however, the drug has a long half-life of 113 hours. Because of the potential for serious adverse reactions to gilteritinib in nursing infants, patients should be advised to discontinue nursing during gilteritinib therapy and for at least 2 months after discontinuance of therapy.

Females and Males of Reproductive Potential

The effect of gilteritinib on fertility in humans is not known. Based on animal studies, gilteritinib may impair male fertility. In male dogs, gilteritinib was associated with degeneration and necrosis of germ cells, formation of spermatid giant cells, and single cell necrosis of the epididymal duct epithelia of the epididymal head.

Advise females of reproductive potential to use effective contraception during treatment and for 6 months after the last dose of gilteritinib. Advise males of reproductive potential to use effective contraception during treatment and for 4 months after the last dose of gilteritinib.

Pediatric Use

Safety and efficacy of gilteritinib have not been established in pediatric patients.

Geriatric Use

In clinical trials evaluating gilteritinib in patients with relapsed or refractory acute myeloid leukemia (AML), 43% of patients receiving gilteritinib were 65 years of age or older, while 13% were 75 years of age or older. No overall differences in safety and efficacy were observed between geriatric patients and younger adults.

Hepatic Impairment

In a hepatic impairment study, systemic exposure of unbound gilteritinib in noncancer patients with mild or moderate hepatic impairment (Child-Pugh class A or B) was similar to that in individuals with normal hepatic function. The effects of severe hepatic impairment (Child-Pugh class C) on the pharmacokinetics of gilteritinib have not been established.

Renal Impairment

Formal pharmacokinetic studies of gilteritinib have not been conducted in patients with renal impairment; however, gilteritinib undergoes minimal renal elimination.

In a population pharmacokinetic analysis, alterations in serum creatinine concentrations did not have a substantial effect on the systemic exposure of gilteritinib in patients with relapsed or refractory AML; therefore, mild or moderate renal impairment (creatinine clearance of 30–80 mL/minute) is not expected to have clinically important effects on the systemic exposure of gilteritinib. The effects of severe renal impairment (creatinine clearance of 29 mL/minute or less) on the pharmacokinetics of gilteritinib have not been established.

● Common Adverse Effects

Adverse effects occurring in 20% or more of patients with relapsed or refractory AML receiving gilteritinib include increased transaminase, myalgia/arthralgia, fatigue/malaise, fever, mucositis, edema, rash, noninfectious diarrhea, dyspnea, nausea, cough, constipation, eye disorders, headache, dizziness, hypotension, vomiting, and renal impairment.

DRUG INTERACTIONS

Gilteritinib is metabolized principally by cytochrome P-450 (CYP) isoenzyme 3A4. In vitro studies indicate that gilteritinib is a weak inhibitor of CYP3A4.

In vitro, gilteritinib is a substrate of P-glycoprotein (P-gp) and breast cancer resistance protein (BCRP). In vitro studies indicate that gilteritinib is a potent inhibitor of multidrug and toxin extrusion (MATE) transporter 1 and organic cation transporter (OCT) 2 and inhibits BCRP, P-gp, and OCT 1 at clinically relevant concentrations.

● Drugs Affecting Hepatic Microsomal Enzymes and/or Efflux Transport Systems

Inhibitors of CYP3A

Concomitant use of gilteritinib with potent inhibitors of CYP3A may result in increased systemic exposure to gilteritinib. When the potent CYP3A4 and P-gp inhibitor itraconazole (200 mg twice daily on day 1 followed by 200 mg once daily on days 2–28) was administered concomitantly with gilteritinib (single 10-mg dose on day 6) in healthy individuals, peak plasma concentrations and area under the serum concentration-time curve (AUC) of gilteritinib were increased by approximately 20 and 120%, respectively. When the moderate CYP3A4 inhibitor fluconazole (400 mg on day 1 followed by 200 mg once daily on days 2–28) was administered concomitantly with gilteritinib (single 10-mg dose on day 6) in healthy individuals, peak plasma concentrations and AUC of gilteritinib were increased by approximately 16 and 40%, respectively.

Concomitant use of gilteritinib with potent inhibitors of CYP3A (e.g., itraconazole) should be avoided, and selection of an alternative drug with less CYP3A inhibition potential should be considered. If concomitant use of a potent CYP3A inhibitor cannot be avoided, patients should be monitored more frequently for signs of gilteritinib toxicity. If serious or life-threatening toxicity occurs, temporary interruption of gilteritinib therapy followed by dosage reduction may be necessary.

Inducers of CYP3A and Efflux Transport Systems

Concomitant use of gilteritinib with drugs that are combined P-gp and potent CYP3A inducers may result in decreased systemic exposure to gilteritinib and reduced gilteritinib efficacy. When the P-gp and potent CYP3A4 inducer rifampin (600 mg once daily for 21 days) was administered concomitantly with gilteritinib (single 20-mg dose on day 8) in healthy individuals, peak plasma concentrations and AUC of gilteritinib were decreased by approximately 30 and 70%, respectively.

Concomitant use of gilteritinib with drugs that are combined P-gp and potent CYP3A inducers (e.g., rifampin) should be avoided.

● Drugs Metabolized by Hepatic Microsomal Enzymes

When gilteritinib was administered concomitantly with the CYP3A substrate midazolam (single 2-mg dose on day 15) in patients with relapsed or refractory acute myeloid leukemia (AML), peak plasma concentrations and AUC of midazolam were increased by approximately 10%.

● Drugs Affected by Multidrug and Toxin Extrusion Transporter

When gilteritinib (200 mg once daily) was administered concomitantly with the MATE1 substrate cephalexin (single 500-mg dose on day 15) in patients with relapsed or refractory AML, peak plasma concentrations and AUC of cephalexin were decreased by less than 10%.

● Drugs that Interact with Serotonin Type 2B Receptor or Nonspecific σ-receptors

In vitro, gilteritinib is an inhibitor of type 2B serotonergic receptors ($5\text{-}HT_{2B}$) and nonspecific σ-receptors. Concomitant use of gilteritinib with drugs that bind to $5\text{-}HT_{2B}$ or nonspecific σ-receptors (e.g., escitalopram, fluoxetine, sertraline) may result in reduced efficacy of such drugs. Concomitant use of gilteritinib with drugs that bind to $5\text{-}HT_{2B}$ or nonspecific σ-receptors should be avoided unless use of the drugs that interact with $5\text{-}HT_{2B}$ or nonspecific σ-receptors is considered necessary.

Substrates of P-gp, BCRP, and OCT1

Coadministration of gilteritinib may increase the exposure of P-gp, BCRP, and OCT1 substrates. For P-gp, BCRP, or OCT1 substrates where small concentration changes may lead to serious adverse reactions, decrease the dose or modify the dosing frequency of the substrate and monitor for adverse reactions as recommended in the respective prescribing information.

DESCRIPTION

Gilteritinib, an inhibitor of multiple receptor tyrosine kinases including fms-like tyrosine kinase-3 (Flt-3), is an antineoplastic agent. Receptor tyrosine kinases are involved in the initiation of various cascades of intracellular signaling events that lead to cell proliferation and/or influence processes critical to cell survival and tumor progression (e.g., angiogenesis, metastasis, inhibition of apoptosis), based on the respective kinase. Gilteritinib has been shown to inhibit Flt-3 signaling resulting in inhibition of cell proliferation induced by Flt-3 mutations (i.e., internal tandem duplications [ITD] and/or tyrosine kinase domain [TKD] point mutations in codon D835Y). The drug also has demonstrated apoptosis in leukemic cells harboring Flt-3-ITD mutations in the presence or absence of Flt-3-TKD

point mutations. In vitro, gilteritinib has demonstrated potent inhibitory activity against AXL, an oncogenic tyrosine kinase commonly overexpressed in patients with acute myeloid leukemia (AML). AXL promotes Flt-3 signaling and may contribute to the development of resistance to receptor tyrosine kinase inhibitors; therefore, inhibitory activity against AXL may counteract a mechanism of resistance to the drug. The drug also has demonstrated inhibition of wild-type Flt-3, anaplastic lymphoma kinase (ALK), leukocyte receptor tyrosine kinase (LTK), and stem cell factor receptor (c-Kit). In patients with relapsed or refractory AML receiving gilteritinib 120 mg daily, greater than 90% inhibition of Flt-3 phosphorylation occurred within 24 hours of the initial dose. Inhibition above 90% also has been demonstrated on day 8 of cycle 1 in patients with relapsed or refractory AML receiving a gilteritinib dosage of at least 80 mg daily.

Peak plasma concentrations and area under the serum concentration-time curve (AUC) of gilteritinib are dose proportional over the gilteritinib dosage range of 20–450 mg daily in patients with relapsed or refractory AML. Following oral administration in a fasted state, the median time to peak plasma concentrations of gilteritinib is 4–6 hours. Steady-state concentrations of gilteritinib are reached within 15 days of once-daily dosing and the accumulation ratio is approximately tenfold. Administration of a single 40-mg dose of gilteritinib with a high-fat, high-calorie meal (800–1000 calories with 500–600 calories from fat) decreased peak plasma concentrations and AUC of gilteritinib by 26 and less than 10%, respectively, compared with administration in the fasted state. Following oral administration with a high-fat meal, the median time to peak plasma concentrations of gilteritinib was delayed by 2 hours.

Gilteritinib is metabolized principally by cytochrome P-450 (CYP) isoenzyme 3A4, via N-dealkylation and oxidation to the metabolites M17, M16, and M10; however, pharmacologic activity of these metabolites has not been established. The metabolites M17, M16, and M10 account for 10% or less of the total drug exposure. Gilteritinib is extensively distributed to tissues. Gilteritinib is highly bound (approximately 94%) to plasma proteins in vivo. In vitro, the drug is primarily bound to albumin. The estimated half-life of gilteritinib is 113 hours. Following administration of a radiolabeled dose of gilteritinib, 64.5% of the recovered dose is excreted in feces and 16.4% is eliminated in urine (10% or less as unchanged drug).

The pharmacokinetics of gilteritinib do not appear to be affected by age (20–87 years), gender, or ethnicity (Japanese versus non-Japanese).

ADVICE TO PATIENTS

- Advise patients to swallow gilteritinib tablets whole with a cup of water and not to break, crush, or chew the tablets.

- If a dose of gilteritinib is missed by 12 hours or less, importance of administering the missed dose on the same day as soon as it is remembered and taking the next dose at the regularly scheduled time on the following day. If a dose of gilteritinib is missed by more than 12 hours, importance of administering the next dose at the regularly scheduled time; an additional dose should not be administered to replace the missed dose. Patients should be advised not to take 2 doses within a 12-hour period.

- Risk of differentiation syndrome. Importance of informing clinician immediately of any symptoms suggestive of differentiation syndrome (e.g., fever, cough, dyspnea, rapid weight gain or peripheral edema, hypotension, rash, decreased urinary output).

- Risk of posterior reversible encephalopathy syndrome. Importance of informing clinician immediately if manifestations of posterior reversible encephalopathy syndrome (e.g., seizure; altered mental status; rapidly worsening headache, decreased alertness, confusion, or visual disturbances) occur.

- Risk of QT interval prolongation. Importance of informing clinician immediately if an abnormal heartbeat, loss of consciousness, or feelings of dizziness, lightheadedness, or faintness occur. Importance of monitoring electrolytes in patients with a history of electrolyte abnormalities (i.e., hypokalemia, hypomagnesemia).

- Risk of pancreatitis. Importance of informing clinician immediately if manifestations of pancreatitis (e.g., severe and persistent abdominal pain, with or without nausea and vomiting) occur.

- Risk of fetal harm. Necessity of advising women of reproductive potential that they should use effective methods of contraception while receiving the drug and for at least 6 months after discontinuance of therapy; necessity of advising men who are partners of such women that they should use effective methods of contraception while receiving the drug and for at least 4 months after discontinuance of therapy. Importance of women informing clinicians if they are or plan to become pregnant. If pregnancy occurs, advise pregnant women of potential risk to the fetus.

- Importance of advising women to avoid breast-feeding while receiving the drug and for at least 2 months after discontinuance of therapy.

- Importance of informing clinicians of existing or contemplated concomitant therapy, including prescription and OTC drugs and dietary or herbal supplements, as well as any concomitant illnesses (e.g., hypokalemia, hypomagnesemia).

- Importance of informing patients of other important precautionary information.

PREPARATIONS

Gilteritinib fumarate can only be obtained through designated specialty pharmacies and distributors. Clinicians may contact the manufacturer (Astellas) at 844-632-9272 or consult the Xospata® website (https://xospata.com/) for specific ordering and availability information.

Excipients in commercially available drug preparations may have clinically important effects in some individuals; consult specific product labeling for details.

Gilteritinib Fumarate

Oral

Tablets, film-coated	40 mg (of gilteritinib)	Xospata®, Astellas

† Use is not currently included in the labeling approved by the US Food and Drug Administration.

Selected Revisions August 28, 2023, © Copyright, December 17, 2018, American Society of Health-System Pharmacists, Inc.

Ibrutinib

10:00 • ANTINEOPLASTIC AGENTS

■ Ibrutinib, a selective irreversible inhibitor of Bruton's tyrosine kinase (BTK), is an antineoplastic agent.

USES

Ibrutinib is used for the treatment of certain B-cell malignancies (chronic lymphocytic leukemia [CLL]/small lymphocytic leukemia [SLL] with or without 17p deletion, Waldenstrom macroglobulinemia) and for the treatment of chronic graft-versus-host disease (GVHD).

● Chronic Lymphocytic Leukemia (CLL)/Small Lymphocytic Lymphoma (SLL)

Ibrutinib is used for the treatment of CLL and SLL, including those with CLL/SLL harboring the 17p13.1 deletion (17p deletion) chromosomal abnormality. Ibrutinib has been designated an orphan drug by FDA for the treatment of these conditions.

Clinical Experience

Safety and efficacy of ibrutinib in the treatment of CLL and SLL are based principally on favorable results of an uncontrolled, open-label, multicenter study (Study 1102) and 5 randomized, controlled phase 3 studies (RESONATE, RESONATE-2, HELIOS, ILLUMINATE, E1912); patients in Study 1102, RESONATE, and HELIOS had received at least one prior therapy for their disease and patients in the RESONATE-2, ILLUMINATE, and E1912 studies were treatment-naïve. Following initiation of single-agent ibrutinib therapy, lymphocytosis (i.e., absolute lymphocyte count exceeding 5000/mm³ and an increase of at least 50% from baseline) occurred in 66% of patients, generally during the initial month of therapy; lymphocytosis resolved in a median of 14 weeks. However, lymphocytosis occurred in 7% of patients receiving ibrutinib in combination with bendamustine and rituximab and also in those receiving the drug in combination with obinutuzumab.

In Study 1102, the median age of patients was 67 years; all patients in the study had a baseline Eastern Cooperative Oncology Group (ECOG) performance status of 0 or 1. Patients enrolled in the study had received a median of 4 prior therapies for their disease. In this study, 48 patients received ibrutinib 420 mg orally once daily until disease progression or unacceptable toxicity occurred. The overall response rate (as assessed by an independent review committee) was 58.3%; none of the patients achieved a complete response. At the time of data analysis, median duration of response had not been reached.

In the RESONATE study, 391 patients with CLL or SLL who were at risk for a poor outcome were treated with ibrutinib or the anti-CD20 antibody ofatumumab. Ibrutinib 420 mg was given orally once daily until disease progression or unacceptable toxicity occurred; ofatumumab was given by IV infusion at an initial dose of 300 mg (dose 1), followed by 2 g weekly for 7 doses (doses 2–8), then 2 g every 4 weeks for 4 doses (doses 9–12). The primary efficacy end point was progression-free survival as assessed by an independent review committee. The median age of patients in the study was 67 years (range: 30–88 years); all patients had a baseline ECOG performance status of 0 or 1 and 32% of patients harbored the 17p deletion chromosomal abnormality. Patients enrolled in the study had received a median of 2 (range: 1–13) prior therapies for their disease. Progression-free survival and overall survival had not been reached at the time of the initial data analysis; however, patients receiving ibrutinib had a median reduction of 78% (range: 68–85%) in the risk of death or disease progression and a median reduction of 57% (range: 21–76%) in the risk of death compared with those receiving ofatumumab. The overall response rates with ibrutinib and ofatumumab were 42.6 and 4.1%, respectively; there were no complete responses in either group. In patients with CLL harboring the 17p deletion chromosomal abnormality, a similar reduction in the risk of death or progression (75%) and a higher overall response rate compared with those receiving ofatumumab (47.6 versus 4.7%) were observed. In an updated analysis with a follow-up of 63 months, prolonged median investigator-assessed progression-free survival (44.1 versus 8.1 months) and a higher overall response rate (87.2 versus 22.4%) were observed in patients receiving ibrutinib compared with those receiving ofatumumab; prolonged median investigator-assessed progression-free survival (40.6 versus 6.2 months) and a higher overall response rate (88.9 versus 18.8%) also were observed in patients with CLL harboring the 17p deletion chromosomal abnormality receiving ibrutinib compared with those receiving ofatumumab.

In the HELIOS study, 578 patients with previously treated CLL or SLL received ibrutinib or placebo until disease progression or unacceptable toxicity in addition to therapy with bendamustine and rituximab (bendamustine/rituximab) for a maximum of six 28-day cycles. Ibrutinib 420 mg was given orally once daily; bendamustine 70 mg/m² was given IV on days 2 and 3 of cycle 1 and on days 1 and 2 of cycles 2–6; and rituximab 375 mg/m² was given IV on day 1 of cycle 1 followed by 500 mg/m² on day 1 of cycles 2–6. The primary efficacy end point was progression-free survival as assessed by an independent review committee. The median age of patients in the study was 64 years (range: 31–86 years); all patients had a baseline ECOG performance status of 0 or 1, 56% of patients had at least one tumor 5 cm or greater in size, and 26% of patients harbored the 11q22.3 deletion chromosomal abnormality. In this study, patients with CLL or SLL harboring the 17p deletion chromosomal abnormality were excluded because of known poor responses of such patients to bendamustine/rituximab. Patients enrolled in the study had received a median of 2 (range 1–11) prior therapies for their disease. At a median follow-up of 17 months, progression-free survival had not been reached in patients receiving ibrutinib in combination with bendamustine/rituximab; these patients had a median reduction of 80% (range: 72–85%) in the risk of death or disease progression. The overall response rates with ibrutinib in combination with bendamustine/rituximab or placebo in combination with bendamustine/rituximab were 82.7 or 67.8%, respectively; 8.3% of patients receiving ibrutinib in combination with bendamustine/rituximab achieved a complete response. At the final analysis (median follow-up of 63.7 months), median progression-free survival with ibrutinib plus bendamustine/rituximab was 65.1 months compared to 14.3 months for placebo plus bendamustine/rituximab. At 60 months, the progression-free survival rate was 52.7 or 8.2% for ibrutinib or placebo, respectively. Median overall survival at 60 months was 75.7 or 61.2% for ibrutinib or placebo, respectively.

In the RESONATE-2 study, 269 geriatric patients with treatment-naïve CLL or SLL were treated with ibrutinib or chlorambucil. Ibrutinib 420 mg was given orally once daily until disease progression or unacceptable toxicity occurred; chlorambucil was given orally at an initial dosage of 0.5 mg/kg (dose escalation up to 0.8 mg/kg was permitted if tolerated) on days 1 and 15 of each 28-day cycle for a maximum of 12 cycles. The primary efficacy end point was progression-free survival as assessed by an independent review committee. The median age of patients in the study was 73 years (range: 65–90 years); 91% patients had a baseline ECOG performance status of 0 or 1, 45% had Rai stage III or IV disease, and 20% of patients harbored the 11q22.3 deletion chromosomal abnormality. At a median follow-up of 28.1 months, progression-free survival and overall survival had not been reached; however, patients receiving ibrutinib had a median reduction of 84% (range: 72–91%) in the composite risk of death or disease progression and a median reduction of 84% (range: 44–95%) in the risk of death compared with those receiving chlorambucil. The overall response rates with ibrutinib and chlorambucil were 82.4 and 35.3%, respectively; complete responses were achieved in 3.7 and 1.5% of patients receiving ibrutinib and chlorambucil, respectively. Approximately one-half of the patients (41%) randomized to chlorambucil had therapy switched to ibrutinib; however, based on intent-to-treat analysis, patients receiving ibrutinib had a median reduction of 56% (range: 8–79%) in the risk of death compared with those receiving chlorambucil and a higher rate of 2-year overall survival (94.7 versus 84.3%). At a follow-up of 55 months, median progression-free survival had not been reached in patients receiving ibrutinib. At up to 8 years of follow-up (median 82.7 months), treatment with ibrutinib was associated with an 85% reduction in risk of progressive disease or death compared to chlorambucil. Median progression-free survival was not reached for ibrutinib and was 15 months for chlorambucil.

In the ILLUMINATE study, 229 patients with treatment-naïve CLL or SLL were treated with obinutuzumab in combination with either ibrutinib or chlorambucil. Patients were randomized to receive ibrutinib 420 mg once daily continuously or chlorambucil 0.5 mg/kg on days 1 and 15 of each 28-day cycle for 6 cycles; all patients received obinutuzumab 1 g by IV infusion once weekly for 3 doses during cycle 1, followed by 1 g by IV infusion every 4 weeks for an additional 5 cycles. Patients enrolled in the study were 65 years of age or older or less than 65 years of age with coexisting medical conditions (i.e., creatinine clearance less than 70 mL/minute). The primary efficacy end point was progression-free survival as assessed by an independent review committee (IRC). The median age of patients in the study was 71 years (range: 40–87 years); all patients had a baseline ECOG performance status of 0–2, 96% were white, and 65% of patients presented with CLL/SLL with high risk factors (presence of 17p or 11q22.3 deletion chromosomal abnormality or unmutated immunoglobulin heavy chain variable region). At a median follow-up of 31 months, progression-free survival had not been reached; however, the risk of death or disease progression was reduced by 77% in patients receiving ibrutinib and obinutuzumab compared with those receiving chlorambucil and obinutuzumab. Higher overall response rates were observed in patients receiving ibrutinib in combination with obinutuzumab compared with those receiving chlorambucil in combination with obinutuzumab (88.5 versus 73.3%); complete responses were achieved in 19.5 or 7.8% of patients receiving the respective treatments. In the cohort of patients with high risk CLL or SLL, the risk of death or disease progression was reduced by 85%. At the final analysis of the ILLUMINATE study (median follow-up of 45 months), progression-free survival was longer with ibrutinib plus obinutuzumab compared to chlorambucil plus obinutuzumab (median not reached versus 22 months, respectively) for a 75% reduction in risk of disease progression or death.

In the E1912 study, 529 adults with previously untreated CLL or SLL (without 17p deletion) were treated with ibrutinib in combination with rituximab, and compared with patients who received standard combination therapy with fludarabine, cyclophosphamide, and rituximab (FCR). Ibrutinib was administered at a dosage of 420 mg daily until disease progression or unacceptable toxicity occurred. Fludarabine was administered at a dose of 25 mg/m^2 and cyclophosphamide was administered at a dose of 250 mg/m^2 on days 1, 2, and 3 of cycles 1–6. When given with ibrutinib, rituximab was administered at 50 mg/m^2 on day 1 of cycle 2, 325 mg/m^2 on day 2 of cycle 2, and 500 mg/m^2 on day 1 of cycles 3–7 for a total of six 28-day cycles. When given with fludarabine and cyclophosphamide, rituximab was administered at 50 mg/m^2 on day 1 of cycle 1, 325 mg/m^2 on day 2 of cycle 1, and 500 mg/m^2 on day 1 of cycles 2–6 for a total of six 28-day cycles. Patients enrolled in the study were 70 years of age or older and had a creatinine clearance less than 40 mL/minute at baseline. The primary efficacy end point was progression-free survival. The median age of patients in the study was 58 years (range: 28–70 years); 98% had a baseline ECOG performance status of 0–1, 90% were white, and 59% presented with high risk factors (presence of TP53 mutation, 11q chromosome deletion [del11q], or unmutated immunoglobulin heavy change variable region). At a median follow-up of 37 months, progression-free survival had not been reached, but ibrutinib reduced the risk of disease progression or death by 66% compared to FCR. At a median follow-up of 49 months, median overall survival was not reached; 11 deaths (3%) occurred with ibrutinib plus rituximab and 12 deaths (7%) occurred with FCR. Long term outcomes for study E1912 have also been reported; at a median follow-up of 5.8 years, progression-free survival was greater with ibrutinib plus rituximab compared to FCR, with 5-year progression-free survival rates of 78 or 51%, respectively.

Clinical Perspective

Guidelines for CLL are available from the National Cancer Institute, with treatment individualized based on disease stage and behavior Observation may be an option for asymptomatic or minimally symptomatic patients. For symptomatic patients or patients with progressive CLL, first line agents include the BTK inhibitors acalabrutinib, ibrutinib, and zanubrutinib; venetoclax with initial use of obinutuzumab or rituximab; bendamustine and rituximab; fludarabine, cyclophosphamide, and rituximab; a BTK inhibitor (acalabruntinib or ibrutinib) plus venetoclax; or R-CHOP (rituximab, cyclophosphamide, doxorubicin, vincristine, and prednisone).

● Waldenstrom's Macroglobulinemia (WM)

Ibrutinib is used for the treatment of Waldenstrom's macroglobulinemia (WM); the drug has been designated an orphan drug by FDA for the treatment of this condition.

Clinical Experience

Evidence of safety and efficacy of ibrutinib in the treatment of WM is based principally on the results of an open-label, multicenter study (Study 1118) in patients who had received prior therapy for this disease and a randomized, double-blind, placebo-controlled study (INNOVATE) in patients with treatment-naïve or previously treated WM.

In Study 1118, 63 patients received single-agent ibrutinib 420 mg orally once daily until disease progression or unacceptable toxicity occurred. The median age of patients enrolled in the study was 63 years (range: 44–86 years); all patients had a baseline ECOG performance status of 0 or 1. Patients in the study received a median of 2 (range: 1–11) prior therapies for their disease. Response to ibrutinib treatment was assessed by investigators and an independent review committee (IRC) based on criteria from the International Workshop on WM. The IRC-assessed response rate, consisting of complete plus very good partial plus partial responses, was 61.9%; there were no complete responses. At the time of data analysis, responses were ongoing. The median time to response was 1.2 (range: 0.7–13.4) months. Substantial reductions from baseline in serum IgM concentration and bone marrow involvement and increases in hemoglobin concentration occurred with ibrutinib treatment, and overall toxicity (e.g., neutropenia, thrombocytopenia, bleeding, infection) was reported to be moderate. In addition, 31 patients with previously treated WM who failed prior rituximab-containing therapy in the INNOVATE study received single-agent ibrutinib (420 mg once daily). At a median follow-up of 34 months, the response rate was 71% in patients receiving single-agent ibrutinib; there were no complete responses. At the time of analysis, the median duration of response had not been reached.

In the INNOVATE study, 150 patients were randomized to receive ibrutinib 420 mg orally once daily or placebo in combination with rituximab; rituximab 375 mg/m^2 was given IV once weekly for 4 consecutive weeks during weeks 1–4 and weeks 17–20. The median age of patients enrolled in the study was 69 years (range: 36–89 years); 93% had a baseline ECOG performance status of 0 or 1, 79% were white, 77% of patients had disease harboring MYD88 L265P mutation, 55% of patients had previously treated disease, 45% were treatment-naïve, and median baseline serum IgM concentration was 3.2 g/dL. Patients who had received prior therapy for their disease received a median of 2 (range: 1–6) prior therapies. At a follow-up of 30 months, progression-free survival had not been reached in patients receiving ibrutinib and rituximab; however, the risk of death or disease progression was reduced by 80% in patients receiving ibrutinib and rituximab compared with those receiving placebo and rituximab. Response to ibrutinib treatment was assessed by an IRC. The IRC-assessed response rate, consisting of complete plus very good partial plus partial responses, was 72% in patients receiving combination therapy with ibrutinib and rituximab and 32% in those receiving placebo and rituximab; complete responses were achieved in 3 or 1% of patients receiving combination therapy with ibrutinib and rituximab or placebo and rituximab, respectively. At the time of data analysis, responses were ongoing in patients receiving combination therapy with ibrutinib and rituximab. Increases in hemoglobin concentration (increase of 2 g/dL or more from baseline) for at least 8 weeks without RBC transfusions or hematopoietic growth factor support occurred in 65% of patients receiving ibrutinib in combination with rituximab and in 39% of those receiving placebo and rituximab. At final data analysis (median 50 months follow-up), progression-free survival was longer with ibrutinib plus rituximab compared to placebo plus rituximab, for a 75% reduction in risk of disease progression or death (median progression-free survival not reached for ibrutinib and 20.3 months for placebo). Overall response rate was also substantially higher with ibrutinib (92%) compared to placebo (44%).

Clinical Perspective

A recent consensus statement outlined treatment options for WM. For treatment-naïve patients with symptomatic WM, first-line therapy options include chemoimmunotherapy (e.g., dexamethasone, cyclophosphamide plus rituximab; bendamustine plus rituximab), ibrutinib alone or plus rituximab, or zanubrutinib, with selection based on patient factors such as comorbidities, tumor burden, and risks of toxicity. For patients with relapsed or refractory disease, selection of therapy depends on initial treatment used and can include chemoimmunotherapy and/or a covalent BTK inhibitor (e.g., acalabrutinib, ibrutinib, or zarubrutinib). Additional factors to consider when selecting treatment for relapsed or refractory disease include patient age, comorbidities, hematopoietic reserve, and type of relapse.

● Graft-versus-host Disease (GVHD)

Ibrutinib is used for the treatment of chronic GVHD following failure of at least 1 prior systemic therapy in adults and pediatric patients 1 year of age or greater; the drug has been designated an orphan drug by FDA for the treatment of this condition.

Clinical Experience

The current indication for ibrutinib in the treatment of chronic GVHD in adults is based principally on the results of an open-label, multicenter study (Study 1129) in patients who required additional therapy following failure of first-line corticosteroid therapy. The median age of patients enrolled in the study was 56 (range: 19–74) years; 88% of patients had at least 2 organs involved at baseline, and 60% of patients had a baseline Karnofsky performance status of 80 or less. The most common underlying malignancies resulting in stem cell transplantation were acute lymphocytic leukemia (ALL), acute myeloid leukemia (AML), and CLL. Patients in the study received a median of 2 (range: 1–3) prior therapies for chronic GVHD. Approximately 50% of patients were receiving immunosuppressants and systemic corticosteroids (median daily prednisone [or equivalent] dosage was 0.3 mg/kg) at baseline. In this study, 42 patients received ibrutinib 420 mg orally once daily. Response to ibrutinib treatment was assessed by investigators based on criteria from the National Institutes of Health (NIH) Consensus Panel.

In this study, the overall response rate was 67%; 21% of patients receiving the drug achieved a complete response. At the time of data analysis, 48% of patients had sustained responses of 20 weeks or more. Responses in all organs affected by chronic GVHD (i.e., skin, mouth, GI tract, liver) were observed. The median time to response was 12.3 (range: 4.1–42.1) weeks. Exploratory analysis of patient-reported symptoms based on the Lee Symptom Scale showed at least a 7-point decrease in overall summary score in 24% of patients on at least 2 consecutive assessments (visits). After a follow-up of 26 months, the best overall response rate in patients treated with ibrutinib was 69%, with 31% of patients achieving a complete response and 38% achieving a partial response.

Efficacy of ibrutinib in pediatric (1 year of age and greater) and young adult (less than 22 years) patients with moderate to severe chronic GVHD was evaluated in the IMAGINE study, an open-label, phase 1/2, single arm trial. A total of 47 patients (median 13 years of age) who failed 1 or more prior lines of therapy were treated with ibrutinib 420 mg once daily (12 years of age and greater) or 240 mg/m^2 once daily (1 year of age and greater to less than 12 years of age). Supportive therapies for chronic GVHD were allowed. At week 25, the overall response rate (primary outcome) was 60%, with a complete response seen in 4% of patients and a partial response in 55% of patients. The median time to first response was 0.9 months, with a median duration of response of 5.3 months. The median time to death or new systemic therapies for chronic GVHD after first response was 14.8 months.

DOSAGE AND ADMINISTRATION

● General

Pretreatment Screening

- Assess cardiac history and cardiac function at baseline.
- Assess baseline risk for tumor lysis syndrome.
- Verify pregnancy status in females of reproductive potential.
- Evaluate bilirubin and transaminases at baseline.

Patient Monitoring

- Monitor CBCs monthly.
- Monitor for signs and symptoms of bleeding. Concomitant use of antiplatelet or anticoagulant therapy increases risk of major hemorrhage.
- Monitor for signs and symptoms of infection, including fever.
- Monitor patients for symptoms of cardiac arrhythmias and cardiac failure.
- Monitor blood pressure.
- Monitor for tumor lysis syndrome.
- Monitor bilirubin and transaminases. Monitor more frequently for patients who develop abnormal liver tests and clinical signs and symptoms of hepatotoxicity during therapy.

Premedication and Prophylaxis

- Consider anti-infective prophylaxis in patients at increased risk of opportunistic infections.

Other General Considerations

- Consider the potential benefits and risks of withholding ibrutinib therapy for 3–7 days or greater prior to and following surgery (based on the type of surgery and bleeding risk).

● Administration

Ibrutinib is available as immediate-release capsules containing 70 mg or 140 mg; immediate-release tablets containing 140 mg, 280 mg, or 420 mg; and as an immediate-release oral suspension containing 70 mg of ibrutinib per mL. The oral suspension bottle is provided in a carton with two 3 mL reusable oral dosing syringes.

Administer ibrutinib orally once daily at approximately the same time each day. Swallow tablets or capsules whole with a glass of water; do not open, break, or chew capsules, and do not cut, crush, or chew tablets. For administration of ibrutinib oral suspension, refer to the full instructions for use in the prescribing information for details.

Store ibrutinib capsules and tablets in the original packaging at 20–25°C; brief exposures to 15–30°C are permitted.

Store ibrutinib oral suspension at 2–25°C; do not freeze. Dispense in original sealed container, and do not use if the carton seal is missing or broken. Discard any unused oral suspension remaining 60 days after first opening the bottle.

If a dose is missed, administer the missed dose on the same day as soon as it is remembered and resume the normal schedule the following day; do not take extra doses to make up for a missed dose.

● Dosage

Adult Dosage

Chronic Lymphocytic Leukemia (CLL)/Small Lymphocytic Lymphoma (SLL)

For the treatment of chronic lymphocytic leukemia (CLL) or small lymphocytic lymphoma (SLL), the recommended dosage of ibrutinib is 420 mg once daily. Continue therapy until disease progression or unacceptable toxicity occurs.

For CLL or SLL, ibrutinib can be administered as a single agent, in combination with bendamustine and rituximab, or in combination with obinutuzumab or rituximab. When ibrutinib is administered on the same day as rituximab or obinutuzumab, consider administering ibrutinib prior to rituximab or obinutuzumab.

Waldenstrom's Macroglobulinemia (WM)

For the treatment of Waldenstrom's macroglobulinemia (WM), the recommended dosage of ibrutinib is 420 mg once daily. Continue therapy until disease progression or unacceptable toxicity occurs.

For WM, ibrutinib can be administered as a single agent or in combination with rituximab. When ibrutinib is administered on the same day as rituximab, consider administering ibrutinib prior to rituximab.

Dosage adjustment is not necessary in patients undergoing plasmapheresis.

Chronic Graft-versus-host Disease (GVHD)

For the treatment of chronic graft-versus-host disease (GVHD) following failure of 1 or more prior systemic therapy, the recommended dosage of ibrutinib is 420 mg once daily. Continue therapy until progression of chronic GVHD, recurrence of the underlying malignancy, or unacceptable toxicity occurs. When treatment for chronic GVHD is no longer necessary, discontinue ibrutinib considering the medical assessment of the individual patient.

Pediatric Dosage

Chronic Graft-versus-host Disease (GVHD)

For the treatment of chronic GVHD following failure of 1 or more prior systemic therapy for patients 12 years of age and greater, the recommended dosage of ibrutinib is 420 mg once daily.

For the treatment of chronic GVHD following failure of 1 or more prior systemic therapy for patients 1 to less than 12 years of age, the recommended dosage of ibrutinib is 240 mg/m^2 once daily (up to a dose of 420 mg). Refer to Table 1 for the recommended dosage to achieve 240 mg/m^2 based on body surface area (BSA) for patients 1 to less than 12 years of age.

Continue therapy until progression of chronic GVHD, recurrence of the underlying malignancy, or unacceptable toxicity occurs. When treatment for chronic GVHD is no longer necessary, discontinue ibrutinib considering the medical assessment of the individual patient.

TABLE 1. Recommended Dosage to Achieve 240 mg/m² Based on Body Surface Area (BSA) for Patients 1 to Less Than 12 Years of Age using Ibrutinib Capsules/Tablets or Oral Suspension.

BSA (m²) range	Dose (mg) of ibrutinib capsules or tablets to administer	Volume (mL) of ibrutinib oral suspension to administer
>0.3–0.4		1.2 mL
>0.4–0.5		1.5 mL
>0.5–0.6		1.9 mL
>0.6–0.7		2.2 mL
>0.7–0.8	210 mg	2.6 mL
>0.8–0.9	210 mg	2.9 mL
>0.9–1	210 mg	3.3 mL
>1–1.1	280 mg	3.6 mL
>1.1–1.2	280 mg	4 mL
>1.2–1.3	280 mg	4.3 mL
>1.3–1.4	350 mg	4.6 mL
>1.4–1.5	350 mg	5 mL
>1.5–1.6	350 mg	5.3 mL
>1.6	420 mg	6 mL

Dosage Modification for Toxicity

Withhold ibrutinib therapy for adverse reactions listed in Table 2. Upon improvement to grade 1 or baseline (recovery), follow the recommended dosage modifications described in Table 2.

TABLE 2. Dosage Modification for Toxicity

Adverse Reaction	Occurrence	Dosage Modification for CLL/SLL, WM, and Patients 12 Years of Age and Greater with Chronic GVHD after Recovery Starting Dose = 420 mg	Dosage Modification for Patients 1 to Less than 12 Years of Age with Chronic GVHD after Recovery Starting Dose = 240 mg/m² a
Grade 2 cardiac failure	First	Restart at 280 mg daily b	Restart at 160 mg/m² daily b
Grade 2 cardiac failure	Second	Restart at 140 mg daily b	Restart at 80 mg/m² daily b
Grade 2 cardiac failure	Third	Discontinue ibrutinib	Discontinue ibrutinib
Grade 3 cardiac arrhythmias	First	Restart at 280 mg daily b	Restart at 160 mg/m² daily b

TABLE 2. Continued

Adverse Reaction	Occurrence	Dosage Modification for CLL/SLL, WM, and Patients 12 Years of Age and Greater with Chronic GVHD after Recovery Starting Dose = 420 mg	Dosage Modification for Patients 1 to Less than 12 Years of Age with Chronic GVHD after Recovery Starting Dose = 240 mg/m² a
Grade 3 cardiac arrhythmias	Second	Discontinue ibrutinib	Discontinue ibrutinib
Grade 3 or 4 cardiac failure, OR Grade 4 cardiac arrhythmias	First	Discontinue ibrutinib	Discontinue ibrutinib
Other grade 3 or 4 nonhematological toxicities c, OR Grade 3 or 4 neutropenia with infection or fever, OR Grade 4 hematological toxicities	First	Restart at 280 mg daily	Restart at 160 mg/m² daily b
Other grade 3 or 4 nonhematological toxicities c, OR Grade 3 or 4 neutropenia with infection or fever, OR Grade 4 hematological toxicities	Second	Restart at 140 mg daily	Restart at 80 mg/m² daily b
Other grade 3 or 4 nonhematological toxicities c, OR Grade 3 or 4 neutropenia with infection or fever, OR Grade 4 hematological toxicities	Third	Discontinue ibrutinib	Discontinue ibrutinib

a See Table 3 for dosage modifications based on BSA.

b Assess the benefit-risk before resuming treatment.

c For grade 4 non-hematologic toxicities, assess the benefit-risk before resuming treatment.

TABLE 3. Recommended Dosage Modifications Based on BSA Using Either ibrutinib Capsules/Tablets or Oral Suspension

BSA (m²) range	Dose (mg) of capsules or tablets to administer to achieve 160 mg/m²	Volume (mL) of ibrutinib oral suspension to administer to achieve 160 mg/m²	Dose (mg) of capsules or tablets to administer to achieve 80 mg/m²	Volume (mL) of ibrutinib oral suspension to administer to achieve 80 mg/m²
>0.3–0.4		0.8 mL		0.4 mL
>0.4–0.5		1 mL		0.5 mL
>0.5–0.6		1.3 mL		0.6 mL
>0.6–0.7		1.5 mL		0.7 mL
>0.7–0.8	140 mg	1.7 mL	70 mg	0.9 mL
>0.8–0.9	140 mg	1.9 mL	70 mg	1 mL

TABLE 3. Continued

BSA (m²) range	Dose (mg) of capsules or tablets to administer to achieve 160 mg/m²	Volume (mL) of ibrutinib oral suspension to administer to achieve 160 mg/m²	Dose (mg) of capsules or tablets to administer to achieve 80 mg/m²	Volume (mL) of ibrutinib oral suspension to administer to achieve 80 mg/m²
>0.9–1	140 mg	2.2 mL	70 mg	1.1 mL
>1–1.1	140 mg	2.4 mL	70 mg	1.2 mL
>1.1–1.2	210 mg	2.6 mL		1.3 mL
>1.2–1.3	210 mg	2.9 mL		1.4 mL
>1.3–1.4	210 mg	3.1 mL		1.5 mL
>1.4–1.5	210 mg	3.3 mL	140 mg	1.7 mL
>1.5–1.6	280 mg	3.5 mL	140 mg	1.8 mL
>1.6	280 mg	4 mL	140 mg	2 mL

Dosage Modification with Concomitant Use of CYP3A Inhibitors

Refer to Table 4 for recommended dosage modifications for use of ibrutinib with cytochrome P-450 (CYP) 3A inhibitors. After discontinuation of a CYP3A inhibitor, resume previous dosage of ibrutinib.

TABLE 4. Recommended Dosage Modifications for Use with CYP3A Inhibitors

Patient Population	Coadministered Drug	Recommended Ibrutinib Dosage
B-cell malignancies (CLL/SLL or WM)	Moderate CYP3A inhibitor	280 mg once daily Modify dosage as recommended for adverse reactions
B-cell malignancies (CLL/SLL or WM)	Voriconazole 200 mg twice daily Posaconazole suspension 100 mg once daily, 100 mg twice daily, or 200 mg twice daily	140 mg once daily Modify dosage as recommended for adverse reactions
B-cell malignancies (CLL/SLL or WM)	Posaconazole suspension 200 mg three times daily or 400 mg twice daily Posaconazole IV 300 mg once daily Posaconazole delayed-release tablets 300 mg once daily	70 mg once daily Interrupt dosage as recommended for adverse reactions
B-cell malignancies (CLL/SLL or WM)	Other strong CYP3A inhibitors	Avoid concomitant use If these inhibitors will be used short-term (e.g., anti-infectives for 7 days or less), interrupt ibrutinib
Patients 12 years of age and greater with chronic GVHD	Moderate CYP3A inhibitor	420 mg once daily Modify dosage as recommended for adverse reactions
Patients 12 years of age and greater with chronic GVHD	Voriconazole 200 mg twice daily Posaconazole suspension 100 mg once daily, 100 mg twice daily, or 200 mg twice daily	280 mg once daily Modify dosage as recommended for adverse reactions

TABLE 4. Continued

Patient Population	Coadministered Drug	Recommended Ibrutinib Dosage
Patients 12 years of age and greater with chronic GVHD	Posaconazole suspension 200 mg three times daily or 400 mg twice daily Posaconazole IV 300 mg once daily Posaconazole delayed-release tablets 300 mg once daily	140 mg once daily Interrupt dosage as recommended for adverse reactions
Patients 12 years of age and greater with chronic GVHD	Other strong CYP3A inhibitors	Avoid concomitant use If these inhibitors will be used short-term (e.g., anti-infectives for 7 days or less), interrupt ibrutinib
Patients 1 to less than 12 years of age with chronic GVHD	Moderate CYP3A inhibitor	240 mg/m² once daily Modify dosage as recommended for adverse reactions
Patients 1 to less than 12 years of age with chronic GVHD	Voriconazole for suspension 9 mg/kg (maximum dose: 350 mg) twice daily	160 mg/m²ᵃ
Patients 1 to less than 12 years of age with chronic GVHD	Posaconazole at any dosage	80 mg/m²ᵃ
Patients 1 to less than 12 years of age with chronic GVHD	Other strong CYP3A inhibitors	Avoid concomitant use If these inhibitors will be used short-term (e.g., anti-infectives for 7 days or less), interrupt ibrutinib

ᵃ See Table 3 for dosage modifications based on BSA.

● Special Populations

Hepatic Impairment

Adults with B-cell Malignancies (CLL/SLL or WM)

For adults with mild hepatic impairment (Child-Pugh class A), the manufacturer recommends an ibrutinib dosage of 140 mg once daily.

For adults with moderate hepatic impairment (Child-Pugh class B), the manufacturer recommends an ibrutinib dosage of 70 mg once daily.

Avoid use of ibrutinib in adults with severe hepatic impairment (Child-Pugh class C).

Patients with Chronic GVHD

For patients 12 years of age and greater with total bilirubin level greater than 1.5–3 times upper limit of normal (ULN) (unless of non-hepatic origin or due to Gilbert's syndrome), the manufacturer recommends an ibrutinib dosage of 140 mg once daily.

For patients 1 to less than 12 years of age with total bilirubin level greater than 1.5–3 times ULN (unless of non-hepatic origin or due to Gilbert's syndrome), the manufacturer recommends an ibrutinib dosage of 80 mg/m² daily.

Avoid use of ibrutinib in patients with total bilirubin level greater than 3 times ULN (unless of non-hepatic origin or due to Gilbert's syndrome).

Renal Impairment

The manufacturer makes no specific dosage recommendations for patients with renal impairment.

Geriatric Patients

The manufacturer makes no specific dosage recommendations for geriatric patients. Certain ibrutinib toxicities may be more frequent in geriatric patients.

CAUTIONS

● **Contraindications**

● None.

● **Warnings/Precautions**

Hemorrhage

Hemorrhage, sometimes fatal, has been reported in patients receiving ibrutinib. Grade 3 or higher bleeding events (i.e., intracranial hemorrhage, subdural hematoma, GI bleeding, hematuria, postprocedural hemorrhage) occurred in 4.2% of patients treated with ibrutinib in clinical trials; fatal cases were reported in 0.4% of patients. Overall, hemorrhagic events of any grade or severity, including bruising and petechiae, occurred in 39% of patients receiving ibrutinib, and events excluding bruising and petechiae occurred in 23% of patients in clinical trials. The mechanism of bleeding with ibrutinib therapy is unclear.

Concomitant use of ibrutinib with antiplatelet or anticoagulant therapies may increase the risk of hemorrhagic events. In clinical trials, major hemorrhagic events were reported in 3.1, 4.4, or 6.1% of patients receiving ibrutinib without antiplatelet or anticoagulant therapy, with concomitant antiplatelet therapy with or without anticoagulant therapy, or with concomitant anticoagulant therapy with or without antiplatelet therapy, respectively.

Consider the potential benefits and risks of concomitant anticoagulant or antiplatelet therapy. Monitor patients for manifestations of bleeding.

Because of the risk of bleeding, consider the potential benefits and risks of withholding ibrutinib therapy for ≥3–7 days prior to and following surgery (based on the type of surgery and bleeding risk).

Infections

Serious infections (bacterial, viral, or fungal), sometimes fatal, have been reported in patients receiving ibrutinib. Grade 3 or higher infections occurred in 21% of patients with B-cell malignancies receiving ibrutinib in clinical trials. Progressive multifocal leukoencephalopathy and *Pneumocystis jirovecii* (formerly *P. carinii*) pneumonia also have been reported.

Monitor patients for signs and symptoms of infection and initiate appropriate anti-infective treatment as clinically indicated. Consider prophylaxis according to current standards of care in patients who are at increased risk for opportunistic infections.

Cytopenias

Cytopenias, including thrombocytopenia, anemia, and neutropenia, have been reported in patients receiving ibrutinib. Grade 3 or 4 neutropenia, thrombocytopenia, or anemia was reported in 23, 8, or 2.8%, respectively, of patients with B-cell malignancies receiving single-agent ibrutinib in clinical trials.

Monitor CBC counts monthly. Temporary interruption of ibrutinib therapy or dosage reduction may be necessary if myelosuppression occurs.

Cardiac Arrhythmias, Cardiac Failure, and Sudden Death

Serious arrhythmias, sometimes fatal, and cardiac failure have been reported in patients receiving ibrutinib. Sudden deaths or deaths due to cardiac causes occurred in 1% of patients who received ibrutinib in clinical trials, including in patients who received ibrutinib in unapproved monotherapy or combination regimens. These events occurred in patients with and without preexisting hypertension or cardiac comorbidities; however, patients with cardiac comorbidities may be at greater risk.

Grade 3 or higher ventricular tachyarrhythmias occurred in 0.2%, grade 3 or higher atrial fibrillation and atrial flutter occurred in 3.7%, and grade 3 or higher cardiac failure occurred in 1.3% of patients receiving ibrutinib in clinical trials, including in patients who received ibrutinib in unapproved monotherapy or combination regimens. These events have occurred particularly in patients with cardiac risk factors (e.g., hypertension, diabetes), acute infections, and a previous history of cardiac arrhythmias.

Assess cardiac history and function at baseline. Monitor patients for cardiac arrhythmias and cardiac function. Obtain further evaluation (e.g., ECG, echocardiogram) as indicated for patients who develop symptoms of arrhythmia (e.g., palpitations, lightheadedness, syncope, angina), new-onset dyspnea, or other cardiovascular issues. Manage cardiac arrhythmias and cardiac failure appropriately, follow dose modification recommendations (refer to "Dosage Modification for Toxicity" section), and consider the risks and benefits of continued ibrutinib therapy.

Hypertension

Hypertension has been reported in 19% of patients with B-cell malignancies receiving ibrutinib in clinical trials. Grade 3 or higher hypertension occurred in 8% of patients. The median time to occurrence of grade 3 or higher hypertension was 5.9 months (range: 0–24 months). In a long-term (5-year) safety study evaluating ibrutinib in patients with B-cell malignancies, the incidence of hypertension increased over time with prolonged ibrutinib therapy; the overall incidence for the 5-year period was 11%.

Monitor blood pressure in patients treated with ibrutinib, and initiate or adjust anti-hypertensive therapy throughout treatment with ibrutinib as appropriate. Follow dosage modification recommendations for grade 3 or higher hypertension (refer to "Dosage Modification for Toxicity" section).

Second Primary Malignancies

Other malignancies (10%), including non-skin carcinomas (3.9%), have been reported in ibrutinib-treated patients with B-cell malignancies in clinical trials. Non-melanoma skin cancer was the most frequent second primary malignancy, occurring in 6% of ibrutinib-treated patients.

Hepatotoxicity, Including Drug-induced Liver Injury

Hepatotoxicity, including severe, life-threatening, and potentially fatal cases of drug-induced liver injury (DILI), has occurred in patients treated with Bruton tyrosine kinase inhibitors, including ibrutinib.

Evaluate bilirubin and transaminases at baseline and throughout treatment. For patients who develop abnormal liver tests after ibrutinib therapy, monitor more frequently for liver test abnormalities and clinical signs and symptoms of hepatic toxicity. If DILI is suspected, withhold ibrutinib. Upon confirmation of DILI, discontinue therapy.

Tumor Lysis Syndrome

Tumor lysis syndrome has been reported infrequently in patients receiving ibrutinib.

Assess the potential for developing tumor lysis syndrome (e.g., large tumor burden) at baseline and take appropriate precautions. Monitor patients closely and treat as clinically indicated.

Fetal/Neonatal Morbidity and Mortality

Based on findings in animals, ibrutinib may cause fetal harm if administered to pregnant females. There are no available data in pregnant females to inform a drug-associated risk. Embryofetal toxicity (i.e., increased fetal resorption, postimplantation loss) and teratogenicity (i.e., visceral and skeletal anomalies) have been demonstrated in animals receiving ibrutinib at exposure levels 3–20 times the human exposure at the maximum recommended dosage (i.e., 420 mg daily).

Avoid pregnancy during ibrutinib therapy. Verify pregnancy status in in females of reproductive potential prior to initiating ibrutinib therapy . If ibrutinib is used during pregnancy or if the patient becomes pregnant while receiving the drug, apprise the patient of the potential fetal hazard. Advise females of reproductive potential, and males with female partners of reproductive potential, to use effective contraception during treatment with ibrutinib and for 1 month after the last dose.

Specific Populations

Pregnancy

Although there are no available data in pregnant females, ibrutinib may cause fetal harm based on animal findings. Verify pregnancy status prior to initiating ibrutinib therapy in females of reproductive potential. If ibrutinib is used during pregnancy or if the patient becomes pregnant while receiving the drug, apprise the patient of the potential fetal hazard.

Lactation

It is not known whether ibrutinib or its metabolites are distributed into human milk or if the drug has any effect on milk production or the nursing infant. Advise females not to breast-feed during treatment with ibrutinib and for 1 week after discontinuing the drug due to the potential for serious adverse reactions in the breast-fed child.

Females and Males of Reproductive Potential

Verify pregnancy status in females of reproductive potential prior to initiating ibrutinib therapy. Advise females of reproductive potential, and males with female partners of reproductive potential, to use effective contraceptive methods during and for 1 month after discontinuance of ibrutinib.

Pediatric Use

Safety and efficacy of ibrutinib have been established for treatment of chronic graft-versus-host-disease (GVHD) after failure of ≥1 lines of systemic therapy in pediatric patients ≥1 year of age. For this indication, the recommended dosage of ibrutinib in children ≥12 years of age is the same as that in adults, and the recommended dosage in children 1 to <12 years of age is based on body surface area. Safety and efficacy of ibrutinib have not been established for treatment of chronic GVHD in pediatric patients <1 year of age.

Safety and efficacy of ibrutinib have not been established in pediatric patients with chronic lymphocytic leukemia (CLL)/small lymphocytic lymphoma (SLL), CLL/SLL with 17p deletion, or Waldenstrom's macroglobulinemia.

Geriatric Use

In clinical trials of ibrutinib for B-cell malignancies or chronic GVHD, 62% of patients were ≥65 years of age and 22% were ≥75 years of age. No overall differences in efficacy were observed between geriatric and younger patients, but some adverse effects (e.g., anemia, grade 3 or higher pneumonia, thrombocytopenia, hypertension, atrial fibrillation) occurred more frequently in geriatric patients.

Hepatic Impairment

Adults with B-cell malignancies: Avoid use of ibrutinib in patients with severe hepatic impairment (Child-Pugh class C). The safety of ibrutinib has not been evaluated in mild to severe hepatic impairment by Child-Pugh criteria. Reduce the recommended dosage of ibrutinib in patients with mild or moderate hepatic impairment (Child-Pugh class A or B), and monitor patients more frequently for adverse reactions of ibrutinib.

Patients with chronic GVHD: Avoid use of ibrutinib in patients with total bilirubin level >3 times upper limit of normal (ULN) (unless of non-hepatic origin or due to Gilbert's syndrome). Reduce the recommended dosage of ibrutinib in patients with total bilirubin level >1.5–3 times ULN (unless of non-hepatic origin or due to Gilbert's syndrome).

In a single-dose study, systemic exposure of ibrutinib was increased 2.7-, 8.2-, or 9.8-fold in patients with mild (Child-Pugh class A), moderate (Child-Pugh class B), or severe (Child-Pugh class C) hepatic impairment, respectively, compared with that in individuals with normal hepatic function. In addition, peak plasma concentration of ibrutinib was increased 5.2-, 8.8-, or 7-fold in patients with mild, moderate, or severe hepatic impairment, respectively, compared with that in individuals with normal hepatic function.

Renal Impairment

Systemic exposure of ibrutinib does not appear to be altered in patients with mild or moderate renal impairment (creatinine clearance >25 mL/minute). The manufacturer states that there is no experience with ibrutinib in patients with severe renal impairment (creatinine clearance <25 mL/minute) or in patients undergoing dialysis.

● Common Adverse Effects

Adverse effects reported in ≥30% of patients with B-cell malignancies include thrombocytopenia, diarrhea, fatigue, musculoskeletal pain, neutropenia, rash, anemia, bruising, and nausea.

Adverse effects reported in ≥20% of adult or pediatric patients with chronic graft versus host disease include fatigue, anemia, bruising, diarrhea, thrombocytopenia, musculoskeletal pain, pyrexia, muscle spasms, stomatitis, nausea, hemorrhage, abdominal pain, headache, and pneumonia.

DRUG INTERACTIONS

Metabolism of ibrutinib to several metabolites is mediated principally by cytochrome P-450 (CYP) isoenzyme 3A and, to a lesser extent, by CYP2D6.

In vitro studies indicate that ibrutinib and PCI-45227 (active metabolite) are not expected to inhibit CYP isoenzymes 1A2, 2B6, 2C8, 2C9, 2C19, 2D6, or 3A or induce CYP isoenzymes 1A2, 2B6, or 3A at clinically relevant concentrations.

In vitro studies indicate that ibrutinib may inhibit P-glycoprotein (P-gp) and breast cancer resistance protein (BCRP) transport at clinically relevant concentrations. In vitro studies suggest that ibrutinib is not a substrate of P-gp or BCRP.

● Drugs and Foods Affecting Hepatic Microsomal Enzymes

Inhibitors of CYP3A

Concomitant use of ibrutinib with strong or moderate inhibitors of CYP3A may result in increased plasma concentrations of ibrutinib and an increased risk of drug-related toxicity.

When the strong CYP3A inhibitor ketoconazole was administered concomitantly with ibrutinib, the peak plasma concentration and AUC of ibrutinib were increased by 29- and 24-fold, respectively.

With multiple dosing of the strong CYP3A inhibitor voriconazole concomitantly with ibrutinib, the peak plasma concentration and AUC of ibrutinib were increased by 6.7- and 5.7-fold, respectively.

Simulations suggest that the strong CYP3A inhibitor posaconazole may increase the AUC of ibrutinib by threefold to tenfold under fed conditions.

With repeated dosing of the moderate CYP3A inhibitor erythromycin concomitantly with ibrutinib, the peak plasma concentration and AUC of ibrutinib were increased by 3.4- and 3-fold, respectively.

If concomitant use of the strong CYP3A inhibitor posaconazole or voriconazole or a moderate CYP3A inhibitor is required, reduce the daily dosage of ibrutinib as recommended in Table 4 in the "Dosage" section. Avoid concomitant use of other strong CYP3A inhibitors; interrupt ibrutinib therapy if these inhibitors will be used short-term (e.g., anti-infectives for ≤7 days).

Avoid grapefruit products and Seville oranges during ibrutinib therapy since they are known to contain strong or moderate inhibitors of CYP3A.

Inducers of CYP3A

Concomitant use of ibrutinib with strong inducers of CYP3A may result in decreased plasma concentrations of ibrutinib.

Administration of the strong CYP3A inducer rifampin concomitantly with ibrutinib reduced the peak plasma concentration and AUC of ibrutinib by more than 13- and 10-fold, respectively. Other simulations suggest that the moderate CYP3A inducer efavirenz may decrease the AUC of ibrutinib by threefold.

Avoid concomitant use of ibrutinib with strong CYP3A inducers.

● Substrates of Efflux Transport Systems

Concomitant use of ibrutinib with oral drugs that are substrates of P-gp or BCRP (e.g., digoxin, methotrexate) may result in increased concentrations of the substrate drug.

● Anticoagulants and Antiplatelet Agents

Use of anticoagulant or antiplatelet agents concomitantly with ibrutinib increases risk of hemorrhagic events. Monitor patients for bleeding manifestations.

DESCRIPTION

Ibrutinib is a selective, irreversible inhibitor of Bruton's tyrosine kinase (BTK); the drug is an antineoplastic agent. BTK, a member of the tyrosine protein kinase (Tec) family of kinases, is positioned early within the B-cell antigen receptor (BCR) signaling pathway. BCR is involved in the initiation of various cascades of intracellular signaling events, including activation of BTK, which leads to cell proliferation, differentiation, apoptosis, and cell migration essential for the development and survival of normal and malignant B-cells. Ibrutinib binds covalently to the active site of the tyrosine kinase BTK and irreversibly inhibits phosphorylation of tyrosine kinase, resulting in inhibition of downstream effector activity within the BCR signaling pathway.

In vitro kinase assays also have shown that ibrutinib inhibits (with up to tenfold less activity) the activity of several other receptor tyrosine kinases, including Bmx/Etk, epidermal growth factor receptor (EGFR), and members of the Src family of tyrosine kinases (e.g., Hck, Yes). In vivo, ibrutinib inhibits the proliferation and survival of malignant B-cells. The drug also has demonstrated cell migration and substrate adhesion in vitro; the mobilization of cells from tissues to peripheral blood results in a transient increase in absolute lymphocyte count (lymphocytosis) in the peripheral blood.

When given in a single dose of 1680 mg (3 times the maximum recommended daily dosage), ibrutinib did not prolong the QT interval to any clinically relevant extent. In vitro, the 50% inhibitory concentration of ibrutinib for collagen-induced platelet aggregation is 2026 ng/mL in blood samples from healthy donors, 1321 ng/mL in those with severe renal dysfunction, and 352 ng/mL in those taking warfarin. Clinically meaningful inhibition of adenosine diphosphate (ADP), arachidonic acid, ristocetin, and thrombin receptor agonist peptide-6 (TRAP-6) by ibrutinib have not been demonstrated.

Following oral administration of ibrutinib in healthy, fasting individuals, the absolute bioavailability of the drug was 2.9%. Ibrutinib is absorbed after oral administration with a median time to peak plasma concentration of 1–2 hours. Systemic exposure of ibrutinib increases with doses up to 840 mg in patients with B-cell malignancies. Following repeated doses of ibrutinib 420 mg daily, steady-state concentrations of the drug were achieved in 1 week and the accumulation ratio for the drug was 1–1.6. Administration of ibrutinib with a high-fat, high-calorie meal (800–1000 calories with fat accounting for approximately 50% of caloric content) resulted in an approximately twofold to fourfold increase in peak plasma concentrations and an approximately twofold increase in systemic exposure, compared with administration following overnight fasting.

Ibrutinib is metabolized to several metabolites by the cytochrome P-450 (CYP) microsomal enzyme system, principally by the isoenzyme 3A and to a minor extent by isoenzyme 2D6. The active metabolite, PCI-45227 (a dihydrodiol metabolite), has demonstrated BTK inhibition approximately 15 times less than that of ibrutinib. In vitro, ibrutinib is 97.3% bound to plasma proteins. Following administration of a single radiolabeled dose of ibrutinib, 80% of the dose was recovered in feces and <10% was recovered in urine; unchanged drug accounted for 1% of the dose recovered in feces. The elimination half-life of ibrutinib is 4–6 hours. The pharmacokinetics of ibrutinib do not appear to be affected by age or sex.

ADVICE TO PATIENTS

- Advise patients and caregivers to read the FDA-approved patient labeling (patient information and instructions for use).

- Advise patients to take ibrutinib as directed by their clinician and at approximately the same time each day. If a dose is missed, administer missed dose on the same day as soon as it is remembered, and resume normal schedule the following day. Advise patients not to take extra doses on the same day to make up for a missed dose.

- Instruct patients or caregivers to read and follow the instructions for use for proper preparation, administration, storage, and disposal of ibrutinib oral suspension.

- Advise patients to take ibrutinib capsules or tablets orally with a glass of water; do not open, break, or chew capsules or cut, crush, or chew tablets.

- Advise patients of the risk of bleeding. Inform clinician of any episodes of unusual bleeding (e.g., severe headache, blood in stool or urine, prolonged or uncontrolled bleeding). Notify clinician of any planned surgeries, including dental procedures.

- Advise patients of the risk of serious infection. Report signs or symptoms of possible infection (e.g., chills, fever, weakness, confusion).

- Advise patients of the risk of cardiac arrhythmias, cardiac failure, and sudden death. Inform clinician if palpitations, lightheadedness, dizziness, fainting, shortness of breath, edema, or chest discomfort occurs.

- Advise patients of the risk of hypertension, which may require antihypertensive therapy.

- Advise patients of the possible risk of developing a second primary malignancy (e.g., skin cancer).

- Advise patients of the risk of tumor lysis syndrome. Report signs or symptoms of tumor lysis syndrome (e.g., arrhythmia, seizure).

- Advise patients of the risk of diarrhea. Advise patients to maintain adequate hydration during ibrutinib therapy. Inform clinician if diarrhea persists.

- Inform patients that liver problems may develop during therapy. Advise patients to contact their clinician immediately if they experience abdominal discomfort, dark urine, or jaundice.

- Advise patients of the risk of fetal harm. Advise females to inform their clinician if they are or plan to become pregnant or plan to breast-feed. Apprise patients of potential hazard to the fetus if ibrutinib is used during pregnancy. Advise females of reproductive potential, and males with female partners of reproductive potential, to use effective contraception during ibrutinib therapy and for 1 month after discontinuance of therapy.

- Due to potential adverse events to the breast-fed child, advise females to not breast-feed during ibrutinib treatment and for 1 week after discontinuation of therapy.

- Inform clinicians of existing or contemplated concomitant therapy, including prescription and OTC drugs and dietary or herbal supplements, as well as any concomitant illnesses. Advise patients not to consume grapefruit or Seville oranges.

- Inform patients of other important precautionary information.

PREPARATIONS

Ibrutinib can only be obtained through designated specialty pharmacies. Contact the manufacturer or consult the Imbruvica website (https://www.imbruvicahcp .com/cll/support-and-resources/prescribing-resources) for specific availability information.

Excipients in commercially available drug preparations may have clinically important effects in some individuals; consult specific product labeling for details.

Ibrutinib

Oral		
Capsules	70 mg	Imbruvica®, Pharmacyclics (comarketed by Janssen Biotech)
	140 mg	Imbruvica®, Pharmacyclics (comarketed by Janssen Biotech)
Tablets	140 mg	Imbruvica®, Pharmacyclics (comarketed by Janssen Biotech)
	280 mg	Imbruvica®, Pharmacyclics (comarketed by Janssen Biotech)
	420 mg	Imbruvica®, Pharmacyclics (comarketed by Janssen Biotech)
Oral Suspension	70 mg/mL	Imbruvica®, Pharmacyclics (comarketed by Janssen Biotech)

† Use is not currently included in the labeling approved by the US Food and Drug Administration.

Selected Revisions July 10, 2024, © Copyright, September 28, 2015, American Society of Health-System Pharmacists, Inc.

Imatinib Mesylate

10:00 • ANTINEOPLASTIC AGENTS

■ Imatinib mesylate, an inhibitor of Bcr-Abl tyrosine kinase, is an antineo-plastic agent.

USES

• Philadelphia Chromosome-Positive Chronic Myelogenous Leukemia

Imatinib is used for the treatment of Philadelphia chromosome-positive (Ph⁺) chronic myelogenous leukemia (CML) in adult and pediatric patients. Imatinib is designated an orphan drug by FDA for use in this condition.

Adult Patients

First-line Therapy for Chronic Phase CML

Imatinib is used for the first-line treatment of chronic phase Ph⁺ CML in adult patients.

The indication for this use is based on the results of an open-label, multicenter, randomized phase 3 trial in 1,106 patients receiving either imatinib or combination therapy with interferon alfa and cytarabine for newly diagnosed chronic phase Ph⁺ CML. Single-agent therapy consisted of imatinib at an initial dose of 400 mg daily with dose escalations to 600 mg daily and 800 mg daily as tolerated. Combination therapy consisted of interferon alfa 5 million units/m² given subcutaneously daily with cytarabine 20 mg/m² given subcutaneously daily for 10 days every month. Crossover therapy was permitted if treatment failure or unacceptable toxicity occurred. The patients were mostly Caucasian (59% males and 41% females) with a median age of 51 years.

At the time of data cut-off, the median duration of first-line therapy with imatinib or combination therapy with interferon alfa and cytarabine was 82 or 8 months, respectively. The primary efficacy endpoint was progression-free survival, and progression was defined as death, progression to accelerated phase or blast phase CML, loss of complete hematologic response, loss of major cytogenetic response, or increasing WBC count in patients who did not achieve complete hematologic response. According to the intention-to-treat analysis, the estimated rate of progression-free survival at 84 months was higher in patients receiving imatinib (81.2%) than in those receiving interferon alfa and cytarabine (60.6%). The estimated rate of patients free of progression to accelerated phase CML or blast crisis at 84 months was higher in patients receiving imatinib (92.5%) than in those receiving interferon alfa and cytarabine (85.1%); however, no statistically significant difference in overall survival was observed (hazard ratio: 0.75 with 95% confidence interval of 0.547–1.028).

In patients who achieved complete cytogenetic response and major molecular response (a reduction of at least 3 logarithms in the amount of Bcr-Abl transcripts measured by quantitative reverse transcriptase polymerase chain reaction) at 12 months, the probability of remaining progression free at 60 months was 95%. In patients who achieved complete cytogenetic response, but not major molecular response, the probability of remaining progression free at 60 months was 89% and for those who did not achieve complete cytogenetic response, the probability was 70%. Secondary endpoints, including complete hematologic response and major cytogenetic response, were higher in patients receiving imatinib than in those receiving interferon alfa and cytarabine.

Second-line Therapy for CML

Imatinib mesylate is used for the treatment of Ph⁺ CML in patients who are in blast crisis, in the accelerated phase, or in the chronic phase of the disease after failure of interferon alfa therapy.

The current indication of imatinib is based principally on the results of 3 international, open-label, single-arm studies in more than 1000 patients with Ph⁺ CML. The first study enrolled patients in the chronic phase of CML previously treated with interferon alfa therapy (i.e., inadequate hematologic response following 6 months of treatment, inadequate cytogenetic response following 1 year of treatment, hematologic or cytogenetic relapse, or intolerance to interferon). The

second study enrolled patients who were in the accelerated phase of CML, while the third study enrolled patients in myeloid blast crisis. Patients chronic phase of CMLpreviously treated with interferon alfa received an initial imatinib dosage of 400 mg daily (increased to 600 mg daily as necessary), while those in accelerated phase or blast crisis received either 400 or 600 mg of the drug daily. The median duration of therapy with imatinib in patients in chronic phase, accelerated phase, or blast crisis was 29, 18, or 4 months, respectively. Among 532 patients with chronic phase CML following failure of interferon alfa therapy, hematologic response rate was 95% and major cytogenetic response rate was 60%. Among 235 patients with CML in accelerated phase, hematologic response rate was 71% and major cytogenetic response rate was 21%. Among 260 patients in myeloid blast crisis, hematologic response rate was 31% and major cytogenetic response was 7%.

Hematologic response (i.e., complete hematologic response and, in patients in accelerated phase or blast crisis, no evidence of leukemia or return to chronic phase of CML) was reported in 95, 71, or 31% of patients in the chronic phase, accelerated phase, or blast crisis, respectively; complete hematologic response was achieved in approximately 95, 38, or 7% of these patients, respectively. Major cytogenetic response (i.e., complete or partial suppression of Ph⁺ cells) occurred in 60, 21, or 7% of patients in the chronic phase, accelerated phase, or blast crisis, respectively, while complete cytogenetic response (i.e., no Ph⁺ cells in metaphase) was achieved in 39, 16, or 2% of these patients, respectively. The rates of hematologic response and major cytogenetic response were higher in patients in accelerated phase or blast crisis who received an initial dosage of 600 mg of imatinib daily compared with those who received an initial dosage of 400 mg daily.

Median time to hematologic response in patients receiving imatinib was 1 month; median duration of hematologic response was 10 months in patients in blast crisis and 29 months in those with accelerated phase CML receiving an initial dosage of imatinib 600 mg daily. About 88% of patients with late chronic phase CML and 64% of patients with accelerated phase CML maintained major cytogenetic response for 2 years. About 27% of patients with blast crisis who achieved an initial hematologic response to imatinib therapy maintained hematologic response for 2 years. In patients with late chronic phase CML who received imatinib therapy for 2 years, the estimated overall survival was 91%. In patients with accelerated CML, median survival was 21 months in patients receiving an initial imatinib dosage of 400 mg daily; median survival had not been reached in those receiving an initial imatinib dosage of 600 mg daily. In patients with blast crisis, median survival was 7 months.

Resistance to imatinib, particularly in patients with advanced stage CML, has developed during therapy with the drug. In patients with myeloid blast crisis, development of imatinib resistance was observed as early as 42 days following initiation of therapy. Resistance to imatinib has not been evaluated in all patient groups; however, limited data from several open-label studies indicate a relapse rate of 4 or 43–80% in patients in chronic phase or blast crisis, respectively. Although the mechanism(s) of resistance to imatinib has not been fully determined to date, mutation and/or amplification of the *Bcr-Abl* gene (resulting in increased expression of Bcr-Abl tyrosine kinase) may be associated with decreased efficacy of the drug.

Pediatric Patients

First-line Therapy for Chronic Phase CML

Imatinib is used for the first-line treatment of chronic phase Ph⁺ CML in pediatric patients.

Efficacy and safety for this indication are based on the results of an open-label, uncontrolled phase 2 trial in 51 pediatric patients receiving imatinib 340 mg/m² daily for newly diagnosed chronic phase Ph⁺ CML. After 8 weeks of imatinib therapy, complete hematologic response was observed in 78% of patients. The complete cytogenetic response rate (typically achieved between months 3 and 10) was 65%, which is comparable to the rate observed in adult patients; the majority of these patients achieved a complete cytogenetic response between month 3 and 10 with an estimated median time to response of 6.74 months. Patients were allowed to withdraw from protocol therapy to undergo alternative therapy, including hematopoietic stem cell transplantation; 31 children withdrew from protocol therapy and underwent stem cell transplantation. Among 25 patients who withdrew from protocol therapy to undergo stem cell transplantation following a median of 9 treatment cycles, 52 or 20% achieved complete or partial cytogenetic response, respectively.

Second-line Therapy for Chronic Phase CML

Imatinib is used for the second-line treatment of pediatric patients with chronic phase Ph[+] CML that has recurred following stem cell transplantation or is resistant to interferon alfa therapy.

The indication for this use is based on the results of 2 small uncontrolled studies in pediatric patients receiving imatinib as second-line therapy for chronic phase CML. In the first study, which involved 14 pediatric patients ranging in age from 3 to 20 years of age, a complete cytogenetic response was observed in 7 patients. In the second study, which involved 3 patients, a complete cytogenetic response was observed in 2 patients.

Clinical Perspective
Adult Patients: Chronic Phase CML

Some experts recommend dasatinib, imatinib, or nilotinib for the first-line treatment of chronic phase CML; selection of the tyrosine kinase inhibitor should be based on patient preference and factors such as age, comorbidities, and expected tolerability of therapy. Following confirmation of Bcr-Abl positivity, therapy with a tyrosine kinase inhibitor should be initiated immediately. The risk of transformation to advanced or blast phase disease is lower in Sokal non-low risk patients treated with dasatinib or nilotinib.

If treatment failure occurs during tyrosine kinase inhibitor therapy, a bone marrow biopsy should be performed to evaluate CML phase and clonal changes; therapy may be switched to an alternative tyrosine kinase inhibitor (e.g., bosutinib, dasatinib, imatinib, nilotinib, ponatinib), or stem cell transplantation may be considered.

● Philadelphia Chromosome-Positive Acute Lymphocytic Leukemia

Imatinib is used for the treatment of Ph[+] acute lymphocytic (lymphoblastic) leukemia (ALL) in adults following failure (secondary to resistance or intolerance) of prior therapy; the drug also is used in combination with chemotherapy for the treatment of pediatric patients at least 1 year of age with newly diagnosed Ph[+] ALL. Imatinib is designated an orphan drug by FDA for use in this condition.

Adult Patients
Relapsed or Refractory Ph[+] ALL

Imatinib is used for the treatment of adult patients with relapsed or refractory Ph[+] ALL. Safety and efficacy of imatinib for the treatment of ALL is based on 43 patients with relapsed or refractory Ph[+] ALL who received imatinib 600 mg daily in a phase 2 or study. Complete hematologic response was achieved in 19% of patients. Complete cytogenetic response and major cytogenetic response was achieved in 35 and 21%, respectively, of patients. No evidence of leukemia was observed in 12% of patients.

Pediatric Patients
Newly Diagnosed Ph[+] ALL

Imatinib is used in combination with chemotherapy for the treatment of newly diagnosed Ph[+] ALL in pediatric patients. Safety and efficacy of imatinib for the treatment of newly diagnosed Ph[+] ALL in pediatric patients is based principally on a multicenter, nonrandomized pilot study in pediatric and young adult patients with very high-risk ALL (defined as those with an expected 5-year event-free survival of less than 45%). Patients were enrolled in the study following induction therapy.

Pediatric patients in the Ph[+] ALL cohort who had an appropriate HLA-matched family donor received a minimum of 2 cycles of consolidation therapy followed by imatinib 340 mg/m[2] per day in combination with intensive chemotherapy and hematopoietic stem cell transplantation. The median age of 92 patients with Ph[+] ALL was 9.5 years (range of 1–21 years). In 5 successive cohorts of patients, imatinib exposure was systematically increased by earlier introduction and prolonged duration. Cohort 1 received the lowest intensity and cohort 5 received the highest intensity of imatinib exposure. Among 50 patients with Ph[+] ALL in cohort 5, 30 patients received chemotherapy and imatinib and 20 patients received chemotherapy and imatinib therapy followed by hematopoetic stem cell transplantation and imatinib maintenance therapy. Patients in cohort 5 received chemotherapy and imatinib continuously beginning on cycle 1 of post-induction chemotherapy; imatinib was continued through cycles 1–4 of maintenance

therapy. During cycles 5–12 of maintenance therapy, imatinib was administered for 28 days of a 56-day treatment cycle. Patients who underwent hematopoietic stem cell transplantation received 42 days of imatinib prior to transplantation, and 28 weeks (196 days) of imatinib after the immediate post-transplant period. At a median follow-up duration of 40.5 months, the estimated 4-year event-free survival was 70%.

Efficacy of imatinib also was evaluated in a phase 3, open-label trial in 189 pediatric patients with Ph[+] ALL. In this study, patients were randomized to receive imatinib or dasatinib as soon as diagnosis was made, usually on day 8 of remission induction. In this study, the median age of patients was 7.8 years (range of 5.2–11.3 years). Both 4-year event-free survival and overall survival rates were higher in patients receiving dasatinib compared with those receiving imatinib.

Clinical Perspective
Adult Patients: Relapsed or Refractory Ph[+] ALL

Although there is no universally accepted treatment protocol for the treatment of relapsed or refractory ALL and evidence based on randomised, controlled trials is lacking, there is consensus on the general approach to managing patients with relapsed or refractory ALL. Some experts recommend prolonged monitoring of Bcr-Abl transcript levels and resistance mutation screening in patients with persistent minimal residual disease or re-increasing minimal residual disease level; therapy with a second- or third-generation tyrosine kinase inhibitor should be offered to high risk patients with Ph[+] ALL. Patients with imatinib-refractory Ph[+] ALL may respond to nilotinib or dasatinib while patients with T315I Bcr-Abl mutation-positive Ph[+] ALL may respond to ponatinib therapy. Tyrosine kinase inhibitors have been shown to have a more favorable toxicity profile in elderly patients compared to repeated cycles of conventional myelosuppressive chemotherapy. Long-term survival has not been demonstrated with tyrosine kinase inhibitor therapy post-relapse; the majority of patients undergo allogeneic stem cell transplantation.

● Myelodysplastic/Myeloproliferative Diseases

Imatinib is used for the treatment of adult patients with myelodysplastic/myeloproliferative diseases (MDS/MPD) associated with platelet-derived growth factor receptor (PDGFR) gene rearrangements. Imatinib is designated an orphan drug by FDA for use in this condition.

Efficacy and safety of imatinib in patients with MDS/MPD is based principally on the results of an open-label, multicenter, phase 2 trial in patients with life-threatening diseases associated with Abl, c-Kit, or PDGFR protein tyrosine kinases. Seven patients with MDS/MPD received imatinib 400 mg daily. The age range of the 7 patients enrolled in this study was 20–86 years. The primary efficacy analysis also included published case reports and a clinical study of 24 patients with MDS/MPD between 2–79 years of age; most of these patients received imatinib 400 mg daily. In a pooled analysis of the 31 patients, complete hematologic response was reported in 45% of patients and major cytogenetic response was achieved in 39%. Among 16 patients with PDFGR gene rearrangement, 13 patients achieved complete hematologic response. Among 12 patients with PDGFR gene rearrangement evaluated for cytogenetic response, 10 patients achieved complete cytogenetic response. Among 14 patients without a chromosome translocation associated with PDGFR gene rearrangement, 1 patient achieved complete hematologic response.

● Systemic Mastocytosis

Imatinib is used for the treatment of adult patients with aggressive systemic mastocytosis (ASM) with unknown c-Kit mutation status or absence of a c-Kit D816V mutation. Imatinib is designated an orphan drug by FDA for use in this condition.

Efficacy and safety of imatinib in patients with ASM are based principally on the results of an open-label, multicenter, phase 2 trial in patients with life-threatening diseases associated with Abl, c-Kit, or PDGFR protein tyrosine kinases. Five patients with ASM were treated with imatinib 100–400 mg daily. The age range of the 5 patients enrolled in this study was 49–74 years. The primary efficacy analysis also included published literature and case reports of 23 patients with ASM who received imatinib 100–400 mg daily. In a combined analysis of the 28 patients, complete hematologic response was reported in 29% of patients. All 7 patients with FIP1L1-PDGFRα fusion kinase positive status achieved complete hematologic response while only 25% of those with a D816V mutation achieved a complete hematologic response.

Imatinib has not been shown to be effective in patients with less aggressive forms of systemic mastocytosis (SM); therefore, the manufacturer does *not* recommend imatinib for the treatment of cutaneous mastocytosis, indolent systemic mastocytosis (smoldering SM or isolated bone marrow mastocytosis), SM with an associated clonal hematological nonmast cell lineage disease, mast cell leukemia, mast cell sarcoma or extracutaneous mastocytoma.

Patients with SM harboring a *c-Kit* D816V mutation are not sensitive to imatinib; the manufacturer states that such patients should *not* receive imatinib.

Hypereosinophilic Syndrome and/or Chronic Eosinophilic Leukemia

Imatinib is used for the treatment of adult patients with hypereosinophilic syndrome (HES) and/or chronic eosinophilic leukemia (CEL) who have *FIP1L1-PDGFRα* fusion kinase (as detected by mutational analysis or CHIC2 allele deletion on FISH); the drug also is used in patients with HES and/or CEL with unknown or negative *FIP1L1-PDGFRα* fusion kinase status. Imatinib is designated an orphan drug by FDA for use in this condition.

Efficacy and safety of imatinib in patients with HES/CEL are based principally on the results of an open-label, multicenter, phase 2 trial in patients with life-threatening diseases associated with Abl, c-Kit, or PDGFR protein tyrosine kinases. Fourteen patients with HES/CEL were treated with imatinib 100 mg to 1 g daily. The age range of the 14 patients enrolled in this study was 16–64 years. The primary efficacy analysis also included published case reports and case series of 162 patients with HES/CEL who received imatinib 75–800 mg daily. In a combined analysis of the 176 patients, complete hematologic response was reported in 61% of patients. All 61 patients with *FIP1L1-PDGFRα* fusion kinase positive status achieved complete hematologic response.

Soft Tissue Sarcoma

Imatinib is used for the treatment of adult patients with unresectable, recurrent and/or metastatic dermatofibrosarcoma protuberans. Imatinib is designated an orphan drug by FDA for use in this condition.

Efficacy and safety of imatinib in patients with dermatofibrosarcoma protuberans are based principally on the results of an open-label, multicenter, phase 2 trial in patients with severe diseases associated with Abl, c-Kit, or PDGFR protein tyrosine kinases. Twelve patients with dermatofibrosarcoma protuberans were treated with imatinib 800 mg daily. The age range of the 12 patients enrolled in this study was 23–75 years. The primary efficacy analysis also included published case reports of 6 patients with dermatofibrosarcoma protuberans who received varying dosages of imatinib. In a combined analysis of the 18 patients, complete response was achieved in 39% of patients. Among 10 patients with *PDGF-β* gene rearrangement, 4 patients achieved complete responses. The median duration of response in the phase 2 study was 6.2 months, with a maximum duration of 24.3 months, while the duration of response was 4 weeks to more than 20 months in published literature.

Gastrointestinal Stromal Tumors

Adjuvant Therapy

Imatinib is used for the adjuvant treatment of *c-Kit* (CD117) positive gastrointestinal stromal tumors (GIST) following complete resection. Imatinib is designated an orphan drug by FDA for use in this condition. The indication for this use is based on the results of 2 multicenter, randomized studies.

In a multicenter, double-blind, placebo-controlled, randomized study, 713 patients were randomized to receive imatinib 400 mg daily or placebo for 12 months. Patients were included in the study if they had a histologic diagnosis of primary GIST expressing c-Kit protein by immunochemistry and complete gross resection (tumor size ≥3 cm in maximum dimension) 14–70 days prior to study enrollment. At median follow-up duration of 15 months in patients without a recurrence-free survival event, the risk of recurrence or death from any cause was decreased by 61%. After the interim analysis, 72 of 354 patients initially randomized to placebo crossed over to the imatinib treatment group. In an updated analysis at a median follow-up duration of 50 months, the risk of recurrence or death was decreased by 28%. At a median follow-up duration of 61 months, the risk of death was decreased by 19%; however, statistical significance was not reached.

In another randomized, multicenter, open-label, phase 3 trial, imatinib 400 mg daily was evaluated in 397 adult patients with *c-Kit* (CD117) positive GIST following surgical resection. At a median follow-up duration of 42 months in patients without a recurrence-free survival event, imatinib therapy for a duration of 36 months significantly prolonged recurrence-free survival compared with 12 months of therapy (hazard ratio 0.46). At a median follow-up duration of 48 months for living patients, imatinib therapy for a duration of 36 months significantly prolonged overall survival compared 12 months of therapy (hazard ratio 0.45).

Advanced GIST

Imatinib is used for the treatment of malignant GIST in patients with unresectable tumor or metastatic disease that is *c-Kit* (CD117) positive. This indication is based on objective response rate; there currently are no controlled trials demonstrating a clinical benefit (e.g., reduced disease-related symptoms, increased survival).

Efficacy and safety of this indication are based on the results of 2 open-label, multinational, phase 3 studies and a phase 2 study.

In the phase 3 studies, 1640 patients received either imatinib 400 mg daily or imatinib 800 mg daily continuously until disease progression or unacceptable toxicity occurred. Patients randomized to imatinib 400 mg daily were permitted to crossover to receive imatinib 800 mg daily upon disease progression. All patients enrolled in the studies had *c-Kit* (CD117) positive unresectable and/or metastatic malignant GIST. At a combined median follow-up duration of 37.5 months, median progression-free survival was 18.9 or 23.2 months in patients receiving imatinib 400 or 800 mg daily, respectively. No difference in overall survival was observed between the treatment groups.

In the phase 2 study, 147 patients received either imatinib 400 or 600 mg daily for up to 36 months for unresectable or metastatic malignant GIST. The objective response rate was 68.5 or 67.6% in patients who received imatinib 400 mg daily or 600 mg daily, respectively. The median time to response was 12 weeks and the estimated median duration of response was 118 weeks. The study was not designed with adequate power to detect a statistically significant difference in response rates between the dose groups.

Other Uses

Imatinib has also been evaluated for the treatment of bone cancer†, desmoid tumors†, AIDS-related Kaposi sarcoma†, melanoma†, pigmented villonodular synovitis/tenosynovial giant cell tumor†.

DOSAGE AND ADMINISTRATION

General

Pretreatment Screening

- Complete blood cell count (CBC).
- Baseline liver and renal function.
- Consider performing an echocardiogram and determining serum troponin concentrations in patients with hypereosinophilic syndrome (HES) and/or chronic eosinophilic leukemia (CEL), and in patients with myelodysplastic/myeloproliferative diseases or aggressive systemic mastocytosis associated with high eosinophil levels. If results of the echocardiogram or serum troponin concentrations are abnormal, consider prophylactic use of systemic corticosteroids.
- Verify pregnancy status in females of reproductive potential.

Patient Monitoring

- Monitor for signs or symptoms of fluid retention (e.g., weight gain) regularly during therapy.
- Monitor CBC weekly for the first month of therapy, every other week during the second month, and periodically (e.g., every 2–3 months) thereafter as clinically indicated.
- Carefully monitor patients with cardiac disease or risk factors for cardiac disease for signs and symptoms of cardiac toxicity or renal failure.
- Carefully monitor patients with a history of renal failure for signs and symptoms of cardiac toxicity or renal failure.
- Monitor liver function monthly or as clinically indicated during therapy.
- Monitor renal function during therapy.

- Monitor serum TSH concentrations in patients receiving levothyroxine replacement therapy following thyroidectomy.
- In pediatric patients, monitor bone growth and development.
- Monitor patients with high tumor burden or those with a high proliferative rate for tumor lysis syndrome.

Premedication and Prophylaxis

- In patients with HES and/or CEL, myelodysplastic/myeloproliferative diseases, or aggressive systemic mastocytosis associated with high eosinophil levels, and an abnormal echocardiogram or serum troponin concentrations, consider prophylaxis with systemic corticosteroids (1–2 mg/kg) for 1–2 weeks concomitantly with imatinib therapy at the time of initiation of therapy to reduce risk of hypereosinophilic cardiac toxicity.

Dispensing and Administration Precautions

Handling and Disposal

- Consult specialized references for procedures for proper handling (e.g., use of gloves) and disposal of antineoplastics.
- Avoid direct contact of crushed tablets with the skin or mucous membranes. If such contact occurs, wash affected area thoroughly according to specialized references for procedures for proper handling of antineoplastics.

● Administration

Administer imatinib mesylate orally.

In adults, an imatinib dosage of 400 or 600 mg should be administered once daily and a dosage of 800 mg daily should be administered as 400 mg twice daily using the 400-mg tablet to reduce exposure to iron.

In children or adolescents, imatinib may be given as a once-daily dose or, alternatively, divide the daily dose equally in the morning and the evening.

Administer imatinib mesylate with a meal and a large glass of water to minimize gastric irritation. Alternatively, for patients unable to swallow tablets, imatinib tablets may be dispersed in a glass of water or apple juice. The required number of tablets should be dispersed in 50 mL of beverage for each 100-mg tablet or 200 mL of beverage for each 400-mg tablet. Administer suspension immediately after complete disintegration of the tablet(s).

The manufacturer states that imatinib therapy may be continued as indicated in the absence of progressive disease or unacceptable toxicity.

If a dose of imatinib is missed, the prescribed dose should be taken at the next scheduled time; an additional dose should not be administered to replace the missed dose.

Store imatinib capsules at 20–25°C; excursions between 15–30°C are permitted.

● Dosage

Dosage of imatinib mesylate is expressed in terms of imatinib.

Chronic Myelogenous Leukemia

Adult Patients

First- or second-line treatment of Ph⁺ chronic phase CML: The recommended initial adult dosage of imatinib for the first-line treatment of Ph⁺ chronic phase CML is 400 mg daily. If there is inadequate hematologic response after at least 3 months of therapy, failure to achieve a cytogenetic response after 6–12 months of therapy, loss of a previously achieved hematologic or cytogenetic response, or evidence of disease progression, the manufacturer states that, in the absence of severe adverse drug or hematologic effects, adult dosage of imatinib may be increased to 600 mg daily.

Second-line treatment of Ph⁺ CML in accelerated phase or blast crisis: The recommended adult dosage of imatinib for the second-line treatment of Ph⁺ CML in accelerated phase or blast crisis is 600 mg daily. If there is inadequate hematologic response after at least 3 months of therapy, failure to achieve a cytogenetic response after 6–12 months of therapy, loss of a previously achieved hematologic or cytogenetic response, or evidence of disease progression, the manufacturer states that, in the absence of severe adverse drug or hematologic effects, adult

dosage of imatinib may be increased to 800 mg daily (administered as 400 mg twice daily).

Pediatric Patients

The recommended pediatric dosage of imatinib for the first-line treatment of Ph⁺ chronic phase CML is 340 mg/m² daily; the daily dose should not exceed 600 mg. Imatinib may be administered as a once-daily dose or twice-daily in 2 equally divided doses.

Safety and efficacy of imatinib therapy has not been established in pediatric patients less than 1 year of age with Ph⁺ chronic phase CML.

Acute Lymphocytic Leukemia

Adult Patients

For the treatment of relapsed or refractory Ph⁺ ALL, the recommended adult dosage of imatinib is 600 mg daily.

Pediatric Patients

For the treatment of newly diagnosed Ph⁺ ALL in combination with chemotherapy in children 1 year of age or older, the recommended pediatric dosage of imatinib is 340 mg/m² daily; the daily dose should not exceed 600 mg. Imatinib may be administered as a once-daily dose or twice-daily in 2 equally divided doses.

Myelodysplastic Syndrome/Myeloproliferative Diseases

For the treatment of myelodysplastic syndrome or myeloproliferative disease associated with gene rearrangements of *PDGFR*, the recommended adult dosage of imatinib is 400 mg daily.

Aggressive Systemic Mastocytosis

For the treatment of aggressive systemic mastocytosis (ASM) without the D816V *c-Kit* mutation, the recommended adult dosage of imatinib is 400 mg daily. For ASM with unknown status of the D816V *c-Kit* mutation that is not responding satisfactorily to other therapies, treatment with an adult imatinib dosage of 400 mg daily may be considered. For ASM without the D816V *c-Kit* mutation or of unknown D816V *c-Kit* mutational status that is associated with eosinophilia (a clonal hematologic disease related to the *FIP1L1-PDGFRα* fusion kinase), the recommended initial adult dosage of imatinib is 100 mg daily; if therapeutic response is insufficient, the dosage may be escalated from 100 mg to 400 mg as tolerated.

Hypereosinophilic Syndrome/Chronic Eosinophilic Leukemia

For the treatment of hypereosinophilic syndrome (HES) or chronic eosinophilic leukemia (CEL) in patients without *FIP1L1-PDGFRα* fusion kinase expression or in patients in whom expression of *FIP1L1-PDGFRα* fusion kinase is unknown, the recommended adult dosage of imatinib is 400 mg daily. For HES or CEL with *FIP1L1-PDGFRα* fusion kinase expression, the recommended initial adult dosage of imatinib is 100 mg daily; if therapeutic response is insufficient, the dosage may be escalated from 100 to 400 mg as tolerated.

Dermatofibrosarcoma Protuberans

For unresectable, recurrent, and/or metastatic dermatofibrosarcoma protuberans, the recommended adult dosage of imatinib is 800 mg daily.

Gastrointestinal Stromal Tumors

Unresectable and/or metastatic malignant GIST: The recommended adult dosage of imatinib is 400 mg daily for the treatment of unresectable and/or metastatic malignant GIST; if therapeutic response is insufficient, the dosage may be increased to 800 mg daily as tolerated.

Adjuvant therapy: The recommended adult dosage of imatinib is 400 mg daily for the adjuvant treatment of GIST following complete gross resection.

Dosage Modification for Toxicity

Hepatic Toxicity

Adults: In patients who exhibit substantial increases in bilirubin (more than 3 times the upper limit of normal [ULN]) or aminotransferase concentrations (more than 5 times the ULN), the manufacturer recommends withholding imatinib therapy until bilirubin concentrations decrease to less than 1.5 times the ULN or aminotransferase concentrations decrease to less than 2.5 times the ULN. Imatinib therapy may then be resumed at a reduced daily dosage (e.g., 400 mg to 300 mg, 600 mg to 400 mg, or 800 mg to 600 mg).

Pediatric patients: In pediatric patients who exhibit substantial increases in bilirubin (more than 3 times the ULN) or hepatic aminotransferase concentrations (more than 5 times the ULN), the manufacturer recommends that therapy with imatinib be withheld until bilirubin concentrations decrease to less than 1.5 times the ULN or aminotransferase concentrations decrease to less than 2.5 times the ULN. Imatinib therapy may then be resumed at a dosage reduced from 340 mg/m^2 daily to 260 mg/m^2 daily.

Hematologic Toxicity

If hematologic toxicity occurs, dosing interruption, dosage reduction, or discontinuance of imatinib therapy may be necessary in adults (see Table 1) and pediatric patients (see Table 2).

TABLE 1. Adults: Dosage Adjustments for Hematologic Toxicity

Use (Initial Dosage)	Hematologic Measurements	Dosage Modification
Aggressive systemic mastocytosis (initial starting dosage = 400 mg daily)	ANC <1000/mm³ and/or platelets <50,000/mm³	First occurrence: Withhold therapy until ANC ≥1500/mm³ and platelet count ≥75,000/mm³, then resume at original starting dosage (400 mg daily) Second occurrence: Withhold therapy until ANC ≥1500/mm³ and/or platelet count ≥75,000/mm³, then resume at a reduced dosage of 300 mg daily
Aggressive systemic mastocytosis associated with eosinophilia (initial starting dosage = 100 mg daily)	ANC <1000/mm³ and/or platelets <50,000/mm³	Withhold therapy until ANC ≥1500/mm³ and platelet count ≥75,000/mm³, resume at same dosage
Hypereosinophilic syndrome/chronic eosinophilic leukemia without FIP1L1-PDGFRα fusion kinase expression or unknown FIP1L1-PDG-FRα status (initial starting dosage = 400 mg)	ANC <1000/mm³ and/or platelets <50,000/mm³	First occurrence: Withhold therapy until ANC ≥1500/mm³ and platelet count ≥75,000/mm³, then resume at original starting dosage (400 mg daily) Second occurrence: Withhold therapy until ANC ≥1500/mm³ and/or platelet count ≥75,000/mm³, then resume at a reduced dosage of 300 mg daily
Hypereosinophilic syndrome/chronic eosinophilic leukemia with FIP1L1-PDGFRα fusion kinase (initial starting dosage = 100 mg daily)	ANC <1000/mm³ and/or platelets <50,000/mm³	Withhold therapy until ANC ≥1500/mm³ and platelet count ≥75,000/mm³, resume at same dosage
Chronic phase CML (initial starting dosage = 400 mg daily)	ANC <1000/mm³ and/or platelets <50,000/mm³	First occurrence: Withhold therapy until ANC ≥1500/mm³ and platelet count ≥75,000/mm³, then resume at original starting dosage (400 mg daily) Second occurrence: Withhold therapy until ANC ≥1500/mm³ and/or platelet count ≥75,000/mm³, then resume at a reduced dosage of 300 mg daily

TABLE 1. Continued

Use (Initial Dosage)	Hematologic Measurements	Dosage Modification
Myelodysplastic syndrome/myeloproliferative Diseases (initial starting dosage = 400 mg daily)	ANC <1000/mm³ and/or platelets <50,000/mm³	First occurrence: Withhold therapy until ANC ≥1500/mm³ and platelet count ≥75,000/mm³, then resume at original starting dosage (400 mg daily) Second occurrence: Withhold therapy until ANC ≥1500/mm³ and/or platelet count ≥75,000/mm³, then resume at a reduced dosage of 300 mg daily
GIST (initial starting dosage = 400 mg daily)	ANC <1000/mm³ and/or platelets <50,000/mm³	First occurrence: Withhold therapy until ANC ≥1500/mm³ and platelet count ≥75,000/mm³, then resume at original starting dosage (400 mg daily) Second occurrence: Withhold therapy until ANC ≥1500/mm³ and/or platelet count ≥75,000/mm³, then resume at a reduced dosage of 300 mg daily
Ph⁺ CML in accelerated phase or blast crisis (initial starting dosage = 600 mg daily)	ANC <500/mm³ and/or platelets <10,000/mm³ and unrelated to CML	Reduce dosage to 400 mg daily If cytopenia persists for 2 weeks, further reduce dosage to 300 mg daily If cytopenia persists for 4 weeks, withhold subsequent doses until ANC ≥1000/mm³ and platelet counts ≥20,000/mm³, then resume therapy at a reduced dosage of 300 mg daily
Ph⁺ ALL (initial starting dosage = 600 mg daily)	ANC <500/mm³ and/or platelets <10,000/mm³ and unrelated to ALL	Reduce dosage to 400 mg daily If cytopenia persists for 2 weeks, reduce dosage further to 300 mg daily If cytopenia persists for 4 weeks, withhold subsequent doses until ANC ≥1000/mm³ and platelet counts ≥20,000/mm³, then resume therapy at a reduced dosage of 300 mg daily
Dermatofibrosarcoma protuberans (initial starting dosage = 800 mg daily)	ANC <1000/mm³ and/or platelets <50,000/mm³	First occurrence: Withhold therapy until ANC ≥1500/mm³ and platelet count ≥75,000/mm³, then resume therapy at a reduced dosage of 600 mg Second occurrence: Withhold therapy until ANC ≥1500/mm³ and platelet count ≥75,000/mm³, then resume at a reduced dosage of 400 mg daily

TABLE 2. Pediatric Patients ≥1 Year of Age: Dosage Modification for Hematologic Toxicity

Use	Absolute Neutrophil Count (ANC) and/or Platelet Count	Dosage Modification
Newly diagnosed chronic phase CML (initial starting dosage = 340 mg/m²)	ANC <1000/mm³ and/or platelets <50,000/mm³	First occurrence: Withhold therapy until ANC ≥1500/mm³ and platelet count ≥75,000/mm³, then resume at same dosage
		Second occurrence: Withhold therapy until ANC ≥1500/mm³ and platelet count ≥75,000/mm³, then resume at a reduced dosage of 260 mg/m²

Nonhematologic Toxicity

If severe nonhematologic toxicity (e.g., severe fluid retention) develops, withhold therapy until the toxicity resolves, then resume therapy as appropriate.

Concomitant Use of Drugs Affecting Hepatic Microsomal Enzymes

Avoid concomitant use with potent CYP3A4 inducers. If concomitant use of a potent CYP3A4 inducer cannot be avoided, the manufacturer recommends increasing the imatinib dosage by at least 50%. Carefully monitor clinical response.

● Special Populations

Hepatic Impairment

In patients with mild to moderate hepatic impairment, no dosage adjustment is necessary.

In patients with severe hepatic impairment, the manufacturer recommends reducing the dosage by 25%.

Renal Impairment

In patients with mild renal impairment (creatinine clearance 40–59 mL/minute), the daily dosage should not exceed 600 mg.

In patients with moderate renal impairment (creatinine clearance 20–39 mL/minute), decrease initial dosage by 50%; subsequent dosage may be increased as tolerated up to a maximum dosage of 400 mg.

In patients with severe renal impairment, use imatinib with caution. An imatinib dosage of 100 mg daily has been tolerated in 2 patients with severe renal impairment.

Geriatric Patients

The manufacturer makes no specific dosage recommendations for geriatric patients.

CAUTIONS

● Contraindications

● None.

● Warnings/Precautions

Fluid Retention and Edema

Edema, occasionally serious, may occur in patients receiving imatinib. The risk of edema was increased in patients older than 65 years of age and those receiving higher imatinib dosages. Severe superficial edema was reported in 1.5% of patients with newly diagnosed CML and in 2–6% of other adult patients with CML. Other types of severe fluid retention were reported (e.g., pleural effusion, pericardial effusion, pulmonary edema, ascites) in imatinib-treated patients with newly diagnosed CML (1.3%), and in other adult patients with CML (2–6%). In patients with

GIST, severe fluid retention was reported in 9–13% of imatinib-treated patients. In a randomized trial, severe (grade 3 or 4) fluid retention occurred in 2.5% of patients with newly diagnosed Ph⁺ chronic phase CML receiving imatinib and in 3.9% of patients receiving nilotinib 300 mg twice daily. Effusions (i.e., pleural effusion, pericardial effusion, ascites) or pulmonary edema have been observed in 2.1% of patients receiving imatinib and in 2.2% of those receiving nilotinib 300 mg twice daily.

Monitor signs (e.g., body weight) and symptoms of fluid retention regularly during imatinib therapy; provide appropriate treatment as necessary.

Hematologic Effects

Cytopenias, including neutropenia, thrombocytopenia, and anemia, have occurred in patients receiving imatinib. In patients with CML, the frequency of cytopenias is dependent on the stage of disease (higher incidence in patients with accelerated phase or blast crisis CML). In pediatric patients receiving imatinib for the treatment of CML, grade 3 or 4 neutropenia, thrombocytopenia, and anemia were the most common toxicities. Monitor complete blood cell counts (CBCs) weekly during the first month of therapy, every other week during the second month, and periodically (e.g., every 2–3 months) thereafter as clinically indicated.

Cardiovascular Effects

● Congestive Heart Failure and Left Ventricular Dysfunction

Congestive heart failure and left ventricular dysfunction have been reported during imatinib therapy, mostly in geriatric patients or patients with a history of cardiac disease. In an international randomized phase 3 study in 1106 patients with newly diagnosed Ph⁺ chronic phase CML, severe cardiac failure and left ventricular dysfunction were observed in 0.7% of patients receiving imatinib compared to 0.9% of patients receiving interferon alfa and cytarabine. In another randomized trial evaluating imatinib in patients with newly diagnosed chronic phase Ph⁺ CML, cardiac failure was observed in 1.1% of patients receiving imatinib and 2.2% of patients receiving nilotinib 300 mg twice daily; severe (grade 3 or 4) cardiac failure occurred in 0.7% of patients in each treatment group.

Carefully monitor patients with cardiac disease, risk factors for cardiac disease, or a history of renal failure. Evaluate and treat any patient with manifestations of cardiac or renal failure.

● Hypereosinophilic Cardiac Toxicity

In patients with hypereosinophilic syndrome (HES) with occult infiltration of hypereosinophilic syndrome cells within the myocardium, cases of cardiogenic shock/left ventricular dysfunction, cardiogenic shock have been associated with HES cell degranulation upon initiation of imatinib therapy. The condition has been reversed following administration of systemic corticosteroids, circulatory support measures, and temporary interruption of imatinib therapy.

Patients with elevated eosinophil concentrations are at increased risk for hypereosinophilic cardiac toxicity associated with imatinib. Test patients with myelodysplastic syndrome (MDS)/myeloproliferative disease (MPD) or aggressive systemic mastocytosis (ASM) for elevated eosinophil concentrations. Perform an echocardiogram and measure serum troponin concentrations in patients with elevated eosinophil concentrations, including patients with hypereosinophilic syndrome/chronic eosinophilic leukemia, MDS/MPD, or ASM associated with high eosinophil concentrations. If the results of the echocardiogram or serum troponin concentrations are abnormal, consider the use of prophylactic therapy with systemic corticosteroids upon initiation of imatinib therapy.

Hepatic Effects

Hepatotoxicity, sometimes severe, has been reported in patients receiving imatinib. Fatal hepatic failure and severe hepatic injury requiring transplant have been reported with short- and long-term use. When imatinib is used in combination with chemotherapy, elevations in aminotransferase concentrations, hyperbilirubinemia, and acute hepatic failure have been reported.

Monitor liver function tests (i.e., aminotransferase, bilirubin, alkaline phosphatase) prior to initiation of therapy and monthly thereafter or as clinically indicated. If liver function test results are elevated, withhold imatinib and/or reduce dosage of the drug.

Hemorrhage

Grade 3 or 4 hemorrhage has occurred in 1.8% of patients receiving imatinib for first-line treatment of CML. The incidence of hemorrhage is higher in patients receiving imatinib for the treatment of GIST (12.9%). In patients with GIST, hemorrhagic events included GI bleeds, intratumoral bleeds, or both; GI tumor sites may have been the source of GI bleeds. In a randomized trial in patients with newly diagnosed Ph+ chronic phase CML, GI hemorrhage occurred in 1.4% of patients receiving imatinib and in 2.9% of patients receiving nilotinib 300 mg twice daily. Postmarketing reports have also identified gastric antral vascular ectasia in patients receiving imatinib.

GI Effects

Nausea, vomiting, and diarrhea occur frequently in patients receiving imatinib. Administration with food and a large glass of water may minimize GI irritation. Gastrointestinal perforation, sometimes fatal, has occurred rarely in patients receiving imatinib.

Dermatologic Effects

Bullous skin reactions, including erythema multiforme and Stevens-Johnson syndrome, have been reported in patients receiving imatinib. Some cases of bullous dermatologic reactions, including erythema multiforme and Stevens-Johnson syndrome, have recurred upon rechallenge of imatinib. Following resolution or lessening of the bullous skin reaction, imatinib therapy has been reinitiated in some patients at a reduced dosage with or without concomitant administration of corticosteroids or antihistamines.

Hypothyroidism

Hypothyroidism has been reported in imatinib-treated patients receiving levothyroxine replacement therapy after thyroidectomy; monitor serum TSH concentrations in such patients.

Fetal/Neonatal Morbidity and Mortality

May cause fetal harm; teratogenicity and embryolethality demonstrated in animals. No adequate and well-controlled studies to date in humans; however, spontaneous abortions and congenital anomalies have been reported in women exposed to imatinib during pregnancy in postmarketing reports. Avoid pregnancy during therapy. Prior to initiation of imatinib therapy, verify pregnancy status of females of reproductive potential and advise such patients to use an effective contraceptive method during imatinib and for 14 days after discontinuation. If used during pregnancy, apprise patients of potential fetal hazard.

Effects on Growth of Pediatric Patients

Imatinib may be associated with adverse reactions related to growth in children or pre-adolescents receiving the drug. The long-term effects of imatinib treatment on growth in children is unknown. Growth should be monitored during imatinib therapy in pediatric patients.

Tumor Lysis Syndrome

Tumor lysis syndrome, sometimes fatal, has been reported in patients with CML, GIST, ALL, and eosinophilic leukemia receiving imatinib. Patients with high tumor burden or those with a high proliferative rate are at an increased risk of developing tumor lysis syndrome; monitor such patients and take appropriate precautions (e.g, adequate hydration, correct uric acid levels).

Impaired Driving/Machinery Operation

Motor vehicle accidents have been reported in patients receiving imatinib. Dizziness, blurred vision, or somnolence may occur in patients receiving imatinib. Advise patients to use caution when driving or operating machinery.

Renal Toxicity

Reduced renal function has been observed in patients receiving imatinib therapy. Monitor renal function prior to initiation of and during imatinib therapy, with close attention to patients with risk factors for renal dysfunction (e.g., preexisting renal impairment, diabetes mellitus, hypertension, congestive heart failure).

Specific Populations

Pregnancy

Can cause fetal harm based on human postmarketing reports and animal studies.

Lactation

Imatinib and its metabolites are distributed into human milk; discontinue breastfeeding during therapy and for 1 month after the last dose.

Pediatric Use

Safety and efficacy of imatinib in children younger than 1 years of age have not been established.

Safety and efficacy in pediatric patients with newly diagnosed Ph+ chronic phase CML and Ph+ ALL have been demonstrated.

Imatinib may be associated with adverse reactions related to growth in children or pre-adolescents receiving the drug. The long-term effects of imatinib treatment on growth in children is unknown. Growth should be monitored during imatinib therapy in pediatric patients.

Geriatric Use

In clinical trials in patients with CML, approximately 20% of patients were over 65 years of age. With the exception of a higher incidence of edema, no substantial differences in safety and efficacy relative to younger adults were observed.

In the trial in patients with unresectable or metastatic GIST, 16% of patients were over 65 years of age. No substantial differences in safety and efficacy relative to younger adults were observed, but data are limited. In the adjuvant GIST study, 31% were over 65 years of age. With the exception of a higher incidence of edema, no substantial differences in safety and efficacy relative to younger adults were observed.

Hepatic Impairment

Pharmacokinetics of imatinib are not significantly affected by mild or moderate hepatic impairment.

In patients with severe hepatic impairment, peak plasma concentrations and AUC of imatinib are increased by 63 and 45%, respectively, compared with patients with normal hepatic function; peak plasma concentrations and AUC of CGP74588 are increased by 56 and 55%, respectively, compared with patients with normal hepatic function. In patients with severe hepatic impairment, the manufacturer recommends reducing the imatinib dosage by 25%.

Renal Impairment

Mild and moderate renal impairment increases mean exposure to imatinib by 1.5- to 2-fold compared with patients with normal renal function. Data in patients with severe renal impairment are insufficient. The manufacturer recommends adjusting the dosage of imatinib in patients with moderate or severe renal impairment.

● Common Adverse Effects

Adverse effects reported in at least 30% of patients were edema, nausea, vomiting, muscle cramps, musculoskeletal pain, diarrhea, rash, fatigue, and abdominal pain.

DRUG INTERACTIONS

Metabolized in the liver, principally by CYP3A4 and to a lesser degree by CYP1A2, CYP2D6, CYP2C9, and CYP2C19. Imatinib is a potent competitive inhibitor of CYP isoenzymes 2C9, 2D6, and 3A4/5.

● Drugs Affecting or Metabolized by Hepatic Microsomal Enzymes

CYP3A4 Inhibitors

Cytochrome P-450 (CYP) isoenzyme 3A4 (CYP3A4) inhibitors (e.g., atazanavir, clarithromycin, indinavir, itraconazole, ketoconazole, nefazodone, nelfinavir, ritonavir, saquinavir, telithromycin, voriconazole): Potential pharmacokinetic interaction causing increased serum imatinib concentrations.

Grapefruit juice may increase imatinib plasma concentrations and should be avoided.

CYP3A4 Inducers

CYP3A4 inducers (e.g., carbamazepine, dexamethasone, fosphenytoin, oxcarbamazepine, phenobarbital, phenytoin, primidone, rifabutin, rifampin, St. John's wort): Potential pharmacokinetic interaction causing substantially decreased serum imatinib concentrations; alternative agents with less enzyme induction potential should be considered. For patients receiving a potent CYP3A4 inducer, such as rifampin or phenytoin, imatinib dosage should be increased by at least 50%, and clinical response should be monitored carefully.

CYP3A4 Substrates

Imatinib inhibits CYP3A4. Potential pharmacokinetic interaction (increased plasma CYP3A4-substrate concentrations) when imatinib is used with CYP3A4 substrates (e.g., alfentanil, cyclosporine, dihydroergotamine, ergotamine, fentanyl, pimozide, quinidine, triazolo-benzodiazepines, dihydropyridine calcium-channel blockers, certain HMG-CoA reductase inhibitors, sirolimus, tacrolimus).

● *Warfarin*

Imatinib inhibits CYP2C9 and CYP3A4. Potential pharmacokinetic and pharmacologic interaction (enhanced anticoagulant effect). Patients requiring anticoagulation therapy should receive heparin or low molecular weight heparin.

● *CYP2D6 Substrates*

Imatinib appears to inhibit CYP2D6. Potential pharmacokinetic interaction (increased CYP2D6 substrate plasma concentrations); use caution with CYP2D6 substrates with a narrow therapeutic window (e.g., alfentanil, cyclosporine, dihydroergotamine, ergotamine, fentanyl, pimozide, quinidine, sirolimus, tacrolimus).

● *Acetaminophen*

Potential pharmacokinetic interaction (increased serum acetaminophen concentrations). No pharmacokinetic or safety data on concomitant use of acetaminophen and imatinib at doses exceeding 400 mg daily or with concomitant long-term use of imatinib and acetaminophen; caution is recommended.

PHARMACOKINETICS

The pharmacokinetics of imatinib are similar in CML and GIST patients.

● *Absorption*

Bioavailability

Well absorbed following oral administration. Mean absolute bioavailability is 98%.

Following oral administration, peak plasma concentrations are attained within 2–4 hours in adult and pediatric patients. When dosed once daily, accumulation is 1.5–2.5-fold at steady state.

Administration of 260 mg/m^2 or 340 mg/m^2 in pediatric patients achieved an AUC similar to that attained with a 400-mg dose in adults. Mean imatinib AUC increases proportionally with dose in adults but not in pediatric patients.

● *Distribution*

Extent

Distributed into human milk.

Plasma Protein Binding

Approximately 95% (mainly albumin and α_1-acid glycoprotein).

● *Elimination*

Metabolism

Metabolized in the liver, principally by CYP3A4 and to a lesser degree by CYP1A2, CYP2D6, CYP2C9, and CYP2C19. The major active metabolite is the *N*-desmethyl derivative, which has an in vitro potency and plasma protein binding similar to the parent drug.

Elimination Route

Predominantly in feces, mostly as metabolites. Following oral administration of a single radiolabeled dose of imatinib, approximately 81% of the dose was eliminated within 7 days (68% of the dose in feces and 13% of the dose in urine); unchanged drug accounted for 25% of the dose (20% in feces, 5% in urine), the remainder being metabolites.

Half-life

Approximately 18 hours for imatinib and 40 hours for its major active metabolite in adults; the elimination half-lives in pediatric patients appear to be similar to those in adults.

Special Populations

Apparent oral clearance appears to be similar in adults and pediatric patients.

Clearance appears to increase with increasing body weight.

DESCRIPTION

Imatinib mesylate, an inhibitor of Bcr-Abl tyrosine kinase, is an antineoplastic agent.

The Philadelphia chromosome, characteristic of chronic myelogenous leukemia (CML), is created by a reciprocal translocation between chromosomes 9 and 22. Translocation between these chromosomes results in production of an abnormal protein (Bcr-Abl tyrosine kinase) that exhibits enhanced tyrosine kinase activity (i.e., increased phosphorylation of tyrosine residues); phosphorylation of tyrosine residues on growth factor receptors is thought to be important in stimulating cell proliferation and inhibiting cell death (apoptosis). Imatinib competitively inhibits Bcr-Abl tyrosine kinase, thereby inhibiting tyrosine phosphorylation of proteins involved in Bcr-Abl signal transduction. The drug has been shown to inhibit proliferation and induce apoptosis of Bcr-Abl-positive cells as well as fresh leukemic cells from Ph$^+$ CML.

Imatinib also inhibits receptor tyrosine kinases for platelet-derived growth factor (PDGF) and stem cell factor (SCF), c-Kit, and PDGF-mediated and SCF-mediated cellular events. Data from in vitro studies shows that imatinib inhibits proliferation and induces apoptosis in gastrointestinal stromal tumor (GIST) cells, which express an activating c-kit mutation.

Imatinib is metabolized by the cytochrome P-450 (CYP) microsomal enzyme system, principally by the isoenzyme 3A4 (CYP3A4) and, to a lesser extent, by CYP1A2, CYP2D6, CYP2C9, and CYP2C19. The active metabolite, an *N*-demethylated piperazine derivative, formed principally by CYP3A4, accounts for approximately 15% of total plasma concentrations of the drug. Approximately 68 and 13% of an oral dose of imatinib is excreted in feces and urine, respectively, as active and inactive metabolites within 7 days.

ADVICE TO PATIENTS

- Advise patients to take imatinib exactly as prescribed with a full glass of water. If a dose is missed, take the next dose at its regular time; do not take 2 doses at the same time.
- Advise patients of the possibility of fluid retention/edema and the importance of informing their clinician if rapid weight gain occurs.
- Advise patients that hepatic toxicity may occur and the importance of contacting their clinician if signs of liver dysfunction (e.g., jaundice, anorexia, bleeding, bruising) occur.
- Advise women to inform their clinician if they are or plan to become pregnant or plan to breastfeed. Advise women to avoid becoming pregnant while taking imatinib; advise women to use highly effective contraception while taking imatinib and for 2 weeks after stopping treatment.
- Advise patients to inform their clinician of existing or contemplated concomitant therapy, including prescription and OTC drugs and dietary and

herbal supplements, as well as any concomitant illnesses. Avoid grapefruit juice. Advise patients to inform their clinician if they plan to take iron supplements.

- Advise patients that growth should be monitored in pediatric patients receiving imatinib.

- Advise patients that blurred vision, dizziness, or somnolence may occur while receiving imatinib and caution is advised while driving or operating machinery.

- Importance of advising women to avoid breast-feeding while receiving imatinib and for 1 month after discontinuance of therapy.

- Importance of informing clinicians of existing or contemplated concomitant therapy, including prescription and OTC drugs and dietary or herbal supplements (e.g., St. John's wort), as well as any concomitant illnesses.

- Importance of informing patients of other important precautionary information.

For further information on the handling of antineoplastic agents, see the ASHP Guidelines on Handling Hazardous Drugs at http://www.ahfsdrug information.com.

PREPARATIONS

Excipients in commercially available drug preparations may have clinically important effects in some individuals; consult specific product labeling for details.

Imatinib Mesylate

Oral

Tablets, film-coated	100 mg (of imatinib)*	**Gleevec®**, Novartis
		Imatinib Tablets
	400 mg (of imatinib)*	**Gleevec®**, Novartis
		Imatinib Tablets

† Use is not currently included in the labeling approved by the US Food and Drug Administration.

* available from one or more manufacturer, distributor, and/or repackager by generic (nonproprietary) name

Ipilimumab

10:00 • ANTINEOPLASTIC AGENTS

- Ipilimumab, a recombinant, fully human monoclonal antibody that binds to cytotoxic T-lymphocyte-associated antigen 4 (CTLA-4), is an antineoplastic agent.

REMS

FDA approved a REMS for ipilimumab to ensure that the benefits outweigh the risk. However, FDA later rescinded REMS requirements. See the FDA REMS page (https://www.accessdata.fda.gov/scripts/cder/rems/index.cfm).

USES

● Melanoma

Ipilimumab is used for the treatment of unresectable or metastatic melanoma. Ipilimumab is designated an orphan drug by the US Food and Drug Administration (FDA) for the treatment of this cancer.

Efficacy of ipilimumab is based principally on observed survival benefits from a randomized, phase 3, double-blind, controlled study in 676 adults with previously treated (e.g., aldesleukin [23% of patients], dacarbazine, temozolomide, fotemustine [not commercially available in the US], carboplatin) unresectable or metastatic melanoma. Eligible patients (59% male, median 57 years of age, 71% with TNM metastasis stage M1c, 98% with Eastern Cooperative Oncology Group [ECOG] performance status of 0 or 1, positive for human leukocyte antigen [HLA]-A2*0201 allele) were randomized (3:1:1) to receive ipilimumab with glycoprotein 100 (gp100) melanoma peptide vaccine (an investigational vaccine), ipilimumab monotherapy, or gp100 vaccine monotherapy. Patients received induction regimens of ipilimumab (or placebo, as assigned) as a 90-minute IV infusion of 3 mg/kg followed by gp100 vaccine (or placebo, as assigned) as 2 separate 1-mg subcutaneous injections every 3 weeks for 4 doses. This study excluded patients with autoimmune disease, primary ocular melanoma or untreated active CNS metastasis, and those receiving immunosuppressive agents (including long-term corticosteroids). Assessment of tumor response occurred at 12 and 24 weeks and every 3 months thereafter. Median survival in patients receiving ipilimumab (with or without gp100 vaccine) was 10 months versus 6 months in patients receiving gp100 vaccine monotherapy. After a median follow-up of 28 months, rates of overall survival at 12, 18, and 24 months in patients receiving ipilimumab monotherapy were 45.6, 33.2, and 23.5%, respectively, compared with 25.3, 16.3, and 13.7%, respectively, in patients receiving gp100 vaccine monotherapy. Based on investigator assessment, best overall response rate was 10.9 or 1.5% in those receiving ipilimumab monotherapy or gp100 vaccine monotherapy, respectively.

Another phase 3 study evaluated ipilimumab as part of a combination chemotherapy regimen with dacarbazine in 502 adults with previously untreated, unresectable or metastatic melanoma. Patients were randomized to receive either ipilimumab and dacarbazine or dacarbazine and placebo. Treatment consisted of ipilimumab at higher than recommended doses (i.e., 10 mg/kg) and dacarbazine at doses of 850 mg/m². Patients received induction regimens of ipilimumab and dacarbazine or dacarbazine and placebo IV at 1, 4, 7, and 10 weeks followed by dacarbazine alone every 3 weeks for 22 weeks. Patients with stable disease or an objective response during induction therapy were eligible to receive a maintenance regimen of ipilimumab or placebo every 12 weeks until disease progression, development of adverse effects, or study completion. This study excluded patients receiving any prior treatment for metastatic disease or concomitant therapy with immunosuppressive agents (including long-term corticosteroids), or those with brain metastasis, primary ocular or mucosal melanoma, or autoimmune disease. Patients receiving ipilimumab and dacarbazine had increased median overall survival (11.2 months) compared with those receiving dacarbazine and placebo (9.1 months) with higher 1-year (47.3 versus 36.3%), 2-year (28.5 versus 17.9%), and 3-year (20.8 versus 12.2%) survival rates, respectively.

Ipilimumab therapy has shown variable patterns of clinical response that differ from the patterns observed with conventional chemotherapeutic agents. While disease regression shortly after initiation of ipilimumab therapy has been reported in some patients, durable stable disease (potentially with small decreases in total tumor burden over a long period of time), response after apparent disease progression, and reduced total tumor burden despite development of new lesions also have been observed. These variable response patterns to ipilimumab have all been associated with improved survival. Utilization of conventional response criteria for measurement of disease progression (e.g., Response Evaluation Criteria in Solid Tumors [RECIST], modified World Health Organization [WHO] criteria) may identify progressive disease before the full benefits of immunotherapy have been realized and may not detect all clinical responses to ipilimumab. Response criteria specific for immunotherapeutic agents that account for total tumor burden and uniquely define progressive disease have been proposed, but have not been prospectively validated. While there is some evidence that development of immune-mediated adverse events correlates with antitumor response to ipilimumab, the occurrence of high-grade immune-mediated adverse events is not required for a clinical response to ipilimumab, nor does this type of adverse reaction ensure a clinical response to the drug. Definitive criteria (e.g., biomarkers, genetic polymorphisms, preexisting antitumor immune response) to reliably identify patients who are likely to respond favorably to ipilimumab have not been established to date.

DOSAGE AND ADMINISTRATION

● Administration

Ipilimumab is administered by IV infusion.

Ipilimumab is available as a 5-mg/mL, preservative-free, injection concentrate in single-use vials containing 50 or 200 mg of the drug.

Ipilimumab injection concentrate should be protected from light, stored at 2–8°C, and should not be frozen.

Ipilimumab injection concentrate must be diluted prior to administration. Prior to dilution, the appropriate number of vials containing ipilimumab injection concentrate should stand at room temperature for approximately 5 minutes. For IV infusion, the appropriate dose should be withdrawn from the vial(s) and injected into an IV bag. The injection concentrate should then be diluted with 0.9% sodium chloride or 5% dextrose injection to achieve a final ipilimumab concentration of 1–2 mg/mL. This diluted solution should be mixed by gentle inversion. Vials containing ipilimumab injection concentrate and diluted solutions of the drug should not be shaken. The diluted solution may be refrigerated or stored at controlled room temperature for no more than 24 hours. Any partially used vials, including unused diluted solution, should be discarded.

Ipilimumab injection concentrate should not be admixed or infused with other drugs. Final diluted ipilimumab solutions should be infused IV over 90 minutes using an in-line, sterile, nonpyrogenic, low-protein-binding filter. The IV line should be flushed with 0.9% sodium chloride or 5% dextrose injection after each dose.

● Dosage

The recommended adult dosage of ipilimumab for the treatment of unresectable or metastatic melanoma is 3 mg/kg given by IV infusion once every 3 weeks for a total of 4 doses.

Dosage Modification for Toxicity

Ipilimumab therapy should be permanently discontinued in patients experiencing any severe or life-threatening immune-mediated adverse reactions. (See Warnings under Cautions: Warnings/Precautions.)

Ipilimumab therapy should be temporarily withheld in patients experiencing any moderate immune-mediated adverse reactions or symptomatic endocrinopathy. (See Warnings under Cautions: Warnings/Precautions.) If the adverse reaction completely or partially resolves to grade 0 or 1 and the patient is receiving 7.5 mg or less of prednisone per day (or equivalent), ipilimumab may be resumed at a dosage of 3 mg/kg every 3 weeks until all 4 planned doses have been administered or 16 weeks have elapsed since the first dose, whichever occurs first.

Ipilimumab therapy should be permanently discontinued in patients experiencing persistent moderate immune-mediated adverse reactions and in those unable to reduce corticosteroid dosage to 7.5 mg or less of prednisone per day (or equivalent).

Ipilimumab therapy should be permanently discontinued in patients unable to complete the full treatment course within 16 weeks after receiving the first dose.

● Special Populations

No special population dosage recommendations at this time.

CAUTIONS

● Contraindications

The manufacturer states that there are no known contraindications to the use of ipilimumab.

● Warnings/Precautions

Warnings

Severe, sometimes fatal, immune-mediated adverse reactions have occurred with ipilimumab treatment. These reactions are a result of T-cell activation and proliferation, and may involve any organ system. The most common, severe immune-mediated adverse reactions are enterocolitis, hepatitis, dermatitis (including toxic epidermal necrolysis), neuropathy, and endocrinopathy. These reactions have usually manifested during ipilimumab treatment, but also have occurred weeks or months after discontinuing the drug.

Patients should be evaluated for manifestations of enterocolitis, dermatitis, neuropathy, and endocrinopathy using appropriate laboratory tests (e.g., liver function and thyroid function tests) prior to each dose of ipilimumab. If severe immune-mediated adverse reactions occur, the drug should be discontinued and high-dose systemic corticosteroid therapy should be initiated. (See REMS and also see Dosage Modification for Toxicity under Dosage and Administration: Dosage.)

Immune-mediated GI Effects

Immune-mediated enterocolitis, sometimes fatal, has occurred with ipilimumab therapy. Among patients receiving ipilimumab for unresectable or metastatic melanoma in a phase 3 clinical trial, severe or life-threatening (grade 3–5) immune-mediated enterocolitis (i.e., diarrhea [7 or more stools per day above baseline], fever, ileus, peritoneal signs) occurred in 7% of patients. Moderate (grade 2) immune-mediated enterocolitis (i.e., diarrhea [up to 6 stools per day above baseline], abdominal pain, mucus or blood in stool) occurred in 5% of patients. In addition, intestinal perforation occurred in 1% and fatal immune-mediated enterocolitis occurred in 0.8% of patients receiving ipilimumab. The incidence and severity of enterocolitis appear to be dose dependent.

The majority of patients experiencing severe, life-threatening, or fatal (grade 3–5) enterocolitis required hospitalization and the median time to onset was 7.4 weeks (range 1.6–13.4 weeks) after initiation of ipilimumab. Treatment with high-dose corticosteroids (40 mg or more of prednisone per day [or equivalent]) was used in 85% of these patients (median daily dosage of 80 mg of prednisone [or equivalent], median duration of 2.3 weeks [up to 13.9 weeks] followed by tapering of the corticosteroid dosage). Infliximab was administered to 8% of patients experiencing moderate, severe, or life-threatening immune-mediated enterocolitis following an inadequate response to corticosteroid therapy. The majority (74%) of patients experiencing grade 3–5 enterocolitis had complete resolution, while 3% improved to grade 2 enterocolitis, and 24% did not report improvement.

Among the 5% of patients experiencing moderate (grade 2) enterocolitis, the median time to onset was 6.3 weeks (range 0.3–18.9 weeks) after initiation of ipilimumab; 54% of such patients were treated with corticosteroids. High-dose corticosteroid therapy (40 mg or more of prednisone per day [or equivalent], median duration of 10 days) was administered in 25% of patients followed by tapering of the corticosteroid dosage, while 29% were treated with less than 40 mg of prednisone per day [or equivalent] for a median duration of 5.1 weeks. The majority (79%) of patients experiencing grade 2 enterocolitis had complete resolution, while 11% reported improvement, and 11% did not report improvement.

Patients should be monitored for manifestations of enterocolitis, including diarrhea, abdominal pain, and mucus or blood in the stool with or without fever, and for manifestations of bowel perforation, including peritoneal signs and ileus. Infectious etiologies should be ruled out in symptomatic patients; for severe or persistent symptoms, endoscopic evaluation should be considered.

Ipilimumab should be permanently discontinued in patients experiencing severe or life-threatening adverse GI reactions, including colitis with abdominal pain, fever, ileus, or peritoneal signs; an increase in stool frequency of 7 or more per day above baseline; stool incontinence; a need for IV hydration exceeding 24 hours; or GI hemorrhage or perforation. Once bowel perforation has been ruled out, systemic corticosteroid therapy should be initiated at a dosage of 1–2 mg/kg per day of prednisone (or equivalent). Once symptoms have resolved or severity of symptoms is reduced, corticosteroid dosage should be tapered over at least

1 month. Dosage tapering schedules less than 1 month in duration have resulted in recurrence or worsening of enterocolitis in some patients. If symptoms persist, patients should continue to be monitored for GI perforation or peritonitis. Repeating the endoscopic evaluation and initiating alternative immunosuppressive therapy (e.g., infliximab) may be considered.

In cases of moderate enterocolitis, ipilimumab should be temporarily withheld and antidiarrheal therapy initiated. If symptoms persist for longer than 1 week, systemic corticosteroid therapy should be initiated at a dosage of 0.5 mg/kg per day of prednisone (or equivalent). Therapy with ipilimumab may be resumed once symptoms have resolved or improved to mild severity and daily prednisone dosage is 7.5 mg or less (or equivalent). Ipilimumab should be permanently discontinued in patients unable to reduce corticosteroid dosage to 7.5 mg or less of prednisone per day (or equivalent) or in those unable to complete the full ipilimumab treatment course within 16 weeks after receiving the first dose. (See Dosage Modification for Toxicity under Dosage and Administration: Dosage.)

Symptomatic treatment with antidiarrheal agents (e.g., diphenoxylate and atropine, loperamide) is used by some clinicians for grade 1 or 2 diarrhea associated with ipilimumab therapy. Treatment guidelines from some experts recommend the use of budesonide for treatment of grade 2 diarrhea and high-dose corticosteroid therapy for treatment of grade 3 or 4 diarrhea. Prophylactic use of budesonide also has been investigated to reduce the frequency of grade 2 or greater diarrhea associated with ipilimumab. However, in one randomized, double-blind study, prophylactic therapy with budesonide during ipilimumab therapy did *not* result in a decreased frequency of grade 2 or greater diarrhea.

Immune-mediated Hepatic Effects

Severe, sometimes fatal, hepatotoxicity, including immune-mediated hepatitis, has occurred with ipilimumab therapy. Among patients receiving ipilimumab for unresectable or metastatic melanoma in a phase 3 clinical trial, severe, life-threatening, or fatal (grade 3–5) hepatotoxicity (i.e., serum AST or ALT concentrations exceeding 5 times the upper limit of normal [ULN] or total bilirubin concentrations exceeding 3 times the ULN) occurred in 2% of patients. In addition, moderate (grade 2) hepatotoxicity (i.e., serum AST or ALT concentrations 2.5–5 times the ULN or total bilirubin concentrations 1.5–3 times the ULN) occurred in 2.5% of patients. Of patients receiving ipilimumab during clinical trials, 0.4% of patients required hospitalization for hepatotoxicity and 0.2% experienced fatal hepatotoxicity. Mycophenolate therapy has been used in patients with persistent, severe hepatitis despite treatment with high-dose corticosteroids. The incidence and severity of hepatitis appear to be dose dependent.

Patients should be assessed for manifestations of hepatotoxicity using appropriate laboratory tests (e.g., AST, ALT, and bilirubin concentrations) prior to each dose of ipilimumab. Infectious and malignant etiologies should be ruled out and liver function tests should be evaluated more frequently in patients experiencing hepatotoxicity until resolution of the toxicity.

Ipilimumab should be permanently discontinued in patients experiencing severe or life-threatening hepatotoxicity. In such patients, systemic corticosteroid therapy should be initiated at a dosage of 1–2 mg/kg per day of prednisone (or equivalent). Once liver function tests indicate a sustained improvement or have returned to baseline levels, corticosteroid therapy should be tapered over at least 1 month. If severe or life-threatening hepatotoxicity persists, alternative immunosuppressive therapy may be considered.

In cases of moderate (grade 2) hepatotoxicity, ipilimumab therapy should be temporarily withheld. Ipilimumab may be resumed once serum ALT and AST concentrations are less than 2.5 times the ULN and total bilirubin is less than 1.5 times the ULN or these values have returned to baseline. (See Dosage Modification for Toxicity under Dosage and Administration: Dosage.)

Ipilimumab should be permanently discontinued if the patient is unable to complete the full treatment course within 16 weeks after receiving the first dose.

Immune-mediated Dermatologic Effects

Immune-mediated dermatitis, sometimes fatal, has occurred with ipilimumab therapy. Among patients receiving ipilimumab for unresectable or metastatic melanoma in a phase 3 clinical trial, severe, life-threatening, or fatal (grade 3–5) immune-mediated dermatitis (e.g., Stevens-Johnson syndrome; toxic epidermal necrolysis; rash complicated by full thickness dermal ulceration; or necrotic, bullous, or hemorrhagic manifestations) occurred in 2.5% of patients. One patient required hospitalization for severe dermatitis, and one death occurred as a result of toxic epidermal necrolysis. In addition, moderate (grade 2) immune-mediated dermatitis occurred in 12% of patients. Among patients experiencing moderate, severe, or life-threatening immune-mediated dermatitis, the median onset was 3.1 weeks (up to 17.3 weeks) following initiation of ipilimumab therapy.

Treatment of severe dermatitis with high-dose corticosteroids was utilized in 54% of these patients (median daily dosage of 60 mg of prednisone [or equivalent], duration up to 14.9 weeks followed by tapering of the corticosteroid dosage). The majority (86%) of these patients had complete resolution occurring in up to 15.6 weeks.

Among patients experiencing moderate dermatitis during ipilimumab treatment in the clinical study, 40% were treated with systemic corticosteroids (median daily dosage of 60 mg of prednisone [or equivalent], median duration of 2.1 weeks), 11% were treated with topical corticosteroids, and 49% did not receive treatment with either systemic or topical corticosteroids. The majority (70%) of patients experiencing moderate dermatitis had complete resolution, while 11% reported improvement, and 19% did not report improvement.

Patients should be monitored for manifestations of dermatitis, (e.g., rash, pruritus). Dermatitis should be considered immune mediated unless another etiology can be identified.

Ipilimumab should be permanently discontinued in patients experiencing severe or life-threatening dermatitis. In such patients, systemic corticosteroid therapy should be initiated at a dosage of 1–2 mg/kg per day of prednisone (or equivalent). Once dermatitis is controlled, corticosteroid dosage should be tapered over at least 1 month.

Ipilimumab should be withheld for moderate (diffuse, 50% or less of skin surface) signs and symptoms of dermatitis. Topical or systemic corticosteroids should be administered if there is no symptomatic improvement within 1 week. Ipilimumab may be resumed once dermatitis is resolved or severity is reduced (i.e., localized rash) and daily prednisone dosage is 7.5 mg or less (or equivalent).

For mild dermatitis (including localized rash and pruritus), the patient should be treated symptomatically. Topical or systemic corticosteroid therapy should be administered if there is no symptomatic improvement within 1 week. (See Dosage Modification for Toxicity under Dosage and Administration: Dosage.)

Immune-mediated Neurologic Effects

Severe or fatal immune-mediated neurologic reactions, including sensory neuropathy, motor neuropathy, Guillain-Barré syndrome, and myasthenia gravis, have occurred with ipilimumab therapy. Among patients receiving ipilimumab for unresectable or metastatic melanoma in a phase 3 clinical trial, one death attributed to Guillain-Barré syndrome and one case of severe (grade 3) peripheral motor neuropathy were reported. Additional cases of Guillain-Barré syndrome and myasthenia gravis have been reported in other clinical studies with the drug.

Patients should be monitored for symptoms of motor or sensory neuropathy (e.g., unilateral or bilateral weakness, sensory alterations, paresthesia). Unless an alternative etiology is identified, such symptoms should be considered immune mediated.

Ipilimumab should be permanently discontinued in patients experiencing severe neurologic reactions, including new or worsening severe neuropathy (interfering with daily activities), Guillain-Barré syndrome, or myasthenia gravis. Severe neuropathy should be appropriately managed and consideration given to initiating systemic corticosteroids at a dosage of 1–2 mg/kg per day of prednisone (or equivalent).

Ipilimumab should be withheld in patients experiencing moderate neuropathy that does not interfere with daily activities and appropriate medical intervention should be initiated. Therapy with ipilimumab may be resumed once symptoms have resolved or returned to baseline. Ipilimumab should be permanently discontinued in patients unable to complete the full treatment course within 16 weeks after receiving the first dose. (See Dosage Modification for Toxicity under Dosage and Administration: Dosage.)

Immune-mediated Endocrine Effects

Immune-mediated endocrinopathies have occurred with ipilimumab therapy and were most frequently manifested as hypopituitarism, adrenal insufficiency, adrenal crisis, hyperthyroidism, or hypothyroidism. Among patients receiving ipilimumab for unresectable or metastatic melanoma in a phase 3 clinical trial, severe or life-threatening (grade 3–4) immune-mediated endocrinopathies (i.e., requiring hospitalization and/or urgent medical intervention, interfering with activities

of daily living) occurred in 1.8% of patients. While all of these patients developed hypopituitarism, some developed other concomitant endocrinopathies that included adrenal insufficiency, hypogonadism, and hypothyroidism; 66% of these patients required hospitalization. In addition, moderate (grade 2) immune-mediated endocrinopathies (requiring hormone replacement or medical intervention) occurred in 2.3% of patients and included hypothyroidism, adrenal insufficiency, hypopituitarism, hyperthyroidism, and Cushing's syndrome. In patients experiencing moderate to severe immune-mediated endocrinopathies, the median onset was 11 weeks (up to 19.3 weeks) after the initiation of ipilimumab. Long-term hormone replacement therapy (including adrenal or thyroid hormones) was necessary in 81% of these patients experiencing moderate or severe endocrinopathies associated with ipilimumab therapy.

Patients should be monitored for manifestations of hypophysitis, adrenal insufficiency, adrenal crisis, hyperthyroidism, and hypothyroidism. Clinical presentation may consist of fatigue, headache, mental status change, abdominal pain, unusual bowel habits, hypotension, or nonspecific symptoms that may resemble other causes (including brain metastasis, underlying disease). Such signs and symptoms of endocrinopathy should be considered immune mediated unless another etiology can be identified. Thyroid function tests and clinical chemistry values should be evaluated prior to the first dose of ipilimumab and each subsequent dose of the drug, and as clinically indicated throughout treatment. In a limited number of patients, imaging studies that revealed enlargement of the pituitary gland were used to diagnose hypophysitis.

Ipilimumab therapy should be withheld in patients with symptoms of endocrinopathy. In such patients, systemic corticosteroid therapy should be initiated at a dosage of 1–2 mg/kg per day of prednisone (or equivalent) in conjunction with appropriate hormone replacement therapy. Ipilimumab may be resumed once symptoms have resolved or returned to baseline, the patient is stable on hormone replacement therapy (if indicated), and corticosteroid dosage does not exceed 7.5 mg of prednisone daily (or equivalent). (See Dosage Modification for Toxicity under Dosage and Administration: Dosage.) Ipilimumab should be permanently discontinued in patients unable to reduce corticosteroid dosage to 7.5 mg or less of prednisone daily (or equivalent) or in those unable to complete the full ipilimumab treatment course within 16 weeks after receiving the first dose of drug.

Other Warnings/Precautions
Other Immune-mediated Effects

Other immune-mediated adverse reactions, including nephritis, pneumonitis, meningitis, pericarditis, uveitis, iritis, and hemolytic anemia have occurred with ipilimumab therapy. Among patients receiving ipilimumab for unresectable or metastatic melanoma in a phase 3 clinical trial, such immune-mediated reactions were observed in less than 1% of patients. In addition, immune-mediated reactions such as myocarditis, angiopathy, temporal arteritis, vasculitis, polymyalgia rheumatica, conjunctivitis, blepharitis, episcleritis, scleritis, leukocytoclastic vasculitis, erythema multiforme, psoriasis, pancreatitis, arthritis, and autoimmune thyroiditis were reported in less than 1% of patients in clinical trials of the drug.

Ipilimumab should be permanently discontinued in patients experiencing clinically important or severe immune-mediated adverse reactions. In patients experiencing severe immune-mediated reactions, systemic corticosteroid therapy should be initiated at a dosage of 1–2 mg/kg per day of prednisone (or equivalent). Ipilimumab should be permanently discontinued in patients unable to reduce corticosteroid dosage to 7.5 mg or less of prednisone daily (or equivalent) or in those unable to complete the full ipilimumab treatment course within 16 weeks after receiving the first dose of drug.

In patients experiencing uveitis, iritis, or episcleritis, therapy with an ophthalmic corticosteroid preparation should be administered. Ipilimumab should be permanently discontinued in patients experiencing immune-mediated ocular disease unresponsive to topical corticosteroid therapy.

Immunogenicity

There is a potential for immunogenicity with ipilimumab therapy. Development of binding antibodies to ipilimumab were detected by electrochemiluminescence (ECL) in 1.1% of patients receiving the drug during clinical trials. Among these patients, infusion-related reactions consistent with hypersensitivity or anaphylaxis were not observed. Neutralizing antibodies to ipilimumab also were not detected in these patients. The ability of the ECL assay to detect anti-ipilimumab antibodies is limited by the presence of circulating drug. In a cohort of patients with the lowest trough concentrations of ipilimumab after receiving 0.3 mg/kg of drug, 6.9% tested positive for ipilimumab-binding antibodies.

Because the observed incidence of antibody positivity may be influenced by several factors including assay methodology, sample handling, timing of sample collection, concomitant drug therapy, and underlying disease, comparison of the incidence of antibodies to ipilimumab to that of other drugs may be misleading.

Specific Populations

Pregnancy

Category C. (See Users Guide.)

Lactation

It is not known whether ipilimumab is distributed into milk. A decision should be made whether to discontinue nursing or the drug, taking into account the importance of the drug to the woman.

Pediatric Use

Safety and efficacy of ipilimumab have not been established in pediatric patients younger than 18 years of age.

Geriatric Use

No substantial difference in safety and efficacy relative to younger adults have been observed.

Hepatic Impairment

Ipilimumab has not been studied in patients with hepatic impairment.

Renal Impairment

Ipilimumab has not been studied in patients with renal impairment.

● Common Adverse Effects

Adverse effects reported in 5% or more of patients receiving ipilimumab include fatigue, diarrhea, pruritus, rash, and colitis.

DRUG INTERACTIONS

No formal drug interaction studies have been performed to date.

DESCRIPTION

Ipilimumab, a recombinant, fully human monoclonal antibody that binds to cytotoxic T-lymphocyte-associated antigen 4 (CTLA-4), is an antineoplastic agent. The drug is an IgG_1 kappa immunoglobulin that is produced in mammalian (Chinese hamster ovary) cell culture.

Ipilimumab has high affinity and specificity for CTLA-4, an inducible receptor expressed on the surface of T-cells after activation. CTLA-4 competes with CD28, a costimulatory T-cell receptor, for the ligands CD80 (B7-1) and CD86 (B7-2) on antigen-presenting cells. The interaction between CTLA-4 and CD80 or CD86 results in inhibition of T-cell activation and proliferation. Anti-CTLA-4 antibodies block the interaction with CD80 and CD86, and allow for prolonged T-cell activation and enhanced immune response. The antineoplastic effects of the drug are indirect and appear to result from augmented T-cell-mediated anti-tumor immune response. An initial increase in total tumor burden (e.g., enlargement of baseline lesions, development of new lesions) observed in the absence of substantial clinical deterioration during ipilimumab therapy may not indicate treatment failure, but may be a result of lymphocytic infiltration of the lesions or tumor growth prior to complete immune system activation.

The pharmacokinetics of ipilimumab following IV administration is characterized by a 2-compartment model with first-order elimination and dose-dependent clinical effects. Plasma concentrations and area under the serum concentration-time curve (AUC) reportedly are dose proportional in the ipilimumab dosage range of 0.3–10 mg/kg with minimal systemic accumulation when administered every 3 weeks. Steady-state concentrations are reached by the third infusion dose and terminal half-life is approximately 14.7 days. Systemic clearance of ipilimumab increases with increasing body weight, but this is not considered clinically important when the drug is dosed based on body weight. Clearance of the drug is not affected by age, gender, anti-ipilimumab antibody status, previous antineoplastic therapy, baseline lactate dehydrogenase concentrations, human leukocyte antigen (HLA)-A2*0201 allele status, performance status, or concomitant use of budesonide. Renal impairment (i.e., baseline creatinine clearance of 29 mL/min or greater) did not have a clinically important effect on the pharmacokinetics of ipilimumab. In patients with various degrees of hepatic impairment, baseline serum ALT, AST, and total bilirubin concentrations also did not have a clinically important effect on the pharmacokinetics of the drug.

ADVICE TO PATIENTS

Risk of severe, and potentially fatal, immune-mediated adverse reactions, including enterocolitis, hepatitis, dermatitis, neuropathy, and endocrinopathy. (See REMS.)

Importance of promptly contacting clinician if signs or symptoms of immune-mediated reactions (e.g., changes in bowel movements or diarrhea, rash or pruritus, weakness or paresthesia, fatigue, headache, mental status changes, abdominal pain, hypotension) occur.

Importance of advising patient to read the manufacturer's medication guide before beginning treatment and each time the drug is administered.

Importance of women informing clinicians if they are or plan to become pregnant or plan to breast-feed. Ipilimumab may cause fetal harm. Importance of advising nursing women not to breast-feed during therapy with the drug.

Importance of informing clinicians of existing or contemplated concomitant therapy, including prescription and OTC drugs, as well as any concomitant illnesses, including autoimmune disease, history of organ transplantation, or liver damage.

Importance of informing patients of other important precautionary information. (See Cautions.)

PREPARATIONS

Excipients in commercially available drug preparations may have clinically important effects in some individuals; consult specific product labeling for details.

Ipilimumab (recombinant)

Parenteral

Injection concentrate, for IV infusion only	5 mg/mL (50 or 200 mg)	Yervoy®, Bristol-Myers Squibb

Selected Revisions April 6, 2016, © Copyright, November 2, 2011, American Society of Health-System Pharmacists, Inc.

Irinotecan Hydrochloride

10:00 · ANTINEOPLASTIC AGENTS

■ Irinotecan, a type I DNA topoisomerase inhibitor, is an antineoplastic agent.

USES

Irinotecan is commercially available in 2 types of formulations: conventional (nonencapsulated) and liposomal irinotecan hydrochloride. The efficacy and safety of irinotecan for each indication is based on research and clinical experience using a specific formulation.

● GI Cancers

Combination Therapy for Colorectal Cancer

Conventional irinotecan hydrochloride is used as a component of first-line therapy in combination with fluorouracil and leucovorin for the treatment of metastatic carcinoma of the colon or rectum.

The current indication for use of conventional irinotecan in combination therapy for advanced colorectal cancer is based principally on data from 2 phase 3, multinational, randomized, controlled trials evaluating the combination of conventional irinotecan with fluorouracil and leucovorin compared with fluorouracil and leucovorin alone. In both studies, the addition of irinotecan to fluorouracil and leucovorin prolonged survival and increased objective response rate and time to tumor progression.

In a randomized trial involving 3 treatment arms, combination therapy with conventional irinotecan and rapid IV ("bolus") fluorouracil/leucovorin weekly for 4 weeks every 6 weeks was compared with a standard regimen of rapid IV ("bolus") fluorouracil/leucovorin daily for 5 consecutive days every 4 weeks and with conventional irinotecan alone weekly for 4 weeks every 6 weeks. Higher confirmed objective response rate (39 vs 21%), longer median time to disease progression (7 vs 4.3 months), and prolonged median survival (14.8 vs 12.6 months) were observed in patients receiving combination therapy with irinotecan and fluorouracil/leucovorin compared with fluorouracil/leucovorin alone. This difference in survival with the triple-drug regimen was noted even though 56% of the patients receiving fluorouracil/leucovorin received an irinotecan-based regimen after the conclusion of the study. Outcome was similar for patients receiving irinotecan alone compared with fluorouracil/leucovorin. Grade 3 diarrhea and grade 3 or 4 vomiting occurred more frequently in patients receiving the irinotecan-containing combination regimen, whereas grade 3 or 4 mucositis, grade 4 neutropenia, and neutropenic fever were more common in patients receiving fluorouracil/leucovorin. No difference between the irinotecan-combination and fluorouracil/leucovorin treatment groups was observed in a quality-of-life analysis, and the incidence of treatment-related mortality was approximately 1% in each of the 3 groups.

In another randomized trial, the addition of conventional irinotecan to infusional fluorouracil/leucovorin increased objective response rate (35 vs 22%), median time to disease progression (6.7 vs 4.4 months) and median survival (17.4 vs 14.1 months). Diarrhea, neutropenia, leukopenia, and asthenia occurred with greater frequency and severity in patients receiving irinotecan-based combination chemotherapy compared with those receiving fluorouracil/leucovorin alone.

Higher rates of hospitalization, neutropenic fever, thromboembolism, treatment discontinuance during the first cycle, and early deaths were associated with a baseline performance status of 2 (vs 0 or 1) regardless of treatment regimen. Diarrhea and neutropenia occurred frequently and were often severe in patients receiving irinotecan-based combination therapy or fluorouracil/leucovorin alone; comparison of data from the randomized trial including a group of patients receiving irinotecan alone reveals that nausea, vomiting, and alopecia each occurs at a higher incidence or with greater severity in patients receiving irinotecan, whereas neutropenic fever and mucositis are more commonly associated with fluorouracil/leucovorin.

The optimal dosage regimen for conventional irinotecan-based combination therapy has not been established. An unexpectedly high rate of death associated with use of the conventional irinotecan and rapid IV ("bolus") fluorouracil/leucovorin regimen (3 times the rate of death in the comparative regimens) resulted in the suspension of enrollment in 2 randomized trials (one for metastatic colon cancer and one for adjuvant treatment of resectable colon cancer). Most of the deaths occurred during or immediately after the first 6-week cycle of treatment, particularly during the first 3–4 weeks, and were attributed to the combined effect of several moderate or severe toxicities described either as a GI syndrome or as a vascular syndrome. (See GI Toxicity and Cardiovascular Toxicity under Dosage: Dosage Modification for Toxicity and Contraindications for Continued Therapy, in Dosage and Administration.) A direct comparison of the safety and efficacy of the 2 regimens has not been performed; however, lower rates of treatment-related mortality have been reported when fluorouracil was administered by IV infusion.

Monotherapy for Colorectal Cancer

Conventional irinotecan hydrochloride is used as a single agent for the treatment of metastatic carcinoma of the colon or rectum in patients whose disease has recurred or progressed following initial therapy with fluorouracil-based antineoplastic regimens. The drug originally became commercially available in the US under the principles and procedures of the FDA's accelerated review policy that allows approval based on effects on a clinical endpoint (e.g., tumor shrinkage) other than survival, irreversible morbidity, or quality of life pending completion of studies to establish and define the degree of clinical benefit. Conventional irinotecan received full approval following the completion of randomized trials demonstrating prolonged survival in patients receiving the drug for this use.

Evidence of clinical benefit of conventional irinotecan is based principally on data from 2 randomized trials in which conventional irinotecan 300–350 mg/m² was administered once every 3 weeks and in 3 phase 2 trials in which conventional irinotecan 125 mg/m² was administered once weekly for 4 weeks followed by a 2-week rest period. In 2 randomized trials involving a total of 535 patients with metastatic carcinoma of the colon or rectum that recurred or progressed following fluorouracil-containing chemotherapy, survival was prolonged in those receiving conventional irinotecan compared with those receiving fluorouracil or supportive care.

In a randomized trial of patients with metastatic colorectal cancer that progressed within 6 months following treatment with fluorouracil, patients receiving conventional irinotecan 300–350 mg/m² as a single 90-minute infusion once every 3 weeks and supportive care had longer median survival (9.2 vs 6.5 months) than those receiving supportive care alone. Patients receiving irinotecan had longer time to development of pain (6.9 vs 2 months), longer time to deterioration of performance status (5.7 vs 3.3 months), and longer time to weight loss of 5% or greater (6.4 vs 4.2 months) compared with those receiving supportive care alone; although patients receiving irinotecan had a higher rate of diarrhea than those receiving supportive care alone, other quality-of-life measures were comparable or better for patients receiving the drug. In addition, patients with a baseline performance status of 1 or 2 receiving irinotecan and supportive care or supportive care alone showed an improvement in performance status of 33.3 or 11.3%, respectively. Supportive care included the use of anti-infectives, analgesics, corticosteroids, transfusions, psychotherapy, or any other symptomatic therapy as clinically indicated, including palliative radiation therapy. Approximately 21% of patients treated with irinotecan and supportive care also received other chemotherapy regimens, and 31% of patients treated with supportive care also received various chemotherapy regimens.

In another randomized trial, patients with recurrent or refractory metastatic colorectal cancer receiving conventional irinotecan 300–350 mg/m² as a single 90-minute IV infusion once every 3 weeks had longer median survival (10.8 vs 8.5 months) than those receiving fluorouracil by continuous IV infusion. The rate of survival at 1 year was higher in patients receiving irinotecan compared with those receiving fluorouracil (45 vs 32%); the quality of life as assessed by the European Organization of Research and Treatment of Cancer Quality of Life Questionnaire (EORTC QLQ-C30) was similar and both treatments were equally well tolerated.

In an open-label, single-agent, multicenter study involving 132 patients with metastatic cancer of the colon or rectum that recurred or progressed following therapy with fluorouracil-containing regimens, the intent-to-treat response rate was 12% in patients receiving conventional irinotecan at a starting dose of 350 mg/m² administered by 30-minute IV infusion once every 3 weeks. In 3 phase 2 clinical trials, 304 patients with metastatic colorectal cancer who previously had been treated with a fluorouracil-containing antineoplastic regimen received conventional irinotecan 125 mg/m² once weekly. These open-label, single-agent trials evaluated the surrogate endpoint of tumor response rate and did *not* provide information on actual clinical benefit (e.g., decrease in disease-related symptoms, increase in survival) of irinotecan therapy. Patients received irinotecan in repeated 6-week cycles, each cycle consisting of once-weekly, 90-minute IV infusions of irinotecan for 4 weeks followed by a 2-week drug-free period. In one trial, an initial weekly irinotecan hydrochloride dose of 150 mg/m^2 was administered to a few patients; however, these patients developed unacceptably high rates of severe diarrhea, dehydration, and febrile neutropenia, and subsequent patients in the trial received an initial dose of 125 mg/m^2. In another trial, the initial dose of irinotecan hydrochloride was reduced from 125 to 100 mg/m^2 to evaluate the therapeutic ratio of this initial dose. In these trials, 34, 63, or 3% of patients received initial irinotecan hydrochloride doses of 100, 125, or 150 mg/m^2, respectively.

Intent-to-treat analysis of the pooled data from the 3 trials revealed an overall response rate of 15% (2 complete and 27 partial responses) among patients who received the recommended initial conventional irinotecan hydrochloride dose of 125 mg/m^2; however, the response rate was only 7.8% among patients who received an initial dose of 100 mg/m^2. More than 50% of patients responding to irinotecan in these trials had failed to respond to previous fluorouracil-based regimens administered for colorectal cancer with metastases. The median response duration for patients receiving an initial irinotecan hydrochloride dose of 125 mg/m^2 was 5.8 months (range: 2.6–15.1 months). Among patients with disease responding to irinotecan, all but 2 patients achieved responses by the second 6-week cycle of irinotecan therapy; one response was observed by the fourth and one after the eighth cycle of therapy.

Among patients receiving irinotecan on a weekly dosage schedule in phase 2 trials, response rates were similar regardless of gender, age (greater than or less than 65 years), primary cancer site (colon or rectum), history of previous pelvic radiation therapy, or number of metastatic lesions (single or multiple). The response rate among patients with a performance status of zero (i.e., fully active; able to perform all predisease activities without restriction) was 18.5%, while the response rate among those with a performance status of 1 (i.e., restricted in physically strenuous activity but ambulatory and able to perform work of a light or sedentary nature [e.g., light housework, office work]) or 2 (i.e., ambulatory and capable of all self-care but unable to carry out any work activities; up and about more than 50% of waking hours) was 8.2%. Patients with a performance status of 3 or 4 have not been studied.

● Pancreatic Cancer

Liposomal irinotecan hydrochloride is used in combination with fluorouracil and leucovorin for the treatment of metastatic adenocarcinoma of the pancreas in patients whose disease has progressed following gemcitabine-based chemotherapy; liposomal irinotecan is designated an orphan drug by FDA for the treatment of this cancer.

The current indication for use of liposomal irinotecan in combination therapy with fluorouracil and leucovorin for the treatment of metastatic adenocarcinoma of the pancreas in patients whose disease has progressed following gemcitabine-based chemotherapy is based principally on data from a randomized, controlled, open-label phase 3 study (NAPOLI-1). In patients with previously treated metastatic adenocarcinoma of the pancreas, liposomal irinotecan has been shown to prolong overall survival compared with fluorouracil and leucovorin alone.

In this study, 417 patients were randomized in a 1:1:1 ratio to receive liposomal irinotecan (70 mg/m^2 by IV infusion over 90 minutes) in combination with fluorouracil and leucovorin (leucovorin 400 mg/m^2 by IV infusion over 30 minutes followed by fluorouracil 2.4 g/m^2 by IV infusion over 46 hours) administered every 2 weeks, liposomal irinotecan (100 mg/m^2 by IV infusion over 90 minutes) administered every 3 weeks, or fluorouracil and leucovorin (leucovorin 200 mg/m^2 by IV infusion over 30 minutes followed by fluorouracil 2 g/m^2 by IV infusion over 24 hours) administered on days 1, 8, 15, and 22 of each 6-week cycle. The initial dosage of liposomal irinotecan was reduced by 20 mg/m^2 in patients who were homozygous for the UGT1A1*28 allele; however, the dose was increased to the full dosage following the first cycle if adverse events did not occur. Treatment was continued until disease progression or unacceptable toxicity occurred. The primary measure of efficacy was overall survival. The median age of patients was 63 years; 53% had a baseline Karnofsky performance status of 90–100, 67% had liver metastasis, and 31% had lung metastasis. All patients enrolled in the study had received prior therapy with gemcitabine; 54% had received prior therapy with gemcitabine in combination with another agent, and 13% had received prior therapy with gemcitabine in combination with albumin-bound paclitaxel.

In this study, patients randomized to receive liposomal irinotecan in combination with fluorouracil and leucovorin had longer median overall survival

(6.1 versus 4.2 months) and progression-free survival (3.1 versus 1.5 months) compared with patients receiving fluorouracil and leucovorin alone; however, improvement in overall survival was not demonstrated in patients receiving liposomal irinotecan alone compared with those receiving fluorouracil and leucovorin (4.9 versus 4.2 months, respectively). In addition, patients receiving liposomal irinotecan in combination with fluorouracil and leucovorin had a higher overall response rate compared with those receiving fluorouracil and leucovorin alone (7.7 versus 0.8%, respectively). Results of a subgroup analysis (based on age, disease stage, Karnofsky performance status, baseline albumin concentration, previous lines of therapy for metastatic disease, prior exposure to radiation therapy or surgery, prior exposure to fluorouracil-, irinotecan-, or platinum-based chemotherapy) suggested that the drug's effect on overall survival was consistent across most subgroups.

● Small Cell Lung Cancer

Conventional irinotecan is used in combination with cisplatin for the initial treatment of extensive small cell lung cancer†.

A phase 3, randomized trial was terminated early when interim analysis of the data showed that median overall survival was prolonged (12.8 versus 9.4 months) and the rate of survival at 2 years was higher (19.5 versus 5.2%) in patients receiving irinotecan and cisplatin versus etoposide and cisplatin for extensive small cell lung cancer. Patients received a regimen of conventional irinotecan 60 mg/m^2 on days 1, 8, and 15 and cisplatin 60 mg/m^2 on day 1 during a 4-week cycle for 4 cycles; or a regimen of etoposide 100 mg/m^2 on days 1, 2, and 3 and cisplatin 80 mg/m^2 on day 1 during a 3-week cycle for 4 cycles. Severe or life-threatening diarrhea occurred more frequently in patients receiving irinotecan and cisplatin, whereas severe or life-threatening myelosuppression occurred more frequently in those receiving etoposide and cisplatin. Interim analysis of another randomized trial using a modified irinotecan-containing regimen suggests that overall survival is similar in patients receiving a regimen of either irinotecan and cisplatin or etoposide and cisplatin.

In phase 2 studies, objective response rates of 16–47% have been observed in patients receiving conventional irinotecan alone, typically at initial doses of 100–125 mg/m^2 infused IV over a period of 90 minutes once weekly, for refractory or relapsed small cell lung cancer. Higher doses of irinotecan are associated with increased frequency and severity of adverse effects, particularly neutropenia.

Because the current prognosis for small cell lung cancer is unsatisfactory regardless of stage and despite considerable diagnostic and therapeutic advances, all patients with this cancer are candidates for inclusion in clinical trials at the time of diagnosis.

● Cervical Cancer

Conventional irinotecan is being investigated as an active agent in the treatment of metastatic or recurrent cervical cancer†. Objective response rates of 13–21% have been reported with use of irinotecan as a single agent for advanced squamous cell carcinoma of the cervix. Although no responses to irinotecan were observed in one small uncontrolled phase 2 study of patients with platinum-resistant advanced squamous cell carcinoma of the cervix, responses to the drug have been reported in similar patients in another phase 2 study. The benefit of combination chemotherapy regimens vs single-agent therapy (e.g., cisplatin alone) has not been fully established, and further study is needed to determine the role of irinotecan in the treatment of advanced cervical cancer. (See Uses: Cervical Cancer in Cisplatin 10:00 for an overview of therapy for cervical cancer.)

DOSAGE AND ADMINISTRATION

Irinotecan is commercially available in 2 types of formulations: conventional (nonencapsulated) and liposomal irinotecan hydrochloride. The properties of irinotecan may differ according to formulation, and the dosage and reconstitution instructions for irinotecan are specific to formulation. Liposomal irinotecan hydrochloride may *not* be substituted for other formulations of irinotecan hydrochloride.

Dosage of liposomal irinotecan hydrochloride is expressed in terms of anhydrous irinotecan, whereas dosage of conventional irinotecan hydrochloride is expressed in terms of the hydrated salt.

In addition to GI and hematologic toxicity, other severe adverse effects have occurred in patients receiving conventional or liposomal irinotecan. Hypersensitivity reactions, including severe anaphylactic or anaphylactoid reactions, have been reported. Renal impairment and acute renal failure have occurred, usually in patients who became volume-depleted from severe vomiting and/or diarrhea. Cardiovascular and thromboembolic events also have been reported in patients receiving conventional irinotecan. (See Cardiovascular Toxicity under Dosage: Dosage Modification for Toxicity and Contraindications for Continued Therapy, in Dosage and Administration.)

The manufacturer of conventional irinotecan recommends close monitoring in patients older than 65 years of age because of increased risk of treatment-related toxicity, such as early and late diarrhea, during therapy with conventional irinotecan. Patients receiving conventional irinotecan/fluorouracil/leucovorin therapy should be monitored closely (e.g., weekly assessment), particularly during the first cycle of treatment, since most of the treatment-related toxicities leading to early death occurred within the first 3–4 weeks. Changes in serum electrolytes and/or acid-base balance, including hyponatremia or hypernatremia, hypokalemia, and/or metabolic acidosis, may be an early indication of treatment-related toxicity; patients with abnormalities in serum sodium, potassium, and/or bicarbonate concentrations, with or without concomitant elevations in BUN or serum creatinine concentrations, should be evaluated carefully for dehydration and receive aggressive medical management, including fluid and electrolyte replacement.

Liposomal irinotecan hydrochloride can only be obtained through select specialty distributors. Clinicians may consult the Onivyde® website for specific availability information (https://www.onivyde.com).

• Administration

Conventional or liposomal irinotecan hydrochloride is administered by IV infusion. Care should be taken to avoid extravasation of conventional irinotecan, and the infusion site should be monitored for signs of inflammation. Should manifestations of extravasation appear, the infusion should immediately be stopped and restarted in another vein. The manufacturer of conventional irinotecan recommends that extravasation of the drug be treated by flushing the infusion site promptly with sterile water and applying an ice pack.

Procedures for proper handling and disposal of antineoplastic drugs (e.g., use of protective clothing and gloves) should be used to avoid exposure to conventional or liposomal irinotecan during preparation of IV solutions. If conventional irinotecan hydrochloride for injection concentrate or a solution of the drug comes in contact with the skin or mucous membranes, the skin should be washed immediately and thoroughly with soap and water or the mucosa should be flushed with copious amounts of water.

Conventional Irinotecan Hydrochloride

Commercially available conventional irinotecan hydrochloride for injection concentrate must be diluted prior to IV administration. For IV infusion, the manufacturer recommends diluting the drug in 5% dextrose injection to a final irinotecan hydrochloride concentration of 0.12–2.8 mg/mL. In most clinical trials, the dose of conventional irinotecan hydrochloride was diluted in 250–500 mL of 5% dextrose injection. The manufacturer states that although 5% dextrose injection is the preferred diluent, 0.9% sodium chloride injection also may be used for dilution of conventional irinotecan. The diluted solution of conventional irinotecan should be infused over a period of 90 minutes; more rapid infusion rates may increase the likelihood of cholinergic symptoms (e.g., early diarrhea, diaphoresis, flushing, abdominal cramping, rhinitis, increased salivation, miosis, lacrimation).

Solutions of conventional irinotecan hydrochloride prepared in 5% dextrose injection are physically and chemically stable for up to 24 hours when stored at room temperature (approximately 25°C) under ambient fluorescent lighting or for up to 48 hours when protected from light and refrigerated at 2–8°C. For conventional irinotecan hydrochloride solutions prepared in 5% dextrose injection, the manufacturer recommends administration of such drug solutions within 24 hours if refrigerated or within 4 hours if maintained at room temperature because of the potential for microbial contamination during preparation of the admixtures; however, if dilution is performed under strict aseptic conditions (e.g., under laminar airflow conditions), administration of solutions prepared in 5% dextrose injection and stored at room temperature should be completed within 12 hours. Solutions of conventional irinotecan hydrochloride prepared in 0.9% sodium chloride are stable for up to 24 hours when stored at room

temperature (approximately 25°C) under ambient fluorescent lighting. The manufacturer states that solutions of conventional irinotecan hydrochloride prepared in 0.9% sodium chloride may occasionally develop visible particulates when refrigerated at 2–8°C; therefore, solutions prepared in sodium chloride injection should *not* be refrigerated but should be stored at room temperature and used within 4 hours. However, if dilution is performed under strict aseptic conditions (e.g., under laminar airflow conditions), administration of solutions prepared in 0.9% sodium chloride injection and stored at room temperature should be completed within 12 hours. Freezing of commercially available conventional irinotecan hydrochloride for injection concentrate or IV admixtures of the drug may result in formation of a precipitate and should be avoided.

Conventional irinotecan hydrochloride for injection concentrate should be inspected visually for particulate matter in the vial and again in the syringe when transferring the drug solution to prepare admixtures of the drug. The manufacturer states that other drugs should not be added to IV solutions of conventional irinotecan hydrochloride.

Liposomal Irinotecan Hydrochloride

Liposomal irinotecan hydrochloride for injection concentrate must be diluted prior to IV infusion. The concentrate should be diluted in 500 mL of 5% dextrose injection or 0.9% sodium chloride injection. The diluted solution of liposomal irinotecan should be infused over a period of 90 minutes. The manufacturer states that in-line filters should *not* be used during administration of liposomal irinotecan hydrochloride. Any unused solution should be discarded.

Solutions of liposomal irinotecan hydrochloride should be administered within 24 hours of preparation when stored under refrigeration at 2–8°C or within 4 hours when stored at room temperature. The diluted drug should be protected from light and should *not* be frozen. Prior to administration, the diluted solution should be allowed to come to room temperature.

• Dosage

Because irinotecan often causes neutropenia, leukopenia, and anemia, which can be severe, the drug should *not* be used in patients with severe bone marrow failure. In addition, concurrent radiation therapy has not been adequately studied and is not recommended. Because conventional irinotecan hydrochloride for injection concentrate contains sorbitol, the drug should *not* be given to patients with hereditary fructose intolerance. Treatment with conventional or liposomal irinotecan should *not* be initiated until resolution of bowel obstruction.

Irinotecan is considered an antineoplastic agent of *moderate emetic risk* (i.e., incidence of emesis without antiemetics exceeds 30% but does not exceed 90%). Because nausea and/or vomiting occur frequently in patients receiving irinotecan therapy and may be severe, effective antiemetic therapy (e.g., dexamethasone 8 mg and a 5-HT$_3$ serotonin receptor antagonist such as palonosetron) should be administered orally or IV at least 30 minutes prior to irinotecan therapy. Additional oral antiemetic therapy also should be considered for subsequent home use by the patient as needed. Unless clinically contraindicated, clinicians should consider prophylactic or therapeutic administration of antimuscarinic therapy (e.g., 0.25–1 mg of atropine sulfate by IV or subcutaneous injection) for patients experiencing rhinitis, increased salivation, miosis, lacrimation, diaphoresis, flushing, bradycardia, abdominal cramping, or early diarrhea (i.e., diarrhea with an onset during or shortly after [within 24 hours of] administration of irinotecan); such symptoms are expected to occur more frequently in patients receiving higher doses of irinotecan.

Dosage adjustment may be required according to the patient's status for activity of UGT1A1, a uridine diphosphate-glucuronosyltransferase (UGT) enzyme involved in the metabolism of SN-38, an active metabolite of irinotecan. In patients who are homozygous for the UGT1A1*28 allele, UGT1A1 activity is reduced, and the risk of irinotecan-induced neutropenia is increased; reduction in the initial dosage of conventional irinotecan by at least one dose level should be considered in such patients. The optimal dosage reduction for conventional irinotecan has not been established, and subsequent dosage adjustment may be necessary according to patient tolerance. The recommended initial dose of liposomal irinotecan in patients with metastatic adenocarcinoma of the pancreas who are homozygous for the UGT1A1*28 allele is 50 mg/m²; the dose may be increased to 70 mg/m² as tolerated during subsequent cycles. In patients who are heterozygous for the UGT1A1*28 allele, UGT1A1 activity is intermediate, and the risk of irinotecan-induced neutropenia may be increased. Clinical results have been variable with conventional irinotecan.

Inadvertent overdosage of conventional irinotecan has occurred in several patients, including at least one fatal case, because the manufacturer's label on the vial was misread. Therefore, particular care should be taken to ensure that the correct dose of the drug is administered, including careful attention to the concentration of conventional irinotecan for injection concentrate present in the vial and the appropriate volume needed to provide the prescribed dose.

Patients should be instructed to contact their clinician if any of the following occur during irinotecan therapy: diarrhea for the first time during treatment; black or bloody stools; symptoms of dehydration, such as lightheadedness, dizziness, or faintness; inability to take fluids by mouth because of nausea or vomiting; inability to control diarrhea within 24 hours; new-onset cough or dyspnea; manifestations of severe hypersensitivity reactions; or fever or evidence of infection. Patients should be warned about the potential for dizziness or visual disturbances that may occur within 24 hours following the administration of conventional irinotecan and be advised not to drive or operate machinery if these symptoms occur. Patients also should be alerted to the possibility of alopecia during conventional or liposomal irinotecan therapy.

Colorectal Cancer
Combination Therapy

For use in a combination regimen as first-line therapy for metastatic carcinoma of the colon or rectum, conventional irinotecan is administered with leucovorin and fluorouracil. For all regimens, the dose of leucovorin should be administered immediately following conventional irinotecan, and then followed immediately by administration of fluorouracil. The optimal dosage regimen for conventional irinotecan-based combination therapy has not been established; an unexpectedly high rate of death has been reported in 2 clinical trials using irinotecan with fluorouracil given by rapid IV injection ("bolus"), and some clinicians prefer administration of fluorouracil by IV infusion in this regimen. (See Combination Therapy for Colorectal Cancer in Uses: GI Cancers.)

In regimen 1, the initial dose of conventional irinotecan hydrochloride is 125 mg/m² infused IV over a period of 90 minutes followed by leucovorin 20 mg/m² given by rapid IV injection and then fluorouracil 500 mg/m² given by rapid IV injection ("bolus"). Treatment is given weekly for 4 weeks on days 1, 8, 15, and 22 during a 6-week cycle; the next cycle begins on day 43.

In regimen 2, the initial dose of conventional irinotecan hydrochloride is 180 mg/m² infused IV over a period of 90 minutes followed by leucovorin 200 mg/m² infused IV over 2 hours, then fluorouracil 400 mg/m² by rapid IV injection ("bolus"), and then fluorouracil 600 mg/m² infused IV over 22 hours. Treatment is given during a 6-week cycle with administration of conventional irinotecan on days 1, 15, and 29, and administration of the leucovorin and fluorouracil (rapid IV injection ["bolus"] and infusional) component of the regimen on days 1, 2, 15, 16, 29, and 30, with the next cycle beginning on day 43.

Patients who have received prior pelvic or abdominal radiation therapy, who have a performance status of 2, or who have modestly elevated baseline total serum bilirubin concentrations (i.e., 1–2 mg/dL) are at increased risk for irinotecan-induced toxicity such as grade 3 or 4 neutropenia; the manufacturer states that reduction of the initial dose of conventional irinotecan hydrochloride by one dose level (e.g., to 100 mg/m² for regimen 1 or to 150 mg/m² for regimen 2) should be considered in such patients. The manufacturer states that specific dosage recommendations for conventional irinotecan for patients with baseline total serum bilirubin concentrations exceeding 2 mg/dL currently are not available.

During a cycle of therapy or when initiating a subsequent cycle of therapy, the dose level should be reduced as necessary based on modification for toxicity. (See Table 1 and Table 2.) Further reductions in dose level in decrements of 20% may be warranted in patients who continue to experience toxicity. Unless intolerable toxicity develops, treatment with additional cycles may be administered every 6 weeks in patients who continue to experience clinical benefit.

TABLE 1. Dosage Regimens and Dosage Modifications for Conventional Irinotecan-based Combination Therapy for Metastatic Colon or Rectal Cancer

Regimen/Agent	Initial Dosage and Dosage Modifications for Combination Therapy (mg/m²)		
	Initial Dosage	Reduced Dosage Level 1	Reduced Dosage Level 2
Regimen 1 [a]			
Irinotecan hydrochloride	125	100	75
Leucovorin	20	20	20
Fluorouracil	500	400	300
Regimen 2 [b]			
Irinotecan hydrochloride	180	150	120
Leucovorin	200	200	200
Fluorouracil bolus	400	320	240
Fluorouracil infusion	600	480	360

[a] Treatment on days 1, 8, 15, and 22.

[b] Administration of irinotecan on days 1, 15, and 29, and administration of leucovorin, bolus fluorouracil, and infusional fluorouracil on days 1, 2, 15, 16, 29, and 30.

Outside of a well-designed clinical trial, irinotecan should not be used in combination with the "Mayo clinic" regimen of rapid IV injection ("bolus") fluorouracil/leucovorin (i.e., administration for 4–5 consecutive days every 4 weeks) because of increased toxicity, including deaths.

Monotherapy

For the treatment of metastatic carcinoma of the colon or rectum in patients whose disease has recurred or progressed following fluorouracil-based antineoplastic therapy, conventional irinotecan may be administered on a weekly dosage schedule or once every 3 weeks with doses specific to the selected dosage schedule.

The recommended initial dose of conventional irinotecan hydrochloride as a single agent for the treatment of metastatic carcinoma of the colon or rectum in patients receiving the drug on a *weekly dosage schedule* is 125 mg/m² infused IV over a period of 90 minutes. The dose of conventional irinotecan is administered once weekly for 4 weeks followed by a 2-week rest period. Additional cycles (i.e., weekly doses for 4 weeks followed by a 2-week rest period) may be administered every 6 weeks in patients who attain a response or whose disease remains stable, provided intolerable toxicity does not develop.

The recommended initial dose of conventional irinotecan hydrochloride for the treatment of metastatic carcinoma of the colon or rectum in patients receiving the drug *once every 3 weeks* is 350 mg/m² infused IV over a period of 90 minutes. The dose of conventional irinotecan is administered once every 3 weeks for as long as intolerable toxicity does not occur and the patient continues to experience clinical benefit.

Patients who have received prior pelvic or abdominal radiation therapy, who have a performance status of 2, or who have modestly elevated baseline total serum bilirubin concentrations (i.e., 1–2 mg/dL) are at increased risk for irinotecan-induced toxicity such as grade 3 or 4 neutropenia; the manufacturer states that reduction of the initial dose of conventional irinotecan hydrochloride by one dose level (e.g., to 100 mg/m² for the weekly dosage schedule or to 300 mg/m² for the once-every-3-weeks dosage schedule) should be considered in such patients. A reduced initial dose of 300 mg/m² also is recommended for patients 70 years of age or older who are receiving the once-every-3-weeks dosage schedule of conventional irinotecan hydrochloride; however, the manufacturer states that geriatric patients receiving the weekly dosage schedule of conventional irinotecan may receive the usual initial dose of the drug. Reduction in the initial dose of conventional irinotecan may be considered in patients with baseline total serum bilirubin concentrations exceeding 2 mg/dL; the manufacturer states that specific dosage recommendations for conventional irinotecan for such patients currently are not available.

Pancreatic Cancer

For use in a combination regimen for metastatic adenocarcinoma of the pancreas that has progressed following gemcitabine-based therapy, liposomal irinotecan is administered with leucovorin and fluorouracil. Liposomal irinotecan is *not* indicated as a single agent for the treatment of metastatic adenocarcinoma of the pancreas.

The recommended initial dose of liposomal irinotecan is 70 mg/m^2 infused IV over a period of 90 minutes followed by leucovorin 400 mg/m^2 infused IV over 30 minutes and then fluorouracil 2.4 g/m^2 infused IV over 46 hours. Treatment is repeated every 2 weeks.

The manufacturer makes no specific dosage recommendations for liposomal irinotecan for patients with total serum bilirubin concentrations exceeding the upper limit of normal (ULN).

Dosage Modification for Toxicity and Contraindications for Continued Therapy

Dosage of conventional or liposomal irinotecan should be modified as necessary based on individual patient tolerance; the patient should be monitored carefully to obtain optimum therapeutic response with minimum adverse effects. Among those receiving conventional or liposomal irinotecan-based combination therapy, doses of fluorouracil also should be modified as necessary based on individual patient tolerance.

The manufacturer states that a new cycle of conventional irinotecan therapy should not be undertaken until the granulocyte count has recovered to at least 1500/mm^3, the platelet count has recovered to at least 100,000/mm^3, and treatment-related diarrhea has fully resolved. If the patient experiences multiple toxicities, adjustment of conventional irinotecan hydrochloride dose within a cycle of therapy and prior to starting a new cycle of therapy should be based on the preceding toxicity requiring the largest dose reduction. Treatment should be delayed for 1–2 weeks to allow for recovery from treatment-related toxicities. If the patient experiences an irinotecan-induced toxicity that does not resolve after delaying drug administration for 2 weeks, discontinuance of the drug should be considered.

Among patients receiving conventional irinotecan as a single agent, initial doses of conventional irinotecan hydrochloride are based on body surface area alone, but subsequent doses within a cycle of therapy or for a new cycle of therapy in patients receiving the drug on a *weekly dosage schedule* should be adjusted in increments of 25–50 mg/m^2 to a dose within the range of 50–150 mg/m^2 based on the worst toxicity encountered with the previous dose of conventional irinotecan; subsequent doses for a new cycle of therapy in patients receiving the drug *once every 3 weeks* should be decreased in increments of 50 mg/m^2 to a dose as low as 200 mg/m^2 based on the worst toxicity encountered with the previous dose of conventional irinotecan. If the patient experiences no toxicity within a cycle of therapy using the once-every-3-weeks dosage schedule, the current conventional irinotecan hydrochloride dose should be maintained for the subsequent cycle of therapy. If the patient experiences no toxicity during an entire 6-week cycle of therapy using the weekly dosage schedule, the dose of conventional irinotecan hydrochloride may be increased by 25 mg/m^2 at the start of the next cycle; however, the dose should not exceed 150 mg/m^2.

The Recommended Dosage Modifications tables (Tables 2–4) describe recommended modifications in conventional irinotecan hydrochloride dose based on commonly observed toxicities of the drug for patients receiving combination or single-agent therapy with the drug. The dose-limiting toxicities of conventional irinotecan are diarrhea and neutropenia.

Recommended dosage modifications for liposomal irinotecan based on observed toxicities of the drug are described in the following sections on specific types and severities of toxicity.

For a more complete discussion of dosage modifications, cautions, and precautions associated with conventional or liposomal irinotecan therapy, the respective manufacturer's labeling should be consulted.

GI Toxicity

Conventional or liposomal irinotecan may induce both early and late forms of diarrhea, both of which may be severe. Early diarrhea (occurring during or within 24 hours of administration of conventional or liposomal irinotecan) is cholinergic in nature and generally is transient; diarrhea may be accompanied by diaphoresis, flushing, rhinitis, increased salivation, miosis, lacrimation, bradycardia, and abdominal cramping and may be prevented or ameliorated by administration of atropine sulfate (e.g., 0.25–1 mg by IV or subcutaneous injection) unless administration of the drug is clinically contraindicated. Late diarrhea (occurring more than 24 hours after administration of conventional or liposomal irinotecan) can be life-threatening since it may be prolonged and may lead to dehydration, electrolyte imbalance, or sepsis.

Patients receiving conventional irinotecan in combination with rapid IV ("bolus") fluorouracil/leucovorin have experienced early death induced or exacerbated by treatment-related GI toxicity, typically during or immediately following the first cycle of treatment. This GI syndrome is manifested by diarrhea, nausea, vomiting, anorexia, and abdominal cramping, and is often associated with severe dehydration, neutropenia, fever, and electrolyte abnormalities. Radiographic findings include dilated bowel, air-fluid levels without anatomic obstruction, and thickened bowel wall. An independent panel of clinicians that reviewed the causes of these early deaths has recommended close monitoring and prompt, aggressive treatment of toxicity in conjunction with treatment discontinuance in patients experiencing unresolved drug-related toxicity.

Late diarrhea, as an isolated event or as part of the GI syndrome, should be treated promptly with intensive oral loperamide hydrochloride therapy (e.g., 4 mg at the onset of diarrhea, then 2 mg every 2 hours until the patient is diarrhea-free for 12 hours). Use of loperamide at these doses should not exceed 48 consecutive hours because of the risk of paralytic ileus. The efficacy of other antiperistaltic agents in the management of irinotecan-induced diarrhea is unclear. During the night, the patient may take loperamide hydrochloride 4 mg every 4 hours. Baseline bowel patterns should be documented prior to initiation of irinotecan therapy, and any increase in the frequency of bowel movements or change in stool consistency should prompt initiation of loperamide therapy. Premedication with loperamide is not recommended. If diarrhea persists for more than 24 hours despite loperamide therapy, or if diarrhea occurs with fever, some clinicians recommend a 7-day course of oral fluoroquinolone therapy. If diarrhea persists for longer than 48 hours, some clinicians advise discontinuance of loperamide and hospitalization of the patient for parenteral hydration. Prophylactic treatment with an oral fluoroquinolone also should be initiated in patients with an absolute neutrophil count below 500/mm^3, even in the absence of fever or diarrhea.

Cases of late diarrhea complicated by colitis, ulceration, bleeding, ileus, and infection have occurred in patients receiving conventional irinotecan; megacolon and intestinal perforation also have been reported. Anti-infective therapy should be initiated promptly in patients who develop ileus.

Patients with bowel obstruction should *not* receive conventional or liposomal irinotecan.

Patients with diarrhea should be monitored carefully and given fluid and electrolyte replacement if they become dehydrated or anti-infective therapy if they develop ileus, fever, or severe neutropenia. Some clinicians recommend appropriate anti-infective therapy in any patient with prolonged diarrhea, regardless of neutrophil count, with treatment continued until resolution. Delayed initiation of anti-infective therapy, premature discontinuance of anti-infective therapy, or selection of inappropriate anti-infectives probably contributed to early deaths among patients receiving conventional irinotecan with rapid IV ("bolus") fluorouracil/leucovorin. Patients experiencing severe diarrhea that does not resolve to baseline bowel function for at least 24 hours without the use of antidiarrheal medications or anti-infectives should *not* receive further treatment with the conventional irinotecan/fluorouracil/leucovorin regimen.

Following the first treatment with conventional irinotecan-based 3-drug combination therapy, subsequent weekly chemotherapy treatments should be delayed until pretreatment bowel function has been restored for at least 24 hours without the need for antidiarrhea medication. If NCI grade 2, 3, or 4 late diarrhea occurs, administration of conventional irinotecan should be interrupted until the patient recovers, and subsequent doses of the drug should be reduced within the current treatment cycle. An independent panel of clinicians that reviewed the causes of early deaths in patients receiving the 3-drug regimen has recommended that the same guidelines for dosage modification be followed for abdominal cramping; if grade

2 or higher abdominal cramping occurs, treatment should be interrupted until the cramping has fully resolved, and subsequent doses of the drug should be reduced within the current treatment cycle. Among patients receiving conventional irinotecan as a single agent, subsequent doses within the treatment cycle should be reduced in those experiencing grade 2 diarrhea. If severe (NCI grade 3 or 4) diarrhea occurs, administration of conventional irinotecan should be interrupted until the patient recovers, and subsequent doses of the drug should be reduced.

If grade 2–4 diarrhea occurs in patients receiving liposomal irinotecan, therapy with the drug should be withheld until diarrhea resolves to grade 1 or less. Liposomal irinotecan therapy may then be resumed at a reduced dosage (i.e., 70 mg/m² reduced to 50 mg/m² or 50 mg/m² reduced to 43 mg/m²). If grade 2–4 diarrhea recurs following dosage reduction, therapy should be withheld again until diarrhea resolves to grade 1 or less; therapy may then be resumed at a further reduced dosage (i.e., 50 mg/m² reduced to 43 mg/m² or 43 mg/m² reduced to 35 mg/m²). If grade 2–4 diarrhea recurs at this reduced dosage, treatment with liposomal irinotecan should be discontinued.

Hematologic Toxicity

Conventional or liposomal irinotecan can induce severe myelosuppression, particularly neutropenia, and deaths caused by sepsis have been reported in patients treated with the drug. In studies using the weekly dosage schedule for conventional irinotecan monotherapy, patients with even modestly elevated (i.e., 1–2 mg/dL) total serum bilirubin concentrations and those who had received prior pelvic or abdominal radiation therapy were at increased risk of grade 3 or 4 neutropenia associated with the drug. The risk of myelosuppression also may be greater in patients with deficient glucuronidation of bilirubin (e.g., Gilbert's syndrome) who are receiving conventional irinotecan. Complications of neutropenia should be managed promptly with anti-infective therapy.

Therapy with conventional irinotecan should be interrupted during a treatment cycle if neutropenic fever occurs or if the absolute neutrophil count (ANC) drops below 1000/mm³. Following recovery to an ANC of at least 1000/mm³, subsequent doses of conventional irinotecan should be reduced according to the level of neutropenia observed (see the Recommended Dosage Modifications tables [Tables 2–4]). Blood tests should be obtained no sooner than 48 hours before scheduled treatment and trends in the ANC as well as absolute values should be considered; in patients with a rapidly falling ANC, conventional irinotecan therapy should be interrupted even if the current ANC is considered adequate to permit treatment.

The manufacturer of liposomal irinotecan recommends that complete blood cell (CBC) counts be obtained on days 1 and 8 of each cycle and more frequently if clinically indicated. Therapy with liposomal irinotecan should be interrupted if neutropenic fever occurs or if the ANC drops below 1500/mm³. Following recovery to an ANC of at least 1500/mm³, subsequent doses of liposomal irinotecan should be reduced if grade 3 or 4 neutropenia or neutropenic fever was observed.

Cardiovascular Toxicity

Patients receiving conventional irinotecan in combination with rapid IV ("bolus") fluorouracil/leucovorin have experienced early death induced or exacerbated by treatment-related cardiovascular toxicity, typically during or immediately following the first cycle of treatment. This vascular syndrome is characterized by an acute, fatal myocardial infarction, pulmonary embolus, or cerebrovascular accident that occurs during or shortly after receiving chemotherapy. An underlying cardiovascular or thromboembolic condition, if present, was considered stable or well-compensated at the time of treatment. Vascular syndrome may occur as an isolated event or in association with GI or other toxicities of conventional irinotecan-based therapy. Cardiovascular and thromboembolic events also have been reported in patients receiving conventional irinotecan with fluorouracil administered as an IV infusion.

Pulmonary Toxicity

Interstitial lung disease (ILD), sometimes fatal, has been reported in patients receiving conventional irinotecan-based therapy. Patients who have preexisting lung disease or those who have received pneumotoxic drugs, radiation therapy, or hematopoietic agents (i.e., granulocyte or granulocyte-macrophage colony-stimulating factors [G-CSF, GM-CSF]) may be at greater risk for ILD. Patients at risk for developing ILD should be closely monitored for respiratory symptoms before and during irinotecan-based therapy. If manifestations of ILD (i.e., new or progressive dyspnea, cough, or fever) occur, therapy with conventional or liposomal irinotecan should be withheld pending results of clinical investigation. Conventional or liposomal irinotecan should be discontinued in patients who are diagnosed with treatment-related ILD.

Hypersensitivity Reactions

If severe hypersensitivity reactions, including anaphylaxis, occur, therapy with conventional or liposomal irinotecan should be permanently discontinued.

Grade 3 or 4 Toxicity

If grade 3 or 4 adverse events occur in patients receiving liposomal irinotecan, therapy with the drug should be withheld until the toxicity resolves to grade 1 or less. Liposomal irinotecan therapy may then be resumed at a reduced dosage (i.e., 70 mg/m² reduced to 50 mg/m² or 50 mg/m² reduced to 43 mg/m²). If grade 3 or 4 adverse events recur following dosage reduction, therapy should be withheld again until the toxicity resolves to grade 1 or less; therapy may then be resumed at a further reduced dosage (i.e., 50 mg/m² reduced to 43 mg/m² or 43 mg/m² reduced to 35 mg/m²). If grade 3 or 4 adverse events recur at this reduced dosage, treatment with liposomal irinotecan should be discontinued.

TABLE 2. Recommended Dosage Modifications for Conventional Irinotecan in Combination Therapy with Fluorouracil and Leucovorin

The administration of chemotherapy treatments should be delayed until pretreatment bowel function has been restored for at least 24 hours without the need for antidiarrhea medication. A new cycle of conventional irinotecan-based combination therapy should not begin until the granulocyte count has recovered to ≥1500/mm³, the platelet count has recovered to ≥100,000/mm³, and treatment-related diarrhea is fully resolved. Treatment should be delayed 1–2 weeks to allow for recovery from treatment-related toxicities. If the patient has not recovered after a 2-week delay, consideration should be given to discontinuing conventional irinotecan.

Toxicity – NCI Grade (Value) [a]	During a Cycle of Therapy [b]	At the Start of Subsequent Cycles of Therapy [b]
No toxicity	Maintain dose level	Maintain dose level
Neutropenia		
1 (1500 to 1999/mm³)	Maintain dose level	Maintain dose level
2 (1000 to 1499/mm³)	Decrease by 1 dose level	Maintain dose level
3 (500 to 999/mm³)	Omit dose until resolved to ≤ grade 2, then decrease by 1 dose level	Decrease by 1 dose level
4 (<500/mm³)	Omit dose until resolved to ≤ grade 2, then decrease by 2 dose levels	Decrease by 2 dose levels
Neutropenic fever	Omit dose until resolved, then decrease by 2 dose levels	
Other hematologic toxicities	Dose modifications for leukopenia or thrombocytopenia during a cycle of therapy and at the start of subsequent cycles of therapy are also based on NCI toxicity criteria and are the same as recommended for neutropenia above	
Diarrhea		
1 (2–3 stools/day > pretreatment)	Delay dose until resolved to baseline, then resume the same dose	Maintain dose level
2 (4–6 stools/day > pretreatment)	Omit dose until resolved to baseline, then decrease by 1 dose level	Maintain dose level
3 (7–9 stools/day > pretreatment)	Omit dose until resolved to baseline, then decrease by 1 dose level	Decrease by 1 dose level
4 (≥10 stools/day > pretreatment)	Omit dose until resolved to baseline, then decrease by 2 dose levels	Decrease by 2 dose levels

TABLE 2. Continued

Toxicity – NCI Grade (Value) [a]	During a Cycle of Therapy [b]	At the Start of Subsequent Cycles of Therapy [b]
Other nonhematologic toxicities [c]		
1	Maintain dose level	Maintain dose level
2	Omit dose until resolved to ≤ grade 1, then decrease by 1 dose level	Maintain dose level
3	Omit dose until resolved to ≤ grade 2, then decrease by 1 dose level	Decrease by 1 dose level
4	Omit dose until resolved to ≤ grade 2, then decrease by 2 dose levels	Decrease by 2 dose levels
	Note: For mucositis/stomatitis, decrease only fluorouracil, not conventional irinotecan	*Note:* For mucositis/stomatitis, decrease only fluorouracil, not conventional irinotecan

[a] National Cancer Institute Common Toxicity Criteria (version 1.0).

[b] All dose modifications should be based on the worst preceding toxicity.

[c] Excluding alopecia, anorexia, asthenia.

TABLE 3. Recommended Dosage Modifications for Single-Agent *Weekly* Dosage Schedule of Conventional Irinotecan [a]

A new cycle of conventional irinotecan therapy should not begin until the granulocyte count has recovered to ≥1500/mm³, the platelet count has recovered to ≥100,000/mm³, and treatment-related diarrhea is fully resolved. Treatment should be delayed 1–2 weeks to allow for recovery from treatment-related toxicities. If the patient has not recovered after a 2-week delay, consideration should be given to discontinuing conventional irinotecan.

Toxicity – NCI Grade [b]	During a Cycle of Therapy [a]	At the Start of the Next Cycle of Therapy [a]
No toxicity	Maintain dose level	Increase dose by 25 mg/m² up to a maximum dose of 150 mg/m²
Neutropenia		
1 (1500 to 1999/mm³)	Maintain dose level	Maintain dose level
2 (1000 to 1499/mm³)	Decrease dose by 25 mg/m²	Maintain dose level
3 (500 to 999/mm³)	Omit dose until resolved to ≤ grade 2, then decrease dose by 25 mg/m²	Decrease dose by 25 mg/m²
4 (<500/mm³)	Omit dose until resolved to ≤ grade 2, then decrease dose by 50 mg/m²	Decrease dose by 50 mg/m²
Neutropenic fever	Omit dose until resolved, then decrease dose by 50 mg/m²	Decrease dose by 50 mg/m²
Other hematologic toxicities	Dose modifications for leukopenia, thrombocytopenia, and anemia during a cycle of therapy are also based on NCI toxicity criteria and are the same as recommended for neutropenia above	Dose modifications for leukopenia, thrombocytopenia, and anemia at the start of subsequent cycles of therapy are also based on NCI toxicity criteria and are the same as recommended for neutropenia above

TABLE 3. Continued

Toxicity – NCI Grade [b]	During a Cycle of Therapy [a]	At the Start of the Next Cycle of Therapy [a]
Diarrhea		
1 (2–3 stools/day > pretreatment)	Maintain dose level	Maintain dose level
2 (4–6 stools/day > pretreatment)	Decrease dose by 25 mg/m²	Maintain dose level
3 (7–9 stools/day > pretreatment)	Omit dose until resolved to ≤ grade 2, then decrease dose by 25 mg/m²	Decrease dose by 25 mg/m²
4 (≥10 stools/day > pretreatment)	Omit dose until resolved to ≤ grade 2, then decrease dose by 50 mg/m²	Decrease dose by 50 mg/m²
Other nonhematologic toxicities [c]		
1	Maintain dose level	Maintain dose level
2	Decrease dose by 25 mg/m²	Decrease dose by 25 mg/m²
3	Omit dose until resolved to ≤ grade 2, then decrease dose by 25 mg/m²	Decrease dose by 25 mg/m²
4	Omit dose until resolved to ≤ grade 2, then decrease dose by 50 mg/m²	Decrease dose by 50 mg/m²

[a] All dose modifications should be based on the worst preceding toxicity.

[b] National Cancer Institute Common Toxicity Criteria (version 1.0).

[c] Excluding alopecia, anorexia, asthenia.

TABLE 4. Recommended Dosage Modifications for Single-Agent *Once-Every-3-Weeks* Schedule of Conventional Irinotecan [a]

A new cycle of conventional irinotecan therapy should not begin until the granulocyte count has recovered to ≥1500/ mm³, the platelet count has recovered to ≥100,000/ mm³, and treatment-related diarrhea is fully resolved. Treatment should be delayed 1–2 weeks to allow for recovery from treatment-related toxicities. If the patient has not recovered after a 2-week delay, consideration should be given to discontinuing conventional irinotecan.

Toxicity – NCI Grade [b]	At the Start of the Next Cycle of Therapy [a]
No toxicity	Maintain dose level
Neutropenia	
1 (1500 to 1999/mm³)	Maintain dose level
2 (1000 to 1499/mm³)	Maintain dose level
3 (500 to 999/mm³)	Decrease dose by 50 mg/m²
4 (<500/mm³)	Decrease dose by 50 mg/m²
Neutropenic fever	Decrease dose by 50 mg/m²
Other hematologic toxicities	Dose modifications for leukopenia, thrombocytopenia, and anemia at the start of subsequent cycles of therapy are also based on NCI toxicity criteria and are the same as recommended for neutropenia above

TABLE 4. Continued

Toxicity – NCI Grade [b]	At the Start of the Next Cycle of Therapy [a]
Diarrhea	
1 (2–3 stools/day > pretreatment)	Maintain dose level
2 (4–6 stools/day > pretreatment)	Maintain dose level
3 (7–9 stools/day > pretreatment)	Decrease dose by 50 mg/m²
4 (≥10 stools/day > pretreatment)	Decrease dose by 50 mg/m²
Other nonhematologic toxicities[c]	
1	Maintain dose level
2	Decrease dose by 50 mg/m²
3	Decrease dose by 50 mg/m²
4	Decrease dose by 50 mg/m²

[a] All dose modifications should be based on the worst preceding toxicity.

[b] National Cancer Institute Common Toxicity Criteria (version 1.0)

[c] Excluding alopecia, anorexia, asthenia

● *Dosage in Renal and Hepatic Impairment*

Conventional Irinotecan Hydrochloride

Safety and efficacy of conventional irinotecan hydrochloride have not been evaluated systematically in patients with renal impairment. The manufacturer makes no specific recommendations regarding dosage adjustment in patients with renal impairment, but states that use of conventional irinotecan in patients requiring dialysis is not recommended.

In patients with hepatic impairment, clearance of conventional irinotecan is decreased and exposure to the SN-38 active metabolite is increased. In clinical trials for GI cancer using either dosage schedule, conventional irinotecan was not administered to patients with serum bilirubin concentrations exceeding 2 mg/dL; specific dosage recommendations are not available for such patients. The drug also was *not* administered to patients who had serum aminotransferase concentrations exceeding 3 times the ULN in the absence of hepatic metastases or to those with hepatic metastases who had serum aminotransferase concentrations exceeding 5 times the ULN. The manufacturer states that reduction of the initial dose of conventional irinotecan hydrochloride by one dose level (e.g., to 100 mg/m² for regimen 1 or to 150 mg/m² for regimen 2 as first-line combination therapy; to 100 mg/m² for the weekly dosage schedule or to 300 mg/m² for the once-every-3-weeks dosage schedule as monotherapy) should be considered for patients with modestly elevated serum bilirubin concentrations (i.e., 1–2 mg/dL). (See Colorectal Cancer under Dosage and Administration: Dosage.)

Liposomal Irinotecan Hydrochloride

In a population pharmacokinetic analysis of liposomal irinotecan hydrochloride, systemic exposure to the SN-38 active metabolite in patients with mild (creatinine clearance of 60–89 mL/minute) or moderate (creatinine clearance of 30–59 mL/minute) renal impairment was similar to that in patients with normal renal function. Pharmacokinetic data in patients with severe renal impairment (creatinine clearance less than 30 mL/minute) are limited. The manufacturer makes no specific dosage recommendations for patients with renal impairment.

Formal pharmacokinetic studies with liposomal irinotecan hydrochloride have not been conducted in patients with hepatic impairment. Data from a population pharmacokinetic analysis indicate that average steady-state concentrations of total SN-38 are increased by 37% in patients with baseline serum bilirubin concentrations of 1–2 mg/dL compared with patients with baseline serum bilirubin concentrations of less than 1 mg/dL; however, elevated concentrations of serum aminotransferases (ALT or AST) did not affect total SN-38 concentrations. The drug has not been studied in patients with serum bilirubin concentrations exceeding 2 mg/dL, and patients with bilirubin concentrations exceeding the ULN were not included in the pivotal clinical trial evaluating liposomal irinotecan therapy for metastatic pancreatic cancer. The manufacturer makes no specific recommendations regarding dosage adjustment in patients with hepatic impairment.

DESCRIPTION

Irinotecan (CPT-11), a semisynthetic derivative of camptothecin, is an antineoplastic agent. Camptothecins are alkaloids with antitumor activity that are extracted from plants such as *Camptotheca acuminata*. Conventional and liposomal preparations of irinotecan hydrochloride are commercially available as the trihydrate. Each mL of conventional irinotecan hydrochloride for injection concentrate contains 20 mg of the drug in terms of the hydrated salt. Each mL of liposomal irinotecan hydrochloride for injection concentrate contains 4.3 mg of the drug in terms of the anhydrous base.

Irinotecan is a type I DNA topoisomerase inhibitor. DNA topoisomerases (i.e., types I and II) are enzymes in the cell nucleus that regulate DNA topology (3-dimensional conformation) and facilitate nuclear processes such as DNA replication, recombination, and repair. During these processes, type I DNA topoisomerase creates transient (reversible) single-stranded breaks in double-stranded DNA, allowing intact single DNA strands to pass through the break and relieve the topologic constraints (e.g., torsional strain) inherent in supercoiled DNA. The 3'-DNA terminus of the broken DNA strands bind covalently with the topoisomerase enzyme to form a catalytic intermediate, termed a cleavable complex. After the DNA is sufficiently relaxed and the strand passage reaction is complete, DNA topoisomerase reattaches the broken DNA strands to form the chemically unaltered topoisomers that allow transcription to proceed. Irinotecan is a water-soluble precursor to the lipophilic active metabolite SN-38 (7-ethyl-10-hydroxycamptothecin), which is 1000 times as potent as irinotecan in vitro as an inhibitor of type I DNA topoisomerase. However, the precise contribution of SN-38 to the pharmacologic activity of administered irinotecan is unknown because of the variable in vitro cytotoxic potency reported for SN-38 relative to the parent drug and differences in the area under the plasma concentration-time curve and plasma protein binding of SN-38 compared with irinotecan.

Irinotecan, its active metabolite SN-38, and other type I topoisomerase inhibitors are believed to exert their cytotoxic effects during the S-phase of DNA synthesis through an interaction with the DNA–DNA topoisomerase cleavable complex. The cleavable complex is bound and stabilized by irinotecan and/or SN-38, preventing the topoisomerase from religating the single-strand breaks. The ternary complex of irinotecan/SN-38, DNA, and DNA topoisomerase interferes with the moving replication fork, inducing replication arrest and lethal double-stranded breaks in DNA. This DNA damage is not efficiently repaired and apparently leads to apoptosis (programmed cell death).

For further information on the handling of antineoplastic agents, see the ASHP Guidelines on Handling Hazardous Drugs at http://www.ahfsdrug information.com.

PREPARATIONS

Distribution of liposomal irinotecan hydrochloride is restricted. (See Dosage and Administration.)

Excipients in commercially available drug preparations may have clinically important effects in some individuals; consult specific product labeling for details.

Irinotecan Hydrochloride (Trihydrate)

Parenteral

Concentrate, for injection, for IV infusion only	20 mg/mL (40 and 100 mg)*	**Camptosar®**, Pfizer

* available from one or more manufacturer, distributor, and/or repackager by generic (nonproprietary) name

Irinotecan Hydrochloride Liposomal (Trihydrate)

Parenteral

Concentrate, for injection, for IV infusion only	4.3 mg (of irinotecan) per mL (43 mg)	**Onivyde®**, Merrimack

† Use is not currently included in the labeling approved by the US Food and Drug Administration.

Lapatinib Ditosylate

10:00 • ANTINEOPLASTIC AGENTS

- Lapatinib, an inhibitor of human epidermal growth factor receptor type 2 (HER2/ERBB2) and epidermal growth factor receptor (HER1/EGFR/ERBB1) tyrosine kinases, is an antineoplastic agent.

USES

● Breast Cancer

Advanced or Metastatic Breast Cancer

Lapatinib ditosylate is used in combination with letrozole (an aromatase inhibitor) for the treatment of hormone receptor-positive metastatic breast cancer that overexpresses the HER2 protein in postmenopausal women who are candidates for hormonal therapy. Lapatinib also is used in combination with capecitabine for the treatment of advanced or metastatic breast cancer that overexpresses the HER2 protein in patients who have received prior therapy including an anthracycline, a taxane, and trastuzumab. Lapatinib plus capecitabine should only be initiated in patients with a history of disease progression on trastuzumab.

Combination Therapy with Lapatinib and Letrozole

Lapatinib is used in combination with letrozole for the treatment of hormone receptor-positive metastatic breast cancer that overexpresses the HER2 protein in postmenopausal women who are candidates for hormonal therapy. Safety and efficacy of lapatinib for this indication are supported by 2 randomized phase 3 trials. In patients with hormone receptor-positive, HER2-positive breast cancer, guidelines generally recommend HER2-targeted therapy plus chemotherapy, endocrine therapy plus trastuzumab or lapatinib (in selected cases), or endocrine therapy alone (in selected cases).

Safety and efficacy of lapatinib in combination with letrozole for this indication have been evaluated in a phase 3, randomized, double-blind, controlled clinical study in postmenopausal women with hormone receptor-positive (estrogen- and/or progesterone-positive) metastatic breast cancer; 17% of patients enrolled in this study had HER2-positive tumors. Patients were randomized to receive lapatinib (1.5 g once daily) and letrozole (2.5 mg once daily) or letrozole (2.5 mg once daily) and placebo. Patients who had received prior therapy for advanced or metastatic disease were excluded from the study. However, prior adjuvant or neoadjuvant chemotherapy, radiation therapy, or antiestrogen therapy was allowed; adjuvant use of aromatase inhibitors and trastuzumab was allowed if such treatment was completed at least one year prior to study entry. Approximately one-half of the 219 patients with HER2-positive tumors had previously received antiestrogens and/or chemotherapy, approximately one-third had received adjuvant antiestrogen therapy within 6 months of study entry, and less than 1% had received prior trastuzumab therapy.

In the subgroup of patients with HER2-positive tumors, those receiving combined therapy with lapatinib and letrozole had longer median progression-free survival (35.4 versus 13 weeks) and a higher objective response rate (28 versus 15%) compared with those receiving letrozole alone. However, in the subgroup of patients with HER2-negative tumors, combined therapy with lapatinib and letrozole did not improve progression-free survival or response rate over that observed with letrozole alone.

The efficacy and safety of combination therapy with lapatinib and an aromatase inhibitor were confirmed in another randomized, phase 3 trial (ALTERNATIVE) in postmenopausal women with hormone receptor-positive/HER2-positive metastatic breast cancer that had progressed after prior treatment with trastuzumab-containing chemotherapy and endocrine therapies in the metastatic setting. Patients were randomized to one of the following regimens: lapatinib (1 g once daily) plus trastuzumab and an aromatase inhibitor, trastuzumab plus an aromatase inhibitor, or lapatinib 1.5 g once daily plus an aromatase inhibitor. In all trastuzumab-containing arms, trastuzumab was administered with a loading dose of 8 mg/kg IV followed by a maintenance dosage of 6 mg/kg IV every 3 weeks; patients receiving an aromatase inhibitor were administered letrozole

2.5 mg once daily, exemestane 25 mg once daily, or anastrozole 1 mg once daily based on the investigator's choice.

The primary efficacy endpoint was progression-free survival comparing lapatinib plus trastuzumab and an aromatase inhibitor to trastuzumab plus an aromatase inhibitor. The median duration of treatment was 53.6 weeks across all arms. At the time of data cutoff, patients receiving lapatinib plus trastuzumab and an aromatase inhibitor had longer median progression-free survival (11 versus 5.6 months) and a higher overall response rate (22.5 versus 8.5%) compared with those receiving trastuzumab plus an aromatase inhibitor. Median overall survival had not been reached at the time of the efficacy analysis.

Combination Therapy with Lapatinib and Capecitabine

Lapatinib is used in combination with capecitabine for the treatment of advanced or metastatic breast cancer that overexpresses the HER2 protein in patients who have received prior therapy including an anthracycline, a taxane, and trastuzumab. Safety and efficacy of lapatinib for this indication are supported by a single randomized controlled trial. Guidelines generally recommend lapatinib among several potential third-line treatment options in patients with advanced, HER2-positive breast cancer who have trialed 2 previous anti-HER2 regimens.

Safety and efficacy of lapatinib (in combination with capecitabine) in the treatment of HER2-positive advanced or metastatic breast cancer have been evaluated in a phase 3, open-label, randomized, controlled clinical study. The study enrolled patients with locally advanced or metastatic breast cancer that had progressed following treatment with regimens that included an anthracycline, a taxane, and trastuzumab. Patients were randomized to receive lapatinib (1.25 g once daily, continuously) in conjunction with capecitabine (2 g/m² daily on days 1–14 every 21 days) or capecitabine monotherapy (2.5 g/m² daily on days 1–14 every 21 days).

Enrollment in this study was terminated early when a planned interim analysis indicated that patients receiving lapatinib in combination with capecitabine had a longer median time to progression (8.4 versus 4.4 months) and longer median progression-free survival (8.4 versus 4.4 months) than did those receiving capecitabine alone. At the time of the interim analysis, overall survival and overall response rates did not differ substantially between the 2 treatment groups. Overall response rates were 22% for patients receiving lapatinib in combination with capecitabine and 14% for those receiving capecitabine monotherapy. Two efficacy analyses performed 4 months later (one an independent assessment and the other an investigator assessment that incorporated updated tumor assessment data) indicated that response rates were higher in patients receiving lapatinib in combination with capecitabine than in those receiving capecitabine alone (23.7 versus 13.9%, respectively [independent analysis]; 31.8 versus 17.4%, respectively [investigator analysis]). These analyses, like the interim analysis, indicated that median time to progression was longer in patients receiving lapatinib in combination with capecitabine than in those receiving capecitabine alone (27.1 versus 18.6 weeks, respectively [independent analysis]; 23.9 versus 18.3 weeks, respectively [investigator analysis]). Based on these results, the study was unblinded and combination therapy with lapatinib and capecitabine was offered to all patients who had been receiving capecitabine alone. Early termination of the study and patient crossover resulted in insufficient power to detect a survival benefit with the combination regimen; at 2 years after the independent and investigator analyses, median overall survival was 75 weeks for patients receiving lapatinib in combination with capecitabine compared with 65.9 weeks for those receiving capecitabine alone.

A randomized, open-label, active-controlled multicenter study (NALA) compared oral neratinib plus capecitabine to oral lapatinib plus capecitabine in patients with HER2-positive metastatic breast cancer who had previously received 2 or more anti-HER2-based regimens. In this trial, neratinib was associated with longer progression-free survival than lapatinib (median 5.6 versus 5.5 months, respectively). At the time of follow-up, median overall survival was similar with neratinib plus capecitabine and lapatinib plus capecitabine (21 or 18.7 months, respectively).

Clinical Perspective

In the 2022 ASCO guidelines on systemic treatment for advanced HER2-positive breast cancer, first-line recommended treatment includes a combination of trastuzumab, pertuzumab, and a taxane. Trastuzumab deruxtecan is recommended for second-line treatment of patients whose breast cancer progresses after initial

HER2-targeted treatment. Multiple potential treatment options are recommended for third-line treatment, including lapatinib in combination with trastuzumab and lapatinib in combination with capecitabine. Selection of an appropriate regimen should be made after discussing treatment schedules, routes of administration, and adverse effects with the patient. In patients with hormone receptor-positive, HER2-positive breast cancer, the guidelines recommend HER2-targeted therapy plus chemotherapy, endocrine therapy plus trastuzumab or lapatinib (in selected cases), or endocrine therapy alone (in selected cases).

DOSAGE AND ADMINISTRATION

● General

Pretreatment Screening

- Measure liver function tests, including serum concentrations of transaminases, bilirubin, and alkaline phosphatase, prior to initiation of lapatinib.

- Monitor serum electrolytes and correct hypokalemia or hypomagnesemia prior to treatment with lapatinib.

- Evaluate left ventricular ejection fraction (LVEF) prior to initiation of lapatinib.

- Perform pregnancy testing in females of reproductive potential prior to starting lapatinib.

Patient Monitoring

- Monitor liver function tests, including serum concentrations of transaminases, bilirubin, and alkaline phosphatase, every 4–6 weeks during therapy, and as clinically indicated.

- Monitor for pulmonary symptoms of interstitial lung disease or pneumonitis during treatment with lapatinib.

- Evaluate LVEF during treatment with lapatinib to ensure that it does not fall below the institution's normal limits.

● Administration

Lapatinib is administered orally once daily. Administer the drug at least 1 hour before or 1 hour after meals. Do not divide the daily dosage because such administration may increase systemic exposure to the drug (by approximately twofold). Advise patients not to double the next dose if a dose is missed. Store lapatinib tablets at 20–25°C (excursions permitted between 15–30°C).

● Dosage

Dosage of lapatinib ditosylate monohydrate is expressed in terms of lapatinib.

Advanced or Metastatic Breast Cancer

For use in combination with letrozole for the treatment of hormone receptor-positive, HER2-positive metastatic breast cancer in postmenopausal women, the recommended dosage of lapatinib is 1.5 g orally once daily, given continuously in combination with letrozole 2.5 mg once daily. In a clinical trial evaluating this regimen, treatment was continued until disease progression occurred or the patient withdrew from the study.

For use in combination with capecitabine for the treatment of HER2-positive advanced or metastatic breast cancer in patients who have received prior therapy including an anthracycline, a taxane, and trastuzumab, the recommended adult dosage of lapatinib is 1.25 g orally once daily on days 1–21 in combination with capecitabine 2 g/m^2 daily (administered orally in 2 divided doses approximately 12 hours apart) on days 1–14 of each 21-day cycle. Continue treatment until disease progression or unacceptable toxicity occurs.

Dosage Modification

Dosage Modification for Toxicity

If adverse reactions occur during lapatinib therapy, temporary interruption of therapy, dosage reduction, and/or permanent discontinuance of the drug may be necessary. If dosage reduction is required, the dosage of lapatinib should be reduced as described in Table 1.

TABLE 1. Recommended Dosage Reduction for Lapatinib Toxicity

Adverse Reaction	Recommended Dosage Reduction of Lapatinib when Used in Combination with Letrozole for Hormone Receptor-positive, HER2-positive Metastatic Breast Cancer	Recommended Dosage Reduction of Lapatinib when Used in Combination with Capecitabine for HER2-positive, Advanced or Metastatic Breast Cancer
Cardiac events	1.25 g once daily	1 g once daily
Diarrhea	1.25 g once daily in patients previously receiving 1.5 g once daily	1.25 g once daily in patients previously receiving 1.5 g once daily
	1 g once daily in patients previously receiving 1.25 g once daily	1 g once daily in patients previously receiving 1.25 g once daily
Other toxicity	1.25 g once daily	1 g once daily

Table 2 indicates the recommended dosage modification (i.e., temporary interruption of therapy, dosage reduction, discontinuance of therapy) for adverse effects according to severity.

TABLE 2. Dosage Modification for Lapatinib Toxicity.

Adverse Reaction and Severity[a]	Modification
Cardiac Events	
Grade ≥2 decreased LVEF or LVEF that decreases below institution's lower limit of normal (LLN)	Discontinue lapatinib; may restart at a reduced dosage (see Table 1) after ≥2 weeks if LVEF returns to normal and the patient is asymptomatic
Diarrhea	
Grade 3 or Grade 1–2 with complicating features[b]	Withhold therapy; may restart at a reduced dosage (see Table 1) once diarrhea resolves to ≤grade 1
Grade 4	Permanently discontinue lapatinib
Interstitial Lung Disease/Pneumonitis	
Grade ≥3	Discontinue lapatinib
Other Toxicity	
Grade ≥2	Consider interruption or discontinuance of lapatinib
	May restart at the standard dosage of 1.25 or 1.5 g once daily once the toxicity improves to grade ≤1; If the toxicity recurs, restart lapatinib at a reduced dosage (see Table 1)

[a] Severity is defined by the National Cancer Institute Common Terminology Criteria for Adverse Events (NCI CTCAE)

[b] Complicating features include moderate to severe abdominal cramping, nausea or vomiting of grade ≥2, decreased performance status, sepsis, fever, neutropenia, frank bleeding, or dehydration

Dosage Modification with Concomitant Therapy

Avoid concomitant use of lapatinib with potent *inhibitors* of cytochrome P-450 (CYP) isoenzyme 3A4. If concomitant therapy cannot be avoided, consider reduction of the lapatinib dosage to 500 mg daily. This recommendation is based on pharmacokinetic considerations; no clinical data on this dosage adjustment are available. If the potent CYP3A4 inhibitor is discontinued, a period of approximately 1 week should elapse before lapatinib dosage is increased to the usual recommended dosage.

Avoid concomitant use of lapatinib with potent CYP3A4 *inducers*. If concomitant therapy cannot be avoided, consider an increase in lapatinib dosage. Lapatinib dosage should be increased gradually as tolerated from a dosage of 1.5 g daily up to 5.5 g daily when given in combination with letrozole for the treatment of hormone receptor-positive, HER2-positive metastatic breast cancer and from a dosage of 1.25 g daily up to 4.5 g daily when given in combination with capecitabine for the treatment of HER2-positive, advanced or metastatic breast cancer. These recommendations are based on pharmacokinetic considerations; no clinical data on these dosage adjustments in these patient populations are available. If the potent CYP3A4 inducer is discontinued, reduce the lapatinib dosage to the usual recommended dosage.

● **Special Populations**

Hepatic Impairment

In patients with severe preexisting hepatic impairment (Child-Pugh class C), consider a reduced dosage of lapatinib based on pharmacokinetic considerations. Consider a reduced dosage of 1 g once daily when lapatinib is given in combination with letrozole for the treatment of hormone receptor-positive, HER2-positive metastatic breast cancer; consider a reduced dosage of 750 mg once daily when lapatinib is given in combination with capecitabine for the treatment of HER2-positive, advanced or metastatic breast cancer. These dosage reductions in patients with severe hepatic impairment have been predicted to adjust AUC to the normal range. However, no clinical data on these dosage adjustments in these patient populations are available.

Renal Impairment

The manufacturer makes no specific dosage recommendations for patients with renal impairment. However, renal impairment is unlikely to affect the pharmacokinetics of lapatinib since less than 2% of the dose is eliminated renally.

Geriatric Patients

The manufacturer makes no specific dosage recommendations for geriatric patients.

CAUTIONS

● **Contraindications**

- Known hypersensitivity (e.g., anaphylaxis) to the drug or any ingredient in the formulation.

● **Warnings/Precautions**

Warnings

Hepatotoxicity

A boxed warning about the risk of hepatotoxicity is included in the prescribing information for lapatinib. Hepatotoxicity may be severe and deaths have been reported in patients receiving lapatinib. The cause of the deaths is uncertain.

Hepatotoxicity indicated by abnormal liver function test results, including serum concentrations of ALT or AST >3 times the upper limit of normal and serum concentrations of total bilirubin >2 times the upper limit of normal, have been observed in <1% of patients receiving lapatinib in clinical trials and in postmarketing experience. Hepatotoxicity may occur within days to several months following initiation of lapatinib therapy.

Monitor liver function tests (serum concentrations of transaminases, bilirubin, and alkaline phosphatase) before initiation of lapatinib therapy, every 4–6 weeks during therapy, and as clinically indicated. If severe changes in liver function occur, discontinue lapatinib therapy permanently.

Pharmacogenomics of Lapatinib-induced Hepatotoxicity

In a genetic substudy of a trial evaluating lapatinib monotherapy, the human leukocyte antigen (HLA) alleles DQA1*02:01 and DRB1*07:01 were associated with hepatotoxicity reactions. Severe liver injury (ALT >5 times the upper limit of normal, National Cancer Institute Common Terminology Criteria for Adverse Events [NCI-CTCAE] grade 3) occurred in 2% of patients overall; the incidence of severe liver injury was 8 versus 0.5% among carriers of the DQA1*02:01 or DRB1*07:01 alleles versus non-carriers, respectively. The DQA1*02:01 and DRB1*07:01 alleles are present in approximately 15–25% of Caucasian, Asian, African, and Hispanic populations and in 1% of Japanese populations. Monitor liver function in all patients receiving lapatinib regardless of genotype.

Other Warnings/Precautions

Decreased Left Ventricular Ejection Fraction

Lapatinib has been reported to cause decreased LVEF. Clinical studies indicate that the majority (more than 57%) of decreases in LVEF associated with the drug occur within the first 12 weeks of lapatinib treatment. Data on long-term exposure are limited. Caution should be exercised if lapatinib is administered to patients with conditions that could impair LVEF. Evaluate LVEF in patients prior to the initiation of lapatinib and periodically during treatment.

Discontinue lapatinib in patients with decreased LVEF of NCI-CTCAE grade 2 or greater and in patients with an LVEF that drops below the institution's lower limit of normal.

Diarrhea

Diarrhea, including severe diarrhea and deaths, have been reported in patients receiving lapatinib. Diarrhea typically occurs early in the course of treatment, with approximately half of patients in clinical trials experiencing diarrhea within the first 6 days of lapatinib therapy. Diarrhea associated with lapatinib therapy typically lasts 4–5 days and is low-grade; severe diarrhea of grade 3 or 4 occurred in less than 10 or 1% of patients, respectively, in clinical trials.

Early identification and intervention is crucial for optimal management of diarrhea. Instruct patients to report any change in bowel habits immediately and treat diarrhea promptly with antidiarrheal agents (e.g., loperamide) after the first unformed stool. Management of severe diarrhea may include oral or IV electrolytes and fluids, administration of antibiotics (especially for diarrhea that persists beyond 24 hours or when there is a fever or grade 3–4 neutropenia), and interruption or discontinuance of lapatinib therapy.

Interstitial Lung Disease/Pneumonitis

Lapatinib therapy (alone or in combination with other antineoplastics) has been associated with interstitial lung disease and pneumonitis. Monitor patients for pulmonary symptoms, and discontinue the drug if symptoms suggestive of grade 3 or higher interstitial lung disease or pneumonitis develop.

QT Interval Prolongation

QT interval prolongation has been reported in patients receiving lapatinib. Monitor patients taking lapatinib who have or may develop prolongation of the corrected QT (QT$_c$) interval (e.g., patients with hypokalemia, hypomagnesemia, or congenital long QT syndrome; those receiving concomitant drugs that may prolong the QT$_c$ interval, or are associated with torsades de pointes; those with cumulative high-dose anthracycline therapy). Prior to administration of lapatinib, correct hypokalemia or hypomagnesemia.

Severe Cutaneous Reactions

Severe cutaneous reactions have been reported in patients receiving lapatinib. Discontinue treatment if life-threatening cutaneous reactions (erythema multiforme, Stevens-Johnson syndrome, or toxic epidermal necrolysis) are suspected.

Fetal/Neonatal Morbidity and Mortality

Lapatinib can cause fetal harm if administered to pregnant women based on its mechanism of action and animal findings; fetal anomalies, abortion, and death of offspring within days after birth have been demonstrated in animals. A significant decrease in the number of live fetuses or fetal body weights was seen in female rats given oral doses of lapatinib at exposure levels approximately 6.4 or 3.3 times the human exposure at the recommended dosage, respectively.

Pregnancy should be avoided during therapy. (See Females and Males of Reproductive Potential under Cautions.) Perform a pregnancy test prior to initiation of lapatinib in females of reproductive potential. Inform pregnant women and females of reproductive potential of the potential hazard to the fetus.

Specific Populations

Pregnancy

Lapatinib can cause fetal harm if administered to pregnant women based on its mechanism of action and animal findings. (See Fetal/Neonatal Morbidity and Mortality under Cautions.) Inform pregnant women and females of reproductive potential of the potential hazard to the fetus. (See Females and Males of Reproductive Potential under Cautions.)

Lactation

It is not known whether lapatinib is distributed into human milk. Because of the potential for serious adverse reactions to lapatinib in nursing infants, advise women to discontinue nursing while receiving lapatinib and for at least 1 week after the drug is discontinued. The effects of the drug on nursing infants or on the production of milk are unknown.

Females and Males of Reproductive Potential

The effect of lapatinib on human fertility is not known. In animal studies, no effects on male or female fertility were found in rats receiving lapatinib at exposure levels approximately 2.6–6.4 times the human exposure at the recommended dosage. However, a significant decrease in the number of live fetuses or fetal body weights was seen in female rats given oral doses of lapatinib at exposure levels approximately 6.4 or 3.3 times the human exposure at the recommended dosage, respectively.

Lapatinib may cause fetal harm. Advise females of childbearing potential to use effective contraceptive methods while receiving lapatinib and for at least 1 week after discontinuance of the drug. In addition, advise males with such female partners to use effective methods of contraception while receiving lapatinib and for 1 week after discontinuance of the drug.

Pediatric Use

Safety and efficacy have not been established in children.

Geriatric Use

No substantial differences in safety or efficacy have been observed in geriatric patients relative to younger adults, but increased sensitivity cannot be ruled out.

Hepatic Impairment

Use lapatinib with caution in patients with severe preexisting hepatic impairment (Child-Pugh class C); systemic exposure to the drug may be increased. Consider dosage reduction in such patients. Permanently discontinue lapatinib in patients who develop severe hepatotoxicity while on therapy.

Renal Impairment

Safety and efficacy have not been established in patients with renal impairment or in patients undergoing hemodialysis. However, renal impairment is unlikely to affect lapatinib pharmacokinetics since less than 2% of the drug and its metabolites are eliminated by the kidneys.

● Common Adverse Effects

Adverse effects reported in ≥20% of patients receiving lapatinib in combination with capecitabine include diarrhea, palmar-plantar erythrodysesthesia, nausea, vomiting, rash, and fatigue.

Adverse effects reported in ≥20% of patients receiving lapatinib in combination with letrozole include diarrhea, rash, nausea, and fatigue.

DRUG INTERACTIONS

Lapatinib is metabolized by cytochrome P-450 (CYP) isoenzymes, principally by CYP3A4 and 3A5. Lapatinib inhibits CYP3A4 and CYP2C8, but does not substantially inhibit CYP isoenzymes 1A2, 2C9, 2C19, and 2D6 or uridine 5′-diphospho-glucuronosyltransferase (UGT) enzymes in vitro.

Lapatinib is a substrate and inhibitor of efflux transporter P-glycoprotein (P-gp).

● Drugs Affecting or Metabolized by Hepatic Microsomal Enzymes

Potent inhibitors of cytochrome CYP3A4: Avoid concomitant use of lapatinib with potent inhibitors of CYP3A4 (e.g., atazanavir, clarithromycin, indinavir, itraconazole, ketoconazole, nefazodone, nelfinavir, ritonavir, saquinavir, telithromycin, voriconazole). In drug interaction studies with ketoconazole (200 mg twice daily for 7 days), systemic lapatinib exposure increased approximately 3.6-fold, and lapatinib half-life increased 1.7-fold. If concomitant use of lapatinib with a potent CYP3A4 inhibitor cannot be avoided, consider reducing the dosage of lapatinib.

Potent inducers of CYP3A4: Avoid concomitant use of lapatinib with potent CYP3A4 inducers (e.g., carbamazepine, dexamethasone, phenobarbital, phenytoin, rifabutin, rifampin, rifapentine, St. John's wort [Hypericum perforatum]). In drug interaction studies, carbamazepine (100 mg twice daily for 3 days and 200 mg twice daily for 17 days) decreased systemic lapatinib exposure approximately 72%. If concomitant use of lapatinib with a potent CYP3A4 inducer cannot be avoided, adjust the dosage of lapatinib.

Substrates of CYP isoenzymes: Lapatinib inhibits CYP2C8 in vitro at clinically relevant concentrations and is a weak inhibitor of CYP3A4 in vivo, but does not appear to substantially inhibit CYP isoenzymes 1A2, 2C9, 2C19, and 2D6, or UGT enzymes in vitro. Concomitant administration of lapatinib with oral or IV midazolam (a CYP3A4 substrate) increased midazolam exposure (as measured by AUC over 24 hours) by 45 or 22%, respectively. Exercise caution and consider a dosage reduction of the substrate drug when lapatinib is administered concomitantly with a CYP2C8 or CYP3A4 substrate with a narrow therapeutic index.

● Drugs that are Substrates or Inhibitors of P-glycoprotein Transport System

Lapatinib is both a substrate and an inhibitor of the efflux transporter P-gp, ABCB1. Exercise caution if lapatinib is administered with drugs that are substrates or inhibitors of P-gp; increased plasma concentrations of the substrate drug or lapatinib are likely. When lapatinib is used concomitantly with a P-gp substrate with a narrow therapeutic index, consider reducing the dosage of the P-gp substrate drug.

● Drugs that Prolong the QT Interval

Because lapatinib may cause prolongation of the QT interval, use lapatinib with caution in patients receiving concomitant therapy with other drugs (e.g., antiarrhythmic agents) known to prolong the QT interval.

● Drugs Affecting Gastric Acidity

Concomitant use of lapatinib with drugs affecting gastric acidity may decrease the solubility of lapatinib. However, concomitant administration of lapatinib and esomeprazole, a proton pump inhibitor, did not result in a clinically meaningful reduction in lapatinib exposure.

● Digoxin

Concomitant administration of lapatinib and oral digoxin (a P-gp substrate) increased systemic exposure (AUC) of digoxin by approximately 2.8-fold. In patients receiving digoxin, measure serum digoxin concentrations prior to initiation of lapatinib therapy and monitor concentrations throughout concomitant therapy. If serum digoxin concentrations exceed 1.2 ng/mL, reduce the digoxin dosage by 50%.

● Paclitaxel

In patients receiving lapatinib and paclitaxel (a CYP2C8 and P-gp substrate) concomitantly, systemic exposure (AUC over 24 hours) of paclitaxel was increased by 23%. However, the manufacturer states that because of limitations of the study design, these data may underestimate the potential increase in paclitaxel exposure during concomitant use.

● Grapefruit

Avoid grapefruit products because of the potential for increased plasma lapatinib concentrations.

DESCRIPTION

Lapatinib, a tyrosine kinase inhibitor, is an antineoplastic agent. The drug inhibits the intracellular tyrosine kinase domains of both epidermal growth factor receptor (HER1/EGFR/ERBB1) and human epidermal growth factor receptor type 2 (HER2/ERBB2). Lapatinib has been shown to inhibit ERBB-driven tumor cell growth in vitro and in various animal models. The drug also has exhibited additive antineoplastic activity with fluorouracil (the active metabolite of capecitabine) in vitro. Lapatinib has been shown in vitro to retain significant antineoplastic activity against breast cancer cell lines selected for long-term growth in trastuzumab-containing medium, suggesting a lack of cross-resistance between lapatinib and trastuzumab.

Hormone receptor-positive breast cancer cells that overexpress EGFR and HER2 tend to be resistant to endocrine (antiestrogen) therapies. Similarly, hormone receptor-positive breast cancer cells that initially lack EGFR or HER2 may upregulate these receptor pathways as the tumor becomes resistant to endocrine therapy. In vitro data indicate that complex interactions between pathways involving the estrogen receptor and epidermal growth factor receptors (e.g., EGFR, HER2) may result in enhanced signal transduction and eventually lead to sustained tumor growth. Therefore, combined use of endocrine therapy (e.g., letrozole) and therapy targeting EGFR/HER2 (e.g., lapatinib) in women with hormone receptor-positive, HER2-positive breast cancer may delay or prevent the emergence of acquired endocrine resistance resulting from increased EGFR and HER2 signaling.

Steady-state concentrations of lapatinib are reached in approximately 6–7 days, indicating an effective half-life of 24 hours. Systemic exposure of lapatinib is increased threefold or fourfold when the drug is administered with a low-fat or high-fat meal, respectively, and is increased approximately twofold when the total daily dose is administered in divided doses instead of once daily. Lapatinib is highly bound (greater than 99%) to plasma proteins (mainly to albumin and α1-acid glycoprotein). Lapatinib is metabolized principally by cytochrome P-450 (CYP) isoenzymes 3A4 and 3A5 and, to a lesser extent, by CYP2C19 and 2C8 to several oxidated metabolites. Following oral administration of lapatinib, a median of 27% (range; 3–67%) of the oral dose is excreted unchanged in feces; less than 2% of the drug is eliminated via renal excretion.

ADVICE TO PATIENTS

- Inform patients about the importance of taking the total daily dose of lapatinib as a single dose; dividing the total daily dose is not recommended.
- Advise patients to take lapatinib at least 1 hour before or at least 1 hour after food.
- Inform patients to not eat or drink grapefruit products while taking lapatinib.
- If a dose of lapatinib is missed, inform patients to take the next dose at the regularly scheduled time; do not double the dose.

- Inform patients of symptoms of decreased left ventricular ejection fraction (e.g., shortness of breath, palpitations, fatigue) and advise them to inform their clinician if such symptoms occur during treatment with lapatinib.
- Advise patients that periodic laboratory testing will be performed while taking lapatinib.
- Inform patients of symptoms of liver dysfunction (e.g., itching, yellow eyes or skin, dark urine, pain or discomfort in the right upper area of the abdomen) and advise them to immediately contact their clinician if such symptoms occur.
- Risk of severe diarrhea with lapatinib use; advise patients about appropriate countermeasures to prevent and/or manage diarrhea and advise them to inform their clinician if a change in bowel pattern or severe diarrhea occurs while taking lapatinib.
- Advise patients to report pulmonary signs or symptoms indicative of interstitial lung disease or pneumonitis.
- Advise patients to report severe cutaneous reactions to their clinician if they develop these symptoms while taking lapatinib.
- Advise patients to inform their clinician of existing or contemplated concomitant therapy, including prescription and OTC drugs and herbal supplements, as well as any concomitant illnesses.
- Inform female patients of the risk to a fetus. Advise females to inform their clinician if they are or plan to become pregnant or plan to breast-feed.
- Advise females of reproductive potential to use effective contraception during treatment with lapatinib and for at least 1 week after discontinuance of therapy. Advise males who are partners of such females to use effective contraception during treatment with lapatinib and for 1 week after discontinuance of therapy.
- Advise females to avoid breast-feeding while receiving the drug and for at least 1 week after discontinuance of therapy.
- Advise patients of other important precautionary information. (See Cautions.)

PREPARATIONS

Excipients in commercially available drug preparations may have clinically important effects in some individuals; consult specific product labeling for details.

Lapatinib Ditosylate

Oral

Tablets, film-coated	250 mg (of lapatinib)	Tykerb®, Novartis

† Use is not currently included in the labeling approved by the US Food and Drug Administration.

Selected Revisions October 14, 2022, © Copyright, November 1, 2007, American Society of Health-System Pharmacists, Inc.

Larotrectinib Sulfate

10:00 • ANTINEOPLASTIC AGENTS

■ Larotrectinib, a potent and selective inhibitor of tropomyosin receptor kinase (TRK) A, TRK-B, and TRK-C, is an antineoplastic agent.

USES

● Solid Tumors with Neurotrophic Receptor Tyrosine Kinase Gene Fusion

Larotrectinib sulfate is used for the treatment of solid tumors harboring a neurotrophic receptor tyrosine kinase (*NTRK*) gene fusion (without a known acquired mutation for resistance) in adults and pediatric patients who have metastatic disease or are not candidates for surgical resection because of the likelihood of severe morbidity; the drug is indicated in such patients who have no satisfactory alternative treatments or have disease that has progressed following prior treatments. The presence of *NTRK* gene fusion in tumor specimens should be confirmed prior to initiation of therapy. In clinical studies, presence of *NTRK* fusion was determined by fluorescence in situ hybridization (FISH), reverse transcription-polymerase chain reaction (RT-PCR), or next-generation sequencing (NGS). Larotrectinib has been designated an orphan drug by FDA for the treatment of solid tumors with NTRK-fusion proteins. The accelerated approval of larotrectinib for this indication is based on overall response rate and duration of response. Continued approval for this indication may be contingent on verification and description of clinical benefit of larotrectinib in confirmatory studies.

Clinical Experience

The current indication for larotrectinib in the treatment of solid tumors harboring *NTRK* fusion is based principally on data from 3 open-label noncomparative studies (LOXO-TRK-14001, SCOUT, and NAVIGATE) evaluating larotrectinib in patients with unresectable or metastatic solid tumors harboring *NTRK* fusion. The primary efficacy population consisted of the initial 55 adult and pediatric patients enrolled in the LOXO-TRK-14001, SCOUT, and NAVIGATE studies with solid tumors harboring an *NTRK* fusion. Patients were eligible for these studies if they experienced disease progression following prior systemic therapy, if available, or if severe morbidity following surgical resection for locally advanced disease was expected. In these studies, adult patients received larotrectinib 100 mg orally twice daily and pediatric patients (18 years of age or younger) received larotrectinib 100 mg/m^2 (maximum dose of 100 mg) orally twice daily. Therapy was continued until the occurrence of unacceptable toxicity or disease progression. The primary efficacy end points were overall response rate and duration of response (as evaluated by a blinded independent review committee) according to Response Evaluation Criteria in Solid Tumors (RECIST). In the primary efficacy population, the median age of patients was 45 years (range: 4 months to 76 years); 78% of patients were 18 years of age or older, 22% were younger than 18 years of age, 93% had an Eastern Cooperative Oncology Group (ECOG) performance status of 0 or 1, 67% were white, 7% were Hispanic or Latino, 4% were Asian, and 4% were black. Most patients (82%) had metastatic disease (including brain metastases) and 18% had unresectable locally advanced disease. The majority (98%) of patients in the primary efficacy population had received prior surgery, radiation therapy, or systemic therapy for their disease; 82% of these patients had received a median of 2 prior systemic therapies and 35% had received at least 3 prior systemic therapies. The most common cancers in the primary efficacy population were salivary gland tumors (22%), soft tissue sarcoma (20%), infantile fibrosarcoma (13%), and thyroid cancer (9%).

At the time of data analysis, the overall response rate in the primary efficacy population was 75%; complete response was achieved in 25% of patients. The estimated median duration of response was 32.9 months; 63 or 49% of patients had durable responses exceeding 12 or 24 months, respectively. The overall response rate in patients with infantile fibrosarcoma, thyroid carcinoma, gastrointestinal stromal tumor (GIST), soft tissue sarcoma, salivary gland cancer, lung cancer, melanoma, or colon cancer was 100, 100, 100, 91, 83, 75, 50, or 25%, respectively.

Stable disease was reported in patients with cholangiocarcinoma, appendix cancer, or pancreatic cancer while progressive disease was reported in one patient with breast cancer. The most common *NTRK* fusion was *ETV6-NTRK3*; however, *NTRK* fusions were inferred in 3 patients with infantile fibrosarcoma with documented *ETV6* translocation as detected by FISH. The overall response rate in patients with tumors harboring inferred *ETV6-NTRK3*, *IRF2BP2-NTRK1*, *SQSTM1-NTRK1*, documented *ETV6-NTRK3*, *TPM3-NTRK1*, or *LMNA-NTRK1* fusion was 100, 100, 100, 84, 56, or 40%, respectively. Although *PDE4DIP-NTRK1*, *PPL-NTRK1*, *STRN-NTRK2*, *TPM4-NTRK3*, *TPR-NTRK1*, and *TRIM63-NTRK1* fusions were detected in one patient each, patients with tumors harboring these *NTRK* fusions achieved complete or partial responses.

Clinical Perspective

The incidence of solid tumors harboring activating *NTRK* fusions is low (present in approximately 0.28% of cancers). Although a relatively small subset (less than 1%) of patients with common solid tumors (e.g., lung, colon, or prostate cancer) harbor *NTRK* fusions, such fusions have been frequently reported in certain rare cancers (i.e., 91–100% of mammary analogue secretory carcinomas, secretory breast carcinomas, or infantile fibrosarcomas; 61% of congenital mesoblastic nephromas; 12–15% of papillary thyroid cancers). Although *NTRK* fusions are rare in colorectal cancer, patients with *RAS/BRAF* wild-type colorectal cancer and high microsatellite instability and/or mismatch repair deficiency are more likely to exhibit *NTRK* fusions.

Testing for *NTRK* fusions is recommended in patients with metastatic or advanced solid tumors who may be candidates for tropomyosin receptor kinase (TRK) inhibitor therapy; American Society of Clinical Oncology (ASCO) states that clinicians should consider the prevalence of *NTRK* fusions in individual tumor types when deciding whether to perform *NTRK* fusion testing. International experts have published consensus statements on the treatment of *TRK* fusion cancers in adults and pediatric patients.

Adults

Treatment with a selective TRK inhibitor (e.g., entrectinib, larotrectinib) should be considered in adult patients with *TRK* fusion-positive cancers including radioactive iodine-refractory thyroid carcinoma, colorectal cancer (if alternative treatments are not suitable, but also may be considered in the first-line setting), non-small cell lung cancer, soft tissue sarcoma, salivary gland carcinoma, and other *TRK* fusion-positive cancers where no other effective or suitable treatment options are available.

Pediatric Patients

Because *NTRK* gene fusions are pathognomonic in infantile fibrosarcoma, international experts recommend considering a selective TRK inhibitor as first-line systemic therapy in patients with unresectable or metastatic infantile fibrosarcoma. TRK inhibitors have demonstrated high response rates in infantile fibrosarcoma with the potential to prevent disfiguring surgery, such as limb amputations, and to avoid cytotoxic chemotherapy in very young patients. Selective TRK inhibitors should also be considered in pediatric patients with other *TRK* fusion-positive cancers, including unresectable/metastatic non-rhabdomyosarcoma soft tissue sarcoma, differentiated thyroid carcinoma (if standard therapy is not effective or suitable), unresectable/metastatic glioma, and other *TRK* fusion-positive cancers without other effective or suitable treatment options.

DOSAGE AND ADMINISTRATION

● General

Pretreatment Screening

- Confirm presence of a neurotrophic receptor tyrosine kinase (*NTRK*) gene fusion in tumor specimens. Information on FDA-approved tests are available at https://www.fda.gov/companiondiagnostics.

- Verify pregnancy status prior to initiating larotrectinib therapy in females of reproductive potential.

- Obtain liver function tests (ALT, AST, alkaline phosphatase, bilirubin) prior to initiation of therapy.

Patient Monitoring

- Monitor liver function tests every 2 weeks for the first 2 months of therapy and then monthly thereafter or more frequently following the occurrence of grade 2 or greater AST or ALT elevation.

- Promptly evaluate patients with signs or symptoms of potential fracture (e.g., pain, changes in mobility, deformity).

● *Administration*

Larotrectinib is administered orally (as capsules or oral solution) twice daily without regard to meals. The capsules should be swallowed whole with water; they should *not* be chewed or crushed. The oral solution should be administered using an oral dosing syringe according to the manufacturer's directions.

If a dose of larotrectinib is missed, the dose may be taken up to 6 hours prior to the next dose; do not take within 6 hours of the next scheduled dose. If vomiting occurs following administration of larotrectinib, a replacement dose should not be administered; take the next dose at the regularly scheduled time.

Larotrectinib capsules should be stored at room temperature of 20–25°C (excursions permitted between 15–30°C).

Larotrectinib 20 mg/mL oral solution (packaged in one bottle containing 100 mL) should be stored in a refrigerator at 2–8°C; the oral solution should not be frozen. Unused portions of this larotrectinib oral solution should be discarded after 90 days of opening the bottle.

Larotrectinib 20 mg/mL oral solution (packaged in two bottles each containing 50 mL) should be stored in a refrigerator at 2-8°C; the oral solution should not be frozen. Unused portions of this larotrectinib oral solution should be discarded after 31 days of opening the bottles.

● *Dosage*

Dosage of larotrectinib sulfate is expressed in terms of larotrectinib.

Solid Tumors with Neurotrophic Receptor Tyrosine Kinase Gene Fusion

For the treatment of solid tumors harboring *NTRK* fusion (without a known acquired mutation for resistance) in patients who have metastatic disease or may experience severe morbidity following surgical resection and whose disease progressed following prior therapy or those who are not candidates for other treatment options, the recommended dosage of larotrectinib in *adult and pediatric patients with a body surface area (BSA) of at least 1 m²* is 100 mg twice daily. In *pediatric patients with a BSA less than 1 m²*, the recommended dosage of larotrectinib is 100 mg/m² twice daily.

Larotrectinib therapy should be continued until disease progression or unacceptable toxicity occurs.

Dosage Modification for Toxicity

If a grade 2 or higher liver function test abnormalities occur, refer to Table 2. For all other grade 3 or 4 adverse reactions, larotrectinib therapy should be withheld. If the grade 3 or 4 adverse reaction resolves to grade 1 or baseline within 4 weeks of withholding larotrectinib, the drug should be resumed at a reduced dosage (or discontinued) as described in Table 1. If the grade 3 or 4 adverse reaction does not resolve within 4 weeks of withholding larotrectinib, the drug should be permanently discontinued.

TABLE 1. Recommended Dosage Reductions for Larotrectinib Toxicity.

Dosage Modification	Dosage Modification after Recovery from Toxicity Adult and Pediatric Patients with BSA ≥1 m² (Starting Dosage = 100 mg twice daily)	Dosage Modification after Recovery from Toxicity Pediatric Patients with BSA <1 m² (Starting Dosage = 100 mg/m² twice daily)
First	Restart at 75 mg twice daily	Restart at 75 mg/m² twice daily
Second	Restart at 50 mg twice daily	Restart at 50 mg/m² twice daily

TABLE 1. Continued

Dosage Modification	Dosage Modification after Recovery from Toxicity Adult and Pediatric Patients with BSA ≥1 m² (Starting Dosage = 100 mg twice daily)	Dosage Modification after Recovery from Toxicity Pediatric Patients with BSA <1 m² (Starting Dosage = 100 mg/m² twice daily)
Third	Restart at 100 mg once daily	Restart at 25 mg/m² twice daily[a]
Fourth	Permanently discontinue larotrectinib	Permanently discontinue larotrectinib

[a] If BSA increases to >1 m² in pediatric patients following dosage reduction to 25 mg/m² twice daily, do not increase dosage. Maximum dose should be 25 mg/m² twice daily at the third dosage modification

TABLE 2. Dosage Modifications for Hepatotoxicity

Severity	Dosage Modification
AST or ALT ≥5 times ULN with bilirubin ≤2 times ULN	Withhold until recovery to grade 1 or baseline then resume therapy at the next lower dose level
	Permanently discontinue if grade 4 AST and/or ALT elevation occurs after resuming therapy
AST or ALT >3 times ULN with total bilirubin >2 times ULN in the absence of alternative etiologies	Permanently discontinue therapy

Concomitant Use with CYP3A4 Inhibitors or Inducers

Concomitant use of larotrectinib with *strong inhibitors of cytochrome P-450 (CYP) isoenzyme 3A4* should be avoided; however, if such concomitant use cannot be avoided, reduce dosage of larotrectinib by 50% (e.g., dosage of 100 mg twice daily reduced to 50 mg twice daily; dosage of 100 mg/m² twice daily reduced to 50 mg/m² twice daily). After the CYP3A4 inhibitor has been discontinued for 3–5 elimination half-lives, resume the larotrectinib dosage that was used prior to initiation of the strong CYP3A4 inhibitor.

Concomitant use of larotrectinib with *strong inducers of CYP3A4* should be avoided; however, if such concomitant use cannot be avoided, the dosage of larotrectinib should be doubled (e.g., dosage of 100 mg twice daily increased to 200 mg twice daily; dosage of 100 mg/m² twice daily increased to 200 mg/m² twice daily). In addition, for concurrent use with a *moderate CYP3A4 inducer*, the manufacturer recommends doubling the dosage of larotrectinib. After the strong or moderate CYP3A4 inducer has been discontinued for 3–5 elimination half-lives, resume the larotrectinib dosage that was used prior to initiating the CYP3A4 inducer.

● *Special Populations*

Hepatic Impairment

For patients with moderate or severe hepatic impairment (Child-Pugh class B or C), the manufacturer recommends reducing the initial dosage of larotrectinib by 50% (e.g., dosage of 100 mg twice daily reduced to 50 mg twice daily; dosage of 100 mg/m² twice daily reduced to 50 mg/m² twice daily). No initial dosage adjustment is necessary in patients with mild hepatic impairment (Child-Pugh class A).

Renal Impairment

The manufacturer states that no adjustment to the dosage of larotrectinib is necessary in patients with renal impairment.

Geriatric Patients

The manufacturer makes no specific dosage recommendations for geriatric patients.

CAUTIONS

● *Contraindications*

● None.

● *Warnings/Precautions*

CNS Effects

Larotrectinib can cause a variety of adverse neurologic effects including dizziness, cognitive impairment, mood disorders, and sleep disturbances. In studies of larotrectinib, adverse CNS effects occurred in 42% of patients receiving the drug and were grade 3 or 4 in 3.9% of patients.

Cognitive impairment occurred in 11% of patients receiving larotrectinib, with grade 3 cognitive adverse reactions occurring in 2.5% of patients. The most common types of cognitive impairment reported were memory impairment, confusional state, disturbance in attention, delirium, and cognitive disorders; these occurred in 3.6, 2.9, 2.9, 2.2, and 1.4% of patients, respectively. The median time to onset of cognitive impairment, which was reported in 11% of patients (grade 3 in 2.5%), was 5.6 months (range: 2 days to 41 months). Temporary interruption or dosage reduction of larotrectinib was necessary because of cognitive impairment in 20 or 7% of patients, respectively.

Mood disorders occurred in 14% of patients receiving larotrectinib, with grade 3 mood disorders occurring in 0.4% of patients. The most common types of mood disorders reported were anxiety, depression, agitation, and irritability; these occurred in 5, 3.9, 2.9, and 2.9% of patients, respectively The median time to onset of mood disorders, which were reported in 14% of patients (grade 3 in 0.4%), was 3.9 months (range: 1 day to 40.5 months).

Dizziness was reported in 27% of patients and was grade 3 in 1.1% of patients; temporary interruption and dosage reduction of larotrectinib because of dizziness each were necessary in 5% of patients.

Sleep disturbances were reported in 10% of patients and included insomnia, somnolence, or sleep disorder in 7, 2.5, or 0.4% of patients, respectively. Temporary interruption and dosage reduction of larotrectinib because of sleep disturbances each were necessary in 3.6% of patients.

Temporary interruption of larotrectinib therapy followed by dosage reduction or permanent discontinuance of therapy may be necessary in patients experiencing neurologic events during therapy with the drug, and such patients should be advised not to drive or operate machinery.

Skeletal Fractures

Skeletal fractures have been reported in patients receiving larotrectinib. Among 187 adult patients receiving larotrectinib in clinical trials, fractures were reported in 7% of patients; fractures were reported in 9% of 92 pediatric patients receiving the drug. The median time to onset of fracture was 11.6 months (range: 0.9–45.8 months). Fractures of the femur, hip, or acetabulum were reported in four patients (three adults and one pediatric patient). Most fractures were associated with minimal or moderate trauma, and some fractures were associated with radiologic abnormalities suggestive of local tumor involvement. Interruption of larotrectinib therapy due to fracture occurred in 1.4% of patients.

Promptly evaluate patients with signs or symptoms of potential fracture (e.g., pain, changes in mobility, deformity). Data on the effects of larotrectinib on the healing of known fractures or risk of future fractures are not available.

Hepatotoxicity

Hepatotoxicity, including drug-induced liver injury, has been reported in patients receiving larotrectinib. In studies of larotrectinib, elevations in serum concentrations of ALT or AST occurred in 45 or 52% of patients, respectively, receiving the drug and were grade 3–4 in 2.5 or 3.1%, respectively, of patients. The median time to occurrence of elevated ALT or AST concentration was 2.1–2.3 months (range: 1 day to 4.3 years). Dosage reduction of larotrectinib was necessary because of elevated AST or ALT concentrations in 1.4 or 2.2%, respectively, of patients receiving the drug. Therapy was permanently discontinued because of elevations in ALT or AST concentrations in 1.1% of patients receiving the drug.

There have also been reports of grade ≥2 increases in ALT and/or AST with increases in bilirubin ≥2 times the upper limit of normal in adult patients.

Obtain liver function tests (ALT, AST, alkaline phosphatase, bilirubin) before larotrectinib initiation. Monitor liver function tests every 2 weeks for the first 2 months of therapy and then monthly thereafter or more frequently following the occurrence of grade 2 or greater AST or ALT elevation. Temporary interruption of larotrectinib therapy followed by dosage reduction or permanent discontinuance of therapy may be necessary if hepatotoxicity occurs.

Embryo-fetal Toxicity

Larotrectinib may cause fetal harm in humans based on its mechanism of action and animal findings; embryofetal toxicity and teratogenicity have been demonstrated in animals. There are no available data regarding use of larotrectinib in pregnant women. Larotrectinib has been shown to cross the placenta in animals. In animal reproduction studies, fetal anasarca and omphalocele were observed in rats and rabbits receiving larotrectinib at exposure levels approximately 11 and 0.7 times the human exposure, respectively, at the recommended dosage. Literature reports in individuals with congenital mutations in the tropomyosin receptor kinase (TRK) pathway suggest an association between decreased TRK-mediated signaling and obesity, developmental delays, cognitive impairment, insensitivity to pain, and anhidrosis.

Pregnancy should be avoided during larotrectinib therapy. The manufacturer recommends confirmation of pregnancy status prior to initiation of larotrectinib in females of reproductive potential and states that such females should be advised to use effective contraceptive methods while receiving larotrectinib and for at least 1 week after discontinuance of the drug. In addition, males with such female partners should use effective methods of contraception while receiving larotrectinib and for at least 1 week after discontinuance of the drug. Patients should be apprised of the potential hazard to the fetus if larotrectinib is used during pregnancy.

Specific Populations

Pregnancy

Larotrectinib may cause fetal harm if administered to pregnant women based on its mechanism of action and animal findings.

Possible association between decreased TRK-mediated signaling and obesity, developmental delays, cognitive impairment, insensitivity to pain, and anhidrosis based on data from individuals with congenital mutations in the TRK pathway.

Lactation

It is not known whether larotrectinib or its metabolites are distributed into human milk. Because of the potential for serious adverse reactions to larotrectinib in breast-fed infants, females should be advised not to breast-feed while receiving the drug and for 1 week after the last dose. The effects of the drug on breast-fed infants or on the production of milk are unknown.

Females and Males of Reproductive Potential

The manufacturer recommends verifying pregnancy status prior to initiation of larotrectinib in females of reproductive potential and states that such patients should be advised to use effective contraceptive methods while receiving larotrectinib and for at least 1 week after discontinuance of the drug. In addition, males with such female partners should use effective methods of contraception while receiving larotrectinib and for at least 1 week after discontinuance of the drug.

Based on animal studies, larotrectinib may impair female fertility; however, the effect of the drug on fertility in humans is not known. In a repeat-dose toxicity study, decreased uterine weight, uterine atrophy, decreased corpora lutea, and increased incidence of anestrus were observed in female rats receiving larotrectinib at exposure levels approximately 10–45 times the human exposure at the recommended dosage.

Pediatric Use

Safety and efficacy of larotrectinib have not been established in pediatric patients younger than 28 days. Efficacy of larotrectinib in pediatric patients with solid tumors harboring a neurotrophic receptor tyrosine kinase (*NTRK*) gene fusion has been established in 3 noncomparative studies that included 12 pediatric patients 28 days of age or older. Based on limited safety data in 92 pediatric patients receiving larotrectinib, some adverse effects and laboratory abnormalities (i.e., pyrexia, vomiting, diarrhea, rash, upper respiratory tract infection, nasopharyngitis, otitis media, rhinitis, increased AST concentrations, neutropenia, leukopenia, hyperkalemia, increased lymphocyte count) occurred more frequently in pediatric patients compared with adults; however, because the studies were uncontrolled, it is unclear whether this effect was related to larotrectinib or to other confounding factors (e.g., differences in susceptibility to infection).

No differences in pharmacokinetics were observed between pediatric patients and adults.

Geriatric Use

In clinical trials evaluating larotrectinib, 19% of patients receiving larotrectinib were 65 years of age or older, while 5% were 75 years of age or older. There is insufficient experience in patients 65 years of age or older to determine whether geriatric patients respond differently than younger patients.

Hepatic Impairment

Following administration of a single 100-mg dose of larotrectinib, the area under the plasma concentration-time curve (AUC) in individuals with mild, moderate, or severe hepatic impairment (Child-Pugh class A, B, or C) was increased by 1.3-, 2-, or 3.2-fold, respectively, compared with individuals with normal hepatic function; peak plasma concentrations were increased by 1.5-fold in individuals with severe hepatic impairment compared with individuals with normal hepatic function. Initial dosage adjustment is required in patients with moderate or severe hepatic impairment.

Renal Impairment

Following administration of a single 100-mg dose of larotrectinib to individuals with end-stage renal disease requiring dialysis, AUC and peak plasma concentrations were increased by 1.5- and 1.3-fold, respectively, compared with individuals with normal renal function (creatinine clearance of 90 mL/minute or greater). Larotrectinib has not been studied in patients with moderate or severe renal impairment (creatinine clearance of 60 mL/minute or less).

No dosage adjustment is necessary in patients with renal impairment of any severity.

● Common Adverse Effects

Adverse effects reported in >20% of patients receiving larotrectinib include increased AST concentrations, increased ALT concentrations, anemia, musculoskeletal pain, fatigue, hypoalbuminemia, neutropenia, increased alkaline phosphatase concentrations, cough, leukopenia, constipation, diarrhea, dizziness, hypocalcemia, nausea, vomiting, pyrexia, lymphopenia, and abdominal pain.

DRUG INTERACTIONS

Larotrectinib is metabolized principally by cytochrome P-450 (CYP) isoenzyme 3A4.

In vitro studies indicate that larotrectinib is an inhibitor of CYP3A4. In vitro, larotrectinib does not inhibit or induce CYP isoenzymes 1A2, 2B6, 2C8, 2C9, 2C19, or 2D6 at clinically relevant concentrations.

In vitro, larotrectinib is a substrate of the efflux transporters P-glycoprotein (P-gp) and breast cancer resistance protein (BCRP), but is not a substrate for organic anion transporter (OAT) 1, OAT3, organic cation transporter (OCT) 1, OCT2, organic anion transport protein (OATP) 1B1, or OATP1B3. In vitro studies indicate that larotrectinib does not inhibit P-gp, BCRP, OAT1, OAT3, OCT1, OCT2, OATP1B1, OATP1B3, bile salt export pump (BSEP), multidrug and toxin extrusion (MATE) transporter 1, and MATE2K at clinically relevant concentrations.

● Drugs and Foods Affecting Hepatic Microsomal Enzymes

Inhibitors of CYP3A4

Concomitant use of larotrectinib with strong or moderate inhibitors of CYP3A4 may increase systemic exposure to larotrectinib and possible toxicity. When the strong CYP3A inhibitor itraconazole (200 mg once daily for 7 days) was administered concomitantly with larotrectinib (single 100-mg dose), peak plasma concentration and area under the plasma concentration-time curve (AUC) of larotrectinib were increased by 2.8- and 4.3-fold, respectively. The potential for

weak CYP3A inhibitors to alter larotrectinib pharmacokinetics has not been established.

Concomitant use of larotrectinib with strong inhibitors of CYP3A4 (e.g., itraconazole, grapefruit juice) should be avoided. If concomitant use of a strong CYP3A4 inhibitor cannot be avoided, the manufacturer recommends reducing the dosage of larotrectinib by 50% (e.g., dosage of 100 mg twice daily reduced to 50 mg twice daily; dosage of 100 mg/m² twice daily reduced to 50 mg/m² twice daily). After the CYP3A4 inhibitor has been discontinued for 3–5 elimination half-lives, resume the larotrectinib dosage used prior to initiation of the strong CYP3A4 inhibitor.

If concomitant use of a moderate CYP3A4 inhibitor with larotrectinib occurs, patients should be monitored more frequently for adverse reactions and the dosage of larotrectinib should be reduced based on the severity of the adverse reaction.

Inducers of CYP3A4

Concomitant use of larotrectinib with strong or moderate inducers of CYP3A4 may decrease systemic exposure to larotrectinib and reduce larotrectinib efficacy. When the strong CYP3A inducer rifampin (600 mg once daily for 11 days) was administered concomitantly with larotrectinib (single 100-mg dose), peak plasma concentration and AUC of larotrectinib were decreased by 71 and 81%, respectively. The potential for weak CYP3A inducers to alter larotrectinib pharmacokinetics has not been established.

Concomitant use of larotrectinib with strong inducers of CYP3A4 (e.g., rifampin, St. John's wort [*Hypericum perforatum*]) should be avoided. If concomitant use of a strong CYP3A4 inducer cannot be avoided, the manufacturer recommends doubling the dosage of larotrectinib (e.g., dosage of 100 mg twice daily increased to 200 mg twice daily; dosage of 100 mg/m² twice daily increased to 200 mg/m² twice daily). In addition, for concurrent use with a moderate CYP3A4 inducer, the manufacturer recommends doubling the dosage of larotrectinib. After the strong or moderate CYP3A4 inducer has been discontinued for 3–5 elimination half-lives, resume the larotrecrinib dosage used prior to initiation of the CYP3A4 inducer.

● Drugs Metabolized by Hepatic Microsomal Enzymes

Substrates of CYP3A4

Larotrectinib may increase systemic exposure and risk of adverse effects of other drugs metabolized by CYP3A4. When the sensitive CYP3A4 substrate midazolam (single 2-mg dose) was administered concomitantly with larotrectinib (100 mg twice daily for 10 days) in healthy individuals, peak plasma concentration and AUC of midazolam were both increased by 1.7-fold; peak plasma concentration and AUC of the major metabolite of midazolam (1-hydroxymidazolam) were both increased by 1.4-fold. Concomitant use with sensitive substrates of CYP3A4 (e.g., midazolam) should be avoided. If concomitant use of a sensitive CYP3A4 substrate cannot be avoided, the patient should be monitored for CYP3A4 substrate-related toxicity.

● Drugs Affecting the P-glycoprotein Transport System

When the P-gp inhibitor rifampin (single 600-mg dose) was administered concomitantly with larotrectinib (single 100-mg dose) in healthy individuals, peak plasma concentration and AUC of larotrectinib were increased by 1.8- and 1.7-fold, respectively.

DESCRIPTION

Larotrectinib, a potent and selective inhibitor of tropomyosin receptor kinase (TRK) A, TRK-B, and TRK-C, is an antineoplastic agent. The TRK family of tyrosine kinases (encoded by the neurotrophic receptor tyrosine kinase genes *NTRK1*, *NTRK2*, and *NTRK3*) are involved in the initiation of various cascades of intracellular signaling events (i.e., Ras/MAPK/ERK, PI3K/Akt, and PLCγ1/Pkc signal transduction pathways), which leads to cell proliferation, differentiation, apoptosis, and regulation of processes critical to neuron survival in the central and peripheral nervous systems. Chromosomal rearrangements of the *NTRK1*, *NTRK2*, and *NTRK3* genes result in fusions with an unrelated gene. These *NTRK* gene fusions encode a constitutively active chimeric TRK oncogenic fusion protein resulting in dysregulation of TRK signaling and subsequent tumorigenesis. In vitro biochemical assays have shown that larotrectinib inhibits the activity of wild-type TRK-A, TRK-B, and TRK-C. In vitro and in vivo, larotrectinib has demonstrated antitumor activity in cell lines with TRK expression from constitutive activation, deletion of a protein regulatory domain, or overexpression of wild-type TRK. Larotrectinib also has demonstrated inhibition of tyrosine kinase nonreceptor 2 (TNK2).

Clinical resistance to larotrectinib has been attributed to secondary point mutations of the NTRK kinase domain in 90% of cases. Larotrectinib has shown minimal activity in cell lines with point mutations in the TRK-A kinase domain, including the acquired resistance mutation G595R. Acquired resistance to larotrectinib also has been identified in cell lines with G623R, G696A, or F617L point mutations in the TRK-C kinase domain.

Following oral administration of larotrectinib capsules, systemic exposure to larotrectinib increases in a dose-proportional manner over a dose range of 100–400 mg and increases in a slightly more than dose-proportional manner over a dose range of 600–900 mg. Following oral administration of larotrectinib capsules at a dosage of 100 mg twice daily, peak plasma concentrations of the drug were achieved in approximately 1 hour and steady-state concentrations were achieved within 3 days. The mean absolute oral bioavailability of larotrectinib capsules was 34%. The area under the plasma-concentration time curve (AUC) for larotrectinib oral solution was similar to the AUC for larotrectinib capsules; peak plasma concentrations were 36% higher for larotrectinib oral solution compared with larotrectinib capsules. Administration of larotrectinib capsules (single 100-mg dose) with a high-fat meal decreased peak plasma concentrations by 35% and delayed the time to peak plasma concentrations by 2 hours compared with administration in the fasted state, but did not substantially affect the extent of absorption. Larotrectinib is metabolized principally by cytochrome P-450 (CYP) isoenzyme 3A4. Larotrectinib is 70% bound to plasma proteins, and binding is independent of larotrectinib concentration. Following oral administration of a single 100-mg radiolabeled dose of larotrectinib, 58% of the dose was recovered in feces (5% as unchanged drug) and 39% was recovered in urine (20% as unchanged drug). The terminal half-life of larotrectinib is 2.9 hours.

The pharmacokinetics of larotrectinib do not appear to be affected by age (range of 28 days to 82 years), sex, or body weight (range of 3.8–179 kg).

ADVICE TO PATIENTS

- Instruct patients to read the manufacturer's patient information.

- Advise patients to take larotrectinib exactly as prescribed and to not alter the dosage or discontinue therapy unless advised to do so by their clinician. Advise patients to swallow larotrectinib capsules whole and to not chew or crush the capsules.

- Advise patients to take a missed dose as soon as it is remembered unless the dose was missed by more than 6 hours, in which case they should not take the missed dose. If a dose is vomited, administer the next dose at the regularly scheduled time.

- Risk of adverse neurologic effects. Importance of informing clinician if new or worsening manifestations of neurologic events (e.g., confusion; dizziness; problems with concentration, attention, or memory; mood changes; sleep disturbance) occur. Advise patients to avoid driving or operating hazardous machinery if they experience neurologic events.

- Risk of skeletal fractures. Importance of informing clinician if signs or symptoms of skeletal fractures (e.g., pain, changes in mobility, deformity) occur.

- Risk of hepatotoxicity; importance of regular liver function test monitoring. Importance of immediately informing clinician if signs or symptoms of hepatotoxicity (e.g., loss of appetite, nausea, vomiting, abdominal pain [especially right upper quadrant pain]) occur.

- Risk of fetal harm. Advise females of reproductive potential to avoid pregnancy and to use effective contraceptive methods while receiving larotrectinib and for ≥1 week following discontinuance of therapy. Advise males who are partners of such females that they should use effective methods of contraception while receiving the drug and for ≥1 week after the drug is discontinued. Importance of females informing their clinicians if they become pregnant during therapy or think they may be pregnant. Advise males and females of reproductive potential of potential risk to the fetus.

- Advise females to avoid breast-feeding while receiving larotrectinib and for 1 week after discontinuance of therapy.

- Risk of impaired female fertility.

- Importance of informing clinicians of existing or contemplated concomitant therapy, including prescription and OTC drugs and dietary or herbal supplements (e.g., St. John's wort [*Hypericum perforatum*], grapefruit, grapefruit juice), as well as any concomitant illnesses (e.g., hepatic impairment).

- Inform patients of other important precautionary information.

For further information on the handling of antineoplastic agents, see the ASHP Guidelines on Handling Hazardous Drugs at https://www.ahfsdruginformation.com.

PREPARATIONS

Larotrectinib sulfate can only be obtained through designated specialty pharmacies and distributors. Clinicians may contact the manufacturer (Bayer) at 844-634-8725 or consult the Vitrakvi® website (https://www.vitrakvi.com) for specific ordering and availability information.

Excipients in commercially available drug preparations may have clinically important effects in some individuals; consult specific product labeling for details.

Larotrectinib Sulfate

Oral		
Capsules	25 mg (of larotrectinib)	**Vitrakvi®**, Bayer
	100 mg (of larotrectinib)	**Vitrakvi®**, Bayer
Solution	20 mg (of larotrectinib) per mL	**Vitrakvi®** available in a package containing one 100-mL bottle or a package of 2 bottles each containing 50 mL, Bayer

† Use is not currently included in the labeling approved by the US Food and Drug Administration.

Lenalidomide

10:00 • ANTINEOPLASTIC AGENTS

REMS

FDA approved a REMS for lenalidomide to ensure that the benefits outweigh the risks. The REMS may apply to one or more preparations of lenalidomide and consists of the following: elements to assure safe use and implementation system. See the FDA REMS page (https://www.accessdata.fda.gov/scripts/cder/rems/index .cfm).

■ Lenalidomide, a thalidomide analog, is an immunomodulatory agent with antineoplastic and antiangiogenic activity.

USES

● Multiple Myeloma

Lenalidomide is used in combination with dexamethasone for the treatment of multiple myeloma and as maintenance therapy in patients with multiple myeloma after autologous hematopoietic stem cell transplantation. Lenalidomide is designated an orphan drug by the FDA for use in multiple myeloma.

Newly Diagnosed Multiple Myeloma

Safety and efficacy of lenalidomide in patients with newly diagnosed multiple myeloma who are ineligible for stem-cell transplantation are based principally on the results of a randomized, multicenter, open-label clinical trial (MM-020; FIRST) in 1623 patients. Patients were randomized to receive one of the following treatment groups: continuous lenalidomide (25 mg once daily on days 1–21 of a 28-day cycle) in combination with dexamethasone (40 mg once daily on days 1, 8, 15, and 22 of a 28-day cycle; patients older than 75 years of age received reduced doses [i.e., 20 mg] of dexamethasone) until disease progression; the same dosage of lenalidomide and dexamethasone for 72 weeks (eighteen 28-day cycles); or melphalan, prednisone, and thalidomide (MPT) for up to 72 weeks (twelve 42-day cycles). All patients received appropriate thromboprophylaxis (e.g., aspirin). Median progression-free survival at a median follow-up duration of 45.5 months was 25.5, 20.7, or 21.2 months in patients receiving continuous lenalidomide-dexamethasone, lenalidomide-dexamethasone for 18 cycles, or MPT, respectively. Median progression-free survival was significantly prolonged in patients receiving continuous lenalidomide-dexamethasone compared with those receiving MPT (hazard ratio: 0.72 with a 95% confidence interval of 0.61–0.85). Median progression-free survival also was prolonged in patients receiving continuous lenalidomide-dexamethasone compared with lenalidomide-dexamethasone for 18 cycles (hazard ratio: 0.70 with a 95% confidence interval of 0.60–0.82); however, statistical significance was not reached. Median overall survival was 58.9, 56.7, or 48.5 months in patients receiving continuous lenalidomide-dexamethasone, lenalidomide-dexamethasone for 18 cycles, or MPT, respectively. The overall response rate (as assessed by an independent committee) in patients receiving continuous lenalidomide-dexamethasone, lenalidomide-dexamethasone for 18 cycles, or MPT was 75.1, 73.4, or 62.3%, respectively; complete response was achieved in 15.1, 14.2, or 9.3% of patients in the respective groups.

Previously Treated Multiple Myeloma

Safety and efficacy of lenalidomide in patients with multiple myeloma previously treated with at least 1 prior therapy are based principally on 2 randomized, double-blind, placebo-controlled, multicenter studies (MM-009 and MM-010) involving a total of 704 patients. Patients were randomized to receive lenalidomide and placebo (25 mg once daily on days 1–21 of a 28-day cycle and placebo once daily on days 22–28 of each 28-day cycle) or placebo alone (on days 1–28 of each 28-day cycle); all patients received oral dexamethasone 40 mg once daily on days 1–4, 9–12, and 17–20 of each 28-day cycle for the first 4 cycles of therapy, followed by dexamethasone 40 mg once daily on days 1–4 of each subsequent 28-day cycle. In both studies, treatment was continued until disease progression. Time to progression was substantially longer in patients receiving lenalidomide

and dexamethasone compared with those receiving dexamethasone and placebo in both studies (12.1–13.9 months versus 4.7 months). Patients receiving lenalidomide and dexamethasone also experienced substantially higher overall (59–61 versus 19–23%), complete (13–15 versus 1–4%), and partial (44–48 versus 19%) response rates compared with those receiving dexamethasone and placebo, respectively.

Maintenance Therapy Following Autologous Hematopoietic Stem Cell Transplantation

Safety and efficacy of maintenance therapy with lenalidomide in patients with multiple myeloma who have undergone autologous HSCT is based principally on the results of 2 randomized, double-blind, multicenter, placebo-controlled studies (CALGB 100104 and IFM 2005-02). In these studies, patients with at least stable disease were randomized to receive lenalidomide (10 mg once daily on days 1–28 of a 28-day cycle; a dosage increase to 15 mg once daily was permitted if dose-limiting toxicities did not occur during the initial 3 months of maintenance therapy) or placebo within 90–100 days of autologous HSCT. Treatment was continued until disease progression or withdrawal from the study for other reasons. The primary endpoint of progression-free survival was prolonged in patients receiving lenalidomide compared with those receiving placebo in both studies; however, the trials were unblinded at the time of the interim analysis at the request of data monitoring committees after surpassing the threshold for preplanned interim analyses of progression-free survival. At the time of analysis, median progression-free survival was significantly prolonged in patients receiving lenalidomide compared with those receiving placebo in both trials (hazard ratio of 0.38 and 0.50). Longer-term follow-up data from these studies demonstrated prolonged median progression-free survival in patients receiving lenalidomide; median progression-free survival in patients receiving lenalidomide was 68.6 or 46.3 months in the CALGB 100104 or IFM 2005-02 study, respectively, compared with 22.5 or 23.8 months, respectively, in patients receiving placebo.

Clinical Perspective

The American Society of Clinical Oncology (ASCO) and Cancer Care Ontario (CCO) state that treatment recommendations for patients with multiple myeloma should be individualized based on factors such as stage, cytogenetic abnormalities, age, comorbidities, functional status, frailty status, and patient preferences.

Newly Diagnosed Multiple Myeloma

Transplant eligible: ASCO and CCO state that the optimal regimen and number of cycles for the treatment of multiple myeloma remain unestablished; however, at least 3–4 cycles of induction therapy including an immunomodulatory drug, proteasome inhibitor, and corticosteroid is advised prior to stem cell collection. Drugs associated with stem cell toxicity (e.g., melphalan) and/or prolonged exposure to immunomodulatory drugs (more than four cycles) should be avoided in patients who are potential candidates for SCT. Because prolonged exposure to oral melphalan or immunomodulatory drugs (e.g., lenalidomide beyond 4–6 cycles) may compromise stem-cell yield, the manufacturer of lenalidomide states that stem cell mobilization should occur within 4 cycles of lenalidomide-containing therapy in patients who will undergo autologous HSCT.

Transplant ineligible: ASCO and CCO also state that initial treatment of patients with multiple myeloma who are transplant ineligible should at least include a corticosteroid in combination with an immunomodulatory drug or proteasome inhibitor; however, triplet combination therapy including bortezomib, lenalidomide, and dexamethasone† should be considered. Continuous therapy should be offered instead of a fixed duration in patients receiving an immunomodulatory drug or proteasome inhibitor-based regimen. Continuous therapy in transplant-ineligible patients generally refers to treatment administered until progression or intolerance occurs or a prolonged but finite time frame (e.g., 2–3 years).

Previously Treated Multiple Myeloma

ASCO and CCO state that prior therapies should be taken into consideration when selecting the treatment at first relapse. Treatment options include triplet combination therapy (two novel agents and a corticosteroid) or doublet combination therapy (one novel agent and a corticosteroid); novel agents include immunomodulatory drugs, proteasome inhibitors, and monoclonal antibodies (e.g., daratumumab, elotuzumab). For patients who are fit, triplet combination therapy is generally recommended over doublet combination therapy due to improved clinical outcomes. In patients with genetic high-risk disease, a triplet combination regimen with a proteasome inhibitor, immunomodulatory drug, and a corticosteroid should be the initial treatment, followed by one or two autologous HSCT, followed by proteasome inhibitor-based maintenance therapy until disease progression occurs.

Treatment of relapsed multiple myeloma may be continued until disease progression. There are not enough data to recommend risk-based versus response-based duration of treatment.

Maintenance Therapy Following Autologous Hematopoietic Stem Cell Transplantation

ASCO and CCO state that maintenance therapy with lenalidomide should be routinely offered to standard-risk patients starting at approximately day 90–110 following autologous HSCT. A minimum of 2 years of maintenance therapy in such patients has been associated with improved survival, and efforts to maintain therapy for at least this duration are recommended by ASCO and CCO.

Because survival benefit has not been demonstrated in high-risk patients (i.e., ISS stage III disease, adverse cytogenetic features such as t(4;14) or del(17p), elevated lactate dehydrogenase, low creatinine clearance) receiving maintenance therapy with lenalidomide alone, bortezomib-based therapy in high-risk patients may be preferred.

● Myelodysplastic Syndrome

Lenalidomide is used in the management of transfusion-dependent anemia associated with low-risk or intermediate-1-risk myelodysplastic syndrome (MDS) in individuals with a cytogenetic deletion abnormality involving the long arm of chromosome 5 (a deletion 5q abnormality), with or without additional cytogenetic abnormalities. Lenalidomide is designated an orphan drug by FDA for use in MDS.

The current indication for lenalidomide is based principally on results from an uncontrolled, open-label, multicenter trial (MDS-003) in 148 patients with transfusion-dependent anemia (i.e., requiring at least 2 units of red blood cells within 8 weeks prior to study treatment) secondary to MDS; all patients enrolled in the trial had a cytogenetic abnormality involving a deletion between bands 31 and 33 of the long (q) arm of chromosome 5, designated as del(5)(q31-33), either in isolation or in association with additional cytogenetic abnormalities. Most (81%) of the patients in this trial had low-risk or intermediate-1-risk MDS, as determined by the International Prognosis Scoring System (IPSS), a method for evaluating MDS prognosis (i.e., survival and risk of transformation to acute myeloid leukemia [AML]) based on the karyotype, percentage of blast cells in the bone marrow, and number of cytopenias. Patients received lenalidomide at a dosage of either 10 mg once daily or 10 mg once daily for 21 days of each 28-day period. Sequential dosage reductions (to 5 mg daily or 5 mg every other day) as well as interruptions in the dosage regimen were allowed for management of toxicity. Transfusion independence, defined as the absence of red blood cell transfusions during any period of 56 consecutive days (8 weeks) during therapy, was achieved in 67% of patients; the transfusion-free period was sustained for a median of 44 weeks (range: 0 to more than 67 weeks) following the end of this 56-day period of transfusion independence. Response to lenalidomide was rapid; the median time to response was 4.6 weeks, and 90% of patients who achieved a transfusion benefit with therapy did so within 3 months.

Lenalidomide also has been studied for the management of transfusion-dependent low-risk or intermediate-1-risk MDS in patients *without* the deletion 5q (del[5q]) chromosomal abnormality (non-del[5q])†. In a multicenter, phase 2, noncomparative clinical trial (MDS-002), 214 patients with transfusion-dependent anemia (i.e., requiring at least 2 units of red blood cells within 8 weeks prior to study treatment) secondary to low-risk or intermediate-1-risk MDS without the deletion 5q chromosomal abnormality received lenalidomide 10 mg once daily on days 1–21 of a 28-day cycle or 10 mg once daily continuously. Treatment was administered cyclically upon initiation of the study, but the schedule was amended when data from a prior study in MDS suggested a faster onset of response to lenalidomide, with no apparent increase in toxicity, with continuous administration; patients were permitted to switch from cyclic to continuous treatment. Sustained (for at least 8 weeks) hematologic improvement involving the erythroid cell line was reported in 43% of patients in this study, with 26% of patients achieving transfusion independence accompanied by an increase in hemoglobin concentration of at least 1 g/dL after a median of 4.8 weeks of

treatment; the median duration of transfusion independence was 41 weeks. An additional 17% of patients had a 50% or greater reduction in transfusions. When the study data were analyzed to exclude minor responses and to use a more stringent definition of baseline transfusion dependence (transfusion of 4 or more units of red blood cells in response to a hemoglobin concentration of 9 g/dL or less within 8 weeks prior to study treatment), 62% of patients had baseline transfusion dependence and 30% of those patients achieved a reduction in transfusion requirements equaling 4 or more units during any 8-week period during therapy. In the subset of patients without baseline transfusion dependence, 37% achieved a sustained (for at least 8 weeks) increase in hemoglobin concentration of at least 1.5 g/dL during therapy. Overall, 17 or 33% of patients achieved sustained (for at least 8 weeks) transfusion independence or hematologic improvement involving the erythroid cell line. Grade 3/4 neutropenia and thrombocytopenia occurred in 30 and 25% of patients, respectively. There were no apparent differences in response and few differences in adverse effects between those who initiated therapy with cyclic administration and those who received only continuous daily dosing. Efficacy of lenalidomide is being evaluated in a phase 3, placebo-controlled, clinical trial (MDS-005) in patients with low-risk or intermediate-1-risk MDS without the deletion 5q chromosomal abnormality who have transfusion-dependent anemia and are unresponsive to therapy with erythropoiesis-stimulating agents or have endogenous erythropoietin concentrations exceeding 500 mU/mL.

A post-hoc analysis of the MDS-002 and MDS-003 clinical trials demonstrated a correlation between treatment-related cytopenias and likelihood of achieving transfusion independence in patients with the deletion 5q chromosomal abnormality; however, no relationship between the development of treatment-related cytopenias and response could be established for lower-risk MDS patients without the deletion 5q abnormality.

Use of lenalidomide for the treatment of transfusion-dependent low-risk or intermediate-1-risk MDS without the deletion 5q chromosomal abnormality is a reasonable choice (accepted, with possible conditions). However, randomized controlled studies in adequate numbers of patients are lacking; additional data are needed to further elucidate clinical benefit (i.e., hematologic improvement-erythroid response) and to assess the relevance of prognostic factors (e.g., transfusion requirement, baseline platelet count, duration of MDS, serum lactate dehydrogenase concentration) to lenalidomide response.

● Mantle Cell Lymphoma

Lenalidomide is used for the treatment of mantle cell lymphoma in patients who have progressed or relapsed after 2 prior therapies including bortezomib. Lenalidomide has been designated an orphan drug by the FDA for use in mantle cell lymphoma.

Safety and efficacy of lenalidomide in patients with mantle cell lymphoma are based principally on the results of an open-label, multicenter, single-arm phase 2 trial (MCL-001; EMERGE). In this study, patients received lenalidomide 25 mg once daily for 21 days of each 28-day cycle; therapy was continued until disease progression or unacceptable toxicity occurred. Approximately one-third (29%) of patients had undergone autologous stem cell or bone marrow transplantation and 60% of patients had bortezomib-refractory disease. The overall response rate in 133 evaluable patients who received at least one dose of lenalidomide was 26% with a duration of response of 16.6 months (range: 7.7–26.7 months); 7% achieved a complete response or unconfirmed complete response. The median time to response was 2.2 months (range: 1.8–13 months).

Use of lenalidomide for the treatment of mantle cell lymphoma also was evaluated in an open-label, randomized phase 2 trial (mantle cell lymphoma-002; SPRINT). In this study, 254 patients with relapsed or refractory mantle cell lymphoma who were ineligible for intensive chemotherapy or stem cell transplantation were randomized to receive lenalidomide (25 mg on days 1–21 of a 28-day cycle) or investigator's choice of standard monotherapy (i.e., rituximab, gemcitabine, fludarabine, chlorambucil, cytarabine). At a median follow-up duration of 15.9 months, median progression-free survival was prolonged in patients receiving lenalidomide compared with those receiving an investigator's choice of therapy (8.7 versus 5.2 months; hazard ratio of 0.61 with a 95% confidence interval of 0.44–0.84).

● Follicular Lymphoma and Marginal-zone Lymphoma

Lenalidomide is used in combination with rituximab for the treatment of previously treated follicular lymphoma and marginal-zone lymphoma. Lenalidomide has been designated an orphan drug by the FDA for these uses.

The use of lenalidomide with rituximab in patients with previously treated follicular lymphoma or marginal-zone lymphoma is based principally on a randomized, double-blind, multicenter study (AUGMENT) and an open-label, multicenter study (MAGNIFY).

In the AUGMENT study, 358 patients with relapsed or refractory follicular lymphoma or marginal-zone lymphoma were randomized to receive the combination of lenalidomide (20 mg once daily on days 1–21 for up to 12 cycles or until unacceptable toxicity occurred) and rituximab (375 mg/m² on days 1, 8, 15, and 22 of cycle 1, followed by 375 mg/m² on day 1 during cycles 2–5) or the same dosage of rituximab in combination with placebo. Treatment cycles were repeated every 28 days. At a median follow-up of 28.3 months, median progression-free survival was prolonged in patients receiving lenalidomide in combination with rituximab compared with rituximab and placebo (39.4 versus 14.1 months (hazard ratio: 0.46 with a 95% confidence interval of 0.34–0.62). In a subgroup of 295 patients with follicular lymphoma, objective response rate (as assessed by an independent review committee) in patients receiving lenalidomide in combination with rituximab was 80% compared with 55% in those receiving rituximab and placebo. In the subgroup of patients with marginal-zone lymphoma, the objective response rate in patients receiving lenalidomide in combination with rituximab was 65% compared with 44% in those receiving rituximab and placebo.

In the MAGNIFY study, 232 patients with relapsed or refractory follicular lymphoma, marginal-zone lymphoma, or mantle cell lymphoma received lenalidomide (20 mg once daily on days 1–21 of each 28-day cycle for up to 12 cycles or until unacceptable toxicity or disease progression occurred) in combination with rituximab (375 mg/m² on days 1, 8, 15, and 22 of cycle 1, followed by 375 mg/m² on day 1 of every other cycle [cycles 3, 5, 7, 9, and 11]). In the subgroup of patients with follicular lymphoma or marginal-zone lymphoma, investigator-assessed objective response rate in patients receiving lenalidomide in combination with rituximab was 59 or 51%, respectively. At a median follow-up duration of 7.9 or 11.5 months in patients with follicular lymphoma or marginal-zone lymphoma, respectively, median duration of response had not been reached.

DOSAGE AND ADMINISTRATION

● General

Pretreatment Screening

- Tests to exclude pregnancy must be performed within 10–14 days and again within 24 hours immediately prior to treatment initiation.

- Baseline absolute neutrophil count (ANC) and platelet counts.

- Thyroid function.

- Assess risk factors for thromboembolism.

Patient Monitoring

- *Multiple myeloma*: Complete blood cell counts (CBCs) weekly during the first 2 cycles, on days 1 and 15 of cycle 3, and then every 28 days thereafter.

- *Myelodysplastic syndrome*: CBCs weekly during first 8 weeks of therapy, and at least monthly thereafter.

- *Mantle cell lymphoma*: CBCs weekly during the first cycle, every 2 weeks during cycles 2–4, and then monthly thereafter.

- *Follicular lymphoma or marginal-zone lymphoma*: CBCs weekly for the first 3 weeks of cycle 1, every 2 weeks during cycles 2–4, and then monthly thereafter.

- Signs or symptoms of neutropenia or thrombocytopenia (e.g., bleeding, bruising, infection).

- Pregnancy tests weekly during the first month of therapy, then every 2 or 4 weeks in women with irregular or regular menstrual cycles, respectively.

- Development of second primary malignancies.

- Liver function tests periodically.

- Tumor lysis syndrome in patients with a high tumor burden.

- Thyroid function.

- Manifestations of tumor flare reaction.

Premedication and Prophylaxis

- Manufacturer recommends thromboprophylaxis; select an appropriate prophylactic regimen based on assessment of patient risk factors.

Thromboprophylaxis in Patients with Multiple Myeloma

- International Myeloma Working Group (IMWG) recommends thromboprophylaxis with aspirin for multiple myeloma patients receiving thalidomide with 1 or no underlying individual and/or myeloma-related risk factors for venous thromboembolism.

- IMWG recommends thromboprophylaxis with a low molecular weight heparin (LMWH) for those with 2 or more individual and/or myeloma-related risk factors.

- IMWG recommends thromboprophylaxis with a LMWH should be considered in thalidomide-treated patients receiving high-dose dexamethasone, doxorubicin, or multiple antineoplastic agents, independent of additional risk factors.

- IMWG states that full-dose warfarin (international normalized ratio [INR] 2–3) is an alternative to LMWH; however, there is limited clinical experience with this approach.

- American Society of Clinical Oncology (ASCO) recommends pharmacologic thromboprophylaxis for multiple myeloma patients receiving lenalidomide in conjunction with dexamethasone or antineoplastic agents, and states that those at lower risk for thromboembolism may receive either aspirin or a LMWH, while those at higher risk should receive a LMWH.

Dispensing and Administration Precautions
Handling and Disposal

- Consult specialized references for procedures for proper handling and disposal of antineoplastics.

- Avoid contact of capsule contents with skin or mucous membranes. If such contact occurs, wash affected areas of skin thoroughly with soap and water and rinse affected mucosa thoroughly with water.

REMS

- *Because lenalidomide is an analog of thalidomide (a known human teratogen that can cause severe, life-threatening birth defects if administered during pregnancy), commercially available lenalidomide must be obtained through a restricted distribution program, the Lenalidomide Risk Evaluation and Mitigation Strategy (REMS) program, designed to help ensure that fetal exposure to the drug does not occur.*

- Clinicians, pharmacists, and patients must be registered in the Lenalidomide REMS program before they can prescribe, dispense, and receive lenalidomide, and compliance with all terms outlined in the program is mandatory.

- The Lenalidomide REMS program controls access to lenalidomide; educates program participants (clinicians, pharmacists, patients) about the risks associated with lenalidomide and the procedural requirements for safe use of the drug; and monitors compliance with the registration, education, and safety requirements of the program. Clinicians may contact the REMS Call Center at 888-423-5436 or visit https://www.lenalidomiderems.com/ for additional information and to enroll in the program.

- No more than a 28-day supply of lenalidomide should be dispensed at one time.

● Administration

Lenalidomide capsules should be administered orally with water, with or without food, once daily. The capsules should be swallowed intact and should not be broken, chewed, or opened.

● Dosage

Multiple Myeloma

Combination Therapy for the Treatment of Multiple Myeloma

For the treatment of multiple myeloma in adults, the recommended initial dosage of lenalidomide is 25 mg once daily on days 1–21 of repeated 28-day cycles in combination with dexamethasone. Clinicians should consult published protocols for dexamethasone dosing. (See Multiple Myeloma under Uses.) In clinical studies, lenalidomide was continued until disease progression or unacceptable toxicity occurred in patients who were not candidates for autologous hematopoietic stem cell transplantation (HSCT). In patients who are undergoing autologous HSCT, stem cell mobilization should occur within 4 cycles of lenalidomide-containing therapy.

Temporary interruption of lenalidomide therapy followed by dosage reduction may be necessary in patients experiencing hematologic adverse effects (see Table 1).

TABLE 1. Dosage Modification for Hematologic Adverse Effects in Patients with Multiple Myeloma Receiving Lenalidomide in Combination with Dexamethasone

Adverse Reaction and Severity	Lenalidomide Dosage Modification (Lenalidomide Starting Dosage = 25 mg daily on days 1–21 of each 28-day cycle)
Thrombocytopenia	
Platelet count <30,000/mm³	First occurrence: Withhold therapy and monitor CBCs weekly; when platelet count ≥30,000/mm³, then resume next lower dosage (do not administer dosages lower than 2.5 mg daily)
	Subsequent occurrences: Withhold therapy until platelet count ≥30,000/mm³, then resume at next lower dosage (do not administer dosages lower than 2.5 mg daily)
Neutropenia	
Absolute neutrophil count (ANC) <1000/mm³	First occurrence (neutropenia is only toxicity): Withhold therapy and monitor CBCs weekly; when ANC ≥1000/mm³, then resume at 25 mg daily or initial starting dosage
	First occurrence (in presence of other toxicity): Withhold therapy and monitor CBCs weekly; when ANC ≥1000/mm³, then resume at next lower dosage (do not administer dosages lower than 2.5 mg daily)
	Subsequent occurrence: Withhold therapy until ANC ≥1000/mm³, then resume at next lower dosage (do not administer dosages lower than 2.5 mg daily)

Maintenance Therapy Following Autologous HSCT

In adults who have undergone autologous HSCT, maintenance therapy with lenalidomide at an initial dosage of 10 mg once daily on days 1–28 of a 28-day cycle should be started when the ANC reaches 1000/mm³ or more and/or platelet count reaches 75,000/mm³ or more. Therapy should be continued until disease progression or unacceptable toxicity occurs. (See Maintenance Therapy Following Autologous Hematopoietic Stem Cell Transplantation under Uses.) Following 3 cycles of maintenance therapy, the dosage of lenalidomide may be increased to 15 mg once daily, if tolerated.

Temporary interruption of lenalidomide therapy followed by dosage reduction may be necessary in patients experiencing hematologic adverse effects (see Table 2).

TABLE 2. Dosage Modification for Hematologic Adverse Effects in Patients with Multiple Myeloma Receiving Lenalidomide Maintenance Therapy

Adverse Reaction and Severity	Lenalidomide Dosage Modification (Lenalidomide Dosage = 10 or 15 mg daily on days 1–28 of each 28-day cycle)
Thrombocytopenia	
Platelet count <30,000/mm³	First occurrence: Withhold therapy and monitor CBCs weekly; when platelet count ≥30,000/mm³, resume at next lower dosage and administer continuously (for 28 days of each 28-day cycle)
	For subsequent occurrences in patients receiving a reduced dosage of 5 mg daily: Withhold therapy; when platelet count ≥30,000/mm³, resume therapy at 5 mg daily on days 1–21 of each 28-day cycle (do not administer dosages lower than 5 mg daily)

TABLE 2. Continued

Adverse Reaction and Severity	Lenalidomide Dosage Modification (Lenalidomide Dosage = 10 or 15 mg daily on days 1–28 of each 28-day cycle)
Neutropenia	
ANC <500/mm³	First occurrence: Withhold therapy and monitor CBCs weekly; when ANC ≥500/mm³, resume at next lower dosage and administer continuously (for 28 days of each 28-day cycle)
	For subsequent occurrences in patients receiving a reduced dosage of 5 mg daily: Withhold therapy; when ANC ≥500/mm³, resume therapy at 5 mg daily on days 1–21 of each 28-day cycle (do not administer dosages lower than 5 mg daily)

Myelodysplastic Syndrome

For the management of myelodysplastic syndrome (MDS), the recommended initial dosage in adults is 10 mg once daily. Treatment is continued until disease progression or unacceptable toxicity occurs. (See Myelodysplastic Syndrome under Uses.)

For the management of transfusion-dependent low-risk or intermediate-1-risk MDS in patients *without* the deletion 5q (del[5q]) chromosomal abnormality (non-del[5q])†, lenalidomide 10 mg once daily has been used.

Dosage Modification for Hematologic Toxicity in Patients with Myelodysplastic Syndromes

Temporary interruption of lenalidomide therapy followed by dosage reduction may be necessary in patients experiencing thrombocytopenia (see Table 3) or neutropenia (see Table 4).

TABLE 3. Dosage Modification for Thrombocytopenia in Patients with MDS

Severity	Lenalidomide Dosage Modification (Lenalidomide Starting Dosage = 10 mg daily)
Platelet count <50,000/mm³ occurs *within* 4 weeks of therapy	
Baseline platelet count ≥100,000/mm³	Withhold therapy until platelet count ≥50,000/mm³, then resume at 5 mg daily
Platelet count decreases to 50% of baseline value within 4 weeks of therapy	
Baseline platelet count ≥60,000/mm³ to <100,000/mm³	Withhold therapy until platelet count ≥50,000/mm³, then resume at 5 mg daily
Platelet count decreases to 50% of baseline value within 4 weeks of therapy	
Baseline platelet count <60,000/mm³	Withhold therapy until platelet count ≥30,000/mm³, then resume at 5 mg daily
Thrombocytopenia occurring after 4 weeks of therapy	
Platelet count <30,000/mm³ or <50,000/mm³ and requiring platelet transfusions	Withhold therapy until platelet count ≥30,000/mm³ (without hemostatic failure), then resume at 5 mg daily
Thrombocytopenia recurs on a reduced dosage of 5 mg daily	
Platelet count <30,000/mm³ or <50,000/mm³ and requiring platelet transfusions	Withhold therapy until platelet count ≥30,000/mm³ (without hemostatic failure), then resume at 2.5 mg daily

TABLE 4. Dosage Modification for Neutropenia in Patients with MDS

Severity	Lenalidomide Dosage Modification (Lenalidomide Starting Dosage = 10 mg daily)
ANC <750/mm³ occurs *within* 4 weeks of therapy	
Baseline ANC ≥1,000/mm³	Withhold therapy until ANC ≥1000/mm³, then resume at 5 mg daily
ANC <500/mm³ *within* 4 weeks of therapy	
Baseline ANC is <1,000/mm³	Withhold therapy until ANC ≥500/mm³, then resume at 5 mg daily
Neutropenia occurring after 4 weeks of therapy	
ANC <500/mm³ for ≥7 days or <500/mm³ with fever (≥38.5°C)	Withhold therapy until ANC ≥500/mm³, then resume at 5 mg daily
Neutropenia recurs on a reduced dosage of 5 mg daily	
ANC <500/mm³ for ≥7 days or <500/mm³ with fever (≥38.5°C) on a reduced dosage of 5 mg daily	Withhold therapy until ANC ≥500/mm³, then resume at 2.5 mg daily

Mantle Cell Lymphoma

For the treatment of relapsed or refractory mantle cell lymphoma, the recommended initial adult dosage of lenalidomide is 25 mg once daily on days 1–21 of a 28-day cycle until disease progression or unacceptable toxicity occurs. (See Mantle Cell Lymphoma under Uses.)

Dosage Modification for Hematologic Toxicity in Patients with Mantle Cell Lymphoma

Temporary interruption of lenalidomide therapy followed by dosage reduction may be necessary in patients experiencing hematologic adverse effects (see Table 5).

TABLE 5. Dosage Modification for Hematologic Adverse Effects in Patients with Mantle Cell Lymphoma

Adverse Reaction and Severity	Lenalidomide Dosage Modification (Lenalidomide Starting Dosage = 25 mg daily)
Thrombocytopenia	
Platelet count <50,000/mm³	Withhold therapy and monitor CBC weekly; when platelet count ≥50,000/mm³, resume at dosage reduced by 5 mg (do not administer dosages lower than 5 mg daily)
Neutropenia	
ANC <1000/mm³ for ≥7 days, or <1000/mm³ with fever (≥38.5°C), or <500/mm³	Withhold therapy and monitor CBC weekly; when ANC ≥1000/mm³, resume at dosage reduced by 5 mg (do not administer dosages lower than 5 mg daily)

Follicular Lymphoma or Marginal-zone Lymphoma

For the treatment of follicular lymphoma or marginal-zone lymphoma, the recommended initial adult dosage of lenalidomide is 20 mg once daily on days 1–21 of a 28-day cycle in combination with rituximab. In the AUGMENT and MAGNIFY studies, lenalidomide was administered for up to 12 cycles. (See Follicular Lymphoma and Marginal-zone Lymphoma under Uses.)

In the AUGMENT study, rituximab 375 mg/m² was administered on days 1, 8, 15, and 22 of cycle 1, followed by 375 mg/m² on day 1 during cycles 2–5.

Dosage Modification for Hematologic Toxicity in Patients with Follicular Lymphoma or Marginal-zone Lymphoma

Temporary interruption of lenalidomide therapy followed by dosage reduction may be necessary in patients experiencing hematologic adverse effects (see Table 6).

TABLE 6. Dosage Modification for Hematologic Adverse Effects in Patients with Follicular Lymphoma or Marginal-zone Lymphoma

Adverse Reaction and Severity	Lenalidomide Dosage Modification (Lenalidomide Starting Dosage = 20 mg daily)
Thrombocytopenia	
Platelet count <50,000/mm³	Withhold therapy and monitor CBC weekly; when platelet count ≥50,000/mm³, resume at dosage reduced by 5 mg (do not administer dosages lower than 5 mg daily; if initial dosage was 10 mg daily, do not administer dosages lower than 2.5 mg daily)
Neutropenia	
ANC <1000/mm³ for ≥7 days, or <1000/mm³ with fever (≥38.5°C), or <500/mm³	Withhold therapy and monitor CBC weekly; when ANC ≥1000/mm³, resume at dosage reduced by 5 mg (do not administer dosages lower than 5 mg daily; if initial dosage was 10 mg daily, do not administer dosages lower than 2.5 mg daily)

Dosage Modification for Nonhematologic Adverse Reactions

If angioedema, anaphylaxis, grade 4 rash, skin exfoliation, bullae, or any other severe dermatologic reaction occurs, lenalidomide therapy should be permanently discontinued. (See Hypersensitivity Reactions and also Cutaneous Reactions under Cautions.)

If grade 3 or 4 nonhematologic toxicities occur, temporarily interrupt lenalidomide therapy; when the toxicity resolves or improves to grade 2 or less, lenalidomide therapy may be resumed at the next lower dosage level.

● *Special Populations*

Hepatic Impairment

The manufacturer makes no specific dosage recommendations for patients with hepatic impairment.

Renal Impairment

Initial dosage reduction may be necessary in patients with renal impairment (see Table 7).

TABLE 7. Recommended Initial Dosage of Lenalidomide in Patients with Renal Impairment

Cl$_{cr}$ (mL/minute)	Multiple Myeloma (Combination Therapy with Dexamethasone)	Mantle Cell Lymphoma	Follicular Lymphoma and Marginal-zone Lymphoma (Combination Therapy with Rituximab)	Multiple Myeloma (Maintenance Therapy) and MDS
30–60	10 mg once daily If reduced dosage is tolerated, consider increasing dosage to 15 mg once daily after 2 cycles	10 mg once daily[a]	10 mg once daily If reduced dosage is tolerated, consider increasing dosage to 15 mg once daily after 2 cycles	5 mg once daily[a]
<30 (not requiring dialysis)	15 mg every other day	15 mg every other day[a]	5 mg once daily	2.5 mg once daily[a]
<30 (requiring dialysis)	5 mg once daily[b]	5 mg once daily[b]	5 mg once daily[b]	2.5 mg once daily[b]

[a] Subsequent dosage adjustments should be based on patient tolerance
[b] Administer lenalidomide after dialysis

Geriatric Patients

Because lenalidomide is excreted substantially by the kidneys and geriatric patients are more likely to have decreased renal function, careful dosage selection and monitoring of renal function are advised in such patients.

CAUTIONS

● Contraindications

- Lenalidomide is contraindicated in women who are pregnant. The drug should be used in women of childbearing potential only when alternative therapies are not available and adequate precautions are taken to avoid pregnancy. (See REMS under Dosage and Administration and also see Fetal/Neonatal Morbidity and Mortality under Cautions.)

- Lenalidomide is contraindicated in patients with known hypersensitivity (e.g., angioedema, Stevens-Johnson syndrome [SJS], toxic epidermal necrolysis [TEN]) to the drug.

● Warnings/Precautions

Warnings

Fetal/Neonatal Morbidity and Mortality

Lenalidomide may cause fetal toxicity; the drug is a structural analog of thalidomide, a known human teratogen, and teratogenic and other fetotoxic effects have been demonstrated in animals.

All females of reproductive potential and all sexually mature males receiving lenalidomide must use effective contraceptive measures (which may include abstinence) to help ensure that fetal exposure to lenalidomide does not occur. Contraceptive measures are indicated even in females with a history of infertility. The only females who do not need to observe mandatory contraceptive measures are those who have undergone hysterectomy, bilateral oophorectomy, or who are postmenopausal and have had no menses for at least 24 consecutive months. All female patients of reproductive potential must use 2 reliable forms of contraception simultaneously (unless the patient chooses to remain continuously abstinent from engaging in heterosexual sexual contact) beginning at least 4 weeks prior to initiation of therapy, during therapy or interruptions of therapy, and continue such contraception for at least 4 weeks after lenalidomide therapy is discontinued. The patient must use at least 2 birth control methods, preferably one should be a highly effective birth control method (intrauterine device [IUD], hormonal

contraceptives, tubal ligation, vasectomized partner) and one additional effective barrier method (latex condom, diaphragm, cervical cap). Sexually mature males (including those who have successfully undergone vasectomy) receiving lenalidomide must completely avoid unprotected sexual contact with women of reproductive potential because lenalidomide is present in semen. While receiving lenalidomide and for at least 4 weeks after discontinuing the drug, sexually mature males must use a latex or synthetic condom each time they have sexual contact with a woman of reproductive potential and must not donate sperm. All females of reproductive potential must be tested for pregnancy within 10–14 days prior and again within the 24 hours immediately prior to the first dose of lenalidomide.

The prescribing clinician should not provide the woman with a prescription for lenalidomide until a written report of the pregnancy test is available indicating that results are negative. Pregnancy tests must then be repeated at regular intervals during lenalidomide therapy (i.e., weekly during the first month, then every 2 or 4 weeks in women with irregular or regular menstrual cycles, respectively). Pregnancy tests and counseling also should be performed if a patient misses her period or if there is any abnormality in menstrual bleeding. The drug should be discontinued during the evaluation period. If lenalidomide is inadvertently administered during pregnancy or if the patient becomes pregnant while receiving the drug, lenalidomide should be immediately discontinued and the patient informed of the potential hazard to the fetus; the patient should be referred to an obstetrician/gynecologist experienced in reproductive toxicity, and the clinician should notify Bristol Myers Squibb's REMS Call Center (888-423-5436) and the FDA via the MedWatch program (800-FDA-1088). (See REMS under Dosage and Administration.)

Because lenalidomide may cause fetal harm and because of the possibility that the drug may be present in blood and be transfused into a woman who is pregnant, patients receiving lenalidomide must not donate blood during therapy and for at least 1 month following discontinuance of the drug.

Hematologic Effects

Lenalidomide is associated with substantial neutropenia and thrombocytopenia. Periodic monitoring of CBCs is recommended. Patients should be monitored for signs or symptoms of neutropenia or thrombocytopenia (e.g., bleeding, bruising, infection).

In the principal efficacy studies evaluating maintenance therapy with lenalidomide in patients with multiple myeloma, grade 3 or 4 neutropenia or thrombocytopenia occurred in up to 59 or 38% of lenalidomide-treated patients, respectively. When lenalidomide is used as maintenance therapy or in combination with dexamethasone in patients with multiple myeloma, CBCs should be monitored weekly for the first 2 cycles, then on days 1 and 15 of cycle 3, and then every 4 weeks thereafter. If hematologic toxicity occurs, dosage interruption and/or reduction may be required. (See Multiple Myeloma under Dosage and Administration.)

In the principal efficacy study evaluating lenalidomide therapy in patients with MDS, grade 3 or 4 hematologic toxicity was reported in 80% of patients with myelodysplastic syndromes receiving lenalidomide. Median time to onset of grade 3 or 4 neutropenia (occurring in 48% of patients) was 42 days (range: 14–411 days), and median time to documented recovery was 17 days (range: 2–170 days). Median time to onset of grade 3 or 4 thrombocytopenia (occurring in 54% of patients) was 28 days (range: 8–290 days) and median time to documented recovery was 22 days (range: 5–224 days). CBCs should be monitored weekly for the first 8 weeks of therapy and at least monthly thereafter. If hematologic toxicity occurs, dosage interruption and/or reduction may be required. (See Dosage Modification for Hematologic Toxicity in Patients with Myelodysplastic Syndrome under Dosage and Administration.)

In the principal efficacy study evaluating lenalidomide therapy in patients with mantle cell lymphoma, grade 3 or 4 neutropenia or thrombocytopenia was reported in 43 or 28% of patients receiving the drug, respectively. CBCs should be monitored weekly for the first cycle, every 2 weeks during cycles 2–4, and then monthly thereafter. If hematologic toxicity occurs, dosage interruption and/or reduction may be required. (See Dosage Modification for Hematologic Toxicity in Patients with Mantle Cell Lymphoma under Dosage and Administration.)

In the principal efficacy studies evaluating lenalidomide in combination with rituximab in patients with follicular lymphoma or marginal-zone lymphoma, grade 3 or 4 neutropenia occurred in 50% or 33%, respectively, of patients receiving combination therapy. Grade 3 or 4 thrombocytopenia was reported in 2% or 8% of lenalidomide-treated patients, respectively. CBCs should be monitored weekly for the first 3 weeks of cycle 1 (28 days), every 2 weeks during cycles 2–4, and then monthly thereafter. If hematologic toxicity occurs, dosage interruption and/or reduction may be required. (See Dosage Modification for Hematologic Toxicity in Patients with Follicular Lymphoma or Marginal-zone Lymphoma.)

Thromboembolic Events

Lenalidomide increases the risk of venous and arterial thromboembolic events (e.g., DVT, PE, myocardial infarction, stroke). Patients with known risk factors, including prior thrombotic events, may be at greater risk and actions should be taken to minimize all modifiable factors (e.g., hyperlipidemia, hypertension, smoking).

In clinical trials that did not use concomitant thromboprophylaxis in patients with refractory and relapsed multiple myeloma receiving lenalidomide and dexamethasone, thrombotic events occurred in 21.5% of lenalidomide-treated patients compared with 8.3% of those treated with dexamethasone. The median time to first thrombotic event was 2.8 months. In the principal efficacy study evaluating lenalidomide in combination with dexamethasone in patients with newly diagnosed multiple myeloma, nearly all patients received thromboprophylaxis; thrombotic events occurred in 17.4% of lenalidomide-treated patients compared with 11.6% of patients receiving melphalan, prednisone, and thalidomide combination therapy.

In the principal efficacy study evaluating lenalidomide in patients with follicular lymphoma or marginal-zone lymphoma, venous or arterial thromboembolic events occurred in 3.4 or 0.6% of patients receiving lenalidomide in combination with rituximab, respectively.

The manufacturer recommends thromboprophylaxis; selection of an appropriate prophylactic regimen (e.g., aspirin, anticoagulant) should be based on assessment of patient risk factors. The risk of thrombosis may be increased with concomitant use of erythropoietin-stimulating agents or estrogens. The International Myeloma Working Group (IMWG) currently recommends thromboprophylaxis with aspirin for multiple myeloma patients receiving lenalidomide with 1 or no underlying individual and/or myeloma-related risk factors for venous thromboembolism and thromboprophylaxis with a low molecular weight heparin for those with 2 or more individual and/or myeloma-related risk factors. The IMWG also recommends that thromboprophylaxis with a low molecular weight heparin be considered in lenalidomide-treated patients receiving high-dose dexamethasone, doxorubicin, or multiple antineoplastic agents, independent of additional risk factors. The IMWG states that although full-dose warfarin (international normalized ratio [INR] 2–3) is an alternative to low molecular weight heparin, there is limited clinical experience with this approach. American Society of Clinical Oncology (ASCO) currently recommends pharmacologic thromboprophylaxis for multiple myeloma patients receiving lenalidomide in conjunction with dexamethasone or antineoplastic agents, and states that those at lower risk for thromboembolism may receive either aspirin or a low molecular weight heparin, while those at higher risk should receive a low molecular weight heparin.

Other Warnings and Precautions
Treatment-related Mortality

A prospective clinical trial evaluating single-agent lenalidomide therapy in patients with newly diagnosed chronic lymphocytic leukemia (CLL) was terminated prematurely following revelation of a substantial increase in risk of death in patients receiving lenalidomide compared with those receiving single-agent chlorambucil (hazard ratio of 1.92 with 95% confidence interval 1.08–3.41). Serious adverse cardiovascular reactions (e.g., atrial fibrillation, myocardial infarction, cardiac failure) occurred more frequently in patients receiving lenalidomide. The manufacturer states that lenalidomide should not be used in patients with CLL outside of a controlled clinical trial.

Increased mortality also has been reported in clinical trials in patients with multiple myeloma receiving pembrolizumab in combination with a thalidomide analog and dexamethasone. The manufacturer of lenalidomide states that an anti-programmed death receptor-1 (anti-PD-1) or anti-programmed-death ligand-1 (anti-PD-L1) antibody should not be used in combination with a thalidomide analog and dexamethasone in patients with multiple myeloma outside of a controlled clinical trial. FDA recommends that ongoing clinical trials evaluating an anti-PD-1 or anti-PD-L1 agent in combination with an immunomodulatory agent (e.g., lenalidomide) be evaluated for permanent discontinuance or protocol amendments.

In patients with mantle cell lymphoma, an increase in early deaths (within 20 weeks) was reported in patients receiving lenalidomide compared with those in the control group (12.9 versus 7.1%) in a clinical trial. High tumor burden, baseline mantle cell lymphoma International Prognostic Index (MIPI) score, and high white blood cell count (10,000/mm³ or greater) at baseline were factors associated with early death.

Development of Second Primary Malignancy

In clinical trials, the risk of hematologic and solid second primary malignancies was increased in patients with multiple myeloma receiving lenalidomide. The trials suggested an increased risk of second primary malignancies with lenalidomide compared to other therapies or placebo in patients with newly diagnosed multiple myeloma, those with relapsed or refractory multiple myeloma, and those receiving lenalidomide after autologous hematopoietic stem cell transplantation (HSCT). Patients who received lenalidomide therapy until disease progression did not demonstrate an increased risk of invasive second primary malignancy compared with those who received lenalidomide for a fixed duration.

In patients with newly diagnosed multiple myeloma, 5.3% of patients receiving lenalidomide in combination with oral melphalan developed a hematologic malignancy, including acute myeloid leukemia (AML) and MDS, compared with 1.3% of patients receiving melphalan alone. When lenalidomide was used in combination with dexamethasone without melphalan in patients with newly diagnosed multiple myeloma, MDS and AML were reported in 0.4% of patients.

In patients receiving lenalidomide maintenance therapy after high-dose IV melphalan and autologous HSCT, hematologic second primary malignancy occurred in 7.5% of lenalidomide-treated patients compared with 3.3% of patients receiving placebo. Hematologic and solid malignancy (excluding squamous cell carcinoma and basal cell carcinoma) occurred in 14.9% of patients treated with lenalidomide compared with 8.8% of those receiving placebo at a median follow-up duration of 91.5 months. Nonmelanoma skin carcinoma, including squamous cell carcinoma and basal cell carcinoma, was reported in 3.9% of patients receiving lenalidomide maintenance therapy compared with 2.6% of those receiving placebo.

In patients with relapsed or refractory multiple myeloma receiving lenalidomide and dexamethasone, hematologic or solid malignancy (excluding squamous cell carcinoma and basal cell carcinoma) occurred in 2.3% of lenalidomide-treated patients compared with 0.6% of those receiving dexamethasone. Nonmelanoma skin carcinoma, including squamous cell carcinoma and basal cell carcinoma, was reported in 3.1% of patients receiving lenalidomide and dexamethasone compared with 0.6% of those treated with dexamethasone alone.

In patients with follicular lymphoma or marginal-zone lymphoma, AML occurred in 0.6% of patients receiving lenalidomide in combination with rituximab. Hematologic or solid malignancy (excluding nonmelanoma skin carcinoma) occurred in 1.7% of patients receiving lenalidomide in combination with rituximab at a median follow-up duration of 29.8 months.

Patients treated with lenalidomide should be monitored for development of second primary malignancies. The risk of second primary malignancies should be considered along with the potential benefit of lenalidomide.

Hepatotoxicity

Hepatic failure, sometimes fatal, has occurred in patients treated with lenalidomide in combination with dexamethasone. The exact mechanism of lenalidomide-induced hepatotoxicity is not known. In clinical trials, hepatotoxicity (with hepatocellular, cholestatic and mixed characteristics) occurred in 15% of lenalidomide-treated patients; serious hepatotoxic events occurred in 2 or 1% of patients with multiple myeloma or myelodysplastic syndrome (MDS), respectively.

Patients with pre-existing liver disease of viral etiology, elevated baseline liver enzymes, and those receiving concomitant medications may be at increased risk. Liver function tests should be monitored periodically. If elevations in liver enzymes occur, lenalidomide therapy should be interrupted or discontinued. When liver enzymes return to baseline values, resumption of lenalidomide therapy may be considered at a reduced dosage. (See Dosage Modification for Nonhematologic Adverse Reactions under Dosage and Administration.)

Cutaneous Reactions

Severe cases of cutaneous reactions (i.e., SJS, TEN, and drug reaction with eosinophilia and systemic symptoms [DRESS]) have been reported in patients receiving lenalidomide. DRESS may present with a cutaneous reaction (such as rash or exfoliative dermatitis), eosinophilia, fever, and/or lymphadenopathy with systemic complications such as hepatitis, nephritis, pneumonitis, myocarditis, and/or pericarditis. These reactions can be fatal. Lenalidomide should not be used in patients with a prior history of grade 4 rash with thalidomide. For grade 2 or 3 skin rash, temporary interruption or discontinuance of lenalidomide should be considered. If grade 4 rash, exfoliative or bullous rash, or other severe cutaneous reactions (SJS, TEN, or DRESS) occurs, lenalidomide therapy should be permanently discontinued.

Tumor Lysis Syndrome

Fatal tumor lysis syndrome has been reported in patients receiving lenalidomide. Patients with high tumor burden at baseline are at risk for tumor lysis syndrome, and should be monitored closely; appropriate precautions also should be instituted. In the principal efficacy studies in patients with follicular lymphoma or marginal-zone lymphoma, tumor lysis syndrome occurred in 0.5–1.1% of patients receiving lenalidomide in combination with rituximab; serious (grade 3) adverse reactions occurred in 1 patient receiving lenalidomide and rituximab during the induction phase.

Tumor Flare Reaction

Tumor flare reaction, including fatalities, has been reported in clinical trials in patients with CLL and lymphoma receiving lenalidomide. Tumor flare reactions (i.e., tender lymph node swelling, low grade fever, pain, rash) may mimic disease progression. The manufacturer states that lenalidomide should not be used in patients with CLL outside of a controlled clinical trial.

In the principal efficacy study in patients with mantle cell lymphoma (MCL), grade 1 or 2 tumor flare reaction occurred in 10% of patients receiving lenalidomide. All reactions occurred during the first cycle; tumor flare reaction recurred in one patient in cycle 11. In the principal efficacy studies in patients with follicular lymphoma or marginal-zone lymphoma, tumor flare reaction was reported in 4.1–10.8% of patients receiving lenalidomide in combination with rituximab; 2 events were considered serious. In a separate MCL phase 2 trial, one case of tumor flare reaction resulted in a fatal outcome.

Patients with MCL, follicular lymphoma, or marginal-zone lymphoma should be monitored for signs or symptoms of tumor flare reaction. In patients experiencing grade 1 or 2 tumor flare reaction, lenalidomide may be continued without dosage adjustment or interruption of therapy. In patients with grade 3 or 4 tumor flare reaction, lenalidomide should be withheld until tumor flare reaction resolves to grade 1 or less. Symptomatic treatment for tumor flare reaction may include corticosteroids, non-steroidal anti-inflammatory drugs, and/or opiate analgesics.

Impaired Stem Cell Mobilization

A decrease in collection of CD34+ peripheral blood progenitor cells (PBPCs) has been reported following lenalidomide therapy for more than 4 cycles. (See Multiple Myeloma under Dosage and Administration.) Patients who are eligible for autologous HSCT should be promptly referred to a transplant center to optimize timing of stem cell collection. In patients who have received more than 4 cycles of lenalidomide-containing therapy or those who previously failed to achieved adequate PBPC collection following mobilization with a granulocyte-colony stimulating factor (G-CSF) alone, hematopoietic stem cell mobilization combination regimens such as G-CSF and cyclophosphamide or a G-CSF and a CXCR4 chemokine-receptor antagonist may be used.

Thyroid Disorders

Hyperthyroidism and hypothyroidism have been reported in patients receiving lenalidomide. Thyroid function should be monitored before initiating lenalidomide and during therapy.

Hypersensitivity Reactions

Hypersensitivity reactions such as angioedema, anaphylaxis, and anaphylactic reactions have been reported in patients receiving lenalidomide. If angioedema or anaphylaxis occurs, lenalidomide should be permanently discontinued.

Specific Populations

Pregnancy

Lenalidomide is a thalidomide analog and is contraindicated for use during pregnancy. (See REMS under Dosage and Administration and also see Fetal/Neonatal Morbidity and Mortality under Cautions.)

Females or Males of Reproductive Potential

Pregnancy must be excluded prior to treatment initiation and throughout therapy. Pregnancy must be prevented for ≥4 weeks prior to and during therapy, during dosage interruptions, and for 4 weeks after completion of therapy. (See Fetal/Neonatal Morbidity and Mortality under Cautions.)

Lenalidomide has been shown to be present in semen at 2 and 24 hours following administration of the drug at a dosage of 25 mg daily. Therefore, males must always use a latex or synthetic condom during any sexual contact with females of reproductive potential while taking lenalidomide and for up to 4 weeks after discontinuing therapy, even if they have undergone a successful vasectomy. Male patients taking lenalidomide must not donate sperm and for up to 4 weeks after discontinuing the drug.

Lactation

Not known whether lenalidomide is distributed into human milk; discontinue nursing or the drug, taking into account the importance of the drug to the woman.

Pediatric Use

Safety and efficacy of lenalidomide have not been established in pediatric patients.

Geriatric Use

In clinical trials of lenalidomide in patients with newly diagnosed multiple myeloma, 94% of patients were 65 years of age or older and 35% of patients were over 75 years of age. Overall, patients over 75 years of age experienced more adverse reactions (including serious adverse reactions) than younger adults regardless of treatment arm.

In clinical trials evaluating maintenance therapy with lenalidomide in patients with multiple myeloma, 10% of patients were 65 years of age or older and no patients were over 75 years of age. Grade 3 or 4 adverse reactions occurred more frequently in patients 65 years of age or older receiving lenalidomide maintenance therapy than in younger patients. Experience in patients 65 years of age or older receiving lenalidomide maintenance therapy is insufficient to determine whether they respond differently to the drug than younger adults.

In clinical trials in patients with previously treated multiple myeloma, 45% of patients were 65 years of age or older and 12% patients were over 75 years of age. In the studies of previously treated patients, deep-vein thrombosis (DVT), pulmonary embolism (PE), atrial fibrillation, and renal failure were more common in patients over 65 years of age than younger adults treated with lenalidomide.

In clinical trials in patients with MDS or mantle cell lymphoma, 38 or 63% of patients, respectively, were 65 years of age or older. In patients with MDS or mantle cell lymphoma, 33 or 22% of patients, respectively, were 75 years of age or older. All patients with MDS experienced an adverse reaction; however, the frequency of serious adverse reactions was higher in patients over 65 years of age (54%) compared with younger adults (33%). In patients with mantle cell lymphoma, the frequency of overall adverse events was similar among patients over 65 years of age than in younger patients; however, serious adverse reactions were more common among patients over 65 years than in younger patients (55% versus 41%).

In clinical trials in patients with follicular lymphoma or marginal-zone lymphoma, 48% of patients were 65 years of age or older and 14% patients were over 75 years of age. The overall frequency of adverse reactions was 98% in both patients 65 years of age or older and younger adults. Serious adverse reactions were higher among lenalidomide-treated patients 65 years of age or older versus younger adults (37% versus 18%).

Renal Impairment

In a single-dose (25-mg) pharmacokinetic study, the elimination half-life of lenalidomide increased and clearance of the drug decreased as creatinine clearance decreased from mild to severe renal impairment. Patients with moderate and severe renal impairment had a threefold increase in half-life and a 66–75%

decrease in drug clearance compared with healthy individuals. In patients on hemodialysis, an approximate 4.5-fold increase in elimination half-life and an 80% decrease in clearance have been observed following single-dose administration of lenalidomide compared with healthy individuals. Approximately 30% of an administered dose of the drug was removed during a single hemodialysis session.

The initial dosage of lenalidomide should be adjusted in patients with renal impairment. (See Renal Impairment under Dosage and Administration.)

Hepatic Impairment

The pharmacokinetics of lenalidomide were not altered in patients with mild hepatic impairment (total bilirubin exceeding 1–1.5 times the upper limit of normal [ULN] or any aspartate aminotransferase concentration exceeding the ULN). Lenalidomide has not been studied in patients with moderate to severe hepatic impairment. (See Hepatic Impairment under Dosage and Administration.)

● Common Adverse Effects

Adverse effects reported in at least 20% of patients with multiple myeloma receiving lenalidomide include diarrhea, fatigue, anemia, constipation, neutropenia, leukopenia, peripheral edema, insomnia, muscle cramp/spasms, abdominal pain, back pain, nausea, asthenia, pyrexia, upper respiratory tract infection, bronchitis, nasopharyngitis, gastroenteritis, cough, rash, dyspnea, dizziness, decreased appetite, thrombocytopenia, and tremor.

Adverse effects reported in more than 15% of patients with MDS receiving lenalidomide include thrombocytopenia, neutropenia, diarrhea, pruritus, rash, fatigue, constipation, nausea, nasopharyngitis, arthralgia, pyrexia, back pain, peripheral edema, cough, dizziness, headache, muscle cramp, dyspnea, pharyngitis, and epistaxis.

Adverse effects reported in at least 15% of patients with mantle cell lymphoma, follicular lymphoma, or marginal-zone lymphoma receiving lenalidomide include neutropenia, thrombocytopenia, anemia, leukopenia, diarrhea, constipation, nausea, fatigue, pyrexia, cough, upper respiratory tract infection, and rash.

DRUG INTERACTIONS

Lenalidomide does not inhibit or induce cytochrome P-450 (CYP) isoenzymes in vitro.

Lenalidomide does not inhibit P-glycoprotein (P-gp), bile salt export pump (BSEP), breast cancer resistance protein (BCRP), multidrug resistance-associated protein (MRP) 2, organic anion transporter (OAT) 1 or 3, organic anion transport protein (OATP) 1B1 or 1B3, or organic cation transporter (OCT) 2.

Lenalidomide is a substrate, but not an inhibitor, of P-gp.

● Drugs Affecting or Metabolized by Hepatic Microsomal Enzymes

CYP-mediated drug interactions with lenalidomide unlikely.

● Drugs Affecting Efflux Transport Systems

Administration with P-gp inhibitors did not significantly increase the concentration of lenalidomide.

● Drugs Associated with an Increased Risk of Thrombosis

Erythropoietic agents, estrogen-containing therapies, or other agents that increase the risk of thrombosis should be used with caution in patients receiving lenalidomide, only if the potential benefits of concomitant therapy outweigh the risks.

● Digoxin

When digoxin was coadministered with lenalidomide (10 mg daily), the peak plasma concentration and AUC of digoxin increased by 14%. Manufacturer recommends periodic monitoring of plasma digoxin concentrations in patients receiving lenalidomide and digoxin concurrently.

● Warfarin

When warfarin was used concomitantly with lenalidomide, the pharmacokinetics of lenalidomide and R- and S-warfarin were unchanged. Manufacturer recommends close monitoring of PT and INR in patients with multiple myeloma receiving concomitant lenalidomide and warfarin.

DESCRIPTION

Lenalidomide, a thalidomide analog, is an immunomodulatory agent with antineoplastic and antiangiogenic activity. Cellular activities of lenalidomide are mediated through its target cereblon, a component of a cullin ring E3 ubiquitin ligase enzyme complex. In vitro, lenalidomide induces direct cytotoxic and immunomodulatory effects following ubiquitination and degradation of substrate proteins such as Aiolos, Ikaros, and CK1α. In vitro, lenalidomide also has been shown to inhibit proliferation and induce apoptosis of certain hematopoietic tumor cells including multiple myeloma, mantle cell lymphoma, myelodysplastic syndrome (MDS), follicular lymphoma, and marginal-zone lymphoma. In vivo, lenalidomide has been shown to delay tumor growth in some nonclinical hematopoietic tumor models including multiple myeloma. The drug has been shown to increase count and activation of T cells and natural killer (NK) cells resulting in direct and enhanced antibody-dependent cell-mediated cytotoxicity (ADCC) via inhibition of production of proinflammatory cytokines (e.g., tumor necrosis factor [TNF; TNF-α], interleukin-6 [IL-6]), increased secretion of IL-2 and interferon gamma, and increased NK cells.

Concomitant use of lenalidomide and dexamethasone results in synergistic inhibition of cell proliferation and induction of apoptosis in multiple myeloma cells. In vitro, the combination of lenalidomide and rituximab increased ADCC and direct tumor apoptosis in follicular lymphoma cells and increased ADCC in marginal-zone lymphoma cells compared with rituximab alone.

Lenalidomide is principally eliminated by the kidneys. After administration of a single 25-mg radiolabeled dose of lenalidomide, approximately 90 or 4% was eliminated in the urine or feces, respectively, within 10 days, and approximately 82% was excreted as unchanged drug in urine within 24 hours. Lenalidomide is rapidly absorbed after oral administration with maximum plasma concentrations occurring between 0.5 and 6 hours post-dose. The mean half-life of lenalidomide is 3 hours in healthy subjects and 3–5 hours in patients with multiple myeloma, MDS, or mantle cell lymphoma. Lenalidomide is minimally metabolized to 5-hydroxy-lenalidomide and N-acetyl-lenalidomide.

Clearance of lenalidomide is not affected substantially by age (39–85 years), weight (33–135 kg), sex, race, or type of hematologic malignancy.

ADVICE TO PATIENTS

- Importance of educating patients regarding the Lenalidomide® Risk Evaluation and Mitigation Strategy (REMS) restricted distribution program for obtaining lenalidomide. (See REMS under Dosage and Administration.)

- Importance of informing patients of Pregnancy Exposure Registry that monitors pregnancy outcomes in females exposed to lenalidomide during pregnancy.

- Importance of advising patients to swallow capsules intact and not to break, chew, or open capsules.

- Importance of advising patients that a missed dose may be taken up to 12 hours after the scheduled administration time; if more than 12 hours have elapsed, the missed dose should be omitted, and the regular dosing schedule resumed the following day. Importance of not taking 2 doses at the same time to make up for a missed dose.

- Risk of fetal harm. Necessity of advising women of reproductive potential to use effective methods of contraception beginning at least 4 weeks prior to initiation of therapy, throughout therapy, during dosage interruptions, and for at least 4 weeks after discontinuance of therapy (see Fetal/Neonatal Morbidity and Mortality under Cautions); importance of obtaining pregnancy tests at appropriate intervals during therapy and of immediately discontinuing therapy and contacting their clinician if pregnancy is suspected. Advise patient that if their healthcare provider is not available, they should call the REMS Call Center at 1-888-423-5436.

- Advise men (including those who have successfully undergone vasectomy) to use a latex or synthetic condom during sexual encounters with women of reproductive potential; these contraceptive measures are required during and for at least 4 weeks after discontinuance of lenalidomide therapy.

- Importance of advising women to avoid breast-feeding while receiving lenalidomide therapy.

- Importance of advising men to avoid donating semen while receiving lenalidomide and for 4 weeks after discontinuing the drug.

- Necessity of monitoring CBCs for neutropenia and thrombocytopenia during lenalidomide therapy.

- Risk of venous and arterial thromboembolic events; importance of advising patients to seek medical care if they develop symptoms of shortness of breath, chest pain, or swelling of the arms or legs. (See Thromboembolic Events under Cautions.)

- Possible increased mortality and risk of serious adverse cardiovascular reactions, including atrial fibrillation, myocardial infarction, and cardiac failure in patients with CLL.

- Risk of developing a second primary malignancy.

- Risk of hepatotoxicity, including hepatic failure and death; importance of advising patients to report signs and symptoms of hepatotoxicity to their clinician for evaluation.

- Risk of severe skin reactions; importance of advising patients to seek medical care for signs and symptoms of SJS, TEN, or DRESS. Lenalidomide therapy should be avoided in patients with a history of grade 4 rash associated with thalidomide. (See Cutaneous Reactions under Cautions.)

- Risk of tumor lysis syndrome. Importance of informing clinician if signs and symptoms of tumor lysis syndrome occur.

- Risk of tumor flare reaction. Importance of informing clinician of signs and symptoms of tumor flare reaction.

- Importance of informing patients with mantle cell lymphoma of the risk of early death.

- Risk of severe hypersensitivity reactions; importance of advising patients to seek medical care for signs and symptoms of hypersensitivity reactions.

- Importance of informing clinicians of existing or contemplated concomitant therapy, including prescription and OTC drugs and dietary or herbal supplements, as well as any concomitant illnesses.

- Importance of informing patients of other important precautionary information. (See Cautions.)

PREPARATIONS

Because lenalidomide is an analog of thalidomide (a known human teratogen that can cause severe, life-threatening birth defects if administered during pregnancy), distribution of lenalidomide is restricted. (See REMS under Dosage and Administration.)

Excipients in commercially available drug preparations may have clinically important effects in some individuals; consult specific product labeling for details.

Lenalidomide

Oral		
Capsules	2.5 mg	**Revlimid®**, Bristol Myers Squibb
	5 mg	**Revlimid®**, Bristol Myers Squibb
	10 mg	**Revlimid®**, Bristol Myers Squibb
	15 mg	**Revlimid®**, Bristol Myers Squibb
	20 mg	**Revlimid®**, Bristol Myers Squibb
	25 mg	**Revlimid®**, Bristol Myers Squibb

† Use is not currently included in the labeling approved by the US Food and Drug Administration.

Selected Revisions December 17, 2023, © Copyright, April 1, 2007, American Society of Health-System Pharmacists, Inc.

Lenvatinib Mesylate

10:00 • ANTINEOPLASTIC AGENTS

■ Lenvatinib, an inhibitor of multiple receptor tyrosine kinases, is an antineoplastic agent.

USES

● Differentiated Thyroid Cancer

Lenvatinib mesylate is used for the treatment of locally recurrent or metastatic, progressive, radioactive iodine (iodine-131)-refractory differentiated thyroid cancer (DTC) in adults. The drug has been designated an orphan drug by the FDA for the treatment of follicular, medullary, anaplastic, and metastatic or locally advanced papillary thyroid cancer. Currently available evidence indicates that lenvatinib therapy is associated with significantly prolonged progression-free survival and improved response rates compared with placebo in patients with locally recurrent or metastatic, radioactive iodine-refractory DTC.

Efficacy and safety of lenvatinib for the treatment of DTC are based principally on the results of a randomized, multicenter, double-blind, placebo-controlled, phase 3 study (SELECT) conducted in patients with locally recurrent or metastatic, radioactive iodine-refractory DTC and radiographic evidence of progressive disease within 12 months prior to randomization. Patients in the study were considered refractory to radioactive iodine if at least one of the following occurred: uptake of radioactive iodine did not occur in at least 1 measurable lesion on any iodine-131 scan, progression of at least 1 measurable lesion with iodine uptake within 12 months of radioactive iodine therapy, or cumulative iodine-131 activity exceeding 600 mCi with the last dose administered at least 6 months prior to study entry. In this study, 392 patients were randomized in a 2:1 ratio to receive either lenvatinib (24 mg) or placebo orally once daily in 28-day cycles until disease progression or intolerable toxicity occurred. The primary efficacy end point of this study was progression-free survival (as evaluated by a blinded independent review committee) according to Response Evaluation Criteria in Solid Tumors (RECIST); secondary endpoints included objective response rate and overall survival.

The median age of patients enrolled in the SELECT study was 63 years; 24% of the patients had received one prior therapy with a vascular endothelial growth factor (VEGF) or vascular endothelial growth factor receptor (VEGFR) inhibitor. Most patients (66%) had papillary thyroid cancer and 34% had follicular thyroid cancer; of the patients with follicular histology, 44 and 11% had Hürthle and clear cell subtypes, respectively. Most patients (67%) in the lenvatinib treatment arm did not demonstrate uptake of radioactive iodine on any scan and 59% of the patients in the lenvatinib treatment arm had progressed within 12 months of prior radioactive iodine therapy. The median cumulative radioactive iodine activity administered prior to study entry was 350 mCi.

The median progression-free survival was substantially longer in patients receiving lenvatinib (18.3 months) compared with those receiving placebo (3.6 months) in the SELECT study. Improved progression-free survival was observed in the lenvatinib-treated patients regardless of gender, age, ethnicity, previous therapy with a tyrosine kinase inhibitor, geographic region, histologic findings, and baseline thyrotropin concentrations. The objective response rate was 65% for patients receiving lenvatinib and 2% for those receiving placebo; partial response was achieved in 63% and complete response was achieved in 2% of the lenvatinib-treated patients. Median overall survival had not been reached at the time of the analysis. Upon radiographic confirmation of progression, 83% of patients previously randomized to receive placebo crossed over to receive open-label lenvatinib treatment; the median progression-free survival among evaluable patients entering the open-label phase was 10.1 months and the objective response rate was 52.3%.

● Renal Cell Carcinoma

Lenvatinib mesylate is used in combination with pembrolizumab for the treatment of previously untreated advanced renal cell carcinoma (RCC), or in combination with everolimus for the treatment of advanced RCC following therapy with an anti-angiogenic agent.

Clinical Experience

First-line Treatment of Advanced Renal Cell Carcinoma

Efficacy and safety of lenvatinib in combination with pembrolizumab for the first-line treatment of advanced RCC are based primarily on results from the multicenter, open-label, randomized, phase 3 CLEAR trial. Patients enrolled in the study were adults with treatment-naive advanced RCC with clear-cell histology and at least one measurable lesion. Patients were enrolled regardless of programmed-death ligand-1 (PD-L1) tumor expression; however, patients with active autoimmune disease or a medical condition that required immunosuppression were ineligible. In this study, 1069 patients were randomized in a 1:1:1 ratio (stratified by geographic region and prognostic risk group) to receive lenvatinib 20 mg orally once daily on days 1–21 and pembrolizumab 200 mg IV on day 1 of each 21-day cycle, lenvatinib 18 mg orally once daily in combination with everolimus 5 mg orally once daily of each 21-day cycle, or sunitinib 50 mg orally once daily for 4 consecutive weeks followed by a 2-week period without treatment. Treatment was continued until disease progression or unacceptable toxicity occurred; however, clinically stable patients with disease progression receiving lenvatinib in combination with pembrolizumab could continue treatment if they were considered to be deriving clinical benefit. The maximum duration of therapy for pembrolizumab was 24 months; however, lenvatinib therapy could continue beyond 24 months. The primary endpoint of the CLEAR trial was progression-free survival (as determined by an independent review committee); overall survival and objective response rate were key secondary endpoints. All of these endpoints were evaluated by an independent review committee.

The median age of patients enrolled in the study was 62 years; 75% were male, 74% were white, 21% were Asian, 1% were Black, 82% had a baseline Karnofsky performance status score of 90 to 100. Memorial Sloan Kettering Cancer Center (MSKCC) risk categories were favorable, intermediate, and poor risk in 27, 64, and 9% of patients, respectively. Common sites of metastases in patients were lung (68%), lymph node (45%), and bone (25%). At the protocol-specified interim analysis, median progression-free survival was substantially longer in patients receiving lenvatinib in combination with pembrolizumab (23.9 months) and those receiving lenvatinib in combination with everolimus (14.7 months) compared with those receiving sunitinib alone (9.2 months). Results of a subgroup analysis (based on age, sex, geographic region, MSKCC prognostic risk group, International Metastatic Renal Cell Carcinoma Database Consortium [IMDC] risk group, baseline Karnofsky performance status score, number of organs with metastases, and PD-L1 combined positive score) suggested that the effect of pembrolizumab on progression-free survival was evident across all subgroups. Median overall survival had not been reached at the time of interim analysis; however, the risk of death was decreased by 34% in patients receiving lenvatinib in combination with pembrolizumab compared with those receiving sunitinib. Overall survival was not substantially longer in patients receiving lenvatinib in combination with everolimus compared with those receiving sunitinib. Objective response rate was observed in 71, 53.5, or 36.1% of patients receiving lenvatinib in combination with pembrolizumab, lenvatinib in combination with everolimus, or sunitinib alone, respectively.

A final overall survival analysis was performed after approximately 304 deaths had been observed. The median follow-up at the time of final overall survival analysis was 49.8 months in the lenvatinib plus pembrolizumab group and 49.4 months in the sunitinib group. Median overall survival was 53.7 months in the lenvatinib plus pembrolizumab group and 54.3 months in the sunitinib group (hazard ratio 0.79).

Previously Treated Advanced Renal Cell Carcinoma

Efficacy and safety of lenvatinib in combination with everolimus for the treatment of adults with advanced RCC following one prior anti-angiogenic therapy are based primarily on results from a multicenter, open-label, randomized, phase 2 study (Study 205). Patients enrolled in the study had clear cell histology and radiographic evidence of progressive advanced or metastatic RCC within 9 months of discontinuing prior therapy. Patients also were enrolled if they had measurable disease and previous disease progression with anti-angiogenic therapy. In this study, 153 patients were randomized (stratified by hemoglobin level and corrected serum calcium concentration) to receive lenvatinib (18 mg orally once daily) in combination with everolimus (5 mg orally once daily), lenvatinib (24 mg orally once daily) alone, or everolimus (10 mg orally once daily) alone. Treatment cycles were repeated every 28 days and continued until disease progression or unacceptable toxicity occurred. The primary endpoint was investigator-assessed progression-free survival; overall survival and objective response rate were key secondary efficacy endpoints.

The median age of patients randomized to receive lenvatinib in combination with everolimus or everolimus alone was 60 years; 72% were male, 96% were white, and 95% had metastatic disease. All patients had a baseline Eastern Cooperative Oncology Group (ECOG) performance status of 0 (54%) or 1 (46%). MSKCC favorable, intermediate, and poor risk categories were observed in 24, 37, and 39%, respectively, of patients receiving lenvatinib in combination with everolimus, and 24, 38, and 38%, respectively, of patients receiving everolimus alone. Median progression-free survival was substantially improved in patients receiving the combination of lenvatinib and everolimus (14.6 months) compared with those receiving everolimus alone (5.5 months). At the time of analysis, median overall survival was 25.5 months in patients receiving lenvatinib in combination with everolimus and 15.4 months in those receiving everolimus alone (hazard ratio 0.64). An objective response was observed in 37% of patients receiving lenvatinib in combination with everolimus compared with 6% of those receiving everolimus monotherapy; complete response was achieved in one patient receiving lenvatinib in combination with everolimus and none of the patients receiving everolimus monotherapy.

Clinical Perspective

Prognosis is generally poor in patients with metastatic RCC, including those who have undergone complete tumor resection. First-line therapy with vascular endothelial growth factor receptor (VEGFR) inhibitors has been shown to provide benefits in patients with advanced RCC; however, relapsed or refractory RCC eventually develops in most patients. Combination regimens (e.g., immune checkpoint inhibitor in combination with a tyrosine kinase inhibitor) have become a standard for the treatment of advanced RCC.

The American Society of Clinical Oncology (ASCO) recommends that all patients with metastatic RCC who require systemic therapy in the first-line setting undergo risk stratification. Patients with intermediate- or poor-risk disease should be offered combination treatment with 2 immune checkpoint inhibitors (i.e., ipilimumab and nivolumab) or an immune checkpoint inhibitor in combination with a VEGFR tyrosine kinase inhibitor (e.g., pembrolizumab plus axitinib, nivolumab plus cabozantinib, avelumab plus axitinib, pembrolizumab plus lenvatinib). Treatment selection should be based on adverse events, comorbid conditions, provider experience, and treatment cost. Patients with favorable-risk disease who require systemic therapy may be offered an immune checkpoint inhibitor in combination with a VEGFR tyrosine kinase inhibitor.

● *Hepatocellular Carcinoma*

Lenvatinib mesylate is used for the first-line treatment of patients with unresectable hepatocellular carcinoma (HCC). The drug has been designated an orphan drug by the FDA for the treatment of this cancer.

Clinical Experience

Efficacy and safety of lenvatinib for the first-line treatment of unresectable HCC are principally based on results from a multicenter, open-label, randomized, non-inferiority, phase 3 study (REFLECT) in patients with previously untreated unresectable HCC who were ineligible for local liver-directed therapy and had at least one measurable target lesion according to modified RECIST for HCC. In this study, 954 patients were randomized in a 1:1 ratio (stratified by geographic region, presence of macroscopic portal vein invasion or extrahepatic spread, ECOG performance status, body weight) to receive lenvatinib (12 mg orally once daily in patients weighing 60 kg or more, or 8 mg orally once daily in those weighing less than 60 kg) or sorafenib (400 mg orally twice daily). Treatment cycles were repeated every 28 days until disease progression or unacceptable toxicity occurred. The primary endpoint was overall survival; secondary endpoints included progression-free survival, time to progression, and objective response rate.

The median age of patients enrolled in the study was 62 years; 84% of patients were male, 69% were Asian, 29% were white, and 63% had an ECOG performance status score of 0. The majority (62%) of patients had at least one site of documented distant metastatic disease; 52, 45, or 16% of patients had lung, lymph node, or bone metastases, respectively. Macroscopic portal vein invasion, extra-hepatic spread, or both were present in 70% of patients. HCC was categorized as Child-Pugh class A and Barcelona Clinic Liver Cancer (BCLC) stage C in 79% of patients and Child-Pugh class A and BCLC stage B in 21% of patients.

The majority (75%) of patients had radiographic evidence of cirrhosis at baseline. Chronic hepatitis B virus (HBV), chronic hepatitis C virus (HCV) infection, or alcohol consumption was the cause of HCC in 50, 23, or 6% of patients, respectively. At a median duration of 27 months, lenvatinib demonstrated non-inferiority to sorafenib for overall survival. Median overall survival was 13.6 or 12.3 months for lenvatinib-treated or sorafenib-treated patients, respectively. Median progression-free survival (7.3 versus 3.6 months) was prolonged in patients receiving lenvatinib compared with those receiving sorafenib. Objective response rate was 19 or 7% in patients receiving lenvatinib or sorafenib, respectively; complete response was achieved in 0.4 or 0.2% of patients receiving these respective treatments.

Clinical Perspective

For the treatment of early stage HCC, liver transplantation, surgical resection, and ablation offer a potential cure and high rates of complete response; however, survival is usually less than 6 months in patients with untreated advanced stage HCC.

The ASCO guideline on systemic therapy for advanced HCC states that lenvatinib, sorafenib, or durvalumab may be offered as first-line therapy for patients with advanced HCC, Child-Pugh class A, and an ECOG performance status of 0 or 1 if therapy with atezolizumab plus bevacizumab or durvalumab plus tremelimumab is contraindicated. ASCO also states that tyrosine kinase inhibitors (i.e., cabozantinib, lenvatinib, sorafenib) may be used as second-line therapy† following therapy with atezolizumab plus bevacizumab or durvalumab plus tremelimumab. The decision to pursue second-line therapy and choice of treatment should be based on patient and clinician preferences and other factors (i.e., comorbidities, liver function, performance status, potential for benefit and risk of harm).

Guideline recommendations from the American Gastroenterological Association (AGA) and the American Association for the Study of Liver Diseases (AASLD) are generally similar to the ASCO guidelines. The AGA guideline suggests either lenvatinib or sorafenib over no systemic therapy for first-line treatment of patients with HCC and preserved liver function who are not eligible for locoregional therapy or resection or who have metastatic disease and are not eligible for treatment with atezolizumab plus bevacizumab. The AASLD guideline recommends sorafenib or lenvatinib as first-line therapy for advanced HCC patients with Child-Pugh class A cirrhosis in whom atezolizumab plus bevacizumab and durvalumab plus tremelimumab are contraindicated.

● *Endometrial Carcinoma*

Lenvatinib mesylate is used in combination with pembrolizumab for the treatment of advanced endometrial carcinoma that is mismatch repair proficient (pMMR), as determined by an FDA-approved test, or *not* microsatellite instability-high (MSI-H), in patients who have disease progression following prior systemic therapy and who are not candidates for curative surgery or radiation.

Clinical Experience

Efficacy and safety of lenvatinib in combination with pembrolizumab for the treatment of advanced endometrial carcinoma are based on results from a multicenter, open-label, randomized, phase 3 trial (KEYNOTE-775; Study 309). Patients with endometrial sarcoma, including carcinosarcoma, and patients with a history of active autoimmune disease or a medical condition that requires immunosuppression were ineligible for the study. In this study, 697 patients with cancer that was pMMR or not MSI-H were randomized (stratified by ECOG performance status, geographic region, and history of pelvic radiation) to receive lenvatinib 20 mg orally once daily continuously in combination with pembrolizumab 200 mg IV every 3 weeks or an investigator's choice chemotherapy (doxorubicin hydrochloride 60 mg/m^2 IV every 3 weeks or paclitaxel 80 mg/m^2 IV on days 1, 8, and 15 of each 28-day cycle).

Among the cohort of patients with advanced endometrial carcinoma that was pMMR or not MSI-H, the median age of patients was 65 years; 62% were white, 22% were Asian, 3% were Black, and 60% had an ECOG performance status of 0. The histologic subtypes were endometrioid carcinoma (55%), serous (30%), clear-cell carcinoma (7%), mixed (4%), and other (3%). All patients received prior systemic therapy for endometrial carcinoma; 67, 30, or 3% of patients previously received 1, 2, or ≥3 systemic therapies, respectively. Approximately one-third (37%) of patients received prior neoadjuvant or adjuvant therapy. The primary endpoints were progression-free survival and overall survival; objective response rate was a key secondary efficacy endpoint. In the cohort of patients with advanced endometrial carcinoma that was pMMR or not MSI-H, median progression-free survival was 6.6 months in patients receiving lenvatinib in combination with pembrolizumab and 3.8 months in those receiving an investigator's choice chemotherapy. Median overall survival was prolonged (17.4 versus 12.0 months) and objective response rate was higher (30 versus 15%) in patients receiving lenvatinib in combination with pembrolizumab compared with those receiving an investigator's choice of chemotherapy. A final overall survival analysis and updated progression-free survival analysis was performed at a median follow-up of 14.7 months. Among patients with cancer that was pMMR, the median overall survival in this analysis was 18 months for the combination of lenvatinib and pembrolizumab and 12.2 months for chemotherapy. The median progression-free survival was 6.7 months for the combination of lenvatinib and pembrolizumab and 3.8 months for chemotherapy.

Clinical Perspective

Endometrial cancer is usually diagnosed at an early stage that can be treated with surgery alone. Options for advanced endometrial cancer may include surgery followed by chemotherapy or radiation therapy; chemotherapy and radiation therapy; hormone therapy; biological therapy; or immunotherapy (e.g., pembrolizumab plus lenvatinib). A panel of international experts recommends pembrolizumab plus lenvatinib for the second-line treatment of patients with pMMR or microsatellite stable advanced or recurrent endometrial cancer.

DOSAGE AND ADMINISTRATION

● General

Pretreatment Screening

- Obtain blood pressure; control blood pressure prior to initiating therapy.
- Evaluate proteinuria on urine dipstick.
- Assess thyroid and liver function.
- Assess serum electrolytes; correct electrolyte abnormalities prior to initiating therapy.
- Perform oral examination.
- Perform pregnancy test in females of reproductive potential.
- For advanced endometrial carcinoma, select patients for treatment based on mismatch repair (MMR) or microsatellite instability (MSI) status in tumor specimens. See information on FDA-approved tests for patient selection at https://www.fda.gov/companiondiagnostics. FDA-approved test for MSI-H not currently available.

Patient Monitoring

- Monitor blood pressure following 1 week of therapy, every 2 weeks for the first 2 months of therapy, and then at least monthly thereafter.
- Monitor liver function every 2 weeks for the first 2 months, and at least monthly thereafter during treatment.
- Monitor for proteinuria with dipstick urinalysis periodically during therapy.
- Monitor patients for clinical symptoms or signs of cardiac dysfunction.
- Monitor ECGs in patients with congenital long QT syndrome, congestive heart failure, bradyarrhythmias, or those taking drugs known to prolong the QT interval.
- Monitor serum calcium concentrations at least monthly during therapy.
- Monitor thyroid function at least monthly during therapy.
- Assess serum electrolytes periodically during therapy.
- Perform oral examination periodically during therapy.
- In patients with hepatocellular carcinoma (HCC), closely monitor for signs of hepatic failure, including hepatic encephalopathy.

Other General Considerations

- Clinicians should consult published protocols for information on the dosage, method of administration, and administration sequence of other antineoplastic agents used in combination regimens with lenvatinib.

- Withhold therapy for at least 1 week prior to elective surgery. Do not administer for ≥2 weeks following major surgery and until adequate wound healing has occurred.

● Administration

Administer lenvatinib mesylate orally without regard to meals at the same time each day. Swallow the capsules whole; do not crush or chew the capsules.

If lenvatinib capsules cannot be swallowed whole, an oral suspension may be prepared from the capsules using water or apple juice. If preparing a suspension for feeding tube administration, use water. To prepare a suspension from the capsules, place the required amount of unopened capsules (up to a maximum of 5), into a small container or oral syringe (approximately 20 mL capacity). For doses that require 6 capsules, prepare 3 capsules at a time according to instructions. Add 3 mL of liquid to the small container or oral syringe without breaking or crushing the capsules. Allow the capsules to remain in the liquid for at least 10 minutes to allow the capsule shell to disintegrate, and then stir or shake for at least 3 minutes. After the mixture has been consumed, add an additional 2 mL of liquid to the container or syringe, swirl and shake, then administer. Repeat this step at least once and until no residue is visible to ensure all of the dose is consumed. If the suspension cannot be used immediately, it may be stored under refrigeration (2–8°C) for 24 hours in a covered container. After 24 hours, discard any remaining suspension.

For feeding tube administration, lenvatinib suspension is compatible with polypropylene syringes, with polyvinyl chloride (PVC) and polyurethane feeding tubes of at least 5 French diameter, and with silicone feeding tubes of at least 6 French diameter.

If a dose of lenvatinib is missed and cannot be taken within 12 hours, skip the missed dose and take the next dose at the regularly scheduled time.

Store lenvatinib capsules at controlled room temperature (20–25°C). Excursions are permitted to 15–30°C.

● Dosage

Dosage of lenvatinib mesylate is expressed in terms of lenvatinib.

Differentiated Thyroid Cancer

The recommended adult dosage of lenvatinib for the treatment of locally recurrent or metastatic, progressive, radioactive iodine-refractory differentiated thyroid cancer (DTC) is 24 mg once daily. Therapy should be continued until disease progression or unacceptable toxicity occurs.

Renal Cell Carcinoma

First-line Treatment of Advanced Renal Cell Carcinoma

The recommended adult dosage of lenvatinib for the treatment of previously untreated advanced renal cell carcinoma (RCC) is 20 mg once daily in combination with pembrolizumab 200 mg by IV infusion over 30 minutes every 3 weeks. Lenvatinib in combination with pembrolizumab should be continued for up to 2 years or until disease progression or unacceptable toxicity occurs. Following completion of 2 years of combination therapy with pembrolizumab, lenvatinib monotherapy may be continued until disease progression or unacceptable toxicity occurs.

The prescribing information for pembrolizumab should be consulted for detailed information on dosage modifications for this drug. If adverse effects occur, modify the dosage of lenvatinib and/or pembrolizumab as appropriate.

Previously Treated Advanced Renal Cell Carcinoma

The recommended adult dosage of lenvatinib for the treatment of advanced RCC following therapy with an anti-angiogenic agent is 18 mg once daily in combination with everolimus 5 mg orally once daily. Therapy should be continued until disease progression or unacceptable toxicity occurs.

The prescribing information for everolimus should be consulted for detailed information on dosage modifications for this drug. If adverse effects associated with both lenvatinib and everolimus occur during combination therapy, withhold lenvatinib therapy or reduce the dosage of lenvatinib first, and then reduce the dosage of everolimus.

Hepatocellular Carcinoma

The recommended adult dosage of lenvatinib for the first-line treatment of unresectable hepatocellular carcinoma (HCC) is based on actual body weight. For patients weighing ≥60 kg, the recommended dosage is 12 mg once daily. For patients weighing <60 kg, the recommended dosage is 8 mg once daily. Therapy should be continued until disease progression or unacceptable toxicity occurs.

Endometrial Carcinoma

The recommended adult dosage of lenvatinib for the treatment of advanced endometrial carcinoma that is mismatch repair proficient (pMMR) or *not* microsatellite instability-high (MSI-H) is 20 mg once daily in combination with pembrolizumab 200 mg by IV infusion over 30 minutes every 3 weeks. Therapy should be continued until disease progression or unacceptable toxicity occurs.

Dosage Modification for Toxicity

If adverse effects occur during lenvatinib therapy, temporary interruption of therapy, dosage reduction, and/or permanent discontinuance of the drug may be necessary. If dosage modification is required, the dosage of lenvatinib should be reduced as described in Table 1 in patients with DTC, RCC, or endometrial carcinoma and in Table 2 in patients with HCC.

TABLE 1. Recommended Dosage Reduction for Lenvatinib Toxicity in Patients with DTC, RCC, or Endometrial Carcinoma.

Dosage Reduction Level	DTC (Starting Dosage = 24 mg daily)	RCC (Starting Dosage = 20 mg daily in combination with pembrolizumab or 18 mg in combination with everolimus)	Endometrial Carcinoma (Starting Dosage = 20 mg daily)
First	Restart at 20 mg once daily	Restart at 14 mg once daily	Restart at 14 mg once daily
Second	Restart at 14 mg once daily	Restart at 10 mg once daily	Restart at 10 mg once daily
Third	Restart at 10 mg once daily	Restart at 8 mg once daily	Restart at 8 mg once daily

TABLE 2. Recommended Dosage Reduction for Lenvatinib Toxicity in Patients with HCC.

Dosage Reduction Level	Patients Weighing ≥60 kg (Starting Dosage = 12 mg daily)	Patients Weighing <60 kg (Starting Dosage = 8 mg daily)
First	Restart at 8 mg once daily	Restart at 4 mg once daily
Second	Restart at 4 mg once daily	Restart at 4 mg every other day
Third	Restart at 4 mg every other day	Discontinue therapy

Temporary interruption of therapy, dosage reduction, and/or permanent discontinuance of lenvatinib may be necessary in patients experiencing certain adverse effects (see Table 3).

TABLE 3. Recommended Dosage Modification for Lenvatinib Toxicity.

Adverse Reaction and Severity	Modification
Hypertension	
Grade 3 (despite optimal antihypertensive therapy)	Withhold therapy; when toxicity improves to ≤ grade 2, resume at reduced dosage (see Table 1)
Grade 4	Permanently discontinue therapy

TABLE 3. Continued

Adverse Reaction and Severity	Modification
Cardiac Dysfunction	
Grade 3	Withhold therapy; when toxicity resolves or improves to grade 0 or 1, resume at reduced dosage (see Table 1) or discontinue therapy depending on severity and persistence of the toxicity
Grade 4	Permanently discontinue therapy
Arterial Thromboembolic Events	
Any grade	Permanently discontinue therapy
Hepatotoxicity	
Grade 3 or 4	Withhold therapy; when toxicity resolves or improves to grade 0 or 1, resume at reduced dosage (see Table 1) or discontinue therapy depending on severity and persistence of hepatotoxicity
Hepatic Failure	Permanently discontinue therapy
Nephrotoxicity	
Grade 3 or 4 (including renal failure)	Withhold therapy; when toxicity resolves or improves to grade 0 or 1, resume at reduced dosage (see Table 1) or discontinue therapy depending on severity and persistence of renal impairment
Proteinuria	
≥2 g proteinuria per 24 hours	Withhold therapy; when proteinuria improves to ≤2 g per 24 hours, resume at reduced dosage (see Table 1)
Nephrotic syndrome	Permanently discontinue therapy
GI Perforation	
Any grade	Permanently discontinue therapy
Fistula Formation	
Grade 3 or 4	Permanently discontinue therapy
QT Prolongation	
>500 msec or >60 msec increase from baseline	Withhold therapy; when toxicity resolves or improves to ≤480 msec, resume at a reduced dosage (see Table 1)
Reversible Posterior Leukoencephalopathy Syndrome (RPLS)	
Any grade	Withhold therapy; when RPLS fully resolves, resume at reduced dosage (see Table 1) or discontinue therapy depending on severity and persistence of neurologic symptoms
Other Adverse Effects	
Grade 2 or 3 (persistent or intolerable)	Withhold therapy; when toxicity resolves or improves to grade 0 or 1, resume at reduced dosage (see Table 1)
Grade 4 adverse effect	Permanently discontinue therapy
Grade 4 laboratory abnormality	Withhold therapy; when the laboratory abnormality resolves or improves to grade 0 or 1, resume at reduced dosage (see Table 1)

Special Populations

Hepatic Impairment

No dosage adjustment is recommended for patients with HCC and pre-existing mild hepatic impairment. The manufacturer makes no specific dosage recommendations for patients with HCC and pre-existing moderate or severe hepatic impairment.

No dosage adjustment is recommended for patients with DTC, RCC, or endometrial carcinoma and mild or moderate hepatic impairment; however, reduced dosages are recommended in such patients with severe hepatic impairment.

For patients with DTC, RCC, or endometrial carcinoma and pre-existing severe hepatic impairment (Child-Pugh class C), the manufacturer recommends reducing the lenvatinib dosage as described in Table 4.

TABLE 4. Recommended Dosage Modifications for Pre-existing Severe Hepatic Impairment in Patients with DTC, RCC, or Endometrial Carcinoma.

Indication	Reduced Initial Dosage
DTC	14 mg once daily
RCC	10 mg once daily
Endometrial carcinoma	10 mg once daily

Renal Impairment

Dosage adjustment is not necessary in patients with pre-existing mild (creatinine clearance of 60–89 mL/minute) or moderate (creatinine clearance of 30–59 mL/minute) renal impairment.

Use of lenvatinib in patients with end-stage renal disease has not been studied, and the manufacturer provides no specific dosage recommendations for such patients.

There is no recommended dosage of lenvatinib in patients with HCC and severe renal impairment.

For patients with RCC, DTC, or endometrial carcinoma and pre-existing severe renal impairment (creatinine clearance <30 mL/minute), the manufacturer recommends reducing the lenvatinib dosage as described in Table 5.

TABLE 5. Recommended Dosage Modifications for Pre-existing Severe Renal Impairment in Patients with DTC, RCC, and Endometrial Carcinoma.

Indication	Reduced Initial Dosage
DTC	14 mg once daily
RCC	10 mg once daily
Endometrial carcinoma	10 mg once daily

Geriatric Patients

The manufacturer makes no specific dosage recommendations for geriatric patients.

CAUTIONS

Contraindications
- None.

Warnings/Precautions

Hypertension

In the SELECT study evaluating lenvatinib in patients with differentiated thyroid cancer (DTC), hypertension occurred in 73% of patients receiving lenvatinib 24 mg once daily. Grade 3 hypertension was reported in 44% and grade 4 hypertension was reported in less than 1% of the lenvatinib-treated patients. In the REFLECT study evaluating lenvatinib in patients with hepatocellular carcinoma (HCC), hypertension occurred in 45% of patients receiving lenvatinib 8 or 12 mg once daily, with grade 3 and grade 4 hypertension reported in 24 and 0% of patients, respectively. In Study 205 evaluating lenvatinib in combination with everolimus in patients with renal cell carcinoma (RCC), hypertension occurred in 42% of patients receiving lenvatinib 18 mg once daily in combination with everolimus, with grade 3 hypertension reported in 13% of patients.

In the SELECT and REFLECT trials, the median time to onset of new or worsening hypertension was 16 or 26 days, respectively, after initiating the drug. Hypertension necessitated discontinuance of therapy in approximately 1% of lenvatinib-treated patients.

Blood pressure should be assessed and controlled, if necessary, prior to initiating lenvatinib therapy. Blood pressure should be monitored following 1 week of therapy, every 2 weeks for the first 2 months of therapy, and then at least monthly thereafter. If hypertension occurs, temporary interruption of lenvatinib therapy, dosage reduction, or discontinuance of therapy may be necessary.

Cardiac Dysfunction

Lenvatinib may cause serious and fatal cardiac dysfunction. In clinical trials evaluating lenvatinib in patients with DTC, RCC, or HCC, grade 3 or higher cardiac dysfunction (i.e., cardiomyopathy, left or right ventricular dysfunction, congestive heart failure, ventricular hypokinesia, decrease in left or right ventricular ejection fraction of >20% from baseline) occurred in 3% of lenvatinib-treated patients.

Patients receiving lenvatinib should be monitored for manifestations of cardiac dysfunction. If cardiac dysfunction occurs, temporary interruption of lenvatinib therapy, dosage reduction, or discontinuance of therapy may be necessary.

Arterial Thromboembolic Events

In the SELECT, REFLECT, and Study 205 trials, arterial thromboembolic events occurred in 5, 2, and 2% of patients, respectively. Across all trials, the occurrence of grade 3 to 5 thromboembolic events ranged from 2–3%. In the CLEAR trial evaluating lenvatinib in combination with pembrolizumab in patients with RCC, arterial thrombotic events of any severity occurred in 5% of patients. These events included myocardial infarction (3.4%) and cerebrovascular accident (2.3%).

Lenvatinib therapy should be permanently discontinued if an arterial thromboembolic event occurs. The safety of resuming lenvatinib therapy following such an event has not been established, and the drug has not been evaluated in patients who have had an arterial thromboembolic event within the previous 6 months.

Hepatotoxicity

In clinical studies evaluating lenvatinib in patients with malignancies other than HCC, serious hepatic adverse effects occurred in 1.4% of lenvatinib-treated patients and were fatal in 0.5% of patients. In the REFLECT trial, hepatic encephalopathy was reported in 8% of lenvatinib-treated patients versus 3% of sorafenib-treated patients. Among lenvatinib- and sorafenib-treated patients in the REFLECT trial, grade 3 to 5 hepatic encephalopathy occurred in 5% versus 2% of patients, respectively, and grade 3 to 5 hepatic failure occurred in 3% of patients in both treatment groups. Discontinuation of lenvatinib therapy due to hepatic encephalopathy occurred in 2% of lenvatinib-treated patients versus 0.2% of sorafenib-treated patients. Overall, 1% of patients in both treatment groups discontinued therapy due to hepatic failure.

Liver function tests should be evaluated prior to initiation of therapy and monitored every 2 weeks for the first 2 months of therapy and then at least monthly thereafter during therapy. Patients with HCC should be monitored closely for signs of hepatic failure. If hepatotoxicity occurs, temporary interruption of lenvatinib therapy, dosage reduction, or discontinuance of therapy may be necessary.

Proteinuria

In the SELECT and REFLECT trials, proteinuria occurred in 34 and 26% of lenvatinib-treated patients, respectively, with grade 3 proteinuria occurring in 11 and 6% of patients, respectively. In Study 205, 31% of patients administered lenvatinib in combination with everolimus experienced proteinuria compared to 14% of patients administered everolimus alone; grade 3 proteinuria occurred in 8% of patients receiving combination therapy compared with 2% of those receiving everolimus alone.

Patients should be monitored for proteinuria prior to initiation of lenvatinib and periodically during treatment with the drug. In patients with a 2+ or greater urine dipstick reading for proteinuria, a 24-hour urine protein measurement should be obtained. If proteinuria occurs, temporary interruption of lenvatinib therapy, dosage reduction, or discontinuance of therapy may be necessary.

Renal Failure or Impairment

In the SELECT and REFLECT trials, renal impairment occurred in 14 and 7% of lenvatinib-treated patients, respectively, with grade 3 to 5 renal failure or impairment occurring in 3 and 2% of patients, respectively. In Study 205, 18% of patients administered lenvatinib in combination with everolimus developed renal impairment or renal failure; grade 3 renal impairment was observed in 10% of patients.

In patients experiencing diarrhea or dehydration/hypovolemia, appropriate management should be promptly initiated. If nephrotoxicity occurs, temporary interruption of lenvatinib therapy, dosage reduction, or discontinuance of therapy may be necessary.

Diarrhea

In the SELECT and REFLECT trials, diarrhea occurred in 49% of lenvatinib-treated patients, with grade 3 diarrhea observed in 6% of patients. In Study 205, 81% of patients administered lenvatinib in combination with everolimus experienced diarrhea; grade 3 diarrhea was observed in 19% of patients. In this trial, diarrhea was the most frequent cause of dose interruption or reduction. Diarrhea recurred despite dosage reduction.

Prompt management of diarrhea should be initiated if necessary. If diarrhea occurs, temporary interruption of lenvatinib therapy, dosage reduction, or discontinuance of therapy may be necessary.

Fistula Formation and GI Perforation

GI perforation and fistula formation have been reported in patients receiving lenvatinib or other tyrosine kinase inhibitors. In most cases, GI perforation and fistula occurred in patients with risk factors (e.g., prior surgery, recent sigmoidoscopy or colonoscopy, radiotherapy, underlying tumor, diverticulitis, bowel obstruction). In the SELECT, REFLECT, and Study 205 trials, GI perforation or fistula formation was reported in 2% of lenvatinib-treated patients.

Lenvatinib should be permanently discontinued in patients who develop GI perforation of any severity or grade 3 or 4 fistula.

QT Interval Prolongation

Prolongation of the QT interval has been reported in patients receiving lenvatinib. In the SELECT study, prolongation of the QT interval or the corrected QT (QT_c) interval was reported in 9% of lenvatinib-treated patients and QT interval prolongation (>500 msec) occurred in 2% of patients. In the REFLECT and Study 205 trials, QT_c interval increases of >60 msec occurred in 11 and 8% of lenvatinib-treated patients, respectively; QT_c interval >500 msec occurred in 6 and 2% of lenvatinib-treated patients, respectively.

Monitor serum electrolyte concentrations (e.g., potassium, magnesium, calcium) at baseline and periodically during lenvatinib therapy, and correct any abnormalities. ECGs should be monitored during lenvatinib therapy in patients with congenital long QT syndrome, congestive heart failure, bradyarrhythmias, and/or in those concurrently receiving other drugs known to prolong the QT interval. If QT interval prolongation occurs, temporary interruption of lenvatinib therapy, dosage reduction, or discontinuance of therapy may be necessary.

Hypocalcemia

In the SELECT and Study 205 trials, grade 3 to 4 hypocalcemia occurred in 9 and 6% of lenvatinib-treated patients, respectively. In the REFLECT trial, grade 3 hypocalcemia occurred in 0.8% of lenvatinib-treated patients. Among patients with grade 3 to 4 hypocalcemia in the SELECT trial, hypocalcemia improved or resolved in 65% of patients following calcium replacement therapy, with or without lenvatinib dose interruption or reduction.

Blood calcium concentrations should be monitored at least monthly during lenvatinib therapy. If hypocalcemia occurs, calcium replacement therapy should be administered as necessary; temporary interruption of lenvatinib therapy, dosage reduction, or discontinuance of therapy may be necessary.

Reversible Posterior Leukoencephalopathy Syndrome

Reversible posterior leukoencephalopathy syndrome (RPLS) occurred rarely (0.3%) in patients treated with lenvatinib as a single agent in clinical studies. Magnetic resonance imaging (MRI) is necessary to confirm the diagnosis of RPLS.

If RPLS occurs, temporary interruption of lenvatinib therapy, dosage reduction, or discontinuance of therapy may be necessary.

Hemorrhagic Events

In the SELECT, REFLECT, and Study 205 trials, hemorrhagic events of any grade occurred in 29% of patients receiving lenvatinib. The incidence of grade 3–5 hemorrhage (including fatal hemorrhagic events) occurred in 2, 5, and 8% of lenvatinib-treated patients in the SELECT, REFLECT, and Study 205 trials, respectively. The most common hemorrhagic event in these studies occurring in ≥5% of patients were epistaxis and hematuria. In lenvatinib-treated patients in clinical trials and in postmarketing surveillance, serious tumor related bleeds, including fatal hemorrhagic events, have been reported. In postmarketing surveillance, serious and fatal carotid artery hemorrhagic events occurred more frequently in patients with anaplastic thyroid carcinoma than in other tumor types. The safety and efficacy of lenvatinib in patients with anaplastic thyroid carcinoma have not been demonstrated in clinical trials.

The risk of severe or fatal hemorrhagic events associated with tumor invasion or infiltration of major blood vessels (e.g., carotid artery) should be considered during lenvatinib therapy. If hemorrhagic events occur, temporary interruption of lenvatinib therapy, dosage reduction, or discontinuance of therapy may be necessary.

Impairment of Thyroid-stimulating Hormone Suppression/Thyroid Dysfunction

Lenvatinib impairs exogenous thyroid suppression. Among patients with a normal thyroid-stimulating hormone (TSH) concentration at baseline in the SELECT study, elevated TSH concentrations (exceeding 5 microunits/L) were observed in 57% of patients treated with lenvatinib. In the REFLECT and Study 205 trials, grade 1 or 2 hypothyroidism occurred in 21 and 24% of lenvatinib-treated patients, respectively. An increase in TSH levels from normal or low at baseline was observed in 70 and 60% of lenvatinib-treated patients in REFLECT and Study 205 trials, respectively.

Thyroid function should be monitored prior to initiation and at least monthly during lenvatinib therapy. Hypothyroidism should be treated according to standard medical practice.

Impaired Wound Healing

Lenvatinib may impair wound healing and this adverse effect has been reported among patients treated with the drug.

Lenvatinib should be withheld for at least 1 week prior to an elective surgery and should not be administered for at least 2 weeks following major surgery and until adequate wound healing has occurred. The safety of resuming lenvatinib therapy after resolution of wound healing complications has not been established.

Osteonecrosis of the Jaw

Lenvatinib therapy is associated with the occurrence of osteonecrosis of the jaw. The risk of osteonecrosis of the jaw may be increased by concomitant exposure to other risk factors (e.g., bisphosphonate or denosumab therapy, dental disease, or invasive dental procedures).

An oral examination should be performed prior to, and periodically during, lenvatinib therapy. Patients should be advised to regularly practice good oral hygiene practices.

Invasive dental procedures should be avoided, particularly in patients at higher risk for osteonecrosis of the jaw, during lenvatinib therapy, if possible. Lenvatinib therapy should be withheld for at least 1 week before a scheduled dental surgery or invasive dental procedure, if possible. In patients receiving concomitant bisphosphonate therapy, discontinuance of bisphosphonate therapy may reduce the risk of osteonecrosis of the jaw in patients requiring invasive dental procedures. If osteonecrosis of the jaw occurs, withhold lenvatinib therapy and resume based on clinical judgment of adequate resolution.

Fetal/Neonatal Morbidity and Mortality

Lenvatinib may cause fetal harm in humans based on its mechanism of action and animal findings; the drug has been shown to be teratogenic, embryotoxic, and fetotoxic in animals. There are no available data regarding the risk of lenvatinib use in pregnant women to date. In animal reproduction studies, dose-related decreases in mean fetal body weight; delayed fetal ossifications; and dose-related increases in fetal external, visceral, and skeletal anomalies were observed in rats at daily lenvatinib doses ≥0.3 mg/kg (approximately 0.14 times the recommended clinical dose of 24 mg based on body surface area). Postimplantation loss was observed in more than 80% of pregnant rats at a lenvatinib dosage of 1 mg/kg per day (approximately 0.5 times the recommended human dosage based on body surface area). Fetal external, visceral, and skeletal anomalies and postimplantation loss (including one fetal death) also were observed in rabbits receiving dosages below the recommended human dosage; the drug also was abortifacient.

Pregnancy should be avoided during lenvatinib therapy. Verify the pregnancy status of females of reproductive potential before initiating lenvatinib. Females of reproductive potential should be advised to use an effective method of contraception while receiving lenvatinib and for 30 days after discontinuance of therapy. If lenvatinib is used during pregnancy or if the patient becomes pregnant while receiving the drug, the patient should be apprised of the potential fetal hazard.

Specific Populations

Pregnancy

Lenvatinib may cause fetal harm if administered to pregnant women based on its mechanism of action and animal findings. In animal reproduction studies, oral lenvatinib administered during organogenesis at doses below the recommended human doses resulted in embryotoxicity, fetotoxicity, and teratogenicity in rats and rabbits.

Verify the pregnancy status of females of reproductive potential before initiating lenvatinib. If lenvatinib is used during pregnancy or if the patient becomes pregnant while receiving the drug, the patient should be apprised of the potential fetal hazard.

Lactation

Lenvatinib and its metabolites are distributed into milk in rats at concentrations higher than maternal plasma; it is not known whether the drug is distributed into milk in humans. Because of the potential for serious adverse reactions to lenvatinib in breast-fed infants, women should be advised to discontinue nursing during lenvatinib therapy and for at least 1 week after the last dose.

Females and Males of Reproductive Potential

Prior to initiation of lenvatinib therapy, verify pregnancy status of females of reproductive potential and such females should be advised to use effective contraceptive methods during lenvatinib therapy and for 30 days after the last dose.

Lenvatinib may impair fertility in males and females of reproductive potential.

Pediatric Use

Safety and efficacy of lenvatinib have not been established in pediatric patients.

Growth retardation (decreased weight gain, food consumption, and femur and tibia width and/or length), secondary delays in physical development, and reproductive organ immaturity have been observed in juvenile rats receiving daily oral administration of lenvatinib for 8 weeks.

Safety and efficacy of lenvatinib were investigated but not established in pediatric patients 2 to <17 years of age with relapsed or refractory solid tumors, including osteosarcoma, Ewing sarcoma, rhabdomyosarcoma, and high-grade glioma. Hypothyroidism and pneumothorax were observed at a higher rate in pediatric patients compared to adult patients.

Geriatric Use

In the SELECT, REFLECT, CLEAR, Study 205, and Study 309 trials, 45, 44, 45, 36, and 50% of lenvatinib-treated patients, respectively, were 65 years of age or older. The percentages of patients receiving lenvatinib who were 75 years of age or older in the SELECT, REFLECT, and CLEAR trials, were 11, 12, and 13%, respectively. No overall differences in safety and efficacy were observed between these geriatric patients and younger adults.

In a pharmacokinetic population analysis, age did not have a substantial effect on the clearance of lenvatinib.

Hepatic Impairment

Following administration of a single 10-mg dose of lenvatinib, dose-adjusted total exposure to the drug in individuals with pre-existing mild or moderate hepatic impairment (Child-Pugh class A or B) was 119 or 107% higher, respectively, compared with individuals with normal hepatic function; no dosage adjustment is required in patients with DTC, RCC, or endometrial carcinoma and pre-existing mild or moderate hepatic impairment. In patients with HCC and pre-existing mild hepatic impairment, no dosage adjustment is necessary; however, the manufacturer makes no specific recommendations for patients with HCC and pre-existing moderate hepatic impairment.

Following administration of a single 5-mg dose of lenvatinib, dose-adjusted total exposure to the drug was 180% in individuals with pre-existing severe hepatic impairment (Child-Pugh class C) compared with that in individuals with normal hepatic function; therefore, dosage adjustment is necessary in patients with DTC, RCC, or endometrial carcinoma and pre-existing severe hepatic impairment. The manufacturer makes no specific dosage recommendations for patients with HCC and pre-existing severe hepatic impairment.

Renal Impairment

Pre-existing renal impairment (creatinine clearance 15–89 mL/minute) does not significantly impact oral clearance of lenvatinib. No dosage adjustment is recommended in patients with mild (creatinine clearance 60–89 mL/minute) or moderate (creatinine clearance 30–59 mL/minute) renal impairment.

The manufacturer recommends dosage adjustment in patients with DTC, RCC, and endometrial carcinoma and severe renal impairment (creatinine clearance 15–29 mL/minute). The manufacturer makes no specific dosage recommendations for patients with HCC and severe renal impairment.

Lenvatinib has not been studied in patients with end-stage renal disease.

● Common Adverse Effects

Adverse effects reported in ≥30% of patients receiving lenvatinib for the treatment of DTC include hypertension, fatigue, diarrhea, arthralgia/myalgia, decreased appetite and weight, nausea, stomatitis, headache, vomiting, proteinuria, palmar-plantar erythrodysesthesia syndrome, abdominal pain, and dysphonia.

Adverse effects reported in ≥20% of patients receiving lenvatinib in combination with pembrolizumab for the treatment of RCC include fatigue, diarrhea, musculoskeletal pain, hypothyroidism, hypertension, stomatitis, decreased appetite, rash, nausea, decreased weight, dysphonia, proteinuria, palmar-plantar erythrodysesthesia syndrome, abdominal pain, hemorrhagic events, vomiting, constipation, hepatotoxicity, headache, and acute kidney injury.

Adverse effects reported in ≥30% of patients receiving lenvatinib in combination with everolimus for the treatment of RCC include diarrhea, fatigue, stomatitis/oral inflammation, hypertension, peripheral edema, cough, abdominal pain, dyspnea, decreased weight, hemorrhagic events, and proteinuria.

Adverse effects reported in ≥20% of patients receiving lenvatinib for the treatment of HCC include hypertension, fatigue, diarrhea, arthralgia/myalgia, decreased appetite and weight, abdominal pain, palmar-plantar erythrodysesthesia syndrome, proteinuria, dysphonia, hemorrhagic events, hypothyroidism, and nausea.

Adverse effects reported in ≥20% of patients receiving lenvatinib for the treatment of endometrial carcinoma include hypothyroidism, hypertension, fatigue, diarrhea, musculoskeletal disorders, nausea, decreased appetite and weight, vomiting, stomatitis, abdominal pain, urinary tract infection, proteinuria, constipation, headache, hemorrhagic events, palmar-plantar erythrodysesthesia syndrome, dysphonia, and rash.

DRUG INTERACTIONS

Lenvatinib is metabolized principally by cytochrome P-450 (CYP) isoenzyme 3A4. In vitro studies indicate that lenvatinib inhibits CYP isoenzymes 2C8, 1A2, 2B6, 2C9, 2C19, 2D6, and 3A, and also uridine diphosphate-glucuronosyl transferases (UGT) 1A1, 1A4, and 1A9, but does not inhibit CYP isoenzymes 2A6 or 2E1. The drug also does not inhibit UGT 1A6 or 2B7 or aldehyde oxidase. Lenvatinib induces CYP3A, but does not induce CYP isoenzymes 1A1, 1A2, 2B6, or 2C9, and UGT 1A1, 1A4, 1A6, 1A9, or 2B7.

In vitro, the drug is a substrate for P-glycoprotein (P-gp) and breast cancer resistance protein (BCRP), but is not a substrate for organic anion transporter (OAT)1, OAT3, organic cation transporter (OCT)1, OCT2, organic anion transport protein (OATP)1B1, OATP1B3, multidrug and toxin extrusion (MATE) 1, MATE2-K, or the bile salt export pump (BSEP). Lenvatinib does not have the potential to inhibit MATE1, MATE2-K, OCT1, OCT2, OAT1, OAT3, BSEP, OATP1B1, or OATP1B3 in vivo.

● Drugs Affecting Hepatic Microsomal Enzymes and/or Efflux Transport Systems

Inhibitors of CYP3A and Efflux Transport Systems

When ketoconazole (a CYP3A4, P-gp, and BCRP inhibitor) 400 mg was administered once daily for 18 days with a single 5-mg dose of lenvatinib on day 5, peak plasma concentrations and systemic exposure of lenvatinib were increased by 19 and 15%, respectively.

When the P-gp inhibitor, rifampin (single 600-mg dose), was administered concomitantly with lenvatinib (single 24-mg dose), peak plasma concentrations and systemic exposure of lenvatinib were increased by 33 and 31%, respectively.

Inducers of CYP3A and Efflux Transport Systems

When rifampin (a CYP3A and P-gp inducer) 600 mg was administered once daily for 21 days with a single 24-mg dose of lenvatinib on day 15, systemic exposure of lenvatinib was decreased by 18% and peak plasma concentrations were unchanged.

● Drugs Metabolized by Hepatic Microsomal Enzymes

Substrates of CYP3A4

Clinically important pharmacokinetic interactions between drugs that are substrates of CYP3A4 (e.g., midazolam) and lenvatinib are not expected during concurrent use.

Substrates of CYP2C8

Clinically important pharmacokinetic interactions between drugs that are substrates of CYP2C8 (e.g., repaglinide) and lenvatinib are not expected during concurrent use.

● Drugs that Prolong the QT Interval

Avoid concurrent administration of lenvatinib with drugs that are known to prolong the QT/QT$_c$ interval. Because lenvatinib has been associated with QT-interval prolongation, the manufacturer recommends ECG monitoring in lenvatinib-treated patients concurrently receiving other drugs known to prolong the QT interval, including class IA antiarrhythmics (e.g., quinidine, procainamide) and class III antiarrhythmics (e.g., amiodarone, sotalol). In addition, electrolyte monitoring and correction of any electrolyte abnormalities are recommended in all patients receiving lenvatinib at baseline and periodically during treatment.

DESCRIPTION

Lenvatinib, an inhibitor of multiple receptor tyrosine kinases, is an antineoplastic agent. Receptor tyrosine kinases (RTKs) are involved in the initiation of various cascades of intracellular signaling events that lead to cell proliferation and/or influence processes critical to cell survival and tumor progression (e.g., angiogenesis, metastasis, inhibition of apoptosis), based on the respective kinase. Lenvatinib inhibits the kinase activities of vascular endothelial growth factor (VEGF) receptors VEGFR-1, VEGFR-2, and VEGFR-3. The drug also inhibits other RTKs involved in pathogenic angiogenesis, tumor growth, and cancer progression, including fibroblast growth factor (FGF) receptors (FGFR1, FGFR2, FGFR3, and FGFR4), the platelet-derived growth factor receptor (PDGFR), stem cell factor receptor (c-Kit), and ret proto-oncogene (RET). Lenvatinib also demonstrates

antiproliferative activity in hepatocellular carcinoma (HCC) cell lines dependent on FGFR signaling with concurrent inhibition of FGF-receptor substrate 2 α(FRS2α) phosphorylation.

In syngeneic mouse tumor models, the combination of lenvatinib and an anti-PD-1 monoclonal antibody demonstrated greater antitumor activity compared to either agent alone. The combination of lenvatinib and an anti-PD-1 monoclonal antibody also decreased tumor-associated macrophages and increased activated cytotoxic T cells. The combination of lenvatinib and everolimus demonstrated greater antiangiogenic and antitumor activity in mouse xenograft models of human renal cell cancer compared to either agent alone.

In a randomized study of patients with radioactive iodine-refractory differentiated thyroid cancer (DTC), a dose-response relationship for overall response rate (ORR) was observed over the oral dose range of 18 mg (less than the recommended dose) to 24 mg (recommended dose), with a higher ORR reported in patients receiving the recommended dose of 24 mg once daily. No dose-response relationship was observed over the oral dose range of 18—24 mg for adverse reactions (including serious adverse reactions), or adverse reactions leading to discontinuation or treatment interruption.

Following oral administration, lenvatinib is rapidly absorbed with peak plasma concentrations usually occurring within 1–4 hours. Peak plasma concentrations and systemic exposure to lenvatinib are proportional to dose following single or repeated administration of the drug over the dosage range of 3.2–32 mg once daily. Administration of lenvatinib with food delayed the rate of absorption (time to reach peak concentrations delayed by 2 hours), but did not affect the extent of absorption. Lenvatinib is metabolized in the liver principally by cytochrome P-450 (CYP) 3A4, aldehyde oxidase, and nonenzymatic processes. Lenvatinib is highly bound (97–99%) to plasma proteins. The elimination half-life of the drug is approximately 28 hours. Following oral administration of a single radiolabeled dose of lenvatinib, approximately 64% of the dose is recovered in the feces and approximately 25% of the dose is recovered in urine within 10 days.

ADVICE TO PATIENTS

- Advise patients to read the manufacturer's patient information before starting lenvatinib therapy and each time their prescription is refilled.

- If a dose is missed by more than 12 hours, advise patients to skip that dose and take the next dose at the regularly scheduled time.

- Risk of hypertension developing or worsening during therapy. Stress importance of regular monitoring of blood pressure during treatment and informing clinician if hypertension occurs.

- Risk of cardiac dysfunction. Stress importance of immediately informing clinician if symptoms of cardiac dysfunction (e.g., shortness of breath, peripheral edema) occur.

- Risk of arterial thromboembolic events. Advise patients to seek immediate medical attention for new onset chest pain or acute neurologic symptoms consistent with myocardial infarction or stroke (e.g., severe chest pain or pressure, shortness of breath, unilateral numbness or weakness, difficulty talking, severe headache, vision changes, arm, back, neck, or jaw pain).

- Risk of hepatotoxicity. Stress importance of liver function test monitoring before and during lenvatinib therapy and immediately reporting any possible manifestations of hepatotoxicity (e.g., jaundice, dark or "tea-colored" urine, light-colored stools).

- Risk of proteinuria and renal impairment or failure. Advise patients that they will be monitored regularly for renal function and proteinuria during lenvatinib therapy.

- Inform patients when to initiate anti-diarrheal medication and to maintain adequate hydration. Instruct patients to contact a clinician if they cannot maintain adequate hydration.

- Increased risk of GI perforation or fistula formation. Stress importance of seeking immediate medical attention if severe abdominal pain occurs.

- Increased risk of hemorrhagic events. Advise patients to contact their clinician if bleeding or symptoms of severe bleeding occur.

- Risk of QT-interval prolongation. Inform patients that ECGs and/or serum electrolytes may be monitored during lenvatinib therapy.

- Risk of hypocalcemia. Stress importance of monitoring calcium concentrations during therapy.

- Risk of reversible posterior leukoencephalopathy syndrome (RPLS). Stress importance of contacting clinician promptly if severe headache, seizures, weakness, confusion, or visual disturbances occur during therapy.

- Advise patients that lenvatinib therapy may cause hypothyroidism and regular monitoring of thyroid function during therapy may occur.

- Instruct patients that lenvatinib therapy may impair wound healing and to inform a clinician of any planned surgical procedure.

- Advise patients to employ good oral hygiene practices and attend regular dental checkups before and throughout treatment with lenvatinib. Instruct patients, particularly those at high risk for osteonecrosis of the jaw, to avoid invasive dental procedures, if possible. Advise patients to inform a clinician of any planned dental procedures and immediately contact a clinician if they have signs or symptoms of osteonecrosis of the jaw (e.g., pain or swelling in the mouth, loosening of teeth, poor healing or infection of the gums, or an area of exposed bone in the mouth).

- Risk of impairment of exogenous thyroid suppression. Stress importance of monitoring thyroid-stimulating hormone (TSH) during therapy.

- Risk of fetal harm. Advise women of childbearing potential to avoid pregnancy and to use an effective method of contraception during therapy and for 30 days after the last dose. Advise women to inform their clinicians if they are or plan to become pregnant. If pregnancy occurs, advise pregnant women of potential risk to the fetus.

- Advise women to avoid breast-feeding during lenvatinib therapy and for at least 1 week after the last dose. Advise women to inform their clinicians if they are or plan to breast-feed.

- Advise patients to inform their clinicians of existing or contemplated concomitant therapy, including prescription and OTC drugs, as well as any concomitant illnesses (e.g., cardiovascular disease [including congenital long QT syndrome]).

- Inform patients of other important precautionary information.

For further information on the handling of antineoplastic agents, see the ASHP Guidelines on Handling Hazardous Drugs at https://www.ahfsdrug information.com.

PREPARATIONS

Lenvatinib is obtained through designated specialty pharmacies. Contact the manufacturer or consult the Lenvima® website for specific availability information.

Excipients in commercially available drug preparations may have clinically important effects in some individuals; consult specific product labeling for details.

Lenvatinib Mesylate

Oral

Capsules	4 mg (of lenvatinib)	Lenvima®, Eisai
	10 mg (of lenvatinib)	Lenvima®, Eisai

† Use is not currently included in the labeling approved by the US Food and Drug Administration.

Selected Revisions July 10, 2024, © Copyright, October 30, 2015, American Society of Health-System Pharmacists, Inc.

Lorlatinib

10:00 • ANTINEOPLASTIC AGENTS

■ Lorlatinib, an inhibitor of multiple receptor tyrosine kinases including anaplastic lymphoma kinase (ALK) and c-ros oncogene-1 (ROS-1), is an antineoplastic agent.

USES

● Non-small Cell Lung Cancer

Lorlatinib is used for the treatment of anaplastic lymphoma kinase (*ALK*)-positive metastatic non-small cell lung cancer (NSCLC). The drug has been designated an orphan drug by the FDA for the treatment of *ALK*-positive or c-ros oncogene-1 (*ROS-1*)-positive NSCLC.

Efficacy and safety of lorlatinib in the treatment of *ALK*-positive NSCLC is supported by several randomized controlled trials. Lorlatinib has demonstrated substantial overall and intracranial activity in treatment-naive and previously treated patients with *ALK*-positive NSCLC. Guidelines generally support the use of lorlatinib in the second- or third-line setting in patients with NSCLC previously treated with an ALK inhibitor in the first-line setting.

The efficacy of lorlatinib in treatment-naive patients with NSCLC harboring an *ALK* rearrangement was evaluated in an open-label, randomized, active-controlled trial (CROWN study). The primary end point was progression-free survival. In this study, 296 patients were randomized to receive lorlatinib 100 mg orally once daily or crizotinib 250 mg orally twice daily. The median age of patients enrolled in the study was 59 years; 35% of patients were 65 years or older, 59% were female, 49% were white, 44% were Asian, and 0.3% were Black. The Eastern Cooperative Oncology Group (ECOG) performance status at baseline was 0 or 1 in 96% of patients. The majority of patients had adenocarcinoma (95%) and had never smoked (59%). CNS metastases were present in 26% of patients: 30 of these patients had measurable CNS lesions. The median duration of follow-up was 18.3 and 14.8 months in patients receiving lorlatinib and crizotinib, respectively. At the time of data analysis, median progression-free survival had not been reached in patients receiving lorlatinib; however, the risk of disease progression or death was reduced by 72% in patients receiving lorlatinib compared with those receiving crizotinib (hazard ratio: 0.28; 95% confidence interval 0.19–0.41). Objective response and intracranial response rate also was substantially improved in patients who received lorlatinib compared with those who received crizotinib. The overall response rate was 76% in patients who received lorlatinib and 58% in those who received crizotinib. The median duration of response had not been reached in patients receiving lorlatinib and was 11 months in patients receiving crizotinib; response duration of ≥6, ≥12, and ≥18 months was 89, 70, and 30% in patients receiving lorlatinib, respectively, and 62, 27, and 11% in patients receiving crizotinib, respectively. Among patients with measurable CNS metastases at baseline, complete intracranial response was observed in 71 and 8% of patients who received lorlatinib and crizotinib, respectively.

The efficacy of lorlatinib in patients previously treated with an ALK inhibitor is based on the results of a subgroup of 215 patients enrolled in a multicenter, nonrandomized, open-label, dose-ranging, phase 2 study (Study B7461001). Prior therapy included crizotinib or 1–3 non-crizotinib ALK inhibitors, all with or without chemotherapy. Patients received lorlatinib 100 mg orally once daily until disease progression, unacceptable toxicity, death, or study withdrawal occurred. The primary efficacy end points were overall response rate and intracranial overall response rate according to the Response Evaluation Criteria in Solid Tumors (RECIST 1.1) as evaluated by a central independent review committee (IRC); additional outcome measures included duration of response and intracranial duration of response. The median age of patients included in the study analysis was 53 years (range: 29–85 years), 51% of patients were white and 34% were Asian, and 59% were female. All patients had metastatic disease and 95% had adenocarcinoma histology. Approximately 30% of patients evaluated had disease progression during crizotinib therapy, and 13, 35, or 22% had disease progression during prior therapy with 1 (non-crizotinib), 2, or 3 ALK inhibitors, respectively. CNS metastases were present in 69% of patients and 60% of such patients had previously received radiation to the brain. The IRC-assessed overall response rate

with lorlatinib was 48%; partial responses were achieved in 44% of patients and 4% had a complete response. The median duration of response was 12.5 months. In the subgroup of 89 patients with measurable brain metastases at baseline, the IRC-assessed intracranial overall response rate was 60% (38% partial responses and 21% complete responses) and the median duration of intracranial response was 19.5 months.

Clinical Perspective

A relatively small subset of patients with NSCLC (approximately 3–7%) have *ALK*-positive disease, which indicates potential responsiveness to ALK inhibitor therapy (e.g., alectinib, brigatinib, ceritinib, crizotinib). Patients with this form of lung cancer typically are nonsmokers or have a history of light smoking, and are younger in age and often have adenocarcinoma histology. Although crizotinib is highly active in patients with *ALK*-positive NSCLC, most patients treated with the drug eventually experience disease progression, limiting the drug's long-term therapeutic potential. Disease progression in patients receiving ALK inhibitors (e.g., alectinib, ceritinib, crizotinib) can result from acquired resistance mutations in *ALK*, amplification of gene expression, activation of alternate signaling pathways, and/or progression of brain metastases (e.g., because of poor distribution of crizotinib into the CSF).

The American Society of Clinical Oncology (ASCO) and Ontario Health (OH; formerly known as Cancer Care Ontario) 2021 joint guideline specifically addresses treatment of stage IV NSCLC harboring driver alterations such as *ALK* mutations. ASCO/OH state that alectinib or brigatinib should be offered in the first-line setting in patients with stage IV NSCLC and driver alterations in *ALK*; however, if alectinib or brigatinib are not available, ceritinib or crizotinib should be offered in the first-line setting. In patients with a performance status of 0–2 who received prior therapy with alectinib or brigatinib in the first-line setting, lorlatinib may be offered in the second-line setting. In patients with a performance status of 0–2 who received prior therapy with crizotinib in the first-line setting, and alectinib, brigatinib, or ceritinib in the second line-setting, lorlatinib may be offered in the third-line setting.

ASCO/OH state that in patients with previously untreated NSCLC harboring driver alterations in *ROS-1* who have a performance status of 0–2, ceritinib or lorlatinib may be offered.

DOSAGE AND ADMINISTRATION

● General

Pretreatment Screening

- Confirm presence of *ALK*-positivity in tumor specimens in patients with metastatic NSCLC.
- Verify pregnancy status in females of reproductive potential prior to initiating therapy.
- Assess serum cholesterol and triglyceride concentrations prior to initiating therapy; initiate or optimize antilipemic therapy as clinically indicated.
- Perform ECG prior to initiating therapy.
- Assess blood pressure prior to initiating therapy; blood pressure must be controlled prior to initiation of the drug.
- Assess fasting serum glucose concentrations prior to initiation of the drug.
- Assess concomitant therapy, including prescription drug, OTC drugs, and dietary or herbal supplements. Concomitant use of lorlatinib with *potent inducers* of CYP3A is contraindicated

Patient Monitoring

- Monitor blood pressure after 2 weeks of therapy and then at least monthly during therapy.
- Monitor serum cholesterol and triglyceride concentrations 1 and 2 months after initiating therapy, and then periodically thereafter. Initiate or optimize antilipemic therapy as clinically indicated.
- Monitor ECG periodically during therapy.
- Monitor fasting serum glucose concentration periodically during therapy.

● Administration

Lorlatinib is administered orally once daily at the same time each day without regard to food. The tablets should be swallowed whole and should *not* be crushed, chewed, or split. The manufacturer states that lorlatinib tablets should not be taken if they are broken, cracked, or otherwise not intact.

If a dose of lorlatinib is missed, the dose should be taken as soon as it is remembered unless the next dose is due within 4 hours. Two doses should not be taken at the same time to make up for a missed dose. If vomiting occurs after taking a dose, the next dose should be taken at the regularly scheduled time; an additional dose should not be taken.

● Dosage

Non-small Cell Lung Cancer

For the treatment of anaplastic lymphoma kinase (*ALK*)-positive metastatic non-small cell lung cancer (NSCLC), the recommended adult dosage of lorlatinib is 100 mg once daily. Therapy with the drug should be continued until disease progression or unacceptable toxicity occurs.

Dosage Modification for Toxicity

Dosing interruption and/or dosage reduction of lorlatinib may be necessary based on individual safety and tolerability.

In the CROWN study, dosage reduction because of adverse reactions was necessary in approximately 21% of patients treated with lorlatinib (most commonly for edema, hypertriglyceridemia, and peripheral neuropathy). Among previously-treated patients with *ALK*-positive NSCLC, approximately 48% required dosage interruption and 24% of patients required at least one dosage reduction, most commonly for edema, peripheral neuropathy, cognitive effects, and mood effects. Treatment interruption due to adverse effects was required in 49% of patients, most commonly for hypertriglyceridemia, edema, pneumonia, cognitive effects, mood effects, or hypercholesterolemia.

If dosage reduction is necessary, an initial dosage reduction to 75 mg once daily is recommended. If further dosage reduction is necessary, the dosage should be reduced to 50 mg once daily. If a dosage of 50 mg once daily is not tolerated, lorlatinib should be permanently discontinued.

CNS Effects

If grade 1 adverse CNS effects occur, lorlatinib therapy may be continued at the same dosage or therapy may be interrupted until recovery to baseline. Therapy may then be resumed at the same dosage or at the next lower dosage.

If grade 2 or 3 adverse CNS effects occur, lorlatinib therapy should be interrupted until recovery to grade 0 or 1. Therapy may then be resumed at the next lower dosage.

If grade 4 adverse CNS effects occur, lorlatinib therapy should be permanently discontinued.

Hyperlipidemia

If grade 4 hypercholesterolemia (serum cholesterol concentration exceeding 500 mg/dL) and/or grade 4 hypertriglyceridemia (serum triglyceride concentration exceeding 1000 mg/dL) occurs, lorlatinib therapy should be interrupted and appropriate antilipemic therapy should be initiated, the dosage of existing antilipemic therapy should be increased, or the existing antilipemic regimen should be changed to a new lipid-lowering therapy. Lorlatinib therapy may be resumed at the same dosage upon recovery of hypercholesterolemia and/or hypertriglyceridemia to grade 2 or less.

If severe hypercholesterolemia and/or hypertriglyceridemia *recurs* despite optimal antilipemic therapy, therapy should then be resumed at the next lower dosage of lorlatinib.

Atrioventricular Block

If second-degree atrioventricular (AV) block occurs, lorlatinib therapy should be interrupted until the PR interval is less than 200 msec. Lorlatinib should then be resumed at the next lower dosage.

If complete AV block occurs, lorlatinib therapy should be interrupted until a pacemaker is placed *or* the PR interval is less than 200 msec. If a pacemaker is placed, lorlatinib therapy may be resumed at the same dosage. If a pacemaker is *not* placed, lorlatinib therapy should be resumed at the next lower dosage.

If complete AV block *recurs*, a pacemaker should be placed or lorlatinib therapy should be permanently discontinued.

Interstitial Lung Disease/Pneumonitis

If treatment-related interstitial lung disease/pneumonitis of any grade occurs, lorlatinib therapy should be permanently discontinued.

Hypertension

If grade 3 hypertension (defined as systolic blood pressure [SBP] ≥160 mm Hg, diastolic blood pressure [DBP] ≥100 mm Hg, or elevation requiring medical intervention, more than one antihypertensive drug, or more intensive therapy than previously indicated) occurs, withhold lorlatinib therapy; when hypertension improves to grade 1 or less (SBP <140 mm Hg and DBP <90 mm Hg), may then resume lorlatinib at the same dosage. If grade 3 hypertension recurs, withhold lorlatinib therapy until hypertension improves to grade 1 or less, and then resume lorlatinib at a reduced dosage. If adequate control of hypertension cannot be achieved with optimal medical management, lorlatinib should be permanently discontinued.

If grade 4 (life-threatening or requires urgent intervention) hypertension occurs, withhold lorlatinib; when hypertension improves to grade 1 or less, may then resume lorlatinib at a reduced dosage or permanently discontinue drug. If grade 4 hypertension recurs, permanently discontinue lorlatinib.

Hyperglycemia

If grade 3 hyperglycemia (serum glucose concentration >250 mg/dL) occurs despite optimal antihyperglycemic therapy or if grade 4 hyperglycemia occurs, withhold lorlatinib until adequate glycemic control is achieved; may then resume lorlatinib at the next lower dosage. Lorlatinib should be permanently discontinued if glycemic control cannot be achieved.

Other Toxicity

If any other grade 1 or 2 adverse reaction occurs, lorlatinib therapy may be continued at the same dosage or reduced to the next lower dosage.

If any other grade 3 or 4 adverse reaction occurs, lorlatinib therapy should be interrupted until recovery to grade 2 or less, or to baseline. Lorlatinib therapy may then be resumed at the next lower dosage.

Concomitant Use of Drugs Affecting Hepatic Microsomal Enzymes

Concomitant use of lorlatinib with *potent inducers* of cytochrome P-450 (CYP) isoenzyme 3A is contraindicated. Potent CYP3A inducers should be discontinued for 3 plasma half-lives of the potent CYP3A inducer prior to initiating lorlatinib therapy.

Concomitant use of lorlatinib with *moderate inducers* of CYP3A should be avoided. If concomitant use of a moderate CYP3A inducer cannot be avoided, increase lorlatinib dosage to 125 mg once daily.

Concomitant use of lorlatinib with *potent inhibitors* of CYP3A should be avoided. If concomitant use of a potent CYP3A inhibitor cannot be avoided, the initial dosage of lorlatinib should be reduced from 100 mg once daily to 75 mg once daily. In patients who have had a dosage reduction to 75 mg once daily because of adverse reactions, the dosage of lorlatinib should be reduced to 50 mg once daily during concomitant use of a potent CYP3A inhibitor. If concomitant use of the potent CYP3A inhibitor is discontinued, the lorlatinib dosage should be increased (after 3 plasma half-lives of the CYP3A inhibitor) back to the dosage that was used prior to initiation of the potent CYP3A inhibitor.

Concomitant use of lorlatinib with *fluconazole* should be avoided. If concomitant use with fluconazole cannot be avoided, the initial dosage of lorlatinib should be reduced from 100 mg once daily to 75 mg once daily.

● Special Populations

Hepatic Impairment

No dosage adjustment is necessary in patients with mild hepatic impairment (total bilirubin concentrations not exceeding the upper limit of normal [ULN] with AST concentrations exceeding the ULN, or total bilirubin concentrations exceeding 1 but not exceeding 1.5 times the ULN with any AST concentration).

The recommended dosage of lorlatinib has not been established in patients with moderate or severe hepatic impairment.

Renal Impairment

In patients with severe renal impairment (creatinine clearance 15 to <30 mL/minute), the dosage of lorlatinib should be reduced from 100 mg to 75 mg once daily.

No dosage adjustment is necessary in patients with mild or moderate renal impairment (creatinine clearance of 30–89 mL/minute).

Geriatric Patients

The manufacturer makes no specific dosage recommendations for geriatric patients.

CAUTIONS

● Contraindications

Lorlatinib is contraindicated in patients receiving potent cytochrome P-450 (CYP) isoenzyme 3A inducers because of the potential for serious hepatotoxicity.

● Warnings/Precautions

Serious Hepatotoxicity with Concurrent Use of Potent CYP3A Inducers

Severe hepatotoxicity occurred in 10 of 12 healthy individuals receiving a single dose of lorlatinib with multiple daily doses of rifampin (a potent CYP3A inducer) during a drug interaction study. Grade 3 or 4 elevations in ALT or AST concentrations occurred in 83% and grade 2 elevations occurred in 8% of individuals who received the drugs concomitantly during the study. ALT or AST elevations occurred within 3 days of concomitant administration and returned to within normal limits after a median of 15 days (range: 7–34 days). The median time to recovery was 18 days following grade 3 or 4 elevations in ALT or AST concentrations and 7 days following grade 2 elevations. Concomitant use of lorlatinib with drugs that are *potent* CYP3A inducers is contraindicated. Potent CYP3A inducers should be discontinued for 3 plasma half-lives of the potent CYP3A inducer prior to initiating lorlatinib therapy.

Concomitant use of lorlatinib with drugs that are *moderate* CYP3A inducers should be avoided.

CNS Effects

Lorlatinib can cause a wide variety of adverse CNS effects, including seizures, psychotic effects, and changes in cognitive function (including memory impairment, cognitive disorder, and amnesia), mood (including suicidal ideation/suicidality, irritability, anxiety, depression, and labile affect), speech, mental status, and sleep. Although adverse CNS effects associated with lorlatinib therapy generally are mild in severity and intermittent and improve or resolve upon dosage modification, treatment interruption, dosage reduction, or drug discontinuance may be required depending on their severity.

In clinical trials, CNS effects occurred in 52% of 476 patients who received lorlatinib 100 mg once daily. Cognitive, mood, speech, sleep, and psychotic effects were observed in 28, 21, 11, 12, and 7% of patients, respectively. Grade 3 or 4 cognitive, mood, speech, and psychotic effects were reported in 2.9, 1.7, 0.6, and 0.6% of patients, respectively. Mental status changes occurred in 1.3% of patients; 1.1% of these events were grade 3 or 4 in severity. Seizures occurred in 1.9% of patients, sometimes in conjunction with other neurologic findings. The median time to onset of any CNS effect was 1.4 months (range 1 day to 3.4 years).

Hyperlipidemia

Increases in serum cholesterol and triglyceride concentrations may occur in patients receiving lorlatinib. Hypercholesterolemia or hypertriglyceridemia occurred in 90% or more of patients receiving the recommended dosage of lorlatinib in Study B7461001 and the CROWN study; 83% of patients receiving lorlatinib required initiation of antilipemic therapy. Grade 3 or 4 elevations in serum total cholesterol or triglyceride concentrations occurred in 18 or 19% of patients treated with lorlatinib, respectively. Treatment interruption or dosage reduction of lorlatinib was required in approximately 7 or 3% of patients, respectively, due to hypercholesterolemia or hypertriglyceridemia. The median time to onset of hypercholesterolemia or hypertriglyceridemia was 15 days; the median time to initiation of antilipemic therapy was 17 days.

Serum cholesterol and triglycerides should be assessed prior to initiating lorlatinib therapy, 1 and 2 months after initiating therapy, and periodically thereafter. Antilipemic therapy should be initiated or the dosage of existing antilipemic therapy should be increased in patients with hyperlipidemia. Temporary interruption followed by resumption of lorlatinib therapy at the same dosage or at a reduced dosage may be necessary, depending on the severity of the hyperlipidemia.

Atrioventricular Block

PR-interval prolongation and atrioventricular (AV) block may occur in patients receiving lorlatinib. AV block has been reported in 1.9% of 476 patients who received lorlatinib at the recommended dosage who had a baseline ECG; 0.2% of these patients experienced grade 3 AV block and underwent pacemaker placement. ECG monitoring is recommended prior to initiating lorlatinib and periodically during therapy. If AV block occurs, lorlatinib therapy should be interrupted; dosage reduction may be necessary unless a pacemaker is placed. If complete AV block recurs in patients without a pacemaker, lorlatinib should be permanently discontinued.

Interstitial Lung Disease/Pneumonitis

Severe or life-threatening adverse pulmonary reactions consistent with interstitial lung disease (ILD)/pneumonitis may occur in patients receiving lorlatinib. ILD or pneumonitis has been reported in 1.9% of patients receiving lorlatinib 100 mg once daily, including grade 3 or 4 ILD or pneumonitis in 0.6% of patients. One patient (0.3%) discontinued the drug because of ILD/pneumonitis.

Patients receiving lorlatinib who present with worsening of respiratory symptoms indicative of ILD or pneumonitis (e.g., dyspnea, cough, fever) should be promptly evaluated. Lorlatinib therapy should be immediately interrupted in patients with suspected ILD/pneumonitis. The drug should be permanently discontinued in patients with treatment-related ILD or pneumonitis of any severity.

Hypertension

Hypertension has occurred in 13% of patients who received lorlatinib. Grade 3 or 4 hypertension has been reported in 6% of patients. The median time to onset of hypertension was 6.4 months. Temporary interruption of lorlatinib therapy was necessary in 2.3% of patients experiencing hypertension.

Blood pressure should be monitored after 2 weeks of treatment and at least monthly thereafter. Blood pressure must be controlled prior to initiation of lorlatinib therapy.

Hyperglycemia

Hyperglycemia has occurred in 9% of patients who received lorlatinib. Grade 3 or 4 hyperglycemia has been reported in 3.2% of patients. The median time to onset of hyperglycemia was 4.8 months. Temporary interruption of lorlatinib therapy was necessary in 0.8% of patients experiencing hyperglycemia.

Fasting serum glucose should be assessed prior to initiation of lorlatinib and periodically thereafter. If hyperglycemia occurs, temporary interruption of therapy, dosage reduction, or permanent discontinuance of therapy may be necessary based on severity of hyperglycemia.

Fetal/Neonatal Morbidity and Mortality

Lorlatinib may cause fetal harm if administered to pregnant women based on its mechanism of action and animal findings. There are no clinical data on the use of lorlatinib in pregnant women. Malformations, increased post-implantation loss, and abortion were observed when the drug was administered to pregnant animals during the period of organogenesis at maternal exposures that were equal to or less than human exposure at the recommended dosage of 100 mg once daily based on area under the concentration-time curve (AUC).

Pregnancy should be avoided during lorlatinib therapy. The manufacturer recommends confirmation of pregnancy status prior to initiation of lorlatinib in females of reproductive potential; such females should use effective nonhormonal contraception during lorlatinib therapy and for at least 6 months after the drug is discontinued. In addition, males with female partners of reproductive potential should use effective methods of contraception while receiving lorlatinib and for at least 3 months after the drug is discontinued. Pregnant females and females of reproductive potential should be apprised of the potential fetal hazard.

Specific Populations

Pregnancy

Although there are no clinical data in pregnant females to date, animal studies and its mechanism of action suggest that lorlatinib may cause fetal harm.

Lactation

It is not known whether lorlatinib or its metabolites are distributed into either human or animal milk or if the drug has any effect on milk production or the nursing infant. Because of the potential for adverse reactions to lorlatinib in breast-fed infants, females should be advised not to breast-feed while receiving the drug and for 7 days after the drug is discontinued.

Females and Males of Reproductive Potential

Based on findings in male reproductive organs in animal studies, lorlatinib may transiently impair male fertility.

Verify pregnancy status prior to initiation of lorlatinib in females of reproductive potential; such females should use effective nonhormonal contraception during lorlatinib therapy and for at least 6 months after the drug is discontinued.

Males with female partners of reproductive potential should use effective methods of contraception while receiving lorlatinib and for at least 3 months after the drug is discontinued. Pregnant females and females of reproductive potential should be apprised of the potential fetal hazard.

Pediatric Use

Safety and efficacy of lorlatinib have not been established in pediatric patients.

Geriatric Use

In Study B7461001 and the CROWN study evaluating lorlatinib in patients with NSCLC, approximately 18 and 40%, respectively, of patients receiving lorlatinib at the recommended dosage were 65 years of age or older. Although data are limited, no clinically important differences in safety or efficacy were observed between geriatric patients and younger adults in this study.

Age (19–85 years) does not appear to have clinically important effects on the pharmacokinetics of lorlatinib.

Hepatic Impairment

Mild hepatic impairment (total bilirubin concentrations not exceeding the upper limit of normal [ULN] with AST concentrations exceeding the ULN, or total bilirubin concentrations exceeding 1 but not exceeding 1.5 times the ULN with any AST concentration) did not have clinically important effects on the pharmacokinetics of lorlatinib; dosage adjustment in patients with mild hepatic impairment is therefore not necessary.

Pharmacokinetics of lorlatinib have not been studied to date in patients with moderate or severe hepatic impairment.

Renal Impairment

Mild to moderate renal impairment (creatinine clearance of 30–89 mL/minute) did not have clinically important effects on the pharmacokinetics of lorlatinib; dosage adjustment in patients with mild or moderate renal impairment is therefore not necessary.

Dosage reduction is recommended in patients with creatinine clearance 15 to <30 mL/minute. In patients with creatinine clearance 15 to <30 mL/minute, systemic exposure of lorlatinib was increased by 42% compared with patients with normal renal function. Effects of end-stage renal disease or dialysis on the pharmacokinetics of lorlatinib are not known.

● Common Adverse Effects

Adverse effects reported in ≥20% of patients who received lorlatinib 100 mg once daily for the treatment non-small cell lung cancer (NSCLC) included edema, peripheral neuropathy, weight gain, cognitive effects, fatigue, dyspnea, arthralgia, diarrhea, mood effects, and cough. The most commonly reported grade 3 or 4 laboratory abnormalities (occurring in ≥20% of patients) included hypercholesterolemia and hypertriglyceridemia.

DRUG INTERACTIONS

Lorlatinib is metabolized principally by cytochrome P-450 (CYP) isoenzyme 3A4 and uridine diphosphate-glucuronosyltransferase (UGT) 1A4, with minor contributions by CYP isoenzymes 2C8, 2C19, and 3A5 and UGT1A3. In vitro studies indicate that lorlatinib inhibits P-glycoprotein (P-gp), organic cation transporter (OCT) 1, organic anion transporter (OAT) 3, multidrug and toxin extrusion (MATE) 1, and intestinal breast cancer resistance protein (BCRP).

In vitro studies indicate that lorlatinib is a time-dependent inhibitor as well as an inducer of CYP3A and that it activates the pregnane X receptor (PXR); the net effect in vivo is induction. Lorlatinib induces CYP2B6 and activates the human constitutive androstane receptor (CAR). Lorlatinib and its major metabolite M8 do not inhibit CYP isoenzymes 1A2, 2B6, 2C8, 2C9, 2C19, or 2D6 nor UGT isoenzymes 1A1, 1A4, 1A6, 1A9, 2B7, or 2B15. M8 does not inhibit CYP3A nor induce CYP isoenzymes 1A2, 2B6, and CYP3A.

Lorlatinib does not inhibit organic anion transporting polypeptide (OATP) 1B1, OATP1B3, OAT1, OCT2, MATE2K, and systemic BCRP. M8 does not inhibit P-gp, BCRP, OATP1B1, OATP1B3, OAT1, OAT3, OCT1, OCT2, MATE1, and MATE2K.

● Drugs Affecting Hepatic Microsomal Enzymes

Inducers of CYP3A

Concomitant use of lorlatinib with *potent* CYP3A inducers may result in severe hepatotoxicity. Grade 3 or 4 elevations in serum ALT or AST concentrations occurred in 83% and grade 2 elevations occurred in 8% of healthy individuals who received the potent CYP3A inducer rifampin (600 mg daily on days 1–8) and lorlatinib (single 100-mg dose on day 8) in a drug interaction study. Grade 2–4 elevations in hepatic enzymes (ALT or AST) occurred within 3 days of concomitant administration. In addition, peak plasma concentrations and area under the concentration-time curve (AUC) of lorlatinib were decreased by 76 and 85%, respectively. The mechanism of hepatotoxicity is thought to be through activation of the PXR by lorlatinib and rifampin, which are both PXR agonists.

Concomitant use of lorlatinib with *potent* CYP3A inducers is contraindicated. Potent CYP3A inducers must be discontinued and 3 plasma half-lives of the potent CYP3A inducer must elapse prior to initiation of lorlatinib therapy.

Concomitant use of lorlatinib with *moderate* CYP3A inducers may decrease serum concentrations of lorlatinib and reduced efficacy of the drug. Concomitant use of lorlatinib with drugs that are *moderate* CYP3A inducers should be avoided. If concomitant use of *moderate* CYP3A inducers cannot be avoided, the dosage of lorlatinib should be increased to 125 mg once daily.

Inhibitors of CYP3A

Concomitant use of lorlatinib with potent inhibitors of CYP3A may increase plasma concentrations of lorlatinib, which may increase the incidence and severity of adverse effects. Concurrent administration of itraconazole (200 mg daily) and lorlatinib (single 100-mg dose) in healthy individuals increased peak plasma concentrations and AUC of lorlatinib by 24 and 42%, respectively.

Concomitant use of lorlatinib with potent CYP3A inhibitors should be avoided. If concomitant use cannot be avoided, the initial lorlatinib dosage should be reduced from 100 mg daily to 75 mg daily. In patients who have had a dosage reduction to 75 mg daily, the dosage of lorlatinib should be reduced to 50 mg daily during concomitant use with a potent CYP3A inhibitor. If concomitant use of the potent CYP3A inhibitor is discontinued, the lorlatinib dosage should be increased back to the dosage that was tolerated prior to initiation of the potent CYP3A inhibitor after 3 plasma half-lives of the potent CYP3A inhibitor have elapsed.

Concomitant use of lorlatinib with fluconazole may also increase plasma concentrations of lorlatinib, which may increase the incidence and severity of adverse effects. Concomitant use of lorlatinib with fluconazole should be avoided. If concomitant use cannot be avoided, the initial lorlatinib dosage should be reduced from 100 mg daily to 75 mg daily.

● Drugs Metabolized by Hepatic Microsomal Enzymes

Lorlatinib is a moderate inducer of CYP3A. Concomitant use of lorlatinib and drugs metabolized by CYP3A may result in decreased concentrations and reduced efficacy of the CYP3A substrate. When lorlatinib (150 mg daily for 15 days) was administered concurrently with midazolam (single 2-mg oral dose), peak plasma concentrations and AUC of midazolam decreased by 50 and 64%, respectively. When lorlatinib (100 mg once daily) was administered concomitantly with bupropion (CYP2B6 substrate) and tolbutamide (CYP2C9 substrate), peak plasma concentration and AUC of the substrate drugs were decreased.

Concomitant use of lorlatinib and CYP3A substrates where minimal concentration changes may result in serious therapeutic failure should be avoided. If concomitant use cannot be avoided, dosage adjustment of the CYP3A substrate may be required; specific product labeling for the CYP3A substrate should be consulted.

● **Drugs Affected by Transport Systems**

Concomitant use of lorlatinib and P-gp or UGT1A substrates may result in decreased concentrations and reduced efficacy of the P-gp or UGT1A substrate. When lorlatinib (100 mg once daily) was administered concomitantly with fexofenadine (P-gp substrate) and acetaminophen (UGT1A substrate), peak plasma concentration and AUC of the substrate drugs were decreased.

Avoid concomitant use of lorlatinib and P-gp substrates with a narrow therapeutic index. If concomitant use cannot be avoided, consult the manufacturer's labeling of the P-gp substrate for dosage recommendations.

● **Drugs Affecting Gastric pH**

Concomitant administration of lorlatinib and the proton-pump inhibitor rabeprazole did not have a clinically important effect on the pharmacokinetics of lorlatinib.

● **Hormonal Contraceptives**

Concomitant use of lorlatinib and hormonal contraceptives may result in reduced efficacy of the hormonal contraceptive. Women of childbearing potential should therefore use effective nonhormonal contraception during lorlatinib therapy and for at least 6 months after the drug is discontinued.

● **Fluconazole**

Concomitant use of lorlatinib with fluconazole may increase plasma concentrations of lorlatinib, which may increase the incidence and severity of adverse effects.

Concomitant use of lorlatinib with fluconazole should be avoided. If concomitant use with fluconazole cannot be avoided, the initial dosage of lorlatinib should be reduced from 100 mg once daily to 75 mg once daily.

DESCRIPTION

Lorlatinib, an inhibitor of multiple tyrosine kinases, including anaplastic lymphoma kinase (ALK) and c-ros oncogene-1 (ROS1) as well as TYK1, FER, FPS, TRKA, TRKB, TRKC, FAK, FAK2, and ACK, is an antineoplastic agent. The drug inhibits phosphorylation of ALK and ALK-mediated signal transduction, specifically STAT3, AKT, ERK, and S6.

Activating mutations or translocations of the ALK gene have been identified in several malignancies and can result in the expression of oncogenic fusion proteins (e.g., echinoderm microtubule-associated protein-like 4 [EML4]-ALK). Such ALK gene rearrangements have been identified in approximately 3–7% of patients with non-small cell lung cancer (NSCLC). Formation of ALK fusion proteins such as EML4-ALK results in activation and dysregulation of the gene's expression and signaling, which can contribute to increased cell proliferation and survival in tumors expressing these proteins.

Although the ALK inhibitor crizotinib has demonstrated improved outcomes in patients with NSCLC harboring ALK mutations, secondary resistance to crizotinib eventually develops, generally within the first 1–2 years of treatment. Clinical resistance to crizotinib has been attributed to several possible mechanisms, including acquired resistance mutations of ALK, amplification of gene expression, and activation of alternate signaling pathways. More potent ALK inhibitors (e.g., alectinib, ceritinib) were developed to overcome resistance to crizotinib; however, resistance to these drugs also develops over time. Secondary mutations of ALK are responsible for about 30% of cases of acquired crizotinib resistance while about 50% of cases of acquired resistance to other ALK inhibitors are attributed to ALK

mutations, with G1202R predominating. The CNS is a common site of disease progression in crizotinib-treated patients because of poor distribution of the drug into CSF; development and/or progression of brain metastases occurs in approximately one-third to one-half of patients during crizotinib treatment.

In vitro, lorlatinib demonstrates greater potency than alectinib, ceritinib, and crizotinib in its activity against wild-type ALK and is active against cell lines expressing ALK mutations that confer resistance to crizotinib, including G1202R (which also confers resistance to alectinib and ceritinib), G1269A, and L1196M. Lorlatinib also demonstrated dose-dependent antitumor activity in mice bearing NSCLC tumor xenografts that expressed EML4-ALK fusions with either ALK variant 1 or ALK mutations, including G1202R and I1171T mutations that were detected in tumors of patients at the time of disease progression in patients receiving therapy with other ALK inhibitors. Lorlatinib also demonstrated antitumor activity and prolonged survival in mice bearing intracranial EML4-ALK-positive tumor xenografts and antitumor activity in patients with CNS metastases who had received prior treatment with other ALK inhibitors (e.g., alectinib, ceritinib, crizotinib).

Peak plasma concentration of lorlatinib is dose proportional and systemic exposure to lorlatinib is slightly less than dose proportional at steady state over the oral dosage range of 10–200 mg once daily. Following oral administration, peak plasma concentrations of lorlatinib are achieved at a median of 1.2 hours. The mean absolute bioavailability of lorlatinib is 81%. Administration of lorlatinib with a high-fat, high-calorie meal has no clinically important effect on the pharmacokinetics of lorlatinib. Lorlatinib is 66% bound to plasma proteins in vitro and is distributed into CSF at a CSF-to-plasma ratio of 0.75. Lorlatinib is metabolized principally by cytochrome P-450 (CYP) isoenzyme 3A4 and uridine diphosphate-glucuronosyltransferase (UGT) 1A4, with minor contributions by CYP isoenzymes 2C8, 2C19, and 3A5, and UGT1A3. The major metabolite, M8, is pharmacologically inactive. Following oral administration of a single dose of radiolabeled lorlatinib, 48% of the dose is eliminated in urine (less than 1% as unchanged drug) and 41% of the dose is eliminated in feces (about 9% as unchanged drug). Oral clearance of lorlatinib is higher at steady state than following a single dose, suggesting that autoinduction occurs. The mean plasma half-life of lorlatinib is 24 hours. Age (19–85 years), sex, race/ethnicity, body weight, and CYP3A5 or CYP2C19 metabolizer phenotypes do not have clinically important effects on the pharmacokinetics of lorlatinib.

ADVICE TO PATIENTS

- Importance of reading the manufacturer's patient information.
- Importance of advising patients to take lorlatinib exactly as prescribed and of not altering the dosage or discontinuing therapy unless advised to do so by their clinician. Importance of advising patients to swallow lorlatinib tablets whole without regard to food and not to crush, chew, or split the tablets. If a dose is missed, the missed dose should be taken as soon as possible unless it is within 4 hours of the next dose, in which case the missed dose should not be taken. Inform patients to not take 2 doses at the same time to make up for a missed dose. If vomiting occurs after taking a dose, the next dose should be taken at the regularly scheduled time; an additional dose should not be taken.
- Risk of severe hepatotoxicity when used concomitantly with potent CYP3A inducers.
- Importance of informing clinicians of existing or contemplated concomitant therapy, including prescription drugs (e.g., antilipemic agents, rifampin, oral contraceptives), OTC drugs, and dietary or herbal supplements (e.g., St. John's wort), as well as any concomitant illnesses (e.g., history of depression or other mood disorders, hyperlipidemia, cardiac arrhythmias, pulmonary disease).
- Risk of adverse CNS effects. Patients should notify their clinician if they experience new or worsening CNS symptoms such as changes in cognitive function or mood, suicidal ideation, hallucinations, or seizures.
- Risk of hyperlipidemia. Importance of informing patients about the need for monitoring serum cholesterol and triglyceride concentrations during therapy. Advise patients that initiation of antilipemic therapy or an increase in the dosage of existing antilipemic agents may be required.
- Risk of AV block. Importance of patients immediately contacting their clinician if they experience new or worsening cardiac symptoms such as dizziness, faintness, or arrhythmia during therapy.

- Risk of severe or life-threatening ILD/pneumonitis. Importance of advising patients that symptoms may be similar to those of lung cancer and to contact their clinician immediately if they experience any new or worsening respiratory symptoms (e.g., dyspnea or shortness of breath, cough, fever).
- Risk of hypertension. Importance of advising patients to monitor blood pressure regularly. Advise patients that initiation or optimization of blood pressure medications may be necessary during lorlatinib therapy. Importance of immediately informing clinician if signs or symptoms of hypertension, including headaches, dizziness, blurred vision, chest pain, or shortness of breath occur.
- Risk of hyperglycemia. Importance of advising patients that regular monitoring of blood glucose may be needed prior to and during treatment with lorlatinib. Patients should be advised of the possible need to change or start medications for hyperglycemia. Importance of informing clinician of new or worsening signs and symptoms of hyperglycemia, including increased thirst, increased need to urinate, increased hunger, nausea, weakness or tiredness, or confusion.
- Risk of fetal harm. Necessity of advising females of reproductive potential that they should use effective, nonhormonal methods of contraception while receiving lorlatinib and for ≥6 months after discontinuance of therapy and of also advising such females that oral contraceptives and other hormonal forms of contraception may not be effective during lorlatinib therapy. Importance of advising males with female partners of reproductive potential to use effective methods of contraception while receiving the drug and for ≥3 months after the drug is discontinued. Importance of also advising males of reproductive potential that lorlatinib may transiently impair fertility and to discuss any concerns about fertility with their clinician.
- Importance of females informing their clinicians if they are or plan to become pregnant. Advise of potential fetal risk.

- Importance of advising females to avoid breast-feeding while receiving lorlatinib and for 7 days after discontinuance of therapy.
- Importance of informing patients of other important precautionary information. (See Cautions.)

For further information on the handling of antineoplastic agents, see the ASHP Guidelines on Handling Hazardous Drugs at http://www.ahfsdruginformation.com.

PREPARATIONS

Lorlatinib is available through specialty pharmacies. Clinicians may consult the Lorbrena® website for specific information regarding distribution of the drug.

Excipients in commercially available drug preparations may have clinically important effects in some individuals; consult specific product labeling for details.

Lorlatinib

Oral

Tablets, film-coated	25 mg	Lorbrena®, Pfizer
	100 mg	Lorbrena®, Pfizer

Selected Revisions June 29, 2022, © Copyright, November 26, 2018, American Society of Health-System Pharmacists, Inc.

Methotrexate, Methotrexate Sodium

10:00 • ANTINEOPLASTIC AGENTS

■ Methotrexate, a folic acid antagonist, is an antineoplastic agent and immunosuppressant.

USES

• Trophoblastic Neoplasms

Methotrexate is used in the treatment of trophoblastic neoplasms (choriocarcinoma, chorioadenoma destruens, and hydatidiform mole) in women except in those with impaired renal or hepatic function or who have failed to respond to previous therapy with methotrexate. These latter patients may be treated with dactinomycin. Methotrexate therapy is most effective in patients who have had the disease for only a short period prior to initiation of chemotherapy, who have low initial gonadotropin concentrations, and who do not have metastases. Complete remissions have been attained in about 75% of patients with metastases and in a higher percentage of patients without metastases. Methotrexate has also been used prophylactically against malignant trophoblastic disease in patients with hydatidiform mole.

In contrast to uterine choriocarcinoma, testicular choriocarcinomas are usually resistant to methotrexate alone. In patients with metastatic tumors of the testes, combination therapy utilizing methotrexate, dactinomycin, and chlorambucil has produced objective responses, as evidenced by decrease in size of metastases and tumor masses and/or lowered urinary chorionic gonadotropin concentrations in approximately 33–50% or more of patients treated. Following initial treatment, repeated courses of therapy at 1- to 3-month intervals for several years appear to be necessary in order to suppress tumor growth. In a few patients there has been an apparently permanent remission but control of tumor growth is often of only short duration.

• Leukemias

Methotrexate also is used as a component of various chemotherapeutic regimens in the palliative treatment of acute leukemias. Present regimens are most effective in the treatment of acute lymphocytic (lymphoblastic) leukemia and have been reported to produce remissions in 90% of patients treated. Methotrexate has been used with corticosteroids to induce remissions, but the drug is now most frequently used alone or in combination with other antineoplastic agents for maintenance therapy following induction of remission with vincristine sulfate and prednisone. Combination chemotherapy usually produces longer remissions than use of a single drug. Methotrexate alone rarely is effective in the treatment of acute myeloblastic leukemia; remissions are short with relapses common and resistance develops rapidly. Methotrexate, however, may produce remissions in adults who have responded initially to mercaptopurine and who have become resistant to this drug. In addition, methotrexate has been used in combination regimens in induction of remissions of acute myeloblastic leukemia.

Leukemic infiltration into the meninges and CSF has been relieved temporarily by intrathecal administration of methotrexate. The drug may be effective in patients whose systemic disease has become resistant to methotrexate since leukemic cells in the CNS usually retain their original degree of sensitivity to methotrexate; however, poor responses generally occur in patients with initial methotrexate resistance. Focal leukemic involvement of the CNS may not respond to intrathecal methotrexate and usually responds best to radiation therapy. Methotrexate is also used prophylactically against meningeal leukemia.

• Osteosarcoma

High-dose methotrexate, followed by rescue therapy with either leucovorin or levoleucovorin, is used in combination chemotherapy regimens as an adjunct to surgical resection or amputation of the primary tumor in patients with nonmetastatic osteosarcoma. These regimens appear to prolong the relapse-free survival in such patients. Methotrexate is designated an orphan drug by the US Food and Drug Administration (FDA) for use in osteogenic sarcoma.

• Breast Cancer

Methotrexate has been used alone or, more commonly, in combination chemotherapy for the treatment of breast cancer.

Combination chemotherapy used as an adjunct to surgery has been shown to increase both disease-free (i.e., decreased recurrence) and overall survival in premenopausal and postmenopausal women with node-negative or -positive early (TNM stage I or II) breast cancer. Adjuvant combination chemotherapy in early breast cancer has produced overall reductions in the annual rates of recurrence and death of 28 and 16%, respectively, with overall 5-year disease-free survival rates of 58.8 versus 49.6% for patients receiving combination chemotherapy versus those who did not. Adjuvant combination chemotherapy that includes methotrexate, cyclophosphamide, and fluorouracil has been used most extensively and is considered a regimen of choice. Although adjuvant hormonal therapy with tamoxifen (with or without combination chemotherapy) generally is used for node-positive, estrogen-receptor-positive postmenopausal women, adjuvant combination chemotherapy (with or without tamoxifen) also can be used in such patients, but differences in toxicity profiles may influence the choice of regimen. For node-positive premenopausal women, adjuvant combination chemotherapy (with or without tamoxifen) generally is used. Adjuvant therapy with combination chemotherapy and/or tamoxifen has been used in women with node-negative disease.

Controversy currently exists regarding which patients with node-negative and estrogen-receptor-negative breast cancer are most likely to benefit from such adjuvant therapy following surgery (see Uses: Breast Cancer, in Fluorouracil 10:00), but such patients with poor prognosis are reasonable candidates for adjuvant chemotherapy with an effective regimen (e.g., 6–12 months of methotrexate, cyclophosphamide, and fluorouracil initiated within 6 weeks of surgery); other node-negative patients also may be suitable candidates, but toxicities, costs, and other quality-of-life considerations should be weighed in assessing potential benefit. All patients with node-negative breast cancer are at some risk of recurrence, and effective adjuvant combination chemotherapy can increase both disease-free and overall survival, albeit less markedly than in patients with node-positive disease.

In patients with node-positive early breast cancer (i.e., stage II), an effective regimen of adjuvant combination chemotherapy (e.g., methotrexate, cyclophosphamide, and fluorouracil; cyclophosphamide, doxorubicin, and fluorouracil; cyclophosphamide and doxorubicin with or without tamoxifen) is used to reduce the rate of recurrence and improve survival in both premenopausal and postmenopausal patients once treatment to control local disease (surgery, with or without radiation therapy) has been undertaken. These combinations have been tested and established as providing therapeutic benefit, and are superior to single-agent therapy with conventional agents; numerous other combination regimens providing apparently similar outcomes also have been used but are less common or have been studied less extensively. Although long-term (e.g., 6 months or longer) chemotherapy with adjuvant regimens is clinically superior to short-term (e.g., preoperative and perioperative) adjuvant regimens, clinical superiority between 6- versus 12-month regimens has not been demonstrated. There is some evidence that the addition of doxorubicin to a regimen of methotrexate, cyclophosphamide, and fluorouracil can improve outcome further in patients with more than 3 positive axillary lymph nodes, and that sequential (i.e., administering several courses of doxorubicin first) regimens are more effective than alternating regimens in such patients; in patients with fewer positive nodes, no additional benefit from doxorubicin has been demonstrated. The dose intensity of adjuvant combination chemotherapy also appears to be an important factor influencing clinical outcome in patients with early node-positive breast cancer, with response increasing with increasing dose intensity; therefore, arbitrary reductions in dose intensity should be avoided. In women with stage II disease and more than 10 positive lymph nodes, high-dose chemotherapy and autologous bone marrow transplant is an option currently being evaluated.

In stage III (locally advanced) breast cancer, combination chemotherapy (with or without hormonal therapy) is used sequentially following surgery and radiation therapy for operable disease and following biopsy and radiation therapy for inoperable disease; commonly employed effective regimens include methotrexate, cyclophosphamide, and fluorouracil; cyclophosphamide, doxorubicin, and fluorouracil; and methotrexate, cyclophosphamide, fluorouracil, and prednisone.

These and other regimens also have been used in the treatment or more advanced (stage IV) and recurrent disease.

Lymphoma

Methotrexate may also be useful in the treatment of Burkitt's lymphoma, advanced stages (III and IV, Peters' Staging System) of lymphosarcoma, especially in children when used with other drugs, and in advanced cases of mycosis fungoides (cutaneous T-cell lymphoma). Although radiation therapy is generally used for treatment of localized histiocytic lymphoma, lymphosarcoma, and mycosis fungoides, chemotherapy may be useful in the treatment of generalized stages of these diseases. Hodgkin's disease responds poorly to methotrexate therapy.

Psoriasis

Methotrexate is used in carefully selected patients in the symptomatic control of severe, recalcitrant, disabling psoriasis that is not adequately responsive to other forms of therapy; however, the drug is not curative. Methotrexate should be used in the treatment of psoriasis only after the diagnosis has been definitely established, as by biopsy and/or after dermatologic consultation. Although methotrexate has been reported to produce beneficial effects in up to 75% of patients with psoriasis, there has been only one brief controlled study and the long-term effects of the drug and optimal dosage have not been established. Prior to initiation of methotrexate therapy, patients should be carefully screened to exclude pregnant women and patients with renal, hepatic or hematopoietic disease, or infections. The potential benefit to the patient must be carefully weighed against the possible risks involved and patients should be informed of potential toxicity.

Methotrexate has also been used topically in the treatment of psoriasis; however, results of one study indicated that the drug had little visible effect on the psoriatic lesions and another reported that the usefulness of topical methotrexate was limited by adverse effects on the surrounding skin.

Rheumatoid Arthritis

Methotrexate is used for the management of rheumatoid arthritis in adults whose symptoms progress despite an adequate regimen of nonsteroidal anti-inflammatory agents (NSAIAs). Methotrexate is one of several disease-modifying antirheumatic drugs (DMARDs) that can be used when DMARD therapy is appropriate.

Pharmacologic therapy for rheumatoid arthritis usually consists of combinations of nonsteroidal anti-inflammatory agents (NSAIAs), DMARDs, and/or corticosteroids. The ultimate goal in managing rheumatoid arthritis is to prevent or control joint damage, prevent loss of function, and decrease pain. Although NSAIAs may be useful for initial symptomatic treatment of rheumatoid arthritis, these drugs do not alter the course of the disease or prevent joint destruction. DMARDs have the potential to reduce or prevent joint damage, preserve joint integrity and function, and reduce total health care costs, and all patients with rheumatoid arthritis are candidates for DMARD therapy. DMARDs should be initiated early in the disease course and should not be delayed beyond 3 months in patients with active disease (i.e., ongoing joint pain, substantial morning stiffness, fatigue, active synovitis, persistent elevation of erythrocyte sedimentation rate [ESR] or C-reactive protein [CRP], radiographic evidence of joint damage) despite an adequate regimen of NSAIAs. DMARDs commonly used in the treatment of rheumatoid arthritis include methotrexate, etanercept, hydroxychloroquine, infliximab, leflunomide, and sulfasalazine. Less frequently used DMARDs include azathioprine, cyclosporine, minocycline, penicillamine, and/or oral or injectable gold compounds. The role of anakinra, a recombinant human interleukin-1 (IL-1) receptor antagonist, in the management of rheumatoid arthritis remains to be established.

While many factors influence the choice of a DMARD, methotrexate has substantially greater long-term efficacy than other DMARDs and is used as the initial or anchor DMARD in many patients with rheumatoid arthritis. Because residual inflammation generally persists in patients receiving maximum dosages of a single DMARD, many rheumatoid arthritis patients are candidates for combination therapy to achieve optimum control. Although the most effective combination regimen of DMARDs has not been determined, regimens that have been found efficacious in clinical studies include combinations of methotrexate and cyclosporine, etanercept, hydroxychloroquine, infliximab, leflunomide, or sulfasalazine.

Low-dose oral corticosteroids and local injection of corticosteroids are effective in relieving symptoms in patients with active rheumatoid arthritis. In addition, limited evidence indicates that low-dose corticosteroids slow the rate of joint damage.

Several international groups of rheumatologists have issued consensus reports that address the role of tumor necrosis factor (TNF) blocking agents (e.g., etanercept, infliximab) in the management of rheumatoid arthritis. These groups state that use of TNF blocking agents is most appropriate in patients with active disease (5 swollen joints and elevated acute-phase response [ESR of 28 mm/hour or greater, or CRP level of 2 mg/dL or greater]) despite adequate exposure to methotrexate or other effective DMARD. A course of methotrexate in a dosage of at least 20 mg weekly (or lower dosage if toxicity develops) for 3 months is considered an adequate course of DMARD therapy, and failure with such a course should prompt consideration of modification of the therapeutic regimen (e.g., initiation of a TNF blocking agent). Other factors to consider when deciding whether to use a TNF blocking agent in the treatment of rheumatoid arthritis are differences in the aggressiveness of the disease, extent of structural damage, effects of the disease on quality of life, and toxicity of previously used DMARDs.

Once therapy with a TNF blocking agent has been started, patients should be assessed for therapeutic response (e.g., a 20% reduction in swollen joint count with a 20% reduction in acute-phase response). While therapy should be continued indefinitely in those who have responded to therapy and are not experiencing substantial adverse effects, therapy with the TNF blocking agent should be discontinued in patients who have not responded after 12 weeks.

Administration of methotrexate alone is not a complete treatment for rheumatoid arthritis, and the drug should be used only as part of a comprehensive treatment program, including nondrug therapies such as rest and physical therapy. Most patients with active rheumatoid arthritis will show some benefit from methotrexate therapy, although improvement often plateaus during the first 6 months of therapy with the drug (occasionally being maintained for 2 years or longer) and may wane during continued use. There is no substantial evidence that methotrexate permanently arrests or reverses the underlying disease process, although the drug slows its progression in some patients. NSAIA and/or low-dose corticosteroid therapy may be continued when methotrexate therapy is initiated; however, the possible increased risk of toxicity with concomitant use of methotrexate and NSAIAs should be considered. (See Drug Interactions: Protein Bound Drugs and Weak Organic Acids, and also Nonsteroidal Anti-inflammatory Agents.) Depending on the patient's response to methotrexate, corticosteroid dosage may be gradually reduced. The manufacturer of methotrexate states that combined use of methotrexate and gold compounds, penicillamine, hydroxychloroquine, sulfasalazine, or other antirheumatic cytotoxic or immunosuppressive agents has not been adequately studied to date and may increase the risk of adverse effects.

Head and Neck Cancer

Methotrexate is used alone and in combination therapy for the palliative treatment of recurrent or metastatic head and neck carcinoma. When used alone, at a dosage of 40–60 mg/m^2 once weekly, methotrexate produces an average objective response rate of 30%. Duration of response is short at an average of 4 months.

In a randomized study, patients with recurrent or metastatic squamous cell carcinoma of the head and neck who received cisplatin and fluorouracil, carboplatin and fluorouracil, or methotrexate alone had objective response rates of 32, 21, or 10%, respectively. Although the objective response rate achieved with cisplatin and fluorouracil was greater than that observed with methotrexate alone, combination chemotherapy was associated with increased toxicity and no difference in survival was observed. In patients with recurrent or metastatic head and neck cancer who cannot tolerate combination therapy with cisplatin and fluorouracil, weekly low-dose methotrexate may be used.

Methotrexate frequently is used in combination regimens with other antineoplastic agents (e.g., bleomycin, fluorouracil, vincristine). Combination therapy with cisplatin, methotrexate, bleomycin, and vincristine has been used for the treatment of recurrent or metastatic squamous cell carcinoma of the head and neck. Further study is needed to establish the comparative benefit of methotrexate-containing regimens in the treatment of advanced head and neck cancer.

Crohn's Disease

Methotrexate has been used for its anti-inflammatory effects in the management of Crohn's disease†. Results of several open-label, and double-blind, placebo-controlled studies in adults indicate that use of methotrexate can result in clinical response (including clinical remission) in patients with chronically active Crohn's disease who have not responded to prior therapies (e.g., corticosteroids, other immunosuppressants), although efficacy of orally administered methotrexate has not been consistently reported in placebo-controlled clinical studies.

Safety and efficacy of parenteral methotrexate in the management of active Crohn's disease was evaluated in a double-blind placebo-controlled multicenter 16-week study that included 141 adults with chronically active Crohn's disease who had inadequate response to a corticosteroid (i.e. , prednisone). To be included in the study, patients had to have a chronically active disease unresponsive to a minimum of 3-months of therapy with prednisone (12.5 mg daily) with at least one attempt to discontinue the corticosteroid. At baseline, patients had a median Crohn's Disease Activity Index (CDAI) of 181–190. The CDAI score is based on subjective observations by the patient (e.g., the daily number of liquid or very soft stools, severity of abdominal pain, general well-being) and objective evidence (e.g., number of extraintestinal manifestations, presence of an abdominal mass, use or nonuse of antidiarrheal drugs, the hematocrit, body weight). Patients were randomized to receive IM methotrexate (94 patients; 25 mg once weekly) or placebo (47 patients). Patients continued to receive prednisone, which was tapered over 10 weeks (starting 2 weeks after randomization), unless their condition worsened; however, no other drugs used for management of Crohn's disease (e.g., oral or topical derivatives of 5-aminosalicylic acid, budesonide, other immunosuppressive agents, topical corticosteroids) were allowed. The primary outcome was clinical remission (defined as a CDAI index of 150 points or less and discontinuance of prednisone) at the end of the trial (16 weeks). Clinical remission at the end of the study was reported in 39 or 19% of patients receiving methotrexate or placebo, respectively. In addition, patients receiving methotrexate used less prednisone overall and had a lower mean average CDAI score than those receiving placebo (170 points for methotrexate versus 193 points for placebo). Many patients in this study who entered remission after 16–24 weeks of treatment with IM methotrexate (25 mg weekly) were enrolled in a new trial which evaluated the safety and efficacy of parenteral methotrexate for maintenance therapy of Crohn's disease. In this multicenter, double-blind, placebo-controlled trial, 76 patients with chronically active Crohn's disease in remission were randomized to receive 15 mg of IM methotrexate once weekly (40 patients) or placebo (36 patients) for 40 weeks; no other treatment for Crohn's disease was allowed. After 40 weeks, a greater proportion of patients receiving methotrexate were free of relapse (defined as an increase of baseline CDAI of 100 points or more, or the need to initiate therapy for active disease) than those receiving placebo (65% for methotrexate versus 39% for placebo); in addition, a smaller proportion of patients receiving methotrexate required prednisone therapy for relapse when compared with those receiving placebo (28% for methotrexate versus 58% for placebo).

Safety and efficacy of oral methotrexate in the management of chronically active Crohn's disease was evaluated in 2 other randomized double-blind, placebo-controlled trials in 59 corticosteroid-dependent adults. Patients received a weekly oral methotrexate dosage of 12.5 mg for 9 months in one trial and 15–22.5 mg for up to 1 year in the other. Efficacy (measured by reduction of dosage of corticosteroids, reduction in CDAI, or reduction in Harvey Bradshaw index) of oral methotrexate was similar to that of oral mercaptopurine (50 mg daily) in one of the studies and to placebo in both studies.

Some clinicians state that pediatric patients† with corticosteroid-dependent or corticosteroid-resistant, moderately to severely active Crohn's disease† who had an inadequate response to or were intolerant of azathioprine or mercaptopurine, may receive methotrexate (10–15 mg/m² weekly) for the management of such disease. (See Cautions: Pediatric Precautions.)

For further information on the management of Crohn's disease, see Uses: Crohn's Disease, in Mesalamine 56:36.

● **Other Uses**

Methotrexate is used in combination regimens with cisplatin and vinblastine, with or without doxorubicin, for the treatment of invasive and advanced bladder cancer. (See Uses: Bladder Cancer, in Cisplatin 10:00.) Because methotrexate is absorbed through the ileum, placement of a Foley catheter or frequent emptying of the reservoir is advised in patients with long ileal loops or internal reservoirs during administration of methotrexate-containing regimens for the treatment of advanced or metastatic bladder cancer. Because elimination of methotrexate may be impaired and risk of toxicity increased in patients with renal dysfunction, edema, pleural fluid collections, or ascites, use of leucovorin rescue or deletion of methotrexate is advised if methotrexate-containing regimens are being considered for the treatment of advanced or metastatic bladder cancer in such patients.

Methotrexate has been used in second-line therapy for the treatment of recurrent small cell lung cancer. Although methotrexate is labeled for use in the treatment of the squamous cell type of non-small cell lung cancer, other agents are preferred for the treatment of this neoplasm.

Methotrexate has been used in treating a variety of solid tumors†. In some studies, the drug has been administered by intra-arterial infusion alone or in conjunction with IM leucovorin calcium in the palliative management of carcinomas capable of being infused via a single artery. Low-dose oral methotrexate has been used in patients with chronic progressive multiple sclerosis†. Results of several clinical studies indicate that low-dose methotrexate (7.5 mg weekly for up to 2 years) reduces both disease activity (as assessed by magnetic resonance imaging [MRI]) and sustained progression of disability (as assessed by the Expanded Disability Status Scale, the Ambulation Index, and standardized tests of upper extremity function). Patients with secondary progressive multiple sclerosis benefited the most from methotrexate therapy.

Methotrexate has been used for its immunosuppressive and/or anti-inflammatory effects in the treatment of psoriatic arthritis†, systemic lupus erythematosus†, vasculitis†, dermatomyositis†, polymyositis†, Wegener's granulomatosis†, and a variety of dermatologic and chronic refractory ocular diseases†. Controlled studies have shown that oral or parenteral methotrexate therapy is effective in the short-term management of psoriatic arthritis; however, because of its potential toxicities, methotrexate is generally used in the management of this condition only in patients whose disease is severe and/or unresponsive to conventional therapy.

DOSAGE AND ADMINISTRATION

● **Reconstitution and Administration**

Methotrexate is administered orally. Methotrexate sodium is administered by IM, IV, or intrathecal injection; the drug may also be administered intra-arterially.

Methotrexate sodium injection and powder for injection should be reconstituted according to the manufacturers' directions.

For the treatment of meningeal leukemia, methotrexate must be administered intrathecally since passage of the drug from the blood to CSF is minimal. Prior to intrathecal administration of methotrexate, a volume of CSF approximately equivalent to the volume of methotrexate solution to be injected (e.g., 5–15 mL) is usually removed. If a lumbar puncture is traumatic, methotrexate should not be administered intrathecally. Two days should elapse before again attempting the injection. Methotrexate should be injected intrathecally only if there is easy flow of blood-free spinal fluid. Some clinicians recommend that the entire volume of methotrexate injection be injected intrathecally in 15–30 seconds. Aspiration should not be performed. *For intrathecal injection, preservative-free methotrexate solutions containing 1 mg/mL are used*; solutions may be prepared using preservative-free 0.9% sodium chloride injection as a diluent. *Methotrexate formulations or diluents containing preservatives must not be used for intrathecal administration or high-dose methotrexate therapy.*

Methotrexate sodium solutions should be inspected visually for particulate matter and discoloration whenever solution and container permit.

● **Dosage**

Methotrexate should only be used under the supervision of a clinician who is experienced in cancer chemotherapy and in the use of antimetabolites. (See Cautions: Precautions and Contraindications.) Dosage of methotrexate sodium is expressed in terms of methotrexate. Various dosage schedules for methotrexate therapy alone and in combination with other antineoplastic agents and/or radiation therapy have appeared in the literature; dosage, route of administration, and duration of therapy must be individualized according to the disease being treated, other therapy being employed, and the condition, response, and tolerance of the patient. In patients in whom discontinuance of methotrexate has been required, therapy should be reinstituted with caution, giving complete consideration to further need for the drug and the possibility of recurrence of toxicity. Clinicians should consult published protocols for additional dosages of methotrexate and other chemotherapeutic agents and the method and sequence of administration.

Careful review of the intended use for methotrexate should be undertaken to ensure that inadvertent overdosage (e.g., administering antineoplastic rather than anti-inflammatory dosages) does not occur. Dosages used in rheumatic conditions (e.g., rheumatoid arthritis, psoriasis) and certain inflammatory GI conditions (e.g., Crohn's disease†) are substantially lower than those used to treat cancer, and intermittent dosing rather than daily dosing is used for such inflammatory conditions. It is essential that any order for daily dosing of the drug be reviewed carefully to ensure that the intended use is an antineoplastic one. Inadvertent daily administration of the drug for non-cancer uses can prove fatal. Regimens for rheumatic conditions and certain inflammatory GI conditions employ intermittent dosing, usually once weekly as a single dose or once weekly as 3-divided doses at 12-hour intervals. Clinicians also should ensure that printed materials (e.g., discharge instructions) patients and/or their caregivers receive describe the correct dosing regimen for their condition, and they should be instructed carefully about their prescribed regimen, paying particular attention to the frequency of administration.

Trophoblastic Neoplasms

For the treatment of trophoblastic neoplasms, the usual dosage of methotrexate is 15–30 mg daily, administered orally or IM for 5 days. A repeat course may be given after a period of one or more weeks provided all signs of residual toxicity have disappeared. Three to five courses of therapy are usually employed. Therapy is usually evaluated by 24-hour quantitative analysis of urinary chorionic gonadotropin which should return to normal or less than 50 IU/24 hours, usually after the third or fourth course. Complete resolution of measurable lesions usually occurs 4–6 weeks later. One or two courses of methotrexate therapy are usually given after normalization of urinary chorionic gonadotropin hormone concentrations is achieved. In the treatment of trophoblastic disease in women, regimens alternating courses of methotrexate therapy and dactinomycin therapy or combining administration of methotrexate and mercaptopurine or methotrexate, dactinomycin, and chlorambucil have also been used. In the treatment of trophoblastic disease in women, 10–15 mg of methotrexate daily has also been administered via the hypogastric artery† until toxicity or therapeutic response occurred. Combination chemotherapy with methotrexate, chlorambucil, and dactinomycin has been used in the treatment of metastatic testicular tumors in men.

Leukemia

Although methotrexate is not generally a drug of choice for induction of remission of lymphoblastic leukemia, oral methotrexate dosage of 3.3 mg/m² daily and prednisone 60 mg/m² daily for 4–6 weeks have been used. After a remission is attained, maintenance therapy with methotrexate is administered twice weekly, orally or by IM injection, for a total weekly dose of 30 mg/m². Administration of the drug in twice-weekly doses appears to be more effective than daily drug administration. Alternatively, 2.5 mg/kg has been administered IV every 14 days.

For the treatment of meningeal leukemia, an intrathecal methotrexate dosage of 12 mg/m² or an empiric dose of 15 mg, administered at 2- to 5-day intervals until CSF cell counts return to normal, has been suggested; this is then followed by one additional dose of the drug. Alternatively, 12 mg/m² has been administered once weekly for 2 weeks and then once monthly thereafter. For prophylaxis against meningeal leukemia, a methotrexate dose of 12 mg/m² or 15 mg has been used; the intervals for administration differ from the regimen used in the treatment of meningeal leukemia, and specialized references and the medical literature should be consulted for specific recommendations. However, because the volume of CSF is related to age and not body surface area, dosage regimens based on body surface area may result in inadequate CSF concentrations in children and high, potentially neurotoxic CSF concentrations in adults; therefore, some clinicians recommend that intrathecal dosage be based on the patient's age. Clinical studies indicate that intrathecal methotrexate dosage regimens based on age may be more effective and less neurotoxic than dosage regimens based on body surface area. The suggested intrathecal doses based on age are 6 mg for children younger than 1 year of age, 8 mg for children 1 year of age, 10 mg for children 2 years of age, and 12 mg for children 3 years of age or older and for adults; geriatric patients may require reduced doses because of reduced CSF turnover and decreasing brain volume. *Regardless of the method used to determine intrathecal methotrexate dosage, the dose should be carefully checked prior to administration to minimize the risk of inadvertent intrathecal overdosage.* Because methotrexate appears in systemic circulation following intrathecal administration, systemic administration of the drug should be appropriately adjusted, reduced, or discontinued. Systemic administration of leucovorin calcium simultaneously with intrathecal methotrexate may prevent systemic toxicity without abolishing the activity of the antimetabolite in the CNS. The manufacturers state that focal leukemic involvement of the CNS may not respond to intrathecal methotrexate therapy and may be best treated with radiation therapy.

Osteosarcoma

The recommended initial dose for high-dose methotrexate treatment of nonmetastatic osteosarcoma is 12 g/m² administered by IV infusion over 4 hours (followed by leucovorin or levoleucovorin rescue) on postoperative weeks 4, 5, 6, 7, 11, 12, 15, 16, 29, 30, 44, and 45, on a schedule in combination with other chemotherapy agents (e.g., doxorubicin, cisplatin, the combination of bleomycin, cyclophosphamide, and dactinomycin [BCD regimen]). If the initial dosage is not sufficient to produce peak serum methotrexate concentrations of 454 mcg/mL (1000 µM [10⁻³ mol/L]) at the end of the infusion, the dose may be increased to 15 g/m² in subsequent treatments.

Leucovorin and levoleucovorin are used as rescue therapy following a high-dose methotrexate regimen to prevent acute toxicity. Leucovorin is administered orally, IM, or by IV injection starting 24 hours after the beginning of the methotrexate infusion. If the patient experiences GI toxicity (e.g., nausea, vomiting), leucovorin should be administered parenterally. The usual dosage of leucovorin is 15 mg (approximately 10 mg/m²) orally, IM, or by IV injection every 6 hours for a total of 60 hours or a total of 10 doses. (See Leucovorin Calcium 92:12.)

Levoleucovorin is administered as an IV infusion at a rate no faster than 160 mg of levoleucovorin per minute every 6 hours for a total of 60 hours or a total of 10 doses, starting 24 hours after the beginning of the methotrexate infusion. (See Levoleucovorin Calcium 92:12.)

Patients receiving high-dose methotrexate regimens must be well hydrated and carefully monitored. (See Cautions: Precautions and Contraindications.) For specific information on dosage modifications, cautions, and precautions associated with high-dose methotrexate therapy, the manufacturer's prescribing information should be consulted.

Breast Cancer

Various methotrexate-containing combination chemotherapy regimens have been used in the treatment of breast cancer, and published protocols should be consulted for dosages and the method and sequence of administration. The dose intensity of adjuvant combination chemotherapy appears to be an important factor influencing clinical outcome in patients with early node-positive breast cancer, with response increasing with increasing dose intensity; therefore, *arbitrary* reductions in dose intensity should be avoided.

One commonly employed regimen for the treatment of early breast cancer includes a methotrexate dosage of 40 mg/m² (administered IV) on days 1 and 8 of each cycle combined with cyclophosphamide 100 mg/m² on days 1 through 14 of each cycle and fluorouracil 600 mg/m² on days 1 and 8 of each cycle. In patients older than 60 years of age, the initial methotrexate dosage was reduced to 30 mg/m² and the initial fluorouracil dosage was reduced to 400 mg/m². Dosage also was reduced if myelosuppression developed. Cycles generally were repeated monthly (i.e., allowing a 2-week rest period between cycles) for a total of 6–12 cycles (i.e., 6–12 months of therapy). Clinical superiority between 6- versus 12-month regimens has not been demonstrated.

There is some evidence that the addition of doxorubicin to a regimen of cyclophosphamide, methotrexate, and fluorouracil can improve outcome further in patients with early breast cancer and more than 3 positive axillary lymph nodes, and that sequential (i.e., administering several courses of doxorubicin first) regimens are more effective than alternating regimens in such patients; in patients with fewer positive nodes, no additional benefit from doxorubicin has been demonstrated. In the sequential regimen, 4 doses of doxorubicin hydrochloride 75 mg/m² were administered initially at 3-week intervals followed by 8 cycles of methotrexate 40 mg/m², cyclophosphamide 600 mg/m², and fluorouracil 600 mg/m² at 3-week intervals for a total of approximately 9 months of therapy. If myelosuppression developed with this sequential regimen, the subsequent cycle generally was delayed rather than reducing dosage.

Burkitt's Lymphoma and Lymphosarcoma

The usual dosage of methotrexate for the treatment of stages I or II of Burkitt's lymphoma is 10–25 mg/day orally for 4–8 days. Methotrexate is commonly given concomitantly with other antineoplastic agents in the treatment of stage III

Burkitt's lymphoma and lymphosarcomas. In all stages, several courses of drug therapy are usually administered interposed with 7- to 10-day rest periods. Stage III lymphosarcomas may respond to combined drug therapy with methotrexate given in doses of 0.625–2.5 mg/kg daily.

Mycosis Fungoides

Clinical response occurs in up to 50% of patients receiving single-agent therapy with methotrexate for mycosis fungoides (cutaneous T-cell lymphoma). In early stages of the disease, the usual dosage is 5–50 mg orally once weekly. The need for dosage reduction or discontinuance of therapy is determined by response to therapy and hematologic monitoring. Methotrexate also has been administered twice weekly in doses of 15–37.5 mg in patients with disease that has responded poorly to once-weekly dosing. In patients with advanced stages of mycosis fungoides, combination chemotherapy regimens that include IV methotrexate in higher doses followed by leucovorin rescue have been used.

Psoriasis

For the management of psoriasis, a single 5- to 10-mg dose of methotrexate should be given 1 week prior to initiation of methotrexate therapy to detect idiosyncratic reactions. Optimum dosage has not been established and dosage must be based on individual requirements and response. Dosage must be constantly supervised by a physician who is experienced in the use of antineoplastic agents.

There are 2 dosage schedules suggested by the manufacturers. To avoid potentially lethal overdosage, patients should be instructed carefully about their dosage regimen, paying particular attention to the frequency of administration.

The divided oral dosage schedule, which is based on cellular kinetic studies, consists of 2.5 mg of methotrexate administered orally at 12-hour intervals for 3 doses each week; in this regimen, dosage may be increased gradually by 2.5 mg/week, but weekly dosage should usually not exceed 25 mg and should *not* exceed 30 mg.

In the weekly single-dosage schedule, the manufacturers suggest that 10–25 mg may be administered orally, IM, or IV as a single dose once weekly. The usual oral dose in the weekly single-dosage schedule is 7.5–25 mg, with an occasional patient requiring up to 37.5 mg; dosage may be increased gradually by 2.5–5 mg/week. The usual IM or rapid IV dose in the weekly single-dosage schedule is 7.5–50 mg, with an occasional patient requiring up to 100 mg; dosage may be increased gradually. The manufacturers state that the oral, IM, or IV dose in the weekly single-dosage schedule should usually not exceed 50 mg.

In most patients, substantial improvement usually occurs within 4 weeks and optimum results occur in 2–3 months. Cessation of methotrexate usually results in a recurrence of symptoms in 2 weeks to 6 months. After optimal response is achieved, each schedule should be reduced to the lowest possible dose with the longest possible rest period. Conventional topical therapy should be resumed as soon as possible.

Psoriatic Arthritis

The optimum dosage of methotrexate in the management of psoriatic arthritis† has not been clearly established, although oral and parenteral dosage regimens similar to those used in the management of psoriasis have been employed. Clinicians should consult specialized references for detailed information on specific dosage regimens.

Rheumatoid Arthritis

For the management of rheumatoid arthritis, a single test dose of methotrexate may be given prior to initiation of therapy to detect possible sensitivity to adverse effects associated with the drug. Optimum dosage has not been fully established and dosage must be based on individual requirements and response. Patients receiving methotrexate therapy for rheumatoid arthritis must be constantly supervised by a physician who is experienced in the use of antineoplastic agents. The mnemonic dispensing packages (Rheumatrex® Dose Pack) may be used for initial methotrexate therapy and are suitable for maintenance therapy in patients receiving weekly methotrexate doses of 5–20 mg; however, use of these dispensing packages is *not* recommended for titration to weekly doses higher than 20 mg. To avoid potentially lethal overdosage, patients should be instructed carefully about their dosage regimen, paying particular attention to the frequency of administration.

For the management of rheumatoid arthritis, methotrexate is administered in low-dose, intermittent (i.e., weekly rather than daily) regimens. The usual initial dosage in adults is 7.5 mg orally once weekly. This dosage may be administered either in a single-dosage schedule consisting of a single 7. 5-mg oral dose once weekly or in a divided-dosage schedule consisting of 2.5 mg of methotrexate administered orally at 12-hour intervals for 3 doses each week. Dosage in either the single- or divided-dosage schedule may be gradually increased until an optimum therapeutic response is achieved. However, dosage usually should not exceed 20 mg weekly, since higher dosages have been associated with a substantially increased incidence and severity of serious adverse reactions (e.g., bone marrow suppression). After an optimum response to the drug is achieved, the weekly dosage should be reduced to the lowest possible effective level. Therapeutic response in patients with rheumatoid arthritis usually is apparent within 3–6 weeks, but optimum response may not be achieved for another 3 or more months of therapy. The optimum duration of therapy is unknown; however, limited data from long-term clinical studies indicate that initial clinical improvement may be maintained for prolonged periods (e.g., 2 years or longer) with continued methotrexate therapy. Following discontinuance of the drug, rheumatoid arthritis usually worsens within 3–6 weeks.

Parenteral methotrexate regimens in the management of rheumatoid arthritis are variable, but have often consisted of 7.5–15 mg given IM once weekly in adults†.

Crohn's Disease

For the management of Crohn's disease†, methotrexate has been administered in low-dose, intermittent (i.e., weekly rather than daily) regimens. For the management of chronically active, refractory Crohn's disease, methotrexate has been administered once weekly either IM in a dosage of 25 mg for 16 weeks or orally in a dosage of 12.5–22.5 mg for up to 1 year. For maintenance therapy of Crohn's disease, an IM methotrexate dosage of 15 mg weekly has been used.

CAUTIONS

The major toxic effects of methotrexate are on normal, rapidly proliferating tissues, particularly of the bone marrow and lining of the GI tract. These adverse effects generally are dose related and are reversible if detected early. Ulcerations of the oral mucosa are usually the earliest signs of toxicity, but in some patients bone marrow depression coincides with or precedes the appearance of mouth lesions.

● *Hematologic Effects*

Leukopenia, thrombocytopenia, anemia, and hemorrhage from various sites may result from methotrexate therapy and may develop rapidly. In one study using single IV doses of methotrexate, the nadir of hemoglobin concentrations occurred in 6–13 days and was followed by recovery; reticulocytes reached their nadir in 2–7 days followed by recovery with rebound between 9 and 19 days. Leukocytes generally had two periods of depression; the first occurred in 4–7 days with recovery in 7–13 days and the second in 12–21 days with recovery in 15–29 days. Platelets reached their minimum in 5–12 days and recovered in number in 15–27 days.

Thrombocytopenia has been reported in approximately 5%, leukopenia and pancytopenia in approximately 1.5%, and decreased hematocrit and epistaxis in less than 1% of patients receiving 12–18 weeks of methotrexate for the management of rheumatoid arthritis.

● *GI Effects*

Toxic effects of methotrexate on oral and GI mucosa are manifested by gingivitis, glossitis, pharyngitis, stomatitis, enteritis, ulcerations and bleeding of the mucous membranes of the mouth or other portions of the GI tract, abdominal distress, anorexia, nausea, vomiting, hematemesis, diarrhea, and melena. If ulcerative stomatitis or diarrhea occurs, methotrexate therapy must be interrupted in order to prevent hemorrhagic enteritis and death from intestinal perforation.

Pancreatitis also has been reported in patients receiving methotrexate.

● *Hepatic Effects*

Methotrexate therapy has been associated with both acute and chronic hepatotoxicity. Acutely, elevations in serum aminotransferase (transaminase) concentrations frequently occur 1–3 days after a dose of the drug. Such elevations generally are transient, asymptomatic, and do not appear to be predictive of subsequent hepatic damage. Elevated liver function test results reportedly occurred in approximately 15% of patients receiving 12–18 weeks of methotrexate for the management of rheumatoid arthritis.

Hepatotoxicity manifested as hepatic fibrosis or cirrhosis or other histologic changes in the liver has occurred during long-term methotrexate therapy; such hepatotoxicity may require hepatic allotransplantation and can be fatal. In patients with psoriasis, when such changes occur, they often may *not* be preceded by symptoms of hepatotoxicity or abnormal liver function test results; in patients with rheumatoid arthritis, prolonged, substantial abnormalities in liver function test results may precede appearance of hepatic fibrosis or cirrhosis. Chronic hepatotoxicity generally has been associated with prolonged (2 years or longer) methotrexate therapy and cumulative doses of 1.5 g or more. Although accurate estimates of the incidence of chronic hepatotoxicity currently are not available, the incidence appears to be greater in patients receiving frequent (e.g., daily), small doses of the drug (such as the daily-dosage regimen used for psoriasis) than in those receiving intermittent regimens (such as those used for neoplastic disease and possibly rheumatoid arthritis). The risk of developing chronic hepatotoxicity in patients receiving methotrexate therapy for the management of psoriasis appears to be related to the cumulative dose of the drug, and presence of concurrent conditions such as alcoholism, obesity, or diabetes as well as advanced age appear to contribute to this risk. Although clinical experience is limited, these risk factors also may apply to patients receiving methotrexate therapy for the management of rheumatoid arthritis. In one retrospective analysis in a limited number of patients with rheumatoid arthritis who underwent periodic percutaneous liver biopsy as routine monitoring for potential hepatotoxicity while receiving intermittent methotrexate regimens for an average of 32 months, progressive hepatic changes, principally progression to mild to moderate fatty infiltration with portal inflammation, occurred in about 20% of these patients; alterations in liver function test results were not predictive of such changes. In this study, fibrosis that developed in patients with rheumatoid arthritis was considered mild and no patient with rheumatoid arthritis developed cirrhosis; however, the drug was discontinued in most patients when fibrosis was evident and additional study and experience are necessary to better elucidate the potential risk of hepatotoxicity associated with methotrexate therapy for arthritis.

Although various pathologic hepatic changes including atrophy, necrosis, fatty changes, fibrosis, and cirrhosis have been observed in patients with methotrexate-induced hepatotoxicity, no specific pathologic finding appears to be characteristic of methotrexate hepatotoxicity. The rate of progression of hepatic lesions with continued therapy and the potential reversibility of such lesions following discontinuance of the drug currently are not known. (See Cautions: Precautions and Contraindications.)

● **Respiratory Effects**

Pulmonary toxicity, which can progress rapidly and is potentially fatal, has been associated with methotrexate therapy. Adverse pulmonary effects, including pulmonary fibrosis and acute or chronic interstitial pneumonitis, appear to occur at any time during therapy at any dosage of the drug, including low dosages. Although the clinical presentation of methotrexate-induced pulmonary toxicity is variable, manifestations commonly include fever, cough (especially one that is dry and nonproductive), dyspnea, chest pain, hypoxemia (which can be severe), and/or radiographic evidence of pulmonary infiltrates (usually diffuse and/or alveolar). Lung biopsies have revealed variable degrees of interstitial inflammation, granulomatous inflammation, and/or fibrosis. Because patients with rheumatoid arthritis may have underlying interstitial pulmonary changes associated with their disease, it may be difficult to differentiate such changes from potential methotrexate-induced changes; however, rheumatoid changes generally progress more slowly. In addition, a potential association between preexisting rheumatoid pulmonary changes and susceptibility to methotrexate-induced pulmonary toxicity has been suggested but requires further elucidation.

The possibility of methotrexate-induced pulmonary toxicity should be considered in any patient who develops pulmonary manifestations (e.g., dry, nonproductive cough; dyspnea) while receiving the drug. If such manifestations occur, methotrexate should be discontinued and careful clinical evaluation of the patient performed, including exclusion of possible infectious causes. Management of methotrexate-induced pulmonary toxicity mainly is supportive and may include mechanical ventilation; limited evidence suggests that administration of relatively high dosages of corticosteroids may provide some benefit, but additional experience is necessary. In addition, pulmonary toxicity induced by the drug may not be fully reversible and fatalities have been reported.

● **Dermatologic and Sensitivity Reactions**

Severe, occasionally fatal cutaneous or sensitivity reactions (e.g., toxic epidermic necrolysis, Stevens-Johnson syndrome, exfoliative dermatitis, skin necrosis, erythema multiforme) have been reported in pediatric and adult patients within days of receiving single or multiple oral, IM, IV, or intrathecal doses of methotrexate. These reactions occurred following high-, intermediate-, or low-dose methotrexate therapy in patients with neoplastic or non-neoplastic diseases. Recovery has been reported after discontinuance of the drug. Other adverse dermatologic effects of methotrexate include erythematous rashes, pruritus, dermatitis, urticaria, folliculitis, photosensitivity, depigmentation, hyperpigmentation, petechiae, ecchymoses, telangiectasia, acne, and furunculosis. Alopecia occasionally occurs. Regrowth of hair usually occurs after methotrexate is discontinued but may require several months. Burning and erythema may occur in psoriatic areas for 1–2 days following each dose of the drug and psoriatic lesions may be aggravated by concomitant exposure to ultraviolet radiation. In addition, painful plaque erosions rarely have been reported in patients receiving methotrexate for the treatment of psoriasis.

● **Effects following Intrathecal Administration**

Following intrathecal administration of methotrexate, acute chemical arachnoiditis manifested by headache, back pain, nuchal rigidity, and/or fever; subacute myelopathy manifested by paraparesis/paraplegia involving one or more spinal nerve roots; chronic leukoencephalopathy (which may be progressive and even fatal) manifested by confusion, irritability, somnolence, ataxia, dementia, and occasionally seizures and coma; and increased CSF pressure have occurred. Systemic toxicity also may occur following intrathecal and intra-arterial administration. Leukoencephalopathy, manifested by mental confusion, tremors, ataxia, irritability, somnolence, and seizures, and rarely progressing to coma and death, has been reported in patients receiving simultaneous oral and intrathecal methotrexate therapy. Leukoencephalopathy also has occurred following IV administration of methotrexate to patients who had received craniospinal irradiation. In addition, chronic leukoencephalopathy also has been reported in patients receiving repeated high doses of methotrexate with leucovorin rescue, but without cranial irradiation. Discontinuance of methotrexate may not be associated with complete recovery.

Inadvertent intrathecal overdosage of methotrexate has occurred rarely. In cases in which the inadvertent intrathecal dose was less than 100 mg and the error was usually rapidly recognized and appropriate therapy promptly instituted, the patients experienced no or only mild neurotoxicity. In cases in which the dose exceeded 100 mg, severe neurotoxicity occurred, manifested as prompt burning or numbness in the lower extremities, stupor, agitation, seizures, and/or respiratory insufficiency; in some cases, brain damage or fatal necrotizing leukoencephalopathy resulted despite prompt treatment, but complete recovery following prompt and aggressive therapy has been reported.

Inadvertent intrathecal overdosage of methotrexate constitutes a medical emergency, requiring prompt treatment and management. Although data are limited, management may be guided by the dose administered, time elapsed since administration, and anticipated severity of neurotoxicity. Regardless of the dose administered, as soon as the overdose is recognized, a repeat lumbar puncture should be performed immediately and CSF allowed to drain to gravity.

The efficacy of CSF drainage alone as a means for removing the drug is a function of the dose administered and time elapsed since administration, and decreases as these factors increase. If the dose exceeds 100 mg, prompt neurosurgical intervention with ventriculolumbar perfusion following immediate CSF drainage should be considered; continuous CSF drainage or multiple CSF exchanges may also be considered but are not likely to be as effective.

Other treatment measures may include high-dose parenteral leucovorin calcium therapy to minimize systemic toxicity, corticosteroids to minimize CNS inflammatory reactions, and other supportive therapy as necessary. Efficacy of carboxypeptidase G2 (glucarpidase) has not been established in the management of severe overdoses of intrathecal methotrexate; however, successful use of the drug in this setting has been reported. Successful treatment with intrathecal glucarpidase in a 6-year-old patient who received a 600-mg dose of methotrexate intrathecally has been reported; the patient also was treated with CSF drainage, ventriculolumbar perfusion, IV dexamethasone, IV leucovorin calcium, and hydration and alkalinization. While the addition of leucovorin to the ventriculolumbar perfusion fluid has been suggested and employed, its value is not known and the possibility that it may be epileptogenic via this route of administration should be considered. Intrathecal administration of leucovorin is contraindicated, and the drug has contributed to at least one death when administered by this route. The possible benefits of prophylactic anticonvulsant therapy are probably outweighed by the potential for obscuring acute neurologic symptoms and causing additional adverse effects.

● Cardiovascular Effects

Pericarditis, pericardial effusion, hypotension, and thromboembolic complications (e.g., thrombophlebitis; pulmonary embolism; arterial, cerebral, deep vein, or retinal vein thrombosis) have been reported in patients receiving methotrexate therapy.

● Other Adverse Effects

Headaches, drowsiness, blurred vision, eye discomfort, conjunctivitis, severe visual changes of unknown etiology, tinnitus, malaise, undue fatigue, and dizziness may occur in patients receiving methotrexate. A transient acute neurologic syndrome manifested by confusion, hemiparesis, seizures, and coma has been reported in patients receiving high-dose methotrexate therapy. The exact cause of this stroke-like encephalopathy is not known; however, it has been suggested that the syndrome may have been related to hemorrhage or complications from intra-arterial catheterization. Other reported complications from intra-arterial infusion techniques include arterial spasm, thrombosis, hemorrhage, infection at the catheter site, and thrombophlebitis. Transient subtle cognitive dysfunction, mood alteration, unusual cranial sensations, leukoencephalopathy, or encephalopathy have been reported in some patients receiving low-dose methotrexate therapy.

Other reported adverse effects of methotrexate include chills and fever, sweating, arthralgia, myalgia, decreased resistance to infection, septicemia, upper respiratory infection, osteoporosis including aseptic necrosis of the femoral head, hypogammaglobulinemia, cystitis, dysuria, vaginal discharge, gynecomastia, loss of libido, impotence, diabetes, abnormal tissue cell changes, and even sudden death.

Severe nephropathy manifested by azotemia, hematuria, and renal failure may occur in patients receiving methotrexate; fatalities have been reported. In one study, postmortem examination revealed extensive necrosis of the epithelium of the convoluted tubules. In patients with renal impairment, methotrexate accumulation and increased toxicity or additional renal damage may occur.

Soft tissue necrosis and osteonecrosis have been reported rarely in patients receiving methotrexate. The risk of soft tissue necrosis and osteonecrosis associated with methotrexate may be elevated in patients receiving concomitant radiotherapy.

Elevations in serum uric acid concentrations may occur in patients receiving methotrexate as a result of cell destruction and hepatic and renal damage. In some patients, uric acid nephropathy and acute renal failure may result. Tumor lysis syndrome associated with other cytotoxic drugs (e.g., fludarabine, cladribine), also has been reported in patients with rapidly growing tumors who were receiving methotrexate. Pharmacologic and appropriate supportive treatment may prevent or alleviate this complication. Methotrexate also was reported to precipitate acute gouty arthritis in two patients being treated for psoriasis. Administration of large volumes of fluids, alkalinization of the urine, and/or administration of allopurinol may be useful in preventing acute attacks of hyperuricemia and uric acid nephropathy.

Nodulosis, vasculitis, and reversible lymphomas (see Precautions and Contraindications) have been reported rarely in patients receiving methotrexate. Sometimes fatal opportunistic infections have been reported in patients receiving methotrexate for neoplastic or non-neoplastic diseases. The most frequent infection was Pneumocystis carinii pneumonia; however, other infections (e.g., nocardiosis, histoplasmosis, cryptococcosis, herpes zoster, herpes simplex hepatitis, disseminated herpes simplex) also were reported.

● Precautions and Contraindications

Methotrexate is a highly toxic drug with a very low therapeutic index and a therapeutic response is not likely to occur without some evidence of toxicity. The drug can produce hepatotoxicity, severe hematologic toxicity, and GI hemorrhage; severe infection and even death may result. When methotrexate is used in combination with other antineoplastic agents and/or radiation therapy, toxic reactions may be more severe than would occur with methotrexate therapy

alone. Concomitant use of methotrexate and radiation therapy may result in an increased risk of soft tissue necrosis and osteonecrosis (see Cautions: Other Adverse Effects). Although doses of methotrexate used in the management of psoriasis and rheumatoid arthritis are usually lower than those used in antineoplastic chemotherapy, severe toxicity may occur in any patient receiving the drug and deaths have been reported with the use of methotrexate in the management of malignancy, psoriasis, and rheumatoid arthritis.

Since methotrexate may produce severe toxicity, which may be fatal, the manufacturer states that the drug should only be used in patients with life-threatening neoplastic diseases or in those with severe, recalcitrant, disabling psoriasis or rheumatoid arthritis that is not adequately responsive to other forms of therapy.

The use of high-dose methotrexate regimens employed in the adjunctive treatment of osteosarcoma requires a meticulous understanding of the risks associated with such therapy and of leucovorin rescue. Particular attention to leukocyte counts, serum bilirubin and ALT (SGPT) concentrations, presence of mucositis or persistent pleural effusions, renal function, hydration, urinary alkalinization, fluid and electrolyte balance, and pharmacokinetic monitoring must be ensured when such regimens are used. The manufacturer's labeling and published protocols should be consulted for specific recommendations, including dosage guidelines based on these findings.

Methotrexate must be used only under constant supervision by a clinician who is experienced in the use of antimetabolites. Patients should be fully informed of the risks involved and should be instructed to report promptly any symptoms of toxicity. Because methotrexate is a highly toxic drug, the manufacturers recommend that patients be given no more than a 7-day supply of the drug at one time or, if an intermittent regimen is used (i.e., weekly rather than daily doses), no more than a 1-month supply (e.g., using a mnemonic dispensing package); refills should be only by direct order (i.e., written or oral) of the prescribing clinician. In addition, patients receiving intermittent regimens consisting of weekly rather than daily doses of the drug for the management of rheumatic conditions (e.g., rheumatoid arthritis, psoriasis) and certain inflammatory GI conditions (e.g., Crohn's disease†) should be carefully instructed about their regimen and the frequency of methotrexate administration since mistaken daily use of the drug has resulted in fatalities; patients should be provided with and encouraged to read a copy of the patient instructions supplied by the manufacturer.

Patients receiving methotrexate should be closely monitored for hematologic, renal, hepatic, and pulmonary toxicities, with complete hematologic studies, urinalysis, renal function tests, liver function tests, and chest radiographs. Liver biopsy and bone marrow aspiration studies may be advisable, especially in patients receiving high-dose or prolonged methotrexate therapy. Particular attention to close monitoring is recommended for patients with renal impairment or with pleural effusions or other third-space compartments (e.g., ascites) since elimination of the drug may be impaired. In addition, consideration should be given to evacuating accumulated fluid if possible in patients with substantial compartmental third-spacing prior to methotrexate therapy; monitoring serum concentrations of the drug, reducing drug dosage, or, occasionally, discontinuance of methotrexate also is recommended. Dehydrated patients also are at risk of increased serum methotrexate concentrations. The patient's bleeding time, coagulation time, blood group, and blood type should be on record in case the need for transfusion or surgery arises. If toxic effects or adverse reactions occur, dosage should be reduced or the drug discontinued and appropriate corrective measures taken; however, it should be considered that serious toxic reactions may occur in the absence of abnormal laboratory test results. Severe, occasionally fatal cutaneous reactions have been reported in patients receiving single or multiple oral, IM, IV, or intrathecal doses of methotrexate. These reactions usually occur within days of administration of the drug and recovery has been reported after discontinuance of methotrexate. (See Cautions: Dermatologic and Sensitivity Reactions.)

Hematologic studies must be performed prior to and at frequent intervals during methotrexate therapy. Complete blood cell counts, including differential and platelet counts, generally should be determined at least once weekly in patients receiving the drug for the treatment of neoplastic disease, and at least once monthly in patients receiving the drug for psoriasis or rheumatoid arthritis. If a profound drop in blood cell count occurs, the drug must be immediately discontinued and appropriate alternative therapy instituted. If profound leukopenia and fever occur, the patient should be closely observed and antibiotic therapy should be initiated if there are signs of infection. Blood or platelet transfusions may be necessary in patients with severe bone marrow depression.

There is poor correlation between liver function test results and chronic hepatotoxicity in patients receiving methotrexate, and liver scans are of minimal value in detecting methotrexate hepatotoxicity; liver biopsy is currently the only reliable measure of hepatotoxicity. Nonetheless, hepatic function must be determined prior to initiation of methotrexate and liver function tests, including serum albumin concentrations, should be repeated periodically throughout therapy (at 1- to 2-month intervals in patients treated for psoriasis or rheumatoid arthritis). In patients being treated for psoriasis, liver biopsy should be performed before instituting methotrexate or shortly thereafter (i.e., 2–4 months after). Repeat liver biopsies are recommended after a total cumulative dose of 1.5 g and after additional cumulative doses of 1–1.5 g. In patients with psoriasis, a relationship between abnormal liver function test results and hepatic fibrosis or cirrhosis has not been established, and prolonged, substantial abnormalities in liver function test results may *not* precede appearance of hepatic fibrosis or cirrhosis in such patients. When a pre-methotrexate liver biopsy is not feasible, a liver scan might be useful to detect occult liver disease. Because some patients may discontinue methotrexate after 2–4 months of therapy (due to adverse effects or lack of efficacy), pre-methotrexate liver biopsy might be postponed in patients with psoriasis until this initial period is completed; if long-term methotrexate therapy is anticipated, liver biopsy should then be performed. Abnormal liver function test results frequently occur 1–2 days following a dose of methotrexate, and it is recommended that liver function tests be performed at least 1 week after the last dose of the drug. Because these tests generally return to normal within a few days, repeat tests should be done before performing a liver biopsy. If substantial abnormal liver function test results develop and persist, methotrexate therapy should be withheld for 1–2 weeks and liver function tests repeated. Liver function test results should generally return to normal within 1–2 weeks following discontinuance of the drug; however, if substantial abnormal liver function test results persist, a liver biopsy is recommended.

The decision to perform liver biopsies during methotrexate therapy for rheumatoid arthritis must be carefully individualized. Age at first use of methotrexate and duration of therapy reportedly are risk factors for methotrexate-induced hepatotoxicity. Although unconfirmed to date, it is not known if other risk factors similar to those observed in patients with psoriasis also are present in patients with rheumatoid arthritis. In patients with a history of excessive alcohol consumption, those with prolonged, substantial abnormal liver function test results, or those with chronic hepatitis B or C, liver biopsy should be performed before instituting methotrexate therapy. In patients with rheumatoid arthritis, prolonged, substantial abnormal liver function test results may precede appearance of fibrosis or cirrhosis. In patients with normal liver function, history and physical examination, and no other risk factors (obesity, diabetes mellitus, impaired renal function, history of liver disease, history of IV drug abuse, family history of inheritable liver disease, history of significant exposure to known hepatotoxic drugs), a liver biopsy is recommended after a cumulative methotrexate dosage of approximately 1.5 g. In addition, a liver biopsy should be performed during therapy in patients with prolonged, substantial abnormal liver function test results or with serum albumin concentration below normal values (but whose rheumatoid arthritis is under control). If pre-methotrexate and the first post-methotrexate therapy biopsies show no serious abnormalities and the patient has no risk factors, repeat liver biopsies are recommended every 2–3 years or after additional cumulative dosages of 1–1.5 g. Patients with grade I, II, or IIIA pathologic changes may continue to receive methotrexate therapy, but some clinicians state that those with grade IIIA changes should have a repeat liver biopsy after approximately 6 months of continuous methotrexate therapy. Patients with prolonged, substantial abnormal liver function test results who refuse liver biopsy or those with grade IIIB or IV pathologic changes should not receive further methotrexate therapy; however, occasional patients may require additional therapy with careful follow-up liver biopsies. Concomitant administration of methotrexate and other drugs with hepatotoxic potential including alcohol should be avoided.

Renal function tests should be performed prior to and periodically during methotrexate therapy (at 1- to 2-month intervals in patients with psoriasis or rheumatoid arthritis; more frequent monitoring usually is necessary in patients receiving methotrexate for the treatment of neoplastic disease). If renal impairment develops during methotrexate therapy, dosage should be reduced or the drug discontinued until renal function is improved or restored. In addition, tumor lysis syndrome associated with other cytotoxic drugs (e.g., fludarabine, cladribine) also has been reported in patients with rapidly growing tumors who were receiving methotrexate. Pharmacologic and appropriate supportive treatment may prevent or alleviate this complication.

Malignant lymphomas may occur in patients receiving low-dose methotrexate therapy; such lymphomas may regress following withdrawal of the drug and therefore may not require cytotoxic therapy. However, if lymphomas do not regress following discontinuance of methotrexate, appropriate therapy should be instituted. The manufacturers state that the potential benefits of methotrexate therapy (alone or in combination with other drugs) should be weighed against these potential risks, especially in children or young adults.

Since potentially fatal opportunistic infections (e.g., *Pneumocystis carinii* pneumonia) have been reported in patients receiving methotrexate therapy, the possibility of *P. carinii* pneumonia should be considered in patients who develop pulmonary symptoms. In addition, pulmonary function tests may be useful if methotrexate-induced pulmonary toxicity is suspected, particularly if baseline values are available. For other precautions associated with the potential toxic effects of the drug on the lungs, see Cautions: Pulmonary Effects.

The immunosuppressive action of methotrexate must be considered when evaluating use of the drug in patients in whom immune responses may be important or essential. In patients at high risk for acquired immunodeficiency syndrome (AIDS), an HIV antibody determination should be considered because of the potential for additive immunosuppression and increased risk of opportunistic infections. Two psoriatic patients developed tuberculosis while receiving methotrexate and it has been suggested that, in addition to a chest radiograph, a tuberculin skin test should be performed prior to initiation of methotrexate therapy. If the initial tuberculin test is positive, isoniazid preventive therapy (see 8:16.04) should be initiated concomitantly with methotrexate therapy. Since an accurate evaluation of the tuberculin test is not possible in patients receiving methotrexate, chest radiographs should be repeated every 6 months during therapy in these patients.

Methotrexate should be used with extreme caution in patients with infection, peptic ulcer, ulcerative colitis, or debility, and in very young or geriatric patients. Methotrexate should be used with extreme caution, if at all, in patients with malignant disease who have preexisting liver damage or impaired hepatic function, preexisting bone marrow depression, aplasia, leukopenia, thrombocytopenia, or anemia; the drug is usually contraindicated in patients with impaired renal function. In the management of psoriasis or rheumatoid arthritis, methotrexate is contraindicated in patients with preexisting blood dyscrasias such as bone marrow hypoplasia, leukopenia, thrombocytopenia, or clinically important anemia; those with overt or laboratory evidence of immunodeficiency syndromes; and those with excessive alcohol consumption, alcoholic liver disease, or chronic liver disease.

● Pediatric Precautions

The manufacturer states that safety and efficacy of methotrexate in pediatric patients for the management of any conditions other than cancer chemotherapy or polyarticular-course juvenile rheumatoid arthritis have not been established. Severe neurotoxic effects, manifested mainly by focal or generalized seizures, have been reported with increased frequency in pediatric patients with acute lymphoblastic leukemia who were receiving intermediate-dose IV methotrexate (1 g/m²). Leukoencephalopathy and/or microangiopathic calcifications usually were observed in diagnostic imaging procedures of symptomatic patients.

● Mutagenicity and Carcinogenicity

Methotrexate has been reported to cause chromosome damage. Although patients who had previously received methotrexate have conceived and borne normal children, both men and women should be advised to avoid conception during and immediately following methotrexate therapy so that normal production of germinal cells may be reestablished. (See Cautions: Pregnancy, Fertility, and Lactation.) It has been suggested that methotrexate may be carcinogenic; however, extensive epidemiologic studies are required before its carcinogenicity can be confirmed or refuted. Malignant lymphomas (e.g., non-Hodgkin's lymphoma) may occur in patients receiving low-dose oral methotrexate therapy; such lymphomas may regress following withdrawal of the drug and, therefore, may not require cytotoxic therapy. However, if lymphomas do not regress following discontinuance of methotrexate, appropriate therapy should be instituted. Therefore, the manufacturers state that the potential benefits of methotrexate therapy (alone or in combination with other drugs) should be weighed against these potential risks, especially in children or young adults.

• Pregnancy, Fertility, and Lactation

Pregnancy

Abortion, fetal death, and/or congenital anomalies have occurred in pregnant women receiving methotrexate, especially during the first trimester of pregnancy. Methotrexate is contraindicated in the management of psoriasis or rheumatoid arthritis in pregnant women. Women of childbearing potential should not receive methotrexate until pregnancy is excluded. For the management of psoriasis or rheumatoid arthritis, methotrexate therapy in women should be started immediately following a menstrual period and appropriate measures should be taken in men or women to avoid conception during and for at least 12 weeks following methotrexate therapy. Both men and women receiving methotrexate should be informed of the potential risk of adverse effects on reproduction. Women of childbearing potential should be fully informed of the potential hazard to the fetus should they become pregnant during methotrexate therapy. In cancer chemotherapy, methotrexate should not be used in pregnant women or women of childbearing potential who might become pregnant unless the potential benefits to the mother outweigh the possible risks to the fetus.

Fertility

Defective oogenesis or spermatogenesis, transient oligospermia, menstrual dysfunction, and infertility have been reported in patients receiving methotrexate.

Lactation

Methotrexate is distributed into breast milk. Because of the potential for serious adverse reactions to methotrexate in nursing infants, the drug is contraindicated in nursing women.

DRUG INTERACTIONS

• Protein-bound Drugs and Weak Organic Acids

Because methotrexate is partly bound to serum proteins, its toxicity may be increased as a result of displacement by certain drugs such as salicylates, sulfonamides, sulfonylureas, phenytoin, phenylbutazone, tetracyclines, chloramphenicol, and aminobenzoic acid. Until the clinical importance of these findings is established, these drugs should be given cautiously in patients receiving methotrexate. In addition, the possibility that weak organic acids, including salicylates, may delay renal excretion of methotrexate and increase accumulation should be considered.

• Nonsteroidal Anti-inflammatory Agents

Severe, sometimes fatal, toxicity (including hematologic and GI toxicity) has occurred following administration of a NSAIA (e.g., indomethacin, ketoprofen) concomitantly with methotrexate (particularly with high-dose therapy) in patients with various malignant neoplasms, psoriasis, or rheumatoid arthritis. The toxicity was associated with elevated and prolonged serum concentrations of methotrexate. The exact mechanism of the interaction remains to be established, but it has been suggested that NSAIAs may inhibit renal elimination of methotrexate, possibly by decreasing renal perfusion via inhibition of renal prostaglandin synthesis or by competing for renal elimination.

NSAIAs should be avoided in patients receiving relatively high dosages of methotrexate (e.g., those used in the treatment of neoplastic disease). The risk of concomitant low-dose, intermittent (e.g., 5–15 mg weekly) methotrexate therapy and NSAIAs has not been fully elucidated, but the drugs have been used concomitantly in many patients receiving methotrexate for the management of rheumatoid arthritis. However, in clinical studies in which the drugs were used concomitantly, the patients often were monitored closely and were receiving relatively stable dosages of NSAIAs; in addition, those with conditions that might predispose to methotrexate toxicity generally were excluded from the studies. NSAIAs should be used with caution in patients receiving low-dose methotrexate regimens such as those employed in the management of rheumatoid arthritis, and the possibility of increased and prolonged serum methotrexate concentrations and resultant toxicity should be considered. Although intermittent regimens also are used in the management of psoriasis, methotrexate dosages in such regimens usually are higher than those used in the management of rheumatoid arthritis and therefore are more likely to result in toxicity during concomitant NSAIA therapy; serious toxicity, including at least one death, has been reported in several patients with psoriasis receiving combined therapy with the drugs. Further study is needed to evaluate the interaction between NSAIAs and methotrexate.

• Penicillins

Concomitant use of penicillins (e.g., amoxicillin, carbenicillin) may decrease renal clearance of methotrexate, presumably by inhibiting renal tubular secretion of the drug. Increased serum concentrations of methotrexate, resulting in GI or hematologic toxicity, have been reported in patients receiving low- or high-dose methotrexate therapy concomitantly with penicillins, and patients receiving the drugs concomitantly should be carefully monitored.

• Proton-Pump Inhibitors

Although no formal drug interaction studies have been conducted with methotrexate and proton-pump inhibitors, data from case reports, population pharmacokinetic studies, and retrospective analyses suggest that concomitant use of methotrexate (particularly at high dosages) with proton-pump inhibitors (e.g., esomeprazole, omeprazole, pantoprazole) may decrease methotrexate clearance, resulting in elevated and prolonged serum concentrations of methotrexate and/or its metabolite hydroxymethotrexate and possibly leading to methotrexate toxicities. Increased concentrations of methotrexate and/or hydroxymethotrexate with or without associated adverse effects (e.g., renal toxicity, adverse hematologic effects, severe mucositis, myalgia) have been reported when methotrexate dosages ranging from 300 mg/m^2 to 12 g/m^2 were administered concomitantly with proton-pump inhibitors. Although the majority of reported cases occurred in patients receiving high dosages of methotrexate, methotrexate toxicity also has been reported following concomitant administration of *low* dosages of methotrexate (15 mg per week) with a proton-pump inhibitor. Therefore, the manufacturers of proton-pump inhibitors state that temporary discontinuance of proton-pump inhibitor therapy may be considered in some patients receiving high-dose methotrexate. Some clinicians specifically recommend withholding proton-pump inhibitor therapy for several days before, during, and for several days after methotrexate administration; in patients in whom acid suppression is clinically indicated during methotrexate therapy, substitution of a histamine H$_2$-receptor antagonist (e.g., ranitidine) for the proton-pump inhibitor may be considered. Pending further evaluation, some clinicians state that these recommendations should extend to patients receiving low-dose methotrexate.

• Other Drugs

Drugs with similar pharmacologic activity such as pyrimethamine should not be given to patients receiving methotrexate.

Concomitant use of other potentially hepatotoxic drugs (e.g., retinoids, azathioprine, sulfasalazine) and methotrexate may increase the risk of hepatotoxicity; patients receiving concomitant therapy with these drugs should be closely monitored.

Although concomitant use of methotrexate with cisplatin exhibits possible synergistic antineoplastic effects, cisplatin may alter renal elimination of methotrexate. Caution is advised if high-dose methotrexate is administered in conjunction with cisplatin for the treatment of osteosarcoma.

Co-trimoxazole should be used with caution in patients receiving methotrexate, since sulfonamides can displace methotrexate from plasma protein-binding sites resulting in increased free methotrexate concentrations.

It has been suggested that folic acid preparations including vitamin products may decrease the effectiveness of methotrexate therapy and should not be given to patients receiving methotrexate; however, there have been no clinical studies to support or refute this hypothesis.

Methotrexate increases plasma mercaptopurine concentrations; dosage adjustment may be necessary.

Probenecid diminishes renal tubular transport of methotrexate; patients should be carefully monitored during concomitant use of these agents.

Methotrexate may decrease clearance of theophylline; serum theophylline concentrations should be monitored in patients receiving theophylline concomitantly with methotrexate.

Vaccination with live virus vaccines generally should not be performed in patients receiving methotrexate. Disseminated vaccinia infection has been reported following smallpox vaccination in at least one patient receiving methotrexate. Although the antibody response to killed virus vaccines is not normal, partial or complete protection may still be attained and these vaccines may be used if necessary in patients receiving methotrexate.

ACUTE TOXICITY

● Treatment

Treatment of toxicity resulting from impaired elimination or an inadvertent overdosage of methotrexate consists of administration of a folic acid antidote (i.e., leucovorin, levoleucovorin) with or without a carboxypeptidase G2 (i.e., glucarpidase); however, glucarpidase is indicated only for the treatment of toxic plasma methotrexate concentrations (exceeding 0.454 mcg/mL [1 μM]) in patients with delayed methotrexate clearance due to renal impairment. Because of the potential for subtherapeutic concentrations of methotrexate, glucarpidase should not be used in patients who exhibit the expected clearance of methotrexate or in those with normal or mildly impaired renal function.

In cases of inadvertent overdosage of methotrexate, leucovorin or levoleucovorin should be administered as soon as possible. In patients with impaired elimination of methotrexate, leucovorin or levoleucovorin should be administered within 24 hours of methotrexate administration when there is delayed methotrexate excretion. Leucovorin or levoleucovorin should *not* be administered intrathecally. As the time interval between methotrexate administration and rescue therapy with leucovorin or levoleucovorin increases, the effectiveness of either drug in counteracting methotrexate toxicity may decrease. Serum creatinine and methotrexate concentrations should be determined at 24-hour intervals. The optimal dose of leucovorin or levoleucovorin should be determined based on serum methotrexate concentrations. (See Leucovorin Calcium 92:12 and Levoleucovorin Calcium 92:12.)

If glucarpidase is used, rescue therapy with leucovorin or levoleucovorin should be continued following administration of the drug; however, because leucovorin is a substrate for glucarpidase (and the pharmacokinetics of levoleucovorin and leucovorin are comparable), leucovorin and levoleucovorin should not be administered within 2 hours before or after a dose of glucarpidase. During the first 48 hours following administration of glucarpidase, leucovorin or levoleucovorin should be administered at the dose utilized prior to administration of glucarpidase. After 48 hours, the dose of leucovorin or levoleucovorin should be determined based on plasma methotrexate concentrations. (See Glucarpidase 92:12.)

For specific information on dosage modifications, cautions, and precautions associated with impaired methotrexate elimination or an inadvertent overdosage, the manufacturer's prescribing information should be consulted.

If accidental overdosage of intrathecal methotrexate occurs, intensive systemic supportive therapy (e.g., administration of high-dose leucovorin calcium, alkaline diuresis, rapid CSF drainage, ventriculolumbar perfusion) may be required (see Cautions: Effects following Intrathecal Administration).

In case of severe overdosage of methotrexate, hydration and urinary alkalinization may be needed to prevent precipitation of the drug and/or its metabolites in the renal tubules. Hemodialysis and peritoneal dialysis generally have been ineffective in improving the elimination of methotrexate. However, effective clearance of methotrexate has been reported with the use of acute, intermittent hemodialysis with a high-flux polysulfone dialyzer (the F-80B Fresenius Dialyzer) in a small number of patients with acute renal failure secondary to methotrexate or with end-stage renal disease unrelated to methotrexate therapy.

For additional information on the treatment of intrathecal methotrexate overdosage, see Cautions: Effects following Intrathecal Administration.

PHARMACOLOGY

Methotrexate and its polyglutamate metabolites reversibly inhibit dihydrofolate reductase, the enzyme that reduces folic acid to tetrahydrofolic acid. Inhibition of tetrahydrofolate formation limits the availability of one-carbon fragments necessary for synthesis of purines and the conversion of deoxyuridylate to thymidylate in the synthesis of DNA and cell reproduction. The affinity of dihydrofolate reductase for methotrexate is far greater than its affinity for folic acid or dihydrofolic acid and, therefore, even very large doses of folic acid given simultaneously will not reverse the effects of methotrexate. Leucovorin calcium, a derivative of tetrahydrofolic acid, may block the effects of methotrexate if given shortly

after the antineoplastic agent. Results of one study indicate that methotrexate also causes an increase in intracellular deoxyadenosine triphosphate, which is thought to inhibit ribonucleotide reduction, and polynucleotide ligase, an enzyme concerned in DNA synthesis and repair. Tissues with high rates of cellular proliferation such as neoplasms, psoriatic epidermis, bone marrow, the lining of the GI tract, hair matrix, and fetal cells are most sensitive to the effects of methotrexate.

Resistance to methotrexate may develop and has been associated with decreased cellular uptake of the drug, increased dihydrofolate reductase activity (associated with increased synthesis of the enzyme), decreased binding of methotrexate to dihydrofolate reductase (because of mutated dihydrofolate reductase protein), and decreased intracellular concentrations of polyglutamylated metabolites of methotrexate; however, the precise mechanism of this resistance development has not been established.

Methotrexate also has immunosuppressive activity, in part possibly as a result of inhibition of lymphocyte multiplication. The mechanism(s) of action in the management of rheumatoid arthritis of the drug is not known, although suggested mechanisms have included immunosuppressive and/or anti-inflammatory effects.

PHARMACOKINETICS

● Absorption

Oral absorption of methotrexate appears to be highly variable and dose dependent. While older studies demonstrated good absorption from the GI tract with relatively low oral doses of methotrexate, more recent studies indicate that the oral bioavailability of the drug may be below 50% even at relatively low doses (i.e., 15 mg/m^2 or lower). The bioavailability of methotrexate decreases with increasing oral doses (suggesting the presence of a saturable absorption process) and absorption is substantially reduced at doses exceeding 80 mg/m^2. Studies investigating the use of divided doses of methotrexate in an attempt to improve the oral bioavailability of the drug have shown conflicting results. It has been suggested that poor bioavailability should be assumed with oral methotrexate doses of 100 mg/m^2 or greater, regardless of the dosage schedule used. Food delays absorption and decreases peak serum concentrations of the drug. Peak serum concentrations of methotrexate generally are achieved in 1–2 hours following oral administration in adults.

Oral administration of methotrexate in pediatric patients with leukemia reportedly results in wide variability in the rate and extent of oral absorption. Oral bioavailability of 23–95%, with a 20-fold difference between the highest and lowest peak serum concentration measurements (range: 0.11–2.3 μM), has been reported in pediatric patients receiving oral methotrexate 20 mg/m^2 for the treatment of leukemia. Substantial variability in the time to peak serum concentration also has been observed; in patients receiving methotrexate at an oral dose of 15 mg/m^2, the time to peak serum concentration ranged from 0.67–4 hours.

Methotrexate appears to be completely absorbed following IM administration at doses of up to at least 100 mg. Peak serum concentrations are achieved 30–60 minutes after IM administration of the drug. Serum concentrations following intra-arterial administration are similar to those achieved following IV administration.

● Distribution

Methotrexate is actively transported across cell membranes. At serum methotrexate concentrations exceeding 0.1 μmol/mL, passive diffusion becomes a major means of intracellular transport of the drug. The drug is widely distributed into body tissues with highest concentrations in the kidneys, gallbladder, spleen, liver, and skin. Following systemic administration of a single dose of methotrexate, the drug inhibits DNA synthesis in psoriatic epidermis for 12–16 hours. Following oral or IV administration of the drug to animals, synovial fluid methotrexate concentrations are higher in inflamed than in uninflamed joints; concurrent administration of salicylates did not affect distribution of methotrexate into joints, but pretreatment with prednisone reduced the amount of drug distributed into inflamed joints relative to that into normal joints. In patients receiving long-term, oral methotrexate therapy for rheumatoid arthritis, the ratio of synovial fluid to serum concentrations of methotrexate ranged from 0.9–1.2. Methotrexate distributes into third space fluids, and the presence of pleural effusions or ascites can substantially alter the disposition of the drug (see Pharmacokinetics: Elimination). Slow release of methotrexate from third space accumulations may prolong the terminal half-life and may increase the risk of drug toxicity with high doses (i.e., exceeding 250 mg/m^2).

Methotrexate is retained for several weeks in the kidneys and for months in the liver. Sustained serum concentrations and tissue accumulation of methotrexate may result from repeated daily doses. Following IV administration, an initial volume of distribution of approximately 0.18 L/kg and a steady-state volume of distribution of approximately 0.4–0.8 L/kg have been reported. According to the manufacturer, the drug does not reach therapeutic concentrations in the CSF when given orally or parenterally. However, high-dose systemic methotrexate therapy can result in peak CSF concentrations above the therapeutic threshold of 0.001 μmol/mL and has been used to prevent meningeal leukemia and lymphoma. Following IV administration of methotrexate, CSF drug concentrations are dose related; a CSF concentration of 0.0001 μmol/mL was reported after a dose of 500 mg/m^{2}y 24-hour IV infusion, and CSF concentrations exceeding 0.01 μmol/mL were observed following an IV bolus dose of 7500 mg/m^2. Intrathecal administration of methotrexate may result in potentially cytotoxic serum drug concentrations that can persist for 24–48 hours.

Methotrexate crosses the placental barrier. Methotrexate is distributed into breast milk; the highest reported breast milk plasma concentration ratio, which occurred 10 hours after administration of a 22.5-mg oral dose, was 0.08:1. (See Cautions: Pregnancy, Fertility, and Lactation.)

At serum concentrations of 0.001–0.1 μmol/mL, about 50% of the drug is bound to plasma proteins (primarily albumin).

● Elimination

In patients receiving methotrexate for the treatment of psoriasis or rheumatoid arthritis, or as low-dose antineoplastic therapy (i.e., less than 30 mg/m^2), a terminal half-life of about 3–10 hours has been reported. Higher doses of methotrexate have been associated with a longer elimination half-life of about 8–15 hours.

Plasma concentrations of methotrexate following high-dose IV infusion appear to decline in a biphasic manner. The half-life of the initial phase (t$_{½α}$) averages 1.5–3.5 hours in patients with normal total body clearance and the half-life in the terminal phase (t$_{½β}$) is about 8–15 hours.

After absorption, methotrexate undergoes hepatic and intracellular metabolism to form methotrexate polyglutamates, metabolites which by hydrolysis may be converted back to methotrexate. Methotrexate polyglutamates inhibit dihydrofolate reductase and thymidylate synthetase. Small amounts of these polyglutamate metabolites may remain in tissues for extended periods; the retention and prolonged action of these active metabolites vary among different cells, tissues, and tumors. In addition, small amounts of methotrexate polyglutamates may be converted to 7-hydroxymethotrexate; accumulation of this metabolite may become substantial following administration of high doses of methotrexate, since the aqueous solubility of 7-hydroxymethotrexate is threefold to fivefold lower than that of the parent compound. Following oral administration of methotrexate, the drug also is partially metabolized by the intestinal flora.

The drug is excreted primarily by the kidneys via glomerular filtration and active transport. Small amounts are excreted in the feces, probably via the bile. Methotrexate has a biphasic excretion pattern. Up to 92% of a single dose is excreted within 24 hours following IV administration followed by excretion of 1–2% of the retained dose daily. In one study, 58–92% of an IV methotrexate dose of 0.1–10 mg/kg was excreted in the urine within 24 hours. Only slightly less urinary excretion occurred following oral administration of 0.1 mg/kg. Following oral administration of 10 mg/kg, however, only 15% of the dose was excreted in the urine within 24 hours and 48% within 5 days. About 39% of the larger oral dose was recovered in the feces as compared to 7–9% following 0.1 mg/kg administered orally and 2–5% of 0.1–10 mg/kg administered IV. Enterohepatic recirculation of methotrexate may occur. Methotrexate excretion is impaired and accumulation occurs more rapidly in patients with impaired renal function, pleural effusions, or those with other third-space compartments (e.g., ascites). In addition, simultaneous administration of other weak organic acids such as salicylates may suppress methotrexate clearance.

CHEMISTRY AND STABILITY

● Chemistry

Methotrexate is a mixture containing at least 85% 4-amino-10-methylfolic acid, calculated on the anhydrous basis, and small amounts of related compounds. Methotrexate is a folic acid antagonist. Structurally, the primary constituent of methotrexate differs from folic acid in the substitution of an amino group for a hydroxyl group in the pteridine nucleus and in the addition of a methyl group on the amino nitrogen between the pteroyl and benzoyl groups. Methotrexate is a weak acid that occurs as an orange-brown, crystalline powder and is practically insoluble in water and in alcohol. Great care should be taken to prevent inhaling particles of the chemical and exposing the skin to it. Methotrexate sodium occurs as a yellow powder and is soluble in water. Methotrexate sodium injection has a pH of 7.5–9. Commercially available injections of methotrexate sodium are available with benzyl alcohol as a preservative or without a preservative.

● Stability

Methotrexate sodium tablets should be protected from light and stored in well-closed containers at 20–25°C. Methotrexate sodium injection and powder for injection should be protected from light and stored at 20–25°C. Stability and compatibility of methotrexate sodium solutions depend on several factors including the formulation of methotrexate sodium used, presence of preservatives, concentration of drug(s), specific diluents used, resulting pH, and temperature; the manufacturers' labeling and specialized references should be consulted for specific information.

For further information on the handling of antineoplastic agents, see the ASHP Guidelines on Handling Hazardous Drugs at https://www.ahfsdrug information.com.

PREPARATIONS

Excipients in commercially available drug preparations may have clinically important effects in some individuals; consult specific product labeling for details.

Methotrexate Sodium

Oral		
Tablets	2.5 mg (of methotrexate)*	**Methotrexate Sodium Tablets** (scored)
		Rheumatrex® Dose Pack (scored), Dava
Tablets, film coated	5 mg (of methotrexate)	**Trexall®** (scored), Duramed
	7.5 mg (of methotrexate)	**Trexall®** (scored), Duramed
	10 mg (of methotrexate)	**Trexall®** (scored), Duramed
	15 mg (of methotrexate)	**Trexall®** (scored), Duramed

Parenteral		
For injection	1 g (of methotrexate)*	**Methotrexate Sodium for Injection**
Injection	10 mg (of methotrexate) per mL*	**Methotrexate Sodium Injection Isotonic**
	25 mg (of methotrexate) per mL*	**Methotrexate Sodium Injection Isotonic**

* available from one or more manufacturer, distributor, and/or repackager by generic (nonproprietary) name

† Use is not currently included in the labeling approved by the US Food and Drug Administration.

Neratinib Maleate

10:00 • ANTINEOPLASTIC AGENTS

- Neratinib, a potent, selective, and irreversible inhibitor of human epidermal growth factor receptor type 2 (HER2), HER4, and epidermal growth factor receptor (EGFR) tyrosine kinases, is an antineoplastic agent.

USES

● Breast Cancer

Extended Adjuvant Therapy for Early-stage Breast Cancer

Neratinib is used as extended adjuvant therapy in adults with human epidermal growth factor receptor type 2 (HER2)-positive, early-stage breast cancer who have received adjuvant trastuzumab therapy. Safety and efficacy of neratinib for this indication are supported by a single randomized controlled trial. Guidelines generally suggest that neratinib may be used for extended adjuvant therapy in patients with early-stage, HER2-positive breast cancer after receiving treatment with trastuzumab plus chemotherapy.

Clinical Experience

This indication for neratinib is based principally on the results of a randomized, double-blind, placebo-controlled phase 3 study (ExteNET) in women with HER2-positive early-stage breast cancer who completed neoadjuvant and adjuvant trastuzumab therapy within 2 years of randomization. In this study, 2840 patients were randomized (stratified by hormone receptor status, nodal status, and adjuvant trastuzumab regimen) to receive either neratinib (240 mg orally once daily) or placebo. Treatment was continued for 12 months unless disease progression, new breast cancer, or unacceptable toxicity occurred, or treatment was discontinued for other reasons. The primary measure of efficacy was invasive disease-free survival. The median age of patients enrolled in the study was 52 years; 81% of the patients were white, 99.7% had an ECOG (Eastern Cooperative Oncology Group) performance status of 0 or 1, 57% had hormone receptor-positive disease, and 30% had 4 or more positive nodes. Most patients (81%) were enrolled within 1 year of completion of adjuvant trastuzumab therapy; the median time from completion of adjuvant trastuzumab therapy to randomization was 4.4 or 4.6 months in patients randomized to neratinib or placebo, respectively.

At a follow-up of 2 years, invasive disease-free survival rates were 94.2 or 91.9% in patients receiving neratinib or placebo, respectively. Subgroup analysis suggested that neratinib had a greater effect on invasive disease-free survival relative to placebo in patients with hormone receptor-positive disease than in those with hormone receptor-negative disease (hazard ratio: 0.49 and 0.93, respectively), in those who received sequential adjuvant trastuzumab therapy than in those who received adjuvant trastuzumab concurrently with chemotherapy (hazard ratio: 0.46 and 0.80, respectively), and in those who completed adjuvant trastuzumab therapy within 1 year of randomization than in those who completed adjuvant trastuzumab therapy 1-2 years prior to randomization (hazard ratio: 0.63 and 0.92, respectively). Median overall survival had not been reached at the time of the efficacy analysis. A final analysis of the ExteNET study separately reported 5-year rates of invasive disease-free survival among patients who were hormone receptor-positive and received neratinib within 1 year of completion of trastuzumab or in those who received neratinib more than 1 year after completion of trastuzumab. In patients who were hormone receptor-positive who received treatment within 1 year of completion of trastuzumab, 5-year rates of invasive disease-free survival were 90.8% in patients treated with neratinib and 85.7% in patients treated with placebo. In patients who were hormone receptor-positive who received treatment more than 1 year after completion of trastuzumab, 5-year rates of invasive disease-free survival were 93% in patients treated with neratinib and 91.7% in patients treated with placebo. After a median of 8 years of follow-up (median duration of study treatment 11.5 and 11.9 months with neratinib and placebo, respectively), estimated overall survival rates were 91.5% in patients receiving neratinib and 89.4% in those receiving placebo; this difference was not found to be statistically significant.

Clinical Perspective

In the 2020 American Society of Clinical Oncology (ASCO) guidelines on selection of optimal adjuvant chemotherapy and targeted therapy for early breast cancer, adjuvant trastuzumab emtansine is recommended for patients with HER2-positive breast cancer with pathologic invasive residual disease at surgery after receiving standard preoperative chemotherapy and HER2-targeted therapy. In this setting, trastuzumab is recommended in combination with chemotherapy for all patients with HER2-positive, node-positive breast cancer and for patients with HER2-positive, node-negative breast cancer with tumors greater than 1 cm. Neratinib is suggested as an option for extended adjuvant therapy in patients with early-stage, HER2-positive breast cancer; the greatest potential benefit appears to be derived when neratinib is administered within 1 year of completion of trastuzumab treatment. The guideline further notes that use of neratinib is preferred in hormone receptor-positive and node-positive patients.

Advanced or Metastatic Breast Cancer

Neratinib is used in combination with capecitabine to treat advanced or metastatic HER2-positive breast cancer in adults who have received at least 2 prior anti-HER2 treatment regimens in the metastatic setting. Safety and efficacy of neratinib for this indication are supported by a single randomized controlled trial. Guidelines generally recommend neratinib among several potential third-line treatment options in patients whose advanced, HER2-positive breast cancer has progressed during or after 2 previous anti-HER2 regimens.

Clinical Experience

This indication for neratinib is based principally on the results of a randomized, open label, active-controlled multicenter study (NALA) in adults with HER2-positive metastatic breast cancer who had previously received 2 or more anti-HER2-based regimens. In this study, 621 patients were randomized (stratified by hormone receptor status, number of previous HER2-directed treatments for metastatic breast cancer, geographic region, and visceral disease) to receive oral administration of either neratinib 240 mg once daily on cycle days 1-21 plus capecitabine 750 mg/m^2 twice daily on days 1-14 of each 21-day cycle or lapatinib 1250 mg daily on cycle days 1-21 plus capecitabine 1000 mg/m^2 twice daily on days 1-14 of each 21-day cycle. Treatment was continued until disease progression or unacceptable toxicity occurred. The co-primary measures of efficacy were independently adjudicated progression-free survival and overall survival. At baseline, 59% of enrolled patients were hormone receptor-positive, 69% had received 2 prior anti-HER2 based regimens, and 31% had received 3 or more previous anti-HER2 based regimens; 81% of patients had visceral disease.

At a median follow-up of 29.9 months, median progression-free survival was 5.6 months in the neratinib plus capecitabine group compared with 5.5 months in the lapatinib plus capecitabine group. These results were generally consistent across subgroups based on disease location, hormone receptor status, and previous HER2 regimens. At the time of follow-up, median overall survival was similar with neratinib plus capecitabine versus lapatinib plus capecitabine (21 or 18.7 months, respectively).

Clinical Perspective

In the 2022 ASCO guidelines on systemic treatment for advanced HER2-positive breast cancer, first-line recommended treatment includes a combination of trastuzumab, pertuzumab, and a taxane. Trastuzumab deruxtecan is recommended for second-line treatment of patients whose breast cancer progresses after initial HER2-targeted treatment. Multiple potential treatment options are recommended for third-line treatment, including neratinib in combination with capecitabine. Selection of an appropriate regimen should be made after discussing treatment schedules, routes of administration, and adverse effects with the patient.

DOSAGE AND ADMINISTRATION

● General

Pretreatment Screening

- Measure total bilirubin, AST, ALT, and alkaline phosphatase prior to initiating treatment with neratinib.

- Perform pregnancy testing in females of reproductive potential prior to starting neratinib.

Patient Monitoring

- Measure liver function tests monthly for the first 3 months of treatment with neratinib, then every 3 months during treatment and as clinically indicated.

- Monitor patients for diarrhea during treatment with neratinib and administer antidiarrheal therapy as needed.

Premedication and Prophylaxis

- To minimize the incidence and severity of treatment-related diarrhea, antidiarrheal prophylaxis with loperamide (initiated with the first dose of neratinib and continued during the first 56 days of treatment) is recommended in patients not using a dose escalation approach. The manufacturer recommends taking loperamide hydrochloride 4 mg 3 times daily during weeks 1–2 (days 1–14), followed by 4 mg twice daily during weeks 3–8 (days 15–56), and then 4 mg as needed from week 9 until discontinuation of neratinib; the daily dosage of loperamide hydrochloride should not exceed 16 mg. After the first 56 days of therapy, dosage of loperamide should be adjusted to maintain a bowel movement frequency of 1–2 per day.

● Administration

Neratinib maleate is administered orally with food. The drug should be taken at approximately the same time each day.

Neratinib tablets should be swallowed whole; tablets should *not* be chewed, crushed, or split.

Store neratinib tablets at a controlled room temperature of 20–25°C (excursions permitted between 15–30°C).

● Dosage

Dosage of neratinib maleate is expressed in terms of neratinib.

Breast Cancer

Extended Adjuvant Therapy for Early-stage Breast Cancer

For extended adjuvant treatment of human epidermal growth factor receptor type 2 (HER2)-positive early-stage breast cancer following adjuvant trastuzumab-based therapy, the recommended adult dosage of neratinib is 240 mg (6 tablets) orally once daily, given continuously for up to one year or until disease recurrence.

A 2-week dose escalation may be considered to minimize the risk of diarrhea (see Table 1):

TABLE 1. Neratinib Dose Escalation Schedule

Time on Neratinib	Dose
Week 1 (days 1–7)	120 mg daily (three 40-mg tablets)
Week 2 (days 8–14)	160 mg daily (four 40-mg tablets)
Week 3 and onwards	240 mg daily (six 40-mg tablets)[a]

[a] Recommended dosage

Advanced or Metastatic Breast Cancer

For use in combination with capecitabine in the treatment of HER2-positive advanced or metastatic breast cancer, the recommended adult dosage of neratinib is 240 mg (6 tablets) once daily given orally on days 1–21 of a 21-day cycle. Capecitabine 750 mg/m² is administered orally twice daily on days 1–14 of a 21-day cycle. Continue therapy until disease progression or unacceptable toxicity occurs.

A 2-week dose escalation may be considered to minimize the risk of diarrhea (see Table 2):

TABLE 2. Neratinib Dose Escalation Schedule

Time on Neratinib	Dose
Week 1 (days 1–7)	120 mg daily (three 40-mg tablets)
Week 2 (days 8–14)	160 mg daily (four 40-mg tablets)
Week 3 and onwards	240 mg daily (six 40-mg tablets)[a]

[a] Recommended dosage

Dosage Modification for Toxicity

Dosage interruption and/or reduction or discontinuance of neratinib therapy may be necessary based on severity of adverse reactions. Dosage adjustment of neratinib is recommended based on individual safety and tolerability.

Discontinue neratinib in patients with persistent grade 2 or greater adverse effects that do not recover to grade 0–1 or baseline and patients with any toxicity that requires a treatment delay of greater than 3 weeks; discontinuance of therapy is also recommended in those who cannot tolerate a dosage of 120 mg daily.

Monotherapy

If dosage modification of neratinib monotherapy is required for toxicity, reduce the dosage of neratinib as described in Table 3.

TABLE 3. Recommended Dosage Modification for Toxicity with Neratinib Monotherapy

Dose Reduction Level	Neratinib Dosage (Starting Dosage = 240 mg once daily)
First	Restart at 200 mg daily (five 40-mg tablets)
Second	Restart at 160 mg daily (four 40-mg tablets)
Third	Restart at 120 mg daily (three 40-mg tablets)

If an adverse reaction occurs, modify dosage accordingly (see Table 4).

TABLE 4. Recommended Dosage Modification for Toxicity with Neratinib Monotherapy

Adverse Reaction and Severity	Modification
Diarrhea	
Grade 1 (<4 stools per day over baseline) or	Adjust antidiarrheal treatment, modify diet, and maintain fluid intake of about 2 L/day to avoid dehydration
Grade 2 (4–6 stools per day over baseline) lasting ≤5 days or	Once diarrhea resolves to ≤ grade 1, initiate loperamide hydrochloride 4 mg with each subsequent administration of neratinib
Grade 3 (≥7 stools per day over baseline, fecal incontinence, need for hospitalization, limiting self-care activities of daily living) lasting ≤2 days	
Any grade with additional complicating features[a] or	Withhold therapy; modify diet, and maintain fluid intake of about 2 L/day to avoid dehydration
Grade 2 lasting >5 days despite treatment with optimal medical therapy or	If diarrhea resolves to ≤grade 1 within 1 week, resume neratinib at same dosage
Grade 3 lasting >2 days despite treatment with optimal medical therapy	If diarrhea resolves to ≤grade 1 in longer than 1 week, resume neratinib at a reduced dosage (see Table 3)
	Once event resolves to ≤ grade 1 or baseline, initiate loperamide hydrochloride 4 mg with each subsequent administration of neratinib

TABLE 4. Continued

Adverse Reaction and Severity	Modification
Grade 4 (life-threatening diarrhea or need for urgent intervention)	Permanently discontinue therapy
Recurrence of grade 2 or higher diarrhea at a dosage of 120 mg daily	Permanently discontinue therapy
Hepatotoxicity	
Grade 3 ALT or AST (>5–20 × ULN) or Grade 3 bilirubin (>3–10 × ULN)	Withhold therapy until recovery to ≤grade 1 and evaluate for alternative causes
	If recovery to ≤grade 1 occurs within 3 weeks, resume neratinib at the next lower dose level (see Table 3)
	If grade 3 hepatotoxicity recurs after one dose reduction, permanently discontinue therapy
Grade 4 ALT or AST (>20 × ULN) or Grade 4 bilirubin (>10 × ULN)	Permanently discontinue therapy and evaluate for alternative causes
Other Adverse Effects	
Grade 3	Withhold therapy; if adverse effect resolves to ≤ grade 1 or baseline within 3 weeks, resume at next dose level (see Table 3)
Grade 4	Permanently discontinue therapy

a Additional complicating features include dehydration, pyrexia, hypotension, renal failure, or grade 3–4 neutropenia

Combination Therapy with Capecitabine

If an adverse reaction occurs when neratinib is used in combination with capecitabine, refer to the prescribing information for capecitabine for dosage modifications of capecitabine and reduce the dosage of neratinib as described in Table 5.

TABLE 5. Recommended Dosage Modification for Toxicity with Neratinib in Combination with Capecitabine

Dose Reduction Level	Neratinib Dosage (Starting Dosage = 240 mg once daily)
First	Restart at 160 mg daily (four 40-mg tablets)
Second	Restart at 120 mg daily (three 40-mg tablets)

If an adverse reaction occurs when neratinib is used in combination with capecitabine, modify the dosage accordingly (see Table 6).

TABLE 6. Recommended Dosage Modification for Toxicity with Neratinib in Combination with Capecitabine

Adverse Reaction and Severity	Modification
Diarrhea	
Grade 1 (<4 stools per day over baseline) or	Continue neratinib and capecitabine at full doses
Grade 2 (4–6 stools per day over baseline) lasting ≤5 days or	Adjust antidiarrheal treatment, modify diet, and maintain fluid intake of about 2 L/day to avoid dehydration
Grade 3 (≥7 stools per day over baseline, fecal incontinence, need for hospitalization, limiting self-care activities of daily living) lasting ≤2 days	Once diarrhea resolves to grade ≤1 or baseline, initiate loperamide hydrochloride 4 mg with each subsequent administration of neratinib

TABLE 6. Continued

Adverse Reaction and Severity	Modification
Persistent/intolerable grade 2 lasting >5 days or Grade 3 lasting >2 days Grade 4 (life-threatening diarrhea or need for urgent intervention)	Withhold neratinib and capecitabine until recovery to grade ≤1 or baseline; if recovered within 1 week, resume both drugs at same dosage; if recovered in 1–3 weeks, resume neratinib at reduced dosage and continue capecitabine at same dosage (see Table 5)
	Adjust antidiarrheal treatment, modify diet, and maintain fluid intake of about 2 L/day to avoid dehydration[b]
	If recovery occurs within 1 week of withholding treatment, resume both drugs at same dosage; if recovery occurs within 1–3 weeks of withholding treatment, reduce neratinib dose to 160 mg and maintain same dose of capecitabine
	If event occurs a second time and the dosage of neratinib has not already been decreased, reduce neratinib dose to 160 mg and maintain same dose of capecitabine; if the dosage of neratinib has already been reduced, reduce the dosage of capecitabine to 550 mg/m² twice daily[a] and maintain the same dosage of neratinib
	If subsequent events occur, reduce the dose of neratinib or capecitabine to the next lower dose level in an alternating fashion
	Once the event resolves to grade ≤1 of baseline, initiate loperamide hydrochloride 4 mg with each subsequent administration of neratinib
Hepatotoxicity	
Grade 3 ALT or AST (>5–20 × ULN) or Grade 3 bilirubin (>3–10 × ULN)	Withhold neratinib until recovery to grade ≤1 and evaluate for alternative causes
	If recovery to grade ≤1 within 3 weeks, resume neratinib at next lower dose level (see Table 5)
	If grade 3 hepatotoxicity recurs after dosage reduction, permanently discontinue neratinib
Grade 4 ALT or AST (>20 × ULN) or Grade 4 bilirubin (>10 × ULN)	Permanently discontinue neratinib and evaluate for alternative causes
Other Adverse Effects	
Grade 3	Withhold neratinib; if adverse effect resolves to grade≤1 or baseline within 3 weeks, resume therapy at the next lower dose level (see Table 5)
Grade 4	Permanently discontinue neratinib

a Since capecitabine is provided as 150-mg or 500-mg tablets, it is recommended to round the dose reduction down to the nearest 500 mg or multiple of 150 mg for the twice daily dose. If the patient's body surface area is >2 m², the standard of care for the study center can be utilized for capecitabine mg/m² dosing.

b Fluid intake should be maintained intravenously, if needed

● Special Populations

Hepatic Impairment

For patients with severe preexisting hepatic impairment (Child-Pugh class C), reduce the initial neratinib dosage to 80 mg once daily. No dosage adjustment is necessary in patients with mild or moderate hepatic impairment (Child-Pugh class A or B).

Renal Impairment

No dosage adjustment is necessary in patients with renal impairment.

Geriatric Patients

There are currently no specific dosage recommendations for geriatric patients.

CAUTIONS

● *Contraindications*

- None.

● *Warnings/Precautions*

Diarrhea

Severe diarrhea associated with dehydration, hypotension, and renal impairment has been reported in patients receiving neratinib. In the ExteNET study in patients with human epidermal growth factor receptor type 2 (HER2)-positive early-stage breast cancer, diarrhea was reported in 95% of patients receiving neratinib and was grade 3 in severity in 40% of patients. The majority (93%) of patients experienced diarrhea during the first month of therapy; the median time to onset of grade 3 or greater diarrhea was 8 days. The median cumulative duration of grade 3 or greater diarrhea was 5 days. In a small study, the incidence and time to onset of grade 1 or greater diarrhea were not ameliorated by administering the total daily dosage of neratinib in 2 divided doses (120 mg twice daily) instead of the recommended 240 mg once daily.

In the NALA study of patients with metastatic breast cancer treated with neratinib plus capecitabine, diarrhea was reported in 83% of patients; all patients received anti-diarrheal prophylaxis in the first 21-day cycle. The majority of patients (70%) had diarrhea within the first 21 days of treatment. Grade 3 or greater diarrhea occurred in 24% of patients with a median time to first onset of 11 days and a median duration of 3 days.

The manufacturer recommends antidiarrheal prophylaxis with loperamide during the first 56 days of treatment with neratinib in patients not using a dose escalation approach. After day 56, dosage of loperamide should be adjusted to maintain 1–2 bowel movements per day; consider addition of other antidiarrheal agents as clinically indicated. As an alternate approach to diarrhea management, a 2-week dosage escalation of neratinib can be considered. In patients managed with this approach, grade 3 or greater diarrhea occurred in 13% of patients with a median time to onset of 45 days and a median duration of 2.5 days.

Patients receiving neratinib should be monitored for development of diarrhea and treated as necessary with appropriate therapy (e.g., antidiarrheal agents, fluid replacement). Stool cultures should be performed as clinically indicated to exclude infectious causes in patients experiencing grade 3 or 4 diarrhea or diarrhea of any severity associated with dehydration, pyrexia, or neutropenia. Liver function tests also should be evaluated in patients experiencing grade 3 or greater diarrhea. Temporary interruption followed by dosage reduction or discontinuance of neratinib may be necessary depending on the severity of the diarrhea.

Hepatic Toxicity

Elevations in aminotransferase (ALT or AST) concentrations have been reported in patients receiving neratinib. In the ExteNET study, elevations in ALT or AST concentrations ≥2 times the upper limit of normal (ULN) occurred in 10 or 5% of patients of patients receiving neratinib, respectively; severe (grade ≥3) elevations occurred in 1.7% of patients. Hepatotoxicity or elevations in ALT or AST concentrations led to discontinuance of neratinib in 1.7% of patients.

In the NALA study in patients treated with neratinib and capecitabine, 7% of patients experienced elevations in ALT or AST to >3 times the ULN, and 2% of patients experienced elevations in ALT or AST to >5 times the ULN; 7 and 1.3% of patients experienced bilirubin elevations >1.5 and >3 times the ULN, respectively. Hepatotoxicity or increases in liver enzymes led to treatment discontinuance in 0.3% of patients treated with neratinib and capecitabine.

Evaluate liver function tests (i.e., serum ALT, AST, total bilirubin, alkaline phosphatase concentrations) prior to initiation of therapy, monthly for the first 3 months of therapy, every 3 months thereafter during therapy, and as clinically indicated. Liver function tests should also be evaluated in patients experiencing

grade 3 or greater diarrhea or manifestations of hepatotoxicity (e.g., worsening fatigue, nausea, vomiting, right upper quadrant pain or tenderness, pyrexia, rash, eosinophilia).

Fetal/Neonatal Morbidity and Mortality

There are no adequate and well-controlled studies of neratinib in pregnant women; however, based on its mechanism of action and animal findings, neratinib may cause fetal harm. Embryofetal toxicity (i.e., increased fetal resorption, abortion) and teratogenicity (i.e., external, visceral, and skeletal anomalies) have been demonstrated in animals receiving neratinib at exposure levels approximately 0.2 times the human exposure at the maximum recommended dosage. Effects on long-term memory have been observed in male pups when pregnant rats received the drug from day 7 of gestation through day 20 of lactation at a dosage approximately 0.2 times the maximum recommended human dosage based on body surface area.

Pregnancy should be avoided during neratinib therapy. Apprise patients of the potential hazard to the fetus if neratinib is used during pregnancy. (See Females and Males of Reproductive Potential under Cautions.)

Specific Populations

Pregnancy

Neratinib may cause fetal harm if administered to pregnant women based on its mechanism of action and animal findings. (See Fetal/Neonatal Morbidity and Mortality under Cautions.)

Lactation

It is not known whether neratinib or its metabolites are distributed into milk. Because of the potential for serious adverse reactions to neratinib in nursing infants, women should be advised to discontinue nursing while receiving neratinib and for at least 1 month after the drug is discontinued. The effects of the drug or its metabolites on nursing infants or on the production of milk are unknown.

Females and Males of Reproductive Potential

Advise females of childbearing potential to use effective contraceptive methods while receiving neratinib and for at least 1 month after discontinuance of the drug. In addition, advise male patients with such female partners to use effective methods of contraception while receiving neratinib and for 3 months after discontinuance of the drug.

Pediatric Use

Safety and efficacy of neratinib have not been established in pediatric patients.

Geriatric Use

In the ExteNET study, 12% of patients receiving neratinib in the safety population were ≥65 years of age and 1.8% were ≥75 years of age. Patients ≥65 years of age had higher incidences of discontinuance of neratinib due to adverse reactions but similar incidences of serious adverse reactions (e.g., vomiting, diarrhea, renal failure, dehydration) compared with younger adults.

In the NALA study, 20% of patients receiving neratinib plus capecitabine in the safety population were ≥65 years of age and 4% were ≥75 years of age. The incidence of serious adverse reactions was similar between patients ≥65 years of age and younger patients; the most commonly reported serious adverse events in geriatric patients were diarrhea, acute kidney injury, and dehydration. No overall differences in efficacy were noted between patients ≥65 years of age and those <65 years of age.

Hepatic Impairment

Systemic exposures of neratinib in individuals with mild or moderate hepatic impairment (Child-Pugh class A or B) were similar to those in individuals with normal hepatic function but were increased in those with severe hepatic impairment (Child-Pugh class C); therefore, dosage adjustment is necessary in patients with severe hepatic impairment.

Renal Impairment

Renal function does not have a clinically significant effect on the pharmacokinetics of neratinib. No dosage adjustment is necessary in such patients.

● *Common Adverse Effects*

Adverse effects reported in ≥5% of patients receiving neratinib monotherapy include diarrhea, nausea, abdominal pain, abdominal distension, fatigue, vomiting, rash, stomatitis, decreased appetite, nail disorders, dry skin, muscle spasms, epistaxis, decreased weight, increased AST or ALT, urinary tract infections, and dyspepsia.

Adverse effects reported in ≥5% of patients receiving neratinib in combination with capecitabine include diarrhea, nausea, vomiting, decreased appetite, constipation, fatigue, decreased weight, dizziness, back pain, arthralgia, urinary tract infection, upper respiratory tract infection, abdominal distension, renal impairment, and muscle spasms.

DRUG INTERACTIONS

Neratinib is primarily metabolized by cytochrome P-450 (CYP) isoenzyme 3A4 and, to a lesser extent, by flavin-containing monooxygenase (FMO).

● *Drugs and Foods Affecting Hepatic Microsomal Enzymes*

Inhibitors of CYP3A4

Concomitant use of neratinib with potent or moderate inhibitors of CYP3A4 may result in increased systemic exposure to neratinib and an increased incidence of adverse effects. Concomitant administration of the potent CYP3A4 inhibitor ketoconazole increased the peak plasma concentration and AUC of neratinib by 221 and 381%, respectively. Concomitant administration of the moderate CYP3A4 inhibitor fluconazole with neratinib increased the peak plasma concentration and AUC of neratinib by 30 and 68%, respectively.

Avoid concomitant use of neratinib with potent inhibitors of CYP3A4 (e.g., clarithromycin; cobicistat; conivaptan; diltiazem; *ritonavir-boosted* elvitegravir; grapefruit products; idelalisib; *ritonavir-boosted* indinavir; itraconazole; ketoconazole; the fixed combination of lopinavir and ritonavir [lopinavir/ritonavir]; nefazodone; nelfinavir; the fixed combination of ombitasvir, paritaprevir, and ritonavir [with or without dasabuvir]; posaconazole; ritonavir; *ritonavir-boosted* saquinavir; *ritonavir-boosted* tipranavir; voriconazole) or moderate (e.g., aprepitant, cimetidine, ciprofloxacin, clotrimazole, crizotinib, cyclosporine, dronedarone, erythromycin, fluconazole, fluvoxamine, imatinib, verapamil).

Inducers of CYP3A4

Concomitant use of neratinib with potent or moderate inducers of CYP3A4 may result in decreased systemic exposure to neratinib and its active *N*-desmethyl (M6) and dimethylamine *N*-oxide (M7) metabolites, resulting in reduced neratinib efficacy. When the potent CYP3A4 inducer rifampin was administered concomitantly with neratinib, the AUCs of neratinib and its active metabolites (M6 and M7) were decreased by 87 and 37–49%, respectively, and the peak plasma concentration of neratinib was decreased by 76%. When the moderate CYP3A4 inducer efavirenz was administered concomitantly with neratinib, the peak plasma concentration and AUC of neratinib were decreased by 36 and 52%, respectively.

Avoid concomitant use with potent CYP3A4 inducers (e.g., carbamazepine, enzalutamide, mitotane, phenytoin, rifampin, St. John's wort [*Hypericum perforatum*]) or moderate (e.g., bosentan, efavirenz, etravirine, modafinil).

● *P-Glycoprotein and Moderate CYP3A4 Dual Inhibitors*

Concomitant use of neratinib with P-glycoprotein (P-gp) and moderate CYP3A4 dual inhibitors may result in increased systemic exposure of neratinib and an increased incidence of adverse effects. When the P-gp and moderate CYP3A4 dual inhibitor verapamil was administered concomitantly with neratinib, peak plasma concentrations and AUC of neratinib increased by 203 and 299%, respectively.

Avoid concomitant use of neratinib with P-gp and moderate CYP3A4 dual inhibitors.

● *Substrates of P-Glycoprotein Transport Systems*

Concomitant use of neratinib with P-gp substrates (e.g., digoxin, dabigatran, fexofenadine) may result in increased systemic exposure of the substrate drug. When the P-gp substrate digoxin was administered concomitantly with neratinib, peak plasma concentrations and AUC of digoxin increased by 54 and 32%, respectively.

Monitor for adverse reactions of certain P-gp substrates for which minimal concentration changes may lead to serious adverse reactions when used concomitantly with neratinib.

● *Drugs Affecting Gastric Acidity*

Concomitant use of neratinib with drugs affecting gastric acidity may decrease the solubility of neratinib and subsequently reduce its bioavailability and efficacy. Concomitant administration of the proton-pump inhibitor lansoprazole with neratinib in healthy individuals decreased the peak plasma concentration and AUC of neratinib by 71 and 65%, respectively. Administration of the histamine H_2-receptor antagonist ranitidine 2 hours prior to neratinib decreased the peak plasma concentration and AUC of neratinib by 57 and 48%, respectively; administration of ranitidine 2 hours after neratinib reduced the peak plasma concentration and AUC of neratinib by 44 and 32%, respectively.

Avoid concomitant use of neratinib with proton-pump inhibitors. Administer neratinib at least 2 hours before or 10 hours after histamine H_2-receptor antagonists. Separate administration of neratinib by at least 3 hours after administration of antacids.

DESCRIPTION

Neratinib, a potent, selective, and irreversible inhibitor of human epidermal growth factor receptor type 2 (HER2), HER4, and epidermal growth factor receptor (EGFR) tyrosine kinases, is an antineoplastic agent. In vitro, neratinib and its active metabolites (M3, M6, M7, M11) exhibit inhibitory activity against EGFR, HER2, and HER4. In vitro, the drug has been shown to reduce phosphorylation of EGFR and HER2 resulting in inhibition of downstream signaling of the mitogen-activated protein kinase (MAPK) and phosphoinositide 3-kinase (PI3K/Akt) pathways. Neratinib has demonstrated antitumor activity in mice bearing tumor xenografts that expressed EGFR and HER2.

Neratinib exhibits nonlinear pharmacokinetics. Peak plasma concentrations and areas under the serum concentration-time curve (AUCs) of neratinib are less than dose proportional over the dosage range of 40–400 mg once daily. Peak plasma concentrations of neratinib and its major active metabolites (M3, M6, and M7) are achieved about 2–8 hours following oral administration of the drug. Following repeated doses of neratinib 240 mg once daily, the mean accumulation ratio for the drug was 1.14. Oral administration of neratinib with a high-fat meal increased peak plasma concentrations and AUC by 70 and 120%, respectively, compared with administration in the fasting state. Oral administration of neratinib with a standard breakfast increased peak plasma concentrations and AUC by 20 and 10%, respectively, compared with administration in the fasting state. In vitro, neratinib is highly bound (greater than 99%) to plasma proteins (mainly to albumin and α_1-acid glycoprotein), independent of concentration. Neratinib is metabolized principally by cytochrome P-450 (CYP) isoenzyme 3A4 and, to a lesser extent, by flavin-containing monooxygenase (FMO). Major metabolites of the drug include active pyridine *N*-oxide (M3), *N*-desmethyl (M6), dimethylamine *N*-oxide (M7), and bis-*N*-oxide (M11) derivatives which account for 15, 33, 22, and 4%, respectively, of total plasma concentrations of the drug. Following repeated administration of neratinib, the mean elimination half-lives of neratinib, M3, M6, and M7 are 14.6, 21.6, 13.8, and 10.4 hours, respectively. Following oral administration of a single radiolabeled dose of neratinib, approximately 97% of the recovered dose is excreted in feces and 1.1% is eliminated in urine.

Age, sex, and race do not have clinically important effects on the pharmacokinetics of neratinib.

ADVICE TO PATIENTS

- Importance of reading the manufacturer's patient information.

- If a dose is missed, importance of administering the next dose at the regularly scheduled time; an additional dose should *not* be administered to make up for a missed dose.

- For patients undergoing extended adjuvant treatment for early-stage breast cancer, instruct patients to take neratinib with food at approximately the same time each day consecutively until disease recurrence or for up to 1 year.

- For patients undergoing treatment for metastatic breast cancer, instruct patients to take neratinib with food on days 1–21 of a 21-day cycle, with capecitabine on days 1–14 of a 21-day cycle until disease progression or unacceptable toxicities occur.

- Risk of diarrhea. Importance of informing patients how to manage diarrhea (e.g., dietary modification, antidiarrheal agents) to maintain 1–2 bowel movements per day. Instruct patients who are not using dose escalation to initiate antidiarrheal prophylaxis with the first dose of neratinib. Instruct patients who are using dose escalation to initiate 2 weeks of lower-dose neratinib prior to receiving the recommended full dose. Importance of informing clinician if severe diarrhea or diarrhea associated with weakness, dizziness, or fever occurs.

- Risk of hepatotoxicity. Importance of advising patients to immediately report possible signs and symptoms of hepatotoxicity (e.g., worsening fatigue, nausea, vomiting, right upper quadrant pain, jaundice, fever, rash, pruritus) to their clinician.

- Risk of fetal harm. Necessity of advising females of childbearing potential to use effective methods of contraception while receiving neratinib and for at least 1 month after the drug is discontinued. Importance of advising male patients who are partners of females of childbearing potential to use effective methods of contraception while receiving the drug and for 3 months after discontinuance of therapy. Importance of women informing clinicians if they are or plan to become pregnant. If pregnancy occurs, advise pregnant women of potential risk to the fetus.

- Neratinib may interact with gastric acid reducing agents. Advise patients to avoid concomitant use of proton pump inhibitors. When patients require gastric acid reducing agents, use an H_2-receptor antagonist or antacid. Advise patients to separate the dosing of neratinib by 3 hours after antacid medicine, and to take neratinib at least 2 hours before or 10 hours after a H_2-receptor antagonist.

- Neratinib may interact with grapefruit. Advise patients to avoid taking neratinib with grapefruit products.

- Importance of advising females to avoid breast-feeding while receiving the drug and for at least 1 month after discontinuance of therapy.

- Advise patients to inform their clinician of existing or contemplated concomitant therapy, including prescription and OTC drugs, as well as any concomitant illnesses.

- Advise patients of other important precautionary information. (See Cautions.)

For further information on the handling of antineoplastic agents, see the ASHP Guidelines on Handling Hazardous Drugs at http://www.ahfsdrug information.com.

PREPARATIONS

Neratinib is available only from designated specialty distributors and pharmacies. Consult the manufacturer for additional information.

Excipients in commercially available drug preparations may have clinically important effects in some individuals; consult specific product labeling for details.

Neratinib Maleate

Oral

| Tablets, film-coated | 40 mg (of neratinib) | Nerlynx®, Puma Biotechnology |

Nilutamide

10:00 • ANTINEOPLASTIC AGENTS

■ Nilutamide is a nonsteroidal antiandrogen.

USES

● Prostate Cancer

Nilutamide is used in combination with orchiectomy in the treatment of metastatic prostate cancer (stage D2). For maximum benefit, nilutamide must begin on the same day as or on the day after surgical castration. Overall, results of controlled clinical studies in patients with metastatic prostate cancer indicate that nilutamide in combination with orchiectomy slows progression of the disease, relieves bone pain associated with metastatic disease, and improves overall survival rate after long-term therapy (8.5 years). Use of nilutamide in combination with androgen deprivation therapy (including orchiectomy) for metastatic prostate cancer is not supported by current guidelines in light of the strong evidence available for alternative therapies.

Clinical Experience

The indication for nilutamide in metastatic prostate cancer is based principally on the results of a double-blind, randomized, multicenter study in 457 patients with prostate cancer and distant metastases. Patients were randomized to undergo treatment with orchiectomy plus nilutamide (300 mg daily for 1 month followed by 150 mg daily thereafter) or orchiectomy plus placebo. The assigned oral treatment was initiated on the day after orchiectomy. The mean age was 71 years in the nilutamide group and 72 years in the placebo group; the majority of patients were white. The median months of stage D2 diagnosis was 0.50 (range: 0–90) in the nilutamide group and 0.53 (range: 0–59) in the placebo group. Patients who received nilutamide had a median survival of 27.3 months, while patients who received placebo had a median survival of 23.6 months. Progression-free survival was also prolonged among patients receiving nilutamide compared with placebo (median 21.2 months versus 14.9 months). Complete or partial regression of the cancer was observed in 41% of patients receiving nilutamide and 24% of patients receiving placebo. More patients receiving nilutamide indicated improvement in bone pain than those receiving placebo (54% versus 37%). Nilutamide was also associated with improvement or delayed worsening in subjective parameters such as metastasis-related pain and urinary symptoms. At 8.5 years of follow-up, nilutamide combined with orchiectomy continued to demonstrate improvements in overall survival and progression-free survival compared with placebo plus orchiectomy.

Meta-analyses of randomized controlled trials comparing nilutamide plus orchiectomy to placebo plus orchiectomy in metastatic prostate cancer have found that nilutamide plus orchiectomy is associated with reduced disease progression and potential survival benefits.

Clinical Perspective

A joint guideline from the American Urological Association (AUA), American Society for Radiation Oncology (ASTRO), and Society of Urologic Oncology (SUO) states that, in light of the compelling evidence to support use of docetaxel, abiraterone acetate plus prednisone, apalutamide, or enzalutamide in combination with androgen deprivation therapy in men with newly diagnosed metastatic hormone-sensitive prostate cancer, long-term use of first-generation antiandrogens (i.e., bicalutamide, flutamide, nilutamide) in lieu of these agents cannot be supported. Androgen pathway-directed therapy (e.g., abiraterone plus prednisone, apalutamide, bicalutamide, darolutamide, enzalutamide, flutamide, nilutamide) should not be offered without concomitant androgen deprivation therapy in metastatic hormone-sensitive prostate cancer.

DOSAGE AND ADMINISTRATION

● General

Pretreatment Screening

- Perform a routine chest radiograph prior to initiation of treatment with nilutamide. Consider obtaining baseline pulmonary function tests.

- Measure serum transaminase levels prior to treatment with nilutamide.

● Patient Monitoring

- Monitor for any new or worsening shortness of breath during treatment with nilutamide. If symptoms occur, immediately discontinue nilutamide until it is determined if symptoms are drug related.

- Monitor serum transaminase levels at regular intervals for the first 4 months of treatment, and then periodically thereafter. Obtain liver function tests if symptoms of nausea, vomiting, abdominal pain, fatigue, anorexia, jaundice, dark urine, "flu-like" symptoms, or right upper quadrant tenderness occurs. If at any time jaundice is present, or the ALT rises above 2 times the upper limit of normal (ULN), immediately discontinue nilutamide and closely monitor liver function tests until resolved.

- Monitor prostate specific antigen (PSA) concentrations periodically and consider conventional imaging during treatment to monitor therapeutic response.

● Administration

Nilutamide is administered orally without regard to meals.

Store tablets between 20–25°C (excursions permitted between 15–30°C) and protect from light.

● Dosage

Prostate Cancer

For use in combination with orchiectomy in the management of metastatic (stage D2) prostate cancer, the usual dosage of nilutamide is 300 mg once daily for 30 days, followed by 150 mg once daily thereafter. For maximum benefit, treatment with nilutamide should be initiated on the day of or the day after orchiectomy.

● Special Populations

Hepatic Impairment

The use of nilutamide is contraindicated in patients with severe hepatic impairment.

Renal Impairment

The manufacturer makes no specific dosage recommendations for patients with renal impairment.

Geriatric Patients

The manufacturer makes no specific dosage recommendations for geriatric patients.

CAUTIONS

● Contraindications

- Severe hepatic impairment.
- Severe respiratory insufficiency.
- History of hypersensitivity to nilutamide or any ingredient in the formulation.

● Warnings/Precautions

Warnings

Interstitial Pneumonitis

A boxed warning about the risk of interstitial pneumonitis is included in the prescribing information for nilutamide. Interstitial pneumonitis was reported in 2% of patients receiving the drug in controlled clinical trials and in 17% (8/47) of patients in a small Japanese study. Interstitial changes, including pulmonary fibrosis leading to hospitalization and death, have been reported rarely during post-marketing experience with the drug. Symptoms of interstitial pneumonitis included exertional dyspnea, cough, chest pain, and fever; chest radiographs showed interstitial or alveolo-interstitial changes, and pulmonary function tests showed a restrictive pattern with decreased carbon monoxide diffusing capacity. In most patients, interstitial pneumonitis occurred within the first 3 months of nilutamide therapy and resolved following discontinuation of the drug.

Perform chest radiograph prior to initiation of nilutamide therapy. Baseline pulmonary function tests also may be considered. Nilutamide therapy should be discontinued immediately if symptoms occur until it can be determined if symptoms are drug related.

Other Warnings/Precautions
Hepatitis

Severe liver injury, in some cases leading to hospitalization and/or death, has been reported rarely in association with nilutamide therapy. Hepatotoxicity generally occurred within the first 3–4 months of nilutamide therapy. Hepatitis or a marked increase in serum concentrations of hepatic transaminases leading to discontinuation of nilutamide therapy was reported in 1% of patients receiving the drug in controlled clinical trials.

Serum transaminase concentrations should be measured prior to initiation of nilutamide therapy, at regular intervals during the first 4 months of treatment, and periodically thereafter. If clinical signs or symptoms suggestive of liver dysfunction (e.g., nausea, vomiting, abdominal pain, fatigue, anorexia, "flu-like" symptoms, dark urine, jaundice, right upper quadrant tenderness) occur, immediately measure serum transaminase concentrations. Immediately discontinue nilutamide in any patient who develops jaundice or an increase in serum ALT concentration to greater than 2 times the ULN, and closely monitor liver function.

Use in Women

Nilutamide is not intended for use in women and should not be used in women, particularly for nonserious or nonlife-threatening conditions.

Hematologic Effects

Post-marketing cases of aplastic anemia have been reported with nilutamide, although a causal relationship has not been determined.

Withdrawal Syndrome

Patients whose disease progresses while being treated with an antiandrogen, such as nilutamide, may experience clinical improvement with discontinuation of the antiandrogen.

Specific Populations
Pregnancy

There are no available data on the use of nilutamide in pregnant women to evaluate the drug-associated risk in pregnancy. It is unknown whether nilutamide can cause fetal harm when administered to a pregnant patient. Administer nilutamide to a pregnant patient only if clearly needed.

Nilutamide is not intended for use in women.

Lactation

There are no available data on use during lactation.

Pediatric Use

The safety and efficacy of nilutamide in pediatric patients have not been established.

Geriatric Use

The safety and efficacy of nilutamide in geriatric patients have not been established.

Hepatic Impairment

Nilutamide is contraindicated for use in severe hepatic impairment. Evaluate serum transaminase levels prior to starting nilutamide, at regular intervals for the first 4 months of treatment, and then periodically thereafter. Additionally, obtain liver function tests if symptoms of nausea, vomiting, abdominal pain, fatigue, anorexia, jaundice, dark urine, "flu-like" symptoms, or right upper quadrant tenderness are present. If at any time jaundice is present, or the ALT rises to above 2 times the ULN, immediately discontinue nilutamide and closely monitor liver function tests until resolution.

Renal Impairment

In a pharmacokinetic study, only a small quantity of nonmetabolized nilutamide was found in the urine. Renal impairment is likely to have little effect on the pharmacokinetics of nilutamide.

● Common Adverse Effects

Adverse effects reported in ≥5% of patients in clinical trials receiving nilutamide with surgical castration include hypertension, nausea, constipation, hot flushes, increased ALT, increased AST, dizziness, dyspnea, impaired adaptation to the dark, abnormal vision, and urinary tract infection.

Adverse effects reported in ≥10% of patients in clinical trials receiving nilutamide with leuprolide include pain, headache, asthenia, back pain, abdominal pain, nausea, constipation, anorexia, hot flushes, impotence, decreased libido, increased AST, peripheral edema, insomnia, dizziness, dyspnea, impaired adaptation to the dark, testicular atrophy, and gynecomastia.

DRUG INTERACTIONS

In vitro studies indicate that nilutamide inhibits the activity of cytochrome P-450 (CYP) isoenzymes in the liver, and may therefore reduce their metabolism.

● Drugs with Low Therapeutic Margin

Monitor drugs with a narrow therapeutic window such as warfarin, phenytoin, and theophylline while on nilutamide. These drugs could have a delayed elimination and increased serum half-life leading to a toxic level. Adjust the dosage of these drugs if necessary. Monitor prothrombin time carefully and adjust the dosage of warfarin, if necessary, when warfarin is used concomitantly with nilutamide.

● Alcohol

Since nilutamide may cause an intolerance to alcohol (reported in 5% of patients) resulting in facial flushes, malaise and hypotension, it is recommended that patients who experience this reaction avoid alcoholic beverages while taking nilutamide.

DESCRIPTION

Nilutamide is a nonsteroidal antiandrogen that is structurally and pharmacologically related to bicalutamide and flutamide.

Nilutamide is a pure antiandrogen, possessing no intrinsic hormonal activity; the antiandrogenic mechanism of action of the drug is via androgen-receptor antagonism. Nilutamide inhibits the action of androgens by competitively blocking nuclear androgen receptors in target tissues such as the prostate, seminal vesicles, and adrenal cortex; blockade of androgen receptors in the hormone-sensitive tumor cells may result in growth arrest or transient tumor regression through inhibition of androgen-dependent DNA and protein synthesis. Nilutamide is a selective antiandrogen with no estrogenic, antiestrogenic, progestational, antiprogestational, or adrenocortical activity in various animal models. The relative binding affinity of nilutamide at the androgen receptor is less than that of bicalutamide, but similar to that of hydroxyflutamide, the active metabolite of flutamide.

Common pharmacologic therapies for prostate cancer (i.e., gonadotropin-releasing hormone [GnRH] analogs, nonsteroidal antiandrogens) when used as monotherapy initially result in increased serum testosterone concentrations, which may limit the effects of the drugs. Androgen receptors in the hypothalamus are blocked by nilutamide, which disrupts the inhibitory feedback of testosterone on luteinizing hormone (LH) release, resulting in a temporary increase in secretion of LH; the increase in LH stimulates an increase in the production of testosterone. As GnRH analogs have potent GnRH agonist properties, testicular steroidogenesis continues during the first few weeks after initiating therapy. However, the combination of orchiectomy or GnRH analog therapy to suppress testicular androgen production and an antiandrogen to block response of remaining adrenal androgens provides maximal androgen blockade. Concomitant administration of antiandrogens such as nilutamide in patients initiating therapy with a GnRH analog can inhibit initial androgenic stimulation and potential exacerbation of symptoms (e.g., bone pain, urinary obstruction, liver pain, impending spinal cord compression) that may occur during the first month of GnRH analog therapy.

Following multiple doses of 150 mg nilutamide twice daily, steady state is attained in most patients within 2–4 weeks. After multiple doses, the AUC was shown to be 110% higher than the AUC obtained from a single 150 mg dose, indicating that with multiple doses, metabolic enzyme inhibition may occur. Based on blood, urine, and fecal samples in patients with metastatic prostate cancer, nilutamide has been shown to be rapidly and completely absorbed. Nilutamide moderately binds to plasma proteins, and exhibits low binding to erythrocytes. Studies indicate that nilutamide does not exhibit nonlinear pharmacokinetics. Nilutamide undergoes extensive metabolism in the liver and lungs by CYP isoenzymes, with less than 2% of radiolabeled drug excreted unchanged in the urine after 5 days. Five metabolites of nilutamide have been isolated from human urine; however, the pharmacokinetics and pharmacodynamics of these metabolites have not been fully investigated. Following oral administration of a single 150 mg radiolabeled dose of nilutamide, 62% of the dose is eliminated in the urine during the first 5 days; however, excretion of radioactivity in the urine likely extends beyond this period. After 4–5 days, 1.4%–7% of the nilutamide dose is eliminated in the feces. The mean elimination half-life of nilutamide based on a single dose of 100–300 mg ranged from 38–59.1 hours, with most values ranging from 41–49 hours; however, the half-life of one metabolite of nilutamide ranges from 59–126 hours.

ADVICE TO PATIENTS

- Importance of reading the manufacturer's patient information prior to starting nilutamide.
- Risk of interstitial pneumonitis. Inform patients to notify their clinicians if dyspnea or worsening of pre-existing dyspnea occurs.
- Risk of hepatic toxicity. Inform patients to notify their clinicians if nausea, vomiting, abdominal pain, fatigue, anorexia, "flu-like" symptoms, dark urine, jaundice, or right upper quadrant pain occurs.

- Risk of delay in visually adapting to changes from light to dark. Inform patients who experience this effect to wear tinted glasses during exposure to bright light and to exercise caution when driving at night or through tunnels.
- Risk of alcohol intolerance (e.g., facial flushing, malaise, hypotension). Instruct patients to avoid alcohol consumption if such intolerance occurs.
- Inform patients that nilutamide should be started the day of or on the day after surgical castration, and that dosing should not be interrupted or stopped without consulting the prescriber.
- Advise patients to inform their clinicians of existing or contemplated concomitant therapy, including prescription and OTC drugs and dietary or herbal supplements as well as any concomitant illnesses (eg, hepatic impairment).
- Inform patients of other important cautionary information.

PREPARATIONS

Excipients in commercially available drug preparations may have clinically important effects in some individuals; consult specific product labeling for details.

Nilutamide

Oral		
Tablets	150 mg	**Nilandron®**, Sanofi-Aventis

† Use is not currently included in the labeling approved by the US Food and Drug Administration.

Niraparib Tosylate

10:00 · ANTINEOPLASTIC AGENTS

■ Niraparib tosylate, an inhibitor of poly (adenosine diphosphate [ADP]-ribose) polymerase (PARP), is an antineoplastic agent.

USES

● Ovarian Cancer

First-line Maintenance Treatment of Platinum-sensitive Advanced Ovarian Cancer

Niraparib is used as maintenance therapy for the treatment of advanced epithelial ovarian, fallopian tube, or primary peritoneal cancer in adults who are in complete or partial response following first-line platinum-based chemotherapy. The drug has been designated an orphan drug by the FDA for the treatment of this cancer.

This indication for niraparib is based principally on the results of a randomized, double-blind, placebo-controlled, phase 3 study (PRIMA).

In the PRIMA study, 733 patients with stage 3 or 4 high grade serous or endometrioid tumors were randomized in a 2:1 ratio to receive niraparib or placebo within 12 weeks of the last dose of platinum-based chemotherapy. In the initial trial protocol, niraparib was given at a dosage of 300 mg once daily; however, the trial protocol was amended when predictive modeling of the NOVA study indicated that patients with a body weight less than 77 kg or platelet count less than 150,000/mm³ should receive an initial niraparib dosage of 200 mg once daily and those with a body weight of 77 kg or greater and platelet count of 150,000/mm³ or greater should receive an initial niraparib dosage of 300 mg once daily. Approximately 35% of patients enrolled in the study received an initial niraparib dosage of 200 or 300 mg according to baseline body weight and platelet count. Treatment cycles were repeated every 28 days and continued for 36 months or until disease progression occurred. Patients randomized to receive placebo were not permitted to cross over to niraparib therapy upon disease progression. Patients were stratified by best response during the front-line platinum-based regimen, neoadjuvant chemotherapy, and homologous recombination deficiency (HRD) status.

The primary endpoint of the PRIMA study was progression-free survival as assessed by a blinded independent central review (BICR) committee according to Response Evaluation Criteria in Solid Tumors (RECIST) v1.1 and, in some cases, additional criteria (e.g., increasing serum cancer antigen-125 [CA-125] concentration, clinical signs and symptoms) were applied. In the overall study population, the median age of patients was 62 years; 89% of patients were white, 71% had a baseline Eastern Cooperative Oncology Group (ECOG) performance status of 0, 65% had stage III disease, 67% had received neoadjuvant chemotherapy, and 69% had a complete response to first-line platinum-based chemotherapy. Approximately one-half of patients enrolled in the study were HRD-positive (defined as the presence of a BRCA mutation and/or a genomic instability score of 42 or greater as determined by the Myriad myChoice CDx assay).

Patients receiving niraparib had a substantially longer median progression-free survival than those receiving placebo in the HRD-positive cohort (21.9 versus 10.4 months; hazard ratio: 0.43; 95% confidence interval, 0.31–0.59) and overall study population (13.8 versus 8.2 months; hazard ratio: 0.62; 95% confidence interval, 0.50–0.76). Results of subgroup analyses (based on response to platinum-based chemotherapy, receipt of neoadjuvant chemotherapy, and presence/absence of BRCA mutation or HRD) suggested that the effect of niraparib on progression-free survival was generally consistent across subgroups. In an exploratory analysis of patients who received a weight- and platelet count-based starting dosage of niraparib, the hazard ratio for progression-free survival was 0.39 (95% confidence interval of 0.22–0.72) in the HRD cohort and 0.68 (95% confidence interval of 0.48–0.97) in the overall study population. At the time of analysis, overall survival data were immature; however, estimated overall survival at 24 months was 84% in patients receiving niraparib compared with 77% in those receiving placebo (hazard ratio: 0.70; 95% confidence interval, 0.44–1.11) in the overall study population and 91 or 85% (hazard ratio: 0.61; 95% confidence interval, 0.27–1.39), respectively, in the HRD-positive cohort.

Recurrent Ovarian Cancer

Maintenance Treatment of Platinum-sensitive Germline BRCA-mutated Recurrent Ovarian Cancer

Niraparib is used as maintenance therapy for the treatment of deleterious or suspected deleterious germline BRCA-mutated recurrent epithelial ovarian, fallopian tube, or primary peritoneal cancer in adults in complete or partial response following platinum-based chemotherapy. The drug has been designated an orphan drug by the FDA for the treatment of this cancer.

The initial approved indication for niraparib as maintenance therapy for adults with recurrent epithelial ovarian, fallopian tube, or primary peritoneal cancer in complete or partial response following platinum-based chemotherapy was based principally on the results of a randomized, double-blind, placebo-controlled phase 3 study (NOVA). Patients in the NOVA study were enrolled into 1 of 2 cohorts based on BRCA mutation status (confirmed or suspected deleterious); those with germline BRCA mutations were assigned to the germline BRCA-mutated (gBRCA-mutation) cohort and those without germline BRCA mutations were assigned to the non-gBRCA-mutation cohort (including those with wild-type gBRCA using the BRACAnalysis CDx diagnostic test). The non-gBRCA-mutation cohort included patients with HRD-positive tumors, including those with somatic BRCA mutations and other defects, as well as patients with HRD-negative tumors.

In the NOVA study, 553 patients were randomized in a 2:1 ratio to receive either niraparib (300 mg once daily) or placebo within 8 weeks following the last dose of platinum-based chemotherapy. Treatment was continued until disease progression or unacceptable toxicity occurred or the patient withdrew from the study. Patients randomized to receive placebo were not permitted to cross over to niraparib therapy upon disease progression. Patients were stratified according to time to progression following the penultimate platinum-based regimen, concomitant use of bevacizumab with the penultimate or last platinum-based regimen, and best response following the most recent platinum-based regimen.

The primary end point of the NOVA study was progression-free survival as assessed by a BICR according to RECIST v1.1 and, in some cases, additional criteria (e.g., increasing serum CA-125 concentrations, clinical signs and symptoms) were considered. The median age of patients ranged from 57–64 years in those receiving niraparib and 58–67 years in those receiving placebo; 86% of all patients were White and 67 and 69% of patients in the niraparib and placebo groups, respectively, had a baseline ECOG performance status of 0. All enrolled patients had previously received at least 2 platinum-based regimens; approximately 40% of all patients had received 3 or more previous lines of therapy, 26% of the niraparib-treated patients had previously received bevacizumab therapy, 51% of all patients were in complete response following platinum-based chemotherapy, and 6–12 months had elapsed since penultimate platinum-based chemotherapy in 39% of patients in both the niraparib and placebo groups. In the initial NOVA analysis, patients receiving niraparib had a substantially longer median progression-free survival than those receiving placebo in both the gBRCA-mutation (21 versus 5.5 months; hazard ratio: 0.26) and non-gBRCA-mutation cohorts (9.3 versus 3.9 months; hazard ratio: 0.45). Median progression-free survival also was significantly longer in niraparib-treated patients with HRD-positive epithelial ovarian, fallopian tube, or primary peritoneal cancer in the non-gBRCA-mutation cohort compared with those receiving placebo (12.9 versus 3.8 months; hazard ratio: 0.38). A subgroup analysis of patients 70 years of age or older suggested that progression-free survival benefit and the incidence of adverse effects in patients receiving niraparib were comparable to those observed in younger adults. In a post-hoc analysis, significant progression-free survival benefit was observed regardless of the best response to the last platinum-based chemotherapy in patients receiving niraparib compared with those receiving placebo. At the time of the progression-free survival analysis, limited overall survival data were available; deaths were reported in 17% of patients across the 2 cohorts.

In 2022, an FDA review of the final overall survival analysis of the NOVA trial revealed that, in the non-gBRCA-mutation cohort only, median overall survival (a secondary endpoint) was substantially reduced among patients administered niraparib versus those administered placebo (31 versus 35.8 months; hazard ratio: 1.06). This resulted in the FDA requesting restriction of the second-line maintenance indication for niraparib to only the patient population with deleterious or suspected gBRCA mutations.

In a long-term safety analysis, hematologic adverse events generally decreased in incidence over time, with dosage reductions due to hematologic adverse events occurring most frequently during the first 3 months of niraparib therapy. Quality of life (measured with the Functional Assessment of Cancer Therapy–Ovarian Symptoms Index [FOSI], European quality of life (QOL) five-dimension five-level questionnaire [EQ-5D-5L], and European QOL-visual analog scale [EQ-VAS]) did not change substantially from baseline during the maintenance period, and were similar between both treatment groups.

Treatment of Previously Treated Advanced Ovarian Cancer

Niraparib was previously indicated, based on the QUADRA study, for the treatment of adults with homologous recombination deficiency (HRD)-positive advanced ovarian, fallopian tube, or primary peritoneal cancer previously treated with 3 or more chemotherapy regimens; however, the manufacturer voluntarily withdrew this indication in September 2022 based on the totality of information from PARP inhibitors in the late line treatment setting in ovarian cancer. A potential detrimental effect on overall survival was observed with other PARP inhibitors in 2 independent randomized, active-controlled clinical trials conducted in a BRCA mutant 3L+ advanced ovarian cancer population..

Clinical Perspective

Newly Diagnosed Ovarian Cancer

Substantial progression-free survival benefit has been observed in patients with newly diagnosed advanced ovarian cancer who have achieved complete or partial response to first-line platinum-based chemotherapy receiving maintenance therapy with a PARP inhibitor.

The American Society of Clinical Oncology (ASCO) recommends that olaparib, niraparib, or rucaparib should be offered based on identification of deleterious germline or somatic mutations in BRCA1 or BRCA2 in patients with platinum-sensitive disease. ASCO recommends olaparib or rucaparib maintenance therapy for a duration of 2 years and niraparib maintenance therapy for a duration of 3 years. A longer treatment duration may be considered in selected individuals after a discussion of risks. For patients who are HRD-positive, rucaparib and niraparib are options. Niraparib or rucaparib may be offered for non-BRCAmut/HRD-negative patients.

ASCO strongly encourages clinicians and patients to consider the full life cycle of advanced ovarian cancer against current data (i.e., lack of overall survival benefit to date and the unknown short-term and late risks) and development of collateral resistance to other drugs (e.g., platinum agents) in determining when to use PARP inhibitors for individual care.

Recurrent Ovarian Cancer

In the recurrent ovarian cancer setting, ASCO states that PARP inhibitor maintenance (second-line or more) monotherapy may be offered to patients who have not already received a PARP inhibitor and who have responded to platinum-based therapy regardless of BRCA mutation status. Treatment may be continued until disease progression or unacceptable toxicity; options include olaparib, rucaparib, or niraparib. ASCO notes that maintenance treatment with niraparib for patients without germline or somatic BRCA mutation should weigh the potential progression-free survival benefit against the potential negative effect on overall survival.

ASCO also states that PARP inhibitor monotherapy should not be routinely offered to patients for the treatment of recurrent platinum-sensitive disease and that PARP inhibitor monotherapy is not recommended for the treatment of patients with either BRCA wild-type or platinum-resistant recurrent ovarian cancer.

DOSAGE AND ADMINISTRATION

● General

Pretreatment Screening

- Complete blood count (CBC).
- Delay initiation until hematologic toxicity caused by previous chemotherapy resolves to grade 1 or less.
- Verify pregnancy status for females of reproductive potential.

- Confirm presence of a confirmed or suspected deleterious BRCA mutation prior to initiation of niraparib therapy for maintenance treatment of recurrent germline BRCA-mutated ovarian cancer. Consult FDA website for list of FDA-approved or cleared companion diagnostic tests (https://www.fda.gov/companiondiagnostics).

Patient Monitoring

- CBC weekly for the first month of therapy, monthly for the next 11 months, and then periodically thereafter.
- Blood pressure and heart rate at least weekly for the first 2 months of therapy, then monthly for first year and periodically thereafter.
- Signs and symptoms of posterior reversible encephalopathy syndrome (e.g., seizure, headache, altered mental status, visual disturbance, and cortical blindness with or without associated hypertension).

● Administration

Niraparib tosylate is administered orally without regard to meals at approximately the same time each day. The manufacturer states that bedtime administration may help relieve nausea.

ASCO also states that a light meal or snack prior to each dose of a PARP inhibitor may mitigate nausea. According to ASCO, many patients will have tachyphylaxis of nausea symptoms during the first cycle of PARP inhibitor therapy, often without antiemetic therapy or dose reduction. If persistent nausea/vomiting, weight loss exceeding 5%, and/or reduction in performance status occurs, patients should be evaluated to rule out other causes, such as bowel obstruction. In the absence of other causes, ASCO recommends temporarily withholding therapy followed by dosage reduction.

The capsules should be swallowed whole and should not be chewed, crushed, or split.

If a dose of niraparib is missed or vomited, patients should *not* take an extra dose. The next dose should be taken at the regularly scheduled time.

● Dosage

Dosage of niraparib tosylate monohydrate is expressed in terms of niraparib.

Ovarian Cancer

First-line Maintenance Treatment of Platinum-sensitive Advanced Ovarian Cancer

The recommended adult dosage of niraparib for the maintenance treatment of advanced epithelial ovarian, fallopian tube, or primary peritoneal cancer in patients who are in complete or partial response following first-line platinum-based chemotherapy is based on body weight and platelet count.

For patients weighing less than 77 kg or platelet count less than 150,000/mm³, the recommended dosage is 200 mg (two 100-mg capsules) once daily.

For patients weighing 77 kg or greater and a platelet count of 150,000/mm³ or greater, the recommended dosage is 300 mg (three 100-mg capsules) once daily.

Niraparib therapy should be initiated no later than 12 weeks following the most recent platinum-based chemotherapy regimen. Therapy should be continued until disease progression or unacceptable toxicity occurs.

Maintenance Treatment of Platinum-sensitive Germline BRCA-mutated Recurrent Ovarian Cancer

The recommended adult dosage of niraparib for maintenance treatment of recurrent germline BRCA-mutated epithelial ovarian, fallopian tube, or primary peritoneal cancer in patients who are in complete or partial response to platinum-containing chemotherapy is 300 mg (three 100-mg capsules) once daily.

Niraparib therapy should be initiated no later than 8 weeks following the most recent platinum-based chemotherapy regimen. Therapy should be continued until disease progression or unacceptable toxicity occurs.

Dosage Modification for Toxicity

Dosing interruption and/or dosage reduction or discontinuance of niraparib therapy may be necessary based on severity and persistence of an adverse effect. If dosage reduction from *an initial dose of 300 mg once daily* is necessary, the dosage should be reduced to 200 mg once daily. If the toxicity recurs on a dosage of 200 mg once daily, the dosage should be reduced to 100 mg once daily. If the toxicity recurs on a dosage of 100 mg once daily, niraparib therapy should be discontinued.

If dosage reduction from *an initial dose of 200 mg once daily* is necessary, the dosage should be reduced to 100 mg once daily; if the toxicity recurs on this dose, niraparib therapy should be discontinued.

Hematologic Toxicity

For platelet counts less than 100,000/mm³, niraparib therapy should be withheld for no more than 28 days and CBCs should be monitored weekly until platelet counts reach or exceed 100,000/mm³. For the first occurrence of a platelet count less than 100,000/mm³, niraparib therapy may then be resumed at the same dosage or at a reduced dosage. For subsequent occurrences of a platelet count less than 100,000/mm³, the daily dosage of niraparib should be reduced in decrements of 100 mg; however, if a dosage of 100 mg once daily requires further reduction or if platelet counts do not return to acceptable levels within 28 days of withholding the drug, niraparib should be discontinued.

For platelet counts less than 75,000/mm³, niraparib therapy should be withheld for no more than 28 days and CBCs should be monitored weekly until platelet counts reach or exceed 100,000/mm³. Upon resumption of therapy, the daily dosage of niraparib should be reduced. If platelet counts do not return to acceptable levels within 28 days of withholding the drug or if a platelet count less than 75,000/mm³ recurs on a reduced dosage of 100 mg once daily, niraparib therapy should be discontinued.

For platelet counts of 10,000/mm³ or less, niraparib therapy should be withheld for no more than 28 days and platelet transfusion should be considered; however, the manufacturer states that if there are other risk factors such as concomitant use of anticoagulants or antiplatelet agents, withholding these drugs and/or a platelet transfusion may be considered at a higher platelet count. Upon completion of platelet transfusion, CBCs should be monitored weekly for 1 month. Niraparib therapy may be resumed at a reduced dosage once platelet counts reach or exceed 100,000/mm³ and 7 or more days have elapsed since platelet transfusion. Upon resumption of therapy, CBCs should be monitored weekly for an additional month to ensure the platelet count is stable.

For neutropenia (absolute neutrophil count [ANC] less than 1,000/mm³) or anemia (hemoglobin concentration less than 8 g/dL), niraparib therapy should be withheld for no more than 28 days and CBCs should be monitored weekly. Niraparib therapy may be resumed when ANC reaches or exceeds 1,500/mm³ or hemoglobin concentrations reach or exceed 9 g/dL. Upon resumption of therapy, the daily dosage of niraparib should be reduced. If ANC and/or hemoglobin concentrations do not return to acceptable levels within 28 days of withholding the drug or if the dosage has already been reduced to 100 mg once daily, niraparib therapy should be discontinued.

If MDS/AML is confirmed, niraparib therapy should be discontinued.

Nonhematologic Toxicity

For grade 3 or greater nonhematologic toxicity that persists despite medical management, niraparib therapy should be withheld until the toxicity resolves, but for no longer than 28 days. Upon resumption of therapy, the daily dosage of niraparib should be reduced; however, if a dosage of 100 mg once daily requires further reduction, the drug should be discontinued.

If prolonged grade 3 or greater nonhematologic toxicity (lasting more than 28 days) occurs on a dosage of 100 mg once daily, niraparib should be discontinued.

● Special Populations

Hepatic Impairment

For patients with moderate hepatic impairment (total bilirubin 1.5–3 times the upper limit of normal [ULN] with any AST), the manufacturer recommends an initial niraparib dosage of 200 mg once daily. These patients should be monitored for hematologic toxicity, and the dosage reduced further if necessary. No initial dosage adjustment of niraparib is necessary in patients with mild hepatic impairment (total bilirubin not exceeding the ULN with AST exceeding ULN, or total bilirubin exceeding the ULN, but less than 1.5 times the ULN with any AST). Niraparib has not been studied in patients with severe hepatic impairment (total

bilirubin greater than 3 times the ULN with any AST), and the manufacturer makes no specific dosage recommendations for such patients.

Renal Impairment

No initial dosage adjustment of niraparib is necessary in patients with mild (creatinine clearance 60–89 mL/minute) or moderate (creatinine clearance 30–59 mL/minute) renal impairment. Niraparib has not been studied in patients with severe renal impairment (creatinine clearance less than 30 mL/minute) or end-stage renal disease requiring hemodialysis, and the manufacturer provides no specific dosage recommendations for such patients.

Geriatric Patients

The manufacturer makes no specific dosage recommendations for geriatric patients.

CAUTIONS

● Contraindications

● None.

● Warnings/Precautions

Myelodysplastic Syndrome/Acute Myeloid Leukemia

Myelodysplastic syndrome (MDS) and acute myeloid leukemia (AML), including fatal cases, have been reported in niraparib-treated patients. Overall, MDS/AML have been reported in 16 of 620 patients receiving niraparib versus 5 of 309 patients treated with placebo in clinical studies (PRIMA and NOVA). All of these patients had received previous chemotherapy with platinum-containing agents and/or other DNA-damaging antineoplastic agents and radiotherapy. The duration of niraparib therapy in patients who developed MDS/AML varied from 3.6 months to 5.9 years.

Complete blood cell (CBC) counts should be monitored in patients receiving niraparib. If MDS/AML is confirmed, niraparib should be discontinued.

Hematologic Effects

Adverse hematologic effects (e.g., thrombocytopenia, anemia, neutropenia) have been reported in patients receiving niraparib therapy. In the PRIMA study, grade 3 or greater thrombocytopenia, anemia, and neutropenia occurred in 39, 31, and 21%, respectively, of patients receiving niraparib. Discontinuance of therapy was necessary in 4, 2, and 2% of patients experiencing thrombocytopenia, anemia, and neutropenia, respectively. In patients who received a weight- or platelet count-based initial dose of niraparib, grade 3 or greater thrombocytopenia, anemia, and neutropenia occurred in 22, 23, and 15%, respectively. Discontinuance of therapy was necessary in 3, 3, and 2% of patients experiencing thrombocytopenia, anemia, and neutropenia, respectively. In the NOVA study, grade 3 or greater thrombocytopenia, anemia, and neutropenia occurred in 29, 25, and 20%, respectively, of patients receiving niraparib. Discontinuance of therapy was necessary in 3, 1, and 2% of patients experiencing thrombocytopenia, anemia, and neutropenia, respectively.

Niraparib therapy should not be initiated until patients have recovered from hematologic toxicity caused by previous chemotherapy (to grade 1 or less). CBC counts should be monitored weekly for the first month of therapy, monthly for the next 11 months, and then periodically thereafter. If hematologic toxicity develops and persists for more than 28 days following interruption of niraparib therapy, patients should be referred to a hematologist for further evaluation, including bone marrow analysis and cytogenetic testing of a blood sample.

Cardiovascular Effects

Hypertension and hypertensive crisis have been reported in niraparib-treated patients.

In the PRIMA study, grade 3 or greater hypertension occurred in 6% of niraparib-treated patients compared with 1% of those receiving placebo; discontinuance of therapy was not necessary in any patient. Median time to onset was 43 days (range: 1–531 days), and median duration of hypertension was 12 days (range: 1–61 days). Maximum mean increases from baseline in pulse rate, systolic blood pressure, and diastolic blood pressure were 22.4 beats per minute, 24.4 mm Hg, and 15.9 mm Hg, respectively, in patients receiving niraparib compared with 14 beats per minute, 19.6 mm Hg, and 13.9 mm Hg, respectively, in those receiving placebo.

In the NOVA study, grade 3 or greater hypertension occurred in 9% of niraparib-treated patients compared with 2% of those receiving placebo; discontinuance of therapy was necessary in less than 1% of patients receiving niraparib or placebo. Median time to onset was 77 days (range: 4–504 days), and median duration of hypertension was 15 days (range: 1–86 days). Maximum mean increases from baseline in pulse rate, systolic blood pressure, and diastolic blood pressure were 24.1 beats per minute, 24.5 mm Hg, and 16.5 mm Hg, respectively, in patients receiving niraparib compared with 15.8 beats per minute, 18.3 mm Hg, and 11.6 mm Hg, respectively, in those receiving placebo.

In a randomized, placebo-controlled study in patients with cancer, substantial changes in the mean QT interval corrected for rate (QT_c) (i.e., greater than 20 msec) were not observed when niraparib 300 mg was administered once daily.

Blood pressure and heart rate should be monitored at least weekly for the first 2 months of niraparib therapy, then monthly for the first year and periodically thereafter. Patients with cardiovascular disorders, particularly those with coronary insufficiency, cardiac arrhythmias, and/or hypertension, should be closely monitored. Hypertension should be managed with antihypertensive therapy and adjustment of the niraparib dosage, if necessary.

Posterior Reversible Encephalopathy Syndrome

In clinical trials, posterior reversible encephalopathy syndrome occurred in 0.1% of 2165 patients; it has also been described in postmarketing reports.

Patients should be monitored for signs and symptoms of posterior reversible encephalopathy syndrome, including seizure, headache, altered mental status, visual disturbance, and cortical blindness with or without associated hypertension. The diagnosis of posterior reversible encephalopathy syndrome requires confirmation by brain imaging (preferably magnetic resonance imaging). If posterior reversible encephalopathy syndrome is suspected, niraparib should be discontinued promptly, and appropriate treatment should be initiated. The safety of restarting niraparib in patients who previously experienced posterior reversible encephalopathy syndrome is not known.

Fetal/Neonatal Morbidity and Mortality

Based on its mechanism of action, niraparib may cause fetal harm (e.g., teratogenicity, embryofetal death) in humans. There are no data regarding use of niraparib in pregnant women to inform the drug-associated risk. Niraparib has the potential to cause teratogenicity and/or embryofetal death since the drug is genotoxic and targets actively dividing cells in animals and patients (e.g., bone marrow). Due to the potential risk to the fetus based on its mechanism of action, animal developmental and reproductive toxicology studies have not been conducted with niraparib.

Pregnancy should be avoided during niraparib therapy. Pregnancy status should be verified prior to starting niraparib therapy. Females of reproductive potential should be advised to use effective contraceptive methods while receiving niraparib and for at least 6 months after discontinuance of therapy. If niraparib is used during pregnancy or if the patient becomes pregnant while receiving the drug, the patient should be apprised of the potential risk to the fetus and the potential risk for loss of the pregnancy.

Sensitivity Reactions

Niraparib capsules contain the dye tartrazine (FD&C Yellow No. 5), which may cause allergic-type reactions including bronchial asthma in susceptible individuals. Although the incidence of tartrazine sensitivity is low, it frequently occurs in individuals who are sensitive to aspirin.

Specific Populations

Pregnancy

Although there are no available data in pregnant women, niraparib may cause fetal harm based on its mechanism of action. If niraparib is used during pregnancy or if the patient becomes pregnant while receiving the drug, the patient should be apprised of the potential fetal hazard and potential for loss of the pregnancy.

In females of reproductive potential, the manufacturer recommends a pregnancy test prior to initiating niraparib therapy.

Lactation

It is not known whether niraparib or its metabolites are distributed into human milk or if the drug has any effect on milk production or the breast-fed infant. Because of the potential for serious adverse reactions to niraparib in breast-fed infants, women should be advised to discontinue breast-feeding while receiving the drug and for 1 month after last dose.

Females and Males of Reproductive Potential

Females of reproductive potential should be advised to use effective contraceptive methods while receiving niraparib and for at least 6 months after discontinuance of therapy. If niraparib is used during pregnancy or if the patient becomes pregnant while receiving the drug, the patient should be apprised of the potential risk to the fetus and the potential risk for loss of the pregnancy.

Results of animal studies suggest that niraparib may impair male fertility. The effect of the drug on fertility in humans is not known.

Fertility studies have not been conducted with niraparib in animals. In a general toxicity study, reduced sperm, spermatids, and germ cells in epididymides and testes were observed in male animals receiving niraparib at exposure levels approximately 0.3 and 0.012 times the human exposure at a dose of 300 mg daily. A trend toward reversibility of these findings 4 weeks after discontinuance of therapy was observed.

Pediatric Use

Safety and efficacy of niraparib have not been established in pediatric patients.

Geriatric Use

In the PRIMA study, 39% of patients were 65 years of age or older and 10% were 75 years of age or older. In the NOVA study, 35% of patients were 65 years of age or older and 8% were 75 years of age or older. No overall differences in safety and efficacy were observed between geriatric patients and younger adults. However, the possibility of increased sensitivity to the drug in some geriatric patients cannot be ruled out.

Hepatic Impairment

In pharmacokinetic studies, mild hepatic impairment (total bilirubin not exceeding the ULN with AST exceeding ULN, or total bilirubin exceeding the ULN, but less than 1.5 times the ULN with any AST) had no clinically significant effect on the pharmacokinetics of niraparib; therefore, no initial dosage adjustment of niraparib is necessary in such patients.

In patients with moderate hepatic impairment (total bilirubin 1.5–3 times the ULN with any AST), the niraparib area under the serum concentration-time curve (AUC) was 1.56 times higher than the AUC observed in patients with normal hepatic function. Therefore, a reduction in the initial dosage of niraparib is recommended for such patients.

Pharmacokinetics and safety of niraparib in patients with severe hepatic impairment (total bilirubin greater than 3 times the ULN with any AST) have not been evaluated to date.

Renal Impairment

Population pharmacokinetic analyses indicate that the pharmacokinetics of niraparib in patients with mild or moderate renal impairment (creatinine clearance 30–90 mL/minute) are similar to those in patients with normal renal function; therefore, no initial dosage adjustment of the drug is necessary in such patients.

Pharmacokinetics and safety of niraparib in patients with severe renal impairment (creatinine clearance less than 30 mL/minute) or end-stage renal disease requiring hemodialysis have not been established to date.

● Common Adverse Effects

Adverse effects reported in 10% or more of patients receiving niraparib include nausea, thrombocytopenia, anemia, fatigue, constipation, musculoskeletal pain, abdominal pain, vomiting, neutropenia, decreased appetite, leukopenia, insomnia, headache, dyspnea, rash, diarrhea, hypertension, cough, dizziness, acute kidney injury, urinary tract infection, and hypomagnesemia.

DRUG INTERACTIONS

Niraparib is principally metabolized by carboxylesterases to form a major inactive metabolite, M1, which subsequently undergoes glucuronidation by uridine diphosphate-glucuronosyltransferases (UGT) to form the M10 metabolite. In vivo, niraparib is a substrate of carboxylesterases and UGT. In vitro studies indicate that niraparib is not an inhibitor of UGT1A1, UGT1A4, UGT1A9, or UGT2B7.

In vitro studies indicate that neither niraparib nor its major metabolite (M1) are inhibitors of cytochrome P-450 (CYP) isoenzymes 1A2, 2B6, 2C8, 2C9, 2C19, 2D6, and 3A4 or inducers of CYP3A4. The drug is a weak inducer of CYP1A2 in vitro.

Niraparib is an inhibitor of multidrug and toxin extrusion (MATE) 1 and 2 in vitro, but is not a substrate of MATE1 or 2. The M1 metabolite is a substrate but not an inhibitor of MATE1 and 2. In vitro studies indicate that niraparib is a substrate, but not an inhibitor, of P-glycoprotein (P-gp). Niraparib is also a substrate and a weak inhibitor of breast cancer resistance protein (BCRP). In vitro, neither niraparib nor M1 is a substrate or inhibitor of bile salt export pump (BSEP), organic anion transport protein (OATP) 1B1, OATP1B3, organic cation transporter (OCT) 1, OCT2, organic anion transporter (OAT) 1, and OAT3. In vitro studies also show that M1 is not a substrate or inhibitor of P-gp and BCRP. Neither niraparib nor M1 is a substrate or inhibitor of multidrug resistance-associated protein (MRP) 2.

● Drugs Affecting Gastric Acidity

Although not specifically studied in drug interaction studies to date, clinically important pharmacokinetic interactions between niraparib and drugs affecting gastric acidity (e.g., histamine H_2-receptor antagonists, proton-pump inhibitors) appear unlikely based on the drug's solubility in an acidic pH range.

● Drugs Affected by Transport Systems

Niraparib is an inhibitor of multidrug and toxin extrusion (MATE) 1 and 2; therefore, increased plasma concentrations of coadministered drugs that are substrates of MATE1 or 2 (e.g., metformin) cannot be excluded.

● Anticoagulants and Antiplatelet Agents

There is a potential for increased risk of adverse hematologic effects and hemorrhagic events in patients concurrently receiving niraparib and anticoagulants or antiplatelet agents.

DESCRIPTION

Niraparib, an inhibitor of mammalian poly(adenosine diphosphate [ADP]-ribose) polymerase (PARP) enzymes PARP-1 and PARP-2, is an antineoplastic agent. The drug is a highly selective inhibitor of PARP-1 and PARP-2, which are involved in detection of DNA damage and its repair. In vitro studies have demonstrated that niraparib-induced cytotoxicity may involve inhibition of PARP enzymatic activity and increased formation of PARP-DNA complexes, which result in DNA damage, apoptosis, and cell death. In vitro, niraparib exhibits cytotoxic activity in tumor cell lines with or without deficiencies in *BRCA1/2*. In addition, niraparib reduced tumor growth in xenograft models of human cancer cell lines with BRCA1/2 deficiencies in mice and in patient-derived xenograft tumor models with HRD expressing either mutated or wild-type *BRCA1/2*.

Following oral administration, the absolute bioavailability of niraparib is approximately 73%. Peak plasma concentrations and AUCs of niraparib are proportional to dose following repeated administration of the drug over the dosage range of 30–400 mg once daily. Following oral administration, niraparib is rapidly absorbed with peak plasma concentrations occurring within 3 hours. Repeated administration of niraparib 30–400 mg daily resulted in a twofold niraparib accumulation ratio. Oral administration of niraparib with a high-fat meal (800–1000 calories with fat accounting for approximately 50% of the caloric content) resulted in a decrease in peak plasma concentrations of approximately 22% and an increase in AUC of approximately 7%; however, these effects were not considered clinically important. The drug is 83% bound to plasma proteins.

Following oral administration of multiple doses of niraparib (300 mg once daily), the mean terminal half-life of niraparib was 36 hours. Niraparib is metabolized to inactive metabolites principally by amide hydrolysis followed by glucuronidation. Following oral administration of a single radiolabeled dose of niraparib, 47.5% of the radioactivity was recovered in urine (11% of the dose as unchanged drug) and 38.8% was recovered in feces (19% of the dose as unchanged drug). Population pharmacokinetic analyses indicate that age (18–65 years), gender, and race/ethnicity do not have clinically important effects on the pharmacokinetics of niraparib.

ADVICE TO PATIENTS

- Instruct patients to read the manufacturer's patient information.

- Advise patients to take niraparib capsules once daily at approximately the same time each day, either with or without food, and to swallow the capsules whole. Advise patients that administration of the drug at bedtime may help alleviate any nausea symptoms.

- If a dose is missed or vomited, advise patients not to take an extra dose and to take the next normal dose at the regularly scheduled time.

- Risk of myelodysplastic syndrome and acute myeloid leukemia. Stress importance of informing clinician if weakness, fatigue, fever, weight loss, frequent infections, bruising, unusual bleeding (including hematuria or bloody stool), or shortness of breath occurs.

- Risk of bone marrow suppression. Stress importance of periodic hematologic monitoring during therapy and informing clinician if new onset of bleeding, fever, or symptoms of infection occur.

- Risk of adverse cardiovascular effects, including hypertension and increased heart rate. Advise patients to undergo at least weekly blood pressure and heart rate monitoring during the first 2 months of treatment, followed by monthly monitoring during the first year of treatment and periodic monitoring thereafter. Advise patients to contact their clinician if elevated blood pressure occurs.

- Risk of posterior reversible encephalopathy syndrome. Advise patients to contact their clinician if seizure, headaches, altered mental status, or vision changes occur.

- Risk of fetal harm and pregnancy loss. Advise females of reproductive potential to avoid pregnancy and to use effective contraception while receiving niraparib and for at least 6 months following discontinuance of therapy. Stress importance of women informing clinicians immediately if they become pregnant during therapy or think they may be pregnant. If pregnancy occurs, advise pregnant women of potential risk to the fetus.

- Advise women to avoid breast-feeding while receiving niraparib and for 1 month following discontinuance of therapy.

- Advise patients that niraparib capsules contain FD&C Yellow No. 5 (tartrazine), which may cause allergic-type reactions (including bronchial asthma) in susceptible individuals or in those who also have aspirin hypersensitivity.

- Stress importance of informing clinicians of existing or contemplated concomitant therapy, including prescription and OTC drugs and dietary or herbal supplements, as well as any concomitant illnesses (e.g., cardiovascular disease, including hypertension, coronary insufficiency, or cardiac arrhythmias).

- Inform patients of other important precautionary information.

For further information on the handling of antineoplastic agents, see the ASHP Guidelines on Handling Hazardous Drugs at https://www.ahfsdrug information.com.

PREPARATIONS

Excipients in commercially available drug preparations may have clinically important effects in some individuals; consult specific product labeling for details.

Niraparib Tosylate

Oral

Capsules	100 mg (of niraparib)	Zejula®, GlaxoSmithKline

† Use is not currently included in the labeling approved by the US Food and Drug Administration.

Selected Revisions August 10, 2024, © Copyright, May 08, 2017, American Society of Health-System Pharmacists, Inc.

Nivolumab

10:00 · ANTINEOPLASTIC AGENTS

■ Nivolumab, a fully human anti-programmed-death receptor-1 (anti-PD-1) monoclonal antibody, is an antineoplastic agent. The drug is an IgG$_4$ kappa immunoglobulin.

USES

● *Melanoma*

Unresectable or Metastatic Melanoma

Nivolumab is used as monotherapy or in combination with ipilimumab for the treatment of unresectable or metastatic melanoma; nivolumab is designated an orphan drug by FDA for the treatment of this cancer.

The current indications for nivolumab as monotherapy or in combination with ipilimumab for the treatment of unresectable or metastatic melanoma are based principally on the results of an open-label, multicenter, randomized phase 3 study (CheckMate-037) and results of 2 multicenter, double-blind, randomized phase 3 studies (CheckMate-066 and CheckMate-067).

The CheckMate-037 study included 405 adults with unresectable or metastatic melanoma that had progressed during or following therapy with ipilimumab and, in those with tumors bearing the b-Raf serine-threonine kinase (BRAF) V600 mutation, therapy with a BRAF inhibitor. Patients were randomized (stratified by programmed-death ligand-1 [PD-L1] expression status, BRAF mutation status, and response to prior ipilimumab therapy) in a 2:1 ratio to receive either nivolumab (3 mg/kg administered by IV infusion every 2 weeks) or investigator's choice of chemotherapy (either dacarbazine 1 g/m^2 every 3 weeks or carboplatin at the dose required to obtain an area under the plasma concentration-time curve [AUC] of 6 mg/mL per minute in combination with paclitaxel 175 mg/m^2 every 3 weeks) until disease progression or unacceptable toxicity occurred. However, clinically stable patients with disease progression could continue treatment if they were considered to be deriving clinical benefit. In a planned noncomparative interim analysis, efficacy in the initial 120 patients randomized to receive nivolumab was evaluated based on overall response rate (as evaluated by a blinded independent central review committee) and duration of response. The median age of patients in the initial nivolumab-treated cohort was 58 years; all patients in this cohort had an Eastern Cooperative Oncology Group (ECOG) performance status of 0 or 1. Most patients (76%) in this cohort had TNM metastasis stage M1c disease, 68% had received 2 or more prior systemic therapies for their disease, 56% had elevated LDH concentrations, 22% had tumors bearing the BRAF V600 mutation, and 18% had a history of brain metastasis. Demographic characteristics of the entire study population were similar to those of the initial nivolumab-treated cohort. This study excluded patients receiving immunosuppressive agents and those with autoimmune disease, ocular melanoma, active brain metastasis, or a history of immune-mediated adverse effects with prior ipilimumab therapy (i.e., any grade 4 immune-mediated adverse effect [except for endocrinopathies] or grade 3 immune-mediated adverse effect that persisted for more than 12 weeks).

After a minimum follow-up of 6 months in the CheckMate-037 study, the overall response rate in the initial cohort of nivolumab-treated patients was 32%; complete response was achieved in 4 patients. At the time of analysis, the median duration of response had not been reached; most (87%) of the patients who responded to nivolumab had ongoing responses. Exploratory analysis suggested higher objective response rates for nivolumab compared with investigator's choice of chemotherapy regardless of BRAF mutation status or prior ipilimumab benefit; although a response benefit was observed for nivolumab compared with chemotherapy in patients with negative PD-L1 expression, the benefit of nivolumab relative to that of chemotherapy appeared to be greater in those with positive PD-L1 expression (defined as PD-L1 expression of any intensity on at least 5% of tumor cells as detected by immunohistochemistry assay). In the entire study population, median overall survival was 15.7 or 14.4 months in patients receiving nivolumab or investigator's choice of chemotherapy, respectively.

In the CheckMate-066 study, 418 patients with previously untreated unresectable or metastatic BRAF wild-type melanoma were randomized (stratified by PD-L1 expression status and stage of metastasis) to receive either nivolumab (3 mg/kg administered by IV infusion every 2 weeks) or dacarbazine (1 g/m^2 every

3 weeks) until disease progression or unacceptable toxicity occurred. However, patients with disease progression could continue receiving treatment if they were considered to be deriving clinical benefit. The primary measure of efficacy was overall survival; additional outcome measures were progression-free survival and overall response rate. The median age of patients was 65 years; 99.5% were Caucasian and 59% were male. Most patients (99%) enrolled in the study had an ECOG performance status of 0 or 1; however, a larger proportion of patients receiving nivolumab had an ECOG performance status of 0 compared with those receiving dacarbazine (71 versus 58%). Most patients (61%) had TNM metastasis stage M1c disease, 74% had cutaneous melanoma, 11% had mucosal melanoma, 37% had elevated LDH concentrations, 35% had positive PD-L1 expression (defined as PD-L1 expression of any intensity on at least 5% of tumor cells as detected by immunohistochemistry assay), and 4% had a history of brain metastasis. Patients with a history of serious autoimmune disease, ocular/uveal melanoma, or active brain or leptomeningeal metastasis were excluded from the study.

In the CheckMate-066 study, median overall survival in patients receiving nivolumab had not been reached at the time of the interim analysis; however, nivolumab reduced the risk of death by 58% compared with dacarbazine. At the time of the initial interim analysis, patients receiving nivolumab had a higher overall response rate (34 versus 9%) and longer median progression-free survival (5.1 versus 2.2 months) compared with patients receiving dacarbazine. After a minimum follow-up of 38.4 or 38.5 months in patients receiving nivolumab or dacarbazine, respectively, median overall survival was 37.5 months in patients receiving nivolumab compared with 11.2 months in those receiving dacarbazine. Progression-free survival for nivolumab- and dacarbazine-treated patients at the time of the updated analysis remained similar to the initial interim results. At the time of the updated analysis, overall response rates in nivolumab- and dacarbazine-treated patients were 42.9 and 14.4%, respectively; complete responses were achieved in 19 and 1.4% of nivolumab- and dacarbazine-treated patients, respectively. Median duration of response had not been reached in those receiving nivolumab and was 6 months in those receiving dacarbazine. The median time to complete or partial response was 2.1 months in nivolumab-treated patients and 2.9 or 2.2 months, respectively, in dacarbazine-treated patients. A planned subgroup analysis indicated that the effect of nivolumab on progression-free survival and overall survival was consistent regardless of PD-L1 expression (less than 5% versus 5% or more of tumor cells).

In the CheckMate-067 study, 945 patients with previously untreated unresectable or metastatic melanoma were randomized (stratified by PD-L1 expression status, BRAF V600 mutation status, and stage of metastasis) to receive one of 3 regimens: nivolumab (1 mg/kg by IV infusion) in combination with ipilimumab (3 mg/kg by IV infusion) every 3 weeks for 4 doses, followed by nivolumab monotherapy (3 mg/kg by IV infusion every 2 weeks); nivolumab (3 mg/kg by IV infusion every 2 weeks) and placebo; or ipilimumab (3 mg/kg by IV infusion every 3 weeks for 4 doses) and placebo. Treatment was continued until disease progression or unacceptable toxicity occurred; however, patients with disease progression could continue receiving treatment if they were considered to be deriving clinical benefit. The primary measures of efficacy were progression-free survival and overall survival; additional outcome measures were overall response rate and duration of response. In this study, the median age of patients was 61 years; 97% were Caucasian, 65% were male, 46% had positive PD-L1 expression (defined as PD-L1 expression of any intensity on at least 5% of tumor cells as detected by immunohistochemistry assay), 36% had elevated LDH concentrations, 32% had BRAF V600 mutation-positive melanoma, 22% had received prior adjuvant therapy, and 4% had a history of brain metastasis. All patients enrolled in the study had an ECOG performance status of 0 or 1. Most patients (93%) had metastatic disease; 58% of patients had TNM metastasis stage M1c disease. Patients with autoimmune disease, conditions requiring therapy with immunosuppressive agents, ocular melanoma, or active brain metastasis were excluded from the study.

After a minimum follow-up of 28 months in the CheckMate-067 study, overall survival rate was higher in patients receiving nivolumab in combination with ipilimumab and in those receiving nivolumab compared with those receiving ipilimumab (59 and 55%, respectively, versus 37%). Progression-free survival also was prolonged in patients receiving nivolumab in combination with ipilimumab and in those receiving nivolumab compared with those receiving ipilimumab (11.7 and 6.9 months, respectively, versus 2.9 months). In addition, patients receiving nivolumab in combination with ipilimumab and those receiving nivolumab had higher overall response rates compared with those receiving ipilimumab (50 and 40%, respectively, versus 14%); complete responses were achieved in 8.9, 8.5, or 1.9% of patients receiving combination therapy with nivolumab and ipilimumab, nivolumab, or ipilimumab, respectively. After a minimum follow-up of

28 months, 55, 56, or 39% of patients receiving these respective treatments had durable responses of 24 months or more. After a minimum follow-up of 48 months, median overall survival was 36.9 or 19.9 months in patients receiving nivolumab or ipilimumab, respectively, but had not been reached in those receiving nivolumab in combination with ipilimumab. Progression-free survival at a minimum follow-up of 48 months in patients receiving combination therapy with nivolumab and ipilimumab, nivolumab, or ipilimumab remained similar to the initial interim results. The study was not designed to assess whether combination therapy with nivolumab and ipilimumab results in improved survival relative to nivolumab alone. Results of a subgroup analysis (based on age, geographic region, ECOG performance status, PD-L1 expression status, BRAF V600 mutation status, stage of metastasis, tumor burden, and number of lesions) suggested that the progression-free survival and overall survival benefit of nivolumab or nivolumab in combination with ipilimumab versus ipilimumab was consistent across all subgroups.

Adjuvant Therapy for Locally Advanced or Metastatic Melanoma

Nivolumab is used as adjuvant therapy of locally advanced or metastatic melanoma following complete resection.

The current indication for nivolumab as adjuvant therapy for locally advanced or metastatic melanoma is based principally on the results of a randomized, double-blind phase 3 study (CheckMate-238) in patients with completely resected stage IIIB, IIIC, or IV melanoma. In this study, 906 patients were randomized (stratified by disease stage and PD-L1 expression status) to receive either nivolumab (3 mg/kg administered by IV infusion every 2 weeks) or ipilimumab (10 mg/kg by IV infusion every 3 weeks for 4 doses then every 12 weeks beginning at week 24) for up to 1 year or until disease recurrence or unacceptable toxicity occurred. The primary measure of efficacy was recurrence-free survival. The median age of patients enrolled in the study was 55 years; 95% were Caucasian, 90% had a baseline ECOG performance status of 0, 58% were male, 81% had stage IIIB or IIIC disease, 42% had BRAF V600 mutation-positive melanoma, 48% had macroscopic lymph node involvement, 34% had positive PD-L1 expression (defined as PD-L1 expression of any intensity on at least 5% of tumor cells as detected by a clinical trial assay), 32% had tumor ulceration, and 8% had elevated LDH concentrations. Patients were eligible for enrollment in the study following complete resection of melanoma within 12 weeks prior to randomization. The study excluded patients with a history of autoimmune disease, ocular/uveal melanoma, or any condition requiring therapy with systemic corticosteroids or immunosuppressive agents; those who had received prior therapy for melanoma other than surgery; those who had received adjuvant radiation therapy following neurosurgical resection; and those who had received adjuvant therapy with interferon alfa 6 months or more prior to randomization.

After a minimum follow-up of 18 months, median recurrence-free survival had not been reached in either group; however, nivolumab reduced the risk of recurrence or death by 35% compared with ipilimumab. At 18 months, the recurrence-free survival rate was 66.4 or 52.7% in patients receiving nivolumab or ipilimumab, respectively. Results of a subgroup analysis (based on age, gender, disease stage, PD-L1 status, BRAF mutation status, presence of tumor ulceration, lymph node involvement, and disease subtype) suggested that the effect of nivolumab on recurrence-free survival was consistent across most subgroups; however, a recurrence-free survival benefit for nivolumab versus ipilimumab was not apparent in patients with stage IV M1c disease, those with microscopic lymph node involvement and ulceration of the primary tumor, or those with a mucosal subtype.

● Non-small Cell Lung Cancer

Nivolumab is used for the treatment of metastatic non-small cell lung cancer (NSCLC) that has progressed during or following therapy with platinum-based chemotherapy and, in those with epidermal growth factor receptor (EGFR) mutation- or anaplastic lymphoma kinase (ALK)-positive tumors, therapy with an EGFR or ALK inhibitor. The current indication for use of nivolumab for the treatment of previously treated metastatic NSCLC is based principally on the results of 2 randomized open-label studies (CheckMate-017 and CheckMate-057) and a supportive multicenter, noncomparative phase 2 study (CheckMate-063).

In the CheckMate-017 study, 272 patients with metastatic squamous NSCLC that had progressed during or following therapy with one platinum-containing, 2-drug combination regimen were randomized to receive either nivolumab (3 mg/kg administered by IV infusion every 2 weeks) or docetaxel (75 mg/m² administered by IV infusion every 3 weeks). The primary measure of efficacy was

overall survival. The median age of patients enrolled in the study was 63 years; all patients enrolled in the study had an ECOG performance status of 0 or 1. Patients were eligible for enrollment in the study regardless of tumor expression of PD-L1. This study excluded patients with autoimmune disease, any condition requiring therapy with immunosuppressive agents, symptomatic interstitial lung disease, or untreated brain metastasis.

At the time of data analysis in the CheckMate-017 study, median overall survival (9.2 versus 6 months) and progression-free survival (3.5 versus 2.8 months) were prolonged and overall response rates (20 versus 9%) were higher in patients receiving nivolumab compared with those receiving docetaxel; complete response was achieved in 1 patient receiving nivolumab and none of those receiving docetaxel. Median overall survival, median progression-free survival, and overall response rates remained similar at the time of a 24-month analysis. Among patients with evaluable PD-L1 expression, there were no clear differences in overall survival based on PD-L1 expression.

In the CheckMate-057 study, 582 patients with metastatic nonsquamous NSCLC that had progressed during or following therapy with one platinum-containing, 2-drug combination regimen were randomized to receive either nivolumab (3 mg/kg administered by IV infusion every 2 weeks) or docetaxel (75 mg/m² administered by IV infusion every 3 weeks) until disease progression or unacceptable toxicity occurred. The primary measure of efficacy was overall survival; additional outcome measures were overall response rate and progression-free survival. The median age of patients enrolled in the study was 62 years; all patients enrolled in the study had an ECOG performance status of 0 or 1, 93% had adenocarcinoma histology, 14% had EGFR mutation-positive disease, 3.6% had ALK-positive disease, and 40% had received maintenance therapy as part of their first-line regimen. This study excluded patients with autoimmune disease, symptomatic interstitial lung disease, untreated brain metastasis, or any condition requiring therapy with immunosuppressive agents.

At the time of the interim analysis in the CheckMate-057 study, patients receiving nivolumab had longer median overall survival compared with those receiving docetaxel (12.2 versus 9.4 months). Although not statistically significant, progression-free survival appeared to be shorter in patients receiving nivolumab compared with those receiving docetaxel (2.3 versus 4.2 months). Patients receiving nivolumab had a higher overall response rate compared with those receiving docetaxel (19 versus 12%); complete responses were achieved in 1.4 or 0.3% of patients receiving nivolumab or docetaxel, respectively. At the time of analysis, the median duration of response was 17 months in patients receiving nivolumab and 6 months in those receiving docetaxel; however, responses were ongoing in nivolumab-treated patients. Median overall survival, median progression-free survival, and overall response rates remained similar at the time of a 24-month analysis. Subgroup analysis based on relevant patient characteristics (prior maintenance therapy, line of therapy, age, gender, ECOG performance status, smoking status, EGFR mutation status, KRAS mutation status) suggested that nivolumab had a greater effect on overall survival relative to docetaxel in most patient subgroups; however, a survival benefit for nivolumab versus docetaxel was not apparent for patients receiving the drug as third-line therapy, those who had never smoked, and those with EGFR mutation-positive disease. Subgroup analysis also indicated that increasing levels of PD-L1 expression were associated with overall survival and progression-free survival benefits for nivolumab compared with docetaxel.

In the CheckMate-063 study, 117 patients with advanced squamous NSCLC that had progressed following therapy with a platinum-based regimen and at least one additional systemic therapy received nivolumab 3 mg/kg administered by IV infusion every 2 weeks. The primary measure of efficacy was overall response rate (as evaluated by an independent central review committee); an additional outcome measure was duration of response. The median age of patients enrolled in the study was 65 years; all patients enrolled in the study had an ECOG performance status of 0 or 1. Patients were eligible for enrollment in the study regardless of their PD-L1 status. This study excluded patients with autoimmune disease, symptomatic interstitial lung disease, or untreated brain metastasis. After a minimum follow-up of 10 months, the overall response rate was 15%; there were no complete responses. At the time of analysis, 76% of the responders had ongoing responses; 59% of these patients had durable responses of 6 months or more.

● Small Cell Lung Cancer

Nivolumab is used for the treatment of metastatic small cell lung cancer (SCLC) that has progressed following therapy with platinum-based chemotherapy and at least one other line of therapy; nivolumab has been designated an orphan drug by FDA for the treatment of this cancer. The accelerated approval of nivolumab for the treatment of metastatic SCLC that has progressed following therapy with platinum-based chemotherapy and at least one other line of therapy is based on objective response rate and duration of response; continued approval for this indication may be contingent on verification and description of clinical benefit of nivolumab in confirmatory studies.

The current indication for nivolumab in the treatment of previously treated metastatic SCLC is based principally on the results for a cohort of patients with metastatic SCLC who received nivolumab monotherapy in an ongoing, multicenter, open-label phase ½ study (CheckMate-032). This cohort of patients included 109 adults with metastatic SCLC that had progressed following therapy with platinum-based chemotherapy and at least one other line of therapy who received nivolumab (3 mg/kg administered by IV infusion over 60 minutes every 2 weeks). The primary measure of efficacy was objective response rate (as evaluated by a blinded independent central review committee according to RECIST). The median age of patients enrolled in this SCLC cohort was 64 years (6% of patients were 75 years of age or older); 99% had a baseline ECOG performance status of 0 or 1, 94% were Caucasian, 93% were former or current smokers, 56% were male, and 7% had brain metastases. Approximately 65% had platinum-sensitive disease (defined as disease progression 90 days or more following the last dose of platinum-containing therapy). All patients enrolled in the cohort had received 2 or more prior lines of therapy; 94% had received 2 or 3 lines of therapy and 6% had received 4 or 5 lines of therapy. Patients were eligible for enrollment in the study regardless of tumor expression of PD-L1. This study excluded patients with autoimmune disease, any condition requiring therapy with immunosuppressive agents, symptomatic interstitial lung disease, or untreated brain metastasis.

The overall response rate in the CheckMate-032 study for patients receiving nivolumab monotherapy for treatment of metastatic SCLC that had progressed following treatment with platinum-based chemotherapy and at least one other line of therapy was 12%; complete responses were achieved in 0.9% of patients. At the time of analysis, 77, 62, or 39% of the responders had durable responses of at least 6, 12, or 18 months, respectively.

● Renal Cell Carcinoma
Previously Treated Advanced Renal Cell Carcinoma

Nivolumab is used as monotherapy for the treatment of advanced renal cell carcinoma previously treated with antiangiogenic therapy. In patients with advanced renal cell carcinoma, nivolumab therapy has been shown to prolong overall survival and increase response rate compared with everolimus.

The current indication for nivolumab as monotherapy in the treatment of advanced renal cell carcinoma is based principally on the results of a randomized, open-label phase 3 study (CheckMate-025) in adults with advanced renal cell carcinoma that had progressed during or following treatment with 1 or 2 prior antiangiogenic therapies. In this study, 821 patients were randomized (stratified by geographic region, Memorial Sloan-Kettering Cancer Center [MSKCC] risk category, number of prior therapies including an antiangiogenic agent) to receive either nivolumab (3 mg/kg administered by IV infusion every 2 weeks) or everolimus (10 mg orally once daily). The primary measure of efficacy was overall survival. The median age of patients enrolled in the study was 62 years (9% of patients were 75 years of age or older); 88% were Caucasian, 75% were male, 81% had MSKCC favorable- or intermediate-risk disease, and 77% had received one prior antiangiogenic therapy. All patients enrolled in the study had a baseline Karnofsky performance status of 70 or greater. Patients were eligible for enrollment in the study regardless of tumor expression of PD-L1. This study excluded patients with active autoimmune disease, any history of or active brain metastasis, or any condition requiring therapy with immunosuppressive agents, and those previously treated with a mammalian target of rapamycin (mTOR) inhibitor.

After a minimum follow-up of 14 months, patients receiving nivolumab had longer median overall survival compared with those receiving everolimus (25 versus 19.6 months). Results of a subgroup analysis suggested that the effect of nivolumab on overall survival was consistent regardless of MSKCC risk category, number of prior therapies including an antiangiogenic agent, and geographic region; however, an overall survival benefit for nivolumab versus everolimus was not apparent in the small group of patients 75 years of age or older. Patients receiving nivolumab also had higher objective response rates (21.5 versus 3.9%), with a median response duration of 23 months for those receiving nivolumab and 13.7 months for those receiving everolimus. The median time to response was 3

months (range: 1.4–13 months) for nivolumab-treated patients. This study was terminated prematurely at the request of the independent data monitoring committee because of improved overall survival observed during the prespecified interim analysis in patients receiving nivolumab.

First-line Therapy for Advanced Renal Cell Carcinoma

Nivolumab is used in combination with ipilimumab for the treatment of intermediate- or poor-risk, previously untreated, advanced renal cell carcinoma. In patients with intermediate- or poor-risk, previously untreated, advanced renal cell carcinoma, nivolumab in combination with ipilimumab has been shown to prolong overall survival and increase response rate compared with sunitinib. Efficacy of nivolumab in combination with ipilimumab in patients with favorable-risk†, previously untreated, advanced renal cell carcinoma has not been established.

The current indication for nivolumab in combination with ipilimumab in the treatment of intermediate- or poor-risk, previously untreated, advanced renal cell carcinoma is based principally on the results of a randomized, open-label phase 3 study (CheckMate-214) in adults with previously untreated advanced renal cell carcinoma. In this study, 1082 patients were randomized (stratified by geographic region and International Metastatic Renal Cell Carcinoma Database Consortium [IMDC] risk score) to receive either nivolumab (3 mg/kg by IV infusion) in combination with ipilimumab (1 mg/kg by IV infusion) every 3 weeks for 4 doses, followed by nivolumab monotherapy (3 mg/kg by IV infusion every 2 weeks), or sunitinib (50 mg orally once daily for 4 consecutive weeks of each 6-week cycle). Treatment was continued until disease progression or unacceptable toxicity occurred. The primary measures of efficacy were overall survival, progression-free survival (as evaluated by an independent review committee according to RECIST), and objective response rate (as evaluated by an independent review committee according to RECIST) in patients with intermediate- or poor-risk disease (defined as patients with at least one prognostic risk factor according to IMDC criteria). The median age of patients enrolled in the study was 61 years (8% of patients were 75 years of age or older); 87% were Caucasian and 73% were male. All patients enrolled in the study had a baseline Karnofsky performance status of 70 or greater. Patients were eligible for enrollment in the study regardless of tumor expression of PD-L1. This study excluded patients with active autoimmune disease, any history of or active brain metastasis, or any condition requiring therapy with immunosuppressive agents.

At a median follow-up of 25.2 months, median overall survival for patients with intermediate- or poor-risk disease receiving nivolumab in combination with ipilimumab had not been reached; however, nivolumab in combination with ipilimumab reduced the risk of death by 37% compared with sunitinib. Progression-free survival was 11.6 months in patients receiving nivolumab in combination with ipilimumab and 8.4 months in those receiving sunitinib; however, the difference was not statistically significant. Patients with intermediate- or poor-risk disease receiving nivolumab in combination with ipilimumab also had higher objective response rates (41.6 versus 26.5%); complete response was achieved in 9.4% of patients receiving nivolumab in combination with ipilimumab and 1.2% of those receiving sunitinib. At the time of analysis, the median duration of response had not been reached in patients receiving nivolumab in combination with ipilimumab and was 18.2 months in those receiving sunitinib. Results of a subgroup analysis (based on age, gender, geographic region, IMDC risk category, prior nephrectomy, baseline level of PD-L1 expression, and site of metastases) in patients with intermediate- or poor-risk disease suggested a survival benefit for nivolumab in combination with ipilimumab relative to sunitinib across subgroups. In an exploratory analysis, an overall survival benefit for the nivolumab-ipilimumab combination regimen compared with sunitinib was not apparent in the subgroup of patients who had favorable-risk disease (hazard ratio: 1.45).

● Hodgkin Lymphoma

Nivolumab is used for the treatment of classical Hodgkin lymphoma (cHL) that has relapsed or progressed following autologous stem cell transplantation and subsequent therapy with brentuximab vedotin or following failure of at least 3 systemic therapies (including autologous stem cell transplantation); nivolumab has been designated an orphan drug by FDA for the treatment of this cancer. The accelerated approval of nivolumab for this indication is based on objective response rate. Continued approval for this indication may be contingent on verification and description of clinical benefit of nivolumab in confirmatory studies.

The current indication for nivolumab in the treatment of cHL is based principally on analysis of combined data from a cohort of patients in an open-label, multicenter, noncomparative phase 2 study (CheckMate-205) and an open-label, multicenter phase 1 dose-escalation study (CheckMate-039); 95 patients with cHL that had relapsed or progressed following autologous stem cell transplantation and subsequent therapy with brentuximab vedotin and 258 patients with cHL that had relapsed or progressed following autologous stem cell transplantation were included in the pooled analysis. The primary measure of efficacy was objective response rate as assessed by an independent review committee; an additional outcome measure was duration of response. Patients in both studies received nivolumab 3 mg/kg administered by IV infusion every 2 weeks. Treatment was continued until disease progression, maximum clinical benefit, or unacceptable toxicity occurred. Patients were eligible for enrollment in these studies regardless of tumor expression of PD-L1. The studies excluded patients with an ECOG performance status of 2 or greater, autoimmune disease, or symptomatic interstitial lung disease; those who had received an allogeneic stem cell transplant; those who had received radiation therapy to the chest area within 24 weeks prior to enrollment; and those with a history of pulmonary toxicity who had an adjusted diffusion lung capacity for carbon monoxide (DLCO) of 60% or less.

In the cohort of patients who had relapsed or had experienced disease progression following autologous stem cell transplantation and subsequent therapy with brentuximab vedotin, the median age of patients was 37 years; 87% were Caucasian and 64% were male. The median number of previous systemic therapies for patients in this cohort was 5 (range: 2–15). The overall response rate for patients in this cohort was 66%; complete response was achieved in 6% of patients in this cohort. At a median follow-up of 9.9 months, the estimated median duration of response was 13.1 months for patients in this cohort. The median time to response was 2 months (range: 0.7–11.1 months).

In the cohort of patients who had relapsed or had experienced disease progression following autologous stem cell transplantation, the median age of patients was 34 years; 86% were Caucasian and 59% were male. Most patients (85%) in this cohort had received at least 3 prior therapies; the median number of previous therapies was 4 (range: 2–15). Most patients (76%) in this cohort had received prior therapy with brentuximab vedotin; 78% of patients received brentuximab vedotin following stem cell transplantation, 17% received the drug prior to stem cell transplantation, and 5% received the drug prior to and following stem cell transplantation. The overall response rate for patients in this cohort was 69%; complete response was achieved in 14% of patients in this cohort. At a median follow-up of 6.7 months, the median duration of response had not been reached. The median time to response was 2 months (range: 0.7–11.1 months).

● Head and Neck Cancer

Nivolumab is used for the treatment of metastatic or recurrent squamous cell carcinoma of the head and neck that has progressed during or following therapy with platinum-based chemotherapy. In patients with metastatic or recurrent squamous cell carcinoma of the head and neck, nivolumab therapy has been shown to prolong overall survival compared with standard chemotherapy.

The current indication for nivolumab in the treatment of metastatic or recurrent squamous cell carcinoma of the head and neck is based principally on the results of a randomized, open-label phase 3 study (CheckMate-141) in adults with metastatic or recurrent squamous cell carcinoma of the head and neck that had progressed during or within 6 months following platinum-based chemotherapy in the neoadjuvant, adjuvant, primary (unresectable locally advanced), or metastatic setting. In this study, 361 patients were randomized (stratified by prior cetuximab use) to receive either nivolumab (3 mg/kg administered by IV infusion every 2 weeks) or investigator's choice of standard chemotherapy (cetuximab 400 mg/m² by IV infusion followed by cetuximab 250 mg/m² by IV infusion weekly; methotrexate 40–60 mg/m² by IV infusion weekly; or docetaxel 30–40 mg/m² by IV infusion weekly) until disease progression or unacceptable toxicity occurred. However, nivolumab therapy could be continued in patients with disease progression if they were considered to be deriving clinical benefit. The primary measure of efficacy was overall survival; additional outcome measures were overall response rate and progression-free survival. The median age of patients enrolled in the study was 60 years; most patients (98%) had an ECOG performance status of 0 or 1, 90% had metastatic disease, 83% were Caucasian, 83% were male, 76% were former or current smokers, 55% had received at least 2 prior therapies, 51% had unknown human papillomavirus (HPV) status, and 25% had HPV-positive disease (as assessed by p16 immunohistochemistry assay). This study excluded patients with autoimmune disease, untreated brain metastasis, conditions requiring therapy with immunosuppressive agents, human immunodeficiency virus

(HIV) infection, hepatitis B virus (HBV) or hepatitis C virus (HCV) infection, recurrent or metastatic carcinoma of the nasopharynx, squamous cell carcinoma of unknown primary histology, or salivary gland or nonsquamous histology (e.g., mucosal melanoma).

A planned interim analysis indicated that patients receiving nivolumab had longer overall survival compared with patients receiving standard chemotherapy (7.5 versus 5.1 months). The median follow-up at the time of the interim analysis was 5.1 months. Results of the interim analysis suggested a numerical, but not statistically significant, increase in overall response rate with nivolumab compared with standard chemotherapy; progression-free survival was similar in both groups. Results of a subgroup analysis (based on age, ECOG performance status, prior cetuximab therapy, lines of prior therapy, investigator's choice of standard chemotherapy, site of primary tumor, and platinum-refractory disease in the primary setting) suggested that the effect of nivolumab on overall survival was consistent across all subgroups. A planned exploratory analysis indicated a survival benefit for nivolumab compared with standard chemotherapy regardless of PD-L1 expression or p16 tumor status; although the survival benefit appeared to be more pronounced in patients with PD-L1 expression on 1% or more of tumor cells compared with those with PD-L1 expression levels of less than 1% (hazard ratios: 0.55 and 0.89, respectively) and in patients with p16-positive tumors compared with those with p16-negative tumors (hazard ratios: 0.56 and 0.73, respectively), these interactions were not statistically significant.

● Urothelial Carcinoma

Nivolumab is used for the treatment of locally advanced or metastatic urothelial carcinoma that has progressed during or following platinum-containing therapy or within 12 months of platinum-containing therapy in the neoadjuvant or adjuvant setting. The accelerated approval of nivolumab for this indication is based on objective response rate and duration of response. Continued approval for this indication may be contingent on verification and description of clinical benefit of nivolumab in confirmatory studies.

The current indication for nivolumab in the treatment of locally advanced or metastatic urothelial carcinoma is based principally on the results of a multicenter, noncomparative phase 2 study (CheckMate-275) in adults with locally advanced or metastatic urothelial carcinoma that had progressed during or following platinum-containing therapy for metastatic disease or within 12 months of platinum-containing therapy in the neoadjuvant or adjuvant setting. The primary measure of efficacy was objective response rate as assessed by a blinded independent review committee according to Response Evaluation Criteria in Solid Tumors (RECIST 1.1). In this study, the median age of patients was 66 years; 86% were Caucasian, 84% had visceral metastases, 78% were male, and 27% had nonbladder urothelial carcinoma. All patients enrolled in the study had an ECOG performance status of 0 or 1. Approximately one-third (29%) of patients had received at least 2 prior therapies for metastatic disease and 34% had disease progression following platinum-containing therapy in the neoadjuvant or adjuvant setting; 36, 23, or 7% of patients had received prior treatment with cisplatin-, carboplatin-, or both cisplatin- and carboplatin-based regimens, respectively, for metastatic disease. Patients received nivolumab 3 mg/kg administered by IV infusion every 2 weeks until disease progression or unacceptable toxicity occurred; however, patients with disease progression could continue treatment if they were considered to be deriving clinical benefit. Patients with active brain or leptomeningeal metastases, autoimmune disease, or any condition requiring therapy with immunosuppressive agents were excluded from the study. Patients were eligible for enrollment in the study regardless of their PD-L1 status.

At a minimum follow-up of 6 months, the objective response rate was 19.6%; complete responses were achieved in 2.6% of patients. Among patients who had received prior therapy only in the neoadjuvant and adjuvant setting, the objective response rate was 23.4%. At the time of analysis, the estimated median duration of response was 10.3 months; however, 77% of the patients who responded to nivolumab had ongoing responses. The median time to response was 1.9 months (range: 1.6–7.2 months). In the planned subgroup analysis based on PD-L1 expression (as detected by an immunohistochemistry assay [Dako PD-L1 IHC 28-8 pharmDx]), the objective response rate with nivolumab therapy was 15.1% in patients with PD-L1 expression on less than 1% of tumor cells and 25% in those with PD-L1 expression on 1% or more of tumor cells; complete responses were achieved in 0.7 or 4.8% of patients in these respective subgroups. The median progression-free survival as assessed by the blinded independent review committee was 2 months. At a median follow-up of 7 months, median overall survival was

8.7 months in the overall population, 11.3 months in those with PD-L1 expression of 1% or more, and 6 months in those with PD-L1 expression of less than 1%. Results of a subgroup analysis (based on site of metastasis, ECOG performance status, Bellmunt risk factors, baseline hemoglobin concentration, baseline creatinine clearance, site of primary tumor, and prior therapy for advanced or metastatic disease) suggested that the drug's effect on tumor response was consistent across most subgroups; however, the effect on tumor response appeared to be reduced in patients with increasing number of Bellmunt risk factors.

• Colorectal Cancer

Nivolumab is used as monotherapy or in combination with ipilimumab for the treatment of metastatic colorectal cancer with high microsatellite instability (MSI-H) or mismatch repair deficiency (dMMR) that has progressed following fluoropyrimidine-, oxaliplatin-, and irinotecan-containing therapy. The accelerated approval of nivolumab as a single agent or in combination with ipilimumab for this indication is based on objective response rate and duration of response. Continued approval for this indication may be contingent on verification and description of clinical benefit of nivolumab in confirmatory studies.

Although some solid tumors, such as colorectal cancer, are generally unresponsive to anti-PD-1 therapy, a subpopulation of patients with solid tumors with MSI-H or dMMR has been shown to be particularly responsive to anti-PD-1 therapy. Deficiencies in the DNA mismatch repair pathway as a result of germline or somatic mutations in mismatch repair genes subsequently result in elevated levels of DNA instability in regions of short tandem repeat sequences (microsatellites) that are prone to replication errors (MSI-H). It has been postulated that the increased mutational burden in tumors with microsatellite instability produces tumor-specific neoantigens responsible for elevated levels of tumor-infiltrating lymphocytes and upregulation of immune checkpoint proteins such as PD-1 and PD-L1, suggesting that patients with solid tumors with MSI-H or dMMR are good candidates for immune checkpoint therapy. Clinical studies have demonstrated increased response rates in patients with solid tumors, particularly colorectal cancer, with MSI-H or dMMR receiving anti-PD-1 therapy. In a phase 2 study evaluating pembrolizumab, an anti-PD-1 antibody, in patients with solid tumors with dMMR or proficient mismatch repair (pMMR), the objective response rate (40 versus 0%) and progression-free survival rate (78 versus 11%) were substantially higher in patients with colorectal cancer with dMMR compared with those with pMMR colorectal cancer; response rates in patients with noncolorectal cancers with dMMR were similar to those in patients with colorectal cancer with dMMR.

The current indication for nivolumab as a single agent or in combination with ipilimumab is based principally on the results of an open-label, multicenter, noncomparative phase 2 study (CheckMate-142) in adults with MSI-H or dMMR metastatic colorectal cancer who had experienced disease progression during or following at least one prior therapy, including fluoropyrimidine- and oxaliplatin- or irinotecan-containing therapy, or who had not tolerated such therapies. Objective response rate was assessed by a blinded independent review committee according to RECIST 1.1. In this study, patients assigned to the monotherapy cohort received nivolumab 3 mg/kg administered as an IV infusion every 2 weeks until disease progression or unacceptable toxicity occurred, and patients assigned to the combination therapy cohort received nivolumab 3 mg/kg administered as an IV infusion and ipilimumab 1 mg/kg administered as an IV infusion on day 1 of each 21-day cycle for 4 doses, followed by single-agent nivolumab therapy (3 mg/kg administered as an IV infusion every 2 weeks) until disease progression or unacceptable toxicity occurred; however, patients in both cohorts could continue single-agent nivolumab beyond initial disease progression if they were considered to be deriving clinical benefit. Patients with active autoimmune disease, active brain metastasis, any condition requiring therapy with immunosuppressive agents, history of HIV infection, or HBV or HCV infection were excluded from the study.

In the cohort of 74 patients who received single-agent nivolumab, the median age of patients was 53 years; 98% had an ECOG performance status of 0 or 1, 88% were Caucasian, 59% were male, and 36% had a history of Lynch syndrome. Most patients (72%) had previously received fluoropyrimidine-, oxaliplatin-, and irinotecan-containing therapy and 42% of patients had previously received anti-EGFR therapy; 30, 28, 19, or 16% of patients had received 1, 2, 3, or 4 or more prior lines of therapy for metastatic disease, respectively. At a median follow-up of 12 months, the objective response rate was 32%; complete responses were achieved in 2.7% of patients. At the time of analysis, 63 or 38% of patients had durable responses of at least 6 or 12 months, respectively. Among patients previously treated with fluoropyrimidine-, oxaliplatin-, and irinotecan-containing therapy,

the objective response rate was 28%; complete responses were achieved in 1.9% of patients who had received such prior therapy; and 67 or 40% of the responders had durable responses of at least 6 or 12 months, respectively. Objective responses were observed regardless of PD-L1 expression (on tumor cells or tumor-infiltrating immune cells), presence of mutated or wild-type BRAF or KRAS, or history of Lynch syndrome.

In the cohort of 119 patients who received nivolumab in combination with ipilimumab, the median age of patients was 58 years; 92% were Caucasian, 59% were male, and 29% had a history of Lynch syndrome. All patients enrolled in the combination therapy cohort had a baseline ECOG performance status of 0 or 1. Most patients (69%) had previously received fluoropyrimidine-, oxaliplatin-, and irinotecan-containing therapy and 29% of patients had previously received anti-EGFR therapy; 10, 40, 24, or 15% of patients had received 1, 2, 3, or 4 or more prior lines of therapy for metastatic disease, respectively. At a median follow-up of 13.4 months, the objective response rate was 49%; complete responses were achieved in 4.2% of patients. At the time of analysis, 83 or 19% of patients had durable responses of at least 6 or 12 months, respectively. Among patients previously treated with fluoropyrimidine-, oxaliplatin-, and irinotecan-containing therapy, the objective response rate was 46%; complete responses were achieved in 3.7% of patients who had received such prior therapy; and 89 or 21% of the responders had durable responses of at least 6 or 12 months, respectively.

• Hepatocellular Carcinoma

Nivolumab is used for the treatment of hepatocellular carcinoma previously treated with sorafenib; nivolumab has been designated an orphan drug by FDA for the treatment of this cancer. The accelerated approval of nivolumab for this indication is based on objective response rate and duration of response. Continued approval for this indication may be contingent on verification and description of clinical benefit of nivolumab in confirmatory studies.

The current indication for nivolumab in the treatment of previously treated hepatocellular carcinoma is based principally on the results for a cohort of patients with hepatocellular carcinoma in an open-label, multicenter, noncomparative, phase ½ study (CheckMate-040); the cohort included 154 adults with advanced hepatocellular carcinoma who had experienced disease progression during sorafenib therapy or who had not tolerated such therapy. The primary measure of efficacy was objective response rate according to RECIST 1.1 and modified RECIST for hepatocellular carcinoma as assessed by a blinded independent review committee. The median age of patients in the hepatocellular carcinoma cohort was 63 years; 99% had Child-Pugh class A hepatic impairment, 77% were male, 71% had extrahepatic spread, 46% were Caucasian, 31% had active HBV infection, 37% had α-fetoprotein concentrations of 0.4 mg/L or more, 29% had macrovascular invasion, 21% had active HCV infection, and 19% had received at least 2 prior systemic therapies. All patients enrolled in the hepatocellular carcinoma cohort had an ECOG performance status of 0 or 1 and previously had received sorafenib therapy; sorafenib was discontinued because of intolerable toxicity in 23% of patients. Alcohol consumption or nonalcoholic liver disease was the cause of hepatocellular carcinoma in 18 or 6.5% of patients, respectively. Prior therapies included surgical resection, locoregional therapy, and radiation therapy in 66, 58, and 24% of patients, respectively. Patients received nivolumab 3 mg/kg administered as an IV infusion every 2 weeks until disease progression or unacceptable toxicity occurred. The study excluded patients with autoimmune disease, brain metastasis, a history of hepatic encephalopathy, current or prior episodes of clinically important ascites, HIV infection, active HBV and HCV coinfection, or active HBV and hepatitis D virus (HDV) coinfection.

At the time of analysis, the objective response rate according to RECIST 1.1 or modified RECIST for patients in the hepatocellular carcinoma cohort of this study was 14.3 or 18.2%, respectively; according to these response criteria, complete response was achieved in 1.9 or 3.2%, respectively, of patients. The median duration of response had not been reached; however, 91% of patients who responded to the drug had durable responses of 6 months or more and 55% had durable responses of 12 months or more.

DOSAGE AND ADMINISTRATION

• Administration

Nivolumab is administered by IV infusion over 30 minutes. *The drug should not be administered by rapid IV injection, such as IV push or bolus.* Following nivolumab administration, the IV administration line should be flushed with 0.9% sodium chloride injection or 5% dextrose injection.

For IV infusion over 30 minutes, the appropriate dose of nivolumab injection (containing 10 mg/mL) should be diluted with an appropriate volume of 0.9% sodium chloride or 5% dextrose injection to a final concentration of 1–10 mg/mL. The total volume of the infusion solution must not exceed 160 mL; for adults and pediatric patients weighing less than 40 kg, the total volume of the infusion solution must not exceed 4 mL per kg of body weight. Prior to dilution, the injection should be inspected visually for particulate matter and discoloration. The solution should be clear to opalescent and colorless to pale yellow; the solution should not be used if it is cloudy or discolored or if foreign particles other than translucent to white proteinaceous particles are present. The diluted solution should be mixed by gentle inversion and should *not* be shaken. Nivolumab should be administered through a sterile, nonpyrogenic, low-protein-binding 0.2- to 1.2-μm inline filter.

Diluted solutions of the drug are stable for up to 8 hours after dilution (including infusion time) when stored at room temperature or up to 24 hours after dilution when stored under refrigeration (2–8°C); diluted solutions of the drug should *not* be frozen.

Any unused portion in the vial or infusion bag should be discarded since nivolumab injection contains no preservative.

Nivolumab should *not* be administered simultaneously through the same IV line with any other drug or admixed with ipilimumab in the same infusion bag. When nivolumab is used in combination with ipilimumab, separate inline filters should be used for each infusion.

● Dosage

Clinicians should consult published protocols for information on the dosage, method of administration, and administration sequence of other antineoplastic agents used in combination regimens with nivolumab.

Melanoma
Monotherapy for Unresectable or Metastatic Melanoma

When used as monotherapy for the treatment of unresectable or metastatic melanoma, the recommended adult dosage of nivolumab is 240 mg administered every 2 weeks or 480 mg administered every 4 weeks as a 30-minute IV infusion. Therapy should be continued until disease progression or unacceptable toxicity occurs.

Combination Therapy for Unresectable or Metastatic Melanoma

When used in combination with ipilimumab for the treatment of unresectable or metastatic melanoma, the recommended adult dosage of nivolumab is 1 mg/kg administered as a 30-minute IV infusion in combination with ipilimumab 3 mg/kg administered as a 90-minute IV infusion every 3 weeks for up to 4 doses or until unacceptable toxicity occurs, followed by single-agent nivolumab therapy at a dosage of 240 mg administered every 2 weeks or 480 mg administered every 4 weeks as a 30-minute IV infusion until disease progression or unacceptable toxicity occurs. Nivolumab should be administered before ipilimumab.

If nivolumab therapy is temporarily interrupted for toxicity, ipilimumab should also be withheld.

Adjuvant Therapy for Locally Advanced or Metastatic Melanoma

For the adjuvant therapy of completely resected locally advanced or metastatic melanoma, the recommended adult dosage of nivolumab is 240 mg administered every 2 weeks or 480 mg administered every 4 weeks as a 30-minute IV infusion. Therapy should be continued for up to 1 year or until disease recurrence or unacceptable toxicity occurs.

Non-small Cell Lung Cancer

For the treatment of metastatic non-small cell lung cancer (NSCLC) that has progressed during or following therapy with platinum-based chemotherapy and, in those with epidermal growth factor receptor (EGFR) mutation- or anaplastic lymphoma kinase (ALK)-positive tumors, therapy with an FDA-labeled EGFR or ALK inhibitor, the recommended adult dosage of nivolumab is 240 mg administered every 2 weeks or 480 mg administered every 4 weeks as a 30-minute IV infusion. Therapy should be continued until disease progression or unacceptable toxicity occurs.

Small Cell Lung Cancer

For the treatment of metastatic small cell lung cancer (SCLC) that has progressed following therapy with platinum-based chemotherapy and at least one other line

of therapy, the recommended adult dosage of nivolumab is 240 mg administered every 2 weeks as a 30-minute IV infusion. Therapy should be continued until disease progression or unacceptable toxicity occurs.

Renal Cell Carcinoma
Monotherapy for Advanced Renal Cell Carcinoma

When used as monotherapy for the treatment of advanced renal cell carcinoma previously treated with antiangiogenic therapy, the recommended adult dosage of nivolumab is 240 mg administered every 2 weeks or 480 mg administered every 4 weeks as a 30-minute IV infusion. Therapy should be continued until disease progression or unacceptable toxicity occurs.

Combination Therapy for Advanced Renal Cell Carcinoma

When used in combination with ipilimumab for the treatment of intermediate- or poor-risk, previously untreated, advanced renal cell carcinoma, the recommended adult dosage of nivolumab is 3 mg/kg administered as a 30-minute IV infusion in combination with ipilimumab 1 mg/kg administered as a 30-minute IV infusion every 3 weeks for 4 doses, followed by single-agent nivolumab therapy at a dosage of 240 mg administered every 2 weeks or 480 mg administered every 4 weeks as a 30-minute IV infusion until disease progression or unacceptable toxicity occurs. Nivolumab should be administered before ipilimumab.

If nivolumab therapy is temporarily interrupted for toxicity, ipilimumab should also be withheld.

Hodgkin Lymphoma

For the treatment of classical Hodgkin lymphoma (cHL) that has relapsed or progressed following autologous stem cell transplantation and subsequent therapy with brentuximab vedotin or following failure of at least 3 systemic therapies (including autologous stem cell transplantation), the recommended adult dosage of nivolumab is 240 mg administered every 2 weeks or 480 mg administered every 4 weeks as a 30-minute IV infusion. Therapy should be continued until disease progression or unacceptable toxicity occurs.

Head and Neck Cancer

For the treatment of metastatic or recurrent squamous cell carcinoma of the head and neck that has progressed during or following therapy with platinum-based chemotherapy, the recommended adult dosage of nivolumab is 240 mg administered every 2 weeks or 480 mg administered every 4 weeks as a 30-minute IV infusion. Therapy should be continued until disease progression or unacceptable toxicity occurs.

Urothelial Carcinoma

For the treatment of locally advanced or metastatic urothelial carcinoma that has progressed during or following platinum-containing therapy or within 12 months of platinum-containing therapy in the neoadjuvant or adjuvant setting, the recommended adult dosage of nivolumab is 240 mg administered every 2 weeks or 480 mg administered every 4 weeks as a 30-minute IV infusion. Therapy should be continued until disease progression or unacceptable toxicity occurs.

Colorectal Cancer
Monotherapy for Metastatic Colorectal Cancer

When used as monotherapy for the treatment of metastatic colorectal cancer with high microsatellite instability (MSI-H) or mismatch repair deficiency (dMMR) that has progressed following fluoropyrimidine-, oxaliplatin-, and irinotecan-containing therapy in adults and adolescents (12 years of age and older), the recommended dosage of nivolumab is 240 mg administered as a 30-minute IV infusion every 2 weeks. Therapy should be continued until disease progression or unacceptable toxicity occurs.

Combination Therapy for Metastatic Colorectal Cancer

When used in combination with ipilimumab for the treatment of metastatic colorectal cancer with MSI-H or dMMR that has progressed following fluoropyrimidine-, oxaliplatin-, and irinotecan-containing therapy in adults and adolescents (12 years of age and older), the recommended dosage of nivolumab is 3 mg/kg administered as a 30-minute IV infusion in combination with ipilimumab 1 mg/kg administered as a 30-minute IV infusion every 3 weeks for 4 doses, followed by single-agent nivolumab therapy at a dosage of 240 mg administered every 2 weeks as a 30-minute IV infusion until disease progression or unacceptable toxicity occurs. Nivolumab should be administered before ipilimumab.

If nivolumab therapy is temporarily interrupted for toxicity, ipilimumab should also be withheld.

Hepatocellular Carcinoma

For the treatment of hepatocellular carcinoma previously treated with sorafenib, the recommended adult dosage of nivolumab is 240 mg administered every 2 weeks or 480 mg administered every 4 weeks as a 30-minute IV infusion. Therapy should be continued until disease progression or unacceptable toxicity occurs.

Therapy Interruption for Toxicity

If immune-mediated adverse effects occur, temporary or permanent discontinuance of nivolumab may be required based on severity of the reaction.

Nivolumab should be permanently discontinued in patients experiencing persistent grade 2 or 3 immune-mediated adverse effects lasting 12 weeks or longer and in those requiring a corticosteroid dosage of 10 mg or more of prednisone daily (or equivalent) for more than 12 weeks. (See Cautions: Warnings/Precautions.)

Nivolumab should be permanently discontinued in patients experiencing any life-threatening or grade 4 immune-mediated adverse effect. Therapy with the drug also should be permanently discontinued if grade 3 immune-mediated adverse effects recur.

Immune-mediated Pneumonitis

If grade 2 immune-mediated pneumonitis occurs, nivolumab therapy should be interrupted until the toxicity resolves to grade 0 or 1. (See Immune-mediated Pneumonitis under Cautions: Warnings/Precautions.)

If grade 3 or 4 immune-mediated pneumonitis occurs, nivolumab therapy should be permanently discontinued.

Immune-mediated GI Effects

If grade 2 or 3 immune-mediated colitis or diarrhea occurs, nivolumab therapy should be interrupted until the toxicity resolves to grade 0 or 1; however, if grade 3 immune-mediated colitis or diarrhea occurs in patients receiving nivolumab in combination with ipilimumab, nivolumab therapy should be permanently discontinued. If colitis recurs upon reinitiation of therapy, nivolumab therapy should be permanently discontinued. (See Immune-mediated GI Effects under Cautions: Warnings/Precautions.)

If grade 4 immune-mediated colitis or diarrhea occurs, nivolumab therapy should be permanently discontinued.

Immune-mediated Hepatic Effects

For serum aminotransferase (ALT or AST) elevations exceeding 3 times but not more than 5 times the upper limit of normal (ULN) or total bilirubin concentrations exceeding 1.5 times but not more than 3 times the ULN (i.e., grade 2) in patients *without* hepatocellular carcinoma, nivolumab therapy should be interrupted until the toxicity resolves to grade 0 or 1. (See Immune-mediated Hepatic Effects under Cautions: Warnings/Precautions.)

For ALT or AST elevations exceeding 5 times the ULN or total bilirubin concentrations exceeding 3 times the ULN (i.e., grade 3 or greater) in patients *without* hepatocellular carcinoma, nivolumab therapy should be permanently discontinued.

For ALT or AST elevations exceeding 3 times but not more than 5 times the ULN in patients *with* hepatocellular carcinoma and baseline ALT and AST concentrations within normal limits, nivolumab therapy should be interrupted until the toxicity resolves to baseline.

For ALT or AST elevations exceeding 5 times but not more than 10 times the ULN in patients *with* hepatocellular carcinoma and baseline ALT or AST concentrations exceeding the ULN but not more than 3 times the ULN, nivolumab therapy should be interrupted until the toxicity resolves to baseline.

For ALT or AST elevations exceeding 8 times but not more than 10 times the ULN in patients *with* hepatocellular carcinoma and baseline ALT or AST concentrations exceeding 3 times but not more than 5 times the ULN, nivolumab therapy should be interrupted until the toxicity resolves to baseline.

For ALT or AST elevations exceeding 10 times the ULN or total bilirubin concentrations exceeding 3 times the ULN in patients *with* hepatocellular carcinoma, nivolumab therapy should be permanently discontinued.

Immune-mediated Endocrine Effects

If grade 2 or 3 immune-mediated hypophysitis, grade 2 immune-mediated adrenal insufficiency, or grade 3 immune-mediated hyperglycemia occurs, nivolumab

therapy should be interrupted until the toxicity resolves to grade 0 or 1. (See Immune-mediated Endocrine Effects under Cautions: Warnings/Precautions.)

If grade 4 immune-mediated hypophysitis, grade 3 or 4 immune-mediated adrenal insufficiency, or grade 4 immune-mediated hyperglycemia occurs, nivolumab therapy should be permanently discontinued.

The manufacturer states that there are no recommended dosage modifications of nivolumab for patients with immune-mediated hypothyroidism or hyperthyroidism.

Immune-mediated Renal Effects

For serum creatinine elevations exceeding 1.5 times but not more than 6 times the ULN or exceeding 1.5 times baseline values (i.e., grade 2 or 3), nivolumab therapy should be interrupted until the toxicity resolves to grade 0 or 1. (See Immune-mediated Renal Effects under Cautions: Warnings/Precautions.)

For elevated serum creatinine concentrations exceeding 6 times the ULN (i.e., grade 4), nivolumab therapy should be permanently discontinued.

Immune-mediated Dermatologic Effects

If grade 3 immune-mediated rash occurs or Stevens-Johnson syndrome or toxic epidermal necrolysis is suspected, nivolumab therapy should be interrupted until the toxicity resolves to grade 0 or 1. (See Immune-mediated Dermatologic Effects under Cautions: Warnings/Precautions.)

If grade 4 immune-mediated rash occurs or Stevens-Johnson syndrome or toxic epidermal necrolysis is confirmed, nivolumab therapy should be permanently discontinued.

Immune-mediated CNS Effects

If new-onset moderate or severe neurologic signs or symptoms occur, nivolumab therapy should be interrupted until the toxicity resolves to grade 0 or 1. (See Immune-mediated CNS Effects under Cautions: Warnings/Precautions.)

If immune-mediated encephalitis occurs, nivolumab therapy should be permanently discontinued.

Other Immune-mediated Adverse Effects

If grade 3 immune-mediated myocarditis occurs, nivolumab therapy should be permanently discontinued.

If any other grade 3 immune-mediated adverse effects occur, nivolumab therapy should be interrupted until the toxicity resolves to grade 0 or 1. If the grade 3 adverse effect recurs, nivolumab therapy should be permanently discontinued. (See Other Immune-mediated Effects under Cautions: Warnings/Precautions.)

Infusion-related Reactions

If mild or moderate infusion-related reactions occur, the infusion should be interrupted or the infusion rate should be reduced. (See Infusion-related Effects under Cautions: Warnings/Precautions.)

If severe or life-threatening infusion-related reactions occur, nivolumab therapy should be permanently discontinued.

● Special Populations

No dosage adjustment is necessary in patients with mild or moderate preexisting hepatic impairment. Nivolumab has not been studied in patients with severe preexisting hepatic impairment, and the manufacturer provides no specific dosage recommendations for such patients. (See Hepatic Impairment under Warnings/Precautions: Specific Populations, in Cautions.)

No dosage adjustment is necessary in patients with mild, moderate, or severe preexisting renal impairment. (See Renal Impairment under Warnings/Precautions: Specific Populations, in Cautions.)

The manufacturer makes no special dosage recommendations for geriatric patients. (See Geriatric Use under Warnings/Precautions: Specific Populations, in Cautions.)

CAUTIONS

● Contraindications

The manufacturer states there are no known contraindications to the use of nivolumab.

● *Warnings/Precautions*

Immune-mediated Pneumonitis

Immune-mediated pneumonitis (defined as pneumonitis of no clear alternate etiology requiring corticosteroid therapy), sometimes fatal, has occurred in patients receiving nivolumab therapy.

In clinical studies evaluating single-agent nivolumab, immune-mediated pneumonitis occurred in 3.1% of patients receiving nivolumab; the median time to onset of immune-mediated pneumonitis was 3.5 months (range: 1 day to 22.3 months). Nivolumab was temporarily interrupted or permanently discontinued because of immune-mediated pneumonitis in 1.3 or 1.1%, respectively, of patients receiving the drug. Most patients (89%) experiencing immune-mediated pneumonitis received high-dose corticosteroid therapy (40 mg or more of prednisone daily [or equivalent]) for a median duration of 26 days (range: 1 day to 6 months). Following tapering of the corticosteroid dosage, complete resolution of immune-mediated pneumonitis occurred in 67% of patients. Following reinitiation of nivolumab therapy, immune-mediated pneumonitis recurred in approximately 8% of patients.

In clinical studies evaluating nivolumab 1 mg/kg in combination with ipilimumab 3 mg/kg, immune-mediated pneumonitis occurred in 6% of patients with melanoma receiving combination therapy; the median time to onset of immune-mediated pneumonitis was 1.6 months (range: 24 days to 10.1 months). Combination therapy with nivolumab 1 mg/kg and ipilimumab 3 mg/kg was temporarily interrupted or permanently discontinued because of immune-mediated pneumonitis in 3.7 or 2.2%, respectively, of patients receiving the drug combination. Most patients (84%) experiencing immune-mediated pneumonitis received high-dose corticosteroid therapy (40 mg or more of prednisone daily [or equivalent]) for a median duration of 30 days (range: 5 days to 11.8 months). Complete resolution of immune-mediated pneumonitis occurred in 68% of patients. Following reinitiation of combination therapy with nivolumab 1 mg/kg and ipilimumab 3 mg/kg, immune-mediated pneumonitis recurred in approximately 13% of patients.

In clinical studies evaluating nivolumab 3 mg/kg in combination with ipilimumab 1 mg/kg, immune-mediated pneumonitis occurred in 4.4 or 1.7% of patients with renal cell carcinoma or colorectal cancer, respectively, receiving combination therapy; the median time to onset of immune-mediated pneumonitis was 2.6 months (range: 8 days to 9.2 months) in patients with renal cell carcinoma and 1.9 months (range: 27 days to 3 months) in patients with colorectal cancer. Combination therapy with nivolumab 3 mg/kg and ipilimumab 1 mg/kg was temporarily interrupted or permanently discontinued because of immune-mediated pneumonitis in 1.7 or 1.8%, respectively, of patients receiving the drug combination. All patients experiencing immune-mediated pneumonitis received systemic corticosteroid therapy. The majority (92%) of patients experiencing immune-mediated pneumonitis received high-dose corticosteroid therapy (40 mg or more of prednisone daily [or equivalent]) for a median duration of 19 days (range: 4 days to 3.2 months); however, adjunctive therapy with infliximab was required in approximately 8% of patients. Complete resolution of immune-mediated pneumonitis occurred in 81% of patients. Following reinitiation of combination therapy with nivolumab 3 mg/kg and ipilimumab 1 mg/kg, immune-mediated pneumonitis recurred in one patient with colorectal cancer.

Patients receiving nivolumab should be monitored clinically and by radiographic imaging for manifestations of pneumonitis. In patients who develop grade 2 or greater immune-mediated pneumonitis, systemic corticosteroid therapy should be initiated at a dosage of 1–2 mg/kg of prednisone daily (or equivalent) followed by tapering of the corticosteroid dosage. Temporary interruption or discontinuance of nivolumab may be necessary if immune-mediated pneumonitis occurs during therapy with the drug. (See Therapy Interruption for Toxicity under Dosage and Administration: Dosage.)

Immune-mediated GI Effects

Immune-mediated colitis (defined as colitis of no clear alternate etiology requiring corticosteroid therapy), sometimes fatal, has occurred in patients receiving nivolumab therapy.

In clinical studies evaluating single-agent nivolumab, immune-mediated colitis occurred in 2.9% of patients receiving nivolumab; the median time to onset of immune-mediated colitis was 5.3 months (range: 2 days to 20.9 months). Nivolumab was temporarily interrupted or permanently discontinued because of immune-mediated colitis in 1 or 0.7%, respectively, of patients receiving the drug. Most (approximately 91%) of the 58 patients experiencing immune-mediated colitis received high-dose corticosteroid therapy (40 mg or more of prednisone daily [or equivalent]) for a median duration of 23 days (range: 1 day to 9.3

months); however, adjunctive therapy with infliximab was required in 4 patients. Complete resolution of immune-mediated colitis occurred in 74% of patients. Following reinitiation of nivolumab therapy, immune-mediated colitis recurred in approximately 16% of patients.

In clinical studies evaluating nivolumab 1 mg/kg in combination with ipilimumab 3 mg/kg, immune-mediated colitis occurred in 26% of patients with melanoma receiving combination therapy and was fatal in 3 patients; the median time to onset of immune-mediated colitis was 1.6 months (range: 3 days to 15.2 months). Combination therapy with nivolumab 1 mg/kg and ipilimumab 3 mg/kg was temporarily interrupted or permanently discontinued because of immune-mediated colitis in 7 or 16%, respectively, of patients receiving the drug combination. Most patients (96%) experiencing immune-mediated colitis received high-dose corticosteroid therapy (40 mg or more of prednisone daily [or equivalent]) for a median duration of 1.1 months (range: 1 day to 12 months); however, adjunctive therapy with infliximab was required in approximately 23% of patients. Complete resolution of immune-mediated colitis occurred in 75% of patients. Following reinitiation of combination therapy with nivolumab 1 mg/kg and ipilimumab 3 mg/kg, immune-mediated colitis recurred in approximately 28% of patients.

In clinical studies evaluating nivolumab 3 mg/kg in combination with ipilimumab 1 mg/kg, immune-mediated colitis occurred in 10 or 7% of patients with renal cell carcinoma or colorectal cancer, respectively, receiving combination therapy; the median time to onset of immune-mediated colitis was 1.7 months (range: 2 days to 19.2 months) in patients with renal cell carcinoma and 2.4 months (range: 22 days to 5.2 months) in patients with colorectal cancer. Combination therapy with nivolumab 3 mg/kg and ipilimumab 1 mg/kg was temporarily interrupted or permanently discontinued because of immune-mediated colitis in 3.9 or 3.2%, respectively, of patients receiving the drug combination. All patients experiencing immune-mediated colitis received systemic corticosteroid therapy. Most patients (80%) experiencing immune-mediated colitis received high-dose corticosteroid therapy (40 mg or more of prednisone daily [or equivalent]) for a median duration of 21 days (range: 1 day to 27 months); however, adjunctive therapy with infliximab was required in approximately 23% of patients with immune-mediated colitis. Complete resolution of immune-mediated colitis occurred in 88% of patients. Following reinitiation of combination therapy with nivolumab 3 mg/kg and ipilimumab 1 mg/kg, immune-mediated colitis recurred in 2 patients with renal cell carcinoma.

Patients receiving nivolumab should be monitored for manifestations of colitis. In patients who develop grade 3 or 4 immune-mediated colitis, systemic corticosteroid therapy should be initiated at a dosage of 1–2 mg/kg of prednisone daily (or equivalent) followed by tapering of the corticosteroid dosage. In patients who experience grade 2 immune-mediated colitis for more than 5 days, systemic corticosteroid therapy should be initiated at a dosage of 0.5–1 mg/kg of prednisone daily (or equivalent) followed by tapering of the corticosteroid dosage; if immune-mediated colitis worsens or fails to improve, the systemic corticosteroid dosage should be increased to 1–2 mg/kg of prednisone daily (or equivalent). Temporary interruption or discontinuance of nivolumab may be necessary if immune-mediated colitis occurs during therapy with the drug. (See Therapy Interruption for Toxicity under Dosage and Administration: Dosage.)

Immune-mediated Hepatic Effects

Immune-mediated hepatitis (defined as hepatitis of no clear alternate etiology requiring corticosteroid therapy) has occurred in patients receiving nivolumab therapy.

In clinical studies evaluating single-agent nivolumab, immune-mediated hepatitis occurred in 1.8% of patients receiving nivolumab; the median time to onset of immune-mediated hepatitis was 3.3 months (range: 6 days to 9 months). Nivolumab was temporarily interrupted or permanently discontinued because of immune-mediated hepatitis in 1 or 0.7%, respectively, of patients receiving the drug. All 35 patients experiencing immune-mediated hepatitis received high-dose corticosteroid therapy (40 mg or more of prednisone daily [or equivalent]) for a median duration of 23 days (range: 1 day to 2 months); however, adjunctive therapy with mycophenolic acid was required in 2 patients. Complete resolution of immune-mediated hepatitis occurred in 74% of patients. Following reinitiation of nivolumab therapy, immune-mediated hepatitis recurred in approximately 29% of patients.

In clinical studies evaluating nivolumab 1 mg/kg in combination with ipilimumab 3 mg/kg, immune-mediated hepatitis occurred in 13% of patients with melanoma receiving combination therapy; the median time to onset of immune-mediated hepatitis was 2.1 months (range: 15 days to 11 months). Combination therapy with nivolumab 1 mg/kg and ipilimumab 3 mg/kg was temporarily interrupted or permanently discontinued because of immune-mediated hepatitis in 5 or 6%, respectively, of patients receiving the drug combination. Most patients (92%) experiencing immune-mediated hepatitis received high-dose corticosteroid therapy (40 mg or more of prednisone daily [or equivalent]) for a median duration of 1.1 months (range: 1 day to 13.2 months). Complete resolution of immune-mediated hepatitis occurred in 75% of patients. Following reinitiation of combination therapy with nivolumab 1 mg/kg and ipilimumab 3 mg/kg, immune-mediated hepatitis recurred in approximately 11% of patients.

In clinical studies evaluating nivolumab 3 mg/kg in combination with ipilimumab 1 mg/kg, immune-mediated hepatitis occurred in 7 or 8% of patients with renal cell carcinoma or colorectal cancer, respectively, receiving combination therapy; the median time to onset of immune-mediated hepatitis was 2 months (range: 14 days to 26.8 months) in patients with renal cell carcinoma and 2.2 months (range: 22 days to 10.5 months) in patients with colorectal cancer. Combination therapy with nivolumab 3 mg/kg and ipilimumab 1 mg/kg was temporarily interrupted or permanently discontinued because of immune-mediated hepatitis in 3.5 or 3.6%, respectively, of patients receiving the drug combination. All patients experiencing immune-mediated hepatitis received systemic corticosteroid therapy. The majority (94%) of patients experiencing immune-mediated hepatitis received high-dose corticosteroid therapy (40 mg or more of prednisone daily [or equivalent]) for a median duration of 1 month (range: 1 day to 7 months); however, adjunctive therapy with mycophenolate was required in approximately 19% of patients with immune-mediated hepatitis. Complete resolution of immune-mediated hepatitis occurred in 83% of patients; upon resumption of combination therapy with nivolumab 3 mg/kg and ipilimumab 1 mg/kg, no patients had recurrence of immune-mediated hepatitis.

Liver function tests should be performed prior to initiation of nivolumab therapy and periodically during therapy. If grade 3 or 4 elevations of serum ALT or AST concentrations (with or without concomitant elevations of total bilirubin concentrations) occur in patients *without* hepatocellular carcinoma, systemic corticosteroid therapy should be initiated at a dosage of 1–2 mg/kg of prednisone daily (or equivalent) followed by tapering of the corticosteroid dosage. If grade 2 elevations of serum ALT or AST concentrations occur in patients *without* hepatocellular carcinoma, systemic corticosteroid therapy should be initiated at a dosage of 0.5–1 mg/kg of prednisone daily (or equivalent). In patients who develop immune-mediated hepatitis, temporary interruption of therapy or drug discontinuance may be required. (See Therapy Interruption for Toxicity under Dosage and Administration: Dosage.) Whenever nivolumab therapy is temporarily interrupted or discontinued because of immune-mediated hepatitis in patients *with* hepatocellular carcinoma, systemic corticosteroid therapy should be initiated at a dosage of 1–2 mg/kg of prednisone daily (or equivalent) followed by tapering of the corticosteroid dosage.

Immune-mediated Endocrine Effects

Immune-mediated endocrinopathies, such as hypophysitis, thyroid dysfunction (i.e., hypothyroidism, hyperthyroidism), adrenal insufficiency, and diabetes mellitus (including diabetic ketoacidosis), have occurred in patients receiving nivolumab therapy.

Hypophysitis

In clinical studies evaluating single-agent nivolumab, immune-mediated hypophysitis occurred in 0.6% of patients receiving nivolumab; the median time to occurrence was 4.9 months (range: 1.4–11 months). Nivolumab was temporarily interrupted or permanently discontinued because of immune-mediated hypophysitis in 0.2 or 0.1%, respectively, of patients receiving the drug. Approximately 67% of patients experiencing immune-mediated hypophysitis received hormone replacement therapy and 33% received high-dose corticosteroid therapy (40 mg or more of prednisone daily [or equivalent]) for a median duration of 14 days (range: 5–26 days).

In clinical studies evaluating nivolumab 1 mg/kg in combination with ipilimumab 3 mg/kg, immune-mediated hypophysitis occurred in 9% of patients with melanoma receiving combination therapy; the median time to occurrence was 2.7 months (range: 27 days to 5.5 months). Combination therapy with nivolumab 1 mg/kg and ipilimumab 3 mg/kg was temporarily interrupted or permanently discontinued because of immune-mediated hypophysitis in 3.9 or 1%, respectively, of patients receiving the drug combination. Approximately 75% of patients experiencing immune-mediated hypophysitis received hormone replacement therapy and 56% received high-dose corticosteroid therapy (40 mg or more of prednisone daily [or equivalent]) for a median duration of 19 days (range: 1 day to 2 months).

In clinical studies evaluating nivolumab 3 mg/kg in combination with ipilimumab 1 mg/kg, immune-mediated hypophysitis occurred in 4.6 or 3.4% of patients

with renal cell carcinoma or colorectal cancer, respectively, receiving combination therapy; the median time to onset of immune-mediated hypophysitis was 2.8 months (range: 1.3–7.3 months) in patients with renal cell carcinoma and 3.7 months (range: 2.8–5.5 months) in patients with colorectal cancer. Combination therapy with nivolumab 3 mg/kg and ipilimumab 1 mg/kg was temporarily interrupted or permanently discontinued because of immune-mediated hypophysitis in 2.6 or 1.2%, respectively, of patients receiving the drug combination. Approximately 72% of patients experiencing immune-mediated hypophysitis received hormone replacement therapy and 55% received high-dose corticosteroid therapy (40 mg or more of prednisone daily [or equivalent]) for a median duration of 13 days (range: 1 day to 1.6 months).

Patients receiving nivolumab should be monitored for manifestations of hypophysitis. If grade 2 or greater hypophysitis occurs, hormone replacement therapy should be administered as clinically indicated and systemic corticosteroid therapy should be initiated at a dosage of 1 mg/kg of prednisone daily (or equivalent) followed by tapering of the corticosteroid dosage. If immune-mediated hypophysitis occurs, temporary interruption or discontinuance of nivolumab may be necessary. (See Therapy Interruption for Toxicity under Dosage and Administration: Dosage.)

Adrenal Insufficiency

In clinical studies evaluating single-agent nivolumab, immune-mediated adrenal insufficiency occurred in 1% of patients receiving nivolumab; the median time to occurrence was 4.3 months (range: 15 days to 21 months). Nivolumab was temporarily interrupted or permanently discontinued because of immune-mediated adrenal insufficiency in 0.5 or 0.1%, respectively, of patients receiving the drug. Most patients (85%) experiencing immune-mediated adrenal insufficiency received hormone replacement therapy and 25% received high-dose corticosteroid therapy (40 mg or more of prednisone daily [or equivalent]) for a median duration of 11 days (range: 1 day to 1 month).

In clinical studies evaluating nivolumab 1 mg/kg in combination with ipilimumab 3 mg/kg, immune-mediated adrenal insufficiency occurred in 5% of patients with melanoma receiving combination therapy; the median time to occurrence was 3 months (range: 21 days to 9.4 months). Combination therapy with nivolumab 1 mg/kg and ipilimumab 3 mg/kg was temporarily interrupted or permanently discontinued because of immune-mediated adrenal insufficiency in 1.7 or 0.5%, respectively, of patients receiving the drug combination. Approximately one-half (57%) of patients experiencing immune-mediated adrenal insufficiency received hormone replacement therapy and 33% received high-dose corticosteroid therapy (40 mg or more of prednisone daily [or equivalent]) for a median duration of 9 days (range: 1 day to 2.7 months).

In clinical studies evaluating nivolumab 3 mg/kg in combination with ipilimumab 1 mg/kg, immune-mediated adrenal insufficiency occurred in 7 or 5.9% of patients with renal cell carcinoma or colorectal cancer, respectively, receiving combination therapy; the median time to onset of immune-mediated adrenal insufficiency was 3.4 months (range: 2–22.3 months) in patients with renal cell carcinoma and 3.7 months (range: 2.5–13.4 months) in patients with colorectal cancer. Combination therapy with nivolumab 3 mg/kg and ipilimumab 1 mg/kg was temporarily interrupted or permanently discontinued because of immune-mediated adrenal insufficiency in 2.6 or 1.2%, respectively, of patients receiving the drug combination. Approximately 94% of patients experiencing immune-mediated adrenal insufficiency received hormone replacement therapy and 27% received high-dose corticosteroid therapy (40 mg or more of prednisone daily [or equivalent]) for a median duration of 12 days (range: 2 days to 5.6 months).

Patients receiving nivolumab should be monitored for manifestations of adrenal insufficiency. If grade 3 or 4 adrenal insufficiency occurs, systemic corticosteroid therapy should be initiated at a dosage of 1–2 mg/kg of prednisone daily (or equivalent) followed by tapering of the corticosteroid dosage. If immune-mediated adrenal insufficiency occurs, temporary interruption or discontinuance of nivolumab may be necessary. (See Therapy Interruption for Toxicity under Dosage and Administration: Dosage.)

Thyroid Dysfunction

In clinical studies evaluating single-agent nivolumab, immune-mediated hypothyroidism or thyroiditis-associated hypothyroidism occurred in 9% of patients receiving nivolumab; the median time to occurrence was 2.9 months (range: 1 day to 16.6 months). Most patients (79%) experiencing immune-mediated hypothyroidism received thyroid hormone replacement therapy with levothyroxine and 4% also required therapy with corticosteroids. Resolution of immune-mediated hypothyroidism or thyroiditis-associated hypothyroidism occurred in 35% of patients. In addition, immune-mediated hyperthyroidism has been reported in 2.7% of patients receiving single-agent nivolumab in clinical studies; the median time to occurrence was 1.5 months (range: 1 day to 14.2 months). Approximately one-half of patients (48%) experiencing immune-mediated hyperthyroidism received therapy with antithyroid agents or corticosteroids; 26, 9, 4 or 9% of patients received methimazole, carbimazole (not commercially available in the US), propylthiouracil, or corticosteroids, respectively. Resolution of immune-mediated hyperthyroidism occurred in 76% of patients.

In clinical studies evaluating nivolumab 1 mg/kg in combination with ipilimumab 3 mg/kg, immune-mediated hypothyroidism or thyroiditis-associated hypothyroidism occurred in 22% of patients with melanoma receiving combination therapy; the median time to occurrence was 2.1 months (range: 1 day to 10.1 months). Most patients (73%) experiencing immune-mediated hypothyroidism received thyroid hormone replacement therapy with levothyroxine. Resolution of immune-mediated hypothyroidism or thyroiditis-associated hypothyroidism occurred in 45% of patients. In addition, immune-mediated hyperthyroidism has been reported in 8% of patients receiving nivolumab 1 mg/kg in combination with ipilimumab 3 mg/kg in clinical studies; the median time to occurrence was 23 days (range: 3 days to 3.7 months). Approximately one-half of patients (53%) experiencing immune-mediated hyperthyroidism received therapy with antithyroid agents; 29% of patients received methimazole and 24% received carbimazole. Resolution of immune-mediated hyperthyroidism occurred in 94% of patients.

In clinical studies evaluating nivolumab 3 mg/kg in combination with ipilimumab 1 mg/kg, immune-mediated hypothyroidism or thyroiditis-associated hypothyroidism occurred in 22 or 15% of patients with renal cell carcinoma or colorectal cancer, respectively, receiving combination therapy; the median time to occurrence was 2.2 months (range: 1 day to 21.4 months) in patients with renal cell carcinoma and 2.3 months (range: 22 days to 9.8 months) in patients with colorectal cancer. Approximately 81 or 78% of patients with renal cell carcinoma or colorectal cancer, respectively, who were experiencing immune-mediated hypothyroidism received thyroid hormone replacement therapy with levothyroxine. In addition, immune-mediated hyperthyroidism has been reported in 12% of patients with renal cell carcinoma or colorectal cancer who were receiving nivolumab 3 mg/kg in combination with ipilimumab 1 mg/kg; the median time to occurrence was 1.4 months (range: 6 days to 14.2 months) in patients with renal cell carcinoma and 1.1 months (range: 21 days to 5.4 months) in patients with colorectal cancer. Approximately 15% of patients experiencing immune-mediated hyperthyroidism received therapy with methimazole and 2% received carbimazole.

Thyroid function should be evaluated prior to initiation of nivolumab therapy and periodically during therapy. In patients who develop immune-mediated hypothyroidism, thyroid hormone replacement therapy should be initiated. If immune-mediated hyperthyroidism occurs, appropriate medical therapy should be initiated.

Diabetes Mellitus

Immune-mediated type 1 diabetes mellitus and diabetic ketoacidosis have occurred in patients receiving nivolumab therapy.

In clinical studies evaluating single-agent nivolumab, immune-mediated type 1 diabetes mellitus occurred in 0.9% of patients receiving nivolumab; the median time to occurrence was 4.4 months (range: 15 days to 22 months). Two of 17 patients with immune-mediated type 1 diabetes mellitus experienced diabetic ketoacidosis.

In clinical studies evaluating nivolumab 1 mg/kg in combination with ipilimumab 3 mg/kg, immune-mediated type 1 diabetes mellitus occurred in 1.5% of patients with melanoma receiving combination therapy; the median time to occurrence was 2.5 months (range: 1.3–4.4 months). Combination therapy with nivolumab 1 mg/kg and ipilimumab 3 mg/kg was temporarily interrupted or permanently discontinued in 2 of the 6 patients with immune-mediated type 1 diabetes mellitus.

In clinical studies evaluating nivolumab 3 mg/kg in combination with ipilimumab 1 mg/kg, immune-mediated type 1 diabetes mellitus occurred in 2.7% of patients with renal cell carcinoma receiving combination therapy; the median time to occurrence was 3.2 months (range: 19 days to 16.8 months). Combination therapy with nivolumab 3 mg/kg and ipilimumab 1 mg/kg was temporarily interrupted or permanently discontinued in 33 or 20%, respectively, of patients with immune-mediated type 1 diabetes mellitus.

Patients receiving nivolumab should be monitored for hyperglycemia. If grade 3 immune-mediated hyperglycemia occurs, nivolumab therapy should be temporarily interrupted until blood glucose concentrations have stabilized. If grade 4 immune-mediated hyperglycemia occurs, nivolumab therapy should be permanently discontinued. (See Therapy Interruption for Toxicity under Dosage and Administration: Dosage.)

Immune-mediated Renal Effects

Immune-mediated nephritis (defined as renal dysfunction or grade 2 or greater elevations in serum creatinine concentrations with no clear alternate etiology and requiring corticosteroid therapy) has occurred in patients receiving nivolumab therapy.

In clinical studies evaluating single-agent nivolumab, immune-mediated nephritis and renal dysfunction occurred in 1.2% of patients receiving nivolumab; the median time to onset of immune-mediated nephritis and renal dysfunction was 4.6 months (range: 23 days to 12.3 months). Nivolumab was temporarily interrupted or permanently discontinued because of immune-mediated nephritis and renal dysfunction in 0.8 or 0.3%, respectively, of patients receiving the drug. All patients experiencing immune-mediated nephritis and renal dysfunction received high-dose corticosteroid therapy (40 mg or more of prednisone daily [or equivalent]) for a median duration of 21 days (range: 1 day to 15.4 months). Complete resolution of immune-mediated nephritis and renal dysfunction occurred in 48% of patients; upon resumption of nivolumab, no patients had recurrence of immune-mediated nephritis or renal dysfunction.

In clinical studies evaluating nivolumab 1 mg/kg in combination with ipilimumab 3 mg/kg, immune-mediated nephritis and renal dysfunction occurred in 2.2% of patients with melanoma receiving combination therapy; the median time to onset of immune-mediated nephritis and renal dysfunction was 2.7 months (range: 9 days to 7.9 months). Combination therapy with nivolumab 1 mg/kg and ipilimumab 3 mg/kg was temporarily interrupted or permanently discontinued because of immune-mediated nephritis and renal dysfunction in 0.5 or 0.7%, respectively, of patients receiving the drug combination. Approximately 67% of patients experiencing immune-mediated nephritis and renal dysfunction received high-dose corticosteroid therapy (40 mg or more of prednisone daily [or equivalent]) for a median duration of 13.5 days (range: 1 day to 1.1 months). Complete resolution of immune-mediated nephritis and renal dysfunction occurred in all patients. Following reinitiation of combination therapy with nivolumab 1 mg/kg and ipilimumab 3 mg/kg in 2 patients, neither patient had recurrence of immune-mediated nephritis or renal dysfunction.

In clinical studies evaluating nivolumab 3 mg/kg in combination with ipilimumab 1 mg/kg, immune-mediated nephritis and renal dysfunction occurred in 4.6 or 1.7% of patients with renal cell carcinoma or colorectal cancer, respectively, receiving combination therapy; the median time to onset of immune-mediated nephritis and renal dysfunction was 3 months (range: 1 day to 13.2 months) in these patients. Combination therapy with nivolumab 3 mg/kg and ipilimumab 1 mg/kg was temporarily interrupted or permanently discontinued because of immune-mediated nephritis and renal dysfunction in 2.3 or 1.2%, respectively, of patients receiving the drug combination. Most patients (78%) experiencing immune-mediated nephritis and renal dysfunction received high-dose corticosteroid therapy (40 mg or more of prednisone daily [or equivalent]) for a median duration of 17 days (range: 1 day to 6 months). Complete resolution of immune-mediated nephritis and renal dysfunction occurred in 63% of patients. Following reinitiation of combination therapy with nivolumab 3 mg/kg and ipilimumab 1 mg/kg, immune-mediated nephritis and renal dysfunction recurred in one patient with renal cell carcinoma.

Renal function should be evaluated prior to initiation of nivolumab therapy and periodically during therapy. In patients who develop grade 4 elevations in serum creatinine concentrations, systemic corticosteroid therapy should be initiated at a dosage of 1–2 mg/kg of prednisone daily (or equivalent) followed by tapering of the corticosteroid dosage. In patients who develop grade 2 or 3 elevations in serum creatinine concentrations, systemic corticosteroid therapy should be initiated at a dosage of 0.5–1 mg/kg of prednisone daily (or equivalent); if renal function worsens or fails to improve, the systemic corticosteroid dosage should be increased to 1–2 mg/kg of prednisone daily (or equivalent). Temporary interruption or discontinuance of nivolumab may be necessary if elevations in serum creatinine concentrations occur during therapy with the drug. (See Therapy Interruption for Toxicity under Dosage and Administration: Dosage.)

Immune-mediated Dermatologic Effects

Immune-mediated rash has occurred in patients receiving nivolumab therapy. Severe, sometimes fatal, skin reactions (including Stevens-Johnson syndrome and toxic epidermal necrolysis) have been reported with the drug.

In clinical studies evaluating single-agent nivolumab, immune-mediated rash occurred in 9% of patients receiving nivolumab; the median time to onset of immune-mediated rash was 2.8 months (range: less than 1 day to 25.8 months). Nivolumab was temporarily interrupted or permanently discontinued because of immune-mediated rash in 0.8 or 0.3%, respectively, of patients receiving the drug. Most patients (85%) experiencing immune-mediated rash received topical corticosteroid therapy and approximately 16% of patients received high-dose corticosteroid therapy (40 mg or more of prednisone daily [or equivalent]) for a median duration of 12 days (range: 1 day to 8.9 months). Complete resolution of immune-mediated rash occurred in 48% of patients. Following reinitiation of nivolumab therapy, immune-mediated rash recurred in approximately 1.4% of patients.

In clinical studies evaluating nivolumab 1 mg/kg in combination with ipilimumab 3 mg/kg, immune-mediated rash occurred in 22.6% of patients with melanoma receiving combination therapy; the median time to onset of immune-mediated rash was 18 days (range: 1 day to 9.7 months). Combination therapy with nivolumab 1 mg/kg and ipilimumab 3 mg/kg was temporarily interrupted or permanently discontinued because of immune-mediated rash in 3.9 or 0.5%, respectively, of patients receiving the drug combination. Approximately 17% of patients experiencing immune-mediated rash received high-dose corticosteroid therapy (40 mg or more of prednisone daily [or equivalent]) for a median duration of 14 days (range: 2 days to 4.7 months). Complete resolution of immune-mediated rash occurred in 47% of patients. Following reinitiation of combination therapy with nivolumab 1 mg/kg and ipilimumab 3 mg/kg, immune-mediated rash recurred in approximately 6% of patients.

In clinical studies evaluating nivolumab 3 mg/kg in combination with ipilimumab 1 mg/kg, immune-mediated rash occurred in 16 or 14% of patients with renal cell carcinoma or colorectal cancer, respectively, receiving combination therapy; the median time to onset of immune-mediated rash was 1.5 months (range: 1 day to 20.9 months) in patients with renal cell carcinoma and 26 days (range: 5 days to 9.8 months) in patients with colorectal cancer. Combination therapy with nivolumab 3 mg/kg and ipilimumab 1 mg/kg was temporarily interrupted or permanently discontinued because of immune-mediated rash in 2.6 or 0.5%, respectively, of patients receiving the drug combination. All patients experiencing immune-mediated rash received systemic corticosteroid therapy; 19% of patients received high-dose corticosteroid therapy (40 mg or more of prednisone daily [or equivalent]) for a median duration of 22 days (range: 1 day to 23 months). Complete resolution of immune-mediated rash occurred in 66% of patients. Following reinitiation of combination therapy with nivolumab 3 mg/kg and ipilimumab 1 mg/kg, immune-mediated rash recurred in approximately 3% of patients.

In patients who develop grade 3 or 4 immune-mediated rash, systemic corticosteroid therapy should be initiated at a dosage of 1–2 mg/kg of prednisone daily (or equivalent) followed by tapering of the corticosteroid dosage. Temporary interruption or discontinuance of nivolumab may be necessary if immune-mediated rash occurs during therapy with the drug. (See Therapy Interruption for Toxicity under Dosage and Administration: Dosage.) If Stevens-Johnson syndrome or toxic epidermal necrolysis is suspected, nivolumab therapy should be temporarily interrupted and the patient should be referred for evaluation and treatment by a specialist. If Stevens-Johnson syndrome or toxic epidermal necrolysis is confirmed, nivolumab should be permanently discontinued.

Immune-mediated CNS Effects

Immune-mediated encephalitis of no clear alternate etiology, sometimes fatal, has occurred in patients receiving nivolumab therapy.

In clinical studies evaluating single-agent nivolumab, immune-mediated encephalitis occurred in 0.2% of patients receiving nivolumab. Following 7.2 months of nivolumab therapy, fatal limbic encephalitis occurred in one patient despite discontinuance of nivolumab therapy and administration of systemic corticosteroid therapy. Immune-mediated encephalitis occurred following allogeneic stem cell transplantation in 2 patients.

In clinical studies evaluating nivolumab 1 mg/kg in combination with ipilimumab 3 mg/kg, immune-mediated encephalitis occurred in one patient with melanoma receiving the drug combination after 1.7 months of exposure.

In clinical studies evaluating nivolumab 3 mg/kg in combination with ipilimumab 1 mg/kg, immune-mediated encephalitis occurred in one patient with renal cell carcinoma receiving the drug combination after approximately 4 months of exposure and one patient with colorectal cancer receiving the drug combination

after 15 days of exposure. One patient received high-dose corticosteroid therapy (40 mg or more of prednisone daily [or equivalent]) and adjunctive therapy with infliximab.

In patients with new moderate to severe neurologic manifestations suggestive of encephalitis (e.g., headache, pyrexia, confusion, memory loss, hallucinations, fatigue/asthenia, somnolence, drowsiness, seizures, stiff neck), nivolumab should be withheld and adequate evaluation (e.g., consultation with a neurologist, brain magnetic resonance imaging [MRI] scan, lumbar puncture) should be performed to exclude other causes (e.g., infection). If immune-mediated encephalitis is confirmed, nivolumab should be permanently discontinued and systemic corticosteroid therapy should be initiated at a dosage of 1–2 mg/kg of prednisone daily (or equivalent) followed by tapering of the corticosteroid dosage.

Other Immune-mediated Effects

Other immune-mediated adverse effects, including myocarditis, rhabdomyolysis, myositis, uveitis, iritis, pancreatitis, facial and abducens nerve paresis, demyelination, polymyalgia rheumatica, autoimmune neuropathy, Guillain-Barré syndrome, hypopituitarism, systemic inflammatory response syndrome, gastritis, duodenitis, sarcoidosis, histiocytic necrotizing lymphadenitis (Kikuchi lymphadenitis), motor dysfunction, vasculitis, aplastic anemia, pericarditis, and myasthenic syndrome, have occurred rarely in patients receiving nivolumab as a single agent or in combination with ipilimumab. Some cases have resulted in death. Immune-mediated adverse effects may occur following discontinuance of nivolumab therapy.

If an immune-mediated adverse effect is suspected, adequate evaluation should be performed to exclude other causes. Depending on the severity of the immune-mediated adverse effect, nivolumab therapy should be interrupted or permanently discontinued and high-dose corticosteroid therapy and, if indicated, hormone replacement therapy should be initiated. Once the toxicity has resolved to grade 0 or 1, the corticosteroid dosage should be tapered over at least 1 month. If clinically appropriate, nivolumab may be restarted following completion of the corticosteroid taper. (See Therapy Interruption for Toxicity under Dosage and Administration: Dosage.)

If uveitis occurs in conjunction with other immune-mediated adverse effects, a Vogt-Koyanagi-Harada-like syndrome (which has been observed in patients receiving nivolumab as a single agent or in combination with ipilimumab) should be considered. Systemic corticosteroid therapy may be required to reduce the risk of permanent vision loss.

Infusion-related Effects

Infusion-related reactions have occurred in patients receiving nivolumab therapy. Severe infusion-related reactions have been reported rarely in patients receiving nivolumab in clinical studies.

In clinical studies evaluating single-agent nivolumab, infusion-related reactions occurred in 6.4% of patients receiving nivolumab as a 60-minute IV infusion.

In clinical studies evaluating nivolumab 1 mg/kg in combination with ipilimumab 3 mg/kg, infusion-related reactions occurred in 2.5% of patients with melanoma receiving combination therapy.

In clinical studies evaluating nivolumab 3 mg/kg in combination with ipilimumab 1 mg/kg, infusion-related reactions occurred in 5.1 or 4.2% of patients with renal cell carcinoma or colorectal cancer, respectively, receiving combination therapy.

In a pharmacokinetic and safety comparison of 30- and 60-minute IV nivolumab infusions, infusion-related reactions occurred in 2.7 or 2.2% of patients receiving the drug over 30 or 60 minutes, respectively, and resulted in dose delay, temporary interruption of therapy, or permanent drug discontinuance in 1.4 or 0.5%, respectively, of patients.

In patients experiencing mild or moderate infusion-related reactions, interruption of the infusion or a reduction in the infusion rate may be necessary. For patients experiencing severe or life-threatening infusion-related reactions, nivolumab therapy should be permanently discontinued.

Allogeneic Stem Cell Transplantation-related Complications

Patients who undergo allogeneic stem cell transplantation either before or after receiving therapy with an anti-programmed-death receptor-1 (anti-PD-1) monoclonal antibody, including nivolumab, may experience serious or fatal transplant-related complications, including hyperacute, acute, or chronic graft-versus-host disease (GVHD); hepatic veno-occlusive disease following allogeneic stem cell transplantation with a reduced-intensity conditioning regimen; and corticosteroid-requiring febrile syndrome with no identified infectious cause. These complications may occur despite other intervening therapy between administration of the anti-PD-1 monoclonal antibody and transplantation.

In clinical studies evaluating nivolumab in patients with classical Hodgkin lymphoma (cHL), 17 patients underwent allogeneic stem cell transplantation following discontinuance of nivolumab. Fatal transplant-related complications occurred in 6 of the 17 patients (35%); 5 of the fatal cases occurred in the setting of severe or refractory GVHD. Hyperacute GVHD occurred in 2 patients (12%), and grade 3 or greater GVHD occurred in 5 patients (29%). Hepatic veno-occlusive disease occurred in one patient following allogeneic stem cell transplantation with a reduced-intensity conditioning regimen; death occurred following development of GVHD and multiorgan failure.

Potential benefits and risks of anti-PD-1 monoclonal antibody therapy administered either before or after allogeneic stem cell transplantation should be considered. Patients who receive nivolumab should be monitored closely for early manifestations of stem cell transplantation-related complications and such conditions should be managed promptly if they occur.

Fetal/Neonatal Morbidity and Mortality

Nivolumab may cause fetal harm if administered to pregnant women. Blockade of signaling of the programmed death 1 (PD-1) and ligand 1 (PD-L1) pathway in animals has been shown to disrupt maternal immune tolerance to the fetus and has been associated with increased fetal loss and immune-mediated disorders. Therefore, inhibition of this pathway by nivolumab may increase the risk of fetal loss (e.g., abortion, stillbirth) or neonatal death. In cynomolgus monkeys receiving nivolumab (at exposure levels of 9 and 42 times the human exposure at a dose of 3 mg/kg), the incidence of fetal loss during the first and third trimesters was higher compared with concurrent or historical controls. Human immunoglobulin G_4 (IgG$_4$) has been shown to cross the placenta; therefore, fetal exposure to nivolumab may occur. The effects of nivolumab may be greater during the second and third trimesters of pregnancy.

Pregnancy should be avoided during nivolumab therapy. Women of childbearing potential should be advised to use an effective method of contraception while receiving nivolumab and for at least 5 months after the last dose of the drug. If nivolumab is used during pregnancy or if the patient becomes pregnant while receiving the drug, the patient should be apprised of the potential fetal hazard.

Treatment-related Mortality

Increased mortality has been reported in clinical trials in patients with multiple myeloma who received an anti-PD-1 monoclonal antibody, including nivolumab, in combination with an immunomodulatory agent (i.e., lenalidomide, pomalidomide) and dexamethasone; nivolumab is *not* currently FDA-labeled for use in patients with multiple myeloma. The manufacturer of nivolumab states that use of an anti-PD-1 or anti-PD-L1 antibody in combination with a thalidomide analog and dexamethasone in patients with multiple myeloma is *not* recommended outside of a controlled clinical trial.

Immunogenicity

There is a potential for immunogenicity with nivolumab therapy. Development of anti-nivolumab antibodies was detected by electrochemiluminescence (ECL) in 11.2, 37.8, or 23.8–26% of patients receiving nivolumab monotherapy, nivolumab 1 mg/kg in combination with ipilimumab 3 mg/kg, or nivolumab 3 mg/kg in combination with ipilimumab 1 mg/kg, respectively. Neutralizing antibodies to nivolumab were detected in 0.7, 4.6, or 0.5–1.9% of patients receiving these respective treatments. No effects on safety (including infusion-related reactions) or efficacy were observed in the presence of anti-nivolumab antibodies. No effects on nivolumab pharmacokinetics were observed in patients receiving single-agent nivolumab; however, clearance of nivolumab increased by 20% in the presence of anti-nivolumab antibodies in patients receiving nivolumab in combination with ipilimumab.

Specific Populations

Pregnancy

Nivolumab may cause fetal harm if administered to pregnant women based on its mechanism of action and animal findings. The effects of nivolumab may be greater during the second and third trimesters of pregnancy. (See Fetal/Neonatal Morbidity and Mortality under Cautions: Warnings/Precautions.)

Lactation

It is not known whether nivolumab is distributed into human milk. Because many drugs are distributed into human milk and because of the potential for serious adverse reactions to nivolumab in nursing infants, women should be advised to discontinue nursing during nivolumab therapy.

Pediatric Use

Safety and efficacy of nivolumab for the treatment of melanoma, non-small cell lung cancer (NSCLC), small cell lung cancer (SCLC), renal cell carcinoma, cHL, squamous cell carcinoma of the head and neck, urothelial carcinoma, and hepatocellular carcinoma have not been established in pediatric patients younger than 18 years of age.

Safety and efficacy of nivolumab as monotherapy or in combination with ipilimumab for the management of metastatic colorectal cancer with high microsatellite instability (MSI-H) or mismatch repair deficiency (dMMR) have not been established in pediatric patients younger than 12 years of age. Because the clinical course of MSI-H or dMMR metastatic colorectal cancer is similar in adults and pediatric patients, safety and efficacy of nivolumab as monotherapy or in combination with ipilimumab for the treatment of MSI-H or dMMR metastatic colorectal cancer in adolescents 12 years of age or older are supported by extrapolation of data from clinical studies evaluating nivolumab in adults, population pharmacokinetic analyses indicating that age and body weight do not have clinically important effects on systemic exposure to the drug, and evidence that exposure to monoclonal antibodies generally is similar in adults and adolescents.

Geriatric Use

Some clinical studies of nivolumab monotherapy in patients with melanoma (CheckMate-037), cHL (CheckMate-205 and CheckMate-039), squamous cell carcinoma of the head and neck (CheckMate-141), MSI-H or dMMR metastatic colorectal cancer (CheckMate-142), hepatocellular carcinoma (CheckMate-040), or SCLC (CheckMate-032) did not include sufficient numbers of patients 65 years of age and older to determine whether geriatric patients respond differently than younger adults; however, no clinically important differences in safety or efficacy were observed between patients 65 years of age and older and younger adults in other clinical studies in patients with melanoma (CheckMate-066, CheckMate-067, and CheckMate-238), NSCLC (CheckMate-017 and CheckMate-057), renal cell carcinoma (CheckMate-025), or urothelial carcinoma (CheckMate-275).

In the CheckMate-067 study, 41% of patients with unresectable or metastatic melanoma receiving nivolumab 1 mg/kg in combination with ipilimumab 3 mg/kg were 65 years of age or older, and 11% were 75 years of age or older. No overall differences in safety and efficacy were observed between geriatric patients and younger adults.

In the CheckMate-214 study, 38% of patients with advanced renal cell carcinoma receiving nivolumab 3 mg/kg in combination with ipilimumab 1 mg/kg were 65 years of age or older, and 8% were 75 years of age or older. No overall difference in safety was observed between geriatric patients and younger adults. In addition, no overall difference in efficacy was observed between geriatric patients with intermediate- or poor-risk disease and younger adults.

Hepatic Impairment

Analysis of population pharmacokinetic data indicates that nivolumab clearance in patients with hepatocellular carcinoma or other malignancies and mild hepatic impairment (total bilirubin concentration not exceeding the ULN *with* AST concentration exceeding the ULN, or total bilirubin concentration more than 1 times but no more than 1.5 times the ULN *with* any AST concentration) and those with hepatocellular carcinoma and moderate hepatic impairment (total bilirubin concentration more than 1.5 times but not more than 3 times the ULN *with* any AST concentration) is similar to that in patients with normal hepatic function. Data are not available for patients with severe hepatic impairment (total bilirubin concentration exceeding 3 times the ULN *with* any AST concentration).

Renal Impairment

Analysis of population pharmacokinetic data indicates that nivolumab clearance in patients with mild, moderate, or severe renal impairment (estimated glomerular filtration rate [GFR] 15–89 mL/minute per 1.73 m²) is similar to that in patients with normal renal function.

● Common Adverse Effects

Adverse effects reported in 10% or more of patients receiving nivolumab as a single agent for the treatment of unresectable or metastatic melanoma and at an incidence that is at least 5% higher than that reported with the comparator chemotherapy regimen(s) in either the CheckMate-037 or CheckMate-066 study include fatigue, musculoskeletal pain, rash, pruritus, cough, upper respiratory infection, edema, vitiligo, and erythema. Laboratory abnormalities reported in 10% or more of patients receiving nivolumab for the treatment of unresectable or metastatic melanoma and at an incidence that is at least 5% higher than that reported with chemotherapy include elevated concentrations of hepatic aminotransferase enzymes (i.e., ALT, AST), hyponatremia, elevated concentrations of alkaline phosphatase,hyperkalemia, and elevated concentrations of bilirubin.

Adverse effects reported in 10% or more of patients receiving nivolumab as a single agent for the treatment of unresectable or metastatic melanoma and at an incidence that is at least 5% higher than that reported with ipilimumab in the CheckMate-067 study include fatigue, musculoskeletal pain, cough, upper respiratory infection, arthralgia, hypothyroidism, and vitiligo. Laboratory abnormalities reported in 20% or more of patients receiving nivolumab as a single agent for the treatment of unresectable or metastatic melanoma and at an incidence that is at least 5% higher than that reported with ipilimumab include hyperglycemia, lymphopenia and elevated concentrations of lipase.

Adverse effects reported in 10% or more of patients receiving nivolumab in combination with ipilimumab for the treatment of unresectable or metastatic melanoma and at an incidence that is at least 5% higher than that reported with ipilimumab in the CheckMate-067 study include fatigue, diarrhea, rash, nausea, pyrexia, vomiting, decreased appetite, cough, dyspnea, upper respiratory infection, arthralgia, hypothyroidism, weight loss, and hyperthyroidism. Laboratory abnormalities reported in 20% or more of patients receiving nivolumab in combination with ipilimumab for the treatment of unresectable or metastatic melanoma and at an incidence that is at least 5% higher than that reported with ipilimumab include elevated concentrations of hepatic aminotransferase enzymes (i.e., ALT, AST), hyperglycemia, anemia, hyponatremia, elevated concentrations of pancreatic enzymes (i.e., lipase, amylase), elevated concentrations of alkaline phosphatase, lymphopenia, hypocalcemia, and elevated concentrations of serum creatinine.

Adverse effects reported in 10% or more of patients receiving nivolumab for the adjuvant therapy of locally advanced or metastatic melanoma following complete resection and at an incidence that is at least 5% higher than that reported with ipilimumab in the CheckMate-238 study include musculoskeletal pain, upper respiratory infection, and arthralgia. Laboratory abnormalities reported in 10% or more of patients receiving nivolumab for the adjuvant therapy of locally advanced or metastatic melanoma following complete resection and at an incidence that is at least 5% higher than that reported with ipilimumab include lymphopenia, leukopenia, and neutropenia.

Adverse effects reported in 10% or more of patients receiving nivolumab as a single agent for the treatment of metastatic NSCLC and at an incidence that is at least 5% higher than that reported with docetaxel in the CheckMate-017 and CheckMate-057 studies combined include cough, decreased appetite, and pruritus. Laboratory abnormalities reported in 10% or more of patients receiving nivolumab for the treatment of metastatic NSCLC and at an incidence that is at least 5% higher than that reported with docetaxel include elevated concentrations of hepatic aminotransferase enzymes (i.e., ALT, AST), alkaline phosphatase, serum creatinine, and thyroid-stimulating hormone (TSH).

Adverse effects reported in patients receiving nivolumab as a single agent for the treatment of metastatic SCLC in the CheckMate-032 study were generally similar to those observed in patients with other malignancies. Adverse effects reported in 20% or more of patients receiving nivolumab as a single agent for the treatment of metastatic SCLC include fatigue, decreased appetite, musculoskeletal pain, dyspnea, nausea, diarrhea, constipation, and cough.

Adverse effects reported in more than 15% of patients receiving nivolumab as a single agent for the treatment of advanced renal cell carcinoma previously treated with antiangiogenic therapy and at an incidence that is at least 5% higher than that reported with everolimus in the CheckMate-025 study include constipation, back pain, arthralgia, pruritus, and upper respiratory infection. Laboratory abnormalities reported in more than 15% of patients receiving nivolumab for the treatment of advanced renal cell carcinoma and at an incidence that is at least 5% higher than that reported with everolimus include hyponatremia, hyperkalemia, and hypercalcemia.

Adverse effects reported in more than 15% of patients receiving nivolumab in combination with ipilimumab for the treatment of intermediate- or poor-risk, previously untreated, advanced renal cell carcinoma and at an incidence that is at least 5% higher than that reported with sunitinib in the CheckMate-214 study include rash, pruritus, and pyrexia. Laboratory abnormalities reported in more than 15% of patients receiving nivolumab in combination with ipilimumab for the treatment of intermediate- or poor-risk, previously untreated, advanced renal cell carcinoma and at an incidence that is at least 5% higher than that reported with sunitinib include elevated concentrations of amylase.

Adverse effects reported in 10% or more of patients receiving nivolumab as a single agent for the treatment of cHL in the CheckMate-205 and CheckMate-039 studies combined include upper respiratory infection, fatigue, cough, diarrhea, pyrexia, musculoskeletal pain, rash, nausea, pruritus, vomiting, headache, abdominal pain, arthralgia, dyspnea, constipation, infusion-related reactions, pneumonia, hypothyroidism/thyroiditis, peripheral neuropathy, and nasal congestion. Laboratory abnormalities reported in 10% or more of patients receiving nivolumab for the treatment of cHL include leukopenia, neutropenia, thrombocytopenia, elevated concentrations of hepatic aminotransferase enzymes (i.e., ALT, AST), lymphopenia, anemia, elevated concentrations of pancreatic enzymes (i.e., lipase, amylase), elevated concentrations of alkaline phosphatase, hyponatremia, hypokalemia, elevated concentrations of serum creatinine, hypocalcemia, hyperkalemia, hypomagnesemia, and elevated concentrations of bilirubin.

Adverse effects reported in 10% or more of patients receiving nivolumab as a single agent for the treatment of recurrent or metastatic squamous cell carcinoma of the head and neck and at an incidence higher than that reported with the comparator chemotherapy regimens in the CheckMate-141 study include cough and dyspnea. Laboratory abnormalities reported in 10% or more of patients receiving nivolumab for the treatment of recurrent or metastatic squamous cell carcinoma of the head and neck and at an incidence higher than that reported with chemotherapy include elevated concentrations of alkaline phosphatase, elevated concentrations of amylase, hypercalcemia, hyperkalemia, and elevated concentrations of TSH.

Adverse effects reported in 10% or more of patients receiving nivolumab as a single agent for the treatment of locally advanced or metastatic urothelial carcinoma in the CheckMate-275 study include asthenia/fatigue/malaise, musculoskeletal pain, decreased appetite, nausea, cough, diarrhea, pyrexia, urinary tract infection, constipation, rash, thyroid disorders, dyspnea, abdominal pain, edema, pruritus, vomiting, and arthralgia. Laboratory abnormalities reported in 10% or more of patients receiving nivolumab for the treatment of locally advanced or metastatic urothelial carcinoma include hyperglycemia, lymphopenia, hyponatremia, anemia, elevated concentrations of serum creatinine, elevated concentrations of alkaline phosphatase, hypocalcemia, elevated concentrations of hepatic aminotransferase enzymes (i.e., ALT, AST), elevated concentrations of pancreatic enzymes (i.e., lipase, amylase), hyperkalemia, hypomagnesemia, thrombocytopenia, and leukopenia.

Adverse effects reported in 10% or more of patients receiving nivolumab as a single agent for the treatment of metastatic colorectal cancer with MSI-H or dMMR in the CheckMate-142 study include fatigue, diarrhea, abdominal pain, nausea, musculoskeletal pain, vomiting, cough, pyrexia, rash, constipation, upper respiratory infection, arthralgia, hyperglycemia, pruritus, headache, decreased appetite, dizziness, and edema. Laboratory abnormalities reported in 10% or more of patients receiving nivolumab as a single agent for the treatment of metastatic colorectal cancer with MSI-H or dMMR include anemia, elevated concentrations of alkaline phosphatase, lymphopenia, elevated concentrations of hepatic aminotransferase enzymes (i.e., ALT, AST), elevated concentrations of pancreatic enzymes (i.e., lipase, amylase), hyponatremia, neutropenia, hypocalcemia, hypomagnesemia, thrombocytopenia, elevated concentrations of bilirubin, hypokalemia, elevated concentrations of serum creatinine, and hyperkalemia.

Adverse effects reported in 10% or more of patients receiving nivolumab in combination with ipilimumab for the treatment of metastatic colorectal cancer with MSI-H or dMMR in the CheckMate-142 study include fatigue, diarrhea, musculoskeletal pain, pyrexia, abdominal pain, pruritus, nausea, rash, decreased appetite, vomiting, cough, headache, constipation, arthralgia, hypothyroidism, dyspnea, insomnia, hyperthyroidism, dizziness, dry skin, and decreased weight. Laboratory abnormalities reported in 10% or more of patients receiving nivolumab in combination with ipilimumab for the treatment of metastatic colorectal cancer with MSI-H or dMMR include anemia, elevated concentrations of hepatic aminotransferase enzymes (i.e., ALT, AST), elevated concentrations of pancreatic enzymes (i.e., lipase, amylase), elevated concentrations of alkaline phosphatase, hyponatremia, thrombocytopenia, elevated concentrations of serum creatinine, lymphopenia, hyperkalemia, elevated concentrations of bilirubin, hypomagnesemia, neutropenia, hypocalcemia, and hypokalemia.

Adverse effects reported in patients receiving nivolumab as a single agent for the treatment of advanced hepatocellular carcinoma in the CheckMate-040 study were generally similar to those observed in patients with other malignancies; however, a higher incidence of elevated concentrations of hepatic aminotransferase enzymes (i.e., ALT, AST) and bilirubin were reported in these patients.

DRUG INTERACTIONS

No formal drug interaction studies have been performed to date.

● *Ipilimumab*

Concomitant administration of nivolumab 1 mg/kg and ipilimumab 3 mg/kg increased nivolumab clearance by 29% but did not alter clearance of ipilimumab; however, concomitant administration of nivolumab 3 mg/kg and ipilimumab 1 mg/kg did not alter clearance of either drug.

DESCRIPTION

Nivolumab, a fully human anti-programmed-death receptor-1 (anti-PD-1) monoclonal antibody, is an antineoplastic agent. The drug is an IgG₄ kappa immunoglobulin.

Nivolumab is selective for PD-1, an immune-checkpoint receptor expressed on activated T cells, monocytes, B cells, natural killer (NK) T cells, and dendritic cells. Overexpression of PD-1 ligands on the surface of tumor cells results in activation of PD-1 and suppression of cytotoxic T-cell activity. Nivolumab blocks the interaction between PD-1 and its ligands, resulting in enhanced immune response, including enhanced antitumor immune response. The drug also has been shown to reduce tumor growth in syngeneic mouse tumor models. The combination of nivolumab and an anti-cytotoxic T-lymphocyte-associated antigen 4 (anti-CTLA-4) antibody (i.e., ipilimumab) also has demonstrated enhanced T-cell function, including enhanced antitumor immune response, compared with either drug alone. Combined blockade of PD-1 and CTLA-4 also has been shown to enhance antitumor activity in syngeneic mouse tumor models.

Systemic exposure to nivolumab is proportional to dose over the dosage range of 0.1–10 mg/kg every 2 weeks. Following repeated 3-mg/kg doses of nivolumab every 2 weeks, steady-state concentrations are reached by 12 weeks; systemic accumulation of the drug is 3.7-fold. Based on dose-exposure relationships, no clinically important differences in safety and efficacy have been observed between nivolumab 240 mg every 2 weeks and nivolumab 3 mg/kg every 2 weeks in patients with melanoma, non-small cell lung cancer (NSCLC), renal cell carcinoma, urothelial carcinoma, metastatic colorectal cancer with high microsatellite instability (MSI-H), or hepatocellular carcinoma. In addition, the predicted exposure to nivolumab administered as a 30-minute IV infusion is comparable to that observed following administration as a 60-minute IV infusion. Although nivolumab clearance decreases over time (by about 25% from baseline to steady state) in patients with metastatic tumors, the decrease in clearance is not considered clinically important. Nivolumab clearance does not decrease over time in patients with completely resected melanoma; clearance in this patient population is 24% lower than that observed at steady state in patients with metastatic melanoma. The mean terminal half-life of nivolumab is approximately 25 days.

Clearance of nivolumab does not appear to be affected by age (range of 29–87 years), body weight (35–160 kg), gender, race, baseline LDH concentration, programmed death ligand 1 (PD-L1) expression, solid tumor type, tumor burden, renal impairment, or mild hepatic impairment.

ADVICE TO PATIENTS

Importance of advising patients to read the manufacturer's medication guide before beginning treatment and each time nivolumab is administered.

Risk of immune-mediated pneumonitis. Importance of informing clinician immediately if new or worsening cough, chest pain, or shortness of breath occurs.

Risk of immune-mediated colitis. Importance of informing clinician immediately if diarrhea, severe abdominal pain, or changes in stool occur.

Risk of immune-mediated hepatitis. Importance of informing clinician immediately if signs and symptoms of liver damage (e.g., jaundice, severe nausea or vomiting, abdominal pain [particularly in the right upper quadrant], lethargy, easy bruising or bleeding, lack of appetite, dark urine, drowsiness) occur.

Risk of immune-mediated endocrine effects. Importance of informing clinician immediately if manifestations of hypophysitis, hyperthyroidism, hypothyroidism, adrenal insufficiency, or diabetes mellitus occur.

Risk of immune-mediated nephritis or renal dysfunction. Importance of informing clinician immediately if signs and symptoms of nephritis (e.g., decreased urine output, hematuria, peripheral edema, lack of appetite) occur.

Risk of immune-mediated rash. Importance of informing clinician immediately if a rash develops.

Risk of immune-mediated encephalitis. Importance of informing clinician immediately if signs and symptoms of encephalitis (e.g., headache, fever, confusion, memory loss, hallucinations, fatigue, asthenia, somnolence, drowsiness, seizures, stiff neck) occur.

Risk of infusion-related reactions. Importance of informing clinician immediately if signs and symptoms of such reactions, including dizziness, chills, fever, breathing difficulty, pruritus, flushing, and feeling of faintness, occur.

Risk of allogeneic stem cell transplantation-related complications.

Risk of fetal harm. Necessity of advising women of childbearing potential that they should use an effective method of contraception while receiving nivolumab and for at least 5 months after the last dose of the drug. Importance of women informing clinicians if they are or plan to become pregnant. If pregnancy occurs, advise pregnant women of potential risk to the fetus.

Importance of advising women to avoid breast-feeding while receiving nivolumab therapy.

Importance of informing clinicians of existing or contemplated concomitant therapy, including prescription and OTC drugs, as well as any concomitant illnesses (e.g., autoimmune disorders, history of organ transplantation, liver damage, pulmonary disorders).

Importance of informing patients of other important precautionary information. (See Cautions.)

For further information on the handling of antineoplastic agents, see the ASHP Guidelines on Handling Hazardous Drugs at http://www.ahfsdruginformation.com.

PREPARATIONS

Excipients in commercially available drug preparations may have clinically important effects in some individuals; consult specific product labeling for details.

Nivolumab

Parenteral		
Injection, for IV infusion only	10 mg/mL (40, 100, and 240 mg)	Opdivo®, Bristol-Myers Squibb

† Use is not currently included in the labeling approved by the US Food and Drug Administration.

Selected Revisions October 7, 2019, © Copyright, June 29, 2015, American Society of Health-System Pharmacists, Inc.

Osimertinib Mesylate

10:00 · ANTINEOPLASTIC AGENTS

■ Osimertinib mesylate, a third-generation inhibitor of receptor tyrosine kinases, is an antineoplastic agent.

USES

● Non-small Cell Lung Cancer

Osimertinib mesylate is used for the treatment of non-small cell lung cancer (NSCLC) harboring epidermal growth factor receptor (*EGFR*) exon 19 deletions (del19), exon 21 (L858R) substitution, or T790M mutations; the drug is used as adjuvant treatment of early stage NSCLC harboring del19 and L858R mutations following tumor resection, as first-line therapy for metastatic NSCLC harboring del19 and L858R mutations, and for the treatment of T790M mutation-positive metastatic NSCLC in patients refractory to previous EGFR tyrosine kinase therapy. Osimertinib has been designated an orphan drug by FDA for the treatment of *EGFR* mutation-positive NSCLC. Information on FDA-approved companion diagnostic tests for the detection of EGFR mutations in NSCLC is available at https://www.fda.gov/CompanionDiagnostics.

EGFR-activating mutations are present in approximately 15–22% of NSCLC cases in North America and Europe and are present in up to 30–50% of cases in patients of East Asian descent. The majority of *EGFR* mutations are exon 19 deletions or an L858R substitution in exon 21, which together account for about 90% of *EGFR* mutations in patients with NSCLC.

Adjuvant Treatment for Non-small Cell Lung Cancer

Osimertinib mesylate is used for adjuvant treatment after tumor resection in patients with non-small cell lung cancer (NSCLC) harboring epidermal growth factor receptor (*EGFR*) exon 19 deletions (del19) or exon 21 (L858R) substitution mutations as detected by an FDA-approved diagnostic test (e.g., cobas® EGFR Mutation Test). Disease-free survival benefit has been observed in adults receiving osimertinib in the adjuvant setting compared with those receiving placebo.

The current indication for osimertinib as adjuvant treatment of early stage (IB-IIIA) *EGFR* mutation-positive NSCLC following complete tumor resection is based principally on the results of an ongoing randomized, multicenter, double-blind, placebo-controlled phase 3 study (ADAURA). In this study, 682 patients were randomized (stratified by disease stage, *EGFR* mutation, and Asian or non-Asian race) in a 1:1 ratio to receive either osimertinib 80 mg daily or placebo following recovery from surgery or standard adjuvant chemotherapy. Patients were randomized within 10 or 26 weeks of surgery based on receipt of adjuvant chemotherapy. Therapy was continued for 3 years or until disease recurrence or unacceptable toxicity occurred. The primary measure of efficacy was disease-free survival (as evaluated by the investigator) in patients with stage II to IIIA NSCLC; additional measures of efficacy were disease-free survival in the overall population and overall survival in patients with stage II to IIIA disease. Preoperative, postoperative, or planned radiation therapy was not permitted. The median age of patients was 63 years (range: 30–86 years); approximately 72% had never smoked, 70% were female, 64% were of Asian ancestry, and 60% had received adjuvant chemotherapy. All enrolled patients had a World Health Organization (WHO) performance status of 0 or 1; 55% of patients had an *EGFR* del19 mutation, 45% had exon 21 (L858R) substitution mutations, and 1% had T790M mutations. At the time of an interim analysis, enrollment was complete and enrolled patients had been followed for at least 1 year; at the time of this analysis, the independent data monitoring committee recommended unblinding the treatment groups because of evidence of benefit.

At the time of the interim analysis, the median follow-up for disease-free survival in 470 patients with stage II to IIIA disease was 22.1 or 14.9 months in patients receiving osimertinib or placebo, respectively. Median disease-free survival had not been reached in patients receiving osimertinib, but was 19.6 months in those receiving placebo. At 24 months, osimertinib decreased the risk of disease progression or death by 83% in the subgroup of patients with stage II to IIIA disease. In the overall study population, median disease-free survival had not been reached in patients receiving osimertinib, but was 27.5 months in those receiving placebo. At 24 months, osimertinib decreased the risk of disease progression or death by 80% in the overall study population. Results of subgroup analyses (based on age, gender, race, smoking status, *EGFR* mutation, disease stage, or use of adjuvant chemotherapy) suggested that the effect of osimertinib on disease-free survival was consistent across all subgroups. Overall survival data were immature at the time of the interim analysis. In an exploratory analysis, 5 osimertinib-treated patients and 34 placebo-recipients had CNS involvement at the time of disease recurrence.

First-line Therapy for Metastatic Non-small Cell Lung Cancer

Osimertinib mesylate is used for the first-line treatment of metastatic NSCLC in patients whose tumors harbor *EGFR* exon 19 deletions (del19) or exon 21 (L858R) substitution mutations as detected by an FDA-approved diagnostic test (e.g., cobas® EGFR Mutation Test). A progression-free survival benefit has been observed in adults with previously untreated *EGFR* mutation-positive metastatic NSCLC receiving osimertinib compared with patients receiving erlotinib or gefitinib.

The current indication for osimertinib in the first-line treatment of metastatic NSCLC is based principally on the results of a randomized, multicenter, double-blind phase 3 study (FLAURA) in adults with previously untreated locally advanced or metastatic NSCLC. In this study, 556 patients were randomized (stratified by race and *EGFR* mutation) in a 1:1 ratio to receive either osimertinib (80 mg orally once daily) or investigator's choice of gefitinib (250 mg orally once daily) or erlotinib (150 mg orally once daily) until disease progression or unacceptable toxicity occurred. The primary measure of efficacy was progression-free survival (as evaluated by the investigator). Patients with CNS metastases not requiring corticosteroid therapy and whose condition was neurologically stable for at least 2 weeks following completion of surgery or radiation therapy were eligible for this study. The median age of patients was 64 years (range: 26–93 years); most patients (95%) had metastatic disease, 64% had never smoked, 63% were female, 62% were of Asian ancestry, and 7% had received prior adjuvant or neoadjuvant chemotherapy. All enrolled patients had a World Health Organization (WHO) performance status of 0 or 1 and were required to have evidence of an EGFR mutation (confirmed by the cobas® EGFR Mutation Test or a clinical trial assay); 63% of patients had exon 19 deletions, 37% had exon 21 (L858R) substitution mutations, and less than 1% also had T790M mutations. Approximately 20% of the patients randomized to investigator's choice of erlotinib or gefitinib received osimertinib therapy following disease progression.

At a median follow-up of 15 or 9.7 months in patients receiving osimertinib or investigator's choice of erlotinib or gefitinib, respectively, patients receiving osimertinib had a longer median progression-free survival than those receiving erlotinib or gefitinib (18.9 versus 10.2 months; hazard ratio of 0.46). Effects of osimertinib on investigator-assessed progression-free survival and progression-free survival as assessed by a blinded independent central review committee (BICR) were comparable. The objective response rate in osimertinib-treated patients was 77% compared with 69% in those receiving erlotinib or gefitinib; complete responses were achieved in 2 or 1% of patients, respectively. Patients receiving osimertinib had a longer median duration of response (17.6 versus 9.6 months) compared with those receiving erlotinib or gefitinib. Results of subgroup analyses (based on age, gender, WHO performance status, race, smoking status, *EGFR* mutation, or presence of brain metastases) suggested that the effect of osimertinib on progression-free survival was consistent across all subgroups. In the subgroup of 41 patients with baseline measurable CNS metastases, BICR-assessed CNS objective response rates were 77 or 63% in the osimertinib or investigator's choice of EGFR tyrosine kinase inhibitor groups, respectively, with durable responses of 6 months or more in 47 or 33% of patients, respectively, or 12 months or more in 47 or 33% of patients, respectively; complete responses were achieved in 18% of patients receiving osimertinib and none of those receiving erlotinib or gefitinib. At a median duration of follow-up of 35.8 or 27 months in patients receiving osimertinib or investigator's choice of an EGFR tyrosine kinase inhibitor, respectively, median overall survival was prolonged in patients receiving osimertinib compared with those receiving erlotinib or gefitinib (38.6 versus 31.8 months; hazard ratio of 0.80). Results of subgroup analyses (based on age, gender, WHO performance status, race, smoking status, *EGFR* mutation, or presence of brain metastases) suggested that the effect of osimertinib on overall survival was consistent across subgroups.

Previously Treated Metastatic Non-small Cell Lung Cancer

Osimertinib mesylate is used for the treatment of metastatic NSCLC in patients with the EGFR T790M mutation (as detected by an FDA-approved diagnostic test) who experienced disease progression during or following EGFR tyrosine kinase inhibitor therapy.

The current indication for osimertinib in the treatment of metastatic NSCLC following failure of prior EGFR tyrosine kinase inhibitor therapy is based principally on the results of a randomized, multicenter, open-label, active-controlled study (AURA3) in 419 adults with metastatic EGFR T790M mutation-positive NSCLC (confirmed by the cobas® EGFR Mutation Test) whose disease had progressed while receiving prior systemic therapy, including a first-line EGFR tyrosine kinase inhibitor (e.g., gefitinib, erlotinib, afatinib). Patients were randomized in a 2:1 ratio to receive osimertinib (80 mg orally once daily) or platinum-based chemotherapy (pemetrexed 500 mg/m^2 in combination with either cisplatin 75 mg/m^2 or carboplatin dosed to a target area under the plasma concentration-time curve [AUC] of 5 mg/mL per minute by IV infusion once every 3 weeks for a maximum of 6 cycles); patients receiving platinum-based chemotherapy whose disease had not progressed after 4 cycles were permitted to receive maintenance pemetrexed therapy. Treatment was continued until disease progression, unacceptable toxicity, or study withdrawal occurred. The primary efficacy end point of the study was progression-free survival as assessed by the investigator according to Response Evaluation Criteria in Solid Tumors (RECIST 1.1); secondary end points included objective response rate, duration of response, and overall survival. The median age of patients was 62 years; the majority of patients were female (64%), of Asian ancestry (65%), had never smoked (68%), and had adenocarcinoma histology (84%). Thirty-four percent of the patients had CNS metastases at baseline, among which 11% had measurable disease.

At a median follow-up of 8.3 months, patients receiving osimertinib in the AURA3 study had a longer median investigator-assessed progression-free survival compared with patients receiving platinum-based chemotherapy (10.1 versus 4.4 months). Analysis of progression-free survival according to BICR resulted in similar findings as the investigator assessment. Patients receiving osimertinib also had a higher objective response rate (65 versus 29%) and a longer median duration of response (11 versus 4.2 months) compared with those receiving platinum-based chemotherapy. Complete response was achieved in 1% of patients in both treatment groups. In the subgroup of patients with baseline measurable CNS metastases, BICR-assessed CNS objective response rates were 57 or 25% in the osimertinib or platinum-based chemotherapy groups, respectively, with durable responses of 6 months or more in 47 or 0% of patients receiving these respective treatments, or 9 months or more in 12 or 0% of patients receiving these respective treatments; complete responses were achieved in 7% of patients receiving osimertinib and none of those receiving platinum-based chemotherapy. At a median follow-up 23.5 or 20.3 months in patients receiving osimertinib or platinum-based chemotherapy, respectively, no substantial difference in median overall survival was observed between the treatment groups (26.8 versus 22.5 months; hazard ratio 0.87).

Osimertinib has been studied in *EGFR* T790M mutation-positive NSCLC in patients with brain or leptomeningeal metastases† who previously received an EGFR tyrosine kinase inhibitor.

DOSAGE AND ADMINISTRATION

● General

Pretreatment Screening

● *Adjuvant therapy of NSCLC*: Confirm presence of epidermal growth factor receptor (*EGFR*) exon 19 deletions (del19) or exon 21 (L858R) substitution mutations in tumor specimens using an FDA-approved companion diagnostic test (e.g., cobas® EGFR Mutation Test).

● *First-line treatment of metastatic NSCLC*: Confirm presence of *EGFR* del19 or L858R substitution mutations in tumor or plasma specimens using an FDA-approved diagnostic test (e.g., cobas® EGFR Mutation Test). Patients with a negative plasma del19 or L858R mutation result should be reevaluated for feasibility of a tumor biopsy.

● *Previously treated metastatic NSCLC*: Confirm presence of *EGFR* T790M mutation in tumor or plasma specimens by an FDA-approved diagnostic test (e.g., cobas® EGFR Mutation Test). Because of the high rate of false-negative results, plasma testing is recommended only when a tumor biopsy cannot be obtained; patients with a negative plasma result should be reevaluated for feasibility of a tumor biopsy.

● Baseline left ventricular ejection fraction (LVEF) in patients with cardiac risk factors.

● Perform a complete blood count (CBC) with differential before initiating therapy.

● Verify pregnancy status in females of reproductive potential.

Patient Monitoring

● Monitor for symptoms of interstitial lung disease and pneumonitis during therapy.

● Monitor for corrected QT (QT$_c$) interval prolongation in patients with congenital long QT$_c$ syndrome, congestive heart failure, or electrolyte abnormalities, and those receiving concomitant drugs known to prolong the QT$_c$ interval.

● Periodic monitoring of electrolyte concentrations recommended in patients with congenital long QT$_c$ syndrome, congestive heart failure, or electrolyte abnormalities, and those receiving concomitant drugs known to prolong the QT$_c$ interval.

● *Patients with cardiac risk factors*: Monitor for signs and symptoms of cardiomyopathy during therapy; assess LVEF in patients with cardiac risk factors at baseline and in those who develop signs or symptoms of cardiomyopathy during therapy.

● Perform a CBC with differential periodically during therapy, and more frequently if clinically indicated.

Dispensing and Administration Precautions

● Based on the Institute for Safe Medication Practices (ISMP), osimertinib is a high-alert medication that has a heightened risk of causing significant patient harm when used in error.

● Administration

Osimertinib is administered orally once daily without regard to meals. The tablets should be swallowed whole and should *not* be crushed.

For patients unable to swallow solids, osimertinib tablets may be dispersed in a container with 60 mL (2 ounces) of noncarbonated water and immediately swallowed; no other liquids should be used. When preparing the drug dispersion, the water should be stirred (without crushing, heating, or ultrasonicating) until the tablet is dispersed (the tablet will not completely dissolve). Following administration, the container should be rinsed with an additional 120–240 mL (4–8 ounces) of water and the contents swallowed immediately to ensure that the full dose is given.

Alternatively, if administration through a nasogastric tube is required, the tablet should be dispersed in a container with 15 mL of noncarbonated water and drawn into a syringe; the container should then be rinsed with an additional 15 mL of water to transfer any residue to the syringe. The resulting 30-mL drug dispersion should be administered through the nasogastric tube, and the tube should be flushed with appropriate volumes of water (approximately 30 mL).

If a dose of osimertinib is missed, the next dose should be taken at the regularly scheduled time; the missed dose should not be taken.

● Dosage

Dosage of osimertinib mesylate is expressed in terms of osimertinib.

Non-small Cell Lung Cancer

Adjuvant Treatment for Non-small Cell Lung Cancer

The recommended adult dosage of osimertinib for adjuvant therapy of *EGFR* del19 or L858R mutation-positive non-small cell lung cancer (NSCLC) after tumor resection is 80 mg once daily. Osimertinib therapy should be continued for up to 3 years or until disease recurrence or unacceptable toxicity occurs.

First-line Therapy for Metastatic Non-small Cell Lung Cancer

The recommended adult dosage of osimertinib for the initial treatment of *EGFR* del19 or L858R mutation-positive metastatic NSCLC is 80 mg once daily. Osimertinib therapy should be continued until disease progression or unacceptable toxicity occurs.

Previously Treated Metastatic Non-small Cell Lung Cancer

The recommended adult dosage of osimertinib for the treatment of *EGFR* T790M mutation-positive metastatic NSCLC following failure of prior EGFR tyrosine kinase inhibitor therapy is 80 mg once daily. Osimertinib therapy should be continued until disease progression or unacceptable toxicity occurs.

Dosage Modification

Pulmonary Effects

If interstitial lung disease or pneumonitis occurs, osimertinib therapy should be permanently discontinued.

Cardiac Effects

If corrected QT (QT_c) interval exceeds 500 msec on at least 2 separate ECGs, osimertinib therapy should be withheld until the QT_c interval is less than 481 msec or returns to baseline (if baseline QT_c interval is 481 msec or more). Osimertinib therapy may then be resumed at a reduced dosage of 40 mg daily. If QT_c-interval prolongation is accompanied by signs and/or symptoms of life-threatening arrhythmia, the drug should be permanently discontinued.

If symptomatic congestive heart failure occurs, osimertinib should be permanently discontinued.

Cutaneous Toxicity

If Stevens-Johnson syndrome or erythema multiforme major is suspected, osimertinib therapy should be withheld. Permanently discontinue osimertinib therapy if Stevens-Johnson syndrome or erythema multiforme major is confirmed.

If cutaneous vasculitis is suspected, osimertinib should be withheld and the patient should be evaluated for systemic involvement; consider consultation with a dermatologist. Consider permanent discontinuance of osimertinib based on severity when no other etiology is identified.

Other Toxicity

If any other grade 3 or higher adverse reaction occurs, osimertinib therapy should be interrupted for up to 3 weeks. If the adverse reaction improves to grade 2 or less within this time period, the drug may be resumed at the original dosage or at a reduced dosage of 40 mg daily. If there is no improvement within 3 weeks of withholding osimertinib, the drug should be permanently discontinued.

Concomitant Use with CYP3A Inducers

If osimertinib is used concomitantly with a potent inducer of cytochrome P-450 (CYP) isoenzyme 3A, osimertinib dosage should be increased to 160 mg daily. The usual dosage of 80 mg daily should be resumed 3 weeks after the potent CYP3A inducer is discontinued. No dosage adjustment is required when osimertinib is used concomitantly with moderate and/or weak CYP3A inducers.

● Special Populations

The manufacturer makes no specific dosage recommendations for geriatric patients.

No dosage adjustment is necessary in patients with mild to severe renal impairment (creatinine clearance 15–89 mL/minute). Insufficient data are available to provide dosage recommendations for patients with end-stage renal disease (creatinine clearance less than 15 mL/minute).

No dosage adjustment is necessary in patients with mild to moderate hepatic impairment (Child-Pugh class A or B; total bilirubin concentration not exceeding the upper limit of normal [ULN] with AST concentration exceeding the ULN; or total bilirubin concentration 1–3 times the ULN with any AST concentration). Insufficient data are available to provide dosage recommendations for patients with severe hepatic impairment.

CAUTIONS

● Contraindications

● The manufacturer states that there are no known contraindications to the use of osimertinib mesylate.

● Warnings/Precautions

Interstitial Lung Disease/Pneumonitis

Severe or fatal interstitial lung disease/pneumonitis may occur in patients receiving osimertinib. Across all clinical studies, interstitial lung disease or pneumonitis occurred in 3.7% of 1479 osimertinib-treated patients and was fatal in 0.3% of patients receiving the drug.

Osimertinib therapy should be withheld in patients who experience any respiratory manifestations suggestive of interstitial lung disease (e.g., dyspnea, cough, fever). If a diagnosis of interstitial lung disease is confirmed, the drug should be permanently discontinued.

Prolongation of QT Interval

Prolongation of the corrected QT (QT_c) interval has been reported in patients receiving osimertinib. The prolongation appears to occur in a concentration-dependent manner. Across all clinical studies, QT_c-interval prolongation exceeding 500 msec or an increase from baseline QT_c interval of greater than 60 msec occurred in 0.8 or 3.1%, respectively, of 1479 osimertinib-treated patients. Patients with baseline QT_c interval exceeding 470 msec were excluded from these studies.

The manufacturer recommends periodic monitoring of ECG and serum electrolytes during osimertinib therapy in patients at risk for QT-interval prolongation, including those with congenital long QT syndrome, congestive heart failure, or electrolyte abnormalities, and in those receiving concomitant drugs known to prolong the QT interval with known risk of torsades de pointes. If QT-interval prolongation occurs, dosage reduction, temporary interruption, or permanent discontinuance of therapy may be necessary. If QT_c-interval prolongation is accompanied by signs and/or symptoms of life-threatening arrhythmia, osimertinib therapy should be permanently discontinued.

Cardiomyopathy

Cardiomyopathy has been reported in patients receiving osimertinib. Across all clinical studies, cardiomyopathy (defined as acute or chronic cardiac failure, congestive heart failure, pulmonary edema, or decreased ejection fraction) was reported in 3% of 1479 osimertinib-treated patients; fatal cardiomyopathy occurred in 0.1% of patients receiving the drug. Across all clinical studies, decreases in left ventricular ejection fraction (LVEF) to less than 50% with a decline of ≥10% from baseline was reported in 3.2% of 1233 osimertinib-treated patients who had baseline and follow-up LVEF assessments. In the primary clinical study evaluating osimertinib for the adjuvant treatment of NSCLC, decreases in LVEF of ≥10% and to <50% were reported in 1.5% of 325 osimertinib-treated patients.

In patients with cardiac risk factors, cardiac function (including LVEF) should be assessed prior to initiating osimertinib and periodically during therapy; LVEF should be assessed in any patient who develops cardiac complications during osimertinib therapy. Osimertinib should be permanently discontinued in patients who develop symptomatic congestive heart failure.

Keratitis

Keratitis has been reported in 0.7% of 1479 patients receiving osimertinib in clinical studies.

Patients who develop manifestations suggestive of keratitis (e.g., eye inflammation, lacrimation, photosensitivity, blurred vision, eye pain, red eye) should be referred promptly to an ophthalmologist for evaluation.

Erythema Multiforme and Stevens-Johnson Syndrome

In postmarketing surveillance, erythema multiforme major and Stevens-Johnson syndrome have been reported in patients receiving osimertinib.

Osimertinib should be withheld if erythema multiforme major or Stevens-Johnson syndrome is suspected; if diagnosis is confirmed, permanently discontinue osimertinib.

Cutaneous Vasculitis

In postmarketing surveillance, cutaneous vasculitis (e.g., leukocytoclastic vasculitis, urticarial vasculitis, and IgA vasculitis) have been reported in patients receiving osimertinib.

If cutaneous vasculitis is suspected, osimertinib should be withheld and the patient should be evaluated for systemic involvement; consultation with a dermatologist should be considered. Permanent discontinuation of osimertinib should be considered based on severity when no other etiology is identified.

Aplastic Anemia

Aplastic anemia has been reported in patients recieving osimertinib in clinical trials (0.7%) and in postmarketing surveillance; some cases have resulted in fatal outcomes. Patients should be advised of the signs and symptoms of aplastic anemia (e.g., new or persistent fevers, bruising, bleeding, pallor). If aplastic anemia is suspected, osimertinib should be withheld and a hematology consultation should be obtained. If an aplastic anemia diagnosis is confirmed, permanently discontinue osimertinib. Perform a complete blood count with differential before initiating therapy, periodically throughout treatment, and more frequently if indicated.

Fetal/Neonatal Morbidity and Mortality

Osimertinib may cause fetal harm if administered to pregnant women based on its mechanism of action and animal findings. Embryofetal toxicity (e.g., postimplantation loss, early embryonic death, decreased fetal weight) has been demonstrated in animals at exposures approximately 1.5 times those observed in humans at the recommended dosage. There are no adequate and well-controlled studies in pregnant women.

Pregnancy should be avoided during therapy. The manufacturer states that pregnancy status should be verified prior to initiation of osimertinib therapy in females of reproductive potential and that such females should be advised to use effective contraception during osimertinib therapy and for 6 weeks after the drug is discontinued. In addition, males with female partners of reproductive potential should use effective methods of contraception while receiving the drug and for 4 months after the drug is discontinued.

Impairment of Fertility

Results of animal studies suggest that osimertinib may impair female and male fertility. In female rats, administration of osimertinib at a dosage of 20 mg/kg daily (producing peak plasma osimertinib concentrations approximately 1.5 times those observed with the recommended human dosage) from 2 weeks before mating to pregnancy day 8 had no effect on estrus cycles or pregnancy rates, but caused early embryonic deaths; the effects of osimertinib on fertility appeared to be reversible when female rats were mated 1 month after discontinuance of the drug.

Increased preimplantation embryonic loss was observed in untreated female rats mated to osimertinib-treated male rats; it is not known whether these effects are reversible.

Specific Populations

Pregnancy

Although there are no available data in pregnant women, animal studies suggest that osimertinib may cause fetal harm. If osimertinib is used during pregnancy or if the patient becomes pregnant while receiving the drug, the patient should be apprised of the potential fetal hazard.

Lactation

It is not known whether osimertinib is distributed into human milk or if the drug has any effect on milk production or the nursing infant. Adverse effects (e.g., reduced growth rates, neonatal deaths) have been observed in the offspring of rats administered osimertinib during gestation and early lactation. Because of the potential for serious adverse reactions to osimertinib in nursing infants, women should be advised to discontinue nursing while receiving the drug and for 2 weeks after the drug is discontinued.

Pediatric Use

Safety and efficacy of osimertinib have not been established in pediatric patients.

Geriatric Use

In clinical studies of osimertinib, 43% of patients were 65 years of age or older. No overall differences in efficacy were observed based on age; however, an exploratory analysis suggests a higher incidence of grade 3 or 4 adverse reactions (35 versus 27%) and more frequent dosage modifications (32 versus 21%) for adverse reactions in geriatric patients compared with younger adults.

Hepatic Impairment

Population pharmacokinetic analysis suggests that the pharmacokinetics of osimertinib are not substantially altered in patients with mild to moderate hepatic impairment (Child-Pugh class A or B; total bilirubin concentration not exceeding the upper limit of normal [ULN] with AST concentration exceeding the ULN; or total bilirubin concentration 1–3 times the ULN with any AST concentration). The drug has not been studied in patients with severe (total bilirubin concentration 3–10 times the ULN with any AST concentration) hepatic impairment.

Renal Impairment

Population pharmacokinetic analysis suggests that the pharmacokinetics of osimertinib are not substantially altered in patients with mild to severe renal impairment (creatinine clearance of 15–89 mL/minute). The drug has not been studied in patients with end-stage renal disease (creatinine clearance less than 15 mL/minute).

● Common Adverse Effects

Adverse effects reported in more than 20% of patients receiving osimertinib include diarrhea, rash, musculoskeletal pain, dry skin, nail toxicity, stomatitis, fatigue, and cough. Laboratory abnormalities reported in at least 20% of patients receiving osimertinib include leukopenia, lymphopenia, anemia, thrombocytopenia, and neutropenia.

DRUG INTERACTIONS

Osimertinib mesylate is metabolized principally by cytochrome P-450 (CYP) isoenzyme 3A. In vitro studies indicate that osimertinib induces CYP1A2; the drug does not inhibit CYP1A2, 2A6, 2B6, 2C8, 2C9, 2C19, 2D6, or 2E1.

Osimertinib is a substrate of P-glycoprotein (P-gp) and breast cancer resistance protein (BCRP), but not a substrate of organic anion transport protein (OATP) 1B1 or OATP1B3. Osimertinib inhibits BCRP but does not inhibit organic anion transporter (OAT) 1, OAT3, OATP1B1, OATP1B3, multidrug and toxin extrusion transporter (MATE) 1, MATE2K, or organic cation transporter (OCT) 2.

● Drugs Affecting Hepatic Microsomal Enzymes

When the potent CYP3A4 inhibitor itraconazole (200 mg twice daily) was administered concomitantly with osimertinib, peak plasma concentrations of osimertinib decreased by 20% and area under the plasma concentration-time curve (AUC) increased by 24%; however, these changes were not considered to be clinically important.

Concomitant use of osimertinib with potent inducers of CYP3A may decrease plasma concentrations of osimertinib. When the potent CYP3A4 inducer rifampin (600 mg daily for 21 days) was administered concomitantly with osimertinib (80 mg once daily) in patients with epidermal growth factor receptor (EGFR) mutation-positive non-small cell lung cancer (NSCLC), peak plasma concentrations and AUC of osimertinib decreased by 73 and 78%, respectively. Because of the potential for reduced efficacy of osimertinib, concomitant administration of osimertinib and potent CYP3A inducers (e.g., rifampin) should be avoided. If concomitant use cannot be avoided, dosage of osimertinib should be increased.

● Drugs Metabolized by Hepatic Microsomal Enzymes

When the CYP3A4 substrate simvastatin (single 40-mg dose) was administered concomitantly with osimertinib (80 mg daily) in patients with EGFR mutation-positive NSCLC, peak plasma concentrations and (AUC) of simvastatin were not substantially affected.

● Drugs Transported by Breast Cancer Resistance Protein

Concomitant use of osimertinib and drugs that are substrates of BCRP (e.g., rosuvastatin) may increase exposure and toxicity of the BCRP substrate. When the BCRP substrate rosuvastatin (single 20-mg dose) was administered concomitantly with osimertinib (80 mg daily) in patients with EGFR mutation-positive NSCLC, peak plasma concentrations and AUC of rosuvastatin were increased by 72 and 35%, respectively. Patients receiving BCRP substrates concomitantly with osimertinib should be monitored for adverse effects of the substrate drug, unless otherwise specified in the manufacturer's labeling for the substrate.

● Drugs Affected by the P-glycoprotein Transport System

Concomitant use of osimertinib and drugs that are substrates of P-gp (e.g., fexofenadine) may increase exposure and toxicity of the P-gp substrate. When the P-gp substrate fexofenadine was administered concomitantly with osimertinib, peak plasma concentrations and AUC of fexofenadine were increased by 76 and 56%, respectively, following a single dose, and by 25 and 27%, respectively, at steady state. Patients receiving P-gp substrates concomitantly with osimertinib should be monitored for adverse effects of the substrate drug, unless otherwise specified in the manufacturer's labeling for the substrate drug.

● Drugs that Prolong the QT Interval

Concomitant use of osimertinib and drugs that prolong the QT interval may result in additive effects on QT-interval prolongation. Concomitant use of drugs known to prolong the QT interval with known risk of torsades de pointes should be avoided when possible. If concomitant use of drugs known to prolong the QT interval with known risk of torsades de pointes cannot be avoided, the manufacturer recommends periodic monitoring of ECG and electrolytes.

● Drugs Affecting Gastric Acidity

Concomitant administration of a single 80-mg dose of osimertinib with omeprazole (40 mg daily for 5 days) did not affect systemic exposure to osimertinib.

DESCRIPTION

Osimertinib mesylate, a third-generation inhibitor of receptor tyrosine kinases, is an antineoplastic agent. The drug binds irreversibly and selectively to certain mutant forms of the epidermal growth factor receptor (EGFR), including EGFR-sensitizing mutations (e.g., exon 19 deletion [del19], exon 21 substitution [L858R]) and the secondary T790M mutation.

Although first- and second-generation EGFR tyrosine kinase inhibitors (e.g., afatinib, erlotinib, gefitinib) have demonstrated improved outcomes in patients with non-small cell lung cancer (NSCLC) harboring EGFR mutations (e.g., del19, L858R), secondary resistance eventually develops following approximately 9–13 months of treatment. Clinical resistance to EGFR tyrosine kinase inhibitors has been attributed to the development of a secondary mutation, EGFR T790M, in approximately 50–60% of cases; this mutation results in production of a bulky methionine side chain in the receptor kinase domain of EGFR that is thought to sterically hinder the binding of first-generation (reversible) EGFR tyrosine kinase inhibitors to EGFR. Second-generation (irreversible) EGFR tyrosine kinase inhibitors (e.g., afatinib, dacomitinib) were developed to overcome this resistance; however, their clinical use has been limited by dose-limiting toxicities (e.g., skin rash, GI toxicity) possibly due to activity against wild-type EGFR. Osimertinib, a third-generation EGFR tyrosine kinase inhibitor, exhibits approximately ninefold greater affinity for mutant forms of EGFR than wild-type EGFR. In vitro studies and studies in animal tumor xenograft models indicate that the drug has antitumor activity against NSCLC cell lines expressing EGFR mutations L858R/T790M, L858R, T790M/del19, and del19 and, to a lesser extent, wild-type EGFR. Osimertinib also inhibits the activity of HER2/ErbB2, HER3/ErbB3, HER4/ErbB4, ACK1, and BLK at clinically relevant concentrations in vitro.

Following oral administration, median time to peak plasma osimertinib concentrations is approximately 6 hours (range 3–24 hours) with steady-state concentrations achieved within approximately 15 days. Dose-proportional increases in area under the plasma concentration-time curve (AUC) and peak plasma

concentration of osimertinib are observed over a dose range of 20–240 mg. Administration of osimertinib with a high-fat meal slightly increased the AUC and peak plasma concentration of the drug by 19 and 14%, respectively, compared with the fasted state. Limited data in animals suggest that osimertinib distributes into the brain. Osimertinib is predominantly metabolized by the cytochrome P-450 (CYP) isoenzyme 3A. Two active metabolites (AZ7550 and AZ5104) have been identified, each accounting for approximately 10% of total drug exposure; AZ7550 has a similar potency to osimertinib, but AZ5104 exhibits higher potency against mutant EGFR and wild-type EGFR. Osimertinib is 95% bound to plasma proteins. Osimertinib is principally eliminated in feces (68%) and to a lesser extent in urine (14%); approximately 2% of an administered dose is eliminated as unchanged drug. The mean elimination half-life of osimertinib is 48 hours.

The pharmacokinetics of osimertinib do not appear to be affected by age, gender, or race (Asian versus non-Asian), body weight, baseline albumin concentration, line of therapy, or smoking status.

ADVICE TO PATIENTS

- Risk of severe or fatal interstitial lung disease/pneumonitis. Importance of immediately informing clinician if new or worsening respiratory symptoms (e.g., difficulty breathing, shortness of breath, cough, fever) occur.

- Risk of QT_c-interval prolongation. Importance of immediately informing clinician if any possible symptoms of QT-interval prolongation (e.g., dizziness, lightheadedness, syncope) occur.

- Risk of cardiomyopathy. Importance of immediately informing clinician if manifestations of heart failure (e.g., palpitations, shortness of breath, edema) occur.

- Risk of keratitis. Importance of informing clinician if manifestations of keratitis (e.g., eye inflammation, lacrimation, photosensitivity, eye pain, red eye, changes in vision) occur.

- Risk of erythema multiforme and Stevens-Johnson syndrome. Importance of promptly informing clinician if target lesions or severe blistering/peeling of the skin occur.

- Risk of cutaneous vasculitis. Importance of informing clinician if they develop multiple, non-blanching red papules on their extremities or buttocks, or large hives on their trunk that do not resolve within 24 hours and develop a bruised appearance.

- Risk of aplastic anemia. Importance of informing clinician if signs and symptoms develop such as new or persistent fevers, bruising, bleeding, or pallor

- Risk of fetal harm. Necessity of advising females of reproductive potential to use effective methods of contraception while receiving osimertinib and for 6 weeks after the drug is discontinued. Necessity of advising males with female partners of reproductive potential to use effective methods of contraception while receiving the drug and for 4 months after the drug is discontinued. Importance of females informing their clinician if they are pregnant or think they may be pregnant. If pregnancy occurs, the patient should be advised of the potential risk to the fetus.

- Importance of advising females to avoid breast-feeding while receiving osimertinib therapy and for 2 weeks after the drug is discontinued.

- Importance of informing clinicians of existing or contemplated concomitant therapy, including prescription and OTC drugs and dietary or herbal supplements, as well as any concomitant illnesses.

- Importance of informing patients of other important precautionary information.

For further information on the handling of antineoplastic agents, see the ASHP Guidelines on Handling Hazardous Drugs at https://www.ahfsdrug information.com.

PREPARATIONS

Osimertinib mesylate can only be obtained through a limited network of specialty distributors. Consult manufacturer's website for additional information.

Excipients in commercially available drug preparations may have clinically important effects in some individuals; consult specific product labeling for details.

Osimertinib Mesylate

Oral

Tablets, film-coated	40 mg (of osimertinib)	**Tagrisso®**, AstraZeneca
	80 mg (of osimertinib)	**Tagrisso®**, AstraZeneca

† Use is not currently included in the labeling approved by the US Food and Drug Administration.

Oxaliplatin

10:00 · ANTINEOPLASTIC AGENTS

■ Oxaliplatin is a platinum-containing antineoplastic agent.

USES

● Colorectal Cancer

Oxaliplatin, in combination with fluorouracil and leucovorin, is used as adjuvant therapy for stage III cancer of the colon in patients who have undergone complete resection of the primary tumor. Oxaliplatin also is used in combination with fluorouracil and leucovorin in the treatment of advanced cancer of the colon and rectum.

Oxaliplatin also has been used in combination with capecitabine† (a prodrug of fluorouracil) as adjuvant therapy following the complete resection of the primary tumor in patients with stage III colon cancer.

Adjuvant Therapy for Stage III Colon Cancer

Oxaliplatin in Combination with Fluorouracil and Leucovorin

Oxaliplatin, in combination with fluorouracil and leucovorin, is used as adjuvant therapy for stage III cancer of the colon in patients who have undergone complete resection of the primary tumor. This indication is based on survival benefit observed with the combination of oxaliplatin, fluorouracil, and leucovorin compared with the combination of fluorouracil and leucovorin.

Use of oxaliplatin, in combination with fluorouracil and leucovorin, as adjuvant therapy for stage III colon cancer is based principally on evidence of improved disease-free and overall survival from a multicenter, open-label, randomized study (Multicenter International Study of Oxaliplatin/5-Fluorouracil/Leucovorin in the Adjuvant Treatment of Colon Cancer [MOSAIC]) in 2246 patients with stage II or III colon cancer who had undergone complete resection of the primary tumor. Eligible patients were randomized to receive a 2-day combination regimen of oxaliplatin, fluorouracil, and leucovorin (leucovorin 200 mg/m^2 administered by IV infusion over 2 hours, followed by fluorouracil 400 mg/m^2 administered by IV injection and fluorouracil 600 mg/m^2 administered by IV infusion over 22 hours, administered for 2 consecutive days; oxaliplatin 85 mg/m^2 was administered by IV infusion over 2 hours concurrently with leucovorin on the first day only) or a 2-day combination regimen of fluorouracil and leucovorin (leucovorin 200 mg/m^2 administered by IV infusion over 2 hours, followed by fluorouracil 400 mg/m^2 administered by IV injection and fluorouracil 600 mg/m^2 administered by IV infusion over 22 hours). Treatment with both regimens was repeated at intervals of 2 weeks for a total of 12 cycles.

Among patients with stage III colon cancer, treatment with the oxaliplatin/fluorouracil/leucovorin regimen was associated with higher rates of disease-free survival at 5 years and overall survival at 6 years (66 and 73%, respectively) compared with the fluorouracil/leucovorin regimen (59 and 69%, respectively). At a median follow-up of 9.5 years, the disease-free and overall survival benefit of oxaliplatin/fluorouracil/leucovorin in patients with stage III colon cancer was maintained (10-year disease-free and overall survival rates of 62 and 67%, respectively, with oxaliplatin/fluorouracil/leucovorin compared with 54 and 59%, respectively, with fluorouracil/leucovorin). Among patients with stage II disease, 5-year disease-free survival rates and 6-year overall survival rates with the 2 regimens were similar. Likewise, 10-year disease-free and overall survival rates failed to show a benefit for oxaliplatin/fluorouracil/leucovorin compared with fluorouracil/leucovorin in patients with stage II disease. Grade 3 and 4 hematologic toxicity (neutropenia, thrombocytopenia, anemia) occurred more commonly with oxaliplatin/fluorouracil/leucovorin than with fluorouracil/leucovorin, although the incidence of febrile neutropenia was low with both regimens. Grade 3 and 4 GI toxicity (nausea, vomiting, diarrhea) also occurred more commonly with oxaliplatin/fluorouracil/leucovorin. Peripheral sensory neuropathy was reported in 92% of patients receiving oxaliplatin/fluorouracil/leucovorin compared with 16% of those receiving fluorouracil/leucovorin (see Neuropathy under Warnings/Precautions: Other Warnings and Precautions, in Cautions).

Oxaliplatin and Capecitabine

Efficacy and safety of oxaliplatin in combination with capecitabine† (CapeOx, CapOx, XELOX) as adjuvant therapy in patients with stage III colon cancer have been evaluated in an open-label, randomized phase 3 study (NO16968; XELOXA). In this study, 1886 patients were randomized to receive either combination therapy with oxaliplatin (130 mg/m^2 administered by IV infusion over 2 hours on day 1) and capecitabine (1 g/m^2 administered orally twice daily on days 1–14) on a 3-week cycle for 8 cycles or combination therapy with IV fluorouracil and leucovorin (Mayo Clinic or Roswell Park regimen). The Mayo Clinic regimen consisted of fluorouracil 425 mg/m^2 administered by rapid IV injection ("bolus") and leucovorin 20 mg/m^2 administered by rapid IV infusion on days 1–5 of each 4-week cycle for a total of 6 cycles (24 weeks), and the Roswell Park regimen consisted of fluorouracil 500 mg/m^2 administered by rapid IV injection ("bolus") and leucovorin 500 mg/m^2 administered as a 2-hour IV infusion on day 1 of weeks 1–6 of each 8-week cycle for a total of 4 cycles (32 weeks). Patients were enrolled no more than 8 weeks following surgery with curative intent, by which time full recovery from surgery was required. The median age of patients was 61–62 years. Most patients (99%) enrolled in the study had a baseline ECOG performance status of 0 or 1. The primary measure of efficacy was disease-free survival.

At a median follow-up of 74 months, patients who received oxaliplatin in combination with capecitabine had higher disease-free (66.1 versus 59.8%; hazard ratio: 0.8) and relapse-free (69.3 versus 62.2%; hazard ratio: 0.78) survival rates compared with patients who received fluorouracil and leucovorin. At a median follow-up of 83 months, patients who received oxaliplatin in combination with capecitabine also had a higher overall survival rate (74.4 versus 69.6%; hazard ratio: 0.83) compared with those who received fluorouracil and leucovorin. Subgroup analysis based on prognostic factors (e.g., age, regional lymph node involvement, baseline carcinoembryonic antigen [CEA] concentration) suggested that the effect of capecitabine in combination with oxaliplatin on disease-free and overall survival was consistent across the subgroups, including those 70 years of age or older; however, the effect size appeared to be reduced in patients 70 years of age or older compared with younger patients. Neurosensory toxicity (any grade: 78 versus 8%; grade 3 or 4: 11 versus less than 1%), grade 3 or 4 hand-foot syndrome (5 versus less than 1%), and grade 3 or 4 thrombocytopenia (5% versus less than 1%) occurred more frequently in patients receiving oxaliplatin in combination with capecitabine, while grade 3 or 4 neutropenia (9 versus 16%), febrile neutropenia (less than 1 versus 4%), and stomatitis (less than 1 versus 9%) occurred more frequently in those receiving fluorouracil and leucovorin.

Use of combination therapy with oxaliplatin and capecitabine also was investigated in a randomized, multicenter, phase 3 study in patients with high-risk stage II or stage III colorectal cancer who had undergone complete resection of the primary tumor; however, interpretation of the results is limited by the failure to meet the planned accrual of 800 patients in the study to demonstrate superiority. In this study, 408 patients were randomized to receive either combination therapy with oxaliplatin (130 mg/m^2 on day 1) and capecitabine (1 g/m^2 twice daily on days 1–14) on a 3-week cycle for 8 cycles or combination therapy with an oxaliplatin, fluorouracil, and leucovorin (modified FOLFOX6) regimen on a 2-week cycle for 12 cycles. At a median follow-up of 74.7 months, median disease-free and overall survival had not been reached; however, 3-year disease-free and overall survival rates were similar between patients receiving capecitabine in combination with oxaliplatin (79.5 and 86.9%, respectively) compared with patients receiving modified FOLFOX6 (79.8 and 87.2%, respectively).

Because the duration and severity of peripheral neuropathy appear to increase with increasing cumulative dosage of oxaliplatin, the International Duration Evaluation of Adjuvant Chemotherapy (IDEA) collaboration pooled data from 6 similarly designed prospective, randomized controlled phase 3 studies (Cancer and Leukemia Group B/Southwest Oncology Group [CALGB/SWOG] study 80702, Short Course Oncology Treatment [SCOT], Adjuvant Chemotherapy for Colon Cancer with High Evidence [ACHIEVE], Three or Six Colon Adjuvant [TOSCA], Hellenic Oncology Research Group [HORG], IDEA France) to evaluate noninferiority of a shortened duration (i.e., 3 months) of adjuvant fluoropyrimidine-oxaliplatin doublet therapy compared to the standard duration of 6 months in patients with stage II or III colon cancer. In this pooled analysis, 12,834 patients with stage III colon cancer received fluoropyrimidine-oxaliplatin doublet therapy with FOLFOX (i.e., FOLFOX4, modified FOLFOX6) or capecitabine in combination with oxaliplatin for 3 or 6 months; however, trials conducted in the US and Canada allowed only the use of modified FOLFOX6. Subgroup analysis of the IDEA collaboration demonstrated noninferiority of a shorter duration (i.e., 3 months) of capecitabine in combination with oxaliplatin (particularly in those with low-risk stage III disease [T1-T3 and N1]) and less toxicity compared with 6 months of therapy. (See Duration of Adjuvant Therapy under Colorectal Cancer: Adjuvant Therapy for Stage III Colon Cancer, in Uses.)

Based on current evidence, combination therapy with oxaliplatin and capecitabine is a reasonable choice (accepted, treatment option) for use as adjuvant therapy in patients with stage III colon cancer who have undergone complete resection of the primary tumor. Although the standard duration of adjuvant capecitabine in combination with oxaliplatin has been 6 months, subgroup analysis of the IDEA collaboration demonstrated noninferiority of a shorter duration (i.e., 3 months) of capecitabine in combination with oxaliplatin, particularly in those with low-risk stage III disease (T1-T3 and N1), and less toxicity compared with 6 months of therapy. Some clinicians state that factors that should be considered when selecting the duration of adjuvant fluoropyrimidine-oxaliplatin doublet therapy, such as capecitabine in combination with oxaliplatin, include tolerability, patient preference, patient characteristics, preexisting conditions, and other factors.

Duration of Adjuvant Therapy

In a pooled analysis (IDEA collaboration) of 6 similarly designed prospective randomized controlled phase 3 studies evaluating noninferiority of a shortened duration (i.e., 3 months) of adjuvant fluoropyrimidine-oxaliplatin doublet therapy compared to the standard duration of 6 months in patients with stage II or III colon cancer, 12,834 patients with stage III colon cancer received fluoropyrimidine-oxaliplatin doublet therapy with FOLFOX (i.e., FOLFOX4, modified FOLFOX6) or capecitabine in combination with oxaliplatin for 3 or 6 months. At the time of the initial analysis (median follow-up of 41.8 months), fluoropyrimidine-oxaliplatin doublet therapy for a duration of 3 months did not meet the noninferiority criterion for 3- or 5-year disease-free survival when compared to a duration of 6 months. However, in patients treated with capecitabine in combination with oxaliplatin, 3 months of therapy appeared to be at least equivalent to a treatment duration of 6 months, particularly in patients with low-risk disease. In patients treated with FOLFOX, 6 months of therapy appeared to be superior to the shorter treatment duration of 3 months. (See Tables 1, 2, and 3.) Grade 3 or 4 neurosensory toxicity was substantially lower in patients receiving 3 months of fluoropyrimidine-oxaliplatin doublet therapy compared with those receiving 6 months of therapy (2.5–2.6 versus 8.9–15.9%, respectively). Although the standard duration of adjuvant fluoropyrimidine-oxaliplatin doublet therapy has been 6 months, a shorter duration of therapy may be considered in certain patients based on these data. Some clinicians state that factors that should be considered when selecting the duration of adjuvant fluoropyrimidine-oxaliplatin doublet therapy include tolerability, patient preference, patient characteristics, preexisting conditions, and other factors.

TABLE 1. Efficacy Results for Fluoropyrimidine-oxaliplatin Doublet Regimens for a Duration of 3 versus 6 Months in the IDEA Study

Treatment and Efficacy Measure	Hazard Ratio (3 vs 6 months of therapy)	Absolute Difference
Fluoropyrimidine-oxaliplatin Doublet Therapy		
3-year Disease-free Survival	1.07	0.9%
5-year Disease-free Survival	1.08	1.7%
5-year Overall Survival	1.02	0.4%
FOLFOX		
3-year Disease-free Survival	1.16	2.4%
5-year Disease-free Survival	1.16	...
5-year Overall Survival	1.07	...
Capecitabine in Combination with Oxaliplatin		
3-year Disease-free Survival	0.95	1.1%
5-year Disease-free Survival	0.98	...
5-year Overall Survival	0.96	...

TABLE 2. Efficacy Results for Patients with Low-Risk Disease Receiving Fluoropyrimidine-oxaliplatin Doublet Regimens for a Duration of 3 versus 6 Months

Treatment and Efficacy Measure	Hazard Ratio (3 vs 6 months of therapy)	Absolute Difference
Fluoropyrimidine-oxaliplatin Doublet Therapy		
3-year Disease-free Survival	1.01	0.2%
5-year Disease-free Survival	1.04	...
5-year Overall Survival	0.95	0.7%
FOLFOX		
3-year Disease-free Survival	1.1	1.6%
5-year Disease-free Survival	1.15	2.4%
5-year Overall Survival	1.02	0.3%
Capecitabine in Combination with Oxaliplatin		
3-year Disease-free Survival	0.85	1.9%
5-year Disease-free Survival	0.87	3.2%
5-year Overall Survival	0.85	2.3%

TABLE 3. Efficacy Results for Patients with High-Risk Disease Receiving Fluoropyrimidine-oxaliplatin Doublet Regimens for a Duration of 3 versus 6 Months

Treatment and Efficacy Measure	Hazard Ratio (3 vs 6 months of therapy)	Absolute Difference
Fluoropyrimidine-oxaliplatin Doublet Therapy		
3-year Disease-free Survival	1.12	1.7%
5-year Disease-free Survival	1.13	...
5-year Overall Survival	1.08	2.1%
FOLFOX		
3-year Disease-free Survival	1.2	3.2
5-year Disease-free Survival	1.18	5%
5-year Overall Survival	1.12	2.8%
Capecitabine in Combination with Oxaliplatin		
3-year Disease-free Survival	1.02	0.1%
5-year Disease-free Survival	1.05	2.6%
5-year Overall Survival	1.03	1%

Treatment of Advanced Colorectal Cancer

Oxaliplatin, in combination with fluorouracil and leucovorin, is used in the treatment of advanced cancer of the colon and rectum. The combination regimen has been studied as first-line therapy for unresectable cancer of the colon or rectum and also as second-line therapy in patients whose disease has recurred or progressed during or within 6 months following first-line therapy with the combination of fluorouracil, leucovorin, and irinotecan.

Previously Untreated Advanced Colorectal Cancer

Use of oxaliplatin, in combination with fluorouracil and leucovorin, as first-line therapy for advanced colorectal cancer is based principally on evidence of improved response and survival from a multicenter, open-label, randomized study conducted by the North Central Cancer Treatment Group (NCCTG N9741) in patients with previously untreated unresectable colorectal cancer. The oxaliplatin/fluorouracil/leucovorin regimen was compared with 2 other regimens (oxaliplatin plus irinotecan and the combination of irinotecan, fluorouracil, and leucovorin) in 795 concurrently randomized patients with previously untreated unresectable colorectal cancer.

In this study, the oxaliplatin/fluorouracil/leucovorin combination was administered as a 2-day regimen (leucovorin 200 mg/m^2 administered by IV infusion over 2 hours, followed by fluorouracil 400 mg/m^2 administered by IV injection and fluorouracil 600 mg/m^2 administered by IV infusion over 22 hours, administered for 2 consecutive days; oxaliplatin 85 mg/m^2 was administered by IV infusion over 2 hours concurrently with leucovorin on the first day only); therapy was repeated at intervals of 2 weeks. The irinotecan/oxaliplatin regimen consisted of oxaliplatin 85 mg/m^2 and irinotecan 200 mg/m^2, both administered by IV infusion on day 1 and repeated at 3-week intervals. The irinotecan/fluorouracil/leucovorin regimen consisted of irinotecan 125 mg/m^2 administered by IV infusion, fluorouracil 500 mg/m^2 administered by IV injection, and leucovorin 20 mg/m^2 administered by IV injection on days 1, 8, 15, and 22 and repeated at 6-week intervals.

Overall response rates were higher with oxaliplatin/fluorouracil/leucovorin therapy (45%) compared with irinotecan/fluorouracil/leucovorin (31%) or irinotecan/oxaliplatin (35%) therapy. The median time to disease progression was similar with the irinotecan/oxaliplatin (6.5 months) and irinotecan/fluorouracil/leucovorin (6.9 months) regimens, but was longer (8.7 months) with the oxaliplatin/fluorouracil/leucovorin regimen. Median overall survival of patients receiving oxaliplatin/fluorouracil/leucovorin therapy (19.5 months) was longer than that of patients receiving irinotecan/fluorouracil/leucovorin therapy (15 months) but did not differ from that of patients receiving irinotecan/oxaliplatin (17.4 months). Grade 3 and 4 GI toxicity (nausea, vomiting, diarrhea) and febrile neutropenia were more commonly associated with the irinotecan-containing regimens, whereas grade 3 and 4 paresthesias were more commonly associated with the oxaliplatin/fluorouracil/leucovorin regimen.

Previously Treated Advanced Colorectal Cancer

Use of oxaliplatin, in combination with fluorouracil and leucovorin, as second-line therapy for advanced colorectal cancer is based principally on response rate and an interim analysis showing improved time to radiographic progression of the disease in a multicenter, randomized, open-label, controlled study in over 450 patients (of more than 800 patients enrolled) with advanced colorectal cancer that had recurred or progressed during or within 6 months following first-line therapy with the combination of fluorouracil, leucovorin, and irinotecan. There currently are no data demonstrating a clinical benefit (e.g., improvement in disease-related symptoms, increased survival).

In this study, eligible patients with unresectable, measurable, and histologically proven disease were randomized to receive oxaliplatin alone (85 mg/m^2 administered by IV infusion over 2 hours), a 2-day combination regimen of fluorouracil and leucovorin (leucovorin 200 mg/m^2 administered by IV infusion over 2 hours, followed by fluorouracil 400 mg/m^2 administered by IV injection and fluorouracil 600 mg/m^2 administered by IV infusion over 22 hours), or a 2-day combination regimen of oxaliplatin, fluorouracil, and leucovorin (leucovorin 200 mg/m^2 administered by IV infusion over 2 hours, followed by fluorouracil 400 mg/m^2 administered by IV injection and fluorouracil 600 mg/m^2 administered by IV infusion over 22 hours, administered for 2 consecutive days; oxaliplatin 85 mg/m^2 was administered by IV infusion over 2 hours concurrently with leucovorin on the first day only). Therapy was repeated at intervals of 2 weeks until radiographic progression, toxicity, or 13 months since the first dose had elapsed, whichever occurred first. Patients randomized to receive oxaliplatin monotherapy or fluorouracil/leucovorin received a median of 3 cycles, while those randomized to receive oxaliplatin/fluorouracil/leucovorin received a median of 6 cycles.

Partial response rates were higher in patients receiving oxaliplatin/fluorouracil/leucovorin (9%) than in those who received oxaliplatin monotherapy (1%) or fluorouracil/leucovorin (0%). There were no complete responses in any group. In addition, the median time to radiographic disease progression was longer in patients receiving oxaliplatin/fluorouracil/leucovorin (4.6 months) than in those who received oxaliplatin alone (1.6 months) or fluorouracil/leucovorin (2.7 months).

DOSAGE AND ADMINISTRATION

● Reconstitution and Administration

Oxaliplatin is administered by IV infusion over 2 hours. Commercially available oxaliplatin powder for injection must be reconstituted and diluted prior to administration; the commercially available concentrate for injection must be diluted prior to administration. Reconstitution or final dilution of the drug must *never* be performed with a sodium chloride solution or other chloride-containing solutions. Because aluminum has been reported to cause degradation of platinum compounds (see Chemistry and Stability, in Cisplatin 10:00), the manufacturers state that needles or IV administration sets containing aluminum parts should not be used for the reconstitution or dilution of oxaliplatin.

Oxaliplatin sterile powder for injection is reconstituted by adding 10 mL (to the vial labeled as containing 50 mg of oxaliplatin) or 20 mL (to the vial labeled as containing 100 mg of oxaliplatin) of water for injection or 5% dextrose injection to provide a solution containing 5 mg/mL; the reconstituted drug may be stored in the vial under refrigeration for up to 24 hours. Alternatively, the commercially available concentrate for injection containing oxaliplatin 5 mg/mL can be used. The appropriate dose should be withdrawn and diluted in 250–500 mL of 5% dextrose injection prior to administration; the diluted drug may be stored under refrigeration for up to 24 hours or at room temperature for up to 6 hours. Oxaliplatin solutions should be inspected visually for particulate matter and/or discoloration prior to administration and should be discarded if either is present. The commercially available concentrate for injection must be protected from light and freezing; following dilution, protection from light is not required. Oxaliplatin powder for injection is not sensitive to light.

The manufacturers state that oxaliplatin solutions must not be mixed or administered simultaneously through the same IV line with alkaline drugs or media (e.g., basic solutions of fluorouracil). The infusion line should be flushed with 5% dextrose injection prior to administration of oxaliplatin or any concomitant drug.

Leucovorin is administered by IV infusion over 2 hours concurrently with oxaliplatin but in a separate container using a Y-type administration set. The dose of fluorouracil then is administered by direct IV injection over 2–4 minutes, followed by the maintenance dose administered by IV infusion over 22 hours. The respective manufacturer's prescribing information should be consulted for additional information on the reconstitution and administration of fluorouracil and leucovorin.

The manufacturers of oxaliplatin recommend that procedures for proper handling and disposal of antineoplastic drugs (e.g., use of gloves) be used to avoid exposure to oxaliplatin during preparation of IV solutions. If oxaliplatin solution comes in contact with the skin or mucous membranes, the skin should be washed immediately and thoroughly with soap and water or the mucosa should be flushed with copious amounts of water. Since oxaliplatin is an antineoplastic agent, the manufacturers state that consideration should be given to handling and disposal according to guidelines issued for cytotoxic drugs, although there is no general agreement that all of the procedures recommended in such guidelines are necessary or appropriate. For further information on the handling of antineoplastic agents, see the ASHP Guidelines on Handling Hazardous Drugs at https://www.ahfsdruginformation.com.

● General Dosage

For the treatment of colorectal cancer, an oxaliplatin dosage of 85 mg/m^2 is administered by IV infusion on day 1 as part of a 2-day combination regimen that includes fluorouracil and leucovorin. The 2-day regimen may be repeated at intervals of 2 weeks. Because this regimen may be associated with an increased incidence of grade 3 or 4 nausea and vomiting compared with the combination regimen containing only fluorouracil and leucovorin, the manufacturer of oxaliplatin states that premedication with antiemetics, including selective inhibitors of type 3 serotonergic (5-HT$_3$) receptors (e.g., dolasetron, granisetron, ondansetron) with or without dexamethasone, should be considered prior to each 2-day cycle. According to the manufacturer, hydration prior to administration of oxaliplatin is not necessary.

The combination regimen of oxaliplatin, fluorouracil, and leucovorin (FOLFOX4) is administered over 2 consecutive days. On day 1, oxaliplatin 85 mg/m^2 and leucovorin 200 mg/m^2 (diluted with 5% dextrose injection) are administered concurrently (in separate containers using a Y-type administration set) by IV infusion over 2 hours. Fluorouracil 400 mg/m² then is administered by IV injection over 2–4 minutes followed by fluorouracil 600 mg/m² (diluted with 500 mL of 5% dextrose injection) administered as an IV infusion over 22 hours. On day 2, leucovorin 200 mg/m² is administered by IV infusion over 2 hours, followed by fluorouracil 400 mg/m² administered by IV injection over 2–4 minutes and fluorouracil 600 mg/m² administered as an IV infusion over 22 hours. When this regimen is used as adjuvant therapy for stage III colon cancer, a total of 12 cycles (6 months) of therapy is recommended. In patients with advanced colorectal cancer, treatment with the regimen is recommended until evidence of disease progression or unacceptable toxicity occurs.

An alternative regimen of oxaliplatin, fluorouracil, and leucovorin (i.e., modified FOLFOX6) also has been used for treatment of advanced colorectal cancer and for adjuvant therapy of colon cancer. The modified FOLFOX6 regimen is administered over 2 consecutive days. Oxaliplatin 85 mg/m² and leucovorin 400 mg/m² (or, alternatively, leucovorin 350 mg) (diluted with 5% dextrose injection) are administered concurrently (in separate containers using a Y-type administration set) by IV infusion over 2 hours. Fluorouracil 400 mg/m² then is administered by IV injection over 5 minutes followed by fluorouracil 1200 mg/m² administered as an IV infusion daily for 2 days (i.e., 2400 mg/m² administered as an IV infusion over 46–48 hours [total fluorouracil dosage of 2800 mg/m² per cycle]). Clinicians should consult individual protocols for specific dosage information.

When oxaliplatin has been used in combination with capecitabine† (CapeOx, CapOx, XELOX) as adjuvant therapy following the complete resection of the primary tumor in patients with stage III colon cancer, oxaliplatin 130 mg/m² has been administered by IV infusion over 2 hours on day 1 and capecitabine 1 g/m² has been administered orally twice daily on days 1–14 of each 3-week cycle. Treatment has been continued for 4 or 8 cycles of therapy; however, 4 cycles (for a treatment duration of 3 months) of capecitabine in combination with oxaliplatin has been shown to have comparable efficacy and less toxicity than 8 cycles of therapy (for a treatment duration of 6 months).

● Dose Modification for Toxicity

The management of certain adverse effects (e.g., neurosensory effects, GI or hematologic toxicity) may require modification of oxaliplatin dosage or duration of infusion. Increasing the duration of oxaliplatin infusion from 2 to 6 hours may minimize acute toxicities; adjustment of infusion duration for fluorouracil or leucovorin is not necessary.

Oxaliplatin should be permanently discontinued in patients experiencing a hypersensitivity reaction, posterior reversible encephalopathy syndrome (PRES), interstitial lung disease, pulmonary fibrosis, or rhabdomyolysis.

Adjuvant Therapy for Stage III Colon Cancer

If persistent grade 2 peripheral sensory neuropathy occurs in patients receiving oxaliplatin in the adjuvant setting for the treatment of stage III colon cancer, reduction of oxaliplatin dosage to 75 mg/m² should be considered; in those with persistent grade 3 peripheral sensory neuropathy, discontinuance of oxaliplatin should be considered. If grade 4 peripheral sensory neuropathy occurs, oxaliplatin should be discontinued.

If grade 3 or 4 thrombocytopenia, grade 4 neutropenia, or febrile neutropenia occurs in patients receiving oxaliplatin in the adjuvant setting for the treatment of stage III colon cancer, administration of the next dose of oxaliplatin should be delayed until neutrophil count reaches or exceeds 1500/mm³ and platelet count reaches or exceeds 75,000/mm³; oxaliplatin may then be resumed at a reduced dosage of 75 mg/m².

If grade 3 or 4 GI toxicity occurs in patients receiving oxaliplatin in the adjuvant setting for the treatment of stage III colon cancer, oxaliplatin therapy should be withheld. When GI toxicity resolves, oxaliplatin may be resumed at a reduced dosage of 75 mg/m²; the dosage of fluorouracil should be reduced to 300 mg/m² by IV injection over 2–4 minutes and 500 mg/m² by IV infusion over 22 hours.

Therapy for Advanced Colorectal Cancer

If persistent grade 2 adverse neurosensory effects occur in patients with advanced colorectal cancer, reduction of oxaliplatin dosage to 65 mg/m² should be considered; in those with persistent grade 3 neurosensory effects, discontinuance of oxaliplatin should be considered. If grade 4 peripheral sensory neuropathy occurs, oxaliplatin should be discontinued.

If grade 3 or 4 thrombocytopenia, grade 4 neutropenia, or febrile neutropenia occurs in patients with advanced colorectal cancer, administration of the next dose of oxaliplatin should be delayed until neutrophil count reaches or exceeds 1500/mm³ and platelet count reaches or exceeds 75,000/mm³; oxaliplatin may then be resumed at a reduced dosage of 65 mg/m².

If grade 3 or 4 GI toxicity occurs in patients with advanced colorectal cancer, oxaliplatin therapy should be withheld. When GI toxicity resolves, oxaliplatin may be resumed at a reduced dosage of 65 mg/m²; the dosage of fluorouracil should be reduced to 300 mg/m² by IV injection over 2–4 minutes and 500 mg/m² by IV infusion over 22 hours.

● Special Populations

Renal Impairment

For patients with severe renal impairment (creatinine clearance less than 30 mL/minute), the oxaliplatin dosage should be reduced to 65 mg/m².

No initial dosage adjustment is necessary in patients with mild (creatinine clearance 50–79 mL/minute) or moderate (creatinine clearance 30–49 mL/minute) renal impairment.

CAUTIONS

● Contraindications

History of hypersensitivity reactions to oxaliplatin, any ingredient in the formulation, or other platinum-containing compounds.

● Warnings/Precautions

Warnings

Hypersensitivity Reactions

Serious and fatal hypersensitivity reactions may occur within minutes of administration of oxaliplatin and during any cycle. Grade 3 or 4 hypersensitivity reactions, including anaphylaxis, have been reported in 2–3% of patients with colon cancer receiving oxaliplatin. These hypersensitivity reactions (e.g., rash, urticaria, erythema, pruritus, bronchospasm, hypotension) are similar in nature and severity to those associated with other platinum-containing antineoplastic agents. If hypersensitivity reactions occur, the drug should be immediately and permanently discontinued and appropriate treatment should be initiated.

Other Warnings and Precautions

Because the oxaliplatin therapeutic regimen includes the use of fluorouracil and leucovorin, the usual cautions, precautions, and contraindications of these drugs also should be considered.

Neuropathy

Treatment with oxaliplatin is consistently associated with acute or delayed neuropathy, both of which are principally peripheral neuropathies. The duration and severity of peripheral neuropathy appear to increase with increasing cumulative dosage of oxaliplatin. Peripheral sensory neuropathy occurred in 92% of patients receiving the combination of oxaliplatin, fluorouracil, and leucovorin as adjuvant therapy for colon cancer; grade 3 events occurred in 12% of patients. In patients with advanced colorectal cancer, peripheral sensory neuropathy occurred in 82 or 74% of patients receiving the oxaliplatin/fluorouracil/leucovorin regimen as first- or second-line therapy, respectively; grade 3 or 4 events occurred in 19% of those receiving the regimen as first-line therapy and 7% of those receiving the regimen as second-line therapy. The median onset of grade 3 peripheral sensory neuropathy was cycle 9 of adjuvant therapy and cycle 6 of second-line therapy.

Acute, reversible sensory neuropathy that is principally peripheral has been reported in 56% of patients receiving oxaliplatin/fluorouracil/leucovorin therapy; acute neurotoxicity has been reported in approximately 30% of patients during an individual treatment cycle. Grade 3 or 4 acute neuropathy occurred in 2% of patients receiving the oxaliplatin/fluorouracil/leucovorin regimen as second-line therapy for advanced colorectal cancer. In the adjuvant setting, 12% of patients experienced grade 3 peripheral neuropathy during treatment. Differences among studies in the reporting of oxaliplatin-associated neuropathy reflect the use of different grading scales. In studies in patients with advanced colorectal cancer, neuropathy was graded using a study-specific scale (range of 1–4) for characterizing paresthesias and dysesthesias; in the study of adjuvant therapy, the National Cancer Institute Common Toxicity Criteria (NCI-CTC Version 2.0) scale for grading neuropathy (applicable range of 0–3) was used.

Manifestations of acute peripheral neuropathy include transient paresthesia, dysesthesia, and hypoesthesia in the hands, feet, perioral area, or throat; jaw spasm, abnormal tongue sensation, dysarthria, ocular pain, and a feeling of chest pressure also have been observed. These symptoms may occur within hours or 2 days following administration of oxaliplatin, resolve within 14 days, and frequently recur with further administration of the drug. Because symptoms of acute sensory neuropathy may be precipitated or exacerbated by exposure to cold temperature or cold objects, patients should be advised to refrain from ingesting cold beverages or food, to avoid exposure to cold temperatures, and to use gloves when handling cold or frozen objects; the manufacturer states that ice (e.g., for mucositis prophylaxis) should be avoided during infusion of oxaliplatin. (See Advice to Patients.)

An acute syndrome of pharyngolaryngeal dysesthesia (grade 3 or 4), characterized by subjective sensations of dysphagia or dyspnea without laryngospasm or bronchospasm (i.e., no stridor or wheezing), has been reported in 1–2% of patients with previously untreated advanced colorectal cancer receiving oxaliplatin in clinical studies; symptoms usually resolve within hours of onset. Some evidence indicates that prolonging the duration of oxaliplatin infusion may reduce the incidence of laryngopharyngeal dysesthesia.

Delayed sensory neuropathy that is principally peripheral has been reported in 48% of patients receiving oxaliplatin/fluorouracil/leucovorin therapy. Symptoms of delayed neuropathy usually include paresthesias, dysesthesias, and hypoesthesias; however, impaired proprioception, which can interfere with daily activities (e.g., writing, buttoning clothing, swallowing, walking), also has been observed. Delayed neuropathy can occur without any prior acute neuropathic event and typically persists for more than 14 days following administration of oxaliplatin. Approximately 80% of patients who developed grade 3 persistent neuropathy during clinical studies had progressed from prior grade 1 or 2 neuropathic events. Symptoms of persistent neuropathy may improve in some patients upon discontinuance of oxaliplatin. Long-term follow-up of patients receiving adjuvant therapy with the oxaliplatin/fluorouracil/leucovorin regimen indicated that the incidence of peripheral sensory neuropathy after completion of such therapy was 39% at 6 months with a decline to 21% at 18 months; the incidence of grade 3 neurotoxicity was 1% at 6 and 18 months and 0.7% at 48 months. Grade 3 or 4 neuropathy occurred in 7% of patients receiving the oxaliplatin/fluorouracil/leucovorin regimen as second-line therapy for advanced colorectal cancer.

Preventive strategies, including the use of intermittent oxaliplatin regimens (i.e., "stop and go" schedule) and other potential neuromodulatory regimens (e.g., amifostine, carbamazepine, gabapentin, glutathione), have been evaluated to reduce the incidence and severity of oxaliplatin-induced neurotoxicity; however, due to the lack of adequate data from well-conducted clinical trials, there is insufficient evidence to support the use of any preventive therapy. In a retrospective cohort study in patients with advanced colorectal cancer, the incidence of grade 3 distal paresthesias was lower in those who received IV infusions of calcium gluconate and magnesium sulfate (immediately before and after infusions of oxaliplatin) compared with those who did not receive such infusions (7 versus 26%). Calcium gluconate and magnesium sulfate infusions are being evaluated in randomized, double-blind, placebo-controlled studies in patients receiving oxaliplatin/fluorouracil/leucovorin-based regimens for colorectal cancer. Preliminary data from one of these studies suggest a reduction in neurotoxicity in patients receiving prophylactic calcium and magnesium therapy; however, data from another study suggested that addition of calcium and magnesium to the chemotherapy regimen had a negative effect on clinical response and antitumor activity. Additional data are needed to define the role of prophylactic calcium and magnesium therapy in reducing the severity and duration of acute and chronic oxaliplatin-induced neurotoxicity and to confirm the effects, if any, of such therapy on clinical response to oxaliplatin-based regimens used in the treatment of colorectal cancer.

Hematologic Effects

Grade 3 or 4 neutropenia occurred in 41 or 44%, respectively, of patients receiving oxaliplatin/fluorouracil/leucovorin therapy for colorectal cancer. Febrile neutropenia or documented infection with severe neutropenia occurred in 1.8% of patients receiving this adjuvant regimen. Among patients with advanced colorectal cancer, febrile neutropenia occurred in 4 or 6% of those receiving oxaliplatin/fluorouracil/leucovorin as first- or second-line therapy, respectively, and

neutropenia with infection occurred in 8% of those receiving first-line oxaliplatin/fluorouracil/leucovorin therapy. Sepsis, neutropenic sepsis, and septic shock, sometimes fatal, also have been reported in patients receiving oxaliplatin/fluorouracil/leucovorin therapy for colorectal cancer.

Grade 3 or 4 thrombocytopenia occurred in 2–5% of patients receiving oxaliplatin/fluorouracil/leucovorin therapy for colorectal cancer.

Complete blood cell counts (CBCs) should be monitored at baseline, prior to each cycle of oxaliplatin, and as clinically indicated. The manufacturer states that oxaliplatin should not be administered until neutrophil counts reach 1500/mm^3 or more and platelet counts reach 75,000/mm^3 or more. If sepsis or septic shock occurs, oxaliplatin therapy should be withheld. Temporary interruption followed by dosage reduction may be necessary if neutropenia or thrombocytopenia occurs.

Posterior Reversible Encephalopathy Syndrome

Posterior reversible encephalopathy syndrome (PRES), with or without concomitant hypertension, occurred in less than 0.1% of patients receiving oxaliplatin in clinical trials. Manifestations of PRES include headache, altered mental status, seizure, and visual disturbance (e.g., vision loss, blurred vision). If PRES is suspected, an MRI should be performed for diagnostic evaluation. If PRES is confirmed. therapy with oxaliplatin should be permanently discontinued.

Pulmonary Toxicity

Pulmonary fibrosis, which may be fatal, occurred in less than 1% of patients receiving oxaliplatin in clinical trials. In patients receiving the oxaliplatin/fluorouracil/leucovorin regimen as adjuvant therapy, the combined incidence of grade 3 cough and dyspnea was less than 1% (with no reports of grade 4 pulmonary toxicity); grade 3 or 4 pulmonary toxicity (cough, dyspnea, hypoxia) was reported in 7% of patients receiving first-line oxaliplatin/fluorouracil/leucovorin therapy for advanced colorectal cancer. In the study of adjuvant oxaliplatin/fluorouracil/leucovorin therapy, one death secondary to eosinophilic pneumonia was reported. If unexplained respiratory manifestations (e.g., nonproductive cough, dyspnea, crackles, radiographic evidence of pulmonary infiltrates) develop, the manufacturer states that oxaliplatin should be discontinued temporarily until further pulmonary investigation excludes interstitial lung disease or pulmonary fibrosis. If interstitial lung disease or pulmonary fibrosis is confirmed, therapy with oxaliplatin should be permanently discontinued.

Hepatic Effects

Increased concentrations of aminotransferases (ALT, AST) and alkaline phosphatase occurred in 57 and 42%, respectively, of patients receiving oxaliplatin/fluorouracil/leucovorin as adjuvant therapy compared with 34 and 20%, respectively, of patients receiving fluorouracil/leucovorin; the incidence of hyperbilirubinemia was similar in both treatment groups. Liver biopsy specimens from patients receiving oxaliplatin/fluorouracil/leucovorin therapy have revealed evidence of hepatic vascular conditions (e.g., peliosis hepatis, nodular regenerative hyperplasia or sinusoidal changes, perisinusoidal fibrosis, veno-occlusive lesions). In patients with abnormal liver function test results or portal hypertension that cannot be explained by metastases to the liver, hepatic vascular toxicity should be considered and, if appropriate, investigated.

Liver function tests (e.g., aminotransferases, bilirubin) should be monitored at baseline, prior to each cycle of oxaliplatin, and as clinically indicated.

Cardiac Effects

Prolongation of the QT interval and subsequent ventricular arrhythmia, including torsades de pointes with fatal outcome, have occurred in patients receiving oxaliplatin.

Oxaliplatin should be avoided in patients with congenital long QT syndrome. Electrocardiograms (ECGs) should be monitored in patients with congestive heart failure, bradyarrhythmias, or electrolyte abnormalities and in those who are receiving drugs known to prolong the QT interval (i.e., class IA and III antiarrhythmics). Serum electrolyte abnormalities should be monitored and corrected prior to initiation of oxaliplatin and periodically during therapy.

Rhabdomyolysis

Rhabdomyolysis, which may be fatal, has been reported in patients receiving oxaliplatin.

If manifestations of rhabdomyolysis (e.g., hematuria, anuria) occur, therapy with oxaliplatin should be permanently discontinued.

Hemorrhage

In clinical trials, hemorrhage occurred more frequently in patients receiving oxaliplatin/fluorouracil/leucovorin therapy than in those receiving fluorouracil/leucovorin. Grade 3 or 4 GI bleeding was reported in 0.2% of patients receiving adjuvant oxaliplatin/fluorouracil/leucovorin therapy. Epistaxis was reported in 10% of patients receiving oxaliplatin/fluorouracil/leucovorin compared with 2% of patients receiving irinotecan/fluorouracil/leucovorin and 1% of those receiving irinotecan/oxaliplatin as first-line therapy for advanced colorectal cancer.

Prolongation of the prothrombin time and international normalized ratio (INR), occasionally associated with hemorrhage, has been reported in patients receiving oxaliplatin/fluorouracil/leucovorin therapy concomitantly with anticoagulant therapy. More frequent monitoring is required for patients receiving oxaliplatin/fluorouracil/leucovorin therapy concomitantly with oral anticoagulants (e.g., warfarin).

Thrombocytopenia and immune-mediated thrombocytopenia have occurred in patients receiving oxaliplatin. Rapid onset of thrombocytopenia and increased risk of hemorrhage have been observed in patients experiencing immune-mediated thrombocytopenia; discontinuance of oxaliplatin therapy should be considered if immune-mediated thrombocytopenia occurs. (See Hematologic Effects under Warnings/Precautions: Other Warnings and Precautions, in Cautions.)

Fetal/Neonatal Morbidity and Mortality

Based on its mechanism of action and animal findings, oxaliplatin may cause fetal harm. Embryotoxicity (i.e., increased early resorption, decreased fetal weight, delayed ossification) was observed in pregnant rats receiving oxaliplatin at a dosage equivalent to less than one-tenth the recommended human dose based on body surface area.

Pregnancy should be avoided during therapy. The manufacturer recommends confirmation of pregnancy status prior to initiation of therapy, and women of reproductive potential should be advised to use effective contraceptive methods during therapy and for at least 9 months after the last dose of the drug. In addition, men with female partners of reproductive potential should use effective methods of contraception during therapy and for 6 months after the last dose of the drug. If oxaliplatin is used during pregnancy or if the patient becomes pregnant while receiving the drug, the patient should be apprised of the potential hazard to the fetus.

Impairment of Fertility

Results of animal studies suggest that oxaliplatin may cause impairment of male and female fertility. In these animal studies, degeneration of reproductive tissues (i.e., testicular degeneration, hypoplasia, atrophy) was observed in male dogs given oxaliplatin at doses approximately one-sixth the recommended human dose based on body surface area.

Specific Populations

Pregnancy

Oxaliplatin may cause fetal harm if administered to pregnant women based on its mechanism of action and animal findings. (See Fetal/Neonatal Morbidity and Mortality under Warnings/Precautions: Other Warnings and Precautions, in Cautions.)

Lactation

It is not known whether oxaliplatin or its metabolites are distributed into milk. Because of the potential for serious adverse reactions to oxaliplatin in nursing infants, women should be advised to discontinue nursing during therapy and for 3 months after the last dose of the drug. The effects of oxaliplatin on nursing infants or on milk production are unknown.

Pediatric Use

Safety and efficacy of oxaliplatin have not been established in pediatric patients. No substantial antitumor activity has been reported in clinical trials in 69 pediatric patients with solid tumors.

Geriatric Use

Clearance of ultrafilterable platinum does not appear to be affected substantially by age; however, the incidence of certain adverse effects (i.e., granulocytopenia, leukopenia, grade 3 or 4 neutropenia, diarrhea, dehydration, hypokalemia, fatigue, syncope) was higher in geriatric patients than in younger adults. In the study of adjuvant therapy for colon cancer, the effect on disease-free survival of the oxaliplatin/fluorouracil/leucovorin regimen compared with that of fluorouracil/leucovorin in patients 65 years of age or older was inconclusive. In patients receiving the oxaliplatin/fluorouracil/leucovorin regimen as first-line therapy for advanced colorectal cancer, no differences in efficacy were observed in patients 65 years of age or older compared with the overall study population. In patients receiving the oxaliplatin/fluorouracil/leucovorin regimen for previously treated advanced colorectal cancer, no differences in efficacy were observed in patients 65 years of age or older compared with younger adults.

Renal Impairment

Following administration of oxaliplatin 85 mg/m², mean dose-adjusted area under the plasma concentration-time curve (AUC) of unbound platinum increased by 40 or 95% in patients with mild (creatinine clearance of 50–80 mL/minute) or moderate (creatinine clearance of 30–49 mL/minute) renal impairment, respectively, compared with patients with normal renal function. Mean dose-adjusted peak plasma concentration of unbound platinum appeared to be similar in patients with mild or moderate renal impairment compared with those with normal renal function. Following administration of oxaliplatin 65 mg/m² in patients with severe renal impairment (creatinine clearance less than 30 mL/minute), mean dose-adjusted AUC and peak plasma concentration of unbound platinum increased by 342 or 38%, respectively, compared with patients with normal renal function receiving oxaliplatin 85 mg/m²; dosage adjustment is recommended in patients with severe renal impairment.

• Common Adverse Effects

Adverse effects reported in 20% or more of patients receiving the oxaliplatin/fluorouracil/leucovorin regimen as adjuvant therapy for colon cancer and at an incidence that is at least 5% higher than that reported with fluorouracil/leucovorin alone include peripheral sensory neuropathy, nausea, vomiting, diarrhea, fatigue, anorexia, and pyrexia. Laboratory abnormalities reported in 20% or more of patients receiving the oxaliplatin/fluorouracil/leucovorin regimen and at an incidence that is at least 5% higher than that reported with fluorouracil/leucovorin alone include neutropenia, thrombocytopenia, anemia, elevated aminotransferase concentrations, and elevated alkaline phosphatase concentrations.

Adverse effects reported in 20% or more of patients receiving the oxaliplatin/fluorouracil/leucovorin regimen for previously untreated advanced colorectal cancer include adverse neurologic effects (i.e., neuropathy, including paresthesia, pharyngo-laryngeal dysesthesias), adverse GI effects (i.e., nausea, diarrhea, vomiting, stomatitis, anorexia, constipation, abdominal pain), fatigue, cough, and alopecia. Laboratory abnormalities reported in 20% or more of patients receiving the oxaliplatin/fluorouracil/leucovorin regimen include leukopenia, neutropenia, thrombocytopenia, and anemia.

Adverse effects reported in 20% or more of patients receiving the oxaliplatin/fluorouracil/leucovorin regimen for previously treated advanced colorectal cancer include adverse neurologic effects (i.e., neuropathy, including acute or persistent neuropathy), adverse GI effects (nausea, vomiting, diarrhea, stomatitis, abdominal pain, anorexia), fatigue, pyrexia, dyspnea, and constipation. Laboratory abnormalities reported in 20% or more of patients receiving the oxaliplatin/fluorouracil/leucovorin regimen include anemia, leukopenia, neutropenia, thrombocytopenia, and elevated aminotransferase concentrations.

DRUG INTERACTIONS

• Anticoagulants

Prolongation of prothrombin time and international normalized ratio (INR), occasionally associated with hemorrhage, has been reported in patients receiving oxaliplatin/fluorouracil/leucovorin therapy concomitantly with anticoagulant therapy. More frequent monitoring is required for patients receiving oxaliplatin/fluorouracil/leucovorin therapy concomitantly with oral anticoagulants (e.g., warfarin).

• Fluorouracil

Pharmacokinetic interaction unlikely when recommended dosages and administration schedule (see Dosage and Administration) are used. Potential pharmacokinetic interaction (20% increase in plasma fluorouracil concentrations) during concomitant use of fluorouracil and 130 mg/m^2 of oxaliplatin at intervals of 3 weeks.

● Other Antineoplastic Agents

Pharmacokinetic interaction with irinotecan or topotecan unlikely.

● Nephrotoxic Drugs

Potential pharmacokinetic interaction (decreased clearance of platinum-containing compounds); however, this interaction has not been specifically studied. The manufacturer states that concomitant use of oxaliplatin with other nephrotoxic drugs should be avoided.

● Protein-bound Drugs

In vitro data indicate that erythromycin, granisetron, paclitaxel, salicylates, and valproate sodium are unlikely to displace platinum from plasma proteins.

● Drugs Affecting Hepatic Microsomal Enzymes

Pharmacokinetic interaction with drugs metabolized by cytochrome P-450 (CYP) isoenzymes or those that induce or inhibit these isoenzymes unlikely. However, no studies have been conducted.

● Drugs that Prolong the QT Interval

Because oxaliplatin has been associated with QT-interval prolongation and ventricular arrhythmias, the manufacturer states that concomitant use of oxaliplatin with other drugs known to prolong the QT interval should be avoided. (See Cardiac Effects under Warnings/Precautions: Other Warnings and Precautions, in Cautions.)

PHARMACOKINETICS

Undergoes rapid and extensive nonenzymatic biotransformation to numerous platinum-containing transient reactive intermediates. Pharmacokinetic parameters generally expressed in terms of platinum-containing complexes rather than parent compound.

● Distribution

Extent

Following a 2-hour IV infusion, 85% of administered platinum is rapidly distributed into tissues or eliminated in urine; approximately 15% of administered platinum is present in systemic circulation.

No evidence of accumulation in plasma following usual dosage; possible progressive accumulation in erythrocytes.

Not known whether oxaliplatin or its metabolites are distributed into milk.

Plasma Protein Binding

>90% irreversibly bound to plasma proteins (principally albumin and γ-globulins).

● Elimination

Metabolism

Undergoes rapid and extensive nonenzymatic biotransformation; no evidence of CYP-mediated metabolism in vitro.

Elimination Route

Eliminated principally by renal excretion; renal clearance of ultrafilterable platinum appears to be directly proportional to GFR.

Following 2-hour IV infusion, approximately 54 or 2% of platinum-containing derivatives is excreted in urine and feces, respectively, within 5 days.

Half-life

Distribution and elimination of platinum-containing derivatives appears to be triphasic, with 2 relatively short distribution phases with half-lives of approximately 0.43 and 16.8 hours, respectively, and a long elimination phase with a half-life of approximately 392 hours.

DESCRIPTION

Oxaliplatin is a platinum-containing antineoplastic agent. The drug is an organoplatinum complex, consisting of a platinum atom complexed with 1,2-diaminocyclohexane (DACH) and a labile oxalate ligand. Oxaliplatin must undergo nonenzymatic activation before antineoplastic activity occurs. In physiologic solutions, the labile oxalate ligand of oxaliplatin presumably is displaced, forming several transient reactive complexes (e.g., monoaquo DACH platinum, diaquo DACH platinum) that covalently bind to specific DNA base sequences, producing intrastrand and interstrand DNA cross-links. Cross-links between specific DNA base sequences (i.e., adjacent guanine residues, adjacent adenine and guanine residues, guanine residues separated by an intervening nucleotide) produced by transient reactive intermediates of oxaliplatin are thought to inhibit DNA replication and transcription. Some evidence indicates that the presence of the bulky DACH carrier ligand of oxaliplatin may contribute to a greater degree of inhibition of DNA synthesis and cytotoxicity compared with that observed with cisplatin and may result in the lack of cross-resistance between oxaliplatin and cisplatin. Oxaliplatin is cycle-phase nonspecific.

Oxaliplatin has been shown to exhibit antitumor activity against colon carcinoma in vivo. Synergistic antiproliferative activity of oxaliplatin and fluorouracil has been demonstrated in vitro and in vivo in several tumor models (i.e., HT29 [colon], GR [mammary], L1210 [leukemia]).

Because oxaliplatin undergoes rapid and extensive nonenzymatic biotransformation to numerous platinum-containing transient reactive intermediates, pharmacokinetic parameters of the drug generally are expressed in terms of platinum-containing complexes rather than the parent compound. Following a 2-hour IV infusion of oxaliplatin, approximately 15% of the administered platinum is present in the systemic circulation while the remaining 85% is rapidly distributed into tissues or eliminated in urine. A fraction of the platinum-containing complexes distributed into peripheral tissues is irreversibly bound to and accumulates (approximately twofold) in erythrocytes, where the complexes appear to have no relevant activity. Approximately 90% of the platinum in the systemic circulation is irreversibly bound to plasma proteins, principally albumin and gamma globulins. It is thought that antineoplastic activity of oxaliplatin resides only in platinum-containing species present in the ultrafilterable plasma fraction (biotransformed, nonprotein-bound species); however, the pharmacodynamic relationship between platinum ultrafiltrate concentrations and safety or efficacy of oxaliplatin has not been established. There is no evidence that platinum accumulates in plasma following administration of 85 mg/m^2 dosages of oxaliplatin once every 2 weeks; however, a progressive accumulation of platinum in erythrocytes has been reported.

Oxaliplatin undergoes rapid and extensive nonenzymatic biotransformation; there is no evidence of cytochrome P-450 (CYP)-mediated metabolism in vitro. As many as 17 platinum-containing derivatives, including several cytotoxic species (e.g., monochloro DACH platinum, dichloro DACH platinum, monoaquo DACH platinum, diaquo DACH platinum) and various noncytotoxic species, have been isolated from plasma ultrafiltrate samples from patients receiving oxaliplatin. Distribution of platinum-containing derivatives appears to be triphasic, with the half-lives of the first, second, and third phases averaging approximately 0.43, 16.8, and 391 hours, respectively. Platinum-containing derivatives are eliminated principally by renal excretion; renal clearance of ultrafilterable platinum appears to be directly proportional to glomerular filtration rate (GFR). Following administration of a single 2-hour IV infusion of oxaliplatin, approximately 54 or 2% of platinum-containing derivatives is excreted in urine and feces, respectively, within 5 days.

ADVICE TO PATIENTS

Risk of hypersensitivity reactions. Importance of seeking immediate medical attention if signs of severe hypersensitivity reaction (e.g., chest tightness, shortness of breath, wheezing, dizziness, faintness, angioedema) occur.

Risk of neuropathy. Importance of understanding that symptoms of acute sensory neuropathy may be precipitated or exacerbated by exposure to cold temperature or cold objects; importance of avoiding cold drinks or use of ice and of covering exposed skin prior to exposure to cold temperature or cold objects. Importance of reading manufacturer's patient information for further instructions to minimize exposure to cold temperature or cold objects.

Risk of anemia, leukopenia, neutropenia, and thrombocytopenia; importance of informing a clinician immediately if bleeding, fever (particularly if associated with persistent diarrhea), or evidence of infection develops.

Risk of posterior reversible encephalopathy syndrome and visual abnormalities (e.g., transient vision loss); such effects may affect ability to drive or operate machinery.

Risk of pulmonary toxicity. Importance of promptly informing clinician of any persistent or recurrent respiratory symptoms (e.g., nonproductive cough, dyspnea).

Risk of hepatotoxicity. Importance of informing clinician if symptoms of hepatotoxicity occur.

Risk of QT-interval prolongation. Importance of informing clinician if symptoms of QT-interval prolongation (e.g., syncope) occur.

Risk of rhabdomyolysis. Importance of promptly informing clinician if new or worsening signs or symptoms of rhabdomyolysis (e.g., dark urine, anuria, urinary retention) occur.

Risk of persistent vomiting, diarrhea, or signs of dehydration.

Risk of fetal harm. Necessity of advising women of reproductive potential that they should use effective contraceptive methods while receiving the drug and for 9 months after the last dose of the drug. Importance of advising men who are partners with women of reproductive potential to use effective methods of contraception while receiving the drug and for 6 months after the last dose of the drug. Importance of patients informing their clinicians if they are pregnant or think they may be pregnant. If pregnancy occurs, advise patient of potential risk to fetus.

Importance of advising women to avoid breast-feeding while receiving oxaliplatin therapy and for 3 months after the last dose of the drug.

Risk of impaired male and female fertility.

Importance of informing clinicians of existing or contemplated concomitant therapy, including prescription and OTC drugs, as well as concomitant illness. (See Cautions.)

Importance of informing patients of other important precautionary information. (See Cautions.)

For further information on the handling of antineoplastic agents, see the ASHP Guidelines on Handling Hazardous Drugs at http://www.ahfsdrug information.com.

PREPARATIONS

Excipients in commercially available drug preparations may have clinically important effects in some individuals; consult specific product labeling for details.

Oxaliplatin

Parenteral		
For injection, for IV infusion	50 mg*	Oxaliplatin
	100 mg*	Oxaliplatin
For injection concentrate, for IV infusion	5 mg/mL (50 and 100 mg)	Eloxatin®, Sanofi-Aventis
	5 mg/mL (50, 100, and 200 mg)*	Oxaliplatin

† Use is not currently included in the labeling approved by the US Food and Drug Administration.

* available from one or more manufacturer, distributor, and/or repackager by generic (nonproprietary) name

Selected Revisions October 24, 2022, © Copyright, November 01, 2002, American Society of Health-System Pharmacists, Inc.

PACLitaxel

10:00 • ANTINEOPLASTIC AGENTS

■ Paclitaxel is a natural or semisynthetic diterpene antineoplastic agent extracted from the bark of the Western (Pacific) yew (*Taxus brevifolia*) or the needles and twigs of *Taxus baccata*.

USES

Paclitaxel is commercially available in 2 types of formulations: conventional paclitaxel (in a nonaqueous solution) and albumin-bound paclitaxel. The efficacy and safety of paclitaxel for each indication is based on research and clinical experience using a specific formulation. Albumin-bound paclitaxel currently is labeled for use only in the second-line therapy of metastatic breast cancer, first-line therapy of non-small cell lung cancer in combination with carboplatin, and first-line therapy of metastatic adenocarcinoma of the pancreas in combination with gemcitabine. The functional properties of paclitaxel may differ substantially according to formulation; therefore, albumin-bound paclitaxel may *not* be substituted for or used in combination with other formulations of paclitaxel.

● Ovarian Cancer

Paclitaxel is used alone or in combination therapy for the treatment of ovarian cancer.

Adjuvant Therapy for Early-stage Ovarian Epithelial Cancer

The use of platinum-based therapy, such as carboplatin and paclitaxel, is being investigated for adjuvant treatment following surgery in poor-prognosis early-stage ovarian epithelial cancer†. (See Uses: Ovarian Cancer: Adjuvant Therapy for Early-stage Ovarian Epithelial Cancer in Carboplatin 10:00.)

First-line Therapy for Advanced Ovarian Epithelial Cancer

A platinum-containing agent in combination with paclitaxel is a preferred regimen for the initial treatment of advanced ovarian epithelial cancer.

Carboplatin Versus Cisplatin

Randomized trials have demonstrated that carboplatin is as effective as but less toxic than cisplatin when used in combination with paclitaxel for the initial treatment of advanced ovarian cancer. Carboplatin in combination with paclitaxel† currently is a preferred regimen for the initial treatment of advanced ovarian epithelial cancer. (See Uses: Ovarian Cancer: First-line Therapy for Advanced Ovarian Epithelial Cancer in Carboplatin 10:00.)

Platinum-containing Agent With Paclitaxel Versus Platinum-containing Agent With Cyclophosphamide

Evidence from randomized trials indicates that combined paclitaxel and cisplatin therapy is superior to combined cyclophosphamide and cisplatin therapy for the initial treatment of advanced epithelial ovarian cancer.

The current indication for the use of paclitaxel in combination with cisplatin for the initial treatment of advanced ovarian epithelial cancer is based principally on a comparative study in which 410 patients (386 evaluable patients) with suboptimally debulked (greater than 1 cm residual tumor mass) stage III or IV ovarian cancer who had no prior chemotherapy were randomized to receive paclitaxel 135 mg/m² (administered by 24-hour IV infusion) with cisplatin 75 mg/m² versus cyclophosphamide 750 mg/m² with cisplatin 75 mg/m². Among 216 evaluable patients with measurable disease, those receiving paclitaxel and cisplatin had an overall objective response of 73% (51% complete responses, 22% partial responses) compared with 60% (31% complete responses, 29% partial responses) for those receiving cisplatin and cyclophosphamide; the higher response rate for the combination of paclitaxel and cisplatin was maintained according to intention-to-treat analysis of 240 women with measurable disease (62 versus 48%). Patients receiving paclitaxel and cisplatin also had a longer median time to progression (evaluable patients: 18 versus 13 months; intention-to-treat analysis: 16.6 versus 13 months) and increased median overall survival (evaluable patients: 38 versus 24 months; intention-to-treat analysis: 35.5 versus 24.2 months) than those receiving cyclophosphamide and cisplatin. Higher frequencies of severe neutropenia (81 versus 58%), alopecia (55 versus 37%), asthenia (17 versus 10%), diarrhea (16 versus 8%), febrile neutropenia (15 versus 4%), myalgia/arthralgia (9 versus 2%), and hypersensitivity reactions (8 versus 1%) were observed in patients receiving paclitaxel and cisplatin compared with those receiving cyclophosphamide and cisplatin.

In a confirmatory randomized trial involving 680 patients with advanced ovarian cancer, longer median survival (35.6 versus 25.9 months), longer median time to progression (15.3 versus 11.5 months), and higher response rates (59 versus 45%) were observed for combination therapy with paclitaxel (175 mg/m² administered as a 3-hour IV infusion) and cisplatin versus cyclophosphamide and cisplatin. Limited evidence from subset analysis suggests that the same patterns were observed in patients with non-optimally debulked disease. Higher frequencies of neurotoxicity (87 versus 52%, severe in 21 versus 2%), myalgia/arthralgia (60 versus 27%), and diarrhea (37 versus 29%) were observed in patients receiving paclitaxel and cisplatin compared with those receiving cyclophosphamide and cisplatin.

At a follow-up of 6.5 years, the survival benefit associated with the paclitaxel and cisplatin regimen in both randomized trials has been maintained.

Combination therapy with paclitaxel and cisplatin is preferable to either high-dose cisplatin or paclitaxel alone for the initial treatment of advanced ovarian cancer.

Intraperitoneal Cisplatin and Paclitaxel

Combined IV and intraperitoneal therapy with IV paclitaxel, intraperitoneal cisplatin, and intraperitoneal paclitaxel† has been used for the treatment of optimally debulked stage III epithelial ovarian cancer.

The National Cancer Institute (NCI) recommends use of a combined IV and intraperitoneal regimen for eligible patients with advanced epithelial ovarian cancer because of a substantial survival benefit. Based on clinical trials, NCI recommends that use of a regimen containing intraperitoneal cisplatin (100 mg/m²) and a taxane (either IV only or IV plus intraperitoneal) should be strongly considered following primary surgery in patients with optimally debulked stage III epithelial ovarian cancer. Although an optimal intraperitoneal chemotherapy regimen has not been established, favorable results were observed following sequential administration of IV paclitaxel, intraperitoneal cisplatin, and intraperitoneal paclitaxel in the Gynecologic Oncology Group (GOG)-172 study.

In this randomized, phase 3 trial (GOG-172), 429 patients with previously untreated stage III epithelial ovarian cancer or primary peritoneal cancer, with no residual mass exceeding 1 cm in diameter following surgery, received either combined IV and intraperitoneal therapy or IV therapy. All patients enrolled in this study had good baseline GOG performance status (0–2) and adequate bone marrow, renal, and hepatic function. Most patients (88%) had ovarian cancer, and serous adenocarcinoma was the most common histologic type (79% of patients). The primary end points of the study were progression-free survival and overall survival. Combined IV and intraperitoneal therapy consisted of IV paclitaxel 135 mg/m² by 24-hour infusion on day 1, followed by intraperitoneal cisplatin 100 mg/m² on day 2 and intraperitoneal paclitaxel 60 mg/m² on day 8. IV therapy consisted of IV paclitaxel 135 mg/m² by 24-hour infusion on day 1 followed by IV cisplatin 75 mg/m² on day 2. Both regimens were repeated every 21 days for up to 6 cycles. Patients who received combined IV and intraperitoneal therapy had longer median progression-free (23.8 versus 18.3 months) and overall (65.6 versus 49.7 months) survival compared with patients who received IV therapy.

Most (83%) of the patients receiving IV therapy completed 6 cycles of their assigned chemotherapy regimen; however, only 42% of patients receiving combined IV and intraperitoneal therapy completed 6 cycles of assigned chemotherapy; patients who could not complete the intraperitoneal regimen received IV therapy for the remaining treatment cycles. The most common reason for discontinuance of intraperitoneal therapy was catheter-related complications. Grade 3 or 4 leukopenia (76 versus 64%), GI effects (46 versus 24%), metabolic effects (27 versus 7%), fatigue (18 versus 4%), neurologic effects (19 versus 9%), infection (16 versus 6%), thrombocytopenia (12 versus 4%), and pain (11 versus 1%) occurred more frequently in patients receiving combined IV and intraperitoneal therapy than in those receiving IV therapy. Although patients receiving combined IV and intraperitoneal therapy reported less improvement in abdominal discomfort before cycle 4, improvement in abdominal discomfort was similar in both treatment groups 1 year after completion of therapy. Among patients who received combined IV and intraperitoneal therapy, quality of life was worse during and shortly after completion of therapy (before cycle 4 and at 3–6 weeks following therapy) compared with those who received IV therapy. Quality of life scores were similar for the groups at 1 year after completion of treatment, except for greater persistence of moderate paresthesias in patients receiving combined IV and intraperitoneal therapy.

Retrospective review of baseline data (patient and disease characteristics) from two phase 3 clinical trials (including GOG-172) for patients receiving intraperitoneal therapy for optimally debulked stage III epithelial ovarian cancer suggested that extent of residual tumor mass, histology, and age were important predictors of survival in such patients. Patients with clear cell histology appeared to derive less benefit from intraperitoneal therapy compared with those with serous histology (hazard ratio for progression-free and overall survival of 2.66 and 3.88, respectively). In addition, each additional year of age was associated with a 1% increase in the risk of death. Although patients enrolled in the studies had optimally debulked (1 cm or less residual tumor mass) disease, survival was greater in patients with only microscopic residual disease.

Retrospective analysis of data from patients receiving a modified IV and intraperitoneal regimen suggests that a reduced dosage of intraperitoneal cisplatin administered in conjunction with a shortened IV paclitaxel infusion time may result in less toxicity and produce a survival benefit similar to that reported in the GOG-172 study (67 months versus 65.6 months reported in GOG-172). The modified IV and intraperitoneal regimen consisted of IV paclitaxel 135 mg/m^2 by 3-hour infusion on day 1, followed by intraperitoneal cisplatin 75 mg/m^2 on day 2 and intraperitoneal paclitaxel 60 mg/m^2 on day 8 of each 21-day cycle. Most patients (80%) completed 4 or more cycles of therapy and 55% completed 6 cycles. The frequency of grade 3 or 4 neutropenia (12%), GI effects (8%), metabolic effects (5%), neurologic effects (6%), infection (2%), fatigue (2%), and thrombocytopenia (0%) in this series of patients receiving the modified IV and intraperitoneal regimen appeared to be lower than toxicity rates reported in the GOG-172 study. By shortening the infusion time for IV paclitaxel to 3 hours, the modified regimen also may provide an outpatient alternative to inpatient administration over 24 hours. However, randomized controlled trials are needed to establish comparative safety and efficacy of this modified regimen. The modified IV and intraperitoneal schedule containing the lower intraperitoneal cisplatin dosage and the 3-hour IV paclitaxel infusion also has been studied in conjunction with a third cytotoxic drug, but with evidence of excessive toxicity.

Based on current evidence, combined IV and intraperitoneal therapy with IV paclitaxel, intraperitoneal cisplatin, and intraperitoneal paclitaxel is recommended (accepted) for use as initial adjuvant treatment of optimally debulked stage III epithelial ovarian cancer in patients with good performance status (GOG performance status of 0–2).

Second-line Therapy for Advanced Ovarian Epithelial Cancer

Paclitaxel is used alone or in combination therapy as second-line or subsequent therapy in patients with advanced ovarian epithelial cancer.

Paclitaxel is used alone as second-line or subsequent therapy in patients with advanced ovarian epithelial cancer. In the treatment of advanced ovarian cancer refractory to prior chemotherapy, paclitaxel alone produces an objective response in about 35% (range: 16–48%) of patients. Patients whose cancer is resistant to platinum-containing therapy (defined as tumor progression while on platinum-containing therapy or tumor relapse within 6 months after completion of a platinum-containing regimen) who then receive paclitaxel therapy reportedly have had response rates of 14–35%.

The current indication of paclitaxel monotherapy for recurrent or refractory ovarian cancer was initially based on data from 5 phase I and II clinical studies involving 189 patients, a multicenter randomized phase III study involving 407 patients, and interim analysis of experience from an additional 300 patients who received the drug under a treatment IND protocol. According to the manufacturer, patients in 2 of the phase II clinical studies receiving an initial dose of paclitaxel of 135–170 mg/m^2 administered by 24-hour IV infusion had objective response rates (complete or partial responses) of 22% and 30%. The median duration of overall response in these 2 studies was about 7 months, and the median survival was 8.1 and 15.9 months. Similar responses were observed in other clinical studies using higher initial doses of paclitaxel or concomitant administration of paclitaxel and filgrastim, a recombinant human granulocyte colony-stimulating factor (G-CSF).

The response rates observed in these phase II studies were confirmed in a large case series in which 1000 patients with platinum-refractory ovarian cancer who received paclitaxel 135 mg/m^2 administered by 24-hour IV infusion had an overall objective response rate of 22%. According to the manufacturer, patients in a phase

III study with a bifactorial design receiving paclitaxel 135 or 175 mg/m^2 as a 3- or 24-hour IV infusion had an overall objective response rate of 16.2% with 6 complete responses and 60 partial responses. The duration of response measured from the first day of treatment was 8.3 months (range: 3.2–21.6 months). Median time to disease progression was 3.7 months (range: 0.1 to longer than 25 months), and median survival was 11.5 months (range: 0.2 to longer than 26 months).

Response rates did not differ significantly according to dose or infusion schedule. Patients receiving a paclitaxel dose of either 175 or 135 mg/m^2 had objective (partial or complete) response rates of 20 or 15%, respectively. Patients receiving paclitaxel doses by either 3- or 24-hour IV infusion had objective (partial or complete) response rates of 16 or 19%, respectively. Median time to disease progression was longer in patients receiving 175 mg/m^2 than in those receiving 135 mg/m^2 (4.2 versus 3.1 months) and similar in patients receiving paclitaxel by 3-hour IV infusion or 24-hour IV infusion (4 versus 3.7 months). No difference in survival was observed according to dose or infusion schedule. Median survival was 11.6 or 11 months in patients receiving paclitaxel 175 or 135 mg/m^2, respectively, and 11.7 or 11.2 months in patients receiving paclitaxel by 3- or 24-hour infusion, respectively. Although severity of myelosuppression was affected by dose, the most important factor was duration of infusion; the same paclitaxel doses administered by 24-hour IV infusion were more myelotoxic than those administered by 3-hour IV infusion. The results of this randomized study support the use of paclitaxel doses of 135 or 175 mg/m^2 administered by 3-hour IV infusion, but the power of the study was inadequate to determine whether a particular dosage schedule for paclitaxel produced superior efficacy.

Paclitaxel also has been used in combination therapy with a platinum agent (carboplatin or cisplatin) as second-line or subsequent therapy† for advanced ovarian epithelial cancer. Analysis of combined data for 802 patients involved in parallel randomized, multicenter trials indicates that median survival and median progression-free survival are prolonged in patients receiving combination therapy with paclitaxel and a platinum agent (a regimen of paclitaxel and carboplatin in 80% of patients) rather than platinum-based therapy alone (a regimen of carboplatin alone in 71% of patients) for the treatment of relapsed platinum-sensitive ovarian cancer.

Dosage and Other Considerations

Response rates for paclitaxel therapy vary with tumor histology, volume of residual tumor, and development of resistance to previous platinum-based chemotherapy.

Current evidence suggests that increased dose intensity (amount of paclitaxel per unit time) may affect response to paclitaxel but that paclitaxel doses exceeding 175 mg/m^2 are more toxic and do not improve survival in patients with advanced ovarian cancer. In addition to dose effect, the effect of duration of infusion of paclitaxel has been studied in patients with ovarian cancer. Efficacy was similar but toxicity, particularly myelosuppression, was greater when paclitaxel alone was administered by 24-hour versus 3-hour infusion for the subsequent therapy of advanced ovarian cancer. Limited evidence suggests that subsequent therapy with prolonged infusion of paclitaxel (96-hour IV infusion) does not produce response in patients with advanced ovarian cancer that was resistant to previous therapy with the drug administered by 3-hour or 24-hour IV infusion.

The effect of duration of infusion on the efficacy and toxicity of paclitaxel administered as a component of combination therapy also has not been fully established. Increased incidence and severity of neurotoxicity is associated with administration of paclitaxel by 3-hour IV infusion in combination therapy with cisplatin in patients with gynecologic cancers. In a large randomized trial, patients with advanced ovarian cancer receiving paclitaxel (175 mg/m^2 administered as a 3-hour IV infusion) and cisplatin had an increased incidence of severe neurosensory toxicity compared with those receiving cyclophosphamide and cisplatin. Prolonged paclitaxel infusions do not appear to offer benefit in the treatment of ovarian cancer. In a randomized trial comparing 96-hour infusion of paclitaxel 120 mg/m^2 with 24-hour infusion of paclitaxel 135 mg/m^2 (each in a combination regimen of paclitaxel and cisplatin) for suboptimal stage III or IV ovarian epithelial cancer, median survival rates were similar between the groups but the relative death rate was approximately 5% greater among patients receiving the prolonged infusion of paclitaxel.

Maintenance therapy with paclitaxel for advanced ovarian cancer† is being investigated. In a randomized trial, patients receiving 12 months of single-agent paclitaxel therapy following complete response to induction therapy with platinum/paclitaxel therapy for advanced ovarian cancer experienced longer progression-free survival but greater neurotoxicity than those receiving 3 months of such therapy. Because the trial was terminated according to study design following a planned interim analysis that detected the difference in progression-free survival, and cross-over treatment was allowed, overall survival data may be unavailable. Whether maintenance therapy with paclitaxel is superior to treatment upon progression of disease is unclear, and a confirmatory randomized trial is needed. Until further evidence is available, clinicians should discuss maintenance paclitaxel therapy and offer it as an option for patients with advanced ovarian cancer that has a complete response to induction therapy.

● Breast Cancer

Adjuvant Therapy for Breast Cancer

Adjuvant Therapy for Node-positive Breast Cancer

Paclitaxel is administered sequentially to standard doxorubicin-containing combination chemotherapy as adjuvant therapy for node-positive breast cancer, particularly in patients with hormone receptor-negative disease.

The current indication for paclitaxel as adjuvant therapy is based on data from a multicenter, randomized trial involving 3170 patients with node-positive breast cancer. Following completion of 4 courses of doxorubicin and cyclophosphamide (AC), patients received paclitaxel (175 mg/m^2 as a 3-hour IV infusion once every 3 weeks for 4 courses) or no additional chemotherapy. Patients with hormone receptor-positive disease were assigned to receive tamoxifen, and patients who had received segmental mastectomies were assigned to receive radiation therapy following recovery from treatment-related toxicity. At a median follow-up of 30.1 months, patients receiving AC followed by adjuvant therapy with paclitaxel had a 22% reduction in the risk of disease recurrence and a 26% reduction in the risk of death compared with patients receiving AC alone. Subset analysis according to number of positive nodes, tumor size, menopausal status, and hormone receptor status suggests a similar effect of adjuvant paclitaxel on disease-free or overall survival in all of the larger subsets except for patients with hormone receptor-positive tumors, who experienced a smaller reduction in risk for disease recurrence or death.

The study was also designed to assess the efficacy and toxicity of 3 dose levels of doxorubicin (60, 75, or 90 mg/m^2). No effect on disease-free or overall survival was observed for doxorubicin doses exceeding 60 mg/m^2; higher incidences of severe hematologic toxicities (including severe thrombocytopenia and platelet transfusions), infections, mucositis, and cardiovascular events were observed for higher doses of doxorubicin. Higher frequencies of severe (grade 3 or 4) toxicity, including neurosensory toxicity, myalgia/arthralgia, neurologic pain (5 versus 1%), flu-like symptoms (5 versus 3%), and hyperglycemia (3 versus 1%), were observed in patients receiving AC followed by paclitaxel compared with those receiving AC alone. Two deaths (0.1%) were attributed to treatment with adjuvant paclitaxel.

In another randomized trial, involving 3060 patients with node-positive breast cancer, disease-free survival was longer in patients receiving paclitaxel (versus no additional therapy) following postoperative chemotherapy with doxorubicin and cyclophosphamide.

Differing dosage schedules are being investigated for the use of paclitaxel as adjuvant therapy for node-positive breast cancer (e.g., increased dose density, concurrent versus sequential administration of doxorubicin and cyclophosphamide with paclitaxel). In a randomized trial, increased dose density of the doxorubicin, cyclophosphamide, and paclitaxel regimen with treatment every 2 weeks rather than every 3 weeks was associated with prolonged disease-free and overall survival, but no effect was observed for concurrent administration (doxorubicin/cyclophosphamide followed by paclitaxel) versus sequential administration (doxorubicin followed by paclitaxel and then cyclophosphamide). Further follow-up of this study and a confirmatory trial are needed to establish the effect of dose densification for this regimen.

Adjuvant Therapy for Early-stage HER2-positive Breast Cancer

Paclitaxel-containing adjuvant therapy is used in conjunction with trastuzumab for the treatment of operable HER2-positive breast cancer†. In several large randomized trials, the addition of trastuzumab to standard adjuvant chemotherapy in patients with operable HER2-positive breast cancer reduced the risk of death and/or prolonged disease-free survival. See Adjuvant Therapy for Early-stage Breast Cancer under Uses: Breast Cancer, in Trastuzumab 10:00.

First-line Therapy for Advanced Breast Cancer

Paclitaxel and Gemcitabine

Paclitaxel is used in combination with gemcitabine for the initial treatment of metastatic breast cancer following failure of adjuvant chemotherapy; prior therapy in

such patients should have included an anthracycline antineoplastic agent (e.g., doxorubicin) unless clinically contraindicated.

The current indication for combination therapy with paclitaxel and gemcitabine for the first-line treatment of metastatic breast cancer is based on data from a randomized, multinational, phase III trial involving 529 patients who had prior adjuvant or neoadjuvant anthracycline therapy unless clinically contraindicated. Patients were randomized to receive either combination therapy with paclitaxel and gemcitabine (paclitaxel 175 mg/m^2 by 3-hour IV infusion followed by gemcitabine 1250 mg/m^2 by 30-minute IV infusion on day 1 and then the same dosage of gemcitabine on day 8) or paclitaxel alone (paclitaxel 175 mg/m^2 by 3-hour IV infusion on day 1) in 21-day cycles. Longer median time to disease progression (5.2 versus 2.9 months) and higher response rates (40.8 versus 22.1%) were observed in patients receiving paclitaxel and gemcitabine compared with those receiving paclitaxel monotherapy. In an interim analysis, a trend toward prolonged survival was noted among patients receiving combination therapy with paclitaxel and gemcitabine. Greater toxicity was reported in patients receiving combination therapy with paclitaxel and gemcitabine than in those receiving paclitaxel alone, including neutropenia (all: 69 versus 31%, severe: 48 versus 11%), anemia (69 versus 51%), thrombocytopenia (26 versus 7%), elevated serum ALT (SGPT) concentrations (18 versus 6%), and elevated serum AST (SGOT) concentrations (16 versus 5%).

Paclitaxel With or Without Doxorubicin

Paclitaxel has been used alone or in combination with doxorubicin as first-line chemotherapy for metastatic breast cancer†.

In a randomized trial with crossover, patients with metastatic breast cancer who had no previous chemotherapy with anthracyclines or taxanes received paclitaxel 200 mg/m^2 administered by 3-hour IV infusion or doxorubicin IV 75 mg/m^2 for 7 courses or until disease progression or unacceptable toxicity were observed; patients with disease progression were crossed over to therapy with the alternative agent. Although overall survival did not differ, lower response rates and shorter median progression-free survival were observed among patients receiving initial therapy with paclitaxel versus doxorubicin; arthralgia/myalgia and sensory neurotoxicity were associated with paclitaxel whereas mucositis, gastrointestinal toxicity, grade 4 neutropenia, febrile neutropenia, and cardiotoxicity were more frequently observed with doxorubicin.

In a randomized, phase III, multicenter trial, patients with metastatic breast cancer receiving first-line therapy with doxorubicin and paclitaxel had higher response rates, longer median time to progression, and longer median survival than those receiving cyclophosphamide, doxorubicin, and fluorouracil (CAF). Neutropenia (including grade 3 or 4 neutropenia), arthralgia/myalgia, peripheral neuropathy, and diarrhea occurred more frequently in patients receiving doxorubicin and paclitaxel, whereas nausea and vomiting was more common in those receiving CAF. In another randomized trial, similar response rates, median progression-free survival, and median survival were observed for patients receiving doxorubicin and paclitaxel versus doxorubicin and cyclophosphamide as first-line therapy for metastatic breast cancer.

Results from a phase III trial comparing a combination of paclitaxel and doxorubicin to either agent alone (with subsequent crossover to the alternative agent) as first-line therapy for metastatic breast cancer showed a higher overall response rate and longer time to treatment failure with the combination regimen; however, overall survival and quality of life were similar for combination therapy compared with either agent alone. Results from a randomized study comparing paclitaxel monotherapy to a standard combination chemotherapy regimen (CMFP [cyclophosphamide, methotrexate, fluorouracil, and prednisolone]) showed a similar objective response rate, time to progression, and overall survival duration with the 2 regimens.

The choice of single-agent or combination chemotherapy as first-line therapy for metastatic breast cancer may depend on the rate of disease progression, the presence of comorbid conditions, and clinician and patient preferences.

Paclitaxel and Trastuzumab for HER2-positive Metastatic Breast Cancer

Paclitaxel is used in combination with trastuzumab (Herceptin®, Genentech), a humanized anti-HER2 antibody, for the initial treatment of metastatic breast cancer in patients with tumors that overexpress the HER2 protein. (See First-line Therapy for Advanced Breast Cancer under Uses: Breast Cancer, in Trastuzumab 10:00.)

The current indication for combination therapy with paclitaxel and trastuzumab for the initial treatment of metastatic breast cancer is based on data from a randomized, controlled, multicenter trial involving 469 patients with 2+ or 3+ HER2-overexpressing breast tumors (based on a 0–3+ scale). Patients were randomized to receive chemotherapy alone or chemotherapy combined with trastuzumab (4 mg/kg IV loading dose followed by once-weekly doses of 2 mg/kg IV). Chemotherapy consisted of an anthracycline and cyclophosphamide unless patients had received prior adjuvant chemotherapy with an anthracycline, in which case chemotherapy consisted of paclitaxel 175 mg/m² administered by 3-hour IV infusion every 21 days for at least 6 cycles. Longer median time to disease progression (6.7 versus 2.5 months), higher overall response rate (38 versus 15%), and longer median duration of response (8.3 versus 4.3 months) were reported for combination therapy with paclitaxel and trastuzumab compared with paclitaxel alone in patients with metastatic breast cancer characterized by excess production of the HER2 protein.

Second-line Therapy for Advanced Breast Cancer
Conventional Paclitaxel

Paclitaxel is used as monotherapy for the treatment of breast cancer in patients who have metastatic disease refractory to conventional combination chemotherapy or who have experienced relapse within 6 months of adjuvant chemotherapy; prior therapy in such patients should have included an anthracycline antineoplastic agent (e.g., doxorubicin) unless clinically contraindicated.

The current indication for use of paclitaxel as a single agent in advanced breast cancer is based principally on data from a multicenter, randomized study involving 471 patients who were treated previously with 1 or 2 regimens of chemotherapy. For 454 evaluable patients in the study, overall response rate was 26%, median time to disease progression was 3.5 months, and median survival was 11.7 months. The median duration of response was 8.1 months. Patients receiving a paclitaxel dose of either 175 or 135 mg/m² administered as a 3-hour infusion had similar rates of objective (partial or complete) response of 28 or 22%, respectively. Median time to progression of disease was longer (4.2 versus 3 months) but median survival was similar (11.7 versus 10.5 months) for patients receiving paclitaxel doses of 175 or 135 mg/m², respectively.

In this randomized study, 60% of patients had symptomatic disease with impaired performance status at study entry and 73% had visceral metastases. Overall, 30% of these patients had disease that progressed following adjuvant chemotherapy, 39% had metastatic disease refractory to conventional chemotherapy, and 31% of patients had disease that progressed or failed to respond in both settings. Of the patients in this study, 67% had received an anthracycline antineoplastic agent and 23% had disease considered resistant to this class of agents.

Two uncontrolled phase II studies of paclitaxel therapy were conducted in a total of 53 patients with metastatic breast cancer who had been treated previously with a maximum of one regimen of antineoplastic therapy (including some patients who had received no prior chemotherapy). Treatment consisted of paclitaxel as a 24-hour IV infusion at initial doses of 250 mg/m² (with G-CSF support) or 200 mg/m², and overall objective response rates of 57 and 52% were observed. Dose reductions were required in patients who experienced severe hematologic (e.g., neutropenia) or nonhematologic (e.g., infection, neurotoxicity) toxicity; therefore, the median dose of paclitaxel per course was 203 mg/m² for both studies. Overall, response rates were not influenced by initial dose or dose intensity of paclitaxel or by concomitant administration of filgrastim.

In another phase II study of patients whose disease was refractory to at least 2 regimens of antineoplastic therapy, including anthracycline therapy, an overall response rate of 30% (partial response only) was observed with a paclitaxel dose of 200 mg/m² given as a 24-hour infusion with concomitant administration of filgrastim. In phase II studies that evaluated the use of a 3-hour infusion schedule, patients with metastatic breast cancer that was refractory to previous chemotherapy, including anthracyclines, who received paclitaxel doses of 175–225 mg/m² had overall response rates (partial or complete) of 18–38%.

The optimal dosage regimen of paclitaxel when used as single-agent therapy in patients with metastatic breast cancer has not been established. The effect of dose on the efficacy and toxicity of paclitaxel has been studied in patients with metastatic breast cancer. In patients with metastatic breast cancer receiving paclitaxel administered as a 3-hour IV infusion, paclitaxel doses exceeding 175 mg/m² are associated with greater toxicity, particularly hematologic and neurosensory toxicity, but do not appear to increase response rate or prolong survival. The use of a weekly schedule of paclitaxel to increase dose density is being investigated. In a phase II study, an overall response rate of 53% was observed in patients with metastatic breast cancer receiving paclitaxel 100 mg/m² administered once weekly until disease progression (median of 14 infusions per patient); this regimen was

notable for lack of myelosuppression although peripheral neuropathy prohibited dose escalation above paclitaxel 100 mg/m².

The effect of duration of infusion on the efficacy and toxicity of paclitaxel has been studied in patients with metastatic breast cancer. Evidence from a randomized trial indicates that response rate is higher in patients with advanced breast cancer receiving high-dose paclitaxel (250 mg/m²) by 24- versus 3-hour IV infusion but event-free survival and survival are similar; hematologic toxicity, including febrile neutropenia, occurs more frequently with the 24-hour infusion of paclitaxel whereas severe neurotoxicity is more common with the 3-hour infusion. No difference in response rate, duration of response, or survival was observed in patients with metastatic breast cancer receiving paclitaxel 140 mg/m² by 96-hour IV infusion or paclitaxel 250 mg/m² by 3-hour IV infusion.

Albumin-bound Paclitaxel

Albumin-bound paclitaxel is used as monotherapy for the treatment of breast cancer in patients who have metastatic disease refractory to conventional combination chemotherapy or who have experienced relapse within 6 months of adjuvant chemotherapy; prior therapy in such patients should have included an anthracycline antineoplastic agent (e.g., doxorubicin) unless clinically contraindicated.

The current indication for use of albumin-bound paclitaxel as a single agent in advanced breast cancer is based principally on data from 2 single-arm open-label studies and a randomized trial.

In a randomized trial involving 460 patients with metastatic breast cancer, patients received either albumin-bound paclitaxel 260 mg/m² by 30-minute IV infusion or paclitaxel 175 mg/m² by 3-hour IV infusion. Most patients in the study had visceral metastases, had received prior chemotherapy in the adjuvant and/or metastatic setting, and had received therapy with anthracyclines. Patients with metastatic breast cancer receiving albumin-bound paclitaxel had a higher rate of reconciled target lesion response (21.5%) than those receiving conventional paclitaxel (11.1%). The reconciled target lesion response rate was based on independent radiologic assessment of tumor response reconciled with the investigator assessment of response for the first 6 cycles of therapy. Compared with conventional paclitaxel, albumin-bound paclitaxel was associated with a lower incidence of grade 4 neutropenia (9 versus 22%) and hypersensitivity reactions (all: 4 versus 12%, severe: 0 versus 2%), but a higher frequency of sensory neuropathy (all: 71 versus 56%, severe: 10 versus 2%), asthenia (47 versus 39%), nausea (30 versus 22%), diarrhea (27 versus 15%), and vomiting (18 versus 10%).

Objective responses to albumin-bound paclitaxel were observed in 2 phase II studies in patients with metastatic breast cancer. In one study, patients received albumin-bound paclitaxel 300 mg/m² by 30-minute IV infusion once every 3 weeks. In the other study, patients received albumin-bound paclitaxel 175 mg/m² by 30-minute IV infusion once every 3 weeks.

● Non-small Cell Lung Cancer
Adjuvant Therapy

Platinum-containing therapy, such as paclitaxel and carboplatin, is used in selected patients for the adjuvant treatment of completely resected non-small cell lung cancer†. In a randomized trial, patients receiving 4 cycles of paclitaxel and carboplatin therapy following surgery for stage IB non-small cell lung cancer had a higher overall survival rate at 4 years (71%) than those in an observation group (59%). Analysis of pooled data abstracted from randomized trials suggests that adjuvant chemotherapy prolongs survival in patients with resected non-small cell lung cancer.

Therapy for Advanced Disease

Currently preferred regimens for the initial treatment of advanced non-small cell lung cancer in patients with good performance status include a platinum-containing agent in combination with another cytotoxic agent such as paclitaxel, docetaxel, gemcitabine, pemetrexed, or vinorelbine.

Although the primary objective of treatment in patients with advanced non-small cell lung carcinoma is palliation, small improvements in survival have been demonstrated with the use of platinum-based chemotherapy.

Conventional Paclitaxel and Carboplatin

Paclitaxel and carboplatin is used in the treatment of advanced non-small cell lung cancer†. Similar response rates and median survival were observed in a randomized trial in which patients received paclitaxel and carboplatin versus regimens of cisplatin in combination with paclitaxel, gemcitabine, or docetaxel for advanced non-small cell lung cancer. Paclitaxel and carboplatin (paclitaxel 225 mg/m² by 3-hour IV infusion on day 1 followed on the same day by carboplatin at the dose required to obtain an AUC of 6 mg/mL per minute) was less toxic than the other regimens and was selected as a reference regimen for further studies. However, another randomized trial showed a survival benefit in patients receiving cisplatin/paclitaxel rather than carboplatin/paclitaxel for advanced non-small cell lung cancer. In this study, paclitaxel 200 mg/m² by 3-hour IV infusion was administered with either cisplatin 80 mg/m² or carboplatin at the dose required to obtain an AUC of 6 mg/mL per minute. In another randomized trial, response rates, median survival, and 1- and 2-year survival rates were similar in patients receiving either paclitaxel/carboplatin or vinorelbine/cisplatin for advanced non-small cell lung cancer; grade 3 peripheral neuropathy occurred more frequently in patients receiving paclitaxel and carboplatin whereas grade 3 or 4 leukopenia and grade 3 nausea and vomiting were more frequent in patients receiving vinorelbine and cisplatin. Further study is needed to clarify the comparative efficacy of carboplatin and cisplatin in the treatment of non-small cell lung cancer.

Weekly schedules of paclitaxel and carboplatin for the treatment of advanced non-small cell lung cancer are being investigated.

Conventional Paclitaxel and Cisplatin

Paclitaxel and cisplatin is used in the treatment of advanced non-small cell lung cancer. Combination chemotherapy with paclitaxel and cisplatin is associated with higher response rates and similar survival compared with other cisplatin-containing regimens (e.g., cisplatin with etoposide, cisplatin with teniposide).

The current indication for the use of paclitaxel in combination with cisplatin for the initial treatment of advanced non-small cell lung cancer is based on a comparative study in which 599 patients with stage IIIB or IV non-small cell lung cancer who had not received previous chemotherapy were randomized to receive paclitaxel at a dose of 135 or 250 mg/m² administered by 24-hour IV infusion followed by IV cisplatin 75 mg/m² versus IV cisplatin 75/mg/m² with IV etoposide 100 mg/m². Patients receiving the higher dose of paclitaxel received concomitant administration of granulocyte colony-stimulating factor [G-CSF]). Patients receiving paclitaxel (135 or 250 mg/m²) combined with cisplatin had higher response rates (25 or 23%, respectively, versus 12%) but similar median survival (9.3 or 10 months, respectively, versus 7.4 months) compared with those receiving combination therapy with etoposide and cisplatin. Longer time to progression of disease was observed in patients receiving the higher dose of paclitaxel combined with cisplatin compared with etoposide and cisplatin (4.9 versus 2.7 months). Quality of life assessed by the Functional Assessment of Cancer Therapy-Lung (FACT-L) questionnaire showed a more favorable score in the Lung Cancer Specific Symptoms subscale for patients receiving the lower dose of paclitaxel combined with cisplatin compared with etoposide and cisplatin.

Similar response rates and median survival were observed in patients receiving paclitaxel doses of either 250 or 135 mg/m², but greater toxicity occurred in patients receiving the higher dose, including arthralgia/myalgia (42 versus 21%), severe neurosensory toxicity (28 versus 13%), and severe hypersensitivity reactions (4 versus 1%). Although patients received concomitant administration of G-CSF with the higher dose of paclitaxel, severe neutropenia was common in patients receiving paclitaxel 250 or 135 mg/m² with cisplatin (65 or 74%, respectively) and occurred more frequently than in patients receiving etoposide with cisplatin (55%). Other adverse effects that occurred more frequently in patients receiving paclitaxel 250 or 135 mg/m² by 24-hour IV infusion followed by cisplatin than in those receiving etoposide with cisplatin included arthralgia/myalgia (42 or 21%, respectively, versus 9%) and severe neurosensory toxicity (28 or 13%, respectively, versus 8%).

Conventional Paclitaxel and Gemcitabine

Paclitaxel also is used in non-platinum-based combination regimens for the treatment of advanced non-small cell lung cancer†. In a phase III randomized trial, efficacy and toxicity were similar in patients with advanced non-small cell lung cancer receiving initial treatment with paclitaxel/gemcitabine or paclitaxel/carboplatin. Treatment consisted of paclitaxel 200 mg/m² as a 3-hour IV infusion on day 1 followed by either gemcitabine (1000 mg/m² as a 30-minute IV infusion on days 1 and 8) or carboplatin (at the dose required to obtain an AUC of 6 mg/mL per minute as a 1-hour IV infusion on day 1) with treatment cycles repeated every 3 weeks for up to 6 cycles. Treatment-related toxicity was mild in both groups.

Albumin-bound Paclitaxel and Carboplatin

Albumin-bound paclitaxel in combination with carboplatin is used for the initial treatment of advanced non-small cell lung cancer in patients who are not

candidates for curative surgery or radiation therapy. Combination chemotherapy with albumin-bound paclitaxel and carboplatin is associated with higher response rates and similar survival compared with conventional paclitaxel and carboplatin.

The current indication for albumin-bound paclitaxel in combination with carboplatin is based principally on the results of a randomized, multicenter, open-label trial in patients with previously untreated advanced non-small cell lung cancer. In this study, 1052 patients with stage IIIB or IV non-small cell lung cancer were randomized to receive either albumin-bound paclitaxel (100 mg/m² by 30-minute IV infusion) on days 1, 8, and 15 followed by IV carboplatin (at the dose required to obtain an AUC of 6 mg/mL per minute) on day 1 of each 21-day cycle or conventional paclitaxel (200 mg/m² by 3-hour IV infusion) followed by IV carboplatin (at the dose required to obtain an AUC of 6 mg/mL per minute) on day 1 of each 21-day cycle. Treatment was continued until disease progression or unacceptable toxicity occurred. Patients receiving albumin-bound paclitaxel combined with carboplatin had higher overall response rates (33 versus 25%) but similar median overall survival (12.1 versus 11.2 months) and progression-free survival (6.3 versus 5.8 months) compared with those receiving conventional paclitaxel combined with carboplatin. Albumin-bound paclitaxel therapy was associated with higher overall response rates (41 versus 24%) compared with conventional paclitaxel therapy in patients with squamous cell histology and was as effective as conventional paclitaxel in patients with nonsquamous cell histology (response rate of 26 versus 25% in patients with nonsquamous cell histology receiving therapy with albumin-bound paclitaxel or conventional paclitaxel, respectively). Grade 3 or greater thrombocytopenia (18 versus 9%) and anemia (27 versus 7%) occurred more frequently in patients receiving albumin-bound paclitaxel, whereas grade 3 or greater neutropenia (58 versus 47%) and sensory neuropathy (12 versus 3%) occurred more frequently in those receiving conventional paclitaxel.

Conventional Paclitaxel

Paclitaxel appears to be one of the most active single agents in patients with non-small cell lung carcinoma who have not received prior chemotherapy. In phase II studies of patients with advanced non-small cell lung carcinoma who had not received prior chemotherapy, objective response rates of 21–24% (0–4% complete responses, 20–21% partial responses) and 1-year survival rates of approximately 40% have been observed with paclitaxel alone at doses of 200–250 mg/m² administered by 24-hour infusion every 3 weeks. Response rates of 10–26% have been observed in additional phase II studies of patients who had not received previous chemotherapy for advanced disease with paclitaxel doses of 135–225 mg/m² administered over shorter periods of infusion (i.e., 1 or 3 hours). Limited evidence suggests that paclitaxel is not active against disease refractory to platinum-containing chemotherapy.

Intrapleural injections of paclitaxel have been used for the treatment of malignant pleural effusions† in a limited number of patients with non-small cell lung cancer.

● AIDS-related Kaposi's Sarcoma

Paclitaxel alone is used for the palliative treatment of advanced or refractory AIDS-related (epidemic) Kaposi's sarcoma. Use of a liposomal anthracycline (doxorubicin or daunorubicin) is a first-line therapy of choice for advanced AIDS-related Kaposi's sarcoma (see Uses: AIDS-related Kaposi's Sarcoma in Doxorubicin 10:00 or Daunorubicin 10:00).

Although the comparative efficacy of paclitaxel versus other treatments for advanced AIDS-related Kaposi's sarcoma (e.g., liposomal doxorubicin; liposomal daunorubicin; combination therapy with conventional doxorubicin, bleomycin, and a vinca alkaloid [vinblastine or vincristine]) has not been established, paclitaxel has shown substantial activity in patients with advanced disease (e.g., extensive mucocutaneous disease, lymphedema, symptomatic visceral disease). Objective responses to paclitaxel therapy have been reported in patients with poor prognostic factors, including low baseline helper/inducer (CD4⁺, T4⁺) T-cell counts (less than 200/mm³), visceral involvement (e.g., pulmonary disease), or history of opportunistic infection, as well as in patients who have received prior systemic chemotherapy. However, the depressed immunologic status of the patient limits the therapeutic benefit of systemic chemotherapy, and there currently are no data showing unequivocal evidence of improved survival with any treatment for AIDS-related Kaposi's sarcoma; new therapies are continually being evaluated.

The current indication for use of paclitaxel in advanced AIDS-related Kaposi's sarcoma is based on limited data from 2 uncontrolled phase II studies involving 59 patients who previously had received systemic therapy, including interferon alfa (32%), liposomal daunorubicin (31%), liposomal doxorubicin (2%), and/or conventional doxorubicin-containing chemotherapy (42%); 64% of the patients had received previous chemotherapy with anthracycline agents. Most of these patients experienced progression of disease during, or could not tolerate, previous systemic therapy for AIDS-related Kaposi's sarcoma. According to the manufacturer, the overall objective response rate was 59% (3% complete responses, 56% partial responses). A cutaneous (i.e., objective) response was defined principally as flattening of the size of all previously raised lesions by at least 50%. The median duration of response measured from the first day of treatment was 10.4 months (range: 7–11 months). Median time to disease progression was 6.2 months (range: 4.6–8.7 months).

Retrospective analysis of the data showed that some patients receiving paclitaxel as second-line therapy for AIDS-related Kaposi's sarcoma experienced additional clinical benefits, including improvement of pulmonary function in those with pulmonary involvement, increased ambulation, resolution of ulcers, decreased analgesic requirements for pain caused by foot lesions, and resolution of facial lesions. Rapid, substantial improvement in tumor-associated lymphedema also has been observed in patients receiving paclitaxel for advanced AIDS-related Kaposi's sarcoma.

The optimum dosage regimen for paclitaxel in the treatment of AIDS-related Kaposi's sarcoma has not been established. In the first phase II study, paclitaxel was administered IV over 3 hours at an initial dosage of 135 mg/m² once every 3 weeks. The paclitaxel dose was to be increased by 20 mg/m² for each subsequent cycle of therapy to a maximum dose of 175 mg/m²; however, at least 12 of 29 patients required dose reduction to less than 135 mg/m² because of dose-limiting toxicity, particularly neutropenia. Patients in this study initially did not receive concomitant therapy with granulocyte colony-stimulating factor (i.e., filgrastim), but the study protocol was later modified to allow concomitant administration of filgrastim to reduce the severity of paclitaxel-associated myelosuppression. In the second phase II study, paclitaxel was administered IV over 3 hours at a dosage of 100 mg/m² once every 2 weeks. Concomitant administration of a granulocyte colony-stimulating factor (G-CSF) was initiated as clinically indicated, and most of the patients in this study were already receiving G-CSF prior to the initiation of paclitaxel therapy. The dose intensity of paclitaxel per week was 38–39 mg/m² for both studies.

Although direct comparison of data from these uncontrolled phase II studies is not possible, a higher incidence of hematologic toxicity was reported in patients receiving paclitaxel 135 mg/m² compared with that reported in patients receiving paclitaxel 100 mg/m², including severe neutropenia (76 versus 35%), febrile neutropenia (55 versus 9%), and opportunistic infections (76 versus 54%). The higher incidence of hematologic toxicity in patients receiving paclitaxel 135 mg/m² may have been at least partially secondary to the delayed administration of G-CSF in these patients. The manufacturer recommends concomitant administration of a granulocyte colony-stimulating factor (e.g., filgrastim) as clinically indicated in patients with AIDS-related Kaposi's sarcoma to reduce the severity of myelosuppression associated with paclitaxel therapy.

The incidence of nonhematologic toxicity also appears to be higher in patients receiving higher doses of paclitaxel. Certain adverse effects occurred more frequently in patients receiving the higher dose of paclitaxel (135 versus 100 mg/m²) for AIDS-related Kaposi's sarcoma, including arthralgia and/or myalgia (93 versus 48%), peripheral neuropathy (79 versus 46%), and hypersensitivity reaction (14 versus 9%).

Other schedules of paclitaxel therapy have been investigated in patients with AIDS-related Kaposi's sarcoma. Some responses have been reported in patients with advanced AIDS-related Kaposi's sarcoma receiving paclitaxel administered by continuous 96-hour infusion (initial dosage of 105 mg/m² with or without filgrastim) following progression of disease or absence of response with administration of the drug by 3-hour infusion. Further study is needed to determine the optimal dosage and schedule of paclitaxel for the treatment of advanced AIDS-related Kaposi's sarcoma.

Optimal therapy for the treatment of advanced AIDS-related Kaposi's sarcoma has not been established. The potential effects of systemic chemotherapy on the patient's immune and hematologic status must be considered in the management of AIDS-related Kaposi's sarcoma.

● **Pancreatic Cancer**

Albumin-bound paclitaxel in combination with gemcitabine is used as first-line therapy in patients with metastatic adenocarcinoma of the pancreas. Combination chemotherapy with albumin-bound paclitaxel and gemcitabine is associated with higher response rates and prolonged overall and progression-free survival compared with gemcitabine monotherapy.

The current indication for albumin-bound paclitaxel in combination with gemcitabine is based principally on the results of a randomized, multicenter, open-label trial in patients with previously untreated metastatic adenocarcinoma of the pancreas. In this study, 861 patients with metastatic adenocarcinoma of the pancreas were randomized (stratified according to performance status, presence of liver metastases, and geographic region) to receive either albumin-bound paclitaxel (125 mg/m² administered IV over 30–40 minutes) followed by gemcitabine (1 g/m² administered IV over 30–40 minutes) on days 1, 8, and 15 of each 28-day cycle or gemcitabine (1 g/m² IV over 30–40 minutes) alone once weekly for 7 weeks followed by a treatment-free week, and then once weekly for 3 consecutive weeks (days 1, 8, and 15) of each subsequent 28-day cycle. Median overall survival was prolonged in patients receiving albumin-bound paclitaxel combined with gemcitabine compared with those receiving gemcitabine alone (8.5 versus 6.7 months); 1-year survival was reported in 35% of patients receiving combined therapy and 22% of those receiving gemcitabine alone. Median progression-free survival also was prolonged in patients receiving albumin-bound paclitaxel combined with gemcitabine compared with those receiving gemcitabine alone (5.5 versus 3.7 months). The median time to treatment failure was 5.1 months in patients receiving combined therapy and 3.6 months in those receiving gemcitabine monotherapy. Patients receiving albumin-bound paclitaxel combined with gemcitabine had higher overall response rates (23 versus 7%); one patient receiving combined therapy achieved a complete response compared with none of those receiving gemcitabine alone. Subgroup analysis suggested that combined therapy consistently had a greater effect than gemcitabine monotherapy on overall and progression-free survival in patients with more advanced disease (i.e., those with poor performance status, presence of liver metastasis, more than 3 sites of metastatic disease, or carbohydrate antigen [CA] 19-9 level of 59 or more times the upper limit of normal). Compared with gemcitabine monotherapy, combined therapy was associated with a higher incidence of grade 3 or greater neutropenia (38 versus 27%), leukopenia (31 versus 16%), thrombocytopenia (13 versus 9%), febrile neutropenia (3 versus 1%), fatigue (17 versus 7%), peripheral neuropathy (17 versus 1%), and diarrhea (6 versus 1%).

● **Small Cell Lung Cancer**

Paclitaxel is an active agent in the treatment of small cell lung cancer†.

In phase II studies of patients with previously untreated extensive-stage small cell lung cancer, objective response rates of 35–41% (mostly partial responses) have been observed with paclitaxel alone (using a regimen of paclitaxel 250 mg/m² by 24-hour IV infusion every 3 weeks). Responses to paclitaxel (175 mg/m² by 3-hour IV infusion every 3 weeks) used alone or in combination therapy have been reported in patients with advanced small cell lung cancer that has relapsed following one or more previous chemotherapy regimens. In phase I and II studies, combination therapy with paclitaxel (e.g., cisplatin, etoposide, and paclitaxel; carboplatin, etoposide, and paclitaxel) has produced high response rates in patients with limited- or extensive-stage small cell lung cancer; however, randomized studies to date have not demonstrated a survival benefit from adding paclitaxel to standard combination regimens.

In a randomized trial, response rates and median survival were similar but toxicity was greater when paclitaxel was added to etoposide and cisplatin for previously untreated extensive-stage small cell lung cancer. Another randomized trial was terminated early because excessive toxicity and toxicity-related mortality occurred when paclitaxel was added to etoposide/cisplatin for the initial treatment of limited-stage or extensive-stage small cell lung cancer. Based on experience in these randomized trials, the addition of paclitaxel to standard regimens for the treatment of small-cell lung cancer is *not* recommended.

Concomitant administration of granulocyte colony-stimulating factor (G-CSF) has been used in some patients with small cell lung cancer to reduce the severity of myelosuppression associated with paclitaxel therapy; however, use of G-CSF generally is not required when paclitaxel is administered by short IV infusion (e.g., 1 or 3 hours).

Because the current prognosis for patients with small cell lung cancer is unsatisfactory regardless of stage and despite considerable diagnostic and therapeutic advances, all patients with this cancer are candidates for inclusion in clinical trials at the time of diagnosis.

● **Esophageal Cancer**

Paclitaxel has been used alone or in combination therapy for the treatment of esophageal cancer†. Like cisplatin, paclitaxel is active against both histologic types of esophageal cancer (i.e., squamous cell carcinoma and adenocarcinoma).

In a phase II study of patients with advanced esophageal cancer who had not received prior chemotherapy, an objective response rate of 32% (2% complete responses, 30% partial responses) has been observed with paclitaxel alone using an initial paclitaxel dosage of 250 mg/m² administered as a 24-hour IV infusion every 3 weeks. Response rates did not differ significantly according to histologic type; patients with adenocarcinoma and squamous cell carcinoma of the esophagus had objective response rates of 34 and 28%, respectively. Concomitant administration of granulocyte colony-stimulating factor was used to reduce the severity of myelosuppression associated with paclitaxel therapy, particularly with longer infusion schedules and higher doses of the drug.

The use of paclitaxel in combination with other antineoplastic agents (e.g., cisplatin, fluorouracil) for the treatment of advanced esophageal cancer is being investigated. The use of paclitaxel-containing regimens (with or without radiation therapy) prior to surgical resection is being investigated for the treatment of esophageal cancer. Optimal therapy for esophageal cancer has not been established, and new therapies are continually being evaluated. Because the prognosis for most patients with esophageal cancer remains poor, all newly diagnosed patients should be considered for enrollment in clinical trials comparing various treatment modalities.

● Bladder Cancer

Paclitaxel is an active agent in the treatment of transitional cell bladder cancer†. Paclitaxel has been used alone and in combination therapy for the treatment of advanced or metastatic bladder cancer.

In a phase II study of 26 patients with advanced transitional cell bladder cancer who had not received prior chemotherapy, objective responses occurred in 42% (27% complete responses, 15% partial responses) of patients receiving paclitaxel 250 mg/m² by 24-hour IV infusion every 21 days. Concomitant administration of granulocyte colony-stimulating factor (i.e., filgrastim) was used to reduce the severity of myelosuppression associated with paclitaxel therapy. Only partial responses have been reported in a small number of patients receiving paclitaxel alone or in combination with other antineoplastic agents for advanced or metastatic bladder cancer refractory to previous chemotherapy and/or radiation therapy. A low response rate (10%, partial responses only) was observed in patients receiving paclitaxel 80 mg/m² by 1-hour IV infusion once weekly for 4 weeks for previously treated advanced urothelial cancer.

Because paclitaxel is eliminated principally via hepatic metabolism, it may be a reasonable alternative in patients with advanced transitional cell urothelial cancer who have renal impairment and cannot tolerate the renal toxicity associated with cisplatin-based regimens. Paclitaxel also may be a useful alternative for the treatment of advanced or metastatic bladder cancer in patients with poor performance status who cannot tolerate standard platinum-based regimens.

Combination therapy with paclitaxel followed by carboplatin has been investigated as an active regimen in patients with advanced bladder cancer. Although high response rates were observed in earlier phase II studies of paclitaxel and carboplatin for previously untreated advanced bladder cancer, lower response rates were reported for this combination in a later phase II study and another phase II study involving patients with cisplatin-treated disease. Limited evidence from a small randomized trial that did reach full enrollment suggests that response rates and survival are similar but toxicity is lesser in patients receiving paclitaxel/carboplatin versus cisplatin, methotrexate, vinblastine, and doxorubicin (M-VAC). In this study, paclitaxel 225 mg/m² by 3-hour IV infusion was administered on day 1 followed by carboplatin at the dose required to obtain an AUC of 6 mg/mL per minute administered over 30 minutes; this cycle was administered every 3 weeks for a maximum of 6 cycles. Combination therapy with paclitaxel and carboplatin may be a reasonable option for the treatment of advanced bladder cancer in patients with renal dysfunction. The use of weekly dosing schedules of paclitaxel and carboplatin for patients with advanced bladder cancer is being investigated.

The use of paclitaxel in combination therapy with other antineoplastic agents (e.g., cisplatin, ifosfamide, gemcitabine) is being evaluated for the palliative treatment of advanced or metastatic bladder cancer. New chemotherapy regimens are continually being evaluated for the treatment of bladder cancer.

● Head and Neck Cancer

Paclitaxel is an active agent in the treatment of head and neck cancer†.

Paclitaxel is used in combination with cisplatin for the palliative treatment of advanced head and neck cancer. In a randomized trial involving patients with locally advanced, recurrent, or metastatic head and neck cancer, similar response

rates and survival were observed in those receiving cisplatin and paclitaxel (paclitaxel 175 mg/m² by 3-hour IV infusion on day 1 followed by cisplatin 75 mg/m² IV on day 1) versus those receiving cisplatin and fluorouracil (cisplatin 100 mg/m² on day 1 and fluorouracil 1000 mg/m² per 24 hours by continuous IV infusion day 1 through 4). Hematologic toxicities and stomatitis were more common in the patients receiving cisplatin and fluorouracil, but the frequency of neurotoxicity was similar between the groups. The use of paclitaxel in combination with other antineoplastic agents is being investigated.

Paclitaxel has been used alone for the treatment of advanced head and neck cancer. In phase II studies of patients with advanced or unresectable locally advanced squamous cell carcinoma of the head and neck, objective response rates of 36–40% (7–12% complete responses, 24–33% partial responses) have been observed with paclitaxel alone using a regimen of paclitaxel 250 mg/m² as a 24-hour IV infusion administered every 3 weeks. Long-term follow-up for one of these studies indicates a median survival of 9.2 months with paclitaxel monotherapy in patients with advanced head and neck cancer.

The effect of dose on the efficacy and toxicity of paclitaxel has been studied in patients with advanced head and neck cancer. Results of a randomized clinical trial indicate that response rates and duration of survival are similar when paclitaxel doses of 200 mg/m² (with granulocyte colony-stimulating factor [G-CSF]) or 135 mg/m²(without G-CSF) are administered by 24-hour infusion followed by cisplatin 75 mg/m² with treatment cycles administered every 3 weeks; however, unacceptably high rates of hematologic toxicity occurred and neither regimen is recommended for use in the treatment of advanced head and neck cancer. Concomitant administration of granulocyte colony-stimulating factor has been used in patients with squamous cell carcinoma of the head and neck to reduce the severity of myelosuppression associated with paclitaxel therapy, particularly with high doses of the drug.

Paclitaxel also has been administered by IV infusion over shorter periods (e.g., 1 or 3 hours) in patients with head and neck cancer. The effect of duration of infusion on the efficacy and toxicity of paclitaxel has been studied in patients with advanced head and neck cancer. Interim analysis from a randomized study shows that toxicity is greater in patients with recurrent or metastatic squamous cell carcinoma of the head and neck receiving paclitaxel 175 mg/m² administered by 24-hour IV infusion versus 3-hour IV infusion. Paclitaxel has been administered by IV infusion over longer periods in patients with head and neck cancer; low response rates were observed for a regimen of paclitaxel 120 or 140 mg/m² by 96-hour IV infusion in patients with advanced squamous cell carcinoma of the head and neck.

In addition to its antitumor activity, in vitro studies indicate that paclitaxel is a radiosensitizer, and the use of paclitaxel in combination with radiation therapy is being investigated in patients with advanced head and neck cancer. Paclitaxel-containing therapy has been used with concurrent radiation therapy in the treatment of advanced head or neck cancer. Paclitaxel-containing therapy is being investigated as induction therapy preceding surgery and/or radiation therapy, or concurrent chemotherapy and radiation therapy, in the treatment of locally advanced squamous cell carcinoma of the head and neck. The prognosis for patients with advanced head and neck cancer generally is poor; the optimal timing and regimens of chemotherapy used alone or in the combined modality treatment of advanced head and neck cancer have not been established, and new therapies are continually being evaluated.

● Cervical Cancer

Paclitaxel is an active agent in the treatment of cervical cancer†. (See Uses: Cervical Cancer in Cisplatin 10:00 for an overview of therapy for cervical cancer.)

Paclitaxel and Radiation Therapy for Locally Advanced Cervical Cancer

The use of paclitaxel as a radiation sensitizer is being investigated in patients with locally advanced cervical cancer†. Additional comparative studies are needed to determine the optimum chemotherapy regimens and schedules to be used concurrently with radiation therapy for the treatment of locally advanced cervical cancer.

Paclitaxel for Advanced Cervical Cancer

Paclitaxel is an active agent in the treatment of metastatic or recurrent cervical cancer†. Objective response rates of 17–25% have been observed in patients receiving paclitaxel as a single agent for advanced squamous cell carcinoma of the cervix. An objective response rate of 31% was reported in patients receiving paclitaxel alone for advanced nonsquamous cervical cancer.

Paclitaxel and Cisplatin for Advanced Cervical Cancer

Paclitaxel and cisplatin is used in the treatment of advanced cervical cancer. Objective responses of 40–45% for combination therapy with cisplatin and paclitaxel have been reported in patients who previously had not received chemotherapy for advanced or recurrent cervical cancer. In a randomized trial involving patients with advanced squamous cell cervical cancer, response rate was higher (36 versus 19%) and progression-free survival was longer (4.8 versus 2.8 months) in those receiving paclitaxel and cisplatin than in those receiving cisplatin alone; overall survival was similar between the groups (9.7 versus 8.8 months). In this study, patients received either paclitaxel and cisplatin (paclitaxel 135 mg/m² by 24-hour IV infusion followed immediately by IV cisplatin 50 mg/m²) or single-agent cisplatin (same dosage of cisplatin used for combination therapy) every 3 weeks.

● Endometrial Cancer

Paclitaxel is used in the treatment of endometrial cancer†.

Paclitaxel is an active agent that has been used in the treatment of advanced or recurrent endometrial cancer. Paclitaxel and carboplatin, with or without radiation therapy, is used in the palliative treatment of advanced or recurrent endometrial cancer. In a randomized trial, similar response rates, progression-free survival, and overall survival were observed for patients receiving doxorubicin and cisplatin versus doxorubicin and paclitaxel (with filgrastim) for advanced endometrial cancer. In another randomized trial, higher response rate and prolonged progression-free and overall survival but greater neurotoxicity was observed with the addition of paclitaxel to doxorubicin and cisplatin for advanced endometrial cancer. A phase III randomized trial comparing doxorubicin, cisplatin, paclitaxel and filgrastim (G-CSF) versus carboplatin and paclitaxel for advanced endometrial cancer is under way.

The use of adjuvant radiation therapy and chemotherapy with cisplatin and paclitaxel following surgery for high-risk endometrial cancer confined to the uterus is being investigated.

● Other Uses

Paclitaxel is used in the treatment of gastric cancer†. Paclitaxel is used in the treatment of relapsed or refractory testicular cancer†.

DOSAGE AND ADMINISTRATION

● Reconstitution and Administration

Paclitaxel is administered by IV infusion. Paclitaxel also has been administered intraperitoneally†.

Paclitaxel is commercially available in 2 types of formulations: conventional paclitaxel (in a nonaqueous solution) and albumin-bound paclitaxel. The properties of paclitaxel may differ according to formulation, and the dosage and reconstitution instructions for paclitaxel are specific to formulation. Albumin-bound paclitaxel may *not* be substituted for or used in combination with other formulations of paclitaxel.

Caution should be exercised in handling and preparing solutions of conventional or albumin-bound paclitaxel. Because dermatologic reactions (e.g., tingling, burning, erythema) may occur with accidental exposure to the drug, the manufacturers recommend the use of protective gloves during preparation and administration of paclitaxel. Skin accidentally exposed to the drug should be washed immediately and thoroughly with soap and water. If the drug comes into contact with mucous membranes, thorough flushing with water should be used immediately. Dyspnea, chest pain, ocular burning, sore throat, and nausea have been reported upon inhalation, and inadvertent inhalation should be avoided during preparation and administration of paclitaxel solutions.

Paclitaxel for injection concentrate, diluted solutions of conventional paclitaxel, and reconstituted suspensions of albumin-bound paclitaxel should be inspected visually for particulate matter and discoloration whenever solution and container permit.

Medication errors have occurred that involved confusion between paclitaxel (Taxol®) and docetaxel (Taxotere®). To avoid medication errors, the prescriber should print both the brand and generic names for paclitaxel on the prescription order form. If a handwritten prescription is difficult to read, the pharmacist should confirm the drug name with the prescriber. If the prescription is confirmed verbally, the drug names should be spelled out. Pharmacy labels and preprinted order forms should list both the generic and brand names using upper- and lower-case

fonts (i.e., PACLItaxel and TaxOL). Two pharmacists should provide independent confirmation that the correct drug is being administered before chemotherapy is dispensed, and two nurses should confirm that the correct drug has been dispensed for the correct patient before administering the medication.

IV Administration

Adverse local effects have occurred following extravasation of paclitaxel during administration, and the injection site should be monitored closely during infusion of conventional or albumin-bound paclitaxel for possible infiltration of the drug. (See Cautions: Local Effects.)

Conventional Paclitaxel

Paclitaxel for injection concentrate must be diluted prior to IV infusion. For IV infusion, the manufacturer recommends diluting the concentrate in 0.9% sodium chloride injection, 5% dextrose injection, 5% dextrose and 0.9% sodium chloride injection, or 5% dextrose in Ringer's injection to a final paclitaxel concentration of 0.3–1.2 mg/mL.

Undiluted paclitaxel for injection concentrate should not be placed in plasticized polyvinyl chloride (PVC) equipment or devices used to prepare solutions for infusion. To minimize exposure of the patient to leached DEHP, *diluted* paclitaxel solutions preferably should be stored in glass or polypropylene bottles or in plastic (polypropylene or polyolefin) bags and administered through polyethylene-lined administration sets. Leaching of unacceptable amounts of DEHP has been reported with some administration sets labeled as not containing PVC (probably because of pumping segments made of heavily plasticized PVC); therefore, compatibility of administration sets with paclitaxel solutions should be verified prior to their use. (See Chemistry and Stability: Stability.)

Because a small number of fibers (within acceptable USP limits) have been detected in paclitaxel solutions prepared from the commercially available for injection concentrate, a hydrophilic, microporous inline filter with a pore size not exceeding 0.22 µm is necessary during administration of paclitaxel solutions. The manufacturer reports that use of filter devices such as IVEX-2® filters, which incorporate short inlet and outlet PVC-coated tubing, has not resulted in significant leaching of DEHP. (See Chemistry and Stability: Stability.) The Chemo Dispensing Pin® device or similar devices with spikes should *not* be used with vials of paclitaxel; this type of device can cause the stopper to collapse and contaminate the paclitaxel solution.

Albumin-bound Paclitaxel

Albumin-bound paclitaxel in the form of lyophilized powder must be reconstituted to an injectable suspension prior to IV infusion. Using aseptic technique, 20 mL of 0.9% sodium chloride injection should be injected slowly (over a minimum period of 1 minute) into the vial containing the lyophilized paclitaxel. The flow from the sterile syringe should be injected onto the inside wall of the vial; injection of 0.9% sodium chloride injection directly onto the lyophilized cake should be avoided because it causes foaming. Once injection of the 20 mL of 0.9% sodium chloride injection into the vial is complete, the vial should be allowed to sit for a minimum of 5 minutes to ensure thorough wetting of the lyophilized cake/powder. The vial then should be swirled and/or inverted gently for at least 2 minutes until the cake/powder is completely dissolved; foaming should be avoided. If foaming or clumping occurs, the reconstituted paclitaxel suspension should be allowed to stand for at least 15 minutes until foam subsides.

The reconstituted suspension has a final paclitaxel concentration of 5 mg/mL. The exact dosing volume of the injectable suspension should be calculated using the following formula: dosing volume in mL equals total dose in mg divided by 5 mg/mL. Before the dosing volume is withdrawn from the vial, the suspension should be inspected. The reconstituted paclitaxel suspension should appear milky and homogeneous with no visible particulates. If particulates are visible or settling has occurred, the vial should be inverted *gently* to ensure complete resuspension of the particles in solution. Then the appropriate dosing volume of paclitaxel suspension should be withdrawn from the vial and injected into an empty sterile PVC IV bag. Unlike conventional paclitaxel, DEHP-free containers or administration sets are not required for the preparation or administration of albumin-bound paclitaxel suspension. Unlike conventional paclitaxel, the use of an inline filter is *not* recommended for the IV infusion of albumin-bound paclitaxel suspension.

The injection site should be monitored closely during the infusion for possible infiltration of the drug. According to the manufacturer, limiting the infusion of albumin-bound paclitaxel to 30 minutes as directed reduces the likelihood of infusion-related reactions.

Intraperitoneal Instillation
Conventional Paclitaxel

For intraperitoneal† administration in the Gynecologic Oncology Group (GOG)-172 study in patients with advanced epithelial ovarian cancer, the paclitaxel dose was diluted in 1 L of 0.9% sodium chloride solution that was warmed to 37°C and infused through a surgically implanted peritoneal catheter, followed by intraperitoneal infusion of an additional liter of warmed saline solution. Following peritoneal infusion, the patient was asked to roll into a different position every 15 minutes for the next 2 hours to disperse the drug throughout the peritoneal cavity.

Various implanted access ports and connecting catheters have been used for intraperitoneal administration of chemotherapeutic agents. The intraperitoneal catheter may be placed at the time of primary (cytoreductive) surgery as long as contamination of the peritoneal cavity has not occurred. Timing of placement of the intraperitoneal catheter (at the time of primary surgery versus delayed insertion) does not appear to affect tolerance of intraperitoneal therapy or treatment completion rates. The intraperitoneal catheter should be removed as soon as intraperitoneal therapy is completed to avoid catheter-related complications. Further study is needed to optimize techniques for intraperitoneal therapy to minimize the risk of complications (e.g., infection, catheter obstruction, catheter retraction, bowel perforation, pain, leakage, port access problems). Specialized sources should be consulted for guidance on how to administer intraperitoneal therapy.

Supportive therapy should include premedication to prevent hypersensitivity reactions to paclitaxel.

● Dosage

Paclitaxel is commercially available in 2 types of formulations: conventional paclitaxel (in a nonaqueous solution) and albumin-bound paclitaxel. The functional properties of paclitaxel may differ according to formulation, and the dosage instructions for paclitaxel are specific to formulation. Albumin-bound paclitaxel may *not* be substituted for or used in combination with other formulations of paclitaxel. Clinicians should consult the respective manufacturer's labeling and published protocols for formulation-specific regimens and specific dosages, methods of administration, and administration sequence of other antineoplastic agents used in combination regimens.

Dosage of albumin-bound paclitaxel is expressed in terms of paclitaxel.

Conventional or albumin-bound paclitaxel should not be administered to patients with baseline neutrophil counts less than 1500/mm³. In patients with HIV infection, conventional paclitaxel should not be administered if baseline neutrophil counts are less than 1000/mm³. To monitor the occurrence of paclitaxel-induced bone marrow suppression, mainly neutropenia, which may be severe and result in infection, it is recommended that frequent peripheral blood cell counts be performed in all patients receiving paclitaxel.

Conventional Paclitaxel

All patients should be premedicated before administration of conventional paclitaxel to prevent severe hypersensitivity reactions.

For patients receiving paclitaxel for the treatment of solid tumors, the manufacturer recommends the following premedication regimen: oral dexamethasone 20 mg administered approximately 12 and 6 hours before paclitaxel; IV diphenhydramine hydrochloride (or similar antihistamine) 50 mg administered 30–60 minutes before paclitaxel; and either IV cimetidine hydrochloride (300 mg of cimetidine) or ranitidine hydrochloride (50 mg of ranitidine) administered 30–60 minutes before paclitaxel.

For patients with HIV infection who are receiving conventional paclitaxel for the treatment of AIDS-related Kaposi's sarcoma, the manufacturer recommends the following premedication regimen: oral dexamethasone 10 mg administered approximately 12 and 6 hours before paclitaxel; IV diphenhydramine hydrochloride (or similar antihistamine) 50 mg administered 30–60 minutes before paclitaxel; and either IV cimetidine hydrochloride (300 mg of cimetidine) or ranitidine hydrochloride (50 mg of ranitidine) administered 30–60 minutes before paclitaxel. This is the same premedication regimen as for other patients receiving paclitaxel with the exception of a reduced dose of oral dexamethasone (10 mg).

Concomitant administration of filgrastim is used to reduce the severity of myelosuppression in patients receiving paclitaxel therapy, particularly those who are at high risk for febrile neutropenia. Because of immunosuppression in patients with advanced HIV disease, the manufacturer recommends concomitant administration of a granulocyte colony-stimulating factor (e.g., filgrastim) as clinically indicated to reduce the severity of myelosuppression associated with paclitaxel in patients with AIDS-related Kaposi's sarcoma.

Albumin-bound Paclitaxel

Unlike conventional paclitaxel, which requires premedication prior to administration to prevent severe hypersensitivity reactions, premedication generally is *not* required prior to administration of albumin-bound paclitaxel. However, premedication may be necessary in patients who experienced a hypersensitivity reaction during a previous course of therapy with the drug.

Ovarian Cancer
Conventional Paclitaxel as First-line Therapy for Advanced Ovarian Epithelial Cancer

When used in combination therapy with cisplatin for the initial treatment of advanced ovarian cancer, there are 2 recommended paclitaxel-containing regimens. Differences in toxicity should be considered when selecting the appropriate regimen for a patient. One recommended regimen is conventional paclitaxel 175 mg/m² administered by 3-hour IV infusion followed by cisplatin 75 mg/m² IV with cycles repeated every 3 weeks. Another recommended regimen is conventional paclitaxel 135 mg/m² administered by 24-hour IV infusion followed by cisplatin 75 mg/m² IV with cycles repeated every 3 weeks.

Intraperitoneal Conventional Paclitaxel and Cisplatin as First-line Therapy for Advanced Ovarian Epithelial Cancer

When combined therapy with IV and intraperitoneal conventional paclitaxel and intraperitoneal cisplatin† has been used for the initial adjuvant treatment of optimally debulked stage III epithelial ovarian cancer, IV paclitaxel 135 mg/m² by 24-hour infusion on day 1, followed by intraperitoneal cisplatin 100 mg/m² on day 2 and intraperitoneal paclitaxel 60 mg/m² on day 8, has been administered every 21 days for up to 6 cycles. Modified IV and intraperitoneal regimens are being investigated. (See Uses: Ovarian Cancer.)

Conventional Paclitaxel as Second-line or Subsequent Therapy for Advanced Ovarian Epithelial Cancer

When used as monotherapy in patients with metastatic carcinoma of the ovary that failed to respond to first-line or subsequent chemotherapy, the recommended regimen is conventional paclitaxel 135 or 175 mg/m² infused IV over 3 hours and repeated every 3 weeks as tolerated. Optimal dosage of paclitaxel has not been established in this patient population.

Breast Cancer
Conventional Paclitaxel as Adjuvant Therapy for Node-positive Breast Cancer

For the adjuvant therapy of node-positive breast cancer, conventional paclitaxel 175 mg/m² is administered as a 3-hour IV infusion once every 3 weeks for 4 courses following the completion of doxorubicin-containing combination chemotherapy. In a large randomized trial on which this indication is based, patients received 4 courses of doxorubicin and cyclophosphamide followed by adjuvant therapy with paclitaxel.

Conventional or Albumin-bound Paclitaxel as Second-line Therapy for Advanced Breast Cancer

For metastatic breast cancer that is refractory to initial chemotherapy or breast cancer that has relapsed within 6 months of adjuvant therapy, *conventional* paclitaxel 175 mg/m² is administered as a 3-hour IV infusion once every 3 weeks.

For metastatic breast cancer that is refractory to combination chemotherapy or breast cancer that has relapsed within 6 months of adjuvant therapy, *albumin-bound* paclitaxel 260 mg/m² is administered as a 30-minute IV infusion once every 3 weeks.

Non-small Cell Lung Cancer
Conventional Paclitaxel and Cisplatin

When used in combination therapy with cisplatin for the initial treatment of advanced non-small cell lung cancer in patients who are not candidates for potentially curative surgery and/or radiation therapy, the recommended regimen is conventional paclitaxel 135 mg/m² administered by 24-hour IV infusion followed by cisplatin 75 mg/m² IV with cycles repeated every 3 weeks. A regimen of conventional paclitaxel 175 mg/m² administered by 3-hour IV infusion followed by cisplatin 80 mg/m² IV with cycles repeated every 3 weeks also has been used in patients with advanced non-small cell lung cancer.

Albumin-bound Paclitaxel and Carboplatin

When used in combination therapy with carboplatin for the initial treatment of advanced non-small cell lung cancer in patients who are not candidates for potentially curative surgery and/or radiation therapy, the recommended regimen is albumin-bound paclitaxel 100 mg/m² administered by 30-minute IV infusion on days 1, 8, and 15 and IV carboplatin at the dose required to obtain an area under the concentration-time curve (AUC) of 6 mg/mL per minute on day 1 of each 21-day cycle.

AIDS-related Kaposi's Sarcoma
Conventional Paclitaxel

For patients with advanced HIV infection, paclitaxel therapy should be initiated only if the neutrophil count is at least 1000/mm³.

For patients with AIDS-related Kaposi's sarcoma that has failed to respond to first-line or subsequent chemotherapy, there are 2 recommended paclitaxel regimens. One recommended regimen is conventional paclitaxel 135 mg/m² administered by 3-hour IV infusion once every 3 weeks. Another recommended regimen is conventional paclitaxel 100 mg/m² administered by 3-hour IV infusion once every 2 weeks. Both of these regimens achieve a dose intensity of 45–50 mg/m² per week. In phase II studies, greater toxicity was observed with the higher-dose schedule, and patients with poor performance status were treated with paclitaxel 100 mg/m² once every 2 weeks.

Pancreatic Cancer
Albumin-bound Paclitaxel and Gemcitabine

When used in combination therapy with gemcitabine for the initial treatment of metastatic adenocarcinoma of the pancreas, the recommended regimen is albumin-bound paclitaxel 125 mg/m² administered IV over 30–40 minutes followed by gemcitabine 1 g/m² administered IV over 30–40 minutes on days 1, 8, and 15 of each 28-day cycle.

Dosage Modification for Toxicity and Contraindications for Continued Therapy with Conventional Paclitaxel
Hematologic Toxicity

For patients receiving conventional paclitaxel, repeat cycles of the drug should be withheld until platelet counts exceed 100,000/mm³ *and* neutrophil counts are at least 1500/mm³ in patients with solid tumors or are at least 1000/mm³ in patients with advanced AIDS-related Kaposi's sarcoma.

For patients receiving conventional paclitaxel who experience severe neutropenia (neutrophil count less than 500/mm³ for at least 7 days), a 20% reduction in the dose of conventional paclitaxel is recommended for subsequent courses of therapy.

The incidence and severity of hematologic toxicity (i.e., neutropenia) have been shown to increase with dose and duration of infusion for conventional paclitaxel. The use of supportive therapy, such as G-CSF, with administration of conventional paclitaxel is recommended for patients who have experienced severe neutropenia.

Sensitivity Reactions

Mild symptoms (e.g., flushing, skin reactions, dyspnea, hypotension, tachycardia) do not require interruption of therapy. If signs or symptoms of a severe reaction (e.g., hypotension requiring treatment, dyspnea requiring bronchodilators, angioedema, generalized urticaria) occur during administration of paclitaxel, the infusion should be discontinued immediately and aggressive symptomatic therapy instituted as necessary. Such therapy may include epinephrine, IV fluids, and additional doses of antihistamine (e.g., diphenhydramine) and corticosteroid as clinically indicated.

Further therapy with conventional paclitaxel should *not* be undertaken in any patient who experienced a severe hypersensitivity reaction during a previous course of therapy with the drug. It is not known whether patients who have

exhibited hypersensitivity to conventional paclitaxel can tolerate subsequent therapy with albumin-bound paclitaxel.

Hepatic Toxicity

In patients with preexisting hepatic impairment, dose reduction is recommended depending on the degree of hepatic impairment for the first course of therapy with conventional paclitaxel. Further dose reduction may be required during subsequent courses of paclitaxel therapy based on hepatic toxicity. (See Dosage of Conventional Paclitaxel in Hepatic Impairment under Dosage and Administration: Dosage in Renal and Hepatic Impairment.)

Cardiovascular Toxicity

If a patient develops substantial conduction abnormalities during administration of paclitaxel, appropriate therapy should be initiated and continuous cardiac monitoring should be performed during subsequent therapy with the drug. Paclitaxel infusions occasionally must be interrupted or discontinued because of initial or recurrent hypertension.

Neurologic Toxicity

For patients who experience severe peripheral neuropathy while receiving conventional paclitaxel, the manufacturer recommends a 20% reduction in the dose for subsequent courses of therapy. The incidence and severity of neurotoxicity increase with paclitaxel dose.

Dosage Modification for Toxicity and Contraindications for Continued Therapy with Albumin-bound Paclitaxel for Breast Cancer
Hematologic Toxicity

For patients receiving albumin-bound paclitaxel, repeat cycles of the drug should be withheld until neutrophil counts exceed 1500/mm³ and platelet counts exceed 100,000/mm³.

For patients who experience severe neutropenia (neutrophil count less than 500/mm³ for at least 7 days) while receiving albumin-bound paclitaxel for breast cancer, the manufacturer recommends a reduction in dose to albumin-bound paclitaxel 220 mg/m² for subsequent courses of therapy. For patients who experience recurrence of severe neutropenia, further reduction in dose to albumin-bound paclitaxel 180 mg/m² is recommended.

Sensitivity Reactions

Further therapy with paclitaxel should *not* be undertaken in any patient who experienced a severe hypersensitivity reaction during a previous course of therapy with the drug. It is not known whether patients who have exhibited hypersensitivity to conventional paclitaxel can tolerate subsequent therapy with albumin-bound paclitaxel.

Hepatic Toxicity

In patients with preexisting hepatic impairment, dose reduction is recommended depending on the degree of hepatic impairment for the first course of therapy with albumin-bound paclitaxel. Further dose reduction may be required during subsequent courses of albumin-bound paclitaxel therapy based on hepatic toxicity. (See Dosage of Albumin-bound Paclitaxel in Hepatic Impairment under Dosage and Administration: Dosage in Renal and Hepatic Impairment.)

Neurologic Toxicity

Sensory neuropathy associated with albumin-bound paclitaxel is dose and schedule dependent. In patients with breast cancer, the incidence and severity of sensory neuropathy associated with albumin-bound paclitaxel increased with cumulative dose of the drug.

For patients who experience grade 1 or 2 sensory neuropathy while receiving albumin-bound paclitaxel, dosage modification generally is not required.

For patients with breast cancer who experience severe sensory neuropathy while receiving albumin-bound paclitaxel, treatment should be withheld until resolution to grade 1 or 2 severity followed by reduction in dose to albumin-bound paclitaxel 220 mg/m² for subsequent courses of therapy. For patients who experience recurrence of severe sensory neuropathy, treatment should be withheld until resolution to grade 1 or 2 severity followed by further reduction in dose to albumin-bound paclitaxel 180 mg/m² for subsequent courses of therapy.

Dosage Modification for Toxicity and Contraindications for Continued Therapy with Albumin-bound Paclitaxel for Non-small Cell Lung Cancer

Hematologic Toxicity

For patients receiving albumin-bound paclitaxel, repeat cycles of the drug should be withheld until neutrophil counts are at least 1500/mm³ and platelet counts are at least 100,000/mm³.

For patients who experience severe neutropenia (neutrophil count less than 500/mm³ for at least 7 days) or thrombocytopenia (platelet count less than 50,000/mm³) while receiving albumin-bound paclitaxel for non-small cell lung cancer, the manufacturer recommends dose reduction upon resumption of therapy.

For patients with non-small cell lung cancer who experience severe neutropenia or febrile neutropenia (neutrophil count less than 500/mm³ with fever exceeding 38°C) while receiving albumin-bound paclitaxel and carboplatin, treatment should be delayed until neutrophil counts are at least 1500/mm³ on day 1 or at least 500/mm³ on day 8 or 15 of the cycle; treatment may then be resumed at a permanently reduced dose of albumin-bound paclitaxel 75 mg/m² and a target carboplatin AUC of 4.5 mg/mL per minute. Following a second episode of severe neutropenia or febrile neutropenia, treatment should again be delayed; treatment may be resumed at a permanently reduced dose of albumin-bound paclitaxel 50 mg/m² and a target carboplatin AUC of 3 mg/mL per minute. Albumin-bound paclitaxel and carboplatin should be discontinued following a third episode of severe neutropenia or febrile neutropenia.

If initiation of a repeat cycle of therapy for non-small cell lung cancer is delayed by more than 7 days because the patient's neutrophil count is less than 1500/mm³, permanent dose reduction of albumin-bound paclitaxel to 75 mg/m² and a target carboplatin AUC of 4.5 mg/mL per minute is recommended. Following a second such treatment delay, permanent dose reduction of albumin-bound paclitaxel to 50 mg/m² and a target carboplatin AUC of 3 mg/mL per minute is recommended. Albumin-bound paclitaxel and carboplatin should be discontinued following a third such delay.

For patients with non-small cell lung cancer who experience severe thrombocytopenia while receiving albumin-bound paclitaxel and carboplatin, treatment should be delayed until platelet counts are at least 100,000/mm³ on day 1 or at least 50,000/mm³ on day 8 or 15 of the cycle; treatment may then be resumed at a permanently reduced dose of albumin-bound paclitaxel 75 mg/m² and a target carboplatin AUC of 4.5 mg/mL per minute. Albumin-bound paclitaxel and carboplatin should be discontinued following a second episode of severe thrombocytopenia.

Sensitivity Reactions

Further therapy with paclitaxel should *not* be undertaken in any patient who experienced a severe hypersensitivity reaction during a previous course of therapy with the drug. It is not known whether patients who have exhibited hypersensitivity to conventional paclitaxel can tolerate subsequent therapy with albumin-bound paclitaxel.

Hepatic Toxicity

In patients with preexisting hepatic impairment, dose reduction is recommended depending on the degree of hepatic impairment for the first course of therapy with albumin-bound paclitaxel. Further dose reduction may be required during subsequent courses of albumin-bound paclitaxel therapy based on hepatic toxicity. (See Dosage of Albumin-bound Paclitaxel in Hepatic Impairment under Dosage and Administration: Dosage in Renal and Hepatic Impairment.)

Neurologic Toxicity

Sensory neuropathy associated with albumin-bound paclitaxel is dose and schedule dependent.

For patients who experience grade 1 or 2 peripheral neuropathy while receiving albumin-bound paclitaxel, dosage modification generally is not required.

For patients with non-small cell lung cancer who experience grade 3 or 4 peripheral neuropathy while receiving albumin-bound paclitaxel and carboplatin, treatment should be withheld until resolution to grade 1 or less followed by a permanent reduction in dose to albumin-bound paclitaxel 75 mg/m² and a target carboplatin AUC of 4.5 mg/mL per minute. Following a second episode of grade 3 or 4 peripheral neuropathy, treatment should again be withheld until resolution to grade 1 or less; treatment may then be resumed at a permanently reduced dose of albumin-bound paclitaxel 50 mg/m² and a target carboplatin AUC of 3 mg/mL

per minute. Albumin-bound paclitaxel and carboplatin should be discontinued following a third episode of grade 3 or 4 peripheral neuropathy.

Dosage Modification for Toxicity and Contraindications for Continued Therapy with Albumin-bound Paclitaxel for Pancreatic Cancer

When dosage modification is necessary for patients receiving albumin-bound paclitaxel and gemcitabine for pancreatic cancer, dosage of albumin-bound paclitaxel should be reduced in decrements of 25 mg/m² (i.e., 1 dose level) and dosage of gemcitabine should be reduced in decrements of 200 mg/m² (i.e., 1 dose level); however, if a dose of albumin-bound paclitaxel 75 mg/m² or gemcitabine 600 mg/m² requires further reduction, both drugs should be discontinued.

Hematologic Toxicity

For patients receiving albumin-bound paclitaxel, repeat cycles of the drug should be withheld until neutrophil counts are at least 1500/mm³ and platelet counts are at least 100,000/mm³. See Table 1 for recommended dosage modifications for hematologic toxicity occurring either within a cycle or at the start of a repeat cycle of albumin-bound paclitaxel and gemcitabine therapy in patients with pancreatic cancer.

TABLE 1. Recommended Dosage Modifications for Hematologic Toxicity During or at the Start of a Cycle of Albumin-bound Paclitaxel and Gemcitabine for Pancreatic Cancer

Cycle Day and Cell Counts (cells/mm³)	Albumin-bound Paclitaxel and Gemcitabine Dosage Modification
Day 1:	
Neutrophil count <1500 or platelet count <100,000	Delay start of cycle until recovery
Day 8:	
Neutrophil count 500 to <1000 or platelet count 50,000 to <75,000	Reduce dose of both drugs by 1 dose level
Neutrophil count <500 or platelet count <50,000	Withhold day 8 dose of both drugs
Day 15 (when day 8 doses were reduced or given without modification):	
Neutrophil count 500 to <1000 or platelet count 50,000 to <75,000	Reduce dose of both drugs by 1 dose level from day 8
Neutrophil count <500 or platelet count <50,000	Withhold day 15 dose of both drugs
Day 15 (when day 8 doses were withheld):	
Neutrophil count ≥1000 or platelet count ≥75,000	Reduce dose of both drugs by 1 dose level from day 1
Neutrophil count 500 to <1000 or platelet count 50,000 to <75,000	Reduce dose of both drugs by 2 dose levels from day 1
Neutrophil count <500 or platelet count <50,000	Withhold day 15 dose of both drugs

For patients with pancreatic cancer who experience grade 3 or 4 febrile neutropenia while receiving albumin-bound paclitaxel and gemcitabine, therapy should be withheld until fever resolves and neutrophil count reaches or exceeds 1500/mm³; albumin-bound paclitaxel and gemcitabine may then be resumed at 1 dose level lower than the previous dosage.

Sensitivity Reactions

Further therapy with paclitaxel should *not* be undertaken in any patient who experienced a severe hypersensitivity reaction during a previous course of therapy with the drug. It is not known whether patients who have exhibited hypersensitivity to conventional paclitaxel can tolerate subsequent therapy with albumin-bound paclitaxel.

Hepatic Toxicity

In patients with preexisting hepatic impairment, dose reduction is recommended depending on the degree of hepatic impairment for the first course of therapy with albumin-bound paclitaxel. Further dose reduction may be required during subsequent courses of albumin-bound paclitaxel therapy based on hepatic toxicity. (See Dosage of Albumin-bound Paclitaxel in Hepatic Impairment under Dosage and Administration: Dosage in Renal and Hepatic Impairment.)

Neurologic Toxicity

Sensory neuropathy associated with albumin-bound paclitaxel is dose and schedule dependent.

For patients who experience grade 1 or 2 peripheral neuropathy while receiving albumin-bound paclitaxel, dosage modification generally is not required.

For patients with pancreatic cancer who experience grade 3 or 4 peripheral neuropathy while receiving albumin-bound paclitaxel and gemcitabine, treatment with albumin-bound paclitaxel should be withheld until resolution to grade 1 or less; the drug may then be resumed at 1 dose level lower than the previous dosage. No modification of gemcitabine dosage is required.

Dermatologic Toxicity

For patients with pancreatic cancer who experience grade 2 or 3 cutaneous toxicity while receiving albumin-bound paclitaxel and gemcitabine, the dose of albumin-bound paclitaxel and gemcitabine should be reduced by 1 dose level. If cutaneous toxicity persists, treatment should be discontinued.

GI Toxicity

For patients with pancreatic cancer who experience grade 3 mucositis or diarrhea while receiving albumin-bound paclitaxel and gemcitabine, treatment should be withheld until resolution to grade 1 or less; albumin-bound paclitaxel and gemcitabine may then be resumed at 1 dose level lower than the previous dosage.

Pulmonary Toxicity

For patients with pancreatic cancer who develop signs and symptoms of pneumonitis while receiving albumin-bound paclitaxel and gemcitabine, therapy should be interrupted during evaluation of suspected pneumonitis. Albumin-bound paclitaxel and gemcitabine should be permanently discontinued in patients diagnosed with pneumonitis.

• Dosage in Renal and Hepatic Impairment

The effect of renal impairment on the disposition of paclitaxel has not been fully established. Reduction of paclitaxel dosage in patients with impaired renal function does not appear to be necessary.

Paclitaxel is metabolized mainly in the liver, and increased toxicity may occur in patients with hepatic impairment.

Dosage of Conventional Paclitaxel in Hepatic Impairment

Toxicity associated with paclitaxel, particularly grade 3 or 4 myelosuppression, may be exacerbated in patients with serum total bilirubin concentrations greater than 2 times the upper limit of normal. Paclitaxel should be used with extreme caution in patients with hepatic impairment, and dosage reduction is recommended depending on the degree of hepatic impairment. Such patients should be monitored closely for the development of profound myelosuppression.

For patients receiving conventional paclitaxel as a 24-hour IV infusion for ovarian or non-small cell lung cancer, the usual dose of 135 mg/m^2 may be administered for the first course of therapy in those who have serum transaminase concentrations less than 2 times the upper limit of normal and serum bilirubin concentrations up to 1.5 mg/dL; for patients with elevated serum transaminase concentrations less than 10 times the upper limit of normal and serum bilirubin concentrations up to 1.5 mg/dL, a reduced dose of paclitaxel 100 mg/m^2 is recommended; for patients with elevated serum transaminase concentrations less than 10 times the upper limit of normal and serum bilirubin concentrations of 1.6–7.5 mg/dL, a reduced dose of paclitaxel 50 mg/m^2 is recommended. For patients with elevated serum transaminase concentrations at least 10 times the upper limit of normal or serum bilirubin concentrations exceeding 7.5 mg/dL, paclitaxel therapy is *not* recommended.

For patients receiving conventional paclitaxel as a 3-hour IV infusion for ovarian or breast cancer, the usual dose of 175 mg/m^2 may be administered for the first course of therapy in those who have serum transaminase concentrations less than 10 times the upper limit of normal and serum bilirubin concentrations up to 1.25 times the upper limit of normal; for patients with serum transaminase concentrations less than 10 times the upper limit of normal and serum bilirubin concentrations of 1.26–2 times the upper limit of normal, a reduced dose of paclitaxel 135 mg/m^2 is recommended; for patients with serum transaminase concentrations less than 10 times the upper limit of normal and serum bilirubin concentrations of 2.01–5 times the upper limit of normal, a reduced dose of paclitaxel 90 mg/m^2 is recommended. For patients with elevated serum transaminase concentrations at least 10 times the upper limit of normal or serum bilirubin concentrations exceeding 5 times the upper limit of normal, paclitaxel therapy is *not* recommended.

Further reduction of paclitaxel dosage for subsequent courses of therapy should be based on patient tolerance.

Dosage of Albumin-bound Paclitaxel in Hepatic Impairment

Patients should be monitored closely since toxicity associated with paclitaxel may be exacerbated in patients with hepatic impairment. Paclitaxel should be used with caution in patients with hepatic impairment, and dosage reduction is recommended depending on the degree of hepatic impairment. No adjustment of the initial dosage is required in patients with mild hepatic impairment.

Breast Cancer

For patients receiving albumin-bound paclitaxel for breast cancer, the usual dose of 260 mg/m^2 may be administered for the first course of therapy in those who have mild hepatic impairment (AST concentrations less than 10 times the upper limit of normal and elevated serum bilirubin concentrations up to 1.25 times the upper limit of normal).

For patients with moderate hepatic impairment (AST concentrations less than 10 times the upper limit of normal and serum bilirubin concentrations of 1.26–2 times the upper limit of normal), a reduced initial dose of albumin-bound paclitaxel 200 mg/m^2 is recommended. For patients with severe hepatic impairment (AST concentrations less than 10 times the upper limit of normal and serum bilirubin concentrations of 2.01–5 times the upper limit of normal), a reduced initial dose of albumin-bound paclitaxel 130 mg/m^2 is recommended. If the 130-mg/m^2 dose of albumin-bound paclitaxel is tolerated, the dose may be increased to 200 mg/m^2 in subsequent cycles. For patients with serum AST concentrations exceeding 10 times the upper limit of normal or serum bilirubin concentrations exceeding 5 times the upper limit of normal, albumin-bound paclitaxel therapy is *not* recommended. Further reduction of albumin-bound paclitaxel dosage for subsequent courses of therapy should be based on patient tolerance.

Non-small Cell Lung Cancer

For patients receiving albumin-bound paclitaxel for non-small cell lung cancer, the usual dose of 100 mg/m^2 may be administered for the first course of therapy in those who have mild hepatic impairment (AST concentrations less than 10 times the upper limit of normal and elevated serum bilirubin concentrations up to 1.25 times the upper limit of normal).

For patients with moderate hepatic impairment (AST concentrations less than 10 times the upper limit of normal and serum bilirubin concentrations of 1.26–2 times the upper limit of normal), a reduced initial dose of albumin-bound paclitaxel 75 mg/m^2 is recommended. For patients with severe hepatic impairment (AST concentrations less than 10 times the upper limit of normal and serum bilirubin concentrations of 2.01–5 times the upper limit of normal), a reduced initial dose of albumin-bound paclitaxel 50 mg/m^2 is recommended. If the 50-mg/m^2 dose of albumin-bound paclitaxel is tolerated, the dose may be increased to 75 mg/m^2 in subsequent cycles. For patients with serum AST concentrations exceeding 10 times the upper limit of normal or serum bilirubin concentrations exceeding 5 times the upper limit of normal, albumin-bound paclitaxel therapy is *not* recommended. Patients with serum bilirubin concentrations exceeding the upper limit of normal were excluded from clinical studies evaluating use of the drug in non-small cell lung cancer. Further reduction of albumin-bound paclitaxel dosage for subsequent courses of therapy should be based on patient tolerance.

Pancreatic Cancer

For patients receiving albumin-bound paclitaxel for pancreatic cancer, the usual dose of 125 mg/m² may be administered for the first course of therapy in those who have mild hepatic impairment (AST concentrations less than 10 times the upper limit of normal and elevated serum bilirubin concentrations up to 1.25 times the upper limit of normal). For patients with AST concentrations less than 10 times the upper limit of normal and serum bilirubin concentrations of 1.26–5 times the upper limit of normal, AST concentrations exceeding 10 times the upper limit of normal, or serum bilirubin concentrations exceeding 5 times the upper limit of normal, albumin-bound paclitaxel therapy is *not* recommended. Patients with serum bilirubin concentrations exceeding the upper limit of normal were excluded from clinical studies evaluating use of the drug in pancreatic cancer. Further reduction of albumin-bound paclitaxel dosage for subsequent courses of therapy should be based on patient tolerance.

CAUTIONS

● Hematologic Effects and Infectious Complications

The major and dose-limiting adverse effect of paclitaxel is bone marrow suppression, manifested by neutropenia, leukopenia, thrombocytopenia, and anemia. The frequency and severity of hematologic toxicity increase with higher dose, especially at conventional paclitaxel doses exceeding 190 mg/m². Paclitaxel-induced neutropenia does not appear to increase with cumulative exposure and does not appear to be more frequent or more severe in patients who have received prior radiation therapy. In clinical studies, myelosuppression was more profound when paclitaxel was given after cisplatin rather than with the alternative sequence (i.e., paclitaxel before cisplatin), apparently because plasma clearance of paclitaxel was decreased by approximately 33% when the drugs were administered in this sequence.

Neutropenia and Leukopenia

Paclitaxel-induced neutropenia, which is dose and schedule dependent, generally is rapidly reversible.

Conventional Paclitaxel

Neutropenia (neutrophil count less than 2000/mm³) occurred in 90% of patients with ovarian or breast cancer and in 95–100% of patients with AIDS-related Kaposi's sarcoma receiving paclitaxel as a single agent in clinical trials. Severe neutropenia (neutrophil count less than 500/mm³) occurred in 52% of patients during paclitaxel monotherapy for ovarian or breast cancer. In a phase III clinical trial of patients with metastatic ovarian cancer receiving subsequent therapy with paclitaxel alone at a dose of 135 or 175 mg/m² administered as an infusion over 3 hours, severe neutropenia occurred in 14 or 27%, respectively. In patients with AIDS-related Kaposi's sarcoma receiving paclitaxel 100 or 135 mg/m² by 3-hour IV infusion, severe neutropenia occurred in 35 or 76%, respectively.

In a randomized trial in patients receiving initial treatment for advanced ovarian cancer, grade 4 neutropenia occurred in 81%, and febrile neutropenia occurred in 15%, of patients receiving paclitaxel 135 mg/m² by 24-hour IV infusion followed by cisplatin; episodes of fever associated with grade 4 neutropenia were reported in approximately 3% of courses. In another randomized trial in patients receiving initial treatment for advanced ovarian cancer, grade 4 neutropenia occurred in 33%, and febrile neutropenia occurred in 4%, of patients receiving paclitaxel 175 mg/m² by 3-hour IV infusion followed by cisplatin. In patients with node-positive breast cancer receiving cyclophosphamide and doxorubicin followed by paclitaxel, grade 4 neutropenia was reported in 76% of patients but it occurred during the period of paclitaxel therapy in only 15% of patients. In patients with non-small cell lung cancer receiving initial treatment with paclitaxel 135 mg/m² by 24-hour IV infusion followed by cisplatin, neutropenia occurred in 89% of patients and was severe in 74% of patients.

The onset of neutropenia usually occurs by 8–10 days and neutrophil nadirs generally occur at a median of 10–12 days following paclitaxel administration; neutrophil counts commonly recover by 15–21 days after administration. Subsequent paclitaxel courses of therapy generally do not result in lower neutrophil nadirs than the initial course, suggesting that the drug may not be irreversibly toxic to stem cells. Some data suggest that the addition of filgrastim to paclitaxel therapy may reduce the duration and severity of neutropenia and/or allow dose intensification. There also is some evidence that shorter paclitaxel infusion times (e.g., 3 hours) may result in a lower frequency and severity of neutropenia. In a phase III trial of subsequent therapy for patients with metastatic ovarian cancer,

neutropenia, including severe neutropenia, occurred more frequently in patients receiving paclitaxel doses by 24-hour infusion than in those receiving the drug by 3-hour infusion; duration of infusion had a greater effect on paclitaxel-induced myelosuppression than did the amount of dose (135 versus 175 mg/m²).

Leukopenia (less than 4000/mm³) occurred in 90% of patients with ovarian or breast cancer receiving paclitaxel as a single agent in clinical trials and was severe (less than 1000/mm³) in 17% of patients.

Albumin-bound Paclitaxel

Neutropenia (neutrophil count less than 2000/mm³) occurred in 80%, severe neutropenia (neutrophil count less than 500/mm³) occurred in 9%, and febrile neutropenia occurred in 2% of patients receiving albumin-bound paclitaxel for metastatic breast cancer. In a phase III clinical trial of patients with advanced non-small cell lung cancer receiving therapy with albumin-bound paclitaxel 100 mg/m² by 30-minute IV infusion in combination with carboplatin, grade 3 or 4 neutropenia occurred in 47% of patients. In patients with metastatic pancreatic cancer receiving albumin-bound paclitaxel 125 mg/m² by 30- to 40-minute IV infusion in combination with gemcitabine, grade 3 or 4 neutropenia occurred in 38% of patients.

Infectious Complications
Conventional Paclitaxel

Fever was associated with 12% of all paclitaxel treatment courses in patients with solid tumors receiving the drug as a single agent. Among patients receiving paclitaxel monotherapy for ovarian or breast cancer, at least one episode of infection was reported in 30% of patients, and 9% of all treatment courses were associated with an infectious episode. These infectious episodes, including sepsis, pneumonia, and peritonitis, were fatal in 1% of all patients. In a phase III trial of paclitaxel as subsequent therapy for patients with metastatic ovarian cancer, infectious episodes occurred in 20 or 26% of patients receiving paclitaxel 135 or 175 mg/m², respectively, by 3-hour infusion. Urinary and respiratory tract infections were the most frequently reported infectious complications.

In patients with node-positive breast cancer receiving cyclophosphamide and doxorubicin followed by paclitaxel, severe infection was reported in 14% of patients. In patients with non-small cell lung cancer receiving initial treatment with paclitaxel 135 mg/m² by 24-hour IV infusion followed by cisplatin, infections occurred in 38% of patients.

Among patients receiving paclitaxel for AIDS-related Kaposi's sarcoma, at least one episode of opportunistic infection was reported in 61% of patients. In patients with AIDS-related Kaposi's sarcoma, febrile neutropenia (neutrophil count less than 500/mm³ with fever exceeding 38°C and IV anti-infectives and/or hospitalization required) occurred in 55% of patients receiving paclitaxel 135 mg/m² and in 9% of those receiving paclitaxel 100 mg/m².

Albumin-bound Paclitaxel

Infection was reported in 24% of patients receiving albumin-bound paclitaxel for metastatic breast cancer. Oral candidiasis, respiratory tract infections, and pneumonia were the most frequently reported infectious complications. In patients with metastatic breast cancer, febrile neutropenia occurred in 2% of patients receiving albumin-bound paclitaxel as a single agent.

Among patients receiving albumin-bound paclitaxel combined with gemcitabine for pancreatic cancer, pyrexia was reported in 41% of patients and urinary tract infections were reported in 11% of patients. Other infections reported in less than 10% of patients were oral candidiasis and pneumonia. In patients with pancreatic cancer, sepsis (irrespective of neutrophil count) occurred in 5% of patients receiving albumin-bound paclitaxel combined with gemcitabine; biliary obstruction or the presence of a biliary stent appear to be risk factors for sepsis.

Thrombocytopenia
Conventional Paclitaxel

Thrombocytopenia (platelet count less than 100,000/mm³) developed less frequently than neutropenia, with at least one episode occurring in 20% of patients with ovarian or breast cancer receiving paclitaxel alone as subsequent therapy in clinical trials, and was severe (platelet count less than 50,000/mm³) in 7% of patients. In patients with AIDS-related Kaposi's sarcoma receiving paclitaxel 135 or 100 mg/m², thrombocytopenia occurred in 52 or 27% of patients, and was severe in 17 or 5%, respectively.

In randomized trials for the initial treatment of advanced ovarian cancer, thrombocytopenia (platelet count less than 130,000/mm³) was reported in 21% of patients receiving paclitaxel 175 mg/m² by 3-hour IV infusion followed by cisplatin, and thrombocytopenia (platelet count less than 100,000/mm³) was reported in 26% of patients receiving paclitaxel 135 mg/m² by 24-hour IV infusion followed by cisplatin. In patients with node-positive breast cancer receiving cyclophosphamide and doxorubicin followed by paclitaxel, severe thrombocytopenia (platelet count less than 50,000/mm³) was reported in 25% of patients. In patients with non-small cell lung cancer receiving initial treatment with paclitaxel 135 mg/m² by 24-hour IV infusion followed by cisplatin, thrombocytopenia occurred in 48% of patients and was severe (platelet count less than 50,000/mm³) in 6% of patients.

Platelet nadirs usually occur 8 or 9 days after administration of the drug. Bleeding episodes occurred in 14% of patients with ovarian or breast cancer receiving paclitaxel alone as subsequent therapy and in 4% of all treatment courses, but most episodes were localized, and the frequency of such events was unrelated to paclitaxel dose or schedule; 2% of patients received platelet transfusions. In a phase III clinical trial of subsequent therapy for metastatic ovarian carcinoma, bleeding episodes were reported in 10% of patients receiving paclitaxel (135 or 175 mg/m²) by 3-hour infusion; none of the patients who were treated with the 3-hour infusion received platelet transfusions.

Albumin-bound Paclitaxel

Thrombocytopenia (platelet count less than 100,000/mm³) occurred in 2%, and was severe (platelet count less than 50,000/mm³) in less than 1%, of patients receiving albumin-bound paclitaxel for metastatic breast cancer. Bleeding was reported in 2% of patients. In a phase III clinical trial of patients with advanced non-small cell lung cancer receiving therapy with albumin-bound paclitaxel 100 mg/m² by 30-minute IV infusion in combination with carboplatin, grade 3 or 4 thrombocytopenia occurred in 18% of patients; epistaxis occurred in 7% of patients. In patients with metastatic pancreatic cancer receiving albumin-bound paclitaxel 125 mg/m² by 30- to 40-minute IV infusion in combination with gemcitabine, grade 3 or 4 thrombocytopenia occurred in 13% of patients; epistaxis occurred in 15% of patients.

Anemia
Conventional Paclitaxel

Anemia (hemoglobin less than 11 g/dL) occurred in 78% of patients with ovarian or breast cancer receiving paclitaxel monotherapy in clinical trials and was severe (less than 8 g/dL) in 16% of patients. No consistent relationship between paclitaxel dose or schedule and the frequency of anemia was observed. Anemia occurred in 69% of patients with a baseline hemoglobin of 11 g/dL or higher at study entry, and 7% had severe anemia. Among patients receiving paclitaxel alone as subsequent therapy for ovarian or breast cancer, packed red blood cell transfusions were administered to 25% of all patients and to 12% of patients with a baseline hemoglobin of 11 g/dL or higher. In patients with AIDS-related Kaposi's sarcoma receiving paclitaxel 135 or 100 mg/m², anemia occurred in 86 or 73% of patients, and was severe in 34 or 25%, respectively.

In randomized trials for the initial treatment of advanced ovarian cancer, anemia (hemoglobin less than 12 g/dL) was reported in 96% of patients receiving paclitaxel 175 mg/m² by 3-hour IV infusion followed by cisplatin, and anemia (hemoglobin less than 11 g/dL) was reported in 88% of patients receiving paclitaxel 135 mg/m² by 24-hour IV infusion followed by cisplatin. In patients with node-positive breast cancer receiving cyclophosphamide and doxorubicin followed by paclitaxel, severe anemia (hemoglobin less than 8 g/dL) was reported in 21% of patients. In patients receiving paclitaxel 135 mg/m² by 24-hour IV infusion followed by cisplatin for the initial treatment of advanced non-small cell lung cancer, anemia occurred in 94% of patients and was severe (hemoglobin less than 8 g/dL) in 22% of patients.

Albumin-bound Paclitaxel

Anemia (hemoglobin less than 11 g/dL) occurred in 33%, and was severe (hemoglobin less than 8 g/dL) in 1%, of patients receiving albumin-bound paclitaxel for metastatic breast cancer.

Anemia of grade 3 or 4 severity occurred in 28% of patients receiving albumin-bound paclitaxel combined with carboplatin for non-small cell lung cancer.

Eosinophilia

Eosinophilia was reported in 40% of patients receiving a paclitaxel dose of 135 mg/m² for AIDS-related Kaposi's sarcoma.

• Sensitivity Reactions
Conventional Paclitaxel

Anaphylaxis and severe hypersensitivity reactions have occurred in 2–4% of patients receiving conventional paclitaxel in clinical trials. Paclitaxel frequently causes hypersensitivity reactions, and all patients receiving the conventional formulation of the drug should be premedicated to prevent severe reactions. (See Dosage and Administration: Dosage.) Fatal hypersensitivity reactions have occurred in patients receiving conventional paclitaxel despite premedication.

In clinical trials involving use of paclitaxel alone as subsequent therapy for ovarian or breast cancer, 20% of all courses of paclitaxel therapy were associated with hypersensitivity reactions; reactions occurred in 41% of patients despite premedication and were severe in 2%. The frequency and severity of hypersensitivity reactions were not affected by the dose or schedule of paclitaxel administration in patients receiving the drug alone as subsequent therapy for ovarian cancer. The frequency and severity of hypersensitivity reactions were not affected by dose in patients receiving the drug alone as subsequent therapy for breast cancer. In patients with AIDS-related Kaposi's sarcoma receiving paclitaxel 135 or 100 mg/m², hypersensitivity reactions occurred in 14 or 9% of patients, respectively.

In randomized trials for the initial treatment of advanced ovarian cancer, hypersensitivity reactions were reported in 11% of patients receiving paclitaxel 175 mg/m² by 3-hour IV infusion followed by cisplatin and in 8% of patients receiving paclitaxel 135 mg/m² by 24-hour IV infusion followed by cisplatin. In patients with node-positive breast cancer receiving cyclophosphamide and doxorubicin followed by paclitaxel, severe hypersensitivity reactions were reported in 4% of patients; all patients were designated to receive premedication. In patients with non-small cell lung cancer receiving initial treatment with paclitaxel 135 mg/m² by 24-hour IV infusion followed by cisplatin, hypersensitivity reactions occurred in 16% of patients and were severe in 1%.

The most frequent manifestations of minor hypersensitivity reactions were flushing (28%), rash (12%), hypotension (4%), dyspnea (2%), tachycardia (2%), and hypertension (1%), as observed in patients receiving paclitaxel alone as subsequent therapy for ovarian or breast cancer. Rarely, chills and back pain have been reported in association with hypersensitivity reactions in patients receiving paclitaxel. The frequency of hypersensitivity reactions remained relatively stable during the entire treatment period.

Severe reactions, which generally occur within the first hour of paclitaxel infusion, are characterized by dyspnea and hypotension requiring treatment, flushing, chest pains, tachycardia, angioedema, and generalized urticaria, and are probably histamine mediated. Delayed onset of urticarial rash, 7–10 days following completion of a course of therapy, has been observed in patients receiving paclitaxel for AIDS-related Kaposi's sarcoma. Discontinuance of paclitaxel therapy and aggressive management of symptoms are required in patients experiencing severe hypersensitivity reactions. (See Dosage Modification for Toxicity and Contraindications for Continued Therapy: Sensitivity Reactions in Dosage and Administration: Dosage.)

The exact cause of the hypersensitivity reactions is not known, but they may result from the polyoxyl 35 castor oil (Cremophor® EL, polyethoxylated castor oil) in the paclitaxel for injection concentrate or from paclitaxel itself. (For information on hypersensitivity reactions associated with this vehicle, see Cautions: Sensitivity Reactions, in Cyclosporine 92:44.)

Other cutaneous reactions associated with hypersensitivity to paclitaxel, including acral erythema, generalized pustular dermatosis, and bullous fixed drug eruption, have been reported.

Albumin-bound Paclitaxel

Hypersensitivity reactions occurred in 4% of patients receiving albumin-bound paclitaxel for metastatic breast cancer; no severe hypersensitivity reactions were reported. Hypersensitivity reactions, which were grade 1 or 2 in severity, occurred on the day that albumin-bound paclitaxel was administered and consisted of dyspnea in 1%, and flushing, hypotension, chest pain, or arrhythmia, each in less than 1% of patients. However, severe and sometimes fatal hypersensitivity reactions have been reported during postmarketing experience in patients receiving albumin-bound paclitaxel. The use of albumin-bound paclitaxel in patients who have experienced hypersensitivity reactions to conventional paclitaxel has not been studied.

• Nervous System Effects

The frequency and severity of adverse neurologic effects were dose dependent in patients receiving therapy with conventional or albumin-bound paclitaxel. The frequency and severity of neurologic toxicity in patients receiving paclitaxel were influenced by prior and/or concomitant therapy with neurotoxic agents.

Peripheral Neuropathy

Conventional Paclitaxel

Peripheral neuropathy was reported in 60% of all patients receiving paclitaxel alone as subsequent therapy for ovarian or breast cancer in clinical trials, and in 52% of patients without preexisting neuropathy. Among patients receiving paclitaxel alone as subsequent therapy for ovarian or breast cancer, paclitaxel-induced neuropathy was severe in 3% of patients (2% of patients without preexisting neuropathy) and required discontinuance of the drug in 1% of patients. The frequency and severity of peripheral neuropathy increased with the higher dose but did not appear to be affected by the schedule of paclitaxel administration in patients receiving the drug alone as subsequent therapy for ovarian cancer. The frequency and severity of peripheral neuropathy increased with the higher dose in patients receiving the drug alone as subsequent therapy for breast cancer. In patients with AIDS-related Kaposi's sarcoma receiving paclitaxel 135 or 100 mg/m², peripheral neuropathy occurred in 79 or 46% of patients, and was severe in 10 or 2%, respectively.

Comparison across studies in patients with ovarian cancer suggests that higher incidences of neurotoxicity and severe neurotoxicity occur when paclitaxel 175 mg/m² by 3-hour IV infusion is followed by cisplatin. In randomized trials for the initial treatment of advanced ovarian cancer, neuromotor or neurosensory toxicity was reported in 87% (severe in 21%) of patients receiving paclitaxel 175 mg/m² by 3-hour IV infusion followed by cisplatin, and peripheral neuropathy was reported in 25% (severe in 3%) of patients receiving paclitaxel 135 mg/m² by 24-hour IV infusion followed by cisplatin. In patients with node-positive breast cancer receiving cyclophosphamide and doxorubicin followed by paclitaxel, grade 2 or 3 neurosensory toxicity occurred during the period of paclitaxel therapy in 15% of patients. In patients with advanced non-small cell lung cancer receiving initial treatment with paclitaxel 135 mg/m² by 24-hour IV infusion followed by cisplatin, neuromotor toxicity occurred in 37% of patients and was severe in 6%; neurosensory toxicity occurred in 48% of patients and was severe in 13%. This incidence of severe neurotoxicity in patients with non-small cell lung cancer receiving paclitaxel followed by cisplatin is higher than the incidence (severe peripheral neuropathy in 3%) reported in patients with ovarian or breast cancer receiving paclitaxel alone.

The neuropathy usually is sensory in nature and is characterized by paresthesia with numbness and tingling in a stocking-and-glove distribution. Perioral numbness also has been reported, and many patients experience burning pain (often associated with hyperesthesia), particularly in the feet. The onset may be rapid, occurring within a few days. Pruritus preceding the onset of peripheral neuropathy has been reported in patients receiving high doses of paclitaxel by 3-hour IV infusion; paclitaxel-induced pruritus was relieved by treatment with tricyclic antidepressant therapy. One patient experienced a "recall" reaction of severe peripheral neuropathy following extravasation of paclitaxel.

The frequency and severity of peripheral neuropathy are dose dependent and increase with cumulative dose; toxicity may be dose limiting or require dose modification.

The frequency and severity of paclitaxel-induced neurotoxicity increase with dose, especially at doses exceeding 190 mg/m². Among patients receiving paclitaxel alone as subsequent therapy for ovarian or breast cancer, neurologic manifestations were apparent in 27% of patients following the initial course of therapy and in 34–51% of patients receiving 2–10 courses of therapy; such manifestations tended to worsen with increasing exposure to the drug. Sensory manifestations usually improve or resolve within several months after discontinuance of paclitaxel. Infrequently, motor neuron toxicity also has occurred in patients receiving the drug.

Preexisting neuropathies resulting from previous therapies are not a contraindication to paclitaxel therapy; however, the incidence of paclitaxel-related neurotoxicity appears to be increased in patients with preexisting neuropathy or other risk factors for neuropathy.

Albumin-bound Paclitaxel

Sensory neuropathy occurred in 71%, and was severe in 10%, of patients receiving albumin-bound paclitaxel for metastatic breast cancer. The frequency of sensory neuropathy increased with the cumulative dose of albumin-bound paclitaxel. In the randomized trial comparing albumin-bound paclitaxel with conventional paclitaxel for metastatic breast cancer, 24 (10%) of 229 patients receiving albumin-bound paclitaxel developed grade 3 peripheral neuropathy, and none developed grade 4 peripheral neuropathy. Of these 24 patients, amelioration of symptoms at a median of 22 days was documented in 14 patients; 10 patients resumed treatment at a reduced dose of albumin-bound paclitaxel, and 2 patients discontinued therapy with the drug. Improvement was not documented in the other 10 patients, and 4 of these patients discontinued therapy with albumin-bound paclitaxel.

Peripheral neuropathy occurred in 48%, and was severe in 3%, of patients receiving albumin-bound paclitaxel combined with carboplatin for non-small cell lung cancer. In the randomized trial comparing albumin-bound paclitaxel combined with carboplatin with conventional paclitaxel combined with carboplatin for non-small cell lung cancer, 3% of patients receiving albumin-bound paclitaxel combined with carboplatin developed grade 3 peripheral neuropathy and none developed grade 4 peripheral neuropathy. Grade 3 peripheral neuropathy improved to grade 1 or resolved in 59% of these patients following interruption or discontinuation of albumin-bound paclitaxel therapy. In comparison, severe (grade 3 or 4) peripheral neuropathy occurred in 12% of patients receiving conventional paclitaxel combined with carboplatin.

Peripheral neuropathy occurred in 54%, and was severe in 17%, of patients receiving albumin-bound paclitaxel combined with gemcitabine for metastatic pancreatic cancer. In the randomized trial comparing albumin-bound paclitaxel combined with gemcitabine with gemcitabine monotherapy for pancreatic cancer, 17% of patients receiving albumin-bound paclitaxel developed grade 3 peripheral neuropathy, and none developed grade 4 peripheral neuropathy. The median time to onset of grade 3 peripheral neuropathy was 140 days following albumin-bound paclitaxel administration. Amelioration of grade 3 peripheral neuropathy to grade 1 severity or less at a median of 29 days following discontinuance of the drug was reported. Albumin-bound paclitaxel was resumed at a reduced dosage in 44% of patients with grade 3 peripheral neuropathy.

Other Nervous System Effects

Conventional Paclitaxel

Rarely, seizures (including tonoclonic seizures), syncope, ataxia, and neuroencephalopathy have occurred during or immediately following administration of paclitaxel. Autonomic neuropathy resulting in paralytic ileus has been reported rarely in patients receiving paclitaxel. A case of acute and temporary worsening of parkinsonian syndrome following paclitaxel infusion has been reported in a geriatric patient with Parkinson's disease.

The formulation of conventional paclitaxel contains ethyl alcohol, and some adverse neurologic effects of paclitaxel appear to be related to the effects of alcohol, particularly when high doses of conventional paclitaxel are administered over short infusion periods (e.g., 3 hours). CNS toxicity, rarely fatal, has been reported in pediatric patients receiving high doses of conventional paclitaxel by 3-hour IV infusion. (See Cautions: Pediatric Precautions.) Ethanol intoxication has been reported in a patient receiving high doses of conventional paclitaxel (348 mg/m²) by 3-hour IV infusion.

Albumin-bound Paclitaxel

In patients receiving albumin-bound paclitaxel combined with gemcitabine for pancreatic cancer, depression occurred in 12%, and was severe in less than 1%, of patients. Headache occurred in 14%, and was severe in less than 1%, of patients receiving albumin-bound paclitaxel combined with gemcitabine for pancreatic cancer.

Cranial nerve palsies, vocal cord paresis, and autonomic neuropathy resulting in paralytic ileus have been reported in patients receiving albumin-bound paclitaxel.

● Cardiovascular Effects

Hypotension and Bradycardia

Conventional Paclitaxel

Hypotension and bradycardia are the most common adverse cardiovascular effects of paclitaxel. During the first 3 hours of paclitaxel IV infusion in clinical trials of paclitaxel used alone as subsequent therapy for ovarian or breast cancer, hypotension occurred in 12% of all patients and 3% of all treatment courses, and bradycardia occurred in 3% of all patients and 1% of all treatment courses. In a phase III trial of patients receiving paclitaxel alone as subsequent therapy for metastatic ovarian cancer, the frequency of hypotension or bradycardia did not appear to be influenced by paclitaxel dose or schedule. The frequency of hypotension or bradycardia did not appear to be influenced by prior anthracycline therapy. In a phase II study in patients receiving paclitaxel 135 mg/m^2 by 3-hour IV infusion for AIDS-related Kaposi's sarcoma, hypotension and bradycardia occurred in 17 and 3% of all patients, respectively. Hypotension was reported in 9% of patients receiving paclitaxel 100 mg/m^2 by 3-hour IV infusion for AIDS-related Kaposi's sarcoma.

In patients with advanced non-small cell lung cancer receiving initial treatment with paclitaxel 135 mg/m^2 by 24-hour IV infusion followed by cisplatin, adverse cardiovascular effects occurred in 33% of patients and were severe in 13%.

Most episodes of bradycardia and hypotension associated with paclitaxel were asymptomatic and did not require further treatment or discontinuance of the drug, although hypotension associated with severe hypersensitivity reactions to the drug may require intervention. Chest pain is a frequent manifestation of a severe hypersensitivity reaction. (See Cautions: Sensitivity Reactions.) Atypical chest pain also has been reported during paclitaxel infusion and may be another manifestation of a hypersensitivity reaction.

Albumin-bound Paclitaxel

During the 30-minute IV infusion, hypotension occurred in 5%, and bradycardia occurred in less than 1%, of patients receiving albumin-bound paclitaxel for metastatic breast cancer. Most episodes of hypotension or bradycardia were asymptomatic and did not require treatment or discontinuance of the paclitaxel infusion.

Hypertension

Hypertension, often associated with a hypersensitivity reaction, has been observed in patients during administration of conventional paclitaxel. Hypertension also has been reported in patients receiving albumin-bound paclitaxel.

ECG Abnormalities

ECG abnormalities in patients receiving conventional or albumin-bound paclitaxel generally were asymptomatic, were not dose limiting, and did not require therapeutic intervention.

Conventional Paclitaxel

ECG abnormalities were present in 23% of all paclitaxel-treated patients during clinical trials of the drug as a single agent for the subsequent therapy of ovarian or breast cancer, developing in 14% of patients with normal baseline ECGs during therapy with the drug. The most frequent ECG abnormalities included nonspecific repolarization, sinus bradycardia, sinus tachycardia, and premature beats. Among patients with normal baseline ECGs, prior therapy with anthracyclines did not influence the frequency of ECG abnormalities.

Albumin-bound Paclitaxel

ECG abnormalities were observed in 60% of all patients receiving albumin-bound paclitaxel for metastatic breast cancer and developed in 35% of patients with normal baseline ECGs. The most frequent ECG abnormalities included nonspecific repolarization, sinus bradycardia, and sinus tachycardia.

Arrhythmias, Conduction Abnormalities, and Other Severe Cardiovascular Effects

Conventional Paclitaxel

Severe adverse cardiovascular effects occurred in about 1% of all patients receiving paclitaxel alone as subsequent therapy for ovarian or breast cancer in clinical trials. These effects included arrhythmias (e.g., asymptomatic ventricular tachycardia, bigeminy, syncope, hypertension, and venous thrombosis. In one patient treated with paclitaxel 175 mg/m^2 over 24 hours, syncope was accompanied by progressive hypotension and resulted in death. Severe conduction abnormalities, such as complete atrioventricular (AV) block requiring pacemaker insertion, have occurred in less than 1% of patients receiving paclitaxel. Atrial fibrillation and supraventricular tachycardia have been reported rarely in patients receiving paclitaxel. Junctional tachycardia has been reported in patients receiving paclitaxel. A higher incidence of severe adverse cardiovascular effects (12–13%) was reported in patients with advanced non-small cell lung cancer receiving paclitaxel in combination with cisplatin; difference in the cardiovascular risk factors in this patient population may have contributed to this increase.

Rarely, vascular toxicity, including myocardial infarction, has been reported in patients receiving paclitaxel. In one case, fatal myocardial infarction not preceded by an arrhythmia occurred during paclitaxel infusion in a patient with atherosclerotic cardiovascular disease. A patient with no history of cardiac disease experienced acute myocardial infarction while receiving paclitaxel therapy for metastatic breast cancer and subsequently died; previous radiation therapy to the left breast may have increased the risk of myocardial infarction in this patient. In another patient, sudden death occurred 7 days following completion of paclitaxel infusion; the immediate cause of death was determined to be acute pulmonary edema, which was probably caused by acute heart failure. Cerebrovascular infarction occurred 36 hours following completion of paclitaxel infusion in a patient with metastatic ovarian cancer; although the mechanism is not clear, it has been suggested that administration of paclitaxel precipitated thrombus formation in a patient predisposed to thromboembolic disorder by underlying disease.

Albumin-bound Paclitaxel

Severe adverse cardiovascular effects occurred in about 3% of patients receiving albumin-bound paclitaxel for metastatic breast cancer. These effects included chest pain, cardiac arrest, cardiac ischemia, myocardial infarction, supraventricular tachycardia, edema, thrombosis, pulmonary thromboembolism, pulmonary embolism, and hypertension. Cerebrovascular events (strokes) and transient ischemic attacks also have been reported in patients receiving albumin-bound paclitaxel for metastatic breast cancer. Other adverse cardiovascular effects reported in patients receiving albumin-bound paclitaxel include tachycardia and AV block.

Congestive Heart Failure and Cardiomyopathy

Conventional Paclitaxel

Congestive heart failure, with progressive deterioration and death in at least one patient, has been reported in patients receiving paclitaxel who had also received previous chemotherapy, including anthracyclines. Although congestive heart failure has been associated with anthracycline therapy, suspected paclitaxel-induced myocardial damage detected by electron microscopy has been reported. Cardiomyopathy associated with acute renal failure has been reported in a patient receiving paclitaxel for AIDS-related Kaposi's sarcoma; although this may have been a complication of the underlying disease, a causal relationship with the administration of paclitaxel could not be ruled out.

Albumin-bound Paclitaxel

Congestive heart failure and left ventricular dysfunction have been reported in patients receiving albumin-bound paclitaxel, generally in those who previously received cardiotoxic drugs such as anthracyclines or had a history of cardiac disease.

Edema

Conventional Paclitaxel

In clinical trials of paclitaxel as a single agent for the subsequent therapy of ovarian or breast cancer, edema occurred in 21% of all patients receiving paclitaxel, 17% of patients without baseline edema, and 5% of treatment courses in patients without baseline edema. Severe edema occurred in 1% of patients receiving subsequent therapy with paclitaxel alone for ovarian or breast cancer, and none of these patients required discontinuance of the drug. Edema in patients receiving paclitaxel commonly was focal and disease related; frequency of edema did not increase with length of time spent in the study.

Albumin-bound Paclitaxel

Edema occurred in 10% of patients receiving albumin-bound paclitaxel for metastatic breast cancer, and none had severe edema. Peripheral edema occurred in 10% of patients receiving albumin-bound paclitaxel combined with carboplatin for non-small cell lung cancer, and none had severe edema. In patients receiving albumin-bound paclitaxel combined with gemcitabine for pancreatic cancer, peripheral edema occurred in 46%, and was severe in 3%, of patients.

● GI Effects

The most common GI toxicities associated with paclitaxel therapy are nausea and vomiting, diarrhea, and mucositis; these adverse effects usually are mild to moderate in severity. Intestinal obstruction, intestinal perforation, pancreatitis, ischemic colitis, and dehydration have occurred in patients receiving paclitaxel. Neutropenic enterocolitis (typhlitis) has been reported rarely in patients receiving conventional paclitaxel (alone or in combination therapy) despite concomitant administration of granulocyte colony-stimulating factor.

Conventional Paclitaxel

Nausea and vomiting occurred in 52% of patients with ovarian or breast cancer and in 69% of patients with AIDS-related Kaposi's sarcoma receiving paclitaxel monotherapy in clinical trials. Higher incidences of nausea and vomiting are reported in clinical trials of combination therapy with paclitaxel and cisplatin for the initial treatment of advanced ovarian cancer (65 and 88%) or non-small cell lung cancer (85 and 87%). In patients with node-positive breast cancer receiving cyclophosphamide and doxorubicin followed by paclitaxel, severe nausea and vomiting was reported in 18% of patients.

Diarrhea and mucositis occurred in 38 and 31%, respectively, of patients receiving paclitaxel alone as subsequent therapy for ovarian or breast cancer. In patients with AIDS-related Kaposi's sarcoma receiving paclitaxel, diarrhea and mucositis occurred in 79 and 28% of patients, respectively; one-third of patients with AIDS-related Kaposi's sarcoma reported diarrhea before initiation of paclitaxel therapy. In randomized trials for the initial treatment of advanced ovarian cancer, diarrhea was reported in 37% of patients receiving paclitaxel 175 mg/m² by 3-hour IV infusion followed by cisplatin and in 16% of patients receiving paclitaxel 135 mg/m² by 24-hour IV infusion followed by cisplatin. In patients with node-positive breast cancer receiving cyclophosphamide and doxorubicin followed by paclitaxel, severe mucositis was reported in 4% of patients. In patients with non-small cell lung cancer receiving initial treatment with paclitaxel 135 mg/m² by 24-hour IV infusion followed by cisplatin, mucositis occurred in 18% of patients and was severe in 1%.

Paclitaxel-induced mucositis is characterized by diffuse ulceration of the lips, oral cavity, and pharynx; dysphagia and pain reflecting esophageal involvement may occur. In clinical trials of paclitaxel as a single agent for the subsequent therapy for ovarian or breast cancer, mucositis was schedule dependent and occurred more frequently in patients receiving paclitaxel by 24-hour infusion than in those receiving the drug by 3-hour infusion.

Anorexia and taste perversion have been reported with use of paclitaxel.

Albumin-bound Paclitaxel

Nausea occurred in 30% and was severe in 3%, diarrhea occurred in 26% and was severe in less than 1%, and vomiting occurred in 18% and was severe in 4% of patients receiving albumin-bound paclitaxel for metastatic breast cancer. Mucositis was reported in 7% of patients receiving albumin-bound paclitaxel for metastatic breast cancer and was severe in less than 1%.

In the randomized trial comparing albumin-bound paclitaxel combined with gemcitabine with gemcitabine monotherapy for pancreatic cancer, nausea occurred in 54% and was severe in 6%, diarrhea occurred in 44% and was severe in 6%, and vomiting occurred in 36% and was severe in 6% of patients receiving albumin-bound paclitaxel. Mucositis was reported in 10% of patients receiving albumin-bound paclitaxel combined with gemcitabine for pancreatic cancer and was severe in 1%. Decreased appetite, dehydration, and dysgeusia were reported in 36, 21, and 16%, respectively, of patients receiving albumin-bound paclitaxel combined with gemcitabine.

• Dermatologic Effects

Conventional Paclitaxel

Alopecia occurred in 87% of patients receiving paclitaxel alone as subsequent therapy for ovarian or breast cancer in clinical trials. In randomized trials for the initial treatment of advanced ovarian cancer, alopecia was reported in 96% of patients receiving paclitaxel 175 mg/m² by 3-hour IV infusion followed by cisplatin and in 55% of patients receiving paclitaxel 135 mg/m² by 24-hour IV infusion followed by cisplatin. In patients with node-positive breast cancer receiving cyclophosphamide and doxorubicin followed by paclitaxel, alopecia occurred during the period of paclitaxel therapy in 46% of patients.

Alopecia, which usually is complete, generally occurs 14–21 days after administration of paclitaxel with a sudden onset, often occurring in a single day. In addition, patients often experience a loss of all body hair including axillary, pubic, and extremity hair and eyelashes and eyebrows. Paclitaxel-induced alopecia is reversible, usually within 6–8 weeks after treatment, and patients receiving multiple courses of therapy often experience hair regrowth after 5–7 cycles.

Transient skin changes have been observed in patients with paclitaxel-induced hypersensitivity reactions. (See Cautions: Sensitivity Reactions.) Nail changes (changes in pigmentation, discoloration of nail bed) occurred in 2% of patients receiving paclitaxel monotherapy for ovarian or breast cancer. Severe nail changes, including dark discoloration of hands and/or feet followed by nail raising and paronychia with exudation and subungual hemorrhage, partial or complete loss of nails, or pain in the nail beds, have been reported in patients receiving paclitaxel on a weekly schedule for metastatic breast cancer. Radiation recall dermatitis associated with paclitaxel, resulting in extensive desquamation and necrosis in one patient with metastatic breast cancer, has been reported in several patients.

Maculopapular rash, pruritus, Stevens-Johnson syndrome, and toxic epidermal necrolysis have been reported rarely in patients receiving paclitaxel.

Albumin-bound Paclitaxel

Alopecia occurred in 90% of patients receiving albumin-bound paclitaxel for metastatic breast cancer. Nail changes, such as changes in pigmentation or discoloration of the nail bed, were uncommon in patients receiving albumin-bound paclitaxel.

In a randomized trial comparing albumin-bound paclitaxel combined with gemcitabine with gemcitabine monotherapy for pancreatic cancer, alopecia occurred in 50% of patients receiving albumin-bound paclitaxel. Rash was reported in 30% of patients receiving albumin-bound paclitaxel combined with gemcitabine for pancreatic cancer and was severe in 2%.

Skin abnormalities related to radiation recall, generalized or maculopapular rash, erythema, pruritus, photosensitivity reactions, Stevens-Johnson syndrome, and toxic epidermal necrolysis also have been reported in patients receiving albumin-bound paclitaxel.

• Local Effects

Specific treatment for paclitaxel-induced extravasation reactions currently is unknown, and the injection site should be monitored closely for possible infiltration of the drug during infusion of conventional or albumin-bound paclitaxel.

Conventional Paclitaxel

Injection site reactions occurred in 13% of patients receiving paclitaxel alone as subsequent therapy for ovarian or breast cancer in clinical studies. Injection site reactions, including reactions secondary to extravasation, usually were mild and were characterized by erythema, tenderness, skin discoloration, or swelling at the injection site. Such reactions have been observed more frequently in patients receiving paclitaxel by 24-hour infusion than in those receiving the drug by 3-hour infusion. Recurrence of skin reactions at a previous site of extravasation (i.e., "recall" reactions) following administration of paclitaxel at a different injection site has been reported rarely.

Rarely, severe local effects of paclitaxel, such as phlebitis, cellulitis, induration, skin exfoliation, necrosis, and fibrosis have been reported. In some patients, the onset of injection site reaction occurred during prolonged infusion of paclitaxel; delayed onset of injection site reactions, 3–13 days following completion of paclitaxel infusion, also has been reported.

Albumin-bound Paclitaxel

Injection site reactions occurred in less than 1% of patients receiving albumin-bound paclitaxel for metastatic breast cancer.

• Musculoskeletal Effects

Arthralgia and/or myalgia usually were transient, occurred 2 or 3 days after administration of conventional or albumin-bound paclitaxel, and resolved within a few days.

Conventional Paclitaxel

Arthralgia and/or myalgia occurred in 60% of patients receiving paclitaxel alone as subsequent therapy for ovarian or breast cancer in clinical trials and was severe in 8% of patients. In patients with AIDS-related Kaposi's sarcoma receiving paclitaxel 135 or 100 mg/m², arthralgia and/or myalgia occurred in 93 or 48% of patients, and was severe in 14 or 16%, respectively.

In randomized trials for the initial treatment of advanced ovarian cancer, myalgia or arthralgia was reported in 60% of patients receiving paclitaxel 175 mg/m² by 3-hour IV infusion followed by cisplatin and in 9% of patients receiving paclitaxel 135 mg/m² by 24-hour IV infusion followed by cisplatin. In patients with node-positive breast cancer receiving cyclophosphamide and doxorubicin followed by paclitaxel, grade 2 or 3 myalgias occurred during the period of paclitaxel therapy in 23% of patients. In patients with advanced non-small cell lung cancer receiving initial treatment with paclitaxel 135 mg/m² by 24-hour IV infusion followed by cisplatin, arthralgia/myalgia occurred in 21% of patients and was severe in 3%.

In clinical trials of patients with ovarian or breast cancer, the frequency and severity of arthralgia and/or myalgia did not appear to be dose or schedule dependent and did not vary throughout the treatment period.

Albumin-bound Paclitaxel

Myalgia and/or arthralgia occurred in 44%, and was severe in 8%, of patients receiving albumin-bound paclitaxel for metastatic breast cancer. In a phase III clinical trial of patients with advanced non-small cell lung cancer receiving therapy with albumin-bound paclitaxel 100 mg/m² by 30-minute IV infusion in combination with carboplatin, arthralgia or myalgia occurred in 13 or 10% of patients, respectively, and was severe in less than 1% of patients. In patients with advanced pancreatic cancer receiving albumin-bound paclitaxel 125 mg/m² by 30- to 40-minute IV infusion in combination with gemcitabine, arthralgia, myalgia, or extremity pain occurred in 11, 10, or 11% of patients, respectively, and was severe in 1% of patients.

● Hepatic Effects

Hepatic necrosis and hepatic encephalopathy resulting in death have occurred rarely in patients receiving conventional paclitaxel and may occur in patients receiving albumin-bound paclitaxel. Fatal hepatic coma occurred following administration of conventional paclitaxel in a patient with breast cancer and hepatic metastases.

Conventional Paclitaxel

Abnormalities in liver function test results have occurred in patients receiving paclitaxel for ovarian or breast cancer but do not appear to be dose or schedule related. In patients with normal baseline hepatic function, increased serum alkaline phosphatase concentrations occurred in 22%, increased serum AST (SGOT) concentrations occurred in 19%, and increased serum bilirubin concentrations occurred in 7% of patients receiving paclitaxel monotherapy for ovarian or breast cancer. Prolonged exposure to paclitaxel has not been associated with cumulative hepatic toxicity.

Albumin-bound Paclitaxel

Among patients with normal baseline hepatic function, increased serum AST (SGOT) concentrations occurred in 39%, increased serum alkaline phosphatase concentrations occurred in 36%, and increased serum bilirubin concentrations occurred in 7%, of patients receiving albumin-bound paclitaxel for metastatic breast cancer in a randomized trial. Elevations in serum GGT concentrations (grade 3 or 4) occurred in 14% of patients receiving albumin-bound paclitaxel.

● Renal Effects

Conventional Paclitaxel

Renal toxicity, including acute renal failure, has been reported in patients with HIV infection receiving paclitaxel. In patients with AIDS-related Kaposi's sarcoma receiving paclitaxel 135 or 100 mg/m² by 3-hour IV infusion, elevation of serum creatinine occurred in 34 or 18% of patients, and was severe in 7 or 5%, respectively. Elevations of serum creatinine generally were reversible; however, discontinuance of paclitaxel therapy was required in one patient suspected of having severe HIV nephropathy.

Albumin-bound Paclitaxel

Elevations of serum creatinine occurred in 11%, and were severe in 1%, of patients receiving albumin-bound paclitaxel for metastatic breast cancer. No interruptions, delay, or reductions in dose of albumin-bound paclitaxel were required for renal toxicity.

● Respiratory Effects

Lung fibrosis has been reported rarely in patients receiving conventional paclitaxel and may occur in patients receiving albumin-bound paclitaxel.

Conventional Paclitaxel

Radiation pneumonitis and interstitial pneumonia have been reported in patients receiving paclitaxel and concurrent radiation therapy. Possible radiation recall pneumonitis has been reported in a patient who received paclitaxel 12 days following completion of radiation therapy for metastatic adenocarcinoma of the lung. Adverse respiratory effects associated with hypersensitivity to paclitaxel, including pneumonitis and transient pulmonary infiltrates, also have been reported. Pulmonary embolism has been reported rarely in patients receiving paclitaxel.

Albumin-bound Paclitaxel

Dyspnea was reported in 12%, and cough in 7%, of patients receiving albumin-bound paclitaxel for metastatic breast cancer. Pneumothorax has been reported in less than 1% of patients following treatment with albumin-bound paclitaxel for metastatic breast cancer. Cough was reported in 17% of patients receiving albumin-bound paclitaxel combined with gemcitabine for pancreatic cancer.

Pneumonitis, interstitial pneumonia, pulmonary embolism, and radiation pneumonitis have been reported in patients receiving albumin-bound paclitaxel. Pneumonitis was reported in 4% of patients, and was fatal in 2 of 17 patients, following treatment with albumin-bound paclitaxel combined with gemcitabine for pancreatic cancer.

● Ocular Effects

Conventional Paclitaxel

Optic nerve disturbances and visual disturbances have been reported following administration of paclitaxel, particularly in patients receiving high doses. Rare reports of abnormalities in visual evoked potentials suggest persistent damage of the optic nerve related to paclitaxel. Other visual disturbances reported in association with paclitaxel infusion (e.g., scintillating scotomata, photopsia) generally appear to be reversible. Conjunctivitis and increased lacrimation have been reported rarely in patients receiving paclitaxel.

Albumin-bound Paclitaxel

Ocular or visual disturbances occurred in 13% of 366 patients receiving albumin-bound paclitaxel for metastatic breast cancer in single-arm studies or a randomized trial. Severe ocular or visual disturbances occurred in 1% of patients and consisted of keratitis and blurred vision in patients receiving high doses (300 or 375 mg/m²) of albumin-bound paclitaxel. These adverse ocular effects generally have been reversible; however, rare reports of abnormal visual evoked potentials in patients receiving conventional paclitaxel suggest that persistent damage of the optic nerve may occur. Reduced visual acuity due to cystoid macular edema has been reported in patients receiving albumin-bound paclitaxel or other taxanes; following discontinuance of therapy, cystoid macular edema improves and visual acuity may return to baseline. Conjunctivitis and increased lacrimation have been reported rarely in patients receiving conventional paclitaxel and may occur in patients receiving albumin-bound paclitaxel.

● Otic Effects

Ototoxicity, including hearing loss and tinnitus, has been reported in patients receiving paclitaxel.

● Other Adverse Effects

Conventional Paclitaxel

Asthenia and malaise have been reported in patients receiving paclitaxel. In a randomized trial for the initial treatment of advanced ovarian cancer, asthenia was reported in 17% of patients receiving paclitaxel 135 mg/m² by 24-hour IV infusion followed by cisplatin.

Albumin-bound Paclitaxel

Asthenia was reported in 47%, and was severe in 8%, of patients receiving albumin-bound paclitaxel for metastatic breast cancer. Fatigue and asthenia were reported in 59 and 19%, respectively, of patients receiving albumin-bound paclitaxel combined with gemcitabine for pancreatic cancer, and were severe in 18 or 7%, respectively, of patients. In addition, hypokalemia was reported in 12%, and was severe in 4%, of patients receiving albumin-bound paclitaxel combined with gemcitabine for pancreatic cancer.

● Precautions and Contraindications

Paclitaxel is a toxic drug with a low therapeutic index, and a therapeutic response is not likely to occur without evidence of toxicity. The drug must be used only under constant supervision by clinicians experienced in therapy with cytotoxic agents and only when the potential benefits of paclitaxel therapy are thought to outweigh the possible risks. In addition, appropriate diagnostic and treatment facilities must be readily available in case the patient develops any severe hypersensitivity reactions to paclitaxel therapy (e.g., hypotension, dyspnea requiring bronchodilators, angioedema, generalized urticaria).

Paclitaxel (conventional or albumin-bound paclitaxel) should *not* be used in patients with known severe hypersensitivity to the drug. In addition, paclitaxel for injection concentrate should *not* be used in patients with known severe hypersensitivity to the polyoxyl 35 castor oil vehicle. (See Cautions: Sensitivity Reactions.) To prevent severe hypersensitivity reactions, patients should be pretreated with corticosteroids (e.g., dexamethasone), diphenhydramine, and H₂-receptor antagonists (e.g., cimetidine, ranitidine) before receiving conventional paclitaxel. Premedication generally is not required in patients receiving albumin-bound paclitaxel. (See Dosage and Administration: Dosage.)

At least one commercially available formulation of paclitaxel injection contains metabisulfite, a sulfite that may cause serious allergic-type reactions in certain susceptible individuals. The overall incidence of sulfite sensitivity in the general population is probably low, but in susceptible individuals, exposure to sulfites can result in acute bronchospasm or, less frequently, life-threatening anaphylaxis. The paclitaxel formulation containing metabisulfite should be used with caution in atopic, nonasthmatic individuals.

Paclitaxel therapy (with conventional or albumin-bound paclitaxel) should not be administered to patients with baseline neutrophil counts less than 1500/mm³. In patients with HIV infection, paclitaxel therapy should not be administered if baseline neutrophil counts are less than 1000/mm³. To monitor the occurrence of paclitaxel-induced bone marrow suppression, mainly neutropenia, which may be severe and result in infection, it is recommended that frequent peripheral blood cell counts, including blood cell counts prior to each dose of the drug, be performed in all patients. (See Dosage and Administration: Dosage.) Because sepsis has been reported in patients receiving albumin-bound paclitaxel, administration of a broad-spectrum anti-infective should be initiated if the patient becomes febrile (regardless of neutrophil count).

Reduction in dosage of paclitaxel and close monitoring are required in patients with hepatic impairment. (See Dosage and Administration: Dosage in Renal and Hepatic Impairment.)

Because paclitaxel may cause adverse cardiovascular effects, including hypotension, bradycardia, and hypertension, frequent monitoring of vital signs is recommended, particularly during the first hour of the drug infusion; however, continuous cardiac monitoring is not required except in patients with preexisting serious conduction abnormalities.

Because albumin-bound paclitaxel may cause life-threatening pneumonitis, monitoring for manifestations of pneumonitis is recommended.

Patients should be warned that the alcohol contained in conventional paclitaxel may impair their ability to perform hazardous activities requiring mental alertness (e.g., operating machinery, driving a motor vehicle) following paclitaxel infusion, particularly when high doses of the drug are administered over short infusion periods (e.g., 3 hours), and that CNS depressants (e.g., opiates, sedatives) should be used concomitantly with caution.

Because albumin-bound paclitaxel contains albumin, a derivative of human blood, there is a remote risk of transmission of disease, such as viral disease or Creutzfeldt-Jakob disease, associated with its use. To date, no cases of transmission of bloodborne illness have been associated with use of albumin.

● Pediatric Precautions

Safety and efficacy of conventional or albumin-bound paclitaxel in children have not been established.

The manufacturer reports that CNS toxicity, rarely fatal, has been observed in pediatric patients receiving high doses of conventional paclitaxel (350–420 mg/m²) by 3-hour IV infusion in a clinical trial. Because paclitaxel injection contains dehydrated alcohol, toxicity may have resulted from IV administration of large amounts of alcohol over a short period of time. The use of concomitant antihistamine as a component of the premedication regimen may intensify the toxic effect of the alcohol. However, the possibility of a direct toxic effect of paclitaxel itself cannot be ruled out.

● Geriatric Precautions

When the total number of patients studied in clinical trials of conventional paclitaxel for advanced ovarian, breast, or non-small cell lung cancer and in the study for the adjuvant treatment of breast cancer is considered, 17% were 65 years of age or older, and 1% were 75 years of age or older. Clinical studies of conventional paclitaxel did not include sufficient numbers of patients 65 years of age and older to determine whether geriatric patients respond differently than younger patients. In a study of paclitaxel for the first-line treatment of advanced ovarian cancer, median survival was lower in geriatric patients than in younger patients. Geriatric patients are at increased risk for certain adverse effects of paclitaxel, including severe myelosuppression and severe neuropathy. In 2 clinical studies of conventional paclitaxel for non-small cell lung cancer, geriatric patients had a higher incidence of cardiovascular toxicity than younger patients.

In a randomized trial evaluating albumin-bound paclitaxel for the treatment of metastatic breast cancer, 13% of patients receiving albumin-bound paclitaxel were 65 years of age or older, and less than 2% were 75 years of age or older. No difference in toxicity of albumin-bound paclitaxel was observed between geriatric and younger patients.

In a randomized trial evaluating albumin-bound paclitaxel combined with carboplatin for the treatment of advanced non-small cell lung cancer, 31% of patients receiving albumin-bound paclitaxel combined with carboplatin were 65 years of age or older, and less than 3.5% were 75 years of age or older. Although no overall differences in efficacy were observed between geriatric and younger patients, toxicity (i.e., myelosuppression, peripheral neuropathy, arthralgia) occurred more frequently in patients 65 years of age or older.

In a clinical trial evaluating albumin-bound paclitaxel combined with gemcitabine for the treatment of metastatic pancreatic cancer, 41% of patients receiving albumin-bound paclitaxel combined with gemcitabine were 65 years of age or older, and less than 10% were 75 years of age or older. Although no overall differences in efficacy were observed between geriatric and younger patients, toxicity (i.e., diarrhea, decreased appetite, dehydration, epistaxis) occurred more frequently in patients 65 years of age or older. The clinical trial did not include sufficient numbers of patients older than 75 years of age to determine whether these patients respond differently than younger patients.

● Mutagenicity and Carcinogenicity

Paclitaxel has been shown to induce chromosome aberrations in human lymphocytes in vitro, and the drug was mutagenic in the micronucleus test in mice in vivo; however, paclitaxel was not mutagenic in the Ames test or the CHO/HGPRT gene mutation assay.

Studies to determine the carcinogenic potential of paclitaxel have not been performed to date.

● Pregnancy, Fertility, and Lactation
Pregnancy

Paclitaxel can cause fetal toxicity when administered to pregnant women, but potential benefits may be acceptable in certain conditions despite the possible risks to the fetus.

Reproduction studies in rabbits receiving IV conventional paclitaxel doses of 3 mg/kg daily (approximately 0.2 times the maximum recommended human dose on a mg/m² basis) during organogenesis revealed evidence of maternal toxicity, embryotoxicity, and fetotoxicity. The drug caused intrauterine mortality, increased resorptions, and increased fetal deaths. Reproduction studies in rats receiving IV paclitaxel doses of 1 mg/kg daily (approximately 0.04 times the maximum recommended human dose on a mg/m² basis) during organogenesis resulted in embryotoxicity and fetotoxicity. No teratogenic effects were observed in the offspring of rats receiving daily IV paclitaxel doses of 1 mg/kg; however, the teratogenic potential of higher paclitaxel doses could not be assessed because of extensive fetal mortality.

Reproduction studies in rats receiving albumin-bound paclitaxel at IV doses of 6 mg/m² (approximately 2% of the maximum recommended human dose on a mg/m² basis) on gestation days 7 to 17 resulted in embryotoxicity and fetotoxicity. The drug caused intrauterine mortality, increased resorptions, reduced numbers of litters, increased fetal deaths, reduction in fetal body weight, and increased fetal anomalies including soft tissue and skeletal malformations, such as eye bulge, folded retina, microphthalmia, and dilation of brain ventricles. Fetal anomalies also occurred in the offspring of rats receiving lower doses of albumin-bound paclitaxel (IV doses of 3 mg/m² or approximately 1% of the maximum recommended human dose on a mg/m² basis).

There are no adequate and well-controlled studies to date using paclitaxel in pregnant women. Paclitaxel should be used during pregnancy only in life-threatening situations or for severe disease for which safer drugs cannot be used or are ineffective. When paclitaxel is used during pregnancy or if the patient becomes pregnant while receiving the drug, the patient should be informed of the potential hazard to the fetus. Women of childbearing potential should be advised to avoid becoming pregnant during therapy with paclitaxel. Men receiving albumin-bound paclitaxel should be advised to avoid fathering a child.

Fertility

At an IV dose of 1 mg/kg daily, conventional paclitaxel reduced fertility in rats.

Reduced fertility with decreased pregnancy rates and increased loss of embryos in mated females occurred in male rats given albumin-bound paclitaxel at a dose of 42 mg/m² weekly (approximately 16% of the daily maximum recommended human dose on a mg/m² basis) for 11 weeks prior to mating with untreated female rats. Fetal anomalies, including soft tissue and skeletal malformations, occurred in the offspring of male rats receiving lower doses of albumin-bound paclitaxel

(IV doses of 3 and 12 mg/m² or approximately 1–5% of the maximum recommended human dose on a mg/m² basis). Testicular atrophy/degeneration has been observed with the administration of a single dose of albumin-bound paclitaxel in rats receiving 54 mg/m² and dogs receiving 175 mg/m².

Lactation

It is not known whether paclitaxel is distributed into human milk. However, in lactating rats given radiolabeled paclitaxel, concentrations of radioactivity in milk were higher than those in plasma and declined in parallel with plasma concentrations of the drug. Because of the potential for serious adverse reactions to paclitaxel in nursing infants, a decision should be made whether to discontinue nursing or the drug, taking into account the importance of the drug to the woman.

DRUG INTERACTIONS

• CNS Depressants

Concomitant administration of CNS depressants such as antihistamines or opiates with paclitaxel should be undertaken with caution as these drugs may cause potentiation of CNS depression caused by the alcohol contained in the paclitaxel formulation.

• Drugs Affecting Hepatic Microsomal Enzymes

Although specific studies have not been performed and the clinical importance has not been determined, concomitant administration of drugs that affect cytochrome P-450 (CYP) hepatic microsomal enzymes could alter the metabolism of paclitaxel. Metabolism of paclitaxel is mediated by CYP2C8 and CYP3A4, and the possibility exists that drugs that induce these isoenzymes may reduce plasma paclitaxel concentrations. Conversely, concomitant administration of paclitaxel with drugs that inhibit CYP2C8 and/or CYP3A4 may increase plasma paclitaxel concentrations. In addition, concomitant administration of paclitaxel with other drugs that are metabolized by CYP2C8 and/or CYP3A4 may result in decreased metabolism of the drug(s) because of competition for the enzyme. Caution should be exercised when paclitaxel is used concomitantly with drugs that are substrates, inhibitors, or inducers of CYP2C8 and/or CYP3A4.

Lower steady-state or peak plasma concentrations of paclitaxel, increased rates of clearance, and reduced toxicity have been reported in patients receiving anticonvulsants known to induce CYP enzymes (e.g., phenobarbital, phenytoin). Histamine H₂-receptor antagonists are a component of the premedication regimen used to prevent severe hypersensitivity reactions in patients receiving conventional paclitaxel; no pharmacokinetic, toxicologic, or pharmacologic differences were observed in a prospective, crossover trial in which patients received either cimetidine or famotidine despite the variable effects of these drugs on cytochrome P-450 enzyme activity. In addition, no difference in paclitaxel steady-state concentrations was observed between cycles in a small number of patients who received standard-dose (i.e., 300 mg) versus high-dose (i.e., 2400 mg) cimetidine during subsequent cycles of paclitaxel therapy. The potential interaction between paclitaxel and protease inhibitors (e.g., indinavir, nelfinavir, ritonavir, saquinavir), which are substrates and/or inhibitors of the CYP3A4 isoenzyme, has not been studied in clinical trials.

Results of in vitro studies show that the metabolism of paclitaxel to its principal metabolite, 6α-hydroxypaclitaxel, was inhibited by ketoconazole, verapamil, diazepam, quinidine, dexamethasone, cyclosporine, teniposide, etoposide, or vincristine; however, the concentrations of drugs used in these studies exceeded the plasma concentrations found in vivo following typical therapeutic doses. Other agents that inhibited the metabolism of paclitaxel in vitro include testosterone, 17α-ethinyl estradiol, retinoic acid, or quercetin (a specific inhibitor of CYP2C8).

• Antineoplastic Agents

Sequence-dependent drug interactions have been reported to occur when paclitaxel is administered with other antineoplastic agents, including cisplatin, doxorubicin, and cyclophosphamide. In a phase I trial using escalating doses of IV conventional paclitaxel 110–200 mg/m² sequentially administered with IV cisplatin 50 or 75 mg/m², increased severity of myelosuppression was observed when paclitaxel was administered following cisplatin compared with the alternative sequence (paclitaxel administered preceding cisplatin). Pharmacokinetic studies show that administration of cisplatin followed by conventional paclitaxel decreases paclitaxel clearance by approximately 25–33%. When cisplatin and paclitaxel must be administered sequentially, the sequence of paclitaxel followed by cisplatin is recommended. Increased severity of neutropenia and thrombocytopenia

have been reported when paclitaxel is administered (by 24-hour IV infusion) followed by cyclophosphamide.

Use of paclitaxel in combination therapy with doxorubicin may result in increased plasma concentrations of doxorubicin and its active metabolite doxorubicinol; this interaction may contribute to the antitumor efficacy as well as the increased incidence of cardiac toxicity when paclitaxel is used in conjunction with doxorubicin. Synergistic cytotoxicity with paclitaxel followed by doxorubicin has been observed in in vitro studies and may result from a paclitaxel-induced increase in activity of DNA topoisomerase II, one of the intracellular targets involved in doxorubicin cytotoxicity.

Administration of conventional paclitaxel followed by carboplatin was associated with similar rates of neutropenia but less severe thrombocytopenia compared with carboplatin alone; a pharmacodynamic mechanism for the interaction between the drugs has been postulated since the pharmacokinetics of the agents were unchanged. When administration of albumin-bound paclitaxel was followed immediately by carboplatin, no clinically important changes in paclitaxel exposure occurred; although mean exposure to free carboplatin was about 23% higher than the targeted exposure (6 mg/mL per minute), mean half-life and clearance of carboplatin were consistent with values reported for carboplatin alone.

The potential for pharmacokinetic interactions between paclitaxel and gemcitabine has not been elucidated.

• Protein-bound Drugs

In vitro data indicate that paclitaxel is highly bound (89–98%) to plasma proteins; however, the presence of cimetidine, ranitidine, dexamethasone, or diphenhydramine did not displace paclitaxel from plasma proteins.

ACUTE TOXICITY

• Manifestations

Limited information is available on acute overdosage of paclitaxel. Overdosage with paclitaxel would be expected to produce effects such as myelosuppression, peripheral or sensory neurotoxicity, and mucositis.

Overdosage of conventional paclitaxel in pediatric patients may be associated with acute ethanol toxicity because of the presence of dehydrated alcohol in the formulation. (See Cautions: Pediatric Precautions.)

• Treatment

There is no known specific antidote for paclitaxel overdosage. Management of paclitaxel overdosage consists of discontinuance of the drug and initiation of supportive measures appropriate for the type of toxicity observed. Paclitaxel appears to be minimally removed by hemodialysis.

PHARMACOLOGY

Paclitaxel is an antimicrotubule antineoplastic agent. Unlike some other common antimicrotubule agents (e.g., vinca alkaloids, colchicine, podophyllotoxin), which inhibit microtubule assembly, paclitaxel and docetaxel (a semisynthetic taxoid) promote microtubule assembly.

Microtubules are organelles that exist in a state of dynamic equilibrium with their components, tubulin dimers. They are an essential part of the mitotic spindle and also are involved in maintenance of cell shape and motility, and transport between organelles within the cell.

By binding in a reversible, concentration-dependent manner to the β-subunit of tubulin at the N-terminal domain, paclitaxel enhances the polymerization of tubulin, the protein subunit of the spindle microtubules, even in the absence of factors that are normally required for microtubule assembly (e.g., guanosine triphosphate [GTP]), and induces the formation of stable, nonfunctional microtubules. Paclitaxel promotes microtubule stability even under conditions that typically cause depolymerization in vitro (e.g., cold temperature, the addition of calcium, the presence of antimitotic drugs). While the precise mechanism of action of the drug is not understood fully, paclitaxel disrupts the dynamic equilibrium within the microtubule system and blocks cells in the late G₂ phase and M phase of the cell cycle, inhibiting cell replication.

Evidence suggests that paclitaxel also may induce cell death by triggering apoptosis. In addition, paclitaxel and docetaxel enhance the effects of ionizing radiation, possibly by blocking cells in the G₂ phase, the phase of the cell cycle in which cells are most radiosensitive. Preclinical evidence suggests that cross-resistance between paclitaxel and docetaxel is incomplete.

PHARMACOKINETICS

Conventional paclitaxel exhibits nonlinear, dose-dependent pharmacokinetics, particularly when the drug is administered over shorter periods of infusion (e.g., 3 hours). Both saturable distribution and elimination contribute to the nonlinear disposition of conventional paclitaxel. Although the relevance of these findings in humans is unknown, a study in mice comparing the pharmacokinetic profiles of differing formulations of paclitaxel suggests that the nonlinear distribution of conventional paclitaxel may be related to the formulation vehicle, polyoxyl 35 castor oil (Cremophor® EL, polyoxyethylated castor oil). Because of the nonlinearity of pharmacokinetics for conventional paclitaxel, relatively small changes in dose may lead to large changes in peak plasma concentrations and total drug exposure. The pharmacokinetics of conventional paclitaxel in patients with AIDS-related Kaposi's sarcoma have not been evaluated. In addition, the disposition of conventional paclitaxel and its metabolites has not been evaluated in geriatric patients.

● Absorption
Conventional Paclitaxel

Peak plasma concentrations and areas under the plasma concentration-time curve (AUCs) following IV administration of paclitaxel exhibit marked interindividual variation. Plasma concentrations of paclitaxel increase during continuous IV administration of the drug and decline immediately following completion of the infusion. Following 24-hour IV infusion of paclitaxel at doses of 135 or 175 mg/m² in patients with advanced ovarian cancer, peak plasma concentrations averaged 195 or 365 ng/mL, respectively; the increase in dose (30%) was associated with a disproportionately greater increase in peak plasma concentration (87%), but the increase in AUC was proportional. When paclitaxel was administered by continuous IV infusion over 3 hours at doses of 135 or 175 mg/m² in patients with advanced ovarian cancer, peak plasma concentrations averaged 2.17 or 3.65 mcg/mL, respectively; the increase in dose (30%) was associated with disproportionately greater increases in peak plasma concentration (68%) and AUC (89%).

Albumin-bound Paclitaxel

For the dose range 80–375 mg/m², increase in dose of albumin-bound paclitaxel was associated with a proportional increase in AUC. The duration of infusion did not affect the pharmacokinetic disposition of albumin-bound paclitaxel. Following 30-minute or 3-hour IV infusion of albumin-bound paclitaxel 260 mg/m² in patients with metastatic breast cancer, the peak plasma concentration averaged 18,741 ng/mL.

● Distribution

At plasma concentrations ranging from 0.1–50 mcg/mL, 88–98% of paclitaxel is bound to plasma proteins.

Conventional Paclitaxel

Following IV administration, paclitaxel is widely distributed into body fluids and tissues. Paclitaxel has a large volume of distribution that appears to be affected by dose and duration of infusion. Following administration of paclitaxel doses of 135 or 175 mg/m² by IV infusion over 24 hours in patients with advanced ovarian cancer, the mean apparent volume of distribution at steady state ranged from 227–688 L/m². The steady-state volume of distribution ranged from 18.9–260 L/m² in children with solid tumors or refractory leukemia receiving paclitaxel 200–500 mg/m²by 24-hour IV infusion.

Paclitaxel does not appear to readily penetrate the CNS, but paclitaxel has been detected in ascitic fluid following IV infusion of the drug. It is not known whether paclitaxel is distributed into human milk, but in lactating rats given radiolabeled paclitaxel, concentrations of radioactivity in milk were higher than those in plasma and declined in parallel with plasma concentrations of the drug.

Albumin-bound Paclitaxel

Paclitaxel bound to nanoparticles of the serum protein albumin is delivered via endothelial transport mediated by albumin receptors, and the resulting concentration of paclitaxel in tumor cells is increased compared with that achieved using an equivalent dose of conventional paclitaxel.

Like conventional paclitaxel, albumin-bound paclitaxel has a large volume of distribution. Following 30-minute or 3-hour IV infusion of 80–375 mg/m² albumin-bound paclitaxel, the volume of distribution averaged 632 L/m². The volume of distribution of albumin-bound paclitaxel 260 mg/m² by 30-minute IV infusion was 53% larger than the volume of distribution of conventional paclitaxel 175 mg/m² by 3-hour IV infusion.

● Elimination

Paclitaxel is extensively metabolized in the liver. Metabolism of paclitaxel to its major metabolite, 6α-hydroxypaclitaxel, is mediated by cytochrome P-450 isoenzyme CYP2C8, while metabolism to 2 of its minor metabolites, 3′-p-hydroxypaclitaxel and 6α,3′-p-dihydroxypaclitaxel, is catalyzed by CYP3A4.

Conventional Paclitaxel

Following IV infusion of paclitaxel over periods ranging from 6–24 hours in adults with malignancy, plasma concentrations of paclitaxel appeared to decline in a biphasic manner in some studies, with an average distribution half-life (t½α) of 0.34 hours and an average elimination half-life (t½β) of 5.8 hours. However, additional studies, particularly those in which paclitaxel is administered over shorter periods of infusion, show that the drug exhibits nonlinear pharmacokinetic behavior. In patients receiving paclitaxel 175 mg/m²administered by 3-hour IV infusion, the distribution half-life (t½α) averages 0.27 hours and the elimination half-life (t½β) averages 2.33 hours.

The plasma clearance of paclitaxel was studied in patients with ovarian cancer; the total body clearance averaged 12.2 L/hour per m² in those receiving paclitaxel 175 mg/m² by 3-hour IV infusion, 17.7 L/hour per m² in those receiving paclitaxel 135 mg/m² by 3-hour IV infusion, and 21.7 L/hour per m² in those receiving paclitaxel 135 mg/m² by 24-hour IV infusion.

Paclitaxel and its metabolites are excreted principally in the feces via biliary elimination. Urinary excretion of paclitaxel is minimal, with unchanged drug typically accounting for less than 10% of an administered dose. Following IV administration of paclitaxel over 1, 6, or 24 hours, 1.3–12.6% of the dose was excreted as unchanged drug in the urine. In patients receiving 3-hour IV infusions of radiolabeled paclitaxel, a mean of 71% of the radioactivity (about 5% of which was unchanged drug) was excreted in the feces in 120 hours and 14% was recovered in urine.

Administration of cisplatin followed by paclitaxel decreases paclitaxel clearance by approximately 25–33%. When cisplatin and paclitaxel must be administered sequentially, the sequence of paclitaxel followed by cisplatin is recommended. (See Drug Interaction: Antineoplastic Agents.)

The effect of renal impairment on the elimination of conventional paclitaxel has not been fully established. Paclitaxel is metabolized mainly in the liver, and limited data indicate that clearance of conventional paclitaxel is reduced in patients with hepatic impairment. The frequency and severity of myelotoxicity associated with paclitaxel may be increased in patients with elevated serum total bilirubin concentrations, and dosage reduction is advised. (See Dosage in Renal and Hepatic Impairment.)

Paclitaxel appears to be minimally removed by hemodialysis. In a patient undergoing hemodialysis approximately 24 hours following administration of paclitaxel 135 mg/m² by 3-hour IV infusion, paclitaxel was not detected in the dialysate; AUC and clearance of paclitaxel were within the range of values reported for patients not undergoing dialysis.

Albumin-bound Paclitaxel

Following 30-minute or 3-hour IV infusion of 80–375 mg/m² albumin-bound paclitaxel, plasma concentrations of paclitaxel declined in a biphasic manner with initial rapid distribution to the peripheral compartment and then a slower phase of elimination; the terminal half-life of albumin-bound paclitaxel was about 27 hours. The total body clearance of albumin-bound paclitaxel averaged 15 L/hour per m². The plasma clearance of albumin-bound paclitaxel 260 mg/m² by 30-minute IV infusion was 43% higher than the plasma clearance of conventional paclitaxel 175 mg/m² by 3-hour IV infusion.

Urinary excretion of albumin-bound paclitaxel is minimal. Following 30-minute IV infusion of albumin-bound paclitaxel 260 mg/m², about 4% of the dose was excreted in the urine as unchanged drug and less than 1% was excreted as metabolites. Approximately 20% of the dose was excreted in feces.

Following 30-minute IV infusion of albumin-bound paclitaxel 260 or 200 mg/m² in patients with mild or moderate hepatic impairment, respectively, systemic exposure to the drug was similar to values previously reported for patients with normal hepatic function. In patients with severe hepatic impairment, systemic exposure following 30-minute IV infusion of albumin-bound paclitaxel 130 mg/m^2 was lower than reported exposure levels for patients with normal hepatic function. In addition, mean nadir neutrophil counts in cycle 1 were higher in patients with severe hepatic impairment compared with patients with mild or moderate hepatic impairment. Doses of 200 mg/m^2 have not been evaluated in patients with severe hepatic impairment but are predicted to result in systemic exposure levels similar to those reported for patients with normal hepatic function. Pharmacokinetics of albumin-bound paclitaxel have not been elucidated in patients with AST concentrations exceeding 10 times the upper limit of normal or bilirubin concentrations of 5 or more times the upper limit of normal.

The effect of renal impairment on the elimination of albumin-bound paclitaxel has not been established.

CHEMISTRY AND STABILITY

● Chemistry

Paclitaxel, a natural product extracted from the bark of the Western (Pacific) yew (*Taxus brevifolia*) or produced from the needles and twigs of a more prevalent yew (*Taxus baccata*) using a semisynthetic process, is an antineoplastic agent. Paclitaxel also is obtained from *Taxus media*. The taxanes (paclitaxel and docetaxel) differ structurally from other currently available antineoplastic agents. Because of paclitaxel's complex, unusual chemistry, supplies initially were limited to drug extracted from the slow-growing Western (Pacific) yew. An alternative method allowing preparation of the drug in larger yields (i.e., a semisynthetic method using a precursor extracted from needles and twigs of a more prevalent yew) has been developed; semisynthetic paclitaxel is bioequivalent to the natural drug. Additional sources of the drug (e.g., production of paclitaxel by *Taxomyces andreanae*, an endophytic fungus associated with Pacific yew) continue to be explored.

Paclitaxel is a complex diterpene with a taxane ring system and a four-membered oxetane ring. An ester side chain at position 13 of the taxane ring is essential for the drug's cytotoxic activity. In addition, presence of an accessible hydroxyl group at position 2′ of this ester side chain enhances the drug's activity. Paclitaxel differs structurally from docetaxel by the presence of an acetyl group rather than a hydroxyl group on position 10 of the baccatin III ring and by a benzamide phenyl group instead of a trimethylmethoxy moiety on the 3′ position of the side chain at position 13 of the taxane ring.

Paclitaxel occurs as a white to off-white crystalline powder. Paclitaxel is highly lipophilic and insoluble in water.

Conventional Paclitaxel

Because paclitaxel is extremely hydrophobic, the commercially available injection concentrate is a sterile, nonaqueous solution of the drug in polyoxyl 35 castor oil (Cremophor® EL, polyoxyethylated castor oil) and dehydrated alcohol. Commercially available paclitaxel for injection concentrate is a clear, colorless to slightly yellow, viscous solution. Following dilution of paclitaxel for injection concentrate with 5% dextrose and 0.9% sodium chloride injection or 5% dextrose and Ringer's injection, solutions containing 0.6 or 1.2 mg of paclitaxel per mL maintain a pH of 4.4–5.6 for up to 27 hours.

Albumin-bound Paclitaxel

Paclitaxel is commercially available as protein-bound particles consisting of paclitaxel bound to albumin; the mean particle size of albumin-bound paclitaxel is about 130 nm. Albumin-bound paclitaxel is a sterile, white to yellow lyophilized powder that must be reconstituted for use as an injectable suspension; there are no solvents. Each single-use vial contains 100 mg of paclitaxel and approximately 900 mg of human albumin.

● Stability
Conventional Paclitaxel

Commercially available paclitaxel for injection concentrate should be stored in unopened vials at 20–25°C and retained in the original package for protection from light. Neither freezing nor refrigeration adversely affects paclitaxel for injection concentrate. Refrigeration may result in precipitation of the drug or formulation vehicle; however, the precipitate typically will dissolve at room temperature without loss of potency. If freezing occurs, paclitaxel for injection concentrate may be thawed at room temperature until precipitate dissolves; the manufacturer states that the chemical or physical stability of the injection is not affected. If the solution remains cloudy or if an insoluble precipitate remains at room temperature, the vial should be discarded. When stored under recommended conditions, unopened vials of commercially available paclitaxel for injection concentrate are stable until the date indicated on the package.

The manufacturer states that, when diluted as directed, paclitaxel solutions are stable for up to 27 hours when stored at approximately 25°C under ambient lighting conditions.

Contact of undiluted paclitaxel for injection concentrate with plasticized polyvinyl chloride (PVC) equipment or devices used to prepare solutions for infusion is *not* recommended. Polyoxyl 35 castor oil can cause leaching of diethylhexylphthalate (DEHP) from PVC containers and, following dilution of paclitaxel for injection concentrate in PVC containers, substantial leaching of DEHP occurs in a time- and concentration-dependent manner. To minimize exposure of the patient to leached DEHP, diluted paclitaxel solutions preferably should be stored in glass or polypropylene bottles or in plastic (polypropylene or polyolefin) bags and administered through polyethylene-lined administration sets. Leaching of unacceptable amounts of DEHP has been reported with some administration sets labeled as not containing PVC (probably because of pumping segments made of heavily plasticized PVC); therefore, compatibility of administration sets with paclitaxel solutions should be verified prior to their use.

Solutions of paclitaxel prepared with 5% dextrose injection or 0.9% sodium chloride injection at concentrations of 0.3–1.2 mg/mL reportedly were chemically and physically stable for up to 48 hours when prepared and stored in polyolefin containers at ambient temperature (20–23°C) under normal fluorescent light; however, in this study, physical stability was determined only by the absence of gross precipitation. In another study, paclitaxel solutions of 0.1 and 1 mg/mL in 5% dextrose injection or 0.9% sodium chloride injection were stable for up to 3 days when prepared and stored in polyolefin bags at 4, 22, or 32°C. Extemporaneously compounded admixtures of paclitaxel 1 mg/mL in 5% dextrose solution with addition of dehydrated alcohol injection to achieve a final ethanol concentration of 20 or 25% were chemically and physically stable for up to 7 days when prepared and stored in polyolefin containers at 4, 22, or 32°C.

Solutions of paclitaxel have been reported to be physically incompatible with various drugs, including amphotericin B, chlorpromazine hydrochloride, hydroxyzine hydrochloride, methylprednisolone sodium succinate, and mitoxantrone hydrochloride. The physical and/or chemical compatibility of paclitaxel with other drugs depends on several factors (e.g., concentrations of the drugs, specific diluents used, resulting pH, temperature); studies evaluating the stability of paclitaxel with other drugs, particularly other antineoplastic agents, are ongoing. Specialized references should be consulted for specific information.

Because a small number of fibers (within acceptable USP limits) have been detected in paclitaxel solutions prepared from the commercially available for injection concentrate, a hydrophilic, microporous inline filter with a pore size not exceeding 0.22 μm is necessary during administration of paclitaxel solutions. The manufacturer reports that use of filter devices such as IVEX-2® filters, which incorporate short inlet and outlet PVC-coated tubing, has not resulted in significant leaching of DEHP.

Diluted solutions of paclitaxel may appear hazy. When such solutions are passed through a 0.22-μm filter, no clinically important loss of potency is observed, suggesting that the haze is caused by the formulation vehicle rather than precipitation of the drug.

Albumin-bound Paclitaxel

Commercially available albumin-bound paclitaxel for injectable suspension should be stored in unopened vials at 20–25°C and retained in the original package for protection from bright light. Neither freezing nor refrigeration adversely affects albumin-bound paclitaxel for injectable suspension. When stored under recommended conditions, unopened vials of commercially available albumin-bound paclitaxel for injectable suspension are stable until the date indicated on the package.

Reconstituted suspensions of albumin-bound paclitaxel should be used immediately; if immediate use is not possible, vials of reconstituted albumin-bound paclitaxel suspension may be placed in the original carton to protect them from bright light and refrigerated at 2–8°C for up to 8 hours. After 8 hours, any unused portion of the reconstituted albumin-bound paclitaxel suspension should be discarded.

Before the dosing volume is withdrawn from the vial, the suspension should be inspected. Settling of the reconstituted albumin-bound paclitaxel suspension may occur. Mild agitation of the vial should ensure complete resuspension of the albumin-bound paclitaxel. If particulates are visible after mild agitation of the vial, the suspension should be discarded and another reconstituted albumin-bound paclitaxel suspension should be prepared. When reconstituted as directed, albumin-bound paclitaxel suspension is stable in the IV infusion bag for up to 4 hours when stored at approximately 25°C under ambient lighting conditions.

For further information on the handling of antineoplastic agents, see the ASHP Guidelines on Handling Hazardous Drugs at http://www.ahfsdrug information.com.

PREPARATIONS

Excipients in commercially available drug preparations may have clinically important effects in some individuals; consult specific product labeling for details.

PACLitaxel

Parenteral

For injection, concentrate, for IV infusion	6 mg/mL*	Onxol®, Teva
		Paclitaxel Injection

* available from one or more manufacturer, distributor, and/or repackager by generic (nonproprietary) name

PACLitaxel (albumin-bound)

Parenteral

For injectable suspension, for IV infusion	100 mg (of paclitaxel)	Abraxane®, Celgene

† Use is not currently included in the labeling approved by the US Food and Drug Administration.

Selected Revisions August 10, 2017, © Copyright, June 1, 1993, American Society of Health-System Pharmacists, Inc.

Palbociclib

10:00 • ANTINEOPLASTIC AGENTS

■ Palbociclib, a reversible and selective inhibitor of cyclin-dependent kinase (CDK) 4 and 6, is an antineoplastic agent.

USES

● Breast Cancer

Palbociclib is used in combination with an aromatase inhibitor or fulvestrant for the treatment of hormone receptor-positive, human epidermal growth factor receptor type 2 (HER2)-negative advanced or metastatic breast cancer.

Initial Therapy for Advanced Breast Cancer

Palbociclib is used in combination with an aromatase inhibitor for the initial treatment of hormone receptor-positive, HER2-negative advanced or metastatic breast cancer.

This indication for palbociclib is based principally on the results of a randomized, double-blind, placebo-controlled, phase 3 study (PALOMA-2) in postmenopausal women with previously untreated estrogen receptor-positive, HER2-negative, advanced or metastatic breast cancer. In this study, 666 patients were randomized (stratified according to disease site, disease-free interval, and prior neoadjuvant or adjuvant endocrine therapy) in a 2:1 ratio to receive either palbociclib (125 mg orally once daily for 3 consecutive weeks of each 4-week cycle) in combination with letrozole (2.5 mg orally once daily continuously) or placebo in combination with letrozole. Patients were treated until disease progression, symptomatic deterioration, unacceptable toxicity, death, or withdrawal of patient consent occurred. The primary measure of efficacy was progression-free survival as assessed by the investigator according to Response Evaluation Criteria in Solid Tumors (RECIST) criteria. Additional outcomes included objective response rate, overall survival, median duration of response, and clinical benefit response (complete/partial response or stable disease).

The majority of patients (98%) had an Eastern Cooperative Oncology Group (ECOG) performance status of 0 or 1 and 78% of patients were white. Approximately one-half (48%) of patients received prior chemotherapy, 56% received neoadjuvant or adjuvant endocrine therapy prior to diagnosis of advanced breast cancer, and 37% had not received prior systemic therapy in the neoadjuvant or adjuvant setting. The majority of patients (97%) had metastatic disease and 49 or 23% of patients had visceral or bone-only disease, respectively.

The median follow-up was 23 months. Patients receiving palbociclib in combination with letrozole had a longer median progression-free survival (24.8 versus 14.5 months) compared with patients receiving placebo in combination with letrozole. The objective response rate (for patients with measurable disease) was 55.3 or 44.4% for palbociclib or placebo, respectively. The median overall survival was 53.8 or 49.8 months for palbociclib or placebo, respectively. The median duration of response was 22.5 or 16.8 months, and the rate of clinical benefit response was 84.9 or 70.3% for palbociclib or placebo, respectively. At a median follow-up of 38 months, median progression-free survival was 27.6 or 14.5 months for palbociclib and placebo, respectively. Benefits of palbociclib on progression-free survival were seen across all subgroups evaluated (e.g., visceral, nonvisceral, bone-only or no bone-only disease, measurable or nonmeasurable disease). At a median follow-up of 90.1 months, the median overall survival was 53.9 or 51.2 months for palbociclib or placebo, respectively.

Previously Treated Advanced Breast Cancer

Palbociclib is used in combination with fulvestrant for the treatment of hormone receptor-positive, HER2-negative, advanced or metastatic breast cancer in patients with disease progression following endocrine therapy.

This indication for palbociclib is based principally on the results of a randomized, double-blind, placebo-controlled, phase 3 study (PALOMA-3) in women with hormone receptor-positive, HER2-negative, metastatic breast cancer. A total of 521 patients were randomized (stratified according to sensitivity to endocrine therapy, menopausal status, and presence of visceral metastases) in a 2:1 ratio to receive either palbociclib (125 mg orally once daily for 3 consecutive weeks of each 4-week cycle) in combination with fulvestrant (500 mg IM on days 1 and 15 during cycle 1 and then on day 1 of each 4-week cycle thereafter) or placebo in combination with fulvestrant. Patients were treated until disease progression, symptomatic deterioration, unacceptable toxicity, death, or withdrawal of patient consent occurred. Premenopausal or perimenopausal patients received goserelin acetate for at least 4 weeks prior to and during the study. The primary measure of efficacy was progression-free survival as assessed by the investigator according to RECIST criteria. Additional outcomes included objective response rate, clinical benefit (complete/partial response or stable disease) and overall survival. The median age of patients was 57 years. All patients enrolled in the study had a baseline ECOG performance status of 0 or 1. The majority of patients (80%) were postmenopausal and 60 or 23% of patients had visceral or bone-only disease, respectively. All patients enrolled in the study received prior systemic therapy, 75% of patients received prior chemotherapy, and 25% of patients had not received prior therapy for metastatic disease.

The median follow-up was 8.9 months. Patients receiving palbociclib in combination with fulvestrant had a longer median progression-free survival (9.5 versus 4.6 months) compared with patients receiving placebo in combination with fulvestrant. The objective response rate for patients with measurable disease was 24.6 or 10.9% for palbociclib or placebo, respectively, with a clinical benefit of 67 or 40%, respectively. At a median follow-up of 73.3 months, the median overall survival was 34.8 months with palbociclib and 28 months with placebo. The 6-year overall survival was 19.1 or 12.9% for palbociclib or placebo, respectively.

Clinical Perspective

Guidelines from the American Society of Clinical Oncology (ASCO) provide recommendations for treatment of hormone receptor-positive, HER2-negative, metastatic breast cancer. For patients with hormone receptor-positive, HER2-negative, metastatic breast cancer who have not received any prior treatment, received treatment with tamoxifen only, or who have not recently (within 1 year) been treated with an aromatase inhibitor (i.e., anastrozole, exemestane, letrozole), first-line treatment should be initiated with an aromatase inhibitor plus a CDK4/6 inhibitor. For patients recently exposed to aromatase inhibitor therapy or who experienced recurrence during treatment with an aromatase inhibitor, first-line treatment should be initiated with fulvestrant plus a CDK4/6 inhibitor.

DOSAGE AND ADMINISTRATION

● General

Pretreatment Screening

- Obtain baseline complete blood count (CBC).
- Verify pregnancy status in females of reproductive potential.
- Because palbociclib may impair male fertility, consider sperm preservation prior to initiating therapy.

Patient Monitoring

- Obtain CBC prior to initiation of each cycle, on day 15 of cycles 1 and 2, and as clinically indicated. More frequent monitoring may be required in patients who develop hematologic toxicity during therapy.
- Monitor patients for manifestations of pneumonitis.

Other General Considerations

- Consult respective manufacturers' labelings for information on dosage adjustments, adverse effects, and contraindications of other antineoplastic agents used in combination regimens.

● Administration

Palbociclib is administered orally (as capsules or tablets) with food at approximately the same time each day. The capsules and tablets should be swallowed intact and should not be chewed, crushed, or opened/split.

If a dose of palbociclib is missed or vomited, patients should not double the dose or take extra doses. The next dose should be taken at the regularly scheduled time.

Store palbociclib capsules and tablets at 20–25°C; excursions permitted between 15–30°C. Store tablets in their original blister pack.

● Dosage

Breast Cancer

Initial Therapy for Advanced Breast Cancer

For the initial treatment of hormone receptor-positive, HER2-negative, advanced or metastatic breast cancer, the recommended adult dosage of palbociclib is 125 mg once daily on days 1–21 of each 28-day cycle in combination with an aromatase inhibitor. In the PALOMA-2 study, therapy was continued until disease progression or unacceptable toxicity occurred.

Clinicians should consult the respective manufacturers' labelings for the recommended dosage of the aromatase inhibitor used in combination with palbociclib.

Premenopausal or perimenopausal women receiving combination therapy with palbociclib and an aromatase inhibitor should be treated with a luteinizing hormone-releasing hormone (LHRH) agonist according to current standards of care. Men receiving combination therapy with palbociclib and an aromatase inhibitor should consider treatment with an LHRH agonist according to current standards of care.

Previously Treated Advanced Breast Cancer

For the treatment of hormone receptor-positive, HER2-negative, advanced or metastatic breast cancer in patients with disease progression following endocrine therapy, the recommended adult dosage of palbociclib is 125 mg once daily on days 1–21 of each 28-day cycle in combination with fulvestrant 500 mg IM on days 1 and 15 during cycle 1, and then on day 1 of each 28-day cycle thereafter. In the PALOMA-3 study, therapy was continued until disease progression or unacceptable toxicity occurred.

Premenopausal or perimenopausal patients receiving combination therapy with palbociclib and fulvestrant should be treated with a LHRH agonist according to current standards of care.

Dosage Modification for Toxicity

Management of some adverse effects may require temporary interruption of therapy, dosage reduction, and/or permanent discontinuance of palbociclib therapy. Dosage adjustment of palbociclib is recommended based on individual safety and tolerability. Up to 2 dosage reductions for toxicity may be made. If dosage modification is necessary, an initial dosage reduction to 100 mg once daily is recommended. If further dosage reduction is necessary, the dosage should be reduced to 75 mg once daily. Dosages less than 75 mg once daily are not recommended.

Hematologic Toxicity

For grade 3 febrile neutropenia (absolute neutrophil count [ANC] 500 to less than 1000/mm^3 associated with fever of 38.5°C or more and/or infection), palbociclib therapy should be interrupted until ANC reaches or exceeds 1000/mm^3. Upon resumption of therapy, the dosage of palbociclib should be reduced.

If grade 1 or 2 hematologic toxicity occurs, palbociclib may be continued at the same dosage.

If grade 1 or 2 neutropenia occurs during cycle 1–6, monitoring of CBCs should be repeated every 3 months, prior to subsequent cycles, and as clinically indicated.

If grade 3 hematologic toxicity is reported after CBC monitoring on day 1 of any cycle, therapy with palbociclib should be interrupted; monitoring of CBCs should be repeated within 1 week. The next cycle should be delayed until the toxicity resolves to grade 2 or less; therapy with palbociclib may be continued at the same dosage.

If grade 3 hematologic toxicity is reported after CBC monitoring on day 15 of cycle 1 or 2, palbociclib may be continued at the same dosage; monitoring of CBCs should be repeated on day 22. If grade 4 hematologic toxicity is reported after repeat CBC monitoring on day 22 of the cycle, therapy with palbociclib should be interrupted; therapy may be resumed at a reduced dosage when the toxicity resolves to grade 2 or less.

If prolonged (i.e., lasting longer than 7 days) recovery from grade 3 neutropenia occurs or grade 3 neutropenia recurs on day 1 of subsequent cycles, resumption of therapy at a reduced dosage may then be considered.

For grade 4 hematologic toxicity, therapy with palbociclib should be interrupted; therapy may be resumed at a reduced dosage when the toxicity resolves to grade 2 or less.

An exception is made for patients with grade 3 or 4 lymphopenia presenting without an associated clinical event such as an opportunistic infection; no dosage modification is required in such patients.

Interstitial Lung Disease/Pneumonitis

For severe interstitial lung disease (ILD)/pneumonitis, palbociclib therapy should be permanently discontinued.

Nonhematologic Toxicity

If persistent grade 3 or greater nonhematologic toxicity occurs despite appropriate medical management, palbociclib therapy should be withheld until the toxicity resolves to grade 1 or less, or to grade 2 or less if the toxicity is not considered a safety risk for the patient. Upon resumption of therapy, the palbociclib dosage should be reduced.

Concomitant Use with Drugs or Foods Affecting Hepatic Microsomal Enzymes

Concomitant use of palbociclib with drugs that are strong inhibitors of cytochrome P-450 (CYP) isoenzyme 3A should be avoided; an alternative drug with no or minimal CYP3A inhibition potential should be considered. If concomitant use of a strong CYP3A inhibitor cannot be avoided, the manufacturer recommends reducing the dosage of palbociclib to 75 mg once daily. If concomitant use of the strong CYP3A inhibitor is discontinued, the palbociclib dosage should be returned (after 3–5 terminal half-lives of the CYP3A inhibitor) to the dosage used prior to initiation of the strong CYP3A inhibitor.

● Special Populations

Hepatic Impairment

For patients with severe hepatic impairment (Child-Pugh class C), the manufacturer recommends reducing the initial dosage of palbociclib to 75 mg once daily on days 1–21 of each 28-day cycle. No dosage adjustment is necessary in patients with mild or moderate hepatic impairment (Child-Pugh class A or B).

Renal Impairment

No dosage adjustment is necessary in patients with creatinine clearance >15 mL/minute. Palbociclib has not been studied in patients requiring dialysis.

Geriatric Patients

The manufacturer makes no specific dosage recommendations for geriatric patients.

CAUTIONS

● Contraindications

- None.

● Warnings/Precautions

Neutropenia

Neutropenia is the most commonly occuring adverse reaction in studies of patients receiving palbociclib. In the principal efficacy studies, grade 3 or greater neutropenia occurred in 66% of patients receiving palbociclib in combination with letrozole and those receiving palbociclib in combination with fulvestrant. The median time to occurrence of neutropenia was 15 days. The median duration of grade 3 or greater neutropenia was 7 days. Febrile neutropenia has been observed in 1.8% of patients receiving palbociclib. In the PALOMA-3 study, fatal neutropenic sepsis occurred in one patient.

Monitor complete blood counts (CBC) at baseline, prior to initiation of each cycle, and as clinically indicated; additional monitoring of CBC should be obtained on day 15 of cycles 1 and 2. More frequent monitoring may be necessary in patients who develop hematologic toxicity during therapy. Temporary interruption, dosage reduction, or treatment delay may be necessary if neutropenia occurs during therapy with the drug.

Interstitial Lung Disease/Pneumonitis

Severe, life-threatening, or fatal interstitial lung disease (ILD)/pneumonitis has occurred in patients receiving cyclin-dependent kinases 4 (CDK4) and 6 (CDK6) inhibitors, including palbociclib in combination with endocrine therapy. In the PALOMA-3, PALOMA-2, and PALOMA-1 studies, ILD or pneumonitis occurred in 1% of palbociclib-treated patients, and grade 3 or 4 ILD or pneumonitis occurred in 0.1% of patients receiving the drug. No fatal cases of ILD or pneumonitis were reported in these studies; however, additional cases of ILD or pneumonitis, including fatal cases, have been reported during postmarketing experience in patients receiving palbociclib.

Patients receiving palbociclib should be monitored for symptoms of ILD and pneumonitis. If manifestations suggestive of ILD or pneumonitis (e.g., hypoxia, cough, dyspnea, interstitial infiltrates) occur, palbociclib therapy should be temporarily interrupted and other etiologies (e.g., infection, neoplasm) should be excluded. If severe ILD or pneumonitis occurs, therapy with palbociclib should be permanently discontinued.

Fetal/Neonatal Morbidity and Mortality

There are no adequate and well-controlled studies of palbociclib in pregnant women; however, based on its mechanism of action and animal findings, palbociclib may cause fetal harm. Embryofetal toxicity (i.e., decreased fetal weight) and teratogenicity (i.e., skeletal alterations) have been demonstrated in rats and rabbits receiving palbociclib at exposure levels of approximately 4 and 9 times the human exposure at the recommended dosage, respectively; however, embryofetal toxicity was not observed in the offspring of female rats receiving the drug from 15 days prior to breeding through day 7 of gestation at exposure levels of approximately 4 times the human exposure at the recommended dosage.

Pregnancy should be avoided during palbociclib therapy. The manufacturer recommends confirmation of pregnancy status prior to initiation of palbociclib, and women of childbearing potential should be advised to use an effective method of contraception while receiving palbociclib and for at least 3 weeks after discontinuance of therapy. Male patients should be advised to use an effective method of contraception while receiving palbociclib and for 3 months after discontinuance of therapy each time they have sexual contact with women of childbearing potential. Patients should be apprised of the potential hazard to the fetus if used during pregnancy.

Specific Populations

Pregnancy

Palbociclib may cause fetal harm if administered to pregnant women based on its mechanism of action and animal findings. Pregnancy should be avoided during palbociclib therapy. The manufacturer recommends confirmation of pregnancy status prior to initiation of palbociclib, and women of childbearing potential should be advised to use an effective method of contraception while receiving palbociclib and for at least 3 weeks after discontinuance of therapy.

Lactation

It is not known whether palbociclib is distributed into human milk. Because many drugs are distributed into human milk and because of the potential for serious adverse reactions to palbociclib in nursing infants, women should be advised to discontinue nursing during therapy and for 3 weeks after discontinuance of the drug. The effects of the drug on nursing infants or on milk production are unknown.

Females and Males of Reproductive Potential

Results of animal studies suggest that palbociclib may impair male fertility. Adverse effects on male reproductive organs and sperm (i.e., decreased organ weight, atrophy or degeneration, intratubular cellular debris, hypospermia, low sperm motility and density, decreased secretion) were observed in rats and dogs receiving palbociclib at exposure levels of approximately 10 or more and 0.1

times the human exposure at the recommended dosage, respectively, in a repeat-dose toxicity study; effects on male reproductive organs were partially reversible following a 4- and 12-week nondosing period in rats and dogs, respectively. Decreased fertility also was observed in male rats receiving palbociclib at exposure levels 20 times the human exposure at the recommended dosage.

The manufacturer states that men should consider sperm preservation prior to initiating palbociclib therapy.

Pregnancy should be avoided during palbociclib therapy. The manufacturer recommends confirmation of pregnancy status prior to initiation of palbociclib, and women of childbearing potential should be advised to use an effective method of contraception while receiving palbociclib and for at least 3 weeks after discontinuance of therapy. Male patients should be advised to use an effective method of contraception while receiving palbociclib and for 3 months after discontinuance of therapy each time they have sexual contact with women of childbearing potential. Patients should be apprised of the potential hazard to the fetus if used during pregnancy.

Pediatric Use

Safety and efficacy of palbociclib have not been established in pediatric patients younger than 18 years of age.

Altered glucose metabolism associated with pancreatic islet cell vacuolation, cataracts, ocular lens degeneration, renal tubule vacuolation, chronic progressive nephropathy, and atrophy of adipose tissue have been observed in immature animals receiving palbociclib for 27 weeks (at exposure levels approximately 11 times the AUC in humans at the recommended dosage); tooth abnormalities (i.e., discoloration, ameloblast degeneration or necrosis, mononuclear cell infiltrate) also have been observed in animals receiving palbociclib at exposure levels approximately 15 times the AUC in humans at the recommended dosage.

Geriatric Use

In the PALOMA-2 study, 41% of palbociclib-treated patients were ≥65 years of age and 11% were ≥75 years of age. In the PALOMA-3 study, 25% of palbociclib-treated patients were ≥65 years of age and 8% were ≥75 years of age. No overall differences in safety and efficacy were observed between geriatric and younger patients.

Hepatic Impairment

In individuals with moderate (Child-Pugh class B) or severe (Child-Pugh class C) hepatic impairment, AUC of the unbound fraction of palbociclib was increased by 34 or 77%, respectively, compared with individuals with normal hepatic function. Peak plasma concentrations of the unbound fraction of palbociclib also were increased by 38 or 72% in individuals with moderate or severe hepatic impairment, respectively, compared with individuals with normal hepatic function.

In individuals with mild hepatic impairment (Child-Pugh class A), AUC of the unbound fraction of palbociclib was decreased by 17% and peak plasma concentrations of the unbound fraction of palbociclib were increased by 7% compared with individuals with normal hepatic function. In a population pharmacokinetic analysis, no clinically important differences in systemic exposure of palbociclib were observed between patients with mild hepatic impairment (total bilirubin concentration not exceeding the upper limit of normal [ULN] with AST concentration exceeding the ULN, or total bilirubin concentration exceeding 1 to 1.5 times the ULN with any AST concentration) and those with normal hepatic function.

In vivo, the mean unbound fraction of palbociclib increased incrementally with worsening hepatic function.

Renal Impairment

The AUC of palbociclib was increased by 39, 42, or 31% in individuals with mild (creatinine clearance of 60 to less than 90 mL/minute), moderate (creatinine clearance of 30 to less than 60 mL/minute), or severe (creatinine clearance less than 30 mL/minute) renal impairment, respectively, compared with individuals with normal renal function. Peak plasma concentrations of palbociclib were increased by 17, 12, or 15% in individuals with mild, moderate, or severe renal impairment, respectively, compared with individuals with normal renal function. In a population pharmacokinetic analysis, no clinically important differences in systemic exposure of palbociclib were observed between patients with mild or moderate renal impairment and those with normal renal function.

In vivo, renal impairment does not appear to affect the mean unbound fraction of palbociclib.

Formal pharmacokinetic studies have not been conducted in patients requiring dialysis.

● Common Adverse Effects

Adverse effects and laboratory abnormalities reported in ≥10% of patients receiving palbociclib include neutropenia, infection, leukopenia, fatigue, nausea, stomatitis, anemia, alopecia, diarrhea, thrombocytopenia, rash, vomiting, decreased appetite, asthenia, and pyrexia.

DRUG INTERACTIONS

Palbociclib is metabolized principally by cytochrome P-450 (CYP) isoenzyme 3A and sulfotransferase (SULT) 2A1. In vitro studies indicate that palbociclib does not inhibit CYP isoenzymes 1A2, 2A6, 2B6, 2C8, 2C9, 2C19, and 2D6 or induce CYP isoenzymes 1A2, 2B6, 2C8, and 3A4 at clinically relevant concentrations; however, in vivo studies indicate that the drug is a weak time-dependent inhibitor of CYP3A.

In vitro studies indicate that palbociclib has a low potential for inhibition of organic cation transporter (OCT) 2, organic anion transporter (OAT) 1, OAT 3, organic anion transport protein (OATP) 1B1 and OATP1B3 at clinically relevant concentrations. In vitro studies also indicate that palbociclib has potential to inhibit P-glycoprotein (P-gp) and breast cancer resistance protein (BCRP) at clinically relevant concentrations.

● Drugs Affecting Hepatic Microsomal Enzymes

Inhibitors of CYP3A

Concomitant use of palbociclib with strong inhibitors of CYP3A may result in increased peak plasma concentrations and systemic exposure (AUC) of palbociclib. When the strong CYP3A inhibitor itraconazole (200 mg daily) was administered concomitantly with palbociclib (single 125-mg dose) in healthy individuals, the peak plasma concentrations and AUC of palbociclib were increased by 34 and 87%, respectively.

Concomitant use of palbociclib with strong inhibitors of CYP3A (e.g., clarithromycin, itraconazole, ketoconazole, ritonavir-boosted lopinavir, nefazodone, nelfinavir, posaconazole, ritonavir, saquinavir, verapamil, voriconazole) should be avoided, and selection of an alternative drug with no or minimal CYP3A inhibition potential should be considered. If concomitant use of a strong CYP3A inhibitor cannot be avoided, the manufacturer recommends dosage reduction of palbociclib to 75 mg once daily. If concomitant use of the strong CYP3A inhibitor is discontinued, the palbociclib dosage should be returned (after 3–5 terminal half-lives of the CYP3A inhibitor) to the dosage used prior to initiation of the strong CYP3A4 inhibitor.

Grapefruit products are CYP3A inhibitors and should be avoided because of the potential for increased plasma palbociclib concentrations during concurrent use.

Inducers of CYP3A

Concomitant use of palbociclib with CYP3A inducers may result in decreased peak plasma concentrations and AUC of palbociclib. When the strong CYP3A inducer rifampin (600 mg daily) was administered concomitantly with palbociclib (single 125-mg dose) in healthy individuals, the peak plasma concentrations and AUC of palbociclib were decreased by 70 and 85%, respectively. When the moderate CYP3A inducer modafinil (400 mg daily) was administered concomitantly with palbociclib (single 125-mg dose) in healthy individuals, peak plasma concentrations and AUC of palbociclib were decreased by 11 and 32%, respectively.

Concomitant use of palbociclib with strong inducers of CYP3A (e.g., carbamazepine, phenytoin, rifampin, St. John's wort [Hypericum perforatum]) should be avoided.

● Drugs Metabolized by Hepatic Microsomal Enzymes

Substrates of CYP3A

When the CYP3A substrate midazolam was administered concomitantly with palbociclib in healthy individuals, peak plasma concentrations and AUC of midazolam were increased by 37 and 61%, respectively. If concomitant use of palbociclib with CYP3A substrates with a narrow therapeutic index (e.g., alfentanil, cyclosporine, dihydroergotamine, ergotamine, everolimus, fentanyl, pimozide, quinidine, sirolimus, tacrolimus) cannot be avoided, a dosage reduction of the CYP3A substrate should be considered.

● Drugs Affecting Gastric Acidity

When multiple doses of the proton-pump inhibitor rabeprazole were administered concomitantly with palbociclib (single 125-mg dose) in healthy individuals, peak plasma concentrations and AUC of palbociclib were decreased by 41 and 13%, respectively, under fed conditions and by 80 and 62%, respectively, under fasting conditions. Because effects on gastric pH are less marked with histamine H_2-receptor antagonists or antacids compared with proton-pump inhibitors, decreases in palbociclib exposure are expected to be minimal when H_2-receptor antagonists or antacids are used concomitantly with palbociclib under fed conditions. Clinically important effects on palbociclib exposure were not observed when antacids, histamine H_2-receptor antagonists, or proton-pump inhibitors were used concomitantly with palbociclib under fed conditions.

● Anastrozole

Concomitant use of palbociclib and anastrozole is not expected to have a clinically important effect on the pharmacokinetics of either drug.

● Exemestane

Concomitant use of palbociclib and exemestane is not expected to have a clinically important effect on the pharmacokinetics of either drug.

● Fulvestrant

Concomitant administration of palbociclib and fulvestrant did not affect the pharmacokinetics of either drug.

● Goserelin

Concomitant administration of palbociclib and goserelin did not affect the pharmacokinetics of either drug.

● Letrozole

Concomitant administration of palbociclib and letrozole did not affect the pharmacokinetics of either drug.

DESCRIPTION

Palbociclib, a reversible and selective inhibitor of cyclin-dependent kinase (CDK) 4 and 6, is an antineoplastic agent. Several mechanisms contribute to the dysregulation of the cell cycle during the G1 into S phase, including amplification or overexpression of the cyclin D oncogene or the loss of intrinsic CDK inhibitors (i.e., p16, p15, p18, p19, p21, p27, p57) in breast cancer. Palbociclib specifically inhibits CDK4 and 6 and blocks the interaction of CDK4 and 6 with cyclin D, resulting in inhibition of phosphorylation of the tumor suppressor protein retinoblastoma and inhibition of progression of the cell cycle from the G1 into S phase. In vitro, palbociclib has demonstrated reduced cellular proliferation of estrogen receptor-positive breast cancer cell lines by inhibiting the G1 into S phase of the cell cycle. Decreased phosphorylation of retinoblastoma protein resulting in reduced E2F expression and signaling and increased cell growth arrest have been reported in breast cancer cell lines treated with palbociclib and antiestrogens compared with either drug alone. In vitro, the combination of palbociclib with antiestrogens increased cell senescence for up to 6 days following discontinuance of therapy in estrogen receptor-positive breast cancer cell lines. The combination of palbociclib and letrozole also has demonstrated increased inhibition of retinoblastoma protein phosphorylation, downstream signaling, and tumor growth compared with either drug alone in patient-derived estrogen receptor-positive breast tumor xenografts. In vitro, human bone marrow mononuclear cells treated with palbociclib with or without an antiestrogen did not become senescent and cell proliferation resumed following discontinuance of exposure.

Following oral administration, the mean absolute bioavailability of palbociclib is 46%. AUC and peak plasma concentrations of palbociclib are dose proportional over a dosage range of 25–225 mg. Peak plasma concentrations of palbociclib are achieved about 6–12 hours following oral administration of the capsules. Peak plasma concentrations are attained 4–12 hours following oral administration of the tablets. Following repeated doses of palbociclib administered once daily, steady-state concentrations of the drug were achieved in 8 days and the median accumulation ratio for the drug was 2.4.

Absorption and systemic exposure to palbociclib capsules were decreased in approximately 13% of individuals receiving the drug in a fasting state; systemic exposure to palbociclib increased when the drug was administered with food in these individuals, but administration with food did not alter systemic exposure to a clinically important extent in other individuals. Administration of palbociclib with food reduces the interindividual variability in systemic exposure to palbociclib. Oral administration of palbociclib capsules with a low-fat, low-calorie (approximately 400–500 calories) or high-fat, high-calorie meal (approximately 800–1000 calories) resulted in increases in systemic exposure of 12 or 21%, respectively, and increases in peak plasma concentrations of 27 or 38%, respectively, compared with administration in the fasting state. When an oral dose of palbociclib capsules was administered between 2 moderate-fat, standard-calorie meals (approximately 500–700 calories per meal) (i.e., single dose administered 1 hour after the first meal and 2 hours before the second meal), systemic exposure and peak plasma concentrations of the drug were increased by 13 and 24%, respectively, compared with administration in the fasting state. Oral administration of palbociclib tablets with a high-fat, high-calorie meal (approximately 800–1000 calories per meal) or with a moderate-fat, standard-calorie meal (approximately 500–700 calories per meal) resulted in increases in systemic exposure of 22 or 9%, respectively, and increases in peak plasma concentrations of 26 or 10%, respectively, compared with administration of the tablets in the fasting state.

Palbociclib is metabolized in the liver principally by cytochrome P-450 (CYP) isoenzyme 3A and sulfotransferase (SULT) 2A1. In vitro, palbociclib is approximately 85% bound to plasma proteins. Following oral administration of a single radiolabeled dose of palbociclib, 74.1% of the radioactivity was recovered in feces and 17.5% was recovered in urine; the majority of the dose was excreted as metabolites. The mean plasma elimination half-life of the drug is 29 hours.

Population pharmacokinetic analyses indicate that age (22–89 years), sex, race (Asian versus non-Asian), and body weight do not have clinically important effects on the exposure of palbociclib.

ADVICE TO PATIENTS

- Stress importance of taking palbociclib with food. Avoid grapefruit and grapefruit juice while taking the drug.
- For premenopausal or perimenopausal women, stress importance of receiving concomitant luteinizing hormone-releasing hormone (LHRH) agonist therapy.
- Advise patients to swallow palbociclib capsules and tablets whole and not to chew, crush, or open/split.
- If a dose is missed or vomited, administer the next dose at the regularly scheduled time; an additional dose should not be administered to make up for a missed dose.

- Risk of myelosuppression or infection. Stress importance of informing clinician immediately if signs or symptoms of myelosuppression or infection (e.g., fever, chills, dizziness, shortness of breath, weakness, increased tendency to bleed and/or bruise) occur.
- Risk of severe, life-threatening, or fatal interstitial lung disease/pneumonitis. Stress importance of informing clinician immediately if new or worsening cough (with or without mucus), chest pain, or shortness of breath occurs.
- Risk of fetal harm. Advise women of childbearing potential and men who are partners of such women that they should use an effective method of contraception during treatment and for at least 3 weeks in women or 3 months in men after discontinuance of therapy. Stress importance of women informing clinicians if they are or plan to become pregnant. If pregnancy occurs, advise patients of potential risk to the fetus.
- Risk of serious adverse reactions in nursing infants. Advise women to discontinue nursing during therapy and for 3 weeks after discontinuance of the drug.
- Risk of male infertility. Advise men to consider sperm preservation prior to initiating palbociclib therapy.
- Stress importance of informing clinicians of existing or contemplated concomitant therapy, including prescription and OTC drugs and dietary or herbal supplements (e.g., St. John's wort), as well as any concomitant illnesses.
- Inform patients of other important precautionary information.

For further information on the handling of antineoplastic agents, see the ASHP Guidelines on Handling Hazardous Drugs at https://www.ahfsdruginformation.com.

PREPARATIONS

Palbociclib is obtained from specialty pharmacy providers. Contact manufacturer for additional information.

Excipients in commercially available drug preparations may have clinically important effects in some individuals; consult specific product labeling for details.

Palbociclib

Oral		
Capsules	75 mg	Ibrance®, Pfizer
	100 mg	Ibrance®, Pfizer
	125 mg	Ibrance®, Pfizer
Tablets	75 mg	Ibrance®, Pfizer
	100 mg	Ibrance®, Pfizer
	125 mg	Ibrance®, Pfizer

† Use is not currently included in the labeling approved by the US Food and Drug Administration.

Selected Revisions August 10, 2024, © Copyright, October 14, 2016, American Society of Health-System Pharmacists, Inc.

PAZOPanib Hydrochloride

10:00 · ANTINEOPLASTIC AGENTS

■ Pazopanib hydrochloride, an inhibitor of multiple receptor tyrosine kinases, is an antineoplastic agent.

USES

● Renal Cell Carcinoma

Pazopanib hydrochloride is used for the treatment of advanced renal cell carcinoma in adults. Safety and efficacy of pazopanib for the treatment of advanced renal cell carcinoma are based principally on the results of a randomized, double-blind, placebo-controlled, multicenter, phase 3 study (VEG105192), with supportive data from a long-term extension study. Guidelines generally recommend pazopanib as a first-line treatment option in patients with clear-cell metastatic renal cell carcinoma who cannot receive or tolerate immune checkpoint inhibitors.

The current indication for pazopanib hydrochloride in the treatment of advanced renal cell carcinoma is based principally on the results of a randomized, double-blind, placebo-controlled, multicenter, phase 3 study (VEG105192) in 435 patients 18 years of age and older (median age: 59 years) with locally advanced and/or metastatic clear-cell (or predominantly clear-cell) renal cell carcinoma. This study initially enrolled patients whose disease had progressed following one prior cytokine-based regimen (i.e., aldesleukin, interferon alfa); the study protocol was subsequently amended (after enrollment of 7 patients) to include patients who had received no prior therapy (treatment-naive patients). Because other drugs (e.g., sorafenib, sunitinib) had been approved in the US for treatment of renal cell carcinoma, the US Food and Drug Administration (FDA) expressed concerns about the use of a placebo control, and agreement was not reached on the study design. The VEG105192 study, thus, was conducted outside of the US in countries where patients did not have access to established therapies (e.g., aldesleukin, interferon alfa, sorafenib, sunitinib) or where cytokines were not recognized as standard treatment for renal cell carcinoma.

In this study, 435 patients (233 treatment-naive and 202 cytokine-pretreated patients) were randomized in a 2:1 ratio to receive either pazopanib (800 mg daily) or placebo along with best supportive care. Treatment in both groups was continued until disease progression, unacceptable toxicity, death, or discontinuance of therapy for other reasons occurred; upon disease progression, patients previously randomized to receive placebo were permitted to cross over to open-label pazopanib. The median duration of treatment was 7.4 or 3.8 months in patients randomized to receive pazopanib or placebo, respectively. Enrolled patients had clear cell histology (90%) or predominantly clear cell histology (10%); 88–89% had undergone nephrectomy, and approximately 50% had metastatic disease involving 3 or more organs. Radiographic assessment of efficacy was performed every 6 weeks during the first 24 weeks of therapy and then every 8 weeks thereafter. The primary measure of efficacy was progression-free survival; the secondary end points included overall survival, overall response rate, and duration of response.

The median progression-free survival in the overall population was 9.2 months in patients receiving pazopanib compared with 4.2 months in those receiving placebo; the effect size appeared to be larger in the treatment-naive subgroup (11.1 versus 2.8 months) but also was clinically important in the cytokine-pretreated subgroup (7.4 versus 4.2 months). Improved progression-free survival was observed in patients receiving pazopanib regardless of Memorial Sloan-Kettering Cancer Center (MSKCC) risk category, gender, age, or ECOG performance status. The overall response rate for all patients receiving pazopanib was 30%, and the median duration of response was 58.7 weeks. Response rates were similar among treatment-naive (32%) and cytokine-pretreated (29%) subgroups of patients who received pazopanib. The median time to response was 11.9 weeks. At the time of the final overall survival analysis, median overall survival was 22.9 months in the pazopanib group and 20.5 months in the placebo group (hazard ratio of 0.91; 95% confidence interval: 0.71, 1.16). Although 54% of patients in the placebo group crossed over to receive pazopanib; median progression-free survival and overall survival were 9.2 and 23.5 months, respectively, in these patients which was consistent with the values observed in pazopanib-treated patients in the VEG105192 trial. Use of other subsequent anticancer treatments differed between the treatment arms of the VEG105192 trial as well; 66% of patients in

the placebo group received at least 1 systemic anticancer treatment after disease progression, compared to 30% of pazopanib-treated patients. Although results of the final overall survival analysis may be confounded by the high rate of crossover from placebo to pazopanib and by receipt of subsequent anticancer treatments, a post-hoc analysis adjusting for treatment crossover suggested a benefit for pazopanib in terms of overall survival.

An additional randomized, open-label phase 3 trial (COMPARZ) compared pazopanib to sunitinib in 1110 adults with advanced or metastatic clear-cell renal cell carcinoma. Patients enrolled in the trial had not received any previous systemic therapy. Patients were randomized in a 1:1 ratio (stratified according to Karnofsky performance status score, lactate dehydrogenase level, and history of nephrectomy) to receive pazopanib 800 mg once daily or sunitinib administered in 6-week cycles (sunitinib 50 mg once daily for 4 consecutive weeks followed by a 2-week period without treatment). Treatment cycles were repeated until disease progression, unacceptable toxicity, or withdrawal of consent occurred. The primary efficacy measure was progression-free survival.

Treatment with pazopanib was noninferior to treatment with sunitinib in terms of progression-free survival. The median progression-free survival was 8.4 months in the pazopanib group and 9.5 months in the sunitinib group. Objective response rates were 31 and 25% in the pazopanib and sunitinib groups, respectively. In the final overall survival analysis, no substantial difference in median overall survival was observed (28.3 and 29.1 months in patients receiving pazopanib or sunitinib, respectively).

Clinical Perspective

Prognosis is generally poor in patients with metastatic RCC, including those who have undergone complete tumor resection. First-line therapy with vascular endothelial growth factor receptor (VEGFR) inhibitors has been shown to provide benefits in patients with advanced RCC; however, relapsed or refractory RCC eventually develops in most patients. Combination regimens (e.g., immune checkpoint inhibitor in combination with a tyrosine kinase inhibitor) have generally become a standard for the treatment of advanced RCC. A limited number of randomized controlled trials have compared sunitinib with other treatment options for advanced renal cell carcinoma (e.g., pembrolizumab plus axitinib, avelumab plus axitinib, atezolizumab plus bevacizumab, nivolumab plus ipilimumab, nivolumab plus cabozantinib, or lenvatinib plus pembrolizumab). In clinical trials, combination chemotherapy resulted in longer progression-free survival compared with sunitinib alone in patients with previously untreated advanced renal cell carcinoma.

Some experts also state that subsequent monotherapy with a tyrosine kinase inhibitor (e.g., sunitinib, pazopanib) may be offered as an alternative to programmed death 1 (PD-1) inhibitor-based combinations in the first-line setting when immune checkpoint therapy is contraindicated or not available or as a second-line option following disease progression during immune checkpoint inhibitor-based therapy.

● Soft Tissue Sarcoma

Pazopanib hydrochloride is used for the treatment of advanced soft tissue sarcoma in adults who have received prior chemotherapy. The drug has been designated an orphan drug by the FDA for the treatment of this cancer. Efficacy of pazopanib for the treatment of patients with adipocytic soft tissue sarcoma or GI stomal tumors has not been demonstrated. Safety and efficacy of pazopanib for the treatment of advanced soft tissue sarcoma are based principally on the results of a randomized, double-blind, placebo-controlled study (VEG110727). Guidelines state that pazopanib is an option for second or subsequent line of therapy in non-adipogenic soft tissue sarcoma.

The current indication for pazopanib hydrochloride in the treatment of soft tissue sarcoma is based principally on the results of a randomized, double-blind, placebo-controlled trial (PALETTE [VEG110727]). In this study, 369 adults with metastatic soft tissue sarcoma who were previously treated with at least 1 anthracycline-containing chemotherapy regimen or were not eligible for anthracycline-based chemotherapy were randomized in a 2:1 ratio (stratified by World Health Organization [WHO] performance status and number of prior therapies) to receive pazopanib 800 mg once daily or placebo. Treatment was continued until disease progression, unacceptable toxicity, withdrawal of consent, or death occurred. Enrolled patients had leiomyosarcoma (43%), synovial sarcoma (10%), or other soft tissue sarcomas (47%). Approximately one-half (56%) of patients had received 2 or more previous lines of systemic therapy. The median duration of treatment was 16.4 or 8.1 weeks in patients randomized to receive pazopanib or placebo, respectively. The primary measure of efficacy was progression-free survival as assessed by independent radiological review.

Median progression-free survival was 4.6 months in the pazopanib group and 1.6 months in the placebo group. Improved progression-free survival was observed in patients receiving pazopanib regardless of soft tissue sarcoma type. Overall response rate was 4 and 0% in the pazopanib and placebo groups, respectively. Median duration of response in the pazopanib group was 9 months. Median overall survival did not differ significantly between treatment groups in the final analysis (12.6 or 10.7 months in the pazopanib or placebo group, respectively).

Clinical Perspective

Chemotherapy is standard treatment for soft tissue sarcoma, with single-agent doxorubicin being the treatment of choice. Other agents with clinical activity in soft tissue sarcoma include VEGF tyrosine kinase inhibitors such as pazopanib and regorafenib.

Some experts state that pazopanib is an option for second or subsequent line of therapy in non-adipogenic soft tissue sarcoma.

DOSAGE AND ADMINISTRATION

● General

Pretreatment Screening

- Blood pressure should be adequately controlled prior to initiating therapy. Do not initiate in patients with uncontrolled hypertension.
- Assess ECG and electrolytes at baseline.
- In patients at risk of cardiac dysfunction (including those previously treated with an anthracycline), assess left ventricular ejection fraction (LVEF) at baseline.
- Perform thyroid function tests at baseline.
- Perform urinalysis at baseline.
- Verify pregnancy status of females of reproductive potential prior to initiation of therapy.

Patient Monitoring

- Monitor liver function tests at weeks 3, 5, 7, and 9, and months 3 and 4, and then periodically thereafter as clinically indicated. Increase frequency of monitoring in patients who develop hepatotoxicity.
- Monitor ECG and electrolytes as clinically indicated; correct hypokalemia, hypomagnesemia, and hypocalcemia as needed.
- Monitor for signs and symptoms of congestive heart failure (CHF); in patients at risk of cardiac dysfunction (including those previously treated with an anthracycline), monitor LVEF periodically during therapy.
- Monitor for signs and symptoms of venous thromboembolism (VTE), pulmonary embolism (PE), arterial thromboembolism, thrombotic microangiopathy, GI perforation/fistula, or interstitial lung disease/pneumonitis.
- Monitor blood pressure as clinically indicated.
- Monitor thyroid function during therapy as clinically indicated.
- Perform urinalysis periodically during therapy; assess urine protein levels over a 24-hour period as clinically indicated.
- Monitor for signs and symptoms of infection.

Dispensing and Administration Precautions

- To avoid medication errors, the Institute for Safe Medication Practices (ISMP) recommends that prescribers communicate both the brand and generic names for pazopanib on the prescription order form.

Other General Considerations

- Withhold pazopanib ≥7 days prior to scheduled surgery, and for ≥2 weeks following major surgery and until adequate wound healing has occurred.

● Administration

Pazopanib hydrochloride is administered orally once daily. Administer the drug without food (i.e., at least 1 hour before or 2 hours after a meal). Pazopanib hydrochloride tablets should be swallowed whole and should not be crushed; crushing the tablets has been shown to increase the rate of absorption and systemic exposure to the drug. Store tablets at 20–25°C (excursions permitted between 15–30°C).

Concomitant use of pazopanib with drugs affecting gastric pH may result in decreased pazopanib exposure and should be avoided. If concomitant use with a drug affecting gastric pH cannot be avoided, consider a short-acting antacid rather than a proton-pump inhibitor or histamine H_2-receptor antagonist. The administration of a short-acting antacid and pazopanib should be separated by several hours.

● Dosage

Dosage of pazopanib hydrochloride is expressed in terms of pazopanib.

Renal Cell Carcinoma

For the treatment of advanced renal cell carcinoma, the recommended adult dosage of pazopanib is 800 mg once daily. Continue therapy for as long as the patient derives clinical benefit from the drug or until unacceptable toxicity occurs.

Soft Tissue Sarcoma

For the treatment of advanced soft tissue sarcoma previously treated with chemotherapy, the recommended adult dosage of pazopanib is 800 mg once daily. Continue therapy for as long as the patient derives clinical benefit from the drug or until unacceptable toxicity occurs.

Dosage Modification

If adverse reactions occur, temporary interruption of therapy, dosage reduction, and/or discontinuance of pazopanib may be necessary. If dosage modification is required, reduce the dosage of pazopanib as described in Table 1.

TABLE 1. Recommended Dosage Reduction for Pazopanib Toxicity

Dosage Reduction	Renal Cell Carcinoma (Starting dosage = 800 mg once daily)	Soft Tissue Sarcoma (Starting dosage = 800 mg once daily)
First	400 mg once daily	600 mg once daily
Second	200 mg once daily	400 mg once daily
Third	Permanently discontinue drug	Permanently discontinue drug

Hepatotoxicity

If hepatotoxicity occurs, reduce pazopanib dosage, or interrupt or permanently discontinue therapy. (See Table 2.)

TABLE 2. Recommended Dosage Modifications for Hepatotoxicity

ALT (SGPT) and/or Bilirubin Concentrations	Recommended Action
Serum ALT concentration 3–8 times the upper limit of normal (ULN)	Continue pazopanib; monitor liver function weekly until serum ALT concentration returns to grade 1 or baseline
Serum ALT concentration >8 times the ULN	Interrupt pazopanib therapy until serum ALT concentration returns to grade 1 or baseline; if benefit outweighs risk, reinitiate pazopanib at a reduced dosage of 400 mg or less once daily; following reinitiation, monitor liver function weekly for 8 weeks; if serum ALT concentration rises to >3 times the ULN, discontinue pazopanib *permanently*
Serum ALT concentration >3 times the ULN *and* mild, indirect (unconjugated) hyperbilirubinemia in patients with known Gilbert syndrome	Manage per recommendations for patients with isolated serum ALT elevations
Serum ALT concentration >3 times the ULN *and* serum bilirubin concentration >2 times the ULN	Discontinue pazopanib *permanently*; monitor liver function until hepatotoxicity resolves

Cardiac Dysfunction

If symptomatic or grade 3 left ventricular systolic dysfunction occurs, withhold pazopanib until toxicity improves to grade 2 or less; therapy may be resumed based on clinical judgment.

If grade 4 left ventricular systolic dysfunction occurs, permanently discontinue pazopanib.

Hemorrhage

If a grade 2 hemorrhagic event occurs, withhold pazopanib until toxicity improves to grade 1 or less; therapy may then be resumed at a reduced dosage (see Table 1).

If a grade 3 or 4 hemorrhagic event occurs, permanently discontinue pazopanib.

Thromboembolic Events

If a grade 3 venous thromboembolic event (VTE) occurs, withhold pazopanib; therapy may be resumed at the same dosage after at least 1 week of appropriate therapy for the thromboembolic event.

If an arterial thromboembolic event or grade 4 VTE occurs, permanently discontinue pazopanib.

Thrombotic Microangiopathy

If thrombotic microangiopathy occurs, permanently discontinue pazopanib.

GI Toxicity

If GI perforation occurs, permanently discontinue pazopanib.

If grade 2 or 3 GI fistula occurs, withhold pazopanib; therapy may be resumed based on clinical judgment.

If grade 4 GI fistula occurs, permanently discontinue pazopanib.

Interstitial Lung Disease/Pneumonitis

If interstitial lung disease or pneumonitis of any grade occurs, permanently discontinue pazopanib.

Posterior Reversible Encephalopathy Syndrome

If posterior reversible encephalopathy syndrome of any grade occurs, permanently discontinue pazopanib.

Hypertension

If grade 2 or 3 hypertension occurs, reduce the dosage of pazopanib (see Table 1) and initiate or adjust antihypertensive therapy. If grade 3 hypertension persists despite reducing the dosage of pazopanib and use of antihypertensive therapy, permanently discontinue pazopanib.

If grade 4 hypertension or hypertensive crisis occurs, permanently discontinue pazopanib.

Proteinuria

If urine protein levels 3 grams or greater per 24 hours occurs, withhold pazopanib until urine protein levels improve to grade 1 or less; therapy may then be resumed at a reduced dosage (see Table 1). If urine protein levels over a 24-hour period do not improve or urine protein levels 3 grams or greater per 24 hours recurs despite reducing the dosage of pazopanib, permanently discontinue drug.

If nephrotic syndrome is confirmed, permanently discontinue pazopanib.

Concomitant Use with Drugs Affecting Hepatic Microsomal Enzymes

Concomitant use of pazopanib with potent inhibitors of CYP3A4 may result in increased plasma concentrations of pazopanib and should be *avoided*. If concomitant use with a potent CYP3A4 inhibitor cannot be avoided, reduce the dosage of pazopanib to 400 mg daily.

Concomitant use of pazopanib with potent inducers of CYP3A4 may result in decreased plasma concentrations of pazopanib and should be *avoided*.

● Special Populations

Hepatic Impairment

No dosage adjustment is necessary in patients with mild hepatic impairment (total serum bilirubin concentration not exceeding 1.5 times the ULN with any level of ALT). The manufacturer recommends that dosage of pazopanib be reduced to 200 mg once daily in patients with moderate hepatic impairment (total serum bilirubin concentration exceeding 1.5 times, but not more than 3 times, the ULN with any level of ALT). Safety of pazopanib has not been established in patients with severe hepatic impairment (total serum bilirubin concentration exceeding 3 times the ULN with any level of ALT); therefore, the manufacturer recommends that the drug *not* be used in such patients.

Renal Impairment

Renal impairment is not expected to influence pazopanib exposure; therefore, the manufacturer states that dosage adjustment is not necessary in patients with renal impairment.

Geriatric Patients

The manufacturer makes no specific dosage recommendations for geriatric patients.

CAUTIONS

● Contraindications

● The manufacturer states there are no known contraindications to the use of pazopanib.

● Warnings/Precautions

Warnings

Hepatic Effects

A boxed warning about the risk of hepatotoxicity is included in the prescribing information for pazopanib. Severe or fatal hepatotoxicity, manifested as increases in serum concentrations of aminotransferases (ALT [SGPT], AST [SGOT]) and bilirubin, has been reported in patients receiving pazopanib. Most (92%) cases of aminotransferase elevations (of any grade) occurred during the first 18 weeks of therapy. In the randomized, placebo-controlled study (VEG105192) in patients with renal cell carcinoma, increases in ALT concentrations exceeding 3 or 10 times the upper limit of normal (ULN) were reported in approximately 18 or 4%, respectively, of patients receiving pazopanib. Concurrent increases in concentrations of ALT (exceeding 3 times the ULN) *and* bilirubin (exceeding twice the ULN) in the absence of substantial (exceeding 3 times the ULN) increases in alkaline phosphatase concentrations were reported in approximately 2% of patients receiving pazopanib. Death (resulting from disease progression and hepatic failure) occurred in 2 patients receiving pazopanib. In a randomized, placebo-controlled study (VEG110727) in patients with soft tissue sarcoma, increases in ALT concentrations exceeding 3 or 10 times the ULN were reported in approximately 18 or 5%, respectively, of patients receiving pazopanib. Concurrent increases in ALT (exceeding 3 times the ULN) and bilirubin (exceeding twice the ULN) concentrations in the absence of substantial increases in alkaline phosphatase concentrations (exceeding 3 times the ULN) were reported in approximately 2% of patients receiving pazopanib. Fatal hepatic failure was reported in one patient.

Because pazopanib inhibits uridine diphosphate-glucuronosyltransferase (UGT) 1A1 (an enzyme that catalyzes the glucuronidation of bilirubin for elimination), mild elevations in indirect (unconjugated) bilirubin may occur in patients with deficient glucuronidation of bilirubin (i.e., Gilbert syndrome).

Concomitant use of pazopanib and simvastatin increases the risk of elevations of ALT concentrations. In clinical trials evaluating pazopanib monotherapy, increases in ALT concentrations exceeding 3 times the ULN were reported in 14% of patients who were not receiving a HMG-CoA reductase inhibitor (statin) and in 27% of those receiving concomitant simvastatin. Data are insufficient to assess the risk of other statins administered concomitantly with pazopanib.

Perform liver function tests prior to initiation of pazopanib, during weeks 3, 5, 7, and 9 of therapy, at months 3 and 4, and then periodically thereafter as clinically indicated. If hepatotoxicity occurs, withhold pazopanib and resume at a reduced dosage with continued weekly liver function monitoring for 8 weeks, or permanently discontinue pazopanib and monitor liver function tests weekly until resolution, depending on the severity of hepatotoxicity. If ALT elevations occur in a patient taking concomitant simvastatin, monitor liver function weekly.

Other Warnings and Precautions

Prolongation of QT Interval and Torsades de Pointes

Prolongation of the QT interval and torsades de pointes have been reported in patients receiving pazopanib. In the VEG105192 and VEG110727 studies, prolongation of the QT interval (500–549 msec) was reported in approximately 1 and 0.4%, respectively, of patients receiving pazopanib. In an analysis of pooled data from 3 studies involving 558 patients with renal cell carcinoma, prolongation of the QT interval (500 msec or greater) or torsades de pointes was reported in approximately 2% or less than 1%, respectively, of patients receiving pazopanib.

Avoid concomitant administration of pazopanib and drugs that prolong the QT interval. Monitor patients at significant risk for QT prolongation, including patients with a history of prolongation of the QT interval, patients receiving antiarrhythmic agents or other drugs that cause prolongation of the QT interval, and patients with relevant preexisting cardiac disease. Monitor ECG and serum electrolytes (e.g., calcium, magnesium, potassium) prior to initiation of pazopanib and periodically during treatment. Correct hypokalemia, hypomagnesemia, and hypocalcemia prior to initiation of pazopanib and as necessary during treatment.

Cardiac Dysfunction

Cardiac dysfunction, including decreased left ventricular ejection fraction and congestive heart failure, has been reported in patients receiving pazopanib. In renal cell carcinoma trials, cardiac dysfunction was observed in 0.6% of patients. Among patients who had baseline and post-baseline left ventricular ejection fraction measurement in the COMPARZ trial, cardiac dysfunction occurred in 13% of patients. Congestive heart failure has been reported in 0.5% of patients. In the VEG110727 study in patients with soft tissue sarcoma, cardiac dysfunction occurred in 11% of patients who had baseline and post-baseline left ventricular ejection fraction measurements; congestive heart failure occurred in 1% of patients. Most patients with cardiac dysfunction in the VEG110727 study had concurrent hypertension, which may have exacerbated cardiac dysfunction in patients who had preexisting risk factors for cardiac dysfunction (e.g., those with prior anthracycline therapy).

Monitor patients receiving pazopanib for signs and symptoms of congestive heart failure. Monitor left ventricular ejection fraction in patients at risk of cardiac dysfunction (including those with previous anthracycline exposure) at baseline and periodically during therapy. If cardiac dysfunction occurs, withhold or permanently discontinue pazopanib depending on the severity of the cardiac dysfunction.

Hemorrhage

Hemorrhage, sometimes severe or fatal, has been reported in patients receiving pazopanib. In renal cell carcinoma trials, fatal hemorrhagic events occurred in 0.9% of patients receiving pazopanib, and cerebral/intracranial hemorrhage occurred in <1% of patients receiving pazopanib. In the VEG105192 study, hemorrhage was reported in 13% of patients receiving pazopanib. The most common hemorrhagic events reported with pazopanib in this study included hematuria, epistaxis, hemoptysis, and rectal hemorrhage; severe hemorrhagic events included pulmonary, GI, and genitourinary hemorrhage. Fatal hemorrhage was reported in approximately 1% of patients receiving pazopanib. In the VEG110727 study in patients with soft tissue sarcoma, hemorrhage (most commonly epistaxis and oral or anal hemorrhage) was reported in 22% of patients. Grade 4 hemorrhagic events occurred in 1% of patients and included intracranial, subarachnoid, and peritoneal hemorrhage.

Pazopanib has not been evaluated in patients with a history of hemoptysis or patients with cerebral or clinically important GI hemorrhage within the past 6 months. If a hemorrhagic event occurs, withhold pazopanib and resume at a reduced dosage or permanently discontinue drug depending on the severity of the hemorrhagic event.

Thromboembolic Events

Arterial thromboembolic events, sometimes severe or fatal, have been reported in patients receiving pazopanib. In renal cell carcinoma trials, fatal arterial embolic events occurred in 0.3% of patients. In the VEG105192 study, myocardial infarction/ischemia, cerebrovascular accident, or transient ischemic attack (TIA) was reported in approximately 2, less than 0.3, or 1%, respectively, of patients receiving pazopanib. In the VEG110727 study in patients with soft tissue sarcoma, myocardial infarction/ischemia and cerebrovascular accident were reported in 2 and 0.4% of patients receiving pazopanib, respectively.

Pazopanib has not been evaluated in patients who had experienced an arterial thromboembolic event within the past 6 months. If arterial thromboembolism occurs, permanently discontinue pazopanib.

Venous thromboembolic events (VTE), including venous thrombosis and fatal pulmonary embolism, have been reported in patients receiving pazopanib. In the VEG105192 study in patients with renal cell carcinoma, venous thromboembolism occurred in 1% of patients receiving pazopanib; in the VEG110727 study evaluating pazopanib in patients with soft tissue sarcoma, venous thromboembolism and fatal pulmonary embolism occurred in 5 and 1%, respectively, of patients receiving pazopanib.

Monitor patients receiving pazopanib for signs and symptoms of venous thromboembolism and pulmonary embolism during pazopanib therapy. If venous thromboembolism or pulmonary embolism occurs, withhold pazopanib and resume at the same dosage or permanently discontinue drug depending on the severity of the thromboembolic event.

Thrombotic Microangiopathy

Thrombotic microangiopathy, including thrombotic thrombocytopenic purpura and hemolytic uremic syndrome, has been reported in patients receiving pazopanib as monotherapy, in combination with bevacizumab†, or in combination with topotecan†. Pazopanib is not indicated for use in combination with other agents. Thrombotic microangiopathy generally occurs within 90 days of initiation of pazopanib therapy, and improves following discontinuance of the drug.

Monitor patients receiving pazopanib for signs and symptoms of thrombotic microangiopathy. If thrombotic microangiopathy occurs, permanently discontinue pazopanib.

GI Effects

GI perforation or fistula, sometimes fatal, has been reported in patients receiving pazopanib. In renal cell carcinoma trials and soft tissue sarcoma trials, GI perforation or fistula occurred in 0.9 and 1%, respectively, of patients receiving pazopanib. Fatal GI perforation occurred in 0.3% of patients in renal cell carcinoma and soft tissue sarcoma trials.

Monitor patients receiving pazopanib for manifestations of GI perforation or fistula formation. If GI fistula occurs, withhold pazopanib and resume based on medical judgment or permanently discontinue pazopanib, depending on the severity of the GI fistula. If GI perforation occurs, permanently discontinue pazopanib.

Interstitial Lung Disease/Pneumonitis

Interstitial lung disease/pneumonitis, which can be fatal, has been reported in patients receiving pazopanib. In clinical trials, interstitial lung disease/pneumonitis occurred in 0.1% of patients receiving pazopanib.

Monitor patients receiving pazopanib for pulmonary symptoms indicative of interstitial lung disease/pneumonitis. If interstitial lung disease or pneumonitis occurs, permanently discontinue pazopanib.

Posterior Reversible Encephalopathy Syndrome

Posterior reversible encephalopathy syndrome, which can be fatal, has been reported in patients receiving pazopanib. Symptoms of posterior reversible encephalopathy syndrome may include headache, seizure, lethargy, confusion, blindness, and other visual and neurologic disturbances. Mild to severe hypertension may also be present.

If symptoms of posterior reversible encephalopathy syndrome occur, confirm the diagnosis with MRI. If posterior reversible encephalopathy syndrome occurs, permanently discontinue pazopanib.

Hypertension

Hypertension (systolic blood pressure of 150 mm Hg or greater or diastolic blood pressure of 100 mm Hg or greater) and hypertensive crisis have been reported in patients receiving pazopanib. Most (90%) cases occurred during the first 18 weeks of therapy. Approximately 1% of patients require permanent discontinuation of pazopanib due to hypertension. In the VEG105192 study, hypertension was reported in approximately 40 or 10% of patients receiving pazopanib or placebo, respectively; grade 3 hypertension was reported in approximately 4 or less than 1% of patients receiving pazopanib or placebo, respectively. In the VEG110727 study, hypertension was reported in 42 or 6% of patients receiving pazopanib or placebo, respectively; grade 3 hypertension was reported in 7 or 0% of patients receiving pazopanib or placebo, respectively. The majority of hypertension cases were managed with antihypertensive therapy or by reduction in pazopanib dosage.

Blood pressure must be adequately controlled prior to initiation of pazopanib. Monitor and treat for hypertension as clinically indicated as clinically indicated. If hypertension occurs, withhold pazopanib and resume at a reduced dosage or permanently discontinue pazopanib, depending on the severity of hypertension.

Wound-healing Complications

Because inhibitors of the vascular endothelial growth factor (VEGF) signaling pathway, including pazopanib, may impair wound healing, pazopanib may adversely affect wound healing. Discontinue pazopanib at least 7 days prior to scheduled surgery, and withhold for at least 2 weeks following major surgery and until adequate wound healing has occurred. The safety of resuming pazopanib therapy after resolution of wound healing complications has not been established.

Hypothyroidism

Hypothyroidism has been reported in patients receiving pazopanib. In the VEG105192 study, hypothyroidism was reported in 7% of patients receiving pazopanib; hypothyroidism was reported in 5% of patients receiving pazopanib. In an analysis of pooled data from renal cell carcinoma studies, hypothyroidism was reported in 4% of patients receiving pazopanib; in an analysis of pooled data from soft tissue sarcoma studies, hypothyroidism was reported in 5% of patients receiving pazopanib.

Assess thyroid function at baseline and during therapy as clinically indicated. Manage hypothyroidism as appropriate.

Proteinuria

Proteinuria has been reported in patients receiving pazopanib. In the VEG110727 study, proteinuria was reported in 1% of patients receiving pazopanib; nephrotic syndrome was reported in 1 patient.

Perform urinalysis prior to initiation of pazopanib and periodically during therapy, with follow-up measurement of 24-hour urine protein as clinically indicated. If proteinuria occurs, withhold pazopanib and resume at a reduced dosage or permanently discontinue pazopanib, depending on the severity of proteinuria. If nephrotic syndrome occurs, permanently discontinue pazopanib.

Tumor Lysis Syndrome

Tumor lysis syndrome, sometimes fatal, has been reported in patients receiving pazopanib.

Monitor patients at risk of tumor lysis syndrome (e.g., those with rapidly growing tumors, high tumor burden, renal dysfunction, dehydration) closely during pazopanib therapy; consider prophylactic therapy, and initiate treatment for tumor lysis syndrome as clinically indicated.

Infection

Serious, sometimes fatal, infections (with or without neutropenia) have been reported in patients receiving pazopanib.

Monitor for signs and symptoms of infection. If serious infections occur, consider interruption or discontinuation of pazopanib.

Combination Therapy

Pazopanib is not indicated for use in combination with other agents. Clinical trials of pazopanib in combination with pemetrexed or lapatinib were terminated early due to increased toxicity and mortality. Fatal toxicities included pulmonary hemorrhage, GI hemorrhage, and sudden death.

Increased Toxicity in Developing Organs

Pazopanib is not indicated for use in pediatric patients, as safety and efficacy in this patient population have not been established. Based on animal studies and its mechanism of action, pazopanib may have severe effects on organ growth

and maturation during early postnatal development. In studies of juvenile rats less than 21 days old, organ toxicity (i.e., lungs, liver, heart, kidney) and death occurred following administration of pazopanib at doses significantly lower than the clinically recommended dose or doses tolerated in older animals.

Fetal/Neonatal Morbidity and Mortality

Pazopanib may cause fetal harm; the drug has been shown to cause maternal toxicity, teratogenicity, and abortion in animal studies. There are no adequate and well-controlled studies in pregnant women. Avoid pregnancy during therapy. If used during pregnancy or if the patient becomes pregnant while receiving pazopanib, apprise the patient of the potential fetal hazard. Advise females of reproductive potential to use effective contraception during pazopanib therapy and for at least 2 weeks after the final dose. Advise males with such female partners to use condoms during pazopanib therapy and for at least 2 weeks after the final dose.

Specific Populations

Pregnancy

Based on animal reproduction studies and its mechanism of action, pazopanib may cause fetal harm. There are no adequate and well-controlled studies in pregnant women. In animal studies, administration of pazopanib during organogenesis resulted in teratogenicity and abortion at systemic exposures lower than those observed at the maximum recommended human dose. Avoid pregnancy during therapy. If used during pregnancy or if the patient becomes pregnant while receiving pazopanib, apprise the patient of the potential fetal hazard.

Lactation

It is not known whether pazopanib or its metabolites are distributed into human milk. The effects of pazopanib or its metabolites on a breast-fed infant or milk production are unknown. Because of the potential for serious adverse reactions to pazopanib in breast-fed infants, avoid breast-feeding during pazopanib treatment and for 2 weeks after the final dose of pazopanib.

Females and Males of Reproductive Potential

Prior to initiation of pazopanib therapy, verify pregnancy status of females of reproductive potential. Advise females of reproductive potential to use effective contraception during pazopanib treatment and for at least 2 weeks after the last dose of pazopanib. Advise males with such female partners to use condoms during pazopanib treatment and for at least 2 weeks after the last dose of pazopanib.

Based on animal studies, pazopanib may impair fertility in females and males of reproductive potential.

Pediatric Use

Safety and efficacy have not been established in pediatric patients younger than 18 years of age.

Pazopanib may cause serious adverse effects on organ development in pediatric patients, particularly in those less than 2 years of age. In animal studies conducted in juvenile rats less than 21 days old, organ toxicity (i.e., lungs, liver, heart, kidney) and death occurred following administration of pazopanib at doses significantly lower than the clinically recommended dose or doses tolerated in older animals.

Geriatric Use

In an analysis of pooled clinical trial data from all pazopanib studies, 30% of patients were 65 years of age or older; ALT elevations exceeding 3 times the ULN occurred more frequently in older patients compared to younger adults. ALT elevations exceeding 3 times the ULN occurred in 23% of patients 65 years of age or older and in 18% of patients less than 65 years of age.

In an analysis of pooled data from studies involving 586 patients with renal cell carcinoma, 33% of patients were 65 years of age or older; no overall differences in safety or efficacy were observed between older and younger adults.

In an analysis of pooled data from studies involving 382 patients with soft tissue sarcoma, 24% of patients were 65 years of age or older. Patients 65 years of age or older had a higher incidence of grade 3 or 4 fatigue, hypertension, decreased appetite, ALT elevations, and AST elevations. No overall differences in efficacy were observed between patients 65 years of age or older and younger adults.

Hepatic Impairment

An analysis of pharmacokinetic data indicated that pazopanib clearance in patients with mild hepatic impairment (total bilirubin concentration not exceeding the ULN with ALT exceeding the ULN, or total serum bilirubin concentration not exceeding 1.5 times the ULN with any level of ALT) was similar to that in patients with normal hepatic function. Therefore, the manufacturer states that no dosage adjustment is necessary in patients with mild hepatic impairment.

In a pharmacokinetic study, the maximum tolerated dosage of pazopanib in patients with moderate hepatic impairment (total serum bilirubin concentration exceeding 1.5 times, but not more than 3 times, the ULN with any level of ALT) was 200 mg once daily. The steady-state peak plasma concentration or median AUC was approximately 43 or 29%, respectively, of the corresponding median values after administration of pazopanib 800 mg once daily in patients with normal hepatic function. Pazopanib is not recommended for use in patients with moderate hepatic impairment; if pazopanib is used in such patients, reduce the dosage of pazopanib to 200 mg once daily.

In a pharmacokinetic study of patients with severe hepatic impairment (total serum bilirubin concentration exceeding 3 times the ULN with any level of ALT) receiving pazopanib 200 mg once daily, the median steady-state peak plasma concentration and median AUC were approximately 18 and 15%, respectively, of the corresponding median values after administration of pazopanib 800 mg once daily in patients with normal hepatic function. Avoid the use of pazopanib in patients with severe hepatic impairment.

Renal Impairment

In a population pharmacokinetic analysis involving patients with various cancers, creatinine clearance of 30–150 mL/minute did not substantially affect clearance of pazopanib. Because renal impairment is unlikely to affect the pharmacokinetics (e.g., exposure) of pazopanib (i.e., less than 4% of a radiolabeled oral dose of pazopanib is recovered in urine), the manufacturer states that no dosage adjustment is necessary in patients with renal impairment.

Pazopanib has not been studied in patients with severe renal impairment or in patients undergoing peritoneal dialysis or hemodialysis.

Pharmacogenomics

Pazopanib inhibits UGT1A1, an enzyme that catalyzes the glucuronidation of bilirubin for elimination. Patients who are homozygous for the UGT1A1*28 allele (characterized by a mutation in the promoter region of the UGT1A1 gene) have reduced expression of UGT1A1, which may manifest as mild hyperbilirubinemia (i.e., Gilbert syndrome). Mild elevations of indirect (unconjugated) bilirubin concentrations may occur in patients with Gilbert syndrome receiving pazopanib.

In a pooled pharmacogenomic analysis of data from 31 clinical studies evaluating pazopanib, ALT elevations exceeding 3 times the upper limit of normal (ULN) occurred in 32% of patients who were HLA-B*57:01 allele carriers and in 19% of noncarriers. ALT elevations exceeding 5 times the ULN occurred in 19% of HLA-B*57:01 allele carriers and in 10% of noncarriers.

● Common Adverse Effects

Adverse effects reported in 20% or more of patients receiving pazopanib for renal cell carcinoma include diarrhea, hypertension, hair color changes (depigmentation), nausea, anorexia, and vomiting.

Adverse effects reported in 20% or more of patients receiving pazopanib for soft tissue sarcoma include fatigue, diarrhea, nausea, decreased weight, hypertension, decreased appetite, vomiting, tumor pain, hair color changes, musculoskeletal pain, headache, dysgeusia, dyspnea, and skin hypopigmentation.

DRUG INTERACTIONS

Pazopanib is metabolized principally by cytochrome P-450 (CYP) isoenzyme 3A4 and, to a lesser extent, by CYP isoenzymes 1A2 and 2C8. Results of drug interaction studies in cancer patients suggest that pazopanib is a weak inhibitor of CYP isoenzymes 3A4, 2C8, and 2D6 but has no effect on CYP isoenzymes 1A2, 2C9, or 2C19. In vitro studies indicate that pazopanib may induce and/or inhibit CYP3A4, and inhibit CYP isoenzymes 1A2, 2B6, 2C8, 2C9, 2C19, 2D6, and 2E1.

In vitro studies indicate that pazopanib inhibits uridine diphosphate-glucuronosyltransferase (UGT) 1A1 and organic anion transport protein (OATP) 1B1; the drug appears to be a substrate of P-glycoprotein (P-gp) and breast cancer resistance protein (BCRP).

● Drugs and Foods Affecting Hepatic Microsomal Enzymes

Inhibitors of CYP3A4

Pharmacokinetic interaction (increased peak plasma concentrations and area under the plasma concentration-time curve [AUC] of pazopanib) observed during concomitant use of oral pazopanib with ketoconazole (a potent inhibitor of CYP3A4 and an inhibitor of P-gp) or during concomitant use of pazopanib oral tablets with lapatinib (a substrate and weak inhibitor of CYP3A4, P-gp, and BCRP).

Avoid concomitant use of pazopanib with *potent* CYP3A4 inhibitors; if concomitant use cannot be avoided, reduce pazopanib dosage. Avoid concomitant use with grapefruit or grapefruit juice.

Inducers of CYP3A4

Potential pharmacokinetic interaction (decreased plasma concentrations of pazopanib).

Avoid concomitant use of pazopanib with a potent inducer of CYP3A4; consider selecting an alternative agent with minimal or no enzyme induction potential. If long-term use of a potent CYP3A4 inducer is required, do not initiate therapy with pazopanib.

● Drugs Metabolized by Hepatic Microsomal Enzymes

Substrates of CYP isoenzymes 3A4, 2D6, or 2C8

Pharmacokinetic interaction (increased exposure to substrate) observed during concomitant use with midazolam (a CYP3A4 substrate), dextromethorphan (a CYP2D6 substrate), or paclitaxel (a CYP3A4 and CYP2C8 substrate). Concomitant use with substrates of CYP isoenzymes 3A4, 2D6, or 2C8 that have a narrow therapeutic index is not recommended.

Substrates of CYP isoenzymes 1A2, 2C9, or 2C19

No clinically relevant pharmacokinetic interaction with caffeine (a CYP1A2 substrate), warfarin (a CYP2C9 substrate), or omeprazole (a CYP2C19 substrate).

● Drugs Transported by Organic Anion Transport Protein (OATP)

Potential pharmacokinetic interaction (increased plasma concentration of drugs transported by OATP1B1).

● Drugs Metabolized by Uridine Diphosphate-glucuronosyltransferase (UGT)

Potential pharmacokinetic interaction (increased plasma concentration of drugs metabolized by UGT1A1).

● Drugs Affecting Gastric Acidity

Pharmacokinetic interaction (decreased exposure to pazopanib) has been observed during concomitant use with esomeprazole.

Avoid concomitant use of pazopanib with drugs affecting gastric acidity. If concomitant administration of a drug affecting gastric acidity cannot be avoided, consider short-acting antacids rather than a proton-pump inhibitor or histamine H$_2$-receptor antagonist. Administration of a short-acting antacid and pazopanib should be separated by several hours.

● Drugs that Prolong the QT Interval

Risk of prolonged QT interval and torsades de pointes. Avoid concomitant use of pazopanib and drugs that prolong the QT interval.

● HMG-CoA Reductase Inhibitors (Statins)

Concomitant administration of simvastatin and pazopanib increased the incidence of ALT elevations in clinical trials. If a patient develops ALT elevations while receiving concomitant pazopanib and simvastatin, monitor liver function weekly; depending on the severity of hepatotoxicity, withhold pazopanib and resume pazopanib at a reduced dosage or permanently discontinue pazopanib therapy.

Data are insufficient to assess the risk of other statins administered concomitantly with pazopanib.

DESCRIPTION

Pazopanib hydrochloride, an inhibitor of multiple receptor tyrosine kinases, is an antineoplastic agent. Receptor tyrosine kinases (RTKs) are involved in the initiation of various cascades of intracellular signaling events that lead to cell proliferation and/or influence processes critical to cell survival and tumor progression (e.g., angiogenesis, metastasis, inhibition of apoptosis), based on the respective kinase. Pazopanib inhibits signal transduction pathways involving multiple receptor tyrosine kinases, principally vascular endothelial growth factor receptors (i.e., VEGFR-1, VEGFR-2, VEGFR-3), platelet-derived growth factor receptors (i.e., PDGFR-α, PDGFR-β), and stem cell factor receptor (i.e., c-Kit); the drug has modest inhibitory effects on fibroblast growth factor receptors (i.e., FGFR1, FGFR3), transmembrane glycoprotein receptor tyrosine kinase (c-Fms), leukocyte-specific protein tyrosine kinase (Lck), and interleukin-2 receptor inducible T-cell kinase (Itk). In vitro, pazopanib has been shown to inhibit ligand-induced autophosphorylation of VEGFR-2, PDGFR-β, and c-Kit. In vivo, pazopanib inhibited VEGF-induced VEGFR-2 phosphorylation in mouse lungs and in human umbilical vein endothelial cells (HUVEC), angiogenesis in a mouse model, and the growth of some human tumor xenografts in mice.

Pazopanib appears to be as potent as sorafenib and sunitinib against VEGFR (i.e., VEGFR-1, VEGFR-2, VEGFR-3) and less potent than sunitinib against fms-like tyrosine kinase 3 (Flt-3). Differences in potencies against non-VEGF receptors may account for variabilities in non-VEGFR-related ("off-target") adverse effects observed with pazopanib (e.g., hepatotoxicity, lower incidence of palmar-plantar erythrodysesthesia [hand-foot syndrome] and rash compared with sorafenib or sunitinib [based on indirect cross-study comparison], lower incidence of and less severe myelosuppression compared with sunitinib [based on indirect cross-study comparison]). The relatively lower incidence of and less severe myelosuppressive effects reported with pazopanib may be explained, in part, by the drug's lower potency against Flt-3 (a regulator of hematopoiesis).

Pazopanib is incompletely absorbed from the GI tract, with reported bioavailabilities of 14–39%. Following oral administration, peak plasma concentrations of pazopanib occurred at a median of 2–4 hours. Administration of a single 400-mg crushed tablet increased the peak plasma concentrations and area under the plasma concentration-time curve (AUC) by approximately twofold and 46%, respectively, and decreased the time to peak plasma concentrations by approximately 2 hours, compared with administration of the whole tablet. Administration of pazopanib with food (i.e., low-fat or high-fat meal) resulted in an approximately twofold increase in peak plasma concentrations and AUC of the drug. Pazopanib is more than 99% bound to plasma proteins; in vitro studies suggest that pazopanib is a substrate of P-glycoprotein (Pgp) and breast cancer resistant protein (BCRP). Pazopanib is metabolized by the cytochrome P-450 (CYP) microsomal enzyme system, principally by the isoenzyme 3A4 (CYP3A4) and, to a lesser extent, by CYP1A2 and CYP2C8; in plasma, pazopanib metabolites accounted for less than 10% of the administered dose. The mean half-life of pazopanib is approximately 31 hours. Approximately 82% of a radiolabeled dose of pazopanib is excreted in feces (67% of which is unchanged drug), and less than 4% is eliminated in urine. Hemodialysis is not expected to enhance elimination of pazopanib because the drug is highly bound to plasma proteins and is not substantially excreted renally.

Pazopanib inhibits uridine diphosphate-glucuronosyltransferase (UGT) 1A1, an enzyme that catalyzes the glucuronidation of bilirubin for elimination. Patients who are homozygous for the UGT1A1*28 allele (characterized by a mutation in the promoter region of the UGT1A1 gene) have reduced expression of UGT1A1, which may manifest as mild hyperbilirubinemia (i.e., Gilbert's syndrome). Mild elevations of indirect (unconjugated) bilirubin concentrations may occur in patients with Gilbert's syndrome receiving pazopanib. A pooled pharmacogenetic analysis of 236 Caucasian patients that evaluated the polymorphisms of UGT1A1 and its potential association with hyperbilirubinemia during pazopanib treatment found that the (TA)7/(TA)7 genotype (UGT1A1*28/*28, underlying genetic susceptibility to Gilbert's syndrome) was associated with an increase in the risk of hyperbilirubinemia relative to the (TA)6/(TA)6 and (TA)6/(TA)7 genotypes.

ADVICE TO PATIENTS

- Pazopanib medication guide should be provided to patient each time the drug is dispensed; importance of patient reading the medication guide prior to initiating pazopanib therapy and each time the prescription is refilled.
- Importance of taking pazopanib without food (i.e., ≥1 hour before or 2 hours after a meal). Importance of swallowing tablets whole and not crushing the tablets. Avoid grapefruit or grapefruit juice while taking the drug.
- If a dose is missed by <12 hours, take it as soon as it is remembered, and take the next dose at the regularly scheduled time. Do not take more than one dose at a time.
- Risk of adverse hepatic effects and importance of periodic laboratory testing. Importance of immediately reporting any manifestations of hepatotoxicity (e.g., jaundice, unusual fatigue, unusual darkening of urine, nausea, vomiting, loss of appetite, right-upper quadrant pain, easy bruising).
- Risk of QT prolongation and torsades de pointes. Advise patients to report any concomitant medications. Inform patients that ECG monitoring may be performed.
- Risk of interstitial lung disease/pneumonitis. Importance of reporting any manifestations of interstitial lung disease or pneumonitis (e.g., persistent cough, dyspnea).
- Risk of adverse cardiovascular effects. Importance of monitoring BP regularly during therapy. Importance of immediately reporting irregular or fast heart beat, fainting, or manifestations of a heart attack or stroke (e.g., chest pain or pressure; pain in arms, back, neck, or jaw; shortness of breath; numbness or weakness on one side of body; trouble talking; headache; dizziness).
- Risk of bleeding. Importance of promptly informing clinicians of any unusual bleeding, bruising, or wounds that do not heal.
- Risk of adverse GI effects (e.g., diarrhea, nausea, vomiting, GI perforation). Importance of understanding measures to manage mild diarrhea and of notifying clinician if moderate or severe diarrhea occurs. Importance of immediately reporting any manifestations of GI perforation (e.g., abdominal pain or swelling, vomiting blood, black sticky stools).
- Risk of thromboembolic events. Importance of reporting any manifestations of thromboembolic events.
- Risk of posterior reversible encephalopathy syndrome. Importance of reporting any manifestations of posterior reversible encephalopathy syndrome (e.g., headache, seizure, lethargy, confusion, blindness).
- Risk of GI perforation or fistula. Importance of reporting any manifestations of GI perforation or fistula.
- Risk of impaired wound healing. Importance of informing clinician of any scheduled surgical procedures.
- Risk of hypothyroidism and proteinuria. Importance of thyroid function tests and urinanalysis during therapy.
- Risk of tumor lysis syndrome. Importance of informing clinician of any manifestations of tumor lysis syndrome occur (e.g., abnormal heart rhythm, seizure, confusion, muscle cramps/spasms, decreased urine output).
- Risk of infection. Importance of informing clinician of any manifestations of infection.
- Risk of depigmentation of hair and skin.
- Risk of impaired male or female fertility.
- Importance of females informing clinicians if they are or plan to become pregnant or plan to breast-feed. Apprise patient of potential hazard to the fetus if used during pregnancy; females of reproductive potential should avoid becoming pregnant. Advise females of reproductive potential to use effective contraception during treatment and for at least 2 weeks after the last dose of pazopanib. Advise males with such female partners to use

condoms during treatment and for at least 2 weeks after the last dose of pazopanib.

- Advise women to inform their clinicians if they are or plan to breast-feed. Avoid breast-feeding during pazopanib treatment and for at least 2 weeks after the last dose of pazopanib.

- Importance of informing clinicians of existing or contemplated concomitant therapy, including prescription and OTC drugs and dietary or herbal supplements, as well as any concomitant illnesses (e.g., cardiovascular disease, hepatic impairment).

- Importance of informing patients of other important precautionary information. (See Cautions.)

For further information on the handling of antineoplastic agents, see the ASHP Guidelines on Handling Hazardous Drugs at http://www.ahfsdruginformation.com.

PREPARATIONS

Excipients in commercially available drug preparations may have clinically important effects in some individuals; consult specific product labeling for details.

PAZOPanib Hydrochloride

Oral

Tablets, film-coated	200 mg (of pazopanib)	Votrient®, Novartis

† Use is not currently included in the labeling approved by the US Food and Drug Administration.

Selected Revisions March 30, 2022, © Copyright, December 01, 2010, American Society of Health-System Pharmacists, Inc.

Pembrolizumab

10:00 • ANTINEOPLASTIC AGENTS

■ Pembrolizumab, a humanized anti-programmed-death receptor-1 (anti-PD-1) monoclonal antibody, is an antineoplastic agent.

USES

● *Melanoma*

Unresectable or Metastatic Melanoma

Pembrolizumab is used for the treatment of unresectable or metastatic melanoma; pembrolizumab has been designated an orphan drug by FDA for the treatment of this cancer.

The current indication for pembrolizumab in the treatment of unresectable or metastatic melanoma is based principally on the results of an open-label, randomized phase 3 study (KEYNOTE-006) and a randomized phase 2 study (KEYNOTE-002).

In the KEYNOTE-006 study, 834 patients with ipilimumab-naive unresectable or metastatic melanoma who had received no more than one prior systemic therapy for metastatic disease were randomized (stratified by number of prior therapies, Eastern Cooperative Oncology Group [ECOG] performance status, and programmed-death ligand-1 [PD-L1] expression) in a 1:1:1 ratio to receive pembrolizumab 10 mg/kg administered as a 30-minute IV infusion every 2 or 3 weeks for up to 24 months or ipilimumab 3 mg/kg every 3 weeks administered as a 90-minute IV infusion for a maximum of 4 cycles. Treatment was continued for the specified duration or until the occurrence of unacceptable toxicity or disease progression that was symptomatic, rapidly progressive, associated with a decline in performance status, requiring urgent intervention, or confirmed in 4–6 weeks by repeat radiographic studies. The primary measures of efficacy were overall survival and progression-free survival (as evaluated by a blinded independent central review committee according to Response Evaluation Criteria in Solid Tumors [RECIST] modified to follow no more than 10 target lesions and no more than 5 target lesions per organ); additional outcome measures were objective response rate and duration of response.

The median age of patients enrolled in the KEYNOTE-006 study was 62 years; 98% were Caucasian and 60% were male. All patients enrolled in the study had an ECOG performance status of 0 or 1. Most patients (80%) had positive PD-L1 expression (defined as PD-L1 expression of any intensity on at least 1% of tumor cells as detected by an investigational assay), 65% had stage M1c disease, 66% had not received prior systemic therapies for metastatic disease, 68% had LDH concentrations within normal limits, 36% had tumors bearing the b-Raf serine-threonine kinase (BRAF) mutation, and 9% had a history of brain metastases. Approximately one-half of patients (46%) with BRAF mutation-positive disease had received prior therapy with a BRAF inhibitor. This study excluded patients with ocular melanoma, active brain metastases, autoimmune disease, conditions requiring therapy with immunosuppressive agents, human immunodeficiency virus (HIV) infection, or hepatitis B virus (HBV) or hepatitis C virus (HCV) infection.

In the KEYNOTE-006 study, a planned interim analysis indicated prolonged median progression-free survival in patients receiving pembrolizumab every 3 or 2 weeks compared with those receiving ipilimumab (4.1 or 5.5 months, respectively, versus 2.8 months; hazard ratio for both dosages: 0.58). The median follow-up period at the time of interim analysis was 7.9 months. After a minimum follow-up of 12 months, the risk of death in patients receiving pembrolizumab every 3 or 2 weeks was reduced by 31 or 37%, respectively, compared with those receiving ipilimumab. Patients receiving pembrolizumab every 3 or 2 weeks also had a higher objective response rate compared with those receiving ipilimumab (33 or 34%, respectively, versus 12%); complete responses were achieved in 5–6% of patients treated with pembrolizumab compared with 1% of those treated with ipilimumab. At the time of interim analysis, the median duration of response had not been reached in any group; however, responses were ongoing in 97, 89, or 88% of patients receiving pembrolizumab every 3 weeks, pembrolizumab every 2 weeks, or ipilimumab, respectively. Because of the survival benefit observed at the interim analysis, this study was terminated prematurely at the request of the independent data monitoring committee and patients previously randomized to receive ipilimumab were permitted to cross over to open-label pembrolizumab therapy. Overall survival, progression-free survival, and objective response rates for pembrolizumab- and ipilimumab-treated patients at the time of final analysis (at a median follow-up of 22.9 months) remained similar to the interim results; in the final analysis, no substantial differences in efficacy were observed between the 2 pembrolizumab dosage regimens. Results of a subgroup analysis (based on age, sex, ECOG performance status, serum LDH concentration, BRAF mutation status, number of prior therapies, PD-L1 status, and baseline tumor size) suggested that the effect of pembrolizumab on overall survival was consistent across all subgroups.

In the KEYNOTE-002 study, 540 patients with unresectable or metastatic melanoma were randomized (stratified by ECOG performance status, serum LDH concentrations, and BRAF mutation status) in a 1:1:1 ratio to receive pembrolizumab 2 or 10 mg/kg by IV infusion every 3 weeks or investigator's choice of chemotherapy (dacarbazine 1 g/m² IV every 3 weeks; temozolomide 200 mg/m² orally once daily for 5 days every 28 days; carboplatin at the dose required to obtain an area under the plasma concentration-time curve [AUC] of 6 mg/mL per minute in combination with paclitaxel 225 mg/m² IV every 3 weeks for 4 cycles followed by carboplatin at the dose required to obtain an AUC of 5 mg/mL per minute and paclitaxel 175 mg/m² IV every 3 weeks; paclitaxel 175 mg/m² IV every 3 weeks; or carboplatin at the dose required to obtain an AUC of 5 or 6 mg/mL per minute IV every 3 weeks). Treatment with pembrolizumab was continued until the occurrence of unacceptable toxicity or disease progression that was symptomatic, rapidly progressive, associated with a decline in performance status, requiring urgent intervention, or confirmed in 4–6 weeks by repeat radiographic studies. Patients randomized to receive chemotherapy were permitted to cross over to pembrolizumab therapy following disease progression.

Patients were enrolled in the KEYNOTE-002 study if their disease had progressed within 24 weeks of ipilimumab therapy and was refractory following at least 2 doses of ipilimumab (at a dose of at least 3 mg/kg) and, in those with tumors bearing the BRAF V600 mutation, refractory to therapy with a BRAF or mitogen-activated extracellular signal-regulated kinase (MEK) inhibitor. The primary measures of efficacy were progression-free survival (as evaluated by a blinded independent central review committee according to RECIST modified to follow no more than 10 target lesions and no more than 5 target lesions per organ) and overall survival; additional outcome measures were objective response rate (as evaluated by a blinded independent central review committee according to RECIST modified to follow no more than 10 target lesions and no more than 5 target lesions per organ) and duration of response. The median age of patients enrolled in the study was 62 years; 98% were Caucasian, 61% were male, 40% had elevated LDH concentrations at baseline, and 23% had tumors bearing the BRAF mutation. All patients enrolled in the study had an ECOG performance status of 0 or 1. Most patients (82%) had stage M1c disease and 73% had received at least 2 prior therapies for advanced or metastatic disease. This study excluded patients with uveal melanoma, active brain metastases or carcinomatous meningitis, autoimmune disease, active infection requiring systemic therapy, a history of HIV infection, or active HBV or HCV infection.

In the KEYNOTE-002 study, a planned interim analysis for progression-free survival indicated a 43 or 50% reduction in the risk of disease progression or death in patients receiving pembrolizumab 2 or 10 mg/kg, respectively, compared with those receiving chemotherapy. The median follow-up period at the time of interim analysis was 10 months. Patients receiving pembrolizumab at either dosage also had a higher objective response rate compared with those receiving chemotherapy (21–25% versus 4%); complete responses were achieved in 2–3% of patients treated with pembrolizumab compared with none of those treated with chemotherapy. At the final analysis (at a median follow-up of 28 months), median overall survival was prolonged in patients receiving pembrolizumab 2 or 10 mg/kg compared with those receiving chemotherapy (13.4 or 14.7 months, respectively, versus 11 months). Pembrolizumab 2 or 10 mg/kg reduced the risk of death by 14 or 26%, respectively, compared with chemotherapy; however, the prespecified level of statistical significance was not achieved. At the time of final analysis, the median duration of response was 22.8 months in patients receiving pembrolizumab 2 mg/kg, had not been reached in those receiving pembrolizumab 10 mg/kg, and was 6.8 months in those receiving chemotherapy. Progression-free survival and objective response rates for pembrolizumab- and chemotherapy-treated patients at the time of final analysis remained similar to the interim results; no substantial differences in efficacy were observed between the 2 pembrolizumab dosage regimens. Results of a subgroup analysis (based on ECOG performance status, baseline serum LDH concentration, BRAF mutation status, number of prior therapies, PD-L1 status, baseline tumor size, prior chemotherapy regimen, best response to ipilimumab, and disease stage) suggested that the effect of pembrolizumab on overall survival was consistent across all subgroups.

Adjuvant Therapy for Locally Advanced Melanoma

Pembrolizumab is used as adjuvant therapy of melanoma with lymph node involvement following complete resection.

The current indication for use of pembrolizumab as adjuvant therapy of melanoma with lymph node involvement following complete resection is based principally on the results of a phase 3 randomized, double-blind, placebo-controlled study (KEYNOTE-054). In this study, 1019 adults with completely resected stage III melanoma were randomized (stratified by disease stage and geographic region) in a 1:1 ratio to receive either pembrolizumab (200 mg by IV infusion every 3 weeks) or placebo for up to 18 doses (approximately one year) or until disease progression or unacceptable toxicity occurred. Upon disease recurrence, patients could cross over to pembrolizumab therapy or receive repeat treatment with the drug. Patients were eligible for enrollment in the study following complete regional lymphadenectomy and, if indicated, radiation therapy within 13 weeks prior to initiation of study treatment. The primary measure of efficacy was recurrence-free survival in the entire study population and in the subset of patients with PD-L1-positive tumors (defined as a PD-L1 expression combined positive score of at least 1%, as measured by a clinical trial immunohistochemistry assay).

The median age of patients enrolled in the KEYNOTE-054 study was 54 years; 62% were male, 84% had positive PD-L1 expression, and 50% had tumors bearing the BRAF V600 mutation. Approximately one-half of patients (46%) had stage IIIB melanoma, 20% had stage IIIC disease with 4 or more positive lymph nodes, 18% had stage IIIC disease with 1–3 positive lymph nodes, and 16% had stage IIIA disease. All patients had an ECOG performance status of 0 or 1. The study excluded patients who had received prior systemic therapy for melanoma and those with autoimmune disease, uncontrolled infection, or any condition requiring use of systemic glucocorticoids.

At a median follow-up of 15 months in the KEYNOTE-054 study, median recurrence-free survival had not been reached in patients receiving pembrolizumab; however, pembrolizumab reduced the risk of recurrence or death by 43% compared with placebo. A recurrence-free survival benefit was observed for pembrolizumab regardless of tumor PD-L1 expression. For patients with PD-L1 positive tumors, pembrolizumab reduced the risk of recurrence or death by 46% compared with placebo. Results of an exploratory analysis (based on age, sex, disease stage, number of positive lymph nodes, microscopic versus macroscopic lymph node involvement, presence of tumor ulceration, and BRAF mutation status) suggested that the effect of pembrolizumab on recurrence-free survival was consistent across subgroups.

● Non-small Cell Lung Cancer

First-line Therapy for Metastatic Non-small Cell Lung Cancer

Monotherapy

Pembrolizumab is used as a single agent for the initial treatment of metastatic non-small cell lung cancer (NSCLC) with high PD-L1 expression (defined as PD-L1 expression of any intensity on at least 50% of tumor cells [i.e., tumor proportion score of at least 50%]) and without epidermal growth factor receptor (EGFR) or anaplastic lymphoma kinase (ALK) genomic aberrations. An FDA-approved diagnostic test is required to confirm the presence of high PD-L1 expression prior to initiation of therapy.

The current indication for use of pembrolizumab as a single agent for the initial treatment of metastatic NSCLC in patients with high PD-L1 expression is based principally on the results of an open-label, randomized phase 3 study (KEYNOTE-024). In this study, 305 patients with previously untreated metastatic NSCLC with high PD-L1 expression (tumor proportion score of at least 50%) were randomized (stratified by ECOG performance status, histology, and geographic region) in a 1:1 ratio to receive either pembrolizumab (200 mg by IV infusion every 3 weeks for up to 24 months) or investigator's choice of platinum-based chemotherapy (pemetrexed 500 mg/m^2 IV and carboplatin at the dose required to obtain an AUC of 5–6 mg/mL per minute on day 1 of each 3-week cycle for 4–6 cycles, followed by an option to continue pemetrexed maintenance therapy; pemetrexed 500 mg/m^2 IV and cisplatin 75 mg/m^2 on day 1 of each 3-week cycle for 4–6 cycles, followed by an option to continue pemetrexed maintenance therapy; gemcitabine 1.25 g/m^2 on days 1 and 8 and cisplatin 75 mg/m^2 on day 1 of each 3-week cycle for 4–6 cycles; gemcitabine 1.25 g/m^2 on days 1 and 8 and carboplatin at the dose required to obtain an AUC of 5–6 mg/mL per minute on day 1 of each 3-week cycle for 4–6 cycles; paclitaxel 200 mg/m^2 and carboplatin at the dose required to obtain an AUC of 5–6 mg/mL per minute on day 1 of each

3-week cycle for 4–6 cycles, followed by an option to continue pemetrexed maintenance therapy). Treatment was continued for the specified duration or until disease progression or unacceptable toxicity occurred; however, clinically stable patients with disease progression could continue treatment if they were considered to be deriving clinical benefit. In addition, patients randomized to receive platinum-based chemotherapy were permitted to cross over to pembrolizumab therapy upon disease progression. Approximately 44% of the patients randomized to platinum-based chemotherapy crossed over to pembrolizumab therapy following disease progression. The primary measure of efficacy was progression-free survival (as evaluated by a blinded independent central review committee according to RECIST modified to follow no more than 10 target lesions and no more than 5 target lesions per organ); additional outcome measures were overall survival and objective response rate (as evaluated by a blinded independent central review committee according to RECIST modified to follow no more than 10 target lesions and no more than 5 target lesions per organ).

The median age of patients enrolled in the KEYNOTE-024 study was 65 years; 82% were Caucasian, 82% had nonsquamous histology, 61% were male, 18% had squamous histology, 15% were of Asian ancestry, and 9% had a history of brain metastases. With one exception, all patients had a baseline ECOG performance status of 0 or 1. This study excluded patients with EGFR or ALK genomic aberrations, untreated brain metastases, active autoimmune disease that required systemic therapy within 2 years of randomization, conditions requiring therapy with systemic corticosteroids or immunosuppressive agents, active interstitial lung disease or a history of pneumonitis requiring glucocorticoid therapy, or irradiation of the thoracic region at a dose exceeding 30 Gy within 26 weeks of enrollment.

In the KEYNOTE-024 study, patients receiving pembrolizumab had a longer median progression-free survival (10.3 versus 6 months based on intent-to-treat analysis; hazard ratio: 0.5) and overall survival (30 versus 14.2 months; hazard ratio: 0.6) compared with patients receiving platinum-based chemotherapy. Patients receiving pembrolizumab also had higher objective response rates compared with those receiving platinum-based chemotherapy (45 versus 28%); complete responses were achieved in 4 or 1% of patients receiving pembrolizumab or platinum-based chemotherapy, respectively. At the second interim analysis (at a median follow-up of 11.2 months), the median duration of response had not been reached in patients receiving pembrolizumab. The median time to response was similar in both treatment groups (2.2 months). Results of a subgroup analysis (based on age, sex, geographic region, ECOG performance status, histology, smoking status, presence of brain metastases, and prior use of pemetrexed in combination with platinum-based chemotherapy) suggested that the effect of pembrolizumab on progression-free survival was evident across all subgroups.

Combination Therapy for Metastatic Nonsquamous NSCLC

Pembrolizumab is used in combination with pemetrexed and a platinum-containing antineoplastic agent (carboplatin or cisplatin) for the initial treatment of metastatic nonsquamous NSCLC without EGFR or ALK genomic aberrations.

Efficacy of pembrolizumab in combination with pemetrexed and a platinum-containing antineoplastic agent (carboplatin or cisplatin) for the initial treatment of metastatic nonsquamous NSCLC is based principally on the results of a randomized, double-blind, phase 3 study (KEYNOTE-189). In this study, 616 adults with previously untreated metastatic NSCLC with nonsquamous histology were randomized (stratified by PD-L1 expression, platinum-containing antineoplastic agent, and smoking status) in a 2:1 ratio to receive either pembrolizumab in combination with pemetrexed and investigator's choice of a platinum-containing antineoplastic agent (carboplatin or cisplatin) or placebo in combination with pemetrexed and investigator's choice of a platinum-containing antineoplastic agent; 72% of patients enrolled in the study received carboplatin. Those randomized to the pembrolizumab combination regimen received pembrolizumab (200 mg by IV infusion) in combination with pemetrexed (500 mg/m^2 by IV infusion) and either carboplatin (at the dose required to obtain an AUC of 5 mg/mL per minute by IV infusion) or cisplatin (75 mg/m^2 by IV infusion) on day 1 of each 21-day cycle for 4 cycles followed by pembrolizumab (200 mg by IV infusion) in combination with pemetrexed (500 mg/m^2 by IV infusion) every 3 weeks. Those randomized to the placebo combination regimen received placebo in combination with pemetrexed and either carboplatin or cisplatin at the same dosages for 4 cycles followed by placebo in combination with pemetrexed (500 mg/m^2 by IV infusion) every 3 weeks. Treatment was continued for up to 24 months or until disease progression or unacceptable toxicity occurred; however, clinically stable patients with disease progression could continue treatment if they were considered to be deriving clinical benefit. In addition, patients randomized to receive placebo in combination with pemetrexed and a platinum-containing antineoplastic agent were permitted to cross over to single-agent pembrolizumab upon disease progression. Approximately 41% of patients randomized to receive the placebo combination regimen crossed over to therapy with an anti-programmed-death receptor-1 (PD-1) or anti-programmed-death ligand-1 (PD-L1) antibody following disease progression.

The primary measures of efficacy in the KEYNOTE-189 study were overall survival and progression-free survival (as evaluated by a blinded independent central review committee according to RECIST modified to follow no more than 10 target lesions and no more than 5 target lesions per organ); additional outcome measures were objective response rate (as evaluated by a blinded independent central review committee according to RECIST modified to follow no more than 10 target lesions and no more than 5 target lesions per organ) and duration of response.

The median age of patients enrolled in the KEYNOTE-189 study was 64 years; 94% were Caucasian, 59% were male, 56% had a baseline ECOG performance status of 1, 31% had a PD-L1 expression tumor proportion score of less than 1%, 18% had a history of brain metastases, 12% had never smoked, and 3% were of Asian ancestry. This study excluded patients with EGFR or ALK genomic aberrations, conditions requiring therapy with systemic corticosteroids or immunosuppressive agents, active autoimmune disease requiring systemic therapy within the previous 2 years, symptomatic brain metastases, history of pneumonitis requiring therapy with glucocorticoids, or irradiation of the thoracic region at a dose exceeding 30 Gy within 26 weeks of enrollment.

At a median follow-up of 10.5 months in the KEYNOTE-189 study, patients receiving the pembrolizumab combination regimen had a longer median progression-free survival compared with patients receiving the placebo combination regimen (8.8 versus 4.9 months; hazard ratio: 0.52). Although median overall survival for patients receiving the pembrolizumab combination regimen had not been reached at the time of analysis, median overall survival appeared to be prolonged in patients receiving pembrolizumab in combination with pemetrexed and a platinum-containing antineoplastic agent compared with those receiving placebo in combination with pemetrexed and a platinum-containing antineoplastic agent (hazard ratio: 0.49). Patients receiving the pembrolizumab combination regimen also had higher objective response rates compared with those receiving the placebo combination regimen (48 versus 19%); complete responses were achieved in 0.5% of patients in both treatment groups. At the time of analysis, the median duration of response was 11.2 and 7.8 months in patients receiving the pembrolizumab combination regimen and those receiving the placebo combination regimen, respectively.

Results of a subgroup analysis (based on age, sex, ECOG performance status, smoking status, presence of brain metastases, level of PD-L1 expression, and platinum-containing antineoplastic agent) suggested that the effect of pembrolizumab on overall survival and progression-free survival was evident across all subgroups. Subgroup analysis also indicated that the effect of pembrolizumab on objective response rate was evident regardless of level of PD-L1 expression, but objective response rates were substantially greater in patients with PD-L1 expression of any intensity on at least 50% of tumor cells (i.e., tumor proportion score of at least 50%) who received the pembrolizumab combination regimen compared with those who received the placebo combination regimen (61.4 versus 22.9%).

Combination Therapy for Metastatic Squamous NSCLC

Pembrolizumab is used in combination with carboplatin and paclitaxel (conventional or albumin-bound) for the initial treatment of metastatic squamous NSCLC.

Efficacy of pembrolizumab in combination with carboplatin and paclitaxel (conventional or albumin-bound) for the initial treatment of metastatic squamous NSCLC is based principally on the results of a randomized, double-blind phase 3 study (KEYNOTE-407). In this study, 559 adults with previously untreated metastatic NSCLC with squamous histology were randomized (stratified by PD-L1 expression, geographic region, and paclitaxel formulation) in a 1:1 ratio to receive either pembrolizumab in combination with carboplatin and investigator's choice of paclitaxel formulation (conventional or albumin-bound paclitaxel) or placebo in combination with carboplatin and investigator's choice of paclitaxel formulation; 60% of patients enrolled in the study received conventional paclitaxel. Those randomized to the pembrolizumab-carboplatin-paclitaxel regimen received pembrolizumab (200 mg by IV infusion) in

combination with carboplatin (at the dose required to obtain an AUC of 6 mg/mL per minute by IV infusion) on day 1 of each 21-day cycle for 4 cycles and either conventional paclitaxel (200 mg/m²) on day 1 of each 21-day cycle or albumin-bound paclitaxel (100 mg/m²) on days 1, 8, and 15 of each 21-day cycle for 4 cycles followed by pembrolizumab (200 mg by IV infusion) every 3 weeks. Those randomized to the placebo-carboplatin-paclitaxel regimen received placebo in combination with carboplatin and either conventional or albumin-bound paclitaxel at the same dosages for 4 cycles followed by placebo every 3 weeks. Therapy was continued for up to 24 months or until disease progression or unacceptable toxicity occurred; however, clinically stable patients with disease progression could continue receiving pembrolizumab if they were considered to be deriving clinical benefit. In addition, patients randomized to receive placebo-carboplatin-paclitaxel were permitted to cross over to single-agent pembrolizumab upon disease progression. Approximately 32% of patients randomized to receive placebo-carboplatin-paclitaxel crossed over to therapy with an anti-PD-1 or anti-PD-L1 antibody following disease progression.

The primary measures of efficacy in the KEYNOTE-407 study were progression-free survival and objective response rate (as evaluated by a blinded independent central review committee according to RECIST modified to follow no more than 10 target lesions and no more than 5 target lesions per organ) and overall survival; an additional outcome measure was duration of response (as evaluated by a blinded independent central review committee according to RECIST modified to follow no more than 10 target lesions and no more than 5 target lesions per organ).

The median age of patients enrolled in the KEYNOTE-407 study was 65 years; 81% were male, 77% were Caucasian, 71% had a baseline ECOG performance status of 1, 35% had a PD-L1 expression tumor proportion score of less than 1%, 19% were of East Asian ancestry, and 8% had a history of brain metastases. This study excluded patients with conditions requiring therapy with immunosuppressive agents, active autoimmune disease requiring systemic therapy within the previous 2 years, symptomatic brain metastases, history of pneumonitis requiring therapy with glucocorticoids, or irradiation of the thoracic region at a dose exceeding 30 Gy within 26 weeks of enrollment.

At a median follow-up of 7.8 months in the KEYNOTE-407 study, patients receiving pembrolizumab-carboplatin-paclitaxel had a longer median overall survival (15.9 versus 11.3 months based on intent-to-treat analysis; hazard ratio: 0.64) and progression-free survival (6.4 versus 4.8 months based on intent-to-treat analysis; hazard ratio: 0.56) compared with patients receiving placebo-carboplatin-paclitaxel. In the primary efficacy population (consisting of the initial 204 patients enrolled in the study), patients receiving pembrolizumab-carboplatin-paclitaxel had higher objective response rates compared with those receiving placebo-carboplatin-paclitaxel (58 versus 35%); the median duration of response was 7.2 and 4.9 months in patients receiving these respective treatments.

Results of a subgroup analysis (based on age, sex, ECOG performance status, level of PD-L1 expression, and paclitaxel formulation) suggested that the effect of pembrolizumab on overall survival and progression-free survival was evident across all subgroups. Subgroup analysis also indicated that the effect of pembrolizumab on objective response rate was evident regardless of level of PD-L1 expression, but objective response rates were substantially greater in patients with PD-L1 expression of any intensity on at least 50% of tumor cells (i.e., tumor proportion score of at least 50%) who received pembrolizumab-carboplatin-paclitaxel compared with those who received placebo-carboplatin-paclitaxel (60.3 versus 32.9%).

Previously Treated Metastatic Non-small Cell Lung Cancer

Pembrolizumab is used as a single agent for the treatment of PD-L1-positive (defined as PD-L1 expression of any intensity on at least 1% of tumor cells [i.e., tumor proportion score of at least 1%]) metastatic NSCLC that has progressed during or following platinum-based chemotherapy, and, if the tumor is EGFR- or ALK-positive, during or following an FDA-labeled anti-EGFR or anti-ALK therapy. An FDA-approved diagnostic test is required to confirm the presence of PD-L1 expression prior to initiation of therapy.

The current indication for use of pembrolizumab as a single agent for the treatment of metastatic NSCLC in patients with disease progression during or following platinum-based chemotherapy is based principally on the results of an open-label, randomized phase 2/3 study (KEYNOTE-010). Patients were enrolled in the study if PD-L1 expression of any intensity on at least 1% of tumor cells was detected by immunohistochemistry assay (PD-L1 IHC 22C3 pharmDx). In this study, 1033 patients were randomized (stratified by level of PD-L1 expression,

ECOG performance status, and geographic region) in a 1:1:1 ratio to receive pembrolizumab 2 or 10 mg/kg by IV infusion every 3 weeks or docetaxel 75 mg/m² by IV infusion every 3 weeks. Treatment was continued for up to 24 months or until the occurrence of unacceptable toxicity or disease progression that was symptomatic, rapidly progressive, associated with a decline in performance status, requiring urgent intervention, or confirmed in 4–6 weeks by repeat radiographic studies. The primary measures of efficacy were overall survival and progression-free survival (as evaluated by a blinded independent central review committee according to RECIST modified to follow no more than 10 target lesions and no more than 5 target lesions per organ) in the total population and in patients with high PD-L1 expression (defined as PD-L1 expression of any intensity on at least 50% of tumor cells); additional outcome measures were objective response rate and duration of response.

The median age of patients enrolled in the KEYNOTE-010 study was 63 years; 72% were Caucasian, 70% had nonsquamous histology, 66% had an ECOG performance status of 1, 61% were male, 43% had high PD-L1 expression, 21% were of Asian ancestry, 21% had squamous histology, 15% had a history of brain metastases, 8% had EGFR genomic aberrations, and 1% had ALK genomic aberrations. Most of the patients (91%) had metastatic disease; all patients enrolled in the study had received prior therapy with a platinum-containing, 2-drug combination regimen and 29% had received at least 2 prior therapies for metastatic disease. This study excluded patients with active autoimmune disease requiring systemic corticosteroids, conditions requiring therapy with immunosuppressive agents, active brain metastases or carcinomatous meningitis; interstitial lung disease or a history of pneumonitis requiring corticosteroid therapy, or irradiation of the thoracic region at a dose exceeding 30 Gy within 26 weeks of enrollment.

In the total patient population of the KEYNOTE-010 study, median overall survival was prolonged in patients receiving pembrolizumab 2 or 10 mg/kg compared with those receiving docetaxel (10.4 or 12.7 months, respectively, versus 8.5 months; hazard ratio: 0.71 or 0.61, respectively). Among patients with high PD-L1 expression, median overall survival also was prolonged in patients receiving pembrolizumab 2 or 10 mg/kg compared with those receiving docetaxel (14.9 or 17.3 months, respectively, versus 8.2 months; hazard ratio: 0.54 or 0.5, respectively). In the total patient population, no difference in median progression-free survival was observed between patients receiving pembrolizumab 2 or 10 mg/kg and those receiving docetaxel; however, among those with high PD-L1 expression, median progression-free survival was prolonged in patients receiving pembrolizumab at either dosage compared with those receiving docetaxel (5.2 versus 4.1 months; hazard ratio: 0.58–0.59). Patients receiving pembrolizumab at either dosage also had higher objective response rates compared with those receiving docetaxel in the total patient population (18–19 versus 9%) and in the cohort of patients with high PD-L1 expression (29–30% versus 8%). Complete responses were not achieved in any treatment group. At a median follow-up of 13.1 months, the median duration of response had not been reached in patients receiving pembrolizumab. The median time to response in the cohort of patients with high PD-L1 expression was similar in each treatment group (9 weeks). Results of a subgroup analysis (based on age, sex, ECOG performance status, PD-L1 expression, new or archival tumor sample, EGFR mutation status, and histology) suggested that the effect of pembrolizumab on overall survival was consistent across all subgroups.

● **Head and Neck Cancer**

Pembrolizumab is used for the treatment of recurrent or metastatic head and neck squamous cell carcinoma that has progressed during or following platinum-containing therapy. The accelerated approval of pembrolizumab for this indication is based on objective response rate and duration of response. Continued approval for this indication may be contingent on verification and description of clinical benefit of pembrolizumab in confirmatory studies.

The current indication for pembrolizumab in the treatment of recurrent or metastatic head and neck squamous cell carcinoma is based principally on the results for a cohort of patients with head and neck squamous cell carcinoma in an open-label, multicenter, nonrandomized, phase 1b study (KEYNOTE-012); the cohort of patients with head and neck squamous cell carcinoma included 174 adults with head and neck squamous cell carcinoma that had progressed during or following platinum-containing therapy for recurrent or metastatic disease or following platinum-containing therapy as part of induction, concurrent, or adjuvant therapy. Patients were enrolled in the study if PD-L1 expression of any intensity on at least 1% of tumor cells was detected by immunohistochemistry assay. Patients were eligible for enrollment in the study regardless of their human papillomavirus (HPV) status. Patients received pembrolizumab 10 mg/kg administered as an IV infusion every 2 weeks or 200 mg administered as an IV infusion

every 3 weeks for up to 24 months or until the occurrence of unacceptable toxicity or disease progression that was symptomatic, rapidly progressive, associated with a decline in performance status, requiring urgent intervention, or confirmed after at least 4 weeks by repeat radiographic studies. Reinitiation of pembrolizumab was permitted for subsequent disease progression for up to one additional year.

The median age of patients enrolled in the head and neck squamous cell carcinoma cohort of the KEYNOTE-012 study was 60 years; 87% had metastatic disease, 82% were male, 75% were Caucasian, 63% previously had received cetuximab therapy, 33% had HPV-positive tumors, 16% were of Asian ancestry, and 6% were black. All patients enrolled in the study had an ECOG performance status of 0 or 1. In the cohort of patients with head and neck squamous cell carcinoma, the median number of prior therapies was 2. This study excluded patients with active autoimmune disease, conditions requiring therapy with immunosuppressive agents, interstitial lung disease, brain metastases, infections requiring systemic therapy, HIV infection, or HBV or HCV infection.

At a median follow-up of 8.9 months, the objective response rate for patients in the head and neck squamous cell carcinoma cohort of the KEYNOTE-012 study was 16%; complete response was achieved in 5% of patients. At the time of analysis, the median duration of response had not been reached; however, 82% of patients who responded to pembrolizumab had durable responses of 6 months or more. Objective response rates and duration of response were similar in both dosage groups and those with HPV-negative or HPV-positive disease. Objective response rate was similar in an expansion cohort of patients who received a fixed dosage of pembrolizumab (200 mg administered by IV infusion every 3 weeks). Adverse effects were similar between both dosage regimens.

● **Hodgkin Lymphoma**

Pembrolizumab is used for the treatment of refractory classical Hodgkin lymphoma (cHL) and cHL that has relapsed following at least 3 prior therapies; pembrolizumab has been designated an orphan drug by FDA for the treatment of this cancer. The accelerated approval of pembrolizumab for this indication is based on objective response rate and duration of response. Continued approval for this indication may be contingent on verification and description of clinical benefit of pembrolizumab in confirmatory studies.

The current indication for use of pembrolizumab for the treatment of relapsed or refractory cHL is based principally on the results of an open-label, multicenter, noncomparative phase 2 study (KEYNOTE-087). Patients were enrolled in 3 cohorts: those with disease progression following autologous stem cell transplantation and subsequent therapy with brentuximab vedotin, those with disease progression following salvage chemotherapy and brentuximab vedotin, and those with disease progression following autologous transplantation only. In this study, 210 patients received pembrolizumab 200 mg by IV infusion every 3 weeks for up to 24 months or until disease progression or unacceptable toxicity occurred; however, clinically stable patients were permitted to continue pembrolizumab therapy despite disease progression at the time of the initial assessment. The primary measure of efficacy was objective response rate (as evaluated by a blinded independent central review committee according to revised International Working Group [IWG] criteria).

The median age of patients enrolled in the KEYNOTE-087 study was 35 years; 88% were Caucasian and 9% were 65 years of age or older. With one exception, all patients had a baseline ECOG performance status of 0 or 1. Patients in this study had received a median of 4 prior therapies for cHL; 58% of patients were refractory to their most recent therapy (35% of these patients had primary refractory disease and 14% were refractory to all prior therapies), 61% had undergone prior autologous stem cell transplantation, 83% previously had received brentuximab vedotin, and 36% had received prior radiation therapy. This study excluded patients with active noninfectious pneumonitis; those who had received an allogeneic stem cell transplant within the past 5 years; those who had received an allogeneic stem cell transplant and experienced symptoms of graft-versus-host disease (GVHD); and those with CNS involvement, active autoimmune disease that required systemic therapy in the past 2 years, conditions requiring therapy with immunosuppressive agents, active infection requiring systemic therapy, HIV infection, or active HBV or HCV infection.

At a median follow-up of 9.4 months, the objective response rate was 69% with a median response duration of 11.1 months; complete response was achieved in 22% of patients. Objective response rates were similar in each cohort.

● Primary Mediastinal Large B-cell Lymphoma

Pembrolizumab is used for the treatment of refractory primary mediastinal large B-cell lymphoma (PMBL) and PMBL that has relapsed following at least 2 prior therapies; pembrolizumab has been designated an orphan drug by FDA for the treatment of this cancer. The accelerated approval of pembrolizumab for this indication is based on objective response rate and duration of response. Continued approval for this indication may be contingent on verification and description of clinical benefit of pembrolizumab in confirmatory studies.

The current indication for use of pembrolizumab for the treatment of relapsed or refractory PMBL is based principally on the results of an open-label, multicenter, noncomparative phase 2 study (KEYNOTE-170). In this study, 53 patients received pembrolizumab 200 mg by IV infusion every 3 weeks for up to 24 months or until disease progression or unacceptable toxicity occurred. The primary measures of efficacy were objective response rate (as evaluated by a blinded independent central review committee according to revised IWG criteria) and duration of response.

The median age of patients enrolled in the KEYNOTE-170 study was 33 years; 92% were Caucasian and 43% were male. All patients had a baseline ECOG performance status of 0 or 1. Patients in this study had received a median of 3 prior therapies for PMBL; 49% of patients had relapsed disease refractory to their most recent therapy, 36% had primary refractory disease, 32% had received prior radiation therapy, 26% had undergone prior autologous stem cell transplantation, and 15% had untreated relapsed disease. All patients had received prior therapy with rituximab. This study excluded patients with active noninfectious pneumonitis; those who had received an allogeneic stem cell transplant within the past 5 years; those who had received an allogeneic stem cell transplant and experienced symptoms of graft-versus-host disease (GVHD); those with active autoimmune disease; and those with conditions requiring therapy with immunosuppressive agents or active infection requiring systemic therapy.

At a median follow-up of 9.7 months, the objective response rate was 45% with a median time to response of 2.8 months; complete response was achieved in 11% of patients. At the time of analysis, median duration of response had not been reached.

Pembrolizumab is not recommended for the treatment of PMBL in patients who require urgent cytoreduction.

● Urothelial Carcinoma

Pembrolizumab is used for the treatment of locally advanced or metastatic urothelial carcinoma that has progressed during or following platinum-containing therapy or within 12 months of platinum-containing therapy in the neoadjuvant or adjuvant setting. Pembrolizumab also is used for the treatment of locally advanced or metastatic urothelial carcinoma in patients with high PD-L1 expression (defined as a PD-L1 expression combined positive score of at least 10%) who are not candidates for cisplatin-containing therapy and those who are not candidates for platinum-containing chemotherapy regardless of PD-L1 expression. An FDA-approved diagnostic test is required to confirm the presence of high PD-L1 expression prior to initiation of pembrolizumab therapy in patients who are not candidates for cisplatin. The accelerated approval of pembrolizumab for the treatment of locally advanced or metastatic urothelial carcinoma in patients who are not candidates for cisplatin or platinum-containing therapy is based on objective response rate and duration of response. Continued approval for use of pembrolizumab for this indication may be contingent on verification and description of clinical benefit of pembrolizumab in confirmatory studies.

The current indication for pembrolizumab in the treatment of locally advanced or metastatic urothelial carcinoma that has progressed during or following platinum-containing therapy or within 12 months of platinum-containing therapy in the neoadjuvant or adjuvant setting is based principally on the results of an open-label, multicenter, randomized, phase 3 study (KEYNOTE-045). In this study, 542 patients with locally advanced or metastatic urothelial carcinoma that had progressed following platinum-containing therapy or within 12 months following platinum-containing therapy in the neoadjuvant or adjuvant setting were randomized (stratified by ECOG performance status, presence of liver metastases, baseline hemoglobin concentration, and time elapsed since last dose of chemotherapy) in a 1:1 ratio to receive either pembrolizumab (200 mg by IV infusion) or investigator's choice of chemotherapy (paclitaxel 175 mg/m² IV, docetaxel 75 mg/m² IV, or vinflunine 320 mg/m² IV [not commercially available in the US]) every 3 weeks. Treatment was continued for up to 24 months or until the occurrence of unacceptable toxicity or disease progression that was symptomatic, rapidly progressive, associated with a decline in performance status, requiring urgent

intervention, or confirmed by repeat radiographic studies. The primary measures of efficacy were overall survival and progression-free survival (as evaluated by a blinded independent central review committee according to RECIST modified to follow no more than 10 target lesions and no more than 5 target lesions per organ); additional outcome measures were objective response rate (as evaluated by a blinded independent central review committee according to RECIST modified to follow no more than 10 target lesions and no more than 5 target lesions per organ) and duration of response.

The median age of patients enrolled in the KEYNOTE-045 study was 66 years; 98% had an ECOG performance status of 0 or 1, 96% had metastatic disease, 87% had visceral metastases (including 34% with metastases to the liver), 74% were male, 72% were Caucasian, 23% were of Asian ancestry, and 21% had received at least 2 prior systemic therapies for metastatic disease. The lower or upper urinary tract was the primary site of the tumor in 86 or 14% of patients, respectively. Most patients (76%) had received prior therapy with cisplatin, 23% had received carboplatin, and 1% had received therapy containing other platinum agents; 15% of patients had disease progression following platinum-containing therapy in the neoadjuvant or adjuvant setting. Patients with active brain metastases or carcinomatous meningitis, autoimmune disease, interstitial lung disease, conditions requiring therapy with immunosuppressive agents, active infection requiring systemic therapy, a history of HIV infection, active HBV or HCV infection, or at least one poor prognostic factor for second-line therapy (i.e., hemoglobin concentration less than 10 g/dL, liver metastases, last dose of chemotherapy less than 3 months prior to enrollment) were excluded from the study.

In the KEYNOTE-045 study, median overall survival was prolonged in patients receiving pembrolizumab compared with those receiving chemotherapy (10.3 versus 7.4 months; hazard ratio: 0.73); however, a difference in median progression-free survival was not observed between the treatment groups. Patients receiving pembrolizumab also had higher objective response rates compared with those receiving chemotherapy (21 versus 11%); complete responses were achieved in 7 or 3% of patients receiving pembrolizumab or chemotherapy, respectively. Median duration of response had not been reached in patients receiving pembrolizumab. The median follow-up period at the time of the analysis was 9 months. Results of a subgroup analysis (based on age, sex, ECOG performance status, smoking status, histology, PD-L1 expression, site of primary tumor, site of metastases, presence of liver metastases, baseline hemoglobin concentration, number of risk factors, setting of most recent therapy, time elapsed since most recent therapy, previous platinum therapy, and investigator's choice of chemotherapy) suggested that the effect of pembrolizumab on overall survival was consistent across all subgroups; however, an overall survival benefit for the drug compared with chemotherapy was not apparent in the subgroup of patients who had never smoked (hazard ratio: 1.06).

The current indication for pembrolizumab in the treatment of locally advanced or metastatic urothelial carcinoma in patients who are not candidates for cisplatin-containing therapy is based principally on the results of an open-label, multicenter, noncomparative, phase 2 study (KEYNOTE-052). In this study, 370 patients with locally advanced or metastatic urothelial carcinoma who were not candidates for cisplatin-containing therapy received pembrolizumab 200 mg by IV infusion every 3 weeks. Treatment was continued for up to 24 months or until the occurrence of unacceptable toxicity or disease progression that was symptomatic, rapidly progressive, associated with a decline in performance status, requiring urgent intervention, or confirmed by repeat radiographic studies. The primary measure of efficacy was objective response rate (as evaluated by an independent central review committee according to RECIST modified to follow no more than 10 target lesions and no more than 5 target lesions per organ) and duration of response.

The median age of patients enrolled in the KEYNOTE-052 study was 74 years; 89% were Caucasian, 87% had metastatic disease, 85% had visceral metastases (including 21% with metastases to the liver), and 77% were male. The lower or upper urinary tract was the primary site of the tumor in 81 or 19% of patients, respectively. Most patients (90%) were treatment-naive and 10% had received platinum-containing therapy in the neoadjuvant or adjuvant setting. Approximately one-third (30%) of patients had high expression of PD-L1 (defined as a combined positive score of at least 10% as detected by an immunohistochemistry assay); the median age of these patients was 73 years, 87% were Caucasian, 68% were male, 82% had metastatic disease, 81% had a primary tumor in the lower urinary tract, 18% had a primary tumor in the upper urinary tract, 76% had visceral metastases (including 11% with metastases to the liver), 90% were treatment-naive, and 10% had received platinum-containing therapy in the neoadjuvant or adjuvant setting. Reasons for cisplatin ineligibility included baseline renal impairment (creatinine clearance less than 60 mL/minute), poor performance status (ECOG performance status of 2), poor performance status and baseline renal impairment, or other reasons (i.e., New York Heart Association [NYHA] class III heart failure, peripheral neuropathy or hearing loss of grade 2 or greater severity) in 50, 32, 9, or 9%, respectively, of patients in the total patient population and 45, 37, 10, or 8%, respectively, of patients in the subset of patients with high PD-L1 expression. Patients with active brain metastases and/or carcinomatous meningitis, autoimmune disease, interstitial lung disease, conditions requiring therapy with immunosuppressive agents, active infection requiring systemic therapy, a history of HIV infection, or active HBV or HCV infection were excluded from the study.

In the KEYNOTE-052 study, the objective response rate was 29%; complete response was achieved in 7% of patients. Among patients with high PD-L1 expression, the objective response rate was 47%; complete response was achieved in 15% of patients. At a median follow-up of 7.8 months, median duration of response had not been reached.

Decreased survival with pembrolizumab monotherapy compared with platinum-based therapy has been reported in an ongoing clinical trial (KEYNOTE-361) in patients with previously untreated metastatic urothelial carcinoma with low PD-L1 expression; pembrolizumab monotherapy is *not* currently FDA-labeled for use in such patients. In this trial, patients with previously untreated metastatic urothelial carcinoma who were eligible for platinum-containing therapy were randomized to receive pembrolizumab monotherapy, pembrolizumab in combination with platinum-based therapy (cisplatin or carboplatin in combination with gemcitabine), or platinum-based therapy alone. A preliminary data analysis showed decreased survival of patients with low PD-L1 expression who were receiving pembrolizumab monotherapy compared with those receiving platinum-based therapy. Therefore, at the request of the independent data monitoring committee, enrollment in the pembrolizumab monotherapy group was halted for patients with low expression of PD-L1 (defined as a PD-L1 expression combined positive score of less than 10%).

● Solid Tumors with High Microsatellite Instability or Mismatch Repair Deficiency

Pembrolizumab is used for the treatment of unresectable or metastatic solid tumors with high microsatellite instability (MSI-H) or mismatch repair deficiency (dMMR) that have progressed following prior therapy in patients who are not candidates for other treatment options; in the treatment of unresectable or metastatic MSI-H or dMMR colorectal cancer, pembrolizumab is used in patients who have experienced disease progression following therapy with a fluoropyrimidine, oxaliplatin, and irinotecan. The accelerated approval of pembrolizumab for this indication is based on objective response rate and duration of response. Continued approval for this indication may be contingent on verification and description of clinical benefit of pembrolizumab in confirmatory studies.

Although some solid tumors, such as colorectal cancer, are generally unresponsive to anti-PD-1 therapy, a subpopulation of patients with solid tumors with MSI-H or dMMR has been shown to be particularly responsive to anti-PD-1 therapy. Deficiencies in the DNA mismatch repair pathway as a result of germline or somatic mutations in mismatch repair genes subsequently result in elevated levels of DNA instability in regions of short tandem repeat sequences (microsatellites) that are prone to replication errors (MSI-H). It has been postulated that the increased mutational burden in tumors with microsatellite instability produces tumor-specific neoantigens responsible for elevated levels of tumor-infiltrating lymphocytes and upregulation of immune checkpoint proteins such as PD-1 and PD-L1, suggesting that patients with solid tumors with MSI-H or dMMR are good candidates for immune checkpoint therapy. Clinical studies have demonstrated increased response rates in patients with solid tumors, particularly colorectal cancer, with MSI-H or dMMR receiving anti-PD-1 therapy. In a phase 2 study evaluating pembrolizumab in patients with solid tumors with dMMR or proficient mismatch repair (pMMR), the objective response rate (40 versus 0%) and progression-free survival rate (78 versus 11%) were substantially higher in patients with colorectal cancer with dMMR compared with those with pMMR colorectal cancer; response rates in patients with noncolorectal cancers with dMMR were similar to those in patients with colorectal cancer with dMMR.

The current indication for pembrolizumab in the treatment of unresectable or metastatic MSI-H or dMMR solid tumors, including colorectal cancer, is based principally on pooled results for 149 patients with MSI-H or dMMR solid tumors

across 5 open-label, multicenter, noncomparative trials (KEYNOTE-016, KEYNOTE-164, KEYNOTE-012, KEYNOTE-028, KEYNOTE-158). In these trials, patients received either pembrolizumab 200 mg IV every 3 weeks or pembrolizumab 10 mg/kg IV every 2 weeks for up to 24 months or until the occurrence of unacceptable toxicity or disease progression that was symptomatic, rapidly progressive, associated with a decline in performance status, or requiring urgent intervention. The primary measures of efficacy were objective response rate (as evaluated by a blinded independent central review committee according to RECIST modified to follow no more than 10 target lesions and no more than 5 target lesions per organ) and duration of response.

The median age of patients included in the pooled analysis was 55 years; 98% had metastatic disease, 77% were Caucasian, 19% were of Asian ancestry, and 2% were black. Most patients with metastatic colorectal cancer (84%) and 53% of those with other solid tumors had received at least 2 prior therapies. Patients evaluated in the pooled analysis had received a median of 2 prior therapies for metastatic or unresectable disease. Patients with active autoimmune disease or conditions requiring therapy with immunosuppressive agents were excluded from these trials.

In the pooled cohort of patients with MSI-H or dMMR solid tumors, the objective response rate was 39.6%; complete response was achieved in 7.4% of patients. At the time of analysis, the median duration of response had not been reached; however, 78% of the patients who responded to pembrolizumab had durable responses of 6 months or more. Among patients with colorectal cancer or other solid tumors, the objective response rate was 36 or 46%, respectively.

The safety and efficacy of pembrolizumab in pediatric patients with MSI-H CNS malignancies have not been established; use of pembrolizumab is *not* indicated for use in these patients.

● Gastric Cancer

Pembrolizumab is used for the treatment of recurrent, locally advanced or metastatic, PD-L1-positive (defined as a combined positive score of at least 1%, reflecting the proportion of PD-L1-staining tumor cells, macrophages, and lymphocytes relative to tumor cells in the tumor microenvironment) gastric adenocarcinoma, including adenocarcinoma of the gastroesophageal junction, that has progressed during or following at least 2 prior therapies, including fluoropyrimidine- and platinum-containing chemotherapy, and, if the tumor overexpresses the human epidermal growth factor receptor type 2 (HER2) protein, during or following therapy with an anti-HER2 agent. An FDA-approved diagnostic test is required to confirm the presence of PD-L1 expression prior to initiation of therapy. The accelerated approval of pembrolizumab for this indication is based on objective response rate and duration of response. Continued approval for this indication may be contingent on verification and description of clinical benefit of pembrolizumab in confirmatory studies.

The current indication for pembrolizumab in the treatment of gastric cancer is based principally on the results of an open-label phase 2 trial (KEYNOTE-059) in a cohort of 143 patients with gastric adenocarcinoma, including adenocarcinoma of the gastroesophageal junction, that had progressed during or following at least 2 prior therapies; with a PD-L1-expression combined positive score of at least 1%, as detected by an immunohistochemistry assay (PD-L1 IHC 22C3 pharmDx); and with either microsatellite stable disease or unknown microsatellite instability (MSI) or mismatch repair (MMR) status. Patients enrolled in the study must have received a platinum- and fluoropyrimidine-containing regimen and, in those with tumors overexpressing the HER2 protein, therapy with an anti-HER2 agent. In this study, patients received pembrolizumab 200 mg by IV infusion every 3 weeks. Treatment was continued for up to 24 months or until the occurrence of unacceptable toxicity or disease progression that was symptomatic, rapidly progressive, associated with a decline in performance status, requiring urgent intervention, or confirmed after at least 4 weeks by repeat radiographic studies. The primary measures of efficacy were objective response rate (as evaluated by a blinded independent central review committee according to RECIST modified to follow no more than 10 target lesions and no more than 5 target lesions per organ) and duration of response.

The median age of patients enrolled in the KEYNOTE-059 trial was 64 years; 82% were Caucasian, 77% were male, and 11% were of Asian ancestry. Most patients (85%) had metastatic disease; 51 or 49% had received at least 2 or 3 prior therapies, respectively, for recurrent or metastatic disease. All enrolled patients had a baseline ECOG performance status of 0 or 1. Patients with active autoimmune disease, conditions requiring therapy with immunosuppressive agents, or clinical evidence of ascites were excluded from the trial.

In the KEYNOTE-059 trial, the objective response rate was 13.3%; complete response was achieved in 1.4% of patients. At the time of analysis, the median duration of response had not been reached; however, 58% of the patients who responded to pembrolizumab had durable responses of at least 6 months and 26% had durable responses of at least 12 months. Among 7 patients with MSI-H tumors, 4 patients achieved an objective response, including 1 patient with a complete response; median duration of response had not been reached.

● *Cervical Cancer*

Pembrolizumab is used for the treatment of recurrent or metastatic, PD-L1-positive (defined as a combined positive score of at least 1%) cervical cancer that has progressed during or following chemotherapy. An FDA-approved diagnostic test is required to confirm the presence of PD-L1 expression prior to initiation of therapy. The accelerated approval of pembrolizumab for this indication is based on objective response rate and duration of response. Continued approval for this indication may be contingent on verification and description of clinical benefit of pembrolizumab in confirmatory studies.

The current indication for pembrolizumab in the treatment of recurrent or metastatic cervical cancer is based principally on the results for a subset of 77 patients with PD-L1-positive cervical cancer (part of a cohort of 98 patients with cervical cancer) in an open-label, multicenter, nonrandomized, phase 2 study (KEYNOTE-158). These 77 patients had a PD-L1 combined positive score of at least 1% as detected by an immunohistochemistry assay (PD-L1 IHC 22C3 pharmDx) and had received at least one prior chemotherapy regimen in the metastatic setting. Patients received pembrolizumab 200 mg administered as an IV infusion every 3 weeks. Treatment was continued for up to 24 months or until unacceptable toxicity or disease progression occurred; however, patients with disease progression could receive additional doses of the drug until disease progression was confirmed, unless disease progression was symptomatic, rapidly progressive, associated with a decline in performance status, or requiring urgent intervention.

The median age of the 77 patients in the KEYNOTE-158 study with PD-L1-positive cervical cancer was 45 years; 81% were Caucasian, 14% were of Asian ancestry, 3% were black, 92% had squamous cell carcinoma, 6% had adenocarcinoma, and 1% had adenosquamous histology. Of these 77 patients, 95% had metastatic disease and 65% had received at least 2 prior therapies for recurrent or metastatic disease. All of the patients had an ECOG performance status of 0 or 1. The study excluded patients with autoimmune disease or conditions requiring therapy with immunosuppressive agents.

At a median follow-up of 11.7 months, the objective response rate in the KEYNOTE-158 study for patients with PD-L1-positive cervical cancer who had received at least one prior chemotherapy regimen for metastatic disease was 14.3%; complete response was achieved in 2.6% of patients. At the time of analysis, the median duration of response had not been reached; however, 91% of patients who responded to pembrolizumab had durable responses of 6 months or more. Objective responses were not observed in patients with a PD-L1 combined positive score of less than 1%.

● *Hepatocellular Carcinoma*

Pembrolizumab is used for the treatment of hepatocellular carcinoma previously treated with sorafenib; pembrolizumab has been designated an orphan drug by FDA for the treatment of this cancer. The accelerated approval of pembrolizumab for this indication is based on objective response rate and duration of response. Continued approval for this indication may be contingent on verification and description of clinical benefit of pembrolizumab in confirmatory studies.

The current indication for pembrolizumab in the treatment of previously treated hepatocellular carcinoma is based principally on the results of a phase 2, nonrandomized, noncomparative study (KEYNOTE-224) in 104 adults with hepatocellular carcinoma who had experienced disease progression during or following sorafenib therapy or who had not tolerated such therapy. Patients received pembrolizumab 200 mg administered as an IV infusion every 3 weeks for up to 24 months or until unacceptable toxicity or disease progression occurred; however, clinically stable patients with disease progression could continue treatment if they were considered to be deriving clinical benefit. The primary measures of efficacy were objective response rate (as evaluated by a blinded independent central review committee according to RECIST modified to follow no more than 10 target lesions and no more than 5 target lesions per organ) and duration of response. The study excluded patients with active autoimmune disease, any condition requiring

immunosuppressive therapy, more than one etiology of hepatitis, brain metastasis, clinical evidence of ascites, hepatic encephalopathy, or esophageal or gastric variceal bleeding within the prior 6 months. The study also excluded patients who had received any prior systemic therapy other than sorafenib for advanced hepatocellular carcinoma; sorafenib was discontinued because of intolerable toxicity in 20% of patients.

The median age of patients enrolled in the KEYNOTE-224 study was 68 years; 83% were male, 81% were Caucasian, and 14% were of Asian ancestry. All patients had an ECOG performance status of 0 or 1. Most patients (94%) had Child-Pugh class A hepatic impairment, 64% had extrahepatic disease, 17% had vascular invasion, 9% had both extrahepatic disease and vascular invasion, 38% had α-fetoprotein concentrations of 0.4 mg/L or more, 21% were seropositive for HBV, 25% were seropositive for HCV, and 9% were seropositive for both HBV and HCV. At a median duration of follow-up of 12.3 months, the objective response rate was 17%; complete response was achieved in 1% of patients. The median duration of response had not been reached at the time of analysis; however, 89% of patients who responded to the drug had durable responses of 6 months or more and 56% had durable responses of 12 months or more. Results of a subgroup analysis (based on age, sex, geographic region, performance status, etiology, disease stage, α-fetoprotein concentration, presence of extrahepatic disease, presence of macrovascular invasion, reason for sorafenib discontinuance) suggested that objective response rates were generally similar across subgroups.

● *Merkel Cell Carcinoma*

Pembrolizumab is used for the treatment of recurrent, locally advanced or metastatic Merkel cell carcinoma; pembrolizumab has been designated an orphan drug by FDA for the treatment of this cancer. The accelerated approval of pembrolizumab for this indication is based on objective response rate and duration of response. Continued approval for this indication may be contingent on verification and description of clinical benefit of pembrolizumab in confirmatory studies.

The current indication for pembrolizumab in the treatment of recurrent, locally advanced or metastatic Merkel cell carcinoma is based principally on the results of a phase 2, noncomparative, nonrandomized study (KEYNOTE-017) in 50 adults with recurrent locally advanced or metastatic Merkel cell carcinoma who had not received prior systemic therapy for advanced disease. Patients received pembrolizumab 2 mg/kg administered as an IV infusion every 3 weeks for up to 24 months or until the occurrence of unacceptable toxicity or disease progression that was symptomatic, rapidly progressive, associated with a decline in performance status, requiring urgent intervention, or confirmed in at least 4 weeks with repeat radiographic studies. The primary measures of efficacy were objective response rate (as evaluated by a blinded independent central review committee according to RECIST) and duration of response. The study excluded patients with active autoimmune disease or any condition requiring immunosuppressive therapy. The median age of patients enrolled in the KEYNOTE-017 study was 71 years (80% were 65 years of age or older); 68% were male and 90% were Caucasian. All patients had an ECOG performance status of 0 or 1. Most patients (86%) had stage IV disease; 14% had stage IIIB disease. Prior therapies included surgery or radiation therapy in 84 or 70% of patients, respectively. At a median follow-up of 14.9 months, the objective response rate was 56%; complete response was achieved in 24% of patients. The median duration of response had not been reached at the time of analysis; however, 96% of patients who responded to the drug had durable responses of 6 months or more and 54% had durable responses of 12 months or more.

DOSAGE AND ADMINISTRATION

● *Reconstitution and Administration*

Pembrolizumab is administered by IV infusion over 30 minutes.

Pembrolizumab is commercially available as an injection concentrate and as a lyophilized powder. The lyophilized powder must be reconstituted and then diluted to prepare a final pembrolizumab infusion solution. Pembrolizumab injection concentrate must be diluted prior to IV administration.

Prior to administration, commercially available pembrolizumab powder for injection must be reconstituted and diluted using proper aseptic technique. The powder is reconstituted by adding 2.3 mL of sterile water for injection to a vial labeled as containing 50 mg of the drug to provide a solution containing 25 mg/mL. The diluent should be directed toward the wall of the vial and not directly at the pembrolizumab powder. The vial should be gently swirled and allowed to stand for up to 5 minutes to let the bubbles dissipate; the vial should not be shaken.

The reconstituted pembrolizumab solution or commercially available injection concentrate should be inspected visually for particulate matter and discoloration prior to dilution and administration. The solution should be clear to slightly opalescent and colorless to slightly yellow, and should not be used if visible particles are present.

For preparation of the final diluted pembrolizumab solution for infusion, the required amount of reconstituted pembrolizumab solution or commercially available injection concentrate should be injected into an infusion bag containing a sufficient volume of 0.9% sodium chloride injection or 5% dextrose injection to yield a final solution with a pembrolizumab concentration of 1–10 mg/mL. The final diluted pembrolizumab solution for infusion should be mixed by gentle inversion. Reconstituted and diluted solutions of the drug are stable for up to 6 hours (including infusion time) after reconstitution of the lyophilized powder or dilution of the injection concentrate when stored at room temperature or up to 24 hours when stored under refrigeration (2–8°C); diluted solutions of the drug should be brought to room temperature prior to administration. Reconstituted and diluted solutions of the drug should not be frozen. Pembrolizumab should be administered through a sterile, nonpyrogenic, low-protein-binding 0.2- to 5-μm inline or add-on filter.

Pembrolizumab should *not* be administered simultaneously through the same IV line with any other drug. Commercially available pembrolizumab for injection and pembrolizumab injection concentrate contain no preservatives and are intended for single use only; any unused portions should be discarded.

● Dosage

Clinicians should consult published protocols for information on the dosage, method of administration, and administration sequence of other antineoplastic agents used in combination regimens with pembrolizumab.

Melanoma

Unresectable or Metastatic Melanoma

For the treatment of unresectable or metastatic melanoma, the recommended adult dosage of pembrolizumab is 200 mg administered as a 30-minute IV infusion every 3 weeks. Therapy should be continued until disease progression or unacceptable toxicity occurs.

Adjuvant Therapy for Locally Advanced Melanoma

For the adjuvant therapy of completely resected advanced melanoma with regional nodal involvement, the recommended adult dosage of pembrolizumab is 200 mg administered as a 30-minute IV infusion every 3 weeks. Therapy should be continued for up to 12 months or until disease recurrence or unacceptable toxicity occurs.

Non-small Cell Lung Cancer

Monotherapy for Metastatic Non-small Cell Lung Cancer (NSCLC)

For the initial treatment of metastatic NSCLC in patients with epidermal growth factor receptor (EGFR)- and anaplastic lymphoma kinase (ALK)-negative tumors with high levels of programmed-death ligand-1 (PD-L1) expression (defined as PD-L1 expression of any intensity on at least 50% of tumor cells), the recommended adult dosage of pembrolizumab is 200 mg administered as a 30-minute IV infusion every 3 weeks. Therapy should be continued for up to 24 months or until disease progression or unacceptable toxicity occurs.

For the treatment of PD-L1-positive (defined as PD-L1 expression of any intensity on at least 1% of tumor cells) metastatic NSCLC that has progressed during or following platinum-based chemotherapy and, if the tumor is EGFR- or ALK-positive, during or following therapy with an FDA-labeled anti-EGFR or anti-ALK agent, the recommended adult dosage of pembrolizumab is 200 mg administered as a 30-minute IV infusion every 3 weeks. Therapy should be continued for up to 24 months or until disease progression or unacceptable toxicity occurs.

Selection of single-agent pembrolizumab for the treatment of metastatic NSCLC should be based on the presence of PD-L1 expression. (See Uses: Non-small Cell Lung Cancer.)

Combination Therapy for Metastatic NSCLC

For the initial treatment of metastatic nonsquamous NSCLC without EGFR or ALK genomic aberrations, the recommended adult dosage of pembrolizumab is 200 mg administered as a 30-minute IV infusion every 3 weeks in combination

with pemetrexed and a platinum-containing antineoplastic agent (carboplatin, cisplatin). Pembrolizumab should be administered before pemetrexed and the platinum-containing antineoplastic agent. Therapy should be continued for up to 24 months or until disease progression or unacceptable toxicity occurs.

For the initial treatment of metastatic squamous NSCLC, the recommended adult dosage of pembrolizumab is 200 mg administered as a 30-minute IV infusion every 3 weeks in combination with carboplatin and paclitaxel (conventional or albumin-bound). Pembrolizumab should be administered before carboplatin and paclitaxel. Therapy should be continued for up to 24 months or until disease progression or unacceptable toxicity occurs.

Head and Neck Cancer

For the treatment of recurrent or metastatic head and neck squamous cell carcinoma that has progressed during or following platinum-containing therapy, the recommended adult dosage of pembrolizumab is 200 mg administered as a 30-minute IV infusion every 3 weeks. Therapy should be continued for up to 24 months or until disease progression or unacceptable toxicity occurs.

Hodgkin Lymphoma

For the treatment of refractory classical Hodgkin lymphoma (cHL) and cHL that has relapsed following at least 3 prior therapies, the recommended *adult* dosage of pembrolizumab is 200 mg administered as a 30-minute IV infusion every 3 weeks. The recommended *pediatric* dosage of pembrolizumab for this indication is 2 mg/kg (up to a maximum of 200 mg) administered as a 30-minute IV infusion every 3 weeks. Therapy should be continued for up to 24 months or until disease progression or unacceptable toxicity occurs.

Primary Mediastinal Large B-cell Lymphoma

For the treatment of refractory primary mediastinal large B-cell lymphoma (PMBL) or PMBL that has relapsed following at least 2 prior therapies, the recommended *adult* dosage of pembrolizumab is 200 mg administered as a 30-minute IV infusion every 3 weeks. The recommended *pediatric* dosage of pembrolizumab for this indication is 2 mg/kg (up to 200 mg) administered as a 30-minute IV infusion every 3 weeks. Therapy should be continued for up to 24 months or until disease progression or unacceptable toxicity occurs.

Pembrolizumab is not recommended for the treatment of PMBL in patients who require urgent cytoreduction.

Urothelial Carcinoma

For the treatment of locally advanced or metastatic urothelial carcinoma that has progressed during or following platinum-containing therapy or within 12 months of platinum-containing therapy in the neoadjuvant or adjuvant setting, locally advanced or metastatic urothelial carcinoma in patients with high levels of PD-L1 expression (defined as PD-L1 expression combined positive score of at least 10%) who are not candidates for cisplatin-containing therapy, or locally advanced or metastatic urothelial carcinoma in patients who are not candidates for platinum-containing chemotherapy regardless of PD-L1 expression, the recommended adult dosage of pembrolizumab is 200 mg administered as a 30-minute IV infusion every 3 weeks. Therapy should be continued for up to 24 months or until disease progression or unacceptable toxicity occurs.

Selection of pembrolizumab therapy for the treatment of locally advanced or metastatic urothelial carcinoma in patients who are not candidates for cisplatin-containing therapy should be based on the presence of PD-L1 expression. (See Uses: Urothelial Carcinoma.)

Solid Tumors with High Microsatellite Instability or Mismatch Repair Deficiency

For the treatment of unresectable or metastatic solid tumors with high microsatellite instability (MSI-H) or mismatch repair deficiency (dMMR) that have progressed following prior therapy in patients who are not candidates for other treatment options or for the treatment of unresectable or metastatic MSI-H or dMMR colorectal cancer that has progressed following therapy with a fluoropyrimidine, oxaliplatin, and irinotecan, the recommended *adult* dosage of pembrolizumab is 200 mg administered as a 30-minute IV infusion every 3 weeks. The recommended *pediatric* dosage of pembrolizumab for this indication is 2 mg/kg (up to a maximum of 200 mg) administered as a 30-minute IV infusion every 3 weeks. Therapy should be continued for up to 24 months or until disease progression or unacceptable toxicity occurs.

Gastric Cancer

For the treatment of recurrent, locally advanced or metastatic, PD-L1-positive (defined as a PD-L1 expression combined positive score of at least 1%) gastric adenocarcinoma, including adenocarcinoma of the gastroesophageal junction, that has progressed during or following at least 2 prior therapies, including fluoropyrimidine- and platinum-containing chemotherapy and, if the tumor overexpresses the human epidermal growth factor receptor type 2 (HER2) protein, during or following therapy with an anti-HER2 agent, the recommended adult dosage of pembrolizumab is 200 mg administered as a 30-minute IV infusion every 3 weeks. Therapy should be continued for up to 24 months or until disease progression or unacceptable toxicity occurs.

Initiation of pembrolizumab therapy should be based on the presence of PD-L1 expression; if PD-L1 expression is not detected in an archival tumor specimen, the feasibility of obtaining a new tumor specimen should be considered. (See Uses: Gastric Cancer.)

Cervical Cancer

For the treatment of recurrent or metastatic, PD-L1-positive (defined as a PD-L1 expression combined positive score of at least 1%) cervical cancer that has progressed during or following chemotherapy, the recommended adult dosage of pembrolizumab is 200 mg administered as a 30-minute IV infusion every 3 weeks. Therapy should be continued for up to 24 months or until disease progression or unacceptable toxicity occurs.

Initiation of pembrolizumab therapy should be based on the presence of PD-L1 expression. (See Uses: Cervical Cancer.)

Hepatocellular Carcinoma

For the treatment of hepatocellular carcinoma previously treated with sorafenib, the recommended adult dosage of pembrolizumab is 200 mg administered as a 30-minute IV infusion every 3 weeks. Therapy should be continued for up to 24 months or until disease progression or unacceptable toxicity occurs.

Merkel Cell Carcinoma

For the treatment of recurrent, locally advanced or metastatic Merkel cell carcinoma, the recommended *adult* dosage of pembrolizumab is 200 mg administered as a 30-minute IV infusion every 3 weeks. The recommended *pediatric* dosage of pembrolizumab for this indication is 2 mg/kg (up to a maximum of 200 mg) administered as a 30-minute IV infusion every 3 weeks. Therapy should be continued for up to 24 months or until disease progression or unacceptable toxicity occurs.

Therapy Interruption for Toxicity

If immune-mediated adverse effects occur, temporary or permanent discontinuance of pembrolizumab may be required based on severity of the reaction.

Pembrolizumab should be permanently discontinued in patients experiencing persistent grade 2 or 3 immune-mediated adverse effects (except for endocrinopathies) that do not recover to grade 0 or 1 within 12 weeks of the last dose of pembrolizumab. Therapy with the drug also should be permanently discontinued in patients unable to reduce corticosteroid dosage to less than 10 mg of prednisone daily (or equivalent) within 12 weeks.

Pembrolizumab should be permanently discontinued in patients experiencing any life-threatening immune-mediated adverse effect (except for endocrinopathies or hematologic toxicity in patients with cHL or PMBL). Therapy with the drug also should be permanently discontinued if grade 3 or 4 immune-mediated adverse effects recur.

Hematologic Toxicity

If grade 4 hematologic toxicity occurs in patients with cHL or PMBL, pembrolizumab therapy should be interrupted until the toxicity resolves to grade 0 or 1.

Immune-mediated Pneumonitis

If grade 2 immune-mediated pneumonitis occurs, pembrolizumab therapy should be interrupted until the toxicity resolves to grade 0 or 1 *and* the corticosteroid dosage has been tapered. (See Immune-mediated Pneumonitis under Cautions: Warnings/Precautions.)

If grade 3 or 4 immune-mediated pneumonitis occurs or grade 2 immune-mediated pneumonitis recurs, pembrolizumab therapy should be permanently discontinued.

Immune-mediated GI Effects

If grade 2 or 3 immune-mediated colitis occurs, pembrolizumab therapy should be interrupted until the toxicity resolves to grade 0 or 1 *and* the corticosteroid dosage has been tapered. (See Immune-mediated GI Effects under Cautions: Warnings/Precautions.)

If grade 4 immune-mediated colitis occurs, pembrolizumab therapy should be permanently discontinued.

Immune-mediated Hepatic Effects

For serum aminotransferase (ALT or AST) elevations exceeding 3 times but not more than 5 times the upper limit of normal (ULN) or total bilirubin concentrations exceeding 1.5 times but not more than 3 times the ULN in patients *without* hepatocellular carcinoma, pembrolizumab therapy should be interrupted until the toxicity resolves to grade 0 or 1 *and* the corticosteroid dosage has been tapered. (See Immune-mediated Hepatic Effects under Cautions: Warnings/Precautions.)

For ALT or AST elevations exceeding 5 times the ULN or total bilirubin concentrations exceeding 3 times the ULN in patients *without* hepatocellular carcinoma, pembrolizumab therapy should be permanently discontinued. In addition, in patients with liver metastasis with baseline grade 2 serum aminotransferase elevations, pembrolizumab therapy should be permanently discontinued if ALT or AST concentrations increase by 50% or more from baseline for at least 1 week.

For ALT or AST concentrations that are 5 or more times the ULN in patients *with* hepatocellular carcinoma and baseline ALT and AST concentrations less than 2 times the ULN, pembrolizumab therapy should be interrupted until the toxicity resolves to grade 0 or 1 or the AST and ALT concentrations return to baseline.

For ALT or AST concentrations exceeding 3 times the baseline concentrations in patients *with* hepatocellular carcinoma and baseline ALT or AST concentrations of 2 or more times the ULN, pembrolizumab therapy should be interrupted until the toxicity resolves to grade 0 or 1 or the AST and ALT concentrations return to baseline.

For total bilirubin concentrations exceeding 2 mg/dL in patients *with* hepatocellular carcinoma and baseline total bilirubin concentrations of less than 1.5 mg/dL, pembrolizumab therapy should be interrupted until the toxicity resolves to grade 0 or 1 or the bilirubin concentrations return to baseline.

For total bilirubin concentrations exceeding 3 mg/dL (regardless of the baseline concentration) in patients *with* hepatocellular carcinoma, pembrolizumab therapy should be interrupted until the toxicity resolves to grade 0 or 1 or the bilirubin concentrations return to baseline.

For ALT or AST concentrations exceeding 10 times the ULN in patients *with* hepatocellular carcinoma, pembrolizumab therapy should be permanently discontinued.

For Child-Pugh score of 9 or more in patients *with* hepatocellular carcinoma, pembrolizumab therapy should be permanently discontinued.

If GI bleeding suggestive of portal hypertension, new onset of clinically detectable ascites, or encephalopathy occurs in patients *with* hepatocellular carcinoma, pembrolizumab therapy should be permanently discontinued.

Immune-mediated Endocrine Effects

If grade 2 immune-mediated hypophysitis or severe hyperglycemia occurs, pembrolizumab therapy should be interrupted. (See Immune-mediated Endocrine Effects under Cautions: Warnings/Precautions.)

If grade 3 or 4 immune-mediated endocrinopathies, including hypophysitis and hyperthyroidism, occur, pembrolizumab therapy should be interrupted until the patient is clinically stable or the drug should be discontinued.

Immune-mediated Renal Effects

If grade 2 immune-mediated nephritis occurs, pembrolizumab therapy should be interrupted until the toxicity resolves to grade 0 or 1 *and* the corticosteroid dosage has been tapered. (See Immune-mediated Renal Effects under Cautions: Warnings/Precautions.)

If grade 3 or 4 immune-mediated nephritis occurs, pembrolizumab therapy should be permanently discontinued.

Immune-mediated Dermatologic Effects

If a grade 3 immune-mediated skin reaction occurs or Stevens-Johnson syndrome or toxic epidermal necrolysis is suspected, pembrolizumab therapy should be interrupted until the toxicity resolves to grade 0 or 1. (See Immune-mediated Dermatologic Effects under Cautions: Warnings/Precautions.)

If a grade 4 immune-mediated skin reaction occurs or Stevens-Johnson syndrome or toxic epidermal necrolysis is confirmed, pembrolizumab therapy should be permanently discontinued.

Other Immune-mediated Adverse Effects

If any other grade 2 immune-mediated adverse effects occur, pembrolizumab therapy should be interrupted until the toxicity resolves to grade 0 or 1 *and* the corticosteroid dosage has been tapered. (See Other Immune-mediated Effects under Cautions: Warnings/Precautions.)

If any other grade 3 immune-mediated adverse effects occur, pembrolizumab therapy should be interrupted until the toxicity resolves to grade 0 or 1 *and* the corticosteroid dosage has been tapered, or the drug should be permanently discontinued (depending on the severity and type of reaction).

If any other grade 4 immune-mediated adverse effects occur, pembrolizumab therapy should be permanently discontinued.

Infusion-related Reactions

If grade 1 or 2 infusion-related reactions occur, the infusion should be interrupted or the infusion rate should be slowed.

If grade 3 or 4 infusion-related reactions occur, pembrolizumab therapy should be permanently discontinued.

● Special Populations

The manufacturer makes no special dosage recommendations for patients with preexisting hepatic or renal impairment or for geriatric patients. (See Specific Populations under Cautions: Warnings/Precautions.)

CAUTIONS

● Contraindications

The manufacturer states there are no known contraindications to the use of pembrolizumab.

● Warnings/Precautions

Immune-mediated Pneumonitis

Immune-mediated pneumonitis, sometimes fatal, has occurred in patients receiving pembrolizumab therapy.

In clinical studies evaluating single-agent pembrolizumab, immune-mediated pneumonitis occurred in 3.4% of patients and was grade 3 or greater in approximately 1.3% of patients receiving the drug. The median time to onset of immune-mediated pneumonitis was 3.3 months and the median duration was 1.5 months. Most patients (67%) experiencing immune-mediated pneumonitis received systemic corticosteroid therapy; 79% of these patients received high-dose corticosteroid therapy for a median duration of 8 days followed by tapering of the corticosteroid dosage. Immune-mediated pneumonitis occurred more frequently in patients who had received prior thoracic irradiation compared with those who had not received thoracic irradiation (6.9 versus 2.9%). Pembrolizumab was discontinued because of immune-mediated pneumonitis in 1.3% of patients receiving the drug. Immune-mediated pneumonitis resolved in 59% of patients.

Patients receiving pembrolizumab should be monitored for pulmonary symptoms indicative of pneumonitis. If pneumonitis is suspected, patients should be evaluated for pneumonitis using radiographic imaging. In patients who develop grade 2 or greater pneumonitis, systemic corticosteroid therapy should be initiated (1–2 mg/kg of prednisone daily [or equivalent]) followed by tapering of the corticosteroid dosage. Temporary interruption or discontinuance of pembrolizumab may be necessary if immune-mediated pneumonitis occurs during therapy with the drug. (See Therapy Interruption for Toxicity under Dosage and Administration: Dosage.)

Immune-mediated GI Effects

Immune-mediated colitis has occurred in patients receiving pembrolizumab therapy.

In clinical studies evaluating single-agent pembrolizumab, immune-mediated colitis occurred in 1.7% of patients and was grade 3 or 4 in approximately 1.2% of patients receiving the drug. The median time to onset of immune-mediated colitis was 3.5 months and the median duration was 1.3 months. Most patients (69%) experiencing immune-mediated colitis received systemic corticosteroid therapy; 82% of these patients received high-dose corticosteroid therapy for a median duration of 7 days followed by tapering of the corticosteroid dosage. Pembrolizumab was discontinued because of immune-mediated colitis in 0.5% of patients receiving the drug. Immune-mediated colitis resolved in 85% of patients.

Patients receiving pembrolizumab should be monitored for manifestations of colitis. In patients who develop grade 2 or greater colitis, systemic corticosteroid therapy should be initiated (1–2 mg/kg of prednisone daily [or equivalent]) followed by tapering of the corticosteroid dosage. Temporary interruption or discontinuance of pembrolizumab may be necessary if immune-mediated colitis occurs during therapy with the drug. (See Therapy Interruption for Toxicity under Dosage and Administration: Dosage.)

Immune-mediated Hepatic Effects

Immune-mediated hepatitis has occurred in patients receiving pembrolizumab therapy.

In clinical studies evaluating single-agent pembrolizumab, immune-mediated hepatitis occurred in 0.7% of patients and was grade 3 or 4 in approximately 0.5% of patients receiving the drug. The median time to onset of immune-mediated hepatitis was 1.3 months and the median duration was 1.8 months. Most patients (68%) experiencing immune-mediated hepatitis received systemic corticosteroid therapy; 92% of these patients received high-dose corticosteroid therapy for a median duration of 5 days followed by tapering of the corticosteroid dosage. Pembrolizumab was discontinued because of immune-mediated hepatitis in 0.2% of patients receiving the drug. Immune-mediated hepatitis resolved in 79% of patients.

Patients receiving pembrolizumab should be assessed for changes in liver function. If grade 2 hepatitis occurs, systemic corticosteroid therapy should be initiated at a dosage of 0.5–1 mg/kg of prednisone daily (or equivalent) followed by tapering of the corticosteroid dosage. In patients who develop grade 3 or greater hepatitis, systemic corticosteroid therapy should be initiated at a dosage of 1–2 mg/kg of prednisone daily (or equivalent) followed by tapering of the corticosteroid dosage. In patients who develop elevations of serum aminotransferase or bilirubin concentrations, temporary interruption of therapy or drug discontinuance may be required. (See Therapy Interruption for Toxicity under Dosage and Administration: Dosage.)

Immune-mediated Endocrine Effects

Immune-mediated endocrinopathies, including hypophysitis, thyroid dysfunction (i.e., hyperthyroidism, hypothyroidism, thyroiditis), and diabetes mellitus, have occurred in patients receiving pembrolizumab therapy.

Hypophysitis

In clinical studies evaluating single-agent pembrolizumab, immune-mediated hypophysitis occurred in 0.6% of patients and was grade 3 or 4 in approximately 0.4% of patients receiving pembrolizumab. The median time to onset of immune-mediated hypophysitis was 3.7 months and the median duration was 4.7 months. Most patients (94%) experiencing immune-mediated hypophysitis received systemic corticosteroid therapy; 38% of these patients received high-dose corticosteroid therapy. Pembrolizumab was discontinued because of immune-mediated hypophysitis in 0.1% of patients receiving the drug. Immune-mediated hypophysitis resolved in 41% of patients.

Patients should be monitored for manifestations of hypophysitis (including hypopituitarism and adrenal insufficiency) during pembrolizumab therapy. If hypophysitis occurs, systemic corticosteroid therapy and hormone replacement therapy should be administered as clinically indicated. In patients who develop hypophysitis, temporary interruption or discontinuance of pembrolizumab may be required. (See Therapy Interruption for Toxicity under Dosage and Administration: Dosage.)

Thyroid Dysfunction

In clinical studies evaluating single-agent pembrolizumab, immune-mediated hyperthyroidism occurred in 3.4% of patients and was grade 2 or 3 in 0.9% of patients receiving pembrolizumab. The median time to onset of immune-mediated hyperthyroidism was 1.4 months and the median duration was 2.1 months. Pembrolizumab was discontinued because of immune-mediated hyperthyroidism in less than 0.1% of patients receiving the drug. Immune-mediated hyperthyroidism resolved in 74% of patients.

In clinical studies evaluating single-agent pembrolizumab, immune-mediated hypothyroidism occurred in 8.5% of patients and was grade 2 or 3 in 6.3% of patients receiving pembrolizumab. The median time to onset of immune-mediated hypothyroidism was 3.5 months and the median duration was not reached but ranged from 2 days to more than 27 months. Pembrolizumab was discontinued because of immune-mediated hypothyroidism in less than 0.1% of patients receiving the drug. Immune-mediated hypothyroidism resolved in 20% of patients. In clinical studies evaluating pembrolizumab in patients with squamous cell carcinoma of the head and neck, new-onset or worsening immune-mediated hypothyroidism occurred in 15% of patients and was grade 3 in 0.5% of patients receiving the drug; 54% of patients with immune-mediated hypothyroidism had no history of hypothyroidism.

In clinical studies evaluating single-agent pembrolizumab, immune-mediated thyroiditis occurred in 0.6% of patients and was grade 2 in 0.3% of patients receiving pembrolizumab. The median time to onset of immune-mediated thyroiditis was 1.2 months.

Thyroid function should be evaluated prior to initiation of therapy, periodically during therapy, and as clinically indicated. Patients should be monitored for manifestations of hyperthyroidism, hypothyroidism, or thyroiditis during pembrolizumab therapy. In patients who develop hypothyroidism, thyroid hormone replacement therapy should be initiated as clinically indicated. If hyperthyroidism occurs, antithyroid agents and β-adrenergic blocking agents (β-blockers) should be initiated as clinically indicated. In patients who develop hyperthyroidism, temporary interruption or discontinuance of pembrolizumab may be required. (See Therapy Interruption for Toxicity under Dosage and Administration: Dosage.)

Diabetes Mellitus

In clinical studies evaluating single-agent pembrolizumab, immune-mediated type 1 diabetes mellitus and diabetic ketoacidosis occurred in 0.2% of patients receiving pembrolizumab.

Patients receiving pembrolizumab should be monitored for manifestations of diabetes mellitus (e.g., hyperglycemia). If type 1 diabetes mellitus occurs, insulin should be initiated. If severe hyperglycemia occurs, pembrolizumab therapy should be temporarily interrupted and antidiabetic agents should be initiated. (See Therapy Interruption for Toxicity under Dosage and Administration: Dosage.)

Immune-mediated Renal Effects

Immune-mediated nephritis has occurred in patients receiving pembrolizumab therapy.

In clinical studies evaluating single-agent pembrolizumab, immune-mediated nephritis occurred in 0.3% of patients and was grade 3 or 4 in approximately 0.2% of patients receiving the drug. The median time to onset of immune-mediated nephritis was 5.1 months and the median duration was 3.3 months. Most patients (89%) experiencing immune-mediated nephritis received systemic corticosteroid therapy; 88% of these patients received high-dose corticosteroid therapy for a median duration of 15 days followed by tapering of the corticosteroid dosage. Pembrolizumab was discontinued because of immune-mediated nephritis in 0.1% of patients receiving the drug. Immune-mediated nephritis resolved in 56% of patients.

In clinical studies evaluating pembrolizumab in combination with pemetrexed and a platinum-containing antineoplastic agent, immune-mediated nephritis occurred in 1.7% of patients receiving combination therapy and was grade 3 or 4 in 1.5% of patients receiving combination therapy. The median time to onset of immune-mediated nephritis was 3.2 months and the duration ranged from 1.6–16.8 months or more. Most patients (86%) experiencing immune-mediated nephritis received systemic corticosteroid therapy; all of these patients received high-dose corticosteroid therapy for a median duration of 3 days followed by tapering of the corticosteroid dosage. Pembrolizumab was discontinued because of immune-mediated nephritis in 1.2% of patients receiving pembrolizumab in combination with pemetrexed and a platinum-containing agent. Immune-mediated nephritis resolved in 29% of patients.

Patients receiving pembrolizumab should be monitored for changes in renal function. In patients who develop nephritis, temporary interruption of therapy or drug discontinuance may be required. (See Therapy Interruption for Toxicity under Dosage and Administration: Dosage.) If grade 2 or greater nephritis occurs, systemic corticosteroid therapy should be initiated (1–2 mg/kg of prednisone daily [or equivalent]) followed by tapering of the corticosteroid dosage.

Immune-mediated Dermatologic Effects

Immune-mediated rash, including Stevens-Johnson syndrome, toxic epidermal necrolysis (sometimes fatal), exfoliative dermatitis, and bullous pemphigoid, may occur in patients receiving pembrolizumab therapy.

Patients receiving pembrolizumab should be monitored for severe skin reactions. If an immune-mediated skin reaction is suspected, adequate evaluation should be performed to exclude other causes. Temporary interruption or discontinuance of pembrolizumab may be necessary if immune-mediated rash occurs during therapy with the drug; systemic corticosteroid therapy also should be initiated. (See Therapy Interruption for Toxicity under Dosage and Administration: Dosage.) If Stevens-Johnson syndrome or toxic epidermal necrolysis is suspected, pembrolizumab therapy should be temporarily interrupted and the patient referred for evaluation and treatment by a specialist. If Stevens-Johnson syndrome or toxic epidermal necrolysis is confirmed, pembrolizumab should be permanently discontinued.

Other Immune-mediated Effects

Other immune-mediated adverse effects, which may be severe or fatal and may affect any organ system or tissue, have occurred in patients receiving pembrolizumab therapy.

In clinical studies evaluating single-agent pembrolizumab, uveitis, myositis, pancreatitis, arthritis, hemolytic anemia, sarcoidosis, encephalitis, Guillain-Barré syndrome, myasthenia gravis, and vasculitis have occurred in patients receiving the drug. In these clinical studies, such immune-mediated adverse effects were observed in less than 1% of patients; however, arthritis occurred in 1.5% of patients. In addition, immune-mediated adverse effects such as myelitis and myocarditis have been reported in other clinical trials of the drug and during postmarketing experience. Immune-mediated rejection of solid organ transplants also has been reported during postmarketing experience in patients who received pembrolizumab. Immune-mediated adverse effects generally occur during therapy with an anti-programmed-death receptor-1 (anti-PD-1) or anti-programmed-death ligand-1 (anti-PD-L1) antibody, but also may occur following discontinuance of the drug.

If an immune-mediated adverse effect is suspected, adequate evaluation should be performed to exclude other causes. Depending on the type and severity of the immune-mediated adverse effect, pembrolizumab therapy should be interrupted until the toxicity resolves to grade 0 or 1 or the drug should be discontinued, and systemic corticosteroid therapy should be initiated. (See Therapy Interruption for Toxicity under Dosage and Administration: Dosage.) Once the toxicity has resolved to grade 0 or 1, the corticosteroid dosage should be tapered over at least 1 month. Based on limited data, systemic immunosuppressive therapy may be considered in patients experiencing immune-mediated adverse effects inadequately controlled with systemic corticosteroid therapy. Because pembrolizumab may increase the risk of rejection in solid organ transplant recipients, the risk of possible organ rejection should be weighed against potential benefits of the drug.

Infusion-related Effects

Severe or life-threatening infusion-related reactions, including hypersensitivity reactions and anaphylaxis, have occurred in 0.2% of patients receiving single-agent pembrolizumab.

Patients receiving pembrolizumab should be monitored for signs and symptoms of infusion-related reactions. In patients experiencing grade 3 or 4 infusion-related reactions, the pembrolizumab infusion should be stopped and the drug permanently discontinued.

Allogeneic Stem Cell Transplantation-related Immune-mediated Complications

Immune-mediated complications, including graft-versus-host disease (GVHD) and hepatic veno-occlusive disease, have occurred in patients who underwent allogeneic stem cell transplantation prior to or following therapy with pembrolizumab. Some cases have resulted in death. Immune-mediated complications following allogeneic stem cell transplantation may occur despite other intervening therapy between pembrolizumab administration and transplantation.

In clinical trials evaluating pembrolizumab in patients with classical Hodgkin lymphoma (cHL), 6 of 23 patients (26%) who underwent allogeneic stem cell transplantation following therapy with pembrolizumab developed GVHD; one case resulted in death. Severe hepatic veno-occlusive disease following reduced-intensity conditioning occurred in 2 patients, which resulted in one fatality. Hyperacute GVHD resulting in death also has been reported in patients with lymphoma who received an anti-PD-1 antibody prior to allogeneic stem cell transplantation. In patients with a history of allogeneic stem cell transplantation, acute GVHD (including fatal acute GVHD) has occurred following pembrolizumab therapy. Patients with a history of GVHD following allogeneic stem cell transplantation may be at increased risk for developing GVHD following therapy with pembrolizumab.

In patients who previously underwent allogeneic stem cell transplantation, the potential benefit of pembrolizumab therapy should be weighed against the risks of developing GVHD. Patients who receive pembrolizumab should be monitored closely for early manifestations of stem cell transplantation-related immune-mediated complications (e.g., hyperacute GVHD, grade 3 or 4 acute GVHD, corticosteroid-requiring febrile syndrome, hepatic veno-occlusive disease) and such conditions should be managed promptly if they occur.

Treatment-related Mortality

Increased mortality has been reported in clinical trials in patients with multiple myeloma receiving pembrolizumab in combination with an immunomodulatory agent (i.e., lenalidomide, pomalidomide); pembrolizumab is *not* currently FDA-labeled for use in patients with multiple myeloma. In 2 randomized, controlled phase 3 trials (KEYNOTE-183 and KEYNOTE-185) enrolling 550 patients with multiple myeloma, interim analyses indicated that the risk of death was increased by 61 or 106%, respectively, in patients receiving pembrolizumab in combination with an immunomodulatory agent (pomalidomide or lenalidomide, respectively) and low-dose dexamethasone compared with those receiving the immunomodulatory agent and low-dose dexamethasone. Because of these findings, these trials were terminated at FDA's request.

The manufacturer of pembrolizumab states that an anti-PD-1 or anti-PD-L1 antibody should *not* be used in combination with an immunomodulatory agent and dexamethasone in patients with multiple myeloma outside of a controlled clinical trial. FDA recommends that ongoing clinical trials evaluating an anti-PD-1 or anti-PD-L1 agent in combination with an immunomodulatory agent or in combination with other drugs for use in hematologic malignancies be evaluated for permanent discontinuance or protocol amendments.

Fetal/Neonatal Morbidity and Mortality

Pembrolizumab may cause fetal harm if administered to pregnant women. Blockade of signaling of the PD-1 and PD-L1 pathway in animals has been shown to disrupt maternal immune tolerance to the fetus and has been associated with increased fetal loss and immune-mediated disorders. Therefore, inhibition of this pathway by pembrolizumab may increase the risk of fetal loss (e.g., abortion, stillbirth). Human immunoglobulin G_4 (IgG_4) has been shown to cross the placenta; therefore, fetal exposure to pembrolizumab may occur and increase the risk of immune-mediated disorders or alter normal immune response of the developing fetus.

Pregnancy should be avoided during pembrolizumab therapy. The manufacturer states that pregnancy status should be verified prior to initiation of pembrolizumab therapy in women of childbearing potential and such women should be advised to use a highly effective method of contraception while receiving pembrolizumab and for at least 4 months after the last dose. If pembrolizumab is used during pregnancy or if the patient becomes pregnant while receiving the drug, the patient should be apprised of the potential fetal hazard.

Immunogenicity

There is a potential for immunogenicity with pembrolizumab therapy. The ability of the electrochemiluminescence (ECL) assay to detect anti-pembrolizumab antibodies is limited by the presence of circulating drug. Development of anti-pembrolizumab antibodies was detected in 2.1% of patients receiving pembrolizumab 2 mg/kg every 3 weeks, 200 mg every 3 weeks, or 10 mg/kg every 2 or 3 weeks; neutralizing antibodies to pembrolizumab were detected in 0.5% of patients receiving the drug at these dosages. No effects of antibody formation on pharmacokinetics or safety (i.e., infusion-related reactions) of the drug were observed.

Specific Populations

Pregnancy

Pembrolizumab may cause fetal harm if administered to pregnant women based on its mechanism of action. (See Fetal/Neonatal Morbidity and Mortality under Cautions: Warnings/Precautions.)

Pregnancy status should be verified in women of childbearing potential prior to initiation of pembrolizumab therapy.

Lactation

It is not known whether pembrolizumab is distributed into human milk. The effects of pembrolizumab on nursing infants or on milk production also are unknown. Because of the potential for serious adverse reactions to pembrolizumab in nursing infants, women should be advised to discontinue nursing during pembrolizumab therapy and for 4 months after the last dose.

Pediatric Use

Efficacy of pembrolizumab has not been established in pediatric patients with melanoma, non-small cell lung cancer (NSCLC), squamous cell carcinoma of the head and neck, urothelial carcinoma, gastric cancer, cervical cancer, or hepatocellular carcinoma.

Safety and efficacy of pembrolizumab for the treatment of solid tumors with high microsatellite instability (MSI-H), cHL, or primary mediastinal large B-cell lymphoma (PMBL) in pediatric patients is supported by extrapolation of data from clinical studies evaluating pembrolizumab in adults, safety data in pediatric patients, pharmacokinetic analysis indicating that age (range of 15–94 years) does not have clinically important effects on clearance of the drug, and limited data indicating that exposure to pembrolizumab in pediatric patients is similar to that in adults.

Based on limited data in pediatric patients (range: 2–18 years of age) receiving a median of 3 doses of pembrolizumab (2 mg/kg every 3 weeks), plasma concentrations of pembrolizumab in pediatric patients were similar to those observed in adults receiving the same dosage of the drug. The safety profile of pembrolizumab was generally similar between pediatric patients and adults, but some adverse effects (i.e., fatigue, vomiting, abdominal pain, elevated serum aminotransferase concentrations, hyponatremia) occurred more frequently in pediatric patients.

Geriatric Use

In clinical trials evaluating pembrolizumab for melanoma, NSCLC, squamous cell carcinoma of the head and neck, cHL, and urothelial carcinoma, 46% of patients were 65 years of age or older and 16% were 75 years of age or older. No overall differences in safety and efficacy were observed between geriatric patients and younger adults.

Hepatic Impairment

Analysis of population pharmacokinetic data indicates that clearance of pembrolizumab is not altered in patients with mild hepatic impairment (total bilirubin concentration not exceeding the ULN *with* AST concentration exceeding the ULN, or total bilirubin concentration more than 1 times but not more than 1.5 times the ULN *with* any AST concentration). Insufficient data are available for patients with moderate or severe hepatic impairment.

Renal Impairment

Analysis of population pharmacokinetic data indicates that clearance of pembrolizumab is not altered in patients with renal impairment (estimated glomerular filtration rate [GFR] of 15 mL/minute per 1.73 m² or greater).

● Common Adverse Effects

Adverse effects reported in 10% or more of patients receiving pembrolizumab for the treatment of unresectable or metastatic melanoma and at an incidence that is at least 2% higher than that reported with ipilimumab or chemotherapy in the KEYNOTE-006 or KEYNOTE-002 studies include pruritus, rash, constipation, fatigue, arthralgia, cough, decreased appetite, pyrexia, abdominal pain, vitiligo, back pain, dyspnea, asthenia, hypothyroidism, and nausea. Laboratory abnormalities reported in 20% or more of patients receiving pembrolizumab for the treatment of unresectable or metastatic melanoma and at an incidence that is at least 2% higher than that reported with ipilimumab or chemotherapy include hyperglycemia, hypertriglyceridemia, hypoalbuminemia, hyponatremia, anemia, lymphopenia, elevated concentrations of aminotransferases (i.e., ALT, AST), elevated concentrations of alkaline phosphatase, decreased concentrations of bicarbonate, hypocalcemia, and hypercholesterolemia.

Adverse effects reported in 10% or more of patients receiving pembrolizumab as adjuvant therapy for completely resected advanced melanoma with regional lymph node involvement in the KEYNOTE-054 study include diarrhea, pruritus, nausea, arthralgia, hypothyroidism, cough, rash, asthenia, influenza-like illness, weight loss, and hyperthyroidism. Laboratory abnormalities reported in 20% or more of patients receiving pembrolizumab as adjuvant therapy include elevated concentrations of aminotransferases (i.e., ALT, AST) and lymphopenia.

Adverse effects reported in 20% or more of patients receiving pembrolizumab in combination with pemetrexed and a platinum-containing antineoplastic agent (carboplatin or cisplatin) for the initial treatment of metastatic nonsquamous NSCLC and at an incidence that is at least 2% higher than that reported with placebo plus pemetrexed and a platinum-containing agent in the KEYNOTE-189 study include nausea, fatigue, constipation, diarrhea, rash, and pyrexia. Laboratory abnormalities reported in 20% or more of patients receiving pembrolizumab in combination with pemetrexed and a platinum-containing agent (i.e., carboplatin, cisplatin) for the initial treatment of metastatic nonsquamous NSCLC and at an incidence that is at least 2% higher than that reported with placebo plus pemetrexed and a platinum-containing agent include anemia, hyperglycemia, neutropenia, elevated concentrations of aminotransferases (i.e., ALT, AST), elevated concentrations of serum creatinine, hyponatremia, hypophosphatemia, hypocalcemia, and hyperkalemia.

Adverse effects reported in patients receiving pembrolizumab in combination with carboplatin and paclitaxel (conventional or albumin-bound) for the initial treatment of metastatic squamous NSCLC in the KEYNOTE-407 study were similar to those reported in patients receiving the drug in combination with pemetrexed and a platinum-containing antineoplastic agent (carboplatin, cisplatin) for the initial treatment of metastatic nonsquamous NSCLC in the KEYNOTE-189 study; however, higher incidences of alopecia and peripheral neuropathy were reported in patients receiving pembrolizumab in combination with carboplatin and paclitaxel compared with placebo plus carboplatin and paclitaxel.

Adverse effects reported in 10% or more of patients receiving pembrolizumab as a single agent for the treatment of previously treated, PD-L1-positive metastatic NSCLC and at an incidence that is at least 2% higher than that reported with docetaxel in the KEYNOTE-010 study include decreased appetite, dyspnea, nausea, cough, rash, constipation, vomiting, arthralgia, back pain, and pruritus. Laboratory abnormalities reported in 20% or more of patients receiving pembrolizumab for the treatment of previously treated, PD-L1-positive metastatic NSCLC and at an incidence that is at least 2% higher than that reported with docetaxel include hyponatremia, elevated concentrations of alkaline phosphatase, and elevated concentrations of aminotransferases (i.e., ALT, AST).

Adverse effects reported in 20% or more of patients receiving pembrolizumab for the treatment of recurrent metastatic head and neck squamous cell carcinoma in the KEYNOTE-012 study include fatigue, decreased appetite, and dyspnea. Adverse effects in patients receiving pembrolizumab for the treatment of head and neck squamous cell carcinoma were similar to those reported in patients receiving the drug for the treatment of melanoma or NSCLC; however, a higher incidence of facial edema and new or worsening hypothyroidism were reported in patients with head and neck squamous cell carcinoma.

Adverse effects reported in 10% or more of patients receiving pembrolizumab for the treatment of relapsed or refractory cHL in the KEYNOTE-087 study include fatigue, cough, pyrexia, musculoskeletal pain, diarrhea, rash, vomiting, hypothyroidism, nausea, upper respiratory tract infection, dyspnea, headache, pruritus, arthralgia, and peripheral neuropathy. Laboratory abnormalities reported in 20% or more of patients receiving pembrolizumab for the treatment of relapsed or refractory cHL include elevated concentrations of aminotransferases (i.e., ALT, AST), anemia, thrombocytopenia, and neutropenia.

Adverse effects reported in 10% or more of patients receiving pembrolizumab for the treatment of relapsed or refractory PMBL in the KEYNOTE-170 study include musculoskeletal pain, upper respiratory tract infection, pyrexia, cough, fatigue, dyspnea, abdominal pain, diarrhea, arrhythmia, headache, and nausea. Laboratory abnormalities reported in 15% or more of patients receiving pembrolizumab for the treatment of relapsed or refractory PMBL include anemia, hyperglycemia, leukopenia, lymphopenia, neutropenia, hypophosphatemia, elevated concentrations of aminotransferases (i.e., ALT, AST), hypoglycemia, elevated concentrations of alkaline phosphatase, elevated concentrations of serum creatinine, hypocalcemia, and hypokalemia.

Adverse effects reported in 10% or more of cisplatin-ineligible patients receiving pembrolizumab for the treatment of locally advanced or metastatic urothelial carcinoma in the KEYNOTE-052 study include fatigue, musculoskeletal pain, decreased appetite, constipation, rash, diarrhea, pruritus, urinary tract infection,

abdominal pain, nausea, cough, peripheral edema, hematuria, vomiting, dyspnea, pyrexia, arthralgia, and weight loss. Laboratory abnormalities reported in 10% or more of cisplatin-ineligible patients receiving pembrolizumab for the treatment of locally advanced or metastatic urothelial carcinoma include anemia, elevated concentrations of aminotransferases (i.e., ALT, AST), elevated concentrations of serum creatinine, and hyponatremia.

Adverse effects reported in 10% or more of patients receiving pembrolizumab for the treatment of previously treated locally advanced or metastatic urothelial carcinoma and at an incidence that is at least 2% higher than that reported with chemotherapy in the KEYNOTE-045 study include musculoskeletal pain, pruritus, rash, cough, vomiting, dyspnea, and hematuria. Laboratory abnormalities reported in 20% or more of patients receiving pembrolizumab for the treatment of previously treated locally advanced or metastatic urothelial carcinoma and at an incidence that is at least 2% higher than that reported with chemotherapy include elevated concentrations of alkaline phosphatase, serum creatinine, and AST.

Adverse effects reported in the KEYNOTE-059 study in patients receiving pembrolizumab for the treatment of gastric cancer were similar to those reported in other studies in patients receiving the drug for the treatment of melanoma or NSCLC.

Adverse effects reported in 10% or more of patients receiving pembrolizumab for the treatment of recurrent or metastatic cervical cancer in the KEYNOTE-158 study include fatigue, musculoskeletal pain, diarrhea, abdominal pain, pain, decreased appetite, hemorrhage, nausea, pyrexia, vomiting, infection (including urinary tract infection), rash, peripheral edema, constipation, headache, hypothyroidism, and dyspnea. Laboratory abnormalities reported in 20% or more of patients receiving pembrolizumab for the treatment of recurrent or metastatic cervical cancer include anemia, lymphopenia, hypoalbuminemia, elevated concentrations of alkaline phosphatase, hyperglycemia, hyponatremia, elevated concentrations of aminotransferases (i.e., ALT, AST), elevated concentrations of serum creatinine, hypocalcemia, and hypokalemia.

Adverse effects reported in the KEYNOTE-224 study in patients receiving pembrolizumab for the treatment of hepatocellular carcinoma generally were similar to those reported in other studies in patients receiving the drug for the treatment of melanoma or NSCLC; however, higher incidences of ascites, immune-mediated hepatitis, elevated concentrations of aminotransferases (i.e., ALT, AST), and hyperbilirubinemia were reported in patients with hepatocellular carcinoma.

Adverse effects reported in the KEYNOTE-017 study in patients receiving pembrolizumab for the treatment of Merkel cell carcinoma were similar to those reported in other studies in patients receiving the drug for the treatment of melanoma or NSCLC; however, higher incidences of hyperglycemia and elevated AST concentrations were reported in patients with Merkel cell carcinoma.

DRUG INTERACTIONS

No formal drug interaction studies have been performed to date.

DESCRIPTION

Pembrolizumab, a humanized anti-programmed-death receptor-1 (anti-PD-1) monoclonal antibody, is an antineoplastic agent. The drug is an IgG$_4$ kappa immunoglobulin.

Pembrolizumab is highly selective for PD-1, an immune-checkpoint receptor expressed on activated T-cells, monocytes, B-cells, natural killer (NK) T-cells, and dendritic cells. Overexpression of PD-1 ligands on the surface of tumor cells results in activation of PD-1 and suppression of cytotoxic T-cell activity. Pembrolizumab blocks the interaction between PD-1 and its ligands, resulting in enhanced immune response, including enhanced antitumor immune response. The drug also has been shown to reduce tumor growth in syngeneic mouse tumor models.

Area under the serum concentration-time curve (AUC), peak plasma concentration, and trough concentration of pembrolizumab are proportional to dose over the dosage range of 2–10 mg/kg every 3 weeks. Following repeated doses of pembrolizumab every 3 weeks, steady-state concentrations are reached by 16 weeks; systemic accumulation of the drug is 2.1-fold. Based on dose-exposure safety and efficacy relationships, the manufacturer states that there are no clinically important differences in safety and efficacy between pembrolizumab 200 mg every 3 weeks and pembrolizumab 2 mg/kg every 3 weeks in patients with melanoma or non-small cell lung cancer (NSCLC). Clearance of pembrolizumab is approximately 23% lower at steady state than following the initial dose; however, this difference is not considered clinically important. The mean terminal half-life of pembrolizumab is 22 days.

The pharmacokinetics of pembrolizumab do not appear to be affected by age (range of 15–94 years), gender, race (89% Caucasian), renal impairment, mild hepatic impairment, or tumor burden.

ADVICE TO PATIENTS

Importance of advising patient to read the manufacturer's medication guide before beginning treatment and each time the drug is administered.

Risk of immune-mediated pneumonitis. Importance of informing clinician immediately if new or worsening cough, chest pain, or shortness of breath occurs.

Risk of immune-mediated colitis. Importance of informing clinician immediately if diarrhea, severe abdominal pain, or changes in stool occur.

Risk of immune-mediated hepatitis. Importance of informing clinician immediately if signs and symptoms of liver damage (e.g., jaundice, nausea, vomiting, dark urine, abdominal pain [particularly in the right upper quadrant], easy bruising or bleeding, lack of appetite) occur.

Risk of immune-mediated hypophysitis. Importance of informing clinician immediately if persistent or unusual headache, extreme weakness, dizziness or fainting, or vision changes occur.

Risk of immune-mediated nephritis. Importance of informing clinician immediately if signs and symptoms of renal damage (e.g., decreased urine output, change in color of urine) occur.

Risk of immune-mediated hyperthyroidism or hypothyroidism. Importance of informing clinician immediately if symptoms of abnormal thyroid function occur.

Risk of immune-mediated type 1 diabetes mellitus. Importance of informing clinician immediately if signs and symptoms of diabetes mellitus occur.

Risk of immune-mediated severe skin reactions. Importance of informing clinician immediately if severe skin reactions or signs and symptoms of Stevens-Johnson syndrome or toxic epidermal necrolysis develop.

Risk of other immune-mediated adverse effects. Importance of informing clinician immediately if manifestations of other potential immune-mediated adverse effects occur.

Risk of infusion-related reactions. Importance of informing clinician immediately if signs and symptoms of such reactions (e.g., dizziness, chills, fever, difficulty breathing, pruritus, flushing, feeling of faintness) occur.

Risk of immune-mediated rejection of a solid organ transplant. Importance of informing clinician immediately if signs and symptoms of solid organ transplant rejection occur.

Risk of immune-mediated complications following allogeneic stem cell transplantation.

Importance of laboratory monitoring during pembrolizumab therapy.

Risk of fetal harm. Necessity of advising women of childbearing potential that they should use a highly effective method of contraception while receiving the drug and for 4 months after the last dose. Importance of women informing clinicians if they are or plan to become pregnant. If pregnancy occurs, advise pregnant women of potential risk to the fetus.

Importance of advising women to avoid breast-feeding while receiving pembrolizumab therapy and for 4 months after the last dose.

Importance of informing clinicians of existing or contemplated concomitant therapy, including prescription and OTC drugs, as well as any concomitant illnesses (e.g., autoimmune disorders, history of organ transplantation, liver damage).

Importance of informing patients of other important precautionary information. (See Cautions.)

For further information on the handling of antineoplastic agents, see the ASHP Guidelines on Handling Hazardous Drugs at http://www.ahfsdrug information.com.

PREPARATIONS

Excipients in commercially available drug preparations may have clinically important effects in some individuals; consult specific product labeling for details.

Pembrolizumab

Parenteral

For injection, for IV use	50 mg	Keytruda®, Merck
Concentrate, for injection, for IV use	25 mg/mL (100 mg)	Keytruda®, Merck

Selected Revisions October 7, 2019, © Copyright, May 29, 2015, American Society of Health-System Pharmacists, Inc.

PEMEtrexed Disodium

10:00 • ANTINEOPLASTIC AGENTS

■ Pemetrexed, a folic acid antagonist, is an antineoplastic agent.

USES

• Malignant Pleural Mesothelioma

Pemetrexed is used in combination with cisplatin for the treatment of malignant pleural mesothelioma in adults whose disease is unresectable or who otherwise are not candidates for potentially curative surgery. This malignancy occurs infrequently, is linked to asbestos exposure, and previously was considered unresponsive to chemotherapy, with a median survival of 6–8 months following diagnosis. Pemetrexed is designated an orphan drug by the US Food and Drug Administration (FDA) for use in this condition.

Efficacy of pemetrexed and cisplatin in the treatment of malignant pleural mesothelioma was established in a randomized, phase III, comparative, multicenter study in 448 adults who had not received previous chemotherapy. Patients were randomized to receive pemetrexed (500 mg/m²) in combination with cisplatin (75 mg/m²) on day 1 or cisplatin (75 mg/m²) on day 1; both regimens were administered every 21 days. Patients studied were predominantly older (median age: 61 years) white males; approximately 68% of patients had tumors of epithelial histology, and 78% had stage III or IV disease. After 117 patients were treated, the study protocol was changed and patients started receiving folic acid and vitamin B_{12} supplementation because of hematologic and GI toxicity. The primary outcome measure was survival. Patients receiving the combination regimen had a longer median survival (12.1 versus 9.3 months), a longer time to progression (5.7 versus 3.9 months), a higher overall response rate (41.3 versus 16.7%), and improvement in lung function compared with patients receiving cisplatin alone. Addition of folic acid and vitamin B_{12} supplementation reduced toxicity and did not adversely affect survival.

• Non-small Cell Lung Cancer

Pemetrexed is used alone for the treatment of locally advanced or metastatic non-small cell lung cancer in adults who have received prior chemotherapy. This indication is based on the surrogate end point of tumor response rate; there are no controlled clinical studies to date demonstrating improvement in disease-related symptoms or increased survival with pemetrexed therapy.

Pemetrexed has been evaluated in a randomized, phase III, multicenter study in adults with stage III or IV (25 or 75% of patients, respectively) non-small cell lung cancer not amenable to potentially curative therapy. All patients in this study had received prior chemotherapy for advanced disease. Patients were randomized to receive pemetrexed (500 mg/m²) or docetaxel (75 mg/m²) on day 1; the regimens were administered every 21 days. Patients receiving pemetrexed also received folic acid and vitamin B_{12} supplementation. Response rates and clinical benefit (complete or partial response or stable disease) rates were similar in patients receiving pemetrexed or docetaxel. Overall response rates were 9.1 or 8.8% in patients receiving pemetrexed or docetaxel, respectively. Median survival (the primary end point of the study) was 8.3 or 7.9 months in those receiving pemetrexed or docetaxel, respectively; however, efficacy of pemetrexed in terms of survival could not be established, since a reliable and consistent effect of docetaxel on survival could not be estimated from historical study data, and crossover between treatments at the time of disease progression may have confounded interpretation of the survival data. Median progression-free survival was 2.9 months and 1-year survival rate was 29.7% in both treatment groups.

DOSAGE AND ADMINISTRATION

• Reconstitution and Administration

Pemetrexed is administered by IV infusion over 10 minutes.

The usual precautions for handling and preparing solutions of cytotoxic drugs should be observed with pemetrexed. The manufacturer recommends use of protective gloves when handling the drug. If pemetrexed comes in contact with skin or mucosa, affected skin areas should be washed immediately and thoroughly with soap and water and affected mucosa should be thoroughly rinsed with copious amounts of water.

Pemetrexed is not a vesicant. Extravasation should be managed according to local standard of practice; there is no specific antidote for extravasation of pemetrexed.

Vials labeled as containing 500 mg of pemetrexed should be reconstituted by adding 20 mL of 0.9% sodium chloride injection without preservatives to provide a solution containing 25 mg/mL. The vial should be gently swirled until the powder is completely dissolved. The appropriate volume of reconstituted solution must be further diluted with 0.9% sodium chloride injection without preservatives to a volume of 100 mL prior to administration. Pemetrexed is incompatible with diluents containing calcium (e.g., lactated Ringer's injection, Ringer's injection); pemetrexed should not be diluted with these solutions, diluents other than 0.9% sodium chloride injection without preservatives, or other drugs. Because reconstituted and/or diluted pemetrexed solutions contain no preservatives, any unused portions of these solutions should be discarded. When reconstituted and/or diluted as directed, pemetrexed solutions are stable for 24 hours at controlled room temperature under ambient lighting.

• General Dosage

Dosage of pemetrexed disodium heptahydrate is expressed in terms of anhydrous pemetrexed.

All patients should be premedicated with a corticosteroid before pemetrexed administration to reduce the incidence and severity of cutaneous reactions. A regimen of oral dexamethasone 4 mg twice daily for 3 days, starting 1 day prior to pemetrexed administration, has been used in clinical studies.

All patients should be instructed to take a low-dose oral folic acid preparation or a multivitamin preparation containing folic acid daily to reduce toxicity. At least 5 daily doses of folic acid must be taken during the 7-day period preceding the first dose of pemetrexed; dosing should continue during the full course of therapy and for 21 days after the last dose of pemetrexed. Folic acid dosages ranged from 0.35–1 mg daily in clinical studies; the most commonly used dosage was 0.4 mg daily. Patients also must receive one IM injection of vitamin B_{12} during the week preceding the first dose of pemetrexed and every 3 cycles thereafter; injections administered subsequent to the initial dose may be given the same day as pemetrexed. A dose of 1 mg of vitamin B_{12} was used in clinical studies.

Malignant Pleural Mesothelioma

The recommended adult dosage of pemetrexed is 500 mg/m² infused IV over 10 minutes in conjunction with cisplatin 75 mg/m² infused IV over 2 hours beginning approximately 30 minutes after completion of the pemetrexed infusion on day 1 of a 21-day cycle. Patients should be adequately hydrated before and after administration of cisplatin; clinicians should consult published protocols for information related to specific regimens.

Chemotherapy in subsequent cycles should be delayed until absolute neutrophil counts (ANCs) are at least 1500/mm³, platelet counts are at least 100,000/mm³, and creatinine clearances are at least 45 mL/minute.

Non-small Cell Lung Cancer

The recommended adult dosage of pemetrexed is 500 mg/m² infused IV over 10 minutes on day 1 of a 21-day cycle.

Chemotherapy in subsequent cycles should be delayed until ANCs are at least 1500/mm³, platelet counts are at least 100,000/mm³, and creatinine clearances are at least 45 mL/minute.

Dosage Modification for Toxicity

After the first treatment cycle, subsequent doses of pemetrexed as a single agent or in combination with cisplatin should be adjusted based on nadir hematologic counts (i.e., ANCs, platelet counts) and maximum nonhematologic toxicity.

Treatment may be delayed to allow sufficient time for recovery from hematologic toxicity; if pemetrexed therapy is resumed following such toxicity, subsequent doses should be reduced according to the nadir ANCs and platelet counts observed (see Table 1). Therapy should be discontinued if the patient experiences grade 3 or 4 hematologic toxicity after 2 dose reductions.

TABLE 1. Recommended Dosage Modification for Hematologic Toxicity of Pemetrexed Monotherapy or Pemetrexed and Cisplatin Combination Therapy

Toxicity	Dose of Pemetrexed	Dose of Cisplatin
Nadir ANC <500/mm³ and nadir platelets ≥50,000/mm³	75% of previous dose	75% of previous dose
Nadir platelets <50,000/mm³, regardless of nadir ANC	50% of previous dose	50% of previous dose

If the patient experiences grade 3 or 4 nonhematologic toxicity (except neurotoxicity), therapy should be interrupted until the toxicity resolves or decreases in intensity to at least pretreatment values. If pemetrexed therapy is then resumed, subsequent doses should be reduced according to the type and severity of the toxicity (see Table 2). Therapy should be discontinued if the patient experiences grade 3 or 4 nonhematologic toxicity (except neurotoxicity) after 2 dose reductions. These recommendations for dosage modifications for grade 3 or 4 nonhematologic toxicity apply to grade 4 but not to grade 3 elevations in serum transaminase values; dosage modification is not required for grade 3 elevations in serum transaminase values.

TABLE 2. Recommended Dosage Modification for Nonhematologic Toxicity (Except Neurotoxicity) of Pemetrexed Monotherapy or Pemetrexed and Cisplatin Combination Therapy

Toxicity and National Cancer Institute (NCI) Common Toxicity Criteria Grade	Dose of Pemetrexed	Dose of Cisplatin
Any grade 3 or 4 nonhematologic toxicity (except neurotoxicity), excluding grade 3 or 4 mucositis or grade 3 elevation in serum transaminase values	75% of previous dose	75% of previous dose
Any diarrhea requiring hospitalization (regardless of grade) or grade 3 or 4 diarrhea	75% of previous dose	75% of previous dose
Grade 3 or 4 mucositis	50% of previous dose	100% of previous dose

If the patient experiences grade 2 neurotoxicity, the pemetrexed dose may be maintained at the current level but subsequent doses of cisplatin should be reduced (see Table 3). Therapy should be discontinued immediately if grade 3 or 4 neurotoxicity occurs.

TABLE 3. Recommended Dosage Modifications for Neurotoxicity of Pemetrexed Monotherapy or Pemetrexed and Cisplatin Combination Therapy

NCI Common Toxicity Criteria Grade	Dose of Pemetrexed	Dose of Cisplatin
0–1	100% of previous dose	100% of previous dose
2	100% of previous dose	50% of previous dose

● **Special Populations**

In clinical trials, patients with creatinine clearances of 45 mL/minute and greater did not require dosage reductions other than those recommended for all patients. Information concerning patients with creatinine clearances less than 45 mL/minute is insufficient to date to make dosage recommendations for these patients, and use in such patients currently is *not* recommended.

Dosage reductions other than those recommended for all patients are not needed in geriatric patients 65 years of age or older.

CAUTIONS

● *Contraindications*

Known hypersensitivity to pemetrexed or any ingredient in the formulation.

● *Warnings/Precautions*

Warnings

Hematologic Toxicity

The principal manifestations of hematologic toxicity include neutropenia, thrombocytopenia, and/or anemia; myelosuppression is the most common dose-limiting toxicity. Absolute neutrophil count (ANC) reaches nadir at day 8–10 and returns to baseline approximately 4–8 days after nadir.

Folate and Vitamin B_{12} Supplementation

Patients must receive folic acid and vitamin B_{12} to prevent treatment-related hematologic and GI toxicity. Patients receiving supplemental folic acid and vitamin B_{12} in clinical studies had a reduction in grade 3/4 hematologic and nonhematologic toxicities (i.e., neutropenia, febrile neutropenia, infection with grade 3/4 neutropenia) and an overall reduction in toxicity.

Sensitivity Reactions

Dermatologic Effects

Rash reported. Premedication with a corticosteroid reduces the incidence and severity of cutaneous reactions.

General Precautions

Adequate Patient Evaluation and Monitoring

Pemetrexed should be administered only under the supervision of qualified clinicians experienced in the use of cytotoxic therapy.

Complete blood cell counts, including platelet counts, should be performed in all patients receiving pemetrexed. Patients should be monitored for nadir and recovery; blood cell counts were monitored before each dose and on days 8 and 15 of each treatment cycle in clinical studies.

Renal and hepatic function should be monitored periodically.

Other Considerations

Not known whether pemetrexed accumulates in fluid collections such as pleural effusions or ascites; such accumulations could increase toxicity. Some clinicians suggest that large effusions be drained before pemetrexed therapy.

Specific Populations

Pregnancy

Category D. (See Users Guide.)

Lactation

Not known whether pemetrexed or its metabolites are distributed into human milk. Because of the potential for serious adverse reactions to pemetrexed in nursing infants, nursing should be discontinued prior to therapy.

Pediatric Use

Safety and efficacy not established in children.

Geriatric Use

Age-related differences in the pharmacokinetics of pemetrexed were not observed in adults 26–80 years of age.

Age-based dosage adjustments are not necessary in geriatric patients 65 years of age or older.

Hepatic Impairment

Pemetrexed has not been studied in patients with hepatic impairment. Patients with serum bilirubin concentrations exceeding 1.5 times the upper limit of normal were excluded from clinical studies. Patients with serum transaminase concentrations exceeding 3 times the upper limit of normal who had no evidence of hepatic metastases were excluded from clinical studies; patients with serum transaminase concentrations 3–5 times the upper limit of normal who had hepatic metastases were included in clinical studies.

Pemetrexed is not appreciably metabolized by the liver. Elevated serum transaminase or total bilirubin concentrations do not affect pharmacokinetics of pemetrexed.

Renal Impairment

Pemetrexed is eliminated principally unchanged by renal excretion; renal impairment is associated with reduced clearance of and increased systemic exposure to pemetrexed.

Dosage adjustment is not needed in patients with creatinine clearance of 45 mL/minute or greater. Information concerning patients with creatinine clearance less than 45 mL/minute is insufficient to date to make dosage recommendations for these patients; use of the drug in these patients currently is *not* recommended. Repeat cycles of pemetrexed should be withheld until creatinine clearances are at least 45 mL/minute.

Concomitant use of pemetrexed with cisplatin has not been evaluated in patients with moderate renal impairment.

Caution is advised if nonsteroidal anti-inflammatory agents (NSAIAs) are used concomitantly with pemetrexed in patients with renal impairment. (See Drug Interactions: Nonsteroidal Anti-inflammatory Agents.)

● Common Adverse Effects

Common adverse effects include hematologic effects, fever and infection, stomatitis/pharyngitis, rash/desquamation, nausea, fatigue, dyspnea, vomiting, constipation, chest pain, and anorexia.

DRUG INTERACTIONS

● Drugs Metabolized by Hepatic Microsomal Enzymes

Pharmacokinetic interaction unlikely with drugs metabolized by cytochrome P-450 (CYP) isoenzymes 1A2, 2C9, 2D6, or 3A.

● Cisplatin

Pharmacokinetic interaction unlikely.

● Nonsteroidal Anti-inflammatory Agents

Pharmacokinetic interaction (decreased clearance of pemetrexed; increased pemetrexed AUC) with ibuprofen. The manufacturer states that ibuprofen (up to 400 mg 4 times daily) may be used concomitantly with pemetrexed in patients with normal renal function (creatinine clearance of 80 mL/minute or greater); however, caution is advised if ibuprofen is used concomitantly with pemetrexed in patients with mild to moderate renal impairment (creatinine clearance of 45–79 mL/minute). Patients with mild to moderate renal impairment should not receive nonsteroidal anti-inflammatory agents (NSAIAs) having short half-lives (e.g., ibuprofen) for 2 days before, the day of, and for 2 days after administration of pemetrexed.

Data are not available to date regarding possible interactions with NSAIAs having longer half-lives, and the manufacturer states that all patients receiving such NSAIAs should interrupt therapy with the NSAIA for at least 5 days before, the day of, and for 2 days after administration of pemetrexed. If concomitant use of a NSAIA is necessary, the patient should be closely monitored for toxicity, particularly myelosuppression and renal and GI toxicity.

Pharmacokinetic interaction unlikely with low to moderate aspirin dosage (325 mg every 6 hours). Effect of higher aspirin dosage on pemetrexed pharmacokinetics not known.

● Nephrotoxic Drugs

Possible pharmacokinetic interaction (delayed clearance of pemetrexed).

● Probenecid

Possible pharmacokinetic interaction (delayed clearance of pemetrexed). Pharmacokinetic interaction also possible with other substances secreted at the renal tubule.

● Vitamins

Pharmacokinetic interaction unlikely with oral folic acid and vitamin B_{12} given IM.

DESCRIPTION

Pemetrexed, a folic acid antagonist, exerts its antineoplastic activity by disrupting folate-dependent metabolic processes that are essential for cell replication. Pemetrexed inhibits the folate-dependent enzymes thymidylate synthase, dihydrofolate reductase, and phosphoribosylglycinamide formyltransferase (glycinamide ribonucleotide formyltransferase), enzymes involved in *de novo* biosynthesis of thymidine and purine nucleotides. Pemetrexed enters cells through the reduced folate carrier and membrane folate binding protein transport systems and undergoes extensive intracellular polyglutamation by tetrahydrofolylpolyglutamate synthase (folylpolyglutamate synthase). The polyglutamate forms are retained for long periods in the cells and are inhibitors of thymidylate synthase and phosphoribosylglycinamide formyltransferase. Polyglutamation is a time- and concentration-dependent process that occurs in tumor cells and, to a lesser extent, in normal tissues.

Preclinical studies have shown that pemetrexed inhibits the in vitro growth of mesothelioma cell lines (MSTO-211H, NCI-H2052). Synergistic inhibitory effects have been observed in the MSTO-211H mesothelioma cell line when pemetrexed was combined with cisplatin.

ADVICE TO PATIENTS

Importance of taking folic acid and vitamin B_{12} to reduce the risk of adverse effects. Importance of taking a corticosteroid for 3 days during each treatment cycle to reduce the risk of a skin reaction.

Importance of recognizing and reporting adverse effects of pemetrexed, including myelosuppressive effects, infectious complications, and GI symptoms (i.e., diarrhea, mucositis). Necessity of monitoring blood cell counts and serum creatinine. Necessity of dosage adjustment or delay in treatment if toxicity occurs.

Importance of women informing clinicians if they are or plan to become pregnant or to breast-feed. Apprise patient of potential hazard to the fetus if used during pregnancy; women of childbearing potential should avoid becoming pregnant.

Importance of informing clinicians of existing or contemplated concomitant therapy, including prescription and OTC drugs, especially nonsteroidal anti-inflammatory agents.

PREPARATIONS

Excipients in commercially available drug preparations may have clinically important effects in some individuals; consult specific product labeling for details.

PEMEtrexed Disodium

Parenteral

For injection, for IV infusion only	500 mg (of pemetrexed)	**Alimta®**, Lilly

Selected Revisions © Copyright, November 1, 2004, American Society of Health-System Pharmacists, Inc.

Pertuzumab

10:00 • ANTINEOPLASTIC AGENTS

- Pertuzumab, a recombinant humanized anti-human epidermal growth factor receptor type 2 (anti-HER2/ERBB2) monoclonal antibody, is an antineoplastic agent.

USES

• Breast Cancer

Metastatic Breast Cancer

Pertuzumab is used in combination with trastuzumab and docetaxel for the treatment of human epidermal growth factor receptor type 2 (HER2)-positive metastatic breast cancer in patients who have not received prior anti-HER2 therapy or chemotherapy for metastatic disease.

The current indication for pertuzumab in the treatment of metastatic breast cancer is based principally on the results of a randomized, double-blind, placebo-controlled, phase 3 study (CLEOPATRA) in adults with HER2-positive metastatic breast cancer. Patients were eligible for enrollment in the study if they had disease demonstrating an immunohistochemistry (IHC) assay score of 3+ or a fluorescent in situ hybridization (FISH) amplification ratio of 2 or higher. In addition, patients with prior adjuvant or neoadjuvant chemotherapy were required to have a disease-free interval of more than 12 months before diagnosis of metastatic breast cancer and enrollment into the study; patients may have received one prior hormonal treatment for metastatic disease before study enrollment.

In this study, 808 patients were randomized (stratified according to prior treatment and geographic region) in a 1:1 ratio to receive either pertuzumab (840 mg by IV infusion initially, followed by 420 mg by IV infusion every 3 weeks thereafter) in combination with trastuzumab (8 mg/kg by IV infusion initially, followed by 6 mg/kg by IV infusion every 3 weeks thereafter) and docetaxel (75 mg/m² by IV infusion initially, followed by 75 or 100 mg/m² every 3 weeks thereafter) or placebo in combination with trastuzumab and docetaxel. Patients received pertuzumab and trastuzumab until disease progression, withdrawal of patient consent, or unacceptable toxicity occurred; docetaxel was continued for at least 6 cycles. The primary measure of efficacy was progression-free survival as assessed by an independent review facility (IRF-assessed progression-free survival); secondary end points included overall survival, progression-free survival as assessed by the investigator (investigator-assessed progression-free survival), objective response rate, and duration of response. The median age of patients enrolled in the study was 54 years (range: 22–89 years). Approximately half of the patients had received prior adjuvant or neoadjuvant chemotherapy, including regimens consisting of an anthracycline (39%), taxane (23%), trastuzumab (11%), or hormonal therapy (25%); approximately 11% of patients with hormone receptor-positive tumors had received hormonal therapy for metastatic disease. All except 2 of the enrolled patients were women. Approximately 89% of patients had an IHC score of 3+, and approximately 95% of patients had FISH-positive tumors.

Patients randomized to receive pertuzumab in combination with trastuzumab and docetaxel had a longer median IRF-assessed progression-free survival compared with patients receiving placebo in combination with trastuzumab and docetaxel (18.5 versus 12.4 months, respectively). Effects of pertuzumab on investigator-assessed progression-free survival and IRF-assessed progression-free survival were comparable. Prolonged progression-free survival was observed in pertuzumab-treated patients regardless of age, race, geographic region, or prior adjuvant or neoadjuvant therapy. In addition, patients receiving pertuzumab in combination with trastuzumab and docetaxel appeared to have a higher objective response rate (80.2 versus 69.3%, respectively) and a longer median duration of response (20.2 versus 12.5 months, respectively) compared with those receiving placebo in combination with trastuzumab and docetaxel. The median follow-up period at the time of interim analysis was 19.3 months in both treatment arms; the median duration of treatment was estimated to be 18.1 months for pertuzumab-treated patients and 11.8 months for placebo-treated patients. At the time of interim analysis, pertuzumab- or placebo-treated patients had received a mean of 19.9 or 16.2 treatment cycles, respectively; both groups received a median of 8 docetaxel cycles. In the final analysis of overall survival at a median follow-up of

50 months, median overall survival was prolonged in pertuzumab-treated patients compared with placebo-treated patients (56.5 versus 40.8 months). Results of an exploratory subgroup analysis (based on age, geographic region, race or ethnic group, presence of visceral metastases, hormone receptor status, HER2 status, prior adjuvant or neoadjuvant therapy) suggested that the effect of pertuzumab on overall survival was generally consistent across all subgroups; however, overall survival benefit for pertuzumab-treated patients was not apparent in the subgroup of patients with disease limited to nonvisceral metastasis (hazard ratio 1.11; 95% confidence interval of 0.66–1.85).

Early-stage Breast Cancer

Neoadjuvant Therapy

Pertuzumab is used in combination with trastuzumab and chemotherapy for the neoadjuvant treatment of HER2-positive locally advanced, inflammatory, or early-stage breast cancer (either node-positive or tumor size exceeding 2 cm in diameter) as part of a complete treatment regimen.

The current indication for pertuzumab for the neoadjuvant treatment of HER2-positive early-stage breast cancer is based principally on the results of 2 randomized, open-label, phase 2 studies (NeoSphere, TRYPHAENA) in adults with operable, locally advanced, or inflammatory early-stage HER2-positive breast cancer and a supportive open-label, multicenter, nonrandomized phase 2 study (BERENICE) evaluating the cardiac safety of anthracycline- and taxane-based neoadjuvant chemotherapy regimens in combination with pertuzumab and trastuzumab. In the NeoSphere, TRYPHAENA, and BERENICE studies, HER2 overexpression was defined as a score of 3+ on IHC assay or a FISH amplification ratio of 2 or greater. The primary measure of efficacy was pathological complete response (pCR) in the breast (defined as the absence of invasive cancer in the breast and axillary nodes).

In the NeoSphere study, 417 patients were randomized (stratified according to breast cancer type and hormone receptor status) to 1 of 4 neoadjuvant chemotherapy regimens prior to surgery (trastuzumab and docetaxel; pertuzumab, trastuzumab, and docetaxel; pertuzumab and trastuzumab; or pertuzumab and docetaxel). In this study, pertuzumab 840 mg was administered by IV infusion initially, followed by 420 mg by IV infusion every 3 weeks for 4 cycles; trastuzumab 8 mg/kg was administered by IV infusion initially, followed by 6 mg/kg by IV infusion every 3 weeks for 4 cycles; and docetaxel 75 mg/m² was administered by IV infusion initially, followed by 100 mg/m², if the initial dose was tolerated, every 3 weeks for 4 cycles. Following surgery, all patients received fluorouracil (600 mg/m²), epirubicin hydrochloride (90 mg/m²), and cyclophosphamide (600 mg/m²) (also referred to as FEC) by IV infusion every 3 weeks for 3 cycles and trastuzumab IV every 3 weeks to complete 1 year of therapy; however, patients assigned to the pertuzumab and trastuzumab group received docetaxel every 3 weeks for 4 cycles prior to administration of the FEC regimen.

The median age of patients enrolled in the study was 49–50 years; 71% of the patients were Caucasian, 100% were female, 7% had inflammatory cancer, 32% had locally advanced cancer, and 61% had operable cancer. Approximately one-half of the patients enrolled in the study had estrogen receptor-positive and/or progesterone receptor-positive disease. Patients randomized to receive pertuzumab in combination with trastuzumab and docetaxel had a higher pCR rate compared with patients receiving trastuzumab and docetaxel, pertuzumab and trastuzumab, or pertuzumab and docetaxel (39.3% versus 21.5, 11.2, or 17.7%, respectively). The magnitude of benefit with pertuzumab was lower in the subgroup of patients with hormone receptor-positive tumors compared with those with hormone receptor-negative tumors. At the time of the final analysis at a median follow-up of approximately 60 months, the 5-year progression-free survival rate was 86% in patients receiving pertuzumab in combination with trastuzumab and docetaxel, 81% in those receiving trastuzumab and docetaxel, 73% in those receiving pertuzumab and trastuzumab, and 73% in those receiving pertuzumab and docetaxel. Exploratory analysis suggested prolonged 5-year progression-free survival in patients who achieved a total pCR (defined as the absence of invasive cancer in the breast) compared with those who did not achieve a total pCR (85 versus 76%).

In the TRYPHAENA study, 225 patients were randomized (stratified according to breast cancer type and hormone receptor status) to 1 of 3 neoadjuvant regimens prior to surgery: fluorouracil (500 mg/m² IV), epirubicin hydrochloride (100 mg/m² IV), and cyclophosphamide (600 mg/m² IV) (also referred to as FEC) in combination with pertuzumab (840 mg IV during cycle 1, followed by 420 mg thereafter) and trastuzumab (8 mg/kg IV during cycle 1, followed by

6 mg/kg thereafter) every 3 weeks for 3 cycles, followed by docetaxel (75 mg/m² by IV infusion initially, followed by 100 mg/m² by IV infusion every 3 weeks, if the initial dose was tolerated) in combination with the same dosage of pertuzumab and trastuzumab for 3 cycles; FEC for 3 cycles followed by pertuzumab in combination with trastuzumab and docetaxel for 3 cycles; or pertuzumab in combination with docetaxel (75 mg/m² by IV infusion every 3 weeks), carboplatin (dose required to obtain an area under the plasma concentration-time curve [AUC] of 6 mg/mL per minute by IV infusion), and trastuzumab every 3 weeks for 6 cycles. All patients received trastuzumab every 3 weeks to complete 1 year of therapy following surgery. The median age of patients enrolled in the study was 49–50 years; 76% were Caucasian, 100% were female, 6% of patients had inflammatory cancer, 25% had locally advanced cancer, and 69% had operable cancer. Approximately one-half of patients enrolled in the study had estrogen receptor-positive and/or progesterone receptor-positive disease. Pathological complete response was achieved in 56.2% of patients receiving pertuzumab in combination with trastuzumab and FEC followed by pertuzumab in combination with trastuzumab and docetaxel, 54.7% of those receiving pertuzumab in combination with trastuzumab and docetaxel followed by FEC, and 63.6% of those receiving pertuzumab in combination with docetaxel, carboplatin, and trastuzumab. The pCR rate was lower in the subgroup of patients with hormone receptor-positive tumors compared with those with hormone receptor-negative tumors. At a follow-up of 3 years, similar progression-free survival (87–89%), disease-free survival (87–90%), and overall survival (93–94%) rates were observed in each of the treatment groups. Disease-free survival appeared to be improved in patients who achieved a total pCR compared with those who did not achieve total pCR (hazard ratio: 0.27; 95% confidence interval of 0.11–0.64).

In the BERENICE study, 401 patients with locally advanced, inflammatory, or early-stage HER2-positive breast cancer received an investigator's choice of a neoadjuvant anthracycline- and taxane-based regimen prior to surgery. In this study, patients received either dose-dense doxorubicin hydrochloride (60 mg/m² IV) and cyclophosphamide (600 mg/m² IV) every 2 weeks for 4 cycles, followed by pertuzumab (840 mg by IV infusion during cycle 1, followed by 420 mg by IV infusion every 3 weeks during cycles 2–4) in combination with trastuzumab (8 mg/kg by IV infusion during cycle 1, followed by 6 mg/kg by IV infusion every 3 weeks during cycles 2–4) and paclitaxel (80 mg/m² IV weekly for 12 weeks), or fluorouracil (500 mg/m² IV), epirubicin hydrochloride (100 mg/m² IV), and cyclophosphamide (600 mg/m² IV) every 3 weeks for 4 cycles, followed by pertuzumab in combination with trastuzumab and docetaxel (75 mg/m² by IV infusion initially, followed by 100 mg/m², if the initial dose was tolerated) every 3 weeks for 4 cycles. All patients received pertuzumab and trastuzumab every 3 weeks to complete 1 year of therapy following surgery. In this study, HER2 overexpression was defined as a score of 3+ on IHC assay or a FISH amplification ratio of 2 or greater. The median age of patients enrolled in the study was 49 years; 83% were Caucasian, and all but one patient were female. Pathological complete response was achieved in 61.8% of patients receiving dose-dense doxorubicin and cyclophosphamide followed by pertuzumab in combination with trastuzumab and paclitaxel and 60.7% of those receiving fluorouracil, epirubicin, and cyclophosphamide followed by pertuzumab in combination with trastuzumab and docetaxel. The pCR rate was lower in the subgroup of patients with hormone receptor-positive tumors compared with those with hormone receptor-negative tumors.

Adjuvant Therapy

Pertuzumab is used in combination with trastuzumab and chemotherapy for the adjuvant treatment of early-stage HER2-positive breast cancer at high risk of recurrence.

The current indication for pertuzumab for the adjuvant treatment of breast cancer is based principally on the results of a randomized, double-blind, placebo-controlled trial (APHINITY) in 4804 adults with operable early-stage HER2-positive (defined as an IHC assay score of 3+ or amplification of HER2 by in situ hybridization) breast cancer. In this study, patients were randomized (stratified by nodal status, adjuvant chemotherapy regimen, hormone receptor status, geographic region, and protocol) to receive an investigator's choice of adjuvant chemotherapy (fluorouracil-epirubicin-cyclophosphamide for 3 or 4 cycles or fluorouracil-doxorubicin-cyclophosphamide for 3 or 4 cycles, followed by docetaxel for 3 or 4 cycles or weekly paclitaxel for 12 cycles; doxorubicin-cyclophosphamide or epirubicin-cyclophosphamide for 4 cycles, followed by docetaxel for 4 cycles or weekly paclitaxel for 12 cycles; or docetaxel-carboplatin for 6 cycles) in combination with trastuzumab (8 mg/kg IV initially, followed by 6 mg/kg by IV infusion every 3 weeks) and either pertuzumab (840 mg IV

initially, followed by 420 mg IV every 3 weeks) or placebo for 1 year. The majority of patients (78%) received an anthracycline-containing regimen. Trastuzumab was administered on day 1 of the first taxane-containing cycle and continued for a total of 1 year (up to 18 cycles) or until disease recurrence, withdrawal of consent, or unacceptable toxicity occurred.

In the APHINITY study, the primary measure of efficacy was invasive disease-free survival (DFS), defined as the time from randomization to first occurrence of ipsilateral local or regional invasive breast cancer recurrence, distant recurrence, contralateral invasive breast cancer, or death from any cause. The median age of patients enrolled in the study was 51 years; 71% were Caucasian, over 99% were female, 63% had node-positive disease, and 64% had hormone receptor-positive disease.

At a median follow-up duration of 45.4 months, invasive DFS was higher in pertuzumab-treated patients compared with placebo-treated patients (93 versus 91%). The invasive disease-free survival rate, when defined to include development of a second primary non-breast cancer, was 92% in pertuzumab-treated patients and 90% in placebo-treated patients. An exploratory subgroup analysis suggested that the magnitude of benefit (i.e., invasive DFS) was greater in patients with node-positive disease receiving pertuzumab. At the time of the interim analysis, no difference in overall survival was observed between pertuzumab-treated patients and placebo-treated patients. Pertuzumab-treated patients and those assigned to placebo received a median of 18 cycles of anti-HER2 therapy.

DOSAGE AND ADMINISTRATION

● General

Patients should be selected for pertuzumab therapy based on HER2 protein over-expression or HER2 gene amplification in tumor specimens.

Because infusion or hypersensitivity reactions may occur, patients should be closely observed for 30–60 minutes after each infusion of pertuzumab. Subsequent administration of trastuzumab (IV or subcutaneous) or a taxane should not be started until after the 30- to 60-minute observation period following pertuzumab administration. (See Infusion-related Reactions under Cautions.)

Pertuzumab, trastuzumab, and a taxane should be administered sequentially. Pertuzumab and trastuzumab (IV or subcutaneous) can be given in any order; however, a taxane should be given after pertuzumab and trastuzumab (IV or subcutaneous). In patients receiving an anthracycline-based regimen, pertuzumab and trastuzumab (IV or subcutaneous) should be administered after completion of the anthracycline.

Restricted Distribution

Pertuzumab can only be obtained through select specialty distributors. The manufacturer should be contacted for additional information.

● Administration

Pertuzumab is administered by IV infusion only. Pertuzumab solutions should not be administered by rapid IV injection, such as IV push or bolus.

Prior to administration, pertuzumab injection concentrate must be diluted using proper aseptic technique. Pertuzumab injection concentrate is diluted by adding the appropriate volume of the concentrated pertuzumab 30-mg/mL solution to a polyvinyl chloride (PVC) or non-PVC polyolefin infusion bag containing 250 mL of 0.9% sodium chloride injection; the bag should be inverted gently to mix the solution and should not be shaken. Pertuzumab injection concentrate should not be diluted in 5% dextrose injection. Any unused portion left in the vial should be discarded since the injection concentrate contains no preservative. Pertuzumab solutions should be inspected visually for particulate matter and discoloration prior to dilution and administration. Following dilution, pertuzumab infusion solution may be administered immediately or stored at 2–8°C for up to 24 hours. Diluted pertuzumab solution should not be admixed with any other drug.

Unopened vials of pertuzumab injection concentrate should be protected from light and stored in the original carton at 2–8°C until use; vials should not be frozen or shaken.

Procedures for proper handling (e.g., use of gloves) and disposal of antineoplastic drugs should be followed when preparing or administering pertuzumab.

Rate of Administration

The initial dose of pertuzumab should be administered by IV infusion over 60 minutes; subsequent doses may be administered by IV infusion over 30–60 minutes. (See General under Dosage and Administration.)

Dispensing and Administration Precautions

Single-entity pertuzumab and trastuzumab preparations should *not* be substituted for or used with the fixed combination of pertuzumab, trastuzumab, and hyaluronidase (Phesgo®).

● Dosage

Clinicians should consult published protocols for information on the dosage, method of administration, and administration sequence of other antineoplastic agents used in combination regimens with pertuzumab.

Pertuzumab should be discontinued if trastuzumab is discontinued. If a dose of pertuzumab and trastuzumab is missed or delayed, and the time between 2 sequential infusions of the combination is less than 6 weeks, the maintenance dose of pertuzumab and trastuzumab should be administered as soon as possible; waiting until the next scheduled dose is not recommended. If the time between 2 sequential infusions of the combination is 6 weeks or longer, the initial pertuzumab and trastuzumab (IV only) dose should be re-administered (see Table 1).

TABLE 1. Recommendations for Continuation of Pertuzumab and Trastuzumab Following Treatment Interruption for 6 Weeks or More

Time Between Sequential Doses	Pertuzumab	Trastuzumab (IV)
≥6 weeks	Administer 840 mg by IV infusion over 60 minutes, followed by 420 mg by IV infusion over 30–60 minutes every 3 weeks thereafter	Administer 8 mg/kg by IV infusion over approximately 90 minutes, followed by 6 mg/kg by IV infusion over 30 or 90 minutes every 3 weeks thereafter

Breast Cancer

Metastatic Breast Cancer

For the treatment of HER2-positive metastatic breast cancer, the recommended initial dose of pertuzumab is 840 mg IV in combination with trastuzumab (IV or subcutaneous) and docetaxel (IV), followed by pertuzumab 420 mg IV in combination with trastuzumab (IV or subcutaneous) and docetaxel (IV) every 3 weeks thereafter.

In the CLEOPATRA study, pertuzumab and trastuzumab were continued for a mean of 19.9 cycles, and docetaxel was continued for a median of 8 cycles.

Neoadjuvant Treatment of Early-stage Breast Cancer

For the neoadjuvant treatment of HER2-positive early-stage breast cancer, the recommended initial dose of pertuzumab is 840 mg IV in combination with trastuzumab (IV or subcutaneous), followed by pertuzumab 420 mg IV in combination with trastuzumab (IV or subcutaneous) every 3 weeks for 3–6 cycles as part of one of the following chemotherapy regimens:

- 4 preoperative cycles of pertuzumab in combination with trastuzumab (IV or subcutaneous) and docetaxel, followed by 3 postoperative cycles of fluorouracil, epirubicin, and cyclophosphamide.
- 3 or 4 preoperative cycles of fluorouracil, epirubicin, and cyclophosphamide alone, followed by 3 or 4 preoperative cycles of pertuzumab in combination with docetaxel and trastuzumab (IV or subcutaneous).
- 6 preoperative cycles of pertuzumab in combination with docetaxel (dose escalation above 75 mg/m² is not recommended), carboplatin, and trastuzumab (IV or subcutaneous).
- 4 preoperative cycles of dose-dense doxorubicin and cyclophosphamide alone, followed by 4 preoperative cycles of pertuzumab in combination with paclitaxel and trastuzumab (IV or subcutaneous).

Following surgery, pertuzumab and trastuzumab should be continued to complete 1 year of therapy (up to 18 cycles).

Adjuvant Treatment of Early-stage Breast Cancer

For the adjuvant treatment of HER2-positive early-stage breast cancer, pertuzumab is administered in combination with trastuzumab (IV or subcutaneous) as part of a complete regimen, including standard anthracycline- and/or taxane-based chemotherapy regimens.

The recommended initial dose of pertuzumab is 840 mg IV in combination with trastuzumab (IV or subcutaneous). Pertuzumab and trastuzumab therapy should begin on day 1 of the first taxane-containing cycle. The initial regimen should be followed by pertuzumab 420 mg IV in combination with trastuzumab (IV or subcutaneous) every 3 weeks for a total of 1 year (up to 18 cycles) or until disease recurrence or intolerable toxicity occurs.

Dosage Modification for Toxicity and Contraindications for Continued Therapy

Dosage reductions are not recommended for pertuzumab. If toxicities occur, reduction in infusion rate or temporary or permanent discontinuance of pertuzumab should be considered based on causality. The prescribing information for individual chemotherapy agents used in combination with pertuzumab should be consulted for detailed information on dosage modifications.

Left Ventricular Dysfunction

Metastatic Breast Cancer: Baseline left ventricular ejection fraction (LVEF) should be 50% or higher prior to starting pertuzumab therapy. If LVEF decreases to less than 40% or to 40–45% with an absolute decrease from baseline of 10% or more, pertuzumab and trastuzumab should be withheld for at least 3 weeks. (See Left Ventricular Dysfunction under Cautions.) LVEF should be reassessed within approximately 3 weeks. If LVEF has recovered to greater than 45% *or* to 40–45% with an absolute decrease from baseline of less than 10%, pertuzumab and trastuzumab therapy may be resumed. If LVEF has not improved or has declined further, discontinuance of pertuzumab and trastuzumab should be strongly considered.

Early-stage Breast Cancer: Baseline LVEF should be 55% or higher prior to starting pertuzumab therapy; however, for patients receiving anthracycline-based chemotherapy, an LVEF of 50% or higher is required prior to starting pertuzumab and trastuzumab. If LVEF decreases to less than 50% with an absolute decrease from baseline of 10% or more, pertuzumab and trastuzumab should be withheld for at least 3 weeks. (See Left Ventricular Dysfunction under Cautions.) LVEF should be reassessed within approximately 3 weeks. If LVEF has recovered to greater than 50% or to an absolute decrease from baseline of less than 10%, pertuzumab and trastuzumab therapy may be resumed. If LVEF has not improved or has declined further, discontinuance of pertuzumab and trastuzumab should be strongly considered.

Infusion-related Reactions

If clinically important infusion-related reactions occur, the infusion rate should be slowed or the infusion should be interrupted, and appropriate medical therapy should be initiated. (See Infusion-related Reactions under Cautions.)

Hypersensitivity Reactions

If serious hypersensitivity reactions occur, the pertuzumab infusion should be immediately discontinued, and the drug should be permanently discontinued. (See Hypersensitivity Reactions under Cautions.)

● Special Populations

Dosage adjustment is not necessary based on body weight or baseline albumin concentration. (See Description.)

Hepatic Impairment

The manufacturer makes no specific dosage recommendations for patients with hepatic impairment. (See Hepatic Impairment under Cautions.)

Renal Impairment

No dosage adjustment is necessary in patients with mild (creatinine clearance of 60–90 mL/minute) or moderate (creatinine clearance of 30–60 mL/minute) renal impairment.

The manufacturer makes no specific dosage recommendations for patients with severe renal impairment (creatinine clearance less than 30 mL/minute) because data are limited in this population. (See Renal Impairment under Cautions.)

Geriatric Use

The manufacturer makes no specific dosage recommendations for geriatric patients. (See Geriatric Use under Cautions.)

CAUTIONS

● Contraindications

Pertuzumab is contraindicated in patients with known hypersensitivity to the drug or any ingredients in the formulation.

● Warnings/Precautions

Warnings

Left Ventricular Dysfunction

Decreases in left ventricular ejection fraction (LVEF) have been reported with inhibitors of human epidermal growth factor receptor type 2 (HER2), including pertuzumab. In the CLEOPATRA study evaluating pertuzumab in combination with trastuzumab and docetaxel in patients with metastatic breast cancer, the combination regimen was not associated with an increased incidence of symptomatic left ventricular systolic dysfunction (LVSD) or decreases in LVEF compared with placebo in combination with trastuzumab and docetaxel. LVSD occurred in 4% of pertuzumab-treated patients and in 8% of placebo-treated patients; symptomatic LVSD (congestive heart failure) occurred in 1 and 2% of patients, respectively. Pooled analysis of data from several studies evaluating use of pertuzumab as a single agent or in combination with either chemotherapy or targeted therapy for the treatment of various malignancies demonstrated that the median time to development of LVSD and symptomatic heart failure was around cycle 4, with 87% of the events occurring between cycles 1 and 7. In this pooled analysis, no substantial increases in cardiac dysfunction were observed following use of pertuzumab in combination with trastuzumab or non-anthracycline-based chemotherapy.

In the NeoSphere study evaluating pertuzumab in combination with trastuzumab and docetaxel as neoadjuvant therapy, the combination regimen was associated with an increased incidence of LVSD compared with the trastuzumab- and docetaxel-treated groups. An increased incidence of decreased LVEF also was observed in patients treated with pertuzumab in combination with trastuzumab and docetaxel. The incidence of asymptomatic and symptomatic LVSD and decreases in LVEF varied with each of the neoadjuvant regimens containing pertuzumab in the NeoSphere, TRYPHAENA, and BERENICE studies. (See Tables 2, 3, and 4.) In the TRYPHAENA study, recovery of LVEF to 50% or more occurred in all but one patient.

In the APHINITY study evaluating pertuzumab for the adjuvant treatment of early-stage breast cancer, the incidence of symptomatic heart failure (New York Heart Association [NYHA] class III/IV) with an LVEF less than 50% and an absolute decrease in LVEF of 10% or more was 0.6% in pertuzumab-treated patients and 0.2% in placebo-treated patients. Among the patients who developed symptomatic heart failure, LVEF recovery (defined as 2 consecutive LVEF measurements above 50%) occurred in 47 or 67% of patients receiving pertuzumab or placebo, respectively. The majority of patients who developed symptomatic heart failure (86%) received an anthracycline-based chemotherapy regimen. Asymptomatic or mildly symptomatic (NYHA class II) decreases in LVEF to less than 50% and an absolute decrease in LVEF of 10% or more occurred in 3% of patients in each treatment group.

TABLE 2. Incidence of Left Ventricular Dysfunction in the NeoSphere Study

Findings	Neoadjuvant Chemotherapy Regimen	
	Pertuzumab, Trastuzumab, and Docetaxel	Trastuzumab and Docetaxel
Decreased LVEF [a]	8%	2%
LVSD	3%	0.9%
Symptomatic LVSD	0.9%	0%

[a] LVEF decrease to less than 50% with an absolute decrease from baseline of greater than 10%.

TABLE 3. Incidence of Left Ventricular Dysfunction in the TRYPHAENA Study

Findings	Neoadjuvant Chemotherapy Regimen		
	Pertuzumab, Trastuzumab, and FEC [b] Followed by Pertuzumab, Trastuzumab, and Docetaxel	FEC Followed by Pertuzumab, Trastuzumab, and Docetaxel	Pertuzumab, Docetaxel, Carboplatin, and Trastuzumab
Decreased LVEF [a]	7%	16%	11%
LVSD	6%	4%	3%
Symptomatic LVSD	0%	4%	1%

[a] LVEF decrease to less than 50% with an absolute decrease from baseline of greater than 10%.
[b] Fluorouracil, epirubicin, and cyclophosphamide.

TABLE 4. Incidence of Left Ventricular Dysfunction in the BERENICE Study

Findings	Neoadjuvant Chemotherapy Regimen	
	Dose-dense Doxorubicin and Cyclophosphamide Followed by Pertuzumab, Trastuzumab, and Paclitaxel	FEC [c] Followed by Pertuzumab, Trastuzumab, and Docetaxel
Decreased LVEF [a]	7%	2%
Asymptomatic LVSD	7%	4%
Symptomatic LVSD [b]	2%	0%

[a] LVEF decrease to less than 50% with an absolute decrease from baseline of greater than 10% as measured by echocardiogram or multigated acquisition (MUGA) scan.
[b] New York Heart Association (NYHA) class III/IV congestive heart failure.
[c] Fluorouracil, epirubicin, and cyclophosphamide.

Pertuzumab has not been studied in patients with a baseline LVEF of less than 50%, prior history of congestive heart failure, decreases in LVEF to less than 50% during prior trastuzumab therapy, or conditions that could impair left ventricular function (e.g., uncontrolled hypertension, recent myocardial infarction, serious cardiac arrhythmia requiring treatment, cumulative prior anthracycline exposure greater than 360 mg/m^2 of doxorubicin or its equivalent). However, patients who have received prior anthracycline therapy or who have had prior radiation therapy to the chest area may be at greater risk for development of LVSD.

LVEF should be assessed prior to initiation of pertuzumab and at regular intervals (e.g., every 3 months) during treatment. If substantial decreases in LVEF occur, temporary or permanent discontinuance of pertuzumab may be required. (See Left Ventricular Dysfunction under Dosage and Administration.)

Fetal/Neonatal Morbidity and Mortality

There are no adequate and well-controlled studies to date evaluating pertuzumab in pregnant women; however, pertuzumab may cause embryofetal mortality and/or teratogenicity if administered to pregnant women based on its mechanism of action and animal studies. Oligohydramnios and oligohydramnios sequence manifesting as pulmonary hyperplasia, skeletal abnormalities, and neonatal death have been reported in patients receiving the anti-human epidermal growth factor receptor type 2 (anti-HER2) antibody trastuzumab during pregnancy in postmarketing experience. In pregnant cynomolgus monkeys, exposure to pertuzumab at concentrations 2.5–20 times that of human clinical exposure (based on peak plasma concentrations) resulted in oligohydramnios, delayed fetal kidney development, and embryo-fetal death.

The manufacturer states that a pregnancy test should be performed prior to initiation of pertuzumab, and females of reproductive potential should be advised to use effective contraceptive methods during therapy and for 7 months after discontinuance of the drug.

If pertuzumab is used during pregnancy or if the patient becomes pregnant while receiving the drug, the patient should be apprised of the potential fetal hazard. (See Pregnancy under Cautions.) Patients who become pregnant during pertuzumab therapy should be monitored for development of oligohydramnios; if oligohydramnios occurs, appropriate fetal testing within the standards of care should be performed.

Sensitivity Reactions
Infusion-related Reactions

Infusion-related reactions, including fatal events, have been reported in patients receiving pertuzumab. In the CLEOPATRA study in which the initial dose of pertuzumab was administered one day before trastuzumab and docetaxel during the first cycle (to allow for evaluation of pertuzumab-related infusion reactions), infusion reactions were reported in 13% of patients receiving pertuzumab compared with 10% of those receiving placebo; the most common infusion reactions were pyrexia, chills, fatigue, headache, asthenia, hypersensitivity, and vomiting. During the second cycle when pertuzumab, trastuzumab, and docetaxel were administered on the same day, the most common infusion reactions included fatigue, dysgeusia, hypersensitivity, myalgia, and vomiting.

Patients should be observed closely for 60 minutes after the first infusion of pertuzumab and for 30 minutes after subsequent infusions of the drug. If infusion-related reactions occur, reduction in infusion rate or temporary or permanent discontinuance of pertuzumab may be required. (See Infusion-related Reactions under Dosage and Administration.)

In the APHINITY study, infusion-related reactions occurred in 21 or 18% of patients on the first day of receiving pertuzumab or placebo, respectively. The incidence of grade 3 or 4 infusion-related reactions was 1 or 0.7% in patients receiving pertuzumab or placebo, respectively. In this study, patients randomized to pertuzumab received the drug on the same day as other treatment drugs.

Hypersensitivity Reactions

Severe hypersensitivity, including anaphylaxis and fatal events, has been reported in patients receiving pertuzumab. Angioedema has been reported in postmarketing experience. In the CLEOPATRA study, hypersensitivity or anaphylactic reactions occurred in 11 or 9% of patients receiving pertuzumab or placebo, respectively; grade 3–4 hypersensitivity or anaphylactic reactions occurred in 2 or 3% of patients, respectively. Anaphylaxis occurred in 4 patients receiving pertuzumab and 2 patients receiving placebo.

The frequencies of hypersensitivity or anaphylactic events observed in the NeoSphere, TRYPHAENA, BERENICE, and APHINITY studies were consistent with those observed in the CLEOPATRA study. In the NeoSphere study, anaphylaxis occurred in 2 patients receiving pertuzumab, trastuzumab, and docetaxel. In the APHINITY study, anaphylaxis occurred in 5 or 4% of patients receiving pertuzumab or placebo, respectively. The incidence of hypersensitivity or anaphylaxis was 8% in patients treated with pertuzumab in combination with docetaxel, carboplatin, and trastuzumab (TCH); 1% of these reactions were grade 3 or 4 in severity.

Pertuzumab is contraindicated in patients with known hypersensitivity to the drug or any ingredients in the formulation. Patients should be observed closely for hypersensitivity reactions, including anaphylaxis. If serious hypersensitivity reactions occur, pertuzumab therapy should be discontinued. Pertuzumab should be administered in a setting where emergency equipment and appropriate medical support are available for the management of potential reactions. (See Hypersensitivity Reactions under Dosage and Administration.)

Other Warnings and Precautions
Evaluation of HER2

Patients should be selected for pertuzumab therapy based on HER2 protein overexpression or *HER2* gene amplification. In clinical practice and clinical research studies, the methods of HER2 evaluation most commonly used are immunohistochemistry (IHC) assays, which directly measure overexpression of the HER2 protein, and fluorescent *in situ* hybridization (FISH), which measures amplification of the *HER2* oncogene. (See Evaluation of HER2/neu in Breast Cancer under Uses: Breast Cancer, in Trastuzumab 10:00.) In clinical trials evaluating pertuzumab, patients with breast cancer were required to have disease demonstrating an IHC score of 3+ or a FISH amplification ratio of 2 or higher.

Assessment of HER2 status should be performed using FDA-approved tests specific for breast cancer by laboratories with demonstrated proficiency in the specific technology being used. Improper assay performance, including use of suboptimally fixed tissue, failure to use specified reagents, deviation from specific assay instructions, and failure to include appropriate controls for assay validation, can lead to unreliable results.

Immunogenicity

As with all therapeutic proteins, there is a potential for immunogenicity with pertuzumab. In the CLEOPATRA study, anti-pertuzumab antibodies were detected in 13 of 389 patients (3%) receiving pertuzumab in combination with trastuzumab and docetaxel and in 25 of 372 patients (7%) receiving placebo in combination with trastuzumab and docetaxel. Anaphylactic or hypersensitivity reactions related to the presence of anti-pertuzumab antibodies were not observed in these patients.

During the neoadjuvant period of the BERENICE study, anti-pertuzumab antibodies were detected in 1 of 383 pertuzumab-treated patients (0.3%). Anaphylactic or hypersensitivity reactions were not observed in this patient.

The presence of pertuzumab in the serum sample may interfere with assays used to measure antibodies to the drug. In addition, the assay may be detecting antibodies to trastuzumab. Therefore, data may not accurately reflect the true incidence of anti-pertuzumab antibody formation.

Tumor Lysis Syndrome

Tumor lysis syndrome has occurred in patients receiving pertuzumab during postmarketing experience. The risk may be increased in patients with high tumor burden (e.g., bulky metastases). Manifestations of tumor lysis syndrome may include hyperuricemia, hyperphosphatemia, and acute renal failure. The manufacturer states that additional monitoring and/or treatment should be considered as clinically indicated.

Prolongation of QT Interval

In a subset of 20 patients enrolled in the CLEOPATRA study, no large (i.e., more than 20 msec) increases in the corrected QT (QT_c) interval were observed in patients receiving pertuzumab in combination with trastuzumab and docetaxel. However, smaller increases (i.e., less than 10 msec) in QT_c interval cannot be excluded because of study limitations.

Specific Populations
Pregnancy

Pertuzumab may cause fetal harm if administered to a pregnant female based on its mechanism of action and animal data. (See Fetal/Neonatal Morbidity and Mortality under Cautions.)

If pertuzumab is used during pregnancy or if the patient becomes pregnant while receiving the drug or within 7 months following the last dose of pertuzumab, the patient should be apprised of the potential fetal hazard and the patient and clinician should immediately report pertuzumab exposure to the manufacturer (888-835-2555).

Lactation

It is not known whether pertuzumab is distributed into milk; however, human immunoglobulin G (IgG) is distributed into milk, but does not distribute to neonatal and infant circulation in substantial amounts. (See Description.) The benefit of pertuzumab therapy to the woman as well as the benefits of breast-feeding to the infant should be weighed against the potential risk to the infant from exposure to the drug or from the underlying maternal condition. Clinicians should take into account the long elimination half-life of pertuzumab and the 7-month washout period following therapy with the anti-HER2 antibody trastuzumab.

Pediatric Use

Safety and efficacy of pertuzumab have not been established in children younger than 18 years of age.

Geriatric Use

In the CLEOPATRA, NeoSphere, TRYPHAENA, BERENICE, and APHINITY studies, the incidence of the most common grade 3 or 4 adverse effects (i.e., neutropenia, febrile neutropenia, diarrhea) were similar in patients 65 years of age and older and patients 75 years of age or older. Grade 3 or 4 anemia also occurred frequently in both age groups. Adverse effects that occurred at an incidence that is at least 5% higher in patients 65 years of age or older than that reported in younger adults included decreased appetite, anemia, decreased weight, asthenia, dysgeusia, peripheral neuropathy, and hypomagnesemia. No overall differences in efficacy were observed between geriatric and younger patients; however, the number of patients 75 years of age or older was insufficient to determine whether they respond differently from younger adults. In a population pharmacokinetic analysis, no substantial differences in pharmacokinetics were observed between geriatric and younger adults.

Hepatic Impairment

The pharmacokinetics of pertuzumab have not been studied in patients with hepatic impairment.

Renal Impairment

In a population pharmacokinetic analysis, systemic exposure to pertuzumab was similar between patients with mild (creatinine clearance of 60–90 mL/minute) or moderate (creatinine clearance of 30–60 mL/minute) renal impairment and those with normal renal function. Pharmacokinetic data in patients with severe renal impairment (creatinine clearance less than 30 mL/minute) are limited. (See Dosage and Administration: Special Populations.)

● Common Adverse Effects

Adverse effects occurring in more than 30% of patients receiving pertuzumab in combination with trastuzumab and docetaxel for the treatment of metastatic breast cancer include diarrhea, alopecia, neutropenia, nausea, fatigue, rash, and peripheral neuropathy. Adverse effects occurring in more than 30% of patients receiving pertuzumab in combination with trastuzumab and docetaxel for neoadjuvant treatment of breast cancer include alopecia, diarrhea, nausea, and neutropenia.

Adverse effects occurring in more than 30% of patients receiving pertuzumab in combination with trastuzumab and docetaxel for 3 cycles following combination therapy with fluorouracil, epirubicin, and cyclophosphamide for 3 cycles for the neoadjuvant treatment of breast cancer include fatigue, alopecia, diarrhea, nausea, vomiting, and neutropenia. Asthenia, constipation, mucosal inflammation, myalgia, anemia, fatigue, alopecia, diarrhea, nausea, and vomiting were reported in patients receiving pertuzumab in combination with trastuzumab and docetaxel for 4 cycles following combination therapy with fluorouracil, epirubicin, and cyclophosphamide for 4 cycles in the neoadjuvant setting.

Adverse effects occurring in more than 30% of patients receiving pertuzumab in combination with docetaxel, carboplatin, and trastuzumab for the neoadjuvant treatment of breast cancer include fatigue, alopecia, diarrhea, nausea, vomiting, neutropenia, thrombocytopenia, and anemia. Adverse effects occurring in more than 30% of patient receiving pertuzumab in combination with trastuzumab and paclitaxel following dose-dense doxorubicin and cyclophosphamide for the neoadjuvant treatment of breast cancer include nausea, diarrhea, alopecia, fatigue, constipation, peripheral neuropathy, and headache.

Adverse effects occurring in more than 30% of patient receiving pertuzumab in combination with trastuzumab and chemotherapy for the adjuvant treatment of breast cancer include diarrhea, nausea, alopecia, fatigue, peripheral neuropathy and vomiting. In the APHINITY study, the incidence of diarrhea was higher in patients receiving pertuzumab and trastuzumab in combination with a non-anthracycline-based chemotherapy regimen (85%) compared with pertuzumab and trastuzumab in combination with an anthracycline-based chemotherapy regimen (67%). The incidence of diarrhea was 18% when pertuzumab and trastuzumab were administered without chemotherapy compared with 9% in placebo recipients. In the APHINITY study, the median duration of diarrhea was 8 days; however, the duration of diarrhea was prolonged in patients experiencing grade 3 or higher diarrhea with a median duration of 20 days. Diarrhea requiring hospitalization occurred in more pertuzumab-treated patients compared with placebo-treated patients (2.4 versus 0.7%).

In the CLEOPATRA, NeoSphere, TRYPHAENA, BERENICE, and APHINITY studies, diarrhea was among the most common adverse effects reported

during pertuzumab therapy. In the CLEOPATRA, NeoSphere, TRYPHAENA, and APHINITY studies, diarrhea, generally occurring during the first pertuzumab-containing cycle, was grade 1 or 2 in most patients. In these studies, loperamide was the most frequently prescribed medication for the management of diarrhea. Interruption or discontinuance of therapy due to diarrhea was uncommon. The incidence of diarrhea is higher when pertuzumab and trastuzumab are administered with chemotherapy.

DRUG INTERACTIONS

● Antineoplastic Agents

No drug-drug interactions were observed between pertuzumab and trastuzumab, or between pertuzumab and docetaxel, paclitaxel, or carboplatin.

DESCRIPTION

Pertuzumab, a recombinant humanized anti-human epidermal growth factor receptor type 2 (anti-HER2/ERBB2) monoclonal antibody, is an antineoplastic agent. The drug is an IgG_1 kappa immunoglobulin produced by recombinant DNA technology in mammalian cell (Chinese hamster ovary) culture. Pertuzumab also is referred to as a HER2/neu receptor antagonist.

Pertuzumab binds specifically to the extracellular dimerization domain (subdomain II) of the HER2 protein, blocking heterodimerization of HER2 with other ligand-bound members of the HER/ERBB family (i.e., epidermal growth factor receptor [HER1/EGFR/ERBB1], HER3/ERBB3, HER4/ERBB4). Blockade of HER2 heterodimerization (particularly with HER3) by pertuzumab results in inhibition of ligand-activated intracellular signaling through 2 major signal pathways, mitogen-activated protein kinase (MAPK) and phosphoinositide 3-kinase (PI3K/Akt), potentially causing cell growth arrest and apoptosis, respectively. Similar to trastuzumab, pertuzumab also mediates antibody-dependent cell-mediated cytotoxicity (ADCC).

Pertuzumab binds to a different HER2 domain than trastuzumab and exhibits complementary mechanisms of action with trastuzumab; the combined use of these agents, therefore, may result in more comprehensive inhibition of *HER2* signaling. Pertuzumab alone inhibits proliferation of human tumor cells, while the combination of pertuzumab and trastuzumab has been shown to substantially augment antitumor activity in HER2-overexpressing xenograft models.

The pharmacokinetics of pertuzumab are linear over a dose range of 2–25 mg/kg. Following administration of an initial dose of 840 mg followed by a maintenance dosage of 420 mg every 3 weeks thereafter, steady-state concentrations of pertuzumab were reached after the first maintenance dose. The median half-life of pertuzumab is 18 days.

The pharmacokinetics of pertuzumab do not appear to be affected by age, sex, ethnicity (Japanese versus non-Japanese), or disease status (neoadjuvant or adjuvant early-stage versus metastatic setting). Baseline serum albumin concentration and lean body weight had a minor influence on pharmacokinetic parameters; therefore, the manufacturer states that dosage adjustment based on body weight or baseline albumin concentration is not necessary.

ADVICE TO PATIENTS

Risk of left ventricular dysfunction. Advise patients to contact a health care professional immediately if new-onset or worsening shortness of breath, cough, swelling of the ankles and/or legs, swelling of the face, palpitations, weight gain exceeding 5 pounds in 24 hours, dizziness, or loss of consciousness occurs.

Risk of fetal harm (e.g., embryo-fetal death, birth defects). Necessity of advising women of childbearing potential to use effective contraceptive methods during and for 7 months after discontinuance of pertuzumab. Encourage women who have been exposed to pertuzumab during pregnancy to report exposure to the manufacturer. (See Fetal/Neonatal Morbidity and Mortality under Cautions.)

Risk of infusion or hypersensitivity reactions.

Importance of informing clinicians of existing or contemplated concomitant therapy, including prescription and OTC drugs, as well as any concomitant illnesses.

Importance of informing patients of other important precautionary information. (See Cautions.)

For further information on the handling of antineoplastic agents, see the ASHP Guidelines on Handling Hazardous Drugs at http://www.ahfsdruginformation.com.

PREPARATIONS

Pertuzumab can only be obtained through select specialty distributors. Contact manufacturer for additional information.

Excipients in commercially available drug preparations may have clinically important effects in some individuals; consult specific product labeling for details.

Pertuzumab

Parenteral

Injection concentrate, for IV infusion	30 mg/mL (420 mg)	Perjeta®, Genentech

Selected Revisions September 13, 2021, © Copyright, May 30, 2013, American Society of Health-System Pharmacists, Inc.

Pomalidomide

10:00 • ANTINEOPLASTIC AGENTS

REMS

FDA approved a REMS for pomalidomide to ensure that the benefits outweigh the risk. The REMS may apply to one or more preparations of pomalidomide and consists of the following: elements to assure safe use and implementation system. See the FDA REMS page (https://www.accessdata.fda.gov/scripts/cder/rems/index.cfm).

■ Pomalidomide, a thalidomide analog, is an immunomodulatory agent with antineoplastic and antiangiogenic activity.

USES

● Multiple Myeloma

Pomalidomide is used for the treatment of multiple myeloma in adult patients who have received at least 2 prior therapies including lenalidomide and a proteasome inhibitor and have demonstrated disease progression during or within 60 days following completion of their last therapy. Pomalidomide has been designated an orphan drug by the FDA for use in multiple myeloma.

Clinical Experience

The use of pomalidomide in patients with multiple myeloma is based principally on the results of a randomized, open-label, multicenter, phase 2 trial (MM-002) in adults with relapsed multiple myeloma who previously received lenalidomide and bortezomib. Patients were enrolled if their disease was refractory to their most recent therapy (i.e., disease progression during or within 60 days following completion of their most recent therapy). In this trial, 221 patients were randomized in a 1:1 ratio to receive pomalidomide (4 mg once daily on days 1–21 of a 28-day cycle) alone or in combination with low-dose dexamethasone (40 mg once daily on days 1, 8, 15, and 22 of a 28-day cycle; patients older than 75 years of age received reduced doses [i.e., 20 mg] of dexamethasone); treatment was continued until disease progression or unacceptable toxicity occurred or treatment was discontinued for other reasons. Patients who received pomalidomide alone could add low-dose dexamethasone to their treatment regimen upon disease progression. All enrolled patients were required to receive thromboprophylaxis (i.e., aspirin 81–100 mg once daily or other antithrombotic therapy if aspirin was contraindicated). The primary end point of this study was progression-free survival; secondary end points included objective response rate, duration of response, time to response, and overall survival. The median age of enrolled patients was 63 years, and patients had received a median of 5 prior therapies for multiple myeloma. Most of the patients (approximately 75%) had undergone stem cell transplantation and approximately 60% of patients had disease that was refractory to both bortezomib and lenalidomide. A planned interim analysis indicated that patients receiving pomalidomide in combination with low-dose dexamethasone had a higher overall response rate than patients receiving pomalidomide alone (29.2 versus 7.4%), with a median response duration of 7.4 months; one patient receiving pomalidomide in combination with low-dose dexamethasone achieved a complete response compared with none of those receiving pomalidomide alone. The median follow-up at the time of the interim analysis was 9.6 weeks. At the time of the final analysis at a median follow-up of 14.2 months, median progression-free survival was prolonged in patients receiving pomalidomide in combination with low-dose dexamethasone compared with patients receiving pomalidomide alone (4.6 versus 2.6 months); however, median overall survival was similar in both treatment groups (14.4 and 13.7 months for these respective treatments).

Use of pomalidomide in combination with dexamethasone also was investigated in an open-label, multicenter, phase 3 trial (MM-003) in patients with relapsed or refractory multiple myeloma. In this trial, 455 patients were randomized in a 2:1 ratio to receive pomalidomide (4 mg once daily on days 1–21 of a 28-day cycle) in combination with low-dose dexamethasone (40 mg once daily on days 1, 8, 15, and 22 of a 28-day cycle) or high-dose dexamethasone alone (40 mg daily on days 1–4, 9–12, and 17–20 of a 28-day cycle); patients older than 75 years of age received reduced doses (i.e., 20 mg) of dexamethasone. Patients enrolled in the trial had received a median of 5 prior therapies. Most patients (74%) in this trial had disease that was refractory to both lenalidomide and bortezomib. Patients receiving pomalidomide in combination with low-dose dexamethasone had longer median progression-free survival compared with those receiving high-dose dexamethasone alone (3.6 versus 1.8 months). Median overall survival also was prolonged in patients receiving the combination of pomalidomide with low-dose dexamethasone compared with those receiving high-dose dexamethasone alone (12.4 versus 8.0 months).

Pomalidomide also has been used in 3-drug combination regimens† in patients with relapsed or refractory multiple myeloma.

Clinical Perspective

Previously Treated Multiple Myeloma

ASCO and CCO state that prior therapies should be taken into consideration when selecting the treatment at first relapse. Treatment options include triplet combination therapy (two novel agents and a corticosteroid) or doublet combination therapy (one novel agent and a corticosteroid); novel agents include immunomodulatory drugs, proteasome inhibitors, and monoclonal antibodies (e.g., daratumumab, elotuzumab). For patients who are fit, triplet combination therapy is generally recommended over doublet combination therapy due to improved clinical outcomes. In patients with genetic high-risk disease, a triplet combination regimen with a proteasome inhibitor, immunomodulatory drug, and a corticosteroid should be the initial treatment, followed by one or two autologous hematopoietic stem cell transplantations, followed by proteasome inhibitor-based maintenance therapy until disease progression occurs.

Treatment of relapsed multiple myeloma may be continued until disease progression. There are not enough data to recommend risk-based versus response-based duration of treatment.

● Kaposi Sarcoma

Pomalidomide is used for the treatment of adult patients with acquired immunodeficiency syndrome (AIDS)-related Kaposi sarcoma after failure of highly active antiretroviral therapy (HAART) or Kaposi sarcoma in adult patients who are human immunodeficiency virus (HIV)-negative. Pomalidomide has been designated an orphan drug by the FDA for use in Kaposi sarcoma. This indication is approved under accelerated approval based on overall response rate. Continued approval for this indication may be contingent upon verification of clinical benefit in confirmatory trials.

Clinical Experience

The use of pomalidomide in patients with Kaposi sarcoma is based principally on the results of a single-arm, single-center, open-label clinical trial (Study 12-C-0047) conducted in 28 adults (10 HIV-negative and 18 HIV-positive). In this study, patients received pomalidomide 5 mg orally once daily on days 1–21 of each 28-day cycle; therapy was continued until disease progression or unacceptable toxicity occurred. All patients received thromboprophylaxis with aspirin 81 mg once daily during therapy. The primary efficacy outcome was overall response rate. All patients were male and the median age of these patients was 52.5 years. The majority of patients had advanced disease (75%) and had received prior chemotherapy (75%). Overall response rate was 67% among HIV-positive patients and 80% among HIV-negative patients. The duration of response was 12.5 or 10.5 months in HIV-positive or HIV-negative patients, respectively.

DOSAGE AND ADMINISTRATION

● General

Pretreatment Screening

• Tests to exclude pregnancy must be performed within 10–14 days and again within 24 hours immediately prior to treatment initiation.

- Assess patients with multiple myeloma for risk factors for thromboembolism.

- *Multiple myeloma*: Do *not* begin a new treatment cycle until absolute neutrophil count (ANC) ≥500/mm³ and platelet count ≥50,000/mm³.

- *Kaposi sarcoma*: Do *not* begin a new treatment cycle until ANC ≥1000/mm³ and platelet count ≥75,000/mm³.

Patient Monitoring

- *Multiple myeloma*: CBCs weekly during first 8 weeks of therapy and at least monthly thereafter.

- *Kaposi sarcoma*: CBCs every 2 weeks for the first 3 months and monthly thereafter.

- Pregnancy tests weekly during the first month of therapy, then every 2 or 4 weeks in females with irregular or regular menstrual cycles, respectively.

- Development of second primary malignancies.

- Liver function tests (LFTs) monthly.

- Tumor lysis syndrome in patients with a high tumor burden.

Premedication and Prophylaxis

- Thromboprophylaxis recommended. Carefully assess patients receiving pomalidomide for risk factors for thromboembolism; base decisions regarding use of thromboprophylaxis and appropriate thromboprophylaxis regimens (e.g., aspirin, anticoagulant) on patient's risk.

Dispensing and Administration Precautions
Handling and Disposal

- Consult specialized references for procedures for proper handling and disposal of antineoplastics.

- Avoid contact of capsule contents with skin or mucous membranes. If such contact with the skin or mucous membranes occurs, affected areas of skin should be washed thoroughly with soap and water and affected mucosa should be rinsed thoroughly with water.

REMS

- Distribution of pomalidomide is restricted because it is an analog of thalidomide (a known human teratogen that can cause severe birth defects).

- Must be obtained through a restricted distribution program (Pomalyst Risk Evaluation and Mitigation Strategy [REMS]®) to help ensure that fetal exposure to pomalidomide does not occur. Clinicians, pharmacists, and patients must be registered in the program before they can prescribe, dispense, and receive pomalidomide; compliance with all terms outlined in the program is mandatory.

- The Pomalyst REMS® program controls access to pomalidomide; educates participants (clinicians, pharmacists, patients) about the risks associated with pomalidomide and the procedural requirements for safe use; and monitors compliance with the registration, education, and safety requirements of the program.

- Prescribe and dispense *no* more than a 28-day supply at one time.

- For additional details on program requirements, contact Bristol Myers Squibb at 888-423-5436 or visit https://pomalystrems.com/.

● Administration

Pomalidomide capsules should be administered orally with water once daily. The drug can be administered without regard to food. The capsules should be swallowed intact and should not be broken, chewed, or opened. No more than a 28-day supply of pomalidomide should be prescribed and dispensed at one time.

● Dosage
Multiple Myeloma

For the treatment of multiple myeloma in adults who have received at least 2 prior therapies including lenalidomide and a proteasome inhibitor, the recommended initial dosage of pomalidomide is 4 mg once daily on days 1–21 of each 28-day cycle in combination with dexamethasone. In clinical studies, therapy was continued for as long as the patient derived clinical benefit from the drug or until unacceptable toxicity occurred. New cycles of therapy should *not* be undertaken until neutrophil counts reach or exceed 500/mm³ and platelet counts reach or exceed 50,000/mm³.

Dosage Modification for Toxicity in Patients with Multiple Myeloma

Temporary interruption of therapy, dosage reduction, and/or permanent discontinuance of pomalidomide may be necessary in patients experiencing adverse effects (see Table 1).

If angioedema, anaphylaxis, grade 4 rash, skin exfoliation, bullae, or any other severe dermatologic reaction occurs, pomalidomide should be permanently discontinued.

TABLE 1. Dosage Modifications for Toxicity in Patients with Multiple Myeloma

Adverse Reaction and Severity	Pomalidomide Dosage Modification (Starting Dosage = 4 mg daily on days 1–21 of each 28-day cycle)
Neutropenia: ANC <500/mm³	First occurrence: Withhold therapy and monitor CBCs weekly; when ANC ≥500/mm³, then resume at a dosage reduced by 1 mg
	Subsequent occurrence: Withhold therapy until ANC ≥500/mm³, then resume at a dosage reduced by 1 mg
	If a daily dosage of 1 mg is not tolerated, permanently discontinue pomalidomide
Febrile neutropenia (temperature of ≥38.5°C and ANC <1000/mm³)	Withhold therapy and monitor CBCs weekly; when ANC ≥500/mm³, then resume at a dosage reduced by 1 mg
Thrombocytopenia: Platelet count <25,000/mm³	First occurrence: Withhold therapy and monitor CBCs weekly; when platelet count ≥50,000/mm³, then resume at a dosage reduced by 1 mg
	Subsequent occurrence: Withhold therapy until platelet count ≥50,000/mm³, then resume at a dosage reduced by 1 mg
	If a daily dosage of 1 mg is not tolerated, permanently discontinue pomalidomide
Non-hematologic adverse reactions: Grade 3 or 4 (excluding hypersensitivity or dermatologic reactions)	Withhold therapy; when toxicity resolves or improves to grade 2 or less, then resume at a dosage reduced by 1 mg

Kaposi Sarcoma

For the treatment of Kaposi sarcoma in adult patients, the recommended initial dosage is 5 mg once daily on days 1–21 of each 28-day cycle. Treatment should be continued until disease progression or unacceptable toxicity occurs. In patients with AIDS-related Kaposi sarcoma, highly active antiretroviral therapy (HAART) should be continued. New cycles of pomalidomide should not be undertaken until ANC reaches or exceeds 1000/mm³ and platelet count reaches or exceeds 75,000/mm³.

Dosage Modification for Toxicity in Patients with Kaposi Sarcoma

Temporary interruption of therapy, dosage reduction, and/or permanent discontinuance of pomalidomide may be necessary in patients experiencing adverse effects (see Table 2).

If angioedema, anaphylaxis, grade 4 rash, skin exfoliation, bullae, or any other severe dermatologic reaction occurs, pomalidomide should be permanently discontinued.

TABLE 2. Dosage Modifications for Adverse Effects in Patients with Kaposi Sarcoma

Adverse Reaction and Severity	Pomalidomide Dosage Modification (Starting Dosage = 5 mg daily on days 1–21 of each 28-day cycle)
Neutropenia: ANC 500 to <1000/mm³	Day 1 of cycle: Withhold therapy; when ANC ≥1000/mm³, resume at same dosage
	During cycle: Continue current dosage
ANC <500/mm³	Withhold therapy; when ANC ≥1000/mm³, resume at same dosage
Febrile neutropenia (ANC <1000/mm³ and single temperature of ≥38.3°C or sustained temperature of ≥38°C for >1 hour)	Withhold therapy; when ANC ≥1000/mm³, then resume at a dosage reduced by 1 mg
	If a daily dosage of 1 mg is not tolerated, permanently discontinue pomalidomide
Thrombocytopenia: Platelet count 25,000 to <50,000/mm³	Day 1 of cycle: Withhold therapy; when platelet count ≥50,000/mm³, resume at same dosage
	During cycle: Continue current dosage
Platelet count <25,000/mm³	Permanently discontinue pomalidomide
Non-hematologic adverse reactions: Grade 3 or 4 (excluding hypersensitivity or dermatologic reactions)	Withhold therapy; when toxicity resolves or improves to grade 2 or less, then resume at a dosage reduced by 1 mg

Dosage Modification for Concomitant Use with Cytochrome P-450 (CYP) 1A2 Inhibitors

Concomitant use with strong cytochrome P-450 (CYP) isoenzyme 1A2 inhibitors should be avoided. If concomitant use is necessary, the dosage of pomalidomide should be reduced to 2 mg daily.

● Special Populations

Hepatic Impairment

In patients with hepatic impairment, the manufacturer recommends reducing the initial dosage of pomalidomide as described in Tables 3 and 4.

TABLE 3. Initial Recommended Pomalidomide Dosage in Patients with Multiple Myeloma and Hepatic Impairment

Severity	Dose
Mild (Child-Pugh class A)	3 mg once daily
Moderate (Child-Pugh class B)	3 mg once daily
Severe (Child-Pugh class C)	2 mg once daily

TABLE 4. Initial Recommended Pomalidomide Dosage in Patients with Kaposi Sarcoma and Hepatic Impairment

Severity	Dose
Mild (Child-Pugh class A)	3 mg once daily
Moderate (Child-Pugh class B)	3 mg once daily
Severe (Child-Pugh class C)	3 mg once daily

Renal Impairment

In patients with multiple myeloma and severe renal impairment requiring dialysis, the recommended initial dosage of pomalidomide is 3 mg daily.

In patients with Kaposi sarcoma and severe renal impairment requiring dialysis, the recommended initial dosage of pomalidomide is 4 mg daily.

Pomalidomide should be administered after completion of hemodialysis.

Geriatric Patients

The manufacturer makes no specific dosage recommendations for geriatric patients.

CAUTIONS

● Contraindications

- Pregnancy.
- Known hypersensitivity (e.g., angioedema, anaphylaxis) to the drug or any ingredient in the formulation.

● Warnings/Precautions

Warnings

Fetal/Neonatal Morbidity and Mortality

Pomalidomide may cause fetal toxicity; pomalidomide is a structural analog of thalidomide, a known human teratogen, and teratogenic and other fetotoxic effects of pomalidomide (e.g., musculoskeletal anomalies and deformities; absence of internal organs, including bladder and thyroid; defects of internal organ systems, including cardiovascular, respiratory, renal, hepatic, and CNS abnormalities; increased fetal resorptions) have been demonstrated in animals. Therefore, pomalidomide is contraindicated in women who are pregnant.

All female patients of childbearing potential and all sexually mature males receiving pomalidomide must use effective contraceptive measures (which may include abstinence) to help ensure that fetal exposure to the drug does not occur. Contraceptive measures are indicated even in females with a history of infertility. The only females who do not need to observe mandatory contraceptive measures are those who have undergone hysterectomy or bilateral oophorectomy and those who are postmenopausal and have had no menses for 24 or more consecutive months. All female patients of childbearing potential must use 2 reliable forms of contraception simultaneously (unless the patient chooses to remain continuously abstinent from engaging in heterosexual sexual contact) beginning at least 4 weeks prior to initiation of therapy, during therapy and treatment interruptions, and then for at least 4 weeks following discontinuance of pomalidomide therapy. At least one contraceptive method should be a highly effective method (intrauterine device [IUD], hormonal contraceptives, tubal ligation, vasectomized partner); the other may be an effective barrier method (latex or synthetic condom, diaphragm, cervical cap). Sexually mature males receiving pomalidomide must completely avoid unprotected sexual contact with women of childbearing potential and must not donate semen while receiving pomalidomide and for 4 weeks after discontinuing the drug. While receiving pomalidomide and for up to 28 days after discontinuing the drug, sexually mature males (including those who have successfully undergone vasectomy) must use a latex or synthetic condom each time they have sexual contact with a woman of childbearing potential.

Because pomalidomide may cause fetal harm and because of the possibility that the drug may be present in blood and be transfused into a woman who is pregnant, patients receiving pomalidomide must not donate blood during therapy and for at least 1 month following discontinuance of the drug.

All females of childbearing potential must be tested for pregnancy within 10–14 days and again within 24 hours immediately prior to initiation of pomalidomide therapy. The prescribing clinician should not provide the patient with a prescription for pomalidomide until reports of the pregnancy tests are available indicating that the results are negative. Pregnancy tests must then be repeated at regular intervals during pomalidomide therapy (i.e., weekly during the first month, then every 2 or 4 weeks in women with irregular or regular menstrual cycles, respectively). Pregnancy tests and counseling also should be performed if a patient misses her period or if there is any abnormality in menstrual bleeding. The drug should be discontinued during the evaluation period. If the drug is used during pregnancy or if the patient becomes pregnant while receiving the drug, pomalidomide should be immediately discontinued and the patient informed of the potential hazard to the fetus; the patient should be referred to an obstetrician/gynecologist experienced in reproductive toxicity, and the clinician should notify

Bristol Myers Squibb (888-423-5436) and the US Food and Drug Administration (FDA) via the MedWatch program (800-332-1088).

Thromboembolic Events

Serious venous and arterial thromboembolic events have been reported in patients receiving pomalidomide. Despite required thromboprophylaxis, 8% of patients treated with pomalidomide and low-dose dexamethasone in trial MM-003 had a thromboembolic event compared with 3.3% of patients treated with high-dose dexamethasone. Venous and arterial thromboembolic events occurred more frequently in patients receiving pomalidomide in combination with low-dose dexamethasone (4.7 and 3%, respectively) compared with patients receiving high-dose dexamethasone (1.3 and 1.3%, respectively).

Patients with known risk factors (e.g., history of thrombosis) may be at greater risk and measures should be taken to minimize modifiable factors (e.g., hyperlipidemia, hypertension, smoking). The manufacturer recommends thromboprophylaxis in patients receiving pomalidomide. The manufacturer and some experts state that decisions regarding use of thromboprophylaxis and selection of an appropriate thromboprophylaxis regimen (e.g., aspirin, anticoagulant) should be based on careful assessment of the patient's risk factors for thromboembolism.

Other Warnings and Precautions

Treatment-related Mortality

Increased mortality has been reported in clinical trials in patients with multiple myeloma receiving pembrolizumab in combination with a thalidomide analog and dexamethasone. The manufacturer of pomalidomide states that an anti-programmed death receptor-1 (anti-PD-1) or anti-programmed-death ligand-1 (anti-PD-L1) antibody should not be used in combination with a thalidomide analogue and dexamethasone in patients with multiple myeloma outside of a controlled clinical trial. FDA recommends that ongoing clinical trials evaluating an anti-PD-1 or anti-PD-L1 agent in combination with an immunomodulatory agent (e.g., pomalidomide) be evaluated for permanent discontinuance or protocol amendments.

Hematologic Effects

In the pivotal multiple myeloma trials, neutropenia was the most commonly reported grade 3 or 4 adverse reaction, followed by anemia and thrombocytopenia in patients receiving pomalidomide in combination with low-dose dexamethasone. Neutropenia of any grade occurred in 51% of patients receiving pomalidomide in combination with low-dose dexamethasone. Grade 3 or 4 neutropenia or febrile neutropenia occurred in 46 or 8%, respectively, of patients receiving pomalidomide in combination with low-dose dexamethasone. Complete blood cell counts (CBCs) should be monitored weekly for the first 8 weeks of therapy and monthly thereafter. If hematologic toxicity occurs, dosage interruption and/or reduction may be required.

In the pivotal Kaposi sarcoma trial, the most common adverse reactions were hematologic toxicities. Grade 3 or 4 neutropenia occurred in 50% of patients receiving single-agent pomalidomide. CBCs should be monitored every 2 weeks for the first 3 months and monthly thereafter. If hematologic toxicity occurs, dosage interruption, reduction, or discontinuation may be required.

Hepatotoxicity

Cases of hepatic failure, sometimes fatal, have occurred in patients treated with pomalidomide. Increased serum concentrations of ALT and bilirubin have also been reported in patients receiving pomalidomide. Liver function tests should be monitored monthly. If elevations in liver enzymes occur, temporarily interrupt pomalidomide therapy. When liver enzyme levels return to baseline values, resumption of pomalidomide therapy may be considered at a reduced dosage.

Cutaneous Reactions

Severe cases of cutaneous reactions (i.e., Stevens-Johnson syndrome [SJS], toxic epidermal necrolysis [TEN], drug reaction with eosinophilia and systemic symptoms [DRESS]) have been reported. DRESS may present with a cutaneous reaction (such as rash or exfoliative dermatitis), eosinophilia, fever, and/or lymphadenopathy with systemic complications such as hepatitis, nephritis, pneumonitis, myocarditis, and/or pericarditis. These reactions can be fatal. For grade 2 or 3 skin rash, temporary interruption or discontinuance of pomalidomide should be considered. If grade 4 rash, exfoliative or bullous rash, or other severe cutaneous

reactions (SJS, TEN, or DRESS) occur, pomalidomide should be permanently discontinued.

Dizziness and Confusion

In the pivotal multiple myeloma trials, dizziness or confusion occurred in 14 or 7%, respectively, of patients receiving pomalidomide in combination with low-dose dexamethasone; grade 3 or 4 dizziness occurred in 1% of patients, and grade 3 or 4 confusion occurred in 3% of patients. Instruct patients to avoid situations where dizziness or confusional state may be a problem and avoid other medications that may cause dizziness or confusional state without adequate medical advice.

Neuropathy

In the pivotal multiple myeloma trials, neuropathy was reported in 18% of patients receiving pomalidomide in combination with low-dose dexamethasone, and peripheral neuropathy was reported in approximately 12% of patients. Grade 4 neuropathy occurred in none of the patients; however, grade 3 neuropathy occurred in 2% of patients in the MM-003 study.

Development of Second Primary Malignancy

Acute myelogenous leukemia (AML) has been reported in patients receiving pomalidomide as investigational therapy for uses other than multiple myeloma.

Tumor Lysis Syndrome

Tumor lysis syndrome may occur in patients receiving pomalidomide. Patients treated with pomalidomide with a high tumor burden are at risk for tumor lysis syndrome. Such patients should be monitored closely, and appropriate precautions should be instituted.

Hypersensitivity Reactions

Hypersensitivity reactions such as angioedema, anaphylaxis, and anaphylactic reactions have been reported in patients receiving pomalidomide. If angioedema or anaphylaxis occurs, pomalidomide should be permanently discontinued.

Specific Populations

Pregnancy

Pomalidomide is a thalidomide analogue and is contraindicated for use during pregnancy. Based on animal studies, female fertility may be impaired with pomalidomide treatment.

Lactation

Pomalidomide is distributed into milk in rats; it is not known whether pomalidomide is distributed into milk in humans. Because many drugs are excreted in human milk and because of the potential for serious adverse reactions to pomalidomide in nursing infants, women should not breast-feed during therapy with pomalidomide.

Females and Males of Reproductive Potential

Results of animal studies suggest that pomalidomide may impair female fertility. See Fetal/Neonatal Morbidity and Mortality under Warnings for more information regarding effects of pomalidomide on reproductive potential.

Pediatric Use

Safety and efficacy of pomalidomide have not been established in pediatric patients.

Safety and efficacy of pomalidomide in pediatric patients (4 to less than 17 years of age) were assessed, but not established, in 2 open-label studies. New safety concerns were not observed in pediatric patients in these studies. When pomalidomide was administered at the same dose by body surface area, exposure in patients 4 to <17 years of age was similar to adult patients with multiple myeloma, but higher than exposure observed in adults with Kaposi sarcoma.

Geriatric Use

In clinical trials evaluating pomalidomide in patients with multiple myeloma, 44% of patients were 65 years of age or older and 10% were 75 years of age or older. Although no overall differences in efficacy were observed between geriatric and younger patients, pneumonia occurred more frequently in patients 65 years of age or older compared with younger patients.

In patients with Kaposi sarcoma, experience in patients 65 years of age or older is insufficient to determine whether they respond differently to pomalidomide than younger patients.

Hepatic Impairment

Pomalidomide is primarily metabolized in the liver. Following administration of a single-dose of pomalidomide, the AUC of pomalidomide increased by 51, 58, or 72% in patients with mild, moderate, or severe hepatic impairment, respectively, compared with patients with normal hepatic function.

Renal Impairment

Pomalidomide pharmacokinetic parameters were not significantly affected in patients with moderate (creatinine clearance 30 to less than 60 mL/minute) or severe (creatinine clearance 15 to less than 30 mL/minute) renal impairment relative to patients with normal renal function.

Approximately 73% of a radiolabeled dose of pomalidomide is excreted by the kidneys (primarily as metabolites) in healthy individuals. Following administration of a single-dose of pomalidomide, the AUC of pomalidomide increased by 38% and the rate of serious adverse events increased by 64% in patients with severe renal impairment requiring dialysis compared with patients with normal renal function. In patients with end-stage renal disease (creatinine clearance less than 15 mL/minute), the AUC of pomalidomide increased by 40% on non-dialysis days.

In patients with severe renal impairment requiring dialysis, the estimated dialysis clearance is higher than the total body clearance of pomalidomide, indicating removal of pomalidomide from blood circulation during hemodialysis.

● Common Adverse Effects

Adverse effects reported in at least 30% of patients with multiple myeloma receiving pomalidomide in combination with low-dose dexamethasone include fatigue and asthenia, neutropenia, anemia, constipation, nausea, diarrhea, dyspnea, upper respiratory tract infection, back pain, and pyrexia.

Adverse effects reported in at least 30% of patients with Kaposi sarcoma receiving pomalidomide include decreased absolute neutrophil count (ANC), decreased white blood cell count (WBC), decreased hemoglobin concentrations, decreased platelet count, decreased serum phosphate concentrations, decreased serum albumin concentrations, decreased serum calcium concentrations, increased serum creatinine concentrations, increased serum glucose concentrations, increased serum ALT concentrations, rash, constipation, fatigue, nausea, and diarrhea.

DRUG INTERACTIONS

Metabolism of pomalidomide is mediated primarily by cytochrome P-450 (CYP) isoenzymes 1A2 and CYP3A4, and to a lesser extent by CYP isoenzymes 2C19 and 2D6.

Pomalidomide does not inhibit or induce CYP isoenzymes in vitro.

Pomalidomide is a substrate of P-glycoprotein (P-gp).

Pomalidomide does not inhibit or induce transporters in vitro.

● Drugs Affecting or Metabolized by Hepatic Microsomal Enzymes

Inhibitors of CYP3A

Concomitant use of pomalidomide with the potent CYP3A4 inhibitor and P-gp inhibitor ketoconazole increased the AUC of pomalidomide by 19% in healthy male subjects; however, this is not considered clinically significant.

Inducers of CYP3A

Concomitant use of pomalidomide with the potent CYP3A4 inducer carbamazepine decreased AUC of pomalidomide by 20% in healthy male subjects; however, this is not considered clinically significant.

Concomitant use of pomalidomide with the weak to moderate CYP3A4 inducer dexamethasone did not affect the pharmacokinetics of pomalidomide in patients with multiple myeloma.

Inhibitors of CYP1A2

Concomitant use of pomalidomide with the potent CYP1A2 inhibitor fluvoxamine increased systemic exposure to pomalidomide by 125% in healthy subjects.

Concomitant use with potent CYP1A2 inhibitors (e.g., ciprofloxacin, fluvoxamine) should be avoided; if concomitant use cannot be avoided, the dosage of pomalidomide should be reduced.

Inducers of CYP1A2

Concomitant use of pomalidomide with drugs that induce CYP1A2 has not been studied; however, such concomitant use with CYP1A2 inducers may reduce pomalidomide exposure. Cigarette smoking (a potent CYP1A2 inducer) increased peak plasma concentration of pomalidomide and decreased the AUC of the drug.

● Drugs Affecting Efflux Transport Systems

Concomitant use of pomalidomide with ketoconazole, a potent inhibitor of P-gp did not substantially affect pomalidomide exposure.

● Cigarette Smoking

Cigarette smoking may potentially reduce the AUC and efficacy of pomalidomide. Following a single 4-mg dose of pomalidomide, peak plasma concentrations of pomalidomide increased by 14% and AUC decreased by 32% in healthy male subjects who smoked 25 cigarettes per day compared with healthy nonsmoker male subjects.

DESCRIPTION

Pomalidomide, a thalidomide analog, is an immunomodulatory agent with antineoplastic and antiangiogenic activity. Cellular activities of pomalidomide are mediated through its target cereblon, a component of a cullin ring E3 ubiquitin ligase enzyme complex. In vitro, pomalidomide induces direct cytotoxic and immunomodulatory effects following ubiquitination and degradation of substrate proteins such as Aiolos and Ikaros. The drug has been shown to inhibit production of proinflammatory cytokines (e.g., tumor necrosis factor [TNF], interleukin-6) and increase cytolytic T-cell and natural killer (NK) cell responses. Pomalidomide has been shown to inhibit the growth of hematopoietic tumor cells, including lenalidomide-resistant multiple myeloma cell lines, by inducing apoptosis. The drug has shown synergistic antitumor effects when combined with dexamethasone in lenalidomide-sensitive and lenalidomide-resistant cell lines. Pomalidomide has been shown to inhibit angiogenesis in vitro and in mice bearing tumor xenografts.

Pomalidomide is extensively metabolized in the liver, principally by CYP-450 isoenzymes 1A2 and 3A4, with minor contributions from CYP isoenzymes 2C19 and 2D6. Following multiple-dose oral administration (2 mg once daily for 4 days) in healthy men, pomalidomide concentrations in semen were approximately 67% of plasma concentrations at 4 hours after a dose (near-peak plasma concentrations). Administration of pomalidomide with a high-fat, high-calorie meal decreased the rate of absorption (time to peak concentrations delayed by 2.5 hours), mean peak plasma concentrations (decreased by 27%), and extent of absorption (AUC decreased by 8%). The median terminal half-life of pomalidomide in patients with multiple myeloma or Kaposi sarcoma is 7.5 hours. Following oral administration of a single 2-mg dose of radiolabeled pomalidomide, approximately 73% of the dose was recovered in urine and 15% was recovered in feces; unchanged drug accounted for only 2% of the dose recovered in urine and 8% of the dose recovered in feces.

The pharmacokinetics of pomalidomide are not affected substantially by age (61–85 years), sex, and race.

ADVICE TO PATIENTS

- Educate patients regarding the Pomalyst Risk Evaluation and Mitigation Strategy (REMS)® restricted distribution program for obtaining pomalidomide. (See REMS under Dosage and Administration.)

- Inform patients of the Pregnancy Exposure Registry that monitors pregnancy outcomes in females exposed to pomalidomide during pregnancy.

- Advise patients to swallow capsules intact and not to break, chew, or open capsules.

- Advise patients that a missed dose may be taken up to 12 hours after the scheduled administration time; if more than 12 hours have elapsed, the missed dose should be omitted and the regular dosing schedule resumed the following day. Importance of not taking 2 doses at the same time to make up for a missed dose.

- Risk of fetal harm. Advise women of childbearing potential to use effective methods of contraception beginning at least 4 weeks prior to initiation of therapy, throughout therapy, during dosage interruptions, and for at least 4 weeks after discontinuance of therapy; importance of obtaining pregnancy tests at appropriate intervals during therapy and of immediately discontinuing therapy and contacting their clinician if pregnancy is suspected. Advise men (including those who have successfully undergone vasectomy) to use a latex or synthetic condom during sexual encounters with women of childbearing potential; these contraceptive measures are required during and for at least 28 days after discontinuance of pomalidomide therapy. Availability of information on emergency contraception at 888-668-2528.

- Advise women to avoid breast-feeding while receiving pomalidomide therapy.

- Advise men to avoid donating semen while receiving pomalidomide and for 4 weeks after discontinuing therapy with the drug.

- Advise patients to avoid donating blood while receiving pomalidomide and for 1 month after discontinuing therapy with the drug.

- Risk of neutropenia, thrombocytopenia, and anemia. Importance of regular monitoring of blood cell counts during pomalidomide therapy. Importance of informing clinician if signs and symptoms of neutropenia, thrombocytopenia, or anemia occur.

- Risk of venous and arterial thromboembolic events; advise patients to seek medical care if shortness of breath, chest pain, or swelling of the arms or legs occurs.

- Risk of hepatotoxicity, including hepatic failure; advise patients to report signs and symptoms of hepatotoxicity to their clinician for evaluation.

- Risk of severe skin reactions; advise patients to seek medical care for signs and symptoms of Stevens-Johnson syndrome (SJS), toxic epidermal necrolysis (TEN), or drug reaction with eosinophilia and systemic symptoms (DRESS).

- Risk of dizziness or confusion; importance of avoiding activities where dizziness or confusion could cause serious harm to self or others. Importance of not taking other drugs that may cause dizziness or confusion without consulting their clinician.

- Risk of neuropathy. Importance of informing clinician if signs and symptoms of neuropathy occur.

- Possible risk of developing a second primary malignancy (i.e., acute myelogenous leukemia [AML]).

- Risk of tumor lysis syndrome. Importance of informing clinician if signs and symptoms of tumor lysis syndrome occur.

- Risk of severe hypersensitivity reactions; advise patients to seek medical care for signs and symptoms of hypersensitivity reactions.

- Advise patients that smoking may reduce the drug's efficacy.

- Importance of informing clinicians of existing or contemplated concomitant therapy, including prescription and OTC drugs and dietary or herbal supplements, as well as any concomitant illnesses.

- Inform patients of other important precautionary information.

For further information on the handling of antineoplastic agents, see the ASHP Guidelines on Handling Hazardous Drugs at https://www.ahfsdrug information.com.

PREPARATIONS

Excipients in commercially available drug preparations may have clinically important effects in some individuals; consult specific product labeling for details.

Because pomalidomide is an analog of thalidomide (a known human teratogen that can cause severe, life-threatening birth defects), distribution of pomalidomide is restricted.

Pomalidomide

Oral		
Capsules	1 mg	**Pomalyst®**, Bristol Myers Squibb
	2 mg	**Pomalyst®**, Bristol Myers Squibb
	3 mg	**Pomalyst®**, Bristol Myers Squibb
	4 mg	**Pomalyst®**, Bristol Myers Squibb

† Use is not currently included in the labeling approved by the US Food and Drug Administration.

Selected Revisions June 10, 2024, © Copyright, November 1, 2013, American Society of Health-System Pharmacists, Inc.

Ramucirumab

10:00 · ANTINEOPLASTIC AGENTS

- Ramucirumab, a recombinant human IgG$_1$ monoclonal antibody, is a vascular endothelial growth factor receptor (VEGFR)-2 antagonist.

USES

● Gastric Cancer

Ramucirumab is used alone or in combination with paclitaxel for the treatment of advanced or metastatic gastric adenocarcinoma, including adenocarcinoma of the gastroesophageal junction, that has progressed during or following fluoropyrimidine- or platinum-based chemotherapy; ramucirumab is designated an orphan drug by FDA for the treatment of this cancer.

The current indication for ramucirumab in the treatment of gastric cancer is based principally on the results of 2 randomized, double-blind, placebo-controlled phase 3 studies (REGARD and RAINBOW) in patients with locally advanced or metastatic gastric adenocarcinoma, including adenocarcinoma of the gastroesophageal junction, who had received platinum- and/or fluoropyrimidine-containing regimens. In both studies, the primary measure of efficacy was overall survival.

In the REGARD study, 355 patients were randomized in a 2:1 ratio to receive either ramucirumab (8 mg/kg by IV infusion) or placebo every 2 weeks; all patients received best supportive care. Treatment was continued until disease progression, unacceptable toxicity, or death occurred. The median age of patients was 60 years; all except one of the enrolled patients had a baseline ECOG performance status of 0 or 1. Most patients (81%) enrolled in the study had received prior combined chemotherapy with a platinum compound and a fluoropyrimidine; 15% of patients had received fluoropyrimidine-containing regimens without a platinum compound, and 4% had received platinum-containing regimens without a fluoropyrimidine. At the time of the primary analysis, patients receiving ramucirumab had longer median overall survival (5.2 versus 3.8 months) and progression-free survival (2.1 versus 1.3 months) compared with patients receiving placebo. Results of an exploratory subgroup analysis (based on age, gender, race, and geographic region) suggested a lack of an overall survival benefit in women; patients in North America, Europe, Australia, and New Zealand; and patients categorized as "other" race.

In the RAINBOW study, 665 patients were randomized in a 1:1 ratio to receive either ramucirumab (8 mg/kg by IV infusion over 1 hour on days 1 and 15 of each 28-day cycle) in combination with paclitaxel (80 mg/m^2 by IV infusion over 1 hour on days 1, 8, and 15 of each 28-day cycle) or placebo in combination with paclitaxel. The median age of patients was 61 years; all patients enrolled in the study had a baseline ECOG performance status of 0 or 1. Most patients (81%) enrolled in the study had received prior combined chemotherapy with a platinum compound and a fluoropyrimidine; 15% of patients had received fluoropyrimidine-containing chemotherapy without a platinum compound, and 4% had received platinum-containing regimens without a fluoropyrimidine. Final analysis of overall survival, using derived data, indicated that patients receiving ramucirumab in combination with paclitaxel had longer median overall survival (9.6 versus 7.4 months) and median progression-free survival (4.4 versus 2.9 months) compared with patients receiving placebo in combination with paclitaxel. The objective response rate (complete and partial responses) was 28% for patients receiving ramucirumab in combination with paclitaxel compared with 16% for those receiving placebo in combination with paclitaxel. Data from this study indicate that effects of ramucirumab on survival were consistent across various patient subgroups (including women and patients in Europe, North America, and Australia) and support the hypothesis that results of the exploratory subgroup analysis of the REGARD study were likely limited by small sample size and random effects.

● Non-small Cell Lung Cancer

Ramucirumab is used in combination with docetaxel for the treatment of metastatic non-small cell lung cancer (NSCLC) that has progressed during or following platinum-based chemotherapy. Patients with epidermal growth factor receptor (EGFR)- or anaplastic lymphoma kinase (ALK)-positive tumors also should have documented disease progression during or following an FDA-labeled anti-EGFR or anti-ALK therapy prior to initiating therapy with ramucirumab.

The current indication for ramucirumab in the treatment of metastatic NSCLC is based principally on the results of a randomized, double-blind, placebo-controlled phase 3 study (REVEL) in patients with locally advanced or metastatic NSCLC that had progressed during or following platinum-based chemotherapy. The primary measure of efficacy was overall survival. In this study, 1253 patients were randomized in a 1:1 ratio to receive either ramucirumab (10 mg/kg by IV infusion on day 1 of each 21-day cycle) in combination with docetaxel (75 mg/m^2 by IV infusion on day 1 of each 21-day cycle) or placebo in combination with docetaxel; because an increased incidence of neutropenia and febrile neutropenia was noted in patients in East Asia, these patients received a reduced docetaxel dosage (60 mg/m^2 every 21 days). Treatment was continued until disease progression, death, or unacceptable toxicity occurred, or treatment was discontinued for other reasons. The median duration of treatment was 3.5 months for patients receiving ramucirumab in combination with docetaxel. The median age of patients was 62 years. All patients enrolled in the study had a baseline ECOG performance status of 0 or 1, and 73% had nonsquamous histology. The majority (99%) of patients had received previous platinum-based chemotherapy. In addition to platinum-based chemotherapy, 38% of patients also had received pemetrexed; 25% had received gemcitabine; 24% had received a taxane; and 14% had received bevacizumab.

Patients randomized to receive ramucirumab in combination with docetaxel had a longer median overall survival (10.5 versus 9.1 months) and progression-free survival (4.5 versus 3 months) compared with patients receiving placebo in combination with docetaxel. In addition, patients receiving ramucirumab in combination with docetaxel appeared to have a higher investigator-assessed objective response rate (complete and partial responses) (23 versus 14%) and higher disease control rate (64 versus 53%) compared with those receiving placebo in combination with docetaxel.

● Colorectal Cancer

Ramucirumab is used in combination with fluorouracil, leucovorin (folinic acid), and irinotecan (the combination of fluorouracil, leucovorin, and irinotecan is hereafter referred to as FOLFIRI in this monograph) for the treatment of metastatic colorectal cancer that has progressed during or following combination therapy with oxaliplatin, bevacizumab, and a fluoropyrimidine. Results of a randomized, placebo-controlled study (RAISE) demonstrated improved overall and progression-free survival with such second-line ramucirumab therapy; an increase in the frequency of certain adverse effects with ramucirumab therapy generally was manageable with appropriate dosage adjustments and supportive therapy.

In the RAISE study, 1072 patients were randomly assigned to receive either ramucirumab 8 mg/kg by IV infusion over 1 hour or placebo in combination with FOLFIRI. The FOLFIRI regimen consisted of irinotecan 180 mg/m^2 by IV infusion over 90 minutes concurrent with (or followed by) leucovorin 400 mg/m^2 by IV infusion over 2 hours, followed by fluorouracil 400 mg/m^2 by IV injection over 2–4 minutes, then fluorouracil 2.4 g/m^2 by IV infusion over 46–48 hours. Treatment was repeated every 2 weeks and continued until radiographically confirmed disease progression or unacceptable toxicity occurred; if one or more components of treatment were discontinued for toxicity, patients were permitted to continue therapy with the remaining treatment component(s) until disease progression or unacceptable toxicity occurred. The median duration of treatment was 4.4 months for patients receiving ramucirumab in combination with FOLFIRI. The median age of patients was 62 years; 76% of patients were white, 49% had a baseline ECOG performance status of 0, 49% had KRAS mutations, and 24% had experienced disease progression within less than 6 months after beginning first-line therapy.

Patients receiving the ramucirumab-FOLFIRI regimen had a longer median overall survival (13.3 versus 11.7 months) and a longer progression-free survival (5.7 versus 4.5 months) than patients receiving the placebo-FOLFIRI regimen. In addition, results of a subgroup analysis (based on age, disease stage, ECOG performance status, KRAS mutation status, time to disease progression, number of metastatic sites, presence of metastasis only in the liver, site of primary tumor, and baseline carcinoembryonic antigen [CEA] concentration) suggested that the drug's effect on overall and progression-free survival was consistent across all subgroups. Ramucirumab therapy was associated with a higher incidence of grade 3 or worse treatment-emergent adverse effects (e.g., neutropenia, hypertension). (See Cautions.)

DOSAGE AND ADMINISTRATION

● General

Ramucirumab should be administered only in settings where adequate monitoring can be performed and appropriate medical support is available for management of potential infusion-related reactions. (See Infusion-related Effects under Warnings/Precautions: Other Warnings and Precautions, in Cautions.)

To minimize the risk of infusion-related reactions associated with ramucirumab, premedication with an antihistamine (e.g., IV diphenhydramine hydrochloride) is recommended prior to each infusion. Patients who have experienced a grade 1 or 2 infusion-related reaction also should receive dexamethasone (or equivalent) and acetaminophen prior to subsequent infusions.

Ramucirumab can only be obtained through a limited network of specialty pharmacies. Clinicians may contact the manufacturer (Eli Lilly) by telephone at 800-545-5979 or consult the Cyramza® website for specific ordering and availability information (http://www.cyramzahcp.com).

● Administration

Ramucirumab is administered by IV infusion over 1 hour. *The drug should not be administered by rapid IV injection, such as IV "push" or "bolus."*

Ramucirumab injection concentrate *must* be diluted prior to administration.

Diluted ramucirumab solution should be inspected visually for particulate matter and discoloration prior to administration; if particulate matter or discoloration is evident, the diluted solution should be discarded.

Diluted ramucirumab solution should be administered using an infusion pump. The manufacturer recommends administering the drug through a low-protein-binding 0.22-μm inline filter. Diluted ramucirumab solution should *not* be administered in the same IV line with any other drug or electrolyte solution. The IV line should be flushed with 0.9% sodium chloride injection at the end of the infusion.

Unopened vials of ramucirumab injection concentrate should be protected from light, stored at 2–8°C, and should not be frozen or shaken.

Dilution

Prior to dilution, ramucirumab injection concentrate should be inspected visually for particulate matter and discoloration; if particulate matter or discoloration is evident, the solution should be discarded.

Ramucirumab is diluted by withdrawing the appropriate dose (8 mg/kg) of ramucirumab injection concentrate from the vial labeled as containing 10 mg/mL and diluting in 0.9% sodium chloride injection to yield a final volume of 250 mL. The diluted ramucirumab solution for infusion should be mixed by gentle inversion and should *not* be shaken. Ramucirumab injection concentrate should *not* be diluted in diluents containing dextrose. Ramucirumab should *not* be admixed with any other drug or electrolytes. Commercially available ramucirumab injection concentrate contains no preservatives and is intended for single use; any partially used vials should be discarded.

Diluted ramucirumab solution may be stored at room temperature (below 25°C) for up to 4 hours or under refrigeration (2–8°C) for up to 24 hours; the diluted solution should not be frozen.

● Dosage

Gastric Cancer

For the treatment of advanced or metastatic gastric adenocarcinoma, including adenocarcinoma of the gastroesophageal junction, that has progressed during or following fluoropyrimidine- or platinum-based chemotherapy, the recommended adult dosage of ramucirumab (as a single agent or in combination with paclitaxel) is 8 mg/kg administered by IV infusion every 2 weeks.

When used in combination with paclitaxel, ramucirumab should be administered before administration of paclitaxel. In the RAINBOW study, patients received ramucirumab (8 mg/kg by IV infusion over 1 hour) on days 1 and 15 of each 28-day cycle and paclitaxel (80 mg/m² by IV infusion over 1 hour) on days 1, 8, and 15 of each 28-day cycle.

Treatment with ramucirumab should be continued until disease progression or unacceptable toxicity occurs. In the REGARD study in which ramucirumab was used as a single agent, patients received a median of 4 doses of ramucirumab. In the RAINBOW study in which ramucirumab was used in combination with paclitaxel, patients received a median of 9 doses of ramucirumab.

Non-small Cell Lung Cancer

For the treatment of metastatic non-small cell lung cancer (NSCLC) that has progressed during or following platinum-based chemotherapy, the recommended adult dosage of ramucirumab is 10 mg/kg administered by IV infusion every 3 weeks in combination with docetaxel.

Ramucirumab should be administered before administration of docetaxel.

Treatment with ramucirumab should be continued until disease progression or unacceptable toxicity occurs. In the REVEL study, patients received a median of 4.5 doses of ramucirumab.

Colorectal Cancer

For the treatment of metastatic colorectal cancer that has progressed during or following combination therapy with oxaliplatin, bevacizumab, and a fluoropyrimidine, the recommended dosage of ramucirumab in adults is 8 mg/kg administered by IV infusion every 2 weeks in combination with FOLFIRI (i.e., fluorouracil, leucovorin [folinic acid], and irinotecan).

Ramucirumab should be administered before FOLFIRI.

Treatment with ramucirumab should be continued until disease progression or unacceptable toxicity occurs. In the RAISE study, patients received a median of 8 doses of ramucirumab over a median of 4.4 months.

Dosage Modification for Toxicity

If toxicities occur, temporary or permanent discontinuance of ramucirumab may be required based on causality.

Ramucirumab should be *permanently discontinued* in patients who develop severe (grade 3 or 4) bleeding, arterial thromboembolic events, clinically important hypertension that is not controlled with antihypertensive therapy, hypertensive crisis, hypertensive encephalopathy, grade 3 or 4 infusion-related effects, GI perforation, nephrotic syndrome, proteinuria exceeding 3 g per 24 hours, or reversible posterior leukoencephalopathy syndrome (RPLS). (See Cautions: Warnings/Precautions.)

Ramucirumab therapy should be *temporarily suspended* prior to surgery or if wound healing complications develop during therapy. Therapy also should be temporarily interrupted in patients who develop severe hypertension or proteinuria. (See Hypertension and also Proteinuria under Dosage: Dosage Modification for Toxicity, in Dosage and Administration.)

Infusion-related Effects

If grade 1 or 2 infusion-related reactions occur, the infusion rate should be reduced by 50%. If grade 3 or 4 infusion-related reactions occur, ramucirumab should be permanently discontinued. (See Infusion-related Effects under Warnings/Precautions: Other Warnings and Precautions, in Cautions.)

Hypertension

If severe hypertension occurs, ramucirumab therapy should be interrupted until hypertension is controlled. Ramucirumab should be permanently discontinued in patients with clinically important hypertension that is not controlled with antihypertensive therapy or in patients who develop hypertensive crisis or hypertensive encephalopathy. (See Hypertension under Warnings/Precautions: Other Warnings and Precautions, in Cautions.)

Proteinuria

Ramucirumab therapy should be interrupted for proteinuria of 2 g or more per 24 hours; when proteinuria declines below this level, ramucirumab may be resumed at a reduced dosage of 6 mg/kg every 2 weeks (in patients receiving ramucirumab for advanced or metastatic gastric adenocarcinoma or metastatic colorectal cancer) or 8 mg/kg every 3 weeks (in patients receiving ramucirumab for metastatic NSCLC). If proteinuria recurs, therapy should be withheld again; when proteinuria declines below 2 g per 24 hours, ramucirumab may then be resumed at a reduced dosage of 5 mg/kg every 2 weeks (in patients receiving ramucirumab for advanced or metastatic gastric adenocarcinoma or metastatic colorectal cancer) or 6 mg/kg every 3 weeks (in patients receiving ramucirumab for metastatic NSCLC). If nephrotic syndrome or proteinuria exceeding 3 g per 24 hours occurs, treatment with ramucirumab should be permanently discontinued. (See Proteinuria under Warnings/Precautions: Other Warnings and Precautions, in Cautions.)

● Special Populations

No dosage adjustment is necessary in patients with mild hepatic impairment (total bilirubin concentration within the upper limit of normal [ULN] and AST concentration exceeding the ULN, or total bilirubin concentration ranging from more than 1 to 1.5 times the ULN and any AST concentration). (See Hepatic Impairment under Warnings/Precautions: Specific Populations, in Cautions.)

No dosage adjustment is necessary in patients with renal impairment. (See Renal Impairment under Warnings/Precautions: Specific Populations, in Cautions.)

The manufacturer makes no specific dosage recommendations for geriatric patients. (See Geriatric Use under Warnings/Precautions: Specific Populations, in Cautions.)

CAUTIONS

● Contraindications

The manufacturer states there are no known contraindications to the use of ramucirumab.

● Warnings/Precautions

Warnings

Hemorrhage

Ramucirumab is associated with an increased risk of hemorrhage and GI hemorrhage, including severe and sometimes fatal hemorrhage.

In the REGARD study, severe bleeding was reported in 3.4% of patients receiving ramucirumab compared with 2.6% of those receiving placebo, and red blood cell transfusions were required in 11% of patients receiving ramucirumab compared with 8.7% of those receiving placebo. In the RAINBOW study, severe bleeding was reported in 4.3% of patients receiving ramucirumab in combination with paclitaxel compared with 2.4% of those receiving placebo plus paclitaxel. Patients with gastric cancer receiving nonsteroidal anti-inflammatory agents (NSAIAs) were excluded from the REGARD and RAINBOW studies; therefore, the risk of gastric hemorrhage associated with ramucirumab is unknown in such patients.

In the REVEL study, severe bleeding was reported in 2.4% of patients with metastatic non-small cell lung cancer (NSCLC) receiving ramucirumab in combination with docetaxel compared with 2.3% of those receiving placebo plus docetaxel. Pulmonary hemorrhage was reported in 7% of patients with nonsquamous histology receiving ramucirumab in combination with docetaxel compared with 6% of those receiving placebo plus docetaxel; among patients with squamous histology, pulmonary hemorrhage was reported in 10% of patients receiving ramucirumab in combination with docetaxel compared with 12% of those receiving placebo plus docetaxel. Patients with NSCLC receiving therapeutic anticoagulation, long-term therapy with NSAIAs, or antiplatelet therapy other than once-daily aspirin, and those with radiographic evidence of major airway or blood vessel invasion or intratumor cavitation, were excluded from the REVEL study; therefore, the risk of pulmonary hemorrhage associated with ramucirumab is unknown in such patients.

In the RAISE study, severe bleeding was reported in 2.5% of patients with metastatic colorectal cancer receiving ramucirumab in combination with FOLFIRI (i.e., fluorouracil, leucovorin [folinic acid], and irinotecan) compared with 1.7% of those receiving placebo plus FOLFIRI.

Ramucirumab should be permanently discontinued if severe (grade 3 or 4) hemorrhage occurs during therapy with the drug.

GI Perforation

GI perforation, potentially fatal, has been reported with antiangiogenic agents that are inhibitors of vascular endothelial growth factor receptor (VEGFR), including ramucirumab. In clinical trials, GI perforation was reported in 4 of 570 patients (0.7%) receiving ramucirumab as a single agent. In the RAINBOW study, GI perforation was reported in 1.2% of patients receiving ramucirumab in combination with paclitaxel compared with 0.3% of patients receiving placebo plus paclitaxel. In the REVEL study, GI perforation was reported in 1% of patients receiving ramucirumab in combination with docetaxel compared with 0.3% of patients receiving placebo plus docetaxel. In the RAISE study, GI perforation was reported in 1.7% of patients receiving ramucirumab in combination with FOLFIRI compared with 0.6% of those receiving placebo plus FOLFIRI.

Ramucirumab should be permanently discontinued in patients who develop GI perforation.

Impaired Wound Healing

Data are lacking on the effects of ramucirumab in patients with serious or non-healing wounds; however, inhibitors of VEGFR may impair wound healing. Ramucirumab should be discontinued in patients with impaired wound healing.

The manufacturer recommends that ramucirumab be discontinued prior to scheduled surgery. The decision to resume therapy postoperatively should be based on clinical assessment of the adequacy of wound healing. If wound healing complications develop during ramucirumab therapy, the drug should be discontinued until the wound is fully healed.

Other Warnings and Precautions

Arterial Thromboembolic Events

Severe, sometimes fatal, arterial thromboembolic events (including myocardial infarction, cardiac arrest, cerebrovascular accident, and cerebral ischemia) have been reported in patients receiving ramucirumab. In the REGARD study, arterial thromboembolic events were reported in 1.7% of patients receiving ramucirumab compared with none of those receiving placebo.

Ramucirumab should be permanently discontinued if a severe arterial thromboembolic event occurs during therapy with the drug.

Hypertension

Ramucirumab is associated with an increased risk of severe hypertension. In the REGARD study, grade 3 or 4 hypertension was reported in 8% of patients receiving ramucirumab compared with 3% of those receiving placebo. In the RAINBOW study, grade 3 or greater hypertension was reported in 15% of patients receiving ramucirumab in combination with paclitaxel compared with 3% of those receiving placebo plus paclitaxel. In the REVEL study, grade 3 or greater hypertension was reported in 6% of patients receiving ramucirumab in combination with docetaxel compared with 2% of those receiving placebo plus docetaxel. In the RAISE study, grade 3 or greater hypertension was reported in 11% of patients receiving ramucirumab in combination with FOLFIRI compared with 3% of those receiving placebo plus FOLFIRI.

Hypertension should be controlled prior to initiating therapy with ramucirumab. Blood pressure should be monitored every 2 weeks or more frequently as clinically indicated during therapy with the drug. If severe hypertension occurs, ramucirumab therapy should be interrupted until hypertension is controlled. Ramucirumab should be permanently discontinued in patients with clinically important hypertension that is not controlled with antihypertensive therapy or in patients who develop hypertensive crisis or hypertensive encephalopathy.

Infusion-related Effects

Infusion-related reactions, sometimes severe, have been reported in patients receiving ramucirumab. In clinical studies, infusion-related reactions occurred in 16% of patients receiving ramucirumab without premedication. Infusion-related reactions generally occurred more frequently during or following the first 2 infusions. Infusion-related reactions may include bronchospasm, supraventricular tachycardia, hypotension, rigors/tremors, back pain/spasms, chest pain and/or tightness, chills, flushing, dyspnea, wheezing, hypoxia, and paresthesia.

Premedication with an antihistamine (e.g., IV diphenhydramine hydrochloride) should be administered prior to each infusion of ramucirumab. (See Dosage and Administration: General.) Patients should be monitored during infusions of the drug for manifestations of infusion-related reactions. If infusion-related reactions occur, reduction in the infusion rate or permanent discontinuance of ramucirumab may be required. (See Infusion-related Effects under Dosage: Dosage Modification for Toxicity, under Dosage and Administration.)

Hepatic Effects

New-onset or worsening encephalopathy, ascites, or hepatorenal syndrome has been reported in patients with preexisting Child-Pugh class B or C cirrhosis receiving ramucirumab as a single agent.

Reversible Posterior Leukoencephalopathy Syndrome

Reversible posterior leukoencephalopathy syndrome (RPLS) has been reported in less than 0.1% of patients receiving ramucirumab in clinical studies.

If signs or symptoms of RPLS develop, diagnosis of RPLS should be confirmed by magnetic resonance imaging (MRI), and ramucirumab therapy should be discontinued. Symptoms of RPLS may resolve or improve within days, but some patients can experience ongoing neurologic sequelae or death.

Proteinuria

Proteinuria has been reported in patients receiving ramucirumab. In the RAINBOW study, proteinuria of any grade occurred in 17% of patients receiving ramucirumab in combination with paclitaxel compared with 6% of those receiving placebo plus paclitaxel. In the RAISE study, grade 3 or greater proteinuria occurred in 3% of patients receiving ramucirumab in combination with FOLFIRI compared with 0.2% of those receiving placebo plus FOLFIRI; among these patients, nephrotic syndrome occurred in 0.6% of patients receiving ramucirumab in combination with FOLFIRI versus none of those receiving placebo plus FOLFIRI.

Urine dipstick proteinuria and/or urinary protein-to-creatinine ratio should be monitored for development or worsening of proteinuria during therapy.

Ramucirumab therapy should be interrupted in patients with urine protein levels of 2 g or more per 24 hours and resumed at a reduced dosage when proteinuria declines below this level. If urine protein levels exceed 3 g per 24 hours or if nephrotic syndrome occurs, treatment with ramucirumab should be permanently discontinued. (See Proteinuria under Dosage: Dosage Modification for Toxicity, in Dosage and Administration.)

Thyroid Dysfunction

Hypothyroidism has been reported in patients receiving ramucirumab in combination with FOLFIRI. In the RAISE study, hypothyroidism occurred in 2.6% of patients receiving ramucirumab in combination with FOLFIRI compared with 0.9% of those receiving placebo plus FOLFIRI. Among patients with normal baseline thyroid-stimulating hormone (TSH) concentrations, increases in TSH concentrations were reported in 46% of patients receiving ramucirumab in combination with FOLFIRI compared with 4% of those receiving placebo plus FOLFIRI.

Thyroid function should be monitored during ramucirumab therapy.

Fetal/Neonatal Morbidity and Mortality

There are no adequate and well-controlled studies of ramucirumab in pregnant women; however, based on its mechanism of action, ramucirumab can cause fetal harm. In animals, angiogenesis, vascular endothelial growth factors (VEGF), and vascular endothelial growth factor receptor 2 (VEGFR-2) have a critical role in female reproduction, embryofetal development, and postnatal development. Teratogenicity (i.e., poor development of cranial region, forelimbs, forebrain, heart, blood vessels) has been observed in animals following disruption of VEGF signaling.

Pregnancy should be avoided during ramucirumab therapy. Women of childbearing potential should be advised to use an effective method of contraception while receiving ramucirumab and for at least 3 months after discontinuance of therapy. Patients should be apprised of the potential hazard to the fetus if the drug is used during pregnancy.

Immunogenicity

Antibodies to ramucirumab have been detected in patients receiving the drug. In clinical studies, anti-ramucirumab antibodies were detected in 86 of 2890 patients (3%) receiving ramucirumab. Neutralizing antibodies were detected in 14 of the 86 patients who tested positive for anti-ramucirumab antibodies.

Impairment of Fertility

Results of animal studies suggest that inhibitors of VEGFR, such as ramucirumab, may impair female fertility or ability to maintain pregnancy.

Specific Populations
Pregnancy

Based on its mechanism of action, ramucirumab may cause fetal harm if administered to pregnant women. (See Fetal/Neonatal Morbidity and Mortality under Cautions: Warnings/Precautions.)

Lactation

It is not known whether ramucirumab is distributed into human milk. Human immunoglobulin G (IgG) is distributed into milk; however, published data suggest that antibodies contained in breast milk do not enter the neonatal and infant circulation in substantial amounts. Nevertheless, because of the potential for serious adverse reactions to ramucirumab in nursing infants, the manufacturer states that nursing during ramucirumab therapy is not recommended. Data are lacking on the effects of the drug in nursing infants or on the production of milk.

Pediatric Use

Safety and efficacy of ramucirumab have not been established in pediatric patients younger than 18 years of age.

In animals, exposure to ramucirumab at concentrations 0.2 times that of human clinical exposure resulted in toxicities in bone (i.e., thickening of epiphyseal growth plates, osteochondropathy).

Geriatric Use

In the REGARD and RAINBOW studies, 36% of patients with advanced or metastatic gastric adenocarcinoma receiving ramucirumab were 65 years of age or older, and 7% were 75 years of age or older. No overall differences in safety or efficacy were observed between geriatric and younger adults.

In the REVEL study, 36% of patients with metastatic NSCLC receiving ramucirumab in combination with docetaxel were 65 years of age or older, and 7% were 75 years of age or older. In an exploratory subgroup analysis, survival benefit was not observed in patients 65 years of age or older receiving ramucirumab in combination with docetaxel (hazard ratio 1.10).

In the RAISE study, 40% of patients with metastatic colorectal cancer receiving ramucirumab in combination with FOLFIRI were 65 years of age or older, and 10% were 75 years of age or older. No overall differences in safety or efficacy were observed between geriatric and younger adults in this study.

Hepatic Impairment

In a population pharmacokinetic analysis, no clinically meaningful differences in the average steady-state concentrations of ramucirumab were observed between patients with mild (total bilirubin concentration within the upper limit of normal [ULN] and AST concentration exceeding the ULN, or total bilirubin concentration ranging from more than 1 to 1.5 times the ULN and any AST concentration) or moderate (total bilirubin concentration ranging from 1.5 to 3 times the ULN and any AST concentration) hepatic impairment and those with normal hepatic function. Formal pharmacokinetic studies have not been conducted in patients with severe (total bilirubin concentration exceeding 3 times the ULN and any AST concentration) hepatic impairment. (See Dosage and Administration: Special Populations.)

New-onset or worsening encephalopathy, ascites, or hepatorenal syndrome has been reported in patients with preexisting Child-Pugh class B or C cirrhosis receiving ramucirumab as a single agent. Ramucirumab should be used in patients with Child-Pugh class B or C cirrhosis only if the potential benefit outweighs the risk of clinical deterioration.

Renal Impairment

In a population pharmacokinetic analysis, no clinically meaningful differences in the average steady-state concentrations of ramucirumab were observed between patients with mild (creatinine clearance of 60–89 mL/minute), moderate (creatinine clearance of 30–59 mL/minute), or severe (creatinine clearance of 15–29 mL/minute) renal impairment and those with normal renal function. (See Dosage and Administration: Special Populations.)

● Common Adverse Effects

Adverse effects reported in 5% or more of patients with advanced or metastatic gastric adenocarcinoma receiving ramucirumab as a single agent in the REGARD study and occurring at an incidence at least 2% higher than that reported with placebo include hypertension, diarrhea, bleeding or hemorrhage, headache, proteinuria, and hyponatremia. Clinically important adverse effects reported in less than 5% of patients receiving ramucirumab as a single agent in the REGARD study include neutropenia, epistaxis, rash, anemia, intestinal obstruction, arterial thromboembolic events, GI perforation, and infusion-related reactions.

Adverse effects reported in 5% or more of patients with advanced or metastatic gastric adenocarcinoma receiving ramucirumab in combination with paclitaxel in the RAINBOW study and occurring at an incidence at least 2% higher than that reported with placebo plus paclitaxel include fatigue or asthenia, neutropenia, diarrhea, epistaxis, peripheral edema, hypertension, stomatitis, proteinuria, thrombocytopenia, hypoalbuminemia, and GI hemorrhage. Clinically important adverse effects reported in less than 5% of patients receiving ramucirumab in combination with paclitaxel in the RAINBOW study include sepsis and GI perforation.

Adverse effects reported in 5% or more of patients with metastatic NSCLC receiving ramucirumab in combination with docetaxel in the REVEL study and occurring at an incidence at least 2% higher than that reported with placebo plus docetaxel include neutropenia, fatigue or asthenia, stomatitis or mucosal inflammation, epistaxis, febrile neutropenia, peripheral edema, thrombocytopenia, increased lacrimation, hypertension, diarrhea, decreased appetite, neuropathy, leukopenia, pyrexia, myalgia, arthralgia, back pain, dysgeusia, and insomnia. Clinically important adverse effects reported in less than 5% of patients receiving ramucirumab in combination with docetaxel in the REVEL study include hyponatremia and proteinuria.

Adverse effects reported in the RAISE study in 5% or more of patients with metastatic colorectal cancer receiving ramucirumab in combination with FOLFIRI and at an incidence at least 2% higher than that reported with placebo plus FOLFIRI include diarrhea, neutropenia, fatigue, hemorrhage, decreased appetite, epistaxis, stomatitis, vomiting, constipation, abdominal pain, thrombocytopenia, hypertension, peripheral edema, mucosal inflammation, proteinuria, pyrexia, headache, decreased weight, cough, liver injury or liver failure, palmar-plantar erythrodysesthesia (hand-foot syndrome), GI hemorrhage, venous thromboembolic event, hypoalbuminemia, and infusion-related reactions. Clinically important adverse effects reported in less than 5% of patients receiving ramucirumab in combination with FOLFIRI include GI perforation.

DRUG INTERACTIONS

● Antineoplastic Agents

Docetaxel

Concomitant administration of ramucirumab (10 mg/kg) with docetaxel (75 mg/m²) in patients with solid tumors did not substantially alter systemic exposure to ramucirumab or docetaxel.

Irinotecan

Concomitant administration of ramucirumab with irinotecan in patients with solid tumors did not substantially alter systemic exposure to ramucirumab or irinotecan (including its active metabolite SN-38).

Paclitaxel

Concomitant administration of ramucirumab (8 mg/kg) with paclitaxel (80 mg/m²) in patients with solid tumors did not substantially alter systemic exposure to ramucirumab or paclitaxel.

DESCRIPTION

Ramucirumab, a recombinant human IgG₁ monoclonal antibody, is a vascular endothelial growth factor receptor (VEGFR)-2 antagonist. Ramucirumab binds specifically to VEGFR-2 and blocks the interaction of VEGFR-2 with its ligands (VEGF-A, VEGF-C, and VEGF-D), resulting in inhibition of VEGF-stimulated activation of both VEGFR-2 and downstream signaling pathways. The VEGFR signaling pathway plays an important role in the pathogenesis and progression of several types of tumors since it is a pivotal mediator of tumor angiogenesis; the pathway also regulates tumor growth and metastatic spread. In vitro assays have shown that binding of ramucirumab to VEGFR-2 blocks ligand-induced phosphorylation and activation of the receptor. Ramucirumab has been shown to inhibit VEGF-induced endothelial cell proliferation and migration in vitro. Ramucirumab also has been shown to inhibit angiogenesis in vivo.

Following administration of 8 mg/kg every 2 weeks in patients with advanced or metastatic gastric adenocarcinoma, the mean elimination half-life of ramucirumab was 15 days. Following administration of 10 mg/kg every 21 days in patients with metastatic non-small cell lung cancer [NSCLC]), the mean elimination half-life of ramucirumab was 23 days. Data from a population pharmacokinetic analysis indicate that age, gender, and race do not have clinically important effects on the pharmacokinetics of ramucirumab.

ADVICE TO PATIENTS

Risk of severe bleeding. Importance of informing clinician of any episodes or symptoms of bleeding (e.g., lightheadedness).

Risk of arterial thromboembolic events.

Risk of hypertension. Importance of receiving routine monitoring of blood pressure and informing clinician if blood pressure is elevated or if manifestations of hypertension (e.g., severe headache, lightheadedness, neurologic symptoms) occur.

Importance of informing clinician if severe diarrhea, vomiting, or severe abdominal pain occurs.

Risk of wound healing complications. Importance of informing clinician of any scheduled surgery.

Risk of fetal or neonatal toxicity and miscarriage. Necessity of advising women receiving ramucirumab to use an effective method of contraception during and for at least 3 months after the last dose of ramucirumab. Importance of immediately informing clinician if the patient becomes pregnant during therapy. If pregnancy occurs, apprise patient of potential hazard to the fetus.

Importance of discontinuing nursing while receiving ramucirumab therapy.

Importance of informing clinicians of existing or contemplated concomitant therapy, including prescription and OTC drugs and dietary or herbal supplements (e.g., nonsteroidal anti-inflammatory agents [NSAIAs]), as well as any concomitant illnesses (e.g., hypertension, hepatic disease).

Importance of informing patients of other important precautionary information. (See Cautions.)

For further information on the handling of antineoplastic agents, see the ASHP Guidelines on Handling Hazardous Drugs at http://www.ahfsdrug information.com.

PREPARATIONS

Excipients in commercially available drug preparations may have clinically important effects in some individuals; consult specific product labeling for details.

Ramucirumab (Recombinant)

Parenteral

Concentrate for injection, for IV infusion only	10 mg/mL (100 and 500 mg)	Cyramza®, Eli Lilly

Selected Revisions August 7, 2017, © Copyright, April 6, 2015, American Society of Health-System Pharmacists, Inc.

Regorafenib

10:00 · ANTINEOPLASTIC AGENTS

■ Regorafenib, an inhibitor of multiple receptor tyrosine kinases, is an antineoplastic agent.

USES

● Colorectal Cancer

Regorafenib is used for the treatment of metastatic colorectal cancer in patients who have received fluoropyrimidine-, oxaliplatin-, and irinotecan-containing regimens; a vascular endothelial growth factor inhibitor (anti-VEGF therapy); and, in those with tumors bearing the wild-type (nonmutated) KRAS gene, an epidermal growth factor receptor inhibitor (anti-EGFR therapy).

The current indication for regorafenib in the treatment of metastatic colorectal cancer is based principally on the results of a randomized, double-blind, placebo-controlled phase 3 study (CORRECT) in patients with previously treated metastatic colorectal cancer. The primary measure of efficacy was overall survival. The median age of patients was 61 years. Patients enrolled in the study had received a median of 3 prior therapies for their disease; all patients had received previous treatment with bevacizumab and with fluoropyrimidine-, oxaliplatin-, and irinotecan-containing regimens. With one exception, all patients with tumors bearing the wild-type KRAS gene had previously received panitumumab or cetuximab therapy. In this study, 760 patients were randomized in a 2:1 ratio to receive either regorafenib (160 mg orally once daily) or placebo for 3 consecutive weeks of each 4-week cycle; all patients received best supportive care. Treatment was continued until disease progression, death, or unacceptable toxicity occurred or treatment was discontinued for other reasons. The median duration of treatment was 1.7 months for patients receiving regorafenib. Results of a planned interim analysis indicated that patients receiving regorafenib had a longer median overall survival (6.4 versus 5 months; hazard ratio for death: 0.77) and longer median progression-free survival (2 versus 1.7 months) than those receiving placebo. Overall response rates were low (1 versus 0.4%, respectively) and were not substantially different between regorafenib-treated patients and placebo-treated patients, suggesting that the drug's main effect in this patient population was disease stabilization; none of the patients achieved a complete response. Subgroup analysis according to primary site of disease suggested that regorafenib had a greater effect on overall survival relative to placebo in patients with colon cancer than in those with rectal cancer (hazard ratio: 0.7 and 0.95, respectively); an overall survival benefit for the drug versus placebo was not apparent in the small subgroup of patients with primary disease involving both the colon and rectum (hazard ratio: 1.09). Subgroup analysis suggested that the drug's effect on progression-free survival was uniform across all 3 subgroups.

Clinical Perspective

The American Society of Clinical Oncology (ASCO) guideline for the treatment of patients with late-stage colorectal cancer generally recommends doublet or triplet fluoropyrimidine-based chemotherapy with or without bevacizumab regardless of RAS mutation status; however, patients with wild-type RAS and certain comorbidities or risk factors who are not candidates for chemotherapy may be offered monotherapy with anti-EGFR therapy (e.g., cetuximab, panitumumab). Immune checkpoint inhibitors (e.g., pembrolizumab, nivolumab, nivolumab in combination with ipilimumab) may also be considered in patients with deficient mismatch repair (dMMR) or high microsatellite instability (MSI-H) colorectal cancer (regardless of RAS mutation status) who are not candidates for intensive chemotherapy.

First-line treatment options for patients with late-stage colorectal cancer are the same regardless of whether the intent is curative or palliative. Second-line treatment options for the treatment of metastatic colorectal cancer include immune checkpoint inhibitors or chemotherapy with or without anti-EGFR therapy or ziv-aflibercept, and should be chosen based on the regimen used in the first-line setting (e.g., bevacizumab, oxaliplatin, irinotecan) and disease characteristics (e.g., RAS or BRAF mutation status, dMMR, microsatellite instability [MSI] status). ASCO states that regorafenib or trifluridine/tipiracil may be considered in

the third- or fourth-line setting in patients with any RAS/BRAF status; however, the drugs are recommended in patients with metastatic colorectal cancer harboring wild-type RAS who were previously treated with fluoropyrimidines, oxaliplatin, irinotecan, bevacizumab, and anti-EGFR therapy.

● GI Stromal Tumor

Regorafenib is used for the treatment of locally advanced, unresectable, or metastatic GI stromal tumor (GIST) in patients who previously received imatinib and sunitinib therapy; regorafenib has been designated an orphan drug by FDA for the treatment of this cancer.

The current indication for regorafenib in the treatment of GIST is based principally on the results of a randomized, double-blind, placebo-controlled phase 3 study (GRID) in patients with locally advanced, unresectable, or metastatic GIST following failure of both imatinib and sunitinib therapy. The primary measure of efficacy was progression-free survival based on radiographic evidence. The median age of patients was 60 years; all patients enrolled in the study had a baseline ECOG performance status of 0 or 1. In this study, 199 patients were randomized in a 2:1 ratio to receive either regorafenib (160 mg orally once daily) or placebo for 3 consecutive weeks of each 4-week cycle; all patients received best supportive care. Treatment cycles were continued until disease progression or unacceptable toxicity occurred or treatment was discontinued for other reasons; upon radiographic progression, patients previously randomized to receive placebo were permitted to cross over to open-label regorafenib treatment. The median duration of treatment was 5.7 months for patients receiving regorafenib. A planned interim analysis indicated that patients receiving regorafenib had longer median progression-free survival (4.8 months) compared with those receiving placebo (0.9 months). The overall response rate was 4.5% for patients receiving regorafenib and 1.5% for those receiving placebo; none of the patients achieved a complete response. Median overall survival had not been reached at the time of the interim analysis; however, no significant difference in overall survival was observed between the treatment groups.

In a randomized, open-label phase 3 study, regorafenib was compared with avapritinib for the treatment of patients with unresectable or metastatic GIST previously treated with 2 lines of therapy. Median progression-free survival was not significantly different between regorafenib (5.6 months) and avapritinib (4.2 months). Treatment-related adverse events also were similar between the treatment groups.

Clinical Perspective

Treatment of GIST includes surgical resection and/or the use of tyrosine kinase inhibitors depending on the extent of disease and tumor sensitivity to the tyrosine kinase inhibitor. Approximately 85% of all GIST contain a mutation in KIT and/or platelet-derived growth factor receptor alpha (PDGFRA) which result in constitutive activation of the receptor tyrosine kinase; therefore, inhibition of KIT is a primary therapeutic modality for the treatment of GIST. Imatinib is a selective inhibitor of the KIT protein tyrosine kinase, and is considered standard therapy for the treatment of locally advanced, inoperable or metastatic GIST (including patients who did not relapse during therapy with adjuvant imatinib) in patients with imatinib-sensitive mutations. Following disease progression or intolerance to imatinib, sunitinib is standard second-line therapy in patients with metastatic or recurrent GIST. Regorafenib is generally recommended in the third-line setting in patients with imatinib-sensitive mutations and imatinib-nonsensitive-mutations (e.g., PDGFRA D842V, NTRK-translocated, SDH-deficient).

Although the majority of GIST cases have either a mutation in KIT or PDGFRA, approximately 10–15% of cases do not have a detectable KIT or PDGFRA mutation. Loss-of-function mutations in succinate dehydrogenase (SDH) or loss of SDHB expression have been identified in a majority of KIT/PDGFRA-wild-type GIST (also referred to as SDH-deficient GIST); such tumors are usually resistant to imatinib, but may have some sensitivity to sunitinib and regorafenib.

● Hepatocellular Carcinoma

Regorafenib is used for the treatment of hepatocellular carcinoma in patients who previously received sorafenib therapy; regorafenib has been designated an orphan drug by FDA for the treatment of this cancer.

The current indication for regorafenib in the treatment of hepatocellular carcinoma is based principally on the results of a randomized, double-blind, placebo-controlled phase 3 study (RESORCE) in patients with Barcelona Clinic

Liver Cancer (BCLC) stage B or C hepatocellular carcinoma following failure of sorafenib therapy. Patients were enrolled in the study if they were not eligible for surgical or locoregional therapies; 81% of patients enrolled in the study had macroscopic vascular invasion and/or extrahepatic disease. Patients who permanently discontinued prior therapy with sorafenib because of toxicity or who were unable to tolerate a sorafenib dosage of 400 mg once daily were excluded from the study. The median age of patients was 63 years; 98% had mild (Child-Pugh class A) hepatic impairment, 88% were male, 87% had BCLC stage C disease, 61% had received prior locoregional therapies, and 41% were Asian. All patients enrolled in the study had a baseline ECOG performance status of 0 or 1. Chronic hepatitis B virus (HBV) infection, alcohol consumption, chronic hepatitis C virus (HCV) infection, or nonalcoholic steatohepatitis were risk factors for underlying cirrhosis in 38, 25, 21, or 7% of patients, respectively. The median duration of prior sorafenib treatment was 7.8 months. The primary measure of efficacy was overall survival.

In this study, 573 patients were randomized in a 2:1 ratio to receive either regorafenib (160 mg orally once daily) or placebo for 3 consecutive weeks of each 4-week cycle; all patients received best supportive care. Treatment cycles were continued until disease progression or unacceptable toxicity occurred or treatment was discontinued for other reasons; placebo recipients were permitted to cross over to open-label regorafenib treatment after the primary analysis. The median duration of treatment was 3.5 months for patients receiving regorafenib. Median overall survival was 10.6 months in patients receiving regorafenib compared with 7.8 months in those receiving placebo. In addition, patients receiving regorafenib had prolonged progression-free survival (3.1 versus 1.5 months) and higher objective response rates (11 versus 4%) according to modified Response Evaluation Criteria in Solid Tumors (RECIST) assessment for hepatocellular carcinoma (mRECIST) compared with those receiving placebo; complete responses were achieved in 0.5% of regorafenib-treated patients. Use of either mRECIST or RECIST version 1.1 to assess progression-free survival and objective response rates resulted in comparable findings. Subgroup analysis according to disease etiology (HCV infection, HBV infection, alcohol consumption), tumor burden (presence or absence of macroscopic vascular invasion and/or extrahepatic disease), ECOG performance status (0 or 1), Child-Pugh score (A5 or A6), α-fetoprotein (AFP) concentration, age, gender, and geographic region suggested that regorafenib consistently improved median overall and progression-free survival and time to progression across all subgroups.

Clinical Perspective

Management of early stage hepatocellular carcinoma includes liver transplantation, surgical resection, and ablation. Survival is usually less than 6 months in patients with untreated advanced stage hepatocellular carcinoma. Treatment of hepatocellular carcinoma is complicated by the presence of underlying liver disease, the extent and location of tumor, comorbidities, and performance status. The American Society of Clinical Oncology (ASCO) states that the risk of potential toxicities and benefits of therapy should be considered when selecting therapy.

ASCO guideline on systemic therapy for advanced hepatocellular carcinoma states that lenvatinib or sorafenib may be offered as first-line therapy for patients with advanced hepatocellular carcinoma, Child-Pugh class A, and an ECOG performance status of 0 or 1 if therapy with atezolizumab and/or bevacizumab is contraindicated. ASCO also states that tyrosine kinase inhibitors (i.e., cabozantinib, lenvatinib, regorafenib, sorafenib) may be used as second-line therapy† following therapy with atezolizumab in combination with bevacizumab.

The decision to pursue second-line therapy and choice of treatment should be based on patient and clinician preferences and other factors (i.e., comorbidities, liver function, performance status, and potential for benefit and risk of harm).

● Other Uses

Regorafenib has been studied in patients with gastric cancer†, osteosarcoma†, soft-tissue sarcoma†, and glioblastoma†.

DOSAGE AND ADMINISTRATION

● General

Pretreatment Screening

- Blood pressure; control blood pressure prior to initiating therapy.

- Assess serum aminotransferase (ALT and AST) and bilirubin concentrations prior to initiating therapy.
- Verify pregnancy status in females of reproductive potential.

Patient Monitoring

- Monitor blood pressure weekly during the first 6 weeks of therapy and then every cycle, or more frequently, as clinically indicated.
- Monitor serum aminotransferase (ALT and AST) and bilirubin concentrations at least every 2 weeks for the first 2 months of therapy, and then monthly thereafter or more frequently as clinically indicated.

Other General Considerations

- Withhold therapy for at least 2 weeks prior to elective surgery. Do not administer for ≥2 weeks following major surgery and until adequate wound healing has occurred.
- If regorafenib is used in patients receiving a coumarin-derivative anticoagulant (e.g., warfarin), monitor international normalized ratio (INR) more frequently.

● Administration

Regorafenib is administered orally with water following a low-fat meal containing less than 600 calories and less than 30% fat at the same time each day. The tablets should be swallowed whole.

If a dose of regorafenib is missed, the prescribed dose should be taken as soon as possible on the same day; two doses should *not* be administered on the next day to replace the missed dose.

Store regorafenib in its original container in a dry place at controlled room temperature (20–25ºC); excursions are permitted between 15–30ºC. Discard any unused tablets 7 weeks after first opening the bottle.

● Dosage

Dosage of regorafenib, which is commercially available as the monohydrate, is expressed in terms of anhydrous regorafenib.

Colorectal Cancer

For the treatment of metastatic colorectal cancer in patients who previously received fluoropyrimidine-, oxaliplatin-, and irinotecan-containing regimens, anti-vascular endothelial growth factor (anti-VEGF) therapy, and, in those with tumors bearing the wild-type (nonmutated) KRAS gene, anti-epidermal growth factor receptor (anti-EGFR) therapy, the recommended dosage of regorafenib is 160 mg once daily for 21 days followed by a 7-day rest period; courses of therapy are given in 28-day cycles. Therapy should be continued until disease progression or unacceptable toxicity occurs.

GI Stromal Tumor

For the treatment of locally advanced, unresectable, or metastatic GI stromal tumor (GIST) in patients who previously received imatinib and sunitinib therapy, the recommended dosage of regorafenib is 160 mg once daily for 21 days followed by a 7-day rest period; courses of therapy are given in 28-day cycles. Therapy should be continued until disease progression or unacceptable toxicity occurs.

Hepatocellular Carcinoma

For the treatment of hepatocellular carcinoma in patients who previously received sorafenib therapy, the recommended dosage of regorafenib is 160 mg once daily for 21 days followed by a 7-day rest period; courses of therapy are given in 28-day cycles. Therapy should be continued until disease progression or unacceptable toxicity occurs.

Dosage Modification for Toxicity

When dosage modification is necessary, the daily dosage of regorafenib should be reduced in decrements of 40 mg; however, if a dosage of 80 mg daily is not tolerated, regorafenib should be permanently discontinued.

Grade 3 or 4 Toxicity

If grade 3 or 4 toxicity occurs, regorafenib therapy should be interrupted. If the toxicity is grade 4, the manufacturer states that therapy should be permanently discontinued; the manufacturer states that therapy may be resumed following recovery from grade 4 toxicity *only* if the potential benefits of resuming therapy outweigh the risks. When therapy is resumed following recovery from the first episode of grade 3 or 4 toxicity (except hepatotoxicity or infection), regorafenib should be administered at a reduced dosage of 120 mg daily; if grade 3 or 4 toxicity (except hepatotoxicity or infection) occurs at a dosage of 120 mg daily, therapy should be withheld again until recovery occurs and then may be resumed at a further reduced dosage of 80 mg daily. If the patient does not tolerate a dosage of 80 mg daily, regorafenib therapy should be permanently discontinued.

Dermatologic Toxicity

For the first episode of grade 2 palmar-plantar erythrodysesthesia (hand-foot syndrome) of any duration, dosage of regorafenib should be reduced to 120 mg daily. If grade 2 palmar-plantar erythrodysesthesia does not improve within 7 days of dosage reduction or if it recurs at a dosage of 120 mg daily, therapy should be withheld; when therapy is resumed, the dosage should be further reduced to 80 mg daily. If the patient does not tolerate a dosage of 80 mg daily, regorafenib therapy should be permanently discontinued. (See Dermatologic Effects under Warnings/Precautions: Other Warnings and Precautions, in Cautions.)

If grade 3 palmar-plantar erythrodysesthesia occurs, regorafenib therapy should be withheld for at least 7 days; following recovery, therapy may be resumed at a reduced dosage of 120 mg daily. If grade 3 palmar-plantar erythrodysesthesia recurs at a dosage of 120 mg daily, therapy should be withheld again for at least 7 days; following recovery, therapy may be resumed at a further reduced dosage of 80 mg daily. If the patient does not tolerate a dosage of 80 mg daily, regorafenib therapy should be permanently discontinued.

For recommended dosage modifications in patients experiencing grade 4 palmar-plantar erythrodysesthesia, see Grade 3 or 4 Toxicity under Dosage and Administration.

Hepatotoxicity

In patients who exhibit grade 3 serum aminotransferase (ALT and/or AST) elevations (i.e., exceeding 5 times the upper limit of normal [ULN], but not more than 20 times the ULN), regorafenib therapy should be interrupted; following recovery, therapy may be resumed at a reduced dosage of 120 mg daily *only* if the potential benefits of resuming therapy outweigh the risk of hepatotoxicity. If grade 3 elevations in ALT or AST recur at a dosage of 120 mg daily, treatment with regorafenib should be permanently discontinued.

Following any occurrence of grade 4 ALT and/or AST elevations (i.e., exceeding 20 times the ULN), regorafenib therapy should be permanently discontinued.

Following any occurrence of grade 2 or higher AST and/or ALT elevations (i.e., exceeding 3 times the ULN) *and* bilirubin concentrations exceeding twice the ULN, regorafenib therapy should be permanently discontinued.

Hypertension

If symptomatic grade 2 hypertension occurs, regorafenib therapy should be interrupted. For recommended dosage modifications in patients with grade 3 or 4 hypertension, see Grade 3 or 4 Toxicity under Dosage and Administration.

Infectious Complications

If grade 3 or 4 infection develops or worsening infection of any grade occurs, regorafenib therapy should be interrupted; following resolution of the infection, therapy may be resumed at the same dosage.

● Special Populations

Hepatic Impairment

No dosage adjustment is necessary in patients with mild (total bilirubin concentration not exceeding the ULN with AST concentration exceeding the ULN *or* total bilirubin concentration exceeding the ULN, but no more than 1.5 times the ULN) or moderate (total bilirubin concentration exceeding 1.5 times, but not more than 3 times the ULN with any AST concentration) preexisting hepatic impairment; however, patients with hepatic impairment should be closely monitored for adverse effects. Use of regorafenib in patients with severe preexisting hepatic impairment (total bilirubin concentration exceeding 3 times the ULN) is *not* recommended because safety and efficacy have not been established in these patients.

Renal Impairment

No dosage adjustment is necessary in patients with mild to severe renal impairment. The pharmacokinetics of regorafenib have not been studied in patients with end-stage renal disease requiring dialysis; therefore, the manufacturer states that an appropriate dosage for these patients has not been established.

Geriatric Patients

The manufacturer makes no specific dosage recommendations for geriatric patients.

Race

Although hepatotoxicity and palmar-plantar erythrodysesthesia occur more frequently in Asian patients, the manufacturer states that no initial dosage adjustment is necessary in this population.

CAUTIONS

● Contraindications

- Manufacturer states none known.

● Warnings/Precautions

Warnings

Hepatic Toxicity

A boxed warning about the risk of hepatotoxicity is included in the prescribing information for regorafenib. Severe and sometimes fatal hepatotoxicity has been reported in patients receiving regorafenib, generally during the initial 2 months of therapy; hepatic toxicity is usually characterized by a hepatocellular pattern of injury. In the CORRECT study, fatal hepatic failure was reported more frequently in patients with metastatic colorectal cancer receiving regorafenib compared with those receiving placebo (1.6 versus 0.4%). Among patients receiving regorafenib for GI stromal tumor (GIST) in the GRID study, fatal hepatic failure occurred in 0.8% of patients. In the RESORCE study, the incidence of fatal hepatic failure was not increased in patients with hepatocellular carcinoma receiving regorafenib compared with those receiving placebo. In an analysis of pooled data from 3 trials involving patients with metastatic colorectal cancer, GIST, or hepatocellular carcinoma, liver function test abnormalities were reported more frequently in Asian patients receiving regorafenib compared with Caucasian patients.

Serum aminotransferase (ALT and AST) and bilirubin concentrations should be evaluated prior to initiation of therapy, at least every 2 weeks for the first 2 months of therapy, and then monthly thereafter or more frequently as clinically indicated. If aminotransferase and/or bilirubin concentrations rise above pretreatment levels, liver function tests should be monitored weekly until the elevated concentrations have returned to baseline values or have decreased to less than 3 times the upper limit of normal (ULN). Temporary interruption of therapy followed by dosage reduction or permanent drug discontinuance may be necessary depending on the severity and persistence of the toxicity (i.e., elevated liver function test results or hepatocellular necrosis).

Other Warnings and Precautions

Infectious Complications

Infections, sometimes fatal, have been reported in patients receiving regorafenib. In clinical studies, infection was reported in 32% (grade 3 or greater in 9%) of patients receiving regorafenib compared with 17% of those receiving placebo. Urinary tract infections, nasopharyngitis, mucocutaneous and systemic fungal infections, and pneumonia were the most common infections, occurring in 5.7, 4, 3.3, and 2.6% of patients, respectively. Fatal infections, most commonly respiratory infections, occurred in 1% of regorafenib-treated patients compared with 0.3% of those receiving placebo.

Temporary interruption of therapy may be necessary depending on the severity of the infection.

Hemorrhage

Hemorrhage, sometimes fatal, has been reported in patients receiving regorafenib. In clinical studies, hemorrhage was reported more frequently in regorafenib-treated patients compared with patients receiving placebo (18.2 versus 9.5%); grade 3 or greater hemorrhage occurred in 3% of regorafenib-treated patients. Fatal hemorrhage (CNS bleeding or respiratory, GI, or genitourinary tract bleeding) was reported in 0.7% of patients receiving regorafenib.

If severe or life-threatening hemorrhage occurs, regorafenib should be permanently discontinued. If regorafenib is used in patients receiving a coumarin-derivative anticoagulant (e.g., warfarin), the international normalized ratio (INR) should be monitored more frequently.

GI Perforation and Fistula Formation

GI perforation occurred in 0.6% of 4518 patients receiving regorafenib in clinical trials; 8 deaths were reported. In placebo-controlled trials, GI fistula formation was reported in 0.8 or 0.2% of patients receiving regorafenib or placebo, respectively.

Regorafenib should be permanently discontinued in patients with GI perforation or fistula formation.

Dermatologic Effects

In clinical studies, skin reactions, including palmar-plantar erythrodysesthesia (hand-foot syndrome) and severe rash requiring dosage modification, occurred in 71.9% of patients receiving regorafenib and 25.5% of those receiving placebo. Palmar-plantar erythrodysesthesia was reported in 53% of patients receiving regorafenib and 8% of those receiving placebo; the onset generally occurred during the first cycle of therapy. Grade 3 palmar-plantar erythrodysesthesia, grade 3 rash, severe erythema multiforme, and severe Stevens-Johnson syndrome were reported more frequently in patients receiving regorafenib compared with those receiving placebo. Toxic epidermal necrolysis also occurred in patients receiving regorafenib in clinical trials. In an analysis of pooled data from 3 trials involving patients with metastatic colorectal cancer, GIST, or hepatocellular carcinoma, palmar-plantar erythrodysesthesia was reported more frequently in Asian patients receiving regorafenib compared with Caucasian patients.

Dosage reduction, temporary interruption of therapy, or permanent drug discontinuance may be necessary depending on the severity and persistence of the toxicity; other symptomatic and supportive measures also should be employed.

Cardiovascular Effects

In the CORRECT study, hypertension was reported more frequently in patients with metastatic colorectal cancer receiving regorafenib compared with those receiving placebo (30 versus 8%). In the GRID study, hypertension occurred in 59% of patients with GIST receiving regorafenib compared with 27% of those receiving placebo. In the RESORCE study, hypertension occurred in 31% of patients with hepatocellular carcinoma receiving regorafenib compared with 6% of those receiving placebo. Hypertensive crisis has been reported. Onset of hypertension generally occurred during the first cycle of therapy. Blood pressure should be controlled before regorafenib therapy is initiated. Blood pressure should be monitored weekly during the first 6 weeks of regorafenib therapy and thereafter should be monitored every cycle, or more frequently, as clinically indicated. If hypertension is severe or uncontrolled, temporary or permanent discontinuance of therapy is recommended.

In clinical studies, cardiac ischemia or infarction occurred more frequently in patients receiving regorafenib than in those receiving placebo (0.9 versus 0.2%). Therapy should be interrupted in patients who develop new or acute-onset cardiac ischemia or cardiac infarction. Upon resolution of acute cardiac ischemic events, therapy may be resumed if the potential benefits outweigh the risk of further cardiac ischemia.

Reversible Posterior Leukoencephalopathy Syndrome

Reversible posterior leukoencephalopathy syndrome (RPLS) has occurred in patients receiving regorafenib. This complication occurred in one of 4800 patients treated with regorafenib in clinical trials. RPLS is a syndrome of subcortical vasogenic edema that may manifest with headache, seizures, visual disturbances, confusion, or altered mental function. Magnetic resonance imaging (MRI) is necessary to confirm the diagnosis of RPLS.

The possible diagnosis of RPLS should be considered in any patient receiving regorafenib who presents with neurologic manifestations suggestive of RPLS. Regorafenib should be discontinued in patients who develop RPLS.

Wound Healing Complications

The effect of regorafenib on wound healing has not been specifically studied to date; however, inhibitors of vascular endothelial growth factor receptor (VEGFR) may impair wound healing.

The manufacturer recommends that regorafenib be discontinued at least 2 weeks prior to scheduled surgery. The decision to resume therapy postoperatively should be based on clinical assessment of the adequacy of wound healing. Do not resume regorafenib for at least 2 weeks following major surgery and until adequate wound healing occurs. The safety of resuming regorafenib after resolution of wound healing has not been established.

Fetal/Neonatal Morbidity and Mortality

Regorafenib may cause fetal harm if administered to pregnant females; embryolethality and teratogenicity have been demonstrated in animals. Regorafenib produced developmental toxicity, including cardiovascular, genitourinary, and skeletal abnormalities, when administered to pregnant animals in dosages associated with exposure levels lower than those associated with the recommended human dosage. Pregnancy should be avoided during therapy and for 2 months after drug discontinuance. If regorafenib is used during pregnancy or if the patient becomes pregnant while receiving the drug, the patient should be apprised of the potential fetal hazard.

Specific Populations

Pregnancy

Regorafenib may cause fetal harm if administered to pregnant females based on its mechanism of action and animal findings.

Lactation

Regorafenib and its metabolites are distributed into milk in rats; it is not known whether the drug is distributed into milk in humans. Because of the potential for serious adverse reactions to regorafenib in nursing infants, women should be advised to discontinue nursing during regorafenib therapy. The effects of the drug on nursing infants or on milk production are unknown. Women may begin nursing 2 weeks after discontinuance of therapy.

Females and Males of Reproductive Potential

Females and males of reproductive potential should use effective contraception during therapy and for 2 months after discontinuance of therapy.

Results of animal studies suggest that regorafenib may impair male and female fertility. The effect of regorafenib on fertility in humans is not known.

Pediatric Use

Safety and efficacy of regorafenib have not been established in pediatric patients younger than 18 years of age.

Persistent growth and thickening of the femoral epiphyseal growth plate, as well as dose-dependent angiectasis and dentin alteration, have been observed in animals receiving repeated doses of regorafenib at exposure levels lower than those associated with the recommended human dosage.

Geriatric Use

In clinical studies, 40% of patients were 65 years of age or older and 10% were 75 years of age or older. No overall differences in safety and efficacy were observed between geriatric patients and younger adults, but grade 3 or 4 hypertension occurred more frequently in geriatric patients.

Hepatic Impairment

In a population pharmacokinetic analysis, no clinically meaningful differences in the mean systemic exposure to regorafenib and its active N-oxide (M-2) and N-oxide and N-desmethyl (M-5) metabolites were observed in patients with hepatocellular carcinoma and mild (total bilirubin concentration not exceeding the ULN with AST concentration exceeding the ULN or total bilirubin concentration exceeding the ULN, but no more than 1.5 times the ULN) or moderate (total bilirubin concentration exceeding 1.5 times, but not more than 3 times, the ULN with any AST concentration) hepatic impairment compared with patients with normal hepatic function; no dosage adjustment is required in patients with mild or moderate hepatic impairment. However, patients with mild or moderate hepatic impairment should be monitored closely for adverse effects. Regorafenib has not been studied in patients with severe hepatic impairment (total bilirubin concentration exceeding 3 times the ULN); therefore, use of the drug is not recommended in these patients.

Renal Impairment

Following administration of regorafenib (160 mg daily for 21 days), systemic exposure to regorafenib and its active M-2 and M-5 metabolites in patients with severe renal impairment (creatinine clearance 15–29 mL/minute) was similar to that in patients with normal renal function; no dosage adjustment is recommended in patients with mild to severe renal impairment. However, regorafenib has not been studied in patients with end-stage renal disease requiring dialysis, and an appropriate dosage for these patients has not been established.

Race

In clinical trials, a higher incidence of palmar-plantar erythrodysesthesia (hand-foot syndrome) and liver function abnormalities were observed in Asian patients. No dosage adjustment is recommended based on race.

● Common Adverse Effects

The most common adverse reactions (≥20%) are pain (including GI and abdominal pain), palmar-plantar erythrodysesthesia (hand-foot syndrome), asthenia/fatigue, diarrhea, decreased appetite/food intake, hypertension, infection, dysphonia, hyperbilirubinemia, fever, mucositis, weight loss, rash, and nausea.

DRUG INTERACTIONS

● Drugs and Foods Affecting Hepatic Microsomal Enzymes

Metabolism of regorafenib to M-2 (an active N-oxide metabolite) is mediated by cytochrome P-450 isoenzyme 3A4 (CYP3A4); the enzyme responsible for conversion of M-2 to M-5 (an active N-oxide and N-desmethyl metabolite) has not been established to date. Therefore, concomitant use of regorafenib with potent inhibitors of CYP3A4 may result in increased systemic exposure to the parent drug, decreased systemic exposure to M-2 and M-5, and an increased incidence of adverse effects. In healthy individuals, the potent CYP3A4 inhibitor ketoconazole (400 mg daily for 18 days) increased the area under the concentration-time curve (AUC) of regorafenib (single 160-mg dose administered 5 days after initiation of ketoconazole) by 33% and decreased the AUCs of both M-2 and M-5 by approximately 93%. Concomitant use of regorafenib with potent inhibitors of CYP3A4 (e.g., clarithromycin, grapefruit juice, itraconazole, ketoconazole, nefazodone, posaconazole, telithromycin, voriconazole) should be avoided.

Concomitant use of regorafenib with potent inducers of CYP3A4 may result in decreased systemic exposure to the parent drug, increased systemic exposure to M-5, and reduced regorafenib efficacy. In healthy individuals, the potent CYP3A4 inducer rifampin (600 mg daily for 9 days) decreased the AUC of regorafenib (single 160-mg dose administered 7 days after initiation of rifampin) by 50% and increased the AUC of M-5 by 264%; the AUC of M-2 was not substantially altered. Concomitant use of regorafenib with potent inducers of CYP3A4 (e.g., carbamazepine, phenobarbital, phenytoin, rifampin, St. John's wort [*Hypericum perforatum*]) should be avoided.

● Drugs Metabolized by Hepatic Microsomal Enzymes

In vitro studies have suggested that regorafenib inhibits CYP isoenzymes 2B6, 2C8, 2C9, 2C19, and 3A4; that the active M-2 metabolite inhibits CYP isoenzymes 2C8, 2C9, 2D6, and 3A4; and that the active M-5 metabolite inhibits CYP2C8. In vitro studies also have suggested that regorafenib does not induce CYP isoenzymes 1A2, 2B6, 2C19, or 3A4. However, when patients with advanced solid tumors received a single dose of midazolam (2 mg; a CYP3A4 substrate), rosiglitazone (4 mg; a CYP2C8 substrate), warfarin sodium (10 mg; a CYP2C9 substrate), or omeprazole (40 mg; a CYP2C19 substrate) following 2 weeks of regorafenib administration (160 mg once daily), the AUCs of midazolam and rosiglitazone were not substantially altered, the AUC of warfarin was increased by 25%, and plasma concentrations of omeprazole measured 6 hours after administration were not substantially altered.

● Drugs Affected by Transport Systems

In vitro data indicate that regorafenib is an inhibitor of the efflux transporter breast cancer resistance protein (BCRP). Therefore, concomitant use of regorafenib with drugs that are substrates of BCRP may result in increased systemic exposure to the substrate drug. When regorafenib (160 mg once daily for 14 days) was administered prior to the BCRP substrate rosuvastatin (single 5-mg dose), peak plasma concentration and AUC of rosuvastatin were increased 4.6- and 3.8-fold, respectively. Patients receiving regorafenib concomitantly with BCRP substrates (e.g., atorvastatin, fluvastatin, methotrexate) should be closely monitored for signs of toxicity associated with the substrate drug.

Although in vitro data also indicate that regorafenib is an inhibitor of the efflux transporter P-glycoprotein (P-gp), clinical data indicate that regorafenib does not alter the pharmacokinetics of digoxin (a P-gp substrate). No clinically meaningful interactions between regorafenib and P-gp substrates are expected.

● Drugs Affecting Transport Systems

In vitro studies indicate that the active M-2 and M-5 metabolites of regorafenib are substrates of P-gp and BCRP. Inhibitors or inducers of these efflux transporters may alter M-2 and M-5 exposure; however, the clinical importance of these in vitro findings is not known.

● Drugs Metabolized by Uridine Diphosphate-glucuronosyltransferase (UGT)

In vitro studies indicate that regorafenib and its active metabolites competitively inhibit UGT1A1 and UGT1A9 at clinically relevant concentrations. In patients receiving an irinotecan-containing regimen concomitantly with regorafenib, the AUCs of irinotecan and its active metabolite SN-38 (a UGT1A1 substrate) were increased by 28 and 44%, respectively, when a dose of irinotecan hydrochloride (180 mg/m² as a 1.5-hour IV infusion) was given 5 days after completion of a series of 7 doses of regorafenib (160 mg orally once daily).

● Antibiotics

When regorafenib (single 160-mg dose) was administered concomitantly with neomycin sulfate (1 g orally 3 times daily for 5 days) in healthy individuals, the AUC of regorafenib was not substantially altered; however, the AUCs of M-2 and M-5 were decreased by 76 and 86%, respectively. The effect of other antibiotics on systemic exposure of regorafenib and its active metabolites has not been established.

● Antineoplastic Agents

Fluorouracil

In patients receiving a fluorouracil-containing regimen concomitantly with regorafenib, the pharmacokinetics of fluorouracil were not substantially altered when fluorouracil (400 mg/m² by IV injection, followed by continuous IV infusion of 2400 mg/m² over 46 hours) was given 5 days after completion of a series of 7 doses of regorafenib (160 mg orally once daily).

Irinotecan

In patients receiving an irinotecan-containing regimen concomitantly with regorafenib, the AUCs of irinotecan and its active metabolite SN-38 were increased by 28 and 44%, respectively.

Oxaliplatin

In patients receiving an oxaliplatin-containing regimen concomitantly with regorafenib, the AUCs of total and unbound platinum were increased by 39 and 17%, respectively, when oxaliplatin (85 mg/m² as a 2-hour IV infusion) was given 5 days after completion of a series of 7 doses of regorafenib (160 mg orally once daily).

● Warfarin

When regorafenib is used in patients receiving a coumarin-derivative anticoagulant (e.g., warfarin), international normalized ratio (INR) should be monitored more frequently. When a single dose of warfarin sodium (10 mg; a CYP2C9 substrate) was administered following 2 weeks of therapy with regorafenib (160 mg once daily), the AUC of warfarin was increased by 25%.

DESCRIPTION

Regorafenib, an inhibitor of multiple receptor tyrosine kinases (RTKs), is an antineoplastic agent. Receptor tyrosine kinases are involved in the initiation of various cascades of intracellular signaling events that lead to cell proliferation and/or influence processes critical to cell survival and tumor progression (e.g., angiogenesis, metastasis, inhibition of apoptosis), based on the respective kinase. In vitro, regorafenib or its active metabolites (M-2 and M-5) exhibit inhibitory activity against vascular endothelial growth factor receptors (i.e., VEGFR-1, VEGFR-2, VEGFR-3), platelet-derived growth factor receptors (i.e., PDGFR-α, PDGFR-β), fibroblast growth factor receptors (i.e., FGFR1, FGFR2), and tyrosine kinase with immunoglobulin and epidermal growth factor homology (i.e., TIE-2) at clinically relevant concentrations; the drug also has a broad spectrum of inhibitory effects on other receptor kinases involved in normal cellular functions and pathologic processes (e.g., RET, c-Kit, DDR2, TrkA, EphA-2, Raf-1, b-Raf, mutant b-Raf, SAPK2, Ptk5, Bcr-Abl, CSF-1R). Regorafenib has been shown to inhibit tumor angiogenesis in vivo. The drug also has demonstrated inhibition of tumor growth in mice bearing tumor xenografts, including human colorectal carcinoma, GI stromal tumor (GIST), and hepatocellular carcinoma. In addition, regorafenib has demonstrated inhibition of tumor metastasis in xenograft models of human colorectal carcinoma in mice.

When regorafenib is administered in dosages exceeding 60 mg daily, steady-state exposure to the drug, as measured by area under the serum concentration-time curve (AUC), increases in a less than dose-proportional manner. Regorafenib is metabolized principally by cytochrome P-450 (CYP) isoenzyme 3A4 and uridine diphosphate-glucuronosyl transferase (UGT) 1A9. The main circulating metabolites, M-2 (an N-oxide metabolite) and M-5 (an N-oxide and N-desmethyl metabolite), have been shown to be equipotent to regorafenib in biochemical and cellular assays. Regorafenib and its active metabolites are highly bound (more than 99%) to plasma proteins. Regorafenib undergoes enterohepatic circulation. Following oral administration of a single 160-mg dose of regorafenib, the terminal half-life of regorafenib and M-2 were similar (28 and 25 hours, respectively); however, elimination of M-5 was slower, with a terminal half-life of approximately 51 hours. Following oral administration of 120 mg of radiolabeled regorafenib (as an oral solution), approximately 71% of the dose was recovered in feces (47% of the dose as unchanged drug and 24% as metabolites) and 19% was recovered in urine within 12 days.

Bioavailability of regorafenib and its active metabolites is affected by the presence of food and the fat content of the meal. Administration of a single 160-mg dose of regorafenib with a high-fat meal (945 calories and 54.6 g of fat) increased the AUC of regorafenib by 48% and decreased the AUCs of M-2 and M-5 by 20 and 51%, respectively, compared with administration in the fasted state. When the drug was administered with a low-fat meal (319 calories and 8.2 g of fat), the AUCs of regorafenib, M-2, and M-5 were increased by 36, 40, and 23%, respectively, compared with administration in the fasted state. In clinical trials establishing safety and efficacy, regorafenib was administered with a low-fat meal.

Age, gender, ethnicity, and body weight do not have clinically important effects on the pharmacokinetics of regorafenib.

ADVICE TO PATIENTS

- Importance of taking regorafenib with water at the same time each day following a low-fat meal (<600 calories and <30% fat). Importance of avoiding grapefruit juice while taking the drug.
- If a dose is missed, importance of administering the missed dose on the same day as soon as it is remembered; do not take 2 doses on the same day to make up for a missed dose.
- Risk of severe or life-threatening hepatotoxicity and importance of liver function test monitoring. Importance of promptly informing clinician of signs and symptoms of severe liver damage (e.g., jaundice, nausea, vomiting, dark urine, changes in sleep pattern).

- Risk of infection. Importance of promptly informing clinician of signs and symptoms of infection (e.g., fever, severe cough or sore throat, shortness of breath, burning or pain upon urination, unusual vaginal discharge or irritation).
- Risk of severe bleeding. Importance of informing clinician of signs and symptoms of unusual bleeding (e.g., bruising, lightheadedness).
- Risk of palmar-plantar erythrodysesthesia (hand-foot syndrome) or rash. Importance of informing clinician of skin changes (e.g., redness, pain, blisters, bleeding, swelling).
- Risk of hypertension developing or worsening during therapy. Importance of regular monitoring of BP. Importance of informing clinician of signs and symptoms of hypertension (e.g., severe headache, lightheadedness, neurologic symptoms).
- Risk of myocardial ischemia and infarction. Importance of seeking immediate medical attention if chest pain, shortness of breath, dizziness, or feelings of faintness occur.
- Risk of RPLS. Importance of immediately informing clinician if severe headache, seizure, confusion, or visual and neurologic disturbances occur.
- Risk of GI perforation. Importance of promptly informing clinician if severe abdominal pain, persistent abdominal swelling, chills, nausea, vomiting, dehydration, or high fever occurs.
- Risk of wound healing complications. Importance of informing clinician of any recent or scheduled surgery.
- Risk of fetal harm. Necessity of advising women of childbearing potential and men who are partners of such women to use effective methods of contraception during therapy and for 2 months after drug discontinuance. Importance of patients informing their clinicians if they or their partners are pregnant or think they may be pregnant.
- Importance of advising women to avoid breast-feeding while receiving regorafenib therapy and for 2 weeks after the final dose.
- Importance of informing clinicians of existing or contemplated concomitant therapy, including prescription and OTC drugs and dietary or herbal supplements (e.g., St. John's wort), as well as any concomitant illnesses (e.g., hypertension or other cardiovascular disease, hepatic disease, bleeding disorders).
- Importance of storing regorafenib tablets in the original container, tightly closed, with the desiccant; do not place tablets in daily or weekly pill boxes. Discard any unused tablets 7 weeks after the container is first opened.
- Importance of informing patients of other important precautionary information. (See Cautions.)

For further information on the handling of antineoplastic agents, see the ASHP Guidelines on Handling Hazardous Drugs at http://www.ahfsdrug information.com.

PREPARATIONS

Distribution of regorafenib is restricted. Regorafenib can only be obtained through designated specialty pharmacies. Contact the manufacturer or consult the Stivarga® website for specific information.

Excipients in commercially available drug preparations may have clinically important effects in some individuals; consult specific product labeling for details.

Regorafenib

Oral		
Tablets, film-coated	40 mg	Stivarga®, Bayer

† Use is not currently included in the labeling approved by the US Food and Drug Administration.

riTUXimab

10:00 • ANTINEOPLASTIC AGENTS

■ Rituximab, a chimeric human-murine anti-human antigen CD20 mono-clonal antibody, is an antineoplastic agent.

USES

● *Non-Hodgkin's Lymphoma*

Rituximab is used alone or in combination with other chemotherapy regimens for the treatment of B-cell non-Hodgkin's lymphoma (NHL) and is designated an orphan drug by the US Food and Drug Administration (FDA) for the treatment of this cancer.

Relapsed or Refractory Low-grade or Follicular Non-Hodgkin's Lymphoma

Immunotherapy with Rituximab

Rituximab is used as a single agent for the treatment of relapsed or refractory low-grade or follicular, antigen CD20-positive, B-cell NHL. Treatment of advanced-stage or relapsed low-grade NHL generally is palliative, and many therapeutic options have been employed, including single-agent chemotherapy, combination chemotherapy and/or radiation therapy, and aggressive management with combination chemotherapy and bone marrow or peripheral stem cell transplantation. Although most patients with relapse of low-grade or follicular NHL initially achieve an objective clinical response to treatment, further relapse eventually occurs, and subsequent therapy is associated with lower response rates and shorter durations of remission. The optimal management of indolent recurrent NHL has not been established, and new therapies are continually being evaluated.

The current indication for use of rituximab in the treatment of relapsed or refractory low-grade or follicular NHL is based on data from noncomparative studies. The use of rituximab for the treatment of relapsed or refractory low-grade or follicular B-cell NHL has been investigated in clinical studies including a total of 296 patients receiving rituximab regimens of 4 or 8 once-weekly doses administered as initial treatment, initial treatment of bulky disease, or retreatment.

In a multicenter, open-label, single-arm study, 166 patients with relapsed or refractory low-grade or follicular B-cell NHL who received rituximab 375 mg/m² as an IV infusion once weekly for 4 weeks had an overall response rate of 48% (6% complete responses, 42% partial responses). Patients with bulky disease (tumor masses greater than 10 cm) or with greater than 5000 lymphocytes/mm³ in the peripheral blood were excluded from the study. The median time to onset of response was 50 days, and the median duration of response was 11.2 months (range: 1.9–42.1 or more months). Resolution of disease-related signs and symptoms was reported in 64% (25/39) of patients with such manifestations (including B symptoms) at the time of study entry. According to multivariate analysis, overall response rate was higher in patients with International Working Formulation (IWF) histologic lymphoma subtypes B, C, or D than in those with subtype A (58 versus 12%). In addition, overall response rate was higher in patients whose largest lesion was less than 5 cm versus greater than 7 cm (maximum, 21 cm) in greatest diameter (53 versus 38%), and in patients with chemosensitive versus chemoresistant relapse (defined as duration of response of less than 3 months) (53 versus 36%). Response rates did not differ according to age, presence of extranodal disease or bone marrow involvement, or history of prior anthracycline therapy. The overall response rate in patients receiving rituximab who had been treated previously with autologous bone marrow transplantation was 78%.

Rituximab also has been administered once weekly in an 8-week regimen. In a multicenter, single-arm study, 37 patients with relapsed or refractory low-grade NHL who received rituximab 375 mg/m² as an IV infusion once weekly for 8 weeks had an overall response rate of 57% (14% complete responses, 43% partial responses). The projected median duration of response was 13.4 months (range: 2.5–36.5 or more months). Treatment with 8 weekly doses of rituximab was associated with a higher overall incidence of grade 3 and 4 adverse effects compared with a regimen of 4 weekly doses (70 versus 57%).

Rituximab appears to have activity in patients with relapsed or refractory low-grade NHL who have bulky disease (single lesion exceeding 10 cm in diameter) but is associated with an increased incidence of clinically important adverse events, including neutropenia, anemia, dyspnea, hypotension, and abdominal pain, in such patients. In pooled data from multiple studies, 39 patients with relapsed or refractory, bulky disease, low-grade NHL who received rituximab 375 mg/m² as an IV infusion once weekly for 4 weeks had an overall response rate of 36% (3% complete responses, 33% partial responses) and a median duration of response of 6.9 months (range: 2.8–25 or more months).

Responses also have been observed in patients with NHL receiving additional courses of rituximab for refractory disease or for relapse of disease that initially responded to the drug. In a multicenter, single-arm study, an overall response rate of 38% (10% complete responses, 28% partial responses) and a projected median duration of response of 15 months (range: 3–25.1 or more months) were reported in 60 patients receiving retreatment with rituximab 375 mg/m² once weekly for 4 weeks for relapsed or refractory, low-grade or follicular B-cell NHL following an objective clinical response to one or more prior courses of rituximab at a median of 14.5 months prior to retreatment. Among the 60 patients, 55 patients received their second course of rituximab, 3 patients received their third course, and 2 patients received both their second and third course of rituximab in the study. The incidence of grade 3 or 4 adverse effects was similar in patients retreated with rituximab and patients receiving initial treatment with rituximab (58 and 57%, respectively).

Maintenance therapy with rituximab following induction chemotherapy (with or without rituximab) has been shown to offer benefit in patients with relapsed or refractory indolent NHL. In a phase 3 randomized trial, progression-free survival was prolonged in patients receiving 2 years of maintenance therapy with rituximab following chemotherapy with cyclophosphamide, vincristine, and prednisone (CVP) for advanced indolent NHL compared with those receiving CVP alone. In another randomized trial, duration of response was prolonged in patients receiving maintenance therapy with rituximab following salvage chemotherapy (with or without rituximab) for recurring or refractory follicular or mantle cell lymphoma compared with those receiving induction chemotherapy alone. In a phase 3 randomized trial, median progression-free survival and median overall survival were prolonged in patients receiving maintenance therapy with rituximab following chemotherapy with either cyclophosphamide, doxorubicin, vincristine, and prednisone (CHOP) or rituximab-CHOP for relapsed or resistant follicular NHL compared with those receiving induction chemotherapy alone.

Radioimmunotherapy with Rituximab and Ibritumomab

Rituximab is used as a required component of a therapeutic regimen with ibritumomab tiuxetan (ibritumomab tiuxetan therapeutic regimen) for the treatment of relapsed or refractory low-grade or follicular B-cell NHL, including follicular NHL that is refractory to rituximab therapy. Limited evidence indicates that the overall response rate is higher in such patients receiving the ibritumomab tiuxetan therapeutic regimen compared with standard rituximab immunotherapy; comparative effects on survival have not been established. The regimen consists of an initial rituximab dose (administered on day 1) and a second rituximab dose (administered on day 7, 8, or 9) followed within 4 hours by a therapeutic dose of yttrium Y 90 ibritumomab tiuxetan. For additional information on the use of rituximab as part of the ibritumomab tiuxetan therapeutic regimen for NHL, see Ibritumomab Tiuxetan 10:00.

Rituximab in Combination with Bendamustine

Efficacy and safety of rituximab in combination with bendamustine† for the treatment of relapsed or refractory indolent NHL or relapsed or refractory mantle cell lymphoma† in patients who had received up to 3 prior treatment regimens has been studied in 2 open-label, phase 2 studies.

In both studies, patients received rituximab 375 mg/m² IV on day 1, followed by bendamustine hydrochloride 90 mg/m² daily as an IV infusion on days 2 and 3, administered on a 28-day cycle for a total of 4 cycles. An additional dose of rituximab was administered one week prior to the first rituximab-bendamustine treatment cycle and repeated at 28 days following the last rituximab-bendamustine treatment cycle. Patients achieving a response between the second and fourth treatment cycles were permitted to receive an additional 2 cycles of rituximab-bendamustine treatment in the second study. Overall response rates in the 2 studies were similar (90–92%), with 41–60% of patients exhibiting complete responses. Overall and complete response rates were higher in patients with no prior exposure to rituximab (100 and 48%, respectively) than in those with prior rituximab exposure (86 and 35%, respectively). Median progression-free survival was similar in both studies (24 and 23 months). At the time of the data analysis, median duration of survival had not been reached in the first study; however, the actuarial 48-month survival rate was 55%.

Small numbers of patients in each study (16 and 12, respectively) had relapsed or refractory mantle cell lymphoma. Overall and complete response rates for these patients were 75–92 and 42–50%, respectively. Median progression-free survival was 18 months in the first study; median response duration was 19 months in the second study.

Based on current evidence and because of the favorable toxicity profile, combination therapy with rituximab and bendamustine is recommended (accepted) for use in the treatment of relapsed or refractory indolent NHL or mantle cell lymphoma.

For further information on the use of combination therapy with rituximab and bendamustine for the treatment of relapsed or refractory indolent NHL or mantle cell lymphoma, see Relapsed or Refractory Non-Hodgkin's Lymphoma or Mantle Cell Lymphoma under Uses: Non-Hodgkin's Lymphoma, in Bendamustine 10:00.

Previously Untreated Follicular Non-Hodgkin's Lymphoma
Immunotherapy with Rituximab

Rituximab is used in combination with chemotherapy for the treatment of previously untreated follicular, antigen CD20-positive, B-cell NHL.

In an open-label, multicenter, randomized trial, 322 patients with previously untreated follicular B-cell NHL received either rituximab with cyclophosphamide, vincristine, and prednisone (CVP) or CVP alone. CVP was administered in eight 3-week cycles; in the combined modality regimen, rituximab 375 mg/m^2 was administered on day 1 of each cycle of CVP. Among patients receiving rituximab, 85% received the maximum dosage (a total of 8 doses). The median age of the patients was 52 years, and 26% of the patients were 60 years of age or older. Most of the patients had stage III or IV disease, 50% had an International Prognostic Index score of at least 2, and the diagnosis of follicular NHL was centrally confirmed in 95% of the patients.

Median progression-free survival was prolonged in patients with advanced follicular NHL receiving rituximab with CVP (2.4 years) compared with those receiving CVP alone (1.4 years). The risk of disease progression, relapse, or death was reduced (hazard ratio: 0.44, range: 0.29–0.65) in patients receiving the rituximab-containing regimen. Patients receiving rituximab and CVP experienced higher incidences of neutropenia (8 versus 3%) and infusion-related toxicity, including rash (17 versus 5%), cough (15 versus 6%), flushing (14 versus 3%), rigors (10 versus 2%), pruritus (10 versus 1%), and chest tightness (7 versus 1%) than those receiving CVP alone.

Radioimmunotherapy with Rituximab and Ibritumomab

Rituximab is used as a required component of a therapeutic regimen with ibritumomab tiuxetan (ibritumomab tiuxetan therapeutic regimen) for consolidation treatment of newly diagnosed follicular NHL in patients who have achieved partial or complete response to first-line induction chemotherapy. Data from a phase 3, open-label study indicate that median progression-free survival is longer in such patients receiving consolidation therapy with the ibritumomab tiuxetan therapeutic regimen compared with those receiving no further treatment; comparative effects on survival have not been established. The regimen consists of an initial rituximab dose (administered on day 1) and a second rituximab dose (administered on day 7, 8, or 9) followed within 4 hours by a therapeutic dose of yttrium Y 90 ibritumomab tiuxetan. For additional information on the use of rituximab as part of the ibritumomab tiuxetan therapeutic regimen for NHL, see Ibritumomab Tiuxetan 10:00.

Previously Untreated Indolent Non-Hodgkin's Lymphoma or Mantle Cell Lymphoma

Efficacy and safety of rituximab in combination with bendamustine† for the treatment of previously untreated advanced-stage indolent NHL or previously untreated advanced-stage mantle cell lymphoma† have been studied in two phase 3 studies (Study Group Indolent Lymphomas [StiL] NHL 1-2003 and BRIGHT).

In the StiL NHL 1-2003 study in 514 patients with previously untreated mantle cell lymphoma or CD20-positive indolent NHL, rituximab in combination with bendamustine was noninferior to rituximab in combination with cyclophosphamide, doxorubicin, vincristine, and prednisone (R-CHOP) in terms of progression-free survival; median progression-free survival was 69.5 and 31.2 months in patients receiving rituximab in combination with bendamustine and those receiving R-CHOP, respectively. Overall response rates were similar in patients receiving rituximab in combination with bendamustine and those receiving R-CHOP (93 versus 91%, respectively); however, the complete response rate was higher in the rituximab-bendamustine group (40 versus 30%). Although median overall survival had not been reached in either group at the time of analysis, substantial differences were not observed between the treatment groups.

In the BRIGHT study in 447 patients with previously untreated mantle cell lymphoma or CD20-positive indolent NHL, rituximab in combination with bendamustine was noninferior to standard combination chemotherapy (R-CHOP or rituximab in combination with cyclophosphamide, vincristine, and prednisone [R-CVP]) for attainment of complete response; complete response was achieved in 31% of patients receiving rituximab in combination with bendamustine and 25% of those receiving R-CHOP or R-CVP. Although complete response rates in patients with indolent NHL (mainly follicular lymphoma) tended to favor the rituximab-bendamustine regimen over R-CHOP or R-CVP, subset analysis failed to establish noninferiority of the rituximab-bendamustine regimen in patients with indolent NHL or follicular lymphoma. In the subset of patients with mantle cell lymphoma, complete response rates were higher in patients receiving rituximab in combination with bendamustine compared with those receiving R-CHOP or R-CVP. Overall response rates were higher in patients receiving rituximab in combination with bendamustine compared with those receiving R-CHOP or R-CVP (97 versus 91%).

Based on current evidence, use of rituximab in combination with bendamustine may be considered a reasonable choice (accepted, with possible conditions) for the treatment of previously untreated advanced-stage indolent NHL or mantle cell lymphoma; however, the histologic subtype of NHL should be considered when selecting a combination chemotherapy regimen.

For further information on the use of combination therapy with rituximab and bendamustine for the treatment of previously untreated advanced-stage indolent NHL or mantle cell lymphoma, see Previously Untreated, Indolent Non-Hodgkin's Lymphoma or Mantle Cell Lymphoma under Uses: Non-Hodgkin's Lymphoma, in Bendamustine 10:00.

Nonprogressing Low-grade Non-Hodgkin's Lymphoma

Rituximab is used as a single agent for the treatment of nonprogressing (including stable disease) low-grade, antigen CD20-positive, B-cell NHL following first-line combination chemotherapy with cyclophosphamide, vincristine, and prednisone (CVP). This indication is based on data from an open-label, multicenter, randomized trial in which 322 patients with previously untreated low-grade B-cell NHL (IWF histologic subtype A, B, or C) received 6 or 8 cycles of CVP followed by rituximab or no further treatment.

In the combined modality regimen, patients received rituximab 375 mg/m^2 once weekly for 4 weeks (4 doses total) every 6 months for up to 16 doses total; 59% of the patients received the maximum dosage of rituximab. The median age of patients receiving rituximab was 58 years; 37% of the patients in the study were 60 years of age or older. Most of the patients had stage III or IV disease, 63% had an International Prognostic Index score of at least 2, and the diagnosis of low-grade NHL was centrally confirmed in 62% of the patients.

The risk of disease progression, relapse, or death was reduced (estimated hazard ratio: 0.36–0.49) in patients receiving the rituximab-containing regimen. Patients receiving rituximab following CVP experienced higher incidences of grade 3 or 4 neutropenia (4 versus 1%) than those receiving no further treatment; other adverse effects that occurred more frequently in patients receiving rituximab included fatigue (39 versus 14%), anemia (35 versus 20%), peripheral sensory neuropathy (30 versus 18%), infection (19 versus 9%), pulmonary toxicity (18 versus 10%), hepatobiliary toxicity (17 versus 7%), rash and/or pruritus (17 versus 5%), arthralgia (12 versus 3%), and weight gain (11 versus 4%).

Previously Untreated Diffuse Large B-cell Non-Hodgkin's Lymphoma

Rituximab is used in combination with cyclophosphamide, doxorubicin, vincristine, and prednisone (CHOP) or other anthracycline-based regimens for the treatment of previously untreated diffuse large B-cell, antigen CD20-positive, NHL. This indication is based on data from 3 open-label, multicenter, randomized trials involving a total of 1854 patients who received rituximab with combination chemotherapy (CHOP or other anthracycline-based regimen) or combination chemotherapy alone for previously untreated diffuse large B-cell NHL. The addition of rituximab to chemotherapy was shown to offer benefit in older patients with advanced-stage disease as well as younger patients with early-stage disease.

In the first randomized trial (the NCI-sponsored E4494 trial), 632 patients (60 years of age or older) with diffuse large B-cell NHL (IWF histologic subtype F, G, or H B-cell NHL or diffuse large B-cell NHL including primary mediastinal B-cell lymphoma according to the Revised European-American Lymphoma [REAL] classification) received 6 or 8 cycles of CHOP with or without rituximab 375 mg/m² (2 doses preceding the first 21-day cycle of chemotherapy and then 1 dose preceding cycles 3, 5, and 7 for a total of 4 or 5 doses). Most of the patients (73%) had stage III or IV disease, 30% had extranodal disease in at least 2 sites, 56% had an International Prognostic Index score of at least 2, 86% had an ECOG performance status less than 2, and the diagnosis of diffuse large B-cell NHL was centrally confirmed in 62% of the patients. Median progression-free survival was prolonged in patients with diffuse large B-cell NHL receiving rituximab and CHOP (3.1 years) compared with those receiving CHOP alone (1.6 years). The risk of disease progression, relapse, or death was reduced (hazard ratio: 0.69) in patients receiving the rituximab-containing regimen. Patients with disease that responded to treatment with rituximab and CHOP then received either additional rituximab therapy or no further therapy. The statistical evaluation of the data for induction therapy with rituximab was designed to exclude the effect of additional rituximab therapy; additional rituximab therapy did not affect survival.

In the second randomized trial (the Groupe d'Etude des Lymphomes de l'Adulte trial), 399 patients (60 years of age or older, median age: 69 years) with diffuse large B-cell NHL received up to 8 cycles of CHOP with or without rituximab 375 mg/m² on day 1 of each 21-day cycle. Most of the patients (80%) had stage III or IV disease, 52% had extranodal disease in at least 2 sites, 60% had an age-adjusted International Prognostic Index score of at least 2, and 80% had an ECOG performance status less than 2. Median event-free survival was prolonged in patients with diffuse large B-cell NHL receiving rituximab and CHOP (2.9 years) compared with those receiving CHOP alone (1.1 years). The risk of disease progression, relapse, change in therapy, or death from any cause was reduced (hazard ratio: 0.60) in patients receiving the rituximab-containing regimen. Estimated overall survival at 5 years was 58% for patients receiving rituximab-CHOP versus 46% for patients receiving CHOP alone.

In the third randomized trial (the MabThera International Trial M39045), 823 patients (18–60 years of age) with diffuse large B-cell NHL received an anthracycline-containing chemotherapy regimen with or without rituximab. Among all patients, 28% had stage III or IV disease, 49% had bulky disease, and 34% had extranodal disease; 100% had an International Prognostic Index score of 1 or less, and 99% had an ECOG performance status less than 2. The main end point of the study was time to treatment failure. The risk of disease progression, failure to achieve a complete response, relapse, or death was reduced (hazard ratio: 0.45) in patients receiving the rituximab-containing regimen.

Patients with diffuse large B-cell NHL receiving rituximab and CHOP in clinical trials experienced a higher incidence of certain adverse effects. Grade 3 or 4 thrombocytopenia (9 versus 7%) and grade 3 or 4 lung disorder (6 versus 3%) occurred more frequently in patients receiving rituximab-CHOP than in those receiving CHOP alone. Other adverse effects that occurred more frequently in patients 60 years of age or older who received rituximab and CHOP included pyrexia (56 versus 46%), lung disorder (31 versus 24%), cardiac disorder (29 versus 21%), and chills (13 versus 4%). In the second randomized trial, the higher incidence of cardiac disorders in patients receiving rituximab and CHOP was caused mainly by increased frequency of supraventricular arrhythmias or tachycardia (4.5 versus 1%). Other severe adverse effects that occurred more frequently in patients receiving rituximab and CHOP than in those receiving CHOP alone (in one or more studies) were viral infection, neutropenia, and anemia.

Responses to rituximab therapy have been observed in patients with recurrent aggressive antigen CD20-positive NHL†.

● *Chronic Lymphocytic Leukemia*

Rituximab is used in combination with fludarabine and cyclophosphamide (R-FC) for the treatment of previously untreated and previously treated antigen CD20-positive chronic lymphocytic leukemia (CLL). Rituximab is designated an orphan drug by FDA for the treatment of this cancer.

Previously Untreated Chronic Lymphocytic Leukemia

Rituximab is used in combination with fludarabine and cyclophosphamide (R-FC) for the treatment of previously untreated antigen CD20-positive chronic lymphocytic leukemia (CLL). This indication is based principally on the results of

a multicenter, open-label, randomized study (CLL8) in which 817 adult patients with previously untreated CLL were randomized to receive 6 cycles of either FC (fludarabine 25 mg/m² and cyclophosphamide 250 mg/m², administered IV on days 1–3 of each 28-day cycle) or FC in combination with rituximab (rituximab 375 mg/m² administered by IV infusion on day 0 during the first FC cycle, followed by rituximab 500 mg/m² IV on day 1 during subsequent FC cycles). The median age of patients in this study was 61 years, and 30% of the patients were 65 years of age or older. Approximately 5, 64, or 31% of patients in this study had Binet stage A, stage B, or stage C disease, respectively. More than 99% of patients had an ECOG performance status of 0–1.

At a median follow-up of 37.7 months, patients receiving R-FC experienced prolonged median progression-free survival (51.8 versus 32.8 months), a higher overall response rate (95 versus 88%), a higher complete response rate (44 versus 22%), and a higher overall survival rate (84 versus 79%, although median survival has not been reached) compared with patients receiving FC. In patients receiving R-FC, the largest benefit on progression-free survival, overall response, and complete response was observed in those with Binet stage A or stage B CLL; in addition, only patients with Binet stage A or stage B CLL experienced an improved benefit in overall survival. Based on results of an exploratory analysis (stratified by age), the addition of rituximab to FC resulted in no additional benefit in progression-free survival in patients 70 years of age or older.

Patients receiving R-FC experienced higher incidences of adverse hematologic effects (i.e., neutropenia, leukopenia, febrile neutropenia, pancytopenia) compared with those receiving FC; however, this was not associated with an increase in infection rate. Patients receiving R-FC also experienced a higher incidence of infusion-related effects. The treatment-related mortality rate was similar (2%) in patients receiving R-FC compared with those receiving FC.

Previously Treated Chronic Lymphocytic Leukemia

Rituximab is used in combination with fludarabine and cyclophosphamide (R-FC) for the treatment of previously treated antigen CD20-positive chronic lymphocytic leukemia (CLL). This indication is based principally on the results of a multicenter, open-label, randomized study (REACH) in which 552 adult patients with previously treated CLL were randomized to receive 6 cycles of either FC (fludarabine 25 mg/m² and cyclophosphamide 250 mg/m², administered IV on days 1–3 of each 28-day cycle) or FC in combination with rituximab (rituximab 375 mg/m² administered by IV infusion on day 0 during the first FC cycle, followed by 500 mg/m² IV on day 1 during subsequent FC cycles). The median age in this study was 63 years, and 44% of the patients were 65 years of age or older. Approximately 9, 60, or 31% of patients in this study had Binet stage A, stage B, or stage C disease, respectively. Most patients (82%) had received previous treatment with an alkylating agent (27% alkylator refractory, 55% alkylator sensitive), and 17% had previously received (and demonstrated response to) fludarabine; fludarabine-refractory patients or patients who had received previous treatment with interferon, rituximab, other monoclonal antibodies, or stem-cell transplantation were excluded from the study. All patients had an ECOG performance status of 0–1.

At a median follow-up of 25 months, patients receiving R-FC experienced prolonged median progression-free survival (27 versus 21.9 months), a higher overall response rate (61 versus 49%), and a higher complete response rate (9 versus 3%) compared with patients receiving FC. Among patients receiving R-FC, improved progression-free survival was observed in patients across all Binet stages as well as in patients with high lymphocyte counts, poor renal function, or poor prognostic factors (e.g., del11q, unmutated IgVH, positive ZAP-70). Based on results of an exploratory analysis (stratified by age), the addition of rituximab to FC resulted in no additional benefit in progression-free survival in patients 65 years or older. No difference in overall survival has been observed with the R-FC regimen compared with the FC regimen.

Patients receiving R-FC experienced higher incidences of grade 3 or 4 neutropenia; however, this was not associated with an increase in the overall incidence of infections or grade 3 or 4 infections. Hepatitis B (primary infection and reactivation) was reported in 3% of patients receiving R-FC and in less than 1% of those receiving FC.

● *Rheumatoid Arthritis*

Rituximab in combination with methotrexate is used for the treatment of moderately to severely active rheumatoid arthritis (RA) in adults with disease that has shown an inadequate response to therapy with at least one tumor necrosis factor (TNF; TNF-α) antagonist. This indication is based mainly on data from 2 randomized, double-blind, placebo-controlled studies in patients at least 18 years of age who had a diagnosis of RA according to American College of Rheumatology (ACR) criteria and had active disease (at least 8 swollen joints and 8 tender joints).

In the first randomized study, patients received an IV infusion of either rituximab 1 g or placebo on days 1 and 15 (for a total of 2 doses) in combination with continued therapy with oral or parenteral methotrexate 10–25 mg weekly for 24 weeks. Patients were permitted to receive additional courses of rituximab (given as 2 separate doses of 1 g each) in combination with methotrexate in an open-label extension study at intervals determined by clinical evaluation, but no sooner than 16 weeks after the previous dose of rituximab. IV glucocorticoid was administered prior to each rituximab infusion, and oral glucocorticoid was administered on a tapering schedule from baseline through day 14. At 24 weeks, the number of patients achieving a response measured as a percentage improvement (20%, 50%, or 70%) in disease symptoms according to ACR criteria was higher for those receiving rituximab and methotrexate compared with those receiving placebo and methotrexate (ACR 20: 51 versus 18%, ACR 50: 27 versus 5%, ACR 70: 12 versus 1%). Favorable responses were noted for all components of the ACR response including reduced counts for swollen and tender joints, improvement according to physician and patient global assessments, reduced pain, reduced disability, and reduced serum C-reactive protein (CRP) concentrations. Although all patients experienced similar benefits at week 4 following a brief course of IV and oral glucocorticoids, the number of patients experiencing ACR responses (at all levels) from week 8 through week 24 was higher among those receiving rituximab and methotrexate. Results of the open-label extension study indicate that the combination of rituximab and methotrexate is more effective than methotrexate alone in delaying radiographic progression of structural damage (defined as changes in the Genant-modified total Sharp score [TSS], erosion score [ES], and joint space narrowing [JSN] score) after one year of therapy; progression of structural damage was further delayed following 2 years of therapy. Approximately 57% of patients receiving rituximab in combination with methotrexate had no progression of structural damage after 2 years of therapy.

In the second randomized study, all patients received the first course of rituximab (2 separate doses of 1 g each) in combination with methotrexate. Patients who experienced ongoing disease activity were randomized to receive either a second course of rituximab (2 separate doses of 1 g each) in combination with methotrexate or placebo in combination with methotrexate, generally between weeks 24–28. At week 48, 54, 29, or 14% of patients receiving rituximab in combination with methotrexate achieved ACR 20, ACR 50, or ACR 70, respectively, compared with 45, 26, or 13%, respectively, of those receiving methotrexate alone.

Efficacy of rituximab has been established in 4 controlled studies in patients with RA who had an inadequate response to nonbiologic disease-modifying antirheumatic drugs (DMARDs) and in one controlled study in methotrexate-naive patients; however, a favorable risk-benefit ratio has not been established for the use of rituximab in these patient populations. In one of the 4 controlled studies, 342 adult patients with moderately to severely active RA who had an inadequate response to methotrexate were randomized to receive methotrexate in combination with either rituximab 1 g (given as 2 separate does of 500 mg each), rituximab 2 g (given as 2 separate does of 1 g each), or placebo. At 24 weeks, more patients receiving methotrexate in combination with rituximab 2 g had clinically meaningful improvement in physical function, as reflected by improvement in the Health Assessment Questionnaire Disability Index (HAQ-DI) score, than patients receiving methotrexate with placebo (58 versus 48%). In addition, patients receiving methotrexate in combination with rituximab experienced greater improvement from baseline in HAQ-DI score at 24 weeks than did patients receiving methotrexate with placebo. These improvements were maintained at 48 weeks. Improvements in HAQ-DI score observed with the 2 rituximab dosages (1 g or 2 g) were similar; however, radiographic responses were not assessed. In another randomized study, 161 patients with active RA despite treatment with methotrexate received one of the following regimens: oral methotrexate (at least 10 mg weekly), rituximab (1 g IV on days 1 and 15), rituximab (same dosage) and cyclophosphamide (750 mg IV on days 3 and 17), or rituximab (same dosage) and methotrexate (at least 10 mg weekly). At week 24, the proportion of patients achieving an ACR 50 response was greater in those receiving rituximab-methotrexate (43%) or rituximab-cyclophosphamide (41%) than in those receiving methotrexate alone (13%). Responses at all levels of improvement (i.e., ACR 20, 50, and 70 responses) were maintained at week 48 in the rituximab-methotrexate group.

Efficacy of rituximab also has been established in one randomized, double-blind, placebo-controlled study in methotrexate-naive patients. In this study, patients with moderately to severely active RA were randomized to

receive methotrexate (7.5 mg weekly initially, then titrated up to 20 mg weekly by week 8) in combination with either rituximab 1 g (500 mg IV on days 1 and 15), rituximab 2 g (1 g IV on days 1 and 15), or placebo. After a minimum of 24 weeks, patients with ongoing disease activity were permitted to receive retreatment with additional courses of their assigned treatment. Following one year of therapy, the proportion of patients achieving ACR 20, ACR 50, or ACR 70 was similar among those receiving methotrexate with either dose of rituximab, which was higher than the proportion of patients receiving methotrexate with placebo. However, only the combination of methotrexate with high dose rituximab (2 g) was shown to be more effective than methotrexate alone in delaying radiographic progression of structural damage (as assessed by TSS). Despite the demonstrated efficacy in patients who had an inadequate response to DMARDs and in methotrexate-naive patients, a favorable risk-benefit ratio has not been established for the use of rituximab in these patient populations; therefore, the use of rituximab for RA in patients with disease that has no prior inadequate response to one or more TNF antagonists currently is *not* recommended.

Adverse effects during the 24-hour period following the first infusion, such as acute infusion reactions, occurred more frequently in patients receiving rituximab-methotrexate than in those receiving placebo-methotrexate (overall adverse effects: 32 versus 23%, acute infusion reactions: 27 versus 19%).

● *Other Uses*

Rituximab has been used in the treatment of other forms of NHL, including lymphoplasmacytic lymphoma (Waldenstrom's macroglobulinemia)†. Rituximab also has been used in the treatment of relapsed or refractory hairy cell leukemia†.

Rituximab has been used for the treatment of idiopathic thrombocytopenic purpura (ITP; also known as immune thrombocytopenic purpura)† in adult patients. Results of a meta-analysis indicated an overall response (platelet counts exceeding 50,000/mm³) or complete response (platelet counts exceeding 150,000/mm³) rate of approximately 63 or 46%, respectively; however, because of the lack of controlled randomized studies, efficacy of rituximab compared with standard treatments for ITP cannot be determined, and indiscriminate use of rituximab for the treatment of ITP in adult patients should be *avoided*. Rituximab also has been used in children with severe chronic ITP refractory to standard therapy†. However, because of the low response rate (30–60%) and potentially serious adverse effects (including progressive multifocal leukoencephalopathy [PML]), some experts recommend that rituximab be reserved for pediatric patients with chronic ITP who have failed splenectomy.

Rituximab and immune globulin IV has been used in the treatment of refractory pemphigus vulgaris†.

DOSAGE AND ADMINISTRATION

● *Reconstitution and Administration*

Rituximab is administered by IV infusion. Rituximab solutions should *not* be administered undiluted nor by rapid IV injection.

Rituximab for injection concentrate *must* be diluted prior to IV infusion. For IV infusion, the appropriate dose of rituximab for injection concentrate should be withdrawn and diluted in the appropriate volume of 0.9% sodium chloride or 5% dextrose injection to yield a final rituximab concentration of 1–4 mg/mL. Aseptic technique should be used, and the IV bag should be gently inverted to mix the solution. Any unused solution remaining in the vial should be discarded. No other drug should be added to or administered in the same IV line with rituximab infusion. Prior to administration, rituximab solutions should be inspected visually for particulate matter and discoloration. If particulate matter or discoloration is evident, the solution should not be used.

The initial rituximab dose should be infused at an initial rate of 50 mg/hour; if infusion-related events do not occur, the infusion rate may be increased in increments of 50 mg/hour every 30 minutes to a maximum infusion rate of 400 mg/hour. In patients who tolerate the first infusion well, subsequent rituximab infusions may be administered at an initial infusion rate of 100 mg/hour; the rate of infusion may be increased in increments of 100 mg/hour every 30 minutes as tolerated to a maximum infusion rate of 400 mg/hour.

Patients with previously untreated follicular non-Hodgkin's lymphoma (NHL) or previously untreated diffuse large B-cell NHL who are receiving rituximab in combination with a glucocorticoid-containing chemotherapy regimen may receive the second rituximab dose at an accelerated infusion rate if they tolerate the first dose (administered at the standard rate) without experiencing grade 3 or 4 infusion-related events. In such patients, the second rituximab infusion may be administered over a total infusion time of 90 minutes, with 20% of the total dose administered over the first 30 minutes and the remaining 80% of the total dose administered over the next 60 minutes. Those who tolerate this 90-minute infusion may receive subsequent rituximab doses (through cycle 6 or 8) at the same 90-minute infusion rate. Patients should receive the glucocorticoid component of the chemotherapy regimen prior to each rituximab infusion to reduce the incidence and severity of infusion reactions. Patients with clinically important cardiovascular disease (i.e., uncontrolled hypertension, myocardial infarction [MI], unstable angina, New York Heart Association [NYHA] functional class II or greater congestive heart failure [CHF], ventricular arrhythmia requiring medication within the past year, NYHA class II or greater peripheral vascular disease) or with a high circulating lymphocyte count (5000/mm³ or greater) before cycle 2 should *not* receive rituximab over 90 minutes, as these patients were excluded from the phase 3 noncomparative trial (RATE) evaluating this infusion rate.

● Dosage

To minimize the risk of infusion-related events (see Cautions: Infusion-Related Effects) associated with rituximab, premedication with acetaminophen and an antihistamine is recommended before each infusion of the drug. Because transient hypotension may occur during administration of rituximab, it may be appropriate to withhold antihypertensive therapy during the 12-hour period preceding each rituximab infusion.

Non-Hodgkin's Lymphoma

Immunotherapy for Relapsed or Refractory Low-grade or Follicular Non-Hodgkin's Lymphoma

For the treatment of relapsed or refractory low-grade or follicular, antigen CD20-positive, B-cell NHL, the recommended dosage of rituximab is 375 mg/m² administered by IV infusion once weekly for 4 weeks or 8 weeks. Patients who subsequently develop progressive disease following response to previous rituximab therapy may receive an additional course of rituximab 375 mg/m² by IV infusion once weekly for 4 weeks.

Radiotherapy for Relapsed or Refractory Low-grade or Follicular Non-Hodgkin's Lymphoma

When used in conjunction with ibritumomab as a component of a radioimmunotherapeutic regimen for relapsed or refractory low-grade or follicular B-cell NHL, rituximab 250 mg/m² should be infused on day 1 and then again on day 7, 8, or 9; the second dose of rituximab should be followed within 4 hours by a therapeutic dose of yttrium Y 90 ibritumomab tiuxetan. For additional dosage information regarding the use of rituximab as part of the ibritumomab tiuxetan therapeutic regimen, see Ibritumomab Tiuxetan 10:00.

Combination Therapy for Relapsed or Refractory Indolent Non-Hodgkin's Lymphoma or Mantle Cell Lymphoma

When rituximab has been used in combination with bendamustine† in adults with relapsed or refractory indolent NHL or relapsed or refractory mantle cell lymphoma†, rituximab 375 mg/m² has been administered by IV infusion on day 1, followed by IV infusion (over 30–60 minutes) of bendamustine hydrochloride 90 mg/m² on days 2 and 3. The bendamustine-rituximab regimen has been administered on a 28-day cycle for a total of 4–6 cycles. An additional dose of rituximab has been administered one week prior to the first bendamustine-rituximab treatment cycle and repeated at 28 days following the last bendamustine-rituximab treatment cycle.

Previously Untreated Follicular Non-Hodgkin's Lymphoma

For the treatment of previously untreated follicular, antigen CD20-positive, B-cell NHL, the recommended dosage of rituximab is 375 mg/m² administered by IV infusion on day 1 of each cycle of chemotherapy for up to 8 doses.

When used in conjunction with ibritumomab as a component of a radioimmunotherapeutic regimen for consolidation treatment of follicular NHL in patients who have achieved partial or complete response to first-line induction chemotherapy, rituximab 250 mg/m² should be infused on day 1 and then again on day 7, 8, or 9; the second dose of rituximab should be followed within 4 hours by a therapeutic dose of yttrium Y 90 ibritumomab tiuxetan. For additional

dosage information regarding the use of rituximab as part of the ibritumomab tiuxetan therapeutic regimen, see Ibritumomab Tiuxetan 10:00.

Combination Therapy for Previously Untreated Indolent Non-Hodgkin's Lymphoma or Mantle Cell Lymphoma

When rituximab has been used in combination with bendamustine† in adults with previously untreated advanced-stage indolent NHL or previously untreated advanced-stage mantle cell lymphoma†, rituximab 375 mg/m² has been administered by IV infusion on day 1, followed by IV infusion (over 30–60 minutes) of bendamustine hydrochloride 90 mg/m² on days 1 and 2. The bendamustine-rituximab regimen has been administered on a 28-day cycle for up to 8 cycles.

Nonprogressing, Low-grade Non-Hodgkin's Lymphoma

For the treatment of nonprogressing (including stable disease), low-grade, antigen CD20-positive, B-cell NHL following first-line therapy with 6–8 cycles of chemotherapy with cyclophosphamide, vincristine, and prednisone (CVP), the recommended dosage of rituximab is 375 mg/m² administered by IV infusion once weekly for 4 doses every 6 months for up to 16 doses total.

Previously Untreated Diffuse Large B-cell Non-Hodgkin's Lymphoma

For the treatment of previously untreated diffuse large B-cell NHL, the recommended dosage of rituximab is 375 mg/m² administered by IV infusion on day 1 of each cycle of chemotherapy (such as cyclophosphamide, doxorubicin, vincristine, and prednisone [CHOP]) for up to 8 doses total.

Chronic Lymphocytic Leukemia

For patients receiving rituximab in combination with fludarabine and cyclophosphamide for chronic lymphocytic leukemia, prophylaxis against *Pneumocystis jiroveci* (formerly *Pneumocystis carinii*) pneumonia (PCP) (i.e., co-trimoxazole) and herpes virus infection (i.e., acyclovir/valacyclovir) is recommended during treatment and for up to 12 months following discontinuance of therapy.

Previously Untreated Chronic Lymphocytic Leukemia

For the treatment of previously untreated antigen CD20-positive chronic lymphocytic leukemia, the recommended dosage of rituximab is 375 mg/m² administered by IV infusion on day 0 of the *first* cycle of chemotherapy with fludarabine and cyclophosphamide (FC, administered on days 1–3 of each 28-day cycle), followed by 500 mg/m² administered by IV infusion on day 1 of *subsequent* FC cycles (cycles 2–6, administered every 28 days), for up to 6 doses total.

Previously Treated Chronic Lymphocytic Leukemia

For the treatment of previously treated antigen CD20-positive chronic lymphocytic leukemia, the recommended dosage of rituximab is 375 mg/m² administered by IV infusion on day 0 of the *first* cycle of chemotherapy with fludarabine and cyclophosphamide (FC, administered on days 1–3 of each 28-day cycle), followed by 500 mg/m² administered by IV infusion on day 1 of *subsequent* FC cycles (cycles 2–6, administered every 28 days), for up to 6 doses total.

Rheumatoid Arthritis

For patients receiving rituximab for rheumatoid arthritis, glucocorticoid (methylprednisolone 100 mg IV or its equivalent) should be administered 30 minutes prior to each infusion to reduce the incidence and severity of infusion reactions.

When used in combination with methotrexate to reduce the signs and symptoms of moderately to severely active rheumatoid arthritis (RA) in adults with disease that has shown an inadequate response to therapy with at least one tumor necrosis factor (TNF; TNF-α) antagonist, rituximab 1 g is administered as an IV infusion on days 1 and 15 (for a total of 2 doses per course). Subsequent courses of rituximab and methotrexate may be administered every 24 weeks or based on clinical evaluation, but not sooner than every 16 weeks.

Dosage Modification for Toxicity and Contraindications for Continued Therapy

Depending on the severity of the symptoms, the manufacturer recommends temporary or permanent discontinuance of rituximab when severe adverse effects occur; slower infusion rates should be employed when rituximab therapy is reinitiated following interruption of the infusion because of severe drug-related reactions (e.g., infusion-related effects).

Infusion-related Effects

In patients experiencing signs and symptoms of a severe infusion reaction (e.g., urticaria, hypotension, angioedema, hypoxia, bronchospasm, pulmonary infiltrates, acute respiratory distress syndrome, myocardial infarction, ventricular fibrillation, cardiogenic shock, anaphylactoid events), appropriate medications and supportive care (e.g., epinephrine, glucocorticoids, oxygen, bronchodilators) should be provided as clinically indicated. Depending on the severity of the infusion reaction and the required interventions, rituximab infusion should be temporarily or permanently discontinued. Once manifestations of infusion reactions have resolved, the infusion may be resumed but the rate of infusion should be reduced by at least 50%.

Mucocutaneous Effects

In the event of a severe mucocutaneous reaction, rituximab should be discontinued, and the patient should undergo prompt medical evaluation. (See Cautions: Mucocutaneous and Dermatologic Effects and also see Mucocutaneous and Dermatologic Effects under Cautions: Precautions and Contraindications.) Skin biopsy may be useful to diagnose the mucocutaneous reaction and guide treatment. The safety of readministration of rituximab in patients who have experienced a severe mucocutaneous reaction to the drug has not been determined.

Progressive Multifocal Leukoencephalopathy

In patients who develop progressive multifocal leukoencephalopathy (PML), rituximab therapy should be discontinued and reductions or discontinuance of any concomitant chemotherapy or immunosuppressive therapy should be considered. (See Cautions: Progressive Multifocal Leukoencephalopathy and also see Nervous System Effects under Cautions: Precautions and Contraindications.)

Hepatitis B Virus Reactivation

In patients with reactivation of hepatitis B virus (HBV) infection, rituximab therapy and any concomitant chemotherapy should be discontinued, and appropriate treatment, including antiviral therapy, should be initiated. It has not been established whether rituximab can be safely readministered in patients who develop HBV reactivation. Clinicians with expertise in managing HBV infection should be consulted regarding resumption of rituximab therapy once control of the reactivated infection has been achieved. (See Cautions: Hepatitis B Virus Reactivation and also see Hepatic Effects under Cautions: Precautions and Contraindications.)

Infectious Complications

In patients who develop severe infections, rituximab therapy should be discontinued, and appropriate anti-infective therapy should be initiated. (See Cautions: Infectious Complications and also see Infectious Complications under Cautions: Precautions and Contraindications.)

Cardiovascular Effects

Rituximab infusion should be discontinued in the event of clinically important adverse cardiac events or serious or life-threatening cardiac arrhythmias. In patients who develop serious arrhythmias during rituximab therapy, or who have a history of arrhythmia or angina, cardiac monitoring should be instituted during and following all infusions of rituximab. (See Cautions: Cardiovascular Effects and also see Cardiovascular Effects under Cautions: Precautions and Contraindications.)

Renal Effects

Rituximab therapy should be discontinued in patients who experience oliguria or increases in serum creatinine concentrations. (See Cautions: Renal Effects.)

Respiratory Effects

Some clinicians recommend discontinuance of rituximab if interstitial lung disease is suspected. The manufacturer states the safety of continuing or reinitiating rituximab therapy in patients who have experienced pneumonitis or bronchiolitis obliterans has not been established. (See Cautions: Respiratory Effects and also see Respiratory Effects under Cautions: Precautions and Contraindications.)

CAUTIONS

Serious adverse effects, sometimes fatal, have occurred in patients receiving rituximab. Severe or fatal infusion-related reactions; tumor lysis syndrome associated with fatal renal failure; severe or fatal mucocutaneous reactions; progressive multifocal leukoencephalopathy causing death; hepatitis B reactivation with fulminant hepatitis, hepatic failure, and death; other severe or fatal, bacterial, fungal, and viral infections; serious or life-threatening cardiac arrhythmias; severe or fatal renal toxicity; and fatal bowel obstruction and perforation have occurred in patients receiving rituximab.

Adverse effects, including serious adverse effects, commonly occur with rituximab therapy. In clinical studies of rituximab in patients with relapsed or refractory low-grade or follicular non-Hodgkin's lymphoma (NHL), adverse effects were reported in 99% of patients, and grade 3 or 4 adverse effects were reported in 57% of patients. The most common adverse effects reported in 25% or more of patients in clinical studies are infusion-related reactions, fever, lymphopenia, chills, infection, and asthenia.

The incidence of adverse effects in patients with NHL is based on data collected from clinical trials involving 1606 patients receiving rituximab alone or in combination with chemotherapy, including data collected from 356 patients (median age: 57 years) with relapsed or refractory, low-grade NHL during a 12-month observation period following use of rituximab as a single agent in nonrandomized, single-arm clinical studies. Most patients with NHL received rituximab 375 mg/m^2 IV, given as a single agent weekly for up to 8 doses, in combination with chemotherapy for up to 8 doses, or following chemotherapy for up to 16 doses. Unless otherwise specified for a particular adverse effect in the following discussion, incidence rates for adverse effects in patients with NHL are based mainly on the data for patients receiving single-agent rituximab for relapsed or refractory low-grade or follicular NHL. Many adverse effects of rituximab in patients with NHL generally were mild or moderate in severity; the incidence of grade 3 or 4 adverse effects often was 1% or less with the exception of a smaller subset of certain adverse effects that occurred more frequently with greater severity (e.g., grade 3 or 4 lymphopenia in 40%, grade 3 or 4 neutropenia in 6%).

The incidence of adverse effects in patients with chronic lymphocytic leukemia (CLL) is based on data from clinical trials involving 676 patients receiving rituximab in combination with chemotherapy. The most common adverse effects reported in 25% or more of patients are infusion-related reactions and neutropenia.

Incidence rates for adverse effects in patients with rheumatoid arthritis (RA) are based mainly on data from 2578 patients receiving methotrexate with either rituximab or placebo in phase 2 and 3 studies. The most common adverse effects reported in 10% or more of patients are upper respiratory tract infection, nasopharyngitis, urinary tract infection, and bronchitis; other important adverse effects include infusion-related effects, serious infections, and cardiovascular events.

● Infusion-related Effects

Severe infusion-related effects, sometimes fatal, have been reported in patients receiving rituximab. Severe reactions typically occurred during the first infusion, with time to onset of 30–120 minutes. Fatal reactions have occurred within 24 hours of infusion, approximately 80% of which was associated with the first infusion. Manifestations and sequelae of an infusion-related reaction include urticaria, hypotension, angioedema, hypoxia, bronchospasm, pulmonary infiltrates, acute respiratory distress syndrome, myocardial infarction, ventricular fibrillation, cardiogenic shock, anaphylactoid events, or death. (See Infusion-related Effects under Dosage: Dosage Modification for Toxicity and Contraindications for Continued Therapy, in Dosage and Administration and also see Infusion-related Effects under Cautions: Precautions and Contraindications.) Acute infusion-related reactions observed with rituximab result from the release and/or activation of cytokines during B-cell depletion, often referred to as cytokine-release syndrome. Reported risk factors for cytokine-release syndrome and subsequent infusion-related reactions induced by rituximab include older age, high tumor burden, elevated cytokine or complement levels, and B-lymphocyte aggregation or tumor cell agglutination at baseline.

The manufacturer reports that approximately 70 cases of serious infusion-related events, 8 of which were fatal, have been reported out of an estimated 12,000–14,000 patients worldwide who received rituximab therapy between November 1997 and December 1998. In 7 of the 8 fatal cases, manifestations developed during the initial infusion of rituximab, and death in most cases was preceded by severe bronchospasm, dyspnea, hypotension, and/or angioedema. Severe respiratory events, including hypoxia, pulmonary infiltrates, and adult respiratory distress syndrome, contributed to 6 of the 8 deaths. In some cases, manifestations worsened over time, while in others, initial improvement was followed by clinical deterioration. Therefore, patients experiencing any severe infusion-related manifestation should be monitored closely until complete resolution occurs. (See Infusion-related Effects under Dosage: Dosage Modification for Toxicity and Contraindications for Continued Therapy, in Dosage and Administration and also see Infusion-related Effects under Cautions: Precautions and Contraindications.)

Among patients receiving rituximab for NHL, the incidence of infusion reactions was 77% during the first infusion and decreased with each subsequent infusion. Manifestations of infusion-related reactions in these patients included fever, chills/rigors, nausea, pruritus, angioedema, hypotension, headache, bronchospasm, urticaria, rash, vomiting, myalgia, dizziness, and hypertension. These reactions generally occurred within 30–120 minutes of starting the first rituximab infusion and usually resolved with slowing or interruption of the infusion and administration of supportive care, including diphenhydramine, acetaminophen, and IV sodium chloride injection.

Among patients with previously untreated follicular NHL or previously untreated diffuse large B-cell NHL who did not experience a grade 3 or 4 infusion-related reaction to rituximab during the first treatment cycle and who received rituximab as a 90-minute infusion during subsequent treatment cycles, the incidence of grade 3 or 4 infusion-related reactions was 1.1% during cycle 2 and 2.8% during cycles 2–8. During cycle 2, the incidence of grade 3 or 4 infusion-related reactions was 3.5% among patients with follicular NHL receiving rituximab in combination with cyclophosphamide, vincristine, and prednisone (CVP) and 0% among patients with diffuse large B-cell NHL receiving rituximab in combination with cyclophosphamide, doxorubicin, vincristine, and prednisone (CHOP).

Among patients receiving rituximab in combination with fludarabine and cyclophosphamide (FC) for CLL, grade 3 and 4 infusion reactions (defined as nausea, pyrexia, chills, hypotension, vomiting, or dyspnea occurring during or within 24 hours after initiation of rituximab infusion) occurred in 9 or 7% of previously untreated or previously treated patients, respectively.

Among patients receiving rituximab and methotrexate for RA, adverse effects occurred during the 24-hour period following the infusion in 32% of patients following the first infusion and in 11% of patients following the second infusion. Acute infusion reactions (manifested by fever, chills, rigors, pruritus, urticaria, rash, angioedema, sneezing, throat irritation, cough, and/or bronchospasm, with or without associated hypotension or hypertension) occurred in 27% of patients following the first infusion and in 9% of patients following the second infusion. Serious acute infusion reactions occurred in less than 1% of patients. Dosage modification of rituximab (stopping, slowing, or interrupting the infusion) for infusion-related toxicity was required after the first course of therapy in 10% of patients receiving rituximab and methotrexate. The percentage of patients experiencing acute infusion reactions decreased with subsequent courses of rituximab. Although the administration of IV glucocorticoids prior to rituximab infusions reduced the incidence and severity of acute infusion reactions, the administration of oral glucocorticoids provided no clear benefit in preventing such reactions. Antihistamines and acetaminophen also were administered prior to rituximab infusions to prevent infusion-related effects.

● *Tumor Lysis Syndrome*

Tumor lysis syndrome, consisting of rapid reduction in tumor volume followed by acute renal failure, hyperkalemia, hypocalcemia, hyperuricemia, or hyperphosphatemia, occurring within 12–24 hours of completion of the initial infusion of rituximab, has been reported in patients with NHL and sometimes has been fatal. The risk of tumor lysis syndrome is increased in patients with a high number of circulating malignant cells (25,000/mm³ or greater) or a large tumor burden. (See Tumor Lysis Syndrome under Cautions: Precautions and Contraindications.)

● *Mucocutaneous and Dermatologic Effects*

Severe mucocutaneous reactions, sometimes fatal, have been reported in patients receiving rituximab. Severe mucocutaneous reactions associated with rituximab therapy include paraneoplastic pemphigus (an uncommon disorder which is a manifestation of the underlying malignancy), Stevens-Johnson syndrome, lichenoid dermatitis, vesiculobullous dermatitis, and toxic epidermal necrolysis. The onset of severe mucocutaneous reactions is variable but has occurred as early

as the first day of rituximab administration. (See Mucocutaneous Effects under Dosage: Dosage Modification for Toxicity and Contraindications for Continued Therapy, in Dosage and Administration and also see Mucocutaneous and Dermatologic Effects under Cautions: Precautions and Contraindications.)

Adverse effects involving the skin or appendages were reported in 44% of patients receiving single-agent rituximab for NHL in clinical studies and were grade 3 or 4 in severity in 2% of patients. Rash, night sweats, pruritus, and urticaria were reported in 15, 15, 14, and 8% of patients, respectively.

Among patients receiving rituximab and methotrexate for RA, pruritus occurred in 5%, and urticaria in 2%, of patients.

● *Progressive Multifocal Leukoencephalopathy*

Progressive multifocal leukoencephalopathy (PML) secondary to JC infection, sometimes fatal, has been reported in patients receiving rituximab for hematologic malignancies or autoimmune diseases (e.g., RA, systemic lupus erythematosus [SLE]†). Most patients with hematologic malignancies who were diagnosed with PML had received rituximab in combination with chemotherapy or as part of a hematopoietic stem cell transplantation. Patients with autoimmune diseases who developed PML had received prior or concurrent immunosuppressive therapy. Most cases of PML were diagnosed within 12 months of the last infusion of rituximab. PML usually causes death or severe disability, and no therapy is known to prevent, treat, or cure this condition.

In a report from the Research on Adverse Drug Events and Reports (RADAR) project, 52 cases of PML were identified in patients with B-cell lymphoid malignancy (e.g., CLL, NHL); all of these patients had received prior therapies that affect immune function (e.g., alkylating agents, purine analogs, corticosteroids, drugs that prevent allogeneic stem cell or solid organ graft rejection). Reported manifestations of PML, which progressed over weeks to months, included confusion, mental status changes, focal motor weakness, hemiparesis, loss of motor coordination, and speech and vision changes. According to the report, a median of 6 rituximab doses was administered prior to diagnosis of PML, and the median time to diagnosis of PML was 5.5 months following the last dose of rituximab. The case-fatality rate of PML derived from this report was 90%, with a median time to death of 2 months after diagnosis of PML.

Two fatal cases of PML have been reported in patients with RA receiving rituximab; these patients had possible risk factors for PML (e.g., prior chemotherapy and radiation therapy, long-standing lymphopenia). In addition, at least one case of PML has been reported in a patient with RA receiving rituximab who had *not* received prior therapy with a tumor necrosis factor (TNF) antagonist. The manufacturer states that the reported incidence of PML is rare (3 out of 100,000 patients); however, data suggest that patients with RA who receive rituximab are at increased risk of developing PML. (See Progressive Multifocal Leukoencephalopathy under Dosage: Dosage Modification for Toxicity and Contraindications for Continued Therapy, in Dosage and Administration and also see Nervous System Effects under Cautions: Precautions and Contraindications.)

● *Hepatitis B Virus Reactivation*

Reactivation of hepatitis B virus (HBV) infection has been reported in patients receiving anti-CD20 monoclonal antibodies, including rituximab, and has resulted in fulminant hepatitis, hepatic failure, and death. HBV reactivation has been reported in patients who are hepatitis B surface antigen-positive [HBsAg-positive]; HBsAg-negative and hepatitis B core antibody-positive [anti-HBc-positive]; or HBsAg-negative, anti-HBc-positive, and hepatitis B surface antibody-positive [anti-HBs-positive].

Following review of the Adverse Event Reporting System (AERS) database, the US Food and Drug Administration (FDA) identified 106 cases of fatal HBV-related acute liver injury in patients receiving rituximab (between November 1997 and August 2012) and 3 such cases in patients receiving ofatumumab (between October 2009 and August 2012); 32 of these case reports contained sufficient data to meet the criteria for HBV reactivation. In this review, acute liver injury was attributed to HBV reactivation if seroconversion of HBsAg from negative to positive occurred in those with either anti-HBc or a history of HBV, or if an increase in serum HBV DNA level occurred in those who were HBsAg-positive prior to therapy with an anti-CD20 monoclonal antibody (i.e., rituximab, ofatumumab). HBV reactivation was diagnosed by seroconversion of HBsAg in most (69%) cases. In this review, the duration of rituximab or ofatumumab therapy prior to diagnosis of HBV reactivation was highly variable, ranging from 63 days after initiation of the drug to 12 months following the last dose; however, delayed onset of HBV reactivation (up to 24 months following completion of rituximab therapy) has been reported. All of the patients experiencing HBV reactivation had received recent or concomitant therapy with other immunosuppressive agents. Among patients with HBV reactivation, 10% received HBV antiviral prophylaxis and 28% received antiviral treatment for HBV reactivation. (See Hepatitis B Virus Reactivation under Dosage: Dosage Modification for Toxicity and Contraindications for Continued Therapy, in Dosage and Administration and also see Hepatic Effects under Cautions: Precautions and Contraindications.)

● **Infectious Complications**

Serious, including fatal, bacterial, fungal, and new or reactivated viral infections, have been reported during and following completion of rituximab-based therapy. Infections have been reported in some patients with prolonged hypogammaglobulinemia (i.e., hypogammaglobulinemia lasting longer than 11 months following rituximab therapy). New or reactivated viral infections include cytomegalovirus, herpes simplex virus, parvovirus B19, varicella zoster virus, West Nile virus, and hepatitis B and C. (See Infectious Complications under Dosage: Dosage Modification for Toxicity and Contraindications for Continued Therapy, in Dosage and Administration and also see Infectious Complications under Cautions: Precautions and Contraindications.) An increased incidence of fatal infections has been observed in patients receiving rituximab for HIV-associated lymphoma†.

Infection was reported in 31% of patients receiving rituximab for NHL in clinical studies; severe (grade 3 or 4) infections, including sepsis, occurred in 4% of patients. The incidence of bacterial, viral, and fungal infections was 19, 10, and 1%, respectively; 6% of patients had infections of unknown etiology. In patients with NHL receiving rituximab monotherapy, B-cell depletion occurred in 70–80% of patients with NHL, and reduction in serum concentrations of IgG and IgM occurred in 14% of patients.

Among patients receiving rituximab and methotrexate for RA in clinical studies, 39% of patients experienced an infection; the most common infections were nasopharyngitis, upper respiratory tract infection, urinary tract infection, bronchitis, and sinusitis. Serious infection was reported in approximately 2% of patients with RA receiving rituximab; the most common serious infections were pneumonia, lower respiratory tract infection, cellulitis, and urinary tract infection. Fatal serious infections included pneumonia, sepsis, and colitis. The incidence of serious infection remained stable in patients receiving subsequent courses of rituximab. In 185 patients with active RA receiving rituximab, subsequent treatment with a biologic disease-modifying antirheumatic drug (DMARD) did not appear to increase the incidence of serious infection.

JC virus infection causing progressive multifocal leukoencephalopathy (PML), sometimes fatal, has been reported in patients receiving rituximab. (See Cautions: Progressive Multifocal Leukoencephalopathy.)

● **Cardiovascular Effects**

Myocardial infarction, ventricular fibrillation, cardiogenic shock, and/or hypotension have occurred as severe manifestations and sequelae of infusion-related reactions and sometimes led to death in patients receiving rituximab. (See Cautions: Infusion-related Effects.) Other severe adverse cardiac effects, including rare instances of fatal cardiac failure with onset of manifestations weeks after rituximab therapy, have been reported. Cardiac arrhythmias and angina also have been reported. (See Cardiovascular Effects under Dosage: Dosage Modification for Toxicity and Contraindications for Continued Therapy, in Dosage and Administration and also see Cardiovascular Effects under Cautions: Precautions and Contraindications.)

Adverse cardiovascular effects were reported in about 25% of patients receiving single-agent rituximab for NHL in clinical studies and were grade 3 or 4 in severity in 3% of patients. Hypotension, peripheral edema, and hypertension were reported in 10, 8, and 6% of patients, respectively.

Among patients receiving rituximab and methotrexate for RA, serious adverse cardiovascular effects, sometimes fatal, occurred in about 2% of patients; hypertension was reported in 8% of patients.

● **Renal Effects**

Severe, including fatal, renal toxicity can occur after rituximab administration in patients with NHL. Acute renal failure requiring dialysis and sometimes resulting in death, has occurred in patients who experience tumor lysis syndrome. (See Cautions: Tumor Lysis Syndrome, and see Renal Effects under Dosage: Dosage Modification for Toxicity and Contraindications for Continued Therapy, in Dosage and Administration, and also see Tumor Lysis Syndrome under Cautions: Precautions and Contraindications.)

Renal toxicity associated with rituximab also has occurred in patients with NHL receiving concomitant cisplatin therapy† during clinical studies. Combined therapy with rituximab and cisplatin currently is not approved by the US Food and Drug Administration (FDA).

● **GI Effects**

Abdominal pain, bowel obstruction, and bowel perforation, sometimes fatal, can occur in patients receiving rituximab in combination with chemotherapy. In postmarketing reports in patients with NHL, the mean time to documented GI perforation was 6 days (range: 1–77 days).

Adverse GI effects were reported in about 37% of patients receiving single-agent rituximab for NHL in clinical studies and were grade 3 or 4 in severity in 2% of patients. Nausea and vomiting occurred in 23 and 10% of patients, respectively. Abdominal pain and diarrhea occurred in 14 and 10% of patients, respectively.

Among patients receiving rituximab and methotrexate for RA, nausea occurred in 8%, dyspepsia in 3%, and upper abdominal pain in 2% of patients.

Patients receiving rituximab who have complaints suggestive of bowel obstruction, such as abdominal pain or repeated vomiting, should receive a diagnostic evaluation.

● **Respiratory Effects**

Adverse respiratory effects, including acute respiratory distress syndrome, bronchospasm, dyspnea, hypoxia, and pulmonary infiltrates, have occurred as severe manifestations and sequelae of infusion-related reactions to rituximab and sometimes have been fatal. Patients with preexisting pulmonary conditions should be closely monitored for possible infusion-related toxicity. (See Cautions: Infusion-related Effects and also see Infusion-related Effects under Cautions: Precautions and Contraindications.)

Delayed pulmonary toxicity (e.g., bronchiolitis obliterans [presenting during and up to 6 months following rituximab infusion], pneumonitis [including interstitial pneumonitis]), sometimes fatal, has been reported in patients receiving rituximab alone or in combination with other chemotherapeutic agents. In several reports evaluating cases of interstitial lung disease (i.e., interstitial pneumonitis), the most common manifestations observed included dyspnea, fever, and cough. In these reports, if interstitial lung disease was suspected, immediate discontinuance of rituximab was required, and patients were managed with corticosteroid therapy (e.g., methylprednisolone, prednisolone, prednisone) and other clinically appropriate measures (e.g., antibiotics). The manufacturer states the safety of continuing or reinitiating rituximab therapy in patients experiencing pneumonitis or bronchiolitis obliterans has not been established. Interstitial pneumonitis reportedly recurred in a limited number of patients following rechallenge with rituximab. (See Respiratory Effects under Dosage: Dosage Modification for Toxicity and Contraindications for Continued Therapy, in Dosage and Administration and also see Respiratory Effects under Cautions: Precautions and Contraindications.)

Adverse respiratory effects were reported in about 38% of patients receiving single-agent rituximab for NHL in clinical studies and were grade 3 or 4 in severity in 4% of patients. Increased cough, bronchospasm, and dyspnea were reported in 13, 8, and 7% of patients, respectively. Rhinitis, throat irritation, and sinusitis occurred in 12, 9, and 6% of patients, respectively.

Among patients receiving rituximab and methotrexate for RA, rhinitis occurred in 3%, and throat irritation in 2%, of patients.

● **Metabolic and Electrolyte Effects**

Among patients receiving single-agent rituximab for NHL, hyperglycemia and increases in LDH were reported in 9 and 7% of patients, respectively.

Among patients receiving rituximab and methotrexate for RA in controlled clinical studies, hypophosphatemia and hyperuricemia were reported in 12 and 1.5% of patients, respectively. The majority of cases of hypophosphatemia occurred during the rituximab infusion and was considered transient; hypophosphatemia reportedly occurred more frequently in patients who received glucocorticoids.

● **Hematologic Effects**

Adverse hematologic effects, mainly manifested by lymphopenia, occur frequently in patients receiving rituximab. Adverse hematologic or lymphatic system effects were reported in 67% of patients receiving single-agent rituximab for NHL in clinical studies and were grade 3 or 4 in severity in 48% of patients. Lymphopenia was reported in 48% of patients and was grade 3 or 4 in severity in 40% of patients; the median duration of lymphopenia was 14 days (range: 1–588 days).

Grade 3 and 4 cytopenias occurred in 48% of patients receiving single-agent rituximab for NHL in clinical studies. Neutropenia and leukopenia each were reported in 14% of patients and were grade 3 or 4 in severity in 6 and 4% of patients, respectively. The median duration of neutropenia was 13 days (range: 2–116 days). Thrombocytopenia occurred in 12% of patients and was grade 3 or 4 in severity in 2% of patients. Agranulocytosis has been reported in patients receiving rituximab.

Anemia was reported in 8% of patients receiving single-agent rituximab for NHL and was grade 3 or 4 in severity in 3% of patients. At least one case of transient aplastic anemia (pure red cell aplasia) and two cases of hemolytic anemia have been reported in patients receiving rituximab therapy for NHL.

Prolonged pancytopenia, marrow hypoplasia, late onset neutropenia, and hyperviscosity syndrome in lymphoplasmacytic lymphoma (Waldenstrom's macroglobulinemia) have been reported in patients with hematologic malignancies receiving rituximab.

Complete blood cell counts (CBC) and platelet counts should be monitored regularly during rituximab therapy with more frequent monitoring in patients who develop cytopenias. (See Hematologic Effects under Cautions: Precautions and Contraindications.) Cytopenias associated with rituximab may persist for an extended duration (i.e., months) following discontinuation of the drug.

● Immunologic Effects

Administration of rituximab is associated with rapid and sustained depletion of B cells from the peripheral blood and tissues. (See Pharmacology.)

In patients with NHL, sustained and clinically important reductions in serum IgM and IgG concentrations were observed from 5 through 11 months following rituximab therapy; serum IgM and/or IgG concentrations below the normal range were observed in 14% of patients. In clinical studies of patients receiving rituximab for rheumatoid arthritis, total and individual serum immunoglobulin concentrations were reduced at 6 months with the greatest change observed in IgM concentrations. Following 24 weeks of therapy with rituximab, decreases in serum IgM, IgG, or IgA concentrations to below the lower limit of normal were observed in 10, 2.8, or 0.8% of patients, respectively; following repeated courses of rituximab, decreases in serum IgM, IgG, or IgA concentrations to below the lower limit of normal were observed in 23.3, 5.5, or 0.5% of patients, respectively. The clinical importance of decreased immunoglobulin concentrations in patients receiving rituximab for rheumatoid arthritis is uncertain.

Adverse immunologic and/or autoimmune effects reported in patients receiving rituximab include uveitis, optic neuritis, systemic vasculitis, pleuritis, lupus-like syndrome, serum sickness, polyarticular arthritis, and vasculitis with rash.

Among 356 patients with low-grade or follicular NHL receiving single-agent rituximab in clinical studies, positive human antichimeric antibody (HACA) responses were detected in 4 patients (1.1%), 3 of whom achieved an objective clinical response.

Among 2578 patients with RA receiving rituximab, positive HACA responses were detected in 273 patients (11%). Positive HACA responses typically were detected at any time after administration of rituximab and were not associated with increased infusion reactions or other adverse effects. Upon retreatment, the incidence of infusion reactions was similar between HACA-positive and HACA-negative patients; most infusion reactions were mild to moderate. Four HACA-positive patients with RA experienced serious infusion reactions; however, the temporal relationship between HACA positivity and infusion reaction was variable among these patients. The clinical importance of HACA formation in patients receiving rituximab is unclear.

The immune response to various antigens have been evaluated in a randomized, controlled study in patients with RA receiving either rituximab in combination with methotrexate or methotrexate alone. The proportion of patients demonstrating an immune response to pneumococcal vaccine (i.e., measured as an increase in antibody titers to at least 6 of 12 serotypes) was lower in patients receiving rituximab in combination with methotrexate (19%) than in patients receiving methotrexate alone (61%). In addition, a smaller proportion of patients receiving rituximab in combination methotrexate developed detectable concentrations of anti-keyhole limpet hemocyanin (KLH) antibodies after vaccination compared with patients receiving methotrexate alone (47 versus 93%). The

immune response to tetanus toxoid (a recall antigen) and delayed-type hypersensitivity (DTH) response to a candida skin test, however, were similar in patients receiving rituximab in combination with methotrexate compared with patients receiving methotrexate alone. Most patients receiving rituximab in combination with methotrexate had B-cell counts below the lower limit of normal at the time of immunization; the clinical implications of these findings are not known.

● Nervous System Effects

Adverse nervous system effects were reported in about one-third of patients receiving single-agent rituximab for NHL in clinical studies. Headache, dizziness, and anxiety were reported in 19, 10, and 5% of patients, respectively.

Among patients receiving rituximab and methotrexate for RA, anxiety, migraine, and paresthesia each occurred in 2% of patients.

PML secondary to JC infection, sometimes fatal, has been reported in patients receiving rituximab for hematologic malignancies or autoimmune diseases (e.g., RA, systemic lupus erythematosus [SLE]†). (See Cautions: Progressive Multifocal Leukoencephalopathy.)

● Musculoskeletal Effects

Adverse musculoskeletal effects were reported in about 26% of patients receiving single-agent rituximab for NHL in clinical studies and were grade 3 or 4 in severity in 3% of patients. Back pain, myalgia, and arthralgia, each was reported in 10% of patients.

Among patients receiving rituximab and methotrexate for RA, arthralgia occurred in 6% of patients.

● Other Adverse Effects

Fever occurred in 53% of patients receiving rituximab monotherapy for NHL. Chills were reported in 33% of patients with NHL and were grade 3 or 4 in severity in 3% of patients. Other adverse effects in patients receiving single-agent rituximab for NHL included asthenia in 26%, pain in 12%, angioedema in 11%, and flushing in 5% of patients.

Among patients receiving rituximab and methotrexate for RA, pyrexia occurred in 5%, chills in 3%, and asthenia in 2% of patients.

The incidences and types of adverse effects reported in patients with RA were similar following a single course versus repeated courses of rituximab. In a clinical study in which patients received an initial course of methotrexate in combination with rituximab, followed by a second course of methotrexate in combination with either rituximab or placebo, the safety profile reported in patients receiving methotrexate plus rituximab was similar to that reported in patients receiving methotrexate plus placebo.

● Precautions and Contraindications

The use of rituximab is *not* recommended in patients with severe, active infections. Serious adverse effects, including infusion-related reactions, tumor lysis syndrome, mucocutaneous reactions, progressive multifocal leukoencephalopathy, hepatitis B reactivation with fulminant hepatitis, bacterial/fungal/viral infections, cardiac arrhythmias, renal toxicity, and bowel obstruction and perforation, have occurred in patients receiving rituximab and have sometimes been fatal. (See Cautions for further discussion of adverse effects.)

Interruption or discontinuance of rituximab therapy is required in patients experiencing severe or life-threatening adverse reactions. Reinitiation at a slower infusion rate (minimum of 50% reduction in rate) is required if rituximab therapy is resumed following complete resolution of symptoms. (See Dosage Modification for Toxicity and Contraindications for Continued Therapy under Dosage and Administration: Dosage.)

Rituximab may be administered in an outpatient setting; however, appropriate diagnostic and treatment facilities, including medications for the treatment of severe adverse reactions, such as infusion-related reactions, hypersensitivity reactions, and cardiac arrhythmias, must be readily available.

Infusion-related Effects

To minimize the risk of infusion-related effects associated with rituximab, premedication is recommended before each infusion of the drug. (See Dosage and Administration.) Patients (particularly those with preexisting cardiac or pulmonary conditions, those with a high number of circulating malignant B-cells [i.e., 25,000/mm³ or greater], and patients with a history of a cardiopulmonary reaction to rituximab) should be carefully monitored during rituximab infusions. If an infusion reaction occurs, the rituximab infusion should be interrupted and appropriate medications and supportive care provided as clinically indicated. (See Infusion-related Effects under Dosage and Administration: Dosage Modification for Toxicity and Contraindications for Continued Therapy, in Dosage and Administration.)

Because infusion reactions may occur during or within 24 hours after rituximab infusion, patients should be instructed to notify a clinician if they experience any of the following symptoms during or following rituximab infusion: hives (red itchy welts) or rash; itching; swelling of the lips, tongue, throat, or face; sudden cough; shortness of breath, difficulty breathing, or wheezing; weakness; dizziness or feeling faint; palpitations; or chest pain.

Tumor Lysis Syndrome

Patients receiving rituximab should be closely monitored for development of tumor lysis syndrome, including manifestations of renal failure. The manufacturer states that patients at high risk of tumor lysis syndrome (i.e., patients with a high number of circulating malignant cells [25,000/mm³ or greater] or a high tumor burden) should receive aggressive IV hydration and anti-hyperuricemic therapy. If tumor lysis syndrome develops, patients should receive appropriate medical treatment, including correction of electrolyte abnormalities, monitoring of renal function and fluid balance, and any necessary supportive care (e.g., dialysis) as clinically indicated.

Mucocutaneous and Dermatologic Effects

Severe mucocutaneous reactions, sometimes fatal, have been reported in patients receiving rituximab. Patients should be instructed to notify a clinician or to immediately seek medical attention if they experience any of the following symptoms at any time during rituximab therapy: painful sores or ulcers on the skin, lips, or in the mouth; blisters; peeling skin; rash; or pustules. (See Mucocutaneous Effects under Dosage: Dosage Modification for Toxicity and Contraindications for Continued Therapy, in Dosage and Administration and also see Cautions: Mucocutaneous and Dermatologic Effects.)

Nervous System Effects

Neurologic function should be monitored during rituximab therapy. The possible diagnosis of PML should be considered in any patient receiving rituximab who experiences new onset of neurologic manifestations. Diagnostic evaluation, including consultation with a neurologist, brain magnetic resonance imaging (MRI) scan, and lumbar puncture, should be considered as clinically indicated.

Patients receiving rituximab should be advised to immediately inform a clinician if they experience any of the following symptoms: confusion, trouble thinking, loss of balance, change in walking or talking, decreased strength or weakness on one side of the body, or blurred or loss of vision.

Hepatic Effects

To decrease the risk of HBV reactivation, all patients should be screened for HBV infection by measuring HBsAg and anti-HBc before initiating treatment with rituximab. Hepatitis experts should be consulted regarding monitoring and use of antiviral therapy in those with evidence of HBV infection (HBsAg-positive with any antibody status or HBsAg-negative and anti-HBc-positive); although data are limited, treatment guidelines from some experts recommend the use of prophylactic antiviral therapy in patients who are chronic carriers of HBV. Patients with evidence of current or prior HBV infection should be monitored for clinical and laboratory evidence of hepatitis or HBV reactivation during rituximab therapy and for several months thereafter, since reactivation has occurred more than 12 months following completion of therapy. Rituximab and any concomitant chemotherapy should be discontinued immediately if HBV reactivation occurs, and appropriate treatment for HBV infection should be initiated. Concomitant chemotherapy should be discontinued until the HBV infection has been controlled or has resolved. Clinicians with expertise in managing HBV infection should be consulted regarding resumption of rituximab therapy once control of the reactivated HBV infection has been achieved. It has not been established whether rituximab can be safely readministered in patients who develop HBV reactivation. (See Hepatitis B Virus Reactivation under Dosage: Dosage Modification for Toxicity and Contraindications for Continued Therapy, in Dosage and Administration.)

Infectious Complications

Serious, sometimes fatal, infections, have been reported with rituximab therapy. (See Cautions: Infectious Complications.) The manufacturer states that rituximab should *not* be used in patients with severe, active infections.

Patients receiving rituximab in combination with fludarabine and cyclophosphamide for treatment of CLL should receive prophylaxis against *Pneumocystis jiroveci* (formerly *Pneumocystis carinii*) pneumonia (PCP) (i.e., co-trimoxazole) and herpes virus infection (e.g., acyclovir or valacyclovir) during treatment and for up to 12 months following discontinuance of therapy.

Patients should be advised to inform a clinician before initiating rituximab therapy if they have an infection, a weakened immune system, or a history of severe infections (e.g., hepatitis B or C virus, cytomegalovirus, herpes simplex virus, parvovirus B19, varicella zoster virus [chickenpox or shingles], West Nile virus). Patients also should be advised to immediately inform a clinician if they experience any of the following symptoms: fever; persistent runny nose or sore throat; cough; tiredness; body aches; earache; headache; pain during urination; white patches in the mouth or throat; or cuts, scrapes, or incisions that are red, warm, swollen, or painful. (See Infectious Complications under Dosage: Dosage Modification for Toxicity and Contraindications for Continued Therapy, in Dosage and Administration.)

Cardiovascular Effects

Cardiac monitoring should be performed during and after all infusions of rituximab in patients who develop clinically important arrhythmias or who have a history of arrhythmia or angina. Because patients with RA are at increased risk for cardiovascular toxicity compared with the general population, such patients should be monitored carefully throughout the rituximab infusion. (See Cautions: Cardiovascular Effects and also see Cardiovascular Effects under Dosage: Dosage Modification for Toxicity and Contraindications for Continued Therapy, in Dosage and Administration.)

Patients receiving rituximab should be advised to inform a clinician if they experience chest pain or irregular heart beats.

Vaccination Status

The manufacturer makes no specific recommendations regarding vaccination in patients with NHL receiving rituximab; however, the US Centers for Disease Control and Prevention (CDC) and US Public Health Service Advisory Committee on Immunization Practices (ACIP) have established guidelines on the use of vaccines in individuals with altered immunocompetence.

Prior to administering rituximab therapy for RA, the manufacturer states that clinicians should follow CDC guidelines and administer *non-live* (i.e., inactivated) vaccines at least 4 weeks prior to a course of rituximab. Some experts state that appropriate vaccination (e.g., to prevent influenza) may be given during rituximab therapy when clinically indicated; however, immune responses have been shown to be submaximal.

The manufacturer states that administration of vaccines containing *live* virus is *not* recommended prior to or during rituximab therapy. However, some experts state that live, attenuated vaccines may be administered in patients with RA, but only *before* initiation of rituximab therapy.

Prior to initiation of rituximab therapy, patients should be advised to inform their clinician if they recently received or are scheduled to receive any vaccines. Patients also should be advised to inform their clinician if any household contacts are scheduled to receive vaccines.

Hematologic Effects

In patients with lymphoid malignancies receiving rituximab as a single agent, CBCs and platelet counts should be obtained prior to each rituximab course. In those receiving rituximab in combination with chemotherapy, CBCs and platelet counts should be obtained at weekly to monthly intervals; more frequent monitoring is recommended in patients who develop cytopenias.

In patients with RA receiving rituximab, CBCs and platelet counts should be obtained every 2–4 months during treatment.

Cytopenias associated with rituximab may persist for an extended duration (i.e., months) following discontinuance of the drug.

Respiratory Effects

Patients with preexisting pulmonary conditions should be closely monitored for possible infusion-related toxicity.

Patients presenting with manifestations of delayed pulmonary toxicity (e.g., dyspnea, fever, cough) that are *not* associated with an acute infusion-related reaction should undergo prompt medical evaluation (i.e., pulse oximetry or blood gases, chest CT, pulmonary function tests documenting a restrictive pattern and decreased pulmonary diffusion capacity for carbon monoxide [DL$_{CO}$], other evaluations to rule out an infectious etiology or interstitial fibrosis) for possible interstitial lung disease. If interstitial lung disease is suspected, some clinicians recommend that rituximab be discontinued and corticosteroid (i.e., glucocorticoid) therapy, along with other clinically appropriate measures (e.g., antibiotics), initiated. (See Cautions: Respiratory Effects.)

Other Precautions and Contraindications

Prior to each treatment session, the patient should be given a copy of the manufacturer's patient information (medication guide) and an opportunity to discuss any questions.

The manufacturer states there are no known contraindications to the use of rituximab.

● Pediatric Precautions

Safety and efficacy of rituximab in children have not been established. The pharmacokinetics of rituximab have not been studied in children or adolescents.

● Geriatric Precautions

Clinical studies of rituximab in low-grade or follicular, antigen CD20-positive, B-cell NHL did not include sufficient numbers of patients 65 years of age and older to determine whether geriatric patients respond differently than younger patients. Among patients with diffuse large B-cell NHL in 3 randomized trials, 927 patients received rituximab in combination with chemotherapy; of these, 396 (43%) were 65 years of age or older and 123 (13%) were 75 years of age or older. Although no overall difference in efficacy was observed between geriatric and younger patients, geriatric patients were more likely to experience certain adverse effects, such as supraventricular arrhythmias and severe respiratory effects, including pneumonia and pneumonitis.

Among the 676 patients with previously untreated or previously treated chronic lymphocytic leukemia (CLL) receiving rituximab in 2 randomized studies (CLL8 and REACH studies), 243 (36%) were 65 years of age or older and 100 (15%) were 70 years of age or older. Based on results of an exploratory analysis (stratified by age), the addition of rituximab to fludarabine and cyclophosphamide (FC) resulted in no additional benefit in previously untreated patients 70 years of age or older or in previously treated patients 65 years of age or older. (See Uses: Chronic Lymphocytic Leukemia.) Previously untreated geriatric patients received lower dosages of fludarabine and cyclophosphamide compared with younger patients, while previously treated geriatric patients received lower dosages of fludarabine, cyclophosphamide, and rituximab. Compared with younger patients, patients 70 years of age or older experienced higher incidences of grade 3 or 4 adverse effects, including neutropenia, febrile neutropenia, anemia, and pancytopenia (among patients with previously untreated CLL), and neutropenia, anemia, thrombocytopenia, pancytopenia, and infections (among patients with previously treated CLL).

Among the 2578 patients with RA enrolled in studies worldwide, 12% were 65–75 years of age and 2% were 75 years of age or older. In one clinical trial among patients receiving rituximab and methotrexate for RA, ACR 20 response rates were similar (53 versus 51%) in geriatric (65 years of age or older) and younger patients, respectively. The incidences of adverse effects were similar in older and younger patients; however, the rates of serious adverse effects, including serious infections, malignancies, and cardiovascular events, were higher in older patients.

● Mutagenicity and Carcinogenicity

Long-term animal studies to determine the mutagenic or carcinogenic potential of rituximab have not been performed to date.

● Pregnancy, Fertility, and Lactation
Pregnancy

Although rituximab has been shown to cross the monkey placenta, results of an embryofetal developmental toxicity study in which IV rituximab was administered to pregnant cynomolgus monkeys during early gestation did not indicate teratogenicity. However, a decrease in levels of lymphoid tissue B cells was observed in the offspring of treated dams. In another developmental toxicity study in cynomolgus monkeys receiving rituximab during prenatal and postnatal periods, decreased levels of B cells and immunosuppression were observed in the offspring; levels of B cells and immune function returned to normal within 6 months of birth. There are no adequate and well-controlled studies in pregnant women.

Postmarketing data indicate that B-cell lymphocytopenia generally lasting less than 6 months can occur in infants exposed to rituximab in utero. Rituximab was detected postnatally in the serum of infants exposed to the drug in utero. The manufacturer states that rituximab should be used during pregnancy only if the potential benefit justifies the potential risk to the fetus. Individuals of childbearing potential should use effective contraception during treatment and for up to 12 months following rituximab therapy.

Fertility

Studies have not been conducted to date to determine whether rituximab affects fertility in males or females.

Lactation

Rituximab is distributed into milk in lactating cynomolgus monkeys. It is not known whether rituximab is distributed into milk in humans. IgG is distributed into human milk; however, published data suggest that antibodies in breast milk do not enter the neonatal and infant circulations in substantial amounts. The unknown risks to the infant from oral ingestion of rituximab should be weighed against the known benefits of breastfeeding.

DRUG INTERACTIONS

Formal drug interaction studies of rituximab have not been conducted.

● Antirheumatic Agents

The safety of concomitant use of rituximab with biologic agents or nonbiologic disease-modifying antirheumatic drugs (DMARDs) other than methotrexate in patients with rheumatoid arthritis (RA) exhibiting peripheral B cell depletion following treatment with rituximab has not been established. Such patients should be monitored closely for signs of infection if biologic agents and/or DMARDs are used concomitantly. In clinical trials, concomitant administration of methotrexate or cyclophosphamide did not alter the pharmacokinetic disposition of rituximab in patients with RA.

● Cisplatin

Renal toxicity has been reported in patients receiving cisplatin in combination with rituximab for NHL in clinical studies. If rituximab is administered concomitantly with cisplatin (e.g., in the clinical trial setting), *extreme caution* should be used, and patients should be monitored closely for signs of renal toxicity.

● Cyclophosphamide

Concomitant administration of rituximab with cyclophosphamide in patients with chronic lymphocytic leukemia (CLL) did not alter systemic exposure to cyclophosphamide.

● Fludarabine

Concomitant administration of rituximab with fludarabine in patients with CLL did not alter systemic exposure to fludarabine.

● Live Vaccines

The safety of immunization with live viral vaccines following rituximab therapy has not been established. The manufacturer states that use of vaccines containing live virus is *not* recommended prior to or during rituximab therapy. (See Cautions: Immunologic Effects and also see Vaccination Status under Cautions: Precautions and Contraindications.)

ACUTE TOXICITY

Limited information is available on the acute toxicity of rituximab. Overdosage has not been reported in clinical studies with patients receiving rituximab in single doses of up to 500 mg/m^2.

PHARMACOLOGY

Rituximab is an antineoplastic agent that binds specifically to antigen CD20 (human B-lymphocyte-restricted differentiation antigen, Bp35), a hydrophobic transmembrane protein located on pre-B and mature B lymphocytes. Antigen CD20 also is expressed on greater than 90% of B-cell non-Hodgkin's lymphomas (NHL) but is not found on hematopoietic stem cells, early pre-B cells, normal plasma cells, or other normal tissues. Antigen CD20 is involved in the regulation of cell cycle initiation and differentiation and also may function as a calcium ion channel.

Following binding of the Fab domain of rituximab to antigen CD20 on B lymphocytes, the Fc domain triggers a host immune response causing lysis of normal and malignant B cells; the exact mechanism of cell lysis has not been fully elucidated but is thought to involve complement-dependent cytotoxicity (CDC) and antibody-dependent cell-mediated cytotoxicity (ADCC). Rapid and sustained depletion of circulating and tissue-based B cells occurs as a result of the lysis of B cells induced by rituximab. Depletion of circulating B cells lasted for up to 6–9 months in 83% of patients receiving rituximab for NHL in a clinical study. Antigen CD20 is not shed from the cell surface and does not internalize following antibody binding. Circulation of free CD20 antigen does not occur. Following completion of rituximab therapy, recovery of B cells begins at approximately 6 months, and median levels of B cells return to normal by 12 months.

Inhibition of cellular proliferation and induction of apoptosis by rituximab have been demonstrated in some NHL cell lines. Rituximab also has been shown to increase the in vitro sensitivity of certain chemoresistant human lymphoma cell lines to some cytotoxic agents, including doxorubicin.

B cells may contribute to the pathogenesis of rheumatoid arthritis and associated chronic synovitis by involvement in the production of rheumatoid factor and other autoantibodies, presentation of antigen, activation of T cells, and/or production of inflammatory cytokines. By binding and causing lysis of B cells, rituximab interferes with the autoimmune and inflammatory processes in rheumatoid arthritis. In patients with rheumatoid arthritis, nearly complete depletion of peripheral B lymphocytes (CD19 counts below the lower limit of quantification [20/μL]) occurred within 2 weeks following the first dose of rituximab. In most patients, depletion of circulating B cells lasted for at least 6 months. A small number of patients (approximately 4%) experienced prolonged peripheral B-cell depletion (more than 3 years) after a single course of treatment. Rituximab therapy also was associated with the reduction of certain biologic markers of inflammation, including interleukin-6, C-reactive protein, serum amyloid protein, S100 A8/S100 A9 heterodimer complex, anti-citrullinated peptide, and rheumatoid factor.

PHARMACOKINETICS

The pharmacokinetic disposition of rituximab when administered in conjunction with 6 cycles of combination chemotherapy with CHOP (i.e., cyclophosphamide, doxorubicin, vincristine, and prednisone) is similar to that observed with rituximab alone.

The pharmacokinetics of rituximab have not been studied in children or adolescents. The effects of renal or hepatic impairment on the pharmacokinetic disposition of rituximab have not been formally studied.

● Absorption

In a study of 203 patients with non-Hodgkin's lymphoma (NHL) receiving rituximab 375 mg/m² by IV infusion once weekly for 4 weeks, rituximab was detected in the serum of patients 3–6 months after completion of treatment.

In patients with rheumatoid arthritis (RA) receiving rituximab, the peak serum concentration averaged 183 mcg/mL following two 500-mg doses and 381 mcg/mL following two 1-g doses.

● Distribution

Following IV infusion, binding of rituximab has been observed on lymphoid cells in the thymus, the white pulp of the spleen, and a majority of B lymphocytes in peripheral blood and lymph nodes. Little or no binding has been observed upon examination of non-lymphoid tissues.

Based on a population pharmacokinetic analysis of data in 2005 patients with RA, the volume of distribution of rituximab was 3.1 L.

It is not known whether rituximab crosses the placenta or distributes into milk in humans; however, IgG distributes into milk in humans. (See Cautions: Pregnancy, Fertility, and Lactation.)

● Elimination

Based on a population pharmacokinetic analysis of data in 298 patients with NHL receiving rituximab once weekly or once every 3 weeks, the estimated median terminal elimination half-life was 22 days (range: 6–52 days). Patients with higher CD19-positive cell count or larger measurable tumor lesions at pretreatment had a higher rate of clearance. Age and gender had no effect on the pharmacokinetics of rituximab in patients with NHL.

In 21 patients with chronic lymphocytic leukemia (CLL) receiving rituximab 375 mg/m² approximately every 28 days, the estimated median terminal half-life was 32 days (range: 14–62 days).

Based on a population pharmacokinetic analysis of data in 2005 patients with RA, the estimated clearance of rituximab was 0.335 L/day (approximately 0.014 L/hour), and the mean terminal elimination half-life was 18 days (range: 5–78 days). Age, weight, and gender had no effect on the pharmacokinetics of rituximab in patients with RA.

CHEMISTRY AND STABILITY

● Chemistry

Rituximab, a chimeric human-murine anti-human antigen CD20 monoclonal antibody, is an antineoplastic agent.

The rituximab antibody is an IgG₁ kappa immunoglobulin containing murine light-chain and heavy-chain variable region sequences and human constant region sequences. Because of the presence of human constant region sequences, the chimeric antibody is characterized by lower immunogenicity, longer half-life, and more effective lysis of tumor cells compared with murine monoclonal antibodies.

Rituximab binds specifically to antigen CD20, a hydrophobic transmembrane protein located on pre-B and mature B lymphocytes.

Commercially available rituximab concentrate for injection occurs as a sterile, clear, colorless, preservative-free solution. The product is formulated for IV administration in 9 mg/mL sodium chloride, 7.35 mg/mL sodium citrate dihydrate, 0.7 mg/mL polysorbate 80, and water for injection and has been adjusted to a pH of 6.5.

● Stability

Vials of rituximab should be stored at 2–8°C and should not be frozen or shaken; when stored under recommended conditions, commercially available rituximab liquid concentrate for injection should be stable up to the date of expiration marked on the vial. Vials of rituximab should be protected from direct sunlight.

Following dilution of rituximab as recommended, solutions of the drug may be stored for 24 hours at 2–8°C. Rituximab solutions for infusion have been shown to be stable for an additional 24 hours at room temperature; however, since rituximab solutions do not contain a preservative, diluted solutions should be stored at 2–8°C. No incompatibilities between rituximab and polyvinylchloride or polyethylene bags have been observed.

For further information on the handling of antineoplastic agents, see the ASHP Guidelines on Handling Hazardous Drugs at http://www.ahfsdruginformation.com.

PREPARATIONS

Excipients in commercially available drug preparations may have clinically important effects in some individuals; consult specific product labeling for details.

riTUXimab

Parenteral		
For injection concentrate, for IV infusion	10 mg/mL (100 and 500 mg)	Rituxan®, Biogen Idec (also promoted by Genentech)

† Use is not currently included in the labeling approved by the US Food and Drug Administration.

Selected Revisions June 29, 2016, © Copyright, October 1, 1998, American Society of Health-System Pharmacists, Inc.

Sacituzumab Govitecan-hziy

10:00 • ANTINEOPLASTIC AGENTS

■ Sacituzumab govitecan, a trophoblast antigen-2 (Trop-2)-directed antibody-drug conjugate consisting of a humanized immunoglobulin G1 (IgG₁) kappa monoclonal antibody (sacituzumab) covalently linked to a topoisomerase I inhibitor (SN-38), is an antineoplastic agent.

USES

• Breast Cancer

Sacituzumab govitecan-hziy is used for the treatment of metastatic triple-negative (i.e., estrogen receptor-, progesterone receptor-, and human epidermal growth factor receptor type 2 [HER2]-negative) breast cancer (mTNBC) previously treated with at least 2 therapies for metastatic disease. The accelerated approval of sacituzumab govitecan-hziy is based on tumor response rate and duration of response; continued approval for this indication may be contingent upon verification and description of clinical benefit in confirmatory trials.

The current indication for sacituzumab govitecan-hziy is based principally on the results for a cohort of 108 adults with metastatic triple-negative breast cancer (mTNBC) previously treated with at least 2 therapies for metastatic disease in a multicenter, phase 1/2, single-arm trial (IMMU-132-01). In this study, patients received sacituzumab govitecan-hziy 10 mg/kg as an IV infusion on days 1 and 8 of each 21-day cycle. Treatment was continued until disease progression or unacceptable toxicity occurred. The primary measure of efficacy was objective response rate according to the Response Evaluation Criteria in Solid Tumors (RECIST 1.1); additional outcome measures included duration of response and progression-free and overall survival. The median age of patients in the mTNBC cohort was 55 years; 76% of patients were White, 7% were Black, 99% were female, 76% had visceral disease, 42% had hepatic metastases, 56% had lung/pleura metastases, and 2% had brain metastases. Twelve patients (11%) had Stage IV disease at the time of initial diagnosis. In the mTNBC cohort, patients had received a median of 3 prior systemic therapies in the metastatic setting. Most patients (98%) with mTNBC received prior therapy with taxanes and 86% received anthracyclines either in the neoadjuvant or metastatic setting. This study excluded patients with known Gilbert syndrome. Patients with known brain metastases were initially excluded from the trial; however, the protocol was later amended to allow enrollment of patients with stable brain metastases who did not require high-dose corticosteroid therapy (e.g., more than 20 mg of prednisone or equivalent) for at least 4 weeks. Objective response rate in patients receiving sacituzumab govitecan-hziy was 33%, with a complete response in 2.8% of patients. The median duration of response was 7.7 months and 56% of the patients who responded to sacituzumab govitecan-hziy had durable responses of 6 months or more. Median progression-free survival was 5.5 months and median overall survival was 13 months.

In a confirmatory phase 3 randomized controlled trial (ASCENT), 468 patients with relapsed or refractory mTNBC without brain involvement who had previously received at least 2 chemotherapies (including therapy with a taxane) in the advanced or metastatic setting were randomized to receive sacituzumab govitecan-hziy 10 mg/kg administered by IV infusion on days 1 and 8 of each 21-day cycle or a single-agent treatment of the clinician's choice (i.e., capecitabine, eribulin, vinorelbine, or gemcitabine) until disease progression or unacceptable toxicity occurred. The primary measure of efficacy was progression-free survival according to the RECIST 1.1 as assessed by a central review committee. In this study, the median age of patients was 54 years and patients had received a median of 4 prior therapies. Median progression-free survival (5.6 versus 1.7 months) and overall survival (12.1 versus 6.7 months) were prolonged in patients receiving sacituzumab govitecan-hziy compared with those receiving standard single-agent therapy. Objective response rate also was higher in patients receiving sacituzumab govitecan-hziy compared with those receiving standard single-agent therapy (35 versus 5%).

DOSAGE AND ADMINISTRATION

• General

Sacituzumab govitecan should *not* be substituted for or used with other drugs containing irinotecan or its active metabolite SN-38.

Because infusion or hypersensitivity reactions may occur with sacituzumab govitecan, patients should be closely observed during infusions and for at least 30 minutes following completion of the infusion. Premedication with an antipyretic, a histamine H₁-receptor antagonist, and a histamine H₂-receptor antagonist is recommended prior to each infusion. If an infusion-related reaction occurs, corticosteroids may be considered for subsequent infusions. Sacituzumab govitecan should be administered in settings where emergency equipment and appropriate medical support are available for the management of potential infusion-related or hypersensitivity reactions. (See Hypersensitivity Reactions under Cautions.)

Because sacituzumab govitecan is moderately emetogenic, premedication with a 2- or 3-drug antiemetic regimen (e.g., dexamethasone with either a type 3 serotonin [5-HT₃] receptor antagonist or a neurokinin-1 [NK₁] receptor antagonist, and other drugs as indicated) is recommended prior to each dose of sacituzumab govitecan.

Because neutropenia occurs frequently during sacituzumab govitecan therapy, the manufacturer states that secondary prophylaxis with a granulocyte colony-stimulating factor (G-CSF) should be considered.

• Administration

Procedures for proper handling and disposal of antineoplastic agents should be followed.

Sacituzumab govitecan-hziy is administered by IV infusion only. The drug should not be administered by rapid IV injection, such as IV push or bolus. Following completion of the infusion, the IV line should be flushed with 20 mL of 0.9% sodium chloride injection.

Sacituzumab govitecan-hziy should not be mixed with or administered simultaneously through the same IV line with other drugs.

Unopened vials of sacituzumab govitecan-hziy powder for injection should be stored at 2–8°C and retained in the original carton to protect from light. Vials should not be frozen.

Reconstitution and Dilution

Prior to administration, commercially available sacituzumab govitecan-hziy lyophilized powder for injection must be reconstituted and diluted. The appropriate number of vials containing sacituzumab govitecan-hziy should be removed from the refrigerator and allowed to reach room temperature. The powder for injection is reconstituted by adding 20 mL of 0.9% sodium chloride injection to a vial labeled as containing 180 mg of the drug to provide a solution containing 10 mg/mL. The vial should be gently swirled and allowed to sit until complete dissolution occurs (e.g., up to 15 minutes); the resulting solution should not be shaken. The reconstituted solution should be inspected visually for particulate matter and discoloration prior to dilution. The reconstituted solution should be clear and yellow, and free of visible particulates. The reconstituted solution should be used immediately to prepare a diluted solution for infusion.

Prior to administration, the required amount of reconstituted sacituzumab govitecan-hziy solution must be diluted in *only* 0.9% sodium chloride injection to provide a final solution with a sacituzumab govitecan-hziy concentration of 1.1–3.4 mg/mL in a total volume of no more than 500 mL (i.e., if a 500-mL infusion bag of 0.9% sodium chloride injection is used, a volume of diluent equal to the total required volume of reconstituted sacituzumab govitecan solution should be removed from the infusion bag prior to addition of the reconstituted solution). The manufacturer states that the drug must be diluted in a polypropylene infusion bag. The reconstituted solution should be slowly injected into the infusion bag to minimize foaming. The final diluted solution for infusion should not be shaken. Any unused portions in the vials should be discarded.

For patients weighing more than 170 kg, the total dose of sacituzumab govitecan-hziy should be divided equally between two 500-mL infusion bags and infused sequentially. If immediate administration of the diluted solution is not possible, the solution may be stored at 2–8°C for up to 4 hours; following removal from refrigeration, the diluted solution for infusion must be administered within 4 hours (including infusion time). Diluted solutions of the drug must be protected from light.

Rate of Administration

The initial sacituzumab govitecan-hziy infusion should be administered IV over 3 hours.

Subsequent infusions of the drug should be administered over 1–2 hours if infusion-related reactions did not occur during the previous infusion.

● Dosage

Dosage of sacituzumab govitecan-hziy should be based on the patient's body weight prior to each cycle. If body weight changes by more than 10% compared with the previous dose, the dosage of sacituzumab govitecan-hziy may be adjusted more frequently during treatment cycles.

Breast Cancer

For the treatment of previously treated metastatic triple-negative breast cancer in adults, the recommended adult dosage of sacituzumab govitecan-hziy is 10 mg/kg administered as an IV infusion on days 1 and 8 of each 21-day treatment cycle. Therapy should be continued until disease progression or unacceptable toxicity occurs. Sacituzumab govitecan-hziy should not be administered at a dosage exceeding 10 mg/kg.

Dosage Modification for Toxicity

Temporary interruption of therapy, dosage reduction, and/or permanent discontinuance of sacituzumab govitecan-hziy may be necessary if adverse effects occur. In the IMMU-132-01 study, interruption of therapy was necessary in 45% of patients receiving sacituzumab govitecan-hziy; 1 or 2 dosage reductions were required in 24 or 9% of patients, respectively.

Dosage of sacituzumab govitecan-hziy should not be re-escalated following a dosage reduction.

Hematologic Toxicity

For absolute neutrophil count (ANC) below 1500/mm³ on day 1 of any cycle, ANC below 1000/mm³ on day 8 of any cycle, or febrile neutropenia, sacituzumab govitecan therapy should be withheld.

For the first occurrence of grade 4 neutropenia lasting 7 or more days, grade 3 febrile neutropenia (ANC less than 1000/mm³ and fever 38.5°C or higher), or grade 3 or 4 neutropenia that delays scheduled dosing by 2 or 3 weeks until recovery to grade 1 or less, the dosage of sacituzumab govitecan should be reduced by 25% and G-CSF therapy should be initiated.

If these neutropenic events recur following a 25% reduction in dosage, the dosage of sacituzumab govitecan should be reduced by 50%.

If these neutropenic events recur following a 50% reduction in dosage or if grade 3 or 4 neutropenia delays scheduled dosing beyond 3 weeks until recovery to grade 1 or less, treatment with sacituzumab govitecan should be discontinued.

For other grade 3 or 4 hematologic toxicities that do not recover to grade 1 or less within 3 weeks, treatment with sacituzumab govitecan should be discontinued.

GI Toxicity

If grade 3 or 4 nausea, vomiting, or diarrhea occurs, sacituzumab govitecan therapy should be withheld until the toxicity improves to grade 1 or less.

For the first occurrence of grade 3 or 4 nausea, vomiting, or diarrhea that persists despite antiemetic or antidiarrheal therapy, sacituzumab govitecan therapy should be withheld until the toxicity improves to grade 1 or less, and then may be resumed with a 25% reduction in dosage.

For the second occurrence of grade 3 or 4 nausea, vomiting, or diarrhea that persists despite antiemetic or antidiarrheal therapy, sacituzumab govitecan therapy should be withheld until the toxicity improves to grade 1 or less, and then may be resumed at a dosage reduced by 50%.

For the third occurrence of grade 3 or 4 nausea, vomiting, or diarrhea that persists despite antiemetic or antidiarrheal therapy, treatment with sacituzumab govitecan should be discontinued.

Nonhematologic Toxicity

For the first occurrence of grade 4 nonhematologic toxicity of any duration or grade 3 or 4 nonhematologic toxicity persisting for longer than 48 hours despite optimal medical management, or grade 3 or 4 nonhematologic toxicity that delays scheduled dosing by 2 or 3 weeks until recovery to grade 1 or less, the dosage of sacituzumab govitecan should be reduced by 25%.

If such nonhematologic effects recur following a 25% reduction in dosage, the dosage of sacituzumab govitecan should be reduced by 50%.

If such nonhematologic effects recur following a 50% reduction in dosage, treatment with sacituzumab govitecan should be discontinued.

For grade 3 or 4 nonhematologic toxicity that does not recover to grade 1 or less within 3 weeks, treatment with sacituzumab govitecan should be discontinued.

Infusion-related Reaction

If an infusion-related reaction occurs, the infusion should be interrupted or the infusion rate should be reduced. If life-threatening infusion-related reactions occur, sacituzumab govitecan therapy should be permanently discontinued.

● Special Populations

Hepatic Impairment

In patients with mild hepatic impairment (serum bilirubin concentration not exceeding the upper limit of normal [ULN] and AST concentration exceeding the ULN, or serum bilirubin concentration exceeding the ULN, but no more than 1.5 times the ULN and any AST concentration), no initial dosage adjustment is necessary.

The safety of sacituzumab govitecan-hziy in patients with moderate or severe hepatic impairment has not been established; therefore, the manufacturer makes no specific dosage recommendations for such patients. (See Hepatic Impairment under Cautions.)

Renal Impairment

The manufacturer makes no specific dosage recommendations for patients with renal impairment. (See Renal Impairment under Cautions.)

Geriatric Use

The manufacturer makes no specific dosage recommendations for geriatric patients. (See Geriatric Use under Cautions.)

Pharmacogenomic Dosage Considerations

Patients who are homozygous for the uridine diphosphate-glucuronosyl transferase 1A1 (UGT1A1)*28 allele have an increased risk of neutropenia and other toxicities. The manufacturer states that an appropriate dosage for patients who are homozygous for UGT1A1*28 has not been established; therefore, such patients should be closely monitored for severe neutropenia and managed based on individual patient tolerance. (See Pharmacogenomic Considerations under Cautions.)

In the IMMU-132-01 study, patients with known Gilbert syndrome were excluded since this condition is associated with UGT1A1 deficiency.

CAUTIONS

● Contraindications

Sacituzumab govitecan is contraindicated in patients with known severe hypersensitivity reaction to the drug or any ingredient in the formulation. (See Hypersensitivity Reactions under Cautions.)

● Warnings/Precautions

Warnings

Neutropenia

Severe or life-threatening neutropenia may occur during sacituzumab govitecan therapy. In the IMMU-132-01 study, neutropenia of any grade occurred in 64% of patients with metastatic triple-negative breast cancer (mTNBC) receiving sacituzumab govitecan-hziy and in 54% of the total study population. In the total study population, grade 4 neutropenia was reported in 13% of patients receiving the drug. Febrile neutropenia occurred in 6% of the total study population, including 8% of patients with mTNBC receiving the drug. Permanent discontinuance of therapy due to neutropenia or febrile neutropenia was necessary in less than 1% of the total study population. Neutropenia was the most common reason for treatment interruption and dosage reduction.

Complete blood cell (CBC) counts should be monitored periodically during therapy. The manufacturer states that secondary prophylaxis with a granulocyte colony-stimulating factor (G-CSF) should be considered. If neutropenia occurs, temporary interruption of therapy, dosage reduction, or discontinuance of the drug may be required. (See Dosage Modification for Toxicity under Dosage and Administration.) If febrile neutropenia occurs, anti-infective therapy should be promptly initiated.

Diarrhea

Severe diarrhea may occur during sacituzumab govitecan therapy. Clinical experience suggests diarrhea typically occurs within the first few days of therapy. In the IMMU-132-01 study, diarrhea occurred in 63% of patients with mTNBC receiving sacituzumab govitecan-hziy and in 62% of the total study population. Grade 3 or 4 diarrhea occurred in 9% of patients with mTNBC and in 9% of the total study population. Neutropenic colitis occurred in 2% of patients with mTNBC and in 1% of the total study population. Discontinuance of therapy was necessary because of diarrhea in less than 1% of the total study population.

If diarrhea occurs, patients should receive appropriate therapy (e.g., antidiarrheal agents, fluid replacement) as necessary. If early diarrhea of any severity occurs, the manufacturer recommends therapy with atropine as appropriate. At the onset of late diarrhea, patients should be evaluated for infectious causes; if an infectious etiology is ruled out, loperamide should be initiated at a dosage of 4 mg initially, followed by 2 mg with every episode of diarrhea up to a maximum of 16 mg daily. Loperamide should be discontinued 12 hours after diarrhea resolves. If an excessive cholinergic response (e.g., abdominal cramping, diarrhea, salivation) occurs, premedication with appropriate therapy (e.g., atropine) may be used prior to subsequent infusions. Temporary interruption, dosage reduction, or permanent discontinuance of therapy may be necessary if diarrhea occurs. (See Dosage Modification for Toxicity under Dosage and Administration.)

Other Warnings and Precautions

Hypersensitivity Reactions

Severe or life-threatening hypersensitivity reactions and anaphylaxis have been reported during therapy with sacituzumab govitecan. In the IMMU-132-01 study, grade 3 or 4 hypersensitivity reactions occurred in 3% of patients with mTNBC receiving sacituzumab govitecan-hziy and in 1% of the total study population. Hypersensitivity reactions occurred within 24 hours of sacituzumab govitecan dosing in 37% of the total study population. Permanent discontinuance of sacituzumab govitecan-hziy due to hypersensitivity reactions was necessary in 1% of the total study population.

Patients should be closely observed during infusions and for at least 30 minutes following completion of sacituzumab govitecan infusions. Premedication with an antipyretic, a histamine H_1-receptor antagonist, and a histamine H_2-receptor antagonist is recommended prior to each infusion of sacituzumab govitecan. (See General under Dosage and Administration.)

Nausea and Vomiting

Sacituzumab govitecan has moderate emetogenic potential. In the IMMU-132-01 study, the incidence of nausea in the mTNBC cohort was similar to the incidence in the total study population (69%); grade 3 nausea occurred in 6 or 5% of patients in these respective groups. Vomiting occurred in 49 or 45% of patients in the mTNBC cohort or the total study population, respectively; grade 3 vomiting occurred in 6 or 4% of patients in these respective groups.

Because sacituzumab govitecan is moderately emetogenic, premedication with a 2- or 3-drug antiemetic regimen is recommended prior to each dose of sacituzumab govitecan. (See General under Dosage and Administration.) Temporary interruption of therapy, dosage reduction, or permanent discontinuance of therapy may be necessary if nausea or vomiting occurs. (See Dosage Modification for Toxicity under Dosage and Administration.)

Pharmacogenomic Considerations

Genetic variants of the UGT1A1 gene, such as the UGT1A1*28 allele, may result in reduced UGT1A1 enzyme activity. The small-molecule component (SN-38) of the antibody-drug conjugate is metabolized via UGT1A1; therefore, individuals who are homozygous for the UGT1A1*28 allele are at increased risk for neutropenia and other adverse reactions. Approximately 20, 10, and 2% of Blacks, Whites, and East Asians are homozygous for the UGT1A1*28 allele. Decreased-function alleles other than UGT1A1*28 may be present in certain populations.

Among patients who received sacituzumab govitecan-hziy in the IMMU-132-01 study and had retrospective UGT1A1 genotyping results available, 45, 43, or 11% were heterozygous for the UGT1A1*28 allele, homozygous for the wild-type allele, or homozygous for the UGT1A1*28 allele, respectively; grade 4 neutropenia occurred in 13, 11, or 26% of patients in these respective groups. In a phase 1/2 trial, grade 3 or greater neutropenia occurred more frequently in patients with homozygous UGT1A1*28 allele haplotype compared with those with homozygous wild-type allele or heterozygous UGT1A1*28 allele haplotypes; however, no significant correlation between the 3 haplotypes and severe neutropenia for the combined dose groups (8 or 10 mg/kg on day 1 and 8 of each 21-day cycle) within the first 2 cycles or at any time during treatment was observed.

In the IMMU-132-01 study, patients with known Gilbert syndrome were excluded since this condition is associated with UGT1A1 deficiency.

The manufacturer makes no specific recommendations for screening for UGT1A1 genetic variants prior to initiating therapy with sacituzumab govitecan; however, some clinicians state that management of a neutropenic event is more appropriate than screening for UGT1A1 genetic variants. The appropriate dose for patients who are homozygous for UGT1A1*28 has not been established; therefore, such patients should be closely monitored for severe neutropenia and managed based on individual patient tolerance.

Fetal/Neonatal Morbidity and Mortality

There are no available data regarding the risk of sacituzumab govitecan use in pregnant women; however, based on its mechanism of action, the drug may cause embryofetal mortality and/or teratogenicity. The SN-38 component of sacituzumab govitecan is genotoxic and toxic to rapidly dividing cells.

Pregnancy should be avoided during sacituzumab govitecan therapy. The manufacturer states that a pregnancy test should be performed prior to initiation of sacituzumab govitecan, and females of reproductive potential should be advised to use effective contraceptive methods during therapy and for 6 months after the last dose. In addition, men with such female partners should be advised to use effective methods of contraception during therapy and for 3 months after the last dose. Patients should be apprised of the potential hazard to the fetus if sacituzumab govitecan is used during pregnancy.

Impairment of Fertility

Based on findings in animals, sacituzumab govitecan may impair fertility in females.

Immunogenicity

There is a potential for immunogenicity with sacituzumab govitecan. Persistent anti-sacituzumab govitecan antibodies developed in 2 of 106 patients with mTNBC in the IMMU-132-01 study.

Specific Populations

Pregnancy

Sacituzumab govitecan can cause embryofetal mortality and/or teratogenicity if administered to a pregnant woman based on its mechanism of action. (See Fetal/Neonatal Morbidity and Mortality under Cautions.)

Lactation

It is not known whether sacituzumab govitecan or SN-38 is distributed into human milk. Because of the potential for serious adverse reactions to sacituzumab govitecan in breast-fed infants, women should be advised to discontinue nursing while receiving the drug and for 1 month after the last dose. The effects of the drug on breast-fed infants or on the production of milk are unknown.

Pediatric Use

Safety and efficacy of sacituzumab govitecan-hziy have not been established in pediatric patients.

Geriatric Use

In the IMMU-132-01 study, 18 or 35% of patients who received sacituzumab govitecan-hziy in the mTNBC cohort or total study population, respectively, were 65 years of age or older. No overall differences in safety and efficacy were observed between geriatric patients and younger adults.

Age does not appear to affect the pharmacokinetics of sacituzumab govitecan.

Hepatic Impairment

Exposure to sacituzumab govitecan was similar in patients with mild hepatic impairment (serum bilirubin concentration not exceeding the ULN and AST concentration exceeding the ULN, or serum bilirubin concentration exceeding the ULN, but no more than 1.5 times the ULN with any AST concentration) and those with normal hepatic function.

The pharmacokinetics of sacituzumab govitecan have not been established in patients with moderate or severe hepatic impairment (serum bilirubin concentration exceeding 1.5 times the ULN, or AST and ALT concentration exceeding 3 times the ULN); however, systemic exposure to SN-38 may be elevated in such patients due to decreased hepatic UGT1A1 activity.

Renal Impairment

The pharmacokinetics of sacituzumab govitecan have not been established in patients with renal impairment or end-stage renal disease (creatinine clearance of 30 mL/minute or less); however, renal elimination of SN-38 is minimal.

● Common Adverse Effects

Adverse effects reported in 25% or more of patients with mTNBC treated with sacituzumab govitecan-hziy include nausea, neutropenia, diarrhea, fatigue, anemia, vomiting, alopecia, constipation, rash, decreased appetite, and abdominal pain.

DRUG INTERACTIONS

No formal drug interaction studies have been performed with sacituzumab govitecan or SN-38; however, the small-molecule component of sacituzumab govitecan, SN-38, undergoes conjugation by uridine diphosphate-glucuronosyl transferase 1A1 (UGT1A1) to form a glucuronide metabolite.

● Drugs Affecting Uridine Diphosphate-glucuronosyltransferase (UGT)

Inhibitors of UGT1A1

Concomitant use of sacituzumab govitecan with inhibitors of UGT1A1 may result in increased systemic exposure to SN-38 and an increased risk of adverse reactions. Concomitant use of sacituzumab govitecan with UGT1A1 inhibitors should be avoided.

Inducers of UGT1A1

Concomitant use of sacituzumab govitecan with inducers of UGT1A1 may result in substantially decreased systemic exposure to SN-38. Concomitant use of sacituzumab govitecan with UGT1A1 inducers should be avoided.

DESCRIPTION

Sacituzumab govitecan, a trophoblast antigen-2 (Trop-2)-directed antibody-drug conjugate, is an antineoplastic agent. Trop-2 (also referred to as tumor-associated calcium signal transducer 2; TACS TD2) is an antigen expressed in various epithelial cancers, and has been associated with more aggressive

tumors. The anti-Trop-2 antibody, a humanized immunoglobulin G1 (IgG₁) kappa monoclonal antibody (sacituzumab), is covalently linked by a hydrolyzable linker to a topoisomerase I inhibitor (SN-38). Following binding of the antibody to Trop-2-expressing cancer cells, the resultant complex is internalized by the cell. SN-38 is released via hydrolysis of the maleimide-containing cross-linker CL2A and also may be released extracellularly into the tumor microenvironment. SN-38 interacts with topoisomerase I and prevents re-ligation of topoisomerase I-induced single-strand breaks. The resulting DNA damage leads to apoptosis and cell death.

Sacituzumab govitecan has a high drug-to-antibody ratio (approximately 7–8 molecules of SN-38 are attached to each antibody molecule). Sacituzumab govitecan releases more than 90% of SN-38 over approximately 3 days. Plasma concentrations of sacituzumab govitecan are considerably higher than those of free SN-38, suggesting that the majority of SN-38 remains linked to the antibody while in circulation. SN-38 is metabolized by UGT1A1 to the glucuronide metabolite SN-38G. Because SN-38 is less susceptible to inactivation via glucuronidation when bound to sacituzumab, the antibody-drug conjugate maintains SN-38 in its most active form until the antibody-drug conjugate binds to Trop-2; therefore, sacituzumab govitecan delivers higher concentrations of SN-38 to tumors compared with irinotecan-derived SN-38 therapy. In addition, the substantially lower plasma concentration of SN-38G achieved following administration of sacituzumab govitecan compared with administration of irinotecan may contribute to a lower incidence of severe diarrhea observed with sacituzumab govitecan. The terminal half-lives of the antibody-drug conjugate and free SN-38 are 16 and 18 hours, respectively.

Population pharmacokinetic analyses indicate that age and race do not appear to have clinically important effects on the pharmacokinetics of the antibody-drug conjugate.

ADVICE TO PATIENTS

- Advise the patient to read the FDA-approved patient labeling.
- Advise patients of the risk of neutropenia. Instruct patients to immediately contact their healthcare provider if they experience fever, chills, or other signs of infection.
- Advise patients of the risk of diarrhea. Instruct patients to immediately contact their healthcare provider if they experience diarrhea for the first time during treatment; black or bloody stools; symptoms of dehydration such as lightheadedness, dizziness, or faintness; inability to take fluids by mouth due to nausea or vomiting; or inability to control diarrhea within 24 hours.
- Inform patients of the risk of serious infusion reactions and anaphylaxis. Instruct patients to immediately contact their healthcare provider if they experience facial, lip, tongue, or throat swelling, urticaria, difficulty breathing, lightheadedness, dizziness, chills, rigors, wheezing, pruritus, flushing, rash, hypotension, or fever during or within 24 hours following the infusion.
- Advise patients of the risk of nausea and vomiting. Premedication according to established guidelines with a 2- or 3-drug regimen for prevention of chemotherapy-induced nausea and vomiting (CINV) is recommended. Additional antiemetics, sedatives, and other supportive measures may also be employed as clinically indicated. All patients should receive take-home medications for preventing and treating delayed nausea and vomiting, with clear instructions. Instruct patients to immediately contact their healthcare provider if they experience uncontrolled nausea or vomiting.
- Advise female patients to contact their healthcare provider if they are pregnant or become pregnant. Inform female patients of the risk to a fetus and potential loss of the pregnancy.
- Advise female patients of reproductive potential to use effective contraception during treatment and for 6 months after the last dose of sacituzumab govitecan.
- Advise male patients with female partners of reproductive potential to use effective contraception during treatment and for 3 months after the last dose of sacituzumab govitecan.

- Advise women not to breastfeed during treatment and for 1 month after the last dose of sacituzumab govitecan.
- Advise females of reproductive potential that sacituzumab govitecan may impair fertility.
- Advise patients of the importance of informing clinicians of existing or contemplated concomitant therapy, including prescription and OTC drugs and dietary or herbal supplements, as well as any concomitant illnesses.
- Advise patients of other important precautionary information. (See Cautions.)

For further information on the handling of antineoplastic agents, see the ASHP Guidelines on Handling Hazardous Drugs at http://www.ahfsdrug information.com.

PREPARATIONS

Excipients in commercially available drug preparations may have clinically important effects in some individuals; consult specific product labeling for details.

Sacituzumab Govitecan-hziy

Parenteral

For injection, for IV infusion only	180 mg	**Trodelvy®**, Immunomedics

Selected Revisions July 26, 2021, © Copyright, May 11, 2020, American Society of Health-System Pharmacists, Inc.

SORAfenib Tosylate

10:00 • ANTINEOPLASTIC AGENTS

■ Sorafenib tosylate, an inhibitor of several serine/threonine and receptor tyrosine kinases, is an antineoplastic agent.

USES

● Hepatocellular Carcinoma

Sorafenib tosylate is used for the treatment of unresectable hepatocellular carcinoma and is designated an orphan drug by FDA for the treatment of this cancer.

Efficacy and safety of sorafenib tosylate for the treatment of unresectable hepatocellular carcinoma is based principally on the results of a randomized, double-blind, placebo-controlled phase 3 study (Sorafenib Hepatocellular Carcinoma Assessment Randomized Protocol [SHARP] trial) in patients with previously untreated advanced hepatocellular carcinoma. In this study, 602 patients were randomized in a 1:1 ratio to receive either sorafenib (400 mg orally twice daily) or placebo. Treatment was continued until disease progression, death, or unacceptable toxicity occurred.

Patients were enrolled in the study if they were not eligible for or had disease progression after surgical or locoregional therapies; approximately 70% of patients enrolled in the study had macroscopic vascular invasion, extrahepatic spread, or both. The majority of enrolled patients had mild (Child-Pugh class A) hepatic impairment (97%) and a baseline Eastern Cooperative Oncology Group (ECOG) performance status of 0 (54%) or 1 (38%). Chronic hepatitis C virus (HCV) infection, alcohol consumption, or chronic hepatitis B virus (HBV) infection was the cause of hepatocellular carcinoma in 28, 26, or 18% of patients, respectively. The median duration of treatment was 5.3 months for patients receiving sorafenib and 4.3 months for those receiving placebo.

The primary measure of efficacy was overall survival; secondary end points included time to progression (based on independent radiologic review) and disease control rate. A planned second interim analysis indicated that patients receiving sorafenib had a longer median overall survival than those receiving placebo (10.7 versus 7.9 months; hazard ratio for death: 0.69). Final analysis of the time to disease progression (which occurred at an earlier time point than the survival analysis) indicated that patients receiving sorafenib had a longer median time to progression compared with those receiving placebo (5.5 versus 2.8 months). Patients receiving sorafenib had higher disease control rates compared with those receiving placebo (43 versus 32%). The proportion of patients with disease stabilization was slightly higher among those receiving sorafenib compared with those receiving placebo (71 versus 67%, respectively); however, partial response rates were low (2 versus 1%, respectively) and none of the patients achieved a complete response. Subgroup analysis according to disease etiology (HCV, HBV, alcohol consumption), tumor burden (presence or absence of macroscopic vascular invasion and/or extrahepatic spread), ECOG performance status (0–2), tumor stage (Barcelona Clinic Liver Cancer [BCLC] stage), and prior therapy (resection/ablation or chemoembolization) suggested that sorafenib consistently improved median overall survival across all subgroups; an effect on time to progression was not apparent in the small subgroup of HBV-positive patients.

Efficacy of sorafenib also was demonstrated in a supportive phase 3 study conducted in the Asia-Pacific area (i.e., China, South Korea, Taiwan). In this study, 271 adults with previously untreated advanced hepatocellular carcinoma were randomized in a 2:1 ratio to receive either sorafenib (400 mg orally twice daily) or placebo. In contrast to the SHARP trial, most patients in this study were HBV-positive (73%) and had an ECOG performance status of 1 (69%). Although absolute overall survival, time to progression, and disease control were poorer in this study as compared to the SHARP trial, patients in this study who received sorafenib had a longer median overall survival (6.5 versus 4.2 months), longer median time to progression (2.8 versus 1.4 months), and higher disease control rate (35.3 versus 15.8%) than those who received placebo.

Sorafenib also has been used in combination with transarterial chemoembolization (TACE) in patients with intermediate-advanced hepatocellular carcinoma and as monotherapy following surgical resection†. Additional studies are needed to more fully evaluate the efficacy and safety of sorafenib for the treatment of hepatocellular carcinoma in patients with more severe (i.e., Child-Pugh class B) hepatic impairment as monotherapy or in combination with other therapies and as adjuvant therapy†.

Clinical Perspective

For the treatment of early stage hepatocellular carcinoma, liver transplantation, surgical resection, and ablation offer a potential cure and high rates of complete response; however, survival is usually less than 6 months in patients with untreated advanced stage hepatocellular carcinoma. Treatment of hepatocellular carcinoma is complicated by the presence of underlying liver disease, the extent and location of tumor, comorbidities, and performance status; therefore, the American Society of Clinical Oncology (ASCO) states that the risk of potential toxicities and potential benefits from treatment should be considered when selecting therapy.

The ASCO guideline on systemic therapy for advanced hepatocellular carcinoma states that lenvatinib or sorafenib may be offered as first-line therapy for patients with advanced hepatocellular carcinoma, Child-Pugh class A, and an ECOG performance status of 0 or 1 if therapy with atezolizumab and/or bevacizumab is contraindicated. ASCO also states that tyrosine kinase inhibitors (i.e., cabozantinib, lenvatinib, regorafenib, sorafenib) may be used as second-line therapy† following first-line therapy with atezolizumab in combination with bevacizumab.

The decision to pursue second-line therapy and choice of treatment should be based on patient and clinician preferences and other factors (i.e., comorbidities, liver function, performance status, and potential for benefit and risk of harm).

● Renal Cell Carcinoma

Sorafenib tosylate is used for the treatment of advanced renal cell carcinoma and is designated an orphan drug by FDA for the treatment of this cancer. Safety and efficacy of sorafenib tosylate in the treatment of advanced renal cell carcinoma were established in 2 randomized, controlled clinical trials (one phase 2 and one phase 3).

In the phase 3 trial, patients with unresectable and/or metastatic clear cell renal carcinoma who had received one prior systemic (e.g., cytokine) therapy were randomized to receive sorafenib 400 mg twice daily or placebo. Patients receiving sorafenib had a longer median progression-free survival (167 versus 84 days), an increased rate of progression-free survival at 12 weeks (79 versus 50%), and a decreased risk of progression compared with those receiving placebo. A similar benefit on progression-free survival was observed in patients receiving sorafenib regardless of prior cytokine therapy. In the final overall survival analysis that included patients who crossed over from placebo to sorafenib therapy, survival was similar between sorafenib and placebo (17.8 versus 15.2 months, respectively); however, a significant difference in overall survival (17.8 versus 14.3 months) was observed when crossover data were censored.

The phase 2 trial included patients with metastatic malignancies, including individuals with untreated or previously treated renal cell carcinoma. Following a 12-week run-in induction period during which all patients received sorafenib 400 mg twice daily, tumor response was assessed and those with stable disease (i.e., less than 25% change from baseline in bidimensional tumor measurements) were randomized to receive either sorafenib 400 mg twice daily or placebo for an additional 12 weeks, those with tumor shrinkage (at least 25% reduction from baseline) continued to receive sorafenib in an open-label arm of the study, and those with tumor growth (at least 25% increase from baseline) discontinued therapy with the drug. Of the 202 patients with renal cell carcinoma who were enrolled in the run-in induction phase, 65 were randomized to receive either sorafenib or placebo and 79 were assigned to receive open-label treatment with the drug. Patients in the placebo group who experienced disease progression were allowed to cross over to open-label sorafenib. In the subgroup of patients randomized to receive sorafenib or placebo, those receiving sorafenib had a higher rate of progression-free survival at 24 weeks (50 versus 18%) and a longer median progression-free survival (163 versus 41 days) than did those receiving placebo.

Clinical Perspective

Prognosis is generally poor in patients with metastatic renal cell carcinoma, including those who have undergone complete tumor resection. First-line therapy with vascular endothelial growth factor receptor (VEGFR) inhibitors has been shown to provide benefits in patients with advanced renal cell carcinoma; however, relapsed or refractory renal cell carcinoma eventually develops in most patients. Combination regimens (e.g., immune checkpoint inhibitor in combination with a tyrosine kinase inhibitor) have generally become a standard for the treatment of advanced renal cell carcinoma.

Some experts also state that subsequent monotherapy with a tyrosine kinase inhibitor (e.g., sunitinib, pazopanib) may be offered to patients who experience a treatment-limiting immune-mediated adverse effect following combination therapy with an immune checkpoint inhibitor or as a second-line option following disease progression during immune checkpoint inhibitor-based therapy; however, certain regimens (e.g., nivolumab, lenvatinib and everolimus combination therapy, cabozantinib, axitinib, everolimus) may be recommended over sorafenib in the second-line setting.

● Differentiated Thyroid Carcinoma

Sorafenib tosylate is used for the treatment of locally recurrent or metastatic, progressive, differentiated thyroid carcinoma refractory to radioactive iodine treatment. The drug has been designated an orphan drug by the FDA for the treatment of medullary, anaplastic, and recurrent or metastatic follicular or papillary thyroid cancer.

Differentiated thyroid cancer, specifically papillary and follicular (including Hürthle cell) thyroid cancer, is the most common type of thyroid cancer. Differentiated thyroid cancer is generally treated with surgery and radioactive iodine therapy.

Efficacy and safety of sorafenib tosylate for the treatment of differentiated thyroid carcinoma are based principally on a multicenter, randomized, double-blind, placebo-controlled phase 3 trial (DECISION) in patients with locally advanced or metastatic, progressive differentiated thyroid carcinoma refractory to radioactive iodine treatment. In this study, 417 patients were randomized in a 1:1 ratio to receive either sorafenib (400 mg orally twice daily) or placebo. Treatment was continued until disease progression, unacceptable toxicity, noncompliance, or withdrawal of consent occurred. Crossover to open-label sorafenib occurred in 77% of placebo-treated patients following investigator-determined disease progression.

Patients were enrolled in the study if they had actively progressing disease defined as progression within 14 months of enrollment. Approximately 96% of patients enrolled in the study had metastatic disease; the most common sites of metastases were the lungs (86%) followed by lymph nodes (51%) and bone (27%). The majority of enrolled patients had a baseline ECOG performance status of 0 (62%) or 1 (34%). Histologic subtypes were papillary, follicular, and poorly differentiated carcinoma in approximately 57, 25, and 10% of patients, respectively. The median duration of treatment was 10.6 months in patients receiving sorafenib and 6.5 months in those receiving placebo.

The primary measure of efficacy was progression-free survival. Median progression-free survival was 10.8 or 5.8 months in patients receiving sorafenib or placebo, respectively, which corresponds to a 41% reduction in the risk of disease progression or death (hazard ratio of 0.59). Median time to progression was prolonged in patients receiving sorafenib compared with those receiving placebo (11.1 versus 5.7 months, respectively). No significant difference in overall survival was observed between the treatment groups; median overall survival was 42.8 months in patients receiving sorafenib and 39.4 months in patients receiving placebo. The objective response rate was 12.2 or 0.5% in patients receiving sorafenib or placebo, respectively; none of the patients achieved complete response. In a post-hoc analysis, stable disease for 6 months or more was observed in 41.8 or 33.2% of patients who received sorafenib or placebo, respectively. Results of a subgroup analysis (based on geographic region, age, histology, site of metastases, fluorodeoxyglucose [FDG] uptake, number of target or non-target lesions, target lesion size, sex, cumulative radioactive iodine [RAI] dosage) suggested that the effect of sorafenib on progression-free survival was consistent across all subgroups. Although thyroglobulin concentrations may be a pharmacodynamic biomarker of tumor response or progression, exploratory analyses of the DECISION trial suggested that median progression-free survival was improved in patients receiving sorafenib regardless of baseline thyroglobulin concentrations.

Clinical Perspective

The American Thyroid Association (ATA) published a guideline on the management of patients with thyroid nodules and differentiated thyroid carcinoma in 2015. The basic goals of initial therapy for patients with differentiated thyroid carcinoma are to improve overall and disease-specific survival, reduce the risk of persistent/recurrent disease and associated morbidity, and permit accurate disease staging and risk stratification, while minimizing treatment-related morbidity and unnecessary therapy. In patients with metastatic disease, ATA states that the preferred hierarchy of treatment is surgical excision of locoregional disease in potentially curable patients, iodine I 131 therapy for RAI-responsive disease, directed treatment modalities (e.g., external beam radiation therapy, thermal ablation), TSH-suppressive thyroid hormone therapy for patients with stable or slowly progressive asymptomatic disease, and systemic therapy with kinase inhibitors, especially for patients with significantly progressive macroscopic refractory disease.

At the time of publication of the ATA guideline, limited evidence of efficacy was available for certain kinase inhibitors (e.g., sorafenib, lenvatinib, vandetanib); however, a 2019 guideline published by international experts states that lenvatinib and sorafenib should be considered the standard first-line systemic therapy in patients with radioactive iodine-refractory differentiated thyroid carcinoma.

● Other Uses

Sorafenib also has been studied in patients with acute myeloid leukemia (AML) harboring fms-like tyrosine kinase 3 (FLT3) internal tandem duplication (ITD) mutations who have undergone allogeneic hematopoietic stem cell transplant (HSCT)†, advanced or metastatic GI stromal tumor†, and recurrent or metastatic angiosarcoma†.

DOSAGE AND ADMINISTRATION

● General

Pretreatment Screening

- Verify pregnancy status in females of reproductive potential.

Patient Monitoring

- Monitor electrolytes and ECG in patients with congestive heart failure or bradyarrhythmias and in those receiving concomitant therapy with drugs known to prolong the QT interval (e.g., class Ia and III antiarrhythmics); correct electrolyte abnormalities (magnesium, potassium, calcium).
- Monitor blood pressure weekly during the first 6 weeks of therapy and periodically thereafter.
- Monitor liver function tests regularly.
- In patients with differentiated thyroid carcinoma, monitor TSH levels monthly and adjust thyroid replacement therapy as needed.

Other General Considerations

- Withhold therapy for at least 10 days prior to elective surgery. Do not administer for ≥2 weeks following major surgery and until adequate wound healing has occurred.
- If sorafenib is used in patients receiving a coumarin-derivative anticoagulant (e.g., warfarin), monitor international normalized ratio (INR) more frequently.
- Due to the potential risk of bleeding, treat tracheal, bronchial, and esophageal infiltration with local therapy prior to initiating sorafenib in patients with differentiated thyroid carcinoma.

● Administration

Because administration with a high-fat meal may decrease oral bioavailability of sorafenib, the manufacturer recommends that sorafenib tosylate be administered orally at least 1 hour before or 2 hours after a meal.

If a dose is missed, skip the missed dose and take the next dose at the regularly scheduled time.

Store sorafenib tablets in a dry place at controlled room temperature (20–25ºC). Excursions are permitted to 15–30ºC.

● Dosage

Dosage of sorafenib tosylate is expressed in terms of sorafenib.

Hepatocellular Carcinoma

For the treatment of unresectable hepatocellular carcinoma, the recommended adult dosage of sorafenib is 400 mg twice daily. Therapy should be continued for as long as the patient derives clinical benefit from the drug or until unacceptable toxicity occurs.

Renal Cell Carcinoma

For the treatment of advanced renal cell carcinoma, the recommended adult dosage of sorafenib is 400 mg twice daily. Therapy should be continued for as long as the patient derives clinical benefit from the drug or until unacceptable toxicity occurs.

Differentiated Thyroid Carcinoma

For the treatment of locally recurrent or metastatic, progressive, differentiated thyroid carcinoma refractory to radioactive iodine treatment, the recommended adult dosage of sorafenib is 400 mg twice daily. Therapy should be continued for as long as the patient derives clinical benefit from the drug or until unacceptable toxicity occurs.

Dosage Modification for Toxicity

If dosage modification is required, the dosage of sorafenib should be reduced as described in Table 1 in patients with hepatocellular carcinoma, renal cell carcinoma, or differentiated thyroid carcinoma.

TABLE 1. Recommended Dosage Reduction for Sorafenib Toxicity in Patients with Hepatocellular Carcinoma, Renal Cell Carcinoma, or Differentiated Thyroid Carcinoma.

Dosage Reduction Level	Hepatocellular Carcinoma (Starting Dosage = 400 mg twice daily)	Renal Cell Carcinoma (Starting Dosage = 400 mg twice daily)	Differentiated Thyroid Carcinoma (Starting Dosage = 400 mg twice daily)
First	Restart at 400 mg once daily	Restart at 400 mg once daily	Restart at 400 mg in the morning and 200 mg in the evening (approximately 12 hours apart) or 200 mg in the morning and 400 mg in the evening (approximately 12 hours apart)
Second	Restart at 200 mg once daily or 400 mg every other day	Restart at 200 mg once daily or 400 mg every other day	Restart at 200 mg twice daily
Third	Discontinue drug	Discontinue drug	Restart at 200 mg once daily

Temporary interruption of therapy, dosage reduction, and/or permanent discontinuance of sorafenib may be necessary in patients experiencing certain adverse effects (see Table 2) or cutaneous toxicity (see Table 3).

TABLE 2. Recommended Dosage Modification for Sorafenib Toxicity.

Adverse Reaction and Severity	Modification
Cardiac ischemia and/or infarction	
Grade 2 or higher	Permanently discontinue therapy
Congestive heart failure	
Grade 3	Interrupt therapy; when toxicity resolves or improves to grade 1 or less, resume at dosage reduced by one dose level; however, if recovery does not occur within 30 days of withholding therapy, discontinue sorafenib (unless the patient is deriving clinical benefit). Discontinue therapy if more than 2 dosage reductions are necessary
Grade 4	Permanently discontinue therapy

TABLE 2. Continued

Hemorrhage	
Grade 2 or higher requiring medical intervention	Permanently discontinue therapy
Hypertension	
Grade 2 (symptomatic/persistent)	Interrupt therapy; when diastolic BP resolves or improves to <90 mm Hg, resume at dosage reduced by one dose level; if necessary, reduce dosage by another dose level. Discontinue therapy if more than 2 dosage reductions are necessary
Grade 2 symptomatic increase in diastolic BP by >20 mm Hg or BP >140/90 mm Hg if previously normal	Interrupt therapy; when diastolic BP resolves or improves to <90 mm Hg, resume at dosage reduced by one dose level; if necessary, reduce dosage by another dose level. Discontinue therapy if more than 2 dosage reductions are necessary
Grade 3	Interrupt therapy; when diastolic BP resolves or improves to <90 mm Hg, resume at dosage reduced by one dose level; if necessary, reduce dosage by another dose level. Discontinue therapy if more than 2 dosage reductions are necessary
Grade 4	Permanently discontinue therapy
GI Perforation	
Any grade	Permanently discontinue therapy
QT Prolongation	
>500 msec or ≥60 msec increase from baseline	Interrupt therapy and correct electrolyte abnormalities (e.g., magnesium, potassium, calcium); resume therapy if appropriate
Hepatotoxicity	
Grade 3 or higher ALT concentrations in absence of other etiology[a]	Permanently discontinue therapy
AST/ALT concentrations >3 times the ULN with bilirubin concentrations >2 times the ULN in absence of other etiology[a]	Permanently discontinue therapy
Other Adverse Effects	
Grade 2	Continue therapy at dosage reduced by one dose level
Grade 3	1st occurrence: Interrupt therapy; if toxicity resolves to grade 2 or less within 7 days, resume at dosage reduced by one dose level; if toxicity does not improve to grade 2 or less within 7 days, resume at dosage reduced by two dose levels. 2nd or 3rd occurrence: Interrupt therapy; when toxicity resolves to grade 2 or less, resume at dosage reduced by two dose levels. 4th occurrence: Interrupt therapy; when toxicity resolves to grade 2 or less, resume at dosage reduced by two dose levels in patients with hepatocellular carcinoma or renal cell carcinoma and by 3 dose levels in patients with differentiated thyroid carcinoma
Grade 4	Permanently discontinue therapy

[a] In addition, any grade increased alkaline phosphatase in the absence of known bone pathology and grade 2 or worse increased bilirubin; any one of the following: INR of ≥1.5, ascites and/or encephalopathy in the absence of underlying cirrhosis or other organ failure considered to be due to drug-induced liver injury.

TABLE 3. Recommended Dosage Modification for Cutaneous Toxicity

Cutaneous Toxicity Grade	Occurrence	Recommended Dosage Modification in Patients with Hepatocellular Carcinoma or Renal Cell Carcinoma	Recommended Dosage Modification in Patients with Differentiated Thyroid Carcinoma
Grade 2: Painful erythema and swelling of the hands or feet and/or discomfort affecting the patient's normal activities	1st occurrence	Continue sorafenib therapy and consider topical therapy for symptomatic relief	Decrease sorafenib dosage to 600 mg daily
	No improvement within 7 days at reduced dosage or 2nd or 3rd occurrence	Interrupt therapy until toxicity resolves to grade 0 or 1 When resuming therapy, reduce sorafenib dosage by one dose level	Interrupt therapy until toxicity completely resolves or improves to grade 1 When resuming therapy, reduce sorafenib dosage by one dose level for 2nd occurrence and by 2 dose levels for 3rd occurrence
	4th occurrence	Discontinue therapy	Discontinue therapy
Grade 3: Moist desquamation, ulceration, blistering or severe pain of the hands or feet, or severe discomfort that causes the patient to be unable to work or perform activities of daily living	1st occurrence	Interrupt therapy until toxicity resolves to grade 0 or 1 When resuming therapy, reduce sorafenib dosage by one dose level (e.g., to 400 mg once daily or 400 mg every other day)	Interrupt therapy until toxicity completely resolves or improves to grade 1 When resuming therapy, reduce sorafenib dosage by one dose level
	2nd occurrence	Interrupt therapy until toxicity resolves to grade 0 or 1 When resuming therapy, reduce sorafenib dosage by one dose level (e.g., to 400 mg once daily or 400 mg every other day)	Interrupt therapy until toxicity completely resolves or improves to grade 1 When resuming therapy, reduce sorafenib dosage by 2 dose levels
	3rd occurrence	Discontinue therapy	Discontinue therapy

Following improvement of grade 2 or 3 cutaneous toxicity to grade 0 or 1 for at least 28 days or a reduced sorafenib dosage, the dosage may be increased one dose level from the reduced dosage. Approximately 50% of patients requiring a dosage reduction for cutaneous toxicity are expected to meet the criteria for resumption of the higher dosage and about 50% of patients resuming the previous dosage are expected to tolerate the higher dosage without recurrent grade 2 or higher cutaneous toxicity.

• Special Populations

Hepatic Impairment

No dosage adjustment is necessary in patients with mild (Child-Pugh class A) or moderate (Child-Pugh class B) hepatic impairment. The pharmacokinetics of sorafenib have not been studied in patients with severe (Child-Pugh class C) hepatic impairment.

Renal Impairment

No dosage adjustment is necessary in patients with mild to severe renal impairment who are not receiving dialysis. The pharmacokinetics of sorafenib have not been studied in patients with renal impairment requiring dialysis.

Geriatric Patients

The manufacturer makes no specific dosage recommendations for geriatric patients.

CAUTIONS

• Contraindications

- Known severe hypersensitivity to sorafenib or any ingredient in the formulation.
- In combination with carboplatin and paclitaxel in patients with squamous cell lung cancer.

• Warnings/Precautions

Cardiovascular Effects

In the phase 3 trial of sorafenib in patients with unresectable hepatocellular carcinoma, cardiac ischemia or infarction occurred in 2.7% of patients receiving sorafenib compared with 1.3% of those receiving placebo. In the phase 3 trial in patients with advanced renal cell carcinoma, cardiac ischemia or infarction occurred more frequently in patients receiving sorafenib than in those receiving placebo (2.9 versus 0.4%). In a clinical trial of sorafenib in patients with differentiated thyroid carcinoma, cardiac ischemia or infarction occurred in 1.9% of patients receiving sorafenib and in 0% of those receiving placebo. In multiple clinical trials, congestive heart failure was reported in 1.9% of sorafenib-treated patients. Temporary or permanent discontinuance of sorafenib should be considered in patients who develop cardiovascular events.

In several clinical trials, congestive heart failure was reported in 1.9% of patients receiving sorafenib.

In the phase 3 trial of sorafenib in patients with unresectable hepatocellular carcinoma, hypertension was reported in 9.4% of patients receiving sorafenib compared with 4.3% of those receiving placebo. In the phase 3 trial in patients with advanced renal cell carcinoma, hypertension was reported more frequently in patients receiving sorafenib compared with those receiving placebo (16.9 versus 1.8%). In a clinical trial of sorafenib in patients with differentiated thyroid carcinoma, hypertension was reported in 40.6% of patients receiving sorafenib and in 12.4% of those receiving placebo. Hypertension usually was mild or moderate in severity, occurred early in the course of treatment, and was managed with standard antihypertensive therapy. Permanent discontinuance of sorafenib therapy because of hypertension was necessary in 1 patient in each of the clinical trials. Blood pressure should be monitored weekly during the first 6 weeks of sorafenib therapy and thereafter should be monitored periodically and treated, if required, in accordance with established medical practice. If hypertension is severe or persistent despite initiation of antihypertensive therapy, temporary or permanent discontinuance of sorafenib should be considered.

Sorafenib may prolong the QT interval, which may increase the risk of ventricular arrhythmias. In a small multicenter, open-label, nonrandomized trial evaluating the effects of sorafenib (400 mg twice daily) on the QT interval in patients with advanced cancer, no large (i.e., exceeding 20 msec) increases in the corrected QT (QT_c) interval were observed. Following the first 28-day treatment cycle (cycle 1), the maximum mean change in QT_c interval was 8.5 msec, which was observed at 6 hours following the first dose of cycle 2. Sorafenib should be avoided in patients with congenital long QT syndrome. ECGs and serum electrolytes (potassium, calcium, and magnesium) should be monitored in patients with congestive heart failure, bradyarrhythmias, and in those who are receiving drugs known to prolong the QT interval (e.g., class IA and III antiarrhythmic agents). Electrolyte (magnesium, potassium, calcium) abnormalities should be corrected. Sorafenib therapy should be interrupted if QT interval is >500 msec or an increase of ≥60 msec from baseline occurs.

Hemorrhage

Sorafenib may increase the risk of bleeding. In the phase 3 trial of sorafenib in patients with unresectable hepatocellular carcinoma, the incidence of bleeding from esophageal varices was similar in patients receiving sorafenib compared with those receiving placebo (2.4 versus 4%); similarly, fatal hemorrhage from any site occurred in 2.4% of patients receiving sorafenib and 4% of those receiving placebo. In the phase 3 trial in patients with advanced renal cell carcinoma, bleeding (regardless of causality) was reported in 15.3 or 8.2% of patients receiving sorafenib or placebo, respectively; grade 3 and 4 bleeding were reported in 2 and 0%, respectively, of patients receiving sorafenib compared with 1.3 and 0.2%, respectively, of patients receiving placebo. Fatal hemorrhage occurred in one patient in each treatment group in this study. In a clinical trial of sorafenib in patients with differentiated thyroid carcinoma, hemorrhage occurred in 17.4% of patients receiving sorafenib and in 9.6% of those receiving placebo; the incidence of grade 3 bleeding was 1% and 1.4% in those receiving sorafenib and placebo, respectively.

Permanent discontinuance of sorafenib should be considered if any bleeding episode requires medical intervention. Because of the potential risk of bleeding, treat tracheal, bronchial, and esophageal infiltration with local therapy prior to initiating sorafenib in patients with differentiated thyroid carcinoma.

Patients concurrently receiving sorafenib and warfarin should be regularly monitored for changes in PT or INR and for clinical bleeding episodes.

Dermatologic Effects

Palmar-plantar erythrodysesthesia (commonly referred to as hand-foot syndrome) and rash are common adverse effects of sorafenib. Permanent discontinuance of therapy because of palmar-plantar erythrodysesthesia occurred in 1.3, 0.7, and 5.3% of sorafenib-treated patients with unresectable hepatocellular carcinoma, renal cell carcinoma, and differentiated thyroid carcinoma trials, respectively. Rash and hand-foot syndrome usually are grade 1 or 2 and generally appear during the first 6 weeks of treatment with sorafenib. Management of dermatologic toxicities may include topical therapies for symptomatic relief, temporary interruption of therapy, and/or dosage modification of sorafenib; in severe or persistent cases, permanent discontinuance of sorafenib therapy may be necessary.

Cases of severe and possibly life-threatening dermatologic toxicities, including Stevens-Johnson syndrome and toxic epidermal necrolysis, have been reported in patients receiving sorafenib. If Stevens-Johnson syndrome or toxic epidermal necrolysis is suspected, sorafenib therapy should be discontinued.

GI Effects

GI perforation, sometimes associated with apparent intra-abdominal tumor, has been reported in less than 1% of patients receiving sorafenib. Sorafenib therapy should be permanently discontinued if GI perforation occurs.

Wound-healing Complications

Drugs that inhibit the VEGF signaling pathway, like sorafenib, have the potential to impair wound healing. Sorafenib should be withheld for at least 10 days prior to elective surgery and should not be administered for at least 2 weeks following major surgery and until adequate healing has occurred. The safety of resuming sorafenib therapy after resolution of wound healing complications has not been established.

Increased Mortality in Squamous Cell Carcinoma of the Lung

Subset analysis of data from 2 randomized controlled trials in patients with previously untreated advanced (stage IIIB or IV) non-small cell lung cancer revealed an increased risk of mortality in patients with squamous cell carcinoma receiving sorafenib in combination with carboplatin and paclitaxel (hazard ratio of 1.81) and in those receiving sorafenib in combination with gemcitabine and cisplatin (hazard ratio of 1.22) compared with those receiving the corresponding dual regimen (i.e., therapy with carboplatin and paclitaxel or with gemcitabine and cisplatin, respectively).

Sorafenib in combination with carboplatin and paclitaxel is contraindicated in patients with squamous cell carcinoma of the lung. In addition, the manufacturer states that use of sorafenib in combination with gemcitabine and cisplatin is *not* recommended in patients with squamous cell carcinoma of the lung.

Safety and efficacy of sorafenib in patients with non-small cell lung cancer have not been established.

Hepatic Effects

Serious or fatal drug-induced hepatitis characterized by a hepatocellular pattern of hepatic injury with substantially elevated serum aminotransferase concentrations

may occur; increased serum concentrations of bilirubin and increased INR also may occur. The incidence of severe drug-induced liver injury (aminotransferase concentrations >20 ULN or with significant clinical sequelae such as elevated INR, ascites, fatal, or transplantation) was 0.06% (2 of 3357 patients) in a global monotherapy database.

Liver function tests should be monitored regularly in patients receiving sorafenib. Sorafenib therapy should be discontinued if substantially elevated serum aminotransferase concentrations occur and other possible causes (i.e., viral hepatitis, malignancy progression) have been ruled out.

Fetal/Neonatal Morbidity and Mortality

Sorafenib may cause fetal harm if administered to pregnant women; teratogenicity and embryolethality have been demonstrated in animals. Although there are no adequate and well-controlled studies in humans, sorafenib has been shown to have teratogenic and embryolethal effects (i.e., postimplantation loss, resorptions, skeletal retardation, retarded fetal weight) in rats and rabbits when given in dosages lower than the usual human dosage. Pregnancy should be avoided during therapy. If sorafenib is used during pregnancy or if the patient becomes pregnant while receiving the drug, the patient should be apprised of the potential hazard to the fetus.

Verify pregnancy status of females of reproductive potential prior to initiation of therapy. Females of reproductive potential receiving the drug should use an effective contraceptive method during treatment and for at least 6 months following discontinuance of sorafenib therapy. Male patients with female partners of reproductive potential and pregnant partners should use an effective contraceptive method during treatment and for at least 3 months following discontinuance of sorafenib therapy.

Endocrine Effects

Sorafenib impairs exogenous thyroid suppression. In the differentiated thyroid carcinoma clinical study, elevation of TSH above 0.5 mU/L was observed in 41% of patients who received sorafenib and in 16% of those who received placebo.

Thyroid function should be monitored prior to initiation and at least monthly during sorafenib therapy. Hypothyroidism should be treated according to standard medical practice.

Specific Populations

Pregnancy

Sorafenib may cause fetal harm if administered to a pregnant female based on its mechanism of action and animal findings.

Lactation

Sorafenib is distributed into milk in rats; it is not known whether the drug or its metabolites are distributed into milk in humans. It is also not known if the drug has effects on the breast-fed infant or on milk production. Because of the potential for serious adverse reactions to sorafenib in breast-fed infants, females should not breast-feed during treatment with sorafenib and for 2 weeks following discontinuance of the drug.

Females and Males of Reproductive Potential

Females of reproductive potential should be advised to use effective contraceptive methods while receiving sorafenib and for at least 6 months after discontinuance of the drug.

Male patients with female partners of reproductive potential and pregnant partners should use an effective contraceptive method during sorafenib treatment and for at least 3 months following discontinuance of the drug.

Males should be advised that sorafenib may impair fertility.

Pediatric Use

The pharmacokinetics of sorafenib have not been studied in pediatric patients younger than 18 years of age.

Geriatric Use

In clinical trials evaluating sorafenib in patients with unresectable hepatocellular carcinoma or advanced renal cell carcinoma, 59 or 32%, respectively, of patients were 65 years of age or older, and 19 or 4%, respectively, were 75 years of age or older. No substantial differences in safety and efficacy relative to younger adults have been observed, but increased sensitivity to the drug cannot be ruled out.

Hepatic Impairment

Systemic exposure to sorafenib in patients with mild or moderate (Child-Pugh class A or B) hepatic impairment, including both patients with hepatocellular carcinoma and individuals without such disease, is similar to that observed in individuals with normal hepatic function. In patients with hepatocellular carcinoma, systemic exposure and peak plasma concentrations of the drug were slightly higher in those with moderate (Child-Pugh class B) hepatic impairment compared with those with mild (Child-Pugh class A) hepatic impairment; however, the differences were not clinically meaningful.

Limited safety and efficacy data are available for patients with hepatocellular carcinoma and moderate (Child-Pugh class B) hepatic impairment. In a phase 2 study in patients with hepatocellular carcinoma, median overall survival was shorter in patients with moderate (Child-Pugh class B) hepatic impairment than in those with mild (Child-Pugh class A) hepatic impairment (3.2 versus 9.5 months, respectively). Shorter median overall survival in patients with moderate hepatic impairment also has been reported from several prospective and retrospective studies of sorafenib use for hepatocellular carcinoma.

The pharmacokinetics of sorafenib have not been studied in patients with severe (Child-Pugh class C) hepatic impairment.

Renal Impairment

Mild (creatinine clearance 50–80 mL/minute), moderate (creatinine clearance 30 to <50 mL/minute), and severe (creatinine clearance <30 mL/minute) renal impairment does not affect the pharmacokinetics of sorafenib.

Pharmacokinetic parameters of sorafenib have not been evaluated in patients with renal impairment requiring dialysis.

● Common Adverse Effects

The most common adverse reactions (≥20%) are diarrhea, fatigue, infection, alopecia, palmar-plantar erythrodysesthesia (hand-foot skin reaction), rash, decreased weight, decreased appetite, nausea, GI and abdominal pain, hypertension, and hemorrhage.

DRUG INTERACTIONS

Sorafenib undergoes oxidative metabolism by cytochrome P450 (CYP) 3A4 and glucuronidation by uridine diphosphate-glucuronosyltransferase (UGT) 1A9.

In vitro studies using human hepatic microsomes indicate that sorafenib competitively inhibits CYP isoenzymes 2B6, 2C8, 2C9, 2C19, 2D6, and 3A4. Sorafenib is unlikely to induce CYP1A2 or CYP3A4. Sorafenib also inhibits glucuronidation by UGT1A1 and UGT1A9 in vitro. In vitro data also indicate that sorafenib is an inhibitor of the efflux transporter P-glycoprotein (P-gp).

● Drugs Affecting Hepatic Microsomal Enzymes

Sorafenib is partially metabolized by CYP3A4; however, when the potent CYP3A4 inhibitor ketoconazole (400 mg daily for 7 days) was administered concomitantly with sorafenib (single 50-mg dose) in healthy individuals, mean systemic exposure to sorafenib was unchanged. These data suggest that clinically important interactions with drugs that inhibit CYP3A4 are unlikely.

Concomitant use of sorafenib with inducers of CYP3A4 may result in increased metabolism of and decreased systemic exposure to sorafenib. In healthy individuals, the potent CYP3A4 inducer rifampin (600 mg daily for 5 days) decreased systemic exposure to sorafenib (single 400-mg dose) by 37%. Concomitant use of sorafenib with potent inducers of CYP3A4 (e.g., carbamazepine, dexamethasone, phenobarbital, phenytoin, rifabutin, rifampin, St. John's wort [Hypericum perforatum]) should be avoided when possible.

● Drugs Metabolized by Hepatic Microsomal Enzymes

In vitro studies using human hepatic microsomes indicate that sorafenib competitively inhibits CYP isoenzymes 2B6, 2C8, 2C9, 2C19, 2D6, and 3A4. However, concomitant administration of sorafenib with cyclophosphamide (a CYP2B6 substrate) or paclitaxel (a CYP2C8 substrate) did not result in clinically

important changes in enzyme inhibition, suggesting that sorafenib, when administered at the recommended dosage, may not result in clinically important inhibition of CYP2B6 or CYP2C8. In addition, sorafenib does not appear to alter systemic exposure to dextromethorphan (a CYP2D6 substrate), midazolam (a CYP3A4 substrate), or omeprazole (a CYP2C19 substrate), suggesting that clinically important interactions with drugs that are metabolized by these isoenzymes also are unlikely. When warfarin (a CYP2C9 substrate) was administered concomitantly with sorafenib, mean changes from baseline in prothrombin time (PT)/international normalized ratio (INR) did not appear to be greater in patients receiving sorafenib as compared with placebo, suggesting that the risk for clinically important inhibition of CYP2D6 by sorafenib also may be low (see Warfarin under Drug Interactions).

The manufacturer states that sorafenib is unlikely to induce CYP isoenzymes 1A2 or 3A4.

● Drugs Metabolized by Uridine Diphosphate-glucuronosyltransferase

In vitro studies indicate that sorafenib inhibits glucuronidation by the uridine diphosphate-glucuronosyltransferase (UGT) 1A1 and 1A9 pathways; sorafenib may increase systemic exposure to UGT1A1 or UGT1A9 substrates. Caution is advised when sorafenib is used concomitantly with drugs predominantly metabolized by the UGT1A1 or UGT1A9 pathway.

● Drugs Affecting Gastric Acidity

Because the aqueous solubility of sorafenib is dependent on pH, drugs that increase the pH of the upper GI tract (e.g., proton-pump inhibitors) may potentially decrease the solubility of sorafenib. However, concomitant administration of the proton-pump inhibitor omeprazole (40 mg once daily for 5 days) with a single dose of sorafenib did not result in clinically important changes in systemic exposure to sorafenib. The manufacturer states that dosage adjustment of sorafenib is not necessary when sorafenib is administered concurrently with drugs affecting gastric acidity.

● Substrates of P-Glycoprotein Transport System

In vitro data indicate that sorafenib is an inhibitor of the efflux transporter P-glycoprotein (P-gp). Concomitant use of sorafenib with drugs that are substrates of P-gp (e.g., digoxin) may result in increased systemic exposure to the substrate drug.

● Antibiotics

In healthy individuals, neomycin (1 g orally 3 times daily for 5 days) decreased the mean systemic exposure to sorafenib (single 400-mg dose) by 54%. Bacterial glucuronidases in the GI tract may cleave sorafenib conjugates, allowing reabsorption of unconjugated drug; neomycin interferes with this enterohepatic circulation process, thereby reducing bioavailability of sorafenib. Avoid concomitant use of sorafenib and neomycin.

The effect of other antibiotics on the pharmacokinetics of sorafenib has not been established.

● Antineoplastic Agents

When docetaxel was administered concomitantly with sorafenib, systemic exposure and peak plasma concentration of docetaxel were increased by 36–80 and 16–32%, respectively. Caution is advised.

When irinotecan was administered concomitantly with sorafenib, systemic exposure to irinotecan and its active metabolite SN-38 was increased by 26–42 and 67–120%, respectively. Caution is advised.

When doxorubicin was used concomitantly with sorafenib, systemic exposure to doxorubicin was increased by 21%.

Concomitant use of capecitabine with sorafenib did not substantially alter systemic exposure to sorafenib but increased systemic exposure to capecitabine and its active metabolite fluorouracil by 15–50 and 0–52%, respectively.

Concomitant use of paclitaxel and carboplatin with continuous sorafenib therapy increased systemic exposure to sorafenib and to paclitaxel and its major metabolite 6-hydroxypaclitaxel (a metabolite formed by CYP2C8) by 47, 29, and 50%, respectively, but did not alter the pharmacokinetics of carboplatin.

Sorafenib does not appear to affect the pharmacokinetics of cisplatin, cyclophosphamide, gemcitabine, or oxaliplatin.

● *Drugs that Prolong the QT Interval*

Sorafenib can prolong the QT interval. Avoid concomitant use with other drugs that can prolong the QT interval (e.g., class 1a and III antiarrhythmic agents).

● *Warfarin*

When warfarin (a CYP2C9 substrate) was administered concomitantly with sorafenib, mean changes from baseline in PT/INR did not appear to be greater in patients receiving sorafenib as compared with placebo. However, infrequent bleeding events or elevations in INR have been reported in some patients receiving concomitant therapy with warfarin and sorafenib. Patients concurrently receiving sorafenib and warfarin should be regularly monitored for changes in PT, INR, or clinical bleeding episodes.

DESCRIPTION

Sorafenib tosylate, an inhibitor of several serine/threonine and receptor tyrosine kinases, is an antineoplastic agent. Serine/threonine and receptor tyrosine kinases are involved in various cascades of intracellular signaling events that lead to cell proliferation and/or influence processes critical to cell survival and tumor progression (e.g., angiogenesis, apoptosis, metastasis), based on the respective kinase. Although the exact mechanism of antineoplastic activity of sorafenib has not been fully elucidated, sorafenib appears to inhibit signal transduction pathways involving multiple intracellular (e.g., c-Raf, b-Raf, mutant b-Raf) and cell surface kinases (e.g., c-Kit, Flt-3, RET, RET/PTC, vascular endothelial growth factor receptor [VEGFR]-1, VEGFR-2, VEGFR-3, platelet-derived growth factor receptor [PDGFR]-β) in vitro. In vivo, sorafenib inhibited angiogenesis and/or growth of human hepatocellular carcinoma, renal cell carcinoma, differentiated thyroid carcinoma, and several other human tumor xenografts in immunocompromised mice.

Sorafenib is metabolized mainly in the liver via oxidation by cytochrome P-450 (CYP) isoenzyme 3A4, as well as via glucuronidation by uridine diphosphate-glucuronosyltransferase (UGT) 1A9. At least 8 metabolites of sorafenib have been identified. The main circulating metabolite, a pyridine *N*-oxide derivative, is pharmacologically active and accounts for approximately 9–16% of total plasma concentrations of the drug. Approximately 77% of an oral dose of sorafenib is excreted in feces and 19% is eliminated in urine; unchanged sorafenib, which accounts for 51% of a dose, is recovered in feces but not in urine. The pharmacokinetics of sorafenib do not appear to be affected by age or gender; however, systemic exposure to the drug was 30% lower in Asians than in Caucasians.

ADVICE TO PATIENTS

- Instruct patients to read the manufacturer's patient information before starting sorafenib therapy and each time their prescription is filled.
- If a dose is missed, importance of administering the next dose at the regularly scheduled time; do *not* administer a double dose to make up for a missed dose.
- Importance of females informing clinicians if they are or plan to become pregnant or plan to breast-feed. Necessity of advising females to avoid pregnancy during therapy and for ≥6 months following completion of sorafenib therapy. Necessity of advising females to use effective contraceptive methods during sorafenib therapy and for ≥6 months following completion of therapy. Necessity of advising men with female partners of reproductive potential or who have partners who are pregnant to use effective contraceptive methods during therapy and for at least 3 months following completion of sorafenib therapy. Advise females of the potential risk to the fetus (e.g., birth defects) and/or the potential risk for loss of the pregnancy.

- Advise females to discontinue breast-feeding during sorafenib therapy and for ≥2 weeks following completion of sorafenib therapy.
- Risk of hand-foot syndrome and rash. Importance of advising patient about appropriate countermeasures.
- Risk of hypertension, particularly during the first 6 weeks of sorafenib therapy. Importance of monitoring BP regularly during therapy.
- Risk of bleeding. Importance of patients promptly informing clinicians of any episodes of bleeding.
- Risk of bleeding or INR elevation in patients receiving concomitant therapy with warfarin and sorafenib. Importance of monitoring INR regularly during concomitant therapy.
- Risk of potential GI perforation. Importance of informing clinician immediately if high fever, nausea, vomiting, or severe stomach or abdominal pain occurs.
- Risk of potential cardiac ischemia and/or infarction and congestive heart failure. Importance of patients immediately informing clinicians or to seek emergency medical care if any episodes of chest pain or other symptoms of cardiac ischemia or congestive heart failure occur.
- Risk of wound healing complications. Importance of informing clinician of any scheduled surgery.
- Risk of QT-interval prolongation. Importance of informing clinicians immediately if an abnormal heartbeat or feelings of dizziness or faintness occur. Inform patients with a history of prolonged QT interval that sorafenib can worsen the condition and that ECGs and/or serum electrolytes may be monitored during sorafenib therapy.
- Risk of hepatitis and importance of regular liver function test monitoring. Importance of informing clinician if signs and symptoms of hepatitis (e.g., jaundice, dark tea-colored urine, light-colored stool, worsening nausea or vomiting, abdominal pain) occur.
- Importance of informing clinicians of existing or contemplated concomitant therapy, including prescription and OTC drugs and herbal supplements (e.g., St. John's wort), as well as any concomitant illnesses (e.g., cardiovascular disease [including congenital long QT syndrome]).
- Importance of informing patients of other important precautionary information. (See Cautions.)

For further information on the handling of antineoplastic agents, see the ASHP Guidelines on Handling Hazardous Drugs at http://www.ahfsdruginformation.com.

PREPARATIONS

Sorafenib can only be obtained through designated specialty pharmacies. Contact the manufacturer for more information.

Excipients in commercially available drug preparations may have clinically important effects in some individuals; consult specific product labeling for details.

SORAfenib Tosylate

Oral

Tablets, film-coated	200 mg (of sorafenib)*	NexAVAR®, Bayer (comarketed by Onyx)
		SORAfenib Tosylate Film-coated Tablets

† Use is not currently included in the labeling approved by the US Food and Drug Administration.

* available from one or more manufacturer, distributor, and/or repackager by generic (nonproprietary) name

Selected Revisions July 22, 2022, © Copyright, May 01, 2006, American Society of Health-System Pharmacists, Inc.

SUNItinib Malate

10:00 · ANTINEOPLASTIC AGENTS

■ Sunitinib malate, an inhibitor of multiple receptor tyrosine kinases, is an antineoplastic agent.

USES

● Gastrointestinal Stromal Tumor

Sunitinib malate is used for the treatment of GI stromal tumor (GIST) in adults who are intolerant of or whose disease has progressed during imatinib therapy.

The current indication for sunitinib malate is based principally on the results of 2 studies (one randomized, double-blind, placebo-controlled, phase 3 study and one open-label, single-arm, phase 1/2 dose-escalation study) in patients with GIST who were intolerant of or whose disease had progressed during imatinib therapy. In the phase 3 study, 312 patients were randomized in a 2:1 ratio to receive either sunitinib (50 mg) or placebo given once daily for 4 consecutive weeks followed by a 2-week period without treatment. Treatment cycles were repeated until disease progression or withdrawal from the study for other reasons occurred. A planned interim analysis indicated that patients receiving sunitinib had a longer median time to tumor progression (27.3 versus 6.4 weeks) and a longer median progression-free survival (24.1 versus 6 weeks) than those receiving placebo. Following these favorable results, the study was unblinded, and study investigators permitted patients previously randomized to receive placebo to cross over to open-label sunitinib; those previously randomized to receive sunitinib were permitted to continue therapy based on clinical judgment. After the study was unblinded, 94.3% of patients initially randomized to receive placebo crossed over to receive sunitinib therapy. Updated analysis confirmed that, following administration of a median of 5–6 treatment cycles, patients receiving sunitinib (i.e., those originally randomized to sunitinib and those who switched from placebo to sunitinib) had a longer median time to tumor progression (28.4 weeks) than those who received placebo (8.7 weeks); the time to tumor progression in patients who switched from placebo to sunitinib was not statistically different from that in patients originally randomized to sunitinib therapy. At the planned final analysis, median overall survival was 72.7 weeks in patients receiving sunitinib compared with 64.9 weeks in those receiving placebo.

In the open-label, single-arm, dose-escalation study, treatment with sunitinib given in 6-week cycles at a dosage of 50 mg once daily for 4 consecutive weeks followed by a 2-week drug-free period produced partial responses in 5 of 55 patients (9.1%).

Clinical Perspective

Treatment of GIST includes surgical resection and/or the use of tyrosine kinase inhibitors depending on the extent of disease and tumor sensitivity to the tyrosine kinase inhibitor. Approximately 85% of all GIST contain a mutation in KIT and/or platelet-derived growth factor receptor alpha (PDGFRA) which result in constitutive activation of the receptor tyrosine kinase; therefore, inhibition of KIT is a primary therapeutic modality for the treatment of GIST. Imatinib is a selective inhibitor of the KIT protein tyrosine kinase, and is considered standard therapy for the treatment of locally advanced, inoperable or metastatic GIST (including patients who did not relapse during therapy with adjuvant imatinib) in patients with imatinib-sensitive mutations. Following disease progression or intolerance to imatinib, sunitinib is standard second-line therapy in patients with metastatic or recurrent GIST. Regorafenib is generally recommended in the third-line setting in patients with imatinib-sensitive mutations and imatinib-nonsensitive-mutations (e.g., PDGFRA D842V, NTRK-translocated, SDH-deficient).

Although the majority of GIST cases have either a mutation in KIT or PDGFRA, approximately 10–15% of cases do not have a detectable KIT or PDGFRA mutation. Loss-of-function mutations in succinate dehydrogenase (SDH) or loss of SDHB expression have been identified in a majority of wild type KIT/PDGFRA GIST (also referred to as SDH-deficient GIST); such tumors are usually resistant to imatinib, but may have some sensitivity to sunitinib and regorafenib.

● Renal Cell Carcinoma

Sunitinib malate is used for the adjuvant treatment of renal cell carcinoma in patients at high risk of recurrence following nephrectomy; the drug is also used for the treatment of advanced renal cell carcinoma.

Adjuvant Treatment

Efficacy and safety of sunitinib for the adjuvant treatment of renal cell carcinoma are based principally on the results of a randomized, double-blind, placebo-controlled study (S-TRAC) in adult patients at high risk of disease recurrence following nephrectomy. In this study, 615 patients were randomized to receive either sunitinib 50 mg once daily for 4 consecutive weeks followed by a 2-week period without treatment or placebo. Treatment with sunitinib was continued for 9 cycles until disease recurrence or unacceptable toxicity occurred or withdrawal of consent occurred. The median age of patients enrolled in the study was 58 years; 73% were male, 84% were white, 12% were Asian, and most patients had an ECOG performance status score of 0. The primary efficacy end point was disease-free survival; overall survival was a secondary endpoint.

At the time of analysis, median disease-free survival was substantially improved in patients receiving sunitinib (6.8 years) compared with those receiving placebo (5.6 years). At the time of data cutoff, overall survival data were not mature. In a prespecified subgroup analysis based on disease stage, no substantial difference in median disease-free survival was observed between the treatment arms.

Advanced Renal Cell Carcinoma

Efficacy and safety of sunitinib malate for the treatment of advanced renal cell carcinoma are based principally on the results of a large randomized trial and 2 uncontrolled studies.

In a multicenter randomized trial, 750 patients received either sunitinib or interferon alfa as initial treatment for metastatic renal cell cancer. Treatment consisted of sunitinib 50 mg once daily for 4 consecutive weeks followed by a 2-week period without treatment, or interferon alfa 9 million units subcutaneously 3 times a week, until disease progression, intolerable toxicity, or withdrawal from the study occurred. Progression-free survival was prolonged (47.3 versus 22 weeks) and overall response rate was higher (27.5 versus 5.3%) in patients receiving sunitinib compared with those receiving interferon alfa. At the planned final analysis, median overall survival was 114.6 weeks in patients receiving sunitinib compared with 94.9 weeks in those receiving interferon alfa. The median overall survival for the interferon alfa-treated group included 6.7% of patients who crossed over to treatment with sunitinib and 32% of patients who received post-study therapy with sunitinib.

Patients receiving sunitinib had a greater frequency of ventricular dysfunction, including left ventricular ejection fraction (LVEF) below the lower limit of normal (27 versus 15%) and decline in LVEF (7 versus 2%), than those receiving interferon alfa. Hypertension (34 versus 4%), including grade 3 hypertension (13 versus less than 1%), and bleeding events (37 versus 10%) occurred more frequently in patients receiving sunitinib than in those receiving interferon alfa.

The use of sunitinib also was investigated in 2 single-arm, phase 2 studies in 169 patients with metastatic renal cell carcinoma who were intolerant of cytokine-based therapy (e.g., aldesleukin, interferon alfa, combination of aldesleukin and interferon alfa) and/or whose disease had progressed during or following completion of such therapy. Approximately 95% of enrolled patients had at least some component of clear-cell histology, and 97% had undergone nephrectomy. Metastatic disease present at the time of study entry included lung (82%), liver (23%), and bone (35%) metastases; patients with known brain metastases or leptomeningeal disease were excluded from both studies. All patients in both studies received sunitinib (dosage schedule of 50 mg once daily for 4 consecutive weeks followed by a 2-week period without treatment) until disease progression, intolerable toxicity, or withdrawal from the study occurred. Data analysis from the first study revealed a partial response rate of 34% and a median progression-free survival of 8.3 months; the median overall survival had not been reached at the time of this analysis. Data analysis from the second study revealed a partial response rate of 36.5% and a median time to tumor progression of 8.7 months. In these studies, more than 90% of partial responses were observed during the first 4 cycles of sunitinib therapy, with the latest response observed during cycle 10.

Clinical Perspective

Advanced Renal Cell Carcinoma

Prognosis is generally poor in patients with metastatic RCC, including those who have undergone complete tumor resection. First-line therapy with vascular endothelial growth factor receptor (VEGFR) inhibitors has been shown to provide benefits in patients with advanced RCC; however, relapsed or refractory RCC eventually develops in most patients. Combination regimens (e.g., immune checkpoint inhibitor in combination with a tyrosine kinase inhibitor) have generally become a standard for the treatment of advanced RCC. A limited number of randomized controlled trials have compared sunitinib with other treatment options for advanced renal cell carcinoma (e.g., pembrolizumab plus axitinib, avelumab plus axitinib, atezolizumab plus bevacizumab, nivolumab plus ipilimumab, nivolumab plus cabozantinib, or lenvatinib plus pembrolizumab). In clinical trials, combination chemotherapy resulted in longer progression-free survival compared with sunitinib alone in patients with previously untreated advanced renal cell carcinoma.

Some experts state that subsequent monotherapy with a tyrosine kinase inhibitor (e.g., sunitinib, pazopanib) may be offered as an alternative to programmed death 1 (PD-1) inhibitor-based combinations in the first-line setting when immune checkpoint therapy is contraindicated or not available or as a second-line option following disease progression during immune checkpoint inhibitor-based therapy.

Neuroendocrine Tumors of Pancreatic Origin

Sunitinib malate is used for the treatment of progressive, well-differentiated neuroendocrine tumors (NET) of pancreatic origin in patients with unresectable, locally advanced, or metastatic disease.

Efficacy and safety of sunitinib malate for the treatment of pancreatic NET are based principally on the results of a randomized, double-blind, placebo-controlled, multicenter, phase 3 study in patients with unresectable, locally advanced, or metastatic well-differentiated pancreatic NET that had progressed within the previous 12 months. In this study, 171 patients were randomized in a 1:1 ratio to receive either sunitinib (37.5 mg) or placebo orally once daily; therapy was given continuously (i.e., without a scheduled off-treatment period). Approximately 27 or 29% of patients randomized to receive sunitinib or placebo, respectively, also received concomitant therapy with a somatostatin analog. Treatment with sunitinib or placebo was continued until disease progression, unacceptable toxicity, or death occurred; upon disease progression, patients previously randomized to receive placebo were permitted to cross over to open-label sunitinib therapy in an extension study. The primary end point of this study was progression-free survival; secondary end points included safety, overall response rate, time to tumor response, response duration, and overall survival. Median duration of treatment was approximately 4.6 months in patients receiving sunitinib and 3.7 months in those receiving placebo. This study was terminated prematurely (prior to the prespecified interim analysis) after an independent data monitoring committee found longer median progression-free survival among patients randomized to receive sunitinib and higher incidences of death and severe adverse effects among those randomized to receive placebo. Data analysis revealed a median progression-free survival of 10.2 months in patients receiving sunitinib compared with 5.4 months in patients receiving placebo, although the magnitude of effect on progression-free survival may have been overestimated by early termination of the study. Objective response was observed in 9.3% (25% complete and 75% partial responses) of patients receiving sunitinib compared with none of those receiving placebo. Overall survival had not been reached at the time of this analysis; however, death had occurred in 9 patients receiving sunitinib compared with 21 patients receiving placebo.

Clinical Perspective

Treatment options for grade 1 and 2 (G1 and G2) neuroendocrine tumors (NET) include surgery (primary and cytoreductive), liver-directed therapy, and systemic therapy. Systemic therapy (e.g., lutetium Lu 177 dotatate, somatostatin analog, targeted therapy, cytotoxic chemotherapy) is generally used for disease control and symptom palliation in patients with metastatic disease. Long-acting somatostatin analogs are generally considered first-line therapy for metastatic NET, while sunitinib and everolimus are generally used in the second-line setting. Although the role of chemotherapy in NET is evolving and an optimal chemotherapy regimen for grade 3 (G3) neuroendocrine carcinoma (poorly differentiated tumors) has not been established, several studies have shown promising results with combination therapy with capecitabine and temozolomide (CAPTEM).

Other Uses

Sunitinib also has been studied in nongastrointestinal stromal tumor sarcomas† and thyroid cancer†.

DOSAGE AND ADMINISTRATION

General

Pretreatment Screening

- Monitor liver function tests (ALT, AST, and bilirubin concentrations) prior to initiation of sunitinib.
- Consider monitoring left ventricular ejection fraction (LVEF) at baseline.
- Blood pressure at baseline.
- Perform urinalysis at baseline.
- Perform thyroid function tests at baseline.
- Assess blood glucose levels at baseline.
- Perform an oral examination prior to initiating therapy.
- Verify pregnancy status in females of reproductive potential.

Patient Monitoring

- Monitor liver function tests (ALT, AST, and bilirubin concentrations) during each cycle, and as clinically indicated.
- Consider monitoring LVEF periodically as indicated.
- Carefully monitor for clinical signs or symptoms of CHF.
- Monitor for development of or worsening of proteinuria. Perform urinalysis periodically during therapy; assess urine protein levels over a 24-hour period as clinically indicated.
- Monitor patients at high risk of developing QT interval prolongation (i.e., concomitant antiarrhythmic therapy, preexisting cardiac disease, bradycardia, or electrolyte disturbances). Consider periodic monitoring of ECGs and electrolytes (i.e., magnesium, potassium) during therapy.
- Monitor QT interval more frequently in patients receiving sunitinib concomitantly with a potent cytochrome P-450 (CYP) 3A4 inhibitor or drug known to prolong the QT interval.
- Monitor blood pressure as clinically indicated.
- Monitor for hemorrhagic events (e.g., serial CBCs, physical examinations).
- Monitor for tumor lysis syndrome.
- Monitor for signs or symptoms of thyroid dysfunction. Periodically monitor thyroid function during therapy and as clinically indicated.
- Monitor blood glucose levels regularly during therapy and as clinically indicated; continue monitoring following discontinuance of the drug.
- Perform oral examinations periodically during therapy.

Administration

Sunitinib malate is administered orally without regard to meals.

Store sunitinib at 20–25ºC; excursions are permitted between 15–30ºC.

Dosage

Dosage of sunitinib malate is expressed in terms of sunitinib.

Gastrointestinal Stromal Tumor

For the treatment of gastrointestinal stromal tumor (GIST) in adults who are intolerant of or whose disease has progressed during imatinib therapy, sunitinib is given in 6-week cycles at a recommended dosage of 50 mg once daily for 4 consecutive weeks followed by a 2-week period without the drug. In clinical studies, therapy was continued for as long as the patient derived clinical benefit from the drug or until unacceptable toxicity occurred.

Renal Cell Carcinoma

Adjuvant Therapy

For the adjuvant treatment of renal cell carcinoma in adults, sunitinib is given in 6-week cycles at a recommended dosage of 50 mg once daily for 4 consecutive weeks followed by a 2-week period without the drug. Therapy is continued for 9 cycles.

Advanced Renal Cell Carcinoma

For the treatment of advanced renal cell carcinoma in adults, sunitinib is given in 6-week cycles at a recommended dosage of 50 mg once daily for 4 consecutive weeks followed by a 2-week period without the drug. In clinical studies, therapy was continued for as long as the patient derived clinical benefit from the drug or until unacceptable toxicity occurred.

Neuroendocrine Tumors of Pancreatic Origin

For the treatment of progressive, well-differentiated neuroendocrine tumors (NET) of pancreatic origin in adults with unresectable, locally advanced, or metastatic disease, sunitinib is given continuously (i.e., without an off-treatment period) at a recommended dosage of 37.5 mg once daily. In the principal efficacy study, sunitinib was continued until disease progression, unacceptable toxicity, or death occurred.

Dosage Modification

Dosage of sunitinib should be adjusted in increments or decrements of 12.5 mg daily (i.e., 1 dose level), depending on individual patient safety and tolerability.

If dosage modification is required, the dosage of sunitinib should be reduced as described in Table 1 in patients with GIST, renal cell carcinoma, or NET of pancreatic origin.

TABLE 1. Recommended Dosage Reduction for Sunitinib Toxicity in Patients with GIST, Renal Cell Carcinoma, or NET of Pancreatic Origin.

Dosage Reduction Level	GIST (Starting Dosage = 50 mg daily)	Advanced Renal Cell Carcinoma (Starting Dosage = 50 mg daily)	Adjuvant Treatment of Renal Cell Carcinoma (Starting Dosage = 50 mg daily)	NET of Pancreatic Origin (Starting Dosage = 37.5 mg daily)
First	Restart at 37.5 mg once daily	Restart at 37.5 mg once daily	Restart at 37.5 mg once daily	Restart at 25 mg once daily
Second	Restart at 25 mg once daily	Restart at 25 mg once daily	Not applicable	Not applicable

Hepatotoxicity

If grade 3 hepatotoxicity occurs, withhold therapy; when the toxicity resolves or improves to grade 0 or 1, may then resume therapy at a reduced dosage. If grade 3 hepatotoxicity recurs, permanently discontinue sunitinib.

Permanently discontinue sunitinib in patients who experience grade 4 hepatotoxicity.

Cardiovascular Toxicity

If manifestations of congestive heart failure develop, the drug should be discontinued. In patients without clinical evidence of congestive heart failure but in whom left ventricular ejection fraction (LVEF) is greater than 20%, but less than 50% below baseline, or below the lower limit of normal if LVEF was not assessed at baseline, sunitinib therapy should be withheld; when the toxicity resolves or improves to grade 0 or 1, may then resume therapy at a reduced dosage.

For grade 3 hypertension, withhold sunitinib; when hypertension resolves or improves to grade 0 or 1, may then resume therapy at a reduced dosage. For grade 4 hypertension, permanently discontinue sunitinib.

Hemorrhagic Events

If grade 3 or 4 hemorrhagic events occur, withhold sunitinib therapy; when the toxicity resolves or improves to grade 0 or 1, may then resume therapy at a reduced dosage or discontinue therapy depending on the severity and persistence of the hemorrhagic event. If grade 3 or 4 hemorrhagic events do not resolve, discontinue sunitinib therapy.

Proteinuria

Interrupt sunitinib therapy and reduce dosage if proteinuria ≥3 g per 24 hours (in the absence of nephrotic syndrome) occurs. When proteinuria resolves or improves to grade 0 or 1, may then resume at a reduced dosage. If nephrotic syndrome occurs or if proteinuria recurs despite dosage reduction, permanently discontinue therapy.

Other Toxicity

Permanently discontinue sunitinib in patients who experience any grade thrombotic microangiopathy, dermatologic toxicities (i.e., erythema multiforme, Stevens-Johnson syndrome, toxic epidermal necrolysis, necrotizing fasciitis) or reversible posterior leukoencephalopathy syndrome.

If osteonecrosis of the jaw or impaired wound healing occurs, sunitinib therapy may be resumed at a reduced dosage or discontinued depending on the severity and persistence of the adverse effects; however, safety of resuming sunitinib therapy in patients who experience osteonecrosis of the jaw or impaired wound healing has not been established.

Concomitant Use with Drugs Affecting Hepatic Microsomal Enzymes

Concomitant use of sunitinib with potent inhibitors or inducers of cytochrome P-450 (CYP) isoenzyme 3A4 may alter the combined plasma concentrations of sunitinib and its primary active metabolite.

If concomitant use of sunitinib with a potent CYP3A4 *inhibitor* cannot be avoided, reduction of sunitinib dosage to no less than 37.5 mg daily (in patients receiving sunitinib for GIST or advanced renal cell carcinoma) or no less than 25 mg daily (in patients receiving sunitinib for progressive, well-differentiated NET of pancreatic origin) should be considered.

• Special Populations

Hepatic Impairment

The manufacturer states that initial dosage adjustment is not necessary in patients with mild or moderate hepatic impairment (Child-Pugh class A or B).

Renal Impairment

The manufacturer states that initial dosage adjustment is not necessary in patients with mild, moderate, or severe renal impairment; subsequent dosage modifications should be based on safety and tolerability. Initial dosage adjustment is not necessary in patients with end-stage renal disease receiving hemodialysis; however, subsequent dosages may be increased gradually up to twofold based on safety and tolerability.

Geriatric Patients

The manufacturer makes no specific dosage recommendations for geriatric patients.

CAUTIONS

• Contraindications

The manufacturer states there are no known contraindications to the use of sunitinib.

• Warnings/Precautions

Warnings

Hepatotoxicity

A boxed warning regarding the risk of severe hepatotoxicity is included in the prescribing information for sunitinib. Severe hepatotoxicity, resulting in liver failure or death, has been reported in patients receiving sunitinib. Hepatic failure has been reported in patients receiving sunitinib in clinical trials (<1%). Manifestations of hepatic failure include jaundice, elevated aminotransferase concentrations and/or hyperbilirubinemia in conjunction with encephalopathy, coagulopathy, and/or renal failure.

Monitor liver function tests (ALT, AST, and bilirubin concentrations) prior to initiation of sunitinib, during each cycle, and as clinically indicated. If grade 3 hepatotoxicity occurs, interrupt sunitinib therapy until the toxicity resolves or improves to grade 1 or less, then resume sunitinib at a reduced dosage. If grade 4 hepatotoxicity occurs or grade 3 hepatotoxicity persists, discontinue sunitinib therapy. Sunitinib should not be restarted in patients who subsequently experience severe changes in liver function tests or exhibit other manifestations of hepatic failure.

Safety of sunitinib in patients with AST and/or ALT concentrations exceeding 2.5 times the upper limit of normal or, if caused by liver metastases, exceeding 5 times the upper limit of normal has not been established.

Other Warnings and Precautions

Cardiovascular Effects

Cardiovascular events (including heart failure, myocardial ischemia, myocardial infarction, and cardiomyopathy), sometimes fatal, have been reported in patients receiving sunitinib during postmarketing surveillance.

In a pooled safety population, heart failure was reported in 3% of patients (<1% were fatal); however, heart failure resolved in the majority (71%) of these patients. In a clinical study, 11 patients receiving sunitinib for the adjuvant treatment of renal cell carcinoma experienced grade 2 decreases in left ventricular ejection fraction (LVEF) (defined as LVEF 40–50% with a 10–19% reduction from baseline values). LVEF did not return to ≥50% or baseline by the time of the last measurement in 3 of the 11 patients. None of the patients were diagnosed with congestive heart failure.

Because patients with a history of cardiovascular disease (e.g., myocardial infarction [MI], severe or unstable angina, coronary or peripheral artery bypass graft, symptomatic congestive heart failure, cerebrovascular accident or transient ischemic attack, pulmonary embolism) within 12 months prior to sunitinib administration and patients with prior anthracycline use or cardiac radiation were excluded from clinical studies, it is unknown whether such patients have a higher risk of developing drug-related left ventricular dysfunction.

Consider monitoring LVEF prior to initiating therapy and periodically as clinically indicated. Monitor patients for signs and symptoms of congestive heart failure; if manifestations of congestive heart failure develop, discontinue sunitinib. In patients without clinical evidence of congestive heart failure but in whom LVEF is greater than 20% but less than 50% below baseline or below the lower limit of normal if LVEF was not assessed at baseline, interrupt therapy and/or reduce the dosage.

Prolongation of QT Interval and Torsades de Pointes

Sunitinib prolongs the QT interval in a dose-dependent manner, which may increase the risk of ventricular arrhythmias, including torsades de pointes. Torsades de pointes has been reported in less than 0.1% of patients receiving sunitinib.

Monitor patients at high risk of developing QT interval prolongation, including patients with a history of prolongation of the QT interval, those receiving antiarrhythmic agents, and those with relevant preexisting cardiac disease, bradycardia, or electrolyte disturbances. Periodic monitoring of ECGs and serum magnesium and potassium concentrations should be considered. More frequent QT interval monitoring and reduction of sunitinib dosage should be considered in patients concomitantly receiving potent CYP3A4 inhibitors or drugs known to prolong the QT interval.

Hypertension

Hypertension has been reported in 29% of patients receiving sunitinib in the pooled safety population. Grade 3 hypertension occurred in 7% of patients and grade 4 hypertension was reported in 0.2%.

Monitor blood pressure at baseline and as clinically indicated; treat hypertension as needed with standard antihypertensive therapy. If grade 3 hypertension occurs, interrupt sunitinib until hypertension resolves or improves to grade 1 or less; sunitinib therapy may then be resumed at a lower dosage. If grade 4 hypertension occurs, discontinue sunitinib therapy.

Hemorrhage

Hemorrhagic events (including GI, respiratory, tumor, urinary tract, and brain hemorrhage), sometimes fatal, have been reported in patients receiving sunitinib. Hemorrhagic events were reported in 30% of patients in the pooled safety population (grade 3 or 4 in 4.2% of patients). The most common hemorrhagic event was epistaxis, and the most common grade 3–5 event was GI hemorrhage.

Tumor-related hemorrhage has been reported in patients receiving sunitinib. These events may occur suddenly and, in the case of pulmonary tumors, may present as severe and life-threatening hemoptysis or pulmonary hemorrhage. Pulmonary hemorrhage, sometimes fatal, has been reported in patients receiving sunitinib for GIST, advanced renal cell carcinoma, or metastatic lung cancer†.

Serious, sometimes fatal GI complications, including GI perforation, have occurred rarely in patients with intra-abdominal malignancies treated with sunitinib.

The manufacturer recommends clinically monitoring for hemorrhagic events (i.e., serial CBCs, physical examinations). If grade 3 or 4 hemorrhagic events occur, withhold sunitinib therapy; when the hemorrhagic event resolves or improves to grade 0 or 1, may then resume therapy at a reduced dosage or discontinue therapy depending on the severity and persistence of the hemorrhagic event.

Tumor Lysis Syndrome

Tumor lysis syndrome, sometimes fatal, has been reported principally in patients with GIST or advanced renal cell carcinoma receiving sunitinib in clinical studies and during postmarketing surveillance. The risk of tumor lysis syndrome is increased in patients with a large tumor burden; such patients should be monitored closely and treated as clinically indicated.

Thrombotic Microangiopathy

Thrombotic microangiopathy, including thrombotic thrombocytopenic purpura and hemolytic uremic syndrome, has occurred and sometimes resulted in renal failure or death. These events occurred in clinical trials and postmarketing experience when sunitinib was administered alone or in combination with bevacizumab. If thrombotic microangiopathy occurs, discontinue sunitinib therapy. Reversal of the effects of thrombotic microangiopathy have been observed following discontinuance of sunitinib therapy.

Proteinuria

Proteinuria and nephrotic syndrome, sometimes resulting in renal failure or death, have occurred in patients receiving sunitinib therapy. Monitor patients for the development or worsening of proteinuria. Perform urinalysis prior to initiation of sunitinib and periodically during therapy; further assessment with a 24-hour urine collection should be performed as clinically indicated. Interrupt sunitinib therapy and reduce dosage if proteinuria ≥3 g per 24 hours (in the absence of nephrotic syndrome) occurs. If nephrotic syndrome occurs or if proteinuria recurs despite dosage reduction, permanently discontinue therapy. The safety of continued sunitinib therapy in patients with moderate to severe proteinuria has not been systematically evaluated.

Dermatologic Effects

Severe and sometimes fatal cutaneous reactions, including erythema multiforme, Stevens-Johnson syndrome, and toxic epidermal necrolysis, have been reported. Cases of necrotizing fasciitis, including fatalities, also have been reported in patients receiving sunitinib. Necrotizing fasciitis has occurred secondary to fistula formation and has included sites such as the perineum.

Permanently discontinue sunitinib if erythema multiforme, Stevens-Johnson syndrome, toxic epidermal necrolysis, or necrotizing fasciitis occur.

Reversible Posterior Leukoencephalopathy Syndrome

Reversible posterior leukoencephalopathy syndrome (RPLS), sometimes fatal, has been reported in less than 1% of patients receiving sunitinib. If manifestations of RPLS (e.g., hypertension, headache, decreased alertness, altered mental functioning, visual loss, cortical blindness) occur, discontinue sunitinib therapy. Use magnetic resonance imaging (MRI) to confirm diagnosis of RPLS.

Thyroid Dysfunction

Hyperthyroidism, sometimes followed by hypothyroidism, has been reported in clinical studies and during postmarketing surveillance.

Thyroid function should be measured in all patients at baseline and periodically during treatment. Monitor all patients closely for manifestations of thyroid dysfunction, including hypothyroidism, hyperthyroidism, and thyroiditis during sunitinib therapy; if signs and/or symptoms suggestive of thyroid dysfunction occur, thyroid function tests should be performed and treatment instituted as clinically indicated.

Hypoglycemia

Symptomatic hypoglycemia, including cases associated with loss of consciousness or hospitalization, has been reported in patients receiving sunitinib. Reductions in blood glucose levels may be worse in patients with diabetes. In a pooled safety population, hypoglycemia occurred in 2% of patients receiving sunitinib. In clinical trials, hypoglycemia was reported in 2% of patients with advanced renal cell carcinoma or GIST and in 10% of patients with NET of pancreatic origin. In a clinical trial, patients with NET of pancreatic origin who developed hypoglycemia did not have preexisting glucose abnormalities at baseline.

In patients with diabetes, assess if antidiabetic therapies need to be adjusted to minimize the risk of hypoglycemia.

Monitor blood glucose at baseline, regularly during therapy, as clinically indicated, and after discontinuance of sunitinib therapy.

Osteonecrosis of the Jaw

Osteonecrosis of the jaw (ONJ) has been reported in patients receiving sunitinib. The risk of ONJ may be increased in patients with dental disease or in those receiving concomitant bisphosphonate therapy.

Prior to initiating sunitinib and periodically during therapy, routine oral examinations and appropriate preventive dentistry should be performed. If possible, withhold sunitinib at least 3 weeks before scheduled dental surgery or invasive dental treatments. If osteonecrosis of the jaw occurs, sunitinib therapy may be resumed at a reduced dosage or discontinued depending on the severity and persistence of the adverse effect; however, safety of resuming sunitinib therapy in patients who develop osteonecrosis of the jaw has not been established.

Wound-healing Complications

Impaired wound healing has been reported during sunitinib therapy. Withhold sunitinib at least 3 weeks before elective surgery and for at least 2 weeks after major surgery and until adequate wound healing occurs. If impaired wound healing occurs, sunitinib therapy may be resumed at a reduced dosage or discontinued depending on the severity and persistence of the adverse effect; however, safety of resuming sunitinib therapy in patients who experience impaired wound healing has not been established.

Fetal/Neonatal Morbidity and Mortality

Sunitinib can cause fetal harm because of its inhibitory effects on angiogenesis. Teratogenicity, embryotoxicity, and fetotoxicity have been demonstrated in animals. Pregnancy should be avoided during therapy. Advise females of reproductive potential to use effective methods of contraception during sunitinib therapy and for 4 weeks after the last dose. Males who are partners with females of reproductive potential should use effective contraception during treatment and for at least 7 weeks after the last dose. If sunitinib is used during pregnancy or if the patient becomes pregnant while receiving the drug, the patient should be apprised of the potential fetal hazard.

Specific Populations

Pregnancy

Based on animal data, sunitinib can cause fetal harm when administered during pregnancy. There are no adequate data regarding the developmental risk associated with the use of sunitinib during pregnancy in humans; however, teratogenic and embryolethal effects have been demonstrated in animal studies with doses similar to or less than those used clinically.

If sunitinib is used during pregnancy or if the patient becomes pregnant while receiving the drug, the patient should be apprised of the potential fetal hazard.

Lactation

Sunitinib and/or its metabolites are extensively distributed into milk in rats, with a milk-to-plasma ratio of up to 12:1. It is not known whether sunitinib or its primary active metabolite is distributed into human milk. Because of the potential for serious adverse reactions to sunitinib in nursing infants, females should not breast-feed during sunitinib therapy and for at least 4 weeks after the last dose.

Females and Males of Reproductive Potential

Verify pregnancy status of females of reproductive potential prior to initiating therapy. Advise females of reproductive potential to use effective methods of contraception during sunitinib therapy and for 4 weeks after the last dose. Males who are partners with females of reproductive potential should use effective contraception during treatment and for at least 7 weeks after the last dose.

Sunitinib may impair male and female fertility based on animal studies.

Pediatric Use

Safety and efficacy of sunitinib have not been established in pediatric patients.

Safety and pharmacokinetics of sunitinib have been assessed in 2 open-label studies in 56 pediatric patients 2 years to <17 years of age with refractory solid tumors, high-grade glioma, or ependymoma. The maximum tolerated dose, apparent clearance, and volume of distribution adjusted for body surface area for sunitinib and its major active metabolite were lower in pediatric patients compared to adults. In pediatric patients 2 years to <17 years of age with refractory solid tumors, sunitinib was poorly tolerated; the study also was amended to exclude patients with previous exposure to anthracyclines or cardiac radiation due to the occurrence of dose-limiting cardiotoxicity. The effect of sunitinib on open tibial growth plates in pediatric patients has not been established.

Geriatric Use

Of the 7527 patients receiving sunitinib for GIST, renal cell carcinoma, or NET of pancreatic origin in clinical studies, 32% were 65 years of age or older and 7% were 75 years of age or older. The incidence of grade 3 or 4 adverse effects was higher in patients 65 years of age or older compared to younger adults.

In the clinical studies evaluating sunitinib in patients with GIST or metastatic renal cell carcinoma, 30 or 41% of patients, respectively, were 65 years of age or older. No overall differences in safety and efficacy were observed relative to younger adults.

In the clinical study evaluating sunitinib in patients with NET of pancreatic origin, 27% of patients receiving sunitinib were 65 years of age or older. The study did not include sufficient numbers of patients with NET of pancreatic origin to determine if patients 65 years of age or older respond differently relative to younger patients.

Hepatic Impairment

Following administration of a single dose of sunitinib, systemic exposure in patients with mild or moderate (Child-Pugh class A or B) hepatic impairment was similar to that in individuals with normal hepatic function; no initial dosage adjustment is required in patients with mild or moderate hepatic impairment. Safety and efficacy of sunitinib have not been established in patients with severe (Child-Pugh class C) hepatic impairment.

Clinical studies for cancer that were conducted excluded patients with AST or ALT concentrations exceeding 2.5 times the upper limit of normal or, if caused by liver metastases, exceeding 5 times the upper limit of normal.

Renal Impairment

Following administration of a single dose of sunitinib, systemic exposure in patients with severe renal impairment (creatinine clearance less than 30 mL/minute) was similar to that in individuals with normal renal function (creatinine clearance exceeding 80 mL/minute). In individuals with end-stage renal disease undergoing hemodialysis, systemic exposure to sunitinib was decreased by 47% compared with those with normal renal function. No initial dosage adjustment is required in patients with renal impairment or in those with end-stage renal disease undergoing hemodialysis; however, adjustments to subsequent dosages may be necessary.

● Common Adverse Effects

The most common adverse effects occurring in 25% or more of patients receiving sunitinib include are fatigue/asthenia, diarrhea, mucositis/stomatitis, nausea, decreased appetite/anorexia, vomiting, abdominal pain, hand-foot syndrome, hypertension, bleeding events, dysgeusia/altered taste, dyspepsia, and thrombocytopenia.

DRUG INTERACTIONS

Sunitinib and its primary active metabolite are metabolized principally by cytochrome P-450 (CYP) isoenzyme 3A4. However, in vitro studies indicate that the drug does not inhibit or induce major CYP isoenzymes.

● Drugs and Foods Affecting Hepatic Microsomal Enzymes

Concomitant use of sunitinib with potent inhibitors of CYP3A4 (e.g., atazanavir, clarithromycin, indinavir, itraconazole, ketoconazole, nefazodone, nelfinavir, ritonavir, saquinavir, telithromycin, voriconazole, grapefruit) may result in increased plasma concentrations of sunitinib. When the potent CYP3A4 inhibitor ketoconazole was administered concomitantly with a single dose of sunitinib in healthy individuals, peak plasma concentrations and area under the plasma concentration-time curve (AUC) of sunitinib and its primary active metabolite increased by 49 and 51%, respectively. Selection of an alternative agent with minimal or no enzyme inhibition potential is recommended during sunitinib therapy. If concomitant use of sunitinib with a potent CYP3A4 inhibitor cannot be avoided, reduction of sunitinib dosage to no less than 37.5 mg daily (in patients receiving sunitinib for GIST or advanced renal cell carcinoma) or no less than 25 mg daily (in patients receiving sunitinib for progressive, well-differentiated NET of pancreatic origin) should be considered.

Concomitant use of sunitinib with inducers of CYP3A4 (e.g., carbamazepine, dexamethasone, phenobarbital, phenytoin, rifabutin, rifampin, rifapentine, St. John's wort [*Hypericum perforatum*]) may result in decreased plasma concentrations of sunitinib. When the potent CYP3A4 inducer rifampin was administered concomitantly with a single dose of sunitinib in healthy individuals, peak plasma concentrations and AUC of sunitinib and its primary active metabolite decreased by 23 and 46%, respectively. Selection of an alternative agent with minimal or no enzyme induction potential is recommended during sunitinib therapy. If concomitant use of sunitinib with a CYP3A4 inducer cannot be avoided, an increase in sunitinib dosage up to a maximum of 87.5 mg daily (in patients receiving sunitinib for GIST or advanced renal cell carcinoma) or 62.5 mg daily (in patients receiving sunitinib for progressive, well-differentiated NET of pancreatic origin) should be considered, and the patient should be monitored carefully for toxicity.

● Drugs Metabolized by Hepatic Microsomal Enzymes

In vitro studies indicate that sunitinib and its primary active metabolite are unlikely to have clinically relevant interactions with drugs metabolized by CYP isoenzymes 1A2, 2A6, 2B6, 2C8, 2C9, 2C19, 2D6, 2E1, 3A4/5, or 4A9/11.

● Antiarrhythmics

Sunitinib prolongs the QT interval, which may increase the risk of ventricular arrhythmias, including torsades de pointes. Monitor the QT interval more frequently in patients taking drugs known to prolong the QT interval.

● Bisphosphonates

Concomitant use of sunitinib with bisphosphonates (e.g., alendronate, etidronate, ibandronate, pamidronate, risedronate, zoledronic acid) may increase the risk of developing osteonecrosis of the jaw (ONJ).

DESCRIPTION

Sunitinib malate, an inhibitor of multiple receptor tyrosine kinases, is an antineoplastic agent. Receptor tyrosine kinases (RTKs) are involved in the initiation of various cascades of intracellular signaling events that lead to cell proliferation and/or influence processes critical to cell survival and tumor progression (e.g., angiogenesis, metastasis, inhibition of apoptosis), based on the respective kinase. Although the exact mechanism of antineoplastic activity of sunitinib has not been fully elucidated, data from biochemical and cellular assays indicate that sunitinib may inhibit signal transduction pathways involving multiple receptor (i.e., cell surface) tyrosine kinases, including platelet-derived growth factor receptors (i.e., PDGFR-α, PDGFR-β), vascular endothelial growth factor receptors (i.e., VEGFR-1, VEGFR-2, VEGFR-3), stem cell factor receptor (i.e., c-Kit), fms-like tyrosine kinase 3 (Flt-3), colony stimulating factor receptor type 1 (CSF-1R), and the glial cell line-derived neurotrophic factor receptor (RET). Sunitinib-induced inhibition of signal transduction pathways involving PDGFR-β, VEGFR-2, and c-Kit has been confirmed in tumor xenografts expressing receptor tyrosine kinase targets in vivo. Sunitinib has been shown to inhibit growth of tumor cells expressing dysregulated target receptor tyrosine kinases (i.e., PDGFR, RET, c-Kit) in vitro; the drug also has been shown to inhibit PDGFR-β- and VEGFR-2-dependent tumor angiogenesis in vivo.

Following oral administration, peak plasma concentrations of sunitinib generally occur within 6–12 hours. Food has no effect on bioavailability of sunitinib. Sunitinib is metabolized principally by cytochrome P-450 (CYP) isoenzyme 3A4 to several metabolites. The main circulating metabolite, an *N*-desethyl derivative, has been shown to be equipotent to sunitinib in biochemical and cellular assays; this metabolite accounts for approximately 23–37% of total plasma concentrations of the drug and also is metabolized by CYP3A4. Steady-state concentrations of sunitinib and its primary active metabolite are achieved within 10–14 days. Sunitinib and its primary active metabolite are 95 and 90% bound to human plasma proteins in vitro, respectively. Following oral administration of a single dose in healthy volunteers, the terminal half-life of sunitinib or its primary active metabolite is approximately 40–60 or 80–110 hours, respectively. Approximately 61% of an oral dose of sunitinib is excreted in feces and 16% is eliminated in urine, mainly as sunitinib and the primary metabolite; minor metabolites are recovered in feces and urine but generally are not found in plasma.

Population pharmacokinetic analyses of demographic data indicate that the pharmacokinetics of sunitinib or its primary active metabolite are not substantially affected by age (18–84 years of age), body weight (34–168 kg), race (white, Black, or Asian), sex, or ECOG performance status.

ADVICE TO PATIENTS

- Importance of reading the manufacturer's patient information prior to beginning sunitinib therapy and rereading it each time the prescription is refilled.
- If a dose is missed by less than 12 hours, importance of administering the missed dose right away. If a dose is missed by more than 12 hours, the dose should be skipped and the next dose should be taken at the regularly scheduled time.
- Risk of hepatotoxicity. Importance of contacting clinician if manifestations of hepatotoxicity (e.g., abdominal pain [particularly in the right upper quadrant], dark urine, generalized pruritus, jaundice) occur.
- Risk of cardiovascular events. Importance of promptly informing clinician promptly if symptoms of heart failure develop.
- Risk of QT prolongation and torsades de pointes.
- Risk of hypertension and importance of monitoring blood pressure regularly. Importance of informing clinician if signs or symptoms of hypertension occur.
- Risk of adverse GI effects (e.g., diarrhea, nausea, vomiting, dyspepsia, and constipation). Advise patients to seek medical attention if they experience persistent or severe abdominal pain because there is a risk of GI perforation.
- Risk of adverse dermatologic effects (e.g., skin discoloration due to the drug color [yellow]; hair or skin depigmentation; skin dryness, thickness, or cracking; blisters or rash on the hands and soles of the feet), including severe cutaneous reactions (e.g., Stevens-Johnson syndrome, toxic epidermal necrolysis, erythema multiforme, and necrotizing fasciitis). Importance of informing clinician immediately if severe dermatologic reactions occur.
- Increased risk of bleeding. Importance of promptly informing clinician of any manifestations or episodes of bleeding (e.g., abdominal pain or swelling; hematemesis; black, sticky stools; hematuria; headache; change in mental status).
- Risk of reversible posterior leukoencephalopathy syndrome. Importance of informing clinician if signs or symptoms of reversible posterior leukoencephalopathy syndrome occur.
- Risk of osteonecrosis of the jaw. Importance of advising patient that their clinician should examine their mouth before sunitinib therapy. Importance of informing dentist about sunitinib treatment prior to dental procedures. Importance of informing clinician of any signs or symptoms of osteonecrosis of the jaw.
- Risk of thyroid dysfunction. Importance of informing clinician if symptoms of abnormal thyroid function (e.g., persistent or worsening fatigue, hair loss, weight gain or loss, irregular menstrual cycles, feeling hot or cold) occur.
- Risk of hypoglycemia. Importance of informing clinician if signs or symptoms of hypoglycemia occur.

- Risk of impaired wound healing. Advise patients that sunitinib may impair wound healing. Importance of informing clinician of any planned surgical procedures.
- Importance of females informing clinicians if they are or plan to become pregnant or plan to breast-feed. Importance of advising females not to breast-feed during and for at least 4 weeks after discontinuance of therapy.
- Risk of impaired fertility in females and males.
- Risk of fetal harm. Necessity of advising females to avoid pregnancy while receiving therapy. Necessity of advising females of reproductive potential to use effective contraception during sunitinib therapy and for at least 4 weeks after the last dose of the drug. Necessity of advising males who are partners of such females that they should use effective contraception during sunitinib therapy and for at least 7 weeks after the last dose of the drug.
- Importance of informing clinicians of existing or contemplated concomitant therapy, including prescription and OTC drugs and herbal supplements (e.g., St. John's wort), as well as any concomitant illnesses.
- Importance of informing patients of other important precautionary information. (See Cautions.)

For further information on the handling of antineoplastic agents, see the ASHP Guidelines on Handling Hazardous Drugs at http://www.ahfsdruginformation.com.

PREPARATIONS

Sunitinib can only be obtained through designated specialty pharmacies. Contact the manufacturer or consult the Pfizer website for specific availability information.

Excipients in commercially available drug preparations may have clinically important effects in some individuals; consult specific product labeling for details.

SUNItinib Malate

Oral

Capsules	12.5 mg (of sunitinib)*	Sutent®, Pfizer
	25 mg (of sunitinib)*	Sutent®, Pfizer
	37.5 mg (of sunitinib)*	Sutent®, Pfizer
	50 mg (of sunitinib)*	Sutent®, Pfizer

† Use is not currently included in the labeling approved by the US Food and Drug Administration.

* available from one or more manufacturer, distributor, and/or repackager by generic (nonproprietary) name

Selected Revisions May 20, 2022, © Copyright, January 01, 2007, American Society of Health-System Pharmacists, Inc.

Temozolomide

10:00 • ANTINEOPLASTIC AGENTS

■ Temozolomide, a prodrug that is converted in vivo to a cytotoxic alkylating metabolite, is an alkylating antineoplastic agent.

USES

● Brain Tumors

Temozolomide is used in adults for the treatment of newly diagnosed glioblastoma, concomitantly with radiotherapy and then as maintenance treatment. Temozolomide is also used in adults for the adjuvant treatment of newly diagnosed anaplastic astrocytoma and for the treatment of refractory disease.

Glioblastoma

Temozolomide is used in adults concomitantly with radiation therapy for the treatment of newly diagnosed glioblastoma multiforme and then as maintenance treatment.

Clinical Experience

Efficacy of temozolomide in patients with newly diagnosed glioblastoma is based on a randomized, multicenter, open-label trial (EORTC-NCIC 26981-22981; MK-7365-051) involving 573 patients. Patients were randomized to temozolomide (75 mg/m² once daily) with standard fractionated radiation therapy (total dose of 60 Gy in 30 daily fractions of 2 Gy each) for 42 days (up to a maximum of 49 days) followed by a 4-week rest period and then adjuvant therapy with up to 6 cycles of temozolomide (150 or 200 mg/m²) on days 1–5 of every 28-day cycle or radiation therapy alone. The median age of patients was 56 years and 84% of patients had undergone debulking surgery. Salvage therapy with temozolomide was administered upon disease progression in 22% of patients who received initial therapy with temozolomide and radiation therapy and in 57% of patients who received initial therapy with radiation therapy alone.

Overall survival was prolonged (unadjusted hazard ratio for death: 0.63) and median survival was increased by 2.5 months (14.6 versus 12.1 months) in patients receiving concomitant temozolomide and radiation therapy followed by adjuvant temozolomide compared with those receiving radiation therapy alone as initial therapy for glioblastoma multiforme. At a median follow-up of 61 months, overall survival benefit in patients receiving temozolomide and radiation therapy followed by adjuvant temozolomide compared with radiation therapy alone remained similar to the initial results. A subgroup analysis of tumor specimens in 206 patients for whom adequate tumor specimens were available indicated that methylation status of the MGMT promoter was a strong prognostic biomarker for overall survival benefit. Results of the subgroup analysis also suggested that the effect of temozolomide and radiation therapy followed by adjuvant temozolomide on overall survival was consistent regardless of MGMT promoter methylation status; however, progression-free survival benefit was observed only in temozolomide-treated patients with MGMT promoter methylated disease. Nausea (36 versus 16%), vomiting (20 versus 6%), anorexia (19 versus 9%), constipation (18 versus 6%), and thrombocytopenia (4 versus 1%) occurred more frequently in patients receiving concomitant temozolomide and radiation therapy than in those receiving radiation therapy alone.

Among elderly patients with good performance status, the addition of concomitant and adjuvant temozolomide to hypofractionated radiation therapy appears to be safe and efficacious without impairing quality of life. In a randomized phase 3 study, 562 patients 65 years of age or older with newly diagnosed glioblastoma multiforme received temozolomide 75 mg/m² once daily with hypofractionated radiation therapy (total dose of 40 Gy in 15 daily fractions) over a period of 3 weeks followed by maintenance therapy with up to 12 cycles of temozolomide (150 or 200 mg/m²) on days 1–5 of every 28-day cycle; or hypofractionated radiation therapy alone. Overall survival was prolonged (hazard ratio for death: 0.67; 95% confidence interval 0.56–0.80) and median survival was increased by 1.7 months (9.3 versus 7.6 months) in patients receiving concomitant temozolomide and hypofractionated radiation therapy followed by maintenance therapy with temozolomide compared with those receiving hypofractionated radiation therapy alone as initial therapy for glioblastoma multiforme. Although the magnitude of overall survival benefit was greatest in patients with methylated MGMT promoter receiving concomitant temozolomide and hypofractionated radiation therapy followed by adjuvant temozolomide compared with patients receiving hypofractionated radiation therapy alone, a numerical, but not statistically significant, overall survival benefit was observed in patients with unmethylated MGMT promoter (10.0 versus 7.9 months; hazard ratio of 0.75 with a 95% confidence interval 0.56–1.01).

Clinical Perspective

Malignant gliomas often have inactivated MGMT (also referred to as O6-methylguanine DNA methyltransferase) due to aberrant methylation of its promoter region. The presence of MGMT promoter methylation has been used as a prognostic and predictive marker for response to therapy with alkylating agents. High expression of MGMT in cancer cells, such as glioma cells, account for the predominant mechanism of resistance to alkylating agents. Epigenetic silencing of MGMT by promoter methylation has been associated with improved survival in patients with glioblastoma multiforme receiving temozolomide, with or without radiation therapy. In the European Organisation for Research and Treatment of Cancer (EORTC) and National Cancer Institute of Canada Clinical Trials Group (NCIC) 26981-22981 study, overall survival benefit was observed regardless of MGMT promoter methylation status in patients with glioblastoma receiving concomitant temozolomide and radiation therapy; however, the magnitude of benefit was more pronounced in patients with methylated MGMT promoter.

Lack of standardization in MGMT promoter methylation assays complicates interpretation of the prognostic and predictive impact of MGMT methylation status. Common methods for quantitating methylation status include methylation-specific polymerase chain reaction (MSP) and pyrosequencing (PSQ), both of which evaluate the MGMT promoter region, and immunohistochemistry (IHC), which evaluates MGMT protein expression. In a meta-analysis, MSP and PSQ appeared to be more prognostic for overall survival than IHC in patients with glioblastoma treated with temozolomide. The exact promoter regions (5′-cytosine-phosphate-guanine-3′ [CpG]) and thresholds for interpretation are not well-defined; however, targeting multiple CpG promoter sites is likely to be more prognostic than targeting a single site.

The current standard of treatment for newly diagnosed patients with glioblastoma includes maximum safe surgical resection followed by radiotherapy with concurrent and adjuvant chemotherapy with or without Tumor Treating Fields. Radiation therapy remains a key adjuvant therapy for most patients with glioblastoma given the locally recurrent pattern of disease spread after surgical resection. Temozolomide is the recommended systemic therapy in newly diagnosed glioblastoma due to its demonstrated survival benefit, with the greatest benefit seen in patients who harbor MGMT promoter methylation. Experts recommend conventional radiation therapy with concurrent and adjuvant temozolomide in glioblastoma patients up to 70 years of age with reasonable performance status. In elderly glioblastoma patients ≥70 years of age with reasonable performance status, hypofractionated radiation therapy with concurrent and adjuvant temozolomide may be considered.

Anaplastic Astrocytoma

Temozolomide is used for the adjuvant treatment of adults with newly diagnosed anaplastic astrocytoma and in the treatment of refractory disease.

Clinical Experience

The use of temozolomide as an adjuvant treatment in adults with newly diagnosed anaplastic astrocytoma is based on studies in the published literature in addition to interim results from the ongoing open-label, randomized, multicenter, phase 3 CATNON trial. Enrolled patients in CATNON had newly diagnosed anaplastic glioma without 1p/19q co-deletion, a World Health Organization (WHO) performance status score of 0-2, and adequate hematological, renal, and liver function, and were taking stable or decreasing corticosteroid doses. Patients were randomly assigned to radiotherapy alone, radiotherapy with adjuvant temozolomide (12 four-week cycles of 150-200 mg/m² given on days 1-5), radiotherapy with concurrent temozolomide (75 mg/m² per day), or radiotherapy and concurrent temozolomide plus adjuvant temozolomide. The primary endpoint was overall survival.

At the initial interim analysis, the hazard ratio for overall survival for patients administered adjuvant temozolomide was 0.65 (99.145% confidence interval: 0.45-0.93); the median follow-up was 27 months. Median overall survival was not reached among patients who received adjuvant temozolomide and was 41.1 months in patients who did not receive adjuvant temozolomide. At 5 years, overall survival was 55.9% versus 44.1% in the respective groups. Similar beneficial results with the use of adjuvant temozolomide were observed at a second interim analysis conducted at a median follow-up of 55.7 months. Adjuvant temozolomide significantly improved median overall survival compared with no adjuvant temozolomide therapy (82.3 versus 46.9 months). However, administration of concurrent temozolomide did not result in a significant improvement in median overall survival when compared to no concurrent temozolomide therapy (66.9 months versus 60.4 months).

The use of temozolomide in refractory anaplastic astrocytoma is based on tumor response rates in this population from an uncontrolled phase 2 study. In a single-arm, multicenter study in 162 patients with relapsed anaplastic astrocytoma who had a baseline Karnofsky performance status of 70 or greater, efficacy in a subgroup of 54 patients with refractory disease (i.e., progression following treatment with a nitrosourea and procarbazine) was demonstrated by an overall (complete plus partial) tumor response rate of 22% and a complete response rate of 9%. Median durations of all responses and complete responses were 50 and 64 weeks, respectively. Progression-free survival at 6 and 12 months was 45 and 29%, respectively; median progression-free survival was 4.4 months; 12-month overall survival was 65%; and median overall survival was 15.9 months.

DOSAGE AND ADMINISTRATION

● General

Pretreatment Screening

- Obtain a complete blood count (CBC) and monitor absolute neutrophil count (ANC) and platelet count before initiation of treatment. Withhold dosing until patients have an ANC ≥1500/mm³ and a platelet count ≥100,000/mm³.

- Monitor liver function tests at baseline and prior to each cycle.

- Screen for hepatitis.

- Verify pregnancy status in females of reproductive potential.

Patient Monitoring

- When used in combination with radiotherapy, obtain a CBC weekly during treatment and as clinically indicated.

- Monitor ANC and platelet counts as clinically indicated during treatment.

- For 28-day treatment cycles, obtain a CBC prior to treatment on Day 1 and Day 22 of each cycle. Perform CBCs weekly until recovery if the ANC is <1500/mm³ and the platelet count is <100,000/mm³.

- Closely monitor all patients, particularly those receiving steroids, for the development of lymphopenia or *Pneumocystis jiroveci* (formerly *P. carinii*) pneumonia (PCP).

- Obtain liver function tests half-way through the first treatment cycle and 2–4 weeks following the last dose of temozolomide.

Premedication and Prophylaxis

- Administer prophylaxis for *Pneumocystis jiroveci* (e.g., inhaled pentamidine, oral co-trimoxazole) during concomitant temozolomide and radiation therapy. In patients with lymphopenia, continue *Pneumocystis jiroveci* prophylaxis until lymphocytopenia resolves to grade 1 or less.

- Clinicians should consider antiemetic therapy prior to and following temozolomide administration.

Dispensing and Administration Precautions

Handling and Disposal

- Temozolomide is a hazardous medication. Clinicians and patients should follow applicable special handling and disposal procedures.

- Patients may need to take combinations of temozolomide capsules of different strengths to receive the correct daily dose. To minimize the risk of

inappropriate dosing, the clinician or pharmacist should provide written instructions for the dosage schedule.

Other General Considerations

- Adjust dosage based on nadir platelet and ANC during the previous cycle and ANC and platelet counts on day 1 of the next cycle.

- Consider hepatitis prophylaxis with antiviral agents as clinically indicated.

● Reconstitution and Administration

Temozolomide is administered orally or by IV infusion.

Oral Administration

When given orally, temozolomide capsule is administered once daily at the same time each day and should be swallowed intact with water. Patients should be advised not to open, chew, or dissolve capsule contents. If capsules are accidentally opened or damaged, precautions should be taken to avoid inhalation of capsule contents or contact with the skin or mucous membranes. If contact with skin occurs, the affected area should be washed thoroughly immediately. Because food may decrease the rate and extent of absorption of temozolomide, the drug should be administered in a consistent manner relative to food intake. To reduce nausea and vomiting, administration of temozolomide on an empty stomach or at bedtime may be advisable. Store capsules at 25ºC (excursions permitted between 15-30ºC).

Based on the dose prescribed, the number of each strength capsules needed (e.g., for a dose of 275 mg daily for 5 days, dispense five 250-mg capsules, five 20-mg capsules, and five 5-mg capsules) should be determined. Each strength of capsules should be dispensed in a separate container. Each container should be labeled with the strength per capsule and with the appropriate number of capsules to be taken each day. The patient should be instructed to take the appropriate number of capsules from each container to equal the total daily dose.

IV Administration

Temozolomide for injection should be stored at 2–8°C and must be reconstituted prior to administration. Prior to reconstitution, temozolomide for injection should be brought to room temperature. Temozolomide for injection should be reconstituted by adding 41 mL of sterile water for injection to a vial labeled as containing 100 mg of temozolomide to provide a solution containing 2.5 mg/mL of the drug; reconstituted vials should be gently swirled but not shaken. The reconstituted solution may be stored at room temperature (25°C) for up to 14 hours (including infusion time). Reconstituted temozolomide for injection should be a clear solution free of visible particles; the drug should be discarded if the solution contains visible particulate matter. The reconstituted solution should not be further diluted prior to administration. Using aseptic technique, withdraw up to 40 mL from each reconstituted vial to reach the total dose and discard any unused portion. The reconstituted solution should then be transferred from each vial into an empty 250 mL infusion bag. IV lines should be flushed before and after each temozolomide infusion. The manufacturer states that drugs or solutions other than 0.9% sodium chloride injection should not be infused through the same IV line.

Rate of Administration

Temozolomide for injection should be administered by IV infusion over 90 minutes using an infusion pump.

Infusion of temozolomide over a shorter or longer duration may result in suboptimal dosing.

● Dosage

Glioblastoma

Concomitant Use Phase

During the concomitant use phase of therapy, the initial oral or IV dosage of temozolomide for the treatment of newly diagnosed glioblastoma is 75 mg/m² once daily for 42 to 49 consecutive days. Temozolomide is to be administered concomitantly with focal radiotherapy. Focal radiotherapy includes the tumor bed or resection site with a 2-3 cm margin. Other administration schedules have been used.

Temozolomide dosing should be *interrupted* for any of the following criteria: ANC of ≥500 and <1500/mm³, platelet count of ≥10,000 and <100,000/mm³, or any grade 2 nonhematologic toxicity (except alopecia, nausea, and vomiting). Temozolomide therapy may be resumed at the same dose when ANC ≥1500/mm³, platelet count ≥100,000/mm³, and non-hematological adverse reactions resolve to grade 1 or less.

Temozolomide dosing should be *discontinued* for any of the following criteria: ANC <500/mm³, platelet count <10,000/mm³, or any grade 3 or 4 nonhematologic toxicity (except alopecia, nausea, and vomiting).

Single Agent Maintenance Use Phase

The maintenance phase of therapy is initiated after a 4-week rest period following completion of temozolomide and radiation therapy. The maintenance phase consists of six 28-day cycles of treatment.

During the maintenance phase of therapy, the initial oral or IV dosage of temozolomide is 150 mg/m² once daily on days 1 to 5 of cycle 1. The dosage may be increased to 200 mg/m² once daily on days 1 to 5 before starting cycle 2 if no dosage interruptions or discontinuations are required. If the temozolomide dosage is not increased at cycle 2 onset, do *not* increase the dosage for cycles 3 to 6.

A CBC should be obtained prior to treatment on day 1 and day 22 of each treatment cycle, and then weekly until recovery if ANC <1500/mm³ and platelet count <100,000/mm³. The next cycle should not be initiated until ANC and platelet counts exceed these levels.

Temozolomide dosing should be *interrupted* for any of the following criteria: ANC <1000/mm³, platelet count <50,000/mm³, or any grade 3 nonhematologic toxicity (except alopecia, nausea, and vomiting). Temozolomide therapy may be resumed at a reduced dose (i.e., decreased by 50 mg/m² per day) for the next cycle when ANC is ≥1500/mm³, platelet count is ≥100,000/mm³, and nonhematological adverse reactions resolve to grade 1 or less.

Temozolomide dosing should be *discontinued* for any of the following criteria: inability to tolerate a dose of 100 mg/m² per day, recurrence of the same grade 3 nonhematologic toxicity following dose reduction, or any grade 4 nonhematologic toxicity (except alopecia, nausea, and vomiting).

Anaplastic Astrocytoma

Adjuvant Treatment of Newly Diagnosed Anaplastic Astrocytoma

Temozolomide should be administered orally in a single dose on days 1 to 5 of a 28-day cycle for 12 cycles beginning 4 weeks after the end of radiotherapy. The recommended dosage of temozolomide for cycle 1 is 150 mg/m² once daily on days 1 to 5. The dosage may be increased to 200 mg/m² once daily on days 1 to 5 for cycles 2 to 12 if the patient experienced no or minimal toxicity in cycle 1. If the temozolomide dosage is not increased at cycle 2 onset, do not increase the dosage during subsequent cycles.

A CBC should be obtained prior to treatment on day 1 and day 22 of each treatment cycle, and then weekly until recovery if ANC <1500/mm³ and platelet count <100,000/mm³. The next cycle should not be initiated until ANC and platelet counts exceed these levels.

Temozolomide dosing should be *interrupted* for any of the following criteria: ANC <1000/mm³, platelet count <50,000/mm³, or any grade 3 nonhematologic toxicity (except alopecia, nausea, and vomiting). Temozolomide therapy may be resumed at a reduced dose (i.e., decreased by 50 mg/m² per day) for the next cycle when ANC is ≥1500/mm³, platelet count is ≥100,000/mm³, and nonhematological adverse reactions resolve to grade 1 or less.

Temozolomide dosing should be *discontinued* for any of the following criteria: inability to tolerate a dose of 100 mg/m² per day, recurrence of the same grade 3 nonhematologic toxicity (except alopecia, nausea, and vomiting) following dose reduction, or any grade 4 nonhematologic toxicity (except alopecia, nausea, and vomiting).

Refractory Anaplastic Astrocytoma

The initial oral or IV dosage of temozolomide for the treatment of refractory anaplastic astrocytoma in adults is 150 mg/m² daily on days 1 to 5 of each 28-day treatment cycle.

Subsequent dosage is adjusted based on nadir platelet and ANC during the previous cycle and on ANC and platelet counts on day 1 of the next cycle. A CBC should be obtained prior to treatment on day 1 and day 22 of each treatment cycle, and then weekly until recovery if the ANC and platelet counts are <1500 and <100,000/mm³, respectively. The next cycle should be withheld until these counts

are exceeded. If both nadir and day-of-dosing ANC and platelet counts exceed 1500 and 100,000/mm³, respectively, then temozolomide dosage may be increased to 200 mg/m² daily for days 1 to 5 of the next 28-day cycle. If either the ANC or platelet count declines to <1000 or 50,000/mm³, respectively, during any cycle, the dosage for the next cycle should be reduced *by* 50 mg/m² daily. Permanently discontinue therapy if patients are unable to tolerate a dosage of 100 mg/m² daily.

Temozolomide therapy can be continued until disease progression or unacceptable toxicity occurs.

● Special Populations

Hepatic Impairment

No dosage adjustment is necessary in patients with mild to moderate hepatic impairment (Child-Pugh class A and B).

Temozolomide has not been studied in patients with severe hepatic impairment (Child-Pugh class C), and the manufacturer provides no specific dosage recommendations for such patients.

Renal Impairment

No dosage adjustment is necessary in patients with creatinine clearance of 36–130 mL/minute per m².

Temozolomide has not been studied in patients with creatinine clearance <36 mL/minute per m² and in those with end-stage renal disease requiring dialysis, and the manufacturer provides no specific dosage recommendations for such patients.

Geriatric Patients

The manufacturer makes no specific recommendations regarding dosage adjustment in geriatric patients other than usual adjustment for ANC and platelet counts.

CAUTIONS

● Contraindications

● History of serious hypersensitivity reactions to temozolomide, any other ingredients in temozolomide, and dacarbazine, which is metabolized to the same active metabolite as temozolomide.

● Warnings/Precautions

Myelosuppression

Myelosuppression (e.g., pancytopenia, leukopenia, anemia) has been reported with temozolomide, with fatal outcomes observed in some patients. In certain cases, assessment has been complicated by exposure to concomitant medications (e.g., carbamazepine, phenytoin, co-trimoxazole) which may be associated with aplastic anemia.

In a clinical study (MK-7365-006), myelosuppression with temozolomide usually occurred during the initial cycles of therapy and was not observed to be cumulative in nature. The median nadirs occurred for platelets at 26 days (range: 21 to 40 days) and for neutrophils at 28 days (range: 1 to 44 days). Myelosuppression resulted in hospitalization, blood transfusion, or discontinuation of temozolomide therapy in approximately 10% of patients. In clinical trials, women and geriatric patients have been shown to have an increased risk of developing myelosuppression.

A complete blood count (CBC) should be obtained and absolute neutrophil count (ANC) and platelet count monitored before therapy initiation and as clinically indicated during treatment. When temozolomide is used concurrently with radiotherapy, a CBC should be obtained prior to initiation, weekly during treatment, and as clinically indicated.

Temozolomide should be withheld if severe myelosuppression occurs. Temozolomide may be resumed at the same or reduced dose, or permanently discontinued, based on myelosuppression occurrence.

Hepatotoxicity

Severe hepatotoxicity sometimes fatal, has occurred in patients receiving temozolomide. Reactivation of hepatitis B resulting in death has been reported in a patient receiving temozolomide for glioblastoma. Increased serum aminotransferase concentrations, hyperbilirubinemia, cholestasis, and hepatitis have been reported in postmarketing surveillance. Liver function tests should be evaluated at baseline, half-way through the first treatment cycle, prior to each subsequent cycle, and approximately 2–4 weeks following the last dose of temozolomide. Hepatitis screening and prophylactic therapy with antiviral agents as clinically indicated should be considered in patients receiving temozolomide.

Pneumocystis Pneumonia

Pneumocystis pneumonia has been observed in patients administered temozolomide, with an increased risk seen in patients administered steroids or receiving longer treatment regimens of temozolomide.

Prophylaxis against *Pneumocystis* pneumonia should be provided to all patients with newly diagnosed glioblastoma during the concomitant phase. Prophylaxis should be continued in patients with lymphopenia until resolution to grade 1 or less. All patients should be monitored for lymphopenia and *Pneumocystis* pneumonia development.

Secondary Malignancies

Temozolomide-containing regimens are associated with an increased incidence of secondary malignancies. Myelodysplastic syndrome and secondary malignancies, including myeloid leukemia, have been observed.

Fetal/Neonatal Morbidity and Mortality

May cause fetal harm based on its mechanism of action and animal findings; teratogenicity and embryolethality were demonstrated in animals at doses less than the maximum human dose based on body surface area (200 mg/m²). Spontaneous abortion and congenital malformations, including polymalformations with CNS, facial, cardiac, skeletal, and genitourinary system anomalies have been reported with exposure to temozolomide during pregnancy in postmarketing surveillance.

Pregnancy should be avoided during therapy. The manufacturer states that a pregnancy test should be performed prior to starting temozolomide and females of reproductive potential should be advised to use effective contraceptive methods during and for ≥6 months after the last dose. In addition, male patients with such female partners should be advised to use effective methods of contraception during and for ≥3 months after the last dose. Male patients should not donate semen during therapy and for ≥3 months after the last dose. Patients should be apprised of the potential hazard to the fetus if temozolomide is used during pregnancy.

Exposure to Opened Capsules

Recommended precautions should be observed to avoid exposure to opened capsules of temozolomide. (See Dosage and Administration.)

Specific Populations
Pregnancy

Temozolomide can cause fetal harm.

Lactation

It is not known whether temozolomide or its metabolites are distributed in human milk. The effects of the drug on breast-fed infants or on the production of milk are also unknown. Patients should discontinue breast-feeding during therapy and for at least 1 week after the last dose because of potential risk, including myelosuppression, in breast-fed infants.

Females and Males of Reproductive Potential

Temozolomide can cause fetal harm if administered during pregnancy. Females of reproductive potential should be advised to use effective contraceptive methods during and for ≥6 months after the last temozolomide dose. Male patients with such female partners should also be advised to use effective methods of contraception during and for ≥3 months after the last dose.

Based on limited data, temozolomide may impair fertility in males. Changes in sperm parameters and genotoxic effects on sperm cells have occurred in men receiving temozolomide; however, the duration or reversibility of these effects has not been established. Male patients should not donate semen during therapy and for ≥3 months after the last dose.

Pediatric Use

Safety and efficacy in pediatric patients have not been established. Efficacy was not demonstrated in open-label studies of children 3–18 years of age receiving temozolomide mostly for CNS tumors. Similar toxicity was observed in pediatric patients and adults.

Geriatric Use

Experience in those 65 years of age and older with newly diagnosed glioblastoma is insufficient to determine whether they respond differently than younger adults.

An increased incidence of grade 4 thrombocytopenia and/or neutropenia has been reported in patients 70 years of age or older compared with younger patients receiving temozolomide for refractory anaplastic astrocytoma.

Similar toxicity was observed in patients 65 years of age or older and younger patients receiving temozolomide for newly diagnosed glioblastoma multiforme.

Hepatic Impairment

Pharmacokinetics of temozolomide are not substantially altered in patients with mild to moderate hepatic impairment (Child-Pugh class A and B).

Renal Impairment

Pharmacokinetics of temozolomide are not substantially altered in patients with creatinine clearance of 36–130 mL/minute per m².

● Common Adverse Effects

The most common adverse reactions (≥20%) include: alopecia, fatigue, nausea, vomiting, headache, constipation, anorexia, and convulsions.

DRUG INTERACTIONS

● Drugs Affecting Hepatic Microsomal Enzymes

Temozolomide and 5-(3-methyltriazen-1-yl)imidazole-4-carboxamide (MTIC) are only minimally metabolized by CYP isoenzymes.

● Carbamazepine

Unlikely to affect temozolomide clearance. Possible additive hematologic toxicity (i.e., aplastic anemia); concomitant administration may complicate assessment of hematologic toxicity.

● Co-trimoxazole

Possible additive hematologic toxicity (i.e., aplastic anemia); concomitant administration may complicate assessment of hematologic toxicity.

● Dexamethasone

Unlikely to affect temozolomide clearance.

● Histamine H₂-receptor Antagonists

Unlikely to affect temozolomide clearance.

● Ondansetron

Unlikely to affect temozolomide clearance.

● Phenobarbital

Unlikely to affect temozolomide clearance.

● Phenytoin

Unlikely to affect temozolomide clearance. Possible additive hematologic toxicity (i.e., aplastic anemia); concomitant administration may complicate assessment of hematologic toxicity.

● Prochlorperazine

Unlikely to affect temozolomide clearance.

● *Valproic Acid*

Pharmacokinetic interaction (decreased temozolomide clearance by about 5%). Clinical importance unknown.

DESCRIPTION

Temozolomide, an imidazotetrazine derivative, is an antineoplastic agent. Temozolomide is a prodrug and has little, if any, pharmacologic activity until hydrolyzed in vivo to 5-(3-methyltriazen-1-yl)imidazole-4-carboxamide (MTIC). Following administration of temozolomide, the drug undergoes rapid, nonenzymatic hydrolysis at physiologic pH to MTIC. MTIC is thought to exert its cytotoxic effects by acting as an alkylating agent at the O^6 and N^7 positions of guanine in DNA.

Temozolomide is rapidly and completely absorbed after oral administration, with nearly 100% bioavailability. Peak plasma concentrations usually are attained within 1 hour. The bioequivalence of temozolomide (with respect to both peak plasma concentration and AUC) administered orally or as an IV infusion over 90 minutes at a dosage of 150 mg/m^2 has been demonstrated. Food decreases the rate and extent of absorption after oral administration. A modified high fat breakfast decreased mean peak plasma temozolomide concentrations (32%) and AUC (9%).

Temozolomide efficiently crosses the blood brain barrier. It is not known if temozolomide is distributed into human milk. Plasma protein binding is approximately 15%. MTIC, the main active metabolite, is further hydrolyzed to 5-amino-imidazole-4-carboxamide (AIC) and to methylhydrazine. CYP isoenzymes play only a minor role in metabolism of temozolomide and MTIC. About 38% of an administered dose is recovered over 7 days, principally in urine with <1% in feces. The mean elimination half-life of temozolomide is 1.8 hours. Apparent half-lives for metabolites MTIC and AIC are 2.1 and 2.6 hours, respectively.

In patients with mild to moderate hepatic impairment, the pharmacokinetic profile resembles that in patients with normal hepatic function. Temozolomide has not been studied in patients with severe hepatic impairment. The pharmacokinetic profile of temozolomide is not affected by renal function in patients with creatinine clearance 36–130 mL/minute per m^2. The drug has not been studied in patients with severe renal impairment (creatinine clearance <36 mL/minute per m^2) or in patients with end-stage renal disease receiving dialysis.

ADVICE TO PATIENTS

● Stress importance of adherence to dosage and laboratory appointment schedules.

● Advise patients that there is a risk of developing myelodysplastic syndrome and secondary malignancies.

● Stress importance of *Pneumocystis jiroveci* pneumonia prophylaxis for certain patients with newly diagnosed glioblastoma. Advise patients to inform clinicians of signs and symptoms of PCP infection (e.g., shortness of breath, fever, chills, dry cough).

● Risk of hepatotoxicity. Advise patients to inform clinicians of signs and symptoms of hepatotoxicity.

● Risk of fetal harm. Stress importance of women informing clinicians immediately if they are or plan to become pregnant or plan to breastfeed. Advise females of reproductive potential and men with such female partners to use effective contraceptive methods during and for ≥6 and 3 months after the last dose, respectively.

● Advise females not to breastfeed while receiving temozolomide and for ≥1 week after the last dose.

● Advise patients of the risk of impaired fertility in males.

● Advise male patients not to donate semen while receiving temozolomide and for ≥3 months after the last dose.

● Stress importance of taking temozolomide in a consistent manner relative to food intake to ensure consistent bioavailability and clinical effect. Advise patients to swallow capsules whole, without chewing.

● Inform patients to avoid exposure to capsule contents (carcinogen potential) and to safely store and dispose.

● Advise patients of risk of nausea and vomiting. Premedication with antiemetics and bedtime administration recommended.

● Advise patients of risk of low platelet counts and possible risk of bleeding. Stress importance of patients informing clinicians of any unusual bruising or bleeding.

● Stress importance of informing clinicians of existing or contemplated concomitant therapy, including prescription and OTC drugs, as well as concomitant illnesses.

● Inform patients of other important precautionary information.

For further information on the handling of antineoplastic agents, see the ASHP Guidelines on Handling Hazardous Drugs at https://www.ahfsdruginformation.com.

PREPARATIONS

Excipients in commercially available drug preparations may have clinically important effects in some individuals; consult specific product labeling for details.

Temozolomide

Oral			
Capsules	5 mg*	**Temozolomide Capsules**, Merck	
	20 mg*	**Temozolomide Capsules**, Merck	
	100 mg*	**Temodar®**, Merck	
		Temozolomide Capsules	
	140 mg*	**Temodar®**, Merck	
		Temozolomide Capsules	
	180 mg*	**Temodar®**, Merck	
		Temozolomide Capsules	
	250 mg*	**Temodar®**, Merck	
		Temozolomide Capsules	
Parenteral			
For injection, for IV infusion	100 mg	**Temodar® for Injection**, Merck	

* available from one or more manufacturer, distributor, and/or repackager by generic (nonproprietary) name

† Use is not currently included in the labeling approved by the US Food and Drug Administration.

Trametinib Dimethyl Sulfoxide

10:00 · ANTINEOPLASTIC AGENTS

■ Trametinib, an inhibitor of mitogen-activated extracellular signal-regulated kinase (MEK) 1 and MEK2 in cells with b-Raf serine-threonine kinase (*BRAF*) V600E or V600K mutations, is an antineoplastic agent.

USES

● Melanoma

Trametinib, alone or in combination therapy, is used for the treatment of unresectable or metastatic melanoma in selected patients; the drug also is used in combination therapy for the adjuvant treatment of melanoma in selected patients.

Trametinib, as a single agent, is *not* indicated for use in patients with melanoma who have experienced disease progression following treatment with a b-Raf serine-threonine kinase (BRAF) inhibitor.

Adjuvant Therapy for Melanoma

Trametinib is used in combination with dabrafenib as adjuvant therapy following complete resection of melanoma with *BRAF* V600E or V600K mutation and nodal involvement. An FDA-approved diagnostic test (e.g., THxID® BRAF kit) is required to confirm the presence of the BRAF V600E or V600K mutation prior to initiation of therapy.

The current indication for trametinib in combination with dabrafenib as adjuvant therapy following complete resection of melanoma with BRAF V600E or V600K mutation and nodal involvement is based principally on the results of a randomized, double-blind, placebo-controlled phase 3 study (COMBI-AD) in patients who had undergone complete resection of stage III melanoma with *BRAF* V600E or V600K mutation (as detected by the bioMerieux THxID® BRAF V600 mutation test) and involvement of regional lymph nodes. In this study, 870 patients were randomized (stratified by disease stage and *BRAF* mutation status) in a 1:1 ratio to receive trametinib 2 mg once daily with dabrafenib 150 mg twice daily or placebo for up to 12 months. Patients enrolled in this study had undergone complete resection of melanoma with complete lymphadenectomy within 12 weeks of randomization. The primary measure of efficacy was relapse-free survival. Secondary outcomes included overall survival and freedom from relapse. The median age of patients was 51 years; 99% were white, 55% were male, 91% had a baseline Eastern Cooperative Oncology Group (ECOG) performance status of 0, 65% had macroscopic lymph node involvement, 41% had tumor ulceration, 41% had stage IIIb disease, and 40% had stage IIIc disease. The majority (91%) of patients had a *BRAF* V600E mutation and 9% had a V600K mutation. Patients who had mucosal or ocular melanoma, unresectable in-transit metastases, or distant metastatic disease and those who had previously received systemic therapy (including radiation therapy) were not eligible to enroll in the study.

After a median follow-up of 2.8 years, median relapse-free survival had not been reached in patients receiving trametinib in combination with dabrafenib and was 16.6 months in those receiving placebo. In an updated analysis of this study at a median follow-up of 44 months, 3- or 4-year relapse-free rates were 59 or 54%, respectively, for dabrafenib plus trametinib. At a median of 42 months for those receiving placebo, 3- or 4-year relapse-free survival rates were 40 or 38%, respectively.

Unresectable or Metastatic Melanoma
Monotherapy

Trametinib is used as monotherapy, in BRAF-inhibitor treatment-naive patients, for the treatment of unresectable or metastatic melanoma harboring *BRAF* V600E or V600K mutations. Trametinib has been designated an orphan drug by the FDA as monotherapy for the treatment of this cancer. An FDA-approved diagnostic test (e.g., THxID® BRAF kit) is required to confirm the presence of the *BRAF* V600E or V600K mutation prior to initiation of therapy.

The current indication for trametinib monotherapy in patients with unresectable or metastatic melanoma positive for V600E or V600K *BRAF* mutations is based principally on the results of a randomized, open-label, phase 3 study (METRIC study). Trametinib improved progression-free survival and overall survival when compared with conventional chemotherapy. A total of 322 adults (median 54 years of age, 54% male, more than 99% white, 36% with elevated lactate dehydrogenase [LDH]) were randomized in a 2:1 ratio to receive oral trametinib 2 mg daily or investigator's choice of chemotherapy (dacarbazine 1 g/m² or paclitaxel 175 mg/m²) every 3 weeks. In this study, 87% of patients with unresectable or metastatic melanoma had *BRAF* V600E mutations and 12% had V600K mutations. The majority of patients (66%) had not received prior chemotherapy for advanced melanoma; prior use of MEK inhibitors, BRAF inhibitors, or ipilimumab was not allowed. Once disease progression occurred, patients originally randomized to conventional chemotherapy were allowed to cross over to trametinib treatment. The primary measure of efficacy was progression-free survival. Median progression-free survival was 4.8 months in patients randomized to trametinib versus 1.5 months in patients randomized to conventional chemotherapy. The overall response rate was 22% in the trametinib group and 8% in the conventional chemotherapy group. Complete response was seen in 2 or 0% of patients given trametinib or conventional chemotherapy; partial response rates were 20 or 8%, respectively. Median duration of response was 5.5 months for patients randomized to trametinib and was not reached for those randomized to conventional chemotherapy.

Trametinib is *not* indicated for use in patients with melanoma who have experienced disease progression following treatment with a BRAF inhibitor. In an open-label, phase 2 study in patients with unresectable or metastatic melanoma with BRAF mutations, no confirmed objective responses were observed in the cohort of 40 patients who had previously received treatment with a BRAF inhibitor. The median progression-free survival among these patients was 1.8 months.

Combination Therapy

Trametinib is used in combination with dabrafenib for the treatment of unresectable or metastatic melanoma with *BRAF* V600E or V600K mutation. Trametinib has been designated an orphan drug by the FDA when used in combination with dabrafenib for the treatment of this cancer. An FDA-approved diagnostic test (e.g., THxID® BRAF kit) is required to confirm the presence of the *BRAF* V600E or V600K mutation prior to initiation of therapy.

The current indication for trametinib in combination with dabrafenib in the treatment of unresectable or metastatic melanoma with *BRAF* V600E or V600K mutation is based principally on the results of a randomized phase 3 study (COMBI-d) in patients with previously untreated stage IIIc or IV cutaneous melanoma with *BRAF* V600E or V600K mutation. In this study, 423 patients were randomized in a 1:1 ratio to receive either trametinib (2 mg once daily) in combination with dabrafenib (150 mg twice daily) or dabrafenib in combination with placebo. Treatment was continued until disease progression or unacceptable toxicity occurred, or the patient withdrew from the study; however, patients with disease progression could continue receiving treatment if they met prespecified criteria for continuation.

A total of 423 patients were enrolled, with a median age of 56 years; more than 99% were white, 72% had an ECOG performance status of 0, 66% had stage M1c disease, 65% had normal LDH concentrations, and 2 patients had a history of brain metastases. Most patients (85%) had a *BRAF* V600E mutation and 15% had a V600K mutation. The primary outcome was progression-free survival with secondary outcomes of overall survival, response rate, and response duration.

At a median follow-up of 9 months, median progression-free survival was 9.3 or 8.8 months in patients receiving trametinib plus dabrafenib or placebo plus dabrafenib, respectively. The overall response rates were 67 (10% as complete response) or 51% (9% as complete response) in patients given trametinib plus dabrafenib or placebo plus dabrafenib, respectively. The median duration of response was 9.2 and 10.2 months for trametinib plus dabrafenib versus placebo plus dabrafenib, respectively.

The COMBI-d trial was continued after analysis of the primary outcome to assess the secondary endpoint of overall survival. A final analysis for overall survival estimated a prolonged median overall survival (25.1 versus 18.7 months) and a reduction in the risk of death (29%) in patients receiving trametinib in combination with dabrafenib. The 1-year overall survival estimates were 74 or 68% for trametinib plus dabrafenib versus placebo plus dabrafenib, respectively.

The corresponding 2-year overall survival estimates were 51 or 42%, respectively. In addition, patients receiving trametinib and dabrafenib had higher overall response rates (66 versus 51%) compared with those receiving placebo and dabrafenib; complete responses were achieved in 10 or 8% of patients receiving trametinib in combination with dabrafenib or placebo in combination with dabrafenib, respectively. The median duration of response was 9.2 months in patients receiving trametinib in combination with dabrafenib and 10.2 months in those receiving dabrafenib alone. Results of a subgroup analysis (based on age, gender, disease stage, baseline ECOG performance status, baseline serum LDH concentration, visceral involvement, number of disease sites, and *BRAF* V600 mutation status) suggested that the effects of combination therapy with trametinib and dabrafenib on progression-free survival and overall survival were consistent across all subgroups.

Trametinib in combination with dabrafenib also has been evaluated in 121 adults with melanoma and brain metastases in an open-label, multicohort phase 2 study (COMBI-MB). In this study, patients received dabrafenib 150 mg twice daily in combination with trametinib 2 mg daily until disease progression or unacceptable toxicity occurred. Eligible patients were required to have at least one measurable intracranial lesion. Patients with leptomeningeal disease, parenchymal brain metastases greater than 4 cm in diameter, ocular melanoma, or primary mucosal melanoma were excluded. Previous therapy with up to two systemic therapies (except BRAF or MEK inhibitors) for metastatic melanoma was permitted prior to study entry. The primary efficacy outcome measure was intracranial response rate as assessed by independent review. Intracranial response rate was defined as the percentage of patients with confirmed intracranial complete or partial response (according to a modified Response Evaluation Criteria in Solid Tumors [RECIST] v1.1 to allow up to 5 intracranial target lesions ≥5 mm in diameter). Enrolled patients (N=121) were a median of 54 years of age; 58% were male, 100% were white, 65% had baseline LDH concentrations within normal limits, and 97% had an ECOG performance status of 0 or 1. Most (87%) patients with intracranial metastases were asymptomatic and 13% were symptomatic; 87% of patients had extracranial metastases and 22% of patients had received prior therapy for brain metastases. The intracranial response rate was 50%; complete response was 4.1% and partial response rate was 46%. The median duration of intracranial response was 6.4 months (range 1–31 months). Stable or progressive disease was the best overall intracranial response for 9% of the responders.

Trametinib in combination with dabrafenib has also been compared to immunotherapy (nivolumab and ipilimumab) in patients with unresectable stage III or IV melanoma in a 2-arm, 2-step, open-label, randomized phase 3 trial (DREAMseq). The goal of DREAMseq was to determine whether immunotherapy or the combination of BRAF and MEK inhibition should be preferred as initial therapy in patients with *BRAF*-mutant melanoma. Patients were required to have an ECOG performance status of 0 or 1 and be untreated in the metastatic setting, but were eligible if they had received adjuvant therapy that did not include a programmed death 1 (PD-1), programmed death-ligand 1 (PDL-1), cytotoxic T-cell lymphocyte-4, BRAF, or MEK inhibitor. In step 1 of this study, 265 patients were randomized in a 1:1 ratio to receive either trametinib (2 mg once daily) in combination with dabrafenib (150 mg twice daily) until disease progression or unacceptable toxicity occurred or nivolumab (1 mg/kg) in combination with ipilimumab (3 mg/kg) once every 3 weeks for 4 doses, followed by nivolumab alone (240 mg once every 2 weeks for up to 72 weeks); patients who experienced disease progression by RECIST criteria proceeded to step 2 where they crossed over to the alternate therapy. The primary endpoint of DREAMseq was 2-year overall survival among patients followed for at least 2 years.

Enrolled patients were a median of 61 years of age; 63% were male, 95% were white, and 60% had baseline LDH within normal limits. Most patients had *BRAF* V600E mutations; a higher proportion of patients randomized in step 1 to receive trametinib in combination with dabrafenib had *BRAF* V600K mutations (25%) compared to those randomized to immunotherapy (12%). Study accrual was halted by an independent data safety monitoring committee after an interim analysis, at which time 265 patients were randomized in step 1 and 73 patients had crossed over in step 2 (63% of whom were initially randomized to trametinib in combination with dabrafenib). The median follow-up was 27.7 months.

The 2-year overall survival rate was substantially lower in patients initially randomized to trametinib in combination with dabrafenib compared to those initially randomized to immunotherapy (51.5% versus 71.8%, respectively). The data safety monitoring committee determined that this difference was clinically meaningful and recommended closing the study to accrual, with patients initially

randomized to trametinib in combination with dabrafenib given the option to cross over to immunotherapy without prerequisite disease progression. The overall response rate for patients who received trametinib in combination with dabrafenib in step 1 was 43%, similar to this combination in step 2 (48%). Response rates appeared to be higher in patients who received immunotherapy in step 1 (46%) compared to those who received immunotherapy in step 2 (30%). The median duration of response among responders to step 1 therapy was not reached with immunotherapy and was 12.7 months with the combination of trametinib and dabrafenib.

Clinical Perspective

Adjuvant Therapy for Melanoma

The 2023 American Society of Clinical Oncology (ASCO) guidelines on systemic therapy for melanoma provide recommendations for adjuvant treatment of patients with resected stage IIIA-D melanoma with *BRAF* mutation (V600E/K). For such patients, adjuvant therapy options include nivolumab, pembrolizumab, or dabrafenib plus trametinib, with no preference for one therapy over another, all given for 52 weeks. For patients with resected stage IV melanoma with *BRAF* mutation (V600E/K), dabrafenib plus trametinib can be offered.

Patients with unresectable and/or metastatic mucosal melanoma may be offered the same treatment regimens as those recommended for cutaneous melanoma. However, due to limited data, the ASCO Expert Panel states that these patients should be offered or referred for enrollment in clinical trials whenever possible.

Unresectable or Metastatic Melanoma

The 2023 ASCO guideline on systemic therapy for melanoma recommends one of the following as first-line therapy in patients with unresectable and/or metastatic cutaneous melanoma with *BRAF* mutations (V600): programmed cell death protein (PD-1) inhibitors (nivolumab alone; pembrolizumab alone; nivolumab plus ipilimumab followed by nivolumab; or nivolumab plus relatlimab); or combination BRAF/MEK inhibitor therapy (dabrafenib plus trametinib; encorafenib plus binimetinib; or vemurafenib plus cobimetinib). Per the ASCO guidelines, nivolumab plus ipilimumab is preferred as first-line therapy for patients with unresectable and/or metastatic *BRAF* - mutant (V600) disease over BRAF/MEK inhibitor combination therapy.

For patients with *BRAF* mutation-positive (V600) unresectable/metastatic cutaneous melanoma who progress on first-line PD-1 inhibitor therapy, combination BRAF/MEK inhibitor therapy may be offered. Patients with *BRAF* mutation-positive (V600) unresectable/metastatic cutaneous melanoma who had disease progression following combination BRAF/MEK inhibitor therapy may be offered PD-1 inhibitor therapy.

● Non-small Cell Lung Cancer

Trametinib is used in combination with dabrafenib for the treatment of metastatic non-small cell lung cancer (NSCLC) in patients with *BRAF* V600E mutations. Trametinib has been designated an orphan drug by the FDA when used in combination with dabrafenib for the treatment of this cancer. An FDA-approved diagnostic test (e.g., THxID® BRAF kit) is required to confirm the presence of the *BRAF* V600E mutation prior to initiation of therapy.

Clinical Experience

Efficacy of trametinib in combination with dabrafenib for the treatment of metastatic NSCLC with *BRAF* V600E mutation is based principally on the results of an open-label, multicenter, nonrandomized, 3-cohort, phase 2 study (BRF113928). Patients in the BRF113928 study were enrolled into 2 cohorts: those previously treated with 1–3 systemic therapies with disease progression following at least one platinum-containing regimen and those with treatment-naive metastatic NSCLC. The cohort of patients with previously treated disease received either single-agent dabrafenib (150 mg twice daily) or trametinib (2 mg once daily) in combination with dabrafenib (150 mg twice daily). The cohort of patients with previously untreated disease received trametinib (2 mg once daily) in combination with dabrafenib (150 mg twice daily). Treatment was continued until disease progression or unacceptable toxicity occurred or the patient withdrew from the study. Patients with prior exposure to BRAF or MEK inhibitors were not eligible to enroll in the study; however, prior exposure to epidermal growth factor receptor (EGFR) or anaplastic lymphoma kinase (ALK) inhibitors was permitted in patients with

EGFR- or ALK-positive tumors. The primary measure of efficacy was objective response rate as assessed by an independent review committee according to RECIST and duration of response.

Enrolled patients (N=171) were a median of 66 years of age; 98% had squamous cell histology, 90% had an ECOG performance status of 0 or 1, 48% were male, 81% were white, 60% had a history of smoking, 48% were male, 32% were nonsmokers, 14% were Asian, 11% had received adjuvant chemotherapy, and 8% were current smokers. The majority (99%) of patients had metastatic disease; brain or liver metastases were present in 6 or 14% of these patients, respectively. Among the cohort of patients with previously treated disease, 58% had received only one prior systemic therapy for metastatic disease.

In the cohort of patients with previously treated disease, the objective response rate was 27 or 61% in patients receiving single-agent dabrafenib or combination therapy with trametinib and dabrafenib, respectively, and the median duration of response was 18 or 9 months, respectively. In the cohort of patients receiving trametinib in combination with dabrafenib for treatment-naive disease, the overall response rate was 61%, with a median duration of response of 15.2 months. In an updated 5-year survival analysis of previously treated and treatment-naive patients, the overall response rates with dabrafenib in combination with trametinib were 68.4 or 63.9%, respectively. Median progression-free survival was 10.2 or 10.8 months for previously-treated and treatment-naive patients, respectively. Median overall survival was 18.2 or 17.3 months, respectively.

Clinical Perspective

Approximately 60% of patients with lung cancer have driver alterations (e.g., mutations in *EGFR*, *ALK*, or *BRAF*; *ROS-1* fusions, *RET* fusions, *MET* exon 14 skipping mutations, and *NTRK* fusions). The ASCO and Ontario Health (OH; previously known as Cancer Care Ontario) living guideline specifically addresses treatment of stage IV NSCLC with driver alterations, including *BRAF* gene alterations.

For patients with stage IV NSCLC with a *BRAF* V600E mutation, dabrafenib and trametinib or encorafenib and binimetinib should be offered as first line treatment; however, standard first-line therapy based on the ASCO/OH nondriver mutation guideline may also be offered if these therapies are unavailable.

In the second line setting, standard first-line treatment based on the ASCO/OH nondriver mutation guideline should be offered in patients with stage IV NSCLC harboring *BRAF* V600E driver alterations who were previously treated with BRAF/MEK inhibitor combination therapy. In patients who did not receive BRAF-targeted therapy in the first-line setting, dabrafenib in combination with trametinib or encorafenib in combination with binimetinib may be offered. For patients with stage IV NSCLC with *BRAF* mutations other than V600E, standard treatment based on the ASCO/OH nondriver mutation guideline should be offered.

● Anaplastic Thyroid Cancer

Trametinib is used in combination with dabrafenib for the treatment of locally advanced or metastatic anaplastic thyroid cancer with *BRAF* V600E mutation when no satisfactory locoregional treatment options are available. Trametinib has been designated an orphan drug by the FDA when used in combination with dabrafenib for the treatment of this cancer. Confirmation of the presence of the *BRAF* V600E mutation is necessary prior to initiation of therapy; no FDA-approved diagnostic test for the detection of the *BRAF* V600E mutation in anaplastic thyroid cancer is currently available.

Clinical Experience

Efficacy of trametinib in combination with dabrafenib for the treatment of anaplastic thyroid cancer with *BRAF* V600E mutation is based principally on the results of an open-label, multicenter, nonrandomized, multicohort, phase 2 basket trial (BRF117019, ROAR) in patients with rare BRAF V600E mutation-positive malignancies. In this trial, a cohort of 36 patients with locally advanced, unresectable, or metastatic anaplastic thyroid cancer received trametinib (2 mg once daily) in combination with dabrafenib (150 mg twice daily). Treatment was continued until disease progression or unacceptable toxicity occurred or the patient withdrew from the study. Patients with prior exposure to BRAF or MEK inhibitors, symptomatic or untreated CNS metastases, airway obstruction, or inability to swallow or retain oral drugs were not eligible to enroll in the study. The primary measure of efficacy was overall response rate as assessed by an independent review committee according to RECIST and duration of response.

The median age of patients enrolled in the anaplastic thyroid cancer cohort was 71 years; 44% were male, 50% were white, 44% were Asian, and 94% had an ECOG performance status of 0 or 1. The majority of patients had received prior surgery and external beam radiation therapy (83% each) and 67% had received systemic therapy. The overall response rate in 36 evaluable patients in the anaplastic thyroid cancer cohort was 53%; complete response was achieved in 6% of the evaluable patients. The median duration of response was 13.6 months. Duration of response was ≥6 or ≥12 months in 68 or 53% of patients, respectively. A final analysis of data from the ROAR trial reported a median duration of response of 14.4 months, with a median progression-free survival of 6.7 months. The overall response rate was 56% based on investigator assessment.

Clinical Perspective

Approximately 40–70% of patients with anaplastic thyroid cancer have *BRAF* V600E driver alterations. Mainstays of therapy in addition to surgery involve locoregional approaches (commonly radiotherapy with or without concurrent chemotherapy) or systemic therapy (cytotoxic therapy or targeted therapy).

The 2021 American Thyroid Association (ATA) guidelines for the management of anaplastic thyroid cancer recommend BRAF/MEK inhibitor combination therapy (dabrafenib in combination with trametinib) over other systemic therapies in patients with stage 4C or unresectable stage 4B anaplastic thyroid cancer harboring *BRAF* V600E mutation who decline radiation therapy. If radiotherapy is feasible in patients with *BRAF* V600E mutation-positive unresectable stage 4B anaplastic thyroid cancer, ATA recommends chemoradiotherapy or neoadjuvant dabrafenib-trametinib combination therapy as alternatives to initial treatment.

● BRAF *V600E-mutant Solid Tumors*

Trametinib is used in combination with dabrafenib for the treatment of adult and pediatric patients ≥1 year of age with unresectable or metastatic solid tumors (excluding colorectal cancer) harboring the *BRAF* V600E mutation who have progressed following prior treatment and have no satisfactory alternative treatment. The accelerated approval of the use of trametinib with dabrafenib for this indication is based on overall response rate and duration of response. Continued approval for this indication may be contingent upon verification and description of clinical benefit in confirmatory studies. Trametinib has been designated an orphan drug by the FDA for the treatment of malignant glioma with *BRAF* V600 mutation. Confirmation of the presence of the *BRAF* V600E mutation is necessary prior to initiation of therapy; no FDA-approved diagnostic test for the detection of the *BRAF* V600E mutation in solid tumors other than melanoma and NSCLC is currently available.

Trametinib is *not* indicated for use in patients with *BRAF*-mutant colorectal cancer because of intrinsic resistance to *BRAF* inhibition.

Clinical Experience

Efficacy of trametinib in combination with dabrafenib for the treatment of unresectable or metastatic *BRAF* V600E-mutant solid tumors was shown in trials BRF117019 (ROAR), NCI-MATCH, CTMT212X2101, and CDRB436G2201, and supported by results of the COMBI-d, COMBI-v, and BRF113928 trials.

Adults

In addition to adults with anaplastic thyroid cancer, the ROAR trial enrolled adults with high-grade glioma (N=45), low-grade glioma (N=13), gastrointestinal stromal tumor (N=1), biliary tract cancer (N=43), and adenocarcinoma of the small intestine (N=3).

NCI-MATCH is a precision medicine clinical trial platform with multiple subprotocol cohorts; subprotocol H (EAY131-H) was a multicenter, single-arm, open-label phase 2 basket trial in adult patients with solid tumors, lymphoma, or multiple myeloma with *BRAF* V600 mutations who had received at least 1 prior line of standard therapy. Patients in NCI-MATCH received trametinib (2 mg once daily) and dabrafenib (150 mg twice daily) until disease progression or unacceptable toxicity occurred or the patient withdrew from the study. Patients were excluded from NCI-MATCH if they had melanoma, thyroid cancer, colorectal cancer, or NSCLC (following a protocol amendment), prior exposure to BRAF or MEK inhibitors, history of any RAS-mutant cancer, or left ventricular ejection fraction below the lower limit of normal, or if they did not have measurable disease. The primary endpoint of ROAR and EAY131-H was objective response rate.

A pooled analysis of ROAR and EAY131-H included a total of 131 patients with *BRAF* V600E-mutant solid tumors (excluding patients with NSCLC and anaplastic thyroid cancer). Among patients in the pooled analysis, 37% had biliary tract cancers, 37% had high-grade gliomas, 11% had low-grade gliomas, and 15% had other GI, lung, gynecologic, peritoneal, or various other tumors. In this pooled cohort, patients were a median of 51 years of age; 56% were female, 85% were white, and 93% had an ECOG performance status of 0 (37%) or 1 (56%). Most patients (90%) had received prior systemic therapy.

Among disease groups composed of more than 5 patients, RECIST objective response rate was 33% in those with high-grade gliomas, 46% in those with biliary tract cancers, and 50% in those with low-grade gliomas. Median duration of response was 13.6 months and 9.8 months in patients with high-grade gliomas and biliary tract cancers, respectively.

Pediatric Patients

CTMT212X2101 was a multicenter, multi-cohort, open-label phase 2 trial investigating trametinib monotherapy and trametinib in combination with dabrafenib in pediatric patients 1 to 17 years of age with recurrent or refractory cancers. Part C of this study was a dose escalation of trametinib and dabrafenib in pediatric patients with *BRAF* V600-mutant tumors; part D was an expansion cohort in pediatric patients with *BRAF* V600-mutant low-grade glioma or Langerhans cell histiocytosis. Patients received trametinib and dabrafenib at recommended dosage levels according to weight and age.

A pooled analysis of parts C and D of the CTMT212X2101 trial included a total of 48 pediatric patients with *BRAF* V600E-mutant tumors, including 34 patients with low-grade gliomas and 2 patients with high-grade gliomas. Enrolled patients with gliomas were a median of 10 years of age; 50% were male, 75% were white, and 58% had a Karnofsky/Lansky performance status of 100. Most patients had undergone prior surgical (83%) and/or systemic treatment (92%).

Overall response rate among the pediatric patients with gliomas as assessed by independent review according to Response Assessment in Neuro-Oncology (RANO) criteria for gliomas, the major efficacy outcome in the pooled glioma analysis, was 25%. Among responders, duration of response was ≥6 months in 78% and ≥24 months in 44% of patients.

Study CDRB436G2201 was a multicenter, randomized, open-label, phase 2 trial in chemotherapy-naïve pediatric patients with BRAF V600E-mutant low-grade gliomas and pediatric patients with relapsed or progressive BRAF V600E-mutant high-grade gliomas. Forty-one patients with high-grade gliomas were enrolled and received trametinib plus dabrafenib. Enrolled patients in the cohort with high-grade gliomas were a median of 13 years of age; 56% were female, 61% white, 27% Asian, and 37% had a Karnofsky/Lansky performance status of 100. The primary endpoint was overall response rate, with secondary endpoints of duration of response and progression-free survival. At a median follow-up of 25.1 months, the overall response rate was 56% (29.3% assessed as complete response and 26.8% as partial response), with a median duration of response of 22.2 months. The rate of progression-free survival was 58.5%.

● Low-Grade Glioma

Trametinib in combination with dabrafinib is used for treatment of low-grade glioma with *BRAF* V600E mutation in pediatric patients ≥1 year of age who require systemic therapy. Trametinib has been designated an orphan drug by the FDA when used in combination with dabrafenib for the treatment of this cancer. Confirmation of the presence of the *BRAF* V600E mutation is necessary prior to initiation of therapy; no FDA-approved diagnostic test for the detection of the *BRAF* V600E mutation in low-grade glioma is currently available.

Clinical Experience

Efficacy of trametinib in combination with dabrafenib for treatment of low-grade glioma in pediatric patients was shown in a phase 2, multicenter, open-label trial (CDRB436G2201). Patients 1 to <18 years of age with *BRAF* V600E-mutant low-grade glioma requiring systemic therapy were randomized to treatment at a 2:1 ratio to either trametinib plus dabrafenib or carboplatin plus vincristine. Trametinib and dabrafenib were administered at age- and weight-based dosages until loss of clinical benefit or unacceptable toxicity occurred; carboplatin and vincristine were given as a single 10-week induction course followed by eight 6-week cycles. The primary outcome assessed was overall response rate, with secondary outcomes of progression-free survival and overall survival.

Enrolled patients (N=110) were a median of 9.5 years of age and 60% were female. The overall response rate with trametinib plus dabrafenib was 46.6% (2.7% complete response and 44% partial response) versus 10.8% (2.7% complete response and 8% partial response) with chemotherapy. The median duration of response was 23.7 months with trametinib plus dabrafenib; the median duration of response was not estimable with chemotherapy. The median progression-free survival was 20.1 months with trametinib plus dabrafenib versus 7.4 months with chemotherapy.

DOSAGE AND ADMINISTRATION

● General

Pretreatment Screening

- *Melanoma*: Confirm presence of the b-Raf serine-threonine kinase (*BRAF*) V600E or V600K mutation using an FDA-approved diagnostic test (e.g., THxID® BRAF kit) prior to initiation of trametinib as a single agent or in combination with dabrafenib.

- *Other solid tumors*: Confirm presence of the *BRAF* V600E mutation using an FDA-approved diagnostic test (e.g., THxID® BRAF kit), when available, prior to initiation of combination therapy with trametinib and dabrafenib for the treatment of metastatic non-small cell lung cancer (NSCLC), locally advanced or metastatic anaplastic thyroid cancer, low-grade glioma, or other unresectable or metastatic solid tumors.

- Perform a dermatologic evaluation prior to initiation of therapy when used in combination with dabrafenib.

- Assess left ventricular ejection fraction (LVEF) by echocardiogram or multigated acquisition (MUGA) scan prior to the initiation of trametinib as a single agent or in combination with dabrafenib.

- Monitor serum glucose concentrations upon initiation of combination therapy with trametinib and dabrafenib in patients with preexisting diabetes mellitus or hyperglycemia.

- Perform pregnancy test in females of childbearing age.

Patient Monitoring

- When used in combination with dabrafenib, perform dermatologic evaluations for new cutaneous malignancies every 2 months during therapy and for up to 6 months following discontinuance of combination therapy. In addition, monitor for signs and symptoms of new noncutaneous malignancies.

- Assess LVEF by echocardiogram or MUGA scan 1 month after initiation of therapy, and then every 2–3 months during therapy.

- Perform ophthalmologic examinations periodically during therapy and as clinically indicated for visual disturbances.

- Closely monitor for manifestations of colitis or GI perforation.

- Monitor for symptoms of deep-vein thrombosis or pulmonary embolism (e.g., shortness of breath, chest pain, arm or leg swelling).

- Monitor for new or worsening serious skin reactions during therapy.

- Monitor serum glucose concentrations as clinically appropriate during combination therapy with trametinib and dabrafenib in patients with preexisting diabetes mellitus or hyperglycemia.

Premedication and Prophylaxis

- Administer antipyretics as secondary prophylaxis when resuming trametinib therapy following resolution of a severe febrile reaction or fever associated with complications.

Other General Considerations

- Clinicians should consult published protocols for information on the dosage, method of administration, and administration sequence of other antineoplastic agents used in combination regimens with trametinib. When used in combination with dabrafenib, the usual cautions, precautions, and contraindications associated with dabrafenib must be considered in addition to those associated with trametinib.

● *Administration*

Trametinib is administered orally once daily (approximately every 24 hours), at least 1 hour before or 2 hours after a meal.

If a dose of trametinib is missed by ≤12 hours, the missed dose should be taken as soon as it is remembered.

If a dose of trametinib is vomited, do not take an additional dose; take the next dose at the regularly scheduled time.

Tablets

Do not crush or break trametinib tablets.

Store trametinib tablets in the refrigerator at 2–8°C; dispense the drug in its original bottle, protected from moisture and light, and instruct patients not to remove the desiccant or to repackage the drug in a pill box.

Oral Solution

Trametinib powder for oral solution must be reconstituted prior to use and is intended for administration by a caregiver.

To reconstitute, tap the bottle to loosen the powder. Then, add 90 mL of distilled or purified water to the bottle and invert or shake for up to 5 minutes until powder is dissolved, yielding a clear solution.

Once reconstituted, the solution yields a trametinib concentration of 0.05 mg/mL.

The oral solution may be administered from an oral dosing syringe or feeding tube.

Store unreconstituted powder in the refrigerator at 2–8°C in the original carton to protect from moisture and light. After reconstitution, store oral solution at <25°C and do not freeze. Discard any remaining reconstituted solution after 35 days.

● *Dosage*

Dosage of trametinib dimethyl sulfoxide is expressed in terms of trametinib.

Pediatric Patients

BRAF *V600E-mutant Solid Tumors*

When used in combination with dabrafenib for the treatment of pediatric patients ≥1 year of age with unresectable or metastatic solid tumors (excluding colorectal cancer) harboring the *BRAF* V600E mutation who have progressed following prior treatment and who have no satisfactory alternative treatment, the recommended dosage of trametinib oral solution and tablets is based on body weight (see Table 1 and Table 2). A recommended tablet dosage has not been established for patients weighing <26 kg. Therapy should be continued until disease progression or unacceptable toxicity occurs.

BRAF *V600E-mutant Low-Grade Glioma*

When used in combination with dabrafenib for the treatment of pediatric patients ≥1 year of age with low-grade glioma (LGG) with a *BRAF* V600E mutation who require systemic therapy, the recommended dosage of trametinib oral solution and tablets is based on body weight (see Table 1 and Table 2). A recommended tablet dosage has not been established for patients weighing <26 kg. Therapy should be continued until disease progression or unacceptable toxicity occurs.

TABLE 1. Dosing of Trametinib Oral Solution in Pediatric Patients ≥1 Year of Age

Body Weight	Recommended Oral Dosage
8 kg	0.3 mg (6 mL) once daily
9 kg	0.35 mg (7 mL) once daily
10 kg	0.35 mg (7 mL) once daily
11 kg	0.4 mg (8 mL) once daily

TABLE 1. Continued

Body Weight	Recommended Oral Dosage
12—13 kg	0.45 mg (9 mL) once daily
14—17 kg	0.55 mg (11 mL) once daily
18—21 kg	0.7 mg (14 mL) once daily
22—25 kg	0.85 mg (17 mL) once daily
26—29 kg	0.9 mg (18 mL) once daily
30—33 kg	1 mg (20 mL) once daily
34—37 kg	1.15 mg (23 mL) once daily
38—41 kg	1.25 mg (25 mL) once daily
42—45 kg	1.4 mg (28 mL) once daily
46—50 kg	1.6 mg (32 mL) once daily
≥51 kg	2 mg (40 mL) once daily

a Concentration of trametinib oral solution: 0.05 mg/mL.

TABLE 2. Dosing of Trametinib Tablets in Pediatric Patients ≥1 Year of Age

Body Weight	Recommended Oral Dosage
26—37 kg	1 mg (two 0.5-mg tablets) once daily
38—50 kg	1.5 mg (three 0.5-mg tablets) once daily
≥51 kg	2 mg once daily

Adults

Melanoma

Adjuvant Therapy for Melanoma

When used in combination with dabrafenib as adjuvant treatment following complete resection of melanoma with *BRAF* V600E or V600K mutation and nodal involvement, the recommended adult dosage of trametinib is 2 mg once daily. Therapy should be continued for up to 1 year or until disease progression or unacceptable toxicity occurs.

Unresectable or Metastatic Melanoma

When used for the treatment of unresectable or metastatic melanoma with *BRAF* V600E or V600K mutation, the recommended adult dosage of trametinib (as a single agent or in combination with dabrafenib) is 2 mg once daily. Therapy should be continued until disease progression or unacceptable toxicity occurs.

Non-small Cell Lung Cancer

When used in combination with dabrafenib for the treatment of metastatic NSCLC with *BRAF* V600E mutation, the recommended adult dosage of trametinib is 2 mg once daily. Therapy should be continued until disease progression or unacceptable toxicity occurs.

Anaplastic Thyroid Cancer

When used in combination with dabrafenib for the treatment of locally advanced or metastatic anaplastic thyroid cancer with *BRAF* V600E mutation when no satisfactory locoregional treatment options are available, the recommended adult dosage of trametinib is 2 mg once daily. Therapy should be continued until disease progression or unacceptable toxicity occurs.

BRAF *V600E-mutant Solid Tumors*

When used in combination with dabrafenib for the treatment of unresectable or metastatic solid tumors (excluding colorectal cancer) harboring the *BRAF* V600E mutation when no satisfactory alternative treatment is available, the recommended adult dosage of trametinib is 2 mg once daily. Therapy should be continued until disease progression or unacceptable toxicity occurs.

Dosage Modification for Toxicity

Dosage of trametinib may be reduced or therapy temporarily interrupted in patients who develop adverse effects. Up to 2 dosage reductions for toxicity may be made. Recommended dosage modifications for trametinib tablets and oral solutions are presented in Tables 3 and 4, respectively. Permanently discontinue trametinib if the patient is unable to tolerate a maximum of 2 dosage reductions.

TABLE 3. Trametinib Tablet Dosage Modifications for Toxicity

Recommended Dosage	1 mg orally once daily	1.5 mg orally once daily	2 mg orally once daily
First dose reduction	0.5 mg (one 0.5-mg tablet) orally once daily	1 mg (two 0.5-mg tablets) orally once daily	1.5 mg (three 0.5-mg tablets) orally once daily
Second dose reduction[a]	N/A	0.5 mg (one 0.5-mg tablet) orally once daily	1 mg (two 0.5-mg tablets) orally once daily

[a] Permanently discontinue trametinib if unable to tolerate a maximum of 2 dosage reductions.

TABLE 4. Trametinib Oral Solution[a] Dosage Modifications for Toxicity

Body Weight and Recommended Dosage	First Dose Reduction	Second Dose Reduction[b]
8 kg 0.3 mg (6 mL) once daily	5 mL once daily	3 mL once daily
9 kg 0.35 mg (7 mL) once daily	5 mL once daily	4 mL once daily
10 kg 0.35 mg (7 mL) once daily	5 mL once daily	4 mL once daily
11 kg 0.4 mg (8 mL) once daily	6 mL once daily	4 mL once daily
12—13 kg 0.45 mg (9 mL) once daily	7 mL once daily	5 mL once daily
14—17 kg 0.55 mg (11 mL) once daily	8 mL once daily	6 mL once daily
18—21 kg 0.7 mg (14 mL) once daily	11 mL once daily	7 mL once daily
22—25 kg 0.85 mg (17 mL) once daily	13 mL once daily	9 mL once daily
26—29 kg 0.9 mg (18 mL) once daily	14 mL once daily	9 mL once daily
30—33 kg 1 mg (20 mL) once daily	15 mL once daily	10 mL once daily
34—37 kg 1.15 mg (23 mL) once daily	17 mL once daily	12 mL once daily
38—41 kg 1.25 mg (25 mL) once daily	19 mL once daily	13 mL once daily

TABLE 4. Continued

Body Weight and Recommended Dosage	First Dose Reduction	Second Dose Reduction[b]
42—45 kg 1.4 mg (28 mL) once daily	21 mL once daily	14 mL once daily
46—50 kg 1.6 mg (32 mL) once daily	24 mL once daily	16 mL once daily
≥51 kg 2 mg (40 mL) once daily	30 mL once daily	20 mL once daily

[a] Concentration of trametinib oral solution: 0.05 mg/mL.

[b] Permanently discontinue trametinib if unable to tolerate a maximum of 2 dosage reductions.

Dosage Modification for New Primary Cutaneous Malignancies

If new primary cutaneous malignancies occur, no dosage modification of trametinib is recommended.

Dosage Modification for New Primary Noncutaneous Malignancies

If new noncutaneous malignancies occur during combination therapy with trametinib and dabrafenib, no dosage modification of trametinib is required.

Dosage Modification for Febrile Drug Reactions

If fever (temperature of 38–40°C) or any initial symptom of fever recurrence occurs, interrupt trametinib therapy until the adverse reaction resolves. Once fever resolves, trametinib may be resumed at the same or a reduced dosage.

If fever (temperature exceeding 40°C) or fever complicated by rigors, hypotension, dehydration, or renal failure occurs, interrupt trametinib treatment until the adverse reaction resolves for at least 24 hours. Once fever has resolved, resume trametinib at the same or reduced dosage or permanently discontinue trametinib.

Dosage Modification for Dermatologic Effects

If grade 2 skin toxicity develops and is intolerable, interrupt trametinib for up to 3 weeks. If grade 2 toxicity improves within 3 weeks of withholding trametinib, resume at a reduced dosage. If grade 2 skin toxicity does not improve within 3 weeks of withholding trametinib, permanently discontinue trametinib.

If grade 3 or 4 skin toxicity occurs, interrupt trametinib for up to 3 weeks. If grade 3 or 4 skin toxicity does not improve within 3 weeks of withholding trametinib, permanently discontinue trametinib. If grade 3 or 4 skin toxicity improves within 3 weeks of withholding trametinib, resume at a reduced dosage.

If severe cutaneous adverse reactions (SCARs) occur, permanently discontinue trametinib.

Dosage Modification for Cardiac Effects

If an asymptomatic decrease in left ventricular ejection fraction (LVEF) from baseline of 10% or more and to a level below institution-specific lower limit of normal occurs, interrupt trametinib for up to 4 weeks. If LVEF improves to normal values within 4 weeks of withholding trametinib, resume at a reduced dosage. If LVEF does not improve to normal values within 4 weeks of withholding trametinib, permanently discontinue trametinib.

If symptomatic cardiomyopathy or an absolute decrease in LVEF from baseline exceeding 20% and to a level below institution-specific lower limit of normal occurs, permanently discontinue.

Dosage Modification for Hemorrhage

If grade 3 hemorrhagic events occur, interrupt trametinib treatment. If improvement is observed, resume trametinib at a lower dosage. If grade 3 hemorrhagic events do not improve, permanently discontinue trametinib.

If any grade 4 hemorrhagic events occur, permanently discontinue trametinib.

Dosage Modification for Venous Thromboembolism

If uncomplicated deep-vein thrombosis (DVT) or pulmonary embolism (PE) occurs, interrupt trametinib for up to 3 weeks. If improvement to grade 0 or 1 is observed within 3 weeks, resume trametinib at a lower dosage. If no improvement is observed within 3 weeks, permanently discontinue trametinib.

If life-threatening PE occurs, permanently discontinue trametinib.

Dosage Modification for Ocular Effects

If retinal pigment epithelial detachment occurs, interrupt trametinib for up to 3 weeks. If retinal pigment epithelial detachment improves within 3 weeks of withholding trametinib, resume at the same or a reduced dosage. If retinal pigment epithelial detachment does not improve within 3 weeks of withholding trametinib, resume at a reduced dosage or permanently discontinue trametinib.

If retinal vein occlusion occurs, permanently discontinue trametinib.

If uveitis occurs during combination therapy with trametinib and dabrafenib, no dosage modification of trametinib is necessary.

Dosage Modification for Pulmonary Effects

If treatment-related interstitial lung disease or pneumonitis occurs, permanently discontinue trametinib.

Dosage Modification for Other Toxicity

If an intolerable grade 2 or any grade 3 adverse reaction occurs, interrupt trametinib treatment. If the adverse reaction improves to grade 0 or 1, resume trametinib at a reduced dosage. If the adverse reaction does not improve to grade 0 or 1, permanently discontinue trametinib.

At the first occurrence of any grade 4 adverse reaction, interrupt trametinib until the adverse reaction improves to grade 0 or 1 and then resume at a reduced dosage. If the grade 4 adverse reaction does not improve to grade 0 or 1, permanently discontinue trametinib. If there is a recurrent grade 4 adverse reaction, permanently discontinue trametinib.

• Special Populations

Hepatic Impairment

In patients with mild hepatic impairment (total bilirubin concentration not exceeding the ULN with AST concentration exceeding the ULN or total bilirubin concentration exceeding the ULN, but no more than 1.5 times the ULN, with any AST concentration), dosage adjustment is not necessary.

An appropriate dosage has not been established in patients with moderate (bilirubin concentration >1.5–3 times the ULN and any AST concentration) to severe (bilirubin concentration 3–10 times the ULN and any AST concentration) hepatic impairment. No increase in exposure of trametinib occurred in patients with moderate or severe hepatic impairment compared with patients with normal hepatic function. Consider the potential risks and benefits of the drug when initiating trametinib therapy and when determining the appropriate dosage in patients with moderate or severe hepatic impairment.

Renal Impairment

In patients with renal impairment (estimated glomerular filtration rate [GFR] 15–89 mL/minute per 1.73 m^2), dosage adjustments are not necessary; no clinically important effects on the exposure of trametinib are anticipated.

Geriatric Patients

The manufacturer does not make any specific dosage recommendations for geriatric patients.

CAUTIONS

• Contraindications

- None.

• Warnings/Precautions

Combination Therapy

When combination therapy with trametinib includes the use of dabrafenib, consult the manufacturer's prescribing information for dabrafenib for detailed information on the usual cautions, precautions, and contraindications of this drug.

New Primary Malignancies

New primary cutaneous and noncutaneous malignancies are a known class effect of b-Raf serine-threonine kinase (BRAF) inhibitors (i.e., dabrafenib, encorafenib, vemurafenib). Among adult patients receiving trametinib in combination with dabrafenib, cutaneous squamous cell carcinomas and keratoacanthomas occurred in 2% of patients in the pooled safety population. Basal cell carcinoma and new primary melanoma occurred in approximately 3% and <1% of patients, respectively. Among pediatric patients receiving trametinib in combination with dabrafenib, new primary melanoma was reported in <1% of patients.

Dabrafenib may promote the growth and development of *RAS* mutation-positive noncutaneous malignancies. Among adult patients receiving trametinib in combination with dabrafenib, noncutaneous malignancies occurred in 1% of patients in the pooled safety population.

Perform dermatologic evaluations for new cutaneous malignancies prior to initiation of combination therapy with trametinib and dabrafenib, every 2 months during therapy, and for up to 6 months following discontinuance of combination therapy. Close monitoring for signs and symptoms of new noncutaneous malignancies also is necessary. In patients developing new primary cutaneous malignancies or noncutaneous malignancies during combination therapy, dosage modification of trametinib is not necessary.

Hemorrhage

Hemorrhage, including major hemorrhagic events (i.e., symptomatic bleeding in a critical area or organ), sometimes fatal, has occurred when trametinib is used in combination with dabrafenib. In the pooled safety population of adult patients receiving trametinib in combination with dabrafenib, hemorrhagic events occurred in 17% of patients. GI hemorrhage and intracranial hemorrhage occurred in 3% and 0.6% of patients receiving trametinib in combination with dabrafenib, respectively. Fatal hemorrhagic events (e.g., cerebral or brainstem hemorrhage) occurred in 0.5% of patients receiving trametinib in combination with dabrafenib.

In the pooled safety population of pediatric patients receiving trametinib in combination with dabrafenib, hemorrhagic events occurred in 25% of patients. The most common type of bleeding was epistaxis, which occurrred in 16% of patients. Serious bleeding events developed in 3.6% of pediatric patients, which included GI hemorrhage (1.2%), cerebral hemorrhage (0.6%), uterine hemorrhage (0.6%), post-procedural hemorrhage (0.6%), and epistaxis (0.6%).

If hemorrhagic events occur, dosage modification and/or treatment discontinuance may be necessary. For grade 3 hemorrhagic events, interrupt use of trametinib. If improvement occurs, resume trametinib at a lower dosage level. If improvement does not occur, permanently discontinue trametinib. For grade 4 hemorrhagic events, permanently discontinue trametinib.

Colitis and GI Perforation

Colitis and GI perforation, sometimes fatal, have occurred in patients receiving trametinib as monotherapy or in combination with dabrafenib. In the pooled safety population of adults taking trametinib as monotherapy or in combination with dabrafenib, colitis and GI perforation each occurred in <1% of patients. In the pooled safety population of pediatric patients receiving trametinib in combination with dabrafenib, colitis occurred in <1% of patients.

Patients should be monitored closely for manifestations of colitis and GI perforation.

Venous Thromboembolic Events

Venous thromboembolism (VTE) has occurred when trametinib is used in combination with dabrafenib. In the pooled safety population, deep-vein thrombosis (DVT) and pulmonary embolism (PE) occurred in 2% of adult patients receiving trametinib in combination with dabrafenib. In the pooled safety population of pediatric patients receiving trametinib in combination with dabrafenib, rates of embolism were <1%.

Advise patients to immediately seek medical care if they develop symptoms of DVT or PE such as shortness of breath, chest pain, or arm or leg swelling. Dosage modification or treatment discontinuance may be necessary if DVT or PE occurs.

Cardiomyopathy

Cardiomyopathy, including cardiac failure, has occurred in patients receiving trametinib.

Across the pooled safety population of adult patients receiving trametinib in combination with dabrafenib, cardiomyopathy (defined as an absolute decrease in left ventricular ejection fraction [LVEF] from baseline of ≥10% and to a level below the institution-specific lower limit of normal [LLN]) occurred in 6% of patients. Dosage interruption or discontinuance of trametinib was necessary in 3% or <1 %, respectively. Cardiomyopathy resolved in 45 of 50 patients receiving combination therapy with trametinib and dabrafenib. In the pooled safety population of pediatric patients receiving trametinib in combination with dabrafenib, cardiomyopathy occurred in 9% of patients.

Before initiation of trametinib, as monotherapy or in combination with dabrafenib, assess LVEF using echocardiogram or multigated radionuclide angiography (MUGA). Reassess LVEF 1 month after initiation of trametinib and then every 2–3 months during treatment. Interrupt trametinib treatment for up to 4 weeks in patients experiencing an asymptomatic absolute decrease in LVEF from baseline of 10% or more and to a level below institution-specific lower limit of normal; if LVEF improves to normal values, may resume trametinib at a lower dose, but discontinue permanently if this improvement does not occur. Permanently discontinue trametinib in patients experiencing symptomatic cardiomyopathy or an absolute decrease in LVEF from baseline exceeding 20% and to a level below institution-specific lower limit of normal.

Ocular Toxicities

Retinal pigment epithelial detachment and retinal vein occlusion can occur with trametinib.

Retinal pigment epithelial detachment may be bilateral and multifocal, occurring in the macular region of the retina or other sites in the retina. Routine ophthalmologic examinations were not performed to detect asymptomatic retinal pigment epithelial detachment in clinical trials evaluating trametinib in patients with melanoma or non-small cell lung cancer (NSCLC); therefore, the true incidence of this adverse effect is unknown. In the pooled safety population of pediatric patients receiving trametinib in combination with dabrafenib, retinal pigment epithelial detachment occurred in <1% of patients.

Retinal vein occlusion may lead to macular edema, decreased visual function, neovascularization, and glaucoma. Retinal vein occlusion occurred in 0.6% of adult patients receiving trametinib monotherapy in the pooled safety population; no cases of retinal vein occlusion were reported across the pooled safety population of patients who received trametinib with dabrafenib.

Perform ophthalmologic examinations periodically and as clinically indicated during trametinib therapy. If visual disturbances are reported, urgent ophthalmologic evaluation (within 24 hours) is needed.

If retinal pigment epithelial detachment is diagnosed, interrupt trametinib treatment. If repeat ophthalmologic evaluation confirms resolution of retinal pigment epithelial detachment within 3 weeks, resume trametinib at the same or a reduced dosage. If no improvement is observed within 3 weeks, resume trametinib at a reduced dosage or permanently discontinue trametinib.

If retinal vein occlusion is diagnosed, permanently discontinue trametinib.

If uveitis occurs in patients receiving combination therapy with trametinib and dabrafenib, no dosage modification of trametinib is required.

Interstitial Lung Disease/Pneumonitis

Interstitial lung disease or pneumonitis has been reported in patients receiving trametinib monotherapy or combination therapy with dabrafenib. In the pooled safety population, interstitial lung disease or pneumonitis occurred in 2% of adult patients receiving trametinib monotherapy. Across the pooled safety population, interstitial lung disease or pneumonitis occurred in 1% of adult patients receiving trametinib in combination with dabrafenib.

In patients presenting with new or progressive pulmonary symptoms (including cough, dyspnea, hypoxia, pleural effusion, infiltrates), interrupt trametinib pending results of clinical investigation. Permanently discontinue trametinib in patients diagnosed with treatment-related interstitial lung disease or pneumonitis.

Serious Febrile Reactions

Serious febrile drug reactions (including fever accompanied by hypotension, rigors/chills, dehydration, or renal failure) have occurred in patients receiving combination therapy with trametinib and dabrafenib.

Across the pooled safety population evaluating combination therapy with trametinib and dabrafenib in adult patients, the incidence of pyrexia was 58%. In these studies, serious febrile reactions or fever of any severity complicated by hypotension, severe rigors/chills, dehydration, renal failure, or syncope occurred in 5% of patients receiving combination therapy with trametinib and dabrafenib. Fever was complicated by severe chills/rigors, renal failure, syncope, dehydration, or hypotension in <1, 1, 2, 3, or 4%, respectively, of patients receiving combination therapy with trametinib and dabrafenib. In the pooled safety population of pediatric patients receiving trametinib in combination with dabrafenib, pyrexia occurred in 66% of patients.

Interrupt trametinib, and dabrafenib if used in combination, if the patient's temperature is ≥ 100.4°F (38.0°C). Evaluate for signs and symptoms of infection and monitor renal function (e.g., serum creatinine) during and following severe pyrexia. If the patient has recovered from the febrile reaction for at least 24 hours, restart trametinib, and dabrafenib if used in combination, at the same or reduced dosage. Administer prophylactic antipyretics in patients resuming trametinib following a serious febrile reaction or fever associated with complications. For second or subsequent occurrences of prolonged fever (lasting longer than 3 days) or fever associated with complications (e.g., dehydration, hypotension, renal failure, severe chills/rigors) without evidence of an active infection, administer corticosteroids (e.g., prednisone 10 mg daily) for at least 5 days.

Serious Skin Toxicities

Severe cutaneous adverse reactions (SCARs), including Stevens-Johnson syndrome and drug reaction with eosinophilia and systemic symptoms, have been reported in postmarketing surveillance during therapy with trametinib in combination with dabrafenib. Across the pooled safety population, other serious dermatologic toxicity occurred in <1% of adult patients receiving trametinib in combination with dabrafenib. Across the pooled safety population of pediatric patients receiving trametinib in combination with dabrafenib, serious skin and subcutaneous tissue disorders were reported in 1.8% of patients.

Monitor for new or worsening serious skin toxicities. If dermatologic toxicity occurs, dosage modification or treatment discontinuance may be necessary. Permanently discontinue trametinib if SCARs occur.

Hyperglycemia

Hyperglycemia has occurred in patients receiving combination therapy with trametinib and dabrafenib. Across the pooled safety population, grade 3 or 4 hyperglycemia occurred in 2% of adult patients receiving trametinib in combination with dabrafenib. Among patients with a history of diabetes mellitus, 15% required intensification of antihyperglycemic therapy. In the pooled safety population of pediatric patients receiving trametinib in combination with dabrafenib, grade 3 or 4 hyperglycemia was reported in <1% of patients.

Monitor serum glucose concentrations prior to initiation of therapy and as clinically appropriate in patients with preexisting diabetes mellitus or hyperglycemia. Initiate or optimize antihyperglycemic therapy as clinically indicated.

Hemophagocytic Lymphohistiocytosis

Hemophagocytic lymphohistiocytosis (HLH) has been reported in postmarketing reports from patients receiving trametinib in combination with dabrafenib. If HLH is suspected, treatment interruption is recommended. After confirmation of HLH, discontinue treatment and initiate appropriate management of HLH.

Fetal/Neonatal Morbidity and Mortality

Trametinib may cause fetal harm in humans based on its mechanism of action and animal findings; the drug has been shown to be abortifacient and embryotoxic in rabbits at dosages resulting in exposures as low as 0.3 times the human exposure at recommended adult dosages.

Verify pregnancy status in females of reproductive potential prior to initiating trametinib. Women with reproductive potential should use effective contraceptive methods while receiving trametinib and for 4 months following discontinuance of the drug. If pregnancy is confirmed or suspected during therapy, the patient should contact her clinician. If a woman is or becomes pregnant while taking trametinib, she should be informed of the risk to the fetus.

Specific Populations

Pregnancy

Trametinib may cause fetal harm if administered to pregnant women based on its mechanism of action and animal findings. Verify pregnancy status in females of reproductive potential prior to initiating trametinib.

Lactation

There are no data on the presence of trametinib in human milk, the effects on the breast-fed infant, or the effects on milk production. Because of the potential for serious adverse reactions to trametinib in breast-fed infants, advise women not to breast-feed while receiving the drug and for 4 months after the last dose.

Females and Males of Reproductive Potential

Results of animal studies suggest that trametinib may reduce female fertility. In fertility studies, impairment of fertility (increased follicular cysts and reduced corpora lutea) was observed in female animals receiving trametinib at exposure levels equivalent to 0.3 times the human exposure at the recommended adult dosage.

Verify pregnancy status in females of reproductive potential prior to initiating trametinib. Females of reproductive potential should use effective contraceptive methods during trametinib therapy and for 4 months following discontinuance of the drug.

To avoid potential drug exposure to female partners who are pregnant or of reproductive potential, males should use condoms during trametinib therapy and for at least 4 months after the last dose.

Pediatric Use

Safety and efficacy of trametinib monotherapy have not been established in pediatric patients.

Safety and efficacy of trametinib in combination with dabrafenib have been established in pediatric patients ≥1 year of age with *BRAF* V600E mutation-positive unresectable or metastatic solid tumors who progressed on prior therapy (with no satisfactory treatment options) and *BRAF* V600E mutation-positive low-grade glioma requiring systemic therapy. The use of trametinib for these indications is supported by evidence from a study in pediatric patients with refractory or recurrent solid tumors (CTMT212X2101), and a study in pediatric patients with low-grade glioma (CDRB436G2201).

Safety and efficacy of trametinib in combination with dabrafenib have not been established for these indications in pediatric patients <1 year of age.

Geriatric Use

Clinical experience with trametinib monotherapy in patients 65 years of age or older with melanoma is insufficient to determine whether geriatric patients respond differently than younger adults.

In clinical studies evaluating trametinib in combination with dabrafenib in patients with melanoma, 21% of patients were 65 years of age or older and 5% were 75 years of age or older. No overall differences in efficacy were observed between geriatric patients and younger adults, but some adverse effects (i.e., peripheral edema, anorexia) occurred more frequently in geriatric patients with metastatic melanoma.

Clinical experience with trametinib in patients 65 years of age or older with NSCLC is insufficient to determine whether geriatric patients respond differently than younger adults.

In clinical studies evaluating trametinib in combination with dabrafenib in anaplastic thyroid cancer, 77% of patients were 65 years of age and older and 31% were 75 years of age or older. An insufficient number of younger adults were included in the study to determine if there are differences in response to trametinib.

Hepatic Impairment

In population pharmacokinetic analyses, systemic exposure of trametinib was not affected in patients with mild hepatic impairment (total bilirubin concentration not exceeding the ULN with AST concentration exceeding the ULN or total bilirubin concentration exceeding the ULN, but no more than 1.5 times the ULN, with any AST concentration).

An appropriate dosage has not been established in patients with moderate (bilirubin concentration greater than 1.5–3 times the ULN and any AST concentration) to severe (bilirubin concentration 3–10 times the ULN and any AST concentration) hepatic impairment. No increase in exposure of trametinib occurred in patients with moderate or severe hepatic impairment compared with patients with normal hepatic function. Consider the potential risks and benefits of the drug when initiating trametinib therapy or determining the appropriate dosage in patients with moderate or severe hepatic impairment.

During clinical trials, dose-limiting toxicities were not observed during the first cycle of therapy in 5 patients with moderate hepatic impairment (3 patients received an initial trametinib dosage of 1.5 mg once daily and 2 patients received an initial dosage of 2 mg once daily) and in 3 patients with severe hepatic impairment receiving trametinib (initial trametinib dosage of 1 mg once daily). One patient with severe hepatic impairment who received an initial trametinib dosage of 1.5 mg once daily experienced grade 3 acneiform rash.

Renal Impairment

Systemic exposure of trametinib was not affected by renal impairment in patients with estimated glomerular filtration rate (eGFR) 15–89 mL/minute per 1.73 m².

● Common Adverse Effects

The most common adverse reactions (≥20%) in adults with unresectable or metastatic melanoma receiving trametinib monotherapy are rash, diarrhea, and lymphedema.

The most common adverse reactions (≥ 20%) in adults receiving trametinib in combination with dabrafenib for adjuvant treatment of melanoma include pyrexia, fatigue, nausea, headache, rash, chills, diarrhea, vomiting, arthralgia, and myalgia.

The most common adverse reactions (≥ 20%) in adults receiving trametinib in combination with dabrafenib for unresectable or metastatic melanoma include pyrexia, nausea, rash, chills, diarrhea, vomiting, hypertension, and peripheral edema.

The most common adverse reactions (≥ 20%) in adults receiving trametinib in combination with dabrafenib for metastatic NSCLC include pyrexia, fatigue, nausea, vomiting, diarrhea, dry skin, decreased appetite, edema, rash, chills, hemorrhage, cough, and dyspnea.

The most common adverse reactions (≥ 20%) in adults receiving trametinib in combination with dabrafenib for other solid tumors include pyrexia, fatigue, nausea, rash, chills, headache, hemorrhage, cough, vomiting, constipation, diarrhea, myalgia, arthralgia, and edema.

The most common adverse reactions (≥ 20%) in pediatric patients receiving trametinib in combination with dabrafenib for solid tumors include pyrexia, rash, vomiting, fatigue, dry skin, cough, diarrhea, dermatitis acneiform, headache, abdominal pain, nausea, hemorrhage, constipation, and paronychia.

The most common adverse reactions (≥ 20%) in pediatric patients receiving trametinib in combination with dabrafenib for low-grade glioma (LGG) include pyrexia, rash, headache, vomiting, musculoskeletal pain, fatigue, diarrhea, dry skin, nausea, hemorrhage, abdominal pain, and dermatitis acneiform.

DRUG INTERACTIONS

In vitro studies have indicated that trametinib is an inhibitor of cytochrome P-450 (CYP) isoenzyme 2C8.

Trametinib is a substrate of P-glycoprotein (P-gp) and bile salt export pump (BSEP). Pharmacokinetic interactions are unlikely with drugs that inhibit the P-gp transport system since trametinib exhibits high passive permeability and bioavailability.

Trametinib is not a substrate for CYP isoenzymes, breast cancer resistance protein (BCRP), organic anion transporter polypeptide (OATP) 1B1, OATP1B3, OATP2B1, organic cation transporter (OCT) 1, multidrug resistance-associated protein (MRP) 2, or multidrug and toxic compound extrusion 1 (MATE1). Trametinib is not an inhibitor of CYP 1A2, 2A6, 2B6, 2C9, 2C19, or 2D6, and also is not an inhibitor of OATP1B1, OATP1B3, organic anion transporter (OAT) 1, OAT3, OCT2, P-gp, BCRP, BSEP, MRP2, or MATE1.

● **Drugs Metabolized by Hepatic Microsomal Enzymes**

Concomitant use of trametinib 2 mg once daily with a sensitive CYP3A4 substrate had no clinically relevant effects on the area under the concentration-time curve (AUC) or peak plasma concentration of the sensitive CYP3A4 substrate.

● **Dabrafenib**

Concomitant administration of trametinib 2 mg once daily with dabrafenib resulted in no change in AUC of trametinib.

DESCRIPTION

Trametinib, a selective, reversible inhibitor of mitogen-activated extracellular signal regulated kinase (MEK) 1 and MEK2 activation and kinase activity in cells with b-Raf serine-threonine kinase (BRAF) V600E or V600K mutations, is an antineoplastic agent. MEK proteins are upstream regulators of the extracellular signal-related kinase (ERK) pathway, which promotes cellular proliferation. Approximately 50% of cutaneous melanomas carry a BRAF mutation. The most common BRAF mutation is the substitution of glutamic acid for valine at codon 600 (BRAF V600E); a less frequently occurring BRAF mutation is the substitution of lysine for valine at codon 600 (BRAF V600K). BRAF V600 mutations result in activation of the BRAF pathway that includes MEK 1 and 2. The mutation of BRAF V600E activates the mitogen-activated protein kinase (MAPK) and extracellular signal-regulated kinase (ERK) signal transduction pathway, which enhances cell proliferation and tumor progression (e.g., metastasis). Trametinib inhibits BRAF V600 mutation-positive melanoma cell growth in vitro and in vivo by decreasing cell proliferation, causing cell cycle arrest, and inducing apoptosis. Trametinib inhibits cell growth of various BRAF V600 mutation-positive tumors in vitro and in vivo.

Clinical resistance to monotherapy with a BRAF inhibitor, generally occurring 6–7 months following initiation of therapy, has been attributed to several possible resistance mechanisms mostly relying on reactivation of the MAPK/ERK pathway. Complete inhibition of the MAPK/ERK pathway resulting in durable responses may be achieved with the use of combination therapy with a BRAF inhibitor (i.e., dabrafenib, encorafenib, vemurafenib) and an MEK inhibitor (i.e., binimetinib, cobimetinib, trametinib). Use of trametinib and dabrafenib in combination resulted in greater growth inhibition of tumor cell lines testing positive for BRAF V600 mutations in vitro. In addition, combination therapy was associated with prolonged inhibition of tumor growth in tumor xenografts testing positive for BRAF V600 mutations compared with either drug alone.

Following oral administration, the absolute bioavailability of trametinib tablets and oral solution is 72 and 81%, respectively. Peak plasma concentrations of trametinib occur within 1.5 hours after oral administration. Following single and repeated once-daily doses of 0.125–4 mg as tablets, increases in peak plasma concentrations and AUC are dose proportional. Trametinib is 97.4% bound to plasma proteins. Administration of a single dose of trametinib tablets with a high-fat, high-calorie meal (approximately 1000 calories) decreased peak plasma concentrations and AUC of the drug by 70 and 24%, respectively, and delayed the rate of absorption (time to reach peak concentrations delayed by 4 hours). Trametinib is principally metabolized by deacetylation with or without mono-oxygenation or in combination with glucuronidation in vitro. The estimated terminal half-life of trametinib is 3.9–4.8 days. Following oral administration of a radiolabeled dose of trametinib, more than 80% of the dose is recovered in feces and less than 20% is recovered in urine. Age (18—93 years), sex, body weight (36—170 kg), and renal impairment (estimated glomerular filtration rate 15—89 mL/minute/1.73 m^2) do not have a clinically significant impact on trametinib exposure. Insufficient data are available to assess whether race or ethnicity affect trametinib exposure. In pediatric patients 1—17 years of age, the pharmacokinetic exposures of trametinib at the recommended weight-adjusted dosage were within the range of those observed in adults. In this population, weight (6—156 kg) was shown to have a substantial impact on oral clearance of trametinib.

ADVICE TO PATIENTS

- Advise patients to read the manufacturer's patient information before beginning treatment and each time the prescription is refilled.

- Trametinib oral solution is intended for administration by a caregiver; ensure caregivers receive training on proper dosing and administration of oral solution and provide copy of manufacturer's instructions for use.

- Advise patients to take trametinib at least 1 hour before or 2 hours after a meal.

- Stress importance of taking a missed dose as soon as it is remembered, but only if it can be taken at least 12 hours before the next scheduled dose.

- Risk of new primary cutaneous and noncutaneous malignancies with trametinib/dabrafenib combination therapy. Stress importance of contacting clinician promptly if dermatologic changes (i.e., new lesions, changes to existing lesions) or signs and/or symptoms of other malignancies occur.

- Risk of intracranial and GI hemorrhage with trametinib/dabrafenib combination therapy. Stress importance of contacting clinician promptly if signs and/or symptoms of unusual bleeding or hemorrhage occur.

- Risk of colitis or GI perforation. Stress importance of contacting clinician promptly if unusual bleeding, diarrhea, abdominal pain or tenderness, fever, or nausea occurs.

- Risk of DVT and PE with trametinib/dabrafenib combination therapy. Stress importance of contacting clinician promptly if sudden onset of breathing difficulty, leg pain, or swelling occurs.

- Risk of cardiomyopathy. Stress importance of immediately contacting clinician if manifestations of heart failure occur.

- Risk of visual disturbances that may lead to blindness. Stress importance of contacting clinician if vision changes occur.

- Risk of interstitial lung disease (or pneumonitis). Stress importance of immediately contacting clinician if cough or dyspnea occurs.

- Risk of serious febrile reactions with trametinib/dabrafenib combination therapy. Stress importance of contacting clinician if fever develops.

- Risk of skin toxicities (possibly requiring hospitalization). Stress importance of contacting clinician if progressive or intolerable rash occurs.

- Risk of hypertension. Stress importance of monitoring blood pressure regularly during therapy and of contacting clinician if manifestations of hypertension occur.

- Risk of diarrhea (sometimes severe). Stress importance of contacting clinician if severe diarrhea occurs.

- Risk of fetal harm if taken during pregnancy. Advise female patients to use effective contraception during treatment and for 4 months after discontinuance of trametinib. Advise male patients with female partners of reproductive potential to use condoms during trametinib therapy and for 4 months after discontinuance of the drug. Stress importance of contacting clinician if pregnancy is suspected or confirmed during treatment.

- Risk of serious adverse reactions in nursing infants of women receiving trametinib. Advise patients to discontinue breast-feeding during therapy and for 4 months after the last dose.

- Advise women of reproductive potential that trametinib may reduce female fertility.

- Stress importance of informing clinicians of existing or contemplated concomitant therapy, including prescription and OTC drugs and dietary or herbal supplements, as well as any concomitant illnesses (e.g., cardiovascular disease).

- Inform patients of other important precautionary information.

PREPARATIONS

Excipients in commercially available drug preparations may have clinically important effects in some individuals; consult specific product labeling for details.

Trametinib Dimethyl Sulfoxide

Oral

For solution	0.05 mg/mL	Mekinist®
Tablets	0.5 mg (of trametinib)	Mekinist®, Novartis
	2 mg (of trametinib)	Mekinist®, Novartis

† Use is not currently included in the labeling approved by the US Food and Drug Administration.

Selected Revisions July 10, 2024, © Copyright, January 30, 2014, American Society of Health-System Pharmacists, Inc.

Trastuzumab

10:00 • ANTINEOPLASTIC AGENTS

Special Alerts:

Trastuzumab (Herceptin®) should not be confused with ado-trastuzumab emtansine (Kadcyla®). The latter agent is an anti-human epidermal growth factor receptor type 2 (anti-*HER2*) antibody-drug conjugate; the anti-*HER2* antibody trastuzumab, a humanized immunoglobulin (IgG_1), is conjugated with the microtubule inhibitor DM1 (derivative of maytansine) via the linker MCC (4-[N-maleimidomethyl] cyclohexane-1-carboxylate).

The original generic name for Kadcyla®, as established by the US Adopted Name (USAN) Council in 2009, was trastuzumab emtansine. Because of the similarity between the original generic name (trastuzumab emtansine) and the generic name for Herceptin® (trastuzumab), the US Food and Drug Administration (FDA) approved the addition of the prefix "ado" to the generic name for Kadcyla® (i.e., ado-trastuzumab emtansine); however, the potential exists for dispensing or prescribing errors involving these drugs. The manufacturer of ado-trastuzumab emtansine (Kadcyla®) states that this drug should *not* be substituted for or used with trastuzumab (Herceptin®). Therefore, extra care should be exercised to ensure the accuracy of prescriptions for trastuzumab (Herceptin®) or ado-trastuzumab emtansine (Kadcyla®).

To avoid medication errors, the Institute for Safe Medication Practices (ISMP), the FDA, and the manufacturer of ado-trastuzumab emtansine (Kadcyla®) recommend that prescribers communicate both the brand and generic names for ado-trastuzumab emtansine (Kadcyla®) on the prescription order form. (See Dispensing and Administration Precautions under Dosage and Administration: Reconstitution and Administration and also under Cautions: Precautions and Contraindications.)

■ Trastuzumab, a recombinant DNA-derived humanized anti-*HER2* monoclonal antibody, is an antineoplastic agent.

USES

● Breast Cancer

Overview

Trastuzumab is used as monotherapy for the treatment of metastatic breast cancer that has relapsed following prior chemotherapy in patients with tumors that overexpress the *HER2* protein. Trastuzumab also is used in combination with paclitaxel for the initial treatment of metastatic breast cancer in patients with tumors that overexpress the *HER2* protein. Trastuzumab is used in conjunction with standard adjuvant chemotherapy for the treatment of operable HER2-positive breast cancer. The benefit of combination therapy with trastuzumab and chemotherapy appears to be largely limited to patients with disease testing 3+ for HER2 overexpression. Trastuzumab, the second monoclonal antibody approved for the treatment of cancer and the first monoclonal antibody approved for the treatment of breast cancer, received fast-track and priority review from the US Food and Drug Administration (FDA).

Although the use of trastuzumab in combination with an anthracycline and cyclophosphamide for the initial treatment of *HER2*-overexpressing metastatic breast cancer has been investigated in a large, randomized clinical trial, the clinical benefit obtained with this regimen did not outweigh the increased risk of serious cardiac toxicity, and an indication for the use of trastuzumab with this combination regimen did *not* receive approval from the FDA.

Trastuzumab also is *not* indicated for the treatment of metastatic breast cancer in patients with tumors that do not overexpress the *HER2* protein.

Patients with metastatic breast tumors with 2+ or 3+ overexpression of *HER2* protein (based on a 0–3+ scale with 3+ being the highest degree of overexpression) as determined by an immunohistochemical assay using 4D5 and CB11 murine monoclonal anti-*HER2* antibodies (known as the Clinical Trial Assay [CTA]) were eligible for enrollment in clinical trials of trastuzumab. About 33% of women with metastatic breast cancer screened for eligibility for enrollment in clinical trials of trastuzumab were found to have 2+- or 3+-*HER2*-overexpressing tumors; among patients enrolled in the pivotal clinical trials, about 75% had 3+-overexpressing tumors and 25% had 2+-overexpressing tumors. Although these studies were not designed to include stratification by degree of *HER2* overexpression, and the small number of patients with 2+-overexpressing tumors limits interpretation of the data, retrospective analysis of the data from clinical trials suggests that benefit of trastuzumab (i.e., higher response rates, increased time to progression of disease) may be limited to patients with tumors that have 3+ overexpression of the *HER2* protein. Further study is needed to establish the benefit of trastuzumab in patients with 2+-overexpressing (weakly positive) breast tumors.

Evaluation of HER2/neu in Breast Cancer

The methods of *HER2/neu* evaluation most commonly used in routine clinical practice and clinical research studies are immunohistochemistry (IHC) assays, which directly measure overexpression of the *HER2/neu* protein, and fluorescent *in situ* hybridization (FISH), which measures amplification of the *HER2/neu* oncogene. The presence of HER2 overexpression may be inferred when HER2 gene amplification is detected using the FISH assay. HercepTest® and PATHWAY® (IHC assays) and PathVysion®, INFORM®, and HER2 FISH pharmDx® (FISH assays) are examples of appropriate commercial assays that may be used to identify candidates for trastuzumab therapy.

Findings from small studies show conflicting results for the agreement of IHC and FISH testing, with some studies citing high levels of concordance, while others report levels as low as 49%. Some experts argue for use of a FISH assay as the primary screening tool because of greater accuracy whereas others argue for use of an IHC assay because of lesser time and cost requirements. In addition, overexpression of the *HER2* protein has been observed in the absence of detectable *HER2* gene amplification (i.e., FISH-negative). In a large quality control and quality assurance study in which both FISH and IHC test results were available for 2913 of 2963 breast cancer specimens, the concordance rate was 65% when IHC scores of 2+ and 3+ were grouped together; the concordance rate increased to 96% when results for the IHC 2+ specimens were excluded from the analysis. The FISH assay had a higher failure rate (5 versus 0.08%), higher cost, and longer testing and interpretation times than the IHC assay.

Because of limitations in the accuracy and precision of each of these types of assays, use of a single methodology for the evaluation of HER2 overexpression is not advised. Many experts currently recommend initial screening using an IHC assay followed by confirmation of positive results using a FISH assay, particularly for 2+ HER2-overexpressing tumors. The precision of *HER2/neu* evaluation may vary according to the type of assay and assay procedures used. Further study of these methods, particularly regarding their comparative efficacy in predicting disease prognosis and response to therapy, is needed to establish the optimum procedure for determining the *HER2/neu* status of breast cancer.

The reliability of HER2 testing is improved when performed in large-volume central laboratories compared with local laboratories. Assessment of *HER2* overexpression in breast tumors using IHC or FISH methodology should be performed by laboratories with demonstrated proficiency in the specific technology being used. Improper assay performance, including use of suboptimally fixed tissue, failure to use specified reagents, deviation from specific assay instructions, and failure to include appropriate controls for assay validation, can lead to unreliable results. For full instructions on assay performance, refer to the prescribing information for each assay kit.

Detection of HER2 Protein Overexpression

The IHC assay used to test breast tumors for *HER2* overexpression in the pivotal trials of trastuzumab is a research assay known as the Clinical Trial Assay (CTA). The DAKO HercepTest® is a commercially available immunohistochemical test that is used to measure *HER2* protein in tumors and to help identify patients who may be candidates for treatment with trastuzumab. In the randomized trial involving patients with metastatic breast cancer (study 3), data suggest that benefit of combination therapy with trastuzumab and chemotherapy was largely limited to patients with disease testing 3+ for HER2 overexpression on the CTA.

The HercepTest® has been assessed for concordance with the CTA. The low specificity reported for the HercepTest® when used according to manufacturer guidelines and the FDA-approved scoring system raises concerns about large numbers of false-positive specimens resulting in inappropriate use of trastuzumab. In one study using tissue specimens from 48 cases of invasive breast cancer, consideration of the level of staining of nonneoplastic epithelium in a specimen as an internal control helped compensate for variability in tissue fixation and processing and improved the specificity of the HercepTest® from 42% to 93%.

Detection of HER2 Gene Amplification

Measurement of the number of HER2 gene copies using the FISH assay to detect gene amplification may be used as a surrogate measurement of protein overexpression. PathVysion® is a commercially available FISH assay that is used to identify patients who may be candidates for trastuzumab therapy.

In a retrospective analysis of known CTA 2+ or 3+ tumor specimens from patients with metastatic breast cancer receiving trastuzumab and chemotherapy in a randomized trial (study 3), the data suggest that benefit of treatment was greater in patients with FISH-positive tumors than in those with FISH-negative tumors; however, time to progression of disease was prolonged in patients receiving combination therapy with trastuzumab and chemotherapy for CTA 2+ or 3+ tumors regardless of the FISH test status. This treatment effect was particularly strong among patients receiving trastuzumab and chemotherapy for CTA 3+ tumors even if the tumor was FISH-negative. There are insufficient data to determine whether the FISH assay can be used to identify a subgroup of patients with CTA 2+ tumors who would be unlikely to benefit from trastuzumab therapy.

Adjuvant Therapy for Early-stage Breast Cancer

Trastuzumab is used in conjunction with standard adjuvant chemotherapy (doxorubicin and cyclophosphamide followed by paclitaxel) for the treatment of HER2-overexpressing, node-positive breast cancer.

In several large randomized trials, the addition of trastuzumab to standard adjuvant chemotherapy in patients with operable HER2-positive breast cancer reduced the risk of death and/or prolonged disease-free survival.

The current indication for trastuzumab as adjuvant therapy for HER2-overexpressing, node-positive breast cancer is based on 2 North American randomized clinical trials. In the National Surgical Adjuvant Breast and Bowel Project trial B-31 (study 1), 2043 women were randomly assigned to receive either doxorubicin and cyclophosphamide followed by paclitaxel or the same regimen with trastuzumab given concurrently with paclitaxel. In the North Central Cancer Treatment Group trial N9831 (study 2), 1633 of the 2766 patients enrolled were randomly assigned to receive either doxorubicin and cyclophosphamide followed by paclitaxel or the same regimen with trastuzumab given concurrently with paclitaxel.

A total of 3752 patients were randomly assigned to treatment in the 2 trials prior to a planned interim analysis. In a combined analysis of data from patient groups from the 2 trials at a median follow-up of 2 years, disease-free survival at 3 years was prolonged (hazard ratio: 0.48, absolute disease-free survival rate: 87 versus 75%) and the risk of death at 3 years was decreased (hazard ratio: 0.67, absolute survival rate: 94 versus 92%) in patients receiving trastuzumab in combination with standard adjuvant chemotherapy compared with those receiving standard adjuvant chemotherapy alone. Subgroup analysis of the data from study 2 exploring efficacy according to HER2 overexpression showed a strong effect on disease-free survival (hazard ratio: 0.42) for the addition of trastuzumab to adjuvant chemotherapy in patients with disease that was 3+ HER2-overexpressing and FISH-positive. Because of the small number of events in the other subgroups, it is not known whether adjuvant therapy including trastuzumab would benefit patients with breast tumors that are FISH-positive but lack 3+ HER2 overexpression.

Trastuzumab also was used as adjuvant therapy for operable HER2-positive breast cancer in an international multicenter randomized trial. In the Herceptin Adjuvant (HERA) trial, 5081 women received trastuzumab (1 or 2 years) or underwent observation following neoadjuvant and/or adjuvant chemotherapy for operable HER2-positive breast cancer. At a median follow-up of 1 year among 3387 patients receiving either 1 year of trastuzumab therapy or observation, the rate of disease-free survival was prolonged in patients receiving trastuzumab (hazard ratio for an event: 0.54, absolute difference in disease-free survival at 2 years of 8.4 percentage points). At a median follow-up of 2 years, prolonged survival has been observed in patients receiving 1 year of trastuzumab therapy compared with observation (hazard ratio for death: 0.66, absolute difference in death rate at 3 years of 2.7 percentage points).

Patients were eligible for enrollment in the randomized trials if they had operable breast cancer that was identified as HER2-positive with either 3+ HER2 overexpression according to the IHC assay or positive results for amplification of the HER2 gene according to the FISH assay. HER2 testing was performed at a reference laboratory (study 1) or HER2 test results were confirmed by a central laboratory prior to randomization (study 2). For 1153 tumor specimens in study 2 which tested as IHC 3+ using HercepTest® at a local laboratory, 85% were concordant and 15% were discordant when testing was confirmed by a central laboratory. For

414 tumor specimens in study 2 which tested as FISH-positive using PathVysion® at a local laboratory, 94% were concordant and 6% were discordant when testing was confirmed by a central laboratory.

In the 2 North American trials, most patients (91%) had node-positive disease. The median age of the patients was 49 years (range: 22–80 years), and most were Caucasian (84%). Most patients had intermediate-grade (27%) or high-grade (66%) breast tumors, and 53% had hormone receptor-positive disease. The benefit of trastuzumab appeared to be similar among patients with hormone receptor-positive or hormone receptor-negative breast tumors. Because of the lack of data in these trials, it is unknown whether the addition of trastuzumab to standard adjuvant chemotherapy would benefit patients with node-negative breast cancer. In the international trial, the median age of the patients was 49 years; about one-third of the patients had node-negative breast cancer, and 48% had hormone receptor-negative tumors. In this trial, the benefit of 1 year of trastuzumab therapy did not appear to differ according to nodal or estrogen receptor status.

In both North American trials, for the comparison groups receiving trastuzumab given concurrently with paclitaxel, an initial dose of trastuzumab 4 mg/kg was administered with the first dose of paclitaxel followed by trastuzumab 2 mg/kg once weekly for 51 weeks. The same regimen of adjuvant chemotherapy with doxorubicin and cyclophosphamide was used in both trials (four 21-day cycles of doxorubicin 60 mg/m^2 and cyclophosphamide 600 mg/m^2), but the regimens for paclitaxel differed: 80 mg/m^2 once weekly or 175 mg/m^2 once every 3 weeks for a total of 12 weeks in trial B-31 (study 1) and 80 mg/m^2 once weekly in trial N9831 (study 2). When administered, radiation therapy was initiated following the completion of chemotherapy. Patients with estrogen receptor-positive and/or progesterone receptor-positive tumors also received hormonal therapy.

In trial N9831 (study 2), a third group of patients received adjuvant chemotherapy with doxorubicin and cyclophosphamide, followed by paclitaxel therapy, and then trastuzumab therapy. Further follow-up is needed before the comparative efficacy of concurrent versus sequential paclitaxel and trastuzumab therapy can be assessed, but an interim analysis of the data from this trial suggests that concurrent therapy may be more effective.

In the international trial, differing regimens of neoadjuvant and/or adjuvant chemotherapy (including both anthracyclines and taxanes in about 26% of patients) were followed by an initial dose of trastuzumab 8 mg/kg and then trastuzumab 6 mg/kg once every 3 weeks.

Increased risk of cardiac toxicity was associated with trastuzumab therapy. Among patients receiving adjuvant therapy for breast cancer, those receiving trastuzumab and paclitaxel following completion of doxorubicin and cyclophosphamide therapy experienced a higher incidence of symptomatic, laboratory-confirmed cardiomyopathy compared with those receiving paclitaxel alone (2 versus 0.4%). The cumulative incidence of class III or IV congestive heart failure or death from cardiac causes at 3 years in patients receiving trastuzumab was 4.1% in trial B-31 (study 1) and 2.9% in trial N9831 (study 2). The incidence of class III or IV congestive heart failure in patients receiving trastuzumab was 0.5% at 1 year in the international trial.

Patients were eligible for enrollment in the North American randomized trials if they did not have previous or currently active cardiac disease based on symptoms or test findings (ECG, radiographs, and left ventricular ejection fraction [LVEF]) or uncontrolled hypertension (diastolic blood pressure exceeding 100 mm Hg or systolic blood pressure exceeding 200 mm Hg). Cardiac function was monitored at regular intervals, and trastuzumab therapy was not initiated or was discontinued if clinical manifestations or decline in LVEF indicated cardiac toxicity. Trastuzumab therapy was permanently discontinued in patients who developed congestive heart failure or persistent/recurrent LVEF decline. Similar eligibility criteria, cardiac monitoring, and stopping rules for cardiotoxicity were applied in the international trial. Further follow-up is needed to fully assess the risk of cardiotoxicity associated with trastuzumab as adjuvant therapy for operable HER2-positive breast cancer.

Increased risk of pulmonary toxicity also was associated with trastuzumab therapy. Among patients receiving adjuvant therapy for breast cancer in the 2 North American trials (studies 1 and 2), those receiving trastuzumab and paclitaxel following completion of doxorubicin and cyclophosphamide therapy experienced a higher incidence of dyspnea, the most common pulmonary toxicity, compared with those receiving paclitaxel alone (study 1: 12 versus 4%, study 2: 2.5 versus 0.1%). Pneumonitis/pulmonary infiltrates (0.7 versus 0.3%) and deaths from respiratory failure (3 deaths versus 1 death) also occurred more frequently in patients receiving trastuzumab compared with chemotherapy alone.

For patients with node-positive, HER2-positive operable breast cancer, trastuzumab should be added to standard adjuvant chemotherapy unless contraindicated. For patients with node-negative, HER2-positive operable breast cancer†, the use of trastuzumab in conjunction with standard adjuvant chemotherapy should be considered with careful weighing of possible benefit versus the risk of cardiac toxicity. Careful patient selection and monitoring of cardiac function is required in all patients receiving trastuzumab as adjuvant therapy. Further follow-up of these clinical trials and additional studies are needed to answer other questions, such as the optimal dosing schedule, timing of administration (concurrent versus sequential), and duration of therapy for trastuzumab, and to fully evaluate the nature and risk of cardiotoxicity associated with trastuzumab in this patient population.

A randomized trial is under way comparing the addition of trastuzumab to anthracycline-containing versus non-anthracycline-containing adjuvant chemotherapy to determine whether similar efficacy can be achieved with less cardiac toxicity for HER2-positive operable breast cancer. Other regimens and schedules for adjuvant trastuzumab therapy are being investigated. For a small subgroup of 232 patients with HER2-positive tumors among 1010 women receiving adjuvant chemotherapy for node-positive or high-risk node-negative early breast cancer in a randomized trial, the addition of trastuzumab to chemotherapy with either docetaxel or vinorelbine compared with chemotherapy alone (prior to treatment with an anthracycline-containing regimen) prolonged recurrence-free survival. This shortened schedule for trastuzumab (9 weekly infusions) preceding the use of an anthracycline was not associated with decreased left ventricular ejection fraction or cardiac failure.

First-line Therapy for Advanced Breast Cancer

The current indication for use of trastuzumab in combination with paclitaxel for the initial treatment of metastatic breast cancer is based on data from a randomized, controlled, multicenter clinical trial involving 469 patients with 2+ or 3+ HER2-overexpressing metastatic breast cancer. Patients were randomized to receive combination therapy with trastuzumab (4-mg/kg IV initial dose followed by once-weekly doses of 2 mg/kg IV) and chemotherapy or chemotherapy alone. For patients who had received prior adjuvant therapy with an anthracycline, chemotherapy consisted of paclitaxel 175 mg/m² IV over 3 hours every 21 days for at least 6 cycles; for all other patients, chemotherapy consisted of an anthracycline (doxorubicin hydrochloride 60 mg/m² or epirubicin hydrochloride 75 mg/m² every 21 days) and cyclophosphamide (600 mg/m² every 21 days) for 6 cycles. Trastuzumab therapy was continued until disease progression or intolerable toxicity was observed. The median age of the patients was 52 years (range: 25–77 years) and most (89%) were Caucasian.

Longer time to disease progression (7.2 versus 4.5 months), higher overall response rate (45 versus 29%), longer median duration of response (8.3 versus 5.8 months), and longer median survival (25.1 versus 20.3 months) were reported in patients receiving trastuzumab in combination with chemotherapy compared with those receiving chemotherapy alone. With the exception of overall survival, the magnitude of benefit was greater with the addition of trastuzumab to paclitaxel versus an anthracycline and cyclophosphamide despite the poorer prognosis of patients in the paclitaxel subgroup; in addition, the incidence and severity of cardiac toxicity were greater in patients receiving trastuzumab combined with an anthracycline and cyclophosphamide.

The benefit of adding trastuzumab to conventional chemotherapy was greater in patients with 3+-HER2-overexpressing breast tumors than in those with 2+-HER2-overexpressing breast tumors. Although the study was not designed to include stratification by degree of HER2 overexpression, and the small number of patients with 2+-overexpressing tumors limits interpretation of the data, retrospective analysis suggests that response to trastuzumab is limited to the patients with the highest level of HER2 overexpression (3+). The relative risk for disease progression in patients receiving trastuzumab in combination with chemotherapy versus those receiving chemotherapy alone was lower among patients with 3+ versus 2+ HER2-overexpressing disease (relative risk 0.42 versus 0.76) using the CTA methodology; lower relative risk for disease progression represents longer time to disease progression.

Compared with patients receiving paclitaxel alone, those receiving trastuzumab and paclitaxel experienced a longer median time to disease progression (6.7 versus 2.5 months) and a higher overall response rate (38 versus 15%); median duration of response was 8 versus 4 months and median survival was 22 versus 18 months. Because of the difference in patient characteristics between the groups (i.e., poorer prognosis for patients in the paclitaxel subgroup), the results

of this clinical trial cannot be used to compare the efficacy and safety of combination therapy with trastuzumab and paclitaxel versus standard first-line therapy of an anthracycline and cyclophosphamide for metastatic breast cancer.

Combination therapy with trastuzumab, paclitaxel, and carboplatin† is used in the treatment of HER2-overexpressing metastatic breast cancer. In a phase 3 randomized trial, the addition of carboplatin to trastuzumab and paclitaxel increased response rate and prolonged progression-free survival in patients with HER2-overexpressing metastatic breast cancer. Combination therapy with vinorelbine and trastuzumab† is being investigated as an active regimen for the treatment of HER2-overexpressing metastatic breast cancer. (See Uses: Breast Cancer in Vinorelbine 10:00.) Another ongoing study will compare the efficacy of trastuzumab in combination with paclitaxel for tumors with overexpression versus normal expression of HER2 in patients with recurrent or metastatic breast cancer.

Second-line or Salvage Therapy for Advanced Breast Cancer

The current indication for use of trastuzumab as monotherapy for metastatic breast cancer is based on data from a single-arm, open-label, multicenter clinical trial in 222 patients with 2+ or 3+ HER2-overexpressing metastatic breast cancer that relapsed following 1 or 2 previous chemotherapy regimens. Among patients enrolled in the study, 66% had received prior adjuvant chemotherapy, 68% had received 2 prior chemotherapy regimens for metastatic disease, and 25% had received prior myeloablative therapy with hematopoietic rescue. About 72% of the patients had visceral disease (i.e., lung or liver metastases), and patients with only bone metastases, a characteristic that generally is associated with an indolent course of disease, were ineligible for enrollment in the trial.

Patients received an initial dose of trastuzumab 4 mg/kg IV followed by once weekly doses of 2 mg/kg IV; the overall response rate was 14% (2% complete responses, 12% partial responses), the median duration of response was 9 months, and the median survival was 13 months. Trastuzumab therapy was continued until disease progression or intolerable toxicity was observed. Complete responses to trastuzumab were observed only in patients with metastatic breast disease limited to the skin and the lymph nodes.

Retrospective analysis suggests that response to trastuzumab is related to the degree of HER2 overexpression with an overall response rate of 18% in patients with 3+ overexpressing tumors versus 6% in those with 2+ overexpressing tumors. According to retrospective analysis of the tumor specimens, the overall response rate was 20% in patients with FISH-positive tumors compared with no responses in those with FISH-negative tumors.

Among 352 patients (including 213 patients in the multicenter clinical trial) receiving trastuzumab as monotherapy for metastatic breast cancer, the median age of the patients was 50 years (range: 28–86 years), and most were Caucasian (86%).

DOSAGE AND ADMINISTRATION

● Reconstitution and Administration

Trastuzumab is administered by IV infusion. The initial dose of trastuzumab should be administered as an IV infusion over 90 minutes; if the first infusion is well tolerated, subsequent doses may be administered by IV infusion over 30 minutes. Trastuzumab solutions should *not* be administered by rapid IV injection, such as IV push or bolus. The usual precautions for handling and preparing cytotoxic drugs should be observed when reconstituting or administering trastuzumab.

Commercially available trastuzumab powder for injection must be reconstituted prior to administration. Trastuzumab is supplied with a diluent of bacteriostatic water for injection, which contains 1.1% benzyl alcohol; reconstitution using the 20 mL of supplied diluent results in a solution containing 21 mg/mL of trastuzumab. Alternatively, for patients sensitive to benzyl alcohol, 20 mL of sterile water for injection may be used for reconstitution.

Trastuzumab must be handled carefully during reconstitution; shaking the reconstituted solution of trastuzumab or causing excessive foaming during the addition of diluent may cause problems with dissolution and the amount of the drug that can be withdrawn from the vial. Using a sterile syringe, the 20 mL of supplied diluent should be injected slowly into the vial with the stream of diluent directed into the lyophilized cake of trastuzumab. The vial should be swirled gently to aid reconstitution; because trastuzumab may be sensitive to shear-induced stress (e.g., agitation, rapid expulsion from a syringe), the reconstituted solution of the drug should *not* be shaken. Slight foaming of the reconstituted trastuzumab solution is not unusual, and the vial should be allowed to stand undisturbed for 5 minutes following reconstitution. The reconstituted solution of trastuzumab should be clear to slightly opalescent, colorless to pale yellow, and free of visible particulate matter.

Immediately upon reconstitution with bacteriostatic water for injection, the vial containing trastuzumab solution must be labeled to indicate the date by which the contents should be used (i.e., 28 days from the date of reconstitution); unused portions should be discarded after 28 days. For administration in patients with known hypersensitivity to benzyl alcohol, trastuzumab should be reconstituted using sterile water for injection; the resulting solution must be used *immediately*, and any unused solution should be discarded.

Reconstituted solutions of trastuzumab should be further diluted prior to administration by adding an appropriate volume of trastuzumab 21 mg/mL solution to a polyvinyl chloride or polyethylene infusion bag containing 250 mL of 0.9% sodium chloride injection; the bag should be inverted gently to mix the solution. Trastuzumab solutions for infusion should *not* be diluted in or administered through an IV line containing 5% dextrose injection, and trastuzumab should not be mixed or diluted with other drugs. Prior to administration, trastuzumab solutions should be inspected visually for particulate matter and discoloration.

Dispensing and Administration Precautions

Trastuzumab (Herceptin®) should not be confused with ado-trastuzumab emtansine (Kadcyla®). Because of the similarity between the original generic name of Kadcyla® (trastuzumab emtansine) and the generic name for Herceptin® (trastuzumab), the US Food and Drug Administration (FDA) approved the addition of the prefix "ado" to the generic name for Kadcyla® (i.e., ado-trastuzumab emtansine). However, the potential exists for dispensing or prescribing errors involving these drugs. Extra care should be exercised to ensure the accuracy of prescriptions for trastuzumab (Herceptin®) or ado-trastuzumab emtansine (Kadcyla®). To avoid medication errors, the Institute for Safe Medication Practices (ISMP), the FDA, and the manufacturer of ado-trastuzumab emtansine (Kadcyla®) recommend that prescribers communicate both the brand and generic names for ado-trastuzumab emtansine (Kadcyla®) on the prescription order form. (See Special Alerts.)

● Dosage

Adjuvant Therapy for Early-stage Breast Cancer

For the adjuvant treatment of HER2-overexpressing, node-positive breast cancer, trastuzumab is given concurrently with paclitaxel following adjuvant chemotherapy with doxorubicin and cyclophosphamide; an initial dose of trastuzumab 4 mg/kg is administered (given with the first dose of paclitaxel), followed by trastuzumab 2 mg/kg once weekly for 51 weeks. Trastuzumab should *not* be administered concurrently with doxorubicin and cyclophosphamide. Following the completion of therapy with doxorubicin and cyclophosphamide, trastuzumab is administered weekly for 52 weeks, concurrently with paclitaxel for the first 12 weeks, then as monotherapy.

Therapy for Advanced Breast Cancer

When used for the treatment of metastatic breast cancer that overexpresses the *HER2* protein, either as monotherapy for treatment of disease that has relapsed following prior chemotherapy or in combination therapy with paclitaxel for initial treatment, the manufacturer recommends an initial trastuzumab dose of 4 mg/kg administered by IV infusion over 90 minutes, followed by once-weekly doses of 2 mg/kg IV.

Patients should be observed for fever and chills or other infusion-associated symptoms during trastuzumab infusion. (See Cautions: Infusion-related Effects.) If prior infusions were well tolerated, subsequent weekly doses of trastuzumab 2 mg/kg IV may be administered over 30 minutes. Trastuzumab therapy is administered until disease progression occurs. In clinical trials, once-weekly administration of trastuzumab was continued until disease progression or intolerable toxicity was observed.

Among patients receiving trastuzumab and chemotherapy as first-line therapy for metastatic breast cancer, 58% of patients received trastuzumab for at least 6 months and 9% received trastuzumab for at least 12 months. Among patients receiving trastuzumab monotherapy as second-line or salvage therapy for metastatic breast cancer, 31% of patients received trastuzumab for at least 6 months and 16% received trastuzumab for at least 12 months.

Dosage Modification for Toxicity and Contraindications for Continued Therapy

Respiratory Toxicity

Infusion of trastuzumab should be interrupted in patients experiencing dyspnea, and discontinuance of trastuzumab therapy should be considered strongly in patients who develop pneumonitis or acute respiratory distress syndrome. (Also see Infusion-related Toxicity under Dosage: Dosage Modification for Toxicity and Contraindications for Continued Therapy, in Dosage and Administration.)

Infusion-related Toxicity

Discontinuance of trastuzumab should be strongly considered for infusion reactions manifesting as anaphylaxis, angioedema, pneumonitis, or acute respiratory distress syndrome.

Infusion of trastuzumab should be interrupted in all patients experiencing dyspnea or clinically important hypotension and appropriate medical therapy, which may include epinephrine, corticosteroids, diphenhydramine, bronchodilators, and oxygen, should be instituted. Patients should be evaluated and monitored carefully until signs and symptoms have resolved completely. Permanent discontinuance of trastuzumab therapy should be strongly considered in all patients experiencing severe or life-threatening infusion reactions. For mild or moderate infusion reactions, the rate of infusion of trastuzumab may be slowed.

According to the manufacturer, the most appropriate method for identifying patients who may safely receive additional infusions of trastuzumab following a severe infusion-related reaction to the drug has not been determined. Following complete recovery from a severe infusion-related reaction, some patients have tolerated subsequent infusions of the drug, typically accompanied by prophylactic treatment including antihistamines and/or corticosteroids, but others have experienced severe reactions to additional infusions of trastuzumab despite the use of premedication.

Mild to moderate infusion-related symptoms, such as chills or fever, have been treated with acetaminophen, diphenhydramine, and/or meperidine, and, in some patients, the rate of infusion of trastuzumab was reduced. Permanent discontinuance of the drug because of such infusion-related symptoms was required in less than 1% of patients.

Sensitivity Reactions

Discontinuance of trastuzumab should be strongly considered for infusion reactions manifesting as anaphylaxis or angioedema.

Infusion of trastuzumab should be interrupted in all patients experiencing dyspnea or clinically important hypotension and appropriate medical therapy should be instituted. See Infusion-related Toxicity under Dosage: Dosage Modification for Toxicity and Contraindications for Continued Therapy, in Dosage and Administration.

Cardiovascular Toxicity

Careful assessment of cardiac function and monitoring of clinical condition are required in patients receiving trastuzumab. For cardiac monitoring requirements, see Cardiovascular Effects under Cautions: Precautions and Contraindications. Trastuzumab-induced decline in left ventricular ejection fraction (LVEF) may be asymptomatic. If clinical manifestations of cardiotoxicity or a clinically important decrease in LVEF occurs, trastuzumab therapy should be interrupted or discontinued. Medical management of cardiac dysfunction may result in recovery of LVEF to at least 50% in some patients.

For patients receiving adjuvant therapy, left ventricular function should be assessed before initiation of trastuzumab and frequently during therapy. If LVEF decreases by 16 percentage points or more from the baseline value, or if LVEF decreases by 10 or more percentage points from the baseline value to a value that is below the lower limit of normal, trastuzumab therapy should be discontinued for 4 weeks. After 4 weeks, cardiac function should be reassessed; if there are no clinical manifestations of cardiotoxicity, LVEF returns to normal limits, and the absolute decrease in LVEF from baseline is 15 percentage points or less, trastuzumab therapy can be resumed. If LVEF decline is persistent (greater than 8 weeks) and 2 consecutive holds are placed on therapy, or if therapy has been interrupted on more than 3 occasions for cardiomyopathy, therapy with trastuzumab should be discontinued permanently. Among patients receiving adjuvant trastuzumab in trial B-31 (study 1), 30.5% required at least one dose delay because of asymptomatic decrease in LVEF or cardiac symptoms. In 16% of patients, trastuzumab therapy was discontinued because of substantial decline in LVEF or clinical evidence of myocardial dysfunction.

Patients receiving trastuzumab therapy for advanced or metastatic cancer, particularly those with preexisting cardiac dysfunction, should be monitored closely for signs of cardiotoxicity. Discontinuance of trastuzumab should be considered strongly in patients who develop a clinically important decrease in left ventricular function or congestive heart failure.

An independent committee reviewing cardiac data from clinical trials of trastuzumab used alone or in combination with chemotherapy for metastatic breast cancer found that, in most cases, cardiac dysfunction in patients receiving trastuzumab was similar to anthracycline-induced cardiomyopathy. Others report a lack of anthracycline-like ultrastructural changes and suggest a different mechanism for trastuzumab-induced cardiac toxicity. In clinical trials for metastatic breast cancer, cardiac dysfunction associated with trastuzumab typically responded to appropriate medical therapy, often including discontinuance of the drug. For the treatment of cardiac dysfunction, single-agent therapy with a diuretic or an angiotensin-converting enzyme (ACE) inhibitor often was used in patients receiving trastuzumab and paclitaxel whereas combination therapy with digoxin, a diuretic, and an ACE inhibitor typically was used in patients receiving trastuzumab with an anthracycline and cyclophosphamide.

Among patients for whom trastuzumab therapy is discontinued because of left ventricular dysfunction, close monitoring for evidence of clinical deterioration and further decline in left ventricular function is required. The safety of continuing or restarting treatment with the drug in patients who have developed trastuzumab-induced left ventricular cardiac dysfunction has not been fully evaluated. Some clinicians report reinitiation of therapy in patients with metastatic breast cancer following recovery from trastuzumab-induced cardiac dysfunction.

CAUTIONS

Serious adverse effects, sometimes fatal, have occurred in patients receiving trastuzumab. Serious adverse effects associated with trastuzumab include cardiomyopathy; pulmonary toxicity such as respiratory failure, pneumonitis, and pulmonary infiltrates; infusion reactions such as anaphylaxis or angioedema; febrile neutropenia; and exacerbation of chemotherapy-induced neutropenia. Deaths associated with pulmonary reactions (including acute respiratory distress syndrome), infusion-related reactions, and hypersensitivity reactions (including fatal anaphylaxis) have been reported in patients receiving trastuzumab. Deaths caused by sepsis in patients with severe neutropenia have been reported when trastuzumab is used in combination with myelosuppressive chemotherapy. Another serious adverse effect associated with trastuzumab is cardiotoxicity, including ventricular dysfunction and congestive heart failure, which may be severe and occasionally disabling; the risk of cardiotoxicity increases substantially when the drug is combined with an anthracycline, and such combination therapy for use in metastatic breast cancer is *not* recommended by most experts.

Adverse effects are common with trastuzumab therapy, with the incidence of most effects generally increasing with combination versus monotherapy. The most common adverse effects associated with trastuzumab include fever, nausea, vomiting, infusion reactions, diarrhea, infections, increased cough, headache, fatigue, dyspnea, rash, neutropenia, anemia, and myalgia.

Data regarding serious adverse effects are based on experience in a total of 958 patients receiving trastuzumab alone or in combination with chemotherapy for metastatic breast cancer or other cancers in clinical trials. The incidence of adverse effects that occurred in at least 5% of patients receiving the drug or that occurred at increased incidence among patients receiving trastuzumab and chemotherapy versus chemotherapy alone is derived from data for a total of 586 patients with metastatic breast cancer (352 patients receiving trastuzumab as a single agent and 234 patients receiving trastuzumab in combination with chemotherapy).

Of 213 patients receiving trastuzumab as a single agent, about 3% discontinued the drug because of adverse effects. Of 91 patients receiving trastuzumab and paclitaxel, 6 patients (6.6%) discontinued trastuzumab because of an adverse effect, 3 of which were cardiac in origin. A higher percentage of patients (20/143 or 14%) receiving the drug in combination with an anthracycline and cyclophosphamide discontinued trastuzumab because of adverse effects, mostly cardiovascular in nature.

Limited data were collected for adverse effects in clinical trials of adjuvant trastuzumab for early breast cancer (studies 1 and 2). Unless otherwise noted, the incidence data for noncardiac adverse effects occurring in at least 2% of patients refer to grade 2–5 toxicities for study 1.

● Respiratory Effects

Trastuzumab can cause serious, sometimes fatal, pulmonary toxicity. Severe adverse respiratory effects, including acute respiratory distress syndrome, have been reported in patients receiving trastuzumab and, in some cases, have been fatal. Interstitial pneumonitis, sometimes fatal, was reported rarely in patients receiving adjuvant trastuzumab. Manifestations of severe adverse pulmonary reactions, which may occur as sequelae of infusion-related reactions (see Cautions: Infusion-related Effects), include dyspnea, wheezing, pneumonitis, pulmonary infiltrates, pleural effusions, noncardiogenic pulmonary edema, pulmonary insufficiency and hypoxia requiring supplemental oxygen or ventilatory support, acute respiratory distress syndrome, and pulmonary fibrosis. Patients with symptomatic intrinsic lung disease or extensive tumor involvement of the lungs, resulting in dyspnea at rest, experience more severe pulmonary toxicity associated with trastuzumab. (See Precautions and Contraindications.)

Among patients receiving trastuzumab and paclitaxel as adjuvant therapy for breast cancer, the most common pulmonary toxicity was dyspnea (study 1: 12%, study 2: 2.5%). Pneumonitis/pulmonary infiltrates and respiratory failure, sometimes fatal, also occurred in patients receiving trastuzumab and chemotherapy.

Among patients with metastatic breast cancer, increased cough occurred in 26 or 41% of patients receiving trastuzumab as a single agent or in combination with paclitaxel, respectively. Dyspnea and pharyngitis have been reported in 22 and 12%, respectively, of patients receiving trastuzumab monotherapy for metastatic breast cancer. Rhinitis and sinusitis have been reported in 14 and 9%, respectively, of patients receiving trastuzumab as a single agent and in 22 and 21%, respectively, of patients receiving trastuzumab and paclitaxel for metastatic breast cancer. Other adverse respiratory effects, including apnea, asthma, hypoxia, laryngitis, and pneumothorax, have been reported in patients receiving trastuzumab.

● Infusion-related Effects

Serious infusion-related reactions, sometimes fatal, have been reported infrequently in patients receiving trastuzumab. Severe infusion-related reactions include bronchospasm, hypoxia, and severe hypotension. In most patients experiencing such reactions, manifestations typically occurred with the first dose of trastuzumab, with onset generally occurring during or immediately following the infusion; however, the onset and clinical course were variable. In some patients, symptoms progressively worsened. In some patients, initial improvement was followed by marked clinical deterioration. Delayed adverse events with rapid clinical deterioration occurring following completion of trastuzumab infusion also has been reported. Fatal infusion-related reactions resulted in death within hours or days of the infusion. (See Infusion-related Toxicity under Dosage: Dosage Modification for Toxicity and Contraindications for Continued Therapy, in Dosage and Administration. Also see Infusion-related Effects under Cautions: Precautions and Contraindications.)

Other infusion-related symptoms, typically consisting of chills and/or fever, occurred in approximately 40% of patients with metastatic breast cancer in clinical trials during the first infusion of trastuzumab. Other manifestations of infusion reactions include nausea, vomiting, pain (including pain at tumor sites), rigors, headache, dizziness, dyspnea, hypotension, elevated blood pressure, rash, and asthenia. On second (or subsequent) infusions of trastuzumab administered as monotherapy or in combination with chemotherapy, infusion-related reactions occurred in 21 or 35% of patients, respectively, and were severe in 1.4% or 9% of patients, respectively.

● Sensitivity Reactions

Serious infusion-related reactions may manifest as hypersensitivity reactions, including anaphylaxis, angioedema, bronchospasm, and/or hypotension, in patients receiving trastuzumab. See Cautions: Infusion-related Effects.

Allergic reactions have occurred in 3% of patients receiving trastuzumab monotherapy and 8% of patients receiving trastuzumab and paclitaxel for metastatic breast cancer. Anaphylactoid reactions have been reported in patients receiving trastuzumab.

● Hematologic Effects

Hematologic toxicity occurs infrequently in patients receiving trastuzumab as a single agent. Grade 3 adverse hematologic effects, including leukopenia, anemia, and thrombocytopenia, each occurred in less than 1% of patients receiving trastuzumab monotherapy in clinical trials, and grade 4 hematologic toxicity was not reported.

Deaths caused by sepsis in patients with severe neutropenia have been reported when trastuzumab is used in combination with myelosuppressive chemotherapy for metastatic breast cancer. In controlled clinical trials, the incidence of septic death was not increased in patients receiving trastuzumab in combination with chemotherapy. Although the mechanism is not known, trastuzumab is thought to exacerbate chemotherapy-induced neutropenia. In randomized clinical trials in women with metastatic breast cancer, the incidences of moderate or severe neutropenia and of febrile neutropenia were higher in patients receiving trastuzumab in combination with myelosuppressive chemotherapy than in those receiving chemotherapy alone. In a randomized trial, moderate or severe neutropenia occurred more frequently in patients receiving trastuzumab in combination with myelosuppressive chemotherapy for metastatic breast cancer than in those receiving chemotherapy alone (32 versus 22%). The incidence of febrile neutropenia also was higher in patients receiving trastuzumab in combination with myelosuppressive chemotherapy for metastatic breast cancer than in those receiving chemotherapy alone (23 versus 17%). Among patients receiving adjuvant therapy for breast cancer, neutropenia occurred more frequently in patients receiving trastuzumab and chemotherapy than in those receiving chemotherapy alone (study 1: 7.1 versus 4.5%, grade 4–5 neutropenia in study 2: 2 versus 0.7%).

Leukopenia and anemia occurred in 24 and 14%, respectively, of patients receiving trastuzumab in combination with paclitaxel for metastatic breast cancer in a randomized trial. The incidence of leukopenia was increased in patients receiving trastuzumab combined with chemotherapy compared with those receiving chemotherapy alone (53 versus 37%) for metastatic breast cancer. The incidence of anemia was higher in patients receiving trastuzumab combined with chemotherapy compared with those receiving chemotherapy alone for metastatic breast cancer (30 versus 21%) or as adjuvant therapy for breast cancer (study 1: 13 versus 7%).

Other adverse hematologic effects reported in patients receiving trastuzumab in clinical trials include pancytopenia, acute leukemia (see Mutagenicity and Carcinogenicity), and coagulation disorder.

● Cardiovascular Effects

Deaths from cardiomyopathy have occurred in patients receiving trastuzumab. Trastuzumab can cause left ventricular myocardial dysfunction characterized by a decline in ejection fraction and manifestations of congestive heart failure. Cardiotoxicity manifested by dyspnea, increased cough, paroxysmal nocturnal dyspnea, peripheral edema, S_3 gallop, cardiomyopathy, congestive heart failure, and/or reduced ejection fraction (decrease of greater than 10%) has been observed in patients receiving trastuzumab. Cardiac dysfunction associated with trastuzumab may be severe and in some cases has resulted in disabling heart failure, mural thrombosis and stroke, and/or death. Trastuzumab also can cause asymptomatic decline in left ventricular ejection fraction. Volume overload and congestive heart failure have been reported as complications of nephrotic syndrome in patients receiving trastuzumab. (See Cautions: Renal and Genitourinary Effects.)

In patients receiving trastuzumab monotherapy for metastatic breast cancer in an open-label, phase 2 study, cardiac dysfunction including congestive heart failure occurred in 7% of patients, and class III or IV cardiac dysfunction (according to the New York Heart Association [NYHA] classification system with class IV being the most severe level of cardiac failure) was reported in 5% of patients. Among patients receiving a combination of trastuzumab and paclitaxel for metastatic breast cancer in a randomized, phase 3 trial, cardiac dysfunction including congestive heart failure was reported in 11% of patients, and 4% of patients experienced NYHA class III or IV cardiac dysfunction.

Among patients receiving adjuvant trastuzumab in 2 North American randomized trials, the cumulative incidence of class III or IV congestive heart failure or death from cardiac causes at 3 years was 4.1% in trial B-31 (study 1) and 2.9% in trial N9831 (study 2). The incidence of new-onset left ventricular dysfunction was approximately twofold higher in patients receiving trastuzumab and paclitaxel versus paclitaxel alone following adjuvant chemotherapy with doxorubicin and cyclophosphamide. About 50% of the adverse cardiac events among patients receiving trastuzumab were identified by the completion of paclitaxel therapy and about 90% were identified within 1 year of the completion of paclitaxel therapy. In an international randomized trial, the incidence of class III or IV congestive heart failure in patients receiving adjuvant trastuzumab was 0.5% at 1 year.

In a randomized trial, patients who received trastuzumab in combination with an anthracycline (rather than paclitaxel) for advanced or metastatic breast cancer had the highest incidence of cardiotoxicity; cardiac dysfunction including congestive heart failure occurred in 28% of patients, and 19% of patients developed NYHA class III or IV cardiac dysfunction. Because of the increased frequency and severity of cardiac toxicity, most experts believe that the clinical benefit obtained from the concomitant use of trastuzumab with an anthracycline and cyclophosphamide regimen does *not* outweigh the increased risk of toxicity, and combined therapy with an anthracycline is *not* recommended for the treatment of advanced or metastatic breast cancer.

For discussion of risks of cardiotoxicity, precautions and contraindications, and monitoring requirements in patients receiving trastuzumab therapy, see Cardiovascular Effects under Cautions: Precautions and Contraindications.

Among patients receiving trastuzumab and paclitaxel as adjuvant therapy for breast cancer, hot flushes (flashes) (study 1: 17%) have been reported. Among patients with metastatic breast cancer, tachycardia has been reported in 5% of patients receiving trastuzumab as a single agent and in 12% of patients receiving trastuzumab in combination with paclitaxel. Peripheral edema and edema occurred in 10 and 8%, respectively, of patients receiving trastuzumab alone for metastatic breast cancer. The incidence of thrombosis/embolism was higher in patients receiving trastuzumab and chemotherapy versus chemotherapy alone for metastatic breast cancer (study 3: 2 versus 0%) or as adjuvant therapy for breast cancer (study 1: 3 versus 1%). Other adverse cardiovascular effects reported in patients receiving trastuzumab in clinical trials include pericardial effusion, cardiac arrest, syncope, hemorrhage, shock, and arrhythmia.

● GI Effects

Diarrhea, typically mild to moderate in severity, occurred in 25 or 45% of patients receiving trastuzumab as a single agent or in combination with paclitaxel, respectively, for metastatic breast cancer. An increased incidence of diarrhea was observed in patients receiving trastuzumab in combination with chemotherapy compared with those receiving trastuzumab alone. Among patients with metastatic breast cancer, nausea and vomiting have been reported in 33 and 23%, respectively, of patients receiving trastuzumab as a single agent and in 51 and 37%, respectively, of patients receiving trastuzumab and paclitaxel; nausea in combination with vomiting occurred in 8% of patients receiving trastuzumab as a single agent in clinical trials. Some patients experiencing adverse GI effects of trastuzumab consequently had metabolic complications, such as dehydration and hypokalemia. Anorexia occurred in 14% of patients receiving trastuzumab alone and in 24% of patients receiving trastuzumab and paclitaxel for metastatic breast cancer.

Other adverse GI effects, including gastroenteritis, hematemesis, ileus, intestinal obstruction, colitis, esophageal ulcer, stomatitis, and pancreatitis, have been reported in patients receiving trastuzumab.

● Infectious Complications

Febrile neutropenia and infection with neutropenia resulting in death have been reported in patients receiving trastuzumab in combination with myelosuppressive chemotherapy. (See Cautions: Hematologic Effects.)

Among patients with metastatic breast cancer, infection has been reported in 20 or 47% of patients receiving trastuzumab as a single agent or in combination with paclitaxel, respectively. Among patients receiving trastuzumab and paclitaxel as adjuvant therapy for breast cancer, infection/febrile neutropenia (study 1: 22%, grade 3–5 infection/febrile neutropenia in study 2: 3%) has been reported. Compared with patients receiving chemotherapy alone, patients receiving trastuzumab combined with chemotherapy for metastatic breast cancer or as adjuvant therapy for early breast cancer experienced an increased incidence of infections (study 3: 46 versus 30%, study 1: 22 versus 14%). Upper respiratory tract infections, typically mild, and infections of indwelling catheters were the most commonly reported infectious complications in patients receiving trastuzumab for metastatic breast cancer. Infections of the upper respiratory tract, skin, and urinary tract were the most commonly reported infectious complications in patients receiving trastuzumab as adjuvant therapy for breast cancer. Urinary tract infection occurred in 5% of patients receiving trastuzumab monotherapy for metastatic breast cancer in clinical trials. Lymphangitis and cellulitis also have been reported in patients receiving the drug.

● Musculoskeletal Effects

Back pain has been reported in 22% of patients receiving trastuzumab monotherapy for metastatic breast cancer in clinical trials. Among patients with metastatic breast cancer, bone pain and arthralgia have occurred in 7 and 6%, respectively, of patients receiving trastuzumab as a single agent and in 24 and 37%, respectively, of patients receiving trastuzumab and paclitaxel. Among patients receiving trastuzumab and paclitaxel as adjuvant therapy for breast cancer, arthralgia (study 1: 31%, study 2: 11%) and myalgia (study 2: 10%) have been reported. Bone necrosis, pathologic fractures, and myopathy also have been reported in patients receiving trastuzumab.

● Dermatologic and Immunologic Reactions

Among patients receiving trastuzumab and paclitaxel as adjuvant therapy for breast cancer, rash/desquamation (study 1: 11%) and nail changes (study 2: 9%) have been reported. Among patients with metastatic breast cancer, rash has been reported in 18 or 38% of patients receiving trastuzumab as a single agent or in combination with paclitaxel, respectively. Acne and herpes simplex occurred in 11 and 12%, respectively, of patients receiving trastuzumab and paclitaxel, and each has been reported in 2% of patients receiving trastuzumab alone for metastatic breast cancer. Other adverse dermatologic effects, including herpes zoster and skin ulceration, have been reported in patients receiving trastuzumab.

Of 903 women receiving trastuzumab for metastatic breast cancer, human anti-human antibody (HAHA) to the drug has been detected in one patient, who had no allergic reactions.

● Flu-like Syndrome

Flu-like syndrome has occurred in about 10% of patients receiving trastuzumab alone or in combination with chemotherapy for metastatic breast cancer. Pain, asthenia, and abdominal pain have been reported in 47, 42, and 22%, respectively, of patients receiving trastuzumab monotherapy for metastatic breast cancer.

● Nervous System Effects

Among patients with metastatic breast cancer, paresthesia, which occurred in 48% of patients receiving trastuzumab and paclitaxel, occurred in 9% of patients receiving trastuzumab alone and 39% of those receiving paclitaxel alone. Peripheral neuritis and neuropathy have been reported in 2 and 1%, respectively, of patients receiving trastuzumab as a single agent and in 23 and 13%, respectively, of patients receiving trastuzumab and paclitaxel for metastatic breast cancer. A larger cumulative dose of paclitaxel given in conjunction with trastuzumab (approximately 20% greater than the cumulative dose in patients receiving paclitaxel alone) may have contributed to the increased incidence of paresthesia, peripheral neuritis, and neuropathy in these patients compared with those receiving paclitaxel alone.

Among patients with metastatic breast cancer, headache, insomnia, and dizziness have occurred in 26, 14, and 13%, respectively, of patients receiving trastuzumab monotherapy. Depression has been reported in 6% of patients receiving trastuzumab as a single agent and in 12% of patients receiving trastuzumab and paclitaxel for metastatic breast cancer. Among patients receiving trastuzumab and paclitaxel as adjuvant therapy for breast cancer, headache (study 1: 6%) and insomnia (study 1: 4%) have been reported. Other adverse neurologic effects, including ataxia, confusion, seizures, hydrocephalus, and manic reaction, have been reported in patients receiving trastuzumab.

● Endocrine and Metabolic Effects

Adverse endocrine and metabolic effects, including hypothyroidism, hypercalcemia, hypomagnesemia, hyponatremia, and hypoglycemia, have been reported in patients receiving trastuzumab. Growth retardation and weight loss also occurred in patients receiving the drug.

● Hepatic Effects

Ascites, hepatitis, and hepatic failure have been reported in patients receiving trastuzumab.

● Ocular Effects

Amblyopia has been reported in patients receiving trastuzumab.

● Renal and Genitourinary Effects

Nephrotic syndrome with pathologic evidence of glomerulopathy has been reported rarely in patients receiving trastuzumab. Onset has ranged from 4 to approximately 18 months following initiation of trastuzumab therapy. Pathologic findings have included membranous glomerulonephritis, focal glomerulosclerosis, and fibrillary glomerulonephritis, and complications have included volume overload and congestive heart failure. Renal failure has been reported in patients receiving trastuzumab.

Other adverse genitourinary effects reported in patients receiving trastuzumab include hematuria, hemorrhagic cystitis, hydronephrosis, and pyelonephritis.

● Other Adverse Effects

Among patients with metastatic breast cancer, accidental injury has been reported in 6% of patients receiving trastuzumab as a single agent and in 13% of patients receiving trastuzumab and paclitaxel. Among patients receiving trastuzumab and paclitaxel as adjuvant therapy for breast cancer, fatigue (study 1: 28%) has been reported. Other adverse effects occurring in patients receiving trastuzumab in clinical trials include radiation injury and deafness.

● Precautions and Contraindications

Serious adverse events, rarely fatal, including severe respiratory effects, such as acute respiratory distress syndrome (see Cautions: Respiratory Effects), severe infusion-related reactions (see Cautions: Infusion-related Effects), and severe hypersensitivity reactions, such as anaphylaxis (see Cautions: Sensitivity Reactions), have occurred in patients receiving trastuzumab. In most patients experiencing severe adverse reactions, manifestations typically occurred during or within 24 hours of the infusion of trastuzumab. In some cases, initial improvement in symptoms was followed by marked and delayed clinical deterioration, and a small number of patients died at home. Patients should be informed of the possibility of delayed severe reactions associated with trastuzumab therapy.

Trastuzumab should be administered with extreme caution in patients with pre-existing pulmonary compromise, and the risks and benefits of therapy should be weighed carefully. Most patients experiencing fatal adverse reactions associated with trastuzumab had clinically important preexisting pulmonary compromise secondary to intrinsic lung disease and/or malignant pulmonary involvement.

Interruption or discontinuance of trastuzumab therapy is required in patients experiencing severe or life-threatening adverse reactions. (See Dosage Modification for Toxicity and Contraindications for Continued Therapy under Dosage and Administration: Dosage.)

Respiratory Effects

Patients with either symptomatic intrinsic pulmonary disease (e.g., asthma, COPD) or extensive tumor involvement of the lungs (e.g., lymphangitic spread of tumor, pleural effusions, parenchymal masses) resulting in dyspnea at rest may be at increased risk of serious adverse pulmonary events associated with trastuzumab, and the manufacturer recommends *extreme caution* in such patients.

Infusion-related Effects

Patients with preexisting pulmonary compromise may be at increased risk of serious infusion-related adverse effects associated with trastuzumab.

Sensitivity Reactions

For administration in patients with known hypersensitivity to benzyl alcohol, the preservative in bacteriostatic water for injection (the diluent supplied by the manufacturer), trastuzumab should be reconstituted using sterile water for injection. (See Dosage and Administration: Reconstitution and Administration.)

Trastuzumab should be administered with caution in patients with known hypersensitivity to trastuzumab, Chinese Hamster Ovary (CHO) cell proteins, or any component of the formulation.

Cardiovascular Effects

Because trastuzumab may cause serious adverse cardiovascular effects, including ventricular dysfunction and congestive heart failure, a thorough baseline cardiac evaluation including history, physical examination, and cardiac function tests (i.e., echocardiogram and/or MUGA scan) should be performed prior to initiating trastuzumab therapy.

Among patients with metastatic breast cancer, the risk of cardiac dysfunction including congestive heart failure associated with trastuzumab therapy may be increased with increased age, preexisting cardiac disease, or prior cardiotoxic therapy (e.g., anthracycline therapy or radiation therapy to the chest area). Potential benefit versus the increased risk of cardiac toxicity should be weighed carefully when deciding whether the use of trastuzumab is advisable in patients with preexisting cardiac disease.

Among patients receiving adjuvant therapy for breast cancer, the risk of symptomatic cardiomyopathy associated with trastuzumab may be increased in patients experiencing decline in left ventricular ejection fraction (LVEF) to below the lower limit of normal (following completion of treatment with doxorubicin and cyclophosphamide or during treatment with trastuzumab), patients with previous or concurrent use of antihypertensive medications, and geriatric patients. According to the exclusion criteria applied in the North American randomized trials, use of adjuvant trastuzumab therapy is *not* recommended in patients with angina pectoris requiring medication; arrhythmia requiring medication; a severe conduction abnormality; clinically important valvular disease; cardiomegaly on chest radiography; left ventricular hypertrophy on echocardiography; poorly controlled hypertension; clinically important pericardial effusion; or a history of myocardial infarction, congestive heart failure, or cardiomyopathy. Adjuvant trastuzumab therapy should be initiated only if the measurement of LVEF at baseline is within normal limits (at least 50%) and the decrease from the baseline value is less than 15 points following completion of adjuvant chemotherapy with doxorubicin and cyclophosphamide. Patients who develop clinical manifestations of cardiac toxicity during adjuvant chemotherapy with doxorubicin and cyclophosphamide should *not* receive trastuzumab. In clinical trials of adjuvant therapy for breast cancer, 6% of patients were unable to receive trastuzumab following completion of doxorubicin and cyclophosphamide therapy because of cardiac dysfunction.

Left ventricular function should be monitored frequently in patients receiving trastuzumab. For patients with preexisting cardiac dysfunction, more frequent monitoring is required. Monitoring will not identify all patients who will develop cardiac dysfunction.

In patients receiving adjuvant trastuzumab, cardiac function must be assessed at regular intervals using MUGA scan or echocardiogram performed at baseline (prior to adjuvant therapy with doxorubicin and cyclophosphamide), at the completion of adjuvant chemotherapy with doxorubicin and cyclophosphamide (immediately prior to initiation of trastuzumab therapy), at 3 months following the initiation of concomitant therapy with paclitaxel and trastuzumab, at 3 months following the initiation of trastuzumab monotherapy (upon completion of concomitant therapy with paclitaxel and trastuzumab), and at 3 months following the completion of trastuzumab monotherapy. Age and LVEF following adjuvant chemotherapy with doxorubicin and cyclophosphamide may be risk factors for symptomatic cardiac dysfunction in patients being considered for adjuvant therapy with trastuzumab.

A thorough cardiac assessment, including evaluation of left ventricular function, should be performed in candidates for trastuzumab therapy for advanced or metastatic breast cancer, and cardiac function should be monitored frequently in those receiving the drug. Following baseline echocardiogram or MUGA scan, clinicians recommend cardiac monitoring with either test as indicated by the presence of clinical manifestations of cardiac dysfunction or at regular intervals every 1–4 months according to the patient's age and risk of cardiac toxicity. *Extreme caution is advised during trastuzumab therapy for metastatic disease in patients with preexisting cardiac dysfunction.*

Because of the increased risk of cardiotoxicity, most experts generally do *not* recommend use of trastuzumab in combination with an anthracycline agent for the treatment of metastatic breast cancer.

Dispensing and Administration Precautions

Trastuzumab (Herceptin®) should not be confused with ado-trastuzumab emtansine (Kadcyla®). Because of the similarity between the original generic name of Kadcyla® (trastuzumab emtansine) and the generic name for Herceptin® (trastuzumab), the US Food and Drug Administration (FDA) approved the addition of the prefix "ado" to the generic name for Kadcyla® (i.e., ado-trastuzumab emtansine). However, the potential exists for dispensing or prescribing errors involving these drugs. Such medication errors may be associated with severe toxicity or lack of appropriate therapy in patients who did not receive the intended drug. The manufacturer of ado-trastuzumab emtansine (Kadcyla®) states that this drug should *not* be substituted for or used with trastuzumab (Herceptin®). Therefore, extra care should be exercised to ensure the accuracy of prescriptions for trastuzumab (Herceptin®) and ado-trastuzumab emtansine (Kadcyla®). (See Special Alerts.)

● Pediatric Precautions

Safety and efficacy of trastuzumab in children younger than 18 years of age have not been established.

● Geriatric Precautions

Although safety and efficacy of trastuzumab in geriatric patients 65 years of age or older have not been established specifically, the manufacturer cautions that clinical data currently are insufficient to exclude the possibility of age-related differences during trastuzumab therapy. The risk of cardiotoxicity associated with trastuzumab is increased in geriatric patients compared with younger patients

receiving either adjuvant therapy for early breast cancer or treatment for metastatic breast cancer.

● Mutagenicity and Carcinogenicity

Data from in vitro and in vivo tests of trastuzumab, including Ames tests, the micronucleus assay, and tests in human peripheral blood lymphocytes, have not shown any evidence of mutagenic activity.

The carcinogenicity of trastuzumab has not been evaluated. Acute leukemia and cervical cancer have been reported in patients receiving trastuzumab. Several cases of secondary leukemia have occurred in patients receiving trastuzumab.

● Pregnancy, Fertility, and Lactation

Oligohydramnios has been reported in women receiving trastuzumab during pregnancy. Placental transfer of trastuzumab has been observed in monkeys. Although reproduction studies in cynomolgus monkeys using trastuzumab dosages up to 25 times the weekly human maintenance dosage of 2 mg/kg have not revealed evidence of harm to the fetus, the important role of the *HER2* receptor in embryonic development of the cardiac and central nervous systems raises concerns about possible teratogenic effects of trastuzumab. The *HER2* receptor is expressed at high levels in many embryonic tissues, including cardiac and neural tissues, and death of embryos in early gestation has been observed in mice lacking the *HER2* protein. Further study is needed to determine whether trastuzumab has teratogenic effects in humans. The possibility that trastuzumab may persist in maternal tissues for up to 5–6 months after the last dose should be considered. There are no adequate and controlled studies to date using trastuzumab in pregnant women, and the drug should be used during pregnancy only when the potential benefits justify the possible risks to the fetus.

Reproduction studies in cynomolgus monkeys using trastuzumab dosages up to 25 times the weekly human maintenance dosage of 2 mg/kg have not revealed evidence of impaired fertility.

When trastuzumab was administered in lactating cynomolgus monkeys at dosages 25 times the usual human maintenance dosage of 2 mg/kg weekly, distribution of the drug in milk was demonstrated. No adverse effects on growth or development from birth to 3 months of age were observed in infant monkeys with measurable serum trastuzumab concentrations. It is not known whether trastuzumab is distributed into human milk. Because human IgG is distributed in milk, and because of the potential for absorption of trastuzumab and adverse reactions to the drug in nursing infants, women should be advised to discontinue nursing during trastuzumab therapy and for 6 months following the last dose of the drug.

DRUG INTERACTIONS

Formal drug interaction studies of trastuzumab have not been conducted. However, the incidence of most common adverse effects of the drug has been increased in patients receiving combination chemotherapy. (See Cautions.)

● Anthracycline Antineoplastic Agents

The risk of trastuzumab-induced cardiotoxic effects is increased in patients receiving an anthracycline concomitantly. (See Cautions: Cardiovascular Effects.) Such combined therapy currently is *not* recommended by most experts for use in the treatment of metastatic breast cancer.

● Paclitaxel

In clinical studies, a 1.5-fold increase in mean trough serum concentrations of trastuzumab was reported when the drug was administered concomitantly with paclitaxel versus an anthracycline and cyclophosphamide. In primate studies, administration of trastuzumab in combination with paclitaxel resulted in a two-fold decrease in trastuzumab clearance. The clinical importance of the interaction between trastuzumab and paclitaxel is not known.

ACUTE TOXICITY

Limited information is available on the acute toxicity of trastuzumab. The acute lethal dose of trastuzumab in humans is not known. Overdosage has not been reported in clinical trials with patients receiving single doses of trastuzumab of up to 500 mg.

PHARMACOLOGY

Trastuzumab is an antineoplastic agent that inhibits proliferation of tumor cells that overexpress *HER2*. The *HER2* proto-oncogene (also known as c-*erb*B2 or *neu*) encodes a 185-kd transmembrane tyrosine kinase receptor known as p185^{HER2} or human epidermal growth factor receptor 2 (*HER2*), which has partial homology with other members of the epidermal growth factor receptor family. Trastuzumab, a recombinant humanized murine monoclonal antibody, binds specifically to the extracellular domain of the *HER2* receptor or *HER2/neu* protein. The *HER2* receptor participates in receptor-receptor interactions that regulate cell differentiation, growth, and proliferation. Overexpression of the *HER2* receptor contributes to the process of neoplastic transformation. Results from in vitro assays and animal studies have shown that trastuzumab inhibits the proliferation of human tumor cells that overexpress *HER2/neu* protein. Trastuzumab-mediated antibody-dependent cellular cytotoxicity (ADCC) also has been demonstrated and, according to in vitro studies, occurs preferentially in cells that overexpress the *HER2* protein compared with cells that do not.

Amplification of the *HER2* oncogene and/or overexpression of the *HER2* protein occurs in 25–30% of node-positive or -negative primary breast cancers, and several studies have shown that *HER2* amplification and/or overexpression is an independent predictor of poor prognosis, including more rapid disease progression and shorter overall survival, in patients with node-positive breast cancer. Overexpression of this growth factor receptor also has been shown to be associated with other adverse prognostic factors in breast cancer, including advanced pathologic stage, DNA ploidy, increased S-phase fraction, high nuclear grade, absence of estrogen and progesterone receptors, and number of metastatic axillary lymph nodes.

PHARMACOKINETICS

Data from studies in patients with metastatic breast cancer receiving trastuzumab 10–500 mg once weekly by IV infusion over short periods indicate that the pharmacokinetics of the drug are dose dependent. Limited data suggest that the pharmacokinetics of trastuzumab are not affected by age or increased serum creatinine concentrations up to 2 mg/dL.

● Absorption

In patients with metastatic breast cancer receiving a loading dose of 4 mg/kg IV followed by a weekly maintenance dose of 2 mg/kg IV, peak and trough plasma concentrations of trastuzumab at steady state (between weeks 16 and 32) averaged approximately 123 and 79 mcg/mL, respectively. In patients with metastatic breast cancer receiving trastuzumab 500 mg once weekly by short-duration IV infusion, peak plasma concentrations of the drug averaged 377 mcg/mL.

Measurable serum concentrations of circulating extracellular domain of the *HER2* receptor (i.e., shed antigen) have been detected in some patients with tumors that overexpress *HER2/neu*. Shed antigen in concentrations of up to 1880 ng/mL (median: 11 ng/mL) was detected in baseline serum samples of 64% of patients (286/447) receiving a loading dose of trastuzumab 4 mg/kg IV followed by 2 mg/kg IV once weekly. Higher baseline concentrations of shed antigen were associated with lower trough serum concentrations of trastuzumab; however, with once-weekly dosing of trastuzumab, target serum concentrations of the drug were attained by week 6 in most patients with elevated serum concentrations of shed antigen. Concentration of shed antigen does not appear to affect tumor response to trastuzumab.

● Distribution

Following administration of trastuzumab by short-duration IV infusion, the mean apparent volume of distribution is about 44 mL/kg (approximately equal to serum volume). It is not known whether trastuzumab crosses the blood-brain barrier or distributes into the CSF. It also is not known whether trastuzumab crosses the placenta or distributes into milk in humans; however, placental transfer of trastuzumab and distribution of the drug into milk have been observed in monkeys.

● Elimination

The pharmacokinetics of trastuzumab are nonlinear; increased doses of the drug are associated with increased mean half-life and decreased clearance. In patients receiving a loading dose of trastuzumab 4 mg/kg IV followed by a weekly maintenance dose of 2 mg/kg IV, elimination half-life averaged 5.8 days (range: 1–32 days). Following IV infusion of 10 or 500 mg of trastuzumab, elimination half-life averaged 1.7 or 12 days, respectively. The metabolism of trastuzumab is not fully understood, but it appears that elimination of the drug would involve clearance of IgG through the reticuloendothelial system.

CHEMISTRY AND STABILITY

● Chemistry

Trastuzumab, a recombinant DNA-derived humanized anti-*HER2* monoclonal antibody, is an antineoplastic agent.

Trastuzumab is an IgG$_1$ kappa immunoglobulin containing human framework regions and the complementarity-determining regions of a murine antibody (4D5) that binds to *HER2/neu*, a transmembrane receptor protein that is overexpressed in selected cancer cells. The drug occurs as a sterile, lyophilized, white to pale yellow powder and is soluble in water; trastuzumab powder for injection also contains histidine monohydrochloride, histidine, α,α-trehalose dihydrate, and polysorbate (Tween®) 20. Following reconstitution as recommended with bacteriostatic water for injection containing benzyl alcohol (see Dosage and Administration: Reconstitution and Administration), solutions containing trastuzumab 21 mg/mL are clear to slightly opalescent and colorless to pale yellow and have a pH of about 6.

● Stability

Vials of trastuzumab should be stored at 2–8°C; when stored under recommended conditions, commercially available trastuzumab powder for injection should be stable up to the date of expiration marked on the vial.

Following reconstitution of the sterile powder with bacteriostatic water for injection containing benzyl alcohol (as supplied by the manufacturer), trastuzumab solutions are stable for 28 days when refrigerated at 2–8°C. If trastuzumab powder for injection is reconstituted with sterile water for injection (e.g., in patients with hypersensitivity to benzyl alcohol), the possibility of microbial contamination should be considered, and the manufacturer recommends that such solutions be used immediately and unused portions discarded. The manufacturer states that use of other diluents for the reconstitution of trastuzumab should be avoided. Trastuzumab solutions should not be frozen following reconstitution or dilution.

Reconstituted solutions of trastuzumab diluted in 0.9% sodium chloride injection are stable for no more than 24 hours when prepared and stored in polyvinyl chloride or polyethylene bags at 2–8°C. The manufacturer states that 5% dextrose injection should *not* be used as a diluent for trastuzumab solutions; diluents other than those recommended by the manufacturer may not maintain the stability or sterility of the antibody solution.

For further information on the handling of antineoplastic agents, see the ASHP Guidelines on Handling Hazardous Drugs at http://www.ahfsdrug information.com.

PREPARATIONS

Trastuzumab (Herceptin®) should not be confused with ado-trastuzumab emtansine (Kadcyla®). (See Special Alerts.)

Excipients in commercially available drug preparations may have clinically important effects in some individuals; consult specific product labeling for details.

Trastuzumab

Parenteral		
For injection, for IV infusion	440 mg	Herceptin® (supplied with 20 mL bacteriostatic water for injection containing 1.1% benzyl alcohol;), Genentech

† Use is not currently included in the labeling approved by the US Food and Drug Administration.

Tretinoin (Systemic)

10:00 • ANTINEOPLASTIC AGENTS

■ Tretinoin, a retinoid, is an antineoplastic agent.

USES

● Acute Promyelocytic Leukemia

Tretinoin is used for the induction of remission in adults and pediatric patients 1 year of age and older with acute promyelocytic leukemia (APL) characterized by the presence of certain genetic markers (i.e., 15;17 chromosomal translocation and/or *PML /RAR-α* gene); the drug is FDA-labeled for use in such patients with relapsed or refractory disease following anthracycline-based chemotherapy or in patients for whom anthracycline therapy is contraindicated. Tretinoin also has been used for consolidation and maintenance therapy†.

Tretinoin therapy may be initiated based on the morphologic diagnosis of APL; however, the manufacturer states that the diagnosis should be confirmed with cytogenetic studies to detect the presence of the t(15;17) translocation genetic marker or molecular diagnostic testing for the PML/RAR-α fusion protein. Tretinoin is *not* recommended for use in patients without these genetic markers.

Clinical Experience

Treatment for Relapsed or Refractory Disease

The current indication for tretinoin is based principally on data from an open-label, single-arm trial and from 2 cohorts of compassionate cases treated in multiple centers under the direction of the National Cancer Institute (NCI). All patients received tretinoin 45 mg/m² daily as a divided oral dose for up to 90 days or 30 days beyond attainment of a complete remission. In the clinical trial, tretinoin therapy was associated with a complete remission rate of 80% in the 20 patients with relapsed APL and 73% in the 15 patients with previously untreated APL; median survival was 10.8 months in the patients with relapsed disease. In the 2 cohorts of compassionate cases of APL, complete remission rates of 50–52% in patients with relapsed disease and 36–68% in patients with previously untreated disease were reported. The median time to achieve a complete remission was between 40–50 days (range: 2–120 days) in all patients studied. Most of the patients in these studies also received cytotoxic chemotherapy during the remission phase.

Although tretinoin has been used to induce second remissions in patients with APL that has relapsed following prior treatment with tretinoin, results have been inconsistent; continuous treatment with tretinoin results in resistance to the drug secondary to increased catabolism and decrease in plasma concentrations, and response may be more likely for late relapse occurring after discontinuation of tretinoin therapy.

Limited data on the clinical use of tretinoin in children are available. A complete remission rate of 67% (8 of 10 males and 2 of 5 females) was reported in 15 pediatric patients (age range: 1–16 years) receiving tretinoin induction therapy for APL.

Initial Treatment for Newly Diagnosed Disease

Tretinoin also has been used as initial treatment in patients with newly diagnosed APL†. The NCI includes the combination of tretinoin and arsenic trioxide as an initial treatment option in newly diagnosed patients with low- to intermediate-risk disease.

In early studies, the combination of tretinoin and cytotoxic chemotherapy was shown to be superior over chemotherapy alone in patients with newly diagnosed APL.More recently, the efficacy and toxicity of tretinoin plus arsenic trioxide was compared with tretinoin plus chemotherapy in a phase 3, randomized, open-label study in patients with newly diagnosed low- to intermediate-risk APL. The primary endpoint was event-free survival (defined as no achievement of hematologic complete remission [CR] after induction therapy, no achievement of molecular CR after 3 consolidation courses, molecular relapse, hematologic relapse, or death). The 2-year event-free survival rate was 97% in the tretinoin plus arsenic trioxide group and 86% in the tretinoin plus chemotherapy group.

Clinical Perspective

The treatment of APL has evolved rapidly over the past several decades with the introduction of tretinoin and arsenic trioxide. While traditional cytotoxic chemotherapy is still used in certain patients (e.g., high-risk), it is possible to treat APL without the use of chemotherapy. APL is a distinct subtype of acute myeloid leukemia (AML) that has a specific sensitivity to tretinoin, which acts as a differentiating agent, and to arsenic trioxide, a proapoptotic agent; high complete recovery rates and long-term disease-free survival in APL have been demonstrated with the combination of the 2 drugs. With the inclusion of arsenic trioxide in current treatment regimens, the use of traditional chemotherapy is increasingly restricted to the induction phase for high-risk patients. Current guidelines for APL include various treatment options; selection of an appropriate regimen is determined by the patient's risk category (low, intermediate, or high based on white blood cell [WBC] counts).

Experts currently recommend the use of tretinoin in combination with arsenic trioxide for initial treatment† of APL in patients with low- to intermediate-risk disease (WBC count ≤10,000/mm³). The combination of tretinoin and chemotherapy, followed by arsenic trioxide-based consolidation therapy is recommended for newly-diagnosed patients with high-risk disease (WBC >10,000/mm³).

Because of data indicating that children with APL have a similar response to the combination of tretinoin and arsenic trioxide as adults, experts recommend the use of these 2 agents alone in standard-risk patients, and with short-course chemotherapy during induction in high-risk patients, as the optimal therapeutic approach for children with APL.

Although tretinoin is only FDA-labeled for use in induction therapy, the drug also has been used for consolidation therapy† and is included in current guidelines for this use. For patients who are treated with tretinoin and arsenic trioxide, maintenance therapy is not likely to be necessary.

DOSAGE AND ADMINISTRATION

● General

Pretreatment Screening

- Verify pregnancy status in females of reproductive potential within 1 week prior to initiating tretinoin with a pregnancy test with a sensitivity of at least 50 mIU/mL.
- Monitor fasting triglycerides and cholesterol and liver function at baseline.

Patient Monitoring

- Monitor for signs or symptoms of differentiation syndrome, especially during the first month of treatment.
- Monitor for signs and symptoms of intracranial hypertension, especially in pediatric patients.
- Montor fasting triglycerides and cholesterol periodically during treatment.
- Monitor liver function tests during treatment as clinically indicated.

● Administration

Tretinoin is administered orally in 2 equally divided doses. Take capsules with a meal and swallow the capsules whole with water; do *not* chew, dissolve, or open.

Do not take a missed dose of tretinoin unless it is more than 10 hours until the next scheduled dose.

If vomiting occurs after administration, do not take an additional dose. Continue with the next scheduled dose.

Store at 20-25°C; protect from light.

● Dosage

Acute Promyelocytic Leukemia

Adults

For the induction of remission, the recommended dosage of tretinoin is 45 mg/m² daily administered in 2 evenly divided doses until complete remission is documented. The manufacturer states that tretinoin therapy should be continued until

30 days after complete remission is achieved or 90 days of treatment have elapsed, whichever occurs first.

Although tretinoin is not FDA-labeled for consolidation therapy† in patients with APL, the drug has been used for postremission consolidation at a dosage of 45 mg/m² alternating 7 days on and 7 days off for a total of 28 weeks. An alternative consolidation regimen that has been used is 45 mg/m² daily for 2 weeks every 4 weeks for a total of 7 cycles (28 weeks total).

Pediatric Patients

For the induction of remission in pediatric patients ≥1 year of age with APL, the recommended dosage of tretinoin is 45 mg/m² daily administered in 2 evenly divided doses until complete remission is documented. The manufacturer states that tretinoin therapy should be continued until 30 days after complete remission is achieved, or for a total of 90 days, whichever occurs first.

The maximum tolerated dose is lower in pediatric patients than adults. Dosage reduction may be considered for pediatric patients who experience serious or intolerable drug toxicity. A lower daily dose of 25 mg/m² has been used in the pediatric population, which is thought to decrease the incidence of intracranial hypertension.

Dosage Modification for Toxicity
Differentiation Syndrome

Withholding tretinoin therapy until resolution should be considered in patients experiencing moderate or severe differentiation syndrome.

Hepatotoxicity

Withholding tretinoin therapy until resolution should be considered in patients with liver function test results >5 times the upper limit of normal.

CAUTIONS

- **Contraindications**
  - Known hypersensitivity to tretinoin, any of its components, or other retinoids.

- **Warnings/Precautions**

Warnings
Embryo-Fetal Toxicity

Tretinoin, a retinoid, may cause fetal harm; embryo-fetal loss and malformations occur when administered to pregnant women. A boxed warning about the risk of teratogenic effects has been included in the prescribing information for the drug.

Retinoids are associated with an increased risk of major congenital malformations, spontaneous abortions, and premature births following exposure during human pregnancy. In animals, tretinoin has teratogenic and embryotoxic effects at doses less than the human dose on a mg/m² basis.

Apprise pregnant women of the potential fetal risk. Advise females of reproductive potential to use 2 effective contraceptive methods during treatment and for 1 month following the last tretinoin dose. Advise male patients with female partners of reproductive potential to use effective contraception during treatment and for 1 week following the last dose.

Differentiation Syndrome

Differentiation syndrome, a condition characterized by fever, dyspnea, acute respiratory distress, weight gain, pulmonary infiltrates, pleural and pericardial effusions, edema, and hepatic, renal, and multiorgan failure, has been reported in about 26% of patients with APL treated with tretinoin. A boxed warning about this risk has been included in the prescribing information for tretinoin. The syndrome has been accompanied by impaired myocardial contractility and episodic hypotension, and can occur with or without concomitant leukocytosis. Onset generally occurs within the first month of treatment and can occur after a single dose. Endotracheal intubation and mechanical ventilation were required in some cases due to progressive hypoxemia and several fatalities have occurred due to multi-organ failure. At the first signs or symptoms of differentiation syndrome,

dexamethasone 10 mg IV every 12 hours should be immediately administered and continued until signs and symptoms have abated for at least 3 days. Hemodynamic monitoring should also occur until sign and symptom resolution. Consider withholding tretinoin therapy for moderate and severe disease until resolution.

Other Warnings and Precautions
Leukocytosis

Rapidly evolving leukocytosis has been reported in approximately 40% of patients receiving tretinoin capsules and is associated with an increased risk of life-threatening complications. Patients with a baseline white blood cell (WBC) count >5000 cells/mm³ have an increased leukocytosis risk while those who receive concomitant chemotherapy may be at a reduced risk.

Consider administration of cytoreductive chemotherapy (e.g., an anthracycline if not contraindicated or hydroxyurea) with tretinoin in patients with leukocytosis, as clinically indicated.

Patients Without the t(15;17) Translocation or PML/RARα Fusion

Initiation of therapy with tretinoin may be based on the morphological diagnosis of APL, but the diagnosis should be confirmed with detection of the t(15;17) translocation genetic marker by cytogenetic studies or PML/RARα fusion via molecular diagnostic techniques. Tretinoin is not recommended for use in patients without these genetic markers.

Intracranial Hypertension

Retinoids, including tretinoin, have been associated with intracranial hypertension, especially in pediatric patients. Early signs and symptoms of intracranial hypertension include papilledema, headache, nausea, vomiting, and visual disturbances. Evaluate patients with these symptoms for intracranial hypertension and, if present, perform a neurological assessment and initiate appropriate therapy.

Consider dose reduction, interruption of therapy, or discontinuation of tretinoin as necessary. The concomitant use of other agents known to cause intracranial hypertension, such as tetracyclines, might increase the risk of this condition. Avoid concomitant use of tretinoin with other agents that can cause intracranial hypertension.

Lipid Abnormalities

Up to 60% of patients receiving tretinoin have experienced hypercholesterolemia and/or hypertriglyceridemia, which may be reversible upon completion of treatment. The clinical consequences of elevations of triglycerides and cholesterol are unknown, but venous thrombosis and myocardial infarction (MI) have been reported in patients who ordinarily are at low risk for such complications.

Monitor fasting triglycerides and cholesterol at baseline and periodically during treatment.

Hepatotoxicity

Elevated liver function test results have been reported in 50 to 60% of patients receiving tretinoin. The majority of these abnormalities resolve without interruption of tretinoin or after completion of treatment.

Liver function test results should be carefully monitored at baseline and during tretinoin treatment as clinically indicated. Consider withholding therapy if liver function test results reach >5 times the upper limit of normal (ULN) until resolution.

Thromboembolic Events

Venous and arterial thromboembolic events (e.g., cerebrovascular accident, MI, renal infarct) have occurred with tretinoin therapy. Events may occur during the initial month of treatment and patients administered anti-fibrinolytics may be at an increased risk for their occurrence.

Avoid concomitant use of tretinoin and anti-fibrinolytics (e.g., tranexamic acid, aminocaproic acid).

Specific Populations
Pregnancy

Tretinoin is a retinoid and increased spontaneous abortions and major fetal abnormalities related to the use of retinoids in humans have been documented.

Reported malformations include abnormalities of the CNS, musculoskeletal system, external ear, eye, thymus, and great vessels as well as facial dysmorphia, cleft palate, and parathyroid hormone deficiency. Some of the reported abnomalities resulted in fatalities.

Lactation

It is not known whether tretinoin is distributed into human milk. The effects of tretinoin on the breastfed child or milk production are also unknown. Due to the potential for serious adverse effects in nursing infants, women should not breastfeed during treatment with tretinoin and for 1 week after the last dose.

Females and Males of Reproductive Potential

Tretinoin can cause embryo-fetal loss and malformations when administered to pregnant women.

Verify pregnancy status in females of reproductive potential prior to initiating tretinoin therapy. These females must have a negative pregnancy test within 1 week prior to therapy initiation with a test sensitivity of at least 50 mIU/mL.

Females of reproductive potential should either abstain from sexual intercourse or use 2 effective contraceptive methods during therapy and for 1 month after the last dose. Two contraceptive methods are indicated even in the setting of a history of infertility, unless due to hysterectomy. Male patients with female partners of reproductive potential should use effective contraception during treatment and for 1 week after the last dose.

Based on testicular toxicities in dogs, tretinoin may impair male fertility. The reversibility of this effect is unknown.

Pediatric Use

Safety and efficacy of tretinoin have been established in pediatric patients ≥1 year of age. The maximum tolerated dose is lower in pediatric patients as compared to adults.

Some pediatric patients experience severe headache and intracranial hypertension during therapy, requiring treatment with analgesics and lumbar puncture.

Dosage reduction may be appropriate if serious and/or intolerable adverse effects occur.

Geriatric Use

In clinical studies, 21% of patients were 60 years of age or greater. No overall differences in safety or effectiveness were seen between older and younger patients.

Hepatic Impairment

The manufacturer states that the pharmacokinetics of tretinoin have not been evaluated in individuals with hepatic impairment.

Renal Impairment

The manufacturer states that the pharmacokinetics of tretinoin have not been evaluated in individuals with renal impairment.

● Common Adverse Effects

The most common adverse reactions (≥30%) with tretinoin therapy include headache, fever, skin/mucous membrane dryness, bone pain, malaise, shivering, upper respiratory tract disorders, dyspnea, hemorrhage, infections, nausea/vomiting, rash, peripheral edema, leukocytosis, pain, GI hemorrhage, chest discomfort, and abdominal pain.

DRUG INTERACTIONS

● Drugs Affecting Hepatic Microsomal Enzymes

The concomitant use of tretinoin with a strong CYP3A4 inhibitor (e.g., ketoconazole) increases tretinoin plasma concentrations, which may lead to increased adverse reactions. Avoid concurrent administration of tretinoin with strong CYP3A inhibitors if possible. Monitor these patients more frequently for adverse reactions if concurrent administration cannot be avoided.

The concomitant use of tretinoin with strong CYP3A4 inducers may reduce tretinoin plasma concentrations, which may lead to reduced efficacy. Avoid concurrent administration of tretinoin with strong CYP3A inducers if possible.

● Drugs Known to Cause Intracranial Hypertension

Intracranial hypertension has been reported in patients receiving tretinoin. Concomitant use of other agents known to cause intracranial hypertension, such as tetracyclines, may increase the risk of this condition in patients receiving tretinoin. Avoid coadministration of tretinoin with drugs known to cause intracranial hypertension.

● Antifibrinolytic Agents

Fatal thrombotic complications have been reported in patients receiving tretinoin and concurrent use of fibrinolytic inhibitors, such as tranexamic acid or aminocaproic acid, may increase this risk. Avoid concomitant use of tretinoin with antifibrinolytic agents.

● Hydroxyurea

Concurrent use of hydroxyurea, which is cytotoxic to cells in S phase, and tretinoin, which induces cells to enter the S phase, may cause a synergistic effect leading to massive cell lysis. Bone marrow necrosis, sometimes fatal, has been reported in patients receiving hydroxyurea during tretinoin therapy. Although some clinicians have administered hydroxyurea in conjunction with tretinoin therapy to reduce leukocytosis, the safety and efficacy of this practice have not been established, and caution is recommended in the use of hydroxyurea in patients receiving tretinoin.

● Vitamin A

Like other retinoids, concomitant use of tretinoin with vitamin A should be avoided due to a risk of vitamin A related adverse reactions.

DESCRIPTION

Tretinoin is a retinoid that induces cytodifferentiation and decreased proliferation of acute promyelocytic leukemia (APL) cells in culture and in vivo. The precise mechanism(s) of action of tretinoin has not been fully elucidated. The PML/RAR-α fusion protein resulting from the 15;17 chromosomal translocation appears to block myeloid differentiation at the promyelocyte stage, possibly by complexing and inactivating wild-type PML or by inhibiting the normal retinoic acid signaling pathway. In patients with APL who achieve a complete remission with tretinoin therapy, the drug causes an initial maturation of the primitive promyelocytes derived from the cellular leukemic clone followed by a repopulation of the bone marrow and peripheral blood by normal, polyclonal hematopoietic cells. Observations supporting cellular differentiation effects as a mechanism of tretinoin include the absence of bone marrow hypoplasia during induction, the appearance of immunophenotypically unique "intermediate cells" expressing both mature and immature cell surface antigens, and the presence of both Auer rods and the 15;17 translocation in morphologically mature granulocytes until a late stage of induction. The mechanism by which the population of malignant cells is eliminated is not fully understood but appears to involve apoptosis (programmed cell death). Following induction therapy, the PML/RAR-α fusion protein can be detected in the majority of patients, suggesting that tretinoin alone does not eradicate the leukemic clone.

Following oral administration of tretinoin, the time to reach peak concentrations was 1 to 2 hours. The absolute bioavailability was approximately 50%. The effect of food on absorption has not been evaluated; however, retinoid absorption is generally enhanced with food. Protein binding is >95%, primarily to albumin. The terminal elimination half-life of tretinoin following initial dosing in patients with APL is 0.5 to 2 hours. Tretinoin is metabolized in the liver by cytochrome P-450 (CYP) isoenzymes CYP3A4, 2C8, and 2E and undergoes glucuronidation by UGT2B7; evidence exists that tretinoin induces its own metabolism. Two of its metabolites, 4-oxo retinoic acid and 4-oxo trans retinoic acid glucuronide, have 33% of the pharmacological activity of the parent compound. The drug is excreted in the feces (31% within 6 days) and urine (63% within 72 hours). The effect of age, sex, race, renal impairment, and hepatic impairment on the pharmacokinetics of tretinoin is unknown.

ADVICE TO PATIENTS

- Advise patients to swallow tretinoin capsules whole with water and not to chew, dissolve, or open the capsules.

- Advise patients not to take a missed dose of tretinoin unless it is more than 10 hours until the next scheduled dose. Inform patients that if vomiting occurs after tretinoin administration, they should not take an additional dose, but continue with the next scheduled dose.

- Advise patients that their ability to drive or operate machinery might be impaired, especially if experiencing dizziness or severe headache.

- Advise patients of the risk of differentiation syndrome. Advise patients to immediately report any symptoms of differentiation syndrome, such as fever, cough or difficulty breathing, decreased urinary output, low blood pressure, rapid weight gain, or swelling of their arms or legs, to their clinician.

- Advise patients that tretinoin is not recommended for use in patients without t(15;17) translocation or PML/RAR-α fusion.

- Inform patients of the risk of leukocytosis that can be rapidly evolving and life-threatening.

- Inform patients of the risk of intracranial hypertension, especially in pediatric patients.

- Inform patients of the risk of hypercholesterolemia and/or hypertriglyceridemia during treatment with tretinoin and the need for periodic laboratory monitoring.

- Inform patients of the risk of hepatotoxicity during treatment with tretinoin and the need for periodic laboratory monitoring.

- Inform patients that venous and arterial thromboembolic events, including cerebrovascular accident, myocardial infarction, and renal infarct can occur during treatment.

- Advise females to inform their clinician if they are or plan to become pregnant or plan to breast-feed. Perform pregnancy testing before initiation of tretinoin and advise patients of the potential risk to the fetus.

- Inform women to use effective contraception (i.e., 2 reliable forms of contraception simultaneously unless abstinence is the chosen method) during tretinoin therapy and for 1 month following discontinuance. Advise male patients with female partners of reproductive potential to use effective contraception during tretinoin therapy and for 1 week after the last dose.

- Advise women not to breast-feed during treatment with tretinoin and for 1 week after the final dose.

- Advise patients to inform their healthcare provider about all concomitant medications, including prescription medicine, over the counter (OTC) drugs, vitamins, and herbal products.

- Inform patients of other important precautionary information.

PREPARATIONS

Excipients in commercially available drug preparations may have clinically important effects in some individuals; consult specific product labeling for details.

Tretinoin

Oral

Capsules	10 mg*	Tretinoin Capsules

* available from one or more manufacturer, distributor, and/or repackager by generic (nonproprietary) name

† Use is not currently included in the labeling approved by the US Food and Drug Administration.

Selected Revisions July 10, 2024, © Copyright, February 1, 2005, American Society of Health-System Pharmacists, Inc.

Tucatinib

10:00 · ANTINEOPLASTIC AGENTS

- Tucatinib, a highly selective, reversible tyrosine kinase inhibitor of human epidermal growth factor receptor type 2 (HER2), is an antineoplastic agent.

USES

• Breast Cancer

Combination Therapy with Trastuzumab and Capecitabine

Tucatinib is used in combination with trastuzumab and capecitabine for the treatment of human epidermal growth factor receptor type 2 (HER2)-positive advanced unresectable or metastatic breast cancer in adults, including those with brain metastases, who have previously received at least one anti-HER2-based regimen in the metastatic setting. The drug has been designated an orphan drug by FDA for the treatment of breast cancer patients with brain metastases.

Efficacy of tucatinib for this use is based principally on the results of a randomized, double-blind, placebo-controlled phase 2 study (HER2CLIMB) in adults with HER2-positive, unresectable, locally advanced, or metastatic breast cancer (with or without brain metastases) previously treated with trastuzumab, pertuzumab, or ado-trastuzumab emastine (separately or in combination) in the neoadjuvant, adjuvant, or metastatic setting. In this study, 612 patients were randomized (stratified by presence or history of brain metastases, Eastern Cooperative Oncology Group [ECOG] performance status, and geographic region) in a 2:1 ratio to receive either tucatinib 300 mg orally twice daily in combination with trastuzumab (8 mg/kg IV initially, followed by either 6 mg/kg IV or 600 mg by subcutaneous injection on day 1 of each 21-day cycle) and capecitabine (1 g/m^2 orally twice daily on days 1–14 of each 21-day cycle) or placebo in combination with trastuzumab and capecitabine. Treatment was continued until disease progression or unacceptable toxicity occurred. The primary measure of efficacy was progression-free survival (as assessed by a blinded independent central review committee) according to Response Evaluation Criteria in Solid Tumors (RECIST v1.1). In the primary efficacy population (consisting of the initial 480 patients randomized in the study), the median age of patients was 54 years; 73% of the patients were white, 99% were female, 51% had an ECOG performance status of 1, 60% had estrogen and/or progesterone receptor-positive disease, and 74% had visceral metastases. Approximately one-half (48%) of patients had active brain metastases or a history of brain metastases; 23% of these patients had untreated brain metastases, 40% had previously treated but stable brain metastases, and 37% had previously treated but radiographically progressing brain metastases. Patients had received a median of 4 prior systemic therapies or a median of 3 prior systemic therapies in the metastatic setting; all patients had previously received trastuzumab and ado-trastuzumab emtansine and all but 2 patients had previously received pertuzumab. This study excluded patients with leptomeningeal disease.

In the primary efficacy population, patients receiving tucatinib in combination with trastuzumab and capecitabine had a longer median progression-free survival than those receiving the placebo combination regimen (7.8 versus 5.6 months). In the total patient population, median overall survival also was prolonged in patients receiving the tucatinib combination regimen compared with those receiving the placebo regimen (21.9 versus 17.4 months). Among the patients with a history or presence of parenchymal brain metastases at baseline, median progression-free survival in patients receiving the tucatinib or placebo combination regimen was 7.6 or 5.4 months, respectively. Among patients with measurable disease, patients receiving the tucatinib combination regimen also had higher objective response rates compared with those receiving the placebo combination regimen (40.6% versus 22.8%); complete response was achieved in 0.9 or 1.2% of patients receiving these respective treatments. At the time of analysis, the median duration of response was 8.3 months in patients

receiving the tucatinib combination regimen and 6.3 months in those receiving the placebo combination regimen. Exploratory analyses of the cohort of patients with a history or presence of brain metastases at baseline also suggested prolonged progression-free survival (9.9 versus 4.2 months) and overall survival (18.1 versus 12 months) and higher rates of objective response (47.3 versus 20%) in patients receiving the tucatinib combination regimen compared with those receiving the placebo combination regimen.

• Colorectal Cancer

Combination Therapy with Trastuzumab

Tucatinib is used in combination with trastuzumab for the treatment of adults with RAS wild-type, HER2-positive unresectable or metastatic colorectal cancer that has progressed following treatment with fluoropyrimidine-, oxaliplatin-, and irinotecan-based chemotherapy. Patients should be selected for therapy based on the presence of HER2 overexpression or gene amplification (FDA tests are not currently available) and RAS wild-type mutations (FDA-approved tests are available, see http://www.fda.gov/CompanionDiagnostics). The drug has been designated an orphan drug by the FDA for treatment of HER2-positive colorectal cancer. This indication is approved under accelerated approval based on tumor response rate and durability of response. Continued approval for this indication may be contingent upon verification and description of clinical benefit in confirmatory trials.

Efficacy of tucatinib for this use is based principally on the results of an open-label, multicenter trial (MOUNTAINEER) in 84 patients with HER2-positive, RAS wild-type, unresectable or metastatic colorectal cancer and who received prior treatment (fluoropyrimidines, oxaliplatin, irinotecan, and anti-vascular endothelial growth factor [VEGF] monoclonal antibody). Patients whose disease had deficient mismatch repair (dMMR) proteins or microsatellite instability-high (MSI-H) must have also received an anti-programmed cell death protein-1 (PD-1) monoclonal antibody and patients who received prior anti-HER2 targeting therapy were excluded. The median age of patients was 55 years (range: 24 to 77); 14% of patients were 65 years of age or older, 61% were male, 77% of patients were white, 4% were Black, 4% were Asian, and 4% were Hispanic or Latino. In this study, 70% of patients had lung metastases, 64% had liver metastases, 60% had an ECOG performance status of 0, 37% had an ECOG performance status of 1, and 4% had an ECOG performance status of 2. Prior treatment with fluoropyrimidine, oxaliplatin, and irinotecan occurred in 99% of patients and 83% and 52% of patients received anti-VEGF antibodies and anti-EGFR antibodies, respectively; 23%, 38%, and 39% of patients received 1, 2, or ≥3 prior lines of therapy, respectively. Patients received tucatinib 300 mg orally twice daily with a loading dose of trastuzumab (or a non-US approved trastuzumab product) 8 mg/kg IV on day 1 of cycle 1, followed by a maintenance dose of trastuzumab 6 mg/kg on day 1 of each subsequent 21-day cycle. Patients were treated until disease progression or unacceptable toxicity occurred.

The major efficacy outcome measures were overall response rate and duration of response. At the time of evaluation, the overall response rate was 38%, with 3.6% of patients having a complete response and 35% a partial response. The median duration of response was 12.4 months; 81% of patients had a duration of response ≥6 months and 34% had a duration of response ≥12 months.

DOSAGE AND ADMINISTRATION

• General

Pretreatment Screening

- Serum ALT, AST, and bilirubin concentrations.
- Verify pregnancy status in females of reproductive potential.
- *In patients with unresectable or metastatic colorectal cancer*, confirm presence of specific RAS mutations mutations with an FDA-approved test.
- *In patients with unresectable or metastatic colorectal cancer*, confirm presence of HER2 overexpression or gene amplification with a laboratory assessment of tumor tissue.

Patient Monitoring

- Serum ALT, AST, and bilirubin concentrations every 3 weeks during therapy, and as clinically indicated.

Premedication and Prophylaxis

- Prophylactic use of antidiarrheal agents not required in HER2CLIMB study.

Dispensing and Administration Precautions

- Based on the Institute for Safe Medication Practices (ISMP), tucatinib is a high-alert medication that has a heightened risk of causing significant patient harm when used in error.

● Administration

Tucatinib is administered orally twice daily (approximately every 12 hours), at the same time each day, without regard to meals. Tucatinib tablets should be swallowed intact and should not be chewed, crushed, broken, cracked, or split.

If a dose of tucatinib is missed or vomited, the next dose should be taken at the regularly scheduled time.

● Dosage

Breast Cancer

For use in combination with trastuzumab and capecitabine for the treatment of HER2-positive advanced unresectable or metastatic breast cancer, the recommended adult dosage of tucatinib is 300 mg twice daily. Therapy should be continued until disease progression or unacceptable toxicity occurs.

Clinicians should consult the manufacturers' labelings or published protocols for information on the dosage, method of administration, and administration sequence of other antineoplastic agents used in combination regimens.

Tucatinib and capecitabine may be administered at the same time. In the HER2CLIMB study, capecitabine 1 g/m² twice daily was administered within 30 minutes after a meal on days 1–14 and trastuzumab 8 mg/kg IV initially, followed by either 6 mg/kg IV or 600 mg by subcutaneous injection was administered on day 1 of each 21-day cycle.

Colorectal Cancer

For use in combination with trastuzumab for the treatment of unresectable or metastatic colorectal cancer in adults, the recommended dosage of tucatinib is 300 mg twice daily. Therapy should be continued until disease progression or unacceptable toxicity

Clinicians should consult the manufacturers' labelings or published protocols for information on the dosage, method of administration, and administration sequence of other antineoplastic agents used in combination regimens.

Dosage Modification for Toxicity

If adverse reactions occur during tucatinib therapy, temporary interruption of therapy, dosage reduction, and/or permanent discontinuance of the drug may be necessary. If dosage reduction is required, the dosage of tucatinib should be reduced as described in Table 1.

TABLE 1. Dosage Reduction for Tucatinib Toxicity

Dose Reduction Level	Recommended Dosage Reductions for Adverse Reactions
First	250 mg twice daily
Second	200 mg twice daily
Third	150 mg twice daily
Fourth	Permanently discontinue tucatinib

Table 2 indicates the recommended dosage modification (i.e., temporary interruption of therapy, dosage reduction, discontinuance of therapy) for adverse effects according to severity.

TABLE 2. Dosage Modification for Tucatinib Toxicity

Adverse Reaction and Severity	Modification
Diarrhea (Grade 3 without anti-diarrheal treatment)	Initiate or intensify appropriate medical therapy. Hold tucatinib until recovery to ≤ Grade 1, then resume at the same dose level.
Diarrhea (Grade 3 with anti-diarrheal treatment)	Initiate or intensify appropriate medical therapy. Hold tucatinib until recovery to ≤ Grade 1, then resume at the next lower dose level.
Diarrhea (Grade 4)	Permanently discontinue
Hepatotoxicity (Grade 2 bilirubin [>1.5 to 3 × ULN])	Hold tucatinib until recovery to ≤ Grade 1, then resume at the same dose level.
Hepatotoxicity (Grade 3 ALT or AST [> 5 to 20 × ULN] OR Grade 3 bilirubin [> 3 to 10 × ULN])	Hold tucatinib until recovery to ≤ Grade 1, then resume at the next lower dose level.
Hepatotoxicity (Grade 4 ALT or AST [> 20 × ULN] OR Grade 4 bilirubin [> 10 × ULN])	Permanently discontinue
Hepatotoxicity (ALT or AST > 3 × ULN AND Bilirubin > 2 × ULN)	Permanently discontinue
Other adverse reactions (Grade 3)	Hold tucatinib until recovery to ≤ Grade 1, then resume at the next lower dose level.
Other adverse reactions (Grade 4)	Permanently discontinue

Concomitant Use of Drugs Affecting Hepatic Microsomal Enzymes

Concomitant use of tucatinib with potent inhibitors of cytochrome P-450 (CYP) isoenzyme 2C8 should be avoided. If concomitant use cannot be avoided, the manufacturer recommends reducing the dosage of tucatinib to 100 mg twice daily. If concomitant use of the potent CYP2C8 inhibitor is discontinued, the tucatinib dosage should be returned (after 3 elimination half-lives of the CYP2C8 inhibitor) to the dosage used prior to initiation of the CYP2C8 inhibitor.

● Special Populations

Hepatic Impairment

For patients with severe hepatic impairment (Child-Pugh class C), the manufacturer recommends a tucatinib dosage of 200 mg twice daily.

No dosage adjustment is necessary in patients with mild or moderate hepatic impairment (Child-Pugh class A or B).

Renal Impairment

No dosage adjustment is necessary in patients with mild or moderate renal impairment (creatinine clearance 30–89 mL/minute using Cockcroft-Gault formula).

Because capecitabine is contraindicated in patients with severe renal impairment (creatinine clearance less than 30 mL/minute using Cockcroft-Gault formula), combination therapy with tucatinib, capecitabine, and trastuzumab is not recommended in such patients.

Geriatric Use

The manufacturer makes no specific dosage recommendations for geriatric patients.

CAUTIONS

● Contraindications

None.

• Warnings/Precautions

Diarrhea

Severe diarrhea associated with dehydration, hypotension, acute kidney injury, and death has been reported in patients receiving tucatinib.

Antidiarrheal therapy should be administered as clinically indicated if diarrhea occurs during tucatinib therapy. Diagnostic tests should be performed as clinically indicated to exclude other causes of diarrhea. Temporary interruption, dosage reduction, or permanent discontinuance of tucatinib may be necessary depending on diarrhea severity.

In the HER2CLIMB study where tucatinib was used in combination with trastuzumab and capecitabine, diarrhea was reported in 81% of patients receiving tucatinib and was grade 3 or 4 in severity in 12 or 0.5% of patients, respectively. Death secondary to grade 4 diarrhea occurred in both patients who developed grade 4 diarrhea. The median time to initial onset of diarrhea was 12 days and the median time to resolution was 8 days. Dosage reduction or discontinuance of tucatinib therapy was necessary because of diarrhea in 6 or 1% of patients, respectively. In the HER2CLIMB study, antidiarrheal prophylaxis was not required.

In the MOUNTAINEER study where tucatinib was used in combination with trastuzumab, diarrhea was reported in 64% of patients, including grade 3 (3.5%), grade 2 (10%), and grade 1 (50%).

Hepatic Toxicity

Severe hepatotoxicity has been reported in patients receiving tucatinib.

In the HER2CLIMB study, elevations in ALT or AST concentration exceeding 5 times the upper limit of normal (ULN) occurred in 8 or 6% of patients receiving tucatinib, respectively. In this study, elevations in serum bilirubin concentration exceeding 3 times the ULN occurred in 1.5% of tucatinib-treated patients. Dosage reduction or discontinuance of tucatinib therapy was necessary because of hepatotoxicity in 8 or 1.5% of patients, respectively.

In the MOUNTAINEER study, elevations of ALT or AST concentration exceeding 5 times the ULN occurred in 4.7 or 6% of patients receiving tucatinib, respectively. In this study, elevations in serum bilirubin concentration exceeding 3 times the ULN occurrred in 6% of patients. Dosage reduction or discontinuation of tucatinib therapy was necessary because of hepatotoxicity in 3.5% and 2.3% of of patients, respectively.

Liver function tests (i.e., ALT, AST, bilirubin concentrations) should be evaluated prior to initiation of therapy, every 3 weeks thereafter, and as clinically indicated. Temporary interruption, dosage reduction, or permanent discontinuance of tucatinib may be necessary depending on the severity of hepatotoxicity.

Fetal/Neonatal Morbidity and Mortality

There are no adequate and well-controlled studies of tucatinib in pregnant women; however, based on its mechanism of action and animal findings, tucatinib may cause fetal harm. Embryofetal toxicity (e.g., increased fetal resorption, abortion, decreased fetal weight) and teratogenicity (e.g., skeletal, visceral, external malformations) have been demonstrated in pregnant animals receiving tucatinib at exposure levels 1.3 times or more the human exposure at the recommended dosage.

Pregnancy should be avoided during tucatinib therapy. The manufacturer states that a pregnancy test should be performed prior to initiation of tucatinib therapy in females of reproductive potential and that such women should be advised to use effective contraceptive methods while receiving tucatinib therapy and for at least 1 week after the last dose of the drug. In addition, men with such female partners should use effective contraceptive methods while receiving tucatinib and for at least 1 week after the last dose of the drug. Patients should be apprised of the potential hazard to the fetus if tucatinib is used during pregnancy.

Impairment of Fertility

Results of animal studies suggest that tucatinib may impair male and female fertility.

Specific Populations

Pregnancy

Tucatinib may cause fetal harm if administered to pregnant women based on its mechanism of action and animal findings.

Lactation

It is not known whether tucatinib or its metabolites are distributed into human milk. The effects of the drug on breast-fed infants or on the production of milk also are unknown.

Because of the potential for serious adverse reactions to tucatinib in breast-fed infants, women should be advised not to breast-feed while receiving the drug and for at least 1 week after the last dose.

Pediatric Use

Safety and efficacy of tucatinib have not been established in pediatric patients.

Geriatric Use

In the HER2CLIMB study, 26% of patients receiving tucatinib were 65 years of age or older, while 2.5% were 75 years of age or older. No overall differences in efficacy were observed between geriatric patients and younger adults. Patients 65 years of age or older had a higher incidence of serious adverse reactions (e.g., diarrhea, vomiting, nausea) compared with younger adults (34 or 24%, respectively). In the MOUNTAINEER study, 12 patients were 65 years of age or older; however, there were too few patients in this population to assess differences in effectiveness or safety in this study.

Hepatic Impairment

Following administration of a single 300-mg dose of tucatinib, area under the plasma concentration-time curve (AUC) of tucatinib in individuals with mild or moderate hepatic impairment (Child-Pugh class A or B) was similar to that in individuals with normal hepatic function, but was increased by 1.6-fold in those with severe hepatic impairment (Child-Pugh class C); therefore, the manufacturer recommends a tucatinib dosage of 200 mg twice daily in patients with severe hepatic impairment.

Renal Impairment

In a population pharmacokinetic analysis, mild or moderate renal impairment did not have clinically important effects on the pharmacokinetics of tucatinib; no dosage adjustment is necessary in patients with mild or moderate renal impairment.

The pharmacokinetic profile of tucatinib has not been established in patients with severe renal impairment.

• Common Adverse Effects

Adverse effects reported in at least 20% of patients with metastatic breast cancer receiving tucatinib in combination with trastuzumab and capecitabine include diarrhea, palmar-plantar erythrodysesthesia, nausea, hepatotoxicity, vomiting, stomatitis, decreased appetite, anemia, and rash.

Adverse effects reported in at least 20% of patients with unresectable or metastatic colorectal cancer receiving tucatinib in combination with trastuzumab include diarrhea, fatigue, rash, nausea, abdominal pain, infusion related reactions, and pyrexia.

Tucatinib has been shown to increase serum creatinine concentrations. Tucatinib decreases tubular secretion of creatinine by inhibiting renal organic cation transporter (OCT) 2 and multidrug and toxin extrusion transporter (MATE) 1. The mean increase in serum creatinine was 32%, reported within the initial 21 days of tucatinib therapy. Elevated concentrations of serum creatinine persisted during therapy and reversed in most patients following discontinuance of therapy. The manufacturer states that assessment of alternative markers for renal function may be necessary if elevated serum creatinine concentrations persist.

DRUG INTERACTIONS

Tucatinib is metabolized principally by cytochrome P-450 (CYP) isoenzyme 2C8 and, to a lesser extent, by CYP3A. In vitro, tucatinib demonstrates reversible inhibition of CYP isoenzymes 2C8 and 3A, and time-dependent inhibition of CYP3A. In vitro, the drug is not an inhibitor of CYP isoenzymes 1A2, 2B6, 2C9, 2C19, and 2D6, or uridine diphosphate-glucuronosyltransferase (UGT) 1A1.

In vitro studies indicate that tucatinib is a substrate of P-glycoprotein (P-gp) and breast cancer resistance protein (BCRP), but is not a substrate of organic anion transporter (OAT) 1, OAT3, organic cation transporter (OCT) 1, OCT3, organic anion transporting polypeptide (OATP) 1B1, OATP1B3, multidrug and toxin extrusion (MATE) 1, MATE2K, or bile salt export pump (BSEP).

● Drugs Affecting Hepatic Microsomal Enzymes

Inhibitors of CYP2C8

Concomitant use of tucatinib with potent inhibitors of CYP2C8 may result in increased systemic exposure to tucatinib and an increased incidence of adverse effects. Concomitant administration of the potent CYP2C8 inhibitor gemfibrozil (600 mg twice daily) with tucatinib (single 300-mg dose) increased the area under the concentration-time curve (AUC) and peak plasma concentration of tucatinib by 3- and 1.6-fold, respectively.

Concomitant use of tucatinib with potent inhibitors of CYP2C8 should be avoided. If concomitant use of a potent CYP2C8 inhibitor cannot be avoided, the manufacturer recommends reducing the dosage of tucatinib to 100 mg twice daily. If concomitant use of the potent CYP2C8 inhibitor is discontinued, the tucatinib dosage should be returned (after 3 elimination half-lives of the CYP2C8 inhibitor) to the dosage used prior to initiation of the CYP2C8 inhibitor.

If concomitant therapy with a moderate CYP2C8 inhibitor is required, patients should be monitored closely for signs of tucatinib toxicity.

Inducers of CYP3A or 2C8

Concomitant use of tucatinib with potent CYP3A or moderate CYP2C8 inducers may result in decreased systemic exposure to tucatinib and reduced tucatinib efficacy. Concomitant administration of the potent CYP3A and moderate CYP2C8 inducer rifampin (600 mg once daily) with tucatinib (single 300-mg dose) decreased AUC and peak plasma concentration of tucatinib by 48 and 37%, respectively.

Concomitant use of tucatinib with potent CYP3A or moderate CYP2C8 inducers should be avoided.

Inhibitors of CYP3A

When the potent CYP3A inhibitor itraconazole (200 mg twice daily) was administered concomitantly with tucatinib (single 300-mg dose), both AUC and peak plasma concentration of tucatinib increased by 1.3-fold.

● Drugs Metabolized by Hepatic Microsomal Enzymes

Substrates of CYP3A

Concomitant use of tucatinib with CYP3A substrates may result in increased systemic exposure to the CYP3A substrate and increased incidence of adverse effects of the substrate drug. When the CYP3A substrate midazolam (single 2-mg dose) was administered concomitantly with tucatinib (300 mg twice daily), AUC and peak plasma concentration of midazolam increased 5.7- and 3-fold, respectively.

Concomitant use of tucatinib with CYP3A substrates that have a narrow therapeutic index should be avoided. If concomitant use of CYP3A substrates that have a narrow therapeutic index cannot be avoided, the dosage of the CYP3A substrate should be adjusted as appropriate.

● Drugs Affected by Transport Systems

Substrates of P-gp

Concomitant use of tucatinib with P-gp substrates may result in increased systemic exposure of the P-gp substrate and increased incidence of adverse effects of the substrate drug. When the P-gp substrate digoxin (single 0.5-mg dose) was administered concomitantly with tucatinib (300 mg twice daily), AUC and peak plasma concentrations of digoxin increased 1.5- and 2.4-fold, respectively.

If concomitant use of P-gp substrates that have a narrow therapeutic index is required, the dosage of the P-gp substrate should be adjusted as appropriate.

Substrates of MATE1, MATE2K, and OCT2

When a single 850-mg dose of metformin hydrochloride (a substrate of MATE1, MATE2K, and OCT2) was administered concomitantly with tucatinib (300 mg twice daily for 7 days), AUC and peak plasma concentrations of metformin increased 1.4- and 1.1-fold, respectively. Tucatinib reduced the renal clearance of metformin without any effect on glomerular filtration rate (GFR).

● Omeprazole

Concomitant administration of tucatinib and the proton-pump inhibitor omeprazole did not affect the pharmacokinetics of tucatinib.

● Tolbutamide

Concomitant administration of tucatinib and tolbutamide (sensitive CYP2C9 substrate) did not have a clinically important effect on the pharmacokinetics of tucatinib.

DESCRIPTION

Tucatinib, a highly selective, reversible tyrosine kinase inhibitor of human epidermal growth factor receptor type 2 (HER2), is an antineoplastic agent. In vitro, the drug has been shown to inhibit phosphorylation of HER2 and HER3 resulting in inhibition of downstream signaling of the mitogen-activated protein kinase (MAPK) and phosphoinositide 3-kinase (PI3K/Akt) pathways. In vivo, tucatinib has demonstrated inhibition of cellular proliferation of HER2-expressing tumors. The combination of tucatinib with trastuzumab demonstrated increased antitumor activity compared with either drug alone.

In cell-based assays, tucatinib has demonstrated 500-fold greater selectivity for HER2 than for epidermal growth factor receptor (EGFR), thereby potentially reducing the incidence of adverse effects associated with EGFR inhibition, such as adverse GI and dermatologic effects.

Area under the serum concentration-time curve (AUC) and peak plasma concentrations of tucatinib are dose proportional over a dosage range of 50–300 mg. Following oral administration of tucatinib, peak plasma concentrations of the drug are achieved in a median of approximately 2 hours (range 1–4 hours). With twice-daily administration, steady-state concentrations of the drug are achieved in approximately 4 days and the accumulation based on geometric mean AUC accumulation ratios ranged from 2–2.5-fold. Administration of tucatinib (single 300-mg dose) with a high-fat meal decreased the rate of absorption (time to peak concentrations delayed by 2.5 hours) and increased the mean AUC by 1.5-fold, but did not substantially affect peak plasma concentration; however, these changes are not considered clinically meaningful. Tucatinib is 97.1% bound to plasma proteins at clinically relevant concentrations. Tucatinib is metabolized principally by cytochrome P-450 (CYP) isoenzyme 2C8 and, to a lesser extent, by CYP3A. Following oral administration of a single radiolabeled dose of tucatinib, approximately 86% of the radioactivity was recovered in feces (16% of the dose as unchanged drug) and 4.1% was recovered in urine. The mean elimination half-life of tucatinib is 11.9 hours in patients with metastatic breast cancer and 16.4 hours in patients with metastatic colorectal cancer. Systemic exposure of tucatinib is not affected by age, serum albumin concentration (2.5–5.2 g/dL), body weight (41–138 kg), and race (white, Black, or Asian).

ADVICE TO PATIENTS

- Advise the patient to read the FDA-approved patient labeling (Patient Information).
- Inform patients that tucatinib has been associated with severe diarrhea. Instruct patients on how to manage diarrhea and to inform their healthcare provider immediately if there is any change in bowel patterns.
- Inform patients that tucatinib has been associated with severe hepatotoxicity and that they should report signs and symptoms of liver dysfunction to their healthcare provider immediately.
- Inform pregnant women and females of reproductive potential of the risk to a fetus. Advise women to inform their healthcare provider of a known or suspected pregnancy.
- Advise females of reproductive potential to use effective contraception during treatment with tucatinib and for at least 1 week after the last dose.

- Advise male patients with female partners of reproductive potential to use effective contraception during treatment with tucatinib and for at least 1 week after the last dose.

- Advise women not to breast-feed during treatment with tucatinib and for at least 1 week after the last dose.

- Advise males and females of reproductive potential that tucatinib may impair fertility.

- Inform clinicians of existing or contemplated concomitant therapy, including prescription and OTC drugs and dietary or herbal supplements, as well as any concomitant illnesses.

- Inform patients of other important precautionary information.

For further information on the handling of antineoplastic agents, see the ASHP Guidelines on Handling Hazardous Drugs at https://www.ahfsdrug information.com.

PREPARATIONS

Tucatinib is available only from a designated specialty pharmacy. The manufacturer should be contacted for additional information.

Excipients in commercially available drug preparations may have clinically important effects in some individuals; consult specific product labeling for details.

Tucatinib

Oral

Tablets, film-coated	50 mg	Tukysa®, Seattle Genetics
	150 mg	Tukysa®, Seattle Genetics

Selected Revisions September 28, 2023, © Copyright, May 18, 2020, American Society of Health-System Pharmacists, Inc.

Vandetanib

10:00 • ANTINEOPLASTIC AGENTS

REMS

FDA approved a REMS for vandetanib to ensure that the benefits outweigh the risks. The REMS may apply to one or more preparations of vandetanib and consists of the following: elements to assure safe use and implementation system. See the FDA REMS page (https://www.accessdata.fda.gov/scripts/cder/rems/index.cfm).

■ Vandetanib, an inhibitor of multiple receptor tyrosine kinases, is an antineoplastic agent.

USES

● Medullary Thyroid Cancer

Vandetanib is used for the treatment of symptomatic or progressive medullary thyroid cancer in patients with unresectable locally advanced or metastatic disease; designated an orphan drug by FDA for the treatment of this cancer.

Use vandetanib in patients with indolent, asymptomatic, or slowly progressing disease only after careful consideration of the treatment-related risks of the drug.

Clinical Experience

The current indication for vandetanib is based principally on the results of a randomized, double-blind, placebo-controlled, phase 3 study in patients with unresectable locally advanced or metastatic medullary thyroid cancer. In this study, 331 patients were randomized in a 2:1 ratio to receive either vandetanib (300 mg) or placebo once daily until disease progression occurred. Upon disease progression, patients were eligible to receive open-label vandetanib; 19 or 58% of patients initially randomized to receive vandetanib or placebo, respectively, opted to receive open-label vandetanib. The median duration of treatment during the randomized phase of the study was 90.1 weeks for vandetanib-treated patients and 39.9 weeks for placebo-treated patients. At the time of the primary analysis, patients receiving vandetanib experienced prolonged median progression-free survival (30.5 [predicted via a Weibull model] versus 19.3 months) and a higher overall objective response rate (45 versus 13%) compared with patients receiving placebo. Overall survival data were immature at analysis cutoff.

Clinical Perspective

The American Thyroid Association (ATA) published a guideline on management of medullary thyroid cancer in 2015. Single agent or combination cytotoxic chemotherapy regimens in patients with medullary thyroid cancer is characterized by low response rates and short durations of response; therefore, single agent or combination cytotoxic chemotherapy regimens are not recommended as first-line therapy in patients with persistent or recurrent medullary thyroid cancer. Systemic therapy with tyrosine kinase inhibitors targeting both rearranged during transfection (RET) proto-oncogene and vascular endothelial growth factor receptor (VEGFR) should be considered in patients with significant tumor burden and symptomatic or progressive metastatic disease. The ATA states that cabozantinib or vandetanib can be used as single-agent first-line therapy in patients with advanced progressive disease. Other experts also recommend cabozantinib and vandetanib (both strong recommendations based on high-quality evidence) as first-line systemic therapy in patients with progressive metastatic medullary thyroid cancer.

DOSAGE AND ADMINISTRATION

● General

Pretreatment Screening

- Measure ECG, serum electrolytes (i.e., calcium, magnesium, potassium), and thyroid-stimulating hormone (TSH) concentrations at baseline.

- Verify the pregnancy status of females of reproductive potential prior to initiating treatment with vandetanib.

Patient Monitoring

- Measure ECG, serum electrolytes (i.e., calcium, magnesium, potassium), and TSH concentrations 2–4 weeks and 8–12 weeks after initiating vandetanib, and then every 3 months thereafter.

- Following dosage reduction for QT prolongation or therapy interruption lasting >2 weeks, monitor ECG 2–4 weeks and 8–12 weeks after resuming vandetanib, and then every 3 months thereafter.

- If diarrhea occurs, monitor electrolytes and ECG more frequently.

- In patients with moderate renal impairment, closely monitor ECG.

- If vandetanib is used concomitantly with a drug known to prolong the QT interval, monitor ECG more frequently.

- Monitor for manifestations of heart failure.

- Monitor blood pressure.

- Perform ophthalmologic examination, including slit lamp examinations, in patients who report visual changes.

- Adverse reactions may not resolve quickly because the drug has a long half-life. Monitor patients appropriately.

Dispensing and Administration Precautions
Handling and Disposal

- Consult specialized references for procedures for proper handling and disposal of antineoplastics.

- Avoid direct contact of crushed tablets with skin or mucous membranes. If such contact occurs, wash affected area thoroughly.

REMS

- FDA requires a Risk Evaluation and Mitigation Strategy (REMS) for vandetanib because of risk of QT interval prolongation, torsades de pointes, and sudden death.

- Available only under a restricted distribution program (CAPRELSA® REMS Program). Contact 800-817-2722 or visit https://www.caprelsarems.com for additional information and to enroll in the program for vandetanib.

Other General Considerations

- Discontinue vandetanib ≥1 month prior to scheduled surgery. Do not resume vandetanib for ≥2 weeks following major surgery and until adequate wound healing has occurred.

- Use sun protection during vandetanib therapy and for ≥4 months after discontinuance of the drug.

● Administration

Administer vandetanib orally without regard to meals. Swallow vandetanib tablets whole and do *not* crush.

If a dose is missed, do not take the missed dose if it is ≤12 hours until the next scheduled dose.

If vandetanib tablets cannot be swallowed whole, the manufacturer states that the tablet may be dispersed in a glass containing 60 mL (2 ounces) of noncarbonated water; no other liquids should be used. Stir the water, without crushing the tablet, for approximately 10 minutes until the tablet is dispersed; the tablet will not completely dissolve. Swallow the aqueous dispersion immediately; to ensure the full dose is administered, mix any residue in the glass with an additional 120 mL (4 ounces) of noncarbonated water and swallow. The aqueous dispersion also may be administered through a nasogastric or gastrostomy tube.

Avoid direct contact of crushed tablets with skin or mucous membranes. If such contact occurs, wash the affected area thoroughly.

Follow procedures for proper handling and disposal of antineoplastic drugs when preparing or administering vandetanib.

• Dosage

Medullary Thyroid Cancer

The recommended adult dosage of vandetanib for the treatment of symptomatic or progressive medullary thyroid cancer in patients with unresectable locally advanced or metastatic disease is 300 mg once daily. Continue therapy until disease progression or unacceptable toxicity occurs.

Dosage Modification for Toxicity

If grade 3 or greater toxicity occurs, interrupt vandetanib therapy. When the toxicity resolves or improves to grade 1, vandetanib may be resumed at a reduced dosage. Reduce the dosage of vandetanib in decrements of 100 mg daily (i.e., from 300 to 200 mg daily, from 200 to 100 mg daily).

Dosage Modification for Cardiovascular Toxicity

Interrupt vandetanib therapy if the QT interval (corrected for heart rate using Fridericia's formula [QT$_c$F]) exceeds 500 msec. When QT$_c$F returns to less than 450 msec, vandetanib may be resumed at a reduced dosage.

If hypertension occurs, dosage reduction or temporary interruption of vandetanib therapy may be necessary to control blood pressure. If hypertension cannot be controlled, vandetanib should not be resumed.

Dosage Modification for Dermatologic Toxicity

If severe skin reactions occur, permanently discontinue vandetanib therapy and refer the patient for urgent medical evaluation. Systemic therapy (e.g., corticosteroids) may be required.

Dosage Modification for Diarrhea

If severe diarrhea occurs, interrupt vandetanib therapy. When diarrhea improves, vandetanib may be resumed at a reduced dosage.

• Special Populations

Hepatic Impairment

Vandetanib should not be used in patients with moderate (Child-Pugh class B) or severe (Child-Pugh class C) hepatic impairment.

Renal Impairment

Reduce the initial dosage of vandetanib to 200 mg once daily in patients with moderate (creatinine clearance of 30–49 mL/minute) renal impairment. Vandetanib is not recommended for use in patients with severe (creatinine clearance less than 30 mL/minute) renal impairment. There is no information on use of vandetanib in patients with end-stage renal disease requiring dialysis.

Geriatric Patients

The manufacturer makes no specific dosage recommendations in patients ≥65 years of age.

CAUTIONS

• Contraindications

- Congenital long QT syndrome.

• Warnings/Precautions

Warnings

Prolongation of QT Interval and Torsades de Pointes

The prescribing information of vandetanib contains a boxed warning regarding the risk of QT prolongation, torsade de pointes, and sudden death. Vandetanib prolongs the QT interval in a concentration-dependent manner. Torsades de pointes, ventricular tachycardia, and sudden death have been reported in patients receiving vandetanib. In the phase 3 clinical study, patients randomized to receive vandetanib (300 once daily) had a mean increase in the QT interval (corrected for heart rate using Fridericia's formula [QT$_c$F]) of 35 msec (range: 33–36 msec) from baseline; this increase in QT$_c$F remained above 30 msec for the duration of the study (up to 2 years). In addition, an increase in QT$_c$F of more than 60 msec from baseline occurred in 36% of patients receiving vandetanib, and QT$_c$F exceeded 450 msec or 500 msec in 69 or 7% of patients, respectively.

Vandetanib should not be initiated in patients with QT$_c$F exceeding 450 msec. The drug should not be used in patients who have a history of torsades de pointes, congenital long QT syndrome, bradyarrhythmias, or uncompensated heart failure, or in patients with electrolyte disturbances; hypocalcemia, hypokalemia, and/or hypomagnesemia must be corrected prior to administration of vandetanib. Vandetanib has not been evaluated in patients with ventricular arrhythmias or recent myocardial infarction (MI).

Measure ECG, serum electrolytes (i.e., calcium, magnesium, potassium), and thyroid-stimulating hormone (TSH) concentrations at baseline, at 2–4 weeks and 8–12 weeks after initiating vandetanib, and then every 3 months thereafter. Following dosage reduction for QT prolongation or therapy interruption lasting longer than 2 weeks, monitor ECG as described above. Serum potassium concentrations should be at least 4 mEq/L (within normal range), and serum magnesium and calcium concentrations should be maintained within normal ranges, to reduce the risk of QT interval prolongation. Monitor electrolytes and ECG more frequently in patients who experience diarrhea. Concomitant use of vandetanib with drugs known to prolong the QT interval should be avoided. If a drug known to prolong the QT interval must be administered, more frequent ECG monitoring is recommended.

Vandetanib exposure is increased in patients with impaired renal function. Reduce the initial dose of vandetanib to 200 mg in patients with moderate renal impairment and monitor the QT interval frequently.

Interrupt vandetanib therapy if QT$_c$F exceeds 500 msec. When QT$_c$F returns to less than 450 msec, vandetanib may be resumed at a reduced dosage.

Other Warnings and Precautions

Severe Skin Reactions

Severe skin reactions (including toxic epidermal necrolysis [TEN] and Stevens-Johnson syndrome), some resulting in death, have been reported in patients receiving vandetanib. If severe skin reactions occur, permanently discontinue vandetanib therapy and refer the patient for urgent medical evaluation. Systemic therapy (e.g., corticosteroids) may be required.

Photosensitivity reactions, occurring during therapy and up to 4 months after treatment discontinuation, may also occur.

Interstitial Lung Disease

Interstitial lung disease or pneumonitis, sometimes fatal, has been reported in patients receiving vandetanib. The mechanism of action of this adverse effect is unknown; however, review of available data (including data in patients receiving vandetanib for non-small cell lung cancer†) suggested that Japanese ethnicity, history of smoking, coincidence of interstitial pneumonia, preexisting pulmonary fibrosis, male gender, and previous radiation or chemotherapy may be possible risk factors for developing interstitial lung disease.

Interstitial lung disease should be considered in patients presenting with nonspecific respiratory signs or symptoms. If pulmonary symptoms are acute or worsening, interrupt vandetanib therapy. If interstitial lung disease is confirmed, discontinue vandetanib.

Ischemic Cerebrovascular Events

Ischemic cerebrovascular events, sometimes fatal, have been reported with vandetanib. In the phase 3 clinical study, ischemic cerebrovascular events were observed more frequently with vandetanib compared with placebo (1.3 versus 0%); all ischemic cerebrovascular events reported in this study were grade 3. Vandetanib should be discontinued in patients who experience a severe ischemic cerebrovascular event. The safety of resumption of vandetanib therapy after resolution of an ischemic cerebrovascular event has not been studied.

Hemorrhage

Serious hemorrhagic events, sometimes fatal, have been reported with vandetanib. Vandetanib should not be used in patients with a recent history of hemoptysis (2.5 mL of red blood or more). Vandetanib should be discontinued in patients with severe hemorrhage.

Heart Failure

Heart failure, sometimes fatal, has been reported with vandetanib use. In the phase 3 clinical study, heart failure occurred in 0.9% of patients receiving vandetanib compared with 0% of those receiving placebo. Monitor patients for manifestations of heart failure. If heart failure occurs, discontinuance of vandetanib may be necessary; heart failure may not be reversible following discontinuance of vandetanib.

Hypertension

Hypertension and hypertensive crisis have been reported in 33% of patients receiving vandetanib. Monitor blood pressure in all patients and control as appropriate. Dosage reduction or temporary interruption of vandetanib therapy may be necessary. If hypertension cannot be controlled, vandetanib should *not* be resumed.

Diarrhea

Diarrhea has been reported in patients receiving vandetanib. In the phase 3 clinical study, diarrhea or colitis (all grades) was reported in 57% and grade 3–4 diarrhea or colitis was reported in 11% of patients receiving vandetanib. Because diarrhea may cause electrolyte imbalances, and because QT interval prolongation has been reported in patients receiving vandetanib, the manufacturer recommends careful and more frequent monitoring of serum electrolytes and ECG in patients who develop diarrhea. If severe diarrhea occurs, interrupt vandetanib therapy. When symptoms improve, resume vandetanib at a reduced dosage.

Hypothyroidism

In the phase 3 clinical study in which 90% of enrolled patients had prior thyroidectomy, increases in the dosages of thyroid replacement therapy were required in 49% of patients receiving vandetanib compared with 17% of patients receiving placebo.

Monitor TSH concentrations at baseline, at 2–4 weeks and 8–12 weeks after initiating vandetanib, and then every 3 months thereafter. If manifestations of hypothyroidism occur, examine thyroid hormone concentrations and adjust thyroid replacement therapy accordingly.

Reversible Posterior Leukoencephalopathy Syndrome

Reversible posterior leukoencephalopathy syndrome (RPLS) has been reported in patients receiving vandetanib.

Consider RPLS in any patient presenting with seizures, headache, visual disturbances, confusion, or altered mental function. In clinical studies, 3 of the 4 patients who developed RPLS also had hypertension. Discontinue vandetanib if RPLS occurs.

Renal Failure

Renal failure has been reported in patients administered vandetanib. Withhold, reduce the dose, or permanently discontinue therapy based on severity.

In moderate renal impairment, reduce the starting dose of vandetanib. In severe renal impairment, vandetanib is *not* recommended for use.

Impaired Wound Healing

Impaired wound healing can occur in patients who receive drugs that inhibit the VEGF signaling pathway such as vandetanib.

The manufacturer recommends discontinuing vandetanib at least 1 month prior to scheduled surgery. Do not administer vandetanib for at least 2 weeks following major surgery and until adequate wound healing has occurred.

The safety of resuming vandetanib after resolution of wound healing complications has not been established.

Fetal/Neonatal Morbidity and Mortality

Based on its mechanism of action and animal findings, vandetanib may cause fetal harm if administered to pregnant women; the drug has been shown to be embryotoxic, fetotoxic, and teratogenic in animals.

Advise females of reproductive potential, and males with female partners of reproductive potential, to use effective contraception during treatment with vandetanib and for 4 months following the last dose. If vandetanib is used during pregnancy or if the patient becomes pregnant while receiving the drug, apprise the patient of the potential fetal hazard.

Specific Populations

Pregnancy

Based on its mechanism of action and animal findings, vandetanib can cause fetal harm when administered to a pregnant woman. In animal studies, vandetanib was embryotoxic, fetotoxic, and teratogenic at exposures equivalent to or lower than those expected at the 300-mg clinical dose; adverse effects on female fertility, embryofetal development, and postnatal development of pups also were observed.

Advise patients of the potential hazard to a fetus. Advise females of reproductive potential, and males with female partners of reproductive potential, to use effective contraception during treatment with vandetanib and for 4 months following the last dose.

Lactation

Vandetanib is distributed into milk in rats. It is not known whether vandetanib or its metabolites are distributed into human milk. The effects of vandetanib on the breast-fed child or on milk production are also unknown. Because of the potential for serious adverse reactions to vandetanib in nursing infants, advise females not to breast-feed during vandetanib therapy and for 4 months after the final dose.

Females and Males of Reproductive Potential

Verify the pregnancy status of females of reproductive potential prior to initiating treatment with vandetanib. Advise females of reproductive potential, and males with female partners of reproductive potential, to use effective contraception during treatment with vandetanib and for 4 months after the final dose.

There are no data on the effects of vandetanib on human fertility. Based on animal studies, vandetanib may impair male and female fertility.

Pediatric Use

Safety and efficacy of vandetanib have not been established in pediatric patients.

Geriatric Use

The phase 3 clinical study in patients with medullary thyroid cancer did not include sufficient numbers of patients ≥65 years of age to determine whether they respond differently than younger patients.

Hepatic Impairment

In a pharmacokinetic study in which a limited number of individuals received a single 800-mg dose of vandetanib, mean area under the plasma concentration-time curve (AUC) and clearance of the drug were comparable between individuals with mild (Child-Pugh class A), moderate (Child-Pugh class B), or severe (Child-Pugh class C) hepatic impairment and individuals with normal hepatic function. There are limited data in patients with serum bilirubin concentrations exceeding 1.5 times the upper limit of normal (ULN).

Because safety and efficacy of vandetanib have not been established, use of the drug is not recommended in patients with moderate or severe hepatic impairment.

Renal Impairment

In a pharmacokinetic study in which a limited number of individuals received a single 800-mg dose of vandetanib, mean AUC and clearance of the drug were comparable between individuals with mild renal impairment and individuals with normal renal function; however, in individuals with moderate or severe renal impairment, mean AUC of vandetanib was increased by 39 or 41%, respectively, compared with individuals with normal renal function.

Patients with moderate renal impairment should receive a lower initial dosage of vandetanib; closely monitor ECG in these patients. Vandetanib is not recommended for use in patients with severe renal impairment.

Vandetanib has not been evaluated systematically in patients with end-stage renal disease requiring dialysis.

● Common Adverse Effects

Adverse effects reported in more than 20% of patients receiving vandetanib include diarrhea/colitis, rash, acneiform dermatitis, hypertension, nausea, headache, upper respiratory tract infections, decreased appetite, abdominal pain, hypocalcemia, increased ALT concentrations, and hypoglycemia.

DRUG INTERACTIONS

● *Drugs Affecting Hepatic Microsomal Enzymes*

Concomitant use of vandetanib with a potent inhibitor of cytochrome P-450 (CYP) isoenzyme 3A4 (CYP3A4) (i.e., itraconazole) resulted in no clinically important interaction.

Inducers of CYP3A4 can alter plasma vandetanib concentrations. Concomitant use of vandetanib with potent CYP3A4 inducers (e.g., carbamazepine, dexamethasone, phenobarbital, phenytoin, rifabutin, rifampin, rifapentine) should be *avoided*. In healthy subjects receiving a single oral 300-mg dose of vandetanib on day 1 and day 10 in combination with rifampin 600 mg daily on days 1–31, a 40% decrease in mean AUC of vandetanib, with no clinically meaningful change in mean maximum peak vandetanib concentrations, was observed; in addition, mean AUC and peak plasma concentrations of N-desmethylvandetanib increased by 266% and 414%, respectively. St. John's wort (*Hypericum perforatum*) may unpredictably decrease vandetanib exposure, and concomitant use of vandetanib with this agent also should be avoided.

● *Drugs Metabolized by Hepatic Microsomal Enzymes*

No effects on the mean peak plasma concentration and AUC of midazolam were observed when a single oral 7.5-mg dose of midazolam (a sensitive CYP3A4 substrate) was administered 8 days after a single 800-mg oral dose of vandetanib in healthy subjects.

● *Drugs that Prolong the QT Interval*

Concomitant use of vandetanib with drugs known to prolong the QT interval, including class Ia (e.g., disopyramide, procainamide, quinidine) and class III (e.g., amiodarone, sotalol, dofetilide) antiarrhythmic agents, some anti-infectives (e.g., clarithromycin, moxifloxacin), some antipsychotic agents (e.g., chlorpromazine, thioridazine, haloperidol, olanzapine, pimozide, quetiapine, ziprasidone), some type 3 serotonin (5-HT$_3$) receptor antagonists used as antiemetic agents (e.g., dolasetron, granisetron, ondansetron), chloroquine, and methadone should be *avoided*. If a drug known to prolong the QT interval must be administered, more frequent ECG monitoring is recommended. If a 5-HT$_3$ receptor antagonist is clinically necessary, some clinicians prefer granisetron because its effects on ECG intervals are less pronounced than those observed with dolasetron or ondansetron.

● *Drugs Affecting Organic Cation Transporter Type 2*

Vandetanib increased plasma concentrations of metformin, which is transported by organic cation transporter type 2 (OCT2). An increase of 74 and 50% in the mean AUC and peak plasma concentration, respectively, of metformin was observed when metformin (single 1-g dose) was administered 3 hours after vandetanib (single 800-mg dose) in healthy subjects. Use with caution and closely monitor for toxicities when vandetanib is used concomitantly with drugs that are transported by OCT2.

● *Digoxin*

Vandetanib increased plasma concentrations of digoxin (a P-glycoprotein [P-gp] substrate). Digoxin peak plasma concentrations and mean AUC increased by 29 and 23%, respectively, in healthy subjects receiving digoxin (single 0.25-mg dose) in combination with vandetanib (single 300-mg dose). Use with caution and closely monitor for digoxin toxicity when vandetanib is used concomitantly with digoxin.

● *Omeprazole*

No clinically meaningful effects on the mean AUC and peak plasma concentration of vandetanib were observed when vandetanib (single 300-mg dose) was administered alone and in combination with omeprazole (40 mg once daily for 5 days) in healthy subjects.

DESCRIPTION

Vandetanib, an inhibitor of multiple receptor tyrosine kinases, is an antineoplastic agent. Receptor tyrosine kinases (RTKs) are involved in the initiation of various cascades of intracellular signaling events that lead to cell proliferation and/or influence processes critical to cell survival and tumor progression (e.g., angiogenesis, metastasis, inhibition of apoptosis), based on the respective kinase. Various tyrosine kinases and pathways are abnormally activated in medullary thyroid carcinoma cells (e.g., rearranged during transfection [RET] proto-oncogene signaling is associated with development of hereditary medullary thyroid cancer). *In vitro* studies have shown that vandetanib inhibits the activity of multiple receptor tyrosine kinases, including vascular endothelial growth factor receptors (i.e., VEGFR-1, VEGFR-2, VEGFR-3), members of the epidermal growth factor receptor (EGFR) family, RET, protein tyrosine kinase 6 (BRK), TIE2, members of the EPH receptor kinase family, and members of the Src family of tyrosine kinases. The N-desmethyl metabolite of the drug, which represents 7 to 17.1% of vandetanib exposure, has similar inhibitory activity to the parent compound for VEGF receptors (KDR and Flt-1) and EGFR. *In vivo*, vandetanib has been shown to reduce tumor cell-induced angiogenesis and tumor vessel permeability; the drug also has been shown to inhibit tumor growth and metastasis in mouse models of cancer.

Vandetanib is partially metabolized by cytochrome P-450 (CYP) isoenzyme 3A4. Approximately 44 or 25% of an oral dose of the drug is excreted in feces or urine, respectively, as unchanged drug or metabolites. The terminal half-life of vandetanib is 19 days. Limited data indicate that systemic exposure to vandetanib is higher in Japanese and Chinese patients than in Caucasian patients receiving the same dose.

ADVICE TO PATIENTS

- A copy of the manufacturer's patient information (medication guide) for vandetanib must be provided to all patients with each prescription of the drug. Advise patients to read the medication guide prior to initiation of therapy and each time the prescription is refilled.

- Stress importance of not crushing vandetanib tablets. Avoid direct contact of crushed tablets with the skin or mucous membranes.

- If a dose is missed, do not take the missed dose if it is <12 hours before the next dose.

- Risk of QT interval prolongation, torsades de pointes, ventricular tachycardia, and sudden death. Stress importance of regular monitoring of ECG and serum electrolytes. Contact clinician promptly if feelings of lightheadedness or faintness or an irregular heartbeat occurs.

- Risk of photosensitivity/phototoxicity reactions. Use sunscreen and protective clothing and limit sun exposure during therapy and for at least 4 months after discontinuance of the drug.

- Risk of severe adverse dermatologic effects. Contact clinician promptly if dermatologic manifestations (e.g., rash; acne; dry skin; itching; blisters on skin or in mouth; peeling; fever; muscle or joint aches; redness or swelling of face, hands, or soles of feet) occur.

- Risk of interstitial lung disease. Promptly report new or worsening respiratory manifestations (e.g., shortness of breath, persistent cough, fever).

- Risk of diarrhea. Contact clinician if diarrhea occurs.

- Risk of reversible posterior leukoencephalopathy syndrome (RPLS). Contact clinician promptly if seizures, headache, visual disturbances, confusion, or difficulty thinking occurs.

- Risk of impaired wound healing. Inform clinician of any planned surgical procedure.

- Advise females of reproductive potential, and male partners of females of reproductive potential, to use an effective method of contraception while receiving vandetanib and for 4 months after discontinuance. Advise females to contact their clinician if they become pregnant, or if pregnancy is suspected, during treatment with vandetanib. Discontinue nursing while receiving vandetanib therapy and for 4 months after the final dose.

- Risk of blurred vision. Avoid driving a vehicle or operating machinery if blurred vision occurs.

- Stress importance of informing clinician of existing or contemplated concomitant therapy, including prescription and OTC drugs and herbal supplements, as well as any concomitant illnesses (e.g., hepatic or renal impairment, cardiovascular disease).

- Inform patients of other important precautionary information.

For further information on the handling of antineoplastic agents, see the ASHP Guidelines on Handling Hazardous Drugs at https://www.ahfsdruginformation.com.

PREPARATIONS

Excipients in commercially available drug preparations may have clinically important effects in some individuals; consult specific product labeling for details.

Distribution of vandetanib is restricted. Contact 800-817-2722 or visit https://www.caprelsarems.com for specific availability information.

Vandetanib

Oral

Tablets, film-coated	100 mg	**Caprelsa®**, Genzyme Corporation
	300 mg	**Caprelsa®**, Genzyme Corporation

† Use is not currently included in the labeling approved by the US Food and Drug Administration.

Selected Revisions October 10, 2024, © Copyright, November 3, 2011, American Society of Health-System Pharmacists, Inc.

Vemurafenib

10:00 • ANTINEOPLASTIC AGENTS

■ Vemurafenib, an inhibitor of b-Raf serine-threonine kinase with V600E mutation (*BRAF* V600E), is an antineoplastic agent.

USES

● Melanoma

Vemurafenib is used for the treatment of unresectable or metastatic melanoma with *BRAF* V600E mutation. Vemurafenib is designated an orphan drug by the US Food and Drug Administration (FDA) for the treatment of this cancer. An FDA-approved diagnostic test (e.g., cobas® 4800 BRAF V600 Mutation Test) is required to confirm the presence of the *BRAF* V600E mutation prior to initiation of therapy.

The current indication for vemurafenib is based principally on the results of a randomized, open-label phase 3 study (BRIM-3) in patients with previously untreated, unresectable or metastatic melanoma. All patients in this study tested positive for the *BRAF* V600E mutation detected by the cobas® 4800 BRAF V600 Mutation Test. In this study, 675 patients were randomized in a 1:1 ratio to receive either vemurafenib (960 mg orally twice daily) or dacarbazine (1 g/m^2 IV every 3 weeks). Treatment was continued until disease progression or unacceptable toxicity occurred, or the patient withdrew from the study. The primary endpoints of this study were overall survival and progression-free survival. The median age of patients enrolled in the study was 54 years. Most of the patients had metastatic disease (95%).

A planned interim analysis for overall survival indicated a reduction in the risk of death by 63% and a higher rate of overall survival at 6 months of therapy in patients receiving vemurafenib than in those receiving dacarbazine (84 versus 64%). The median follow-up period at the time of the interim analysis was 3.8 months for those receiving vemurafenib and 2.3 months for those receiving dacarbazine. Because of the survival benefit observed at the interim analysis, study investigators permitted patients previously randomized to receive dacarbazine to cross over to open-label vemurafenib therapy. A final analysis for progression-free survival estimated a prolonged median progression-free survival (5.3 versus 1.6 months) and reduction in risk of either death or disease progression (74%) in patients receiving vemurafenib compared with those receiving dacarbazine. An updated overall survival analysis with a median follow-up of 13.4 months confirmed prolonged median overall survival (13.6 versus 10.3 months; hazard ratio for death: 0.47) in patients receiving vemurafenib compared with those receiving dacarbazine. Patients receiving vemurafenib also had a higher objective response rate (48.4 versus 5.5%) compared with those receiving dacarbazine; complete response was achieved in 0.9% of patients treated with vemurafenib compared with none treated with dacarbazine. A shorter median time to response (1.45 versus 2.7 months) also was observed in patients receiving vemurafenib compared with those receiving dacarbazine.

In a single-arm, multicenter, multinational phase 2 study, treatment with vemurafenib (960 mg orally twice daily) in patients with *BRAF* V600E mutation-positive, metastatic melanoma previously treated with systemic therapy (including interleukin-2 or standard chemotherapy) produced an overall response rate of 53% with a complete response reported in 6% and a partial response reported in 47% of these patients. At the time of the analysis, the median duration of response was 6.7 months and median overall survival was 15.9 months.

In a post-hoc analysis of the BRIM-3 study, median overall and progression-free survival were significantly longer in vemurafenib-treated patients compared with dacarbazine-treated patients in those whose melanoma harbored either the *BRAF* V600E or the less common *BRAF* V600K mutation. Vemurafenib currently is not indicated for the treatment of metastatic melanoma with *BRAF* V600K mutation.

Use of vemurafenib also was investigated in a single-arm, multicenter, open-label phase 2 study in patients with *BRAF* V600E mutation-positive melanoma with symptomatic or asymptomatic brain metastases. Patients in this study were enrolled in 2 cohorts: those with previously untreated brain metastases and those with previously treated brain metastases (i.e., resection, whole brain radiation

therapy, stereotactic radiation therapy) and measurable disease progression. Patients enrolled in this study must have had at least one brain lesion 0.5 cm or greater in size, were receiving a stable or decreasing corticosteroid dosage, and had no history of BRAF or mitogen-activated extracellular signal-regulated kinase (MEK) inhibitor therapy. In this study, 146 patients received vemurafenib 960 mg orally twice daily until disease progression or unacceptable toxicity occurred. The primary measure of efficacy was overall intracranial response rate in the cohort of patients with previously untreated brain metastases (as evaluated by an independent review committee according to Response Evaluation Criteria in Solid Tumors [RECIST]). The median duration of follow-up was 9.6 months. In the cohort of patients with previously untreated brain metastases, the intracranial overall response rate was 18%; complete responses were achieved in 2% of patients. In the cohort of patients with previously treated brain metastases, the overall intracranial response rate was 18%; however, none of the patients in this cohort achieved a complete response. At the time of analysis, the median duration of response was 4.6 or 6.6 months in those with previously untreated or previously treated brain metastases, respectively.

The safety and efficacy of vemurafenib in patients with wild-type *BRAF* melanoma have not been established; use of vemurafenib is *not* indicated for use in these patients.

Clinical Perspective

The American Society of Clinical Oncology (ASCO) guideline for systemic therapy for melanoma published in 2020 states that patients with unresectable or metastatic *BRAF* wild-type cutaneous melanoma should be offered ipilimumab plus nivolumab, nivolumab alone, or pembrolizumab alone. Ipilimumab plus nivolumab, nivolumab alone, pembrolizumab alone, or combination BRAF/MEK inhibitor therapy (e.g., dabrafenib-trametinib, encorafenib-binimetinib, vemurafenib-cobimetinib) may be offered to patients with *BRAF* V600 mutation-positive cutaneous melanoma. For patients who progress on first-line programmed-death receptor-1 (PD-1) inhibitor therapy, combination BRAF/MEK inhibitor therapy may be offered. For patients who progress on first-line combination BRAF/MEK inhibitor therapy, PD-1 inhibitor therapy may be offered. Patients with mucosal melanoma may be offered the same treatment regimens as those recommended for cutaneous melanoma.

ASCO states that switching between BRAF/MEK inhibitor combination regimens may be reasonable if patients experience toxicity since toxicity profiles may differ for each combination; however, no data exist regarding the efficacy of switching to a different BRAF/MEK combination.

For the treatment of melanoma, monotherapy with a BRAF inhibitor is no longer recommended by experts since combination BRAF/MEK inhibition has demonstrated superior outcomes with a similar safety profile.

● Erdheim-Chester Disease

Vemurafenib is used for the treatment of Erdheim-Chester disease with *BRAF* V600 mutation. Vemurafenib is designated an orphan drug by the FDA for the treatment of this condition.

The current indication for vemurafenib in the treatment of Erdheim-Chester disease is based principally on the results of a single-arm, multicenter, open-label phase 2 study in a cohort of 22 patients with *BRAF* V600 mutation-positive Erdheim-Chester disease. In this study, patients received vemurafenib 960 mg orally twice daily. The primary measure of efficacy was overall response rate (as evaluated by the investigator according to RECIST). The median age of patients enrolled in the cohort of patients with Erdheim-Chester disease was 59 years; 55% were male and 68.2% had previously received systemic therapy.

The overall response rate for patients in the Erdheim-Chester disease cohort of this study was 54.5% with a median time to response of 11 months; complete response was achieved in one patient. The median duration of follow-up for the Erdheim-Chester disease cohort was 26.6 months. At the time of analysis, median duration of response had not been reached. At a median follow-up of 28.8 months, median progression-free survival and overall survival had not been reached. The rates of 2-year progression-free survival and overall survival were 83 and 95%, respectively.

Clinical Perspective

Erdheim-Chester disease, which constitutes a rare form of histiocytosis, involves the infiltration of organ systems by myeloid cells with diverse macrophage or dendritic cell phenotypes. Incidence of the *BRAF* V600E mutation has been detected at rates of 50–60% in patients with Erdheim-Chester disease or Langerhans cell histiocytosis.

The most frequent first-line systemic therapies for multiorgan or disseminated forms of Erdheim-Chester disease are interferon alfa-2a and pegylated interferon alfa. Other potential options include anakinra, infliximab, or sirolimus in combination with corticosteroids. BRAF or MEK inhibitors have been used in the first-line setting in patients with life-threatening cases (e.g., CNS or cardiac involvement) of Erdheim-Chester disease. The most frequent second-line systemic therapy or salvage therapy for Erdheim-Chester disease includes BRAF or MEK inhibitors.

DOSAGE AND ADMINISTRATION

● General

Pretreatment Screening

- Presence of the *BRAF* V600E mutation must be confirmed prior to initiation of therapy.
- Obtain ECGs and serum electrolyte concentrations (i.e., potassium, magnesium, calcium) prior to initiation of therapy.
- Evaluate liver enzymes and bilirubin concentrations prior to initiation of therapy.
- Evaluate S_{cr} concentrations at baseline.
- Perform a dermatologic evaluation prior to initiation of therapy.

Patient Monitoring

- Perform a dermatologic evaluation every 2 months during therapy. Consider continuing monitoring for 6 months following discontinuance of vemurafenib. Closely monitor for signs and symptoms of development of new non-cutaneous squamous cell carcinoma or of other primary malignancies.
- Evaluate S_{cr} concentrations periodically during therapy.
- Closely monitor patients receiving vemurafenib concomitantly or sequentially with radiation therapy for signs and symptoms of radiation sensitization or recall.
- Monitor CBC in patients with Erdheim-Chester disease and coexisting myeloid malignancies.
- Monitor for signs and symptoms of uveitis.
- Monitor ECG and serum electrolytes (i.e., potassium, magnesium, calcium) 15 days following initiation of therapy or dosage modification for QT interval prolongation, monthly during the first 3 months of therapy, and then every 3 months thereafter or more often as clinically indicated.
- Monitor liver enzymes and bilirubin monthly during treatment.

Other General Considerations

- Advise patients to avoid sun exposure.

● Administration

Vemurafenib is administered orally twice daily without regard to meals. Vemurafenib tablets should *not* be crushed or chewed.

If a dose of vemurafenib is missed, the dose may be taken up to 4 hours prior to the next dose to maintain the twice-daily dosing regimen. However, 2 doses should not be taken at the same time.

If vomiting occurs following administration of vemurafenib, a replacement dose should *not* be administered, and the next dose should be taken at the regularly scheduled time.

Store at 20–25°C (excursions permitted between 15–30°C).

● Dosage

Melanoma

The recommended adult dosage of vemurafenib for the treatment of unresectable or metastatic melanoma with *BRAF* V600E mutation is 960 mg twice daily. Therapy should be continued until disease progression or unacceptable toxicity occurs.

Erdheim-Chester Disease

The recommended adult dosage of vemurafenib for the treatment of Erdheim-Chester disease with *BRAF* V600 mutation is 960 mg twice daily. Therapy should be continued until disease progression or unacceptable toxicity occurs.

In the principal efficacy study, the initial dosage of vemurafenib was 960 mg twice daily; however, 64 or 36% of patients required dosage reductions to 480 or 720 mg twice daily, respectively. The manufacturer states that efficacy of vemurafenib was maintained in patients requiring dosage reduction. The median duration of exposure to vemurafenib following dosage reduction to 480 or 720 mg twice daily was 236 or 77 days, respectively.

Dosage Modification

General Toxicity

If intolerable grade 2 or any grade 3 toxicity occurs, vemurafenib therapy should be temporarily interrupted. When the toxicity resolves to grade 0 or 1, vemurafenib may be resumed at a reduced dosage of 720 mg twice daily. If the toxicity recurs at a dosage of 720 mg twice daily, therapy should be withheld again until the toxicity resolves to grade 0 or 1; therapy may then be resumed at a reduced dosage of 480 mg twice daily. If toxicity recurs at a dosage of 480 mg twice daily, treatment with vemurafenib should be permanently discontinued.

If grade 4 toxicity occurs, vemurafenib therapy should be permanently discontinued or interrupted until the toxicity resolves to grade 0 or 1; if clinically appropriate, therapy may then be resumed at a reduced dosage of 480 mg twice daily. If toxicity recurs at a dosage of 480 mg twice daily, treatment with vemurafenib should be permanently discontinued.

Dosages less than 480 mg twice daily are not recommended.

Prolongation of QT Interval

Vemurafenib therapy should be temporarily interrupted if the corrected QT interval (QT_c) exceeds 500 msec. When the QT_c interval decreases to 500 msec or less, the drug may be resumed at a reduced dosage. Vemurafenib should be permanently discontinued if the QT_c interval exceeds 500 msec and increases more than 60 msec from baseline despite correction of electrolyte abnormalities and other risk factors for QT prolongation (e.g., congestive heart failure, bradyarrhythmias).

Development of New Primary Cutaneous Malignancies

No dosage adjustment is necessary in patients who develop new primary cutaneous malignancies.

Concomitant Use with Drugs Affecting Hepatic Microsomal Enzymes

Concomitant use of vemurafenib with drugs that are potent inducers of cytochrome P-450 (CYP) isoenzyme 3A4 should be avoided. If concomitant therapy with a potent CYP3A4 inducer cannot be avoided, the manufacturer recommends increasing the dosage of vemurafenib by 240 mg twice daily (e.g., from 960 mg twice daily to 1.2 g twice daily). When concomitant use of the potent CYP3A4 inducer is discontinued, the vemurafenib dosage should be returned (2 weeks after discontinuance of the CYP3A4 inducer) to the dosage used prior to initiation of the potent CYP3A4 inducer.

Concomitant use of vemurafenib with drugs that are potent inhibitors of CYP3A4 should be avoided. If concomitant use cannot be avoided, consider reducing vemurafenib dosage as clinically indicated.

● Special Populations

Hepatic Impairment

No initial dosage adjustment is necessary in patients with mild or moderate hepatic impairment. The manufacturer makes no specific dosage recommendations in patients with severe hepatic impairment because data are limited in this population.

Renal Impairment

No initial dosage adjustment is necessary in patients with mild or moderate renal impairment. The manufacturer makes no specific dosage recommendations in patients with severe renal impairment because data are limited in this population.

Geriatric Patients

The manufacturer makes no specific dosage recommendations for geriatric patients.

CAUTIONS

● Contraindications

● The manufacturer states there are no known contraindications to the use of vemurafenib.

● Warnings/Precautions

Sensitivity Reactions

Hypersensitivity Reactions

Serious hypersensitivity reactions (e.g., anaphylaxis, generalized rash and erythema, hypotension, drug reaction with eosinophilia and systemic symptoms [DRESS syndrome]) may occur during and upon reinitiation of vemurafenib therapy. Vemurafenib should be permanently discontinued in patients who experience a severe hypersensitivity reaction.

Photosensitivity Reactions

Photosensitivity reactions (mild to severe) have been reported in 33–49% of patients receiving vemurafenib in clinical trials. If intolerable grade 2 or greater reaction occurs, the dosage of vemurafenib should be reduced.

Other Warnings and Precautions

Development of New Primary Malignancies

In the phase 3 clinical trial evaluating vemurafenib in patients with unresectable or metastatic melanoma, cutaneous squamous cell carcinoma, keratoacanthoma, and melanoma were reported more frequently in patients receiving vemurafenib compared with those receiving dacarbazine. In this study, cutaneous squamous cell carcinoma and keratoacanthoma occurred in 24% of patients receiving vemurafenib compared with less than 1% of those receiving dacarbazine. In a phase 2 clinical trial in patients receiving the drug for metastatic melanoma, cutaneous squamous cell carcinoma and keratoacanthoma occurred in 24% of patients. In clinical trials, the median time to first appearance of cutaneous squamous cell carcinoma was 7–8 weeks. Approximately 33% of patients in a phase 3 clinical trial who had previously experienced cutaneous squamous cell carcinoma during vemurafenib treatment had more than one subsequent occurrence with median time between occurrences of 6 weeks. In clinical trials, skin lesions were excised and vemurafenib therapy was continued without dosage adjustment. In the phase 3 clinical trial, development of new primary malignant melanoma was reported in 2.1% of patients receiving vemurafenib compared with none of those receiving dacarbazine. In a clinical trial evaluating vemurafenib in patients with Erdheim-Chester disease, cutaneous squamous cell carcinoma and/or keratoacanthoma occurred in 40.9% of patients. In this trial, the median time to first appearance of cutaneous squamous cell carcinoma was 12.1 weeks.

In clinical trials, non-cutaneous squamous cell carcinoma of the head and neck (e.g., oropharyngeal squamous cell carcinoma) has been reported in less than 10% of patients receiving vemurafenib therapy. Progression of a preexisting chronic myelomonocytic leukemia with NRAS mutation also has been reported during postmarketing experience with the drug.

Although the mechanism for development of cutaneous squamous cell carcinoma has not been fully determined, it has been suggested that paradoxical activation of mitogen-activated protein kinase (MAPK) signaling may lead to accelerated growth of such skin lesions as well as development of other primary malignancies. MAPK-mediated events in wild-type BRAF cells have been observed in a study evaluating the pathology and immunohistochemistry of normal and proliferating skin lesions in patients receiving the weak b-Raf kinase inhibitor sorafenib. Another study performed a molecular analysis of DNA extracted from tumor specimens of patients receiving vemurafenib; results indicated that these patients have a secondary mutation (in addition to the BRAF V600E mutation) that appears to be activated by vemurafenib treatment. Some clinicians suggest that advanced age (i.e., 65 years of age or older), history of skin cancer, and chronic sun exposure may be risk factors for developing cutaneous squamous cell carcinoma. Some data suggest that mitogen-activated extracellular signal-regulated kinase (MEK) inhibitors (i.e., binimetinib, cobimetinib, trametinib) block the paradoxical activation of the MAPK pathway induced by BRAF inhibitors (i.e., vemurafenib, dabrafenib, encorafenib); therefore, combination therapy with a BRAF inhibitor and an MEK inhibitor may reduce the risk of developing cutaneous squamous cell carcinoma. Findings from a meta-analysis of randomized controlled studies that assessed the relative risk of development of cutaneous squamous cell carcinoma in cancer patients receiving a BRAF inhibitor indicate that the risk of cutaneous squamous cell carcinoma is higher in patients receiving a BRAF inhibitor than in patients receiving combination therapy with a BRAF inhibitor and an MEK inhibitor.

A dermatologic evaluation should be performed at baseline and every 2 months during therapy. Continued monitoring for 6 months following discontinuance of vemurafenib may be considered. Suspicious cutaneous lesions should be treated as appropriate and excised for pathologic evaluation. Close monitoring for signs and symptoms of development of new non-cutaneous squamous cell carcinoma or of other primary malignancies should be performed.

In clinical trials, myeloid neoplasms have been reported in patients with Erdheim-Chester disease receiving vemurafenib therapy. The manufacturer recommends monitoring complete blood cell (CBC) counts in patients with Erdheim-Chester disease and coexisting myeloid malignancies.

Tumor Promotion in BRAF Wild-Type Melanoma

In vitro, paradoxical activation of MAPK signaling and increased cell proliferation have been observed in wild-type BRAF cells exposed to BRAF inhibitors. Presence of the BRAF V600E mutation must be confirmed prior to initiation of therapy. (See Uses: Melanoma.)

Dermatologic Effects

Severe skin reactions (e.g., Stevens-Johnson syndrome, toxic epidermal necrolysis) have been reported with vemurafenib. If severe skin reactions occur, vemurafenib therapy should be permanently discontinued.

Prolongation of QT Interval

Vemurafenib prolongs the QT interval in a concentration-dependent manner. In a multicenter, open-label, phase 2 study, QT interval prolongation was evaluated in patients with BRAF V600E mutation-positive, metastatic melanoma who were receiving vemurafenib (960 mg twice daily). A maximum mean corrected QT (QT_c) interval change from baseline of 12.8 msec during the first month of treatment and 15.1 msec during the first 6 months of treatment was observed in these patients.

Vemurafenib should not be initiated in patients with electrolyte abnormalities unresponsive to corrective measures, QT_c intervals exceeding 500 msec, or congenital long QT syndrome. In addition, concomitant use of vemurafenib with drugs known to prolong the QT interval (e.g., class Ia and III antiarrhythmic agents) should be avoided.

ECGs and serum electrolyte concentrations, including concentrations of potassium, magnesium, and calcium, should be obtained prior to initiation of therapy or following dosage modification for QT interval prolongation, and monitored 15 days following initiation of therapy, then monthly for the first 3 months of treatment, and then every 3 months thereafter or more often as clinically indicated.

Interruption or discontinuance of vemurafenib may be necessary if increases in the QT_c interval occur during therapy with the drug.

Hepatic Effects

Hepatic injury may occur during therapy with vemurafenib resulting in functional hepatic impairment, including coagulopathy or other organ dysfunction. In clinical trials, grade 3 and 4 elevations in aminotransferase (ALT or AST), bilirubin, and alkaline phosphatase concentrations have been reported in 0.9–2.9% of patients receiving vemurafenib. Serum aminotransferase, bilirubin, and alkaline phosphatase concentrations should be evaluated prior to initiation of therapy and monitored monthly during treatment or as clinically indicated. Laboratory abnormalities should be managed with dosage reduction, treatment interruption, or discontinuance.

The safety and efficacy of vemurafenib used concomitantly with ipilimumab have not been established; however, grade 3 elevations in aminotransferase and bilirubin concentrations have occurred in the majority of patients receiving vemurafenib (720 or 960 mg twice daily) and ipilimumab (3 mg/kg) concurrently. (See Drug Interactions: Ipilimumab.)

Ocular Effects

Uveitis, blurry vision, and photophobia have been reported in patients receiving vemurafenib. In the phase 3 clinical trial evaluating vemurafenib in patients with previously untreated metastatic melanoma, uveitis, including iritis, occurred in 2.1% of patients receiving vemurafenib compared with none of those receiving dacarbazine. Monitoring for signs and symptoms of uveitis should be performed. In patients experiencing uveitis, therapy with ophthalmic corticosteroid and mydriatic preparations may be required. Retinal vein occlusion also has been reported in patients receiving the drug.

Fetal/Neonatal Morbidity and Mortality

Based on its mechanism of action, vemurafenib may cause fetal harm. No evidence of developmental toxicity was observed in pregnant animals receiving vemurafenib at exposure levels equivalent to approximately 0.6–1.3 times the area under the concentration-time curve [AUC] at the recommended human dosage; however, these exposure levels to vemurafenib were not sufficient to fully evaluate its potential toxicity in pregnant women. In animals, fetal plasma concentrations of vemurafenib were 3–5% of maternal plasma concentrations, indicating that vemurafenib has the potential to cross the placenta.

Pregnancy should be avoided during vemurafenib therapy. Women of childbearing potential should be advised to use effective contraception during therapy and for 2 weeks after the last dose. If used during pregnancy or if the patient becomes pregnant while receiving the drug, the patient should be apprised of the potential fetal hazard.

Radiation Sensitization and Recall

Radiation sensitization and recall, sometimes severe or fatal, involving cutaneous and visceral organs have been reported during postmarketing experience in patients receiving vemurafenib prior to, during, or subsequent to radiation therapy. Fatal cases have been reported in patients with radiation sensitization or recall involving visceral organs. Patients receiving vemurafenib concomitantly or sequentially with radiation therapy should be closely monitored for signs and symptoms of radiation sensitization or recall.

Renal Effects

Renal failure, including acute interstitial nephritis and acute tubular necrosis, has been reported in patients receiving vemurafenib.

In the phase 3 clinical trial evaluating vemurafenib in patients with previously untreated metastatic melanoma, grade 1–2 elevations of serum creatinine (exceeding the upper limit of normal [ULN], but no more than 3 times the ULN) occurred in 26% of patients receiving vemurafenib compared with 5% of those receiving dacarbazine; grade 3–4 elevations of serum creatinine (exceeding 3 times the ULN) occurred in 1.2 or 1.1% of patients receiving vemurafenib or dacarbazine, respectively.

In a clinical trial evaluating vemurafenib in patients with Erdheim-Chester disease, grade 1–2 or 3 elevations of serum creatinine occurred in 86 or 9.1% of patients, respectively.

Serum creatinine concentrations should be evaluated at baseline and periodically during therapy.

Dupuytren Contracture and Plantar Fascial Fibromatosis

Dupuytren contracture and plantar fascial fibromatosis have been reported during postmarketing experience in patients receiving vemurafenib. The majority of cases have been mild to moderate in severity, but severe, disabling cases of Dupuytren contracture also have been reported.

Specific Populations

Pregnancy

Vemurafenib may cause fetal harm if administered to pregnant women based on its mechanism of action and animal findings.

Lactation

There are no data on the presence of vemurafenib in human milk, the effects on the breast-fed infant, or the effects on milk production. Because of the potential for serious adverse reactions to vemurafenib in breast-fed infants, women should be advised not to breast-feed while receiving the drug and for 2 weeks after the last dose.

Pediatric Use

Safety and efficacy of vemurafenib in pediatric patients have not been established.

Based on limited data in pediatric patients (range: 15–17 years of age) with unresectable or metastatic melanoma with BRAF V600 mutation, steady-state exposure of vemurafenib in pediatric patients was similar to that observed in adults. The maximum tolerated dosage of the drug has not been established in pediatric patients; however, no new adverse effects were observed in pediatric patients receiving vemurafenib dosages up to 960 mg twice daily.

Geriatric Use

Clinical studies of vemurafenib did not include sufficient numbers of patients 65 years of age or older to determine whether geriatric patients respond differently than younger adults.

Hepatic Impairment

In a population pharmacokinetic analysis, the clearance of vemurafenib was not affected in patients with mild or moderate hepatic impairment. Pharmacokinetic data in patients with severe hepatic impairment are limited; therefore, the drug should be used with caution in these patients.

Renal Impairment

In a population pharmacokinetic analysis, the clearance of vemurafenib was not affected in patients with mild or moderate renal impairment. Pharmacokinetic data in patients with severe renal impairment are limited; therefore, the drug should be used with caution in these patients.

● Common Adverse Effects

Adverse effects reported in 10% or more of patients receiving vemurafenib for the treatment of unresectable or metastatic melanoma include arthralgia, rash, alopecia, fatigue, photosensitivity reaction, nausea, pruritus, cutaneous squamous cell carcinoma, and skin papilloma.

Adverse effects reported in 20% or more of patients receiving vemurafenib for the treatment of Erdheim-Chester disease include arthralgia, maculopapular rash, alopecia, fatigue, QT interval prolongation, skin papilloma, diarrhea, hyperkeratosis, dry skin, palmar-plantar erythrodysesthesia syndrome, photosensitivity reaction, seborrheic keratosis, cough, cutaneous squamous cell carcinoma, hypertension, pruritus, peripheral sensory neuropathy, actinic keratosis, keratosis pilaris, nausea, melanocytic nevus, sunburn, papular rash, and vomiting.

DRUG INTERACTIONS

In vivo studies indicate that vemurafenib is a moderate inhibitor of cytochrome P-450 (CYP) isoenzyme 1A2 and a weak inhibitor of CYP isoenzyme 2D6. In vitro studies suggest that vemurafenib is an inhibitor of CYP isoenzymes 1A2, 2A6, 2B6, 2C8, 2C9, 2C19, 2D6, and 3A4/5. Vemurafenib is an inhibitor and a substrate of CYP isoenzyme 3A4. In vitro studies indicate that vemurafenib is a substrate and an inhibitor of P-glycoprotein (P-gp) and breast cancer resistance protein (BCRP).

● Drugs Affecting Hepatic Microsomal Enzymes

Concomitant use of vemurafenib with potent inhibitors of CYP3A4 may result in increased plasma concentrations of vemurafenib and an increased incidence of adverse effects. When vemurafenib 960 mg twice daily was coadministered with itraconazole 200 mg once daily, systemic exposure to vemurafenib increased by approximately 40% at steady state; the magnitude of effect on peak plasma concentration was similar. Concomitant use with potent CYP3A4 inhibitors (e.g., clarithromycin, indinavir, itraconazole, ketoconazole, nelfinavir, ritonavir, saquinavir, voriconazole) should be avoided. If coadministration of a potent CYP3A4 inhibitor cannot be avoided, consider reducing the dosage of vemurafenib, if clinically indicated.

Concomitant use of vemurafenib with potent inducers of CYP3A4 may result in decreased plasma concentrations of vemurafenib and reduced vemurafenib efficacy. When the potent CYP3A inducer rifampin (600 mg daily) was administered concomitantly with vemurafenib (single 960-mg dose), systemic exposure to vemurafenib was decreased by 40% and peak plasma concentrations were unchanged. Concomitant use with potent CYP3A4 inducers (e.g., carbamazepine, phenytoin, rifampin) should be avoided, and selection of an alternative drug with no or minimal CYP3A4 induction potential is recommended. If concomitant therapy with a potent CYP3A4 inducer cannot be avoided, the manufacturer recommends increasing the dosage of vemurafenib by 240 mg twice daily (e.g., from 960 mg twice daily to 1.2 g twice daily). When concomitant use of the potent CYP3A4 inducer is discontinued, the vemurafenib dosage should be returned (2 weeks after discontinuance of the CYP3A4 inducer) to the dosage used prior to initiation of the potent CYP3A4 inducer.

● Drugs Metabolized by Hepatic Microsomal Enzymes

Concomitant use of vemurafenib with CYP1A2 substrates may result in increased plasma concentrations of the CYP1A2 substrate and possible toxicity. When the CYP1A2 substrate caffeine was administered concomitantly with vemurafenib, the systemic exposure to caffeine increased by 2.6-fold. When the sensitive CYP1A2 substrate tizanidine (single 2-mg dose) was administered concomitantly with vemurafenib (960 mg twice daily), systemic exposure and peak plasma concentrations of tizanidine increased by 4.7- and 2.2-fold, respectively. Concomitant use of vemurafenib with CYP1A2 substrates that have a narrow therapeutic index should be avoided. If concomitant use cannot be avoided, dosage reduction of the CYP1A2 substrate should be considered, and patients should be closely monitored for adverse effects.

When the CYP2D6 substrate dextromethorphan was administered concomitantly with vemurafenib, the systemic exposure of dextromethorphan increased by 47%.

When the CYP3A4 substrate midazolam was administered concomitantly with vemurafenib, the systemic exposure of midazolam decreased by 39%.

When the CYP2C9 substrate warfarin was administered concomitantly with vemurafenib, the systemic exposure of S-warfarin increased by 18%.

When the CYP2C19 substrate omeprazole was administered concomitantly with vemurafenib, the systemic exposure of omeprazole was unchanged.

● Drugs Affected by Efflux Transport Systems

Concomitant use of vemurafenib with P-gp substrates may result in increased plasma concentrations of the P-gp substrate. When the sensitive P-gp substrate digoxin (single 0.25-mg dose) was administered concomitantly with vemurafenib (960 mg twice daily), systemic exposure and peak plasma concentrations of digoxin increased by 1.8- and 1.5-fold, respectively. Concomitant use of vemurafenib with P-gp substrates that have a narrow therapeutic index should be avoided. If concomitant use cannot be avoided, dosage reduction of the P-gp substrate should be considered.

● Drugs that Prolong the QT Interval

Concomitant use of vemurafenib with drugs known to prolong the QT interval, including class Ia (e.g., quinidine, procainamide) and class III (e.g., amiodarone, sotalol) antiarrhythmic agents, some antipsychotic agents (e.g., asenapine, chlorpromazine, haloperidol, olanzapine, paliperidone, pimozide, quetiapine, thioridazine, ziprasidone), some anti-infectives (e.g., gatifloxacin, moxifloxacin), and tetrabenazine, should be avoided.

● Ipilimumab

Concomitant use of vemurafenib with ipilimumab resulted in increased aminotransferase and bilirubin concentrations in a majority of patients.

DESCRIPTION

Vemurafenib, a potent inhibitor of b-Raf serine-threonine kinase with V600E mutation (*BRAF* V600E), is an antineoplastic agent. Approximately 40–60% of cutaneous melanomas carry a BRAF mutation. The most common *BRAF* mutation is the substitution of glutamic acid for valine at codon 600 in exon 15 (*BRAF* V600E); a less frequently occurring *BRAF* mutation is the substitution of lysine

for valine at codon 600 in exon 15 (*BRAF* V600K). The mutation of *BRAF* V600E activates the mitogen-activated protein kinase (MAPK) and extracellular-signal regulated kinase (ERK) signal transduction pathway, which enhances cell proliferation and tumor progression (e.g., metastasis). In vitro studies indicate that vemurafenib also inhibits other kinases such as c-Raf, a-Raf, wild-type b-Raf, SRMS, ACK1, MAP4K5, and FGR at similar concentrations at which inhibition of BRAF V600E occurs.

Clinical resistance to monotherapy with a BRAF inhibitor, generally occurring 6–7 months following initiation of therapy, has been attributed to several possible resistance mechanisms mostly relying on reactivation of the MAPK/ERK pathway. Complete inhibition of the MAPK/ERK pathway resulting in durable responses may be achieved with the use of combination therapy with a BRAF inhibitor (i.e., dabrafenib, encorafenib, vemurafenib) and an MEK inhibitor (i.e., binimetinib, cobimetinib, trametinib).

The bioavailability of vemurafenib is 64% at steady state. Following administration of vemurafenib within the dosage range of 240–960 mg, the drug exhibits linear pharmacokinetics and achieves steady-state concentrations within approximately 15–22 days. The median terminal half-life of vemurafenib in patients with unresectable melanoma is 57 hours. Following oral administration of a radiolabeled dose of vemurafenib, about 94% of the dose is recovered in feces and 1% is recovered in urine.

Systemic exposure to vemurafenib is increased when the drug is administered with a high-fat meal. Administration of a single dose of vemurafenib with a high-fat meal resulted in increases in systemic exposure or peak plasma concentrations of approximately fivefold or 2.5-fold, respectively.

ADVICE TO PATIENTS

- Importance of advising patient to read the manufacturer's medication guide before beginning treatment and each time the prescription is refilled.
- Instruct patients to take a missed dose as soon as it is remembered, but only if it can be taken at least 4 hours before the next scheduled dose.
- If vomiting occurs following administration, take the next dose at the regularly scheduled time. Do *not* take an additional dose.
- Importance of women informing clinicians if they are or plan to become pregnant. Vemurafenib may cause fetal harm. Necessity of advising women of childbearing potential to use effective contraception during therapy and for 2 weeks after the last dose.
- Importance of women informing clinicians if they plan to breast-feed. Necessity of advising women not to breast-feed during therapy and for 2 weeks after the last dose.
- Importance of confirming that patients have melanomas testing positive for the *BRAF* V600E mutation using the cobas® 4800 BRAF V600 Mutation Test or other FDA-approved diagnostic test prior to initiation of therapy.
- Risk of new primary cutaneous malignancies. Importance of contacting clinician promptly if dermatologic changes (e.g., new wart, skin sore or reddish bump that bleeds or does not heal, or mole that changes in size or color) occur.
- Risk of mild to severe photosensitivity reactions. Importance of using sunscreen and lip balm (minimum SPF >30), wearing protective clothing, and avoiding sun exposure during therapy.
- Risk of severe adverse dermatologic effects. Importance of contacting clinician promptly if skin rash occurs with symptoms such as redness or swelling of face, hands, or soles of feet; blisters on skin or in mouth; peeling of skin; fever.
- Risk of QT-interval prolongation, which may result in ventricular arrhythmias. Importance of contacting clinician promptly if an abnormal heartbeat or feelings of dizziness or faintness occur.
- Risk of new primary malignant melanoma. Importance of contacting clinician promptly if skin changes occur.
- Risk of anaphylaxis or other serious hypersensitivity reactions during or upon reinitiation of therapy. Importance of advising patients to promptly notify their clinician if they develop any signs or symptoms of an allergic reaction during therapy (e.g., rash, angioedema, difficulty breathing, tachycardia, throat tightness, hoarseness).

- Risk of hepatic injury resulting in functional hepatic impairment. Importance of advising patients to schedule periodic laboratory monitoring for hepatotoxicity and to report clinically relevant symptoms to their clinician.
- Risk of adverse ocular effects. Importance of monitoring and contacting clinician promptly if ocular pain, swelling, redness, or blurred vision occurs.
- Risk of radiation sensitization and recall in patients receiving vemurafenib prior to, during, or subsequent to radiation therapy. Importance of informing clinician of previous or planned radiation therapy.
- Risk of renal failure. Importance of monitoring S_{cr} concentrations prior to and periodically during therapy.
- Risk of Dupuytren contracture or plantar fascial fibromatosis. Importance of informing clinician if unusual thickening of palms or soles or inward tightening of the fingers occurs.
- Importance of informing clinicians of existing or contemplated concomitant therapy, including prescription and OTC drugs and herbal supplements, as well as any concomitant illnesses (e.g., hepatic, renal, or cardiovascular diseases, electrolyte abnormalities) or planned surgical, dental, or other medical procedures.
- Importance of informing patients of other important precautionary information.

For further information on the handling of antineoplastic agents, see the ASHP Guidelines on Handling Hazardous Drugs at http://www.ahfsdruginformation.com.

PREPARATIONS

Vemurafenib is available only from a designated specialty pharmacies. The manufacturer should be contacted for additional information.

Excipients in commercially available drug preparations may have clinically important effects in some individuals; consult specific product labeling for details.

Vemurafenib

Oral		
Tablets, film-coated	240 mg	Zelboraf®, Genentech

Selected Revisions June 23, 2022, © Copyright, September 01, 2012, American Society of Health-System Pharmacists, Inc.

Venetoclax

10:00 • ANTINEOPLASTIC AGENTS

■ Venetoclax, a selective inhibitor of B-cell lymphoma 2 (BCL-2), is an antineoplastic agent.

USES

● **Chronic Lymphocytic Leukemia and Small Lymphocytic Lymphoma**

Venetoclax is used as monotherapy or as a component of combination therapy for the treatment of chronic lymphocytic leukemia (CLL) or small lymphocytic lymphoma (SLL). Venetoclax has been designated an orphan drug by FDA for the treatment of these cancers. Venetoclax is generally recommended among first-line treatment options for symptomatic CLL.

Clinical Experience as Combination Therapy

Efficacy and safety of venetoclax in combination with obinutuzumab or in combination with rituximab for the treatment of CLL and SLL are based principally on the results of 2 open-label, multicenter, randomized, phase 3 studies (CLL14 and MURANO).

In the CLL14 study, 432 patients with previously untreated CD20+ CLL (Binet stage C or symptomatic disease) and concomitant medical conditions (total Cumulative Illness Rating Scale [CIRS] score exceeding 6 or creatinine clearance less than 70 mL/minute) were randomized in a 1:1 ratio to receive obinutuzumab (1 g by IV infusion on days 1, 8, and 15 during cycle 1, followed by 1 g by IV infusion every 28 days for an additional 5 cycles) in combination with either venetoclax (400 mg orally once daily [after an initial 5-week dose-escalation period] on day 1 of cycle 3) or chlorambucil (0.5 mg/kg orally on days 1 and 15). Treatment cycles were repeated every 28 days for 12 cycles. Patients with Richter transformation or an organ/system impairment score of 4 according to CIRS (except for the eye, ear, nose, or throat) were excluded from the study. The median age of patients was 72 years; 89% were white, 88% had a baseline Eastern Cooperative Oncology Group (ECOG) performance status of 0 or 1, 58% of patients had a creatinine clearance of less than 70 mL/minute, and 36 or 43% of patients had Binet stage B or C disease, respectively. The median CIRS score was 8.0. Presence of a 17p deletion chromosomal abnormality, *TP53* mutation, 11q deletion, or unmutated *IgVH* was detected in 8, 10, 19, or 57% of patients, respectively. The primary efficacy endpoint was progression-free survival as assessed by an independent review committee using the 2008 International Workshop Criteria for CLL (IWCLL) guidelines. At a median follow-up duration of 28 months, median progression-free or overall survival had not been reached; however, progression-free survival was significantly prolonged in patients receiving venetoclax in combination with obinutuzumab compared with those receiving chlorambucil in combination with obinutuzumab (estimated hazard ratio of 0.33 with a 95% confidence interval of 0.22–0.51). The overall response rate was 85% in patients receiving venetoclax in combination with obinutuzumab compared with 71% in patients receiving chlorambucil in combination with obinutuzumab; complete remission or complete remission with incomplete bone marrow recovery was achieved in 50 or 23% of venetoclax- or chlorambucil-treated patients, respectively. In the intent-to-treat population, minimal residual disease negativity (defined as the presence of less than 0.01% CLL cells) in peripheral blood 3 months after completion of therapy was reported in 76 or 35% of patients receiving venetoclax in combination with obinutuzumab or chlorambucil in combination with obinutuzumab, respectively; negative minimal residual disease in the bone marrow was reported in 57 or 17% of patients in the respective treatment groups. Among patients who achieved complete remission, 87 or 69% of these patients receiving venetoclax in combination with obinutuzumab were minimal residual disease negative in peripheral blood or bone marrow, respectively, 3 months after completion of therapy compared with 62 or 45% of those receiving chlorambucil in combination with obinutuzumab, respectively. Twelve months after completion of therapy, minimal residual disease negativity in peripheral blood was reported in 58% in patients receiving venetoclax in combination with obinutuzumab compared with 9% of those receiving chlorambucil in combination with obinutuzumab.

Progression-free survival benefit in patients receiving venetoclax in combination with obinutuzumab compared with those receiving chlorambucil in combination with obinutuzumab at a median follow-up of 39.6 months remained similar to the initial results. Progression-free survival at 3 years was 81.9 or 49.5% in venetoclax- or chlorambucil-treated patients, respectively.

In the MURANO study, 389 patients with CLL previously treated with at least 1 therapy, were randomized in a 1:1 ratio to receive rituximab (375 mg/m² IV on day 1 of cycle 1, followed by 500 mg/m² on day 1 of cycles 2–6) in combination with either venetoclax (400 mg orally once daily [after an initial 5-week dose-escalation period] for 24 months) or bendamustine (70 mg/m² IV on days 1 and 2 of each 28-day cycle for 6 cycles). Patients previously treated with bendamustine were eligible if the duration of response following bendamustine therapy was at least 24 months. The median age of patients was 65 years; 97% were white, 74% were male, and 99% had a baseline ECOG performance status of 0 or 1. Presence of a 17p deletion chromosomal abnormality, *TP53* mutation, 11q deletion, or unmutated *IgVH* was detected in 24, 25, 32, or 63% of patients, respectively. The median number of prior therapies was 1; 59 or 26% of patients had received 1 or 2 prior therapies, respectively. Prior therapies included an alkylating agent, anti-CD20 monoclonal antibodies, B-cell receptor (BCR) pathway inhibitors, and purine analogs. The primary efficacy endpoint was progression-free survival using the 2008 IWCLL guidelines. At a median follow-up 23.4 months, median progression-free survival had not been reached in patients receiving venetoclax in combination with rituximab; however, progression-free survival was significantly prolonged in patients receiving venetoclax in combination with rituximab compared with those receiving bendamustine in combination with rituximab (estimated hazard ratio of 0.19 with a 95% confidence interval of 0.13–0.28). The overall response rate was 92% in patients receiving venetoclax in combination with rituximab compared with 72% in patients receiving bendamustine in combination with rituximab; complete remission or complete remission with incomplete bone marrow recovery was achieved in 8% of venetoclax-treated patients and in 4% of bendamustine-treated patients. Among patients who achieved a partial response or better, 53 or 12% of these patients receiving venetoclax in combination with rituximab or bendamustine in combination with rituximab, respectively, were minimal residual disease negative (defined as the presence of less than 0.01% CLL cells) in peripheral blood 3 months after completion of rituximab combination therapy. Among patients who achieved complete remission or complete remission with incomplete bone marrow recovery, 3 or 2% of these patients receiving venetoclax in combination with rituximab or bendamustine in combination with rituximab, respectively, were minimal residual disease negative (defined as the presence of less than 0.01% CLL cells) in peripheral blood 3 months after completion of rituximab combination therapy. At a median follow-up duration of 22.9 months, median overall survival had not been reached in either group; however, the 24-month overall survival rate was 92 or 87% in patients receiving venetoclax combination therapy or bendamustine combination therapy, respectively. Progression-free and overall survival benefit in patients receiving venetoclax in combination with rituximab compared with those receiving bendamustine in combination with rituximab at 4 years' follow-up remained similar to the initial results. Estimated rates of 4-year progression-free survival were 57.3 and 4.6% for patients receiving venetoclax combination therapy and bendamustine combination therapy, respectively. After an overall follow-up period of 71 months, median progression-free survival was 53.6 months in patients receiving venetoclax in combination with rituximab compared with 17 months in those receiving bendamustine in combination with rituximab; median overall survival had not been reached in either arm.

Clinical Experience as Monotherapy

Efficacy and safety of venetoclax monotherapy for the treatment of CLL and SLL are based principally on the results of 3 open-label, noncomparative, phase 1 and 2 studies (M13-982, M12-175, and M14-032).

In the M13-982 study, 106 adults with relapsed or refractory 17p deletion CLL (confirmed by the Vysis® fluorescent in situ hybridization [FISH] kit) received single-agent venetoclax (400 mg orally once daily [after an initial 5-week dose-escalation period]) until disease progression or unacceptable toxicity occurred. Patients in this study had received a median of 2.5 prior therapies for their disease and had a median time since diagnosis of 6.6 years. The median age of patients was 67 years; 97% were white, 92% had a baseline ECOG performance status of 0 or 1, 50% had an absolute lymphocyte count of 25,000/mm³ or greater, and 53% had one or more lymph nodes measuring 5 cm or greater. The primary end point of this study was overall response rate as assessed by an independent review committee using the 2008 IWCLL guidelines. The overall response rate was 85%; complete remission or complete remission with incomplete bone marrow recovery was achieved in 8% of the patients. Among 8 patients who achieved complete remission, 3 patients were minimal residual disease negative (defined as the presence of less than 0.01% CLL cells) in peripheral blood and bone marrow. At the time of analysis, the median duration of response had not been reached in this study. However, the median time to first response was 0.8 months.

In the M12-175 study, 67 adult patients with previously treated CLL or SLL (59 or 8 patients, respectively) received venetoclax 400 mg once daily (after an initial 5-week dose-escalation period) until disease progression or unacceptable toxicity occurred. The median age of patients was 65 years; 87% were white, 78% were male, 67% had one or more lymph nodes measuring 5 cm or greater, 33% had documented unmutated *IgVH*, and 21% had documented 17p deletion. Baseline absolute lymphocyte count was at least 25,000/mm³ in 30% of patients. The overall response rate was 76% as assessed by an independent review committee using the 2008 IWCLL guidelines; complete remission or complete remission with incomplete bone marrow recovery was achieved in 10% of the patients. The median duration of response was 36.2 months. In the M14-032 study, 127 adult patients with CLL previously treated with and progressed on or after ibrutinib or idelalisib therapy received venetoclax 400 mg once daily (after an initial 3- or 5-week dose-escalation period) until disease progression or unacceptable toxicity occurred. The median age was 66 years; 92% were white, 70% were male, 41% had one or more lymph nodes measuring 5 cm or greater, 57% had documented unmutated *IgVH*, and 39% had documented 17p deletion. Baseline absolute lymphocyte count was at least 25,000/mm³ in 31% of patients, and the median number of prior treatments was 4. The overall response rate was 70% (as assessed by an independent review committee using the 2008 IWCLL guidelines); complete remission or complete remission with incomplete bone marrow recovery was achieved in 5% of patients. At a median follow-up duration of 19.9 months, the median duration of response had not been reached. Among patients previously treated with ibrutinib or idelalisib, investigator-assessed overall response rate was 65 or 67%, respectively. Median progression-free survival and overall survival had not been reached at the time of analysis.

Clinical Perspective

Venetoclax with or without rituximab or obinutuzumab is among one of several recommended treatment options for first-line therapy of CLL. Some experts suggest that choice of a specific agent be based on presence or absence of 17p deletion or *TP53* mutation, *IgHV* mutational status, age, comorbidities, and concomitant medications.

● *Acute Myeloid Leukemia*

Venetoclax is used in combination with azacitidine, decitabine, or low-dose cytarabine for the treatment of newly diagnosed acute myeloid leukemia (AML) in patients who are 75 years of age or older, or those who have comorbidities (e.g., ECOG performance status of 2 or 3, moderate hepatic impairment, creatinine clearance of less than 45 mL/minute, severe cardiac or pulmonary disease) that preclude use of intensive induction chemotherapy. Venetoclax has been designated an orphan drug by FDA for treatment of this cancer.

Clinical Experience for Venetoclax in Combination with Azacitidine or Decitabine

Efficacy and safety of venetoclax in combination with azacitidine or decitabine for the treatment of newly diagnosed AML in patients 75 years of age or older or those with comorbidities are based principally on the results of a randomized, double-blind, multicenter, placebo-controlled, phase 3 study (VIALE-A) and an open-label, noncomparative, phase 1b study (M14-358).

In the VIALE-A study, 431 patients with newly diagnosed AML who were not candidates for standard induction chemotherapy were randomized in a 2:1 ratio to receive either venetoclax 400 mg orally once daily (after a 3-day dose escalation during cycle 1) in combination with azacitidine 75 mg/m² subcutaneously or intravenously on days 1–7 of each 28-day cycle or placebo in combination with the same dosage of azacitidine. If complete remission was achieved following cycle 1 (defined as less than 5% blasts in bone marrow with cytopenia), venetoclax or placebo was interrupted for up to 14 days or until ANC reached

500/mm³ or greater and platelet count reached 50,000/mm³ or greater. If complete remission was not achieved at the end of cycle 1, bone marrow assessment was repeated after cycle 2 or 3 and as clinically indicated. Azacitidine was resumed on the same day as venetoclax or placebo following interruption of therapy. Treatment was continued until disease progression or unacceptable toxicity occurred. The median age of patients was 76 years; 76% were white, 60% were male, 55% had a baseline ECOG performance status of 0 or 1, 29% had a baseline bone marrow blast count below 30%, 25% had secondary AML, and 38% had poor cytogenetic risk factors. Approximately one-half of the patients had at least two reasons for ineligibility for intensive induction chemotherapy. The primary efficacy endpoint of the study was overall survival. Median overall survival was prolonged in patients receiving venetoclax in combination with azacitidine compared with those receiving placebo in combination with azacitidine (14.7 versus 9.6 months, respectively). Complete remission (defined as ANC exceeding 1,000/mm³, platelet count exceeding 100,000/mm³, RBC transfusion independence, and less than 5% blasts in bone marrow) was achieved in 37 or 18% of venetoclax- or placebo-treated patients, respectively. Complete remission and complete remission with partial hematologic recovery (defined as less than 5% blasts in bone marrow without evidence of disease, platelet count exceeding 50,000/mm³, and ANC exceeding 500/mm³) was achieved in 65 or 23% of venetoclax- or placebo-treated patients, respectively. The median time to first complete remission was 1 month in patients receiving venetoclax in combination with azacitidine. The median duration of complete remission, including complete remission with partial hematologic recovery, was 17.8 months in patients receiving the venetoclax combination and 13.9 months in those receiving the placebo combination. Among venetoclax- or placebo-treated patients who were transfusion dependent (RBC and/or platelet) at baseline, 49 or 27%, respectively, became transfusion independent during any consecutive 56 days or more period during the study. Among venetoclax- or placebo-treated patients who were transfusion independent at baseline, 69 or 42%, respectively, remained transfusion independent during any consecutive 56 day or more period during the study.

In the M14-358 study, 80 patients with newly diagnosed AML who were not candidates for intensive induction chemotherapy (i.e., 75 years of age or older, severe cardiac disease, severe pulmonary disease, moderate hepatic impairment, creatinine clearance of less than 45 mL/minute) received venetoclax 400 mg orally once daily (after a dose-escalation period) in combination with either azacitidine (75 mg/m² IV or subcutaneously on days 1–7 of each 28-day cycle) or decitabine (20 mg/m² IV on days 1–5 of each 28-day cycle). If complete remission was achieved following cycle 1 (defined as less than 5% blasts in bone marrow with cytopenia), venetoclax was interrupted for up to 14 days or until ANC reached 500/mm³ or greater and platelet count reached 50,000/mm³ or greater. Therapy was continued until disease progression or unacceptable toxicity occurred. At a median duration of follow-up of 15.9 months in patients receiving venetoclax in combination with azacitidine, complete remission or complete remission with partial hematologic recovery was achieved in 43 or 18%, respectively, of patients; the median time to first complete remission, including complete remission with partial hematologic recovery, was 1 month and the median duration of response was 23.8 months. Among the patients receiving venetoclax in combination with azacitidine, 12% subsequently underwent stem cell transplantation. At a median duration of follow-up of 11 months in patients receiving venetoclax in combination with decitabine, complete remission or complete remission with partial hematologic recovery was achieved in 54 or 7.7% of patients, respectively; the median time to first complete remission, including complete remission with partial hematologic recovery, was 1.9 months and the median duration of response was 12.7 months. In the subgroup of patients 60 to less than 75 years of age without relevant comorbidities who received venetoclax in combination with azacitidine, 35 or 41% of 17 patients achieved complete remission or complete remission with partial hematologic recovery, respectively; 53% of these patients subsequently underwent stem cell transplantation. In the subgroup of patients 65–74 years of age without relevant comorbidities who received venetoclax in combination with decitabine, 56 or 22% of 18 patients achieved complete remission or complete remission with partial hematologic recovery, respectively; 22% of these patients subsequently underwent stem cell transplantation. In the overall study population, which included patients 60 to less than 75 years of age without relevant comorbidities, median overall survival was 16.4 months in patients receiving venetoclax in combination with azacitidine (at a median duration of follow-up of 29 months) and 16.2 months in those receiving venetoclax in combination with decitabine (at a median duration of follow-up of 40 months).

Clinical Experience for Venetoclax in Combination with Low-Dose Cytarabine

Efficacy and safety of venetoclax in combination with low-dose cytarabine for the treatment of newly diagnosed AML in patients 75 years of age or older or those with comorbidities is based principally on the results of a multicenter, randomized, double-blind, placebo-controlled, phase 3 study (VIALE-C) and an open-label, noncomparative, phase 1b/2 study (M14-387).

In the VIALE-C study, 211 patients with newly diagnosed AML who were not candidates for standard induction chemotherapy were randomized in a 2:1 ratio to receive either venetoclax 600 mg orally once daily (after a 4-day dose-escalation period) in combination with low-dose cytarabine 20 mg/m^2 subcutaneously on days 1–10 of each 28-day cycle or placebo in combination with low-dose cytarabine. If complete remission was achieved following cycle 1 (defined as less than 5% blasts in bone marrow with cytopenia), venetoclax or placebo was interrupted for up to 14 days or until ANC reached 500/mm^3 or greater and platelet count reached 50,000/mm^3 or greater. If complete remission was not achieved at the end of cycle 1, bone marrow assessment was repeated after cycle 2 or 3 and as clinically indicated. Low-dose cytarabine was resumed on the same day as venetoclax or placebo following interruption of therapy. Therapy was continued until disease progression or unacceptable toxicity occurred. The primary efficacy endpoint of the study was overall survival. At a median follow-up duration of 12 months, median overall survival was 7.2 months in patients receiving venetoclax in combination with low-dose cytarabine and 4.1 months in patients receiving placebo in combination with low-dose cytarabine; however, the difference was not statistically significant. Complete remission occurred in 27 or 7.4% of patients receiving the venetoclax and placebo combinations, respectively; the median duration of complete remission was 11.1 or 8.3 months in these respective groups. Complete remission or complete remission with partial hematologic recovery was achieved in 47 or 15% of venetoclax- or placebo-treated patients, respectively; the median duration of response was 11.1 or 6.2 months in these respective groups, and the median time to first complete remission or complete remission with partial hematologic recovery was 1 month in patients receiving venetoclax in combination with low-dose cytarabine. Among venetoclax- or placebo-treated patients who were transfusion dependent (RBC and/or platelet) at baseline, 33 or 13%, respectively, became transfusion independent during any consecutive 56 day or more period during the study. Among venetoclax- or placebo-treated patients who were transfusion independent at baseline, 50 or 31%, respectively, remained transfusion independent during any consecutive 56 day or more period during the study. After an additional 6 months of follow-up (median follow-up, 17.5 months), median overall survival was 8.4 months in patients receiving venetoclax in combination with low-dose cytarabine and 4.1 months in patients receiving placebo in combination with low-dose cytarabine.

In the M14-387 study, 82 patients with newly diagnosed AML, including those with prior exposure to a hypomethylating agent for an antecedent hematologic disorder, were treated with venetoclax 600 mg once daily (after a 4- or 5-day dose-escalation period) and cytarabine 20 mg/m^2 on days 1–10 of each 28-day cycle. If complete remission was achieved following cycle 1 (defined as less than 5% blasts in bone marrow with cytopenia), venetoclax was interrupted for up to 14 days or until ANC reached 500/mm^3 or greater and platelet count reached 50,000/mm^3 or greater. Therapy was continued until disease progression or unacceptable toxicity occurred. At a median follow-up of 7.3 months in the subgroup of patients who were 75 years of age or older or had relevant comorbidities, 21 or 21% of these patients achieved complete remission or complete remission with partial hematologic recovery, respectively, with a median time to first complete remission or complete remission with partial hematologic recovery of 1 month; the median duration of complete remission or complete remission with partial hematologic recovery was 22.9 or 14.3 months, respectively. In the subgroup of patients who were 60 to less than 75 years of age without relevant comorbidities receiving venetoclax in combination with low-dose cytarabine, complete remission or complete remission with partial hematologic recovery was achieved in 33 or 24% of patients, respectively; one of these patients subsequently underwent stem cell transplantation. In the overall study population, which included patients 60 to less than 75 years of age without relevant comorbidities, median overall survival was 10.1 months.

Clinical Perspective

Treatment options for newly diagnosed AML include intensive chemotherapy or less-intensive regimens. Although more-intensive therapy is generally recommended over less-intensive regimens when tolerable, decisions should be individualized based on the relative risks and benefits of treatment. In older adults or adults with significant comorbid conditions, venetoclax plus hypomethylating agents (azacitidine and decitabine) or low-dose cytarabine may be used as one of several less-intensive treatment regimens for AML.

DOSAGE AND ADMINISTRATION

● General

Pretreatment Screening

- Prior to initiating first dose, assess patients for risk of tumor lysis syndrome and give appropriate prophylaxis (e.g., adequate hydration and antihyperuricemic agents) based on tumor burden at baseline and other risk factors (e.g., renal impairment, malignancy).
- *In patients with chronic lymphocytic leukemia (CLL) or small lymphocytic lymphoma (SLL)*, assess blood chemistries (i.e., potassium, phosphorus, calcium, uric acid, creatinine); correct any preexisting abnormalities prior to initiation of therapy.
- *In patients with AML*, patients should have a leukocyte count less than 25,000/mm^3 prior to initiation of venetoclax therapy; pretreatment cytoreduction may be necessary. Assess blood chemistries (i.e., potassium, phosphorus, calcium, uric acid, creatinine) and correct any preexisting abnormalities prior to initiation of therapy.
- Perform pregnancy testing prior to initiating treatment in females of reproductive potential.

Patient Monitoring

- Institute appropriate prophylaxis and monitoring for tumor lysis syndrome according to tumor burden at baseline.
- *In patients with CML or SLL*: Assess risk for tumor lysis syndrome and provide prophylaxis and monitoring when starting therapy and prior to resuming therapy following dosage interruption lasting >1 week during initial dose-escalation period or >2 weeks following completion of the dose-escalation period.
- *In patients with AML*: Assess blood chemistries for tumor lysis syndrome (i.e., potassium, phosphorus, calcium, uric acid, creatinine) prior to each dose, at 6–8 hours following each new dose during dosage escalation, and 24 hours after reaching the final dosage. Consider increased laboratory monitoring and reduction of initial dosage for patients with risk factors for tumor lysis syndrome.
- Monitor CBC periodically during therapy.
- Monitor for manifestations of infection during therapy.

Premedication and Prophylaxis

Tumor Lysis Syndrome

- *In patients with AML*, initiate prophylaxis (i.e., hydration and an antihyperuricemic agent) and monitor for tumor lysis syndrome prior to first dose and during dose escalation. Prior to initiation of therapy, leukocyte count should be <25,000/mm^3; pretreatment cytoreduction may be necessary. Assess blood chemistries (i.e., potassium, phosphorus, calcium, uric acid, creatinine) prior to each dose, at 6–8 hours following each new dose during the dose-escalation period, and 24 hours following completion of the dose-escalation period. Consider increased laboratory monitoring and reduction of starting dosage for patients with risk factors for tumor lysis syndrome.
- *In patients with CLL or SLL*, institute appropriate prophylaxis and monitoring as described in Table 1. Assess risk and provide prophylaxis and monitoring when starting therapy and prior to resuming therapy following dosage interruption lasting >1 week during initial dose-escalation period or >2 weeks following completion of the dose-escalation period. Administer initial 20- and 50-mg doses of venetoclax in the hospital in patients with high tumor burden at baseline; may administer subsequent doses in the outpatient setting. Dosage modifications may be necessary if laboratory evidence or clinical manifestations of tumor lysis syndrome occur during therapy.

TABLE 1. Recommended Prophylaxis and Monitoring for Tumor Lysis Syndrome in Patients with CLL/SLL

Tumor Burden	Prophylaxis	Monitoring
Low tumor burden: All lymph nodes with diameter <5 cm AND absolute lymphocyte count <25,000/mm³	Oral hydration (1.5–2 L)[a,b] and allopurinol[c]	Assess blood chemistries (i.e., potassium, phosphorus, calcium, uric acid, creatinine) prior to, at 6–8 and 24 hours following the first 20- and 50-mg doses of venetoclax, and prior to each subsequent escalating dose (100, 200, and 400 mg)
Medium tumor burden: Any lymph node diameter 5 cm to <10 cm OR absolute lymphocyte count ≥25,000/mm³	Oral hydration (1.5–2 L)[a,b] and allopurinol[c] Consider additional IV hydration	Assess blood chemistries (i.e., potassium, phosphorus, calcium, uric acid, creatinine) prior to, at 6–8 and 24 hours following the first 20- and 50-mg doses of venetoclax, and prior to each subsequent escalating dose (100, 200, and 400 mg) In patients with Cl$_{cr}$ <80 mL/minute prior to the first 20- and 50-mg doses, consider hospitalization for drug administration and more intensive hydration and monitoring (see the following recommendations for monitoring in hospital)
High tumor burden: Any lymph node diameter ≥10 cm OR any lymph node diameter ≥5 cm and absolute lymphocyte count ≥25,000/mm³	Oral (1.5–2 L)[a,b] and IV (150–200 mL/hour as tolerated) hydration and allopurinol[c] Consider rasburicase if baseline uric acid concentrations are elevated	Hospitalize patients for administration of the first 20- and 50-mg doses of venetoclax; assess blood chemistries (i.e., potassium, phosphorus, calcium, uric acid, creatinine) prior to and at 4, 8, 12, and 24 hours following each dose Administer subsequent escalating doses (100, 200, and 400 mg) in the outpatient setting; assess blood chemistries prior to and at 6–8 and 24 hours following each dose

[a] Administer IV hydration if oral hydration is not tolerated

[b] Begin oral hydration 2 days prior to initiating venetoclax, on the day of the first dose, and every time the dose is increased

[c] Initiate antihyperuricemic agent (e.g., allopurinol) 2–3 days prior to initiating venetoclax

OTHER GENERAL CONSIDERATIONS

- Consider the usual cautions, precautions, and contraindications associated with drugs used in combination with venetoclax.

● *Administration*

Venetoclax is administered orally once daily with a meal and a full glass of water at approximately the same time each day. Venetoclax tablets should be swallowed intact and should *not* be chewed, crushed, or broken. The recommended dosage of venetoclax may be delivered using any combination of the approved tablet strengths.

Store venetoclax at or below 30°C in its original container to protect from moisture.

● *Dosage*

Chronic Lymphocytic Leukemia or Small Lymphocytic Leukemia

For the treatment of CLL or SLL, the recommended adult dosage of venetoclax is 400 mg once daily; to reduce tumor burden (i.e., debulk) and minimize the risk of tumor lysis syndrome, initiate venetoclax therapy at a low dosage and increase gradually over 5 weeks to the recommended dosage according to the

following schedule: 20 mg daily in the first week, 50 mg daily in the second week, 100 mg daily in the third week, 200 mg daily in the fourth week, and 400 mg daily thereafter.

Venetoclax in Combination with Obinutuzumab

During cycle 1, the recommended dosage of obinutuzumab is 100 mg IV on day 1, followed by 900 mg IV on day 2, and then 1 g on day 8 and day 15. During cycles 2–6, the recommended dosage of obinutuzumab is 1 g IV every 4 weeks (day 1 of each cycle). Do not continue obinutuzumab beyond 6 cycles.

On cycle 1 day 22, initiate venetoclax at a low dosage and titrate over 5 weeks according to the following schedule: 20 mg daily in first week, 50 mg daily in second week, 100 mg daily in third week, 200 mg daily in fourth week, then 400 mg daily thereafter. After completing the dosage escalation phase on cycle 2 day 28, continue venetoclax at a dosage of 400 mg once daily from cycle 3 day 1 until the last day of cycle 12.

Venetoclax in Combination with Rituximab

Initiate venetoclax therapy at a low dosage and increased gradually over 5 weeks to the recommended dosage according to the following schedule: 20 mg daily in the first week, 50 mg daily in the second week, 100 mg daily in the third week, 200 mg daily in the fourth week, and 400 mg daily thereafter. Continue venetoclax 400 mg once daily for 24 months starting from day 1 of cycle 1 of rituximab.

Initiate rituximab after patient has completed the 5-week dose-escalation for venetoclax and has received venetoclax at the recommended dosage of 400 mg once daily for 7 days. The recommended dosage of rituximab is 375 mg/m² IV on day 1 of cycle 1, followed by 500 mg/m² IV on day 1 of cycles 2–6. Treatment cycles are repeated every 28 days. Do not continue rituximab beyond 6 cycles.

Venetoclax Monotherapy

When venetoclax is used as monotherapy for the treatment of CLL or SLL, the recommended adult dosage of venetoclax is 400 mg once daily after the recommended 5-week dose titration; to minimize the risk of tumor lysis syndrome, initiate venetoclax therapy at a low dosage and increase gradually over 5 weeks to the recommended dosage according to the following schedule: 20 mg daily in the first week, 50 mg daily in the second week, 100 mg daily in the third week, 200 mg daily in the fourth week, and 400 mg daily thereafter.

Continue therapy until disease progression or unacceptable toxicity occurs.

Dosage Modification for Toxicity in Patients with CLL/SLL

If adverse reactions occur during venetoclax therapy in patients with CLL or SLL, temporary interruption of therapy, dosage reduction, and/or discontinuance of the drug may be necessary. If dosage reduction is required, the manufacturer recommends reducing the dosage of venetoclax as described in Table 2.

If a dosage reduction occurs during the initial dose-titration period, continue the reduced dosage for 1 week before escalating back to the previous dosage.

If interruption of therapy is necessary for more than 1 week during the initial dose-titration period or for more than 2 weeks while receiving a steady dosage of venetoclax (e.g., 400 mg once daily), reassess patients for risk of tumor lysis syndrome to determine if a reduced dosage is necessary when resuming therapy.

TABLE 2. Recommended Dosage Reduction for Venetoclax Toxicity in Patients with CLL or SLL

Current Venetoclax Dosage	Dosage Reduction after Recovery from Toxicity[a]
400 mg	Restart at 300 mg once daily
300 mg	Restart at 200 mg once daily
200 mg	Restart at 100 mg once daily
100 mg	Restart at 50 mg once daily
50 mg	Restart at 20 mg once daily
20 mg	Restart at 10 mg once daily

[a] Larger dose reductions may be required at the discretion of the clinician

The following Recommended Dosage Modification for Venetoclax Toxicity in Patients with CLL or SLL table indicates the recommended dosage modification (i.e., temporary interruption of therapy, dosage reduction) for adverse effects according to severity.

TABLE 3. Recommended Dosage Modification for Venetoclax Toxicity in Patients with CLL or SLL

Adverse Reaction and Severity	Modification
Tumor Lysis Syndrome	
Blood chemistry abnormalities or symptoms consistent with tumor lysis syndrome	Withhold therapy
	If resolution occurs within 24–48 hours of the last dose, resume therapy at the same dosage; however, if laboratory abnormalities require >48 hours to resolve or if clinical tumor lysis syndrome (clinical sequelae may include acute renal failure, cardiac arrhythmias, sudden death, and/or seizures) occurs, resume therapy at a reduced dosage when resolution occurs (see Table 2)
Hematologic Toxicity	
Grade 3 neutropenia associated with fever or infection	First occurrence: Withhold therapy; when toxicity improves to grade 1 or less, resume at same dosage
	Subsequent occurrences: Withhold therapy, resume therapy at a reduced dosage when the toxicity resolves (see Table 2)
Grade 4 hematologic toxicity (except for lymphopenia)	First occurrence: Withhold therapy; when toxicity improves to grade 1 or less, resume at same dosage
	Subsequent occurrences: Withhold therapy, resume therapy at a reduced dosage when the toxicity resolves (see Table 2)
Nonhematologic Toxicity	
Grade 3 or 4	First occurrence: Withhold therapy; when toxicity improves to grade 1 or less, resume at same dosage
	Subsequent occurrences: Withhold therapy, resume therapy at a reduced dosage when the toxicity resolves (see Table 2)

Dosage Modification for Concomitant Use with CYP3A or P-gp Inhibitors in Patients with CLL/SLL

Concomitant use of venetoclax with a potent or moderate CYP3A inhibitor or a P-gp inhibitor may be contraindicated or reduction of the venetoclax dosage may be necessary in patients with CLL/SLL as described in Table 4. When the potent or moderate CYP3A inhibitor or P-gp inhibitor is discontinued, resume the dosage of venetoclax that was used prior to initiating the CYP3A inhibitor or P-gp inhibitor after 2–3 days.

TABLE 4. Recommended Management of Potential Drug Interactions with Venetoclax in Patients with CLL or SLL

Coadministered Drug	Concomitant Use During Initial Venetoclax Dosage Escalation	Concomitant Use with Steady Daily Dosage of Venetoclax (After Dosage Escalation)
Posaconazole	Contraindicated	Consider using an alternative drug with no or less CYP3A inhibition potential
		If concomitant use cannot be avoided, reduce venetoclax dosage to 70 mg daily; monitor frequently for toxicities

TABLE 4. Continued

Coadministered Drug	Concomitant Use During Initial Venetoclax Dosage Escalation	Concomitant Use with Steady Daily Dosage of Venetoclax (After Dosage Escalation)
Other potent CYP3A inhibitor	Contraindicated	Consider using an alternative drug with no or less CYP3A inhibition potential
		If concomitant use cannot be avoided, reduce venetoclax dosage to 100 mg daily; monitor frequently for toxicities
Moderate CYP3A inhibitor	Reduce venetoclax dosage by at least 50% and monitor frequently for toxicities	Reduce venetoclax dosage by at least 50% and monitor frequently for toxicities
P-gp inhibitor	Reduce venetoclax dosage by at least 50% and monitor frequently for toxicities	Reduce venetoclax dosage by at least 50% and monitor frequently for toxicitie

Acute Myeloid Leukemia

Venetoclax in Combination with Azacitidine

When venetoclax is used in combination with azacitidine for the treatment of newly diagnosed AML in patients 75 years of age or older, or those who are not candidates for intensive induction chemotherapy, initiate venetoclax therapy at a low dosage and increase gradually to the recommended dosage according to the following schedule: 100 mg on day 1, 200 mg on day 2, and 400 mg daily thereafter.

The recommended dosage of azacitidine is 75 mg/m² intravenously or subcutaneously once daily on days 1–7 of each 28-day cycle.

Continue therapy until disease progression or unacceptable toxicity occurs.

Venetoclax in Combination with Decitabine

When venetoclax is used in combination with decitabine for the treatment of newly diagnosed AML in patients 75 years of age or older, or those who are not candidates for intensive induction chemotherapy, initiate venetoclax therapy at a low dosage and increased gradually to the recommended dosage according to the following schedule: 100 mg on day 1, 200 mg on day 2, and 400 mg daily thereafter.

The recommended dosage of decitabine is 20 mg/m² intravenously once daily on days 1–5 of each 28-day cycle.

Continue therapy until disease progression or unacceptable toxicity occurs.

Venetoclax in Combination with Low-Dose Cytarabine

When venetoclax is used in combination with low-dose cytarabine for the treatment of newly diagnosed AML in patients 75 years of age or older, or those who are not candidates for intensive induction chemotherapy, initiate venetoclax therapy at a low dosage and increased gradually to the recommended dosage according to the following schedule: 100 mg on day 1, 200 mg on day 2, 400 mg on day 3, and 600 mg daily thereafter.

The recommended dosage of cytarabine is 20 mg/m² subcutaneously once daily on days 1–10 of each 28-day cycle.

Continue therapy until disease progression or unacceptable toxicity occurs.

Dosage Modification for Toxicity in Patients with AML

If adverse reactions occur during venetoclax therapy in patients with AML, dosage modification or temporary interruption of therapy may be necessary as described in Table 5.

TABLE 5. Recommended Dosage Modification for Venetoclax Toxicity in Patients with AML

Adverse Reaction and Severity	Occurrence	Modification
Hematologic Toxicity		
Grade 4 neutropenia with or without fever or infection	Prior to achieving remission	In most instances, do not interrupt venetoclax in combination with azacitidine, decitabine, or low-dose cytarabine
		Bone marrow evaluation recommended
	First occurrence after achieving remission and lasts ≥7 days	Delay subsequent cycle of venetoclax in combination with azacitidine, decitabine, or low-dose cytarabine and monitor CBCs
		Resume venetoclax at same dosage in combination with azacitidine, decitabine, or low-dose cytarabine when toxicity resolves to grade 1 or 2
	Subsequent occurrences in cycles after achieving remission and lasting ≥7 days	Delay subsequent cycle of venetoclax in combination with azacitidine, decitabine, or low-dose cytarabine and monitor CBCs
		Resume venetoclax at same dosage in combination with azacitidine, decitabine, or low-dose cytarabine when toxicity resolves to grade 1 or 2, and reduce duration of venetoclax therapy by 7 days during each subsequent cycle (e.g., 28 days reduced to 21 days)
Grade 4 thrombocytopenia	Prior to achieving remission	In most instances, do not interrupt venetoclax in combination with azacitidine, decitabine, or low-dose cytarabine
		Bone marrow evaluation recommended
	First occurrence after achieving remission and lasts ≥7 days	Delay subsequent cycle of venetoclax in combination with azacitidine, decitabine, or low-dose cytarabine and monitor CBCs
		Resume venetoclax at same dosage in combination with azacitidine, decitabine, or low-dose cytarabine when toxicity resolves to grade 1 or 2
	Subsequent occurrences in cycles after achieving remission and lasting ≥7 days	Delay subsequent cycle of venetoclax in combination with azacitidine, decitabine, or low-dose cytarabine and monitor CBCs
		Resume venetoclax at same dosage in combination with azacitidine, decitabine, or low-dose cytarabine when toxicity resolves to grade 1 or 2, and reduce duration of venetoclax therapy by 7 days during each subsequent cycle (e.g., 28 days reduced to 21 days)
Nonhematologic Toxicity		
Grade 3 or 4	Any occurrence	If persists despite supportive care, withhold venetoclax therapy; resume venetoclax at same dosage when toxicity resolves to grade 1 or less

Dosage Modification for Concomitant Use with CYP3A or P-gp Inhibitors in Patients with AML

Avoid concomitant use of venetoclax with a potent or moderate cytochrome P-450 (CYP) 3A inhibitor or a P-glycoprotein (P-gp) inhibitor. If concomitant use of potent or moderate CYP3A inhibitors or P-gp inhibitors cannot be avoided, the manufacturer recommends reducing the dosage of venetoclax as described in Table 6. When the potent or moderate CYP3A inhibitor or P-gp inhibitor is discontinued, resume the dosage of venetoclax that was used prior to initiating the CYP3A inhibitor or P-gp inhibitor after 2–3 days. (See Drug Interactions.)

TABLE 6. Recommended Management of Potential Drug Interactions with Venetoclax in Patients with AML

Coadministered Drug	During Dosage Escalation	After Dosage Escalation
Posaconazole	Day 1: 10 mg Day 2: 20 mg Day 3: 50 mg Day 4: 70 mg	Reduce venetoclax dosage to 70 mg daily and monitor frequently for toxicities
Other potent CYP3A inhibitor	Day 1: 10 mg Day 2: 20 mg Day 3: 50 mg Day 4: 100 mg	Reduce venetoclax dosage to 100 mg daily and monitor frequently for toxicities
Moderate CYP3A inhibitor	Reduce venetoclax dosage by at least 50% and monitor frequently for toxicities	Reduce venetoclax dosage by at least 50% and monitor frequently for toxicities
P-gp inhibitor	Reduce venetoclax dosage by at least 50% and monitor frequently for toxicities	Reduce venetoclax dosage by at least 50% and monitor frequently for toxicities

● Special Populations

Hepatic Impairment

No dosage adjustment is necessary in patients with mild (Child-Pugh class A) or moderate (Child-Pugh class B) hepatic impairment. For patients with severe hepatic impairment (Child-Pugh class C), the manufacturer recommends reducing the once-daily dosage of venetoclax by 50% and closely monitoring such patients for adverse reactions.

Renal Impairment

No dosage adjustment is necessary in patients with mild, moderate, or severe renal impairment (creatinine clearance of 15 mL/minute or greater). Venetoclax has not been studied in patients with end-stage renal disease (creatinine clearance of less than 15 mL/minute) or in those requiring dialysis.

Geriatric Patients

The manufacturer makes no specific dosage recommendations for geriatric patients.

CAUTIONS

● Contraindications

Concomitant use of venetoclax and potent cytochrome P-450 (CYP) 3A inhibitors during initiation of therapy and the dose-escalation period is contraindicated in patients with CLL or SLL due to the potential for an increased risk of tumor lysis syndrome.

● Warnings/Precautions

Tumor Lysis Syndrome

Tumor lysis syndrome, sometimes fatal or resulting in renal failure requiring dialysis, has been reported in patients receiving venetoclax. The risk of tumor lysis syndrome generally is greatest when the drug is first administered and during the dose-escalation period in all patients, and, in patients with CLL or SLL, during reinitiation of therapy following a dosage interruption; laboratory abnormalities consistent with tumor lysis syndrome that require prompt medical treatment may occur as early as 6–8 hours following the initial dose of venetoclax and after each dosage increase. Tumor lysis syndrome, including fatal cases, has occurred in patients following a single 20-mg dose of venetoclax.

In clinical studies evaluating venetoclax monotherapy (using a 5-week dose-escalation schedule and following tumor lysis syndrome prophylaxis and monitoring procedures) in patients with CLL/SLL, tumor lysis syndrome occurred in 2% of patients; the incidence of tumor lysis syndrome was similar to that observed in patients receiving venetoclax in combination with obinutuzumab or rituximab. When a higher initial dosage and shorter dose-escalation period (i.e., 2–3 weeks) was used in patients with CLL/SLL, tumor lysis syndrome occurred in 13% of patients, and resulted in death and renal failure in some cases.

In the VIALE-A study evaluating venetoclax in combination with azacitidine in patients with AML, tumor lysis syndrome occurred in 1.1% of patients; this study employed a 3-day dose-escalation schedule along with prophylaxis and monitoring for tumor lysis syndrome. In addition, 3 patients receiving venetoclax in combination with azacitidine developed transient blood chemistry changes consistent with tumor lysis syndrome during the 3-day dose-escalation period; these laboratory abnormalities resolved with uricosuric therapy and supplemental calcium without venetoclax or azacitidine dosage interruption.

In the VIALE-C study evaluating venetoclax in combination with low-dose cytarabine in patients with AML, tumor lysis syndrome occurred in 5.6% of patients, and resulted in death and renal failure in some cases; this study employed a 4-day dose-escalation schedule along with prophylaxis and monitoring for tumor lysis syndrome.

Assess patients for their risk of developing tumor lysis syndrome and administer appropriate interventions (e.g., prophylactic antihyperuricemic therapy, adequate hydration, monitoring) prior to and during venetoclax therapy. The risk is a continuum based on multiple factors (e.g., type of malignancy, tumor burden, renal impairment, splenomegaly). Concomitant use of certain drugs (e.g., inhibitors of CYP3A or P-glycoprotein [P-gp]) may further increase this risk. Perform tumor burden assessments, including radiographic evaluation (e.g., CT scan), and blood chemistries (i.e., potassium, phosphorus, calcium, uric acid, creatinine) and correct any abnormalities prior to initiating venetoclax therapy and during the dose-escalation period. As the overall risk increases, employ more intensive measures (i.e., IV hydration, more frequent monitoring, hospitalization).

If tumor lysis syndrome occurs, temporary interruption of therapy may be necessary. In patients with CLL or SLL, dosage reduction may be necessary when therapy is resumed.

Neutropenia

Grade 3 or 4 neutropenia occurs commonly in patients receiving venetoclax as monotherapy or as a component of combination therapy. In clinical studies evaluating venetoclax as monotherapy or a component of combination therapy in patients with CLL, grade 3 or 4 neutropenia occurred in 63–64% of patients receiving the drug; grade 4 neutropenia occurred in 31–33% of venetoclax-treated patients, and 4–6% of patients developed febrile neutropenia. In patients with AML, baseline neutrophil counts worsened in 95–100% of patients receiving venetoclax in combination with azacitidine, decitabine, or low-dose cytarabine. Neutropenia may recur with subsequent cycles.

Monitor CBC counts periodically during venetoclax therapy. In patients who develop hematologic toxicity, temporary interruption of therapy or dosage modification may be required. Consider supportive therapy with hematopoietic growth factors (e.g., granulocyte colony-stimulating factor [G-CSF]) and/or anti-infective agents.

Infectious Complications

Fatal and serious infections, such as pneumonia and sepsis, have occurred in patients treated with venetoclax.

Monitor patients for manifestations of infection and initiate appropriate treatment promptly. If grade 3 or 4 infection occurs, withhold venetoclax therapy until resolution of the infection occurs; venetoclax dosage reduction may be necessary.

Immunization

Safety and efficacy of immunization with live, attenuated vaccines during or following venetoclax therapy have not been established. Immune response to vaccines may be reduced. The manufacturer recommends that live, attenuated vaccines be avoided prior to, during, and following venetoclax therapy until B-cell counts have recovered.

Fetal/Neonatal Morbidity and Mortality

Based on its mechanism of action and animal findings, venetoclax may cause fetal harm. Embryofetal toxicity (i.e., postimplantation loss, decreased fetal weight) was observed in animals at venetoclax exposure levels equivalent to the human exposure at 400 mg once daily; no evidence of teratogenicity was observed.

Instruct patients to avoid pregnancy during venetoclax therapy. Perform pregnancy testing in females of reproductive potential prior to initiating venetoclax therapy and instruct such patients to use an effective method of contraception while receiving the drug and for at least 30 days after discontinuance of therapy. If venetoclax is used during pregnancy or if the patient becomes pregnant while receiving the drug, apprise the patient of the potential fetal hazard.

Treatment-related Mortality

Increased mortality has been reported in clinical trials in patients with multiple myeloma† receiving venetoclax in combination with bortezomib and dexamethasone; venetoclax is *not* currently FDA-labeled for use in patients with multiple myeloma. The manufacturer recommends against the use of this combination for the treatment of multiple myeloma outside of a controlled clinical trial.

In a randomized, controlled phase 3 trial (BELLINI) that enrolled 291 patients with multiple myeloma, interim analyses indicated that the risk of death was increased by 103% in patients receiving venetoclax in combination with bortezomib and dexamethasone compared with those receiving bortezomib and dexamethasone. Because of these findings, the BELLINI trial was terminated at FDA's request. However, patients experiencing benefit from the drug may continue therapy with venetoclax in combination with bortezomib and dexamethasone, but only after the risks associated with use of the drug combination have been discussed completely with the patient and a new written informed consent has been obtained.

Specific Populations

Pregnancy

There are no adequate and well-controlled studies of venetoclax in pregnant women; however, animal studies suggest that venetoclax may cause fetal harm. (See Females and Males of Reproductive Potential under Cautions.)

Lactation

It is not known whether venetoclax is distributed into human milk. When a single venetoclax 150-mg/kg dose was administered to lactating rats 8 to 10 days after parturition, drug concentrations in milk were 1.6 times lower than in maternal plasma, and were mostly unchanged drug. Because of the potential for serious adverse reactions to venetoclax in nursing infants, advise patients to discontinue nursing during venetoclax therapy and for 1 week after the final dose. The effects of the drug on nursing infants or milk production are unknown.

Females and Males of Reproductive Potential

Results of animal studies suggest that venetoclax may impair male fertility. Testicular toxicity (germ cell loss) was observed in male dogs receiving venetoclax at exposure levels 0.5 times the human exposure at the recommended dosage.

Perform pregnancy testing in females of reproductive potential prior to initiating venetoclax therapy and instruct patients to use an effective method of contraception while receiving the drug and for at least 30 days after discontinuance of therapy.

Pediatric Use

Safety and efficacy of venetoclax have not been established in pediatric patients.

1340 Venetoclax ANTINEOPLASTIC AGENTS 10:00

In a juvenile toxicology study in animals, clinical signs of venetoclax toxicity (i.e., body weight changes, decreased activity, dehydration, hunched posture, skin pallor, death) have been reported in mice receiving venetoclax from 7 to 60 days of age. Reversible decreases in lymphocyte counts also were observed in mice receiving venetoclax at a dosage approximately 0.06 times the human dosage of 400 mg on a mg/m² basis for a 20-kg child.

Geriatric Use

In 3 open-label studies evaluating venetoclax monotherapy in patients with previously treated CLL/SLL, 57% of patients were 65 years of age or older, and 18% were 75 years of age or older. No overall differences in efficacy or safety were observed between geriatric and younger patients when venetoclax was used as monotherapy or as a component of combination therapy.

In the VIALE-A, M14-358, and VIALE-C clinical studies evaluating venetoclax in combination with azacitidine, decitabine, or low-dose cytarabine in patients with AML, 96, 100, and 92%, respectively, of patients were 65 years of age or older, and 60, 62, and 57%, respectively, were 75 years of age or older. Experience in younger adults with AML is insufficient to determine whether they respond differently from patients 65 years of age or older.

Hepatic Impairment

Venetoclax is principally eliminated by the liver. Systemic exposure to venetoclax was similar in patients with mild or moderate hepatic impairment and those with normal hepatic function. Following a single 50-mg dose of venetoclax, systemic exposure to venetoclax increased 2.7-fold in patients with severe hepatic impairment (Child-Pugh class C) compared with those with normal hepatic function.

Renal Impairment

No clinically important differences in the pharmacokinetics of venetoclax have been observed in patients with mild, moderate, or severe renal impairment (creatinine clearance 15–89 mL/minute) compared with patients with normal renal function. The pharmacokinetics of venetoclax have not been evaluated in patients with end-stage renal disease (creatinine clearance less than 15 mL/minute) or those requiring dialysis; however, substantial removal of the drug by dialysis is unlikely because of the drug's large volume of distribution and extensive protein binding.

Patients with reduced renal function (creatinine clearance less than 80 mL/minute) have an increased risk of tumor lysis syndrome; therefore, more intensive prophylaxis and monitoring are necessary during initiation of venetoclax therapy.

● Common Adverse Effects

In patients with CLL/SLL receiving venetoclax in combination with obinutuzumab or rituximab or as monotherapy, adverse effects reported in 20% or more of patients include neutropenia, thrombocytopenia, anemia, diarrhea, nausea, upper respiratory tract infection, cough, musculoskeletal pain, fatigue, and edema.

In patients with AML receiving venetoclax in combination with azacitidine or decitabine or low-dose cytarabine, adverse effects reported in 30% or more of patients include nausea, diarrhea, thrombocytopenia, constipation, neutropenia, febrile neutropenia, fatigue, vomiting, edema, pyrexia, pneumonia, dyspnea, hemorrhage, anemia, rash, abdominal pain, sepsis, musculoskeletal pain, dizziness, cough, oropharyngeal pain, and hypotension.

DRUG INTERACTIONS

Venetoclax is metabolized principally by cytochrome P-450 (CYP) isoenzyme 3A4/5. In vitro studies indicate that venetoclax is a weak inhibitor of CYP isoenzymes 2C8 and 2C9 and uridine diphosphate-glucuronosyltransferase (UGT) 1A1; however, inhibition is not predicted to be clinically relevant because of high plasma protein binding. In vitro, venetoclax does not inhibit or induce CYP isoenzymes 1A2, 2B6, 2C19, 2D6, or 3A4. Venetoclax also does not inhibit UGT1A4, 1A6, 1A9, or 2B7 in vitro.

In vitro, venetoclax is a substrate and inhibitor of P-glycoprotein (P-gp) and breast cancer resistance protein (BCRP) and a weak inhibitor of organic anion transport protein (OATP) 1B1. Venetoclax does not inhibit OATP1B3, organic cation transporter (OCT) 1, OCT2, renal organic anion transporter (OAT) 1, OAT3, multidrug and toxic compound extrusion (MATE) 1, or MATE2K.

● Drugs and Foods Affecting Hepatic Microsomal Enzymes

Inhibitors of CYP3A

Concomitant use of venetoclax with potent or moderate inhibitors of CYP3A may result in increased peak plasma concentrations and systemic exposure (area under the concentration-time curve [AUC]) of venetoclax, and increased risk of tumor lysis syndrome and other toxicities.

In patients with CLL/SLL, concomitant use of venetoclax with potent inhibitors of CYP3A (e.g., ketoconazole, posaconazole, ritonavir) during the initial dose-escalation period of venetoclax is contraindicated. Venetoclax and potent inhibitors of CYP3A may be used concomitantly, if necessary, once the dose titration has been completed and the patient is receiving a steady daily dosage of venetoclax; however, clinicians should consider using an alternative drug with no or minimal CYP3A inhibition potential. If concomitant use with a potent inhibitor is necessary once the dose titration has been completed and the patient is on a steady daily dosage of venetoclax, reduce the dosage of venetoclax, and monitor for toxicity more frequently. If concomitant use of the potent CYP3A inhibitor is discontinued, return the venetoclax dosage to the dosage used prior to initiation of the potent CYP3A inhibitor in 2–3 days. When venetoclax (during or after the initial dose-escalation period) is used in combination with moderate CYP3A inhibitors, reduce the venetoclax dosage by at least 50%.

In patients with AML, reduce the dosage of venetoclax when the drug is used concomitantly with potent inhibitors of CYP3A, and monitor for toxicity more frequently. If concomitant use of the potent CYP3A inhibitor is discontinued, return the venetoclax dosage to the dosage used prior to initiation of the potent CYP3A inhibitor in 2–3 days. When venetoclax (during or after the initial dose-escalation period) is used in combination with moderate CYP3A inhibitors, reduce the venetoclax dosage by at least 50%, and monitor for toxicity more frequently.

Grapefruit products, Seville oranges, and starfruit contain components that inhibit CYP3A; avoid these products during venetoclax therapy.

Inducers of CYP3A

Concomitant use of venetoclax with potent or moderate inducers of CYP3A may result in decreased peak plasma concentrations and AUC of venetoclax, and potentially decrease venetoclax efficacy.

Avoid concomitant use of venetoclax with potent or moderate inducers of CYP3A.

● Drugs Affecting Efflux Transport Systems

Concomitant use of venetoclax with inhibitors of P-gp may result in increased peak plasma concentrations and AUC of venetoclax, and increased risk of tumor lysis syndrome and other toxicities.

Reduce the dosage of venetoclax by 50% when the drug is used concomitantly with inhibitors of P-gp, and monitor for toxicity more frequently. If concomitant use of the P-gp inhibitor is discontinued, return the venetoclax dosage to the dosage used prior to initiation of the P-gp inhibitor in 2–3 days.

● Substrates of Efflux Transport Systems

Concomitant use of venetoclax with substrate drugs of P-gp may result in increased peak plasma concentrations and systemic exposure to the P-gp substrate drug, and increased risk of toxicity. When a single 100-mg dose of venetoclax was administered concomitantly with the P-gp substrate digoxin (0.5 mg), peak plasma concentrations and systemic exposure to digoxin increased by 35 and 9%, respectively. Avoid concomitant use of venetoclax with P-gp substrates. If such concomitant therapy is necessary, the manufacturer recommends administering the substrate drug at least 6 hours prior to venetoclax.

● Drugs Affecting Gastric Acidity

The pharmacokinetics of venetoclax are not substantially altered when used concomitantly with gastric acid-reducing agents. In a population pharmacokinetic analysis, concomitant administration of gastric acid-reducing agents (e.g., antacids, histamine H₂-receptor antagonists, proton-pump inhibitors) with venetoclax did not result in clinically important changes in the bioavailability of venetoclax.

● *Antineoplastic Agents*

The pharmacokinetics of venetoclax are not substantially altered when coadministered with azacitidine, cytarabine, decitabine, obinutuzumab, or rituximab.

● *Azithromycin*

The pharmacokinetics of venetoclax are not substantially altered when coadministered with azithromycin.

● *Ketoconazole*

Ketoconazole is a potent CYP3A, P-gp, and BCRP inhibitor. Concomitant administration of ketoconazole (400 mg daily for 7 days) with venetoclax increased the peak plasma concentration and AUC of venetoclax by 130 and 540%, respectively.

Concomitant use may be contraindicated or reduction in venetoclax dosage may be required.

● *Posaconazole*

Posaconazole is a potent CYP3A and P-gp inhibitor. Concomitant administration of posaconazole (300 mg daily for 7 days) with venetoclax (50 mg daily for 7 days) increased the peak plasma concentration and AUC of venetoclax by 61 and 90%, respectively, compared with venetoclax 400 mg alone; when the dosage of venetoclax was increased to 100 mg daily, peak plasma concentration and AUC of venetoclax increased by 86 and 144%, respectively, compared with venetoclax 400 mg alone.

Concomitant use may be contraindicated or reduction in venetoclax dosage may be required.

● *Rifampin*

Rifampin is a potent CYP3A inducer as well as an OATP1B1/1B3 and P-gp inhibitor. Concomitant administration of a single 600-mg dose of rifampin with venetoclax increased the peak plasma concentration and AUC of venetoclax by 106 and 78%, respectively. Concomitant administration of repeated doses of rifampin as a strong CYP3A inducer (600 mg daily for 13 days) with venetoclax decreased the peak plasma concentration and AUC of venetoclax by 42 and 71%, respectively.

Avoid concomitant use.

● *Ritonavir*

Concomitant administration of the potent CYP3A, P-gp, and OATP1B1/1B3 inhibitor ritonavir (50 mg once daily for 14 days) with venetoclax increased the peak plasma concentration and AUC of venetoclax by 140 and 690%, respectively.

Concomitant use may be contraindicated or reduction in venetoclax dosage may be required.

● *Warfarin*

Concomitant administration of venetoclax (single 400-mg dose) with warfarin sodium (5 mg) in 3 healthy individuals increased peak plasma concentrations and systemic exposure of warfarin by 18–28%. Venetoclax was not dosed to steady state in this study. The manufacturer recommends close monitoring of the international normalized ratio (INR) in patients receiving warfarin.

● *Vaccines*

Live, attenuated vaccines should not be administered prior to, during, and following venetoclax therapy until B-cell recovery occurs. The manufacturer states that vaccinations may be less effective in patients receiving venetoclax.

DESCRIPTION

Venetoclax is a potent and selective inhibitor of B-cell chronic lymphoma 2 (BCL-2); the drug is an antineoplastic agent. BCL-2, an anti-apoptotic protein, is overexpressed in AML and CLL and mediates tumor cell survival and has been associated with resistance to chemotherapy. Following binding of venetoclax to BCL-2, displacement of pro-apoptotic proteins (e.g., BIM), mitochondrial outer membrane permeabilization, and caspase activation occur; these actions result in restoration of the intrinsic apoptotic pathway. In nonclinical studies, venetoclax demonstrated cytotoxic activity in tumor cells overexpressing BCL-2.

Venetoclax exhibits linear pharmacokinetics over a dose range of 150–800 mg. Peak plasma concentrations of the drug are achieved about 5–8 hours following oral administration under fed conditions. Administration of venetoclax with a low-fat or high-fat meal increased systemic exposure by approximately 3.4- or 5.2-fold, respectively, compared with the fasting state. Venetoclax is highly bound (over 99%) to plasma proteins. The mean terminal half-life of venetoclax is approximately 26 hours. Venetoclax is metabolized to its major metabolite (M27) mainly by cytochrome P-450 (CYP) isoenzyme 3A4/5; the AUC for M27 represents 80% of the AUC of venetoclax. The major metabolite has demonstrated inhibitory activity against BCL-2 that is at least 58-fold lower than that of the parent drug. Following oral administration of a single radiolabeled dose of venetoclax, more than 99.9% of the radioactivity was recovered in feces (20.8% as unchanged drug) and less than 0.1% was recovered in urine within 9 days.

Pharmacokinetic analyses indicate that age (19–93 years), sex, and body weight do not have clinically important effects on the pharmacokinetics of venetoclax. No clinically important differences in pharmacokinetics of venetoclax were observed in white, Black, and Asian patients enrolled in clinical studies conducted in the US. Among 771 patients with AML, systemic venetoclax exposure was 63% higher in Asian patients from Asian countries (i.e., China, Japan, South Korea, Taiwan) compared with non-Asian populations.

ADVICE TO PATIENTS

Advise patients to keep venetoclax in its original container, including the titration pack for CLL/SLL. Importance of taking venetoclax exactly as prescribed with food and water. Avoid grapefruit products, Seville oranges, and starfruit while taking the drug.

Importance of advising patients to swallow venetoclax tablets whole and to not chew, crush, or break the tablets.

If a dose is missed, importance of advising patients to take it as soon as they remember and resume the next dose at the regularly scheduled time unless the dose was missed by more than 8 hours, in which case they should not take the missed dose. If a dose is vomited, importance of administering the next dose at the regularly scheduled time; an additional dose should not be administered to make up for a missed dose.

Risk of tumor lysis syndrome, particularly during initiation of therapy, initial dose escalation, and resumption of therapy following dosage interruption. Venetoclax may need to be administered in the hospital or medical office setting to allow monitoring for tumor lysis syndrome. Importance of maintaining scheduled appointments for blood work and other laboratory tests. Importance of immediately reporting any signs or symptoms of tumor lysis syndrome (e.g., fever, chills, nausea, vomiting, confusion, shortness of breath, seizure, arrhythmia, dark or cloudy urine, fatigue, muscle pain, joint discomfort). Importance of advising patients to maintain adequate hydration during venetoclax therapy. The recommended volume is 6–8 glasses (approximately 56 ounces) a day. Patients should start drinking water 2 days before initiating venetoclax, on the day of the first dose, and each time the dose is increased.

Risk of neutropenia. Importance of monitoring complete blood cell (CBC) counts periodically during venetoclax therapy. Importance of immediately reporting any signs or symptoms of infection (e.g., fever).

Risk of infection; importance of immediately reporting any signs or symptoms of infection (e.g., fever).

Importance of avoiding use of live vaccines prior to, during, and following venetoclax therapy until B-cell recovery.

Risk of fetal harm. Necessity of advising females of childbearing potential that they should use an effective method of contraception while receiving the drug and for at least 30 days after discontinuance of therapy. Importance of females informing clinicians if they are or plan to become pregnant. If pregnancy occurs, advise pregnant females of potential risk to the fetus.

Risk of male infertility.

Importance of advising females to avoid breast-feeding while receiving venetoclax and for 1 week after the last dose.

Importance of informing clinicians of existing or contemplated concomitant therapy, including prescription and OTC drugs and dietary or herbal supplements, as well as any concomitant illnesses.

Importance of informing patients of other important precautionary information. (See Cautions.)

For further information on the handling of antineoplastic agents, see the ASHP Guidelines on Handling Hazardous Drugs at http://www.ahfsdrug information.com.

PREPARATIONS

Venetoclax can only be obtained through designated specialty pharmacies and distributors. Contact manufacturer for specific availability information.

Excipients in commercially available drug preparations may have clinically important effects in some individuals; consult specific product labeling for details.

Venetoclax

Oral		
Tablets, film-coated	10 mg	Venclexta®, Genentech
	50 mg	Venclexta®, Genentech
	100 mg	Venclexta®, Genentech
Titration Pack (CLL/SLL)	14 Tablets, Venetoclax 10 mg (Venclexta®)	
	7 Tablets, Venetoclax 50 mg (Venclexta®)	
	7 Tablets, Venetoclax 100 mg (Venclexta®)	
	14 Tablets, Venetoclax 100 mg (Venclexta®)	Venclexta® Starting Pack (CLL/SLL), Genentech

† Use is not currently included in the labeling approved by the US Food and Drug Administration.

Selected Revisions October 13, 2022, © Copyright, October 25, 2016, American Society of Health-System Pharmacists, Inc.

vinCRIStine Sulfate

10:00 • ANTINEOPLASTIC AGENTS

■ Vincristine sulfate, a naturally occurring vinca alkaloid, is an antineoplastic agent.

USES

Vincristine sulfate is commercially available in 2 types of formulations: conventional vincristine sulfate and liposomal vincristine sulfate. The efficacy and safety of vincristine for each indication is based on research and clinical experience using a specific formulation.

● Acute Lymphocytic Leukemia

Conventional Vincristine

Conventional vincristine is used as a component of combination chemotherapeutic regimens for the induction of remissions of childhood or adult acute lymphocytic (lymphoblastic) leukemia (ALL). Various drugs have been used for combination chemotherapy of childhood and adult ALL, and comparative efficacy of these regimens is continually being evaluated. Additional therapy (e.g., intrathecal administration of methotrexate with or without intrathecal cytarabine and hydrocortisone, with or without systemic methotrexate and leucovorin rescue and/or cranial radiation in children; intrathecal methotrexate given alone or in conjunction with cranial radiation or high-dose systemic methotrexate and leucovorin rescue in adults) is needed for prophylaxis of CNS involvement (meningeal leukemia) in patients with ALL. Once remission has been attained, patients generally receive consolidation-intensification therapy and maintenance therapy. Other regimens are preferred in certain subsets of patients with ALL (e.g., B-cell ALL, T-cell ALL, Philadelphia chromosome-positive ALL). Certain patients with a poor prognosis or with a poor response to initial treatment may be candidates for hematopoietic stem cell transplantation. Specialized references and experts should be consulted for additional information.

Although conventional vincristine used with a corticosteroid such as prednisone results in high remission induction rates in children with ALL, addition of an asparaginase preparation and/or an anthracycline (e.g., daunorubicin) can improve both the rate and duration of remission and therefore such 3- or 4-drug regimens generally are preferred. (For additional information on the asparaginase component of ALL regimens, see Asparaginase [Erwinia chrysanthemi] 10:00.) The use of intensive induction regimens with 4 or more drugs, including conventional vincristine, an asparaginase preparation, a corticosteroid (e.g., prednisone), and an anthracycline (e.g., daunorubicin), with or without cyclophosphamide, may improve the rate of event-free survival but is associated with greater toxicity. An induction regimen containing 4 or more drugs does not appear to be necessary to achieve favorable outcomes in patients at low or standard risk of treatment failure provided adequate intensification therapy is provided following achievement of remission. Therefore, some clinicians reserve such regimens for patients with high-risk childhood ALL. However, other clinicians have elected to use a 4- or 5-drug induction regimen for all patients with childhood ALL regardless of presenting features. Maintenance therapy (e.g., methotrexate and mercaptopurine with or without pulses of conventional vincristine and prednisone) is administered for about 2–3 years.

Induction regimens for adult ALL typically include conventional vincristine, prednisone, and an anthracycline; some regimens also add other drugs, such as an asparaginase preparation or cyclophosphamide.

Liposomal Vincristine

Liposomal vincristine is used for the treatment of Philadelphia chromosome-negative (Ph⁻) relapsed or refractory ALL in patients in second or greater relapse or in those whose disease has progressed following at least 2 prior therapies. The drug has been designated an orphan drug by FDA for use in this condition. The accelerated approval of liposomal vincristine for this indication is based on overall response rate; continued approval for this indication may be contingent on verification and description of clinical benefit (e.g., overall survival) of liposomal vincristine in confirmatory studies.

The current indication for liposomal vincristine is based principally on the results of an open-label, noncomparative, phase 2 study in 65 adults with Ph⁻ relapsed or refractory ALL. Patients were enrolled if they were in second or greater relapse or if their disease had relapsed or was refractory following at least 2 prior therapies. Patients enrolled in the study also were required to have achieved complete remission (defined as a leukemia-free interval lasting at least 90 days) after at least one prior therapy. In this study, patients received liposomal vincristine sulfate at a dosage of 2.25 mg/m² of vincristine sulfate by IV infusion over 60 minutes on days 1, 8, 15, and 22 of each 28-day cycle; concomitant therapy with systemic corticosteroids or hydroxyurea was not permitted beyond day 5 or 14, respectively, of the first cycle. The primary measure of efficacy was complete remission (CR) or complete remission with incomplete hematologic recovery (CRi) according to the International Working Group (IWG) response criteria. The median age of patients was 31 years; 85% of the patients had precursor B-cell ALL (pre-B-ALL), 15% had precursor T-cell ALL (pre-T-ALL), 48% had undergone hematopoietic stem cell transplantation prior to study entry, and 80% of the patients had residual neuropathy at baseline following prior therapy with conventional vincristine. Approximately one-half of patients had received 3 or more prior therapies for their disease; all of the enrolled patients received prior therapy with conventional vincristine and 45% were refractory to their most recent therapy prior to study entry. Overall, CR or CRi was reported in 15.4% of patients; 4.6% of patients achieved CR. At the time of analysis, the median duration of response from initial CR or CRi to date of documented relapse, death, or subsequent chemotherapy or stem-cell transplantation was 56 days.

● Acute Myeloid Leukemia

Conventional vincristine is used in various combination regimens for the treatment of acute myeloid (myelogenous, nonlymphocytic) leukemias (AML, ANLL), but the comparative efficacy of these combinations is continually being evaluated. (See Uses: Leukemias, in Cytarabine 10:00.)

● Hodgkin's Disease

Conventional vincristine is used as a component of various chemotherapeutic regimens for the treatment of Hodgkin's disease. Various drugs have been used for combination chemotherapy, and comparative efficacy of these regimens is continually being evaluated. Conventional vincristine is used in combination with bleomycin, etoposide, doxorubicin, cyclophosphamide, procarbazine and prednisone (in the increased-dose BEACOPP regimen) for the treatment of early or advanced Hodgkin's disease. Conventional vincristine also is used in combination with doxorubicin, bleomycin, vinblastine, mechlorethamine, etoposide, and prednisone (Stanford V regimen); mechlorethamine, procarbazine, doxorubicin, bleomycin, and prednisone (MOPP-ABV regimen); and cyclophosphamide, procarbazine, doxorubicin, bleomycin, vinblastine, dacarbazine, and prednisone (COPP-ABVD regimen) for the treatment of Hodgkin's disease.

● Non-Hodgkin's Lymphoma

Conventional vincristine is used as a component of combination chemotherapeutic regimens for the treatment of non-Hodgkin's lymphomas, and the comparative efficacy of various regimens is continually being evaluated. Conventional vincristine generally is used with cyclophosphamide and prednisone with or without doxorubicin (i.e., CHOP or CVP regimen); rituximab usually is administered with these regimens.

● Neuroblastoma

Conventional vincristine is used as a component of various chemotherapeutic regimens for the treatment of neuroblastoma.

● Rhabdomyosarcoma

Conventional vincristine is used as a component of combination chemotherapeutic regimens for the treatment of childhood rhabdomyosarcoma; conventional vincristine is commonly used with dactinomycin, with or without cyclophosphamide, as an adjunct to surgery and/or radiation therapy.

● Wilms' Tumor

Combination chemotherapy is superior to single-drug therapy as an adjunct to surgery and/or radiation therapy in prolonging relapse-free survival and overall survival in children with Wilms' tumor. Conventional vincristine is generally used with dactinomycin (with or without doxorubicin) or in combination with doxorubicin, cyclophosphamide, and etoposide for the treatment of Wilms' tumor.

● Brain Tumors

Conventional vincristine is used for the palliative treatment of various primary brain tumors†. Various regimens that typically include conventional vincristine and lomustine with another antineoplastic agent, such as procarbazine or cisplatin, or a corticosteroid (prednisone) have been used in the treatment of astrocytic tumors (e.g., glioblastoma multiforme and anaplastic astrocytoma), medulloblastoma, and oligodendroglioma. See Uses: Brain Tumors in Lomustine 10:00 for further discussion.

● AIDS-related Kaposi's Sarcoma

Conventional vincristine is used in combination chemotherapy for the palliative treatment of AIDS-related Kaposi's sarcoma†. Combination chemotherapy that includes a vinca alkaloid (vinblastine or conventional vincristine), conventional doxorubicin, and bleomycin has previously been a preferred regimen for the disease, but many clinicians currently consider a liposomal anthracycline (doxorubicin or daunorubicin) the first-line therapy of choice for advanced AIDS-related Kaposi's sarcoma (see Uses: AIDS-related Kaposi's Sarcoma in Doxorubicin 10:00 for overview and further discussion of therapy; also see Daunorubicin 10:00).

Combination chemotherapy with conventional antineoplastic agents (e.g., bleomycin, conventional doxorubicin, etoposide, vinblastine, conventional vincristine) usually has been used for more advanced disease (e.g., extensive mucocutaneous disease, lymphedema, symptomatic visceral disease). However, the results of several randomized, multicenter trials indicate that patients receiving a liposomal anthracycline for the treatment of advanced AIDS-related Kaposi's sarcoma experience similar or higher response rates with a more favorable toxic effects profile than those receiving combination therapy with conventional chemotherapeutic agents.

Conventional vincristine also has been used alone for the palliative treatment of AIDS-related Kaposi's sarcoma. In one study in patients with AIDS-related Kaposi's sarcoma who received a conventional vincristine dosage of 2 mg weekly for 2–5 weeks and then every 2 weeks thereafter as tolerated, partial or minor response was observed in about 61 or 39% of evaluable patients, respectively.

● Small Cell Lung Cancer

Conventional vincristine is used in combination with cyclophosphamide and doxorubicin (CAV) for the treatment of extensive-stage small cell lung cancer†. Survival outcomes are similar in patients with extensive-stage small cell lung cancer receiving CAV or cisplatin/etoposide. Conventional vincristine also has been used in combination with cyclophosphamide and etoposide for the treatment of extensive-stage small cell lung cancer†. Combination chemotherapy regimens have produced response rates of 70–85% and complete response rates of 20–30% in patients with extensive-stage disease; however, comparative efficacy is continually being evaluated. Because the current prognosis for small cell lung carcinoma is unsatisfactory regardless of stage and despite considerable diagnostic and therapeutic advances, all patients with this cancer are candidates for inclusion in clinical trials at the time of diagnosis.

● Other Uses

Conventional vincristine also is used as a component of combination chemotherapy for the treatment of osteosarcoma† (including Ewing's sarcoma†), multiple myeloma†, and choriocarcinoma†. Combination chemotherapy with conventional vincristine, cyclophosphamide, and prednisone, with or without doxorubicin, is used in the treatment of chronic lymphocytic leukemia (CLL)†. Combination chemotherapy with conventional vincristine, cisplatin, and fluorouracil is used in the treatment of hepatoblastoma†. Conventional vincristine combined with cyclophosphamide and dacarbazine is used for the treatment of pheochromocytoma†.

Conventional vincristine has been used in the treatment of immune thrombocytopenic purpura†. IV injections of the drug have also been used with some success for the treatment of thrombotic thrombocytopenic purpura†, and the use of vincristine-loaded platelets has reportedly been useful in some cases for the management of autoimmune hemolytic anemia†.

DOSAGE AND ADMINISTRATION

● Reconstitution and Administration

Vincristine sulfate is commercially available in 2 types of formulations: conventional vincristine sulfate and liposomal vincristine sulfate (Marqibo®). The properties of vincristine may differ according to formulation, and the dosage and preparation for vincristine sulfate are specific to formulation. The manufacturer's instructions for the specific formulation should be consulted to ensure that the correct preparation procedure is followed.

Conventional and liposomal vincristine formulations are for IV use *only* and should be administered by individuals experienced in the administration of the drug. *Conventional and liposomal vincristine sulfate must not be given by other routes (e.g., IM, subcutaneously, intrathecally). Intrathecal administration of vincristine usually results in death.* When dispensed, the infusion bag or syringe holding the individual dose prepared for administration to the patient *must* be labeled with the statement **"For intravenous use only. Fatal if given by other routes."** The syringe *must* be enclosed in an overwrap bearing the statements: **"Do not remove covering until moment of injection. For intravenous use only. Fatal if given by other routes."**

In addition to use of the labels and overwrap, other protective measures to prevent inadvertent intrathecal administration of conventional or liposomal vincristine or other vinca alkaloids include: administration of the diluted drug in small-volume IV bags (i.e., minibags), preparing the medication at the time of administration, attaching a unique filter, dispensing the vinca alkaloid separately from all other medications, dispensing the vinca alkaloid directly to the individual who is administering the drug, conducting an independent check of the dose and route of administration for the drug both at the time of preparation and prior to administration of the drug, and administering the vinca alkaloid in a separate room from rooms where other medications are administered.

Management of patients mistakenly receiving intrathecal conventional or liposomal vincristine is a medical emergency. Unfortunately, the prognosis to date generally has been poor despite immediate efforts at removing spinal fluid and flushing with lactated Ringer's injection as well as other solutions, with such efforts failing to prevent ascending paralysis and death in almost all cases. In one case, progression of paralysis was stopped in an adult patient when the following treatment was initiated immediately after inadvertent intrathecal injection of conventional vincristine. Such treatment consisted of immediate removal of as much CSF as safely possible via lumbar access, followed by flushing of the subarachnoid space with lactated Ringer's solution infused continuously at a rate of 150 mL/hour through a catheter in a cerebral lateral ventricle and removal of fluid through a lumbar access. As soon as available, fresh frozen plasma (25 mL) diluted in 1 L of lactated Ringer's solution was infused through the cerebral ventricular catheter at a rate of 75 mL per hour with removal of fluid through the lumbar access. The rate of infusion was adjusted to maintain a CSF protein concentration of 150 mg/dL. Glutamic acid was administered in a dose of 10 g given IV over 24 hours, followed by 500 mg orally 3 times daily for 1 month or until stabilization of neurologic status. The role of glutamic acid in this treatment is uncertain.

Conventional Vincristine Sulfate

Extra fluid should not be added to the vial containing conventional vincristine sulfate prior to removal of the dose. Conventional vincristine sulfate injection should be withdrawn from the vial into an accurate dry syringe, and the dose should be measured carefully. Extra fluid should not be added to the vial in an attempt to empty it completely.

Preparation of the conventional vincristine dose as a diluted solution in a minibag is recommended as a protective measure to prevent inadvertent intrathecal administration of the drug; however, if the drug is prepared as a diluted solution in a syringe, a 30-mL syringe is recommended. The larger volume of the diluted conventional vincristine solution and incompatible packaging make it less likely that the IV conventional vincristine dose will be confused with a drug that is intended for intrathecal use. For preparation in a minibag, the dose of conventional vincristine sulfate should be diluted with an appropriate volume of 0.9% sodium chloride injection to a final concentration of 0.0015–0.08 mg/mL. If the drug is prepared in a minibag or diluted in a 30-mL syringe, the dose should be administered by IV injection over 5–10 minutes in adults; in children, the dose should be administered at a slower rate. The Oncology Nursing Society (ONS) recommends that if a vesicant drug such as vincristine is administered by short infusion into a peripheral vein, an IV pump *not* be used in order to decrease pressure applied on the veins.

Conventional vincristine also has been diluted in a large volume of IV solution and administered as a slow IV infusion† (e.g., over 4–8 hours); continuous 4- or 5-day IV infusions† have also been used. Specialized references should be consulted for specific information on slow IV infusion of conventional vincristine.

For rapid IV ("bolus") injections, conventional vincristine sulfate injection must be administered through an intact, free-flowing IV needle or catheter. Care should be taken to ensure that the needle or catheter is securely within the vein to avoid extravasation. If leakage or swelling occurs, the injection should be discontinued immediately and the remainder of the dose given through another vein; local treatment of the area of leakage may minimize discomfort and the possibility of cellulitis. (See Cautions: Local Effects.) Conventional vincristine sulfate injection may be injected either directly into a vein or into the tubing of a running IV infusion; injection of the drug should be completed within 1 minute.

When conventional vincristine and asparaginase must be administered sequentially, the sequence of vincristine followed by asparaginase is recommended. (See Drug Interactions: Antineoplastic Agents.)

Liposomal Vincristine Sulfate

Liposomal vincristine sulfate (Marqibo®) is commercially available as a 3-vial kit containing single-use vials of vincristine sulfate solution, sphingomyelin-cholesterol liposome suspension, and dibasic sodium phosphate solution. Preparation of liposomal vincristine sulfate suspension requires 60–90 minutes of dedicated and uninterrupted time because extensive monitoring of temperature and time is required during the process. Deviations from temperature control, timing, and preparation procedures may affect encapsulation of vincristine sulfate into the liposomes. If deviations in the preparation process occur, the components of the kit should be discarded and a new kit should be used to prepare liposomal vincristine sulfate.

Vincristine sulfate solution must be mixed with the sphingomyelin-cholesterol liposome suspension and dibasic sodium phosphate solution provided in the kit; the resultant liposomal vincristine sulfate injection concentrate must be diluted prior to IV infusion. For preparation of liposomal vincristine sulfate injection concentrate, equipment provided by the manufacturer (i.e., water bath or block heater, calibrated thermometer, electronic timer, tongs) must be used. Either the water bath or block heater (but not both) may be used to prepare liposomal vincristine sulfate injection concentrate. All steps required to mix and dilute the drug product should be performed *inside* the sterile area using strict aseptic technique since the injection does not contain any preservative or bacteriostatic agent. Each vial in the kit and the final diluted suspension for infusion should be inspected visually for particulate matter and discoloration prior to preparation and administration whenever solution and container permit; the vials and diluted suspension for infusion should *not* be used if foreign particles or precipitate is present.

Liposomal vincristine is administered by IV infusion over 1 hour. Liposomal vincristine should not be admixed with any other drug and should not be administered using an inline filter. Care should be taken to ensure that the venous access line is secure and free-flowing to avoid extravasation. If extravasation is suspected, the infusion should be discontinued immediately and local treatments considered. (See Cautions: Local Effects.)

Water Bath Preparation Instructions

The water bath should be prepared and maintained *outside* the sterile area. The water in the bath should be maintained at a minimum depth of 8 cm and at a temperature of 63–67°C (measured by the calibrated thermometer) throughout the preparation process. The calibrated thermometer should remain in the water bath throughout the preparation process. All steps required to mix and dilute the drug product should be performed *inside* the sterile area using strict aseptic technique.

For preparation of liposomal vincristine sulfate injection concentrate, a venting needle (or other suitable venting device) with a 0.2-μm filter should be inserted into the vial containing dibasic sodium phosphate solution with the point of the venting needle positioned well above the surface of the solution. A volume of 1 mL of sphingomyelin-cholesterol liposome suspension followed by 5 mL of vincristine sulfate solution should be injected into the vial. The venting needle should then be removed and the vial should be gently inverted 5 times to mix the 3 components; the vial should *not* be shaken. The neck of the vial containing the mixture of the 3 components should be fitted with the manufacturer-provided flotation ring, and then the vial should be placed in the water bath for 10 minutes; the temperature of the water bath and duration of flotation should be closely monitored using the calibrated thermometer and electronic timer. After 10 minutes, the vial should be removed from the water bath using tongs to prevent burns, and the flotation ring should be removed from the vial. The start time and temperature and the end time and temperature should be recorded on the liposomal vincristine sulfate injection concentrate overlabel immediately after the vial is placed into the water bath and upon removal, respectively. The vial exterior should be dried with a clean paper towel upon removal from the water bath, and then the overlabel should be affixed to the vial. The vial should be gently inverted another 5 times to mix the contents; the vial should *not* be shaken. The resultant liposomal vincristine sulfate injection concentrate contains vincristine sulfate 0.16 mg/mL and should be stored at room temperature (15–30°C) for no more than 12 hours. Liposomal vincristine sulfate injection concentrate should be allowed to come to room temperature (i.e., 15–30°C) over at least 30 minutes prior to dilution.

For preparation of the *final* diluted IV infusion of liposomal vincristine sulfate, a volume equivalent to the volume of the appropriate dose of liposomal vincristine sulfate should be withdrawn from an infusion bag containing 100 mL of 5% dextrose or 0.9% sodium chloride injection and discarded; the appropriate dose of liposomal vincristine sulfate injection concentrate is then withdrawn from the vial and added to the infusion bag to yield a final volume of 100 mL. The infusion bag label supplied by the drug's manufacturer should be completed and affixed to the bag. Infusion of the diluted drug should be completed within 12 hours of *initiation* of preparation of liposomal vincristine sulfate injection.

Block Heater Preparation Instructions

When a block heater is used for the preparation of liposomal vincristine sulfate injection concentrate, the block heater should be placed *outside* the sterile area. All steps required to mix and dilute the drug product should be performed *inside* the sterile area using strict aseptic technique.

For preparation of liposomal vincristine sulfate injection concentrate using a block heater, 3 heating blocks should be placed in the block heater with the block that will hold the vial containing the drug components placed between 2 blank blocks. The controller of the block heater should be set to 75°C and the temperature should be allowed to equilibrate to 73–77°C (measured by the calibrated thermometer) for 15 minutes. The temperature of the block heater should be maintained at 73–77°C throughout the preparation process. The calibrated thermometer should remain in the block heater throughout the preparation process.

For preparation of liposomal vincristine sulfate injection concentrate, a venting needle (or other suitable venting device) with a 0.2-μm filter should be inserted into the vial containing dibasic sodium phosphate solution with the point of the venting needle well above the surface of the solution. A volume of 1 mL of sphingomyelin-cholesterol liposome suspension followed by 5 mL of vincristine sulfate solution should be injected into the vial. The venting needle should then be removed and the vial should be gently inverted 5 times to mix the 3 components; the vial should *not* be shaken. The vial containing the mixture of the 3 components should be placed in the block heater for 18 minutes; the temperature of the block heater and duration in the block heater should be closely monitored using the calibrated thermometer and electronic timer. After 18 minutes, the vial should be removed from the block heater using tongs to prevent burns. The start time and temperature and the end time and temperature should be recorded on the liposomal vincristine sulfate injection concentrate overlabel immediately after the vial is placed into the block heater and upon removal, respectively. The vial should be gently inverted another 5 times to mix the contents; the vial should *not* be shaken. The resultant liposomal vincristine sulfate injection concentrate contains vincristine sulfate 0.16 mg/mL and should be stored at room temperature (15–30°C) for no more than 12 hours. Liposomal vincristine sulfate injection concentrate should be allowed to come to room temperature (i.e., 15–30°C) over at least 30 minutes prior to dilution.

For preparation of the *final* diluted IV infusion of liposomal vincristine sulfate, a volume equivalent to the volume of the appropriate dose of liposomal vincristine sulfate should be withdrawn from an infusion bag containing 100 mL of 5% dextrose or 0.9% sodium chloride injection and discarded; the appropriate dose of liposomal vincristine sulfate injection concentrate is then withdrawn from the vial and added to the infusion bag to yield a final volume of 100 mL. The infusion bag label supplied by the drug's manufacturer should be completed and affixed to the bag. Infusion of the diluted drug should be completed within 12 hours of *initiation* of preparation of liposomal vincristine sulfate injection.

● Dosage

Conventional Vincristine Sulfate

Various conventional vincristine sulfate dosages have been used. Clinicians should consult published protocols for the dosage of conventional vincristine sulfate and other chemotherapeutic agents and the method and sequence of administration. The manufacturers of conventional vincristine sulfate recommend a usual adult dose of 1.4 mg/m² and a usual pediatric dose of 1.5–2 mg/m². For children weighing 10 kg or less, the manufacturers of conventional vincristine sulfate recommend that therapy be initiated at 0.05 mg/kg once weekly. Some clinicians recommend that adult doses not exceed 2 mg of conventional vincristine sulfate. Subsequent doses must be determined by the clinical and hematologic response and tolerance of the patient in order to obtain optimum therapeutic results with minimum adverse effects. Conventional vincristine is usually administered at weekly intervals. Small daily doses are not recommended because they produce severe toxicity with no added therapeutic benefit.

Liposomal Vincristine Sulfate

For the treatment of Philadelphia chromosome-negative (Ph⁻) relapsed or refractory ALL in patients in second or greater relapse or in those whose disease has progressed following at least 2 prior therapies, the recommended adult dosage of liposomal vincristine sulfate is 2.25 mg/m² of vincristine sulfate administered IV over 1 hour once weekly.

Dosage Modification for Toxicity

Neurologic Toxicity

Careful monitoring for neurologic toxicity including clinical evaluation (e.g., history, physical examination) is advised, and dosage reduction may be necessary, particularly in patients with preexisting neuromuscular disease or in patients receiving other agents with neurotoxic potential. Adverse neurologic effects, such as neuritic pain or constipation, may lessen or disappear when the dosage of conventional vincristine is reduced.

If grade 3 peripheral neuropathy (severe symptoms resulting in interference with self-care activities of daily living) occurs in patients receiving liposomal vincristine, therapy with the drug should be withheld. If grade 3 peripheral neuropathy persists or worsens despite interruption of therapy, liposomal vincristine therapy should be discontinued. If peripheral neuropathy improves to grade 2 or less, liposomal vincristine therapy may be resumed at a reduced vincristine sulfate dosage (i.e., 2.25 mg/m² reduced to 2 mg/m²).

If persistent grade 2 peripheral neuropathy (moderate symptoms resulting in interference with instrumental activities of daily living) occurs in patients receiving liposomal vincristine, therapy with the drug should be withheld. If grade 2 peripheral neuropathy worsens to grade 3 or 4 despite interruption of therapy, liposomal vincristine therapy should be discontinued. If the toxicity improves, liposomal vincristine therapy may be resumed at a reduced vincristine sulfate dosage (i.e., 2.25 mg/m² reduced to 2 mg/m²).

If the patient has persistent grade 2 peripheral neuropathy at a reduced dosage of 2 mg/m², liposomal vincristine therapy should be withheld again for up to 7 days. If grade 2 peripheral neuropathy worsens despite interruption of therapy, liposomal vincristine therapy should be discontinued. If the toxicity improves to grade 1, liposomal vincristine therapy may be resumed at a further reduced vincristine sulfate dosage (i.e., 2 mg/m² reduced to 1.825 mg/m²). If the patient has persistent grade 2 peripheral neuropathy at a dosage of 1.825 mg/m², liposomal vincristine therapy should be withheld again for up to 7 days. If grade 2 peripheral neuropathy worsens despite interruption of therapy, liposomal vincristine therapy should be discontinued. If the toxicity improves to grade 1, liposomal vincristine therapy may be resumed at a further reduced vincristine sulfate dosage (i.e., 1.825 mg/m² reduced to 1.5 mg/m²).

Hematologic Toxicity

Complete blood cell (CBC) counts should be performed before the administration of each dose of conventional or liposomal vincristine.

Following administration of conventional vincristine, a decrease in leukocyte count or platelet count may occur, particularly in patients for whom previous therapy or disease has reduced bone marrow function. In patients with leukopenia or infectious complications, withholding of the next dose of conventional vincristine should be considered. Leukopenia may lessen or disappear when the dosage of conventional vincristine is reduced.

If grade 3 or 4 neutropenia, thrombocytopenia, or anemia occurs in patients receiving liposomal vincristine, dosage reduction or temporary interruption of liposomal vincristine therapy and supportive care measures should be considered.

Hepatic Toxicity

If hepatotoxicity occurs in patients receiving liposomal vincristine, dosage reduction or temporary interruption of liposomal vincristine therapy should be considered.

Pulmonary Toxicity

Conventional vincristine therapy should be discontinued in patients who develop progressive dyspnea.

Other Nonhematologic Toxicity

If fatigue occurs in patients receiving liposomal vincristine, dosage reduction, temporary interruption, or discontinuance of liposomal vincristine therapy should be considered.

● Dosage in Hepatic Impairment

A 50% reduction in conventional vincristine dose is recommended for patients with a direct serum bilirubin concentration exceeding 3 mg/dL or other evidence of clinically important hepatic impairment.

The manufacturer makes no specific recommendations regarding dosage of liposomal vincristine in patients with hepatic impairment. (See Pharmacokinetics.)

CAUTIONS

In general, adverse reactions to vincristine are dose related and reversible.

The incidence of adverse effects associated with liposomal vincristine is based principally on clinical trial data for 83 patients with Philadelphia chromosome-negative (Ph⁻) relapsed or refractory acute lymphocytic (lymphoblastic) leukemia (ALL) who received the drug at the recommended dosage. The most common adverse effects, each occurring in more than 30% of patients, included constipation, nausea, fever, fatigue, peripheral neuropathy, febrile neutropenia, diarrhea, anemia, decreased appetite, and insomnia. All patients receiving the drug experienced adverse effects; 96% of patients experienced grade 3 or greater adverse effects, and 76% experienced serious adverse effects, most commonly febrile neutropenia (21%), fever (13%), hypotension (7%), respiratory distress (6%), and cardiac arrest (6%). Dose reduction, delay, or omission occurred in 53% of patients, and 28% of patients discontinued therapy because of adverse events, including peripheral neuropathy (10%), leukemia-related effects (7%), and tumor lysis syndrome (2%).

● Nervous System Effects

The major and dose-limiting adverse effect of conventional and liposomal vincristine is neurotoxicity, the severity of which may vary greatly among patients. Adverse neuromuscular effects often occur in a sequence with early development of sensory impairment and paresthesia followed by neuritic pain and motor difficulties as therapy with conventional vincristine is continued. The most frequent neurotoxic manifestation is peripheral (mixed sensorimotor) neuropathy, which occurs in nearly every patient receiving conventional vincristine. In clinical trials in patients with ALL, peripheral neuropathy occurred in 39% of patients receiving liposomal vincristine and was grade 3 or greater in 17% of patients receiving the drug. The earliest and most consistent indication of peripheral neuropathy is asymptomatic depression of the Achilles reflex. Loss of other deep tendon reflexes occurs in most patients after 3 or more weekly doses of conventional vincristine, and peripheral paresthesias, especially numbness, pain, and tingling, are common. If prolonged or high-dose conventional vincristine therapy is given, wrist drop, foot drop, cranial nerve palsy, atrophy, cramps, ataxia, slapping gait, and difficulty in walking or inability to walk may occur. Cranial nerve palsies may account for headaches and jaw pain; jaw pain usually occurs within 24 hours after the first and/or second dose of conventional vincristine and rarely recurs. Pain in other areas, including pharyngeal, parotid gland, bone, back, or limb pain as well as myalgia, has been reported in patients receiving vincristine and may be severe. Cranial nerve palsies and muscular weakness involving the larynx may produce hoarseness and vocal cord paresis, including potentially life-threatening bilateral vocal cord paralysis, while those involving extrinsic eye muscles may cause ptosis, double vision, and optic and extraocular neuropathy. Optic atrophy with blindness or transient cortical blindness has been reported in patients receiving conventional vincristine. Peripheral neuritis (both mononeuritis and polyneuritis) and neuralgia also occur frequently in patients receiving conventional vincristine. Grade 3 or greater asthenia and muscle weakness have been reported during clinical trials in 5 and 1%, respectively, of patients with ALL receiving liposomal vincristine.

Vincristine also produces autonomic and CNS toxicity, although less frequently than peripheral neuropathy. Autonomic effects commonly include severe constipation or obstipation, abdominal cramps, bowel obstruction, and colonic pseudo-obstruction. Adynamic ileus, which mimics "surgical abdomen," is particularly likely to occur in young children. In clinical trials in patients with ALL, grade 3 or greater constipation occurred in 5% of patients receiving liposomal vincristine and grade 3 or greater ileus and colonic pseudo-obstruction occurred in 6% of patients receiving the drug. Constipation may take the form of upper-colon impaction, and a flat abdominal film may be used to facilitate diagnosis so the clinician is not misled by presentation of colicky abdominal pain coupled with an empty rectum. Constipation may be treated with high enemas and laxatives. A routine regimen (e.g., laxatives, enemas) to prevent constipation is recommended for patients receiving conventional or liposomal vincristine. When conventional vincristine is administered in single weekly doses, constipation usually persists less than 7 days; abdominal cramps and adynamic ileus in children usually also disappear in 1 week or less. Urinary tract disturbances including bladder atony, incontinence, urinary retention, nocturia, oliguria, dysuria, and polyuria also have been reported in patients receiving conventional vincristine. Whenever possible, other drugs known to cause urinary retention should be discontinued during the first few days following administration of conventional vincristine, particularly in geriatric patients. Other autonomic effects of vincristine include orthostatic hypotension, abnormal Valsalva response, defective sweating, and myoclonic jerks. CNS effects including episodes of altered consciousness and mental changes such as depression, agitation, insomnia, and hallucinations have been reported. Seizures (frequently accompanied by hypertension), progressive encephalopathy, respiratory difficulties, and coma also have occurred. Seizures followed by coma have been reported in several pediatric patients receiving conventional vincristine.

Neurotoxic effects of conventional or liposomal vincristine may be additive with those of other neurotoxic agents and spinal cord irradiation. Geriatric patients and those with underlying neurologic disease may be more susceptible than other patients to the neurotoxic effects of conventional or liposomal vincristine. No antidote to the neurotoxic effects of vincristine has been found to date. Most experts reduce the dose or discontinue the drug if depression of reflexes, paresthesia, and/or motor weakness develop. Sensory loss, paresthesia, difficulty in walking, slapping gait, loss of deep tendon reflexes, and/or muscle wasting may persist during conventional vincristine therapy. Generalized sensorimotor dysfunction may become increasingly severe with continued therapy with conventional vincristine. Recovery from neurotoxicity usually begins with the discontinuance of conventional vincristine. Paresthesia is the most readily reversible, followed by motor and sensory impairment. Although these symptoms resolve by about the sixth week following discontinuance of conventional vincristine therapy in most patients, some patients may experience neuromuscular problems for prolonged periods. Depressed deep tendon reflexes return slowly, if at all, and some patients experience minor neurologic symptoms up to several months after conventional vincristine has been discontinued.

● **Respiratory Effects**

Acute shortness of breath and bronchospasm, which can be severe or life threatening, have occurred following administration of vinca alkaloids (e.g., vincristine), being reported most frequently when mitomycin was used concomitantly with conventional vincristine. Such reactions may occur a few minutes to several hours after administration of a vinca alkaloid or up to 2 weeks after a dose of mitomycin. Progressive dyspnea, which may require chronic therapy, can occur in patients receiving conventional vincristine; the drug should not be readministered to these patients. In clinical trials in patients with ALL, respiratory distress or failure has been reported in 6 or 5%, respectively, of patients receiving liposomal vincristine.

● **Dermatologic Effects**

Alopecia is reported to occur in 20–70% of patients who receive conventional vincristine. Alopecia is reversible when conventional vincristine is discontinued. Regrowth of hair may occur even when conventional vincristine is continued in therapeutic doses. Rash has occurred occasionally in patients receiving conventional vincristine.

● **Sensitivity Reactions**

Allergic reactions, including anaphylaxis, rash, and edema, that were temporally related to conventional vincristine therapy have been reported in patients receiving the drug as part of combination chemotherapy regimens.

● **Hematologic Effects**

Hematologic toxicity produced by vincristine is less than that produced by most other antineoplastic agents; therefore, the drug is useful in patients with pancytopenia or in combination regimens. Anemia, leukopenia, and thrombocytopenia have been reported. Leukopenia usually persists less than 7 days when conventional vincristine is given in single weekly doses. In clinical trials in patients with ALL, grade 3 or greater anemia, neutropenia, and thrombocytopenia each have been reported in 17–18% of patients receiving liposomal vincristine, and grade 3 or greater febrile neutropenia has occurred in 31% of patients. An increase in the platelet count has been observed in some patients with thrombocytopenia after initiation of therapy with conventional vincristine before evidence of marrow remission is apparent.

● **Local Effects**

Vincristine is a tissue irritant and may cause phlebitis and necrosis. Extravasation results in pain and cellulitis. The manufacturers of conventional vincristine state that local injection of hyaluronidase and application of moderate heat may decrease local reactions resulting from extravasation; however, some clinicians prefer to treat extravasation with cold compresses, dilution with 0.9% sodium chloride injection or infiltration of sodium bicarbonate (5 mL of 8.4% injection), and/or local injection of hydrocortisone. The manufacturer of liposomal vincristine states that the infusion should be discontinued immediately if extravasation is suspected and local treatments should be considered.

● **Cardiovascular Effects**

Hypertension and hypotension have been reported in patients receiving vincristine. In clinical trials in patients with ALL, grade 3 or greater hypotension and cardiac arrest each have been reported in 6% of patients receiving liposomal vincristine. Coronary artery disease and myocardial infarction have occurred in patients receiving conventional vincristine in combination with other antineoplastic agents. Although a causal relationship has not been established, infarction was temporally related to administration of conventional vincristine in several patients, occurring within several hours after injection of the drug. Some conventional vincristine-treated patients who developed myocardial infarction had previously received radiation therapy to the mediastinal area, but infarction also has been reported in patients with no history of mediastinal radiation or risk factors associated with coronary artery disease.

● **GI Effects**

In addition to adverse GI effects of neurogenic origin associated with conventional or liposomal vincristine therapy (see Cautions: Nervous System Effects), local effects including nausea, vomiting, diarrhea, abdominal distention, stomatitis, and oral ulceration occur occasionally in patients receiving conventional vincristine. In clinical trials in patients with ALL, nausea, diarrhea and decreased appetite have been reported in 52, 37, and 33%, respectively, of patients receiving liposomal vincristine. Intestinal necrosis and/or perforation and anorexia also have been reported in patients receiving conventional vincristine.

● **Otic Effects**

Eighth cranial nerve damage, which may be manifested by vestibular manifestations such as dizziness, nystagmus, and vertigo, and by auditory manifestations such as varying degrees of hearing impairment (including partial or total deafness) that may be temporary or permanent, has been reported in patients receiving vinca alkaloids. The manufacturers of conventional vincristine state that the drug should be used concomitantly with other potentially ototoxic drugs such as platinum-containing antineoplastic agents with extreme caution.

● Endocrine Effects

A syndrome of inappropriate secretion of antidiuretic hormone (SIADH) has occurred rarely in patients receiving conventional vincristine therapy. The syndrome may be associated with the neurotoxicity of the drug, possibly resulting from a direct effect on the hypothalamus. In these patients, hyponatremia associated with increased urinary sodium excretion occurs without evidence of renal or adrenal disease, hypotension, dehydration, azotemia, or clinical edema. Fluid restriction produces improvement in sodium balance and facilitates the safe use of repeated courses of conventional vincristine in patients who experience this syndrome.

● Metabolic Effects

Tumor lysis syndrome may occur following rapid lysis of malignant cells. The risk of tumor lysis syndrome is increased in patients with non-Hodgkin's lymphomas or leukemia. Such patients should be monitored closely and appropriate precautions should be taken. In some patients, uric acid nephropathy may result. These effects may be minimized by adequate hydration, alkalinization of the urine, and/or administration of allopurinol.

● Hepatic Effects

Hepatic veno-occlusive disease, sometimes fatal, has been reported in patients receiving conventional vincristine, particularly in pediatric patients receiving conventional vincristine in combination with other chemotherapy agents. Hepatotoxicity, sometimes fatal, also has occurred in patients receiving liposomal vincristine. Grade 3 or greater elevations in AST concentrations have been reported during clinical trials in 6–11% of patients receiving liposomal vincristine.

● Other Adverse Effects

Other occasionally occurring adverse effects of conventional vincristine include fever and, at high doses, weight loss. In clinical trials in patients with ALL, fever and fatigue have occurred in 43 and 41%, respectively, of patients receiving liposomal vincristine and were grade 3 or greater in 15 and 12%, respectively, of patients receiving the drug. In these clinical trials, grade 3 or greater infections (e.g., pneumonia, septic shock, staphylococcal bacteremia) occurred in 40% of patients receiving liposomal vincristine and grade 3 or greater pain and abdominal pain each occurred in 8% of patients.

● Precautions and Contraindications

Vincristine is a highly toxic drug with a low therapeutic index, and a therapeutic response is not likely to occur without some evidence of toxicity. Vincristine must be used only under constant supervision by clinicians experienced in therapy with cytotoxic agents and should only be administered by individuals experienced in administration of the drug. (See Dosage and Administration: Reconstitution and Administration.) Patients and/or their parents or guardians should be advised of the possibility of adverse effects and associated manifestations.

Because of the hepatic metabolism and biliary excretion of vincristine, some clinicians recommend reduced doses in patients with obstructive jaundice or other hepatic impairment. Conventional and liposomal vincristine must be given with care, and dosage and toxicity monitored, particularly in patients receiving other neurotoxic drugs or those with preexisting neuromuscular disease. Complete blood cell (CBC) counts should be performed before the administration of each dose of conventional or liposomal vincristine. Serum concentrations of uric acid should be determined frequently during the first 3–4 weeks of therapy in patients receiving vincristine for the induction of remission in acute leukemia, and appropriate measures should be taken to prevent the occurrence of hyperuricemia related to the rapid lysis of leukemic cells. Because of the potential for hepatotoxicity, liver function tests should be monitored.

The manufacturer states that conventional vincristine is contraindicated in patients with the demyelinating form of Charcot-Marie-Tooth syndrome. Conventional vincristine also should not be administered to patients while they are receiving radiation therapy through ports that include the liver. Liposomal vincristine is contraindicated in patients with demyelinating conditions including Charcot-Marie-Tooth syndrome. Liposomal vincristine also is contraindicated in patients with known hypersensitivity to the conventional or liposomal drug or to any ingredient in the formulation.

Care must be taken to avoid contact of conventional vincristine sulfate solutions with the eye(s), as severe irritation or corneal ulceration (especially if the drug is administered under pressure) may result. If contact with the eye(s) occurs, the eye(s) should be washed immediately with copious amounts of water; patients should consult a clinician if ocular irritation persists.

● Pediatric Precautions

The manufacturer states that safety and efficacy of liposomal vincristine in pediatric patients have not been established.

● Geriatric Precautions

Vincristine should be used with caution in geriatric patients because of the greater frequency of decreased hepatic, renal, and/or cardiac function and of concomitant disease and drug therapy observed in this age group.

● Mutagenicity and Carcinogenicity

Genotoxicity has been demonstrated with conventional vincristine in some in vivo and in vitro studies; however, in vivo and in vitro tests have failed to demonstrate conclusively that vincristine is mutagenic. There was no evidence of carcinogenicity following intraperitoneal administration of conventional vincristine in rats and mice, but the study was limited. Patients receiving chemotherapy that included conventional vincristine and drugs known to be carcinogenic have developed secondary malignancies; however, the contribution of vincristine has not been determined. Formal carcinogenicity studies have not been conducted for conventional or liposomal vincristine.

● Pregnancy, Fertility, and Lactation

Pregnancy

Vincristine can cause fetal toxicity when administered to pregnant women, but potential benefits from use of the drug may be acceptable in certain conditions despite the possible risks to the fetus. The drug can induce teratogenic and embryocidal effects in animals at doses that are not toxic to the pregnant animal. Dosages of conventional vincristine that caused resorption of 23–85% of fetuses in pregnant mice and hamsters produced fetal malformations that were present in surviving offspring. In 5 monkeys receiving single doses of conventional vincristine between days 27–34 of gestation, 3 fetuses were normal at term, while 2 had grossly evident malformations. Administration of liposomal vincristine to pregnant rats during organogenesis caused teratogenicity (skeletal and visceral malformations), decreased fetal weight, increased embryofetal deaths (resorptions, postimplantation losses), and decreased maternal body weight. Fetal malformations were observed in pregnant rats receiving liposomal vincristine at exposure levels that were approximately 20–40% of the human exposure at the recommended dosage. There are no adequate and controlled studies to date using conventional or liposomal vincristine in pregnant women, and the drugs should be used during pregnancy only in life-threatening situations or severe disease for which safer drugs cannot be used or are ineffective. Women of childbearing potential should be advised to avoid becoming pregnant while receiving conventional or liposomal vincristine. When conventional or liposomal vincristine is administered during pregnancy or the patient becomes pregnant while receiving the drug, the patient should be informed of the potential hazard to the fetus.

Fertility

Reproduction studies in animals using conventional vincristine have not been performed to date; however, an animal toxicology study indicates that liposomal vincristine may impair male fertility, which is consistent with literature on conventional vincristine. Azoospermia and increased plasma concentrations of follicle-stimulating hormone have occurred in males who received combination chemotherapy that included conventional vincristine and prednisone with cyclophosphamide or mechlorethamine and procarbazine, and amenorrhea has occurred in females receiving chemotherapy that included conventional vincristine. The manufacturers state that irreversible azoospermia or amenorrhea is less likely when chemotherapy that includes conventional vincristine is administered in prepubertal patients. Epididymal aspermia and testicular degeneration and atrophy have occurred in rats receiving liposomal vincristine.

Lactation

It is not known whether vincristine or its metabolites are distributed into milk. Because of the potential for serious adverse effects in nursing infants, a decision should be made whether to discontinue nursing or conventional or liposomal vincristine, taking into account the importance of the drug to the woman.

DRUG INTERACTIONS

Formal studies of drug interactions have not been conducted for liposomal vincristine; however, liposomal vincristine is expected to interact with drugs known to interact with conventional vincristine.

● Phenytoin

Simultaneous administration of phenytoin (oral or IV) and combination chemotherapy containing conventional vincristine may reduce serum concentrations of phenytoin and increase seizure activity. The mechanism of this interaction may involve reduced absorption of phenytoin and an increase in the rate of its metabolism and elimination. (See Drug Interactions: Drugs Affecting Hepatic Microsomal Enzymes.)

● Antineoplastic Agents

When conventional vincristine and asparaginase must be administered sequentially, the sequence of conventional vincristine followed by asparaginase is recommended. Conventional vincristine should be administered 12–24 hours preceding administration of asparaginase to minimize toxicity; administration of asparaginase first may reduce hepatic clearance of vincristine and increase the severity of adverse effects of the drug.

Concomitant use of mitomycin and conventional vincristine may increase the risk of serious adverse respiratory effects, particularly in patients with preexisting pulmonary dysfunction. (See Cautions: Respiratory Effects.)

● Drugs Affecting Hepatic Microsomal Enzymes

Metabolism of vinca alkaloids is mediated by the cytochrome P-450 (CYP) isoenzyme 3A, and the possibility exists that potent inhibitors of this isoenzyme may impair metabolism of vinca alkaloids. Concomitant use of azole antifungal agents (e.g., itraconazole, ketoconazole, posaconazole, voriconazole) and vincristine may increase plasma concentrations of vincristine and has resulted in serious adverse effects, including neuropathy (peripheral, autonomic, and cranial neuropathy), seizures, hyponatremia or syndrome of inappropriate secretion of antidiuretic hormone (SIADH), and GI toxicity (including paralytic ileus); earlier onset and/or increased severity of adverse neuromuscular effects has occurred. Therefore, concomitant use of vincristine with potent CYP3A inhibitors (e.g., atazanavir, clarithromycin, indinavir, itraconazole, ketoconazole, nefazodone, nelfinavir, posaconazole, ritonavir, saquinavir, telithromycin, voriconazole) should be avoided. Azole antifungal agents should be used concomitantly with vincristine only in patients who have no alternative antifungal treatment options; if concomitant use cannot be avoided, patients should be monitored frequently for toxicity.

Concomitant use of vincristine with potent CYP3A inducers (e.g., carbamazepine, dexamethasone, phenobarbital, phenytoin, rifabutin, rifampin, rifapentine, St. John's wort [Hypericum perforatum]) should be avoided.

● Drugs Affecting or Affected by P-glycoprotein Transport

Vincristine is a P-glycoprotein (P-gp) substrate, and the possibility exists that potent inhibitors or inducers of P-gp may alter the pharmacokinetics or pharmacodynamics of vincristine. Concomitant use of vincristine with potent P-gp inhibitors or inducers should be avoided.

● Ototoxic Drugs

Since varying degrees of permanent or temporary hearing impairment associated with eighth cranial nerve damage have been reported in patients receiving vinca alkaloids, vincristine should be used concomitantly with other potentially ototoxic drugs such as platinum-containing antineoplastic agents with extreme caution.

ACUTE TOXICITY

Overdosage with vincristine produces adverse effects that are mainly extensions of common adverse effects. Doses 10 times the usual recommended doses of conventional vincristine sulfate have been lethal in children younger than 13 years of age, and severe manifestations of toxicity have been apparent following administration of 3–4 mg/m² in this age group. Single doses of 3 mg/m² of conventional vincristine sulfate can be expected to produce severe toxic manifestations in adults. Increased severity of adverse effects may be experienced by patients with hepatic impairment characterized by decreased biliary excretion. Grade 3 motor neuropathy and grade 4 grand mal seizure, elevated concentrations of AST, and hyperbilirubinemia occurred following administration of 2.4 mg/m² of vincristine sulfate as the liposomal drug.

Following vincristine overdosage, supportive and symptomatic treatment should be initiated. Treatment should include the prevention of adverse effects resulting from the syndrome of inappropriate secretion of antidiuretic hormone (SIADH) (e.g., by restricting fluid intake and possibly by use of an appropriate diuretic); prophylactic administration of anticonvulsants; use of enemas to prevent ileus (in some cases, decompression of the GI tract may be necessary); monitoring of the cardiovascular system; and daily blood counts to monitor the hematologic system and guide transfusion requirements. Studies in mice and a few case reports have suggested that administration of leucovorin calcium may be of some value in the management of vincristine overdosage. A suggested regimen is to administer leucovorin calcium 100 mg IV every 3 hours for 24 hours and then every 6 hours for at least 48 hours. Treatment with leucovorin calcium does not preclude the need for the usual treatment measures. Because only small amounts of vincristine are removed by hemodialysis, removal of the drug by this method is not likely to be helpful following overdosage.

In dogs pretreated with cholestyramine, fecal excretion of vincristine was increased; no published data are available regarding the use of cholestyramine as a possible antidote for vincristine overdosage in humans. No published data are available on the clinical outcome of oral ingestion of conventional vincristine. If oral ingestion of vincristine occurs, the stomach should be emptied immediately followed by oral administration of activated charcoal and a cathartic.

PHARMACOLOGY

Although the mechanism of action has not been fully elucidated, vincristine and other vinca alkaloids exert their cytotoxic effects by binding to tubulin, the protein subunit of the microtubules that form the mitotic spindle. The formation of vincristine-tubulin complexes prevents the polymerization of the tubulin subunits into microtubules and induces depolymerization of microtubules resulting in inhibition of microtubule assembly and cellular metaphase arrest. In high concentrations, the drug also exerts complex effects on nucleic acid and protein synthesis. Vincristine exerts some immunosuppressive activity.

PHARMACOKINETICS

● Absorption

Vincristine sulfate is unpredictably absorbed from the GI tract. Following rapid IV injection of a 2-mg dose of conventional vincristine sulfate in patients with normal renal and hepatic function, peak serum drug concentrations of approximately 0.19–0.89 μM occur immediately and the drug is rapidly cleared from serum. The area under the serum vincristine concentration-time curve has been shown to be increased following continuous IV infusion of conventional vincristine compared with rapid IV injection of the drug when comparable doses are administered. Following IV infusion over 1 hour of a 2.25-mg/m² dose of vincristine sulfate as the liposomal drug in patients with acute lymphocytic leukemia (ALL), peak concentrations of total vincristine sulfate average 1220 ng/mL and reflect liposome-encapsulated drug that may not be immediately bioavailable. Because clearance of the drug is slower following administration as liposomal vincristine, systemic exposure of the drug is increased relative to that of conventional vincristine.

Distribution

Distribution of vincristine and its metabolites (and/or decomposition products) into human body tissues and fluids has not been fully characterized, but the drug is rapidly and apparently widely distributed following IV administration of conventional vincristine. Drug that is distributed into tissues is tightly but reversibly bound. Vincristine and its metabolites (and/or decomposition products) are rapidly and extensively distributed into bile, with peak biliary concentrations occurring within 2–4 hours after rapid IV injection of conventional vincristine. Vincristine and its metabolites (and/or decomposition products) cross the blood-brain barrier poorly following rapid IV injection of conventional vincristine and generally do not appear in the CSF in cytotoxic concentrations. It is not known whether vincristine and its metabolites are distributed into milk.

Elimination

Following rapid IV injection of conventional vincristine, serum concentrations of the drug appear to decline in a triphasic manner. The terminal elimination half-life of conventional vincristine has ranged from 19–155 hours. Clearance of the drug is slower following administration as a liposome-encapsulated formulation compared with administration as a conventional formulation (345 versus 11,340 mL/hour).

The metabolic fate of vincristine has not been clearly determined; the drug appears to be extensively metabolized, probably in the liver by the cytochrome P-450 microsomal enzyme system, including CYP3A, but the extent of metabolism is not clear since the drug also apparently undergoes decomposition in vivo. In patients with hepatic impairment, metabolism of vincristine may be decreased. Vincristine and its metabolites (and/or decomposition products) are excreted principally in feces via biliary elimination. Following rapid IV injection of conventional vincristine in adults with normal renal and hepatic function, about 30% of a dose is excreted in feces within 24 hours and 70% within 72 hours; about 10% of a dose is excreted in urine within 24 hours, with very little urinary excretion occurring thereafter. Following IV administration of liposomal vincristine, the extent of urinary excretion (less than 8% of the administered dose within 96 hours) is similar to that of conventional vincristine. The effects of hepatic impairment on the elimination of vincristine and its metabolites (and/or decomposition products) have not been established, but individuals with decreased hepatic function may have impaired elimination. In a limited number of patients with melanoma and moderate hepatic impairment (Child-Pugh class B) secondary to liver metastases, dose-adjusted peak plasma concentrations and systemic exposure of liposomal vincristine were similar to those observed in patients with ALL and normal hepatic function.

Only small amounts of vincristine are removed by hemodialysis.

CHEMISTRY AND STABILITY

Chemistry

Vincristine sulfate, a naturally occurring vinca alkaloid, is an antimicrotubule antineoplastic agent. Vincristine sulfate is the salt of a dimeric alkaloid isolated from *Catharanthus roseus*. Vincristine sulfate occurs as a white, off-white, or slightly yellow, hygroscopic, amorphous or crystalline powder and is freely soluble in water and slightly soluble in alcohol. Sulfuric acid, sodium hydroxide, acetic acid, and/or sodium acetate is added during the manufacture of conventional vincristine sulfate injection to adjust pH to 4–5 or 3.5–5.5 depending on the preparation; the injection also contains mannitol.

Liposomal vincristine sulfate (Marqibo®) is commercially available as a 3-vial kit containing single-use vials of vincristine sulfate solution, sphingomyelin-cholesterol liposome suspension, and dibasic sodium phosphate solution. When prepared as directed, vincristine sulfate liposome injection is a sterile, preservative-free, white to off-white suspension of vincristine sulfate encapsulated in sphingomyelin-cholesterol liposomes. Each mL of vincristine sulfate liposome injection contains 0.16 mg of vincristine sulfate; more than 95% of the drug is encapsulated in liposomes. The liposomes are composed of sphingomyelin and cholesterol in a molar ratio of approximately 60:40; the mean liposome diameter is approximately 100 nm. Vincristine sulfate liposome injection also contains dibasic sodium phosphate, sodium citrate, citric acid, mannitol, sodium chloride, and ethanol.

Stability

Conventional vincristine sulfate solutions are light-sensitive and must be protected from light. Conventional vincristine sulfate injection should be refrigerated at 2–8°C; the vials should be stored in an upright position.

Commercially available liposomal vincristine sulfate (Marqibo®) kits containing single-use vials of vincristine sulfate solution, sphingomyelin-cholesterol liposome suspension, and dibasic sodium phosphate solution should be refrigerated at 2–8°C and should not be frozen. Once the 3 components have been admixed, the resultant liposomal vincristine sulfate injection concentrate may be stored at 15–30°C for up to 12 hours. Administration of the final diluted preparation of the drug should be completed within 12 hours of *initiation* of preparation of vincristine sulfate liposome injection.

When preparing a diluted solution, the manufacturer states that conventional vincristine sulfate injection should be mixed only with 0.9% sodium chloride injection or 5% dextrose injection; the drug should not be diluted in solutions that raise or lower the pH outside the range of 3.5–5.5.

Specialized references should be consulted for specific compatibility information. Doses of 0.5, 1, 2, or 3 mg of conventional vincristine sulfate diluted in 25 or 50 mL of 0.9% sodium chloride solution in small-volume IV bags (i.e., minibags) or in 20 mL of 0.9% sodium chloride solution in a 30-mL syringe remained stable when stored for 7 days at 4°C followed by 2 days at 23°C.

For further information on the handling of antineoplastic agents, see the ASHP Guidelines on Handling Hazardous Drugs at https://www.ahfsdrug information.com.

PREPARATIONS

Excipients in commercially available drug preparations may have clinically important effects in some individuals; consult specific product labeling for details.

vinCRIStine Sulfate

Parenteral

Injection, for IV use only	1 mg/mL (1 and 2 mg)*	Vincristine Sulfate Injection

* available from one or more manufacturer, distributor, and/or repackager by generic (nonproprietary) name

vinCRIStine Sulfate Liposomal

Parenteral

Kit, for suspension, for injection, for IV infusion only	1 Vial, Injection, Vincristine Sulfate 5 mg/5 mL (for preparation of liposome-encapsulated vincristine sulfate suspension, 0.16 mg [of vincristine sulfate] per mL [5 mg]),	Marqibo® available with flotation ring, vial overlabel, and infusion bag label, Spectrum
	1 Vial, For injectable suspension, Sphingomyelin/Cholesterol Liposome 103 mg/mL (Sphingomyelin 73.5 mg/mL and Cholesterol 29.5 mg/mL)	
	1 Vial, Injection, Sodium Phosphate, Dibasic 355 mg/25mL	

† Use is not currently included in the labeling approved by the US Food and Drug Administration.

Selected Revisions October 15, 2018, © Copyright, January 1, 1978, American Society of Health-System Pharmacists, Inc.

Vinorelbine Tartrate

10:00 • ANTINEOPLASTIC AGENTS

■ Vinorelbine, a semisynthetic vinca alkaloid, is an antineoplastic agent.

USES

● Non-small Cell Lung Cancer

Adjuvant Therapy

Cisplatin-containing chemotherapy, such as cisplatin in combination with vinorelbine, is used for the adjuvant treatment of completely resected non-small cell lung cancer†.

The use of cisplatin-containing adjuvant therapy prolongs survival in patients with completely resected non-small cell lung cancer. (Also see Uses: Non-small Cell Lung Cancer in Cisplatin 10:00.) In the International Adjuvant Lung Cancer Trial (IALT), 1867 patients with completely resected stage I, II, or III non-small cell lung cancer were assigned to receive either adjuvant chemotherapy (cisplatin with etoposide, or cisplatin with a vinca alkaloid) or observation. At 5 years, the rate of survival was higher among patients receiving cisplatin-based adjuvant therapy (44.5%) than among those assigned to observation (40.4%). Subset analysis of pooled abstracted data from 11 randomized trials including this one indicates that adjuvant therapy with cisplatin-based therapy prolongs survival in patients with completely resected non-small cell lung cancer.

Vinorelbine is used in combination with cisplatin as adjuvant therapy for completely resected non-small cell lung cancer. In a randomized trial (National Cancer Institute of Canada and Intergroup JBR10 study) involving 482 patients with completely resected stage IB or stage II non-small cell lung cancer, overall survival (94 versus 73 months) and relapse-free survival were prolonged in patients receiving adjuvant therapy with vinorelbine and cisplatin compared with those assigned to observation. Retrospective analysis of the data from this clinical trial showed that, despite receiving lower dose intensities of both drugs, patients older than 65 years experienced a survival benefit similar to that observed for all patients receiving adjuvant therapy with vinorelbine and cisplatin for non-small cell lung cancer. In the Adjuvant Navelbine International Trialist Association (ANITA) trial, which involved 840 patients with stage IB, II, or IIIA non-small cell lung cancer, median survival was prolonged (66 versus 44 months) in patients receiving adjuvant therapy with vinorelbine and cisplatin compared with those assigned to observation.

Analysis of pooled data for individual patients from 5 large randomized trials, including the IALT, JBR10, and ANITA studies, indicates that adjuvant treatment with cisplatin-based therapy prolongs survival in patients with completely resected non-small cell lung cancer. Subgroup analysis showed that survival benefit varies according to stage of disease; cisplatin-based adjuvant chemotherapy prolongs survival in patients with stage II or III disease, may benefit some patients with stage IB disease, and may not benefit patients with stage IA disease.

Therapy for Metastatic Disease

Depending on the stage of disease and the performance status of the patient, vinorelbine is used either alone or in combination with cisplatin as first-line therapy in ambulatory patients for the palliative treatment of unresectable, advanced (stage III or IV) non-small cell lung cancer.

Although the drug is active alone in this cancer, use of vinorelbine in combination with cisplatin is preferred for the treatment of advanced non-small cell lung cancer in patients with good performance status because of improved response and survival. In the American Society of Clinical Oncology (ASCO) practice guidelines for the treatment of unresectable non-small cell lung cancer (NSCLC), an expert panel recommended 2-drug combination chemotherapy for patients with good performance status (ECOG/Zubrod performance status 0 or 1); for patients with ECOG/Zubrod performance status 2, or for geriatric patients, single-agent chemotherapy, such as vinorelbine alone, may be used. A European Experts Panel that convened in April 2003 also stated that single-agent therapy may be used in patients with advanced NSCLC and ECOG performance status 2. In patients with stage IV disease, quality-of-life considerations may prompt monotherapy with vinorelbine, and the manufacturer states that such monotherapy can be used for stage IV but not stage III non-small cell lung cancer.

Age alone should not deter the use of chemotherapy for the treatment of advanced non-small cell lung cancer in geriatric patients. Data from a randomized trial demonstrate a survival benefit among geriatric patients (70 years of age or older) receiving single-agent therapy with vinorelbine compared with those receiving supportive care alone. Subgroup analysis of a phase III randomized trial according to age and performance status indicates that among patients receiving cisplatin-based combination chemotherapy for advanced non-small cell lung cancer, fit older patients (i.e., 70 years of age or older with ECOG performance status of 0 or 1) had similar outcomes for response rate and survival as younger patients; older patients were more likely to have concomitant disease and had a higher incidence rate of certain drug-related toxicities. Results of a large randomized trial among geriatric patients (70 years of age or older) with advanced non-small cell lung cancer showed that combination therapy with vinorelbine and gemcitabine did not improve survival and caused greater toxicity than single-agent therapy with either vinorelbine or gemcitabine. Systemic therapy should be offered to geriatric patients with advanced non-small cell lung cancer; further study is needed to determine optimal therapy with single agents or combination regimens for such patients.

The combination of cisplatin with vinorelbine currently is a preferred regimen for the treatment of advanced non-small cell lung cancer.

In a randomized trial involving 612 patients with advanced non-small cell lung cancer, similar results were noted for response rate, median survival, and time to disease progression between 3 platinum-based regimens; adverse effects occurring more frequently in each group included neutropenia and nausea/vomiting in patients receiving vinorelbine and cisplatin, thrombocytopenia in those receiving gemcitabine and cisplatin, and peripheral neuropathy and alopecia in those receiving paclitaxel followed by carboplatin. In another randomized trial, response rates, median survival, and 1- and 2-year survival rates were similar in patients receiving either cisplatin and vinorelbine or carboplatin and paclitaxel for advanced non-small cell lung cancer; grade 3 or 4 leukopenia and neutropenia and grade 3 nausea and vomiting were more frequent in patients receiving vinorelbine and cisplatin whereas grade 3 peripheral neuropathy occurred more frequently in patients receiving paclitaxel and carboplatin.

In a randomized study, 432 patients with stage IIIb or IV non-small cell lung cancer receiving vinorelbine 25 mg/m² once weekly and cisplatin 100 mg/m² once every 4 weeks had a longer median survival (8 versus 6 months) and higher survival rate at 1 year (38 versus 22%) than those receiving cisplatin 100 mg/m² once every 4 weeks. Objective response rates of 19 and 8% were observed in patients receiving vinorelbine and cisplatin versus cisplatin alone. The incidence and severity of granulocytopenia was substantially higher in patients receiving combination therapy with vinorelbine and cisplatin than in those receiving cisplatin alone. Granulocyte-colony stimulating factor was administered in approximately one-third of patients receiving combination therapy to reduce the severity of myelosuppression associated with vinorelbine. All patients in the study had a WHO performance status of 0 or 1, and none had received prior chemotherapy.

In a randomized study of 612 patients with stage III or IV non-small cell lung cancer who had not received prior chemotherapy, higher response rates and longer survival times (albeit modestly improved) were observed in patients receiving vinorelbine and cisplatin compared with those receiving either vinorelbine alone or vindesine and cisplatin. All patients in this study had a WHO performance status of 0, 1, or 2. Patients were randomized to receive single-agent vinorelbine 30 mg/m² once weekly; vinorelbine 30 mg/m² once weekly and cisplatin 120 mg/m²on days 1 and 29 and then once every 6 weeks; or vindesine 3 mg/m² once weekly for 7 weeks and then once every other week and cisplatin 120 mg/m² on days 1 and 29 then once every 6 weeks. Median survival times of 9.2, 7.4, or 7.2 months were observed in patients with advanced non-small cell lung cancer receiving vinorelbine and cisplatin, vindesine and cisplatin, or vinorelbine alone, respectively. Survival at 1 year was 35% in patients receiving vinorelbine and cisplatin, 27% in those receiving vindesine and cisplatin, and 30% in those receiving single-agent therapy with vinorelbine. The overall objective response rate (all partial responses) was 28% (based on intention-to-treat analysis) in patients receiving vinorelbine and cisplatin, 19% in those receiving vindesine and cisplatin, and 14% in those receiving vinorelbine alone.

Follow-up at 5 years indicates that survival is prolonged for patients receiving vinorelbine and cisplatin compared with either vindesine and cisplatin or vinorelbine alone. However, subgroup analysis suggests that this survival benefit is obtained only among patients with a WHO performance status of 0 or 1. Among patients with nonresectable non-small cell lung cancer who have a WHO performance status of 2, single-agent therapy with vinorelbine may be appropriate.

In a clinical trial in which 211 patients with stage IV non-small cell cancer were randomized on a 2:1 basis to receive vinorelbine 30 mg/m² once weekly or fluorouracil 425 mg/m² IV plus leucovorin 20 mg/m² IV daily for 5 days every 4 weeks, respectively, median survival time was 30 weeks for patients receiving vinorelbine compared with 22 weeks for those receiving fluorouracil with leucovorin. Combination therapy with fluorouracil and leucovorin was chosen as a control treatment because this regimen has a tolerable safety profile and its activity in non-small cell lung cancer is unknown. Because the median survival time in patients with non-small cell lung cancer who received the control treatment was comparable to that usually observed in patients with untreated disease, it appears that combination therapy with fluorouracil and leucovorin did not have a detrimental effect. All patients in the study had a Karnofsky performance status of 70 or higher and none had received prior chemotherapy. Survival at 1 year was 24% in patients receiving vinorelbine and 16% in patients receiving fluorouracil with leucovorin. Overall objective response rates (all partial responses) were 12 and 3% for vinorelbine and fluorouracil with leucovorin, respectively. Measurements of quality of life assessing role functioning, physical functioning, symptom distress, and global quality of life were similar in patients receiving either vinorelbine or combination therapy with fluorouracil and leucovorin.

● Breast Cancer

Vinorelbine and Trastuzumab for HER2-positive Metastatic Breast Cancer

Combination therapy with vinorelbine and trastuzumab is being investigated as an active regimen for the treatment of HER2-overexpressing metastatic breast cancer†.

Monotherapy for Metastatic Breast Cancer

Vinorelbine is used as monotherapy in the first-line or salvage (e.g., second-line or subsequent) treatment of metastatic breast cancer†.

First-line vinorelbine monotherapy produced a median objective response rate (complete and partial responses) of 44% (range: 35–52%) in women with advanced disease. The median duration of response and the median time to treatment failure were 8.5 (range: 4.3–9) and 5 (range: 4.4–6) months, respectively. Patients treated with vinorelbine had a median survival of 16 (range: 9.9–24) months.

Salvage (second-line or subsequent) chemotherapy with vinorelbine alone also has been employed in the treatment of metastatic breast cancer. When administered as salvage therapy, vinorelbine monotherapy produced a median objective response in 28% (range: 16–37%) of patients with advanced/ metastatic breast cancer that failed to respond to a previous cytotoxic chemotherapy regimen. The drug produced a median duration of response, time to treatment failure, and survival of 5 (range: 3.5–8.5), 3.8 (range: 3–4.5), and 11.7 (range: 7–24) months, respectively. Objective responses to vinorelbine have been observed in patients with metastatic breast cancer refractory to anthracyclines or taxanes.

In a randomized, active-control trial involving women with anthracycline-refractory metastatic breast cancer, vinorelbine's antitumor activity appeared superior to that of melphalan. Vinorelbine and melphalan produced objective responses in 16 and 9% of patients, respectively. Differences favoring vinorelbine were noted for median time to disease progression and treatment failure, median survival, and 1-year survival rates. The median time to disease progression and treatment failure was 3 or 2 months for patients receiving vinorelbine or melphalan, respectively, the median survival rate was 8.8 or 7.8 months, respectively, and the 1-year survival rate was 35.7 or 21.7%, respectively.

Vinorelbine has been administered in various regimens for the treatment of metastatic breast cancer, such as a short IV infusion once weekly, or a continuous IV infusion of up to 5 days in duration. The use of oral† vinorelbine (currently not commercially available in the US) also is being investigated in the treatment of metastatic breast cancer.

● Cervical Cancer

Vinorelbine is being investigated as an active agent in the treatment of metastatic or recurrent cervical cancer†. An objective response rate of 18% was reported in a small uncontrolled study of patients receiving vinorelbine as a single agent for advanced or recurrent squamous cell carcinoma of the cervix. The combination of vinorelbine with other antineoplastic agents (e.g., cisplatin) is being evaluated in patients with metastatic or recurrent cervical cancer. (See Uses: Cervical Cancer in Cisplatin 10:00 for an overview of therapy for cervical cancer.)

● Other Uses

Vinorelbine also is used in the treatment of adult soft tissue sarcomas† and esophageal cancer†.

DOSAGE AND ADMINISTRATION

● Administration

Vinorelbine is administered only by IV injection into a free-flowing IV infusion or a large central vein, usually over a period of 6–10 minutes followed by flushing of the vein with a compatible IV solution, by individuals experienced in administration of the drug. The IV needle or catheter must be properly positioned before vinorelbine is injected. Improper administration of vinorelbine may result in extravasation of the drug causing local tissue necrosis and/or thrombophlebitis. Although vinorelbine also has been infused IV over 20–60 minutes via a peripheral vein or by rapid IV injection over 1–2 minutes, such methods of administration are *not* recommended because of the high rate of adverse local effects (e.g., phlebitis, erythema, venous discoloration, ulceration, pain) associated with this infusion rate and reports of severe back pain associated with rapid injection. Continuous IV infusions† of vinorelbine have been well tolerated, but additional study is needed to establish the role of such infusion in treating various cancers.

Vinorelbine tartrate is very irritating and must not be given IM, subcutaneously, or intrathecally. Intrathecal administration of other vinca alkaloids (i.e., vinblastine, vincristine) has resulted in death. When dispensed, the syringe containing the individual dose prepared for administration to the patient *must* be labeled with the statement: **"Warning: For IV use only. Fatal if given intrathecally."** The syringe must be enclosed in an overwrap (e.g., plastic bag or similar wrap with typed label) bearing the statements: **"Do not remove covering until moment of injection. Fatal if given intrathecally. For IV use only."**

In addition to the use of the warning labels and overwrap, other protective measures to prevent inadvertent intrathecal administration of vinorelbine or other vinca alkaloids include: administering diluted vinca alkaloid solutions in minibags, preparing the medication at the time of administration, attaching a unique filter, dispensing the vinca alkaloid separately from all other medications, dispensing the vinca alkaloid directly to the individual who is administering the drug, conducting an independent check of the dose and route of administration for the drug both at the time of preparation and prior to administration of the drug, and administering the vinca alkaloid in a separate room from rooms where other medications are administered.

Management of patients mistakenly receiving intrathecal vinorelbine is a medical emergency. Currently, there are no reports of patients mistakenly receiving intrathecal administration of vinorelbine. Unfortunately, the prognosis to date for patients inadvertently administered vincristine, another vinca alkaloid, intrathecally generally has been poor despite immediate efforts at removing spinal fluid and flushing with lactated Ringer's injection as well as other solutions, with such efforts failing to prevent ascending paralysis and death in almost all cases. In one case, progression of paralysis was stopped in an adult patient when the following treatment was initiated immediately after inadvertent intrathecal injection of vincristine. Such treatment consisted of immediate removal of as much CSF as safely possible via lumbar access, followed by flushing of the subarachnoid space with lactated Ringer's solution infused continuously at a rate of 150 mL/hour through a catheter in a cerebral lateral ventricle and removal of fluid through a lumbar access. As soon as available, fresh frozen plasma (25 mL) diluted in 1 L of lactated Ringer's solution was infused through the cerebral ventricular catheter at a rate of 75 mL/hour with removal of fluid through the lumbar access. The rate of infusion was adjusted to maintain a CSF protein concentration of 150 mg/dL. Glutamic acid was administered in a dose of 10 g given IV over 24 hours, followed by 500 mg orally 3 times daily for 1 month or until stabilization of neurologic status. The role of glutamic acid in this treatment is uncertain. There currently is no experience with this or any other treatment protocol in patients who mistakenly receive vinorelbine intrathecally.

Leakage of vinorelbine into surrounding tissue during IV administration of the drug can cause considerable irritation, local tissue necrosis, and/or thrombophlebitis. If extravasation occurs, the injection should be discontinued immediately, and any remaining portion of the dose should then be administered into another vein. The manufacturer states that there are no established guidelines for the treatment of extravasation injuries caused by vinorelbine and that institutional guidelines for extravasation injuries may be used. (See Cautions: Local Effects.)

Vinorelbine for injection concentrate must be diluted prior to injection into a free-flowing IV infusion or a large central vein. The manufacturer recommends diluting the concentrate in a syringe with 5% dextrose injection or 0.9% sodium chloride injection to a final vinorelbine concentration of 1.5–3 mg/mL *or* in an IV bag with 5% dextrose injection, 0.9% sodium chloride injection, 0.45% sodium chloride injection, 5% dextrose and 0.45% sodium chloride injection, Ringer's injection, or lactated Ringer's injection to a final vinorelbine concentration of 0.5–2 mg/mL. The diluted solution of vinorelbine should then be administered over a period of 6–10 minutes into the side port closest to the IV bag of a free-flowing IV infusion or into a large central vein followed by flushing with at least 75–125 mL of 0.9% sodium chloride injection or 5% dextrose injection over a period of 10 minutes.

Caution should be exercised in handling and preparing solutions of vinorelbine. Because skin reactions may occur with accidental exposure to vinorelbine, the manufacturer recommends the use of latex gloves when handling the drug. If vinorelbine tartrate injection or a solution of the drug comes in contact with the skin or mucosa, the affected area should be washed immediately and thoroughly with soap and water. Care must be taken to avoid contact of vinorelbine tartrate solutions with the eyes since severe irritation of the eye has been reported with accidental exposure to another vinca alkaloid; if contact occurs, the eye should be flushed thoroughly with water immediately.

Vinorelbine tartrate injection or solutions of the drug should be inspected visually for particulate matter and/or discoloration prior to administration.

● *Dosage*

Dosage of vinorelbine tartrate is expressed in terms of the base.

Adjustment of vinorelbine dosage in geriatric patients solely on the basis of age is not necessary.

Non-small Cell Lung Cancer
Combination Therapy

For the treatment of non-small cell lung cancer in adults, IV vinorelbine 25 mg/m² once weekly may be administered in combination with IV cisplatin 100 mg/m² given once every 4 weeks. Dosage reductions for both vinorelbine and cisplatin typically were required (see Dosage Modification for Toxicity and Contraindications for Continued Therapy: Hematologic Toxicity). Another regimen for the treatment of non-small lung cancer in adults is IV vinorelbine 30 mg/m² administered once weekly in combination with cisplatin (120 mg/m² given on days 1 and 29 and then once every 6 weeks).

In a dose-ranging study, 32 patients with non-small cell lung cancer receiving vinorelbine 20, 25, or 30 mg/m² weekly plus cisplatin 120 mg/m² on days 1 and 29 then once every 6 weeks had a median survival of 10 months. No responses were observed in patients receiving the 20 mg/m²dose; a response rate of 33% was observed in patients receiving a vinorelbine dose of either 25 or 30 mg/m².

According to ASCO practice guidelines, patients with unresectable stage III non-small cell lung cancer (NSCLC) who are candidates for combined chemotherapy and radiation should receive 2 to 4 cycles of initial platinum-based chemotherapy; no more than 4 cycles of chemotherapy are recommended. In patients with stage IV NSCLC, a maximum of 4 cycles of first-line chemotherapy should be administered if the disease is not responding to treatment, and a maximum of 6 cycles of chemotherapy should be administered if the disease responds to treatment.

Monotherapy

For the treatment of non-small cell lung cancer in adults, the manufacturer reports a usual initial dosage of single-agent vinorelbine of 30 mg/m² IV administered once weekly.

In clinical studies, dosages of vinorelbine have ranged from 15–30 mg/m² IV once weekly.

The optimum duration of vinorelbine therapy in patients with non-small cell lung cancer has not been determined, and in clinical trials, patients were treated with single-agent vinorelbine until the occurrence of either dose-limiting toxicity or progression of disease. According to ASCO practice guidelines, for patients with stage IV NSCLC, a maximum of 4 cycles of first-line chemotherapy should

be administered if the disease is not responding to treatment, and a maximum of 6 cycles of chemotherapy should be administered if the disease responds to treatment.

Breast Cancer

When used as first-line or salvage (second-line or subsequent) monotherapy in the treatment of advanced/ metastatic breast cancer†, vinorelbine has been infused IV over 20–60 minutes at initial doses of 20–30 mg/m² per week. The drug also has been administered at 30 mg/m² per week as a direct IV injection over 3–5 minutes or as a rapid IV dose. However, because of better local tolerance, the manufacturer currently recommends that vinorelbine usually be infused IV over 6–10 minutes. (See Dosage and Administration: Administration.) During the course of therapy, the dosing regimen generally was modified (e.g., dosing was delayed or doses were reduced) because of vinorelbine-induced toxicity.

Dosage Modification for Toxicity and Contraindications for Continued Therapy
Hematologic Toxicity

Vinorelbine therapy should not be administered to patients with baseline granulocyte counts less than 1000 cells/ mm³. In patients with a granulocyte count less than 1000 cells/ mm³, the granulocyte count should be repeated in 1 week. If it is necessary to withhold vinorelbine doses for 3 consecutive weeks because of persistence of a granulocyte count less than 1000 cells/ mm³, therapy with the drug should be discontinued. In patients with a granulocyte count of 1000–1499 cells/ mm³, the vinorelbine dose should be reduced to 50% of the starting dose.

In patients who have experienced fever and/or sepsis because of granulocytopenia during vinorelbine therapy or in patients in whom the vinorelbine dose has been withheld for 2 consecutive weeks because of granulocytopenia, subsequent doses of vinorelbine should be reduced to 75% of the starting dose in patients with a granulocyte count of at least 1500 cells/ mm³ and to 37.5% of the starting dose in those with a granulocyte count of 1000–1499 cells/ mm³. The vinorelbine dose should be withheld if the granulocyte count is less than 1000 cells/mm³, and the granulocyte count should be repeated in 1 week. If it is necessary to withhold vinorelbine doses for 3 consecutive weeks because of persistence of a granulocyte count less than 1000 cells/mm³, therapy with the drug should be discontinued.

Among patients receiving combination therapy with vinorelbine and cisplatin, blood counts should be checked weekly and dosage of vinorelbine and/or cisplatin should be reduced according to hematologic toxicity. In a large randomized trial, most patients required a 50% dose reduction of vinorelbine at day 15 of each cycle and a 50% dose reduction of cisplatin by cycle 3.

In patients with concurrent hematologic toxicity and hepatic impairment, vinorelbine dosage should be adjusted to the lower dosage advised by these guidelines. (See Dosage and Administration: Dosage in Renal and Hepatic Impairment.)

Hepatic Toxicity

Dosage of vinorelbine should be reduced in patients who develop hyperbilirubinemia. (See Dosage and Administration: Dosage in Renal and Hepatic Impairment.) In patients with concurrent hepatic impairment and hematologic toxicity, vinorelbine dosage should be adjusted to the lower dosage advised by these guidelines.

Renal Toxicity

Reduction of vinorelbine dosage in patients with renal impairment does not appear to be necessary. When vinorelbine is used in combination with cisplatin, appropriate dosage reductions for cisplatin should be made in patients with renal impairment.

Neurologic Toxicity

If manifestations of moderate or severe (grade 2 or higher) neurotoxicity occur in patients receiving vinorelbine, therapy with the drug should be discontinued immediately.

● *Dosage in Renal and Hepatic Impairment*

The effect of renal and/or hepatic impairment on the disposition of vinorelbine has not been fully established. Reduction of vinorelbine dosage in patients with renal impairment does not appear to be necessary.

Because the drug is extensively metabolized in the liver, doses of vinorelbine should be reduced and the drug should be administered with caution in patients with hepatic impairment. In patients with total serum bilirubin concentration of 2 mg/dL or less, no dosage reduction is required. In patients with total serum bilirubin concentration of 2.1–3 mg/dL, vinorelbine dose should be reduced to 50% of the starting dose. In patients with total serum bilirubin concentration exceeding 3 mg/dL, vinorelbine dose should be reduced to 25% of the starting dose. In patients with concurrent hepatic impairment and hematologic toxicity, vinorelbine dosage should be adjusted to the lower dosage advised by these guidelines.

CAUTIONS

A similar pattern of adverse effects is observed in patients receiving vinorelbine as a single agent or in combination therapy. Unless otherwise noted, incidence data for adverse effects are derived from data for 365 patients (222 patients with advanced breast cancer, 143 patients with non-small cell lung cancer) receiving vinorelbine as a single agent in 3 clinical studies. The dosing schedule in each study was vinorelbine 30 mg/m^2 once weekly.

● Hematologic Effects and Infectious Complications

The major and dose-limiting adverse effect of vinorelbine is myelosuppression, manifested principally by granulocytopenia and leukopenia. The incidence of myelosuppression does not appear to be influenced by age or prior exposure to chemotherapy. Granulocyte counts less than 2000 and 500/mm^3 occurred in 90 and 36% of patients, respectively. Leukopenia (less than 4000/mm^3) occurred in 92% of patients, and was severe (less than 1000 cells/mm^3) in 15% of patients. Leukopenia occurred at a similar rate in patients receiving vinorelbine and cisplatin in randomized trials (88 or 94%), but the rate of grade 3 or 4 leukopenia was higher (about 60%). Hospitalization for granulocytopenic complications (e.g., fever, sepsis, infection, pneumonia) occurred in 9% of patients. Hospitalization for documented sepsis was reported in about 4% of patients receiving vinorelbine either alone or with cisplatin. Septic death occurred in approximately 1% of patients.

The manufacturer states that, although the pharmacokinetics of vinorelbine are not influenced by the concurrent administration of cisplatin, the incidence of granulocytopenia is higher when vinorelbine is used in combination with cisplatin than when it is used as a single agent. In a clinical trial in which patients were randomized to receive single-agent vinorelbine or vinorelbine plus cisplatin, grade 3 or 4 granulocytopenia occurred more frequently with the combination (79%) than with single-agent vinorelbine (53%). In another randomized trial, grade 3 or 4 granulocytopenia occurred more frequently in those receiving vinorelbine and cisplatin (82%) than in those receiving cisplatin alone (5%); fever and/or sepsis related to granulocytopenia occurred in 11% of patients receiving combination therapy compared with 0% of patients receiving cisplatin alone, and 4 patients receiving vinorelbine and cisplatin died of granulocytopenia-related sepsis. In the same study, death from febrile neutropenia occurred in 3 patients receiving vinorelbine and cisplatin. Infection (unspecified type) was reported in 11% of patients receiving vinorelbine and cisplatin compared with less than 1% of those receiving cisplatin alone, and severe infection occurred in 6% of patients receiving combination therapy. Respiratory infection was reported in patients receiving vinorelbine and cisplatin (10%) or cisplatin alone (3%).

Vinorelbine-induced myelosuppression generally is reversible and does not appear to increase with cumulative exposure. Granulocyte nadirs generally occur between 7–10 days after dosing, and granulocyte count recovery usually occurs within the following 7–14 days. However, granulocytopenia may require dosage adjustment, treatment delay, or drug discontinuance. Among patients with non-small cell lung cancer receiving vinorelbine and cisplatin who experienced grade 3 or 4 granulocytopenia (1000/mm^3 or less) following the first course of therapy or who developed neutropenic fever between cycles of therapy, the use of granulocyte colony-stimulating factor (G-CSF) was permitted. At 24 hours following completion of chemotherapy, G-CSF 5 mcg/kg daily was initiated and continued until the total granulocyte count exceeded 1000/mm^3 on 2 successive determinations; G-CSF was not administered on the day of treatment. Some data suggest that the addition of filgrastim to vinorelbine therapy may reduce the duration and severity of granulocytopenia and/or allow dose intensification.

Anemia (hemoglobin less than 11 g/dL) was reported in 83% of patients, and was severe (hemoglobin less than 8 g/dL) in 9% of patients. Whole blood and/or packed red blood cells were administered to 18% of patients who received

vinorelbine. Among patients with non-small cell lung cancer in a randomized trial, grade 3 or 4 anemia occurred more frequently in those receiving vinorelbine and cisplatin (24%) than in those receiving cisplatin alone (8%).

Thrombocytopenia (less than 100,000/mm^3) developed less frequently than granulocytopenia, neutropenia, or anemia, occurring in 5% of patients; severe thrombocytopenia (less than 50,000/mm^3) was reported in 1% of patients. In randomized trials, grade 3 or 4 thrombocytopenia was reported in 6% of those receiving vinorelbine and cisplatin compared with 2% of those receiving cisplatin alone, and in 4% of those receiving vinorelbine and cisplatin compared with 0% of those receiving vinorelbine alone.

● Nervous System Effects

Peripheral neuropathy, manifested by paresthesia and hypesthesia, occurred in 25% of patients, and was grade 3 or 4 in 1% and less than 1% of patients, respectively. Painful paresthesia with marked motor loss on the plantar surfaces has been reported rarely. Peripheral neuropathy may be related to cumulative dose and is generally reversible upon drug discontinuance.

In a randomized trial, the incidence of grade 3 or 4 peripheral numbness was higher in patients receiving vinorelbine and cisplatin than in those receiving cisplatin alone (2 versus 1%); paresthesias occurred in 17% of patients receiving combination therapy versus 10% of those receiving cisplatin alone. In another randomized study, the incidence of neurotoxicity (including peripheral neuropathy and constipation) was similar in patients receiving combination therapy with cisplatin and vinorelbine compared with those receiving single-agent vinorelbine (44%).

Loss of deep tendon reflexes occurred in less than 5% of patients. Myasthenia also has been reported. Adverse peripheral nervous system effects, including muscle weakness and gait disturbance, have been observed in patients with and without prior symptoms. Patients with preexisting neuropathy, regardless of etiology, or previous or concomitant exposure to neurotoxic agents (e.g., paclitaxel) may be at increased risk for adverse nervous system effects when receiving vinorelbine. (See Cautions: Precautions and Contraindications.)

Asthenia was reported in 36% of patients, and was grade 3 in 7% of patients. Fatigue occurred in 27% of patients receiving vinorelbine. Fatigue is usually mild to moderate in severity, although the frequency and severity tend to increase with dose or repeated drug administration. Malaise, fatigue, or lethargy was reported in 67% of patients receiving vinorelbine and cisplatin versus 49% of those receiving cisplatin alone. Dizziness, hyperalgesia, confusion, disorientation, hyporeflexia, insomnia, headache, generalized pain, pain in tumor-containing tissue, and back pain also have been reported. In a randomized trial, dizziness/vertigo was reported in patients receiving vinorelbine and cisplatin (9%) or cisplatin alone (3%).

Vestibular and auditory deficits have been reported in patients receiving vinorelbine, principally in those receiving cisplatin concomitantly. Taste alterations occurred at a similar rate among patients receiving vinorelbine and cisplatin versus cisplatin alone (17 versus 15%) in a randomized trial.

● Respiratory Effects

Cases of interstitial pulmonary changes and acute respiratory distress syndrome (ARDS), most of which were fatal, have been reported in patients receiving vinorelbine as monotherapy. The mean time to onset of symptoms was 1 week (range: 3–8 days) after vinorelbine administration. Patients who experience an increase in baseline pulmonary manifestations or the onset of new manifestations (e.g., dyspnea, cough, hypoxia) should undergo prompt evaluation.

Acute shortness of breath and severe bronchospasm have been reported infrequently following the administration of vinorelbine and other vinca alkaloids, usually when administered in combination with mitomycin. These adverse pulmonary events may require treatment with supplemental oxygen, bronchodilators, and/or corticosteroids, particularly in patients with preexisting pulmonary dysfunction.

Dyspnea was reported in 7% of patients, and was severe (grade 3 or 4) in 3% of patients. Shortness of breath was reported in 3% of patients, and was severe in 2% of patients. (See Cautions: Precautions and Contraindications.) Interstitial pulmonary changes, hypoxia, and pneumonia also have been reported. Adverse respiratory effects associated with hypersensitivity to vinorelbine also have been reported. Acute pulmonary reactions to vinorelbine usually resemble an allergic reaction and respond to bronchodilators. Subacute pulmonary reactions generally occur within 1 hour after vinorelbine administration and manifest as cough, dyspnea, hypoxemia, and interstitial infiltration. These reactions usually respond to corticosteroid administration.

● *GI Effects*

A fatal case of neutropenic enterocolitis (typhlitis) occurred in a patient following a single dose of vinorelbine.

Severe constipation (grade 3 or 4), paralytic ileus, and intestinal obstruction, necrosis, and perforation have been reported in patients receiving vinorelbine. In some cases, these events have been fatal.

Nausea was reported in 44% of patients receiving vinorelbine, and was grade 3 in 2% of patients. Antiemetic agents generally were not administered prophylactically in clinical trials, and serotonin type 3 (5-HT$_3$) receptor antagonists generally are not required for management of nausea and vomiting. Vomiting was reported in 20% of patients, and was grade 3 in 2% of patients. Nausea and vomiting usually occur within 24 hours of vinorelbine dosing. Nausea or vomiting each was reported at a similar rate (about 60%) in patients receiving vinorelbine and cisplatin or cisplatin alone in a randomized trial. In another randomized trial, grade 3 or 4 nausea and/or vomiting occurred more frequently in patients receiving vinorelbine and cisplatin (30%) than in those receiving vinorelbine alone (2%).

Constipation occurred in 35% of patients receiving vinorelbine, and was severe in 3% of patients. Constipation may cause treatment delay. Grade 3 or 4 constipation and/or paralytic ileus was reported in 3% of patients receiving vinorelbine and cisplatin and in 1% of patients receiving cisplatin. Diarrhea was reported in 17% of patients, and was grade 3 in 1% of patients. Similar or higher rates of diarrhea (17 or 25%) were reported in patients receiving vinorelbine and cisplatin in randomized trials. Anorexia occurred at a similar rate in patients receiving vinorelbine and cisplatin (46%) or cisplatin alone (37%); anorexia has been reported in patients receiving vinorelbine alone. Stomatitis also has been reported in patients receiving vinorelbine. Vomiting, diarrhea, anorexia, and stomatitis usually were mild or moderate in severity. In a randomized clinical trial, severe nausea and vomiting was reported in 30% of patients receiving vinorelbine concomitantly with cisplatin, compared with less than 2% of patients receiving single-agent vinorelbine. Duration of vinorelbine treatment, previous therapy with emetogenic agents, prior abdominal irradiation, and/or pathology of the abdominal cavity may increase the incidence and severity of GI adverse effects.

Dysphagia, mucositis, dyspepsia, epigastralgia, pancreatitis, esophagitis or radiation recall esophagitis, and abdominal pain also have been reported in patients receiving vinorelbine. Ischemic colitis occurred in a patient receiving vinorelbine and cisplatin.

● *Cardiovascular Effects*

Fatal cardiovascular effects have been reported rarely when vinorelbine was used with cisplatin.

In a randomized trial, 2 deaths related to myocardial ischemia and one death from massive stroke occurred in patients receiving vinorelbine and cisplatin.

Chest pain was reported in 5% of patients receiving vinorelbine in clinical trials. Most patients experiencing chest pain had a history of cardiovascular disease or tumor within the chest. Myocardial ischemia and infarction, and cardiogenic shock have been reported rarely. Flushing, hypertension, hypotension, vasodilation, tachycardia, and pulmonary edema also have been reported.

Thromboembolic adverse effects, including pulmonary embolus and deep venous thrombosis, have been reported in patients receiving vinorelbine, principally in those who were seriously ill and debilitated with known predisposing risk factors for these adverse effects. In a randomized trial, phlebitis/thrombosis/embolism occurred in 10% of those receiving vinorelbine and cisplatin versus less than 1% of those receiving cisplatin alone; these adverse effects were grade 3 or 4 in severity in 3% of those receiving combination therapy versus less than 1% of those receiving cisplatin alone. Central venous catheter thrombosis has been reported in patients receiving vinorelbine by continuous IV infusion.

● *Hepatic Effects*

Fatal hepatic failure has been reported in a patient receiving vinorelbine and gemcitabine.

Increased serum AST (SGOT) concentrations occurred in 67%, and increased serum total bilirubin concentrations occurred in 13% of patients. Increased serum ALT (SGPT) concentrations and increased serum alkaline phosphatase concentrations also have been reported. Transient elevations in hepatic enzymes generally were

not associated with clinical symptoms. However, vinorelbine should be used with caution in patients with hepatic insufficiency, and dosage adjustment may be required. (See Dosage and Administration: Dosage in Renal and Hepatic Impairment.)

● *Dermatologic Effects*

Alopecia, manifested as a gradual thinning of hair, was reported in 12% of patients and was reversible. Total hair loss was uncommon. In a randomized trial, alopecia occurred more frequently in patients receiving vinorelbine and cisplatin (34%) than in those receiving cisplatin alone (14%); in another randomized trial, the incidence of alopecia was higher among patients receiving vinorelbine and cisplatin than in those receiving vinorelbine alone (51 versus 30%), including grade 3 or 4 alopecia (8 versus 2%). Radiation recall dermatitis has been reported.

Hand-foot syndrome, generally manifested as bilateral erythema of both the hands and feet, which responds to corticosteroids, has been reported in patients receiving vinorelbine by prolonged (96-hour) IV infusion; the mechanism of the reaction is unclear, but it appears to be dose related. In vitro, vinorelbine has been shown to stimulate histamine release from mast cells.

● *Local Effects*

Vinorelbine is a moderate vesicant. Injection site reactions and injection site pain occurred in 28 and 16% of patients, respectively. Injection site reactions, including reactions secondary to extravasation, usually were mild and were characterized by erythema, pain at the injection site, and vein discoloration; 5% were severe. Among patients receiving vinorelbine and cisplatin in randomized trials, injection site reactions occurred in 17% and were severe in up to 2% of patients. In clinical practice, injection site reactions also have been characterized by localized rash, urticaria, blister formation, and skin sloughing.

The incidence of injection site reactions may be dose related, and delayed onset of injection site reactions also has been reported. Chemical phlebitis along the vein proximal to the injection site was reported in 10% of patients receiving vinorelbine.

The incidence of adverse local reactions appears to be lower when vinorelbine is administered over 6–10 minutes rather than 20 minutes, and when the veins are flushed with 75–125 mL of IV fluid after the infusion is completed. The incidence of adverse local reactions also may be decreased by flushing the vein with 100 mL of fluid before administering vinorelbine and then flushing with an additional 400 mL of fluid following completion of the vinorelbine infusion. Dexamethasone has been added to the IV fluid used to flush the vein following completion of the vinorelbine infusion to help prevent adverse local reactions. Treatment of injection site reactions has included silver sulfadiazine, local hyaluronidase injection, warm compresses, and central venous catheter placement.

Supravenous hyperpigmentation at the infusion site and a localized necrotizing epidermal reaction each have been reported rarely.

● *Renal Effects*

Elevated serum creatinine concentration was reported in a randomized trial in 13% of patients receiving vinorelbine as a single agent versus 46% of patients receiving vinorelbine and cisplatin; in another randomized trial, elevated serum creatinine concentration occurred at a similar rate among patients receiving vinorelbine and cisplatin (37%) or cisplatin alone (28%).

● *Musculoskeletal Effects*

Jaw pain, myalgia, and arthralgia each have been reported in less than 5% of patients receiving vinorelbine. In a randomized trial, myalgia/arthralgia was reported in 12% of patients receiving vinorelbine and cisplatin versus 3% of patients receiving cisplatin alone. Myalgias generally are controlled with nonopioid analgesics but may require treatment delay until symptoms are relieved.

● *Sensitivity Reactions*

Rash has been reported in less than 5% of patients receiving vinorelbine. Systemic allergic reactions, including anaphylaxis, pruritus, urticaria, and angioedema also have been reported. Drug fever has been reported in patients receiving high doses of vinorelbine as a continuous infusion.

● *Other Effects*

Hemorrhagic cystitis and the syndrome of inappropriate ADH secretion each were reported in less than 1% of patients receiving vinorelbine. Electrolyte abnormalities, including hyponatremia with or without the syndrome of inappropriate ADH secretion, have been reported in seriously ill and debilitated patients receiving vinorelbine. Weight loss has been reported in 34% of patients receiving vinorelbine and cisplatin and in 21% of those receiving cisplatin alone in a randomized trial. Fever without infection occurred more frequently in patients receiving vinorelbine and cisplatin than in those receiving cisplatin alone (20 versus 4%). Hearing loss or impairment occurred at a similar rate (18%) among patients receiving either vinorelbine and cisplatin or cisplatin alone in a randomized trial; in another randomized trial, ototoxicity occurred in 10% of patients receiving vinorelbine and cisplatin versus 1% of patients receiving vinorelbine alone.

● Precautions and Contraindications

Vinorelbine is a toxic drug with a low therapeutic index, and a therapeutic response is not likely to occur without evidence of toxicity. The drug must be used only under constant supervision by clinicians experienced in therapy with cytotoxic agents and only when the potential benefits of vinorelbine therapy are thought to outweigh the possible risks. Most adverse effects of vinorelbine are reversible. When severe adverse effects occur during vinorelbine therapy, the drug should be discontinued or dosage reduced and appropriate measures initiated. Vinorelbine should be reinstituted with caution, if at all, with adequate consideration of further need for the drug, and with awareness of possible recurrence of toxicity. (See Dosage and Administration: Dosage: Dosage Modification for Toxicity and Contraindications for Continued Therapy.)

Administration of vinorelbine is contraindicated in patients with baseline granulocyte counts less than 1000 cells/mm³, and the drug should be administered with extreme caution in patients whose bone marrow reserve may have been compromised by prior irradiation or chemotherapy, or in patients whose marrow function is recovering from the effects of previous chemotherapy. To monitor the occurrence of vinorelbine-induced myelosuppression, mainly granulocytopenia, which may be severe and result in infection, it is recommended that frequent peripheral blood cell counts with differentials be performed before administration of each vinorelbine dose and following discontinuance of therapy with the drug. Vinorelbine therapy should be withheld in patients with granulocyte counts less than 1000 cells/mm³. Patients with severe vinorelbine-induced granulocytopenia should be monitored carefully for evidence of infection and/or fever. For further instructions regarding monitoring and dosage adjustment according to hematologic toxicity, see Dosage Modification for Toxicity: Hematologic Toxicity in Dosage and Administration: Dosage.

Prophylactic colony-stimulating factors have not been used routinely with vinorelbine. However, as clinically indicated, such hematopoietic agents may be used at recommended doses no sooner than 24 hours following completion of the administration of cytotoxic chemotherapy. Growth factors should not be administered in the 24-hour period preceding the administration of chemotherapy. Hematopoietic agents also may be indicated for the treatment of vinorelbine overdosage.

Patients should be informed that the major acute toxicities of vinorelbine are related to bone marrow toxicity, particularly granulocytopenia with increased susceptibility to infection, and should be advised to report fever or chills immediately. Patients also should be advised to contact their clinician if they experience increased shortness of breath, cough, or other new respiratory symptoms, or if they experience abdominal pain or constipation.

Administration of vinorelbine to patients who have received prior radiation therapy may result in radiation recall reactions, such as dermatitis and esophagitis.

Patients who have experienced neuropathy with previous drug therapy (e.g., paclitaxel-associated neuropathy) should be monitored for symptoms of neuropathy while receiving vinorelbine. Patients with a previous or preexisting neuropathy, regardless of etiology, as well as those receiving combination therapy with vinorelbine and paclitaxel, either concomitantly or sequentially, should be monitored for new or worsening signs and symptoms of neuropathy while receiving vinorelbine. For further instructions regarding dosage adjustment according to neurologic toxicity, see Dosage Modification for Toxicity: Neurologic Toxicity in Dosage and Administration: Dosage.

Acute shortness of breath and severe bronchospasm have been reported infrequently following the administration of vinorelbine and other vinca alkaloids, most commonly when these agents were used in combination with mitomycin. If a patient develops these adverse effects during administration of vinorelbine, appropriate therapy (e.g., supplemental oxygen, bronchodilators, corticosteroids) may be required, particularly in patients with preexisting pulmonary dysfunction.

Because severe irritation of the eye has been reported with accidental exposure to another vinca alkaloid, the manufacturer states that care must be taken to avoid contamination of the eyes with concentrations of vinorelbine used clinically. If ocular exposure occurs, the eye(s) should be thoroughly flushed with water immediately.

There is no evidence that the toxicity of vinorelbine is greater in patients with elevated serum hepatic enzyme concentrations, and no data are available regarding the use of the drug in patients with severe baseline cholestasis. Because vinorelbine is metabolized mainly in the liver and clinical experience with the drug in patients with severe liver disease is limited, vinorelbine should be administered with caution in patients with severe hepatic injury or impairment, and dosage reduction may be necessary. (See Dosage and Administration: Dosage in Renal and Hepatic Impairment.)

● Pediatric Precautions

Safety and efficacy of vinorelbine in children younger than 18 years of age have not been established. No meaningful clinical activity was demonstrated among 46 pediatric patients receiving vinorelbine (at dosages similar to those used in adults) for recurrent solid malignant tumors, including rhabdomyosarcoma/undifferentiated sarcoma, neuroblastoma, and CNS tumors; children experienced similar toxicities as adults.

● Geriatric Precautions

When the total number of patients studied in North American clinical trials of vinorelbine is considered, approximately one-third were 65 years of age or older. Although no overall differences in efficacy or safety were observed between geriatric and younger patients, and other clinical experience revealed no evidence of age-related differences, the possibility that some geriatric patients may exhibit increased sensitivity to the drug cannot be ruled out.

● Mutagenicity and Carcinogenicity

In in vivo studies, vinorelbine has been shown to cause chromosomal damage (polyploidy in bone marrow cells from Chinese hamsters and positive results of the micronucleus test in mice). The drug was not mutagenic in the Ames test, and results of the mouse lymphoma TK locus assay were inconclusive.

Studies to determine the carcinogenic potential of vinorelbine have not been performed to date.

● Pregnancy, Fertility, and Lactation
Pregnancy

Vinorelbine can cause fetal toxicity when administered to pregnant women, but potential benefits from use of the drug may be acceptable in certain conditions despite the possible risks to the fetus. Vinorelbine has been shown to be embryotoxic and/or fetotoxic in mice and rabbits at single doses of 9 and 5.5 mg/m², respectively (one-third and one-sixth the usual human dose). At doses that were not toxic to the pregnant animal, fetal weight was reduced and ossification was delayed. Vinorelbine and fluorouracil were administered to 3 women with breast cancer during the second or third trimester of pregnancy. The infants were delivered at 34, 37, and 41 weeks' gestation and no chemotherapy-related adverse effects were observed except for anemia in one infant, which occurred 21 days after delivery. There are no adequate and controlled studies to date using vinorelbine in pregnant women. Vinorelbine should be used during pregnancy only in life-threatening situations or severe disease for which safer drugs cannot be used or are ineffective. When vinorelbine is administered during pregnancy or the patient becomes pregnant while receiving the drug, the patient should be informed of the potential hazard to the fetus. Women of childbearing potential should be advised to avoid becoming pregnant while receiving the drug.

Fertility

Vinorelbine did not affect fertility when administered to rats on either a once-weekly (9 mg/m², approximately one-third the usual human dose) or alternate-day (4.2 mg/m², approximately one-seventh the usual human dose) schedule preceding and during mating. However, studies in rats using biweekly (i.e., once every 2 weeks) administration of vinorelbine for 13 or 26 weeks at doses of 2.1 and 7.2 mg/m² (approximately one-fifteenth and one-fourth the usual human dose, respectively) showed decreased spermatogenesis and prostate/seminal vesicle secretion.

Lactation

It is not known whether vinorelbine is distributed in milk. Because many drugs are distributed in milk and because of the potential for serious adverse reactions to vinorelbine in nursing infants, nursing should be discontinued during vinorelbine therapy.

DRUG INTERACTIONS

● Antineoplastic Agents

Acute pulmonary reactions have been reported in patients receiving vinorelbine or other vinca alkaloids (vinblastine, vincristine) in combination with mitomycin. (See Cautions: Respiratory Effects.) A higher incidence of grade 3 and 4 granulocytopenia has been reported in patients receiving combination therapy with vinorelbine and cisplatin than in those receiving vinorelbine alone. (See Cautions: Hematologic Effects and Infectious Complications.) Concomitant administration of vinorelbine and paclitaxel may be associated with an increased risk of neuropathy. (See Cautions: Nervous System Effects.)

● Drugs Affecting Hepatic Microsomal Enzymes

Metabolism of vinca alkaloids is mediated by the cytochrome P-450 (CYP) isoenzyme CYP3A, and inhibitors of this isoenzyme may impair the metabolism of vinca alkaloids. Caution is advised since concomitant administration of vinorelbine and inhibitors of isoenzyme CYP3A may cause earlier onset and/or increased severity of adverse effects.

Death occurred in a patient following chemotherapy with vinorelbine and cisplatin; an interaction between vinorelbine and itraconazole was cited as possible cause.

Concomitant use of itraconazole, a potent inhibitor of CYP3A, and another vinca alkaloid, vincristine, has been associated with earlier onset and/or increased severity of adverse neuromuscular effects, probably related to inhibition of vincristine metabolism. In vitro studies demonstrate that voriconazole is a less potent inhibitor of CYP3A4 than ketoconazole or itraconazole. Because concomitant use of voriconazole or other azole antifungal agents may increase plasma concentrations of vinca alkaloids, such as vinorelbine, and lead to neurotoxicity, dosage reduction of vinorelbine should be considered.

Caution and careful monitoring are advised during concomitant use of a vinca alkaloid and aprepitant, an antiemetic agent, which may inhibit or induce CYP3A4. In clinical studies, the dosage of vinorelbine was not adjusted during concomitant use of aprepitant.

● Ototoxic Drugs

Because vestibular deficits and varying degrees of permanent or temporary hearing impairment associated with damage of the eighth cranial nerve have been reported in patients receiving vinca alkaloids, vinorelbine should be used concomitantly with other potentially ototoxic drugs, such as platinum-containing antineoplastic agents, with extreme caution.

ACUTE TOXICITY

● Manifestations

Overdosage with vinorelbine produces adverse effects that are mainly extensions of common adverse effects, including paralytic ileus, stomatitis, and esophagitis. Bone marrow aplasia, sepsis, and paresis also have been reported. Overdoses of up to 10 times the recommended dose of 30 mg/m² have been reported, and some fatalities have occurred. Death from multisystem failure caused by an overdose of vinorelbine has been reported in a patient receiving the drug in combination with cisplatin.

● Treatment

There is no known specific antidote for vinorelbine overdosage. Management of vinorelbine overdosage should consist of general supportive measures and symptomatic treatment, including blood transfusions, hematopoietic agents, and anti-infectives, when clinically indicated.

PHARMACOLOGY

Vinorelbine is an antimicrotubule antineoplastic agent. Microtubules are organelles that exist in a state of dynamic equilibrium with their components, tubulin dimers. They form an essential part of the mitotic spindle, participate in intracellular transport, and contribute to the cell's shape, rigidity, and motility.

Vinorelbine and other vinca alkaloids exert their cytotoxic effects by binding to tubulin, the protein subunit of the spindle microtubules. The formation of vinorelbine-tubulin complexes prevents the polymerization of the tubulin subunits into microtubules and induces depolymerization of microtubules resulting in inhibition of microtubule assembly and cellular metaphase arrest.

In addition to the antineoplastic effects of antimicrotubule activity, vinca alkaloids interfere with the microtubule-mediated movement of neurotransmitter substances along neuronal axons resulting in dose-limiting neurotoxicity. Although the depolymerizing action of vincristine, vinblastine, and vinorelbine on axonal microtubules is identical, this action occurs in vitro at higher concentrations of vinorelbine than these other vinca alkaloids, and in vitro studies suggest that vinorelbine has a higher affinity than these drugs for mitotic rather than axonal microtubules. In comparative clinical trials, vinorelbine was shown to be less neurotoxic than vindesine, another vinca alkaloid.

Like other vinca alkaloids, vinorelbine reportedly also interferes with amino acid, cyclic AMP, and glutathione metabolism; calmodulin-dependent Ca^{2+}-transport ATPase activity; cellular respiration; and nucleic acid and lipid biosynthesis.

PHARMACOKINETICS

● Absorption

Following IV administration, plasma concentrations of vinorelbine decline in a triphasic manner with an initial rapid decrease.

● Distribution

The initial rapid decline in plasma vinorelbine concentration following IV administration represents distribution of the drug to peripheral compartments. Following administration of vinorelbine 30 mg/m² IV over 15–20 minutes, a steady-state volume of distribution of 25.4–40.1 L/kg has been reported.

Vinorelbine demonstrates high binding to human platelets and lymphocytes. Binding of the drug to plasma constituents in patients with cancer ranges from 79.6–91.2%, and a free fraction of approximately 0.11 was observed in pooled human plasma over a concentration range of 234–1169 ng/mL. The presence of cisplatin, fluorouracil, or doxorubicin does not affect vinorelbine binding.

● Elimination

The 3 phases of plasma decline of vinorelbine concentrations represent an initial rapid decline in plasma concentrations caused by distribution of the drug to peripheral compartments followed by metabolism and excretion of the drug and a prolonged terminal phase because of relatively slow efflux of drug from peripheral compartments. A mean terminal elimination half-life of 27.7–43.6 hours and a mean plasma clearance of 0.97–1.26 L/hour per kg have been reported for vinorelbine.

Vinorelbine is extensively metabolized in the liver. The metabolism of vinca alkaloids (e.g., vinblastine, vincristine) is mediated by the cytochrome P-450 (CYP) isoenzymes in the CYP3A subfamily. Two metabolites of vinorelbine, vinorelbine N-oxide and deacetylvinorelbine, have been identified in human blood, plasma, and urine. Deacetylvinorelbine, the primary metabolite of vinorelbine in humans, has been shown to possess antitumor activity similar to the parent drug. However, therapeutic doses of vinorelbine result in very small, if any, quantifiable concentrations of either metabolite in blood or urine.

Following IV administration of radiolabeled vinorelbine, approximately 46% of the administered dose was recovered in the feces and 18% in the urine. In another study, approximately 11% of an administered IV dose of vinorelbine was excreted unchanged in the urine.

The effect of renal and/or hepatic impairment on the elimination of vinorelbine has not been evaluated. Limited data from pharmacokinetic studies indicate that the disposition of the drug in geriatric patients is similar to that observed in younger adults.

CHEMISTRY AND STABILITY

● Chemistry

Vinorelbine (didehydrodeoxynorvincaleukoblastine), a semisynthetic vinca alkaloid, is an antineoplastic agent. Like other vinca alkaloids, vinorelbine is a large dimeric asymmetric compound composed of a dihydroindole nucleus (vindoline), which is the major alkaloid present in the periwinkle (*Catharanthus roseus* [Apocynaceae]), and an indole nucleus (catharanthine), which is present in low concentrations in the plant. However, vinorelbine differs structurally from other currently available vinca alkaloids by the presence of substitutions on the catharanthine ring, rather than the vindoline ring, of the molecule.

Vinorelbine tartrate occurs as a white to yellow or light brown amorphous powder. The aqueous solubility of the drug exceeds 1000 mg/mL in distilled water. Commercially available vinorelbine tartrate injection occurs as a clear, colorless to pale yellow solution in water for injection and has a pH of approximately 3.5.

● Stability

Commercially available vinorelbine tartrate injection is stable until the date indicated on the package when stored unopened and refrigerated at 2–8°C and protected from light. Unopened vials of vinorelbine tartrate injection are stable at temperatures up to 25°C for up to 72 hours. Vinorelbine tartrate injection should not be frozen.

For further information on the handling of antineoplastic agents, see the ASHP Guidelines on Handling Hazardous Drugs at http://www.ahfsdrug information.com.

PREPARATIONS

Excipients in commercially available drug preparations may have clinically important effects in some individuals; consult specific product labeling for details.

Vinorelbine Tartrate

Parenteral

For injection concentrate, for IV infusion only	10 mg (of vinorelbine)/mL (10 and 50 mg)	**Navelbine®**, Pierre Fabre
		Vinorelbine Tartrate for Injection

† Use is not currently included in the labeling approved by the US Food and Drug Administration.

Selected Revisions April 6, 2016, © Copyright, September 1, 1995, American Society of Health-System Pharmacists, Inc.

Table of Contents

§ Omitted from the print version of *AHFS Drug Information*® because of space limitations. This monograph is available on the *AHFS Drug Information*® website, http://ahfsdruginformation.com.

Donepezil Hydrochloride

12:04 • PARASYMPATHOMIMETIC (CHOLINERGIC) AGENTS

■ Donepezil hydrochloride is a centrally active, reversible acetylcholinesterase inhibitor.

USES

● Alzheimer's Disease

Donepezil hydrochloride is used for the management of mild, moderate, or severe dementia of the Alzheimer's type (Alzheimer's disease, presenile or senile dementia).

Cholinesterase inhibitors (e.g., donepezil, galantamine, rivastigmine) are used for the symptomatic management of dementia associated with Alzheimer's disease; there is no evidence that these drugs alter the course of the underlying dementing process. The rationale for use of cholinesterase inhibitors in patients with Alzheimer's disease is to increase CNS acetylcholine concentrations, which are deficient in these patients (see Description). Since there is no cure for dementia, the goal of treatment is to improve quality of life and maximize functional ability. The available evidence is modest for the efficacy of cholinesterase inhibitors in the treatment of mild to severe Alzheimer's disease. Randomized controlled studies conducted with these drugs have shown only modest benefits in cognitive and functional measures, and the clinical importance of these effects is not clear. Because of the lack of established alternatives, experts generally recommend a trial with one of the cholinesterase inhibitors in patients with mild to moderate Alzheimer's disease; there is also evidence suggesting that these drugs may have some limited benefits in patients with severe disease. Although few comparative trials have been conducted, the available evidence suggests that efficacy is similar among the various cholinesterase inhibitors, but tolerability may differ. The long-term efficacy of cholinesterase inhibitors in patients with Alzheimer's disease is not clear, and additional studies are needed to determine whether the benefits of these drugs are sustained; however, there is evidence indicating that adverse effects such as anorexia, weight loss, syncope, bradycardia, falls, hip fractures, and increased need for cardiac pacemakers may develop with long-term use.

Efficacy of donepezil in the treatment of *mild to moderate* Alzheimer's disease has been established in 2 short-term (15 or 30 weeks) randomized, double-blind, placebo-controlled studies. Response to treatment in these studies was evaluated using a dual outcome strategy where cognitive performance was assessed by the cognitive subscale of the Alzheimer's Disease Assessment Scale (ADAS cog), and overall clinical effect was assessed by the Clinician's Interview-Based Impression of Change (CIBIC) that required the use of caregiver information (CIBIC plus). The ADAS cog is a multiple-item instrument that has been extensively validated in longitudinal cohorts of patients with Alzheimer's disease for assessing memory, orientation, attention, reasoning, language, and praxis. The CIBIC plus used in the studies of donepezil was a subjective, semistructured instrument intended to measure the patient's ability to function generally, cognitively, behaviorally, and in activities of daily living. In these studies, donepezil was administered for 12 or 24 weeks followed by placebo washout periods of 3 or 6 weeks, respectively, to determine whether rebound effects would occur following discontinuance of the drug. Patients received 5 or 10 mg of donepezil hydrochloride or placebo once daily in these studies; patients who were assigned to receive the 10-mg dosage of donepezil hydrochloride initially received 5 mg daily for 7 days to minimize the likelihood of adverse cholinergic effects.

Both studies demonstrated clinically important but modest and variable improvement in cognitive function and clinician-rated global assessment of observed clinical change with donepezil hydrochloride dosages of 5 or 10 mg daily. However, the improvement was not maintained following discontinuance of therapy. Following the 6-week placebo washout period in the 30-week study, scores on the ADAS cog for patients treated with donepezil or placebo were indistinguishable, indicating no evidence of an effect of donepezil on the underlying disease process in dementia. Results of neuropsychologic tests (i.e., ADAS cog, CIBIC plus, Mini-Mental State Examination [MMSE], and Clinical Dementia Rating [CDR]) performed 6 weeks after discontinuance of donepezil therapy did not show evidence of a rebound deterioration in cognitive symptoms.

Efficacy of donepezil in the treatment of *moderate to severe* Alzheimer's disease has been established in 3 randomized controlled studies using dosages of 10 and 23 mg daily. The primary efficacy outcomes were based on a combination of assessment tools that evaluated cognitive function, daily function, and/or overall clinical effect (i.e., Severe Impairment Battery [SIB], Modified Alzheimer's Disease Cooperative Study Activities of Daily Living Inventory for Severe Alzheimer's Disease [ADCS-ADL-Severe], CIBIC plus). Although these studies demonstrated evidence of benefit with donepezil hydrochloride dosages of 10 and 23 mg daily, a wide range of responses was observed. The 23-mg dosage was more likely to improve cognitive function than the 10-mg dosage, but did not have a significantly greater effect on clinician-rated overall response and was associated with a higher incidence of adverse effects.

Numerous other studies have reported similar findings regarding the modest benefit of donepezil in the management of Alzheimer's disease. In a systematic review of 30 randomized, double-blind, placebo-controlled studies, patients who received donepezil were found to improve only slightly more than those receiving placebo on measures of cognitive function, activities of daily living, and overall clinical state; there was no effect of the drug on quality of life or behavior. The studies were mostly conducted in patients with mild to moderate disease, but a few studies included patients with severe disease. The 23-mg dosage did not provide a greater benefit than the 10-mg dosage, and the 10-mg dosage was only marginally more effective than the 5-mg dosage; withdrawal rates and adverse effects increased with increasing dosage.

Data on long-term use (i.e., beyond 26 weeks) of donepezil in patients with Alzheimer's disease are limited. In patients who received therapy with donepezil for at least 2 years in uncontrolled studies following their participation in placebo-controlled studies of the drug, improvement in cognitive function was maintained for an average of at least 40 weeks, with some benefit still evident after 2 years of follow-up. However, the cognitive abilities of patients receiving donepezil decline over time, although apparently to a lesser degree than in untreated patients.

Donepezil may be used in combination with memantine, an *N*-methyl-D-aspartate (NMDA) receptor antagonist. A fixed-combination preparation containing memantine hydrochloride and donepezil hydrochloride (Namzaric®) is commercially available for the management of moderate to severe dementia of the Alzheimer's type in patients stabilized on a donepezil hydrochloride dosage of 10 mg once daily.

● Mild Cognitive Impairment

Cholinesterase inhibitors including donepezil have been investigated in patients with mild cognitive impairment†; however, evidence of benefit is lacking. Results of a systematic review of 9 randomized, double-blind, placebo-controlled studies of cholinesterase inhibitors in patients with mild cognitive impairment showed no substantial evidence of a beneficial effect on progression to dementia and essentially no effect of these drugs on cognitive test scores. An increased risk of adverse effects, particularly GI effects, was observed with these drugs. These findings do not support the use of cholinesterase inhibitors in individuals presenting with memory complaints who do not meet diagnostic criteria for dementia.

DOSAGE AND ADMINISTRATION

● Administration

Donepezil hydrochloride is administered orally as conventional film-coated or orally disintegrating tablets. The 2 formulations are bioequivalent. The drug is administered once daily, usually in the evening at bedtime. Donepezil hydrochloride orally disintegrating tablets should be allowed to dissolve on the tongue and followed with water. The 23-mg conventional film-coated tablet should not be split, crushed, or chewed.

Because food does not affect the rate or extent of absorption of donepezil when administered as conventional film-coated tablets, the drug may be administered with or without food. The effect of food on absorption of donepezil when administered as orally disintegrating tablets has not been studied. However, the manufacturer states that any effects are expected to be minimal, and the orally disintegrating tablets may be taken without regard to meals.

The fixed-combination preparation containing memantine hydrochloride and donepezil hydrochloride (Namzaric®) may be used in patients receiving a stable dosage of donepezil hydrochloride 10 mg daily. The fixed-combination capsules may be administered with or without food, and should be swallowed intact (and not divided, chewed, or crushed) or may be opened, sprinkled on applesauce, and swallowed without chewing. The entire contents of each capsule should be consumed; the dose should not be divided.

● Dosage
Alzheimer's Disease

For the management of *mild to moderate* dementia of the Alzheimer's type (Alzheimer's disease), the recommended initial dosage of donepezil hydrochloride is 5 mg once daily at bedtime. Dosage may be increased to 10 mg daily as tolerated; although this dosage was not shown in clinical studies to provide substantially greater clinical benefit than a dosage of 5 mg daily, there is evidence suggesting that some patients may derive additional benefit from the higher dosage. Use of the 10-mg daily dosage of donepezil hydrochloride should be based on prescriber and patient preference. Because the rate of dose titration may affect incidence of adverse effects, the manufacturer states that donepezil hydrochloride should be administered at a dosage of 5 mg daily for 4–6 weeks before dosage is increased to 10 mg daily. In clinical studies, increasing dosage from 5 mg daily to 10 mg daily over a 6-week period resulted in a lower rate of adverse effects than did increasing dosage over a period of 1 week.

For the management of *moderate to severe* Alzheimer's disease, the recommended initial dosage of donepezil hydrochloride is 5 mg once daily at bedtime. Dosage may be increased to 10 or 23 mg once daily at bedtime as tolerated. Because the rate of dose titration may affect incidence of adverse effects, the manufacturer states that donepezil hydrochloride should be administered at a dosage of 5 mg daily for 4–6 weeks before dosage is increased to 10 mg daily, and the drug should be administered at a dosage of 10 mg daily for at least 3 months before dosage is increased to 23 mg daily.

Fixed Combination of Memantine Hydrochloride and Donepezil Hydrochloride (Namzaric®)

In patients stabilized on donepezil hydrochloride 10 mg daily who are not currently receiving memantine and who are being switched to the fixed-combination preparation, the recommended initial dosage of the fixed-combination preparation is memantine hydrochloride 7 mg and donepezil hydrochloride 10 mg once daily in the evening. Dosage may be increased after at least 1 week if the previous dosage is tolerated; dosage should be increased in increments of 7 mg of the memantine hydrochloride component up to the maximum recommended maintenance dosage of 28 mg of memantine hydrochloride and 10 mg of donepezil hydrochloride once daily in the evening.

In patients receiving stable dosages of donepezil and memantine as separate preparations (donepezil hydrochloride 10 mg daily; memantine hydrochloride 10 mg twice daily or 28 mg once daily as an extended-release preparation) who are being switched to the fixed-combination preparation, the recommended dosage of the fixed combination is memantine hydrochloride 28 mg and donepezil hydrochloride 10 mg once daily in the evening. Therapy with the fixed-combination preparation should be initiated on the day following the last dose of the individual preparations.

● Dosage in Renal and Hepatic Impairment

The manufacturer of donepezil makes no specific recommendations for dosage adjustment in patients with renal or hepatic impairment.

Fixed Combination of Memantine Hydrochloride and Donepezil Hydrochloride (Namzaric®)

Memantine is eliminated predominately by renal clearance; dosage reduction is therefore recommended in patients with severe renal impairment (creatinine clearance 5–29 mL/minute) receiving the fixed-combination preparation containing memantine hydrochloride and donepezil hydrochloride. If the fixed-combination preparation is being initiated in such patients who are not currently taking memantine, the recommended initial dosage of the fixed-combination preparation is 7 mg of memantine hydrochloride and 10 mg of donepezil hydrochloride once daily in the evening; after 1 week, dosage should be increased to the recommended maintenance dosage of 14 mg of memantine hydrochloride and 10 mg of donepezil hydrochloride once daily in the evening. Patients with severe renal impairment who are receiving stable dosages of memantine and donepezil as separate preparations can be switched to the fixed-combination preparation containing memantine hydrochloride 14 mg and donepezil hydrochloride 10 mg once daily in the evening. No dosage adjustment is required in patients with mild or moderate renal impairment.

CAUTIONS

● Contraindications

Known hypersensitivity to donepezil or piperidine derivatives or any ingredient in the formulation.

● Warnings/Precautions

Use with Anesthesia

Cholinesterase inhibitors can exaggerate the effects of some muscle relaxants (e.g., succinylcholine) during anesthesia.

Cardiac Effects

Cholinesterase inhibitors may produce bradycardia or heart block via vagotonic effects on the sinoatrial or atrioventricular (AV) node. This may occur in patients with or without known cardiac conduction abnormalities. Syncope has been reported in patients receiving donepezil.

Cholinesterase inhibitors should be used with caution in patients with sick sinus syndrome or other conduction defects.

GI Effects

Adverse GI effects associated with cholinesterase inhibitors include diarrhea, nausea, and vomiting. These effects appear to occur in a dose-related manner and are usually mild to moderate in severity. In a controlled clinical trial, nausea and vomiting were reported at a markedly higher rate (9–12 versus 2–3%) in patients receiving a donepezil hydrochloride dosage of 23 mg daily compared with a dosage of 10 mg daily. In most cases, adverse GI effects were transient (lasting 1–3 weeks) and resolved during continued use of the drug without the need for dose modification. Patients should be monitored closely for adverse GI effects during initiation of donepezil therapy and after dosage increases.

Cholinesterase inhibitors such as donepezil may increase gastric acid secretion. Patients should be monitored closely for symptoms of active or occult GI bleeding, especially in those at increased risk for developing ulcers (e.g., those with history of ulcer disease, those receiving concomitant nonsteroidal anti-inflammatory agent [NSAIA] therapy). In clinical studies, the incidence of peptic ulcer disease or GI bleeding was not increased with donepezil hydrochloride dosages of 5 or 10 mg daily compared with placebo; however, these adverse effects occurred at a higher rate with the 23-mg dosage than with the 10-mg dosage of the drug.

Weight Loss

In a controlled clinical trial, weight loss was reported at a higher frequency in patients receiving donepezil hydrochloride 23 mg daily compared with a dosage of 10 mg daily (4.7 versus 2.5%). A decrease of at least 7% from baseline weight occurred in 8.4% of patients receiving the 23-mg dosage compared with 4.9% of patients receiving the 10-mg dosage.

Genitourinary Effects

Although not reported in clinical studies with donepezil, cholinesterase inhibitors may induce or exacerbate urinary obstruction.

Respiratory Effects

Cholinesterase inhibitors should be used with caution in patients with a history of asthma or obstructive pulmonary disease.

Neurologic Effects

Drugs that increase cholinergic activity have the potential for causing seizures; however, seizures also may be a manifestation of Alzheimer's disease. These drugs should be used with caution in patients with seizures.

Use of Fixed Combinations

When donepezil is used in fixed combination with memantine, the usual cautions, precautions, and contraindications associated with memantine should be considered.

Specific Populations

Pregnancy

There are no adequate data to inform the developmental risks associated with the use of donepezil in pregnant women. Animal reproduction studies did not demonstrate any evidence of developmental toxicity when the drug was administered to pregnant rats and rabbits during the period of organogenesis; however, when the drug was administered at clinically relevant doses during later stages of pregnancy and throughout lactation, increased stillbirths and decreased offspring survival were observed.

Lactation

It is not known whether donepezil is distributed into human milk or if the drug has any effects on nursing infants or milk production. The known benefits of breast-feeding should be considered along with the mother's need for the drug and any potential adverse effects on the breast-fed infant from the drug or underlying maternal condition.

Pediatric Use

Safety and efficacy of donepezil have not been established in pediatric patients. Dementia of the Alzheimer's type occurs principally in patients older than 55 years of age.

Geriatric Use

Population pharmacokinetic analysis indicates that clearance of donepezil decreases with increasing age. Compared with patients who were 65 years of age, clearance of donepezil was decreased by 17% in patients 90 years of age and increased by 33% in patients 40 years of age; however, the manufacturer states that these changes may not be clinically important.

Low Body Weight

An increased frequency of some adverse effects (e.g., nausea, vomiting, decreased weight) has been observed in donepezil-treated patients weighing less than 55 kg compared with those with higher body weights; this may be related to higher plasma exposures in patients with lower body weights.

Pharmacogenomic Considerations

Donepezil is metabolized by cytochrome P-450 (CYP) 2D6. Clearance of the drug has been shown to differ based on the patient's CYP2D6 genotype; compared with extensive metabolizers of CYP2D6, clearance of donepezil is decreased by 31.5% in poor CYP2D6 metabolizers and increased by 24% in ultra-rapid metabolizers.

Hepatic Impairment

Clearance of donepezil in a limited number of patients with stable alcoholic cirrhosis was reduced by 20% compared with that in healthy age- and gender-matched individuals; however, the manufacturer makes no specific recommendation for dosage adjustment in patients with hepatic disease.

Renal Impairment

Limited data in a few patients with moderate to severe renal impairment (creatinine clearance less than 18 mL/minute per 1.73 m²) indicate no difference in the clearance of donepezil compared with that in healthy age- and gender-matched individuals.

● Common Adverse Effects

Common adverse effects reported with donepezil in clinical studies include nausea, diarrhea, insomnia, vomiting, muscle cramps, fatigue, and anorexia.

DRUG INTERACTIONS

● Drugs Affecting or Metabolized by Hepatic Enzymes

Donepezil is metabolized by cytochrome P-450 (CYP) isoenzyme 3A4 and CYP2D6. In vitro studies suggest that donepezil is unlikely to alter the clearance of drugs metabolized by CYP3A4 or CYP2D6. In vitro studies show little to no evidence of inhibition of CYP2B6, 2C8, and 2C19 at clinically relevant concentrations. It is not known whether donepezil has any enzyme-inducing potential.

Potent inhibitors of CYP3A (e.g., ketoconazole) or CYP2D6 (e.g., quinidine) can potentially increase plasma concentrations of donepezil. In a study in healthy individuals, ketoconazole increased plasma concentrations of donepezil by about 36%; however, the clinical importance of this change is not known. Population pharmacokinetic analysis indicates that concomitant use of donepezil (10 or 23 mg daily) and CYP2D6 inhibitors may increase systemic exposure of donepezil by 17–20%.

CYP3A inducers (e.g., phenytoin, carbamazepine, dexamethasone, rifampin, phenobarbital) can induce the metabolism of donepezil.

Pharmacokinetic studies indicate that donepezil does not affect the pharmacokinetics of theophylline, cimetidine, warfarin, digoxin, or ketoconazole.

● Protein-bound Drugs

Pharmacokinetic interactions are unlikely with concomitant use of donepezil and highly protein-bound drugs.

DESCRIPTION

Donepezil hydrochloride, a piperidine derivative, is a centrally active, reversible inhibitor of acetylcholinesterase.

Donepezil is an anticholinesterase agent that binds reversibly with and inactivates cholinesterases (e.g., acetylcholinesterase), thus inhibiting hydrolysis of acetylcholine. As a result, the concentration of acetylcholine increases at cholinergic synapses. In vitro data and data in animals indicate that the anticholinesterase activity of donepezil is relatively specific for acetylcholinesterase in the brain compared with butyrylcholinesterase inhibition in peripheral tissues.

A deficiency of acetylcholine caused by selective loss of cholinergic neurons in the cerebral cortex, nucleus basalis, and hippocampus is recognized as one of the early pathophysiologic features of Alzheimer's disease associated with memory loss and cognitive deficits. The deficiency of cholinergic transmission has been associated with the accumulation of β-amyloid peptide and neurofibrillary tangles that is characteristic of Alzheimer's disease. Because synaptic loss has been shown to correlate with cognitive decline in Alzheimer's disease, enhancement of cholinergic function with an anticholinesterase agent such as donepezil is one of the pharmacologic approaches to treatment. However, the potential benefits of anticholinesterase agents may theoretically diminish as the disease process advances and fewer cholinergic neurons remain functioning.

ADVICE TO PATIENTS

Importance of taking donepezil once daily as prescribed.

Importance of informing patients of the potential for adverse effects such as nausea, diarrhea, vomiting, insomnia, fatigue, anorexia, and weight loss.

Importance of informing clinicians of existing or contemplated concomitant therapy, including prescription and OTC drugs, as well as any concomitant illnesses.

Importance of women informing clinicians if they are or plan to become pregnant or plan to breast-feed.

Importance of informing patients of other precautionary information. (See Cautions.)

PREPARATIONS

Excipients in commercially available drug preparations may have clinically important effects in some individuals; consult specific product labeling for details.

Donepezil Hydrochloride

Oral

Tablets, film-coated	5 mg*	Aricept®, Eisai
		Donepezil Hydrochloride Tablets
	10 mg*	Aricept®, Eisai
		Donepezil Hydrochloride Tablets
	23 mg	Aricept®, Eisai
Tablets, orally disintegrating	5 mg*	Aricept® ODT, Eisai
		Donepezil Hydrochloride Orally Disintegrating Tablets
	10 mg*	Aricept® ODT, Eisai
		Donepezil Hydrochloride Orally Disintegrating Tablets

* available from one or more manufacturer, distributor, and/or repackager by generic (nonproprietary) name

Donepezil Hydrochloride Combinations

Oral

Capsules, extended-release	10 mg with Memantine Hydrochloride 7 mg	Namzaric®, Allergan
	10 mg with Memantine Hydrochloride 14 mg	Namzaric®, Allergan
	10 mg with Memantine Hydrochloride 21 mg	Namzaric®, Allergan
	10 mg with Memantine Hydrochloride 28 mg	Namzaric®, Allergan

† Use is not currently included in the labeling approved by the US Food and Drug Administration.

Neostigmine Methylsulfate

12:04 • PARASYMPATHOMIMETIC (CHOLINERGIC) AGENTS

■ Neostigmine methylsulfate is an anticholinesterase agent.

USES

● Reversal of Neuromuscular Blockade

Neostigmine methylsulfate is used for reversal of the effects of nondepolarizing neuromuscular blocking agents (e.g., atracurium, cisatracurium, pancuronium, rocuronium, vecuronium) after surgery. An anticholinergic agent such as atropine sulfate or glycopyrrolate should be used in conjunction with neostigmine to minimize adverse muscarinic effects of the drug (e.g., bradycardia, bradyarrhythmias, increased secretions, bronchoconstriction).

Anticholinesterase agents such as neostigmine are used to reverse the effects of nondepolarizing neuromuscular blocking agents and reduce the risk of postoperative residual neuromuscular blockade. Evidence supporting the efficacy of neostigmine for reversal of neuromuscular blockade is based principally on data from the published literature. In several randomized studies, neostigmine effectively reduced the time to recovery of neuromuscular blockade after surgery when compared with spontaneous recovery or placebo; all of the studies used recovery to a train-of-four (TOF) ratio of 0.9 as the primary measure of response, which is the currently accepted standard for adequate recovery of neuromuscular function.

Anticholinesterase agents are not effective in reversing deep levels of neuromuscular blockade and generally should not be used until some degree of spontaneous recovery occurs (e.g., when there is a detectable twitch response to the first TOF stimulus). However, administration of these drugs to fully recovered patients has resulted in paradoxical neuromuscular effects (e.g., weakness of upper airway muscles, increased airway collapsibility), and some clinicians recommend that this practice be avoided. In contrast to these findings, other investigators have not reported any adverse respiratory effects in patients administered neostigmine at near or full neuromuscular recovery. (See Neuromuscular Dysfunction under Cautions.) Anticholinesterase agents do not antagonize the phase I block of depolarizing neuromuscular blocking agents such as succinylcholine and should not be used to reverse the effects of these drugs.

It is important that the effects of neuromuscular blocking agents are quickly and effectively terminated after surgery to prevent postoperative residual neuromuscular blockade. Incomplete neuromuscular recovery can cause prolonged weakness of the upper airway muscles and associated complications (e.g., airway obstruction, aspiration, hypoxemia, pneumonia, atelectasis, respiratory failure). Risk of postoperative pulmonary complications may be further increased based on certain patient- and procedure-related factors. Therefore, residual neuromuscular block is an important patient safety issue that requires appropriate management. The available data indicate that reversal of neuromuscular blockade should be a standard practice unless there is quantitative evidence that no reversal is needed (TOF >0.9). Anticholinesterase agents such as neostigmine have been traditionally used for reversal of nondepolarizing neuromuscular agents. Sugammadex is another option that may be considered for reversing the effects of rocuronium or vecuronium.

Neostigmine has been compared to sugammadex for the reversal of moderate and deep neuromuscular blockade induced by rocuronium or vecuronium in randomized, active-controlled studies. Results of these studies revealed that time to recovery of neuromuscular function (TOF ratio of 0.9) was substantially faster following administration of sugammadex compared with neostigmine. In a Cochrane meta-analysis which included 41 randomized controlled studies comparing neostigmine and sugammadex for reversal of rocuronium-induced neuromuscular blockade in adults, sugammadex 2 mg/kg was 10.22 minutes (6.6 times) faster than neostigmine 0.05 mg/kg in reversing moderate paralysis, and sugammadex 4 mg/kg was 45.78 minutes (16.8 times) faster than neostigmine 0.07 mg/kg in reversing deep paralysis.

● Myasthenia Gravis

Neostigmine has been used in the symptomatic treatment of myasthenia gravis†, principally to improve muscle strength. The oral preparation (Prostigmin®) previously used for this indication is no longer commercially available in the US, and the currently available parenteral injection is not FDA-labeled for this use.

Anticholinesterase agents are commonly used in the management of myasthenia gravis (both ocular and generalized forms). Although evidence from randomized controlled studies is limited, these drugs have demonstrated marked clinical effects in observational studies, case reports, case series, and during clinical experience. If an anticholinesterase agent is required for symptomatic treatment of myasthenia gravis, pyridostigmine is the preferred drug.

● GI Disorders

Neostigmine has been used for the treatment of acute colonic pseudo-obstruction or Ogilvie syndrome†, a GI motility disorder characterized by marked dilation of the colon in the absence of mechanical obstruction. Conservative therapy is considered the treatment of choice for this condition; however, there is some evidence suggesting that neostigmine may be an effective alternative for patients who fail to respond to conservative management. In several retrospective and prospective studies, IV administration of neostigmine produced rapid colonic decompression and improved symptoms of acute colonic pseudo-obstruction in such patients.

Neostigmine also has been used as a prokinetic agent in patients with postoperative ileus following surgery†; however, the adverse muscarinic effects of the drug (e.g., bradycardia, increased bronchial secretions) may limit its clinical usefulness in this setting.

Limited data suggest that neostigmine may be useful in the management of severe constipation in patients with thoracic spinal cord injury†.

DOSAGE AND ADMINISTRATION

● General

Patient Monitoring

- When used for reversal of neuromuscular blockade, patients must be well ventilated and have a patent airway prior to administration of neostigmine and until complete recovery of normal respiration. Continuous monitoring of neuromuscular function is recommended to ensure adequate reversal from the neuromuscular block. To exclude with certainty the possibility of residual paralysis, use an objective (quantitative) method of monitoring such as peripheral nerve stimulation in conjunction with other clinical assessments (e.g., observation of skeletal muscle tone, respiratory measurements). Adequate recovery of neuromuscular function generally is defined as a train-of-four (TOF) ratio of 0.9 in addition to the patient's ability to maintain satisfactory ventilation and a patent airway. Recovery times may vary based on the patient's medical condition and duration of action of the specific neuromuscular blocking agent used.

Dispensing and Administration Precautions

- Administer only by trained clinicians experienced in the use of neuromuscular blocking agents and their reversal agents.
- Always have atropine and medications to treat anaphylaxis (e.g., epinephrine) readily available in case of hypersensitivity reaction.

Other General Considerations

- Administer IV atropine sulfate or glycopyrrolate immediately prior to or concurrently (in separate syringes) with neostigmine to counteract adverse muscarinic effects. If patient is bradycardic, give IV antimuscarinic before neostigmine.

● Administration

Neostigmine methylsulfate is administered by *slow* IV injection (over a period of at least 1 minute). The drug also has been administered by IM or subcutaneous injection†, but the manufacturer of the currently available injectable preparation labeled for reversal of neuromuscular blocking agents states that the injection is for IV use only.

Neostigmine methylsulfate injection should be stored at controlled room temperature (20–25°C) but may be exposed to temperatures ranging from 15–30°C; the injection should be stored in the original carton until time of use and protected from light.

● Dosage

Reversal of Neuromuscular Block

Dosage of neostigmine methylsulfate should be based on individual patient requirements and response. A peripheral nerve stimulator capable of delivering a

TOF stimulus should be used to determine when neostigmine should be administered and if additional doses are necessary. Neostigmine should be administered only after some degree of spontaneous recovery has occurred (i.e., at least 10% recovery of the first twitch response).

For reversal of the effects of nondepolarizing neuromuscular blocking agents after surgery, the manufacturer states that a neostigmine methylsulfate dose of 0.03–0.07 mg/kg given by slow IV injection usually is sufficient to achieve adequate recovery of neuromuscular function (i.e., TOF ratio of 0.9) within 10–20 minutes of administration. Selection of an appropriate dose should be based on the half-life of the neuromuscular blocking agent being reversed, degree of spontaneous recovery, and the need for rapid reversal. For reversal of neuromuscular blocking agents with a shorter half-life (e.g., rocuronium) or reversal of shallower blocks (i.e., when first twitch response is substantially greater than 10% of baseline or when a second twitch is present), the manufacturer recommends a neostigmine methylsulfate dose of 0.03 mg/kg. The higher dose of 0.07 mg/kg is recommended for reversal of longer-acting neuromuscular blocking agents (e.g., pancuronium, vecuronium), reversal of deeper blocks (i.e., when first twitch response is not substantially greater than 10% of baseline), or when more rapid recovery is needed. Although weight-based dosing of neostigmine methylsulfate is recommended by the manufacturer, the drug also has been administered in fixed IV doses of 0.5–2 mg for reversal of nondepolarizing neuromuscular blockade in adults. The recommended maximum total dose of neostigmine methylsulfate is 0.07 mg/kg or 5 mg, whichever is less; higher doses are unlikely to provide additional clinical benefit. The need for additional doses should be determined by TOF monitoring and the extent of recovery of neuromuscular function.

The manufacturer states that the same dosage recommendations in adults should be applied to pediatric patients since dosing requirements generally are similar between the two populations. Other experts have recommended IV neostigmine methylsulfate doses of 0.025 to 0.07 mg/kg in neonates, 0.025–0.1 mg/kg in infants, and 0.025–0.08 mg/kg in children for reversal of nondepolarizing neuromuscular blocking agents.

To counteract the adverse muscarinic effects of neostigmine methylsulfate, an IV anticholinergic agent (atropine sulfate or glycopyrrolate) should be administered prior to or concomitantly (in separate syringes) with neostigmine. In the presence of bradycardia, the anticholinergic agent should be given before neostigmine.

● Special Populations

Hepatic Impairment

Dosage adjustments do not appear to be necessary in patients with hepatic impairment undergoing reversal of neuromuscular blockade; however, such patients should be carefully monitored if neuromuscular blocking agents with hepatic elimination or active metabolites are administered because the effects of the neuromuscular blocking agent may be prolonged and persist beyond the effects of neostigmine.

Renal Impairment

Dosage adjustments do not appear to be necessary in patients with renal impairment undergoing reversal of neuromuscular blockade; however, such patients should be closely monitored if renally eliminated neuromuscular blocking agents are administered because the effects of the neuromuscular blocking agent may persist beyond the effects of neostigmine.

Geriatric Patients

Although dosage adjustments are not required in geriatric patients undergoing reversal of neuromuscular blockade, a longer period of monitoring is recommended in such patients to ensure that additional doses of neostigmine are not necessary to adequately reverse neuromuscular blockade. (See Geriatric Use under Cautions.)

CAUTIONS

● Contraindications
- Known hypersensitivity to neostigmine.
- Mechanical obstruction of the intestinal or urinary tract.
- Peritonitis.

● Warnings/Precautions

Bradycardia

Bradycardia may occur with neostigmine administration. Atropine sulfate or glycopyrrolate should be administered prior to neostigmine to lessen the risk of bradycardia.

Serious Reactions with Coexisting Conditions

Because of the risk of blood pressure and heart rate complications, neostigmine should be used with caution in patients with certain cardiac conditions such as coronary artery disease, cardiac arrhythmias, or recent acute coronary syndrome. Patients with myasthenia gravis also may be at increased risk of cardiovascular complications. Concomitant use of an anticholinergic agent (e.g., atropine) generally will minimize the risk of adverse cardiovascular effects associated with neostigmine.

Sensitivity Reactions
Hypersensitivity

Neostigmine administration may result in hypersensitivity reactions, including urticaria, angioedema, erythema multiforme, generalized rash, facial swelling, peripheral edema, pyrexia, flushing, hypotension, bronchospasm, bradycardia, and anaphylaxis. Because of the possibility of hypersensitivity, atropine and other drugs for the treatment of anaphylaxis should be readily available during administration.

Neuromuscular Dysfunction

Neostigmine can cause paradoxical neuromuscular effects (e.g., weakness of upper airway muscles and increased airway collapsibility) if used in patients with complete or near complete neuromuscular recovery. Neuromuscular dysfunction and other postoperative respiratory complications have occurred when high doses of neostigmine were administered during minimal neuromuscular blockade. The dose of neostigmine methylsulfate should be reduced if neuromuscular recovery is almost complete.

Cholinergic Crisis

Cholinergic crisis, a condition causing extreme muscle weakness, can occur in patients who receive an overdosage of neostigmine. Manifestations of cholinergic crisis include nausea, vomiting, diarrhea, excessive salivation and sweating, and bradycardia. Increasing muscle weakness can ultimately cause respiratory paralysis and death. Myasthenic crisis, a complication of myasthenia gravis, can also cause extreme muscle weakness and resemble cholinergic crisis. It is extremely important to differentiate between the two conditions since treatment methods differ considerably. Whereas more intensive anticholinesterase therapy is required in patients with myasthenic crisis, administration of higher doses of neostigmine can have serious consequences in patients with cholinergic crisis.

Specific Populations
Pregnancy

It is not known whether neostigmine can cause fetal harm when administered to pregnant women or affect reproductive capacity; the drug should be used during pregnancy only when clearly indicated as no adequate or well-controlled studies of the drug have been conducted in pregnant women. Administration of anticholinesterase drugs such as neostigmine to pregnant women near term may cause uterine irritability and induce premature labor.

There are limited data from animal reproduction studies; in such studies, no teratogenic or other adverse effects were identified; however, drug exposure was well below the predicted exposures in humans.

Lactation

It is not known whether neostigmine is distributed into human milk. Caution should be exercised when the drug is used in nursing women.

Pediatric Use

Neostigmine may be used in pediatric patients of all ages to reverse the effects of nondepolarizing neuromuscular blocking agents after surgery. The available data indicate that efficacy and pharmacokinetics of neostigmine are similar across all pediatric age groups and also similar to those in adults when the same dosing guidelines are applied.

Based on limited data, neostigmine dosing requirements for reversal of neuromuscular blockade may be lower in infants and neonates than in older pediatric patients and adults; however, pediatric patients have a greater risk of incomplete reversal of neuromuscular blockade because of their decreased respiratory reserve. Therefore, the risks of administering higher doses of neostigmine (up to maximum recommended dosage) should not outweigh the risks associated with incomplete reversal in this age group.

Because pediatric patients, particularly neonates and infants, may be more sensitive to changes in heart rate, the effects of anticholinergic agents should be observed prior to administration of neostigmine to lessen the probability of bradycardia and hypotension.

Geriatric Use

Because geriatric patients may have decreased renal function, neostigmine should be used with caution and increased monitoring in this age group. The duration of action of neostigmine is prolonged in geriatric patients; however, such patients also experience slower spontaneous recovery from neuromuscular blocking agents. Geriatric patients should be monitored for longer periods of time to ensure that additional doses of neostigmine are not necessary to adequately reverse neuromuscular blockade. (See Geriatric Patients under Dosage and Administration.)

Hepatic Impairment

The pharmacokinetics of neostigmine methylsulfate in patients with hepatic impairment have not been studied.

Patients with hepatic impairment should be carefully monitored if neuromuscular blocking agents with hepatic elimination or active metabolites are concomitantly administered to patients with hepatic impairment; in such cases, the duration of the neuromuscular blocking agent may be prolonged and persist beyond the effects of neostigmine.

Renal Impairment

Clearance of neostigmine is reduced in patients with renal impairment compared with individuals with normal renal function. In a study in patients with various states of renal function (normal, undergoing renal transplantation, or bilateral nephrectomy), the elimination half-life of neostigmine was prolonged in anephric individuals.

Patients with renal impairment should be carefully monitored if a renally eliminated neuromuscular blocking agent is concomitantly administered; in such cases, the effects of the neuromuscular blocking agent may persist beyond those of neostigmine.

● Common Adverse Effects

The most common adverse effects of neostigmine include bradycardia, nausea, and vomiting. Adverse effects of neostigmine methylsulfate generally are due to exaggerated pharmacologic effects of the drug, particularly at muscarinic-cholinergic receptors.

DRUG INTERACTIONS

Drug interaction studies have not been conducted to date with neostigmine methylsulfate. Clinically important drug interactions are not likely to occur if neuromuscular monitoring is employed and both relaxants and reversal agents are titrated to effect.

● Drugs Affecting Hepatic Microsomal Enzymes

Neostigmine is metabolized by hepatic microsomal enzymes; caution is advised when used concomitantly with drugs that can alter the activity of these enzymes.

● Anticholinergic Agents

Anticholinergic agents such as atropine antagonize the muscarinic effects of neostigmine, and this interaction is utilized to counteract the muscarinic symptoms of neostigmine toxicity.

● Neuromuscular Blocking Agents

Neostigmine does not antagonize, and may in fact prolong, the phase I block of depolarizing muscle relaxants such as succinylcholine. Parenteral neostigmine effectively antagonizes the effect of nondepolarizing muscle relaxants (e.g., atracurium, cisatracurium, pancuronium, rocuronium, vecuronium), and this interaction is used to therapeutic advantage to reverse muscle relaxation after surgery. (See Reversal of Neuromuscular Blockade under Uses.)

DESCRIPTION

Neostigmine is an anticholinesterase agent; the drug inhibits the enzyme acetylcholinesterase, reducing the degradation of acetylcholine. By competing with acetylcholine for binding to acetylcholinesterase, neostigmine slows the rate of hydrolysis of acetylcholine. As a consequence, acetylcholine accumulates in the synaptic cleft, and competes with and reverses the effects of nondepolarizing neuromuscular blocking agents. Neostigmine stimulates both muscarinic and nicotinic receptors, producing generalized cholinergic effects including miosis, increased tonus of intestinal and skeletal musculature, constriction of bronchi and ureters, bradycardia, and stimulation of secretion by salivary and sweat glands. In addition, neostigmine has a direct cholinomimetic effect on skeletal muscle.

Neostigmine does not cross the blood-brain barrier to produce CNS effects. Extremely high doses, however, produce CNS stimulation followed by CNS depression, in addition to a depolarizing neuromuscular blockade, and may result in respiratory depression, paralysis, and death.

Neostigmine is 15–25% bound to serum albumin. Following administration of a single IV dose of neostigmine, the reported elimination half-life of the drug ranged from 24–113 minutes. In a pharmacokinetic study in pediatric patients, the half-life of neostigmine (administered as an IV infusion over 2 minutes) was approximately 39, 48, or 67 minutes in infants 2–10 months of age, children 1–6 years of age, or adults 29–48 years of age, respectively. Neostigmine is metabolized by microsomal enzymes in the liver. Approximately 80% of the drug is excreted in urine within 24 hours (50% as unchanged drug).

ADVICE TO PATIENTS

- Importance of informing clinician of existing or contemplated concomitant therapy, including prescription and OTC drugs and dietary or herbal supplements, as well as any concomitant illnesses.
- Importance of women informing clinicians if they are or plan to become pregnant or plan to breast-feed.
- Importance of informing patients of other important precautionary information. (See Cautions.)

PREPARATIONS

Excipients in commercially available drug preparations may have clinically important effects in some individuals; consult specific product labeling for details.

Neostigmine Methylsulfate

Parenteral		
Injection	0.5 mg/mL*	**Bloxiverz®**, Avadel Legacy
		Neostigmine Methylsulfate Injection
	1 mg/mL*	**Bloxiverz®**, Avadel Legacy
		Neostigmine Methylsulfate Injection

* available from one or more manufacturer, distributor, and/or repackager by generic (nonproprietary) name

† Use is not currently included in the labeling approved by the US Food and Drug Administration.

Atropine
Atropine Sulfate

12:08.08 • ANTIMUSCARINICS/ANTISPASMODICS

■ Atropine (*dl*-hyoscyamine) is a naturally occurring tertiary amine antimuscarinic.

USES

● *Surgery*

Atropine sulfate is used parenterally as a preoperative medication to inhibit salivation and excessive secretions of the respiratory tract (antisialagogue); however, the current surgical practice of using general anesthetics that do not stimulate the production of salivary and tracheobronchial secretions has reduced the need to control excessive respiratory secretions during surgery. Although atropine has been used prophylactically to prevent acid-aspiration pneumonitis during surgery, antimuscarinics, including atropine, have not been shown to be effective for this use.

Atropine also may be used to prevent other cholinergic effects during surgery, such as cardiac arrhythmias, hypotension, and bradycardia, which may result from excessive vagal stimulation, from stimulation of the carotid sinus, or as a pharmacologic effect of some drugs (e.g., succinylcholine). Atropine is administered concurrently with anticholinesterase agents (e.g., neostigmine, pyridostigmine) to block the adverse muscarinic effects of these latter agents when they are used after surgery to reverse the effects of neuromuscular blocking agents.

Atropine has been used prophylactically to prevent reflex bradycardia in pediatric patients undergoing emergency intubation; however, there is no evidence that atropine reduces the risk of cardiac arrest or improves survival in this setting. Because of the lack of supporting evidence, preintubation use of atropine is not routinely recommended, but may be considered in situations where there is an increased risk of bradycardia (e.g., when succinylcholine is used to facilitate intubation).

● *Advanced Cardiovascular Life Support and Bradyarrhythmias*

Atropine sulfate is used in advanced cardiovascular life support (ACLS) for the management of symptomatic bradycardia. The drug reverses cholinergically mediated decreases in heart rate, systemic vascular resistance, and blood pressure, and is considered the initial drug of choice in adults with unstable bradycardia (e.g., that which is accompanied by altered mental status, cardiac ischemia, acute heart failure, hypotension, or other signs of shock). In pediatric advanced life support (PALS), atropine is used for the treatment of bradycardia secondary to increased vagal activity or primary atrioventricular (AV) block when bradycardia persists despite initial management with adequate oxygenation, ventilation, and chest compressions (if indicated).

Atropine was previously included in ACLS guidelines for the treatment of asystole or pulseless electrical activity (PEA) during cardiopulmonary resuscitation (CPR); however, routine use of the drug during cardiac arrest is no longer recommended because of the lack of evidence demonstrating clinical benefit. High-quality CPR and defibrillation are integral components of ACLS and the only proven interventions to increase survival to hospital discharge. Other resuscitative efforts including drug therapy are considered secondary and should be performed without compromising the quality and timely delivery of chest compressions and defibrillation. The principal goal of pharmacologic therapy during cardiac arrest is to facilitate the return of spontaneous circulation (ROSC), and epinephrine is considered the drug of choice for this use. (See Uses: Advanced Cardiovascular Life Support and Cardiac Arrhythmias, in Epinephrine 12:12.12.)

Because atropine can increase conduction through the AV node, the drug also may be beneficial in the management of AV nodal block. However, atropine is not likely to be effective in patients with type II second-degree AV block or third-degree AV block, including third-degree AV block accompanied by a new wide QRS complex when the conduction block is at or below the His-Purkinje level; patients with these bradyarrhythmias are preferably treated with transcutaneous pacing or a rate-accelerating β-adrenergic drug (e.g., dopamine or epinephrine) until transvenous pacing can be performed. Atropine administration should not delay implementation of external pacing for patients with poor perfusion.

Atropine also is used in patients with acute myocardial infarction (MI) who develop symptomatic or hemodynamically unstable sinus bradycardia. Sinus bradycardia caused by increased vagal tone commonly occurs after ST-segment-elevation MI (STEMI), particularly in patients with an inferior infarction. Other uses of atropine in the MI setting include treatment of sustained bradycardia and hypotension associated with nitroglycerin use, and treatment of nausea and vomiting associated with morphine use. Although atropine was previously used for the management of symptomatic type I second- or third-degree AV block associated with MI, the incidence of abnormal conduction in STEMI patients has decreased considerably in the current reperfusion era.

Because heart rate is a major determinant of myocardial oxygen requirements, atropine should be used cautiously in the presence of acute myocardial ischemia or infarction. Excessive rate acceleration in patients with these conditions may worsen ischemia or increase the extent of infarction. In addition, ventricular fibrillation and tachycardia have occurred rarely following IV administration of atropine. Because transplanted hearts lack vagal innervation, atropine may *not* be effective in patients who have undergone cardiac transplantation. Paradoxical slowing of the heart rate and high-degree AV block have been reported in patients who have received atropine after cardiac transplantation.

● *Pesticide Poisoning*

Atropine is used to reverse the muscarinic effects associated with toxic exposure to organophosphate or carbamate anticholinesterase pesticides. For the treatment of toxic exposure to organophosphate pesticides, atropine may be used concomitantly with a cholinesterase reactivator (pralidoxime chloride). Concomitant therapy with pralidoxime chloride may not be necessary in patients with carbamate anticholinesterase pesticide poisoning. Antidotes such as atropine and pralidoxime should not be solely relied upon to provide complete protection against the toxic effects of insecticide poisoning and should be used in conjunction with other protective measures (e.g., decontamination, immediate evacuation, specialized masks and clothing) and treatments (e.g., an anticonvulsant for seizures). Some clinicians have suggested a challenge (test) dose of atropine to aid in the diagnosis of cholinergic poisoning†; failure of the test dose to elicit typical antimuscarinic effects (e.g., mydriasis, tachycardia, dry mucous membranes) strongly suggests the presence of organophosphate or carbamate poisoning.

● *Chemical Warfare Agent Poisoning*

Atropine is used concomitantly with a cholinesterase reactivator (pralidoxime chloride) for the treatment of nerve agent poisoning in the context of chemical warfare or terrorism. The most toxic of the known chemical warfare agents are the nerve agents. Most nerve agents are liquid at room temperature (although most are volatile at ambient temperatures, the term "nerve gas" is a misnomer); nerve agents are readily absorbed after inhalation of aerosols (e.g., following an explosion), ingestion, or dermal contact. Nerve agents (e.g., sarin, soman, tabun, VX [methylphosphonothioic acid]) are chemically similar to the organophosphate pesticides and exert their biologic effects by inhibiting acetylcholinesterase enzymes. Nerve agents alter cholinergic synaptic transmission at neuroeffector junctions (muscarinic effects), at skeletal myoneural junctions and autonomic ganglia (nicotinic effects), and in the CNS. Manifestations of nerve agent exposure include rhinorrhea, chest tightness, pinpoint pupils, dyspnea, excessive salivation and sweating, nausea, vomiting, abdominal cramps, involuntary defecation and/or urination, muscle twitching, confusion, seizures, flaccid paralysis, coma, respiratory failure, and death. While initial effects of nerve agent exposure depend on dose and route of exposure, signs and symptoms generally are similar regardless of the route of exposure. Manifestations may not be apparent until as long as 18 hours following dermal exposure, and CNS effects (e.g., fatigue, irritability, nervousness, memory impairment) may persist as long as 6 weeks following recovery from the acute effects of nerve agent exposure.

Initial management of nerve agent poisoning includes aggressive airway control and ventilation (administration of nebulized β-adrenergic agonist [e.g., albuterol] and antimuscarinics [e.g., ipratropium bromide] may be necessary), and administration of atropine and pralidoxime chloride. Diazepam may be needed for seizure control. Rapid decontamination using standard hazardous materials (HAZMAT) procedures is important to prevent further absorption by the victim and to prevent contamination of others (e.g., emergency personnel, health-care workers) by direct contact or off-gassing of nerve agents from contaminated clothing. Following initial therapy and decontamination, additional treatment with atropine and supportive measures in a hospital setting are likely to be necessary.

● Mushroom Poisoning

Atropine sulfate also is used for the treatment of muscarinic effects associated with toxic ingestion of mushrooms containing muscarine (e.g., certain members of the *Clitocybe* and *Inocybe* genera); however, substantial toxicity is uncommon and supportive symptomatic care (e.g., atropine) rarely is necessary.

● GI Disorders

Atropine sulfate has been used as an adjunct in the treatment of peptic ulcer disease; although synthetic or semisynthetic antimuscarinics, especially quaternary ammonium compounds, have generally replaced atropine in the treatment of peptic ulcer disease, none of these antimuscarinics has been shown to be therapeutically superior to atropine. (See Uses: Peptic Ulcer Disease and GI Hypersecretory States, in the Antimuscarinics/Antispasmodics General Statement 12:08.08) As with other antimuscarinics, there are no conclusive data from well-controlled studies which indicate that, in usually recommended dosage, atropine aids in the healing, decreases the rate of recurrence, or prevents complications of peptic ulcers. In addition, in patients with gastric ulcer, antimuscarinics may delay gastric emptying and result in antral stasis. With the advent of more effective therapies for the treatment of peptic ulcer disease, antimuscarinics have only limited usefulness in this condition. Current epidemiologic and clinical evidence supports a strong association between gastric infection with *Helicobacter pylori* and the pathogenesis of duodenal and gastric ulcers, and the American College of Gastroenterology (ACG), the National Institutes of Health (NIH), and most clinicians currently recommend that all patients with initial or recurrent duodenal or gastric ulcer and documented *H. pylori* infection receive anti-infective therapy for treatment of the infection. For a more complete discussion of *H. pylori* infection, including details about the efficacy of various regimens and rationale for drug selection, see Uses: *Helicobacter pylori* Infection, in Clarithromycin 8:12.12.92.

Atropine has been used in the treatment of functional disturbances of GI motility such as irritable bowel syndrome. As with other antimuscarinics, atropine has limited efficacy in the treatment of these disorders and should be used only if other measures (e.g., diet, sedation, counseling, amelioration of environmental factors) have been of little or no benefit.

Atropine has been used in the treatment of GI hypermotility and diarrhea caused by reserpine, guanethidine, or cholinergic stimulation. Although antimuscarinics have been used in the treatment of diarrhea from other causes (e.g., ulcerative colitis, dysentery, shigellosis, *Clostridium difficile*-associated diarrhea and colitis [also known as antibiotic-associated pseudomembranous colitis]), they should be used with extreme caution, if at all, in patients with these conditions. (See Cautions: Precautions and Contraindications, in the Antimuscarinics/Antispasmodics General Statement 12:08.08.)

● Genitourinary Tract Disorders

Atropine sulfate has been used as adjunctive therapy in the management of hypermotility disorders of the lower urinary tract. Although atropine may provide symptomatic relief, the underlying cause should be determined and specifically treated. Appropriate anti-infective therapy should be initiated whenever urinary tract infection is present. With the exception of uninhibited or reflex neurogenic bladder, there is generally little evidence to support the use of antimuscarinics in the treatment of various genitourinary disorders. (See Uses: Genitourinary Tract Disorders, in the Antimuscarinics/Antispasmodics General Statement 12:08.08.)

● Bronchospasm

Because atropine sulfate is a potent bronchodilator, the drug has been used by oral inhalation for the short-term treatment and prevention of bronchospasm associated with chronic bronchial asthma, bronchitis, and chronic obstructive pulmonary disease; however, a solution of the drug for oral inhalation no longer is commercially available in the US. (See Uses: Bronchospasm, in the Antimuscarinics/Antispasmodics General Statement 12:08.08.) Atropine has also been used as a drying agent in the relief of symptoms of acute rhinitis.

● Other Uses

Atropine sulfate has been used in combination with other drugs (e.g., antihistamines, vasoconstrictors) for the symptomatic relief of cold and cough.

Atropine sulfate has been used to facilitate hypotonic duodenography or contrast examination of the colon by reducing duodenal or colonic motility and spasm; however, glucagon appears to be more effective and is generally preferred in these examinations. Atropine also has been used to increase visualization of the urinary tract in excretion urography.

Atropine sulfate has been used in conjunction with morphine or other opiates for the symptomatic relief of biliary or renal colic; however, since antimuscarinics exert only a weak biliary antispasmodic action, these drugs should not be relied on in the treatment of biliary tract disease. Atropine has also been used to reduce pain and hypersecretion in pancreatitis; however, there is little, if any, evidence that antimuscarinics improve the prognosis of the disease. (See Uses: Other Uses, in the Antimuscarinics/Antispasmodics General Statement 12:08.08.)

For ophthalmic uses of atropine sulfate, see 52:24. For other uses of atropine sulfate, see Uses in the Antimuscarinics/Antispasmodics General Statement 12:08.08.

DOSAGE AND ADMINISTRATION

● Administration

Atropine sulfate is administered by IM, subcutaneous, or direct IV administration. IV administration is preferred for the treatment of severe or life-threatening muscarinic effects.

Atropine also has been administered by intraosseous (IO) injection† in the setting of advanced cardiovascular life support (ACLS), generally when IV access is not readily available; onset of action and systemic concentrations are comparable to those achieved with venous administration.

Atropine may be administered via an endotracheal tube when vascular access (IV or IO) is not possible; however, IV or IO administration is preferred because of more predictable drug delivery and pharmacologic effect. (See Pharmacokinetics: Absorption.)

Atropine sulfate has been administered orally; however, an oral dosage form no longer is commercially available in the US.

Atropine sulfate has been administered by oral inhalation using a nebulizer solution; however, a solution for oral inhalation no longer is commercially available in the US.

Parenteral Administration
IM Administration

Atropine is commercially available in a prefilled auto-injector (e.g., AtroPen®) for IM administration in the treatment of pesticide or nerve agent poisoning. The auto-injector should be used only by individuals who have received proper training in the recognition and treatment of pesticide poisoning. The AtroPen® auto-injector may be self-administered by the patient or caregiver in an out-of-hospital setting to facilitate the initial treatment of muscarinic poisoning (usually breathing difficulty secondary to increased secretions); however, definitive medical care should be sought immediately.

For *self-administration* or administration by a caregiver in an out-of-hospital setting in the event of pesticide or nerve agent poisoning, the appropriate dose of atropine injection (AtroPen®) should be injected IM into the anterolateral aspect of the thigh. For very thin patients and small children, the thigh should be bunched up (to provide a thicker injection area) prior to administration of the drug. For additional instructions on proper use of atropine auto-injectors, the manufacturer's instructions should be consulted.

IV Administration

Although at least one manufacturer recommends that atropine sulfate injection be administered slowly and with caution, the drug generally is given rapidly by direct IV injection since slow injection may cause a paradoxical slowing of the heart rate.

Atropine has occasionally been administered by IV infusion† for the management of muscarinic poisoning (e.g., organophosphate pesticides).

Endotracheal Administration

For endotracheal administration, the appropriate dose of atropine sulfate should be diluted in 5–10 mL of sterile water or 0.9% sodium chloride injection in adults or followed by a flush with 5 mL of 0.9% sodium chloride injection in pediatric patients. Absorption of the drug may be greater when sterile water rather than 0.9% sodium chloride injection is used as the diluent (in adults).

● Dosage

Dosage of atropine sulfate should be individualized based on indication, patient characteristics, and response (e.g., heart rate, blood pressure); pediatric patients tend to be more susceptible than adults to the toxic effects of atropine overdosage.

Parenteral Dosage
Surgery

For antisialagogue or antivagal effects during surgery, the usual initial adult dose of atropine sulfate is 0.5–1 mg by IV, IM, or subcutaneous injection 30–60 minutes prior to surgery; the dose may be repeated in 1–2 hours. Dosing in pediatric patients has not been well studied, but initial doses usually range from 0.01–0.03 mg/kg, administered 30–60 minutes prior to surgery; according to some clinicians, repeat doses may be given every 4–6 hours. Some clinicians recommend a minimum dose of 0.1 mg and maximum dose of 0.4 mg in children; however, doses up to 0.6 mg have been suggested in pediatric patients weighing more than 41 kg.

The American Heart Association (AHA) guidelines for pediatric advanced life support (PALS) recommend a preintubation atropine sulfate dose of 0.02 mg/kg administered IV in infants and children undergoing emergency intubation. Although a minimum dose of 0.1 mg was previously recommended because of concerns about paradoxical bradycardia, current evidence suggests that no minimum dose is necessary.

To block adverse muscarinic effects of anticholinesterase agents (e.g., neostigmine, pyridostigmine) when these agents are used to reverse the effects of neuromuscular blocking agents after surgery, the usual IV dose of atropine sulfate is 0.6–1.2 mg for each 0.5–2.5 mg of neostigmine methylsulfate or 10–20 mg of pyridostigmine bromide administered; atropine is administered concurrently with (but in a separate syringe) or a few minutes before the anticholinesterase agent. In the presence of bradycardia, atropine sulfate should be administered IV before the anticholinesterase agent to increase the pulse rate to about 80 beats/minute. Neonates and infants have been given a 0.02-mg/kg dose of atropine sulfate concomitantly with a 0.04-mg/kg dose of neostigmine methylsulfate. Children have been given a 0.01- to 0.04-mg/kg dose of atropine sulfate concomitantly with each 0.025- to 0.08-mg/kg dose of neostigmine methylsulfate.

Advanced Cardiovascular Life Support and Bradyarrhythmias

For the treatment of symptomatic bradycardia in adults, AHA recommends an initial atropine sulfate dose of 0.5 mg by direct IV injection; the dose may be repeated every 3–5 minutes up to a maximum of 3 mg. Doses less than 0.5 mg may cause paradoxical slowing of the heart rate. In previous ACLS guidelines, an atropine sulfate dosage of 1 mg every 3–5 minutes up to a total of 3 doses by IV or IO injection† was recommended for the treatment of asystole and slow pulseless electrical activity (PEA) in adults; however routine use of atropine during cardiac arrest is no longer recommended. (See Uses: Advanced Cardiovascular Life Support and Bradyarrhythmias.)

In PALS guidelines, an atropine sulfate dose of 0.02 mg/kg by IV or IO injection† (repeated once if needed) is recommended in infants and children with symptomatic bradycardia secondary to increased vagal activity or primary atrioventricular (AV) block; a minimum dose of 0.1 mg and a maximum single dose of 0.5 mg is recommended. Larger doses may be required in special resuscitation situations (e.g., organophosphate toxicity or exposure to nerve gas agents); smaller doses (i.e., less than 0.1 mg) may cause paradoxical bradycardia.

Hypotonic Radiography of the GI Tract

For hypotonic radiography of the GI tract (contrast examination of the duodenum or colon) in adults, the usual IM dose of atropine sulfate is 1 mg.

Pesticide Poisoning

Various atropine sulfate doses and dosing intervals have been recommended for the treatment of muscarinic toxicity resulting from exposure to organophosphate anticholinesterase pesticides; dosage requirements are based on the severity of poisoning and individual patient response.

The usual initial dose of atropine sulfate for the treatment of muscarinic toxicity resulting from exposure to organophosphate anticholinesterase pesticides in adults is 1–2 mg, preferably administered IV. Some clinicians recommend that additional 2-mg doses may be administered IM or IV every 5–60 minutes until muscarinic signs and symptoms subside. In severe cases, 2–6 mg may be given initially, preferably administered IV, and repeated doses given every 5–60 minutes until muscarinic signs and symptoms subside. Mildly symptomatic poisoning may respond to 1–2 mg for reversal of muscarinic toxicity whereas *moderate* poisoning commonly requires total doses up to 40 mg. Some experts state that for *severe* poisoning, 5-mg doses may be repeated every 2–3 minutes for stabilization. Cumulative doses up to 1 g in 24 hours or 11 g over a course of treatment have been used. Atropine sulfate also has been administered by IV infusion† at an initial rate of 0.5–1 mg/hour in adults for muscarinic poisoning; the infusion rate should be adjusted according to response. In severe cases, atropine therapy should be gradually withdrawn to avoid abrupt recurrence of symptoms (e.g., pulmonary edema). Similar doses of atropine sulfate may be used in the treatment of muscarinic toxicity resulting from exposure to carbamate anticholinesterase pesticides.

To facilitate out-of-hospital administration, atropine injection may be administered using the commercially available prefilled auto-injector (e.g., AtroPen®). For *self-administration* or administration by a caregiver, the dose of atropine (AtroPen®) is based on severity of symptoms. Atropine should be administered as soon as symptoms of organophosphate or carbamate poisoning (e.g., tearing, excessive oral secretions, wheezing, muscle fasciculations) appear. For the treatment of adults with 2 or more mild symptoms of pesticide exposure (e.g., miosis or blurred vision, tearing, runny nose, hypersalivation or drooling, wheezing, muscle fasciculations, nausea/vomiting) when such exposure is known or suspected, one 2-mg IM dose of atropine sulfate should be administered. If the patient develops any severe symptoms (behavioral changes, severe breathing difficulty, severe respiratory secretions, severe muscle twitching, involuntary defecation or urination, seizures, unconsciousness), two additional 2-mg IM doses should be administered in rapid succession 10 minutes after the first dose. It is preferable that an individual other than the patient administer the second and third doses. For the treatment of adults who are either unconscious or present with any severe symptoms, three 2-mg doses should be administered IM in rapid succession. Additional treatment (i.e., supportive measures, additional doses of atropine, pralidoxime for organophosphate exposure, an anticonvulsant [e.g., diazepam] for seizures) generally is needed, and such treatment should be carried out under the supervision of trained medical personnel.

In children, the usual IM or IV dose of atropine sulfate for the treatment of muscarinic toxicity resulting from exposure to organophosphate anticholinesterase pesticides is 0.05–0.1 mg/kg every 5–10 minutes until muscarinic signs and symptoms subside. The drug also has been given by IV infusion† at a rate of 0.025 mg/kg per hour; continuous infusions have been maintained for up to several weeks in severe cases. Similar doses of atropine sulfate may be used in the treatment of muscarinic toxicity resulting from exposure to carbamate anticholinesterase pesticides.

To facilitate out-of-hospital administration, atropine injection may be administered using the commercially available prefilled auto-injector (e.g., AtroPen®). The AtroPen® auto-injector containing atropine sulfate 0.25, 0.5, or 1 mg is intended for use in children weighing less than 7, 7–18, or 18–41 kg, respectively. When administered by a caregiver in an out-of-hospital setting, the dose of atropine (AtroPen®) is based on severity of symptoms and body weight. *Mild* symptoms of pesticide exposure include miosis or blurred vision, tearing, runny nose, hypersalivation or drooling, wheezing, muscle fasciculations, and nausea/vomiting. Treatment with atropine is indicated in infants and children with 2 or more mild symptoms of pesticide exposure when such exposure is known or suspected. *Severe* symptoms of pesticide exposure include behavioral changes, severe breathing difficulty, severe respiratory secretions, severe muscle twitching, involuntary defecation or urination, seizures, and unconsciousness. Treatment is indicated in infants and children who are unconscious or have any severe symptoms of pesticide exposure. Atropine should be administered as soon as symptoms of organophosphate or carbamate poisoning (e.g., tearing, excessive oral secretions, wheezing, muscle fasciculations) appear. See Table 1 for specific dosage recommendations. Additional treatment (i.e., supportive measures, additional doses of atropine, pralidoxime for organophosphate exposure, an anticonvulsant [e.g., diazepam] for seizures) generally is needed, and such treatment should be carried out under the supervision of trained medical personnel.

TABLE 1. Pediatric Dosage of Atropine Sulfate Administered by Auto-injector (AtroPen®) for Initial Treatment of Pesticide Poisoning

Child's Weight	Presenting Symptoms	IM Dosage
Less than 7 kg	Mild	0.25 mg initially; if any severe symptoms develop, inject two additional 0.25-mg doses in rapid succession 10 minutes after the first dose
	Severe	Three 0.25-mg doses in rapid succession

TABLE 1. Continued

Child's Weight	Presenting Symptoms	IM Dosage
7–18 kg	Mild	0.5 mg initially; if any severe symptoms develop, inject two additional 0.5-mg doses in rapid succession 10 minutes after the first dose
	Severe	Three 0.5-mg doses in rapid succession
18–41 kg	Mild	1 mg initially; if any severe symptoms develop, inject two additional 1-mg doses in rapid succession 10 minutes after the first dose
	Severe	Three 1-mg doses in rapid succession
Greater than 41 kg	Mild	2 mg initially; if any severe symptoms develop, inject two additional 2-mg doses in rapid succession 10 minutes after the first dose
	Severe	Three 2-mg doses in rapid succession

A cholinesterase reactivator (e.g., pralidoxime) is administered concomitantly with antimuscarinic therapy for the treatment of toxic exposure to organophosphate pesticides. For the treatment of muscarinic toxicity resulting from carbamate exposure, pralidoxime generally is not used unless exposure also included an organophosphate or unless respiratory depression and muscle weakness are severe manifestations of intoxication.

Chemical Warfare Agent Poisoning

Various atropine sulfate doses and dosing intervals have been recommended for the treatment of muscarinic toxicity resulting from exposure to nerve agent poisoning; dosage requirements are based on the severity of poisoning and individual patient response.

The initial dose of atropine for the treatment of nerve agent (e.g., sarin, soman, tabun, VX [methylphosphonothioic acid]) poisoning in the context of chemical warfare or terrorism is based on the severity of symptoms (i.e., mild/moderate or severe) and the victim's age. Mild to moderate symptoms include localized sweating, muscle fasciculations, nausea, vomiting, weakness, dyspnea; severe symptoms include apnea, flaccid paralysis, seizures, and/or coma. When atropine is used for the immediate treatment of nerve agent poisoning in an out-of-hospital setting or in an emergency department, the drug is administered IM. The usual initial adult IM dose of atropine sulfate is 2–4 mg for those with mild to moderate symptoms and 5–6 mg for those with severe symptoms; frail geriatric patients with mild to moderate symptoms may receive atropine sulfate 1 mg and those with severe symptoms may receive atropine sulfate 2–4 mg.

Additional doses of atropine may be administered at 5- to 10-minute intervals until secretions have diminished and breathing is comfortable or airway resistance has returned to near normal. Some patients may require up to 15–20 mg of the drug within the first 3 hours, but most patients respond to less than 20 mg usually during the initial 24 hours. In a report of sarin poisoning, less than 20% of moderately symptomatic patients required more than 2 mg. Pralidoxime chloride is administered concomitantly with atropine. Diazepam may be administered for seizure control.

To facilitate out-of-hospital administration, atropine injection may be administered using the commercially available prefilled auto-injector (e.g., AtroPen®). For *self-administration* or administration by a caregiver in an out-of-hospital setting, the dose of atropine (AtroPen®) is based on severity of symptoms. Atropine should be administered as soon as symptoms of nerve agent poisoning (e.g., tearing, excessive oral secretions, wheezing, muscle fasciculations) appear. For the treatment of adults with 2 or more mild symptoms of exposure (e.g., miosis or blurred vision, tearing, runny nose, hypersalivation or drooling, wheezing, muscle fasciculations,

nausea/vomiting) when such exposure is known or suspected, one 2-mg IM dose of atropine sulfate should be administered. If the patient develops any severe symptoms (behavioral changes, severe breathing difficulty, severe respiratory secretions, severe muscle twitching, involuntary defecation or urination, seizures, unconsciousness), two additional 2-mg IM doses should be administered in rapid succession 10 minutes after the first dose. It is preferable that an individual other than the patient administer the second and third doses. For the treatment of adults who are either unconscious or present with any severe symptoms, three 2-mg doses should be administered IM in rapid succession. Additional treatment (i.e., supportive measures, additional doses of atropine, pralidoxime, an anticonvulsant [e.g., diazepam] for seizures) generally is needed, and such treatment should be carried out under the supervision of trained medical personnel.

The usual initial IM dose of atropine sulfate for the treatment of nerve agent poisoning in children 0–2 years of age, 2–10 years of age, or older than 10 years of age with mild to moderate symptoms is 0.05 mg/kg, 1 mg, or 2 mg, respectively, and the usual initial dose for children 0–2 years of age, 2–10 years of age, or older than 10 years with severe symptoms is 0.1 mg/kg, 2 mg, or 4 mg, respectively. Children 0–2 years of age with mild to moderate or severe symptoms treated in an emergency department may receive atropine sulfate 0.02 mg/kg, administered IV.

To facilitate out-of-hospital administration for infants and children, atropine injection may be administered using the prefilled auto-injector (e.g., AtroPen®). The AtroPen® auto-injector containing atropine sulfate 0.25, 0.5, or 1 mg is intended for use in children weighing less than 7, 7–18, or 18–41 kg, respectively. When administered by a caregiver in an out-of-hospital setting, the dose of atropine (AtroPen®) is based on body weight and severity of symptoms. *Mild* symptoms of nerve agent exposure include miosis or blurred vision, tearing, runny nose, hypersalivation or drooling, wheezing, muscle fasciculations, and nausea/vomiting. Treatment with atropine is indicated in infants and children with 2 or more mild symptoms of nerve agent exposure when such exposure is known or suspected. *Severe* symptoms of nerve agent exposure include behavioral changes, severe breathing difficulty, severe respiratory secretions, severe muscle twitching, involuntary defecation or urination, seizures, and unconsciousness. Treatment is indicated in infants and children who are unconscious or have any severe symptoms of nerve agent exposure. Atropine should be administered as soon as symptoms of nerve agent poisoning (e.g., tearing, excessive oral secretions, wheezing, muscle fasciculations) appear. See Table 2 for specific dosage recommendations. Additional treatment (i.e., supportive measures, additional doses of atropine, pralidoxime, an anticonvulsant [e.g., diazepam] for seizures) generally is needed, and such treatment should be carried out under the supervision of trained medical personnel.

TABLE 2. Pediatric Dosage of Atropine Sulfate Administered by Auto-injector (AtroPen®) for Initial Treatment of Nerve Agent Poisoning

Child's Weight	Presenting Symptoms	IM Dosage
Less than 7 kg	Mild	0.25 mg initially; if any severe symptoms develop, inject two additional 0.25-mg doses in rapid succession 10 minutes after the first dose
	Severe	Three 0.25-mg doses in rapid succession
7–18 kg	Mild	0.5 mg initially; if any severe symptoms develop, inject two additional 0.5-mg doses in rapid succession 10 minutes after the first dose
	Severe	Three 0.5-mg doses in rapid succession
18–41 kg	Mild	1 mg initially; if any severe symptoms develop, inject two additional 1-mg doses in rapid succession 10 minutes after the first dose
	Severe	Three 1-mg doses in rapid succession

TABLE 2. Continued

Child's Weight	Presenting Symptoms	IM Dosage
Greater than 41 kg	Mild	2 mg initially; if any severe symptoms develop, inject two additional 2-mg doses in rapid succession 10 minutes after the first dose
	Severe	Three 2-mg doses in rapid succession

Mushroom Poisoning

If atropine is needed for severe symptoms of mushroom poisoning (i.e., muscarine-containing *Clitocybes* and *Inocybes*) in adults, some experts recommend an IV dose of 1–2 mg (minimum of 0.1 mg), repeated and titrated as needed according to response. If needed for severe symptoms in pediatric patients, an IV dose of 0.02 mg/kg (minimum of 0.1 mg) is recommended, repeated and titrated as needed according to response.

Endotracheal Dosage
Advanced Cardiovascular Life Support and Bradyarrhythmias

When atropine sulfate cannot be administered IV in emergent situations such as during ACLS, the drug may be administered via an endotracheal tube. Although the optimum endotracheal dose of atropine sulfate remains to be established, some experts state that typical doses of drugs administered via this route are 2–2.5 times those administered IV in adults and generally should be diluted in 5–10 mL of 0.9% sodium chloride or sterile water prior to direct injection into the endotracheal tube. One manufacturer recommends an endotracheal atropine sulfate dose of 1–2 mg (diluted in no more than 10 mL of sterile water or 0.9% sodium chloride injection) for the treatment of bradysystolic cardiac arrest in adults.

The optimum dose(s) of atropine sulfate administered via an endotracheal tube in pediatric patients remains to be established; PALS guidelines suggest an endotracheal atropine sulfate dose of 0.04–0.06 mg/kg (repeated once if necessary) for the treatment of pediatric bradycardia, with a minimum dose of 0.1 mg and a maximum single dose of 0.5 mg. Larger doses may be required in special resuscitation situations (e.g., organophosphate toxicity or exposure to nerve gas agents). If cardiopulmonary resuscitation (CPR) is in progress, chest compressions should be interrupted briefly to administer atropine. Following administration, the endotracheal tube should be flushed with 5 mL of 0.9% sodium chloride injection and followed by 5 consecutive positive-pressure ventilations.

Pesticide and Nerve Agent Poisoning

One manufacturer recommends an endotracheal atropine sulfate dose of 1–2 mg (diluted in no more than 10 mL of sterile water or 0.9% sodium chloride injection) in adults.

The recommended endotracheal dose of atropine sulfate for the treatment of insecticide or nerve agent poisoning in pediatric patients is 0.05–0.1 mg/kg given every 5–10 minutes until muscarinic signs and symptoms disappear. The dose should be diluted in 1–2 mL of 0.9% sodium chloride injection for endotracheal administration.

CAUTIONS

For a complete discussion of cautions, precautions, and contraindications associated with atropine, see Cautions in the Antimuscarinics/Antispasmodics General Statement 12:08.08.

PHARMACOLOGY

As the prototype of the antimuscarinics, atropine exhibits the pharmacologic actions associated with this group of drugs. The pharmacologic activity of atropine results almost completely from *l*-hyoscyamine; *d*-hyoscyamine has essentially no antimuscarinic activity. As a racemic mixture, atropine possesses about 50% of the antimuscarinic potency of *l*-hyoscyamine. In terms of central

antimuscarinic activity, *l*-hyoscyamine is 8–50 times as potent as *d*-hyoscyamine. In general, atropine is more potent than scopolamine in its antimuscarinic action on the heart and on bronchial and intestinal smooth muscle, and less potent than scopolamine in its antimuscarinic action on the iris, ciliary body, and certain secretory (salivary, bronchial, sweat) glands. In contrast to scopolamine, atropine stimulates the CNS in usual doses.

For a complete discussion of the pharmacologic effects of atropine, see Pharmacology in the Antimuscarinics/Antispasmodics General Statement 12:08.08.

PHARMACOKINETICS

● Absorption

Atropine is well absorbed from the GI tract. The drug appears to be absorbed principally from the upper small intestine. Atropine is also well absorbed following IM administration, oral inhalation, or endotracheal administration. Following oral administration of a single, radiolabeled, 2-mg dose of atropine in healthy, fasting adults, about 90% of the dose was absorbed. In this study, peak plasma concentrations were reached within 1 hour. Following IM administration, peak plasma concentrations are reached within 30 minutes. Following oral inhalation, atropine appears in serum within 15 minutes and peak concentrations are achieved within 1.5–4 hours. Endotracheal administration of the drug results in lower plasma concentrations than when the drug is given IV.

Atropine-induced inhibition of salivation occurs within 30 minutes or 30 minutes to 1 hour and peaks within 1–1.6 or 2 hours after IM or oral administration, respectively; inhibition of salivation persists for up to 4 hours. Atropine-induced increase in heart rate occurs within 5–40 minutes or 30 minutes to 2 hours and peaks within 20 minutes to 1 hour or 1–2 hours after IM or oral administration, respectively. Following IV administration of the drug, peak increase in heart rate occurs within 2–4 minutes. Low doses of the drug cause a paradoxical decrease in heart rate. The ocular effects of atropine are delayed following systemic administration; in one study, near point of accommodation was increased within 2 or 4 hours after IM administration of a single 3-mg dose or oral administration of a single 4-mg dose, respectively. Bronchodilation (as determined by forced expiratory volume in 1 second [FEV_1]) occurs within 15 minutes and is maximal within 15 minutes to 1.5 hours after oral inhalation of atropine. Based on peak inhibition of salivation in one study, 0.9–1.4 mg of orally administered drug was estimated to be approximately equivalent in effect to 0.6 mg administered IM.

● Distribution

Atropine is well distributed throughout the body. The drug crosses the blood-brain barrier. Following IV administration of a single 0.1 mg/kg dose of radiolabeled atropine in dogs, peak CSF concentrations of the drug were 10.3 ng/mL, about 90% of the peak serum concentration.

Atropine crosses the placental barrier. Following IV administration of a single 12.5 mcg/kg dose of atropine sulfate in pregnant women, mean fetal blood (from the placental side of the cord) concentrations of atropine were 1.2 times those of the mother between 5–15 minutes after administration of the drug. In another study, fetal venous blood (from the cord) concentrations of atropine were 12 and 93% of simultaneous maternal venous concentrations 1 and 5 minutes after administration of the drug, respectively; fetal arterial blood (from the cord) concentrations were approximately 50% of simultaneous fetal venous blood concentrations. Although atropine has been stated to distribute into milk in small quantities, there are minimal data to support this statement.

In one in vitro study, atropine was about 18% bound to serum albumin.

● Elimination

Atropine has a plasma half-life of about 2–3 hours. Following IM administration of atropine in one study, elimination of the drug (determined by urinary excretion of radiolabeled drug) appeared to be biphasic, with a half-life in the initial phase of about 2 hours and a half-life in the terminal phase of 12.5 hours or longer.

Atropine is metabolized in the liver to several metabolites including tropic acid, tropine (or a chromatographically similar compound), and, possibly, esters of tropic acid and glucuronide conjugates. Atropine is excreted mainly in urine. Approximately 77–94% of an IM dose of atropine is excreted in urine within 24 hours. About 30–50% of a dose is excreted in urine unchanged. In one study, about 50% of the dose was excreted in urine unchanged; about 33%

as unknown metabolites, possibly esters of tropic acid; and less than 2% as tropic acid. In another study, tropine or a chromatographically similar compound was the major metabolite in urine. Small amounts of atropine may also be eliminated in expired air as carbon dioxide and in feces.

CHEMISTRY AND STABILITY

● Chemistry

Atropine (*dl*-hyoscyamine) is a naturally occurring tertiary amine antimuscarinic. Atropine is the prototype of the antimuscarinics. The drug may be prepared synthetically but is usually obtained by extraction from various members of the *Solanaceae* genus of plants including *Atropa belladonna* (deadly nightshade), *Datura stramonium* (Jimson weed), or *Duboisia myoporoides*.

Atropine is a racemic mixture of *d*- and *l*-hyoscyamine, a tertiary amine organic ester formed by combining tropine and tropic acid. It is not clear whether atropine occurs naturally as a racemic mixture in plant tissues or is formed during extraction, a process known to cause racemization. Atropine occurs as white crystals, usually needle-like, or a white, crystalline powder; it is optically inactive, but usually contains a slight excess of *l*-hyoscyamine. Atropine has solubilities of approximately 2.17 mg/mL in water and 0.5 g/mL in alcohol at 25°C. The drug has a pK_a of 9.8. Atropine injection is commercially available as a sterile solution of the drug in water for injection and contains a citrate buffer, glycerin, and phenol as a preservative.

Atropine sulfate occurs as colorless crystals or a white, crystalline powder. Atropine sulfate has solubilities of approximately 2 g/mL in water and 0.2 g/mL in alcohol at 25°C. Atropine sulfate injection is commercially available as a sterile solution of the drug in water for injection or 0.9% sodium chloride injection; sulfuric acid may be added to adjust the pH to 3–6.5. The injection may also contain a preservative.

● Stability

Atropine sulfate effloresces on exposure to dry air and is slowly affected by light. Atropine should be stored in tight, light-resistant containers. Atropine sulfate should be stored in tight containers. Atropine injection (AtroPen® Auto-Injector) should be stored at 25°C but may be exposed to temperatures ranging from 15–30°C. Atropine sulfate injections should be stored in single-dose or multiple-dose containers, preferably of USP Type I glass, at a temperature less than 40°C, preferably between 15–30°C; freezing of the injections should be avoided.

When admixed in the same syringe at room temperature, atropine sulfate injection is reported to be physically compatible for at least 15 minutes with the following injections: chlorpromazine hydrochloride, cimetidine hydrochloride, dimenhydrinate, diphenhydramine hydrochloride, droperidol, fentanyl citrate, glycopyrrolate, hydroxyzine hydrochloride, hydroxyzine hydrochloride with meperidine hydrochloride, meperidine hydrochloride, meperidine hydrochloride with promethazine hydrochloride (Mepergan®, no longer commercially available in the US), morphine sulfate, concentrated opium alkaloids hydrochlorides, pentazocine lactate, pentobarbital sodium, prochlorperazine edisylate, promazine hydrochloride, promethazine hydrochloride, propiomazine hydrochloride, or scopolamine hydrobromide. Atropine sulfate injection is also reported to be physically compatible

with butorphanol tartrate injection. Since the compatibility of these and other admixtures with atropine sulfate injection depends on several factors (e.g., concentration of the drugs, resulting pH, temperature), specialized references should be consulted for specific compatibility information.

Atropine sulfate injection is reported to be physically incompatible with norepinephrine bitartrate, metaraminol bitartrate, and sodium bicarbonate injections. A haze or precipitate may form within 15 minutes when atropine sulfate injection is mixed with methohexital sodium solutions.

For further information on the chemistry, pharmacology, pharmacokinetics, uses, cautions, acute toxicity, drug interactions, and dosage and administration of atropine sulfate, see the Antimuscarinics/Antispasmodics General Statement 12:08.08.

PREPARATIONS

Excipients in commercially available drug preparations may have clinically important effects in some individuals; consult specific product labeling for details.

Atropine

Powder

Parenteral

Injection	equivalent to Atropine Sulfate 0.25 mg/0.3 mL	**AtroPen® Auto-Injector** ("yellow label"), Meridian
	equivalent to Atropine Sulfate 0.5 mg/0.7 mL	**AtroPen®Auto-Injector** ("blue label"), Meridian
	equivalent to Atropine Sulfate 1 mg/0.7 mL	**AtroPen®Auto-Injector** ("dark red label"), Meridian
	equivalent to Atropine Sulfate 2 mg/0.7 mL	**AtroPen®Auto-Injector** ("green label"), Meridian

Atropine Sulfate

Powder

Parenteral

Injection	0.05 mg/mL*	**Atropine Sulfate Injection**
	0.1 mg/mL*	**Atropine Sulfate Injection**
	0.4 mg/mL*	**Atropine Sulfate Injection**
	1 mg/mL*	**Atropine Sulfate Injection**

* available from one or more manufacturer, distributor, and/or repackager by generic (nonproprietary) name

† Use is not currently included in the labeling approved by the US Food and Drug Administration.

Ipratropium Bromide

12:08.08 • ANTIMUSCARINICS/ANTISPASMODICS

■ Ipratropium bromide is a synthetic quaternary ammonium antimuscarinic.

USES

● Bronchospasm

Ipratropium bromide is used for the symptomatic treatment of reversible bronchospasm that may occur in association with chronic obstructive pulmonary disease (COPD), including chronic bronchitis and emphysema. Ipratropium bromide in fixed combination with albuterol sulfate is used by oral inhalation for the symptomatic management of bronchospasm associated with COPD in patients who continue to have evidence of bronchospasm despite the regular use of an orally inhaled bronchodilator and who require a second bronchodilator. Ipratropium bromide also is used for the symptomatic treatment of bronchial asthma† and for the prevention of exercise-induced bronchospasm†, and also has been used as a bronchodilator in patients with cystic fibrosis†.

Chronic Obstructive Pulmonary Disease

Ipratropium bromide is used as a bronchodilator for the long-term symptomatic treatment of reversible bronchospasm associated with COPD, including chronic bronchitis and emphysema. Orally inhaled ipratropium is not indicated as a single agent for the initial treatment of acute episodes of bronchospasm or acute exacerbations of COPD; a drug with a more rapid onset of action (e.g., a β_2-adrenergic agonist) may be preferred in such cases. (See Cautions: Precautions and Contraindications.) However, some clinicians consider combined therapy with a β_2-agonist bronchodilator and ipratropium to be useful in selected patients with acute exacerbations of COPD.

The efficacy of ipratropium has been similar to or greater than that of β_2-adrenergic agonists (e.g., albuterol, metaproterenol) in comparative studies in which these drugs were administered via metered-dose inhaler or nebulization. As orally inhaled ipratropium produces fewer adverse effects than these drugs, ipratropium is a first-line maintenance bronchodilator for relief of chronic (e.g., daily) symptoms of bronchospasm in patients with mild COPD. However, in a few long-term studies comparing ipratropium bromide and tiotropium bromide, another long-acting orally inhaled anticholinergic agent, ipratropium bromide (36 mcg 4 times daily) oral inhalation aerosol with chlorofluorocarbon (CFC) propellants (preparation with CFC propellants no longer commercially available in the US) was less effective than tiotropium (18 mcg once daily) in improving lung function (e.g., as determined by changes in forced expiratory volume in 1 second [FEV_1] and peak expiratory flow rate [PEFR]) in patients with COPD. (See Chronic Obstructive Pulmonary Disease under Uses: Bronchospasm, in Tiotropium Bromide 12:08.08.) Short-term (e.g., 3-month) controlled studies indicate that the fixed combination of albuterol and ipratropium results in greater bronchodilation following oral inhalation than either agent given alone in patients with COPD.

The efficacy and safety of ipratropium bromide with a hydrofluoroalkane propellant (Atrovent® HFA) have been shown to be comparable to that of ipratropium bromide with chlorofluorocarbon propellants (Atrovent®, no longer commercially available in the US) in patients with COPD. In 2 randomized, comparative clinical trials in patients with COPD, therapy with ipratropium bromide inhalation aerosol with a hydrofluoroalkane (HFA) propellant (Atrovent® HFA 34 or 68 mcg [dose delivered from the mouthpiece] 4 times daily) produced similar improvements in FEV_1 and forced vital capacity (FVC) over the 12-week study period and had similar adverse effects as therapy with ipratropium bromide with chlorofluorocarbon propellants (Atrovent® 36 mcg [dose delivered from the mouthpiece] 4 times daily). In one of these studies, the mean peak improvement in FEV_1 relative to baseline on day 85 of therapy (one of the primary end points) was 0.295 L after a single dose of Atrovent® HFA (34 mcg or 2 inhalations) compared with 0.14 L observed with placebo (HFA propellant vehicle only).

Administration of nebulized ipratropium generally is reserved for patients with severe disease who do not respond adequately to conventional therapy and for those who find it difficult or are unable to optimally inhale the drug orally via a metered-dose inhaler.

In the stepped-care approach to COPD drug therapy, mild intermittent symptoms and minimal lung impairment (e.g., FEV_1 at least 80% of predicted) can be treated with a short-acting selective inhaled β_2-agonist as needed during acute exacerbations, but use should not exceed 8–12 inhalations daily. Alternatively, some clinicians initiate therapy with ipratropium inhalation aerosol. Patients with COPD who receive orally inhaled ipratropium generally have an increase in FEV_1 (at its peak) of 0.15–0.36 L and a decrease in functional residual capacity of 0.3–0.6 L. Although ipratropium produces objective bronchodilation (i.e., increase in FEV_1 and FVC) in patients with COPD, a beneficial effect on subjective symptom or quality-of-life scores has not been demonstrated in short-term (e.g., 3-month) clinical studies, and current evidence indicates that ipratropium therapy does not alter the disease process (neither accelerates nor slows the age-related decline in FEV_1 associated with COPD).

Low- to high-dose ipratropium bromide (6–16 inhalations daily) can be added to therapy with a selective β_2-agonist in patients with mild to moderate symptoms of COPD, with the frequency of inhalation dosing with either agent not to exceed 4 times daily; the highest dosage of ipratropium bromide included in some guidelines for COPD exceeds the manufacturer's recommended maximum daily dosage (12 inhalations). Therapy with anticholinergic and/or β_2-adrenergic agonist bronchodilators increases airflow and exercise tolerance and reduces dyspnea in patients with symptoms of COPD, and these drugs are used in the long-term management of airflow limitation in such patients. The mean peak FEV_1 increase was 0.37 L following short-term (approximately 3 months) administration of the fixed combination of albuterol sulfate (180 mcg as albuterol base) and ipratropium bromide monohydrate (36 mcg) 4 times daily. The fixed combination of ipratropium and albuterol did not affect morning PEFR after short-term administration (i.e., less than 3 months) in these patients.

Current evidence indicates that concomitant or sequential administration of inhaled ipratropium and an inhaled β_2-adrenergic agonist in patients with COPD generally produces additional bronchodilation compared with that achieved with either agent alone. Although the improvement in bronchodilation produced by combined therapy with ipratropium and a β_2-adrenergic agonist often may not exceed that which could be achieved with larger dosages of either agent alone, the duration of bronchodilation appears to be increased with such concomitant therapy, and the potential for adverse effects also may be minimized. The sequence of administration of ipratropium and a short-acting β_2-agonist generally does not alter the effectiveness of the bronchodilating action.

Home management of COPD exacerbations involves increasing the dose and/or frequency of existing short-acting bronchodilator therapy, preferably with a β_2-adrenergic agonist. If response to a short-acting β_2-adrenergic agonist alone is inadequate, some clinicians recommend the addition of ipratropium. In a severe exacerbation treated at home, administration of these agents by nebulization or metered-dose inhalation with a spacer device may be used as needed for short-term therapy.

Following initiation of oxygen therapy in hospitalized patients with COPD, therapy with a short-acting β_2-adrenergic agonist and/or ipratropium (administered separately or in fixed combination) should be used for acute exacerbations of COPD, although the effectiveness of such combination therapy remains controversial.

Asthma

Orally inhaled ipratropium bromide has been used effectively for the symptomatic treatment of acute or chronic bronchial asthma† and can potentiate the bronchodilatory effects of β_2-adrenergic agonists, but the precise role of the drug in the management of this condition remains to be more fully elucidated. Ipratropium is suggested by some experts as an alternative to short-acting inhaled β_2-agonists for relief of asthma symptoms, particularly in patients who experience adverse effects with β_2-adrenergic agonists. However, the efficacy of ipratropium in the long-term management of asthma has not been established. Because the onset of action of ipratropium is slower than that of β_2-adrenergic agonist bronchodilators and the peak bronchodilator effects generally are less pronounced, β_2-adrenergic agonist bronchodilators generally are preferred initially for the symptomatic relief of bronchospasm in patients with asthma. Current guidelines for the management of asthma and many clinicians recommend concomitant anti-inflammatory therapy with orally inhaled corticosteroids as first-line therapy for long-term management of asthma in adults and children whose symptoms are not controlled by intermittent use of a short-acting β_2-adrenergic agonist alone. For additional information on the stepped-care approach for drug therapy in asthma, see Asthma under Uses: Bronchospasm, in Albuterol 12:12.08.12.

Orally inhaled, selective short-acting β_2-adrenergic agonists currently are recommended by an expert panel of the National Asthma Education and Prevention Program (NAEPP) for prehospital management of asthma exacerbations (e.g., in emergency medicine facilities and/or ambulances). During prolonged emergency transport, NAEPP recommends that other asthma therapies such as ipratropium bromide and oral corticosteroids also be available for use. In patients with acute exacerbations of asthma†, ipratropium generally has been reserved for use as an adjunct to other therapy, usually in combination with a β_2-adrenergic agonist bronchodilator. Because of its delayed onset, ipratropium generally should not be used *alone* for the management of *acute* bronchospasm, particularly if a prompt response is required. Some clinicians suggest that *adjunctive* therapy with ipratropium be considered in the emergency department in patients with moderate or severe exacerbations (peak expiratory flow [PEF] 60–80% or less than 60%, respectively, of predicted or personal best) of asthma who fail to respond adequately to β_2-adrenergic agonists and corticosteroids. NAEPP recommends adjunctive therapy with ipratropium (via nebulization or a metered-dose inhaler) and oral corticosteroids in patients with severe asthma exacerbations (FEV_1 or PEF less than 40% of predicted or personal best) who fail to respond adequately to short-acting, inhaled β_2-agonists. In patients with impending respiratory failure in the emergency department, ipratropium in combination with a short-acting β_2-adrenergic agonist (via nebulization) and an IV corticosteroid is recommended. In certain children with acute exacerbations of asthma, some evidence suggests that orally inhaled ipratropium (via nebulization) in conjunction with an orally inhaled β_2-adrenergic agonist (via nebulization) may be more effective than therapy with the β_2-agonist alone; in one study in children with severe acute asthma, children with the most severe bronchospasm (defined as baseline FEV_1 not exceeding 30% of predicted) who received via nebulization repeated doses of ipratropium in conjunction with albuterol were less likely to require hospitalization or additional bronchodilator therapy than children receiving albuterol alone. However, ipratropium does not appear to confer additional benefit in children once they have been hospitalized and treated with an intensive regimen including a nebulized β_2-agonist and systemic corticosteroids. Based on such data in children, NAEPP recommends discontinuance of ipratropium upon hospitalization for severe asthma exacerbations for patients of all age groups.

The benefit of maintenance therapy with ipratropium in patients with chronic asthma† remains to be elucidated, but the drug may be useful as alternative therapy in adults experiencing adverse effects (e.g., tachycardia, arrhythmia, tremor) with a β_2-adrenergic agonist. Some experts currently consider orally inhaled anticholinergics to have a limited role or no role in the long-term management of asthma in children because of a lack of data on safety and efficacy.

Orally inhaled ipratropium may be particularly useful for preventing or reversing bronchospasm induced by β_2-adrenergic blocking agents† (e.g., propranolol) in asthmatic patients; β_2-adrenergic bronchodilators generally are ineffective for this indication in such patients.

Prevention of Exercise-Induced Bronchospasm

Although orally inhaled ipratropium bromide has been effective in the prevention of exercise-induced asthma† in a limited number of patients, orally inhaled β_2-adrenergic agonists are considered first-line agents in the management of this condition.

Cystic Fibrosis

Orally inhaled ipratropium bromide has produced bronchodilation (i.e., increase in FEV_1) in a limited number of patients with cystic fibrosis†, but additional studies are needed to determine the clinical usefulness of such therapy in these patients.

● Other Uses

Ipratropium also has been used in a limited number of patients to minimize increases in lung resistance following anesthetic induction and tracheal intubation†; to protect against bronchoconstriction in patients undergoing fiberoptic bronchoscopy†; and to improve pulmonary function in ventilator-dependent patients, including preterm infants†. In a few patients with COPD and myasthenia gravis, ipratropium has been used to counteract the bronchoconstriction and the increase in respiratory secretions associated with cholinesterase inhibitor (e.g., pyridostigmine) therapy† in these patients.

Ipratropium bromide is used as a 0.03% nasal spray for the symptomatic relief of rhinorrhea associated with allergic and nonallergic perennial rhinitis in adults and children 6 years of age or older. The drug also is used as a 0.06% nasal spray for the symptomatic relief of rhinorrhea associated with the common cold in adults and children 5 years of age or older.

DOSAGE AND ADMINISTRATION

● Administration

Ipratropium bromide is administered by oral inhalation using an oral aerosol inhaler or via nebulization. Ipratropium bromide is administered in fixed combination with albuterol sulfate via a metered-dose aerosol inhaler or via nebulization. Patients should be advised that ipratropium must be used consistently throughout the course of therapy for maximum benefit. In addition, patients should be advised that the drug will *not* provide immediate symptomatic relief and should *not* be used for the relief of acute bronchospasm.

Oral Inhalation via Metered-Dose Aerosol
Ipratropium Bromide

Patients should be instructed carefully in the use of the ipratropium bromide metered-dose inhaler. To obtain optimum results, patients also should be given a copy of the patient instructions provided by the manufacturer. The aerosol inhaler should be actuated twice prior to the initial use or if it has not been used for more than 3 days. To avoid inadvertent contact of the drug with the eyes and subsequent adverse effects, patients should be advised to close their eyes during inhalation of ipratropium aerosol; it also has been suggested that ipratropium aerosol not be administered using the open-mouth technique in patients at high risk for ocular toxicity. (See Cautions: Precautions and Contraindications and also see Cautions: Ocular Effects.)

After the patient exhales slowly and completely, the inhaler should be held upright and the mouthpiece of the inhaler placed well into the mouth with the lips closed firmly around it. The patient should then inhale slowly and deeply through the mouth while actuating the inhaler. After holding the breath for 10 seconds, the patient should remove the mouthpiece and exhale slowly. If additional inhalations are required, the patient should wait at least 15 seconds and repeat the procedure. The manufacturer recommends that the ipratropium oral inhaler be cleaned at least once a week by removing the canister and dust cap from the mouthpiece and rinsing the mouthpiece in warm water for at least 30 seconds; nothing other than water should be used to wash the mouthpiece. The mouthpiece should be dried by shaking off the excess water and allowing the mouthpiece to air dry. When the mouthpiece is dry, the mouthpiece and the canister should be reassembled; patients should make sure that the canister is fully inserted into the mouthpiece.

Ipratropium Bromide and Albuterol Sulfate

Patients should insert the metal canister into the clear end of the mouthpiece. The aerosol inhaler should be shaken well for at least 10 seconds immediately prior to use and should be actuated 3 times prior to the initial use or if it has not been used for more than 24 hours. The mouthpiece provided for the inhalation aerosol of ipratropium bromide and albuterol sulfate should not be used for other aerosol drugs. Prior to use, the orange dust cap should be removed and the mouthpiece should be checked for foreign objects. Patients should avoid spraying ipratropium bromide and albuterol sulfate inhalation aerosol into their eyes. To avoid inadvertent contact of the drug with the eyes and subsequent adverse effects (e.g., temporary blurred vision, precipitation or worsening of narrow-angle glaucoma, ocular pain), patients should be advised to close their eyes during inhalation of ipratropium bromide and albuterol sulfate aerosol. (See Cautions: Precautions and Contraindications and also see Cautions: Ocular Effects.)

The patient should exhale deeply within 30 seconds of shaking the aerosol inhaler and the mouthpiece of the inhaler should be placed into the mouth with the canister held upright. The patient should then inhale slowly and deeply through the mouth while actuating the inhaler. After holding the breath for 10 seconds, the patient should remove the mouthpiece and exhale slowly. If additional inhalations are required, the patient should wait approximately 2 minutes and repeat the procedure. The manufacturer recommends that the ipratropium bromide and albuterol sulfate oral inhaler mouthpiece be cleaned as needed by rinsing the mouthpiece in hot water. If soap is used, the mouthpiece should be rinsed thoroughly with plain water. When dry, the cap on the mouthpiece should be replaced when the inhaler is not in use.

Oral Inhalation via Nebulization
Ipratropium Bromide

Prior to administration of ipratropium bromide inhalation solution for nebulization, the nebulizer manufacturer's information should be reviewed to ensure thorough familiarity with the use and maintenance of the nebulizer. For administration of ipratropium bromide alone via a nebulizer, the entire contents of the single-use vial of solution should be emptied into the nebulizer reservoir and the reservoir attached to the mouthpiece or face mask and to the compressor according to the manufacturer's instructions. When a face mask is used to deliver the drug during nebulization, care should be taken to avoid leakage around the mask because transient blurred vision and other adverse effects may result if the drug enters the eyes. (See Cautions: Ocular Effects.) To avoid inadvertent entry of drug into the eye, it may be preferable to administer nebulized ipratropium bromide using a mouthpiece rather than a face mask.

The patient should place the mouthpiece of the nebulizer between the teeth and on top of the tongue and close the lips firmly around it, taking care not to block the airflow from the mouthpiece with the tongue. The patient should then breathe through the mouthpiece as calmly, deeply, and evenly as possible until the nebulizer stops producing mist. The duration of treatment for oral inhalation of a full dose of ipratropium usually is about 5–15 minutes. The nebulizer should be cleaned after use according to the manufacturer's instructions.

Ipratropium bromide inhalation solution contains no preservatives; the manufacturer states that once the single-use vial is opened, the entire contents must be used or the remainder discarded. When ipratropium bromide is mixed extemporaneously in a nebulizer with albuterol sulfate, metaproterenol sulfate, or cromolyn sodium solution for oral inhalation, the resulting solutions are stable for 1 hour; the manufacturer states that the drug stability and safety of ipratropium bromide inhalation solution mixed with other drugs in a nebulizer have not been established.

Ipratropium Bromide and Albuterol Sulfate

Prior to administration of ipratropium bromide and albuterol sulfate inhalation solution for nebulization, the nebulizer manufacturer's information should be reviewed to assess any changes in administration. For administration of ipratropium bromide in fixed combination with albuterol sulfate (DuoNeb®) via a nebulizer, the entire contents of the single-use vial of solution should be emptied into the nebulizer reservoir and the reservoir attached to the mouthpiece or face mask and to the compressor according to the manufacturer's instructions.

The patient should place the mouthpiece of the nebulizer into the mouth. Alternatively, patients may put the face mask over the mouth and nose. The patient should then breathe through the mouth as calmly, deeply, and evenly as possible until the nebulizer stops producing mist. The duration of treatment for oral inhalation of a full dose of ipratropium and albuterol sulfate in fixed combination usually is about 5–15 minutes. The nebulizer should be cleaned after use according to the manufacturer's instructions.

● Dosage

Oral Inhalation via Metered-Dose Aerosol

Dosage of ipratropium bromide oral inhalation aerosol (Atrovent® HFA) is expressed in terms of the monohydrate. Dosage of ipratropium bromide in fixed combination with albuterol sulfate is expressed in terms of the monohydrate and dosage of albuterol sulfate is expressed in terms of albuterol.

While some published studies and manufacturers have reported a dose of 20–21 mcg of ipratropium bromide per metered spray, this is the amount released from the valve stem during actuation of the inhaler; the dose of ipratropium bromide alone or in fixed combination with albuterol sulfate delivered to the patient through the mouthpiece (actuator) is approximately 17 or 18 mcg, respectively, per metered spray. The commercially available aerosols deliver 200 metered sprays per canister. The actual amount of drug delivered to the lung via a metered-dose aerosol inhaler may depend on patient factors, such as coordination between actuation of the device and inspiration through the delivery system. The inhaler should be discarded after 200 sprays have been used.

COPD

For the management of bronchospasm associated with COPD, the usual initial dosage of ipratropium bromide administered via a metered-dose aerosol (Atrovent® HFA) in adults is 34 mcg (2 inhalations) 4 times daily. If necessary, additional inhalations of ipratropium bromide may be used. The manufacturer of Atrovent® HFA states that the dosage of ipratropium bromide should not exceed 204 mcg (12 inhalations) in 24 hours, although some clinicians suggest that even higher dosages of ipratropium bromide (up to 6 inhalations 4 times daily) may be used without notable adverse effects. The manufacturer recommends that 15 seconds elapse between successive inhalations of ipratropium.

The usual initial dosage of ipratropium bromide administered in fixed combination with albuterol sulfate (90 mcg of albuterol base per inhalation) via a metered-dose aerosol (Combivent®) in adults is 36 mcg (2 inhalations) 4 times daily. If necessary, additional inhalations of ipratropium bromide combined with albuterol sulfate may be used. The manufacturer recommends that approximately 2 minutes elapse between successive inhalations of ipratropium in fixed combination with albuterol. Since fatalities have been reported in association with excessive use of inhaled β_2-adrenergic agents in patients with asthma, the manufacturer of the fixed combination of ipratropium bromide and albuterol sulfate recommends *not* exceeding 12 inhalations (216 mcg of ipratropium bromide) in 24 hours. (See Cautions: Precautions and Contraindications, in Albuterol Sulfate 12:12.08.12.)

When COPD symptoms are not controlled with ipratropium alone or in fixed combination with albuterol (e.g., if there is a need to increase the dose or frequency of administration of the drug), medical assistance should be sought immediately. The dose or frequency of administration of ipratropium alone or in fixed combination with albuterol should not be increased without consultation with a clinician.

Asthma

For initial management of severe asthma exacerbations† (forced expiratory volume in 1 second [FEV₁] or peak expiratory flow [PEF] of less than 40% of predicted or personal best) in the emergency department in adolescents 12 years of age or older† and adults receiving ipratropium bromide as the metered-dose aerosol (Atrovent® HFA), an expert panel of the National Asthma Education and Prevention Program (NAEPP) recommends a dose of 136 mcg (8 inhalations, 17 mcg per inhalation) every 20 minutes as needed for up to 3 hours, given in conjunction with a short-acting inhaled β_2-adrenergic agonist (administered separately). In children younger than 12 years of age† with severe asthma exacerbations†, NAEPP recommends an ipratropium bromide dose of 68–136 mcg (4–8 inhalations, 17 mcg per inhalation) as the metered-dose aerosol every 20 minutes as needed for up to 3 hours, given in conjunction with a short-acting inhaled β_2-adrenergic agonist (administered separately).

For initial management of severe asthma exacerbations† (FEV₁ or PEF of less than 40% of predicted or personal best) in the emergency department in adolescents 12 years of age or older† and adults receiving the fixed combination of ipratropium bromide and albuterol sulfate (90 mcg of albuterol base per inhalation) as the metered-dose aerosol, NAEPP recommends an ipratropium bromide dose of 144 mcg (8 inhalations, 18 mcg per inhalation) every 20 minutes as needed for up to 3 hours. For initial management of severe asthma exacerbations† in children younger than 12 years of age†, NAEPP recommends an ipratropium bromide dose of 72–144 mcg (4–8 inhalations, 18 mcg per inhalation) every 20 minutes as needed for up to 3 hours.

Oral Inhalation via Nebulization

Dosage of ipratropium bromide inhalation solution for nebulization is expressed in terms of anhydrous drug. Dosage of ipratropium bromide in fixed combination with albuterol sulfate (as albuterol base) for nebulization is expressed as the monohydrate. Using in vitro testing at an average flow rate of 3.6 L per minute for an average of 15 minutes or less, the Pari-LC Plus® nebulizer delivered at the mouthpiece approximately 46 or 42% of the original dosage of albuterol or ipratropium bromide, respectively.

COPD

For administration via a nebulizer, the usual dosage of ipratropium bromide in adults with COPD is 500 mcg 3 or 4 times daily (i.e., every 6–8 hours). To administer 500 mcg of the drug, the contents of a single-use vial (2.5 mL) of the commercially available 0.02% solution of ipratropium bromide may be used.

The usual dosage of ipratropium bromide in fixed combination with albuterol sulfate (as 2.5 mg of albuterol base) for nebulization (DuoNeb®) in adults with COPD is 500 mcg 4 times daily, with up to 2 additional inhalations allowed daily. The flow rate of the nebulizer should be adjusted so that the dose is delivered over a period of approximately 5–15 minutes. The manufacturer of DuoNeb® recommends *not* exceeding 6 inhalations daily since such dosages have not been studied for the treatment of COPD.

Asthma

For initial management of severe asthma exacerbations† in the emergency department, an expert panel of the NAEPP recommends an ipratropium bromide dosage of 500 mcg via nebulization every 20 minutes for 3 doses initially (i.e., for the first hour) in adults and adolescents 12 years of age or older† in conjunction with a short-acting inhaled β_2-adrenergic agonist. For initial management of severe asthma exacerbations† in children younger than 12 years of age†, 250–500 mcg of ipratropium bromide may be given via nebulization every 20 minutes for 3 doses initially (i.e., for the first hour), in conjunction with a short-acting inhaled β₂-adrenergic agonist. Alternatively, ipratropium bromide via nebulization may be used continuously for the first hour after admittance to the emergency department in patients with severe asthma exacerbations. If there is no improvement after the first hour of treatment, ipratropium bromide in conjunction with a short-acting inhaled β₂-adrenergic agonist may be continued for no more than 2 additional hours for a total duration of 3 hours in the emergency department, with the frequency of administration after the first hour based on improvement in airflow obstruction and other symptoms and occurrence of adverse effects. Similarly, if a severe exacerbation develops after the first hour of treatment with a short-acting β₂-adrenergic agonist and an oral corticosteroid, ipratropium bromide in conjunction with a short-acting inhaled β₂-adrenergic agonist may be initiated and continued for no more than 2 additional hours. If the patient is admitted to the hospital, ipratropium bromide should be discontinued since benefit of the drug in conjunction with short-acting inhaled β₂-adrenergic agonist therapy (e.g., albuterol) has not been established once patients with severe asthma exacerbations are hospitalized.

CAUTIONS

Adverse effects reported with orally inhaled ipratropium bromide are similar to those reported with other antimuscarinic drugs; however, because of the drug's limited systemic absorption, oral inhalation of ipratropium bromide produces anticholinergic adverse effects (e.g., increased intraocular pressure, mydriasis, urinary retention) less frequently than systemically administered antimuscarinic drugs. For further information on adverse effects reported with antimuscarinics, see Cautions in the Antimuscarinics/Antispasmodics General Statement 12:08.08. In comparative clinical trials, adverse effects reported with ipratropium inhalation aerosol employing a hydrofluoroalkane (HFA) propellant (ipratropium HFA) were similar to those reported with the drug in a preparation containing chlorofluorocarbon (CFC) propellants (ipratropium CFC aerosol; no longer commercially available in the US).

Unless otherwise stated, adverse effects mentioned in the Cautions section are those reported in patients receiving orally inhaled (via metered-dose inhaler or nebulizer) ipratropium and may or may not be directly attributable to the drug.

Orally inhaled ipratropium therapy generally is well tolerated and has a low incidence of adverse effects. No additive effect on the incidence of adverse effects was observed after short-term oral inhalation therapy with the fixed combination of albuterol and ipratropium as an aerosol. In a large, uncontrolled study in seriously ill patients receiving ipratropium inhalation aerosol, about 7% of patients required discontinuance of the drug because of adverse effects. In controlled clinical studies with nebulized ipratropium, adverse effects resulting in discontinuance of the drug most frequently included respiratory effects such as bronchitis, dyspnea, and bronchospasm. In controlled clinical studies with orally inhaled ipratropium HFA via a metered-dose inhaler, the most frequent drug-related adverse effects included dry mouth and taste perversion.

● Respiratory Effects

Bronchitis or upper respiratory tract infection was reported in 14.6 or 13.2% of patients, respectively, receiving nebulized ipratropium in controlled studies, although these effects may not necessarily be attributable to the drug. Bronchitis or upper respiratory tract infection was reported in 12.3 or 10.9%, respectively, of patients receiving the fixed combination of albuterol and ipratropium inhalation aerosol. Bronchitis was reported in 10–23%, and upper respiratory tract infection in 9–34% of patients receiving ipratropium HFA inhalation aerosol in controlled clinical trials. Cough following inhalation of ipratropium CFC inhalation aerosol (no longer commercially available in the US) has been reported in about 4.6–5.9% of patients with chronic obstructive pulmonary disease (COPD) in controlled clinical studies, and in 4.2% of patients receiving the fixed combination of albuterol and ipratropium inhalation aerosol. Coughing or exacerbation of COPD symptoms has been reported in 3–5 or 8–23%, respectively, of patients receiving ipratropium HFA inhalation aerosol in controlled clinical trials. Exacerbation of respiratory symptoms occurred in about 2.4% of patients receiving ipratropium CFC aerosol (no longer commercially available in the US) in controlled studies and reportedly is more common in patients receiving nebulized dosages of 2 mg or more daily. Dyspnea, pharyngitis, or increase in sputum was reported

in 9.6, 3.7, or 1.4% of patients, respectively, receiving nebulized ipratropium in controlled studies, while bronchospasm, sinusitis, or rhinitis each was reported in 2.3% of such patients. Dyspnea, pharyngitis, sinusitis, bronchospasm, or rhinitis was reported in 4.5, 2.2, 2.3, 0.3, or 1.1%, respectively, of patients receiving the fixed combination of ipratropium and albuterol inhalation aerosol in controlled studies. Dyspnea, rhinitis, or sinusitis has been reported in 7–8, 4–6, or 1–11%, respectively, of patients receiving ipratropium bromide HFA inhalation aerosol in clinical trials. Influenza was reported in 1.4% of patients receiving combined ipratropium and albuterol inhalation aerosol in controlled studies. Influenza-like symptoms occurred in 4–8% of patients receiving ipratropium HFA inhalation aerosol in clinical trials. Irritation from the aerosol occurred in about 2% of patients receiving ipratropium aerosol in controlled studies; drying of secretions or hoarseness was reported in 1% or less of patients receiving the aerosol. As with other inhaled drugs for asthma, paradoxical bronchospasm has been reported in a few patients receiving ipratropium nebulized solution, inhalation aerosol, or the fixed combination (with albuterol) inhalation aerosol, although a causal relationship to the drug has not been definitely established. (See Cautions: Dermatologic and Sensitivity Reactions.) Lower respiratory tract disorders or pneumonia was reported in 2.5 or 1.4% of patients, respectively, receiving orally inhaled albuterol and ipratropium in fixed combination. Nasal congestion or wheezing also has been reported in patients receiving the fixed combination of albuterol and ipratropium inhalation aerosol.

Unlike β₂-adrenergic agonists, inhalation of ipratropium does not aggravate hypoxemia in patients with airway obstruction.

● GI Effects

Dryness of the mouth, throat, or tongue occurred in up to 5% of patients receiving orally inhaled ipratropium CFC inhalation aerosol (no longer commercially available in the US) or ipratropium via nebulization; dry mouth reportedly occurs more frequently with nebulized dosages of 2 mg or more daily. Nausea, GI distress, or constipation has been reported in about 4.1, 2.4, or 0.9% of patients receiving the drug. Nausea has been reported in 2% of patients receiving the fixed combination of albuterol and ipratropium inhalation aerosol. Paralytic ileus, thirst, bad/bitter taste, mucosal ulcers, and reduced appetite have occurred rarely with ipratropium therapy. Diarrhea, dyspepsia, or vomiting has been reported in less than 2% of patients receiving combined albuterol and ipratropium inhalation aerosol. Dyspepsia, dry mouth, or nausea has been reported in 1–5, 2–4, or 4%, respectively, of patients receiving ipratropium HFA inhalation aerosol in clinical trials.

● Ocular Effects

Blurred vision/difficulty in accommodation has been reported in about 1% of patients receiving orally inhaled ipratropium. Burning eyes, mydriasis, temporary blurred vision, ocular pain (sometimes acute), conjunctival or corneal congestion associated with visual halos or colored images, or precipitation or worsening of angle-closure glaucoma also has been reported, probably because of inadvertent contact of the drug with the eyes during administration. Increased intraocular pressure (IOP) has been reported in patients with angle-closure glaucoma receiving nebulized solutions of ipratropium alone or combined with albuterol, apparently as a result of the drug solution escaping from the face mask and entering the eyes. (See Cautions: Precautions and Contraindications.) Increased IOP also has been reported with ipratropium inhalation aerosol and with concomitant administration of ipratropium aerosol (using the open-mouth technique) and nebulized albuterol. While blurred vision has been reported in children given nebulized ipratropium and albuterol via face mask, acute angle-closure glaucoma as a result of environmental exposure to these drugs apparently has not occurred in parents, nurses, or respiratory therapists caring for children undergoing such therapy.

● Cardiovascular Effects

Ipratropium inhalation aerosol and solution for nebulization appear to cause adverse cardiovascular effects less frequently than β₂-adrenergic agonists or theophylline. Palpitation has occurred in up to 3% of patients receiving orally inhaled ipratropium. Chest pain has been reported in 3.2%, and induction or aggravation of hypertension in about 1% of patients receiving nebulized ipratropium in controlled studies. Angina was reported in less than 2% of patients receiving the fixed-combination inhalation aerosol of albuterol and ipratropium in controlled studies. Extrasystole, tachycardia, vasodilation, and hypotension have been reported infrequently with orally inhaled ipratropium therapy. Hospitalizations for supraventricular tachycardia and atrial fibrillation occurred in 0.5% of patients receiving ipratropium inhalation aerosol.

Data from an observational study involving over 32,000 patients and another pooled analysis of 17 studies enrolling almost 15,000 patients have shown an increased risk of mortality and/or cardiovascular events (e.g., myocardial infarction, stroke, transient ischemic attacks) in patients receiving inhaled anticholinergic agents, including ipratropium. (See Cautions: Precautions and Contraindications.)

Nervous System Effects

Because of the drug's low lipid solubility, orally inhaled ipratropium produces adverse nervous system effects less frequently than orally inhaled atropine or β_2-adrenergic agonists. Nervousness, dizziness, and headache have occurred in about 0.5–6.4% of patients receiving orally inhaled ipratropium CFC inhalation aerosol (no longer commercially available in the US). Headache or dizziness occurred in 6–7 or 3%, respectively, of patients receiving ipratropium HFA inhalation aerosol in clinical trials. Headache occurs more frequently in patients receiving nebulized ipratropium bromide in total dosages of 2 mg or more daily. Fatigue or insomnia has been reported in less than 1% of patients receiving the drug. Paresthesia, drowsiness, coordination difficulty, and tremor also have been reported; tremor occurs less frequently with ipratropium than with β_2-adrenergic agonists or theophylline. Weakness or CNS stimulation has been reported in patients receiving albuterol and/or ipratropium inhalation aerosol.

Dermatologic and Sensitivity Reactions

Immediate hypersensitivity reactions, including rash, angioedema of the tongue, lips, and face, urticaria (including giant urticaria), laryngospasm, bronchospasm, oropharyngeal edema, and anaphylactic reaction, have been reported in patients receiving orally inhaled ipratropium, with positive results upon rechallenge in some cases. Many of these patients had a history of allergies to other drugs and/or foods, including peanuts and soybeans (soya lecithin is present as an excipient in the fixed-combination inhalation aerosol containing ipratropium and albuterol sulfate). Paradoxical bronchospasm has occurred occasionally with the use of ipratropium via nebulizer or oral aerosol. While it has been suggested that such bronchospasm may result from hypersensitivity to the active drug or other ingredients in the formulation, altered bronchial reactivity in atopic individuals with asthma, or the acidity of the nebulized solution, such reactions also have occurred following administration of isotonic, pH 7, preservative-free solutions of ipratropium.

Rash was reported in 1.2%, and urticaria in less than 3% of patients receiving orally inhaled ipratropium in controlled studies. Pruritus, flushing, or alopecia has been reported in less than 1% of patients receiving ipratropium aerosol. Contact dermatitis has occurred in at least one patient receiving nebulized ipratropium.

Genitourinary Effects

Although no alteration in micturition function was observed in a controlled study in a small number of geriatric men receiving orally inhaled ipratropium, urinary retention/difficulty has been reported occasionally in patients receiving the drug. Urinary tract infection or dysuria also has been reported in patients receiving ipratropium.

Other Effects

Pain, back pain, or flu-like symptoms have occurred in 4.1, 3.2, or 3.7% of patients, respectively, receiving nebulized ipratropium in controlled studies; arthritis has been reported in 0.9% of such patients. Back pain occurred in 2–7% of patients receiving ipratropium HFA inhalation aerosol in clinical trials. Pain or arthralgia also has been reported in 2.5 or less than 2% of patients, respectively, receiving albuterol and ipratropium in fixed combination in controlled studies. Tinnitus also has occurred with ipratropium therapy. Although a causal relationship has not been established, a slight elevation of serum ALT (SGPT) has been reported during therapy with the drug.

Long-term toxicology studies in monkeys using orally inhaled ipratropium bromide dosages of up to 1.6 mg daily for 6 months did not reveal gross or microscopic changes consistent with systemic anticholinergic activity. Food consumption was reduced and body weight decreased in purebred beagles given oral ipratropium bromide dosages of up to 75 mg/kg daily for 1 year.

Precautions and Contraindications

Although the toxic potential of orally inhaled ipratropium generally is less than that of other antimuscarinics because of its poor systemic absorption, the usual precautions of antimuscarinic therapy should be considered during therapy with ipratropium (e.g., the drug should be used with caution in patients with angle-closure glaucoma, bladder neck obstruction or prostatic hyperplasia). (See Cautions in the Antimuscarinics/Antispasmodics General Statement 12:08.08.)

When the preparation containing ipratropium bromide in fixed combination with albuterol sulfate is used, the cautions, precautions, and contraindications applicable to albuterol sulfate should be considered. Adverse cardiovascular effects (e.g., alterations in heart rate, blood pressure, or other manifestations) have been noted with albuterol in fixed combination with ipratropium as an inhalation aerosol; the combination aerosol should be discontinued if such effects occur.

The manufacturer warns that orally inhaled ipratropium is *not* indicated for the *initial* treatment of acute episodes of bronchospasm when a rapid response is required. For additional information on the use of ipratropium in asthma, see Asthma under Uses: Bronchospasm. In addition, use of orally inhaled ipratropium as a *single* agent for the management of bronchospasm in patients experiencing an acute exacerbation of COPD has not been adequately studied, and an agent with a faster onset of action (e.g., a β_2-adrenergic agonist) may be preferred as *initial* therapy in such patients.

Patients should be reminded that orally inhaled ipratropium is not intended for occasional use; it should be used consistently throughout the course of therapy for maximum effectiveness. Patients should contact their clinician if symptoms of COPD are not relieved by ipratropium or if a previously effective dosage regimen fails to provide the usual relief (i.e., the frequency of administration of the drug needs to be increased). The dosage or frequency of administration of ipratropium inhalation aerosol should not be increased without consultation with a clinician.

Data from an observational study involving over 32,000 patients and another pooled analysis have shown an increased risk of mortality and/or cardiovascular events, including stroke or transient ischemic attacks, in patients receiving inhaled anticholinergic agents, including ipratropium. (See Cautions: Cardiovascular Effects.) While data are conflicting, a possible increased risk of stroke has also been identified from ongoing safety monitoring and pooled analysis of placebo-controlled trials in patients receiving another anticholinergic agent, tiotropium. However, preliminary analysis of a placebo-controlled trial in approximately 6000 patients with COPD did not reveal an increased risk of stroke with tiotropium bromide. FDA has not yet confirmed the results of these analyses and is currently reviewing postmarketing adverse event reports and preliminary results of a recently completed placebo-controlled trial to assess additional long-term safety data and further evaluate the risk of stroke with tiotropium.

As with other inhaled drugs, paradoxical bronchospasm has been reported in a few patients receiving ipratropium nebulized solution, inhalation aerosol, or the fixed-combination (with albuterol) inhalation aerosol, although a causal relationship to the drug has not been definitely established. Ipratropium should be discontinued immediately if bronchoconstriction occurs, and alternative therapy instituted.

Temporary blurred vision, mydriasis, ocular pain, conjunctival or corneal congestion associated with visual halos or colored images, or precipitation or worsening of angle-closure glaucoma may occur following inadvertent contact of ipratropium with the eyes; therefore, when the drug is administered via a nebulizer, procedures to minimize ocular exposure should be employed (e.g., using a mouthpiece rather than a face mask to deliver the drug). In addition, patients should be instructed to close their eyes during oral inhalation of ipratropium aerosol. Patients should contact their clinician immediately if ocular symptoms develop after use of ipratropium inhalation aerosol.

Orally inhaled ipratropium should be used with caution in patients with angle-closure glaucoma, although the drug has been used in patients with open-angle glaucoma without clinically important effects on pupil size, accommodation, visual acuity, or intraocular pressure (IOP). Since the risk of ocular toxicity of ipratropium is associated with local exposure of the eye to aerosolized/nebulized drug, care to avoid such exposure is particularly important in patients who are at increased risk from the ocular consequences of exposure. Therefore, some clinicians suggest that ipratropium aerosol should not be administered using the open-mouth technique in patients at high risk for ocular toxicity (e.g., those with angle-closure glaucoma). It also has been suggested that children with blindness (e.g., marked retinal detachment secondary to retinopathy of prematurity, infantile or childhood glaucoma, traumatic cataracts, or dislocation of the lens) should not receive ipratropium via nebulization.

The manufacturer states that ipratropium should be used with caution in patients with renal or hepatic impairment because the drug has not been evaluated systematically in these patient groups. Albuterol and ipratropium inhalation aerosol should be used with caution in patients with cardiovascular disorders (especially coronary insufficiency, cardiac arrhythmias, or hypertension), seizure disorders, hyperthyroidism, diabetes mellitus, and in those who are unusually responsive to β_2-adrenergic agents.

Ipratropium aerosol and inhalation solution for nebulization are contraindicated in patients with known hypersensitivity to the drug or any other component of the respective formulation, or to atropine or its derivatives. Ipratropium aerosol in fixed combination with albuterol sulfate also is contraindicated in patients with known hypersensitivity to soya lecithin or related food products, including soybeans and peanuts.

● Pediatric Precautions

The manufacturer states that safety and efficacy of orally inhaled ipratropium via a metered-dose inhaler in pediatric patients have not been established, although the drug has been used in such patients (generally in children with asthma) with no unusual risk. The safety and efficacy ipratropium bromide for oral inhalation via nebulization have not been established in patients younger than 12 years of age. The safety and efficacy of albuterol sulfate in fixed combination with ipratropium bromide for oral inhalation via nebulization have not been established in patients younger than 18 years of age.

● Geriatric Precautions

When the total number of patients studied in clinical trials of ipratropium HFA inhalation aerosol is considered, 57% were 65 years of age or older. No overall differences in efficacy or safety were observed between geriatric and younger patients in these studies.

Safety and efficacy of ipratropium bromide in fixed combination with albuterol sulfate inhalation solution in geriatric patients have not been specifically studied to date; however, in clinical studies of the combination for the treatment of bronchospasm, approximately 62% of the patients were 65 years of age or older and 19% were 75 years of age or older. Although no overall differences were observed between geriatric and younger patients in the safety and efficacy of the combination in clinical studies, the possibility that some older patients may exhibit increased sensitivity to the drug cannot be ruled out.

● Mutagenicity and Carcinogenicity

No evidence of mutagenicity was seen with ipratropium in an in vitro microbial mutagen test (Ames test), the mouse micronucleus test, or the mouse dominant lethal assay, nor did the drug induce chromosomal aberrations in the bone marrow of Chinese hamsters.

No evidence of carcinogenic potential was seen in rats or mice receiving oral ipratropium bromide at dosages up to 6 mg/kg daily for 2 years.

● Pregnancy, Fertility, and Lactation

Pregnancy

Reproduction studies in mice, rats, and rabbits receiving oral ipratropium bromide dosages of 10, 1000, and 125 mg/kg daily (approximately 200, 40,000, and 10,000 times the maximum recommended human daily inhalation dosage on a mg/m^2 basis), respectively, and in rats or rabbits receiving orally inhaled ipratropium bromide dosages of 1.5 or 1.8 mg/kg (approximately 60 or 140 times the maximum recommended human daily inhalation dosage on a mg/m^2 basis), respectively, have not revealed evidence of harm to the fetus. There are no adequate and controlled studies to date using orally inhaled ipratropium in pregnant women, and the drug should be used during pregnancy only when clearly needed.

Fertility

Reproduction studies in male and female rats using oral ipratropium bromide dosages up to 50 mg/kg daily have not revealed evidence of impaired fertility; however, the drug was associated with impaired fertility (i.e., increased resorption) when given at an oral dosage exceeding 90 mg/kg in rats (approximately 3600 times the maximum recommended human daily inhalation dosage on a mg/m^2 basis). As these results were not obtained at dosages and a route of administration that were clinically relevant, the manufacturer states that such embryotoxic effects in rats are not considered clinically important.

Lactation

It is not known whether ipratropium is distributed into milk in humans, but highly lipophobic quaternary bases are distributed slowly and at low concentrations into milk. Because ipratropium is not well absorbed systemically following oral inhalation, the manufacturer states that ingestion of substantial amounts of the drug by an infant during breast-feeding is unlikely. The manufacturer recommends that orally inhaled ipratropium be used with caution in nursing women.

DRUG INTERACTIONS

The manufacturer states that because of the limited systemic absorption and low plasma drug concentrations associated with oral inhalation of ipratropium, it is unlikely that the drug would interact with systemically administered drugs. The manufacturer states that patients taking ipratropium bromide in fixed combination with albuterol sulfate should not use other inhaled agents unless directed by a clinician.

Adverse drug interactions have not been reported with concomitant administration of orally inhaled ipratropium and a β-adrenergic agonist bronchodilator (e.g., albuterol, fenoterol [currently not commercially available in the US], isoproterenol, metaproterenol), theophylline derivatives, oral or inhaled corticosteroids, or cromolyn sodium in clinical studies in patients with chronic obstructive pulmonary disease (COPD) or asthma.

While concomitant inhalation of ipratropium and a β$_2$-adrenergic agonist may not always result in substantial additional bronchodilation compared with inhalation of either agent alone, such combined therapy usually increases the duration of bronchodilation. Concomitant administration of ipratropium and albuterol via nebulization has been reported to increase intraocular pressure (IOP) and precipitate acute angle-closure glaucoma in susceptible individuals (i.e., individuals with untreated or undiagnosed angle-closure glaucoma), probably as a result of inadvertent contact of the drugs with the eyes. (See Cautions: Ocular Effects.) Caution is advised if the fixed combination of albuterol and ipratropium inhalation aerosol is used concomitantly with other β$_2$-adrenergic agents since the risk for adverse cardiovascular effects increases.

Although ipratropium inhalation aerosol is minimally absorbed into the systemic circulation, there is some potential for additive interaction with concomitantly used antimuscarinic agents. Therefore, caution is advised when ipratropium aerosol is used concomitantly with other antimuscarinic agents.

For further information on drug interactions reported with antimuscarinics, see Drug Interactions in the Antimuscarinics/Antispasmodics General Statement 12:08.08.

ACUTE TOXICITY

Toxicology studies in animals indicate that ipratropium exhibits a low order of toxicity compared with that of other anticholinergic and bronchospasmolytic agents.

● Pathogenesis

The acute lethal dose of ipratropium bromide in humans is not known. The manufacturer states that ipratropium overdosage as a result of oral inhalation or oral administration is unlikely because systemic absorption of the drug is minimal after inhalation or oral administration of up to 4- or 40-fold the recommended oral inhalation dose, respectively.

The IV LD$_{50}$ of ipratropium bromide in dogs, male rats, female rats, female mice, or male mice is approximately 17.5–20, 16, 15.7, 15, or 12.3 mg/kg, respectively. The oral LD$_{50}$ of ipratropium bromide in rats, mice, or dogs is 1700 mg/kg (approximately 68,000 times the maximum recommended human daily inhalation dosage on a mg/m^2 basis), in excess of 1 g/kg (approximately 20,000 times the maximum recommended human daily inhalation dosage on a mg/m^2 basis), or 400 mg/kg (approximately 53,000 times the maximum human daily inhalation dosage on a mg/m^2 basis), respectively. The subcutaneous LD$_{50}$ of ipratropium bromide in male or female mice is approximately 300 or 340 mg/kg, respectively. The inhalation LD$_{50}$ of ipratropium bromide is about 200 mg/kg in guinea pigs and about 1 mg/kg in monkeys. The oral lethal dose of ipratropium ranges from 1001–2010 mg/kg in mice (approximately 30,000 and 60,000 times the maximum recommended human daily inhalation dose on a mg/m^2 basis), from 1667–4000 mg/kg in rats (approximately 100,000 and 240,000 times the maximum recommended human daily inhalation dose on a mg/m^2 basis), and from 400–1300 mg/kg in dogs (approximately 80,000 and 260,000 times the maximum recommended human daily inhalation dose on a mg/m^2 basis). Death from ipratropium bromide overdosage in animals usually resulted from inhibition of ganglionic transmission, which produced curariform paralysis of skeletal muscle.

● Manifestations

In general, overdosage of ipratropium bromide may be expected to produce effects associated with antimuscarinic administration; however, the manufacturer states that because of the low systemic absorption of orally inhaled ipratropium bromide, acute overdosage of the drug is unlikely following oral administration or oral inhalation.

For further information on acute overdosage reported with antimuscarinics, see Acute Toxicity in the Antimuscarinics/Antispasmodics General Statement 12:08.08.

PHARMACOLOGY

Ipratropium generally exhibits pharmacologic actions similar to those of other antimuscarinics. Similar to atropine, ipratropium is a nonselective competitive antagonist at muscarinic receptors present in airways and other organs. The drug relaxes smooth muscles of bronchi and bronchioles by blocking acetylcholine-induced stimulation of guanyl cyclase and thus reducing formation of cyclic guanosine monophosphate (cGMP), a mediator of bronchoconstriction. Ipratropium generally exhibits greater antimuscarinic activity on bronchial smooth muscle than on secretory (e.g., salivary, gastric) glands.

Following IV administration in animals, the antimuscarinic activity of ipratropium (as measured by mydriasis, inhibition of salivary or gastric secretions, tachycardia, or spasmolysis) is similar to that of atropine; following oral administration, the antimuscarinic activity of ipratropium is only about 10–50% that of atropine. In animals, the relative bronchoselectivity of ipratropium is even more pronounced with oral inhalation of the drug than with IV administration.

• Respiratory Effects

Ipratropium is a potent bronchodilator, particularly in large bronchial airways; however, some evidence suggests that the drug also has bronchodilator activity in small airways. Bronchodilation results from relaxation of smooth muscles of the bronchial tree. The extent of bronchodilation produced by ipratropium appears to be determined by the level of cholinergic parasympathetic bronchomotor tone and by inhibition of bronchoconstriction resulting from neural reflex activation of cholinergic pathways. The importance of cholinergic tone and neural reflexes in producing bronchoconstriction in airway disease remains to be determined; however, limited evidence indicates that cholinergic tone may be increased in patients with chronic obstructive pulmonary disease (COPD). In animals, the bronchodilator activity of ipratropium is similar to or exceeds that of atropine or isoproterenol and exceeds that of albuterol or metaproterenol when these drugs are given via nebulization. In patients with COPD, ipratropium is at least as effective in producing bronchodilation as β-adrenergic agonists. Combined use of ipratropium and a $β_2$-adrenergic agonist (e.g., albuterol) results in greater bronchodilation than either drug alone.

Ipratropium decreases airway resistance as measured by forced expiratory volume in 1 second (FEV_1) and forced expiratory flow during the middle half of forced vital capacity (FEF_{25-75}). Following oral inhalation of ipratropium in patients with pulmonary disease, FVC and specific airway conductance may increase and residual volume (RV) may decrease. In dose-ranging studies with ipratropium bromide inhalation aerosol in patients with chronic bronchitis, maximal bronchodilator effects reportedly were evident with ipratropium bromide doses of 36 mcg. Limited data suggest that in patients with COPD, the optimum dose (as determined by maximal increases in FEV_1 and forced vital capacity [FVC]) of nebulized ipratropium bromide is about 400 mcg. A 36-mcg dose (2 inhalations) of ipratropium bromide administered via a metered-dose inhaler appears to produce bronchodilation (defined as area under the FEV_1 curve) similar to that produced by a 100-mcg dose of ipratropium bromide administered via a nebulizer.

While systemic administration of anticholinergic agents can reduce the volume and fluidity of bronchial secretions, orally inhaled ipratropium has little or no effect on respiratory secretions. Orally inhaled ipratropium does not appear to have any substantial effect on sputum viscosity or, unlike atropine, on mucociliary clearance. Ipratropium decreases ciliary activity in vitro but to a smaller extent than atropine. Volume of sputum usually remains unchanged during ipratropium therapy.

Various mechanisms appear to be involved in irritant-, histamine-, exercise-, or allergen-induced bronchoconstriction, and the protective effect of ipratropium against a bronchoconstrictor stimulus appears to depend in part on the extent to which bronchospasm is mediated by vagal reflexes. As expected, orally inhaled ipratropium reliably prevents bronchospasm induced by cholinergic agonists such as methacholine or acetylcholine in both healthy individuals and asthmatic patients. Ipratropium also prevents bronchospasm induced by irritants such as sulfur dioxide, ozone, or cigarette smoke in healthy individuals, but generally is less effective in asthmatic patients whose airways are more reactive to such stimuli. Although in some asthmatic patients ipratropium may be effective

in preventing bronchospasm provoked by allergens, histamine, exercise, bradykinin, prostaglandin $F_{2α}$, adenosine monophosphate, or substance P (a noncholinergic neurotransmitter), patients with asthma exhibit considerable interindividual variation in their response to ipratropium; asthmatic patients in whom bronchoconstriction is mediated principally by the vagal reflex may respond better to the drug than those in whom other mechanisms predominate. Usual doses of orally inhaled ipratropium bromide in asthmatic patients provide little or no protection against bronchospasm induced by serotonin or leukotrienes. However, the drug does appear to prevent bronchospasm induced by $β_2$-adrenergic blocking agents, pentamidine, or psychogenic stimuli. In patients with COPD, cholinergic bronchomotor tone is the principal determinant of reversible airway constriction. Therefore, while patients with asthma show a variable response to anticholinergic bronchodilators, patients with COPD generally respond to these agents.

Inhalation of ipratropium does not appear to produce clinically important alterations in arterial oxygen or carbon dioxide tension; however, slight increases or decreases in arterial oxygen tension and slight decreases in carbon dioxide tension have been observed in some patients receiving the drug. In a limited number of studies in healthy adults or patients with COPD, no adverse effects on arterial pH, pulmonary blood pressure, or pulmonary diffusing capacity were observed following oral inhalation of ipratropium.

Tolerance to the bronchodilating effect of orally inhaled ipratropium does not appear to develop with prolonged use; the bronchodilator effect has been maintained throughout at least 5 years of continuous use in some patients.

• Cardiovascular Effects

Oral inhalation of ipratropium has not produced appreciable changes in heart rate, blood pressure, or cardiac rhythm in healthy adults, healthy adults with experimentally induced pulmonary hypertension, or patients with COPD or hypertension. Slight decreases in heart rate, accompanied by increases in stroke volume and ejection fraction, have been observed in healthy adults receiving high doses (e.g., up to 2.4 mg) of ipratropium bromide via a metered-dose inhaler; however, cardiac output in these patients remained unchanged, and these cardiovascular effects do not appear to be clinically important.

• GI Effects

Although orally inhaled ipratropium appears to have minimal effect on salivary secretions, the drug has produced inhibition of salivary secretions in animals and in healthy adults when given IV. Following oral administration of 15 mg of ipratropium bromide in healthy adults, basal gastric acid secretion decreased by 50% and gastric pH increased from 2.5 to 5 within 1 hour.

• Ocular Effects

Following IV administration of ipratropium in animals, the mydriatic activity of the drug is similar to that of atropine. When given by oral inhalation, ipratropium does not appear to produce mydriasis, increased intraocular pressure (IOP), or changes in ocular function in children or in adults with normal IOP or open-angle or angle-closure glaucoma. However, increased IOP and other adverse ocular effects have been reported during treatment with the drug, as a result of inadvertent exposure of the eyes during oral inhalation of ipratropium alone or combined with albuterol. (See Cautions: Ocular Effects.) $β_2$-Adrenergic agonists such as albuterol increase production of aqueous humor which, in combination with restricted outflow caused by anticholinergic-associated pupillary dilatation, may increase IOP and lead to acute angle-closure glaucoma in susceptible individuals (i.e., individuals with untreated or undiagnosed angle-closure glaucoma).

• Nervous System Effects

Because of its low lipid solubility, ipratropium, unlike atropine, does not appear to cross the blood-brain barrier. Current evidence indicates that the drug produces little or no CNS stimulation.

PHARMACOKINETICS

• Absorption

Following oral inhalation, ipratropium bromide is only minimally absorbed into systemic circulation from the surface of the lungs or from the GI tract. Following oral inhalation of 2 mg of ipratropium bromide via nebulization in healthy adults, approximately 7% (range: 1.4–16.3%) of the dose was absorbed into systemic circulation. Concomitant oral inhalation of ipratropium and albuterol in a fixed-combination aerosol did not alter the systemic absorption of either component. Following oral inhalation of 555 mcg of radiolabeled ipratropium bromide in healthy adults, radioactivity was detected in blood within 2 minutes, indicating rapid buccal and/or pulmonary absorption; peak plasma concentrations of about 0.06 ng/mL (as total radioactivity) occurred in about 1–3 hours. Following oral inhalation of a single, higher-than-recommended dose (4 inhalations, total dose 68 mcg) of ipratropium bromide (with a hydrofluoroalkane [HFA] propellant), mean peak plasma concentrations of ipratropium in a limited number of adult or geriatric patients with chronic obstructive pulmonary disease (COPD) were 59 or 56 pg/mL, respectively. Following administration of a higher-than-recommended dosage (4 inhalations 4 times daily, 272 mcg total daily dosage) of ipratropium (with HFA propellant) for 1 week, mean peak plasma ipratropium bromide concentrations in adult or geriatric patients increased to 82 or 84 pg/mL, respectively. The trough concentration of ipratropium 6 hours after inhalation in adult and geriatric patients was 28 pg/mL at steady state. Following oral inhalation of the fixed combination of albuterol sulfate (180 mcg as albuterol base) and ipratropium bromide monohydrate (36 mcg), peak plasma concentration of ipratropium bromide remained below detectable limits (less than 100 pg/mL); peak plasma concentrations of albuterol of about 492 pg/mL occurred within 3 hours after administration. Although most of a dose of an orally inhaled drug is actually swallowed, the bronchodilating action of ipratropium appears to result from a local action of the portion of the dose that reaches the bronchial tree.

Following oral aerosol inhalation of 34 mcg of ipratropium bromide (with HFA propellant) in patients with COPD, bronchodilation (as determined by an increase of 15% or more in FEV_1) is evident within 14–17.5 minutes, is maximal within 1–2 hours, and generally persists for 2–4 hours. The onset to a 15% increase in FEV_1 after oral inhalation of albuterol sulfate (180 mcg as albuterol base) and ipratropium bromide monohydrate (36 mcg) in fixed combination in patients with COPD was 15 minutes; median time to peak FEV_1 was 1 hour. The median duration of bronchodilation was 4–5 hours with the fixed combination and 4 hours with ipratropium alone. In dose-ranging studies in patients with bronchospasm, ipratropium bromide doses of 36–72 mcg given via a metered-dose inhaler generally have provided optimal clinical benefit. Because penetration of orally inhaled particles into airways is impaired when airways are severely obstructed, some clinicians suggest that higher doses of ipratropium bromide may be needed for maximal effect in some patients (e.g., those with severe airway disease).

Following oral inhalation via nebulization of 400–600 mcg of ipratropium bromide, bronchodilation (defined as increases of 15% or more in FEV_1) usually is evident within 15–30 minutes with peak effect in approximately 1–2 hours. In a dose-response study in patients with COPD, the optimal dose of nebulized ipratropium bromide was about 400 mcg. Bronchodilation with nebulized ipratropium generally persists for 4–5 hours, but may last up to 7–8 hours in some patients. Following concomitant administration via nebulization of a β_2-adrenergic agonist (i.e., albuterol, metaproterenol) and ipratropium in patients with COPD, bronchodilation persists for 5–7 hours compared with 3–4 hours in patients given a β_2-adrenergic agonist alone.

Following oral administration of a single 30-mg dose of radiolabeled ipratropium bromide in healthy adults, peak plasma ipratropium bromide concentrations of about 25 ng/mL (as total radioactivity) occurred within 2–4 hours. However, peak plasma radioactivity following administration of radiolabeled ipratropium bromide appears to represent both the parent drug and its metabolites. Peak plasma drug concentrations of about 1 ng/mL (determined by a radioreceptor assay that does not measure metabolites of ipratropium bromide) occurred within 2 hours following administration of a single 10-mg oral dose of ipratropium bromide in healthy adults. In these individuals, approximately 3.3% (range: 0.9–6.1%) of the dose of ipratropium bromide was absorbed. Oral administration of 15 mg of ipratropium bromide appears to produce bronchodilation similar to that produced by 36 or 150 mcg of the drug given by oral aerosol inhalation or IV, respectively; plasma concentrations are approximately 1000 times higher following oral administration than following oral inhalation of equipotent doses. Plasma drug concentrations following oral inhalation of ipratropium bromide do not appear to correlate with pharmacologic effects.

● **Distribution**

Distribution of ipratropium bromide into human tissues and body fluids has not been elucidated. Quaternary ammonium antimuscarinics are completely ionized and possess poor lipid solubility; accordingly, they do not readily penetrate the CNS. Following IV administration of ipratropium bromide in rats, the drug is distributed throughout the body with highest concentrations appearing in the stomach, intestines, liver, and kidneys; the drug is minimally distributed into brain,

lung, and muscle. High concentrations of ipratropium bromide in the gut in these animals may indicate biliary elimination or enterohepatic circulation.

Ipratropium bromide reportedly is 0–9% bound to plasma albumin and α_1-acid glycoproteins in vitro.

It is not known whether ipratropium bromide crosses the placenta or is distributed into milk.

● **Elimination**

Following IV administration of ipratropium bromide in healthy adults, plasma drug concentrations appear to decline in a biphasic manner. Using radiolabeled ipratropium bromide, an elimination half-life of about 2–4 hours (determined by measurement of total radioactivity) generally has been reported following administration of the drug orally, IV, or by oral inhalation in animals and healthy adults. However, this method measures both ipratropium bromide and its metabolites. Using a radioreceptor assay that measures only unchanged ipratropium bromide, the initial distribution-phase half-life ($t_{1/2\alpha}$) and the terminal elimination-phase half-life ($t_{1/2\beta}$) following a single 2-mg IV dose of the drug in healthy adults averaged about 0.07 and 1.6 hours, respectively.

The exact metabolic fate of ipratropium bromide has not been fully determined. Following oral or IV administration or oral inhalation, the drug is partially metabolized to at least 8 metabolites. Metabolism appears to involve only the tropic acid moiety and usually consists of hydrolysis and conjugation. The main metabolites appear to be N-isopropylnortropium methobromide, which is formed by enzymatic hydrolysis of the ester; α-phenylacrylic acid-N-isopropylnortropine-ester methobromide, which is formed by enzymatic loss of a water; and phenylacetic acid-N-isopropylnortropine-ester methobromide, which is formed by enzymatic loss of a CH_3OH-group. In vitro, these metabolites have minimal or no antimuscarinic activity.

After oral inhalation, oral administration, or IV injection of radiolabeled ipratropium bromide, unchanged drug recovered in urine within 4 hours (as total radioactivity) averaged 13, 24, or 50% of the dose, respectively. After administration of albuterol sulfate (180 mcg as albuterol base) and ipratropium bromide monohydrate (36 mcg) in fixed combination, 27.1% of the estimated mouthpiece dose is excreted unchanged in urine within 24 hours. Following oral administration or oral inhalation of ipratropium bromide in healthy adults, most of the dose is excreted in feces within 24 hours, principally as unchanged drug. In healthy individuals receiving 555 mcg of radiolabeled ipratropium bromide by oral inhalation, about 69 and 3.2% of the dose was excreted in feces and urine, respectively, within 6–7 days. Following administration of radiolabeled ipratropium bromide in healthy adults, about 9 or 72% of a single oral or IV dose, respectively, was excreted in urine, and about 89 or 6% of the oral or IV dose was excreted in feces within 5–7 days; most excretion occurred within 24 hours. Ipratropium bromide undergoes biliary elimination and/or enterohepatic circulation in animals and appears to undergo some biliary elimination in humans.

CHEMISTRY AND STABILITY

● **Chemistry**

Ipratropium bromide is a synthetic quaternary ammonium antimuscarinic agent. Ipratropium is the quaternary N-methyl isopropyl derivative of noratropine. The drug is commercially available as the monobromide monohydrate (i.e., ipratropium bromide) in an oral aerosol formulation and in a solution for nebulization. Ipratropium bromide is also available in fixed combination with albuterol sulfate in an oral aerosol formulation and in a solution for nebulization. However, potencies of the commercially available preparations differ, the aerosol being expressed in terms of the monohydrate and the solution for nebulization being expressed in terms of anhydrous drug.

Ipratropium bromide, which is hydrated, occurs as a white, bitter-tasting crystalline powder and has solubilities of 90 mg/mL in water and 28 mg/mL in alcohol. Like other quaternary ammonium compounds, ipratropium exists in an ionized state in aqueous solutions and is insoluble in lipophilic solvents such as ether, chloroform, and fluorocarbons. A 1% aqueous solution of ipratropium bromide has a pH of 5–7.5.

Ipratropium bromide inhalation aerosol is commercially available as a solution of the drug in a vehicle containing a hydrofluoroalkane (tetrafluoroethane) propellant, water, dehydrated alcohol, and anhydrous citric acid. For oral inhalation, ipratropium bromide in fixed combination with albuterol sulfate, is commercially available as an aerosol containing a microcrystalline suspension of the drug (as the monohydrate) in a vehicle of chlorofluorocarbon propellants (dichlorodifluoromethane, dichlorotetrafluoroethane, and trichloromonofluoromethane) and soya lecithin. Each actuation of the aerosol inhaler delivers 17 mcg of ipratropium bromide monohydrate from the mouthpiece. Each actuation of the combination aerosol inhaler delivers 18 mcg of ipratropium bromide monohydrate and 103 mcg of albuterol sulfate (equivalent to 90 mcg of albuterol base) from the mouthpiece.

For oral administration by nebulizer, ipratropium bromide is commercially available as a 0.02% solution (expressed in terms of anhydrous drug) in 0.9% sodium chloride; hydrochloric acid may be added to adjust the pH to 3.4 (3–4). Ipratropium bromide also is available in fixed combination with albuterol sulfate as a 0.017% solution (expressed in terms of the anhydrous drug) in sodium chloride; hydrochloric acid may be added to adjust the pH to 4. Each 3-mL unit-dose vial of ipratropium bromide in fixed combination with albuterol sulfate inhalation solution contains 0.5 mg of ipratropium bromide and 2.5 mg of albuterol (equivalent to 3 mg of albuterol sulfate). The commercially available solutions for nebulization are sterile, clear, colorless and do not contain preservatives.

● Stability

Commercially available ipratropium bromide alone or in fixed combination with albuterol sulfate oral inhalation aerosol should be stored at 25 °C but may be exposed to temperatures ranging from 15 to 30°C; exposure to excessive humidity should be avoided. For best results, the aerosol canister should be at room temperature before use; at colder temperatures, cooling of the propellants may decrease the internal pressure of the canister and result in delivery of particles too large to provide full therapeutic effect. Because the contents of ipratropium bromide inhalation aerosol are under pressure, the aerosol container should *not* be punctured, used or stored near heat or an open flame, or placed into a fire or incinerator for disposal; exposure to high temperatures (49°C) may cause the canister to burst. When stored as directed, commercially available ipratropium bromide inhalation aerosol is stable for 18 months from the date of manufacture.

Commercially available ipratropium bromide inhalation solutions for nebulization should be stored at 15–30°C and protected from light, preferably in the manufacturer-supplied foil pouch. The commercially available inhalation solution of ipratropium bromide in fixed combination with albuterol sulfate should be stored at 2–30°C and be protected from light, preferably in the manufacturer-supplied foil pouch. When stored as directed, ipratropium bromide inhalation solution has an expiration date of 18 months following the date of manufacture.

The manufacturer states that solutions containing ipratropium bromide and albuterol sulfate or metaproterenol sulfate for oral inhalation are stable for 1 hour when mixed extemporaneously in a nebulizer prior to administration. Ipratropium

bromide oral inhalation solution also has been reported to be stable for 1 hour when mixed in a nebulizer with cromolyn sodium. The manufacturer states that the stability and safety of ipratropium bromide inhalation solution mixed with other drugs in a nebulizer have not been established.

For further information on the chemistry, pharmacology, pharmacokinetics, uses, cautions, acute toxicity, and drug interactions of ipratropium bromide, see the Antimuscarinics/Antispasmodics General Statement 12.08.08.

PREPARATIONS

Excipients in commercially available drug preparations may have clinically important effects in some individuals; consult specific product labeling for details.

Ipratropium Bromide

Oral Inhalation

Aerosol	17 mcg per metered spray	**Atrovent® HFA** (with hydrofluoroalkane propellant), Boehringer Ingelheim
Solution, for nebulization	0.02%*	**Ipratropium Bromide Inhalation Solution**

* available from one or more manufacturer, distributor, and/or repackager by generic (nonproprietary) name

Ipratropium Bromide Combinations

Oral Inhalation Only

Aerosol	18 mcg with Albuterol Sulfate 90 mcg (of albuterol) per metered spray	**Combivent®** (with chlorofluorohydrocarbon propellants), Boehringer Ingelheim
Solution, for nebulization	0.5 mg with Albuterol Sulfate 2.5 mg (of albuterol) per 3 mL*	**DuoNeb®**, Dey **Ipratropium Bromide and Albuterol Sulfate Inhalation Solution**

* available from one or more manufacturer, distributor, and/or repackager by generic (nonproprietary) name

† Use is not currently included in the labeling approved by the US Food and Drug Administration.

Selected Revisions August 1, 2010, © Copyright, November 1, 1995, American Society of Health-System Pharmacists, Inc.

Tiotropium Bromide

12:08.08 • ANTIMUSCARINICS/ANTISPASMODICS

■ Tiotropium bromide, a synthetic quaternary ammonium antimuscarinic agent, is a long-acting orally inhaled bronchodilator.

USES

● *Bronchospasm*

Chronic Obstructive Pulmonary Disease

Tiotropium bromide is used as a bronchodilator alone or in fixed combination with olodaterol hydrochloride for the long-term maintenance treatment of reversible bronchospasm associated with chronic obstructive pulmonary disease (COPD), including chronic bronchitis and emphysema. Tiotropium bromide alone also is used to reduce exacerbations of COPD in patients with a history of such exacerbations. In patients with moderate to severe COPD (e.g., forced expiratory volume in 1 second [FEV_1] 30 to less than 80% of predicted or, alternatively, less than 60% of predicted) who have persistent symptoms not relieved by as-needed therapy with ipratropium and/or a selective, short-acting inhaled β_2-agonist, maintenance monotherapy with a long-acting bronchodilator (e.g., orally inhaled salmeterol, formoterol, or tiotropium) or an inhaled corticosteroid may be used, and a short-acting, selective inhaled β_2-agonist is used as needed for immediate symptom relief. Maintenance therapy with long-acting bronchodilators in patients with moderate to severe COPD is more effective and more convenient than regular therapy with short-acting bronchodilators. Data are insufficient to favor one maintenance monotherapy over another for use in such patients. Some clinicians recommend therapy with a combination of several long-acting bronchodilators such as tiotropium and a long-acting β-adrenergic agonist in selected patients with inadequate response. In patients with severe to very severe COPD (e.g., FEV_1 less than 30 to less than 50% of predicted), some clinicians recommend addition of an inhaled corticosteroid to maintenance therapy with one or more long-acting bronchodilators given separately or in fixed combination; however, the benefits of combination therapy over monotherapy have not been consistently demonstrated. If symptoms are not adequately controlled with inhaled corticosteroids and a long-acting bronchodilator or if limiting adverse effects occur, addition or substitution of extended-release oral theophylline may be considered. Orally inhaled tiotropium alone or in combination with olodaterol is *not* indicated for treatment of acute episodes of bronchospasm or acute deterioration of COPD; a drug with a more rapid onset of action (e.g., a short-acting β-adrenergic agonist) may be preferred in such cases.

Currently available data indicate that tiotropium improves lung function (e.g., as determined by FEV_1) in patients with COPD compared with ipratropium or placebo. Such improvement in lung function has been maintained throughout the 24-hour dosing interval and for treatment periods of up to 1 year with no evidence of tolerance. In some studies, treatment with tiotropium also has been associated with a reduction in the need for supplemental short-acting β_2 agonists compared with placebo.

In several long-term (e.g., 1-year) comparative studies in patients with COPD, orally inhaled tiotropium (18 mcg once daily) improved lung function (e.g., as determined by mean change in trough FEV_1, morning and evening peak expiratory flow rate [PEFR]) to a greater degree than ipratropium bromide (36 mcg 4 times daily) oral inhalation aerosol. In addition, treatment with tiotropium reduced dyspnea and the number of COPD exacerbations and increased the time to a first exacerbation compared with ipratropium bromide aerosol.

In two 6-month comparative trials in patients with COPD receiving either orally inhaled tiotropium (18 mcg once daily) or salmeterol (50 mcg twice daily), tiotropium was more effective in improving bronchodilation (e.g., FEV_1, evening PEFR) than salmeterol therapy or placebo. In addition, while tiotropium or salmeterol each reduced dyspnea and improved FEV_1 compared with placebo, tiotropium also was more effective than placebo in reducing COPD exacerbations and all-cause hospital admissions and improving quality-of-life scores in these trials.

The efficacy of tiotropium oral inhalation powder for reducing exacerbations in patients with COPD also has been studied in 2 randomized, placebo-controlled clinical trials: a 6-month trial including 1829 patients and a 4-year trial including 5992 patients. In the 4-year study, long-term effects on lung function

and other outcomes also were evaluated. In both studies, patients were allowed to use their prescribed respiratory medications (e.g., short- and long-acting β-agonists, inhaled and systemic corticosteroids, theophyllines) except for inhaled anticholinergic agents. In the 6-month trial, COPD exacerbations were defined as a complex of respiratory symptoms (increase or new onset) including more than one of the following: cough, sputum, wheezing, dyspnea, or chest tightness with a duration of at least 3 days requiring treatment with antibiotics, systemic corticosteroids, or hospitalization. Patients were 40–90 years of age, 99% were male, and 91% were white, with a mean pre-bronchodilator FEV_1 of 36% of predicted (range: 8–93%). The primary end points were the proportion of patients with COPD exacerbations and the proportion of patients with hospitalization due to COPD exacerbations. The proportion of patients with COPD exacerbations was substantially lower in patients receiving tiotropium than in patients receiving placebo (27.9 versus 32.3%). The proportion of patients with hospitalization due to COPD exacerbations (7 or 9.5% in patients receiving tiotropium or placebo, respectively) was not substantially different in the 2 groups.

In the 4-year trial, patients were 40–88 years of age, 75% were male, and 90% were white with a mean pre-bronchodilator FEV_1 of 39% of predicted (range: 9–76%). The primary efficacy end points (i.e., yearly rate of decline in pre- and post-bronchodilator FEV_1) did not differ between the 2 study groups. However, improvements in trough (pre-dose) FEV_1 (adjusted means over time: 87–103 mL) were maintained over the 4 years of the study in patients receiving tiotropium. COPD exacerbations were a secondary end point in this trial and were defined as an increase or new onset of more than one of the following respiratory symptoms: cough, sputum, sputum purulence, wheezing, and dyspnea, with a duration of 3 or more days requiring treatment with antibiotics and/or systemic corticosteroids. The risk of exacerbation and of exacerbation-related hospitalization both were reduced by 14% in patients receiving tiotropium compared with those receiving placebo; in addition, median time to first exacerbation was longer in patients receiving tiotropium compared with placebo (16.7 versus 12.5 months). All-cause mortality was similar in patients receiving tiotropium or placebo.

In a long-term, randomized, double-blind, double-dummy, active-controlled trial (Tiotropium Safety and Performance in Respimat [TIOSPIR]) with an observation period of up to 3 years, all-cause mortality was found to be similar in patients receiving tiotropium oral inhalation powder compared with those receiving tiotropium oral inhalation solution.

Efficacy of tiotropium oral inhalation solution was based principally on 5 confirmatory, placebo- and active-controlled studies of 12–48 weeks' duration. In the randomized, double-blind, placebo- and/or active-controlled trials, efficacy of tiotropium oral inhalation solution was evaluated in 6614 patients with COPD; patients were 40 years of age or older, had a history of smoking greater than 10 pack-years, an FEV_1 of 60% of predicted or less, and a baseline FEV_1/forced vital capacity (FVC) of 0.7 or less. The primary outcome measure was the change from baseline in trough FEV_1. All study medications were administered once daily in the morning via the Respimat® inhaler. In these studies, trough FEV_1 was improved by 100–140 mL with tiotropium compared with placebo. In the 3 trials that evaluated COPD exacerbations, tiotropium oral inhalation solution at a dosage of 5 mcg once daily reduced the rate of exacerbations compared with placebo.

Efficacy of tiotropium in fixed combination with olodaterol hydrochloride was based principally on 2 dose-ranging studies of 4 weeks' duration and 2 confirmatory, active-controlled studies of 52 weeks' duration. In the 2 randomized, double-blind, active-controlled, parallel-group trials, efficacy of tiotropium in combination with olodaterol was evaluated in 5162 patients 40 years of age or older with moderate to very severe COPD. The primary outcome measures were the change from baseline in FEV_1 AUC from 0–3 hours and trough FEV_1 after 24 weeks of therapy. All study medications were administered once daily in the morning via the Respimat® inhaler. In these studies, FEV_1 AUC from 0–3 hours at 24 weeks was improved by 256–268 mL with orally inhaled tiotropium 5 mcg in combination with olodaterol 5 mcg compared with improvements of 139–165 or 133–136 mL with either tiotropium 5 mcg or olodaterol 5 mcg, respectively, alone. Trough FEV_1 at 24 weeks was improved by 136–145 mL with tiotropium in combination with olodaterol compared with improvements of 65–96 or 54–57 mL with either tiotropium or olodaterol, respectively, alone. The increased bronchodilator effects observed with tiotropium in combination with olodaterol were maintained throughout the 52-week studies. Patients receiving the fixed combination of tiotropium and olodaterol required less albuterol as rescue therapy compared with those receiving either tiotropium or olodaterol alone.

For additional information on the treatment of COPD, see Uses: Chronic Obstructive Pulmonary Disease, in Ipratropium Bromide 12:08.08.

Asthma

Tiotropium bromide oral inhalation solution is used for the long-term maintenance treatment of reversible bronchospasm associated with asthma. Orally inhaled tiotropium solution is *not* indicated for the treatment of acute episodes of bronchospasm; a drug with a more rapid onset of action (e.g., a short-acting β-adrenergic agonist) should be used in such cases. Tiotropium bromide in fixed combination with olodaterol hydrochloride is *not* indicated for the treatment of asthma.

Efficacy of tiotropium oral inhalation solution for the treatment of persistent asthma in adults was based principally on 5 randomized, double-blind, placebo-controlled studies of 12–48 weeks' duration. In the randomized, double-blind, placebo- and/or active-controlled trials, efficacy of orally inhaled tiotropium solution was evaluated in 3476 patients 18–75 years of age with a diagnosis of asthma who were receiving baseline therapy with at least inhaled corticosteroids. The primary outcome measure in all of the studies was the change from baseline in peak FEV_1 at 0–3 hours at week 12 or 24. In 2 trials, an additional primary outcome measure was change from baseline in trough FEV_1 at week 24. Patients randomized to receive tiotropium oral inhalation solution received the drug once daily via the Respimat® inhaler. In these studies, peak FEV_1 at 0–3 hours was improved by 160–240 mL with tiotropium compared with placebo. In the 3 trials that evaluated orally inhaled tiotropium dosages of 2.5 or 5 mcg once daily, FEV_1 response was generally lower for the 5-mcg dose compared with the 2.5-mcg dose. Improvement in lung function with tiotropium compared with placebo was maintained for 24 hours. The bronchodilator effects of tiotropium 2.5 mcg once daily were apparent after the first dose; however, maximum bronchodilator effect was not achieved for up to 4–8 weeks.

Efficacy of tiotropium oral inhalation solution for the treatment of persistent asthma in pediatric patients was based on extrapolation of efficacy in adults and on several randomized, double-blind, placebo-controlled studies of 12–48 weeks' duration. The primary outcome measure in these studies was the change from baseline in peak FEV_1 at 0–3 hours at week 12 or 24. In adolescents, 2 clinical studies evaluated efficacy of orally inhaled tiotropium solution in 789 patients 12–17 years of age with a diagnosis of asthma who were receiving baseline therapy with at least inhaled corticosteroids. Patients randomized to receive tiotropium oral inhalation solution were administered 2.5 or 5 mcg of the drug once daily via the Respimat® inhaler. In these studies, peak FEV_1 at 0–3 hours was improved by 110–130 mL with tiotropium 2.5 mcg once daily compared with placebo.

In children, 2 clinical studies evaluated efficacy of tiotropium oral inhalation solution in 801 patients 6–11 years of age with a diagnosis of asthma who were receiving baseline therapy with at least inhaled corticosteroids. Patients randomized to receive tiotropium oral inhalation solution were administered 2.5 or 5 mcg of the drug once daily via the Respimat® inhaler. In the 48-week study, peak FEV_1 at 0–3 hours was improved by 170 mL with tiotropium 2.5 mcg once daily compared with placebo. The efficacy results from the 12-week study were not statistically significant.

DOSAGE AND ADMINISTRATION

● General

Dosage of tiotropium bromide, which is commercially available as the monohydrate, is expressed in terms of anhydrous tiotropium.

Although each capsule under the foil lid of the blister strip contains 18 mcg of tiotropium as an inhalation powder, the precise amount of drug delivered to the lungs with each activation of the HandiHaler® device depends on factors such as the patient's inspiratory flow. Peak inspiratory flow through the HandiHaler® device also varies according to the exposure time of the capsule outside of the blister pack. Using standardized in vitro testing at a flow rate of 39 L/minute for 3.1 seconds, the HandiHaler® inhaler delivered a mean of 10.4 mcg of tiotropium per activation from the mouthpiece.

Each activation of the oral inhalation device containing tiotropium bromide oral inhalation solution (Spiriva® Respimat®) delivers 1.56 or 3.1 mcg of tiotropium bromide monohydrate (equivalent to 1.25 or 2.5 mcg, respectively, of tiotropium) from the mouthpiece. Each activation of the oral inhalation device containing tiotropium and olodaterol in fixed combination (Stiolto® Respimat®) delivers 3.1 mcg of tiotropium bromide monohydrate (equivalent to 2.5 mcg of tiotropium) and 2.7 mcg of olodaterol hydrochloride (equivalent to 2.5 mcg of olodaterol) from the mouthpiece. The precise amount of drug delivered to the lungs with each activation of the inhaler device depends on factors such as the

patient's coordination between actuation of the inhaler and inspiration through the delivery system. Because the Respimat® inhaler mechanically releases the dose, the delivered dose is independent of the patient's inspiratory effort. The commercially available inhalers deliver 60 metered sprays (not including the initial priming actuations) equivalent to 30 doses (2 actuations per dose) of the drug.

● Administration

Oral Inhalation via Dry Powder Inhaler

Tiotropium bromide dry-powder capsules are administered by oral inhalation *only* using a special oral inhalation device (HandiHaler®) that delivers powdered drug from capsules. Tiotropium bromide capsules for oral inhalation must not be taken orally, as the intended effects on the lungs will not be obtained.

To obtain optimal benefit, the patient should be given a copy of the patient instructions provided by the manufacturer. To use the inhaler, the dust cap of the inhaler should be opened by pressing the green piercing button. The dust cap on the side opposite the hinge on the gray base should be pulled upward to expose the mouthpiece. The mouthpiece of the inhaler should be opened by pulling the mouthpiece ridge upward on the side opposite the hinge on the gray base to expose the center chamber. The blister card should be carefully opened to expose only one capsule immediately before use. The capsule contains only a small amount of powder and should not be opened. The capsule should then be placed into the center chamber of the inhaler. After the capsule is loaded, the inhaler mouthpiece should be closed firmly until it snaps (clicks) into position; the dust cap is left open (up). Patients should push down on the mouthpiece ridge to make sure that the mouthpiece is seated in the gray base of the inhaler. While holding the inhaler with the seated mouthpiece upward, the green piercing button on the side of the inhaler should be completely depressed (green button is flush with the gray base of the inhaler) and then released. The button pierces the capsule and disperses the powdered drug upon inspiration; the piercing button should not be pressed more than one time and the Handihaler® device should not be shaken. Piercing the capsule may produce small gelatin pieces, which may pass into the mouth or throat during inhalation of the drug; the gelatin pieces should not cause any harm.

Before inhaling the dose, the patient should exhale as completely as possible, being careful not to exhale into the HandiHaler® device. The inhaler device should be held along the sides of the gray base taking care not to block the air intake vents near the mouthpiece ridge. With the head kept level, the patient should place the mouthpiece of the inhaler between the lips (inhaler is in horizontal position) and inhale deeply and slowly through the inhaler at a rate sufficient to hear or feel the loaded capsule vibrate. Pressure from the inhalation will disperse drug from the center chamber into the air stream created by the patient's inhalation. After a complete inhalation, the patient should remove the inhaler from the mouth and hold their breath for a few seconds, then resume normal breathing. The patient should breathe out completely and inhale once again to ensure full delivery of the powder from the same loaded, pierced capsule. *The green piercing button should not be pressed again.* Upon completion of the second inhalation, the patient should open the mouthpiece and tip the inhaler device to dispose of the used capsule. The mouthpiece and dust cap of the inhaler device should then be closed.

If the patient does not feel or hear the capsule vibrate upon inhalation, the inhaler device should be tapped gently on a table while holding the device in an upright position. The patient then should check to see that the mouthpiece is properly seated in the gray base. The patient should attempt to inhale through the device again. If capsule vibration still cannot be heard or felt during inhalation, the capsule should be discarded and the base of the device should be opened by lifting the green piercing button; the center chamber should be checked for pieces of the capsule. The device should be turned upside down and gently but firmly tapped to remove any capsule pieces, then the clinician should be contacted for instructions. (See Advice to Patients.)

Dry-powder capsules for oral inhalation should be left in foil-sealed blisters until immediately before use. Used or unused dry-powder capsules should not be stored in the inhaler device. The foil of the blister pack should not be cut nor should sharp objects be used to remove the capsule selected for dosing. If additional capsules are inadvertently opened and exposed to air (i.e., not intended for immediate use), they should be discarded since the effectiveness of the drug in those capsules may be reduced.

If patients taking tiotropium do not experience an improvement in control of COPD, a clinician should make sure that the patient is inhaling the drug using the oral inhaler rather than swallowing the dry-powder capsules. (See Accidental Oral Ingestion under Warnings/Precautions, in Cautions.)

The HandiHaler® device should be cleaned as needed. The dust cap and mouthpiece should be opened, and then the base should be opened by lifting the green piercing button. Any capsule pieces or powder buildup in the center chamber should be tapped out. The inhaler should be rinsed with warm water (cleaning agents or detergents should not be used), pressing the green piercing button a few times so that the center chamber and piercing needle are under the running water to remove any remaining powder or capsule pieces. The inhaler should be dried thoroughly and the dust cap, mouthpiece, and gray base left open and fully spread out to air dry for 24 hours. A hair dryer should not be used to dry the device. The inhaler should not be used when wet. If needed, the outside of the mouthpiece may be cleaned with a clean, damp cloth.

Oral Inhalation via Metered-Dose Inhaler

Tiotropium bromide solution is administered by oral inhalation using a specific inhaler (Spiriva® Respimat®) that delivers a metered-dose spray. Tiotropium bromide in fixed combination with olodaterol hydrochloride is administered by oral inhalation using a specific inhaler (Stiolto® Respimat®) that delivers a metered-dose spray. Both inhalers deliver the drugs in an aqueous solution and mechanically produce a fine aerosol mist from the orally inhaled solution. Tiotropium bromide alone or in fixed combination with olodaterol should be administered once daily at the same time every day.

Before first use of either Spiriva® Respimat® or Stiolto® Respimat®, the inhaler cartridge should be placed into the inhaler. The manufacturer's prescribing information should be consulted for detailed information on preparation of the inhalers. The discard date (3 months after the cartridge is inserted into the inhaler) should be written on the inhaler label.

After the cartridge has been inserted into either the Spiriva® Respimat® or the Stiolto® Respimat® inhaler, the unit must be primed prior to first use. Beginning with the inhaler held upright and the cap closed, the clear base should be turned in the direction of the black arrows on the label until a click is heard (one-half turn). The cap should then be flipped until it fully snaps open, the inhaler should be pointed away from the face, the dose release button pressed, and then the cap closed. These steps (turning the clear base until it clicks, opening the cap, actuating the inhaler, and replacing the cap) should be repeated until a spray is visible, and then for 3 additional times. The initial actuation step of the priming process (without the 3 additional repetitions) should be repeated after a period of nonuse (i.e., more than 3 days). If the inhaler is not used for more than 21 days, the entire initial priming process should be repeated.

To administer a dose of tiotropium alone or in fixed combination with olodaterol, the patient should hold the inhaler upright with the cap closed and turn the clear base in the direction of the black arrows on the label until a click is heard (one-half turn). The cap should be flipped until it snaps fully open. Before inhaling the dose, the patient should exhale slowly and completely. The patient should then close the lips around the end of the mouthpiece, without covering the air vents. With the inhaler pointing toward the back of the throat, the patient should press the dose release button while taking a slow, deep inhalation through the mouth; the patient should continue inhaling as long as possible. The patient should then hold the breath for 10 seconds (or as long as comfortable). This procedure should be repeated once more to administer the full dose (2 inhalations) of tiotropium alone or in combination with olodaterol. After the full dose is administered, the cap of the inhaler should be closed.

The mouthpiece of either the Spiriva® Respimat® or the Stiolto® Respimat® inhaler, including the metal part inside, should be cleaned using only a damp tissue or cloth at least once weekly. If the outside of the inhaler gets dirty, it can be wiped with a damp cloth. The function of the inhaler is not affected by minor discoloration in the mouthpiece.

● Dosage

Chronic Obstructive Pulmonary Disease

For the long-term management of reversible bronchospasm associated with chronic obstructive pulmonary disease (COPD), the usual dosage of tiotropium oral inhalation powder in adults is 18 mcg (2 inhalations, the contents of one capsule) once daily via the HandiHaler® device. No more than one dose should be taken in a 24-hour period. Orally inhaled tiotropium powder should not be used for the treatment of acute episodes of bronchospasm.

For the long-term management of reversible bronchospasm associated with COPD, the usual dosage of tiotropium oral inhalation solution in adults is 5 mcg (2 inhalations of the 2.5 mcg per metered-dose spray) once daily via the Respimat® device. No more than one dose should be taken in a 24-hour period.

Orally inhaled tiotropium solution should not be used for the treatment of acute episodes of bronchospasm.

Asthma

For the long-term management of reversible bronchospasm associated with asthma, the usual dosage of tiotropium oral inhalation solution in patients 6 years of age or older is 2.5 mcg (2 inhalations of the 1.25 mcg per metered-dose spray) once daily via the Respimat® device. No more than one dose (2 inhalations) should be taken in a 24-hour period. Orally inhaled tiotropium solution should not be used for the treatment of acute episodes of bronchospasm.

● Special Populations

The manufacturer states that adjustment of tiotropium dosage is not necessary in geriatric patients or patients with hepatic or renal impairment. (See Renal Impairment under Warnings/Precautions: Specific Populations, in Cautions.)

CAUTIONS

● Contraindications

Known hypersensitivity to tiotropium, ipratropium, or any ingredient in the formulation.

● Warnings/Precautions

Sensitivity Reactions

Immediate hypersensitivity reactions, including angioedema (e.g., swelling of the lips, tongue, or throat), urticaria, rash, bronchospasm, anaphylaxis, or itching, may occur after administration of tiotropium. If such a reaction occurs, the drug should be discontinued immediately and alternative therapy considered.

Patients with a history of hypersensitivity reactions to atropine or its derivatives should be closely monitored for hypersensitivity reactions. In addition, tiotropium oral inhalation powder (Spiriva® HandiHaler®) should be used with caution in patients with severe hypersensitivity to milk proteins.

Use of Fixed Combinations

When tiotropium is used in fixed combination with olodaterol, the usual cautions, precautions, contraindications, and interactions associated with olodaterol must be considered. Cautionary information applicable to specific populations (e.g., pregnant or nursing women, individuals with hepatic or renal impairment, geriatric patients) should be considered for each drug in the fixed combination.

Acute Bronchospasm

Tiotropium bromide should not be used for the relief of acute symptoms (i.e., as rescue therapy for the treatment of acute episodes of bronchospasm).

Possible Increased Risk of Stroke, Mortality, and/or Cardiovascular Events

While data are conflicting, a possible increased risk of stroke has been identified by the manufacturer from ongoing safety monitoring and pooled analysis of placebo-controlled trials in patients receiving tiotropium therapy. Other observational data have suggested an increased risk of mortality and/or cardiovascular events in patients receiving the drug.

Analysis of data on approximately 13,500 patients with COPD in 29 studies indicated a stroke case rate of 8 or 6 per 1000 patient-years of exposure in patients receiving tiotropium or placebo, respectively, representing an absolute excess risk of 2 additional strokes per 1000 patient-years. In addition, data from an observational study involving over 32,000 patients and another pooled analysis of 17 studies enrolling almost 15,000 patients have shown an increased risk of mortality and/or cardiovascular events in patients receiving inhaled anticholinergic agents, including tiotropium bromide. However, the results of a placebo-controlled trial (Understanding Potential Long-term Impacts on Function with Tiotropium [UPLIFT]) in approximately 6000 patients with COPD did not reveal an increased risk of stroke, myocardial infarction (MI), or cardiovascular death with tiotropium bromide. Based on a review of the UPLIFT trial, FDA has concluded that the available data do not support an association between the use of tiotropium oral inhalation powder and an increased risk of stroke, MI, or cardiovascular death.

An increased risk of mortality with tiotropium oral inhalation solution compared with placebo has been reported in some meta-analyses and data reviews; however, in a long-term, randomized, double-blind, double-dummy, active-controlled trial (Tiotropium Safety and Performance in Respimat [TIOSPIR]) with an observation period of up to 3 years, all-cause mortality was found to be similar in patients receiving tiotropium oral inhalation powder and those receiving tiotropium oral inhalation solution. In addition, no increased risk of death was observed in patients with a history of cardiac disease (including stable cardiac arrhythmias at baseline) receiving tiotropium oral inhalation solution compared with those receiving tiotropium oral inhalation powder.

Increases in corrected QT (QT$_c$) interval have been reported in patients receiving tiotropium oral inhalation powder. In a multicenter, randomized, double-blind trial in 198 patients with COPD, changes from baseline-corrected QT interval (using either the Bazett or Fridericia corrections) of 30–60 msec occurred in more patients receiving tiotropium compared with those receiving placebo. In other clinical trials, an effect of the drug on QT$_c$ intervals was not observed. In a crossover, placebo-controlled study of tiotropium oral inhalation powder in healthy individuals, the maximum mean change from baseline in study-specific QT$_c$ compared with placebo was 3.2 or 0.8 msec in patients receiving tiotropium 18 or 54 mcg, respectively.

Paradoxical Bronchospasm

Acute paradoxical bronchospasm may occur. If such a reaction occurs, it should be treated immediately with a short-acting inhaled β$_2$-adrenergic agonist; tiotropium should be discontinued and alternative therapy considered.

Ocular Effects

Tiotropium may worsen angle-closure glaucoma. The drug should be used with caution in patients with angle-closure glaucoma. If signs or symptoms of acute angle-closure glaucoma (e.g., ocular pain or discomfort, blurred vision, visual halos, or colored images in association with conjunctival congestion and corneal edema) occur, patients should consult a clinician immediately. (See Advice to Patients.) Miotic eye drops alone are not considered effective treatment for this condition.

Temporary blurring of vision or pupillary dilation may occur following inadvertent contact of tiotropium with the eyes. Care should be taken to avoid contact of the drug with the eyes during oral inhalation. (See Advice to Patients.)

Genitourinary Effects

Urinary retention/difficulty or urinary tract infection has been reported with tiotropium therapy. Tiotropium may worsen symptoms and signs of urinary retention (e.g., dysuria); patients should be carefully monitored for such signs and symptoms, especially those with prostatic hyperplasia or bladder neck obstruction. A clinician should be consulted immediately if such effects occur. Tiotropium should be used with caution in patients with urinary retention.

Accidental Oral Ingestion

Acute intoxication by inadvertent oral ingestion of the dry-powder capsules for oral inhalation is unlikely since tiotropium is not well absorbed systemically. Few patients have reported adverse effects following ingestion of the dry-powder capsules.

Specific Populations

Pregnancy

Category C. (See Users Guide.)

Limited human data regarding use of orally inhaled tiotropium solution during pregnancy are inadequate to inform a drug-associated risk. However, poorly or moderately controlled asthma during pregnancy may increase the maternal risk of preeclampsia and the infant's risk for prematurity, low birth weight, and small size for gestational age. The level of asthma control should be closely monitored in pregnant women and therapy adjusted as needed to maintain optimal control.

Animal studies have not revealed evidence of structural abnormalities at tiotropium dosages of approximately 790 or 8 times the maximum recommended human daily inhalation dosage administered to pregnant rats or rabbits, respectively, during the period of organogenesis. However, tiotropium administration resulted in fetal resorption, fetal loss, decreased number of live pups at birth, decreased mean pup weights, and delays in pup sexual maturation in rats receiving approximately 40 times the maximum recommended human daily inhalation dosage. In pregnant rabbits, tiotropium administration resulted in increased postimplantation fetal loss at dosages of approximately 430 times the maximum recommended human daily inhalation dosage. These adverse fetal effects were not

observed at tiotropium dosages approximately 5 or 95 times the maximum recommended human daily inhalation dosage in pregnant rats and rabbits, respectively.

Lactation

Tiotropium is distributed into milk in rodents. The drug and/or its metabolites are present in milk of lactating rats at concentrations higher than those in plasma. It is not known whether tiotropium is distributed into milk in humans. Effects of the drug on breast-fed infants or milk production also are not known. The benefits of breast-feeding and the woman's clinical need for tiotropium should be considered along with any potential adverse effects on the breast-fed infant from the drug or from the underlying maternal condition. The manufacturer recommends that orally inhaled tiotropium be used with caution in nursing women.

Pediatric Use

Safety and efficacy of orally inhaled tiotropium powder have not been established in children younger than 18 years of age. Tiotropium oral inhalation powder is not indicated for use in pediatric patients.

Safety and efficacy of orally inhaled tiotropium solution for the treatment of asthma have been established in pediatric patients 6–17 years of age in several clinical trials up to 1 years' duration. In 3 of these trials, 327 adolescents 12–17 years of age with asthma received tiotropium oral inhalation solution at a dosage of 2.5 mcg once daily. In 3 additional studies, 345 patients 6–11 years of age with asthma received tiotropium oral inhalation solution at a dosage of 2.5 mcg once daily. Safety and efficacy of the drug in these pediatric patients were similar to the effects in patients 18 years of age or older with asthma receiving the drug.

Safety and efficacy of orally inhaled tiotropium solution have not been established in children younger than 6 years of age.

Geriatric Use

The frequency of dry mouth, constipation, and urinary tract infection increased with age in clinical trials of tiotropium. However, no overall differences in efficacy were observed in geriatric patients relative to younger adults. The manufacturer states that adjustment of tiotropium dosage in geriatric patients is not necessary.

Hepatic Impairment

The pharmacokinetics of tiotropium have not been studied in patients with hepatic impairment.

Renal Impairment

Since tiotropium is excreted predominantly by the kidneys, the manufacturer recommends that patients with moderate to severe renal impairment (creatinine clearance of less than 60 mL/minute) be monitored closely for anticholinergic effects while receiving tiotropium therapy.

● Common Adverse Effects

Adverse reactions occurring in at least 3% of patients with COPD receiving tiotropium oral inhalation powder in long-term clinical trials and at a frequency at least 1% greater than with placebo include upper respiratory tract infection, dry mouth, sinusitis, pharyngitis, urinary tract infection, chest pain (nonspecific), rhinitis, dyspepsia, headache, abdominal pain, edema (dependent), arthralgia, constipation, depression, insomnia, vomiting, infection, moniliasis, epistaxis, myalgia, and rash.

Adverse reactions occurring in more than 3% of patients with COPD receiving tiotropium oral inhalation solution in clinical trials and more frequently than with placebo include pharyngitis, cough, dry mouth, and sinusitis.

Adverse reactions occurring in more than 2% of patients with asthma receiving tiotropium oral inhalation solution in clinical trials and more frequently than with placebo include pharyngitis, headache, bronchitis, and sinusitis.

Adverse effects occurring in more than 3% of patients with COPD receiving tiotropium 5 mcg daily in fixed combination with olodaterol 5 mcg daily and more frequently than in patients receiving either drug alone include nasopharyngitis, cough, and back pain.

DRUG INTERACTIONS

● Histamine H$_2$-Antagonists

Pharmacokinetic interaction (increased area under the concentration-time curve [AUC$_{0-4h}$], decreased renal clearance of IV tiotropium [not currently available in the US]) with concomitant cimetidine but not ranitidine. Pharmacokinetic interactions between tiotropium bromide and histamine H_2-antagonists not considered clinically important.

● **Other Drugs**

Tiotropium has been used concomitantly with sympathomimetic bronchodilators, methylxanthines, oral or inhaled corticosteroids, antihistamines, mucolytics, leukotriene modifiers, mast-cell stabilizers, and anti-IgE monoclonal antibody therapy without apparent increases in adverse effects. Use of tiotropium with other anticholinergic drugs (e.g., ipratropium) may cause increased anticholinergic effects, and is therefore not recommended by the manufacturer.

DESCRIPTION

Tiotropium bromide is a nonselective competitive antagonist at muscarinic (M_1–M_5) receptors. Tiotropium competitively and reversibly inhibits the actions of acetylcholine and other cholinergic stimuli at M_3 receptors in the smooth muscle of the respiratory tract, leading to bronchodilation.

Most of a dose of orally inhaled tiotropium powder is swallowed. The drug is minimally absorbed into systemic circulation from the GI tract (bioavailability administered as an oral solution is 2–3%); the fraction reaching the lungs (about 20%) appears to be readily absorbed. Following administration of the oral inhalation solution, approximately 33% of an inhaled dose reaches the systemic circulation. In a pharmacokinetic study in patients with chronic obstructive pulmonary disease (COPD), similar systemic exposure was observed following once-daily administration of the oral inhalation powder (18 mcg) or the oral inhalation solution (5 mcg). In patients with asthma, peak and total systemic exposure of the drug following oral inhalation of the solution is similar between adults and pediatric patients (6–17 years of age). Maximum bronchodilator effects may take up to 4–8 weeks of therapy in patients with asthma.

Following oral inhalation of tiotropium powder in young healthy individuals, approximately 14% of an administered dose is eliminated in urine, principally as unchanged drug. Urinary excretion of unchanged drug following oral inhalation of tiotropium powder in patients with COPD was 7% over 24 hours. Following oral inhalation of tiotropium solution 5 mcg once daily for 21 days in patients with COPD, approximately 19% of the dose was excreted in urine over 24 hours. Following administration of tiotropium solution 2.5 mcg in patients with asthma, approximately 13% of an inhaled dose was excreted unchanged in urine over 24 hours. Tiotropium is metabolized to a limited extent by the cytochrome P-450 (CYP) microsomal enzyme system, principally by isoenzymes 2D6 and 3A4.

ADVICE TO PATIENTS

Provide a copy of the manufacturer's patient information (medication guide) and instructions for use to all patients each time the drug is dispensed. Importance of instructing patients to read the medication guide prior to initiation of therapy and each time the prescription is refilled.

Importance of informing a clinician of allergies to any medications prior to initiation of tiotropium bromide therapy.

Importance of adequate understanding of proper storage, preparation, and inhalation techniques, including use of the inhalation delivery system (Handi-Haler® or Respimat®).

Importance of instructing caregivers to assist children with use of the Respimat® inhalation device.

Importance of not using the HandiHaler® or Respimat® device to administer other drugs.

Importance of informing a clinician of faulty inhaler performance (i.e., failure to hear or feel capsule vibrate) when certain procedures (i.e., confirming that the mouthpiece is firmly seated in gray base, tapping inhaler gently on a table) do not improve inhaler (Handihaler®) performance.

Importance of storing tiotropium dry-powder capsules in sealed blisters and of removing only one capsule immediately before use; unused additional capsules that are exposed to air should be discarded.

Importance of avoiding contact of the drug with the eyes since this may cause blurred vision and pupillary dilation.

Importance of not using tiotropium therapy to relieve acute symptoms or exacerbations of asthma or chronic obstructive pulmonary disease (COPD).

Importance of advising patients with asthma that maximum benefits may only be apparent after 4–8 weeks of treatment with tiotropium inhalation solution (Spiriva® Respimat®).

Risk of immediate hypersensitivity reactions such as anaphylaxis, angioedema (e.g., swelling of the lips, tongue, or throat), urticaria, rash, bronchospasm, or itching. If such signs and/or symptoms occur, tiotropium should be discontinued immediately and a clinician consulted.

Risk of paradoxical bronchospasm. If paradoxical bronchospasm occurs, tiotropium should be discontinued.

Risk of worsening of angle-closure glaucoma. Importance of immediately informing a clinician if eye pain or discomfort, blurred vision, or visual halos or colored images in association with conjunctival congestion or corneal edema occur.

Importance of advising patients to use caution when engaging in activities (e.g., driving a vehicle, operating appliances or machinery) since the drug may cause dizziness or blurred vision.

Risk of worsening of urinary retention. Importance of immediately informing a clinician if symptoms of urinary retention (e.g., dysuria) occur.

Importance of keeping drug out of reach of children.

Importance of informing clinicians of existing or contemplated therapy, including prescription and OTC drugs (e.g., eye drops) and herbal supplements, as well as any concomitant illnesses (e.g., urinary difficulty, enlarged prostate, narrow angle glaucoma).

Importance of women informing clinicians if they are or plan to become pregnant or plan to breast-feed.

Importance of informing patients of other important precautionary information. (See Cautions.)

PREPARATIONS

Excipients in commercially available drug preparations may have clinically important effects in some individuals; consult specific product labeling for details.

Tiotropium Bromide

Oral Inhalation

Powder for inhalation (contained in capsules)	18 mcg (of anhydrous tiotropium)	Spiriva® HandiHaler®, Boehringer Ingelheim, (comarketed by Pfizer)
Solution for inhalation	1.25 mcg (of tiotropium) per metered spray	Spiriva® Respimat®, Boehringer Ingelheim
	2.5 mcg (of tiotropium) per metered spray	Spiriva® Respimat®, Boehringer Ingelheim

Tiotropium Bromide Combinations

Oral Inhalation

Solution for inhalation	2.5 mcg (of tiotropium) with Olodaterol Hydrochloride 2.5 mcg (of olodaterol) per metered spray	Stiolto® Respimat®, Boehringer Ingelheim

Selected Revisions October 23, 2017, © Copyright, January 1, 2005, American Society of Health-System Pharmacists, Inc.

Lofexidine Hydrochloride

12:12.04 • α-ADRENERGIC AGONISTS

■ Lofexidine hydrochloride is a selective central α₂-adrenergic agonist.

USES

• Opiate Withdrawal

Lofexidine hydrochloride is used for mitigation of opiate withdrawal symptoms to facilitate abrupt opiate discontinuance.

In patients with opiate use disorder, opiate withdrawal management (also referred to as detoxification) generally involves short-term use of tapering dosages of buprenorphine (an opiate partial agonist) or methadone (a full opiate agonist) to reduce withdrawal symptoms. However, prescribing restrictions may limit use of these drugs, and α₂-adrenergic agonists (e.g., lofexidine, clonidine) also have been used for symptomatic relief of noradrenergic-mediated opiate withdrawal symptoms (e.g., lacrimation, sweating, shivering, rhinorrhea) in both inpatient and outpatient settings and may allow for withdrawal over a shorter period of time. The α₂-adrenergic agonists appear to be less effective than buprenorphine or methadone in the management of opiate withdrawal, and some experts suggest that α₂-adrenergic agonists may be most useful in withdrawal management as adjuncts to opiate agonists or partial agonists, to facilitate transition to opiate antagonist (naltrexone) treatment for relapse prevention, or in settings where therapy with opiate agonists or partial agonists is contraindicated, unacceptable, or unavailable. While α₂-adrenergic agonists relieve noradrenergic-mediated symptoms of opiate withdrawal, concomitant supportive therapy for other withdrawal symptoms (e.g., abdominal cramping, diarrhea, nausea and vomiting, muscle spasms, anxiety or restlessness, insomnia) may improve patient comfort, particularly in patients treated principally with an α₂-adrenergic agonist.

Although direct comparisons between lofexidine and clonidine are limited, results of several small comparative studies suggest that lofexidine and clonidine have similar efficacy in managing opiate withdrawal symptoms but lofexidine may be associated with less hypotension. However, the greater cost of lofexidine compared with off-label clonidine use also must be considered.

Because of the potential for hypotension and bradycardia, some experts state that α₂-adrenergic agonists are not drugs of choice for opiate withdrawal management in geriatric patients or patients with coronary insufficiency, ischemic heart disease, bradycardia, or cerebrovascular disease.

Lofexidine is not a treatment for opiate use disorder and should be used for mitigation of opiate withdrawal symptoms in patients with opiate use disorder only in conjunction with a comprehensive treatment program. Opiate withdrawal without subsequent maintenance treatment is associated with high rates of relapse. For most patients with opioid use disorder, maintenance treatment with buprenorphine or methadone or treatment with naltrexone for relapse prevention is superior to opiate withdrawal management.

In patients receiving long-term opiate analgesia, withdrawal symptoms generally are managed by slow tapering of the opiate analgesic dosage.

Clinical Experience

The current indication for lofexidine is based principally on the results of 2 randomized, double-blind, placebo-controlled, phase 3 studies in a total of 866 adults who were physically dependent on short-acting opiates (e.g., heroin, hydrocodone, oxycodone) and receiving inpatient treatment for withdrawal management. In both studies, lofexidine was associated with a reduced severity of opiate withdrawal symptoms (as measured by the Short Opiate Withdrawal Scale of Gossop [SOWS-Gossop]) and higher treatment completion rates compared with placebo. The SOWS-Gossop is a patient-reported outcome instrument used to evaluate the severity of 10 specific opiate withdrawal symptoms; each symptom is evaluated on a scale of 0–3 (corresponding to a rating of none, mild, moderate, or severe), and the total score (range: 0–30) is equal to the sum of the individual item scores. Patients in these studies could receive other concomitant supportive therapy for opiate withdrawal symptoms (e.g., guaifenesin, antacids, docusate, psyllium hydrocolloid suspension, bismuth sulfate, acetaminophen, zolpidem). The studies excluded patients with uncontrolled arrhythmias, corrected QT (QTc) interval prolongation (exceeding

450 msec in males or 470 msec in females), or other clinically important electrocardiographic (ECG) abnormalities; history of myocardial infarction; symptomatic hypotension, systolic blood pressure less than 95 mm Hg (study 1) or 90 mm Hg (study 2), or diastolic blood pressure less than 65 mm Hg (study 1); hypertension with blood pressure exceeding 155/95 mm Hg (study 1) or 160/100 mm Hg (study 2); symptomatic bradycardia or heart rate less than 55 beats/minute (study 1) or 45 beats/minute (study 2); or recent use of antihypertensive or antiarrhythmic agents.

In study 1, 602 patients were randomized to receive lofexidine 0.54 mg given 4 times daily, lofexidine 0.72 mg given 4 times daily, or placebo for 7 days in an inpatient setting. Patients who successfully completed days 1–7 of inpatient treatment were eligible to receive open-label treatment with lofexidine (up to 2.88 mg daily) for an additional 7 days (days 8–14). Mean SOWS-Gossop scores for days 1–7 were 6.5, 6.1, or 8.8 for patients receiving lofexidine 2.16 mg daily, lofexidine 2.88 mg daily, or placebo, respectively; 41, 40, or 28% of patients receiving these respective treatments completed 7 days of treatment.

In study 2, 264 patients were randomized to receive lofexidine 0.72 mg given 4 times daily or placebo for 5 days in an inpatient setting, followed by 2 additional days of placebo prior to discharge. Mean SOWS-Gossop scores for days 1–5 were 7 or 8.9 for patients receiving lofexidine or placebo, respectively; 49 or 33% of patients receiving these respective treatments completed 5 days of treatment.

DOSAGE AND ADMINISTRATION

• General

Vital signs should be assessed prior to lofexidine dosing. Electrocardiographic (ECG) monitoring is recommended in certain patients at risk for QT interval prolongation. (See Hypotension, Bradycardia, and Syncope and also see QT Interval Prolongation under Cautions: Warnings/Precautions.)

• Administration and Preparation

Lofexidine is administered orally 4 times daily (i.e., every 5–6 hours) without regard to meals.

• Dosage

Dosage of lofexidine hydrochloride is expressed in terms of lofexidine. Dosage of the drug also has been expressed in terms of the salt; 0.18 mg of lofexidine is equivalent to 0.2 mg of lofexidine hydrochloride.

The manufacturer states that the usual initial dosage of lofexidine for the mitigation of opiate withdrawal symptoms in adults is 2.16 mg daily administered in 4 divided doses of 0.54 mg every 5–6 hours during the period of peak withdrawal symptoms (generally the first 5–7 days following the last use of opiates), with dosage guided by symptoms and adverse effects. Lofexidine may be administered for up to 14 days, with dosage guided by symptoms. Single adult doses should not exceed 0.72 mg, and the total daily dosage should not exceed 2.88 mg.

Some experts recommend an initial lofexidine dosage of 0.36–0.54 mg twice daily and state that dosage may be increased as necessary and tolerated to a maximum of 2.16 mg daily administered in 2–4 divided doses for 7–10 days.

Dosage of lofexidine should be reduced or therapy with the drug should be interrupted or discontinued in individuals demonstrating greater sensitivity to its adverse effects. As opiate withdrawal symptoms wane, lower dosages of lofexidine may be appropriate.

When lofexidine therapy is discontinued, dosage of the drug should be reduced gradually (e.g., by 0.18 mg per dose every 1–2 days) over 2–4 days to minimize lofexidine withdrawal symptoms and rebound elevations in blood pressure. (See Symptoms Resulting from Abrupt Lofexidine Discontinuance under Cautions: Warnings/Precautions.)

• Special Populations

Hepatic Impairment

In patients with mild hepatic impairment (Child-Pugh score 5–6), the recommended dosage of lofexidine is 0.54 mg 4 times daily. In patients with moderate hepatic impairment (Child-Pugh score 7–9), the recommended dosage of lofexidine is 0.36 mg 4 times daily. In patients with severe hepatic impairment (Child-Pugh score exceeding 9), the recommended dosage of lofexidine is 0.18 mg 4 times daily. (See Hepatic Impairment under Warnings/Precautions: Specific Populations, in Cautions.)

Renal Impairment

The manufacturer provides no specific dosage recommendations for patients with mild renal impairment. In patients with moderate renal impairment (estimated glomerular filtration rate [eGFR] 30–89.9 mL/minute per 1.73 m²), the recommended dosage of lofexidine is 0.36 mg 4 times daily. In patients with severe renal impairment or end-stage renal disease (eGFR less than 30 mL/minute per 1.73 m²) or in patients receiving dialysis, the recommended dosage of lofexidine is 0.18 mg 4 times daily. Supplemental doses are not required following dialysis. Lofexidine may be administered without regard to the timing of dialysis. (See Renal Impairment under Warnings/Precautions: Specific Populations, in Cautions.)

Geriatric Patients

Dosage adjustments similar to those recommended in patients with renal impairment should be considered in geriatric patients.

CAUTIONS

● Contraindications

The manufacturer states there are no known contraindications to the use of lofexidine.

● Warnings/Precautions

Hypotension, Bradycardia, and Syncope

Lofexidine can cause hypotension, bradycardia, and syncope. In a phase 3 study in patients receiving inpatient treatment for opiate withdrawal (study 1), hypotension, orthostatic hypotension, bradycardia, and syncope were reported in approximately 30, 35, 28, and 1%, respectively, of lofexidine-treated patients. The incidence of serious cardiovascular effects was higher in women than in men receiving lofexidine 2.88 mg daily (4 versus 1%); similarly, bradycardia and orthostatic hypotension necessitating drug discontinuance or withholding of doses also occurred more frequently in women than in men receiving lofexidine 2.88 mg daily.

Vital signs should be assessed prior to lofexidine dosing, and patients receiving the drug should be monitored for symptoms of bradycardia and orthostatic hypotension.

Patients receiving lofexidine should be informed of the risk of hypotension. Those receiving the drug in the outpatient setting should be capable of performing self-monitoring for hypotension, orthostasis, bradycardia, and associated symptoms, and should be instructed on measures for reducing the risk of serious consequences should these adverse effects occur. Patients receiving lofexidine in the outpatient setting should be instructed to withhold doses of lofexidine during symptomatic episodes of hypotension or bradycardia and to contact their healthcare provider for guidance on dosage adjustment; following clinically important or symptomatic hypotension and/or bradycardia, the subsequent dose should be reduced in strength, delayed, or omitted. (See Advice to Patients.)

Use of lofexidine should be avoided in patients with severe coronary insufficiency, recent myocardial infarction, cerebrovascular disease, chronic renal failure, or marked bradycardia. To avoid the risk of excessive bradycardia and hypotension, concomitant use of lofexidine with drugs known to decrease heart rate or blood pressure also should be avoided.

QT Interval Prolongation

Lofexidine prolongs the QT interval. In healthy individuals, single 1.44- or 1.8-mg doses of lofexidine produced a maximum mean change from baseline in QT interval (corrected for heart rate using Fridericia's formula [QT_cF]) of 14.4 or 13.6 msec, respectively. In a phase 3, placebo-controlled, dose-response study in opiate-dependent patients, lofexidine 2.16 or 2.88 mg daily was associated with a maximum mean change in QT_cF of 7.3 or 9.3 msec, respectively. Torsades de pointes with cardiac arrest (with successful resuscitation) has been reported during postmarketing experience.

Clinically important QT interval prolongation may occur in patients with hepatic or renal impairment. Administration of lofexidine in patients with hepatic or renal impairment was associated with prolongation of the corrected QT interval; such effects were more pronounced in those with severe impairment.

Electrocardiographic (ECG) monitoring is recommended in patients with heart failure, bradyarrhythmias, or hepatic or renal impairment, and in those receiving other drugs known to prolong the QT interval (e.g., methadone). (See Drug Interactions: Drugs that Prolong the QT Interval.) In patients with electrolyte abnormalities (e.g., hypokalemia, hypomagnesemia), the electrolyte abnormalities should be corrected prior to initiation of lofexidine therapy, and ECG monitoring should be performed upon initiation of lofexidine. Use of lofexidine should be avoided in patients with congenital long QT syndrome.

Concomitant Use of CNS Depressants

Lofexidine potentiates the CNS depressive effects of benzodiazepines and also is expected to potentiate the CNS depressive effects of alcohol and other sedating drugs (e.g., barbiturates). (See Drug Interactions: CNS Depressants.)

Risk of Opiate Overdosage following Relapse to Opiate Use

Patients who complete opiate discontinuance are likely to have a reduced tolerance to opiates and are therefore at an increased risk of fatal opiate overdosage should they resume opiate use. Patients and caregivers should be informed of this increased risk of overdosage. Lofexidine is not a treatment for opiate use disorder and should be used for mitigation of opiate withdrawal symptoms in patients with opiate use disorder only in conjunction with a comprehensive treatment program.

Symptoms Resulting from Abrupt Lofexidine Discontinuance

Abrupt discontinuance of lofexidine can result in marked increases in blood pressure, with peak blood pressure values observed on the second day after abrupt discontinuance. A 50% reduction in lofexidine dosage one day prior to drug discontinuance resulted in a similar incidence and magnitude of blood pressure elevations as compared with abrupt discontinuance. Discontinuance of lofexidine also has been associated with diarrhea, insomnia, anxiety, chills, hyperhydrosis, and extremity pain.

When lofexidine therapy is discontinued, the dosage should be gradually reduced. (See Dosage and Administration: Dosage.) Symptoms related to drug discontinuance can be managed by resuming administration of the previous lofexidine dosage and subsequently tapering the dosage.

Specific Populations

Pregnancy

Safety of lofexidine has not been established in pregnant women. Oral administration of lofexidine during the period of organogenesis in pregnant rats and rabbits resulted in reduced fetal weights, increased fetal resorption, and loss of litters at exposures less than those achieved in humans. When the drug was administered orally from the beginning of organogenesis through lactation, increased stillbirths, loss of litters, and decreased viability and lactation indices resulted, and offspring demonstrated delays in sexual maturation (both males and females), auditory startle, and surface righting.

Experts state that the recommended treatment of opiate dependence in pregnant women is maintenance treatment with buprenorphine or methadone; this approach is superior to medically supervised withdrawal because withdrawal is associated with high relapse rates and poorer outcomes.

Lactation

It is not known whether lofexidine or its metabolites are distributed into milk. The effects of lofexidine or its metabolites on breast-fed infants or on milk production also are unknown. Lofexidine is chemically and pharmacologically related to clonidine, which reaches high concentrations in milk and in breast-fed infants. Caution should be exercised if lofexidine is administered to a nursing woman, especially while breast-feeding a neonate or preterm infant; the developmental and health benefits of breast-feeding and the importance of the drug to the woman should be considered along with the potential adverse effects on the breast-fed child from the drug or from the underlying maternal condition.

Pediatric Use

Safety and efficacy of lofexidine have not been established in pediatric patients.

Geriatric Use

Safety and efficacy of lofexidine have not been established in geriatric patients. Caution should be exercised when lofexidine is used in patients older than 65 years of age. (See Geriatric Patients under Dosage and Administration: Special Populations.)

Hepatic Impairment

Hepatic impairment decreases elimination of lofexidine but has less effect on peak plasma concentrations than on systemic exposure (i.e., area under the plasma concentration-time curve [AUC]) of the drug following a single dose;

dosage adjustment is recommended depending on the degree of hepatic impairment. (See Hepatic Impairment under Dosage and Administration: Special Populations.) Following administration of a single 0.36-mg dose of lofexidine, peak plasma concentration in patients with mild (Class-Pugh class A, score 5–6), moderate (Child-Pugh class B, score 7–9), or severe (Child-Pugh class C, score 10–15) hepatic impairment is 114, 117, or 166%, respectively, and systemic exposure is 117, 185, or 260%, respectively, compared with that in individuals with normal hepatic function. The half-life of the drug in these respective groups is 139, 281, or 401% of that in individuals with normal hepatic function.

Clinically important prolongation of the QT interval may occur in patients with hepatic impairment. QT interval prolongation was more pronounced in patients with severe hepatic impairment. ECG monitoring is recommended in patients with hepatic impairment.

Renal Impairment

Renal impairment decreases elimination of lofexidine but has less effect on peak plasma concentrations than on systemic exposure (AUC) of the drug following a single dose; dosage adjustment is recommended depending on the degree of renal impairment. (See Renal Impairment under Dosage and Administration: Special Populations.) Following administration of a single 0.36-mg dose of lofexidine, peak plasma concentration in patients with mild (estimated glomerular filtration rate [eGFR] 60–89 mL/minute per 1.73 m^2), moderate (eGFR 30–59 mL/minute per 1.73^2), or severe (eGFR 15–29 mL/minute per 1.73 m^2) renal impairment is 124, 117, or 154%, respectively, and systemic exposure is 144, 173, or 243%, respectively, compared with that in individuals with normal renal function (eGFR at least 90 mL/minute per 1.73 m^2). The half-life of the drug in these respective groups is 111, 145, or 157% of that in individuals with normal renal function.

In patients with end-stage renal disease receiving hemodialysis 3 times weekly, mean peak plasma concentration was similar to that in individuals with normal renal function matched for sex, age, and body mass index (BMI). Only a negligible fraction of a lofexidine dose is removed during a typical dialysis session. Decreases in lofexidine plasma concentrations occurring during a 4-hour dialysis session are transient, with a return to near predialysis concentrations within a few hours after completion of the dialysis session.

Clinically important prolongation of the QT interval may occur in patients with renal impairment. QT interval prolongation was more pronounced in patients with severe renal impairment. ECG monitoring is recommended in patients with renal impairment.

Pharmacogenomics and Poor CYP2D6 Metabolizers

Because increased systemic exposure to lofexidine is expected in patients who are poor metabolizers of cytochrome P-450 isoenzyme 2D6 (CYP2D6) substrates, these patients should be monitored for adverse effects (e.g., orthostatic hypotension, bradycardia). Lofexidine exposure in patients with the poor CYP2D6 metabolizer phenotype is expected to be similar to that observed in individuals receiving lofexidine concomitantly with a potent CYP2D6 inhibitor. (See Drug Interactions: Drugs Affecting Hepatic Microsomal Enzymes.)

● Common Adverse Effects

Adverse effects reported in clinical studies in 10% or more of opiate-dependent patients receiving lofexidine for mitigation of opiate withdrawal symptoms and occurring more frequently with lofexidine than with placebo include insomnia, orthostatic hypotension, bradycardia, hypotension, dizziness, somnolence, sedation, and dry mouth.

DRUG INTERACTIONS

In vitro studies indicate that lofexidine is extensively metabolized, principally by cytochrome P-450 (CYP) isoenzyme 2D6 and to a lesser extent by CYP1A2 and CYP2C19. Lofexidine and/or its metabolites cause slight inhibition of CYP2D6, but are unlikely to induce or inhibit major CYP isoenzymes at clinically relevant concentrations. Results from an in vitro study suggest that lofexidine is not a substrate of P-glycoprotein (P-gp).

● Drugs Affecting Hepatic Microsomal Enzymes

Use of lofexidine in combination with CYP2D6 inhibitors may increase lofexidine exposure. When lofexidine is used concomitantly with CYP2D6 inhibitors, patients should be monitored for adverse effects (e.g., orthostatic hypotension, bradycardia).

Paroxetine

Concomitant administration of lofexidine (single 0.36-mg dose) and the potent CYP2D6 inhibitor paroxetine (40 mg daily) in healthy individuals increased peak plasma concentration and systemic exposure of lofexidine by approximately 11 and 28%, respectively.

● Drugs Metabolized by Hepatic Microsomal Enzymes

Clinically important pharmacokinetic interactions of lofexidine with substrates of CYP2D6 are not expected.

● Cardiovascular Drugs

Concomitant use of lofexidine with drugs that are known to cause hypotension or bradycardia should be avoided.

● CNS Depressants

Lofexidine enhances the CNS depressive effects of benzodiazepines and also is expected to enhance the effects of other CNS depressants, such as alcohol, barbiturates, opiate agonists or partial agonists, and other sedating drugs.

● Drugs that Prolong the QT Interval

Lofexidine prolongs the QT interval. Electrocardiographic (ECG) monitoring is recommended when lofexidine is used concomitantly with other drugs that are known to prolong the QT interval.

● Tricyclic Antidepressants

Limited experience suggests that concomitant use of lofexidine with a tricyclic antidepressant may reduce the efficacy of lofexidine, resulting in exacerbation of opiate withdrawal symptoms.

Desipramine

Addition of desipramine hydrochloride (75 mg daily) to lofexidine therapy in a patient with substance (opiate, alcohol, and stimulant) use disorder resulted in exacerbation of opiate withdrawal symptoms (e.g., marked insomnia, feeling cold, twitching, yawning, runny eyes), which was reflected in increasing Short Opiate Withdrawal Scale of Gossop (SOWS-Gossop) scores. Desipramine was discontinued after 2 doses, and opiate withdrawal symptoms abated over the next 24 hours.

● Buprenorphine

In patients receiving maintenance treatment with buprenorphine (16–24 mg daily), concomitant use of lofexidine (up to 2.88 mg daily) resulted in no pharmacokinetic or pharmacodynamic interaction.

In patients receiving maintenance treatment with buprenorphine (16–24 mg daily), concomitant use of lofexidine (2.88 mg daily) resulted in a maximum mean increase from baseline in QT interval (corrected for heart rate using Fridericia's formula [QT_cF]) of 15 msec.

● Methadone

Lofexidine and methadone both prolong the QT interval. (See Drug Interactions: Drugs that Prolong the QT Interval.) In patients receiving maintenance treatment with methadone hydrochloride (80–120 mg daily), concomitant use of lofexidine (2.88 mg daily) resulted in a maximum mean increase from baseline in QT_cF of 9.1 msec.

In patients receiving maintenance treatment with methadone hydrochloride (80–120 mg daily), concomitant use of lofexidine (up to 2.88 mg daily) did not alter the pharmacokinetics of methadone. Lofexidine concentrations may be slightly increased, but the increase in concentration is not expected to be clinically important at recommended dosages.

● Naltrexone

Concomitant administration of oral naltrexone hydrochloride (50 mg daily) with lofexidine (single 0.36-mg dose) in healthy individuals did not result in clinically important changes in lofexidine pharmacokinetics; however, at naltrexone steady state, peak plasma naltrexone and 6-β-naltrexol concentrations were delayed by 2–3 hours and overall exposure to the opiate antagonist was reduced slightly. Administration of oral naltrexone within 2 hours of lofexidine administration may result in reduced efficacy of naltrexone; however, this interaction is not expected if naltrexone is administered via nonoral routes.

DESCRIPTION

Lofexidine hydrochloride, a centrally acting α_2-adrenergic agonist that is structurally and pharmacologically related to clonidine, binds to receptors on adrenergic neurons, reducing the release of norepinephrine and decreasing sympathetic tone. Lofexidine decreases sympathetic neurotransmission from the locus ceruleus, which is responsible for many opiate withdrawal symptoms during acute withdrawal. It has been postulated that lofexidine's greater selectivity for the α_{2A}-adrenergic receptor may be responsible for its improved adverse effect profile (e.g., decreased incidence and severity of hypotension and sedation) compared with structurally similar clonidine. Lofexidine is not an effective antihypertensive agent and does not suppress psychological cravings.

Pharmacokinetics of lofexidine are dose proportional over the dosage range of 0.72–2.88 mg daily. Absolute oral bioavailability of the drug is approximately 72%; approximately 30% of an orally administered dose is converted to inactive metabolites on first pass through the liver. Peak plasma concentrations are achieved 3–5 hours after a single oral dose. Administration of lofexidine with a high-fat, high-calorie meal did not alter peak plasma concentration or area under the concentration-time curve (AUC), and only slightly delayed the median time to peak plasma concentration (from 5 hours to 6 hours). Lofexidine is approximately 55% bound to plasma proteins. The volume of distribution of the drug suggests extensive distribution into tissues. Lofexidine is extensively metabolized, principally by cytochrome P-450 (CYP) isoenzyme 2D6 and to a lesser extent by CYP1A2 and CYP2C19. Lofexidine and its metabolites are eliminated principally by the kidneys; 93.5% of an administered dose is excreted in urine (15–20% as unchanged drug) and 0.9% is excreted in feces. The elimination half-life is approximately 12 hours. The terminal half-life is approximately 11–13 hours following the initial dose and approximately 17–22 hours at steady state. Pharmacokinetics were similar in opiate-dependent patients and healthy individuals.

ADVICE TO PATIENTS

Importance of reading the patient information provided by the manufacturer.

Importance of informing patients that lofexidine may lessen, but not completely prevent, symptoms associated with opiate withdrawal syndrome (e.g., feeling sick, stomach cramps, muscle spasms or twitching, feeling cold, palpitations, muscular tension, aches and pains, yawning, runny eyes, sleep disturbances). Additional supportive measures may be recommended as needed.

Risk of hypotension and bradycardia. Importance of advising patients to be alert for any symptoms of hypotension, orthostasis, or bradycardia (e.g., dizziness, lightheadedness, feelings of faintness at rest or on abrupt standing); to avoid dehydration and overheating; and to rise carefully from a seated or supine position. Importance of instructing patients on how to reduce the risk of serious consequences if hypotension occurs (e.g., by sitting or lying down). Patients experiencing symptomatic episodes of hypotension, orthostasis, or bradycardia in the outpatient setting should be advised to withhold lofexidine and contact their clinician for instructions.

Patients receiving lofexidine in the outpatient setting should be advised to avoid driving, operating heavy machinery, or performing other hazardous activities until they know how the drug will affect them. Risk of increased CNS depression with concomitant use of benzodiazepines, alcohol, barbiturates, or other drugs with sedative effects.

Importance of advising patients to avoid abrupt discontinuance of therapy and to consult a clinician prior to discontinuing therapy.

Risk of opiate overdosage if opiate use is resumed following a period of non-use (i.e., relapse). Importance of informing patients that they may be more sensitive to the effects of opiates and at greater risk of fatal overdosage if they resume opiate use after a period of nonuse.

Importance of women informing their clinicians if they are or plan to become pregnant or plan to breast-feed.

Importance of informing clinicians of existing or contemplated concomitant therapy, including prescription and OTC drugs and dietary or herbal supplements, as well as any concomitant illnesses (e.g., renal or hepatic impairment; cerebrovascular or cardiovascular disease).

Importance of informing patients of other important precautionary information. (See Cautions.)

PREPARATIONS

Excipients in commercially available drug preparations may have clinically important effects in some individuals; consult specific product labeling for details.

Lofexidine Hydrochloride

Oral

Tablets, film-coated	0.18 mg (of lofexidine)	Lucemyra®, US WorldMeds

Selected Revisions October 7, 2019, © Copyright, June 25, 2018, American Society of Health-System Pharmacists, Inc.

Phenylephrine Hydrochloride (Systemic)

12:12.04 • α-ADRENERGIC AGONISTS

■ Phenylephrine hydrochloride is a sympathomimetic amine that predominantly acts by a direct effect on α_1-adrenergic receptors.

USES

● Hypotension

Phenylephrine hydrochloride is used parenterally to increase blood pressure and provide hemodynamic support in the management of certain acute hypotensive states. Phenylephrine hydrochloride injection is labeled by the US Food and Drug Administration (FDA) for use in the setting of anesthesia or septic shock to treat clinically important hypotension resulting principally from vasodilation. Evidence supporting the use of IV phenylephrine is based on studies from the published literature, the majority of which were conducted in the perioperative setting. Only a few clinical studies have evaluated use of the drug in patients with septic shock. The available data clearly indicate that phenylephrine is effective in increasing and maintaining blood pressure in hypotensive patients. In patients who require vasopressor support, individual hemodynamic abnormalities must be identified and monitored so that therapy can be adjusted as necessary. If severe peripheral vasoconstriction exists, phenylephrine may be ineffective and have a deleterious effect by causing further reductions in plasma volume and blood flow to vital organs.

Hypotension During Anesthesia

Phenylephrine hydrochloride is used for the *treatment* of hypotension during anesthesia. Studies performed in a variety of surgical settings have demonstrated that phenylephrine increases systolic and mean arterial blood pressures when administered IV (as a direct "bolus" injection or continuous infusion) following the development of hypotension in patients receiving neuraxial and/or general anesthesia. In many of these studies, the drug was used in low-risk pregnant women undergoing cesarean section with neuraxial anesthesia. Although ephedrine historically has been considered the vasopressor of choice for treatment of hypotension in obstetric anesthesia, phenylephrine is increasingly being used in this setting because of evidence suggesting that the drug may provide a more favorable fetal acid-base balance.

Phenylephrine also has been used for the *prevention* of hypotension in patients undergoing spinal anesthesia. However, routine prophylactic use of vasopressors has been questioned because hypotension does not always occur during spinal anesthesia and treatment can readily be instituted if necessary; some clinicians have suggested that vasopressors be administered prophylactically only in those cases in which a substantial decrease in blood pressure is expected.

Septic Shock

Vasopressors are used in the management of vasodilatory shock, the most common form of which is septic shock, to restore blood pressure and tissue perfusion after initial fluid resuscitation is attempted. The Surviving Sepsis Campaign International Guidelines for Management of Sepsis and Septic Shock recommend norepinephrine as the first-line vasopressor of choice in adults with septic shock; if adequate blood pressure is not achieved, vasopressin or epinephrine may be added. Phenylephrine generally has been considered only in selected situations when norepinephrine cannot be used (e.g., because of tachyarrhythmias) or as salvage therapy when other treatment methods have failed. Although data are limited, studies have shown that phenylephrine increases mean arterial pressure in patients with septic shock; however, the regional hemodynamic effects of the drug (particularly in regards to renal blood flow and possible renal toxicity) have not been completely elucidated. (See Cautions: Adverse Effects.) Because of uncertainty regarding the clinical outcomes of phenylephrine therapy, experts currently state that use of the drug should be limited until more information is available.

Although vasopressors have been used in the management of other types of shock or shock-like states (e.g., hemorrhagic or cardiogenic shock), there is insufficient evidence to support the use of phenylephrine for blood pressure support in general shock settings, particularly those not associated with a vasodilatory component. If a vasopressor is required in these situations, norepinephrine usually is preferred.

● Prolongation of Spinal Anesthesia

Phenylephrine has been used as an additive to solutions of some local anesthetics to decrease the rate of vascular absorption of the anesthetic and prolong the duration of anesthesia†. The risk of systemic toxicity due to the local anesthetic is also decreased. (See Local Anesthetics, Parenteral, General Statement 72:00.) Phenylephrine is not as effective as epinephrine in prolonging local anesthesia but may be preferred when cardiostimulation is undesirable.

● Nasal Congestion

Phenylephrine hydrochloride is administered orally for *self-medication* as a nasal decongestant for temporary relief of nasal congestion associated with upper respiratory allergy (e.g., hay fever) or the common cold; the drug also is used to provide temporary relief of sinus congestion and pressure. Preparations containing phenylephrine in fixed combination with other agents (e.g., acetaminophen, chlorpheniramine, dextromethorphan, diphenhydramine, guaifenesin, pheniramine) are used for temporary relief of nasal/sinus congestion and/or other symptoms (e.g., rhinorrhea, sneezing, lacrimation, itching eyes, oronasopharyngeal itching, cough) associated with seasonal or perennial allergic rhinitis, other upper respiratory allergies, or the common cold. Because of state and federal actions restricting the sale and purchase of nonprescription preparations containing decongestants such as pseudoephedrine, ephedrine, or phenylpropanolamine (no longer commercially available in the US), some manufacturers reformulated various nonprescription pseudoephedrine-containing preparations by substituting phenylephrine for pseudoephedrine. (See Uses: Misuse and Abuse, in Pseudoephedrine 12:12.12.) However, few studies evaluating the efficacy of oral phenylephrine in the treatment of nasal congestion have been published, and efficacy of the drug at currently recommended oral dosages has been questioned by some clinicians.

Nasal decongestants, including phenylephrine, have been used for *self-medication* for the temporary relief of nasal congestion associated with sinusitis. However, prospective studies of nasal decongestants for this use are lacking, and data on their use as adjunctive therapy in the management of sinusitis are limited and controversial. Furthermore, evidence from an animal study indicated that topical nasal decongestants (i.e., oxymetazoline) may *increase* the degree of sinus inflammation, potentially delaying resolution of sinusitis. Because labeling for nonprescription (over-the-counter, OTC) nasal decongestant preparations previously included use for sinusitis, there were concerns that consumers would assume that nasal decongestants were effective in the treatment of sinusitis, thereby choosing *self-medication* over medical evaluation and definitive treatment by a clinician; such delay in medical evaluation could result in a lost opportunity for early diagnosis of another serious medical condition (e.g., bacterial sinusitis). The FDA no longer considers oral or topical nasal decongestants appropriate for *self-medication* of sinusitis. In October 2005, the agency issued a final rule, which was effective in 2007, that amended the final monograph for OTC nasal decongestant preparations to remove the indication for relief of nasal congestion associated with sinusitis from labeling and prohibited use of the term "sinusitis" elsewhere in labeling.

Phenylephrine also is applied topically to the nasal mucosa as a vasoconstrictor to relieve nasal congestion. (See Phenylephrine 52:32.)

● Hemorrhoids

Anorectal preparations (e.g., creams, gels, ointments, suppositories) containing phenylephrine hydrochloride are used *topically* or *rectally* to provide temporary symptomatic relief of external or internal hemorrhoids. When applied topically or rectally to the anorectal area, vasoconstrictors such as phenylephrine stimulate α-adrenergic receptors in the vascular beds with a resultant temporary constriction of arterioles and a modest and transient reduction in congestion (swelling) of hemorrhoidal tissues. Vasoconstrictors also may relieve anorectal pruritus, discomfort, and irritation, possibly in part secondary to some weak local anesthetic action; the mechanism of this local anesthetic effect is unknown. Phenylephrine also may relieve pruritus associated with histamine release. However, vasoconstrictors are expected to provide only partial relief of pruritus associated with hemorrhoids, and there are more effective agents for relief of anorectal itching. The presence of other ingredients in the formulation (e.g., protectants, local anesthetics, astringents, antipruritics, analgesics) may provide additional relief of these and other anorectal symptoms (e.g., discomfort, pain, burning) associated with hemorrhoids. Although locally applied vasoconstrictors have been shown to alter mucosal blood flow, safety and efficacy for *self-medication* control of minor hemorrhoidal bleeding have not been established. If minor bleeding is present, a clinician should be consulted promptly for advice because anorectal bleeding may be a sign of conditions ranging in seriousness from simple abrasions to cancer.

Effectiveness of topical or intrarectal therapy with phenylephrine for relief of symptoms secondary to swollen hemorrhoidal tissues is based on a predicted effect of the drug's vasoconstrictive activity in reducing capillary and arteriovenous congestion in the anorectal area rather than on specific efficacy studies. Effective dosage of anorectal therapy with the drug was based on predictions from established efficacy of local therapy for nasal congestion.

● Other Uses

For the use of phenylephrine as a mydriatic, see Phenylephrine Hydrochloride 52:24. For the use of phenylephrine as a vasoconstrictor in the eye or mucosa, see Phenylephrine Hydrochloride 52:32.

DOSAGE AND ADMINISTRATION

● Administration

Parenteral Administration

Phenylephrine hydrochloride injection concentrate is administered after dilution by direct IV ("bolus") injection or continuous IV infusion. The drug also has been administered by IM† or subcutaneous injection†. The route of administration should be determined by the specific clinical situation and needs of the individual patient. For treatment of hypotension during anesthesia, the manufacturers recommend administration of phenylephrine hydrochloride as an IV injection or continuous infusion; when used in the treatment of septic shock, the drug should be administered as a continuous IV infusion with no initial bolus dose.

Commercially available phenylephrine hydrochloride injection concentrate must be diluted with a compatible IV solution prior to administration as a direct IV ("bolus") injection or continuous infusion. To prepare solutions for direct IV injection, 1 mL of the commercially available phenylephrine hydrochloride injection containing 10 mg/mL should be withdrawn and diluted with 99 mL of 5% dextrose or 0.9% sodium chloride injection to provide a final concentration of 100 mcg/mL. To prepare solutions for continuous IV infusion, 1 mL of the commercially available phenylephrine hydrochloride injection containing 10 mg/mL should be withdrawn and added to 500 mL of 5% dextrose or 0.9% sodium chloride injection to provide a final concentration of 20 mcg/mL. Diluted solutions may be stored at room temperature for up to 4 hours or under refrigeration for up to 24 hours; any unused portions should be discarded.

Commercially available phenylephrine hydrochloride bulk vials are intended for use in a pharmacy admixture program for preparation of single doses to be dispensed to multiple patients. Each vial should be penetrated only one time with a suitable sterile transfer device or dispensing set. The pharmacy bulk vial should be discarded within 4 hours after initial entry.

Prior to administration, phenylephrine hydrochloride solutions should be inspected visually for particulate matter and discoloration; the drug should be discarded if the solution is colored, cloudy, or contains any particulate matter.

During IV administration of phenylephrine, intravascular volume depletion and acidosis should always be corrected if present. Blood pressure should be monitored and dosage of phenylephrine hydrochloride adjusted as necessary to achieve appropriate blood pressure goals. Care should be taken to avoid extravasation and the infusion site should be checked for free flow.

Standardize 4 Safety

Standardized concentrations for phenylephrine have been established through Standardize 4 Safety (S4S), a national patient safety initiative to reduce medication errors, especially during transitions of care. Multidisciplinary expert panels were convened to determine recommended standard concentrations. Because recommendations from the S4S panels may differ from the manufacturer's prescribing information, caution is advised when using concentrations that differ from labeling, particularly when using rate information from the label. For additional information on S4S (including updates that may be available), see https://www .ashp.org/pharmacy-practice/standardize-4-safety-initiative.

TABLE 1. Standardize 4 Safety Continuous IV Infusion Standard Concentrations for Phenylephrine Hydrochloride

Patient Population	Concentration Standards	Dosing Units
Adults	80 mcg/mL	mcg/kg/min
	400 mcg/mL	
Pediatric patients (<50 kg)	80 mcg/mL	mcg/kg/min
	400 mcg/mL	

Oral Administration

As a vasoconstrictor for the management of nasal congestion, phenylephrine is administered orally alone or as a fixed-combination decongestant preparation.

Topical and Rectal Administration

As a vasoconstrictor for the management of hemorrhoidal symptoms, phenylephrine hydrochloride topical preparations are administered externally to the affected perianal area and rectal preparations are administered externally to the affected perianal area and/or intrarectally.

Topical preparations of phenylephrine hydrochloride that are labeled for external use only should be applied externally to the affected area and should *not* be administered inside the rectum by either using fingers or any mechanical device or applicator.

Rectal preparations of phenylephrine hydrochloride are labeled either for rectal use only (e.g., suppositories) or for external and/or intrarectal use only. When a special applicator such as a pile pipe or other mechanical device is used to administer the drug intrarectally, the applicator should be attached to the tube of drug and then the applicator should be lubricated well and gently inserted into the rectum; the applicator should be cleansed thoroughly after each use and stored according to the manufacturer's instructions. Such preparations should *not* be used if introduction of the applicator or device into the rectum causes additional pain; patients should be advised to consult a clinician promptly in such cases. The wrapper should be removed from suppositories prior to insertion into the rectum.

Patients receiving phenylephrine hydrochloride for the local management of hemorrhoids should be advised to cleanse the affected perianal area by patting with warm water and mild soap and rinsing thoroughly or with an appropriate cleansing wipe whenever practical. The area then should be dried by patting or blotting with toilet tissue or a soft cloth before application of the drug.

● Dosage

Phenylephrine hydrochloride should be administered in the lowest effective dosage for the shortest possible time. When used to increase blood pressure in patients with acute hypotensive states, dosage should be individualized based on the pressor response.

Hypotension During Anesthesia

Various phenylephrine hydrochloride dosing regimens have been used for the treatment of hypotension during anesthesia; optimal dosage and method of administration remain to be established. Dosages currently recommended by the manufacturers are based on information from published studies.

For the treatment of hypotension during anesthesia in adults, the manufacturers recommend direct IV ("bolus") doses of phenylephrine hydrochloride ranging from 40–250 mcg; the usual initial dose is 50 or 100 mcg. One manufacturer states that additional IV bolus doses may be administered every 1–2 minutes as needed not to exceed a total dosage of 200 mcg; however, if blood pressure is below the target goal, a continuous IV infusion should be initiated. If phenylephrine hydrochloride is administered by continuous IV infusion, the manufacturers recommend infusion rates of 10–35 mcg/minute or 0.5–1.4 mcg/kg per minute. The infusion generally should be started at a low rate and titrated to effect. Other dosage regimens for phenylephrine hydrochloride have been recommended for the treatment of hypotension; in all situations, dosage should be titrated to effect and the patient should be closely monitored.

Some manufacturers state that total dosage of phenylephrine hydrochloride should not exceed 200 mcg (if given by direct IV injection) or 200 mcg/minute (if given by continuous IV infusion). Higher dosages do not necessarily produce incremental increases in blood pressure and may cause hypertension and reflex bradycardia.

Septic Shock

When used in the treatment of septic shock, phenylephrine hydrochloride is administered by continuous IV infusion without an initial bolus dose. (See Dosage and Administration: Administration.) For the treatment of septic shock or other vasodilatory shock in adults, the manufacturer recommends that phenylephrine hydrochloride therapy be initiated at an infusion rate of 0.5–6 mcg/kg per minute; the rate of infusion should be adjusted to maintain the target blood pressure goal. Infusion rates higher than 6 mcg/kg per minute do not appear to provide substantial incremental increases in blood pressure.

Prolongation of Spinal Anesthesia

To prolong spinal anesthesia†, 2–5 mg of phenylephrine hydrochloride has been added to the anesthetic solution, and has increased the duration of nerve block by as much as approximately 50%.

Vasoconstriction for Regional Anesthesia

To produce vasoconstriction in regional anesthesia†, some clinicians state that the optimum concentration of phenylephrine hydrochloride is 0.05 mg/mL (1:20,000). Solutions have been prepared for regional anesthesia by adding 1 mg of phenylephrine hydrochloride to each 20 mL of local anesthetic solution. Some pressor response can be expected when at least 2 mg is injected.

Nasal Congestion

Phenylephrine is administered orally as a nasal decongestant alone or in fixed combination with other drugs. The usual oral decongestant dosage of phenylephrine hydrochloride for *self-medication* in adults and children 12 years of age or older is 10 mg every 4 hours. The manufacturer states that no more than 6 doses should be administered in a 24-hour period. For *self-medication*, the manufacturer recommends that patients discontinue the drug and consult a clinician if symptoms persist more than 7 days or are accompanied by fever, or if nervousness, dizziness, or insomnia occurs.

Hemorrhoids

When used topically or rectally as a vasoconstrictor for temporary relief of hemorrhoidal symptoms in adults and children 12 years of age and older, phenylephrine hydrochloride is used for *self-medication* as a cream, gel, ointment, or suppository containing 0.25% of the drug alone or in combination with other anorectal agents (e.g., protectants, local anesthetics, astringents, antipruritics, analgesics). Anorectal preparations of the drug usually are administered at bedtime, in the morning, and *after* bowel movements up to 4 times daily.

Patients should be advised not to exceed the recommended dosage of phenylephrine hydrochloride unless otherwise directed by a clinician. Although the systemic bioavailability of phenylephrine hydrochloride following local application to the anorectal area is not known, it is recommended that anorectal dosage for *self-medication* of hemorrhoids *not* exceed 2 mg daily (i.e., 0.5 mg 4 times daily) in order to minimize adverse systemic effects. It currently is not known whether higher dosages would provide additional benefit.

Patients should be advised to consult a clinician if the anorectal condition worsens or does not improve within 7 days or if bleeding occurs.

CAUTIONS

● Adverse Effects

Systemic Use

Phenylephrine hydrochloride may cause restlessness, anxiety, nervousness, weakness, dizziness, precordial pain or discomfort, tremor, respiratory distress, pallor or blanching of the skin, or a pilomotor response. Injections of the drug may be followed by paresthesia in the extremities or a feeling of coolness in the skin. When 2 mg or more of phenylephrine hydrochloride is injected during regional local anesthesia, a pressor response may occur.

Overdosage of phenylephrine may cause a rapid rise in blood pressure and associated manifestations including headache, seizures, cerebral hemorrhage, palpitation, paresthesia, and vomiting. Hypertensive crisis also has been reported.

Hypertension may be relieved by administration of an α-adrenergic blocking agent (e.g., phentolamine).

Phenylephrine can cause severe peripheral and visceral vasoconstriction, reduced blood flow to vital organs, decreased renal perfusion, and possibly reduced urine output and metabolic acidosis. In patients with septic shock, phenylephrine may increase the need for renal replacement therapy. Severe vasoconstrictive effects may be more likely to occur in patients with substantial peripheral vascular disease. In addition, prolonged use of phenylephrine may cause plasma volume depletion that may result in perpetuation or recurrence of hypotension when the drug is discontinued.

Phenylephrine can cause severe bradycardia and decreased cardiac output. Decreased cardiac output may be especially harmful to elderly patients and/or those with initially poor cerebral or coronary circulation. Bradycardia may be treated by administration of atropine. Because of its potent vasoconstricting effects, phenylephrine may precipitate angina in patients with a history of the condition or with severe atherosclerosis. The drug also increases cardiac work by increasing peripheral arterial resistance and may possibly induce or exacerbate heart failure. In addition, phenylephrine may increase pulmonary arterial pressure. In patients with autonomic dysfunction (e.g., those with spinal cord injuries), the blood pressure response to phenylephrine may be increased.

Phenylephrine may cause necrosis or sloughing of tissue if extravasation occurs during IV administration or following subcutaneous administration.

Anorectal Use

When used in recommended dosages for local effect in anorectal disorders (e.g., hemorrhoids), adverse systemic effects of vasoconstrictors such as phenylephrine generally are minimal. Such effects, although unlikely, can include blood pressure elevation, cardiac arrhythmia or irregular heart rate, CNS disturbance or nervousness, tremor, sleeplessness, and aggravation of hyperthyroid symptoms.

Based on observations with local use for nasal congestion, prolonged local use of excessive anorectal dosages of vasoconstrictors will likely lead to rebound vasodilation and congestion. Less commonly, prolonged local use of excessive anorectal dosages of vasoconstrictors can lead to anxiety and paranoia.

Phenylephrine reportedly is less likely than other topical vasoconstrictors (e.g., ephedrine, epinephrine) to cause local irritation. Contact dermatitis has been reported following topical application of certain formulations of vasoconstrictors.

The possibility that topical anorectal application of vasoconstrictors if absorbed systemically in adequate amounts could interact with monoamine oxidase (MAO) inhibitors resulting in potentiated hypertensive effects should be considered. Such hypertensive potentiation could result in serious, potentially fatal effects such as cerebral hemorrhage or stroke. (See Anorectal Precautions and Contraindications under Cautions: Precautions and Contraindications.)

● Precautions and Contraindications

Vasopressor therapy is *not* a substitute for replacement of blood, plasma, fluids, and/or electrolytes. Blood volume depletion should be corrected as fully as possible before or during administration with phenylephrine hydrochloride. In an emergency, the drug may be used as an adjunct to fluid volume replacement or as a temporary supportive measure to maintain coronary and cerebral artery perfusion until volume replacement therapy can be completed, but phenylephrine must *not* be used as sole therapy in hypovolemic patients. Hypoxia and acidosis, which also may reduce the effectiveness of phenylephrine, must be identified and corrected prior to or concurrently with administration of the drug.

Prolonged administration of vasopressors has caused edema, hemorrhage, focal myocarditis, subpericardial hemorrhage, necrosis of the intestine, or hepatic and renal necrosis; these effects have generally occurred in patients with severe shock and it is not clear if the drug or the shock state itself was the cause. Because phenylephrine can cause necrosis of the skin and subcutaneous tissue, care should be taken to avoid extravasation of the drug during IV administration and the infusion site should be checked for free flow.

As with other sympathomimetic drugs, phenylephrine hydrochloride should not be used for *self-medication* of nasal congestion in patients with thyroid disease, diabetes mellitus, hypertension, or heart disease without consulting a clinician. In addition, the drug should not be used for *self-medication* of nasal congestion in patients with difficulty urinating because of prostatic hypertrophy without consulting a clinician. Patients should be advised to discontinue the drug and consult a clinician if symptoms persist more than 7 days or are accompanied by fever, or if nervousness, dizziness, or insomnia develops during therapy. In addition, patients should be advised to avoid phenylephrine if they are currently receiving or have recently received (i.e., within 2 weeks) an MAO inhibitor.

When phenylephrine is used in combination with other drugs, the cautions applicable to all ingredients in the formulations should be kept in mind.

Commercially available formulations of phenylephrine hydrochloride injection may contain sodium metabisulfite, a sulfite that may cause allergic-type reactions, including anaphylaxis and life-threatening or less severe asthmatic episodes, in certain susceptible individuals. The overall prevalence of sulfite sensitivity in the general population is unknown but probably low; such sensitivity appears to occur more frequently in asthmatic than in nonasthmatic individuals. Some manufacturers state that phenylephrine is contraindicated in patients with hypersensitivity to the drug or any of its components.

Some clinicians consider severe coronary disease or cardiovascular disease (including myocardial infarction) to be contraindications to use of phenylephrine. Because of possible renal toxicity in patients with septic shock, renal function should be monitored during phenylephrine use in such patients.

Anorectal Precautions and Contraindications

Unless otherwise directed by a clinician, patients should not receive external or rectal preparations of vasoconstrictors such as phenylephrine hydrochloride for *self-medication* of hemorrhoidal symptoms if they have cardiac disease, high blood pressure, thyroid disease, diabetes mellitus, or difficulty in urination secondary to prostatic hyperplasia. Patients also should be advised to consult a clinician before initiating *self-medication* with an anorectal preparation of the drug if they currently are receiving an antihypertensive agent or antidepressant (e.g., MAO inhibitor). For additional precautions associated with anorectal phenylephrine therapy, see Dosage and Administration.

● Pediatric Precautions

The manufacturers state that safety and efficacy of parenteral preparations of phenylephrine hydrochloride have not been established in pediatric patients; however, the drug has been used in children for the treatment of hypotension during spinal anesthesia.

Overdosage and toxicity (including death) have been reported in children younger than 2 years of age receiving nonprescription (over-the-counter, OTC) preparations containing antihistamines, cough suppressants, expectorants, and nasal decongestants alone or in combination for relief of symptoms of upper respiratory tract infection. There is limited evidence of efficacy for these preparations in this age group, and appropriate dosages (i.e., approved by the US Food and Drug Administration [FDA]) have not been established. Therefore, FDA stated that nonprescription cough and cold preparations should not be used in children younger than 2 years of age; the agency continues to assess safety and efficacy of these preparations in older children. Meanwhile, because children 2–3 years of age also are at increased risk of overdosage and toxicity, some manufacturers of oral nonprescription cough and cold preparations agreed to voluntarily revise the product labeling to state that such preparations should not be used in children younger than 4 years of age. FDA recommends that parents and caregivers adhere to the dosage instructions and warnings on the product labeling that accompanies the preparation if administering to children and consult with their clinician about any concerns. Clinicians should ask caregivers about use of nonprescription cough and cold preparations to avoid overdosage. For additional information on precautions associated with the use of cough and cold preparations in pediatric patients, see Cautions: Pediatric Precautions in Pseudoephedrine 12:12.12.

● Geriatric Precautions

Clinical studies of phenylephrine hydrochloride did not include sufficient numbers of patients 65 years of age and older to determine whether geriatric patients respond differently than younger patients. Clinical experience to date has not identified any differences in response between geriatric and younger patients. If phenylephrine is used in geriatric patients, dosage should be selected carefully, usually starting at the low end of the dosage range, since renal, hepatic, and cardiovascular dysfunction and concomitant disease or other drug therapy are more common in this age group.

● Pregnancy, Fertility, and Lactation

Pregnancy

It is not known whether phenylephrine hydrochloride can cause fetal harm when administered to pregnant women; the drug should be used during pregnancy only if the potential benefit justifies the potential risk to the fetus. Animal studies suggest a potential for adverse cardiovascular effects to the fetus if the drug is administered IV during pregnancy. Administration of phenylephrine to patients in late pregnancy or labor may cause fetal anoxia and bradycardia by increasing contractility of the uterus and decreasing uterine blood flow.

In studies of IV phenylephrine in pregnant women undergoing cesarean delivery with neuraxial anesthesia, common adverse effects reported in the mother included nausea and vomiting, bradycardia, reactive hypertension, and transient arrhythmias. The drug did not appear to affect neonatal Apgar scores or umbilical artery blood-gas status.

If a vasopressor is used in conjunction with oxytocic drugs, the vasopressor effect is potentiated and may result in potentially serious adverse effects. (See Drug Interactions: Oxytocic Drugs.)

Lactation

It is not known whether phenylephrine is distributed into human milk following parenteral administration. The drug should be used with caution in nursing women.

DRUG INTERACTIONS

● α- and β-Adrenergic Blocking Agents

The effects of both phenylephrine and α-adrenergic blocking agents may be blocked when these drugs are administered concomitantly. The vasopressor response to phenylephrine is decreased by prior administration of an α-adrenergic blocking agent such as phentolamine mesylate. Phenothiazine drugs (e.g., chlorpromazine) and amiodarone also have some α-adrenergic blocking effects and can reduce the pressor effect of phenylephrine.

The pressor effects of phenylephrine may be increased with concomitant administration of β-adrenergic blocking drugs.

● Oxytocic Drugs

When a vasopressor (e.g., phenylephrine) is used in conjunction with oxytocic drugs, the pressor effect is potentiated, increasing the risk of hemorrhagic stroke. If phenylephrine is used during labor and delivery to correct hypotension or is added to a local anesthetic solution, the obstetrician should be cautioned that some oxytocic drugs may cause severe persistent hypertension and that rupture of a cerebral blood vessel may occur during the postpartum period.

● General Anesthetics

Rarely, administration of phenylephrine to patients who have received cyclopropane or halogenated hydrocarbon general anesthetics that increase cardiac irritability and seem to sensitize the myocardium to phenylephrine may result in arrhythmias. However, in usual therapeutic doses, phenylephrine is much less likely to produce arrhythmias than is norepinephrine or metaraminol.

● Monoamine Oxidase Inhibitors

The cardiac and pressor effects of phenylephrine are potentiated by prior administration of monoamine oxidase (MAO) inhibitors (e.g., selegiline) because the metabolism of phenylephrine is reduced. The potentiation is greater following oral administration of phenylephrine than after parenteral administration of the drug because reduction of the metabolism of phenylephrine in the intestine results in increased absorption of the drug. Oral administration of phenylephrine to patients receiving a MAO inhibitor should be avoided. Parenteral administration of phenylephrine to these patients, if unavoidable, should be undertaken with extreme caution and with low initial doses. Patients should consult a clinician before initiating anorectal phenylephrine therapy if they are receiving an MAO inhibitor. (See Anorectal Precautions and Contraindications under Cautions: Precautions and Contraindications.)

● Other Drugs

Other drugs that may potentiate the pressor effect of phenylephrine include α₂-adrenergic agonists (e.g., clonidine), tricyclic antidepressants, atropine sulfate, steroids, norepinephrine-reuptake inhibitors (e.g., atomoxetine), and ergot alkaloids (e.g., methylergonovine maleate). Other drugs that can antagonize the pressor effect of phenylephrine include phosphodiesterase (PDE) type 5 inhibitors, benzodiazepines, and antihypertensive agents.

Atropine sulfate blocks the reflex bradycardia caused by phenylephrine and enhances the pressor response to phenylephrine.

An excessive rise in blood pressure may occur if phenylephrine is administered to patients receiving a parenteral injection of an ergot alkaloid such as ergonovine maleate.

The possibility that digitalis can sensitize the myocardium to the effects of sympathomimetic drugs should be considered.

Administration of furosemide or other diuretics may decrease arterial responsiveness to vasopressors such as phenylephrine.

PHARMACOLOGY

Phenylephrine acts predominantly by a direct effect on α_1-adrenergic receptors. In therapeutic doses, the drug has no substantial stimulant effect on the β-adrenergic receptors of the heart (β_1-adrenergic receptors) but substantial activation of these receptors may occur when larger doses are given. Phenylephrine does not stimulate β-adrenergic receptors of the bronchi or peripheral blood vessels (β_2-adrenergic receptors). Phenylephrine also has an indirect effect by releasing norepinephrine from its storage sites. The main effect of phenylephrine at therapeutic doses is vasoconstriction.

Cardiovascular Effects

Phenylephrine constricts both arterial and venous blood vessels, although its effects on arterial vessels are more pronounced. Systemic vascular resistance is increased, resulting in increased systolic blood pressure, diastolic blood pressure, and mean arterial pressure. Vasoconstriction occurs in most vascular beds, including renal, pulmonary, and splanchnic arteries, but minimal to no effect is observed on cerebral blood vessels. In some patients, phenylephrine can substantially reduce cardiac output, presumably due to increased afterload; however, the exact effects of the drug on global cardiac output depend on the dose and contributory effects of the arterial and venous vasculature. Although phenylephrine reduces venous compliance and can potentially increase venous return, accompanying increases in arterial and venous resistance can negate this potential benefit. Phenylephrine may reduce circulating plasma volume (especially with prolonged use) as a result of loss of fluid into the extracellular spaces caused by postcapillary vasoconstriction. In contrast to methoxamine, phenylephrine constricts coronary and pulmonary blood vessels. Pulmonary arterial pressure usually is increased; however, a decrease in pulmonary arterial pressure has occurred in some patients, probably because of decreased cardiac output secondary to reflex bradycardia. At clinically relevant doses, phenylephrine increases myocardial work and oxygen requirements.

Constriction of renal blood vessels by phenylephrine may decrease renal blood flow. In hypotensive patients, phenylephrine may initially decrease urine flow and excretion of sodium and potassium. If the patient is not hypovolemic, renal blood flow and glomerular filtration rate increase as the systemic blood pressure is raised toward normal levels; however, renal blood flow and glomerular filtration rate again decrease if blood pressure is further increased toward hypertensive levels.

Phenylephrine can cause reflex bradycardia because of increased vagal activity. In some patients, phenylephrine has caused a paradoxical increase in heart rate when administered to treat hypotension occurring after spinal anesthesia. Because of some β_1-adrenergic activity, phenylephrine can exert positive inotropic effects on the myocardium at doses greater than those usually used therapeutically. Rarely, the drug may increase myocardial excitability, causing arrhythmias such as atrioventricular nodal rhythm, premature ventricular beats, ventricular tachycardia, or ventricular extrasystoles.

Local vasoconstriction and hemostasis also occur following topical application or infiltration of phenylephrine into tissues. Like epinephrine, phenylephrine probably produces hemostasis in cases of small vessel bleeding but does not control bleeding from larger vessels. Following oral administration or topical application of phenylephrine to the mucosa, constriction of blood vessels in the nasal mucosa may relieve nasal congestion.

Other Effects

In therapeutic doses, phenylephrine causes little if any CNS stimulation but may cause nervousness, restlessness, anxiety, dizziness, and tremor in some patients, especially after overdosage.

As a result of its effects on α-adrenergic receptors, phenylephrine may cause contraction of the pregnant uterus and constriction of uterine blood vessels; however, the vasoconstrictor effect may be overcome by an increase in maternal blood pressure.

PHARMACOKINETICS

Absorption

Phenylephrine is completely absorbed following oral administration and undergoes extensive first-pass metabolism in the intestinal wall. The bioavailability of phenylephrine following oral administration is approximately 38% relative to IV administration. Because of extensive first-pass metabolism, there is considerable interindividual and possibly intraindividual variation in oral bioavailability of the drug. Following oral administration of phenylephrine (1 or 7.8 mg), peak serum concentrations occur at 0.75–2 hours.

To achieve cardiovascular effects, phenylephrine should be given parenterally. After IV administration, a pressor effect occurs almost immediately and persists for 15–20 minutes. After IM administration, a pressor effect occurs within 10–15 minutes and persists for 30 minutes to 1 or 2 hours. Occasionally, enough phenylephrine may be absorbed after oral inhalation to produce systemic effects. Following oral administration, nasal decongestion may occur within 15 or 20 minutes and may persist for 2–4 hours.

Distribution

Phenylephrine undergoes rapid distribution into peripheral tissues; there is some evidence that the drug may be stored in certain organ compartments. The pharmacologic effects of phenylephrine are terminated at least partially by uptake of the drug into tissues. Penetration of phenylephrine into the brain appears to be minimal.

Phenylephrine does not appear to be distributed to any great extent into breast milk.

Elimination

Phenylephrine undergoes extensive metabolism in the intestinal wall (first-pass) and in the liver. The principal routes of metabolism involve sulfate conjugation (primarily in the intestinal wall) and oxidative deamination (by monoamine oxidase [MAO]); glucuronidation also occurs to a lesser extent. The metabolites are not pharmacologically active.

Phenylephrine and its metabolites are excreted mainly in urine. Following oral or IV administration, approximately 80 or 86% of the dose, respectively, is excreted in urine within 48 hours, principally as metabolites; approximately 2.6% of an oral dose or 16% of an IV dose is excreted in urine as unchanged drug. The terminal elimination half-life of phenylephrine averages 2–3 hours following oral or IV administration. The observed effective half-life is approximately 5 minutes following IV infusion of the drug.

Clinical data regarding effects of renal or hepatic impairment on the pharmacokinetics of phenylephrine are limited. Because the majority of an oral dose is metabolized in the intestinal wall and a lower fraction in the liver, hepatic impairment is unlikely to result in major changes following oral administration; however, phenylephrine pharmacokinetics may be substantially altered following IV administration of the drug. Patients with hepatic cirrhosis may have a reduced response to phenylephrine, potentially requiring higher dosages of the drug. Patients with end-stage renal disease may have an increased response to phenylephrine, potentially requiring lower dosages of the drug.

CHEMISTRY AND STABILITY

Chemistry

Phenylephrine is a sympathomimetic amine that is pharmacologically similar to methoxamine hydrochloride. Phenylephrine is commercially available as the hydrochloride. Commercially available phenylephrine hydrochloride injections may contain the antioxidant, sodium metabisulfite.

Stability

Phenylephrine hydrochloride injection should be stored at 20–25°C, but may be exposed to temperatures ranging from 15–30°C; single-dose and pharmacy bulk vials should be kept in their original carton until time of use and protected from light.

Phenylephrine hydrochloride oral tablets should be stored at 15–25°C in a dry place. Phenylephrine hydrochloride injections should be stored at room temperature up to 30°C and protected from light.

PREPARATIONS

Excipients in commercially available drug preparations may have clinically important effects in some individuals; consult specific product labeling for details.

Phenylephrine Hydrochloride

Oral

Tablets	10 mg	Sudafed PE® Congestion, McNeil

Parenteral

Injection	10 mg/mL	Vazculep®, Eclat
		Phenylephrine Hydrochloride Injection

Topical

Cream	0.25% with Glycerin 14.4%, Petrolatum 15%, and Pramokine 1%	Preparation H®, Pfizer
Gel	0.25% with Witch Hazel 50%	Preparation H®, Pfizer
Ointment	0.25% with Mineral Oil 14%, Petrolatum 71.9%	Preparation H®, Pfizer
Suppository	0.25% with Cocoa Butter 85.39%	Preparation H®, Pfizer

Phenylephrine Hydrochloride Combinations

Oral

Capsules, (liquid-filled)	5 mg with Acetaminophen 325 mg and Dextromethorphan Hydrobromide 10 mg	Vicks® DayQuil® Cold & Flu Relief LiquiCaps, Procter & Gamble
For Solution	10 mg/packet with Acetaminophen 325 mg/packet and Pheniramine Maleate 20 mg/packet	Theraflu® Cold & Sore Throat, Novartis
	10 mg/packet with Acetaminophen 650 mg/packet and Dextromethorphan Hydrobromide 20 mg	Theraflu® Daytime Severe Cold & Cough, Novartis
	10 mg/packet with Acetaminophen 650 mg/packet and Pheniramine Maleate 20 mg/packet	Theraflu® Flu & Sore Throat, Novartis
	10mg/packet with Acetaminophen 650 mg/packet and Diphenhydramine Hydrochloride 25 mg	Theraflu® Nighttime Severe Cold & Cough, Novartis
	10 mg/packet with Dextromethorphan Hydrobromide 20 mg/packet and Pheniramine Maleate 20 mg/packet	Theraflu® Cold & Cough, Novartis
Solution	5 mg/15 mL with Acetaminophen 325 mg/15 mL and Dextromethorphan Hydrobromide 10 mg/15 mL	Theraflu Warming Relief® Daytime Severe Cold & Cough, Novartis
		Tylenol® Cold Multi-Symptom Daytime Citrus Burst® Liquid, McNeil
		Vicks® DayQuil® Cold & Flu Relief, Procter & Gamble
	5 mg/15 mL with Acetaminophen 325 mg/15 mL and Diphenhydramine Hydrochloride 12.5 mg/15 mL	Theraflu® Warming Relief® Flu & Sore Throat, Novartis
		Theraflu® Warming Relief® Nighttime Severe Cold & Cough, Novartis
	2.5 mg/5 mL with Acetaminophen 160 mg/5 mL and Chlorpheniramine Maleate 1 mg/5 mL	Children's Tylenol® Plus Cold, McNeil
	2.5 mg/5 mL with Acetaminophen 160 mg/5 mL and Chlorpheniramine Maleate 1 mg/5 mL, and Dextromethorphan Hydrobromide 5 mg/5mL	Children's Tylenol® Plus Multi-Symptom Cold, McNeil
	2.5 mg/5 mL with Acetaminophen 160 mg/5 mL and Diphenhydramine Hydrochloride 12.5 mg/5 mL	Children's Tylenol® Plus Cold & Allergy, McNeil
	2.5 mg/5 mL with Chlorpheniramine Maleate 1 mg/5 mL	Triaminic® Cold & Allergy, Novartis
	2.5 mg/5 mL with Dextromethorphan Hydrobromide 5 mg/5mL	Children's Sudafed PE® Cold & Cough, McNeil
		Triaminic® Day Time Cold & Cough, Novartis
	2.5 mg/5mL with Diphenhydramine Hydrochloride 6.25 mg/5 mL	Triaminic® Night Time Cold & Cough, Novartis
	2.5 mg/5 mL with Guaifenesin 50 mg/5mL	Triaminic® Chest and Nasal Congestion, Novartis
Tablets	5 mg with Acetaminophen 325 mg, Chlorpheniramine Maleate 2 mg, and Dextromethorphan Hydrobromide 10 mg	Theraflu® Warming Relief Caplets® Nighttime Multi-Symptom Cold, Novartis
	5 mg with Acetaminophen 325 mg and Dextromethorphan Hydrobromide 10 mg	Theraflu Warming Relief Caplets® Daytime Multi-Symptom Cold, Novartis
	10 mg with Chlorpheniramine Maleate 4 mg	Sudafed PE® Sinus + Allergy, McNeil
Tablets, film-coated	5 mg with Acetaminophen 325 mg	Excedrin® Sinus Headache, Novartis
		Sudafed PE® Pressure + Pain Caplets, McNeil
	5 mg with Acetaminophen 325 mg, Chlorpheniramine Maleate 2 mg, and Dextromethorphan Hydrobromide 10 mg	Tylenol® Cold Head Congestion Nighttime Cool Burst® Caplets, McNeil
	5 mg with Acetaminophen 325 mg and Dextromethorphan Hydrobromide 10 mg	Tylenol® Cold Head Congestion Daytime Cool Burst® Caplets, McNeil
	5 mg with Acetaminophen 325 mg, Dextromethorphan Hydrobromide 10 mg, and Guaifenesin 100 mg	Sudafed PE® Cold + Cough Caplets, McNeil
	5 mg with Acetaminophen 325 mg, Dextromethorphan Hydrobromide 10 mg, and Guaifenesin 200 mg	Tylenol® Cold Head Congestion Severe Cool Burst® Caplets, McNeil
	5 mg with Acetaminophen 325 mg and Diphenhydramine Hydrochloride 12.5 mg	Sudafed PE® Severe Cold Caplets, McNeil
	5 mg with Guaifenesin 200 mg	Sudafed PE® Non-Drying Sinus Caplets, McNeil

† Use is not currently included in the labeling approved by the US Food and Drug Administration.

Selected Revisions July 10, 2024, © Copyright, September 1, 1976, American Society of Health-System Pharmacists, Inc.

DOBUTamine Hydrochloride

12:12.08.08 • SELECTIVE β₁-ADRENERGIC AGONISTS

■ Dobutamine hydrochloride is a synthetic sympathomimetic that is structurally related to dopamine and generally is considered a relatively selective β₁-adrenergic agonist.

USES

● Cardiac Decompensation

Dobutamine hydrochloride is used for inotropic support in the short-term management of cardiac decompensation caused by depressed contractility from organic heart disease or cardiac surgical procedures. The drug may be ineffective in patients with marked mechanical obstruction such as severe valvular aortic stenosis.

Safety and efficacy of dobutamine or other cyclic AMP (cAMP)-dependent inotropic agents in the long-term (e.g., exceeding 48 hours) treatment of patients with congestive heart failure have not been established, irrespective of their route of administration. In controlled studies in patients with congestive heart failure using chronic oral therapy with cAMP-dependent inotropic agents, symptoms were not consistently alleviated, and an increased risk of hospitalization and death, particularly in patients with New York Heart Association (NYHA) class IV symptoms, was associated with such therapy.

Because positive inotropic agents have not demonstrated improved outcomes in patients with heart failure and can be potentially harmful (e.g., increased risk of arrhythmias), particularly when used long term, the American College of Cardiology Foundation (ACCF) and American Heart Association (AHA) recommend that these drugs be reserved for patients with severe systolic dysfunction who have low cardiac index and evidence of systemic hypoperfusion and/or congestion, or for palliative therapy in those with end-stage heart failure. To minimize the risk of adverse effects, the lowest possible dosage should be used and the patient should be evaluated regularly for the need for continued inotropic therapy.

When used for inotropic support in patients with myocardial dysfunction after cardiac surgery, dobutamine has been shown in clinical studies to effectively increase cardiac output; however, the effects of the drug on clinically important outcomes and survival are not known. Although some data indicate that dobutamine may be preferable to other catecholamines (e.g., dopamine) in the period immediately following cardiopulmonary bypass surgery, additional studies are needed.

Inotropic agents such as dobutamine also are used in the treatment of septic or cardiogenic shock to improve myocardial contractility and maintain systemic perfusion. The Surviving Sepsis Campaign International Guidelines for Management of Severe Sepsis and Septic Shock recommend a trial of dobutamine (alone or in addition to a vasopressor) in patients with septic shock if myocardial dysfunction is present, as evidenced by elevated cardiac filling pressures and low cardiac output, or if there is ongoing hypoperfusion despite adequate intravascular volume and mean arterial pressure. Although the manufacturers of dobutamine hydrochloride state that safety of the drug following myocardial infarction (MI) has not been established (see Cautions: Precautions and Contraindications), dobutamine often is used for temporary inotropic support in patients with cardiogenic shock, a condition caused principally by acute MI. Early revascularization is the standard of care in patients with cardiogenic shock; use of inotropes in this setting should be individualized and guided by hemodynamic monitoring.

● Advanced Cardiovascular Life Support

Inotropic agents such as dobutamine also have been used for postresuscitation stabilization† after cardiac arrest in patients who require additional support of cardiac output and blood pressure.

● Cardiac Diagnostic Testing

Dobutamine has been used as a pharmacologic stress test agent† during echocardiography in patients who are unable to undergo exercise testing. Dobutamine also has been used as an alternative to exercise stress testing in patients undergoing myocardial perfusion imaging†. However, coronary vasodilating agents (e.g., adenosine, dipyridamole, regadenoson) are the drugs of choice for this use; dobutamine generally is recommended only in patients who have contraindications (e.g., bronchospastic airway disease) to these vasodilators.

DOSAGE AND ADMINISTRATION

● Administration

Dobutamine hydrochloride is administered by IV infusion using an infusion pump or other apparatus to control the flow rate. One manufacturer recommends that a precision volume-control IV set be used when administering the drug. Care should be taken to control the rate of infusion to prevent rapid IV ("bolus") administration.

Dobutamine also has been administered by intraosseous (IO) infusion† in the setting of advanced cardiovascular life support (ACLS), generally when IV access is not readily available; onset of action and systemic concentrations are comparable to those achieved with venous administration.

IV Administration

Commercially available dobutamine hydrochloride injection concentrate *must* be further diluted with a compatible IV solution (see Chemistry and Stability: Stability) before IV infusion; 20 mL of concentrate should be diluted in at least 50 mL of diluent and 40 mL of concentrate should be diluted in at least 100 mL of diluent. The concentration of dobutamine hydrochloride administered should be individualized according to dosage and fluid requirements of the patient; concentrations up to 5000 mcg/mL have been administered. Following dilution, solutions of dobutamine should be used within 24 hours.

Commercially available prediluted solutions of dobutamine hydrochloride in 5% dextrose injection should not be administered unless the solution is clear and the container is undamaged; unused portions should be discarded. The flexible containers should not be used in series connections, and additives should not be introduced into the injection containers.

Dobutamine injection should be inspected visually for particulate matter and discoloration prior to administration, whenever solution and container permit. Dobutamine hydrochloride solutions should not be admixed with alkalizing substances (e.g., sodium bicarbonate) since the drug is inactivated in alkaline solution. One manufacturer states that dobutamine hydrochloride should not be used in conjunction with other drugs or solutions containing both sodium bisulfite and ethanol. The manufacturer's labeling should be consulted for proper methods of administration and other associated precautions.

Standardize 4 Safety

Standardized concentrations for dobutamine have been established through Standardize 4 Safety (S4S), a national patient safety initiative to reduce medication errors, especially during transitions of care. Multidisciplinary expert panels were convened to determine recommended standard concentrations. Because recommendations from the S4S panels may differ from the manufacturer's prescribing information, caution is advised when using concentrations that differ from labeling, particularly when using rate information from the label. For additional information on S4S (including updates that may be available), see https://www.ashp.org/pharmacy-practice/standardize-4-safety-initiative.

TABLE 1. Standardize 4 Safety Continuous IV Infusion Standard Concentrations for Dobutamine

Patient Population	Concentration Standards	Dosing Units
Adults	2000 mcg/mL	mcg/kg/min
	4000 mcg/mL	
Pediatric patients (<50 kg)	1000 mcg/mL	mcg/kg/min
	2000 mcg/mL	
	4000 mcg/mL	

● Dosage

Dosage of dobutamine hydrochloride is expressed in terms of dobutamine.

Cardiac Decompensation

Individual response to dobutamine is variable, and infusion rate should be titrated to achieve the desired clinical response.

Dobutamine infusion should be initiated at a slow rate (e.g., 0.5–1 mcg/kg per minute) and carefully adjusted at intervals of a few minutes according to the patient's response as indicated by heart rate, blood pressure, urine flow, presence of ectopic heartbeats, and, whenever possible, by measurement of central venous or pulmonary capillary wedge pressure and cardiac output. Clinical studies have shown that the rate of infusion usually needed to increase cardiac output is 2–20 mcg/kg per minute. Rarely, infusion of doses as great as 40 mcg/kg per minute has been required.

When dobutamine is used in geriatric patients, the initial dosage usually should be at the low end of the dosage range and caution should be exercised since renal, hepatic, and cardiovascular dysfunction and concomitant disease or other drug therapy are more common in this age group than in younger patients.

Advanced Cardiovascular Life Support

If dobutamine is used for postresuscitation stabilization† in adults following cardiac arrest, the usual initial dosage range is 5–10 mcg/kg per minute. In pediatric patients, the usual dosage range is 2–20 mcg/kg per minute by IV or IO infusion. Rate of infusion should be titrated based on cardiac output and blood pressure response.

CAUTIONS

● Cardiovascular Effects

The principal adverse effects of dobutamine hydrochloride include ectopic heartbeats, increased heart rate, angina, chest pain, palpitation, and elevations in blood pressure. In most patients, heart rate increases 5–15 beats per minute and systolic blood pressure increases by 10–20 mm Hg. Occasionally, however, patients experience an increase in heart rate of 30 beats per minute or greater or an increase in systolic blood pressure of 50 mm Hg or greater. Patients with preexisting hypertension may be predisposed to developing an exaggerated pressor response. All of these adverse cardiovascular effects are usually dose related, and dosage should be reduced or temporarily discontinued if they occur. Rarely, dobutamine has caused ventricular tachycardia.

Precipitous decreases in blood pressure also have been described occasionally; blood pressure generally will return to baseline following dosage reduction or discontinuance of the infusion. However, intervention rarely may be required and the effects on pressure may not be readily reversible.

● Dermatologic and Sensitivity Reactions

Manifestations suggestive of hypersensitivity, including skin rash, fever, eosinophilia, and bronchospasm, have been reported occasionally in patients receiving dobutamine hydrochloride.

● Other Adverse Effects

Other less frequent adverse effects include nausea, vomiting, tingling sensation, paresthesia, dyspnea, headache, fever, and mild leg cramps; pruritus of the scalp during IV infusion of dobutamine has been reported in at least one patient. Isolated cases of thrombocytopenia have been reported. Like other drugs with β₂-agonist activity, dobutamine may produce slight decreases in serum potassium concentrations; hypokalemia may occur rarely. Inadvertent overdosage has also reportedly caused nervousness and fatigue. Phlebitis at the site of IV infusion of dobutamine has been reported occasionally. Inadvertent subcutaneous infiltration of dobutamine has caused local inflammatory changes and local pain without local ischemia; however, isolated cases of cutaneous necrosis have been reported.

● Precautions and Contraindications

Before administration of dobutamine, hypovolemia should be corrected with an appropriate plasma volume expander. The ECG, blood pressure and, when possible, cardiac output and pulmonary wedge pressure should be monitored. Because dobutamine increases atrioventricular conduction, patients with atrial fibrillation are at risk of developing a rapid ventricular response and, therefore, should be digitalized prior to administration of dobutamine. Experience with the use of dobutamine following acute myocardial infarction (MI) is limited. The possibility that dobutamine may intensify or extend myocardial ischemia has not been ruled out. Therefore, the drug should be used with extreme caution following MI.

Like other drugs with β₂-agonist activity, dobutamine may produce slight reductions in serum potassium concentrations and hypokalemia may occur rarely. Consideration should be given to monitoring serum potassium concentrations during dobutamine therapy.

Commercially available injections of dobutamine hydrochloride or dobutamine hydrochloride in 5% dextrose may contain sulfites that can cause allergic-type reactions, including anaphylaxis and life-threatening or less severe asthmatic episodes, in certain susceptible individuals. The overall prevalence of sulfite sensitivity in the general population is unknown but probably low; such sensitivity appears to occur more frequently in asthmatic than in nonasthmatic individuals.

Dobutamine is contraindicated in patients with idiopathic hypertrophic subaortic stenosis or with known hypersensitivity to the drug or any ingredient in the formulation.

● Pediatric Precautions

Some manufacturers state that safety and efficacy of dobutamine injection have not been evaluated in pediatric patients. Other manufacturers state that dobutamine increases cardiac output and systemic blood pressure in pediatric patients of all age groups. In premature neonates, however, dobutamine is less effective than dopamine in increasing systemic blood pressure without causing undue tachycardia and has not been shown to provide any additional benefit when administered to such infants who are already receiving optimal dopamine therapy.

● Geriatric Precautions

Clinical studies of dobutamine hydrochloride did not include sufficient numbers of patients 65 years of age and older to determine whether geriatric patients respond differently than younger patients. Clinical experience suggests that substantial hypotension associated with dobutamine therapy may occur more frequently in geriatric patients. One manufacturer of dobutamine hydrochloride in 5% dextrose recommends that if dobutamine is used in geriatric patients, the initial dosage usually should be at the low end of the dosage range, and caution should be exercised since renal, hepatic, and cardiovascular dysfunction and concomitant disease or other drug therapy are more common in this age group than in younger patients.

● Pregnancy, Fertility, and Lactation

Pregnancy

Safe use of dobutamine during pregnancy has not been established. Reproduction studies in rats or rabbits (at up to or 2 times, respectively, the usual human dose on a mg/kg basis) have not revealed evidence of harm to the fetus. Dobutamine should be used in pregnant women only if clearly needed. The effect of dobutamine on labor and delivery is not known.

Fertility

Studies to evaluate the potential of dobutamine to affect fertility have not been performed.

Lactation

It is not known whether dobutamine is distributed into human milk. Because many drugs are distributed into human milk, caution should be exercised when dobutamine is administered to a nursing woman. If a nursing woman requires dobutamine therapy, breast-feeding should be discontinued for the duration of drug therapy.

DRUG INTERACTIONS

In clinical studies, dobutamine hydrochloride was administered concomitantly with atropine, cardiac glycosides (digoxin), furosemide, heparin, lidocaine, morphine, nitroglycerin, isosorbide dinitrate, potassium chloride, folic acid, protamine, acetaminophen, or spironolactone with no evidence of any drug interactions.

● **β-Adrenergic Blocking Agents**

In animals, the cardiac effects of dobutamine are antagonized by β-adrenergic blocking agents such as propranolol and metoprolol, resulting in predominance of α-adrenergic effects and increased peripheral resistance.

● **General Anesthetics**

Ventricular arrhythmias have been reported in animals receiving usual doses of dobutamine during halothane or cyclopropane anesthesia; therefore, caution should be used when administering dobutamine to patients receiving these general anesthetics.

● **Sodium Nitroprusside**

Concomitant use of dobutamine and sodium nitroprusside may potentiate effects on cardiac output and pulmonary wedge pressure.

PHARMACOLOGY

Dobutamine hydrochloride directly stimulates β₁-adrenergic receptors and is generally considered a selective β₁-adrenergic agonist, but the mechanisms of action of the drug are complex. It is believed that the β-adrenergic effects result from stimulation of adenyl cyclase activity. In therapeutic doses, dobutamine also has mild β₂- and α₁-adrenergic receptor agonist effects, which are relatively balanced and result in minimal net direct effect on systemic vasculature. Unlike dopamine, dobutamine does not cause release of endogenous norepinephrine. The main effect of therapeutic doses of dobutamine is cardiac stimulation. While the positive inotropic effect of the drug on the myocardium appears to be mediated principally via β₁-adrenergic stimulation, experimental evidence suggests that α₁-adrenergic stimulation may also be involved and that the α₁-adrenergic activity results mainly from the (-)-stereoisomer of the drug.

The β₁-adrenergic effects of dobutamine exert a positive inotropic effect on the myocardium and result in an increase in cardiac output due to increased myocardial contractility and stroke volume in healthy individuals and in patients with congestive heart failure. Increased left ventricular filling pressure decreases in patients with congestive heart failure. In therapeutic doses, dobutamine causes a decrease in peripheral resistance; however, systolic blood pressure and pulse pressure may remain unchanged or be increased because of augmented cardiac output. With usual doses, heart rate is usually not substantially changed. Coronary blood flow and myocardial oxygen consumption are usually increased because of increased myocardial contractility.

Electrophysiologic studies have shown that dobutamine facilitates atrioventricular conduction and shortens or causes no important change in intraventricular conduction. The tendency of dobutamine to induce cardiac arrhythmias may be slightly less than that of dopamine and is considerably less than that of isoproterenol or other catecholamines. Pulmonary vascular resistance may decrease if it is elevated initially and mean pulmonary artery pressure may decrease or remain unchanged. Unlike dopamine, dobutamine does not seem to affect dopaminergic receptors and causes no renal or mesenteric vasodilation; however, urine flow may increase because of increased cardiac output.

PHARMACOKINETICS

● **Absorption**

Orally administered dobutamine hydrochloride is rapidly metabolized in the GI tract. Following IV administration, the onset of action of dobutamine occurs within 2 minutes. Peak plasma concentrations of the drug and peak effects occur within 10 minutes after initiation of an IV infusion. The effects of the drug cease shortly after discontinuing an infusion.

● **Distribution**

It is not known if dobutamine crosses the placenta or is distributed into milk.

● **Elimination**

The plasma half-life of dobutamine is about 2 minutes. Dobutamine is metabolized in the liver and other tissues by catechol-O-methyltransferase to an inactive compound, 3-O-methyldobutamine, and by conjugation with glucuronic acid. Conjugates of dobutamine and 3-O-methyldobutamine are excreted mainly in urine and to a minor extent in feces.

CHEMISTRY AND STABILITY

● **Chemistry**

Dobutamine is a synthetic sympathomimetic drug which is structurally related to dopamine. Dobutamine hydrochloride occurs as a white to off-white, crystalline powder and is sparingly soluble in water and in alcohol. Dobutamine has a pK$_a$ of 9.4.

Dobutamine hydrochloride is commercially available as a sterile solution of the drug (a racemic mixture) in water for injection. Commercially available concentrates for injection contain sulfites. Hydrochloric acid and/or sodium hydroxide may be added during manufacture of the commercially available concentrate for injection to adjust the pH between 2.5–5.5.

Dobutamine hydrochloride also is commercially available as prediluted solutions of the drug in 5% dextrose. Hydrochloric acid and/or sodium hydroxide may be added during manufacture of dobutamine hydrochloride in 5% dextrose injection to adjust pH to approximately 3 (range: 2.5–5.5); sodium metabisulfite and edetate disodium dihydrate are added as stabilizers. The commercially available injections of the drug in 5% dextrose are sterile, nonpyrogenic solutions of dobutamine hydrochloride; the injections containing 1, 2, or 4 mg/mL of dobutamine have osmolarities of 263, 270, or 284 mOsm/L, respectively.

● **Stability**

Dobutamine hydrochloride for injection concentrate should be stored at 20–25°C.

Commercially available solutions of dobutamine hydrochloride in 5% dextrose should be protected from excessive heat or freezing and stored at room temperature (20–25°C); however, some manufacturers state that brief exposure of the solutions to temperatures up to 40°C does not adversely affect the products. Dobutamine hydrochloride for injection concentrate is compatible with the following IV solutions: 5 or 10% dextrose, 5% dextrose and 0.45 or 0.9% sodium chloride, 5% dextrose in lactated Ringer's, lactated Ringer's, 0.9% sodium chloride, Isolyte®-M with 5% dextrose, Normosol®-M in 5% dextrose, 20% Osmitrol®, or (1/6) M sodium lactate injection. Dobutamine hydrochloride solutions diluted for IV infusion should be used within 24 hours.

Because of potential physical incompatibilities, it is recommended that dobutamine hydrochloride solutions not be admixed with other drugs. Solutions of the drug are incompatible with sodium bicarbonate injection or other strongly alkaline solutions and should not be used in conjunction with other drugs or diluents containing both sodium bisulfite and ethanol. Pink discoloration of solutions of dobutamine hydrochloride indicates slight oxidation of the drug; however, there is no important loss of potency if the drug is administered within the recommended time period. Unused portions of dobutamine hydrochloride solutions should be discarded.

Some commercially available preparations of dobutamine hydrochloride in 5% dextrose injection (e.g., Lifecare®) are provided in plastic containers fabricated from a specially formulated nonplasticized, thermoplastic co-polyester (CR3). Water can permeate from inside the container into the overwrap in amounts insufficient to affect the solution substantially. Solutions in contact with the plastic container also can leach out some of the chemical components in very small amounts; however, safety of the plastic has been confirmed with biological testing.

PREPARATIONS

Excipients in commercially available drug preparations may have clinically important effects in some individuals; consult specific product labeling for details.

DOBUTamine Hydrochloride

Parenteral

For injection concentrate, for IV infusion	12.5 mg (of dobutamine) per mL*	DOBUTamine Hydrochloride Injection,

* available from one or more manufacturer, distributor, and/or repackager by generic (nonproprietary) name

DOBUTamine Hydrochloride in Dextrose

Parenteral

Injection, for IV infusion	1 mg (of dobutamine) per mL (250 or 500 mg) in 5% Dextrose*	DOBUTamine in 5% Dextrose Injection (Lifecare®; Viaflex®)
	2 mg (of dobutamine) per mL (500 mg) in 5% Dextrose*	DOBUTamine in 5% Dextrose Injection (Lifecare®; Viaflex®)
	4 mg (of dobutamine) per mL (1000 mg) in 5% Dextrose*	DOBUTamine in 5% Dextrose Injection (Lifecare®; Viaflex®)

* available from one or more manufacturer, distributor, and/or repackager by generic (nonproprietary) name

† Use is not currently included in the labeling approved by the US Food and Drug Administration.

Selected Revisions June 10, 2024, © Copyright, June 1, 1979, American Society of Health-System Pharmacists, Inc.

Dopamine Hydrochloride

12:12.08.08 • SELECTIVE β₁-ADRENERGIC AGONISTS

■ Dopamine hydrochloride, an endogenous catecholamine that is the immediate precursor of norepinephrine, is a sympathomimetic agent with prominent dopaminergic and β₁-adrenergic effects at low to moderate doses and α-adrenergic effects at high doses.

USES

● Shock

Dopamine hydrochloride is used as adjunctive therapy to correct hemodynamic imbalances (e.g., increase cardiac output and blood pressure) in the treatment of shock. In patients who require vasopressor support, individual hemodynamic abnormalities must be identified and monitored so that therapy can be adjusted as necessary.

Vasopressors such as dopamine are used in the management of shock to restore blood pressure and tissue perfusion after initial fluid resuscitation is attempted. The Surviving Sepsis Campaign International Guidelines for Management of Sepsis and Septic Shock recommend norepinephrine as the first-line vasopressor of choice in adults with septic shock; if adequate blood pressure is not achieved, vasopressin or epinephrine may be added. Although dopamine was used widely in the past as a first-line vasopressor agent in patients with septic shock, more recent evidence indicates that the drug is associated with a greater risk of adverse effects (e.g., arrhythmias) and possibly also an increased risk of death compared with norepinephrine. In a multicenter randomized study (Sepsis Occurrence in Acutely Ill Patients II [SOAP II]) comparing the effects of dopamine and norepinephrine in patients with septic, cardiogenic, or hypovolemic shock, no substantial difference in 28-day mortality was observed between the vasopressors; however, use of dopamine was associated with more arrhythmic events in the overall population and an increased rate of death in the subgroup of patients with cardiogenic shock. In current expert guidelines, dopamine is considered an alternative vasopressor to norepinephrine only in highly selected patients with septic shock (e.g., those with low risk of tachyarrhythmias and bradycardia).

Vasopressors also have been used to provide hemodynamic support in other types of shock (e.g., cardiogenic, hemorrhagic), generally as a temporary measure until the underlying cause can be treated. Some evidence suggests that early use of vasopressors in patients with hemorrhagic shock may be deleterious compared with aggressive fluid resuscitation; however, additional studies are needed to confirm this finding. Dopamine may be particularly useful in the management of cardiogenic shock (including that associated with acute myocardial infarction) because of the drug's net hemodynamic effects; however, some evidence (e.g., from the SOAP II study) suggests an increased risk of mortality compared with norepinephrine when used in patients with this type of shock. Early revascularization is the standard of care in patients with cardiogenic shock; use of vasopressors in this setting should be individualized and guided by hemodynamic monitoring. Some experts state that dopamine may be considered for the treatment of drug-induced hypovolemic shock when the patient is unresponsive to fluid volume expansion and inotropic and/or vasopressor support is required. The use of dopamine in low cardiac output syndrome following open heart surgery has been shown to increase long-term survival. However, because dobutamine lowers peripheral resistance over a wide dosage range, is not dependent on release of endogenous catecholamines for its effects, and is cardioselective, that drug may be preferable in the period immediately following cardiopulmonary bypass surgery.

Dopamine may increase cardiac output, blood pressure, and urine flow in patients with shock; however, the exact effects of the drug are dose related and based on the patient's clinical status at the time of administration. In low or intermediate doses, dopamine usually does not produce sufficient peripheral vasoconstriction to cause a rise in blood pressure; therefore, the dose should be rapidly increased until adequate blood pressure is obtained. If hypotension persists, a more potent vasoconstrictor such as norepinephrine may be required. Dopamine appears to be most effective when therapy is initiated shortly after the signs and symptoms of shock appear and before physiologic parameters such as blood pressure and myocardial function undergo severe deterioration and before urine flow has decreased to less than 0.3 mL/minute. However, the drug may increase urine flow, in some cases to normal levels, in patients with oliguria or anuria. Urine flow may also increase in patients with normal urine output and thereby reduce preexisting fluid accumulation.

An α-adrenergic blocking agent such as phentolamine may be used to counteract the peripheral vasoconstriction produced by high doses of dopamine. Concomitant use of dopamine and a diuretic such as hydrochlorothiazide or furosemide may produce diuresis in patients who do not respond to dopamine or a diuretic alone. However, because dopamine acts as a proximal-tubule diuretic, the increased solute delivery to the distal tubular cells may increase distal oxygen consumption and potentially increase the risk of renal medullary ischemia in patients at risk of renal failure.

● Advanced Cardiovascular Life Support

Dopamine is used in advanced cardiovascular life support (ACLS)† for the treatment of symptomatic bradycardia in adults, particularly if associated with hypotension; although not a first-line drug, dopamine may be considered in patients who are unresponsive to atropine therapy, or as a temporizing measure while awaiting availability of a pacemaker.

Dopamine also has been used during the resuscitation period for management of patients in cardiac arrest. High-quality cardiopulmonary resuscitation (CPR) and defibrillation are integral components of ACLS and the only proven interventions to increase survival to hospital discharge. Other resuscitative efforts, including drug therapy, are considered secondary and should be performed without compromising the quality and timely delivery of chest compressions and defibrillation. The principal goal of pharmacologic therapy during cardiac arrest is to facilitate the return of spontaneous circulation (ROSC), and epinephrine is considered the drug of choice for this use. Vasoactive drugs such as dopamine may be used for hemodynamic support following resuscitation from cardiac arrest. (See Uses: Advanced Cardiovascular Life Support and Cardiac Arrhythmias, in Epinephrine 12:12.12.)

● Acute Renal Failure

Previous data from animal studies and some clinical studies in a limited number of healthy or critically ill adults indicated that low-dose (e.g., less than 5 mcg/kg per minute) infusions of dopamine may increase renal and mesenteric perfusion and improve renal function as a result of selective stimulation of renal dopaminergic receptors and subsequent renal vasodilation. However, more recent studies have failed to demonstrate any benefit from such therapy, and routine use of low-dose ("renal dose") dopamine therapy for the prevention or amelioration of acute renal failure in critically ill patients is no longer recommended. In a randomized, double-blind, placebo-controlled study, adults in an intensive care unit (ICU) at risk for acute renal failure who received dopamine as a continuous, low-dose (2 mcg/kg per minute) infusion had similar peak serum creatinine concentrations during treatment, similar durations of ICU and hospital stay, and similar survival to ICU or hospital discharge compared with those receiving placebo. Other studies in patients at high risk for renal failure receiving low-dose dopamine infusions (generally less than 2–3 mcg/kg per minute) have demonstrated similar findings. In a study in a small number of hemodynamically stable, critically ill patients, infusion of dopamine 3 mcg/kg per minute increased creatinine clearance, diuresis, and fractional excretion of sodium; however, these beneficial effects (except for diuresis) generally diminished after 24 hours, indicating the possibility of tolerance to the effects of dopamine. In addition, alterations in clearance and metabolism in critically ill patients may result in high interindividual variability in plasma dopamine concentrations for a given infusion rate (dosage) of the drug, making it difficult or impossible to guarantee a selective effect of the drug in this patient population. Low-dose infusions of dopamine are not without risk and may be associated with adverse effects such as suppression of respiratory drive, increased cardiac output and myocardial oxygen consumption, arrhythmias, hypokalemia, hypophosphatemia, gut ischemia, and disruption of metabolic and immunologic homeostasis.

● Heart Failure

Dopamine is used for short-term inotropic support in patients with refractory heart failure† to maintain systemic perfusion and preserve end-organ function. Because positive inotropic agents have not demonstrated improved outcomes in patients with heart failure and can be potentially harmful (e.g., increased risk of arrhythmias), particularly when used long term, the American College of Cardiology Foundation (ACCF) and American Heart Association (AHA) recommend that these drugs be reserved for patients with severe systolic dysfunction who have low cardiac index and evidence of systemic hypoperfusion and/or congestion, or for palliative therapy in those with end-stage heart failure. To minimize the risk of adverse effects, the lowest possible dosage should be used and the patient should be evaluated regularly for the need for continued inotropic therapy.

Low-dose dopamine infusion has been used in combination with loop diuretics to augment diuresis and improve renal blood flow in patients with acute decompensated heart failure†; however, the currently available evidence does not support routine use of dopamine for this purpose. Although some studies have suggested that dopamine may prevent worsening of renal function related to diuretic use in patients with acute decompensated heart failure, more recent studies generally have not confirmed this benefit.

DOSAGE AND ADMINISTRATION

● *Administration*

Dopamine hydrochloride is administered by IV infusion using an infusion pump or other apparatus to control the rate of flow. Precise control of the infusion rate is essential to avoid inadvertent administration of a bolus dose. To minimize the risk of necrosis, infusion of dopamine should be given into a large vein, preferably the antecubital vein. Less suitable veins (e.g., hand or ankle vein) should be used only when required, but the site should be switched to a preferred vein as soon as possible. *Care must be taken to avoid extravasation because local necrosis may result.*

Dopamine also has been administered by intraosseous infusion† in the setting of advanced cardiovascular life support (ACLS), generally when IV access is not readily available; onset of action and systemic concentrations are comparable to those achieved with venous administration.

IV Administration

The commercially available dopamine hydrochloride injection concentrate *must* be diluted prior to administration; alternatively, commercially available solutions of dopamine hydrochloride in 5% dextrose may be used without dilution. The concentration of dopamine is dependent upon the dosage and fluid requirements of the individual patient. One suggested solution for infusion may be prepared by diluting 10 mL of the injection concentrate containing 40 mg of dopamine hydrochloride per mL (a total of 400 mg of dopamine hydrochloride) with either 250 or 500 mL of one of the following solutions: 0.9% sodium chloride, 5% dextrose, 5% dextrose with 0.9% sodium chloride, 5% dextrose with 0.45% sodium chloride, lactated Ringer's, 5% dextrose in lactated Ringer's, or (1/6) *M* sodium lactate; dilution with 250 mL of solution will yield a final concentration of 1600 mcg/mL and dilution with 500 mL of solution will yield a final concentration of 800 mcg/mL.

Dopamine hydrochloride injections should be inspected visually for discoloration and/or particulate matter prior to administration whenever solution and container permit. Solutions darker than slightly yellow or that are discolored in any other way should not be used. Dopamine in 5% dextrose should not be infused into an umbilical artery catheter. The drug should be administered via a controlled-infusion device (pump), preferably a volumetric pump; dopamine should not be administered using an ordinary, gravity-controlled IV administration set. Dopamine in 5% dextrose in flexible containers (e.g., LifeCare®) should not be used in series connections.

The manufacturer's prescribing information should be consulted for proper methods of administration and other associated precautions.

Standardize 4 Safety

Standardized concentrations for dopamine have been established through Standardize 4 Safety (S4S), a national patient safety initiative to reduce medication errors, especially during transitions of care. Multidisciplinary expert panels were convened to determine recommended standard concentrations. Because recommendations from the S4S panels may differ from the manufacturer's prescribing information, caution is advised when using concentrations that differ from labeling, particularly when using rate information from the label. For additional information on S4S (including updates that may be available), see https://www.ashp.org/pharmacy-practice/standardize-4-safety-initiative.

TABLE 1. Standardize 4 Safety Continuous IV Infusion Standard Concentrations for Dopamine

Patient Population	Concentration Standards	Dosing Units
Adults[a]	1600 mcg/mL	mcg/kg/min
	3200 mcg/mL	
Pediatric patients (<50 kg)	800 mcg/mL	mcg/kg/min
	1600 mcg/mL	
	3200 mcg/mL	

[a] Consider limiting to 1 bag size for each recommended concentration (e.g., 250 vs 500 mL); this may reduce errors and also reduce inventory needs.

● *Dosage*
Shock

The rate and duration of dopamine hydrochloride infusion should be individualized and carefully adjusted to achieve the desired hemodynamic and renal response as indicated by heart rate, blood pressure, urine flow, and, whenever possible, measurement of central venous or pulmonary wedge pressure and cardiac output.

Dopamine hydrochloride infusion is usually initiated at a rate of 2–5 mcg/kg per minute in patients who are likely to respond to modest increases in cardiac contractility and renal perfusion. The infusion rate may be increased by 1–4 mcg/kg per minute at 10- to 30-minute intervals until the optimal response is attained. In more severely ill patients, dopamine hydrochloride infusion should be initiated at a rate of 5 mcg/kg per minute, and increased gradually in increments of 5–10 mcg/kg per minute, up to 20–50 mcg/kg per minute as needed. Once optimal hemodynamic effects have been achieved, the lowest possible dosage that maintains these effects should be used. In general, most patients can be maintained at an infusion rate less than 20 mcg/kg per minute; however, infusion rates exceeding 50 mcg/kg per minute have been used safely in advanced states of circulatory decompensation.

In patients with occlusive vascular disease, some clinicians recommend that dopamine hydrochloride therapy be initiated with an infusion rate of 1 mcg/kg per minute or less because of the risk of local ischemia. Such patients should be monitored closely for any signs or symptoms of compromised circulation during the infusion; if this occurs, the rate should be decreased or the infusion discontinued.

Patients who have been receiving monoamine oxidase (MAO) inhibitors within the previous 2–3 weeks should receive initial doses of dopamine hydrochloride of no greater than 10% of the usual dose.

At high dosages in patients in whom unnecessary expansion of fluid volume is a concern, administration of a more concentrated solution of dopamine hydrochloride (concentrations as high as 3.2 mg/mL have been used) may be preferable to increasing the flow rate of a dilute solution. Urine output should be measured frequently when doses exceeding 50 mcg/kg per minute are employed. When adjusting dosage to obtain the desired systolic blood pressure, optimal dosage for renal response may be exceeded and urine output may decrease. If urine flow begins to decrease in the absence of hypotension, reduction of the rate of infusion should be considered.

If a disproportionate increase in diastolic pressure (i.e., a marked decrease in pulse pressure) is observed in patients receiving dopamine, the rate of dopamine infusion should be decreased, and the patient observed carefully for further evidence of predominant vasoconstrictor activity, unless such an effect is desired. (See Cautions: Precautions and Contraindications.) Dosage reduction also may be required if a decrease in established urine flow rate, increase in tachycardia, or new dysrhythmia occurs.

Studies have not been conducted to specifically inform dosage recommendations in pediatric patients; however, clinical experience indicates that dosing in pediatric patients is generally similar to that in adults.

The manufacturer states that if dopamine hydrochloride is used in geriatric patients, the initial dosage usually should be at the low end of the dosage range since renal, hepatic, and cardiovascular dysfunction and concomitant disease or other drug therapy are more common in this age group than in younger patients.

When discontinuing an infusion, it may be necessary to gradually decrease the dose of dopamine while expanding blood volume with IV fluids to prevent a recurrence of hypotension. In patients who have been receiving moderate to high doses of dopamine, some clinicians recommend that the final dosage should not be less than 5 mcg/kg per minute in order to avoid hypotension.

Advanced Cardiovascular Life Support

When used in ACLS for the treatment of symptomatic bradycardia in adults†, the usual initial dosage range of dopamine hydrochloride is 2–10 mcg/kg per minute; dosage should be titrated according to patient response. Infusion rates exceeding 10 mcg/kg per minute are associated with vasoconstrictive effects. If used for postresuscitation stabilization in adults, a dopamine hydrochloride infusion rate of 5–10 mcg/kg per minute has been recommended.

If dopamine hydrochloride is used for postresuscitation stabilization in pediatric patients†, the usual IV or intraosseous† infusion rate is 2–20 mcg/kg per minute. Although dosages exceeding 5 mcg/kg per minute stimulate the cardiac β-adrenergic receptors, this effect may be reduced in infants. Infusion rates exceeding 20 mcg/kg per minute may result in excessive vasoconstriction.

Heart Failure

In the short-term treatment of patients with severe, refractory heart failure†, some clinicians recommend that dopamine hydrochloride infusion be initiated at a rate of 0.5–2 mcg/kg per minute. The usual dosage range of dopamine hydrochloride in patients with heart failure is 5–10 mcg/kg per minute. Although dosages exceeding 5 mcg/kg per minute stimulate the cardiac β-adrenergic receptors, this effect may be reduced in patients with congestive heart failure.

To minimize the risk of adverse effects, the lowest possible dosage of dopamine should be used and the patient should be evaluated regularly for the need for continued inotropic therapy.

CAUTIONS

● Adverse Effects

Dopamine hydrochloride may cause ectopic heartbeats, tachycardia, angina, palpitation, vasoconstriction, hypotension, dyspnea, nausea, vomiting, and headache. Other less frequent adverse effects include cardiac conduction abnormalities, widened QRS complex, bradycardia, hypertension, azotemia, anxiety, and piloerection. Ventricular arrhythmias may occur with very high doses. Dopamine may cause elevations in serum glucose although the concentrations usually do not rise above normal limits. A few cases of peripheral cyanosis also have been reported in patients receiving dopamine.

Gangrene of the extremities has occurred when high doses of dopamine were administered for prolonged periods and in patients with occlusive vascular disease receiving low doses of dopamine, and extravasation of dopamine may result in tissue necrosis and sloughing of surrounding tissues. (See Cautions: Precautions and Contraindications.)

● Precautions and Contraindications

Pressor therapy is *not* a substitute for replacement of blood, plasma, fluids, and/or electrolytes. Blood volume depletion should be corrected as fully as possible before dopamine therapy is instituted. In an emergency, the drug may be used as an adjunct to fluid replacement or as a temporary supportive measure to maintain coronary and cerebral artery perfusion until volume replacement can be completed, but dopamine must *not* be used as sole therapy in hypovolemic patients. Additional volume replacement may also be required during or after administration of the drug because of the effects of dopamine on urine flow. Monitoring of central venous pressure or left ventricular filling pressure may be helpful in detecting and treating hypovolemia; in addition, monitoring of central venous or pulmonary arterial diastolic pressure is necessary to avoid overloading the cardiovascular system, diluting serum electrolyte concentrations, and precipitating congestive heart failure or pulmonary edema. Hypoxia, hypercapnia, and acidosis (which may also reduce the effectiveness and/or increase the incidence of adverse

effects of dopamine) must be identified and corrected prior to, or concurrently with, administration of the drug.

During administration of dopamine, blood pressure and urine flow and, when possible, cardiac output and pulmonary wedge pressure should be monitored. If excessive vasoconstriction (as indicated by a disproportionate increase in diastolic blood pressure and a decrease in pulse pressure), decreased urine output, increased heart rate, or an arrhythmia occurs, the rate of infusion of dopamine should be decreased or temporarily suspended and the patient should be observed closely. If blood pressure or urine output fails to respond to discontinuance of the drug, administration of a short-acting α-adrenergic blocking agent such as phentolamine should be considered. If hypotension occurs during dopamine infusion, the infusion rate should be increased rapidly in order to increase blood pressure. If hypotension persists, dopamine should be discontinued and a drug with greater vasoconstricting properties such as norepinephrine should be administered. When discontinuing an infusion, it may be necessary to decrease the dose of dopamine gradually while expanding blood volume with IV fluids to prevent a recurrence of hypotension. *Sudden* cessation of dopamine infusion may result in marked hypotension.

Patients with a history of occlusive vascular disease (e.g., atherosclerosis, arterial embolism, Raynaud's disease, cold injury, diabetic endarteritis, Buerger's disease) should be carefully monitored during dopamine therapy for decreased circulation to the extremities indicated by changes in color or temperature of the skin or pain in the extremities. If such manifestations occur, they may be corrected by decreasing the rate of infusion or discontinuing dopamine; however, these changes occasionally have persisted and progressed after discontinuing the drug. The potential benefits of continuing dopamine should be weighed against the possible risk of necrosis. Some clinicians recommend IV administration of 5–10 mg of phentolamine mesylate if discoloration of the extremities occurs. To reverse ischemia induced by dopamine†, 10 mg of chlorpromazine IV followed by a chlorpromazine infusion of 0.6 mg/minute has been used.

Caution should be used to avoid extravasation of the drug. Dopamine should be administered through a large vein whenever possible, preferably in the antecubital fossa rather than the hand or ankle. One manufacturer states that administration into an umbilical arterial catheter is not recommended. If larger veins are unavailable and the condition of the patient requires that the hand or ankle veins be used to administer dopamine, the injection site should be changed to a larger vein as soon as possible. The site of infusion should be continuously monitored for free flow. If extravasation occurs, 10–15 mL of 0.9% sodium chloride injection containing 5–10 mg of phentolamine mesylate should be infiltrated (using a syringe with a fine hypodermic needle) liberally throughout the affected area. Immediate and conspicuous local hyperemic changes occur if the area is infiltrated within 12 hours; therefore, phentolamine should be administered as soon as possible after extravasation is noted. In children, phentolamine mesylate doses of 0.1–0.2 mg/kg, up to a maximum of 10 mg per dose, may be administered.

Commercially available formulations of dopamine hydrochloride injection may contain sodium metabisulfate, a sulfite that may cause allergic-type reactions, including anaphylaxis and life-threatening or less severe asthmatic episodes, in certain susceptible individuals. The overall prevalence of sulfite sensitivity in the general population is unknown but probably low; such sensitivity appears to occur more frequently in asthmatic than in nonasthmatic individuals.

Dopamine should be used with caution in patients with ischemic heart disease. The drug is contraindicated in patients with pheochromocytoma and in patients with uncorrected tachyarrhythmias or ventricular fibrillation.

● Pediatric Precautions

The manufacturer states that safety and efficacy of IV dopamine infusions have not been established in children; however, the drug has been used in pediatric patients of all age groups from neonate onward. In pediatric patients, dopamine is recommended as an appropriate drug for the treatment of shock when the patient is unresponsive to fluids and systemic vascular resistance is low. Except for vasoconstrictive effects caused by inadvertent infusion of dopamine into the umbilical artery, adverse effects unique to the pediatric population have not been identified, nor have adverse effects identified in adults been found to be more common in pediatric patients. Although dopamine reportedly has been administered at rates as high as 125 mcg/kg per minute in some neonates, the usual dosage in children has been similar to that in adults on a mcg/kg per minute basis.

● Geriatric Precautions

Clinical studies of dopamine hydrochloride did not include sufficient numbers of patients 65 years of age and older to determine whether geriatric patients respond differently than younger patients. Clinical experience to date has not identified any differences in responses between geriatric and younger patients. If dopamine hydrochloride is used in geriatric patients, the initial dosage of the drug usually should be at the low end of the dosage range, and caution should be exercised since renal, hepatic, and cardiovascular dysfunction and concomitant disease or other drug therapy are more common in this age group than in younger patients.

● Mutagenicity and Carcinogenicity

In the Ames microbial (*Salmonella*) mutagen test (with or without metabolic activation), there was a reproducible dose-dependent increase in the number of revertant colonies with strains TA100 and TA98 at dopamine dosages approaching maximal solubility. However, such small increases were considered inconclusive evidence of mutagenicity. In a mammalian mutagenicity assay using L5178Y TK± mouse lymphoma cells, dopamine was associated with toxicity and increases in mutant frequencies at concentrations of 750 mcg/mL without metabolic activation and 3000 mcg/mL with activation. No increases in mutant frequencies occurred at lower concentrations. In the in vivo mouse and male rat bone marrow micronucleus tests, no clear evidence of clastogenic potential was found at IV dosages up to 224 and 30 mg/kg of dopamine hydrochloride, respectively.

Long-term studies in animals have not been performed to date to evaluate the carcinogenic potential of dopamine.

● Pregnancy, Fertility, and Lactation

Pregnancy

Reproduction studies in rats and rabbits using IV dopamine hydrochloride dosages up to 6 mg/kg daily during organogenesis have not revealed evidence of teratogenicity or embryotoxicity; however, maternal toxicity (e.g., decreased body weight gain, death) was observed in rats. In a study in rats, subcutaneous dosages of 10 mg/kg for 30 days markedly prolonged metestrus and increased mean pituitary and ovary weights. After similar administration to pregnant rats, either throughout gestation or for 5 days beginning on day 10 or 15 of gestation, decreased body weight gain, increased mortality, and slight increases in cataract formation occurred in the offspring.

There are no adequate and well-controlled studies to date using dopamine hydrochloride in pregnant women, and the drug should be used during pregnancy only when the potential benefits justify the possible risks to the fetus. It is not known whether dopamine crosses the placenta. When dopamine is administered for advanced cardiovascular life support (ACLS) during cardiopulmonary resuscitation, the drug may decrease blood flow to the uterus; however, the woman must be resuscitated for survival of the fetus. If a vasopressor (e.g., dopamine) is used during labor in conjunction with oxytocic drugs, the vasopressor effect may be potentiated and result in severe hypertension. (See Drug Interactions: Oxytocic Drugs.)

Lactation

It is not known whether dopamine is distributed into human milk. Because many drugs are distributed into milk, the drug should be used with caution in nursing women.

DRUG INTERACTIONS

● Monoamine Oxidase Inhibitors

Because dopamine is metabolized by monoamine oxidase (MAO), the effects of the drug are prolonged and intensified by MAO inhibitors. Patients who have been receiving MAO inhibitors within the previous 2–3 weeks should receive initial doses of dopamine of no greater than 10% of the usual dose.

● α- and β-Adrenergic Blocking Agents

The cardiac effects of dopamine are antagonized by β-adrenergic blocking agents such as propranolol and metoprolol, and the peripheral vasoconstriction caused by high doses of dopamine is antagonized by α-adrenergic blocking agents. Dopamine-induced renal and mesenteric vasodilation is not antagonized by either α- or β-adrenergic blocking agents, but, in animals, is antagonized by haloperidol or other butyrophenones, phenothiazines, and opiates.

● General Anesthetics

Ventricular arrhythmias and hypertension may occur when usual doses of dopamine are administered during halothane (or other halogenated hydrocarbon) or cyclopropane anesthesia. Extreme caution should be used when administering dopamine to patients receiving these general anesthetics which increase cardiac irritability.

● Phenytoin

Administration of IV phenytoin to patients receiving dopamine has resulted in hypotension and bradycardia; some clinicians recommend that phenytoin be used with extreme caution, if at all, in patients receiving dopamine.

● Oxytocic Drugs

When a vasopressor agent (e.g., dopamine) is used in conjunction with oxytocic drugs, the pressor effect may be potentiated and result in severe hypertension.

● Other Drugs

The diuretic effects of low dosages of dopamine may be additive with or potentiated by diuretics (e.g., hydrochlorothiazide or furosemide). The pressor response of dopamine may be potentiated by tricyclic antidepressants. The concomitant use of dopamine with other vasopressors or vasoconstrictors (e.g., ergonovine) may result in severe hypertension.

LABORATORY TEST INTERFERENCES

Dopamine suppresses pituitary secretion of thyrotropin (thyroid-stimulating hormone, TSH), growth hormone, and prolactin.

ACUTE TOXICITY

Acute overdosage of dopamine may result in excessive elevation of blood pressure. The rate of infusion of dopamine should be decreased or the drug should be discontinued temporarily until the patient is stabilized. Because of dopamine's short duration of action, these measures usually provide adequate management of toxicity. In cases of severe toxicity, administration of a short-acting α-adrenergic blocking agent (e.g., phentolamine) should be considered. (See Uses: Other Uses in Phentolamine 12:16.04.04.)

PHARMACOLOGY

Dopamine stimulates adrenergic receptors of the sympathetic nervous system. The drug principally has a direct stimulatory effect on β₁-adrenergic receptors, but also appears to have an indirect effect by releasing norepinephrine from its storage sites. Dopamine also appears to act on specific dopaminergic receptors in the renal, mesenteric, coronary, and intracerebral vascular beds to cause vasodilation. The drug has little or no effect on β₂-adrenergic receptors. In IV doses of 0.5–2 mcg/kg per minute, the drug acts predominantly on dopaminergic receptors; in IV doses of 2–10 mcg/kg per minute, the drug also stimulates β₁-adrenergic receptors. In higher therapeutic doses, α-adrenergic receptors are stimulated and the net effect of the drug is the result of α-adrenergic, β₁-adrenergic, and dopaminergic stimulation. The main effects of dopamine depend on the dose administered. In low doses, cardiac stimulation and renal vascular dilation occur and in larger doses vasoconstriction occurs. It is believed that α-adrenergic effects result from inhibition of the production of cyclic adenosine-3′,5′-monophosphate (cAMP) by inhibition of the enzyme adenyl cyclase, whereas β-adrenergic effects result from stimulation of adenyl cyclase activity.

The β₁-adrenergic effects of dopamine exert a positive inotropic effect on the myocardium and result in an increase in cardiac output because of increased myocardial contractility and stroke volume in healthy individuals and in patients with shock or congestive heart failure. Systolic blood pressure and pulse pressure may be increased as a result of increased cardiac output; however, peripheral vasodilation and the resulting decrease in peripheral resistance may counteract these effects. Blood pressure, therefore, may remain unchanged or be only slightly elevated. Heart rate is usually not substantially changed. Coronary blood flow and myocardial oxygen consumption are usually increased as a result of increased myocardial contractility. Like other catecholamines, dopamine may facilitate atrioventricular conduction and increase myocardial excitability; however, the tendency of dopamine to induce cardiac arrhythmias may be slightly greater than that of dobutamine but is considerably less than that of isoproterenol and other catecholamines. Dopamine has variable effects on pulmonary vascular resistance and pulmonary artery pressure.

In low to moderate doses, dopamine causes renal and mesenteric vasodilation which is not antagonized by either α- or β-adrenergic blocking agents, atropine, or antihistamines and is therefore presumed to be the result of an action on dopaminergic receptors. Renal vasodilation results in increased renal blood flow and glomerular filtration rate. Urine flow is variably affected, but usually increases. Sodium excretion may increase, even in the absence of increased renal blood flow. The renal effects of dopamine may be at least partly due to intrarenal vascular changes and/or an inhibition of renal tubular sodium reabsorption. The osmolality of the urine usually does not decrease with increased urinary output.

In high doses (within and above the therapeutic range), α-adrenergic effects become more prominent and may result in increased peripheral resistance and renal vasoconstriction. This vasoconstriction may decrease previously augmented renal blood flow and urine output. Blood flow to peripheral vascular beds may decrease while mesenteric blood flow is increased because of increased cardiac output; however, with increasing doses of dopamine, mesenteric blood flow also decreases. In the absence of severe volume depletion, both systolic and diastolic blood pressures are increased because of increased cardiac output and increased peripheral resistance. Left ventricular filling pressure may be increased or decreased in patients with congestive heart failure. Heart rate response is variable. Blood pressure may return to normal if hypotension initially existed and may increase to hypertensive levels with excessive doses.

PHARMACOKINETICS

● *Absorption*

Orally administered dopamine is rapidly metabolized in the GI tract. Following IV administration, the onset of action of dopamine occurs within 5 minutes, and the drug has a duration of action of less than 10 minutes.

● *Distribution*

Dopamine is widely distributed in the body but does not cross the blood-brain barrier to a substantial extent. The apparent volume of distribution of the drug in neonates ranges from 0.6–4 L/kg. It is not known if dopamine crosses the placenta.

● *Elimination*

Dopamine has a plasma half-life of about 2 minutes. In neonates, the elimination half-life of dopamine reportedly is 5–11 minutes.

Dopamine is metabolized in the liver, kidneys, and plasma by monoamine oxidase (MAO) and catechol-O-methyltransferase to the inactive compounds homovanillic acid (HVA) and 3,4-dihydroxyphenylacetic acid. In patients receiving MAO inhibitors, the duration of action of dopamine may be as long as 1 hour. About 25% of a dose of dopamine is metabolized to norepinephrine within the adrenergic nerve terminals.

Dopamine is excreted in urine principally as HVA and its sulfate and glucuronide conjugates and as 3,4-dihydroxyphenylacetic acid. A very small fraction of a dose is excreted unchanged. Following administration of radiolabeled dopamine, approximately 80% of the radioactivity reportedly is excreted in urine within 24 hours.

In critically ill infants and children, the clearance rate of dopamine reportedly ranges from 48–168 mL/kg per minute, with the higher values reported in the younger patients.

CHEMISTRY AND STABILITY

● *Chemistry*

Dopamine is an endogenous catecholamine that is the immediate precursor of norepinephrine. Dopamine hydrochloride occurs as a white to off-white, crystalline powder that may have a slight odor of hydrochloric acid. Dopamine

hydrochloride is freely soluble in water and soluble in alcohol. Dopamine hydrochloride concentrate for injection may contain an antioxidant (e.g., sodium metabisulfite) and has a pH of 2.5–5.

Commercially available dopamine hydrochloride in dextrose injections are sterile, nonpyrogenic, isotonic solutions of the drug. Some commercially available dopamine hydrochloride injections containing 200, 400, or 800 mg in 250 mL of 5% dextrose injections have osmolarities of 261–270, 269–275, or 286–295 mOsm/L, respectively; hydrochloric acid and/or sodium hydroxide may have been added to adjust pH to 3.3–3.8 (range: 2.5–4.5).

● *Stability*

Commercially available dopamine hydrochloride injection is sensitive to and should be protected from light. Yellow, brown, or pink to purple discoloration of solutions containing dopamine hydrochloride indicates decomposition of the drug, and solutions that are darker than slightly yellow or discolored in any way should not be used. Commercially available dopamine hydrochloride injections should be stored at 20–25°C; the injections should not be frozen.

Some commercially available preparations of dopamine hydrochloride in 5% dextrose are provided in plastic containers. The amount of water that can permeate from the container into the overwrap is insufficient to significantly affect the injection. Solutions in contact with the plastic can leach out some of the chemical components in very small amounts; however, safety of the plastic has been confirmed during biological testing.

Dopamine hydrochloride is stable for at least 24 hours after dilution with the following solutions: 0.9% sodium chloride, 5% dextrose, 5% dextrose with 0.9% sodium chloride, 5% dextrose with 0.45% sodium chloride, lactated Ringer's, 5% dextrose in lactated Ringer's, or (1/6) *M* sodium lactate. Dopamine hydrochloride is incompatible with alteplase, amphotericin B, iron salts, oxidizing agents, and sodium bicarbonate and other alkaline solutions. In addition, commercially available dopamine hydrochloride injection should not be admixed with alkalinizing substances (e.g., sodium bicarbonate) since the drug is inactivated in alkaline solution. Specialized references should be consulted for specific compatibility information.

PREPARATIONS

Excipients in commercially available drug preparations may have clinically important effects in some individuals; consult specific product labeling for details.

DOPamine Hydrochloride

Parenteral

Concentrate, for injection, for IV infusion	40 mg/mL*	DOPamine Hydrochloride Injection
	80 mg/mL*	DOPamine Hydrochloride Injection
	160 mg/mL*	DOPamine Hydrochloride Injection

* available from one or more manufacturer, distributor, and/or repackager by generic (nonproprietary) name

DOPamine Hydrochloride in Dextrose

Parenteral

Injection, for IV infusion	0.8 mg/mL Dopamine Hydrochloride (200 or 400 mg) in Dextrose 5%*	0.08% DOPamine Hydrochloride in 5% Dextrose Injection (LifeCare®, Viaflex® Plus)
	1.6 mg/mL Dopamine Hydrochloride (400 or 800 mg) in Dextrose 5%*	0.16% DOPamine Hydrochloride in 5% Dextrose Injection (LifeCare®, Viaflex® Plus)
	3.2 mg/mL Dopamine Hydrochloride (800 mg) in Dextrose 5%*	0.32% DOPamine Hydrochloride in 5% Dextrose Injection (LifeCare®, Viaflex® Plus)

* available from one or more manufacturer, distributor, and/or repackager by generic (nonproprietary) name

† Use is not currently included in the labeling approved by the US Food and Drug Administration.

Selected Revisions June 10, 2024, © Copyright, June 1, 1979, American Society of Health-System Pharmacists, Inc.

Formoterol Fumarate

12:12.08.12 • SELECTIVE β₂-ADRENERGIC AGONISTS

■ Formoterol fumarate, a synthetic sympathomimetic amine, is a relatively selective, long-acting β₂-agonist.

USES

● Bronchospasm

Formoterol fumarate is used alone or in fixed combination with budesonide or glycopyrrolate for long-term maintenance treatment of bronchospasm or airflow obstruction associated with chronic obstructive pulmonary disease (COPD), including chronic bronchitis and emphysema. Formoterol fumarate also is used concomitantly with long-term asthma controller therapy, such as inhaled corticosteroids, as a long-acting bronchodilator for the prevention of bronchospasm in patients with reversible obstructive airway disease (e.g., asthma). Monotherapy with long-acting β₂-adrenergic agonists, such as formoterol, increases the risk of asthma-related death and may increase the risk of asthma-related hospitalization in pediatric and adolescent patients. (See Asthma-related Death and Serious Asthma-related Events under Warnings/Precautions: Warnings, in Cautions.) *Because of these risks, the use of formoterol alone for the treatment of asthma without concomitant use of long-term asthma controller therapy, such as inhaled corticosteroids, is contraindicated.* (See Cautions: Contraindications.) The fixed combination of formoterol fumarate and budesonide (formoterol/budesonide; Symbicort®) and fixed combination of formoterol fumarate and mometasone furoate (formoterol/mometasone; Dulera®) are used *only* in patients with asthma who have not responded adequately to long-term asthma controller therapy, such as inhaled corticosteroids, or whose disease severity warrants initiation of treatment with both an inhaled corticosteroid and a long-acting β₂-adrenergic agonist. Once asthma control is achieved and maintained, the patient should be assessed at regular intervals and therapy should be stepped down (e.g., discontinuance of formoterol or formoterol in fixed combination with budesonide), if possible without loss of asthma control, and the patient should be maintained on long-term asthma controller therapy, such as inhaled corticosteroids. Formoterol in fixed combination with budesonide should not be used in patients whose asthma is adequately controlled on a low or medium dosage of inhaled corticosteroids.

Formoterol fumarate alone or in fixed combination with budesonide, glycopyrrolate, or mometasone furoate is *not* indicated for the relief of acute bronchospasm and should *not* be initiated in patients with rapidly deteriorating or potentially life-threatening episodes of asthma or COPD. Use of long-acting β₂-adrenergic agonists with or without inhaled corticosteroids for acute exacerbations of COPD has not been evaluated. A short-acting inhaled β₂-adrenergic agonist should be used intermittently (as needed) for acute symptoms of asthma or COPD. (See Acute Exacerbations of Asthma or Chronic Obstructive Pulmonary Disease under Warnings/Precautions: Warnings, in Cautions.)

Asthma

Considerations in Initiating Antiasthma Therapy

In the stepped-care approach to antiasthmatic drug therapy, asthma is classified according to severity upon initial presentation (intermittent asthma or mild, moderate, or severe persistent asthma) and also by response to treatment (i.e., asthma control). While classification of asthma severity is useful for determining initial treatment, disease severity may vary over time and with treatment; therefore, after therapy is initiated, periodic assessment of asthma control is emphasized for guiding treatment decisions. Asthma management guidelines state that initial therapy for asthma should correspond to disease severity, with subsequent monitoring and adjustments in therapy to achieve and maintain control of asthma according to the goals of treatment. Asthma therapy is aimed at achieving and maintaining control of asthma by reducing ongoing impairment (e.g., prevention of chronic and troublesome symptoms, reducing use of reliever drugs, maintaining normal or near-normal lung function and activity levels) and risk of future events (e.g., exacerbations requiring systemic corticosteroids, treatment-related adverse effects). These 2 components of asthma control (i.e., current impairment and future risk) may respond differently to treatment.

The National Asthma Education and Prevention Program (NAEPP) classifies the levels of asthma control as well controlled, not well controlled, or very poorly controlled. In the stepped-care approach, the treatment step selected for asthma control in patients already receiving asthma therapy is based on the patient's current treatment and level of asthma control. Stepwise therapy is meant to assist, not replace, the clinical decision-making process in selecting therapy for individual patients. Once initiated, treatment is adjusted continuously according to changes in asthma control. Patients should be monitored every 2–6 weeks following initiation of therapy to ensure that asthma control is achieved. If asthma symptoms are not controlled with the current treatment regimen, treatment is stepped up until control is achieved. If an alternative treatment was used and produced an inadequate response, the preferred treatment should be used before stepping up to the next level of therapy. Regular monitoring at 1- to 6-month intervals, depending on the level of control, is recommended to ensure that control of asthma is maintained and that appropriate adjustments in therapy are made. When control has been maintained for at least 3 months, treatment intensity may be stepped down to find the lowest dosage and/or number of drugs required to maintain asthma control, with continued follow-up at 3-month intervals.

Intermittent Asthma

Drugs for asthma may be categorized as relievers (e.g., bronchodilators taken as needed for acute symptoms) or controllers (principally inhaled corticosteroids or other anti-inflammatory agents taken regularly to achieve long-term control of asthma). A reliever drug such as a selective short-acting inhaled β₂-adrenergic agonist (e.g., albuterol, levalbuterol, pirbuterol) is recommended on an as-needed basis to control occasional acute symptoms (e.g., cough, wheezing, dyspnea) of short duration; such use of an inhaled short-acting β₂-agonist alone generally is sufficient as initial treatment for newly diagnosed patients whose asthma severity is initially classified as intermittent (e.g., patients with daytime symptoms of asthma not more than twice weekly and nocturnal symptoms not more than twice a month). Most experts consider short-acting inhaled β₂-adrenergic agonists to be drugs of choice for treating acute asthma symptoms and exacerbations and for preventing exercise-induced bronchospasm. Alternatives to short-acting inhaled β₂-agonists recommended by some clinicians for relief of acute asthma symptoms include an inhaled anticholinergic agent (e.g., ipratropium), a short-acting oral β₂-agonist, or a short-acting theophylline (provided extended-release theophylline is not already used), but these alternatives have a slower onset of action and/or a higher risk for adverse effects. Oral β₂-adrenergic agonist therapy is suggested for use principally in patients unable to use inhaled bronchodilators (e.g., young children). Other experts do not recommend oral β₂-agonists for relief of acute asthma symptoms. Use of short-acting inhaled β₂-agonists in asymptomatic asthma should be limited to pretreatment prior to exercise and, in intermittent asthma, should be limited to providing relief as symptoms develop; some clinicians state that patients requiring symptomatic relief more than twice weekly or repeatedly over 1 or 2 days should be evaluated for possible initiation of long-term controller therapy.

Mild Persistent Asthma

When control of symptoms deteriorates in mild intermittent asthma and symptoms become persistent (e.g., daytime symptoms of asthma more than twice weekly but less than once daily, and nocturnal symptoms of asthma 3–4 times per month), asthma management guidelines and most clinicians recommend initiation of a controller drug such as an anti-inflammatory agent, preferably a low-dose orally inhaled corticosteroid (e.g., 88–264, 88–176, or 176 mcg of fluticasone propionate [or its equivalent] daily via a metered dose inhaler in adults and adolescents, children 5–11 years of age, or children 4 years of age or younger, respectively) as first-line therapy for persistent asthma supplemented by as-needed use of a short-acting, inhaled β₂-agonist. Alternatives to low-dose inhaled corticosteroids for mild persistent asthma include certain leukotriene modifiers (i.e., montelukast, zafirlukast), extended-release theophylline, or mast-cell stabilizers (i.e., cromolyn, nedocromil [preparations for oral inhalation no longer commercially available in the US]), but these therapies are less effective and generally not preferred as initial therapy. Some experts recommend that long-term control therapy be considered in infants and young children who have identifiable risk factors for asthma and who in the previous year have had 4 or more episodes of wheezing that lasted more than 1 day and symptoms that affected sleep. Low-dose inhaled corticosteroids also are recommended as the preferred initial therapy in such children. Cromolyn sodium is suggested (based on extrapolation of data from studies in older children) or montelukast is recommended by some experts as alternative, but not preferred, therapy in children 4 years of age or younger with mild persistent asthma. Other experts do not consider mast cell stabilizers or extended-release theophylline to be acceptable alternatives to inhaled corticosteroids for routine use as initial long-term therapy in such patients.

Moderate Persistent Asthma

According to asthma management guidelines, therapy with a long-acting inhaled β₂-agonist, such as formoterol or salmeterol generally is recommended in adults and adolescents who have moderate persistent asthma and daily asthmatic symptoms that are inadequately controlled following addition of low-dose inhaled corticosteroids to as-needed short-acting inhaled β₂-agonist treatment. However, NAEPP recommends that the beneficial effects of long-acting inhaled β₂-agonists should be weighed carefully against the increased risk (although uncommon) of severe asthma exacerbations and asthma-related deaths associated with daily use of such agents. (See Uses: Bronchospasm and also see Asthma-related Death and Life-threatening Events under Cautions: Respiratory Effects, in Salmeterol 12:12.08.12.) Asthma management guidelines also state that an alternative, but equally preferred option for management of moderate persistent asthma that is not adequately controlled with a low dosage of inhaled corticosteroid is to increase the maintenance dosage to a medium dosage (e.g., exceeding 264 but not more than 440 mcg of fluticasone propionate [or its equivalent] daily via a metered-dose inhaler in adults and adolescents). Alternative less effective therapies that may be added to a low dosage of inhaled corticosteroid include an oral extended-release theophylline or certain leukotriene modifiers (i.e., montelukast, zafirlukast).

Limited data are available in infants and children 11 years of age or younger with moderate persistent asthma, and recommendations of care are based on expert opinion and extrapolation from studies in adults. According to asthma management guidelines, a long-acting inhaled β₂-agonist (e.g., formoterol, salmeterol), a leukotriene modifier (i.e., montelukast, zafirlukast), or extended-release theophylline (with appropriate monitoring) may be added to low-dose inhaled corticosteroid therapy in children 5–11 years of age. Because comparative data establishing relative efficacy of these agents in this age group are lacking, there is no clearly preferred agent for use as adjunctive therapy with a low-dose inhaled corticosteroid for treatment of asthma in these children. In children 5–11 years of age with moderate persistent asthma that is not controlled with a low dosage of an inhaled corticosteroid, another preferred option according to asthma management guidelines is to increase the maintenance dosage of the inhaled corticosteroid to a medium dosage (e.g., exceeding 176 but not more than 352 mcg of fluticasone propionate [or its equivalent] daily via a metered-dose inhaler). In infants and children 4 years of age or younger with moderate persistent asthma that is not controlled by a low dosage of an inhaled corticosteroid, the only preferred option is to increase the maintenance dosage of the inhaled corticosteroid to a medium dosage (e.g., exceeding 176 mcg but not more than 352 mcg of fluticasone propionate [or its equivalent] daily via a metered-dose inhaler).

Severe Persistent Asthma

Maintenance therapy with an inhaled corticosteroid at medium dosages or high dosages (e.g., exceeding 440 mcg of fluticasone propionate in adults and adolescents or 352 mcg in children 5–11 years of age [or its equivalent] daily via a metered-dose inhaler) and adjunctive therapy with a long-acting inhaled β₂-agonist is the preferred treatment according to asthma management guidelines in adults and children 5 years of age or older with severe persistent asthma (i.e., continuous daytime asthma symptoms, nighttime symptoms 7 times per week). Such recommendations in children 5–11 years of age are based on expert opinion and extrapolation from studies in adolescents and adults. Alternatives to a long-acting inhaled β₂-agonist for severe persistent asthma in adults and children 5 years of age or older receiving medium-dose inhaled corticosteroids include extended-release theophylline or certain leukotriene modifiers (i.e., montelukast, zafirlukast), but these therapies are generally not preferred. Omalizumab may be considered in adults and adolescents with severe asthma with an allergic component who are inadequately controlled with high-dose inhaled corticosteroids and a long-acting β₂-agonist. In infants and children 4 years of age or younger with severe asthma, maintenance therapy with an inhaled corticosteroid at medium or high dosages (e.g., exceeding 352 mcg of fluticasone propionate [or its equivalent] daily via a metered-dose inhaler) and adjunctive therapy with either a long-acting inhaled β₂-agonist or montelukast is the only preferred treatment according to asthma management guidelines. Recommendations for care of infants and children with severe asthma are based on expert opinion and extrapolation from studies in older children.

Poorly Controlled Asthma

If asthma symptoms in adults and children 5 years of age or older with moderate to severe asthma are very poorly controlled (i.e., at least 2 exacerbations per year requiring oral corticosteroids) with low to high maintenance dosages of an inhaled corticosteroid and a long-acting inhaled bronchodilator, a short course (3–10 days) of an oral corticosteroid may be added to gain prompt control

of asthma. In infants and children 4 years of age or younger with moderate to severe asthma who are very poorly controlled (more than 3 exacerbations per year requiring oral corticosteroids) with medium to high maintenance dosages of an inhaled corticosteroid with or without adjunctive therapy (i.e., a long-acting inhaled β₂-agonist, montelukast), a short course (3–10 days) of an oral corticosteroid may be added to gain prompt control of asthma.

While clinical efficacy of oral corticosteroids as add-on therapy in adults and children 5 years of age or older with very severe asthma that is inadequately controlled with a high-dose inhaled corticosteroid, intermittent oral corticosteroid therapy, and a long-acting inhaled β₂-agonist bronchodilator has not been established in randomized controlled studies, some experts suggest regular use of oral corticosteroids in such patients, based on consensus and clinical experience. Similarly, some experts, based on consensus and clinical experience, suggest regular use of oral corticosteroid therapy in infants and children 4 years of age or younger with very severe asthma who are not controlled with high-dose inhaled corticosteroid and either a long-acting inhaled β₂-agonist or montelukast and intermittent oral corticosteroid therapy. However, other experts do not consider regular use of oral corticosteroid therapy to be appropriate therapy in children with severely uncontrolled asthma. (See Asthma under Uses: Respiratory Diseases, in the Corticosteroids General Statement 68:04.)

When asthma symptoms at any stage are not controlled with maintenance therapy (e.g., inhaled corticosteroids) plus supplemental short-acting inhaled β₂-agonist bronchodilator therapy as needed (e.g., if there is a need to increase the dose or frequency of administration of the short-acting sympathomimetic agent), prompt reevaluation is required to adjust dosage of the maintenance regimen or institute an alternative maintenance regimen. For additional details on the stepped-care approach to drug therapy in asthma, see Asthma under Uses: Bronchospasm, in Albuterol 12:12.08.12 and also see Asthma under Uses: Respiratory Diseases, in the Corticosteroids General Statement 68:04.

Clinical Experience with Formoterol Fumarate

While formoterol has a more rapid onset of action than salmeterol, the clinical importance of this difference in the treatment of asthma has not been established, and neither formoterol nor salmeterol should be used to relieve symptoms of acute asthma. (See Acute Exacerbations of Asthma or Chronic Obstructive Pulmonary Disease under Warnings/Precautions: Warnings, in Cautions and also see Supplemental Therapy in Acute Asthma under Bronchospasm: Asthma, in Uses in Salmeterol 12:12.08.12.)

Results of several controlled, comparative studies in adolescents and adults with mild to moderate asthma (i.e., requiring daily use of short-acting inhaled β₂-adrenergic bronchodilators with or without orally inhaled corticosteroids or theophylline) indicate that therapy with orally inhaled formoterol fumarate (12 or 24 mcg twice daily) is more effective than therapy with orally inhaled albuterol (180 mcg 4 times daily) or placebo in controlling asthma symptoms (e.g., as determined by days free of asthma symptoms, presence of nocturnal asthma symptoms, nights without nocturnal awakenings), reducing the need for rescue medication (e.g., intermittent use of a short-acting, β₂-agonist bronchodilator to control asthma exacerbations), and improving lung function (e.g., as determined by mean peak expiratory flow rate [PEFR], forced expiratory volume in 1 second [FEV₁]). In a large clinical study in children (5–12 years of age) with persistent asthma who required concomitant therapy with an anti-inflammatory agent (i.e., cromolyn sodium, inhaled corticosteroid) and a daily inhaled bronchodilator (e.g., albuterol) at study entry, usual dosages of orally inhaled formoterol fumarate (12 mcg twice daily) were consistently more effective than placebo in improving pulmonary function (as measured by FEV₁ area under the curve [AUC]) on day 1 of treatment and at 12 weeks and 1 year. Anti-inflammatory agents were continued throughout the study. While regular use of bronchodilators was not permitted during the study, orally inhaled albuterol was used as supplemental therapy for acute symptoms of asthma. While comparative clinical data for formoterol and salmeterol are limited, the drugs appeared to have similar efficacy (in terms of PEFR values, use of rescue medication, and symptom control) and safety in a 6-month, randomized, open-label study in adults with reversible obstructive airways disease who received orally inhaled formoterol fumarate 12 mcg or salmeterol 50 mcg twice daily.

Clinical Experience with Fixed Combination of Formoterol Fumarate and Budesonide

In 2 randomized, double-blind, placebo-controlled clinical studies in patients 12 years of age or older with mild to severe asthma, orally inhaled formoterol/budesonide (9 mcg of formoterol fumarate and 160 or 320 mcg of budesonide twice daily) produced greater improvement in most indices of pulmonary function (e.g., mean percent change from baseline in FEV_1 or morning and evening PEFR) than either drug alone and similar efficacy as concurrent therapy with both drugs given as single-entity preparations.

In one randomized, double-blind, multicenter study, 184 pediatric patients 6 to younger than 12 years of age with asthma received orally inhaled formoterol/budesonide (9 mcg of formoterol fumarate and 160 mcg of budesonide twice daily) or orally inhaled single-entity budesonide 160 mcg twice daily. In patients receiving formoterol/budesonide, there was a substantial change in 1-hour post-dose FEV_1 at 12 weeks, which improved by 0.28 L from baseline in those receiving the fixed combination compared with 0.17 L in those receiving single-entity budesonide.

Clinical Experience with Fixed Combination of Formoterol Fumarate and Mometasone Furoate

In one randomized, double-blind, placebo-controlled, 26-week study in patients with asthma 12 years of age or older, orally inhaled formoterol/mometasone (2 inhalations of preparation containing 5 mcg of formoterol fumarate and 100 mcg of mometasone furoate twice daily) was compared with either mometasone furoate 100 mcg, formoterol fumarate 5 mcg, or placebo (2 inhalations administered twice daily). A co-primary efficacy end point in this study was the change from baseline in FEV_1 AUC from 0–12 hours. In this study, patients receiving formoterol/mometasone had substantially greater increases in FEV_1 AUC 0–12 hours at 12 weeks compared with those receiving single-entity mometasone furoate or placebo; such improvements were maintained over the 26-week study period. Another primary end point in this study was deterioration in asthma or reduction in lung function. Patients who received formoterol/mometasone had fewer reports of asthma deterioration compared with patients receiving single-entity formoterol fumarate.

In a randomized, double-blind, 12-week study in patients with asthma 12 years of age or older, orally inhaled formoterol/mometasone (2 inhalations of preparation containing 5 mcg of formoterol fumarate and 100 or 200 mcg of mometasone furoate administered twice daily) was compared with mometasone furoate 200 mcg (2 inhalations administered twice daily). Patients who received either dosage of the formoterol/mometasone fixed combination had substantially greater increases in mean FEV_1 from baseline and over 12 weeks compared with those receiving single-entity mometasone furoate.

Chronic Obstructive Pulmonary Disease

Orally inhaled formoterol is used alone or in fixed combination with budesonide or glycopyrrolate as a bronchodilator for the long-term symptomatic treatment of airflow obstruction associated with COPD, including chronic bronchitis and emphysema.

In the stepped-care approach to drug therapy for COPD, mild, intermittent symptoms and minimal lung impairment (FEV_1 at least 80% of predicted) can be treated with a short-acting, selective inhaled β₂-adrenergic agonist (e.g., albuterol) as needed for acute symptoms. For the treatment of moderate to severe COPD (e.g., FEV_1 30 to less than 80% of predicted value) who have persistent symptoms despite as-needed therapy with ipratropium or a selective inhaled β₂-agonist, maintenance treatment with one or more long-acting bronchodilators (e.g., orally inhaled formoterol, salmeterol, tiotropium) can be added, and a short-acting, selective inhaled β₂-agonist used as needed for immediate symptom relief. Maintenance therapy with long-acting bronchodilators in patients with moderate to severe COPD is more effective and more convenient than regular use of short-acting bronchodilators.

Maintenance therapy (e.g., 4 times daily) with a short-acting, selective inhaled β₂-agonist is not preferred but may be used in patients with persistent symptoms of COPD; such therapy should not exceed 6–12 inhalations daily. Guidelines for the management of COPD state that low- to high-dose ipratropium (6–16 inhalations daily) can be added to therapy with a short-acting, selective β₂-agonist (as separate inhalations or in fixed combination) in patients with mild to moderate persistent symptoms of COPD, with the frequency of inhalation dosing with either agent not to exceed 4 times daily; the highest dosage of ipratropium included in some guidelines for COPD exceeds the manufacturer's maximum recommended daily dosage (12 inhalations). Combining bronchodilators from different classes and with differing durations of action may increase the degree of bronchodilation with a similar or lower frequency of adverse effects.

For patients not responding adequately to treatment with a long-acting bronchodilator, a combination of several long-acting bronchodilators, such as tiotropium and a long-acting β-adrenergic agonist, may be used. A short-acting bronchodilator may be used as needed for relief of acute symptoms that occur despite regular use of long-acting bronchodilators. For treatment of severe to very

severe COPD (e.g., FEV_1 less than 30 to less than 50% of predicted, history of exacerbations), the addition of an inhaled corticosteroid to one or more long-acting bronchodilators given separately or in fixed combination may be needed. If symptoms are not adequately controlled with inhaled corticosteroids and a long-acting bronchodilator or if limiting adverse effects occur, oral extended-release theophylline may be added or substituted. For additional information on the stepped-care approach to drug therapy in COPD, see Chronic Obstructive Pulmonary Disease under Uses: Bronchospasm, in Ipratropium Bromide 12:08.08.

Clinical Experience with Formoterol Fumarate

In a long-term (12-month) controlled comparative study in patients with COPD, orally inhaled formoterol fumarate (12 mcg twice daily) produced greater bronchodilation (as measured by increases in area under the forced expiratory volume in 1 second [FEV_1]-time curve) than dose-adjusted oral extended-release theophylline (dosage adjusted to maintain plasma drug concentrations within the range of 8–20 mcg/mL) or placebo for a period of 12 hours following the morning dose. Approximately half of the patients in each group were receiving inhaled corticosteroids, which were continued during the study along with as-needed rescue therapy with inhaled albuterol. Therapy with formoterol also decreased mild exacerbations of COPD (defined as the number of days with at least 2 symptom scores of 2 or greater and/or a reduction in peak expiratory flow [PEF] exceeding 20%) and the use of supplemental (rescue) medication compared with oral extended-release theophylline or placebo.

In a similar short-term (12-week) controlled study in patients with COPD, orally inhaled formoterol fumarate (12 mcg twice daily), produced greater improvement in FEV_1 (for 12 hours following the dose), symptoms, and quality of life than inhaled ipratropium bromide (36 mcg 4 times daily) or placebo. Therapy with orally inhaled formoterol also decreased mild exacerbations of COPD (defined as the number of days with at least 2 symptom scores of 2 or greater and/or a reduction in peak expiratory flow [PEF] exceeding 20%) and the need for rescue therapy with a short-acting β₂-agonist (albuterol) compared with orally inhaled ipratropium or placebo. Compared with formoterol fumarate 12 mcg twice daily, a dosage of 24 mcg twice daily did not provide additional benefits on FEV_1 and other end points in these studies.

Clinical Experience with Fixed Combination of Formoterol Fumarate and Budesonide

In 2 randomized, double-blind, placebo-controlled studies of 6 or 12 months' duration in patients with COPD, orally inhaled formoterol/budesonide (9 mcg of formoterol fumarate and 320 mcg of budesonide twice daily) produced greater improvements in the mean percent change from baseline in predose FEV_1 compared with formoterol fumarate alone or placebo and in 1-hour postdose FEV_1 compared with budesonide alone or placebo. The formoterol/budesonide fixed combination given in a dosage of 9 mcg of formoterol fumarate and 160 mcg of budesonide twice daily did not produce greater improvements from baseline in predose FEV_1 than formoterol alone or placebo. Therefore, the higher dosage of formoterol/budesonide is the only recommended dosage for the treatment of airflow obstruction in COPD.

Clinical Experience with Fixed Combination of Formoterol Fumarate and Glycopyrrolate

In 2 randomized, double-blind, placebo-controlled, parallel group studies of 24 weeks' duration in 3699 adults 40 years of age or older with moderate to very severe COPD, orally inhaled formoterol/glycopyrrolate (9.6 mcg of formoterol fumarate and 18 mcg of glycopyrrolate twice daily) resulted in a larger increase in mean change from baseline in trough FEV_1 after 24 weeks compared with either drug alone or placebo. The mean peak FEV_1 improvement from baseline with the formoterol/glycopyrrolate fixed combination compared with placebo after 24 weeks was 291 and 267 mL, respectively. Overall, the need for rescue medication with orally inhaled albuterol also was reduced in patients treated with formoterol/glycopyrrolate compared with those receiving placebo.

DOSAGE AND ADMINISTRATION

● Administration

Oral Inhalation

Formoterol Fumarate

Formoterol fumarate oral inhalation solution (Perforomist®) is administered by oral inhalation using a standard jet nebulizer connected to an air compressor and equipped with a mouthpiece or face mask. Formoterol fumarate oral inhalation solution is available in single-dose vials that should be stored in the foil pouch provided by the manufacturer and removed immediately before use.

For administration of formoterol fumarate oral inhalation solution for nebulization, the entire contents of the 20-mcg vial should be squeezed into the nebulizer reservoir. The nebulizer reservoir should be connected to the mouthpiece or face mask, and then the nebulizer should be connected to the compressor. The patient should be seated in an upright, comfortable position and should inhale the medication as calmly, deeply, and evenly as possible through the mouth using the mouthpiece or face mask of the nebulizer until the nebulizer stops producing mist in the reservoir (average nebulization time is 9 minutes). The nebulizer should be cleaned after use according to the manufacturer's instructions. The safety and efficacy of formoterol fumarate oral inhalation solution delivered from a nebulizer other than the Pari-LC Plus® nebulizer or a compressor other than the PRONEB® Ultra compressor have not been established. Formoterol fumarate oral inhalation solution should *not* be mixed with other inhalation solutions or ingested.

Fixed Combination of Formoterol Fumarate and Budesonide

Formoterol fumarate dihydrate in fixed combination with budesonide (formoterol/budesonide; Symbicort®) is administered by oral inhalation using an oral aerosol inhaler with hydrofluoroalkane (HFA) propellant. Formoterol/budesonide inhalation aerosol should only be used with the actuator supplied with the product.

Before each inhalation of formoterol/budesonide, the inhaler must be shaken well for 5 seconds. The aerosol inhaler should be test sprayed twice into the air (away from the face) before initial use, and shaken well for 5 seconds before each spray. If the inhaler has not been used for more than 7 days or if the inhaler was dropped, the inhaler should be test sprayed twice into the air (away from the face) and shaken well for 5 seconds before each spray. Rinsing the mouth after inhalation of formoterol/budesonide inhalation aerosol and spitting out the water are advised. The mouthpiece of the inhaler should be wiped clean with a dry cloth every 7 days. The inhaler should be discarded when the labeled number of inhalations has been used or within 3 months after removal from the foil pouch. The canister should never be immersed in water to determine the amount of drug remaining in the canister ("float test").

Fixed Combination of Formoterol Fumarate and Glycopyrrolate

Formoterol fumarate in fixed combination with glycopyrrolate (formoterol/glycopyrrolate; Bevespi® Aerosphere®) is administered by oral inhalation using an oral aerosol inhaler with HFA propellant. Formoterol/glycopyrrolate inhalation aerosol should only be used with the actuator supplied with the product.

The aerosol inhaler should be primed by releasing 4 test sprays into the air (away from the face) before initial use, and shaken well before each spray. If the inhaler has not been used for more than 7 days, the priming process should be repeated (using only 2 sprays rather than 4).

To administer a dose of formoterol/glycopyrrolate, the cap should be removed from the mouthpiece. Before each inhalation, the inhaler must be shaken well. The inhaler should be held with the mouthpiece pointing towards the face while the patient exhales through the mouth as fully and comfortably as possible. The lips should be closed around the mouthpiece and the head tilted back, keeping the tongue below the mouthpiece. While inhaling slowly and deeply, the center of the dose indicator should be pressed down until the canister stops moving in the actuator and a spray has been released, then the dose indicator should be released. At the end of inhalation, the mouthpiece should be removed from the mouth and the breath held as long as comfortably possible (up to 10 seconds) then the patient should exhale gently. The process should be repeated for the second inhalation. The cap should be replaced on the mouthpiece immediately after use.

The Bevespi® Aerosphere® inhaler should be cleaned once weekly by removing the canister from the actuator; the canister should not be cleaned or allowed to get wet. The actuator should be held under warm running water for about 30 seconds. The actuator should then be turned upside down and water rinsed through the actuator again for about 30 seconds. The actuator should be allowed to dry overnight. When the actuator is dry, the canister should be pressed gently down into the actuator; the canister should not be pressed down too hard since this may cause drug to be released. Priming of the inhaler should be repeated after each cleaning by shaking well and releasing 2 test sprays into the air away from the face. The inhaler should be discarded 3 months after removal from the foil pouch

or when the dose indicator reads "0," whichever comes first. The canister should never be immersed in water to determine the amount of drug remaining in the canister ("float test").

Fixed Combination of Formoterol Fumarate and Mometasone Furoate

Formoterol fumarate dihydrate in fixed combination with mometasone furoate (formoterol/mometasone; Dulera®) is administered by oral inhalation as an oral inhalation suspension using a metered-dose aerosol inhaler with HFA propellant. Formoterol/mometasone inhalation aerosol should only be used with the actuator supplied with the product.

The aerosol inhaler should be primed by releasing 4 test sprays into the air (away from the face) before initial use, and shaken well before each spray. If the inhaler has *not* been used for more than 5 days, it should be primed again by test spraying 4 times into the air (away from the face) and shaken well before each spray. Before each inhalation, the inhaler must be shaken well. Following each dose, the mouth should be rinsed thoroughly without swallowing. The mouthpiece of the inhaler should be wiped clean with a dry cloth every 7 days; water should not be used to clean the inhaler.

● Dosage

Each 2-mL single-dose vial of formoterol fumarate oral inhalation solution contains 20 mcg of formoterol fumarate. The oral inhalation solution does not require dilution prior to administration by nebulization. The actual amount of drug delivered to the lungs will depend on patient factors and the type of nebulization system used and its performance.

Each actuation of the oral aerosol inhaler containing the fixed combination of formoterol fumarate dihydrate and budesonide delivers 5.1 mcg of formoterol fumarate dihydrate and 91 or 181 mcg of budesonide from the valve and delivers 4.5 mcg of formoterol fumarate dihydrate and 80 or 160 mcg of budesonide from the actuator per metered spray, depending on the preparation used. The strength of formoterol/budesonide preparations and dosage of the fixed combination are expressed in terms of drug delivered from the mouthpiece of the actuator. The actual amount of drug delivered to the lungs depends on factors such as the patient's coordination between the actuation of the inhaler and inspiration through the delivery system. The commercially available formoterol/budesonide aerosol inhaler delivers 60 metered sprays per 6- or 6.9-g canister and 120 metered sprays per 10.2-g canister.

After priming of the oral aerosol inhaler containing the fixed combination of formoterol fumarate and glycopyrrolate, each actuation of the oral aerosol inhaler (Bevespi® Aerosphere®) delivers 5.5 mcg of formoterol fumarate and 10.4 mcg of glycopyrrolate (equivalent to 8.3 mcg of glycopyrronium) from the valve. Dosage is expressed in terms of drug delivered from the mouthpiece; each actuation of the inhaler delivers 4.8 mcg of formoterol fumarate and 9 mcg of glycopyrrolate (equivalent to 7.2 mcg of glycopyrronium) from the actuator. The actual amount of drug delivered to the lungs depends on factors such as the patient's coordination between actuation of the device and inspiration through the delivery system. Commercially available formoterol/glycopyrrolate aerosol inhaler delivers 28 or 120 metered sprays per 5.9- or 10.7-g canister, respectively.

Each actuation of the oral aerosol inhaler containing the fixed combination of formoterol fumarate dihydrate and mometasone furoate delivers 5.5 mcg of formoterol fumarate dihydrate and 115 or 225 mcg of mometasone furoate from the valve and delivers 5 mcg of formoterol fumarate dihydrate and 100 or 200 mcg of mometasone furoate from the actuator per metered spray, depending on the preparation used. The strength of formoterol/mometasone preparations and dosage of the fixed combination are expressed in terms of drug delivered from the mouthpiece of the actuator. The actual amount of drug delivered to the lungs may depend on factors such as the patient's coordination between actuation of the device and inspiration through the delivery system. Commercially available formoterol/mometasone aerosol inhaler delivers 60 or 120 metered sprays per 8.8- or 13-g canister, respectively.

Asthma
Fixed Combination of Formoterol Fumarate and Budesonide

In asthmatic patients 12 years of age or older, the recommended initial dosage of the oral inhalation aerosol containing formoterol fumarate dihydrate in fixed combination with budesonide is based on the patient's asthma severity. The dosage of the formoterol/budesonide fixed combination in this age group is 9 mcg of formoterol fumarate dihydrate and 160 or 320 mcg of budesonide (2 inhalations of preparation containing 4.5 mcg of formoterol fumarate dihydrate and 80 or 160 mcg of budesonide) twice daily, given approximately 12 hours apart (morning and evening). In asthmatic patients 6 to younger than 12 years of age, the recommended initial dosage of formoterol/budesonide is 9 mcg of formoterol fumarate dihydrate and 160 mcg of budesonide (2 inhalations of preparation containing 4.5 mcg of formoterol fumarate dihydrate and 80 mcg of budesonide) twice daily, given approximately 12 hours apart (morning and evening). The maximum recommended dosage of formoterol/budesonide in asthmatic patients 12 years of age or older is 9 mcg of formoterol fumarate dihydrate and 320 mcg of budesonide (2 inhalations of preparation containing 4.5 mcg of formoterol fumarate dihydrate and 160 mcg of budesonide) twice daily. The maximum recommended dosage in asthmatic children 6 to younger than 12 years of age is 9 mcg of formoterol fumarate dihydrate and 160 mcg of budesonide (2 inhalations of preparation containing 4.5 mcg of formoterol fumarate dihydrate and 80 mcg of budesonide) twice daily. The manufacturer states that administration of formoterol/budesonide oral inhalation aerosol more frequently than twice daily or in excess of 2 inhalations twice daily is not recommended. Patients receiving formoterol/budesonide should not use additional long-acting β₂-agonists for any reason.

Improvement in asthma control following oral inhalation of formoterol/budesonide may occur within 15 minutes of initiating treatment, although maximum benefit may not be achieved for 2 weeks or longer after therapy initiation. Individual patients will experience a variable time to onset and degree of symptom relief. If control of asthma is inadequate after 1–2 weeks of therapy at the lower dosage, switching to a higher strength of the fixed combination (higher strengths contain higher dosages of budesonide only) may provide additional asthma control. If acute asthmatic symptoms arise despite therapy with formoterol in fixed combination with budesonide, a short-acting inhaled β₂-adrenergic agonist should be taken for immediate relief. Patients should be advised not to discontinue formoterol/budesonide without medical supervision, as symptoms may recur after treatment discontinuance. If a previously effective dosage of formoterol/budesonide fails to provide adequate asthma control, the therapeutic regimen should be reevaluated and additional therapeutic options should be considered (e.g., switching to a higher strength of the fixed combination [higher strengths contain higher dosages of budesonide only], adding additional inhaled corticosteroids, initiating systemic corticosteroids). (See Acute Exacerbations of Asthma or Chronic Obstructive Pulmonary Disease under Warnings/Precautions: Warnings, in Cautions.)

Fixed Combination of Formoterol Fumarate and Mometasone Furoate

In asthmatic patients 12 years of age or older, the recommended initial dosage of the oral inhalation aerosol containing formoterol fumarate dihydrate in fixed combination with mometasone furoate is based on the patient's asthma severity, previous asthma therapy (including previous inhaled corticosteroid dosage), current control of asthma symptoms, and risk of future asthma exacerbations.

In adults and adolescents 12 years of age or older, the dosage of the formoterol/mometasone fixed combination is 10 mcg of formoterol fumarate dihydrate and 200 or 400 mcg of mometasone furoate (2 inhalations of preparation containing 5 mcg of formoterol fumarate dihydrate and 100 or 200 mcg of mometasone furoate) twice daily. If control of asthma is inadequate after 2 weeks of formoterol/mometasone therapy at the lower dosage, switching to a higher strength of the fixed combination (higher strengths contain higher dosages of mometasone only) may provide additional asthma control. The maximum recommended dosage of formoterol/mometasone in asthmatic adults and adolescents 12 years of age or older is 10 mcg of formoterol fumarate dihydrate and 400 mcg of mometasone furoate twice daily.

Chronic Obstructive Pulmonary Disease
Formoterol Fumarate

For maintenance therapy of airflow obstruction in patients with chronic obstructive pulmonary disease (COPD), the recommended dosage of formoterol fumarate oral inhalation solution is 20 mcg (entire contents of a single-dose vial) every 12 hours (morning and evening) by nebulization. The total daily dosage of formoterol fumarate oral inhalation solution should not exceed 40 mcg. If shortness of breath occurs despite therapy with formoterol oral inhalation solution, a short-acting inhaled β₂-adrenergic agonist should be taken for immediate relief.

Fixed Combination of Formoterol Fumarate and Budesonide

For maintenance therapy of airflow obstruction in patients with COPD, the recommended dosage of the oral inhalation aerosol containing formoterol fumarate

dihydrate in fixed combination with budesonide in adults is 9 mcg of formoterol fumarate dihydrate and 320 mcg of budesonide (2 inhalations of preparation containing 4.5 mcg of formoterol fumarate dihydrate and 160 mcg of budesonide) twice daily (morning and evening). In clinical studies, lower dosages of formoterol/budesonide (i.e., 2 inhalations of preparation containing 4.5 mcg of formoterol fumarate dihydrate and 80 mcg of budesonide twice daily) did not produce greater improvements from baseline in predose FEV₁ than formoterol alone or placebo; therefore, such dosages are not recommended for the treatment of airflow obstruction in COPD.

If shortness of breath occurs despite therapy with the recommended dosage of formoterol/budesonide, a short-acting inhaled β₂-adrenergic agonist should be taken for immediate relief. Patients should be advised not to discontinue formoterol/budesonide without medical supervision, as symptoms may recur after treatment discontinuance. The manufacturer states that administration of formoterol/budesonide inhalation aerosol more frequently than twice daily or in excess of 2 inhalations twice daily is not recommended. Patients receiving formoterol/budesonide should not use additional long-acting β₂-agonists for any reason.

Fixed Combination of Formoterol Fumarate and Glycopyrrolate

For the long-term management of airflow obstruction associated with COPD, the usual dosage of formoterol fumarate in fixed combination with glycopyrrolate in adults is 9.6 mcg of formoterol fumarate and 18 mcg of glycopyrrolate (2 inhalations of preparation containing 4.8 mcg of formoterol fumarate and 9 mcg of glycopyrrolate) twice daily via the Aerosphere® device. More frequent administration or higher dosages are not recommended. Orally inhaled formoterol/glycopyrrolate should *not* be used for the treatment of acute episodes of bronchospasm.

● Special Populations
Hepatic Impairment

The manufacturers of formoterol fumarate and formoterol fumarate in fixed combination with budesonide, glycopyrrolate, or mometasone furoate make no specific dosage recommendations for patients with hepatic impairment at this time. However, since formoterol fumarate, budesonide, and mometasone are cleared predominantly by the liver, impaired liver function theoretically may lead to accumulation of the drugs in plasma. Therefore, the manufacturers of formoterol fumarate in fixed combination with budesonide, glycopyrrolate, or mometasone furoate state that patients with hepatic disease should be closely monitored for signs of increased drug exposure.

Renal Impairment

The manufacturers of formoterol fumarate and formoterol fumarate in fixed combination with budesonide, glycopyrrolate, or mometasone furoate make no specific dosage recommendations for patients with renal impairment at this time.

The manufacturer of formoterol fumarate in fixed combination with glycopyrrolate states that the preparation should be used in patients with severe renal impairment (i.e., creatinine clearance less than 30 mL/minute) or end-stage renal disease requiring dialysis only if expected benefits outweigh potential risks.

Geriatric Patients

The manufacturers of formoterol fumarate and formoterol fumarate in fixed combination with budesonide, glycopyrrolate, or mometasone furoate state that dosage adjustment is not required in geriatric patients.

CAUTIONS

● Contraindications

Formoterol fumarate and fixed combinations containing formoterol fumarate are contraindicated in patients hypersensitive to the drug or any ingredient in the formulation.

Because of the risk of asthma-related death and hospitalization, use of formoterol for the treatment of asthma without concomitant use of long-term asthma controller therapy, such as inhaled corticosteroids, is contraindicated. (See Asthma-related Death and Serious Asthma-related Events under Warnings/Precautions: Warnings, in Cautions and also see Uses: Bronchospasm.)

Formoterol fumarate in fixed combination with budesonide (formoterol/budesonide; Symbicort®) and formoterol fumarate in fixed combination with mometasone furoate (formoterol/mometasone; Dulera®) are contraindicated as primary treatment of status asthmaticus or other acute episodes of asthma or chronic obstructive pulmonary disease (COPD) when intensive measures are required.

Formoterol fumarate in fixed combination with glycopyrrolate (formoterol/glycopyrrolate; Bevespi® Aerosphere®) is not indicated for the treatment of asthma.

● Warnings/Precautions

Warnings

Use of Fixed Combinations

When formoterol fumarate is used in fixed combination with budesonide, glycopyrrolate, or mometasone furoate, the usual cautions, precautions, contraindications, and interactions associated with budesonide, glycopyrrolate, or mometasone furoate must be considered.

Cautionary information applicable to specific populations (e.g., pregnant or nursing women, individuals with hepatic or renal impairment, geriatric patients) should be considered for each drug in the fixed combination.

Asthma-related Death and Serious Asthma-related Events

Monotherapy with long-acting β₂-adrenergic agonists, such as formoterol, increases the risk of asthma-related death. In addition, available data from controlled clinical trials suggest that use of long-acting β₂-adrenergic agonists as monotherapy increases the risk of asthma-related hospitalization in pediatric and adolescent patients. *Because of these risks, the use of long-acting β₂-adrenergic agonists, including formoterol, alone for the treatment of asthma without concomitant use of long-term asthma controller therapy, such as inhaled corticosteroids, is contraindicated.* (See Cautions: Contraindications.) However, FDA has concluded that there is no clinically important increased risk of serious asthma-related events, including hospitalization, intubation, or death, associated with concomitant use of long-acting β₂-adrenergic agonists (e.g., formoterol) and inhaled corticosteroids compared with inhaled corticosteroids alone based on the results of several large clinical studies. In addition, these studies showed that combination therapy with long-acting β₂-adrenergic agonists and inhaled corticosteroids was more effective in reducing the incidence of asthma exacerbations (i.e., events requiring use of systemic corticosteroids for at least 3 outpatient days or an asthma-related hospitalization or emergency department visit requiring use of systemic corticosteroids) compared with use of inhaled corticosteroids alone.

The formoterol/budesonide and formoterol/mometasone fixed combinations should be used *only* in patients with asthma who have not responded adequately to long-term asthma controller therapy, such as inhaled corticosteroids, or whose disease severity warrants initiation of treatment with both an inhaled corticosteroid and a long-acting β₂-adrenergic agonist. Once asthma control is achieved and maintained, the patient should be assessed at regular intervals and therapy should be stepped down (e.g., discontinuance of the long-acting β₂-adrenergic agonist), if possible without loss of asthma control, and the patient should be maintained on long-term asthma controller therapy, such as inhaled corticosteroids. Long-acting β₂-adrenergic agonists, including formoterol alone or in fixed combination with budesonide, should not be used in patients whose asthma is adequately controlled on a low or medium dosage of inhaled corticosteroids. In pediatric and adolescent patients with asthma who require the addition of a long-acting β₂-adrenergic agonist to inhaled corticosteroid therapy, a fixed-combination preparation containing both an inhaled corticosteroid and a long-acting β₂-adrenergic agonist generally should be used to ensure compliance with both drugs. (See Uses: Bronchospasm.)

Data from a large placebo-controlled study (Salmeterol Multi-center Asthma Research Trial ([SMART]) evaluating the safety of another long-acting β₂-adrenergic agonist, salmeterol, in patients with asthma showed an increase in asthma-related deaths in patients receiving salmeterol. (See Asthma-related Death and Life-threatening Events under Cautions: Respiratory Effects, in Salmeterol 12:12.08.12.) The increased risk of asthma-related death with salmeterol is considered a class effect of the long-acting β₂-adrenergic agonists, including formoterol. However, no adequate studies have been conducted to determine whether the rate of asthma-related death is increased with formoterol. Clinical studies with inhalation of formoterol as a dry powder suggest that the incidence of serious asthma exacerbations is increased in patients receiving formoterol compared with those receiving placebo, although the sample sizes in these studies were not adequate to quantify the precise differences between treatment groups.

In 4 randomized, double-blind, active-controlled clinical trials mandated by FDA, the risk of serious asthma-related events from use of inhaled corticosteroids alone compared with combined use of long-acting β₂-adrenergic agonists and inhaled corticosteroids was evaluated over 26 weeks in 41,297 patients with asthma (3 trials in adults and adolescents 12 years of age or older and one trial in children 4–11 years of age). The primary safety end point in all of these trials was serious asthma-related events, including hospitalization, intubation, and death; these events were reviewed by a blinded committee to determine if the events were asthma related. The 3 trials performed in adults and adolescents were designed to rule out a hazard ratio of 2, and the pediatric trial was designed to rule out a hazard ratio of 2.7; this objective was met in all 4 individual trials. The trials were not designed to rule out all risk for serious asthma-related events associated with long-acting β₂-adrenergic agonists in combination with inhaled corticosteroids compared with inhaled corticosteroids alone.

The safety studies in adults and adolescents included one trial comparing salmeterol and fluticasone propionate in fixed combination as the inhalation powder with fluticasone propionate oral inhalation powder alone, one trial comparing formoterol and mometasone furoate in fixed combination with mometasone furoate alone, and one trial comparing formoterol and budesonide in fixed combination with budesonide alone. In a meta-analysis combining data from these 3 trials, a hazard ratio of 1.1 for first serious asthma-related event in patients receiving fixed-combination therapy with long-acting β₂-adrenergic agonists and inhaled corticosteroids compared with patients receiving inhaled corticosteroids alone was reported. Subgroup analyses for gender, adolescents 12–17 years of age, Asian and African-American patients, and obese patients also showed no substantial increase in the risk of serious asthma-related events or asthma exacerbations in these populations.

The safety study in children 4–11 years of age included 6208 patients who were randomized to receive salmeterol and fluticasone propionate in fixed combination as the inhalation powder or fluticasone propionate inhalation powder alone. Serious asthma-related events were reported in 0.9% of patients receiving salmeterol and fluticasone in fixed combination and in 0.7% of patients receiving fluticasone alone, with an estimated hazard ratio for first event of 1.29 for the combination therapy compared with fluticasone alone. No asthma-related deaths or intubations were reported in either group of pediatric patients.

No adequate studies have been conducted to determine whether the rate of death is increased in patients with COPD receiving long-acting β₂-adrenergic agonists.

Acute Exacerbations of Asthma or Chronic Obstructive Pulmonary Disease

Substantially worsening or acutely deteriorating asthma may be a life-threatening condition. Formoterol oral inhalation therapy should not be initiated in patients with substantially worsening or acutely deteriorating asthma. Formoterol in fixed combination with budesonide, glycopyrrolate, or mometasone furoate should not be initiated in patients with rapidly deteriorating or potentially life-threatening episodes of asthma or COPD.

Failure to respond to a previously effective dosage of formoterol may indicate substantially worsening asthma or destabilization of COPD that requires prompt reevaluation. If inadequate control of symptoms persists with supplemental β₂-agonist bronchodilator therapy (i.e., if there is a need to increase the dose or frequency of administration of the short-acting, inhaled bronchodilator), prompt reevaluation of asthma or COPD therapy is required, with special consideration given to the possible need for anti-inflammatory treatment (e.g., corticosteroids); however, extra or increased doses of formoterol should *not* be used in such situations. If asthma deteriorates in patients receiving formoterol in fixed combination with budesonide or mometasone furoate, prompt reevaluation of asthma therapy is required, with special consideration given to the possible need for increasing the strength of the fixed combination (higher strengths contain higher dosages of budesonide or mometasone only), adding additional inhaled corticosteroids, or initiating systemic corticosteroids; patients should not increase the frequency of administration of formoterol/budesonide or formoterol/mometasone. If COPD deteriorates in patients receiving formoterol/glycopyrrolate, prompt reevaluation of COPD therapy is required.

Concomitant Anti-Inflammatory Therapy

The manufacturer states that there are no data demonstrating clinical anti-inflammatory effects of formoterol that could be expected to substitute for or allow reduction in the dosage of corticosteroids. Particular care is needed for patients who have been transferred from systemically active corticosteroids to orally inhaled corticosteroids since death resulting from adrenal insufficiency has occurred in some asthmatic patients during and after such transfer. (See

Withdrawal of Systemic Corticosteroid Therapy under Warnings/Precautions: Warnings, in Cautions in Budesonide 68:04.)

Concomitant Short-Acting Bronchodilators

The manufacturer states that if patients are taking a short-acting, inhaled β₂-agonist bronchodilator on a regular basis (e.g., 4 times daily) at the time formoterol or formoterol in fixed combination with budesonide, glycopyrrolate, or mometasone is initiated, these patients should be instructed to discontinue the *regular* use of the short-acting agent and use it only for relief of acute asthma symptoms. *Regular* (e.g., daily) use of inhaled β₂-agonists does not adequately control asthma symptoms or airway hyperresponsiveness on a long-term basis and is not recommended by current asthma management experts.

Cardiovascular Effects

Formoterol, like other sympathomimetic amines, may increase heart rate or blood pressure. Although such effects are uncommon at recommended dosages, the drug may need to be discontinued if such cardiovascular effects occur.

Excessive Doses

Fatalities have been reported in association with excessive use of inhaled sympathomimetic drugs. (See Cautions, in Albuterol 12:12.08.12.)

Patients receiving formoterol alone or in fixed combination with budesonide, glycopyrrolate, or mometasone furoate should not use additional formoterol or other long-acting β₂-agonists for any reason.

Sensitivity Reactions

Immediate Hypersensitivity Reactions

Anaphylactic reactions, urticaria, angioedema, rash, flushing, allergic dermatitis, and bronchospasm have been reported with oral inhalation therapy with formoterol alone or in fixed combination with budesonide, glycopyrrolate, or mometasone. Orally inhaled formoterol/glycopyrrolate should be discontinued immediately if such allergic reactions occur, particularly angioedema (e.g., difficulties with breathing or swallowing; swelling of the tongue, lips, or face), urticaria, or rash, and alternative therapy considered.

Major Toxicities

Paradoxical Bronchospasm

As with other inhaled β₂-receptor agonists, a patient may develop acute bronchospasm, which may be life-threatening, immediately upon inhalation of formoterol. If paradoxical bronchospasm occurs, formoterol should be discontinued immediately and alternative therapy instituted.

General Precautions

Acute or Worsening Asthma or COPD

Formoterol, alone or in fixed combination with budesonide or mometasone furoate, or other long-acting β₂-adrenergic agonists (e.g., salmeterol) should *not* be used to relieve symptoms of acute asthma. Formoterol alone or in fixed combination with glycopyrrolate should not be used to relieve symptoms of acutely deteriorating COPD.

Failure to respond to a previously effective dosage of formoterol may indicate substantially worsening asthma or destabilization of COPD that requires prompt reevaluation. If inadequate control of symptoms persists with supplemental β₂-agonist bronchodilator therapy (i.e., if there is a need to increase the dose or frequency of administration of the short-acting inhaled bronchodilator or if a substantial decrease in peak expiratory flow or other index of lung function occurs), immediate reevaluation of asthma therapy is required (e.g., adjusting the inhaled corticosteroid dosage or initiating systemic corticosteroids); however, extra or increased doses of formoterol should *not* be used in such situations. If asthma deteriorates in patients receiving formoterol in fixed combination with budesonide or mometasone furoate, prompt reevaluation of asthma therapy is required, with special consideration given to the possible need for increasing the strength of the fixed combination (higher strengths contain higher dosages of budesonide or mometasone only), adding additional inhaled corticosteroids, or initiating systemic corticosteroids; patients should not increase the frequency of administration of formoterol in fixed combination with budesonide or mometasone furoate.

Cardiovascular Effects

Although uncommon at recommended dosages, clinically important changes in systolic and/or diastolic blood pressure, heart rate, and ECG (e.g., flattening of the T wave, prolongation of the QT₍c₎ interval, ST-segment depression) have been associated with formoterol oral inhalation therapy and may necessitate discontinuance of the drug. Cardiovascular effects generally have resolved within a few hours.

Like other sympathomimetic amines, formoterol should be used with caution in patients with cardiovascular disorders, especially coronary insufficiency, cardiac arrhythmias, or hypertension; in patients with seizure disorders or thyrotoxicosis; and in those who are unusually responsive to sympathomimetic amines.

Metabolic and Electrolyte Effects

Clinically important changes in blood glucose and serum potassium have occurred infrequently during clinical studies with formoterol at recommended dosage.

Specific Populations

Pregnancy

Category C. (See Users Guide.) Formoterol may interfere with uterine contractility; carefully weigh benefit versus risk in labor.

There is an increased risk of adverse perinatal outcomes (e.g., preeclampsia, premature birth, low birth weight, and neonates small for gestational age) in women with poorly or moderately controlled asthma. Pregnant women with asthma should be closely monitored and therapy adjusted as necessary to maintain optimal asthma control.

The effects of formoterol fumarate in fixed combination with budesonide, glycopyrrolate, or mometasone furoate during labor and delivery are not known. Because of the potential for β-agonist interference with uterine contractility, use of formoterol in fixed combination with budesonide, glycopyrrolate, or mometasone during labor should be restricted to those patients in whom the benefits clearly outweigh the risk.

Lactation

Formoterol is distributed into milk in rats; it is not known whether formoterol is distributed into human milk. Effects of formoterol fumarate on breast-fed infants or milk production also are not known.

The benefits of breast-feeding and the woman's clinical need for formoterol fumarate alone or in fixed combination with budesonide or mometasone should be considered along with any potential adverse effects on the breast-fed infant from the drug or from the underlying maternal condition.

Because many drugs are distributed into human milk, caution should be exercised when formoterol fumarate in fixed combination with glycopyrrolate is administered to nursing women. Since there are no data from controlled clinical studies, the manufacturer of formoterol/glycopyrrolate states that a decision should be made whether to discontinue nursing or the drug, taking into account the importance of the drug to the woman.

Pediatric Use

Formoterol fumarate oral inhalation solution (Perforomist®) and formoterol fumarate in fixed combination with glycopyrrolate (Bevespi® Aerosphere®) are not indicated for use in children. Safety and efficacy of these preparations in children have not been established.

Safety and efficacy of formoterol fumarate in fixed combination with budesonide (Symbicort®) in pediatric patients 12 years of age or older with asthma have been established in studies of up to 12 months' duration. Safety and efficacy of formoterol/budesonide in pediatric patients 6 to less than 12 years of age with asthma have been established in studies of up to 12 weeks' duration; however, the manufacturer states that safety and efficacy of the fixed-combination preparation in children younger than 6 years of age with asthma have not been established.

Safety and efficacy of formoterol fumarate in fixed combination with mometasone furoate (Dulera®) in pediatric patients 12 years of age or older with asthma have been established in studies of up to 12 months' duration.

Available data from controlled clinical trials suggest that monotherapy with long-acting β₂-adrenergic agonists increases the risk of asthma-related hospitalization in pediatric and adolescent patients. (See Asthma-related Death and Serious Asthma-related Events under Warnings/Precautions: Warnings, in Cautions.)

Geriatric Use

No substantial differences in safety and efficacy of formoterol alone or in fixed combination with budesonide, glycopyrrolate, or mometasone furoate have been observed in geriatric patients relative to younger adults. However, the manufacturers state that the possibility that some geriatric patients may exhibit increased sensitivity to formoterol or fixed combinations containing formoterol cannot be ruled out. (See Dosage and Administration: Special Populations.)

● Common Adverse Effects

Adverse effects occurring in 2% or more of adults in clinical trials receiving formoterol fumarate oral inhalation solution for the treatment of COPD include diarrhea, nausea, vomiting, nasopharyngitis, dry mouth, dizziness, and insomnia.

Adverse effects occurring in 3% or more of patients receiving formoterol fumarate in fixed combination with budesonide for the treatment of asthma include nasopharyngitis, headache, upper respiratory tract infection, pharyngolaryngeal pain, sinusitis, influenza, back pain, nasal congestion, stomach discomfort, vomiting, and oral candidiasis.

Adverse effects occurring in 3% or more of patients receiving formoterol fumarate in fixed combination with budesonide for the treatment of COPD include nasopharyngitis, oral candidiasis, bronchitis, sinusitis, and upper respiratory tract infection.

Adverse effects occurring in 2% or more of patients receiving formoterol fumarate in fixed combination with glycopyrrolate for the treatment of COPD and more frequently than in those receiving placebo include urinary tract infection and cough.

Adverse effects occurring in 3% or more of patients receiving formoterol fumarate in fixed combination with mometasone furoate for the treatment of asthma and more frequently than in those receiving placebo include nasopharyngitis, sinusitis, and headache.

DRUG INTERACTIONS

The following information addresses potential interactions with formoterol fumarate. When formoterol fumarate is used in fixed combination with budesonide, glycopyrrolate, or mometasone furoate, interactions associated with budesonide, glycopyrrolate, and mometasone also should be considered. No formal drug interaction studies have been performed to date with the fixed-combination preparations containing formoterol fumarate and budesonide, glycopyrrolate, or mometasone.

● Drugs that Prolong QT Interval

Potential pharmacologic interaction (increased risk of ventricular arrhythmias and effects of formoterol on the cardiovascular system may be potentiated). Drugs that prolong the QT interval should be used concomitantly with formoterol with extreme caution.

● Sympathomimetic Agents

Potential additive pharmacologic and adverse effects. Additional sympathomimetic agents administered by any route should be used with caution.

● Xanthine Derivatives/Corticosteroids

Potential pharmacologic interaction (increased risk of hypokalemia).

● Non-potassium-sparing Diuretics

Potential additive ECG and/or hypokalemic effects, especially when the recommended dosage of the β-agonist is exceeded; the clinical importance is unknown. Concomitant administration of β-agonists and non-potassium-sparing diuretics should be used with caution.

● Monoamine Oxidase Inhibitors/Tricyclic Antidepressants

Potential pharmacologic interaction (effects of formoterol on the cardiovascular system may be potentiated). Formoterol should be used with extreme caution during concomitant therapy or within 2 weeks following discontinuance of a monoamine oxidase (MAO) inhibitor or tricyclic antidepressant.

● β-Adrenergic Blocking Agents

Potential pharmacologic interaction (antagonism). Cardioselective β-adrenergic blocking agents should be considered if concomitant therapy with formoterol is necessary.

DESCRIPTION

Formoterol fumarate is a synthetic sympathomimetic amine. Like salmeterol, formoterol is a long-acting, selective β₂-receptor agonist, and is structurally and pharmacologically similar to other selective β₂-adrenergic receptor agonists (e.g.,

albuterol, salmeterol). Formoterol occurs as a racemic mixture; only the *R,R* -enantiomer is active.

Formoterol stimulates β₂-adrenergic receptors and apparently has little or no effect on β₁- or α-adrenergic receptors. The drug's β-adrenergic effects appear to result from stimulation of the production of cyclic adenosine-3′,5′-monophosphate (cAMP) by activation of adenyl cyclase. Cyclic AMP mediates numerous cellular responses, and increased concentrations of cAMP are associated with relaxation of bronchial smooth muscle and suppression of some aspects of inflammation, such as inhibition of release of proinflammatory mast-cell mediators (e.g., histamine, leukotrienes). Some studies in patients with mild asthma and in animals suggest that formoterol inhibits allergen-induced infiltration of eosinophils into airways, and reduces extravasation of plasma proteins (e.g., albumin). However, current evidence indicates that formoterol, like salmeterol, does not possess clinically important anti-inflammatory effects.

Tolerance to the bronchoprotective effects of formoterol (diminished effect on FEV1) has been reported after prolonged (2 weeks) dosing at twice the recommended dose (24 mcg), with loss of protection at the end of the 12-hour dosing period.

Limited data suggest that formoterol has a more rapid onset of action than salmeterol but a similar duration of action and similar bronchodilatory effects.

ADVICE TO PATIENTS

When formoterol fumarate is used in fixed combination with budesonide, glycopyrrolate, or mometasone furoate, importance of informing patients of important cautionary information about budesonide, glycopyrrolate, or mometasone furoate.

A copy of the manufacturer's patient information (medication guide) for formoterol alone or in fixed combination with budesonide, glycopyrrolate, or mometasone furoate must be provided to all patients each time the drug is dispensed. Importance of instructing patients to read the medication guide prior to initiation of therapy and each time the prescription is refilled.

Importance of informing patients that monotherapy with long-acting β₂-adrenergic agonists, including formoterol, increases the risk of asthma-related death and may increase the risk of asthma-related hospitalization in pediatric and adolescent patients. Importance of informing patients that long-term asthma controller drugs must be continued when formoterol is added to the treatment regimen.

Importance of pediatric patients receiving therapy under adult supervision.

Importance of adequate understanding of proper storage, preparation, and inhalation techniques, including use of the oral inhalation delivery system.

Importance of correct procedure for administering formoterol alone or in fixed combination with budesonide, glycopyrrolate, or mometasone furoate and any concomitant therapy (e.g., a short-acting β₂-adrenergic agonist). Importance of not breathing into the inhaler.

Importance of adherence to dosing schedules of formoterol alone or in fixed combination with budesonide, glycopyrrolate, or mometasone furoate and any concomitant therapy, including not altering the dose or frequency of use of such drugs unless otherwise instructed by a clinician. Importance of advising patient that if a dose of formoterol alone or in fixed combination with budesonide, glycopyrrolate, or mometasone furoate is missed, the next dose should be taken at the regularly scheduled time; the dose should not be doubled.

Importance of informing patients of adverse effects associated with β₂-adrenergic agonists such as palpitations, chest pain, rapid heart rate, tremor, or nervousness.

Importance of understanding that formoterol-containing therapy does not relieve acute symptoms of asthma or COPD. Importance of all patients being provided with and instructed in the use of a short-acting, inhaled β₂-adrenergic bronchodilator as supplemental therapy for acute asthma or COPD symptoms.

Importance of discontinuing *regular* use of a short-acting, inhaled β-adrenergic bronchodilator when initiating therapy with formoterol and instituting *intermittent* use of a short-acting bronchodilator (*not* formoterol) to relieve acute symptoms of asthma. Importance of contacting a clinician if respiratory symptoms worsen or are not relieved by usual dosage of formoterol fumarate. Importance of contacting a clinician or obtaining medical care right away if 4 or more inhalations of a short-acting β₂-agonist are required daily for 2 or more consecutive days, an entire canister of the short-acting β₂-agonist is used in 8 weeks, peak flow meter results decrease, or asthma symptoms do not improve after 1 week of formoterol therapy.

Importance of instructing patients to seek emergency medical care if breathing problems worsen rapidly and usual doses of a short-acting bronchodilator do not relieve acute asthma or COPD symptoms.

Importance of advising patients who are receiving formoterol-containing preparations not to use additional formoterol or other long-acting inhaled β₂-adrenergic agonists for any reason.

Importance of patients not discontinuing formoterol-containing therapy and not discontinuing or reducing concomitant asthma therapy without medical supervision, since symptoms may worsen.

Importance of promptly contacting clinicians or seeking emergency medical care if symptoms of a serious allergic reaction (e.g., rash, hives, breathing problems, swelling of the face, tongue, or mouth) develop.

Importance of informing clinicians of existing or contemplated concomitant therapy, including prescription and OTC drugs and dietary or herbal supplements, as well as concomitant illnesses (e.g., heart disease, high blood pressure, seizures, thyroid problems, diabetes mellitus, drug or food allergies).

Importance of women informing clinicians if they are or plan to become pregnant or plan to breast-feed.

Importance of informing patients of other important precautionary information. (See Cautions.)

PREPARATIONS

Excipients in commercially available drug preparations may have clinically important effects in some individuals; consult specific product labeling for details.

Formoterol Fumarate (Dihydrate)

Oral Inhalation

Solution, for nebulization	10 mcg (of formoterol fumarate) per mL	**Perforomist®**, Mylan

Formoterol Fumarate Combinations

Oral Inhalation

Aerosol	4.5 mcg (of formoterol fumarate dihydrate) with Budesonide 80 mcg per metered spray	**Symbicort®** (with hydrofluoroalkane propellant), AstraZeneca
	4.5 mcg (of formoterol fumarate dihydrate) with Budesonide 160 mcg per metered spray	**Symbicort®** (with hydrofluoroalkane propellant), AstraZeneca
	4.8 mcg (of formoterol fumarate) with Glycopyrrolate 9 mcg per metered spray	**Bevespi® Aerosphere®** (with hydrofluoroalkane propellant), AstraZeneca
	5 mcg (of formoterol fumarate dihydrate) with Mometasone Furoate 100 mcg per metered spray	**Dulera®** (with hydrofluoroalkane propellant), Merck
	5 mcg (of formoterol fumarate dihydrate) with Mometasone Furoate 200 mcg per metered spray	**Dulera®** (with hydrofluoroalkane propellant), Merck

Selected Revisions January 2, 2020, © Copyright, September 1, 2001, American Society of Health-System Pharmacists, Inc.

Salmeterol Xinafoate

12:12.08.12 • SELECTIVE β₂-ADRENERGIC AGONISTS

■ Salmeterol xinafoate, a synthetic sympathomimetic amine, is a relatively selective, long-acting β₂-adrenergic agonist. The drug is structurally and pharmacologically similar to the short-acting β₂-adrenergic agonist albuterol.

USES

● Bronchospasm

Salmeterol xinafoate is used only with concomitant long-term asthma controller therapy, such as inhaled corticosteroids, as a long-acting bronchodilator for the treatment of asthma and prevention of bronchospasm in patients with reversible obstructive airway disease, including symptoms of nocturnal asthma. Monotherapy with long-acting β₂-adrenergic agonists, such as salmeterol, increases the risk of asthma-related death and may increase the risk of asthma-related hospitalization in pediatric and adolescent patients. (See Asthma-related Death and Life-threatening Events under Cautions: Respiratory Effects.) *Because of these risks, the use of salmeterol for the treatment of asthma without concomitant use of long-term asthma controller therapy, such as inhaled corticosteroids, is contraindicated.* (See Cautions: Precautions and Contraindications.) Salmeterol is used only as additional therapy in patients with asthma who are currently receiving long-term asthma controller therapy, such as inhaled corticosteroids, but whose disease is inadequately controlled with such therapy. The fixed combination of salmeterol and fluticasone propionate is used only in patients with asthma who have not responded adequately to long-term asthma controller therapy, such as inhaled corticosteroids, or whose disease severity warrants initiation of treatment with both an inhaled corticosteroid and a long-acting β₂-adrenergic agonist. Once asthma control is achieved and maintained, the patient should be assessed at regular intervals and therapy should be stepped down (e.g., discontinuance of salmeterol), if possible without loss of asthma control, and the patient should be maintained on long-term asthma controller therapy, such as inhaled corticosteroids. *Salmeterol is not a substitute for corticosteroids; corticosteroid therapy should not be stopped or reduced in dosage when salmeterol is initiated.* (See Cautions: Precautions and Contraindications.) Salmeterol or salmeterol in fixed combination with fluticasone propionate should not be used in patients whose asthma is adequately controlled on a low or medium dosage of inhaled corticosteroids.

In pediatric and adolescent patients with asthma who require the addition of a long-acting β₂-adrenergic agonist to an inhaled corticosteroid, a fixed-combination preparation containing both an inhaled corticosteroid and a long-acting β₂-adrenergic agonist generally should be used to ensure compliance with both drugs. In cases where separate administration of long-term asthma controller therapy (e.g., inhaled corticosteroids) and a long-acting β₂-adrenergic agonist is clinically indicated, appropriate steps must be taken to ensure compliance with both treatment components. If compliance cannot be ensured, a fixed-combination preparation containing both an inhaled corticosteroid and a long-acting β₂-adrenergic agonist is recommended.

Salmeterol also is used for the prevention of exercise-induced bronchospasm. The use of salmeterol as a single agent for the prevention of exercise-induced bronchospasm may be clinically indicated in patients who do not have persistent asthma. In patients with persistent asthma, use of salmeterol for the prevention of exercise-induced bronchospasm may be clinically indicated; however, the treatment of asthma should include long-term asthma controller therapy, such as inhaled corticosteroids.

Salmeterol also is used as a bronchodilator for the long-term symptomatic management of reversible bronchospasm associated with moderate to severe (forced expiratory volume in 1 second [FEV₁] less than 80% predicted) chronic obstructive pulmonary disease (COPD), including chronic bronchitis and emphysema. Salmeterol in fixed combination with fluticasone propionate as the inhalation powder (Advair® Diskus®) is used for the maintenance treatment of airflow obstruction in patients with COPD, including chronic bronchitis and/or emphysema. Salmeterol in fixed combination with fluticasone propionate as the inhalation powder (Advair® Diskus®) also is used to reduce exacerbations of COPD in patients with a history of such exacerbations.

Salmeterol alone or in fixed combination with fluticasone propionate is *not* indicated for the relief of acute bronchospasm. A short-acting inhaled β₂-adrenergic agonist should be used intermittently (as needed) for acute symptoms of asthma or COPD.

Asthma

Considerations in Initiating Antiasthma Therapy

In the current stepped-care approach to antiasthmatic drug therapy, asthma is classified according to severity upon initial presentation (intermittent asthma or mild, moderate, or severe persistent asthma) and also by response to treatment (i.e., asthma control). While classification of asthma severity is useful for determining initial treatment, disease severity may vary over time and with treatment; therefore, after therapy is initiated, periodic assessment of asthma control is emphasized for guiding treatment decisions. Current asthma management guidelines state that initial therapy for asthma should correspond to disease severity, with subsequent monitoring and adjustments in therapy to achieve and maintain control of asthma according to the goals of treatment. Asthma therapy is aimed at achieving and maintaining control of asthma by reducing ongoing impairment (e.g., prevention of chronic and troublesome symptoms, reducing use of reliever drugs, maintaining normal or near-normal lung function and activity levels) and risk of future events (e.g., exacerbations requiring systemic corticosteroids, treatment-related adverse effects). These 2 components of asthma control (i.e., current impairment and future risk) may respond differently to treatment.

The National Asthma Education and Prevention Program (NAEPP) classifies the levels of asthma control as well controlled, not well controlled, or very poorly controlled. In the stepped-care approach, the treatment step selected for asthma control in patients already receiving asthma therapy is based on the patient's current treatment and level of asthma control. Stepwise therapy is meant to assist, not replace, the clinical decision-making process in selecting therapy for individual patients. Once initiated, treatment is adjusted continuously according to changes in asthma control. Patients should be monitored every 2–6 weeks following initiation of therapy to ensure that asthma control is achieved. If asthma symptoms are not controlled with the current treatment regimen, treatment is stepped up until control is achieved. If an alternative treatment was used and produced an inadequate response, the preferred treatment should be used before stepping up to the next level of therapy. Regular monitoring at 1- to 6-month intervals, depending on the level of control, is recommended to ensure that control of asthma is maintained and that appropriate adjustments in therapy are made. When control has been maintained for at least 3 months, treatment intensity may be stepped down to find the lowest dosage and/or number of drugs required to maintain asthma control, with continued follow-up at 3-month intervals.

Intermittent Asthma

Drugs for asthma may be categorized as relievers (e.g., bronchodilators taken as needed for acute symptoms) or controllers (principally inhaled corticosteroids or other anti-inflammatory agents taken regularly to achieve long-term control of asthma). A reliever drug such as a selective short-acting inhaled β₂-adrenergic agonist (e.g., albuterol, levalbuterol, pirbuterol) is recommended on an as-needed basis to control occasional acute symptoms (e.g., cough, wheezing, dyspnea) of short duration; such use of an inhaled short-acting β₂-agonist alone generally is sufficient as initial treatment for newly diagnosed patients whose asthma severity is initially classified as intermittent (e.g., patients with daytime symptoms of asthma not more than twice weekly and nocturnal symptoms not more than twice a month). Most experts consider short-acting inhaled β₂-adrenergic agonists to be drugs of choice for treating acute asthma symptoms and exacerbations and for preventing exercise-induced bronchospasm. Alternatives to short-acting inhaled β₂-agonists recommended by some clinicians for relief of acute asthma symptoms include an inhaled anticholinergic agent (e.g., ipratropium), a short-acting oral β₂-agonist, or a short-acting theophylline (provided extended-release theophylline is not already used), but these alternatives have a slower onset of action and/or a higher risk for adverse effects. Oral β₂-adrenergic agonist therapy is suggested for use principally in patients unable to use inhaled bronchodilators (e.g., young children). Other experts do not recommend oral β₂-agonists for relief of acute asthma symptoms. Use of short-acting inhaled β₂-agonists in asymptomatic asthma should be limited to pretreatment prior to exercise and, in intermittent asthma, should be limited to providing relief as symptoms develop; some clinicians state that patients requiring symptomatic relief more than twice weekly or repeatedly over 1 or 2 days should be evaluated for possible initiation of long-term controller therapy.

Mild Persistent Asthma

When control of symptoms deteriorates in mild intermittent asthma and symptoms become persistent (e.g., daytime symptoms of asthma more than twice weekly but less than once daily, and nocturnal symptoms of asthma 3–4 times per month), current asthma management guidelines and most clinicians recommend initiation of a controller drug such as an anti-inflammatory agent, preferably a low-dose orally inhaled corticosteroid (e.g., 88–264, 88–176, or 176 mcg of fluticasone propionate or equivalent daily via a metered dose inhaler in adults and adolescents, children 5–11 years of age, or children 4 years of age or younger, respectively) as first-line therapy for persistent asthma, supplemented by as-needed use of a short-acting, inhaled β₂-agonist. Alternatives to low-dose inhaled corticosteroids for mild persistent asthma include certain leukotriene modifiers (i.e., montelukast, zafirlukast), extended-release theophylline, or mast-cell stabilizers (i.e., cromolyn, nedocromil [preparations for oral inhalation no longer commercially available in the US]), but these therapies are less effective and not preferred as initial therapy. Some experts recommend that long-term control therapy be considered in infants and young children who have identifiable risk factors for asthma and who in the previous year have had 4 or more episodes of wheezing that lasted more than 1 day and symptoms that affected sleep. Low-dose inhaled corticosteroids also are recommended as the preferred initial therapy in such children. Cromolyn sodium is suggested (based on extrapolation of data from studies in older children) or montelukast is recommended by some experts as alternative, but not preferred, therapy in children 4 years of age or younger with mild persistent asthma. Other experts do not consider mast cell stabilizers or extended-release theophylline to be acceptable alternatives to inhaled corticosteroids for routine use as initial long-term therapy in such patients.

Moderate Persistent Asthma

According to current asthma management guidelines, therapy with a long-acting inhaled β₂-agonist such as salmeterol or formoterol generally is recommended in adults and adolescents who have moderate persistent asthma and daily asthmatic symptoms that are inadequately controlled following addition of low-dose inhaled corticosteroids to as-needed inhaled β₂-agonist treatment. However, NAEPP recommends that the beneficial effects of long-acting inhaled β₂-agonists should be weighed carefully against the increased risk (although uncommon) of severe asthma exacerbations and asthma-related deaths associated with daily use of such agents. (See Asthma-related Death and Life-threatening Events under Cautions: Respiratory Effects and also see Uses: Bronchospasm.) Current asthma management guidelines also state that an alternative, but equally preferred option for management of moderate persistent asthma that is not adequately controlled with a low dosage of inhaled corticosteroid is to increase the maintenance dosage to a medium dosage (e.g., exceeding 264 but not more than 440 mcg of fluticasone propionate [or its equivalent] daily via a metered-dose inhaler in adults and adolescents). Alternative less effective therapies that may be added to a low dosage of inhaled corticosteroid include an oral extended-release theophylline or certain leukotriene modifiers (i.e., montelukast, zafirlukast).

Limited data are available in infants and children 11 years of age or younger with moderate persistent asthma, and recommendations of care are based on expert opinion and extrapolation from studies in adults. According to current asthma management guidelines, a long-acting inhaled β₂-agonist (i.e., salmeterol, formoterol), a leukotriene modifier (i.e., montelukast, zafirlukast), or extended-release theophylline (with appropriate monitoring) may be added to low-dose inhaled corticosteroid therapy in children 5–11 years of age. Because comparative data establishing relative efficacy of these agents in this age group are lacking, there is no clearly preferred agent for use as adjunctive therapy with a low-dose inhaled corticosteroid for treatment of asthma in these children. In children 5–11 years of age with moderate persistent asthma that is not controlled with a low dosage of an inhaled corticosteroid, another preferred option according to current asthma management guidelines is to increase the maintenance dosage of the inhaled corticosteroid to a medium dosage (e.g., exceeding 176 but not more than 352 mcg of fluticasone propionate [or its equivalent] daily via a metered dose inhaler). In infants and children 4 years of age or younger with moderate persistent asthma that is not controlled by a low dosage of an inhaled corticosteroid, the only preferred option is to increase the maintenance dosage of the inhaled

corticosteroid to a medium dosage (e.g., exceeding 176 but not more than 352 mcg of fluticasone propionate [or its equivalent] daily via a metered-dose inhaler).

Severe Persistent Asthma

Maintenance therapy with an inhaled corticosteroid at medium dosages or high dosages (e.g., exceeding 440 mcg of fluticasone propionate in adults and adolescents or 352 mcg in children 5–11 years of age [or its equivalent] daily via a metered-dose inhaler) and adjunctive therapy with a long-acting inhaled β₂-agonist is the preferred treatment according to current asthma management guidelines in adults and children 5 years of age or older with severe persistent asthma (i.e., continuous daytime asthma symptoms, nighttime symptoms 7 times per week). Such recommendations in children 5–11 years of age are based on expert opinion and extrapolation from studies in adolescents and adults. Alternatives to a long-acting inhaled β₂-agonist for severe persistent asthma in adults and children 5 years of age or older receiving medium-dose inhaled corticosteroids include extended-release theophylline or certain leukotriene modifiers (i.e., montelukast, zafirlukast), but these therapies are generally not preferred. Omalizumab may be considered in adolescents and adults with severe asthma with an allergic component who are inadequately controlled with high-dose inhaled corticosteroids and a long-acting β₂-agonist. In infants and children 4 years of age or younger with severe asthma, maintenance therapy with an inhaled corticosteroid at medium or high dosages (e.g., exceeding 352 mcg of fluticasone propionate [or its equivalent] daily via a metered-dose inhaler) and adjunctive therapy with either a long-acting inhaled β₂-agonist or montelukast is the only preferred treatment according to current asthma management guidelines. Recommendations for care of infants and children with severe asthma are based on expert opinion and extrapolation from studies in older children.

Poorly Controlled Asthma

If asthma symptoms in adults and children 5 years of age or older with moderate to severe asthma are very poorly controlled (at least 2 exacerbations per year requiring oral corticosteroids) with low to high maintenance dosages of the inhaled corticosteroid and a long-acting inhaled β₂-agonist bronchodilator, a short course (3–10 days) of an oral corticosteroid may be added to gain prompt control of asthma. In infants and children 4 years of age or younger with moderate to severe asthma who are very poorly controlled (more than 3 exacerbations per year requiring corticosteroids) with medium to high maintenance dosages of an inhaled corticosteroid with or without adjunctive therapy (i.e., a long-acting inhaled β₂-agonist, montelukast), a short course (3–10 days) of an oral corticosteroid may be added to gain prompt control of asthma.

While clinical efficacy of oral corticosteroids as add-on therapy in adults and children 5 years of age or older with very severe asthma that is inadequately controlled with a high-dose inhaled corticosteroid, intermittent oral corticosteroid therapy, and a long-acting inhaled β₂-agonist bronchodilator has not been established in randomized controlled studies, some experts suggest regular use of oral corticosteroids in such patients, based on consensus and clinical experience. Similarly, some experts, based on consensus and clinical experience, suggest regular use of oral corticosteroid therapy in infants and children 4 years of age or younger with very severe asthma who are not controlled with high-dose inhaled corticosteroid and either a long-acting inhaled β₂-agonist or montelukast and intermittent oral corticosteroid therapy. However, other experts do not consider regular use of oral corticosteroid therapy to be appropriate therapy in children with severely uncontrolled asthma. (See Asthma under Uses: Respiratory Diseases, in the Corticosteroids General Statement 68:04.)

When asthma symptoms at any stage are not controlled with maintenance therapy (e.g., inhaled corticosteroids) plus supplemental short-acting inhaled β₂-agonist bronchodilator therapy as needed (e.g., if there is a need to increase the dose or frequency of administration of the short-acting sympathomimetic agent), prompt reevaluation is required to adjust dosage of the maintenance regimen or institute an alternative maintenance regimen. For additional details on the stepped-care approach to drug therapy in asthma, see Asthma under Uses: Bronchospasm, in Albuterol 12:12.08.12 and see also Asthma under Uses: Respiratory Diseases, in the Corticosteroids General Statement 68:04.

Clinical Experience with Salmeterol

The initial studies supporting the indication of salmeterol for the treatment of asthma did not require the regular use of inhaled corticosteroids. However, for the treatment of asthma, salmeterol currently is indicated only as concomitant therapy with long-term asthma controller therapy, such as inhaled corticosteroids. (See Uses: Bronchospasm and also see Asthma-related Death and Life-threatening Events under Cautions: Respiratory Effects.)

Results of a limited number of comparative studies suggest that salmeterol oral inhalation powder is more effective than orally inhaled albuterol or placebo in producing bronchodilation (e.g., as determined by mean peak expiratory flow rate) and reducing nighttime awakenings, and more effective than placebo in reducing the need for rescue medication (e.g., intermittent use of a short-acting, β₂-agonist bronchodilator to control asthma exacerbations). While published studies have reported a salmeterol dose of 25 mcg per inhalation of salmeterol aerosol alone (e.g., 50 mcg per 2 metered sprays) or in fixed combination with fluticasone propionate, this is the amount released during actuation from the valve stem; the dose delivered to the patient through the mouthpiece (actuator) is approximately 21 mcg per inhalation (e.g., 42 mcg per 2 metered sprays). In the Uses section, unless otherwise stated, the dose of salmeterol (as salmeterol xinafoate) administered as the aerosol is expressed in terms of the dose delivered from the mouthpiece.

In a clinical study in patients with mild to moderate asthma, some of whom were receiving concomitant therapy with orally inhaled corticosteroids, inhaled salmeterol powder 50 mcg twice daily was more effective than inhaled albuterol 180 mcg 4 times daily in improving pulmonary function (as measured by forced expiratory volume in 1 second [FEV₁] and PEFR), alleviating respiratory symptoms, and reducing the need for supplemental albuterol oral inhalations. In a 12-week comparative study in patients with mild to moderate persistent asthma who were symptomatic despite receiving low to intermediate dosages of inhaled corticosteroids, salmeterol inhalation powder (50 mcg twice daily) was more effective than montelukast (10 mg daily) in improving lung function (morning PEFR) and asthma symptoms. Data from comparative studies in patients receiving salmeterol inhalation aerosol (no longer commercially available in the US) versus orally inhaled terbutaline, cromolyn sodium, or nedocromil sodium (preparations for oral inhalation no longer commercially available in the US) or individualized oral extended-release theophylline therapy also suggest greater efficacy of salmeterol therapy.

Evidence from a limited number of comparative studies in patients with mild to moderate asthma, including those who did or did not receive concurrent inhaled corticosteroid therapy, suggests similar efficacy and safety of salmeterol oral inhalation powder administered via the Serevent® Diskus® device and orally inhaled salmeterol aerosol (no longer commercially available in the US). However, the manufacturer states that clinical equivalence of salmeterol oral inhalation powder and oral inhalation aerosol should not be assumed in all patient populations. In a short-term (12-week), randomized clinical trial in children 4–11 years of age with mild to moderate asthma who did or did not receive concurrent inhaled corticosteroid therapy, therapy with salmeterol oral inhalation powder (50 mcg twice daily) administered via the Serevent® Diskus® device (with or without concurrent inhaled corticosteroids) produced improvements in peak expiratory flow rate (36–39% postdose increase compared with baseline) and FEV₁ (32–33% postdose increase from baseline).

Prolonged use of some sympathomimetic amines (e.g., albuterol, isoproterenol, terbutaline) in the treatment of chronic asthma or COPD may lead to tolerance to the bronchodilating effects of these drugs, and it has been suggested that prolonged stimulation of β₂-adrenergic receptors by salmeterol may have a greater potential to induce tolerance to bronchodilation than short-acting β₂-agonists. However, in several studies of 1–12 months' duration in patients with mild to moderately severe asthma, salmeterol inhalation aerosol (no longer commercially available) remained effective over the study period as indicated by increases in FEV₁ and PEFR and decreases in diurnal variation in PEFR, asthma symptoms, frequency of asthma exacerbations, and the need for additional relief medication.

Because of its long duration of action, salmeterol may be particularly useful for the management of asthma in patients who have nocturnal symptoms despite maintenance therapy with inhaled or oral corticosteroids, extended-release theophylline, and/or other drug therapy. Comparative studies in patients with moderate asthma and nocturnal symptoms suggest that nocturnal symptoms or the need for nocturnal relief medications was decreased with orally inhaled salmeterol as compared with patients receiving placebo, orally inhaled albuterol, oral montelukast, oral extended-release theophylline, orally inhaled nedocromil sodium (preparations for oral inhalation no longer commercially available in the US), or orally inhaled cromolyn sodium. Combined data from 2 multicenter studies in patients with asthma indicate that the mean percentage of nights with no

awakenings increased from 63 to 85% following 12 weeks of therapy with salmeterol oral inhalation powder and from 68 to 71% following 12 weeks of albuterol oral inhalation therapy.

In patients with moderate to severe asthma, combined therapy with inhaled salmeterol and inhaled corticosteroids has been instituted to promote greater control of asthma symptoms. In one clinical study in patients with mild to moderate asthma, the addition of salmeterol inhalation aerosol (no longer commercially available in the US) to therapy with an orally inhaled corticosteroid and an intermittent, short-acting β₂-agonist allowed a reduction in inhaled corticosteroid use while maintaining adequate asthma control.

In other clinical studies in patients with persistent asthma whose symptoms were not controlled by 336–1000 mcg/day of beclomethasone dipropionate, combined therapy with inhaled beclomethasone dipropionate (336–1000 mcg/day) and orally inhaled salmeterol aerosol with chlorofluorocarbon (CFC) propellant (42–84 mcg/day; CFC preparation no longer commercially available in the US) was more effective in improving lung function and in reducing the need for supplemental albuterol than therapy with higher dosages of beclomethasone dipropionate alone (672–2000 mcg/day).

Results from comparative clinical trials in patients with asthma not adequately controlled by 176 mcg/day of fluticasone propionate indicate that combined therapy with inhaled fluticasone propionate (176 mcg/day) and orally inhaled salmeterol aerosol with CFC propellant (84 mcg/day; CFC preparation no longer commercially available in the US) given separately was more effective in improving lung function and asthma symptoms and in reducing the need for supplemental albuterol than therapy with a higher dosage of fluticasone propionate (440 mcg/day). In addition, fewer patients receiving combined therapy experienced asthma exacerbations in these trials.

In several randomized, double-blind, placebo-controlled clinical trials in patients with mild to severe asthma, fluticasone propionate (100, 250, or 500 mcg) in fixed combination with salmeterol xinafoate (42 mcg as salmeterol) as the inhalation powder produced greater improvement in most indices of pulmonary function (e.g., mean percent change from baseline in FEV₁, morning FEV₁ or PEFR) than either drug alone and similar efficacy as concurrent therapy with both agents given separately. In several randomized, double-blind, comparative trials in patients with mild to moderate persistent asthma who were not optimally controlled on their current antiasthma therapy, the fixed combination of salmeterol (42 mcg twice daily) and fluticasone propionate (90, 230, or 460 mcg twice daily) with hydrofluoroalkane (HFA) propellant for oral inhalation via a metered-dose inhaler (Advair® HFA) produced greater improvement in indices of pulmonary function (e.g., mean percent change from baseline in FEV₁ or morning and evening PEFR) than either drug alone. In a comparative clinical trial in patients with asthma who were not controlled on high dosages of inhaled corticosteroids, salmeterol/fluticasone inhalation aerosol (salmeterol 42 mcg/fluticasone propionate 460 mcg twice daily) produced greater or similar improvement in morning PEFR than fluticasone inhalation aerosol (440 mcg twice daily) with CFC propellants (no longer commercially available in the US) or salmeterol/fluticasone inhalation powder (50 mcg of salmeterol and 500 mcg of fluticasone propionate twice daily), respectively.

Supplemental Therapy in Acute Asthma

Salmeterol has a delayed onset of action, and the drug (alone or in fixed combination with fluticasone propionate) should *not* be used for the relief of acute symptoms (i.e., as rescue therapy for the treatment of acute episodes of bronchospasm). In addition, salmeterol, alone or in fixed combination with fluticasone propionate, should not be *initiated* in patients during rapidly deteriorating or potentially life-threatening episodes of asthma since serious acute respiratory events, including fatalities, have been reported in such situations. (See Cautions: Precautions and Contraindications.)

All patients receiving salmeterol alone or in fixed combination with fluticasone propionate should be provided with and instructed in the use of a short-acting, inhaled β₂-adrenergic agonist (e.g., albuterol) as supplemental therapy for acute symptoms. The manufacturer states that when initiating salmeterol alone or in fixed combination with fluticasone propionate in patients who have been taking short-acting, oral or inhaled β₂-agonists on a regular basis (e.g., 4 times daily), these patients should be instructed to discontinue the *regular* use of the short-acting agent and to use short-acting, inhaled β₂-agonists, not salmeterol (alone or in fixed combination with fluticasone propionate), for relief of acute symptoms, such as shortness of breath. *Regular* (e.g., daily) use of short-acting inhaled β₂-agonists does not adequately control asthma symptoms or airway hyperresponsiveness on a long-term basis and is not recommended by current asthma management guidelines. If such symptoms are not controlled with salmeterol plus supplemental bronchodilator therapy (i.e., if there is a need to increase the dose or frequency of administration of the short-acting sympathomimetic agent), immediate reevaluation with reassessment of the treatment regimen is required, giving special consideration to the possible need for adding additional inhaled corticosteroids or initiating systemic corticosteroids; however, the dosage of salmeterol should *not* be increased in such situations. If asthma deteriorates in patients receiving salmeterol in fixed combination with fluticasone propionate, immediate reevaluation with reassessment of the treatment regimen is required, with special consideration given to the possible need for increasing the strength of the fixed combination (higher strengths contain higher dosages of fluticasone propionate only), adding additional inhaled corticosteroids, or initiating systemic corticosteroids. Patients should not increase the frequency of administration of the fixed combination. Patients receiving salmeterol alone or in fixed combination with fluticasone propionate should not use additional salmeterol or other long-acting inhaled β₂-agonists (e.g., arformoterol, formoterol) for any indication. (See Cautions: Precautions and Contraindications.)

Concerns about the safety of *regular* use of short-acting inhaled β₂-agonist bronchodilators for maintenance therapy of asthma have been raised by evidence from some studies suggesting increased morbidity and mortality in patients receiving long-term therapy with short-acting inhaled β-agonists, particularly fenoterol (currently not commercially available in the US). In a placebo-controlled, cross-over study in which intermittent use of inhaled fenoterol was compared with regularly scheduled use of the drug, regular use over a 24-week period was associated with deterioration in asthma control as determined by peak expiratory flow rate (PEFR), symptoms, and use of additional inhaled bronchodilator. However, the design and interpretation of these study findings suggesting increased morbidity and mortality have been criticized, and reanalysis of these data demonstrated that the differences between treatment periods were small and unlikely to be clinically important. Data from case-control studies have been conflicting and have not demonstrated a causal relationship between inhaled β₂-agonist therapy and asthma mortality. An alternative hypothesis to explain the apparent association between inhaled β-agonist use and asthma mortality is that increased use of β-agonist therapy is a marker of severe asthma. While some studies in patients with mild or moderate asthma suggest that regularly scheduled use of short-acting, inhaled β₂-agonists may not cause harm, such use does not appear to have demonstrable advantages compared with intermittent use and does not adequately control asthmatic symptoms. Regular, daily use of a short-acting, inhaled β₂-agonist generally is not recommended, and increased chronic use of such β₂-agonists more than twice weekly (excluding use for exercise-induced bronchospasm) or acute use (e.g., repeated use over more than 1–2 days) for asthma deterioration may indicate the need to initiate or increase long-term control therapy for asthma.

Monotherapy with long-acting β₂-adrenergic agonists, such as salmeterol, increases the risk of asthma-related death and may increase the risk of asthma-related hospitalization in pediatric and adolescent patients. Data from a large study evaluating the safety of salmeterol in patients with asthma showed an increase in asthma-related deaths in patients receiving salmeterol, particularly in African-American patients. (See Asthma-related Death and Life-threatening Events under Cautions: Respiratory Effects and see Uses: Bronchospasm.)

Exercise-Induced Bronchospasm

Salmeterol is used for the prevention of exercise-induced bronchospasm. However, most experts consider short-acting inhaled β₂-adrenergic agonists to be drugs of choice for prevention of exercise-induced bronchospasm. The manufacturer states that the use of salmeterol as a single agent for the prevention of exercise-induced bronchospasm may be clinically indicated in patients who do not have persistent asthma. The manufacturer also states that in patients with persistent asthma, the use of salmeterol for the prevention of exercise-induced bronchospasm may be clinically indicated; however, the treatment of asthma should include long-term asthma controller therapy, such as inhaled corticosteroids. Experts from the NAEPP state that frequent or chronic use of a long-acting inhaled β₂-agonist for exercise-induced bronchospasm should be discouraged. Such use may disguise poorly controlled persistent asthma, which should be managed with daily anti-inflammatory therapy.

Protection against exercise-induced bronchospasm has been noted in children (4–11 years of age) in controlled trials with salmeterol inhalation powder

(50 mcg 0.5 hour prior to exercise); in 2 single-dose trials, protection against exercise-induced bronchoconstriction (as measured by a decrease in FEV₁ with exercise) lasted up to 11.5 hours following the dose. In 2 single-dose, comparative clinical trials in adults and adolescents, salmeterol inhalation aerosol with CFC propellant (42 mcg; CFC preparation no longer commercially available in the US) and inhalation powder (50 mcg) demonstrated similar efficacy and safety for the prevention of exercise-induced bronchospasm. However, continued dosing with salmeterol oral inhalation aerosol (42 mcg once or twice daily for 4 weeks) has been associated with loss or waning of protection against exercise-induced bronchospasm in some patients or a decreased duration of such protection.

Chronic Obstructive Pulmonary Disease

Salmeterol is used as a bronchodilator for the long-term symptomatic treatment of reversible bronchospasm associated with COPD, including chronic bronchitis and emphysema. Salmeterol in fixed combination with fluticasone propionate as the inhalation powder (Advair® Diskus®) is used for the maintenance treatment of airflow obstruction in patients with COPD, including chronic bronchitis and/or emphysema. Salmeterol in fixed combination with fluticasone propionate as the inhalation powder (Advair® Diskus®) also is used to reduce exacerbations of COPD in patients with a history of such exacerbations. Because of its slow onset of action, orally inhaled salmeterol is *not* indicated as monotherapy for the initial treatment of acute episodes of bronchospasm or acute exacerbations of COPD; a drug with a shorter onset of action (e.g., a short-acting β₂-adrenergic agonist) may be preferred in such cases.

In the stepped-care approach to COPD drug therapy, mild, intermittent symptoms and minimal lung impairment (e.g., FEV₁ at least 80% of predicted) can be treated with a short-acting, selective inhaled β₂-adrenergic agonist (e.g., albuterol) as needed for acute symptoms. For the treatment of persistent symptoms not relieved by as-needed therapy with ipratropium or a short-acting, selective inhaled β₂-agonist in patients with moderate to severe COPD (e.g., FEV₁ 30 to less than 80% of predicted value), a long-acting bronchodilator (e.g., orally inhaled salmeterol, formoterol, tiotropium) can be added and a short-acting, selective inhaled β₂-agonist used as needed for immediate symptom relief. Maintenance therapy with long-acting bronchodilators in patients with moderate to severe COPD is more effective and more convenient than regular use of short-acting bronchodilators.

Maintenance therapy (e.g., 4 times daily) with a short-acting, selective inhaled β₂-agonist is not preferred but may be used in patients with persistent symptoms of COPD; such therapy should not exceed 6–12 inhalations daily. Current guidelines for the management of COPD state that low- to high-dose ipratropium (6–16 inhalations daily) can be added to therapy with a short-acting, selective β₂-agonist (as separate inhalations or in fixed combination) in patients with mild to moderate persistent symptoms of COPD, with the frequency of inhalation dosing with either agent not to exceed 4 times daily; the high dosage of ipratropium included in some guidelines for COPD exceeds the manufacturer's maximum recommended dosage (12 inhalations). Combining bronchodilators from different classes and with differing durations of action may increase the degree of bronchodilation with a similar or lower frequency of adverse effects.

For patients not responding to treatment with a long-acting bronchodilator, a combination of several long-acting bronchodilators such as tiotropium and a long-acting β-adrenergic agonist may be used. A short-acting bronchodilator may be used as needed for relief of acute symptoms that occur despite regular use of long-acting bronchodilators. For treatment of severe to very severe COPD (e.g., FEV₁ less than 30 to less than 50% of predicted value, history of exacerbations), the addition of an inhaled corticosteroid to one or more long-acting bronchodilators given separately or in fixed combination may be needed. If symptoms are not adequately controlled with inhaled corticosteroids and a long-acting bronchodilator or if limiting adverse effects occur, oral extended-release theophylline may be added or substituted. For additional details on the stepped-care approach for drug therapy in COPD, see Chronic Obstructive Pulmonary Disease under Uses: Bronchospasm, in Ipratropium Bromide 12:08.08.

Orally inhaled salmeterol therapy in patients with COPD generally has produced increases in peak FEV₁ averaging 7–20%. In a subset of patients from a short-term (i.e., 24-week) placebo-controlled study in patients with COPD, orally inhaled salmeterol inhalation powder produced improvement in FEV₁ that was apparent on the first day of treatment, sustained over the 12-hour dosing interval, and showed no loss of effectiveness over the study period.

In two 6-month comparative trials in patients with COPD, orally inhaled tiotropium (18 mcg once daily) was more effective in improving FEV₁ than salmeterol (42 mcg twice daily) inhalation aerosol (no longer commercially available in the US) after day 1 of therapy. In addition, while tiotropium or salmeterol each reduced dyspnea and improved FEV₁ compared with placebo, tiotropium also was more effective than placebo in reducing COPD exacerbations and all-cause hospital admissions and improving quality-of-life scores in these trials. In another 6-month, placebo-controlled study in patients with COPD, treatment with tiotropium (18 mcg once daily) was associated with greater improvement in bronchodilation (e.g., FEV₁, evening PEFR), dyspnea, and quality-of-life scores than salmeterol (42 mcg twice daily) oral inhalation aerosol.

In several randomized, double-blind, placebo-controlled studies of 6 or 12 months' duration in patients with COPD, orally inhaled salmeterol (50 mcg twice daily) in fixed combination with fluticasone propionate (250 or 500 mcg twice daily) as the inhalation powder (Advair® Diskus®) produced greater improvement in lung function (defined as predose or postdose FEV₁) than either drug alone or placebo. The improvement in lung function with salmeterol 50 mcg and fluticasone propionate 500 mcg in fixed combination was similar to that observed with salmeterol 50 mcg and fluticasone propionate 250 mcg in fixed combination. In two randomized, double-blind, placebo-controlled studies of 12 months' duration in patients with COPD, orally inhaled salmeterol (50 mcg twice daily) in fixed combination with fluticasone propionate (250 mcg twice daily) as the inhalation powder produced a greater reduction in the annual incidence of moderate/severe COPD exacerbations and exacerbations requiring treatment with oral corticosteroids compared with salmeterol alone. No studies have been conducted to directly compare the efficacy of salmeterol 50 mcg and fluticasone propionate 250 mcg in fixed combination with salmeterol 50 mcg and fluticasone propionate 500 mcg in fixed combination on exacerbations; however, in clinical studies, the reduction in exacerbations observed with salmeterol 50 mcg and fluticasone propionate 500 mcg in fixed combination was not greater than the reduction in exacerbations observed with salmeterol 50 mcg and fluticasone propionate 250 mcg in fixed combination. In a double-blind, placebo-controlled study of 3 years' duration in patients with COPD, orally inhaled salmeterol (50 mcg) in fixed combination with fluticasone propionate (500 mcg) as the inhalation powder did not improve all-cause mortality compared with either drug alone or placebo. Salmeterol 50 mcg and fluticasone propionate 250 mcg in fixed combination twice daily is the only recommended dosage for the treatment of COPD; an efficacy advantage of the higher dosage of the fixed combination containing 50 mcg of salmeterol and 500 mcg of fluticasone propionate over the lower dosage (50 mcg of salmeterol/250 mcg fluticasone propionate) has not been established.

DOSAGE AND ADMINISTRATION

● Administration

Salmeterol xinafoate is administered by oral inhalation using a special preloaded oral inhaler (Serevent® or Advair® Diskus®, or AirDuo® RespiClick®) that delivers powdered drug alone or in fixed combination with fluticasone propionate. The manufacturer of the Diskus® devices states that spacer devices should not be used with Serevent® or Advair® Diskus®. The manufacturer of the RespiClick® device states that spacers or volume holding chambers should not be used with AirDuo® RespiClick®.

Salmeterol/fluticasone propionate inhalation aerosol (Advair® HFA) should only be used with the actuator supplied with the product. Before each inhalation, the inhaler must be shaken well for 5 seconds. The aerosol inhaler should be test sprayed 4 times into the air (away from the face) before initial use, and shaken well for 5 seconds before each spray. If the inhaler has not been used for more than 4 weeks or if the inhaler was dropped, the inhaler should be test sprayed twice into the air (away from the face) and shaken well for 5 seconds before each spray.

The cap covering the mouthpiece should be slipped off the mouthpiece; the strap on the cap will stay attached to the mouthpiece. The patient should look for foreign objects inside the inhaler prior to use, and should check to see that the canister is fully seated within the actuator. After exhaling as completely as possible, the patient should place the mouthpiece of the inhaler well into the mouth and close the lips firmly around it. Then the patient should inhale deeply through the mouth while actuating the inhaler. The patient should remove the mouthpiece from the mouth and hold the breath for as long as possible, up to 10 seconds, and exhale slowly. It is recommended that 30 seconds elapse between inhalations.

Rinsing the mouth after inhalation of salmeterol/fluticasone propionate inhalation aerosol and spitting out the water are advised. The opening for the spray of the metal canister and the mouthpiece should be wiped with a dry cotton swab and dampened tissue, respectively, at least once a week after the evening dose. The actuator should be allowed to air-dry overnight. When the dose counter on the inhaler reads "020," the patient should contact the pharmacy for a refill or consult their clinician to determine whether a refill is needed. The inhaler should be discarded when the dose counter reads "000." The counter should never be altered or removed from the canister.

For administration of salmeterol xinafoate alone (Serevent®) or in combination with fluticasone propionate (Advair®) inhalation powder via the Diskus® device, the patient should hold the device in one hand, put the thumb of the other hand on the thumbgrip, and push the thumbgrip until the mouthpiece appears and snaps into position. The lever on the Diskus® should then be depressed in a direction away from the patient while the inhaler is held in a level, horizontal position; the lever pierces the foil blister and releases the powdered drug into an exit port. To avoid releasing and wasting additional doses of the drug, the patient should not tilt or close the Diskus® device, play with the lever, or advance the lever more than once at this point. A dose counter will advance each time the lever is depressed. Before inhaling the dose, the patient should exhale as completely as possible; the patient should *not* exhale into the Diskus® device because pressure from the exhalation will interfere with proper inhaler operation. The patient should then place the mouthpiece of the inhaler between the lips and inhale deeply and quickly through the inhaler with a steady, even breath; pressure from the inhalation will disperse drug from the exit port into the air stream created by the patient's inhalation. The patient should remove the inhaler from the mouth, hold his or her breath for 10 seconds (or as long as comfortable), and then exhale slowly. While most patients can taste or feel a dose of drug delivered from the Diskus® device, they should be instructed not to use another dose even if they do not perceive that the dose has been delivered. Rinsing the mouth after inhalation of salmeterol in fixed combination with fluticasone propionate is advised. The Diskus® device may be closed and reset for the next dose by sliding the thumbgrip towards the patient as far as it will go. The inhaler should not be washed but should be stored in a dry place away from direct heat or sunlight. The inhaler should be discarded when every blister has been used, or 4 or 6 weeks after removal of the Advair® Diskus® or Serevent® Diskus®, respectively, from its foil overwrap pouch. The inhaler should not be taken apart.

For instructions on use of the AirDuo® RespiClick® oral inhaler, the manufacturer's labeling should be consulted.

To obtain optimal benefit, the patient should be given a copy of the product-specific patient instructions and medication guide provided by the manufacturer. (See Asthma-related Death and Life-threatening Events under Cautions: Respiratory Effects.)

● Dosage

Dosage of salmeterol xinafoate is expressed in terms of salmeterol. Although each blister of the double-foil blister strip in the Serevent® Diskus® device contains 50 mcg of salmeterol as salmeterol xinafoate inhalation powder, the precise amount of drug delivered to the lungs with each activation of the Diskus® device depends on factors such as the patient's inspiratory flow. (See Chemistry and Stability: Chemistry.)

Each blister of the foil blister strip in the Advair® Diskus® device contains 50 mcg of salmeterol as salmeterol xinafoate and 100, 250, or 500 mcg of fluticasone propionate; however, the precise amount of each drug delivered to the lungs with each activation of the Diskus® device depends on factors such as the patient's inspiratory flow. (See Chemistry and Stability: Chemistry.)

Each actuation of the AirDuo® RespiClick® device contains 14 mcg of salmeterol as salmeterol xinafoate and 55, 113, or 232 mcg of fluticasone propionate; however, the precise amount of each drug delivered to the lungs with each actuation of the RespiClick® device depends on factors such as the patient's inspiratory flow.

Each actuation of the oral aerosol inhaler of the fixed combination of salmeterol and fluticasone propionate (Advair® HFA) delivers 50, 125, or 250 mcg of fluticasone propionate and 25 mcg of salmeterol from the valve. Dosages of salmeterol and fluticasone propionate in the fixed-combination inhalation aerosol are expressed in terms of drug delivered from the mouthpiece; each actuation of the inhaler delivers 45, 115, or 230 mcg of fluticasone propionate and 21 mcg of salmeterol from the mouthpiece. The commercially available inhalation aerosol of salmeterol in fixed combination with fluticasone propionate delivers 60 or 120 metered sprays per 8- or 12-g canister, respectively.

The manufacturer states that adjustment of salmeterol dosage alone or in fixed combination with fluticasone propionate is not necessary in geriatric patients.

Asthma

Salmeterol

When salmeterol inhalation powder is administered via the Serevent® Diskus® device, the usual dosage in adults and children 4 years of age or older is 50 mcg (one inhalation) twice daily, given approximately 12 hours apart. If a dose of salmeterol is missed, the next dose should be taken at the regularly scheduled time; the dose should not be doubled. Higher dosages (e.g., 84 mcg of salmeterol twice daily as the inhalation aerosol; no longer commercially available in the US) have been used in some studies in patients with severe asthma, usually in conjunction with corticosteroids, cromolyn sodium, nedocromil sodium (preparations for oral inhalation no longer commercially available in the US), and/or theophylline; however, such dosages are more likely to be associated with adverse effects, and the manufacturer states that patients should not use more than 50 mcg (1 inhalation) twice daily of salmeterol. Patients receiving salmeterol should not use additional long-acting β₂-adrenergic agonists for any reason.

Patients should contact a clinician if asthma symptoms do not improve after 1 week of therapy. Failure to respond to a previously effective dosage of salmeterol may indicate destabilization of asthma that requires immediate medical attention and reevaluation of the therapeutic regimen. If symptoms arise in the period between doses, a short-acting, inhaled β₂-agonist should be used for immediate relief. However, increasing use of short-acting, inhaled β₂-agonists is a marker of deteriorating asthma; patients in this situation require immediate reevaluation with reassessment of the treatment regimen, giving special consideration to the possible need for adding additional inhaled corticosteroids or initiating systemic corticosteroids. Extra/increased doses of salmeterol should *not* be used in such situations. Patients should be advised to contact a clinician immediately if they experience decreasing effectiveness of short-acting, inhaled β₂-agonists, a need for more inhalations than usual of short-acting, inhaled β₂-agonists, or a substantial decrease in lung function as outlined by the clinician. Patients should adhere to dosing schedules, including not altering the dose or frequency of use of salmeterol unless otherwise instructed by a clinician. (See Cautions: Precautions and Contraindications.)

Salmeterol is not a substitute for inhaled or oral corticosteroids, and patients receiving corticosteroid therapy should be advised *not* to discontinue or alter the dosage of corticosteroids without consulting a clinician, even if the patient has subjective improvement after initiating therapy with salmeterol. When initiating therapy and throughout treatment with salmeterol in patients receiving oral or inhaled corticosteroids for treatment of asthma, patients must continue taking a suitable dosage of corticosteroids to maintain clinical stability even if they have subjective improvement as a result of initiation of salmeterol; any change in corticosteroid dosage should be made only after clinical evaluation. In addition, all patients with asthma should be advised that they *must* continue regular maintenance treatment with an inhaled corticosteroid if they are receiving salmeterol. Patients also should be advised not to discontinue salmeterol without medical supervision because symptoms may recur after treatment discontinuance. (See Cautions: Precautions and Contraindications.)

Salmeterol/Fluticasone Propionate Fixed-combination Therapy

In asthmatic patients 4–11 years of age who are inadequately controlled on an inhaled corticosteroid, the recommended dosage of the commercially available inhalation powder preparation containing salmeterol in fixed combination with fluticasone propionate (Advair® Diskus®) is 50 mcg of salmeterol and 100 mcg of fluticasone propionate (1 inhalation) twice daily, given approximately 12 hours apart.

In asthmatic patients 12 years of age or older, the recommended initial dosage of the commercially available inhalation powder preparation containing salmeterol in fixed combination with fluticasone propionate (Advair® Diskus®) is based on the patient's asthma severity and current asthma therapy, including the dosage of inhaled corticosteroids, as well as the patient's current control of asthma symptoms and risk of future exacerbations. The dosage of the inhalation powder fixed-combination preparation is 50 mcg of salmeterol and 100, 250, or 500 mcg

of fluticasone propionate (1 inhalation) twice daily, given approximately 12 hours apart. The maximum recommended dosage of salmeterol in fixed combination is 50 mcg of salmeterol with 500 mcg of fluticasone propionate twice daily. The manufacturer states that administration of the inhalation powder of salmeterol in fixed combination with fluticasone more frequently than twice daily or exceeding 1 inhalation twice daily is not recommended.

When the fixed combination of salmeterol and fluticasone propionate is administered via the AirDuo® RespiClick® device in asthmatic patients 12 years of age or older, the recommended initial dosage is based on the patient's current asthma therapy and asthma severity. For patients with asthma not previously receiving inhaled corticosteroid therapy, the usual recommended initial dosage is 14 mcg of salmeterol and 55 mcg of fluticasone propionate (1 inhalation) twice daily, given approximately 12 hours apart at approximately the same time every day. For patients with asthma switching from another inhaled corticosteroid or fixed-combination therapy, the dosage strength should be selected based on the dosage strength of the previously inhaled corticosteroid alone or in combination as well as disease severity. For patients who do not respond to AirDuo® Respi-Click® containing 14 mcg of salmeterol and 55 mcg of fluticasone propionate after 2 weeks of therapy, increasing the dosage may provide additional asthma control. If the dosage regimen does not provide adequate control of asthma, the regimen should be reevaluated and additional therapeutic options (e.g., replacing the current strength of the fixed combination with a higher strength [higher strengths contain higher dosages of fluticasone propionate only], using additional asthma controller therapy) should be considered. The maximum recommended dosage of salmeterol in fixed combination with fluticasone is 14 mcg of salmeterol and 232 mcg of fluticasone propionate twice daily. The manufacturer states that administration of the inhalation powder of salmeterol in fixed combination with fluticasone more frequently than twice daily or exceeding 1 inhalation twice daily is not recommended.

In asthmatic patients 12 years of age or older, the recommended initial dosage of the inhalation aerosol containing salmeterol in fixed combination with fluticasone propionate (Advair® HFA) is based on the patient's current asthma therapy, including the dosage of inhaled corticosteroids, as well as the patient's current control of asthma symptoms and risk of future exacerbations. The dosage of the inhalation aerosol fixed-combination preparation (Advair® HFA) is 42 mcg of salmeterol and 90, 230, or 460 mcg of fluticasone propionate (2 inhalations) twice daily, given approximately 12 hours apart. The maximum recommended dosage of salmeterol is 42 mcg in fixed combination with 460 mcg of fluticasone propionate (2 inhalations) twice daily. The manufacturer states that administration of salmeterol in fixed combination with fluticasone inhalation aerosol more frequently than twice daily or in excess of 2 inhalations twice daily is not recommended.

If control of asthma is inadequate after 2 weeks of therapy at the initial dosage, replacing the current strength of the fixed combination with a higher strength (higher strengths contain higher dosages of fluticasone propionate only) may provide additional asthma control. Patients receiving the fixed combination of salmeterol and fluticasone propionate twice daily should not use additional salmeterol or other long-acting β₂-adrenergic agonists (e.g., formoterol) for any reason, including the treatment of asthma or prevention of exercise-induced bronchospasm. If a dose of salmeterol in fixed combination with fluticasone is missed, the next dose should be taken at the regularly scheduled time; the dose should not be doubled. Patients also should be advised not to discontinue salmeterol in fixed combination with fluticasone propionate without medical supervision because symptoms may recur after treatment discontinuance. If a previously effective dosage of salmeterol in fixed combination with fluticasone fails to provide adequate improvement in asthma control, the therapeutic regimen should be reevaluated and additional therapeutic options should be considered (e.g., increasing the strength of the fixed combination [higher strengths contain higher dosages of fluticasone only], adding additional inhaled corticosteroids, initiating systemic corticosteroids). (See Cautions: Precautions and Contraindications.)

Exercise-Induced Bronchospasm

For the prevention of exercise-induced bronchospasm, the usual dosage of salmeterol oral inhalation powder in adults and children 4 years of age or older is 50 mcg administered through the Serevent® Diskus® device at least 30 minutes before exercise. *Additional doses of salmeterol should not be used for 12 hours.* In addition, the manufacturer states that patients who are receiving salmeterol oral inhalation powder twice daily should *not* use additional salmeterol for the prevention of exercise-induced bronchospasm. Patients receiving salmeterol alone or in fixed combination with fluticasone propionate should not use additional salmeterol or other long-acting β₂-adrenergic agonists (e.g., formoterol) for any reason, including prevention of exercise-induced bronchospasm.

Chronic Obstructive Pulmonary Disease

Salmeterol

For maintenance therapy of bronchospasm in patients with COPD (including chronic bronchitis and emphysema), the dosage of orally inhaled salmeterol given as the inhalation powder (Serevent® Diskus®) in adults is 50 mcg (1 inhalation) twice daily, given approximately every 12 hours. Higher dosages of salmeterol are more likely to be associated with adverse effects, and more frequent administration or administration of higher dosages (i.e., more than 1 inhalation twice daily) of the drug is not recommended by the manufacturer. Patients should not discontinue salmeterol without medical supervision because symptoms may recur after treatment discontinuance.

Salmeterol/Fluticasone Propionate Fixed-combination Therapy

For maintenance therapy of COPD, the recommended dosage of salmeterol in fixed combination with fluticasone propionate (Advair® Diskus®) in adults is 50 mcg of salmeterol and 250 mcg of fluticasone propionate (1 inhalation) twice daily, given approximately every 12 hours. If shortness of breath occurs between doses, an inhaled, short-acting β₂-adrenergic agonist may be administered for immediate relief. Higher dosages of salmeterol in fixed combination with fluticasone propionate (e.g., 50 mcg of salmeterol and 500 mcg of fluticasone propionate) do not result in additional benefit and are not recommended. Patients receiving salmeterol in fixed combination with fluticasone propionate should not use additional salmeterol or other long-acting β₂-adrenergic agonists (e.g., arformoterol, formoterol, indacaterol) for any reason, including the treatment of COPD. Patients should not discontinue salmeterol in fixed combination with fluticasone propionate without medical supervision because symptoms may recur.

● Dosage in Renal and/or Hepatic Impairment

The pharmacokinetics of salmeterol or salmeterol in fixed combination with fluticasone have not been studied in patients with hepatic impairment. Since salmeterol and fluticasone propionate are cleared predominantly by hepatic metabolism, impaired liver function theoretically may lead to accumulation of the drugs in plasma. Therefore, the manufacturers recommend that patients with hepatic disease be monitored closely while receiving salmeterol therapy.

The pharmacokinetics of salmeterol in fixed combination with fluticasone have not been studied in patients with renal impairment. Therefore, there are no specific dosage recommendations for such patients.

CAUTIONS

Salmeterol xinafoate oral inhalation appears to be well tolerated when administered in recommended doses. However, monotherapy with long-acting β₂-adrenergic agonists, such as salmeterol, increases the risk of asthma-related death and may increase the risk of asthma-related hospitalization in pediatric and adolescent patients. (See Asthma-related Death and Life-threatening Events under Cautions: Respiratory Effects.) In general, adverse effects reported with salmeterol in controlled studies were similar in type and frequency to those reported with other selective β₂-adrenergic agonists (e.g., albuterol) or placebo. The most common adverse effects of salmeterol oral inhalation powder reported in controlled studies in patients with asthma include headache, influenza, nasal/sinus congestion, pharyngitis, rhinitis, and tracheitis/bronchitis. The most common adverse effects of salmeterol oral inhalation powder reported in controlled studies in patients with chronic obstructive pulmonary disease (COPD) include cough, headache, musculoskeletal pain, throat irritation, and viral respiratory infection. In children 4–11 years of age with mild to moderate asthma, currently available data on adverse effects of salmeterol inhalation powder are derived principally from 2 comparative, 12-week clinical trials with salmeterol (50 mcg twice daily) and albuterol inhalation powder (200 mcg 4 times daily). In adolescents and adults with mild to moderate asthma, currently available data on adverse effects of salmeterol inhalation powder are derived principally from 2 large, 12-week comparative trials with salmeterol (50 mcg twice daily) inhalation powder and albuterol (180 mcg 4 times daily) inhalation aerosol. For adverse effects reported

with salmeterol therapy in the Cautions section, a causal relationship to the drug has not always been established.

● Cardiovascular Effects

Usual doses of salmeterol oral inhalation generally produce no apparent cardiovascular effects. However, salmeterol may produce a clinically important cardiovascular effect in some patients as measured by pulse rate, blood pressure, and/or cardiovascular symptoms. Although such effects are uncommon after administration of salmeterol at recommended dosages, if they occur, discontinuance of the drug may be needed. In addition, β₂-agonists have been reported to produce ECG changes, such as flattening of the T wave, prolongation of the QT_c interval, and ST segment depression; the clinical importance of these effects is unknown. Hypertension was reported in 4% of patients with COPD receiving salmeterol inhalation powder during clinical trials and also has been reported during postmarketing surveillance. Supraventricular tachycardia or atrial fibrillation has been reported with salmeterol inhalation powder during postmarketing surveillance. Pallor has been reported in 9% of adults and adolescents with asthma receiving salmeterol inhalation powder in clinical trials.

Nonsustained ventricular tachycardia among patients with COPD receiving salmeterol inhalation powder was reported in an incidence similar to that with placebo and fluticasone propionate. The incidence of clinically important ECG abnormalities indicating myocardial ischemia, ventricular hypertrophy, conduction abnormalities, or arrhythmias was lower in patients with COPD receiving salmeterol inhalation powder alone or in fixed combination with fluticasone propionate than in patients receiving placebo. ECG changes, including extrasystoles (supraventricular and ventricular premature complexes), also have been noted with salmeterol inhalation powder. Clinically important prolongation of the QT_c interval, which potentially can cause ventricular arrhythmias, has been associated with administration of large oral or inhaled doses (about 12–20 times the recommended dose) of salmeterol or other β₂-agonists. Fatalities also have been reported in association with excessive use of inhaled sympathomimetic drugs. (See Cautions: Precautions and Contraindications.) Cardiorespiratory arrest has been reported in a patient with COPD and preexisting alcoholic cardiomyopathy who had received usual dosages of orally inhaled salmeterol in conjunction with orally inhaled ipratropium and albuterol. Salmeterol is a highly selective β₂-agonist, and certain cardiovascular effects (e.g., ventricular or nodal arrhythmias, severe tachycardia, anginal-type pain, myocardial ischemia) reported with less receptor-selective β₂-adrenergic agonists such as isoproterenol theoretically may occur less frequently, or not at all, with salmeterol.

● Nervous System Effects

In clinical trials with salmeterol inhalation powder, headache was reported in 14% of patients with COPD, 13% of adults and adolescents with asthma, and 17% of children with asthma. Migraine has been reported in at least 1% of patients receiving salmeterol inhalation powder for the treatment of COPD. In clinical studies in adults and adolescents 12 years of age or older with asthma, sleep disturbances and paresthesia occurred more frequently in patients receiving salmeterol inhalation powder than those receiving placebo. Dizziness has been reported in 4% of patients receiving salmeterol inhalation powder for the treatment of COPD. Unrest, depression, anxiety, and vertigo also have been reported rarely with salmeterol oral inhalation therapy. Anxiety has been reported in at least 1% of patients receiving salmeterol inhalation powder for the treatment of COPD.

● Respiratory Effects

Asthma-related Death and Life-threatening Events

Monotherapy with long-acting β₂-adrenergic agonists, such as salmeterol, increases the risk of asthma-related death. In addition, available data from controlled clinical trials suggest that monotherapy with long-acting β₂-adrenergic agonists increases the risk of asthma-related hospitalization in pediatric and adolescent patients. *Because of these risks, the use of long-acting β₂-adrenergic agonists, including salmeterol, alone for the treatment of asthma without concomitant use of long-term asthma controller therapy, such as inhaled corticosteroids, is contraindicated.* (See Cautions: Precautions and Contraindications.) However, FDA has concluded that there is no clinically important increased risk of serious asthma-related events, including hospitalization, intubation, or death, associated with concomitant use of long-acting β₂-adrenergic agonists (e.g., salmeterol) and inhaled corticosteroids compared with inhaled corticosteroids alone based on the results of several large clinical studies. In addition, these studies showed that combination therapy with long-acting β₂-adrenergic agonists and inhaled corticosteroids was more effective in reducing the incidence of asthma exacerbations (i.e., events requiring use of systemic corticosteroids for at least 3 outpatient days or an asthma-related hospitalization or emergency department visit requiring use of systemic corticosteroids) compared with use of inhaled corticosteroids alone.

Long-acting β₂-adrenergic agonists, including salmeterol, should only be used as additional therapy in patients with asthma who are currently receiving long-term asthma controller therapy, such as inhaled corticosteroids, but whose disease is inadequately controlled with such therapy. The fixed combination of salmeterol and fluticasone propionate should be used only in patients with asthma who have not responded adequately to long-term asthma controller therapy, such as inhaled corticosteroids, or whose disease severity warrants initiation of treatment with both an inhaled corticosteroid and a long-acting β₂-adrenergic agonist. Once asthma control is achieved and maintained, the patient should be assessed at regular intervals and therapy should be stepped down (e.g., discontinuance of the long-acting β₂-adrenergic agonist), if possible without loss of asthma control, and the patient should be maintained on long-term asthma controller therapy, such as inhaled corticosteroids. Long-acting β₂-adrenergic agonists, including salmeterol alone or in fixed combination with fluticasone propionate, should not be used in patients whose asthma is adequately controlled on a low or medium dosage of inhaled corticosteroids. In pediatric and adolescent patients with asthma who require the addition of a long-acting β₂-adrenergic agonist to inhaled corticosteroid therapy, a fixed-combination preparation containing both an inhaled corticosteroid and a long-acting β₂-adrenergic agonist generally should be used to ensure compliance with both drugs. (See Uses: Bronchospasm.)

Data from a large (approximately 26,000 patients) placebo-controlled study in patients receiving salmeterol xinafoate as part of an asthma treatment regimen showed an increase in asthma-related deaths in patients receiving salmeterol. In the Salmeterol Multi-center Asthma Research Trial (SMART), a 28-week safety study, patients received salmeterol 42 mcg or placebo via metered-dose aerosol with a chlorofluorocarbon (CFC) propellant (CFC preparation no longer commercially available in the US) twice daily in addition to their usual asthma therapy. The primary end point of the SMART study was the combined number of respiratory-related deaths and respiratory-related life-threatening experiences (intubation and mechanical ventilation). Secondary end points included asthma-related deaths and combined asthma-related deaths or life-threatening experiences. The risk of respiratory-related death or life-threatening experience (primary end point) was higher in patients receiving salmeterol versus placebo (relative risk: 1.4) in the SMART trial, although this difference was not statistically significant. However, analysis of secondary end points revealed a statistically significant greater risk for asthma-related death (relative risk: 4.37) or combined asthma-related death or life-threatening experience (relative risk: 1.71) with salmeterol therapy in the overall patient population compared with placebo. Results of a post hoc analysis also revealed a greater risk for asthma-related death (relative risk: 7.26) with salmeterol therapy in African-American patients (18% of study patients) and in patients not receiving concomitant inhaled corticosteroid therapy (53% of study patients) compared with placebo. A greater risk for asthma-related death (relative risk: 5.82) was observed in white patients (71% of the study population) receiving salmeterol therapy compared with placebo; no asthma-related deaths occurred in Hispanic or Asian subpopulations. Factors possibly contributing to the increased numbers of adverse events in African-American patients include the findings that these patients had more severe asthma at baseline than white patients and that fewer African-American than white patients were receiving concomitant inhaled corticosteroid therapy (38 versus 50%, respectively). Results of post hoc analyses in pediatric patients 12–18 years of age (12% of study patients) revealed that the rate of respiratory-related deaths and life-threatening experiences was similar in both the salmeterol and placebo groups (relative risk: 1); however, the rate of all-cause hospitalizations was higher in the salmeterol group compared with the placebo group (relative risk: 2.1). Because of the similar mechanism of action of long-acting β₂-adrenergic agonists, the findings of the SMART study are considered a class effect of these drugs.

A prior 16-week comparative study performed in the United Kingdom (Salmeterol Nationwide Surveillance [SNS] study) also reported a numerically, but not statistically significantly, higher incidence of asthma-related deaths in patients treated with salmeterol (42 mcg twice daily) compared with those receiving albuterol (180 mcg 4 times daily).

The SMART and SNS studies enrolled patients with asthma; no studies have been conducted that were adequate to determine whether the rate of death is increased in patients with COPD receiving long-acting β₂-adrenergic agonists.

In 4 randomized, double-blind, active-controlled clinical trials mandated by FDA, the risk of serious asthma-related events from use of inhaled corticosteroids alone compared with combined use of long-acting β₂-adrenergic agonists and inhaled corticosteroids was evaluated over 26 weeks in 41,297 patients with asthma (3 trials in adults and adolescents 12 years of age or older and one trial in children 4–11 years of age). The primary safety end point in all of these trials was serious asthma-related events, including hospitalization, intubation, and death; these events were reviewed by a blinded committee to determine if the events were asthma related. The 3 trials performed in adults and adolescents were designed to rule out a hazard ratio of 2, and the pediatric trial was designed to rule out a hazard ratio of 2.7; this objective was met in all 4 individual trials. The trials were not designed to rule out all risk for serious asthma-related events associated with long-acting β₂-adrenergic agonists in combination with inhaled corticosteroids compared with inhaled corticosteroids alone.

The safety studies in adults and adolescents included one trial comparing salmeterol and fluticasone propionate in fixed combination as the inhalation powder (Advair® Diskus®) with fluticasone propionate inhalation powder alone, one trial comparing formoterol and mometasone furoate in fixed combination with mometasone furoate alone, and one trial comparing formoterol and budesonide in fixed combination with budesonide alone. In a meta-analysis combining data from these 3 trials, a hazard ratio of 1.1 for serious asthma-related events in patients receiving fixed-combination therapy with long-acting β₂-adrenergic agonists and inhaled corticosteroids compared with patients receiving inhaled corticosteroids alone was reported. Subgroup analyses for gender, adolescents 12–17 years of age, Asian and African-American patients, and obese patients also showed no substantial increase in the risk of serious asthma-related events or asthma exacerbations in these populations.

The trial comparing salmeterol and fluticasone propionate in fixed combination as the inhalation powder (Advair® Diskus) with fluticasone propionate inhalation powder alone included 11,679 adults and adolescents 12 years of age or older with moderate to severe persistent asthma who had a history of asthma-related hospitalization or at least one asthma exacerbation in the previous year requiring treatment with systemic corticosteroids. Patients with a history of life-threatening or unstable asthma were excluded from the study. In this trial, serious asthma-related events were reported in 0.6% of patients in each treatment group, with a hazard ratio for first event for the combination therapy compared with fluticasone alone of approximately 1.

The safety study in children 4–11 years of age included 6208 patients who were randomized to receive salmeterol and fluticasone propionate in fixed combination as the inhalation powder (Advair® Diskus) or fluticasone propionate inhalation powder alone. Patients had a diagnosis of asthma and a history of at least one asthma exacerbation in the previous year requiring treatment with systemic corticosteroids; patients with life-threatening asthma were excluded from the study. Serious asthma-related events were reported in 0.9% of patients receiving salmeterol and fluticasone in fixed combination and in 0.7% of patients receiving fluticasone alone, with an estimated hazard ratio for first event of 1.29 for the combination therapy compared with fluticasone alone. No asthma-related deaths or intubations were reported in either group of pediatric patients.

Other Respiratory Effects

Cough was reported in 5% of patients receiving salmeterol inhalation powder for the treatment of COPD. In clinical studies in adults and adolescents 12 years of age or older with asthma, sinus headache was reported more frequently in patients receiving salmeterol inhalation powder than those receiving placebo. Exacerbations of asthma have been reported in 4% of children and 3% of adults and adolescents receiving salmeterol inhalation powder for the treatment of asthma. Tracheitis/bronchitis or influenza occurred in 7 or 5%, respectively, of adults and adolescents receiving salmeterol inhalation powder. Nasal/sinus congestion or rhinitis occurred in 9 or 5%, respectively, of adults and adolescents with asthma receiving salmeterol inhalation powder. Nasal congestion or blockage, rhinitis, or sinusitis occurred in 4% of patients with COPD receiving salmeterol inhalation powder in clinical trials. Pharyngitis, sinusitis, upper respiratory tract infection, and cough occurred in at least 3% of adults and adolescents receiving salmeterol inhalation powder for the treatment of asthma in clinical trials but occurred less frequently than with placebo. However, throat irritation has been reported in

7% of patients with COPD receiving salmeterol inhalation powder in controlled clinical trials. Pharyngitis was reported in 6% of children with asthma receiving salmeterol inhalation powder in clinical trials. Lower respiratory tract signs and symptoms occurred in greater than 1% of children with asthma receiving salmeterol inhalation powder. Lower respiratory viral infection or lower respiratory tract signs and symptoms occurred in 5% or at least 1% of patients, respectively, receiving salmeterol inhalation powder for the treatment of COPD.

Upper airway symptoms of laryngeal spasm, irritation, or swelling, such as stridor or choking, and oropharyngeal irritation, have been reported during postmarketing experience with salmeterol oral inhalation therapy. As with other inhaled drugs, paradoxical bronchospasm, a potentially life-threatening event, also has occurred with salmeterol therapy. (See Cautions: Dermatologic and Sensitivity Reactions.)

Increased airway reactivity and variability or decreases in pulmonary function (e.g., as measured by PEFR or FEV₁), in some cases progressing to respiratory arrest or death, have been reported with regular use (e.g., 2 inhalations 4 times daily) of short-acting, inhaled β-agonists and also in some patients (generally with severe and/or deteriorating asthma) receiving salmeterol oral inhalation powder. Such detrimental effects may be related to down-regulation of β-adrenergic receptors (tolerance), increased responsiveness of airways to allergens and exercise, genetic changes in β₂-agonist receptor gene, or increased airway accessibility to inhaled allergens, which may lead to increased airway inflammation and reactivity and worsening of asthma symptoms. However, increased airway accessibility to inhaled allergens theoretically also would occur with long-acting bronchodilators such as extended-release theophylline.

● GI Effects

Hyposalivation, dyspepsia, oral (mouth/throat) candidiasis, or GI infections were reported in at least 1% of patients with COPD receiving salmeterol inhalation powder in clinical trials. In clinical studies in adults and adolescents 12 years of age or older with asthma, nausea has been reported more frequently in patients receiving salmeterol inhalation powder than those receiving placebo. Nausea and vomiting have been reported in 3% of patients receiving salmeterol inhalation powder for the treatment of COPD. In clinical studies in patients with asthma, GI signs and symptoms occurred in greater than 1% of children receiving salmeterol inhalation powder, while oral mucosal abnormality was reported more frequently in adults and adolescents 12 years of age or older receiving salmeterol inhalation powder than those receiving placebo.

● Metabolic and Electrolyte Effects

The manufacturer states that large IV doses of the β₂-adrenergic agonist albuterol (IV preparation not currently commercially available in the US) have aggravated preexisting diabetes mellitus and ketoacidosis.

The manufacturer states that clinically important and dose-related changes in blood glucose and/or serum potassium concentrations have been observed infrequently during clinical studies with salmeterol oral inhalation powder at recommended dosages. No clinically important changes in glucose or potassium concentrations were reported in clinical studies in patients with asthma receiving salmeterol oral inhalation powder. In addition, no clinically important changes in serum potassium concentrations were reported in clinical studies in patients with COPD receiving salmeterol oral inhalation powder at recommended dosages. Patients should inform their clinician of the presence of diabetes mellitus prior to initiation of therapy. Salmeterol and other β₂-adrenergic agonists may decrease serum potassium concentrations through increased intracellular uptake of potassium resulting from β₂-receptor mediated Na⁺- K⁺-ATPase activation in liver and skeletal muscle. Although such reductions potentially may cause adverse cardiovascular effects, the decreases usually are transient and supplemental potassium therapy generally is not required. Hyperglycemia occurred in at least 1% of patients receiving salmeterol inhalation powder for the treatment of COPD. The potential for hyperglycemia or hypokalemia with salmeterol therapy appears to be dose related. Tolerance to the hypokalemic effects of albuterol has been demonstrated but has not been reported to date with salmeterol therapy.

● Musculoskeletal Effects

Musculoskeletal pain occurred in 12% of patients receiving salmeterol inhalation powder for the treatment of COPD, and muscle cramps and spasms were reported in 3% of such patients with COPD. In clinical studies in patients with asthma,

joint pain was reported more frequently in adults and adolescents 12 years of age or older receiving salmeterol inhalation powder than those receiving placebo, and arthralgia or arthritis occurred in greater than 1% of children receiving the inhaled powder in such trials. Arthralgia or arthritis; muscle, bone, or skeletal pain; musculoskeletal inflammation; or muscle stiffness, tightness, or rigidity has occurred in at least 1% of patients receiving salmeterol inhalation powder for the treatment of COPD in clinical trials.

● Dermatologic and Sensitivity Reactions

Immediate hypersensitivity reactions, including urticaria, angioedema, rash, and bronchospasm may occur following administration of salmeterol alone or salmeterol and fluticasone propionate in fixed combination. Anaphylactic reactions have been reported very rarely in patients with severe milk protein allergy after inhalation of powder products containing lactose; therefore, patients with severe milk protein allergy should not receive such products containing salmeterol or salmeterol and fluticasone in fixed combination. (See Cautions: Precautions and Contraindications.) Anaphylaxis also has been reported during postmarketing surveillance studies with the drug.

In clinical studies in adults and adolescents 12 years of age or older with asthma, contact dermatitis and eczema were reported more frequently in patients receiving salmeterol inhalation powder than those receiving placebo. Rash, photodermatitis, or urticaria was reported in 4, greater than 1, or 3%, respectively, of children receiving salmeterol inhalation powder in clinical trials. Rash was reported in at least 1% of patients receiving salmeterol inhalation powder for the treatment of COPD.

Although the mechanism(s) has not been fully elucidated, paradoxical bronchospasm (defined as a decrease of 20% or greater in PEFR) has occurred occasionally with repeated or excessive use of orally inhaled sympathomimetic amines (especially isoproterenol). Preliminary results of a controlled study in almost 12,000 patients demonstrated that paradoxical bronchospasm occurred less frequently with salmeterol oral inhalation than with placebo (either lecithin or oleic acid) given via metered-dose inhaler (no longer commercially available), suggesting that orally inhaled ingredients other than the active drug may be more likely to produce paradoxical bronchospasm.

● Other Adverse Effects

Dental discomfort and pain have been reported in at least 1% of patients receiving salmeterol inhalation powder for the treatment of COPD. In clinical studies in patients with asthma, ear symptoms have been reported in 4% of children, and localized aches and pains and fever of unknown origin have been reported more frequently in adults and adolescents 12 years of age or older receiving salmeterol inhalation powder than those receiving placebo. Otic manifestations have been reported in 3% of patients with COPD receiving salmeterol inhalation powder in clinical trials. Edema and swelling have been reported in at least 1% of patients receiving salmeterol inhalation powder for the treatment of COPD. Keratitis and conjunctivitis occurred in at least 1% of patients receiving salmeterol inhalation powder for the treatment of COPD. Pain also has been reported in at least 1% of such patients. Herniated disk has been reported in at least one patient receiving inhaled salmeterol, but a causal relationship to the drug has not been established. A reduction in platelet count has been reported during long-term (1 year) therapy with salmeterol oral inhalation, but platelet count remained within the normal range and the reduction was not associated with sequelae. Elevation of hepatic enzymes was reported in at least 1% of patients with asthma receiving salmeterol oral inhalation powder in clinical studies. However, these elevations were transient and did not lead to discontinuance from the studies.

● Precautions and Contraindications

When salmeterol is used in fixed combination with fluticasone propionate, the usual cautions, precautions, and contraindications associated with fluticasone propionate must be considered in addition to those associated with salmeterol.

Patients should be advised to read the product-specific medication guide, patient information, and/or instructions for use prior to initiating therapy with the drug and each time the prescription is refilled.

Patients should be informed that monotherapy with long-acting β₂-adrenergic agonists, such as salmeterol, increases the risk of asthma-related death and may increase the risk of asthma-related hospitalization in pediatric and adolescent patients. (See Asthma-related Death and Life-threatening Events under Cautions:

Respiratory Effects.) Patients also should be informed that salmeterol should not be the only therapy used for the treatment of asthma and must only be used as additional therapy when long-term asthma controller therapy (e.g., inhaled corticosteroids) does not adequately control asthma symptoms. Patients should be advised that when salmeterol is added to their treatment regimen they must continue to use their long-term asthma controller drugs. (See Uses: Bronchospasm.)

Salmeterol, alone or in fixed combination with fluticasone propionate, should not be initiated in patients during rapidly deteriorating or potentially life-threatening episodes of asthma or COPD. Salmeterol alone or in fixed combination has not been studied in patients with acutely deteriorating asthma or COPD. Initiation of salmeterol in this setting is not appropriate. Serious acute respiratory events, including fatalities, have been reported when salmeterol has been initiated in patients with substantially worsening or acutely deteriorating asthma. In most cases, these adverse events have occurred in patients with severe asthma (e.g., those with a history of corticosteroid dependence, low pulmonary function, intubation, mechanical ventilation, frequent hospitalizations, previous life-threatening acute asthma exacerbations) and in some patients with acutely deteriorating asthma (e.g., patients with substantially increasing symptoms, increasing need for inhaled short-acting β₂-agonists, decreasing response to usual medications, increasing need for systemic corticosteroids, recent emergency room visits, deteriorating lung function). However, such events also have occurred in patients with less severe asthma. It was not possible from these reports to determine whether salmeterol contributed to these events.

Increasing use of short-acting, inhaled β₂-agonists is a marker of deteriorating asthma and failure to respond to a previously effective dosage regimen of salmeterol alone or in fixed combination with fluticasone propionate often is a sign of destabilization of asthma. In this situation in patients receiving salmeterol, the patient requires immediate reevaluation with reassessment of the treatment regimen, giving special consideration to the possible need to add additional inhaled corticosteroids or initiating systemic corticosteroids. If asthma deteriorates in patients receiving salmeterol in fixed combination with fluticasone, immediate reevaluation with reassessment of the treatment regimen is required, with special consideration given to the possible need for increasing the strength of the fixed combination (higher strengths contain higher dosages of fluticasone only), adding additional inhaled corticosteroids, or initiating systemic corticosteroids. However, extra/increased doses of salmeterol alone or in fixed combination with fluticasone propionate should *not* be used in such situations. Patients should be advised to contact a clinician immediately if they experience decreasing effectiveness of short-acting, inhaled β₂-agonists, a need for more inhalations than usual of short-acting, inhaled β₂-agonists, or a substantial decrease in lung function as outlined by the clinician. Patients should be advised not to discontinue therapy with salmeterol alone or in fixed combination with fluticasone without medical supervision since symptoms may recur following discontinuance.

Salmeterol has a delayed onset of action, and the drug alone or in fixed combination with fluticasone propionate should *not* be used for the relief of acute symptoms (i.e., as rescue therapy for the treatment of acute episodes of bronchospasm). A short-acting, inhaled β₂-agonist, not salmeterol (alone or in fixed combination with fluticasone propionate), should be used to relieve acute symptoms such as shortness of breath. All patients receiving salmeterol alone or in fixed combination with fluticasone propionate should be provided with and instructed in the use of a short-acting, inhaled β₂-agonist (e.g,. albuterol) for treatment of acute symptoms. When initiating salmeterol alone or in fixed combination with fluticasone in patients who have been taking short-acting, oral or inhaled β₂-agonists on a regular basis (e.g., 4 times daily), these patients should be instructed to discontinue the *regular* use of the short-acting agent.

Salmeterol is *not* a substitute for inhaled or oral corticosteroids, and patients receiving corticosteroid therapy should be advised *not* to discontinue or alter the dosage of corticosteroids without consulting a clinician, even if the patient has subjective improvement after initiating therapy with salmeterol, since worsening of asthma may occur. In addition, all patients with asthma should be advised that they *must* continue regular maintenance treatment with an inhaled corticosteroid if they are receiving salmeterol. The manufacturer states that there are no data demonstrating that salmeterol has a clinical anti-inflammatory effect such as that associated with corticosteroids. When initiating and throughout therapy with salmeterol in patients receiving oral or inhaled corticosteroids for treatment of asthma, patients must continue taking a suitable dosage of corticosteroids to maintain clinical stability even if they have subjective improvement as a result of

initiation of salmeterol; any change in corticosteroid dosage should be made only after clinical evaluation. Salmeterol in fixed combination with fluticasone as the inhalation aerosol (Advair® HFA) should not be used to transfer patients from systemic corticosteroid therapy. Particular care is needed for patients who have been transferred from systemically active corticosteroids to inhaled corticosteroids since death resulting from adrenal insufficiency has occurred in patients with asthma during and after such transfer. (See Cautions: Precautions and Contraindications, in Beclomethasone Dipropionate 68:04.)

As with other inhaled β₂-adrenergic drugs, salmeterol, alone or in fixed combination with fluticasone propionate, should not be used more often or at higher than recommended dosages, or in conjunction with other preparations containing long-acting β₂-adrenergic agonists, since an overdose may result. Clinically important cardiovascular effects and fatalities have been reported in association with excessive use of inhaled sympathomimetic drugs. Patients receiving salmeterol alone or in fixed combination with fluticasone propionate should not use additional salmeterol or other long-acting β₂-adrenergic agonists (e.g., arformoterol, formoterol, indacaterol) for any reason, including prevention of exercise-induced bronchospasm or treatment of asthma or COPD.

Rarely, a patient may develop acute bronchospasm immediately upon inhalation of a sympathomimetic drug preparation. Acute bronchospasm probably represents a hypersensitivity reaction to the active drug or an ingredient in the formulation. Although it may not be possible to distinguish paradoxical bronchoconstriction or that associated with hypersensitivity to the drug or an ingredient in the formulation from worsening of the asthma, salmeterol alone or in fixed combination with fluticasone propionate should be discontinued immediately if paradoxical bronchospasm occurs. Paradoxical bronchospasm should immediately be treated with a short-acting inhaled bronchodilator, and alternative therapy should be instituted. Patients should inform their clinicians of allergic reactions to salmeterol-containing preparations, other agents, or foods (including milk proteins).

Salmeterol and other β₂-adrenergic agonists may produce substantial hypokalemia in some patients, which has the potential to produce adverse cardiovascular effects (e.g., arrhythmias); however, decreases in serum potassium usually are transient and generally do not require supplementation. (See Cautions: Metabolic and Electrolyte Effects.)

Excessive β₂-adrenergic stimulation has been associated with seizures, angina, hypertension or hypotension, tachycardia with rates up to 200 beats/minute, arrhythmias, nervousness, headache, tremor, palpitation, nausea, dizziness, fatigue, malaise, and insomnia (see Acute Toxicity: Manifestations). Therefore, salmeterol, like all preparations containing sympathomimetic amines, should be used with caution in patients with cardiovascular disorders, especially coronary insufficiency, cardiac arrhythmias, and hypertension; in patients with seizure disorders or thyrotoxicosis; and in those who are unusually responsive to sympathomimetic amines. Patients should be informed of adverse effects associated with β₂-agonists, such as palpitations, chest pain, rapid heart rate, tremor, or nervousness. Patients should inform their clinician of heart problems, hypertension, seizures, thyroid disorders, or diabetes mellitus prior to initiation of salmeterol-containing therapy. Patients receiving salmeterol oral inhalation should use other inhaled medications only as directed by their clinician.

The pharmacokinetics of salmeterol or salmeterol in fixed combination with fluticasone propionate have not been studied in patients with hepatic impairment. Because salmeterol and fluticasone propionate are metabolized predominantly in the liver and potentially may accumulate in the plasma of patients with hepatic impairment, such patients should be monitored closely while receiving such therapy. Patients should inform their clinician of liver dysfunction prior to initiation of therapy.

Clinicians should remain vigilant for the possible development of pneumonia in patients with COPD who are receiving the inhalation powder preparation containing salmeterol in fixed combination with fluticasone propionate (Advair® Diskus®), since the clinical features of pneumonia and COPD exacerbations frequently overlap. Lower respiratory tract infections, including pneumonia, have been reported in patients with COPD following the administration of inhaled corticosteroids, including fluticasone propionate and the inhalation powder preparation containing salmeterol in fixed combination with fluticasone propionate.

Because of the risk of asthma-related death and hospitalization, use of salmeterol for the treatment of asthma without concomitant use of long-term asthma controller therapy, such as inhaled corticosteroids, is contraindicated. (See Asthma-related Death and Life-threatening Events under Cautions: Respiratory Effects and also see Uses: Bronchospasm.) Salmeterol alone or in fixed combination with fluticasone propionate as the inhalation powder (Advair® Diskus®, AirDuo® RespiClick®) is contraindicated in patients with severe hypersensitivity to milk proteins. Salmeterol in fixed combination with fluticasone propionate as the inhalation aerosol (Advair® HFA) is contraindicated in patients with known hypersensitivity to the drugs or any ingredient in the formulation. Patients should inform their clinician of allergies to drugs or food prior to initiation of therapy. Salmeterol alone or in fixed combination with fluticasone propionate is contraindicated in the primary treatment of status asthmaticus or other acute episodes of asthma or COPD where intensive measures are required.

● Pediatric Precautions

Safety and efficacy of salmeterol oral inhalation powder in adolescents 12 years of age or older have been established based on adequate and well-controlled trials conducted in adults and adolescents. However, monotherapy with long-acting β₂-adrenergic agonists, such as salmeterol, increases the risk of asthma-related death. In addition, available data from controlled clinical trials suggest that monotherapy with long-acting β₂-adrenergic agonists increases the risk of asthma-related hospitalization in pediatric and adolescent patients. (See Asthma-related Death and Life-threatening Events under Cautions: Respiratory Effects.) In pediatric and adolescent patients with asthma who require the addition of a long-acting β₂-adrenergic agonist to an inhaled corticosteroid, a fixed-combination preparation containing both an inhaled corticosteroid and a long-acting β₂-adrenergic agonist generally should be used to ensure compliance with both drugs. (See Uses: Bronchospasm.)

Safety and efficacy of salmeterol oral inhalation powder in children 4–11 years of age with asthma have been evaluated for periods not exceeding 1 year, and current data suggest that such children may receive the same dosage as adults for the treatment of asthma or exercise-induced bronchospasm. Pediatric patients should receive salmeterol therapy under adult supervision. Use of salmeterol in fixed combination with fluticasone propionate inhalation powder (Advair® Diskus®) in children 4–11 years of age with asthma is supported by data from one clinical trial and from extrapolation of efficacy data from older patients. Data from a 12-week study in children (4–11 years of age) with persistent asthma who were symptomatic with low dosages of inhaled corticosteroids indicate that the safety profile of salmeterol inhalation powder (50 mcg) in fixed combination with fluticasone propionate (100 mcg) inhalation powder is similar to that of fluticasone propionate monotherapy.

Safety and efficacy of salmeterol in fixed combination with fluticasone propionate inhalation powder (Advair® Diskus®) in children younger than 4 years of age with asthma have not been established. Safety and efficacy of salmeterol in fixed combination with fluticasone propionate inhalation powder (AirDuo® RespiClick®) in children younger than 12 years of age have not been established. Safety and efficacy of salmeterol in fixed combination with fluticasone propionate inhalation aerosol (Advair® HFA) in children younger than 12 years of age have not been established. Data from a limited number of adolescents 12–17 years of age receiving salmeterol and fluticasone propionate inhalation aerosol in fixed combination suggest that safety and efficacy of the fixed combination are similar to those in adults.

● Geriatric Precautions

Data from trials in patients with COPD receiving salmeterol inhalation powder suggested a greater effect on FEV₁ in younger adults compared with geriatric patients. No apparent differences in the type or frequency of adverse effects were noted in geriatric patients with asthma receiving salmeterol alone or in fixed combination with fluticasone inhalation aerosol (Advair® HFA) or in those with COPD receiving salmeterol compared with those in the total population of patients in these studies. No overall differences in safety or efficacy were observed in geriatric patients receiving salmeterol in fixed combination with fluticasone propionate inhalation powder (AirDuo® RespiClick®) compared with younger adults. Clinical studies of salmeterol in fixed combination with fluticasone inhalation powder (Advair® Diskus®) or inhalation aerosol (Advair® HFA) for asthma did not include sufficient numbers of patients 65 years of age or older to determine whether geriatric patients respond differently than younger patients. In clinical studies of salmeterol in fixed combination with fluticasone inhalation powder for COPD, patients 65 years of age or

older experienced a higher incidence of serious adverse effects compared with those younger than 65 years of age, although the distribution of adverse effects was similar in the two groups. The possibility of greater sensitivity of some older patients cannot be ruled out. As with other β₂-agonists, special caution should be observed when using salmeterol alone or in fixed combination with fluticasone in geriatric patients who have concomitant cardiovascular disease that could be adversely affected by this class of drugs. (See Cautions: Precautions and Contraindications.) Adjustment of salmeterol dosage alone or in combination with fluticasone propionate in geriatric patients solely on the basis of age is not necessary.

● Mutagenicity and Carcinogenicity

No evidence of mutagenicity was observed when salmeterol was tested in several in vitro systems, including microbial and mammalian gene mutation tests and in a cytogenic assay of human lymphocytes. In an in vivo rat micronucleus assay, salmeterol did not exhibit evidence of mutagenicity.

Dose-related increases in the incidence of smooth muscle hyperplasia, cystic glandular hyperplasia, uterine leiomyomas, and ovarian cysts occurred in mice given oral salmeterol dosages of at least 1.4 mg/kg (approximately 20 times the maximum recommended daily inhalation dosage for adults and children based on comparisons of the plasma area under the curve [AUC]) in an 18-month carcinogenicity study. In a 24-month study in rats given salmeterol orally and/or by inhalation, mesovarian leiomyomas and ovarian cysts occurred at dosages of at least 0.68 mg/kg (approximately 55 or 25 times the maximum recommended daily inhalation dosage for adults or children respectively, on a mg/m² basis). The findings of these studies in rodents are similar to those reported previously for other β-adrenergic agonist drugs; the relevance of these findings to human use is unknown. No carcinogenic effects were observed in mice given salmeterol in doses of 0.2 mg/kg (approximately 3 times the maximum recommended daily inhalation dosage for adults and children based on AUC comparisons) or in rats given 0.21 mg/kg (approximately 15 or 8 times the maximum recommended daily inhalation dosage for adults or children, respectively, on a mg/m² basis).

● Pregnancy, Fertility, and Lactation
Pregnancy

There are no adequate and well-controlled studies of salmeterol in pregnant women. Because of the potential for β-agonist interference with uterine contractility, use of salmeterol during labor should be restricted to those patients in whom the benefits clearly outweigh the risks. The drug should be used during other stages of pregnancy only if the potential benefit justifies the potential risk to the fetus. Salmeterol in fixed combination with fluticasone propionate inhalation aerosol (Advair® HFA) should be used during pregnancy only if the potential benefit justifies the potential risk to the fetus. In pregnant women with poorly or moderately controlled asthma, there is an increased risk of adverse perinatal events such as preeclampsia in the mother, and prematurity, low birth weight, and small size for gestational age in the neonate. Pregnant women with asthma should be closely monitored and dosage of medications should be adjusted as needed to maintain optimal asthma control.

Reproduction studies in male and female rats using oral salmeterol dosages of up to 2 mg/kg daily (representing 160 times the recommended clinical dosage on a mg/m² basis) have not revealed evidence of harm to the fetus. Dutch rabbit fetuses exposed to oral salmeterol dosages of at least 1 mg/kg (representing 50 times the maximum recommended daily inhalation dosage based on comparison of AUC data) exhibited characteristic effects of β-receptor stimulation, including precocious eyelid openings, cleft palate, sternebral fusion, limb and paw flexures, and delayed ossification of the frontal cranial bones. No teratogenic effects were observed at oral salmeterol doses of 0.6 mg/kg (20 times the maximum recommended daily inhalation dosage based on comparison of AUC data). Delayed ossification of the frontal bones was seen in the fetuses of New Zealand White rabbits given oral salmeterol dosages of 10 mg/kg (representing 1600 times the maximum recommended daily inhalation dosage on a mg/m² basis). Extensive use of other β-agonists has provided no evidence that these class effects in animals are relevant to use in humans.

In reproduction studies in mice and rats, no evidence of an increased toxicity was associated with the use of salmeterol combined with fluticasone propionate when compared with toxicity observed from the components administered separately. Teratogenicity (i.e., cleft palate), fetal death, or increased implantation loss has been observed in mice receiving a subcutaneous dosage of 150 mcg/kg of fluticasone propionate (representing approximately less than the maximum recommended daily inhalation dosage in adults on a mcg/m² basis) combined with a 10 mg/kg oral dosage of salmeterol (representing approximately 410 times the maximum recommended daily inhalation dosage in adults on a mg/m² basis), but these effects did not occur when lower dosages of fluticasone propionate (up to 40 mcg/kg subcutaneously, representing less than the maximum recommended daily inhalation dosage in adults on a mcg/m² basis) were combined with lower dosages of salmeterol (up to 1.4 mg/kg orally, representing approximately 55 times the maximum recommended daily inhalation dosage in adults on a mg/m² basis). Reproduction studies in rats receiving subcutaneous dosages of fluticasone propionate of up to 30 mcg/kg (representing less than the maximum recommended daily inhalation dosage in adults on a mcg/m² basis) combined with dosages of up to 1 mg/kg of salmeterol (approximately 80 times the recommended daily inhalation dosage in adults on a mg/m² basis) did not reveal evidence of teratogenicity. Delayed ossification, changes in the occipital bone, umbilical hernia, decreased placental or fetal weight, and maternal toxicity have been observed in rats receiving subcutaneous dosages of fluticasone propionate 100 mcg/kg (representing less than the maximum recommended daily inhalation dosage in adults on a mcg/m² basis) combined with oral salmeterol dosages of 10 mg/kg (approximately 810 times the maximum recommended daily inhalation dosage in adults on a mg/m² basis).

Fertility

Reproduction studies in rats given oral salmeterol dosages up to 2 mg/kg (approximately 160 times the maximum recommended daily inhalation dosage for adults on a mg/m² basis) have not revealed evidence of impaired fertility.

Lactation

It is not known whether salmeterol xinafoate or fluticasone propionate is distributed into human milk. However, salmeterol is distributed into milk in rats. Corticosteroids, other than fluticasone propionate, are distributed into human milk. Effects of salmeterol xinafoate or fluticasone propionate on breast-fed infants or milk production also are not known. The benefits of breast-feeding and the woman's clinical need for salmeterol xinafoate or fluticasone propionate should be considered along with any potential adverse effects on the breast-fed infant from the drugs or from the underlying maternal condition. Since no data from controlled trials are available on the use of such preparations in nursing women, caution is advised if salmeterol alone or salmeterol in fixed combination with fluticasone propionate is administered in nursing women.

DRUG INTERACTIONS

The following information addresses potential interactions with salmeterol. When salmeterol is used in fixed combination with fluticasone propionate, interactions associated with fluticasone propionate should be considered. No formal drug interaction studies have been performed to date with the fixed-combination preparations containing salmeterol and fluticasone propionate.

● Monoamine Oxidase Inhibitors and Tricyclic Antidepressants

The effects of salmeterol xinafoate on the vascular system may be potentiated in patients receiving concomitant therapy with monoamine oxidase (MAO) inhibitors or tricyclic antidepressants; therefore, salmeterol should be administered with extreme caution to patients being treated with these agents or to patients receiving salmeterol within 2 weeks of discontinuance of these agents.

● Drugs Affecting Hepatic Microsomal Enzymes

Salmeterol and fluticasone propionate are substrates for cytochrome P-450 (CYP) isoenzyme 3A4. The manufacturers state that the use of potent CYP3A4 inhibitors (e.g., atazanavir, clarithromycin, indinavir, itraconazole, ketoconazole, nefazodone, nelfinavir, ritonavir, saquinavir, telithromycin) with salmeterol is not recommended because of the increased potential for systemic adverse effects (e.g., cardiovascular effects such as QT$_c$ prolongation, palpitations, or sinus tachycardia).

● Supplemental Short-Acting β₂-Adrenergic Agonists

In several 3-month clinical trials, adults and adolescents with asthma receiving therapy with salmeterol inhalation powder required an average of approximately 1.5 inhalations daily of a supplemental, short-acting β₂-adrenergic agonist. In patients receiving salmeterol inhalation powder, 26% required 8–24 inhalations daily of a supplemental, short-acting β₂-agonist on at least one occasion. Consistent use of greater than 4 inhalations daily of supplemental, short-acting β₂-agonist therapy was required in 9% of patients receiving orally inhaled salmeterol over the course of these trials. In trials that evaluated salmeterol inhalation powder and as-needed short-acting β₂-agonists, a few patients required an average of 8–11 inhalations of short-acting β₂-agonists daily; no increase in cardiovascular effects were noted. However, the safety of concomitant use of more than 8 inhalations of supplemental, short-acting β₂-agonist therapy daily with salmeterol inhalation therapy has not been established. In a moderate number of patients who experienced a worsening of asthma with salmeterol inhalation powder therapy, administration of albuterol by metered-dose inhaler or nebulizer (one dose in most patients) led to improvement in FEV₁ with no increase in the occurrence of cardiovascular adverse effects.

In two 6-month clinical trials, patients with chronic obstructive pulmonary disease (COPD) receiving therapy with salmeterol inhalation powder alone or in fixed combination with fluticasone propionate required an average of approximately 4 inhalations daily of a supplemental, rapid-acting β₂-adrenergic agonist. In COPD patients receiving salmeterol inhalation powder alone or in fixed combination with fluticasone propionate, 24 or 26%, respectively, required an average of 6 or more inhalations daily of a supplemental, rapid-acting β₂-agonist over the course of these trials; no increase in the frequency of adverse cardiovascular effects was noted.

● Cromolyn Sodium

In clinical studies, inhaled cromolyn sodium did not alter the safety profile of salmeterol oral inhalation when these drugs were administered concurrently.

● Theophyllines

There is some evidence from studies in animals that concomitant administration of sympathomimetic agents (e.g., isoproterenol) and aminophylline may produce increased cardiotoxic effects (e.g., arrhythmias and sudden death, with histologic evidence of myocardial necrosis). Although such an interaction has not been established in humans, a few reports have suggested that such a combination may have the potential for producing cardiac arrhythmias and death. However, in one study in patients receiving theophylline therapy, no evidence of increased cardiotoxic effects was noted when salmeterol aerosol (no longer commercially available) was added to theophylline therapy. In a number of clinical trials in patients with COPD, concurrent therapy with theophylline did not alter the adverse effect profile of salmeterol given alone or in fixed combination with fluticasone propionate.

● β-Adrenergic Blocking Agents

β-Adrenergic blocking agents not only block the pulmonary effects of β-adrenergic agonists (e.g., salmeterol), but also may produce severe bronchospasm in patients with asthma or COPD. Patients with asthma or COPD usually should not be treated with β-adrenergic blocking agents. However, under certain circumstances, there may be no acceptable alternatives to the use of β-adrenergic blocking agents in these patients; the use of cardioselective β-adrenergic blocking agents may be considered but should be used concomitantly with caution.

● Other Drugs

Since salmeterol may decrease serum potassium concentration, care should be taken in patients also receiving other drugs that can lower serum potassium concentration, such as non-potassium-sparing diuretics (loop or thiazide diuretics). ECG changes and/or hypokalemia that may result from the administration of non-potassium-sparing diuretics may be aggravated by concomitant β-agonist therapy, especially when the recommended dosage of the β-agonist is exceeded. Although the clinical importance of these effects is not known, caution is advised when administering salmeterol with non-potassium-sparing diuretics.

ACUTE TOXICITY

● *Pathogenesis*

Rats and dogs survived inhalation doses of 2.9 and 0.7 mg/kg of salmeterol, respectively, representing approximately 240 or 190 times the maximum daily adult inhalation powder dosage, and 110 or 90 times the maximum daily pediatric inhalation powder dosage, respectively, on a mg/m² basis. No deaths occurred in mice and rats given oral salmeterol doses of 150 and 1000 mg/kg, respectively, representing 6100 or 81,000 times the maximum recommended human daily inhalation powder dosage in adults, and 2900 or 38,000 times the maximum recommended daily pediatric inhalation powder dosage, respectively, on a mg/m² basis.

In humans, single orally inhaled doses as high as 400 mcg have been studied and appeared to be relatively safe in short-term use. However, in a dose-response study in healthy men, single orally inhaled 400-mcg doses of salmeterol were associated with tremor, headache, increases in heart rate and blood glucose, and decreases in plasma potassium concentrations. Nonspecific T-wave changes and prolonged QT interval also were observed at this dose; patients receiving lower doses did not display ECG changes.

● *Manifestations*

The expected signs and symptoms associated with overdosage of orally inhaled salmeterol xinafoate are those of excessive β-adrenergic stimulation and/or occurrence or exaggeration of any of the following: tachycardia (with rates up to 200 beats/minute) and/or arrhythmia, nervousness, palpitation, nausea, dizziness, fatigue, malaise, seizures, angina, hypertension or hypotension, insomnia, dry mouth, tremor, headache, hypokalemia, hyperglycemia, and muscle cramps. Large IV doses of albuterol (dosage form currently not commercially available in the US) have been reported to exacerbate preexisting diabetes mellitus and ketoacidosis; the potential for salmeterol to cause such effects has not been determined. Large oral or inhaled doses of salmeterol (12–20 times the recommended dosage) have produced clinically important prolongation of the QT_c interval, which increases the risk for ventricular arrhythmias. Cardiac arrest and fatalities have occurred following excessive use of sympathomimetic pressurized aerosol medications, and may occur with overuse of salmeterol. However, cardiorespiratory arrest has been reported in at least one patient with chronic obstructive pulmonary disease (COPD) and pre-existing alcoholic cardiomyopathy receiving the recommended dosage of inhaled salmeterol in conjunction with usual dosages of ipratropium and albuterol. No cases of overdosage of salmeterol were reported during controlled studies with the orally inhaled drug. The safety of concomitant therapy with salmeterol and more than 8 inhalations per day of a short-acting β₂-agonist has not been established.

● *Treatment*

The manufacturer suggests that in case of salmeterol overdosage, therapy with salmeterol and all other β-adrenergic agonists be discontinued and appropriate symptomatic therapy initiated. The judicious use of a β-adrenergic blocking agent may be considered but only with extreme caution in asthmatic patients because such agents may induce an asthmatic attack. (See Drug Interactions: β-Adrenergic Blocking Agents.) Cardiac monitoring is recommended in cases of overdosage with salmeterol. The manufacturer states that there is insufficient evidence to determine if dialysis is effective for the treatment of salmeterol overdosage.

PHARMACOLOGY

Salmeterol xinafoate has pharmacologic actions similar to those of other selective β₂-adrenergic receptor agonists (e.g., albuterol). Salmeterol stimulates β₂-adrenergic receptors and apparently has little or no effect on α-, β₁-, or β₃-adrenergic receptors. In vitro and in vivo pharmacologic studies indicate that the selectivity of salmeterol for β₂- versus β₁-adrenergic receptors is greater than that of albuterol (e.g., approximately 50–60 times). It is believed that β-adrenergic effects result from stimulation of the production of cyclic adenosine-3′,5′-monophosphate (cAMP) by activation of the enzyme adenyl cyclase. Cyclic AMP appears to mediate numerous cellular responses, and increased concentrations of cAMP are associated with relaxation of bronchial smooth muscle, suppression of some aspects of inflammation, and stimulation of lung ciliary function.

The principal effect following oral inhalation of salmeterol and other β₂-adrenergic agonists is bronchodilation resulting from relaxation of smooth muscles of the bronchial tree. The delayed onset and prolonged duration of action of salmeterol may be the result of its slow cellular uptake and/or membrane translocation to the β₂ receptor, lipophilicity, and protracted binding at the β₂ receptor. Some evidence suggests that salmeterol binds reversibly to an active site on the β₂ receptor and irreversibly to an exosite, which may be a domain adjacent to the active site within the β₂ receptor in the lipid bilayer of the cell membrane. The persistence of salmeterol at the β₂ receptor is thought to be related to the binding of the oxyalkyl side chain of salmeterol to the exosite while the saligenin end of the molecule is free to dissociate from the active receptor site in the presence of β-adrenergic blocking agents. It has been suggested that the slow waning of the bronchodilatory effect of salmeterol is related to slow dissociation from the receptor or to turnover of the occupied β₂-adrenergic receptor protein.

● *Respiratory Effects*

Salmeterol relaxes bronchial smooth muscle by stimulating β₂-adrenergic receptors when administered by oral inhalation. In isolated bronchial smooth muscle tissue in which muscle tone was increased by a spasmogen (e.g., methacholine, prostaglandin F₂ α) or by electrical stimulation, salmeterol generally was more potent than albuterol and at least as potent as isoproterenol in relaxing smooth muscle. In patients with reversible airway obstruction, salmeterol decreases airway resistance (as measured by forced expiratory volume in 1 second [FEV₁], peak expiratory flow rate [PEFR], and vital capacity) and airway reactivity to histamine. Residual elevation of morning PEFR has been maintained for up to at least 1–6 days following completion of salmeterol therapy. In addition to bronchodilator activity, salmeterol and other inhaled β₂-agonists may affect clearance of pulmonary secretions by increasing the ciliary activity of airway epithelial cells.

Salmeterol inhibits the release of proinflammatory mediators associated with early-phase inflammatory response to allergen challenge (e.g., histamine, leukotrienes C₄ and D₄, prostaglandin D₂) in human lung tissue and may thereby attenuate early- and late-phase-associated bronchoconstriction. Salmeterol also attenuates late-phase-associated vascular permeability, and inflammatory cell activation, migration, and recruitment. However, the extent of salmeterol's anti-inflammatory activity is not well characterized, and the lack of a consistent effect of the drug on inflammatory processes suggests that anti-inflammatory effects are of secondary or negligible importance in producing the clinical improvement noted in patients with asthma receiving the drug. Studies in animals and humans indicate that orally inhaled salmeterol inhibits extravasation of plasma proteins, neutrophils, and eosinophils associated with late-phase response to challenge with histamine, leukotriene B₄, antigen, endotoxin, granulocyte-macrophage colony-stimulating factor (GM-CSF), and platelet-activating factor. Some evidence indicates that salmeterol is as potent as isoproterenol and more potent than albuterol in inhibiting the release of these mediators and has a longer duration of anti-inflammatory action, including late-phase response to allergen challenge than either of these drugs. In addition, these anti-inflammatory effects have been reversed by pretreatment with β-adrenergic blocking agents (e.g., propranolol), suggesting that such effects may be mediated by β-adrenergic receptors. As inflammatory changes occur during periods of increased bronchial hyperresponsiveness, the degree of response to bronchoconstrictor stimuli has been used as an indirect measure of inflammation. In a few single-dose, placebo-controlled or comparative studies with albuterol, salmeterol decreased the degree of airway responsiveness to bronchoconstrictor stimuli (e.g., allergens, cold air). Whether these bronchoprotective effects of salmeterol are associated with sustained bronchodilation or anti-inflammatory effects has not been fully determined. The lack of activity of other β-adrenergic agonists on the late-phase response to allergen challenge may be related to their short duration of action.

Current evidence and experience indicate that prolonged therapy with salmeterol does not appear to be associated with development of tolerance to the bronchodilatory effects of the drug. However, conflicting data exist with regard to the development of tolerance to the drug's protective effects against bronchoconstrictor stimuli, and further study is needed to clarify the potential for development of tolerance to these effects of salmeterol.

● *Cardiovascular Effects*

Salmeterol, like other β₂-adrenergic agonists, can produce changes in heart rate and blood pressure. In several studies in asthmatic patients or healthy individuals receiving escalating doses of inhaled salmeterol (up to 84 mcg) or usual doses of inhaled albuterol (180 mcg), dose-related increases in heart rate of 3–16 beats/minute were noted with salmeterol but did not exceed those observed with albuterol therapy. The increase in heart rate observed in patients with asthma with salmeterol or albuterol therapy probably results either indirectly from peripheral vasodilation or directly from a chronotropic effect via β₂-receptors in the heart. In patients with chronic obstructive pulmonary disease (COPD) receiving orally inhaled salmeterol (50 mcg/dose) inhalation powder alone or in combination with fluticasone propionate, pulse rate or systolic or diastolic blood pressure was not affected.

In several studies in patients with asthma in which continuous electrocardiographic monitoring during 12- or 24-hour periods was performed during therapy with orally inhaled salmeterol (42 or 50 mcg twice daily) or albuterol (180 mcg 4 times daily), no clinically important dysrhythmias were noted. In several studies (24 weeks' duration) in patients with COPD in whom electrocardiographic monitoring was performed at weeks 12 and 24 of therapy with orally inhaled salmeterol inhalation powder (50 mcg twice daily) or placebo, the incidence of clinically important dysrhythmias was similar. In a clinical trial in patients with COPD who were receiving salmeterol inhalation powder, fluticasone inhalation powder, salmeterol in fixed combination with fluticasone propionate, or placebo, continuous ECG monitoring for 24 hours (prior to the first dose and after 4 weeks of therapy) did not reveal appreciable differences in ventricular or supraventricular arrhythmias or heart rate. The incidence of ventricular premature complexes with salmeterol, albuterol, or placebo in clinical studies generally has been similar. However at higher dosages, both salmeterol and albuterol administration have been associated with prolongation of the QT꜀ interval. Tolerance to the effects of salmeterol on the QT꜀ interval has been reported in healthy individuals receiving high dosages of the drug.

● *Metabolic Effects*

Administration of salmeterol and other β-adrenergic agonists may cause dose-related increases in blood glucose and/or decreases in serum potassium concentrations. (See Cautions: Metabolic and Electrolyte Effects.) Increases in blood glucose concentration may be caused by stimulation of glycogenolysis or gluconeogenesis through activation of β₂-receptors in skeletal muscle and liver; tolerance to this effect may occur with regular salmeterol treatment. Reductions in serum potassium concentration that occur during therapy with salmeterol and other β-adrenergic agonists may be related to β-adrenergic stimulation of cell membrane Na⁺- K⁺-ATPase, with increased intracellular shunting of potassium from blood into liver, skeletal muscle, and myocardium. Limited data in healthy individuals suggest that tolerance to the hypokalemic effects of high-dose salmeterol does not occur.

● *Other Effects*

Like other sympathomimetic amines, salmeterol may cause CNS stimulation and adverse nervous system effects. (See Cautions: Nervous System Effects.)

PHARMACOKINETICS

Limited data are available on the pharmacokinetics of salmeterol xinafoate after oral inhalation. Salmeterol xinafoate dissociates in solution to salmeterol and xinafoate moieties that are absorbed, distributed, metabolized, and excreted independently. The xinafoate moiety has no intrinsic pharmacologic activity. While commercially available salmeterol is administered as salmeterol xinafoate, dosages and drug concentrations are expressed in terms of salmeterol.

● *Absorption*

The absorption of salmeterol xinafoate from the respiratory tract following oral inhalation has not been fully characterized. Although it has been suggested that most of an orally inhaled drug actually is swallowed, the bronchodilating action of orally inhaled sympathomimetic agents is believed to result from a local action of the portion of the dose that reaches the bronchial tree. Systemic concentrations of salmeterol are low or undetectable after inhalation of the recommended dosage of the powder (50 mcg) twice daily and are not predictive of therapeutic effects. Delayed absorption was noted following oral administration of 1 mg of radiolabeled salmeterol (as salmeterol xinafoate) in a few healthy individuals; peak plasma salmeterol concentrations of about 600–650 pg/mL occurred at 45–75 minutes. Following repeated, twice-daily administration of 50 mcg of

salmeterol as the oral inhalation powder in patients with asthma, salmeterol was detected in the plasma within 5–45 minutes; mean peak plasma concentrations of the drug were 167 pg/mL, and no accumulation was noted with repeated dosing.

Compared with short-acting β-agonists such as albuterol or isoproterenol, the onset and duration of bronchodilation with orally inhaled salmeterol are longer. Following administration of a single dose (50 mcg) of salmeterol oral inhalation powder in patients with asthma, most patients experienced clinically important improvement (as measured by a 15% improvement in FEV₁) within 1 hour. Maximum improvement in FEV₁ generally occurred within 3 hours, and clinically important improvement was maintained for 12 hours in most patients. Following administration of a single dose (50 mcg) of salmeterol oral inhalation powder in patients with chronic obstructive pulmonary disease (COPD), improvement in lung function (as measured by a 12% improvement in FEV₁ and at least 200 mL) occurred in 2 hours. Mean time to maximum improvement in FEV₁ occurred at 4.75 hours, and improvement was maintained for 12 hours. In the prevention of exercised-induced bronchospasm, salmeterol oral inhalation powder provided protection for up to about 9 hours in adolescents and adults and up to about 12 hours in children 4 to 11 years of age following a single 50- mcg dose 30 minutes prior to exercise.

● *Distribution*

Binding of salmeterol averages 96% in vitro to human plasma proteins over the concentration range of 8 ng/mL to 7.7 mcg/mL, which are concentrations greatly exceeding those achieved following usual doses of the drug. Salmeterol is bound to albumin and α₁-acid glycoprotein; the xinafoate moiety also is highly protein bound (exceeding 99%) to albumin.

The distribution of salmeterol into various human organs and tissues following oral inhalation has not been fully characterized. Results of studies in rats indicate that salmeterol crosses the blood-brain barrier in trace amounts.

It is not known if salmeterol and/or its metabolites cross the placenta in humans. Salmeterol crossed the placenta following oral administration in mice and rats. It also is not known if salmeterol is distributed into milk in humans; however the drug is distributed into milk in rats.

● *Elimination*

Salmeterol is extensively metabolized in the liver by hydroxylation and is eliminated predominantly in feces. In a few healthy individuals who received radio-labeled salmeterol 1 mg orally, approximately 25 and 60% of the dose were eliminated in urine and feces, respectively, 1–7 days after administration. Negligible amounts of unchanged salmeterol are detectable in urine or feces. A minor metabolite is formed by *o*-dealkylation of the phenylalkyl side chain. Following oral administration of salmeterol in healthy individuals, the terminal elimination half-lives of salmeterol and the xinafoate moiety are about 5.5 hours and 11–15 days, respectively.

CHEMISTRY AND STABILITY

● *Chemistry*

Salmeterol xinafoate is a long-acting, synthetic, sympathomimetic amine. The drug is structurally and pharmacologically similar to the short-acting β₂-adrenergic agonist albuterol. The pharmacologically active moiety of salmeterol contains a saligenin nucleus identical to that in albuterol. This polar nucleus reversibly attaches to the classic β₂-receptor binding site. Salmeterol differs structurally from albuterol in part by the presence of a long, *N*-substituted, phenylalkyl side chain. This substitution contributes to increased lipophilicity; greater bronchial tissue penetration; increased resistance to metabolism by catechol-*o*-methyltransferase (COMT); prolonged and selective binding to a second, nonpolar domain (exosite) on the β₂-receptor; and decreased clearance from the airways. The ether oxygen on the *N*-substituent facilitates binding of the substituent to the exosite portion of the β₂-adrenergic receptor protein.

Salmeterol is commercially available as the xinafoate salt, the racemic form of the 1-hydroxy-2-naphthoic acid salt of salmeterol. Both the *R*- and *S*- enantiomers of salmeterol are long acting. Available data suggest that the *S*-enantiomer of salmeterol does not antagonize the effects of the *R*-enantiomer and does not have pharmacologic effects that are different from those of the racemic mixture.

Salmeterol xinafoate occurs as an off-white powder and has solubilities of approximately 40 mg/mL in methanol, 7 mg/mL in ethanol, 3 mg/mL in chloroform, 2–3 mg/mL in isopropanol, and 0.07–0.11 mg/mL in water.

Salmeterol xinafoate powder for oral inhalation is a powdered mixture of drug and lactose and is contained in a foil blister strip for use in a special oral inhaler device (Serevent® Diskus®). Salmeterol xinafoate also is commercially available in fixed combination with fluticasone propionate as a powder for oral inhalation (Advair® Diskus® or AirDuo® RespiClick®). With commercially available salmeterol inhalation powder delivered via the Serevent® Diskus®, Advair® Diskus®, or AirDuo® RespiClick® device, the amount of drug delivered to the lungs depends on factors such as the patient's inspiratory flow. Using standardized in vitro testing at a flow rate of 60 L per minute for 2 seconds, the Serevent® Diskus® device delivered 47 mcg of salmeterol per activation. Under similar conditions, the Advair® Diskus® device delivered 93, 233, and 465 mcg of fluticasone propionate and 45 mcg of salmeterol per activation from a Diskus® labeled as containing 100, 250, or 500 mcg of fluticasone propionate and 50 mcg of salmeterol. In adult patients with obstructive lung disease and severely compromised lung function (FEV_1 of 0.65 L or 20–30% of the predicted value), mean peak inspiratory flow through the Diskus® device was 82.4 L per minute for Serevent® and 82.4 L per minute for Advair®. In adults and adolescents with asthma, mean peak inspiratory flow through the Diskus® device was 122.2 L per minute. In a group of children 4 years of age, mean peak inspiratory flow through the Diskus® device averaged 75.5 L per minute; in children 8 years of age, mean peak inspiratory flow averaged 107.3 L per minute. Based on in vitro modeling of these flow rates, a dose of approximately 46 mcg of salmeterol is emitted per activation of the Diskus® device. Results of standardized in vitro testing at a flow rate of 85 L per minute for 1.4 seconds indicated that the AirDuo® RespiClick® device delivered 49, 100, or 202 mcg of fluticasone propionate and 12.75 mcg of salmeterol per actuation from an oral inhaler labeled as containing 55, 113, or 232 mcg of fluticasone propionate and 14 mcg of salmeterol. In adult and adolescent patients with asthma, mean peak inspiratory flow through the RespiClick® device was 108.3 and 106.7 L per minute, respectively.

● **Stability**

The commercially available inhalation powder containing salmeterol xinafoate alone (Serevent®) or in fixed combination with fluticasone propionate (Advair® Diskus®) should be stored at room temperature (20–25°C) in a dry place away from direct heat and sunlight. The Serevent® Diskus® inhaler should be discarded 6 weeks after removal from the foil pouch or when every blister has been used (when the dose counter reads "0"), whichever comes first. The Advair® Diskus® inhaler should be discarded 1 month after removal from the foil pouch or when every blister has been used, whichever comes first.

The commercially available inhalation powder containing salmeterol in fixed combination with fluticasone propionate (AirDuo® RespiClick®) should be stored at 15–25°C in a dry place away from extreme heat, cold, and humidity. The inhaler should be discarded 30 days after opening the foil pouch or when the dose counter reads "0," whichever comes first.

The commercially available inhalation aerosol of salmeterol in fixed combination with fluticasone propionate (Advair® HFA) should be stored (with the mouthpiece down) at 20–25°C but may be exposed to temperatures ranging from 15–30°C. Because the contents of the aerosol oral inhaler are under pressure, the aerosol container should *not* be punctured, used or stored near heat or an open flame, or placed into a fire or an incinerator for disposal. Exposure of the canister to temperatures exceeding 49°C may cause the canister to burst. The inhaler should be discarded when the dose counter reads "0."

Salmeterol xinafoate oral inhalation powder (Serevent® Diskus®) is stable for 18 months from the date of manufacture.

PREPARATIONS

Excipients in commercially available drug preparations may have clinically important effects in some individuals; consult specific product labeling for details.

Salmeterol Xinafoate

Oral-inhalation

| Powder | 50 mcg (of salmeterol) per inhalation | Serevent® Diskus®, GlaxoSmithKline |

Salmeterol Xinafoate Combinations

Oral-inhalation

Aerosol	21 mcg (of salmeterol) with Fluticasone Propionate 45 mcg per metered spray (from the actuator)	Advair® HFA (with hydrofluoroalkane propellant), GlaxoSmithKline
	21 mcg (of salmeterol) with Fluticasone Propionate 115 mcg per metered spray (from the actuator)	Advair® HFA (with hydrofluoroalkane propellant), GlaxoSmithKline
	21 mcg (of salmeterol) with Fluticasone Propionate 230 mcg per metered spray (from the actuator)	Advair® HFA (with hydrofluoroalkane propellant), GlaxoSmithKline
Powder	14 mcg (of salmeterol) with Fluticasone Propionate 55 mcg per inhalation	AirDuo® RespiClick®, Teva
	14 mcg (of salmeterol) with Fluticasone Propionate 113 mcg per inhalation	AirDuo® RespiClick®, Teva
	14 mcg (of salmeterol) with Fluticasone Propionate 232 mcg per inhalation	AirDuo® RespiClick®, Teva
	50 mcg (of salmeterol) with Fluticasone Propionate 100 mcg per inhalation	Advair® Diskus®, GlaxoSmithKline
	50 mcg (of salmeterol) with Fluticasone Propionate 250 mcg per inhalation	Advair® Diskus®, GlaxoSmithKline
	50 mcg (of salmeterol) with Fluticasone Propionate 500 mcg per inhalation	Advair® Diskus®, GlaxoSmithKline

† Use is not currently included in the labeling approved by the US Food and Drug Administration.

Ephedrine Hydrochloride, Ephedrine Sulfate

12:12.12 • α- AND β-ADRENERGIC AGONISTS

■ Ephedrine is a sympathomimetic agent that occurs naturally in plants of the genus *Ephedra*; ephedrine stimulates both α- and β-adrenergic receptors.

USES

● Hypotension During Anesthesia

Ephedrine is used parenterally as a vasopressor for the treatment of hypotension during anesthesia. Ephedrine sulfate injection is labeled by the US Food and Drug Administration (FDA) for the treatment of clinically important hypotension occurring in the setting of anesthesia. Because ephedrine sulfate injection was introduced into the US market before 1962 without an approved new drug application (NDA), some commercially available preparations may not be approved by the FDA.

Evidence supporting the efficacy of ephedrine for this indication is based principally on data from the published literature demonstrating that the drug increases systolic and mean arterial blood pressures when administered as a direct IV ("bolus") injection following the development of hypotension in patients undergoing neuraxial (spinal/epidural) and/or general anesthesia. In these studies, ephedrine was administered as either the sulfate or hydrochloride salt forms of the drug; however, only ephedrine sulfate is commercially available in the US as a parenteral preparation. Although IM use of ephedrine also has been evaluated in this setting, results of studies using IM ephedrine have been equivocal. The majority of patients who received ephedrine for the treatment of hypotension in these clinical studies were pregnant women undergoing cesarean section with neuraxial anesthesia. Although ephedrine historically has been considered the vasopressor of choice for the treatment of hypotension in obstetric anesthesia, there is some evidence suggesting that phenylephrine may provide a more favorable fetal acid-base balance. Experts currently recommend the use of either IV ephedrine or phenylephrine for the treatment of hypotension during neuraxial anesthesia; however, consideration should be given to selection of phenylephrine in the absence of maternal bradycardia because of improved fetal acid-base status in uncomplicated pregnancies.

Ephedrine also has been used with limited success for the prevention of hypotension† in patients undergoing spinal anesthesia; however, routine prophylactic use of vasopressors has been questioned because hypotension does not always occur during spinal anesthesia and treatment can readily be instituted if necessary. In addition, IV ephedrine has been associated with an increased incidence of hypertension when given prophylactically.

● Bronchospasm

Asthma

Ephedrine is used orally as a bronchodilator for the symptomatic treatment of asthma. Preparations containing ephedrine hydrochloride or ephedrine sulfate in fixed-combination with guaifenesin are used as *self-medication* for the temporary relief of mild symptoms of intermittent asthma (e.g., wheezing, chest tightness, shortness of breath). Once a diagnosis of asthma has been confirmed by a clinician, use of a nonprescription (over-the-counter, OTC) bronchodilator may be appropriate in patients with mild symptoms of intermittent asthma; because asthma may be life-threatening, those with more severe asthma (i.e., persistent asthma) or worsening asthma (symptoms not relieved within 60 minutes or with maximum recommended dosages of ephedrine, increasing frequency of asthma attacks) should consult a clinician for other treatment options. A single-ingredient oral ephedrine sulfate preparation no longer is commercially available in the US. Ephedrine sulfate also has been used parenterally for the treatment of bronchial asthma; however, currently available parenteral preparations of the drug are not FDA-labeled for this use.

While oral ephedrine was once widely used for its bronchodilating effects in the management of reversible airway obstruction, the drug generally has been replaced by more selective and rapid-acting agents (e.g., inhaled β₂-adrenergic agonists); ephedrine is not recommended as a drug of choice for the rapid relief of asthma in current asthma management guidelines. In the stepped-care approach to antiasthmatic therapy, most experts currently recommend use of a selective, short-acting inhaled β₂-adrenergic agonist (e.g., albuterol, levalbuterol, pirbuterol) on an intermittent, as-needed basis in all patients with asthma to control acute symptoms (e.g., cough, wheezing, dyspnea). Alternatives to short-acting inhaled β₂-agonists recommended by some clinicians for relief of acute asthma symptoms include an inhaled anticholinergic agent (e.g., ipratropium), a short-acting oral β₂-agonist, or a short-acting theophylline (provided extended-release theophylline is not already used), but these alternatives have a slower onset of action and/or a greater risk of adverse effects.

Expectorants such as guaifenesin are used in combination with ephedrine to help loosen and thin bronchial secretions and facilitate the removal of mucous from bronchial passageways. However, use of expectorants in the management of asthma has been questioned by the FDA because of insufficient evidence supporting their use and inconsistency of such treatment with the pathogenesis of the disease. Increased sputum production is not a common feature of asthma; thus, patients with mild asthma (the population for whom self-medication with OTC drugs may be appropriate) generally do not require expectorant therapy. Furthermore, expectorants are not recommended in current asthma management guidelines. Based on these factors, FDA currently believes that there is no role for expectorants in the routine pharmacologic management of asthma and no longer considers the combination of an oral bronchodilator (i.e., ephedrine) and an expectorant (i.e., guaifenesin) rational therapy for patients with mild asthma.

Ephedrine also has been administered concomitantly with theophylline in the treatment of asthma; however, the combination of ephedrine and theophylline was shown in a study in asthmatic children to be no more effective than theophylline alone and was associated with an increased incidence of adverse effects.

● Nasal Congestion

Ephedrine has been administered orally as a nasal decongestant, but is of doubtful value when used for this condition. Extensive clinical experience indicates that ephedrine produces nasal decongestion when solutions of 0.5–3% (nasal solution no longer commercially available in the US) are applied topically to the nasal mucosa; however, controlled clinical studies supporting its effectiveness are lacking. Rebound congestion and tachyphylaxis may occur within a few days when ephedrine is used topically as a nasal decongestant.

As part of its ongoing review of OTC drug products, FDA has determined that any cough and cold preparation containing an oral bronchodilator active ingredient (e.g., ephedrine, ephedrine hydrochloride, ephedrine sulfate, racephedrine hydrochloride, or any other ephedrine salt) in combination with any analgesic, analgesic/antipyretic, anticholinergic, antihistamine, oral antitussive, or stimulant (e.g., caffeine) active ingredient generally is *not* recognized as safe and effective for *self-medication*. Such a combination is considered by the FDA to be a new drug and misbranded, and cannot be marketed for OTC cough and cold use unless it is the subject of an approved new drug application.

● Obesity

Because of its anorexigenic effects, ephedrine alone or combined with caffeine has been used for *self-medication* in the management of exogenous obesity†. (See Issues and Regulations Associated with Misuse and Abuse of Ephedrine-containing Preparations under Uses: Misuse and Abuse.)

Efficacy and safety of ephedrine and dietary supplements containing ephedra (a plant that contains several ephedrine alkaloids) have been assessed in numerous controlled studies involving several hundred individuals receiving the preparations for exogenous obesity†. Retrospective analysis of pooled data from these studies indicates that short-term (8 weeks up to 4 months) use of ephedrine (high doses), ephedrine combined with caffeine, or dietary supplements containing ephedra with or without herbs containing caffeine was associated with statistically significant, albeit modest, short-term weight loss when compared with placebo. The addition of caffeine to ephedrine moderately increases short-term weight loss. There is no evidence that the effect on short-term (up to 4–6 months) weight loss of dietary supplements containing ephedra combined with caffeine differs from that of ephedrine combined with caffeine; use of both drug combinations was associated with increased weight loss (about 0.9 kg more per month) compared with placebo. Safety and efficacy of *long-term* (i.e., more than 6 months) use of ephedrine for management of obesity have not been established. Because substantial weight loss (5–10% of baseline body weight) *and* long-term weight maintenance are necessary to improve health outcomes and reduce the risk of morbidities associated with obesity, the benefit of short-term weight loss associated with ephedrine or ephedra on health outcomes currently is not known. (See Issues and Regulations Associated with Misuse and Abuse of Ephedrine-containing Preparations under Uses: Misuse and Abuse.)

● **Other Uses**

Ephedrine has reportedly been used orally with good results for the management of peripheral edema secondary to diabetic neuropathy† in a few patients with type 1 diabetes mellitus.

Ephedrine has been used in patients with myasthenia gravis†. Limited data suggest that the drug may improve muscle weakness, fatigue, and quality of life in some patients with myasthenic conditions; however, randomized controlled studies are needed to further evaluate these potential benefits.

Ephedrine also has been used as a CNS stimulant in the treatment of narcolepsy† or depressive states†; however, the cardiovascular effects of the drug limit its usefulness in these conditions, and it has been largely replaced by other CNS stimulants.

Ephedrine sulfate also has been used in the treatment of Stokes-Adams disease†; when used for this condition, ephedrine provides a similar benefit to that of epinephrine.

● **Misuse and Abuse**

Enhancement of Athletic Performance

Because of its stimulant effects, ephedrine has been misused and abused by athletes, bodybuilders, weight lifters, and others, including high school- and college-aged individuals engaged in sports. Evidence from several surveys indicates that about 4% of student athletes and 13–25% of individuals attending a gymnasium use ephedrine. (See Issues and Regulations Associated with Misuse and Abuse of Ephedrine-containing Preparations under Uses: Misuse and Abuse.)

Studies evaluating the safety and efficacy of dietary supplements containing ephedra for enhancement of athletic performance† are lacking. In addition, the few studies evaluating safety and efficacy of ephedrine for this use generally have included only a limited number of fit individuals (i.e., young male military recruits) and have assessed effects of ephedrine only for very short-term use (for immediate performance) rather than for long-term, repeated use as seen in the general population. These data support a modest effect of ephedrine used in combination with caffeine on very short-term athletic performance. Limited data also indicate that addition of caffeine to ephedrine is necessary for the modest enhancement of athletic performance. However, the effect of sustained use of ephedrine on improvement of athletic performance has not been assessed. Therefore, safety and efficacy of dietary supplements containing ephedrine or ephedra, as they have been used in the general population to promote enhancement of athletic performance, have not been established. (See Issues and Regulations Associated with Misuse and Abuse of Ephedrine-containing Preparations under Uses: Misuse and Abuse.)

CNS Stimulation

Over-the-counter ephedrine has been abused by some users including adolescents and young adults for its CNS stimulating action. (See Issues and Regulations Associated with Misuse and Abuse of Ephedrine-containing Preparations under Uses: Misuse and Abuse.) Ephedrine (as the primary precursor) also has been used in the clandestine synthesis of methamphetamine (see Chronic Toxicity in the Amphetamines General Statement 28:20.04) and methcathinone (both potent CNS stimulants with great potential for habituation and physical and/or psychic dependence). Abuse of ephedrine has produced psychic dependence (characterized by compulsion, obsession, and preoccupation) and worsened mental disorders (e.g., depressive anxiety, thought disorders). Acute overdosage of the drug has been associated with tachycardia, difficulty in breathing, and death. (See Acute Toxicity.)

Issues and Regulations Associated with Misuse and Abuse of Ephedrine-containing Preparations

Because use of dietary supplements that contain ephedrine or ephedra, alone or in combination with caffeine, may be associated with substantial adverse health

effects and toxicity (see Dietary Supplements under Cautions: Adverse Effects), FDA issued a final regulation in February 2004 prohibiting the manufacturing, distribution, and sale of all dietary supplements containing ephedrine alkaloids after April 12, 2004. (See Regulations Governing Dietary Supplements under Adverse Effects: Dietary Supplements, in Cautions.) In April 2005, a federal judge in a Utah district court overturned part of the FDA ruling, declaring the agency could not ban the sale of dietary supplements containing ephedrine dosages of 10 mg or less without proving that such low dosages are unsafe; this ruling partially lifted FDA's ban, allowing products with 10 mg or less of active ingredient to return to the US market. However, in August 2006, a 3-judge panel of the US Court of Appeals for the 10th Circuit in Denver reversed the lower Utah district court decision and upheld FDA's final rule declaring all dietary supplements containing ephedrine alkaloids adulterated. FDA then reiterated its position that no dosage of dietary supplements containing ephedrine alkaloids is considered safe, and the sale of these products in the US is illegal and subject to FDA enforcement action.

Transactions (e.g., distribution, receipt, sale, use, importation, exportation) involving ephedrine-containing *drug* products also have been restricted under the Chemical Diversion and Trafficking Act of 1988, the Domestic Chemical Diversion Control Act of 1993, and the Comprehensive Methamphetamine Control Act of 1996 (MCA [US Public Law 104-237]). Under MCA, effective October 1997, 24 g of ephedrine (in terms of the base) was the limit for a single transaction for drug products containing ephedrine in combination with other drugs (regardless of the form in which these drugs are packaged) that could be sold by retail distributors (e.g., grocery stores, general merchandise stores, drug stores). As of October 1997, mail-order distribution of ephedrine-containing drug products must be reported monthly to the US Attorney General according to applicable regulations. In addition, under regulations finalized by the Drug Enforcement Administration (DEA), effective April 2002, nonprescription preparations containing ephedrine had to be stored behind the counter in retail settings that were open to the public to ensure that only employees have access to these products so that their availability to the general public could be more closely controlled.

Despite the enactment of MCA and other stringent laws, methamphetamine abuse remains a serious problem. In March 2006, the Combat Methamphetamine Epidemic Act (CMEA) of 2005 (Title VII of the USA Patriot Act Improvement and Reauthorization Act of 2005) was signed into law, which effectively amends the Federal Controlled Substances Act of 1970 to tighten control over the sale and distribution of nonprescription ephedrine and pseudoephedrine. This law creates a new class of products called "scheduled listed chemical products," which are defined in the law as products containing ephedrine, pseudoephedrine, or phenylpropanolamine (no longer commercially available in the US) or any salt, optical isomer, or salt of an optical isomer of these drugs that are lawful nonprescription products in the US, and sets additional requirements for their sale. Effective September 30, 2006, the law requires pharmacies and other retail distributors to store ephedrine- and pseudoephedrine-containing preparations behind the counter or in locked cabinets; requires purchasers to provide approved photographic identification and sign a written or electronic logbook for each purchase; requires pharmacies and other retail distributors to keep information about the purchasers (e.g., name, address, signature) and purchases (e.g., name of product, quantity sold, date and time of sale) for at least 2 years; and limits the amount of ephedrine that can be purchased to no more than 3.6 g per day or 9 g per month. The law exempts requirements of a written or electronic logbook for any purchase of single-dose packages that contain no more than 60 mg of pseudoephedrine; however, these single-dose packages also must be stored behind the counter. To comply with CMEA, pharmacies and other retail distributors selling preparations containing ephedrine are required to submit to the Attorney General a statement regarding self-certification and employee training on the requirements of this new law and to maintain records relating to such training at their place of operation. Additional information about legal and regulatory requirements under CMEA may be obtained at the website of the Office of Diversion Control of the US Drug Enforcement Administration (DEA) (http://www.deadiversion.usdoj.gov/), including specific requirements for various sellers (e.g., pharmacies, mail-order sellers) and employee training materials developed by DEA. (See Uses: Misuse and Abuse, in Pseudoephedrine 12:12.12.)

Use of ephedrine in some states may be subject to additional controls, since some states had restricted the prescription, dispensing, and distribution of ephedrine (e.g., as a controlled substance or a prescription drug) prior to passage of the federal law. For example, in the state of Oregon, legislation was enacted in August

2005 that required the Oregon State Board of Pharmacy to classify ephedrine, pseudoephedrine, and phenylpropanolamine as schedule III drugs by July 2006, which effectively moved these drugs from the nonprescription to the prescription-only category in that state. Where such state laws are more stringent than the provisions of CMEA, the state requirements also must be followed.

DOSAGE AND ADMINISTRATION

• Administration

Oral Administration

Ephedrine (as the hydrochloride or sulfate salt) is administered orally as fixed-combination preparations containing guaifenesin.

Parenteral Administration

Ephedrine sulfate is administered by IV injection. The drug also has been administered by IM† or subcutaneous† injection.

Ephedrine sulfate injection (Akovaz®) is administered by direct IV ("bolus") injection. Prior to IV administration, the commercially available solution for injection must be diluted. The manufacturer recommends that a 5-mg/mL solution be prepared by diluting 1 mL of the 50-mg/mL injection concentrate with 9 mL of 0.9% sodium chloride injection or 5% dextrose injection. Vials of the drug are for single-use only; unused portions should be discarded.

Ephedrine sulfate injection should be inspected visually for particulate matter and discoloration prior to administration whenever solution and container permit.

• Dosage

Ephedrine is commercially available as ephedrine hydrochloride or ephedrine sulfate; dosage is expressed in terms of the salt.

Oral Dosage

When ephedrine hydrochloride or ephedrine sulfate is administered orally for *self-medication* as a bronchodilator (in fixed combination with guaifenesin) in adults and children 12 years of age and older, the usual oral dosage is 12.5–25 mg every 4 hours as needed, not to exceed 150 mg in 24 hours. Ephedrine should be used in children younger than 12 years of age only under the direction of a clinician.

Parenteral Dosage

When used as a pressor agent, ephedrine should be administered in the lowest effective dosage for the shortest possible time. The recommended initial adult dose of ephedrine sulfate for the treatment of clinically important hypotension during anesthesia is 5–10 mg by IV bolus injection; additional bolus doses should be administered as needed (up to a total dose of 50 mg) to achieve the desired blood pressure response. Other parenteral dosage regimens have been recommended in adults, including a dose of 5–25 mg by slow IV injection (repeated in 5–10 minutes if necessary) and an IM† or subcutaneous† dose of 25–50 mg.

In children†, parenteral ephedrine sulfate doses of 0.5 mg/kg or 16.7 mg/m² have been administered every 4–6 hours by subcutaneous† or IM† injection; however, safety and efficacy of ephedrine sulfate injection have not been established in pediatric patients.

When used parenterally to relieve severe, acute bronchospasm, ephedrine sulfate doses of 12.5–25 mg usually have been given in adults.

CAUTIONS

• Adverse Effects

The CNS-stimulating effects of ephedrine may result in nervousness, anxiety, restlessness, or insomnia, especially with large doses. Vertigo also may occur. Prolonged abuse of ephedrine may cause symptoms of paranoid schizophrenia. Ephedrine also may cause headache, sweating, mild epigastric distress, anorexia, nausea, or vomiting.

Ephedrine increases the work of the heart and probably myocardial oxygen consumption. In patients with coronary insufficiency and/or ischemic heart disease, the drug can induce anginal pain. Ephedrine increases the irritability of the heart muscle and may alter the rhythmic function of the ventricles. Palpitation and tachycardia may result. Extrasystoles and potentially fatal arrhythmias including ventricular fibrillation may occur, especially in patients with organic heart disease or those receiving other drugs that sensitize the heart to arrhythmias including cardiac glycosides, cyclopropane, or halogenated hydrocarbon anesthetics. (See Drug Interactions.) Precordial pain also may occur following administration of ephedrine sulfate injection.

Acute urinary retention may occur in men with prostatism; increased vesicular sphincter tone may cause difficult and painful urination. Some patients may require catheterization.

Ephedrine may cause tachyphylaxis with repeated administration. Although tolerance to ephedrine may develop with prolonged or excessive usage, addiction to the drug does not occur. Temporary cessation of ephedrine and subsequent reinitiation of therapy restores the drug's effectiveness.

Dietary Supplements

Ephedrine alkaloid-containing dietary supplements (frequently combined with caffeine) were previously promoted for various uses (e.g., weight loss, body building, energy enhancement, increased mental concentration, increased sexual sensations, euphoria, alternative to illicit drugs); although these products constituted less than 1% of all dietary supplement sales, they accounted for 64% of adverse events associated with dietary supplements. Use of ephedrine alkaloid-containing dietary supplements has been associated with a twofold to threefold increased risk of nausea, vomiting, adverse psychiatric effects (e.g., anxiety, mood changes), autonomic hyperactivity, and palpitations. Serious adverse effects (e.g., cardiovascular and nervous system effects) and deaths have been reported in individuals receiving ephedrine or ephedra-containing dietary supplements. Such adverse effects, including irregular heart rate, palpitations, increased blood pressure, chest pain, anxiety, nervousness, tremor, hyperactivity, headache, and insomnia, usually were associated with clinically serious conditions (e.g., myocardial infarction, stroke, psychoses, seizures, nephrolithiasis, death) and frequently were reported in young (i.e., 30 years of age or younger) to middle-aged adults (over 70% of whom were females) using the supplements, mainly for weight loss or energy enhancement. Many such adverse effects occurred within 2 weeks of first use, although they were reported on the first day of use in some cases. Most individuals who developed such adverse effects claim that they used the dietary supplements according to labeled instructions.

Source of Ephedrine in Dietary Supplements

The labeled source of ephedrine in dietary supplements varied from raw botanicals to powdered plant material, sometimes pharmaceutical ephedrine alkaloids, but mainly consisted of concentrated extracts of the amphetamine-like *Ephedra* species (usually listed on labels as ma huang, ephedra, Chinese ephedra, Ephedra sinica, ephedra herb powder, epitonin, ephedrine, or ephedrine alkaloids). Small amounts of ephedrine alkaloids also are found in *Sida cordifolia*. Plants of the genus *Ephedra* may contain ephedrine alkaloids as single ingredients; however, ephedrine alkaloids usually are combined with other compounds. Although some dietary supplements contained only *Ephedra* as a labeled ingredient, most dietary supplements contained other ingredients, many of which have known or suspected physiologic and pharmacologic activities that have the potential of interacting with ephedrine alkaloids and thus increasing their effects.

Regulations Governing Dietary Supplements

Although the quality and consistency of prescription and nonprescription drugs in the US generally are ensured by strict FDA regulations concerning drug uniformity, purity, and labeling accuracy, dietary supplements (e.g., herbal preparations, vitamins and minerals, amino acids, tissue extracts) are regulated as *foods* under the Dietary Supplement Health and Education Act (DSHEA) of 1994. Therefore, FDA bears the burden to prove that a marketed dietary supplement is unsafe when used according to the conditions of use on the label or as commonly consumed. These requirements are in contrast to FDA regulations concerning prescription and nonprescription drugs that stipulate that a drug has to be proven safe and effective (for a particular indication) before it is approved for marketing.

Serious adverse effects (e.g., cardiovascular and nervous system effects) and deaths have been reported with ephedrine or ephedra-containing dietary supplements. As a result, FDA has proposed strict regulations for these preparations since 1997 to protect the public health. In 1997, the agency proposed regulations to limit the amount of ephedrine alkaloids that dietary supplement preparations contain and to change labeling and marketing practices for these supplements. In 2001, FDA seized drug products containing synthetic ephedrine hydrochloride labeled as dietary supplements. In 2003, with the emergence of new scientific evidence (including approximately 18,000 adverse event reports received overall by FDA and a comprehensive evaluation of the scientific literature through 2002 conducted by the RAND corporation), FDA proposed additional changes to labeling to emphasize the risks of using ephedrine-containing dietary supplements. In addition, the agency also proposed rules to establish GMPs for all dietary supplements and issued warnings prohibiting manufacturers from making unsubstantiated efficacy claims (e.g., enhancement of athletic performance, street drug alternative) for these preparations.

In February 2004, FDA finally concluded that dietary supplements containing ephedrine alkaloids pose a risk of serious adverse events (e.g., heart attack, stroke, death), and that these risks are unreasonable in light of any benefits that may result from the use of these products. Therefore, the agency issued a final regulation declaring that dietary supplements containing ephedrine alkaloids are *adulterated* under the Federal Food, Drug, and Cosmetic Act. Under this rule, manufacturing, distribution, and sale of all dietary supplements containing ephedrine alkaloids (e.g., *Ephedra* spp. ["ma huang"], *Sida cordifolia*, *Pinellia* spp.) were prohibited after April 12, 2004. This regulation does not apply to traditional Chinese herbal remedies or products regulated as conventional foods (e.g., herbal teas). Ephedra is *not* generally recognized as safe for foods and not approved for use as a food additive.

In April 2005, about one year after issuance of FDA's final ruling, a federal judge in a Utah district court overturned part of the ruling, declaring that the agency cannot ban the sale of dietary supplements containing ephedrine dosages of 10 mg or less without proving that such low dosages are unsafe; this ruling partially lifted FDA's ban, allowing products with 10 mg or less of active ingredient to return to the US market. However, in August 2006, a 3-judge panel of the US Court of Appeals for the 10th Circuit in Denver reversed the lower Utah district court decision and upheld FDA's final rule declaring all dietary supplements containing ephedrine alkaloids adulterated. FDA then reiterated its position that no dosage of dietary supplements containing ephedrine alkaloids is considered safe, and the sale of these products in the US is illegal and subject to FDA enforcement action.

• Precautions and Contraindications

Ephedrine may cause hypertension. The drug should be used with caution in patients with hypertension, cardiovascular disease, angina, diabetes mellitus, hyperthyroidism, or prostatic hyperplasia, and in those receiving digoxin. An increased risk of hypertension has been observed in patients receiving ephedrine sulfate injection for the prevention of hypotension during anesthesia. Serious postpartum hypertension, in some cases resulting in stroke, has been reported in patients receiving a vasopressor (e.g., ephedrine) and an oxytocic agent (e.g., ergonovine, methylergonovine) concomitantly.

Patients considering *self-medication* with ephedrine as a bronchodilator should be advised that the drug be used only if they have been diagnosed by a clinician as having asthma, and that *self-medication* not be undertaken if they ever have been hospitalized for asthma or are currently receiving a prescription drug for the management of this condition unless otherwise directed by a clinician. These patients also should be advised not to use the drug if they have cardiovascular disease, hypertension, diabetes mellitus, thyroid disease, angle-closure (narrow-angle) glaucoma, seizures, a psychiatric or emotional condition, or difficulty urinating because of prostatic hyperplasia unless directed by a clinician. In addition, patients should be advised not to exceed recommended dosages or frequency of administration unless otherwise instructed by a clinician. Patients should contact their clinician if symptoms are not improved within 1 hour or become worse, more than the recommended dosage of ephedrine is required, or asthma attacks become more frequent (i.e., more than 2 asthma attacks in a week). Patients also should be cautioned that ephedrine can cause hypertension and tachycardia, which could increase the risk of cardiovascular disease, stroke, or death. Foods, beverages, and dietary supplements that contain stimulants (e.g., caffeine) should be avoided.

Prolonged use of parenteral ephedrine may produce a syndrome resembling an anxiety state. Tolerance to ephedrine also may develop with repeated administration of the drug; in some cases, effectiveness may return after the drug is temporarily withheld. If ephedrine sulfate injection is used for the treatment of hypotension during anesthesia, clinicians should be aware of the possibility of tachyphylaxis and be prepared to use an alternative vasopressor agent in the event that an unacceptable response to ephedrine occurs.

Because ephedrine is substantially excreted by the kidneys, patients with impaired renal function may eliminate the drug more slowly, consequently prolonging its pharmacologic effect and potentially increasing the risk of adverse effects. Patients with renal impairment should be carefully monitored after administration of the initial IV dose of ephedrine.

Misuse or abuse of ephedrine can result in potentially serious adverse effects. (See Uses: Misuse and Abuse.) Serious adverse effects also have been reported with dietary supplements containing ephedrine alkaloids. In February 2004, FDA issued a final regulation prohibiting the manufacturing, distribution, and sale of all dietary supplements containing ephedrine alkaloids (effective April 12, 2004). Effective August 2006, no dosage of dietary supplements containing ephedrine alkaloids is considered safe, and the sale of these products in the US is illegal and subject to FDA enforcement action. (See Dietary Supplements under Cautions: Adverse Effects.)

Some manufacturers state that ephedrine is contraindicated in patients with known hypersensitivity to the drug or other sympathomimetic agents, although allergic reactions to ephedrine are rare.

• Pediatric Precautions

Ephedrine sulfate injection is not FDA-labeled for use in pediatric patients. Although the drug has been used in children, safety and efficacy have not been established in this patient population.

Overdosage and toxicity (including death) have been reported in children younger than 2 years of age receiving nonprescription (over-the-counter, OTC) preparations containing antihistamines, cough suppressants, expectorants, and nasal decongestants alone or in combination for relief of symptoms of upper respiratory tract infection. There is limited evidence of efficacy for these preparations in this age group, and appropriate dosages (i.e., approved by the FDA) for the symptomatic treatment of cold and cough have not been established. Therefore, FDA stated that nonprescription cough and cold preparations should not be used in children younger than 2 years of age; the agency continues to assess safety and efficacy of these preparations in older children. Meanwhile, because children 2–3 years of age also are at increased risk of overdosage and toxicity, some manufacturers of oral nonprescription cough and cold preparations agreed to voluntarily revise the product labeling to state that such preparations should not be used in children younger than 4 years of age. FDA recommends that parents and caregivers adhere to the dosage instructions and warnings on the product labeling that accompanies the preparation if administering to children and consult with their clinician about any concerns. Clinicians should ask caregivers about use of nonprescription cough and cold preparations to avoid overdosage. For additional information on precautions associated with the use of cough and cold preparations in pediatric patients, see Cautions: Pediatric Precautions, in Pseudoephedrine 12:12.12.

• Geriatric Precautions

Clinical studies of ephedrine sulfate did not include sufficient numbers of patients 65 years of age and older to determine whether geriatric patients respond differently than younger patients. Clinical experience to date has not identified any differences in response between geriatric and younger patients. If ephedrine is used in geriatric patients, dosage should be selected carefully, usually starting at the low end of the dosage range, since renal, hepatic, and cardiovascular dysfunction and concomitant disease or other drug therapy are more common in this age group.

Ephedrine is known to be substantially excreted by the kidneys and the risk of ephedrine-induced adverse effects may be increased in patients with impaired renal function; because geriatric patients may have decreased renal function, it may be useful to monitor renal function in such patients.

• Pregnancy, Fertility, and Lactation
Pregnancy

Animal reproduction studies have not been performed to date with ephedrine sulfate injection; it is not known whether the drug can cause fetal harm or miscarriage when administered during pregnancy. However, ephedrine has been used in pregnant women for the treatment of hypotension during spinal anesthesia, and the available data support the efficacy and safety of ephedrine sulfate injection for such use. There is some evidence indicating that fetal acidosis is more likely to occur with maternal administration of ephedrine compared with phenylephrine. Low umbilical artery pH (7.2 or less) has been reported at the time of delivery in neonates whose mothers were exposed to ephedrine. Newborn infants with such maternal exposure should be assessed for their acid-base status and monitored for signs and symptoms of metabolic acidosis.

Lactation

Limited data indicate that ephedrine is distributed into human milk; however, there is no information regarding the effects of the drug on the breast-fed infant or on milk production. The known benefits of breast-feeding should be considered along with the mother's clinical need for ephedrine and any potential adverse effects of the drug or underlying maternal condition on the infant.

DRUG INTERACTIONS

• α- and β-Adrenergic Blocking Agents

Administration of an α-adrenergic blocking drug reduces the vasopressor response to ephedrine. Phentolamine, by blocking the α-adrenergic effects of ephedrine, can cause vasodilation. However, because of the cardiac stimulating effects of ephedrine, a pressor response may be achieved if sufficient doses are administered.

As with other sympathomimetic drugs having cardiostimulating effects, administration of a β-adrenergic blocking drug such as propranolol may block the cardiac and bronchodilating effects of ephedrine.

Blood pressure should be monitored in patients receiving ephedrine concomitantly with an α- or β-adrenergic blocking agent.

• Cardiac Glycosides

Cardiac glycosides (e.g., digoxin) can sensitize the myocardium to the effects of sympathomimetic drugs and increase the risk of arrhythmias; patients receiving such concomitant therapy should be carefully monitored.

• Diuretics

Administration of furosemide or other diuretics may decrease arterial responsiveness to pressor drugs such as ephedrine.

• Epidural Anesthesia

Ephedrine may decrease efficacy of epidural blockade by facilitating the regression of sensory analgesia. Patients should be monitored for this effect and treated accordingly.

• General Anesthetics

Some manufacturers state that concurrent use of ephedrine with general anesthetics, especially cyclopropane or halogenated hydrocarbons, can sensitize the myocardium to the effects of ephedrine and possibly increase the risk of arrhythmias.

• Monoamine Oxidase Inhibitors

By increasing the quantity of norepinephrine in adrenergic nervous tissue, monoamine oxidase (MAO) inhibitors may potentiate the pressor effects of indirectly acting sympathomimetic drugs such as ephedrine. Potentiation is approximately the same following IV or oral administration of ephedrine. A hypertensive crisis and subarachnoid hemorrhage occurred in a patient receiving an MAO inhibitor after 50 mg of ephedrine was administered orally.

Blood pressure should be carefully monitored in patients receiving ephedrine and an MAO inhibitor concomitantly. Some manufacturers recommend that ephedrine not be used in patients currently receiving, or for 2 weeks after discontinuance of, an MAO inhibitor.

• Oxytocic Drugs

Concomitant use of a vasopressor (e.g., ephedrine) with an oxytocic drug (e.g., ergonovine, methylergonovine) may increase the pressor effect and cause severe postpartum hypertension, which may lead to stroke. Blood pressure should be carefully monitored in patients receiving such concomitant therapy.

• Rocuronium

Ephedrine may reduce the onset time of rocuronium-induced neuromuscular blockade for intubation when administered simultaneously with anesthetic induction.

• Theophylline

Concomitant use of ephedrine and theophylline may increase the frequency of nausea, nervousness, and insomnia. Patients receiving such concomitant therapy should be monitored for these symptoms and treated accordingly.

• Other Drugs

Other drugs that may potentiate the pressor effect of ephedrine include clonidine, propofol, and atropine. Other drugs that can antagonize the pressor effect of ephedrine include reserpine and quinidine. Blood pressure should be carefully monitored in patients receiving such concomitant therapy.

ACUTE TOXICITY

• Manifestations

Overdosage of ephedrine can cause a rapid increase in blood pressure. Hypertension may develop initially, followed later by hypotension accompanied by anuria. Careful monitoring of blood pressure is recommended in the event of an overdosage. Another principal manifestation of ephedrine overdosage is the development of seizures. Acute overdosage of ephedrine also may result in nausea, vomiting, chills, cyanosis, irritability, nervousness, fever, suicidal behavior, tachycardia, dilated pupils, blurred vision, opisthotonos, spasms, pulmonary edema, gasping respirations, coma, and respiratory failure.

• Treatment

If respirations are shallow or cyanosis is present, one manufacturer recommends initiation of assisted respiration. In the presence of cardiovascular collapse, blood pressure should be maintained; however, vasopressors are contraindicated.

Parenteral antihypertensives may be administered at the discretion of the clinician for the management of severe hypertension. One manufacturer recommends administration of 5 mg of phentolamine mesylate diluted in 0.9% sodium chloride injection and administered slowly by IV injection; alternatively, 100 mg of the drug may be given orally (an oral dosage form of phentolamine is not commercially available in the US). Seizures may be controlled with diazepam; pyrexia may be managed with external cooling and IV dexamethasone (1 mg/kg administered slowly).

PHARMACOLOGY

Ephedrine stimulates both α- and β-adrenergic receptors through direct and indirect mechanisms. It is believed that β-adrenergic effects result from stimulation of the production of cyclic adenosine 3′,5′-monophosphate (cAMP) by activation of the enzyme adenyl cyclase, whereas α-adrenergic effects result from inhibition of adenyl cyclase activity. Ephedrine also exerts an indirect effect by releasing norepinephrine from its storage sites. With prolonged or excessive use, ephedrine may deplete norepinephrine stores in sympathetic nerve endings and tachyphylaxis may develop. Tachyphylaxis to the bronchial effects of the drug may also occur, but it is not the result of norepinephrine depletion. The main effects of therapeutic doses of ephedrine are relaxation of the smooth muscle of the bronchial tree, and when norepinephrine stores are not depleted, cardiac stimulation and increased systolic and usually increased diastolic blood pressure. Unlike epinephrine and norepinephrine, ephedrine produces bronchodilation and possibly increased blood pressure and has pronounced CNS activity following oral administration.

• Respiratory Effects

Ephedrine relaxes bronchial smooth muscle by stimulation of β₂-adrenergic receptors. Bronchodilation produced by oral ephedrine occurs more slowly, is less pronounced, and is more prolonged than that achieved with epinephrine administered subcutaneously or by oral inhalation.

• Cardiovascular Effects

The cardiovascular effects of ephedrine are mediated by its α- and β-adrenergic properties and the overall clinical response is based on the balance between α_1-mediated vasoconstriction, β_2-mediated vasoconstriction, and β_2-mediated vasodilation. Ephedrine increases heart rate, increases cardiac output, and variably increases peripheral vascular resistance, resulting in an increase in systemic blood pressure.

Ephedrine acts on β_1-adrenergic receptors in the heart, producing a positive inotropic effect on the myocardium when single low doses are administered. This effect contributes to, and may be principally responsible for, the pressor effects of the drug when venous return to the heart is adequate. Although the drug also produces a positive chronotropic effect through the sinoatrial node, this effect may be overcome by increased vagal activity occurring as a reflex to increased arterial blood pressure. Bradycardia, tachycardia, or unchanged heart rate has been reported. Cardiac output usually is increased, especially after IV administration. Because of its positive inotropic effects, ephedrine increases cardiac work and probably myocardial oxygen consumption, and usually increases pulmonary arterial pressure.

Ephedrine increases the irritability of the heart muscle and may alter the rhythmic function of the ventricles, especially when the heart has been sensitized to this action by other drugs including digitalis glycosides or certain anesthetics. Arrhythmias including ventricular tachycardia, extrasystoles, and fibrillation may result. As with epinephrine, arrhythmias may be more likely to occur if large doses are given or if the patient has acute myocardial infarction.

Ephedrine may dilate coronary blood vessels. As with epinephrine, coronary artery vasodilation may be indirect, caused by enhanced cardiac metabolism due to direct cardiac stimulation. Ephedrine may increase coronary artery blood flow; as with other sympathomimetic drugs, increased coronary blood flow may result from increased systemic blood pressure as well as indirect coronary artery vasodilation. However, decreased coronary artery blood flow has also been reported and the effects of the drug on coronary circulation may be dose dependent.

Like epinephrine, ephedrine can produce both vasodilation by its effect on β_2-adrenergic receptors and vasoconstriction by its effect on α-adrenergic receptors. The drug constricts arterioles in the skin, mucous membranes, and viscera, and dilates arterioles in the skeletal muscle. Either constriction or dilation of pulmonary and cerebral vessels may occur. Peripheral vascular resistance may be increased, decreased, or unchanged after administration of the drug. Conditions causing an increase or decrease in vascular resistance have not been identified. Pressor responses to parenteral ephedrine occur more slowly but are more prolonged than those achieved with epinephrine or norepinephrine. Increased blood pressure may be caused by vasoconstriction as well as by cardiac stimulation; however, when peripheral vascular resistance is decreased, elevation of blood pressure is due entirely to increased cardiac output. Ephedrine may constrict both arterial and venous blood vessels; peripheral venous pressure also is increased. Ephedrine may decrease circulating plasma volume. This may result from loss of fluid into extracellular spaces caused by postcapillary vasoconstriction.

Constriction of renal blood vessels by parenteral ephedrine decreases renal blood flow. In hypotensive patients, ephedrine may initially decrease urine flow and excretion of sodium and potassium. If the patient is not hypovolemic, renal blood flow and glomerular filtration rate increase as the systemic blood pressure is raised toward normal levels; however, renal blood flow and glomerular filtration rate again decrease if blood pressure is further increased toward hypertensive levels.

Ephedrine may constrict dilated blood vessels in the nasal mucosa and produce nasal decongestion following topical application; however, rebound congestion may occur. There is insufficient evidence that the drug is effective as a nasal decongestant when administered orally in usual doses.

• Other Effects

Ephedrine has CNS stimulating effects similar to those of amphetamines but less pronounced. (See Cautions: Adverse Effects.)

Ephedrine generally relaxes smooth muscles of the GI tract. Ephedrine contracts the urinary bladder trigone and sphincter; relaxation of the detrusor muscle is not prominent. (See Cautions: Adverse Effects.) The drug usually decreases the activity of the uterus; however, an excitatory effect has also been reported. Use

of ephedrine during delivery to correct maternal hypotension resulting from spinal anesthesia may result in improved uterine blood flow. In experimental animals, the drug has corrected fetal hypoxia, hypercapnia, acidosis, and bradycardia resulting from maternal hypotension.

Blood glucose concentrations are not increased as much by ephedrine as by epinephrine, and usual doses of ephedrine are not likely to produce hyperglycemia. Ephedrine increases oxygen consumption and metabolic rate, probably as a result of central stimulation.

Administration of ephedrine to patients with myasthenia gravis may result in increased muscle strength. The mechanism by which ephedrine acts in these patients is not known.

PHARMACOKINETICS

• Absorption

Bronchodilation occurs within 15–60 minutes after oral administration of the drug and appears to persist for 2–4 hours. The duration of pressor and cardiac responses to ephedrine is 1 hour after IV administration of 10–25 mg or IM or subcutaneous administration of 25–50 mg and up to 4 hours after oral administration of 15–50 mg of the drug.

There appears to be a wide variation in ephedrine plasma concentrations associated with bronchodilation. In one study, therapeutic plasma concentrations were reported to range from 20 ng/mL to more than 80 ng/mL.

Following oral administration of ephedrine as conventional ephedrine hydrochloride capsules containing 25 mg of ephedrine base (no longer commercially available in the US) or as 3 dietary supplement preparations of *Ephedra* (a botanical source of ephedrine alkaloids referred to as ma huang, no longer commercially available in the US) assayed as containing the equivalent of 23.6, 25.6, or 27 mg of ephedrine base in a randomized, crossover pharmacokinetic study in healthy fasting adults, the absorption rate and area under the serum concentration-time curve (AUC) were similar among the 4 preparations, although the absorption of one of the dietary supplements and AUC of another differed substantially from the remaining preparations. Mean peak serum ephedrine concentrations of about 73.4, 86, and 100 ng/mL were achieved in about 3, 2.6, and 2.7 hours following oral administration of the 23.6-, 25.6-, or 27-mg dose of ephedrine, respectively, compared with a mean peak serum concentration of 86.5 ng/mL at about 2.81 hours with the 25-mg dose of ephedrine administered as the conventional capsules (no longer commercially available in the US). Most of these dietary supplements contained other ingredients besides ephedrine and these ingredients may have increased the rate but not the extent of absorption of ephedrine from the GI tract.

• Distribution

Ephedrine is presumed to cross the placenta and distribute into milk.

In one study in healthy fasting adults comparing oral administration of conventional ephedrine hydrochloride capsules (no longer commercially available in the US) with botanical preparations (ma huang, *Ephedra*, no longer commercially available in the US) containing the drug, the apparent steady-state volume of distribution ranged from about 220–240 L.

• Elimination

The metabolic pathway of ephedrine has not been completely elucidated. However, some data suggest that small quantities of ephedrine are slowly metabolized in the liver by oxidative deamination, demethylation, aromatic hydroxylation, and conjugation. The metabolites have been identified as *p*-hydroxyephedrine, *p*-hydroxynorephedrine, norephedrine, and conjugates of these compounds.

Ephedrine and its metabolites are excreted in urine. Most of the drug is excreted unchanged. The rate of urinary excretion of the drug and its metabolites is dependent upon urinary pH. In one study, 74–92% of an oral dose and 87–99% of an IV dose of 25 mg of ephedrine hydrochloride were excreted as ephedrine and 8–10% of the oral dose and 3–7% of the IV dose were excreted as norephedrine within 24 hours when the urine was acidified to pH 5 by administration of ammonium chloride. When the urine was alkalinized to pH 8 by administration of sodium bicarbonate, 22–35% of a 25-mg oral dose of ephedrine hydrochloride was excreted as ephedrine and 11–24% of this dose was excreted as norephedrine within 24 hours. Approximately 70–80% of a 25-mg oral dose of ephedrine sulfate was excreted in urine within 48 hours when the urine pH averaged 6.3. The ratio of ephedrine to norephedrine excreted in this study was not determined.

The elimination half-life of ephedrine has been reported to be about 3 hours when the urine is acidified to pH 5 and about 6 hours when urinary pH is about 6.3. In a study in healthy fasting adults comparing oral administration of conventional ephedrine hydrochloride capsules (no longer commercially available in the US) with botanical preparations (ma huang, *Ephedra*, no longer commercially available in the US) containing the drug, elimination half-life ranged from 4.85–6.47 hours, with apparent clearances of 25.5–34.1 L/hour; urinary pH was not reported.

CHEMISTRY AND STABILITY

● Chemistry

Ephedrine is a sympathomimetic drug that occurs naturally in plants of the genus *Ephedra*, most commonly *E. sinica*. *Ephedra* spp., known in traditional Chinese medicine as "ma huang," contains 6 ephedrine alkaloids (sometimes collectively referred to as "ephedra"), including ephedrine, pseudoephedrine, norephedrine, methylephedrine, norpseudoephedrine, and methylpseudoephedrine. The total ephedrine alkaloid content of *E. sinica* is approximately 1–2%, with ephedrine being the most abundant alkaloid. Although the content may vary between samples, ephedrine and pseudoephedrine together generally constitute more than 80% of the alkaloid content of the dried herb. In dietary supplements, the ephedrine alkaloid content was typically expressed as a standardized percentage of total herb content. However, results of one study evaluating the content of 20 dietary supplements labeled as containing botanical sources of ephedrine alkaloids indicate that considerable discrepancies exist between the labeled amount of ephedrine alkaloid content and the assayed amount, and that ephedrine alkaloid contents vary from lot to lot. (See Dietary Supplements under Cautions: Adverse Effects.) FDA issued a final regulation in February 2004 prohibiting the manufacturing, distribution, and sale of all dietary supplements containing ephedrine alkaloids after April 12, 2004. (See Regulations Governing Dietary Supplements under Adverse Effects: Dietary Supplements, in Cautions.)

Ephedrine is commercially available as the hydrochloride or sulfate salt. Ephedrine hydrochloride and ephedrine sulfate occur as fine, white, odorless crystals or powders. Ephedrine hydrochloride has solubilities of approximately 0.33 g/mL in water and 71 mg/mL in alcohol at 25°C. Ephedrine sulfate has solubilities of approximately 0.77 g/mL in water and 11 mg/mL in alcohol at 25°C. Ephedrine sulfate injection has a pH of 4.5–7.

● Stability

Ephedrine sulfate injection should be stored at 20–25°C but may be exposed to temperatures of 15–30°C. Ephedrine salts and preparations containing the drugs gradually decompose and darken on exposure to light and must be stored in light-resistant containers.

Ephedrine injections have been reported to be incompatible with various drugs, but the compatibility depends on several factors (e.g., concentration of the drugs, resulting pH, temperature). Specialized references should be consulted for specific compatibility information.

PREPARATIONS

Excipients in commercially available drug preparations may have clinically important effects in some individuals; consult specific product labeling for details.

ePHEDrine Hydrochloride*

ePHEDrine Sulfate

Parenteral		
Injection	50 mg/mL*	**Akovaz®**, Eclat
		ePHEDrine Sulfate Injection

* available from one or more manufacturer, distributor, and/or repackager by generic (nonproprietary) name

ePHEDrine Hydrochloride Combinations

Oral		
Tablets	12.5 mg with Guaifenesin 200 mg	**Ephed Plus®**, DMD
		Primatene®, Pfizer
	25 mg with Guaifenesin 200 mg	**Ephed Plus®**, DMD

ePHEDrine Sulfate Combinations

Oral		
Tablets	25 mg with Guaifenesin 400 mg	**Bronkaid® Caplets**, Bayer

† Use is not currently included in the labeling approved by the US Food and Drug Administration.

Selected Revisions May 15, 2017, © Copyright, September 1, 1976, American Society of Health-System Pharmacists, Inc.

EPINEPHrine, racEPINEPHrine

12:12.12 • α- AND β-ADRENERGIC AGONISTS

■ Epinephrine is an endogenous catecholamine that is the active principle of the adrenal medulla; epinephrine acts directly on both α- and β-adrenergic receptors.

USES

● Sensitivity Reactions

Epinephrine is the drug of choice in the emergency treatment of severe acute anaphylactic reactions, including anaphylactic shock. The drug is used to relieve clinical manifestations such as urticaria, pruritus, angioedema, hypotension, and respiratory distress, which may result from reactions to drugs, contrast media, latex, insect stings, foods (e.g., milk, eggs, fish, shellfish, peanuts, tree nuts), or other allergens, as well as from idiopathic or exercise-induced anaphylaxis. Epinephrine should be given to all patients with signs of systemic reactions, particularly hypotension, airway swelling, or breathing difficulty. Recommendations for the use of epinephrine in anaphylaxis are largely based on clinical pharmacology studies, observational studies, retrospective studies, and animal models; however, the available data provide compelling evidence to support the prompt use of epinephrine in patients with anaphylaxis. When administered at the recommended dosages and routes of administration, beneficial pharmacologic effects mediated by both the α- and β-adrenergic properties of the drug (e.g., increased blood pressure, increased force and rate of cardiac contraction, bronchodilation, decreased airway mucosal edema, and suppression of mediator release) are observed. Patients with anaphylactic shock may require rapid volume resuscitation and vasopressor therapy; epinephrine also is used for its vasopressor effects for the treatment of anaphylactic shock and cardiac arrest associated with anaphylaxis.

Epinephrine should be administered immediately by IM injection as soon as anaphylaxis is diagnosed or strongly suspected. Initial administration by IM injection is preferred, mainly because of safety considerations. Serious adverse effects have occurred after IV administration of epinephrine, in part because of confusion regarding correct dosages and routes of administration for the different indications (e.g., treatment of anaphylaxis versus treatment of cardiac arrest). (See Dosage and Administration: Administration.) However, IV administration of epinephrine may be necessary in extreme situations such as in anaphylactic shock, cardiac arrest, or in unresponsive or severely hypotensive patients who have failed to respond to multiple IM injections; close hemodynamic monitoring is critical during IV administration of the drug. Epinephrine also may be administered subcutaneously, but absorption and subsequent achievement of peak plasma concentrations after subcutaneous injection are slower and may be substantially delayed in patients with shock. Although oral inhalation has been recommended, the drug may be absorbed too slowly and/or inadequately to be effective in treating allergic manifestations other than laryngeal angioedema.

Cardiac arrest secondary to anaphylaxis should be managed with standard advanced cardiovascular life support (ACLS) measures; alternative vasoactive drugs (e.g., vasopressin, norepinephrine) may be considered in patients who do not respond to epinephrine, and other therapeutic agents such as antihistamines, inhaled β$_2$-adrenergic agents, and IV corticosteroids also may be useful. (See Uses: Advanced Cardiovascular Life Support and Cardiac Arrhythmias.)

Patients receiving β-adrenergic blocking agents have an increased incidence and severity of anaphylaxis, and may develop a paradoxical response to epinephrine; glucagon or ipratropium may be considered for the treatment of anaphylaxis in these patients.

● Advanced Cardiovascular Life Support and Cardiac Arrhythmias

Epinephrine is used for its α-adrenergic effects to increase blood flow and facilitate return of spontaneous circulation (ROSC) in patients with cardiac arrest. The drug may be administered by IV, intraosseous (IO)†, endotracheal, or intracardiac injection during cardiopulmonary resuscitation (CPR). The principal benefits of epinephrine in patients with cardiac arrest result from increases in aortic diastolic blood pressure and in coronary and cerebral perfusion pressure during resuscitation. The value and safety of the β-adrenergic effects of epinephrine are controversial because they may increase myocardial work and reduce subendocardial perfusion.

High-quality CPR and defibrillation are integral components of ACLS and the only proven interventions to increase survival to hospital discharge. Other resuscitative efforts, including drug therapy, are considered secondary and should be performed without compromising the quality and timely delivery of chest compressions and defibrillation. The principal goal of pharmacologic therapy during cardiac arrest is to facilitate ROSC, and epinephrine is considered the drug of choice for this use.

Despite epinephrine's widespread use in ACLS and evidence of beneficial physiologic effects in both animals and humans, there currently is no evidence demonstrating that the drug improves survival to hospital discharge. The current evidence does, however, support that the drug improves survival to hospital admission (when the arrest occurs outside of the hospital setting) and the potential for achieving ROSC. The American Heart Association (AHA) states that it is reasonable to administer epinephrine 1 mg IV/IO every 3–5 minutes during adult cardiac arrest. Although higher doses of epinephrine may increase the rate of ROSC, numerous studies comparing standard (1 mg) versus high-dose (e.g., 0.1–0.2 mg/kg) epinephrine have not demonstrated any advantage of the higher doses with regards to survival (i.e., survival to discharge with or without good neurologic recovery, survival to hospital admission). While high-dose epinephrine may improve coronary perfusion and increase vascular resistance to promote initial ROSC during cardiac resuscitation, these same effects may result in increased myocardial dysfunction and occasionally a severe hyperadrenergic state in the postresuscitation period. AHA does not recommend the routine use of high-dose epinephrine in cardiac arrest; however, high-dose epinephrine may be considered in certain circumstances (e.g., overdosage of β-adrenergic or calcium-channel blocking agents).

Management of cardiac arrest is based on the patient's arrest rhythm (i.e., ventricular fibrillation, pulseless ventricular tachycardia, pulseless electrical activity [PEA], or asystole). As the rhythm is likely to evolve over the course of resuscitation, the appropriate management strategy should be adapted accordingly. In adults with ventricular fibrillation or pulseless ventricular tachycardia resistant to initial CPR attempts and at least one defibrillation shock, epinephrine may be administered with the goal of increasing myocardial blood flow during CPR and achieving ROSC; however, the optimal timing of epinephrine administration, particularly in relation to defibrillation, is not known and may vary based on patient-specific factors and resuscitation conditions. In adults with asystole or PEA, epinephrine may be given as soon as feasible after the onset of cardiac arrest based on studies demonstrating improved survival to hospital discharge and increased ROSC when the drug was administered early during the course of treatment for a nonshockable rhythm. In previous ACLS guidelines, vasopressin was recommended as an alternative to epinephrine in the treatment of adult cardiac arrest; however, vasopressin has been removed from the current ACLS guideline because of equivalence of effect with epinephrine and efforts to simplify the management approach when therapies are found to be equivalent.

Once a patient achieves ROSC, appropriate postcardiac arrest care should be initiated immediately because of evidence indicating that systematic postresuscitation care can improve the likelihood of patient survival with good quality of life. Because hemodynamic instability is common after cardiac arrest, epinephrine infusion may be used in the postresuscitation period to optimize blood pressure, cardiac output, and systemic perfusion after ROSC. Epinephrine also may be used during the periarrest period in adults who require inotropic or vasopressor support, in particular for the treatment of symptomatic bradycardia; although not a first-line drug, epinephrine may be considered in patients who are unresponsive to atropine therapy, or as a temporizing measure while awaiting availability of a pacemaker.

In contrast to adults, cardiac arrest in infants and children is not usually precipitated by a primary cardiac cause, but is more often the result of progressive respiratory failure or shock. In addition to high-quality CPR, ventilation is extremely important in pediatric advanced life support (PALS) because of the high percentage of asphyxial arrests that occur in pediatric patients. Similar to adults, vasopressors are used during pediatric cardiac arrest to restore spontaneous circulation although no specific pediatric studies have demonstrated the effectiveness of any vasopressor in this setting. AHA states that it is reasonable to administer epinephrine during pediatric cardiac arrest. The drug also may be used for hemodynamic support during the postresuscitation period. Epinephrine also is used in the emergency treatment of infants and children with bradycardia and cardiopulmonary compromise (with a palpable pulse) and is included in current PALS guidelines for this use; epinephrine is recommended in this situation when bradycardia persists despite ventilation, oxygenation, and chest compressions. Drugs are rarely needed during the resuscitation of neonates; because hypoxemia and inadequate lung inflation are common causes of bradycardia in the newborn infant, establishing adequate ventilation is the most important corrective measure in these patients.

Epinephrine also has been used in the treatment of syncope resulting from atrioventricular (AV) nodal block. However, permanent pacemaker implantation is the treatment of choice for third-degree and advanced second-degree AV nodal block (complete heart block).

● Septic Shock

Epinephrine is used for the treatment of hypotension associated with septic shock, generally as a second-line agent.

Vasopressors such as epinephrine are used in the management of shock to restore blood pressure and tissue perfusion after initial fluid resuscitation is attempted. The Surviving Sepsis Campaign International Guidelines for Management of Sepsis and Septic Shock recommend norepinephrine as the vasopressor of choice in adults with septic shock; if adequate blood pressure is not achieved, epinephrine may be added. Epinephrine is a potent vasoconstrictor with predominantly β-adrenergic effects at low doses and α-adrenergic effects at higher doses. Epinephrine administration can be associated with an increased rate of arrhythmias, decreased splanchnic blood flow, and increased blood lactate concentrations. Despite these adverse effects, there is no clinical evidence indicating that the drug is associated with worse outcomes than norepinephrine, and therefore, some experts suggest that epinephrine should be considered when an additional agent is needed to maintain adequate blood pressure during septic shock. In a double-blind, randomized controlled study comparing the effects of epinephrine and norepinephrine in intensive care patients, including a subgroup with septic shock, no substantial difference in 28- or 90-day mortality or time to achieve mean arterial pressure (MAP) goals was observed between the treatment groups; however, 13% of patients who received epinephrine were withdrawn from the study as a result of lactic acidosis or tachycardia. In another study in patients with septic shock, there was no difference in all-cause mortality, hemodynamic stabilization, resolution of organ dysfunction, or adverse events between patients receiving epinephrine and those receiving norepinephrine plus dobutamine.

Epinephrine should not be used in cardiogenic shock because it increases myocardial oxygen demand, nor should it be used in hemorrhagic or traumatic shock.

● Local Vasoconstriction

Epinephrine may be added to solutions of some local anesthetics to decrease the rate of vascular absorption of the anesthetic, thereby localizing anesthesia and prolonging the duration of anesthesia; the risk of systemic toxicity from the local anesthetic is also decreased.

Epinephrine has been applied topically to control superficial bleeding from arterioles or capillaries in the skin, mucous membranes, or other tissues. Bleeding from larger vessels is not controllable by topical application of epinephrine.

● Premature Labor

Epinephrine has been used to relax uterine musculature and inhibit uterine contractions in premature labor; however, the cardiovascular effects and other adverse effects limit the usefulness of the drug for this purpose. (See Cautions: Pregnancy.) Other β-agonists (e.g., terbutaline) are preferred. Some manufacturers state that epinephrine injection should be avoided during the second stage of labor.

● Bronchospasm

Asthma

Epinephrine and racepinephrine hydrochloride are used for the symptomatic treatment of asthma. Racepinephrine is commercially available as an oral bronchodilator for *self-medication* for the temporary relief of mild symptoms of

intermittent asthma (e.g., wheezing, chest tightness, shortness of breath). Once a diagnosis of asthma has been confirmed by a clinician, use of a nonprescription (over-the-counter, OTC) bronchodilator may be appropriate in patients with mild intermittent asthma; because asthma may be life-threatening, those with more severe asthma (i.e., persistent asthma) or worsening asthma (symptoms not relieved within 20 minutes or with maximum recommended dosages, increasing frequency of asthma attacks) should consult a clinician for other treatment options. An epinephrine preparation for oral inhalation use no longer is commercially available in the US.

While orally inhaled epinephrine was once widely used for its bronchodilating effects in the management of reversible airway obstruction, the drug has been replaced by more selective and rapid-acting agents (e.g., inhaled β₂-adrenergic agonists), and epinephrine is not recommended as a drug of choice for the rapid relief of asthma in current asthma management guidelines. In the stepped-care approach to antiasthmatic therapy, most experts currently recommend use of a selective short-acting inhaled β₂-adrenergic agonist (e.g., albuterol, levalbuterol, pirbuterol) on an intermittent, as-needed basis to control acute symptoms (e.g., cough, wheezing, dyspnea). Less β₂-selective bronchodilators such as epinephrine generally are not recommended because of their potential to cause excessive cardiac stimulation (e.g., increased heart rate, myocardial irritability, increased oxygen demand), particularly at high doses. For information on the stepped-care approach for drug therapy in asthma, see Asthma under Uses: Bronchospasm, in Albuterol 12:12.08.12.

Epinephrine also has been used parenterally for the treatment of severe asthma. Subcutaneous or IM epinephrine is the drug of choice for acute asthma attacks potentially associated with anaphylaxis but otherwise is reserved for severe asthma exacerbations when inhaled or parenteral β₂-selective agents are not readily available or are ineffective. Subcutaneous administration of epinephrine also may be useful when tachypnea and low tidal volume may prevent effective therapy with an orally inhaled β₂-adrenergic agonist or when orally inhaled therapy is not effective. Epinephrine also has been used IV for the treatment of severe asthma exacerbations; however, there is no evidence that the drug improves outcomes when compared with the selective inhaled β₂-adrenergic agonists.

● Upper GI Hemorrhage

Epinephrine injection has been used as an endoscopic treatment modality for the management of acute nonvariceal upper GI bleeding†; when used for this purpose, a dilute solution of epinephrine (in 0.9% sodium chloride injection) is injected into and around the ulcer base during endoscopy to produce tamponade and achieve hemostasis. Such therapy should not be used alone and should be combined with an additional endoscopic hemostatic modality (e.g., clips, thermocoagulation).

For uses of epinephrine in the treatment of glaucoma or as a mydriatic, see 52:24. For use of epinephrine as a vasoconstrictor and hemostatic in the eye and mucosa, see 52:24.

DOSAGE AND ADMINISTRATION

● Administration

USP has changed its labeling standard for single-entity drug products to no longer allow the use of ratios to express drug concentrations. This labeling change was prompted by numerous reports of serious medication errors caused by confusion with different ratio expressions. Effective May 1, 2016, all single-entity preparations of epinephrine injection, USP should be labeled only in terms of strength per mL (i.e., mg/mL). While concentrations of some epinephrine preparations were historically expressed in ratios (e.g., 1:1000 or 1:10,000), such designation is no longer acceptable because of the risk of dosing errors.

Epinephrine usually is administered by IM, subcutaneous, or IV injection, or by continuous IV infusion. Epinephrine also has been administered by intraosseous (IO) injection† in the setting of advanced cardiovascular life support (ACLS), generally when IV access is not readily available; onset of action and systemic concentrations are comparable to those achieved with venous administration. If vascular access (IV or IO) cannot be established during cardiac arrest, epinephrine may be administered endotracheally; however, this method of administration results in lower plasma concentrations compared with the same dose given intravascularly. Epinephrine also has been administered by intracardiac injection (into the left ventricular chamber) during cardiac arrest; however, this route of administration is not recommended in current ACLS guidelines.

The appropriate concentration and route of administration of epinephrine should be selected carefully; serious adverse effects (e.g., cerebral hemorrhage) have occurred after concentrated solutions of epinephrine intended for IM administration were administered IV. Because of the risks associated with IV use, epinephrine generally should be administered by the IV route only in extreme situations (such as in the treatment of septic or anaphylactic shock, cardiac arrest, or when the patient is unresponsive to multiple IM injections). Dilute solutions of epinephrine (e.g., 0.1 mg/mL) should always be used when administering the drug IV. Commercially available epinephrine solutions for IM or subcutaneous injection are tenfold more concentrated (1 mg/mL) and should not be administered IV without dilution.

Solutions of epinephrine should be inspected visually for particulate matter and discoloration prior to administration. Epinephrine injection must not be used if it is discolored or cloudy or contains any particulate matter.

Parenteral Administration

IM or Subcutaneous Administration

Epinephrine injection solution containing epinephrine 1 mg/mL may be administered IM or subcutaneously, but IM injection into the buttock should be avoided. (See Cautions: Adverse Effects.) When used for the treatment of anaphylaxis, epinephrine should be administered by IM (preferred) or subcutaneous injection into the anterolateral aspect of the thigh; injection into or near smaller muscles (i.e., deltoid muscle) is not recommended because of possible differences in absorption. Following subcutaneous administration, absorption and subsequent achievement of peak plasma concentrations may be slower and substantially delayed if shock is present. Repeated injections of epinephrine should not be administered at the same site because of the risk of possible tissue necrosis due to vasoconstriction.

Epinephrine is commercially available in a prefilled auto-injector for the emergency treatment of allergic reactions. When IM or subcutaneous epinephrine is used for *self-medication*, patients and their caregivers should be instructed about proper administration techniques using the auto-injector provided by the manufacturer. Patients should seek immediate medical or hospital care in conjunction with self-administration of the drug. First aid providers should be familiar with auto-injectors in order to assist patients experiencing an anaphylactic reaction, and they should be able to administer epinephrine using an auto-injector if a patient is unable to self-administer the drug, provided that state law permits it and a valid prescription exists. When using the auto-injector, the appropriate weight-based dose should be injected IM or subcutaneously into the anterolateral aspect of the thigh. The injection may be administered through clothing if necessary. Some manufacturers recommend massaging the injection area for several seconds after the drug is administered. The auto-injectors are overfilled and most of the solution will remain in the device after injection of the appropriate dose; however, the auto-injector cannot be reused. The respective manufacturer's prescribing information should be consulted for additional instructions on use of prefilled epinephrine auto-injectors.

IV Administration

For IV administration, epinephrine is commercially available as a 0.1-mg/mL solution. This concentration also may be prepared by diluting the commercially available 1-mg/mL epinephrine injection with a suitable diluent. Various methods have been described for diluting epinephrine solutions for IV administration. Commercially available epinephrine 1-mg/mL injection should not be administered IV unless the solution is further diluted.

In emergency situations, diluted solutions of epinephrine may be administered by slow IV injection or as a continuous IV infusion. Extreme caution is recommended when epinephrine is administered by direct IV injection since the risk of overdosage and adverse cardiovascular effects is substantially higher with such administration; the drug should be administered slowly with close hemodynamic monitoring.

During cardiac resuscitation, epinephrine may be administered IV into a central or peripheral line. IV access should be established and the drug administered without interrupting chest compressions. To ensure delivery of the drug into the central compartment, each dose of epinephrine given by *peripheral* injection should be followed by a 20-mL flush of IV fluid and the extremity should be elevated during and after drug administration. Although central venous access is

advantageous because higher plasma drug concentrations can be achieved and physiologic monitoring for return of spontaneous circulation (ROSC) can be performed, placement of a central line can potentially interrupt cardiopulmonary resuscitation (CPR). Central line placement should be avoided in patients who are candidates for pharmacologic reperfusion (e.g., with thrombolytic therapy).

During resuscitation in infants and children, a peripheral IV line may be established if it can be done rapidly. Central venous access is not recommended as the initial route of vascular access during an emergency because of the expertise and time required for establishing a central line. If, however, both central and peripheral lines are available, the central venous route is preferred. Whereas venous access can be challenging in critically ill infants and children, IO access can be achieved rapidly with minimal complications.

To minimize the risk of necrosis, continuous IV infusions of epinephrine should be infused into a large vein. A catheter tie-in technique should be avoided because obstruction to blood flow around the tubing may cause stasis and increase local concentration of the drug. *Care must be taken to avoid extravasation because local necrosis may result.*

Standardize 4 Safety

Standardized concentrations for epinephrine have been established through Standardize 4 Safety (S4S), a national patient safety initiative to reduce medication errors, especially during transitions of care. Multidisciplinary expert panels were convened to determine recommended standard concentrations. Because recommendations from the S4S panels may differ from the manufacturer's prescribing information, caution is advised when using concentrations that differ from labeling, particularly when using rate information from the label. For additional information on S4S (including updates that may be available), see https://www.ashp.org/pharmacy-practice/standardize-4-safety-initiative.

TABLE 1. Standardize 4 Safety Continuous IV Infusion Standard Concentrations for Epinephrine

Patient Population	Concentration Standards[a]	Dosing Units
Adults	20 mcg/mL	mcg/kg/min
	40 mcg/mL	
Pediatric patients (<50 kg)	10 mcg/mL[b]	mcg/kg/min
	20 mcg/mL	
	40 mcg/mL	

[a] The concentrations for epinephrine and norepinephrine are intentionally different to avoid confusion as recommended by the S4S panel and ISMP.

[b] Babies under 500 g may require a lower concentration

Endotracheal Administration

If vascular access (IV or IO) is not possible during cardiac resuscitation, lipid-soluble drugs such as epinephrine may be administered via an endotracheal tube. However, studies have shown conflicting results regarding the effectiveness of endotracheal versus vascular administration of the drug. Epinephrine administered via an endotracheal tube should be diluted in 5–10 mL of 0.9% sodium chloride or sterile water in adults or flushed with a minimum of 5 mL of 0.9% sodium chloride injection in pediatric patients. Absorption of epinephrine, administered via endotracheal tube, may be increased by diluting the drug in sterile water instead of 0.9% sodium chloride.

Oral Inhalation

Epinephrine and racepinephrine also have been administered via oral inhalation using a nebulizer, aerosol, or intermittent positive-pressure breathing (IPPB) apparatus for the treatment of asthma. However, an oral inhalation preparation of epinephrine is no longer commercially available in the US.

Topical Administration

Solutions of epinephrine hydrochloride also are applied topically as a spray or on cotton or gauze to the skin, mucous membranes, or other tissues.

● *Dosage*

Dosage of epinephrine salts is expressed in terms of epinephrine. Dosage of racepinephrine hydrochloride is expressed in terms of racepinephrine; racepinephrine is about one-half as active as epinephrine.

Sensitivity Reactions

Adult Dosage

For the emergency treatment of allergic reactions, including anaphylaxis, the usual adult dose of epinephrine is 0.2–0.5 mg (0.2–0.5 mL of a 1-mg/mL solution) administered IM or subcutaneously; the dose may be repeated every 5–15 minutes as necessary. A maximum single dose of 0.5 mg in adults is recommended. IM administration is preferred since absorption and subsequent achievement of peak plasma concentrations may be slower and substantially delayed following subcutaneous administration of the drug if shock is present.

For *self-administration* of epinephrine using a prefilled auto-injector (e.g., EpiPen®), an IM or subcutaneous dose of 0.3 mg is recommended. For severe persistent anaphylaxis, repeated doses may be needed; if more than 2 sequential doses are needed, subsequent doses should be administered under direct medical supervision.

In extreme circumstances (e.g., anaphylactic shock, cardiac arrest, or no response to initial IM injections), IV administration may be necessary since absorption of epinephrine may be impaired with subcutaneous or IM administration. The usual adult IV dose of epinephrine for the treatment of anaphylaxis ranges from 0.1 to 0.25 mg (1–2.5 mL of a 0.1-mg/mL solution); the dose may be repeated every 5–15 minutes as needed. Although there is no established dosage for continuous IV infusions of epinephrine, some studies have demonstrated efficacy at IV infusion rates of 2–15 mcg/minute, titrated based on severity of the reaction and clinical response.

Patients with anaphylaxis who respond to therapy require observation for possible recurrence even if there is an intervening asymptomatic period; length of observation time has not been established. Symptoms may recur within 1–36 hours after the initial reaction. The duration of direct observation and monitoring after an episode of anaphylaxis should be individualized based on the severity and duration of the anaphylactic event as well as other factors (e.g., response to treatment, pattern of previous anaphylactic reactions, comorbidities, patient reliability, access to medical care). Some experts suggest that patients with moderate to severe anaphylaxis should be observed for a minimum of 4–8 hours after treatment.

Pediatric Patients

For the treatment of anaphylaxis in pediatric patients, the recommended dose of epinephrine is 0.01 mg/kg (0.01 mL/kg of a 1-mg/mL solution) by IM or subcutaneous injection. Single IM or subcutaneous doses should not exceed 0.3–0.5 mg (depending on the patient's weight). The dose may be repeated every 5–15 minutes as necessary. Some clinicians state that doses may be repeated at 20-minute to 4-hour intervals depending on the severity of the condition and patient response.

For *self-administration* of epinephrine in children using a prefilled auto-injector, a dose of 0.15 or 0.3 mg, depending on body weight, should be injected IM or subcutaneously; 0.3 mg is recommended for patients weighing at least 30 kg and 0.15 mg is recommended for patients weighing 15–30 kg. If doses less than 0.15 mg are considered more appropriate, alternative injectable forms of the drug should be used. For severe persistent anaphylaxis, repeat doses may be needed; however, if more than 2 sequential doses of epinephrine are needed, subsequent doses should only be administered under direct medical supervision.

If IV administration is necessary for the treatment of anaphylaxis in pediatric patients, some clinicians recommend an initial IV epinephrine dose of 0.01 mg/kg (0.1 mL/kg of a 0.1-mg/mL solution). If repeated doses are required, a continuous IV infusion should be initiated at a rate of 0.1 mcg/kg per minute, and increased gradually to 1.5 mcg/kg per minute to maintain blood pressure. A slow, continuous, low-dose infusion is preferred to repeat IV injections because the drug may be titrated to effect.

Advanced Cardiovascular Life Support and Cardiac Arrhythmias

For ACLS during cardiac arrest, epinephrine preferably is administered IV but also may be instilled directly into the tracheobronchial tree via an endotracheal tube or administered by IO injection or intracardially. (See Dosage and Administration: Administration.) Although endotracheal administration of epinephrine is possible, IV or IO administration is preferred because of more predictable drug delivery and pharmacologic effect. IO administration of epinephrine may be particularly useful in children when IV access is not readily available.

Adult Dosage

When used for cardiac resuscitation in adults, epinephrine doses ranging from 0.1–1 mg have been used. In ACLS guidelines, a standard dosage of epinephrine (defined as 1 mg every 3–5 minutes by IV/IO injection) is recommended during adult cardiac arrest. Current evidence indicates that higher doses (e.g., 0.1–0.2 mg/kg) do not provide any benefits in terms of survival or neurologic outcomes compared with the standard dose and may be harmful.

The optimum dose of epinephrine during cardiac resuscitation has been a subject of controversy. Many clinicians had questioned the commonly used doses of 0.5–1 mg because of concern that these doses were not based on body weight, and thus may be lower than necessary for optimum cardiovascular effects. Interest in high doses of epinephrine was stimulated by animal studies indicating that such doses (e.g., 0.045–0.2 mg/kg) provided optimal improvement in hemodynamics, including ROSC, and timely achievement of successful cardiopulmonary resuscitation (CPR). Results of several clinical studies, including randomized controlled studies, found no substantial improvement in survival rates to hospital discharge nor trend for improved neurologic outcomes in patients with cardiac arrest receiving higher than usual doses of epinephrine, despite evidence of increased rates of ROSC and higher initial resuscitation rates with high-dose therapy. A retrospective study of functional neurologic outcomes (assessed by measurement of cerebral performance category) of patients with ventricular fibrillation who received high IV dosages of epinephrine during cardiac resuscitation found that such dosages were independently associated with unfavorable neurologic outcomes. Patients with unfavorable neurologic outcomes after resuscitation had received substantially higher median cumulative doses (i.e., 4 mg [range: 2–8 mg]) of epinephrine than those with favorable neurologic outcomes who received a median cumulative dose of 1 mg (range: less than 1–3 mg). These findings persisted after neurologic outcomes were stratified by duration of CPR and other potentially confounding conditions were considered. Based on the currently available evidence, the American Heart Association (AHA) states that it is reasonable to administer standard-dose epinephrine (1 mg every 3–5 minutes) during cardiac arrest in adults; high-dose epinephrine should not be used routinely, but may be considered in certain situations (e.g., overdosage of β-adrenergic or calcium-channel blocking agents).

The optimal timing of epinephrine administration, particularly in relation to defibrillation, is not known and may vary based on patient-specific factors and resuscitation conditions. In adults with asystole or pulseless electrical activity (PEA), epinephrine may be given as soon as feasible after the onset of cardiac arrest based on studies demonstrating improved survival to hospital discharge and increased ROSC when the drug was administered early during the course of treatment for a nonshockable rhythm.

If IV or IO access cannot be established during cardiac arrest, epinephrine may be administered via the endotracheal route. Although the optimal dose of epinephrine administered via an endotracheal tube remains to be established, some experts state that typical doses should be 2–2.5 times those administered IV.

If epinephrine is used for hemodynamic support following cardiac resuscitation, the usual IV dosage in adults is 0.1–0.5 mcg/kg per minute; the infusion rate should be titrated to patient response.

If epinephrine is used for the treatment of symptomatic bradycardia in adults, an initial infusion rate of 2–10 mcg/minute has been recommended and should be titrated to patient response. Intravascular volume and support should be assessed as needed.

Pediatric Dosage

When used for pediatric advanced life support (PALS), the usual IV or IO dose of epinephrine is 0.01 mg/kg (0.1 mL/kg of a 0.1-mg/mL solution), up to a maximum single dose of 1 mg, and the usual dose of epinephrine administered via an endotracheal tube is 0.1 mg/kg (0.1 mL/kg of a 1-mg/mL solution), up to a maximum single dose of 2.5 mg. The same IV, IO, or endotracheal dose should be repeated every 3–5 minutes if needed. Higher doses are not recommended because of the potential for harm, particularly in cases of asphyxia, and lack of survival benefit. AHA states, however, that high-dose epinephrine may be considered in exceptional circumstances (e.g., β-adrenergic blocking agent overdose).

In a prospective, randomized, double-blind study of 68 children who received either 0.01 mg/kg (standard dose) or 0.1 mg/kg (high dose) of epinephrine as rescue therapy for in-hospital cardiac arrest after failure of CPR and an initial dose of 0.01 mg/kg (standard dose) of epinephrine, high-dose rescue therapy was not associated with any benefits. High-dose epinephrine rescue therapy did not improve the survival rate at 24 hours compared with standard-dose therapy, and appeared to be harmful in children with asphyxia-precipitated cardiac arrest. In addition, a trend toward reduced rate of survival at 24 hours was observed among children who received high-dose therapy as compared with standard-dose therapy. Also, the rates of ROSC or survival to hospital discharge were not significantly different between the 2 groups.

For postresuscitation stabilization in pediatric patients, epinephrine may be administered by IV or IO infusion at a rate of 0.1–1 mcg/kg per minute; the rate of infusion should be adjusted based on patient response. Although low-dose IV infusions (less than 0.3 mcg/kg per minute) generally produce predominantly β-adrenergic effects, while higher-dose IV infusions (exceeding 0.3 mcg/kg per minute) generally result in α-adrenergic vasoconstriction, there is substantial interindividual variation in response, and infusion dosage should be titrated to the desired effect.

The usual neonatal IV dose of epinephrine is 0.01–0.03 mg/kg (0.1–0.3 mL/kg of a 0.1-mg/mL solution). AHA states that higher IV doses are not recommended; in pediatric and animal studies, administration of IV doses in the range of 0.1 mg/kg have been associated with exaggerated hypertension, decreased myocardial function, and worsening neurologic function. In addition, the sequence of hypotension followed by hypertension is likely to increase the risk of intracranial hemorrhage, especially in neonates. IV administration of epinephrine (0.01–0.03 mg/kg per dose) is the preferred route in neonates, since there are limited data available on endotracheal administration of epinephrine. If the endotracheal route is used, doses of 0.01 or 0.03 mg/kg will likely be ineffective. Although safety and efficacy have not been established, endotracheal administration of a higher dose (0.05–0.1 mg/kg) while IV access is being obtained may be considered.

In one retrospective study in children and neonates who received either mean doses of 0.01 mg/kg (standard dose) or 0.12 mg/kg (high dose) of epinephrine administered IV, via an endotracheal tube, or by IO infusion during CPR after cardiac arrest occurring during a hospital stay, high doses of the drug were not associated with improvements in rates of ROSC, short- or long-term survival rates, or overall outcome scores. In this study, the time to ROSC was substantially shorter in patients receiving standard doses of epinephrine than in those receiving higher doses. In addition, high-dose epinephrine may be associated with adverse effects such as increased myocardial oxygen consumption during cardiac resuscitation, a postarrest hyperadrenergic state with tachycardia, hypertension and ventricular ectopy, myocardial necrosis, and worse postarrest myocardial dysfunction. Additional clinical studies are needed to evaluate fully the optimum dosage regimen of epinephrine in pediatric patients.

For the emergency treatment of infants and children with bradycardia and cardiorespiratory compromise (with a palpable pulse), epinephrine may be given at a dose of 0.01 mg/kg (0.1 mL/kg of a 0.1-mg/mL solution) by IV/IO injection, and repeated every 3–5 minutes as needed; alternatively, an endotracheal dose of 0.1 mg/kg (0.1 mL/kg of a 1-mg/mL solution) may be given if IV/IO access is not available.

Septic Shock

For the treatment of hypotension during septic shock in adults, the manufacturer suggests an IV infusion rate of 0.05–2 mcg/kg per minute. The infusion rate may be increased in increments of 0.05–0.2 mcg/kg per minute every 10–15 minutes to achieve the desired blood pressure goal. The duration of therapy or total dose required is not known; continuous epinephrine infusion may be necessary for several hours or days until the patient's hemodynamic status improves. If epinephrine is used in pediatric patients with septic shock, some clinicians have recommended an IV infusion rate of 0.05–0.3 mcg/kg per minute, titrated to effect.

When therapy is discontinued, the infusion rate should be decreased gradually (e.g., by reducing the infusion rate every 30 minutes over a 12- to 24-hour period).

Bronchospasm

Parenteral Dosage

For the treatment of severe asthma exacerbations when orally inhaled, selective short-acting β₂-adrenergic agonists are not available, an expert panel of the National Asthma Education and Prevention Program (NAEPP) states that epinephrine 0.3–0.5 mg may be given subcutaneously every 20 minutes for 3 doses in adults and adolescents older than 12 years of age. Alternatively, some clinicians recommend a subcutaneous epinephrine dose of 0.01 mg/kg (using a 1-mg/mL solution), divided into 3 doses of approximately 0.3 mg each, administered at 20-minute intervals. For the treatment of severe asthma exacerbations in children 12 years of age or younger, 0.01 mg/kg of epinephrine (0.01 mL/kg using a 1-mg/mL solution), but no more than 0.3–0.5 mg per dose, may be administered by subcutaneous injection at 20-minute intervals for 3 doses.

For the treatment of bronchospasm in adults, some manufacturers recommend an epinephrine dose of 0.1–0.25 mg (1–2.5 mL of a 0.1-mg/mL solution) by slow IV injection. If IV administration of epinephrine is required for the management of asthma attacks in pediatric patients, some clinicians recommend a slow IV injection of 0.01 mg/kg in neonates and an initial IV dose of 0.05 mg (which may be repeated at 20- to 30-minute intervals) in infants.

Oral Inhalation Dosage

For the temporary relief of mild symptoms of intermittent asthma, the usual dose of 2.25% racepinephrine inhalation solution (equivalent to 1% epinephrine) in adults and children 4 years of age or older is 1–3 inhalations; doses should not be repeated more often than every 3 hours. Patients should be advised to seek medical assistance immediately if symptoms are not relieved within 20 minutes or become worse.

Local Vasoconstriction

As a topical hemostatic, solutions containing epinephrine in concentrations of 0.002–0.1% have been sprayed or applied with cotton or gauze to the skin, mucous membranes, or other tissues. In conjunction with local anesthetics, epinephrine may be used in concentrations of 0.002–0.02 mg/mL. The most frequently used concentration is 0.005 mg/mL.

CAUTIONS

• Adverse Effects

Epinephrine may cause fear, anxiety, tenseness, restlessness, headache, tremor, dizziness, lightheadedness, nervousness, sleeplessness, excitability, and weakness. In patients with parkinsonian syndrome, the drug increases rigidity and tremor. Patients with diabetes mellitus may experience transient increases in blood glucose concentrations. Epinephrine may aggravate or induce psychomotor agitation, disorientation, impaired memory, assaultive behavior, panic, hallucinations, suicidal or homicidal tendencies, and psychosis characterized by clear consciousness with schizophrenic-like thought disorder and paranoid delusions in some patients. Nausea, vomiting, sweating, pallor, respiratory difficulty, or respiratory weakness and apnea may also occur. It may be advisable to warn patients of possible adverse effects.

Epinephrine causes ECG changes including a decrease in T-wave amplitude in all leads in normal persons. Disturbances of cardiac rhythm and rate may result in palpitation and tachycardia. In patients with a perfusing rhythm, epinephrine may cause tachycardia, ventricular ectopy, tachyarrhythmias, hypertension, and vasoconstriction. In patients with coronary insufficiency and/or ischemic heart disease, epinephrine may aggravate or precipitate angina pectoris by increasing cardiac work and accentuating the insufficiency of the coronary circulation. Epinephrine can cause potentially fatal ventricular arrhythmias including fibrillation, especially in patients with organic heart disease or those receiving other drugs that sensitize the heart to arrhythmias. (See Drug Interactions.)

Epinephrine hydrochloride injection has been reported to cause syncope characterized by pallor, unconsciousness, and tachycardia in 4 children in doses varying from 0.05–0.2 mg subcutaneously. One of the children was later treated with 0.75 mg (0.15 mL of the longer-acting 5 mg/mL aqueous suspension, which is no longer commercially available in the US) subcutaneously with no such complication.

Overdosage or inadvertent IV injection of usual subcutaneous doses of epinephrine may cause hypertension. (See Acute Toxicity.) Subarachnoid hemorrhage and hemiplegia have resulted from hypertension, even following subcutaneous administration of usual doses. To avoid the possibility of dangerously high blood pressure from epinephrine therapy, blood pressure should be monitored closely during IV administration of the drug.

Epinephrine can cause tissue necrosis and sloughing at the site of injection as a result of local vasoconstriction. (See Cautions: Precautions and Contraindications.) Repeated injections of epinephrine can increase the risk of necrosis. Tissue necrosis may also occur in the extremities, kidneys, and liver. Fatal gas gangrene has occurred in patients receiving IM injection of epinephrine oil suspension (no longer available) in the buttocks. Gangrene of the lower extremities also may occur if epinephrine is infused into an ankle vein. It has been postulated that epinephrine-induced vasoconstriction reduces the oxygen tension of tissues, enabling anaerobic *Clostridium welchii* which may be present in the patient's feces and on the buttocks to multiply. IM injection of the drug into the buttocks should be avoided. If gas gangrene is suspected after epinephrine administration, treatment should be instituted immediately.

Prolonged use or overdosage of epinephrine can result in severe metabolic acidosis because of elevated blood concentrations of lactic acid. It has been proposed that epinephrine may cause hyperuricemia by its vasoconstrictor action in the kidneys; however, elevated BUN has been reported only rarely in cases of overdosage. IV use of epinephrine may initially constrict renal blood vessels and decrease urine formation.

Absorption of epinephrine from the respiratory tract following large doses by oral inhalation may result in adverse effects similar to those occurring after parenteral administration. Rarely, bronchial irritation and edema may occur. In some patients, severe prolonged asthma attacks may be precipitated. Rebound bronchospasm may occur when the effects of epinephrine end. Arterial oxygen tension, already reduced during asthmatic attacks, may be further reduced following oral inhalation of epinephrine. Dryness of pharyngeal membranes may follow oral inhalation and may be prevented by rinsing the mouth with water immediately after use of the drug. If epinephrine inhalation is inadvertently swallowed, epigastric pain may occur.

● Precautions and Contraindications

Vasopressor therapy is *not* a substitute for replacement of blood, plasma, fluids, and/or electrolytes. Blood volume depletion should be corrected as fully as possible before epinephrine therapy is instituted.

Because severe local adverse effects (e.g., tissue necrosis) may occur, extravasation of epinephrine infusions must be avoided. *The site of infusion should be checked frequently for free flow and the infused vein should be observed for blanching.* Infusion into leg veins, especially in geriatric patients or those with occlusive vascular diseases (e.g., atherosclerosis, arteriosclerosis, diabetic endarteritis, Buerger's disease) should be avoided. If blanching is observed in the infused vein, changing the infusion site periodically may be advisable. If extravasation occurs, 10–15 mL of sodium chloride solution containing 5–10 mg of phentolamine mesylate should be infiltrated (using a syringe with a fine hypodermic needle) liberally throughout the affected area, which is identified by a cold, hard, and pallid appearance. Immediate and conspicuous local hyperemic changes occur if the area is infiltrated within 12 hours; therefore, phentolamine should be administered as soon as possible after extravasation is noted.

Epinephrine should not be administered in the digits, hands, or feet. Accidental injection into the digits, hands, or feet may result in loss of blood flow to the affected area and has been associated with tissue necrosis.

Particular attention should be paid to the appropriate concentration and route of administration of epinephrine since serious adverse effects (e.g., cerebral hemorrhage) have occurred after concentrated solutions of epinephrine intended for IM administration were administered IV. Because of the risks associated with IV use, epinephrine generally should be administered by the IV route only in extreme situations (such as in the treatment of septic or anaphylactic shock, cardiac arrest, or when the patient is unresponsive to multiple IM injections). (See Dosage and Administration: Administration.)

Racepinephrine, a racemic mixture of epinephrine, shares the toxic potentials of epinephrine, and the usual precautions of epinephrine therapy should be observed. Adverse reactions to epinephrine may be most likely to occur in hypertensive or hyperthyroid patients, and the drug must be administered with extreme caution, if at all, to such patients. Epinephrine should be administered with caution to geriatric patients, patients with diabetes mellitus, hyperthyroidism, Parkinson's disease, pheochromocytoma, or cardiovascular diseases (including cardiac arrhythmias, coronary artery disease, and organic heart disease), and/or those with a history of sensitivity to sympathomimetic amines.

Coronary insufficiency is usually considered to be a contraindication to parenteral use of the drug. The drug must be used cautiously in patients with bronchial asthma and emphysema who may also have degenerative heart disease. Epinephrine injection should be used with caution in patients with psychoneurotic disorders.

Some commercially available formulations of epinephrine hydrochloride or racepinephrine hydrochloride contain sulfites that can cause allergic-type reactions, including anaphylaxis and life-threatening or less severe asthmatic episodes, in certain susceptible individuals. The overall prevalence of sulfite sensitivity in the general population is unknown but probably low; such sensitivity appears to occur more frequently in asthmatic than in nonasthmatic individuals. The presence of sulfites in a parenteral epinephrine preparation and the possibility of allergic-type reactions should *not* deter use of the drug when indicated for the treatment of serious allergic reactions or for other emergency situations. Epinephrine is the preferred treatment for such conditions, and currently available alternatives to epinephrine may not be optimally effective. The possibility of adverse reactions to sulfite(s) contained in the preparation should be considered in asthmatic patients who show paradoxical worsening of respiratory function following use of the drug or whose symptoms worsen or in whom bronchodilatory response decreases with increasing use of the drug.

Patients considering *self-medication* with racepinephrine as a bronchodilator should be advised to use the drug only if they have been diagnosed by a clinician as having asthma; patients also should be advised that the drug should not be used for *self-medication* if they ever have been hospitalized for asthma or are currently receiving a prescription drug for the management of this condition unless otherwise directed by a clinician. These patients also should be advised not to use the drug if they have cardiovascular disease, hypertension, diabetes mellitus, thyroid disease, angle-closure (narrow-angle) glaucoma, seizures, a psychiatric or emotional condition, or difficulty urinating because of prostatic hypertrophy unless directed by a clinician. In addition, patients should be advised not to exceed recommended dosages or frequency of administration unless otherwise instructed by a clinician. Patients should contact their clinician if their symptoms are not relieved within 20 minutes or become worse, more than the recommended dosage is required, or asthma attacks become more frequent (i.e., more than 2 asthma attacks in a week). Patients should be cautioned that racepinephrine can cause hypertension and tachycardia, which could increase the risk of cardiovascular disease, stroke, or death. Foods, beverages, and dietary supplements that contain stimulants (e.g., caffeine) should be avoided.

There are no absolute contraindications to the use of epinephrine in life-threatening conditions. Relative contraindications to epinephrine include shock (other than anaphylactic and septic shock), known hypersensitivity to sympathomimetic amines, coronary insufficiency, and cardiac dilatation, as well as use in most patients with angle-closure glaucoma or organic brain damage. The drug is contraindicated for use during general anesthesia with agents such as cyclopropane and halogenated hydrocarbon anesthetics (e.g., halothane). (See Drug Interactions: General Anesthetics.) In conjunction with local anesthetics, epinephrine is contraindicated for use in certain areas (e.g., fingers, toes, ears).

● Pregnancy, Fertility, and Lactation

Pregnancy

Epinephrine usually inhibits spontaneous or oxytocin-induced contractions of the pregnant human uterus and may delay the second stage of labor. In dosages sufficient to reduce uterine contractions, the drug may cause a prolonged period of uterine atony with hemorrhage. If used during pregnancy, epinephrine may cause anoxia to the fetus and/or spontaneous abortion. When administered in advanced cardiovascular life support (ACLS) during cardiac resuscitation, epinephrine may decrease blood flow to the uterus; however, the woman must be resuscitated for survival of the fetus. Some manufacturers state that epinephrine should be avoided during the second stage of labor; parenteral administration of the drug to maintain blood pressure during spinal anesthesia for delivery can cause acceleration of fetal heart rate and should not be used in obstetric patients when maternal systolic/diastolic blood pressure exceeds 130/80 mm Hg. Epinephrine should be administered cautiously by oral inhalation to pregnant patients. Epinephrine should be used during pregnancy only if the potential benefits justify the possible risks to the fetus. There is some evidence to support that epidural administration of some local anesthetics (e.g., lidocaine) with epinephrine during labor is safe.

DRUG INTERACTIONS

• Sympathomimetic Agents

Epinephrine must not be administered concomitantly with other sympathomimetic agents (e.g., isoproterenol) because of the possibility of additive effects and increased toxicity.

• α- and β-Adrenergic Blocking Agents

The cardiac and bronchodilating effects of epinephrine are antagonized by β-adrenergic blocking drugs such as propranolol, and the vasoconstriction and hypertension caused by high doses of epinephrine are antagonized by α-adrenergic blocking agents such as phentolamine. Because of their α-adrenergic blocking properties, ergot alkaloids can reverse the pressor response to epinephrine. Concomitant use of β-adrenergic blocking drugs (e.g., propranolol) may also potentiate the pressor effects of epinephrine.

• Cardiac Glycosides

Epinephrine should not be used in patients receiving excessive dosages of other drugs (e.g., cardiac glycosides) that can sensitize the heart to arrhythmias.

• Diuretics

Concomitant use of diuretics may antagonize the pressor effect and potentiate the arrhythmogenic effects of epinephrine. Some diuretics also may potentiate the hypokalemic effects of epinephrine.

• General Anesthetics

Administration of epinephrine in patients receiving cyclopropane or halogenated hydrocarbon general anesthetics that increase cardiac irritability and seem to sensitize the myocardium to epinephrine may result in arrhythmias including PVCs, tachycardia, or fibrillation. Epinephrine is contraindicated for use with chloroform, trichloroethylene, or cyclopropane and should be used cautiously, if at all, with other halogenated hydrocarbon anesthetics such as halothane. Epinephrine may not be absorbed rapidly enough to cause serious adverse effects when applied topically as a hemostatic in patients undergoing short surgical procedures such as tonsillectomy and adenoidectomy using halothane anesthesia. Prophylactic administration of lidocaine or prophylactic IV administration of propranolol 0.05 mg/kg may protect against ventricular irritability if epinephrine is used during anesthesia with a halogenated hydrocarbon anesthetic. In one study, arrhythmias occurring after parenteral use of epinephrine during general anesthesia responded promptly to IV propranolol 0.05 mg/kg.

• Hypotensive Agents

Epinephrine may antagonize the neuronal blockade produced by guanethidine (not commercially available in the US), resulting in loss of antihypertensive effectiveness. The vasopressor effect of epinephrine also may be antagonized by rapidly acting vasodilators (e.g., nitrates) and other antihypertensive agents.

• Monoamine Oxidase Inhibitors

Monoamine oxidase (MAO) is one of the enzymes responsible for epinephrine metabolism. The manufacturer states that epinephrine should be administered with caution in patients receiving an MAO inhibitor because severe, prolonged hypertension may result.

• Oxytocic Drugs

Concomitant use of epinephrine with oxytocics may result in severe, persistent hypertension.

• Other Drugs

Tricyclic antidepressants such as imipramine, some antihistamines (especially diphenhydramine, tripelennamine, and dexchlorpheniramine), and thyroid hormones may potentiate the effects of epinephrine, especially on heart rhythm and rate. Potentiation by tricyclic antidepressants or antihistamines may result from inhibition of tissue uptake of epinephrine or norepinephrine or by increased adrenoreceptor sensitivity to epinephrine. Concomitant use of catechol-O-methyltransferase (COMT) inhibitors (e.g., entacapone), clonidine, or doxapram

also may potentiate the pressor effects of epinephrine and quinidine may potentiate the arrhythmogenic effects of epinephrine.

Concomitant use of corticosteroids or theophylline also may potentiate the hypokalemic effects of epinephrine.

Epinephrine should not be used to counteract circulatory collapse or hypotension caused by phenothiazines; a reversal of epinephrine's pressor effects resulting in further lowering of blood pressure may occur.

Because epinephrine may cause hyperglycemia, patients with diabetes mellitus receiving epinephrine may require increased dosage of insulin or oral hypoglycemic agents.

ACUTE TOXICITY

• Pathogenesis

Autopsy findings in patients who died of epinephrine overdosage revealed evidence of circulatory collapse, and most organs and veins were congested with blood. In test animals, there is evidence that death is the result of respiratory arrest caused by hypertension. Death resulting from epinephrine overdosage may partially depend on factors other than the dose received; some patients have died following IV doses not exceeding 10 mg while others have survived doses as high as 30 mg IV or 110 mg subcutaneously.

• Manifestations and Treatment

After overdosage or inadvertent IV administration of usual subcutaneous doses of epinephrine, systolic and diastolic blood pressure rise sharply; venous pressure also rises. Cerebrovascular or other hemorrhage and hemiplegia may result, especially in geriatric patients. Because epinephrine is rapidly inactivated in the body, treatment of acute toxicity is mainly supportive. If necessary, the pressor effects of the drug may be counteracted by rapidly acting α-adrenergic blocking drugs such as phentolamine. Prolonged hypotension may follow, and another pressor agent such as norepinephrine may be required. Pulmonary edema may result from pulmonary arterial hypertension; administration of a rapidly acting α-adrenergic blocking drug and/or intermittent positive-pressure respiration may be required if pulmonary edema interferes with respiration. Respiratory difficulties including hyperventilation sometimes preceded by a brief period of apnea may also occur. Epinephrine overdosage causes transient bradycardia followed by tachycardia and may cause other potentially fatal cardiac arrhythmias. PVCs may appear within 1 minute after injection and may be followed by multifocal ventricular tachycardia (prefibrillation rhythm). Atrial tachycardia, occasionally accompanied by atrioventricular block, may occur after the drug's effects on the ventricles subside. Prolonged ECG changes and substantial changes in serum AST (SGOT) concentration were considered evidence of possibly permanent myocardial injury caused by overdosage of epinephrine in 2 patients. Arrhythmias, if they occur, may be counteracted by a β-adrenergic blocking drug such as propranolol. Kidney failure, metabolic acidosis, and cold, white skin may also occur.

PHARMACOLOGY

Epinephrine acts directly on both α- and β-adrenergic receptors of tissues innervated by sympathetic nerves except the sweat glands and arteries of the face. It is believed that β-adrenergic effects result from stimulation of the production of cyclic adenosine-3′,5′-monophosphate (AMP) by activation of the enzyme adenyl cyclase, whereas α-adrenergic effects result from inhibition of adenyl cyclase activity. The main effects of therapeutic parenteral doses of epinephrine are relaxation of smooth muscle of the bronchial tree, cardiac stimulation, and dilation of skeletal muscle vasculature.

• Respiratory Effects

Epinephrine relaxes bronchial smooth muscle by stimulation of β_2-adrenergic receptors and constricts bronchial arterioles by stimulation of α-adrenergic receptors when administered parenterally or by oral inhalation. In patients with bronchial constriction, the drug relieves bronchospasm, reduces congestion and edema, and increases tidal volume and vital capacity. However, decreased arterial oxygen tension may not be increased and may be further reduced. Respiration rate is increased briefly, but epinephrine has no clinical value as a respiratory stimulant. In some patients receiving the drug IV, respiratory stimulation may be preceded by a brief period of apnea, probably caused by a direct inhibition of the respiratory center.

Epinephrine inhibits histamine release and antagonizes the effect of the mediator on end organs. As a result, the drug may reverse bronchiolar constriction, vasodilation, and edema produced by this mediator.

● Cardiovascular Effects

Systemically absorbed epinephrine acts on β_1-adrenergic receptors in the heart producing a positive chronotropic effect through the sinoatrial node and a positive inotropic effect on the myocardium. Cardiac output, oxygen consumption, and the work of the heart are increased, and cardiac efficiency is decreased. Epinephrine increases the irritability of the heart muscle and often alters the rhythmic function of the ventricles, especially after large doses or when the heart has been sensitized to this action by other drugs including digitalis and certain anesthetics or by acute myocardial infarction. Arrhythmias including ventricular extrasystoles and fibrillation may result. In patients with cardiopulmonary arrest, epinephrine can convert asystole to sinus rhythm. Epinephrine has a direct constricting effect on coronary arteries, but this effect is overcome by indirect vasodilation caused by enhanced cardiac metabolism secondary to cardiac stimulation. As a result, coronary blood flow is increased. Cardiac stimulation produced by epinephrine increases left atrial pressure, and peripheral vasoconstriction causes redistribution of blood from the systemic to the pulmonary circulation. Pulmonary arterial hypertension and increased pulmonary capillary filtration pressure may occur; pulmonary edema may result.

Epinephrine constricts arterioles in the skin, mucous membranes, and viscera after parenteral administration by its effect on α-adrenergic receptors and reduces cutaneous blood flow, especially in the hands and feet. Topically applied epinephrine produces local vasoconstriction and hemostasis in bleeding from small vessels but does not control bleeding from larger vessels. Small doses of parenterally administered epinephrine dilate arterioles of the skeletal muscles as a result of stimulation of β-adrenergic receptors, whereas larger doses stimulate α-adrenergic receptors and cause constriction of these arterioles. With usual therapeutic doses of the drug, the dilator effects predominate; blood flow to the skeletal muscle is increased and total peripheral resistance is decreased. Systolic blood pressure is moderately increased, mainly because of increased cardiac output; however, diastolic blood pressure may be decreased as a result of vasodilation. Doses of epinephrine large enough to constrict blood vessels in the skeletal muscle, however, cause an increase in peripheral resistance and elevate both systolic and diastolic blood pressure. When the drug's effects on α-adrenergic receptors end, the effect on β-adrenergic receptors persists and hypotension may result.

Constriction of renal blood vessels by epinephrine, especially after IV administration, initially reduces renal blood flow and increases renal vascular resistance. Urine flow and excretion of sodium, potassium, and chloride are decreased. Renal blood flow and urine flow may then increase as a result of elevated blood pressure. Glomerular filtration rate is not greatly altered by the drug; alterations in electrolyte and water excretion may be caused by renal vascular changes, a direct tubular action, or an indirect effect through the posterior pituitary. Very large IV or intra-arterial doses of epinephrine may cause total renal shutdown which may be prolonged by trapping of the drug in the vessels as a result of vasoconstriction.

● Metabolic Effects

Epinephrine increases glycogenolysis in the liver, reduces glucose uptake by tissues, and inhibits insulin release in the pancreas, resulting in hyperglycemia. Muscle glycogenolysis also increases, and lactic acid blood concentrations are elevated. Transient hyperkalemia may also occur and may be followed by more prolonged hypokalemia. Epinephrine has calorigenic activity; oxygen consumption may increase by as much as 20–30% after parenteral administration of usual doses. Body temperature may be elevated, partly because of cutaneous vasoconstriction. Blood concentrations of free fatty acids are increased as a result of increased lipolysis in adipose tissue, and plasma concentrations of cholesterol, phospholipids, and low-density lipoproteins are also generally elevated. Fat may be deposited in muscles and liver.

● Other Effects

Epinephrine has no direct effect on cerebral arterioles or cerebral blood flow. However, elevations in cerebral blood flow and oxygen consumption may occur secondary to increased blood pressure. The drug is not a powerful CNS stimulant but may cause restlessness, apprehension, headache, and tremor, probably resulting from peripheral effects. In patients with parkinsonian syndrome, epinephrine increases rigidity and tremor by an unknown mechanism.

Epinephrine generally relaxes smooth muscles of the GI tract by stimulation of either α- or β-adrenergic receptors but contracts the pyloric and ileocecal sphincters by stimulation of α-adrenergic receptors. Because these effects are transient, inconsistent, and usually occur only with doses causing marked cardiovascular response, they have no therapeutic application.

The effects of epinephrine on the uterus are probably mediated through both α- and β-adrenergic receptors in the myometrium and vary with hormonal influences, the route of administration, and the dose given. The drug usually inhibits spontaneous or oxytocin-induced contractions of the pregnant human uterus and may delay the second stage of labor. Transient uterine hyperactivity frequently occurs after the drug is discontinued. In dosage sufficient to reduce uterine contractions, epinephrine may cause prolonged uterine atony with hemorrhage. Use of the drug during pregnancy may cause anoxia in the fetus.

PHARMACOKINETICS

● Absorption

Orally ingested epinephrine is rapidly metabolized in the GI tract and liver; pharmacologically active concentrations are not reached when the drug is given orally. Epinephrine is well absorbed after subcutaneous or IM injection; absorption can be hastened by massaging the injection site. Both rapid and prolonged absorption occur after subcutaneous injection of the longer-acting aqueous suspension (no longer commercially available in the US). Epinephrine also is absorbed following endotracheal administration, although serum concentrations achieved may be only 10% of those with an equivalent IV dose. After oral inhalation of epinephrine absorption is slight and the effects of the drug are restricted mainly to the respiratory tract. Absorption increases somewhat when larger doses are inhaled, and systemic effects may occur.

Epinephrine has a rapid onset and short duration of action when solutions of the drug are administered parenterally or by oral inhalation. Subcutaneous administration of epinephrine hydrochloride injection in patients with asthmatic attacks may produce bronchodilation within 5–10 minutes and maximal effects in about 20 minutes. Following subcutaneous injection of the longer-acting aqueous epinephrine suspension, the onset of action is as rapid as that occurring after subcutaneous administration of epinephrine hydrochloride aqueous injection; however, the effects are more prolonged and may persist for several hours. After oral inhalation of epinephrine, bronchodilation usually occurs within 1 minute.

● Distribution

Epinephrine crosses the placenta but not the blood-brain barrier. The drug is distributed into milk.

● Elimination

The pharmacologic actions of epinephrine are terminated mainly by uptake and metabolism in sympathetic nerve endings. Circulating drug is metabolized in the liver and other tissues by a combination of reactions involving the enzymes catechol-O-methyltransferase (COMT) and monoamine oxidase (MAO). The major metabolites are metanephrine and 3-methoxy-4-hydroxymandelic acid (vanillylmandelic acid, VMA) both of which are inactive. About 40% of a parenteral dose of epinephrine is excreted in urine as metanephrine, 40% as VMA, 7% as 3-methoxy-4-hydroxyphenolglycol, 2% as 3,4-dihydroxymandelic acid, and the remainder as acetylated derivatives. These metabolites are excreted mostly as the sulfate conjugates and, to a lesser extent, the glucuronide conjugates. Only small amounts of the drug are excreted unchanged.

CHEMISTRY AND STABILITY

● Chemistry

Epinephrine is an endogenous catecholamine which is the active principle of the adrenal medulla. Both the endogenous substance and the official preparation are the levorotatory isomer which is 15 times more active than is the dextrorotatory isomer. The drug is also commercially available as racepinephrine hydrochloride, which is a racemic mixture of the hydrochlorides of the enantiomorphs of epinephrine. Racepinephrine is about one-half as active as the levorotatory isomer.

Epinephrine may be obtained from the adrenal glands of animals or prepared synthetically; that obtained from animals may contain up to 4% norepinephrine. Epinephrine occurs as a white to nearly white, microcrystalline powder or granules. Epinephrine is only very slightly soluble in water and in alcohol but readily forms water soluble salts (such as the hydrochloride and bitartrate) with acids.

Racepinephrine hydrochloride occurs as a fine, white powder and is freely soluble in water and sparingly soluble in alcohol. Racepinephrine hydrochloride oral inhalation has a pH of 2–3.5.

● *Stability*

Epinephrine, epinephrine salts, racepinephrine hydrochloride, and preparations containing the drugs gradually darken on exposure to light and air and must be stored in tight, light-resistant containers. Epinephrine injection should be stored at room temperature (approximately 25°C). Freezing of racepinephrine hydrochloride oral inhalation should be avoided. In some commercially available injections, the air has been replaced with nitrogen to avoid oxidation. Withdrawal of doses from multiple-dose vials introduces air into the vials, subjecting the remaining epinephrine to oxidation. Oxidation of the drug imparts first a pink, then a brown color; epinephrine preparations must not be used if they have a pinkish or darker than slightly yellow color or contain a precipitate. Racepinephrine hydrochloride solutions must not be used if they are brown or contain a precipitate. Commercially available epinephrine preparations may contain a variety of preservatives including the antioxidants, sodium bisulfite or sodium metabisulfite, and bacteriostatic agents. Commercially available preparations vary in stability, depending on the form in which epinephrine is present and on the preservatives used. The manufacturer's directions should be followed with respect to storage requirements for each product.

Epinephrine is readily destroyed by oxidizing agents or alkalies including sodium bicarbonate, halogens, permanganates, chromates, nitrates, nitrites, and salts of easily reducible metals such as iron, copper, and zinc. Epinephrine injection has been reported to be physically incompatible with many drugs, but the compatibility depends on several factors (e.g., concentration of the drugs, specific diluents used, resulting pH, temperature). Specialized references should be consulted for specific compatibility information. Epinephrine may be mixed with 0.9% sodium chloride injection but is incompatible with 5% sodium chloride injection. Stability of epinephrine in 5% dextrose injection decreases when the pH exceeds 5.5.

PREPARATIONS

Effective May 1, 2016, a new USP labeling standard for Epinephrine Injection, USP has been implemented. Single-entity preparations of epinephrine injection will be expressed only in terms of strength per mL; use of ratios (e.g., 1:1000 or 1:10,000) to express concentrations is no longer acceptable. Epinephrine injection 1:1000 is equivalent to 1 mg/mL and epinephrine injection 1:10,000 is equivalent to 0.1 mg/mL.

Excipients in commercially available drug preparations may have clinically important effects in some individuals; consult specific product labeling for details.

EPINEPHrine

Parenteral		
Injection	0.1 mg/mL*	**EPINEPHrine Injection** (available in prefilled syringes)
	0.5 mg/mL	**EpiPen® Jr. Auto-Injector** (delivers a single 0.15-mg [0.3 mL] dose), Meridian
	1 mg/mL*	**Adrenaclick® Auto-Injector** (available in dose of 0.15 mg [0.15 mL] or 0.3 mg [0.3 mL]), Amedra
		Adrenalin®, Par
		Auvi-Q® Auto-Injector (available in dose of 0.15 mg [0.15 mL] or 0.3 mg [0.3 mL]), Sanofi-Aventis
		EPINEPHrine Injection
		EpiPen® Auto-Injector (delivers a single 0.3-mg [0.3 mL] dose), Meridian

* available from one or more manufacturer, distributor, and/or repackager by generic (nonproprietary) name

racEPINEPHrine Hydrochloride

Oral-inhalation		
Solution, for nebulization	2.25% (of racepinephrine)	S2®, Nephron Pharmaceuticals

† Use is not currently included in the labeling approved by the US Food and Drug Administration.

Selected Revisions September 10, 2024, © Copyright, March 1, 1976, American Society of Health-System Pharmacists, Inc.

Norepinephrine Bitartrate

12:12.12 · α- AND β-ADRENERGIC AGONISTS

■ Norepinephrine bitartrate is an endogenous catecholamine vasopressor that predominantly acts by a direct effect on α-adrenergic receptors and to a lesser extent on β-adrenergic receptors.

USES

● Acute Hypotensive States

Norepinephrine bitartrate is used to raise blood pressure in the management of adults with severe, acute hypotension. Studies evaluating safety and efficacy of norepinephrine for this use have generally found that compared with other vasopressors, norepinephrine was associated with similar hemodynamic and mortality outcomes and lower risk for arrhythmia. Guidelines for the treatment of sepsis and septic shock generally recommend norepinephrine as a first-line vasopressor for hemodynamic management. The American Heart Association (AHA) states that in the management of cardiogenic shock, norepinephrine may be the vasopressor of choice in many patients, although the optimal first-line vasopressor in this setting remains unclear.

Although not FDA-labeled for use in pediatric patients, norepinephrine also has been used for blood pressure management in pediatric patients with fluid-refractory septic shock†.

Clinical Experience

Norepinephrine in the management of sepsis and septic shock has been evaluated in various studies. One meta-analysis of 11 randomized controlled trials, which included a total of approximately 4800 patients, evaluated the efficacy and safety of norepinephrine compared with other vasopressors, including dopamine, epinephrine, phenylephrine, and vasopressin. Analysis of the primary outcomes revealed no substantial differences between norepinephrine and other vasopressors in the number of patients achieving target mean arterial pressure [MAP] (based on data from 2 trials rated as low-quality) or in all-cause 28-day mortality (based on data from 7 high-quality trials). However, norepinephrine was associated with substantially lower risk for arrhythmia compared with other vasopressors (based on data from 6 trials rated as moderate-quality). Another meta-analysis of 11 trials comparing norepinephrine with dopamine found that norepinephrine was associated with a substantially reduced risk of all-cause mortality as well as reduced risk of major adverse events and cardiac arrhythmias. No other substantial differences in mortality were identify in other comparisons of norepinephrine with epinephrine, phenylephrine, and vasopressin.

Safety and efficacy of norepinephrine in the treatment of cardiogenic shock have also been evaluated in various studies. One meta-analysis of 9 trials comparing norepinephrine with dopamine found that norepinephrine was associated with substantially lower risks of 28-day mortality, arrhythmic events, and GI effects. Another meta-analysis, which identified only one trial that compared norepinephrine with epinephrine in the treatment of cardiogenic shock, found no substantial difference in the risk of all-cause 28-day mortality.

Clinical Perspective

Vasopressors such as norepinephrine are used in the management of shock to restore blood pressure and tissue perfusion after initial fluid resuscitation is attempted. Norepinephrine is a potent vasoconstrictor that increases MAP with minimal change in heart rate and cardiac output, and has been shown to preserve tissue perfusion when titrated to effect (i.e., MAP of at least 65 mm Hg). The Surviving Sepsis Campaign provides recommendations on the management of sepsis and septic shock, which includes guidance on resuscitation and hemodynamic management in this setting. Initial management involves administration of IV crystalloid fluid within the first 3 hours of resuscitation in patients with sepsis-induced hypoperfusion or septic shock. The guideline recommends norepinephrine as the first-line vasopressor of choice in adults with septic shock over other vasopressors; in settings where norepinephrine is not available, epinephrine or dopamine may be used as alternatives. For adults with inadequate MAP response

to norepinephrine, the guideline suggests adding vasopressin instead of escalating the dose of norepinephrine. For adults with continued inadequate MAP response despite norepinephrine and vasopressin, the guideline suggests adding epinephrine. For adults with cardiac dysfunction and persistent hypoperfusion despite adequate volume status and arterial blood pressure, addition of dobutamine to norepinephrine or use of epinephrine alone is recommended. Vasopressor therapy in adults should initially target a MAP of 65 mm Hg.

The American Heart Association (AHA) guideline for pediatric basic and advanced life support provides recommendation for resuscitation in infants and children with septic shock. In those with fluid-refractory septic shock, the guideline states that it is reasonable to use either norepinephrine or epinephrine as an initial vasopressor infusion; if these are unavailable, dopamine may be considered.

AHA published a scientific statement on the contemporary management of cardiogenic shock, offering insight on the medical management of hemodynamic instability. Initial management with vasopressors is directed by the cause and presentation of cardiogenic shock. Norepinephrine is generally listed as an option for management of cardiogenic shock with presentation that is classic wet and cold, euvolemic cold and dry, vasodilatory warm and wet or mixed cardiogenic and vasodilatory, right ventricular shock, mitral regurgitation, and pericardial tamponade. Norepinephrine is associated with lower risk of arrhythmia and may be the vasopressor of choice in many patients, although the optimal first-line vasopressor in cardiogenic shock remains unclear.

● Prolongation of Anesthesia

Norepinephrine has been added to solutions of some local anesthetics to decrease the rate of vascular absorption of the anesthetic and prolong the duration of anesthesia†. Because norepinephrine is less potent than epinephrine and must be used in higher concentrations potentially causing greater risk of adverse effects, epinephrine is more commonly used for this purpose.

DOSAGE AND ADMINISTRATION

● General

Pretreatment Screening

● Correct hypovolemia prior to initiating norepinephrine.

Patient Monitoring

● Monitor blood pressure every 2 minutes until the desired hemodynamic effect is achieved, and then monitor blood pressure every 5 minutes throughout the infusion.

● Monitor for changes to the skin or the extremities in patients susceptible to tissue ischemia.

● Monitor for signs of extravasation.

● Perform continuous cardiac monitoring in patients with arrhythmias.

● Monitor cardiac rhythm in patients treated with halogenated anesthetics.

● Monitor for hypertension in patients receiving concomitant treatment with drugs that can cause hypertension (e.g., monoamine oxidase inhibitors, tricyclic antidepressants).

● Monitor glucose concentration in patients treated with antidiabetic agents.

Dispensing and Administration Precautions

● Based on the Institute for Safe Medication Practices (ISMP), norepinephrine is a high-alert medication that has a heightened risk of causing significant patient harm when used in error.

● Administration

Norepinephrine bitartrate is administered by IV infusion. To minimize the risk of necrosis, infusion of the drug should be given into a large vein; avoid infusions into the veins of the leg in elderly patients or in patients with occlusive vascular disease of the legs. Care must be taken to avoid extravasation because local necrosis may result; check the infusion site frequently for free flow and monitor for signs of extravasation.

Visually inspect solutions of norepinephrine for particulate matter and discoloration prior to administration whenever solution and container permit. Do not use the drug if it is discolored (e.g., pink, dark yellow) or contains any particulate matter.

Store norepinephrine bitartrate at 20–25°C (excursions permitted to 15–30°C) in the original carton until the time of administration and protect from light. Discard any unused portion. Avoid contact of the drug with iron salts, alkalies, or oxidizing agents. Administer whole blood or plasma, if indicated during therapy with norepinephrine, separately.

Norepinephrine bitartrate injection concentrate must be diluted prior to administration; alternatively, commercially available solutions of norepinephrine in 5% dextrose or norepinephrine in 0.9% sodium chloride may be used without dilution.

Dilution

Prior to administration, the commercially available concentrate for injection must be diluted with a dextrose-containing solution (5% dextrose injection, with or without 0.9% sodium chloride injection); the manufacturer states that dilution with 0.9% sodium chloride injection alone is not recommended because of possible loss of potency due to oxidation. The concentration of norepinephrine and the infusion rate depend on the drug and fluid requirements of the individual patient; use higher concentration solutions in patients requiring fluid restriction. The infusion solution is usually prepared by adding 4 mg of norepinephrine (4 mL of the commercially available injection) to 1 liter of a 5% dextrose-containing solution; the resultant solution contains 4 mcg/mL. The diluted norepinephrine solution may be stored for up to 24 hours at room temperature prior to use.

Standardize 4 Safety

Standardize 4 safety (S4S) is a national patient safety initiative to standardize drug concentrations to reduce medication errors, especially during transitions of care. Multidisciplinary expert panels were convened to determine recommended standard concentrations. Because recommendations from the S4S panels may differ from the manufacturer's prescribing information, caution is advised when using concentrations that differ from labeling, particularly when using rate information from the label. For additional information on S4S (including updates that may be available), see http://www.ashp.org/standardize4safety.

TABLE 1. Standardize 4 Safety Continuous Infusion Standards for Norepinephrine

Patient Population	Concentration Standard[a]	Dosing Units
Adults	16 mcg/mL	mcg/kg/min
	32 mcg/mL	
	128 mcg/mL	
Pediatric patients (<50 kg)	16 mcg/mL[b]	mcg/kg/min
	32 mcg/mL	
	64 mcg/mL	

[a] The concentrations for epinephrine and norepinephrine are intentionally different to avoid confusion as recommended by the S4S panel and ISMP

[b] Babies under 500 g may require a lower concentration

Dosage

Avoid abrupt withdrawal of norepinephrine infusion; discontinue by reducing the flow rate gradually.

Acute Hypotensive States

Pediatric Patients

If norepinephrine is used in pediatric patients†, some clinicians have recommended an infusion rate ranging from 0.05–2.5 mcg/kg per minute, titrated to effect.

Adults

For restoration of blood pressure in adults with acute hypotensive states, the usual initial dosage of norepinephrine is 8–12 mcg/minute. The typical maintenance IV

dosage is 2–4 mcg/minute. Other experts have described common dosage ranges of norepinephrine as 0.01–0.5 mcg/kg per minute. Adjust the dosage to maintain the desired hemodynamic effect.

● Special Populations

Hepatic Impairment

The manufacturer makes no specific dosage recommendations for patients with hepatic impairment.

Renal Impairment

The manufacturer makes no specific dosage recommendations for patients with renal impairment.

Geriatric Patients

The manufacturer makes no specific dosage recommendations for geriatric patients. In general, dose selection for an elderly patient should be cautious, usually starting at the low end of the dosing range, reflecting the greater frequency of decreased hepatic, renal, or cardiac function, and of concomitant disease or other drug therapy.

CAUTIONS

● Contraindications
- None.

● Warnings/Precautions

Tissue Ischemia

In patients who have hypovolemia-related hypotension, norepinephrine can cause severe peripheral and visceral vasoconstriction, decreased renal perfusion and reduced urine output, tissue hypoxia, lactic acidosis, and reduced systemic blood flow, even in patients with "normal" blood pressure. Address hypovolemia prior to initiating norepinephrine. Avoid norepinephrine in patients with mesenteric or peripheral vascular thrombosis, which may increase ischemic risk and extend the area of infarction.

Extravasation may occur with administration of norepinephrine. To prevent sloughing and necrosis in areas in which extravasation has occurred, infiltrate the extravasated area with 10–15 mL of sodium chloride solution containing 5–10 mg of phentolamine mesylate using a syringe with a fine hypodermic needle. Immediate and conspicuous local hyperemic changes occur if the area is infiltrated within 12 hours; therefore, administer phentolamine as soon as possible after extravasation is noted.

Hypotension After Abrupt Discontinuation

Abrupt cessation of norepinephrine infusion can cause marked hypotension. When discontinuing the infusion, gradually reduce the infusion rate while expanding blood volume with intravenous fluids.

Cardiac Arrhythmias

Norepinephrine increases intracellular calcium concentrations, which may cause arrhythmias, particularly in patients with hypoxia or hypercarbia. Perform continuous cardiac monitoring of patients with arrhythmias.

Allergic Reactions Associated with Sulfite

Norepinephrine bitartrate injection concentrate (e.g., Levophed®) contains sodium metabisulfite, a sulfite that may cause allergic-type reactions, including anaphylaxis and life-threatening or less severe asthmatic episodes, in certain susceptible individuals. The overall prevalence of sulfite sensitivity in the general population is unknown; such sensitivity appears to occur more frequently in asthmatic than in nonasthmatic individuals.

Specific Populations

Pregnancy

Limited data on the use of norepinephrine in pregnant women at the time of delivery have not identified an increased risk of major birth defects, miscarriage, or adverse maternal or fetal outcomes. There are risks to the mother and fetus from acute hypotensive states that are medical emergencies in pregnancy (e.g., in septic shock, myocardial infarction, and stroke); these can be fatal if untreated. Delaying necessary treatment may increase the risk of maternal and fetal morbidity and mortality. Life-sustaining therapy for the pregnant woman should not be withheld due to potential concerns regarding the effects of norepinephrine on the fetus.

In animal reproduction studies, high doses of IV norepinephrine resulted in lowered maternal placental blood flow; however, the clinical relevance to changes in the human fetus is unknown. Studies of norepinephrine administration to pregnant animals demonstrated decreases in fetal oxygenation, urine and lung liquid flow, production of cataracts, fetal microscopic liver abnormalities, and delayed skeletal ossification.

Lactation

There are no data on the presence of norepinephrine in either human or animal milk, the effects on the breastfed infant, or the effects on milk production. Because of its short half-life and poor oral bioavailability, clinically relevant exposure of norepinephrine in the infant is unlikely.

Pediatric Use

Safety and effectiveness in pediatric patients have not been established.

Geriatric Use

Clinical studies of norepinephrine bitartrate did not include sufficient numbers of patients 65 years of age and older to determine whether geriatric patients respond differently than younger patients. Clinical experience to date has not identified any differences in responses between geriatric and younger patients. If norepinephrine is used in geriatric patients, dosage should be selected carefully, usually starting at the low end of the dosage range, since renal, hepatic, and cardiovascular dysfunction and concomitant disease or other drug therapy are more common in this age group. Do not infuse into the leg veins of geriatric patients.

● Common Adverse Effects

The most common adverse reactions associated with norepinephrine are ischemic injury, bradycardia, anxiety, transient headache, respiratory difficulty, and extravasation necrosis at injection site.

DRUG INTERACTIONS

● Monoamine Oxidase-Inhibiting Drugs

Coadministration of norepinephrine with inhibitors of monoamine oxidase (MAO) or other drugs with MAO-inhibiting properties (e.g., linezolid) can cause severe and prolonged hypertension. If coadministration cannot be avoided in patients who recently have received MAO-inhibiting drugs and in patients who have not yet experienced sufficient recovery of MAO activity following discontinuation of the MAO-inhibiting drug, monitor for hypertension.

● Tricyclic Antidepressants

Coadministration of norepinephrine with tricyclic antidepressants (e.g., amitriptyline, nortriptyline, protriptyline, clomipramine, desipramine, imipramine) can cause severe and prolonged hypertension. Monitor for hypertension if coadministration cannot be avoided.

● Antidiabetics

Norepinephrine can decrease insulin sensitivity and raise blood glucose concentrations. Monitor glucose and consider dosage adjustment of antidiabetic drugs.

● Halogenated Anesthetics

Concomitant use of norepinephrine with halogenated anesthetics (e.g., cyclopropane, desflurane, enflurane, isoflurane, and sevoflurane) may cause ventricular tachycardia or ventricular fibrillation. Monitor cardiac rhythm in patients receiving concomitant halogenated anesthetics.

DESCRIPTION

Norepinephrine acts predominantly by direct effects on α-adrenergic receptors to cause peripheral vasoconstriction and to a lesser extent acts on β-adrenergic receptors to cause inotropic stimulation of the heart, dilation of coronary arteries,

and substantially increased coronary blood flow. Norepinephrine generally does not affect cardiac output, although it can be decreased. Norepinephrine primarily increases systolic, diastolic, and pulse pressures and has minimal effects on chronotropy. The elevations in resistance and blood pressure cause reflex vagal activity, slowing heart rate and increasing stroke volume. The elevation in vascular tone or resistance reduces blood flow to major abdominal organs and skeletal muscle. The pressor response following IV administration of norepinephrine occurs rapidly and reaches steady state within 5 minutes. The pharmacologic actions of norepinephrine are terminated primarily by uptake and metabolism in sympathetic nerve endings. The pressor action stops within 1–2 minutes after the infusion is discontinued.

ADVICE TO PATIENTS

- Advise the patient, family, or caregiver to report signs of extravasation urgently.

- Advise patient to inform their clinician of existing or contemplated concomitant therapy, including prescription and OTC drugs and dietary or herbal supplements, as well as any concomitant illnesses.

- Advise women to inform their clinician if they are or plan to become pregnant or plan to breast-feed.

- Inform patients of other important precautionary information.

PREPARATIONS

Excipients in commercially available drug preparations may have clinically important effects in some individuals; consult specific product labeling for details.

Norepinephrine Bitartrate

Parenteral		
Injection concentrate, for IV infusion	1 mg (of norepinephrine) per mL*	Levophed®, Hospira
		Norepinephrine Bitartrate Injection

* available from one or more manufacturer, distributor, and/or repackager by generic (nonproprietary) name

Norepinephrine Bitartrate in Dextrose

Parenteral		
Injection, for IV infusion	16 mcg/mL norepinephrine (4 mg) in 5% dextrose*	Norepinephrine Bitartrate in Dextrose 5%
	32 mcg/mL norepinephrine (8 mg) in 5% dextrose*	Norepinephrine Bitartrate in Dextrose 5%
	64 mcg/mL norepinephrine (16 mg) in 5% dextrose*	Norepinephrine Bitartrate in Dextrose 5%

* available from one or more manufacturer, distributor, and/or repackager by generic (nonproprietary) name

Norepinephrine Bitartrate in Sodium Chloride

Parenteral		
Injection, for IV infusion	16 mcg/mL norepinephrine (4 mg) in 0.9% sodium chloride*	Norepinephrine Bitartrate in Sodium Chloride Injection
	32 mcg/mL norepinephrine (8 mg) in 0.9% sodium chloride*	Norepinephrine Bitartrate in Sodium Chloride Injection
	64 mcg/mL norepinephrine (16 mg) in 0.9% sodium chloride*	Norepinephrine Bitartrate in Sodium Chloride Injection

* available from one or more manufacturer, distributor, and/or repackager by generic (nonproprietary) name

† Use is not currently included in the labeling approved by the US Food and Drug Administration.

Selected Revisions June 10, 2024, © Copyright, July 1, 1976, American Society of Health-System Pharmacists, Inc.

Phentolamine Mesylate

12:16.04.04 • NONSELECTIVE α-ADRENERGIC BLOCKING AGENTS

■ Phentolamine is an imidazoline α-adrenergic blocking agent.

USES

Phentolamine is used mainly in the diagnosis of pheochromocytoma and to control or prevent paroxysmal hypertension immediately prior to or during pheochromocytomectomy.

● Diagnosis of Pheochromocytoma

Although no single chemical or pharmacological test is completely reliable, determinations of blood concentrations of catecholamines and/or urinary excretion of catecholamines or their metabolites are the safest and most reliable methods for the diagnosis of pheochromocytoma. The phentolamine test may be used when additional confirmatory evidence of pheochromocytoma is required and the potential benefits of the test outweigh the possible risks. (See Cautions: Adverse Effects.) The phentolamine test is more reliable in detecting pheochromocytomas in patients with sustained hypertension than in those with paroxysmal hypertension and is of no value in patients who are not hypertensive at the time of the test. Sudden and marked reduction in blood pressure following parenteral administration of phentolamine to a hypertensive patient suggests the presence of a pheochromocytoma. However, false-negative and false-positive responses to the phentolamine test occur frequently. (See Cautions: Precautions and Contraindications.)

● Hypertension in Pheochromocytoma

In patients with pheochromocytomas, phentolamine may be administered immediately prior to or during pheochromocytomectomy to prevent or control paroxysmal hypertension resulting from anesthesia, stress, or operative manipulation of the tumor. For information regarding pheochromocytoma crisis, see Uses: Hypertensive Crises.

Although phentolamine has also been used for the medical management of patients with pheochromocytomas until surgery is performed and for prolonged treatment of hypertension caused by a pheochromocytoma not amenable to surgery, most clinicians consider phenoxybenzamine the drug of choice because it has a longer duration of action.

● Hypertensive Crises

Phentolamine mesylate also has been used to treat hypertensive crises or emergencies† (severe elevations in blood pressure exceeding 180/120 mm Hg accompanied by new or worsening target organ dysfunction) induced by catecholamine excess (e.g., pheochromocytoma, drug interactions with a monoamine oxidase [MAO] inhibitor, amphetamine overdosage, cocaine toxicity, clonidine withdrawal)†.

Phentolamine is not used in the treatment of essential hypertension because most patients become refractory to the antihypertensive effect of the drug and because of the high incidence of adverse GI effects. Although phentolamine has been used as adjunctive therapy in the treatment of peripheral vasospastic disorders†, the efficacy of the drug has not been established and the frequency of adverse effects limits its usefulness.

● Extravasation of Catecholamines

Phentolamine mesylate is used for the prevention and treatment of dermal necrosis and sloughing following IV administration or extravasation of norepinephrine. Phentolamine mesylate has also been used to prevent necrosis after extravasation of dopamine†.

● Myocardial Infarction

Phentolamine mesylate has been used IV to decrease the impedance to left ventricular ejection and the size of infarction in patients with myocardial infarction (MI) associated with left ventricular failure†. However, the manufacturers state that the drug is contraindicated in patients with MI and investigators do not recommend this therapy for routine use, since left ventricular function and the ECG must be monitored continuously.

● Erectile Dysfunction

Self-injection of small doses of phentolamine mesylate combined with papaverine hydrochloride into a corpus cavernosum of the penis has been effective for the treatment of erectile dysfunction† (impotence). Injection into a single cavernosum can increase tumescence (in both cavernosa because of cross circulation) and produce erection probably secondary to drug-induced increased arterial inflow and sinusoidal relaxation and decreased venous outflow (from increased venous resistance). The goal of such therapy is to provide an erection of adequate rigidity and duration to be sexually functional while avoiding prolonged erection or priapism. Intracavernosal papaverine (alone or combined with phentolamine and/or alprostadil) is one of the most effective and well-studied agents for the treatment of erectile dysfunction and has been in widespread clinical use. The combination has been effective in patients with neurogenic and/or limited vasculogenic impotence or with psychogenic impotence, but efficacy in those with a vasculogenic component of their impotence may be variable depending on the extent and type of vascular dysfunction. Erection, which can be potentiated by sexual arousal, usually occurs within 10 minutes after injection of the drugs and may persist for one to several hours; tolerance to the beneficial vascular effects of the drugs may occur during long-term use and may require an increase in dosage. Occasionally, priapism may occur. (See Cautions: Adverse Effects.)

Because of their convenience (e.g., ease of administration, patient and partner acceptance, and effectiveness in a broad range of patients), most experts (e.g., the American Urological Association [AUA]) currently recommend that selective phosphodiesterase (PDE) type 5 inhibitor therapy (sildenafil, tadalafil, vardenafil) be offered as first-line treatment of erectile dysfunction unless contraindicated. Intracavernosal therapy with papaverine and/or phentolamine generally is reserved for patients who do not respond to psychotherapy/behavioral therapy, vacuum constriction devices, and/or selective PDE type 5 inhibitors, and in whom attempts at identifying and modifying any drug-related (e.g., certain antihypertensive agents) or other potential reversible medical cause of erectile dysfunction have proved inadequate. Intracavernosal therapy or vacuum constriction devices generally are considered or attempted before resorting to more invasive (e.g., surgical) therapies. Ultimately, the choice of therapy for erectile dysfunction should be individualized, taking into account differences in response, tolerability and safety, administration considerations, cost and patient reimbursement factors, experience and judgment of the clinician, and individual patient and partner preference, expectations, and satisfaction.

Intracavernosal vasoactive therapy (e.g., papaverine, papaverine and phentolamine, alprostadil) is the most effective treatment for erectile dysfunction; however, it is invasive and associated with the highest risk of priapism. Clinician preference and experience often guide the initial treatment choice when intracavernosal therapy is indicated.

Additional study of the long-term safety and efficacy of intracavernous injection of vasoactive drugs for the treatment of erectile dysfunction is necessary and ongoing, particularly regarding the relative efficacy of single- versus multiple-drug therapy and the relative complications (e.g., penile scarring, penile fibrosis) and safety of each approach. Additional study also is needed to identify optimal patient education and follow-up support that might improve compliance and decrease dropout rates. Patients should be instructed to visit their clinician regularly (e.g., at 3-month intervals) for assessment of therapeutic benefit, including the need for possible dosage adjustment, and of potential adverse effects of their therapy.

Vasoactive therapy for erectile dysfunction should *not* be used in patients who might have conditions predisposing to priapism (e.g., sickle cell anemia or trait, multiple myeloma, leukemia), in those with anatomic deformation of the penis (e.g., angulation, cavernosal fibrosis, Peyronie's disease), or in men for whom sexual activity is inadvisable or contraindicated. In addition, vasoactive therapy should be discontinued in any patient who develops penile angulation, cavernosal fibrosis, or Peyronie's disease during therapy with the drug. One manufacturer also states that patients with penile implants should *not* be treated with vasoactive therapy for impotence.

Because of the risk of priapism and other potential complications (e.g., adverse morphologic penile effects such as fibrosis) associated with intercavernosal vasoactive therapy, such therapy is *not* recommended for simply enhancing erections in men who are not impotent†.

● Cocaine-induced Acute Coronary Syndrome

Phentolamine has been used as an adjunct in the management of cocaine overdose† to reverse coronary vasoconstriction.

● Other Uses

IV phentolamine has been used effectively to treat ventricular or supraventricular premature contractions†.

DOSAGE AND ADMINISTRATION

● *Reconstitution and Administration*

Phentolamine mesylate may be administered by IM or IV injection. Phentolamine mesylate injection is reconstituted by adding 1 mL of sterile water for injection to the vial containing 5 mg of lyophilized drug. The resulting solution contains 5 mg of phentolamine mesylate per mL.

Phentolamine mesylate also has been administered by intracavernous injection† for the treatment of erectile dysfunction. (See Uses: Erectile Dysfunction.) Patients receiving the drug via intracavernosal injection should be advised of the potential for prolonged erections (priapism) and advised of steps to take in the event that this potentially serious adverse effect occurs. (See Adverse Effects: Adverse Intracavernosal Effects, in Cautions.)

● *Dosage*

Diagnosis of Pheochromocytoma

For the diagnosis of pheochromocytoma, phentolamine mesylate may be administered IM or preferably IV. The usual adult IV or IM dose is 5 mg. Children may receive 1 mg IV or 3 mg IM. Alternatively, some clinicians have recommended an IV pediatric dose of 0.1 mg/kg or 3 mg/m². Before the drug is injected, the patient should rest in a supine position (preferably in a quiet, darkened room) until the blood pressure is stabilized and a basal level is established by blood pressure readings taken every 10 minutes for at least 30 minutes. When phentolamine mesylate is administered IV, injection of the drug should be delayed until the effect of the venipuncture on the blood pressure has passed; the drug should then be rapidly injected. In patients with a pheochromocytoma which is secreting epinephrine or norepinephrine, the response to IV injection of phentolamine mesylate is an immediate, marked decrease in both systolic and diastolic blood pressure. The maximum effect is usually obtained within 2 minutes after IV injection of the drug, and the blood pressure usually returns to pretest levels within 15–30 minutes. Therefore, blood pressure should be recorded immediately after the injection, at 30-second intervals for the first 3 minutes, and at 1-minute intervals for the next 7 minutes. Following IM injection, the maximum effect usually occurs within 20 minutes and persists for about 30–45 minutes. Blood pressure returns to pretest levels after 3–4 hours. After IM injection of phentolamine mesylate, blood pressure determinations should be made at 5-minute intervals for 30–45 minutes.

In the phentolamine test, a typical blood pressure response in patients with pheochromocytomas is a decrease in blood pressure of 60 mm Hg systolic and 25 mm Hg diastolic within 2 minutes after IV administration of the drug or within 20 minutes after IM administration. A blood pressure decrease of at least 35 mm Hg systolic and 25 mm Hg diastolic is considered a positive response and a positive test for pheochromocytoma. A negative response is indicated when the blood pressure is unchanged, elevated, or lowered less than 35 mm Hg systolic and 25 mm Hg diastolic.

Hypertension in Pheochromocytoma

To reduce elevated blood pressure prior to surgical removal of a pheochromocytoma, 5 mg of phentolamine mesylate is given IM or IV 1–2 hours preoperatively to adults or 1 mg, 0.1 mg/kg, or 3 mg/m² is given IM or IV to children; the dose may be repeated if necessary. During surgery for pheochromocytoma, 5 mg of phentolamine mesylate may be given IV to adults as needed to prevent or control paroxysms of hypertension, tachycardia, respiratory depression, convulsions, or other effects of excessive epinephrine secretion due to manipulation of the tumor. For children, the IV dose of phentolamine mesylate during surgery is 1 mg, 0.1 mg/kg, or 3 mg/m². Postoperatively, norepinephrine may be administered to control hypotension which commonly follows removal of a pheochromocytoma; however, this hypotension is more often prevented by administration of blood, plasma, or 5% albumin in 0.9% sodium chloride injection to correct the reduced blood volume which may occur.

Hypertensive Crisis

For hypertensive crisis resulting from catecholamine excess†, some experts recommend 5 mg administered as a rapid IV ("bolus") injection. Experts state that this dosage may be repeated every 10 minutes as necessary to achieve the desired blood pressure target.

If IV phentolamine is used in the management of a hypertensive crisis, patients who have hypertensive crisis *with* a compelling condition (e.g., aortic dissection, severe preeclampsia or eclampsia, pheochromocytoma crisis) should have their systolic blood pressure reduced to less than 140 mm Hg during the first hour and,

in patients with acute aortic dissection, to less than 120 mm Hg within the first 20 minutes. The initial goal of such therapy in adults *without* a compelling condition is to reduce systolic blood pressure by no more than 25% within the first hour, followed by further blood pressure reduction *if stable* to 160/110 or 160/100 mm Hg within the next 2–6 hours, avoiding excessive declines in pressure that could precipitate renal, cerebral, or coronary ischemia. If this blood pressure is well tolerated and the patient is clinically stable, further gradual reductions toward normal can be implemented in the next 24–48 hours.

Extravasation of Catecholamines

To treat dermal necrosis and sloughing following IV administration or extravasation of norepinephrine, 5–10 mg of phentolamine mesylate diluted in 10 mL of 0.9% sodium chloride injection is injected into the affected area within 12 hours. Immediate and conspicuous local hyperemic changes occur if the area is infiltrated within 12 hours, but such treatment is ineffective when given more than 12 hours after extravasation.

To prevent dermal necrosis and sloughing from IV administration or extravasation of norepinephrine, 10 mg of phentolamine mesylate may be added to each liter of IV fluids containing norepinephrine (the pressor effect of norepinephrine is unaffected).

To prevent tissue necrosis and sloughing following extravasation of dopamine injection, 10–15 mL of 0.9% sodium chloride injection containing 5–10 mg of phentolamine mesylate should be infiltrated (using a syringe with a fine hypodermic needle) liberally throughout the affected area, which is identified by coldness, hardness, and a pallid appearance. In children, phentolamine mesylate dosages of 0.1–0.2 mg/kg, up to a maximum of 10 mg per dose, may be administered. Immediate and conspicuous local hyperemic changes occur if the area is infiltrated within 12 hours.

Myocardial Infarction

For the treatment of left ventricular failure secondary to acute myocardial infarction (MI)†, the adult IV dosage of phentolamine mesylate as an infusion has ranged from 0.17–0.4 mg/minute. Left ventricular function and the ECG must be monitored continuously.

Erectile Dysfunction

When used for the treatment of erectile dysfunction† (impotence), self-injection into the corpus cavernosum of the penis of small doses of phentolamine mesylate (0.08–1.25 mg, but usually 0.5–1 mg) combined with papaverine hydrochloride (2.5–37.5 mg, but usually titrated up to 30 mg) have been effective. Erection, which can be potentiated by sexual arousal, usually occurs within 10 minutes after injection of the drugs and may persist for one to several hours; tolerance to the beneficial vascular effects of the drugs may occur during long-term use and may require an increase in dosage. Occasionally, priapism may occur. (See Cautions: Adverse Effects.)

CAUTIONS

● *Adverse Effects*

Phentolamine may cause acute and prolonged hypotension, tachycardia, cardiac arrhythmias, and angina, especially after parenteral administration. Myocardial infarction (MI) and cerebrovascular spasm or occlusion, usually in association with marked hypotension and a shock-like state, have been reported occasionally following parenteral administration of phentolamine. Deaths have occurred after IV administration of phentolamine for the diagnosis of pheochromocytoma.

Weakness, dizziness, flushing, orthostatic hypotension, and nasal congestion have been reported in patients receiving phentolamine. Adverse GI effects are common and include abdominal pain, nausea, vomiting, diarrhea, and exacerbation of peptic ulcer; these adverse effects generally prevent long-term administration of phentolamine.

Adverse Intracavernosal Effects

Intracavernous injection† of combined phentolamine and papaverine for the treatment of impotence occasionally has caused priapism. Priapism is a medical emergency that could result in penile tissue damage and permanent loss of potency if not treated immediately, and therefore, patients should be advised to report promptly to their physician or, if unavailable, to seek alternative immediate medical attention if an erection that persists longer than 4 hours or that is extremely painful occurs. Management of priapism should be according to established medical practice, and has included aspiration of cavernosal blood and/or intracavernous injection of small doses of an α-adrenergic agonist (e.g., metaraminol, phenylephrine), or dopamine. Rarely, more radical therapy for priapism (e.g., cavernospongiosus or Winter's shunt) may be necessary, such as in patients with persistent priapism (e.g., for longer than 24 hours).

Other complications of intracavernous injection of combined phentolamine and papaverine have included transient pain, including referred pain to the glans, burning, and paresthesia. Penile ecchymosis has occurred in many patients, and superficial hematoma and bruising of the penis also have occurred. Fibrotic changes (e.g., induration, lumpy areas of the penis but not necessarily at the injection site), including bilateral fibrosis of the corpora cavernosa, also have been reported. Embolus in the glans has been reported rarely, and the development of priapism, deep vein thrombosis, and fatal pulmonary embolus occurred in one patient. Adverse systemic effects of the drugs (e.g., facial flushing, dizziness, decreased systemic blood pressure, metallic taste) also have occurred.

The risk of priapism, although reportedly uncommon, can be reduced by careful patient instruction and dosage titration. Alternatively, switching to another therapy (e.g., alprostadil) may provide better patient tolerance. Some clinicians also have used alprostadil in combination with papaverine and phentolamine in an attempt to potentiate their therapeutic activity, reduce the dose of each drug required, and decrease the risk of local pain, penile corporal fibrosis, fibrotic nodules, hypotension, and priapism associated with higher dosages. However, additional study is needed to elucidate the long-term safety and benefits of such combined therapy.

● Precautions and Contraindications

If severe hypotension or other signs and symptoms of shock occur following administration of phentolamine, treatment must be vigorous and prompt. Therapy should include supportive measures and norepinephrine may be administered if necessary; epinephrine should not be given since it may cause a paradoxical fall in blood pressure. The manufacturer states that if cardiac arrhythmias occur during therapy with phentolamine, administration of digitalis glycosides should be deferred until the cardiac rhythm returns to normal.

False-negative responses to the phentolamine test may occur, especially in patients with paroxysmal hypertension or with a pheochromocytoma which is not secreting enough epinephrine or norepinephrine to elevate the blood pressure or to sustain an elevation. False-positive reactions occur more commonly than do false-negative responses and have occurred in patients with essential hypertension, in patients who have received sedatives, opiates, or antihypertensive drugs, and in patients with uremia. When practical, sedatives, analgesics, and all other medication should be withdrawn at least 24 hours (but preferably 48–72 hours) prior to the phentolamine test. Antihypertensive drugs should be withdrawn and the test should not be performed until blood pressure returns to pretreatment hypertensive levels; rauwolfia drugs (no longer commercially available in the US) should be withdrawn at least 4 weeks prior to testing.

The possibility that intracavernosal therapy for impotence could result in persistent priapism requiring medical and/or surgical intervention should be considered. (See Cautions: Adverse Effects.) Patients should be advised to contact their clinician if they develop a persistent (e.g., longer than 4 hours) erection during such therapy. The possibility that intracavernosal therapy may be problematic in patients receiving anticoagulants or who cannot tolerate transient hypotension and, because of the self-injection techniques involved, in those with poor manual dexterity, poor vision, or severe psychiatric disease also should be considered. For additional precautions and contraindications associated with vasoactive therapy in impotence, see Uses.

Phentolamine should be used with caution in patients with gastritis or peptic ulcer. Although the manufacturer states that phentolamine is contraindicated in patients with MI or a history of MI, coronary insufficiency, angina, or other evidence suggestive of coronary artery disease, results of some studies indicate that the drug may have a beneficial effect in patients with MI. (See Uses: Other Uses.) The drug is contraindicated in patients who are hypersensitive to phentolamine or to related drugs.

● Mutagenicity and Carcinogenicity

Studies to determine the mutagenic and carcinogenic potentials of phentolamine mesylate have not been performed to date.

● Pregnancy, Fertility, and Lactation
Pregnancy

Reproduction studies in rats and mice using oral phentolamine mesylate dosages 24–30 times the usual daily human dosage (based on a 60-kg individual) have shown slightly decreased fetal growth and slight fetal skeletal immaturity (manifested by an increased incidence of incomplete or unossified calcanei and

phalangeal nuclei of the hind limb and of incompletely ossified sternebrae). In rats receiving oral dosages 60 times the usual human daily dosage (based on a 60-kg individual), a slightly decreased rate of implantation occurred. In rabbits receiving oral dosages 20 times the usual human daily dosage (based on a 60-kg individual), embryonic and fetal development were not affected. No teratogenic or embryotoxic effects were observed in reproduction studies in rats, mice, and rabbits. At least one human death has been reported following the phentolamine test during pregnancy. There are no adequate and well-controlled studies using phentolamine in pregnant women, and the drug should be used during pregnancy only when the potential benefits outweigh the possible risks to the fetus.

Fertility

Studies to determine the potential effects of phentolamine mesylate on fertility have not been performed to date.

Lactation

It is not known whether phentolamine mesylate is distributed into milk. Because of the potential for serious adverse reactions to phentolamine mesylate in nursing infants, a decision should be made whether to discontinue nursing or the drug, taking into account the importance of the drug to the woman.

PHARMACOLOGY

Phentolamine inhibits responses to adrenergic stimuli by competitively blocking α-adrenergic receptors (primarily excitatory responses of smooth muscle and exocrine glands), but the action of the drug is relatively transient and α-adrenergic blockade is incomplete. Phentolamine has greater α-adrenergic blocking effects than does tolazoline. Phentolamine is more effective in antagonizing responses to circulating epinephrine and/or norepinephrine than in antagonizing responses to mediator released at the adrenergic nerve ending. The drug causes peripheral vasodilation and decreases peripheral resistance, primarily by direct relaxation of vascular smooth muscle, but α-adrenergic blockade also contributes to vasodilation. Phentolamine also stimulates β-adrenergic receptors and produces a positive inotropic and chronotropic effect on the heart and increases cardiac output.

Blood pressure response to phentolamine depends on the relative contributions of its vasodilating and cardiac stimulating effects. IV infusion of phentolamine mesylate 0.3 mg/minute may increase blood pressure because of a predominant inotropic effect, but with higher rates of administration vasodilation may predominate, decreasing blood pressure and masking the inotropic effect. Pulmonary vascular resistance and pulmonary arterial pressure are decreased. Cerebral blood flow is generally maintained. Usual doses of phentolamine lower blood pressure when it is maintained by circulating epinephrine or norepinephrine, but have little effect on the blood pressure of healthy individuals or patients with essential hypertension.

When phentolamine is administered IV to patients with acute myocardial infarction (MI) associated with hypertension and/or left ventricular failure, improvement in left ventricular performance results, with cardiac output, stroke index, heart rate, and cardiac index being increased and left ventricular filling pressure being decreased. In one study, IV phentolamine increased coronary blood flow in patients with recent MI. In animal studies, the drug prolonged the action potential duration and the effective refractory period and decreased conduction velocity.

Phentolamine dilates bronchial smooth muscle, presumably through stimulation of β-adrenergic receptors. The drug stimulates the smooth muscle of the GI tract, an effect which is blocked by atropine, and has a histamine-like effect which stimulates gastric secretion of both acid and pepsin. Large IV doses (40–50 mg) cause relaxation of the ureters.

PHARMACOKINETICS

The pharmacokinetics of phentolamine have not been determined. Phentolamine is only about 20% as active after oral administration as after parenteral administration. About 10% of a parenteral dose can be recovered in the urine as active drug; the fate of the remainder is not known. It is not known whether the drug crosses the placenta or appears in milk.

CHEMISTRY AND STABILITY

● Chemistry

Phentolamine is an imidazoline α-adrenergic blocking agent that is related structurally to tolazoline. Phentolamine mesylate occurs as a white or off-white, crystalline powder and has solubilities of approximately 1 g/mL in water and 250 mg/mL in alcohol at 25°C. The pK_a of phentolamine mesylate is 8.01. Following reconstitution of the commercially available lyophilized powder with sterile water for injection to a concentration of 5 mg/mL, phentolamine mesylate injection has a pH of 4.5–6.5.

● *Stability*

Phentolamine mesylate powder for injection should be stored at 15–30°C.

Following reconstitution of the commercially available lyophilized powder with sterile water for injection to a concentration of 5 mg/mL, phentolamine mesylate injection is stable for 48 hours at room temperature or 1 week at 2–8°C; however, the manufacturer recommends that the reconstituted injection be used immediately and not stored.

Following reconstitution of phentolamine mesylate lyophilized powder with 2 mL of commercially available papaverine hydrochloride injection (containing 30 mg/mL) and further dilution in 8 mL of the papaverine injection to provide an admixture containing 0.5 mg of phentolamine mesylate per mL and 30 mg of papaverine hydrochloride per mL, the resultant admixture had a pH of 3.6 and was stable for at least 30 days when stored in the papaverine vial at 5 or 25°C. It should be noted, however, that the manufacturer of papaverine hydrochloride injection recommends that the injection not be refrigerated since solubility of the drug is reduced at cold temperatures, possibly resulting in precipitation or crystallization. In addition, the possibility of microbial contamination of such admixtures during prolonged storage should be considered.

PREPARATIONS

Excipients in commercially available drug preparations may have clinically important effects in some individuals; consult specific product labeling for details.

Phentolamine Mesylate

Parenteral		
For injection	5 mg*	Phentolamine Mesylate for Injection

* available from one or more manufacturer, distributor, and/or repackager by generic (nonproprietary) name

† Use is not currently included in the labeling approved by the US Food and Drug Administration.

Selected Revisions January 27, 2020, © Copyright, September 1, 1977, American Society of Health-System Pharmacists, Inc.

Tamsulosin Hydrochloride

12:16.04.12 • SELECTIVE α₁-ADRENERGIC BLOCKING AGENTS

■ Tamsulosin hydrochloride is an α₁-adrenergic blocking agent with selectivity for α₁ₐ-adrenergic receptors, which are mainly located in nonvascular smooth muscle (e.g., prostate).

USES

● Benign Prostatic Hyperplasia

Tamsulosin is used to reduce urinary obstruction and relieve associated manifestations in hypertensive or normotensive patients with symptomatic benign prostatic hyperplasia (BPH, benign prostatic hypertrophy). Tamsulosin relieves mild to moderate obstructive manifestations (e.g., hesitancy, terminal dribbling of urine, interrupted or weak stream, impaired size and force of stream, sensation of incomplete bladder emptying or straining) and improves urinary flow rates in a substantial proportion of patients and may be a useful alternative to surgery, particularly in those who are awaiting or are unwilling to undergo surgical correction of the hyperplasia (e.g., via transurethral resection of the prostate [TURP]) or who are not candidates for such surgery. Therapy with α₁-adrenergic blocking agents appears to be less effective in relieving irritative (e.g., nocturia, daytime frequency, urgency, dysuria) than obstructive symptomatology, although tamsulosin also has been shown to be effective in relieving irritative symptoms. In addition, therapy with α₁-adrenergic blocking agents generally can be expected to produce less subjective and objective improvement than prostatectomy, and periodic monitoring (e.g., performance of digital rectal examinations, serum creatinine determinations, serum prostate specific antigen [PSA] assays) is indicated in these patients to detect and manage other potential complications of or conditions associated with BPH (e.g., obstructive uropathy, prostatic carcinoma).

Results of several controlled studies indicate that tamsulosin is more effective than placebo and limited data suggest that the drug is at least as effective as other α₁-adrenergic blocking agents (e.g., doxazosin, prazosin, terazosin) in the management of BPH. While symptomatic improvement has been maintained for up to at least 60 weeks of tamsulosin therapy in some patients, the long-term effects of α-blockers on the need for surgery and on the frequency of developing BPH-associated complications such as acute urinary obstruction remain to be established. Although tamsulosin appears to be associated with a decreased incidence of adverse cardiovascular effects including hypotension, dizziness, and syncope, patients should be warned of the possibility of tamsulosin-induced postural dizziness and measures to take if it develops (e.g., sitting, lying down). During initiation of tamsulosin therapy, patients should be cautioned to avoid situations where injury could result if syncope occurs. If syncope occurs, the patient should be placed in a recumbent position and treated supportively as necessary.

Combination therapy with an α₁-blocker and 5α-reductase inhibitor (e.g., finasteride) has been more effective than therapy with either drug alone in preventing long-term BPH symptom progression; combined therapy also can reduce the risks of long-term acute urinary retention and the need for invasive therapy compared with α-blocker monotherapy.

For additional information on the use of α₁-blockers in the management of BPH, see Uses: Benign Prostatic Hyperplasia, in Doxazosin 24:20.

Allergic-type reactions, including skin rash, pruritus, urticaria, and angioedema of the tongue, lips, and face, have been reported in some patients with positive rechallenge of tamsulosin therapy.

The possibility of carcinoma of the prostate and other conditions associated with manifestations that mimic those of BPH should be excluded in any patient for whom tamsulosin therapy for presumed BPH is being considered.

The manufacturer states that tamsulosin should *not* be used in the management of hypertension.

DOSAGE AND ADMINISTRATION

● Administration

Tamsulosin is administered orally. Because food may decrease peak plasma concentrations of tamsulosin and lengthen the time to achievement of peak plasma concentrations and decrease oral bioavailability of the drug, the manufacturer recommends that tamsulosin be taken 30 minutes after a meal; it is recommended that the drug be taken after the same meal each day. Patients should be advised that the capsules must be swallowed intact and *not* be opened, chewed, or crushed.

Risk of Intraoperative Floppy Iris Syndrome

A condition termed intraoperative floppy iris syndrome (IFIS) has been observed during phacoemulsification cataract surgery in some patients receiving α₁-adrenergic blocking agents, including tamsulosin. IFIS is a variant of small pupil syndrome and is characterized by the combination of a flaccid iris that billows in response to intraoperative irrigation currents, progressive intraoperative miosis despite preoperative dilation with mydriatics, and potential prolapse of the iris toward the phacoemulsification incisions. Most reported cases of IFIS were in patients who continued α₁-blocker therapy at the time of cataract surgery. A few cases also were reported in patients who had discontinued such therapy prior to surgery, generally 2–14 days prior to surgery but occasionally 5 weeks to 9 months prior to surgery. The manufacturer of tamsulosin recommends that male patients being considered for cataract surgery be specifically questioned to ascertain whether they have received tamsulosin or other α₁-blockers. If a patient has received such agents, the ophthalmologist should be prepared to modify the surgical technique (e.g., through use of iris hooks, iris dilator rings, or viscoelastic substances) to minimize complications of IFIS. The benefit of discontinuing α₁-blockers, including tamsulosin, prior to cataract surgery has not been established.

● Dosage

The manufacturer states that safety and efficacy of tamsulosin in children younger than 18 years of age have not been established, and clinical experience in these patients is not available.

Benign Prostatic Hyperplasia

For the management of benign prostatic hyperplasia (BPH), the usual initial adult dosage of tamsulosin is 0.4 mg once daily. About 2–4 weeks may be needed to adequately assess the response at this dosage. To achieve the desired improvement in symptoms and/or urinary flow rates, subsequent dosage may be increased to 0.8 mg daily as needed. If tamsulosin is discontinued for several days at either dosage (i.e., 0.4 or 0.8 mg daily), therapy with the drug should be reinstituted at the lower daily dosage. Although the elimination half-life may be slightly prolonged and intrinsic clearance of tamsulosin may be decreased in patients 55 years of age and older, the manufacturer makes no specific recommendations for dosage adjustment in such patients.

The manufacturer states that tamsulosin should not be used concomitantly with other α-adrenergic blocking agents.

● Dosage in Renal and Hepatic Impairment

Although protein binding of tamsulosin may be altered in patients with mild to moderate (i.e., creatinine clearance of 30–70 mL/minute per 1.73 m²) or severe (i.e., creatinine clearance of 10 to less than 30 mL/minute per 1.73 m²) renal impairment and in patients with moderate hepatic impairment resulting in changes of overall plasma concentrations of the drug, alterations in intrinsic clearance and concentrations of unbound tamsulosin do not appear to be substantial. Therefore, the manufacturer states that dosage adjustment in such patients is not necessary. However, tamsulosin has not been studied in patients with end-stage (i.e., creatinine clearance of less than 10 mL/minute per 1.73 m²) renal disease.

CAUTIONS

● Contraindications

Known hypersensitivity to tamsulosin or any ingredient in the formulation.

● Warnings/Precautions

Warnings

Postural Hypotension

Potential for postural hypotension, dizziness, or vertigo; syncope may occur.

Priapism

Priapism reported rarely; treat promptly.

Sensitivity Reactions

Allergic Reactions

Rash, pruritus, urticaria, and angioedema of the tongue, lips, and face reported; positive rechallenge in some patients.

Sulfa Sensitivity

Allergic reaction to tamsulosin reported rarely in patients with sulfa sensitivity. Use with caution in patients with serious or life-threatening sulfa sensitivity.

General Precautions

Prostate Cancer

Exclude possibility of prostate cancer prior to initiation of therapy.

Intraoperative Floppy Iris Syndrome

Intraoperative floppy iris syndrome (IFIS) observed during phacoemulsification cataract surgery in some patients receiving α₁-adrenergic blocking agents, including tamsulosin. Most reported cases were in patients who continued such therapy at the time of cataract surgery.

Manufacturer recommends that male patients being considered for cataract surgery be specifically questioned to ascertain whether they have received tamsulosin or other α₁-blockers. If the patient has received α₁-blockers, the ophthalmologist should be prepared to modify the surgical technique (e.g., through use of iris hooks, iris dilator rings, or viscoelastic substances) to minimize complications of IFIS.

Benefit of discontinuing α₁-blockers prior to cataract surgery not established.

Specific Populations

Pregnancy

Category B. Not indicated for use in women.

Lactation

Not indicated for use in women.

Pediatric Use

Not indicated for use in children.

Geriatric Use

No substantial differences in safety and efficacy relative to younger adults, but increased sensitivity cannot be ruled out.

● Common Adverse Effects

Headache, infection, asthenia, back pain, chest pain, dizziness, somnolence, insomnia, decreased libido, rhinitis, pharyngitis, increased cough, sinusitis, diarrhea, nausea, tooth disorder, abnormal ejaculation, blurred vision.

DESCRIPTION

Tamsulosin hydrochloride is a sulfamoylphenethylamine-derivative α₁-adrenergic blocking agent. Commercially available tamsulosin hydrochloride is a racemic mixture of 2 isomers. The drug is pharmacologically related to doxazosin, prazosin, and terazosin; however, unlike these drugs, tamsulosin has higher affinity and selectivity for α₁ₐ-adrenergic receptors, which are mainly located in nonvascular smooth muscle (e.g., prostate), than for α₁ᵦ-adrenergic receptors located in vascular smooth muscle (e.g., internal iliac artery). Results of in vitro studies indicate that tamsulosin has 7–38 times greater affinity for α₁ₐ-adrenoceptors than for α₁ᵦ-adrenoceptors; the drug has about 12 times greater affinity for α₁-adrenergic receptors in the prostate than for those in the aorta. Such selectivity of tamsulosin for α₁ₐ-receptors may result in a reduced incidence of adverse cardiovascular effects (e.g., syncope, dizziness, hypotension). On a molar basis, the α₁-adrenergic receptor affinity of tamsulosin is about 6 times that of prazosin when tested in human prostatic tissue.

Because of the prevalence of α-receptors on the prostate capsule, prostate adenoma, and bladder trigone and the relative absence of these receptors on the bladder body, α-adrenergic blocking agents decrease urinary outflow resistance in men.

PREPARATIONS

Excipients in commercially available drug preparations may have clinically important effects in some individuals; consult specific product labeling for details.

Tamsulosin

Oral		
Capsules	0.4 mg	Flomax®, Boehringer Ingelheim

Selected Revisions June 9, 2011, © Copyright, June 1, 1998, American Society of Health-System Pharmacists, Inc.

Cyclobenzaprine Hydrochloride

12:20.04 • CENTRALLY ACTING SKELETAL MUSCLE RELAXANTS

■ Cyclobenzaprine is a centrally acting skeletal muscle relaxant.

USES

● Muscular Conditions

Cyclobenzaprine hydrochloride is used as an adjunct to rest and physical therapy for the relief of muscular spasm associated with acute, painful musculoskeletal conditions.

Evidence supporting the efficacy of skeletal muscle relaxants is generally low to moderate in quality; while these agents appear to be more effective than placebo in providing short-term relief of acute low back pain, they are associated with a high incidence of adverse effects (e.g., sedation). Although comparative studies are limited, available data suggest that various skeletal muscle relaxants generally have similar efficacy for such use. Acute low back pain usually is a benign and self-limiting condition that improves spontaneously over time; therefore, nonpharmacologic treatment strategies (e.g., heat, massage) are recommended. If pharmacologic therapy is required, experts state that a nonsteroidal anti-inflammatory agent (NSAIA) or a skeletal muscle relaxant may be used; however, these drugs have been shown to result in only small improvements in pain relief and can increase the risk of adverse effects. In general, skeletal muscle relaxants should be used with caution after weighing the potential risks against the benefits in individual patients. Although skeletal muscle relaxants are often used in combination with NSAIAs for the treatment of acute low back pain, randomized controlled studies generally have not demonstrated any additional improvement in pain or functional outcomes with such combination therapy compared with use of an NSAIA alone.

Efficacy of cyclobenzaprine hydrochloride 10 mg immediate-release tablets was established in 8 controlled clinical studies comparing cyclobenzaprine, diazepam, and placebo for their effect on muscle spasm, local pain and tenderness, limitation of motion, and restriction in activities of daily living. Improvement in patients receiving cyclobenzaprine was substantially greater than in those receiving diazepam in 3 studies and was comparable to diazepam in the remaining 5 studies.

Efficacy of cyclobenzaprine hydrochloride 5 mg immediate-release tablets was evaluated in 2 controlled clinical studies; in one study patients received cyclobenzaprine hydrochloride 5 or 10 mg or placebo 3 times daily, and in the second study patients received 2.5 or 5 mg of the drug or placebo 3 times daily. In both studies, efficacy of cyclobenzaprine hydrochloride 5 mg was substantially greater than placebo for patient-assessed primary end points (i.e., global impression of change, medication helpfulness, and relief from starting backache) by the seventh day of treatment. In addition, cyclobenzaprine 5 mg was substantially more effective than placebo for a physician-assessed secondary end point (reduction in presence and extent of palpable muscle spasm). In the study comparing cyclobenzaprine 5 or 10 mg 3 times daily with placebo, both dosages of the drug were substantially more effective than placebo by the third or fourth day (48–72 hours after the first dose of medication) of treatment. The only efficacy-related difference between the 2 dosages was in onset of patient-rated relief from starting backache, which occurred after the third or fourth dose in patients receiving 5 mg but after the first 2 doses in patients receiving 10 mg. In the second study, the 2.5-mg dosage of cyclobenzaprine hydrochloride was no more effective than placebo. A subanalysis of data from patients in both studies who received either cyclobenzaprine hydrochloride (5 mg 3 times daily as tablets) or placebo and did not report somnolence demonstrated a meaningful treatment effect for all primary efficacy variables for the 5-mg dose despite the absence of somnolence in these patients.

Efficacy of cyclobenzaprine hydrochloride extended-release capsules was evaluated in 2 controlled clinical studies in patients with acute painful musculoskeletal conditions. Both dosages of cyclobenzaprine hydrochloride evaluated in these studies (15 and 30 mg once daily) were more effective than placebo for the primary efficacy end point (patient-rated medication helpfulness). In one of the studies, patients receiving the 30-mg once-daily dosage also experienced improvements in other patient-rated outcomes (relief from local pain due to muscle spasm, restriction of movement, and global impression of change). However, no substantial differences were observed between cyclobenzaprine and placebo for physician-rated global assessment, patient-rated restriction in activities of daily living, and quality of sleep.

No well-controlled clinical studies have been performed to determine whether cyclobenzaprine will enhance the clinical effects of aspirin or other analgesics or vice versa when such combinations are used to manage acute musculoskeletal conditions. Analysis of data from controlled studies indicates that an effective dosage of cyclobenzaprine may produce clinical improvement whether or not sedation occurs.

Cyclobenzaprine is ineffective in the treatment of spasticity associated with cerebral or spinal disease or in children with cerebral palsy.

DOSAGE AND ADMINISTRATION

● Administration

Cyclobenzaprine is administered orally (as immediate-release tablets or extended-release capsules).

The extended-release capsules should be swallowed intact. Alternatively, the capsules may be opened and the contents sprinkled onto a tablespoon of applesauce and consumed immediately without chewing; foods other than applesauce have not been tested and should not be used. Following administration, patients should rinse their mouth to ensure that all the capsule contents have been swallowed. Any unused portion of the capsules should be discarded.

● Dosage

Muscular Conditions

Cyclobenzaprine should be used only for short periods (e.g., up to 2–3 weeks) because adequate evidence of effectiveness for more prolonged use is not available and because muscle spasm associated with acute, painful musculoskeletal conditions generally is of short duration and specific therapy for longer periods seldom is warranted.

Immediate-release Tablets

The recommended dosage of cyclobenzaprine hydrochloride immediate-release tablets for most adults and adolescents 15 years of age and older is 5 mg 3 times daily. Depending on response, dosage may be increased to 10 mg 3 times daily.

Extended-release Capsules

The usual adult dosage of cyclobenzaprine hydrochloride extended-release capsules is 15 mg once daily (administered at approximately the same time each day). Some patients may require a dosage of up to 30 mg once daily.

Dosage in Hepatic Impairment

The manufacturer of cyclobenzaprine hydrochloride tablets states that less frequent dosing should be considered in patients with mild hepatic impairment, beginning with a 5-mg dose and slowly titrating upward. Use of the drug is not recommended in patients with moderate or severe hepatic impairment.

Because of limited dosing flexibility, the manufacturer of the extended-release capsules states that this dosage form is not recommended for use in patients with hepatic impairment.

Dosage in Geriatric Patients

The manufacturer of cyclobenzaprine hydrochloride immediate-release tablets states that less frequent dosing should be considered in geriatric patients, initiating cyclobenzaprine hydrochloride with a 5-mg dose and titrating upward slowly.

Cyclobenzaprine extended-release capsules are not recommended for use in geriatric patients.

CAUTIONS

The most common adverse effects reported in patients receiving cyclobenzaprine in clinical studies were drowsiness, dry mouth, dizziness, fatigue, and headache. Cyclobenzaprine is closely related to the tricyclic antidepressants, and the possibility that cyclobenzaprine may cause adverse effects similar to those of the tricyclic antidepressants should be considered.

● Nervous System Effects

Drowsiness occurred in 29 or 38% of patients receiving cyclobenzaprine 5 or 10 mg, respectively, compared with 10% of those receiving placebo in controlled studies; drowsiness also was reported in 39 or 16% of patients receiving cyclobenzaprine 10 mg in controlled studies or during postmarketing surveillance, respectively. Dizziness occurred in 1–3% of patients receiving cyclobenzaprine 5 or 10 mg in controlled studies, and in 11 or 3% of patients receiving cyclobenzaprine 10 mg in clinical studies or during postmarketing surveillance, respectively. Fatigue occurred in 6% of patients receiving either 5 or 10 mg of cyclobenzaprine compared with 3% of those receiving placebo in controlled studies; fatigue or tiredness occurred in 1–3% of patients receiving 10 mg of the drug in controlled studies and in postmarketing surveillance.

Headache occurred in 5% of those receiving 5 or 10 mg of cyclobenzaprine and in 8% of those receiving placebo in controlled studies; headache occurred in 1–3% of patients receiving 10 mg of the drug in controlled studies and postmarketing surveillance. Irritability, decreased mental acuity, nervousness, asthenia, and confusion occurred in 1–3% of patients receiving 5 or 10 mg of cyclobenzaprine in controlled studies or during postmarketing surveillance in patients receiving 10 mg of the drug.

Malaise, seizures, ataxia, vertigo, dysarthria, hypertonia, tremors, disorientation, insomnia, depressed mood, abnormal sensations, anxiety, agitation, psychosis, abnormal thinking, abnormal dreaming, hallucinations, excitement, paresthesia, and diplopia were reported during postmarketing surveillance or in less than 1% of patients receiving 10 mg of the drug in controlled studies. Other adverse nervous system effects that have been reported in patients receiving other tricyclic drugs or rarely with cyclobenzaprine but for which a causal relationship with the drug could not be established include decreased or increased libido, abnormal gait, delusions, aggressive behavior, paranoia, peripheral neuropathy, Bell's palsy, alterations in EEG patterns, and extrapyramidal manifestations.

● GI Effects

Dry mouth occurred in 21 or 32% of patients receiving 5 or 10 mg, respectively, of cyclobenzaprine and in 7% of those receiving placebo in controlled studies. Dry mouth also occurred in 27 or 7% of patients receiving 10 mg of the drug in clinical studies or during postmarketing surveillance, respectively. Abdominal pain, acid regurgitation, dyspepsia, constipation, diarrhea, nausea, and unpleasant taste occurred in 1–3% of patients receiving 5 or 10 mg of cyclobenzaprine in controlled studies or during postmarketing surveillance in patients receiving 10 mg of the drug. Vomiting, anorexia, GI pain, gastritis, thirst, edema of the tongue, and flatulence were reported during postmarketing surveillance or in less than 1% of patients receiving 10 mg of the drug in controlled studies. Paralytic ileus, tongue discoloration, stomatitis, and parotid swelling were reported in patients receiving other tricyclic drugs or rarely with cyclobenzaprine, but a causal relationship with cyclobenzaprine could not be established.

● Respiratory Effects

Upper respiratory infection and pharyngitis occurred in 1–3% of patients receiving cyclobenzaprine 5 or 10 mg in controlled studies. Dyspnea was reported in patients receiving other tricyclic drugs or rarely with cyclobenzaprine, but a causal relationship with cyclobenzaprine could not be established.

● Cardiovascular Effects

Syncope, tachycardia, arrhythmia, vasodilation, palpitation, and hypotension were reported during postmarketing experience or in less than 1% of patients receiving cyclobenzaprine 10 mg in clinical studies; hypertension, myocardial infarction, heart block, and stroke have been reported in patients receiving other tricyclic drugs or rarely with cyclobenzaprine, but a causal relationship with cyclobenzaprine could not be established.

● Dermatologic and Sensitivity Reactions

Anaphylaxis, angioedema, pruritus, facial edema, urticaria, rash, and sweating occurred during postmarketing experience or in less than 1% of patients receiving cyclobenzaprine 10 mg in clinical studies; photosensitivity, and alopecia have been reported in patients receiving other tricyclic drugs or rarely with cyclobenzaprine, but a causal relationship with cyclobenzaprine could not be established.

● Musculoskeletal Effects

Local weakness and muscle twitching were reported during postmarketing experience or in less than 1% of patients receiving cyclobenzaprine 10 mg in clinical studies; myalgia was reported in patients receiving other tricyclic drugs or rarely with cyclobenzaprine, but a causal relationship with cyclobenzaprine could not be established.

● Genitourinary Effects

Urinary frequency and/or urinary retention were reported during postmarketing experience or in less than 1% of patients receiving cyclobenzaprine 10 mg in clinical studies; impaired urination, dilatation of the urinary tract, impotence, testicular swelling, gynecomastia, breast enlargement, and galactorrhea have been reported in patients receiving other tricyclic drugs or rarely with cyclobenzaprine, but a causal relationship with cyclobenzaprine could not be established.

● Hematologic Effects

Purpura, bone marrow depression, leukopenia, eosinophilia, and thrombocytopenia have been reported in patients receiving other tricyclic drugs or rarely with cyclobenzaprine, but a causal relationship with cyclobenzaprine could not be established.

● Hepatic Effects

Abnormal liver function and rarely, hepatitis, jaundice, and cholestasis were reported during postmarketing experience or in less than 1% of patients receiving cyclobenzaprine 10 mg in clinical studies.

● Other Adverse Effects

Blurred vision was reported in 1–3% of patients receiving cyclobenzaprine 10 mg in controlled studies or in postmarketing surveillance. Tinnitus and ageusia each have been reported during postmarketing surveillance or in less than 1% of patients receiving cyclobenzaprine 10 mg in controlled studies.

Elevation or reduction of blood glucose, weight gain or loss, syndrome of inappropriate antidiuretic hormone (SIADH), chest pain, and edema have been reported in patients receiving other tricyclic drugs or rarely with cyclobenzaprine, but a causal relationship with cyclobenzaprine could not be established.

● Precautions and Contraindications

Cyclobenzaprine shares the toxic and drug interaction potentials of the tricyclic antidepressants, and the usual precautions of tricyclic antidepressant therapy should be observed. (See Cautions and see Drug Interactions in the Tricyclic Antidepressants General Statement 28:16.04.28.) The possibility that cyclobenzaprine may cause other adverse effects similar to those of the tricyclic antidepressants should be kept in mind, especially when the dosage for musculoskeletal conditions is exceeded.

Cyclobenzaprine immediate-release tablets should be used with caution in patients with mild hepatic impairment, and should not be used in patients with moderate or severe hepatic impairment. Use of the extended-release capsule formulation is not recommended in any patient with hepatic impairment. Plasma concentrations of cyclobenzaprine are increased in patients with hepatic impairment, and such patients generally are more susceptible to sedation caused by the drug. (See Dosage and Administration: Dosage in Hepatic Impairment.)

Because cyclobenzaprine has anticholinergic effects, it should be used with caution in patients with a history of urinary retention, angle-closure glaucoma, or increased intraocular pressure or in patients receiving anticholinergic drugs. Patients should be warned that cyclobenzaprine may impair their ability to perform hazardous activities requiring mental alertness or physical coordination such as operating machinery or driving a motor vehicle, particularly when the drug is used with alcohol or other CNS depressants.

Serotonin syndrome has occurred in patients receiving cyclobenzaprine in combination with serotonergic drugs. (See Drug Interactions: Serotonergic Drugs.) Serotonin syndrome is characterized by mental status and behavioral changes (e.g., agitation, confusion, hallucinations), altered muscle tone or neuromuscular activity (e.g., tremor, ataxia, hyperreflexia, clonus, rigidity), autonomic instability (e.g., diaphoresis, tachycardia, labile blood pressure, hyperthermia), and GI symptoms (e.g., nausea, vomiting, diarrhea). Patients should be advised of the symptoms of serotonin syndrome and instructed to seek immediate medical care if they develop any such symptoms. Cyclobenzaprine and any concomitant serotonergic agents should be discontinued immediately if serotonin syndrome is suspected and supportive treatment should be initiated.

Cyclobenzaprine is contraindicated in patients with hyperthyroidism, congestive heart failure, arrhythmias, heart block or conduction disorders, known hypersensitivity to the drug or any ingredient in the formulation, and in the acute recovery phase following myocardial infarction. Cyclobenzaprine also is contraindicated in patients receiving monoamine oxidase inhibitors and should not be used within 14 days following discontinuance of these agents.

Pediatric Precautions

Safety and efficacy of cyclobenzaprine immediate-release tablets in children and adolescents younger than 15 years of age have not been established.

Safety and efficacy of cyclobenzaprine extended-release capsules have not been established in pediatric patients.

Geriatric Precautions

Plasma concentrations of cyclobenzaprine and the frequency and severity of adverse effects, with or without other concomitantly used drugs, are increased in the elderly. Geriatric patients receiving cyclobenzaprine may be at increased risk for adverse CNS effects (e.g., hallucinations, confusion, sedation), adverse cardiovascular effects resulting in falls or other sequelae, and interactions with other drugs or diseases. Because of the risk of injury, skeletal muscle relaxants should generally be avoided in geriatric patients. If cyclobenzaprine is used in a geriatric patient, reduced dosages should be used. (See Dosage and Administration: Dosage in Geriatric Patients.)

Pregnancy, Fertility, and Lactation

Pregnancy

Reproduction studies in animals using cyclobenzaprine doses up to 20 times the human dose have not revealed evidence of harm to the fetus. There are no adequate and controlled studies to date using cyclobenzaprine in pregnant women, and the drug should be used during pregnancy only when clearly needed.

Fertility

Reproduction studies in animals receiving cyclobenzaprine have not revealed evidence of impaired fertility.

Lactation

It is not known whether cyclobenzaprine is distributed into milk; however, the drug is distributed into milk in rats. Because some related tricyclic antidepressants are distributed into milk, cyclobenzaprine should be used with caution in nursing women.

DRUG INTERACTIONS

Cyclobenzaprine is structurally and pharmacologically related to tricyclic antidepressants and shares the drug interaction potentials of these drugs. For additional information on potential drug interactions of tricyclic antidepressants, see Drug Interactions in the Tricyclic Antidepressants General Statement 28:16.04.28.

Monoamine Oxidase Inhibitors

Concomitant use of cyclobenzaprine and monoamine oxidase (MAO) inhibitors has resulted in hyperpyretic crisis, seizures, and death. Cyclobenzaprine is contraindicated in patients receiving MAO inhibitors and should not be used within 14 days following discontinuance of these drugs. (See Drug Interactions: Serotonergic Drugs.)

CNS Depressants

Cyclobenzaprine may be additive with or may potentiate the action of other CNS depressants (e.g., alcohol, barbiturates). Cyclobenzaprine, especially when used concomitantly with alcohol or other CNS depressants, may impair the patient's ability to perform activities requiring mental alertness or physical coordination (e.g., operating machinery, driving a motor vehicle).

Serotonergic Drugs

Concomitant use of cyclobenzaprine with serotonergic agents has been reported to cause serotonin syndrome. (See Cautions: Precautions and Contraindications.) Examples of serotonergic agents include selective serotonin-reuptake inhibitors (SSRIs), serotonin- and norepinephrine-reuptake inhibitors (SNRIs), tricyclic antidepressants, tramadol, meperidine, and MAO inhibitors.

If concomitant use of cyclobenzaprine with a serotonergic agent is necessary, the patient should be carefully monitored, particularly during treatment initiation and dosage adjustments. Cyclobenzaprine and any concomitant serotonergic agents should be discontinued if serotonin syndrome is suspected.

Tramadol

Cyclobenzaprine may enhance the risk of seizures in patients receiving tramadol.

Nonsteroidal Anti-inflammatory Agents

Concomitant use of cyclobenzaprine with diflunisal or naproxen reportedly was well tolerated and did not appear to result in any unexpected adverse effects. However, concomitant use of cyclobenzaprine with naproxen has been associated with an increased incidence of drowsiness. Plasma concentrations of aspirin or cyclobenzaprine were unaffected when the drugs were administered concomitantly.

ACUTE TOXICITY

Because the management of overdose is complex and changing, clinicians should consult a poison control center for additional information on the management of cyclobenzaprine overdosage. Cyclobenzaprine is structurally related to and shares the toxic potentials of the tricyclic antidepressants. For additional information about pathogenesis, manifestations, and treatment of toxic doses of structurally similar tricyclic antidepressants, see Acute Toxicity in the Tricyclic Antidepressants General Statement 28:16.04.28.

Pathogenesis

The manufacturer states that the acute oral LD_{50} of cyclobenzaprine is about 338 and 425 mg/kg in mice and rats, respectively.

Manifestations

Manifestations of toxicity may develop rapidly after a cyclobenzaprine overdose, and rarely, death may occur. The most common toxic effects associated with cyclobenzaprine overdose are drowsiness and tachycardia; less frequent manifestations include tremor, agitation, coma, ataxia, hypertension, slurred speech, confusion, dizziness, nausea, vomiting, and hallucinations. Rarely, potentially serious effects may include cardiac arrest, chest pain, cardiac dysrhythmias, severe hypotension, seizures, and neuroleptic malignant syndrome.

Treatment

Treatment of cyclobenzaprine overdosage, as in that of structurally similar tricyclic antidepressants, generally involves symptomatic and supportive care. Because of the potential for rapid clinical deterioration, cardiac function should be monitored, and IV access should be established; early endotracheal intubation and maintenance of an adequate airway are advised in patients with CNS depression and/or substantial ECG changes (e.g., wide-complex tachycardia).

The manufacturer states that all patients suspected of an overdose with cyclobenzaprine should receive GI decontamination, including gastric lavage followed by activated charcoal; induction of emesis is contraindicated if consciousness is impaired. However, the management of overdose is complex and changing, and clinicians should consult a poison control center for additional information on the management of cyclobenzaprine overdosage, particularly in pediatric patients. For additional information about specific treatment of cardiovascular and CNS disturbances associated with toxic doses of tricyclic compounds, including cyclobenzaprine, see Acute Toxicity: Treatment, in the Tricyclic Antidepressants General Statement 28:16.04.28.

PHARMACOLOGY

Cyclobenzaprine is a CNS depressant that has sedative and skeletal muscle relaxant effects. The precise mechanism of action of the drug is not known. Cyclobenzaprine does not directly relax skeletal muscle and, unlike neuromuscular blocking agents, does not depress neuronal conduction, neuromuscular transmission, or muscle excitability.

Like the tricyclic antidepressants, cyclobenzaprine potentiates the effects of norepinephrine and has anticholinergic effects.

PHARMACOKINETICS

Absorption

Orally administered cyclobenzaprine is well absorbed. Cyclobenzaprine undergoes enterohepatic circulation, and appears to be metabolized during its first pass through the GI tract and/or liver. Mean oral bioavailability of the drug following administration of the immediate-release tablet formulation is estimated to range from 33–55%. Following oral administration of a single 5- or 10-mg dose of cyclobenzaprine hydrochloride (as immediate-release tablets), peak plasma concentrations of 4.3 or 8.5 ng/mL, respectively, are attained in about 4 hours. When cyclobenzaprine is administered 3 times daily (as immediate-release tablets), steady-state plasma concentrations are attained within 3–4 days that are about fourfold greater than those after a single dose. In healthy individuals receiving the drug 3 times daily (as immediate-release tablets), mean steady-state peak plasma cyclobenzaprine concentrations of 14.9 or 25.9 ng/mL were achieved at 4 or 3.9 hours after administration of a 5 or 10 mg dose, respectively.

Following administration of a single 15- or 30-mg dose of cyclobenzaprine hydrochloride (as the extended-release capsule formulation) in healthy adults, peak plasma concentrations of the drug were achieved in 7–8 hours. Administration of a single 30-mg capsule with food increased peak plasma concentrations by 35% and systemic exposure of the drug by 20%, but did not affect time to peak plasma concentration. Following multiple-dose administration (30 mg once daily for 7 days as extended-release capsules), accumulation of cyclobenzaprine was observed (2.5-fold increase in steady-state plasma concentrations).

In a study evaluating the pharmacokinetics of cyclobenzaprine hydrochloride immediate-release tablets in geriatric individuals, values for steady-state mean area under the cyclobenzaprine concentration time curve (AUC) were about 1.7 times greater in individuals 65 years of age and older than in younger adults; mean AUCs in geriatric males were about 2.4 times greater than in younger males, and those in elderly females were about 1.2 times greater than in younger females. In geriatric patients older than 65 years of age receiving the extended-release capsules, AUC was increased by 40% and half-life of the drug was prolonged compared with younger adults. (See Cautions: Geriatric Precautions.)

Peak plasma concentrations and AUC of cyclobenzaprine (administered as immediate-release tablets) in 15 patients with mild hepatic impairment (and one with moderate hepatic impairment) were twice those observed in healthy individuals. Insufficient data exist to establish the safety of cyclobenzaprine use in patients with moderate or severe hepatic impairment. (See Cautions: Precautions and Contraindications.)

Distribution

Cyclobenzaprine is widely distributed into body tissues. It is not known if cyclobenzaprine is distributed into milk in humans; however, the drug is distributed into milk in rats. The drug is extensively (about 93%) bound to plasma protein.

Elimination

Cyclobenzaprine is extensively metabolized by both oxidative and conjugative pathways. Hepatic cytochrome P-450 (CYP) 3A4, 1A2, and (to a lesser extent) 2D6 isoenzymes are responsible for oxidative *N*-demethylation of the drug. Orally administered cyclobenzaprine is excreted in urine principally as inactive glucuronide metabolites; less than 1% of the drug is excreted renally as unchanged drug. Elimination of the drug is slow; plasma clearance is 700 mL/minute per 1.73 m^2 and the effective elimination half-life is about 18 hours (range: 8–37 hours). Decreased clearance and increased plasma concentrations of the drug occur in the elderly and those with hepatic impairment. (See Cautions: Precautions and Contraindications and see Cautions: Geriatric Precautions.)

CHEMISTRY AND STABILITY

Chemistry

Cyclobenzaprine is a centrally acting skeletal muscle relaxant that is structurally and pharmacologically related to the tricyclic antidepressants. Cyclobenzaprine hydrochloride occurs as a white crystalline powder and is freely soluble in water and in alcohol. The drug has a pK_a of 8.47.

Stability

Commercially available cyclobenzaprine hydrochloride immediate-release tablets should be stored at a controlled room temperature of 20–25°C; the extended-release capsules should be stored in tight, light-resistant containers at 25°C, but may be exposed to temperatures ranging from 15–30°C.

For further information on cautions, acute toxicity, and drug interactions of cyclobenzaprine hydrochloride, see the Tricyclic Antidepressants General Statement 28:16.04.28.

PREPARATIONS

Excipients in commercially available drug preparations may have clinically important effects in some individuals; consult specific product labeling for details.

Cyclobenzaprine Hydrochloride

Oral		
Capsules, extended-release	15 mg*	Amrix®, Teva
		Cyclobenzaprine Hydrochloride Extended-release Capsules
	30 mg*	Amrix®, Teva
		Cyclobenzaprine Hydrochloride Extended-release Capsules
Tablets, film-coated, immediate-release	5 mg*	Cyclobenzaprine Hydrochloride Tablets
	7.5 mg*	Cyclobenzaprine Hydrochloride Tablets
	10 mg*	Cyclobenzaprine Hydrochloride Tablets

* available from one or more manufacturer, distributor, and/or repackager by generic (nonproprietary) name

tiZANidine Hydrochloride

12:20.04 • CENTRALLY ACTING SKELETAL MUSCLE RELAXANTS

■ Tizanidine hydrochloride, a centrally acting α_2-adrenergic agonist, is a skeletal muscle relaxant.

USES

● Spasticity

Tizanidine is used alone or in conjunction with other standard therapies (e.g., baclofen) for the management of spasticity associated with cerebral or spinal injury. In these patients, tizanidine decreases the number and severity of spasms, alleviates clonus, and improves mobility to a greater extent than does placebo. Some evidence from comparative studies suggests that tizanidine may produce muscle weakness less frequently than other antispastic agents (e.g., baclofen, diazepam). The manufacturer states that because of its short duration of effect, tizanidine should be reserved for those daily activities and times when relief of spasticity is most important.

Efficacy for the management of spasticity has been demonstrated in 2 placebo-controlled, randomized studies in patients with multiple sclerosis or spinal cord injury. In these studies, patients 18–75 years of age received initial tizanidine hydrochloride dosages of 2 or 4 mg daily, which were titrated according to response and tolerance to a maximum of 36 mg (in up to 3 divided doses) daily over a 3-week period. Following initial dosage titration, tizanidine hydrochloride dosages averaged 30.7–31.1 mg daily. Based on changes in Ashworth scores (a 5-point rating scale for assessing muscle tone, with 0 representing normal muscle tone and 4 representing immobilization of the muscle by spasticity), reductions in muscle tone were greater with tizanidine than with placebo during dosage titration, plateau, and/or study end point assessments. Mean reductions from baseline in Ashworth scores at the end point assessment were 4.41 and 0.44 for the tizanidine and placebo groups, respectively, in one study and 4.4 and 1.2, respectively, in the other study. However, in the larger of these studies, reductions in muscle tone (primary outcome measure) with tizanidine were not associated with comparable improvements in secondary outcome measures such as muscle strength, the frequency of daytime muscle spasms, pain, or deep tendon reflex activity. Improvement in muscle tone with tizanidine therapy was not consistently associated with improvements in quality of life as determined by activities of daily living (ADL) assessment scores.

In comparative studies in patients with spasticity associated with multiple sclerosis or cerebrovascular disorders, principally stroke, tizanidine's ability to improve muscle tone has been shown to be similar to that of baclofen or diazepam. Combined analysis of data from studies of 4–8 weeks' duration indicated improvements in muscle tone, spasms, and clonus in about 50–67% of patients treated with any of these drugs, while improvement in muscle strength was noted in about 33% of such patients. In these studies, patients receiving tizanidine exhibited better retention of muscle strength than those receiving baclofen or diazepam, and the incidence of somnolence was somewhat lower with tizanidine than with diazepam.

Concomitant therapy with tizanidine and another antispastic agent (e.g., baclofen) reportedly may allow control of spasticity with lower dosages of each agent. However, it should be kept in mind that such concomitant therapy may cause additive sedative effects (see Drug Interactions: Alcohol and Other CNS Depressants); some clinicians suggest that tizanidine not be given concomitantly with benzodiazepines (e.g., diazepam).

DOSAGE AND ADMINISTRATION

● General

Tizanidine hydrochloride is administered orally. Food has complex effects on the pharmacokinetics of tizanidine, and these effects differ between the commercially available capsule and tablet formulations. Clinically important differences (e.g., increased adverse effects, delayed or more rapid onset of activity) may be apparent when switching administration of capsules or tablets between fed and/or fasting states, switching between capsules and tablets in the fed state, or switching between administration of intact capsules and sprinkling capsule contents on applesauce. Clinicians should be thoroughly familiar with possible pharmacokinetic changes associated with these conditions. (See Description.)

Dosage of tizanidine hydrochloride is expressed in terms of tizanidine.

The dosage of tizanidine should be individualized according to the patient's requirements and response using the lowest dosage that produces optimum response without adverse effects. While single doses of tizanidine smaller than 8 mg have not been shown to be effective in controlled clinical studies, initiation of tizanidine therapy with single doses of 4 mg is recommended to minimize the incidence of common dose-related adverse effects (e.g., orthostatic hypotension). The dose can be repeated every 6–8 hours as needed for a maximum of 3 doses in 24 hours. Dosage of tizanidine may be increased gradually in increments of 2–4 mg daily until optimum therapeutic effects are obtained with tolerable adverse effects; optimum dosage generally can be attained over a period of 2–4 weeks.

Clinical experience is limited with single doses exceeding 8 mg or total daily dosages exceeding 24 mg, and the manufacturer states that there is essentially no experience with repeated single or total daily dosages exceeding 12 or 36 mg, respectively. The dosage of tizanidine in adults should not exceed 36 mg in any 24-hour period.

● Special Populations

Initiate with caution in patients with renal impairment (creatinine clearance less than 25 mL/minute). In these patients, the manufacturer recommends using smaller individual doses during dosage titration. If higher doses are needed, the manufacturer recommends increasing the amount of each individual dose rather than increasing the frequency of dosing.

Pharmacokinetics not studied in patients with hepatic impairment; however, tizanidine is known to undergo extensive first-pass hepatic metabolism. Therefore, the manufacturer recommends that the drug be avoided or used only with extreme caution in patients with hepatic impairment.

Although use of tizanidine ordinarily should be avoided in women taking oral contraceptives, if the drug is considered clinically necessary in such women, the initial dosage and rate of titration should be reduced. (See Drug Interactions: Oral Contraceptives.)

CAUTIONS

● Contraindications

Concomitant therapy with ciprofloxacin or fluvoxamine. (See Drug Interactions.)

Known hypersensitivity to tizanidine hydrochloride or any ingredient in the formulation.

● Warnings/Precautions

Warnings

Limited Experience with Long-term Use of Higher Dosages

Clinical experience with long-term use of tizanidine at single doses of 8–16 mg or total daily dosages of 24–36 mg is limited. Therefore, only adverse effects with a relatively high incidence are likely to have been identified in long-term clinical studies. (See Dosage and Administration.)

Hypotension

Hypotension was reported in two-thirds of patients treated with 8 mg of tizanidine in a single-dose study. Patients in the study had a 20% reduction in either diastolic or systolic blood pressures within 1 hour after dosing; hypotensive effects peaked 2–3 hours after dosing and were occasionally associated with bradycardia, orthostatic effects, dizziness, and, rarely, syncope. Tizanidine's hypotensive effect is dose related. The risk of marked hypotension may therefore be minimized by careful dosage titration; patients should be observed for manifestations of hypotension prior to dosage adjustment. (See Advice to Patients.)

Tizanidine should be used with caution in patients receiving concomitant antihypertensive therapy. (See Drug Interactions: Hypotensive Agents.) Concomitant use of tizanidine and other α_2-adrenergic agonists (e.g., clonidine) is not recommended.

Because clinically important hypotension has been reported with concurrent use of either fluvoxamine or ciprofloxacin, these drugs are contraindicated in patients receiving tizanidine. (See Drug Interactions.)

Risk of Liver Injury

Liver injury (most often hepatocellular in type) has been reported occasionally. Elevations (i.e., exceeding 3 times the upper limit of normal, or 2 times the upper limit of normal if baseline levels were elevated) of ALT or AST have occurred in approximately 5% of patients receiving tizanidine in controlled clinical studies. Nausea, vomiting, anorexia, and jaundice occasionally have been reported in patients with elevated aminotransferase concentrations. Death associated with liver failure has been reported rarely.

Monitoring of serum aminotransferase concentrations should be performed prior to and during the first 6 months of treatment (e.g., at baseline and at 1, 3, and 6 months) and periodically thereafter based on clinical status. Tizanidine should be avoided or used only with extreme caution in patients with impaired hepatic function. (See Hepatic Impairment under Warnings/Precautions: Specific Populations, in Cautions.)

Sedation

Sedation was reported in 48% of patients receiving any dose of tizanidine in multiple-dose, controlled clinical studies. Sedation was rated as severe by 10% of these tizanidine-treated patients compared with less than 1% of patients receiving placebo. Risk of sedation appears to be dose related. Sedation may interfere with daily activity. During multiple-dose studies, the prevalence of sedation peaked following the first week of dosage titration, then remained stable for the duration of the maintenance treatment phase. In comparative studies with baclofen or diazepam, the incidence of somnolence/drowsiness in patients receiving tizanidine or baclofen (15–67%) was slightly lower than that in patients receiving diazepam (44–82%).

Hallucinations/Psychotic-like Symptoms

Hallucinations (formed, visual) or delusions were reported in 5 of 170 patients (3%) receiving tizanidine in 2 North American controlled studies. All of these cases occurred within the first 6 weeks of therapy. Psychoses associated with hallucinations have been reported in at least one patient.

Potential Interaction with Fluvoxamine or Ciprofloxacin

In pharmacokinetic studies, substantial increases in serum tizanidine concentrations were observed during concurrent administration of fluvoxamine or ciprofloxacin; potentiated hypotensive and sedative effects also were observed. Concurrent administration of tizanidine with either fluvoxamine or ciprofloxacin is contraindicated. (See Drug Interactions.)

Potential Interaction with Other CYP1A2 Inhibitors

Because of potential drug interactions, concurrent administration of tizanidine with other cytochrome P-450 (CYP) isoenzyme 1A2 (CYP1A2) inhibitors should ordinarily be avoided. However, if their concomitant use is considered clinically necessary, the drugs should be used with caution. (See Drug Interactions: Drugs Affecting or Metabolized by Hepatic Microsomal Enzymes.)

General Precautions
Cardiovascular Effects

Prolongation of the QT interval and bradycardia were reported in chronic toxicity studies in animals at dosages equal to the maximum recommended human daily dosage on a mg/m^2 basis. ECG evaluation was not included in controlled clinical studies, but pulse rate reduction in association with decreases in blood pressure has been reported in patients receiving single doses of tizanidine.

Ocular Effects

Evidence of dose-related retinal degeneration and corneal opacities has been reported in animal studies at tizanidine dosages equivalent to approximately the maximum recommended human daily dosage on a mg/m^2 basis. Retinal degeneration and corneal opacities have not been reported to date in clinical studies.

Use in Women Taking Oral Contraceptives

Because drug interaction studies have demonstrated that concurrent use of tizanidine and oral contraceptives may substantially reduce the clearance of tizanidine, concomitant use should ordinarily be avoided. However, if the drug is considered clinically necessary, tizanidine dosage adjustment is recommended. (See Dosage and Administration: Special Populations and also see Drug Interactions: Oral Contraceptives.)

Discontinuance of Therapy

Tizanidine is pharmacologically related to clonidine, and rebound manifestations similar to those reported with abrupt withdrawal of clonidine therapy, including hypertension, tachycardia, hypertonia, tremor, and anxiety, have been reported upon sudden withdrawal of tizanidine therapy.

If tizanidine therapy is to be discontinued, dosage of the drug should be decreased gradually, particularly in patients who have been receiving high dosages for prolonged periods, to minimize the risk of withdrawal and rebound symptoms.

Specific Populations
Pregnancy

Category C. (See Users Guide.)

Lactation

It is not known whether tizanidine is distributed into milk in humans. However, because it is lipid-soluble, tizanidine might be expected to pass into milk in humans. Tizanidine should be used with caution in nursing women.

Pediatric Use

Safety and efficacy not established in children.

Geriatric Use

The manufacturer states that clearance is decreased fourfold in this patient population. Tizanidine should be used with caution in geriatric patients.

Hepatic Impairment

Although the pharmacokinetics of tizanidine have not been evaluated in patients with hepatic impairment, the drug undergoes extensive first-pass metabolism in the liver. Therefore, hepatic impairment would be expected to have substantial effects on tizanidine pharmacokinetics. The manufacturer states that tizanidine ordinarily should be avoided or used only with extreme caution in patients with impaired hepatic function. (See Risk of Liver Injury under Warnings/Precautions: Warnings, in Cautions.)

Renal Impairment

Clearance of tizanidine reportedly is reduced by greater than 50% in patients with a creatinine clearance less than 25 mL/minute. Tizanidine should be used with caution in patients with renal impairment. Patients should be monitored closely for onset or increased severity of common adverse effects (e.g., dry mouth, somnolence, asthenia, dizziness) that may indicate potential overdosage. (See Special Populations under Dosage and Administration.)

● Common Adverse Effects

Adverse effects reported in greater than 2% of patients receiving tizanidine in multiple-dose, controlled clinical studies include dry mouth, somnolence, asthenia (weakness, fatigue, and/or tiredness), dizziness, urinary tract infection, infection, constipation, abnormal liver function test results (e.g., elevated ALT), vomiting, speech disorder, amblyopia (blurred vision), urinary frequency, flu symptoms, dyskinesia, nervousness, pharyngitis, and rhinitis. In addition, hypotension and bradycardia also have been reported in single-dose, placebo-controlled studies.

DRUG INTERACTIONS

● Drugs Affecting or Metabolized by Hepatic Microsomal Enzymes

Potential pharmacokinetic interaction; decreased plasma clearance of tizanidine may occur when tizanidine is given concurrently with other inhibitors of cytochrome P-450 (CYP) isoenzyme 1A2, including acyclovir, antiarrhythmics (e.g., amiodarone, mexiletine, propafenone, verapamil), cimetidine, famotidine, fluvoxamine (see Drug Interactions: Fluvoxamine), fluoroquinolones (e.g., ciprofloxacin [see Drug Interactions: Ciprofloxacin]), oral contraceptives (see Drug Interactions: Oral Contraceptives), ticlopidine, and zileuton. Concomitant use ordinarily should be avoided; if considered clinically necessary, the drugs should be used with caution.

Tizanidine and its major metabolites are not likely to affect the metabolism of other drugs metabolized by CYP isoenzymes.

● Hypotensive Agents

Potential pharmacologic interaction (additive hypotensive effects) when used concomitantly with antihypertensive agents; should not be used with other α_2-adrenergic agonists (e.g., clonidine).

● **Acetaminophen**

Potential pharmacokinetic interaction (delayed time to peak plasma concentration of acetaminophen). Acetaminophen does not affect pharmacokinetics of tizanidine.

● **Alcohol and Other CNS Depressants**

Alcohol increased the areas under the plasma concentration-time curve (AUCs) and peak concentrations of tizanidine by approximately 20 and 15%, respectively; these changes were associated with an increase in adverse effects of tizanidine.

Potential pharmacologic interaction (additive CNS depression) with alcohol or other CNS depressants (e.g., baclofen, dantrolene, diazepam).

● **Ciprofloxacin**

Potential pharmacokinetic interaction; significantly increased plasma concentrations and AUCs of tizanidine have been observed with concomitant administration, resulting in increased risk of adverse cardiovascular (including substantial hypotension) and CNS (e.g., drowsiness, psychomotor impairment) effects associated with tizanidine use. Concomitant use of tizanidine and ciprofloxacin is contraindicated.

● **Fluvoxamine**

Potential pharmacokinetic interaction; significantly increased plasma concentrations, elimination half-life, and AUCs of tizanidine have been observed with concomitant administration, resulting in increased risk of adverse cardiovascular (including substantial hypotension) and CNS (e.g., drowsiness, psychomotor impairment) effects associated with tizanidine use. Concomitant use of tizanidine and fluvoxamine is contraindicated.

● **Oral Contraceptives**

Potential pharmacokinetic interaction; decreased plasma clearance (by up to 50%) of tizanidine reported with concomitant use. Although use of tizanidine ordinarily should be avoided in women taking oral contraceptives, if the drug is considered clinically necessary in such women, tizanidine dosage adjustment is recommended. (See Dosage and Administration: Special Populations.)

DESCRIPTION

Tizanidine hydrochloride, an imidazoline derivative, is a centrally acting α_2-adrenergic agonist with myotonolytic effects on skeletal muscle. Tizanidine is structurally and pharmacologically related to clonidine and other α_2-adrenergic agonists, but studies in animals indicate that tizanidine has one-tenth to one-fiftieth the potency of clonidine in lowering blood pressure. The exact mechanism of tizanidine in reducing muscle tone and spasm frequency is not clear. However, tizanidine reportedly decreases the frequency and amplitude of muscle spasms (tonic reflexes) that arise in response to muscle stretching in patients with various spinal cord lesions. The drug appears to reduce spasticity by increasing presynaptic inhibition of motor neurons, leading to reduced facilitation of spinal motor neurons and a resultant decrease in muscle tone. Tizanidine has its greatest effects on polysynaptic pathways, with no important effect on monosynaptic spinal reflexes. The drug does not have direct effects on skeletal muscle fibers or the neuromuscular junction. Tizanidine has been shown to have antinociceptive effects in animals, and some reports have suggested that it may improve pain associated with muscle spasm.

Tizanidine undergoes extensive first-pass hepatic metabolism. In fasting healthy individuals, peak plasma tizanidine concentrations are attained about 1 hour after administration of the commercially available capsules and tablets. The half-life of tizanidine averages about 2.5 hours. When tizanidine is administered as two 4-mg tablets with food, the mean peak plasma concentration is increased by about 30%, the median time to peak plasma concentration is increased from about 60 to about 85 minutes, and the extent of absorption is increased by about 30%.

When tizanidine is administered as the commercially available capsules, food decreases the mean peak plasma concentration by 20%, increases the median time

to peak plasma concentration from about 1 hour to 3 hours, and increases the extent of absorption by about 10%. When given with food, the amount of tizanidine absorbed from the capsule is about 80% of the amount absorbed from the tablet. Administration of the capsule contents sprinkled on applesauce is not bioequivalent to administration of the intact capsule under fasting conditions and results in a 15–20% increase in peak plasma concentration and AUC and a 15-minute decrease in median lag time and time to achieve peak plasma concentration compared with administration of intact capsules while fasting.

ADVICE TO PATIENTS

Importance of advising patients of limited clinical experience with tizanidine with respect to both duration of therapy and the higher dosages necessary to reduce muscle tone.

Risk of marked orthostatic hypotension; importance of exercising caution when moving from a supine to a fixed upright position.

Risk of sedation, which may be additive when taken in conjunction with alcohol or other CNS depressants; importance of exercising caution when performing activities requiring alertness, including driving a motor vehicle or operating machinery.

Importance of not discontinuing tizanidine abruptly because of potential for rebound hypertension and tachycardia.

Importance of advising patients of potential changes in absorption profile and resulting changes in efficacy and adverse effect profile when taken with food.

Importance of informing clinicians of existing or contemplated concomitant therapy, including prescription and OTC drugs and herbal supplements, as well as any concomitant illnesses, and of informing clinicians or pharmacists whenever any drug is added or discontinued. Importance of not taking tizanidine concomitantly with either ciprofloxacin or fluvoxamine.

Importance of women informing clinicians if they are or plan to become pregnant or plan to breast-feed.

Importance of informing patients of other important precautionary information. (See Cautions.)

PREPARATIONS

Excipients in commercially available drug preparations may have clinically important effects in some individuals; consult specific product labeling for details.

tiZANidine Hydrochloride

Oral			
Capsules	2 mg (of tizanidine)	Zanaflex®, Acorda
	4 mg (of tizanidine)	Zanaflex®, Acorda
	6 mg (of tizanidine)	Zanaflex®, Acorda
Tablets	2 mg (of tizanidine)*	Tizanidine Hydrochloride Tablets
		Zanaflex® (scored), Acorda
	4 mg (of tizanidine)*	Tizanidine Hydrochloride Tablets
		Zanaflex® (scored), Acorda

* available from one or more manufacturer, distributor, and/or repackager by generic (nonproprietary) name

Selected Revisions August 25, 2011, © Copyright, March 1, 2003, American Society of Health-System Pharmacists, Inc.

Baclofen

12:20.12 · GABA-DERIVATIVE SKELETAL MUSCLE RELAXANTS

■ Baclofen, a γ-aminobutyric acid (GABA) derivative, is a skeletal muscle relaxant and antispastic agent.

USES

● Spasticity

Baclofen is used orally in the management of spasticity and its sequelae secondary to severe chronic disorders such as multiple sclerosis and other types of spinal cord lesions. For the drug to be beneficial, patients must have presumably reversible spasticity where relief of spasticity will aid in restoring residual function. In these patients, baclofen decreases the number and severity of spasms (particularly flexor spasms); alleviates associated pain, clonus, and muscle rigidity; and improves mobility to a greater extent than does placebo. In patients with multiple sclerosis, the drug produces little improvement in residual muscle function, but patient comfort is improved when the painful spasms are reversible. In one uncontrolled study, less than one-third of multiple sclerosis patients with urinary retention caused by bladder spasm showed decrease in urinary retention.

Although few controlled studies have been conducted comparing efficacy and tolerability of the various antispastic agents, available data suggest that oral baclofen appears to have similar efficacy to other commonly used oral agents (e.g., diazepam, tizanidine). In studies comparing doses of about 60 mg of baclofen daily to 30 mg of diazepam daily in patients with multiple sclerosis or spinal cord lesions, the drugs were equally effective in reducing the number and severity of muscle spasms; however, baclofen produced a lower incidence of sedation than did diazepam. In comparative studies in patients with spasticity associated with cerebral or spinal disorders, improvement in muscle tone occurred in a similar proportion of patients receiving baclofen, diazepam, or tizanidine. When spasticity cannot be adequately managed with oral antispastic agents, other interventions such as botulinum toxin injection, intrathecal baclofen, intrathecal injection of sclerosing agents (e.g., phenol), or surgery (e.g., rhizotomy, chordotomy) may be necessary.

Baclofen crosses the blood-brain barrier in only small amounts following oral administration. It has been suggested that administration of the drug at the spinal cord level (i.e., intrathecally) would increase drug efficacy while decreasing the dosage required and possibly the toxicity profile in patients with spasticity of spinal cord origin. While baclofen may be effective at relatively high *oral* dosages in some patients with spasticity of spinal cord origin, many other patients, particularly those with severe spasticity, do not respond adequately to and/or do not tolerate such therapy. Therefore, *intrathecal* baclofen may be a suitable alternative to ablative surgical or chemical procedures in patients who do not tolerate or respond adequately to oral therapy with the drug. (See Uses: Severe Spasticity.)

● Severe Spasticity

Baclofen usually is used *intrathecally* in the management of severe spasticity of *spinal cord origin* in patients who do not tolerate or respond adequately to oral therapy with the drug. Baclofen also is used intrathecally in the management of intractable spasticity secondary to severe chronic disorders such as multiple sclerosis and other types of spinal diseases such as spinal ischemia, spinal tumor, transverse myelitis, cervical spondylosis, and degenerative myelopathy. Baclofen is designated an orphan drug by the FDA for use in these conditions. The clinical goal of such therapy is to maintain muscle tone as close to normal as possible and to minimize the frequency and severity of spasms without inducing intolerable adverse effects. In controlled studies in patients with severe spasticity and spasms secondary to spinal cord injury or multiple sclerosis, single doses or 3-day continuous infusions of intrathecal baclofen were more effective than placebo in improving the Ashworth (rigidity) rating of spasticity and in reducing the frequency of spasms. During chronic intrathecal baclofen therapy, many patients experience improvement in activities associated with daily living, especially in self-care, transferring, bowel function, and urinary continence.

Baclofen also is used *intrathecally* in patients with spasticity of *cerebral origin*, including those with cerebral palsy and acquired brain injury. Baclofen injection is designated an orphan drug by the FDA for the management of spasticity in patients with cerebral palsy. The clinical goal of such therapy is to maintain muscle tone as close to normal as possible and to minimize the frequency and severity of spasms without inducing intolerable adverse effects or to titrate dosage of baclofen to the desired degree of muscle tone for optimal function. Results of one randomized, controlled, crossover study in patients with cerebral palsy indicate that intrathecal baclofen was more effective than placebo in reducing spasticity as measured by the Ashworth scale. In addition, results of a small (11 patients) controlled study in patients with brain injury indicate that intrathecal baclofen was more effective than placebo in reducing spasticity.

Patients with spasticity secondary to brain injury should wait at least one year after the injury before considering long-term intrathecal baclofen therapy.

● Other Uses

Baclofen has been used orally to reduce choreiform movements in patients with Huntington's chorea†, to reduce rigidity in patients with parkinsonian syndrome†, and to reduce spasticity in patients with cerebral lesions†, cerebral palsy†, or rheumatic disorders†; however, the drug has not been shown to produce a substantial degree of improvement in these patients. Oral baclofen also has been used to reduce spasticity in patients with cerebrovascular stroke†; however, therapy with the drug generally did not provide substantial improvement and was poorly tolerated. The manufacturer states oral baclofen is *not* indicated for use in patients with rheumatic disorders; use of oral baclofen also is not recommended in patients with stroke, cerebral palsy, or Parkinson's disease.

Although in one study oral baclofen reportedly improved behavior in patients with schizophrenic disorder† receiving other drugs concomitantly (e.g., phenothiazines), schizophrenic behavior worsened in other patients when baclofen was used alone. Preliminary data indicate that oral baclofen has beneficial effects in the treatment of trigeminal neuralgia† and may be synergistic with carbamazepine and phenytoin.

DOSAGE AND ADMINISTRATION

● Administration

Baclofen is administered orally or intrathecally. Abrupt discontinuance of the drug, including inadvertent discontinuance of the intrathecal infusion, should be avoided because of the risk of precipitating withdrawal.

Intrathecal Administration

For intrathecal use, baclofen is administered as an additive-free injection by direct intrathecal injection (via lumbar puncture or catheter) over a period of at least 1 minute employing barbotage or by continuous intrathecal infusion into a lumbar intrathecal space via an implantable controlled-infusion device (pump). The manufacturer's labeling should be consulted for specialized administration techniques.

In the preparation of test doses of the drug for the purposes of drug-response screening prior to initiation of chronic intrathecal baclofen therapy, 1-mL ampuls containing 50 mcg of baclofen should be used without further dilution. For maintenance therapy in patients receiving concentrations of the drug other than the commercially available strengths (i.e., 0.5 or 2 mg/mL), baclofen for injection concentrate for intrathecal administration *must* be diluted. The concentrate *must* only be diluted with sterile, preservative-free 0.9% sodium chloride injection. The specific concentration that should be used depends on the total daily dosage required and the delivery rate of the pump. The manufacturer's manual should be consulted for specific recommendations.

As with other parenteral drug products, baclofen for injection concentrate and diluted solutions of the drug should be inspected visually for particulate matter and/or discoloration prior to administration, whenever solution and container permit.

Patients receiving intrathecal baclofen therapy must be monitored closely in a fully equipped and staffed environment during the initial test for responsiveness and dosage-titration period immediately following implantation of the pump. Resuscitative equipment should be immediately available for use in case of life-threatening or intolerable adverse effects.

Extemporaneously Compounded Oral Suspension

An extemporaneously compounded 5 mg/mL oral suspension of baclofen has been prepared using the commercially available 20-mg tablets and Simple Syrup, NF.

Standardize 4 Safety

Standardized concentrations for an extemporaneously prepared oral liquid formulation of baclofen have been established through Standardize 4 Safety (S4S), a national patient safety initiative to reduce medication errors, especially during transitions of care. Multidisciplinary expert panels were convened to determine recommended standard concentrations. Because recommendations from the S4S panels may differ from the manufacturer's prescribing information, caution is advised when using concentrations that differ from labeling, particularly when using rate information from the label. For additional information on S4S (including updates that may be available), see https://www.ashp.org/pharmacy-practice/standardize-4-safety-initiative.

TABLE 1. Standardize 4 Safety Compounded Oral Liquid Standards for Baclofen

Concentration Standards
5 mg/mL

● Dosage

Spasticity

Oral Dosage

Oral dosage of baclofen should be individualized according to the patient's requirements and response using the lowest dosage that produces optimum response. Initially, low oral dosages of the drug should be administered.

For the management of spasticity, the initial oral dosage of baclofen is 5 mg 3 times daily. Oral daily dosage may be increased by 15 mg at 3-day intervals (i.e., 5 mg 3 times daily for 3 days, then 10 mg 3 times daily for 3 days, then 15 mg 3 times daily for 3 days, then 20 mg 3 times daily for 3 days) until optimum effect is achieved (usually at dosages of 40–80 mg daily). In patients with psychiatric or brain disorders and in geriatric patients, oral dosage should be increased more gradually. In some patients, a smoother antispastic effect is obtained by administering the oral daily dosage in 4 divided doses. Some clinicians suggest that daily oral dosages of up to 150 mg are well tolerated and provide additional therapeutic benefit in some patients; however, the manufacturers state that total dosage should not exceed 80 mg daily (i.e., 20 mg 4 times daily). Some patients require 1–2 months of treatment for full benefit; however, the length of baclofen trial should be determined by the clinical state of the patient. If benefits are not evident after a reasonable trial, baclofen therapy should be discontinued by slowly reducing the daily dosage.

Severe Spasticity

Intrathecal Dosage

Prior to implantation of the controlled-infusion device (e.g., Medtronic SynchroMed® pump) and initiation of chronic intrathecal baclofen therapy, the patient must exhibit a positive response (defined as a clinically important decrease in muscle tone and/or frequency and/or severity of spasms over a 4- to 8-hour observation period) to initial intrathecal baclofen test dose(s). Initially, a dose containing 50 mcg (1 mL of a 50-mcg/mL solution) of baclofen is administered into the intrathecal space by barbotage over a period of at least 1 minute. If response observed at 4–8 hours after the initial test dose is less than desired, a second injection containing 75 mcg (1.5 mL of a 50-mcg/mL solution) of baclofen may be administered 24 hours after the first dose. If response observed at 4–8 hours after the second test dose remains inadequate, a final injection containing 100 mcg (2 mL of a 50-mcg/mL solution) of baclofen may be administered 24 hours after the second dose. In pediatric patients, the initial test dose is the same as in adults (i.e., 50 mcg); however, in very small children, an initial dose of 25 mcg may be considered. Patients not responding to the 100-mcg intrathecal test dose of the drug are not considered candidates for chronic intrathecal baclofen therapy.

Following establishment of responsiveness to intrathecal baclofen and implantation of a compatible pump (e.g., SynchroMed® infusion system), the initial intrathecal dose of baclofen for the management of spasticity is twice the test dose that produced a positive response with a duration not exceeding 8 hours; this dose is infused intrathecally over 24 hours. For patients in whom a positive response to the test dose persisted for longer than 8 hours, the initial intrathecal dose is the same as the test dose that produced a positive response; this dose also is infused intrathecally over 24 hours. Dosage should not be increased within 24 hours after the initial intrathecal dose (i.e., until steady state is achieved). Following the initial infusion dose in adults with spasticity of *spinal cord origin*, the daily dose can be increased slowly by 10–30% increments at 24-hour intervals until the desired clinical response is achieved; in pediatric patients with spasticity of *spinal cord origin* and adult and pediatric patients with spasticity of *cerebral origin*, the daily dose can be increased slowly by 5–15% increments at 24-hour intervals until the desired clinical response is achieved. If no substantive increase in response is observed with upward titration of intrathecal baclofen dosage, the function of the pump and patency of the catheter should be checked.

Adjustment of maintenance dosage often is needed during the initial months of intrathecal baclofen therapy as the patient adjusts to changes in life-style secondary to relief of spasticity. During periodic refills of the pump, the 24-hour dose may be increased by up to 10–40% or up to 5–20% in patients with spasticity of spinal cord origin or those with spasticity of cerebral origin, respectively, as necessary to maintain adequate control of symptoms. In patients who develop intolerable adverse effects, the 24-hour maintenance dose can be decreased by 10–20%. During chronic therapy, gradual increases in dosage will be required in most patients to maintain optimal response. A sudden increase in dosage requirement should suggest the possibility of pump and/or catheter malfunction (i.e., catheter kink or dislodgement). In patients with spasticity of *spinal cord origin*, maintenance dosage during chronic intrathecal therapy has ranged from 12–2003 mcg daily, with most patients responding adequately to 300–800 mcg daily. There is only limited experience with intrathecal baclofen dosages of 1000 mcg daily or greater in these patients. In patients with spasticity of *cerebral origin*, maintenance dosage during chronic intrathecal therapy has ranged from 22–1400 mcg daily, with most patients responding adequately to 90–703 mcg daily. In clinical studies in patients with spasticity of cerebral origin, only about 2% of patients required daily dosages exceeding 1000 mcg daily.

Maintenance dosage recommendations for pediatric patients are similar to those for patients with spasticity of cerebral origin. Pediatric patients younger than 12 years of age may require lower daily dosages; in clinical trials, the maintenance daily dosage averaged 274 mcg daily (range: 24–1199 mcg daily). Dosage requirements for pediatric patients older than 12 years of age does not appear to be different from that for adult patients. Determination of optimum therapy requires individual titration. The lowest possible dosage that produces optimum response should be employed.

During prolonged intrathecal baclofen therapy for spasticity, approximately 5% of patients become refractory to increasing dosages of the drug. While experience currently is insufficient to make firm recommendations regarding amelioration of such tolerance, patients occasionally have been hospitalized and subjected to a "drug holiday" in which intrathecal dosage was decreased gradually over a 2- to 4-week period, during which baclofen therapy was alternated with other methods of spasticity management. After a few days, sensitivity to baclofen may return and continuous intrathecal baclofen therapy may be resumed at the previously effective initial dosage.

For patients achieving relatively satisfactory relief via continuous intrathecal infusion employing an implantable pump, further benefit may be possible with more complex dosing schedules. For example, patients who commonly experience an exacerbation of spasticity at night that disrupts sleep may require a 20% increase in the hourly infusion rate; such changes should be programmed to begin approximately 2 hours before the time of desired clinical benefit.

The manual provided by the manufacturer of the implantable infusion device (i.e., pump) must be consulted for additional information, including specific instructions and precautions for programming the pump and/or refilling the reservoir. Various pumps (with different reservoir volumes) and refill kits are available; clinicians must be familiar with these products in order to select the appropriate refill kit for the particular pump in use.

● Dosage in Renal Impairment

Because baclofen is excreted principally in urine as unchanged drug, it may be necessary to reduce either oral or intrathecal dosage in patients with impaired renal function. (See Cautions: Precautions and Contraindications.)

CAUTIONS

● Adverse Effects

The most common adverse effect of *oral* baclofen therapy is transient drowsiness (10–63%); other common adverse effects of oral baclofen therapy include dizziness (5–15%), weakness (5–15%), and fatigue (2–4%).

The most common adverse effects of *intrathecal* baclofen therapy in patients with spasticity of *spinal cord origin* include somnolence, dizziness, nausea, hypotension, headache, seizures, and hypotonia. The most common adverse effects of *intrathecal* baclofen therapy in patients with spasticity of *cerebral origin* include agitation, constipation, somnolence, leukocytosis, chills, urinary retention, and hypotonia.

The incidence of adverse effects during oral administration of baclofen can be minimized by slowly increasing dosage to therapeutic levels. If adverse effects occur, they can be reduced by decreasing dosage. Psychiatric disturbances, including hallucinations, euphoria, mental excitation, depression, confusion or anxiety, occur most commonly in patients with psychiatric or brain disorders, including stroke, and in geriatric patients; any increase in oral dosage should be made slowly in these patients. Many adverse CNS and genitourinary effects also are symptoms of the underlying disease (i.e., multiple sclerosis, spinal cord lesions) and may not be related to baclofen therapy.

CNS Effects

Neuropsychiatric disturbances reported during oral baclofen treatment include confusion, headache, insomnia, and, rarely, euphoria, excitement, depression, hallucinations, paresthesia, muscle pain, tinnitus, slurred speech, coordination disorder, tremor, rigidity, dystonia, ataxia, blurred vision, nystagmus, strabismus, miosis, mydriasis, diplopia, dysarthria, and seizures. Neuropsychiatric disturbances or adverse CNS effects reported during intrathecal baclofen treatment include hypotonia, somnolence, dizziness, paresthesia, hypertonia, headache, seizures, asthenia, confusion, speech disorder, coma, insomnia, anxiety, depression, abnormal thinking, tremor, agitation, dysautonomia, hallucinations, abnormal gait, amnesia, twitching, vasodilation, cerebrovascular accident, nystagmus, personality disorder, psychotic depression, cerebral ischemia, emotional lability, euphoria, ileus, drug dependence, incoordination, paranoid reaction, ptosis, akathisia, ataxia, opisthotonos, hysteria, insomnia, decreased reflexes, and vasodilation.

Genitourinary Effects

Urinary frequency and, rarely, enuresis, urinary retention, dysuria, impotence, inability to ejaculate, nocturia, and hematuria have occurred during oral baclofen therapy. During intrathecal baclofen therapy, urinary retention or incontinence, impotence, urinary frequency, impaired urination, hematuria, kidney failure, abnormal ejaculation, kidney calculus, oliguria, and vaginitis have been reported.

In female rats, chronic administration of oral baclofen has caused a dose-related increase in the incidence of ovarian cysts and a less marked increase in enlarged or hemorrhagic adrenal glands. Ovarian cysts have been found by palpation in about 4% of multiple sclerosis patients receiving oral baclofen for up to 1 year, but these cysts spontaneously disappeared despite continued use of the drug in most patients. It should be noted, however, that ovarian cysts are estimated to occur spontaneously in approximately 1–5% of healthy females.

Cardiovascular Effects

Adverse cardiovascular effects such as hypotension and, rarely, dyspnea, palpitation, chest pain, and syncope have occurred during oral baclofen therapy. Hypotension (including orthostatic hypotension), hypertension, dyspnea, bradycardia, palpitations, syncope, ventricular arrhythmia, deep thrombophlebitis, pallor, and tachycardia have been reported during intrathecal baclofen therapy.

GI Effects

Adverse GI effects of oral baclofen therapy include nausea and constipation and, rarely, dry mouth, anorexia, taste disorders, abdominal pain, vomiting, diarrhea, and positive tests for occult blood in the stool. Nausea, vomiting, constipation, dry mouth, diarrhea, anorexia, increased salivation, flatulence, dysphagia, dyspepsia, gastroenteritis, fecal incontinence, GI hemorrhage, tongue disorder, and abdominal pain have been reported during intrathecal baclofen therapy.

Abrupt Withdrawal

Abrupt discontinuance of oral baclofen therapy, regardless of the cause, has resulted in hallucinations and seizures. Abrupt discontinuance of intrathecal baclofen therapy has resulted in high fever, altered mental status, exaggerated rebound spasticity, and muscle rigidity that, in rare cases, have progressed to rhabdomyolysis, multisystem organ failure, and death. In most cases, manifestations of withdrawal appeared within hours to a few days following discontinuance of baclofen therapy. All patients receiving intrathecal baclofen therapy are potentially at risk for withdrawal. Early manifestations of intrathecal baclofen withdrawal may include return of baseline spasticity, pruritus, hypotension, and paresthesias. Clinical presentation of advanced intrathecal baclofen withdrawal syndrome may resemble autonomic dysreflexia, infection (sepsis), malignant hyperthermia, neuroleptic malignant syndrome (NMS), or other conditions associated with a hypermetabolic state or widespread rhabdomyolysis. (See Cautions: Precautions and Contraindications.) Baclofen therapy should be slowly discontinued to minimize the risk of withdrawal.

Death

Although fatalities, including one case of unexpected death after administration of 3 test doses and 2 cases of sudden and unexpected death occurring within 2 weeks of pump implantation, have been reported rarely during the use of intrathecal baclofen therapy, the manufacturer states that a causal relationship to the drug could not be established.

Other Adverse Effects

Rash, pruritus, ankle edema, excessive perspiration, weight gain, and nasal congestion have been reported during oral baclofen therapy. Increases in blood glucose concentration and serum AST (SGOT) and alkaline phosphatase concentrations also have been reported during oral therapy. During intrathecal baclofen therapy, accidental injury, death, pain, amblyopia, hypoventilation, peripheral edema, fever, pneumonia, urticaria, diplopia, back pain, pruritus, rash, sweating, alopecia, contact dermatitis, skin ulcer, chills, respiratory disorder, aspiration pneumonia, hyperventilation, apnea, pulmonary embolus, rhinitis, weight loss, albuminuria, dehydration, hyperglycemia, abnormal vision, abnormality of accommodation, photophobia, taste loss, tinnitus, suicide, hypothermia, neck rigidity, chest pain, chills, face edema, flu syndrome, anemia, carcinoma, malaise, leukocytosis, and petechial rash have been reported.

● Precautions and Contraindications

Deteriorations in seizure control and EEG occasionally have been noted in epileptic patients receiving the drug; the epileptic patient's clinical state and EEG should be monitored at regular intervals during baclofen treatment.

Because baclofen may cause sedation and/or drowsiness, patients should be warned that therapy with the drug may impair their ability to perform hazardous activities requiring mental alertness or physical coordination such as operating machinery or driving a motor vehicle. In addition, additive CNS depression may occur when the drug is administered concomitantly with other CNS depressants, including alcohol. Oral or intrathecal baclofen should be used with caution, and it may be necessary to reduce dosage in patients with impaired renal function. The drug should be used with caution, with careful dosage titration, in patients who must use spasticity to maintain upright posture and balance in moving or when spasticity is used to obtain increased or optimal body function.

Patients with psychotic disorders, schizophrenia, or confusional states should be treated cautiously and kept under careful surveillance during intrathecal baclofen therapy, as exacerbations of these conditions have been reported following oral administration of the drug.

Intrathecal baclofen therapy should be instituted with caution in patients with a history of autonomic dysreflexia, since the presence of nociceptive stimuli or the abrupt withdrawal of therapy may precipitate an episode of dysreflexia.

The clinical goal of baclofen therapy is to maintain muscle tone as close to normal as possible and to minimize the frequency and severity of spasms without inducing intolerable adverse effects. It may be important to maintain some degree of muscle tone and allow occasional spasms to help support circulatory function, minimize the risk of development of deep-vein thrombosis, and optimize activities of daily living and ease of care.

If intrathecal baclofen therapy is to be employed, an attempt should be made to discontinue concomitant oral antispasmodic drugs, including oral baclofen, to avoid possible overdose and drug interactions, either prior to the screening phase or following implantation of the infusion device. Dosage reduction and discontinuance of concomitant oral antispasmodics should be employed slowly, and the patient should be monitored carefully; abrupt dosage reduction or discontinuance of concomitant antispasmodics should be avoided.

Patients undergoing pump implantation for the initiation of intrathecal baclofen therapy should be without concurrent infection, as the presence of infection may interfere with assessment of the patient's response to the baclofen test dose(s), increase surgical complications after pump implantation, and complicate attempts to adjust dosage.

Development of intrathecal mass at the tip of the implanted catheter, usually involving pharmacy compounded analgesic admixtures, has been reported in patients receiving long-term intrathecal baclofen therapy. The most common sequelae or manifestations associated with intrathecal mass include decreased therapeutic response (i.e., worsening spasticity, return of spasticity despite previous response, withdrawal symptoms, poor response to escalating doses, frequent or large dosage increases), pain, and neurologic deficit or dysfunction. Patients receiving intraspinal therapy should be carefully monitored for any new neurologic manifestations. If new neurologic manifestations suggestive of an intrathecal mass occur, a neurosurgical consultation should be considered, since many of the symptoms of inflammatory mass are similar to those observed in patients with severe spasticity. In some cases, performance of an imaging procedure may be appropriate to confirm or rule out the diagnosis of an intrathecal mass.

Because of the possibility of potentially life-threatening CNS depression, cardiovascular collapse, and/or respiratory failure, baclofen should be administered intrathecally only by qualified individuals familiar with the techniques of administration and patient management problems. When an implantable pump is used, familiarization with the device is essential, including specific instructions and precautions for programming the pump and refilling the reservoir. The patient, their caregivers, and health-care providers must receive adequate information regarding the risks of such therapy, including information on recognition and management of potential overdosage and proper care of the pump and catheter insertion site. Because of the risks involved, the initial test for responsiveness to intrathecal baclofen, implantation of the pump, and subsequent periods of dosage titration must be performed in a medically supervised setting that is adequately equipped for the management of potential complications; resuscitative equipment should be readily available. Filling of the drug reservoir of the device should be performed under aseptic conditions (to avoid bacterial contamination and serious infection) and only by fully trained and qualified personnel, following the directions provided by the device's manufacturer. The pump should be filled with extreme caution and should be refilled only through the reservoir refill septum of the device. If the reservoir refill septum is not properly accessed, inadvertent injection into the subcutaneous tissue can occur, possibly resulting in life-threatening overdosage or early depletion of the reservoir. Some pumps also are equipped with a catheter access port that allows direct access to the intrathecal catheter; direct injection into this catheter may cause life-threatening overdosage of the drug. During chronic therapy, care should be taken in employing the proper refill frequency so that depletion of the drug reservoir during use is avoided; symptoms of spasticity (e.g., rigidity) usually return within a few days if dosing is discontinued, and manifestations of withdrawal (e.g., hallucinations, seizures) could emerge. Careful patient monitoring is particularly important during the initial phase of pump use, dosage titration, and reservoir refilling so that an acceptable, reasonably stable response is ensured.

Abrupt discontinuance of oral baclofen therapy, regardless of the cause, has resulted in hallucinations and seizures. Abrupt discontinuance of intrathecal baclofen therapy has resulted in high fever, altered mental status, exaggerated rebound spasticity, and muscle rigidity that, in rare cases, have progressed to rhabdomyolysis, multisystem organ failure, and death. Common reasons for abrupt interruption of intrathecal baclofen therapy include malfunction of the catheter (particularly disconnection), low volume in the pump reservoir, end of pump battery life, and, possibly, human error. Cases of intrathecal mass at the tip of the implanted catheter (most of which involved pharmacy compounded analgesic admixtures) also have reportedly resulted in withdrawal symptoms. Therefore, the manufacturer states that careful attention to programming and monitoring of the infusion system, refill scheduling and procedures, and pump alarms is necessary to prevent abrupt discontinuance of intrathecal baclofen therapy. Patients and caregivers should be advised of the importance of keeping scheduled refill visits and should be informed of the early signs and symptoms of baclofen withdrawal. (See Abrupt Withdrawal under Cautions: Adverse Effects.) Special attention should be given to patients at apparent risk for withdrawal (e.g., spinal cord injury at the T6 level or above, communication difficulties, history of withdrawal symptoms from oral or intrathecal baclofen). Rapid, accurate diagnosis and treatment in an emergency room or intensive care setting are important in order to prevent the potentially life-threatening CNS and systemic effects of intrathecal baclofen withdrawal. Treatment of intrathecal baclofen withdrawal includes restoration of intrathecal baclofen at or near the dosage used prior to interruption of therapy. However, if reinstitution of intrathecal delivery is delayed, therapy with drugs that enhance GABA effects (e.g., oral or enteral baclofen; oral, enteral, or IV benzodiazepines) may prevent potentially fatal sequelae. However, the manufacturer states that oral or enteral baclofen alone should not be relied upon to halt the progression of intrathecal baclofen withdrawal.

Oral and intrathecal baclofen are contraindicated in patients with a history of hypersensitivity to the drug. Baclofen injection for intrathecal administration is not recommended or intended for IV, IM, subcutaneous, or epidural administration.

● Pediatric Precautions

The manufacturers state that safety of oral or intrathecal baclofen therapy in pediatric patients younger than 12 or 4 years of age, respectively, has not been established. Pediatric patients undergoing pump implantation for the initiation of intrathecal baclofen therapy should have sufficient body mass to accommodate the pump. Directions provided by the device's manufacturer should be consulted.

● Pregnancy, Fertility, and Lactation

Pregnancy

Reproduction studies in rats receiving oral baclofen at a dosage approximately 13 or 3 times the maximum recommended human oral dosage on a mg/kg or mg/m² basis, respectively, demonstrated an increased incidence of omphaloceles (ventral hernias) in the fetuses; substantial reductions in food intake and weight gain occurred in pregnant rats receiving this dosage. An increased incidence of omphaloceles did not occur in mice or rabbit fetuses. An increased incidence of incomplete sternebral ossification occurred in the fetuses of rats receiving approximately 13 times the maximum recommended human dosage, and an increased incidence of unossified phalangeal nuclei of the forelimbs and hindlimbs occurred in the fetuses of rabbits receiving approximately 7 times the maximum recommended dosage. No teratogenic effects occurred in mice, although reduction in mean fetal weight with consequent delay in skeletal ossification occurred in offspring of mice receiving 17 or 34 times the human daily dosage of baclofen. There are no adequate and controlled studies using baclofen in pregnant women, and the drug should be used during pregnancy only when the potential benefits justify the possible risks to the fetus.

Lactation

Baclofen is distributed into milk following oral administration; it not known whether the drug distributes into milk following intrathecal administration. At least one manufacturer states that nursing should not be undertaken by women receiving oral baclofen. Nursing should be undertaken by women receiving intrathecal baclofen only if the potential benefit justifies the potential risks to the infant.

DRUG INTERACTIONS

Experience with concomitant use of intrathecal baclofen with other drugs is insufficient to predict specific drug-drug interactions.

● CNS Depressants

Concomitant use of baclofen with other CNS depressants (e.g., alcohol) may result in additive CNS depression.

● Morphine

Concomitant use of intrathecal baclofen with epidural morphine reportedly has resulted in hypotension and dyspnea.

ACUTE TOXICITY

● Manifestations

Following ingestion of about 1 g of baclofen by a patient attempting suicide, reflexes were absent, and vomiting, muscle hypotonia, marked salivation, drowsiness, visual accommodation disorders, coma, respiratory depression, and seizures occurred. Serum lactic dehydrogenase and AST (SGOT) concentrations were also elevated. Supportive treatment consisted of endotracheal intubation and positive-pressure ventilation; after 3 days, some signs of muscle flaccidity still persisted. If oral baclofen overdosage occurs, the manufacturer recommends that the stomach be emptied promptly (i.e., by inducing emesis followed by gastric lavage) if the patient is alert. If the patient is obtunded, the airway should be secured with a cuffed endotracheal tube before beginning lavage, and adequate respiratory exchange should be maintained; induction of emesis and use of respiratory stimulants should be avoided.

Signs of intrathecal baclofen overdose may appear suddenly or over a period of time. Special attention must be given to recognizing the signs and symptoms of overdosage, particularly during the initial test for responsiveness, dosage titration, and reintroduction of therapy following temporary interruption. Acute, massive overdose may present as coma; in reports of coma resulting from overdose of intrathecal baclofen, the coma generally has been reversible following discontinuance of the infusion. Less sudden and/or less severe forms of overdose may present with drowsiness, lightheadedness, dizziness, somnolence, respiratory depression, hypothermia, seizures, rostral progression of hypotonia, and loss of consciousness progressing to coma persisting up to 72 hours. Should overdose appear likely, the patient should be taken immediately to a hospital for assessment and emptying of the pump reservoir. The manufacturer states that in cases reported to date, overdose generally has been related to pump malfunction, inadvertent subcutaneous injection, or dosing error; however, symptoms of overdose were reported in a baclofen-sensitive adult patient following intrathecal injection of a 25-mcg dose.

● Treatment

In the treatment of oral baclofen overdosage, immediate removal of the drug from the GI tract by emesis (if patient is conscious) or gastric lavage and maintenance of adequate respiratory exchange are recommended. If the patient is comatose, gastric lavage may be performed if an endotracheal tube with cuff inflated is in place to prevent aspiration of gastric contents. Respiratory stimulants should not be used.

There is no specific antidote for treating overdoses of baclofen intrathecal injection; however, any remaining baclofen solution in the pump should be removed as soon as possible and patients exhibiting respiratory depression should be intubated as necessary until the drug is eliminated.

If lumbar puncture is not contraindicated, consideration should be given to withdrawing 30-40 mL of CSF in order to reduce CSF baclofen concentration.

PHARMACOLOGY

Baclofen decreases the frequency and amplitude of muscle spasms (tonic reflexes) that arise in response to muscle stretching in patients with various spinal cord lesions. The drug simultaneously and equally suppresses cutaneous reflexes and muscle tone but only slightly depresses the amplitude of tendon jerks (phasic reflexes). The mechanism of action of baclofen is not completely understood, but the drug appears to act primarily at the spinal cord level. Apparently, baclofen predominantly inhibits spinal polysynaptic afferent pathways but may also inhibit monosynaptic afferent pathways to a lesser extent. The drug may inhibit monosynaptic and polysynaptic reflexes by acting as an inhibitory neuronal transmitter or by blocking excitatory synaptic transmission through hyperpolarization of afferent terminals. Because baclofen contains both GABA and phenylethylamine moieties, it has been postulated, but not proven, that the drug activates one of these putative inhibitory neurotransmitters. Baclofen has been shown to increase the metabolism of dopamine in animals but, in humans, CSF concentrations of 5-hydroxyindole acetic acid or dopamine metabolites are not altered by the drug. Because baclofen produces generalized CNS depression (e.g., sedation with tolerance, somnolence, ataxia, respiratory and cardiovascular depression), it has also been suggested that the drug may act at supraspinal sites.

Intrathecal administration of the drug in animals has been shown to increase antinociception and decrease muscle rigidity and spasticity.

PHARMACOKINETICS

● Absorption

Studies with radiolabeled baclofen have shown oral doses of 40 mg to be rapidly and almost completely absorbed from the GI tract, but there is relatively large intersubject variation in absorption and/or elimination. GI absorption of baclofen is reduced as dosage is increased. Serum concentrations required for therapeutic effects reportedly range from 80-395 ng/mL. Following oral administration of 40 mg of baclofen to healthy patients, peak blood concentrations of 500-600 ng/mL are reached in 2-3 hours and concentrations remain above 200 ng/mL for 8 hours. Beneficial effects of oral baclofen may not be immediately apparent; onset of therapeutic effect may vary from hours to weeks.

Following intrathecal administration of the drug, concurrent plasma baclofen concentrations are expected to be low (0-5 ng/mL); plasma concentrations of baclofen following intrathecal administration are 100 times lower than those achieved following oral administration. In pediatric patients 8-18 years of age who were receiving a continuous intrathecal infusion of baclofen at dosages of 77-400 mcg daily, plasma baclofen concentrations were near or below 10 mg/mL.

When baclofen is administered via intrathecal injection, the onset of action in adult patients generally is 0.5-1 hour following injection; peak spasmolytic effect is seen approximately 4 hours after dosing and effects may last 4-8 hours, although onset, peak, and duration of action are subject to interindividual variation, depending on the dose and severity of symptoms. Onset and duration of action and peak effects of baclofen in pediatric patients are similar to those reported in adult patients.

Following continuous intrathecal infusions of the drug, initial spasmolytic action is seen within 6-8 hours in adult patients; peak spasmolytic effect is observed within 24-48 hours. Pharmacokinetic data following continuous intrathecal infusion in pediatric patients currently are not available.

● Distribution

In animals, orally administered baclofen is widely distributed throughout the body, but only small amounts of the drug cross the blood-brain barrier.

Limited data suggest that a lumbar-cisternal gradient of approximately 4:1 is established along the neuroaxis during infusion of baclofen injection, based on simultaneous CSF sampling via lumbar and cisternal taps in a limited number of patients receiving continuous lumbar infusion of the drug at doses associated with therapeutic efficacy; however, there was wide interindividual variation. This gradient was not affected by patient position.

Baclofen crosses the placenta. Baclofen is distributed into milk following oral administration; it is not known whether the drug is distributed into milk following intrathecal administration.

At blood concentrations of 10 ng to 300 mcg/mL, 30% of baclofen is bound to serum proteins.

● Elimination

Baclofen has a serum half-life of 2.5-4 hours.

CSF clearance of baclofen following intrathecal administration via injection or continuous infusion approximates CSF turnover, suggesting that elimination of the drug occurs via bulk-flow removal of CSF. Following lumbar injection of the drug in doses of 50 or 100 mcg in a limited number of patients, the mean CSF elimination half-life was 1.51 hours for the first 4 hours following injection; mean CSF clearance of the drug was 30 mL/hour. Mean CSF clearance of the drug also was 30 mL/hour in a limited number of patients receiving the drug via continuous intrathecal infusion.

Only about 15% of a dose of the drug is metabolized in the liver, mostly by deamination. Baclofen is almost completely excreted within 72 hours following oral administration; 70-80% of the drug is excreted in urine unchanged or as metabolites and the remainder is excreted in the feces.

CHEMISTRY AND STABILITY

● *Chemistry*

Baclofen, the *p*-chlorophenyl derivative of γ-aminobutyric acid (GABA) containing a phenylethylamine moiety, is a skeletal muscle relaxant. Baclofen occurs as white to off-white crystals and is slightly soluble in water, very slightly soluble in methanol, and insoluble in chloroform. The drug has pK$_a$ values of 5.4 and 9.5.

● *Stability*

Baclofen tablets should be stored in well-closed containers at 20–25°C.

Baclofen for injection concentrate for intrathecal administration is a sterile, nonpyrogenic, isotonic solution of the drug in water for injection. Each mL of the concentrate contains 0.39 mEq of sodium. Baclofen concentrate does not require refrigeration and is stable in solution at 37°C; however, the concentrate should not be stored at a temperature that exceeds 30°C and should not be frozen or autoclaved. The pH of the concentrate is 5–7. Because baclofen for injection concentrate contains no preservatives, each vial is intended for single use only; any unused solution should be discarded. Baclofen for injection concentrate is compatible with CSF, and must *only* be diluted with sterile, preservative-free 0.9% sodium chloride for injection.

PREPARATIONS

Excipients in commercially available drug preparations may have clinically important effects in some individuals; consult specific product labeling for details.

Baclofen

Oral		
Tablets	10 mg*	**Baclofen Tablets** (scored)
	20 mg*	**Baclofen Tablets** (scored)
Parenteral		
For injection concentrate, for intrathecal administration via compatible infusion device or for intrathecal injection	50 mcg/mL	**Gablofen®**, CNS Therapeutics
		Lioresal® Intrathecal, Medtronic
	0.5 mg/mL	**Gablofen®**, CNS Therapeutics
		Lioresal® Intrathecal, Medtronic
	2 mg/mL	**Gablofen®**, CNS Therapeutics
		Lioresal® Intrathecal, Medtronic

* available from one or more manufacturer, distributor, and/or repackager by generic (nonproprietary) name

† Use is not currently included in the labeling approved by the US Food and Drug Administration.

Selected Revisions June 10, 2024, © Copyright, January 1, 1979, American Society of Health-System Pharmacists, Inc.

Cisatracurium Besylate

12:20.20 • NEUROMUSCULAR BLOCKING AGENTS

■ Cisatracurium besylate, a benzylisoquinolone nondepolarizing neuromuscular blocking agent, is an isomer of atracurium.

USES

● Skeletal Muscle Relaxation

Cisatracurium besylate is used to produce skeletal muscle relaxation during surgery after general anesthesia has been induced. The drug also is used to facilitate endotracheal intubation; however, a neuromuscular blocking agent with a rapid onset of action (e.g., succinylcholine, rocuronium) generally is preferred in emergency situations when rapid intubation is required. Cisatracurium is *not* recommended for rapid sequence intubation because of its intermediate onset of action.

Cisatracurium also is used to facilitate mechanical ventilation in the intensive care unit (ICU). The drug has been given as a continuous IV infusion for up to 6 days in this setting; longer durations of use have not been evaluated. Whenever neuromuscular blocking agents are used in the ICU, the benefits versus risks of such therapy must be considered and patients should be assessed frequently to determine the need for continued paralysis.

Compared with other neuromuscular blocking agents, cisatracurium has an intermediate onset and duration of action. In clinical studies, cisatracurium was administered at a rate of infusion one-third that of atracurium and exhibited a similar time to spontaneous recovery. Studies comparing cisatracurium with vecuronium showed a longer duration of action and faster time to spontaneous recovery with cisatracurium. Cisatracurium has minimal, if any, cardiovascular effects and causes less histamine release than atracurium. Because cisatracurium (and atracurium) undergo Hofmann degradation and are not dependent on renal or hepatic pathways for elimination, these neuromuscular blocking agents may be particularly useful in patients with hepatic or renal impairment; some experts prefer the use of cisatracurium or atracurium if prolonged therapy is necessary in ICU patients with multiple organ dysfunction.

For additional information on uses and treatment principles of neuromuscular blocking agents, see Uses in the Neuromuscular Blocking Agents General Statement 12:20.20.

DOSAGE AND ADMINISTRATION

● Administration

Cisatracurium is administered IV only.

Commercially available 20-mL single-dose vials of cisatracurium besylate containing 10 mg/mL are intended for intensive care unit (ICU) use *only*.

IV Administration

The initial (intubating) dose of cisatracurium is administered by rapid IV injection; maintenance doses may be administered by intermittent IV injection or continuous IV infusion.

For continuous IV infusion, cisatracurium besylate injection should be diluted to the desired concentration (e.g., 0.1–0.4 mg/mL) in a compatible IV solution (5% dextrose, 0.9% sodium chloride, or 5% dextrose and 0.9% sodium chloride injection). Continuous IV infusions of cisatracurium have been administered for up to 3 hours without evidence of cumulative neuromuscular blocking effects; such administration has no effect on duration of blockade, provided partial recovery is allowed to occur between doses. The rate of spontaneous neuromuscular recovery following discontinuance of the infusion is likely to be comparable to the rate of recovery following administration of a single IV injection of the drug.

Cisatracurium besylate injection should be stored at 2–8°C and protected from light prior to use; the drug should not be frozen. Once removed from refrigeration, the injection should be used within 21 days, regardless of whether it was subsequently returned to refrigeration. Following dilution, the infusion solution should be used within 24 hours.

Standardize 4 Safety

Standardized concentrations for cisatracurium have been established through Standardize 4 Safety (S4S), a national patient safety initiative to reduce medication errors, especially during transitions of care. Multidisciplinary expert panels were convened to determine recommended standard concentrations. Because recommendations from the S4S panels may differ from the manufacturer's prescribing information, caution is advised when using concentrations that differ from labeling, particularly when using rate information from the label. For additional information on S4S (including updates that may be available), see https://www.ashp.org/pharmacy-practice/standardize-4-safety-initiative.

TABLE 1. Standardize 4 Safety Continuous IV Infusion Standard Concentrations for Cisatracurium

Patient Population	Concentration Standards	Dosing Units
Adults[b c]	2 mg/mL	mcg/kg/min[a]
Pediatric patients (<50 kg)	1 mg/mL	mg/kg/hour
	2 mg/mL	

[a] dosing units differ from concentration units

[b] Paralytics are recommended to be administered as straight drug. This provides consistency between operating room and the ICU, and eliminates potential compounding errors.

[c] This is a concentration that differs from the package insert, therefore infusion-related calculations will differ from the prescribing information.

Rate of Administration

Initial (intubating) doses of cisatracurium are administered by direct IV injection, usually over 5–10 seconds.

Continuous IV infusion rates should be individualized based on patient requirements and response to peripheral nerve stimulation. (See Tables 2 and 3 for recommended rates of infusion.) Accurate dosage is best achieved using a precision infusion device.

TABLE 2. Infusion Rates Required to Deliver Selected Dosages of Cisatracurium from Solutions Containing 0.1 mg/mL of the Drug

Weight (kg)	Drug Delivery Rate (mcg/kg per minute) 1 — Infusion Delivery Rate (mL/hr)	Drug Delivery Rate (mcg/kg per minute) 1.5 — Infusion Delivery Rate (mL/hr)	Drug Delivery Rate (mcg/kg per minute) 2 — Infusion Delivery Rate (mL/hr)	Drug Delivery Rate (mcg/kg per minute) 3 — Infusion Delivery Rate (mL/hr)	Drug Delivery Rate (mcg/kg per minute) 5 — Infusion Delivery Rate (mL/hr)
10	6	9	12	18	30
45	27	41	54	81	135
70	42	63	84	126	210
100	60	90	120	180	300

TABLE 3. Infusion Rates Required to Deliver Selected Dosages of Cisatracurium from Solutions Containing 0.4 mg/mL of the Drug

Weight (kg)	Drug Delivery Rate (mcg/kg per minute) 1 / Infusion Delivery Rate (mL/hr)	Drug Delivery Rate (mcg/kg per minute) 1.5 / Infusion Delivery Rate (mL/hr)	Drug Delivery Rate (mcg/kg per minute) 2 / Infusion Delivery Rate (mL/hr)	Drug Delivery Rate (mcg/kg per minute) 3 / Infusion Delivery Rate (mL/hr)	Drug Delivery Rate (mcg/kg per minute) 5 / Infusion Delivery Rate (mL/hr)
10	1.5	2.3	3	4.5	7.5
45	6.8	10.1	13.5	20.3	33.8
70	10.5	15.8	21	31.5	52.5
100	15	22.5	30	45	75

Dispensing and Administration Precautions

Neuromuscular blocking agents should be administered only by individuals who are adequately trained in their use and complications. For specific procedures and techniques of administration, specialized references should be consulted. Facilities and personnel necessary for intubation, administration of oxygen, and respiratory support should be immediately available whenever these drugs are used. In addition, a reversal agent should be readily available in the event of a failed intubation or to accelerate neuromuscular recovery after surgery.

Because neuromuscular blocking agents can cause respiratory arrest, precautions (e.g., storage segregation, warning labels, access limitations) should be taken to ensure that these drugs are not administered without adequate respiratory support. Affixing warning labels to storage containers and final administration containers is recommended to clearly communicate that respiratory paralysis can occur and ventilator support is required. The Institute for Safe Medication Practices (ISMP) recommends the following wording for these containers: "Warning: Paralyzing agent—causes respiratory arrest—patient must be ventilated."

Neuromuscular blocking agents have no known effect on consciousness, pain, or cerebration, and should therefore be used in conjunction with adequate levels of anesthesia, and only after appropriate analgesics and sedatives are administered. To avoid distress to the patient, cisatracurium should be administered only after unconsciousness has been induced.

● Dosage

Dosage of cisatracurium besylate is expressed in terms of cisatracurium.

Dosage of cisatracurium must be carefully adjusted according to individual requirements and response. The use of a peripheral nerve stimulator is recommended to accurately monitor the degree of neuromuscular blockade and recovery, determine the need for additional doses, and minimize the possibility of overdosage.

Skeletal Muscle Relaxation in Pediatric Patients

Initial (Intubating) Dose

The recommended initial intubating dose of cisatracurium in infants 1–23 months of age when used concomitantly with halothane or opiate anesthesia is 0.15 mg/kg. This dose generally produces maximum neuromuscular blockade in about 2 minutes and clinically effective blockade for about 43 minutes.

The recommended initial intubating dose of cisatracurium in children 2–12 years of age when used concomitantly with halothane or opiate anesthesia is 0.1–0.15 mg/kg. A dose of 0.1 mg/kg administered under these conditions can be expected to produce maximum neuromuscular blockade in about 2.8 minutes and clinically effective blockade for about 28 minutes, and a dose of 0.15 mg/kg can be expected to produce maximum neuromuscular blockade in about 3 minutes and clinically effective blockade for about 36 minutes.

The manufacturer makes no specific dosage recommendations for adolescents 13 years of age or older.

Maintenance Dosage During Prolonged Surgical Procedures

After the initial intubating dose is administered, children 2 years of age or older may receive a continuous IV infusion of cisatracurium to maintain neuromuscular blockade during prolonged surgical procedures. The infusion should be initiated only after early spontaneous recovery from the initial dose is evident. The rate of infusion should be individualized based on patient response to peripheral nerve stimulation. An initial rate of 3 mcg/kg per minute may be necessary to rapidly counteract spontaneous neuromuscular recovery; thereafter, a rate of 1–2 mcg/kg per minute generally is sufficient to maintain neuromuscular blockade in the range of 89–99% in most pediatric patients receiving balanced anesthesia.

A reduction in the cisatracurium infusion rate by up to 30–40% may be necessary if steady-state anesthesia has been induced with enflurane or isoflurane; greater reductions may be required with prolonged durations of enflurane or isoflurane administration.

Skeletal Muscle Relaxation in Adults

Initial (Intubating) Dose

The recommended initial (intubating) dose of cisatracurium in adults is 0.15 or 0.2 mg/kg depending on the desired time to intubation and duration of the procedure. When used concomitantly with balanced anesthesia, good to excellent intubating conditions generally occur within 2 minutes following a dose of 0.15 mg/kg or 1.5 minutes following a dose of 0.2 mg/kg. A dose of 0.15 mg/kg generally produces maximum neuromuscular blockade in approximately 3.5 minutes and clinically sufficient neuromuscular blockade for about 55 minutes, and a dose of 0.2 mg/kg generally produces maximum neuromuscular blockade in approximately 2.9 minutes and clinically sufficient neuromuscular blockade for about 65 minutes.

Maintenance Dosage During Prolonged Surgical Procedures

For maintenance of neuromuscular blockade during prolonged surgical procedures, additional cisatracurium doses of 0.03 mg/kg may be administered by intermittent IV injection in adults. The first maintenance dose generally is required within 40–50 or 50–60 minutes following an initial dose of 0.15 or 0.2 mg/kg, respectively. Each 0.03-mg/kg dose can provide approximately 20 minutes of additional neuromuscular blockade. Smaller or larger doses may be needed to provide shorter or longer durations of action.

Less frequent or lower doses of cisatracurium may be necessary when administered concomitantly with enflurane or isoflurane anesthesia during prolonged surgical procedures. No dosage adjustment appears to be necessary when the drug is administered shortly (e.g., within 15–30 minutes) after initiation of the inhalation anesthetic.

Alternatively, after the initial intubating dose is administered, patients may receive a continuous IV infusion of cisatracurium to maintain neuromuscular blockade during prolonged surgical procedures; the infusion should be initiated only after early spontaneous recovery from the initial dose is evident. Infusion rates should be individualized and adjusted based on patient response to peripheral nerve stimulation. An initial rate of 3 mcg/kg per minute may be necessary to rapidly counteract spontaneous recovery from neuromuscular blockade. Thereafter, a maintenance infusion rate of 1–2 mcg/kg per minute generally is sufficient to maintain neuromuscular blockade in the range of 89–99% in most patients receiving balanced anesthesia.

A reduction in the cisatracurium infusion rate by up to 30–40% may be necessary if steady-state anesthesia has been induced with enflurane or isoflurane; greater reductions may be required with prolonged durations of enflurane or isoflurane administration.

Maintenance Dosage in Intensive Care Setting

Cisatracurium may be administered by continuous IV infusion for maintenance of neuromuscular blockade during mechanical ventilation in the intensive care unit (ICU). The degree of neuromuscular blockade should be monitored with a peripheral nerve stimulator; additional doses should not be given before there is a definite response to nerve stimulation.

In clinical studies, an average cisatracurium infusion rate of approximately 3 mcg/kg per minute was required for maintenance of neuromuscular blockade in mechanically ventilated adults in the ICU; however, dosage requirements may vary widely among patients and also may increase or decrease with time. In these studies, patients received up to 6 days of cisatracurium infusion; longer durations of use in the ICU have not been evaluated. Recovery of neuromuscular function (train-of-four [TOF] ratio of at least 0.7) generally occurred within approximately 50–55 minutes after the infusion was discontinued. Following neuromuscular recovery, administration of an IV ("bolus") dose of cisatracurium may be necessary to reestablish neuromuscular blockade prior to reinstitution of the infusion.

Reversal of Neuromuscular Blockade

Neuromuscular blockade induced by cisatracurium can be reversed by administering a cholinesterase inhibitor (e.g., neostigmine, pyridostigmine, edrophonium) in conjunction with an anticholinergic agent such as atropine or glycopyrrolate to block the adverse muscarinic effects of the cholinesterase inhibitor. *For specific information on the uses and dosage and administration of these other drugs, see the individual monographs.*

To minimize the risk of residual neuromuscular blockade, reversal should only be attempted after some degree of spontaneous recovery has occurred; patients should be closely monitored until adequate recovery of normal neuromuscular function is assured (i.e., ability to maintain satisfactory ventilation and a patent airway). Time to recovery of neuromuscular function is dependent upon the strength of neuromuscular blockade at the time of reversal.

● Special Populations

Renal Impairment

Since onset of complete neuromuscular blockade may be slower in patients with renal impairment, it may be necessary to extend the interval between administration of cisatracurium and the intubation attempt in such patients.

Geriatric Patients

Since onset of complete neuromuscular blockade may be slower in geriatric patients, it may be necessary to extend the interval between administration of cisatracurium and the intubation attempt in such patients.

Burn Patients

Substantially increased doses of cisatracurium may be required in burn patients due to the development of resistance. *However, there are no clinical studies to date in these patients, and no specific doses are recommended.*

Cardiopulmonary Bypass Patients with Induced Hypothermia

The infusion rate of atracurium required to maintain adequate surgical relaxation during hypothermia (i.e., 25–28°C) is approximately 50% of the infusion rate necessary in normothermic patients; a similar reduction in the infusion rate of cisatracurium may be expected.

Other Populations

A cisatracurium dose of 0.02 mg/kg or less is recommended along with monitoring of subsequent dosage adjustments in patients in whom potentiation of neuromuscular blockade or difficulties with reversal of blockade may occur (e.g., neuromuscular disease, carcinomatosis).

CAUTIONS

● Contraindications

Cisatracurium besylate is contraindicated in patients with known hypersensitivity to the drug or any of its components.

Multiple-dose vials of cisatracurium containing benzyl alcohol are contraindicated in premature infants.

● Warnings/Precautions

Warnings

Cisatracurium shares the toxic potentials of the nondepolarizing neuromuscular blocking agents, and the usual precautions of neuromuscular blocking agent administration should be observed. (See Cautions in the Neuromuscular Blocking Agents General Statement 12:20.20.)

Administration Precautions

When used inappropriately, neuromuscular blocking agents can severely compromise respiratory function and induce respiratory paralysis; special precautions should be taken during and after administration of these drugs. The degree of neuromuscular blockade produced by cisatracurium should be monitored with a peripheral nerve stimulator, particularly in patients with conditions that may potentiate (e.g., neuromuscular diseases) or cause resistance to (e.g., burns) the neuromuscular blocking effects of the drug.

Sensitivity Reactions

Hypersensitivity Reactions

Serious hypersensitivity reactions, including anaphylaxis, have been reported rarely with all neuromuscular blocking agents; such reactions were life-threatening or fatal in some cases. Appropriate emergency treatment should be readily available whenever these drugs are administered. Because of the possibility of cross-sensitivity, cisatracurium should be used with caution in patients who have experienced previous anaphylactic reactions to other neuromuscular blocking agents (depolarizing or nondepolarizing).

General Precautions

Neuromuscular Diseases

Patients with neuromuscular diseases (e.g., myasthenia gravis, Eaton-Lambert syndrome) may have an exaggerated response to cisatracurium. In such patients, the degree of neuromuscular blockade should be monitored with a peripheral nerve stimulator and dosage reduction is recommended.

Burn Patients

Resistance to nondepolarizing neuromuscular blocking agents, including atracurium, can develop in burn patients, particularly those with burns over 25–30% or more of body surface area.

Cisatracurium has not been studied in this population; however, based on its similarity to atracurium, the possible need for substantially increased doses should be considered in such patients.

Intensive Care Setting

Although the manufacturer states that continuous IV infusion of cisatracurium for up to 6 days in the intensive care unit (ICU) has been safely used in several studies, prolonged paralysis and/or muscle weakness have been reported with long-term administration of neuromuscular blocking agents.

Continuous monitoring of neuromuscular transmission with a peripheral nerve stimulator is recommended whenever cisatracurium is used in the ICU. Additional doses of cisatracurium or any other neuromuscular blocking agent should not be administered before there is a definite response to nerve stimulation tests. If no response is elicited, administration of the drug should be discontinued until a response returns.

Seizures have been reported rarely in patients receiving continuous IV infusions of atracurium for facilitation of mechanical ventilation in the ICU; these patients usually had predisposing factors (e.g., head trauma, cerebral edema, hypoxic encephalopathy, viral encephalitis, uremia). It is unclear whether laudanosine (a metabolite of atracurium and cisatracurium that produces CNS excitation at higher doses) contributes to CNS excitation.

Cardiovascular Effects

Cisatracurium has no clinically important effects on heart rate at recommended doses and exhibits minimal, if any, cardiovascular effects; therefore, the drug will not counteract the bradycardia induced by many anesthetic agents or by vagal stimulation.

Electrolyte Disturbances

Acid-base and/or serum electrolyte abnormalities may potentiate or antagonize the action of cisatracurium.

Hemiparesis and Paraparesis

Resistance to cisatracurium may develop in the affected limbs of patients with hemiparesis or paraparesis. To avoid inaccurate dosing, neuromuscular monitoring in the nonparetic limb is recommended.

Malignant Hyperthermia

Malignant hyperthermia is rarely associated with the use of neuromuscular blocking agents and/or potent inhalation anesthetics. In an animal study in susceptible swine, cisatracurium did not trigger malignant hyperthermia; however, the drug has not been studied in patients with increased susceptibility to this condition. Because malignant hyperthermia can occur even in the absence of a recognized precipitating factor, clinicians should be vigilant for its possible development and prepared to manage the condition in any patient undergoing general anesthesia.

Carcinomatosis

Because of possible exaggerated response to cisatracurium in patients with carcinomatosis, the degree of neuromuscular blockade should be monitored carefully with a peripheral nerve stimulator; dosage reduction is recommended.

Specific Populations

Pregnancy

Category B.

It is not known whether use of cisatracurium during labor, delivery, or cesarean section has any effects on the fetus.

Lactation

It is not known whether cisatracurium is distributed into milk. Because many drugs are distributed into human milk, caution is advised if the drug is used in nursing women.

Pediatric Use

Safety and efficacy of cisatracurium have not been established in neonates (younger than 1 month of age).

Each mL of cisatracurium besylate injection in multiple-dose vials contains 9 mg of benzyl alcohol. Although a causal relationship has not been established, administration of injections preserved with benzyl alcohol has been associated with toxicity in neonates. Toxicity appears to have resulted from administration of large amounts (i.e., 100–400 mg/kg daily) of benzyl alcohol in these neonates. Although use of drugs preserved with benzyl alcohol should be avoided in neonates whenever possible, the American Academy of Pediatrics (AAP) states that the presence of small amounts of the preservative in a commercially available injection should not proscribe its use when indicated in neonates.

Pediatric patients may exhibit faster clearance of cisatracurium than adults. Onset of the drug is faster and duration is longer in pediatric patients compared with adults, and in infants compared with older children.

In clinical studies, tracheal intubation was facilitated more reliably in children 1–4 years of age when cisatracurium was used in conjunction with halothane than when used in conjunction with opiates and nitrous oxide.

Geriatric Use

No overall differences in safety and efficacy have been observed in geriatric patients relative to younger adults, but increased sensitivity of some older patients cannot be ruled out.

Minor alterations in cisatracurium pharmacokinetics (e.g., prolonged half-life, slower onset of action) have been observed in geriatric patients compared with younger individuals; however, these changes were not associated with substantial differences in recovery profile.

Cisatracurium half-life may be slightly prolonged in geriatric patients.

Hepatic Impairment

Minor alterations in cisatracurium pharmacokinetics have been observed in patients with end-stage liver disease compared with healthy adults; however, these changes were not associated with substantial differences in recovery profile.

Concentrations of cisatracurium metabolites may be increased after prolonged administration in patients with hepatic disease.

Renal Impairment

The pharmacokinetic/pharmacodynamic and recovery profile of cisatracurium in patients with renal impairment is similar to that in healthy adults. Concentrations of cisatracurium metabolites may be increased after prolonged administration in patients with renal failure.

● Common Adverse Effects

Adverse effects were uncommon in clinical trials in patients who received cisatracurium in conjunction with anesthetic agents or other drugs (e.g., opiates, propofol) during surgery; no adverse effects were reported with an incidence exceeding 1% in these studies.

Similarly, adverse effects were uncommon in ICU patients receiving cisatracurium, but several cases of prolonged recovery were reported.

DRUG INTERACTIONS

Concurrent administration of some drugs, including general anesthetics (e.g., enflurane, isoflurane), antibiotics (e.g., aminoglycosides, polymyxins), lithium, succinylcholine, magnesium salts, procainamide, and quinidine, may affect the neuromuscular blocking activity of cisatracurium besylate. *For additional information on potential drug interactions of cisatracurium, see Drug Interactions in the Neuromuscular Blocking Agents General Statement 12:20.20.*

● Anticonvulsants

Resistance to the neuromuscular blocking effects of cisatracurium may occur in patients receiving long-term phenytoin or carbamazepine therapy. Because this may result in a shorter duration of neuromuscular block, higher infusion rates of cisatracurium may be required.

● Anti-infective Agents

The possibility that some anti-infective agents (e.g., aminoglycosides, bacitracin, clindamycin, lincomycin, polymyxins, tetracyclines) may enhance the neuromuscular blocking effects of cisatracurium should be considered.

● General Anesthetics

Inhalation anesthetics (enflurane and isoflurane) are known to potentiate the effects of neuromuscular blocking agents. A reduction in cisatracurium dose and/or infusion rate may be necessary depending on the duration of administration of the inhalation anesthetic.

● Lithium

The neuromuscular blocking effects of cisatracurium may be enhanced by lithium.

● Local Anesthetics

The neuromuscular blocking effects of cisatracurium may be enhanced by local anesthetics.

● Magnesium Salts

The neuromuscular blocking effects of cisatracurium may be enhanced by magnesium salts. Caution is advised and a reduction in cisatracurium dosage may be necessary.

● Nondepolarizing Neuromuscular Blocking Agents

Potency and duration of nondepolarizing neuromuscular blocking agents may be altered by concurrent or prior administration of other nondepolarizing agents. In clinical studies, vecuronium, pancuronium, or atracurium was administered following various degrees of recovery from cisatracurium-induced neuromuscular blockade without any evidence of interaction.

● Procainamide

The neuromuscular blocking effects of cisatracurium may be enhanced by procainamide.

● Propofol

Propofol has no apparent effect on the duration of neuromuscular blockade induced by cisatracurium. No dosage adjustment of cisatracurium is required.

• *Quinidine*

The neuromuscular blocking effects of cisatracurium may be enhanced by quinidine.

• *Succinylcholine*

Cisatracurium has been used safely following various degrees of recovery from succinylcholine-induced neuromuscular blockade. Prior administration of succinylcholine may decrease the time to maximum neuromuscular blockade with cisatracurium by about 2 minutes. Prior administration of succinylcholine does not appear to alter the duration of blockade induced by intermittent injections of cisatracurium; prior administration resulted in no change or only a slight increase in cisatracurium infusion requirements.

DESCRIPTION

Cisatracurium besylate is a nondepolarizing neuromuscular blocking agent that produces pharmacologic effects similar to those of other nondepolarizing neuromuscular blocking agents. (See Pharmacology in the Neuromuscular Blocking Agents General Statement 12:20.20.) Cisatracurium produces skeletal muscle relaxation by causing a decreased response to acetylcholine (ACh) at the myoneural (neuromuscular) junction of skeletal muscle. The drug exhibits a high affinity for ACh receptor sites and competitively blocks access of ACh to the motor end-plate of the myoneural junction, and may affect ACh release. Cisatracurium blocks the effects of both the small quantities of ACh that maintain muscle tone and the large quantities of ACh that produce voluntary skeletal muscle contraction. The drug does not alter the resting electrical potential of the motor end-plate or cause muscular contractions. The neuromuscular blocking potency of cisatracurium is approximately threefold that of atracurium. Cisatracurium exhibits minimal, if any, cardiovascular effects. The drug exhibits little histamine-releasing activity at usual therapeutic doses.

Cisatracurium has an intermediate onset and duration of action. Cisatracurium is rapidly metabolized via Hofmann elimination (independent of the liver) to form a monoquaternary acrylate metabolite (which undergoes nonspecific plasma esterase hydrolysis and subsequent Hofmann elimination) and laudanosine (which is demethylated and glucuronidated). Both metabolites lack neuromuscular blocking activity; laudanosine may have CNS excitatory

activity when present in large amounts. Cisatracurium is eliminated principally by Hofmann elimination (77–80%) and to lesser extent by renal and hepatic elimination (20%). Metabolites of the drug are eliminated principally by renal and hepatic elimination. The elimination half-life of cisatracurium is approximately 22–30 minutes.

ADVICE TO PATIENTS

Importance of women informing clinicians if they are or plan to become pregnant or plan to breast-feed.

Importance of informing clinician of existing or contemplated concomitant therapy, including prescription and OTC drugs, as well as any concomitant illnesses (e.g., cardiovascular disease, neuromuscular disease).

Importance of informing patients of other important precautionary information. (See Cautions.)

PREPARATIONS

Excipients in commercially available drug preparations may have clinically important effects in some individuals; consult specific product labeling for details.

Cisatracurium Besylate

Parenteral		
Injection, for IV use only	2 mg (of cisatracurium) per mL	Cisatracurium Besylate Injection Nimbex®, Abbvie
	10 mg (of cisatracurium) per mL	Cisatracurium Besylate Injection Nimbex®, Abbvie

† Use is not currently included in the labeling approved by the US Food and Drug Administration.

Selected Revisions June 10, 2024, © Copyright, January 1, 2009, American Society of Health-System Pharmacists, Inc.

Succinylcholine Chloride

12:20.20 • NEUROMUSCULAR BLOCKING AGENTS

■ Succinylcholine chloride is a depolarizing neuromuscular blocking agent.

USES

● Skeletal Muscle Relaxation

Succinylcholine chloride is used to produce skeletal muscle relaxation during procedures of short duration such as endotracheal intubation after general anesthesia has been induced.

Because of its short duration of action, succinylcholine is generally considered the neuromuscular blocking agent of choice for procedures lasting less than 3 minutes. In addition, because of its rapid onset (less than 1 minute after IV administration) and short duration of action (approximately 4–6 minutes), succinylcholine traditionally has been considered the neuromuscular blocking agent of choice in emergency situations when rapid intubation (e.g., rapid sequence intubation) is required. However, the drug is associated with serious adverse effects (e.g., hyperkalemia, bradycardia, malignant hyperthermia), which can limit its use. Because of the risk of hyperkalemic rhabdomyolysis, cardiac arrest, and death, use of succinylcholine in pediatric patients should be restricted to those who require emergency intubation, those in whom an airway should be secured immediately (e.g., patients with laryngospasm, difficult airway, or full stomach), or those in whom a suitable vein is not accessible and IM administration is needed. (See Cautions: Pediatric Precautions.) If succinylcholine cannot be used, rocuronium (a nondepolarizing neuromuscular blocking agent with the most similar pharmacokinetic profile) generally is recommended as an acceptable alternative. Clinical studies have shown that rocuronium can produce similar intubating conditions to succinylcholine when given in sufficient doses (e.g., at least 1 mg/kg); however, succinylcholine is more likely to achieve excellent intubating conditions and remains clinically superior to rocuronium with respect to its shorter duration of action.

Succinylcholine also is used to provide skeletal muscle relaxation during mechanical ventilation; however, the drug is not used for prolonged neuromuscular blockade in the intensive care unit (ICU).

For additional information on uses and treatment principles of neuromuscular blocking agents, see Uses in the Neuromuscular Blocking Agents General Statement 12:20.20.

DOSAGE AND ADMINISTRATION

● Reconstitution and Administration

Succinylcholine chloride usually is administered IV. For infants or older patients in whom a suitable vein is not accessible, the drug may be administered by IM injection. Because of a slower onset of effect (which can potentially compromise respiratory function), some clinicians recommend that IM administration be reserved for life-threatening situations.

For prolonged procedures, the manufacturer states that succinylcholine may be given by continuous IV infusion or intermittent IV injection. Continuous IV infusion of the drug is preferable to administration of repeated fractional doses because the latter method of dosing may lead to tachyphylaxis and prolonged apnea which may be difficult to reverse. However, some clinicians state that continuous IV infusion of succinylcholine also is limited clinically because of tachyphylaxis, potential conversion from phase I to phase II block, and the uncertain nature and prolongation of the blockade.

For continuous IV infusion, succinylcholine chloride usually is diluted to a concentration of 1–2 mg/mL (0.1–0.2%) with a compatible IV solution such as 5% dextrose injection or 0.9% sodium chloride injection. The 1-mg/mL concentration is usually used for optimum dosage control, but in patients in whom the amount of fluid should be limited, the 2-mg/mL concentration may be preferred. To provide a solution containing 1 or 2 mg/mL, 1 g of succinylcholine chloride injection may be added to 1 L or 500 mL of diluent, respectively. The infusion solution should be used within 24 hours of preparation. Use of a controlled-infusion device is recommended to ensure precise control of the flow rate during continuous IV infusion of the drug. Succinylcholine injections should not be admixed with alkaline (having a pH exceeding 8.5) solutions (e.g., barbiturates).

Dispensing and Administration Precautions

Neuromuscular blocking agents should be administered only by individuals who are adequately trained in their use and complications. For specific procedures and techniques of administration, specialized references should be consulted. Facilities and personnel necessary for intubation, administration of oxygen, and respiratory support should be immediately available whenever these drugs are used.

Because neuromuscular blocking agents can cause respiratory arrest, precautions (e.g., storage segregation, warning labels, access limitations) should be taken to ensure that these drugs are not administered without adequate respiratory support. Affixing warning labels to storage containers and final administration containers is recommended to clearly communicate that respiratory paralysis can occur and ventilator support is required. The Institute for Safe Medication Practices (ISMP) recommends the following wording for these containers: "Warning: Paralyzing agent—causes respiratory arrest—patient must be ventilated".

Neuromuscular blocking agents have no known effect on consciousness, pain, or cerebration, and should therefore be used in conjunction with adequate levels of anesthesia and only after appropriate analgesics and sedatives are administered. To avoid distress to the patient, succinylcholine generally should be administered after unconsciousness has been induced; however, in emergency situations, the drug may be administered before a sedative has been given.

● Dosage

Dosage of succinylcholine must be carefully adjusted according to individual requirements and response. The use of a peripheral nerve stimulator is recommended during continuous IV infusion of the drug to accurately monitor the degree of neuromuscular blockade and recovery, detect the development of phase II block, and minimize the possibility of overdosage.

Test Dose

To evaluate sensitivity to succinylcholine in patients with reduced plasma cholinesterase activity, a test dose of 5–10 mg of succinylcholine chloride is recommended; alternatively, a 1-mg/mL solution of the drug may be cautiously administered by slow IV infusion. In patients who metabolize succinylcholine normally, respiratory depression rarely occurs and, if it does, is transient and usually disappears in less than 5 minutes. Patients unable to metabolize the drug develop paralysis sufficient to permit endotracheal intubation; recovery generally occurs in 30–60 minutes. Apnea or prolonged muscle paralysis should be treated with controlled respiration.

Adult Dosage

For short procedures, the manufacturer states that the usual adult IV dose of succinylcholine chloride is 0.6 mg/kg (range 0.3–1.1 mg/kg); following administration of this dose, neuromuscular blockade generally is attained in approximately 1 minute and persists for about 4–6 minutes. Because there is a wide variation in individual patient response, a test dose of succinylcholine chloride may be administered to determine the individual patient's sensitivity and recovery time. (See Test Dose under Dosage and Administration: Dosage.)

For rapid sequence intubation, the usual dose of succinylcholine chloride is 1.5 mg/kg; this dose generally produces an onset of effect within 45 seconds and a duration of paralysis of about 10 minutes.

For maintenance of neuromuscular blockade during prolonged procedures, succinylcholine chloride may be administered by continuous IV infusion, generally at a rate of 2.5–4.3 mg/minute in adults; the rate may range from 0.5–10 mg/minute depending on the response and requirements of the patient. Succinylcholine also may be administered by intermittent IV injection for maintenance of neuromuscular blockade during prolonged procedures; a dose of 0.3–1.1 mg/kg may be given initially in adults, followed by additional doses of 0.04–0.07 mg/kg as necessary to maintain adequate relaxation.

If IM administration is necessary, a succinylcholine chloride dose of up to 3–4 mg/kg may be given, but the total dose should not exceed 150 mg.

Pediatric Dosage

The manufacturer states that the usual pediatric IV dose of succinylcholine chloride is 1–2 mg/kg (2 mg/kg for infants and small pediatric patients, and 1 mg/kg for older pediatric patients and adolescents). The possibility that succinylcholine may produce profound bradycardia or, rarely, asystole when administered by rapid IV injection in infants and children should be considered; as in adults, the risk of these effects increases with repeated doses, and pretreatment with atropine should be considered to reduce the risk of bradyarrhythmias.

Because of the risk of malignant hyperthermia, continuous IV infusions of succinylcholine are considered unsafe in neonates and children.

If IM administration is necessary, a succinylcholine chloride dose of up to 3–4 mg/kg may be given, but the total dose should not exceed 150 mg.

CAUTIONS

● Adverse Effects

Succinylcholine may produce initial muscle fasciculation which may result in postoperative pain; jaw rigidity also has been reported.

Patients with decreased concentrations and/or activity of plasma pseudocholinesterase are especially sensitive to the action of succinylcholine and may experience prolonged respiratory depression and apnea after receiving the drug. (See Cautions: Precautions and Contraindications.) About 1 individual in 2800 has a genetic abnormality that causes the production of an atypical pseudocholinesterase which is incapable of rapidly hydrolyzing succinylcholine. These individuals are homozygous for this trait and invariably respond to administration of succinylcholine by prolonged muscle relaxation. Several other genetic variants also exist, some producing enzymes that hydrolyze succinylcholine at slower than normal rates than others that hydrolyze succinylcholine more rapidly than normal. Plasma pseudocholinesterase concentrations may also be decreased in patients with hepatocellular disease, malnutrition, severe anemia, severe dehydration, burns, cancer, collagen diseases, myxedema, or abnormal body temperature and in pregnant women. (See also Drug Interactions.)

While succinylcholine does not have a direct effect on the myocardium, the drug stimulates autonomic ganglia and muscarinic receptors. Bradycardia accompanied by hypotension and cardiac arrhythmias ranging from nodal rhythms and extrasystoles to bigeminy, atrioventricular block, and cardiac arrest may occur after succinylcholine administration. Cardiac effects also may result from vagal stimulation or from hyperkalemia, and are most common during halothane anesthesia, with repeated administration of succinylcholine, in children, or in patients with pheochromocytoma. Prior administration of atropine may inhibit vagal stimulation. Succinylcholine has also been reported to cause sinus tachycardia with hypertension and sympathetic ganglion stimulation.

Succinylcholine causes an increase in intraocular pressure which may be hazardous in patients with glaucoma or in those undergoing eye surgery and in patients with penetrating wounds of the eye. Although administration of a small dose of a nondepolarizing neuromuscular blocking agent prior to succinylcholine can prevent the rise in intraocular pressure, it may be preferable to use a nondepolarizing blocking agent alone in patients with these conditions of the eye. An increase in intragastric pressure secondary to fasciculation of the abdominal muscles has been reported. An increase in intragastric pressure may be prevented by the administration of a small dose of a nondepolarizing agent prior to succinylcholine. Enlargement of the salivary glands, excessive salivation, rash, hypersensitivity reactions (e.g., anaphylaxis) and, rarely, bronchospasm have also been reported in patients receiving succinylcholine. Premedication with a parasympatholytic agent such as atropine or scopolamine may be used to prevent excessive salivation.

Rarely, myoglobinuria and myoglobinemia have been reported after succinylcholine administration, particularly in children. These symptoms have sometimes been reported in conjunction with malignant hyperthermia and muscle rigidity. Administration of succinylcholine has been associated with acute onset of malignant hyperthermia; the risk of developing such hyperthermia increases with concomitant administration of inhalation anesthetics. (See Cautions: Adverse Effects in the Neuromuscular Blocking Agents General Statement 12:20.20.) Manifestations associated with histamine release also can occur. Hyperkalemia has been reported in several catabolic patients who had either massive tissue destruction or CNS injury with muscle wasting (e.g., those with extensive or severe burns, severe abdominal infections, tetanus, massive trauma, spinal cord injury, neuromuscular disease) who received succinylcholine. The precise time of onset and duration of the risk period are not known. It has been reported that skeletal muscle denervation hypersensitivity usually develops over several weeks; however, it can occur as early as 1–2 days after injury. Results of an animal study indicate that hyperkalemia developed 7 days after denervation when receiving succinylcholine. In humans, succinylcholine-associated hyperkalemia can persist for over 6 months after neural injury. The risk of

hyperkalemia depends on the extent and location of injury, increases over time, and usually peaks 7–10 days after the injury.

Serious hypersensitivity reactions, including anaphylaxis, have been reported rarely with all neuromuscular blocking agents; such reactions have been life-threatening or fatal in some cases. Although uncommon, succinylcholine has the potential to release histamine and cause histamine-related manifestations (e.g., bronchospasm, flushing, hypotension).

● Precautions and Contraindications

Succinylcholine chloride shares the toxic potentials of the depolarizing neuromuscular blocking agents, and the usual precautions of neuromuscular blocking agent administration should be observed. (See Cautions in the Neuromuscular Blocking Agents General Statement 12:20.20.)

When used inappropriately, neuromuscular blocking agents can severely compromise respiratory function and induce respiratory paralysis. Special precautions should be taken during and after administration of these drugs. (See Dispensing and Administration Precautions under Dosage and Administration: Reconstitution and Administration.)

Immediately after administration of succinylcholine and during the fasciculation phase, slight increases in intracranial pressure may occur.

Some clinicians suggest that plasma pseudocholinesterase activity should be determined prior to administration of succinylcholine. The drug should be administered with extreme caution and in reduced doses, if at all, to patients with abnormally low pseudocholinesterase concentrations including those who are homozygous for the genetic trait that causes the production of an atypical pseudocholinesterase. If low pseudocholinesterase activity is suspected, a small test dose (5–10 mg) may be administered or relaxation may be produced by cautious IV infusion of a 0.1% solution of the drug. Apnea or prolonged muscle paralysis should be treated with controlled respiration. Administration of fresh whole blood or plasma has been reported to be of benefit in restoring pseudocholinesterase concentrations.

Succinylcholine should be used with extreme caution in patients with electrolyte imbalance, those receiving quinidine or cardiac glycosides, or those with suspected cardiac glycoside toxicity, since succinylcholine may induce serious cardiac arrhythmias or cardiac arrest in such patients. Succinylcholine should be used with extreme caution, if at all, during ocular surgery or in patients with glaucoma. The drug also should be used with extreme caution in patients with preexisting hyperkalemia or paraplegia and those with chronic abdominal infection, subarachnoid hemorrhage, degenerative or dystrophic neuromuscular disease, or conditions that may cause degeneration of central and peripheral nervous systems, since the potential of developing severe hyperkalemia is increased in such patients. Succinylcholine is contraindicated in patients with upper motor neuron injury, multiple trauma, extensive or severe burns, extensive denervation of skeletal muscle because of disease or injury to the CNS, since such patients tend to become severely hyperkalemic following succinylcholine administration which may result in cardiac arrest. (See Cautions: Adverse Effects.)

Since neuromuscular blocking agents have been reported to cause severe anaphylactic reactions, appropriate emergency treatment should be readily available whenever these drugs are administered. Because of potential cross-sensitivity, succinylcholine should be used with caution in patients who have experienced previous anaphylactic reactions to other neuromuscular blocking agents (depolarizing or nondepolarizing).

Succinylcholine is contraindicated in patients with known hypersensitivity to the drug, personal or familial history of malignant hyperthermia, or skeletal muscle myopathies.

● Pediatric Precautions

Acute rhabdomyolysis with hyperkalemia followed by ventricular dysrhythmias, cardiac arrest, and death has been reported rarely in apparently healthy children and adolescents receiving succinylcholine; subsequently it was observed that these children had undiagnosed skeletal muscle myopathy, most frequently Duchenne type muscular dystrophy. Peaked T-waves and sudden cardiac arrest within minutes of administration of succinylcholine may occur in apparently healthy children, usually males 8 years of age or younger, although this syndrome has been reported in some adolescents. Therefore, when an apparently healthy infant or child develops cardiac arrest shortly after administration of succinylcholine (supposedly not associated with inadequate ventilation, oxygenation, or overdosage of an anesthetic), treatment for hyperkalemia should be initiated immediately. Emergency measures for the treatment of hyperkalemia should include hyperventilation and IV administration of calcium, sodium bicarbonate, glucose, and insulin. Since this syndrome is characterized by an abrupt onset, standard resuscitative measures may be unsuccessful. Prolonged or unusual resuscitative measures have been successful in some patients. If signs of malignant hyperthermia are present, appropriate therapy should be instituted concurrently. Since it is difficult to identify which children and adolescents may be at risk of developing such a syndrome, it is recommended that a nondepolarizing neuromuscular blocking agent be used in these patients and succinylcholine be reserved for children and adolescents undergoing emergency intubation, for those in whom an airway should be secured immediately (e.g., those with laryngospasm, difficult airway, full stomach), or for those in whom a suitable vein is not accessible and IM administration is needed.

The possibility that succinylcholine may produce profound bradycardia or, rarely, asystole when administered by rapid IV injection in infants and children should be considered; as in adults, the risk of these effects increases with repeated doses, and pretreatment with atropine should be considered to reduce the risk of bradyarrhythmias.

● **Geriatric Precautions**

Clinical studies of succinylcholine did not include sufficient numbers of patients 65 years of age and older to determine whether geriatric patients respond differently than younger patients. While other clinical experience has not revealed age-related differences in response or tolerance, drug dosage generally should be titrated carefully in geriatric patients, usually initiating therapy at the low end of the dosage range. The greater frequency of decreased hepatic, renal, and/or cardiac function and of concomitant disease and drug therapy observed in the elderly also should be considered.

● **Pregnancy, Fertility, and Lactation**

Pregnancy

Animal reproduction studies have not been performed to date with succinylcholine chloride. It is also not known whether the drug can cause fetal harm when administered to pregnant women. Pseudocholinesterase concentrations are decreased during pregnancy and for several days postpartum, and a higher proportion of patients may be expected to show sensitivity to succinylcholine when pregnant. Succinylcholine may be used to provide muscle relaxation during delivery by cesarean section. Although succinylcholine generally crosses the placenta in small amounts, residual neuromuscular blockade (apnea, flaccidity) may occur in the neonate after repeated administration of high doses to the mother or in the presence of atypical pseudocholinesterase in the mother. Succinylcholine should be used during pregnancy only when clearly needed.

Lactation

It is not known whether succinylcholine is distributed into human milk, and the manufacturers recommend that the drug be used with caution in nursing women.

DRUG INTERACTIONS

Cholinesterase inhibitors, particularly the irreversible organophosphate type, can substantially reduce the activity of plasma pseudocholinesterase. Prolonged apnea and death have occurred following administration of succinylcholine to patients who had received prolonged therapy with echothiophate iodide ophthalmic drops (no longer commercially available in the US). The possibility of reactions should be considered in patients receiving isofluorophate or demecarium bromide and in those who have recently been exposed to organophosphate insecticides. In high blood concentrations, procaine competes with succinylcholine for hydrolysis by pseudocholinesterase, and procaine should not be given IV concurrently with succinylcholine because prolonged apnea may result. In addition, promazine, oxytocin, certain anti-infective agents (excluding penicillins), chloroquine, quinine, terbutaline, β-adrenergic blocking agents, lidocaine, procainamide, quinidine, lithium carbonate, magnesium salts, metoclopramide, and inhalation anesthetics (e.g., isoflurane) may potentiate the neuromuscular blocking effect of succinylcholine. Several other drugs, including cyclophosphamide, oral contraceptives, corticosteroids, some monoamine oxidase inhibitors (e.g., phenelzine), pancuronium, neostigmine, phenothiazines, and thiotepa, have been reported to reduce plasma pseudocholinesterase concentrations and possibly enhance the neuromuscular blocking effects of succinylcholine. Although most of these reports are poorly documented and the clinical importance of their interaction with succinylcholine is unknown, caution should be used when administering these drugs simultaneously with succinylcholine.

ACUTE TOXICITY

● **Manifestations**

The duration of neuromuscular blockade produced by an overdose of succinylcholine may be longer than that following usual doses, and skeletal muscle weakness, decreased respiratory reserve, low tidal volume, or apnea beyond the period of surgery and anesthesia may occur.

● **Treatment**

In succinylcholine overdosage, supportive and symptomatic treatment should be initiated. Maintenance of an adequate, patent airway and respiratory support are necessary until recovery of normal respiration is assured. Depending on the dose and duration of succinylcholine administration, the characteristic phase I depolarizing neuromuscular block may change to a superficially resembling, phase II nondepolarizing neuromuscular block.

PHARMACOLOGY

Succinylcholine produces pharmacologic effects similar to those of other depolarizing neuromuscular blocking agents. The drug possesses histamine-releasing properties. It has been reported that succinylcholine stimulates the cardiac vagus and subsequently sympathetic ganglia.

Succinylcholine causes a slight, transient increase in intraocular pressure immediately after injection and during the fasciculation phase, and the increase may persist after the onset of complete paralysis.

PHARMACOKINETICS

● **Absorption**

Succinylcholine has a rapid onset and a short duration of action. Following IV administration of 10–30 mg of succinylcholine chloride in healthy adults, complete muscle relaxation occurs within 0.5–1 minute, persists for about 2–3 minutes, and gradually dissipates within 10 minutes. The duration of action following a single IV dose appears to be determined by the rate of diffusion of the drug away from the motor end-plate rather than the elimination of the drug by enzymatic hydrolysis. After relatively stable blood concentrations are achieved, however, as with continuous infusion or multiple injections, the short duration of action of succinylcholine results from its rapid hydrolysis. Following IM administration the onset of action occurs in about 2–3 minutes and the duration of action ranges from 10–30 minutes. The duration of action is prolonged in patients with low plasma pseudocholinesterase concentrations.

● **Distribution**

Succinylcholine crosses the placenta, generally in small amounts.

● **Elimination**

Succinylcholine (succinyldicholine) is metabolized rapidly, mainly by plasma pseudocholinesterase, to succinylmonocholine and choline. Succinylmonocholine has only about one-twentieth the activity of succinylcholine and produces a nondepolarizing rather than a depolarizing block.

Succinylmonocholine is excreted partly in urine; the remainder of the metabolite is further broken down in the plasma, principally by alkaline hydrolysis to succinate and choline, which are inactive. Since hydrolysis of succinylmonocholine occurs relatively slowly, succinylmonocholine may occasionally accumulate and cause prolonged apnea, especially in patients with impaired renal function. Up to 10% of a dose of succinylcholine is excreted unchanged in urine.

CHEMISTRY AND STABILITY

● **Chemistry**

Succinylcholine chloride is a depolarizing neuromuscular blocking agent. The drug occurs as a white, odorless, crystalline powder and has solubilities of approximately 1 g/mL in water and 2.9 mg/mL in alcohol at 25°C. Succinylcholine chloride usually contains about 2 molecules of water of hydration, but its potency is labeled in terms of its anhydrous equivalent. Commercially available succinylcholine chloride injections are adjusted to pH 3–4.5 with hydrochloric acid or sodium hydroxide and may contain methylparaben and propylparaben as preservatives.

● Stability

Succinylcholine decomposes in solutions with pH greater than 4.5. Succinylcholine chloride injection is incompatible with alkaline solutions such as barbiturates; decomposition of succinylcholine chloride and precipitation of the barbiturate may occur if the drugs are mixed.

Succinylcholine chloride undergoes hydrolysis in aqueous solutions and the commercially available injections should be stored at 2–8°C to retard loss of potency. Multiple-dose vials of the injection are stable for up to 14 days at room temperature without substantial loss of potency.

For further information on chemistry, pharmacology, pharmacokinetics, uses, cautions, drug interactions, and dosage and administration of succinylcholine chloride, see the Neuromuscular Blocking Agents General Statement 12:20.20.

PREPARATIONS

Excipients in commercially available drug preparations may have clinically important effects in some individuals; consult specific product labeling for details.

Succinylcholine Chloride

Parenteral

Injection	20 mg/mL	Anectine®, Sandoz
		Quelicin®, Hospira

Vecuronium Bromide

12:20.20 • NEUROMUSCULAR BLOCKING AGENTS

■ Vecuronium bromide is an aminosteroid nondepolarizing neuromuscular blocking agent.

USES

● Skeletal Muscle Relaxation

Vecuronium bromide is used to produce skeletal muscle relaxation during surgery after general anesthesia has been induced. The drug also is used to facilitate endotracheal intubation; however, a neuromuscular blocking agent with a more rapid onset of action (e.g., succinylcholine, rocuronium) generally is preferred in emergency situations when rapid intubation is required.

Vecuronium has produced adequate neuromuscular blockade in patients undergoing cesarean section, vagotomy, and other types of surgery, including otolaryngologic, cardiovascular (e.g., coronary artery bypass), facial, dental and oral, ophthalmic, orthopedic, abdominal (i.e., gynecologic, splenic, pancreatic, exploratory, and hernia procedures, as well as adrenalectomy, colostomy, sigmoidectomy, laparotomy, cholecystectomy, and gastrectomy), and routine minor procedures. The drug has also produced adequate blockade with minimal adverse effects in patients with renal or hepatic failure, critically ill or high-risk patients, and children 7 weeks of age and older.

Vecuronium also has been used to facilitate mechanical ventilation in the intensive care unit (ICU); however, the manufacturer states that insufficient data are available to support dosage recommendations for such use. Whenever neuromuscular blocking agents are used in the ICU, the benefits versus risks of such therapy must be considered and patients should be assessed frequently to determine the need for continued paralysis. (See Cautions: Precautions and Contraindications.)

Compared with other neuromuscular blocking agents, vecuronium has an intermediate onset and duration of action, and exhibits minimal cardiovascular effects. Because of its slow onset of paralysis, vecuronium is not suitable for rapid sequence intubation, but may be used for procedures requiring profound muscle relaxation for short durations (e.g., laryngoscopy, bronchoscopy) or for maintenance of neuromuscular blockade during the postintubation period. Although vecuronium is mostly metabolized, cumulative effects attributed to its active 3-desacetyl metabolite may occur in patients with renal or hepatic dysfunction. Because vecuronium has minimal effects on the heart, it may be a suitable neuromuscular blocking agent during surgery.

For additional information on uses and treatment principles of neuromuscular blocking agents, see Uses in the Neuromuscular Blocking Agents General Statement 12:20.20.

DOSAGE AND ADMINISTRATION

● Reconstitution and Administration

Vecuronium bromide is administered IV only. The initial (intubating) dose is administered by rapid IV injection; maintenance doses may be administered by intermittent IV injection or by continuous IV infusion. *Vecuronium should not be administered by IM injection*, since there are no clinical data to support this route of administration.

While reactions associated with histamine release are unlikely with vecuronium, if the drug is used in patients in whom substantial histamine release would be particularly hazardous (e.g., patients with clinically important cardiovascular disease) or in patients with any history suggesting a greater risk of histamine release (e.g., a history of severe anaphylactoid reactions or asthma), it may be prudent to administer the drug slowly over a period of 1–2 minutes or longer and discontinue administration if any signs of histamine release occur.

For IV injection, commercially available vecuronium bromide for injection should be reconstituted with a compatible IV solution (e.g., 5% dextrose, 5% dextrose and 0.9% sodium chloride, 0.9% sodium chloride, lactated Ringer's, bacteriostatic water for injection). When reconstituted with bacteriostatic water for injection, the solution should be used within 5 days; when reconstituted with other compatible solutions, the solution should be used within 24 hours and any unused portions should be discarded. (See Chemistry and Stability: Stability.)

For continuous IV infusion, the reconstituted vecuronium solution should be further diluted to the desired concentration (usually 0.1 or 0.2 mg/mL) in a compatible IV infusion solution such as 5% dextrose, 5% dextrose and 0.9% sodium chloride, 0.9% sodium chloride, or lactated Ringer's. Use of a controlled-infusion device is recommended to ensure precise control of the flow rate during continuous IV infusion of the drug.

Reconstituted solutions of vecuronium and diluted solutions of the drug should be inspected visually for particulate matter and discoloration prior to administration whenever solution and container permit. Vecuronium should not be mixed in the same syringe nor administered simultaneously through the same needle as an alkaline solution (e.g., barbiturate solution). (See Chemistry and Stability: Stability.)

Dispensing and Administration Precautions

Neuromuscular blocking agents should be administered only by individuals who are adequately trained in their use and complications. For specific procedures and techniques of administration, specialized references should be consulted. Facilities and personnel necessary for intubation, administration of oxygen, and respiratory support should be immediately available whenever these drugs are used. In addition, a reversal agent should be readily available in the event of a failed intubation or to accelerate neuromuscular recovery after surgery. (See Dosage and Administration: Reversal of Neuromuscular Blockade.)

Because neuromuscular blocking agents can cause respiratory arrest, precautions (e.g., storage segregation, warning labels, access limitations) should be taken to ensure that these drugs are not administered without adequate respiratory support. Affixing warning labels to storage containers and final administration containers is recommended to clearly communicate that respiratory paralysis can occur and ventilator support is required. The Institute for Safe Medication Practices (ISMP) recommends the following wording for these containers: "Warning: Paralyzing agent—causes respiratory arrest—patient must be ventilated."

Neuromuscular blocking agents have no known effect on consciousness, pain threshold, or cerebration, and should therefore be used in conjunction with adequate levels of anesthesia, and only after appropriate analgesics and sedatives are administered. To avoid distress to the patient, vecuronium should be administered only after unconsciousness has been induced.

Standardize 4 Safety

Standardized concentrations for vecuronium have been established through Standardize 4 Safety (S4S), a national patient safety initiative to reduce medication errors, especially during transitions of care. Multidisciplinary expert panels were convened to determine recommended standard concentrations. Because recommendations from the S4S panels may differ from the manufacturer's prescribing information, caution is advised when using concentrations that differ from labeling, particularly when using rate information from the label. For additional information on S4S (including updates that may be available), see https://www.ashp.org/pharmacy-practice/standardize-4-safety-initiative.

TABLE 1. Standardize 4 Safety Continuous IV Infusion Standard Concentrations for Vecuronium

Patient Population	Concentration Standards	Dosing Units
Adults[a]	1 mg/mL	mcg/kg/min[b]
Pediatric patients (<50 kg)	1 mg/mL[c]	mg/kg/hr

[a] Paralytics are recommended to be administered as straight drug. This provides consistency between operating room and the ICU, and eliminates potential compounding errors.

[b] dosing units differ from concentration units

[c] Babies under 500 g may require a lower concentration.

● **Dosage**

Dosage of vecuronium bromide must be carefully adjusted according to individual requirements and response. The use of a peripheral nerve stimulator is recommended to accurately monitor the degree of neuromuscular blockade and recovery, determine the need for additional doses, and minimize the possibility of overdosage.

The possible need for substantially increased doses of vecuronium bromide in burn patients should be considered. (See Cautions: Precautions and Contraindications.)

Initial Dose

The usual initial (intubating) adult dose of vecuronium bromide is 0.08–0.1 mg/kg (1.4–1.75 times the dose necessary to induce 90% neuromuscular blockade). Following administration of this initial dose, endotracheal intubation for nonemergency surgical procedures can be performed within 2.5–3 minutes in most patients and maximum neuromuscular blockade generally occurs within 3–5 minutes. When used concomitantly with balanced anesthesia, this initial dose usually results in clinically sufficient neuromuscular blockade for about 25–30 minutes; spontaneous recovery to about 25% of baseline generally occurs within 25–40 minutes and is usually 95% complete 45–65 minutes after administration. When used concomitantly with inhalation anesthesia, this initial dose usually results in clinically sufficient neuromuscular blockade for 30–40 minutes. When administration of a larger initial dose is considered necessary, the manufacturer states that vecuronium bromide has been administered in initial doses ranging from 0.15–0.28 mg/kg in patients undergoing halothane anesthesia with minimal adverse cardiovascular effects as long as ventilation was adequately maintained. Although onset of action may be delayed with usual initial doses in patients with impaired circulation or in whom volume of distribution of the drug may be increased (e.g., patients with cardiovascular disease or edema), larger than usual initial doses are not recommended for these patients.

When vecuronium is used concomitantly with general anesthetics (e.g., enflurane, isoflurane, halothane) that potentiate its neuromuscular blocking activity, dosage of vecuronium bromide may need to be reduced. The manufacturer states that the initial adult dose of vecuronium bromide may be reduced by about 15% (i.e., to 0.06–0.085 mg/kg) when the drug is administered more than 5 minutes after administration of enflurane, isoflurane, or halothane has been initiated or after steady-state anesthesia has been achieved.

When used following succinylcholine, vecuronium bromide should be administered at a reduced initial dose and its administration should be delayed until the patient begins recovering from the neuromuscular blockade induced by succinylcholine. Following use of succinylcholine for endotracheal intubation in adults, a reduced initial vecuronium bromide dose of 0.05–0.06 mg/kg with balanced anesthesia or 0.04–0.06 mg/kg with inhalation anesthesia may be necessary.

Because even small doses of vecuronium may cause profound neuromuscular blockade in patients with neuromuscular diseases (e.g., myasthenia gravis, Eaton-Lambert syndrome), response should be monitored carefully with a peripheral nerve stimulator; use of a small test dose of vecuronium bromide (e.g., 0.005–0.02 mg/kg) may be of value in monitoring the response to administration of skeletal muscle relaxants in these patients.

Maintenance Dosage

Intermittent IV Injection

For maintenance of neuromuscular blockade during prolonged surgical procedures in adults receiving balanced anesthesia, additional vecuronium bromide doses of 0.01–0.015 mg/kg may be administered by intermittent IV injection as necessary. In patients receiving inhalation anesthesia, the usual maintenance dose is 0.008–0.012 mg/kg, administered as necessary. The manufacturer states that a maintenance dose of 0.01 mg/kg during enflurane anesthesia is approximately equivalent to a dose of 0.015 mg/kg during balanced anesthesia. In patients undergoing balanced or inhalation anesthesia, the first maintenance dose of vecuronium bromide generally is necessary 25–40 minutes after administration of the initial dose. Because the drug lacks clinically important cumulative effects at usual doses, the manufacturer states that repeated maintenance doses of vecuronium bromide may be administered at relatively regular intervals, generally ranging from 12–15 minutes in patients undergoing balanced anesthesia and at slightly longer intervals in patients undergoing enflurane or isoflurane anesthesia. When longer intervals between doses are desirable, the size of each maintenance dose may be increased (i.e., to greater than 0.01–0.015 mg/kg).

Continuous IV Infusion

After the initial intubating dose is administered, patients may receive a continuous IV infusion of vecuronium to maintain neuromuscular blockade during prolonged surgical procedures; the infusion should be initiated approximately 20–40 minutes after administration of the initial dose when early spontaneous recovery from this dose is evident. The wide interindividual range in dosage requirements of vecuronium with continuous IV infusions requires that patients be very closely monitored to avoid excessive dosage when this method of administration is employed. Following rapid IV injection of an initial dose of vecuronium, required infusion rates of the drug initially decrease progressively and become relatively constant within 30–50 minutes. When administered by continuous IV infusion in adults, an initial vecuronium bromide infusion rate of 1 mcg/kg per minute is recommended by the manufacturer. Subsequently, the infusion rates should be adjusted to maintain 90% neuromuscular blockade; maintenance infusion rates of 0.8–1.2 mcg/kg per minute usually are adequate to maintain continuous neuromuscular blockade in most patients. Following rapid IV administration of an initial 0.1-mg/kg dose in a limited number of patients undergoing general surgery with nitrous oxide and halothane anesthesia, the rate of continuous IV infusion necessary to maintain 95% neuromuscular blockade at steady state ranged from approximately 0.55–1.67 mcg/kg per minute (mean: 1 mcg/kg per minute).

The rate of spontaneous recovery from vecuronium-induced neuromuscular blockade following discontinuance of the infusion is likely to be comparable to that following administration of a single IV injection of the drug.

When vecuronium is administered by IV infusion in patients receiving general anesthetics that potentiate its neuromuscular blocking activity, a reduction in the infusion rate of vecuronium bromide may be required. The manufacturer states that the infusion rate may need to be reduced by about 25–60% approximately 45–60 minutes following the initial IV dose when the drug is administered in the presence of steady-state anesthesia with enflurane or isoflurane. However, a reduction in the vecuronium bromide infusion rate may not be necessary in the presence of steady-state anesthesia with halothane.

The manufacturer states that prolonged use of continuous IV infusions of vecuronium during mechanical ventilation in the ICU has not been adequately studied to date to establish dosage recommendations for this use.

Pediatric Dosage

Recommendations for initial and maintenance doses of vecuronium bromide administered by intermittent IV injection in pediatric patients 10–16 years of age and older are the same as those for adults. (See Initial Dose and Maintenance Dosage: Intermittent IV Injection under Dosage and Administration: Dosage.) Slightly higher initial doses of vecuronium bromide and more frequent administration of maintenance doses may be necessary in children 1–9 years of age than in older children and adults. Infants older than 7 weeks but less than 1 year of age appear to be more sensitive than adults to the neuromuscular blocking effects of vecuronium and may experience a longer period of time (about 1.5 times longer) to neuromuscular recovery; although these children may receive doses comparable to those used in adults, less frequent administration of maintenance doses may be necessary.

Safety and efficacy of vecuronium in children younger than 7 weeks of age have not been established. In addition, the manufacturer states that administration of the drug by continuous IV infusion has not been adequately studied to date to establish dosage recommendations for this route of administration in any pediatric age group.

● **Dosage in Renal and Hepatic Impairment**

The manufacturer states that vecuronium is well tolerated and neuromuscular blockade induced by the drug is not substantially prolonged in patients with renal failure who are optimally prepared with dialysis prior to surgery; although experience with these patients is limited, most clinicians use the usual initial and maintenance doses of the drug, with the interval between doses based on careful monitoring of the patient. Since prolongation of blockade may occur in patients with severe renal failure (i.e., creatinine clearance less than 10 mL/minute) who are not optimally prepared with dialysis, the manufacturer cautions that a lower than usual initial dose of vecuronium bromide should be considered if emergency surgery is necessary in these patients; however, most clinicians believe that the usual initial dose can be administered, anticipating that the duration of blockade may be prolonged, with maintenance dosing adjusted carefully according to the patient's response.

Data currently are insufficient for specific dosage recommendations in patients with hepatic impairment. The duration of and rate of recovery from vecuronium-induced neuromuscular blockade appear to be prolonged in these patients. If vecuronium is used in patients with impaired hepatic function, some clinicians suggest that the usual initial dose of the drug may be given while others suggest giving a reduced initial dose; maintenance dosing (probably with reduced doses) would be adjusted carefully according to the patient's response.

● Reversal of Neuromuscular Blockade

Neuromuscular blockade induced by vecuronium can be reversed by administering a cholinesterase inhibitor (e.g., neostigmine, pyridostigmine, edrophonium) in conjunction with an anticholinergic agent such as atropine or glycopyrrolate to block the adverse muscarinic effects of the cholinesterase inhibitor. Alternatively, sugammadex may be used for the reversal of vecuronium-induced neuromuscular blockade after surgery. *For specific information on the uses and dosage and administration of these other drugs, see the individual monographs.*

To minimize the risk of residual neuromuscular blockade, reversal should only be attempted after some degree of spontaneous recovery has occurred; patients should be closely monitored until adequate recovery of normal neuromuscular function is assured (i.e., ability to maintain satisfactory ventilation and a patent airway).

CAUTIONS

● Adverse Effects

Adverse effects of vecuronium bromide generally are manifestations of the usual pharmacologic actions of the nondepolarizing neuromuscular blocking agents, including skeletal muscle weakness or paralysis and respiratory insufficiency or apnea. However, the respiratory depression that occurs during or following anesthesia that includes vecuronium bromide may also result at least in part from concomitantly administered drugs, including opiate agonists, barbiturates, and other CNS depressants.

Prolonged to profound extensions of paralysis and/or muscle weakness as well as muscle atrophy have been reported after long-term use of the drug to support mechanical ventilation in intensive care settings. Prolonged paralysis has been associated with electrolyte disturbances (e.g., increased plasma magnesium concentrations), metabolic acidosis, and renal failure (which may result in high plasma concentrations of 3-desacetyl vecuronium); limited data indicate that prolonged paralysis may occur more frequently in female patients. (See Cautions: Precautions and Contraindications, in the Neuromuscular Blocking Agents General Statement 12:20.20.)

Following intradermal administration of vecuronium in several healthy individuals, minimal induration, redness, and itching, which are characteristic manifestations of cutaneous histamine release, have been observed, but these effects were less severe than those seen with other neuromuscular blocking agents. Rarely, hypersensitivity reactions associated with histamine release (e.g., bronchospasm, flushing, erythema, acute urticaria, hypotension, tachycardia) have been reported following IV administration of usual doses of the drug. Redness (flare) in skin proximal to the injection site, with subsequent urticaria, occurred in one patient following IV injection of vecuronium; subsequent intradermal testing with the drug produced a wheal and flare. In another patient, bronchospasm occurred following IV injection of the drug; subsequent intradermal testing with the drug was positive, although other immunologic studies, including basophil degranulation tests, revealed no evidence that the reaction was mediated by IgE or direct histamine release.

Cardiovascular effects, including changes in heart rate, cardiac index, cardiac output, filling pressure of the heart, mean systolic blood pressure, mean arterial pressure, and systemic vascular resistance, have been observed occasionally following administration of vecuronium; however, these effects appear to be minimal and transient. Some cardiovascular effects may be associated with endotracheal intubation rather than with the drug. Systolic blood pressure, diastolic blood pressure, and/or mean arterial pressure reportedly did not change substantially in healthy patients following administration of doses of vecuronium bromide up to 0.15 mg/kg (up to 3 times the doses necessary for clinical relaxation); heart rate remained unchanged or decreased by an average of up to 8% from baseline values. The drug did not produce changes in heart rate or rhythm, mean arterial pressure, central venous pressure, or pulmonary wedge pressure when administered in a dose of 0.28 mg/kg in patients undergoing preparation for coronary artery bypass surgery; systemic vascular resistance decreased 12% and cardiac output increased 9% in these patients. Vecuronium did not produce tachycardia or changes in blood pressure in several patients undergoing surgery for pheochromocytoma. In comatose patients not receiving anesthesia who were administered vecuronium bromide doses of 0.1 mg/kg, the drug did not increase heart rate or cardiac output; in doses of 0.3 mg/kg, the drug caused only a very slight, transient increase in heart rate and cardiac output.

Serious hypersensitivity reactions, including anaphylaxis, have been reported rarely with all neuromuscular blocking agents; such reactions were life-threatening or fatal in some cases.

● Precautions and Contraindications

Vecuronium bromide shares the toxic potentials of the nondepolarizing neuromuscular blocking agents, and the usual precautions of neuromuscular blocking agent administration should be observed. (See Cautions in the Neuromuscular Blocking Agents General Statement 12:20.20.)

When used inappropriately, neuromuscular blocking agents can severely compromise respiratory function and cause respiratory paralysis; special precautions should be taken during and after administration of these drugs. (See Dispensing and Administration Precautions under Dosage and Administration: Reconstitution and Administration.) The degree of neuromuscular blockade produced by vecuronium should be monitored with a peripheral nerve stimulator, particularly in patients with conditions that may potentiate (e.g., neuromuscular diseases) or cause resistance to (e.g., burns) the neuromuscular blocking effects of the drug.

Data from some clinical studies and intradermal skin testing indicate that histamine-like hypersensitivity reactions, including bronchospasm, flushing, redness, hypotension, and tachycardia, are *not* likely to occur following administration of vecuronium; however, this does not preclude the rare development of a hypersensitivity reaction and the possibility of histamine release should be considered. (See Pharmacology: Effects on Histamine.)

Since vecuronium exhibits minimal effects on heart rate, especially at recommended doses, the drug will not counteract the bradycardia induced by many anesthesia agents (e.g., high-dose fentanyl) or by vagal stimulation; as a result, bradycardia may be more common when vecuronium is used concomitantly during anesthesia with agents that may cause bradycardia than when certain other neuromuscular blocking agents are used concomitantly.

Many drugs administered during anesthesia are suspected of being capable of initiating the development of malignant hyperthermia. The manufacturer states that data from screening in susceptible animals are insufficient to determine whether vecuronium is capable of initiating the development of this condition. However, because malignant hyperthermia can occur even in the absence of a recognized precipitating factor, clinicians should be vigilant for its possible development and prepared for its management in any patient undergoing general anesthesia.

Resistance to nondepolarizing neuromuscular blocking agents, including vecuronium, can develop in burn patients and may be substantial. The magnitude of resistance depends on the extent of thermal injury and elapsed time since the burn. The possible need for substantially increased doses of vecuronium bromide in burn patients should be considered.

Vecuronium is well tolerated and neuromuscular blockade induced by the drug is not substantially prolonged in patients with renal dysfunction who have undergone adequate dialysis prior to surgery. Since blockade may be prolonged in patients with severe renal failure (i.e., creatinine clearance less than 10 mL/minute) who are undergoing emergency surgery and cannot be adequately prepared with dialysis preoperatively, the manufacturer cautions that a lower than usual initial dose of vecuronium bromide be considered in these patients. (See Dosage and Administration: Dosage in Renal and Hepatic Impairment.) The manufacturer also cautions that inadvertent overdosage in patients with renal dysfunction may be avoided by careful monitoring with a peripheral nerve stimulator.

Since the onset of neuromuscular blockade and maximum effect of vecuronium may be delayed secondary to impaired circulation or an increased volume of distribution of the drug, larger than usual doses of the drug are not recommended in patients with these conditions (e.g., patients with cardiovascular disease or edema) and caution should be used when administering a subsequent dose of the drug in such patients before the maximum effect of the initial dose is attained.

Vecuronium should be administered with caution in patients with hepatic dysfunction (e.g., cirrhosis, cholestasis), since the drug appears to be eliminated principally via bile and recovery from neuromuscular blockade may be prolonged in these patients. The manufacturer cautions that inadvertent overdosage in patients with impaired circulation or hepatic dysfunction may be avoided by careful monitoring with a peripheral nerve stimulator.

Vecuronium should be administered with caution in severely obese patients; maintenance of an adequate airway and ventilation support prior to, during, and following administration of neuromuscular blocking agents may require particular care in these patients.

Patients with neuromuscular diseases (e.g., myasthenia gravis, Eaton-Lambert syndrome) may have an exaggerated response to vecuronium. In patients with neuromuscular diseases, the degree of neuromuscular blockade induced by vecuronium should be monitored with a peripheral nerve stimulator; use of a small test dose of the drug (e.g., 0.005–0.02 mg/kg) may be of value in monitoring the response to administration of skeletal muscle relaxants in these patients. The degree of neuromuscular blockade produced by vecuronium should also be monitored with a peripheral nerve stimulator in patients with severe electrolyte disturbances (i.e., hypermagnesemia, hypokalemia, hypocalcemia) or diseases that result in electrolyte disturbances (e.g., adrenal cortical insufficiency) and in patients with severe debilitation or carcinomatosis. *For other conditions associated with increased response to neuromuscular blocking agents, see* Cautions: Precautions and Contraindications, in the Neuromuscular Blocking Agents General Statement 12:20.20.

Long-term use of neuromuscular blocking agents to support mechanical ventilation in the intensive care unit (ICU) has been associated with prolonged paralysis and/or skeletal muscle weakness. Although confounding factors were present and a causal relationship has not been definitively established, the risks versus benefits of neuromuscular blockade should be considered whenever there is a need for long-term mechanical ventilation. Continuous monitoring of neuromuscular transmission with a peripheral nerve stimulator is recommended whenever vecuronium is used in the ICU. Additional doses of vecuronium or any other neuromuscular blocking agent should not be administered before there is a definite response to nerve stimulation tests. If no response is elicited, administration of the drug should be discontinued until a response returns.

Since neuromuscular blocking agents have been reported to cause severe anaphylactic reactions, appropriate emergency treatment should be readily available whenever these drugs are administered. Vecuronium is contraindicated in patients with known hypersensitivity to the drug. Because of the possibility of cross-sensitivity, vecuronium should be used with caution in patients who have experienced previous anaphylactic reactions to other neuromuscular blocking agents (depolarizing or nondepolarizing).

● Pediatric Precautions

Safety and efficacy of vecuronium in children younger than 7 weeks of age have not been established. The drug has been used safely and effectively in children older than 7 weeks of age who were undergoing surgery. Vecuronium bromide that has been reconstituted with bacteriostatic water for injection containing benzyl alcohol should *not* be used in neonates.

● Mutagenicity and Carcinogenicity

Long-term animal studies to determine the mutagenic and carcinogenic potentials of vecuronium bromide have not been performed to date.

● Pregnancy, Fertility, and Lactation

Pregnancy

Animal reproduction studies have not been performed to date with vecuronium. It is not known whether administration of neuromuscular blocking agents during vaginal delivery has immediate or delayed adverse effects on the fetus or whether it increases the likelihood that resuscitation of the neonate will be necessary. Vecuronium should be used with caution and dosage reduced as necessary in pregnant women receiving magnesium sulfate during delivery, since the neuromuscular blockade may be potentiated and its reversal impeded. When vecuronium was administered to pregnant women during delivery by cesarean section, no adverse effects attributed to the drug were observed in neonates born to these women. In 2 limited studies, Apgar scores were 9 or greater at 5 minutes after birth in neonates born to women who received vecuronium bromide 0.04 or 0.06–0.08 mg/kg (after

tracheal intubation with succinylcholine) during cesarean delivery. However, the drug crosses the placenta minimally, and the possibility of respiratory depression in neonates should be considered following cesarean section in which a neuromuscular blocking agent is administered to the mother. It is not known whether vecuronium can cause fetal harm when administered to pregnant women. The drug should be used during pregnancy only when clearly needed.

Fertility

It is not known if vecuronium affects fertility.

Lactation

Since it is not known if vecuronium is distributed into milk, the drug should be administered with caution to nursing women. However, since animal studies suggest that GI absorption of vecuronium is negligible, any drug that may be present in milk is not likely to be of any clinical importance to a nursing infant.

DRUG INTERACTIONS

Concurrent administration of some drugs, including general anesthetics (i.e., enflurane, isoflurane, halothane), antibiotics (e.g., aminoglycosides, tetracyclines, bacitracin, polymyxins, clindamycin), skeletal muscle relaxants (e.g., succinylcholine, pancuronium), magnesium salts, and quinidine, may affect the neuromuscular blocking activity of vecuronium bromide. Concurrent administration of barbiturates, opiate agonists, nitrous oxide, or droperidol appears to have little effect on the intensity or duration of the neuromuscular blockade induced by vecuronium. For additional information on potential drug interactions of vecuronium, see Drug Interactions in the Neuromuscular Blocking Agents General Statement 12:20.20.

● General Anesthetics

Enflurane and isoflurane reportedly increase the potency and prolong the duration of the neuromuscular blockade induced by vecuronium by about 30–50%; halothane appears to have only a marginal effect on the potency and duration of neuromuscular blockade induced by vecuronium, prolonging the duration by about 20%. In a study comparing concomitant administration of vecuronium and either enflurane, isoflurane, or halothane with 60% nitrous oxide anesthesia, the ED_{50} (dose required to produce 50% suppression of the control twitch response) of vecuronium decreased by about 50, 33, or 18% when the MAC (minimal alveolar anesthetic concentration) of enflurane, isoflurane, or halothane anesthesia, respectively, was increased from 1.2 to 2.2. When the MAC of the inhalation anesthetic was increased to 2.2 in this study, the duration of neuromuscular blockade was increased twofold by enflurane but only minimally by isoflurane or halothane; the potentiating effect of an increasing MAC is markedly less for vecuronium than for pancuronium.

● Skeletal Muscle Relaxants

Administration of succinylcholine prior to vecuronium appears to increase the potency and prolong the duration of neuromuscular blockade induced by vecuronium. In one study, when a 0.04-mg/kg dose of vecuronium bromide was given 15 or 30 minutes after complete recovery from the blockade of a 1-mg/kg dose of succinylcholine, the duration of neuromuscular blockade to 90% recovery was about 26 minutes compared with 12 minutes when vecuronium was administered alone; the onset of blockade was more rapid in patients receiving vecuronium subsequent to succinylcholine. In another study, a 1-mg/kg dose of succinylcholine followed 9–14 minutes later by a 0.036-mg/kg dose of vecuronium bromide induced a 91% neuromuscular blockade compared with a 72–78% blockade when vecuronium was administered alone; the time for recovery from 25% to 75% of the control twitch tension was about 10 or 8 minutes in patients who received both succinylcholine and vecuronium or vecuronium alone, respectively. If succinylcholine is administered prior to vecuronium, the manufacturer states that administration of vecuronium should be delayed until the effects of succinylcholine begin to dissipate. The manufacturer states that the administration of vecuronium prior to succinylcholine in order to attenuate some of the adverse effects of succinylcholine has not been fully evaluated.

Concomitant use of vecuronium and other nondepolarizing neuromuscular blocking agents (e.g., pancuronium bromide) may result in additive or synergistic effects. The manufacturer states that data are insufficient to support concomitant administration of vecuronium and other nondepolarizing neuromuscular blocking agents. In healthy adults in one study, concomitant administration of vecuronium and pancuronium did not result in potentiation, whereas in another study concomitant administration of vecuronium and tubocurarine (no longer commercially available in the US) did result in potentiation.

● Anti-infective Agents

IV and/or intraperitoneal injection of high doses of certain anti-infective agents, including aminoglycosides, metronidazole, tetracyclines, bacitracin, clindamycin, lincomycin, and polymyxins (i.e., polymyxin B sulfate, colistin, sodium colistimethate), has been shown to induce neuromuscular blockade. If these anti-infective agents are used before, during, or after surgical procedures in which vecuronium is administered, the possibility of prolonged duration of neuromuscular blockade (or recurarization, particularly postoperatively) should be considered. For additional information, see see Drug Interactions: Anti-Infective Agents, in the Neuromuscular Blocking Agents General Statement 12:20.20.

Intraoperative administration of acylaminopenicillins, including piperacillin, reportedly prolongs vecuronium-induced neuromuscular blockade, increasing the duration of skeletal muscle relaxation by an average of 40–55%. Acylaminopenicillins should be used perioperatively with caution in patients receiving vecuronium and the possibility of prolonged neuromuscular blockade should be considered.

● Other Drugs

When magnesium sulfate is administered for the management of toxemia of pregnancy, the neuromuscular blockade induced by vecuronium may be potentiated and its reversal impeded. If used in pregnant women receiving magnesium sulfate, vecuronium should be used with caution and its dosage reduced as necessary.

Experience with skeletal muscle relaxants other than vecuronium suggests that recurrence of paralysis may occur in patients following parenteral administration of quinidine during recovery from neuromuscular blockade. The manufacturer states that the possibility of recurrence of paralysis following parenteral administration of quinidine during recovery from vecuronium-induced neuromuscular blockade should be considered.

Although further documentation is needed, a difficult and prolonged recovery from vecuronium-induced neuromuscular blockade in a patient receiving IV verapamil suggests that calcium-channel blocking agents may be capable of prolonging the duration of neuromuscular blockade induced by vecuronium. Similarly, a prolonged duration of vecuronium-induced blockade was reported in a patient who received oral dantrolene preoperatively, but further evaluation of a potential interaction is needed.

ACUTE TOXICITY

The manufacturer states that there has been no experience to date with overdosage following parenteral administration of vecuronium bromide. The possibility of overdosage can be minimized by assessing the vecuronium-induced effect on the response to peripheral nerve stimulation.

Overdosage of vecuronium is likely to produce symptoms that are mainly extensions of the usual pharmacologic effects of the drug. The duration of neuromuscular blockade produced by an overdose of vecuronium may be longer than that following usual doses and skeletal muscle weakness, decreased respiratory reserve, low tidal volume, or apnea beyond the period of surgery and anesthesia may occur. A peripheral nerve stimulator should be used to monitor recovery from blockade and may be used to differentiate prolonged neuromuscular blockade from other causes of diminished respiratory reserve.

In vecuronium overdosage, supportive and symptomatic treatment should be initiated. An adequate, patent airway should be maintained, using assisted or controlled respiration as necessary. The possibility that other drugs (e.g., general anesthetics, opiate agonists, barbiturates) used during the surgical procedure may be wholly or partially responsible for respiratory depression should be considered. If cardiovascular support is necessary, treatment should include proper patient positioning, IV fluid administration, and, if necessary, use of vasopressors. Reversal of the neuromuscular blockade produced by vecuronium may be achieved by administration of a cholinesterase inhibitor such as neostigmine, pyridostigmine, or edrophonium. (See Dosage and Administration: Reversal of Neuromuscular Blockade.)

PHARMACOLOGY

● Neuromuscular Blockade

Vecuronium bromide is a nondepolarizing neuromuscular blocking agent that produces pharmacologic effects similar to those of other nondepolarizing neuromuscular blocking agents. (See Pharmacology in the Neuromuscular Blocking Agents General Statement 12:20.20). On a weight basis, vecuronium bromide is about 1.2–1.7 or 4–5 times as potent as pancuronium bromide or atracurium besylate, respectively. The duration of neuromuscular blockade induced by initially equipotent doses of vecuronium bromide is about 33–50% or 25–33% that induced by pancuronium bromide or tubocurarine chloride (no longer commercially available in the US), respectively, and about 70–100% that induced by atracurium besylate. The neuromuscular blocking activity of vecuronium is enhanced in the presence of some inhalation general anesthetics (e.g., enflurane, isoflurane). (See Drug Interactions: General Anesthetics.)

The effects of patient age on vecuronium-induced neuromuscular blockade in adults remain to be clearly determined. The time of onset of neuromuscular blockade appears to be increased and the dose of vecuronium bromide necessary to maintain steady-state neuromuscular blockade and the rate of recovery appear to be decreased in older adults compared with younger adults. In one study in anesthetized patients younger than 40, 40–60, and older than 60 years of age, mean steady-state vecuronium bromide dosage requirements were approximately 3, 2.4, and 1.8 mg/m^2 per hour, respectively, and the mean times for the recovery of twitch height to 75% of the original twitch height were approximately 25, 31, and 60 minutes, respectively. However, other preliminary data suggest that vecuronium dosage requirements and the rate of recovery from neuromuscular blockade are similar in young and older adults. Further studies are needed to fully evaluate the effects of age on vecuronium-induced neuromuscular blockade in adults. Young (1–10 years of age) children may require slightly larger doses of vecuronium bromide than adolescents and adults, when calculated on a weight basis, to achieve the same degree of neuromuscular blockade during comparable techniques of anesthesia; however, children younger than 1 year of age may require smaller doses of the drug or doses similar to adults, administered at longer time intervals. (See Pediatric Dosage in Dosage and Administration: Dosage.)

The ED$_{50}$ (dose required to produce 50% suppression of the control twitch response) of vecuronium bromide in patients undergoing balanced or nitrous oxide and halothane anesthesia reportedly ranges from 0.015–0.036 mg/kg. The manufacturer states that the ED$_{90}$ (dose required to produce 90% suppression of the control twitch response) of the drug in patients undergoing balanced anesthesia averages 0.057 mg/kg; in several studies in patients undergoing balanced anesthesia, the ED$_{90}$ has ranged from 0.043–0.062 mg/kg. The ED$_{95}$ (dose required to produce 95% suppression of the control twitch response) of vecuronium bromide in patients undergoing balanced anesthesia has ranged from 0.037–0.065 mg/kg.

The ED$_{50}$ in children 7–45 weeks, 1–9 years, and 10–17 years of age undergoing nitrous oxide and halothane anesthesia has reportedly averaged 0.0165, 0.019–0.033, and 0.023 mg/kg, respectively; the ED$_{95}$ in children 2–9 and 10–17 years of age undergoing nitrous oxide and halothane anesthesia has reportedly averaged 0.06 and 0.045 mg/kg, respectively.

In animals, metabolic or respiratory acidosis substantially increases and metabolic alkalosis substantially decreases the intensity of vecuronium-induced neuromuscular blockade; respiratory alkalosis only slightly decreases the intensity of neuromuscular blockade. The effects of acid-base balance on vecuronium-induced neuromuscular blockade in humans have not been fully determined. In anesthetized patients receiving vecuronium by an infusion sufficient to produce a continual 50% depression of the control twitch tension, induced hypercapnia or hypocapnia decreased or increased twitch tension, respectively; however, changes in Paco$_2$ induced prior to administration of vecuronium had little effect on the maximal depression of twitch tension induced by the drug or the time necessary for spontaneous recovery from 25% to 75% of control twitch tension.

● Effects on Histamine

Vecuronium appears to have little histamine-releasing activity when administered at usual clinical doses. In studies comparing vecuronium bromide, atracurium besylate, metocurine iodide (no longer commercially available in the US), pancuronium bromide, and tubocurarine chloride (no longer commercially available in the US), vecuronium was the least potent stimulator of histamine release as determined by cutaneous reaction (i.e., induration, redness, itching) to intradermal injection of the drugs. While the risk of a histamine-induced sensitivity reaction to vecuronium appears to be low, anaphylaxis and anaphylactoid reactions have been reported rarely in patients receiving the drug. (See Cautions: Precautions and Contraindications.)

● Other Effects

Despite its steroidal structure, vecuronium apparently exhibits no hormonal activity.

The effect of vecuronium on intraocular pressure (IOP) in patients undergoing elective ophthalmic surgery has not been clearly determined. In one study, a 0.12-mg/kg dose of vecuronium bromide caused an additional reduction in IOP following an initial anesthesia-induced reduction, while in another study, a 0.1-mg/kg dose of the drug appeared to slightly reverse the initial anesthesia-induced reduction in IOP.

Vecuronium is about 10 times less potent than pancuronium bromide and about 1000 times more potent than succinylcholine chloride in its ability to inhibit plasma pseudocholinesterase; vecuronium's activity appears to be of no clinical importance. Although probably of no clinical relevance, vecuronium is also about 5 times more potent than pancuronium bromide or atracurium besylate in its ability to inhibit erythrocyte cholinesterase.

In animals, the effects of vecuronium on adrenergic receptors, cardiac muscarinic receptors, or norepinephrine reuptake mechanisms are minimal and occur only at dosages many times in excess of those required for neuromuscular blockade.

Unlike most other nondepolarizing neuromuscular blocking agents, vecuronium exhibits minimal cardiovascular effects. The drug does not appear to substantially affect heart rate or rhythm, systolic or diastolic blood pressure, mean arterial pressure, cardiac output, systemic vascular resistance, or pulmonary capillary wedge pressure. (See Cautions: Adverse Effects.) In animals, 50% vagal blockade occurs only at vecuronium bromide doses 50–80 times greater than those required for 50% neuromuscular blockade.

PHARMACOKINETICS

● Absorption

The onset and duration of and the rate of recovery from neuromuscular blockade induced by vecuronium bromide vary among individuals, are dose dependent, and may be altered by the anesthetic agent (e.g., enflurane, isoflurane, halothane) employed. (See Drug Interactions: General Anesthetics.) The onset and duration of and rate of recovery from neuromuscular blockade generally do not appear to be substantially altered by renal dysfunction; however, the duration of blockade may be prolonged in patients with severe renal impairment who have not undergone dialysis prior to surgery. The duration of and rate of recovery from neuromuscular blockade appear to be prolonged by hepatic dysfunction (i.e., cirrhosis, cholestasis). The duration of blockade may also be prolonged in patients undergoing cardiopulmonary bypass surgery under induced hypothermia.

As with other nondepolarizing neuromuscular blocking agents, the time from injection to maximum blockade decreases as the dose of vecuronium bromide increases. The manufacturer states that following IV administration of a vecuronium bromide dose of 0.08–0.1 mg/kg, neuromuscular blockade begins within 1 minute and is maximal at 3–5 minutes. Following concomitant administration of vecuronium bromide and halothane or nitrous oxide in adults, the time from injection to maximum blockade ranges from 3.3–6.7 minutes with doses of 0.01–0.05 mg/kg and 2.2–5.9 minutes with doses of 0.06–0.2 mg/kg. Following concomitant administration of a vecuronium bromide dose of 0.07 mg/kg and halothane and nitrous oxide anesthesia in children 7–45 weeks and 1–8 years of age, the time from injection to maximum blockade has reportedly averaged 1.5 and 2.4 minutes, respectively.

The duration of neuromuscular blockade increases as the dose of vecuronium bromide increases. In animals, the intensity of vecuronium-induced neuromuscular blockade has been shown to be increased by acidosis; however, the effects of acid-base balance on vecuronium-induced blockade in humans have not been fully determined. (See Pharmacology: Neuromuscular Blockade.) The duration of neuromuscular blockade induced by initially equipotent doses of vecuronium bromide is about 33–50% or 25–33% of that induced by pancuronium bromide or tubocurarine chloride (no longer commercially available in the US), respectively, and about 70–100% of that induced by atracurium besylate. The manufacturer states that the duration of clinically sufficient neuromuscular blockade

(i.e., time from injection to 25% spontaneous recovery of control twitch response) induced by initial vecuronium bromide doses of 0.08–0.1 mg/kg under balanced (e.g., thiopental [no longer commercially available in the US], nitrous oxide, fentanyl) or halothane anesthesia is about 25–30 or 30–40 minutes, respectively. Following intubation with succinylcholine, the duration of clinically sufficient neuromuscular blockade of initial vecuronium bromide doses of 0.05–0.06 mg/kg under balanced anesthesia is 20–25 minutes and the duration of initial doses of 0.03–0.06 mg/kg under inhalation anesthesia is 25–30 minutes. In various studies, the duration of vecuronium-induced blockade (time from injection to 90% spontaneous recovery of control twitch response) under nitrous oxide, halothane, or enflurane anesthesia has reportedly averaged from 14–32 minutes with initial doses of approximately 0.01–0.05 mg/kg and 34–60 minutes with initial doses of approximately 0.06–0.12 mg/kg. In children 7–45 weeks and 1–8 years of age, the duration of blockade (time from injection to 90% spontaneous recovery of control twitch response) under halothane and nitrous oxide anesthesia has reportedly averaged 73 and 35 minutes, respectively, following administration of a vecuronium bromide dose of 0.07 mg/kg. The prolonged duration of action in children younger than 1 year of age appears to be related to the larger volume of distribution of, and possibly an increased sensitivity to, the drug in this age group. Repeated administration of maintenance doses of vecuronium bromide appears to have little, if any, cumulative effect on duration of the neuromuscular blockade. In addition, since the time necessary to recover from maintenance doses of the same size generally does not change with each additional dose, doses may be administered at relatively regular intervals with predictable neuromuscular blocking results; however, the interval between maintenance doses depends on the size of the dose and concomitant anesthesia.

Recovery from the neuromuscular blocking effects of vecuronium bromide occurs more rapidly than recovery from those of pancuronium bromide or tubocurarine chloride. Recovery from neuromuscular blockade may be enhanced slightly by alkalosis and prolonged by acidosis. The manufacturer states that the recovery time (the time necessary for spontaneous recovery of the twitch response from 25% to 75% of the control response) following administration of vecuronium bromide doses of 0.08–0.1 mg/kg under balanced or halothane anesthesia is about 15–25 minutes; the recovery time following initial doses of vecuronium bromide appears to be dose dependent. In children 7–45 weeks and 1–8 years of age, the recovery time following administration of a vecuronium bromide dose of 0.07 mg/kg under halothane and nitrous oxide anesthesia has reportedly averaged 20 and 9 minutes, respectively. Following administration of a single vecuronium bromide dose of 0.2 mg/kg in patients with cirrhosis, the recovery time reportedly averaged 44 minutes. Repeated administration of maintenance doses of vecuronium bromide appears to have little, if any, cumulative effect on the rate of recovery from neuromuscular blockade. The rate of recovery from vecuronium-induced blockade is more rapid than that from pancuronium-induced blockade and is similar to that from atracurium-induced blockade.

Good to excellent conditions for performing endotracheal intubation generally are present within 2.5–3.7 minutes after administration of a 0.08- to 0.1-mg/kg dose of vecuronium bromide in most patients; however, intubation has been performed successfully within 1.5–2.5 minutes in some patients after administration of 0.07- to 0.2-mg/kg doses of the drug.

In adults, mean plasma vecuronium concentrations of 0.09–0.14 and 0.2 mcg/mL at steady-state are reportedly associated with 50% and 90% neuromuscular blockade, respectively.

● Distribution

Distribution of vecuronium into human body tissues and fluids has not been fully characterized. Following IV administration, vecuronium appears to rapidly distribute into the extracellular space. Limited data indicate that the drug undergoes rapid and extensive hepatic extraction. Following administration of a single 0.025- to 0.28-mg/kg dose in adults with normal renal and hepatic function, the volume of distribution of vecuronium in the central compartment (V_c) and at steady-state (V_{ss}) reportedly ranges from 50–120 and 179–400 mL/kg, respectively. The V_c and V_{ss} averaged 50 and 200–210 mL/kg, respectively, following an initial 0.06-mg/kg dose and continuous infusion at 1 mcg/kg per minute in adults with normal renal and hepatic function undergoing inhalation or balanced anesthesia. The volume of distribution of vecuronium is increased in children younger than 1 year of age and may be decreased in geriatric patients; although not clearly established, the volume of distribution may be slightly increased in patients with renal failure.

Vecuronium is approximately 60–90% bound to plasma proteins; however, in one study, the drug was reportedly 30 and 24% bound to serum proteins in healthy patients and patients with cirrhosis, respectively. The wide range in reported values may have resulted from the different methods used to determine the extent of protein binding. Vecuronium crosses the placenta minimally; placental transfer of the drug appears to be about 50% that of pancuronium. Umbilical venous plasma concentrations of vecuronium were 11% of maternal concentrations at delivery in 2 limited studies in women undergoing cesarean section who received 0.04 or 0.06–0.08 mg/kg of vecuronium bromide after tracheal intubation with succinylcholine. It is not known if vecuronium distributes into milk.

● Elimination

Plasma concentrations of vecuronium generally appear to decline in a biphasic manner. In adults with normal renal function, the plasma half-life in the distribution phase ($t_{\frac{1}{2}a}$) averages 3.3–9 minutes and in the terminal elimination phase ($t_{\frac{1}{2}\beta}$) averages 31–80 minutes. Some pharmacokinetic data indicate that plasma concentrations of vecuronium decline in a triphasic manner, with the drug undergoing a very rapid initial distribution. In adults with normal renal function, the plasma half-life in the initial distribution phase reportedly averages 1.1–3 minutes, the plasma half-life in the redistribution phase ($t_{\frac{1}{2}a}$) reportedly averages 9–14 minutes, and the plasma half-life in the terminal elimination phase ($t_{\frac{1}{2}\beta}$) reportedly averages 58–103 minutes. In a few children 3–11 months or 1–5 years of age, the $t_{\frac{1}{2}\beta}$ of vecuronium reportedly averaged 65 or 41 minutes, respectively. The $t_{\frac{1}{2}a}$ and $t_{\frac{1}{2}\beta}$ of vecuronium are not substantially altered in patients with renal failure, the $t_{\frac{1}{2}a}$ averaging 4–11 minutes and the $t_{\frac{1}{2}\beta}$ averaging 68–97 minutes. In one study in patients with cirrhosis, the $t_{\frac{1}{2}\beta}$ averaged 84 minutes. The $t_{\frac{1}{2}\beta}$ is reportedly decreased to about 35–40 minutes during late pregnancy.

The metabolic fate of vecuronium in humans has not been fully characterized. In aqueous solution in vitro, vecuronium undergoes spontaneous deacetylation at the 3α- and/or 17β-positions to form the hydroxy derivatives. The neuromuscular blocking activity of the 3α-hydroxy derivative appears to be at least 50% that of the unchanged drug; in animals, equipotent doses of vecuronium bromide and the 3α-hydroxy derivative induce neuromuscular blockade of similar duration. In vitro, the 3α-hydroxy derivative undergoes rapid conversion to the 3α,17β-dihydroxy derivative. The 17β-hydroxy and 3α,17β-dihydroxy derivatives appear to have about 5 and 2% of the neuromuscular blocking activity of the unchanged drug, respectively. The extent of spontaneous deacetylation and/or metabolism of vecuronium in vivo in humans remains to be clearly determined.

Vecuronium and its metabolite(s) appear to be excreted principally in feces via biliary elimination; the drug and its metabolite(s) are also excreted in urine. Although only unchanged drug has been detected in plasma in patients receiving the drug as an adjunct to surgical anesthesia, up to 10% of a dose of vecuronium has been excreted in urine and 5–25% in bile as the 3α-hydroxy derivative in some patients. Another metabolite, 3-desacetyl vecuronium, has been detected rarely in plasma following prolonged clinical use of the drug in an intensive care setting. Studies in rabbits with orally administered drug indicate that enterohepatic circulation of vecuronium and its active metabolites probably does not occur. Approximately 20–30% (range: 3–36%) of an IV dose of vecuronium bromide is excreted in urine within 24 hours after administration in humans, principally as unchanged drug and to a lesser extent as the 3α-hydroxy derivative; most urinary excretion occurs within the first 4–6 hours. In patients with a T-tube in the common bile duct, 12–45% of an IV dose of vecuronium was reportedly excreted in bile within 18–42 hours after administration, almost completely as unchanged drug, with most biliary excretion occurring within the first 4–6 hours. Since excretion of the drug occurs mainly via biliary elimination, temporary or permanent exclusion of the liver in animals results in increased intensity and duration of the neuromuscular blockade induced by vecuronium bromide and prolongs recovery.

Total body clearance of vecuronium reportedly averages 2.9–6.4 mL/minute per kg in patients with normal renal function. Total body clearance reportedly averages 2.5–4.5 mL/minute per kg in patients with renal dysfunction and 0.97–2.7 mL/minute per kg in patients with hepatic dysfunction (i.e., cirrhosis, biliary obstruction).

The manufacturer states that the effect of hemodialysis or peritoneal dialysis on plasma concentrations of vecuronium and its metabolite(s) is unknown.

CHEMISTRY AND STABILITY

● Chemistry

Vecuronium bromide is a synthetic, nondepolarizing neuromuscular blocking agent. Vecuronium bromide differs structurally from pancuronium bromide only by the absence of an *N*-methyl group on the piperidine ring at position 2, resulting in a monoquaternary rather than bisquaternary compound. Vecuronium, like pancuronium bromide, contains the steroid or androstane nucleus.

Vecuronium bromide occurs as white to off-white or slightly pink crystals or crystalline powder and has solubilities of 9 and 23 mg/mL in water and in alcohol, respectively. The drug has a pK_a of 8.97 in distilled water at 25°C. The commercially available powders for injection occur as a lyophilized cake of very fine microscopic crystals. Anhydrous citric acid, anhydrous dibasic sodium phosphate, sodium hydroxide, and/or phosphoric acid are added during manufacture of the powders for injection to buffer and adjust the pH. Mannitol is also added during manufacture of the powders for injection to adjust tonicity. Following reconstitution with sterile water for injection, vecuronium bromide solutions containing 2 mg/mL are clear, colorless, and isotonic and have a pH of 4.

● Stability

Vecuronium bromide is unstable in the presence of bases and undergoes gradual hydrolysis in aqueous solutions, alcohol, and chlorinated hydrocarbons. Vecuronium bromide solutions should not be administered in the same syringe as an alkaline solution nor should vecuronium bromide and an alkaline solution be administered simultaneously through the same needle.

Commercially available vecuronium bromide powder for injection should be stored at 20–25°C and protected from light.

When reconstituted with 5% dextrose, 5% dextrose and 0.9% sodium chloride, 0.9% sodium chloride, or lactated Ringer's, resulting vecuronium bromide solutions are stable for 24 hours when refrigerated. Since vials of the drug do not contain a preservative and are designed for single use only, unused portions of the reconstituted solution should be discarded. Following reconstitution with bacteriostatic water for injection, vecuronium bromide solutions are stable for 5 days at room temperature or when refrigerated. Vecuronium bromide solutions are stable for 48 hours after reconstitution with sterile water for injection when stored in plastic or glass syringes at 2–8°C or 15–30°C, but the manufacturer recommends that they be used within 24 hours.

Vecuronium bromide is physically and chemically compatible with the following IV solutions: 5% dextrose, 0.9% sodium chloride, 5% dextrose and 0.9% sodium chloride, or lactated Ringer's.

PREPARATIONS

Excipients in commercially available drug preparations may have clinically important effects in some individuals; consult specific product labeling for details.

Vecuronium Bromide

Parenteral

For injection, for IV use only	10 mg*	Vecuronium Bromide for Injection,
	20 mg*	Vecuronium Bromide for Injection,

* available from one or more manufacturer, distributor, and/or repackager by generic (nonproprietary) name

† Use is not currently included in the labeling approved by the US Food and Drug Administration.

Selected Revisions September 10, 2024, © Copyright, May 1, 1985, American Society of Health-System Pharmacists, Inc.

16:00 BLOOD DERIVATIVES

Albumin Human   *p. 1483*   alpha-1-Proteinase Inhibitor   Plasma Protein Fraction §   Plasminogen, Human-tmvh §
                                    (Human) §

§ Omitted from the print version of *AHFS Drug Information*® because of space limitations. This monograph is available on the *AHFS Drug Information*® web site, http://www.ahfsdrug
information.com.

Albumin Human

16:00 • BLOOD DERIVATIVES

■ Albumin human, a protein colloid, is a sterile solution of serum albumin prepared by fractionating pooled plasma from healthy human donors.

USES

● Hypovolemia

Albumin human solutions are used for plasma volume expansion and maintenance of cardiac output (fluid resuscitation) in the emergency treatment of hypovolemia (with or without shock) when urgent restoration of blood volume is indicated.

The goal of fluid resuscitation is to restore intravascular volume and preserve organ perfusion while minimizing fluid overload complications (e.g., pulmonary edema). Albumin human, a protein colloid, is one of several options that can be used to restore effective circulating volume. Other options include nonprotein colloids (e.g., hetastarch, dextran) and large volume crystalloids (e.g., lactated Ringer's, various sodium chloride-containing solutions). When used for fluid resuscitation, the beneficial effects of albumin human are thought to result principally from its contribution to colloid osmotic pressure (i.e., oncotic pressure).

Ongoing controversy exists regarding the optimum choice of fluid (i.e., crystalloids, albumin human, nonprotein colloids) for fluid resuscitation in emergency situations. Protocols used for fluid resuscitation, including the type of replacement fluid, vary widely among health-care facilities and may depend on the geographic area (e.g., country) where the patient is being treated. Some clinicians state that colloids such as albumin human are preferred because they offer therapeutic advantages over crystalloids, while others recommend use of crystalloids based on cost considerations and lack of established superiority of colloids. The potential advantages of colloids include greater retention in the intravascular space, more rapid and effective plasma volume expansion, and a reduced risk of pulmonary edema. However, such benefits are theoretical and have not been proven; in addition, the favorable oncotic gradients that colloids provide may be diminished in situations where there is endothelial damage and transcapillary leakage (e.g., in septic shock or burns). Clinical studies generally have not shown colloids to be more effective than crystalloids for fluid resuscitation, and costs associated with colloid administration are substantially higher than those associated with crystalloid administration.

Previous pooled analyses of randomized controlled clinical studies have questioned the role and safety of albumin human relative to other colloids and crystalloids in the management of critically ill patients, including those with hypovolemia. In a pooled analysis of 30 randomized, controlled clinical studies involving 1419 critically ill patients receiving albumin human or plasma protein fraction (with or without crystalloids) that was performed by the Cochrane Injuries Group Albumin Reviewers in 1998, there was no evidence that albumin human reduced mortality compared with control (crystalloid solution alone or no albumin human) in patients with hypovolemia, burns, or hypoproteinemia (hypoalbuminemia). Instead, this analysis revealed evidence suggesting that mortality risk actually may be increased by 6% overall with use of albumin human in these patients. An increased risk of mortality also was observed in each patient population, reaching statistical significance for patients with burns or hypoproteinemia. As a result of this analysis, the authors and others cautioned that recommendations for the use of albumin human in critically ill patients should be reevaluated, and such use should be undertaken only after careful consideration, weighing the potential benefits and risks. However, the findings of this study have been criticized for methodologic problems that limit clinical interpretation, and the clinical studies that were evaluated used many different end points, making it difficult to determine comparative efficacy and safety. In a larger, subsequent

meta-analysis of 55 randomized, controlled trials comparing albumin human to crystalloid therapy, no albumin, or lower dosages of albumin in 3504 patients from a broad population (e.g., patients with trauma, burns, hypoalbuminemia, or ascites; high-risk neonates; surgery patients), there was no evidence of increased risk of death associated with use of albumin human.

To resolve conflicting evidence from meta-analyses, a large, multicenter randomized controlled study (the Saline versus Albumin Fluid Evaluation [SAFE] trial) was conducted comparing the effects of normal saline (0.9% sodium chloride) with albumin human in approximately 7000 adults in intensive care units (ICUs) who required fluid resuscitation. Pediatric patients, burn patients, and those who had undergone liver transplantation or cardiac surgery were excluded from the study. Eligible patients who had at least one objective sign of hypovolemia were randomized to receive either albumin human 4% solution (not commercially available in the US) or normal saline for 28 days in addition to maintenance fluids, specific replacement fluids, blood products, or other concurrent interventions as required. There was no difference in 28-day mortality (primary outcome), development of organ failure, length of hospital or ICU stay, duration of mechanical ventilation, or duration of renal replacement therapy between patients who received albumin human and those who received normal saline. Results generally were consistent across subgroups of patients with severe sepsis, trauma, and acute respiratory distress syndrome (ARDS; previously known as adult respiratory distress syndrome), although there was a slight trend towards increased mortality in patients with head trauma who received albumin human and a trend towards reduced mortality in those with severe sepsis who received albumin human. However, the study was not specifically designed to detect any clinically important differences between subgroups and results of such analysis should be interpreted with caution. Based on findings from the SAFE study, the US Food and Drug Administration (FDA) Blood Products Advisory Committee concluded in 2005, that the prior safety issues raised by the Cochrane Injuries Group had been resolved. In an updated meta-analysis performed by the Cochrane Albumin Reviewers, there was no difference in overall mortality between albumin human and normal saline in critically ill patients with hypovolemia, burns or hypoalbuminemia. There was a suggestion of a higher risk of death with albumin human in patients with burns and hypoalbuminemia (relative risk of 2.4 and 1.38, respectively), but not in patients with hypovolemia (relative risk of 1.01). The authors note that the estimate in hypovolemic patients was heavily influenced by results of the SAFE study.

Based on current evidence, albumin human appears to offer no advantage in terms of survival over crystalloids for fluid resuscitation, although the possibility of a modest benefit or harm cannot be excluded. Although results of a meta-analysis suggest that albumin human may provide a protective effect in reducing morbidity among acutely ill hospitalized patients, additional study is needed to substantiate these findings and more fully evaluate the effect of albumin human on other clinically important outcomes. Additional studies also are needed to evaluate the use of albumin human in specific groups who were excluded from the SAFE study (e.g., pediatric, burn, liver transplant, cardiac surgery patients).

Hemorrhagic Shock

Albumin human is used for fluid resuscitation in patients with hemorrhagic shock.

Guidelines on use of albumin, nonprotein colloids, and crystalloids issued by the US University Health System (formerly Hospital) Consortium (UHC) in 2000 state that crystalloid solutions are preferred for initial fluid resuscitation in adults with hemorrhagic shock, but that nonprotein colloids may be considered if crystalloids (4 L) fail to produce an adequate response within 2 hours. These guidelines state that albumin human 5% solution may be used if nonprotein colloids are contraindicated.

Crystalloids and colloids should *not* be considered substitutes for blood or blood components when oxygen-carrying capacity is reduced and/or when replenishment of clotting factors or platelets is necessary. Transfusion with whole blood or packed red blood cells (RBCs) should be initiated as soon as possible when there is active hemorrhage and/or substantial anemia.

Nonhemorrhagic (Maldistributive) Shock

Albumin human has been used for fluid resuscitation in patients with nonhemorrhagic (maldistributive) shock, including septic shock. Severe sepsis or septic shock with hypotension or signs of hypoperfusion requires early, vigorous fluid resuscitation to restore tissue perfusion and normalize oxidative metabolism.

The UHC guidelines state that crystalloids should be considered first-line treatment in adults with nonhemorrhagic (maldistributive) shock and that nonprotein colloids and albumin human should be used with caution in those with systemic sepsis. These guidelines also state that, in the presence of capillary leak with pulmonary and/or severe peripheral edema, use of up to 4 L of crystalloid solution is appropriate before using colloids. If albumin human is used for acute management of nonhemorrhagic shock, the possibility that it may have a potentially detrimental effect on edema in patients with increased capillary permeability or capillary leak should be considered.

Other experts state that either crystalloids or colloids can be used for fluid resuscitation in patients with septic shock. However, additional study is needed since there is no evidence-based support from prospective, randomized studies to clearly identify which type of fluid is superior for fluid resuscitation in patients with septic shock. Although there is some evidence that adult or pediatric patients with severe infection and shock who receive albumin human for fluid resuscitation have lower mortality compared with those who receive crystalloids, most studies to date comparing the relative efficacy of crystalloids, albumin human, and nonprotein colloids in patients with septic shock are hampered by difficulties in controlling the effects of concomitant therapy and were not designed or adequately powered to examine mortality as a primary outcome.

Thermal Injury

Albumin human has been used for fluid resuscitation in burn patients.

Fluid resuscitation is an essential component of burn therapy; however, the optimum regimen of crystalloids, colloids, electrolytes, and fluid for the management of patients with thermal (burn) injuries has not been clearly established. There is ongoing controversy regarding the role of and most appropriate time to initiate colloids for fluid resuscitation in burn patients. Some clinicians believe that use of colloids during the initial hours after a burn is inappropriate because much of the volume is drawn into the interstitial space secondary to increased permeability of surrounding unburned tissue; others believe that colloids should be administered from the beginning of fluid resuscitation. In patients with thermal injury, crystalloids generally are recommended during the first 24 hours to reverse acute hypovolemia and maintain hemodynamic stability. Beyond 24 hours, use of colloids also may be employed to prevent hemoconcentration, combat electrolyte imbalances, and counteract the protein deficit that occurs in severe burns. To avoid complications of over-resuscitation ("fluid creep"), such as abdominal compartment syndrome and ARDS, the least amount of fluid necessary to maintain adequate organ perfusion should be used.

The UHC guidelines recommend that crystalloids be used for initial fluid resuscitation in adults with thermal injury, but state that nonprotein colloids may be added if burns extend over more than 30% of body surface area and more than 4 L of crystalloid solution has been administered 18–26 hours following initial injury. These guidelines state that albumin human may be considered if nonprotein colloids are contraindicated. Guidelines issued by the American Burn Association state that the addition of colloids to burn resuscitation protocols may be beneficial in terms of decreasing total fluid volume requirements, but randomized, controlled trials are needed to clearly establish other benefits.

Additional study is needed to determine the acute-phase and short-term differences between albumin human, crystalloids, and nonprotein colloids for fluid resuscitation in pediatric burn patients. Albumin human does not appear to decrease morbidity and mortality when used in pediatric burn patients and, depending on the preparation used, may result in aluminum accumulation in infants. (See Aluminum Content under Cautions: Precautions and Contraindications.)

● Kidney Disease
Nephrosis and Nephrotic Syndrome

Albumin human is used as an adjunct to diuretic therapy to treat edema in patients with acute nephrosis refractory to cyclophosphamide and steroid therapy.

Cardinal features of nephrotic syndrome include albuminuria, hypoalbuminemia, and edema. Urinary albumin loss, with a resultant decrease in plasma oncotic pressure, was thought to be associated with the development of edema and secondary renal sodium retention. Additional evidence indicates that decreased hepatic production and increased renal catabolism are responsible for

hypoalbuminemia, while renal sodium retention is responsible for edema. The principal goal of therapy for nephrotic syndrome is treatment of the underlying cause; when the cause does not respond to therapy, alleviation of pathophysiologic manifestations, including sodium retention and edema, is important.

Diuretic therapy is the treatment of choice for symptomatic management of nephrotic syndrome. The UHC guidelines recommend short-term adjunctive use of albumin human with diuretics in adults with nephrotic syndrome who have acute, severe peripheral and/or pulmonary edema that is unresponsive to diuretics alone; however, the possibility of a potentially detrimental effect on edema should be considered.

Albumin human has no role in the management of chronic nephrosis since parenteral albumin is rapidly excreted renally with no relief of the chronic edema or effect on the underlying renal lesion.

Hemodialysis

Albumin human has been used as an adjunct to hemodialysis in long-term hemodialysis patients with oncotic or volume deficits or in those experiencing shock or hypotension who cannot tolerate substantial volumes of sodium chloride solutions.

Intradialytic hypotension, a complication of hemodialysis (especially in long-term hemodialysis patients), usually is managed by volume expansion through the use of crystalloids (e.g., 0.9% sodium chloride solutions, hypertonic sodium chloride solutions), nonprotein colloids, or albumin human. Some experts state that colloids may be preferred to crystalloids for dialysis-related hypotension and maintenance of hemodynamics in chronic dialysis patients. Others recommend 0.9% sodium chloride solution as first-line therapy if treatment of intradialytic hypotension is indicated in maintenance hemodialysis patients. This recommendation is based on results of a randomized, controlled study that indicated that albumin human 5% solution is not superior to 0.9% sodium chloride solution for treatment of symptomatic hypotension in maintenance hemodialysis patients with a previous history of intradialytic hypotension.

The UHC guidelines state that albumin human should not be used for intradialytic blood pressure support. If adults undergoing hemodialysis experience shock symptoms, the UHC guidelines state that crystalloid solutions are preferred for initial fluid resuscitation, but that nonprotein colloids may be considered if crystalloids (4 L) fail to produce an adequate response within 2 hours. These guidelines state that albumin human 5% solution may be used if nonprotein colloids are contraindicated.

Kidney Transplantation

Albumin human has been used intraoperatively in conjunction with crystalloids for volume expansion in kidney transplant patients. However, there is no conclusive evidence from controlled, randomized studies that albumin human given during and/or after renal transplant surgery improves outcome.

● Liver Disease
Cirrhotic Ascites and Paracentesis

Albumin human is used to prevent central volume depletion following paracentesis in adults with cirrhosis who require removal of large volumes of ascitic fluid.

Diet modification (e.g., sodium restricted to 2 g daily) combined with oral diuretic therapy is the first-line therapy for adults with cirrhosis and ascites. An initial large-volume paracentesis may be necessary in addition to sodium restriction and oral diuretic therapy if tense ascites is present in new-onset disease. In patients with refractory ascites (fluid overload unresponsive to sodium restriction and high-dose oral diuretic therapy or that recurs rapidly after paracentesis), serial therapeutic paracentesis may be indicated to control ascites. A single paracentesis involving removal of no more than 4–5 L of fluid usually can be performed safely without postparacentesis colloid support; however, when larger volumes (greater than 5 L) are removed, use of albumin human may be considered and usually is recommended to decrease the risk of postparacentesis circulatory dysfunction and maintain arterial blood volume. Nonprotein colloids also have been used for plasma expansion following paracentesis and have been recommended as alternatives to albumin human; however, some clinicians state that albumin human may be preferred since there is some evidence that the incidence of postparacentesis circulatory dysfunction following large-volume paracentesis may be less with albumin human than with some nonprotein colloids. The UHC guidelines and some clinicians state that when less than 3–5 L of ascites fluid has been removed and repletion of intravascular volume is of concern, adjunctive use of a crystalloid (e.g., sodium chloride solution) should be considered following paracentesis.

Although albumin human has been used alone (without large-volume paracentesis) in patients with cirrhosis in an attempt to control or prevent recurrence of ascites, guidelines issued by the American Association for the Study of Liver Diseases (AASLD) and UHC state that such use is not recommended. In addition, the UHC guidelines state that albumin human should not be used for the treatment of noncirrhotic postsinusoidal portal hypertension.

Despite the presence of hypoalbuminemia, albumin human has no role in the management of *chronic* cirrhosis†.

Hepatorenal Syndrome

Albumin human has been used in conjunction with vasoconstrictors for the treatment of type I hepatorenal syndrome† in patients with cirrhosis. Type I hepatorenal syndrome is characterized by acute, rapidly progressing renal failure caused by intrarenal vasoconstriction and usually requires liver transplantation if not reversed. There is some evidence that use of regimens that include albumin human to expand intravascular volume and vasoconstrictors to increase vascular tone (e.g., terlipressin [not commercially available in the US], octreotide and midodrine, norepinephrine) in patients with rapidly progressing type I hepatorenal syndrome may improve renal function and delay the need for or improve outcomes after liver transplantation. Although additional study is needed, the AASLD and other experts state that a regimen of albumin human used in conjunction with vasoconstrictors (e.g., terlipressin, octreotide and midodrine) should be considered in the treatment of type I hepatorenal syndrome.

Data are limited regarding the use of albumin human alone or in conjunction with vasoconstrictors in the management of type II hepatorenal syndrome† (characterized by moderate and slowly progressive renal failure and typically associated with refractory ascites), and additional study is needed to determine if albumin human has a role in this form of the disease.

Spontaneous Bacterial Peritonitis

Albumin human has been used as an adjunct to anti-infectives in the treatment of spontaneous bacterial peritonitis† in patients with cirrhosis and ascites.

Spontaneous bacterial peritonitis is a complication that can occur in patients with cirrhosis and ascites, develops without a contiguous source of infection (e.g., intestinal perforation, intra-abdominal abscess), requires prompt empiric anti-infective treatment, and may result in potentially fatal, progressive renal impairment or hepatorenal syndrome. There is some evidence that adjunctive use of albumin human for volume expansion in addition to appropriate anti-infective treatment in patients with spontaneous bacterial peritonitis may decrease the risk of renal impairment and death. Such use is controversial and additional study is needed. The AASLD recommends that albumin human be used in addition to appropriate anti-infective treatment (e.g., cefotaxime) in patients who have ascitic fluid polymorphonuclear (PMN) counts of 250 cells/mm³ or higher and also have serum creatinine concentrations greater than 1 mg/dL, BUN greater than 30 mg/dL, or total bilirubin concentrations greater than 4 mg/dL.

Acute Liver Failure

Albumin human has been used in patients with acute liver failure. In such patients, albumin human may provide a stabilizing effect and serve the dual purpose of supporting plasma colloid osmotic pressure as well as binding excess plasma bilirubin in the uncommon situation of rapid loss of liver function, with or without coma. Use of albumin human in patients with acute liver failure should be individualized based on the clinical situation. When fluid resuscitation is indicated in patients with acute liver failure, some experts recommend use of colloids (e.g., albumin human) instead of crystalloids.

Hepatic Resection

Albumin human has been used for postoperative fluid support in patients undergoing hepatic resection†. Surgical resection of the liver results in substantial blood loss and, depending on the preoperative functional status of the liver, decreased albumin production capacity. The UHC guidelines state that crystalloids should be considered first-line therapy for maintenance of effective circulating volume following hepatic resection in adults and, if crystalloids have no effect and anemia and/or coagulopathy are present, then packed RBCs and fresh frozen plasma should be considered before use of albumin human. However, the UHC guidelines state that albumin human is appropriate to maintain effective circulation volume following major hepatic resection (more than 40%) in adults and also is indicated if clinically important edema develops secondary to use of crystalloids.

Liver Transplantation

Albumin human has been used to control ascites and severe pulmonary and peripheral edema in liver transplant recipients†. Because of excessive blood loss, volume expanders such as crystalloids, blood products, nonprotein colloids, and albumin human may be required intraoperatively during liver transplantation. The UHC guidelines state that albumin human may be used in adult liver transplant recipients when serum albumin is less than 2.5 g/dL, pulmonary capillary wedge pressure is less than 12 mm Hg, and hematocrit exceeds 30%.

● *Hypoproteinemia*

Albumin human has been used in the management of severe hypoalbuminemia (with or without edema) in an attempt to restore serum albumin concentrations to within the normal range. However, in the absence of clinically important hypovolemia, albumin human should not be used to correct temporary protein deficits resulting from redistribution of albumin.

The principal goal of therapy in hypoproteinemia (hypoalbuminemia) is treatment of the underlying cause; albumin human may be used to provide symptomatic relief and prevent acute complications. Hypoproteinemia can occur in association with various clinical conditions (e.g., surgery, sepsis, chronic liver failure, chronic renal impairment) and is a result of inadequate production, increased catabolism, redistribution, and/or excessive loss of albumin. Use of albumin human in patients with severe hypoalbuminemia simply in an attempt to increase serum albumin concentrations to within the normal range (i.e., the patient does not exhibit manifestations of hypovolemia) cannot be recommended based on current evidence; instead, the cause of the underlying hypoalbuminemia should be identified and treated. To varying degrees, albumin human may relieve edema associated with hypoproteinemia by increasing colloid osmotic pressure and producing diuresis. However, if albumin human is administered to hypoproteinemic patients who do not have an accompanying volume deficit, there is a potential risk of fluid overload.

Albumin human should not be used for the treatment of hypoproteinemia associated with chronic cirrhosis, chronic nephrosis, malabsorption, protein-losing enteropathies, pancreatic insufficiency, or malnutrition, unless there is a concomitant indication that warrants use.

Although albumin human has been used to treat neonatal hypoalbuminemia†, data are insufficient to determine whether routine use of albumin human reduces mortality or morbidity in preterm neonates with hypoalbuminemia.

● *Nutritional Support*

Although there is some evidence suggesting that serum albumin concentration is an accurate measure of patient prognosis using indicators of morbidity and mortality, and that albumin concentrations can be safely and effectively restored using total parenteral nutrition (TPN) supplemented with albumin human, other evidence has led many clinicians to question the importance of albumin supplementation. Serum albumin concentration is a poor indicator of nutritional status and it may take several weeks to months to see an increase in the serum albumin concentration following adequate nutritional support. Albumin human is not recommended for use as a supplemental caloric protein source in patients requiring nutritional support. Iatrogenic elevation of serum albumin concentrations above 4 g/dL may increase the overall catabolic rate. In general, oral, enteral, and/or parenteral nutrition with amino acids and treatment of underlying disorders will restore plasma protein concentrations more effectively than albumin human. However, patients with diarrhea associated with enteral feeding intolerance may benefit from parenteral administration of albumin human if they have severe diarrhea (more than 2 L daily) and a serum albumin concentration less than 2 g/dL or if diarrhea occurs despite a trial of short-peptide and elemental formulas and other causes of diarrhea have been excluded.

● *Neonatal Hyperbilirubinemia*

In the treatment of neonatal hyperbilirubinemia, including hemolytic disease of the newborn (erythroblastosis fetalis), albumin human (20 or 25% solution) is used as an adjunct to exchange transfusions in an attempt to bind unconjugated bilirubin and decrease the risk of kernicterus. Albumin human has been administered prior to exchange transfusion (as a primer) or during the procedure (as a substitute for a portion of the blood) in infants with severe hemolytic disease of the newborn. Because there is some evidence that administration of albumin human prior to exchange transfusion is less efficient in bilirubin removal and may increase the risk of volume overload, the UHC guidelines recommend that albumin human be administered during the procedure if it is used as an adjunct to exchange transfusion. Albumin human should be used with caution in hypervolemic infants. (See Hypervolemia/Hemodilution under Cautions: Precautions and Contraindications.)

Albumin human should *not* be used if neonatal hyperbilirubinemia is treated using phototherapy without exchange transfusion.

Crystalloids and nonprotein colloids do not share the bilirubin-binding properties of albumin human and should *not* be considered alternatives for adjunctive treatment of hyperbilirubinemia in neonates.

● *Ovarian Hyperstimulation Syndrome*

Albumin human (20 or 25% solution) is used as a plasma expander for fluid management in the treatment of severe ovarian hyperstimulation syndrome (OHSS). Severe OHSS is a life-threatening complication of gonadotropin treatment characterized by growth of multiple large ovarian follicles with massive extravascular protein-rich fluid shift; this can lead to hypovolemia, hemoconcentration, ascites, oliguria, and electrolyte disturbances and may result in potentially fatal thromboembolic complications and acute respiratory distress syndrome. Albumin human 20 or 25% solution has been recommended in the treatment of severe OHSS if 0.9% sodium chloride solutions fail to achieve or maintain hemodynamic stability and adequate urine output.

Albumin human also has been investigated for prevention of severe OHSS in high-risk women undergoing ovulation induction†. However, additional study is needed to more fully evaluate the benefits and risks of albumin human for prevention of OHSS. One meta-analysis of 5 randomized, controlled clinical studies in high-risk women (i.e., younger than 35 years of age, multifollicular development, high serum estradiol concentrations, nonobesity, polycystic ovary disease) indicated that administration of a single IV infusion of albumin human 20 or 25% immediately before or after oocyte retrieval appeared to reduce the risk of severe OHSS in such patients. This meta-analysis indicated that use of albumin human in women at high risk may prevent 1 case of severe OHSS in every 18 women who receive such prophylaxis. However, other studies and meta-analyses evaluating use of albumin human for prevention of OHSS in high-risk women failed to demonstrate a statistically significant reduction in the occurrence of severe OHSS in those receiving albumin human.

● *Acute Respiratory Distress Syndrome and Acute Lung Injury*

Albumin human (20 or 25% solution) has been used in conjunction with a diuretic in the management of acute respiratory distress syndrome (ARDS, previously known as adult respiratory distress syndrome). However, use of albumin human in patients with ARDS is controversial because of the risk of aggravating interstitial fluid accumulation and other possible detrimental pulmonary effects. Although uncertainty exists regarding the precise indication for albumin human in patients with ARDS, some manufacturers state that albumin human may have a therapeutic effect if used in conjunction with a diuretic in patients with pulmonary overload accompanied by hypoalbuminemia.

Albumin human has been used in conjunction with furosemide in the management of hypoproteinemic patients with acute lung injury† (ALI) and has resulted in improved oxygenation and hemodynamic stability in some patients. Some experts state that conservative fluid management or restriction is appropriate for most patients with hemodynamically stable ALI/ARDS; however, although conclusive data are lacking, a regimen of colloids and diuretics may be considered in those with hypo-oncotic ALI/ARDS.

● *Sequestration of Protein Rich Fluids*

Albumin human has been used for volume and oncotic replacement in conditions associated with sequestration of protein rich fluid or third-spacing (e.g., acute peritonitis, pancreatitis, mediastinitis, extensive cellulitis).

Albumin human has been used as an adjunct to anti-infectives in the treatment of spontaneous bacterial peritonitis† in patients with cirrhosis and ascites. (See Spontaneous Bacterial Peritonitis under Uses: Liver Disease.)

Albumin human may be useful in the early treatment of shock associated with acute hemorrhagic pancreatitis or peritonitis.

The UHC guidelines state that albumin human is not recommended in the treatment of acute or chronic pancreatitis.

● *Cardiac Surgery*

Albumin human has been used as a pump prime for preoperative dilution of blood prior to cardiopulmonary bypass procedures, usually in conjunction with a crystalloid. However, studies generally have shown only marginal or no additional benefit when colloids were added to crystalloids in the preoperative regimen. The UHC guidelines state that crystalloids alone usually are the regimen of choice for priming cardiopulmonary bypass pumps, although use of nonprotein colloids in addition to crystalloids may be preferable in cases in which it is extremely important to avoid pulmonary shunting.

Albumin human also has been used in cardiac surgery patients to restore fluid balance during surgery and in the postoperative period. Although albumin human has been recommended prior to or during cardiopulmonary bypass and there is some evidence that use of albumin human in cardiopulmonary bypass patients is associated with less postoperative bleeding than use of hetastarch (a nonprotein colloid), there are no data establishing a clear benefit for use of albumin human over use of crystalloids alone. For postoperative volume expansion after cardiac surgery, the UHC guidelines state that crystalloids are preferred, followed in descending order of preference by nonprotein colloids and then albumin human.

● *Neurosurgery and Cerebral Injury*

Albumin human has been used for hemodilution to maintain or improve cerebral perfusion in the treatment of subarachnoid hemorrhage†, acute ischemic stroke†, traumatic brain injury†, and in other neurosurgical patients†. Various fluid protocols have been used in an attempt to prevent secondary ischemia after subarachnoid hemorrhage, severe ischemic stroke, or severe traumatic brain injury. Although improved clinical outcomes have been reported in some patients, results have been conflicting and there is no clear evidence to date from adequately controlled, randomized studies that hemodilution decreases mortality or improves functional outcome in survivors of acute ischemic stroke.

The UHC guidelines state that crystalloids are preferred for maintenance of cerebral perfusion pressure in the treatment of cerebral vasospasm associated with subarachnoid hemorrhage, cerebral ischemia, or head trauma in adults; however, if cerebral edema is a concern, albumin human 25% solution should be used. These guidelines state that patients with elevated hematocrits should receive crystalloids first to increase intravascular volume, creating a state of hypervolemia and hemodilution, and that those with hematocrits less than 30% should receive packed RBCs to increase the intravascular volume and maintain cerebral perfusion pressure. If volume therapy alone is inadequate to maintain cerebral perfusion pressure, vasopressor therapy may be necessary.

● *Plasmapheresis*

Albumin human is used in conjunction with large-volume plasma exchange as protein volume replacement in plasmapheresis† procedures involving exchange of more than 20 mL of plasma per kg in one session or more than 20 mL/kg weekly in multiple sessions. The UHC guidelines state that nonprotein colloids and crystalloids may substitute for some of the albumin human in therapeutic plasmapheresis procedures and should be considered cost-effective exchange media. Some evidence indicates that nonprotein colloids (e.g., hetastarch 3%) are comparably effective and tolerated relative to albumin for small- or large-volume plasma exchange.

● *Erythrocyte Resuspension*

Albumin human has been used to resuspend large volumes of previously frozen or washed RBCs prior to administration or during certain types of exchange transfusion to provide sufficient volume and/or avoid excessive hypoproteinemia during the transfusion.

DOSAGE AND ADMINISTRATION

● *Administration*

Albumin human solutions are administered by IV infusion.

The concentration of albumin human administered (i.e., albumin human 5, 20, or 25% solution) depends on the fluid and protein requirements of the patient and is determined in part by whether there is a greater need for volume or oncotic replacement.

Albumin human 5% solutions usually are preferred in the treatment of acute blood volume deficits in the *absence* of adequate or excessive hydration.

Albumin human 20 or 25% solutions may be preferred when there is an oncotic deficit or when hypovolemia is long standing (e.g., due to treatment delay) and hypoalbuminemia exists in the *presence* of adequate or excessive hydration. Albumin human 20 or 25% solutions also are preferred when the drug is being used for its binding rather than oncotic effects (e.g., in the treatment of neonatal hyperbilirubinemia).

When used for the treatment of hypovolemia, albumin human solutions are most effective in well-hydrated patients. If the patient is dehydrated, albumin human 5% solution usually is preferred; if albumin human 20 or 25% solutions are used in dehydrated patients, additional crystalloids or other fluids should be administered.

IV Infusion

Depending on the indication, protein and fluid requirements, sodium restrictions, and availability, commercially available albumin human solutions can be administered *undiluted* or can be further diluted in a compatible IV solution (e.g., 0.9% sodium chloride, 5% dextrose).

Whenever dilution of albumin human is considered necessary (e.g., to prepare a 5% solution from a 25% solution), **the oncotic and osmotic properties as well as the tonicity of the resultant dilution must be considered**.

Because of the risk of potentially life-threatening hemolysis, **albumin human must not be diluted using hypotonic solutions such as sterile water for injection.** (See Oncotic, Osmotic, and Tonicity Considerations under Cautions: Precautions and Contraindications.)

If necessary, albumin human 5% solutions may be prepared from albumin human 25% solutions by adding 1 volume of the 25% solution to 4 volumes of 0.9% sodium chloride injection or 5% dextrose injection. Since albumin human 25% solution diluted with 0.9% sodium chloride or 5% dextrose results in 5% dilutions that are approximately isotonic and iso-oncotic with citrated plasma, these diluents are preferred for such dilutions.

When sodium restriction is necessary, albumin human solutions should be administered either undiluted or diluted in a sodium-free carbohydrate solution such as 5% dextrose. However, because administration of large volumes of albumin human 5% prepared by diluting 25% solutions with 5% dextrose could result in hyponatremia and potentially serious adverse effects (e.g., cerebral swelling), 0.9% sodium chloride generally should be used as the preferred diluent when administration, particularly rapid administration, of large volumes is anticipated (e.g., during plasmapheresis or plasma exchange) and the fluid and electrolyte status of the patient permits.

Prior to administration, albumin human solution should be inspected visually for particulate matter and discoloration and should not be used if it appears turbid or contains sediment.

Albumin human should be used immediately after the vial or container is opened. Albumin human solutions should be discarded if more than 4 hours have elapsed since the container was first entered.

The manufacturers' prescribing information should be consulted for specific directions regarding use of IV administration sets and filters. Some manufacturers state that adequate filtration is required; other manufacturers state that filtration is not required.

Albumin human may be administered in conjunction with whole blood, plasma, or dextrose, sodium lactate, or sodium chloride injections. Albumin human should *not* be mixed with parenteral nutrient solutions, protein hydrolysates, amino acid solutions, or solutions containing alcohol. (See Chemistry and Stability: Stability.)

Rate of Administration

The rate of IV infusion of albumin human should be individualized based on the indication, concentration of albumin human solution used, and clinical status and response of the patient. The manufacturers' information should be consulted for specific information regarding recommended rates of administration.

When albumin human 5% solution is used for the treatment of hypovolemic shock in patients with greatly reduced blood volume, a rapid IV infusion rate may be necessary *initially* to provide clinical improvement and restore normal blood volume. However, in patients with a history of cardiac or vascular disease, some manufacturers suggest a slow infusion rate (e.g., 5–10 mL/minute) to avoid an increase in blood pressure that is too rapid. In patients with normal or slightly low blood volume, some manufacturers suggest that albumin human 5% solution should be administered at a rate of 1–2 mL/minute.

When albumin human 20 or 25% solution is used for the treatment of hypovolemic shock in patients with greatly reduced blood volume, a rapid IV infusion rate may be necessary *initially* to provide clinical improvement and restore normal blood volume. However, in patients with normal or slightly low blood

volume, some manufacturers state that the IV infusion rate should not exceed 1 mL/minute since more rapid infusion rates may result in circulatory overload or pulmonary edema. A slower infusion rate also is recommended in patients with hypertension. When albumin human 20 or 25% solution is used in hypoproteinemic patients with approximately normal blood volume, a maximum infusion rate of 2 mL/minute (Plasbumin®-20, Plasbumin®-25) or 2–3 mL/minute (Albuminar®-25) has been recommended.

When albumin human solutions are used in pediatric patients, some manufacturers recommend that the IV infusion rate should be reduced to 25% of the usual adult rate.

● *Dosage*

Dosage of albumin human is variable and should be individualized based on the specific indication, concentration of albumin human solution used, and clinical status and response of the patient. The manufacturers' information should be consulted for specific dosage recommendations.

Predetermined formulas for dosage calculation generally are avoided since they assume that the same dose is appropriate for all patients. In the absence of active hemorrhage, total daily albumin dosage should not exceed the theoretical amount present in normal plasma volume (i.e., 2 g/kg body weight).

Response to therapy should be determined by factors such as hemodynamic response (e.g., blood pressure), degree of pulmonary congestion, and hematocrit. Serum protein concentrations usually do not need to be monitored during albumin human therapy, but may be useful in some cases of hypoproteinemia to estimate the total body albumin deficit and guide selection of dosage.

OSMOTIC EQUIVALENCE OF COMMERCIALLY AVAILABLE ALBUMIN HUMAN INJECTIONS FOR IV INFUSION

Albumin human injection for IV infusion	Osmotic equivalence
100 mL of 5% solution (5 g)	100 mL of normal human plasma
100 mL of 20% solution (20 g)	400 mL of normal human plasma
100 mL of 25% solution (25 g)	500 mL of normal human plasma

Hypovolemia

Adults

When albumin human is used for the treatment of hypovolemic shock in adults, some manufacturers recommend the following initial dose. The dose may be repeated in 15–30 minutes if the response is inadequate.

Albumin human 5% solution: 12.5–25 g (250–500 mL of a 5% solution).

Albumin human 20% solution: 25 g (125 mL of a 20% solution).

Albumin human 25% solution: 25–50 g (100–200 mL of a 25% solution).

Pediatric Patients

Some manufacturers recommend that 25–50% of the usual initial adult dosage be used and adjusted according to the child's weight and clinical condition. The manufacturers' prescribing information should be consulted for specific dosing recommendations in children.

If albumin human is used for the treatment of hypovolemic shock in pediatric patients, some clinicians recommend a dose of 0.5–1 g/kg (maximum of 6 g/kg in 24 hours or 250 g in 48 hours).

Albumin human 5% solution: Some manufacturers recommend an initial dose of 0.5–1 g/kg or 2.5–12.5 g for the treatment of hypovolemia in pediatric patients. One manufacturer recommends a dose of 12–20 mL/kg for infants and young children and 250–500 mL for older children. The dose may be repeated after 15–30 minutes if the response is inadequate.

Albumin human 20% solution: One manufacturer recommends an initial dose of 0.5–1 g/kg or 2.5–12.5 g for the treatment of hypovolemia in pediatric patients. The dose may be repeated after 15–30 minutes if the response is inadequate.

Albumin human 25% solution: Some manufacturers recommend an initial dose of 0.5–1 g/kg or 2.5–12.5 g for the treatment of hypovolemia in pediatric patients. The dose may be repeated after 15–30 minutes if the response is inadequate.

Thermal Injury

The optimum regimen of crystalloids, colloids, electrolytes, and fluid for the management of patients with thermal (burn) injuries has not been clearly established. In addition, the duration of replacement therapy in burn patients varies, depending on such factors as the extent of protein loss from renal excretion, denuded skin areas, and decreased albumin production.

A suggested goal of burn therapy is to maintain a plasma albumin concentration of 2–3 g/dL and plasma oncotic pressure of 20 mm Hg (equivalent to a total plasma protein concentration of 5.2 g/dL).

If albumin human is used in burn patients, one manufacturer recommends that large volumes of crystalloids be given initially to maintain plasma volume; after 24 hours, albumin human may be added using an initial dose of 25 g with dosage adjusted thereafter to maintain a plasma protein concentration of 2.5 g/dL or a serum protein concentration of 5.2 g/dL.

Kidney Disease

Acute Nephrosis

If albumin human 20 or 25% solution is used as an adjunct to treat edema in the management of acute nephrosis, some manufacturers recommend a dosage of 20 or 25 g once daily for 7–10 days (in conjunction with an appropriate diuretic).

Hemodialysis

If albumin human 20 or 25% solution is used for the treatment of a volume or oncotic deficit in patients undergoing long-term hemodialysis or for the treatment of shock or hypotension in these patients, some manufacturers state that the usual dose is about 100 mL (the initial dose should not exceed 100 mL). Patients must be carefully monitored for signs of circulatory overload.

Liver Disease

Cirrhotic Ascites and Paracentesis

If albumin human is used to prevent central volume depletion following large-volume paracentesis in adults with cirrhosis and ascites, the usual dose is 6–8 g per liter of ascitic fluid removed. A single paracentesis involving removal of no more than 4–5 L of fluid usually can be performed safely without colloid support; however, use of albumin human may be considered when larger volumes (greater than 5 L) are removed.

Hepatorenal Syndrome

Although albumin human used in conjunction with vasoconstrictors has been recommended for the treatment of type I hepatorenal syndrome† in patients with cirrhosis (see Hepatorenal Syndrome under Uses: Liver Disease), optimum regimens have not been identified.

If albumin human is used in conjunction with vasoconstrictors in adults with type I hepatorenal syndrome†, some experts recommend a dosage regimen that includes an initial dose of 1 g/kg (up to 100 g) of albumin human on day 1, followed by 20–40 g once daily. If a response is obtained, treatment should be continued until serum creatinine concentrations are less than 1.5 mg/dL. Albumin human may be discontinued if serum albumin concentrations exceed 4.5 g/dL and should be discontinued if pulmonary edema is present.

Spontaneous Bacterial Peritonitis

Although albumin human has been used as an adjunct to anti-infectives in the treatment of spontaneous bacterial peritonitis† in patients with cirrhosis and ascites, optimum regimens have not been identified.

The American Association for the Study of Liver Diseases (AASLD) recommends that adults with ascitic fluid polymorphonuclear (PMN) counts of 250 cells/mm³ or higher and clinical suspicion of spontaneous bacterial peritonitis who also have serum creatinine concentrations greater than 1 mg/dL, BUN greater than 30 mg/dL, or total bilirubin concentrations greater than 4 mg/dL receive 1.5 g/kg of albumin human within 6 hours of detection and another dose of 1 g/kg on day 3.

Hypoproteinemia

Adults

If albumin human 5% solution is used for the treatment of hypoproteinemia in adults, one manufacturer recommends a dose of 50–75 g.

If albumin human 20 or 25% solution is used for the treatment of hypoproteinemia in adults, some manufacturers recommend a daily dosage of 50–75 g (e.g., 250–375 mL of a 20% solution or 200–300 mL of a 25% solution). Larger amounts may be required in patients with severe hypoproteinemia who continue to lose albumin. Some manufacturers recommend a maximum dosage of 2 g/kg daily.

The total body albumin deficit (including hidden extravascular albumin deficiency) should be considered when determining the dosage of albumin human necessary to reverse hypoalbuminemia. When using serum albumin concentrations to estimate the protein deficit in hypoproteinemia, some manufacturers recommend that the body albumin compartment be calculated based on 80–100 mL/kg body weight to account for any hidden extravascular albumin deficits.

Pediatric Patients

If albumin human is used for the treatment of hypoproteinemia in pediatric patients, some clinicians recommend a dosage of 0.5–1 g/kg given by IV infusion over 0.5–2 hours and repeated once every 1–2 days as needed (maximum of 6 g/kg in 24 hours or 250 g in 48 hours).

For the treatment of hypoproteinemia in children, one manufacturer recommends that albumin human 20 or 25% be given in a dosage of 25 g daily. Larger amounts may be required in patients with severe hypoproteinemia who continue to lose albumin.

Neonatal Hyperbilirubinemia

If albumin human 20 or 25% solution is used as an adjunct to exchange transfusions for the treatment of neonatal hyperbilirubinemia, including hemolytic disease of the newborn (erythroblastosis fetalis), the recommended dose is 1 g/kg. The dose of albumin human has been given prior to exchange transfusion (as a primer) or during the procedure (as a substitute for a portion of the blood). (See Uses: Neonatal Hyperbilirubinemia.)

Ovarian Hyperstimulation Syndrome

If albumin human 20 or 25% solution is used for fluid management in the treatment of severe ovarian hyperstimulation syndrome (OHSS), one manufacturer recommends that 50–100 g be given by IV infusion over 4 hours every 4–12 hours as necessary.

Acute Respiratory Distress Syndrome

If albumin human 20 or 25% solution is used in conjunction with a diuretic in the management of fluid overload in adults with acute respiratory distress syndrome (ARDS; previously known as adult respiratory distress syndrome), one manufacturer recommends that 25 g be given by IV infusion over 30 minutes and repeated at 8-hour intervals for 3 days, if necessary.

Cardiac Surgery

The optimum fluid regimen to ensure adequate blood volume during cardiopulmonary bypass is unclear. (See Uses: Cardiac Surgery.) Some manufacturers recommend that albumin human and crystalloid pump prime solutions be adjusted to achieve a plasma albumin concentration of 2.5 g/dL and a hematocrit of 20%.

Erythrocyte Resuspension

If albumin human 20 or 25% solution is used to resuspend red blood cells (RBCs) during certain types of exchange transfusion or to resuspend large volumes of previously frozen or washed RBCs, some manufacturers recommend that approximately 20–25 g of albumin be added per liter of isotonic suspended RBCs immediately prior to transfusion. Greater amounts may be required in patients with preexisting hepatic impairment or hypoproteinemia.

CAUTIONS

● Adverse Effects

Although adverse effects occur infrequently in patients receiving albumin human, serious adverse effects (e.g., anaphylaxis, circulatory failure, cardiac failure, pulmonary edema), including some fatalities possibly related to albumin human, have been reported rarely.

The most common adverse effects reported in patients receiving albumin human include anaphylactoid reactions, fever, chills, rash, nausea, vomiting, tachycardia, and hypotension.

Anaphylaxis, urticaria, pruritus, angioneurotic edema, erythema or flushing, dysgeusia, increased salivation, hyperhidrosis, headache, confusion, loss of consciousness, pulmonary edema, dyspnea, and bronchospasm have been reported during postmarketing surveillance.

Albumin human has variable effects on respiration, blood pressure, and heart rate. Hypotension, hypertension, circulatory failure, tachycardia, bradycardia, congestive heart failure, and cardiac failure have been reported. Rapid IV infusion of albumin human may cause vascular overload with resultant pulmonary edema. (See Hypervolemia/Hemodilution under Cautions: Precautions and Contraindications.)

Several cases of hemolysis (e.g., during or after plasmapheresis) and at least one death probably related to hemolysis have been reported following administration of as little as 270 mL of an albumin human 5% solution that had been prepared extemporaneously by diluting albumin human 25% with sterile water. Such dilutions are markedly hypotonic with respect to blood, with calculated resultant sodium concentrations of 26–32 mEq/L. (See Oncotic, Osmotic, and Tonicity Considerations under Cautions: Precautions and Contraindications.)

● **Precautions and Contraindications**

Albumin human is contraindicated in patients hypersensitive to albumin, any ingredient in the formulation, or any component of the container. (See Sensitivity Reactions under Cautions: Precautions and Contraindications.)

Albumin human is contraindicated in patients with severe anemia or with cardiac failure in the presence of normal or increased intravascular volume. Certain individuals are at particular risk of circulatory overload, including those with stabilized chronic anemia, congestive heart failure, or renal insufficiency. (See Hypervolemia/Hemodilution under Cautions: Precautions and Contraindications.)

Because of the risk of aluminum accumulation, the manufacturer states that Buminate® 25% should not be used in patients with chronic renal impairment. (See Aluminum Content under Cautions: Precautions and Contraindications.)

Use of sterile water for injection for dilution of commercially available albumin human solutions is contraindicated because of the risk of potentially life-threatening hemolysis and acute renal failure. (See Oncotic, Osmotic, and Tonicity Considerations under Cautions: Precautions and Contraindications.)

Risk of Transmissible Agents in Plasma-derived Preparations

Because albumin human is prepared using pooled human plasma, it is a potential vehicle for transmission of human viruses (e.g., hepatitis A virus [HAV], hepatitis B virus [HBV], hepatitis C virus [HCV], human immunodeficiency virus [HIV]) and theoretically may carry a risk of transmitting the causative agent of Creutzfeldt-Jakob disease (CJD) or related agents such as variant CJD (vCJD). Although donor plasma is screened for certain viruses and all currently available albumin human preparations undergo viral elimination/inactivation processes (e.g., pasteurization) to further reduce the risk of transmission of infectious agents, a potential for transmission of infectious agents still remains.

Because no purification method has been shown to be totally effective in removing the risk of viral infectivity from plasma-derived preparations and because new blood-borne viruses or other disease agents may emerge that may not be removed or inactivated by the manufacturing processes currently used, clinicians should discuss the risks and benefits of albumin human with the patient. Any infection believed to have been transmitted by albumin human should be reported to the manufacturer.

Risk of Hepatitis and Human Immunodeficiency Virus Infection

Although albumin human is prepared from human plasma and is a potential vehicle for transmission of the causative agents of viral hepatitis and HIV infection, the risk of transmission of viral diseases with plasma-derived albumin human is considered extremely remote.

Studies using plasma-derived coagulation factor preparations indicate that improved donor screening practices and viral elimination/inactivation procedures (e.g., pasteurization) have resulted in plasma-derived preparations with greatly reduced risk for transmission of HBV, HCV, and HIV viruses. There have been no documented cases of transmission of enveloped viruses (including HBV, HCV, and HIV) or nonenveloped viruses (including HAV and parvovirus B19) associated with commercially available albumin human. However, transmission of nonenveloped viruses (HAV, parvovirus B19) has been documented following administration of plasma-derived coagulation factors. (See Risk of Transmissible

Agents in Plasma-derived Preparations under Cautions: Precautions and Contraindications, in Antihemophilic Factor [Human] 20:28.16.)

Risk of Creutzfeldt-Jakob Disease or Variant Creutzfeldt-Jakob Disease

Because albumin human is prepared from human blood, it theoretically may carry a risk of transmitting the causative agent of Creutzfeldt-Jakob disease (CJD) or other related agents such as variant CJD (vCJD). CJD is a rare, but invariably fatal, degenerative disease of the CNS associated with a poorly understood transmissible agent. The nature of this agent is not completely known, but it is highly resistant to current methods of viral inactivation applied to plasma-derived products; the effect, if any, of fractionation procedures on the agent is not known. CJD may be acquired by exogenous (usually iatrogenic) exposure to infectious material or may be familial, caused by a genetic mutation of the prion protein gene. There is some evidence that infected individuals may harbor the causative agent for up to 30 years before becoming symptomatic. A variant of CJD (vCJD) was first identified in the United Kingdom in 1996. The clinical presentation and neuropathologic changes associated with vCJD are different than those of CJD and include an earlier age of onset, absence of diagnostic EEG changes, and detectable abnormal prion protein in lymphoid tissue.

There are no documented cases of CJD or vCJD transmitted through plasma-derived preparations (including plasma-derived albumin human) and the theoretical risk for transmission of CJD with commercially available albumin human is considered extremely remote. However, there have been 3 probable cases of vCJD acquired through transfusion of human red blood cells (RBCs) identified by an ongoing epidemiologic review being conducted in the United Kingdom. One of these patients developed symptoms of vCJD 6.5 or 7.8 years, respectively, after receiving non-leukodepleted RBCs from 2 different donors; the donors developed clinical symptoms approximately 40 and 21 months after donating. The third probable case of transfusion-associated vCJD had no clinical symptoms of the disease prior to death, but abnormal prion protein was found in postmortem lymphoid tissue (5 years after RBC transfusion); the donor involved in this case had made the RBC donation 18 months before the onset of their clinical symptoms. Although attempts to transmit CJD to nonhuman primates via blood transfusion have failed, bovine spongiform encephalopathy (BSE) has been transmitted to at least one sheep through blood transfusion.

CJD has been transmitted in humans by transplantation of cornea or dura mater from infected individuals, injection of growth hormone (somatropin) derived from human pituitary of infected individuals, or the reuse of surface EEG electrodes contaminated by use on an infected individual. The disease also has been transmitted experimentally in rodents and primates by intracerebral injection of the buffy coat cell portion of blood, homogenates of brain or cornea, whole blood, or untreated CSF from a known infected individual.

Certain lots of plasma products, including coagulation factors, albumin human, plasma protein fraction, and immune globulin IV (IGIV), produced from blood derived from donors with probable CJD were withdrawn from the market during 1995. Withdrawal of the implicated products was seen by the US Food and Drug Administration (FDA) as a prudent interim measure pending further analysis of the relative risks and benefits of such plasma products. A similar withdrawal of certain lots of Buminate® 25% was made by the manufacturer in 1997 when it was discovered that a healthy plasma donor who contributed to the plasma pools from which these lots of albumin human were derived had a history of having received a dura mater transplant; this was done as a precautionary measure only, since there was no evidence of CJD in the transplant donor and no cases of CJD associated with products derived from the transplant recipient's plasma.

Tests are being developed to detect CJD and vCJD infection in blood and plasma donors. Until such donor screening tests are available for these diseases, the FDA has recommended interim preventive measures that include specific guidelines for deferral of blood and plasma donors with possible exposure to CJD and vCJD that are based on geographic considerations and guidelines for product retrieval, quarantine, and disposition that are based on consideration of risk in the donor and product and the effect that withdrawals and deferrals might have on the supply of blood, blood components, and plasma derivatives.

For further information on CJD and vCJD precautions related to blood and blood products, the FDA's guidance for industry on this topic should be consulted (http://www.fda.gov/downloads/BiologicsBloodVaccines/GuidanceCompliance-RegulatoryInformation/Guidances/UCM213415.pdf).

Risk of West Nile Virus

It is unlikely that West Nile Virus (WNV) could be transmitted through commercially available plasma-derived preparations since WNV is an enveloped virus, like HCV, which is known to be inactivated by the purification and viral elimination/inactivation procedures used in the manufacture of these preparations. However, there is evidence that WNV can be transmitted in transplanted organs (e.g., heart, liver, kidney) and blood products (e.g., whole blood, packed RBCs, fresh frozen plasma). WNV has been isolated from frozen plasma obtained from a blood donor subsequently found to have WNV, indicating that the virus can survive in frozen blood components.

Beginning in 2003, specific tests to screen donated blood for WNV became available in the US. The FDA also recommends additional measures to assess donor suitability to help screen out potential blood donors who have past or present manifestations that suggest WNV illness. These recommendations apply to whole blood and blood components intended for transfusion and blood components, including recovered plasma, source leukocytes, and source plasma intended for use in further manufacturing into injectable or noninjectable products.

Because of the possible transmission of WNV through organ transplants and blood transfusions, any case of WNV that occurs in a patient who received organs, blood, or blood products within the 8 weeks preceding onset of the illness should be reported to CDC through state and local health authorities and serum or tissue samples should be retained for later studies. In addition, cases of WNV infection occurring in blood or organ donors within 2 weeks after their donation should be reported to CDC.

For further information on WNV precautions related to blood and blood products, the FDA's guidance for industry on this topic should be consulted (http://www.fda.gov/downloads/BiologicsBloodVaccines/GuidanceCompliance-RegulatoryInformation/Guidances/Blood/ucm080286.pdf).

Sensitivity Reactions

If an allergic or hypersensitivity reaction (e.g., anaphylaxis) occurs or is suspected, albumin human should be discontinued immediately and appropriate therapy initiated as indicated. Epinephrine should be readily available in case acute hypersensitivity occurs.

Patients should be advised that albumin human should be discontinued immediately if allergic symptoms (e.g., rash, hives, itching, breathing difficulties, coughing, nausea, vomiting, decrease in blood pressure, increased heart rate) occur.

Latex Sensitivity

Some packaging components of certain albumin human preparations (e.g., Buminate® 5%, Buminate® 25%) contain natural latex proteins in the form of natural rubber latex. Health-care personnel should take appropriate precautions if these albumin human preparations are administered to individuals with a history of latex sensitivity.

Some individuals may be hypersensitive to natural latex proteins found in a wide range of medical devices, including packaging components, and the level of sensitivity may vary depending on the form of natural rubber present; rarely, hypersensitivity reactions to natural latex proteins have been fatal.

Hypervolemia/Hemodilution

Hypervolemia may occur if the dosage and IV infusion rate of albumin human are not adjusted based on the patient's volume status. Rapid IV infusion of albumin human solutions may cause vascular overload.

Albumin human should be used with caution in conditions where hypervolemia and its consequences or hemodilution could represent a special risk for the patient (e.g., decompensated cardiac insufficiency, hypertension, esophageal varices, pulmonary edema, hemorrhagic diathesis, severe anemia, renal and postrenal anuria).

Albumin human should be administered with caution in patients with low cardiac reserve (e.g., cardiac disease) and in those who do not have albumin deficiency. Albumin human should be administered with great caution in patients with chronic anemia, hypertension, or renal insufficiency.

Patients should be closely observed for signs of increased venous pressure such as pulmonary edema.

At the first clinical sign of possible cardiovascular overload (e.g., headache, dyspnea, increased blood pressure, jugular venous distention, elevated central venous pressure, pulmonary edema), albumin human infusion should be immediately stopped and the patient reevaluated.

Hemodynamic Monitoring

Hemodynamic performance should be monitored closely during albumin human therapy, and the patient evaluated for evidence of cardiac, respiratory, or renal failure or increasing intracranial pressure.

Arterial blood pressure and pulse rate, central venous pressure, pulmonary artery occlusion pressure, urine output, electrolytes, hemoglobin, and hematocrit should be monitored frequently.

In postoperative or injured patients, a rapid rise in blood pressure following administration of albumin human may reveal bleeding points that were not apparent at lower blood pressure. To prevent hemorrhage and shock, such patients should be observed carefully and treated appropriately.

Anemia and Coagulation Abnormalities

If hemorrhage has occurred in a patient receiving albumin human, relative anemia may be present and should be controlled by supplemental administration of compatible whole blood or RBCs.

If comparatively large volumes of fluid are being replaced with albumin human, coagulation parameters and hematocrit must be monitored and adequate substitution of other blood constituents (coagulation factors, electrolytes, platelets, erythrocytes) ensured.

Electrolyte Imbalance

Compared with albumin human 5% solution, albumin human 20 or 25% solutions are relatively low in electrolytes.

Electrolyte status should be monitored in patients receiving albumin human, and appropriate steps taken to restore or maintain electrolyte balance.

Commercially available albumin human preparations contain 130–160 mEq of sodium per liter.

Oncotic, Osmotic, and Tonicity Considerations

When dilution of albumin human is necessary (e.g., to prepare a 5% solution from a 25% solution), **the oncotic and osmotic properties as well as the tonicity of the resultant dilution must be considered.** Because the membrane of erythrocytes is not perfectly semipermeable, it can permit the passage of water (solvent) molecules and solutes; as a result, solutions that are iso-osmotic with blood are not necessarily isotonic with blood. Substantially hypotonic solutions when admixed with erythrocytes result in the inward passage of water causing the cells to swell and finally burst (hemolyze), releasing hemoglobin. Such hemolysis occurs when erythrocytes are admixed in vitro with albumin human solutions containing less than 90 mEq of sodium per L; the risk of such hemolysis depends on the sodium concentration, not on the suspending medium (albumin) or cell concentration.

When albumin human 25% is diluted with 0.9% sodium chloride injection or 5% dextrose injection, resulting 5% dilutions are approximately isotonic and iso-oncotic with citrated plasma; therefore, these diluents are preferred if such dilutions are considered necessary (e.g., if commercially available albumin human 5% solution cannot be obtained). Although sterile water occasionally was used in the past to dilute albumin human solutions (e.g., to adjust the sodium content when restriction of intake of the electrolyte was considered necessary), sterile water must *not* be used to dilute albumin human. Depending on the relative proportions of albumin human and diluent, dilutions with sterile water may be dangerously hypotonic, carrying the risk of life-threatening hemolysis, particularly if large volumes of markedly hypotonic dilutions are inadvertently administered. Several cases of hemolysis (e.g., during or after plasmapheresis) and at least one death probably related to the hemolysis have been reported following administration of as little as 270 mL of an albumin human 5% solution that had been prepared by inappropriately diluting a 25% solution with sterile water. Such dilutions are markedly hypotonic with respect to blood, with calculated resultant sodium concentrations of 26–32 mEq/L. In the hypotonic environment, shearing forces produced by the plasmapheresis procedures may have contributed to hemolysis in these cases. Potentially life-threatening acute renal failure can result from the toxic effects of hemoglobin (released from hemolyzed erythrocytes) in the renal tubules.

Albumin human dilutions with substantially reduced tonicity should *not* be used as replacement fluids in plasmapheresis procedures or other situations where administration of large volumes and resultant replacement of a significant fraction of the patient's blood volume could result. When sodium restriction is necessary, 5% dextrose injection is the diluent of choice for albumin human solutions. However, because administration of large volumes of albumin human 5% solution prepared by diluting 25% solutions with 5% dextrose could result in hyponatremia and potentially serious adverse effects (e.g., cerebral swelling), 0.9% sodium chloride generally should be used as the preferred diluent when administration of large volumes is anticipated (e.g., during plasmapheresis or plasma exchange) and the fluid and electrolyte status of the patient permits, particularly if rapid infusion is expected. The use of more physiologic diluents (e.g., those closely resembling plasma) also has been suggested as an alternative for diluting albumin human for use in plasmapheresis or plasma exchange.

If sterile water is used for other situations to dilute albumin human (e.g., when only small volumes are to be infused) and unless other diluents are used concomitantly to raise the final tonicity to a clinically acceptable level, the resultant tonicity of the solution must be considered and any potential risks (e.g., hemolysis, acute renal failure) weighed carefully.

Aluminum Content

Aluminum has been detected as a contaminant in albumin human solutions, and aluminum accumulation and associated toxicity (e.g., hypercalcemia, osteodystrophy with associated fracturing osteomalacia, severe progressive encephalopathy) have been reported in some patients with renal failure receiving albumin human (e.g., via plasmapheresis procedures).

The possibility that aluminum could accumulate in patients with impaired renal function should be considered.

Aluminum concentrations in albumin human solutions have varied widely from brand to brand and lot to lot, and reportedly may range up to 323–1830 mcg/L.

Because of the risk of aluminum accumulation, the manufacturer states that Buminate® 25% should not be used in patients with chronic renal impairment.

Certain commercially available albumin human preparations are labeled as containing no more than 200 mcg/L of aluminum (AlbuRx® 5 or 25%, Albutein® 5 or 25%, Plasbumin® 5, 20, or 25% [low aluminum formulations]). It has been suggested that preparations containing no more than 200 mcg/L of aluminum may be preferred in patients at high risk for aluminum toxicity (e.g., neonates, premature infants, geriatric adults, dialysis patients and others with impaired renal function, patients receiving total parenteral nutrition, burn patients).

● Pediatric Precautions

The manufacturers of Albuminar® and Plasbumin® state that safety and efficacy of albumin human have not been established in pediatric patients.

The manufacturers of Buminate® and Flexbumin® state that, although specific pediatric safety studies have not been performed, the safety of albumin human has been demonstrated in children receiving dosages appropriate for the child's body weight.

Some manufacturers state that data regarding use of albumin human in pediatric patients, including premature infants, are limited. Clinicians should weigh the benefits and risks and use albumin human in pediatric patients only when clearly needed.

Albumin human has been used as an adjunct to exchange transfusions in the treatment of neonatal hyperbilirubinemia, including hemolytic disease of the newborn (erythroblastosis fetalis), but should *not* be used if neonatal hyperbilirubinemia is treated using phototherapy without exchange transfusion. (See Uses: Neonatal Hyperbilirubinemia.) Albumin human should be used with caution in hypervolemic infants .

Some clinicians state that albumin human 25% solution is contraindicated in preterm infants because of the risk of intraventricular hemorrhage.

If albumin human is used in neonates or premature infants, a preparation with low aluminum may be preferred because of the risk of aluminum accumulation and associated toxicity. (See Aluminum Content under Cautions: Precautions and Contraindications.)

● Geriatric Precautions

Clinical studies of albumin human did not include sufficient numbers of geriatric patients 65 years of age or older to determine whether they respond differently than younger patients.

● Pregnancy, Fertility, and Lactation

Pregnancy

Animal reproduction studies have not been performed with albumin human. It is not known whether albumin human can cause fetal harm when administered during pregnancy or during labor or delivery. Potential risks and benefits for the specific patient should be considered, and albumin human should be used in pregnant women or during labor and delivery only if clearly needed. One manufacturer states that there is no evidence for any contraindications specifically associated with reproduction, pregnancy, or the fetus.

Fertility

It is not known whether albumin human can affect reproductive capacity.

Lactation

It is not known whether albumin human is distributed into milk. Albumin human should be used with caution in breast-feeding women and only when clearly needed.

DRUG INTERACTIONS

Specific drug interaction studies have not been performed using albumin human.

● Angiotensin-converting Enzyme Inhibitors

Patients receiving angiotensin-converting enzyme (ACE) inhibitors are at increased risk of atypical reactions (e.g., flushing, hypotension) to the drugs if they undergo therapeutic plasma exchange with albumin human replacement. It has been suggested that this interaction may result from prekallikrein activator (PKA, a metabolite of factor XII) present in albumin human, which activates prekallikrein to bradykinin; metabolism of bradykinin is inhibited by ACE inhibitors, thus resulting in accumulation of this naturally occurring vasoactive peptide. Because of the risk of atypical reactions, ACE inhibitors should be withheld for at least 24 hours prior to plasma exchange in which large volumes of albumin human are administered.

PHARMACOLOGY

Serum albumin is an important factor in the regulation of plasma volume and tissue fluid balance through its contribution to the colloid oncotic pressure of plasma. Albumin, a highly soluble globular protein with a relatively low molecular weight (66,500), exerts 70–80% of the colloidal oncotic pressure of normal plasma.

Albumin human 5% solution is iso-oncotic with normal human plasma and will expand circulating blood volume by an amount approximately equal to the volume infused. IV administration of concentrated albumin human solutions causes a shift of fluid from the interstitial spaces into the circulation. When used for the treatment of hypovolemia, albumin human solutions are most effective in well-hydrated patients. When administered IV to a well-hydrated patient, each volume of albumin human 20 or 25% solution draws about 2.5 or 3.5 volumes of additional fluid, respectively, into the circulation within 15 minutes, reducing hemoconcentration and blood viscosity. The extent and duration of volume expansion produced by albumin human is dependent on the initial blood volume. In patients with reduced circulating blood volumes (as from hemorrhage or loss of fluid through exudates or into extravascular spaces), hemodilution persists for many hours, but in patients with normal blood volume, excess fluid and protein are lost from the circulation within a few hours.

Although albumin is a protein, it provides only modest nutritive effect.

Albumin binds and functions as a carrier of intermediate metabolites (including bilirubin), trace metals, some drugs, dyes, fatty acids, hormones, and enzymes, thus affecting the transport, inactivation, and/or exchange of tissue products.

CHEMISTRY AND STABILITY

● Chemistry

Albumin human, a protein colloid, is a sterile solution of serum albumin prepared by fractionating pooled plasma from healthy human donors. Albumin human commercially available in the US meets standards established by the US Food and Drug Administration (FDA). No less than 96% of the total protein in the product is albumin.

Depending on the manufacturer, albumin human solutions occur as clear to slightly opalescent, pale straw to amber or brownish fluids which may have a slight greenish tint. The pH of albumin human solutions is adjusted to 6.4–7.4 with sodium carbonate, sodium bicarbonate, sodium hydroxide, and/or acetic acid. The commercially available preparations contain no preservatives or antimicrobial agents, but do contain stabilizers (e.g., caprylic acid, sodium caprylate, sodium acetyltryptophanate).

In the US, albumin human is commercially available as 5, 20, or 25% solutions; other concentrations (e.g., 4% solutions) are commercially available in other countries. Because of the risks associated with administration of hypotonic solutions, commercially available 5, 20, and 25% solutions of albumin human contain 130–160 mEq of sodium per liter. (See Oncotic, Osmotic, and Tonicity Considerations under Cautions: Precautions and Contraindications.) Albumin human 5% solutions are approximately isotonic and iso-oncotic with normal human plasma; albumin human 20 and 25% solutions are oncotically equivalent to approximately 4 and 5 times the volume of normal human plasma, respectively.

Plasma used for preparation of albumin human undergoes viral screening procedures, and albumin human is pasteurized at 60°C for 10–11 hours to reduce the viral infectious potential of the preparation. However, no method has been shown to be totally effective in removing the risk of viral infectivity from plasma-derived preparations. (See Risk of Transmissible Agents in Plasma-derived Preparations under Cautions: Precautions and Contraindications.)

● *Stability*

Albumin human solutions should be stored in tight containers at the temperature recommended by the manufacturer or indicated on the label and should be protected from light. Most commercially available 5, 20, or 25% solutions of albumin human should be stored at 30°C or less.

Albumin human solutions should not be frozen; solutions that have been frozen should not be used. Albumin human solutions should not be used if they appear turbid or contain sediment. The solutions do not contain preservatives and should not be used if more than 4 hours have elapsed since the vial or container was first entered.

Albumin human solutions may be used in conjunction with whole blood or plasma, or with dextrose, sodium lactate, or sodium chloride injections. However, albumin human solutions should not be mixed with parenteral nutrient solutions, protein hydrolysates, amino acid solutions, or solutions containing alcohol since protein precipitates may occur.

When albumin human 25% is diluted with 0.9% sodium chloride injection or 5% dextrose injection, resulting 5% dilutions are approximately isotonic and iso-oncotic with citrated plasma; therefore, these diluents are preferred for such dilutions. Sterile water for injection must *not* be used to dilute albumin human solutions. Depending on the relative proportions of albumin human and

diluent, dilutions prepared with sterile water may be dangerously hypotonic, carrying the risk of life-threatening hemolysis, particularly if large volumes of markedly hypotonic dilutions are inadvertently administered. (See Oncotic, Osmotic, and Tonicity Considerations under Cautions: Precautions and Contraindications.) Sterile water is compatible with albumin human and can be a suitable diluent in *non*-clinical situations (e.g., for preparing dilutions to be used in *in vitro* laboratory procedures).

There are conflicting reports of the compatibility of albumin human with other IV infusion fluids; specialized references should be consulted for specific compatibility information.

PREPARATIONS

Excipients in commercially available drug preparations may have clinically important effects in some individuals; consult specific product labeling for details.

Albumin Human

Parenteral		
Injection, for IV infusion	50 mg/mL*	Albuminar®-5, CSL Behring
		AlbuRx®-5, CSL Behring
		Albumin Human 5%
		Albutein® 5%, Grifols
		Buminate® 5%, Baxter
		Plasbumin®-5, Talecris
	200 mg/mL*	Albumin Human 20%
		Plasbumin® -20, Talecris
	250 mg/mL*	Albuminar®-25, CSL Behring
		Albumin Human 25%
		Albutein® 25%, Grifols
		AlbuRx® 25, CSL Behring
		Buminate® 25%, Baxter
		Flexbumin® 25%, Baxter
		Plasbumin®-25, Talecris

* available from one or more manufacturer, distributor, and/or repackager by generic (nonproprietary) name

† Use is not currently included in the labeling approved by the US Food and Drug Administration.

Selected Revisions September 28, 2011, © Copyright, May 1, 1978, American Society of Health-System Pharmacists, Inc.

Table of Contents

20:00 BLOOD FORMATION, COAGULATION, AND THROMBOSIS

§ Omitted from the print version of *AHFS Drug Information*® because of space limitations. This monograph is available on the *AHFS Drug Information*® web site, http://www.ahfsdruginformation.com. See the Preface for details on accessing this site.

Iron Dextran

20:04.04 • IRON PREPARATIONS

■ Iron dextran injection, a sterile, colloidal solution of ferric hydroxide or ferric oxyhydroxide in a complex with partially hydrolyzed low molecular weight dextran, corrects the erythropoietic abnormalities that are due to a deficiency of iron.

USES

● *Iron Deficiency Not Amenable to Oral Iron Therapy*

Iron dextran is used in the treatment of iron deficiency when oral iron preparations are ineffective or cannot be used. There are relatively few indications for parenteral iron therapy. Occasionally, however, parenteral administration may be required in iron-deficient patients in whom oral administration of iron is infeasible or ineffective because of intolerance, poor absorption, GI disease, refusal or inability to take the oral medication, or when rapid replenishment of iron stores is necessary as in hypochromic anemia of infancy or the last trimester of pregnancy. In addition, most chronic kidney disease patients who receive therapy with erythropoiesis-stimulating agents (ESAs) (e.g., epoetin alfa, darbepoetin alfa) will require oral or parenteral iron therapy because of the dramatic decrease in iron stores associated with erythrocyte formation. In several randomized controlled studies comparing IV and oral administration of iron in patients with chronic kidney disease on hemodialysis, IV iron was superior to orally administered iron in increasing hemoglobin concentrations and/or minimizing the dosage of ESA required to maintain target hemoglobin levels; guidelines from the National Kidney Foundation Kidney Disease Outcomes Quality Initiative (NKF-KDOQI) state that the IV route is preferred for administration of iron in patients with chronic kidney disease undergoing hemodialysis. (See Uses: Anemia of Chronic Kidney Disease, in Epoetin Alfa 20:16.) The response to iron dextran is quantitatively similar to that produced by other iron preparations administered parenterally.

Since parenteral use of complexes of iron and carbohydrates has resulted in fatal anaphylactoid reactions, iron dextran should be used only in patients in whom a clearly established indication for parenteral iron therapy exists, confirmed by appropriate laboratory tests.

For additional information on the prevention and treatment of iron deficiency, including anemia, see Uses in Iron Preparations, Oral, 20:04.04.

DOSAGE AND ADMINISTRATION

● *Administration*

Iron dextran injection is administered undiluted by *slow* (50 mg/minute or less if undiluted) IV injection; some preparations (i.e., INFeD®) also are FDA-labeled for IM injection. Iron dextran injection also has been diluted in 0.9% sodium chloride injection and administered by IV infusion† (e.g., over 1–6 hours).

Before administration of the first therapeutic dose of iron dextran, a test dose of iron should be given by the chosen route and appropriate method of administration. If iron dextran is to be administered IV, the manufacturer of INFeD® recommends that a test dose of 25 mg (0.5 mL) of iron dextran be given IV over at least 30 seconds; the manufacturer of Dexferrum® recommends a 25-mg (0.5 mL) test dose given IV over at least 5 minutes. If administered IM, a test dose of 25 mg (0.5 mL) of iron dextran (InFeD®) should be administered into the buttock using the IM injection technique recommended by the manufacturer. It has been recommended that the test dose and subsequent doses of iron dextran be administered by individuals trained to provide emergency treatment of serious allergic reactions should they occur and that immediate access to drugs and resuscitation equipment needed to treat such reactions be available. Although anaphylactic reactions usually are evident within a few minutes when they occur, it is recommended that a period of 1 hour or longer elapse before the remaining portion of the initial dose is given.

IV administration may be preferred to IM administration when there is insufficient muscle mass for IM administration, when there is impaired absorption from the muscle because of stasis or edema, when there is a possibility of uncontrolled IM bleeding (as in hemophilia), or when massive and prolonged parenteral therapy is indicated (as in chronic substantial blood loss), and to avoid the pain, irritation, and staining of the skin at the injection site secondary to IM administration. IM administration may be preferred when venous access is difficult or infeasible (e.g., in infants or in adults with poor veins).

For IM administration, the manufacturer of INFeD® recommends that iron dextran be injected deeply with a 2- or 3-inch, 19- or 20-gauge needle into the upper outer quadrant of the buttock only; the drug should never be administered into the arm or any other exposed area. When the drug is administered IM, if the patient is standing, the injection should be made in the buttock of the leg opposite the patient's weight-bearing leg; if supine, the patient should be in a lateral position with the injection site uppermost. To avoid injection or leakage into subcutaneous tissue, the Z-track technique of injection in which the subcutaneous tissue over the site of injection is firmly pushed aside before inserting the needle is recommended.

The manufacturers state that iron dextran should not be mixed with other drugs or added to parenteral nutrition solutions for IV infusion. Iron dextran solutions should be inspected visually for particulate matter and discoloration prior to administration whenever solution and container permit.

● *Dosage*

Dosage of iron dextran is expressed in terms of mg of elemental iron. Iron dextran injection contains the equivalent of 50 mg of elemental iron per mL.

Iron Deficiency Anemia

Before initiating therapy for *iron deficiency anemia*, total iron requirements (allowing for storage iron) are calculated by using a dose formula or table. Calculations are based on the amount of iron needed to restore hemoglobin concentration to normal or near normal plus an additional amount to provide adequate replenishment of iron stores in most individuals with moderately or severely reduced levels of hemoglobin. In the formula recommended by the manufacturers, the total dose of iron dextran injection (in mL) containing the equivalent of 50 mg/mL of iron is calculated as follows:

$$[0.0442 \times (Hb_d - Hb_o) \times Wt] + (0.26 \times Wt) = \text{total dose of iron dextran injection (mL)}$$

Where Wt is the patient's lean body weight in kg, Hb_d is the *desired* hemoglobin concentration in g/dL (14.8 for patients weighing more than 15 kg and 12 for patients weighing 15 kg or less), Hb_o is the patient's *observed* hemoglobin concentration in g/dL, and (0.26 × lean body weight) is a factor that accounts for storage iron.

In patients with chronic kidney disease who are receiving supplemental therapy with an erythropoiesis-stimulating agent (ESA), sufficient iron should be administered to maintain certain indices of iron therapy (i.e., transferrin saturation and serum ferritin concentrations) at target levels; periodic monitoring of these iron indices is recommended, and the results should be used (in conjunction with hemoglobin concentrations and ESA dosage) to guide iron therapy.

Iron Replacement Secondary to Blood Loss

For *iron replacement secondary to blood loss* (e.g., in patients with hemorrhagic diatheses or patients on long-term renal hemodialysis), total iron requirements are based on estimates of the amount of iron represented in the blood loss; the formula above for iron deficiency anemia is *not* applicable. Instead, the following formula, based on the approximation that 1 mL of normocytic, normochromic erythrocytes contains 1 mg of elemental iron, may be used to calculate the required total dosage in mL of iron dextran injection containing the equivalent of 50 mg of iron per mL:

$$0.02 \times \text{blood loss (in mL)} \times \text{hematocrit (expressed as a decimal fraction)} = \text{total dosage of iron dextran injection in mL}$$

IV Dosage

Iron dextran may be injected IV, undiluted, at a slow, gradual rate not exceeding 50 mg of iron per minute (1 mL/minute). If adverse reactions to the test dose do not occur, subsequent IV doses may be increased to up to 100 mg of iron daily until the total calculated dose has been administered. The manufacturers recommend that the maximum daily IV dosage of *undiluted* iron dextran not exceed 25 mg (0.5 mL) of iron in infants weighing less than 5 kg; 50 mg (1 mL) of iron in children weighing less than 10 kg; and 100 mg (2 mL) of iron in other patients.

Although the manufacturers do not recommend dilution of iron dextran injection† or administration of the drug in single IV doses exceeding 100 mg†, numerous reports have been made in which the total dose of an iron dextran preparation was administered as a single dose either by direct IV injection or as an IV infusion. Large IV doses of iron dextran, such as those used in total-dose infusions†, reportedly have been associated with an increased frequency of adverse effects, especially delayed reactions (e.g., arthralgia, myalgia, fever). In the total-dose infusion technique, the total calculated dose of iron dextran is diluted in 250–1000 mL of 0.9% sodium chloride injection. The use of 5% dextrose injection instead of 0.9% sodium chloride injection has been reported to be associated with a higher incidence of local pain and phlebitis. With the total-dose infusion technique, if no reaction occurs after administration of a 25-mg IV test dose over 5 minutes, the remainder of the dose may be infused (e.g., over 1–6 hours). After the infusion is completed, the vein is often flushed with 0.9% sodium chloride injection.

IM Dosage

Iron dextran labeled for IM use (i.e., INFeD®) may be injected IM daily or less frequently until the calculated amount has been given. If adverse reactions to the test dose do not occur, subsequent doses may be given. The manufacturer of INFeD® recommends that the maximum daily IM dosage of *undiluted* iron dextran not exceed 25 mg (0.5 mL) of iron in infants weighing less than 5 kg, 50 mg (1 mL) of iron in children weighing less than 10 kg, and 100 mg (2 mL) of iron in other patients.

CAUTIONS

Sensitivity (e.g., anaphylactoid or anaphylactic) reactions appear to be the most common adverse effects of iron dextran, occurring with either IV or IM administration, and such reactions vary widely in severity and can be immediate or delayed. Incidences of such reactions are difficult to ascertain since some studies only reported severe or potentially serious reactions whereas others reported a wide range of severity. Sensitivity reactions may be severe enough to require discontinuance of iron dextran therapy and can be fatal. (See Cautions: Sensitivity Reactions.) Local reactions associated with IV or IM administration also appear to be relatively common. Adverse reactions associated with IV administration of the drug generally resemble those associated with IM administration. Large IV doses of iron dextran, such as those used in total-dose infusions, have been associated with an increased incidence of adverse effects, and such adverse effects frequently have been delayed (1–2 days).

● Sensitivity Reactions

Anaphylactic or anaphylactoid reactions to iron dextran, including fatal anaphylaxis, have been reported. These reactions occur most frequently within the first several minutes of administration and are generally characterized by sudden onset of respiratory difficulty (e.g., wheezing, bronchospasm, rigor, dyspnea, cyanosis), tachycardia, hypotension, respiratory arrest, and/or cardiovascular collapse. The manufacturers state that concomitant use of angiotensin-converting enzyme (ACE) inhibitors may increase the risk for reactions to iron dextran. The level of risk for anaphylactic-type reactions following exposure to specific iron dextran preparations is not known and may vary. Iron dextran preparations differ in chemical characteristics and may differ in clinical effects; the manufacturers state that such preparations are not clinically interchangeable.

Acute hypersensitivity reactions to iron dextran have been estimated to occur in 0.2–3% of patients. These reactions have been reported after administration of uneventful test doses of iron dextran as well as after therapeutic doses of the drug. Although it has been suggested that severe systemic reactions, including anaphylactoid reactions, are more common following IV rather than IM administration of iron dextran, the risk of severe systemic reactions following IV or IM administration has not been directly compared and there appears to be no well-substantiated evidence of a difference in the frequency of anaphylactoid reactions following either route of administration. The National Kidney Foundation Kidney Disease Outcomes Quality Initiative (NKF-KDOQI) guidelines state that direct observation of the patient after IV administration of an iron agent permits the most reliable assessment of the frequency of associated adverse drug reactions. Relatively large IV doses such as those employed with total-dose infusions have been associated with an increased risk of adverse effects, mainly delayed effects. The risk of

anaphylactic or anaphylactoid reactions to iron dextran appears to be increased in patients with a positive history of drug allergy, particularly those with multiple drug allergies. Other hypersensitivity reactions may include sweating, dyspnea, urticaria, other rashes and pruritus, arthralgia, myalgia, and febrile episodes.

The mechanism of anaphylactic/anaphylactoid reactions to iron dextran has not been elucidated, but because of the rapid nature of their onset and similarity to anaphylactoid reactions observed with radiographic contrast media they probably result from a direct effect on mast cells and basophils leading to their degranulation and release of mediators (e.g., histamine). An immunoglobulin E-mediated reaction appears unlikely.

● Musculoskeletal and Delayed Adverse Effects

Large IV doses of iron dextran, such as those used in total-dose infusions†, may be associated with an increased frequency of adverse effects, especially delayed (1–2 days) reactions manifested by arthralgia, backache, myalgia, adenopathy, moderate to high fever, backache, chills, dizziness, headache, malaise, nausea, and/or vomiting. The onset of these adverse effects is usually 24–48 hours after administration of the drug, and the effects generally subside within 3–4 days. Delayed adverse effects have also occurred following IM administration and usually subsided within 3–7 days. The etiology of delayed adverse effects is not known, but the symptom complex resembles that of a serum sickness reaction. Patients with rheumatoid arthritis and possibly other inflammatory diseases (e.g., ankylosing spondylitis, lupus erythematosus) may be at particular risk for delayed reactions. IV administration of iron dextran has caused fever and exacerbation or reactivation of joint pain and swelling in patients with rheumatoid arthritis; in addition, exacerbation of ankylosing spondylitis in one patient and arthralgia, myalgia, erythema nodosum, and fever in a patient with lupus erythematosus have been reported. Such exacerbations of underlying inflammatory conditions may respond to nonsteroidal anti-inflammatory agent (NSAIA) therapy and may be prevented with corticosteroid pretreatment.

● Local Effects

Local reactions may occur at the injection site of iron dextran and are more common following IM administration. Local reactions at the injection site following IM injection include soreness or pain (in rare cases persisting longer than a year), inflammation, sterile abscesses, necrosis, atrophy, fibrosis, cellulitis, swelling, and harmless but persistent brown staining of the skin and/or underlying tissue. Phlebitis, pain along the course of the vein, and venospasm may occur following IV injection. Inadvertent intra-arterial injection of a 1-g undiluted dose over 20 minutes resulted in marked erythema, warmth, and tingling in the hand and arm distal to the brachial artery injection site during infusion.

● Cardiovascular Effects

Chest pain, chest tightness, shock, hypotension, hypertension, tachycardia, bradycardia, flushing, edema, cardiac arrest, thrombophlebitis, pulmonary embolus, and arrhythmias have occurred in patients receiving iron dextran. Flushing and hypotension may occur when the drug is administered IV too rapidly.

● GI Effects

Abdominal pain, dyspepsia, nausea, vomiting, diarrhea, metallic taste in the mouth, altered taste, and transient loss of taste perception have occurred in patients receiving iron dextran.

● Nervous System Effects

Headache, transient paresthesia, weakness, dizziness, faintness, syncope, unresponsiveness, disorientation, numbness, malaise, and seizures (which may accompany anaphylaxis) have been reported in patients receiving iron dextran.

● Hematologic Effects

Latent folic acid deficiency may occasionally become apparent in patients receiving iron dextran. Leukocytosis, frequently with fever, may occur. One case of leukocytosis was reported in a severely iron-deficient infant who received the drug. Purpura has also occurred.

● Other Adverse Effects

Other adverse effects of iron dextran include chills, shivering, regional lymphadenopathy (generally inguinal and associated with IM injection of the drug), and hematuria.

● Precautions and Contraindications

Because anaphylactic reactions to iron dextran, including fatal anaphylaxis, have been reported, an initial test dose should be administered prior to administration of the first therapeutic dose of the drug and the patient should be observed for manifestations of anaphylactic-type reactions. Because anaphylaxis and other hypersensitivity reactions have been reported after administration of uneventful test doses of iron dextran as well as after therapeutic doses of the drug, the manufacturers state that administration of subsequent test doses should be considered during iron dextran therapy. (See Dosage and Administration: Administration.) It is recommended that the test dose and subsequent doses of iron dextran be administered by personnel trained to provide emergency treatment and that appropriate resuscitation equipment and drugs for the treatment of a severe allergic or anaphylactic reaction (e.g., epinephrine) be readily available when iron dextran is administered. Patients receiving β-adrenergic blocking agents may not respond adequately to epinephrine, and use of isoproterenol or a similar β-adrenergic agonist may be required in these patients.

The fact that large IV doses of iron dextran, such as those used in total-dose infusions, have been associated with an increased incidence of adverse effects, especially delayed reactions, should be considered when evaluating the benefits and risks of such therapy. Patients should be advised of potential effects associated with the use of iron dextran.

Iron dextran should be used with caution in patients with a history of serious allergies and/or asthma. Iron dextran should be used with extreme caution in patients with serious impairment of hepatic function. Adverse effects following administration of iron dextran may exacerbate cardiovascular complications in patients with preexisting cardiovascular disease.

Extreme caution should also be used in administering the drug IV in patients with rheumatoid arthritis, since IV administration may cause fever and exacerbation or reactivation of joint pain and swelling in these patients; the possibility of an increased risk of delayed reactions (e.g., arthralgia, myalgia, fever) should also be considered in patients with other inflammatory diseases (e.g., ankylosing spondylitis, lupus erythematosus). (See Cautions: Musculoskeletal and Delayed Adverse Effects.)

Unwarranted administration of parenteral iron preparations may cause excess storage of iron and a syndrome similar to hemosiderosis in patients whose anemia is not attributable to iron deficiency (e.g., those with hemoglobinopathies and other refractory anemias that might be erroneously diagnosed as iron deficiency anemias).

Because iron can increase the pathogenicity of certain microorganisms and has been postulated as potentially adversely affecting prognosis in certain HIV-infected individuals, some clinicians recommend that HIV-infected individuals who do not have documented iron-deficiency anemia avoid iron supplementation for the management of HIV-associated anemia. *Iron dextran should not be administered concomitantly with oral iron preparations.* Determinations of hematologic response, such as serum ferritin, blood hemoglobin concentration, hematocrit, and reticulocyte count, should be performed periodically during the course of therapy with iron dextran. Serum ferritin has been shown to correlate with iron stores, at least in nonuremic patients; while a correlation between serum ferritin and iron stores has been reported in hemodialysis patients, other data suggest that elevated serum ferritin can result from hepatosplenic siderosis in some of these patients, and may not reliably indicate bone marrow iron stores.

Iron dextran should not be used during the acute phase of infectious renal disease. The drug is contraindicated in patients with any anemia other than iron deficiency anemia and in patients who are hypersensitive to iron dextran.

● Pediatric Precautions

The manufacturers state that the use of iron dextran in children younger than 4 months of age is not recommended. Use of IM iron dextran in neonates† in other countries (e.g., New Zealand) reportedly has been associated with an increased incidence of gram-negative sepsis, principally infections caused by *Escherichia coli*. However, the drug has been administered IV in a limited number of neonates in the US without evidence of unusual adverse effect or risk of sepsis.

● Mutagenicity and Carcinogenicity

IM administration of iron-carbohydrate complexes may be associated with a risk of carcinogenesis. Subcutaneous injection of very large doses of iron dextran or small doses injected repeatedly at the same site have been shown to produce sarcomas in mice, rats, rabbits, and possibly hamsters. Such tumors have not been produced in guinea pigs. Animal studies suggest that sarcomas may result from high tissue concentrations of iron remaining at the site of injection and that the latent period between administration of the drug and appearance of the tumor may be one-quarter to one-third of the life span of the particular species. Sarcoma at the site of injection has been reported rarely in patients approximately 4–14 years after receiving IM iron dextran or other complexes of iron and carbohydrates; however, a causal relationship has not been proven. Although the carcinogenic potential of iron dextran is generally considered remote by most authorities, it may require years before the carcinogenic potential in humans can be clearly defined.

● Pregnancy, Fertility, and Lactation

Pregnancy

Reproduction studies in mice, rats, rabbits, dogs, and monkeys using iron dextran doses about 3 times the maximum human dose have shown the drug to be teratogenic and embryocidal. At doses equivalent to 50 mg/kg or less of iron, no consistent adverse fetal effects were observed in mice, rats, rabbits, dogs, or monkeys. At a total IV dose equivalent to 90 mg/kg of iron given over a 14-day period, fetal and maternal toxicity has been reported in monkeys; similar effects were observed in mice and rats with a single dose equivalent to 125 mg/kg of iron. In dogs and rats, fetal abnormalities were observed at doses equivalent to 250 mg/kg or higher of iron. The animals used in reproduction studies were not iron deficient. The effect of iron dextran on the human fetus is not known. Results of various studies in pregnant animals and humans have been inconclusive regarding placental transfer of intact iron dextran. Small amounts of iron apparently cross the placenta (the form in which it crosses the placenta has not been clearly established) and increase neonatal serum iron concentrations when iron dextran is administered within 2 weeks of delivery; however, no adverse effects on the neonate have been reported. There are no adequate and well-controlled studies using iron dextran in pregnant women, and the drug should be used during pregnancy only when the potential benefits justify the possible risks to the fetus.

Lactation

Only traces of unmetabolized iron dextran are distributed into milk, but the drug should be used with caution in nursing women.

LABORATORY TEST INTERFERENCES

Large IV doses (250 mg or more of iron) of iron dextran may cause serum from blood samples obtained 4 hours after administration of the drug to have a brown color. The drug may cause falsely elevated values of serum bilirubin and falsely decreased values of serum calcium. Serum iron determinations (especially colorimetric assays) may not be meaningful for 3 weeks following the administration of iron dextran. Results of serum iron measurements obtained within 1–2 weeks of administration of large doses of the drug should be interpreted with caution. Serum ferritin concentrations peak approximately 7–9 days following an IV dose of iron dextran and slowly return to baseline over a period of about 3 weeks. Examination of the bone marrow for iron stores may not be meaningful for prolonged periods following iron dextran therapy because residual iron dextran may remain in the reticuloendothelial cells.

Prolongation of the partial thromboplastin time has been reported to occur after IV administration of iron dextran when the blood sample for the test is mixed with anticoagulant citrate dextrose solution. This interference apparently does not occur when anticoagulant sodium citrate solution is used. Blood typing and cross-matching are not affected by iron dextran.

Bone scans involving technetium Tc 99m diphosphonate have been reported to exhibit dense, crescentic areas of activity along the contour of the iliac crest, visualized 1–6 days after IM injections of iron dextran. Bone scans using imaging agents labeled with technetium Tc 99m, in the presence of high serum ferritin concentrations or following IV infusions of iron dextran, have been reported to show reduced bone uptake, marked renal activity, and excessive blood pool and soft tissue accumulation.

ACUTE TOXICITY

The LD$_{50}$ of iron dextran in mice is 500 mg/kg or greater. Overdosage of iron dextran is unlikely to be associated with any acute manifestations; however, dosage of the drug in excess of that required for restoration of hemoglobin and replenishment of iron stores may lead to hemosiderosis. Periodic monitoring of serum ferritin concentrations may be useful in recognizing a deleterious, progressive accumulation of iron resulting from impaired iron uptake from the reticuloendothelial system that may occur in some patients (e.g., those with chronic kidney disease, Hodgkin's disease, rheumatoid arthritis). Only negligible amounts of iron dextran are removed by hemodialysis.

PHARMACOLOGY

Iron is a constituent of hemoglobin, and administration of iron dextran corrects the erythropoietic abnormalities that are due to a deficiency of iron. Some iron also may be utilized for synthesis of myoglobin or nonhemoglobin heme units. In iron-deficient patients, reticulocytosis may begin by the fourth day following an IV infusion of the total calculated dose of iron dextran and reaches a maximum by about the tenth day. Iron does not stimulate erythropoiesis nor does it correct hemoglobin disturbances not caused by iron deficiency.

Administration of iron may reverse esophageal, gastric, and other tissue changes associated with iron deficiency. Iron therapy also relieves other symptoms associated with iron deficiency such as soreness of the tongue, cheilosis, dysphagia, and dystrophy of the nails and skin. Some of the toxic effects of iron dextran may be due to a pharmacologic or allergenic effect of dextran; however, conclusive studies have not been performed to establish the importance of this effect.

PHARMACOKINETICS

● Absorption

Following IM injection, iron dextran is absorbed from the site of injection principally through the lymphatic system. Absorption takes place in two stages. In the initial phase lasting about 3 days, a local inflammatory reaction facilitates passage of the drug from the site of IM injection into the lymphatic system. In the second, slower phase, iron dextran is ingested by macrophages, which then enter the lymphatic system and eventually the blood. Results of studies using radiolabeled iron dextran have shown that about 60% of an IM dose of iron dextran is absorbed after 3 days and up to 90% is absorbed after 1–3 weeks; the remainder is gradually absorbed over a period of several months or longer. Absorption of iron dextran from subcutaneous tissue is very slow, and the skin may be stained brown for up to 2 years if the drug is deposited in this tissue.

● Distribution

Following IM or IV injection, iron dextran is gradually cleared from the plasma by the reticuloendothelial cells of the liver, spleen, and bone marrow. Results of several studies indicate that a variable portion of an IV dose of iron dextran may be stored in an unusable form in bone marrow. Following IV doses containing more than 500 mg of elemental iron, the uptake of iron dextran by the reticuloendothelial system appears to be constant and amounts to 10–20 mg per hour. Reticuloendothelial cells separate iron from the iron dextran complex and the iron becomes a part of the body's total iron stores.

Ferric iron is gradually released into the plasma where it rapidly combines with transferrin and is carried to the bone marrow and incorporated into hemoglobin. Rate of incorporation of iron into hemoglobin is determined by the extent of iron deficiency, with greater rates of hemoglobin synthesis occurring in iron deficient patients than in normal or mildly anemic patients. Following an IV infusion of the total calculated dose of iron dextran in iron-deficient patients, the rate of increase in hemoglobin concentration appears to be most rapid during the first 1–2 weeks and ranges from 1.5–2.2 g/dL per week. Subsequently, hemoglobin concentration increases at a rate of 0.7–1.6 g/dL per week until normal hemoglobin concentrations are attained.

Small amounts of iron apparently reach the fetus following administration of iron dextran during pregnancy, but the form in which it crosses the placenta is not clearly established. Only traces of unmetabolized iron dextran are distributed into breast milk.

For additional information on the distribution of iron, see Pharmacokinetics: Distribution, in Iron Preparations, Oral, 20:04.04.

● Elimination

In doses of 500 mg or less, iron dextran plasma concentrations decrease exponentially with a half-life of about 6 hours. In studies in iron-deficient patients with coexistent end-stage renal disease and other clinical problems, the serum elimination half-life of iron averaged 58.9 hours (range: 9.4–87.4 hours) following IV administration of iron dextran; these studies measured the total serum iron directly as well as transferrin bound iron non-radioisotopically. It should be recognized that elimination of iron from serum, including elimination half-life, does *not* correspond to clearance of the mineral from the body.

Dextran, a polyglucose, is either metabolized or excreted. Only traces of unmetabolized iron dextran are excreted in urine, bile, or feces.

Iron dextran is negligibly removed by hemodialysis. Several dialyzer membranes have been studied (e.g., polysulphone, cuprophane, cellulose acetate, cellulose triacetate, polymethylmethacrilate, polyacrylonitrile), including those considered high efficiency and high flux.

CHEMISTRY AND STABILITY

● Chemistry

Iron dextran injection is a sterile, colloidal solution of ferric hydroxide or oxyhydroxide in a complex with partially hydrolyzed low molecular weight dextran. During the manufacture of iron dextran, polymerization occurs resulting in a complex with a molecular weight estimated to be approximately 165,000. Approximately 98–99% of the iron in iron dextran is present as a stable ferric-dextran complex; the remainder is present as a weak ferrous complex. Iron dextran injection occurs as a dark brown, slightly viscous liquid that is completely miscible with water and 0.9% sodium chloride injection. The commercially available injection of InFed® or Dexferrum® has a pH of 5.2–6.5 or 4.5–7, respectively; sodium hydroxide and/or hydrochloric acid may have been added to adjust pH.

● Stability

Iron dextran injection should be stored at a controlled room temperature of 20–25°C, with excursions permitted to 15–30°C.

Iron dextran injection has been reported to be physically incompatible with oxytetracycline and with sulfadiazine sodium in IV infusions.

PREPARATIONS

Excipients in commercially available drug preparations may have clinically important effects in some individuals; consult specific product labeling for details.

Iron Dextran

Parenteral		
Injection, for IV use	equivalent to 50 mg of elemental iron per mL	Dexferrum®, American Regent
Injection, for IV or IM use	equivalent to 50 mg of elemental iron per mL	INFeD®, Watson

† Use is not currently included in the labeling approved by the US Food and Drug Administration.

Iron Preparations, Oral

20:04.04 • IRON PREPARATIONS

■ Ferrous fumarate, ferrous gluconate, ferrous sulfate, carbonyl iron, and polysaccharide-iron complex are iron preparations that are commercially available in the US for oral administration in the prevention and treatment of iron deficiency.

USES

● Iron Deficiency

Iron preparations are used for the prevention and treatment of iron deficiency. Iron will not correct hemoglobin disturbances caused by conditions other than iron deficiency but may cause iron toxicity or iron storage disease if used in these conditions. Iron also is not indicated for the treatment of anemia resulting from causes other than iron deficiency.

Ensuring adequate dietary iron intake is the principal means for primary prevention of iron deficiency in all age groups, reserving iron supplementation for individuals and groups at high risk of deficiency and/or in whom adequate dietary intake is unlikely to be achieved and iron therapy for those with presumed or established iron-deficiency anemia. Oral administration is the route of choice for iron therapy in most patients and for iron supplementation. Because they appear to be the most readily absorbed, ferrous salts are the iron preparations of choice. Since absorption of iron salts occurs maximally in the duodenum and proximal jejunum, extended-release or enteric-coated preparations should be used only if objective bioavailability data have shown the preparation to be effective and if the potential benefits outweigh the disadvantage of added cost.

Iron deficiency is the most common known nutritional deficiency. Deficiency of iron may result from inadequate ingestion, decreased absorption or utilization, abnormal blood losses (including menstruation), or increased requirements. When a diagnosis of iron deficiency is confirmed, a cause must be identified. Iron deficiency represents a spectrum ranging from iron depletion, which results in no physiologic impairment, to anemia, which affects the functioning of several organ systems. In depletion, the amount of stored iron is reduced but the amount of functional iron (e.g., in hemoglobin) may not be affected; if body requirements increase in depleted individuals, there are no stores from which to mobilize iron. Erythropoiesis in iron deficiency depletes iron stores and reduces transport iron further; GI absorption of iron is insufficient to replace the amount depleted or to provide the amount needed for growth and function. As a result, erythrocyte production is limited and erythrocyte protoporphyrin concentration increases secondarily. In iron-deficiency anemia, the most severe form of deficiency, the iron shortage results in inadequate production of iron-containing functional compounds, including hemoglobin; erythrocytes are microcytic and hypochromic. In the treatment of iron deficiency, administration of iron in combination with other minerals and/or vitamins has not been established as being superior to iron alone.

Risks and Prevalence of Iron Deficiency

Despite recent improvements (e.g., secondary to increased use of iron-fortified formulas in nonbreast-fed infants), iron deficiency remains relatively prevalent in the US in adolescent girls and women of childbearing age and in infants. Considerable morbidity, particularly among young children and pregnant women, can result from iron deficiency, and efforts to prevent, detect, and treat iron deficiency should be heightened in the US, especially among such individuals and females of childbearing age. Because some developmental deficits in young children may not be fully reversible, the importance of primary prevention in this age group is particularly important.

Infants and Young Children

Iron-deficiency anemia can result in considerable morbidity in young children. In infants and preschool children up to 5 years of age, iron-deficiency anemia results in developmental delays and behavioral disturbances (e.g., decreased motor activity, social interaction, and attention to tasks). Such developmental delays may persist beyond 5 years of age into the school years if the iron deficiency is not reversed fully, and some developmental deficits may not be fully reversible even with iron therapy. The effects of *mild* iron-deficiency anemia on infant and early childhood development and behavior remain to be further elucidated. Iron-deficiency

anemia also may enhance the risk of lead toxicity in children by increasing GI absorption of heavy metals, including lead. Iron-deficiency anemia in young children also may be associated with conditions (e.g., low birthweight, undernutrition, poverty, high blood lead concentrations) that independently affect development, and such potential confounding factors should be considered when interventions aimed at managing iron-deficiency anemia are developed and evaluated.

Rapid growth rate combined with frequently inadequate dietary iron intake places children younger than 2 years of age, particularly those 9–18 months of age, at the highest risk of any age group for iron deficiency. Iron stores of full-term infants generally meet iron requirements until 4–6 months of age, and iron-deficiency anemia generally does not become evident until about 9 months of age. However, iron stores can be depleted by 2–3 months of age in premature or low-birthweight infants secondary to lower iron stores at birth and more rapid growth during infancy, placing such infants at greater risk for iron deficiency than full-term infants with normal or high birthweight.

In the US, iron deficiency occurs in about 9% of children 12–36 months of age, in about one-third of whom the deficiency has progressed to anemia. The prevalence of iron deficiency is greater in children living at or below the poverty line than in those living above the poverty line and also is greater in blacks and Mexican-Americans than in white children.

The iron content and absorption efficiency of various milk sources and feeding practices are a strong predictor of iron nutritional status during the first year of life.

Breast milk has the highest percentage of bioavailable iron (about 50%), and breast milk and iron-fortified formula can provide adequate iron to meet an infant's iron requirements. However, the relatively high iron bioavailability of breast milk does not completely compensate for the relatively low iron content. Although iron-fortified formula has a relatively low iron bioavailability (about 4%), it has a substantially higher iron concentration than breast milk, which can compensate for differences in bioavailability. Nonfortified-formulas and whole cow's milk have an iron bioavailability of about 10% but relatively low iron concentrations (especially cow's milk).

Although most nonbreast-fed infants in the US appear to receive the recommended dietary allowance of iron through diet, 20–40% of infants fed nonfortified formula or whole cow's milk are at risk for iron deficiency by 9–12 months of age, while those fed mainly iron-fortified formula are unlikely to have deficiency (e.g., about an 8% risk). In addition, 15–25% of US breast-fed infants are at risk for iron deficiency by 9–12 months of age, and more than 50% of US children 1–2 years may not be receiving adequate dietary iron. Consumption of iron-fortified cereal can reduce the risk of iron deficiency in infants. Although the effect of prolonged exclusive breast-feeding on iron status remains unclear, limited evidence suggests that exclusive breast-feeding for longer than 7 months minimizes the risk of iron deficiency relative to breast-feeding that is supplemented by nonfortified foods beginning at 7 months of age or younger. Introduction of whole cow's milk before 1 year of age or consumption of more than 720 mL (24 oz) after the first year of life increases the risk of iron deficiency because such milk has little bioavailable iron, may displace the desire for foods with higher iron content, and may cause occult GI bleeding; goat's milk is likely to carry a similar risk because of similar iron composition to whole cow's milk, and soy milk (not iron-fortified soy-based formula) also should be avoided for the milk-based part of the diet before 12 months of age. Because iron-fortified formulas are readily available, do not cost much more than nonfortified formulas, and have few proven adverse effects other than dark stools, they are preferred for primary prevention of iron deficiency in nonbreast-fed or partially breast-fed infants younger than 1 year old as well as for weaning breast-fed infants in this age group; no common medical indication exists for the use of low-iron formulas.

The risk of iron deficiency declines after 24 months of age because growth velocity slows, the diet becomes more diversified, and iron stores start to accumulate. After 36 months of age, dietary iron and iron status usually are adequate. However, iron deficiency can develop in either age group as a result of limited access to food (e.g., because of low income or migrant or refugee status), a low-iron or other specialized diet, or a medical condition that affects iron status (e.g., inflammatory or bleeding disorders).

Females of Childbearing Age and Adolescents

In adolescents 12 up to 18 years of age, iron requirements and the risk of iron deficiency increase because of rapid growth. Among boys, the risk subsides after the peak pubertal growth period. However, among girls and women, menstruation increases the risk of iron deficiency throughout childbearing years. In addition, heavy menstrual blood loss (80 mL or more monthly) is an important risk factor for iron-deficiency anemia in women, affecting about 10% of such women in the US. Other risk factors for iron deficiency include use of an intrauterine device (secondary to increased menstrual blood loss), high parity, previous diagnosis of iron-deficiency anemia, and low iron intake. Oral contraceptive use is associated with a decreased risk of iron deficiency. Only about 25% of adolescent girls and women of childbearing age (12–49 years old) achieve the recommended dietary allowance of iron through diet, and 11% of nonpregnant women 16–49 years of age experience iron deficiency, in about 25–50% of whom the deficiency has progressed to anemia.

Pregnancy

During the first and second trimester of pregnancy, iron-deficiency anemia is associated with a twofold increased risk of premature delivery and a threefold increased risk of a low-birthweight delivery. Although iron supplementation during pregnancy has been shown to decrease the incidence of anemia, evidence on the effect of routine iron supplementation during pregnancy on adverse maternal and infant outcomes is inconclusive. Blood volume expands by about 35% during pregnancy, and growth of the fetus, placenta, and other maternal tissues increases the iron requirement threefold during the second and third trimesters of pregnancy to about 5 mg of iron daily. Although menstruation ceases and iron absorption increases during pregnancy, most pregnant women who do not use iron supplements to meet increased iron requirements cannot maintain adequate iron stores, particularly during the last 2 trimesters. Following delivery, iron in the fetus and placenta are lost to the woman, although some of the iron in the expanded blood volume may return to blood stores. Among low-income pregnant women enrolled in health programs in the US, the prevalence of iron-deficiency anemia is 9, 14, and 37% during the first, second, and third trimesters, respectively. While similar data currently are not available for all pregnant women in the US, the low dietary iron intake among US women of childbearing age, the high prevalence of iron deficiency and associated anemia among such women, and the increased iron requirements during pregnancy suggest that anemia during pregnancy may extend beyond low-income women. In addition, use of prenatal multivitamin and mineral supplements among African-Americans, native American and Alaskan Indians, women younger than 20 years of age, and those having less than a high school education is substantially lower than in the general US pregnant population.

The principal reasons for the current lack of widespread adoption of a recommended iron supplementation regimen during pregnancy in US women may include lack of health-care provider and patient perceptions that iron supplements improve maternal and infant outcomes, complicated dose schedules, and adverse effects (e.g., constipation, nausea, vomiting). However, adequate dietary iron intake and iron supplementation generally are recommended for primary prevention of iron deficiency during pregnancy. By employing low-dose (i.e., 30 mg of iron daily) regimens with simplified dose schedules (i.e., once-daily dosing), patient compliance may be improved; low-dose regimens have been shown to increase patient tolerance and are as effective as higher dosages (e.g., 60–120 mg iron daily) in preventing iron-deficiency anemia.

Other Adults

In adults 18 years of age and older, effects of iron-deficiency anemia on daily functioning may be less overt than in children. Such anemia in laborers (e.g., tea pickers, latex tappers, cotton mill workers) in developing countries can impair work capacity, which appears to be at least partially reversible with iron therapy. Whether iron-deficiency anemia in adults affects the capacity to perform less physically demanding labor that depends on sustained cognitive or coordinated motor function remains to be elucidated. Iron-deficiency anemia also can manifest as impaired exercise capacity, lethargy, and dyspnea. Skin, nail, and other epithelial changes of chronic iron deficiency include atrophic changes of the skin, nail changes such as koilonychia (spoon-shaped nails) that manifest as brittle flattened nails, angular stomatitis (i.e., painful fissuring at the angles of the lips), glossitis, and esophageal and pharyngeal webs with associated dysphagia.

Iron-deficiency anemia is uncommon in the US among males 18 years of age and older and among postmenopausal women. The incidence of this anemia in the US is 2% or less among males 20 years of age and older and 2% among postmenopausal women. Most adults in the US with iron-deficiency anemia have GI bleeding secondary to lesions (e.g., ulcers, tumors), and about two-thirds of anemia cases among men and postmenopausal women were attributable to chronic disease or inflammatory conditions; therefore, iron-deficiency anemia in adults, unlike that in children or women of childbearing age, appears to be caused principally by an underlying disease rather than by low iron intake.

● Prevention and Treatment of Iron Deficiency

Primary prevention of iron deficiency involves ensuring adequate dietary intake of the mineral in all age groups, and selective use of iron supplementation (e.g., in individuals or groups at high risk or when adequate dietary intake is unlikely to be achieved). Primary prevention of iron deficiency is particularly important in children younger than 2 years of age and in women (including adolescents) of childbearing age, including those who are or who are not pregnant. Secondary prevention involves screening for, diagnosing, and treating iron deficiency.

Prevention of Deficiency

The normal US diet, which provides about 12 mg of iron per 2000 calories, is usually sufficient to maintain iron equilibrium in normal adult men and postmenopausal women. Fish, meat (especially liver), and fortified cereals and bread are the best dietary sources of iron. Dietary intake of iron is inadequate and prophylactic iron is required during the first year of life in infants whose diet consists largely of milk and in pregnant women; dietary iron may be marginal in menstruating women. Prophylactic iron therapy may also be required in chronic blood donors. Hemodialysis patients who are receiving therapy with an erythropoiesis-stimulating agent (ESA) (e.g., epoetin alfa, darbepoetin alfa) for anemia of chronic kidney disease may not respond adequately to oral iron therapy and may require parenteral (IV) iron replacement therapy. (See Treatment of Anemia, under Uses: Prevention and Treatment of Iron Deficiency.)

Infants and Young Children

Primary prevention of iron deficiency is most important in children younger than 2 years of age because this age group is at greatest risk for deficiency secondary to inadequate iron intake. To minimize the risk of iron deficiency in infants, exclusive breast feeding (without supplemental liquid, formula, or food) should be encouraged for 4–6 months after birth. In premature or low birthweight (less than 2.5 kg) breast-fed infants, prophylactic iron supplementation with 2–4 mg/kg (not exceeding 15 mg) daily should be initiated by at least 2 months, preferably at 1 month, of age.

When exclusive breast-feeding is stopped in full-term infants, an additional source of iron should be used (about 1 mg/kg daily of iron), preferably from supplementary foods (e.g., iron-fortified formula and/or cereals). In normal full-term infants, iron stores are usually adequate during the first few months of life, but prophylactic iron should be initiated when the infant is about 4–6 months of age. Infants who are not breast-fed or who are only partially breast-fed should receive prophylactic iron, preferably as iron-fortified formula, usually beginning at birth and continuing during the first year of life; iron-fortified formula should be the only type of infant formula used during this period, regardless of when formula-feeding is started. For breast-fed infants who receive insufficient iron from supplementary foods by 6 months of age (i.e., less than 1 mg/kg daily), iron supplementation (e.g., 1 mg/kg daily) is suggested. If breast-feeding is not possible, only iron-fortified formulas should be used during the first year of life, supplementing the formula with foods beginning at 4–6 months of age or once the extrusion reflex disappears.

To improve iron absorption, one feeding daily preferably should include foods rich in ascorbic acid (vitamin C) (e.g., fruits, vegetables, juices), by approximately 6 months of age, given with meals if possible. Plain pureed meats can be introduced to the diet after 6 months of age or when the infant is developmentally ready to consume such food. (See Cautions: Adverse Effects.) Although infants' iron requirements may be provided by use of iron-containing infant formulas or cereals, these preparations should not be relied upon to *treat* iron deficiency if it occurs. Consumption of regular cow's, goat's, or soy milk should be limited to 720 mL (24 oz) daily in children 1–5 years of age.

Older Children and Adolescents

Because of slight increases in iron requirements associated with increases in iron mass related to growth in body size, children and adolescents approximately 10 years of age and older may require prophylactic iron during the pubertal growth spurt and with the start of menstruation in females. However, most adolescents, including menstruating girls, do not require iron supplementation; instead, consumption of iron-rich foods and foods that enhance GI iron absorption should be encouraged.

Pregnant Women

Primary prevention of iron deficiency in pregnant women requires adequate dietary iron intake and iron supplementation. Although conclusive evidence of the benefits of *routine* iron supplementation for all women currently is lacking, routine prophylactic iron supplementation currently is recommended for all *pregnant* women because a large proportion of such women experience difficulty in maintaining iron stores during pregnancy, iron-deficiency anemia during pregnancy is associated with adverse outcomes, and such supplementation during pregnancy is not associated with important health risks.

Prophylactic iron supplementation during pregnancy should be initiated with oral, low-dose (30 mg daily) iron at the initial prenatal visit. Pregnant women also should be encouraged to consume iron-rich foods and foods that enhance GI iron absorption. Pregnant women with low-iron diets should be counseled about optimizing dietary iron intake. If no risk factors for iron deficiency are present at delivery, iron supplementation should be discontinued. Iron supplementation is particularly important for pregnant women who are vegetarians. Women at risk for anemia should be screened postpartum and treated as necessary.

Patients with Anemia of Chronic Kidney Disease

Almost all patients with chronic kidney disease who receive therapy with an ESA (e.g., epoetin alfa, darbepoetin alfa) will require iron therapy because of the dramatic decrease in iron stores associated with erythrocyte formation. Although chronic kidney disease patients with iron overload prior to starting ESA therapy may not require iron supplementation initially, profound iron deficiency may develop subsequently, so monitoring of serum and tissue iron stores is essential during therapy with the drug. Supplemental iron should be administered to prevent iron deficiency and to maintain adequate iron stores in patients with chronic kidney disease who are receiving ESA therapy. (See Uses: Anemia of Chronic Kidney Disease and also see Cautions: Precautions and Contraindications, in Epoetin Alfa 20:16.)

Most hemodialysis patients receiving ESAs require IV iron to maintain iron stores. (See Treatment of Anemia, under Uses: Prevention and Treatment of Iron Deficiency.) Even though a temporary improvement in hematocrit may occur with oral iron therapy, iron depletion resulting from blood loss exceeds the absorption of iron from oral supplements in most ESA-treated hemodialysis patients, and iron stores eventually decrease (as indicated by decreasing serum ferritin concentrations). As negative iron balance continues, iron stores decrease and become inadequate. Although GI absorption of iron does not appear to be impaired in patients with chronic kidney disease, only a small fraction of orally administered iron is absorbed even in individuals without the disease. Consequently, 200 mg of elemental iron (approximately two 325-mg tablets of ferrous fumarate or three 325-mg tablets of ferrous sulfate) ingested daily usually cannot meet the demands of epoetin alfa-induced erythropoiesis in hemodialysis-associated blood losses. Inadequate absorption of oral iron is exacerbated by the fact that patient compliance with oral iron regimens is often poor due to the inconvenience of dosing (i.e., 1 hour before or 2 hours after meals for optimal absorption), adverse effects such as GI irritation and constipation, and costs of therapy.

Some clinicians state that a small percentage of hemodialysis patients, and many predialysis or peritoneal dialysis patients, are able to maintain adequate iron stores using only oral iron supplements, perhaps as a result of augmented intestinal iron absorption, smaller blood losses, and/or lower epoetin alfa requirements.

Other Adults

Most nonpregnant women of childbearing age also do not require iron supplementation, but instead primary prevention of iron deficiency should be through dietary means, encouraging the consumption of iron-rich foods and foods that increase GI iron absorption. Although women with low-iron diets are at additional risk for iron deficiency, counseling such women about optimizing dietary iron intake can be sufficient. Men 18 years of age and older and postmenopausal women usually do not require iron supplementation.

Screening for Anemia

Routine screening currently is recommended by the US Centers for Disease Control (CDC) and American Academy of Pediatrics (AAP) for all infants and children from populations at high risk of iron-deficiency anemia (e.g., those from low-income families, children eligible for the Special Supplemental Nutrition program for Women, Infants, and Children [WIC], recently arrived refugees) beginning at 9–12 months of age and then 6 months later (i.e., at 15–18 months of age) and annually thereafter from 2–5 years of age. AAP also considers *routine* screening an option for all full-term infants, regardless of risk, beginning at 9–12 months of age and repeated 6 months later at 15–18 months of age; continued routine screening beyond this period is not recommended for the general pediatric population because few children older than 2 years of age develop iron deficiency.

Selective screening is recommended by CDC and AAP for selected individuals who reside in communities or under circumstances where the incidence of anemia is low (e.g., 5% or less) and there generally are good dietary practices relative to iron intake but who nonetheless are at risk for iron deficiency. Selective screening is targeted at subsets of children who have a less than satisfactory diet or have special health-care needs and should follow the same schedule as routine screening. Selective screening is recommended for premature or low-birthweight infants, infants fed a diet of nonfortified formula for longer than 2 months, infants introduced to cow's milk before 12 months of age, breast-fed infants whose supplementary diet does not provide adequate iron after 6 months of age, children who consume more than 720 mL (24 oz) of cow's milk daily, and those with special health-care needs such as conditions that interfere with iron absorption, chronic infection, inflammatory disorders, restricted (e.g., nonmeat) diets, or excessive blood loss from a wound, accident, or surgery. Although anemia screening before 6 months of age generally is of little value for detecting iron deficiency because iron stores are adequate for most infants, premature or low-birthweight infants who are not fed iron-fortified formula may benefit from beginning screening before 6 months of age. Children 2–5 years of age not previously identified as being at risk for iron deficiency should be assessed annually for risk factors (e.g., low-iron diet, limited access to food because of poverty or neglect, special health-care needs), screening those who have any such identifiable risk.

Because preadolescent school-age children 5 years of age and older in the US, other than those receiving a very restrictive diet, are at lower risk for iron deficiency than are younger children, *routine* screening for anemia in this age group is not recommended. Instead, anemia screening should be employed *selectively*. Children in this age group who consume a strict vegetarian diet should be screened for iron-deficiency anemia as should those with a history of iron-deficiency anemia, special health-care needs, or low iron intake. Likewise, adolescent males 12 up to 18 years of age generally should be screened selectively, although screening also can be considered during a routine physical examination that coincides with the peak growth period. Iron deficiency is particularly common in children consuming vegan diets, but is less common in lacto-ovo vegetarians.

All nonpregnant females should be screened for iron-deficiency anemia during all routine adolescent physical examinations and every 5–10 years throughout their childbearing years as part of routine health examinations. In addition, women with risk factors for anemia (e.g., extensive menstrual or other blood loss, low iron intake, history of iron-deficiency anemia) should be screened annually.

Pregnant women should be screened for iron-deficiency anemia during the initial prenatal visit. Postpartum women at risk for anemia also should be screened 4–6 weeks postpartum.

Routine screening for iron-deficiency anemia is not recommended for males 18 years of age and older or for postmenopausal women. Iron deficiency or anemia suspected or detected during routine medical examinations should be evaluated fully.

Treatment of Anemia

Presumed or confirmed iron-deficiency anemia should be treated with iron, preferably with oral preparations in most patients. However, hemodialysis patients with anemia of chronic kidney disease who are receiving epoetin alfa may have an inadequate response to oral iron and may require parenteral (IV) iron supplementation. (See Patients with Anemia of Chronic Kidney Disease, under Prevention and Treatment of Iron Deficiency: Treatment of Anemia, in Uses.)

Infants and Young Children

Iron-deficiency anemia can be treated presumptively in infants and preschool-age children with 3 mg/kg daily of iron; the parent or guardian should be counseled about adequate diet to correct the underlying problem of low iron intake. If anemia is confirmed by a repeat screening 4 weeks later, dietary counseling should be reinforced and iron treatment should continue for 2 more months, at which time testing should be repeated. Hemoglobin and hematocrit should be reassessed 6 months after completion of successful iron treatment. If iron deficiency is not corrected after 4 weeks of iron treatment in the absence of acute illness (e.g., otitis, diarrhea, upper respiratory tract infection), further diagnostic measures (e.g., mean corpuscular volume [MCV], erythrocyte distribution width [RDW], serum ferritin concentration) should be performed to determine whether the anemia is secondary to iron deficiency.

Older Children and Adolescents

Preadolescent school-age children and adolescent boys up to 18 years of age can be treated presumptively for iron-deficiency anemia with a trial of iron; school-age children 5 up to 12 years of age can receive 60 mg of iron daily and adolescent boys can receive 120 mg daily. Follow-up and laboratory evaluation are the same as those for infants and preschool children. Menstruating adolescent girls 12 up to

18 years of age also can be treated presumptively for anemia with a trial of 60–120 mg of iron daily. Follow-up and laboratory evaluation are the same as those for infants and preschool children, except that iron treatment should continue for 2–3 months longer if anemia is confirmed. If iron deficiency is not corrected after 4 weeks of iron treatment in the absence of acute illness, further diagnostic measures (e.g., mean corpuscular volume [MCV], erythrocyte distribution width [RDW], serum ferritin concentration) should be performed to determine whether the anemia is secondary to iron deficiency.

Pregnant Women

Iron-deficiency anemia can be treated presumptively in pregnant women with 60–120 mg of iron daily. However, if the hemoglobin concentration is less than 9 g/dL or hematocrit is less than 27%, the woman should be referred for further evaluation to a clinician familiar with anemia during pregnancy. If after 4 weeks the anemia does not respond to iron treatment to a level appropriate for the stage of pregnancy despite compliance with an iron treatment regimen in the absence of an acute illness, further diagnostic measures (e.g., mean corpuscular volume [MCV], erythrocyte distribution width [RDW], serum ferritin concentration) should be performed to determine whether the anemia is secondary to iron deficiency. When hemoglobin concentration becomes normal for the stage of pregnancy, iron treatment should be decreased to 30 mg daily. If hemoglobin concentration exceeds 15 g/dL or hematocrit exceeds 45% during the second or third trimester, the woman should be evaluated for potential pregnancy complications related to poor blood volume expansion.

Iron-deficiency anemia in postpartum women should be treated the same as that in nonpregnant women of childbearing age.

Patients with Anemia of Chronic Kidney Disease

Iron supplementation is required in virtually all patients with chronic kidney disease who are undergoing hemodialysis, particularly those receiving ESAs, because of the blood losses associated with hemodialysis and the increased demands for iron resulting from ESA-induced erythropoiesis. While some clinicians state that a trial of oral iron therapy is acceptable in hemodialysis patients, orally administered iron has been reported to be ineffective in maintaining adequate iron stores in such patients. To maintain and achieve adequate hemoglobin concentrations in hemodialysis patients, most of these patients receiving ESAs will require IV iron on a regular basis. (See Uses: Anemia of Chronic Kidney Disease and also see Cautions: Precautions and Contraindications, in Epoetin Alfa 20:16.) Oral iron therapy is not indicated for chronic kidney disease patients who requires maintenance doses of IV iron.

In predialysis and peritoneal dialysis patients with minimal daily iron losses, provision of 200 mg of elemental oral iron per day may be sufficient to replace ongoing losses and support erythropoiesis.

If oral iron is used, some experts state that use of one of the ionic iron salts, such as iron sulfate, fumarate, or gluconate, is preferable since these salts are inexpensive and provide known amounts of elemental iron. Well-controlled studies have not documented that iron polysaccharide is better tolerated (i.e., the incidence of nausea, vomiting, or abdominal discomfort leading to discontinuance is not reduced) than other iron salts.

Other Adults

Nonpregnant women of childbearing age also can be treated presumptively for anemia with a trial of 60–120 mg of iron daily. Follow-up and laboratory evaluation are the same as those for infants and preschool children, except that iron treatment should continue for 2–3 months longer if anemia is confirmed. If iron deficiency is not corrected after 4 weeks of iron treatment in the absence of acute illness, further diagnostic measures (e.g., mean corpuscular volume [MCV], erythrocyte distribution width [RDW], serum ferritin concentration) should be performed to determine whether the anemia is secondary to iron deficiency. In women of African, Mediterranean, or Southeast Asian descent, mild anemia may be secondary to thalassemia minor or sickle-cell trait.

Dietary Requirements

The National Academy of Sciences (NAS) has issued a comprehensive set of Recommended Dietary Allowances (RDAs) as reference values for dietary nutrient intakes since 1941. In 1997, the NAS Food and Nutrition Board (part of the Institute of Medicine [IOM]) announced that they would begin issuing revised nutrient recommendations that would replace RDAs with Dietary Reference Intakes (DRIs). DRIs are reference values that can be used for planning and assessing diets for healthy populations and for many other purposes and that encompass the Estimated Average Requirement (EAR), the Recommended Dietary Allowance (RDA), the Adequate Intake (AI), and the Tolerable Upper Intake Level (UL).

The NAS has established an EAR and RDA for iron for adults, children and adolescents 1–18 years of age, and infants 7–12 months of age based on the need to maintain a normal functional iron concentration but only minimal stores. Physiologic requirements for absorbed iron were calculated by factorial modeling of the components of iron requirement. Components used as factors in the modeling include basal iron losses, menstrual losses, fetal requirements in pregnancy, increased requirement during growth for expansion of blood volume, and/or increased tissue and storage iron. An AI has been established for infants through 6 months of age based on the observed mean iron intake of infants fed principally human milk. (For a definition of Estimated Average Intake, Recommended Dietary Allowance, Adequate Intake, and other reference values for dietary nutrient intakes, see Uses: Dietary Requirements in Folic Acid 88:08.)

The principal goal of maintaining an adequate intake of iron in the US and Canada is to prevent the functional consequences of iron deficiency such as impaired physical work performance, developmental delay, cognitive impairment, or adverse pregnancy outcome. Adequate intake of iron usually can be accomplished through consumption of foodstuffs; however, women usually need iron supplementation during pregnancy. Iron is present in food as part of heme (meat, poultry, fish) or as nonheme iron (vegetables, fruits, milk, cereals). Most grain products in the US are fortified with iron, and about one-half of ingested iron is supplied by iron-fortified breads, cereals, and breakfast bars.

For specific information on currently recommended AI and RDAs of iron for various life-stage and gender groups, see Dosage: Dietary and Replacement Requirements, under Dosage and Administration.

DOSAGE AND ADMINISTRATION

● Administration

Oral iron preparations generally should be taken between meals (e.g., 1 hour before or 2 hours after a meal) for maximum absorption but may be taken with or after meals, if necessary, to minimize adverse GI effects. Patients who have difficulty tolerating oral iron supplements also may benefit from smaller, more frequent doses, starting with a lower dose and increasing slowly to the target dose, trying a different form or preparation, or taking the supplement at bedtime.

● Dosage

Dosage of oral iron preparations should be expressed in terms of elemental iron. The elemental iron content of the various preparations is approximately:

TABLE 1.

Drug	Elemental Iron
ferric pyrophosphate	120 mg/g
ferrous gluconate	120 mg/g
ferrous sulfate	200 mg/g
ferrous sulfate, dried	300 mg/g
ferrous fumarate	330 mg/g
ferrous carbonate, anhydrous	480 mg/g
carbonyl iron	1000 mg/g [a]

[a] carbonyl iron is elemental iron, not an iron salt.

Treatment of Iron Deficiency

In general, large oral doses of iron, based on calculated deficiency, must be given because of the incomplete and variable absorption of these preparations. The usual therapeutic dosage of elemental iron for adults is 50–100 mg 3 times daily. Smaller dosages (e.g., 60–120 mg daily) also have been recommended, and may be particularly useful for minimizing GI intolerance, but the possibility that iron stores will be replenished at a slower rate should be considered. Iron-deficient children should receive elemental iron in a dosage of 3–6 mg/kg daily given in

3 divided doses. In patients with chronic kidney disease undergoing hemodialysis and receiving epoetin alfa therapy, some experts currently recommend oral iron in a daily dosage of at least 200 mg of elemental iron for adults and 2–3 mg/kg for children and state that the daily dosage should be given in 2 or 3 divided doses. For additional information, see Prevention and Treatment of Iron Deficiency: Treatment of Anemia, in Uses.

With usual oral therapeutic dosages of iron salts, symptoms of iron deficiency usually improve within a few days, peak reticulocytosis occurs in 5–10 days, and the hemoglobin concentration rises after 2–4 weeks. Hemoglobin production usually increases at a rate of 100–200 mg/dL of blood daily; normal hemoglobin values are usually attained in 2 months unless blood loss continues. Because iron stores remain depleted, recurrence of anemia may result if iron therapy is discontinued at this time. In the treatment of severe deficiencies, iron therapy should be continued for approximately 6 months.

If a satisfactory response is not noted after 3 weeks of oral iron therapy, consideration should be given to the possibilities of patient noncompliance, simultaneous blood loss, additional complicating factors, or incorrect diagnosis.

Prevention of Iron Deficiency

To prevent iron deficiency, pregnant women generally should receive daily iron supplementation sufficient to maintain the daily dietary iron intake at 30 mg. Normal full-term infants who are not breast-fed or are only partially breast-fed should receive supplemental iron, preferably as iron-fortified formula, in a dosage of 1 mg/kg daily starting at birth and continuing during the first year of life. Premature or low-birthweight infants require 2–4 mg/kg daily starting by at least 2 months, preferably at 1 month, of age. Infants of normal or low birthweight should not receive iron supplementation exceeding 15 mg daily. Children approximately 10 years of age and older who have begun their pubertal growth spurt may require daily iron supplementation of 2 and 5 mg daily in males and females, respectively. For additional information, see Prevention and Treatment of Iron Deficiency: Prevention of Deficiency, in Uses.

Dietary and Replacement Requirements

The Adequate Intake (AI) (see Uses: Dietary Requirements) of iron currently recommended by the National Academy of Sciences (NAS) for healthy infants through 6 months of age is 0.27 mg daily. The Recommended Dietary Allowance (RDA) of iron currently recommended by NAS for healthy children 7–12 months of age, 1–3 years, 4–8 years, or 9–13 years of age is 11, 7, 10, or 8 mg daily, respectively. The RDA of iron for boys 14–18 years of age is 11 mg daily, and the RDA for girls 14–18 years of age is 15 mg daily. The RDA for healthy men of all ages (19–70 years of age and those older than 70 years of age) is 8 mg of iron daily. The RDA for healthy women 19–50 years of age is 18 mg of iron daily, and the RDA for healthy women 51–70 years of age and those older than 70 years of age is 8 mg daily.

The RDA of iron recommended by the NAS for pregnant women 14–50 years of age is 27 mg daily. The NAS recommends an RDA of 10 or 9 mg of iron daily for lactating women 14–18 or 19–50 years of age, respectively.

CAUTIONS

• GI Effects

Usual oral therapeutic dosages of iron preparations produce constipation, diarrhea, dark stools, nausea, and/or epigastric pain in approximately 5–20% of patients. GI intolerance of all iron preparations is mainly a function of the total amount of elemental iron per dose and of psychological factors. Adverse GI effects usually subside within a few days. If necessary, they can be reduced or eliminated by ingesting iron after meals instead of between meals, by reducing the daily dosage for a few days, or by decreasing the size of the individual dose and increasing the number of doses daily.

Claims for prolonged action and reduced incidence of adverse effects with extended-release and enteric-coated preparations are not well substantiated. The low incidence of adverse effects associated with these preparations may reflect the small amount of iron released or the low total dose of elemental iron.

Large amounts of iron exert a strong corrosive action on the GI mucosa. Administration of Fero-Gradumet® has resulted in a perforated jejunal diverticulum in at least one patient and a Meckel's diverticulum with localized gangrene in

at least one other patient. Liquid iron preparations may temporarily stain dental enamel or the membrane covering the teeth of infants.

• Hemosiderosis

Long-term administration of large amounts of iron may cause hemosiderosis clinically resembling hemochromatosis, which is a genetic condition characterized by excessive iron absorption, excess tissue iron stores, and potential tissue injury. Iron overload is particularly likely to occur in patients given excessive amounts of parenteral iron, in those taking both oral and parenteral preparations, and in patients with hemoglobinopathies or other refractory anemias that might be erroneously diagnosed as iron deficiency anemia. Iron overload is associated with an increased susceptibility to certain infections (e.g., those caused by *Vibrio vulnificus*, *Yersinia enterocolitica*, or *Y. pseudotuberculosis*). Iron overload also may adversely affect prognosis in patients infected with human immunodeficiency virus (HIV). Since there is no excretory mechanism for iron, therapeutic removal by repeated phlebotomy or long-term administration of deferoxamine is necessary to prevent or reverse tissue damage if hemosiderosis occurs.

• Other Adverse Effects

Administration of iron preparations to premature infants who normally have low serum vitamin E concentrations may cause increased red cell hemolysis and hemolytic anemia. Therefore, vitamin E deficiency should also be corrected if possible. Because vitamin E may not be well absorbed from the GI tract in these infants and oral iron may reduce vitamin E absorption, IM administration of the vitamin may be advisable.

• Precautions and Contraindications

Administration of iron for longer than 6 months should be avoided except in patients with continued bleeding, menorrhagia, or repeated pregnancies. Iron should not be used to treat hemolytic anemias unless an iron-deficient state also exists, since excess storage of iron with possible secondary hemochromatosis can result. Iron should not be administered to patients receiving repeated blood transfusions, since there is a considerable amount of iron in the hemoglobin of transfused erythrocytes. Some manufacturers state that iron preparations usually are contraindicated in patients with peptic ulcer, regional enteritis, or ulcerative colitis. Parenteral iron should not be administered concomitantly with oral iron therapy.

Although primary hemochromatosis has been considered a contraindication to iron preparations, there currently is no evidence that iron fortification of foods or the use of a recommended low-dose iron supplementation regimen during pregnancy is associated with increased risk for hemochromatosis-associated clinical disease. Even when dietary iron intake is approximately average, individuals with hemochromatosis-associated iron overload will require phlebotomy to reduce their iron stores.

Because accidental overdosage of iron-containing preparations is a leading cause of fatal poisoning in children younger than 6 years of age, patients should be advised to keep such preparations out of reach of children. If accidental overdosage occurs, a poison control center or clinician should be contacted immediately.

Because iron can increase the pathogenicity of certain microorganisms and has been postulated as potentially adversely affecting prognosis in certain HIV-infected individuals, some clinicians recommend that HIV-infected individuals who do not have documented iron-deficiency anemia avoid iron supplementation for the management of HIV-associated anemia.

Fergon® 225-mg tablets contain the dye tartrazine (FD&C yellow No. 5), which may cause allergic reactions including bronchial asthma in susceptible individuals. Although the incidence of tartrazine sensitivity is low, it frequently occurs in patients who are sensitive to aspirin.

DRUG INTERACTIONS

• Antacids and Other GI Drugs

Concurrent administration of antacids or aluminum-containing phosphate binders with oral iron preparations may decrease iron absorption. Antacids and oral iron preparations should be administered as far apart as possible.

Drugs such as H_2-receptor antagonists and proton-pump inhibitors increase gastric pH and possibly may decrease the GI absorption of oral iron preparations that depend on gastric acidity for dissolution and absorption. The clinical importance of this potential interaction has not been fully determined. Some clinicians recommend that oral iron preparations be given at least 1 hour prior to these drugs if concomitant therapy is necessary.

Methyldopa

Results of one crossover study in healthy adults indicate that concomitant administration of a single oral dose of ferrous sulfate (325 mg) or ferrous gluconate (600 mg) can decrease oral absorption of methyldopa (500 mg) by 61–73%. In addition, concomitant administration of either oral iron preparation appears to affect metabolism of methyldopa since there was a 79–88% decrease in urinary excretion of free methyldopa and an increase in urinary excretion of the sulfate conjugate of the drug. When oral ferrous sulfate therapy (325 mg every 8 hours) was initiated in hypertensive patients receiving chronic methyldopa therapy (250 mg 1–3 times daily or 500 mg 3 times daily), there was an increase in blood pressure during concomitant therapy and an decrease in blood pressure when the oral iron preparation was discontinued. Although further study is needed to evaluate the clinical importance of this drug interaction, the fact that oral iron preparations apparently can decrease the hypotensive effect of methyldopa probably should be considered in situations when the drugs might be used concomitantly (e.g., pregnant women being treated for hypertension, geriatric patients with hypertension).

Quinolones

Concomitant administration of oral preparations containing iron may interfere with oral absorption of some quinolone anti-infective agents (e.g., ciprofloxacin, norfloxacin, ofloxacin) resulting in decreased serum and urine concentrations of the quinolones. Therefore, oral preparations containing iron should not be ingested concomitantly with or within 2 hours of a dose of an oral quinolone. In one crossover study, concomitant administration of a single dose of oral ferrous sulfate complex with ofloxacin decreased the area under the concentration-time curve (AUC) of the anti-infective agent by 36%.

Tetracyclines

Oral administration of iron preparations inhibits absorption of tetracyclines from the GI tract and vice versa, leading to decreased serum concentrations of both the antibiotic and iron. If simultaneous administration of the drugs is necessary, patients should receive the tetracycline 3 hours after or 2 hours before oral iron administration.

Thyroid Agents

Concomitant administration of ferrous sulfate (300 mg once daily) in patients with primary hypothyroidism receiving thyroxine replacement therapy (0.075–0.15 mg of l-thyroxine daily) resulted in an increase in serum concentrations of thyrotropin (thyroid-stimulating hormone, TSH) and increased signs and symptoms of hypothyroidism. Although the free thyroxine index (FTI) was decreased in some patients after 12 weeks of concomitant therapy, the extent of this reduction was not clinically important; free serum thyroxine concentration and resin triiodothyronine uptake (RT_3U) were not substantially affected by concomitant therapy. It has been suggested that thyroxine and ferrous sulfate (and possibly other oral iron preparations) may form an insoluble ferric-thyroxine complex in vivo resulting in decreased absorption of thyroxine. If concomitant administration of oral iron preparations and thyroxine replacement therapy is necessary (e.g., geriatric patients, premature infants, pregnant women), doses of the drugs probably should be administered at least 2 hours apart and thyroid function should be monitored.

Vitamin C

Concurrent administration of more than 200 mg of ascorbic acid per 30 mg of elemental iron increases absorption of iron from the GI tract. However, most individuals are able to absorb orally ingested iron adequately without concurrent administration of ascorbic acid, and preparations containing iron and ascorbic acid may not contain sufficient quantities of ascorbic acid to substantially affect iron absorption. Inclusion of foods rich in vitamin C in the diet of infants has been suggested as a possible means of increasing GI iron absorption.

Chloramphenicol

Response to iron therapy may be delayed in patients receiving chloramphenicol. Therefore, chloramphenicol therapy should be avoided, if possible, in patients with iron-deficiency anemia receiving iron therapy.

Penicillamine

Orally administered iron decreases the cupruretic effect of penicillamine, probably by decreasing its absorption. Therefore, at least 2 hours should elapse between administration of penicillamine and iron.

LABORATORY TEST INTERFERENCES

Iron preparations color the feces black, and large amounts may interfere with tests used for detection of occult blood in the stools. The guaiac test occasionally yields false-positive tests for blood, whereas results with the benzidine test are not likely to be affected by iron medication.

ACUTE TOXICITY

Pathogenesis

Following acute overdosage, most iron preparations are probably equally toxic per unit of elemental iron. Some studies in animals suggest that carbonyl iron may be less toxic than iron salts because of the mechanism of absorption of carbonyl iron, but comparative studies between these formulations in humans generally are lacking. The acute lethal dose of elemental iron in humans is estimated to be 180–300 mg/kg. However, a dose of elemental iron as low as 30 mg/kg may be toxic in some individuals, and ingestion of doses as low as 60 mg/kg have resulted in death.

Iron is the most common cause of pediatric poisoning deaths reported to US poison control centers. In 1991, there were 5144 cases of accidental ingestion of oral iron preparations reported; 11 of these were fatal. Although many reported fatalities in children have been associated with accidental ingestion of 30 or more tablets of an oral iron preparation containing 60 mg of elemental iron per tablet (total dose 1.8 g or more of elemental iron), ingestion of as few as 5 or 6 tablets of a high-potency preparation could be fatal for a 10-kg child. Serious toxicity and/or death have occurred after accidental ingestion of oral iron preparations as well as multivitamin preparations (including prenatal vitamins) containing iron.

Toxicity occurring with acute iron overdosage results from a combination of the corrosive effects on the GI mucosa and the metabolic and hemodynamic effects caused by the presence of excessive elemental iron.

Manifestations

The clinical course of acute iron poisoning has 4 distinct phases. Signs and symptoms may occur within 10–60 minutes or may be delayed several hours.

During the first phase, which may last 6–8 hours after ingestion, the patient experiences acute GI irritation including epigastric pain, nausea, vomiting, diarrhea of green and subsequently tarry stools, melena, and hematemesis which may be associated with drowsiness, pallor, cyanosis, lassitude, seizures, shock, and coma. Local erosion of the stomach and small intestine may result in increased iron absorption.

If death does not occur during the first phase, there may be a transient period of apparent recovery which may last up to 24 hours after ingestion (second phase). CNS abnormalities, metabolic acidosis, hepatic dysfunction or necrosis, renal failure, and bleeding diathesis occur during the third phase from 4–48 hours after ingestion and may progress to cardiovascular collapse, coma, and death.

Late complications of iron intoxication (fourth phase) occurring 2–6 weeks after overdosage include intestinal obstruction, pyloric stenosis, hepatic cirrhosis, or severe gastric scarring.

Treatment

Careful assessment of the severity of acute iron poisoning (the patient's clinical status, based on the estimated amount of iron ingested, abdominal radiographs, and measurement of serum iron concentrations and iron binding capacity) is necessary to determine appropriate management of the patient and to avoid unnecessary treatment. Patients who develop vomiting, diarrhea, leukocytosis (leukocyte count exceeding 15,000/mm³), hyperglycemia (blood glucose concentration exceeding 150 mg/dL), and/or an abdominal radiograph positive for iron within 6 hours of iron ingestion are likely to have a serum iron concentration exceeding 300 mcg/dL and to be at risk of serious toxicity, while those who do not develop any of these signs are unlikely to have a serum iron concentration exceeding 300 mcg/dL or to be at risk of toxicity requiring treatment. A negative deferoxamine challenge (see Deferoxamine Mesylate 64:00) or iron screening test obtained within 2 hours of ingestion also indicates that the patient has not ingested a clinically important amount of iron and probably does not require further assessment or treatment.

If ingestion exceeding 10 mg/kg of elemental iron has occurred within the previous 4 hours, the stomach should be emptied immediately by ipecac-induced emesis or, preferably, by lavage with a large bore tube. If the patient has had multiple episodes of vomiting, and especially if the vomitus contains blood, ipecac syrup should not be administered. Gastric lavage should be performed with tepid water or 1–5% sodium bicarbonate solution. Gastric lavage with disodium phosphate solution has also been used; however, administration of large volumes of this lavage solution has produced life-threatening hyperphosphatemia and hypocalcemia in some children. Although some clinicians suggest that use of sodium bicarbonate solution for gastric lavage generally appears to have no advantage compared with water for the treatment of iron overdose, the value of sodium bicarbonate solution in reducing iron absorption via formation of insoluble iron complexes remains to be established. Deferoxamine has also been used as an additive to gastric lavage solutions to chelate elemental iron in the GI tract; however, the efficacy of this procedure has not been clearly established. (See Deferoxamine Mesylate 64:00.) The possibility that gastric lavage may not remove enteric-coated and/or extended-release preparations should be considered. Whole gut lavage with 0.9% sodium chloride solution, administration of a saline cathartic, or surgical removal of iron tablets (which are visible in abdominal radiographs) may be required if other methods of removing the drug are unsuccessful. Hemodialysis is of little value in the treatment of iron intoxication.

When a potentially lethal dose of iron (180–300 mg/kg or more of elemental iron) has been ingested, serum iron concentrations exceed 400–500 mcg/dL or serum iron concentrations exceed total iron binding capacity, and/or the patient has severe symptoms of iron intoxication such as coma, shock, or seizures, chelation therapy with deferoxamine should be initiated. (See Deferoxamine Mesylate 64:00.) Supportive treatment including suction and maintenance of airway, correction of acidosis, and control of shock and dehydration with IV fluids or blood, oxygen, and vasopressors should be administered as required.

PHARMACOLOGY

Iron is present in all cells and has several vital functions. Ionic iron is a component of a number of enzymes necessary for energy transfer (e.g., cytochrome oxidase, xanthine oxidase, succinic dehydrogenase) and is also present in compounds necessary for transport and utilization of oxygen (e.g., hemoglobin, myoglobin). Cytochromes serve as a transport medium for electrons within cells. Hemoglobin is a carrier of oxygen from the lungs to tissues and myoglobin facilitates oxygen use and storage in muscle. Iron deficiency can interfere with these vital functions and lead to morbidity and mortality.

Administration of iron preparations corrects erythropoietic abnormalities caused by a deficiency of iron. Iron does not stimulate erythropoiesis nor does it correct hemoglobin disturbances not caused by iron deficiency. Administration of iron also relieves other manifestations of iron deficiency such as soreness of the tongue, dysphagia, dystrophy of the nails and skin, and fissuring of the angles of the lips.

Iron is vital for microorganisms such as bacteria, and the mineral plays a role both in bacterial pathogenicity and in host defense mechanisms. (See Cautions: Hemosiderosis.)

PHARMACOKINETICS

● Absorption

Regulation of iron balance occurs mainly in the GI tract through absorption. When GI absorption is normal, functional iron is maintained and there is a tendency to establish iron stores.

Absorption of iron is complex and is influenced by many factors including the form in which it is administered, the dose, iron stores, the degree of erythropoiesis, and diet. Oral bioavailability of iron can vary from less than 1% to greater than 50%, and the principal factor controlling GI iron absorption is the amount of iron stored in the body. GI absorption of iron increases when body iron stores are low and decreases when stores are sufficient or large. Increased erythrocyte production also can stimulate GI absorption of iron by severalfold.

Approximately 5–13% of dietary iron is absorbed in healthy individuals and about 10–30% in iron-deficient individuals. Among adults, dietary iron absorption averages approximately 6% for males and 13% for nonpregnant females of childbearing potential; the higher GI absorption efficiency in these women principally results from lower body stores secondary to menstruation and pregnancy. GI absorption of iron increases during pregnancy to compensate for tissue growth and blood loss at delivery and postpartum, but the extent of this increase is not well defined; as iron stores become replenished postpartum, GI iron absorption decreases. GI iron absorption also is increased in iron-deficient individuals. As much as 60% of a therapeutic dose of an iron salt may be absorbed in iron-deficient patients; however, absorption of inorganic iron is decreased when it is administered with many foods and with some drugs. (See Drug Interactions.)

Inorganic iron reportedly is absorbed up to twice as well as dietary iron. Although the precise form in which iron is absorbed has not been elucidated, ferrous iron appears to be most readily absorbed. Oral bioavailability of iron also depends on dietary composition. Heme iron, which is present in meat, poultry, and fish, is absorbed 2–3 times more readily than non-heme iron, which is present in plant-based and iron-fortified foods. GI absorption of iron can be enhanced by dietary heme iron and vitamin C and can be inhibited by polyphenols (e.g., from certain vegetables), tannins (e.g., from tea), phytates (e.g., from bran), and calcium (e.g., from dairy products). Vegetarian diets are low in heme iron, but iron bioavailability can be increased by including other sources of iron and enhancers of GI iron absorption. Prior to the introduction of solid foods into the diet, the amount of iron absorbed in infants depends on the amount of iron present in breast milk or formula.

Although absorption of iron can occur along the entire length of the GI tract, it is greatest in the duodenum and proximal jejunum and becomes progressively less distally. Enteric-coated and some extended-release preparations may transport iron past the duodenum and proximal jejunum, thus reducing iron absorption.

Following oral administration, carbonyl iron is dissolved in gastric secretions (i.e., hydrochloric acid) and converted to the hydrochloride salt prior to absorption from the stomach. The rate of absorption is affected by gastric acid production and the equilibrium between the formation of ionized iron and passage of the ionized iron to the intestine. Also affecting absorption is the particle size of carbonyl iron; a smaller particle size will be ionized more rapidly and thus absorbed more rapidly than formulations with a larger particle size.

The mechanisms involved in iron absorption have not been completely elucidated; however, two mechanisms, which are believed to operate simultaneously, appear to be involved. An active transport process with enzymatic or carrier characteristics occurs principally with normal dietary concentrations of iron; a first-order passive transport process occurs principally with doses of iron exceeding those in a normal diet.

● Distribution

Ferrous iron passes through GI mucosal cells directly into the blood and is immediately bound to transferrin. Transferrin, a glycoprotein β_1-globulin, transports iron to the bone marrow where it is incorporated into hemoglobin. When sufficient iron is present to meet the body's needs, most iron (greater than 70%) in the body is present as functional iron, with greater than 80% of functional iron existing in erythrocytes as hemoglobin and the rest existing in myoglobin and intracellular respiratory enzymes (e.g., cytochromes); less than 1% of total body iron is present in enzymes. The remainder of body iron is present as storage or transport iron. Total body iron is determined by intake, loss, and storage of the mineral.

Small excesses of iron within the villous epithelial cells are oxidized to the ferric state. Ferric iron combines with the protein apoferritin to yield ferritin and is stored in mucosal cells, which are exfoliated at the end of their life span and excreted in the feces. Ferritin, a soluble protein complex, is the principal storage form of iron (about 70% in men and 80% in women), with smaller amounts being stored in hemosiderin, an insoluble protein complex. Ferritin and hemosiderin are present principally in the liver, reticuloendothelial system, bone marrow, spleen, and skeletal muscle; small amounts of ferritin also circulate in plasma. When long-term negative iron balance occurs, iron stores are depleted before hemoglobin concentration is reduced or iron deficiency ensues. In women, the iron storage reserve tends to be substantially less than that in men (about 0.2–0.4 g versus 1–4 g of iron), and is even less in children. Total body iron in full-term infants with normal or high birthweight is relatively high (averaging 75 mg/kg), to which iron stores contribute about 25%. Premature or low-birthweight infants are born with the same ratio of total body iron to body weight, but the amount of stored iron is low because of low body weight.

The body of a healthy adult man contains approximately 3.8 g total or 50 mg/kg; that of an adult woman contains about 2.3 g total or 35–42 mg/kg. Iron exists in humans almost exclusively complexed to protein or in heme molecules. Approximately 70% is in hemoglobin, 25% in iron stores as ferritin and hemosiderin, 4% in myoglobin, 0.5% in heme enzymes, and 0.1% in transferrin. Erythrocyte formation and destruction is responsible for most iron turnover in the body. In adult males, about 95% of the iron required for erythropoiesis is recycled from the breakdown of erythrocytes and only 5% comes from oral intake. In infants, about 70% of iron required for erythropoiesis is recycled from the breakdown of erythrocytes and about 30% from oral intake.

About 0.15–0.3 mg of iron is distributed into milk daily.

Transfer of iron across the placenta is believed to be an active process since it occurs against a concentration gradient. The total iron requirement for pregnancy may be 440 mg to 1.05 g.

● Elimination

Iron metabolism occurs in a virtually closed system. Most of the iron liberated by destruction of hemoglobin is conserved and reused by the body. Daily excretion of iron in healthy men amounts to only 0.5–2 mg. This excretion occurs principally through feces and as desquamation of cells such as skin, GI mucosa, nails, and hair; only trace amounts of iron are excreted in bile and sweat.

Blood loss greatly increases iron loss. The average monthly loss of iron in normal menstruation is 12–30 mg, increasing the average iron requirement by 0.3–0.5 mg daily to compensate for this loss. The increased requirement secondary to pregnancy-associated tissue growth and blood loss at delivery and postpartum averages 3 mg daily over 280 days of gestation. In healthy individuals, trace amounts of blood are lost through physiologic GI loss secondary to normal turnover of intestinal mucosa. Pathologic GI blood loss occurs in infants and children sensitive to cow's milk and in adults secondary to peptic ulcer disease, inflammatory bowel syndrome, and GI cancer. Hookworm infections also are associated with blood loss.

CHEMISTRY AND STABILITY

● Chemistry

Ferrous fumarate, ferrous gluconate, ferrous sulfate, carbonyl iron, and polysaccharide-iron complex are commercially available in the US for oral administration in the prevention and treatment of iron deficiency. Ferric pyrophosphate and ferrous carbonate are available only as components of combination products.

Ferrous Fumarate

Ferrous fumarate occurs as a reddish-orange to red-brown, odorless powder. It may contain soft lumps that produce a yellow streak when crushed. The drug is slightly soluble in water and very slightly soluble in alcohol.

Ferrous Gluconate

Ferrous gluconate occurs as a yellowish-gray or pale greenish-yellow fine powder or granules with a slight odor of burned sugar. The drug is soluble in water with slight heating and practically insoluble in alcohol.

Ferrous Sulfate

Ferrous sulfate occurs as pale bluish-green, odorless crystals or granules which have a saline, styptic taste. The drug is efflorescent in dry air. Ferrous sulfate is freely soluble in water and insoluble in alcohol. Dried ferrous sulfate, which contains 86–89% anhydrous ferrous sulfate, occurs as a grayish-white to buff-colored powder which dissolves slowly in water and is insoluble in alcohol. Ferrous sulfate contains 7 molecules of water of hydration; dried ferrous sulfate consists mainly of the monohydrate with varying amounts of the tetrahydrate.

Carbonyl Iron

Carbonyl iron consists of microparticles of elemental iron; it is not an iron salt. Carbonyl iron is produced by a manufacturing process involving the controlled heating of vaporized iron pentacarbonyl, which is designed to result in the deposition of unchanged elemental iron as microscopic spheres of less than 5 μm in diameter. Carbonyl iron prepared for pharmaceutical or nutritional use in the US reportedly has an average particle size of 5–6 μm.

Polysaccharide-Iron Complex

Polysaccharide-iron complex occurs as an amorphous brown powder and is very soluble in water and insoluble in alcohol.

● Stability

Ferrous Sulfate

In moist air, ferrous sulfate rapidly oxidizes and becomes coated with brownish-yellow ferric sulfate which must not be used medicinally. The rate of oxidation is increased by the addition of alkali or by exposure to light.

PREPARATIONS

Excipients in commercially available drug preparations may have clinically important effects in some individuals; consult specific product labeling for details.

Carbonyl Iron

Oral		
Suspension	15 mg (of iron) per 1.25 mL	**Icar® Pediatric**, Hawthorn
Tablets	45 mg (of iron)	**Feosol® Caplets**, GlaxoSmithKline
Tablets, chewable	15 mg (of iron)	**Icar® Pediatric**, Hawthorn

Ferrous Fumarate

Oral		
Tablets	200 mg (66 mg iron)	**Ircon®**, Kenwood
	324 mg (106 mg iron)*	**Hemocyte®**, US Pharmaceutical
	325 mg (107 mg iron)*	**Ferrous Fumarate Tablets**
	350 mg (115 mg iron)	**Nephro-Fer®**, R&D Labs
Tablets, chewable	100 mg (33 mg iron)	**Feostat®**, Forest

* available from one or more manufacturer, distributor, and/or repackager by generic (nonproprietary) name

Ferrous Fumarate Combinations

Oral		
Capsules, extended-release	150 mg (50 mg iron) with Docusate Sodium 100 mg*	**Ferrous Fumarate with DSS® Timed Capsules**, Vita-Rx
Tablets, extended-release, film-coated	150 mg (50 mg iron) with Docusate Sodium 100 mg	**Ferro-DSS® Caplets®**, Time-Caps
		Ferro-Sequels®, Inverness

* available from one or more manufacturer, distributor, and/or repackager by generic (nonproprietary) name

Ferrous Gluconate

Powder		
Oral		
Tablets	225 mg (27 mg iron)	**Fergon®**, Bayer
		Ferrous Gluconate Tablets
	300 mg (35 mg iron)	**Ferrous Gluconate Tablets**
	320 mg (37 mg iron)*	
	325 mg (38 mg iron)*	

* available from one or more manufacturer, distributor, and/or repackager by generic (nonproprietary) name

Ferrous Sulfate

Powder

Oral

Solution	220 mg (44 mg iron) per 5 mL*	Ferrous Sulfate Elixir
	300 mg (60 mg iron) per 5 mL	Ferrous Sulfate Solution
	125 mg (25 mg iron) per mL*	Fer-Gen-Sol® Drops, Teva
		Fer-In-Sol® Drops, Mead Johnson
Tablets	195 mg (39 mg iron)*	Mol-Iron®, Schering-Plough
	300 mg (60 mg iron)*	Feratab®, Upsher-Smith
	325 mg (65 mg iron)*	
Tablets, enteric-coated	325 mg (65 mg iron)*	Ferrous Sulfate Tablets EC
Tablets, film-coated	325 mg (65 mg iron)	Ferrous Sulfate Tablets

* available from one or more manufacturer, distributor, and/or repackager by generic (nonproprietary) name

Ferrous Sulfate, Dried

Oral

Capsules	190 mg (60 mg iron)	
Tablets	200 mg (65 mg iron)	Feosol®, GlaxoSmithKline
Tablets, extended-release	160 mg (50 mg iron)	Slow FE®, Novartis

Polysaccharide-iron Complex

Oral

Capsules	150 mg (of iron)	Ferrex®-150, Breckenridge
		Fe-Tinic® 150, Ethex
		Hytinic®, Hyrex
		Niferex®-150, Ther-Rx
Solution	100 mg (of iron) per 5 mL	Niferex® Elixir, Ther-Rx
Tablets, film-coated	50 mg (of iron)	Niferex®, Ther-Rx

Oral iron preparations are also commercially available in combination with vitamins and minerals and oral contraceptives.

Iron Sucrose

20:04.04 • IRON PREPARATIONS

■ Iron sucrose, a polynuclear iron (III)-hydroxide sucrose complex, is used to replenish and maintain the total body content of iron and has pharmacologic actions similar to those of other parenteral iron preparations.

USES

● Iron Deficiency Anemia in Patients with Chronic Kidney Disease

Iron sucrose injection is used for the treatment of iron deficiency anemia in patients with chronic kidney disease, including those who are undergoing dialysis (hemodialysis or peritoneal) and those who do not require dialysis. In several randomized controlled studies comparing IV and oral administration of iron in patients with chronic kidney disease undergoing hemodialysis, IV iron was superior to orally administered iron in increasing hemoglobin concentrations and/or minimizing the dosage of an erythropoiesis-stimulating agent (ESA) (e.g., epoetin alfa) required to maintain target hemoglobin levels; guidelines for the treatment of anemia of chronic kidney disease from the National Kidney Foundation Kidney Disease Outcomes Quality Initiative (NKF-KDOQI) state that the IV route is preferred for administration of iron in patients with chronic kidney disease undergoing hemodialysis. (See Uses: Iron Deficiency Anemia in Hemodialysis Patients Receiving Epoetin Alfa Therapy, in Sodium Ferric Gluconate 20:04.04.) Although published clinical studies do not permit a reliable comparison of iron sucrose with other parenteral iron preparations (e.g., iron dextran, sodium ferric gluconate), it has been suggested that these iron preparations may have comparable efficacy but different safety profiles. Available data suggest that iron sucrose and sodium ferric gluconate may be associated less frequently with serious adverse effects (e.g., hypersensitivity reactions) than iron dextran. (See Sensitivity Reactions under Warnings/Precautions: Warnings, in Cautions and also see Cautions: Sensitivity Reactions, in Sodium Ferric Gluconate 20:04.04.)

Efficacy and safety of iron sucrose injection for the treatment of iron deficiency anemia have been established in several open-label, multicenter clinical trials in patients with chronic kidney disease, both in dialysis-dependent (hemodialysis or peritoneal dialysis) adults and in adults who did not require dialysis (non-dialysis dependent). In dialysis-dependent patients, increases in mean hemoglobin, hematocrit, serum ferritin, and transferrin saturation (TSAT) from baseline were observed following iron sucrose therapy (e.g., consisting of 100-mg doses given at consecutive dialysis treatment sessions for a cumulative elemental iron dosage of 1 g); most patients in these studies were receiving an ESA prior to study enrollment and continued to receive such therapy at either the same dosage or an adjusted dosage based on study protocol or the investigator's discretion. In one of these studies, 66% of hemodialysis patients receiving iron sucrose therapy achieved a target hemoglobin concentration exceeding 11 g/dL within 5 weeks of completing iron sucrose therapy (the primary study end point); 78% of patients attained this target hemoglobin level at one or more intervals after the treatment period. Compared with a historical control group of patients with similar ferritin levels who were receiving epoetin alfa but who had not received IV iron for at least 2 weeks, patients receiving iron sucrose therapy in this study achieved greater increases in hemoglobin and hematocrit; the mean change in hemoglobin concentration at the 5-week follow-up evaluation was 1.2 or –0.1 g/dL for the iron sucrose or historical control group, respectively. In another study in patients with hemodialysis-dependent chronic kidney disease, substantial increases from baseline in mean hemoglobin (1.7 g/dL), hematocrit (5%), serum ferritin (434.6 ng/mL), and TSAT (14%) were observed by week 2 of the observation period and maintained at week 4 (the final evaluation). Results of a study comparing IV iron and an ESA with ESA therapy alone in patients undergoing peritoneal dialysis demonstrated superiority of the iron sucrose/ESA regimen compared with ESA alone in increasing mean hemoglobin concentrations from baseline. In a study conducted in non-dialysis-dependent chronic kidney disease patients, treatment with iron sucrose (with or without ESA therapy) was more effective than an oral iron preparation (i.e., ferrous sulfate) in increasing hemoglobin concentrations. Response to IV iron appears to be more vigorous in patients with TSATs less than 20% compared with those having higher TSATs.

Iron sucrose injection also is used as iron *maintenance* therapy in children with dialysis-dependent (hemodialysis or peritoneal dialysis) or non-dialysis-dependent chronic kidney disease. (See Pediatric Use under Warnings/Precautions: Specific Populations, in Cautions.)

DOSAGE AND ADMINISTRATION

● General

Iron sucrose is administered by slow IV injection or IV infusion.

When given by IV injection, the drug is administered undiluted at a slow rate (e.g., over 2–5 minutes). (See Cardiovascular Effects under Warnings/Precautions: Warnings, in Cautions.)

When given by IV infusion, iron sucrose should be diluted in 0.9% sodium chloride injection; specific recommendations for dilution and administration of the drug by IV infusion vary depending on the intended patient population (e.g., hemodialysis-dependent adults, peritoneal dialysis-dependent adults, non-dialysis-dependent adults, pediatric patients). (See Dosage and Administration: Dosage.) Iron sucrose injection should not be mixed with other drugs or added to parenteral nutrition solutions for IV infusion. Iron sucrose injection and diluted solutions of the drug should be inspected visually for particulate matter and discoloration prior to administration whenever solution and container permit.

Although the manufacturer does not make any specific recommendations regarding a test dose of iron sucrose, test doses of 20–25 or 50 mg have been administered in some clinical trials. (See Sensitivity Reactions under Warnings/Precautions: Warnings, in Cautions.) The manufacturer states that personnel trained to provide emergency treatment and appropriate agents for the treatment of a severe allergic or anaphylactic reaction should be immediately available whenever iron sucrose is administered.

● Dosage

Dosage of iron sucrose is expressed in terms of mg of elemental iron. Iron sucrose injection contains the equivalent of 20 mg of elemental iron per mL.

For the treatment of iron deficiency anemia in hemodialysis-dependent adults with chronic kidney disease, the recommended dosage of iron sucrose is 100 mg administered by slow IV injection (over 2–5 minutes) or by IV infusion (diluted in a maximum of 100 mL of 0.9% sodium chloride injection) over at least 15 minutes during each consecutive hemodialysis session. Doses should be administered early during the dialysis procedure. A cumulative dose of 1 g of iron sucrose usually is required to achieve a favorable response in these patients.

In peritoneal dialysis-dependent adults with chronic kidney disease, a series of 3 doses of iron sucrose should be administered by IV infusion (diluted in a maximum of 250 mL of 0.9% sodium chloride injection) 14 days apart over a 28-day period. Patients should receive 300 mg of iron sucrose by IV infusion over 1.5 hours for the first 2 doses, followed by a dose of 400 mg administered over 2.5 hours.

For the treatment of iron deficiency anemia in adults with non-dialysis-dependent chronic kidney disease, the recommended dosage of iron sucrose is 200 mg administered by slow IV injection (over 2–5 minutes) or by IV infusion (diluted in a maximum of 100 mL of 0.9% sodium chloride injection and administered over 15 minutes) for a total of 5 doses; doses should be administered on 5 different occasions over a 14-day period. Iron sucrose also has been administered as a 2-dose regimen in a limited number of patients with non-dialysis-dependent chronic kidney disease; in this regimen, 500 mg of iron sucrose is administered by IV infusion (diluted in a maximum of 250 mL of 0.9% sodium chloride injection and administered over 3.5–4 hours) on days 1 and 14.

For iron *maintenance* therapy in children 2 years of age or older with hemodialysis-dependent chronic kidney disease, the recommended dosage of iron sucrose is 0.5 mg/kg (not to exceed 100 mg per dose) every 2 weeks for 12 weeks; doses may be administered undiluted by slow IV injection over 5 minutes or diluted in 25 mL of 0.9% sodium chloride injection and administered over 5–60 minutes.

For iron *maintenance* therapy in children 2 years of age or older with non-dialysis-dependent chronic kidney disease or peritoneal dialysis-dependent chronic kidney disease who are receiving supplemental erythropoiesis-stimulating agent (ESA) therapy, the recommended dosage of iron sucrose is 0.5 mg/kg (not to exceed 100 mg per dose) every 4 weeks for 12 weeks; doses may be administered undiluted by slow IV injection over 5 minutes or diluted in 25 mL of 0.9% sodium chloride injection and administered over 5–60 minutes.

If necessary, iron sucrose treatments may be repeated.

Special Populations

Dosage should be selected carefully for geriatric patients 65 years of age and older because of limited experience with iron sucrose in these patients and the greater frequency of decreased hepatic, renal, and cardiac function and of concomitant disease and/or other drug therapies.

CAUTIONS

Contraindications

Known hypersensitivity to iron sucrose or any ingredient in the formulation.

Warnings/Precautions

Warnings

Sensitivity Reactions

Hypersensitivity reactions, including anaphylactic shock, loss of consciousness, collapse, hypotension, dyspnea, and seizures, have been reported in patients receiving iron sucrose therapy. In some cases, serious or fatal reactions have occurred. If hypersensitivity reactions or signs of intolerance develop during iron sucrose therapy, immediate drug discontinuance and medical intervention is required. Since hypersensitivity reactions associated with IV iron preparations tend to occur within 30 minutes after completion of an infusion, patients should be observed for at least this period of time until they are clinically stable. (See Dosage and Administration: General.)

Cardiovascular Effects

Iron sucrose may cause clinically important hypotension. Patients should be observed closely for signs and symptoms of hypotension during and following administration of the drug. Hypotension associated with IV administration of iron sucrose may be minimized by adhering to recommended total doses and rates of administration. (See Dosage and Administration.)

General Precautions

Iron Toxicity

Because body iron excretion is limited and excessive iron in tissues can be hazardous, iron sucrose should not be administered to patients with evidence suggesting iron overload. Periodic monitoring of laboratory values indicative of iron storage in the body (e.g., transferrin saturation, serum ferritin concentrations, hemoglobin, hematocrit) may assist in the recognition of iron accumulation. Because transferrin saturation values increase rapidly after IV administration of iron sucrose, serum iron measurements should not be performed until at least 48 hours after the drug is administered.

Specific Populations

Pregnancy

Category B. (See Users Guide.)

Lactation

It is not known whether iron sucrose is distributed into milk. Caution is advised if the drug is administered in nursing women.

Pediatric Use

Efficacy and safety of iron sucrose for iron maintenance therapy have been established in children 2 years of age or older with dialysis-dependent or non dialysis-dependent-chronic kidney disease. In a 12-week open-label, dose-ranging study in pediatric patients with chronic kidney disease (dialysis-dependent or non-dialysis dependent) who were receiving stable dosages of an erythropoiesis-stimulating agent (ESA), treatment with iron sucrose maintained hemoglobin concentrations between 10.5 and 14 g/dL in approximately 45–59% of the patients receiving 0.5, 1, or 2 mg/kg of the drug; a dose-response relationship was not demonstrated. Safety and efficacy of iron sucrose for iron *replacement* therapy in pediatric patients with chronic kidney disease have not been established.

Experience principally in another country revealed that 5 premature neonates (each weighing less than 1250 g) who received iron sucrose developed necrotizing enterocolitis; 2 of the 5 infants died during or following a period during which they received epoetin alfa, iron sucrose, and several other drugs concomitantly. A causal relationship to iron sucrose or any of the drugs could not be established.

Geriatric Use

Experience in those 65 years of age and older insufficient to determine whether they respond differently from younger adults; use caution in selecting and adjusting dosage. (See Dosage and Administration: Special Populations.)

Concomitant Disease States

Clinicians should consider that clinical studies in which the effects of iron sucrose were established generally excluded patients with serious underlying disease, inflammatory conditions, or active infections.

Common Adverse Effects

Adverse effects occurring in 2% or more of patients receiving iron sucrose injection include diarrhea, nausea, vomiting, headache, dizziness, hypotension, pruritus, extremity pain, arthralgia, back pain, muscle cramp, injection site reactions, chest pain, and peripheral edema.

DRUG INTERACTIONS

Oral Iron Preparations

Potential pharmacokinetic interaction (reduced absorption of concomitantly administered oral iron).

DESCRIPTION

Iron sucrose (iron sucrose complex) is a polynuclear iron(III)-hydroxide sucrose complex with a molecular weight of approximately 34,000–60,000. Iron sucrose is used to replenish and maintain the total body content of iron and has pharmacologic actions similar to those of other parenteral iron preparations (e.g., iron dextran, sodium ferric gluconate). Unlike iron dextran, however, iron sucrose is free of ferrous ions and dextran polysaccharides, which are believed to be antigenic stimuli for anaphylactic reactions.

Following IV administration of iron sucrose, the drug is dissociated into iron and sucrose by the reticuloendothelial system. It has been suggested that the release of iron from iron sucrose is more rapid than that from iron dextran but less rapid than that from sodium ferric gluconate. In a limited number of hemodialysis patients receiving iron sucrose dosages equivalent to 100 mg of elemental iron 3 times weekly for 3 weeks, substantial increases in serum iron and serum ferritin and decreases in total iron binding capacity occurred within 4 weeks from initiation of iron therapy.

ADVICE TO PATIENTS

Risk of potentially fatal sensitivity (e.g., anaphylactoid) reactions. (See Sensitivity Reactions under Warnings/Precautions: Warnings, in Cautions.) Risk of hypotension. Importance of informing clinicians of existing or contemplated concomitant therapy, including prescription and OTC drugs.

PREPARATIONS

Excipients in commercially available drug preparations may have clinically important effects in some individuals; consult specific product labeling for details.

Iron Sucrose

Parenteral

For injection, for IV infusion	equivalent to 20 mg of elemental iron per mL	Venofer®, American Regent

Selected Revisions November 4, 2013, © Copyright, September 1, 2001, American Society of Health-System Pharmacists, Inc.

Sodium Ferric Gluconate

20:04.04 • IRON PREPARATIONS

■ Sodium ferric gluconate, a stable macromolecular complex composed of ferric oxide hydrate directly bonded to sucrose and chelated with gluconate, is used to replenish and maintain the total body content of iron and has pharmacologic actions similar to those of other parenteral iron preparations.

USES

Iron Deficiency Anemia in Hemodialysis Patients Receiving Epoetin Alfa Therapy

Sodium ferric gluconate is used for the treatment of iron deficiency anemia in adults and children 6 years of age or older with chronic kidney disease who are undergoing hemodialysis and receiving supplemental epoetin alfa therapy. Patients undergoing hemodialysis lose an estimated 1–3 g of iron annually as a result of blood loss from repeated laboratory tests, blood retention in the dialyzer equipment, and the bleeding diathesis associated with anticoagulants used during dialysis. In addition, epoetin alfa therapy results in an increased demand for iron by stimulating erythroid marrow; virtually all patients receiving epoetin alfa therapy will require supplemental iron therapy. (See Uses: Anemia of Chronic Kidney Disease, in Epoetin Alfa 20:16.) Orally administered iron has been reported to be ineffective in maintaining adequate iron stores in hemodialysis patients during epoetin alfa therapy. In several randomized controlled studies comparing IV and oral administration of iron in patients with chronic kidney disease undergoing hemodialysis, IV iron was found to be superior to orally administered iron in increasing hemoglobin concentrations and/or minimizing the dosage of an erythropoiesis-stimulating agent (ESA) (e.g., epoetin alfa) required to maintain target hemoglobin levels; guidelines for the treatment of anemia of chronic kidney disease from the National Kidney Foundation Kidney Disease Outcomes Quality Initiative (NKF-KDOQI) state that the IV route is preferred for administration of iron in patients with chronic kidney disease undergoing hemodialysis. The goal of iron therapy is achievement of the target hematocrit/hemoglobin with the lowest dosage of epoetin alfa necessary to stimulate erythropoiesis.

One of the most important factors in patient response to epoetin alfa therapy is iron status. Current evidence indicates that regular administration of parenteral iron improves the erythroid response to epoetin alfa and generally allows attainment of the target hematocrit at lower epoetin alfa dosages. In addition, appropriate use of iron therapy may minimize the fluctuation of hematocrit/hemoglobin concentrations compared with manipulation of epoetin alfa dosage as the principal means of managing anemia. (See Uses: Anemia of Chronic Kidney Disease, in Epoetin Alfa 20:16.)

The current FDA-labeled indication for sodium ferric gluconate in the treatment of iron deficiency anemia in hemodialysis patients receiving epoetin alfa is based principally on 2 clinical trials of approximately 50 days' duration in adults and one clinical trial in pediatric patients.

In a randomized, open-label study, patients undergoing chronic hemodialysis and receiving stable dosages of epoetin alfa were given an IV test dose of sodium ferric gluconate equivalent to 25 mg of elemental iron. Patients then received sodium ferric gluconate IV in either a low-dose (62.5 mg in 50 mL of 0.9% sodium chloride injection over 30 minutes) or high-dose (125 mg in 100 mL of 0.9% sodium chloride injection over 60 minutes) regimen for 8 doses during sequential dialysis sessions over a period of 16–17 days (cumulative dosage equivalent to 500 or 1000 mg, respectively, of elemental iron). Efficacy of iron replacement therapy in this study was evaluated based on a primary end point of change in hemoglobin from baseline to the last available observation through day 40. Patients receiving high-dose sodium ferric gluconate therapy had greater increases in hemoglobin, hematocrit, and iron saturation at all time points during the study than patients receiving low-dose sodium ferric gluconate or oral iron therapy. Fourteen days after completion of iron therapy, the mean change in hematocrit and hemoglobin in patients receiving high-dose sodium ferric gluconate therapy was 3.6% and 1.1 g/dL, respectively. Increases in hematocrit and hemoglobin in patients receiving low-dose sodium ferric gluconate therapy (1.4% and 0.3 g/dL, respectively) were similar to those in patients who received oral iron therapy (0.8% and 0.4 g/dL, respectively).

A smaller, nonrandomized study in iron-deficient hemodialysis patients receiving variable, cumulative doses of sodium ferric gluconate IV also demonstrated appreciable increases in hematocrit and hemoglobin compared with those produced by oral iron therapy. In this study, a total of 14 patients (37%) completed the study protocol (receiving at least 8 doses of either low- or high-dose IV sodium ferric gluconate); the remainder received less than 8 doses (32%) or had incomplete information on the sequence of dosing (32%). An unspecified number of patients also failed to receive the drug at consecutive dialysis sessions, and many received oral iron during the study.

In a randomized, open-label study in iron-deficient pediatric patients 6–15 years of age (mean age: 12 years) who were undergoing chronic hemodialysis and receiving stable dosages of epoetin alfa, sodium ferric gluconate in doses equivalent to 1.5 or 3 mg/kg of elemental iron (maximum dose of elemental iron not exceeding 125 mg) was administered IV in 25 mL of 0.9% sodium chloride injection over 1 hour during each of 8 sequential dialysis sessions. The primary end point in this study was change in hemoglobin from baseline to 2 weeks after the last dose of sodium ferric gluconate. Two weeks after completion of iron therapy, the mean change in hemoglobin in patients receiving 1.5 mg/kg or 3 mg/kg of elemental iron was 0.8 or 0.9 g/dL, respectively; increased hemoglobin concentrations were maintained at 4 weeks after the final dose of sodium ferric gluconate in both treatment groups. Patients receiving either dosage of sodium ferric gluconate had similar increases in hematocrit, iron saturation, serum ferritin levels, and reticulocyte hemoglobin content 2 weeks after completion of iron therapy.

Because of a lack of randomized, comparative studies, the relative efficacy of sodium ferric gluconate and other parenteral iron preparations (e.g., iron dextran) for the treatment of iron deficiency anemia in hemodialysis patients has not been clearly established. However, limited data suggest that sodium ferric gluconate may be associated with less frequent serious adverse effects (e.g., hypersensitivity reactions) than iron dextran. (See the introductory discussion under Cautions and see also Cautions: Sensitivity Reactions.)

Iron Deficiency Anemia

Data regarding the safety and efficacy of sodium ferric gluconate injection for the prevention and/or treatment of iron deficiency anemia not associated with chronic kidney disease (e.g., anemia in HIV or cancer patients) generally are lacking. In a study in a limited number of pregnant women with iron deficiency anemia who did not benefit from or could not tolerate oral iron therapy, IV sodium ferric gluconate (mean cumulative dosage: 1 g) produced appreciable improvement in hematocrit, hemoglobin, and other indices of iron status; reported adverse effects (sinus tachycardia, palpitation, shortness of breath, hot flushes) generally were mild and transient.

For additional information on the prevention and treatment of iron deficiency anemia, see Uses in Iron Preparation, Oral, 20:04.04.

DOSAGE AND ADMINISTRATION

Administration

Sodium ferric gluconate is administered by IV infusion. The drug should be diluted in 0.9% sodium chloride injection and administered by slow IV infusion (e.g., over 1 hour). Sodium ferric gluconate also may be administered undiluted by slow IV injection at a rate of up to 12.5 mg/minute at the end of dialysis. Sodium ferric gluconate should be administered immediately after dilution; any unused portion of the diluted solution should be discarded.

A test dose equivalent to 25 mg of elemental iron, which has been diluted in 50 mL of 0.9% sodium chloride injection and given IV over 60 minutes, was recommended in the past by the manufacturer prior to administration of the first therapeutic dose of sodium ferric gluconate.

It has been suggested that administration of sodium ferric gluconate even at recommended dosage and infusion rates may result in adverse effects (e.g., hypotension, flushing) that have been attributed to oversaturation of transferrin and accompanying adverse effects. (See Acute Toxicity.) Although the cause of such adverse effects has not been fully elucidated, reducing the dose to 62.5 mg and infusing the drug over 4 hours has been shown to reduce the occurrence of adverse effects.

Dosage

The dosage of sodium ferric gluconate is expressed in terms of mg of elemental iron. Sodium ferric gluconate injection contains the equivalent of 12.5 mg of elemental iron per mL.

For the treatment of iron deficiency in adults undergoing chronic hemodialysis who are receiving supplemental epoetin alfa therapy, the recommended dosage of sodium ferric gluconate is 125 mg administered by IV infusion over 1 hour. Most adults will require a minimum cumulative dose of 1 g of elemental iron, administered over 8 sessions at or during sequential dialysis treatments, to achieve a favorable hemoglobin or hematocrit response.

In patients with chronic kidney disease who are receiving supplemental therapy with an erythropoiesis-stimulating agent (ESA), sufficient iron should be administered to maintain selected indices of iron therapy (i.e., transferrin saturation [TSAT] and serum ferritin concentrations) at target levels; periodic monitoring of these iron indices is recommended, and the results should be used (in conjunction with hemoglobin concentrations and ESA dosage) to guide iron therapy. Once patients achieve TSAT levels of 20% or greater or serum ferritin concentrations of 100 ng/mL or greater, IV iron therapy with sodium ferric gluconate or other IV iron preparations should be continued at the lowest dose necessary to maintain target hematocrit/hemoglobin levels and iron stores within acceptable limits.

For the treatment of iron deficiency in children undergoing chronic hemodialysis who are receiving supplemental epoetin alfa therapy, the recommended dosage of sodium ferric gluconate is 1.5 mg/kg (up to 125 mg/dose) diluted in 25 mL 0.9% sodium chloride and administered by IV infusion over 1 hour during 8 sequential dialysis sessions.

CAUTIONS

Current evidence suggests that sodium ferric gluconate is well tolerated. In a single-dose, post-marketing safety study, 11% of patients who received sodium ferric gluconate and 9.4% of patients who received placebo reported adverse reactions. The most frequent adverse reactions following sodium ferric gluconate were hypotension (2%); nausea, vomiting, and/or diarrhea (2%); pain (0.7%); hypertension (0.6%); allergic reaction (0.5%); chest pain (0.5%); pruritus (0.5%); and back pain (0.4%). Similar adverse reactions were seen following placebo administration. However, because of the high baseline incidence of adverse events in the hemodialysis patient population, insufficient number of exposed patients, and limitations inherent to the crossover, single-dose study design, no comparison of event rates between sodium ferric gluconate and placebo treatments can be made at this time.

Clinical experience with sodium ferric gluconate has been documented in over 1400 adults on hemodialysis, including 1097 treatment-naive individuals who received a single 125-mg dose of undiluted sodium ferric gluconate over 10 minutes during a postmarketing safety study. No test dose was used in this postmarketing study. From a total of 1498 adults in medical reports, North American trials, and postmarketing studies who received sodium ferric gluconate therapy, 12 patients (0.8%) experienced serious reactions that precluded further therapy with the drug.

In iron-deficient pediatric patients undergoing chronic hemodialysis and receiving stable dosages of epoetin alfa who received 1.5 or 3 mg/kg of sodium ferric gluconate IV during 8 sequential dialysis sessions, the most common adverse effects (whether or not drug related) occurring in at least 5% of patients were hypotension (35%), headache (24%), hypertension (23%), tachycardia (17%), vomiting (11%), fever (9%), nausea (9%), abdominal pain (9%), pharyngitis (9%), diarrhea (8%), infection (8%), rhinitis (6%), and thrombosis (6%). The incidences of the following adverse effects were higher with the 3-mg/kg versus the 1.5-mg/kg dosage of sodium ferric gluconate: hypotension (41 or 28%, respectively), tachycardia (21 or 13%, respectively), fever (15 or 3%, respectively), headache (29 or 19%, respectively), abdominal pain (15 or 3%, respectively), nausea (12 or 6%, respectively), vomiting (12 or 9%, respectively), pharyngitis (12 or 6%, respectively), and rhinitis (9 or 3%, respectively).

IV iron dextran preparations are associated with idiopathic sensitivity reactions. Although the mechanism of sensitivity reactions is unknown, it has been suggested that dextran polymers may be the antigenic stimulus for these reactions. (See Cautions: Sensitivity Reactions, in Iron Dextran 20:04.04.) Published clinical studies do not permit a reliable comparison of IV sodium ferric gluconate with IV iron dextran, but limited data suggest that sodium ferric gluconate, a compound devoid of dextran, may be associated with fewer sensitivity reactions than IV iron dextran. Sensitivity (e.g., anaphylactoid or anaphylactic) reactions appear to occur rarely with sodium ferric gluconate injection, and no fatalities associated with the use of sodium ferric gluconate have been reported. In addition, sodium ferric gluconate has been administered without incident to a limited number of hemodialysis patients who had experienced severe sensitivity reactions to iron dextran. However, sensitivity reactions to sodium ferric gluconate severe enough to require discontinuance of the drug have occurred. (See Cautions: Sensitivity

Reactions.) In addition, rapid IV infusion of the drug has been associated with an increased incidence of acute iron toxicity manifested by flushing; pain in the chest, back, flank, or groin; and hypotension. (See Acute Toxicity.)

Unless otherwise stated in the Cautions section, adverse effects reported during therapy with sodium ferric gluconate may or may not be directly attributable to the drug.

• Sensitivity Reactions

The risk of acute anaphylactic reactions following administration of sodium ferric gluconate has been estimated to be 3.3 cases per million doses versus 8.7 cases per million doses for iron dextran based on retrospective analysis of adverse events data from use of sodium ferric gluconate in Germany and Italy or iron dextran in the United States. Although fatal hypersensitivity reactions did not occur during therapy with sodium ferric gluconate in clinical studies, the number of patients exposed to the drug during such studies may not have been sufficient to observe such reactions.

Of 88 patients in a randomized, controlled clinical trial of sodium ferric gluconate therapy, 3 patients (3.4%) experienced type III sensitivity reactions manifested by rash, pruritus, nausea, fatigue, and/or pain in the chest, abdomen, and flank that resulted in premature study discontinuance. These events were not dose-dependent and occurred in 2 cases following the first dose of sodium ferric gluconate and immediately after the IV test dose in the other incident. In addition, one case of a life-threatening hypersensitivity reaction, consisting of diaphoresis, nausea, vomiting, severe lower back pain, dyspnea, and wheezing, for 20 minutes, out of 1097 patients who received a single dose of sodium ferric gluconate has been observed in a postmarketing safety study, and 3 serious hypersensitivity reactions have been reported from the spontaneous reporting system in the US.

Serious adverse events that precluded further therapy with sodium ferric gluconate have been reported in 6 of 387 patients (1.6%) treated with the drug in clinical studies and in 9 of 1097 patients (0.8%) treated with the drug in a postmarketing safety study. During the postmarketing safety study, adverse reactions that, in the view of the investigator, precluded further administration of the drug because of drug intolerance included one life-threatening reaction, 6 allergic reactions (e.g., pruritus [2 cases], facial flushing, chills, dyspnea/chest pain, rash), and 2 other reactions (hypotension and nausea). Another 2 patients (0.2%) experienced allergic reactions not deemed to represent drug intolerance (nausea/malaise and nausea/dizziness) following administration of the drug. Anaphylactoid reaction, characterized by severe hypotension and paresthesias in the lips, fingers, and genitalia, also has been reported immediately following initiation of a slow infusion of sodium ferric gluconate in at least one patient; the reaction subsided completely within 1 hour. In clinical studies conducted in Europe, 2 of 226 hemodialysis patients (0.9%) experienced adverse events (malaise, heat, vomiting, loin pain, and/or intense epigastric pain lasting 3–4 hours) when treated with sodium ferric gluconate. These reactions recurred when patients were rechallenged with the drug and precluded further therapy. Since allergy histories of patients who experienced sensitivity reactions to sodium ferric gluconate were not reported in the literature, it is not known whether patients with a history of multiple drug allergies are at increased risk for adverse sensitivity reactions with sodium ferric gluconate as they are with iron dextran. The manufacturer states that the incidence of both drug intolerance and suspected allergic events following the first dose of sodium ferric gluconate administration in the postmarketing study was 2.8% in patients with prior iron dextran sensitivity and 0.8% in patients without prior iron dextran sensitivity. The one patient who experienced a life-threatening adverse event following administration of sodium ferric gluconate during the postmarketing study did have a previous severe anaphylactic reaction to both commercially available preparations of iron dextran (INFeD® and Dexferrum®).

Clinical studies of sodium ferric gluconate included 9 patients undergoing chronic hemodialysis who had a history of allergic reactions to iron dextran; 5 of these patients had a history of anaphylaxis to iron dextran. All patients were treated successfully with sodium ferric gluconate (1000 mg) given IV during each of 8 consecutive dialysis treatments, although one patient reported paresthesias within 1 hour of completing a full course of therapy with the drug.

For additional information on sensitivity reactions to sodium ferric gluconate, including that pertaining to this drug versus iron dextran, see the introductory discussion under Cautions.

• Cardiovascular Effects

The most common adverse cardiovascular effect associated with sodium ferric gluconate is hypotension, occurring in 29% of patients receiving the drug in clinical trials. Serious hypotensive events, accompanied by flushing in 2 cases, reportedly occurred in 3 of 226 hemodialysis patients (1.3%) treated with IV sodium ferric gluconate. Hypotensive episodes reported in clinical studies were not thought to be dose dependent since they occurred in 34 versus 36% of patients receiving 62.5 mg of sodium ferric gluconate IV over 30 minutes versus 125 mg IV over 60 minutes, respectively, and were comparable to those occurring in patients receiving oral iron therapy. However, rapid IV administration of sodium ferric gluconate has been associated with hypotensive episodes accompanied by flushing, lightheadedness, malaise, fatigue, weakness, or severe pain in the chest, back, flanks, or groin, which are unrelated to sensitivity reactions. These hypotensive episodes usually resolved within 1–2 hours following clinical interventions ranging from observation to volume expansion as warranted by the severity of the symptoms. Such hypotension and flushing have been attributed to oversaturation of transferrin and excessive free iron in the serum. Alternatively, it has been suggested that such transferrin oversaturation is unlikely because of the high binding coefficient of ferric iron in the sodium ferric gluconate complex; such adverse effects may instead result from direct chemical or mechanical stimulation of mast cells. Sodium ferric gluconate is intended to be administered during dialysis, during which many patients may experience transient hypotension. Administration of sodium ferric gluconate may augment hypotension caused by dialysis.

Hypertension, chest pain, syncope, tachycardia, and generalized edema have been reported in 13, 6, 5, and 5% of patients in clinical trials, respectively. In addition, bradycardia, angina pectoris, leg edema, myocardial infarction, vasodilation, or pulmonary edema occurred in more than 1% of patients receiving sodium ferric gluconate in clinical trials.

● Nervous System Effects

Dizziness, asthenia, headache, fatigue, and paresthesias are the most common adverse nervous system effects of sodium ferric gluconate, occurring in 13, 7, 7, 6, and 6% of patients, respectively. In addition, agitation, insomnia, or somnolence occurred in more than 1% of patients receiving sodium ferric gluconate in clinical trials. Lightheadedness, diplopia, malaise, and/or weakness have been reported rarely during therapy with sodium ferric gluconate in North American clinical trials and hypertonia and nervousness rarely were reported during postmarketing surveillance. Transient decreased level of consciousness without hypotension has been reported in at least one patient receiving the drug.

● Respiratory Effects

Dyspnea, coughing, and upper respiratory infection are the most common adverse respiratory effects of sodium ferric gluconate, occurring in 11, 6, and 6% of patients, respectively. Rhinitis or pneumonia occurred in more than 1% of patients receiving sodium ferric gluconate.

● GI Effects

Vomiting, nausea, and/or diarrhea are the most common adverse GI effects of sodium ferric gluconate, each occurring in 35% of patients. In addition, abdominal pain occurred in 6% of patients and nausea, rectal disorder, dyspepsia, eructation, GI disorder, flatulence, or melena occurred in more than 1% of patients receiving sodium ferric gluconate in clinical trials. Dry mouth was reported rarely during postmarketing surveillance.

● Musculoskeletal Effects

Generalized cramps and leg cramps are the most common adverse musculoskeletal effects of sodium ferric gluconate, occurring in 25 and 10% of patients, respectively. Myalgia, back pain, arm pain, or arthralgia occurred in more than 1% of patients receiving sodium ferric gluconate in clinical trials. Whether these events were dose dependent or delayed reactions similar to those observed with iron dextran has not been determined.

● Renal and Electrolyte Effects

Hyperkalemia occurred in 6% of patients receiving sodium ferric gluconate in clinical trials. In addition, hypokalemia or hypervolemia has been reported in more than 1% of patients receiving sodium ferric gluconate.

● Hematologic Effects

Abnormal erythrocytes occurred in 11% of patients receiving sodium ferric gluconate in clinical trials. In addition, anemia, leukocytosis, or lymphadenopathy occurred in more than 1% of patients receiving sodium ferric gluconate in clinical trials. Hemorrhage was reported rarely during postmarketing surveillance.

● Other Adverse Effects

Injection site reaction and fever have been reported in 33 and 5% of patients receiving sodium ferric gluconate in clinical trials, respectively. Other adverse effects reported in more than 1% of patients receiving sodium ferric gluconate in clinical trials include pain, otic disorder, increased sweating, conjunctivitis, abnormal vision, hypoglycemia, urinary tract infection, infection, rigors, chills, flu-like syndrome, sepsis, and carcinoma.

● Precautions and Contraindications

Unwarranted administration of parenteral iron preparations may cause excess storage of iron and possibly result in a syndrome similar to hemosiderosis, particularly in patients whose anemia is not attributable to iron deficiency (e.g., those with hemoglobinopathies or other refractory anemias that might be erroneously diagnosed as iron deficiency anemia). Periodic monitoring of laboratory values indicative of iron storage in the body (e.g., transferrin saturation, serum ferritin concentrations) may assist in the recognition of iron accumulation. Sodium ferric gluconate should not be administered to patients with iron overload.

Potentially fatal sensitivity (e.g. anaphylactic or anaphylactoid) reactions characterized by cardiovascular collapse, cardiac arrest, bronchospasm, oral or pharyngeal edema, dyspnea, angioedema, urticaria, or pruritus sometimes associated with pain and muscle spasm of the chest or back have been reported rarely in patients receiving sodium ferric gluconate; fatal immediate hypersensitivity reactions have been reported with other iron carbohydrate complexes. Serious anaphylactoid reactions require appropriate resuscitative measures. Although fatal reactions have not been observed with sodium ferric gluconate in clinical studies, insufficient numbers of patients may have been enrolled to observe such events. (See Caution: Sensitivity Reactions.) Although sodium ferric gluconate has been used successfully to treat iron deficiency anemia in a few hemodialysis patients with a history of allergic reactions to iron dextran, sodium ferric gluconate should be used with extreme caution in such patients (especially those who experienced life-threatening anaphylaxis or anaphylactoid reactions) since the drug itself is known to cause potentially life-threatening sensitivity reactions and the incidence of cross-reactivity between iron dextran and sodium ferric gluconate is unknown.

Hypotension not associated with sensitivity and accompanied by flushing, lightheadedness, malaise, fatigue, weakness, or severe pain in the chest, back, flanks, or groin has been associated with rapid IV administration of iron. Such reactions usually have resolved within 1–2 hours. Successful treatment of these reactions may include observation or, if symptoms are present, volume expansion.

Sodium ferric gluconate should not be used in patients with serum ferritin concentrations exceeding 1000 ng/mL. In addition, clinicians should consider that clinical studies in which the effects of sodium ferric gluconate were established excluded patients with serious underlying disease or inflammatory conditions. Sodium ferric gluconate is contraindicated in patients with any anemia not associated with iron deficiency, in patients who are hypersensitive to sodium ferric gluconate or any ingredients in the formulation, and in patients with evidence of iron overload.

● Pediatric Precautions

The safety and efficacy of sodium ferric gluconate in children younger than 6 years of age has not been established.

Sodium ferric gluconate contains benzyl alcohol, and the manufacturer states that the drug should not be used in neonates. Although a causal relationship has not been established, administration of injections preserved with benzyl alcohol has been associated with toxicity in neonates. Toxicity appears to have resulted from administration of large amounts (i.e., about 100–400 mg/kg daily) of benzyl alcohol in these neonates. Although use of drugs preserved with benzyl alcohol should be avoided in neonates whenever possible, the American Academy of Pediatrics (AAP) states that the presence of small amounts of the preservative in a commercially available injection should not proscribe its use when indicated in neonates.

● Geriatric Precautions

Clinical studies of sodium ferric gluconate did not include sufficient numbers of patients aged 65 years and older to determine whether they respond differently to the drug than do younger patients. Although other reported clinical experience has not revealed age-related differences in response or tolerance, drug dosage should be titrated carefully in geriatric patients, usually initiating therapy at the low end of the dosage range. The greater frequency of decreased hepatic, renal, and/or cardiac function and of concomitant disease and drug therapy observed in the elderly also should be considered.

● Mutagenicity and Carcinogenicity

No evidence of mutagenicity was seen when sodium ferric gluconate was evaluated in in vitro test systems (Ames test and rat micronucleus test). Long-term studies in animals to evaluate the carcinogenic potential of sodium ferric gluconate are ongoing.

● Pregnancy, Fertility, and Lactation

Pregnancy

Reproductive studies in mice and rats using sodium ferric gluconate dosages up to 100 or 20 mg/kg daily, respectively, have not revealed evidence of harm to the fetus. These dosages were 1.3 or 3.24 times, respectively, the recommended human daily dosage of 125 mg or 92.5 mg/m² (based on a patient of average height weighing 50 kg and having a body surface area of 1.46 m²). In a study involving 21 pregnant women who were treated with sodium ferric gluconate as an alternative to blood transfusions, dose-dependent adverse events occurred; these adverse events included sinus tachycardia, palpitations, shortness of breath, and hot flushes (flashes), which were transient and resolved spontaneously without treatment after a few minutes. There are no adequate and controlled studies to date using sodium ferric gluconate in pregnant women, and the drug should be used during pregnancy only when clearly needed.

Fertility

Studies to assess the effects of sodium ferric gluconate on fertility in animals have not been conducted. However, the drug produced a clastogenic effect in an in vitro chromosomal aberration assay in Chinese hamster ovary cells.

Lactation

Since it is not known whether sodium ferric gluconate is distributed into milk, the drug should be used with caution in nursing women.

DRUG INTERACTIONS

● Angiotensin-converting Enzyme Inhibitors

Limited data suggest that concomitant administration of IV sodium ferric gluconate and oral enalapril may potentiate adverse effects associated with IV iron therapy. During a postmarketing safety study, one patient who was already receiving an ACE inhibitor had facial flushing immediately following exposure to sodium ferric gluconate. No hypotension occurred in this patient, and the event resolved rapidly and spontaneously without intervention other than drug withdrawal. However, hypotension (systolic blood pressure of 80 mm Hg), diffuse erythema, nausea, vomiting, and abdominal cramps have been reported in a few patients who received IV sodium ferric gluconate while receiving enalapril therapy. The onset of these adverse effects varied from immediately after administration of IV iron to a couple of hours or days following infusion of the drug. These reactions subsided within 20–30 minutes following prompt discontinuance of the IV iron infusion and IV administration of hydrocortisone. One patient, who agreed to discontinue enalapril therapy while on sodium ferric gluconate, was successfully treated again with sodium ferric gluconate; the other patients were not treated with IV iron therapy again but were able to continue enalapril therapy without further incident.

It has been suggested that Angiotensin-converting enzyme (ACE) inhibitors potentiate sensitivity reactions by decreasing the breakdown of kinins. In a postmarketing safety study in which 28% of the patients received concomitant ACE inhibitor therapy, the incidences of both drug intolerance or suspected allergic events following first dose administration of sodium ferric gluconate were 1.6% in patients with concomitant ACE inhibitor use compared with 0.7% in patients without concomitant ACE inhibitor use. The patient with a life-threatening event during the postmarketing study was not on ACE inhibitor therapy. Although this interaction appears to occur rarely, the potential seriousness of the interaction warrants caution when IV iron and ACE inhibitors are used together.

ACUTE TOXICITY

Dosage of sodium ferric gluconate in excess of that required for restoration of hemoglobin and replenishment of iron stores may lead to hemosiderosis. Serum iron concentrations exceeding 300 mcg/dL (combined with transferrin oversaturation) may indicate iron toxicity, which is characterized by abdominal pain, diarrhea, or vomiting that progresses to pallor or cyanosis, lassitude, drowsiness, hyperventilation secondary to acidosis, and cardiovascular collapse. Symptoms following rapid IV infusion of sodium ferric gluconate have been reported rarely; such symptoms include flushing; chest, back, and loin pain; and hypotension. (See Cautions: Cardiovascular Effects.) Periodic monitoring of laboratory indices of iron storage (e.g., serum ferritin, transferrin saturation [TSAT]) may assist in recognition of iron accumulation. Sodium ferric gluconate should not be administered to patients with iron overload. Sodium ferric gluconate is not dialyzable.

Overdosage of sodium ferric gluconate in animals produced symptoms such as decreased activity, staggering, ataxia, increases in the respiratory rate, tremor, and convulsions. Deaths occurred with sodium ferric gluconate at elemental iron doses of 125, 78.8, 62.5, or 250 mg/kg in mice, rats, rabbits, or dogs, respectively.

PHARMACOLOGY

Sodium ferric gluconate is used to replenish and maintain the total body content of iron and has pharmacologic actions similar to those of iron dextran. Iron is essential for normal hemoglobin synthesis to maintain oxygen transport; iron also is necessary for the metabolism and synthesis of DNA and functions as a cofactor in various enzymatic processes.

The total body iron content of an adult ranges from 2–4 g with approximately two-thirds in hemoglobin and one-third in reticuloendothelial storage (liver, spleen, and bone marrow) and bound to tissue ferritin. The human body avidly conserves iron so that only about 1 mg (about 0.03% of total body stores) is excreted daily in healthy, nonmenstruating adults.

Iron deficiency anemia in patients with chronic kidney disease undergoing hemodialysis may result from various factors, including increased iron utilization (e.g., in patients receiving exogenous erythropoietin [epoetin alfa]), blood loss (e.g., from fistula, retention in dialyzer, hematologic testing, menses), decreased dietary intake or absorption, surgery, iron sequestration related to inflammatory processes, and malignancy. In addition, transferrin concentrations reportedly may be depressed in chronic kidney disease, resulting in subnormal iron uptake by cells. Administration of epoetin alfa increases red blood cell production and iron utilization, which may lead to absolute or functional iron deficiency.

Functional iron deficiency in patients with chronic kidney disease receiving epoetin alfa or in other patients with chronic blood loss refers to the condition where the body's demand for iron to maintain erythropoiesis exceeds the rate at which iron can be released from the reticuloendothelial system. Iron-replete hemodialysis patients reportedly have been shown to have decreased iron stores within 3 months of beginning epoetin alfa therapy. Because there is no widely available hematologic indicator of functional iron deficiency, the only way to determine its presence is to monitor the erythroid response to iron administration. Iron administration in hemodialysis patients with functional iron deficiency will result in an increase in hematocrit and/or hemoglobin levels despite a stable dose of epoetin alfa or can maintain a stable hematocrit and/or hemoglobin while allowing a reduction in epoetin alfa dosage. (See Uses: Iron Deficiency Anemia in Hemodialysis Patients Receiving Epoetin Alfa Therapy.)

Administration of iron may reverse esophageal, gastric, and other tissue changes associated with iron deficiency. Iron therapy also relieves other symptoms associated with iron deficiency, such as soreness of the tongue, cheilosis, dysphagia, and dystrophy of the nails and skin. Iron does not stimulate erythropoiesis nor does it correct hemoglobin disturbances not caused by iron deficiency.

Iron is vital for microorganisms such as bacteria, and the mineral plays a role both in bacterial pathogenicity and host defense mechanisms. (See Cautions: Hemosiderosis, in Iron Preparations, Oral.)

PHARMACOKINETICS

● Distribution

Following administration of IV iron, the metal is taken up by the reticuloendothelial system. Subsequently, ferric iron is gradually released into the plasma where it rapidly combines with transferrin and is carried to the bone marrow and incorporated into hemoglobin. Plasma transferrin is normally 30–40% saturated by iron; in iron deficiency, elevated transferrin concentrations maintain circulating iron concentrations despite a reduction in transferrin saturation (TSAT). In a limited number of healthy iron-deficient individuals who received multiple sequential single doses of either 125 mg/hour or 62.5 mg over 30 minutes of undiluted sodium ferric gluconate IV, approximately 80% of drug-bound iron was delivered to transferrin as a mononuclear ionic iron species within 24 hours of administration in each dosage regimen. Direct movement of iron from sodium ferric gluconate to transferrin, however, was not observed. In addition, mean peak transferrin saturation did not exceed 100% in these studies and returned to near baseline by 40 hours after administration of each dose regimen.

Preliminary pharmacokinetic data in a single hemodialysis patient and in a limited number of healthy iron-deficient individuals who received IV sodium ferric gluconate suggest an initial volume of distribution consistent with the vascular compartment, approximately 6 L.

● **Elimination**

Following IV injection of sodium ferric gluconate, the terminal elimination half-life of drug-bound iron varied by dose but not by rate of administration and was approximately 1 hour in healthy iron-deficient adults. The shortest terminal half-life (0.85 hours) occurred in adults administered 62.5 mg of the drug over 4 minutes and the longest terminal half-life (1.45 hours) occurred in adults administered 125 mg of the drug over 7 minutes. In addition, total clearance of sodium ferric gluconate was 3.02–5.35 L/hour and did not substantially vary by rate of administration. The terminal half-life following IV injection of 1.5 or 3 mg/kg sodium ferric gluconate in iron-deficient pediatric patients undergoing chronic hemodialysis was 2.0 or 2.5 hours, respectively. Pharmacokinetic studies in renally competent adults suggest that urinary excretion is not an important route of elimination of the drug in humans. In in vitro studies conducted with sodium ferric gluconate either undiluted or diluted in 0.9% sodium chloride injection or distilled water, less than 1% of the iron species in a dose of sodium ferric gluconate was removed during hemodialysis periods of up to 270 minutes using membranes with pore sizes corresponding to 12,000–14,000 daltons.

Iron metabolism occurs in a virtually closed system. Most of the iron liberated by destruction of hemoglobin is conserved and reused by the body. Daily excretion of iron in healthy men amounts to only 0.5–2 mg. This excretion occurs principally through feces and as desquamation of cells such as skin, GI mucosa, nails, and hair; only trace amounts of iron are excreted in bile and sweat. For additional information on the distribution of iron, see Pharmacokinetics: Elimination, in Iron Preparations, Oral 20:04.04.

CHEMISTRY AND STABILITY

● **Chemistry**

Sodium ferric gluconate is a stable macromolecular complex composed of ferric oxide hydrate directly bonded to sucrose and chelated with gluconate, which has a high affinity for ferric ions and enables the bridging of adjacent ferric oxide centers. Unlike iron dextran, sodium ferric gluconate is free of ferrous ion and dextran polysaccharides. The sodium ferric gluconate complex exists as a 2:1 molar ratio of iron to gluconate and has an apparent molecular weight of approximately 350,000.

Sodium ferric gluconate injection occurs as a deep-red, viscous solution that is completely miscible in water and 0.9% sodium chloride injection. The drug is negatively charged at alkaline pH and is present in solution with sodium cations. The commercially available injection is an alkaline aqueous solution with approximately 20% sucrose w/v in water for injection at a pH of 7.7–9.7. Each mL of sodium ferric gluconate injection contains 9 mg of benzyl alcohol as a preservative.

● **Stability**

Sodium ferric gluconate injection should be stored at 20–25°C, but may be exposed to temperatures ranging from 15–30°C. Sodium ferric gluconate injection should not be frozen. Sodium ferric gluconate injection should not be frozen.

The compatibility of sodium ferric gluconate injection with IV solutions other than 0.9% sodium chloride injection has not been evaluated. The manufacturer states that sodium ferric gluconate injection should not be mixed with other drugs or added to parenteral nutrition solutions for IV infusion.

PREPARATIONS

Excipients in commercially available drug preparations may have clinically important effects in some individuals; consult specific product labeling for details.

Sodium Ferric Gluconate

Parenteral

Injection, for IV use	equivalent to 12.5 mg of elemental iron per mL	Ferrlecit®, Sanofi-Aventis

Selected Revisions November 4, 2013, © Copyright, January 1, 1999, American Society of Health-System Pharmacists, Inc.

Warfarin Sodium

20:12.04.08 • COUMARIN DERIVATIVES

■ Warfarin sodium is a coumarin-derivative anticoagulant that alters the synthesis of vitamin-K dependent blood coagulation factors II, VII, IX, X, and the anticoagulants protein C and protein S.

USES

Warfarin is used for prophylaxis and/or treatment of venous thrombosis and its extension, pulmonary embolism, and prophylaxis and treatment of thromboembolic complications associated with atrial fibrillation and/or cardiac valve replacement. The drug also is used to reduce the risk of death, reinfarction, and thromboembolic events such as stroke or systemic embolization following myocardial infarction (MI).

Warfarin generally is used for follow-up anticoagulant therapy after the effects of an initial parenteral anticoagulant have been established and/or when long-term anticoagulant therapy is indicated. Therapy with warfarin and a parenteral anticoagulant should be overlapped for a short period of time until the therapeutic effects of warfarin are achieved for appropriate indications for use.

● Treatment of Venous Thromboembolism

Adults

Warfarin is used for the treatment of acute proximal deep-vein thrombosis (DVT) or pulmonary embolism (PE) (i.e., venous thromboembolism [VTE]) in adults. Because the effects of warfarin are delayed and early full-dose anticoagulant therapy reduces the risk of extension or recurrence of venous thrombosis, the American College of Chest Physicians (ACCP) recommends a rapid-acting parenteral anticoagulant (e.g., unfractionated heparin, low molecular weight heparin [LMWH], fondaparinux) for the initial treatment of VTE. Therapy with warfarin and the parenteral anticoagulant should be overlapped for a short period of time until the therapeutic effects of warfarin are achieved.

Warfarin should be initiated on the same day that the parenteral anticoagulant is started, and such therapy should be overlapped for at least 5 days and until a stable international normalized ratio (INR) of at least 2 has been maintained for 24 hours or longer. ACCP recommends a moderate intensity of warfarin anticoagulation (target INR of 2.5 [range 2–3]) for most patients. While use of either a lower (INR <2) or higher (INR 3–5) intensity of anticoagulation has been evaluated, both appear to be less optimal than moderate-intensity warfarin; low-intensity warfarin is no safer than moderate-intensity warfarin, and high-intensity warfarin is associated with an increased incidence of bleeding complications.

A systematic review with meta-analysis assessed the efficacy and safety of warfarin compared to direct oral anticoagulants (DOACs; apixaban, edoxaban, dabigatran, rivaroxaban) in patients with acute VTE. The review included 5 good quality trials with a total of 24,455 patients. Patients who received dabigatran or edoxaban were treated with an initial 5–10 days of parenteral anticoagulant therapy. Warfarin patients initially received overlapping parenteral anticoagulation therapy for a minimum of 6 days and were treated to a goal INR of 2–3; the reported time in therapeutic range during warfarin therapy was 58–64%. Efficacy outcomes included recurrent VTE, fatal PE, and overall mortality. Recurrent VTE occurred in 2% and 2.2% of DOAC- and warfarin-treated patients, respectively. Fatal PE (0.07%) and overall mortality rates (2.4%) were not different between the treatment groups. The safety outcome of major bleeding occurred in 1.1% and 1.7% of DOAC- and warfarin-treated patients, respectively. When compared to DOAC-treated patients, overall results of this study showed that warfarin had similar efficacy, but a higher rate of major bleeding.

Pediatric Patients

Although warfarin therapy can be problematic in children for several reasons (e.g., dietary differences, compliance issues, monitoring difficulty, lack of a commercially available liquid preparation), the drug has been used in selected pediatric patients† with VTE. Data are primarily derived from observational studies that do not include a comparator group. Experience with warfarin in the pediatric population is mostly based on use of the drug in children ≥3 months of age; there is little efficacy or safety information in neonates. Unfractionated heparin or LMWH generally is recommended in children for initial VTE treatment for at least 5 days; ongoing therapy may occur with heparin, LMWH, or warfarin. Transition to warfarin therapy is the same in children as in adults where warfarin is initiated on the same day that the parenteral anticoagulant is started, and such therapy is overlapped for at least 5 days and until a stable INR ≥2 has been maintained for ≥24 hours. Duration of therapy decisions should be based on an evaluation of clinical risk factors (e.g., location of thrombi, presence or absence of precipitating factors, presence of cancer, patient's risk of bleeding).

Warfarin has been used in children with central venous catheter-related thromboembolism†. In these situations, ACCP recommends that the catheter be removed if no longer functioning or required; at least 3–5 days of therapeutic anticoagulation is suggested prior to removal. If the central venous access device is required, ACCP suggests that anticoagulants be given until the catheter is removed. After the initial 3 months of therapy, use of prophylactic dosages of warfarin (target INR 1.5–1.9) or a LMWH is suggested until the catheter is removed; however, if recurrent thromboembolism occurs, therapeutic-dose anticoagulation may be necessary.

Clinical Perspective

Warfarin remains an option for the treatment of VTE; however, the DOACs (e.g., dabigatran, rivaroxaban, apixaban, edoxaban) are preferred in most cases by experts such as the American College of Chest Physicians (ACCP), American Society of Hematology (ASH), and the Anticoagulation Forum. DOACs have similar efficacy to warfarin for treatment of VTE, but reduced bleeding (particularly intracranial hemorrhage) and greater convenience for patients and healthcare providers. In addition to relative efficacy and safety, factors that should be considered when selecting an appropriate anticoagulant include convenience of administration, need for INR monitoring, drug-drug or drug-food interactions, cost, patient preference, presence of renal impairment, and cancer or other comorbid conditions.

Warfarin can be recommended in clinical situations where DOACs are generally not used. These include settings with high bleeding risk (e.g., hemorrhagic lesion, renal/hepatic impairment, thrombocytopenia, GI or genitourinary malignancy, mucosal lesion, CNS malignancy or bleeding, recent surgery), or in patients with morbid obesity (body weight >120 kg or body mass index [BMI] ≥40 mg/m²), drug-drug interactions (e.g., potent dual inducers of p-glycoprotein [P-gp] and cytochrome P-450 [CYP]3A4 [e.g., carbamazepine, phenytoin, rifampin]), or GI complications affecting oral therapy (e.g., poor absorption, nausea and vomiting). Warfarin is also preferred in patients with antiphospholipid syndrome and those with significant valvular heart disease, including patients with mechanical heart valves.

In patients with cancer and established VTE, LMWHs or oral factor Xa inhibitors are generally recommended over warfarin for long-term anticoagulation.

In patients with acute VTE, therapy should be continued beyond the acute treatment period for at least 3 months, and possibly longer depending on the individual clinical situation (e.g., location of thrombi, presence or absence of precipitating factors, presence of cancer, patient's bleeding risk). While several randomized, controlled studies indicate that recurrence of VTE is less frequent with longer periods of anticoagulation (exceeding 6 months) compared with shorter periods (3–6 months), particularly in patients with idiopathic (i.e., unprovoked) VTE, prolonged therapy with warfarin (in addition to increased intensity of anticoagulation) is associated with an increased risk of bleeding complications.

The incidence of VTE in pediatric patients is very low. Several organizations (ACCP, ASH) have published guidelines on the use of antithrombotic therapy in pediatric patients.

● Prophylaxis of Venous Thromboembolism

Major Orthopedic Surgery

Warfarin is used for the prevention of VTE in adults undergoing major orthopedic surgery (hip- or knee-replacement surgery or hip-fracture surgery).

Clinical Perspective

Several major guidelines for thromboprophylaxis following hip- or knee-replacement surgery have been published, including guidelines from the

American Academy of Orthopedic Surgeons (AAOS), ACCP, and ASH. Routine thromboprophylaxis is recommended in all patients undergoing major orthopedic surgery, including total hip-replacement, total knee-replacement, and hip-fracture surgery, because of the high risk for postoperative VTE. According to ACCP, thromboprophylaxis with an appropriate antithrombotic agent or an intermittent pneumatic compression device should be continued for at least 10–14 days and possibly for up to 35 days after surgery. Although ACCP suggests that a LMWH generally is preferred because of its relative efficacy and safety and extensive clinical experience, alternative agents such as warfarin may be a reasonable choice in situations in which a LMWH is not available or cannot be used (e.g., in patients with heparin-induced thrombocytopenia [HIT] or in those who refuse or are uncooperative with subcutaneous injections). AAOS guidelines do not recommend any specific thromboprophylaxis agent. The ASH guidelines suggest the use of DOACs over LMWH if anticoagulants are used; however, this recommendation is considered conditional based on moderate certainty in the evidence of harms versus benefits.

Drug selection and duration of therapy should be individualized based on type of surgery, patient risk factors for embolism and bleeding, as well as costs, patient compliance, preference, tolerance, and comorbidities, and other clinical factors such as renal function.

Thromboprophylaxis in Pediatric Patients

Warfarin also has been used for primary thromboprophylaxis in children with ventricular assist devices† or with an arteriovenous fistula undergoing hemodialysis† and in children with certain medical conditions associated with a high risk of thrombosis (e.g., moderate or giant coronary aneurysms following Kawasaki disease†, primary pulmonary hypertension†).

● *Embolism Associated with Atrial Fibrillation*

Warfarin is used for the prevention of stroke and systemic embolism in patients with atrial fibrillation. In several randomized controlled studies in patients with nonvalvular atrial fibrillation, the incidence of thromboembolic events (e.g., transient ischemic attack [TIA], ischemic stroke) in patients anticoagulated with warfarin was substantially reduced compared with that in patients receiving placebo.

Pooled analysis of data from a number of comparative studies evaluating therapy with warfarin and aspirin in patients with chronic atrial fibrillation demonstrate that warfarin therapy is more effective than aspirin (e.g., 75–325 mg daily) in reducing thromboembolic complications. In addition, warfarin therapy appears to have a therapeutic advantage over aspirin in preventing nonfatal stroke. Nonfatal extracranial bleeding occurred more frequently in warfarin patients.

Dual antiplatelet therapy with clopidogrel and aspirin was evaluated as a potential alternative to warfarin in a randomized controlled study in patients with atrial fibrillation at high risk of stroke. The study was terminated early because of clear evidence of superiority of warfarin over antiplatelet therapy for the primary outcome of stroke, systemic embolism, MI, or vascular death. Results of another study comparing dual antiplatelet therapy (clopidogrel and aspirin) with aspirin monotherapy in patients with atrial fibrillation who had an increased risk of stroke but were unable to take warfarin showed that the combination of clopidogrel and aspirin was more effective than aspirin in reducing the risk of nonfatal stroke; however, dual antiplatelet therapy was associated with an increased risk of bleeding. Because the risk of bleeding with combination aspirin and clopidogrel therapy is similar to the risk of bleeding with warfarin, such combination therapy is not recommended in patients with a hemorrhagic contraindication to warfarin.

Warfarin therapy with a goal INR of 2–3 was compared to a DOAC for stroke prevention in atrial fibrillation in 4 phase 3 randomized controlled trials (dabigatran in RE-LY, rivaroxaban in ROCKET-AF, apixaban in ARISTOTLE, and edoxaban in ENGAGE AF-TIMI 48). In these trials, the DOAC was noninferior or superior to warfarin for the primary efficacy endpoint of the occurrence of stroke and systemic embolism and was associated with significantly less intracranial hemorrhage and similar or less frequent major bleeding. A meta-analysis of the studies combined endpoints from 42,411 DOAC- and 29,272 warfarin-treated patients. Stroke or systemic embolism was substantially reduced by 19% with DOAC therapy; this endpoint was primarily driven by a reduction in hemorrhagic stroke. There was also a nonsignificant 14% reduction in major bleeding and a significant 52% reduction in intracranial hemorrhage with DOAC therapy.

While randomized clinical trials evaluating warfarin anticoagulation in patients with atrial fibrillation and prosthetic heart valves or rheumatic mitral valve disease have not been conducted, long-term warfarin therapy is strongly recommended in such patients based on results of studies in patients who have atrial fibrillation *without* these coexisting conditions. The intensity of anticoagulation in patients with prosthetic heart valves should be based on the particular type of prosthesis but should not be less than that required to maintain an INR of 2.5; patients with prosthetic mechanical heart valves should have a target INR of at least 2.5.

The risk of stroke in patients with atrial flutter is similar to the risk in those with atrial fibrillation. Experts state that antithrombotic therapy in patients with atrial flutter generally should be managed in the same manner as in patients with atrial fibrillation.

Clinical Perspective

ACCP, the American College of Cardiology (ACC), the American Heart Association (AHA), the American Stroke Association (ASA), and other experts currently recommend that antithrombotic therapy be administered to all patients with nonvalvular atrial fibrillation (i.e., atrial fibrillation in the absence of rheumatic mitral stenosis, a prosthetic heart valve, or mitral valve repair) who are considered to be at increased risk of stroke, unless such therapy is contraindicated. Although many risk stratification methods have been used, current guidelines recommend the use of the CHA_2DS_2-VAS_c risk stratification tool for assessing a patient's risk of stroke and need for anticoagulant therapy. Established clinical risk factors for stroke include prior ischemic stroke or transient ischemic attack (TIA), advanced age (e.g., ≥65 years of age), history of hypertension, diabetes mellitus, vascular disease, and congestive heart failure; in addition, female sex has been identified as a factor that can modify the risk of stroke. The presence of stroke or TIA places a patient in the high-risk category regardless of other risk factors. Experts state that antithrombotic therapy generally is not necessary in low-risk patients (CHA_2DS_2-VAS_c score of 0 in males, or 1 in females), but should be considered in patients with one or more non-sex CHA_2DS_2-VAS_c stroke risk factors (CHA_2DS_2-VAS_c score of ≥1 in males, or ≥2 in females). Patients also should be assessed for their bleeding risk; those with a high risk of bleeding should be monitored more closely.

In patients with nonvalvular atrial fibrillation who are eligible for oral anticoagulant therapy, DOACs are recommended over warfarin based on improved safety and similar or improved efficacy in clinical trials and meta-analyses. A substantially greater safety benefit of DOACs versus warfarin has been observed when the INR is in the therapeutic range <66% of the time. A DOAC is also recommended in patients unable to achieve optimal warfarin management. Because of limited data on the use of DOACs in obese patients, some experts have discouraged the use of these agents in the morbidly obese population (those with a BMI ≥40 kg/m² or body weight >120) and recommend considering warfarin instead in such patients with nonvalvular atrial fibrillation.

If warfarin is used, patients should be optimally managed with well-controlled INRs (e.g., INR in therapeutic range >70% of the time). The therapeutic range for atrial fibrillation without a mechanical heart valve is 2–3. Factors influencing individual time in the therapeutic range include age, sex, diet, ethnicity, socioeconomic status, medical comorbidities, genetics, length of time on warfarin, nonadherence, polypharmacy, frequency of INR monitoring, and how therapy is managed (e.g., physician practice, anticoagulation clinic, home INR testing). ACCP suggests use of the SAMe-TT_2R_2 tool to identify patients who are likely to do well on warfarin; the tool generates a score based on clinical factors known to influence time in therapeutic range. One point is generated for sex (female), age (<60 years old), medical history (≥2 from hypertension, diabetes mellitus, coronary artery disease/MI, peripheral arterial disease, congestive heart failure, previous stroke, pulmonary disease, and hepatic or renal disease), and treatment with interacting drugs (e.g., amiodarone), and 2 points for tobacco use (current or within 2 years) and race (non-white) for a maximum score of 8. Patients with scores of 0–2 are more likely to achieve an appropriate time in the therapeutic range; scores >2 suggest the patient will need more frequent INR monitoring, frequent follow-ups, and additional education.

● *Cardioversion of Atrial Fibrillation†*

Use of warfarin is recommended to decrease the risk of embolization in patients undergoing pharmacologic or electrical cardioversion of atrial fibrillation.

Because the risk of thromboembolism appears to be greatest when atrial fibrillation has been present for ≥48 hours, recommendations for the use of anticoagulant therapy in such patients vary based on the duration of the arrhythmia. ACCP and other experts recommend that patients with atrial fibrillation of unknown or ≥48 hours' duration who are to undergo elective cardioversion receive therapeutic anticoagulation (e.g., warfarin, apixaban, dabigatran, edoxaban, rivaroxaban) for at least 3 weeks prior to cardioversion; alternatively, a transesophageal echocardiography (TEE)-guided approach with abbreviated anticoagulation before cardioversion may be used. In patients who have atrial fibrillation of short duration (e.g., ≤48 hours), cardioversion usually is performed with full dose heparin or LMWH, without prolonged warfarin anticoagulation or TEE prior to the procedure. After successful cardioversion to sinus rhythm, all patients should receive therapeutic anticoagulation for at least 4 weeks.

Experts suggest that patients with atrial flutter undergoing cardioversion be managed according to the same approach as that used in patients with atrial fibrillation.

● Embolism Associated with Valvular Heart Disease

Warfarin is used for the prevention of thromboembolic complications in patients with valvular heart disease, including those with mechanical and bioprosthetic heart valves.

Clinical Experience in Patients with Prosthetic Heart Valves

In a prospective, randomized, open-label study in 254 patients with mechanical prosthetic heart valves, thromboembolic events occurred significantly less frequently in patients treated with warfarin than in those treated with dipyridamole/aspirin or pentoxifylline/aspirin. In a prospective, open-label study, moderate-intensity warfarin therapy was compared with high-intensity warfarin in 258 patients with mechanical prosthetic heart valves. There was no difference in incidence of thromboembolism, but a higher rate of major bleeding was reported in the high-intensity group. In another study that compared 2 different intensities of warfarin therapy (INR 2–2.25 versus INR 2.5–4), thromboembolism occurred with similar frequency, but major hemorrhage occurred more frequently in the higher-intensity INR group.

Dabigatran was compared to warfarin following mechanical valve replacement in the RE-ALIGN trial. In this study, selection of the initial dabigatran dosage (150, 220, or 300 mg twice daily) was based on kidney function with dosages adjusted to a trough level of at least 50 ng/mL. Warfarin dosage was adjusted to an INR of 2–3 or 2.5–3.5 based on thromboembolic risk. Bridging anticoagulation was allowed based on investigator discretion. In population A (adults undergoing implantation of a mechanical bileaflet valve in the aortic or mitral position or both), the first dose of study drug was administered in 6 days and 5 days following surgery in patients randomly assigned to dabigatran and warfarin, respectively. The trial was terminated early due to an excess rate of thromboembolic and bleeding events in the dabigatran group. The thromboembolic composite endpoint, defined as the occurrence of death, stroke, systemic embolism, or MI, occurred in 8% of dabigatran-treated patients compared to 3% of patients in the warfarin group. Major bleeding with a pericardial location occurred in 5% versus 3% of dabigatran and warfarin patients, respectively; the rate of any bleeding was also higher (26% versus 12%).

Clinical Experience in Patients with other Valvular Heart Conditions

Among the common types of valvular heart disease, rheumatic mitral valve disease is associated with the greatest risk of systemic thromboembolism, and the risk is further increased in patients with concurrent atrial fibrillation, left atrial thrombus, or a history of systemic embolism.

Vitamin K antagonist therapy was compared with a DOAC (rivaroxaban) in INVICTUS, a prospective, open-label study that was conducted in 4531 adults with echocardiographically confirmed rheumatic heart disease and documented atrial fibrillation or atrial flutter and at least one additional criteria (e.g., mitral stenosis, CHA$_2$DS$_2$VASc ≥2); patients with a mechanical heart valve or need for one within the next 6 months were excluded. The primary efficacy outcome was the composite of stroke, systemic embolism, MI, or death from vascular or unknown causes. The primary safety outcome was the occurrence of International Society of Thrombosis and Hemostasis (ISTH)-defined major bleeding. Patients received rivaroxaban 20 mg daily (15 mg daily if creatinine clearance <50 mL/minute) or a vitamin K antagonist (predominantly warfarin) with dosage adjusted to maintain an INR of 2–3. The mean age of patients enrolled in the study was 50.5 years, 72.3% were female, 85.3% had mitral-valve stenosis, and 39.5% had both moderate to severe mitral stenosis and a CHA$_2$DS$_2$VAS$_c$ score ≥2. Time in therapeutic

range of vitamin K antagonist therapy ranged from 56.1 to 65.3% at various study time points; mean rivaroxaban adherence was 83.7%. The primary composite outcome occurred significantly more frequently in the rivaroxaban group than in the vitamin K antagonist group (8.21% versus 6.49% per year). There was no significant difference in major bleeding between the treatment groups (0.67% per year with rivaroxaban and 0.83% per year with the vitamin K antagonist).

Antithrombotic therapy generally should not be initiated in patients with infective endocarditis involving a native valve because of the risk of serious hemorrhage, including intracerebral hemorrhage, and lack of documented efficacy in such patients. In patients with a prosthetic valve who are already receiving warfarin therapy, ACCP suggests temporary discontinuance of the drug if infective endocarditis develops, and reinitiation of therapy once invasive procedures no longer are required and the patient is stabilized without signs of neurologic complications.

Clinical Perspective

All patients with mechanical heart valves require long-term warfarin therapy because of the high risk of thromboembolism with these valves. The risk of systemic embolism is higher with mechanical than with bioprosthetic heart valves, higher with first-generation mechanical (e.g., caged ball, caged disk) valves than with newer mechanical (e.g., bileaflet, Medtronic Hall tilting disk) heart valves, higher with more than one prosthetic valve, and higher with prosthetic mitral than with aortic valves; risk also is higher in the first few days and months after valve insertion (before full endothelialization) and increases in the presence of atrial fibrillation. In patients with mechanical aortic valve replacement who have additional risk factors (e.g., older generation valve, atrial fibrillation, previous thromboembolism, hypercoagulable state, left ventricular systolic dysfunction), a target INR of 3 (range 2.5–3.5) is recommended; in the absence of these risk factors, a target INR of 2.5 (range 2–3) is recommended. In patients with mechanical mitral valve replacement, a target INR of 3 (range 2.5–3.5) is recommended. Due to the increased risk of major bleeding, the addition of aspirin 75–100 mg is no longer routinely recommended in patients with mechanical valve replacement; the decision to add aspirin should be based on thromboembolism risk, bleeding risk, and presence of an indication for antiplatelet therapy.

Warfarin is recommended during the initial 3–6 months following surgical bioprosthetic valve replacement, regardless of position, aortic or mitral. Following transcatheter aortic valve implantation, the decision to select antiplatelet therapy or warfarin during the first 3–6 months should be individualized. The target INR is 2.5 (range 2–3) following either valve replacement approach. Following the initial period of warfarin prophylaxis, patients may be switched to aspirin 75–100 mg provided they are in normal sinus rhythm and have no other indication for therapeutic anticoagulation (e.g., atrial fibrillation, previous thromboembolism, hypercoagulable state, left ventricular dysfunction).

In prosthetic valve patients who experience a thromboembolic event despite achievement of target INR or while adhering to aspirin therapy, antithrombotic therapy may be escalated after a thorough investigation of other causative factors (e.g., medication adherence, new onset atrial fibrillation or other hypercoagulable state, infective endocarditis) and after an assessment of the patient's bleeding risk. Aspirin 75–100 mg daily may be added in patients with mechanical aortic or mitral valves, or warfarin therapy may be adjusted to a target INR of 3 (range 2.5–3.5) for aortic and 4 (range 3.5–4.5) for mitral positions. Patients with a bioprosthetic valve who experience a thromboembolic event on antiplatelet therapy may be converted to warfarin.

The 2020 AHA/ACC guideline for the management of patients with valvular heart disease states that patients with valvular heart disease and atrial fibrillation should be evaluated for risk of thromboembolic events and treated with oral anticoagulation if at high risk. Vitamin K antagonists are the anticoagulants of choice for patients with rheumatic mitral stenosis and mechanical heart valves. DOACs are an alternative to vitamin K antagonists in patients with atrial fibrillation and with bioprosthetic valves >3 months after implantation or with native valvular heart disease, excluding rheumatic mitral stenosis.

● ST-Segment Elevation Myocardial Infarction
Secondary Prevention

Warfarin has been used for secondary prevention to reduce the risk of death, recurrent MI, and thromboembolic events such as stroke or systemic embolism after an acute ST-segment-elevation MI (STEMI). The manufacturer of warfarin states that following an acute STEMI in high-risk patients (e.g., those with a large anterior STEMI, substantial heart failure, intracardiac thrombus visible on transthoracic echocardiography, atrial fibrillation, history of previous thromboembolic event), the use of warfarin (target INR 2–3) in conjunction with low-dose aspirin (not exceeding 100 mg daily) for at least 3 months is recommended. However, antiplatelet therapy is preferred over warfarin for secondary prevention and risk reduction in patients with atherosclerosis, including those with acute STEMI unless there is a separate indication (e.g., atrial fibrillation, prosthetic heart valve, left ventricular thrombus or high risk for such thrombi, concomitant venous thromboembolic disease).

Results of a few prospective studies and analysis of pooled data from other controlled trials suggest that long-term therapy (1–2 years or longer) with a coumarin derivative (e.g., warfarin) may be useful in selected patients for *secondary prevention* of death and/or nonfatal recurrent STEMI. In a randomized, placebo-controlled study in patients with acute STEMI, therapy with warfarin, initiated 2–4 weeks postinfarction and continued for an average of 37 months, was associated with reductions in the risk of death (24% reduction), nonfatal or fatal reinfarction (34% reduction), and total cerebrovascular events (55% reduction). In an open-label, randomized, comparative study in hospitalized patients with recent acute STEMI, long-term (approximately 4 years) therapy with warfarin alone or in combination with aspirin was more effective than aspirin therapy alone in reducing the incidence of the composite end point of death, nonfatal reinfarction, or thromboembolic stroke. The benefit of warfarin (dosage adjusted to achieve an INR of 2–2.5) in combination with aspirin (75 mg daily) or warfarin alone (dosage adjusted to achieve an INR of 2.8–4.2) compared with aspirin alone (160 mg daily) was restricted to reduction of nonfatal reinfarction and thromboembolic stroke; overall mortality was similar among the treatment groups.

Clinical Perspective

An AHA Scientific Statement on the management of patients at risk for and with left ventricular thrombus was published in 2022. Due to the lack of data supporting routine prophylactic anticoagulation in the current era of reperfusion, coronary stenting, and dual antiplatelet therapy (DAPT), prophylactic anticoagulation to prevent left ventricular thrombus post-STEMI is not routinely recommended for all patients, but may be considered on an individual basis. Therapeutic anticoagulation (e.g., with warfarin, DOACs) for the treatment of left ventricular thrombus after acute MI is appropriate.

● *Cerebral Embolism*

Antiplatelet agents are considered preferable to oral anticoagulation for secondary prevention of noncardioembolic stroke in patients with a history of ischemic stroke or TIA. However, oral anticoagulation with warfarin or a DOAC (e.g., apixaban, dabigatran, rivaroxaban, edoxaban) is recommended for secondary prevention in patients with TIAs or ischemic stroke and concurrent atrial fibrillation, provided no contraindications to therapy exist. Warfarin anticoagulation also is recommended for the prevention of recurrent stroke in patients at high risk for recurring cerebral embolism from other cardiac sources (e.g., prosthetic mechanical heart valves, anterior MI, and left ventricular thrombus).

For arterial ischemic stroke associated with dissection or a cardioembolic cause in children†, ACCP suggests the use of warfarin as an option for long-term anticoagulation.

The American Heart Association Stroke Council states that warfarin is recommended following initial therapy with heparin or a LMWH in patients with acute cerebral venous thrombosis (CVT)†. Target INR is 2–3 and the recommended duration of therapy is based on known or unknown provocation and the presence or absence of thrombophilia. One randomized, open-label, prospective study (RE-SPECT CVT) and one retrospective cohort study (ACTION-CVT) compared the use of DOACs (e.g., dabigatran, apixaban, rivaroxaban) with warfarin in adults with CVT following the acute treatment phase. Similar rates of VTE recurrence, bleeding, and recanalization were observed between warfarin and the DOACs; additional prospective studies are in progress (NCT04660747, NCT03178864).

● *Heparin-Induced Thrombocytopenia*

While warfarin should not be used for initial treatment of heparin-induced thrombocytopenia (HIT)†, the manufacturers and other clinicians state that therapy with the drug may be considered after platelet counts have normalized. Cases of venous limb ischemia, necrosis, and gangrene, sometimes resulting in amputation or death, have occurred in patients with HIT when heparin was discontinued

and warfarin was initiated or continued. ACCP and ASH recommend against initiating warfarin in patients with strongly suspected or confirmed HIT until substantial platelet recovery occurs (e.g., platelet count of at least 150,000/mm³); for patients already receiving warfarin at the time of diagnosis of HIT, use of vitamin K is suggested.

ACCP and ASH state that HIT should be treated initially with a parenteral nonheparin anticoagulant (e.g., argatroban, bivalirudin, fondaparinux). Conversion to warfarin therapy should be initiated with low dosages (maximum 5 mg daily) and only after substantial recovery from acute HIT has occurred. To avoid prothrombotic effects and ensure continuous anticoagulation, ACCP recommends that therapy with the parenteral nonheparin anticoagulant and warfarin be administered concurrently for at least 5 days and until the desired INR has been achieved.

● *Thrombotic Antiphospholipid Syndrome†*

The International Society of Thrombosis and Hemostasis (ISTH) recommends the use of warfarin over DOACs in patients with high-risk antiphospholipid syndrome (APS), including those with triple-positive APS and patients non-adherent to warfarin or with recurrent thrombosis while on therapeutic intensity warfarin.

DOSAGE AND ADMINISTRATION

● *General*

Pretreatment Screening

● Obtain baseline international normalized ratio (INR).

● Obtain baseline complete blood count (CBC).

● Verify pregnancy status in females of reproductive potential.

● Perform other relevant baseline laboratory tests as needed based upon the patient's clinical condition (e.g., liver function tests [LFTs]).

● Assess patient for active bleeding and bleeding risk.

● Assess patient for comorbid conditions (e.g., heart failure, diarrhea) and drug-drug interactions (e.g., amiodarone, metronidazole) that may influence warfarin dose selection.

● Pharmacogenomic testing for cytochrome P-450 (CYP)2C9 and vitamin K epoxide reductase (VKORC)1 genotypes is available and recommended, but not required.

Patient Monitoring

● Perform INR assessments regularly during therapy.

● Perform an INR assessment daily after warfarin initiation until the INR stabilizes in the therapeutic range.

● The American College of Chest Physicians (ACCP) states that INR assessments usually are performed daily in hospitalized patients until the INR is in the therapeutic range for at least 2 consecutive days; in nonhospitalized patients, initial INR assessments may be reduced from daily to every few days until a stable response has been achieved.

● The frequency of INR assessments should be based on clinical judgment and patient response, but generally are performed every 1–4 weeks. In patients with consistently stable INRs, ACCP has suggested an INR testing interval of up to 12 weeks.

● Monitor for signs and symptoms of bleeding (e.g., bruising, gum or nose bleeding, blood in stool).

● Monitor for signs and symptoms of thrombosis (e.g., leg swelling).

● Monitor CBC regularly and other laboratory tests based upon the patient's clinical condition.

● Monitor comorbid conditions (e.g., heart failure, diarrhea) for clinical changes that may influence the patient's INR response to warfarin (e.g., diarrhea, resolved or decompensated heart failure).

● Monitor for drug-drug interactions and drug therapy that is added, discontinued, or taken irregularly, that may influence the patient's INR response.

● Perform additional INR assessments when differing warfarin preparations (e.g., proprietary versus nonproprietary [generic]) are interchanged.

Dispensing and Administration Precautions

- Personnel who are pregnant should avoid exposure to crushed or broken tablets.
- Procedures for proper handling and disposal of potentially hazardous drugs should be considered.
- Per the Institute for Safe Medication Practices (ISMP), warfarin is a high-alert medication that has a heightened risk of causing significant patient harm when used in error.

Other General Considerations

- In patients managed by anticoagulation clinics, compared with patients receiving usual monitoring by their primary care clinician, available data indicate that the proportion of time in the therapeutic INR range and patient satisfaction is increased, but clinical outcomes such as bleeding, thrombosis, and mortality are not significantly different.
- Self-testing with or without self-monitoring may be an option for some patients. A Cochrane systematic review with meta-analysis reported no difference in bleeding or mortality, and reduced thromboembolic events, when patient self-testing or self-monitoring was compared to standard therapy; however, the risk of bias downgraded the quality of evidence.
- Self-management of warfarin therapy is suggested by ACCP as an alternative to outpatient INR monitoring in patients who are motivated and can demonstrate competency in self-management strategies, including the use of self-testing equipment.

● *Administration*

Administer warfarin sodium orally as a single daily dose without regard to food. Adhere strictly to the prescribed dosage and schedule of warfarin. Take warfarin tablets at the same time each day.

If a dose of warfarin is missed at the intended time of day, take the dose as soon as possible on the *same* day. A double dose of warfarin should not be taken the next day to make up for the missed dose.

Warfarin is discolored by light; warfarin preparations should be stored at controlled room temperature (20–25°C) in tight, light-resistant containers.

● *Dosage*

Warfarin dosage is expressed in terms of warfarin sodium.

Nonproprietary (generic) preparations of warfarin sodium are available, and the manufacturers warn that patients should be carefully instructed about the preparation they are receiving so that overdosage from inadvertent simultaneous use of equivalent preparations is avoided.

Warfarin sodium dosage requirements vary greatly among individual patients, and dosage must be carefully individualized based on the patient's INR in order to obtain optimum therapeutic effects while minimizing the risk of hemorrhage. Factors influencing initial dose selection include clinical factors (e.g., age, sex, comorbidities, concomitant medications) and genetic factors (e.g., CYP2C9 and VKORC1 genotypes).

Duration and intensity of anticoagulation (i.e., INR) is based on the indication for use. Pharmacogenomic factors (e.g., genetic variations in enzymes that metabolize warfarin or modulate its effect on clotting factor synthesis) also may be considered in determining the warfarin dosage.

Initial Dosage

The appropriate initial dosage of warfarin varies widely among different patients; dosage must be individualized taking into account factors such as age, race, body weight, sex, genotype, concomitant drugs, and the specific indication for use.

Routine use of warfarin loading doses is not recommended as such practice may increase the risk of hemorrhage or other complications and does not offer more rapid protection against clot formation. However, there is some evidence suggesting that use of a 10-mg loading dose may be a safe and effective approach in reducing the time to therapeutic INR. ACCP therefore suggests that in sufficiently healthy, nonhospitalized patients, an initial dosage of 10 mg daily for the first 2 days may be administered, with subsequent dosing based on INR determinations.

Smaller initial dosages (e.g., 2–5 mg of warfarin sodium daily) result in less fluctuation in the degree of anticoagulation and decrease the risk of hemorrhage. Low initial dosages should be considered for geriatric and/or debilitated patients. Lower initial dosages also should be considered in patients with certain genetic variations in CYP2C9 and/or VKORC1 gene(s), which are associated with reduced warfarin clearance or altered pharmacodynamic response. Individuals of Asian descent also appear to require lower initial dosages than white patients, resulting in part from such genetic variations.

In patients whose CYP2C9 and VKORC1 genotypes are not known, the usual initial dosage of warfarin sodium is 2–5 mg daily or the expected maintenance dosage, adjusted based on patient factors (e.g., age, race).

For patients with known CYP2C9 and VKORC1 genotypes, the manufacturers suggest that *initial* dosage may be determined by expected *maintenance* dosages observed in clinical studies of patients with various combinations of these gene variants. (See Pharmacogenomic Considerations in Dosing under Dosage and Administration.)

Maintenance Dosage

Maintenance dosage of warfarin varies greatly among patients and should be based on INR assessments. The manufacturer states that the usual maintenance dosage of warfarin is 2–10 mg daily for patients in whom CYP2C9 and VKORC1 genotypes are not known.

For patients with known CYP2C9 and VKORC1 genotypes, the manufacturer suggests expected maintenance dosages observed in clinical studies of patients with various combinations of these gene variants. Lower maintenance dosages should be considered for geriatric and/or debilitated patients. Because of inherited increased sensitivity and/or reduced metabolism of warfarin, individuals of Asian descent also appear to require lower maintenance dosages of warfarin than white patients.

Acquired or inherited warfarin resistance is rare but should be suspected if large daily dosages are required to maintain INR within a normal therapeutic range. Changes in anticoagulant dosage should be made in small increments, and patient response should be carefully monitored with clinical observation and INR determinations; warfarin dosing nomograms may be utilized.

If a previously stable patient presents with a single subtherapeutic or supratherapeutic INR, consider transient risk factors (e.g., missed dose, acute alcohol ingestion) before making a dosage change; ACCP suggests that the current dosage of warfarin may be continued and the INR retested within 1–2 weeks for outlier INR results not exceeding 0.5 above or below the therapeutic range. If an unexpected result that does not fit the patient's clinical picture occurs, consider repeating the INR.

Warfarin maintenance dosages were analyzed prospectively and retrospectively in atrial fibrillation and venous thromboembolism (VTE) cohorts with a target INR of 2–3. Analysis was performed based on indication, sex, and age. Warfarin dosage in the prospective cohort was higher in younger patients compared to older patients. The median (25th, 75th percentile) daily warfarin dosage in male patients with atrial fibrillation was 5.4 mg (4, 6.4 mg) in those 50–59 years of age and 3.9 mg (2.5, 5 mg) in those 80–89 years of age compared to females of the same age (5 mg [3.9, 6 mg] and 3.2 mg [2.5, 4.3 mg], respectively). The weekly warfarin dosage declined by 0.4 mg per year of age, and women required 4.5 mg less per week than men. The weekly warfarin dosage was 7.3 mg per week lower among those taking amiodarone and was also lower in patients with coronary artery disease or heart failure, but higher in those with diabetes. Based on these results, initial warfarin doses >5 mg per day would be expected to be too high for a majority of women over the age of 60 and men over the age of 70.

The manufacturer states that warfarin dosage in pediatric patients varies based on age, with infants generally having the highest, and adolescents having the lowest dosage requirements to maintain therapeutic INRs.

Target INR and Duration of Therapy

Duration and intensity of warfarin anticoagulation (i.e., INR) is based on the indication for use.

Table 1 contains the indication-based target INR and duration of therapy for adults as described by manufacturers and experts.

Patients with more than 1 indication for warfarin should have a target INR consistent with the greatest thrombotic risk. For example, a patient with atrial fibrillation and mechanical heart valve in the mitral position would have a target INR of 3 (2.5–3.5).

Patients with more than 1 indication for warfarin should have a duration consistent with the greatest thrombotic risk. For example, a patient with a provoked VTE due to surgery and atrial fibrillation would receive long-term warfarin therapy rather than 3 months of treatment.

Targeting an INR >4 appears to provide no additional therapeutic benefit in most patients and is associated with a higher risk of bleeding complications.

When warfarin is used in pediatric patients†, a target INR range of 2–3 generally is suggested by ACCP for most indications except in the setting of prosthetic cardiac valves where adherence to adult recommendations is suggested.

Consensus statements specific to pediatric patients treated with ventricular assist devices†, large or giant coronary aneurysms following Kawasaki disease†, and primary pulmonary hypertension† should be consulted for further information regarding target INR and duration of warfarin therapy.

TABLE 1. Indication-based Target INR and Duration of Therapy Recommendations

Indication	Target INR (Range)	Duration
VTE treatment	2.5 (2–3)	At least 3 months; reevaluate therapy based on risk-benefit and transience of provocation (e.g., provoked due to surgery)
VTE prophylaxis against recurrent VTE	2.5 (2–3)	Extended prophylaxis beyond 3 months is individualized and based on factors such as bleeding risk, cancer status, number of prior VTE events, transience of provocation (e.g., provoked due to surgery, unprovoked)
VTE prophylaxis, major orthopedic surgery	2.5 (2–3)	At least 10–14 days and possibly for up to 35 days after surgery.
Atrial fibrillation	2.5 (2–3)	Long-term
Atrial flutter	2.5 (2–3)	Long-term
Cardioversion	2.5 (2–3)	At least 3 weeks before and at least 4 weeks after pharmacologic or electrical cardioversion
Valvular heart disease	2.5 (2–3)	Long-term
Valve replacement, bioprosthetic	2.5 (2–3)	3–6 months following surgical replacement, regardless of position, aortic or mitral.
Valve replacement, mechanical, aortic bileaflet	2.5 (2–3)	Long-term
Valve replacement, mechanical, aortic, other	3 (2.5–3.5)	Long-term
Valve replacement, mechanical, mitral, all	3 (2.5–3.5)	Long-term
Myocardial infarction (STEMI)	2.5 (2–3)	At least 3 months
Cardioembolic stroke	2.5 (2–3)	Long-term
Left ventricular dysfunction +/- left ventricular thrombus	2.5 (2–3)	Long-term
Heparin-induced thrombocytopenia	2.5 (2–3)	3 months

Pharmacogenomic Considerations in Dosing

Variations in the genes responsible for warfarin metabolism or pharmacodynamic response may affect warfarin dosage requirements. Over 30% of European and white populations have one or more variant alleles encoding CYP2C9, the enzyme principally responsible for metabolism of S-warfarin, and such alleles are associated with reduced clearance of warfarin. Patients with one or more variant CYP2C9 alleles (e.g., CYP2C9*2, CYP2C9*3) are at increased risk of excessive anticoagulation (e.g., INR exceeding 3) and bleeding and require lower dosages of warfarin, particularly during initiation of therapy.

Warfarin inhibits vitamin K epoxide reductase, which is a vitamin K-cycle enzyme complex controlling the regeneration of reduced vitamin K from vitamin K epoxide. Reduced vitamin K is an essential cofactor involved in the formation of vitamin K-dependent clotting factors. Limited evidence suggests that variations in the gene that encodes vitamin K epoxide reductase, VKORC1, may have an even larger impact on warfarin dosage than CYP2C9 genetic variations, and differing average dosage requirements between patients of white, Black, and Asian ancestry may be explained by VKORC1 variant frequency.

The availability and reliability of genetic tests vary, and clinicians should check with their local or reference clinical laboratory to obtain more information about specific tests. Additional information about pharmacogenetic testing can be found at the Genetic Testing Registry (https://www.ncbi.nlm.nih.gov/gtr/). Genetic information does not replace regular INR monitoring and results of genetic testing should not delay initiation of warfarin therapy.

The 2017 update of the Clinical Pharmacogenetics Implementation Consortium (CPIC) guideline for pharmacogenetics-guided warfarin dosing suggests use of pharmacogenetic algorithm-based warfarin dosing over the genetics-based dosing (Table 2) found in the FDA-approved warfarin label.

The 2 recommended pharmacogenetic algorithms (Gage and International Warfarin Pharmacogenetics Consortium [IWPC]) consider age, sex, race or self-identified ancestry, weight, height, smoking status, warfarin indication, target INR, interacting drugs (e.g., amiodarone, phenytoin) and genetic variables (e.g., CYP2C9, VKORC1 genotypes). CPIC recommends the Gage over the IWPC algorithm because it can adjust for CYP4F2, CYP2C9*5 and *6, if those genotypes are known.

CPIC considers initial use of a loading dose to be controversial. If a loading dose is used, a genetically informed approach is suggested with an understanding of the limitations of the loading dose trials (e.g., majority of experience in those of European ancestry).

In patients whose CYP2C9 and VKORC1 genotypes are known, the manufacturer suggests that *initial* warfarin dosage may be determined based on expected maintenance dosages observed in clinical studies of patients with various combinations of these gene variants. (See Table 2.)

TABLE 2. Expected Daily *Maintenance* Dosages of Warfarin Sodium Based on CYP2C9 and VKORC1 Genotypes[a]

VKORC1	CYP2C9					
	*1/*1	*1/*2	*1/*3	*2/*2	*2/*3	*3/*3
GG	5–7 mg	5–7 mg	3–4 mg	3–4 mg	3–4 mg	0.5–2 mg
AG	5–7 mg	3–4 mg	3–4 mg	3–4 mg	0.5–2 mg	0.5–2 mg
AA	3–4 mg	3–4 mg	0.5–2 mg	0.5–2 mg	0.5–2 mg	0.5–2 mg

[a] Manufacturer suggests using these expected *maintenance* dosage ranges to estimate *initial* daily dosage of warfarin sodium in patients with known CYP2C9 and VKORC1 genotypes. Dosage ranges are derived from multiple published clinical studies. VKORC1-1639G > A (rs9923231) variant is used in this table; other co-inherited VKORC1 variants also may be important determinants of warfarin sodium dosage.

Transferring from Parenteral Anticoagulation to Warfarin

When warfarin is indicated for follow-up therapy after initial treatment with a parenteral anticoagulant (e.g., heparin, LMWH, fondaparinux), therapy with the parenteral anticoagulant is usually continued until an adequate response to warfarin is obtained as indicated by INR determinations. The manufacturer recommends that heparin and warfarin be used concurrently for at least 4–5 days until the desired INR has been attained, after which the parenteral anticoagulant may be discontinued. In adults with acute deep-vein thrombosis (DVT) or pulmonary embolism (PE), ACCP and ASH recommend that heparin, LMWH, or fondaparinux be used concurrently with warfarin for at least 5 days and until the INR is ≥2 for 24 hours or longer.

In children with VTE in whom long-term warfarin therapy is being considered, warfarin should be initiated on the same day as heparin or LMWH, and such therapy should be overlapped for ≥5 days and until the INR is therapeutic.

Heparin prolongs the INR, and caution should be observed in evaluating the INR in patients receiving concomitant therapy with warfarin and heparin. Valid INR determinations can usually be made during concurrent heparin therapy if blood samples for the test are drawn at least 5 hours after an IV injection of heparin, 4 hours after cessation of a continuous heparin IV infusion, or 24 hours after a subcutaneous injection of heparin. Warfarin may prolong the activated partial thromboplastin time (aPTT), even in the absence of heparin. However, during initial therapy with warfarin, the interference with heparin anticoagulation is of minimal clinical importance.

When warfarin is indicated for follow-up therapy after a nonheparin anticoagulant (e.g., argatroban, fondaparinux, bivalirudin) in the treatment of heparin-induced thrombocytopenia (HIT), therapy with warfarin and the nonheparin anticoagulant should be overlapped for a minimum of 5 days until an adequate response to warfarin is obtained as indicated by INR determinations. Warfarin therapy should be initiated only after substantial recovery from acute HIT has occurred (i.e., stable platelet counts ≥150,000/mm³ or platelet recovery >50% of baseline). Do not use a warfarin loading dose in HIT patients.

Conversion from anticoagulation with argatroban to warfarin is more complex than with other anticoagulants since combined therapy with argatroban and warfarin prolongs the INR beyond that produced by warfarin alone. The INR should be determined daily during concurrent argatroban and warfarin therapy. For an argatroban infusion rate of 2 mcg/kg per minute, argatroban therapy should be temporarily discontinued when the INR on combined therapy is >4. Overshooting the target INR should be avoided, as supratherapeutic INRs during concomitant therapy with direct thrombin inhibitors and warfarin have been associated with necrosis or gangrene of the skin or limbs. The INR should be determined 4–6 hours after discontinuance of argatroban infusion during warfarin monotherapy. If INR is below the desired therapeutic range, argatroban infusion should be resumed. Attempts to discontinue argatroban should be repeated daily and until the INR (4–6 hours after discontinuance of argatroban) on warfarin alone is in therapeutic range.

For argatroban infusion rates exceeding 2 mcg/kg per minute, the infusion rate should be reduced temporarily to 2 mcg/kg per minute, and the INR should be repeated 4–6 hours later. If the INR is >4, temporarily discontinue argatroban and repeat the INR 4–6 hours later. If the INR is below the desired therapeutic range, the argatroban infusion should be resumed. Attempts to discontinue argatroban should be repeated daily and until the INR on warfarin alone is in therapeutic range.

Transferring from Other Anticoagulants to Warfarin

The manufacturer suggests consulting the labeling of other anticoagulants for instructions on conversion to warfarin.

Managing Anticoagulation in Patients Requiring Invasive Procedures

Temporary interruption of long-term warfarin therapy may be required in patients undergoing surgical or other invasive procedures to minimize the risk of perioperative bleeding. The decision whether to interrupt therapy should be based on an assessment of the patient's risk for thromboembolism versus risk of perioperative bleeding, taking into account individual patient- and surgery-related factors. ACCP issued clinical practice guidelines that include recommendations for standardized surgical bleed and thromboembolic risk assessments, discontinuance and resumption of warfarin therapy, and bridging anticoagulation (e.g., heparin, LMWH). Temporary discontinuance of warfarin usually is required for major surgical or invasive procedures. Warfarin discontinuance for minor procedures associated with a low risk of bleeding (e.g., minor dental procedures, minor dermatologic procedures, cataract surgery) may not be necessary; however, the manufacturer recommends targeting the low end of the INR therapeutic range in these situations.

In patients who require temporary interruption of warfarin prior to surgery, ACCP recommends that the drug be discontinued ≥5 days prior to surgery; elderly patients with comorbidities, patients with low dose warfarin requirements, and those with a higher target INR range are among those who may require >5 days of warfarin interruption prior to surgery. Determine the INR immediately prior to any invasive procedure. Routine use of pre-operative vitamin K when the INR is >1.5 1 to 2 days before the elective surgery or procedure is not recommended. ACCP recommends warfarin resumption within 24 hours, usually on the evening of the surgery or procedure; warfarin resumption may be delayed in those with inadequate hemostasis, need for additional procedures, or those unable to receive enteral medications. Warfarin should be resumed at the patient's established maintenance dosage; loading doses (e.g., double the established maintenance dose) are not recommended.

Heparin bridging is defined as administration of LMWH or IV heparin during the period of interruption of warfarin therapy. The decision to administer heparin bridging should be individualized based on the patient's risk of thromboembolism versus risk of bleeding. ACCP recommends *against* heparin bridging in patients with mechanical heart valves, atrial fibrillation, or VTE who are not classified as high-risk for thromboembolism when warfarin is interrupted for an elective surgery or procedure. ACCP states that heparin bridging is *recommended* for patients at the highest risk for thromboembolism (e.g., patients with older-generation [e.g., tilting-disc] mechanical heart valves, any mechanical mitral valve, thromboembolic event within the last 3 months, atrial fibrillation patients with a CHA₂DS₂VASc score ≥7 or CHADS₂ score ≥5). During the early postoperative period following insertion of a mechanical heart valve, ACCP suggests bridging anticoagulation with heparin or a LMWH until the patient is stable on warfarin therapy.

● Special Populations

Hepatic Impairment

The manufacturer makes no specific dosage recommendations for patients with hepatic impairment; however, more frequent monitoring for bleeding is recommended.

Renal Impairment

The manufacturer makes no specific dosage recommendations for patients with renal impairment; however, more frequent INR monitoring may be required.

Geriatric Patients

In patients >60 years of age, the manufacturer recommends considering lower initial and maintenance warfarin dosages and more frequent monitoring for bleeding.

Asian Patients

A lower initiation and maintenance warfarin dosage may be required in Asian patients. Asian patients appear to be more sensitive than white patients to the anticoagulant effect of warfarin and may require lower initial and maintenance dosages. In an uncontrolled study in Chinese patients receiving warfarin for various indications and on a stable warfarin sodium dosage for at least 1 month, the average daily dosage required to maintain an INR of 2–2.5 was 3.3 mg. Age also was an important determinant of warfarin dosage (inverse correlation) in these patients, as were body weight and underlying disease (positive correlations). A single nucleotide polymorphism of VKORC1 that identifies a low-dose and a high-dose warfarin phenotype has been found to associate with optimal warfarin dosage in both European and Asian patients. The reduced average warfarin maintenance dosage requirement in Asian individuals is largely related to the relatively rare occurrence of the high-dose allele in this ethnic group.

Black Patients

The CYP2C9 *5, *6, *8, and *11 alleles associated with reduced enzymatic activity and warfarin metabolism occur in 45–50% of patients with self-reported African ancestry.

The 2017 update of the CPIC guideline for pharmacogenetics-guided warfarin dosing suggests a 15–30% warfarin dosage reduction when CYP2C9 *5, *6, *8, and *11 variant alleles are detected, regardless of self-reported ancestry.

CAUTIONS

● *Contraindications*

- Pregnancy, except in patients with mechanical heart valves.
- Patients with hemorrhagic tendencies or blood dyscrasias.
- Recent or contemplated surgery of the eye or CNS and in those undergoing traumatic surgery resulting in large open surfaces.
- Bleeding tendencies associated with active ulceration or overt bleeding of the GI, respiratory, or genitourinary tract; CNS hemorrhage; aneurysms (cerebral, dissecting aorta); pericarditis and pericardial effusions; bacterial endocarditis.
- Threatened abortion, eclampsia, and preeclampsia.
- Unsupervised patients with conditions associated with a potential high level of non-compliance with therapy (e.g., dementia/senility).
- Known hypersensitivity (e.g., anaphylaxis).
- Spinal puncture and other diagnostic or therapeutic procedures associated with the potential for uncontrollable bleeding.
- Major regional or lumbar block anesthesia.
- Malignant hypertension.

● *Warnings/Precautions*

Warnings

Bleeding Risk

Warfarin increases bleeding risk and can cause serious, potentially fatal, bleeding. A boxed warning about the risk of major or fatal bleeding is included in the prescribing information for warfarin. Patients should be promptly evaluated if any manifestations of blood loss occur during therapy; discontinue warfarin if active pathological bleeding occurs.

Bleeding is more likely to occur within the first month during the initiation of warfarin therapy. Risk factors for bleeding include higher dosages, high intensity of anticoagulation (INR >4), age ≥65 years, highly variable INRs, history of GI bleeding, hypertension, cerebrovascular disease, anemia, malignancy, trauma, renal or liver impairment, alcohol abuse, prior stroke, certain genetic factors, concomitant drugs that may increase INR response, and a long duration of warfarin therapy. Regular monitoring of INR should be performed in all patients receiving warfarin therapy. Perform more frequent INR monitoring when starting or stopping other drugs, including botanicals, or when changing dosages of other drugs, or when significant dietary changes occur. Patients at high risk of bleeding may benefit from more frequent monitoring, use of lower dosages with careful dosage adjustment to the desired INR, and a shorter duration of therapy appropriate for the clinical condition. Bleeding may still occur when INR is maintained in the therapeutic range.

Patients should be instructed to immediately report any signs and symptoms of bleeding (e.g., pain, swelling or discomfort, prolonged bleeding from cuts, increased menstrual flow or vaginal bleeding, nosebleeds, bleeding of gums from brushing, unusual bleeding or bruising, red or dark brown urine, red or tar black stools, headache, dizziness, or weakness). Bleeding from the GI or urinary tract may warrant investigation of underlying malignancy or other correctable lesions.

Warfarin-induced anticoagulation may be reversed by discontinuing the drug, administering oral or parenteral vitamin K, and/or administering replacement factors with fresh frozen plasma (FFP) or 4-factor prothrombin complex concentrate (PCC). Several hours are usually required for the effects of vitamin K to occur whether the drug is administered orally or parenterally. FFP and 4-factor PCC will result in more rapid warfarin reversal; 4-factor PCC may be administered in a smaller volume and at a more rapid infusion rate and is therefore preferred. In patients with a significantly elevated INR and no evidence of bleeding, the American College of Chest Physicians (ACCP) states that use of vitamin K is not recommended for INR values of 4.5–10 but may be used when the INR >10.

In warfarin patients with a bleed, regardless of INR, therapy should be determined following assessment of bleed severity (e.g., hemodynamic instability, critical site [e.g., intracranial], nonmajor [e.g., not in a critical site, hemodynamically stable, stable hemoglobin]), the urgency of the need to restore normal hemostasis, and whether or not therapy with the anticoagulant is to be maintained, temporarily held, or discontinued.

In patients with major bleeding requiring urgent warfarin reversal, ACCP and the Expert Consensus Decision Pathway from the American College of Cardiology (ACC) suggest the use of IV 4-factor PCC (INR-based dose [e.g., 25, 35, or 50 units/kg] or fixed dose [e.g., 1000 units, 1500 units]) rather than FFP 10–15 mL/kg, with additional use of vitamin K administered at a dosage of 5–10 mg by slow IV infusion. Activated factor VII reversal is not recommended; FFP may be used when 4-factor PCC is not available.

Other Warnings and Precautions

Tissue Necrosis

Tissue necrosis and/or gangrene of skin or other tissues have occurred rarely (<0.1%). This reaction, which can occur on the first exposure to warfarin or during a subsequent course of therapy, usually appears within 1–10 days after initiation of therapy; tissue damage occurs principally at sites of fat tissue such as the abdomen, breasts, buttocks, hips, and thighs. Cases of warfarin-induced necrosis have been reported more frequently in women.

Patients with hereditary or acquired deficiencies of protein C, or its cofactor protein S, appear to have an increased risk of developing necrosis during warfarin therapy; however, necrosis can occur in the absence of this deficiency. Concomitant heparin for 5–7 days during warfarin initiation may minimize the incidence of tissue necrosis in these patients.

The necrotic lesions generally begin as painful, erythematous patches on the skin that progress rapidly to dark, hemorrhagic areas. In severe cases, surgical debridement of the affected tissue, skin grafting, or amputation of the affected tissue, limb, breast, or penis has been required.

To determine whether necrosis is caused by underlying disease, careful clinical evaluation is required. Discontinue warfarin if necrosis occurs; although guidelines do not exist, suggested treatments include supportive care, surgical debridement, aggressive wound care, and topical bactericidal agents. Alternative anticoagulants should be considered.

Patients should be instructed to immediately inform their clinician if they experience pain, temperature change, or discoloration of the skin (a purple bruise-like rash), especially on areas of the body with a high fat content, such as breasts, thighs, buttocks, hips, and abdomen.

Systemic Atheroemboli and Cholesterol Microemboli

Some evidence suggests that warfarin anticoagulation may enhance the release of atheromatous plaque emboli and increase the risk of complications; some cases have progressed to necrosis and death. The most common visceral organs involved are the kidneys, followed by the pancreas, spleen, and liver. Signs and symptoms will vary depending on the site of embolization.

A distinct syndrome resulting from microemboli to the feet is known as "purple toes syndrome". Purple toes syndrome usually occurs 3–10 weeks or later following warfarin initiation or related compounds (e.g., dicumarol [no longer commercially available in the US]) This syndrome typically is characterized by a purplish or mottled discoloration of the plantar surfaces and sides of the toes, which blanches on moderate pressure and fades with elevation of the legs; other characteristics may include pain and tenderness of the toes and waxing and waning of the color over time.

Patients should be instructed to immediately inform their clinician if they experience sudden cool, painful, purple discoloration of the toe(s) or forefoot, or any unusual symptom (e.g., pain, color, or temperature change to any other area of the body). If signs and symptoms are observed, discontinue warfarin and consider an alternative anticoagulant.

Calciphylaxis

Potentially serious and/or fatal calciphylaxis or calcium uremic arteriolopathy has been reported in warfarin-treated patients with and without end stage renal disease. The time course and presentation differ from warfarin-induced necrosis. Warfarin-induced necrosis occurs typically within the first 10 days, whereas warfarin-associated calciphylaxis results after a prolonged duration of warfarin therapy.

If calciphylaxis occurs during therapy, discontinue warfarin, treat the patient as appropriate, and consider alternative anticoagulants.

Acute Kidney Injury

Warfarin-induced acute kidney injury may occur in patients with altered glomerular integrity or with a history of kidney disease, possibly in relation to episodes of excessive anticoagulation and hematuria. Monitor patients with compromised renal function more frequently.

Limb Ischemia, Necrosis, and Gangrene in Patients with HIT and HITTS

Do not use warfarin as initial therapy for heparin-induced thrombocytopenia (HIT) or heparin-induced thrombocytopenia with thrombosis syndrome (HITTS). Cases of limb ischemia, necrosis, and gangrene have occurred in patients with HIT and HITTS when warfarin was initiated or continued after heparin discontinuance. In some patients, amputation of the involved area and/or death have occurred. Delay warfarin initiation until thrombin generation is adequately controlled and thrombocytopenia has resolved (i.e., platelet counts ≥150,000/mm³ and stable).

Use in Pregnant Women with Mechanical Heart Valves

Warfarin can cause fetal harm when administered to a pregnant woman and is contraindicated during pregnancy. If warfarin is used during pregnancy, or if the patient becomes pregnant while taking this drug, the patient should be apprised of the potential hazard to a fetus.

Major congenital malformations (warfarin embryopathy and fetotoxicity), fatal fetal hemorrhage, and an increased risk of spontaneous abortion and fetal mortality may occur as a result of warfarin exposure during pregnancy.

In women with mechanical heart valves at high risk of thromboembolism, the potential benefits of using warfarin may outweigh the fetal risks. The manufacturer states that the decision to initiate or continue warfarin should be reviewed with the patient, taking into consideration the specific risks and benefits pertaining to the individual patient's situation, as well as the most current medical guidelines.

Other Clinical Settings with Increased Risks

The decision to use warfarin in patients with the following conditions should be based on clinical judgment after weighing the increased risks against the benefits: moderate to severe hepatic or renal impairment, infectious diseases (e.g., patients receiving antibiotic therapy) or disturbances of intestinal flora (e.g., sprue), patients with indwelling catheters, moderate to severe hypertension, acquired or hereditary protein C or protein S deficiencies, polycythemia vera, diabetes mellitus, eye surgery, and vasculitis. Although diabetes mellitus is also included in the list of conditions, this should be interpreted with caution because diabetes is a prominent factor in stroke scoring tools (e.g., CHA_2DS_2-VASc, ATRIA), but is a less consistent risk factor for bleeding. With the exception of the modified Outpatient Bleeding Risk Index (mOBRI), diabetes is not included in contemporary bleeding scoring tools (e.g., HAS-BLED, HEMORR2HAGES).

The manufacturer states that cataract surgery in patients taking warfarin has resulted in minor complications of sharp needle and local anesthesia block but has not been associated with potentially sight-threatening operative hemorrhagic complications. The decision to discontinue or reduce the warfarin dosage prior to less invasive or less complex eye surgery (e.g., lens surgery) should be based on the patient's risk of thromboembolism.

Endogenous Factors Affecting INR

Endogenous factors such as diarrhea, hepatic disorders, poor nutritional state, steatorrhea, or vitamin K deficiency may be responsible for an increased INR response. Other factors have been reported in the literature (e.g., decompensated heart failure, non-euthyroid hyperthyroidism).

Endogenous factors that may result in a decreased INR response include increased vitamin K intake or hereditary warfarin resistance. Other factors have been reported in the literature (e.g., alcoholism following chronic ingestion, non-euthyroid hypothyroidism).

Specific Populations

Pregnancy

Warfarin can cause fetal harm and is contraindicated during pregnancy except in women with mechanical heart valves who are at high risk of thromboembolism and for whom the benefits of warfarin may outweigh the risks.

Major congenital malformations (warfarin embryopathy and fetotoxicity), fatal fetal hemorrhage, and an increased risk of spontaneous abortion and fetal mortality may occur as a result of warfarin exposure during pregnancy. Warfarin embryopathy is characterized by nasal hypoplasia with or without stippled epiphyses (chondrodysplasia punctata) and growth retardation (including low birth weight). CNS and eye abnormalities have also been reported, including dorsal midline dysplasia characterized by agenesis of the corpus callosum, Dandy-Walker malformation, midline cerebellar atrophy, and ventral midline dysplasia characterized by optic atrophy. Mental retardation, blindness, schizencephaly, microcephaly, hydrocephalus, and other adverse pregnancy outcomes have been reported following warfarin exposure during the second and third trimesters. Teratogenicity risk is highest during the first trimester, at 6–12 weeks of gestation. However, risk of pregnancy loss or fetal hemorrhage still exists for warfarin exposure in the second and/or third trimester.

The risk of valve thrombosis is much higher with mechanical heart valves because of the hypercoagulable state. Pregnant women with mechanical heart valves should receive therapeutic anticoagulation with frequent monitoring during pregnancy. Despite the risks of warfarin to the fetus, the drug has been used in pregnant women with prosthetic heart valves who are at an increased risk for valve thrombosis. The manufacturer states in these situations, the decision to initiate or continue warfarin should be reviewed with the patient, taking into consideration the specific risks and benefits pertaining to that individual patient's medical situation, as well as the most current medical guidelines. If warfarin is used during pregnancy, or if the patient becomes pregnant while taking warfarin, the patient should be apprised of the potential hazard to a fetus.

The American College of Cardiology/American Heart Association (ACC/AHA) issued guidelines for the management of patients with valvular heart disease, which includes recommendations for the management of women with mechanical heart valves who are pregnant or plan to become pregnant. Multiple strategies to reduce, as well as balance, the maternal (e.g., valve thrombosis, death) and fetal risks (e.g., fetal loss, teratogenicity) are based on factors such as daily warfarin dosage (≤ or >5 mg/day), ability to utilize heparin or low molecular weight heparin (LMWH), ability to conduct frequent laboratory monitoring (e.g., INR, anti-Xa levels), and the patient's values and priorities. No single anticoagulation strategy is optimally safe for both the mother and the fetus; maternal and fetal risks can be reduced, but not eliminated. Options include warfarin continuation throughout pregnancy, dose-adjusted heparin or LMWH with frequent anti-Xa level monitoring throughout pregnancy, or sequential therapy with dose-adjusted heparin or LMWH with frequent anti-Xa level monitoring during the first trimester and warfarin during the second and third trimesters. Heparin and LMWH therapy have been associated with an increased maternal risk for valve thrombosis, death, and major bleeding complications in women with prosthetic heart valves.

Other guidance documents (e.g., American College of Obstetricians and Gynecologists [ACOG], American Society of Hematology [ASH]) should be consulted for the management of other warfarin indications in the context of pregnancy.

The timing of anticoagulation discontinuance in anticipation of labor and delivery is important to reduce the risk of maternal and fetal bleeding; women should have an individualized plan that addresses obstetrical, anesthetic, and thrombotic concerns.

Lactation

Limited data suggest that warfarin is not significantly distributed into human milk, is not detectable in plasma of nursing infants, and has not produced substantial coagulation abnormalities in such infants. Based on limited available data, it is considered unlikely that maternal warfarin therapy would pose a substantial risk to healthy, full-term infants receiving human milk, and ACOG, ASH, American Academy of Pediatrics (AAP), ACCP, and other experts consider maternal warfarin therapy to be compatible with breast-feeding. Women should inform their clinician if they are breast-feeding or plan to breast-feed. The manufacturers state that the decision to breast-feed while receiving warfarin anticoagulation should be made only after careful consideration of the mother's clinical need for warfarin, the developmental and health benefits of breastfeeding, and potential adverse effects.

Neonates are particularly sensitive to the effects of warfarin as a result of vitamin K deficiency; monitor infants receiving human milk for bruising and bleeding. The effects of warfarin in premature infants have not been evaluated.

Females and Males of Reproductive Potential

Females of reproductive potential who are receiving warfarin therapy should be counseled on effective contraception, about the risks of therapy before pregnancy occurs, as well as pre- and post-conception strategies to reduce the risks to the mother and the fetus. Continue effective contraception during treatment and for at least 1 month after the final warfarin dose in such patients.

Pediatric Use

The manufacturer of warfarin states that the optimum dosing, safety, and efficacy in pediatric patients are unknown due to a lack of adequate, well-controlled studies. Pediatric use of warfarin is based on adult data and recommendations, as well as limited pediatric data from observational studies and patient registries. However, the drug has been used in pediatric patients for prevention and treatment of thromboembolic events.

Difficulty achieving and maintaining therapeutic INRs has been reported in pediatric patients, and more frequent assessments of INR are recommended in such patients because of possible changing warfarin requirements due to age, concomitant medications, diet, and comorbid conditions. Variable bleeding rates have been observed in pediatric patients; therefore, such patients should avoid activities or sports that may result in traumatic injury.

Infants may have the highest and adolescents the lowest mg per kg dosage requirements. Human milk-fed children may be more sensitive to warfarin compared to those receiving vitamin-K supplemented nutrition.

Geriatric Use

Age does not appear to substantially affect the pharmacokinetics of racemic warfarin, and the manufacturer states that the clearance of S-warfarin is similar in geriatric versus younger individuals. However, the clearance of R-warfarin appears to be slightly reduced in geriatric patients compared with that in younger individuals. Patients >60 years of age appear to exhibit a greater than expected INR response to warfarin, and a lower dosage is required to produce a therapeutic level of anticoagulation. Increasing age has been shown to confer a greater risk for bleeding outcomes, and advanced age has been included as a risk factor in both disease and bleeding risk stratification tools. The cause for increased sensitivity in geriatric patients is unknown but may be due to a combination of pharmacokinetic and pharmacodynamic factors. Consider lower initial and maintenance doses for elderly and/or debilitated patients. Conduct more frequent monitoring for bleeding in any situation or with any physical condition where added risk of hemorrhage is present.

A systematic review with meta-analysis of 11 clinical trials involving warfarin and direct oral anticoagulants (DOACs; e.g., dabigatran, apixaban, rivaroxaban, edoxaban) for atrial fibrillation and venous thromboembolism (VTE) compared the benefits and harms of these therapies in patients ≥75 years of age. Of the 102,479 patients within the 11 trials, 31,418 were ≥75 years of age. In these patients, DOACs were shown to be at least as effective as warfarin in reducing the recurrence of stroke, systemic embolism, and VTE; however, DOAC therapy was associated with a significantly lower risk of intracranial bleeding. When stratified by major bleeding, GI bleeding, and clinically relevant bleeding, comparisons were limited due to trial design and data availability; warfarin or a specific DOAC was favored depending upon the specific bleeding outcome.

Hepatic Impairment

Patients with hepatic impairment should be monitored more frequently for bleeding due to impaired synthesis of clotting factors and decreased warfarin metabolism that can potentiate the anticoagulation response.

Renal Impairment

No dosage adjustment is necessary in patients with renal impairment; renal clearance is considered a minor determinant of anticoagulant response to warfarin. The manufacturer suggests increased INR monitoring in warfarin patients with renal impairment.

● Common Adverse Effects

Most common adverse effects: fatal and nonfatal hemorrhage from any tissue or organ.

DRUG INTERACTIONS

Concurrent administration of numerous drugs or dietary or herbal supplements has been reported to affect patient response to warfarin.

Drugs may *increase* patient sensitivity to warfarin by decreasing intestinal synthesis or absorption of vitamin K or affecting distribution of the vitamin; decreasing the rate of anticoagulant metabolism by competing for sites of metabolism or inhibiting the function or synthesis of metabolic enzymes; increasing affinity of the anticoagulant for receptor sites; decreasing synthesis and/or increasing catabolism of functional blood coagulation factors II, VII, IX, and X; interfering with other components of normal hemostasis such as platelet function or fibrinolysis; and by producing ulcerogenic effects.

Certain drugs may *decrease* patient response to warfarin by decreasing absorption of the anticoagulant; increasing the rate of metabolism of the anticoagulant by enzyme induction; or by increasing synthesis of functional blood coagulation factors II, VII, IX, and X.

Some dietary or herbal supplements contain naturally occurring coumarins or salicylates that may have anticoagulant, antiplatelet, or fibrinolytic effects; these supplements would be expected to increase the anticoagulant effects of concomitantly administered warfarin.

Certain dietary or herbal supplements also may decrease response to warfarin, possibly as a result of induction of hepatic microsomal enzymes (e.g., St. John's wort) or because of procoagulant effects (e.g., coenzyme Q10).

● Drugs Affecting Hepatic Microsomal Enzymes

Warfarin is metabolized by cytochrome P-450 (CYP) isoenzymes CYP2C9, 2C19, 2C8, 2C18, 1A2, and 3A4; the S-enantiomer is metabolized principally by CYP2C9, while the R-enantiomer is metabolized by CYP1A2 and 3A4. Because the S-enantiomer of warfarin is about 2–5 times more potent than R-warfarin, drugs that preferentially increase or decrease the metabolism of S-warfarin are more likely to be associated with alterations in INR. Drugs that *inhibit* CYP2C9, CYP1A2, or CYP3A4 can potentially *increase* exposure and response to warfarin; conversely, drugs that *induce* CYP2C9, CYP1A2, or CYP3A4 can potentially *decrease* exposure and response to warfarin. (See Table 3.) INR should be closely monitored in patients who initiate, discontinue, or change dosages of concomitant drugs that affect these CYP isoenzymes.

TABLE 3. CYP Interactions with Warfarin

Enzyme	Inhibitors*	Inducers*
CYP2C9	amiodarone, capecitabine, co-trimoxazole, etravirine, fluconazole, fluvastatin, fluvoxamine, metronidazole, miconazole, oxandrolone, tigecycline, voriconazole, zafirlukast	aprepitant, bosentan, carbamazepine, phenobarbital, rifampin
CYP1A2	acyclovir, allopurinol, caffeine, cimetidine, ciprofloxacin, disulfiram, enoxacin, famotidine, fluvoxamine, methoxsalen, mexiletine, oral contraceptives, propafenone, propranolol, terbinafine, thiabendazole, ticlopidine, verapamil, zileuton	montelukast, moricizine, omeprazole, phenobarbital, phenytoin, cigarette smoking
CYP3A4	alprazolam, amiodarone, amlodipine, aprepitant, atorvastatin, atazanavir, bicalutamide, cilostazol, cimetidine, ciprofloxacin, clarithromycin, conivaptan, cyclosporine, darunavir/ritonavir, diltiazem, erythromycin, fluconazole, fluoxetine, fluvoxamine, fosamprenavir, imatinib, indinavir, isoniazid, itraconazole, ketoconazole, lopinavir/ritonavir, nefazodone, nelfinavir, nilotinib, oral contraceptives, posaconazole, ranitidine, ranolazine, ritonavir, tipranavir, voriconazole, zileuton	armodafinil, amprenavir, aprepitant, bosentan, carbamazepine, efavirenz, etravirine, modafinil, nafcillin, phenytoin, pioglitazone, prednisone, rifampin, rufinamide

* list of drugs is not all-inclusive

● Protein-bound Drugs

Drugs may competitively or noncompetitively interfere with protein binding of warfarin, producing increased concentrations of unbound drug and potentiation of anticoagulant effects. In most instances, this is only a temporary effect with marginally increased INR and the INR may return to therapeutic levels after several days of concomitant therapy.

● Drugs That Can Increase Bleeding Risk

Risk of bleeding may be increased when warfarin is used concomitantly with other drugs that can also increase bleeding risk. (See Table 4.) The interacting drug should be initiated only after weighing the risk-benefit of the combination, including other risk factors which may impact bleeding risk (e.g., advanced age, history of bleeding), and should be used for the shortest duration possible; patients should be monitored closely whenever such drugs are used concomitantly with warfarin.

Nonsteroidal anti-inflammatory agents (NSAIAs) can inhibit platelet aggregation and cause GI bleeding and peptic ulceration and/or perforation, in addition to specific drug interactions that may affect the INR. While the manufacturer of warfarin suggests close monitoring in those receiving NSAIAs, including selective cyclooxygenase-2 (COX-2) inhibitors, and others recommend the use of gastroprotective agents when the combination cannot be avoided, some experts (e.g., the American College of Chest Physicians [ACCP]) suggest that such concomitant therapy be avoided.

Concomitant administration of warfarin and antiplatelet agents should be avoided unless the benefit is known or is highly likely to be greater than the potential harm from bleeding; patients in whom benefit may potentially outweigh risk include those with mechanical heart valves, acute coronary syndrome, or patients who have undergone recent coronary artery stent placement or bypass surgery.

TABLE 4. Drugs that Can Increase Bleeding Risk*

Drug Class	Specific Drugs
Anticoagulants	argatroban, dabigatran, bivalirudin, heparin, fondaparinux, apixaban, dabigatran, edoxaban, rivaroxaban, enoxaparin
Antiplatelet agents	aspirin, cilostazol, clopidogrel, dipyridamole, prasugrel, ticlopidine, ticagrelor, vorapaxar
Nonsteroidal anti-inflammatory agents	celecoxib, diclofenac, diflunisal, fenoprofen, ibuprofen, indomethacin, ketoprofen, ketorolac, mefenamic acid, naproxen, oxaprozin, piroxicam, sulindac
Serotonin-reuptake inhibitors	citalopram, desvenlafaxine, duloxetine, escitalopram, fluoxetine, fluvoxamine, milnacipran, paroxetine, sertraline, venlafaxine, vilazodone

* list of drugs is not all-inclusive

● Antibiotics and Antifungals

Changes in INR have been reported in patients receiving certain antibiotics or antifungal agents concomitantly with warfarin; however, clinical pharmacokinetic studies have not shown consistent effects of these drugs on plasma concentrations of warfarin. The manufacturer states that INR should be monitored closely whenever any antibiotic or antifungal agent is initiated or discontinued in patients receiving warfarin.

● Cholestyramine

Concurrent administration of cholestyramine with warfarin results in decreased absorption of the anticoagulant. In addition, cholestyramine has been shown to decrease the plasma half-life of warfarin by interfering with enterohepatic circulation of the drug. However, because vitamin K absorption may also be decreased by cholestyramine, the net effect of concurrent anticoagulant and cholestyramine

therapy is difficult to predict. If concurrent use of cholestyramine and warfarin cannot be avoided, administer warfarin 1 hour before or at least 4 to 6 hours after cholestyramine.

● Acetaminophen

Chronic ingestion of large doses of acetaminophen has been reported to potentiate the effects of coumarin-derivative anticoagulants (e.g., warfarin). Conflicting data exist and the clinical importance of such an interaction has been questioned. Large dosages of acetaminophen (exceeding 1.5 g per day) may augment the anticoagulant effect of warfarin. In addition, results of an observational study in patients stabilized on warfarin therapy indicate an association between ingestion of even low to moderate dosages of acetaminophen (7 or more 325-mg tablets weekly) and excessively high INR values. In a 4-week, randomized controlled trial comparing the addition of placebo, acetaminophen 2 g/day, or acetaminophen 4 g/day in stable chronic warfarin-treated patients, both groups of acetaminophen patients experienced significantly elevated INR values. The average weekly change in INR from baseline was -0.1 to 0.1, 0.1 to 0.3, and 0 to 0.6 for the placebo, 2 g/day, and 4 g/day groups, respectively; 54% of patients in the acetaminophen groups had an INR of 0.3 or more above the upper limit of their therapeutic range. Some clinicians suggest that additional monitoring of INR values may be prudent in patients receiving warfarin therapy following initiation of, and during sustained therapy with, large doses of acetaminophen.

● Miconazole

Concomitant administration of vaginal miconazole creams or suppositories with acenocoumarol or warfarin for approximately 3 days has resulted in an increased PT/INR and/or bleeding. Additional monitoring of INR values and appropriate dosage adjustments may be required in patients receiving concomitant intravaginal miconazole therapy.

● Alcohol

Some clinicians state that alcohol ingestion should be avoided in patients receiving warfarin. However, other clinicians suggest that patients receiving warfarin therapy may consume alcohol in small amounts (e.g., 1–2 drinks occasionally) but that chronic heavy consumption (e.g., defined as greater than 720 mL of beer, 300 mL of wine, or 60 mL of liquor daily) should be avoided. The effects of moderate alcohol consumption (e.g., 1–2 drinks daily) on adverse events or anticoagulation control in patients receiving long-term therapeutic anticoagulation with warfarin has not been well studied. In 2 studies in a small number of healthy young men, daily ingestion of 300-600 mL of wine in the fasting or unfasting state on a short-term basis (21 days) did not affect plasma warfarin concentrations or therapeutic hypoprothrombinemia (maintained at 25–35% of normal prothrombin activity as measured by one-stage prothrombin time). However, numerous patient-specific factors affect response to warfarin, including age, vitamin K status, concomitant disease (e.g., hepatic dysfunction, fat malabsorption, hyperthyroidism, fever), and hereditary resistance; therefore, lack of evidence of a warfarin-alcohol interaction in healthy individuals may not preclude such interactions in individual patients. Acute ingestion of alcohol has been reported to enhance hypoprothrombinemia and prolong INR by inhibiting warfarin metabolism, reducing its clearance, and/or displacing it from plasma proteins, while long-term use of alcohol (e.g., chronic alcoholism) may reduce anticoagulant effects by inducing CYP isoenzymes (e.g., CYP2E1, CYP3A4, CYP1A2) and warfarin metabolism. Alcohol also has antiplatelet effects that may increase bleeding risk with warfarin without affecting INR.

● Dietary or Herbal Supplements

Dietary and herbal supplements also have been reported to increase or decrease the effects of warfarin, in some cases through CYP-mediated interactions (e.g., echinacea, grapefruit juice, gingko, goldenseal, St. John's wort). (See Tables 5 and 6.) In general, caution should be exercised when dietary or herbal supplements are used in patients receiving warfarin, and additional INR monitoring is recommended whenever these products are initiated or discontinued; limited information is available regarding the interaction potential of these products with warfarin.

TABLE 5. Dietary or Herbal Supplements that May *Increase* Response to Coumarin Derivatives (e.g., Warfarin)

agrimony	chamomile (German and Roman)	parsley
alfalfa	clove	passion flower
aloe gel	*cranberry	pau d'arco
Angelica sinensis (dong quai)	dandelion	policosanol
aniseed	fenugreek	poplar
arnica	feverfew	prickly ash (Northern)
asa foetida	garlic	quassia
aspen	German sarsaparilla	red clover
black cohosh	ginger	senega
black haw	*Ginkgo biloba*	sweet clover
bladder wrack (*Fucus*)	ginseng (*Panax*)	sweet woodruff
bogbean	horse chestnut	tamarind
boldo	horseradish	tonka beans
bromelains	inositol nicotinate	wild carrot
buchu	licorice	wild lettuce
capsicum	meadowsweet	willow
cassia	nettle	wintergreen
celery	onion	

TABLE 6. Dietary or Herbal Supplements that May *Decrease* Response to Coumarin Derivatives (e.g., Warfarin)

agrimony	goldenseal	St. John's wort
coenzyme Q_{10} (ubidecarenone)	mistletoe	yarrow
ginseng (*Panax*)		

● Cranberry Products

Several case reports have suggested a possible interaction between warfarin and cranberry juice; in these reports, the effects of warfarin appeared to be potentiated by cranberry juice or a cranberry product, in some cases resulting in clinically important bleeding events. However, confounding factors were present in many of these cases and prospective controlled studies generally have not been able to confirm this interaction. Results of several studies, including a randomized, double-blind trial evaluating the effects of daily consumption of 240 mL of cranberry juice over a 2-week period in 30 patients stabilized on warfarin therapy, showed no evidence of any clinically important pharmacokinetic or pharmacodynamic interaction. The amounts of cranberry juice ingested varied among these studies, but generally were lower than those described in the case reports. It is possible that this interaction may be dose dependent, with response elicited by ingestion of large quantities (approximately 1–2 L) of cranberry juice. In a study of healthy volunteers who were administered concentrated cranberry extract (3 g/day) and warfarin 25 mg daily, the area under the INR-time curve was increased by approximately 30% compared to warfarin treatment alone, a result that was both statistically and clinically significant. Although available data do not appear to support a clinically important interaction between warfarin and moderate amounts of cranberry juice (240–480 mL) or cranberry extract (≤1350 mg/day)

consumption, clinicians should be aware of the possibility of such an interaction and monitor closely for changes in INR and manifestations of bleeding.

DESCRIPTION

● Pharmacology

Warfarin sodium is a coumarin-derivative anticoagulant that alters the synthesis of vitamin-K dependent blood coagulation factors II, VII, IX, X, and the anticoagulant proteins C and protein S.

The mechanism of vitamin-K interference is thought to be inhibition of the C1 subunit of vitamin K epoxide reductase (VKORC1) enzyme complex and reduction of vitamin K1 epoxide regeneration. Reduced vitamin K is an essential cofactor involved in the formation of vitamin K-dependent clotting factors.

Warfarin decreases clotting factor synthesis by inhibiting the regeneration of reduced vitamin K from vitamin K epoxide via inhibition of warfarin's target enzyme, vitamin K epoxide reductase. Without reduced vitamin K as a cofactor for γ-glutamyl carboxylase, carboxylation of glutamic acid residues on coagulation factors II, VII, IX, and X cannot proceed and these proteins do not become fully functional coagulation factors. Certain variations in the gene VKORC1 that encodes vitamin K epoxide reductase may be associated with lower hepatic expression of the gene and lower concentrations of reduced vitamin K. Patients with such variant genes are at increased risk of excessive anticoagulation (e.g., supratherapeutic INRs) and/or bleeding and require lower dosages of warfarin. Other genetic variations in the VKORC1 gene may contribute to warfarin resistance and increased warfarin dosage requirements. (See Pharmacogenomics under Description.)

Because warfarin does not alter catabolism of blood coagulation factors, depletion of circulating functional vitamin K-dependent coagulation factors must occur before effects of the drug become apparent. Depletion of functional coagulation factor II, factor VII, Protein C, factor IX, Protein S, and factor X occurs in a sequential manner; the rate of depletion of these coagulation factors depends on their individual rates of degradation.

Warfarin therapy inhibits thrombus formation when stasis is induced and may prevent extension of existing thrombi. The drug has no direct effect on established thrombi and appears to have little if any effect on the pathogenesis of arterial thrombi that result from interaction of platelets with an abnormal vessel wall. Because warfarin affects synthesis of blood coagulation factors that are involved in both extrinsic and intrinsic coagulation, the drug prolongs both the prothrombin time (PT), which measures the integrity of the extrinsic system, and the activated partial thromboplastin time (aPTT), which measures the integrity of the intrinsic system.

Commercially available warfarin sodium is a racemic mixture of the *R*- and *S*-enantiomers of the drug. The enantiomers have different half-lives, potencies, routes of administration, and rates of elimination. The *S*-enantiomer of warfarin has 2–5 times the anticoagulant activity of the *R*-enantiomer. An anticoagulant effect generally occurs within 24 hours following administration of warfarin, but peak anticoagulant effects may be delayed for 72–96 hours. Antithrombogenic effects of warfarin generally occur only after concentrations of functional coagulation factors IX and X are diminished, which may not occur until 5–10 days following initiation of therapy.

Plasma concentrations of vitamin K-dependent coagulation factors are physiologically decreased in neonates compared with adults, and the capacity of plasma from children receiving warfarin to generate thrombin is delayed and reduced compared with adults.

● Pharmacokinetics

Warfarin sodium is rapidly and extensively absorbed from the GI tract. Peak plasma concentrations of warfarin usually are attained within 4 hours. Following initiation of warfarin therapy, blood concentrations of functional coagulation factor VII (plasma half-life of 4–6 hours) are depressed first, followed by those of factors IX (plasma half-life of 24 hours) and X (plasma half-life of 48–72 hours), and finally factor II (plasma half-life of 60 hours). When warfarin therapy is discontinued or phytonadione is administered, blood concentrations of functional vitamin K-dependent coagulation factors return to pretreatment concentrations.

Warfarin is 99% bound to plasma proteins, principally albumin. Warfarin crosses the placenta, and fetal plasma drug concentrations may be equal to maternal plasma concentrations. The estimated volumes of distribution for R- and S-warfarin and racemic warfarin are similar. Limited data suggest that warfarin is not significantly distributed into milk in humans. In one study, warfarin was not detected in the milk of 15 nursing women; prothrombin times measured in 6 of the infants (PT not obtained in the other 9) were within the expected range.

The effective elimination half-life of warfarin averages about 40 hours and shows considerable interindividual variation (range: 20–60 hours). The clearance of the R-enantiomer of warfarin is about 50% that of the S-enantiomer; since the volumes of distribution of the enantiomers are similar, the half-life of R-warfarin (e.g., 37–89 hours) is longer than that of S-warfarin (e.g., 21–43 hours). Up to 92% of the drug is excreted in the urine and very little is unchanged drug. Racemic warfarin is stereoselectively metabolized by hepatic cytochrome P-450 (CYP) microsomal enzymes to inactive metabolites. The CYP isoenzymes involved in warfarin metabolism include CYP2C9, CYP2C19, CYP2C8, CYP2C18, CYP1A2, and CYP3A4.

● *Pharmacogenomics*

Variations in the genes responsible for warfarin metabolism or pharmacodynamic response may affect warfarin dosage requirements. The enzyme principally responsible for metabolism of S-warfarin is CYP2C9; the degree of activity of the CYP2C9 isoenzyme is under genetic control and is subject to individual variation. Patients who are homozygous for the CYP2C9*1 (wild-type) allele (about 80% of white patients) have normal enzyme activity (i.e., extensive metabolizers). However, approximately 11 or 7% of white patients are intermediate (e.g., CYP2C9*2 allele) or poor (e.g., CYP2C9*3 allele) metabolizers of warfarin, respectively; clearance of S-warfarin, the predominant active form of the drug, is reduced in such patients. Therefore, patients with variant CYP2C9 alleles are at increased risk of bleeding and excessive anticoagulation (e.g., INR exceeding 3) and require lower dosages of warfarin, particularly during initiation of therapy. The CYP2C9*2 and CYP2C9*3 alleles reduce metabolism of warfarin by about 30–50 and 90%, respectively. Other CYP2C9 variant alleles associated with reduced enzymatic activity occur less frequently, including CYP2C9*5, CYP2C9*6, and CYP2C9*11 alleles in African populations and CYP2C9*5, CYP2C9*9, and CYP2C9*11 alleles in white patients.

Warfarin inhibits vitamin K epoxide reductase, which is a vitamin K-cycle enzyme complex controlling the regeneration of reduced vitamin K from vitamin K epoxide. Limited evidence suggests that variations in the gene that encodes vitamin K epoxide reductase, vitamin K epoxide reductase complex subunit 1 (VKORC1), may have an even larger impact on warfarin dosage than CYP2C9 genetic variations, and differing average dosage requirements between patients of white, Black, and Asian ancestry may be explained by VKORC1 variant frequency. Common polymorphisms in non-coding regions of the VKORC1 gene contribute substantially to warfarin dosage variability across the normal dosage range. Asian patients appear to be more sensitive than white patients to the anticoagulant effect of warfarin and may require lower initial and maintenance dosages. A single nucleotide polymorphism of VKORC1 that identifies a low-dose and a high-dose warfarin phenotype has been found to associate with optimal warfarin dosage in both European and Asian patients. The reduced average warfarin maintenance dosage requirement in Asian individuals is largely related to the relatively rare occurrence of the high-dose allele in this ethnic group.

Several dosing algorithms for warfarin have been developed that take into account genetic variations in CYP2C9 and VKORC1 genes and individual clinical factors (e.g., age, height, body weight, interacting drugs, indication for warfarin therapy).

The 2017 update of the Clinical Pharmacogenetics Implementation Consortium (CPIC) guideline for pharmacogenetics-guided warfarin dosing suggests pharmacogenetic algorithm-based warfarin dosing over the genetics-based dosing table found in the FDA approved warfarin label. The two recommended algorithms (Gage or International Warfarin Pharmacogenetics Consortium [IWPC]) consider age, sex, race or self-identified ancestry, weight, height, smoking status, warfarin indication, target INR, interacting drugs (e.g., amiodarone, phenytoin) and genetic variables (e.g., CYP2C9, VKORC1 genotypes). CPIC recommends

the Gage over the IWPC algorithm because it can adjust for CYP4F2, CYP2C9*5, and *6, if those genotypes are known. The availability and reliability of genetic tests vary, and clinicians should check with their local or reference clinical laboratory to obtain more information about specific tests.

ADVICE TO PATIENTS

- Inform patients to strictly adhere to the prescribed dosage schedule and to not discontinue therapy without first consulting a healthcare provider.

- Inform patients that if a dose is missed, it should be taken as soon as possible on the same day; resume the regular dosing schedule the following day. Do not double a dose to make up for a missed dose.

- Inform patients that INR tests must be obtained based on their healthcare provider's recommendations and regular visits are necessary. Instruct patients that their healthcare provider will decide what INR goal is appropriate and adjust the warfarin dosage based on the INR results.

- Advise patients that if warfarin is discontinued, the anticoagulant effects may persist for 2–5 days.

- Inform patients that they may bruise and/or bleed more easily and that a longer than normal time may be required to stop bleeding when taking warfarin. Instruct patients to tell their healthcare provider about any unusual bleeding (e.g., nose bleeds, bleeding gums, heavier than normal menstrual bleeding, unexpected vaginal bleeding, pink or brown urine, red or black stools, coughing up blood, vomiting blood or material that looks like coffee grounds) or bruising during therapy.

- Advise patients to avoid any activity or sport that may result in traumatic injury and to tell their healthcare provider if they fall often as this may increase their risk for complications.

- Advise patients to eat a normal, balanced diet to maintain a consistent intake of vitamin K. Avoid drastic changes in dietary habits, such as eating large amounts of leafy, green vegetables.

- Advise patients to report any serious illness, such as severe diarrhea, infection, or fever to their healthcare provider.

- Advise patients to inform all healthcare providers, including dentists, about their warfarin therapy including before scheduling any medical, surgical, dental, or other invasive procedure.

- Advise patients to carry identification notifying others of their current warfarin therapy.

- Advise patients to immediately contact their healthcare provider if they experience pain and discoloration of the skin (a purple bruise-like rash) that primarily occurs on areas of the body with high fat content, such as breasts, thighs, buttocks, hips, and abdomen.

- Advise patients to immediately contact a healthcare provider if they experience any unusual symptoms or pain since warfarin may cause small cholesterol or atheroemboli. When this occurs in the feet, symptoms may include sudden cool, painful, purple discoloration of the toe(s) or forefoot.

- Advise patients to immediately contact a healthcare provider if any of the following occur: pain, swelling, discomfort, headache, dizziness, weakness, and fall or injury, especially if they hit their head.

- Advise women to inform their clinician if they are or plan to become pregnant or plan to breast-feed. Effective measures to avoid pregnancy should be used while taking warfarin and for 1 month after the last dose.

- Advise patients to inform their clinician of existing or contemplated concomitant therapy, including prescription and OTC drugs and dietary and herbal supplements, as well as any concomitant illnesses. Instruct patients not to take or discontinue any other drug, including salicylates (e.g., aspirin and topical analgesics), other OTC drugs, and botanical (herbal) products except on advice of a healthcare provider.

- Advise patients of other important precautionary information.

PREPARATIONS

Coumadin® (warfarin sodium), Bristol-Myers Squibb was the innovator brand of warfarin sodium from 1954 until its discontinuation in 2020.

Excipients in commercially available drug preparations may have clinically important effects in some individuals; consult specific product labeling for details.

Warfarin Sodium

Oral

Tablets	1 mg*	**Jantoven®** (scored), Upsher-Smith Laboratories
		Warfarin Sodium Tablets (scored)
	2 mg*	**Jantoven®** (scored), Upsher-Smith Laboratories
		Warfarin Sodium Tablets (scored)
	2.5 mg*	**Jantoven®** (scored), Upsher-Smith Laboratories
		Warfarin Sodium Tablets (scored)
	3 mg*	**Jantoven®** (scored), Upsher-Smith Laboratories
		Warfarin Sodium Tablets (scored)
	4 mg*	**Jantoven®** (scored), Upsher-Smith Laboratories
		Warfarin Sodium Tablets (scored)
	5 mg*	**Jantoven®** (scored), Upsher-Smith Laboratories
		Warfarin Sodium Tablets (scored)
	6 mg*	**Jantoven®** (scored), Upsher-Smith Laboratories
		Warfarin Sodium Tablets (scored)
	7.5 mg*	**Jantoven®** (scored), Upsher-Smith Laboratories
		Warfarin Sodium Tablets (scored)
	10 mg*	**Jantoven®** (scored), Upsher-Smith Laboratories
		Warfarin Sodium Tablets (scored)

* available from one or more manufacturer, distributor, and/or repackager by generic (nonproprietary) name

† Use is not currently included in the labeling approved by the US Food and Drug Administration.

Selected Revisions March 24, 2023, © Copyright, May 01, 1981, American Society of Health-System Pharmacists, Inc.

Argatroban

20:12.04.12 · DIRECT THROMBIN INHIBITORS

■ Argatroban, a synthetic piperidinecarboxylic acid derivative of L-arginine that acts as a direct thrombin inhibitor, is an anticoagulant.

USES

● Heparin-induced Thrombocytopenia

Argatroban is used for the prevention and treatment of thrombosis in patients with heparin-induced thrombocytopenia (HIT).

Clinical Perspective

In patients with acute HIT or HIT and thrombosis syndrome (HITTS), all forms of heparin (e.g., unfractionated heparin, low molecular weight heparin [LMWH]) should be discontinued and a nonheparin anticoagulant initiated. When selecting an appropriate nonheparin anticoagulant in patients with HIT/HITTS, the American Society of Hematology (ASH) suggests the use of argatroban, bivalirudin, danaparoid [not commercially available in the US], fondaparinux, or a direct oral anticoagulant (DOAC), but states that due to the low certainty of evidence, these recommendations are considered conditional. An earlier guideline on treatment of acute HIT/HITTS from the American College of Chest Physicians (ACCP) also includes argatroban as a nonheparin anticoagulant that may be used in such patients. Choice of therapy should be determined by drug-related factors (e.g., availability, cost, ability for monitoring, route of administration, pharmacokinetics) and patient-related factors (e.g., kidney function, liver function, bleeding risk, clinical stability). Due to their shorter duration of action, argatroban or bivalirudin may be preferred in patients who are critically ill, have an increased risk of bleeding, or increased risk of needing urgent procedures. For continued anticoagulation following argatroban therapy, patients may be converted to oral anticoagulant therapy.

Clinical Experience

Use of argatroban for the management of HIT is based principally on the results of 2 studies in patients with HIT or HITTS; in these studies, efficacy and safety comparisons were made with a historical control group of patients who did not receive the drug. Patients receiving argatroban were given an initial IV infusion of 2 mcg/kg per minute, with titration up to 10 mcg/kg per minute to achieve an activated partial thromboplastin time (aPTT) of 1.5–3 times the baseline value (not to exceed 100 seconds). The historical control group consisted of patients who had been treated for HIT/HITTS according to the local standard of medical practice (i.e., discontinuance of heparin therapy and/or oral anticoagulation with warfarin) since no other therapy was available for HIT/HITTS at that time. Patients received argatroban therapy until clinical resolution of their underlying condition, appropriate anticoagulation with another drug, or for a maximum of 14 days. In the first study, patients received argatroban for an average of 6 days; patient follow-up averaged 30 days. Most patients in the studies were transitioned to oral anticoagulant therapy with warfarin, and argatroban was continued concurrently with warfarin for 3–4 days.

In both studies, argatroban therapy was associated with a reduction in the incidence of the composite end point (all-cause death, all-cause amputation, or new thrombosis during the 37-day study period) as well as the individual end points (time to first end point event) in patients with HIT, HITTS, or combined HIT/HITTS. A target aPTT of at least 1.5 times the baseline value was achieved in 76% of patients with HIT (following treatment with a mean argatroban dosage of 2 mcg/kg per minute) and in 81% of patients with HITTS (following treatment with a mean argatroban dosage of 1.9 mcg/kg per minute) at the first assessment in one of the studies. Recovery of platelet count (defined as an increase in platelet count to greater than 100,000/mm³ or at least 1.5 times greater than the baseline aPTT) occurred in greater than 69% of argatroban-treated patients overall (53% of patients with HIT and 58% of those with HITTS by study day 3) in this study.

The manufacturers state that safety and effectiveness of argatroban have not been established in pediatric patients. However, the drug has been used in a limited number of seriously ill pediatric patients with HIT†. ACCP states that argatroban may be used as an alternative to heparin in children with HIT.

● Heparin-induced Thrombocytopenia in Patients Undergoing Percutaneous Coronary Intervention

Argatroban is used as an anticoagulant in patients with or at risk for HIT undergoing percutaneous coronary intervention (PCI).

Clinical Perspective

Several nonheparin anticoagulants (e.g., bivalirudin, argatroban, danaparoid, fondaparinux) have been evaluated in patients with or at risk of HIT who require PCI. Among the different options, experts generally suggest the use of bivalirudin or argatroban; factors such as availability, cost, and ease of monitoring may influence choice of a particular agent . ASH suggests bivalirudin as the preferred nonheparin anticoagulant in this setting because of more extensive experience with the drug in general in patients undergoing PCI; argatroban may be used as an appropriate substitute when bivalirudin cannot be used (e.g., because of availability issues or other constraints).

Clinical Experience

Efficacy and safety of argatroban for this indication are based principally on the results of several prospective, historically controlled studies evaluating therapy with the drug in patients with current or prior HIT (with or without thrombosis) or heparin-dependent antibodies who were undergoing PCI. The historical control group (selected by retrospective review of patient records) consisted of patients without HIT undergoing PCI who had been treated with heparin. The rates of procedural success (defined as lack of death, emergency coronary artery bypass grafting, Q-wave myocardial infarction) were similar in patients receiving argatroban (98.2%) versus the control group (94.3%); no deaths were reported in either group. Patients received argatroban 350 mcg/kg as an IV loading dose followed by a maintenance infusion of 25 mcg/kg per minute to achieve a target activated clotting time (ACT) of 300–450 seconds; additional IV loading doses of 150 mcg/kg or adjustments in the maintenance infusion rate over the range of 15–40 mcg/kg per minute to achieve the target ACT were allowed. All patients also received oral aspirin 325 mg 2–24 hours before PCI. Patients requiring anticoagulation following PCI could receive additional argatroban via a maintenance infusion at 2.5–5 mcg/kg per minute, adjusted (but not exceeding 10 mcg/kg per minute) to achieve an aPTT of 1.5–3 times control (not exceeding 100 seconds).

● Other Uses

Argatroban also has been used as an alternative to heparin in other situations where an anticoagulant is needed (e.g., percutaneous ventricular assist devices†, extracorporeal membrane oxygenation [ECMO]†). Argatroban is also suggested as an option in patients with HIT undergoing hemodialysis† as an alternative to unfractionated heparin to prevent clotting in the hemodialysis circuit..

The manufacturers state that safety and efficacy of argatroban for cardiac indications other than PCI in patients with HIT have not been established. Intracranial hemorrhage has been reported with investigational use of argatroban in patients with acute myocardial infarction (MI) receiving concomitant argatroban and thrombolytic therapy and also in patients with stroke.

DOSAGE AND ADMINISTRATION

Administration

Argatroban is administered by continuous IV infusion. The drug is commercially available as a 100-mg/mL injection concentrate, and also available as 1-mg/mL ready-to-use preparations.

The commercially available injection concentrate (100 mg/mL) *must* be diluted 100-fold in 0.9% sodium chloride injection, 5% dextrose injection, or lactated Ringer's injection to a final concentration of 1 mg/mL prior to administration. The solution should be mixed by repeated inversion of the IV container for 1 minute. The argatroban IV solution may be slightly hazy just after preparation because of the formation of microprecipitates that rapidly dissolve upon further mixing. Exposure to cold temperatures may slow the rate of dissolution. The solution should be clear prior to use. Properly prepared diluted solutions of argatroban are stable for 24 hours at room temperature when exposed to ambient indoor light, or for 96 hours at room temperature or under refrigeration when protected from light. Argatroban solutions should not be exposed to direct sunlight.

Commercially available 1-mg/mL ready-to-use preparations of argatroban are available in single-dose 50 mL or 125 mL vials; dilution of these preparations is not required. The vials may be inverted for use with a medical infusion set. The drug should not be used if the solution is cloudy or contains visible particulates.

Before administering argatroban, all parenteral anticoagulants must be discontinued and a baseline activated partial thromboplastin time (aPTT) obtained.

Standardize 4 Safety

Standardize 4 safety (S4S) is a national patient safety initiative to standardize drug concentrations to reduce medication errors, especially during transitions of care. Multidisciplinary expert panels were convened to determine recommended standard concentrations. Because recommendations from the S4S panels may differ from the manufacturer's prescribing information, caution is advised when using concentrations that differ from labeling, particularly when using rate information from the label. For additional information on S4S (including updates that may be available), see http://www.ashp.org/pharmacy-practice/standardize-4-safety-initiative.

TABLE 1. Standardize 4 Safety Continuous IV Infusion Standard Concentrations for Argatroban

Patient Population	Concentration Standard	Dosing Units
Adults	1 mg/mL	mcg/kg/min[a]
Pediatric patients (<50 kg)	1 mg/mL	mcg/kg/min[a]

[a] Dosing units differ from concentration units

Dosage

Heparin-induced Thrombocytopenia

For prevention or treatment of thrombosis in adults with heparin-induced thrombocytopenia (HIT) or HIT and thrombosis syndrome (HITTS), the recommended initial dosage of argatroban in patients without hepatic impairment is 2 mcg/kg per minute by continuous IV infusion.

In patients receiving argatroban for the prevention or treatment of thrombosis associated with HIT, therapy with the drug generally is monitored using activated partial thromboplastin time (aPTT). A steady-state anticoagulant effect generally is achieved 1–3 hours after initiation of the argatroban infusion in patients with normal hepatic function. The aPTT should be determined 2 hours after initiation of the infusion and/or following each dosage adjustment to confirm that a target aPTT of 1.5–3 times the initial baseline aPTT (not to exceed 100 seconds) has been achieved. The infusion rate can be adjusted as clinically indicated to achieve the desired aPTT range but should not exceed 10 mcg/kg per minute.

To minimize the risk of thrombotic events (e.g., limb gangrene) during the transition to oral anticoagulant therapy in patients with HIT/HITTS, the American College of Chest Physicians (ACCP), American Society of Hematology (ASH) and other clinicians recommend that treatment with argatroban or other nonheparin anticoagulant be continued until platelet counts have recovered substantially to near-normal levels (i.e., to at least 150,000/mm³) and are stable.

HIT in Pediatric Patients

The safety and efficacy of argatroban in pediatric patients have not been fully established. However, dosing recommendations have been suggested based on limited pharmacokinetic data in 15 seriously ill pediatric patients (<16 years of age) who received argatroban as an alternative to unfractionated heparin for conditions such as HIT/HITTS or suspected HIT. Reduced dosages are recommended in such patients due to the potential for decreased clearance of the drug. When used as an alternative to heparin in seriously ill pediatric patients with HIT or HITTS, an initial argatroban dosage of 0.75 mcg/kg per minute has been suggested in patients with normal hepatic function and a dosage of 0.2 mcg/kg per minute has been suggested in those with hepatic impairment. The aPTT should be determined 2 hours after initiation of the infusion and the dosage adjusted to achieve a target aPTT 1.5–3 times that of the initial baseline value (not exceeding 100 seconds). Subsequent dosage may be adjusted in increments of 0.1–0.25 mcg/kg per minute in pediatric patients without hepatic impairment, or in increments

of ≤0.05 mcg/kg per minute in those with hepatic impairment; however, dosage adjustments should be individualized based on patient's clinical status, current dosage, and current and target aPTT.

HIT in Patients Undergoing Percutaneous Coronary Intervention

In patients with HIT undergoing percutaneous coronary intervention (PCI), the recommended initial loading dose of argatroban is 350 mcg/kg administered by slow IV injection (over 3–5 minutes) followed by continuous IV infusion at 25 mcg/kg per minute. Some experts suggest a lower initial dosage for patients undergoing PCI who have received prior anticoagulant therapy (200 mcg/kg by slow IV injection followed by continuous IV infusion at 15 mcg/kg per minute).

Argatroban therapy prior to and during PCI generally is monitored using the activated clotting time (ACT). An ACT determination should be obtained 5–10 minutes after infusion of the loading dose; the procedure may proceed once an ACT of >300 seconds has been achieved. If ACT is <300 seconds, an additional IV loading dose of 150 mcg/kg should be administered and the infusion rate increased to 30 mcg/kg per minute. If ACT is >450 seconds, the infusion rate should be decreased to 15 mcg/kg per minute. If dissection, impending abrupt closure, or thrombus of the coronary artery occurs during the procedure, or if an ACT >300 seconds cannot be maintained, additional direct IV injections of 150 mcg/kg may be administered and the infusion rate increased to 40 mcg/kg per minute. ACT values should be determined 5–10 minutes after each additional direct injection or change in the infusion rate, and at the completion of the procedure. Once the target ACT (300–450 seconds) is achieved, the infusion should continue for the duration of the procedure; additional ACT values should be determined every 20–30 minutes during a prolonged procedure.

If a patient requires anticoagulation after PCI, argatroban may be continued, but at the infusion rate used in patients not undergoing PCI (2 mcg/kg per minute).

Transitioning to Warfarin Therapy

For continued anticoagulation, an oral anticoagulant may be initiated after beginning argatroban therapy. If warfarin therapy is planned, ACCP and other clinicians recommend that the drug be initiated only after substantial recovery from acute HIT has occurred (i.e., as indicated by platelet counts that have increased to at least 150,000/mm³ and are stable). Warfarin therapy should be initiated using the expected daily dosage, and a loading dose should not be administered. To avoid prothrombotic effects and ensure continuous anticoagulation when initiating warfarin, argatroban and warfarin therapy should be overlapped. The manufacturer states there are insufficient data to recommend a standard duration of this overlap. Daily international normalized ratio (INR) determinations are recommended during concomitant argatroban and warfarin therapy.

Combined therapy with argatroban and warfarin results in prolongation of the prothrombin time (PT) and INR beyond that produced by warfarin alone; the relationship between the INR on warfarin alone and that on combined warfarin-argatroban therapy depends on the dosage of argatroban and the international sensitivity index (ISI) of the thromboplastin reagent used for INR determinations. The expected INR on warfarin alone (INR$_W$) may be calculated from the INR on combined warfarin-argatroban therapy (INR$_{WA}$). The manufacturer's labeling should be consulted for detailed information regarding calculation of INR$_W$ and conversion from combined warfarin-argatroban therapy to warfarin alone. However, with an argatroban infusion rate of up to 2 mcg/kg per minute, argatroban therapy generally can be discontinued when the INR on combined therapy (INR$_{WA}$) exceeds 4. However, overshooting the target INR should be avoided, as supratherapeutic INRs during concomitant therapy with direct thrombin inhibitors and warfarin have been associated with necrosis or gangrene of the skin or limbs. The INR on warfarin alone should then be determined 4–6 hours after discontinuance of the argatroban infusion; if it is not within the desired therapeutic range for warfarin, the argatroban infusion should be resumed. This procedure (discontinuance of argatroban infusion, checking the INR on warfarin alone, and resumption of argatroban infusion) should be continued on a daily basis until the INR on warfarin alone (i.e., 4–6 hours after discontinuance of argatroban) is in the therapeutic range.

With argatroban infusions at rates exceeding 2 mcg/kg per minute, the relationship between INR on warfarin alone versus that on combined warfarin-argatroban therapy is less predictable. Therefore, the manufacturer states that the argatroban infusion rate should be temporarily reduced to 2 mcg/kg per minute and the INR on combined therapy calculated again 4–6 hours after such dosage reduction in order to predict the INR on warfarin therapy alone.

Transitioning to Direct Oral Anticoagulants (DOACs)

The manufacturer of dabigatran etexilate recommends starting dabigatran at the time of discontinuance of the parenteral anticoagulant.

The manufacturer of apixaban recommends starting apixaban at the time of the next dose of parenteral anticoagulant; no specific recommendations are given for anticoagulants administered by continuous infusion.

The manufacturer of rivaroxaban does not provide specific recommendations for switching patients from argatroban to rivaroxaban; recommendations given for other continuous infusion anticoagulants (e.g., unfractionated heparin) are to discontinue the infusion and start rivaroxaban at the same time.

The manufacturer of edoxaban does not provide specific recommendations for switching patients from argatroban to edoxaban; recommendations given for other continuous infusion anticoagulants (e.g., unfractionated heparin) are to discontinue the infusion and start edoxaban 4 hours later.

• Special Populations

Dosage in Hepatic Impairment

Use of argatroban in patients with hepatic impairment requires dosage reduction and careful monitoring of the aPTT. For adults with HIT/HITTS and moderate or severe hepatic impairment (based on Child-Pugh classification), an initial dosage of 0.5 mcg/kg per minute is recommended based on an approximate four-fold decrease in argatroban clearance relative to that in individuals with normal hepatic function. Subsequent dosage may then be adjusted as clinically indicated. Patients with hepatic impairment may require a longer time and more dosage adjustments to achieve steady-state aPTT concentrations. Use of high dosages of argatroban should be avoided in patients undergoing PCI who have clinically important hepatic disease or serum AST or ALT elevations 3 times the upper limit of normal or higher because such patients have not been studied in clinical trials with the drug.

Dosage in Renal Impairment

No dosage adjustment is necessary in patients with impaired renal function.

Dosage in Geriatric Patients

No dosage adjustment is necessary in geriatric patients.

Dosage in Critically Ill Patients

ACCP suggests a reduced dosage of argatroban for the treatment of HIT/HITTS in patients with heart failure, multiple organ system failure, or severe anasarca, and for patients following cardiac surgery. ACCP suggests an initial infusion rate of 0.5–1.2 mcg/kg per minute due to an increased risk of bleeding in these patient populations.

Dosage in Obese Patients

The manufacturer does not make any dosing recommendations specific to obesity. Argatroban dosing requirements in obese versus nonobese patients were evaluated in a small, single-center, retrospective study; the study included 121 patients with suspected HIT who received argatroban for at least 12 hours. Patients with a body mass index (BMI) >30 kg/m² were compared with patients with a BMI ≤30 kg/m². No meaningful differences were observed in median maintenance dosage requirements, thrombosis events, or in-hospital major bleeding between the patients. Based on these findings, the authors suggest that argatroban dosing be based on actual body weight in obese patients.

CAUTIONS

• Contraindications

- Major bleeding.
- History of hypersensitivity to argatroban or any ingredient(s) in the formulation.

• Warnings/Precautions

Bleeding

Like other anticoagulants, argatroban should be used with extreme caution in disease states or circumstances where there is an increased risk of hemorrhage (e.g., severe hypertension; postlumbar puncture; spinal anesthesia; major surgery,

particularly of the brain, spinal cord, or eye; GI ulceration; congenital or acquired bleeding disorders). All parenteral anticoagulants should be discontinued and a baseline activated thromboplastin time (aPTT) obtained before initiation of argatroban therapy in patients with heparin-induced thrombocytopenia (HIT) or HIT and thrombosis syndrome (HITTS).

Hemorrhage in patients receiving argatroban can occur at any site in the body. Unexplained decreases in hematocrit, hemoglobin, or blood pressure may indicate hemorrhage. Major hemorrhage (defined as overt and associated with a hemoglobin decrease of ≥2 g/dL [in nonsurgical patients] or ≥5 g/dL [in patients undergoing percutaneous coronary intervention (PCI)], transfusion of ≥2 units, or bleeding that was intracranial, retroperitoneal, or into a major prosthetic joint) occurred in 5.3% of patients receiving argatroban in 2 clinical studies and in 6.7% of those (based on retrospective analysis) in a historical control group. Major hemorrhage (i.e., retroperitoneal or GI hemorrhage) occurred in 1.8% of patients with current or prior HIT/HITTS who received argatroban and underwent PCI. Intracranial hemorrhage did not occur in clinical studies of argatroban in nonsurgical patients with HIT/HITTS but has been reported with argatroban therapy for other conditions (e.g., patients with acute myocardial infarction [MI] receiving concomitant thrombolytic therapy, patients with stroke).

In the event of overdose or excessive anticoagulation, discontinue or reduce the dose of the argatroban infusion, monitor aPTT and other coagulation tests (prothrombin time [PT], international normalized ratio [INR]), and provide symptomatic and supportive treatment. Reversal of anticoagulation may be prolonged in patients with hepatic impairment. No specific antidote to argatroban is currently available. Argatroban is partially removed by hemodialysis; approximately 20% of the drug is cleared during a 4-hour period of hemodialysis (when given as a continuous infusion at 2 mcg/kg per minute prior to and during hemodialysis).

Laboratory Monitoring

aPTT is well correlated with the anticoagulant effects of argatroban at therapeutic dosages; following discontinuance of the drug, aPTT generally returns to normal values within 2–4 hours. PT, INR, and thrombin time (TT) are also prolonged by argatroban, but therapeutic ranges for these tests have not been identified.

Specific Populations

Pregnancy

Available data do not support an association between argatroban and adverse fetal outcomes. Women with underlying thromboembolic disease and certain high-risk pregnancy conditions have an increased risk of thromboembolism during pregnancy. Data show that women with a history of venous thrombosis have a high risk for recurrence during pregnancy. The risk of untreated thromboembolism in the mother should be assessed against the risk of hemorrhage in the mother and fetus when considering the use of anticoagulants, including argatroban.

Lactation

Argatroban is distributed into milk in rats; it is not known whether the drug is distributed into human milk. It is not known whether argatroban affects the breast-fed child or affects milk production. The benefits of breast-feeding should be considered along with the importance of the drug to the woman and any potential adverse effects on the breast-fed child from the drug or underlying maternal condition.

Pediatric Use

Safety and efficacy of argatroban have not been fully established in pediatric patients; however, the drug has been evaluated in a limited number of seriously ill pediatric patients <16 years of age with HIT or HITTS. In a small, multi-center open-label study, 18 seriously ill pediatric patients with a clinical condition requiring alternative nonheparin anticoagulation received argatroban at an initial dosage of 1 mcg/kg per minute titrated to maintain a target aPTT of 1.5–3 times the baseline value. During the 30-day study period, thrombotic events occurred in 5 patients and major bleeding (intracranial hemorrhage) was reported in 2 patients. All of the patients had serious comorbid conditions and were receiving multiple concomitant medications; most were diagnosed with documented or suspected HIT. In a pharmacokinetic/pharmacodynamic analysis model using data from 15 seriously ill pediatric patients, argatroban clearance was reduced by 50% in these patients compared with healthy adults and by approximately 80% in pediatric patients with elevated bilirubin concentrations compared to pediatric patients with normal bilirubin concentrations. Based on these findings and an aPTT goal of 1.5–3 times the baseline value (without exceeding aPTT of 100 seconds), a dosage regimen has been suggested for seriously ill pediatric patients with HIT/HITTS who require an alternative to heparin.

Geriatric Use

About one-third of patients in clinical studies of argatroban were ≥65 years of age. No substantial differences in efficacy or safety have been observed relative to younger adults. A safety analysis suggested an increased trend for adverse events in older patients, but it was unclear whether this was due to the greater prevalence of underlying conditions predisposing these patients to adverse reactions or to a different safety profile of argatroban in older patients.

Hepatic Impairment

Caution is advised in patients with hepatic dysfunction. A longer period of time may be required to achieve steady-state anticoagulation and reversal of the anticoagulant effect because of the decreased clearance and increased elimination half-life of argatroban in such patients.

Hepatic impairment decreases the clearance and increases the half-life of argatroban; dosage reductions are recommended.

● Common Adverse Effects

In patients receiving argatroban for the treatment of HIT/HITTS, the most common adverse effects (occurring in >5% of patients) were dyspnea, hypotension, fever, diarrhea, sepsis, and cardiac arrest.

In patients receiving argatroban for PCI, the most common adverse effects (occurring in >5% of patients) were chest pain, hypotension, back pain, nausea, vomiting, and headache.

DRUG INTERACTIONS

● Warfarin

Increased prothrombin time (PT) and international normalized ratio (INR) have been observed when argatroban is administered concurrently with warfarin relative to when warfarin is administered alone. There is no evidence of a pharmacokinetic interaction between warfarin and argatroban. Concurrent administration of argatroban and warfarin did not have additive effects on vitamin K-dependent factor Xa activity compared with warfarin alone. The interaction is dependent on the argatroban dose and the thromboplastin reagent used for the INR lab.

● Heparin

Prior to initiation of argatroban therapy, allow sufficient time for effect of heparin on activated partial thromboplastin time (aPTT) to decrease.

● Other Drugs Affecting Coagulation

Potential pharmacologic interaction (increased risk of hemorrhage) with concomitant use of thrombolytics, antiplatelet agents, or other anticoagulants. No pharmacokinetic or pharmacodynamic interaction demonstrated with low-dose oral aspirin (162.5 mg given 26 and 2 hours prior to argatroban infusion) or oral acetaminophen (1 g given every 6 hours for 5 doses beginning 12 hours prior to argatroban infusion). The manufacturer states that the safety and efficacy of concomitant therapy with argatroban and platelet glycoprotein (GP) IIb/IIIa-receptor antagonists has not been established.

● Other Drugs

No drug interactions have been observed between argatroban and digoxin or erythromycin, a potent inhibitor of cytochrome P-450 (CYP) 3A4/5.

DESCRIPTION

Argatroban, a synthetic piperidinecarboxylic acid derivative of L-arginine, is an anticoagulant. Commercially available argatroban is a racemic mixture of the *R*- and *S*-diastereoisomers in a ratio of approximately 65 to 35, with the *S*-isomer having about twice the thrombin-inhibitory potency of the *R*-isomer.

Argatroban is a highly selective and reversible, small-molecule direct thrombin inhibitor that binds rapidly to the catalytic site/apolar region of both circulating (free) and clot-bound thrombin. Inhibition of thrombin prevents various steps in the coagulation process (e.g., activation of factors V, VIII, and XIII and of protein C; conversion of fibrinogen to fibrin; platelet activation and aggregation). At infusion rates up to 40 mcg/kg per minute, argatroban produces dose-dependent increases in activated partial thromboplastin time (aPTT) and several other coagulation assays (activated clotting time [ACT], prothrombin time [PT], and thrombin time [TT]).

Argatroban is metabolized principally by the liver via hydroxylation and aromatization of the 3-methyltetrahydroquinoline ring. Argatroban does not appear to induce antibody formation to itself nor does it interact with heparin-induced antibodies. Age or gender does not appear to substantially influence the pharmacokinetics and pharmacodynamics of argatroban.

ADVICE TO PATIENTS

- Importance of reporting any signs of bleeding (e.g., bruising, petechiae, hematuria) to clinician immediately.
- Importance of patients informing clinician of history of bleeding disorders.
- Importance of reporting signs of allergic reactions (e.g., airway reactions, skin reactions, vasodilation reactions).
- Importance of women informing clinician if they are or plan to become pregnant or plan to breast-feed.
- Importance of informing clinician of existing or contemplated concomitant therapy, including prescription (e.g., anticoagulants) and OTC drugs.
- Importance of informing patients of other important precautionary information.

PREPARATIONS

Excipients in commercially available drug preparations may have clinically important effects in some individuals; consult specific product labeling for details.

Argatroban

Parenteral

Injection concentrate, for IV infusion	100 mg/mL (250 mg)*	Argatroban Injection
Injection, for IV infusion	1 mg/mL (50 mg)*	Argatroban Injection

* available from one or more manufacturer, distributor, and/or repackager by generic (nonproprietary) name

Argatroban in Sodium Chloride

Parenteral

Injection, for IV infusion	1 mg/mL (125 mg) in 0.9% Sodium Chloride*	Argatroban in 0.9% Sodium Chloride Injection

* available from one or more manufacturer, distributor, and/or repackager by generic (nonproprietary) name

† Use is not currently included in the labeling approved by the US Food and Drug Administration.

Bivalirudin

20:12.04.12 • BIVALIRUDIN

■ Bivalirudin trifluoroacetate, a synthetic analog of hirudin that acts as a direct thrombin inhibitor, is an anticoagulant.

USES

● Percutaneous Coronary Intervention

Bivalirudin is used as an anticoagulant in patients undergoing percutaneous coronary intervention (PCI), including those with heparin-induced thrombocytopenia (HIT) or heparin-induced thrombocytopenia and thrombosis syndrome (HITTS). Bivalirudin has been studied only in patients receiving concomitant aspirin.

Use of a parenteral anticoagulant is recommended in all patients undergoing PCI to prevent thrombus formation at the site of arterial injury, the coronary guidewire, and in the catheters used for the procedure. Bivalirudin (with or without prior unfractionated heparin treatment) is recommended by the American College of Cardiology Foundation (ACCF), the American Heart Association (AHA), and the Society for Cardiovascular Angiography and Interventions (SCAI) as an appropriate choice of anticoagulant for this use; other options include unfractionated heparin, enoxaparin, fondaparinux, and argatroban. In the subset of patients with acute HIT who require PCI, experts generally suggest the use of bivalirudin or argatroban. The American Society of Hematology (ASH) suggests the use of bivalirudin over other nonheparin anticoagulants in these patients because of more extensive experience in general with the drug in patients undergoing PCI; however, argatroban may be considered when bivalirudin cannot be used (e.g., due to availability issues or other constraints). Factors such as availability, cost, experience with the drug, and anticoagulation monitoring capabilities may influence choice of drug.

Efficacy and safety of bivalirudin as an anticoagulant for PCI are primarily based on the results of 2 identical randomized, double-blind, multicenter studies (Bivalirudin Angioplasty [BAT] trials) in adults 29–90 years of age with unstable angina undergoing PCI; results of these studies demonstrated that bivalirudin is as effective as high-dose unfractionated heparin in such patients. In the BAT trials, patients received either bivalirudin (1 mg/kg by direct IV injection followed by IV infusion of 2.5 mg/kg per hour for 4 hours and then 0.2 mg/kg per hour for 14–20 hours) or heparin sodium (175 units/kg by direct IV injection followed by IV infusion of 15 units/kg per hour for 18–24 hours). If activated clotting time (ACT) was below 350 seconds, additional heparin could be administered. All patients also received oral aspirin 300–325 mg before PCI and daily thereafter. The rates of procedural failure (defined as death, MI, or clinical deterioration of cardiac origin requiring revascularization or placement of an aortic balloon pump or angiographic evidence of abrupt vessel closure) were similar in both treatment groups. In a subgroup of patients with postinfarction angina undergoing percutaneous transluminal coronary angioplasty (PTCA), bivalirudin was more effective than heparin in decreasing procedural failures.

In an open-label study (AT-BAT trial) in patients with a history of HIT or HITTS or active HIT/HITTS who were undergoing PCI, 48 of 51 patients receiving bivalirudin therapy (0.75 or 1 mg/kg by direct IV injection followed by continuous IV infusion of 1.75 or 2.5 mg/kg per hour, respectively) had successful PCI outcomes (i.e., TIMI grade 3 flow and stenosis less than 50%). Most patients received concomitant aspirin and/or clopidogrel, and some patients received concomitant GP IIb/IIIa-receptor inhibitors.

Early studies of bivalirudin compared the drug with unfractionated heparin plus a GP IIb/IIIa-receptor inhibitor in patients undergoing PCI. In one such study (REPLACE-2 trial), bivalirudin (with provisional use of a GP IIb/IIIa receptor inhibitor) was noninferior to unfractionated heparin plus planned use of a GP IIb/IIIa inhibitor; the primary composite end point of death, MI, urgent repeat revascularization, or in-hospital bleeding was similar in both treatment groups and bivalirudin was associated with substantially lower rates of bleeding compared with heparin. In other randomized controlled studies (e.g., ACUITY, ISAR-REACT, HORIZONS-AMI) in which bivalirudin was compared with heparin plus a GPIIb/IIIa inhibitor in patients with acute coronary syndrome (ACS) undergoing PCI, similar findings were reported; when bivalirudin was used alone (without a GP IIb/IIIa inhibitor), the drug was associated with similar rates of ischemic events but substantially reduced rates of bleeding compared with heparin plus a GPIIb/IIIa inhibitor. Routine use of GPIIb/IIIa inhibitors has decreased in the current era of dual antiplatelet therapy, and more recent studies have compared bivalirudin with heparin alone in this setting. Results of meta-analyses comparing these anticoagulant strategies have demonstrated that bivalirudin and heparin are associated with similar rates of ischemic events following PCI; although major bleeding tended to be less frequent in patients receiving bivalirudin compared with heparin, this benefit was modulated by avoiding routine use of a GPIIb/IIIa inhibitor with heparin or by concurrent use of P2Y12 inhibitors.

● Non-ST-Segment-Elevation Acute Coronary Syndrome

Bivalirudin also has been used as an initial anticoagulant in patients with non-ST-segment-elevation ACS (NSTE-ACS)† who are being managed with an early invasive strategy. In this setting, bivalirudin is continued until the time of diagnostic angiography or PCI. (See Percutaneous Coronary Intervention under Uses.)

The spectrum of NSTE-ACS includes unstable angina and non-ST-segment-elevation MI (NSTEMI); because these conditions are part of a continuum of acute myocardial ischemia and have indistinguishable clinical features upon presentation, the same initial treatment strategies are recommended. The American Heart Association (AHA)/American College of Cardiology (ACC) guideline for the management of patients with NSTE-ACS recommends an early invasive strategy (angiographic evaluation with the intent to perform revascularization procedures such as PCI with coronary artery stent implantation or coronary artery bypass grafting [CABG]) or an ischemia-guided strategy (initial medical management followed by cardiac catheterization and revascularization if indicated) in patients with definite or likely NSTE-ACS; standard medical therapies for all patients should include an anticoagulant agent regardless of the initial management approach. Initial parenteral anticoagulants with established efficacy in patients with NSTE-ACS include enoxaparin, unfractionated heparin, bivalirudin (only in patients who are being managed with an early invasive strategy), and fondaparinux.

● Cardiac Surgery in Patients with HIT

Bivalirudin also has been used for anticoagulation during cardiovascular surgery in patients with HIT†. Both the American Society of Hematology (ASH) and the American College of Chest Physicians (ACCP) consider bivalirudin to be a treatment option in this setting. In patients with acute HIT or subacute HIT A (platelet count has recovered but functional assay is not yet negative), ASH recommends delaying cardiovascular surgery until the patient has subacute HIT B (functional assay is negative but immunoassay is not yet negative) or remote HIT, if possible. However, if surgery cannot be delayed, ASH conditionally suggests intraoperative anticoagulation with bivalirudin, intraoperative heparin after preoperative or intraoperative plasma exchange, or intraoperative heparin combined with a potent antiplatelet agent (e.g. prostacyclin analog or glycoprotein IIb/IIIa inhibitor). Choice of therapy should be determined by drug availability and cost, and experience of the clinician. ACCP suggests the use of bivalirudin in patients with HIT or subacute HIT (platelets have recovered, but HIT antibodies are still present) who require urgent cardiac surgery; bivalirudin is suggested over other nonheparin anticoagulant options mainly because of direct supporting evidence from prospective, multicenter studies. ACCP recommends delaying nonurgent cardiac surgery until HIT has resolved and HIT antibodies are negative.

● Prevention of Thrombosis During Renal Replacement Therapy

Bivalirudin also has been used as an anticoagulant to prevent thrombosis of dialysis circuitry during renal replacement therapy in patients with acute HIT†. When selecting an appropriate nonheparin anticoagulant in patients with acute HIT while on renal replacement therapy, ASH suggests the use of argatroban, danaparoid (not commercially available in the US), or bivalirudin over other nonheparin anticoagulants, but states that due to the low certainty of evidence, these recommendations are considered conditional. Choice of therapy should be determined by drug-related factors (e.g., availability and cost), patient-related factors (e.g., liver function), and clinician experience.

● Treatment of Acute HIT/HITTS

Bivalirudin has been used in the treatment of acute HIT/HITTS†. In patients with acute HIT/HITTS, all forms of heparin (e.g., unfractionated heparin, low molecular weight heparin [LMWH]) should be discontinued and a nonheparin anticoagulant initiated. When selecting an appropriate nonheparin anticoagulant in patients with HIT/HITTS, ASH suggests the use of argatroban, bivalirudin, danaparoid (not commercially available in the US), fondaparinux, or a direct oral anticoagulant (DOAC), but states that due to the low certainty of evidence, these recommendations are considered conditional. Choice of therapy should be determined by drug-related factors (e.g., availability, cost, monitoring ability, route of administration, pharmacokinetics) and patient-related factors (e.g., kidney function, liver function, bleeding risk, clinical stability). Due to their shorter duration of action, argatroban or bivalirudin may be preferred in patients who are critically ill, at an increased risk of bleeding, or at increased risk of needing urgent procedures. Supporting data cited by ASH for the use of bivalirudin in acute HIT/HITTS management included a retrospective chart review of 461 patients with suspected, confirmed, or prior HIT who were treated with bivalirudin. In an earlier ACCP guideline on treatment of acute HIT/HITTS, bivalirudin was not recommended by ACCP in this setting due to a lack of quality evidence at the time. Notably, the retrospective chart review cited by ASH was not available at the time of the ACCP recommendation.

DOSAGE AND ADMINISTRATION

● Reconstitution and Administration

Bivalirudin is administered by direct IV injection followed by IV infusion. The drug should *not* be administered IM.

Bivalirudin is commercially available as a lyophilized powder that must be reconstituted and diluted prior to administration. The drug is also available in ready-to-use formulations with a concentration of 5 mg/mL (e.g., bivalirudin ready-to-use [RTU] injection, bivalirudin in 0.9% sodium chloride injection).

Bivalirudin Powder for Injection

Commercially available bivalirudin powder for injection must be reconstituted and diluted before administration. The drug should be reconstituted by adding 5 mL of sterile water for injection to a vial labeled as containing 250 mg of bivalirudin to provide a solution containing 50 mg/mL. The vial should be gently swirled to aid reconstitution and inspected for any evidence of particulate matter. The reconstituted solution may be stored at 2–8°C for up to 24 hours. A 5 mL volume should be withdrawn from a 50 mL infusion bag of 5% dextrose or 0.9% sodium chloride injection, and discarded; the contents of the bivalirudin vial should then be added to the infusion bag to yield a final concentration of 5 mg/mL. This diluted solution may be used to administer the appropriate bivalirudin dose as a direct IV injection or 4-hour IV infusion. The manufacturer states that bivalirudin solutions with concentrations of 0.5–5 mg/mL are stable at room temperature for up to 24 hours. Reconstituted or diluted bivalirudin solutions should not be frozen. Any unused reconstituted solution remaining in the vial should be discarded.

Bivalirudin lyophilized powder should be stored at 20–25°C but may be exposed to temperatures ranging from 15–30°C.

Bivalirudin RTU Injection

Vials of bivalirudin RTU injection should be stored at 2–8°C until time of use, but may be exposed to temperatures ranging from 20–25°C; the vials should not be exposed to excessive heat. Prior to administration, each vial should be inspected for discoloration or particulate matter. Once the vials are removed from the refrigerator, the drug should be used immediately; any unused portions should be discarded.

Bivalirudin in 0.9% Sodium Chloride Injection

Commercially available frozen premixed bivalirudin injection in 0.9% sodium chloride should be stored at or below -20°C, and thawed at room temperature (25°C) or under refrigeration (5°C) prior to use. The injection should not be thawed by warming in a water bath or by exposure to microwave radiation. The container may be fragile in the frozen state and should be handled with care. Precipitates that may have formed in the frozen injection usually will dissolve with little or no agitation when the injection reaches room temperature; potency is not affected. After thawing at room temperature, the injection should be agitated and the container checked for minute leaks by firmly squeezing the bag. The injection should be discarded if container seals or outlet ports are not intact or leaks are found or if the solution is cloudy or contains an insoluble precipitate. Additives should not be introduced into the injection container. Upon thawing, premixed bivalirudin solution is stable at room temperature (25°C) for up to 24 hours or under refrigeration (5°C) for up to 14 days; the premixed solution should not be refrozen after thawing. Any unused solution remaining in the bag should be discarded.

● Dosage

Dosage of bivalirudin trifluoroacetate is expressed in terms of bivalirudin.

Percutaneous Coronary Intervention

For use as an anticoagulant in patients undergoing percutaneous coronary intervention (PCI), the recommended dosage of bivalirudin is 0.75 mg/kg by direct IV injection followed by a continuous IV infusion of 1.75 mg/kg per hour for the duration of the procedure. Activated clotting time (ACT) should be assessed 5 minutes after the initial loading dose and an additional direct IV injection of 0.3 mg/kg given if needed. Continued infusion of bivalirudin for up to 4 hours should be considered in patients with ST-segment-elevation MI (STEMI).

In patients with non-ST-segment-elevation acute coronary syndrome (NSTE-ACS) who have received prior treatment with unfractionated heparin therapy, the American Heart Association (AHA)/American College of Cardiology (ACC) recommends waiting 30 minutes and then administering the initial 0.75-mg/kg IV loading dose of bivalirudin followed by continuous IV infusion of bivalirudin at 1.75 mg/kg per hour. In patients with NSTE-ACS who have been receiving bivalirudin for initial anticoagulation, AHA/ACC recommends administering an additional loading dose of 0.5 mg/kg, followed by an increased infusion rate of 1.75 mg/kg per hour during PCI.

The manufacturer states that bivalirudin has only been studied in combination with aspirin. Guidelines also recommend the use of aspirin in combination with bivalirudin, with or without concomitant therapy with a P2Y12 platelet adenosine diphosphate (ADP)-receptor antagonist (e.g., clopidogrel, prasugrel, ticagrelor) depending on the clinical scenario (e.g., stenting).

Initial Anticoagulation in Patients with NSTE-ACS

If bivalirudin is used as an initial anticoagulant in patients with NSTE-ACS† who are being managed with an early invasive strategy, a loading dose of 0.1 mg/kg, followed by continuous IV infusion of 0.25 mg/kg per hour until diagnostic angiography or PCI has been recommended. Combination treatment with aspirin and a P2Y12 inhibitor is recommended in this setting. If PCI is performed while the patient is on bivalirudin, an additional loading dose of 0.5 mg/kg followed by an increased continuous IV infusion rate of 1.75 mg/kg per hour is recommended during PCI.

Cardiac Surgery in Patients with HIT

For patients with acute HIT who undergo cardiac surgery† without the use of cardiopulmonary bypass (i.e., "off-pump"), a bivalirudin dosage of 0.75 mg/kg by direct IV injection followed by 1.75 mg/kg per hour by continuous IV infusion to maintain an ACT exceeding 300 seconds has been used.

During cardiopulmonary bypass, an initial bivalirudin dosage of 1 mg/kg given by direct IV injection followed by continuous IV infusion at a rate of 2.5 mg/kg per hour has been used; additional direct IV doses of 0.1–0.5 mg/kg have been given if needed to maintain a 2.5-fold or greater prolongation of the baseline ACT. In addition, 50 mg of bivalirudin is added to the recirculating priming fluid of the cardiopulmonary bypass circuit. As bivalirudin is metabolized by proteolytic cleavage by thrombin in the blood, special maneuvers are needed to avoid stasis within the cardiopulmonary bypass circuit during and after surgery.

Prevention of Thrombosis During Renal Replacement Therapy

For the prevention of extracorporeal thrombosis in ambulatory dialysis patients with HIT†, a bivalirudin treatment protocol with initial dose and dosage adjustments based on aPTT, risk of bleeding, and risk of thrombosis has been used. Based on this protocol, an initial bivalirudin continuous IV infusion of 0.02 mg/kg per hour is administered; dosage is then subsequently adjusted based on aPTT. In patients considered to be at high bleeding risk, a target aPTT of 1.5–2.5 times the normal value is used; in patients considered to be at high risk of clotting or active HITTS, a target aPTT of 2–2.5 times the normal value is used.

Treatment of Acute HIT/HITTS

If bivalirudin is used for the treatment of acute HIT/HITTS†, a continuous IV infusion of 0.15 mg/kg per hour adjusted to aPTT 1.5–2.5 times the baseline value has been used without an initial direct IV injection. A reduced rate of infusion may be warranted in patients with renal or hepatic impairment.

● Special Populations

Hepatic Impairment

The manufacturers make no specific dosage recommendations for patients with hepatic impairment.

Renal Impairment

Close monitoring of anticoagulation status (e.g., ACT results) is recommended in patients with renal impairment. Total body clearance is reduced by approximately 21% in patients with moderate or severe renal impairment and by 70% in dialysis-dependent patients; approximately 25% of the drug is removed by hemodialysis. The manufacturers state that reduction of the initial loading dose of bivalirudin is not necessary in patients with renal impairment undergoing PCI. However, patients with severe renal impairment (creatinine clearance less than 30 mL/minute) who are undergoing PCI should have their continuous IV infusion rate reduced to 1 mg/kg per hour, and dialysis-dependent patients should have their infusion rate reduced to 0.25 mg/kg per hour (off dialysis).

Geriatric Patients

The manufacturers make no specific dosage recommendations for geriatric patients.

CAUTIONS

● Contraindications

- Active major bleeding.
- Known hypersensitivity to bivalirudin or any ingredient in the formulation.

● Warnings/Precautions

Warnings

Bleeding

Risk of bleeding is increased with bivalirudin; the drug should be used with caution, particularly in patients with an increased risk of hemorrhage. In clinical trials, bleeding risk was higher when bivalirudin was used in combination with heparin, warfarin, thrombolytics, or glycoprotein IIb/IIIa receptor inhibitors. Major hemorrhage (e.g., intracranial or retroperitoneal bleeding, clinically overt bleeding with a hemoglobin concentration decrease of at least 3 g/dL or requiring transfusion of at least 2 units of blood) occurred in 3.7% of bivalirudin-treated patients with unstable angina undergoing percutaneous coronary intervention (PCI); fatal bleeding has been reported.

Unexplained decreases in hematocrit, hemoglobin, or blood pressure may indicate hemorrhage. If severe hemorrhage occurs, bivalirudin should be discontinued.

Acute Stent Thrombosis

In studies of patients with ST-segment-elevation myocardial infarction (STEMI) undergoing primary PCI, a higher rate of acute stent thrombosis (within 4 hours) has been observed in patients receiving bivalirudin than in patients receiving heparin (1.2 versus 0.2%). Patients who developed acute stent thrombosis were treated using target vessel revascularization. Acute stent thrombosis was fatal in 0.03% of patients in both the bivalirudin and heparin treatment groups.

Patients should be closely monitored for signs and symptoms of myocardial ischemia in a setting capable of managing acute ischemic events for at least 24 hours after PCI. Thrombotic Risk with Brachytherapy Procedures

Bivalirudin has been associated with thrombus formation, sometimes fatal, when used in gamma brachytherapy. Caution is advised if bivalirudin is used during vascular brachytherapy procedures. Catheter function should be assessed frequently by attempting to aspirate blood, and patency should be ensured by repeated flushing. Conditions promoting stasis within the catheter or circulatory system should be minimized.

Immunogenicity

In clinical studies of bivalirudin, 2 of 494 patients had positive bivalirudin antibody tests, but neither patient developed clinically apparent allergic or anaphylactic reactions. Nine additional patients who had positive antibody test results were negative on repeat testing.

Specific Populations

Pregnancy

There are no adequate and well-controlled studies of bivalirudin in pregnant women; bivalirudin has not been studied in the perinatal period due to risk of hemorrhage during delivery. Animal findings do not suggest fetal harm at exposure levels equivalent to 1.6 and 3.2 times the maximum human dose; however, at exposure levels equivalent to 5.4 times the maximum human dose, some skeletal abnormalities and a reduction in live births were observed, possibly due to maternal toxicity.

Lactation

It is not known whether bivalirudin is distributed into milk; effects of the drug on milk production and the breast-fed infant have not been studied.

Administration of bivalirudin to lactating rats was not associated with developmental harm to the pups. The benefits of breast-feeding should be considered along with the importance of the drug to the woman and any potential adverse effects on the breast-fed child from the drug or underlying maternal condition.

Pediatric Use

Safety and efficacy of bivalirudin have not been established in pediatric patients.

Geriatric Use

In clinical trials of bivalirudin, geriatric patients experienced more bleeding complications than younger adults.

Renal Impairment

Clearance of bivalirudin is reduced in patients with renal impairment; dosage adjustment may be necessary.

● Common Adverse Effects

The most common adverse effect of bivalirudin is bleeding. Major bleeding occurred in 3.7% of patients in the BAT trials, and included intracranial bleeding, retroperitoneal bleeding, overt bleeding with a reduction in hemoglobin concentration of more than 3 g/dL, and blood transfusions of more than 2 units of blood.

DRUG INTERACTIONS

● Drugs Affecting Hemostasis

There is a potential for increased risk of bleeding when bivalirudin is used concomitantly with drugs affecting hemostasis (e.g., aspirin, heparin, warfarin, GP IIb/IIIa-receptor inhibitors, thrombolytics). Bivalirudin increases the international normalized ratio (INR), and may interfere with therapeutic monitoring and dosage adjustments for warfarin.

DESCRIPTION

Bivalirudin, a synthetic 20-amino acid peptide analog of naturally occurring hirudin, is an anticoagulant. Hirudin is the polypeptide that is responsible for the anticoagulant properties of the saliva of the medicinal leech (Hirudo medicinalis).

Bivalirudin is a specific and reversible direct thrombin inhibitor that binds to the catalytic site and the anion-binding exosite of circulating and clot-bound thrombin. Inhibition of thrombin prevents various steps in the coagulation process (e.g., activation of factors V, VIII, and XIII; conversion of fibrinogen to fibrin; platelet activation and aggregation). These effects of bivalirudin are reversed as thrombin slowly cleaves the bivalirudin-Arg_3-Pro_4 bond, resulting in recovery of thrombin active site function.

The onset of anticoagulant effect is immediate following direct IV injection of bivalirudin. Bivalirudin therapy prolongs several coagulation assays, including the activated clotting time (ACT), activated partial thromboplastin time (aPTT), thrombin time (TT), and prothrombin time (PT). Coagulation times return to the normal range approximately 1–2 hours after discontinuance of the drug.

ADVICE TO PATIENTS

- Importance of patients reporting any signs of bleeding (e.g., bruising, petechiae, hematuria) to clinicians immediately.
- Importance of patients informing clinicians of history of bleeding disorders or impaired renal function.
- Importance of women informing clinicians if they are or plan to become pregnant or plan to breast-feed.
- Importance of patients informing clinicians of existing or contemplated concomitant therapy, including prescription and OTC drugs as well as any concomitant diseases.
- Importance of informing patients of other important precautionary information. (See Cautions.)

Overview® (see Users Guide). For additional information until a more detailed monograph is developed and published, the manufacturer's labeling should be consulted. It is *essential* that the manufacturer's labeling be consulted for more detailed information on usual cautions, precautions, contraindications, potential drug interactions, laboratory test interferences, and acute toxicity.

PREPARATIONS

Excipients in commercially available drug preparations may have clinically important effects in some individuals; consult specific product labeling for details.

Bivalirudin Trifluoroacetate

Parenteral

| For injection, for IV infusion | 250 mg (of bivalirudin) | Angiomax®, SandozBivalirudin for Injection |
| Injection, for IV infusion | 5 mg (of bivalirudin) per mL (250 mg) | Angiomax® RTU, Maia Pharmaceuticals Bivalirudin RTU Injection |

Bivalirudin Trifluoroacetate in Sodium Chloride

Parenteral

| Injection (frozen), for IV infusion | 5 mg (of bivalirudin) per mL (250 or 500 mg) in 0.9% sodium chloride* | Bivalirudin in 0.9% Sodium Chloride Injection Galaxy® [Baxter] |

† Use is not currently included in the labeling approved by the US Food and Drug Administration.

* available from one or more manufacturer, distributor, and/or repackager by generic (nonproprietary) name

Selected Revisions December 15, 2021, © Copyright, March 1, 2001, American Society of Health-System Pharmacists, Inc.

Dabigatran Etexilate Mesylate

20:12.04.12 • DIRECT THROMBIN INHIBITORS

■ Dabigatran etexilate mesylate, a synthetic reversible direct thrombin inhibitor, is an anticoagulant.

USES

● Embolism Associated with Atrial Fibrillation

Nonvalvular Atrial Fibrillation

Dabigatran etexilate mesylate is used to reduce the risk of stroke and systemic embolism in adults with nonvalvular atrial fibrillation. The direct oral anticoagulants (DOACs; apixaban, dabigatran, edoxaban, rivaroxaban) have been shown in randomized controlled studies to be noninferior, and in some trials, superior to warfarin in reducing thromboembolic risk in patients with nonvalvular atrial fibrillation (i.e., atrial fibrillation in the absence of moderate-to-severe mitral stenosis or a mechanical heart valve), and are associated with reduced risk of serious bleeding.

Clinical Experience

Efficacy and safety of dabigatran in patients with nonvalvular atrial fibrillation were established in a multinational, randomized controlled study (Randomized Evaluation of Long-term Anticoagulation Therapy [RE-LY]); the study demonstrated that therapy with dabigatran 150 or 110 mg twice daily was noninferior to adjusted-dose warfarin (target INR 2–3) with respect to the primary efficacy outcome of stroke or systemic embolism. In addition, the 150-mg dosage of dabigatran was superior to warfarin with regard to occurrence of stroke or systemic embolism, and the 110-mg dosage was superior to warfarin with regard to incidence of major bleeding. The net clinical benefit outcome, a measure of overall benefit to risk, was similar for both dosages of dabigatran.

In the RE-LY study, 18,113 adults with paroxysmal, persistent, or permanent atrial fibrillation and at least one additional risk factor for stroke (i.e., history of stroke, transient ischemic attack, or systemic embolism; left ventricular ejection fraction <40%; symptomatic heart failure as defined by New York Heart Association [NYHA] class ≥2; age ≥75 years; age ≥65 years with diabetes mellitus, coronary artery disease, or hypertension) received dabigatran (110 or 150 mg twice daily) in a blinded fashion or adjusted-dose warfarin (target INR 2–3) in an unblinded fashion. The study population was principally white (70%) and male (64%), with a mean age of 71 years and a Congestive Heart Failure, Hypertension, Age, Diabetes, Stroke (doubled) (CHADS$_2$) score of 2.1. Approximately 20% of patients in each group continued aspirin throughout a median of 2 years of follow-up. Study exclusions included, but were not limited to, patients with valvular heart disease, recent stroke, increased risk of hemorrhage, renal impairment (creatinine clearance <30 mL/minute), or active liver disease.

The primary efficacy outcome of stroke (hemorrhagic or ischemic) or systemic embolism occurred substantially less frequently in patients receiving dabigatran 150 mg twice daily compared with adjusted-dose warfarin therapy (annualized rate of 1.11 and 1.69%, respectively; relative risk reduction of 35%). In addition, compared with warfarin, therapy with dabigatran 150 mg twice daily was associated with reductions in ischemic and hemorrhagic stroke (relative risk reductions of 24 and 74%, respectively). Major bleeding occurred at a similar rate with dabigatran 150 mg twice daily and warfarin.

In patients receiving dabigatran 110 mg twice daily, stroke or systemic embolism occurred with a frequency similar to that with warfarin (annualized rate of 1.53 and 1.69% in patients receiving dabigatran and warfarin, respectively). However, hemorrhagic stroke and major hemorrhage each occurred less frequently in those receiving dabigatran 110 mg compared with warfarin (relative risk reductions of 69 and 20%, respectively). Stroke or systemic embolism occurred less frequently with dabigatran 150 mg twice daily than with dabigatran 110 mg twice daily (annualized rate of 1.1 and 1.53%, respectively; relative risk reduction of 28%). Rates of hemorrhagic stroke and major hemorrhage were similar in the

2 dabigatran groups. In patients receiving warfarin, the mean percentage of time within the therapeutic range (INR 2–3) was 64%.

The rate of myocardial infarction (MI) was higher with dabigatran 150 or 110 mg than with warfarin (0.81, 0.82, and 0.64% per year, respectively; relative risk of 1.27 or 1.29 for the 150- or 110-mg dosages, respectively, versus warfarin), but these differences were not statistically significant.

While both a 150- and a 110-mg dosage of dabigatran were evaluated in the RE-LY study, the FDA approved only the 150-mg dosage of dabigatran for stroke risk reduction in patients with nonvalvular atrial fibrillation. Prior to FDA approval, some clinicians expressed interest in using the 110-mg dosage in specific patient populations, such as those that may be at greater risk of bleeding or, at lower risk of embolic events, or those who experienced bleeding when receiving the 150-mg dosage. FDA concluded that in patients who experienced major bleeding during the RE-LY study and who continued or resumed study medication, the risk of a repeat major bleeding event was similar among all 3 treatment groups. According to FDA, the appropriate population for the 110-mg dosage has not been identified. Because of superior efficacy with the 150-mg dosage and concern that a 110-mg dosage could potentially be overused and subsequently result in underdosing of many patients, FDA approved only the 150-mg dosage for stroke risk reduction in patients with nonvalvular atrial fibrillation. Approval of the 75-mg dosage for patients with severe renal impairment (creatinine clearance 15–30 mL/minute) was based on pharmacokinetic (PK) modeling using PK data from RE-LY and a smaller study in individuals with renal impairment.

The risk of stroke in patients with atrial flutter is similar to the risk in those with atrial fibrillation. Experts state that antithrombotic therapy in patients with atrial flutter generally should be managed in the same manner as in patients with atrial fibrillation.

DOACs including dabigatran have been used for pharmacologic cardioversion† in patients with atrial fibrillation or atrial flutter of >48 hours' duration or of unknown duration; DOACs are recommended as a safe and effective alternative to warfarin in this setting.

Clinical Perspective

The American College of Chest Physicians (ACCP), the American College of Cardiology (ACC), the American Heart Association (AHA), the American Stroke Association (ASA), and other experts currently recommend that antithrombotic therapy be administered to all patients with nonvalvular atrial fibrillation who are considered to be at increased risk of stroke, unless such therapy is contraindicated. Although many risk stratification methods have been used, current guidelines recommend the use of the CHA$_2$DS$_2$-VASc risk stratification tool for assessing a patient's risk of stroke and need for anticoagulant therapy. Established clinical risk factors for stroke include prior ischemic stroke or transient ischemic attack (TIA), advanced age (e.g., ≥65 years), hypertension, diabetes mellitus, vascular disease, and congestive heart failure; in addition, female sex has been identified as a factor that can modify the risk of stroke. The presence of stroke or TIA places a patient in the high-risk category regardless of other risk factors. Experts state that antithrombotic therapy generally is not necessary in low-risk patients (CHA$_2$DS$_2$-VASc score of 0 in males, or 1 in females), but should be considered in patients with one or more non-sex CHA$_2$DS$_2$-VASc stroke risk factors (CHA$_2$DS$_2$-VASc score of ≥1 in males, or ≥2 in females). Patients also should be assessed for their risk of bleeding; those with a high risk of bleeding should be monitored more closely.

In patients with nonvalvular atrial fibrillation who are eligible for oral anticoagulant therapy, DOACs are recommended over warfarin based on improved safety and similar or improved efficacy in clinical trials and meta-analyses. A substantially greater benefit of DOACs versus warfarin has been observed when the INR was in the therapeutic range less than 66% of the time. If warfarin is used, patients should be optimally managed with well-controlled INRs (e.g., INR in therapeutic range more than 70% of the time). A DOAC is recommended in patients unable to achieve optimal warfarin management.

Patient age, body weight, and renal and hepatic function should be considered prior to treatment with DOACs. There are limited data on the use of DOACs in obese patients and some experts have discouraged the use of these agents in the morbidly obese population (those with a body mass index [BMI] >40 kg/m^2 or body weight >120 kg). However, the various DOAC agents may have different outcomes. Because of limited data with DOACs in patients with morbid obesity, guidelines recommend considering warfarin over DOACs in morbidly obese patients with nonvalvular atrial fibrillation.

Because of the lack of direct, comparative studies, the relative efficacy and safety of dabigatran compared to other DOACs for the prevention of stroke in patients with nonvalvular atrial fibrillation remain to be fully elucidated. Some evidence from indirect comparisons suggests that there may be important differences (e.g., bleeding risk) between these agents; however, results of such analyses should be interpreted with caution because of possible confounding factors (e.g., differences in study design and methods, patient populations, and anticoagulation control). Selection of an appropriate anticoagulant for patients with nonvalvular atrial fibrillation should be individualized based on the absolute and relative risks of stroke and bleeding; costs; patient compliance, preference, tolerance, and comorbidities; and other clinical factors such as renal function and degree of INR control if the patient has been taking warfarin.

Valvular Heart Disease

Based on the results of a randomized, open-label trial (RE-ALIGN), dabigatran should not be used for the prevention of stroke or other major thromboembolic events in patients with mechanical prosthetic heart valves. In RE-ALIGN, patients received dabigatran (150, 220, or 300 mg twice daily) or adjusted-dose warfarin therapy (target INR of 2–3 or 2.5–3.5 depending on risk factors and position [aortic or mitral] of the mechanical heart valve). The trial was terminated early because of a substantially increased rate of stroke, MI, and valve thrombosis in patients receiving dabigatran compared with those receiving warfarin; dabigatran-treated patients also had a higher risk of major bleeding, predominantly after valve surgery.

The 2020 AHA/ACC guideline for the management of patients with valvular heart disease states that patients with valvular heart disease and atrial fibrillation† should be evaluated for risk of thromboembolic events and treated with oral anticoagulation if at high risk. Vitamin K antagonists are the anticoagulants of choice for patients with rheumatic mitral stenosis and mechanical heart valves. Dabigatran and other DOACs are an alternative to vitamin K antagonists in patients with atrial fibrillation and a bioprosthetic valve more than 3 months after implantation or with native valvular heart disease excluding rheumatic mitral stenosis.

● *Venous Thromboembolism - Treatment and Secondary Prevention*

Dabigatran is used for the treatment of acute deep-vein thrombosis (DVT) and/or pulmonary embolism (PE) in adults following initial treatment with a parenteral anticoagulant for 5–10 days. The drug also is used to reduce the risk of recurrent DVT and PE in adult patients who have been treated previously for an acute venous thromboembolic event (VTE).

Dabigatran is also used for the treatment of VTE in pediatric patients 3 months to <18 years of age after at least 5 days of initial parenteral anticoagulant treatment and to reduce the risk of recurrent VTE in such patients who have been previously treated. Although studied in all age groups <18 years of age, the FDA indication for dabigatran is product-specific. Dabigatran capsules are specifically indicated for children at least 8 years of age who can swallow the dabigatran capsule whole. Dabigatran oral pellets are specifically indicated for children 3 months to <12 years of age.

Clinical Experience in Adults

Efficacy and safety of dabigatran for the acute treatment and secondary prevention of DVT and/or PE in adults have been established principally in 4 randomized, double-blind studies. In 2 identically designed studies (RE-COVER and RE-COVER II) in more than 5000 patients with symptomatic acute proximal DVT or PE who were treated initially with a parenteral anticoagulant (e.g., unfractionated heparin, low molecular weight heparin [LMWH]) for 5–10 days, dabigatran was shown to be noninferior to warfarin in preventing recurrent thromboembolic events over a mean treatment period of approximately 6 months (based on similar rates of the primary composite outcome of fatal or symptomatic nonfatal PE or symptomatic recurrent DVT) and was associated with a lower risk of clinically relevant bleeding. In both studies, patients received either dabigatran 150 mg twice daily or adjusted-dose warfarin (target INR 2–3). Patients who received warfarin in the RE-COVER and RE-COVER II studies had INRs within the therapeutic range (2–3) an average of 60 and 57% of time, respectively, which

improved over the course of treatment from 53 or 51%, respectively, in the first month to 66 or 62%, respectively, in the last month.

Efficacy and safety of extended use of dabigatran for reducing the risk of recurrent DVT and/or PE (secondary prevention) in adults have been established principally in an active-controlled (RE-MEDY) and a placebo-controlled (RE-SONATE) study. Dabigatran was shown to be noninferior to warfarin and superior to placebo in reducing the risk of recurrent DVT and PE in these studies. Patients in the studies had completed at least 3 months of initial anticoagulant therapy for an acute VTE prior to enrollment; the studies included some patients who previously received dabigatran in the RE-COVER and RE-COVER II studies. In the RE-MEDY study, patients received either dabigatran (150 mg twice daily) or warfarin (with dose adjusted to achieve a target INR of 2–3) for a median duration of approximately 17.8 months; in the RE-SONATE study, patients received either dabigatran (150 mg twice daily) or placebo for a median duration of approximately 6 months. In patients receiving warfarin in the RE-MEDY study, the average time in therapeutic INR range was 62%. Although the criteria for noninferiority of dabigatran compared with warfarin was met in this study, there were some limitations associated with the statistical analysis (e.g., large noninferiority margin, upper limit of confidence interval close to noninferiority margin). With respect to safety, dabigatran was associated with a lower risk of major or clinically relevant nonmajor bleeding compared with warfarin, but a higher risk of bleeding compared with placebo.

Clinical Experience in Pediatric Patients

Efficacy and safety of dabigatran for the treatment of acute VTE in pediatric patients were evaluated in a randomized, open-label, multicenter, non-inferiority trial (DIVERSITY). The study compared dabigatran to standard of care (SOC) anticoagulation consisting of a vitamin K antagonist, unfractionated heparin, LMWH, or fondaparinux. Patients <18 years of age with a documented diagnosis of acute VTE, initially treated (5 to 21 days) with parenteral anticoagulation and requiring anticoagulation for at least 3 months were eligible. Exclusion criteria included conditions associated with an increased bleeding risk, hepatic disease, and an estimated glomerular filtration rate (eGFR) <50 mL/minute per 1.73 m². Dabigatran (capsules, pellets, or oral solution) was dosed based on an age- and weight-adjusted nomogram. The treatment period was 3 months, with additional patient follow-up for another month.

The primary endpoint of the DIVERSITY study was a composite of complete thrombus resolution, freedom from recurrent VTE, and freedom from VTE-related mortality. Freedom from major bleeding was a secondary endpoint with major bleeding defined as either fatal bleeding, clinically overt bleeding with a hemoglobin reduction of ≥2 g/dL in a 24-hour period, retroperitoneal, pulmonary, intracranial or CNS bleeding, or bleeding requiring surgical intervention. Results revealed that the composite of complete thrombus resolution, freedom from recurrent VTE, and freedom from VTE-related mortality occurred more frequently in the dabigatran group than in the SOC group (46% versus 42%, respectively), meeting the predefined noninferiority margin. Major bleeding occurred in 2.3% of patients who received dabigatran and 2.2% of those who received SOC; clinically relevant non-major bleeding occurred in 1.1% in each group.

An open-label, single-arm safety study included pediatric patients who required further anticoagulation due to the presence of a clinical risk factor after completing the initial treatment for confirmed VTE (for at least 3 months) or after completing the DIVERSITY study. At 12 months, the overall probability of being free from recurrence of VTE during the treatment period was 0.98 and the probability of being free from bleeding events during the on-treatment period was 0.72.

Clinical Perspective

The DOACs are among several anticoagulants that can be used for the treatment of VTE. DOACs have similar efficacy to warfarin, but reduced bleeding (particularly intracranial hemorrhage) and greater convenience for patients and healthcare providers. In addition to relative efficacy and safety, factors that should be considered when selecting an appropriate anticoagulant include convenience of administration, cost, patient preference, presence of renal impairment, and cancer or other comorbid conditions.

Dabigatran is recommended by the ACCP, American Society of Hematology (ASH), and the Anticoagulation Forum as an acceptable option for initial and long-term anticoagulant therapy in patients with acute proximal DVT of the leg and/or PE. In patients with acute VTE, therapy should be continued beyond the acute treatment period for at least 3 months, and possibly longer depending on the individual clinical situation (e.g., location of thrombi, presence or absence of precipitating factors, presence of cancer, patient's risk of bleeding). Dabigatran may offer some advantages over parenteral or vitamin K antagonist anticoagulants for the treatment of VTE (e.g., oral administration, no requirement for routine coagulation monitoring, minimal drug and food interactions) and guidelines recommend DOACs over vitamin K antagonist anticoagulants with a few exceptions based on risk factors (e.g., antiphospholipid syndrome). The relative efficacy and safety of dabigatran versus other DOACs (e.g., rivaroxaban, apixaban, edoxaban) for the treatment of VTE remains to be fully elucidated due to the lack of head-to-head trials. ACCP does not recommend one DOAC over another as there are very limited published studies directly comparing these agents and indirect comparisons have not shown substantially different outcomes.

DOACs generally should not be used in settings with high risk of bleeding (e.g., hemorrhagic lesion, renal/hepatic impairment, thrombocytopenia, GI or genitourinary malignancy, mucosal lesion, CNS malignancy or bleeding, recent surgery), or in patients with morbid obesity (body weight >120 kg or BMI ≥40 mg/m²), drug-drug interactions, or GI complications affecting oral therapy (e.g., poor absorption, nausea and vomiting) because of the lack of safety data. There is some experience with the use of apixaban and rivaroxaban in patients with morbid obesity.

In patients with cancer and established VTE, LMWHs or oral factor Xa inhibitors (e.g., apixaban, rivaroxaban, edoxaban) are generally recommended over warfarin for long-term anticoagulation. ACCP and ASH recommend the use of an oral factor Xa inhibitor over LMWH for the initiation and treatment phases of therapy in patients with cancer-associated thrombosis.

• Prophylaxis of Venous Thromboembolism

Major Orthopedic Surgery

Dabigatran is used for the prevention of DVT and PE in adults undergoing hip-replacement surgery. Dabigatran has also been used for the prevention of VTE in adult patients undergoing total knee-replacement surgery†.

Clinical Experience

Efficacy and safety of dabigatran for the prevention of postoperative DVT and PE in patients undergoing hip-replacement surgery are based principally on the results of 2 randomized, double-blind, active-controlled studies (RE-NOVATE and RE-NOVATE II). In these studies, dabigatran was noninferior to enoxaparin in preventing VTE in patients undergoing elective total hip-replacement surgery (based on similar rates of the primary composite end point of confirmed VTE [proximal or distal DVT on venogram, confirmed symptomatic DVT, or confirmed PE] and all cause death) and was associated with similar rates of bleeding. Patients in these studies received a single dose of dabigatran 75 mg (administered 1–4 hours after surgery) followed by dabigatran 150 mg daily; a single dose of dabigatran 110 mg (administered 1–4 hours after surgery) followed by dabigatran 220 mg daily; or subcutaneous enoxaparin 40 mg daily starting the evening before surgery for a median duration of 33 days. For efficacy evaluation, all patients underwent bilateral venography of the lower extremities within 24 hours after the last dose of the study drug unless an end point event occurred earlier in the trial. The primary composite end point occurred in 6% (RE-NOVATE) and 7.7% (RE-NOVATE II) of patients receiving dabigatran 220 mg daily and 6.7% (RE-NOVATE) and 8.8% (RE-NOVATE II) of patients receiving enoxaparin therapy. Dabigatran was generally well tolerated across all studies, and rates of major bleeding or any bleeding event were generally similar between treatment groups.

Clinical Perspective

Several major guidelines for thromboprophylaxis following hip- or knee-replacement surgery have been published, including guidelines from the American Academy of Orthopedic Surgeons (AAOS), ACCP, and ASH. Although dabigatran use following knee replacement surgery is not a FDA-labeled indication, the major guidelines make no distinction in their recommendations for thromboprophylaxis following hip versus knee arthroplasty. Routine

thromboprophylaxis is recommended in all patients undergoing major orthopedic surgery, including total hip- or knee-replacement surgery, because of the high risk of postoperative VTE. According to ACCP, thromboprophylaxis with an appropriate antithrombotic agent or an intermittent pneumatic compression device should be continued for at least 10–14 days and possibly for up to 35 days after surgery.

AAOS guidelines do not recommend any specific thromboprophylaxis agent, while the ACCP guidelines favor LMWHs over DOACs. The ASH guidelines suggest the use of DOACs over LMWHs if anticoagulants are used; however, this recommendation is considered conditional based on moderate certainty in the evidence of harms versus benefits.

Drug selection and duration of therapy should be individualized based on type of surgery, patient risk factors for embolism and bleeding, as well as costs, patient compliance, preference, tolerance, and comorbidities; and other clinical factors such as renal function.

DOSAGE AND ADMINISTRATION

• General

Pretreatment Screening

- Prior to initiating therapy with dabigatran, assess renal function in all patients. In children, estimate the glomerular filtration rate (eGFR) using the Schwarz formula as follows: eGFR = (0.413 × height in cm)/serum creatinine in mg/dL. Avoid use of dabigatran in pediatric patients with eGFR <50 mL/minute per 1.73 m².

- When used in pediatric patients for treatment and secondary prevention of venous thromboembolism (VTE), obtain body weight for dosing.

Patient Monitoring

- Periodically assess renal function as clinically indicated (i.e., more frequently in situations that may be associated with a decline in renal function) and adjust therapy accordingly.

- When used in pediatric patients for treatment and secondary prevention of VTE, periodically assess body weight and adjust doses and dosage forms accordingly.

- If dabigatran is administered in an epidural or spinal anesthesia/analgesia or lumbar puncture setting, frequently monitor for signs or symptoms of neurological impairment (e.g., numbness, tingling, weakness in lower limbs, bowel and/or bladder dysfunction).

- Monitor patients for any signs or symptoms of bleeding (e.g., unusual bruising) during therapy.

- Routine monitoring of coagulation status is not required in patients receiving dabigatran. When necessary, the manufacturer states that the ecarin clotting time (ECT) or the activated partial thromboplastin time (aPTT) may be used to assess the anticoagulant effects of dabigatran; however, results of such tests should be interpreted with caution. Use of the prothrombin time (PT)/international normalized ratio (INR) should be avoided since this test is relatively insensitive to the effects of dabigatran and results may be unreliable.

Dispensing and Administration Precautions

- Dabigatran is available in different dosage forms and not all forms are approved for the same indications and age groups. Dabigatran dosage forms are not interchangeable due to bioavailability differences. Avoid substituting different dosage forms on a mg-to-mg basis and do not combine more than one dosage form to achieve the total dose.

- Based on the Institute for Safe Medication Practices (ISMP), dabigatran is a high-alert medication that has a heightened risk of causing significant patient harm when used in error.

• Administration

Administer dabigatran orally (as capsules or oral pellets).

Capsules

Administer dabigatran capsules orally without regard to meals; consider administration with food, if GI distress occurs.

Swallow capsules whole with a full glass of water; do not chew, break, or open the capsules as this may result in increased systemic exposure to the drug.

Take a missed dose as soon as it is remembered on the same day. If a missed dose cannot be taken at least 6 hours before the next scheduled dose, skip the dose; do not double doses.

Dabigatran capsules can be used in pediatric patients ≥8 years of age who are able to swallow capsules whole. The oral pellets should be used in pediatric patients younger than 8 years of age. The capsules should be dosed twice daily, one dose in the morning and one in the evening, at approximately the same time each day, as close to a 12-hour dosing interval as possible.

Dispense dabigatran capsules only in the manufacturer's original bottle or blister package in order to minimize potential product breakdown and loss of potency due to moisture. Do not repackage the capsules. If more than one bottle is dispensed, advise the patient to open only one bottle at a time. The manufacturer recommends that capsules in the bottle be used within 4 months after first opening the bottle. Store bottles and blisters at 20–25°C; excursions permitted to 15–30°C.

Oral Pellets

Dabigatran oral pellets can be used in children 3 months to <12 years of age as soon as they are able to swallow soft food. The oral pellets should be dosed twice daily, one dose in the morning and one in the evening, at approximately the same time each day, as close to a 12-hour dosing interval as possible. Administer the prepared dose before meals to ensure that the child takes the full dose.

If a dose is missed, take the dose as soon as it is remembered on the same day. If a missed dose cannot be taken at least 6 hours before the next scheduled dose, skip the dose; do not double doses. If a partial dose has been taken, do not administer a second dose at that time. Administer the next dose as scheduled approximately 12 hours later.

Dabigatran oral pellets should be administered with only specific soft foods or apple juice. The oral pellets may be mixed with 2 teaspoons of the following foods at room temperature: baby rice cereal prepared with water, mashed carrots, apple sauce, or mashed banana. Alternatively, the oral pellets may be spooned directly into the child's mouth and swallowed with apple juice or added to 1–2 ounces of apple juice for drinking.

Administer prepared pellets immediately after mixing or within 30 minutes following mixing. Discard any dose not administered within 30 minutes and prepare a new dose as necessary. Do not use milk, milk products, or soft foods containing milk to prepare the dose. Do not administer the pellets via syringe or feeding tubes.

The commercially available dabigatran oral pellet packets are provided in an aluminum bag. Store the drug in the original package to protect from moisture. Use the oral pellets within 6 months of opening the aluminum bag. Do not open the pellet packet dose until ready for use. Store at 20–25°C with excursions permitted to 15–30°C.

● *Dosage*

Dosage of dabigatran, which is commercially available as dabigatran etexilate mesylate, is expressed in terms of the prodrug, dabigatran etexilate.

Pediatric Patients

Venous Thromboembolism-Treatment and Secondary Prevention

Pediatric patients 3 months to <12 years of age with eGFR (Schwartz) >50 mL/minute per 1.73 m² (oral pellets): for the treatment and reduction in the risk of recurrence (secondary prevention) of acute deep-vein thrombosis (DVT) and/or pulmonary embolism (PE), the recommended dosage of dabigatran pellets is age- and weight-based. Table 1 provides dosing recommendations for the oral pellets in patients <2 years of age and Table 2 provides dosage recommendations for the oral pellets in patients 2 to <12 years of age.

Treatment with dabigatran should be initiated following treatment with a parenteral anticoagulant for at least 5 days. For reduction in the risk of recurrence of VTE, treatment with dabigatran should be initiated following previous treatment.

TABLE 1. Dosage of Dabigatran Etexilate Oral Pellets in Patients <2 Years of Age

Actual body weight	Age	Dose given twice daily	Number of packets needed
3 kg to <4 kg	3 to <6 months	30 mg	One 30 mg packet twice daily
4 kg to <5 kg	3 to <10 months	40 mg	One 40 mg packet twice daily
5 kg to <7 kg	3 to <5 months	40 mg	One 40 mg packet twice daily
	5 to <24 months	50 mg	One 50 mg packet twice daily
7 kg to <9 kg	3 to <4 months	50 mg	One 50 mg packet twice daily
	4 to <9 months	60 mg	Two 30 mg packets twice daily
	9 to <24 months	70 mg	One 30 mg plus one 40 mg packet twice daily
9 kg to <11 kg	5 to <6 months	60 mg	Two 30 mg packets twice daily
	6 to <11 months	80 mg	Two 40 mg packets twice daily
	11 to <24 months	90 mg	One 40 mg plus one 50 mg packet twice daily
11 kg <13 kg	8 to <18 months	100 mg	Two 50 mg packets twice daily
	18 to <24 months	110 mg	One 110 mg packet twice daily
13 kg to <16 kg	10 to <11 months	100 mg	Two 50 mg packets twice daily
	11 to <24 months	140 mg	One 30 mg plus one 110 mg packet twice daily
16 kg to <21 kg	12 to <24 months	140 mg	One 30 mg plus one 110 mg packet twice daily
21 kg to <26 kg	18 to <24 months	180 mg	One 30 mg plus one 150 mg packet twice daily

TABLE 2. Dosage of Dabigatran Etexilate Oral Pellets in Patients 2 to < 12 Years of Age

Actual body weight	Dose given twice daily	Number of packets needed
7 kg to <9 kg	70 mg	One 30 mg plus one 40 mg packet twice daily
9 kg to <11 kg	90 mg	One 40 mg plus one 50 mg packet twice daily
11 kg to <13 kg	110 mg	One 110 mg packet twice daily
13 kg to <16 kg	140 mg	One 30 mg plus one 110 mg packet twice daily
16 kg to <21 kg	170 mg	One 20 mg plus one 150 mg packet twice daily
21 kg to <41 kg	220 mg	Two 110 mg packets twice daily
≥41 kg	260 mg	One 110 mg plus one 150 mg packet twice daily

Pediatric patients 8 to <18 years of age with eGFR (Schwartz) >50 mL/minute per 1.73 m² (capsules): for the treatment and reduction in the risk of recurrence (secondary prevention) of acute DVT and/or PE, the recommended dosage of dabigatran capsules is weight-based. Table 3 provides dosage recommendations for the capsules in pediatric patients 8 to <18 years of age.

TABLE 3. Dosage of Dabigatran Etexilate Capsules in Patients 8 to <18 Years of Age

Actual body weight	Dose twice daily	Number of capsules needed
11 kg to <16 kg	75 mg twice daily	One 75 mg capsule twice daily
16 kg to <26 kg	110 mg twice daily	One 110 mg capsule twice daily
26 kg to <41 kg	150 mg twice daily	One 150 mg capsule twice daily Or Two 75 mg capsules twice daily
41 kg to <61 kg	185 mg twice daily	One 110 mg plus one 75 mg capsule twice daily
61 kg to <81 kg	220 mg twice daily	Two 110 mg capsules twice daily
≥81 kg	260 mg twice daily	One 150 mg plus one 110 mg capsule twice daily Or One 110 mg plus two 75 mg capsules twice daily

Adults

Embolism Associated with Atrial Fibrillation

For reducing the risk of stroke and systemic embolism in patients with nonvalvular atrial fibrillation, the recommended dosage of dabigatran etexilate in adults with a creatinine clearance >30 mL/minute is 150 mg orally twice daily. Reduce dosage to 75 mg twice daily in patients with creatinine clearance 15–30 mL/minute. Dosing recommendations are unavailable in patients with creatinine clearance <15 mL/minute or in dialysis patients.

If the patient is taking a specific P-glycoprotein inhibitor (i.e., dronedarone, systemic ketoconazole), reduce dabigatran dosage to 75 mg twice daily when creatinine clearance is 30–50 mL/minute. Avoid coadministration of dabigatran with P-glycoprotein inhibitors when creatinine clearance <30 mL/minute.

Venous Thromboembolism-Treatment and Secondary Prevention

For the treatment and reduction in the risk of recurrence (secondary prevention) of acute DVT and/or PE in adults, the recommended dosage of dabigatran etexilate in patents with creatinine clearance >30 mL/minute is 150 mg orally twice daily, after 5–10 days of parenteral anticoagulation.

Dosing recommendations are unavailable when creatinine clearance is ≤30 mL/minute or in dialysis patients. Avoid coadministration of dabigatran with P-glycoprotein inhibitors when creatinine clearance <50 mL/minute.

The optimum duration of anticoagulant therapy in patients with venous thromboembolism (VTE) should be determined by the individual clinical situation (e.g., location of thrombi, presence or absence of precipitating factors for thrombosis, presence of cancer, risk of bleeding). In general, the American College of Chest Physicians (ACCP) states that anticoagulant therapy for VTE should be continued beyond the acute treatment period for at least 3 months and possibly longer in patients with a high risk of recurrence and low risk of bleeding.

Thromboprophylaxis in Hip-Replacement Surgery

For the prevention of DVT and PE in patients who have undergone hip-replacement surgery, the recommended dosage of dabigatran etexilate in adults with a creatinine clearance > 30 mL/minute is 110 mg administered as a single dose 1–4 hours after surgery (provided hemostasis has been achieved), followed by 220 mg once daily. If dabigatran therapy is not initiated on the day of surgery, dabigatran treatment should be initiated at a dosage of 220 mg once daily after

hemostasis has been achieved. Dosing recommendations are unavailable when creatinine clearance ≤30 mL/minute or in dialysis patients. Avoid coadministration of dabigatran with P-glycoprotein inhibitors when creatinine clearance is <50 mL/minute.

The manufacturer recommends a duration of 28–35 days for patients who have undergone hip-replacement surgery. ACCP recommends at least 10–14 days of antithrombotic therapy, possibly up to 35 days, for patients undergoing major orthopedic surgery.

Transitioning from Other Anticoagulant Therapy

When switching to dabigatran therapy from warfarin, dabigatran should be initiated after warfarin has been discontinued and the INR is <2.

When switching to dabigatran therapy in those receiving intermittently dosed parenteral anticoagulants (e.g., enoxaparin), the first dose of dabigatran should be administered within 2 hours prior to what would have been the time of the next scheduled intermittent parenteral dose.

When switching to dabigatran therapy in those receiving parenteral anticoagulants by continuous infusion, dabigatran should be initiated at the time the infusion is discontinued.

Transitioning to Other Anticoagulant Therapy

Because assessment of INR is unreliable in those receiving dabigatran, the therapeutic effects of warfarin are more accurately reflected by INR measurements taken 2 or more days after dabigatran discontinuance.

Pediatric Patients

When switching from dabigatran to warfarin therapy, warfarin should be initiated prior to dabigatran discontinuance. For pediatric patients with an eGFR (Schwartz) ≥50 mL/minute per 1.73 m², warfarin should be started 3 days prior to dabigatran discontinuance.

When switching from dabigatran to therapy with a parenteral anticoagulant, dabigatran should be discontinued prior to initiating the parenteral therapy; the parenteral anticoagulant should be started 12 hours after the last dose of dabigatran.

Adults

When switching from dabigatran to warfarin therapy, warfarin should be initiated prior to dabigatran discontinuance. For patients with a creatinine clearance ≥50 mL/minute, warfarin should be started 3 days prior to dabigatran discontinuance. For patients with a creatinine clearance of 30–50 mL/minute, warfarin should be started 2 days prior and for patients with a creatinine clearance of 15–30 mL/minute, warfarin should be started 1 day prior to discontinuance of dabigatran. Dosing recommendations are not available for patients with a creatinine clearance <15 mL/minute.

When switching from dabigatran to therapy with a parenteral anticoagulant, dabigatran should be discontinued prior to initiating parenteral therapy. For patients with a creatinine clearance ≥30 mL/minute, the parenteral anticoagulant should be started 12 hours after the last dose of dabigatran. If the creatinine clearance is <30 mL/minute, the parenteral anticoagulant should be started 24 hours after the last dose of dabigatran. Dosing recommendations are not available for patients with a creatinine clearance <15 mL/minute.

Managing Anticoagulation in Patients Requiring Invasive Procedures

Pediatric Patients

When possible, dabigatran therapy should be withheld prior to invasive or surgical procedures because of the increased risk of bleeding. Discontinue dabigatran pellets or capsules 24 hours before elective surgery in pediatric patients with eGFR (Schwartz) >80 mL/minute per 1.73 m² or 48 hours in pediatric patients with eGFR (Schwartz) 50–80 mL/minute per 1.73 m². Withholding therapy for longer periods should be considered in patients who may require complete hemostasis (e.g., prior to major surgery, spinal puncture, placement of spinal or epidural catheter or port). When surgery cannot be delayed, the increased risk of bleeding with dabigatran therapy should be weighed against the urgency of the intervention. Idarucizumab, a specific reversal agent for dabigatran, can be used in case of emergency surgery or procedures when reversal of dabigatran's anticoagulant effect is needed; however, efficacy and safety in pediatric patients have not been established. Resumption of anticoagulant therapy should be considered as soon as medically appropriate.

Adults

When possible, dabigatran therapy should be withheld prior to invasive or surgical procedures because of the increased risk of bleeding. For adults with a creatinine clearance ≥50 mL/minute, the manufacturer recommends withholding therapy beginning 1–2 days prior to the procedure. For adults with a creatinine clearance <50 mL/minute, dabigatran should be withheld beginning 3–5 days prior to the procedure. However, withholding therapy for longer periods should be considered in patients who may require complete hemostasis (e.g., prior to major surgery, spinal puncture, placement of spinal or epidural catheter or port). When surgery cannot be delayed, the increased risk of bleeding with dabigatran therapy should be weighed against the urgency of the intervention. Idarucizumab, a specific reversal agent for dabigatran, can be used in case of emergency surgery or procedures when reversal of dabigatran's anticoagulant effect is needed. Dabigatran therapy can be reinitiated 24 hours after administration of idarucizumab; resumption of anticoagulant therapy should be considered as soon as medically appropriate.

● Special Populations

Hepatic Impairment

The manufacturer makes no specific dosage recommendations for patients with hepatic impairment.

Renal Impairment

Embolism Associated with Atrial Fibrillation

Reduce dosage to 75 mg orally twice daily in adult patients with severe renal impairment (creatinine clearance of 15–30 mL/minute). Patients with severe renal impairment were not included in the RE-LY study; therefore, dosage recommendations in this population are based on pharmacokinetic modeling. For patients with a creatinine clearance <15 mL/minute or who are receiving hemodialysis, dosage recommendations cannot be provided. Discontinue dabigatran in patients who develop acute renal failure while on therapy; consider an alternative anticoagulant.

Concomitant use of the P-glycoprotein (P-gp) inhibitors dronedarone and ketoconazole (systemic) in patients with moderate renal impairment (creatinine clearance of 30–50 mL/minute) is expected to increase dabigatran exposure to a similar extent as that observed in patients with severe renal impairment; therefore, the manufacturer recommends that the dosage of dabigatran be reduced to 75 mg twice daily in patients with moderate renal impairment receiving such concomitant therapy. Dosage adjustments are not necessary when dabigatran is administered concomitantly with the P-gp inhibitors verapamil, amiodarone, quinidine, clarithromycin, and ticagrelor in patients with moderate renal impairment. The manufacturer states that these results should not be extrapolated to other P-gp inhibitors. Avoid concomitant use of P-gp inhibitors in patients with a creatinine clearance <30 mL/minute.

Venous Thromboembolism-Treatment and Secondary Prevention

Pediatric Patients: Avoid use in children with an eGFR (Schwartz) <50 mL/minute per 1.73 m^2 due to risk of increased drug exposure. Discontinue in patients who develop acute renal failure while on therapy; consider an alternative anticoagulant.

Adults: The manufacturer states that dosage recommendations cannot be provided for patients with a creatinine clearance ≤30 mL/minute or for those receiving dialysis. Discontinue in patients who develop acute renal failure while on therapy; consider an alternative anticoagulant.

Avoid concomitant use of P-gp inhibitors in patients with a creatinine clearance <50 mL/minute.

Thromboprophylaxis in Hip-Replacement Surgery

Dosage recommendations cannot be provided for adult patients with a creatinine clearance ≤30 mL/minute or for those receiving dialysis. Discontinue in patients who develop acute renal failure while on therapy; consider an alternative anticoagulant.

Avoid concomitant use of P-gp inhibitors in patients with a creatinine clearance <50 mL/minute.

Geriatric Patients

The manufacturer makes no specific dosage recommendations for geriatric patients.

CAUTIONS

● Contraindications

- Active pathologic bleeding.
- History of serious hypersensitivity reaction.
- Mechanical prosthetic heart valve.

● Warnings/Precautions

Warnings

Risk of Thrombosis Following Premature Discontinuance of Anticoagulation

Premature discontinuance of any oral anticoagulant, including dabigatran, in the absence of adequate alternative anticoagulation increases the risk of thrombotic events. A boxed warning about this risk is included in the prescribing information for dabigatran. If discontinuance of dabigatran is required for reasons other than pathologic bleeding or completion of a course of therapy, administration of an alternative anticoagulant should be considered. When transitioning patients from one anticoagulant therapy to another, it is important to ensure continuous anticoagulation while minimizing the risk of bleeding. Particular caution is advised when switching patients from a direct oral anticoagulant (DOAC) to warfarin therapy because of the slow onset of action of warfarin.

Spinal/Epidural Hematoma

Patients receiving anticoagulants are at risk of developing an epidural or spinal hematoma when concomitant neuraxial (epidural/spinal) anesthesia or spinal puncture is employed; such complications can result in long-term or permanent paralysis. A boxed warning about this risk is included in the dabigatran prescribing information. The risk of these complications is increased by postoperative use of indwelling epidural catheters for administration of analgesia or by concomitant use of drugs affecting hemostasis, such as nonsteroidal anti-inflammatory agents (NSAIAs), platelet-aggregation inhibitors, or other anticoagulants. Risk also may be increased in patients with spinal deformity, spinal surgery, or a history of traumatic or repeated epidural or spinal punctures.

To reduce the risk of bleeding with concurrent use of dabigatran and neuraxial anesthesia or spinal puncture procedures, clinicians should carefully consider the pharmacokinetic (PK) profile of dabigatran in relation to timing of such procedures. Insertion or removal of an epidural catheter or lumbar puncture is best performed when the anticoagulant effect of dabigatran is minimal; however, the optimal timing to achieve a sufficiently low anticoagulant effect in individual patients is not known.

Patients receiving dabigatran in the setting of epidural or spinal anesthesia should be monitored frequently for signs and symptoms of neurologic impairment (e.g., midline back pain; numbness, tingling, or weakness in lower limbs; bowel or bladder dysfunction). If spinal hematoma is suspected, urgent diagnosis and treatment is necessary; spinal cord decompression should be considered even though it may not prevent or reverse neurologic sequelae. Clinicians should consider the potential benefits versus risks of spinal/epidural anesthesia or spinal puncture in patients receiving or being considered for anticoagulant therapy.

Other Warnings and Precautions

Bleeding

Dabigatran increases the risk of hemorrhage and may cause serious, sometimes fatal bleeding. The drug should be discontinued if active pathological hemorrhage occurs. However, minor or "nuisance" bleeding is a common occurrence in patients receiving any anticoagulant and should not readily lead to treatment discontinuance.

In the Randomized Evaluation of Long-term Anticoagulation Therapy (RE-LY) study, life-threatening bleeding (i.e., fatal bleeding, symptomatic intracranial bleeding, hemoglobin decrease of ≥5 g/dL, hypotension requiring IV inotropic agents, transfusion of ≥4 units of packed red blood cells, bleeding requiring surgical intervention) occurred at a rate of 1.5% per year in patients receiving dabigatran 150 mg twice daily versus 1.8% per year with adjusted-dose (target international normalized ratio [INR] 2–3) warfarin therapy. Major bleeding (i.e., hemoglobin decrease of ≥2 g/dL, transfusion of ≥2 units of packed red blood cells, bleeding into a critical organ/area, and/or fatal outcome) was similar in patients receiving dabigatran 150 mg twice daily compared with those receiving adjusted-dose warfarin therapy (approximately 3.5 or 3.6% per year, respectively); however, there was a trend towards a higher incidence of major bleeding with dabigatran therapy for patients ≥75 years of age. Dabigatran therapy was associated with substantially lower rates of life-threatening bleeding, intracranial bleeding, and combined major or minor bleeding compared with warfarin in the RE-LY study. However, the rate of GI bleeding, including major GI bleeding, was substantially higher with dabigatran 150 mg twice daily compared with warfarin. Rates of major bleeding or clinically relevant bleeding with dabigatran were lower or similar to those with warfarin in the randomized, controlled studies in patients with acute deep-vein thrombosis (DVT) and/or pulmonary embolism (PE) (RE-COVER and RE-COVER II). In these studies, GI bleeding occurred in 3.1% of patients receiving dabigatran 150 mg twice daily versus 2.4% of those receiving warfarin. In the RE-NOVATE and RE-NOVATE II studies in patients undergoing hip-replacement surgery, major bleeding occurred in 1.4 and 2%, respectively, of patients receiving dabigatran 220 mg daily and 0.9 and 1.6%, respectively, of patients receiving enoxaparin therapy. The rate of major GI bleeding in patients receiving dabigatran and enoxaparin was the same (0.1%) and the rate of any GI bleeding was 1.4% for dabigatran-treated patients and 0.9% for enoxaparin-treated patients. In longer-term studies in which patients received extended treatment with dabigatran for acute venous thromboembolism (VTE; RE-MEDY, RE-SONATE), major or clinically relevant bleeding occurred less frequently with dabigatran than with warfarin, but more frequently with dabigatran than with placebo. The rate of any GI bleeding with dabigatran therapy in these studies was 0.7–3.1%. In the pediatric VTE DIVERSITY trial, major bleeding occurred in 2.3% of dabigatran and 2.2% of standard of care (SOC) patients; clinically relevant non-major bleeding occurred in 1.1% of patients in each group. Minor bleeding was reported in 19% of dabigatran patients and 23% of SOC patients. GI bleeding occurred more frequently in dabigatran versus SOC patients (5.7% versus 1.8%); all other site-specific bleeding rates were considered comparable.

Risk factors for hemorrhage include concomitant use of other drugs that generally increase bleeding risk (e.g., antiplatelet agents, heparin, thrombolytic therapy, chronic use of NSAIAs) and renal impairment. Overdosage also may lead to hemorrhagic complications. Ecarin clotting time (ECT) or activated partial thromboplastin time (aPTT) may be used when necessary to assess the degree of anticoagulation from dabigatran therapy. Management of bleeding complications should be individualized according to the severity and location of hemorrhage. Idarucizumab, a recombinant humanized monoclonal antibody fragment, is a specific reversal agent that is used to neutralize the anticoagulant effect of dabigatran in patients with life-threatening or uncontrolled bleeding or a need to undergo an emergency surgery/urgent procedure. Idarucizumab has been shown to reverse the anticoagulant effects of dabigatran within minutes after administration. Idarucizumab can be used in conjunction with supportive measures (e.g., maintenance of adequate diuresis, mechanical compression, surgical hemostasis, volume replacement, blood products), which should be considered as medically appropriate. Idarucizumab efficacy and safety in pediatric patients have not been established. While clinical experience supporting the use of hemodialysis is limited, dabigatran is dialyzable and approximately 49 and 57% of the drug is removed over 4 hours using a high-flux dialyzer at blood flow rates of 200 and 300 mL/minute, respectively; however, redistribution of the drug may occur after completion of dialysis, and the individual response to dialysis is likely to vary based on patient-specific characteristics.

Limited experimental (in vitro and animal) data and case studies support the administration of anti-inhibitor coagulant complex (e.g., Feiba®; also known as activated prothrombin complex concentrate [aPCC]), factor VIIa (recombinant), or concentrates of coagulation factors II, IX, or X for their anticoagulant reversal effects, but the efficacy and safety of these agents have not been evaluated in clinical studies of patients receiving dabigatran. In a study in a limited number of healthy individuals, use of a nonactivated 4-factor prothrombin complex concentrate (PCC) failed to reverse the anticoagulant effect of dabigatran as measured by aPTT, ECT, or thrombin time (TT). When aPCC was administered to 14 patients with dabigatran-associated major bleeding, good or moderate hemostasis was achieved in 9 (64%) or 5 (36%) patients, respectively. The median initial dose of aPCC was 44 units/kg (range 24–98 units/kg); 4 patients received a second dose. Based on guidance from the Anticoagulation Forum, an IV dose of aPCC 50 units/kg is suggested when idarucizumab is unavailable for the treatment of patients with dabigatran-associated major bleeding in whom a reversal agent is warranted.

Protamine sulfate and vitamin K are not expected to affect the anticoagulant activity of dabigatran. Administration of platelet concentrates may also be considered in cases of thrombocytopenia or when long-acting antiplatelet drugs have been used. In the event of an overdosage, activated charcoal may be used if administered early (e.g., within 1–2 hours) after ingestion.

Patients with Prosthetic Heart Valves

Findings from a randomized controlled study (RE-ALIGN) indicate an increased risk of thromboembolic events (valve thrombosis, stroke, transient ischemic attack, myocardial infarction) and major bleeding (principally postoperative pericardial effusions) with dabigatran compared with warfarin therapy in patients with mechanical prosthetic heart valves. Such thromboembolic and bleeding events were observed in patients with recently implanted as well as older (implanted > 3 months prior to study entry) prosthetic valves. Based on these findings, the FDA and manufacturer state that dabigatran is contraindicated in patients with prosthetic mechanical heart valves. Patients with a mechanical heart valve who are currently receiving dabigatran therapy should be promptly transitioned to another anticoagulant. Dabigatran should not be discontinued without guidance from a healthcare professional as sudden discontinuance may increase the risk of stroke and thromboembolism.

Data are lacking in patients with other forms of valvular heart disease, such as those with bioprosthetic heart valves, and dabigatran is generally not recommended in such patients.

Drugs Affecting P-glycoprotein Transport

Concomitant use of agents that induce P-glycoprotein transport (e.g., rifampin) reduces systemic exposure to dabigatran and generally should be avoided during dabigatran therapy.

Concomitant use of agents such as dronedarone and ketoconazole (systemic) that inhibit P-glycoprotein transport in patients with renal impairment may increase systemic exposure to dabigatran; therefore, dosage reduction or avoidance of such concomitant therapy is recommended in these situations.

Thrombosis Risk in Triple Positive Antiphospholipid Syndrome

Dabigatran and other DOACs are not recommended for use in patients with triple-positive antiphospholipid syndrome (APS) (i.e., positive for lupus anticoagulant, anticardiolipin, and anti-beta 2-glycoprotein I antibodies). Treatment with DOACs has been associated with increased rates of recurrent thrombotic events compared with warfarin treatment in patients with APS, especially those with triple-positive disease. The International Society on Thrombosis and Haemostasis recommends the use of vitamin K antagonists over DOACs in patients with high-risk APS, including those with triple-positive disease.

Specific Populations

Pregnancy

There is insufficient data to inform the associated risks for adverse developmental outcomes following use of dabigatran during pregnancy. In animal studies, decreased implantation, fetal loss, and excess vaginal/uterine bleeding close to parturition have been observed. When administered to rats in maternally toxic doses during organogenesis, abnormal fetal skull bone and vertebrae ossification was observed, but no other major malformations were induced.

Dabigatran use during labor or delivery in women receiving neuraxial anesthesia may result in epidural or spinal hematomas. Consider discontinuation of dabigatran or use of a shorter acting anticoagulant agent as delivery approaches. Based on the pharmacologic activity of anticoagulants, bleeding risk may be increased in the fetus and neonate. Monitor neonates for signs/symptoms of bleeding.

The American College of Chest Physicians (ACCP) and the American College of Obstetricians and Gynecologists (ACOG) recommend avoiding dabigatran in pregnant women due to insufficient safety data; the American Society of Hematology (ASH) states that more data are necessary in their most recent guidelines for the management of VTE in the context of pregnancy.

Lactation

It is not known whether dabigatran is distributed into human milk; dabigatran and/or its metabolites are found in rat milk. The manufacturer does not recommend breastfeeding during dabigatran treatment. ACCP, ACOG, and ASH recommend that anticoagulants other than dabigatran be used in nursing women.

Females and Males of Reproductive Potential

Dabigatran can cause significant uterine bleeding. Females of reproductive potential and those with abnormal uterine bleeding should be assessed for increased risk of clinically significant uterine bleeding, potentially requiring gynecologic surgical intervention.

Pediatric Use

Safety and efficacy of dabigatran for treatment of venous thromboembolism (VTE) and reduction in the risk of recurrent VTE have been established in pediatric patients <12 years of age (oral pellets) and 8 to <18 years of age (oral capsules).

Safety and efficacy of dabigatran have not been established in pediatric patients for other indications.

Geriatric Use

In the RE-LY study, 82% of patients were ≥65 years of age, and 40% were ≥75 years of age. Risk of bleeding increases with age, but the risk-benefit profile is favorable in all age groups.

Hepatic Impairment

In adults with moderate hepatic impairment (Child-Pugh class B), large interpatient variability was apparent, but no consistent change in exposure or pharmacodynamic response was observed. Patients with active liver disease were excluded from the RE-LY study. Pediatric patients with active liver disease were excluded from the DIVERSITY trial.

Renal Impairment

Dabigatran exposure and anticoagulant effects are increased in patients with renal impairment. Renal function should be assessed prior to initiation of dabigatran therapy and periodically thereafter as clinically appropriate. Dosage adjustments in adults may be necessary depending on the patient's degree of renal impairment and indication for use. Dabigatran has not been evaluated in pediatric patients with an estimated glomerular filtration rate (eGFR) <50 mL/minute per 1.73 m²; avoid use in these patients. Concomitant use of dabigatran and P-glycoprotein inhibitors is expected to further increase exposure to dabigatran in patients with renal impairment. In patients who develop acute renal failure during dabigatran therapy, the drug should be discontinued and alternative anticoagulants considered. Hemodialysis can remove dabigatran.

● Common Adverse Effects

Adverse effects reported in >15% of patients receiving dabigatran in clinical studies include GI adverse reactions and bleeding.

DRUG INTERACTIONS

Dabigatran is not a substrate, inducer, or inhibitor of cytochrome P-450 (CYP) isoenzymes. Dabigatran is a substrate for the P-glycoprotein (P-gp) transport system.

The manufacturer states no clinical drug interaction studies have been conducted in pediatric subjects.

● Drugs Affecting or Metabolized by Hepatic Microsomal Enzymes

Concomitant use of a CYP3A4 isoenzyme substrate (atorvastatin) and dabigatran did not have clinically relevant effects on the pharmacokinetics of either drug. In addition, concomitant use of a CYP2C9 substrate (diclofenac) and dabigatran did not have clinically relevant effects on the pharmacokinetics of either drug.

● Drugs Affecting P-glycoprotein Transport

Inducers of P-glycoprotein Transport

Concomitant use of dabigatran with P-gp inducers (e.g., rifampin) may reduce systemic exposure to dabigatran. Concomitant use generally should be avoided.

Rifampin

Administration of rifampin 600 mg daily for 7 days followed by a single dose of dabigatran resulted in decreases of 66 and 67% in dabigatran AUC and peak plasma concentration, respectively. Within 7 days of rifampin discontinuance, dabigatran exposure approached levels expected without concurrent use of rifampin. Concomitant use should be avoided.

Inhibitors of P-glycoprotein Transport

Concomitant use of P-gp transport inhibitors and dabigatran in patients with renal impairment is expected to increase systemic exposure to dabigatran compared with that resulting from either factor alone. Recommendations regarding such concomitant therapy are based on the degree of renal impairment and clinical situation (e.g., stroke prophylaxis in patients with nonvalvular atrial fibrillation versus treatment of venous thromboembolism [VTE]). In patients with atrial fibrillation, the Anticoagulation Forum recommends avoiding use of dabigatran in patients with a creatinine clearance <30 mL/minute who are taking P-gp inhibitors. In the VTE setting, the Anticoagulation Forum recommends avoiding use of dabigatran in patients with a creatinine clearance <50 mL/minute who are taking P-gp inhibitors.

Amiodarone

Administration of a single 600-mg oral dose of amiodarone with dabigatran resulted in increases in dabigatran AUC and peak plasma concentration, respectively. This increase in systemic exposure was accompanied by an increase in renal clearance of dabigatran. Because of the long half-life of amiodarone, increased renal clearance of dabigatran may persist after amiodarone discontinuance. Pharmacokinetics (PK) of amiodarone were not altered. Analysis of patient data from the Randomized Evaluation of Long-term Anticoagulation Therapy (RE-LY) study did not identify important changes in dabigatran trough concentrations in patients receiving dabigatran and amiodarone concurrently.

Clarithromycin

Concomitant use of clarithromycin and dabigatran had no effect on systemic exposure to either drug.

Dronedarone

Concomitant use of dronedarone and dabigatran resulted in an increase in systemic exposure to dabigatran. Administration of dronedarone 2 hours after dabigatran was associated with a smaller increase in systemic exposure to dabigatran. In patients with a creatinine clearance ≥50 mL/minute receiving dabigatran for thromboprophylaxis following hip-replacement surgery, it may be helpful to separate the timing of administration of dabigatran and dronedarone by several hours. Dosage reduction is recommended in patients with nonvalvular atrial fibrillation and moderate renal impairment receiving such concomitant therapy.

Ketoconazole

Administration of a single oral 400-mg dose of ketoconazole or multiple oral doses of ketoconazole (400 mg daily) with dabigatran resulted in increases in dabigatran AUC and peak plasma concentration. In patients with a creatinine clearance ≥50 mL/minute receiving dabigatran for thromboprophylaxis following hip-replacement surgery, it may be helpful to separate the timing of administration of dabigatran and ketoconazole by several hours. Dosage reduction is recommended in patients with nonvalvular atrial fibrillation and moderate renal impairment receiving such concomitant therapy.

Quinidine

Concomitant use of quinidine (200 mg every 2 hours for 5 doses) on the third day of dabigatran administration resulted in increases in dabigatran AUC and peak plasma concentration.

Ticagrelor

Concomitant administration of ticagrelor and dabigatran modestly increases plasma concentrations of dabigatran; the magnitude of increase is dependent on the dosage and timing of dabigatran administration. When dabigatran (110 mg twice daily) was administered concurrently with ticagrelor (90 mg twice daily), the steady-state AUC and peak plasma concentration of dabigatran increased by 26% and 29%, respectively. Concurrent administration of dabigatran with a 180 mg-loading dose of ticagrelor resulted in an increase of 49 and 65% in steady-state dabigatran AUC and peak plasma concentration, respectively. However, when ticagrelor 180 mg was given 2 hours after dabigatran, the AUC and peak plasma concentration of dabigatran at steady state increased by only 27 and 24%, respectively.

Verapamil

Concomitant administration of verapamil and dabigatran may result in increased dabigatran AUC and peak plasma concentration. The extent of interaction depends on the verapamil formulation and timing of administration. The greatest increase in these parameters was observed when a single dose of immediate-release verapamil was given 1 hour prior to dabigatran, resulting in a 2.4-fold increase in dabigatran AUC. Administration of verapamil 2 hours after dabigatran administration resulted in negligible changes in dabigatran AUC. Analysis of data from the RE-LY study did not identify important changes in dabigatran trough concentrations in patients receiving dabigatran and verapamil concurrently.

● *Drugs Affecting Gastric pH*

Dabigatran is available in a capsule formulation containing drug pellets with a tartaric acid core that provides a microacidic environment for enhanced drug absorption. Because the absorption of dabigatran is dependent on an acidic gastric pH, concurrent use with drugs that increase gastric pH may decrease systemic exposure to dabigatran. Clinical studies indicate that ranitidine does not alter the PK parameters of dabigatran but that pantoprazole has the potential to decrease systemic exposure to dabigatran by up to 30%. However, the PK of pantoprazole or ranitidine were not altered by concomitant use with dabigatran. Analysis of PK data from the RE-LY study indicates that concurrent use with histamine H_2-receptor antagonists or proton-pump inhibitors does not appreciably alter trough dabigatran plasma concentrations.

● *Drugs Affecting Hemostasis*

The risk of bleeding may be increased when other agents that increase bleeding risk (e.g., antiplatelets, thrombolytics, heparin, chronic nonsteroidal anti-inflammatory agents) are used in patients receiving dabigatran. Patients should be monitored for manifestations of bleeding (e.g., decrease in hemoglobin/hematocrit, hypotension), and such manifestations should be promptly evaluated.

When a single dose of dabigatran was administered 24 hours after completion of 3 days of therapy with enoxaparin sodium (40 mg subcutaneously once daily), dabigatran exposure and pharmacodynamic assessments (effects on activated partial thromboplastin time [aPTT], ecarin clotting time [ECT], or diluted thrombin time [dTT]) were not altered.

Concurrent administration of clopidogrel (as a 300- or 600-mg loading dose) and dabigatran resulted in increases of 30 and 40% in dabigatran AUC and peak plasma concentration, respectively. Pharmacokinetics of clopidogrel were not affected. The pharmacodynamic effects of clopidogrel (i.e., prolongation of capillary bleeding times, inhibition of platelet aggregation) or dabigatran (i.e., effects on aPTT, ECT, thrombin time) were not altered with concurrent administration when compared with monotherapy.

In the RE-LY trial, the risk of bleeding was increased approximately 2-fold when dabigatran was used concomitantly with either aspirin or clopidogrel compared with dabigatran monotherapy. The observed increase in risk was similar to that observed in patients randomized to warfarin and concomitantly receiving aspirin or clopidogrel when compared with warfarin alone.

Dabigatran has the potential to increase INR. When switching from dabigatran therapy to warfarin, the INR is more reflective of warfarin's effects when dabigatran has been discontinued for at least 2 days.

● *Digoxin*

Pharmacokinetic interaction is unlikely. No meaningful alterations in PK of digoxin or dabigatran were observed with concurrent use.

DESCRIPTION

Dabigatran etexilate mesylate is a selective, competitive, reversible direct thrombin inhibitor. Dabigatran prevents thrombus formation by binding the catalytic site of free and clot-bound thrombin, thereby inhibiting conversion of fibrinogen to fibrin. Dabigatran also inhibits thrombin-mediated platelet aggregation.

Dabigatran is commercially available as capsules and oral pellets as dabigatran etexilate mesylate, an inactive ester prodrug that is rapidly and incompletely absorbed and subsequently hydrolyzed by esterases to dabigatran, the principal active moiety. The indications and intended age groups of the oral capsules and pellets differ, oral absorption and subsequent bioavailability are not the same, and the relative bioavailability between the two formulations is age-dependent. Dabigatran exhibits linear, dose-dependent pharmacokinetics (PK). Following oral administration of dabigatran etexilate, the absolute bioavailability of dabigatran is approximately 3–7%. Peak plasma concentrations are attained within 2 hours of oral administration and correlate with peak pharmacodynamic (PD) effects. The oral pellet formulation is 37% more bioavailable in healthy adults compared to the capsule. The manufacturer states that the relative bioavailability observed in adults cannot be translated to pediatric patients.

Dabigatran undergoes conjugation to several acyl glucuronides that exhibit similar activity to dabigatran and account for approximately 20% of total plasma dabigatran concentrations. Dabigatran is approximately 35% protein bound in plasma. Systemically available dabigatran is primarily (80%) eliminated unchanged in the urine and the terminal half-life of dabigatran capsules administered to healthy adult subjects averages 12–17 hours. The manufacturer states that population PK simulation shows a 12–14 hour elimination half-life in pediatric patients for the capsule dosage form and an elimination half-life of 9–11 hours in pediatric patients receiving the oral pellet formulation. Steady state is achieved within 3 days when the drug is given 3 times daily. Dabigatran AUC and peak plasma concentrations are increased and half-life is prolonged in patients with renal impairment.

Dabigatran prolongs thrombin time (TT) and ecarin clotting time (ECT) linearly over the range of therapeutic plasma concentrations and prolongs activated partial thromboplastin time (aPTT) in a curvilinear manner. The manufacturer states that similar PK/PD relationships for aPTT, ECT, and diluted thrombin time (dTT) were observed across age groups of pediatric patients (ages 26 days to <18 years) and between pediatric and adult patients with venous thromboembolism. This similarity in PK/PD relationship suggests that a similar exposure-response relationship is expected for dabigatran etexilate treatment across the pediatric age groups and adult patients. While dabigatran may contribute to an elevated international normalized ratio (INR), this is a relatively insensitive measure of dabigatran activity. Routine laboratory monitoring of anticoagulation status is not required during dabigatran therapy; however, the preferred and more sensitive method for assessing anticoagulation status is ECT. Alternatively, aPTT may be used as a qualitative measure of anticoagulation when ECT is unavailable. In healthy individuals, plasma dabigatran concentrations did not correlate linearly with aPTT, but were extremely low when aPTT was <1, while an aPTT exceeding 1 indicated the presence of dabigatran in plasma. In the RE-LY study, the median trough aPTT and ECT in patients receiving dabigatran etexilate 150 mg twice daily were 52 and 63 seconds, respectively.

ADVICE TO PATIENTS

- Instruct patients to take dabigatran exactly as prescribed and to not discontinue therapy without first consulting a clinician.

- Inform patients that the oral capsule and pellets are not interchangeable; do not substitute different dosage forms on a mg-to-mg basis. Consult with a health care provider to make sure the proper dosage form and dosage are used.

- Advise patients of the importance of having an adult caregiver administer dabigatran to pediatric patients.

- Instruct patients to take a missed dose (capsules or oral pellets) as soon as it is remembered on the same day, but only if it can be taken at least 6 hours prior to the next scheduled dose. Do not take 2 doses at the same time to make up for a missed dose.

- Inform patients that they may bruise and/or bleed more easily and that a longer than normal time may be required to stop bleeding when taking dabigatran; advise patients on how to recognize signs and symptoms of bleeding.

- Advise patients to inform their clinicians immediately if any unusual bleeding or bruising, including menstrual or vaginal bleeding that is heavier than normal, occurs during therapy.

- Dabigatran is not for patients with artificial heart valves; advise patients to inform their health care provider if they had or will have heart valve surgery.

- Dabigatran is not recommended for use in patients with antiphospholipid syndrome (APS), especially with positive triple antibody testing; advise patients to inform their health care provider if they have APS.

- Inform patients about the risk of adverse GI reactions. Advise patients to consult their healthcare provider if they experience dyspepsia, burning, nausea, abdominal pain/discomfort, epigastric discomfort, or indigestion.

- Advise patients who have had neuraxial anesthesia or spinal puncture to monitor for manifestations of spinal or epidural hematoma (e.g., numbness or weakness of legs, bowel or bladder dysfunction), particularly if they are receiving concomitant nonsteroidal anti-inflammatory agents (NSAIAs), platelet inhibitors, or other anticoagulants; inform patients to seek emergency medical attention if any of these symptoms occur.

- Advise patients to inform their clinicians (e.g., physicians, dentists) that they are receiving dabigatran therapy before scheduling any surgery or invasive procedures, including dental procedures.

- Advise patients to swallow dabigatran capsules whole with a full glass of water, without opening, chewing, or otherwise emptying the contents of the capsule. Advise patients to inform their health care provider if they are unable to swallow the capsule whole. Do not sprinkle contents of capsules on food or into a beverage.

- Inform patients of special storage and handling requirements for dabigatran capsules. Store the drug capsules only in the original container (bottle or blister package) and protect from moisture; do not store capsules in pill boxes or organizers. Remove only one capsule from the bottle at a time, right before use, and close the bottle tightly immediately after use. When more than one bottle is dispensed, advise the patient to open only one bottle at a time. For blister packages of capsules, do not open or puncture the blister until time of use. The manufacturer states that dabigatran capsules should be used within 4 months after the bottle is first opened.

- Advise the adult caregiver on the proper administration of dabigatran oral pellets. The oral pellets should be sprinkled on baby rice cereal (prepared with water), mashed carrots, apple sauce, or mashed bananas, or taken with apple juice. Do not mix with any other food or liquid. Do not mix the oral pellets with milk, milk products, or foods that contain milk. The oral pellets should be administered before meals to help ensure that the full dose is taken.

- Advise the caregiver to administer the oral pellets right away or within 30 minutes after mixing; discard oral pellets that have been in contact with soft food or apple juice for more than 30 minutes. If the child only takes part of their oral pellet dose, do not give another dose at that time; administer the next dose at the regularly scheduled time, about 12 hours later.

- Advise caregivers to not use an oral syringe or feeding tube to administer the oral pellets.

- Inform caregivers of special storage and handling requirements for dabigatran oral pellets. Oral pellet packets are dispensed in an aluminum bag with a desiccant. Keep the oral pellet packets in the original aluminum bag to keep them dry. Remove only one packet at a time. Do not open the oral pellet packet until ready to administer the dose. After opening the aluminum bag, oral pellets must be used within 6 months.

- Advise females to inform their clinician if they are or plan to become pregnant or plan to breast-feed.

- Advise patients to inform their clinician of existing or contemplated concomitant therapy, including prescription and OTC drugs and dietary and herbal supplements, as well as any concomitant illnesses.

- Advise patients of other important precautionary information. (See Cautions.)

PREPARATIONS

Excipients in commercially available drug preparations may have clinically important effects in some individuals; consult specific product labeling for details.

Dabigatran Etexilate Mesylate

Oral		
Capsules	75 mg (of dabigatran etexilate)	**Pradaxa®**, Boehringer Ingelheim
	110 mg (of dabigatran etexilate)	**Pradaxa®**, Boehringer Ingelheim
	150 mg (of dabigatran etexilate)	**Pradaxa®**, Boehringer Ingelheim
Pellets	20 mg (of dabigatran etexilate)	**Pradaxa®**, Boehringer Ingelheim
	30 mg (of dabigatran etexilate)	**Pradaxa®**, Boehringer Ingelheim
	40 mg (of dabigatran etexilate)	**Pradaxa®**, Boehringer Ingelheim
	50 mg (of dabigatran etexilate)	**Pradaxa®**, Boehringer Ingelheim
	110 mg (of dabigatran etexilate)	**Pradaxa®**, Boehringer Ingelheim
	150 mg (of dabigatran etexilate)	**Pradaxa®**, Boehringer Ingelheim

† Use is not currently included in the labeling approved by the US Food and Drug Administration.

Selected Revisions March 22, 2023, © Copyright, November 10, 2011, American Society of Health-System Pharmacists, Inc.

Apixaban

20:12.04.14 • DIRECT FACTOR Xa INHIBITORS

■ Apixaban, an oral, reversible, direct activated factor X (factor Xa) inhibitor, is an anticoagulant.

USES

● Embolism Associated with Atrial Fibrillation

Nonvalvular Atrial Fibrillation

Apixaban is used to reduce the risk of stroke and systemic embolism in patients with nonvalvular atrial fibrillation. The direct oral anticoagulants (DOACs; apixaban, dabigatran, edoxaban, rivaroxaban) have been shown in randomized controlled studies to be noninferior, and in some trials, superior to warfarin in reducing thromboembolic risk in patients with nonvalvular atrial fibrillation (i.e., atrial fibrillation in the absence of moderate-to-severe mitral stenosis or a mechanical heart valve), and are associated with reduced risk of serious bleeding.

Clinical Experience

Efficacy and safety of apixaban for the prevention of stroke and systemic embolism in patients with nonvalvular atrial fibrillation were evaluated in a multinational, randomized, double-blind study (Apixaban for Reduction in Stroke and Other Thromboembolic Events in Atrial Fibrillation [ARISTOTLE]) that was designed to demonstrate noninferiority of apixaban compared with warfarin. The study included a total of 18,201 adults with nonvalvular atrial fibrillation and at least one additional risk factor for stroke (i.e., prior stroke, transient ischemic attack [TIA], or systemic embolism; age ≥75 years; arterial hypertension requiring treatment; diabetes mellitus; symptomatic heart failure as defined by New York Heart Association [NYHA] class ≥2; left ventricular ejection fraction of ≤40%). At baseline, patients had a mean Congestive Heart Failure, Hypertension, Age, Diabetes, Stroke (doubled) (i.e., CHADS$_2$) score of 2.1; 19% had a history of a previous embolic event (stroke, TIA, or non-CNS systemic embolism), and 57% had been treated with warfarin or another vitamin K antagonist prior to study entry. Patients received apixaban at a dosage of 5 mg orally twice daily (or a reduced dosage of 2.5 mg twice daily in patients with at least 2 of the following characteristics: ≥80 years of age, body weight of ≤60 kg, serum creatinine concentration of ≥1.5 mg/dL) or warfarin in a dosage adjusted to achieve an international normalized ratio (INR) of 2–3. Approximately 5% of patients in the apixaban group received the reduced dosage of the drug. The primary efficacy outcome of the study was a composite of stroke (ischemic or hemorrhagic) or systemic embolism, and the primary safety end point was major bleeding as defined by the International Society of Thrombosis and Hemostasis (ISTH) criteria; all-cause mortality was evaluated as a secondary outcome. Although the study was designed principally to test for noninferiority of apixaban compared with warfarin in reducing the rate of stroke or systemic embolism, a sequential testing strategy was employed where superiority testing was performed on the key outcome measures if noninferiority was achieved; all efficacy analyses were conducted in the intent-to-treat (per randomization) population.

Results of the study indicated that apixaban was not only noninferior, but also was superior to warfarin in reducing the risk of stroke and systemic embolism. After a median follow-up of 1.8 years, the rate of the primary outcome of stroke or systemic embolism was substantially lower in patients receiving apixaban than in those receiving warfarin (annual rate of 1.27 and 1.6%, respectively; relative risk reduction of 21%). Superiority of apixaban over warfarin was largely attributed to a reduction in the risk of hemorrhagic stroke and ischemic stroke with hemorrhagic conversion; there was no difference in the incidence of purely ischemic strokes between the treatment groups. With respect to the primary safety outcome, apixaban also demonstrated superiority over warfarin; major bleeding, including intracranial hemorrhage, occurred at a substantially lower rate in patients receiving apixaban than in those receiving warfarin (annual rate of 2.13 and 3.09%, respectively; relative risk reduction of 31%). In addition, a significant reduction in all-cause mortality was observed with apixaban versus warfarin therapy (annual rate of 3.52 and 3.94%, respectively), which was primarily due to a reduction in cardiovascular-related deaths. The beneficial effects of apixaban over warfarin on stroke risk reduction, major bleeding, and all-cause mortality were consistent across a variety of patient subgroups defined by geographic region, prior warfarin use, age, baseline body weight, CHADS$_2$ scores, renal function, apixaban dosage, type of atrial fibrillation, history of stroke or TIA, and aspirin use at randomization.

Patients who received warfarin in the ARISTOTLE study had an INR within therapeutic range 62% of the time, which is comparable to or better than that reported in other trials of non-vitamin K antagonist oral anticoagulants (e.g., dabigatran, rivaroxaban). Some clinicians have criticized this level of INR control as not being reflective of current practice and suggest that the benefits of apixaban may be less pronounced when compared with patients who achieve better warfarin control (e.g., INR in therapeutic range at least 70% of the time). However, in a subanalysis of the ARISTOTLE study, the benefits of apixaban relative to warfarin appeared to be consistent regardless of the quality of INR control (based on center-level comparison).

Apixaban was evaluated in another randomized double-blind study (Apixaban Versus Acetylsalicylic Acid to Prevent Stroke [AVERROES]) for the prevention of stroke in patients with atrial fibrillation and at least one additional risk factor for stroke (i.e., prior stroke or TIA; ≥75 years of age; arterial hypertension requiring treatment; diabetes mellitus requiring treatment; symptomatic heart failure as defined by NYHA class ≥2; left ventricular ejection fraction ≤35%; documented peripheral arterial disease); the study compared apixaban (5 mg twice daily or 2.5 mg twice daily in selected patients) with aspirin (81–324 mg daily) in such patients who had failed or were considered unsuitable for vitamin K antagonist therapy by their clinician. Approximately 5600 patients were included; a major reason for warfarin unsuitability in these patients was difficulty or anticipated difficulty maintaining therapeutic INRs. The AVERROES study was terminated early after a planned interim analysis demonstrated a clear benefit of apixaban over aspirin in reducing the risk of stroke without substantially increasing the risk of bleeding. After a mean follow-up of 1.1 years, the rate of the primary outcome of stroke (ischemic or hemorrhagic) or systemic embolism was substantially lower in patients receiving apixaban than in those receiving aspirin (annual rate of 1.6 and 3.7%, respectively; relative risk reduction of 55%). Although a modest increase in the risk of major bleeding was observed with apixaban versus aspirin, the difference was not statistically significant. The observed benefits of apixaban over aspirin in this study were consistent across major subgroups of patients.

The risk of stroke in patients with atrial flutter is similar to the risk in those with atrial fibrillation. Experts state that antithrombotic therapy in patients with atrial flutter generally should be managed in the same manner as in patients with atrial fibrillation.

DOACs including apixaban have been used for pharmacologic cardioversion† in patients with atrial fibrillation or atrial flutter of >48 hours' duration or of unknown duration; DOACs are recommended as a safe and effective alternative to warfarin in this setting.

Clinical Perspective

The American College of Chest Physicians (ACCP), the American College of Cardiology (ACC), the American Heart Association (AHA), the American Stroke Association (ASA), and other experts currently recommend that antithrombotic therapy be administered to all patients with nonvalvular atrial fibrillation (i.e., atrial fibrillation in the absence of rheumatic mitral stenosis, a prosthetic heart valve, or mitral valve repair) who are considered to be at increased risk of stroke, unless such therapy is contraindicated. Although many risk stratification methods have been used, current guidelines recommend the use of the CHA$_2$DS$_2$-VASc risk stratification tool for assessing a patient's risk of stroke and need for anticoagulant therapy. Established clinical risk factors for stroke include prior ischemic stroke or TIA, advanced age (e.g., ≥65 years), history of hypertension, diabetes mellitus, vascular disease, and congestive heart failure; in addition, female sex has been identified as a factor that can modify the risk of stroke. The presence of stroke or TIA places a patient in the high-risk category regardless of other risk factors. Experts state that antithrombotic therapy generally is not necessary in low-risk patients (CHA$_2$DS$_2$-VASc score of 0 in males, or 1 in females), but should be considered in patients with one or more non-sex CHA$_2$DS$_2$-VASc stroke risk factors (CHA$_2$DS$_2$-VASc score of ≥1 in males, or ≥2 in females). Patients also should be assessed for their risk of bleeding; those with a high risk of bleeding should be monitored more closely.

In patients with nonvalvular atrial fibrillation who are eligible for oral anti-coagulant therapy, DOACs are recommended over warfarin based on improved safety and similar or improved efficacy in clinical trials and meta-analyses. A substantially greater benefit of DOACs versus warfarin has been observed when the INR was in the therapeutic range less than 66% of the time. If warfarin is used, patients should be optimally managed with well-controlled INRs (e.g., INR in therapeutic range more than 70% of the time). A DOAC is recommended in patients unable to achieve optimal warfarin management.

Patient age, body weight, and renal and hepatic function should be considered prior to treatment with DOACs. There are limited data on the use of DOACs in obese patients and some experts have discouraged the use of these agents in the morbidly obese population (those with a body mass index [BMI] >40 kg/m² or body weight >120 kg). However, the various DOAC agents may have different outcomes. Because of limited data with DOACs in patients with morbid obesity, guidelines recommend considering warfarin over DOACs in morbidly obese patients with nonvalvular atrial fibrillation.

Because of the lack of direct, comparative studies, the relative efficacy and safety of apixaban compared to other DOACs for the prevention of stroke in patients with nonvalvular atrial fibrillation remain to be fully elucidated. Some evidence from indirect comparisons suggests that there may be important differences (e.g., bleeding risk) between these agents; however, results of such analyses should be interpreted with caution because of possible confounding factors (e.g., differences in study design and methods, patient populations, and anticoagulation control). Selection of an appropriate anticoagulant for patients with nonvalvular atrial fibrillation should be individualized based on the absolute and relative risks of stroke and bleeding; costs; patient compliance, preference, tolerance, and comorbidities; and other clinical factors such as renal function and degree of INR control if the patient has been taking warfarin.

Valvular Heart Disease

Safety and efficacy of apixaban have not been established in patients with prosthetic heart valves and the manufacturer states that use of apixaban is not generally recommended in such patients.

A subgroup of 156 patients with a history of bioprosthetic valve replacement or native valve repair from the ARISTOTLE trial was analyzed to assess safety and efficacy of apixaban compared with warfarin with regard to the occurrence of stroke/systemic embolism and major bleeding in these patients. Results revealed overall clinical event rates to be low with no significant differences between apixaban and warfarin for any outcomes.

The 2020 AHA/ACC guideline for the management of patients with valvular heart disease states that patients with valvular heart disease and atrial fibrillation† should be evaluated for risk of thromboembolic events and treated with oral anticoagulation if at high risk. Vitamin K antagonists are the anticoagulants of choice for patients with rheumatic mitral stenosis and mechanical heart valves. Apixaban and other DOACs are an alternative to vitamin K antagonists in patients with atrial fibrillation and a bioprosthetic valve more than 3 months after implantation or with native valvular heart disease excluding rheumatic mitral stenosis.

● *Prophylaxis of Venous Thromboembolism*

Major Orthopedic Surgery

Apixaban is used for the prevention of postoperative deep-vein thrombosis (DVT), which may lead to pulmonary embolism (PE), in patients who have undergone total hip- or knee-replacement surgery.

Clinical Experience

Apixaban was evaluated for the prevention of venous thromboembolism (VTE) following total hip- or knee-replacement surgery in 3 multicenter, randomized, double-blind studies known as the ADVANCE (Apixaban Dose Orally versus Anticoagulation with Enoxaparin) studies. In these studies, apixaban was compared with subcutaneous enoxaparin therapy in patients undergoing elective total knee-replacement (ADVANCE 1 and 2) or total hip-replacement surgery (ADVANCE 3). The primary efficacy end point in all 3 studies consisted of a composite of asymptomatic and symptomatic DVT, nonfatal PE, and all-cause mortality; the primary safety outcome was bleeding. These studies were designed principally to test for noninferiority of apixaban compared with enoxaparin in reducing the rate of the primary efficacy end point; superiority testing was performed if noninferiority was achieved. In all 3 studies, apixaban was

administered orally at the same dosage (2.5 mg twice daily, initiated 12–24 hours after surgery), but dosage and timing of enoxaparin sodium administration varied between the studies. In ADVANCE 1, enoxaparin sodium was administered at a dosage of 30 mg twice daily (initiated 12–24 hours after surgery), while in ADVANCE 2 and 3, enoxaparin sodium was administered at a dosage of 40 mg once daily (initiated 12 hours before surgery and continued after surgery according to the investigator's standard of care). Anticoagulant prophylaxis (with apixaban or enoxaparin) was continued postoperatively for 10–14 days in the knee-replacement studies and for 32–38 days in the hip-replacement study. These studies demonstrated that apixaban was more effective than enoxaparin sodium 40 mg once daily in reducing the risk of VTE without increasing the risk of bleeding; the improved efficacy of apixaban over enoxaparin was due principally to a reduction in asymptomatic proximal DVT. When compared with enoxaparin sodium 30 mg twice daily (the approved US regimen for enoxaparin thromboprophylaxis after knee-replacement surgery) in the ADVANCE 1 study, apixaban did not meet the noninferiority criteria for the primary efficacy outcome, although apixaban was associated with lower rates of clinically relevant bleeding.

Clinical Perspective

Several major guidelines for thromboprophylaxis following hip- or knee-replacement surgery have been published, including guidelines from the American Academy of Orthopedic Surgeons (AAOS), American College of Chest Physicians (ACCP), and the American Society of Hematology (ASH). Routine thromboprophylaxis is recommended in all patients undergoing major orthopedic surgery, including total hip- or knee-replacement surgery, because of the high risk of postoperative VTE. According to ACCP, thromboprophylaxis with an appropriate antithrombotic agent or an intermittent pneumatic compression device should be continued for at least 10-14 days and possibly for up to 35 days after surgery.

AAOS guidelines do not recommend any specific thromboprophylaxis agent, while the ACCP guidelines favor low molecular weight heparins (LMWHs) over DOACs. The ASH guidelines suggest the use of DOACs over LMWHs if anticoagulants are used; however, this recommendation is considered conditional based on moderate certainty in the evidence of harms versus benefits.

Drug selection and duration of therapy should be individualized based on type of surgery, patient risk factors for embolism and bleeding, as well as costs, patient compliance, preference, tolerance, and comorbidities and other clinical factors such as renal function.

Acute Medical Illness

Apixaban has been used for VTE prevention in acutely ill medical patients†. Evidence suggests that extended treatment with apixaban is not superior to short-term treatment with subcutaneous enoxaparin for thromboprophylaxis in such patients and is associated with a small but statistically significant increase in the risk of major bleeding.

Clinical Experience

In a randomized, double-dummy, placebo-controlled study (Apixaban Dosing to Optimize Protection from Thrombosis [ADOPT]), patients with an acute medical illness (e.g., congestive heart failure, respiratory failure) and moderately to severely restricted mobility received apixaban 2.5 mg twice daily for 30 days or subcutaneous enoxaparin sodium 40 mg once daily for 6–14 days or until hospital discharge; treatment was initiated within 72 hours of hospital admission. The primary efficacy outcome was the 30-day composite of death related to VTE, PE, symptomatic DVT, or asymptomatic proximal-leg DVT (determined by systematic bilateral compression ultrasonography on day 30); the primary safety outcome was major bleeding. In approximately 4500 evaluable patients, the primary efficacy outcome occurred in 2.71% of those receiving apixaban and 3.06% who received enoxaparin; although this represented a 13% relative risk reduction with apixaban, the difference was not statistically significant. However, the rapid increase in the rate of thromboembolic events following discontinuance of enoxaparin treatment suggests the benefits of some type of extended thromboprophylaxis in this patient population; additional study and experience are needed. In the ADOPT study, apixaban therapy was associated with an increased risk of major bleeding; by day 30, major bleeding had occurred in 0.47% of patients in the apixaban group and 0.19% of enoxaparin-treated patients, representing a 2.58-fold increased risk with apixaban.

Clinical Perspective

Use of apixaban during hospitalization and post-discharge in acutely ill medical patients increases bleeding risk with no significant reduction in DVT, PE, and VTE death.

Clinical trials evaluating extended-duration thromboprophylaxis in medically ill patients were carefully designed with strict patient inclusion and exclusion criteria and data suggesting a sufficient risk of VTE, based on a validated assessment tool, to offset the increased risk of bleeding. However, these trials have varied in design, enrollment criteria, and patient selection, and therefore evidence from these trials is inconclusive. Some clinicians suggest that decisions regarding extended-duration thromboprophylaxis should be based on the inclusion and exclusion criteria used in studies that provide available data.

The American Society of Hematology (ASH) issued a strong recommendation to use LMWHs instead of DOACs for VTE prophylaxis in acutely ill hospitalized medical patients, and also strongly recommends inpatient VTE prophylaxis with LMWH only rather than inpatient and extended-duration outpatient VTE prophylaxis with DOACs.

Cancer

Apixaban has been used for VTE prophylaxis in patients with active cancer†. Such patients are at an increased risk for VTE, and primary thromboprophylaxis with apixaban may be beneficial but carries a bleeding risk.

Clinical Experience

The randomized, double-blind Apixaban for the Prevention of Venous Thromboembolism in High-Risk Ambulatory Cancer Patients (AVERT) trial compared the safety and efficacy of apixaban 2.5 mg twice daily with placebo for primary thromboprophylaxis in ambulatory cancer patients at intermediate-to-high risk for VTE. The treatment period was 180 days with the initial dose of apixaban or placebo administered within 24 hours after chemotherapy initiation. Cancer patients who were initiating a new course of chemotherapy with a minimum treatment intent of 3 months and a Khorana score ≥2 were eligible. Patients with a sole diagnosis of skin carcinoma, acute leukemia or myeloproliferative neoplasm, hepatic disease associated with coagulopathy, conditions associated with an increased bleeding risk, creatinine clearance <30 mL/minute per 1.73 m², planned stem-cell transplantation, or a life expectancy <6 months were excluded.

The primary efficacy outcome was the initial occurrence of objectively confirmed symptomatic or incidentally detected proximal DVT of the lower or upper limbs, any nonfatal symptomatic or incidental PE, or fatal PE within the initial 180 (±3) days after randomization. The main safety outcome, ISTH major bleeding, was defined as overt bleeding associated with a decrease in hemoglobin of ≥2 g/dL, transfusion of ≥2 units of packed red blood cells (or whole blood), bleeding in a critical site (e.g., intracranial, intraspinal, retroperitoneal), or bleeding contributing to a fatal outcome. Results revealed the primary efficacy outcome occurred substantially less frequently in apixaban- versus placebo-treated patients (4.2% versus 10.2%). Major bleeding occurred in more patients who received apixaban than those who received placebo (3.5% versus 1.8%). The difference in the rate of major bleeding complications observed between the treatment groups was mainly due to higher rates of GI bleeding, hematuria, and gynecologic bleeding with apixaban.

Clinical Perspective

Patients with cancer are substantially more likely to develop VTE than patients without cancer. Most hospitalized patients with cancer and an acute medical condition require thromboprophylaxis throughout hospitalization; however, routine pharmacologic thromboprophylaxis is not recommended for all outpatients with cancer. The patient's individual risk for thrombosis and risk of bleeding should be considered for all cancer patients when deciding whether to administer thromboprophylaxis.

The American Society of Clinical Oncology (ASCO) and American Society of Hematology (ASH) have published guidelines for the management of VTE in cancer patients. The ASCO guideline states that high-risk outpatients with cancer (Khorana score ≥2 prior to starting a new systemic chemotherapy regimen) may be offered thromboprophylaxis with apixaban, rivaroxaban, or a LMWH provided there are no significant risk factors for bleeding and no drug interactions. The ASH guideline suggests thromboprophylaxis with a DOAC (apixaban or rivaroxaban) in ambulatory cancer patients at intermediate to high risk for

thrombosis; the decision to administer thromboprophylaxis versus no thromboprophylaxis should be based on the level of risk.

● Venous Thromboembolism – Treatment and Secondary Prevention

Apixaban is used for the treatment of acute DVT and/or PE and to reduce the risk of recurrent DVT and PE (secondary prevention) following initial anticoagulant therapy.

The manufacturer states that apixaban is not recommended as initial therapy (as an alternative to heparin) in patients with PE who have hemodynamic instability or who may receive thrombolytic therapy or undergo pulmonary embolectomy.

Clinical Experience

Efficacy and safety of apixaban for the treatment of acute DVT and/or PE have been established in a randomized, controlled study (Apixaban for the Initial Management of Pulmonary Embolism and Deep-Vein Thrombosis as First-Line Therapy [AMPLIFY]) in more than 5000 adults with symptomatic proximal DVT and/or PE. In this study, therapy with apixaban (10 mg orally twice daily for 7 days, followed by 5 mg twice daily for 6 months) was noninferior to conventional anticoagulant therapy (subcutaneous enoxaparin sodium 1 mg/kg every 12 hours for at least 5 days with overlapping warfarin therapy until therapeutic INR ≥2, followed by daily warfarin therapy adjusted to maintain INR of 2–3 and continued for 6 months) in reducing the incidence of the primary efficacy outcome (composite of symptomatic recurrent VTE [defined as fatal or nonfatal PE and DVT] or death related to VTE) and superior to the conventional regimen in reducing the incidence of major bleeding. The primary efficacy outcome occurred in 2.3% of patients receiving apixaban and 2.7% of those receiving the conventional regimen, and major bleeding occurred in 0.6 and 1.8% of patients in these respective groups (relative risk reduction of 69%).

Efficacy and safety of apixaban for reducing the risk of recurrent DVT and PE (i.e., secondary prevention) have been established in another randomized, placebo-controlled study (AMPLIFY-EXT) in approximately 2500 patients who had received 6–12 months of anticoagulant therapy for VTE. Some patients in the AMPLIFY-EXT study (approximately one-third) were participants in the AMPLIFY study who had received apixaban or enoxaparin and warfarin therapy and in whom clinicians were uncertain about the need for continuing anticoagulation. In the AMPLIFY-EXT study, extended treatment with apixaban 2.5 or 5 mg twice daily for 1 year reduced the incidence of the primary efficacy outcome (composite of symptomatic recurrent VTE [defined as fatal and nonfatal PE and DVT] or death from any cause) without increasing the rate of major bleeding. The 2.5-mg (thromboprophylactic) and 5-mg (treatment) dosages of apixaban used in the extension study showed similar efficacy, and rates of adverse events in the 2 treatment groups were similar to those with placebo. The incidence of thromboembolism in the placebo group was 8.8%, indicating an appreciable continuing risk of recurrent VTE in the study population following an initial 6–12 months of anticoagulant therapy. Patients with provoked VTE related to a transient risk factor (e.g., surgery) were not enrolled in the AMPLIFY and AMPLIFY-EXT studies unless they had another irreversible risk factor requiring 6 months of anticoagulant treatment (e.g., prior VTE, immobilization, history of or active cancer, known prothrombotic genotype). In addition, these studies included relatively few patients with cancer, low body weight (< 60 kg), or renal insufficiency (creatinine clearance <50 mL/minute); additional data on efficacy and safety of apixaban therapy in such patients with VTE are needed.

Patients with Cancer
Clinical Experience

In the open-label, noninferiority CARAVAGGIO trial, the efficacy and safety of apixaban for the prevention of recurrent VTE were evaluated in cancer patients with newly diagnosed symptomatic or incidental proximal lower limb DVT or PE. Patients were randomized to apixaban 10 mg twice daily for the first 7 days, then 5 mg twice daily thereafter or dalteparin 200 units/kg once daily for the first 30 days, followed by 150 units/kg once daily. The maximum dalteparin dosage was 18,000 units daily. Both groups were treated for a total of 6 months. Approximately 97% of patients had active cancer at baseline, and two-thirds of patients had recurrent locally advanced or metastatic lesions. Approximately 60% of patients in both groups were receiving cancer treatment at enrollment.

The primary outcome was objectively confirmed recurrent VTE, which included symptomatic upper limb DVT, symptomatic or incidental proximal DVT of the lower limbs, or symptomatic, incidental, or fatal PE. Major bleeding, the principal safety outcome, was defined as clinically overt bleeding associated with at least one of the following: a decrease in hemoglobin ≥2 g/dL, transfusion of ≥2 units of packed red blood cells, bleeding that occurs at a critical site (e.g., intracranial, intraspinal, retroperitoneal), bleeding that necessitates surgical intervention, or fatal bleeding.

The primary outcome occurred less frequently in the apixaban versus dalteparin group (5.6% versus 7.9%), meeting the criteria for noninferiority. Major bleeding was not substantially different between the groups: 3.8% for apixaban- and 4% for dalteparin-treated patients.

In the randomized, open-label, investigator-initiated ADAM VTE study, the efficacy and safety of apixaban were evaluated in the treatment of patients with active cancer and confirmed acute VTE. In ADAM VTE, patients were randomized to apixaban 10 mg twice daily for the first 7 days, then 5 mg twice daily thereafter or dalteparin 200 units/kg once daily for the first 30 days, followed by 150 units/kg once daily. Both groups were treated for 6 months. At baseline, approximately 73% of patients were receiving concurrent systemic cancer treatment and two-thirds of patients had distant metastases.

The primary safety outcome was the occurrence of major bleeding defined as overt bleeding plus a decrease in hemoglobin ≥2 g/dL, transfusion of ≥2 units of packed red blood cells, bleeding that occurs in at least one critical site (e.g., intracranial, intraspinal, retroperitoneal), or fatal bleeding. VTE recurrence (defined as DVT, PE, fatal PE, or arterial thromboembolism) comprised the secondary efficacy endpoint. Major bleeding was reported in 2 (1.4%) of 142 dalteparin-treated patients and 0 (0%) of 145 apixaban-treated patients. In addition, VTE recurred in 0.7% of apixaban-treated patients and 6.3% of dalteparin-treated patients.

Clinical Perspective

The DOACs are among several anticoagulants that can be used for the treatment of VTE. DOACs have similar efficacy to warfarin, but reduced bleeding (particularly intracranial hemorrhage) and greater convenience for patients and healthcare providers. In addition to relative efficacy and safety, factors that should be considered when selecting an appropriate anticoagulant include convenience of administration, cost, patient preference, presence of renal impairment, and cancer or other comorbid conditions.

Apixaban is recommended by ACCP, ASH, and the Anticoagulation Forum as an acceptable option for initial and long-term anticoagulant therapy in patients with acute proximal DVT of the leg and/or PE. In patients with acute VTE, therapy should be continued beyond the acute treatment period for at least 3 months, and possibly longer depending on the individual clinical situation (e.g., location of thrombi, presence or absence of precipitating factors, presence of cancer, patient's risk of bleeding). Apixaban may offer some advantages over parenteral or vitamin K antagonist anticoagulants for the treatment of VTE (e.g., oral administration, no requirement for routine coagulation monitoring, minimal drug and food interactions) and guidelines recommend DOACs over vitamin K antagonist anticoagulants with a few exceptions based on risk factors (e.g., antiphospholipid syndrome). The relative efficacy and safety of apixaban versus other DOACs (e.g., rivaroxaban, dabigatran edoxaban) for the treatment of VTE remains to be fully elucidated due to the lack of head-to-head trials. ACCP does not recommend one DOAC over another as there are no published trials directly comparing these agents and indirect comparisons have not shown substantially different outcomes.

DOACs generally should not be used in settings with high risk of bleeding (e.g., hemorrhagic lesion, renal/hepatic impairment, thrombocytopenia, GI or genitourinary malignancy, mucosal lesion, CNS malignancy or bleeding, recent surgery), or in patients with morbid obesity (body weight >120 kg or body mass index [BMI] ≥40 mg/m²), drug-drug interactions, or GI complications affecting oral therapy (e.g., poor absorption, nausea and vomiting) because of the lack of safety data. There is some experience with the use of apixaban and rivaroxaban in patients with morbid obesity.

In patients with cancer and established VTE, LMWHs or oral factor Xa inhibitors (e.g., apixaban, rivaroxaban, edoxaban) are generally recommended over warfarin for long-term anticoagulation. ACCP and ASH recommend the use of an oral factor Xa inhibitor over LMWH for the initiation and treatment phases

of therapy in patients with cancer-associated thrombosis. Additional studies and experience are needed to further evaluate the efficacy and safety of apixaban for the treatment of cancer-related VTE.

DOSAGE AND ADMINISTRATION

● General

Pretreatment Screening

- Prior to initiating therapy with apixaban, assess renal function.
- Obtain body weight and serum creatinine to determine dosage in patients with nonvalvular atrial fibrillation.

Patient Monitoring

- Periodically assess serum creatinine concentration as clinically indicated in patients with nonvalvular atrial fibrillation and adjust therapy accordingly.
- Periodically assess body weight in patients with nonvalvular atrial fibrillation who are at risk of decreasing to ≤60 kg.
- If apixaban is administered in an epidural or spinal anesthesia/analgesia or lumbar puncture setting, frequently monitor for signs or symptoms of neurological impairment (e.g., numbness, tingling, weakness in lower limbs, bowel and/or bladder dysfunction).
- Monitor patients for any signs or symptoms of bleeding (e.g., unusual bruising) during therapy.
- Routine coagulation monitoring (e.g., prothrombin time [PT], activated partial thromboplastin time [aPTT], international normalized ratio [INR]) is not necessary with apixaban therapy because of the drug's predictable pharmacokinetic (PK) and pharmacodynamic (PD) effects. However, in certain situations, such as in the case of overdosage or in patients with hemorrhagic or thromboembolic complications or those requiring emergency surgery, it may be useful to assess the degree of anticoagulation. Although apixaban produces concentration-dependent increases in aPTT, PT, INR, and the Heptest (used to measure inhibition of exogenous activated factor X [factor Xa]), these tests generally are not useful for monitoring the anticoagulant effects of apixaban because of a high degree of inconsistency and variability in results. A chromogenic anti-factor Xa assay (Rotachrom® Heparin chromogenic assay) was used during the apixaban development program to measure the effect of apixaban on factor Xa activity. Although the chromogenic assay appears to correlate well with apixaban activity and may produce less variable results than other coagulation tests, a standardized assay specifically calibrated for apixaban currently is not available in most healthcare facilities. The manufacturer does not recommend use of this chromogenic assay for assessing the anticoagulant effects of apixaban.

Dispensing and Administration Precautions

- Based on the Institute for Safe Medication Practices (ISMP), apixaban is a high-alert medication that has a heightened risk of causing significant patient harm when used in error.

● Administration

Oral Tablets

Administer orally twice daily without regard to food.

In patients who are unable to swallow whole tablets, crush apixaban 2.5- or 5-mg tablets and suspend in water, 5% dextrose in water, or apple juice, or mix with applesauce and promptly administer orally. Alternatively, crush apixaban tablets and suspend in 60 mL of water or 5% dextrose in water and promptly deliver through a nasogastric feeding tube. Crushed apixaban tablets are stable in water, dextrose 5% in water, apple juice, or applesauce for up to 4 hours.

If a dose is missed, take the missed dose as soon as possible on the same day, followed by resumption of the regular twice-daily dosing schedule; do not double the dose to make up for the missed dose.

Store apixaban tablets at 20°C to 25°C (excursions permitted to 15°C to 30°C).

● *Dosage*

Embolism Associated with Atrial Fibrillation

For reducing the risk of stroke and systemic embolism in adult patients with non-valvular atrial fibrillation, the recommended dosage of apixaban for most patients is 5 mg orally twice daily.

Reduce dosage to 2.5 mg twice daily in patients with at least 2 of the following characteristics that can increase drug exposure and thus, increase the risk of bleeding: age ≥80 years, body weight ≤60 kg, or serum creatinine concentration ≥1.5 mg/dL.

Thromboprophylaxis in Orthopedic Surgery

Hip or Knee-replacement Surgery

For the prevention of deep-vein thrombosis (DVT), which may lead to pulmonary embolism (PE), in adult patients who have undergone hip- or knee-replacement surgery, the recommended dosage of apixaban is 2.5 mg orally twice daily. Administer the initial dose at least 12–24 hours after surgery, provided hemostasis has been established. The recommended duration of apixaban therapy is 35 days for patients undergoing hip-replacement surgery and 12 days for patients undergoing knee-replacement surgery. In clinical studies, the initial dose of apixaban was administered 12–24 hours after wound closure, and treatment was continued postoperatively for 10–14 days after knee-replacement surgery and for 32–38 days after hip-replacement surgery.

Venous Thromboembolism – Treatment and Secondary Prevention

For the treatment of acute DVT and/or PE in adults, the recommended dosage of apixaban is 10 mg orally twice daily for 7 days, followed by 5 mg orally twice daily; in the principal efficacy trial, apixaban therapy was administered for 6 months. For reduction in the risk of recurrent DVT and PE (secondary prevention) in adult patients who have received at least 6 months of initial anticoagulant therapy, the recommended dosage of apixaban is 2.5 mg orally twice daily.

The optimum duration of anticoagulant therapy in patients with venous thromboembolism (VTE) should be determined by the individual clinical situation (e.g., location of thrombi, presence or absence of precipitating factors for thrombosis, presence of cancer, risk of bleeding). In general, the American College of Chest Physicians (ACCP) states that anticoagulant therapy for VTE should be continued beyond the acute treatment period for at least 3 months and possibly longer in certain patients with a high risk of recurrence and low or moderate risk of bleeding.

Coadministration with Dual Inhibitors of Cytochrome P-450 Isoenzyme 3A4 and P-glycoprotein

In patients receiving apixaban dosages of 5 mg or 10 mg twice daily who are on concomitant therapy with drugs that are potent inhibitors of both cytochrome P-450 (CYP) isoenzyme 3A4 and P-glycoprotein (P-gp) (e.g., ketoconazole, itraconazole, ritonavir), the dosage of apixaban should be reduced by 50% (e.g., from 5 mg twice daily to 2.5 mg twice daily). Patients who are already receiving an apixaban dosage of 2.5 mg twice daily should avoid concomitant use with such potent dual inhibitors of CYP3A4 and P-gp.

Transitioning from Other Anticoagulant Therapy

When transitioning from warfarin to apixaban therapy, the manufacturer states that warfarin should be discontinued and apixaban initiated as soon as the INR is <2.

When transitioning from therapy with anticoagulants other than warfarin, the manufacturer recommends discontinuing the current anticoagulant and initiating apixaban at the time of the next scheduled dose of the current anticoagulant.

Transitioning to Other Anticoagulant Therapy

When transitioning from apixaban to warfarin therapy, INR measurements may not be useful for determining an appropriate dose of warfarin because apixaban also can prolong the INR. The manufacturer suggests that apixaban be discontinued and a parenteral anticoagulant and warfarin initiated simultaneously at the time of the next scheduled dose of apixaban; the parenteral anticoagulant can then be discontinued once an acceptable INR is achieved with warfarin. Some clinicians have suggested other strategies for transitioning from non-vitamin K antagonist oral anticoagulants (e.g., apixaban, rivaroxaban) to warfarin based on the patient's creatinine clearance and the warfarin start date.

When transitioning from apixaban to anticoagulants other than warfarin, including parenteral anticoagulants or other direct oral anticoagulants (DOACs), apixaban should be discontinued and the other anticoagulant initiated at the time of the next scheduled apixaban dose. In patients taking apixaban or other factor Xa inhibitors (e.g., rivaroxaban), heparin anti-Xa assay accuracy may be affected; elevated heparin anti-Xa levels have been reported, which may impact monitoring of the transition from apixaban to IV heparin.

Managing Anticoagulation in Patients Requiring Invasive Procedures

If temporary discontinuance of anticoagulation is necessary prior to surgery or other invasive procedures, the timing of discontinuance should be based upon procedural bleeding risk, the patient's thromboembolic risk, and renal function.

To reduce the bleeding risk, the manufacturer recommends that apixaban be discontinued at least 48 hours prior to elective surgery or invasive procedures with a moderate or high risk of unacceptable or clinically significant bleeding and at least 24 hours prior to elective surgery or invasive procedures with a low risk of bleeding or bleeding in a non-critical location that can be easily controlled.

Bridging anticoagulation generally is not required prior to the procedure or during the 24–48 hours after stopping apixaban. Apixaban therapy should be resumed postoperatively as soon as adequate hemostasis has been established.

● *Special Populations*

Hepatic Impairment

No dosage adjustment is necessary in patients with mild hepatic impairment (Child-Pugh class A). Because of limited experience, the manufacturer states that dosage recommendations cannot be provided in patients with moderate hepatic impairment (Child-Pugh class B). Data are lacking on the use of apixaban in patients with severe hepatic impairment (Child-Pugh class C), and the manufacturer states that use of apixaban is not recommended in this population.

Renal Impairment

The manufacturer states that dosage adjustment of apixaban based solely on renal impairment (including patients with end-stage renal disease [ESRD] who are maintained on intermittent hemodialysis) is not necessary in patients with nonvalvular atrial fibrillation; however, a reduced dosage of 2.5 mg twice daily is recommended in those with at least 2 of the following characteristics: an elevated serum creatinine concentration ≥1.5 mg/dL, age ≥80 years, and/or weight ≤60 kg. The manufacturer states that this recommendation is based on PK and PD (anti-factor Xa activity) data in ESRD patients maintained on hemodialysis; such patients were not studied in clinical efficacy and safety trials of apixaban.

No dosage adjustments are necessary in patients with renal impairment (including ESRD patients maintained on hemodialysis) who are receiving apixaban for the prevention of DVT and associated PE following hip- or knee-replacement surgery or for the treatment or secondary prevention of DVT or PE. The manufacturer states this recommendation is based on PK and PD (anti-factor Xa activity) data in ESRD patients maintained on hemodialysis; patients with ESRD on dialysis or with a creatinine clearance <15 mL/minute were not studied in apixaban clinical efficacy and safety trials.

Geriatric Patients

The manufacturer states that dosage adjustment based solely on age is not necessary in geriatric patients ≥65 years of age; however, a reduced dosage of 2.5 mg twice daily is recommended in patients ≥80 years of age with nonvalvular atrial fibrillation if they also weigh ≤60 kg and/or have a serum creatinine concentration ≥1.5 mg/dL.

Body Weight

The manufacturer states that dosage adjustment based solely on body weight is not necessary; however, a reduced dosage of 2.5 mg twice daily is recommended in patients with nonvalvular atrial fibrillation who weigh ≤60 kg if they also are ≥80 years of age and/or have a serum creatinine concentration ≥1.5 mg/dL.

In the principal efficacy study, patients with high body weight (>120 kg) had decreased drug exposure (approximately 25% lower), but this did not result in loss of efficacy.

The International Society on Thrombosis and Haemostasis (ISTH) Subcommittee on Control of Anticoagulation issued consensus recommendations on VTE prevention and treatment with DOACs in patients with obesity. Based upon the available PK/PD and clinical outcome data, apixaban at the standard dosage is an acceptable treatment and primary prevention option regardless of high body mass index (BMI) and body weight. ISTH does not recommend regularly following peak or trough apixaban levels as there are insufficient data to influence management decisions. Following surgical intervention for obesity, apixaban absorption may be reduced depending on the procedure. Due to limited data, ISTH does not recommend the use of apixaban or other DOACs (e.g., rivaroxaban, edoxaban, dabigatran) for treatment or prevention of VTE in the acute setting after bariatric surgery due to concerns for decreased absorption. In the early postsurgical phase, patients should be initiated on parenteral anticoagulation. The use of a vitamin K antagonist or DOAC following at least 4 weeks of parenteral treatment may be considered and obtaining a DOAC trough level is suggested to check drug absorption.

CAUTIONS

● **Contraindications**

● Active pathologic bleeding.

● Severe hypersensitivity reaction (e.g., anaphylactic reactions) to apixaban.

● **Warnings/Precautions**

Warnings

Risk of Thrombosis Following Premature Discontinuance of Anticoagulation

Premature discontinuance of any oral anticoagulant, including apixaban, in the absence of adequate alternative anticoagulation increases the risk of thrombotic events (e.g., stroke). A boxed warning about this risk is included in the prescribing information for apixaban. An increased incidence of stroke was observed during the transition from apixaban to warfarin in clinical trials in patients with atrial fibrillation. If discontinuance of apixaban is required for reasons other than pathologic bleeding or completion of a course of therapy, anticoagulant coverage with an alternative anticoagulant should be considered. When transitioning patients from one anticoagulant therapy to another, it is important to ensure continuous anticoagulation while minimizing the risk of bleeding. Particular caution is advised when switching patients from a factor Xa inhibitor to warfarin therapy because of the slow onset of action of warfarin.

Spinal/Epidural Hematoma

Patients receiving anticoagulants are at risk of developing an epidural or spinal hematoma when concomitant neuraxial (epidural/spinal) anesthesia or spinal puncture is employed; such complications can result in long-term or permanent paralysis. A boxed warning about this risk is included in the prescribing information for apixaban. The risk of these complications is increased by postoperative use of indwelling epidural catheters for administration of analgesia or by concomitant use of drugs affecting hemostasis, such as nonsteroidal anti-inflammatory agents (NSAIAs), platelet-aggregation inhibitors, or other anticoagulants. Risk also may be increased in patients with a history of traumatic or repeated epidural or spinal punctures, spinal deformity, or spinal surgery.

Removal of an indwelling epidural or intrathecal catheter should be delayed for at least 24 hours after a dose of apixaban, and at least 5 hours should elapse following removal of the catheter prior to administration of the next apixaban dose. If traumatic puncture occurs, the administration of apixaban should be delayed for 48 hours.

Patients receiving apixaban in the setting of epidural or spinal anesthesia should be monitored frequently for manifestations of neurologic impairment (e.g., numbness or weakness of the legs, bowel or bladder dysfunction). If neurologic compromise is noted, urgent diagnosis and treatment are necessary. Clinicians should consider the potential benefits versus risks of neuraxial

intervention in patients who are currently receiving or will receive anticoagulant prophylaxis.

Other Warnings and Precautions

Bleeding

Apixaban increases the risk of hemorrhage and can cause serious, potentially fatal, bleeding. The drug should be discontinued if active pathological hemorrhage occurs. However, minor or "nuisance" bleeding is a common occurrence in patients receiving any anticoagulant and should not readily lead to treatment discontinuance.

In the principal efficacy study of apixaban in patients with nonvalvular atrial fibrillation (ARISTOTLE), major bleeding occurred at an annual rate of 2.13% (327 out of 9088 patients) in patients who received the drug, although the rate was substantially lower with apixaban than with warfarin therapy (rate of 2.13% per year versus 3.09% per year). In this study, bleeding was assessed according to the International Society on Thrombosis and Hemostasis (ISTH) criteria, which defines major bleeding as clinically overt bleeding that is accompanied by one or more of the following events: decrease in hemoglobin ≥ 2 g/dL, transfusion of ≥ 2 units of packed red blood cells, bleeding at a critical site (i.e., intracranial, intraspinal, intraocular, pericardial, intraarticular, intramuscular with compartment syndrome, or retroperitoneal) or resulting in death. Concomitant use of aspirin increased the risk of bleeding in patients receiving apixaban from 1.8 to 3.4% per year, and concomitant use of aspirin and warfarin increased the bleeding risk from 2.7 to 4.6% per year.

Risk of bleeding may be increased in patients with renal impairment and in those receiving concomitant therapy with drugs that affect hemostasis (e.g., aspirin or other antiplatelet drugs, fibrinolytics, heparin or other anticoagulants, selective serotonin reuptake inhibitors, serotonin norepinephrine reuptake inhibitors, chronic use of NSAIAs) or drugs that are inhibitors of both P-glycoprotein (P-gp) and cytochrome P-450 (CYP) isoenzyme 3A4.

Apixaban therapy should be temporarily interrupted prior to any elective surgery or other invasive procedure to reduce the risk of bleeding.

Factor Xa (recombinant), inactivated-zhzo (also known as andexanet alfa), a recombinant modified human factor Xa protein, is a specific reversal agent for the anticoagulant effects of apixaban. Data from clinical trials indicate that factor Xa (recombinant), inactivated-zhzo is effective in rapidly reversing the anticoagulant effects of apixaban (as measured by anti-factor Xa activity, unbound anticoagulant concentration, and thrombin generation). The safety of factor Xa (recombinant), inactivated-zhzo has not been established in patients who have experienced a thromboembolic event or disseminated intravascular coagulation (DIC) within 2 weeks prior to the life-threatening bleeding event requiring treatment with the drug or in those who have received prothrombin complex concentrate (PCC), recombinant factor VIIa, or whole blood products within 7 days prior to the bleeding event. If a serious bleeding event occurs during therapy, apixaban should be discontinued and appropriate supportive measures provided.

Procoagulant reversal agents such as 4-factor PCC may be considered for immediate reversal of the anticoagulant effect of apixaban, when factor Xa (recombinant), inactivated-zhzo is not available. In 2 prospective cohort studies, fixed dose 4-factor PCC was administered to patients with major bleeding due to factor Xa inhibitors. In one study the dose of 4-factor PCC was weight-based (2000 units for patients weighing >65 kg and 1500 units for patients weighing <65 kg). In the second study, the dose of 4-factor PCC was 2000 units. Good or effective hemostasis was achieved in at least 65% of patients in both studies. Embolic complications including ischemic stroke and thromboembolic events were reported in some patients who received the reversal agent.

When PCCs are used, monitoring for the anticoagulation effect of apixaban using a clotting test (prothrombin time [PT], international normalized ratio [INR], activated partial thromboplastin time [aPTT]) or anti-factor Xa activity is not useful and is not recommended.

Protamine sulfate and vitamin K are not expected to affect the anticoagulant activity of apixaban. There is no experience with antifibrinolytic agents (tranexamic acid, aminocaproic acid) or systemic hemostatics (desmopressin) in patients receiving apixaban, and such drugs are not expected to be effective as reversal agents. Because of high plasma protein binding, apixaban is not expected to be dialyzable. In the event of an overdosage, activated charcoal may be used to decrease plasma concentrations of apixaban more rapidly.

Patients with Prosthetic Heart Valves

Safety and efficacy of apixaban have not been established in patients with prosthetic heart valves and use of apixaban is not generally recommended in such patients.

Patients with Pulmonary Embolism

Apixaban is not recommended as initial therapy (as an alternative to unfractionated heparin) in patients with pulmonary embolism (PE) who have hemodynamic instability or who may receive thrombolytic therapy or undergo pulmonary embolectomy.

Thrombosis Risk in Triple Positive Antiphospholipid Syndrome

Apixaban and other DOACs are not recommended for use in patients with triple-positive antiphospholipid syndrome (APS) (i.e., positive for lupus anticoagulant, anticardiolipin, and anti-beta 2-glycoprotein I antibodies). Treatment with DOACs has been associated with increased rates of recurrent thrombotic events compared with warfarin treatment in patients with APS, especially those with triple-positive disease. The International Society of Thrombosis and Hemostasis (ISTH) recommends the use of vitamin K antagonists over DOACs in patients with high-risk APS, including those with triple-positive disease.

Specific Populations

Pregnancy

The manufacturer states the limited available data on apixaban use in pregnant women are insufficient to inform drug-associated risks of major birth defects, miscarriage, or adverse developmental outcomes. Animal studies have not demonstrated any evidence of fetotoxic effects; however, increased maternal bleeding was observed when apixaban was administered to pregnant animals at doses ranging from 1–19 times the human exposure at the maximum recommended dose. All patients receiving anticoagulants, including pregnant women, are at risk for bleeding.

Consider use of a shorter acting anticoagulant as delivery approaches. Based on the pharmacologic activity of factor Xa inhibitors, bleeding may occur at any site in the fetus and/or neonate. Apixaban use during labor or delivery in women who are receiving neuraxial anaesthesia may result in epidural or spinal hematomas.

The American College of Chest Physicians (ACCP) and the American College of Obstetricians and Gynecologists (ACOG) recommend avoiding apixaban in pregnant women due to insufficient safety data; the American Society of Hematology (ASH) states that more data involving the DOACs are necessary in their most recent guidelines for the management of VTE in the context of pregnancy.

Lactation

Apixaban is distributed into milk in rats; it is not known whether the drug is distributed into human milk. The effects of apixaban on the breast-fed infant or on milk production are unknown. The manufacturer states that breast-feeding is not recommended during treatment with apixaban. ACCP, ACOG, and ASH recommend that anticoagulants other than apixaban be used in nursing women.

Females and Males of Reproductive Potential

Apixaban can cause significant uterine bleeding. Females of reproductive potential and those with abnormal uterine bleeding should be assessed for increased risk of clinically significant uterine bleeding, potentially requiring gynecologic surgical intervention.

Pediatric Use

Safety and efficacy of apixaban have not been established in pediatric patients.

Geriatric Use

No substantial differences in efficacy and safety were observed in geriatric patients ≥65 years relative to younger adults in clinical trials. In clinical trials of apixaban in patients with nonvalvular atrial fibrillation or DVT/PE, no clinically important differences in efficacy or safety were observed among different age groups. Pharmacokinetic effects (systemic exposure and peak plasma concentrations) of apixaban were similar in patients ≥65 years and younger adults (18–40 years of age) receiving the drug.

Hepatic Impairment

Pharmacokinetic (systemic exposure and peak plasma concentrations) and pharmacodynamic (inhibition of factor Xa activity) effects of apixaban do not appear to be substantially altered in patients with mild or moderate hepatic impairment. Patients with moderate hepatic impairment may have intrinsic coagulation abnormalities that can affect response to apixaban therapy; there are limited data and dosing recommendations cannot be provided. Data are lacking in patients with severe hepatic impairment, and the manufacturer recommends that apixaban not be used in such patients.

Renal Impairment

Pharmacokinetic (systemic exposure and peak plasma concentrations) and pharmacodynamic (inhibition of factor Xa activity) effects of apixaban do not appear to be substantially altered in patients with renal impairment (mild, moderate, or severe) compared with those with normal renal function.

Although results of a pharmacokinetic study showed an approximate 44% increase in systemic exposure to apixaban in patients with severe renal impairment (i.e., creatinine clearance <15 mL/minute) compared with those with normal renal function, this degree of change was considered to be modest.

In the principal clinical study of the drug, patients with moderate to severe renal impairment had higher rates of bleeding regardless of treatment (apixaban or warfarin).

End-stage renal disease (ESRD) patients on dialysis were not enrolled in apixaban clinical trials. The manufacturer states administration of apixaban in these patients at the usually recommended dosage results in concentrations of apixaban and pharmacodynamic activity similar to those observed in the ARISTOTLE study. It is not known whether these concentrations will lead to similar stroke reduction and bleeding risk.

In the settings of DVT prophylaxis following orthopedic surgery or VTE treatment and reduction in risk of recurrence, no dosage adjustment is recommended for patients with renal impairment including those with ESRD on dialysis. Clinical studies for these indications did not enroll patients with ESRD on dialysis or patients with a creatinine clearance <15 mL/minute. Dosing recommendations are based on pharmacokinetic and pharmacodynamic (anti-FXa activity) data from subjects with ESRD maintained on dialysis.

Dosage adjustment based on renal function alone does not appear to be necessary but is recommended in patients with nonvalvular atrial fibrillation and renal impairment who meet additional criteria for dosage modification.

Race/Ethnicity

Pharmacokinetics of apixaban do not appear to be substantially altered by race or ethnicity. In several studies in which healthy individuals of different ethnic or racial origins (Caucasian, Asian, and African-American) received apixaban, pharmacokinetic parameters (e.g., peak plasma concentrations, half-life, time to steady state) were similar regardless of race or ethnicity.

● Common Adverse Effects

The most common adverse reactions reported with apixaban (>1%) are related to bleeding.

DRUG INTERACTIONS

Apixaban is a substrate of cytochrome P-450 (CYP) 3A4, P-glycoprotein (P-gp), and breast cancer resistance protein (BCRP).

● Drugs Affecting or Metabolized by Hepatic Microsomal Enzymes

Apixaban is metabolized principally by CYP isoenzyme 3A4/5, and to a lesser extent by CYP isoenzymes 1A2, 2C8, 2C9, 2C19, and 2J2. Although pharmacokinetic interactions are possible with drugs that inhibit or induce CYP3A4/5, in vitro studies indicate that the potential may be low because of apixaban's multiple routes of elimination.

In vitro studies indicate that apixaban does not inhibit CYP isoenzymes 1A2, 2A6, 2B6, 2C8, 2C9, 2D6, 3A4/5, or 2C19 nor induce CYP isoenzymes 1A2, 2B6, or 3A4/5; therefore, pharmacokinetic interactions are not expected with drugs that are metabolized by these isoenzymes.

● Drugs Affecting P-glycoprotein Transport

Apixaban is a substrate of the efflux transporter P-gp; inhibitors or inducers of this transport protein may potentially alter apixaban exposure. Apixaban does not substantially inhibit P-gp.

● Drugs Affecting P-glycoprotein Transport and CYP3A4

Since apixaban is a substrate of both P-gp and CYP3A4, concomitant use of drugs that inhibit P-gp and CYP3A4 can increase exposure (peak plasma concentrations and AUC) of apixaban and increase the risk of bleeding. In patients receiving apixaban dosages exceeding 2.5 mg twice daily (e.g., 5 mg twice daily), the dosage of apixaban should be reduced by 50% (e.g., from 5 mg twice daily to 2.5 mg twice daily) if concomitant therapy with potent dual inhibitors of P-gp and CYP3A4 (e.g., itraconazole, ketoconazole, ritonavir) is administered. In patients already receiving apixaban 2.5 mg twice daily, concomitant administration of potent dual inhibitors of P-gp and CYP3A4 should be avoided. While clarithromycin is an inhibitor of P-gp and a strong CYP3A4 inhibitor, pharmacokinetic data suggest that no dosage adjustment is necessary with concomitant use of apixaban and clarithromycin. Concomitant administration of other, less potent inhibitors of CYP3A4 and P-gp (e.g., diltiazem, naproxen) also may increase exposure to apixaban.

Conversely, drugs that induce P-gp and CYP3A4 can reduce plasma concentrations of apixaban and increase the risk of stroke. Concomitant use of apixaban and potent dual inducers of P-gp and CYP3A4 (e.g., carbamazepine, phenytoin, rifampin, St. John's wort [*Hypericum perforatum*]) should be avoided.

Diltiazem

Concomitant administration of apixaban and diltiazem (a moderate CYP3A4 and weak P-gp inhibitor) increased AUC and peak plasma concentrations of apixaban by 1.4- and 1.3-fold, respectively.

Ketoconazole

Concomitant administration of apixaban and ketoconazole (a strong inhibitor of both P-gp and CYP3A4) substantially increased the AUC and peak plasma concentration of apixaban by 2- and 1.6-fold, respectively. Dosage of apixaban should be reduced to 2.5 mg twice daily with such concomitant therapy. Concomitant use of apixaban and ketoconazole should be avoided in patients who have 2 or more of the following characteristics: age ≥80 years, body weight ≤60 kg, serum creatinine concentration ≥1.5 mg/dL or in patients already requiring a 2.5 mg twice daily dosage regimen (e.g., prevention of VTE recurrence).

Naproxen

Concomitant administration of apixaban and naproxen (a P-gp inhibitor) increased AUC and peak plasma concentrations of apixaban by 1.5- and 1.6-fold, respectively.

Apixaban did not substantially alter the pharmacokinetics of naproxen; however, a 50–60% increase in anti-factor Xa activity was observed with such concomitant therapy.

Rifampin

Concomitant administration of apixaban and rifampin (a strong inducer of both P-gp and CYP3A4) decreased AUC and peak plasma concentrations of apixaban by 54 and 42%, respectively; concomitant use of these drugs should be avoided.

● Drugs Affecting Hemostasis

Concomitant use of apixaban and drugs that affect hemostasis (e.g., aspirin or other antiplatelet drugs, heparin or other anticoagulants, fibrinolytics, selective serotonin-reuptake inhibitors [SSRIs], selective serotonin- and norepinephrine-reuptake inhibitors [SNRIs], nonsteroidal anti-inflammatory agents [NSAIAs]) increases the risk of bleeding.

● Amiodarone

Efficacy and safety end points for apixaban compared with warfarin did not appear to be altered by concomitant administration of amiodarone in the principal efficacy study of apixaban in patients with nonvalvular atrial fibrillation.

● Aspirin

In the principal efficacy study of apixaban, bleeding risk was increased in patients who received concomitant apixaban and aspirin therapy. Additionally, a placebo-controlled study of patients with acute coronary syndromes was terminated early after an increased risk of bleeding was observed in patients receiving apixaban in combination with aspirin and clopidogrel.

In drug interaction studies in healthy individuals, apixaban did not substantially alter the pharmacokinetics of aspirin, and a pharmacodynamic interaction was not observed with such concomitant therapy.

● Atenolol

Concomitant administration of apixaban and atenolol in healthy individuals did not appreciably alter the pharmacokinetics of either drug.

● Clopidogrel

No pharmacodynamic interactions (e.g., anti-factor Xa activity) were observed with concomitant apixaban and clopidogrel therapy. However, a placebo-controlled study (APPRAISE-2) of patients with acute coronary syndromes was terminated early after an increased risk of bleeding was observed in patients receiving apixaban in combination with aspirin and clopidogrel.

● Digoxin

In drug interaction studies conducted in healthy individuals, apixaban did not substantially alter the pharmacokinetics of digoxin.

● Enoxaparin

In a study in healthy individuals, concomitant administration of apixaban and enoxaparin had no effect on the pharmacokinetics of apixaban, but had an additive effect on anti-factor Xa activity. The increased pharmacodynamic effect was considered to be modest. When administration of apixaban and enoxaparin was separated by 6 hours in this study, the additive effect on anti-factor Xa activity was attenuated.

● Famotidine

Famotidine did not substantially alter the pharmacokinetics of apixaban in healthy individuals.

● Prasugrel

Concomitant administration of apixaban and prasugrel in healthy individuals did not appreciably alter the pharmacokinetics of either drug.

DESCRIPTION

Apixaban is an oral, reversible, direct activated factor X (factor Xa) inhibitor. Factor Xa plays a central role in the blood coagulation cascade by serving as the convergence point for the intrinsic and extrinsic pathways; inhibition of coagulation factor Xa prevents conversion of prothrombin to thrombin, resulting in decreased thrombin generation and thrombus development. Unlike fondaparinux, heparin, and the low molecular weight heparins, apixaban binds directly to the active site of factor Xa with high affinity and selectivity, and does not require a cofactor (antithrombin III) for its antithrombotic activity. Apixaban inhibits free and clot-bound factor Xa and prothrombinase activity.

Apixaban exhibits linear, dose-proportional pharmacokinetics for oral doses up to 10 mg. The absolute bioavailability of the drug is approximately 50%, and peak plasma concentrations are reached approximately 3–4 hours after oral administration. Following oral administration of 10 mg of apixaban as 2 crushed 5-mg tablets suspended in 30 mL of water, bioavailability was similar to that after 2 intact 5-mg tablets taken orally. Following oral administration of 10 mg of apixaban as 2 crushed 5-mg tablets mixed with 30 g of applesauce, the peak plasma concentration and bioavailability of apixaban were decreased by 20 and 16%, respectively. Following administration via a nasogastric feeding tube of a single crushed 5-mg tablet suspended in 60 mL of 5% dextrose in water, bioavailability of the drug is similar to that of a whole tablet taken orally.

Apixaban has a total clearance of approximately 3.3 L/hour. Despite a short clearance half-life of about 6 hours, the apparent half-life of apixaban is longer (about 12 hours) following repeated administration because of prolonged absorption. Absorption of apixaban occurs throughout the GI tract, with about 55% of the drug absorbed in the distal small intestine and ascending colon. Food does not appear to affect the pharmacokinetics (systemic exposure and peak plasma concentrations) or pharmacodynamics of apixaban.

Apixaban is eliminated via multiple pathways, including hepatic metabolism by the cytochrome P-450 (CYP) enzyme system and through intestinal, biliary, and renal excretion; approximately 25% of an administered dose is eliminated renally. No active circulating metabolites have been identified. Approximately 87% of the drug is bound to plasma proteins. QT-interval prolongation has not been observed with apixaban doses up to 50 mg. Apixaban inhibits factor Xa activity, and prolongs prothrombin time (PT), activated partial thromboplastin time (aPTT), and the international normalized ratio (INR) in a concentration-dependent manner.

ADVICE TO PATIENTS

- Take apixaban exactly as prescribed and do not discontinue therapy without first consulting a clinician.

- Advise patients on how to take the drug if they cannot swallow whole tablets or if they require a nasogastric tube.

- Instruct patients that if a dose is missed, to take it as soon as possible on the same day and then resume the regular twice-daily dosing schedule; do not take 2 doses at the same time.

- Inform patients that they may bruise and/or bleed more easily and that a longer than normal time may be required to stop bleeding when taking apixaban; advise patients on how to recognize signs and symptoms of bleeding.

- Inform clinicians immediately about any unusual bleeding or bruising during therapy, including menstrual or vaginal bleeding that is heavier than normal.

- Apixaban is generally not for patients with artificial heart valves; advise patients to inform their health care provider if they have had or will have heart valve surgery.

- Apixaban is not recommended for use in people with antiphospholipid syndrome (APS), especially with positive triple antibody testing; advise patients to inform their healthcare provider if they have APS.

- Advise patients who have had neuraxial anesthesia or spinal puncture to monitor for manifestations of spinal or epidural hematoma (e.g., numbness or weakness of legs, bowel or bladder dysfunction), particularly if they are receiving concomitant nonsteroidal anti-inflammatory agents (NSAIAs), platelet inhibitors, or other anticoagulants; inform the patient to seek emergency medical attention if any of these symptoms occur.

- Advise patients to inform clinicians (e.g., physicians, dentists) that they are receiving apixaban therapy before scheduling any surgery or invasive procedures, including dental procedures.

- Advise women to inform their clinician if they are or plan to become pregnant or plan to breast-feed.

- Advise patients to inform their clinician of existing or contemplated concomitant therapy, including prescription and OTC drugs and dietary and herbal supplements, as well as any concomitant illnesses.

- Advise patients of other important precautionary information. (See Cautions.)

PREPARATIONS

Excipients in commercially available drug preparations may have clinically important effects in some individuals; consult specific product labeling for details.

Apixaban

Oral

| Tablets | 2.5 mg | Eliquis®, Bristol-Myers Squibb |
| | 5 mg | Eliquis®, Bristol-Myers Squibb |

† Use is not currently included in the labeling approved by the US Food and Drug Administration.

Selected Revisions March 23, 2023, © Copyright, January 01, 2014, American Society of Health-System Pharmacists, Inc.

Edoxaban Tosylate

20:12.04.14 • DIRECT FACTOR Xa INHIBITORS

■ Edoxaban tosylate, an oral, direct, activated factor X (Xa) inhibitor, is an anticoagulant.

USES

● Embolism Associated with Atrial Fibrillation

Edoxaban is used to reduce the risk of stroke and systemic embolism in patients with nonvalvular atrial fibrillation. The direct oral anticoagulants (DOACs; apixaban, dabigatran, edoxaban, rivaroxaban) have been shown in randomized controlled studies to be noninferior, and in some trials, superior to warfarin in reducing thromboembolic risk in patients with nonvalvular atrial fibrillation (i.e., atrial fibrillation in the absence of moderate-to-severe mitral stenosis or a mechanical heart valve), and are associated with reduced risk of serious bleeding. Edoxaban should not be used in patients with creatinine clearance exceeding 95 mL/minute because of possible reduced efficacy in such patients. (See Reduced Efficacy in Nonvalvular Atrial Fibrillation Patients with Creatinine Clearance Exceeding 95 mL/minute under Cautions.)

The American College of Chest Physicians (ACCP), the American College of Cardiology (ACC), the American Heart Association (AHA), the American Stroke Association (ASA), and other experts currently recommend that antithrombotic therapy be administered to all patients with nonvalvular atrial fibrillation who are considered to be at increased risk of stroke, unless such therapy is contraindicated. Although many risk stratification methods have been used, current guidelines recommend the use of the CHA_2DS_2-VASc risk stratification tool for assessing a patient's risk of stroke and need for anticoagulant therapy. Established clinical risk factors for stroke include prior ischemic stroke or transient ischemic attack (TIA), advanced age (e.g., ≥65 years), hypertension, diabetes mellitus, vascular disease, and congestive heart failure; in addition, female sex has been identified as a factor that can modify the risk of stroke. The presence of stroke or TIA places a patient in the high-risk category regardless of other risk factors. Experts state that antithrombotic therapy generally is not necessary in low-risk patients (CHA_2DS_2-VASc score of 0 in males or 1 in females), but should be considered in patients with one or more non-sex CHA_2DS_2-VASc stroke risk factors (CHA_2DS_2-VASc score of at least 1 in males or at least 2 in females). Patients also should be assessed for their risk of bleeding; those with a high risk of bleeding should be monitored more closely.

In patients with nonvalvular atrial fibrillation who are eligible for oral anticoagulant therapy, DOACs are recommended over warfarin based on improved safety and similar or improved efficacy in clinical trials and meta-analyses. A substantially greater benefit of DOACs versus warfarin has been observed when the international normalized ratio (INR) was in the therapeutic range less than 66% of the time. If warfarin is used, patients should be optimally managed with well-controlled INRs (e.g., INR in therapeutic range more than 70% of the time). A DOAC is recommended in patients unable to achieve optimal warfarin management.

Patient age, body weight, and renal and hepatic function should be considered prior to treatment with DOACs. Edoxaban is not recommended in patients with end-stage chronic kidney disease or on dialysis; warfarin or apixaban may be considered in these patients. There are limited data on the use of DOACs in obese patients and some experts have discouraged the use of these agents in the morbidly obese population (body mass index [BMI] >40 kg/m² or body weight >120 kg). However, treatment with the various DOAC agents may result in different outcomes. A post-hoc analysis of the principal efficacy study of edoxaban in patients with atrial fibrillation suggests the pharmacokinetic and pharmacodynamic profile of edoxaban remains consistent across extremes of body weight from low body weight (≤55 kg) to high body weight (≥120 kg). Because of limited data with DOACs in patients with morbid obesity, some experts recommend considering the use of warfarin over DOACs in such patients.

Because of the lack of direct, comparative studies, the relative efficacy and safety of the DOACs for the prevention of stroke in patients with nonvalvular atrial fibrillation remain to be fully elucidated. Some evidence from indirect comparisons suggests that there may be important differences (e.g., bleeding risk) between these agents; however, results of such analyses should be interpreted with caution because of possible confounding factors (e.g., differences in study design and methods, patient populations, and anticoagulation control). Selection of an appropriate anticoagulant for patients with nonvalvular atrial fibrillation should be individualized based on the absolute and relative risks of stroke and bleeding; costs; patient compliance, preference, tolerance, and comorbidities; and other clinical factors such as renal function and degree of INR control if the patient has been taking warfarin.

The risk of stroke in patients with atrial flutter is similar to the risk in those with atrial fibrillation. Experts state that antithrombotic therapy in patients with atrial flutter generally should be managed in the same manner as in patients with atrial fibrillation.

Efficacy and safety of edoxaban for the prevention of stroke and systemic embolism in patients with nonvalvular atrial fibrillation have been established in a randomized, double-blind, double-dummy trial (Effective Anticoagulation with Factor Xa Next Generation in Atrial Fibrillation-Thrombolysis in Myocardial Infarction 48 [ENGAGE AF-TIMI 48]). In this trial, edoxaban was compared with warfarin in 21,105 patients with nonvalvular atrial fibrillation who were at moderate-to-high risk of stroke (Congestive Heart Failure, Hypertension, Age, Diabetes, Stroke [doubled] [i.e., CHADS₂] score of at least 2). Patients received one of 2 fixed dosages of edoxaban (30 or 60 mg daily) or warfarin (dosage-adjusted to achieve therapeutic INR of 2–3) for a median of 2.5 years; for those in the edoxaban treatment groups, dosage was reduced by 50% (from 60 to 30 mg or 30 to 15 mg) if any of the following conditions anticipated to increase drug exposure, and thus bleeding, were present: estimated creatinine clearance of 30–50 mL/minute, body weight of 60 kg or less, or concomitant use of the potent P-glycoprotein inhibitors verapamil, quinidine, or dronedarone.

Edoxaban was noninferior to warfarin in preventing stroke and systemic embolism and was associated with lower rates of bleeding. At a median follow-up of 2.8 years, both dosage regimens of edoxaban demonstrated noninferiority to warfarin for the primary composite outcome of time to first occurrence of stroke (ischemic or hemorrhagic) or a systemic embolic event; annualized rates of the primary end point were 1.5% with warfarin, 1.61% with edoxaban 30 mg, and 1.18% with edoxaban 60 mg. The effect of edoxaban on the primary outcome was attributable principally to a marked reduction in hemorrhagic stroke; the rate of ischemic stroke was similar between edoxaban 60 mg and warfarin, and substantially higher with edoxaban 30 mg than with warfarin. The primary efficacy analysis was performed on the modified intent-to-treat population, which included all patients who underwent randomization and received at least one dose of study drug during the treatment period. In a prespecified superiority analysis that was subsequently conducted on the intent-to-treat population, both dosage regimens of edoxaban failed to demonstrate superiority over warfarin in reducing the rate of stroke or systemic embolism. With regard to the primary safety end point in this trial, major bleeding was substantially reduced with edoxaban (at both dosage levels) compared with warfarin. Other bleeding end points (i.e., intracranial bleeding, life-threatening bleeding, clinically relevant nonmajor bleeding) also favored edoxaban, with the exception of GI bleeding, which occurred at a higher rate in patients receiving the 60-mg dose of edoxaban compared with warfarin. The reduction in major bleeding with edoxaban compared with warfarin was even greater in patients who required a reduction in edoxaban dosage, and no apparent loss of efficacy was observed.

The comparison between edoxaban and warfarin in the ENGAGE AF-TIMI 48 trial was based on well-controlled warfarin therapy; patients who received warfarin achieved a mean time in the therapeutic INR range (2–3) of 65%, which is higher than that reported with warfarin anticoagulation in other trials of DOACs (e.g., dabigatran, apixaban, rivaroxaban) in patients with nonvalvular atrial fibrillation (e.g., 55–64%).

At the end of the ENGAGE AF-TIMI 48 trial, patients were switched to open-label anticoagulant therapy with the use of a transition plan that was specifically incorporated into the protocol to minimize the risk of stroke due to inadequate anticoagulation. (See Risk of Thrombosis Following Premature Discontinuance of Therapy under Cautions.) The transition plan included a period of overlap between edoxaban (at half the initial dosage used in the controlled trial) and warfarin until a therapeutic INR of 2 was achieved or for 14 days (whichever occurred first) in patients who switched from edoxaban to warfarin therapy. Similar rates of stroke and bleeding were observed across all treatment groups during the 30-day period following the end of the trial.

A strong relationship between plasma concentrations of edoxaban and the drug's effectiveness was observed in the ENGAGE AF-TIMI 48 trial. Patients who received the low dosage of edoxaban (30 mg daily) had a 64% higher rate of ischemic stroke compared with those who received the high dosage of the drug (60 mg daily). Because plasma edoxaban concentrations are affected by renal function, patients with good renal function are likely to have a lesser response to edoxaban due to lower plasma concentrations at a given dosage than those with mildly impaired renal function. When results of the ENGAGE AF-TIMI 48 trial were evaluated based on creatinine clearance, the relative benefits of edoxaban versus warfarin in reducing the rate of ischemic stroke decreased as renal function improved to the point where warfarin was more effective than edoxaban at creatinine clearances exceeding 95 mL/minute. Based on these findings, edoxaban should not be used in patients with creatinine clearance exceeding 95 mL/minute. (See Reduced Efficacy in Nonvalvular Atrial Fibrillation Patients with Creatinine Clearance Exceeding 95 mL/minute under Cautions.)

DOACs including edoxaban also have been used for therapeutic anticoagulation prior to and after cardioversion in patients with atrial fibrillation of greater than 48 hours' duration or of unknown duration; DOACs are recommended as a safe and effective alternative to warfarin in this setting.

Safety and efficacy of edoxaban have not been established in patients with mechanical heart valves or moderate to severe mitral stenosis; the drug is not recommended in such patients. (See Patients with Prosthetic Heart Valves or Mitral Stenosis under Cautions.)

● Venous Thromboembolism

Treatment

Edoxaban is used for the treatment of deep-vein thrombosis (DVT) and/or pulmonary embolism (PE) following initial treatment with a parenteral anticoagulant for 5–10 days.

The direct oral anticoagulants (DOACs) are among several anticoagulants that can be used for the treatment of venous thromboembolism (VTE). In addition to relative efficacy and safety, factors that should be considered when selecting an appropriate anticoagulant include convenience of administration, cost, patient preference, presence of renal impairment, and cancer or other comorbid conditions. The American College of Chest Physicians (ACCP) suggests the use of DOACs over warfarin for VTE treatment in patients without cancer. DOACs have similar efficacy to warfarin in these patients, but reduced bleeding (particularly intracranial hemorrhage) and greater convenience for patients and healthcare providers. In patients with cancer and established VTE, low molecular weight heparins (LMWHs) or DOACs are generally recommended over warfarin for long-term anticoagulation. ACCP suggests the use of LMWHs in these patients because of possible greater efficacy and reliability (in those who may have difficulty with oral therapy). DOACs generally should not be used in settings with high risk of bleeding (e.g, hemorrhagic lesion, renal/hepatic impairment, thrombocytopenia, GI or genitourinary malignancy, mucosal lesion, CNS malignancy or bleeding, recent surgery), or in patients with morbid obesity (body weight >120 kg or body mass index [BMI] >40 mg/m²), drug-drug interactions, or GI complications affecting oral therapy (e.g., poor absorption, nausea and vomiting) because of the lack of safety data.

In patients with acute VTE, ACCP recommends that anticoagulant therapy be continued beyond the acute treatment period for at least 3 months, and possibly longer depending on whether the VTE event was unprovoked or provoked by a transient risk factor (e.g., surgery), the presence of cancer, and the patient's risk of bleeding. In patients with cancer, anticoagulation therapy is recommended for at least 6 months; treatment beyond 6 months may be considered for selected patients.

The relative efficacy and safety of edoxaban versus other DOACs for the treatment of VTE remain to be established. ACCP does not recommend one DOAC over another as there are no published trials directly comparing these agents and indirect comparisons have not shown substantially different outcomes.

There is limited data on the use of DOACs in obese patients and some experts recommend that these drugs be used with caution for the treatment of VTE in the morbidly obese population (those with BMI >40 kg/m² or body weight >120 kg). While there is some experience with the use of apixaban and rivaroxaban in this patient population, data are insufficient with edoxaban.

Efficacy and safety of edoxaban for the treatment of VTE have been established in a randomized, double-blind noninferiority trial (Hokusai VTE) in more than 8000 adults with acute venous thromboembolism. In this trial, edoxaban demonstrated noninferiority to warfarin in reducing the risk of recurrent venous thromboembolism and was associated with substantially reduced rates of clinically important bleeding. The Hokusai VTE trial was conducted in a broad population of patients with acute venous thromboembolism, including those with provoked (i.e., associated with a temporary risk factor) or unprovoked venous thromboembolism, and those with severe PE. All patients received initial therapy with heparin (enoxaparin or unfractionated heparin) on an open-label basis for at least 5 days; blinded treatment consisted of either edoxaban (60 mg daily, initiated after the heparin regimen was discontinued) or warfarin (initiated concurrently with heparin and dose-adjusted to achieve a therapeutic INR of 2–3), which was continued for a total of 3–12 months depending on the clinical situation. For those in the edoxaban treatment group, dosage was reduced to 30 mg daily if any of the following conditions anticipated to increase drug exposure, and thus bleeding, were present: estimated creatinine clearance of 30–50 mL/minute, body weight of 60 kg or less, or concomitant use of the potent P-glycoprotein inhibitors verapamil, quinidine, azithromycin, clarithromycin, erythromycin, oral itraconazole, or oral ketoconazole. The primary composite end point of DVT or nonfatal or fatal PE occurred in 3.2% of patients receiving edoxaban and 3.5% of those receiving warfarin during the 12-month trial period. The primary efficacy analysis was performed on a modified intent-to-treat population, which included all patients who underwent randomization and received at least one dose of study drug during the treatment period. With respect to the primary safety outcome, clinically relevant major or nonmajor bleeding occurred less frequently in patients receiving edoxaban than those receiving warfarin (8.5 versus 10.3%). Among patients who required a dosage reduction of edoxaban, bleeding rates were decreased without an apparent loss of efficacy. Patients who received warfarin in the trial achieved a median time in therapeutic INR range (2–3) of 65.6%.

Use of edoxaban in patients with cancer and acute VTE was evaluated in a randomized, open-label, noninferiority trial (Hokusai VTE Cancer). In this study, 1050 patients were randomized to receive oral edoxaban (60 mg daily) or subcutaneous dalteparin (200 units/kg daily [maximum of 18,000 units/day] for 30 days, followed by 150 units/kg daily) for a total of 6–12 months. All patients received initial therapy with therapeutic-dose LMWH for at least 5 days. Dosage of edoxaban was reduced to 30 mg daily if any of the following conditions anticipated to increase drug exposure, and thus bleeding, were present: estimated creatinine clearance of 30–50 mL/minute, body weight ≤60 kg, or concomitant use of the potent P-glycoprotein inhibitors ketoconazole, itraconazole, erythromycin, azithromycin, or clarithromycin. Nearly all randomized patients had active cancer; however, patients with basal cell or squamous cell carcinoma were excluded. Previous VTE was reported in 9.4 and 12% of patients in the edoxaban and dalteparin groups, respectively. Edoxaban was noninferior to dalteparin in reducing the risk of recurrent VTE or major bleeding. The primary efficacy analysis was performed on a modified intent-to-treat population, which included all patients who underwent randomization and received at least one dose of study drug during the treatment period. The primary composite end point of recurrent VTE or major bleeding occurred in 12.8% of patients receiving edoxaban and 13.5% of patients receiving dalteparin. When evaluated separately, recurrent VTE occurred in 7.9% of patients receiving edoxaban and 11.3% of patients receiving dalteparin; however, major bleeding was substantially increased with edoxaban (6.9%) compared with dalteparin (4%). This difference was primarily due to the higher rate of upper GI bleeding with edoxaban.

DOSAGE AND ADMINISTRATION

● General

Pretreatment Screening

Prior to initiating therapy with edoxaban, renal function should be assessed. Creatinine clearance should be calculated using the Cockcroft-Gault method as dosage recommendations for edoxaban are based on estimated creatinine clearance. Patients with nonvalvular atrial fibrillation who have creatinine clearance exceeding 95 mL/minute should not be treated with edoxaban. (See Reduced Efficacy in Nonvalvular Atrial Fibrillation Patients with Creatinine Clearance Exceeding 95 mL/minute under Cautions.)

Patient Monitoring

Routine coagulation monitoring (e.g., prothrombin time [PT], activated partial thromboplastin time [aPTT], international normalized ratio [INR]) is not necessary during edoxaban therapy because of the drug's predictable pharmacokinetic and pharmacodynamic effects. However, in certain situations, such as in the case of overdosage or in patients with hemorrhagic or thromboembolic complications or those requiring emergency surgery, it may be useful to assess the degree of anticoagulation. Although edoxaban has been shown to produce concentration-dependent increases in aPTT, PT, and INR, these tests are not useful for monitoring the anticoagulant effects of edoxaban because of a high degree of inconsistency, insensitivity, and variability in results.

● *Administration*

Edoxaban is administered orally without regard to food. (See Description.)

Edoxaban can be crushed and mixed with 2–3 ounces of water and immediately administered orally or through a gastric tube in patients unable to swallow whole tablets. Crushed tablets can also be mixed into applesauce and immediately administered orally.

If a dose of edoxaban is missed, the missed dose should be taken as soon as possible on the same day, followed by resumption of the regular schedule; the dose should not be doubled to make up for the missed dose.

● *Dosage*

Dosage of edoxaban tosylate monohydrate is expressed in terms of edoxaban.

Embolism Associated with Atrial Fibrillation

For the prevention of stroke and systemic embolism in adults with nonvalvular atrial fibrillation who have a creatinine clearance of 51–95 mL/minute, the recommended initial dosage of edoxaban is 60 mg once daily. Dosage should be reduced to 30 mg daily in patients with creatinine clearance of 15–50 mL/minute. (See Renal Impairment under Dosage and Administration.) The drug should *not* be used in patients with creatinine clearance exceeding 95 mL/minute.

Venous Thromboembolism

Treatment

The recommended dosage of edoxaban for the treatment of deep-vein thrombosis (DVT) and/or pulmonary embolism (PE) is 60 mg once daily following 5–10 days of initial therapy with a parenteral anticoagulant.

Dosage should be reduced to 30 mg once daily in patients with creatinine clearance of 15–50 mL/minute, body weight ≤60 kg, and/or in those receiving concomitant therapy with certain drugs that are potent P-glycoprotein inhibitors. In the Hokusai VTE trial, dosage of edoxaban was reduced in patients receiving concomitant therapy with verapamil or quinidine, or short-term treatment with azithromycin, clarithromycin, erythromycin, oral ketoconazole, or oral itraconazole. (See P-glycoprotein Inhibitors under Drug Interactions.)

The optimum duration of anticoagulant therapy in patients with venous thromboembolism (VTE) should be determined by the individual clinical situation (e.g., location of thrombi, presence or absence of precipitating factors for thrombosis, presence of cancer, risk of bleeding). In general, the American College of Chest Physicians (ACCP) states that anticoagulant therapy for VTE should be continued beyond the acute treatment period for at least 3 months and possibly longer in patients with a high risk of recurrence and low risk of bleeding.

Transitioning from Other Anticoagulant Therapy

When transitioning from warfarin to edoxaban therapy, the manufacturer states that warfarin should be discontinued and edoxaban initiated as soon as the INR is ≤2.5. When transitioning from other oral anticoagulants, the current anticoagulant should be discontinued and edoxaban initiated at the time of the next scheduled dose of the other anticoagulant.

When transitioning from low molecular weight heparin (LMWH) therapy to edoxaban, the LMWH should be discontinued and edoxaban initiated at the time of the next scheduled dose of the LMWH. In patients currently receiving unfractionated heparin by continuous IV infusion, the heparin infusion should be discontinued and edoxaban initiated 4 hours later.

Transitioning to Other Anticoagulant Therapy

When transitioning from edoxaban to warfarin therapy, a parenteral or oral conversion strategy can be used. In the parenteral method, edoxaban is discontinued and a parenteral anticoagulant and warfarin are initiated simultaneously at the time of the next scheduled dose of edoxaban; the parenteral anticoagulant is then discontinued once a stable INR of at least 2 is reached. The oral conversion strategy is similar to the end-of-trial transition plan that was used in the ENGAGE AF-TIMI trial and involves the use of a half-dose edoxaban bridging regimen with overlapping warfarin therapy. In this method, the current dose of edoxaban is decreased by 50% (60 to 30 mg or 30 to 15 mg) and warfarin is initiated simultaneously. The 2 drugs are administered concomitantly until a stable INR of at least 2 is achieved; once this occurs, edoxaban should be discontinued and warfarin continued. INR values should be monitored at least once a week, with testing performed just prior to the daily dose of edoxaban to minimize the effect of the drug on the INR.

When transitioning from edoxaban to other anticoagulants, including parenteral anticoagulants or other direct oral anticoagulants (DOACs), edoxaban should be discontinued and the other anticoagulant initiated at the time of the next scheduled dose of edoxaban.

Managing Anticoagulation in Patients Requiring Invasive Procedures

To minimize the risk of bleeding, edoxaban should be temporarily discontinued at least 24 hours prior to surgery or other invasive procedure. If surgery cannot be delayed, the potential increased risk of bleeding should be weighed against the urgency of the intervention. Edoxaban may be resumed postoperatively as soon as adequate hemostasis has been established; decisions regarding when to restart therapy should take into account the onset of the drug's pharmacodynamic effects (1–2 hours). If oral administration is not possible, a parenteral anticoagulant should be administered in the interim until edoxaban therapy can be resumed. (See Risk of Thrombosis Following Premature Discontinuance of Therapy under Cautions.)

● *Special Populations*

Hepatic Impairment

No dosage adjustment is necessary in patients with mild (Child-Pugh class A) hepatic impairment. Use of edoxaban is not recommended in patients with moderate (Child-Pugh class B) or severe (Child-Pugh class C) hepatic impairment. (See Hepatic Impairment under Cautions.)

Renal Impairment

Dosage of edoxaban should be reduced to 30 mg once daily in patients with creatinine clearance of 15–50 mL/minute, regardless of indication. The drug is not recommended in patients with creatinine clearance of less than 15 mL/minute. (See Renal Impairment under Cautions.)

Body Weight

Edoxaban exposure is increased in patients with low body weight (<60 kg), which may increase the risk of bleeding. The manufacturer makes no dosage adjustment recommendations based on weight in patients with nonvalvular atrial fibrillation. When used for the treatment of VTE, dosage of edoxaban should be reduced to 30 mg once daily in patients who weigh ≤60 kg.

CAUTIONS

● *Contraindications*

- Active pathologic bleeding.

● *Warnings/Precautions*

Warnings

Reduced Efficacy in Nonvalvular Atrial Fibrillation Patients with Creatinine Clearance Exceeding 95 mL/minute

The prescribing information for edoxaban has a boxed warning regarding reduced efficacy in patients with nonvalvular atrial fibrillation who have a creatinine clearance exceeding 95 mL/minute. The benefit of edoxaban in reducing ischemic stroke appears to be strongly dose and plasma-concentration dependent. Approximately half of a dose of edoxaban is eliminated by the kidneys, and plasma concentrations of the drug are lower in patients with better renal function (about 30% lower in patients with creatinine clearance >80 mL/minute and 40% lower in patients with creatinine clearance >95 mL/minute) compared to patients with creatinine clearance >50 to ≤80 mL/minute. Reduced antithrombotic efficacy was observed with edoxaban compared with warfarin in the ENGAGE AF-TIMI 48 study in patients with creatinine clearance exceeding 95 mL/minute. (See Embolism Associated with Atrial Fibrillation under Uses.)

Edoxaban should not be used in patients with creatinine clearance exceeding 95 mL/minute; in these patients, an alternative anticoagulant should be used.

Risk of Thrombosis Following Premature Discontinuance of Therapy

Premature discontinuance of any anticoagulant therapy, including edoxaban, in the absence of adequate alternative anticoagulation increases the risk of thromboembolic events. A boxed warning about this risk is included in the prescribing information for edoxaban. When transitioning patients from one anticoagulant therapy to another, it is important to ensure continuous anticoagulation while minimizing the risk of bleeding. Particular caution is advised when switching patients from a factor Xa inhibitor to warfarin therapy because of the slow onset of action of warfarin.

If discontinuance of edoxaban is required for reasons other than pathologic bleeding or completion of a course of therapy, coverage with an alternative anticoagulant should be considered. (See Dosage under Dosage and Administration.) Patients should be advised about the importance of adhering to the therapeutic regimen and instructed on steps to take if doses are missed. (See Advice to Patients.)

Spinal/Epidural Hematoma

Patients receiving anticoagulants are at risk of developing an epidural or spinal hematoma when concomitant neuraxial (epidural/spinal) anesthesia or spinal puncture is employed; such complications can result in long-term or permanent paralysis. A boxed warning about this risk is included in the prescribing information for edoxaban. The risk of these adverse events may be increased by use of indwelling epidural catheters or by concomitant use of drugs affecting hemostasis, such as nonsteroidal anti-inflammatory agents (NSAIAs), platelet inhibitors, or other anticoagulants. Risk also may be increased in patients with a history of traumatic or repeated epidural or spinal punctures or a history of spinal deformity or spinal surgery.

Although optimal timing between the administration of edoxaban and neuraxial procedures is not known, the manufacturer states that removal of an indwelling epidural or intrathecal catheter should be delayed for at least 12 hours after the last administered dose of edoxaban, and at least 2 hours should elapse following removal of the catheter prior to administration of the next edoxaban dose.

Patients receiving edoxaban in the setting of epidural or spinal anesthesia should be monitored frequently for manifestations of neurologic impairment (e.g., numbness or weakness of the legs, bowel or bladder dysfunction). If neurologic compromise is noted, urgent diagnosis and treatment are necessary. Clinicians should consider the potential benefits versus risks of neuraxial intervention in patients who are currently receiving or will receive anticoagulants.

Other Warnings and Precautions

Bleeding

Edoxaban increases the risk of hemorrhage and can cause serious, potentially fatal, bleeding. Patients should be promptly evaluated if any manifestations of blood loss occur during therapy. The drug should be discontinued if active pathological bleeding occurs. (See Contraindications under Cautions.) However, minor or "nuisance" bleeding is a common occurrence in patients receiving any anticoagulant and should not readily lead to treatment discontinuance. (See Risk of Thrombosis Following Premature Discontinuance of Therapy under Cautions.)

Bleeding complications were the most common adverse effects of edoxaban in clinical trials. In the principal efficacy trial of edoxaban in patients with nonvalvular atrial fibrillation (ENGAGE AF-TIMI 48), major bleeding (i.e., clinically overt bleeding at a critical organ/site or accompanied by a hemoglobin decrease of at least 2 g/dL when adjusted for transfusions or fatal bleeding) occurred at a rate of 2.75% per year with edoxaban 60 mg and 1.61% per year with edoxaban

30 mg; these rates were substantially lower than the rate of major bleeding in patients who received warfarin (3.43% per year). The rate of major GI bleeding was substantially higher with edoxaban 60 mg compared with warfarin (1.51 versus 1.23%), but the lower dosage of edoxaban (30 mg) was associated with the lowest rate of major GI bleeding (0.82%). In a dose-ranging study in patients with atrial fibrillation receiving edoxaban daily in 1 or 2 divided doses (twice-daily dosing currently not FDA-labeled), trough edoxaban concentrations and the frequency of bleeding complications were higher with 30 mg twice daily than with 60 mg once daily. In the Hokusai VTE trial in patients with acute venous thromboembolism (VTE), clinically relevant bleeding (major or nonmajor) occurred in 8.5% of patients receiving edoxaban 60 mg, which was substantially lower than the rate in patients receiving warfarin (10.3%). In the Hokusai VTE Cancer study in patients with cancer and VTE, rates of major, clinically relevant nonmajor, and GI bleeding were substantially higher with edoxaban (6.1, 13.4, and 4.2%, respectively) compared with dalteparin (3.1, 9.2, and 0.8%, respectively). However, the difference in bleeding between these agents appeared to occur primarily in patients with GI cancer. In patients without GI cancer, major bleeding occurred in 3.6 and 3.3% of patients receiving edoxaban and dalteparin, respectively.

Risk of bleeding may be increased in patients with renal impairment, low body weight (e.g., <60 kg), or in those receiving concomitant drugs that affect hemostasis (e.g., aspirin or other antiplatelet drugs, other anticoagulants, chronic use of NSAIAs). (See Drug Interactions.) Edoxaban therapy should be temporarily interrupted prior to surgery or other invasive procedure to minimize the risk of bleeding. (See Managing Anticoagulation in Patients Requiring Invasive Procedures under Dosage and Administration.)

There is no specific reversal agent for edoxaban; anticoagulant effects can be expected to persist for approximately 24 hours after the drug is discontinued. Although coagulation factor Xa (recombinant) inactivated-zhzo (also referred to as andexanet alfa) is not FDA-labeled for reversal of edoxaban, the North American Anticoagulation Forum suggests that the drug may be used if needed in patients with life-threatening bleeding or need for emergent invasive procedures; use of a high dose (800 mg administered IV at a rate of 30 mg/minute followed by a continuous infusion of 8 mg/minute for up to 120 minutes) is recommended. In a phase 2 study in 26 healthy individuals, andexanet alfa rapidly reversed edoxaban-induced anti-factor Xa activity and inhibition of thrombin generation. The use of prothrombin complex concentrates (PCCs), activated prothrombin complex concentrate (aPCC), or recombinant factor VIIa may be considered for reversal of edoxaban; however, clinical outcomes studies have not been conducted. Preliminary findings from a study in healthy individuals suggest that PCC may be an effective reversal agent for edoxaban. In this study, administration of a 4-factor PCC reversed the effects of edoxaban 60 mg in a dose-dependent manner. At the highest dose studied (50 unit/kg), the PCC completely reversed bleeding duration and endogenous thrombin potential and partially reversed PT. Mean endogenous thrombin potential continued to increase and exceeded the pre-edoxaban baseline by approximately 40% at 22 hours following PCC administration. The clinical relevance of this increase in endogenous thrombin potential is unknown. When PCCs are used, monitoring for anticoagulation effect of edoxaban using PT, INR, aPTT, or anti-factor Xa activity is not useful and is not recommended. Protamine sulfate, vitamin K, and tranexamic acid are not expected to be effective in reversing the anticoagulant effects of edoxaban. Edoxaban is not appreciably removed by dialysis.

Patients with Prosthetic Heart Valves or Mitral Stenosis

Safety and efficacy of edoxaban have not been evaluated in patients with mechanical heart valves or moderate to severe mitral stenosis; use of the drug is not recommended in such patients.

● Increased Risk of Thrombosis in Patients with Triple-Positive Antiphospholipid Syndrome

Edoxaban and other DOACs are not recommended for use in patients with triple-positive antiphospholipid syndrome (APS) (i.e., positive for lupus anticoagulant, anticardiolipin antibodies, and anti-beta 2-glycoprotein I antibodies). Treatment with DOACs has been associated with increased rates of recurrent thrombotic events compared with warfarin treatment in patients with APS, especially those with triple-positive APS. The International Society of Thrombosis and Haemostasis recommends the use of warfarin over DOACs in patients with high-risk APS, including those with triple-positive APS.

Specific Populations

Pregnancy

There are no adequate or well-controlled studies of edoxaban in pregnant women; use of the drug in pregnant women is not recommended. In animal studies, edoxaban was not teratogenic at exposure levels 49 times the maximum recommended human dose based on BSA; however, fetotoxic effects, including gallbladder abnormalities, postimplantation pregnancy loss, spontaneous abortion, decreased live fetuses, and decreased fetal weight, occurred at maternally toxic doses. Edoxaban use during labor or delivery in women receiving neuraxial anesthesia may result in epidural or spinal hematomas. (See Spinal/Epidural Hematoma under Cautions.) Use of a shorter-acting anticoagulant should be considered as delivery approaches. Edoxaban should be used during pregnancy only if the potential benefits justify the potential risks to the fetus. Edoxaban may increase the risk of bleeding in the fetus or neonate. Careful monitoring for bleeding is recommended.

Lactation

Edoxaban is distributed into milk in rats; it is not known whether the drug is distributed into human milk. Because of the potential for serious adverse reactions to edoxaban in nursing infants, including hemorrhage, the manufacturer states that breast-feeding is not recommended during treatment with edoxaban.

Females of Reproductive Potential

Edoxaban can cause significant uterine bleeding. Females of reproductive potential and those with abnormal uterine bleeding should be assessed for increased risk of clinically significant uterine bleeding, potentially requiring gynecologic surgical intervention. (See Advice to Patients.)

Pediatric Use

Safety and efficacy of edoxaban have not been established in pediatric patients.

Geriatric Use

No substantial differences in efficacy and safety have been observed in geriatric patients ≥65 years of age relative to younger adults in clinical trials of edoxaban. In the ENGAGE AF-TIMI 48 trial, 74% of patients were ≥65 years of age, and 41% were ≥75 years of age. In the Hokusai VTE trial, 32% of patients were ≥65 years of age, and 14% were ≥75 years of age. In the Hokusai VTE Cancer study, 52% of patients were ≥65 years of age, and 17% were ≥75 years of age.

Hepatic Impairment

Mild (Child-Pugh class A) or moderate (Child-Pugh class B) hepatic impairment does not appear to affect pharmacokinetics or pharmacodynamics of edoxaban. Data on the drug are lacking in patients with severe hepatic impairment (Child-Pugh class C). (See Hepatic Impairment under Dosage and Administration.)

Edoxaban should not be used in patients with moderate or severe hepatic impairment because of the possibility of intrinsic coagulation abnormalities in such patients.

Renal Impairment

Edoxaban is eliminated renally. (See Description.) Clearance of edoxaban is decreased, and consequently, plasma concentrations are increased in patients with renal impairment. In a dedicated pharmacokinetic study in individuals with various degrees of renal dysfunction, systemic exposure of edoxaban was increased by 32, 74, and 72% in those with creatinine clearances of 51–79 mL/minute, 30–50 mL/minute, and <30 mL/minute, respectively, compared with that in individuals with normal renal function (creatinine clearance of ≥80 mL/minute). Systemic exposure of edoxaban was increased by 93% in patients undergoing peritoneal dialysis. Patients with creatinine clearance <15 mL/minute were not evaluated.

Renal function should be evaluated prior to initiating edoxaban therapy and periodically thereafter when clinically indicated. Assessment of renal function should include calculation of estimated creatinine clearance using the Cockcroft-Gault method. Recommendations regarding use and dosage of edoxaban are based on creatinine clearance. (See Dosage and Administration.) As renal function improves, plasma concentrations of edoxaban may decrease and potentially decrease efficacy of the drug. (See Reduced Efficacy in Nonvalvular Atrial Fibrillation Patients with Creatinine Clearance Exceeding 95 mL/minute under Cautions.)

Hemodialysis does not substantially contribute to clearance of edoxaban. Following a 4-hour hemodialysis session, total drug exposure was reduced by <7%.

● Common Adverse Effects

In studies in patients with nonvalvular atrial fibrillation, the most common adverse effects of edoxaban were bleeding and anemia. In studies in patients with acute venous thromboembolism, the most common adverse effects of the drug were bleeding, rash, abnormal liver function tests, and anemia.

DRUG INTERACTIONS

● Drugs Affecting or Metabolized by Hepatic Microsomal Enzymes

Edoxaban is minimally metabolized by cytochrome P-450 (CYP) 3A4; drug interactions are unlikely with inhibitors or inducers of this isoenzyme.

In vitro studies indicate that edoxaban does not inhibit the major CYP isoenzymes (CYP1A2, 2A6, 2B6, 2C8/9, 2C19, 2D6, 2E1, or 3A4) nor induce CYP1A2 or CYP3A4; drug interactions involving these pathways are unlikely.

● Drugs Affecting Efflux Transport Systems

Edoxaban is a substrate of the efflux transporter P-glycoprotein, but does not appear to be a substrate of other major uptake transporters such as organic anion transporters OAT1 and OAT3, organic cation transporter OCT2, or organic anion transporting polypeptide OATP1B1. In vitro studies indicate that edoxaban does not induce the P-glycoprotein transporter. In addition, the drug does not substantially inhibit P-glycoprotein, OAT1, OAT3, OCT1, OCT2, OATP1B1, or OATP1B3.

P-glycoprotein Inhibitors

Concomitant use of edoxaban with P-glycoprotein inhibitors may potentially increase edoxaban exposure; the potential for clinically important effects depends on the degree of P-glycoprotein inhibition. Drug interaction studies have demonstrated substantially increased peak plasma concentrations and systemic exposure of edoxaban when coadministered with the following potent P-glycoprotein inhibitors: ketoconazole, quinidine, verapamil, erythromycin, cyclosporine, and dronedarone. Concomitant administration of edoxaban with amiodarone, also a potent P-glycoprotein inhibitor, increased systemic exposure of edoxaban to a more modest extent. When coadministered with drugs with weaker affinity for the P-glycoprotein transporter (e.g., atorvastatin, digoxin), pharmacokinetics of edoxaban were only slightly altered.

The manufacturer states that based on criteria used in clinical studies, dosage of edoxaban should be reduced in patients with acute venous thromboembolism (VTE) who are receiving certain P-glycoprotein inhibitors; in the Hokusai VTE and Hokusai VTE Cancer trials, dosage of edoxaban was reduced for concomitant therapy with verapamil, quinidine, azithromycin, clarithromycin, erythromycin, oral itraconazole, and oral ketoconazole. (See Dosage under Dosage and Administration.) In patients with nonvalvular atrial fibrillation, no edoxaban dosage adjustment is necessary for concomitant P-glycoprotein inhibitors since patients in whom such dosages were adjusted in the ENGAGE AF-TIMI 48 trial had lower plasma edoxaban concentrations than those who received the full dosage of the drug.

P-glycoprotein Inducers

Concomitant use of edoxaban with P-glycoprotein inducers may potentially decrease edoxaban exposure. Systemic exposure of edoxaban was substantially reduced when the drug was coadministered with rifampin, a known P-glycoprotein inducer; the manufacturer states that concomitant use of edoxaban and rifampin should be avoided.

● Drugs Affecting Hemostasis

Concomitant use of drugs that affect hemostasis (e.g., aspirin or other antiplatelet agents, other anticoagulants, fibrinolytics, nonsteroidal anti-inflammatory agents [NSAIAs]), selective serotonin-reuptake inhibitors [SSRIs], selective norepinephrine-reuptake inhibitors [SNRIs]) can increase the risk of bleeding associated with edoxaban. (See Bleeding under Cautions.)

Anticoagulant Agents

When edoxaban was administered concomitantly with enoxaparin, no substantial changes in the pharmacokinetics of either drug were observed.

Because of the risk of bleeding, long-term concomitant use of edoxaban and other anticoagulants is not recommended; however, short-term concomitant therapy may be necessary in patients transitioning from one anticoagulant to another.

Antiplatelet Agents

In a study in healthy individuals, bleeding time was increased by approximately twofold from baseline when edoxaban and aspirin (100 or 325 mg) were administered concomitantly relative to administration of either drug alone. The higher dose of aspirin (325 mg) increased peak plasma concentrations and systemic exposure of edoxaban, but the lower aspirin dose did not affect pharmacokinetics of edoxaban. The anticoagulant effects of edoxaban (i.e., activated partial thromboplastin time [aPTT], prothrombin time [PT], international normalized ratio [INR], anti-factor Xa activity, intrinsic factor Xa activity) were not altered by aspirin.

In clinical studies, patients who received edoxaban and aspirin concurrently had increased rates of clinically relevant bleeding; patients requiring chronic treatment with aspirin during edoxaban therapy should be carefully monitored for bleeding.

NSAIAs

In a study in healthy individuals, concomitant administration of edoxaban and naproxen (500 mg) increased bleeding time by approximately twofold from baseline relative to administration of either drug alone. Naproxen did not alter the pharmacokinetics or anticoagulant effects (i.e., as indicated by aPTT, PT, INR, anti-factor Xa activity, intrinsic factor Xa activity) of edoxaban.

In clinical studies, patients who received edoxaban and NSAIAs concurrently had increased rates of clinically relevant bleeding; patients requiring long-term treatment with an NSAIA during edoxaban therapy should be carefully monitored for bleeding.

SSRIs/SNRIs

SSRIs and SNRIs have antiplatelet effects that may increase the risk of bleeding when used in combination with anticoagulants, including edoxaban. Patients requiring concomitant treatment with edoxaban and SSRIs or SNRIs should be carefully monitored for bleeding.

● Amiodarone

Peak plasma concentrations and systemic exposure of edoxaban increased by approximately 66 and 40%, respectively, when the drug was administered concomitantly with amiodarone. (See Drugs Affecting Efflux Transport Systems under Drug Interactions.)

● Atorvastatin

Peak plasma concentrations of edoxaban were decreased by 14.2% and systemic exposure increased by 1.7% when the drug was administered concomitantly with atorvastatin. (See Drugs Affecting Efflux Transport Systems under Drug Interactions.)

● Azole Antifungals

Peak plasma concentrations and systemic exposure of edoxaban were substantially increased with concomitant administration of ketoconazole. Dosage of edoxaban should be reduced when the drug is administered concomitantly with oral itraconazole or oral ketoconazole in patients with VTE. (See Drugs Affecting Efflux Transport Systems under Drug Interactions.)

● Cyclosporine

Peak plasma concentrations and systemic exposure of edoxaban were substantially increased with concomitant administration of cyclosporine. (See Drugs Affecting Efflux Transport Systems under Drug Interactions.)

● Digoxin

In healthy individuals, concomitant administration of edoxaban and digoxin did not substantially affect peak plasma concentrations or systemic exposure of edoxaban. Although peak plasma concentrations of digoxin were increased by 28%, such concentrations remained within the established therapeutic range. Clinically important changes in the pharmacodynamics of either drug were not observed.

● Dronedarone

Dronedarone increased peak plasma concentrations and systemic exposure of edoxaban by approximately 46 and 85%, respectively. (See Drugs Affecting Efflux Transport Systems under Drug Interactions.)

● Esomeprazole

Peak plasma concentrations of edoxaban were decreased with concomitant administration of esomeprazole; however, systemic exposure of edoxaban was not substantially affected.

● Macrolide Antibiotics

Peak plasma concentrations and systemic exposure of edoxaban were substantially increased with concomitant administration of erythromycin. Dosage of edoxaban should be reduced when the drug is administered concomitantly with erythromycin, azithromycin, or clarithromycin in patients with VTE. (See Drugs Affecting Efflux Transport Systems under Drug Interactions.)

● Quinidine

Quinidine increased peak plasma concentrations and systemic exposure of edoxaban by approximately 85 and 77%, respectively, but edoxaban did not affect pharmacokinetics of quinidine. Dosage of edoxaban should be reduced when the drug is administered concomitantly with quinidine in patients with VTE. (See Drugs Affecting Efflux Transport Systems under Drug Interactions.)

● Verapamil

Verapamil increased peak plasma concentrations and systemic exposure of edoxaban by approximately 53%; pharmacokinetic parameters of verapamil were altered to only a slight extent. Dosage of edoxaban should be reduced when the drug is administered concomitantly with verapamil in patients with VTE. (See Drugs Affecting Efflux Transport Systems under Drug Interactions.)

DESCRIPTION

Edoxaban, an oral, direct activated factor X (Xa) inhibitor, is an anticoagulant. Factor Xa plays a central role in the blood coagulation cascade by serving as the convergence point for the intrinsic and extrinsic pathways; inhibition of coagulation factor Xa by edoxaban prevents conversion of prothrombin to thrombin and subsequent thrombus formation. The drug binds directly and selectively to factor Xa without the need for a cofactor (e.g., antithrombin III), and inhibits both free and prothrombinase-bound factor Xa as well as thrombin-induced platelet aggregation.

Edoxaban inhibits factor Xa activity, and prolongs prothrombin time (PT), activated partial thromboplastin time (aPTT), and the international normalized ratio (INR) in a dose-dependent manner. A rapid and predictable anticoagulant effect is demonstrated by linear correlations between plasma edoxaban concentrations and coagulation parameters.

Edoxaban exhibits dose-proportional pharmacokinetics over the dosage range of 10–150 mg daily. The drug is rapidly absorbed following oral administration, with peak plasma concentrations occurring within 1–3 hours. The absolute bioavailability of the drug is approximately 62%. The bioavailability is not altered when edoxaban 60-mg tablets are crushed and mixed in either applesauce or suspended in water and given orally or through a nasogastric tube. Food delays absorption, but does not substantially alter systemic exposure of edoxaban. Approximately 50% of edoxaban is excreted unchanged in urine; the remainder is metabolized (minimally by hydrolysis, conjugation, and cytochrome P-450 [CYP] 3A4) and eliminated through biliary and intestinal routes. The terminal half-life of edoxaban is approximately 10–14 hours. Edoxaban is approximately 55% bound to plasma proteins. Systemic exposure of the drug is increased in patients with renal impairment and low body weight, but does not appear to be affected by age, gender, or race/ethnicity.

ADVICE TO PATIENTS

- Importance of taking the drug exactly as prescribed and not discontinuing therapy without first consulting clinician.
- Importance of advising patients who cannot swallow edoxaban tablets whole to crush the tablets and combine with 2–3 ounces of water or applesauce and ingest immediately.
- Importance of advising patients with a gastric tube to crush edoxaban tablets and mix with 2–3 ounces of water and administer immediately via gastric tube.
- Importance of informing patients that they may bruise and/or bleed more easily and that a longer than normal time may be required to stop bleeding when taking edoxaban. Importance of patient informing clinicians about any unusual bleeding or bruising during therapy.
- Importance of advising patients that if a dose is missed, it should be taken as soon as possible on the same day; the regular dosing schedule should be resumed the following day. A dose should not be doubled to make up for a missed dose.
- Importance of advising patients undergoing neuraxial anesthesia or spinal puncture procedures to immediately report manifestations of spinal or epidural hematoma (e.g., tingling or numbness in lower limbs, muscle weakness, back pain, stool or urine incontinence) to clinician.

- Importance of patients informing clinicians that they are receiving edoxaban therapy before scheduling any medical, surgical, or invasive procedure, including dental procedures.
- Importance of women immediately informing clinicians if they are or plan to become pregnant. Importance of informing patients not to breast-feed while taking edoxaban.
- Importance of informing clinicians of existing or contemplated concomitant therapy, including prescription and OTC drugs and herbal supplements, as well as any concomitant illnesses.
- Importance of informing patients of other important precautionary information. (See Cautions.)

PREPARATIONS

Excipients in commercially available drug preparations may have clinically important effects in some individuals; consult specific product labeling for details.

Edoxaban Tosylate

Oral		
Tablets	15 mg (of edoxaban)	**Savaysa®**, Daiichi Sankyo
	30 mg (of edoxaban)	**Savaysa®**, Daiichi Sankyo
	60 mg (of edoxaban)	**Savaysa®**, Daiichi Sankyo

Rivaroxaban

20:12.04.14 • DIRECT FACTOR Xa INHIBITORS

■ Rivaroxaban, an oral, direct activated factor X (Xa) inhibitor, is an anticoagulant.

USES

● Embolism Associated with Atrial Fibrillation

Nonvalvular Atrial Fibrillation

Rivaroxaban is used to reduce the risk of stroke and systemic embolism in adults with nonvalvular atrial fibrillation. The direct oral anticoagulants (DOACs; apixaban, dabigatran, edoxaban, rivaroxaban) have been shown in randomized controlled studies to be noninferior, and in some trials, superior to warfarin in reducing thromboembolic risk in patients with nonvalvular atrial fibrillation (i.e., atrial fibrillation in the absence of moderate-to-severe mitral stenosis or a mechanical heart valve), and are associated with reduced risk of serious bleeding. Current evidence suggests that rivaroxaban is no less effective than warfarin for prevention of stroke and systemic embolism in patients with nonvalvular atrial fibrillation and does not increase the risk of major bleeding relative to warfarin. However, there are limited data on the relative efficacy of rivaroxaban and warfarin for the reduction of stroke and systemic embolism when warfarin anticoagulation is well controlled.

Clinical Experience

Efficacy and safety of rivaroxaban for the prevention of stroke and systemic embolism in patients with nonvalvular atrial fibrillation were evaluated in a randomized, double-blind, noninferiority study (ROCKET AF) in approximately 14,000 adults with nonvalvular atrial fibrillation who were considered to be at moderate to high risk of stroke (defined as having a history of stroke, transient ischemic attack (TIA), non-CNS systemic embolism, or at least 2 of the following additional risk factors: age ≥75 years, hypertension, heart failure or left ventricular ejection fraction of ≤35%, or diabetes mellitus). The study population consisted principally of Caucasian men with a mean age of 71 years and a mean Congestive Heart Failure, Hypertension, Age, Diabetes, Stroke (doubled) (i.e., $CHADS_2$) score of 3.5; approximately 55% of patients had a history of stroke, TIA, or non-CNS systemic embolism. Patients received either rivaroxaban (20 mg once daily for those with a creatinine clearance of at least 50 mL/minute or 15 mg once daily for those with a creatinine clearance of 30–49 mL/minute) or adjusted-dose warfarin (titrated to an international normalized ratio [INR] of 2-3) for a median duration of 590 days; median follow-up was 707 days.

The primary composite end point of the study was the incidence of stroke (hemorrhagic or ischemic) and non-CNS systemic embolism. The primary efficacy analysis was performed in the per-protocol (as-treated) population, which included all patients who received at least one dose of a study drug, did not have a major protocol violation, and were followed for events while receiving a study drug or within 2 days after discontinuance of the drug. Outcome analyses also were performed in the intent-to-treat (per-randomization) population, which included all patients who underwent randomization and were followed for events during treatment or following premature discontinuance, and the safety population, which included all patients who received at least one dose of a study drug and were followed for events while they were receiving study drug or within 2 days after discontinuation, regardless of protocol adherence. Testing for superiority was performed if noninferiority was achieved.

Rivaroxaban was noninferior to warfarin for the primary composite outcome of first occurrence of stroke or non-CNS systemic embolism; noninferiority was demonstrated in both the per-protocol and intent-to-treat populations. Efficacy of rivaroxaban was consistent across a variety of patient subgroups, including in those with renal insufficiency, different $CHADS_2$ scores, prior warfarin use, and history of stroke. Superiority of rivaroxaban over warfarin was not demonstrated in the intent-to-treat population in this study; the rate of stroke or non-CNS systemic embolism with rivaroxaban therapy was no different than

that observed with warfarin therapy (annualized event rate of 2.1 and 2.4% of patients, respectively). However, superiority of rivaroxaban over warfarin was shown in the as-treated safety population. This difference in the results of superiority testing may be explained by the inclusion of embolic events in patients who discontinued drug treatment prematurely as well as those occurring during study drug treatment in the intent-to-treat population, while analysis of the per-protocol population only included events that occurred during drug treatment and for 2 days after drug discontinuance. In addition, a requirement for anticoagulation following study drug discontinuation was not specified in the ROCKET AF protocol; however, patients in the warfarin group generally continued to receive warfarin after the treatment portion of the study, while those who had received rivaroxaban during the treatment portion were switched to warfarin without a period of overlap and therefore were not adequately anticoagulated until a therapeutic INR with warfarin was obtained. During the 28 days following the end of the study, a higher incidence of stroke was observed in patients who had received rivaroxaban compared with those who had received warfarin. There was no statistically significant difference in the risk of major and nonmajor clinically important bleeding between the treatment groups, although intracranial and fatal bleeding occurred less frequently in patients receiving rivaroxaban.

Patients who received warfarin in the ROCKET AF study had INRs within the therapeutic range of 2–3 only 55% of the time on average, which is lower than that reported with warfarin anticoagulation in other trials of DOACs (e.g., dabigatran, apixaban, edoxaban) in patients with atrial fibrillation (e.g., 62–64%). It has been suggested that this difference may be explained in part by the inclusion of a higher-risk patient population in the ROCKET AF trial or to geographic variations among the study sites with respect to warfarin anticoagulation management skills. Therefore, data currently are insufficient to establish the relative efficacy of rivaroxaban and warfarin for the reduction of stroke and systemic embolism when warfarin therapy is well controlled.

The risk of stroke in patients with atrial flutter is similar to the risk in those with atrial fibrillation. Experts state that antithrombotic therapy in patients with atrial flutter generally should be managed in the same manner as in patients with atrial fibrillation or atrial flutter.

DOACs including rivaroxaban also have been used for therapeutic anticoagulation prior to and after cardioversion in patients with atrial fibrillation† of greater than 48 hours' duration or of unknown duration; DOACs are recommended as a safe and effective alternative to warfarin in this setting.

Clinical Perspective

The American College of Chest Physicians (ACCP), the American College of Cardiology (ACC), the American Heart Association (AHA), the American Stroke Association (ASA), and other experts currently recommend that antithrombotic therapy be administered to all patients with nonvalvular atrial fibrillation (i.e., atrial fibrillation in the absence of rheumatic mitral stenosis, a prosthetic heart valve, or mitral valve repair) who are considered to be at increased risk of stroke, unless such therapy is contraindicated. Although many risk stratification methods have been used, current guidelines recommend the use of the CHA_2DS_2-VASc risk stratification tool for assessing a patient's risk of stroke and need for anticoagulant therapy. Established clinical risk factors for stroke include prior ischemic stroke or TIA, advanced age (e.g., ≥65 years), history of hypertension, diabetes mellitus, vascular disease, and congestive heart failure; in addition, female sex has been identified as a factor that can modify the risk of stroke. The presence of stroke or TIA places a patient in the high-risk category regardless of other risk factors. Experts state that antithrombotic therapy generally is not necessary in low-risk patients (CHA_2DS_2-VASc score of 0 in males, or 1 in females), but should be considered or recommended in patients with one or more non-sex CHA_2DS_2-VASc stroke risk factors (CHA_2DS_2-VASc score of ≥1 in males, or ≥2 in females). Patients also should be assessed for their risk of bleeding; those with a high risk of bleeding should be monitored more closely.

In patients with nonvalvular atrial fibrillation who are eligible for oral anticoagulant therapy, DOACs are recommended over warfarin based on improved safety and similar or improved efficacy in clinical trials and meta-analyses. A substantially greater benefit of DOACs versus warfarin has been observed when the INR was in the therapeutic range less than 66% of the time. If warfarin is used, patients should be optimally managed with well-controlled INRs (e.g., INR in therapeutic range more than 70% of the time). A DOAC is recommended in patients unable to achieve optimal warfarin management.

Patient age, body weight, and renal and hepatic function should be considered prior to treatment with DOACs. There are limited data on the use of DOACs in obese patients and some experts have discouraged the use of these agents in the morbidly obese population (those with a body mass index [BMI] >40 kg/m^2 or body weight >120 kg). However, the various DOAC agents may have different outcomes. Because of limited data with DOACs in patients with morbid obesity, guidelines recommend considering warfarin over DOACs in morbidly obese patients with nonvalvular atrial fibrillation.

Because of the lack of direct, comparative studies, the relative efficacy and safety of rivaroxaban compared to other DOACs for the prevention of stroke in patients with nonvalvular atrial fibrillation remain to be fully elucidated. Some evidence from indirect comparisons suggests that there may be important differences (e.g., bleeding risk) between these agents; however, results of such analyses should be interpreted with caution because of possible confounding factors (e.g., differences in study design and methods, patient populations, and anticoagulation control). Selection of an appropriate anticoagulant for patients with nonvalvular atrial fibrillation should be individualized based on the absolute and relative risks of stroke and bleeding; costs; patient compliance, preference, tolerance, and comorbidities; and other clinical factors such as renal function and degree of INR control if the patient has been taking warfarin.

Valvular Heart Disease

Use of rivaroxaban is not recommended in patients with prosthetic heart valves. In the GALILEO study, patients with transcatheter aortic valve replacement who received rivaroxaban experienced higher rates of death and bleeding compared to patients randomized to an antiplatelet regimen. Safety and efficacy of rivaroxaban have not been established in patients with other prosthetic heart valves or other valve procedures.

The 2020 AHA/ACC guideline for the management of patients with valvular heart disease states that patients with valvular heart disease and atrial fibrillation† should be evaluated for risk of thromboembolic events and treated with oral anticoagulation if at high risk. Vitamin K antagonists are the anticoagulants of choice for patients with rheumatic mitral stenosis and mechanical heart valves. Rivaroxaban and other DOACs are an alternative to vitamin K antagonists in patients with atrial fibrillation and a bioprosthetic valve more than 3 months after implantation or with native valvular heart disease excluding rheumatic mitral stenosis.

• Venous Thromboembolism – Treatment and Secondary Prevention

Rivaroxaban is used for the initial treatment of acute deep-vein thrombosis (DVT) and/or pulmonary embolism (PE) in adults. The drug is also used beyond the initial 6 months of treatment to reduce the risk of recurrent venous thromboembolic events (secondary prevention) in adults with DVT and/or PE.

Rivaroxaban is also used for the treatment of venous thromboembolism (VTE) and reduction in the risk of recurrent VTE in pediatric patients (from birth to <18 years of age) after at least 5 days of initial parenteral anticoagulant therapy.

The manufacturer states that rivaroxaban is not recommended acutely (as an alternative to unfractionated heparin) in patients with PE who have hemodynamic instability or who may receive thrombolytic therapy or undergo pulmonary embolectomy.

Clinical Experience in Adults

Use of rivaroxaban for the treatment of DVT and PE in adults was evaluated in 2 randomized, open-label, noninferiority studies (EINSTEIN DVT and EINSTEIN PE); in these studies, rivaroxaban was noninferior to therapy with enoxaparin and a vitamin K antagonist in preventing recurrent thromboembolic events. A total of 8281 patients were included; the mean age was approximately 57 years, 55% of the patients were male, and 70% were Caucasian. Patients received either rivaroxaban (15 mg twice daily for 3 weeks, followed by 20 mg once daily) or a standard anticoagulant regimen consisting of enoxaparin sodium (1 mg/kg subcutaneously twice daily for at least 5 days) with a vitamin K antagonist (warfarin or acenocoumarol adjusted to maintain an INR of 2–3). The average duration of therapy in both treatment groups was

approximately 200 days. The primary efficacy outcome in these studies was a composite of symptomatic recurrent DVT or nonfatal or fatal PE. The primary efficacy outcome (based on the intent-to-treat population) occurred in 2.1 and 3% of patients receiving rivaroxaban and standard therapy, respectively, in the EINSTEIN DVT study, and in 2.1 and 1.8% of patients receiving rivaroxaban and standard therapy, respectively, in the EINSTEIN PE study. The incidence of major and clinically relevant nonmajor bleeding was similar between the treatment groups.

In a double-blind, placebo-controlled extension study (EINSTEIN EXT) in patients who had already completed a course of anticoagulant therapy with rivaroxaban or a vitamin K antagonist, continued treatment with rivaroxaban was substantially more effective than placebo in reducing the rate of recurrent DVT, nonfatal PE, or fatal PE. Patients in the extension study received rivaroxaban 20 mg daily or placebo for an additional 6 or 12 months (average duration of 190 days). Recurrent thromboembolism occurred in 1.3% of patients receiving rivaroxaban compared with 7.1% of those receiving placebo. Major bleeding occurred in 0.7% of patients in the rivaroxaban group and in none of the patients in the placebo group.

Use of rivaroxaban for reduction in the recurrence of DVT and PE was evaluated in the EINSTEIN CHOICE study, a multinational, double-blind, superiority study in patients requiring extended anticoagulation following an acute VTE. The study demonstrated that continued treatment with a prophylactic dose of rivaroxaban (10 mg once daily) was substantially more effective than low-dose aspirin (100 mg once daily) in reducing the risk of a recurrent thromboembolic event (DVT or PE), without a substantial increase in bleeding. Patients had been treated previously with a vitamin K antagonist or a DOAC (e.g., dabigatran, rivaroxaban, apixaban, edoxaban) for a provoked or unprovoked VTE (51% DVT only, 33% PE only, 16% combined DVT and PE). In the study, patients received 10 or 20 mg of rivaroxaban or 100 mg of enteric-coated aspirin once daily for up to 1 year following the initial 6–12 months of anticoagulant therapy. Patients who required extended anticoagulation therapy at therapeutic doses or antiplatelet therapy were excluded from the study. The primary efficacy outcome was a composite of symptomatic, recurrent fatal or nonfatal VTE and unexplained death, and the main safety outcome was major bleeding. Compared with low-dose aspirin, rivaroxaban 10 or 20 mg once daily reduced the relative risk of recurrent VTE or unexplained death by approximately 70%. A primary efficacy outcome event occurred in 13 of 1127 patients (1.2%) who received the 10-mg daily dosage of rivaroxaban compared with 50 of 1131 patients (4.4%) who received aspirin. An increased incidence of bleeding, including major and clinically important nonmajor bleeding, was observed in patients who received continued treatment with rivaroxaban at a treatment dosage (20 mg once daily) compared with those who received a prophylactic dosage of rivaroxaban (10 mg once daily) or aspirin (100 mg once daily). Major bleeding occurred in 5 or 6 patients (0.4 or 0.5%) in the 10- or 20-mg rivaroxaban group compared with 3 patients (0.3%) in the aspirin group.

The SELECT-D study was an open-label pilot trial that evaluated rivaroxaban in active cancer patients with symptomatic VTE or symptomatic or incidental PE. Patients ≥18 years of age weighing ≥40 kg with active cancer (defined as a diagnosis of cancer other than basal-cell or squamous-cell skin carcinoma) in the previous 6 months, any treatment for cancer within the previous 6 months, recurrent or metastatic cancer, or cancer not in complete remission (hematologic malignancy) were eligible for the study. Patients were required to have a performance status of ≤2 based on Eastern Cooperative Oncology Group scoring and adequate hematologic, hepatic, and renal function. Exclusion criteria included a history of VTE, active or high risk of bleeding, and uncontrolled hypertension. Patients were assigned to rivaroxaban (15 mg twice daily for the initial 21 days, followed by 20 mg once daily) or dalteparin (200 units/kg once daily for the initial 30 days, followed by 150 units/kg once daily). The maximum dalteparin dose was 18,000 units per day. Both groups received a total of 6 months of treatment.

The primary outcome of SELECT-D was VTE recurrence (symptomatic or incidental). The secondary outcomes were International Society on Thrombosis and Hemostasis (ISTH) major bleeding and clinically relevant nonmajor bleeding. Baseline characteristics were comparable between treatment groups; 69% of the patients were receiving active cancer treatment, of which about 85% were receiving chemotherapy. VTE recurrence occurred in 8 (3.9%) rivaroxaban and 18 (8.9%) dalteparin patients within the initial 6 months. PE accounted for 50% of cases in each group (4 in the rivaroxaban arm and 9 in the dalteparin arm). Symptomatic PE occurred in 2 patients in each treatment arm, and fatal PE occurred in 1 patient in each treatment arm. Incidental PE was found in 6 patients who received dalteparin and 1 patient who received rivaroxaban. Major bleeding occurred in 11 (5.4%) patients who received rivaroxaban and in 6 (3%) patients who received dalteparin; clinically relevant non-major bleeding occurred in 25 (12.3%) and 7 (3.4%) patients in these respective treatment groups. Overall survival at 6 months was 75% for rivaroxaban and 70% for dalteparin patients; however, SELECT-D was not powered to detect a survival difference.

Clinical Experience in Pediatric Patients

Use of rivaroxaban for the treatment of VTE and reduction in the risk of recurrent VTE in pediatric patients was evaluated in an open-label, active-controlled, randomized study (EINSTEIN-Jr). The study compared rivaroxaban to standard anticoagulation in pediatric patients up to 18 years of age with an objectively confirmed VTE. Patients who had active or high risk of bleeding, coagulopathy due to hepatic disease, or estimated glomerular filtration rate (eGFR) <30 mL/minute per 1.73 m^2 were excluded from the study. Children <6 months of age were excluded if their gestational age at birth was <37 weeks or if they had less than 10 days of oral feeding or a body weight <2.6 kg.

All children received initial therapy with unfractionated heparin, low molecular weight heparin (LMWH), or fondaparinux for a minimum of 5 days, and were then randomized to rivaroxaban (in weight-adjusted dosages) or a comparator arm (unfractionated heparin, LMWH, fondaparinux, or vitamin K antagonist). Vitamin K antagonist therapy could be initiated at any time in children not randomized to rivaroxaban and initial parenteral therapy could be discontinued after a minimum of 5 days and when the target INR was reached; alternatively, these patients could be maintained on parenteral therapy for the entire treatment period. Rivaroxaban dose, frequency, and dosage form were based on the patient's body weight. Duration of treatment was 3 months in all patients except for children <2 years of age with catheter-related thrombosis who were treated for 1 month. After the main treatment period, a decision was made to extend treatment up to a total of 12 months (or up to a total of 3 months in children <2 years of age with catheter-related thrombosis).

The primary efficacy outcome was symptomatic recurrent VTE and the principal safety outcome was the composite of overt major or clinically relevant non-major bleeding. The study included 276 children 12 to <18 years of age, 101 children 6 to <12 years of age, 69 children 2 to <6 years of age, and 54 children <2 years of age. Only 34% of patients in the comparator arm were transitioned to a vitamin K antagonist. The number of patients receiving extended duration treatment was not reported. Recurrent symptomatic VTE occurred in 1.2% of rivaroxaban-treated patients and 3% of patients in the comparator group. Major bleeding did not occur in the rivaroxaban group, but occurred in 2 patients (1.2%) in the comparator group. Clinically relevant non-major bleeding occurred in 1 patient in the comparator group (0.6%) and 10 patients in the rivaroxaban group (3%).

Clinical Perspective

The DOACs are among several anticoagulants that can be used for the treatment of VTE. DOACs have similar efficacy to warfarin, but reduced bleeding (particularly intracranial hemorrhage) and greater convenience for patients and healthcare providers. In addition to relative efficacy and safety, factors that should be considered when selecting an appropriate anticoagulant include convenience of administration, cost, patient preference, presence of renal impairment, and cancer or other comorbid conditions.

Rivaroxaban is recommended by the ACCP, ASH, and the Anticoagulation Forum as an acceptable option for initial and long-term anticoagulant therapy in patients with acute proximal DVT of the leg and/or PE. In patients with acute VTE, therapy should be continued beyond the acute treatment period for at least 3 months, and possibly longer depending on the individual clinical situation (e.g., location of thrombi, presence or absence of precipitating factors, presence of cancer, patient's risk of bleeding). Rivaroxaban may offer some advantages over parenteral or vitamin K antagonist anticoagulants for the treatment of VTE (e.g., oral administration, no requirement for routine coagulation monitoring, minimal drug and food interactions), and guidelines recommend DOACs over vitamin K antagonist anticoagulants with a few exceptions based on patient risk factors (e.g., antiphospholipid syndrome). The relative efficacy and safety of rivaroxaban versus other DOACs (e.g., apixaban, dabigatran, edoxaban) for the

treatment of VTE remains to be fully elucidated due to the lack of head-to-head trials. ACCP does not recommend one DOAC over another as there are very limited published studies directly comparing these agents and indirect comparisons have not shown substantially different outcomes.

DOACs generally should not be used in settings with high risk of bleeding (e.g., hemorrhagic lesion, renal/hepatic impairment, thrombocytopenia, GI or genitourinary malignancy, mucosal lesion, CNS malignancy or bleeding, recent surgery), or in patients with morbid obesity (body weight >120 kg or body mass index [BMI] ≥40 mg/m^2), drug-drug interactions, or GI complications affecting oral therapy (e.g., poor absorption, nausea and vomiting) because of the lack of safety data. There is some experience with the use of apixaban and rivaroxaban in patients with morbid obesity.

In patients with cancer and established VTE, LMWHs or oral factor Xa inhibitors (e.g., apixaban, rivaroxaban, edoxaban) are generally recommended over warfarin for long-term anticoagulation. ACCP and ASH recommend the use of an oral factor Xa inhibitor over LMWH for the initiation and treatment phases of therapy in patients with cancer-associated thrombosis. Additional studies and experience are needed to further evaluate the efficacy and safety of rivaroxaban for the treatment of cancer-related VTE.

● *Prophylaxis of Venous Thromboembolism*

Major Orthopedic Surgery

Rivaroxaban is used for the prevention of postoperative DVT, which may lead to PE, in adults undergoing total hip- or knee-replacement surgery.

Clinical Experience

Efficacy and safety of rivaroxaban for the prevention of postoperative VTE after major orthopedic surgery are based principally on the results of 4 randomized, double-blind, double-dummy trials known as the RECORD (Regulation of Coagulation in Orthopedic Surgery to Prevent Deep-vein Thrombosis and Pulmonary Embolism) trials. In these trials, rivaroxaban was more effective than subcutaneous enoxaparin in preventing VTE in patients undergoing elective total hip-replacement (RECORD 1 and 2) or total knee-replacement (RECORD 3 and 4) surgery and was associated with similar rates of bleeding. The primary efficacy and safety end points in all 4 trials were identical; however, there were differences with respect to dosage and duration of enoxaparin therapy. Patients received oral rivaroxaban (10 mg once daily initiated at least 6–8 hours after surgery) or subcutaneous enoxaparin sodium (40 mg once daily initiated 12 hours before surgery and resumed 6–8 hours after wound closure in RECORD 1, 2, and 3, or 30 mg twice daily initiated 12 hours before surgery and resumed 12–24 hours after wound closure in RECORD 4). Treatment generally was continued for 31–39 days in the hip-replacement trials and for 10–14 days in the knee-replacement trials. However, in RECORD 2, the duration of active drug treatments was different; rivaroxaban was administered for 31–39 (mean 33.5) days (with placebo injection for 10–14 days) while enoxaparin was administered for 10–14 (mean 12.4) days (with placebo tablets for 31–39 days).

In all 4 RECORD trials, the incidence of the composite primary outcome of DVT (symptomatic or venographic), nonfatal PE, and all-cause mortality was substantially lower in patients receiving rivaroxaban than in those receiving enoxaparin. Treatment with rivaroxaban resulted in relative risk reductions for VTE of 70 and 79%, respectively, in patients undergoing hip replacement in RECORD 1 and 2, and relative risk reductions of 49 and 31%, respectively, in patients undergoing knee replacement in RECORD 3 and 4. Rivaroxaban was generally well tolerated across all trials and rates of major bleeding or any bleeding event were generally similar between treatment groups.

Some clinicians have suggested that the observed differences in outcome between the rivaroxaban and enoxaparin groups in the RECORD trials were influenced by differences in dosage and/or duration of enoxaparin therapy. In RECORD 1–3, an enoxaparin sodium dosage of 40 mg once daily was used, while the preferred dosage for thromboprophylaxis after hip-replacement surgery and the only recommended dosage for knee-replacement surgery in the US is 30 mg every 12 hours (i.e., twice daily), which was used only in the RECORD 4 trial. In addition, enoxaparin was given for an average of approximately 2 weeks versus approximately 5 weeks for rivaroxaban in the RECORD 2 trial. It has been suggested that use of a potentially suboptimal enoxaparin sodium dosage of 40 mg daily in RECORD 1–3 and an unequal (shorter) duration of enoxaparin therapy in RECORD 2 may have contributed to the increased risk of the primary efficacy end point with enoxaparin in these trials. In addition, in RECORD 3, which employed the 40-mg once-daily dosage of enoxaparin sodium in patients undergoing total knee replacement, there was an absolute risk difference of 9.2% favoring rivaroxaban for the primary end point (any DVT, nonfatal PE, and all-cause mortality in the modified intent-to-treat population), while in RECORD 4, which employed the US FDA-labeled enoxaparin sodium dosage of 30 mg every 12 hours for the same indication, the absolute risk difference favoring rivaroxaban for the same primary end point was only 3.2%. In an attempt to account for differences in study design among the RECORD trials, an analysis of pooled data that used only the period of active treatment common to all 4 trials (the 12 ± 2 days in which enoxaparin was administered) as the primary efficacy end point was performed; results of this analysis supported those of the individual trials with regard to the greater efficacy of rivaroxaban versus enoxaparin for reduction of total VTE.

In the RECORD trials, use of a definition of major bleeding that did not include surgical site bleeding unless it necessitated reoperation or resulted in death may have resulted in a more conservative estimate of bleeding risk in these trials than in other comparative studies of other DOACs (e.g., apixaban, dabigatran) and enoxaparin. Differences in the timing of initiation of rivaroxaban and enoxaparin therapy (preoperatively in RECORD 1–3; 6–8 hours postoperatively for rivaroxaban versus 12–24 hours postoperatively for enoxaparin in RECORD 4) potentially could have affected relative bleeding risk. The overall incidence of major bleeding in the RECORD trials was low (less than 1%), and these trials were not designed with enough statistical power to demonstrate differences in the end point of major bleeding. However, there was a trend toward increased bleeding events (numerically more frequent) with rivaroxaban in the RECORD trials. In a pooled analysis of data from all 4 trials, a small but statistically significant increase in the end point of major plus clinically relevant nonmajor bleeding was demonstrated for rivaroxaban versus enoxaparin in the total treatment duration pool; however, analysis of the active treatment pool at day 12±2 (i.e., the enoxaparin-controlled period common to all 4 RECORD studies) did not reveal a statistically significant difference in bleeding between the 2 groups.

Clinical Perspective

Several major guidelines for thromboprophylaxis following hip- or knee-replacement surgery have been published, including guidelines from the American Academy of Orthopedic Surgeons (AAOS), ACCP, and ASH. Routine thromboprophylaxis is recommended in all patients undergoing major orthopedic surgery, including total hip- or knee-replacement surgery, because of the high risk of postoperative VTE. According to ACCP, thromboprophylaxis with an appropriate antithrombotic agent or an intermittent pneumatic compression device should be continued for at least 10-14 days and possibly for up to 35 days after surgery.

AAOS guidelines do not recommend any specific thromboprophylaxis agent, while the ACCP guidelines favor LMWHs over DOACs. The ASH guidelines suggest the use of DOACs over LMWHs if anticoagulants are used; however, this recommendation is considered conditional based on moderate certainty in the evidence of harms versus benefits.

Drug selection and duration of therapy should be individualized based on type of surgery, patient risk factors for embolism and bleeding, as well as costs, patient compliance, preference, tolerance, and comorbidities and other clinical factors such as renal function.

Acute Medical Illness

Rivaroxaban is used for the prophylaxis of VTE and VTE-related death during hospitalization and post hospital discharge in adults admitted for an acute medical illness who are at risk for thromboembolic complications due to moderate or severe restricted mobility and other risk factors for VTE, and are not at high risk of bleeding.

Clinical Experience

Efficacy and safety of rivaroxaban for this indication were evaluated in 2 randomized, double-blind trials (MAGELLAN and MARINER) and a pooled analysis investigating the benefits and risks of rivaroxaban 10 mg daily for the prevention of VTE in acutely ill medical patients requiring hospitalization who continued therapy after discharge. The MAGELLAN trial compared

rivaroxaban to enoxaparin, and included adults ≥40 years of age who were hospitalized for an acute medical illness and had a risk of VTE due to moderate or severe immobility in addition to other VTE risk factors (e.g., age ≥75 years, BMI ≥35 kg/m², history of cancer, history of VTE, history of heart failure, thrombophilia, acute infectious disease contributing to the hospitalization).

Patients were randomized to subcutaneous enoxaparin 40 mg once daily for 10±4 days and oral placebo for 35±4 days or to subcutaneous placebo for 10±4 days and oral rivaroxaban 10 mg once daily for 35±4 days. The primary efficacy outcome was a composite of asymptomatic proximal DVT, symptomatic proximal or distal DVT, symptomatic nonfatal PE, or death related to VTE. The analysis of results included events occurring from day 1 to day 10 (i.e., Day 10 analysis) and from day 1 to day 35 time (i.e., Day 35 analysis). The safety outcome was clinically relevant bleeding, a composite of major bleeding or clinically relevant nonmajor bleeding events observed no later than 2 days after administration of the last dose of double-blind study medication. Major bleeding was defined as any bleeding leading to a ≥2 g/dL fall in hemoglobin or a transfusion of ≥2 units of packed red blood cells or whole blood, bleeding into a critical site (intracranial, intraspinal, intraocular, retroperitoneal, intra-articular, pericardial, or intramuscular with compartment syndrome), or bleeding leading to death.

For the Day 10 analysis, rivaroxaban met the noninferiority criteria with a primary efficacy outcome in both treatment groups of 2.7%. For the Day 35 analysis, rivaroxaban met superiority criteria with a primary efficacy outcome of 4.4% for rivaroxaban versus 5.7% for enoxaparin/placebo. Clinically relevant bleeding was significantly higher in the rivaroxaban group than in the enoxaparin group. The safety composite outcome occurred in 2.8% and 4.1% of rivaroxaban patients at the Day 10 and Day 35 analysis, respectively, compared to 1.2% and 1.7% of enoxaparin patients. For the Day 35 analysis, the number needed to treat to prevent the efficacy outcome was 77 and the number needed to harm was 42. Patients with bronchiectasis/pulmonary cavitation, active cancer, dual antiplatelet therapy, active gastroduodenal ulcer, or any bleeding in the previous 3 months experienced an excess of bleeding with rivaroxaban compared with enoxaparin/placebo. In a post-hoc analysis of MAGELLAN which excluded these patients, the incidence of major bleeding was 0.7% in the rivaroxaban group and 0.5% in the enoxaparin/placebo group.

The results of the MAGELLAN trial (reduced incidence of mostly asymptomatic VTE at the cost of increased bleeding) informed the design of the MARINER trial. In this trial, hospitalized patients ≥40 years of age with several conditions (e.g., heart failure with left ventricular ejection fraction ≤45%, acute respiratory insufficiency or exacerbation of chronic obstructive pulmonary disease, acute ischemic stroke, or acute infectious or inflammatory disease including rheumatic diseases) were included if they had additional VTE risk factors as indicated by a total modified International Medical Prevention Registry on Venous Thromboembolism (IMPROVE) risk score of 4 or higher or a risk score of 2 or 3 plus a plasma D-dimer level of more than twice the upper limit of the normal range. Enrolled patients must have also received thromboprophylaxis with a LMWH or unfractionated heparin during the index hospitalization.

Patients in the MARINER study were randomized on either the day of or the day after hospital discharge to either rivaroxaban or placebo daily for 45 days. Dosage of rivaroxaban was based on creatinine clearance as follows: 10 mg daily in patients with a creatinine clearance ≥50 mL/minute or 7.5 mg daily in patients with a creatinine clearance ≥30 but <50 mL/minute. The primary efficacy outcome differed from that of the MAGELLAN study and was defined as a composite of any symptomatic VTE (i.e., DVT in the legs or nonfatal PE) or death related to VTE (i.e., death due to PE or death in which PE could not be ruled out as the cause). The principal safety outcome, ISTH major bleeding, was defined as overt bleeding associated with one or more of the following criteria: fall in hemoglobin level of ≥2 g/dL; transfusion of ≥2 units of packed red blood cells or whole blood; bleeding in a critical site (e.g., intracranial, intraspinal, intraocular, pericardial, intra-articular, intramuscular with compartment syndrome, retroperitoneal); a fatal outcome. The primary efficacy outcome occurred in 0.83% of rivaroxaban and 1.1% of placebo patients, not meeting the criteria for superiority. Major bleeding occurred in 0.28% of patients who received rivaroxaban and 0.15% of those who received placebo.

In an effort to separate events (i.e., mortality, bleeding, or thromboembolic) that occurred during hospitalization and to focus only on significant events occurring during the post hospitalization phase, a post hoc pooled analysis of the MAGELLAN and MARINER trials was conducted. Patient level data from the outpatient portion of both trials were analyzed for the primary composite outcome of symptomatic DVT, nonfatal PE, myocardial infarction (MI), non-hemorrhagic stroke, and all-cause mortality. Critical site or fatal bleeding was the main safety outcome. In this analysis, approximately 31% of patients were ≥75 years of age and 91% had a creatinine clearance ≥50 mL/minute. Other notable characteristics included the presence of heart failure (36%), active infectious disease (29%), history of cancer (12%), acute ischemic stroke (16%), and a D-dimer >2 times the upper limit of normal (58%). The primary efficacy outcome occurred in 1.8% of rivaroxaban and 2.3% of placebo patients. Fatal or critical site bleeding was infrequent in both groups (rivaroxaban 0.09% and placebo 0.04%). Rivaroxaban reduced major or fatal thromboembolic events with a low risk of fatal or critical site bleeding. These results should be considered exploratory and interpreted with caution as the analysis had some limitations.

Clinical Perspective

Use of rivaroxaban during hospitalization and post-discharge in acute medically ill patients should only occur after an adequate assessment of thromboembolic and bleeding risk. The manufacturer states that rivaroxaban should not be used for VTE prophylaxis in acutely ill hospitalized medical patients under the following conditions due to the high risk of bleeding: history of bronchiectasis, pulmonary cavitation or pulmonary hemorrhage, active cancer (i.e., patients undergoing acute, in-hospital cancer treatment), active gastroduodenal ulcer in the 3 months prior to treatment, history of bleeding in the 3 months prior to treatment, or dual antiplatelet therapy.

Clinical trials evaluating extended-duration thromboprophylaxis in medically ill patients were carefully designed with strict patient inclusion and exclusion criteria and data suggesting a sufficient risk of VTE, based on a validated assessment tool, to offset the increased risk of bleeding. However, these trials have varied in design, enrollment criteria, and patient selection, and therefore evidence from these trials is inconclusive. Some clinicians suggest that decisions regarding extended-duration thromboprophylaxis should be based on the inclusion and exclusion criteria used in studies that provide available data.

The American Society of Hematology (ASH) issued a strong recommendation to use LMWHs instead of DOACs for VTE prophylaxis in acutely ill hospitalized medical patients, and also strongly recommends inpatient VTE prophylaxis with LMWH only rather than inpatient and extended-duration outpatient VTE prophylaxis with DOACs.

Cancer

Rivaroxaban has been used for VTE prophylaxis in cancer patients†.

Clinical Experience

The CASSINI trial was designed to evaluate efficacy and safety of rivaroxaban for primary VTE prevention in ambulatory cancer patients with solid tumors or lymphoma who had a moderate to high risk of VTE (Khorana score ≥2) and an expected survival of >6 months. Patients with primary brain tumor or brain metastases, active or high risk of bleeding, and poor performance status defined by the Eastern Cooperative Oncology Group were excluded. In the CASSINI trial, patients without thrombosis, based on venous duplex compression ultrasonography of both legs, were randomized to rivaroxaban 10 mg or placebo daily for 180 days. The primary efficacy outcome was the composite of objectively confirmed symptomatic or asymptomatic proximal DVT in a lower limb, symptomatic DVT in an upper limb or distal DVT in a lower limb, symptomatic or incidental PE, and death from VTE. ISTH major bleeding was the primary safety endpoint. The most common primary tumor types were pancreatic, GI, and lung. The primary efficacy endpoint occurred in 6% of rivaroxaban-treated patients and 8.8% of placebo recipients at 6 months. The primary safety endpoint occurred in 2% of patients who received rivaroxaban and 1% of those who received placebo. The difference between rivaroxaban and placebo for the primary efficacy or primary safety outcomes was not statistically significant.

Clinical Perspective

Patients with cancer are substantially more likely to develop VTE than patients without cancer. Most hospitalized patients with cancer and an acute medical condition require thromboprophylaxis throughout hospitalization; however, routine pharmacologic thromboprophylaxis is not recommended for all outpatients with cancer. The patient's individual risk for thrombosis and risk of bleeding should be considered for all cancer patients when considering the use of thromboprophylaxis.

The American Society of Clinical Oncology (ASCO) and American Society of Hematology (ASH) have published guidelines for the management of VTE in patients with cancer. The ASCO guideline states that high-risk outpatients with cancer (Khorana score ≥2 prior to starting a new systemic chemotherapy regimen) may be offered thromboprophylaxis with apixaban, rivaroxaban, or a LMWH provided there are no significant risk factors for bleeding and no drug interactions. The ASH guideline suggests thromboprophylaxis with a DOAC (apixaban or rivaroxaban) in ambulatory cancer patients at intermediate to high risk for thrombosis; the decision to administer thromboprophylaxis versus no thromboprophylaxis should be based on the level of risk.

● Coronary Artery Disease

Rivaroxaban is used in conjunction with aspirin to reduce the risk of major cardiovascular events (e.g., cardiovascular death, MI, stroke) in patients with coronary artery disease (CAD).

Clinical Experience

Efficacy and safety of rivaroxaban for this indication are based principally on the results of a randomized, double-blind study known as the COMPASS (Cardiovascular Outcomes for People using Anticoagulation Strategies) study. In this study, adults (mean age 68 years) with established CAD and/or peripheral artery disease (PAD) (91% had CAD [referred to as the COMPASS CAD population]; 27% had PAD [referred to as the COMPASS PAD population]; 18% had both) who received rivaroxaban (2.5 mg orally twice daily) in conjunction with aspirin (100 mg once daily) had better cardiovascular outcomes at the cost of an increase in major bleeding events compared with those receiving aspirin alone. Treatment with rivaroxaban 5 mg twice daily alone was not superior to aspirin alone in terms of cardiovascular outcomes and was associated with an increase in major bleeding.

Patients in COMPASS CAD received rivaroxaban 2.5 mg orally twice daily plus aspirin 100 mg once daily, rivaroxaban 5 mg orally twice daily, or aspirin 100 mg once daily. The primary efficacy end point was the composite of cardiovascular death, stroke, or MI, and the primary safety outcome included fatal bleeding, symptomatic bleeding into a critical organ, bleeding into a surgical site requiring reoperation, and bleeding resulting in hospitalization. Secondary efficacy end points included the composite of ischemic stroke, MI, acute limb ischemia, or death from coronary heart disease; the composite of ischemic stroke, MI, acute limb ischemia, or cardiovascular death; and death from any cause.

The incidence of the composite primary outcome of cardiovascular death, stroke, or MI was approximately 25% lower in COMPASS CAD patients receiving rivaroxaban 2.5 mg twice daily in conjunction with aspirin than in those receiving aspirin alone (event rate 4.2 versus 5.6% per year). The beneficial effects of rivaroxaban plus aspirin therapy were observed early and the study was terminated early; the mean duration of follow-up was 23 months. Major bleeding, reported for all COMPASS patients (i.e., CAD, PAD, CAD and PAD), occurred in substantially more patients receiving rivaroxaban 2.5 mg twice daily in conjunction with aspirin compared with aspirin alone (event rate 1.6 versus 0.9% per year). The secondary composite outcome of ischemic stroke, MI, acute limb ischemia, or death from coronary heart disease occurred in fewer patients who received rivaroxaban 2.5 mg twice daily in conjunction with aspirin than in those who received aspirin alone (event rate 3.6 versus 5%). All-cause mortality was higher among those who received aspirin alone compared with those who received rivaroxaban 2.5 mg twice daily in conjunction with aspirin (event rate 4.1 versus 3.2% per year).

A systematic review explored a pooled analysis of randomized controlled trials of rivaroxaban plus antiplatelet therapy in patients with CAD, including symptomatic CAD and acute coronary syndrome. Studies that included patients requiring therapeutic anticoagulation, those with a sample size of <500 patients, and those with a follow-up period <6 months were excluded from the analysis. Five randomized controlled studies including a total of 43,650 patients were evaluated. The primary efficacy and safety endpoints were those adopted by the original studies. Results revealed that the primary efficacy endpoint (e.g., thrombotic event or death) occurred less frequently with rivaroxaban, but the primary safety endpoint (e.g., major bleeding) occurred more frequently.

Clinical Perspective

The use of rivaroxaban in CAD patients may be considered after weighing the patient's risk of ischemic events against the risk of bleeding.

The European Society of Cardiology (ESC) guideline provides perspective on the role of rivaroxaban 2.5 mg twice daily in addition to daily aspirin in CAD patients with normal sinus rhythm. The guideline breaks down the recommendations based on ischemic event and bleeding risk. Rivaroxaban 2.5 mg twice daily is a treatment option for dual antithrombotic therapy in combination with aspirin 75 to 100 mg daily in patients who have a high or moderate risk of ischemic events *without* a high bleeding risk (e.g., history of intracerebral hemorrhage or ischemic stroke, history of intracranial pathology, recent GI bleeding or anemia due to GI blood loss, other GI pathology associated with increased bleeding risk, liver failure, bleeding diathesis or coagulopathy, extreme old age or frailty, or renal failure requiring dialysis or eGFR <15 mL/minute per 1.73 m²).

● *Peripheral Artery Disease*

Rivaroxaban is used in conjunction with aspirin to reduce the risk of major thrombotic vascular events (MI, ischemic stroke, acute limb ischemia, and major amputation of a vascular etiology) in adults with peripheral artery disease (PAD), including patients who have recently undergone a lower extremity revascularization procedure due to symptomatic PAD.

Clinical Experience

Efficacy and safety of rivaroxaban for this indication are based on the results of COMPASS PAD and the VOYAGER PAD trial. COMPASS PAD included prespecified outcomes important to PAD such as acute limb ischemia, chronic limb ischemia, and amputation, and key composite outcomes involving major adverse limb events. Major bleeding, utilizing modified ISTH criteria, was defined as a composite of fatal bleeding, symptomatic bleeding into a critical organ, surgical site bleeding requiring reoperation, or bleeding requiring hospitalization. In the COMPASS PAD study, patients who received rivaroxaban 2.5 mg twice daily plus aspirin 100 mg daily experienced the same rate of acute limb ischemia (1%) and chronic limb ischemia (1%) as patients who received aspirin 100 mg daily alone; composite major adverse limb events occurred in 1% and 2% of patients in these respective treatment groups. Major bleeding occurred less frequently in the aspirin only group (2% versus 3%).

Patients included in the VOYAGER PAD study were ≥50 years of age with documented PAD (e.g., functional limitations in walking activity, ischemic rest pain or ulceration, ankle-brachial index ratio abnormalities) and a successful revascularization procedure performed in the previous 10 days. Patients requiring dual antiplatelet therapy for >6 months or any antiplatelet other than aspirin and clopidogrel, or any oral anticoagulant were excluded from the study. Patients with a history of intracranial hemorrhage, stroke, TIA, medical history of or active clinically significant bleeding, or eGFR <15 mL/minute were also excluded. Patients were randomized to rivaroxaban 2.5 mg twice daily or placebo. All patients received aspirin 100 mg daily. The primary efficacy outcome was a composite of acute limb ischemia, major amputation for vascular causes, MI, ischemic stroke, or death from cardiovascular causes. The primary safety outcome was major bleeding defined according to the Thrombolysis in Myocardial Infarction (TIMI) classification. The median age of patients was 67 years; 40% had diabetes, 35% were active smokers, and 20% had an eGFR <60 mL/minute per 1.73 m². Endovascular procedures were performed in 65% of patients and 35% were treated surgically. The primary composite outcome occurred less frequently in the rivaroxaban group compared to the placebo group (15.5% versus 17.8%) over a median follow-up of 28 months. The primary safety outcome of TIMI major bleeding events occurred in 1.9% of rivaroxaban patients and 1.35% of placebo patients; the most common type of bleeding was GI. This difference in TIMI major bleeding was not statistically significant; however, when the bleeding data were analyzed using ISTH major bleeding criteria, events occurred in significantly more patients in the rivaroxaban group than in the placebo group (4.3% versus 3.08%).

Fifty-one percent of VOYAGER patients also received clopidogrel for a median duration of 29 days. The primary efficacy and safety outcomes of VOYAGER were also analyzed in the context of clopidogrel utilization. Overall, a short course of clopidogrel did not modify any of the primary or secondary efficacy parameters for rivaroxaban. Concomitant use of clopidogrel, particularly with durations >30 days, was associated with numerically increased major bleeding.

● *Congenital Heart Disease*

Rivaroxaban is used for thromboprophylaxis following the Fontan procedure in pediatric patients ≥2 years of age with congenital heart disease. The Fontan surgical procedure is utilized for the management of single ventricle cardiac disorder and results in a predisposition to both bleeding and thrombotic events.

Clinical Experience

Efficacy and safety of rivaroxaban for this use were evaluated in the UNIVERSE study, a prospective, open-label trial that was conducted in 2 parts. Part A was designed to collect initial safety and tolerability data as well as evaluate pharmacokinetic (PK) and pharmacodynamic (PD) data for twice-daily rivaroxaban oral suspension administration. Part B was the randomized, open-label arm of the study that evaluated safety (ISTH major bleeding) and efficacy (any thrombotic event or the occurrence of a clinical event known to be strongly associated with thrombus) of rivaroxaban oral suspension twice daily compared to standard care with aspirin 5 mg/kg daily. Patients were not eligible if they had evidence of thrombosis during the screening period or active bleeding or high risk of bleeding contraindicating antiplatelet or anticoagulant therapy.

In part A of the trial, 12 children received rivaroxaban; in part B, 66 patients received rivaroxaban and 34 patients received aspirin. Results from part A revealed that rivaroxaban oral suspension dosed twice daily, based on body weight, resulted in PK/PD data similar to adults who received rivaroxaban 10 mg daily for thromboprophylaxis. Rivaroxaban PK/PD data analyzed for part B participants showed similar results. The primary efficacy outcome occurred in 3 (3%) rivaroxaban patients (1 in part A and 2 in part B) compared to 3 (9%) aspirin patients in part B. ISTH major bleeding occurred in a single patient who received rivaroxaban during part B. Clinically relevant non-major bleeding occurred in 5 rivaroxaban patients (1 in part A and 4 in part B) compared to 3 aspirin patients in part B.

DOSAGE AND ADMINISTRATION

● *General*

Pretreatment Screening

- Assess renal function in all patients prior to initiating rivaroxaban therapy.

- In adults, calculate creatinine clearance using actual body weight and the Cockcroft-Gault method.

- In children <1 year of age, determine renal function using serum creatinine (S_{cr}) as follows based on the 97.5th percentile of creatinine: 0.52 mg/dL in children 2 weeks of age; 0.46 mg/dL in children 3 weeks of age; 0.42 mg/dL in children 4 weeks of age; 0.37 mg/dL in children 2 months of age; 0.34 mg/dL in children 3 to 9 months of age; 0.36 mg/dL in children 10 to 12 months of age.

- In children ≥1 year of age, avoid use when eGFR <50 mL/minute per 1.73 m². If S_{cr} is measured by an enzymatic creatinine method that has been calibrated to be traceable to isotope dilution mass spectrometry (IDMS), eGFR can be calculated using the updated Schwartz formula as follows: eGFR (Schwartz) = (0.413 × height in cm)/S_{cr} in mg/dL. If S_{cr} is measured with routine methods not recalibrated to be traceable to IDMS, the eGFR should be obtained from the original Schwartz formula as follows: eGFR (mL/minute per 1.73 m²) = k × height in cm/S_{cr} in mg/dL where k is the proportionality constant (k = 0.55 in children 1 to 13 years of age; k = 0.55 in girls >13 and <18 years of age; k=0.70 in boys >13 and <18 years of age).

Patient Monitoring

- Periodically assess renal function as clinically indicated (i.e., more frequently in situations in which renal function may decline or improve, the elderly) and adjust therapy accordingly.

- When used in children for treatment of VTE or thromboprophylaxis after the Fontan procedure, monitor body weight as dosage is based on body weight.

- If rivaroxaban is administered in an epidural or spinal anesthesia/analgesia or lumbar puncture setting, frequently monitor for signs or symptoms of neurological impairment (e.g., numbness, tingling, weakness in lower limbs, bowel and/or bladder dysfunction).

- Monitor patients for any signs or symptoms of bleeding (e.g., unusual bruising) during therapy.

- Routine monitoring of coagulation status is not necessary during rivaroxaban therapy because of the drug's predictable pharmacokinetic and pharmacodynamic effects. However, in certain situations, such as in the case of overdosage or in patients with hemorrhagic or thromboembolic complications, it may be useful to assess the degree of anticoagulation. It has been suggested that the prothrombin (PT) test may be used to assess rivaroxaban plasma concentrations since the drug prolongs PT in a concentration-dependent manner; however, PT test results may vary depending on the type of reagent and may not be a reliable indicator of the degree of anticoagulation with rivaroxaban. The international normalized ratio (INR) is calibrated specifically for vitamin K antagonists (e.g., warfarin) and should not be used to monitor the effects of rivaroxaban.

Dispensing and Administration Precautions

- Based on the Institute for Safe Medication Practices (ISMP), rivaroxaban is a high-alert medication that has a heightened risk of causing significant patient harm when used in error.

● Administration

Rivaroxaban is administered orally (as tablets or oral suspension).

Store rivaroxaban tablets, granules for oral suspension, and reconstituted oral suspension at 20–25°C with excursions permitted to 15–30°C. Do not freeze the granules or reconstituted suspension.

Absorption of rivaroxaban is dependent on the site of drug release in the GI tract. Because of the possibility of reduced absorption and thereby reduced drug exposure, do not administer rivaroxaban by a method that could deposit the drug distal to the stomach.

Administration in Adults

In adults, administer the 15- or 20-mg tablets with food; administer the 2.5- or 10-mg tablets with or without food.

Missed dose instructions in adults are based on the dose and/or frequency of dosing. If a 2.5-mg dose of rivaroxaban is missed, take a single 2.5-mg dose as recommended at the next scheduled time. If a dose is missed in patients receiving a dosage of 10, 15, or 20 mg once daily, take the missed dose immediately. Do not double the dose within the same day to make up for a missed dose. If a dose is missed in patients receiving a dosage of 15 mg twice daily, take a dose of rivaroxaban immediately upon remembering; if necessary, take two 15-mg tablets at the same time to ensure full intake of the 30-mg daily dose. Resume the regular twice-daily dosing schedule the following day.

In adult patients who are unable to swallow whole tablets, crush rivaroxaban tablets and mix with applesauce immediately before administration. When given orally as a crushed 15- or 20-mg tablet, immediately follow the dose of rivaroxaban with food. In patients requiring a nasogastric (NG) or gastric feeding tube (GT), after confirming placement of the tube, administer rivaroxaban tablets by crushing and suspending the drug in 50 mL of water; enteral feeding via the tube should immediately follow administration of a 15- or 20-mg tablet. Crushed rivaroxaban tablets are stable in water or in applesauce for up to 4 hours.

Administration in Pediatric Patients

In pediatric patients, rivaroxaban 10, 15, or 20 mg tablets or the oral suspension may be used. Splitting tablets or administration of the 2.5 mg tablets is not recommended.

In pediatric patients treated for venous thromboembolism (VTE), administer all doses with feeding or food to increase absorption.

For thromboprophylaxis after the Fontan procedure in pediatric patients with congenital heart disease, administer rivaroxaban with or without food.

Missed dose instructions in children are based on the frequency of dosing. If administered once daily, take the missed dose as soon as possible, but only on the same day; skip the dose if this is not possible. If administered twice daily, take the missed morning dose as soon as possible or take together with the evening dose. Take a missed evening dose as soon as possible, but only during that evening. If administered three times a day, skip the missed dose and resume the regular dosing schedule when the next dose is due, without compensating for the missed dose.

If the child vomits or spits up the dose within 30 minutes, administer a new dose. Beyond 30 minutes, do not repeat the dose and administer the next dose at its scheduled time.

Preparation of Oral Suspension

Reconstitute granules for oral suspension at the time of dispensing to provide a suspension containing 1 mg rivaroxaban per 1 mL. Tap the bottle to loosen the granules and then add 150 mL purified water; shake the bottle for 60 seconds until the suspension is uniform and all of the granules have dissolved.

Rivaroxaban oral suspension may be administered via NG or GT; after administration, flush the feeding tube with water. Immediately follow administration with an enteral feeding when the dose and/or indication (e.g., pediatric VTE treatment) requires administration with food. There is no need to follow administration with enteral feeding if the dose may be administered without regard to meals (e.g., Fontan procedure thromboprophylaxis). Rivaroxaban oral suspension is compatible with PVC, polyurethane, and silicone NG tubing.

Use reconstituted rivaroxaban oral suspension within 60 days.

● Dosage
Pediatric Dosage
Venous Thromboembolism – Treatment and Secondary Prevention

Do not administer rivaroxaban until the patient has completed at least 5 days of an initial parenteral anticoagulant (e.g., unfractionated heparin, low molecular weight heparin [LMWH]).

Rivaroxaban use is not recommended in children <6 months of age with any of the following characteristics: <37 weeks' gestation at birth; <10 days of oral feeding; or body weight <2.6 kg.

The recommended dosage *and frequency* of rivaroxaban for the treatment of VTE and reduction in risk of recurrent VTE in pediatric patients (from birth to <18 years of age) is based on patient body weight.

Total daily doses ≤9 mg per day are divided and administered 3 times day (approximately 8 hours apart); a 10 mg total daily dose is administered as 5 mg twice daily (approximately 12 hours apart), and a 15 or 20 mg total daily dose is administered once daily (approximately 24 hours apart).

Table 1 provides dosing recommendations in pediatric patients for treatment of and reduction in risk of recurrent VTE.

TABLE 1. Pediatric Dosage (Birth to <18 Years of Age) for Treatment and Reduction of Recurrent VTE

Dosage form	Body weight	Dosage	Total daily dose
Oral suspension only	2.6 to 2.9 kg	0.8 mg 3 times a day	2.4 mg
Oral suspension only	3 to 3.9 kg	0.9 mg 3 times a day	2.7 mg
Oral suspension only	4 to 4.9 kg	1.4 mg 3 times a day	4.2 mg
Oral suspension only	5 to 6.9 kg	1.6 mg 3 times a day	4.8 mg
Oral suspension only	7 to 7.9 kg	1.8 mg 3 times a day	5.4 mg

TABLE 1. Continued

Dosage form	Body weight	Dosage	Total daily dose
Oral suspension only	8 to 8.9 kg	2.4 mg 3 times a day	7.2 mg
Oral suspension only	9 to 9.9 kg	2.8 mg 3 times a day	8.4 mg
Oral suspension only	10 to 11.9 kg	3 mg 3 times a day	9 mg
Oral suspension only	12 to 29.9 kg	5 mg twice daily	10 mg
Oral suspension OR tablets	30 to 49.9 kg	15 mg once daily	15 mg
Oral suspension OR tablets	≥50 kg	20 mg once daily	20 mg

Duration of therapy in children with thrombosis is at least 3 months and may be continued up to 12 months following an individualized assessment of risk of recurrent thrombosis versus the potential risk of bleeding. The exception is pediatric patients <2 years old with catheter-related thrombosis, where therapy should be administered for at least 1 month, with continuation up to 3 months based on risks versus benefits.

Congenital Heart Disease

The recommended dosage and frequency of rivaroxaban for thromboprophylaxis following the Fontan procedure in pediatric patients ≥2 years of age with congenital heart disease is based on body weight.

Total daily doses ≤5 mg per day are divided and administered 2 times a day (approximately 12 hours apart), and the 7.5 or 10 mg total daily dose is administered once daily (approximately 24 hours apart).

Table 2 provides dosing recommendations in pediatric patients with congenital heart disease.

TABLE 2. Pediatric Dosage for Thromboprophylaxis in Congenital Heart Disease

Dosage form	Body weight	Dosage	Total daily dose
Oral suspension only	7 to 7.9 kg	1.1 mg twice daily	2.2 mg
Oral suspension only	8 to 9.9 kg	1.6 mg twice daily	3.2 mg
Oral suspension only	10 to 11.9 kg	1.7 mg twice daily	3.4 mg
Oral suspension only	12 to 19.9 kg	2 mg twice daily	4 mg
Oral suspension only	20 to 29.9 kg	2.5 mg twice daily	5 mg
Oral suspension only	30 to 49.9 kg	7.5 mg once daily	7.5 mg
Oral suspension OR tablets	≥50 kg	10 mg once daily	10 mg

Adults

Embolism Associated with Atrial Fibrillation

For reduction of the risk of stroke and systemic embolism in patients with nonvalvular atrial fibrillation, the recommended adult dosage of rivaroxaban is 20 mg once daily with the evening meal. Reduce dosage to 15 mg once daily in patients with a creatinine clearance ≤50 mL/minute.

Venous Thromboembolism - Treatment and Secondary Prevention

For the *treatment* of acute DVT and/or PE, the recommended adult dosage of rivaroxaban is 15 mg orally twice daily for the first 21 days, followed by 20 mg once daily taken at approximately the same time every day with food. The initial twice-daily dosing regimen provides higher trough drug concentrations and may be associated with improved thrombus regression compared with a once-daily regimen.

For reduction in the risk of recurrent VTE (secondary prevention) in patients at continued risk for DVT/PE with a creatinine clearance ≥15 mL/minute, the recommended dosage is 10 mg once daily with or without food after an initial ≥6 months of standard anticoagulant (e.g., warfarin, direct oral anticoagualant [DOAC]) treatment.

The optimum duration of anticoagulant therapy should be determined by the individual clinical situation (e.g., location of thrombi, presence or absence of precipitating factors for thrombosis, presence of cancer, risk of bleeding). In general, the American College of Chest Physicians (ACCP) suggest that anticoagulant therapy should be continued beyond the acute treatment period for at least 3 months and possibly longer in certain patients with a high risk of recurrence and low or moderate risk of bleeding.

Thromboprophylaxis in Hip- or Knee-Replacement Surgery

For the prevention of DVT and associated PE in adults who have undergone hip- or knee-replacement surgery, the recommended dosage of rivaroxaban is 10 mg once daily. The initial dose should be administered at least 6–10 hours after surgery, provided hemostasis has been established. The recommended duration of rivaroxaban therapy is 35 days for patients undergoing hip-replacement surgery and 12 days for patients undergoing knee-replacement surgery.

Thromboprophylaxis in Acutely Ill Medical Patients

For the prevention of VTE in acutely ill medical patients at risk for thrombotic complications (not at a high risk of bleeding) with a creatinine clearance ≥15 mL/minute, the recommended dosage is 10 mg once daily, initiated in hospital and following discharge for a recommended total duration of 31 to 39 days.

Coronary Artery Disease

To reduce the risk of major cardiovascular events (e.g., cardiovascular death, myocardial infarction [MI], stroke) in patients with coronary artery disease (CAD), the recommended dosage of rivaroxaban is 2.5 mg twice daily in conjunction with aspirin 75–100 mg once daily with or without food.

Peripheral Artery Disease

To reduce the risk of major thrombotic vascular events (e.g., MI, ischemic stroke, acute limb ischemia, and major amputation of a vascular etiology) in patients with peripheral artery disease (PAD), including patients with a recent lower extremity revascularization procedure due to symptomatic PAD, the recommended dosage of rivaroxaban is 2.5 mg twice daily in conjunction with aspirin 75–100 mg once daily with or without food. The initial dose should be administered after surgery, provided hemostasis has been established.

Transitioning from Other Anticoagulant Therapy

When switching from warfarin to rivaroxaban therapy, the manufacturer states that warfarin should be discontinued and rivaroxaban initiated as soon as the INR is <3 in adults and <2.5 in pediatric patients to avoid periods of inadequate anticoagulation.

For adult or pediatric patients, when transitioning to rivaroxaban from therapy with another non-warfarin anticoagulant (e.g., LMWH, DOACs), the initial dose of rivaroxaban should be administered within 2 hours of the next scheduled evening dose of the other anticoagulant, and the other anticoagulant should be discontinued. When transitioning to rivaroxaban from heparin given by continuous IV infusion, the heparin infusion should be discontinued and rivaroxaban initiated at the same time.

Transitioning to Other Anticoagulant Therapy

The manufacturer states that adult data from clinical trials currently are not available to guide conversion from rivaroxaban to warfarin therapy. Because rivaroxaban may affect INR, INR measurements may not be useful in determining an appropriate dose of warfarin during conversion. A suggested approach is to discontinue rivaroxaban and simultaneously initiate a parenteral anticoagulant and warfarin at the time the next scheduled dose of rivaroxaban would have been administered.

In pediatric patients, continue rivaroxaban for at least 2 days after the first dose of warfarin. After 2 days and prior to the next rivaroxaban dose, obtain an INR; continue coadministration of rivaroxaban and warfarin until the INR is ≥2. INR testing may be done reliably 24 hours after the last rivaroxaban dose.

For adult or pediatric patients, when converting from rivaroxaban to an oral or parenteral anticoagulant with a rapid onset of action, rivaroxaban should be discontinued and the first dose of the other anticoagulant should be administered at the time of the next scheduled dose of rivaroxaban.

In patients taking rivaroxaban or other factor Xa inhibitors (e.g., apixaban), heparin anti-Xa assay accuracy may be affected; elevated heparin anti-Xa levels have been reported. which may impact the monitoring of the transition from rivaroxaban to IV heparin.

Managing Anticoagulation in Patients Requiring Invasive Procedures

If temporary discontinuance of anticoagulation is necessary prior to surgery or other invasive procedures to reduce the risk of bleeding, the manufacturer recommends that rivaroxaban be discontinued at least 24 hours prior to the procedure. In deciding whether a procedure should be delayed until 24 hours after the last dose of rivaroxaban, the increased risk of bleeding should be weighed against the urgency of the intervention. If rivaroxaban is discontinued prior to surgery or other invasive procedure, the drug should be resumed postoperatively as soon as adequate hemostasis has been established; if oral anticoagulation is not possible, use of a parenteral anticoagulant should be considered.

• Special Populations

Hepatic Impairment

No clinical data are available for pediatric patients with hepatic impairment and adult patients with severe hepatic impairment. Use of rivaroxaban should be avoided in patients with moderate (Child-Pugh class B) or severe (Child-Pugh class C) hepatic impairment or with any hepatic disease associated with coagulopathy; systemic exposure and risk of bleeding may be increased in such patients.

Renal Impairment

Embolism Associated with Atrial Fibrillation

For adults with a creatinine clearance of ≤50 mL/minute, the recommended dosage of rivaroxaban is 15 mg once daily with the evening meal. Assess renal function periodically as clinically indicated (i.e., more frequently in situations where renal function may decline) and adjust therapy accordingly. Consider discontinuance of rivaroxaban if acute renal failure develops.

In the ROCKET AF trial, serum concentrations of rivaroxaban and clinical outcomes were similar in patients with moderate renal impairment (creatinine clearance of 30–50 mL/minute) receiving rivaroxaban 15 mg once daily compared with those with normal renal function receiving rivaroxaban 20 mg once daily. Although patients with creatinine clearance ≤30 mL/minute were not studied, the manufacturer states that a rivaroxaban dosage of 15 mg once daily in such patients is expected to result in serum concentrations similar to those observed in patients with moderate renal impairment.

Venous Thromboembolism - Treatment and Secondary Prevention

Pediatric Patients: The manufacturer states to avoid use in patients ≥1 year of age with moderate or severe renal impairment (eGFR <50 mL/minute per 1.73 m^2) due to limited clinical data. Avoid use in patients <1 year of age with serum creatinine above the 97.5th percentile due to a lack of clinical data.

Adults: Avoid rivaroxaban in patients with severe renal impairment (creatinine clearance <15 mL/minute). Rivaroxaban exposure and pharmacodynamic effects are increased in patients with creatinine clearance <30 mL/minute as compared to those with normal renal function. Observe patients with a creatinine clearance of 15 to <30 mL/minute closely and promptly evaluate any signs or symptoms of bleeding. Discontinue rivaroxaban if acute renal failure develops.

Thromboprophylaxis in Hip- or Knee-Replacement Surgery

Avoid rivaroxaban in adults with severe renal impairment (creatinine clearance <15 mL/minute). Rivaroxaban exposure and pharmacodynamic effects are increased in patients with creatinine clearance <30 mL/minute as compared to those with normal renal function. Observe patients with a creatinine clearance of 15 to <30 mL/minute closely and promptly evaluate any signs or symptoms of bleeding. Discontinue rivaroxaban if acute renal failure develops.

Thromboprophylaxis in Acutely Ill Medical Patients

Avoid rivaroxaban in adults with severe renal impairment (creatinine clearance <15 mL/minute). Rivaroxaban exposure and pharmacodynamic effects are increased in patients with creatinine clearance <30 mL/minute as compared to those with normal renal function. Observe patients with a creatinine clearance of 15 to <30 mL/minute closely and promptly evaluate any signs or symptoms of bleeding. Discontinue rivaroxaban if acute renal failure develops.

Coronary Artery Disease

The manufacturer states that dosage adjustments based on creatinine clearance are not needed when rivaroxaban is used to reduce the risk of major cardiovascular events in patients with CAD.

Peripheral Artery Disease

The manufacturer states that dosage adjustments based on creatinine clearance are not needed when rivaroxaban is used to reduce the risk of major thrombotic vascular events in adult patients with PAD.

Congenital Heart Disease

The manufacturer states to avoid use in pediatric patients ≥1 year of age with moderate or severe renal impairment (eGFR <50 mL/minute per 1.73 m^2) due to limited clinical data. Avoid use in patients <1 year of age with serum creatinine above the 97.5th percentile due to a lack of clinical data.

Body Weight

Pediatric Patients

Monitor body weight; review the dose and frequency regularly to ensure an appropriate indication-based dose is maintained.

Adults

Dosage adjustments based on weight are not likely to be necessary. Extremes in body weight in patients weighing ≤50 kg or >120 kg did not influence rivaroxaban exposure.

The International Society on Thrombosis and Haemostasis (ISTH) Subcommittee on Control of Anticoagulation issued consensus recommendations on VTE prevention and treatment with DOACs in patients with obesity. Based upon the available PK/PD and clinical outcome data, rivaroxaban at standard doses is an acceptable option regardless of high body mass index (BMI) and body weight. ISTH does not recommend regularly following peak or trough rivaroxaban levels as there are insufficient data to influence management decisions. Following surgical intervention for obesity, rivaroxaban absorption may be reduced depending on the procedure. Due to limited data, ISTH does not recommend the use of rivaroxaban or other DOACs (e.g., apixaban, edoxaban, dabigatran) for treatment or prevention of VTE in the acute setting after bariatric surgery setting due to concerns for decreased absorption. In the early post-surgical phase, patients should be initiated on parenteral anticoagulation. The use of a vitamin K antagonist or a DOAC following at least 4 weeks of parenteral treatment may be considered and obtaining a DOAC trough level is suggested to check drug absorption.

CAUTIONS

● *Contraindications*

● Active pathologic bleeding.

● Severe hypersensitivity reaction to rivaroxaban.

● *Warnings/Precautions*

Warnings

Risk of Thrombosis Following Premature Discontinuance of Anticoagulation

Premature discontinuance of any oral anticoagulant, including rivaroxaban, in the absence of adequate alternative anticoagulation increases the risk of thrombotic events (e.g., stroke). A boxed warning about this risk is included in the prescribing information for rivaroxaban. An increased incidence of stroke was observed during the transition from rivaroxaban to warfarin in clinical trials (e.g., ROCKET AF) in patients with atrial fibrillation. In the ROCKET AF trial, rivaroxaban-treated patients generally were switched to warfarin without a period of concurrent administration of warfarin and rivaroxaban, so that they were not adequately anticoagulated until attaining a therapeutic international normalized ratio (INR).

If discontinuance of rivaroxaban is required for reasons other than pathologic bleeding or completion of a course of therapy, anticoagulant coverage with an alternative anticoagulant should be considered. When transitioning patients from one anticoagulant therapy to another, it is important to ensure continuous anticoagulation while minimizing the risk of bleeding. Particular caution is advised when switching patients from a factor Xa inhibitor to warfarin therapy because of the slow onset of action of warfarin.

Spinal/Epidural Hematoma

Patients receiving anticoagulants are at risk of developing an epidural or spinal hematoma when concomitant neuraxial (epidural/spinal) anesthesia or spinal puncture is employed; such complications can result in long-term or permanent paralysis. A boxed warning about this risk is included in the prescribing information for rivaroxaban. Epidural and subdural hematomas have been reported during postmarketing experience in patients receiving rivaroxaban. The risk of these adverse events is increased by use of indwelling epidural catheters or by concomitant use of drugs affecting hemostasis, such as nonsteroidal anti-inflammatory agents (NSAIAs), platelet-aggregation inhibitors, or other anticoagulants. Risk also may be increased in patients with a history of traumatic or repeated epidural or spinal punctures, spinal deformity, or spinal surgery.

To reduce the risk of bleeding with concurrent use of rivaroxaban and neuraxial anesthesia or spinal puncture procedures, clinicians should carefully consider the pharmacokinetic profile of the anticoagulant. Insertion or removal of an epidural catheter or lumbar puncture is best performed when the anticoagulant effect of rivaroxaban is minimal. Although the optimal timing between the administration of rivaroxaban and neuraxial procedures is not known, the following recommendations should be considered. At least 2 half-lives of the drug (i.e., 18 hours in patients 20–45 years of age and 26 hours in patients 60–76 years of age) should elapse following administration of a rivaroxaban dose prior to removal of an indwelling epidural or intrathecal catheter, and at least 6 hours should elapse following removal of the catheter before the next dose is administered. If traumatic puncture occurs, administration of rivaroxaban should be delayed for 24 hours.

Patients receiving rivaroxaban in the setting of epidural or spinal anesthesia or lumbar puncture should be monitored frequently for manifestations of neurologic impairment (e.g., midline back pain; numbness, tingling, or weakness in lower limbs; bowel or bladder dysfunction). If spinal hematoma is suspected, urgent diagnosis and treatment are necessary; spinal cord decompression should be considered even though it may not prevent or reverse neurologic sequelae. Clinicians should consider the potential benefits versus risks of neuraxial intervention in patients who are currently receiving or will receive anticoagulant prophylaxis.

Other Warnings and Precautions

Bleeding

Rivaroxaban increases the risk of hemorrhage and can cause serious or fatal bleeding. Bleeding complications were the most common adverse effects of rivaroxaban reported in clinical trials. In the ROCKET AF trial in patients with nonvalvular atrial fibrillation, bleeding that required permanent drug discontinuance occurred in 4.3% of patients receiving rivaroxaban and 3.1% of those receiving warfarin. The rate of major bleeding (defined as clinically overt bleeding that resulted in death, involved a critical site [i.e., intracranial, intraspinal, intraocular, pericardial, intraarticular, intramuscular with compartment syndrome, or retroperitoneal], was associated with a fall in hemoglobin of at least 2 g/dL or required transfusion of at least 2 units of whole blood or packed red blood cells, or resulted in permanent disability) was similar between the rivaroxaban and warfarin treatment groups in the ROCKET AF trial (5.6 and 5.4%, respectively); however, decreases in hemoglobin concentration of at least 2 g/dL, bleeding requiring transfusion, and major bleeding from a GI site were more common in patients receiving rivaroxaban.

In the RECORD trials in patients undergoing orthopedic surgery, major bleeding (defined as fatal bleeding, bleeding into a critical organ, bleeding requiring reoperation, or extra-surgical site bleeding that was clinically overt and was associated with a fall in hemoglobin of at least 2 g/dL or that required transfusion of at least 2 units of whole blood or packed red blood cells) was reported in 0.3% of patients who received rivaroxaban 10 mg once daily and 0.2% of those who received enoxaparin. Although bleeding rates were comparable between rivaroxaban and enoxaparin in these trials, comparison of bleeding rates in the RECORD trials with those of other trials involving non-vitamin K antagonist oral anticoagulants and enoxaparin may be confounded by the use of different definitions for major bleeding. In the EINSTEIN DVT and EINSTEIN PE studies evaluating rivaroxaban for the treatment of venous thromboembolism (VTE), rates of major bleeding and clinically relevant nonmajor bleeding were similar between patients receiving rivaroxaban and those receiving enoxaparin plus a vitamin K antagonist; in the EINSTEIN EXT study in which rivaroxaban was compared with placebo, there was a slight increase in major and clinically relevant nonmajor bleeding with rivaroxaban therapy.

In the MAGELLAN trial of daily rivaroxaban for inpatient and postdischarge VTE prophylaxis in patients with acute medical illness, fatal bleeding occurred in 7 rivaroxaban patients compared to 1 enoxaparin/placebo patient. In the rivaroxaban group, bleeding sites were pulmonary, intracranial, GI, and retroperitoneal. The manufacturer states rivaroxaban should not be used for VTE prophylaxis in acutely ill medical patients under the following conditions due to the high risk of bleeding: history of bronchiectasis, pulmonary cavitation or pulmonary hemorrhage, active cancer (i.e., undergoing acute, in-hospital cancer treatment), active gastroduodenal ulcer in the 3 months prior to treatment, history of bleeding in the 3 months prior to treatment, or dual antiplatelet therapy.

When deciding whether to use rivaroxaban in patients with an increased risk of bleeding (e.g., congenital or acquired bleeding disorders; active ulceration, hemorrhagic stroke, uncontrolled arterial hypertension, diabetic retinopathy; recent brain, spinal, or ophthalmic surgery), clinicians should weigh the risk of bleeding against the risk of thrombotic events. Patients with any manifestations of blood loss during rivaroxaban therapy should be promptly evaluated. Rivaroxaban should be discontinued if active pathologic hemorrhage occurs. However, minor or "nuisance" bleeding is a common occurrence in patients receiving any anticoagulant and should not readily lead to treatment discontinuance.

Risk of bleeding may be increased in patients with renal impairment and in those receiving concomitant therapy with drugs that affect hemostasis (e.g., aspirin or other NSAIAs, fibrinolytics, selective serotonin- and norepinephrine-reuptake inhibitors [SNRIs], selective serotonin-reuptake inhibitors [SSRIs], thienopyridines, other antithrombotic agents) or drugs that are inhibitors of both P-glycoprotein (P-gp) and cytochrome P-450 (CYP) isoenzyme 3A4 (e.g., ketoconazole, ritonavir). Patients with renal impairment taking P-gp inhibitors and weak to moderate CYP3A4 inhibitors may have substantial increases in exposure to rivaroxaban, which may increase bleeding risk.

Because of the risk of pregnancy-related hemorrhage and/or emergent delivery, rivaroxaban should be used with caution in pregnant women. Pregnant women who receive rivaroxaban should be promptly evaluated if any manifestations of blood loss occur, such as a decline in hemoglobin and/or hematocrit, hypotension, or fetal distress.

Factor Xa (recombinant), inactivated-zhzo (also known as andexanet alfa), a recombinant modified human factor Xa protein, is a specific reversal agent for the anticoagulant effects of rivaroxaban. Data from clinical trials indicate that factor Xa (recombinant), inactivated-zhzo is effective in rapidly reversing the anticoagulant effects of rivaroxaban (as measured by anti-factor Xa activity, unbound anticoagulant concentration, and thrombin generation). The safety of factor Xa (recombinant), inactivated-zhzo has not been established in patients who have experienced a thromboembolic event or disseminated intravascular coagulation (DIC) within 2 weeks prior to the life-threatening bleeding event requiring treatment with the drug, or in those who have received prothrombin complex concentrate (PCC), recombinant factor VIIa, or whole blood products within 7 days prior to the bleeding event. The manufacturer states that rivaroxaban should be discontinued and appropriate treatment initiated if bleeding associated with overdosage occurs. Because of high plasma protein binding, rivaroxaban is not expected to be dialyzable.

Procoagulant reversal agents such as 4-factor PCC may be considered for immediate reversal of the anticoagulant effect of rivaroxaban when factor Xa (recombinant), inactivated-zhzo is not available. In 2 prospective cohort studies, fixed dose 4-factor PCC was administered to patients with major bleeding due to factor Xa inhibitors. In one study, the dose was weight-based (2000 units for patients weighing >65 kg and 1500 units for patients weighing <65 kg). In the second study, the dose was 2000 units. Good or effective hemostasis was achieved in at least 65% of patients in both studies. Embolic complications (e.g., ischemic stroke, thromboemolic event) were reported in some of the patients.

Protamine sulfate and vitamin K are not expected to affect the anticoagulant activity of rivaroxaban, and there is no experience with antifibrinolytic agents (tranexamic acid, aminocaproic acid) or systemic hemostatics (desmopressin, aprotinin [no longer commercially available in the US]) in patients receiving rivaroxaban.

Patients with Prosthetic Heart Valves

Use of rivaroxaban is not recommended in patients with prosthetic heart valves. The GALILEO trial investigated rivaroxaban as an alternative to antiplatelet therapy following successful transcatheter aortic valve replacement (TAVR). Rivaroxaban 10 mg daily plus daily aspirin for 3 months followed by rivaroxaban 10 mg daily was compared to dual antiplatelet therapy (clopidogrel 75 mg daily plus daily aspirin for 3 months, followed by aspirin monotherapy). Over a median trial duration of 17 months, death occurred in 7.7% of patients who received rivaroxaban and 4.6% of those who received antiplatelet therapy; ISTH-defined major bleeding occurring in 5.9% and 3.7% of the respective treatment groups.

The manufacturer states that rivaroxaban is not recommended in TAVR patients. Safety and efficacy of rivaroxaban have not been established in patients with other prosthetic heart valves or other valve procedures.

Patients with Pulmonary Embolism

The manufacturer states that rivaroxaban is not recommended *as initial therapy* (as an alternative to unfractionated heparin) in patients with pulmonary embolism (PE) who have hemodynamic instability or who may receive thrombolytic therapy or undergo pulmonary embolectomy.

Thrombosis Risk in Triple Positive Antiphospholipid Syndrome

Rivaroxaban and other DOACs are not recommended for use in patients with triple-positive antiphospholipid syndrome (APS) (i.e., positive for lupus anticoagulant, anticardiolipin, and anti-beta 2-glycoprotein I antibodies). Treatment with DOACs has been associated with increased rates of recurrent thrombotic events compared with warfarin treatment in patients with APS, especially those with triple-positive disease. ISTH recommends the use of vitamin K antagonists over DOACs in patients with high-risk APS, including those with triple-positive disease.

Specific Populations

Pregnancy

There are no adequate or well-controlled studies of rivaroxaban in pregnant women; the manufacturer states post-marketing experience is currently insufficient to determine any rivaroxaban-associated risk for major birth defects or miscarriage. In animal reproduction studies, pronounced maternal bleeding, postimplantation pregnancy loss, and fetotoxic effects have been observed. Because of the risks associated with rivaroxaban during pregnancy (e.g., hemorrhage, emergent delivery), the manufacturer states that the drug should be used with caution in pregnant women and only if the potential benefits justify the potential risks to the mother and fetus.

Unbound rivaroxaban was found to rapidly transfer across the human placenta in an in vitro placenta perfusion model. Based on the pharmacologic activity of factor Xa inhibitors, bleeding may occur at any site in the fetus and/or neonate.

The American College of Chest Physicians (ACCP) and the American College of Obstetricians and Gynecologists (ACOG) recommend that rivaroxaban be avoided in pregnant women due to insufficient safety data; the American Society of Hematology (ASH) states that more data are necessary in their most recent guidelines for the management of VTE in the context of pregnancy. Women of childbearing potential should discuss pregnancy planning with their clinician prior to initiating rivaroxaban therapy. Rivaroxaban dosing in pregnancy has not been studied.

Lactation

Rivaroxaban is distributed into human milk. The effects of rivaroxaban on the breast-fed infant or on milk production are unknown. The benefits of breast-feeding and the clinical need for rivaroxaban in the woman should be considered along with any potential adverse effects on the breast-fed infant from the drug or underlying maternal condition. ACCP, ACOG, and ASH recommend that anticoagulants other than rivaroxaban be used in nursing women.

Females and Males of Reproductive Potential

Rivaroxaban can cause significant uterine bleeding. Females of reproductive potential and those with abnormal uterine bleeding should be assessed for increased risk of clinically significant uterine bleeding, potentially requiring gynecologic surgical intervention.

Pediatric Use

Safety and efficacy of rivaroxaban for VTE treatment and the reduction in risk of recurrent VTE in children from birth to <18 years of age are supported by controlled clinical trials in adults with additional pharmacokinetic, safety, and efficacy data from a multicenter, prospective, open-label, active-controlled randomized study in 500 pediatric patients. Children <6 months who were <37 weeks of gestation at birth, had <10 days of oral feeding, or had a body weight of <2.6 kg were not studied and rivaroxaban is not recommended in these patients because dosing cannot be reliably determined.

Safety and efficacy of rivaroxaban for thromboprophylaxis following the Fontan procedure in children ≥2 years old with congenital heart disease are supported by evidence from adequate controlled studies of rivaroxaban in adults with additional data from a multicenter, prospective, open-label, active-controlled study in 112 pediatric patients; the study evaluated the single- and multiple dose pharmacokinetic properties and safety and efficacy of rivaroxaban when used for thromboprophylaxis for 12 months in children with single ventricle physiology who had the Fontan procedure.

The 10 mg, 15 mg, and 20 mg rivaroxaban tablets may be used in children due to clinical studies that evaluated safety, efficacy, pharmacokinetic, and pharmacodynamic data in this patient population. Safety, efficacy, pharmacokinetic, and pharmacodynamic data do not exist for rivaroxaban 2.5 mg tablets and they are not recommended for use in children.

Although the manufacturer states that not all adverse reactions identified in the adult population have been observed in clinical trials of children and adolescent patients, the same warnings and precautions for adults should be considered for children and adolescents.

Geriatric Use

No substantial differences in efficacy were observed in geriatric patients ≥65 years of age relative to younger adults in clinical trials. The manufacturer states that thrombotic and bleeding event rates were higher in older patients.

Hepatic Impairment

Results of a pharmacokinetic study indicate that rivaroxaban exposure (AUC and peak plasma concentrations) and pharmacodynamic effects (inhibition of factor Xa activity and prolongation of prothrombin time [PT]) are increased in patients with moderate hepatic impairment (Child-Pugh class B). Clinically important changes in pharmacokinetics or pharmacodynamics of rivaroxaban were not observed in patients with mild hepatic impairment (Child-Pugh class A). The safety and pharmacokinetics of rivaroxaban in patients with severe hepatic impairment (Child-Pugh class C) have not been established. Patients with substantial liver disease (hepatitis or cirrhosis) were excluded from the major efficacy trials of rivaroxaban.

Rivaroxaban should not be used in patients with moderate or severe hepatic impairment or with any hepatic disease associated with coagulopathy. The manufacturer states that no clinical data are available in pediatric patients with hepatic impairment.

Renal Impairment

Clearance of rivaroxaban is decreased in patients with renal impairment, resulting in increased systemic exposure and pharmacodynamic effects. Rivaroxaban should be discontinued in patients who develop acute renal failure.

In a study in individuals with various degrees of renal function, rivaroxaban AUC was increased by 44, 52, or 64% in those with mild (creatinine clearance of 50–79 mL/minute), moderate (creatinine clearance of 30–49 mL/minute), or severe (creatinine clearance of 15–29 mL/minute) renal impairment, respectively, compared with individuals with normal renal function (creatinine clearance of at least 80 mL/minute). Increased pharmacodynamic effects (PT prolongation, factor Xa inhibition) also were observed with decreasing renal function.

In an end stage renal disease (ESRD) hemodialysis study, rivaroxaban AUC increased by 56% in patients with ESRD compared to subjects with normal renal function following administration of a single 15-mg dose taken 3 hours after completion of a 4-hour hemodialysis session. When rivaroxaban is administered 2 hours prior to a 4-hour hemodialysis session with a dialysate flow rate of 600 mL/min and a blood flow rate in the range of 320 to 400 mL/min, the AUC was 47% higher compared to those with normal renal function. The manufacturer states that the extent of increase is similar to the increase in patients with a creatinine clearance of 15 to 50 mL/minute taking rivaroxaban 15 mg and therefore, hemodialysis had no significant impact on rivaroxaban exposure.

The manufacturer states that in patients with ESRD maintained on intermittent hemodialysis, administration of rivaroxaban 2.5 mg twice daily will result in rivaroxaban concentrations and pharmacodynamic activity similar to those observed in patients with moderate renal impairment in the COMPASS study. It is not known whether these concentrations will lead to similar cardiovascular risk reduction and bleeding risk as was seen during the COMPASS study.

In patients with a creatinine clearance of 30 mL/minute or less but not on dialysis, a rivaroxaban dosage of 2.5 mg twice daily is expected to result in rivaroxaban exposure similar to that observed in patients with moderate renal impairment whose efficacy and safety outcomes were similar to those with preserved renal function.

In patients with nonvalvular atrial fibrillation, renal function should be assessed periodically and dosage of rivaroxaban adjusted accordingly. More frequent monitoring may be necessary in situations in which renal function may be expected to decline. Patients with moderate renal impairment (creatinine clearance of 30–50 mL/minute) who received a reduced dosage of rivaroxaban (15 mg once daily) had clinical outcomes similar to those in patients with normal renal function who received a dosage of 20 mg once daily. The manufacturer states that in patients with ESRD maintained on intermittent dialysis, a rivaroxaban dosage of 15 mg once daily will result in rivaroxaban concentrations and pharmacodynamic activity similar to those observed in the ROCKET AF trial. It is unknown whether these concentrations will lead to similar stroke reduction and bleeding risk as was seen in the ROCKET AF trial.

In an analysis of pooled data from RECORD trials 1–3, bleeding risk was not increased in patients with creatinine clearance of 30–50 mL/minute, but a possible increase in total VTE was observed in this population. Patients with creatinine clearance of 30–50 mL/minute receiving rivaroxaban therapy for prophylaxis of DVT following hip- or knee-replacement surgery should be observed closely and promptly evaluated if any manifestations of bleeding occur. Rivaroxaban administered 10 mg once daily when creatinine clearance is <30 mL/minute is expected to result in serum concentrations similar to those in patients with moderate renal impairment (creatinine clearance 30 to <50 mL/minute); observe patients closely and promptly evaluate any signs or symptoms of blood loss.

Patients with renal impairment receiving concomitant therapy with drugs that are combined P-gp and moderate CYP3A4 inhibitors may experience a substantial increase in rivaroxaban exposure, which may increase risk of bleeding. Rivaroxaban should not be used in patients with creatinine clearance 15 to <80 mL/minute who are receiving a combined P-gp and moderate CYP3A inhibitor (e.g., erythromycin) concomitantly unless the potential benefit justifies the potential risk.

There are limited clinical data in pediatric patients ≥1 year of age with moderate or severe renal impairment (estimated glomerular filtration rate [eGFR] <50 mL/min per 1.73 m²); avoid the use of rivaroxaban in these patients. There are no clinical data in pediatric patients < 1 year of age with serum creatinine results above the 97.5th percentile; avoid the use of rivaroxaban in these patients.

• Common Adverse Effects

The most common adverse effect (>5%) of rivaroxaban in adults is bleeding. The most common adverse effects (>10%) of rivaroxaban in pediatric patients are bleeding, cough, vomiting, and gastroenteritis.

DRUG INTERACTIONS

• Drugs Affecting or Metabolized by Hepatic Microsomal Enzymes

Rivaroxaban is metabolized by cytochrome P-450 (CYP) isoenzymes 3A4/5 and 2J2; inhibitors or inducers of these enzymes may potentially alter rivaroxaban exposure.

In vitro studies indicate that rivaroxaban does not inhibit CYP1A2, 2C8, 2C9, 2C19, 2D6, 2J2, and 3A4 nor induce CYP1A2, 2B6, 2C19, and 3A4; therefore, drug interactions involving these pathways are unlikely.

• Drugs Affecting Efflux Transport Systems

Rivaroxaban is a substrate of the efflux transporter P-glycoprotein (P-gp); inhibitors or inducers of this transport protein may potentially alter rivaroxaban exposure. In vitro data indicate a low inhibitory potential of rivaroxaban for this transport protein.

Rivaroxaban is a substrate of the efflux transporter ABCG2 (breast cancer resistance protein [BCRP]); inhibitors or inducers of this transport protein may potentially alter rivaroxaban exposure. In vitro data indicate a low inhibitory potential of rivaroxaban for this transporter.

• Drugs Affecting P-glycoprotein Transport and CYP3A4

Concomitant use of rivaroxaban with drugs that inhibit both P-gp and CYP3A4 (e.g., erythromycin, ketoconazole, ritonavir) increases exposure to rivaroxaban and may increase the risk of bleeding. A substantial increase in rivaroxaban exposure may increase risk of bleeding; however, the extent of this interaction appears to be related to the degree of P-gp or CYP3A4 inhibition, and in some cases the increased exposure may not have a substantial effect on bleeding.

Concomitant use of rivaroxaban and combined P-gp and potent CYP3A4 inhibitors such as ketoconazole, itraconazole, lopinavir/ritonavir, ritonavir, and conivaptan should be avoided. When clinical data suggest that increased rivaroxaban exposure is unlikely to affect bleeding, such as in the case of concomitant clarithromycin, no special precautions are necessary for concomitant use with drugs that are combined P-gp and CYP3A4 inhibitors.

Combined P-gp and potent CYP3A4 inducers (e.g., carbamazepine, phenytoin, rifampin, St. John's wort [*Hypericum perforatum*]) may decrease exposure to rivaroxaban, resulting in possible reduced efficacy; such concomitant use should be avoided.

The manufacturer states that rivaroxaban should not be used in patients with creatinine clearances of 15 to <80 mL/minute who are receiving concomitant therapy with a combined P-gp and moderate CYP3A4 inhibitor unless the potential benefits justify the potential risks.

• Drugs Affecting Gastric Acidity

Concomitant administration of a single 30-mg dose of rivaroxaban with ranitidine (150 mg twice daily) or an antacid containing aluminum hydroxide and magnesium hydroxide (10 mL) did not affect bioavailability of or exposure to rivaroxaban. Concomitant administration of a single 20-mg dose of rivaroxaban and omeprazole (40 mg once daily for 5 days) also did not affect the pharmacokinetics of rivaroxaban. The COMPASS trial evaluated clinical outcomes in patients who were initially not receiving a proton pump inhibitor at baseline and were subsequently randomized to pantoprazole 40 mg daily or placebo in addition to rivaroxaban with aspirin, rivaroxaban alone, or aspirin alone. Compared to placebo, pantoprazole therapy had no impact on the primary or secondary composite or individual efficacy outcomes (e.g., myocardial infarction, stroke, cardiovascular death).

• Drugs Affecting Hemostasis

Concomitant use of rivaroxaban and drugs that affect hemostasis (e.g., platelet-aggregation inhibitors, other antithrombotic agents, fibrinolytics, aspirin or other nonsteroidal anti-inflammatory agents [NSAIAs], selective serotonin- and norepinephrine-reuptake inhibitors [SNRIs], selective serotonin-reuptake inhibitors [SSRIs]) increases risk of bleeding. Patients receiving such concomitant therapy should be promptly evaluated if manifestations of bleeding occur.

Anticoagulants

Because of an increased risk of bleeding, use of other anticoagulants should be avoided in patients receiving rivaroxaban unless the benefits outweigh the risks.

Concomitant administration of a single 40-mg dose of enoxaparin sodium with rivaroxaban 10 mg resulted in an additive effect on antifactor Xa activity; enoxaparin did not affect the pharmacokinetics of rivaroxaban. Administration of a single 15-mg dose of warfarin sodium with rivaroxaban 5 mg resulted in additive effects on factor Xa inhibition and prothrombin time; warfarin did not affect the pharmacokinetics of rivaroxaban.

Nonsteroidal Anti-inflammatory Agents

Patients receiving concomitant therapy with rivaroxaban and NSAIAs, including aspirin, should be promptly evaluated if any manifestations of blood loss occur.

In a single-dose drug interaction study in healthy men, concomitant administration of rivaroxaban 15 mg and naproxen (500 mg daily for 2 days) did not result in any substantial pharmacokinetic or pharmacodynamic interaction; although bleeding time was slightly increased, this was not considered clinically important.

In a single-dose study in healthy men, concurrent administration of aspirin and rivaroxaban 15 mg resulted in a slightly increased bleeding time compared with administration of aspirin alone, but did not affect the inhibitory effects of aspirin on platelet aggregation. No substantial change in pharmacokinetics or pharmacodynamics of rivaroxaban was observed. In the ROCKET AF trial, concomitant use of aspirin was identified as an independent risk factor for major bleeding.

Platelet-aggregation Inhibitors

Patients receiving concomitant therapy with rivaroxaban and clopidogrel or other platelet-aggregation inhibitors should be promptly evaluated if any manifestations of blood loss occur. In 2 drug interaction studies in which healthy individuals received clopidogrel (300-mg loading dose followed by 75 mg daily) and a single 15-mg dose of rivaroxaban concomitantly, bleeding time was increased to 45 minutes (approximately twice the maximum increase observed with either

drug alone) in approximately 30–45% of these individuals; no change in pharmacokinetics of either drug was observed.

• Antiarrhythmic Agents

Concomitant administration of rivaroxaban and amiodarone (a combined P-gp and weak CYP3A4 inhibitor) did not increase the risk of bleeding in patients with mild renal impairment. Concomitant administration of rivaroxaban and dronedarone (a combined P-gp and moderate CYP3A4 inhibitor) may increase rivaroxaban exposure in patients with renal impairment.

• Atorvastatin

A substantial pharmacokinetic interaction was not observed with concomitant administration of rivaroxaban (20 mg) and atorvastatin (20 mg once daily) in a study in healthy individuals. However, in the RECORD trials, the incidence of major or nonmajor clinically relevant bleeding was increased in patients receiving the combination of rivaroxaban and a statin compared with those receiving enoxaparin and a statin (23 or 18%, respectively).

• Azole Antifungals

Concomitant administration of rivaroxaban and ketoconazole (400 mg once daily) (a combined P-gp and potent CYP3A4 inhibitor) increased steady-state exposure (AUC) and peak plasma concentrations of rivaroxaban by 160 and 70%, respectively. Concomitant use of ketoconazole should be avoided in patients receiving rivaroxaban. Because of the potential for substantially increased rivaroxaban exposure which may increase risk of bleeding, concomitant use of rivaroxaban and itraconazole (a combined P-gp and potent CYP3A4 inhibitor) also should be avoided.

Concomitant administration of a single dose of rivaroxaban and fluconazole (a moderate CYP3A4 inhibitor) increased AUC and peak plasma concentrations of rivaroxaban by 40 and 30%, respectively.

• Digoxin

A substantial pharmacokinetic interaction was not observed with concomitant administration of rivaroxaban (20 mg) and digoxin (0.375 mg once daily) in healthy individuals.

• HIV Protease Inhibitors

AUC and peak plasma concentrations of rivaroxaban were increased substantially (by 150 and 60%, respectively) when administered concurrently with ritonavir; similar increases in pharmacodynamic effects also were observed.

Because of the potential for substantially increased rivaroxaban exposure which may increase risk of bleeding, concomitant use of rivaroxaban with ritonavir, lopinavir/ritonavir, or indinavir should be avoided.

• Macrolide Antibiotics

Concomitant administration of a single dose of rivaroxaban with clarithromycin increased AUC and peak plasma concentrations of rivaroxaban by 50 and 40%, respectively. Both single-dose AUC and peak plasma concentrations of rivaroxaban were increased by 30% when administered concomitantly with erythromycin. The manufacturer states the increase in rivaroxaban exposure with concomitant clarithromycin use is not expected to increase risk of bleeding; therefore, no special precautions are necessary with concomitant administration of clarithromycin and rivaroxaban. In a pharmacokinetic trial, administration of a single dose of rivaroxaban in conjunction with multiple doses of erythromycin (a combined P-gp and moderate CYP3A4 inhibitor) to patients with mild (creatinine clearance of 50–79 mL/minute) and moderate (creatinine clearance of 30–49 mL/minute) renal impairment resulted in a 76 and 99% increase in drug exposure and a 56 and 64% increase in peak plasma concentrations, respectively. Similar trends in pharmacodynamic effects also were observed. The manufacturer states that erythromycin should not be used concomitantly with rivaroxaban in patients with moderate renal impairment.

• Midazolam

A substantial pharmacokinetic interaction was not observed with concomitant administration of rivaroxaban (20 mg) and midazolam (single dose of 7.5 mg) in healthy individuals.

● **Nondihydropyridine Calcium Channel Blockers**

In a post hoc analysis of the ROCKET AF trial, concomitant use of verapamil or diltiazem (combined P-gp and moderate CYP3A inhibitors) with rivaroxaban was not associated with an increased risk of stroke or non-CNS embolism or the composite outcome of nonmajor clinically relevant or major bleeding; however, there was an increased risk of major bleeding and intracranial hemorrhage. In a case-cohort analysis, coadministration of rivaroxaban with diltiazem did not result in an increased rate of bleeding.

● **Protein-bound Drugs**

Interactions between rivaroxaban and other highly protein-bound drugs such as phenytoin or aspirin are likely.

● **Rifampin**

Concomitant administration of rifampin (a combined P-glycoprotein and potent CYP3A4 inducer) titrated up to a dosage of 600 mg once daily and a single 20-mg dose of rivaroxaban (with food) decreased AUC and peak plasma concentrations of rivaroxaban by 50 and 22%, respectively; similar decreases in pharmacodynamic effects also were observed. Because of the potential for reduced efficacy of rivaroxaban, concomitant use of rifampin should be avoided.

DESCRIPTION

Rivaroxaban, an oral, direct activated factor X (Xa) inhibitor, is an anticoagulant. Factor Xa plays a central role in the blood coagulation cascade by serving as the convergence point for the intrinsic and extrinsic pathways; inhibition of coagulation factor Xa by rivaroxaban prevents conversion of prothrombin to thrombin and subsequent thrombus formation. Rivaroxaban inhibits both free and prothrombinase-bound factor Xa. Unlike fondaparinux, heparin, and the low molecular weight heparins, rivaroxaban binds directly to the active site of factor Xa without the need for a cofactor (e.g., antithrombin III). Rivaroxaban inhibits factor Xa with more than 100,000-fold greater selectivity than other biologically important serine proteases (e.g., thrombin, trypsin, plasmin, factor VIIa, factor IXa, urokinase [no longer commercially available in the US], activated protein C).

Rivaroxaban exerts predictable pharmacokinetic and pharmacodynamic effects over a dose range of 5–80 mg. The drug inhibits factor Xa activity and prolongs prothrombin time (PT), activated partial thromboplastin time (aPTT), and HepTest (an indirect measure of factor Xa activity) in a dose-dependent manner.

Rivaroxaban is rapidly and well absorbed following oral administration in adults, with an estimated bioavailability of about 80–100% for the 2.5- and 10-mg doses and 66% for the 20-mg dose. Peak plasma concentrations of rivaroxaban are obtained 2–4 hours following oral administration. The presence of food delays time to peak concentration and increases systemic exposure to rivaroxaban 20 mg but does not appear to have a substantial effect on systemic exposure to the 2.5- or 10-mg dose. Absorption of rivaroxaban is dependent on the site of release in the GI tract; exposure to the drug is reduced when the drug is released into the proximal small intestine (e.g., via feeding tube) and further reduced in the distal small intestine or ascending colon.

When administered as crushed tablets orally or via a nasogastric or gastric feeding tube, rivaroxaban is stable in applesauce or water for up to 4 hours. In vitro data indicate that the drug is not adsorbed to PVC or silicone nasogastric tubing when administered as a suspension in water. Following oral administration of a crushed 20-mg tablet in applesauce to healthy individuals, mean AUC and mean peak plasma concentrations of rivaroxaban were comparable to those following administration of whole tablets; however, after administration of the crushed tablet in water via nasogastric tube followed by a liquid meal, mean AUC was comparable to that with a whole oral tablet but mean peak plasma concentrations were 18% lower.

Rivaroxaban undergoes oxidative degradation by cytochrome P-450 (CYP) isoenzymes 3A4/5 and 2J2 and hydrolysis; metabolites are subsequently eliminated through renal and fecal/biliary routes. No major circulating metabolites have been identified in plasma. Rivaroxaban is extensively bound (approximately 92–95%) to plasma proteins, mainly to albumin. Terminal elimination half-life of the drug is about 5–9 hours in healthy individuals 20–45 years of age. Following oral administration, approximately one-third of an absorbed dose of rivaroxaban is excreted unchanged in urine, with the remaining two-thirds excreted as inactive metabolites in both urine and feces. In a phase 1 study, approximately 66% of a radiolabeled dose of rivaroxaban was eliminated renally (36% as unchanged drug) and 28% was eliminated in feces (7% as unchanged drug). No substantial accumulation of the drug occurs with repeated dosing. QT-interval prolongation has not been observed with rivaroxaban.

The correlation between anti-factor Xa to plasma concentrations is linear with a slope close to 1 in children treated with rivaroxaban. In pediatric patients, the rate and extent of absorption were similar between the tablet and suspension; the maximum serum concentration was observed at a median time of 1.5 to 2.2 hours. Mean half-life increased with increasing age. Plasma protein binding is approximately 90% in children 6 months to 9 years of age.

ADVICE TO PATIENTS

- Advise patients to take rivaroxaban exactly as prescribed and to not discontinue therapy without first consulting a clinician.

- Advise patients to not split tablets to provide a fraction of a tablet dose.

- Advise patients to use the provided oral syringes when administering the reconstituted oral suspension.

- Advise patients regarding whether the dose needs to be taken with or without food.

- Inform patients who cannot swallow tablets whole to crush the tablets and combine with a small amount of applesauce followed by food. The oral suspension may be used for children unable to swallow whole tablets or for doses not available as a tablet.

- Advise patients with a nasogastric or gastric tube to crush rivaroxaban tablets, mix with a small amount of water, and administer immediately via the tube.

- Advise patients to administer a new dose if a child vomits or spits up the dose within 30 minutes after receiving the dose. However, if the child vomits more than 30 minutes after the dose is taken, do not re-administer the dose and take the next dose as scheduled. If a child vomits or spits up the dose repeatedly, contact the child's doctor right away.

- Advise patients of the importance of having an adult caregiver administer the dose to pediatric patients.

- Advise patients that if a dose is missed, management is based upon the indication for use, dose, and dosage frequency.

- Inform patients that they may bruise and/or bleed more easily and that a longer than normal time may be required to stop bleeding when taking rivaroxaban. Advise patients to inform clinicians about any unusual bleeding or bruising during therapy.

- Advise patients undergoing neuraxial anesthesia or spinal puncture procedures to monitor for manifestations of spinal or epidural hematoma (e.g., tingling or numbness in lower limbs, muscle weakness, back pain, stool or urine incontinence); immediately contact a clinician if any of these symptoms occur.

- Advise patients to inform clinicians that they are receiving rivaroxaban therapy before scheduling any medical, surgical, or invasive procedure, including dental procedures.

- Advise females to inform their clinician if they are or plan to become pregnant or plan to breast-feed.

- Advise patients to inform their clinician of existing or contemplated concomitant therapy, including prescription and OTC drugs and dietary and herbal supplements, as well as any concomitant illnesses.

- Advise patients of other important precautionary information. (See Cautions.)

PREPARATIONS

Excipients in commercially available drug preparations may have clinically important effects in some individuals; consult specific product labeling for details.

Rivaroxaban

Oral

For Suspension	1 mg/mL after reconstitution	**Xarelto®**, Janssen

Tablets	2.5 mg	**Xarelto®**, Janssen
	10 mg	**Xarelto®**, Janssen
	15 mg	**Xarelto®**, Janssen
	20 mg	**Xarelto®**, Janssen

† Use is not currently included in the labeling approved by the US Food and Drug Administration.

Enoxaparin Sodium

20:12.04.16 • HEPARINS

■ Enoxaparin, a low molecular weight heparin (LMWH) prepared by alkaline degradation of unfractionated benzylated heparin of porcine intestinal mucosa origin, is an anticoagulant.

USES

Enoxaparin is used for the prevention of venous thromboembolism (VTE) in patients undergoing orthopedic surgery or general (e.g., abdominal, gynecologic, urologic) surgery, and in medical patients with severely restricted mobility during acute illness. Enoxaparin also is used for the treatment of VTE in hospitalized patients with acute deep-vein thrombosis (DVT) with or without pulmonary embolism (PE) and in outpatients with acute DVT *without* accompanying PE.

Enoxaparin also is used in the management of acute coronary syndrome (ACS), both in patients with non-ST-segment-elevation acute coronary syndrome (NSTE-ACS) and those with acute ST-segment-elevation MI (STEMI) undergoing conservative (medical) management or revascularization strategies (e.g., percutaneous coronary intervention [PCI]).

Other uses of LMWHs include VTE prophylaxis in patients with major trauma† (e.g., brain injury, acute spinal injury), selected patients undergoing intracranial surgery† (e.g., craniotomy for malignant disease), selected cancer patients, and patients with acute ischemic stroke†. Therapy with an LMWH also has been recommended for the prevention and treatment of thromboembolism during pregnancy and for prevention of embolism in selected patients with atrial fibrillation or atrial flutter† who require temporary interruption of oral anticoagulant therapy for diagnostic or surgical procedures. Enoxaparin also has been used to reduce the risk of thromboembolism in pregnant women with mechanical prosthetic heart valves†; however, cases of valve thrombosis resulting in death (including maternal and fetal deaths) and/or requiring surgical intervention have been reported with such use. (See Patients with Mechanical Prosthetic Heart Valves under Cautions.)

● Venous Thromboembolism

Prophylaxis

General/Abdominal Surgery

Enoxaparin is used for the prevention of postoperative deep-vein thrombosis (DVT), which may lead to pulmonary embolism (PE), in patients undergoing general (abdominal) surgery who are at risk for thromboembolic complications. The manufacturer states that risk factors in abdominal surgery patients include age >40 years, obesity, use of general anesthesia for more than 30 minutes, malignancy, and history of venous thromboembolism (VTE). While enoxaparin is specifically labeled for use in the abdominal surgery setting, the scope of general and abdominal surgery in clinical practice guidelines include GI, urologic, gynecologic, bariatric, vascular, plastic, and reconstructive surgeries.

Decisions regarding use of thromboprophylaxis in patients undergoing general surgery should be based on the patient's level of risk for thromboembolism and bleeding. The American College of Chest Physicians (ACCP) guidelines state that no additional thromboprophylaxis measures other than ambulation are necessary in patients with very low VTE risk. Pharmacologic prophylaxis (with low molecular weight heparin [LMWH] or low-dose unfractionated heparin) is generally recommended in patients with moderate to high risk of VTE who do not have a high risk of bleeding. The risk of VTE remains elevated for at least 12 weeks following surgery. Extended VTE prophylaxis (generally considered as beyond 3 weeks) may be considered in selected patients undergoing major surgery. Because the risk of VTE is particularly high in patients undergoing major abdominal or pelvic surgery for cancer, extended (up to 4 weeks) prophylaxis with an LMWH is recommended in such patients.

Use of enoxaparin for VTE prophylaxis in patients undergoing abdominal surgery was established in a randomized, double-blind multicenter trial (ENOX-ACAN) comparing enoxaparin sodium (40 mg subcutaneously once daily) with unfractionated heparin sodium (5000 units subcutaneously every 8 hours) administered 2 hours prior to initiation of GI, urologic, or gynecologic surgery in cancer patients and continuing for a maximum of 12 days after surgery. Enoxaparin and unfractionated heparin demonstrated similar efficacy in preventing thromboembolic events (DVT, PE, or death associated with thromboembolism); these events occurred in 10.1 or 11.3% of patients receiving enoxaparin or unfractionated heparin, respectively (based on intent-to-treat analysis). Data from another randomized double blind trial (Canadian Colorectal DVT Prophylaxis trial) of similar design and treatment duration in patients undergoing colorectal surgery (one-third of whom had cancer) also indicated similar efficacy for enoxaparin sodium (40 mg daily given subcutaneously) and unfractionated heparin sodium (5000 units subcutaneously every 8 hours); thromboembolic events occurred in 7.1 or 6.7% of patients receiving enoxaparin or unfractionated heparin, respectively (based on intent-to-treat analysis).

Orthopedic Surgery

Enoxaparin is used for the prevention of postoperative DVT, which may lead to PE, in patients undergoing hip-replacement surgery. The drug also is used for the prevention of postoperative DVT and/or PE in patients undergoing knee-replacement surgery. Although enoxaparin is not FDA-labeled for thromboprophylaxis in patients undergoing hip-fracture surgery†, the drug also has been used in such patients.

The risk of VTE in major orthopedic surgery is among the highest of all surgical specialties. ACCP recommends routine thromboprophylaxis (with a pharmacologic and/or mechanical method [e.g., intermittent pneumatic compression]) in all patients undergoing major orthopedic surgery, including total hip-replacement, total knee-replacement, and hip-fracture surgery; thromboprophylaxis should be continued for at least 10–14 days. Among the various antithrombotic agents (e.g., LMWHs, fondaparinux, direct oral anticoagulants [DOACs], low-dose unfractionated heparin, warfarin, aspirin), ACCP states that LMWHs are generally preferred because of their relative efficacy and safety and extensive clinical experience; alternative agents may be considered in situations in which an LMWH is not available or cannot be used (e.g., in patients with heparin-induced thrombocytopenia [HIT] or in those who refuse or are uncooperative with subcutaneous injections). More recent guidelines issued by the American Society of Hematology (ASH) include additional evidence from studies with DOACs (e.g., apixaban, rivaroxaban). In patients undergoing total hip or total knee arthroplasty, the ASH guideline panel suggests the use of aspirin or an anticoagulant for VTE prophylaxis. If an anticoagulant is used, DOACs are suggested over LMWHs; if DOACs are not used, LMWHs are generally preferred to warfarin or unfractionated heparin. For patients undergoing hip fracture repair, ASH suggests the use of either LMWHs or unfractionated heparin for VTE prophylaxis. When selecting an appropriate thromboprophylaxis regimen, factors such as relative efficacy and bleeding risk as well as logistics and compliance issues should be considered.

Efficacy of enoxaparin for prevention of VTE in orthopedic patients has been established in several studies. In one study in patients undergoing hip-replacement surgery in whom thromboprophylaxis was initiated 12–24 hours postoperatively and continued for 10–14 days, DVT occurred in 10% of patients treated with enoxaparin sodium 30 mg twice daily versus 46% of placebo-treated patients. Limited data from comparative studies suggest that enoxaparin has efficacy similar to or exceeding that of unfractionated heparin in preventing DVT in patients undergoing hip-replacement surgery. In a large dose-ranging study in patients undergoing hip-replacement surgery and receiving prophylactic enoxaparin sodium 10 mg once daily, 30 mg twice daily (every 12 hours), or 40 mg once daily 24–48 hours following surgery and continuing for 7–11 days, the incidence of DVT was 25, 11, or 14%, respectively. Thus, a prophylactic enoxaparin sodium dosage of 40 mg once daily is an alternative to 30 mg twice daily in patients undergoing hip-replacement surgery.

In a double-blind study in patients undergoing knee-replacement surgery in whom prophylaxis was initiated 12–24 hours postoperatively and continued for up to 15 days, DVT occurred in 11% of patients treated with enoxaparin sodium 30 mg twice daily versus 62% of placebo-treated patients. Limited data from an unblinded comparative study suggest that enoxaparin sodium (30 mg subcutaneously every 12 hours) has efficacy similar to or exceeding that of unfractionated heparin sodium (5000 units subcutaneously every 8 hours) in preventing DVT in patients undergoing knee-replacement surgery.

Some evidence suggests that extended prophylaxis (i.e., up to 35 days post-surgery) with LMWHs may provide additional protection against thromboembolism in patients undergoing total-hip or total-knee replacement surgery. The risk of DVT is greater for the first several months following hip- or knee-replacement surgery compared with general surgery. While the manufacturer states that the usual duration of enoxaparin therapy following hip- or knee-replacement surgery is 7–10 days, with up to 14 days administered in clinical trials, ACCP suggests extended prophylaxis for up to 35 days in patients undergoing major orthopedic surgery and the ASH guidelines state that extended VTE prophylaxis (generally considered as beyond 3 weeks) may be considered in selected patients undergoing major surgery. Results from several placebo-controlled trials that included an extended treatment phase in outpatients with a hip prosthesis who had received short-term prophylaxis with enoxaparin sodium (40 mg once daily initiated 12 hours prior to surgery and continued for 10–15 days) while hospitalized indicate that extended prophylaxis with enoxaparin sodium (40 mg once daily for 3 additional weeks) decreased the incidence of DVT, including asymptomatic thrombosis (as determined by venography), compared with placebo. In one controlled trial in outpatients who had a normal phlebogram at study entry, DVT occurred in 7% of patients receiving extended therapy with enoxaparin compared with 20% of patients receiving placebo; PE was not detected. In another placebo-controlled trial in patients who had no clinical evidence of VTE at study entry, DVT (as determined by venography) occurred in 16% of patients receiving extended enoxaparin therapy versus 34% of those receiving placebo; most thromboembolic events were asymptomatic. Broader inclusion criteria of one trial may have contributed to the relatively greater incidence of later thromboembolic events in these patients with a hip prosthesis receiving extended enoxaparin therapy.

Other Surgical Settings

Enoxaparin also has been used for VTE prophylaxis in patients undergoing other types of surgery including neurosurgery, cardiac, and vascular surgery.

LMWHs have been used for the prevention of VTE in patients undergoing neurosurgery†; however, the benefits of pharmacologic thromboprophylaxis in patients undergoing neurosurgery may be outweighed by the possible increased risk of intracranial hemorrhage. Experts generally suggest the use of a mechanical method of prophylaxis (preferably intermittent pneumatic compression) in neurosurgery patients; for patients considered to be at very high risk for thromboembolism, such as those undergoing craniotomy for malignant disease, a pharmacologic method may be added once adequate hemostasis has been established and the risk of bleeding decreases. For patients in whom pharmacologic prophylaxis is warranted, the ASH guidelines suggest use of LMWHs over unfractionated heparin.

LMWHs also have been used for prevention of VTE in patients undergoing cardiac or major vascular surgery†. Because the risk of VTE in most patients undergoing cardiac surgery is considered to be moderate, ACCP generally recommends mechanical methods of prophylaxis (preferably with an intermittent pneumatic compression device) over pharmacologic prophylaxis. If pharmacologic prophylaxis is used, the ASH guidelines suggest LMWHs or unfractionated heparin.

Acutely Ill Medical Patients

Enoxaparin is used for the prevention of DVT, which may lead to PE in patients who are at risk of thromboembolic complications due to severely restricted mobility during acute illness.

Efficacy of enoxaparin for this use was established in a placebo-controlled trial in hospitalized patients with acute illness (e.g., congestive heart failure, acute or chronic respiratory failure/insufficiency, acute infection, acute rheumatic disorder, acute arthritic episodes involving the lower extremities) who were considered to be at moderate risk for thromboembolism. In this study, VTE events (DVT, PE, and death associated with thromboembolism) between days 1 and 14 (the primary outcome) occurred in 4.4% of patients treated with enoxaparin sodium (40 mg daily given subcutaneously for 6–14 days) versus 11.9% of patients receiving placebo (based on intent-to-treat analysis). Therapy with enoxaparin sodium at a dosage of 20 mg daily was no more effective than placebo in these patients.

Treatment decisions regarding the use of prophylactic anticoagulants in acutely ill hospitalized patients should include an assessment of the patient's individual risk of VTE and risk of bleeding. In general, pharmacologic thromboprophylaxis is recommended only in patients who are considered to be at high risk of VTE because the risk-to-benefit trade-off between the reduction in VTE events and bleeding is considered to be more favorable in such patients. Factors that should be considered when choosing an appropriate anticoagulant include patient preference, compliance, ease of administration, and costs associated with

the individual agents. LMWHs are recommended in clinical practice guidelines as one of several anticoagulant options for thromboprophylaxis in acutely ill, hospitalized medical patients (including those in the ICU) with an increased risk of thrombosis who are not actively bleeding and do not have an increased risk of bleeding. The ASH guideline panel suggests the use of unfractionated heparin, LMWHs, or fondaparinux for VTE prophylaxis in acutely ill medical patients, and unfractionated heparin or LMWHs in critically ill patients. When considering whether to use an LMWH or DOAC, ASH recommends LMWHs over DOACs unless the patient is receiving a DOAC for other reasons.

The manufacturer states that the usual duration of enoxaparin therapy in acute ill hospitalized patients is 6–11 days. ACCP guidelines suggest continued thromboprophylaxis for 6–21 days until full mobility is restored or hospital discharge, whichever comes first, and generally does not recommend extended prophylaxis beyond this period. Several studies have evaluated the effects of extended thromboprophylaxis after hospital discharge in acutely ill medical patients; findings with regard to efficacy and bleeding have varied depending on the anticoagulants used. Additional study is required to provide guidance on extended VTE prophylaxis in medical patients.

Because risk of VTE is particularly high in acutely ill hospitalized patients with cancer, thromboprophylaxis is generally recommended. ASH suggests the use of LMWHs over unfractionated heparin for thromboprophylaxis in these patients. Routine pharmacologic thromboprophylaxis generally is not recommended in cancer patients in the outpatient setting who have no additional risk factors for VTE. However, thromboprophylaxis with an LMWH may be considered in selected outpatients with cancer who have a high risk of thrombosis (e.g., patients with multiple myeloma receiving lenalidomide-, pomalidomide-, or thalidomide-based regimens).

Trauma

LMWHs also have been used for VTE prophylaxis in trauma patients†. In general, some form of thromboprophylaxis (with LMWHs, low-dose unfractionated heparin, or a mechanical method) is suggested by ACCP in all major trauma patients. For patients at high risk of VTE, including those with acute spinal cord injury, traumatic brain injury, or spinal surgery for trauma, ACCP suggests the use of both a pharmacologic and mechanical method of prophylaxis, unless contraindications exist.

Treatment and Secondary Prevention

VTE Treatment in Adults

Enoxaparin is used for the treatment of DVT with or without PE in hospitalized patients and also in outpatients for the treatment of acute DVT *without* PE.

The labeled indication includes the use of warfarin in conjunction with enoxaparin for the treatment of VTE; however, anticoagulants other than warfarin (e.g., the direct oral anticoagulants [DOACs]) have been used for long-term anticoagulation following initial treatment with enoxaparin. In the principal efficacy studies, enoxaparin was used in conjunction with warfarin (starting within 72 hours of initiating enoxaparin and continuing for 90 days). When warfarin therapy is being considered for the long-term treatment of VTE, the drug should be initiated concurrently with enoxaparin, and such therapy should be continued for at least 5 days and until the international normalized ratio (INR) is at least 2 for 24 hours or longer.

LMWHs are recommended by ACCP as one of several parenteral anticoagulant options for initial treatment of VTE. However, initial treatment with a parenteral anticoagulant may not always be necessary since oral anticoagulant options are available. For patients treated with initial parenteral anticoagulation, ACCP generally recommends fondaparinux or LMWHs over unfractionated heparin because of more convenient administration and less risk of HIT. LMWHs and fondaparinux are considered to be comparable; therefore, the choice between these agents should be dictated by local considerations such as cost, availability, and familiarity of use. In cancer patients with VTE, ASH suggests use of either an LMWH or DOAC for initial treatment.

In patients with VTE, ACCP recommends that anticoagulant therapy be continued beyond the acute treatment period for at least 3 months, and possibly longer depending on whether the VTE event was unprovoked or provoked by a transient risk factor (e.g., surgery), the presence of cancer, and the patient's risk of bleeding. In patients with cancer, anticoagulation therapy is recommended for at least 6 months; treatment beyond 6 months may be considered in selected patients.

DOACs are generally preferred for long-term treatment of VTE in patients without cancer. In patients with cancer and established VTE, LMWHs or DOACs are generally recommended over warfarin for long-term anticoagulation. ACCP suggests the use of LMWHs in these patients because of possibly greater efficacy and reliability (in those who may have difficulty with oral therapy). LMWHs are preferred to DOACs in settings with an increased risk of bleeding (e.g, hemorrhagic lesion, renal/hepatic impairment, thrombocytopenia, GI or genitourinary malignancy, mucosal lesion, CNS malignancy or bleeding, recent surgery), and also may be preferred in patients with obesity (body weight greater than 120 kg or BMI greater than 40 mg/m²), drug-drug interactions, or GI complications affecting oral therapy (e.g., poor absorption, nausea and vomiting). Recurrent VTE while on therapeutic anticoagulation is unusual and should prompt investigation of causative factors (e.g., noncompliance, underlying malignancy). In patients experiencing recurrent VTE during therapy with an LMWH, ACCP suggests increasing the dosage (by about one-quarter to one-third).

Data from numerous randomized studies comparing enoxaparin sodium (1 mg/kg twice daily or 1.5 mg/kg daily for a minimum of 5 days) to unfractionated heparin sodium (dosage adjusted to prolong the aPTT between 55 and 85 seconds) in patients with acute lower extremity DVT with or without PE indicate that enoxaparin is as effective as unfractionated heparin in the treatment and secondary prevention of recurrent thromboembolic events. In these studies, warfarin was initiated within 72 hours of initiation of enoxaparin or unfractionated heparin and was continued for 90 days. Other randomized controlled studies have compared LMWHs with warfarin or other oral anticoagulants in the treatment of VTE.

VTE Treatment in Pediatric Patients

LMWHs also have been used for the treatment and secondary prevention of VTE in pediatric patients†. Unlike adults, most episodes of VTE in children are secondary to an identifiable risk factor such as the presence of a central venous access device. Recommendations regarding the use of antithrombotic therapy in children generally are extrapolated from adult guidelines.

● Acute Coronary Syndrome

Enoxaparin is used (in conjunction with aspirin) to reduce the risk of ischemic complications in patients with non-ST-segment-elevation acute coronary syndrome (NSTE-ACS), including those managed with conservative (medical) therapies or revascularization strategies (e.g., percutaneous coronary intervention [PCI] with coronary stent implantation, coronary artery bypass grafting [CABG]); the drug is also used (in conjunction with aspirin) in patients with acute ST-segment-elevation myocardial infarction (STEMI) who are being managed medically (with fibrinolytic therapy) or with subsequent PCI.

● Non-ST-Segment-Elevation Acute Coronary Syndrome

The spectrum of patients with NSTE-ACS includes those with unstable angina and non-ST-segment-elevation MI (NSTEMI); because these conditions are part of a continuum of acute myocardial ischemia and have indistinguishable clinical features upon presentation, the same initial treatment strategies are recommended. The American Heart Association/American College of Cardiology (AHA/ACC) guideline for the management of patients with NSTE-ACS recommends an early invasive strategy (angiographic evaluation with the intent to perform revascularization procedures such as PCI with coronary artery stent implantation or CABG) or an ischemia-guided strategy (initial medical management followed by cardiac catheterization and revascularization if indicated) in patients with definite or likely NSTE-ACS; standard medical therapies for all patients should include an anticoagulant agent regardless of the initial management approach. Initial parenteral anticoagulants with established efficacy in patients with NSTE-ACS include enoxaparin, unfractionated heparin, bivalirudin (only in patients who are being managed with an early invasive strategy), and fondaparinux. In patients with NSTE-ACS who are subsequently undergoing PCI, an additional IV dose of enoxaparin may be required depending on the timing of the last administered subcutaneous dose. (See Non-ST-Segment-Elevation Acute Coronary Syndrome under Dosage and Administration.) Anticoagulation therapy is necessary during PCI to prevent thrombus formation at the site of arterial injury, on the coronary guidewire, and in the catheters used for the procedure.

Data from several trials comparing an LMWH (e.g., enoxaparin, dalteparin) with unfractionated heparin in patients with NSTE-ACS indicate that LMWHs are at least as effective as unfractionated heparin in preventing MI and death during the acute phase (e.g., first week) of therapy. While some patients with unstable angina in these trials had a low risk of further ischemic complications (e.g., effort angina only, no ECG changes indicative of myocardial ischemia), most patients studied were at intermediate to high risk of further ischemic complications.

In the acute phase (first 14 days after hospitalization) of a large comparative trial (Efficacy and Safety of Subcutaneous Enoxaparin in Non-Q-wave Coronary Events [ESSENCE]) evaluating short-term therapy with aspirin and enoxaparin sodium (1 mg/kg twice daily) or unfractionated heparin sodium (loading dose of 5000 units, then a continuous infusion adjusted to maintain the aPTT between 55 and 85 seconds) for a median duration of 2.6 days (range: 2–8 days) in patients with NSTE-ACS, the frequency of the combined outcome of death, nonfatal MI, or recurrent angina was reduced in patients receiving enoxaparin compared with unfractionated heparin. Combined end points in this study occurred in about 16.5 or 19.8% of patients receiving enoxaparin or unfractionated heparin, respectively, at 14 days. The incidence of these end points increased to about 19.8 or 23.4% in those receiving enoxaparin or unfractionated heparin, respectively, at 30 days and to about 32 or 35.7% of those receiving enoxaparin or unfractionated heparin, respectively, at 1 year: differences in these combined end points were statistically significant at all these time points evaluated. Urgent revascularization procedures were performed less frequently in patients receiving enoxaparin (6.3%) than unfractionated heparin (8.2%) at 30 days after initiation of treatment. Of the combined end points, reduction of recurrent angina was most striking with enoxaparin therapy. When the incidence of death or MI was considered separately, the effect of enoxaparin on these remaining end points was similar to unfractionated heparin.

In another comparative trial (Thrombolysis in Myocardial Infarction [TIMI] 11B) evaluating enoxaparin sodium (30 mg loading dose followed by 1 mg/kg twice daily for approximately 5 days) and unfractionated heparin sodium (70 units/kg loading dose followed by an infusion with dosage adjusted to maintain the aPTT between 1.5–2.5 times the control value for 3 days), the combined incidence of death, nonfatal MI, or need for urgent revascularization was 12.4% in those receiving enoxaparin and 14.5% in those receiving unfractionated heparin at 8 days; the relative risk reduction in these end points was 14.6%. The effect of trial therapies of unequal duration on the observed outcome is uncertain.

In a randomized, open-label comparative study (SYNERGY) in approximately 10,000 high-risk patients with NSTE-ACS, therapy with enoxaparin was noninferior to therapy with unfractionated heparin in terms of the incidence of the combined outcome of all-cause death or nonfatal MI at 30 days (primary efficacy end point). The primary efficacy end point occurred in 14% of patients receiving enoxaparin sodium (1 mg/kg subcutaneously every 12 hours) versus 14.5% of patients receiving unfractionated heparin sodium (60 units/kg by direct IV ["bolus"] injection followed by initial infusion of 12 units/kg per hour with subsequent dosage adjustment to achieve an aPTT of 1.5–2 times the upper limit of normal or 50–70 seconds). Patients were intended to be treated with an early invasive strategy, and most received concomitant therapy with aspirin (162–325 mg daily) and GP IIb/IIIa-receptor inhibitors. Approximately 47% of total patients underwent PCI and 19% had surgical revascularization procedures. Major bleeding (defined as intracranial bleeding or a decrease of at least 5 g/dL in hemoglobin or at least 15% in hematocrit, according to TIMI criteria) occurred more frequently in enoxaparin-treated patients and was related principally to CABG.

● ST-Segment-Elevation Myocardial Infarction

The current standard of care in patients with STEMI is timely reperfusion (with primary PCI or thrombolytic therapy). Adjunctive therapy with anticoagulant and antiplatelet agents should be used during and after successful coronary artery reperfusion for the prevention of early reocclusion and death, unless contraindicated. Adjunctive use of an LMWH in patients with STEMI has been associated with improvement in short-term clinical outcomes (e.g., death, reinfarction, recurrent ischemia) with generally similar rates of bleeding complications compared with unfractionated heparin or placebo. When used in conjunction with aspirin, enoxaparin has been shown to reduce the rate of a composite end point of recurrent MI or death in such patients.

The American College of Cardiology Foundation (ACCF) and AHA guidelines state that patients with STEMI undergoing thrombolytic therapy should receive an anticoagulant (e.g., unfractionated heparin, enoxaparin, fondaparinux) for a minimum of 48 hours, and preferably for the duration of the index hospitalization, up to 8 days or until revascularization is performed. Enoxaparin is preferred over unfractionated heparin if extended anticoagulation is necessary beyond 48 hours. In patients with STEMI who are subsequently undergoing PCI, an additional IV dose of enoxaparin may be required depending on the timing of the last administered subcutaneous dose. (See ST-Segment-Elevation Myocardial Infarction under Dosage and Administration.) Anticoagulation therapy is necessary during PCI to prevent thrombus formation at the site of arterial injury, on the coronary guidewire, and in the catheters used for the procedure.

Efficacy of enoxaparin as adjunctive therapy in the management of acute STEMI has been established in more than 20,000 patients with acute STEMI who were scheduled to undergo thrombolytic therapy with tenecteplase, alteplase, reteplase, or streptokinase. In a multicenter, randomized, double-blind, double-dummy, parallel-group study (Enoxaparin and Thrombolysis Reperfusion for Acute Myocardial Infarction treatment-Thrombolysis in myocardial infarction 25 [EXTRACT-TIMI 25]), adjunctive treatment with enoxaparin was more effective than unfractionated heparin (17% relative risk reduction) in reducing the rate of the composite efficacy end point of death from any cause or nonfatal recurrent MI at 30 days; the treatment benefit of enoxaparin emerged after 48 hours and was observed both in patients who were managed medically as well as those managed with PCI. The benefit of enoxaparin on the primary efficacy end point during the first 30 days of treatment was maintained over a 12-month follow-up period; however, there was no additional reduction in recurrent MI after 30 days and no mortality reduction at 1 year. In addition, an increased risk of major bleeding (including intracranial hemorrhage) was observed in patients receiving enoxaparin compared with those receiving unfractionated heparin. Careful patient selection is needed to ensure that the benefits of enoxaparin outweigh the increased risk of bleeding associated with the drug.

In the EXTRACT-TIMI 25 study, enoxaparin was given in an initial dose of 30 mg by direct IV injection in conjunction with a 1-mg/kg subcutaneous dose, followed by 1 mg/kg every 12 hours by subcutaneous injection for patients younger than 75 years of age, or in a dosage of 0.75 mg/kg every 12 hours by subcutaneous injection without an initial direct IV dose for patients 75 years of age or older; unfractionated heparin was administered in an initial dose of 60 units/kg (maximum 4000 units) by direct IV injection followed by continuous IV infusion of 12 units/kg per hour. All patients received aspirin (150–325 mg initially, then 75–325 mg daily) for at least 30 days. Enoxaparin was administered throughout the index hospitalization period (mean treatment duration of 6.6 days), while unfractionated heparin was administered for at least 48 hours (mean duration of 54 hours). The relatively longer duration of enoxaparin treatment compared with that of unfractionated heparin and a possible rebound increase in thrombotic events following discontinuance of heparin therapy may have contributed to the treatment differences in this study.

● *Acute Ischemic Stroke*

Although therapeutic-dose anticoagulation has been used in patients with acute ischemic stroke†, there is strong evidence that such treatment is associated with worse outcomes than aspirin therapy in terms of increased mortality and rates of nonfatal major extracranial bleeding. Therefore, the American College of Chest Physicians (ACCP) recommends early treatment (within 48 hours) with aspirin over therapeutic anticoagulation to prevent recurrent cerebral thromboembolism in patients with acute ischemic stroke or TIA.

Low molecular weight heparins (LMWHs) have been used for thromboprophylaxis in patients with acute ischemic stroke; those with additional risk factors for venous thromboembolism (VTE) (e.g., restricted mobility) are more likely to benefit from such prophylaxis.

LMWHs also have been used in the management of acute arterial ischemic stroke in children† until dissection and embolic causes have been excluded.

● *Thromboembolism During Pregnancy*

Low molecular weight heparins (LMWHs) are used for prevention and treatment of venous thromboembolism (VTE) during pregnancy† and also for prevention of thrombotic complications associated with prosthetic mechanical heart valves in pregnant women†. LMWHs also may be used in combination with aspirin for the prevention of recurrent pregnancy loss in women with antiphospholipid antibodies†. Pregnancy is associated with a hypercoagulable state and an increased risk of thromboembolism, and pregnant women with thromboembolic disease or hereditary or acquired thrombophilias are at greater risk for fetal loss as a result of stillbirth, spontaneous abortion, or premature delivery. (See Thromboembolism Associated with Prosthetic Heart Valves under Uses.)

The American College of Chest Physicians (ACCP) states that LMWHs are the anticoagulant of choice for prevention and treatment of thromboembolism during pregnancy; there is a potential for other agents to cross the placenta. In pregnant women with acute VTE†, LMWHs are recommended for initial *treatment* and *secondary prevention* throughout the remainder of the pregnancy. Anticoagulant therapy should be continued for at least 6 weeks postpartum and a minimum total duration of 3 months to prevent recurrence of VTE.

Recommendations regarding the use of anticoagulant prophylaxis during the antepartum period in pregnant women who have a history of thromboembolism† are based on the patient's risk for recurrent events. In general, thromboprophylaxis (e.g., with LMWHs) is suggested only in patients with moderate to high risk of recurrent thromboembolism (e.g., unprovoked VTE, pregnancy- or estrogen-related VTE, history of multiple unprovoked events).

The presence of hereditary thrombophilias and a family history of VTE substantially increases the risk of pregnancy-related VTE. Homozygous genetic mutations for factor V Leiden or prothrombin G20210A are associated with the highest risks of thromboembolism in pregnant women. ACCP therefore suggests antepartum prophylaxis with LMWHs (in prophylactic or intermediate dosages) in selected pregnant women with these genetic mutations.

To avoid an unwanted anticoagulant effect on the fetus during delivery, therapy with LMWHs should be discontinued prior to induction of labor or cesarean section (or expected time of neuraxial anesthesia). (See Dosage under Dosage and Administration.)

● *Cardioversion of Atrial Fibrillation/Flutter*

Low molecular weight heparins (LMWHs) also have been used for the prevention of stroke and systemic embolism in patients with atrial fibrillation undergoing electrical or pharmacologic cardioversion†. Because the risk of thromboembolism appears to be greatest when atrial fibrillation has been present for >48 hours, recommendations for the use of anticoagulant therapy in such patients vary based on the duration of the arrhythmia. The American College of Chest Physicians (ACCP) and other experts recommend that patients with atrial fibrillation of ≥48 hours' duration or of an unknown duration who are to undergo elective cardioversion receive therapeutic anticoagulation (with warfarin or a direct oral anticoagulant [DOAC]) for at least 3 weeks prior to cardioversion; an alternative strategy is to perform transesophageal echocardiography (TEE) to exclude thrombus and then administer therapeutic anticoagulation with an LMWH or unfractionated heparin prior to cardioversion. Patients with atrial fibrillation of <48 hours' duration and a high risk of stroke (e.g., CHA_2DS_2-VASc score of 2 or more for males or 3 or more for females) usually do not require prolonged anticoagulation or TEE prior to cardioversion; such patients may receive therapeutic anticoagulation (e.g., with an LMWH, unfractionated heparin, or DOAC) at presentation, followed by immediate cardioversion and long-term anticoagulant therapy. In patients with atrial fibrillation of <48 hours' duration and a low risk of stroke (e.g., CHA_2DS_2-VASc score of 0 for males and 1 for females), the same therapeutic anticoagulation strategies or no anticoagulation therapy may be considered for cardioversion. After successful cardioversion in patients with atrial fibrillation of ≥48 hours' duration, experts recommend that patients receive therapeutic anticoagulation for at least 4 weeks; patients with atrial fibrillation of <48 hours' duration who have a low risk of stroke generally do not need oral anticoagulation postcardioversion. In all patients, the decision to administer long-term anticoagulation following cardioversion should be based on the patient's risk of thromboembolism and risk of bleeding.

In patients undergoing cardioversion for atrial flutter†, the same approach to thromboprophylaxis should be used as for those with atrial fibrillation.

● *Thromboembolism Associated with Prosthetic Heart Valves*

Low molecular weight heparins (LMWHs) have been used to reduce the risk of thromboembolism (e.g., stroke) during conversion to maintenance oral anticoagulant therapy (e.g., warfarin) in patients with prosthetic mechanical heart valves†. (See Bridging Anticoagulation under Uses.) In the absence of a bleeding risk, the American College of Chest Physicians (ACCP) suggests bridging therapy (e.g., administration of an LMWH in either prophylactic or therapeutic dosages) during the early postoperative period after insertion of a mechanical heart valve until an adequate response to the oral anticoagulant is obtained. (See Dosage under Dosage and Administration.)

In patients with a mechanical heart valve in whom therapy with an oral anti-coagulant must be temporarily discontinued (e.g., those undergoing major surgery), bridging anticoagulation† with an LMWH has been used in selected patients (e.g., those at high risk of thromboembolism).

Pregnant women with prosthetic mechanical heart valves† may be at even higher risk for thromboembolism; thrombosis of prosthetic heart valves has occurred in some pregnant women receiving enoxaparin prophylaxis and in some cases has resulted in maternal and/or fetal death. (See Patients with Mechanical Prosthetic Heart Valves under Cautions.) Pregnant women with prosthetic mechanical heart valves should receive therapeutic anticoagulation with frequent monitoring during pregnancy. No anticoagulation strategy is optimal in terms of safety to the mother and fetus. While warfarin is safest for the mother, the drug crosses the placenta and can cause adverse fetal effects; although unfractionated heparin and LMWHs do not cross the placenta, both are associated with higher rates of maternal complications than warfarin. There is evidence indicating that fixed-dose LMWHs or adjusted-dose, poorly controlled unfractionated heparin therapy is *not* effective in preventing systemic embolism in pregnant women with prosthetic mechanical heart valves. Strategies using LMWHs include an option where dose-adjusted LMWH (i.e., given twice daily and adjusted to maintain peak anti-factor Xa concentration of 0.8–1.2 units/mL at 4–6 hours postinjection) is used throughout pregnancy and an alternative option where dose-adjusted LMWH is used for the first trimester followed by warfarin for the second and third trimesters.

If enoxaparin is used for anticoagulation in pregnant women with mechanical prosthetic heart valves, frequent monitoring of peak and trough anti-factor Xa levels and dosage adjustments may be required to ensure consistent anticoagulation. (See Pregnancy under Cautions.)

● Cerebral Venous Sinus Thrombosis

Low molecular weight heparins (LMWHs) have been used for the treatment of acute cerebral venous sinus (sinovenous) thrombosis† in adults and pediatric patients.

● Bridging Anticoagulation

Low molecular weight heparins (LMWHs) have been used for bridging anticoagulation† during temporary interruption of long-term oral anticoagulant therapy in patients undergoing surgery or other invasive procedures†. Perioperative use of LMWHs has been recommended during the period of interruption of oral anticoagulant therapy in some patients with venous thromboembolism (VTE), atrial fibrillation, or mechanical prosthetic heart valves depending on the patient's risk of thromboembolism and risk of bleeding. Bridging anticoagulation has been associated with an increased risk of major bleeding without a significant effect on arterial thromboembolism in some settings and therefore should be considered on an individual basis. (See Thromboembolism Associated with Prosthetic Heart Valves under Uses.)

DOSAGE AND ADMINISTRATION

● General

Patient Monitoring

- The possibility of an underlying bleeding disorder should be ruled out before initiating enoxaparin therapy. Since prothrombin time (PT) and activated partial thromboplastin time (aPTT) are insensitive for monitoring enoxaparin activity, routine monitoring of coagulation parameters generally is not required. In pregnant patients, patients at extremes of weight, or if abnormal coagulation parameters, appreciable renal impairment, or bleeding should occur, anti-factor Xa levels may be used to monitor the anticoagulant effects of enoxaparin. (See Special Populations under Dosage and Administration.)
- If enoxaparin is used for anticoagulation in pregnant women with mechanical prosthetic heart valves, frequent monitoring of peak and trough anti-factor Xa concentrations is recommended to assess anticoagulation, and dosage should be adjusted as necessary. (See Patients with Mechanical Prosthetic Heart Valves under Cautions.) The American College of Chest Physicians (ACCP) and other clinicians recommend twice-daily dosing of LMWHs in pregnant women, at least initially, because of altered pharmacokinetics during pregnancy.

● Administration

Enoxaparin sodium is administered by deep subcutaneous injection; *it must not be given IM.* The drug also is administered IV (as a direct IV injection) in certain situations. (See ST-Segment-Elevation Myocardial Infarction and also see Non-ST-Segment-Elevation Acute Coronary Syndrome under Dosage and Administration.)

Patients should be supine during administration of the drug.

To avoid loss of drug when using the prefilled syringes, the manufacturer states that air should not be expelled from the syringe prior to injection. If the prescribed dose is less than the full syringe volume, the excess syringe volume should be ejected until only the prescribed dose remains in the syringe.

Subcutaneous Administration

When injecting enoxaparin subcutaneously, the entire length of the needle should be inserted into a skin fold created by the thumb and the forefinger; the skin fold should be held until the needle is withdrawn. Injections should be made into the left and right anterolateral and posterolateral abdominal wall; injection sites should be alternated frequently. To minimize bruising, injection sites should not be massaged after injection.

IV Administration

When enoxaparin is administered IV, the multiple-dose vial preparation should be used. Enoxaparin should not be mixed with other drugs. The IV line should be flushed before and after enoxaparin administration with either 0.9% sodium chloride injection or 5% dextrose injection.

● Dosage

Dosages for enoxaparin sodium or other low molecular weight heparins (LMWHs) or unfractionated heparin sodium cannot be used interchangeably on a unit-for-unit (or mg-for-mg) basis. Enoxaparin sodium has an approximate anti-factor Xa activity of 100 units/mg according to the World Health Organization (WHO) First International Low Molecular Weight Heparin Reference Standard.

If an LMWH is used for anticoagulation in children, ACCP suggests that dosage of the drug be adjusted to a target anti-factor Xa level of 0.5–1 units/mL based on a sample taken 4–6 hours, or 0.5–0.8 units/mL based on a sample taken 2–6 hours, following subcutaneous administration.

Prevention of Venous Thromboembolism
General/Abdominal Surgery

For venous thromboembolism (VTE) prophylaxis in patients undergoing general (abdominal) surgery who are at risk for thromboembolic complications, the manufacturer recommends an enoxaparin sodium dosage of 40 mg once daily by subcutaneous injection. The initial dosage should be given 2 hours prior to surgery. Enoxaparin should be administered throughout the postoperative period, generally for 7–10 days; however, the manufacturer states that treatment with enoxaparin has been well tolerated for up to 12 days in patients undergoing abdominal surgery in clinical trials. Extended VTE prophylaxis (generally considered as beyond 3 weeks) may be considered in selected patients undergoing major general surgery. Because the risk of VTE is particularly high in patients undergoing abdominal or pelvic surgery for cancer, the American College of Chest Physicians (ACCP) recommends that therapy with LMWHs be continued for up to 4 weeks in such patients.

Hip- or Knee-Replacement Surgery

For VTE prophylaxis in patients undergoing hip-replacement or knee-replacement surgery, the manufacturer recommends an enoxaparin sodium dosage of 30 mg twice daily (every 12 hours) by subcutaneous injection beginning 12–24 hours postoperatively, provided hemostasis has been established. Alternatively, in patients undergoing hip-replacement surgery, the manufacturer states that an enoxaparin sodium dosage of 40 mg once daily (every 24 hours) by subcutaneous injection beginning 12 (±3) hours preoperatively may be considered, based on dose-comparison data indicating that a dosage of 40 mg once daily may be as effective as 30 mg twice daily (every 12 hours) in preventing DVT in such patients. ACCP states that risk of bleeding is closely associated with the timing of initiation of thromboprophylaxis around surgery and recommends that LMWHs be initiated at least 12 hours preoperatively or at least 12 hours postoperatively in patients undergoing major orthopedic surgery.

Enoxaparin should be administered throughout the postoperative period, generally for 7–10 days, until the risk of DVT has diminished; ACCP recommends a minimum of 10–14 days of thromboprophylaxis, with extended prophylaxis suggested for up to 35 days on an outpatient basis. Treatment with enoxaparin for up to 14 days has been well tolerated in clinical trials. Following the initial phase of thromboprophylaxis during the acute postoperative period in patients undergoing hip-replacement surgery, the manufacturer recommends continued prophylaxis with subcutaneous enoxaparin sodium 40 mg once daily for 3 weeks.

Medical Conditions Associated with Thromboembolism

For VTE prophylaxis in patients at increased risk of thromboembolism due to severely restricted mobility during acute illness (e.g., cancer, heart failure, severe lung disease, those confined to bedrest), the manufacturer recommends an enoxaparin sodium dosage of 40 mg daily, usually given for 6–11 days; treatment with the drug for up to 14 days has been well tolerated in clinical trials. ACCP suggests against the use of extended thromboprophylaxis beyond the period of patient immobilization or acute hospitalization in acutely ill medical patients because of an increased risk of bleeding and the burden and costs of daily injections. However, extended thromboprophylaxis has been used in selected patients after hospital discharge.

Treatment of Venous Thromboembolism

For the outpatient treatment of uncomplicated deep-vein thrombosis (DVT) without pulmonary embolism (PE), the usual dosage of enoxaparin sodium is 1 mg/kg twice daily given subcutaneously.

In hospitalized patients with venous thromboembolism (VTE), the usual dosage of enoxaparin sodium is 1 mg/kg twice daily or 1.5 mg/kg once daily administered subcutaneously at the same time every day.

The manufacturer states that the average duration of therapy is 7 days. In patients with VTE, the American College of Chest Physicians (ACCP) recommends that anticoagulant therapy be continued beyond the acute treatment period for at least 3 months, and possibly longer depending on whether the VTE event was unprovoked or provoked by a transient risk factor (e.g., surgery), the presence of cancer, and the patient's risk of bleeding.

Transitioning from Enoxaparin to Oral Anticoagulants

In patients transitioning to warfarin for long-term anticoagulant therapy, warfarin should be initiated when appropriate (usually within 72 hours of enoxaparin initiation) and continued for a minimum of 5 days and until a therapeutic international normalized ratio (INR of 2–3) has been achieved. Enoxaparin may be discontinued after this period of overlap with warfarin, generally after a total of 7 days of enoxaparin treatment.

In patients transitioning to dabigatran for long-term anticoagulant therapy, enoxaparin should be administered for 5–10 days. Enoxaparin should then be discontinued, and dabigatran initiated 0–2 hours prior to the time of the next scheduled dose of enoxaparin.

In patients transitioning to edoxaban for long-term anticoagulant therapy, enoxaparin should be administered for 5–10 days. Enoxaparin should then be discontinued and edoxaban initiated at the time of the next scheduled dose of enoxaparin.

In patients transitioning to apixaban for long-term anticoagulant therapy, enoxaparin should be discontinued and apixaban initiated at the time of the next scheduled dose of enoxaparin.

In patients transitioning to rivaroxaban for long-term anticoagulant therapy, enoxaparin should be discontinued and rivaroxaban initiated 0–2 hours prior to the time of the next scheduled dose of enoxaparin.

Non-ST-Segment-Elevation Acute Coronary Syndrome

In patients with non-ST-segment-elevation acute coronary syndrome (NSTE-ACS) who are receiving concurrent therapy with aspirin (e.g., 75–325 mg once daily), the usual dosage of enoxaparin sodium is 1 mg/kg every 12 hours by subcutaneous injection. Anticoagulant therapy should be administered as soon as possible after hospital admission. Treatment with enoxaparin should continue for a minimum of 2 days until the patient is clinically stabilized, generally for 2–8 days;

the manufacturer states that treatment with enoxaparin for up to 12.5 days has been well tolerated in clinical trials.

The American College of Cardiology Foundation (ACCF), American Heart Association (AHA), and the Society for Cardiovascular Angiography and Interventions (SCAI) state that it is reasonable to administer enoxaparin sodium (e.g., 0.5–0.75 mg/kg *by direct IV injection*†) for prevention of thrombus formation during percutaneous coronary intervention (PCI) in patients with NSTE-ACS who have not received prior anticoagulant therapy. In patients with NSTE-ACS in whom subcutaneous enoxaparin has been initiated prior to PCI ("upstream"), ACCF/AHA/SCAI state that an additional 0.3-mg/kg dose of enoxaparin sodium should be given *by direct IV injection* at the time of PCI if fewer than 2 prior therapeutic (e.g., 1 mg/kg) subcutaneous doses of enoxaparin sodium have been given or if the last subcutaneous dose of the drug was administered 8–12 hours before PCI†. To minimize the possibility of bleeding associated with vascular (e.g., vascular access sheath) instrumentation (e.g., PCI) during treatment of NSTE-ACS, strict adherence to dosage intervals of subcutaneous enoxaparin and precautions in the removal of the vascular access sheath should be observed. The next dose of enoxaparin sodium should be given no sooner than 6–8 hours after removal of the vascular access sheath; ACCF/AHA/SCAI suggest removal of femoral sheaths when the activated clotting time (ACT) falls to less than 150–180 seconds or when the activated partial thromboplastin time (aPTT) falls to less than 50 seconds. Careful monitoring of vascular access sites for signs of bleeding or hematoma formation should be undertaken after removal of the vascular sheath and during treatment with enoxaparin.

ST-Segment-Elevation Myocardial Infarction

In patients with acute ST-segment-elevation myocardial infarction (STEMI) who are younger than 75 years of age, an initial direct IV injection of enoxaparin sodium 30 mg plus a 1-mg/kg subcutaneous dose is recommended by the manufacturer, followed by subcutaneous injections of enoxaparin sodium 1 mg/kg every 12 hours; a maximum of 100 mg is recommended for each of the first 2 subcutaneous doses. For the treatment of acute STEMI in patients 75 years of age or older, the recommended dosage of enoxaparin sodium is 0.75 mg/kg every 12 hours (not to exceed 75 mg per dose for the first 2 doses) by subcutaneous injection; an initial IV dose should not be given. Aspirin (75–325 mg once daily) should be administered in conjunction with enoxaparin therapy unless contraindicated. When used with thrombolytic therapy, enoxaparin therapy should be initiated between 15 minutes before and 30 minutes after the start of thrombolytic therapy. The manufacturer states that the usual duration of enoxaparin treatment is 8 days or until hospital discharge.

In patients with acute STEMI undergoing percutaneous coronary intervention (PCI), the manufacturer recommends administration of an additional 0.3-mg/kg dose of enoxaparin sodium by direct IV injection during PCI if the last subcutaneous dose of enoxaparin sodium was administered more than 8 hours before balloon inflation; otherwise, no additional dose is recommended.

Treatment and Prevention of Thromboembolism During Pregnancy

In pregnant women with acute venous thromboembolism (VTE)†, enoxaparin sodium 1 mg/kg twice daily is recommended by the American College of Chest Physicians (ACCP) for initial treatment and should be continued throughout the remainder of the pregnancy. Anticoagulation should be continued postpartum for at least 6 weeks (for a minimum total duration of 3 months).

If enoxaparin sodium is used for postpartum prophylaxis in pregnant women with a prior VTE†, a prophylactic (e.g., 40 mg once daily) or intermediate dosage (e.g., 40 mg every 12 hours) is suggested.

In pregnant women with mechanical prosthetic heart valves receiving long-term warfarin anticoagulation†, if the decision is made to switch to an LMWH-based strategy, dose-adjusted LMWH is recommended. The LMWH may be administered throughout all 3 trimesters or, alternatively, the LMWH may be administered during the first trimester, followed by warfarin during the second and third trimesters. The LMWH should be administered at least 2 times daily with close monitoring of anti-factor Xa levels. Dosage should be adjusted to target factor Xa levels of 0.8–1.2 units/mL 4–6 hours after dosing. (See Patients with Mechanical Prosthetic Heart Valves under Cautions.)

If enoxaparin sodium is used for primary prevention of VTE in pregnant women with certain high-risk thrombophilias†, a prophylactic (e.g., 40 mg once daily) or intermediate (e.g., 40 mg every 12 hours) subcutaneous dosage is suggested. (See Pregnant Patients under Dosage and Administration.)

Cardioversion of Atrial Fibrillation/Flutter

If enoxaparin sodium is used for the prevention of stroke and systemic embolism in patients undergoing cardioversion for atrial fibrillation or atrial flutter†, administration of full-treatment dosages used for venous thromboembolism (VTE) is recommended.

Bridging Anticoagulation

In patients who are receiving bridging anticoagulation† with therapeutic-dose subcutaneous enoxaparin, the American College of Chest Physicians (ACCP) suggests administering the last preoperative dose of enoxaparin sodium approximately 24 hours prior to surgery to allow sufficient time for anticoagulant effects to dissipate. Postoperative anticoagulation should be administered with caution and only when hemostasis has been achieved because of the potential for bleeding at the surgical site. In patients undergoing procedures associated with a high risk of bleeding, ACCP suggests delaying the resumption of therapeutic-dose enoxaparin until 48–72 hours after surgery when adequate hemostasis has been achieved.

● Special Populations

Renal Impairment

Caution is advised when using enoxaparin in patients with renal impairment since elimination of the drug may be delayed. Patients with renal impairment should be carefully monitored for signs and symptoms of bleeding. In addition, anti-factor Xa levels may be used to monitor the anticoagulant effect of enoxaparin in patients with substantial renal impairment. No dosage adjustment is recommended in patients with mild (creatinine clearance 50–80 mL/minute) or moderate (creatinine clearance 30–50 mL/minute) renal impairment. However, dosage should be adjusted in patients with severe renal impairment (creatinine clearance < 30 mL/minute). (See Table 1.)

TABLE 1. Enoxaparin Sodium Dosage Recommendations for Patients with Severe Renal Impairment (Creatinine Clearance <30 mL/minute)

Indication	Dosage Regimen
VTE prophylaxis in abdominal surgery	30 mg administered subcutaneously once daily
VTE prophylaxis in hip- or knee-replacement surgery	30 mg administered subcutaneously once daily
VTE prophylaxis in medical patients during acute illness	30 mg administered subcutaneously once daily
Treatment of acute VTE in hospitalized patients (when administered in conjunction with warfarin)	1 mg/kg administered subcutaneously once daily
Outpatient treatment of acute VTE (when administered in conjunction with warfarin)	1 mg/kg administered subcutaneously once daily
Prophylaxis of ischemic complications of NSTE-ACS (when administered concurrently with aspirin)	1 mg/kg administered subcutaneously once daily
Treatment of acute STEMI in patients <75 years of age (when administered in conjunction with aspirin)	30 mg as a single direct IV injection plus a 1-mg/kg subcutaneous dose; follow with subcutaneous injections of 1 mg/kg once daily (maximum of 100 mg per dose for each of the first 2 subcutaneous doses)
Treatment of acute STEMI in patients ≥75 years of age (when administered in conjunction with aspirin)	1 mg/kg administered subcutaneously once daily (maximum of 75 mg per dose for each of the first 2 doses); do not administer an initial IV dose

VTE = venous thromboembolism, NSTE-ACS = non-ST-segment-elevation acute coronary syndrome, STEMI = ST-segment-elevation myocardial infarction

Pregnant Patients

Low molecular weight heparins (LMWHs) have lower peak plasma concentrations and shorter half-lives in pregnant women, which often requires higher doses and/or more frequent administration. Adjusted-dose anticoagulation is recommended for all women with acute venous thromboembolism (VTE) during pregnancy. For adjusted-dose LMWH, the American College of Obstetricians and Gynecologists (ACOG) recommends targeting anti-factor Xa levels of 0.6–1 units/mL 4 hours after the last injection of a twice-daily regimen; slightly higher doses may be need for once-daily regimens.

If enoxaparin is used in pregnant women with mechanical prosthetic heart valves, anti-factor Xa levels should be used to monitor the anticoagulant effect of enoxaparin, and enoxaparin sodium dosage should be adjusted as needed. The American College of Cardiology (ACC) and the American Heart Association (AHA) suggest that if an LMWH is used in pregnant women with a mechanical prosthetic heart valve, the dosage should be adjusted to maintain anti-factor Xa levels of 0.8–1.2 units/mL 4–6 hours after administration.

To avoid an unwanted anticoagulant effect on the fetus during delivery, therapy with LMWHs should be discontinued at least 24 hours (or at least 12 hours if using prophylactic-dose LMWH) prior to induction of labor or cesarean section. The American College of Chest Physicians (ACCP) states that if an at-term woman is at very high risk for recurrent VTE (e.g., occurrence of proximal deep-vein thrombosis [DVT] within the past 2 weeks), IV unfractionated heparin may be initiated at this time and then discontinued 4–6 hours prior to the expected time of delivery. Pregnant women with mechanical heart valves who are receiving LMWHs should switch to unfractionated heparin at least 36 hours prior to planned delivery.

Low Body Weight

Increased exposure to enoxaparin has been observed in patients with low body weight (<45 kg in women or <57 kg in men); all such patients should be carefully monitored for signs and symptoms of bleeding.

Obese Patients

Safety and efficacy of thromboprophylactic dosages of enoxaparin in patients with body mass index (BMI) >30 kg/m² have not been established and there is no consensus on how dosage should be adjusted in such patients; these patients should be closely observed for signs and symptoms of thromboembolism during therapy. The American Society of Hematology (ASH) suggests that enoxaparin should be dosed according to the patient's actual body weight when the drug is used for treatment of acute venous thromboembolism (VTE) and does not recommend monitoring anti-factor Xa concentrations to guide dosage adjustments.

CAUTIONS

● Contraindications

- Active major bleeding.
- Immune-mediated heparin-induced thrombocytopenia within the prior 100 days or associated with circulating antiplatelet antibodies.
- Known hypersensitivity to enoxaparin sodium (e.g., pruritus, urticaria, anaphylactic/anaphylactoid reactions), heparin, pork products, benzyl alcohol, or any ingredient in the formulation.

● Warnings/Precautions

Warnings

Spinal/Epidural Hematomas

Concurrent use of low molecular weight heparins (LMWHs) or heparinoids with neuraxial (spinal/epidural) anesthesia or spinal puncture procedures has been associated with epidural or spinal hematomas. The prescribing information for enoxaparin has a boxed warning regarding the risk of spinal/epidural hematomas. Hematomas occurring in such patients have resulted in neurologic injury, including long-term or permanent paralysis. The risk of these adverse events is increased by the use of indwelling epidural catheters for administration of analgesia or by the concomitant use of drugs that affect hemostasis, such as nonsteroidal anti-inflammatory agents (NSAIAs), platelet-aggregation inhibitors, or other anticoagulants. The risk also appears to be increased by a history of traumatic or repeated epidural or spinal puncture, spinal surgery, or spinal deformity. It is important to note that the risk of spinal hematoma applies to all anticoagulants when used in conjunction with neuraxial anesthesia or spinal puncture.

FDA states that cases of epidural or spinal hematomas continue to be reported in patients receiving enoxaparin in the setting of neuraxial procedures. Between July 20, 1992 and January 31, 2013, at least 100 confirmed or probable cases of spinal/epidural hematoma associated with the concurrent use of enoxaparin thromboprophylaxis and neuraxial anesthesia were reported to FDA by the manufacturer. Risk factors that were present in many of these cases included female gender, older age (≥65 years of age), concomitant use of drugs affecting hemostasis, indwelling epidural catheter, epidural technique, twice-daily versus once-daily administration of enoxaparin, and underlying medical conditions with increased risk of hemorrhage. To address this safety concern, the FDA has recommended additional safety measures.

Prior to performing a spinal or epidural procedure, healthcare professionals should determine as part of a preprocedure checklist whether a patient is receiving anticoagulants. In addition, clinicians should carefully consider the timing of spinal catheter placement and removal in relation to anticoagulant use, considering both the dosage and pharmacokinetic properties (e.g., elimination half-life) of the anticoagulant. Insertion or removal of a epidural catheter or lumbar puncture is best performed when the anticoagulant effect of enoxaparin is minimal. Although the optimal timing between the administration of enoxaparin and neuraxial procedures is not known, the following guidelines are recommended. In patients receiving low (prophylactic) dosages of enoxaparin sodium (30 mg once or twice daily or 40 mg once daily), insertion or removal of a spinal catheter should be delayed for at least 12 hours after a dose of enoxaparin. In patients receiving higher (treatment) dosages of enoxaparin sodium (0.75 mg/kg twice daily, 1 mg/kg twice daily, or 1.5 mg/kg once daily), a delay of at least 24 hours is recommended between the enoxaparin dose and catheter placement/removal; if the patient is receiving a twice-daily treatment regimen, the second dose should be omitted to allow for a longer delay. In patients with renal impairment (creatinine clearance less than 30 mL/minute), a doubling of the recommended time delays is recommended to account for possible prolonged elimination of enoxaparin in such patients. The manufacturer suggests that clinicians consider delaying administration of enoxaparin for at least 4 hours after catheter removal, taking into account the patient's risk of bleeding versus thrombosis.

Patients receiving LMWHs or heparinoids in the setting of epidural or spinal anesthesia or lumbar puncture should be monitored frequently for manifestations of neurologic impairment (e.g., midline back pain, numbness or weakness in lower limbs, bowel or bladder dysfunction). If spinal hematoma is suspected, urgent diagnosis and treatment is necessary; spinal cord decompression should be considered even though it may not prevent or reverse neurologic sequelae. Some experts recommend against the concomitant use of a low molecular weight heparin with other drugs affecting hemostasis (e.g., aspirin, NSAIAs, platelet-aggregation inhibitors, other anticoagulants) in patients receiving spinal anesthesia. Clinicians should fully consider the potential benefits versus risks of spinal or epidural anesthesia or spinal puncture in patients receiving or being considered for thromboprophylaxis with anticoagulants.

Bleeding

Major hemorrhage (e.g., intracranial or retroperitoneal bleeding) has occurred in patients receiving enoxaparin, and sometimes resulted in fatalities. Bleeding can occur at any site during therapy. Women treated with LMWHs prior to percutaneous coronary intervention (PCI) appear to experience more bleeding complications than do men.

Enoxaparin should be used with extreme caution in patients with an increased risk of hemorrhage (e.g., bacterial endocarditis; congenital or acquired bleeding disorders; active ulceration and angiodysplastic GI disease; hemorrhagic stroke; recent brain, spinal, or ophthalmic surgery; concomitant platelet inhibitor therapy). The manufacturer states that the drug also should be used with care in patients with a bleeding diathesis, uncontrolled arterial hypertension, history of recent GI ulceration, diabetic retinopathy, or hemorrhage. Patients with low body weight or renal impairment should be monitored carefully for signs and symptoms of bleeding; dosage adjustment may be necessary in such patients. Periodic complete blood cell counts, including platelet counts, and stool occult blood tests are recommended during use of

enoxaparin. Hemorrhage should be seriously considered in anticoagulated patients with unexplained decreases in hematocrit or blood pressure. Protamine sulfate may be used to neutralize the anticoagulant effect of LMWHs in patients with bleeding. Because fatal reactions resembling anaphylaxis have been reported with protamine sulfate administration, the drug should be used only when resuscitation techniques and treatment for anaphylactic shock are readily available.

To minimize risk of bleeding following percutaneous revascularization procedures (i.e., PCI), clinicians should adhere precisely to the recommended dosing intervals for enoxaparin. (See Dosage under Dosage and Administration.) Recommendations for the timing of sheath removal is based on the method of post-PCI arterial closure. If a closure device is used, the sheath may be removed immediately; however, if manual compression is used, the sheath should be removed 6 hours after the last dose of enoxaparin. In patients in whom enoxaparin therapy will be continued, the next scheduled dose should be given no sooner than 6–8 hours after sheath removal. The site of the procedure should be closely monitored for signs of bleeding or hematoma formation; it is important that hemostasis be achieved at the puncture site after PCI.

Thrombocytopenia

Moderate thrombocytopenia (platelet counts between 50,000 and 100,000/mm³) was reported in 1.3% of patients in clinical studies, and severe thrombocytopenia (platelet counts less than 50,000/mm³) was reported in 0.1% of patients. Thrombocytopenia of any degree should be monitored closely, and enoxaparin should be discontinued if platelet counts fall below 100,000/mm³. (See Contraindications under Cautions.)

Heparin-induced thrombocytopenia (HIT) or heparin-induced thrombocytopenia with thrombosis (HITTS) can occur with the administration of enoxaparin; some cases of thrombocytopenia have been complicated by organ infarction with secondary organ dysfunction or limb ischemia, and deaths have resulted. Enoxaparin should be used with extreme caution in patients with a history of HIT/HITTS. In patients with a history of HIT/HITTS, enoxaparin should only be used if more than 100 days have elapsed since the prior episode and the patient has no circulating antiplatelet antibodies. Because of the possibility of HIT/HITTS recurrence in these patients, a careful risk-benefit assessment should occur and nonheparin anticoagulants should be considered.

Interchangeability with Other Heparins

Enoxaparin should not be used interchangeably with other LMWHs or unfractionated heparin because of differences in manufacturing process, molecular weight distribution, anti-factor Xa and anti-factor II_a activities, dosage units, and dosage.

Patients with Mechanical Prosthetic Heart Valves

The use of enoxaparin for prophylaxis of thromboembolism in patients with mechanical prosthetic heart valves has not been adequately studied, and a clinical consensus regarding optimal therapy remains to be established. Valve thrombosis that was fatal (including maternal and fetal death) or potentially fatal and/or required surgical intervention has been reported during prophylaxis with enoxaparin in some patients (including pregnant women) with mechanical prosthetic heart valves. (See Thromboembolism During Pregnancy under Uses.) Insufficient data, the presence of underlying conditions, and the possibility of inadequate anticoagulation complicate the evaluation of these events in such patients. However, women with mechanical prosthetic heart valves may be at higher risk for thromboembolism during pregnancy.

The manufacturer and some clinicians currently state that if enoxaparin is used in pregnant women with mechanical prosthetic heart valves, frequent monitoring of peak and trough anti-factor Xa concentrations and adjustment of enoxaparin sodium dosage may be necessary. The American College of Chest Physicians (ACCP) recommends use of aggressive, adjusted-dose subcutaneous LMWH (i.e., given twice daily and adjusted to maintain the manufacturer-recommended peak anti-factor Xa concentrations 4 hours postinjection) in pregnant women with mechanical prosthetic heart valves. Although empiric, the therapeutic monitoring recommendation for anti-factor Xa concentrations is based on differences in the pharmacokinetics of LMWHs that occur during pregnancy and is aimed at attempting to ensure that dosage is adjusted appropriately to ensure consistent anticoagulation.

Specific Populations

Pregnancy

There are no adequate and well-controlled studies of enoxaparin in pregnant women. Animal studies indicate that enoxaparin crosses the placenta; however, available data in humans indicate that low molecular weight heparins (LMWHs) do not cross the placenta. Available human data also have not shown evidence of teratogenicity or fetotoxicity. In a review of approximately 600 retrospectively followed pregnancies in women exposed to enoxaparin, the incidences of congenital anomalies did not exceed what would be expected in the general population. Maternal and neonatal hemorrhage did occur in some of the followed pregnancies. The American College of Obstetricians and Gynecologists (ACOG) considers LMWHs to be generally safe in pregnancy.

Pregnancy alone is associated with an increased risk of thromboembolism, which is even higher in women with a history of thromboembolism and certain high-risk pregnancy conditions, including hereditary or acquired thrombophilias and the presence of a mechanical prosthetic heart valve. The pharmacokinetics of LMWHs differ in pregnant versus nonpregnant women because of changes in volume of distribution resulting in increased plasma volume, decreased half-life, and changes in renal clearance. Some clinicians recommend frequent monitoring of anti-factor Xa concentrations and adjustment of enoxaparin sodium dosage in pregnant women with mechanical prosthetic heart valves to ensure a consistent anticoagulant effect.

All patients receiving anticoagulants such as enoxaparin, including pregnant women, are at risk for bleeding. Hemorrhage can occur at any site and may lead to death of mother and/or fetus. Pregnant women receiving enoxaparin should be apprised of the potential hazards to the mother and fetus associated with enoxaparin use during pregnancy, and such women should be carefully monitored for evidence of bleeding or excessive anticoagulation. Use of enoxaparin may result in epidural or spinal hematomas in women receiving neuraxial anesthesia during labor and delivery. Pregnant women receiving enoxaparin should be monitored for bleeding and for any unexpected changes in coagulation parameters. As delivery approaches, use of a shorter-acting anticoagulant should be considered.

Use of enoxaparin in pregnant women with mechanical prosthetic heart valves may result in valve thrombosis. (See Patients with Mechanical Prosthetic Heart Valves under Cautions.)

Lactation

It is not known whether enoxaparin is distributed into milk; studies in lactating rats demonstrated very limited distribution of enoxaparin into milk. It is not known whether enoxaparin affects the breast-fed child or affects milk production. The benefits of breast-feeding should be considered along with the importance of the drug to the woman and any potential adverse effects on the breast-fed child from the drug or underlying maternal condition.

The American College of Obstetricians and Gynecologists (ACOG) considers low molecular weight heparins (LMWHs) to be compatible with lactation. The American College of Chest Physicians (ACCP) recommends that LMWHs be continued in nursing women who are already receiving such therapy; the small amounts of drug detected in the milk of nursing women are not likely to be clinically important.

Pediatric Use

Safety and efficacy of enoxaparin have not been established in children younger than 18 years of age.

Each mL of enoxaparin sodium injection in multiple-dose vials contains 15 mg of benzyl alcohol as a preservative. Although a causal relationship has not been established, administration of injections preserved with benzyl alcohol has been associated with toxicity in neonates, including fatal reactions and the "gasping syndrome". Toxicity appears to have resulted from administration of large amounts (i.e., about 100–400 mg/kg daily) of benzyl alcohol in these neonates. Because benzyl alcohol may cross the placenta, the manufacturer states that the preservative-free formulations of enoxaparin should be used in pregnant women whenever possible.

Geriatric Use

No substantial differences in efficacy have been observed in geriatric patients relative to younger adults. In geriatric patients, a higher incidence of bleeding complications has been observed following administration of enoxaparin sodium at a dosage of 1.5 mg/kg once daily or 1 mg/kg every 12 hours, and the risk of bleeding complications increases with age. Enoxaparin should be used with care in geriatric patients, and careful attention to dosing intervals and concomitant medications (particularly antiplatelet drugs) is advised. Monitoring (e.g., using anti-factor Xa assay) of geriatric patients with low body weight (<45 kg) and those predisposed to decreased renal function should be considered.

Renal Impairment

Patients with renal impairment may have increased exposure to enoxaparin; such patients should be closely observed for signs of bleeding. Dosage adjustment is required in patients with severe renal impairment (creatinine clearance <30 mL/minute). (See Renal Impairment under Dosage and Administration.)

● Common Adverse Effects

The most common adverse effects of enoxaparin (i.e., occurring in at least 1% of patients receiving the drug in clinical studies) include bleeding, anemia, ecchymosis, thrombocytopenia, elevation of serum aminotransferase concentrations, fever, nausea, diarrhea, peripheral edema, dyspnea, injection site pain, and confusion.

DRUG INTERACTIONS

● Drugs Affecting Hemostasis

Concomitant use of drugs that affect hemostasis (e.g., anticoagulants, platelet aggregation inhibitors [e.g., salicylates or other nonsteroidal anti-inflammatory agents, dipyridamole, sulfinpyrazone]) can increase the risk of bleeding associated with enoxaparin. The manufacturer recommends that such drugs be discontinued prior to initiating enoxaparin therapy; if concomitant use is essential, careful clinical and laboratory monitoring is advised.

DESCRIPTION

Enoxaparin, a depolymerized heparin prepared by alkaline degradation of benzylated heparin of porcine intestinal mucosa origin, is an anticoagulant. Enoxaparin is commercially available as the sodium salt. The average molecular weight of enoxaparin is approximately one-third that of unfractionated heparin (4500 vs 12,000 daltons); therefore, enoxaparin is referred to as a low molecular weight heparin (LMWH).

Enoxaparin has an approximate anti-factor Xa activity of 100 units/mg according to the World Health Organization (WHO) First International Low Molecular Weight Heparin Reference Standard. At a given level of anti-factor Xa activity, enoxaparin has less effect on thrombin than does unfractionated heparin. However, enoxaparin administration has been associated with a prolongation of some global clotting function tests (i.e., thrombin time, activated partial thromboplastin time [aPTT]) by up to 1.8 times the control value. In patients receiving enoxaparin sodium (1 mg/kg of the 100 mg/mL concentration subcutaneously every 12 hours) in a large clinical trial, the aPTT was 45 seconds or less in most treated patients. The manufacturer states that enoxaparin sodium in a concentration of 150 mg/mL is projected to produce anticoagulant activities similar to those of 100 or 200 mg/mL concentrations of the drug, although the 150 mg/mL concentration has not been studied clinically. Compared with unfractionated heparin, enoxaparin has greater bioavailability (based on anti-factor Xa activity) after subcutaneous administration and a longer half-life, allowing less frequent administration.

The molecular weight, pharmacokinetics, and in vitro and in vivo activity of enoxaparin differ from those of unfractionated heparin or other LMWHs; therefore, the drugs are not interchangeable on a unit-for-unit (or mg-for-mg) basis.

ADVICE TO PATIENTS

- Importance of advising patients who have had neuraxial anesthesia or spinal puncture to monitor for manifestations of spinal or epidural hematoma (e.g., tingling or numbness in lower limbs, muscle weakness), particularly if they are receiving concomitant NSAIAs, platelet-aggregation inhibitors (e.g., clopidogrel), or other anticoagulants; importance of immediately contacting a clinician if any of these symptoms occur.

- If therapy is to continue after hospital discharge, importance of instructing patient on proper injection technique of enoxaparin.

- Importance of informing patients that they may bruise and/or bleed more easily and that a longer than normal time may be required to stop bleeding when taking enoxaparin. Importance of patients reporting any unusual bleeding, bruising, or signs of thrombocytopenia (e.g., dark red spots under skin) to clinician.

- Importance of patients informing clinicians (including dentists) that they are receiving enoxaparin therapy before scheduling any invasive procedures.

- Importance of informing clinicians of existing or contemplated concomitant therapy, including prescription and OTC drugs, as well as any concomitant illnesses.

- Importance of women informing clinicians if they are or plan to become pregnant or plan to breast-feed.

- Importance of informing patients of other important precautionary information. (See Cautions.)

Overview® (see Users Guide). For additional information until a more detailed monograph is developed and published, the manufacturer's labeling should be consulted. It is *essential* that the labeling be consulted for detailed information on the usual cautions, precautions, contraindications, potential drug interactions, and acute toxicity.

PREPARATIONS

Excipients in commercially available drug preparations may have clinically important effects in some individuals; consult specific product labeling for details.

Enoxaparin Sodium (Porcine)

Parenteral

Injection, for subcutaneous and IV use	100 mg/mL*	**Enoxaparin Sodium Injection** Lovenox® (available in single dose of 30, 40, 60, 80, or 100 mg as prefilled syringes or in a 3-mL multiple-dose vial) Sanofi-Aventis
	150 mg/mL*	**Enoxaparin Sodium Injection** Lovenox® (available in single dose of 120 or 150 mg as prefilled syringes) Sanofi-Aventis

* available from one or more manufacturer, distributor, and/or repackager by generic (nonproprietary) name

† Use is not currently included in the labeling approved by the US Food and Drug Administration.

Selected Revisions October 4, 2021, © Copyright, June 1, 1993, American Society of Health-System Pharmacists, Inc.

Heparin Sodium

20:12.04.16 • HEPARINS

■ Heparin, an anionic, sulfated glycosaminoglycan anticoagulant present in mast cells, acts as a catalyst to markedly accelerate the rate at which antithrombin III (heparin cofactor) neutralizes thrombin and activated coagulation factor X (factor Xa). Unless otherwise specified in this monograph, the term "heparin" refers to unfractionated heparin, not low molecular weight heparin or both types of heparin.

USES

Heparin is used for prophylaxis and treatment of venous thrombosis and its extension; prophylaxis of postoperative deep-vein thrombosis and pulmonary embolism in patients undergoing major abdominal or thoracic surgery who are at risk for thromboembolism; prophylaxis and treatment of pulmonary embolism; treatment of embolization associated with atrial fibrillation or atrial flutter and/or prosthetic heart valve replacement; treatment of acute and chronic consumptive coagulopathies (disseminated intravascular coagulation [DIC]); and prophylaxis and treatment of peripheral arterial embolism. Heparin is also used to prevent activation of the coagulation mechanism as blood passes through an extracorporeal circuit in dialysis procedures and during arterial and cardiac surgery. In addition, the drug is used as an in vitro anticoagulant in blood transfusions. Heparin also has been used as adjunctive antithrombotic therapy in patients with unstable angina, non-ST-segment-elevation myocardial infarction (NSTEMI), or ST-segment-elevation myocardial infarction (STEMI).

Heparin or a low molecular weight heparin is used when a rapid anticoagulant effect is required. A coumarin anticoagulant (e.g., warfarin) is generally used for follow-up anticoagulant therapy after the effects of therapy with full-dose heparin or a low molecular weight heparin have been established and when long-term anticoagulant therapy is appropriate. When warfarin is administered for follow-up treatment after full-dose heparin, therapy with warfarin and heparin should be overlapped for a short period of time.

● Deep-Vein Thrombosis and Pulmonary Embolism

Treatment

Heparin is used for the treatment of deep-vein thrombosis or pulmonary embolism. For the initial treatment of proximal deep-vein thrombosis or pulmonary embolism in adults, full-dose heparin generally is administered by continuous IV infusion; alternatively, subcutaneous heparin (given initially in a weight-based dosage) may be used, with or without monitoring. If warfarin is being considered for long-term anticoagulant therapy, the drug should be initiated on the same day as heparin, and such therapy should be overlapped for a minimum of 5 days and until the international normalized ratio (INR) is at least 2 for 24 hours or longer.

The American College of Chest Physicians (ACCP) recommends the use of heparin as an appropriate choice of anticoagulant for the initial treatment of acute proximal deep-vein thrombosis or pulmonary embolism; other options include a low molecular weight heparin or fondaparinux. Among the different anticoagulant options, fondaparinux or a low molecular weight heparin generally is preferred to heparin because of more convenient administration and less risk of heparin-induced thrombocytopenia (HIT). Heparin may be preferred in patients with renal impairment. In addition, ACCP states that IV heparin should be considered over subcutaneous therapies in patients with pulmonary embolism in whom thrombolytic therapy is being considered or if there is a concern about the adequacy of subcutaneous absorption.

After full-dose heparin therapy, warfarin or a low molecular weight heparin generally is administered as follow-up anticoagulant therapy for at least 3 months in patients with venous thromboembolism.

Heparin also may be used for the treatment of venous thromboembolism in pediatric patients. Unlike in adults, most episodes of venous thromboembolism in children are secondary to an identifiable risk factor such as the presence of a central venous access device. Recommendations regarding the use of antithrombotic therapy in children generally are based on extrapolation from adult guidelines.

Heparin or a low molecular weight heparin is recommended by ACCP for both the initial and ongoing treatment of venous thromboembolism in children. In children with central venous catheter-related thromboembolism, ACCP recommends that the catheter be removed if no longer functioning or required; at least 3–5 days of therapeutic anticoagulation is suggested prior to its removal. If the central venous access device is required, ACCP suggests that anticoagulants be given until the catheter is removed.

Prophylaxis

General Surgery

Fixed low-dose subcutaneous heparin therapy is used for prevention of postoperative deep-vein thrombosis and pulmonary embolism in patients undergoing general (e.g., abdominal) surgery who are at risk of thromboembolism.

ACCP recommends pharmacologic (e.g., low-dose heparin) and/or nonpharmacologic/mechanical (e.g., intermittent pneumatic compression) methods of thromboprophylaxis in patients undergoing general surgery, including abdominal, GI, gynecologic, and urologic surgery, according to the patient's level of risk for thromboembolism and bleeding. In general, pharmacologic prophylaxis is recommended in patients with high (and possibly moderate) risk of venous thromboembolism who do not have a high risk of bleeding, while mechanical methods are suggested in patients who require thromboprophylaxis but have a high risk of bleeding. If pharmacologic thromboprophylaxis is used in patients undergoing general surgery, ACCP states that low-dose heparin or a low molecular weight heparin is preferred, but when these agents are contraindicated or not available, aspirin or fondaparinux may be considered. ACCP states that the same recommendations for the use of antithrombotic agents in general surgery patients can be applied to patients undergoing bariatric surgery, vascular surgery, and plastic and reconstructive surgery.

Cardiac Surgery

Because the risk of venous thromboembolism in most patients undergoing cardiac surgery is considered to be moderate, mechanical methods of prophylaxis generally are recommended over pharmacologic prophylaxis in such patients. However, ACCP states that use of a pharmacologic method (e.g., low-dose heparin) may be considered in cardiac surgery patients with a complicated postoperative course.

Thoracic Surgery

Heparin is used for the prevention of postoperative venous thromboembolism in patients undergoing major thoracic surgery. Pharmacologic thromboprophylaxis with low-dose heparin or a low molecular weight heparin is recommended by ACCP in patients undergoing thoracic surgery who are at high risk of venous thromboembolism, provided risk of bleeding is low.

Neurosurgery

Patients undergoing craniotomy, especially for malignant disease, are considered to be at high risk of venous thromboembolism. Although low-dose heparin has been used for the prevention of venous thromboembolism in such patients, the benefits of pharmacologic prophylaxis may be outweighed by the possible increased risk of intracranial hemorrhage. ACCP suggests the use of a mechanical method of prophylaxis (preferably intermittent pneumatic compression) in craniotomy patients; for patients considered to be at *very* high risk for thromboembolism, such as those undergoing craniotomy for malignant disease†, a pharmacologic method (e.g., low-dose heparin) may be added once adequate hemostasis has been established and the risk of bleeding decreases.

In patients undergoing spinal surgery, a mechanical method of thromboprophylaxis (preferably intermittent pneumatic compression) also is suggested, with possible addition of pharmacologic prophylaxis (e.g., heparin) in high-risk patients (e.g., those with malignancy or those undergoing surgery with a combined anterior-posterior approach) once adequate hemostasis is established and risk of bleeding decreases.

Trauma

In general, some form of thromboprophylaxis (with low-dose heparin, a low molecular weight heparin, or a mechanical method) is suggested by ACCP in all patients with major trauma†. For major trauma patients at high risk of venous thromboembolism, including those with acute spinal cord injury, traumatic brain injury, or spinal surgery for trauma, ACCP suggests the use of both a pharmacologic and mechanical method of prophylaxis, unless contraindications exist.

Orthopedic Surgery

Low-dose heparin has been used for the prevention of venous thromboembolism in patients undergoing major orthopedic surgery (total hip-replacement†, total knee-replacement†, or hip-fracture surgery†). ACCP recommends routine thromboprophylaxis (with a pharmacologic and/or mechanical method) in all patients undergoing major orthopedic surgery because of the high risk for postoperative venous thromboembolism; thromboprophylaxis should be continued for at least 10–14 days, and possibly for up to 35 days after surgery. Several antithrombotic agents (e.g., low molecular weight heparins, fondaparinux, low-dose heparin, warfarin, aspirin) are recommended by ACCP for pharmacologic thromboprophylaxis in patients undergoing major orthopedic surgery. Although ACCP suggests that a low molecular weight heparin generally is preferred because of its relative efficacy and safety and extensive clinical experience, alternative agents may be considered in situations in which a low molecular weight heparin is not available or cannot be used. ACCP states that when selecting an appropriate thromboprophylaxis regimen, factors such as relative efficacy and bleeding risk as well as logistics and compliance issues should be considered.

Perioperative Management of Antithrombotic Therapy

Heparin is used in the perioperative management of patients who require temporary interruption of long-term warfarin therapy for surgery or other invasive procedures. Perioperative use of IV heparin or a low molecular weight heparin (bridging anticoagulation) is recommended by ACCP in some patients with venous thromboembolism, atrial fibrillation, or mechanical prosthetic heart valves depending on their risk of developing thromboembolism during temporary interruption of oral anticoagulant therapy. Long-term therapy with warfarin should be resumed postoperatively when adequate hemostasis is achieved.

Medical Conditions Associated with Thromboembolism

Heparin has been used for the prevention of deep-vein thrombosis and pulmonary embolism in acutely ill hospitalized medical patients and in those with medical conditions associated with a high risk of thromboembolism (e.g., cancer). Treatment decisions regarding the use of prophylactic anticoagulants in such patients should include an assessment of the patient's individual risk of venous thromboembolism and risk of bleeding. In general, pharmacologic thromboprophylaxis is recommended only in patients who are considered to be at high risk of venous thromboembolism because the risk-to-benefit trade-off between the reduction in venous thromboembolic events and bleeding is considered to be more favorable in such patients. Factors that should be considered when choosing an appropriate anticoagulant include patient preference, compliance, ease of administration, and local cost considerations. ACCP recommends the use of anticoagulant thromboprophylaxis (e.g., low-dose heparin) in acutely ill, hospitalized medical patients at increased risk of thrombosis who are not actively bleeding and do not have an increased risk of bleeding. Continued thromboprophylaxis is suggested for 6–21 days until full mobility is restored or hospital discharge, whichever comes first; extended prophylaxis beyond these periods generally is not recommended. Risk of venous thromboembolism in critically ill patients in an intensive care unit (ICU) varies depending on their acute or chronic conditions (e.g., sepsis, congestive heart failure) and ICU-specific exposures and events (e.g., surgery, immobilization, mechanical ventilation, central venous catheters). Low-dose heparin is suggested by ACCP as an option for pharmacologic thromboprophylaxis in critically ill patients who are not actively bleeding and do not have risk factors for bleeding.

Risk of venous thromboembolism is particularly high in patients with cancer. Routine pharmacologic thromboprophylaxis generally is not recommended in cancer patients in the outpatient setting who have no additional risk factors for venous thromboembolism; however, ACCP suggests the use of low-dose heparin or a low molecular weight heparin for prophylaxis in cancer outpatients with solid tumors who have additional thromboembolic risk factors and are at low risk of bleeding.

Thromboembolism During Pregnancy

Heparin has been used for the prevention and treatment of venous thromboembolism during pregnancy. Because of a more favorable safety profile, ACCP generally recommends the use of a low molecular weight heparin (rather than heparin or warfarin) for the prevention and treatment of thromboembolism during pregnancy. If adjusted-dose subcutaneous heparin is used during pregnancy, ACCP states that the drug should be discontinued at least 24 hours prior to induction of labor or cesarean section to avoid an unwanted anticoagulant effect on the fetus during delivery. Women at very high risk for recurrent venous thromboembolism (e.g., occurrence of proximal deep-vein thrombosis or pulmonary embolism within 2 weeks of delivery) may have therapy switched to therapeutic dosages of IV heparin, which should then be discontinued 4–6 hours prior to the expected time of delivery.

Prophylaxis for Other Conditions

Heparin (in therapeutic dosages), followed by warfarin, is recommended by ACCP as an option for thromboprophylaxis in children following Fontan surgery†.

● Cardioversion of Atrial Fibrillation/Flutter

Heparin has been used to reduce the risk of stroke and systemic embolism in patients with atrial fibrillation undergoing electrical or pharmacologic cardioversion. Therapeutic anticoagulation with heparin or a low molecular weight heparin may be used in patients in whom prolonged anticoagulation (e.g., with warfarin for at least 3 weeks) prior to cardioversion is not necessary or not possible; in these situations, heparin or a low molecular weight heparin generally is administered at the time of transesophageal echocardiography (TEE) or at presentation (for those with atrial fibrillation of 48 hours or less), followed by cardioversion. In patients requiring urgent cardioversion because of hemodynamic instability, initiation of IV heparin or a low molecular weight heparin also is suggested, if possible; however, such therapy should not delay any emergency intervention.

In patients undergoing cardioversion for atrial flutter, experts state that the same approach to thromboprophylaxis should be used as for those with atrial fibrillation.

● Thromboembolism Associated with Prosthetic Heart Valves

Overview

Heparin is used during conversion to maintenance therapy with warfarin to reduce the incidence of thromboembolism (e.g., stroke) in patients with prosthetic mechanical heart valves, including in pregnant women. In the absence of a bleeding risk, ACCP suggests bridging anticoagulation (administration of a low molecular weight heparin in either prophylactic or therapeutic dosages or IV heparin in prophylactic dosages) during the early postoperative period after insertion of a mechanical heart valve until the patient is stable on warfarin therapy. In patients with a mechanical heart valve in whom therapy with warfarin must be temporarily discontinued (e.g., those undergoing major surgery), substitution with a low molecular weight heparin or heparin is recommended in selected patients (e.g., those at high risk of thromboembolism).

Patients with Prosthetic Heart Valves Undergoing Surgical Procedures

In patients with a prosthetic heart valve receiving long-term oral antithrombotic therapy (e.g., warfarin) who require surgical procedures, the risk of perioperative bleeding should be weighed against the increased risk of thromboembolism that may occur as a result of discontinuance of oral antithrombotic therapy. The American College of Cardiology (ACC) and American Heart Association (AHA) state that perioperative use of heparin should be considered for noncardiac surgery, invasive procedures, or dental procedures in patients with prosthetic heart valves who are at high risk for thrombosis without oral antithrombotic therapy; such patients include those with any mechanical mitral valve or a mechanical aortic valve with additional risk factors. In such high-risk patients, heparin should be initiated after discontinuance of warfarin therapy when the INR is below 2 (approximately 48 hours before surgery). Heparin should be discontinued 4–6 hours before the procedure and then reinitiated as early as possible after surgery once hemostasis has been established. Therapy with heparin should then be continued until the patient has achieved therapeutic anticoagulation on warfarin therapy (as assessed by the INR).

Pregnant Women with Prosthetic Heart Valves

Heparin has been used for thromboprophylaxis in pregnant women with prosthetic mechanical heart valves.†

The risk of valve thrombosis in pregnant women with prosthetic mechanical heart valves is lowest with the use of warfarin. However, warfarin crosses the placenta and is associated with adverse embryopathic and fetopathic effects, prematurity, stillbirths, and spontaneous abortions, with the risk of embryopathy being highest during weeks 6–12 of gestation. Heparin does not cross the placenta and is considered safer to the fetus than warfarin; however, use of heparin has been associated with an increased maternal risk for valve thrombosis, death, and major bleeding complications. In addition, thrombosis of prosthetic heart valves, resulting in maternal and/or fetal death in some cases, has occurred in some pregnant women receiving prophylaxis with a low molecular weight heparin (enoxaparin).

The American College of Cardiology/American Heart Association (ACC/AHA) issued guidelines for the management of patients with valvular heart disease, which includes recommendations for the management of women with mechanical heart valves who are pregnant or plan to become pregnant. Multiple strategies are recommended to reduce, as well as balance, the maternal (e.g., valve thrombosis, death) and fetal risks (e.g., fetal loss, teratogenicity). No single anticoagulation strategy is optimally safe for both the mother and the fetus; maternal and fetal risks can be reduced, but not eliminated. Options include warfarin continuation throughout pregnancy, dose-adjusted heparin or low molecular weight heparin with frequent anti-Xa level monitoring throughout pregnancy, or sequential therapy with dose-adjusted heparin or with frequent anti-Xa level monitoring during the first trimester and warfarin during the second and third trimesters.

● **Arterial Thromboembolism**

Full-dose heparin therapy has been used to reduce the extent of ischemic injury in patients with acute arterial emboli or thrombosis; however, ACCP states that formal studies demonstrating improved outcomes have not been conducted. In patients with limb ischemia secondary to arterial emboli or thrombosis, immediate systemic anticoagulation with heparin to prevent thrombotic propagation is suggested by ACCP.

For neonates and children requiring cardiac catheterization via an artery, thromboprophylaxis with IV heparin is recommended. If femoral artery thrombosis occurs following cardiac catheterization, initial treatment with therapeutic-dose IV heparin is recommended, followed by subsequent conversion to a low molecular weight heparin or continued treatment with heparin to complete 5–7 days of therapeutic anticoagulation.

● **Disseminated Intravascular Coagulation**

Heparin is used for the diagnosis and treatment of acute and chronic consumptive coagulopathies, including DIC. The use of heparin in patients with DIC is controversial. Generally, the underlying cause of the DIC episode should be determined and corrected. However, if the underlying cause is not evident or cannot readily be corrected, some clinicians recommend the use of heparin. Heparin appears to be most effective in the treatment of DIC when gross thrombosis or purpura fulminans is present; however, the drug appears to have little effect on the overall mortality associated with acute DIC.

● **Thrombosis Associated with Indwelling Venous or Arterial Devices**

Heparin lock flush solution is used to maintain patency of indwelling peripheral or central venipuncture devices designed for intermittent injections and/or blood sampling; the flush solution should not be used for anticoagulant therapy. Although such flush solutions generally contain low concentrations of heparin sodium (e.g., 10 or 100 units/mL) in 0.9% sodium chloride injection or other IV fluid, the optimum concentration of heparin sodium, and whether the drug is even needed in all circumstances, for maintaining patency of indwelling venipuncture devices have not been established. Since the optimum concentration of heparin sodium for maintaining patency in indwelling venipuncture devices has not been established, use of the lowest concentration shown to be effective (e.g., 10 units/mL) has been suggested when such heparin-containing flush solutions are deemed necessary. Heparin has no fibrinolytic activity and will not lyse existing clots; therefore, thrombolytic agents (e.g., urokinase [no longer commercially available in the US]) rather than heparin would be appropriate for catheters with preexisting obstruction with blood or fibrin.

Evidence principally in adults and to a limited extent in children, including pooled analysis of data from various studies, indicates that heparin-containing solutions are *no more effective* than 0.9% sodium chloride injection *alone* for maintaining patency of venipuncture devices in *peripheral veins when blood is not aspirated into the device*, and some clinicians state that *routine* use of heparin-containing flush solutions may not be advisable because of heparin-associated drug-drug incompatibilities, laboratory test interferences, and rare but potentially serious adverse effects. It also has been suggested that the type of solution used to maintain venipuncture device patency may not be as important as the positive pressure maintained in the IV line by the capped (sealed) injection device, which appears to prevent blood reflux and clot formation in the device. In several randomized, double-blind studies in which peripherally placed venipuncture devices composed of fluoroethylene propylene (FEP-Teflon®) principally were used, use of 0.9% sodium chloride injection for flushing indwelling venipuncture devices was associated with patency rates similar to those achieved with flush solutions containing 10 or 100 units/mL of heparin sodium, and the frequency of phlebitis with the use of these solutions also was similar. Therefore, some clinicians state that the use of 0.9% sodium chloride injection alone is sufficient to maintain patency of venipuncture devices, at least those made of FEP-Teflon® when such devices are placed in peripheral veins and used for intermittent IV access. Limited data in children also suggest no difference between 0.9% sodium chloride injection alone or with heparin sodium 10 units/mL in maintaining peripheral IV catheter patency, although additional controlled studies in larger numbers of patients are needed to evaluate more fully the potential risks and benefits of using heparinized versus non-heparinized flush solutions routinely for peripheral venipuncture devices in children and infants.

There is some evidence suggesting that heparin-containing flush solutions *are more effective* than 0.9% sodium chloride injection alone in maintaining patency of *indwelling venipuncture devices used to obtain blood specimens* and of *catheters used for arterial access* (arterial lines). Therefore, pending further study, it has been suggested that flush solutions containing heparin be used for maintaining catheter patency in these situations.

For primary thromboprophylaxis of central venous access devices in children, ACCP states that intermittent or continuous infusions of heparin or 0.9% sodium chloride injection generally are used.

Neonates and children with peripheral arterial catheters should receive thromboprophylaxis with continuous infusions of low concentrations of heparin. If arterial thrombosis of the catheter occurs, ACCP suggests immediate removal of the catheter; anticoagulant therapy with heparin may be considered as an option for the treatment of symptomatic catheter-related thromboembolism. ACCP also suggests that neonates with umbilical arterial catheters receive thromboprophylaxis with low-dose heparin infusion through the catheter to maintain patency.

● **Acute Ischemic Complications of ST-Segment Elevation Myocardial Infarction**

Heparin is used as adjunctive therapy in the management of acute ST-segment-elevation MI (STEMI). The current standard of care in patients with STEMI is timely reperfusion (with primary percutaneous coronary intervention [PCI] or thrombolytic therapy). Adjunctive therapy with anticoagulant (e.g., heparin) and antiplatelet (e.g., aspirin and clopidogrel) agents should be used during and after successful coronary artery reperfusion for the prevention of early reocclusion and death. The American College of Cardiology Foundation (ACCF) and AHA state that patients with STEMI undergoing thrombolytic therapy should receive an anticoagulant (e.g., heparin, enoxaparin, fondaparinux) for a minimum of 48 hours, and preferably for the duration of the index hospitalization, up to 8 days or until revascularization is performed. Enoxaparin is preferred over heparin if extended anticoagulation is necessary beyond 48 hours. Heparin also is used for anticoagulation therapy during PCI.

Combined analysis of results from 3 large, randomized comparative studies in patients with suspected acute MI who received thrombolytic therapy (i.e., anistreplase [no longer commercially available in the US], recombinant tissue-type plasminogen activator [rt-PA], or streptokinase [no longer commercially available in the US]) plus low-dose aspirin with or without subcutaneous heparin sodium (12,500 units initiated approximately 4 or 12 hours after thrombolytic therapy and usually continued for 1 week or until hospital discharge) indicated that adjunctive therapy with heparin reduced early (i.e., during heparin treatment) reinfarction and death; however, mortality at long-term follow-up (e.g., at 7 weeks or 6 months) was not different in these studies, and the addition of heparin was associated with an increased risk of bleeding, including cerebral hemorrhage. It should be noted that therapy with heparin in most patients in these studies was not given IV nor was it initiated as early in the course of treatment as was the case in most other studies in which mortality with rt-PA (e.g., alteplase) therapy was examined.

Current evidence from studies in which IV heparin has been administered *simultaneously* with thrombolytic therapy, including results of a multicenter study in more than 41,000 patients with acute MI (GUSTO-1), suggests that conjunctive therapy with IV heparin, in addition to aspirin, is effective in reducing reocclusion following thrombolytic therapy for acute MI. In addition, results of a pooled analysis of data from 300 studies of thrombolytic treatment for acute MI indicated a reduction in mortality for thrombolytic regimens including rt-PA but not for those including streptokinase (no longer commercially available in the US) or anistreplase (no longer commercially available in the US) when regimens in which early conjunctive heparin (initiated before or with thrombolytic agents) was used were compared with those in which late therapy with heparin (initiated after termination of thrombolytic therapy) was used; these data are consistent with results of the GUSTO-1 study demonstrating a mortality benefit for IV alteplase plus simultaneous IV heparin compared with streptokinase-heparin regimens. However, some evidence suggests a narrow margin of safety for upward adjustment of heparin dosage, and the need for serial monitoring of aPTT, in patients receiving heparin concurrently with thrombolytic therapy for acute MI. In 2 multicenter, randomized studies designed to compare IV heparin with IV hirudin (an antithrombin inhibitor) as early (within 1 hour following thrombolysis) adjunctive therapy to thrombolytic agents (rt-PA or streptokinase) and aspirin in patients with acute MI, administration of IV heparin in weight-adjusted dosages approximately 20% higher than the dosages used in the GUSTO-1 study was associated with a marked increase in the risk of hemorrhagic stroke, and recruitment of patients into the studies was halted prematurely. In addition, major hemorrhage appeared to be associated with prolonged aPTT values (i.e., those above the target aPTT range of 60–90 seconds [generally 2–3 times the control value]), especially during the first 12 hours following thrombolysis.

● Acute Ischemic Complications of Percutaneous Coronary Intervention

Heparin also is used to reduce the risk of ischemic complications in patients undergoing PCI. Adjunctive therapy with heparin is recommended in addition to aspirin, a GP IIb/IIIa-receptor inhibitor (i.e., abciximab, eptifibatide) and/or a P2Y12 receptor-antagonist (e.g., clopidogrel) for patients undergoing such procedures. Use of a parenteral anticoagulant is recommended in patients undergoing PCI to prevent thrombus formation at the site of arterial injury, the coronary guidewire, and in the catheters used for the procedure. IV heparin is recommended by the ACCF, AHA, and the Society for Cardiovascular Angiography and Interventions (SCAI) as an appropriate choice of anticoagulant for use during PCI. The activated clotting time (ACT) generally has been used to assess the degree of heparin anticoagulation in patients undergoing PCI; however, the utility of ACT monitoring recently has been questioned because a clear relationship between ACT values and clinical outcomes has not been demonstrated.

Heparin used in conjunction with GP IIb/IIIa-receptor inhibitors has further reduced the incidence of ischemic complications of PCI compared with heparin alone. Since GP IIb/IIIa-receptor inhibitors may have additive effects on ACT in patients receiving one of these drugs with heparin, the dosage of heparin required to maintain an appropriate ACT during such concurrent therapy may be lower than with heparin monotherapy. Full-dose anticoagulation is no longer used after successful PCI procedures. In most cases, the femoral sheath is removed when the ACT falls to less than 150–180 seconds or when the aPTT decreases to less than 50 seconds.

Results of clinical trials indicate that direct thrombin inhibitors (e.g., argatroban) are at least as effective as heparin in reducing the risk of acute ischemic complications (e.g., death, MI, need for urgent revascularization procedures) in patients undergoing PCI. For patients with HIT or a history of HIT undergoing urgent PCI, ACCF, AHA, and ACCP state that bivalirudin or argatroban may be used in place of heparin.

● Cardiac and Arterial Vascular Surgery

Heparin is used for the prevention of blood clotting in arterial and cardiac surgery.

During cardiac surgery, heparin is commonly used to prevent coagulation in the cardiopulmonary bypass circuit and in the operative field. ACCP states that a nonheparin anticoagulant (e.g., bivalirudin) may be used in place of heparin in patients with acute HIT or subacute HIT (platelets have recovered, but HIT antibodies are still present) who require urgent cardiac surgery. Because HIT antibodies are transient, patients with a history of HIT may be re-exposed to heparin in special circumstances. ACCP states that short-term use of heparin may be appropriate in patients with a remote (more than 3 months) history of HIT and no detectable antibodies who require cardiac surgery.

● Acute Ischemic Complications of Non-ST-Segment-Elevation Acute Coronary Syndromes

Heparin is used in the management of non-ST-segment-elevation acute coronary syndromes (NSTE ACS)†. Patients with NSTE ACS have either unstable angina or non-ST-segment-elevation MI (NSTEMI); because these conditions are part of a continuum of acute myocardial ischemia and have indistinguishable clinical features upon presentation, the same initial treatment strategies are recommended. The AHA/ACC guideline for the management of patients with NSTE ACS recommends an early invasive strategy (angiographic evaluation with the intent to perform revascularization procedures such as PCI with coronary artery stent implantation or coronary artery bypass grafting [CABG]) or an ischemia-guided strategy (initial medical management followed by cardiac catheterization and revascularization if indicated) in patients with definite or likely NSTE ACS; standard medical therapies for all patients should include a β-adrenergic blocking agent (β-blocker), antiplatelet agents, anticoagulant agents, nitrates, and analgesic agents regardless of the initial management approach.

All patients with NSTE ACS should receive immediate antiplatelet therapy (e.g., aspirin, clopidogrel) unless contraindicated or not tolerated. An anticoagulant agent should be added to antiplatelet therapy as soon as possible after presentation. Initial parenteral anticoagulants with established efficacy in patients with NSTE ACS include enoxaparin, heparin, bivalirudin (only in patients who are being managed with an early invasive strategy), and fondaparinux. Fondaparinux is preferred over heparin therapy in patients with an increased risk of bleeding. Heparin anticoagulation should be continued for 48 hours or until PCI is performed. In patients who will undergo CABG and who are already receiving heparin, the drug should be continued during surgery. Patients receiving other anticoagulants (enoxaparin, fondaparinux, or bivalirudin) in whom CABG is to be performed should discontinue the anticoagulant and initiate heparin during the surgery.

In patients in whom conservative medical therapy is selected as a postangiographic management strategy, recommendations for continued antiplatelet and anticoagulant therapy generally are based on the presence of coronary artery disease. ACC, AHA, and ACCF state that the optimum duration of heparin therapy has not been established; in clinical trials, the drug generally was administered for 2–5 days.

Current evidence indicates that heparin given by continuous IV infusion can reduce the incidence of acute MI, death, and recurrent refractory angina pectoris in patients with NSTE ACS†.

Early initiation of therapy with IV heparin appears to be necessary for beneficial effects in patients with unstable angina since initiation of the drug more than 24 hours following onset of symptoms has failed to reduce the incidence of adverse coronary events (e.g., angina, MI). In clinical studies in patients with acute unstable angina, data suggest that continuous IV infusion of heparin is more effective than intermittent IV administration, possibly because of inadequate anticoagulation achieved with the latter method.

● Cerebral Thromboembolism

Although therapeutic-dose anticoagulation has been used in patients with acute ischemic stroke, there is strong evidence that such treatment is associated with worse outcomes than aspirin therapy in terms of increased mortality and rates of nonfatal major extracranial bleeding. Therefore, ACCP recommends early treatment (within 48 hours) with aspirin over therapeutic anticoagulation to prevent recurrent cerebral thromboembolism in patients with acute ischemic stroke or transient ischemic attacks (TIA). However, heparin anticoagulants (i.e., low molecular weight heparins or heparin) may be used in prophylactic dosages for thromboprophylaxis in some patients with acute ischemic stroke; those with additional risk factors for venous thromboembolism are more likely to benefit from such therapy. ACCP suggests that thromboprophylaxis with a low molecular weight heparin (in prophylactic dosages), subcutaneous heparin, or an intermittent pneumatic compression device be used in patients with acute ischemic stroke and restricted mobility. Among the anticoagulant options, ACCP suggests the use of a low molecular weight heparin over heparin. Prophylactic-dose heparin or a low molecular weight heparin usually is initiated within 48 hours of the onset of stroke and is continued throughout the hospital stay until the patient regains mobility; such heparin therapy should not be given within the first 24 hours after administration of thrombolytic therapy.

Heparin is recommended by ACCP as an option for the initial treatment of acute arterial ischemic stroke in children† until dissection and embolic causes have been excluded. When dissection or cardioembolic causes have been excluded, daily aspirin therapy (in prophylactic dosages) is suggested for a minimum of 2 years. In children with acute arterial ischemic stroke secondary to non-Moyamoya vasculopathy†, ACCP recommends ongoing antithrombotic therapy (e.g., with heparin) for 3 months. In neonates, antithrombotic therapy generally is not recommended for a first occurrence of arterial ischemic stroke in the absence of a cardioembolic origin; however, ACCP states that heparin may be considered in neonates with a first episode of arterial ischemic stroke associated with a documented cardioembolic source.

Heparin or a low molecular weight heparin is suggested for the treatment of acute cerebral venous sinus thrombosis† in adults. Heparin or a low molecular weight heparin also is recommended for the initial treatment of cerebral venous sinus thrombosis without substantial intracranial hemorrhage in children†, followed by continued treatment with a low molecular weight heparin or warfarin for at least 3 months; another 3 months of anticoagulation is suggested if symptoms persist or there is continued occlusion of the cerebral venous sinuses. Although the evidence is not as compelling as for children without substantial hemorrhage, ACCP also suggests that anticoagulation may be used for the treatment of cerebral venous sinus thrombosis in children with substantial hemorrhage.

Renal Vein Thrombosis

Renal vein thrombosis† is the most common cause of spontaneous venous thromboembolism in neonates. Although use of anticoagulant therapy for this condition remains controversial, heparin is suggested by ACCP as a possible treatment option for neonates with renal vein thrombosis.

Complications of Pregnancy

Heparin should be used during pregnancy† only when clearly needed, weighing carefully the potential benefits versus the possible risks to the mother (e.g., bleeding, osteopenia/osteoporosis) and fetus (e.g., bleeding at the uteroplacental junction [heparin does not cross the placenta], complications secondary to maternal bleeding). Heparin has been used in combination with aspirin for the prevention of complications of pregnancy† (e.g., pregnancy loss in women with a history of antiphospholipid syndrome and recurrent fetal loss). The presence of maternal antiphospholipid antibodies is associated with an increased risk of thrombosis and pregnancy loss. Data from several small comparative studies indicate that combined prophylaxis with heparin and low-dose aspirin is more effective than aspirin alone or aspirin combined with a corticosteroid in preventing recurrent pregnancy loss (fetal death, miscarriage), preeclampsia, or premature delivery in women with antiphospholipid syndrome (Hughes syndrome). A systematic review in more than 800 pregnant women with antiphospholipid antibodies and a history of fetal loss supports the finding that combined prophylaxis with heparin and aspirin is superior to aspirin alone in reducing incidence of pregnancy loss. The beneficial effect of such prophylactic therapy may result from aspirin-induced suppression of thromboxane A_2-mediated vasospasm, ischemia, and thrombosis in the placental vasculature and by heparin-induced anticoagulation combined with binding to phospholipid antibodies that protects the trophoblast from antibody attack and thus promotes successful implantation in early pregnancy.

ACCP recommends that women with antiphospholipid antibody (APLA) syndrome in whom recurrent (3 or more) pregnancy loss has occurred should receive antepartum prophylactic or intermediate dosages of subcutaneous heparin in conjunction with low-dose aspirin. Alternatively, therapy with a low molecular weight heparin instead of heparin may be considered.

Because of experience in women with antiphospholipid syndrome, heparin and aspirin (often combined with immune globulin) also have been used to prevent venous thromboembolism and early pregnancy loss in women who have undergone in vitro fertilization†. However, current evidence suggests that the overall absolute risk of symptomatic thrombosis appears to be low in women undergoing in vitro fertilization. Therefore, ACCP recommends against routine thromboprophylaxis in most women undergoing assisted reproduction.

Anticoagulation in Blood Transfusions, Blood Samples, and Other Procedures

Heparin is used as an in vitro anticoagulant in blood transfusions, extracorporeal circulation, and dialysis procedures.

DOSAGE AND ADMINISTRATION

Administration

USP has changed its labeling standard for Heparin Sodium Injection, USP and Heparin Lock Flush Solution, USP to require that carton and container labels for these products clearly state the strength of the entire container (amount of heparin per total volume of container), followed in close proximity by the strength per mL in parentheses. The labeling change eliminates the need to calculate the total amount of heparin in a product containing more than 1 mL and thus reduces the chance of a dosing error. The new labeling standard for heparin was effective as of May 1, 2013. Clinicians should check the label on all heparin products to confirm the correct formulation and strength prior to dispensing and administering the drug.

For full-dose therapy, heparin is administered by IV infusion, intermittent IV injection, or deep subcutaneous (intrafat) injection. For fixed low-dose therapy, heparin usually is administered by deep subcutaneous injection. *Heparin should not be administered IM because of the frequency of irritation, pain, and hematoma at the injection site.*

IV Administration

Heparin lock flush solution is *not* intended for systemic anticoagulation. Conversely, heparin injection should not be used as a catheter lock flush solution.

For full-dose therapy, many clinicians advocate continuous IV infusion of heparin rather than intermittent IV injection because of a more constant degree of anticoagulation and a lower incidence of bleeding complications. To avoid fluctuations in the rate of administration and minimize the risk of overdosage, IV infusions of full doses of heparin should be administered with a constant-rate infusion pump if possible.

Heparin solutions for IV infusion may be prepared by diluting the drug in a compatible IV solution; when heparin is added to an IV solution, it is recommended that the container be inverted at least 6 times to ensure adequate mixing and prevent pooling of the drug in the solution. Alternatively, commercially available solutions of heparin in 0.45 or 0.9% sodium chloride injection or in 5% dextrose injection may be used. When one of the commercially available IV infusion solutions of heparin is used, accompanying labeling should be consulted for proper methods of administration and associated precautions.

Intermittent IV injections of heparin may be given undiluted or diluted with 50–100 mL of 0.9% sodium chloride injection.

Heparin injections and solutions for infusion and heparin lock flush solutions should be inspected visually for particulate matter and discoloration prior to administration whenever solution and container permit; the injection or solution should not be used if it is discolored, unclear, or contains a precipitate. However, slight discoloration does not alter potency.

Standardize 4 Safety

Standardized concentrations for heparin have been established through Standardize 4 Safety (S4S), a national patient safety initiative to reduce medication errors, especially during transitions of care. Multidisciplinary expert panels were convened to determine recommended standard concentrations. Because recommendations from the S4S panels may differ from the manufacturer's prescribing information, caution is advised when using concentrations that differ from labeling, particularly when using rate information from the label. For additional information on S4S (including updates that may be available), see https://www.ashp.org/pharmacy-practice/standardize-4-safety-initiative.

TABLE 1. Standardize 4 Safety Continuous IV Infusion Standard Concentrations for Heparin

Patient Population	Concentration Standards	Dosing Units
Adults	100 units/mL	units/hour or units/kg/hour[a]
Pediatric patients (<50 kg)	50 units/mL or 100 units/mL for anticoagulant therapy	units/kg/hour
	2 units/mL for arterial line maintenance	

[a] The S4S panel recommends trying to standardize dosing units but understands that some protocols may use "flat" dosing while others may require weight-based dosing

Subcutaneous Administration

Deep subcutaneous injections of heparin should be made with a 25- or 26-gauge ½- or (5/8)-inch needle above the iliac crest or into the abdominal fat layer to minimize tissue trauma; abdominal injections should not be made within 2 inches of the umbilicus. The tissue around the injection site should be grasped creating a tissue roll and the needle inserted quickly into the elevated tissue perpendicular to the skin surface. Finger pressure on the tissue roll should be reduced slightly and the solution fully injected. The needle should be rapidly withdrawn while simultaneously releasing the tissue roll and gentle pressure should be applied to the area for 5–10 seconds. Injection sites should not be massaged before or after injection, and sites should be changed for each dose to prevent the development of a massive hematoma. It has been recommended that the plunger of the syringe not be pulled back to see if a vessel has been entered; however, most clinicians state that although it is not necessary, there is no reason why aspiration cannot be performed to determine if a blood vessel has been entered prior to injection of the solution.

Laboratory Monitoring of Therapy

The activated partial thromboplastin time (aPTT) is the most commonly used laboratory method for monitoring full-dose heparin therapy. The activated coagulation time (ACT) may also be used and is especially convenient for monitoring the degree of anticoagulation in patients undergoing extracorporeal circulation because the test can be performed at bedside. Although the whole blood clotting time (Lee-White clotting time) was used in the past to monitor full-dose heparin therapy, the test is rarely used now because it is less convenient and less reproducible than are other available coagulation tests. The generally accepted therapeutic range for the aPTT during full-dose IV or subcutaneous heparin therapy is 1.5–2 times the control value in seconds, and the generally accepted therapeutic range for the ACT is 2.5–3 times the control value in seconds. However, in some patients at high risk for thromboembolic events (e.g., pregnant women with mechanical heart valves) an aPTT of at least 2 times the control value has been used. When full-dose heparin therapy is administered by continuous IV infusion, coagulation tests should be performed prior to initiation of therapy, approximately every 4 hours during the early stages of therapy, and daily thereafter. When full-dose heparin therapy is administered by intermittent IV injection or deep subcutaneous injection, coagulation tests should be performed prior to each dose (or 4–6 hours following the dose for deep subcutaneous injection) during the early stages of therapy, and at appropriate intervals thereafter. Laboratory monitoring of coagulation tests is not usually performed when fixed low-dose subcutaneous heparin therapy is used because currently available coagulation tests are generally unaffected or only minimally prolonged. Regardless of the route of administration, it is recommended that platelet counts and hematocrit be monitored and tests for occult blood in the stool be performed periodically during the entire course of heparin therapy.

● *Dosage*

Dosage of heparin sodium is expressed in USP units. USP units and international units (IU, units) for heparin sodium are equivalent.

Dosage requirements for full-dose heparin sodium therapy vary greatly among individual patients, and dosage should be carefully individualized based on clinical and laboratory findings in order to obtain optimum therapeutic effects without incurring hemorrhage. (See Laboratory Monitoring of Therapy under

Dosage and Administration: Administration.) Because of a lack of adequate and well-controlled studies of heparin in pediatric patients, dosage recommendations in this population generally are based on clinical experience. Geriatric patients (older than 60 years of age) may require a lower dosage of heparin sodium. (See Cautions: Geriatric Precautions.)

The optimum duration of heparin therapy for thrombotic disorders has not been definitely established and must be determined by the condition being treated and its severity. Full-dose heparin is generally continued for at least 5 days in patients with acute venous thrombosis or pulmonary embolism, and for 2 days in patients with myocardial infarction (MI)†. A coumarin anticoagulant (e.g., warfarin) generally is administered for follow-up treatment after full-dose heparin, and therapy with the 2 drugs is usually overlapped for 4–5 days until an adequate response to the coumarin derivative is obtained (e.g., as indicated by INR values exceeding 2 on two consecutive days).(See Laboratory Test Interferences: Prothrombin Time.) Several manufacturers recommend abrupt discontinuance of heparin without tapering in patients who have an adequate therapeutic response to a coumarin derivative. However, concern exists that abrupt discontinuance of heparin may result in a high-risk period for rebound thrombosis, although recommendations to reduce this risk remain to be established. In the absence of such recommendations, some clinicians recommend that heparin infusions be reduced in a gradual fashion such as by reducing the rate by 50% over 6 hours and then discontinuing over the next 12 hours.

Treatment of Venous Thromboembolism

Adults

For *full-dose continuous IV infusion therapy* for the treatment of venous thrombosis and pulmonary embolism in a 68-kg adult, some manufacturers recommend an initial heparin sodium loading dose of 5000 units given by IV injection, followed by a continuous infusion of 20,000–40,000 units in 1 L of 0.9% sodium chloride injection or other compatible IV solution over 24 hours. The American College of Chest Physicians (ACCP) suggests that therapy with IV heparin sodium may be initiated in a weight-adjusted dosage (loading dose of 80 units/kg followed by a continuous infusion of 18 units/kg per hour) or a fixed dosage (loading dose of 5000 units, followed by a continuous IV infusion of 1000 units/hour). Although the aPTT can be used to monitor either dosage regimen, ACCP states that there is no evidence suggesting that monitoring improves clinical outcomes.

For *full-dose intermittent IV therapy* in a 68-kg adult for the treatment of venous thromboembolism and pulmonary embolism, some manufacturers recommend an initial loading dose of 10,000 units of heparin sodium (either undiluted or diluted in 50 or 100 mL of 0.9% sodium chloride injection), followed by 5000–10,000 units every 4–6 hours.

For *full-dose subcutaneous therapy* in a 68-kg adult, some manufacturers recommend an initial heparin sodium dose of 5000 units by IV injection, then 10,000–20,000 units in a concentrated solution injected subcutaneously for 1 dose, followed by subcutaneous injection of 8000–10,000 units as a concentrated solution every 8 hours or 15,000–20,000 units as a concentrated solution every 12 hours. In patients receiving subcutaneous heparin sodium for the treatment of venous thromboembolism in the outpatient setting, ACCP and some manufacturers suggest the use of weight-based dosing (initial dose of 333 units/kg, followed by a dosage of 250 units/kg twice daily) without monitoring rather than a fixed dosage or a weight-adjusted dosage with monitoring.

In patients in whom long-term warfarin therapy will subsequently be prescribed, ACCP recommends initiating warfarin and heparin together on the first treatment day and overlapping therapy with the 2 drugs for a minimum of 5 days and until the international normalized ratio (INR) is at least 2 for 24 hours or longer.

When converting to oral dabigatran therapy in patients currently receiving heparin therapy by continuous IV infusion, the first dose of dabigatran should be administered, followed immediately by discontinuance of the heparin infusion; for patients currently receiving intermittently dosed IV heparin therapy, oral dabigatran should be initiated within 2 hours prior to what would have been the time of the next scheduled heparin dose.

Pediatric Patients

Dosage recommendations in the pediatric population generally are based on clinical experience because of a lack of adequate and well-controlled studies of heparin in these patients. In children receiving full-dose (therapeutic) heparin therapy, ACCP suggests that dosage be titrated to achieve an anti-factor Xa concentration of 0.35–0.7 units/mL or to prolong the aPTT to a corresponding anti-factor Xa range or to a protamine titration range of 0.2–0.4 units/mL. Because clinical outcome studies have not been conducted in children, the therapeutic range for heparin in neonates and children is mostly derived from experience in adults. Following initial heparin therapy in children with an acute venous thromboembolic event, a low molecular weight heparin or a coumarin anticoagulant (e.g., warfarin) may be initiated, or the patient may continue to receive heparin for ongoing therapy. In children with venous thromboembolism in whom warfarin therapy will subsequently be prescribed, ACCP recommends initiating warfarin on the first treatment day and overlapping therapy with warfarin and heparin for a minimum of 5 days and until the INR is at least 2 for 24 hours or longer.

An initial heparin sodium loading dose of 75–100 units/kg (by direct IV injection over 10 minutes) has been suggested in children based on some data indicating that such doses may be more likely to result in therapeutic aPTT values. Following the initial loading dose, a maintenance IV infusion of 25–30 units/kg per hour in infants or 18–20 units/kg per hour in children older than 1 year of age is suggested. The appropriate maintenance dosage of heparin sodium appears to be age dependent, with infants under the age of 2 months having the highest requirements (e.g., average of 28 units/kg per hour) and older children having lower requirements (e.g., average of 20 units/kg per hour in children older than 1 year of age); some experts suggest using a dosage of 18 units/kg per hour in older children. Although not preferred, a maintenance heparin sodium dosage of 75–100 units/kg every 4 hours by intermittent IV administration has been used. ACCP states that the initial dosing strategy in children should be individualized based on consideration of risk factors for bleeding and thrombosis; in general, loading doses should be withheld or reduced if there are substantial bleeding risks, and long-term use of heparin should be avoided in children.

Thromboprophylaxis in General Surgery

For *fixed low-dose prophylaxis* of postoperative deep-vein thrombosis in general surgery patients, the most widely used dosage of heparin sodium has been 5000 units administered subcutaneously 2 hours prior to surgery and every 8–12 hours after surgery for 7 days or until the patient is fully ambulatory, whichever is longer. If clinical evidence of thromboembolism develops despite fixed low-dose prophylaxis, full-dose IV or subcutaneous heparin should be initiated.

Acute Ischemic Complications of ST-Segment-Elevation Myocardial Infarction

As adjunctive therapy with fibrin-selective thrombolytic agents (e.g., alteplase, tenecteplase, reteplase) in patients with ST-segment-elevation MI (STEMI)†, the American College of Cardiology Foundation (ACCF) and the American Heart Association (AHA) recommend IV heparin sodium given in an initial loading dose of 60 units/kg (maximum 4000 units) followed by a continuous infusion of 12 units/kg per hour (maximum 1000 units/hour), adjusted to maintain a therapeutic aPTT of 1.5–2 times the control value or 50–70 seconds for 48 hours or until revascularization.

In patients with acute MI and concurrent atrial fibrillation, ACCF, AHA, and the Heart Rhythm Society (HRS) recommend continuous IV infusion or intermittent subcutaneous injection of heparin sodium in a dosage sufficient to prolong the aPTT to 1.5–2 times the control value.

Acute Ischemic Complications of Percutaneous Coronary Intervention

In patients undergoing percutaneous coronary intervention (PCI) who are *not* receiving concurrent antiplatelet therapy with a GP IIb/IIIa-receptor inhibitor and who have not received prior anticoagulant therapy, ACCF, AHA, and the Society for Cardiovascular Angiography and Interventions (SCAI) suggest administration of a loading dose of 70–100 units/kg of heparin sodium by direct IV injection to achieve an ACT of 250–300 seconds with the HemoTec device or 300–350 seconds with the Hemochron device. If prior anticoagulant therapy has been administered in such patients, additional heparin sodium doses (e.g., 2000–5000 units) should be given as needed to achieve an ACT of 250–300 seconds with the HemoTec device or 300–350 seconds with the Hemochron device. In patients undergoing PCI who are receiving concurrent therapy with a GP IIb/IIIa-receptor inhibitor and who have not received prior anticoagulant therapy, use of a lower dose of concurrent heparin sodium (50–70 units/kg IV loading dose) targeted

to an ACT of 200–250 seconds is suggested. If prior anticoagulant therapy has been administered in such patients, additional heparin sodium doses (e.g., 2000–5000 units) should be given as needed to achieve an ACT of 200–250 seconds. Lower dosages of heparin may be used in women and geriatric patients undergoing PCI, particularly when heparin is combined with GP IIb/IIIa-receptor inhibitors. Heparin sodium should be discontinued after successful PCI procedures; in most cases, the femoral sheath is removed when the ACT falls to less than 150–180 seconds or when the aPTT decreases to less than 50 seconds.

Acute Ischemic Complications of Non-ST-Segment-Elevation Acute Coronary Syndromes

Adjusted-dose heparin sodium (e.g., 60 units/kg [maximum 4000 units] loading dose followed by continuous IV infusion of 12 units/kg per hour [maximum 1000 units/hr]) is recommended by ACCF, AHA, and ACC to maintain the aPTT between 1.5–2 times the control value in patients with non-ST-segment-elevation acute coronary syndromes (NSTE ACS; unstable angina or non-ST-segment-elevation MI [NSTEMI]) in addition to aspirin and/or clopidogrel. Therapy should be initiated as soon as possible upon presentation. Optimum duration of therapy has not been established; in clinical trials, heparin was continued for 2–5 days.

Disseminated Intravascular Coagulation

When heparin is used for the treatment of disseminated intravascular coagulation (DIC), some clinicians recommend heparin sodium doses of 50–100 units/kg for adults and 25–50 units/kg for children given by IV infusion or IV injection every 4 hours. If there is no improvement after 4–8 hours, the drug should be discontinued.

Cardiac Surgery

The initial dose of heparin sodium recommended by the manufacturers for adults undergoing total body perfusion for open-heart surgery is not less than 150 units/kg. A heparin sodium dose of 300 units/kg is frequently used for procedures estimated to last less than 1 hour and 400 units/kg for those procedures estimated to last longer than 1 hour. Some clinicians recommend that heparin sodium dosage during cardiopulmonary bypass procedures be adjusted to prolong the ACT to 480–600 seconds. In extracorporeal dialysis procedures, the equipment manufacturer's operating instructions should be followed carefully; if manufacturer's instructions are not available, an initial heparin sodium dose of 25–30 units/kg, followed by an infusion of 1500–2000 units/hour is suggested based on pharmacodynamic data.

Cardioversion of Atrial Fibrillation

If heparin is used for the prevention of stroke and systemic embolism in patients undergoing cardioversion for atrial fibrillation or atrial flutter†, the use of full venous thromboembolism treatment dosages is recommended.

Thromboembolism During Pregnancy

When heparin is used for thromboprophylaxis during pregnancy†, the drug is usually administered 2–3 times daily in a prophylactic dosage (fixed-dose) or intermediate dosage (dosage adjusted to target a specific anti-factor Xa level). When used in therapeutic dosages, heparin usually is administered by continuous IV infusion with doses adjusted to achieve a target therapeutic aPTT or by twice-daily subcutaneous injection in doses sufficient to achieve a therapeutic aPTT 6 hours after injection.

In women with antiphospholipid antibody (APLA) syndrome and a history of multiple pregnancy losses, antepartum administration of subcutaneous heparin sodium in a prophylactic or intermediate dosage has been recommended; low-dose aspirin (75–100 mg daily) should be administered in conjunction with heparin.

ACCF/AHA/HRS state that administration of heparin may be considered during the first trimester and last month of pregnancy in patients with atrial fibrillation and additional risk factors for thromboembolism. Heparin sodium may be administered by continuous IV infusion in a dosage sufficient to maintain the aPTT at least 1.5–2 times the control value. Alternatively, 10,000–20,000 units of heparin sodium may be given subcutaneously every 12 hours with dosage adjusted to maintain the mid-interval aPTT (6 hours after the dose) at 1.5–2 times the control value. Coumarin anticoagulant therapy (e.g., warfarin) may be considered during the second trimester in pregnant women with atrial fibrillation who have a high risk for thromboembolism.

If subcutaneous heparin sodium is used for the prevention of thromboembolism in pregnant women with prosthetic mechanical heart valves, the drug should be initiated in high dosages (17,500–20,000 units every 12 hours) and adjusted to maintain the mid-interval aPTT at least twice the control value or an anti-factor Xa concentration of 0.35–0.7 units/mL throughout pregnancy. Alternatively, 17,500–20,000 units of heparin sodium may be administered every 12 hours and adjusted to maintain the mid-interval aPTT at least twice the control value or an anti-factor Xa concentration of 0.35–0.7 units/mL until week 13 of pregnancy; subsequently, therapy is switched to warfarin until close to delivery when heparin may be resumed.

Perioperative Management of Antithrombotic Therapy

If heparin is used for bridging anticoagulation in patients who require temporary interruption of warfarin therapy during surgery or other invasive procedure, ACCP recommends the use of therapeutic dosages (e.g., continuous infusion of heparin adjusted to maintain an aPTT of approximately 1.5–2 times the control value) because of more extensive data and experience; however, other dosage regimens have been used. ACCP suggests that heparin be discontinued approximately 4–6 hours prior to surgery to allow sufficient time for anticoagulant effects to dissipate. Postoperative anticoagulation should be administered with caution and only when hemostasis has been achieved because of the potential for bleeding at the surgical site.

Anticoagulation in Blood Transfusions and Blood Samples

When heparin sodium is used as an in vitro anticoagulant in blood transfusions, 7500 units of the drug is usually added to 100 mL of 0.9% sodium chloride injection and 6–8 mL of this solution is added to each 100 mL of whole blood. When heparin sodium is used as an in vitro anticoagulant for blood samples, 70–150 units is added to each 10–20 mL of whole blood.

Thrombosis Associated with Indwelling Venous or Arterial Devices

When a heparin-containing flush solution is used to maintain patency of indwelling venipuncture devices, a quantity of heparin lock flush solution (e.g., containing 10 or 100 units of heparin sodium per mL) sufficient to fill the device is injected into the lumen of the device after each use, after designated intervals (if the device is not used in the interim), or as necessary. While it has been reported that each dose of the solution will maintain anticoagulation within the lumen of the device for up to 4 hours, longer intervals between instillations of the flush solution (generally every 8–12 hours) are commonly employed when the device is not being used more frequently, and flushing with 0.9% sodium chloride injection alone at such intervals also appears to be effective in maintaining patency in venipuncture devices into which blood is not aspirated, at least those placed peripherally.

When a drug that is incompatible with heparin is to be administered via a venipuncture device in which a heparin-containing flush solution is used, the entire device should be flushed with 0.9% sodium chloride injection prior to and immediately after the incompatible drug is administered. Another dose of heparin lock flush solution may be injected into the device after the second saline flush. When the indwelling venipuncture device is used for repeated withdrawal of blood samples for laboratory analysis and the presence of heparin or 0.9% sodium chloride is likely to interfere with or alter results of the analysis, heparin lock flush solution should be cleared from the device by aspirating and discarding it from the device before withdrawing the blood sample. After the blood sample is drawn, another dose of heparin lock flush solution should be injected into the device.

Following injection of heparin lock solution from a single-dose vial into an indwelling venipuncture device, unused portions of the solutions should be discarded. The device manufacturer's instructions should be consulted for specific directions. Multiple-dose vials are available for repeated use. Since repeated injections of small doses of heparin sodium can alter aPTT results, it is recommended that a baseline aPTT value be obtained prior to insertion of an indwelling venipuncture device.

In neonates and children requiring cardiac catheterization via an artery†, ACCP recommends a heparin sodium dose of 100 units/kg as a direct IV injection. Additional doses may be required in prolonged procedures.

For thromboprophylaxis in neonates with a central venous access device†, ACCP recommends the use of heparin sodium 0.5 units/kg per hour as a continuous infusion.

For thromboprophylaxis of umbilical arterial catheters in neonates†, ACCP suggests the use of low-dose heparin sodium infusion (0.25–1 unit/mL) for a total dosage of 25–200 units/kg per day.

For thromboprophylaxis in neonates and children with peripheral arterial catheters, administration of heparin sodium by continuous IV infusion in low dosages (5 units/mL at 1 mL/hour) is recommended by ACCP.

CAUTIONS

● Hematologic Effects

Hemorrhage, the major adverse effect of heparin, is an extension of the pharmacologic action of the drug and may range from minor local ecchymoses to major hemorrhagic complications. Rarely, hemorrhagic complications may result in death. Bleeding complications occur in approximately 1.5–20% of patients receiving heparin. Major bleeding episodes occur more frequently with full-dose than with low-dose heparin and have been reported more frequently with intermittent IV injection than with continuous IV infusion of the drug. The incidence of major bleeding appears to be similar among patients receiving heparin by continuous IV infusion or subcutaneously. Pooled data from a number of clinical trials evaluating IV heparin for the treatment of venous thromboembolism indicate that the rates of major bleeding range from 0–7% and fatal bleeding from 0–2%. In patients with ischemic coronary syndromes, the incidence of major bleeding ranges from 0–6.3% during the initial 8 days of treatment and from 0.3–3.2% during subsequent long-term therapy (approximately 0.25–3 months). Hemorrhage also has been reported occasionally with repeated administration of heparin lock flush solutions containing low concentrations of heparin sodium (e.g., 10–100 units/mL).

Patients with renal failure or with a history of recent surgery or trauma may be at increased risk of bleeding complications during therapy with heparin. There is some evidence that the risk of heparin-induced hemorrhage may be higher in patients older than 60 years of age, especially in women. Bleeding may occur at any site, and some hemorrhagic complications may be difficult to detect. GI or urinary tract bleeding during therapy with heparin may indicate the presence of occult lesions. Adrenal hemorrhage with acute adrenal insufficiency has occurred during therapy with heparin. Retroperitoneal hemorrhage has been reported in patients receiving anticoagulant therapy, and potentially fatal ovarian (corpus luteum) hemorrhage has also occurred in some women of reproductive age who received short- or long-term anticoagulant therapy. The frequency and severity of heparin-associated hemorrhage may be minimized by careful clinical management of the patient. (See Cautions: Precautions and Contraindications.)

Pooled analyses of data from comparative clinical trials evaluating heparin and low molecular weight heparins for the treatment of venous thromboembolism or ischemic coronary syndromes indicate that use of low molecular weight heparin does not result in an increased risk of major bleeding compared with heparin.

Two forms of acute thrombocytopenia have been reported with heparin. In some patients, thrombocytopenia appears to be caused by a direct, nonimmunologic effect on circulating platelets. In others, the reaction is immune mediated (heparin-induced thrombocytopenia [HIT]) and caused by the development of IgG antibodies to an immune complex that forms between heparin and platelet factor 4; these antibody-bound immune complexes bind to IgG receptors on the surface of platelets, resulting in platelet activation and increased thrombin generation. Thrombocytopenia has been reported with both low-dose and full-dose heparin therapy and does not appear to be dose related. Thrombocytopenia, including accompanying intracranial bleeding and GI hemorrhage, has been reported in patients receiving less than 500 units of heparin sodium daily via heparin lock flush solution. Although the reported incidences are variable (e.g., 0–30%), thrombocytopenia has occurred in about 15% of patients treated with heparin sodium prepared from bovine lung tissue and in about 5% of those treated with heparin sodium prepared from porcine intestinal mucosa. Thrombocytopenia, if it occurs, usually develops 1–20 days after initiation of therapy. Immune-mediated HIT usually is evident 5–10 days after exposure to heparin, but can occur more rapidly (e.g., within 24 hours) in patients with recent exposure (e.g., within the previous 3 months) to the drug or appear as late as several weeks after discontinuance of therapy. Mild thrombocytopenia (platelet count greater than 100,000/mm³) may remain stable or even reverse with continued heparin therapy. However, thrombocytopenia of any degree should be monitored closely since HIT can sometimes lead to the development of serious, sometimes fatal, thrombotic events. Heparin therapy should generally be discontinued if substantial thrombocytopenia (platelet count less than 100,000/mm³) or HIT (with or without thrombosis) occurs.

HIT is a serious complication of heparin therapy that can lead to life- or limb-threatening venous and arterial thrombosis (e.g., cerebral vein thrombosis, limb ischemia, acute myocardial infarction [MI], stroke, gangrene of the extremities [possibly requiring amputation], mesenteric thrombosis). Localized or disseminated thromboses associated with HIT have occurred in patients receiving heparin, even in the low concentrations used in heparin lock flush solution. HIT-associated thrombosis develops as a result of in vivo platelet aggregation induced by heparin and can occur at almost any vascular location. (See Cautions: Precautions and Contraindications.)

● **Sensitivity Reactions**

Allergic reactions to heparin occur rarely. Hypersensitivity, which can be generalized, may be manifested by chills, fever, pruritus, urticaria, asthma, rhinitis, lacrimation, headache, nausea, vomiting, and anaphylactoid reactions including shock. Allergic vasospastic reactions have been reported with heparin. These reactions, if they occur, generally develop 6–10 days after initiation of heparin and last 4–6 hours. The reactions frequently occur in a limb where an artery has been recently catheterized. The affected limb is painful, ischemic, and cyanosed. If heparin is continued, generalized vasospasm with cyanosis, tachypnea, feelings of oppression, and headache may occur. Protamine sulfate has no effect on these reactions.

Itching and burning, especially of the plantar side of the feet, has occurred during heparin therapy and may be caused by a similar allergic vasospastic reaction. Chest pain, hypertension, arthralgia, and/or headache have also been reported in the absence of definite peripheral vasospasm.

● **Local Effects**

Deep subcutaneous injection of heparin may rarely cause local irritation, erythema, mild pain, hematoma, ulceration, or cutaneous and subcutaneous necrosis (sometimes requiring skin grafts). Local irritation and erythema also have been reported with heparin lock flush solution. Histamine-like reactions have also been reported at the site of injection. A slightly lower incidence of local reactions has been reported following deep subcutaneous injection of heparin calcium (no longer commercially available in the US) than that reported following deep subcutaneous injection of equal doses of heparin sodium; this may be due to the smaller volume of heparin calcium required.

● **Hepatic Effects**

Increased serum concentrations of AST (SGOT) and ALT (SGPT), without increased serum concentrations of bilirubin or alkaline phosphatase, have been reported in a high percentage of patients following subcutaneous or IV administration of heparin; transient increases in serum LDH concentrations have also occurred in some patients receiving the drug. Increased concentrations of AST and ALT have also been reported following administration of heparin to healthy individuals. A reversible cholestatic reaction without jaundice, manifested by increased serum aminotransferase (ALT, AST) and alkaline phosphatase concentrations, also has been reported in a few patients receiving heparin therapy. It is not known whether elevated serum aminotransferases in patients receiving heparin represent hepatic toxicity, drug-induced laboratory test interference, or nonspecific stimulation of hepatic enzymes. (See Laboratory Test Interferences.) Since aminotransferase determinations are important in the differential diagnosis of MI, liver disease, and pulmonary emboli, elevation of these enzymes during heparin therapy should be interpreted with caution.

● **Other Adverse Effects**

Osteoporosis and spontaneous fractures of the vertebral column have been reported rarely in patients receiving large daily dosages (10,000 units or more) of heparin sodium for 3 months or longer. Suppression of aldosterone synthesis; priapism; delayed, transient alopecia; and rebound hyperlipemia following

discontinuance of heparin therapy have also been reported rarely in patients receiving the drug.

● **Precautions and Contraindications**

All patients should be screened prior to initiation of heparin therapy to rule out bleeding disorders. In preoperative patients, the prothrombin time (PT), activated partial thromboplastin time (aPTT), hematocrit, and platelet count should be determined prior to surgery; coagulation tests should be normal or only slightly elevated before low-dose heparin therapy is instituted. Although monitoring of blood coagulation tests is useful for assuring adequate dosage during full-dose heparin therapy, coagulation test results do not always correlate with the frequency of bleeding complications. Heparin should be used with extreme caution whenever there is an increased risk of hemorrhage. Factors reported to increase the risk of hemorrhage during heparin therapy include concurrent administration of some drugs (see Drug Interactions); subacute bacterial endocarditis; arterial sclerosis; dissecting aneurysm; increased capillary permeability; presence of inaccessible ulcerative GI lesions; diverticulitis; ulcerative colitis; hemorrhagic blood dyscrasias (e.g., hemophilia, some vascular purpuras, thrombocytopenia); menstruation; ovulation; threatened abortion; severe renal, hepatic, or biliary disease; hypertension; indwelling catheters; eye, brain, or spinal cord surgery; continuous tube drainage of the stomach or small intestine; and spinal tap or spinal anesthesia.

If hemorrhage occurs, heparin should be discontinued immediately. Nosebleed, hematuria, or tarry stools may be noted as the first sign of bleeding or overdosage; easy bruising or petechiae may precede frank bleeding. Discontinuance of heparin will usually correct minor bleeding or overdosage within a few hours. If severe hemorrhage or overdosage occurs, protamine sulfate should be administered immediately. Blood transfusions may also be required in patients with massive blood loss. If signs and symptoms of acute adrenal hemorrhage and insufficiency occur, plasma cortisol concentrations should be measured and vigorous therapy with IV corticosteroids should be initiated after discontinuing heparin. Initiation of corrective therapy should not depend on laboratory confirmation of the diagnosis, since any delay in an acute situation may be fatal.

Heparin is contraindicated in patients with severe thrombocytopenia or a history of HIT or HIT with thrombosis. If HIT with or without thrombosis is diagnosed or strongly suspected during heparin therapy, all sources of heparin (including heparin flushes) should be discontinued and an alternative (nonheparin) anticoagulant (e.g., argatroban, bivalirudin) substituted. Conversion to warfarin therapy (for longer-term anticoagulation) should be initiated only after substantial recovery from acute HIT has occurred (i.e., platelet counts at least 150,000/mm³) with a nonheparin anticoagulant. The manufacturer recommends against future use of heparin in patients who experience HIT, particularly within 3–6 months following the event and if HIT antibodies are still present. HIT with or without thrombosis also can occur up to several weeks following discontinuance of heparin therapy. Patients who are found to have thrombocytopenia or thrombosis after discontinuance of heparin should be evaluated for HIT and HIT with thrombosis. Although there is some uncertainty regarding the risk-to-benefit ratio of platelet count monitoring in patients receiving heparin, the American College of Chest Physicians (ACCP) suggests that platelet counts may be monitored in those who are considered to be at high risk (higher than 1%) of developing HIT; for those considered to be at low risk (less than 1%), platelet count monitoring generally is not recommended.

Patients with familial antithrombin III deficiency may appear to be resistant to the effects of heparin, since adequate levels of antithrombin III are necessary for the drug's anticoagulant effect. Increased resistance to the antithrombotic effects of heparin has been reported in febrile patients, in postoperative patients, and in some patients with MI, pulmonary embolism, thrombophlebitis, infections with thrombosing tendencies, or extensive thrombotic disorders, especially in conjunction with malignant neoplasms. This phenomenon appears to be caused by alterations in the physiology of the patient and pharmacokinetics of the drug, and larger doses of heparin may be required during initial therapy to achieve an anticoagulant response in these patients.

Fatal medication errors have occurred as a result of confusion between different formulations of heparin, in particular with heparin sodium injection and catheter lock flush vials. At least 3 infant deaths have been reported following inadvertent administration of heparin sodium injection 10,000 units/mL instead of HEP-LOCK U/P (heparin lock flush solution) 10 units/mL. Heparin sodium injection should not be used as a catheter lock flush product. To minimize the risk of medication errors, clinicians should take appropriate measures to carefully distinguish between heparin formulations and review all labels for correct drug name, strength, and volume prior to dispensing and administering the drug. Dispensing errors involving heparin sodium injection and HEP-LOCK U/P should be reported to the manufacturer (800-ANA-Drug or 800-262-3784) or the FDA MedWatch program by phone (800-FDA-1088 or online at https://www.accessdata.fda.gov/scripts/medwatch/medwatch-online.htm.

Heparin is generally contraindicated in patients who are hypersensitive to the drug or to pork products. Patients with documented hypersensitivity to heparin should be given the drug only in clearly life-threatening situations.

Heparin is contraindicated in patients with uncontrollable bleeding, unless such bleeding is secondary to disseminated intravascular coagulation. The drug is also contraindicated whenever suitable blood coagulation tests cannot be performed at required intervals; however, this is not generally a contraindication for fixed low-dose heparin therapy, since monitoring of coagulation tests is not usually required when fixed low-dose therapy is used in patients with normal coagulation parameters.

Some commercially available formulations of heparin sodium injection contain sodium metabisulfite, a sulfite that can cause allergic-type reactions, including anaphylaxis and life-threatening or less severe asthmatic episodes, in certain susceptible individuals. The overall prevalence of sulfite sensitivity in the general population is unknown but probably low; such sensitivity appears to occur more frequently in asthmatic than in nonasthmatic individuals.

When heparin is used in combination with dihydroergotamine, the usual cautions, precautions, and contraindications associated with dihydroergotamine must be considered in addition to those associated with heparin. The potential risk of arterial vasospasm should be considered in patients receiving combined therapy with these drugs.

● Pediatric Precautions

There are no adequate and well-controlled studies evaluating the use of heparin in pediatric patients.

Some commercially available heparin sodium injections and heparin lock flush solutions contain benzyl alcohol as a preservative. Although a causal relationship has not been established, administration of injections preserved with benzyl alcohol has been associated with serious toxicity (e.g., "gasping syndrome") in pediatric patients. Toxicity appears to result from administration of large amounts (i.e., about 100–400 mg/kg daily) of benzyl alcohol in these patients, and may be more likely to occur in neonates and low-birthweight infants. When heparin sodium injection is required in neonates and infants, the manufacturer states that a preservative-free formulation should be used. When heparin lock flush is required in neonates, a preservative-free formulation should be used. The American Academy of Pediatrics (AAP) states that use of preservative-containing flush solutions (i.e., with benzyl alcohol) clearly should be avoided in neonates; however, the AAP further states that the presence of small amounts of the preservative in a commercially available injection should not proscribe its use in neonates. Although the recommended dosage range for heparin includes amounts of benzyl alcohol well below that associated with the "gasping syndrome," the minimum amount of benzyl alcohol at which toxicity may occur is unknown. If other benzyl alcohol-containing preparations are to be used in a patient, clinicians should take into account the total daily metabolic load of benzyl alcohol from all sources.

Fatalities have occurred in pediatric patients, including neonates, as a result of medication dispensing errors. Clinicians should take appropriate precautions when dispensing and administering the drug. (See Cautions: Precautions and Contraindications.)

The use of heparin to maintain patency of umbilical-artery catheters reportedly has been associated with an increased risk of germinal matrix-intraventricular hemorrhage in low-birthweight neonates; however, a causal relationship has not been definitely established, and well-controlled studies are needed to further evaluate this finding. Because of the potential risk of systemic anticoagulation, heparin lock flush solutions containing heparin sodium 100 units/mL should be avoided in neonates and in infants who weigh less than 10 kg. Caution also is advised when using heparin lock flush solutions containing 10 units/mL in premature infants who weigh less than 1 kg and are receiving frequent flushes.

● Geriatric Precautions

A higher incidence of bleeding has been reported in patients older than 60 years of age, especially women. Clinical studies indicate that lower dosages of heparin may be appropriate in these patients. (See Dosage and Administration: Dosage.)

● Pregnancy, Fertility, and Lactation

Pregnancy

Increased fetal resorptions have been observed in animals when heparin was administered during the period of organogenesis in dosages higher than the maximum human dosage; there are no adequate and well-controlled studies to date using heparin in pregnant women. Published reports have not shown any evidence of a teratogenic potential or other adverse fetal effects when the drug is used during pregnancy; because heparin does not cross the human placenta, any fetal complications that may occur are likely to be related to other indirect factors (e.g., severe maternal disease).

Long-term (e.g., longer than 1 month) heparin therapy during pregnancy can result in maternal osteopenia and osteoporosis, and prophylactic calcium and vitamin D supplementation has been suggested to reduce this risk. At least one case of fatal cerebral hemorrhage has occurred in a woman receiving heparin and aspirin to prevent pregnancy loss following in vitro fertilization. (See Uses: Complications of Pregnancy.)

Heparin should be used during pregnancy only if the potential benefits justify the potential risks to the fetus; if needed, use of a preservative (benzyl alcohol)-free formulation is recommended. When anticoagulant therapy is required in pregnant women, ACCP generally recommends the use of a low molecular weight heparin because of a more favorable adverse effect profile. For information on the prophylactic use of heparin to improve pregnancy outcomes in certain women at risk (e.g., those with antiphospholipid syndrome), see Uses: Complications of Pregnancy.

Lactation

Because of its high molecular weight, heparin is not likely to be distributed into human milk; any heparin that is ingested during breastfeeding would not be absorbed by a nursing infant. However, if benzyl alcohol is present in maternal serum, it is likely to distribute into human milk and be absorbed by a nursing infant. The manufacturer recommends caution if heparin is used in nursing women. ACCP recommends that heparin be continued in nursing women who are already receiving such therapy.

If heparin therapy is required in nursing women, use of a preservative (benzyl alcohol)-free formulation is recommended.

DRUG INTERACTIONS

● Drugs Affecting Platelet Function

Drugs that affect platelet function (e.g., aspirin and other nonsteroidal anti-inflammatory agents, dextran, dipyridamole, phenylbutazone [no longer commercially available in the US], hydroxychloroquine, GP IIb/IIIa-receptor inhibitors such as abciximab, eptifibatide, and tirofiban) may increase the risk of hemorrhage and should be used with caution in patients receiving heparin.

● Thrombolytic Agents

Concomitant therapy with heparin and/or platelet-aggregation inhibitors has been used with thrombolytic agents to prevent reocclusion following lysis of coronary artery thrombi. However, since such therapy has not been shown to be of unequivocal benefit and may increase the risk of bleeding complications, use of anticoagulants concomitantly with thrombolytic therapy should be individualized and careful monitoring is advised. Some evidence suggests a narrow margin of safety for upward adjustment of heparin dosage, and the need for serial monitoring of activated partial thromboplastin time (aPTT), in patients receiving heparin concurrently with thrombolytic therapy for acute myocardial infarction (MI). (See Uses: Acute Ischemic Complications of ST-Segment-Elevation Myocardial Infarction.)

● *Dihydroergotamine Mesylate*

When used in combination with heparin, dihydroergotamine appears to potentiate the antithrombogenic effects of heparin by helping to reduce factors that contribute to venous thrombus formation. As a result of its vasoconstrictor effect, dihydroergotamine accelerates venous return, reduces venous stasis and pooling, and may also indirectly help to prevent damage to venous endothelium caused by excessive dilation. Therefore, concomitant use of dihydroergotamine and heparin may help to prevent deep-vein thrombosis.

Concomitant subcutaneous administration of dihydroergotamine mesylate with heparin sodium does not appear to affect the pharmacokinetics of heparin. Concomitant subcutaneous administration of the drugs reportedly decreases peak plasma concentrations of dihydroergotamine and decreases the rate of absorption of dihydroergotamine compared with administration of dihydroergotamine alone; however, the area under the concentration-time curve of dihydroergotamine is generally unaffected.

● *Other Drugs*

Although some reports suggest that IV nitroglycerin may antagonize the anticoagulant effect of heparin when these drugs are administered concomitantly, such antagonism has not been confirmed in other studies. Limited data suggest that nitroglycerin-induced heparin resistance, if it occurs, may be manifested only at high nitroglycerin dosages or infusion rates (e.g., greater than 350 mcg/minute) and may possibly be related to a nitroglycerin-induced abnormality in antithrombin III (heparin cofactor). Further study is required to confirm possible IV nitroglycerin-induced heparin resistance in patients receiving these drugs concomitantly and, if confirmed, to elucidate the potential clinical importance of such an interaction. Meanwhile, it has been suggested that patients receiving heparin and IV nitroglycerin concomitantly be monitored closely to avoid inadequate anticoagulation.

Cardiac glycosides, nicotine, quinine, tetracyclines, and antihistamines reportedly may interfere with the anticoagulant effect of heparin. Although there is some experimental evidence that heparin may antagonize the action of corticosteroids, corticotropin, and insulin, these effects have not been definitely established.

The anticoagulant effect of heparin is enhanced by concurrent treatment with antithrombin III (human) in patients with familial antithrombin III deficiency. To avoid bleeding, at least one manufacturer recommends a reduced dosage of heparin during concurrent treatment with antithrombin III.

LABORATORY TEST INTERFERENCES

● *Prothrombin Time*

Heparin prolongs the prothrombin time (PT), and caution should be observed in evaluating the test in patients receiving a coumarin or indandione derivative and heparin. Valid PT determinations can usually be made during concurrent therapy if blood samples for the test are drawn at least 4–6 hours after an IV dose or 12–24 hours after a subcutaneous dose of heparin. The PT may not be significantly prolonged by heparin when the drug is administered by continuous IV infusion and blood samples for the test can usually be obtained at any time during the infusion.

● *Other Laboratory Tests*

Heparin reportedly interferes with the sulfobromophthalein test by increasing the color intensity of the dye in serum and causing a shift in the absorption peak from 580 to 595 nm.

Heparin interferes with competitive protein binding methods for serum thyroxine determinations resulting in falsely elevated concentrations. Radioimmunoassay and protein bound iodine methods do not appear to be affected by heparin.

When heparin is used as an in vitro anticoagulant, leukocyte counts should be done within 2 hours after addition of heparin. Heparinized blood should not be used for erythrocyte sedimentation rates, platelet counts, or erythrocyte fragility tests and is unsuitable for tests involving complement or isoagglutinins.

Heparin may cause false elevations in plasma AST (SGOT) concentrations using an Ektachem dry-chemistry system analyzer. Since aminotransferase determinations are important in the differential diagnosis of myocardial infarction (MI), liver disease, and pulmonary emboli, elevation of these enzymes during heparin therapy should be interpreted with caution.

PHARMACOLOGY

● *Anticoagulant Effect*

Heparin acts as a catalyst to markedly accelerate the rate at which antithrombin III (heparin cofactor) neutralizes thrombin and activated coagulation factor X (Xa). Antithrombin III generally neutralizes these coagulation factors by slowly and irreversibly complexing stoichiometrically with them; however, in the presence of heparin, it neutralizes these factors almost instantaneously. Although the exact mechanism of action has not been fully elucidated, heparin apparently binds to antithrombin III and induces a conformational change in the molecule which promotes its interaction with thrombin and factor Xa. In the presence of heparin, antithrombin III also neutralizes activated coagulation factors IX, XI, XII, and plasmin.

With low-dose heparin therapy (see Dosage and Administration: Dosage), anticoagulation appears to result from neutralization of factor Xa which prevents the conversion of prothrombin to thrombin. Low doses of heparin have very little effect on thrombin and exert a measurable antithrombogenic effect only if thrombin formation has not already occurred. With full-dose heparin therapy (see Dosage and Administration: Dosage), anticoagulation appears to result primarily from neutralization of thrombin which prevents the conversion of fibrinogen to fibrin. Full-dose heparin therapy also prevents the formation of a stable fibrin clot by inhibiting activation of fibrin stabilizing factor. In contrast to coumarin and indandione derivatives, heparin has an anticoagulant effect both in vitro and in vivo. Low-dose or full-dose heparin therapy inhibits thrombus formation when stasis is induced, and full-dose therapy may prevent extension of existing thrombi. Heparin has no fibrinolytic activity and cannot lyse established thrombi.

In adequate dosage, protamine sulfate neutralizes the anticoagulant effect of heparin. Although there is no significant difference in the anticoagulant effectiveness between heparin derived from porcine intestinal mucosa or bovine lung tissue, slightly different amounts of protamine sulfate are required to neutralize one unit of heparin calcium (no longer commercially available in the US) derived from porcine intestinal mucosa or one unit of heparin sodium derived from bovine lung tissue or porcine intestinal mucosa.

Because heparin acts on blood coagulation factors that are involved in both extrinsic and intrinsic coagulation, full-dose heparin therapy produces prolongation of several coagulation assays including the activated coagulation time (ACT), activated partial thromboplastin time (aPTT), plasma recalcification time, prothrombin time (PT), thrombin time, and whole blood clotting time. Coagulation test results are generally unaffected or only minimally prolonged by low-dose heparin therapy. Heparin sodium lock flush solution does not induce systemic anticoagulant effects when administered in single doses of 10 or 100 units/mL to maintain the patency of IV injection devices.

● *Other Effects*

In vivo, heparin clears lipemic plasma by stimulating the release and/or activation of lipoprotein lipase which hydrolyzes triglycerides to free fatty acids and glycerol. This effect may occur following doses of heparin that are smaller than those required to produce anticoagulant effects. Rebound hyperlipemia has been reported following a period of heparin-induced plasma clearing. Protamine sulfate inhibits the plasma-clearing effect of heparin.

Heparin has been reported to increase, decrease, or have no effect on platelet adhesiveness, aggregation, and release reaction. Many reports are based on in vitro studies that were performed under various conditions, and results do not necessarily correspond to in vivo effects of heparin on platelets. (See Cautions: Hematologic Effects.) Various other pharmacologic actions including antiinflammatory, diuretic, antimetastatic, antiviral, and antienzymatic effects have been attributed to heparin; however, most of these reports are based on animal studies and their clinical importance has not been established.

PHARMACOKINETICS

● Absorption

Heparin is not absorbed from the GI tract and must be administered parenterally. The onset of anticoagulant activity is immediate following direct IV injection or the start of continuous IV infusion of full doses of heparin. There may be considerable interpatient variation in the extent of absorption following deep subcutaneous injection of heparin; however, onset of activity usually occurs within 20–60 minutes. Results of preliminary studies indicate that the rate and extent of absorption are lower following deep subcutaneous injection of heparin calcium (no longer commercially available in the US) than following deep subcutaneous injection of equal doses of heparin sodium.

Plasma heparin concentrations may be increased and activated partial thromboplastin times (aPTTs) may be more prolonged in geriatric adults (older than 60 years of age) compared with younger adults.

● Distribution

Heparin appears to be extensively bound to low-density lipoprotein, globulins, and fibrinogen. The drug does not cross the placenta and is not distributed into milk.

● Elimination

The plasma half-life of heparin averages 1–2 hours in healthy adults. However, the half-life of the drug increases with increasing doses. Following IV administration of heparin sodium 100, 200, or 400 units/kg, the plasma half-life of the drug averages 56, 96, and 152 minutes, respectively. Several studies using heparin sodium have shown that the drug has a shorter plasma half-life in patients with pulmonary embolism than in healthy individuals or patients with other thrombotic disorders. The plasma half-life of the drug is also decreased in patients with liver impairment but may be prolonged in cirrhotic patients. In anephric patients or patients with severe renal impairment, the half-life of heparin may be slightly prolonged.

The metabolic fate of heparin has not been fully elucidated, but the drug appears to be removed from the circulation mainly by the reticuloendothelial system and may localize on arterial and venous endothelium. Although there is no reproducible evidence, it has been suggested that heparin may be partially metabolized in the liver to uroheparin, which is partially desulfated heparin. A small fraction of each dose of heparin appears to be excreted in urine as unchanged drug. Heparin is not removed by hemodialysis.

CHEMISTRY AND STABILITY

● Chemistry

Heparin is an anionic, sulfated glycosaminoglycan present in mast cells. Heparin is a heterogeneous molecule with an average molecular weight of about 12,000. Heparin is commercially available as the sodium salt. Heparin sodium is prepared from either porcine intestinal mucosa or bovine lung tissue.

In most countries, potency of heparin is determined using a World Health Organization (WHO) reference standard and is expressed in international units. In the US, the potency of heparin previously was standardized according to a USP reference standard that was expressed in USP Heparin Units and required a potency of not less than 140 units/mg of heparin. On October 1, 2009, USP implemented a new reference standard for heparin to ensure the purity, consistency, and safety of heparin-containing products in the US supply chain. This new compendial standard was developed largely in response to a heparin contamination problem that occurred in 2007–2008. Included in the updated standard is a new potency test method (chromogenic anti-Factor IIa test) that can detect impurities in heparin preparations and a new potency reference standard that will harmonize the USP Heparin Unit with the WHO international unit. As a result of these changes, heparin produced under the new USP standard is approximately 10% less potent, unit for unit, than heparin prepared under the previous USP standard. (See Dosage and Administration: Dosage.) A revised potency limit of not less than 180 Heparin Units per mg also has been established by USP.

Heparin sodium (the calcium salt of heparin is no longer commercially available in the US) occurs as a white or pale-colored, amorphous, hygroscopic powder that may have a faint odor and is soluble in water and practically insoluble in alcohol. Heparin sodium injection is a clear, colorless to slightly yellow solution with a pH of 5–8; sodium hydroxide and/or hydrochloric acid may have been added to adjust the pH. Heparin lock flush solution is a sterile isotonic or hyperosmotic solution of heparin sodium injection adjusted to a pH of 5–7.5 with sodium hydroxide and/or hydrochloric acid. Some commercially available heparin sodium injections or flush solutions have been made isotonic by the addition of sodium chloride and may contain benzyl alcohol or methylparaben and propylparaben as preservatives.

Commercially available solutions of heparin sodium in 0.45% sodium chloride, 0.9% sodium chloride, or 5% dextrose injection have osmolalities of 155, 378, or 287 mOsm/L, respectively.

● Stability

Most commercially available heparin sodium injections and lock flush solutions should be stored at a temperature of 20–25°C. Commercially available injections of heparin sodium in 5% dextrose or in 0.45 or 0.9% sodium chloride should be stored at 20–25°C and protected from freezing.

Commercially available premixed IV solutions with heparin sodium injection are provided in containers fabricated from specially formulated PVC. Water can permeate from inside the containers into the overwrap, but not in amounts sufficient to substantially affect the solution. Solutions in contact with the plastics can leach out some of their chemical components in very small amounts within the expiration period of the injection; however, safety of the plastics has been confirmed in animals according to USP biological tests for plastic containers.

Heparin is strongly acidic and reacts with certain basic compounds resulting in a loss of pharmacologic activity. Although results of some compatibility studies are conflicting, heparin has been reported to be stable for 24 hours at room temperature in lactated Ringer's injection. Heparin should not be mixed with ciprofloxacin, doxorubicin, droperidol, or mitoxantrone since a precipitate may be formed. Heparin is potentially physically and/or chemically incompatible with other drugs, but the compatibility depends on several factors (e.g., concentration of the drugs, specific diluents used, resulting pH, temperature). Specialized references should be consulted for specific information on the stability and compatibility of heparin.

PREPARATIONS

Effective May 1, 2013, a new USP labeling standard for Heparin Sodium Injection, USP and Heparin Lock Flush Solutions, USP was implemented. The labels for these products now state the strength of the entire container (amount of heparin per total volume of container), followed in close proximity by the strength per mL in parentheses.

Excipients in commercially available drug preparations may have clinically important effects in some individuals; consult specific product labeling for details.

Heparin Sodium

Parenteral		
Injection (porcine intestinal mucosa)	1000 units/mL*	Heparin Sodium Injection
	5000 units/mL*	Heparin Sodium Injection
	10,000 units/mL*	Heparin Sodium Injection
	20,000 units/mL*	Heparin Sodium Injection
Solution, lock flush (porcine intestinal mucosa)	10 units/mL (10, 20, 30, 50, 100, 300 units)*	Heparin Lock Flush Solution
	100 units/mL (100, 200, 300, 500, 1000, 3000 units)*	Heparin Lock Flush Solution

* available from one or more manufacturer, distributor, and/or repackager by generic (nonproprietary) name

Heparin Sodium (Preservative-free)

Parenteral

Injection (porcine intestinal mucosa)	1000 units/mL*	Heparin Sodium Injection, Pfizer
	10,000 units/mL*	Heparin Sodium Injection
Solution, lock flush (porcine intestinal mucosa)	10 units/mL (10, 30, 50, or 100 units)*	HepFlush®-10, APP Pharmaceuticals
		Heparin Lock Flush Solution
	100 units/mL (100, 300 or 500 units)*	Heparin Lock Flush Solution

* available from one or more manufacturer, distributor, and/or repackager by generic (nonproprietary) name

Heparin Sodium in Dextrose

Parenteral

Injection, for IV infusion (porcine intestinal mucosa)	40 units/mL (20,000 units) Heparin Sodium in 5% Dextrose*	Heparin Sodium 20,000 units in 5% Dextrose Injection
	50 units/mL (12,500 units) Heparin Sodium in 5% Dextrose*	Heparin Sodium 12,500 units in 5% Dextrose Injection
	50 units/mL (25,000 units) Heparin Sodium in 5% Dextrose*	Heparin Sodium 25,000 units in 5% Dextrose Injection
	100 units/mL (10,000 units) Heparin Sodium in 5% Dextrose*	Heparin Sodium 10,000 units in 5% Dextrose Injection
	100 units/mL (25,000 units) Heparin Sodium in 5% Dextrose*	Heparin Sodium 25,000 units in 5% Dextrose Injection

* available from one or more manufacturer, distributor, and/or repackager by generic (nonproprietary) name

Heparin Sodium in Sodium Chloride

Parenteral

Injection, for IV infusion (porcine intestinal mucosa)	2 units/mL (1000 units) Heparin Sodium in 0.9% Sodium Chloride*	Heparin Sodium 1000 units in 0.9% Sodium Chloride Injection
	2 units/mL (2000 units) Heparin Sodium in 0.9% Sodium Chloride*	Heparin Sodium 2000 units in 0.9% Sodium Chloride Injection
	50 units/mL (12,500 units) Heparin Sodium in 0.45% Sodium Chloride*	Heparin Sodium 12,500 units in 0.45% Sodium Chloride Injection
	50 units/mL (25,000 units) Heparin Sodium in 0.45% Sodium Chloride*	Heparin Sodium 25,000 units in 0.45% Sodium Chloride Injection
	100 units/mL (25,000 units) Heparin Sodium in 0.45% Sodium Chloride*	Heparin Sodium 25,000 units in 0.45% Sodium Chloride Injection

* available from one or more manufacturer, distributor, and/or repackager by generic (nonproprietary) name

† Use is not currently included in the labeling approved by the US Food and Drug Administration.

Selected Revisions September 10, 2024, © Copyright, May 1, 1981, American Society of Health-System Pharmacists, Inc.

Clopidogrel Bisulfate

20:12.18 · CLOPIDOGREL

■ Clopidogrel bisulfate, a thienopyridine P2Y12 platelet adenosine diphosphate (ADP)-receptor antagonist, is a platelet-aggregation inhibitor.

USES

● Acute Coronary Syndrome

Clopidogrel is used in combination with aspirin to reduce the risk of myocardial infarction (MI) and stroke in patients with acute coronary syndrome (ACS), including those with non-ST-segment-elevation ACS (NSTE-ACS) being managed medically or with revascularization strategies (e.g., percutaneous coronary intervention [PCI] with coronary stent implantation, coronary artery bypass grafting [CABG]) and those with acute ST-segment-elevation MI (STEMI) managed medically.

The American College of Cardiology (ACC)/American Heart Association (AHA) has issued guidelines for treatment options and duration of dual antiplatelet therapy in patients with ACS. Recommendations are similar for patients with NSTE-ACS and those with STEMI since both are part of the spectrum of ACS. Decisions about the duration of dual antiplatelet therapy should be individualized based on the risks of bleeding versus benefits of ischemic reduction, clinical judgment, and patient preference. Aspirin should almost always be continued indefinitely; therefore, recommendations are given for the duration of P2Y12 inhibitor therapy in patients treated with dual antiplatelet therapy. While the addition of a P2Y12 inhibitor to aspirin therapy reduces ischemic complications, this occurs at the expense of increased bleeding; a similar risk-benefit trade-off should be considered when determining whether to use a prolonged versus shorter duration of dual antiplatelet therapy. ACC/AHA generally recommends considering shorter duration dual antiplatelet therapy for patients at reduced ischemic, but high bleeding, risk and longer duration dual antiplatelet therapy for patients at high ischemic, but reduced bleeding, risk.

The AHA/ACC guideline recommends that in patients with ACS who are managed medically (without revascularization or reperfusion therapy) or with PCI and stent implantation (bare-metal or drug-eluting), P2Y12 inhibitor therapy should be given for at least 12 months; in such patients who have tolerated dual antiplatelet therapy without bleeding complications and who do not have a high risk of bleeding, continuation of dual antiplatelet therapy for longer than 12 months may be reasonable. With regard to the specific P2Y12 inhibitor, evidence supports the use of clopidogrel or ticagrelor in medically-managed ACS patients; clopidogrel, prasugrel, or ticagrelor may be used in ACS patients treated with PCI. Use of more potent P2Y12 inhibitors such as ticagrelor or prasugrel over clopidogrel results in a greater reduction in ischemic events and stent thrombosis, but increases the risk of bleeding. In some clinical guidelines, ticagrelor or prasugrel is preferred or suggested for maintenance P2Y12 inhibitor therapy in ACS patients while clopidogrel is considered an alternative when the more potent P2Y12 inhibitors cannot be used.

The efficacy of pretreatment with clopidogrel prior to diagnostic cardiac catheterization is controversial; while some studies have suggested a benefit in terms of decreased platelet aggregation and lower rates of periprocedural MI with clopidogrel pretreatment, other studies have found no such benefit compared with administration of the drug in the catheterization laboratory. The potential benefit of pretreatment with clopidogrel should be balanced against the increased risk of bleeding should emergency CABG be needed. If clopidogrel is given at hospital admission or diagnosis of ACS and the patient is subsequently scheduled for CABG, the drug should be temporarily discontinued for at least 5 days prior to the procedure; if the need for CABG is urgent, clopidogrel should be discontinued for at least 24 hours. In patients undergoing CABG, P2Y12 inhibitor therapy (clopidogrel, prasugrel, or ticagrelor) should be resumed after surgery to complete 12 months of dual antiplatelet therapy after ACS.

Non-ST-Segment-Elevation Acute Coronary Syndrome

Efficacy of clopidogrel for the long-term reduction of cardiovascular events in patients with NSTE-ACS has been established in a randomized controlled study (the Clopidogrel in Unstable Angina to Prevent Recurrent Ischemic Events

[CURE] trial) in patients who received clopidogrel (75 mg once daily) or placebo in addition to aspirin (75–325 mg daily) and other standard therapy (e.g., heparin) for 3–12 months. In the CURE study, the combined incidence of cardiovascular death, nonfatal MI, or stroke, and the combined incidence of these events plus refractory ischemia in the clopidogrel group were reduced compared with these outcomes in the placebo group. Clopidogrel therapy also was associated with reductions in the incidences of refractory or severe ischemia, heart failure, and revascularization procedures (during the initial period of hospitalization). In this study, aspirin and clopidogrel or placebo were administered to patients within 24 hours of symptom onset and for 3–12 months (mean: 9 months) thereafter. Although no substantial increase in life-threatening bleeding episodes occurred with clopidogrel and aspirin therapy, major bleeding (principally GI hemorrhage and bleeding at recent arterial puncture sites) was more common in patients receiving clopidogrel and aspirin (3.7%) than in patients receiving aspirin and placebo (2.7%).

ST-Segment-Elevation Myocardial Infarction

Results of randomized, controlled studies indicate that clopidogrel reduces mortality and vascular events beyond those of low-dose aspirin and other standard therapy (e.g., thrombolytic agents, heparin) in patients with acute STEMI, including those undergoing subsequent PCI.

In a randomized, controlled study in approximately 3500 patients with STEMI who were scheduled to receive therapy with a thrombolytic agent, unfractionated heparin or a low molecular weight heparin when appropriate, and aspirin (Clopidogrel as Adjunctive Reperfusion Therapy [CLARITY] study), addition of clopidogrel (300-mg loading dose followed by 75 mg once daily) was associated with a 36% reduction in the risk of the primary composite end point (occluded infarct-related artery at angiography 2–8 days later or death or recurrent MI prior to angiography); at 30 days, clopidogrel therapy had reduced the composite end point of cardiovascular death, recurrent MI, or recurrent ischemia requiring urgent revascularization by 20%. Rates of major bleeding, including intracranial hemorrhage, were similar with or without adjunctive clopidogrel therapy. In a prospective analysis of a subset of patients from the CLARITY study who underwent PCI after angiography (PCI-Clopidogrel as Adjunctive Reperfusion Therapy [CLARITY] study), pretreatment before PCI with clopidogrel (300-mg loading dose followed by 75 mg once daily) in addition to initial standard therapy (e.g., thrombolytic agents, aspirin) during hospitalization for acute STEMI was associated with a reduction of 38% in recurrent MI and stroke compared with standard therapy; considering cardiovascular events before and after PCI through 30 days after randomization in patients undergoing coronary artery stenting, adjunctive clopidogrel therapy reduced cardiovascular death, MI, and stroke by 41%.

In the Clopidogrel and Metoprolol in Myocardial Infarction Trial (COMMIT) in approximately 45,000 patients with acute STEMI, treatment with clopidogrel (75 mg once daily without a loading dose) in addition to aspirin (162 mg daily) beginning at hospital admission and continuing during hospitalization for up to 4 weeks (mean treatment duration: 14.9 days) was associated with a 9% reduction in death, reinfarction, or stroke (the primary composite end point) compared with aspirin therapy. In addition, death from any cause was reduced by 7%, and fatal or nonfatal reinfarction by 14%, in patients receiving adjunctive clopidogrel. Clopidogrel treatment was associated with a small increase in minor bleeding but no excess in major (i.e., transfused, cerebral, or fatal) bleeding complications.

● Peripheral Arterial Disease or History of MI or Stroke

Clopidogrel is used to reduce the risk of MI and stroke in patients with established peripheral arterial disease (PAD) or a history of recent MI or recent stroke.

Both aspirin and clopidogrel have been used for secondary prevention in patients with stable ischemic heart disease (SIHD). Results of a large, randomized study (Clopidogrel versus Aspirin in Patients at Risk of Ischemic Events [CAPRIE] study) showed that clopidogrel was more effective than aspirin in reducing the risk of cardiovascular events in a population of patients with symptomatic atherosclerotic vascular disease and had a similar overall safety profile. However, because of cost considerations, many clinicians recommend aspirin as the antiplatelet drug of choice for most patients requiring long-term antiplatelet therapy for SIHD, and consider clopidogrel an alternative when aspirin is contraindicated.

Antiplatelet therapy also is recommended for secondary prevention of stroke in patients with a history of noncardioembolic ischemic stroke or transient ischemic attack (TIA). In such patients, experts recommend aspirin, clopidogrel, or aspirin in combination with extended-release dipyridamole for antiplatelet therapy. The American Heart Association (AHA) and American Stroke Association (ASA) guidelines recommend that in patients with recent stroke or TIA (within 30 days) attributable to severe stenosis (70-99%) of a major intracranial artery, the addition of clopidogrel to aspirin for 90 days may be reasonable. Oral anticoagulation (e.g., warfarin, direct oral anticoagulants [DOACs]) rather than antiplatelet therapy is recommended for the secondary prevention of cardioembolic stroke in patients with a history of ischemic stroke or TIA and concurrent atrial fibrillation. (See Embolism Associated with Atrial Fibrillation under Uses.)

Recommendations on antiplatelet therapy in patients with lower extremity PAD are provided in guidelines from AHA/ACC. Antiplatelet therapy with either aspirin or clopidogrel is recommended to reduce the risk of cardiovascular events in patients with symptomatic PAD. AHA/ACC states that the effectiveness of dual antiplatelet therapy to reduce the risk of ischemic events in patients with symptomatic PAD is uncertain, but may be reasonable in certain situations.

Efficacy of clopidogrel in patients with recent MI, recent stroke, or established PAD has been established in a multicenter, randomized, controlled study (the CAPRIE trial) in patients with atherosclerotic disease (recent [within 6 months] ischemic stroke, recent [within 35 days] MI, or symptomatic peripheral arterial disease); in this study, patients received clopidogrel 75 mg once daily or aspirin 325 mg daily for an average of 1.6 years (maximum 3 years). The primary analysis of efficacy was based on the first occurrence of a new cardiovascular event (i.e., fatal or nonfatal ischemic stroke or MI, other vascular death) in all patients receiving clopidogrel or aspirin. The annual cardiovascular event rate in patients receiving clopidogrel was 5.32% compared with 5.83% in those receiving aspirin, representing an 8.7% decrease in the annual risk of a new cardiovascular event for clopidogrel-treated patients. The difference in overall risk of cardiovascular events was apparent early in the study and was maintained throughout the 3-year follow-up period. While the study was not designed to evaluate relative benefit of clopidogrel versus aspirin among patients in specific disease subgroups, most of the risk reduction associated with clopidogrel therapy occurred in patients with PAD, who experienced a statistically significant 23.8% decrease in risk compared with those in the same subgroup who received aspirin. Patients in the stroke subgroup who received clopidogrel experienced a relative risk reduction of 7.3%, while those in the MI subgroup experienced a relative risk reduction of −3.7% (*increased* relative risk compared with aspirin); neither of these relative-risk reductions was statistically significant.

Therapy with clopidogrel plus aspirin for prevention of ischemic events in a broad population of patients with established cardiovascular disease or multiple risk factors for atherosclerosis was evaluated in the CHARISMA (Clopidogrel for High Atherothrombotic Risk and Ischemic Stabilization, Management, and Avoidance) trial. In this large, randomized, double-blind, parallel-group study, therapy with clopidogrel (75 mg daily) and low-dose aspirin (75–162 mg daily) for approximately 2 years was not significantly more effective than low-dose aspirin alone in reducing the rate of the composite primary end point of MI, stroke, or death from cardiovascular causes. In addition, the combination of clopidogrel and aspirin was associated with an increased rate of moderate to severe bleeding.

• Prevention of Stent Thrombosis

Clopidogrel has been used in combination with aspirin (dual antiplatelet therapy) to prevent stent thrombosis following implantation of coronary artery stents†.

Compared with bare-metal stents (BMS), implantation of drug-eluting stents (DES) has been associated with a reduction in the frequency of restenosis and repeat revascularization without evidence of excess MI or death in randomized controlled trials. Various drug-eluting stents are available; however, newer-generation (e.g., everolimus- or zotarolimus-eluting) stents have demonstrated lower risk of stent thrombosis and MI compared with first-generation (e.g., sirolimus- and paclitaxel-eluting) stents, which are rarely, if ever, used in current practice. Therefore, current recommendations for duration of dual antiplatelet therapy apply principally to the use of newer-generation stents.

The current ACC/AHA guideline states that patients with ACS who receive a BMS or DES should be treated with dual antiplatelet therapy for at least 12 months. Continuation of dual antiplatelet therapy beyond 12 months may be reasonable in patients who have tolerated such therapy without a bleeding complication and who are not at high bleeding risk. (See Acute Coronary Syndrome under Uses.) A shorter duration of dual antiplatelet therapy may be reasonable in patients with a newer-generation DES. If patients with a DES develop a high risk of bleeding or have a high risk of severe bleeding, discontinuation of a P2Y12 inhibitor after 3 months may be reasonable.

Recommendations are also provided by ACC/AHA for patients with stable ischemic heart disease (SIHD) who undergo stent implantation. Dual antiplatelet therapy with aspirin and clopidogrel should be given for a minimum of 1 month to patients with SIHD who receive a BMS, and for a minimum of 6 months to patients who receive a DES. Continuation of dual antiplatelet therapy beyond these periods may be reasonable in patients who have tolerated dual antiplatelet therapy without a bleeding complication and who are not at high bleeding risk. If patients treated with DES develop a high risk of bleeding or have a high risk of severe bleeding, discontinuation of a P2Y12 inhibitor after 3 months may be reasonable. In patients with SIHD who undergo CABG, treatment with dual antiplatelet therapy for 12 months may be reasonable to improve vein graft patency. In patients treated for an MI that occurred 1 to 3 years earlier who have tolerated dual antiplatelet therapy and are not at high bleeding risk, continuation of dual antiplatelet therapy may be reasonable.

In a randomized, placebo-controlled, double-blind study (Dual Antiplatelet Therapy [DAPT] study), patients who received 30 months of dual antiplatelet therapy (aspirin plus clopidogrel or prasugrel) following placement of a DES had substantially reduced rates of stent thrombosis and major adverse cardiovascular and cerebrovascular events compared with those who received 12 months of dual antiplatelet therapy. Preliminary data from the study indicated that a longer duration of therapy was associated with a higher incidence of moderate to severe bleeding and also an unexpected finding of an increased rate of noncardiovascular mortality (principally related to trauma or cancer); however, these adverse mortality findings were not observed during FDA's final review of the DAPT study and other randomized, controlled clinical studies. FDA review of the DAPT study and additional long-term studies of clopidogrel, including meta-analyses conducted by FDA, concluded that there is no evidence of either a harmful or beneficial effect of clopidogrel on all-cause mortality or cancer-related deaths in a population with, or at risk for, coronary artery disease. The results of the FDA-conducted meta-analyses indicated that long-term (12 months or longer) dual antiplatelet therapy with clopidogrel and aspirin does not appear to change the overall risk of death when compared to short-term (6 months or less) clopidogrel and aspirin therapy, or aspirin alone. Additionally, there was no apparent increase in the risk of cancer-related deaths or cancer-related adverse effects with such long-term treatment.

• Embolism Associated with Atrial Fibrillation

Clopidogrel has been used in combination with aspirin for the prevention of stroke and systemic embolism in patients with atrial fibrillation†. Because of the superiority of warfarin over antiplatelet therapy in reducing the risk of stroke in patients with atrial fibrillation, clopidogrel and aspirin have been used generally as an alternative to warfarin anticoagulation. Dual antiplatelet therapy with clopidogrel and aspirin was evaluated as a potential alternative to warfarin in a randomized controlled study (ACTIVE-W) in patients with atrial fibrillation at high risk of stroke. The study was terminated early because of clear evidence of superiority of warfarin over antiplatelet therapy for the primary outcome of stroke, systemic embolism, MI, or vascular death. Results of another study (ACTIVE-A) comparing dual antiplatelet therapy (clopidogrel and aspirin) with aspirin monotherapy in patients with atrial fibrillation who had an increased risk of stroke but were unable to take warfarin showed that the combination of clopidogrel and aspirin was more effective than aspirin in reducing the risk of stroke; however, dual antiplatelet therapy was also associated with an increased risk of bleeding. These studies were conducted prior to contemporary use of oral anticoagulation in patients with atrial fibrillation. With the availability of direct oral anticoagulants (DOACs) and evidence demonstrating that these drugs are at least as safe and effective as warfarin for preventing stroke and systemic embolism in patients with atrial fibrillation, DOACs are generally recommended over warfarin in patients with atrial fibrillation. Based on the current evidence, oral anticoagulants are currently recommended for antithrombotic therapy in patients with atrial fibrillation; antiplatelet therapy should not be used alone for stroke prevention, but may be added if the patient has other indications for use (e.g., ACS, PCI with stenting).

Clopidogrel has been used in patients with atrial fibrillation and ACS. These patients have an indication for treatment with both antiplatelet and anticoagulant agents. Selecting the optimal antithrombotic regimen in such patients can be challenging. Current guidelines from AHA/ACC/Heart Rhythm Society and other experts provide recommendations regarding the use of P2Y12 inhibitors in patients with atrial fibrillation who present with ACS and/or undergo PCI. Because of the high risk of bleeding associated with triple antithrombotic therapy (aspirin, a P2Y12 inhibitor, and an oral anticoagulant), experts generally recommend against this approach for most patients. Studies have shown similar or lower rates of bleeding and similar rates of thrombotic events with dual antithrombotic therapy compared with triple therapy. Therefore, the preferred strategy in patients with atrial fibrillation who have undergone recent PCI is to use dual antithrombotic therapy (an oral anticoagulant and a P2Y12 inhibitor); if triple therapy is considered in patients with high thrombotic risk and low bleeding risk, such therapy should be given over the shortest possible duration. Clopidogrel is generally recommended over the more potent P2Y12 inhibitors (prasugrel, ticagrelor) when combination antithrombotic therapy is needed because of a lower risk of bleeding. Clopidogrel has also been used in combination with low-dose rivaroxaban (15 mg daily) instead of triple therapy to reduce the risk of bleeding in patients with atrial fibrillation who have undergone PCI with stenting.

DOSAGE AND ADMINISTRATION

● Administration

Clopidogrel is administered orally. Food does not affect systemic exposure to the active metabolite of clopidogrel; therefore, the drug may be administered without regard to meals.

● Dosage

Dosage of clopidogrel bisulfate is expressed in terms of clopidogrel.

Acute Coronary Syndrome

In patients with acute coronary syndrome (ACS) who need an antiplatelet effect within hours, an initial clopidogrel loading dose of 300 mg is recommended by the manufacturer, followed by 75 mg once daily given concomitantly with aspirin (75–325 mg once daily).

The American College of Cardiology (ACC)/American Heart Association (AHA) guidelines recommend a clopidogrel loading dose of 300 or 600 mg followed by a dosage of 75 mg daily in patients with non-ST-segment-elevation ACS (NSTE-ACS) who are treated with an early invasive or ischemia-guided strategy.

In patients with ST-segment-elevation MI (STEMI) who are receiving thrombolytic therapy (e.g., alteplase), experts recommend a clopidogrel loading dose of 300 mg in patients 75 years of age or younger; a loading dose is not recommended in patients older than 75 years of age. Clopidogrel therapy should be initiated prior to or with the thrombolytic agent and continued for at least 14 days and up to 1 year at a maintenance dosage of 75 mg daily.

In patients undergoing percutaneous coronary intervention (PCI), ACC/AHA recommends a loading dose of 600 mg, administered before the procedure; clopidogrel should then be continued at a maintenance dosage of 75 mg once daily for at least 12 months in those who receive a coronary stent.

In patients who are scheduled to undergo CABG, clopidogrel should be temporarily discontinued at least 5 days prior to surgery and resumed as soon as possible after the procedure.

Recommendations for duration of dual antiplatelet therapy can be found in the ACC/AHA guideline. (See Acute Coronary Syndrome under Uses.)

Peripheral Arterial Disease or History of MI or Stroke

In patients with established peripheral arterial disease or a history of recent myocardial infarction (MI) or stroke, the recommended dosage of clopidogrel for reducing the risk of fatal or nonfatal MI, stroke, or vascular death in adults is 75 mg once daily.

● Special Populations

No dosage adjustments are necessary in geriatric patients or in those with hepatic impairment.

CAUTIONS

● Contraindications

- Active pathological bleeding (e.g., peptic ulcer, intracranial hemorrhage).
- Known hypersensitivity to clopidogrel or any ingredient in the formulation.

● Warnings/Precautions

Warnings

Reduced Efficacy in Poor CYP2C19 Metabolizers

The prescribing information for clopidogrel has a boxed warning regarding diminished antiplatelet effects in patients with 2 loss-of-function alleles of CYP2C19. Clopidogrel is a prodrug that requires conversion by the cytochrome P-450 (CYP) enzyme system, principally by CYP2C19, to its pharmacologically active metabolite. (See Description.) Production of the active metabolite and response to clopidogrel may be reduced in patients who are poor metabolizers of CYP2C19. Genetic tests are available to identify a patient's CYP2C19 genotype and can be used to help individualize and optimize clopidogrel therapy. Use of an alternative P2Y12 inhibitor (e.g., prasugrel, ticagrelor) should be considered in patients who are identified as poor metabolizers of CYP2C19.

Specific variant alleles of CYP2C19 (e.g., CYP2C19*2, CYP2C19*3) have been associated with reduced metabolism of and diminished antiplatelet response to clopidogrel; higher rates of major adverse cardiovascular events (e.g., death, MI, stroke, stent thrombosis) have been reported in patients receiving recommended dosages of clopidogrel who possess such variant alleles compared with those who have normal CYP2C19 activity. (See Pharmacogenomics under Description.) The impact of CYP2C19 metabolizer status on the pharmacokinetic and antiplatelet response to clopidogrel was evaluated in a study in healthy individuals. Results showed that exposure to the active metabolite of clopidogrel was decreased and inhibition of platelet response was diminished in poor metabolizers compared with other CYP2C19 metabolizer groups (intermediate, extensive, ultrarapid). The relationship between CYP2C19 genotype and clopidogrel response is particularly evident in ACS patients undergoing PCI. An increased risk of major cardiovascular events and stent thrombosis has been observed in such patients who are CYP2C19*2 heterozygotes or homozygotes. The Clinical Pharmacogenetics Implementation Consortium (CPIC) has issued guidelines for CYP2C19 genotype and clopidogrel therapy. When considering the use of clopidogrel in patients with ACS being managed with PCI, these experts strongly recommend the use of an alternative antiplatelet agent (e.g., prasugrel, ticagrelor) in those who are poor metabolizers of CYP2C19. CPIC gives a moderate recommendation for alternative anticoagulation therapy in patients with an intermediate CYP2C19 phenotype.

Reduced Efficacy with Concomitant Use of Omeprazole or Esomeprazole

Concurrent use of clopidogrel and omeprazole, a potent inhibitor of CYP2C19, can reduce the antiplatelet effects of clopidogrel and should be avoided. Although the clinical importance of this interaction has not been fully elucidated, some evidence suggests that concurrent use of clopidogrel and omeprazole may result in reduced efficacy of clopidogrel in preventing cardiovascular events. A similar reduction in antiplatelet activity has been observed when esomeprazole was used concurrently with clopidogrel. The manufacturer states that concomitant use of clopidogrel and omeprazole or esomeprazole should be avoided. (See Drugs Affecting or Metabolized by Hepatic Microsomal Enzymes under Drug Interactions.)

Other Warnings and Precautions

Bleeding

Clopidogrel increases the risk of bleeding. In patients undergoing surgical procedures with a low or high risk of bleeding, the American College of Surgeons recommends that clopidogrel be held for 5–7 days and resumed when bleeding risk has diminished. The drug should be discontinued at least 5 days prior to elective coronary artery bypass grafting (CABG) and at least 24 hours prior to urgent CABG to reduce the risk of bleeding. If bleeding occurs, hemostasis may be restored with exogenous administration of platelets; however, platelet transfusions within 4 hours of a loading dose of clopidogrel or within 2 hours of a maintenance dose may have reduced effectiveness. Withholding a dose is unlikely to resolve a bleeding episode or prevent bleeding associated with an invasive procedure because of clopidogrel's prolonged effects on platelet inhibition.

In patients with transient ischemic attack (TIA) or stroke who are at high risk for recurrent ischemic events, the combination of clopidogrel and aspirin has *not* been shown to be more effective than clopidogrel alone but has been associated with an increase in major bleeding.

Thienopyridines do not appear to cause GI ulcers or erosions, but their antiplatelet effects may promote bleeding at the site of preexisting lesions associated with use of aspirin or nonsteroidal anti-inflammatory agents or *H. pylori* infection. Current American College of Cardiology Foundation (ACCF)/American College of Gastroenterology (ACG)/American Heart Association (AHA) guidelines recommend prophylactic use of a proton-pump inhibitor to reduce the risk of ulcer complications and GI bleeding in patients receiving clopidogrel and aspirin therapy who have additional GI risk factors. However, the possibility of reduced antiplatelet effects should be considered when clopidogrel is used concomitantly with a proton-pump inhibitor (e.g., omeprazole, esomeprazole). (See Proton-Pump Inhibitors under Drug Interaction.)

Risks of Premature Discontinuance of Therapy

In general, treatment with a thienopyridine derivative should not be discontinued prematurely because of the increased risk of cardiovascular events. If clopidogrel must be temporarily discontinued (e.g., prior to surgery), therapy should be reinitated as soon as possible. Patients should be advised not to discontinue clopidogrel therapy without first consulting the prescribing clinician. Prior to scheduling an invasive procedure, patients should inform their clinicians (including dentists) that they are currently taking clopidogrel, and clinicians performing the invasive procedure should consult with the prescribing clinician before advising patients to discontinue therapy.

Premature discontinuance of dual antiplatelet therapy (a P2Y12 inhibitor and aspirin) in patients with coronary artery stents has been associated with stent thrombosis, often leading to myocardial infarction (MI) and/or death. Before implantation of a drug-eluting stent, patients should be carefully assessed regarding the likelihood of compliance with dual antiplatelet therapy; some experts recommend that PCI with coronary stenting should not be performed in patients not likely to tolerate or comply with dual antiplatelet therapy for the appropriate duration of treatment based on the type of stent implanted. Superficial or "nuisance" bleeding is common in patients receiving dual antiplatelet therapy after drug-eluting stent implantation and may be a reason for premature discontinuation of clopidogrel. In a single-center observational study in 2360 patients who underwent drug-eluting stent implantation, 11.1% of patients who were receiving dual antiplatelet therapy discontinued clopidogrel prematurely as a result of superficial bleeding. The American College of Cardiology Foundation/American College of Gastroenterology/American Heart Association (ACCF/ACG/AHA) states that concomitant use of proton-pump inhibitors may reduce GI symptoms (e.g., dyspepsia) associated with antiplatelet agents and thereby prevent patients from discontinuing their antiplatelet treatment. (See Proton-Pump Inhibitors under Drug Interactions.)

AHA/ACC guidelines provide recommendations for timing of elective surgical procedures in patients with coronary stents. For patients treated with dual antiplatelet therapy after coronary implantation who must undergo surgical procedures that mandate discontinuance of P2Y12 inhibitor therapy, aspirin should be continued if at all possible and the P2Y12 inhibitor restarted as soon as possible after the procedure because of concerns about late stent thrombosis.

Thrombotic Thrombocytopenic Purpura

Thrombotic thrombocytopenic purpura (TTP) has been reported rarely with clopidogrel, sometimes after short exposure (less than 2 weeks) to the drug. TTP is characterized by thrombocytopenia, microangiopathic hemolytic anemia (schistocytes on peripheral blood smear), neurologic findings, renal dysfunction, and fever. TTP is a potentially fatal condition that requires urgent referral to a hematologist for prompt treatment (e.g., plasmapheresis).

Cross-Reactivity Among Thienopyridines

Patients with a history of hypersensitivity or hematologic reaction to other thienopyridines have experienced hypersensitivity, including rash, angioedema, or hematologic reaction, after receiving clopidogrel.

Specific Populations

Pregnancy

Available data from case reports and postmarketing surveillance have not suggested any risks of major birth defects, miscarriage, or adverse fetal outcomes with clopidogrel use in pregnant women. In animal studies, no evidence of fetotoxicity was observed when clopidogrel was administered to pregnant rats and rabbits during organogenesis at doses up to 78 times to recommended daily human dose.

MI and stroke present risks to both the pregnant woman and fetus. Use of clopidogrel during labor or delivery increases the risk of maternal bleeding and hemorrhage. Neuraxial blockade during clopidogrel use should be avoided because of the risk of spinal hematoma. When possible, clopidogrel should be discontinued 5–7 days prior to labor, delivery, or neuraxial blockade.

Lactation

Clopidogrel is distributed into milk in rats; it is not known whether the drug is distributed into milk in humans. The benefits of breast-feeding should be considered along with the importance of the drug to the mother and any potential adverse effects on the infant from the drug or underlying maternal condition.

Pediatric Use

Safety and efficacy of clopidogrel have not been established in pediatric patients. However, the drug has been used in neonates and infants† with certain cardiac conditions that predispose them to arterial thrombosis.

Geriatric Use

No difference in platelet aggregation has been observed in patients 75 years of age or older compared with younger healthy individuals. In the CURE trial, geriatric patients (65 years of age or older) were at greater risk for thrombotic events and major bleeding compared with younger patients. However, in the COMMIT study evaluating patients with ST-segment-elevation MI (STEMI), the efficacy and safety of clopidogrel in preventing ischemic events was independent of age. Dosage adjustment based solely on age does not appear to be necessary in geriatric patients.

Hepatic Impairment

Inhibition of ADP-induced platelet aggregation in patients with severe hepatic impairment appears to be similar to that observed in healthy individuals.

Renal Impairment

Experience is limited in patients with moderate (creatinine clearance of 30–60 mL/minute) or severe (creatinine clearance of 5–15 mL/minute) renal impairment. Inhibition of ADP-induced platelet aggregation may be decreased by 25% in such patients.

● Common Adverse Effects

Bleeding, including life-threatening and fatal bleeding, is the most commonly reported adverse effect of clopidogrel.

DRUG INTERACTIONS

● Drugs Affecting or Metabolized by Hepatic Microsomal Enzymes

Clopidogrel is converted to its active metabolite in part by cytochrome P-450 (CYP) isoenzyme 2C19.

Drugs that induce CYP2C19 (e.g., rifampin) are expected to result in increased concentrations of the active metabolite of clopidogrel and increase its antiplatelet effects. Concomitant use should be avoided.

Drugs that inhibit CYP2C19 are expected to decrease plasma concentrations of the active metabolite of clopidogrel and reduce its antiplatelet effects. (See Proton-Pump Inhibitors under Drug Interactions.) Concomitant use of drugs that are known to be potent inhibitors of CYP2C19 activity (e.g., omeprazole, esomeprazole) should be avoided in patients receiving clopidogrel.

● Nonsteroidal Anti-inflammatory Agents

Potential pharmacodynamic interaction (increased risk of bleeding).

● Opiate Agonists

Concomitant use of opioids may delay and reduce absorption of and exposure to the active metabolites of clopidogrel because of slowed gastric emptying. The use of a parenteral antiplatelet should be considered in patients with ACS who require coadministration of opioid agonists.

● Proton-Pump Inhibitors

Decreased systemic exposure to clopidogrel's active metabolite and reduced antiplatelet effects may occur when clopidogrel is used concomitantly with certain proton-pump inhibitors. Because the antiplatelet activity of clopidogrel (a prodrug) is dependent on biotransformation, principally by CYP2C19, of the prodrug to an active metabolite, concurrent use of drugs such as omeprazole or esomeprazole that inhibit CYP2C19 reduces plasma concentrations of the active metabolite and potentially could reduce clinical efficacy. (See Reduced Efficacy with Concomitant Use of Omeprazole or Esomeprazole under Cautions.) Some experts state that additional data from large, prospective trials are needed to fully elucidate the clinical consequences, if any, of the observed interaction between clopidogrel and certain proton-pump inhibitors. The American College of Cardiology Foundation (ACCF) and the American Heart Association (AHA) state that although proton-pump inhibitors (e.g., omeprazole) can affect clopidogrel metabolism and result in diminished antiplatelet activity in vitro, these pharmacokinetic effects do not appear to be associated with worse clinical outcomes. If concomitant proton-pump inhibitor therapy is considered necessary, use of an agent with little or no CYP2C19-inhibitory activity should be considered.

Proton-pump inhibitors vary in their potency for inhibiting CYP2C19. In pharmacokinetic and pharmacodynamic studies in healthy individuals, dexlansoprazole, lansoprazole, or pantoprazole had less effect on the antiplatelet activity of clopidogrel than did omeprazole or esomeprazole. In these studies, the observed effects of dexlansoprazole, lansoprazole, or pantoprazole on exposure to the active metabolite of clopidogrel and on clopidogrel-induced platelet inhibition were not considered clinically important, and the manufacturers of dexlansoprazole, lansoprazole, and pantoprazole state that no adjustment of clopidogrel dosage is required if clopidogrel is used concomitantly with FDA-labeled dosages of these proton-pump inhibitors. Omeprazole and esomeprazole substantially reduce the antiplatelet activity of clopidogrel; therefore, concomitant use of omeprazole or esomeprazole with clopidogrel should be avoided. When administration of clopidogrel and omeprazole (at the same dosages) was separated by 12 hours, the amounts of reduced exposure to the active clopidogrel metabolite and reduced platelet inhibition were similar to when the drugs were administered at the same time.

The decision to use any proton-pump inhibitor concomitantly with clopidogrel should be based on the assessed risks and benefits in individual patients. The American College of Cardiology Foundation/American College of Gastroenterology/American Heart Association (ACCF/ACG/AHA) states that use of a proton-pump inhibitor concomitantly with dual antiplatelet therapy may provide the optimal balance of risk and benefit in patients with ACS who have a history of upper GI bleeding since such a history is the strongest and most consistent risk factor for GI bleeding in patients receiving antiplatelet therapy. Among stable patients with a history of GI bleeding who undergo coronary revascularization and receive a coronary stent, ACCF/ACG/AHA states that the risk/benefit tradeoff may favor concomitant use of dual antiplatelet therapy and a proton-pump inhibitor. ACCF/ACG/AHA also states that the risk reduction with proton-pump inhibitors is substantial in patients with risk factors for GI bleeding (e.g., advanced age; concomitant use of warfarin, corticosteroids, or nonsteroidal anti-inflammatory agents [NSAIAs]; *H. pylori* infection) and may outweigh any potential reduction in the cardiovascular efficacy of antiplatelet treatment associated with a drug–drug interaction. In contrast, patients without these risk factors for GI bleeding receive little if any absolute risk reduction from proton-pump inhibitor therapy, and the risk/benefit balance may favor use of antiplatelet therapy without a concomitant proton-pump inhibitor.

Results of several large observational studies suggest that concomitant therapy with clopidogrel and omeprazole (or potentially other proton-pump inhibitors) can reduce the effectiveness of clopidogrel in preventing cardiovascular events. However, conflicting data have been reported, including results of a prematurely discontinued randomized controlled trial suggesting no effect of concomitant clopidogrel–proton-pump inhibitor therapy on cardiovascular outcomes; given the limitations of observational studies (possibility of confounding factors such as comorbid conditions, unreported use of aspirin or OTC proton-pump inhibitors), the clinical importance of this interaction has been questioned.

Some clinicians suggest that an antacid or a histamine H_2-receptor antagonist (ranitidine, famotidine, nizatidine) may be considered as an alternative to therapy with a proton-pump inhibitor, although such agents may not be as effective as a proton-pump inhibitor in providing gastric protection. However, cimetidine should *not* be used as alternative therapy since it is a potent CYP2C19 inhibitor.

There currently is no evidence that histamine H_2-receptor antagonists (other than cimetidine) or other drugs that reduce gastric acid (e.g., antacids) interfere with the antiplatelet effects of clopidogrel.

Several observational studies involving large numbers of patients suggest that proton-pump inhibitors reduce the effectiveness of clopidogrel in preventing cardiovascular events. In a case-control study in patients 66 years of age or older, concomitant use of clopidogrel and a proton-pump inhibitor that inhibits CYP2C19 (omeprazole, lansoprazole, rabeprazole) was associated with a 40% greater risk of recurrent myocardial infarction within 90 days of hospital discharge; this effect was not seen with pantoprazole, which does not inhibit CYP2C19. In 2 retrospective cohort studies involving more than 30,000 patients, the incidence of major adverse cardiovascular events (e.g., hospitalization for stroke, angina, myocardial infarction, coronary artery bypass grafting, urgent target vessel revascularization, death) in patients receiving clopidogrel for 12 months following stent placement was higher in those who were also prescribed a proton-pump inhibitor than in those who did not receive a proton-pump inhibitor. A subgroup analysis in one of these studies revealed that each proton-pump inhibitor (omeprazole, esomeprazole, pantoprazole, lansoprazole) was individually associated with an increased risk of cardiovascular events. In other retrospective cohort studies in patients with acute coronary syndrome (ACS), concomitant use of clopidogrel and a proton-pump inhibitor was associated with a significantly higher rate of adverse cardiovascular events (e.g., death or rehospitalization for ACS, coronary stent placement) versus administration of clopidogrel alone.

Data discounting the clinical importance of a clopidogrel–proton-pump inhibitor interaction also have been reported. In a study evaluating health insurance records of more than 18,500 patients 65 years of age or older who had received clopidogrel with or without proton-pump inhibitor therapy, a slightly increased risk of myocardial infarction or death was observed in patients receiving clopidogrel concurrently with a proton-pump inhibitor, but the finding was not statistically significant. In a post hoc analysis of a large randomized study evaluating a clopidogrel loading dose in patients prior to PCI (Clopidogrel for the Reduction of Events During Observation [CREDO]), use of a proton-pump inhibitor was independently associated with an increased risk of a cardiovascular event (e.g., death, myocardial infarction, stroke) regardless of whether patients received clopidogrel therapy. Post-hoc analysis of another large randomized controlled study (Trial to Assess Improvement with Prasugrel-Thrombolysis in Myocardial Infarction [TRITON-TIMI 38]) also found no clinically meaningful interaction between clopidogrel and a proton-pump inhibitor. In the only randomized, placebo-controlled trial (Clopidogrel Optimization of Gastrointestinal EveNTs [COGENT] trial) to date evaluating potential clinical outcomes of the clopidogrel–proton-pump inhibitor interaction, no effect of such concomitant therapy on the rate of cardiovascular events was found in patients receiving an investigational fixed-dose combination of clopidogrel and omeprazole or clopidogrel without a proton-pump inhibitor; however, interpretation of the data is limited due to premature termination of the study, insufficient statistical power, and incomplete follow-up.

● Repaglinide

A metabolite of clopidogrel is a strong inhibitor of CYP2C8, and can increase systemic exposure to drugs cleared by CYP2C8, including repaglinide. Avoid concomitant use or initiate repaglinide at 0.5 mg before each meal and do not exceed total daily dose of 4 mg.

● Selective Serotonin Reuptake Inhibitors and Serotonin-Norepinephrine Reuptake Inhibitors

Potential pharmacodynamic interaction (increased risk of bleeding).

● Warfarin

Potential pharmacodynamic interaction (increased risk of bleeding). Caution is advised.

DESCRIPTION

Clopidogrel bisulfate, a thienopyridine derivative structurally and pharmacologically related to ticlopidine, is a platelet-aggregation inhibitor. Clopidogrel is a prodrug with its platelet-aggregation inhibitory activity dependent on hepatic transformation to an active thiol metabolite.

Biotransformation occurs through a 2-step process where clopidogrel is initially oxidized to a 2-oxo-clopidogrel intermediate metabolite, then subsequently metabolized to the active thiol metabolite. This metabolic pathway has been shown to be mediated by several cytochrome P-450 isoenzymes (e.g., CYP2C19, CYP3A, CYP2B6, CYP1A2). In particular, the CYP2C19 isoenzyme is involved in the formation of both the active metabolite and the 2-oxo-clopidogrel intermediate.

Clopidogrel is an ADP-receptor antagonist; the active metabolite of clopidogrel binds selectively and noncompetitively to a low-affinity, P2Y12 ADP-receptor binding site on the surface of platelets, thereby inhibiting ADP binding to the receptor and subsequent activation of the platelet glycoprotein (GP IIb/IIIa) complex necessary for fibrinogen-platelet binding. Clopidogrel also inhibits ADP-mediated release of platelet dense granule (e.g., ADP, calcium, and serotonin) and alpha granule (e.g., fibrinogen and thrombospondin) contents that augment platelet aggregation. The low-affinity ADP receptor is irreversibly modified by the drug, so platelets exposed to clopidogrel remain affected for the remainder of their lifespan (about 7–10 days). Unlike aspirin, thienopyridine platelet-aggregation inhibitors such as clopidogrel and ticlopidine do not inactivate platelet cyclooxygenase to prevent synthesis of prostaglandin endoperoxides and thromboxane A.

Clopidogrel is rapidly absorbed after oral administration; at least 50% of an oral dose is absorbed. Peak plasma concentrations of the active metabolite occur approximately 30–60 minutes following an oral dose. When clopidogrel 75 mg is administered daily, inhibition of platelet aggregation is apparent on the first day of therapy, with 40–60% inhibition being achieved at steady state between days 3–7. Following discontinuance of the drug, platelet aggregation and bleeding time generally return to baseline values within about 5 days.

● *Pharmacogenomics*

Genetic polymorphism of CYP2C19 can affect the pharmacokinetic and pharmacodynamic response to clopidogrel. Patients with at least one loss-of-function variant CYP2C19 allele (e.g., CYP2C19*2, CYP2C19*3) are described as poor or intermediate metabolizers of clopidogrel and have been shown to have lower plasma concentrations of active metabolite and diminished antiplatelet response, which in turn can lead to a higher incidence of major adverse cardiovascular events. (See Reduced Efficacy in Poor CYP2C19 Metabolizers under Cautions.) The prevalence of reduced-function CYP2C19 genotypes in the general population differs according to race and ethnicity; an estimated 2% of Whites, 4% of Black, and 14% of Chinese individuals are poor CYP2C19 metabolizers.

ADVICE TO PATIENTS

- Importance of counseling patients about potential risks versus benefits of clopidogrel.

- Importance of informing patients that they may bleed more easily and that a longer than normal time will be required to stop bleeding when taking clopidogrel.
- Importance of informing patient not to discontinue therapy without consulting their prescribing clinician.
- Importance of patient informing clinician about any unanticipated, prolonged, or excessive bleeding, or blood in urine or stool.
- Importance of patient informing clinician about clopidogrel therapy before any surgery is scheduled.
- Advise patients not to take omeprazole or esomeprazole while taking clopidogrel.
- Importance of patient informing clinician of existing or contemplated concomitant therapy, including prescription and OTC drugs, particularly omeprazole or esomeprazole and drugs that affect bleeding (e.g., warfarin, NSAIAs).
- Importance of women informing clinicians if they are or plan to become pregnant or plan to breast-feed.
- Importance of informing patients of other important precautionary information. (See Cautions.)

PREPARATIONS

Excipients in commercially available drug preparations may have clinically important effects in some individuals; consult specific product labeling for details.

Clopidogrel Bisulfate

Oral		
Tablets	75 mg (of clopidogrel)*	Clopidogrel Tablets
		Plavix®, Sanofi-Aventis (also promoted by Bristol-Myers Squibb)
	300 mg (of clopidogrel)*	Clopidogrel Tablets
		Plavix®, Sanofi-Aventis (also promoted by Bristol-Myers Squibb)

† Use is not currently included in the labeling approved by the US Food and Drug Administration.

* available from one or more manufacturer, distributor, and/or repackager by generic (nonproprietary) name

Eptifibatide

20:12.18 • PLATELET-AGGREGATION INHIBITORS

■ Eptifibatide, a selective platelet-aggregation inhibitor, has been referred to as a platelet glycoprotein (GP) IIb/IIIa-receptor inhibitor.

USES

● Non-ST-Segment-Elevation Acute Coronary Syndromes

Eptifibatide is used with anticoagulant therapy (e.g., heparin [referring throughout this monograph to unfractionated heparin], low molecular weight heparin), aspirin, and a P2Y12 platelet adenosine diphosphate (ADP)-receptor antagonist (e.g., clopidogrel, prasugrel, ticagrelor) to reduce the risk of acute cardiac ischemic events (death and/or myocardial infarction [MI]) in patients with unstable angina or non-ST-segment-elevation MI (NSTEMI) (i.e., non-ST-segment-elevation acute coronary syndromes [NSTE ACS]), both in patients who are to receive medical management and those undergoing percutaneous coronary intervention (PCI). In clinical trials of eptifibatide, NSTE ACS was defined by prolonged symptoms of cardiac ischemia (at least 10 minutes' duration within the previous 24 hours) that were associated with *transient* ST-segment changes (ST elevation of 0.6–1 mm or ST depression exceeding 0.5 mm), T-wave inversion (exceeding 1 mm), or increased cardiac (MB) fraction of creatine kinase (CK, creatine phosphokinase, CPK); patients who had MI associated with Q waves or *persistent* (30 minutes' duration or longer) ST-segment elevation exceeding 1 mm were not included in these studies. NSTEMI and unstable angina clinically may be indistinguishable at initial presentation and are managed similarly. Almost all patients in clinical trials of eptifibatide received concomitant therapy with aspirin and IV heparin, and the efficacy and safety of eptifibatide without adjunctive aspirin and/or heparin therapy have not been established.

Platelet glycoprotein (GP) IIb/IIIa-receptor inhibitors are used as an adjunct to standard therapeutic measures for managing NSTE ACS. These measures include therapy with aspirin and a P2Y12-receptor antagonist (e.g., clopidogrel, prasugrel, ticagrelor), nitrates (e.g., nitroglycerin), anticoagulant therapy (e.g., low molecular weight heparins, heparin), and β-blockers followed by either conservative medical management or early aggressive management, such as angiographic evaluation and revascularization procedures (e.g., PCI, coronary artery bypass grafting [CABG], coronary artery stent implantation) as required. Several meta-analyses of studies indicate that adjunctive therapy with a GP IIb/IIIa-receptor inhibitor can reduce the incidence of cardiac ischemic events, including subsequent MI and death in patients with NSTE ACS. Benefits of GP IIb/IIIa-receptor inhibitors on mortality principally occur early during therapy (i.e., the first 48–96 hours).

The benefit of aspirin for secondary prevention of ischemic events in patients with unstable angina has been demonstrated in several studies and pooled analyses. Many clinicians recommend that all patients with NSTE ACS receive aspirin as soon as possible after hospital admission and then continued indefinitely unless they have documented hypersensitivity or other definite contraindication (e.g., active or recent major bleeding, peptic ulcer disease). (See Non-ST-Segment-Elevation Acute Coronary Syndromes under Thrombosis: Coronary Artery Disease and Myocardial Infarction, in Uses, in Aspirin 28:08.04.24.) The American College of Cardiology Foundation (ACCF) and the American Heart Association (AHA) state that in patients with NSTE ACS in whom an initial invasive management strategy is planned, an additional antiplatelet agent (either clopidogrel or a GP IIb/IIIa-receptor inhibitor given IV) should be administered prior to diagnostic angiography ("upstream") as an adjunct to aspirin therapy. Eptifibatide or tirofiban is the preferred GP IIb/IIIa-receptor inhibitor for this use; abciximab is indicated only if there is no appreciable delay before angiography and PCI is likely to be performed. The American College of Chest Physicians (ACCP) states that a clear risk-benefit ratio has not been established for the use of GP IIb/IIIa-receptor inhibitors in patients with ACS who are not routinely scheduled for early revascularization.

In patients with NSTE ACS with elevated troponin concentrations who were managed with conservative medical therapy, GP IIb/IIIa-receptor inhibitors were equally effective in men and women. However, in women with NSTE ACS who are not at high risk for acute cardiac ischemic events (e.g., no elevated troponin concentrations) and are managed with a conservative strategy, eptifibatide and tirofiban appear to show little benefit and may possibly have detrimental effects; these agents are not recommended by AHA in women at lower risk for adverse cardiac events.

The current labeled indication for eptifibatide in patients with NSTE ACS is based principally on the results of a large, international, placebo-controlled study, the Platelet Glycoprotein IIb/IIIa in Unstable Angina: Receptor Suppression Using Integrilin Therapy (PURSUIT) study. In the PURSUIT study, therapy with eptifibatide (180-mcg/kg IV loading dose followed by continuous IV infusion of 2 mcg/kg per minute until hospital discharge or initiation of CABG, up to 72 hours or a maximum of 96 hours in patients undergoing PCI) reduced the combined incidence of death or nonfatal MI at 30 days (the primary composite clinical end point).

Beneficial effects of eptifibatide in the PURSUIT study were evident within 72 hours of initiating the infusion and persisted for up to 6 months (based on ischemic events evaluated by a blinded clinical events committee for the first 30 days and on investigator-reported events thereafter up to 6 months). The combined incidence of death or nonfatal MI in the overall study was reduced from 7.6% to 5.9% at 3 days, from 11.6% to 10.1% at 7 days, from 15.7% to 14.2% at 30 days, and from 13.6% to 12.1% at 6 months. This absolute reduction of approximately 1.5% in clinical events was maintained at all time points measured, while relative reductions in risk declined from 22% at 3 days to 12.9 and 9.6% at 7 and 30 days, respectively. The decline in relative benefit over time is related to the continued random occurrence of ischemic events in both placebo and treatment groups after achievement of a constant absolute risk reduction with eptifibatide therapy. The incidences of the individual end points of death or new MI for eptifibatide or placebo were not different at 30 days, although MI was less frequent with eptifibatide therapy at 96 hours.

Most patients in the PURSUIT study received adjunctive therapy with oral aspirin (75–325 mg once daily) and IV or subcutaneous heparin. In patients receiving medical management alone (i.e., those not undergoing PCI), heparin sodium (generally an IV loading dose of 5000 units followed by IV infusion of 1000 units per hour) was given to maintain a target activated partial thromboplastin time (aPTT) of 50–70 seconds. Patients undergoing PCI were given IV heparin (loading dose followed by IV infusion) to maintain an activated clotting time (ACT) of 300–350 seconds. (See Dosage and Administration: Dosage.)

The efficacy of eptifibatide in the PURSUIT study varied according to use of concomitant therapy or procedures and by gender, age, and geographic region. In this study, about 13% of patients underwent PCI during infusion of eptifibatide, while the remainder received medical management alone. For patients who underwent early PCI (within 72 hours after randomization) during eptifibatide infusion, the reduction in adverse ischemic events (nonfatal MI only) was evident prior to the procedure (i.e., during medical management). Patients undergoing early PCI experienced a 5.1% absolute reduction (31% relative reduction) in the combined clinical end point of death or nonfatal MI at 30 days; reduction in this clinical end point also was maintained over 6 months. Of those who received medical management alone, the incidence of clinical events was not appreciably reduced (1.1% absolute reduction, 7% relative reduction).

Subgroup analyses in the PURSUIT study suggested that patients who used aspirin prior to (within 2 weeks of) study entry were less likely to have had a MI (versus unstable angina) at study enrollment but more likely to have worse long-term outcomes (death or MI) than patients who reported no prior aspirin use; however, there was no evidence that prior aspirin use influenced the efficacy of eptifibatide.

The effects of eptifibatide therapy in the PURSUIT study did not appear to be influenced by patient age, but in patients outside North America the drug appeared less beneficial in women than in men. Results were heterogenous among patients in the various geographic regions (US and Canada, Western Europe, Eastern Europe, Latin America) of the study, possibly because of the practice-based nature of the study and the diverse pharmacologic and regional interventional strategies used to manage NSTE ACS. Patients treated in the US, who were the most homogeneous large subgroup in the study with regard to baseline characteristics (except ethnic background) and approach to patient management, achieved greater benefit than the overall study population. Eptifibatide therapy was associated with less benefit than placebo in women in Latin America and Eastern and Western Europe, while in the US and Canada men and women achieved similar benefit. These findings may reflect genuine biologic interactions between eptifibatide and gender, interactions between eptifibatide and international differences in concomitant therapy (e.g., timing and rate of interventions employed) given to men and women, or chance occurrences; the relative contributions of these possible factors are unknown.

● Acute Ischemic Complications of Percutaneous Coronary Intervention

Eptifibatide also is used with anticoagulant therapy (e.g., heparin, low molecular weight heparin), aspirin, and a P2Y12-receptor antagonist (e.g., clopidogrel, prasugrel, ticagrelor) to reduce the risk of acute ischemic complications (death,

MI, and/or the need for urgent revascularization procedures) in patients undergoing PCI, including coronary artery stenting. Despite advances in percutaneous revascularization techniques, abrupt closure of a coronary vessel that occurs during PCI still is associated with substantial morbidity (e.g., MI). GP IIb/IIIa-receptor inhibitors such as eptifibatide are used to minimize PCI-related ischemic complications and improve the risk-benefit ratio of these procedures. Studies involving eptifibatide or another GP IIb/IIIa-receptor inhibitor (i.e., abciximab) have demonstrated consistent reductions in the risk of composite ischemic events (death, MI, need for revascularization procedures) at 30 days in patients with or without NSTE ACS undergoing PCI.

The current labeled indication for eptifibatide in patients undergoing PCI is based principally on the results of large, multicenter, placebo-controlled studies in patients undergoing PCI alone in the Integrilin to Minimize Platelet Aggregation and Coronary Thrombosis-II (IMPACT-II) study or with coronary artery stenting in the Enhanced Suppression of the Platelet IIb/IIIa receptor with Integrilin Therapy (ESPRIT) study. In the IMPACT-II study, therapy with eptifibatide (135-mcg/kg IV loading dose immediately before PCI, followed by 0.5–0.75 mcg/kg per minute by continuous IV infusion for 20–24 hours after PCI) reduced the combined incidence of death, nonfatal MI, or the need for urgent intervention at 30 days (the primary composite clinical end point) in patients undergoing elective, urgent, or emergency PCI (e.g., balloon angioplasty, directional atherectomy, transluminal extraction catheter atherectomy, rotational ablation angioplasty, excimer-laser angioplasty). All patients received adjunctive therapy with aspirin (75–325 mg given 1–24 hours prior to the procedure), and IV heparin sodium (an IV loading dose of 100 units/kg prior to initiation of the study drug followed by up to 2000 units of heparin sodium every 15 minutes by IV injection) was given to achieve and maintain an ACT of 300–350 seconds. The primary clinical end point of death, nonfatal MI (defined as an increase in the cardiac MB fraction of creatine kinase to 3 times the upper limit of normal or development of Q waves of at least 0.04 seconds' duration in 2 or more contiguous ECG leads), or urgent intervention (e.g., abrupt closure of a coronary artery followed by CABG, coronary artery stent implantation, repeat PCI) occurred in approximately 6.6% of patients receiving the lower-dose regimen of eptifibatide (135-mcg/kg IV loading dose and 0.5 mcg/kg per minute by IV infusion) versus 9.6% of placebo recipients (31% relative reduction in clinical events) at 24 hours, and in 9.1 or 11.6% of patients receiving the lower-dose regimen of eptifibatide or placebo, respectively, at 30 days (22% relative reduction in clinical events). However, for patients receiving any amount of study drug (excluding those who did not receive study drug or coronary intervention), the decrease in ischemic complications at 30 days was statistically significant only in the low-dose group (those receiving the 135-mcg/kg IV loading dose and 0.5 mcg/kg per minute infusion). There was no clustering of ischemic events in the 24–48 hours after discontinuance of the eptifibatide infusion, indicating no rebound effect associated with termination of eptifibatide therapy. Most clinical end-point events (63%) reported in the IMPACT-II study occurred within the first 6 hours after coronary intervention.

Unexpected findings in the IMPACT-II study include the inability to prospectively determine outcome according to risk (i.e., the beneficial effect of eptifibatide was more pronounced in low-risk than in high-risk patients) and the lack of a dose-response effect with eptifibatide therapy (i.e., no improvement in clinical efficacy with the higher-dose compared with the lower-dose regimen, and no reduction in bleeding risk with the lower-dose regimen). Because the assay used to determine inhibition of platelet aggregation and adjust eptifibatide dosage in the IMPACT-II study involved anticoagulation with citrate (which binds calcium), binding of eptifibatide to the GP IIb/IIIa-receptor was exaggerated relative to that occurring at physiologic concentrations of calcium. Use in subsequent studies (e.g., PURSUIT) of the anticoagulant D-phenylalanyl-L-propyl-L-arginine chloromethyl ketone (PPACK), which does not affect extracellular calcium concentrations in ex vivo platelet-aggregation assays, indicates that inhibition of platelet aggregation may not have been optimal at the eptifibatide dosages employed in the IMPACT-II study. (See Pharmacology.) An alternative explanation for the lack of improved outcome with the higher infusion rate of eptifibatide in the IMPACT-II trial may be the likelihood that the IV loading dose, rather than the infusion rate, was the principal determinant of plasma eptifibatide concentration at the time of greatest risk of ischemic events (within 6 hours after initiation of therapy).

In a subsequent multicenter placebo-controlled study (ESPRIT) in which the dosage of eptifibatide (2 IV loading doses of 180 mcg/kg given 10 minutes apart with a continuous infusion of 2 mcg/kg per minute initiated after the first loading dose) was 3–4 times higher than that in the IMPACT-II study in patients undergoing non-urgent coronary artery stenting, therapy with the drug reduced the primary end point (the combined incidences of death, nonfatal MI, and urgent

target-vessel revascularization or rescue therapy with open-label drug for thrombotic complications of PCI) at 30 days and 1 year. All patients received adjunctive therapy with aspirin, clopidogrel, or ticlopidine, and IV heparin sodium (60 units/kg) was given as an IV loading dose followed by additional doses (10–40 units/kg) to achieve and maintain an ACT of 200–300 seconds. The combined clinical end point occurred in 7.5% of patients receiving eptifibatide versus 11.7% of placebo recipients, respectively, at 30 days. However, use of rescue therapy for threatened thrombotic complications (e.g., abrupt vessel closure, no reperfusion, coronary thrombosis) is likely to have reduced composite clinical end-point events in the placebo group. Benefits of eptifibatide appeared to be maintained during long-term follow-up as indicated by attainment of the primary end point in 14.3 or 18.5% of eptifibatide or placebo recipients, respectively, at 6 months and in 17.5 or 22.1% of eptifibatide or placebo recipients, respectively, at 1 year.

Randomized controlled studies, including a meta-analysis of 16 randomized trials involving approximately 10,000 patients with ST-segment-elevation MI (STEMI) undergoing primary PCI, generally have failed to demonstrate benefits of GP IIb/IIIa-receptor blockade similar to those observed in patients with NSTE ACS. ACCF, AHA, the Society for Cardiovascular Angiography and Interventions (SCAI), and other experts currently do not recommend the *routine* use of GP IIb/IIIa-receptor inhibitors in patients with STEMI undergoing PCI; however, selective use of these drugs as an adjunct to heparin may be reasonable in certain high-risk patients (e.g., those with large anterior MI and/or large thrombus). Studies evaluating the use of GP IIb/IIIa-receptor inhibitors in patients with NSTE ACS undergoing PCI have demonstrated reductions in ischemic outcomes, particularly in patients with high-risk features (e.g., elevated troponin); therefore, ACCF/AHA/SCAI states that it may be useful to administer a GP IIb/IIIa-receptor inhibitor at the time of PCI as an adjunct to heparin therapy in such high-risk patients who are not receiving bivalirudin and who are not adequately pretreated with a P2Y12-receptor antagonist. Regarding the choice of GP IIb/IIIa-receptor inhibitor in patients undergoing PCI, abciximab, "double-bolus" eptifibatide (i.e., two 180-mcg/kg direct IV injections given 10 minutes apart), and high-dose tirofiban (25 mcg/kg given by direct IV injection) all have been shown to produce a high degree of platelet inhibition and reduce ischemic complications.

● **Adjunctive Therapy During Thrombolysis to Prevent Reocclusion**

Eptifibatide has been administered concomitantly with a thrombolytic agent (e.g., alteplase, tenecteplase) in a limited number of patients to prevent coronary artery reocclusion† after an acute MI. However, the appropriate dosage of adjunctive eptifibatide therapy in terms of efficacy and bleeding complications (see Drug Interactions: Thrombolytic Therapy) in such patients has not been established, and studies to date have not been of sufficient size to detect differences in clinical outcomes such as survival.

DOSAGE AND ADMINISTRATION

● **Administration**

Eptifibatide is administered by IV injection followed by IV infusion using a controlled-infusion device (e.g., pump). For IV injection, the appropriate dose of eptifibatide is withdrawn from the 10-mL vial containing the drug solution and administered undiluted IV over 1–2 minutes. The solution for continuous IV infusion should be administered directly from the 100-mL vial after spiking the vial with a vented infusion set. Care should be taken to center the spike within the circle on the stopper top. Any drug solution remaining after IV injection or infusion of the appropriate dose of eptifibatide should be discarded.

Parenteral eptifibatide solutions should be inspected visually for particulate matter and discoloration prior to administration whenever solution and container permit.

● **Dosage**

In clinical trials of eptifibatide therapy, most patients received adjunctive antithrombotic therapy with aspirin (75–325 mg daily) and IV heparin sodium. The safety and efficacy of eptifibatide therapy without concomitant aspirin and heparin remains to be established.

Non-ST-Segment-Elevation Acute Coronary Syndromes

For reducing the risk of death and/or myocardial infarction (MI) in patients with unstable angina or non-ST-segment-elevation myocardial infarction (NSTEMI) (i.e., non-ST-segment-elevation acute coronary syndromes [NSTE ACS]) who have normal renal function, the recommended initial adult dosage of eptifibatide is 180 mcg/kg given as an IV loading dose over 1–2 minutes as soon as possible following diagnosis, followed by continuous IV infusion of 2 mcg/kg per minute until hospital discharge or initiation of coronary artery bypass grafting (CABG), or for up to 72 hours. In the PURSUIT study, bleeding occurred more frequently in both the placebo and treatment groups in patients undergoing CABG, and the incidence of major bleeding was not different between the groups. However, the manufacturer states that eptifibatide therapy should be discontinued prior to CABG.

The manufacturer states that if a patient with NSTE ACS is to undergo percutaneous coronary intervention (PCI) while receiving eptifibatide, the infusion should be continued at the same rate either up to hospital discharge or for up to 18–24 hours after the procedure, whichever comes first, for a maximum of 96 hours of therapy.

Adjunctive Antithrombotic Therapy

Adjunctive antithrombotic therapy with aspirin and heparin was used in most patients with NSTE ACS receiving eptifibatide therapy in clinical trials. The manufacturer of eptifibatide recommends an initial aspirin dosage of 160–325 mg daily in patients with NSTE ACS. For additional details regarding aspirin dosage regimens in patients with ACS, see Non-ST-Segment-Elevation Acute Coronary Syndromes under Dosage: Thrombosis, in Dosage and Administration in Aspirin 28:08,04.24.

In patients *not* undergoing PCI, the initial dosage of heparin sodium is based on patient weight and subsequently adjusted to a target activated partial thromboplastin time (aPTT) of 50–70 seconds. The manufacturer states that if patient weight is 70 kg or greater, an IV loading dose of 5000 units of heparin sodium should be administered followed by continuous IV infusion of 1000 units per hour. In patients weighing less than 70 kg, an IV loading dose of heparin sodium 60 units/kg should be given followed by infusion of 12 units/kg per hour.

In patients with NSTE ACS who undergo PCI, multiple IV injections of heparin sodium are administered based on activated clotting time (ACT) determinations during PCI to achieve and maintain an ACT of at least 200 seconds. Since eptifibatide and other GP IIb/IIIa-receptor inhibitors may have additive effects on ACT in patients receiving one of these drugs concomitantly with heparin, the dosage of heparin required to maintain an appropriate ACT during such concomitant therapy may be lower than with heparin monotherapy.

Clinical experience from other studies with GP IIb/IIIa-receptor inhibitors (e.g., abciximab) and current American College of Cardiology Foundation (ACCF)/ American Heart Association (AHA)/Society for Cardiovascular Angiography and Interventions (SCAI) guidelines suggest that use of lower dosages of concomitant IV heparin sodium (e.g., 50–70 units/kg) given 6 hours prior to PCI and targeted to an ACT of at least 200 seconds may provide similar reductions in ischemic coronary events as dosages for higher target ACTs with less risk of major bleeding.

Percutaneous Coronary Intervention

For reducing the risk of acute ischemic complications (death, MI, and/or the need for urgent revascularization procedures) in patients undergoing PCI, the manufacturer and some clinicians state that the initial adult dosage of eptifibatide in patients with normal renal function consists of an IV loading dose of 180 mcg/kg given immediately before PCI, followed in 10 minutes by a second 180-mcg/kg IV dose; in addition, a continuous IV infusion of 2 mcg/kg per minute should be initiated immediately after the first loading dose. The IV infusion should be continued until hospital discharge or for up to 18–24 hours, whichever comes first. A minimum infusion period of 12 hours is recommended in patients undergoing PCI. The manufacturer states that eptifibatide therapy should be discontinued prior to CABG.

Adjunctive Antithrombotic Therapy

Adjunctive antithrombotic therapy with aspirin and heparin was used in most patients receiving eptifibatide in clinical trials. In the IMPACT-II study, aspirin was given in a dosage of 75–325 mg 1–24 hours prior to PCI. In patients undergoing PCI, ACCF/AHA/SCAI recommends that aspirin 325 mg be given prior to PCI in patients not already receiving maintenance therapy with aspirin. Patients already receiving maintenance therapy with aspirin should receive a dose of 81–325 mg of aspirin before the procedure. For additional details regarding aspirin dosage regimens in patients undergoing PCI, see Percutaneous Coronary Intervention and Revascularization Procedures under Dosage: Thrombosis, in Dosage and Administration, in Aspirin 28:08.04.24.

In patients undergoing PCI with stent placement, a loading dose of a P2Y12 platelet adenosine diphosphate (ADP)-receptor antagonist (clopidogrel, prasugrel, or ticagrelor) also is recommended.

Since eptifibatide and other GP IIb/IIIa-receptor inhibitors may have additive effects on ACT in patients receiving one of these drugs concomitantly with heparin, the dosage of heparin sodium required to maintain an appropriate ACT during such concomitant therapy may be lower than with heparin monotherapy. The manufacturer recommends a heparin sodium dose of 60 units/kg given by direct ("bolus") IV injection within 6 hours prior to PCI. Additional injections of heparin sodium should be given during PCI to maintain an ACT of 200–300 seconds. In patients who have received prior therapy with heparin before PCI, ACCF/AHA/SCAI states that additional heparin sodium injections should be administered during the procedure as needed.

Postprocedural use of heparin generally is not recommended while GP IIb/ IIIa-receptor inhibitor therapy is given.

● Dosage in Renal and Hepatic Impairment

Results of a small pilot study in patients with mild to moderate renal impairment (as determined by a reduction in creatinine clearance of 30 mL/minute from normal) revealed no apparent differences in mean pharmacokinetic parameters between renally impaired patients and healthy individuals. However, other data in patients with moderate to severe renal impairment (creatinine clearance less than 50 mL/minute) indicate a reduction of approximately 50% in eptifibatide clearance and a doubling of plasma drug concentrations. In vitro studies indicate that eptifibatide may be removed from plasma by dialysis.

Dosage adjustment is not necessary in patients with mild to moderate renal impairment (i.e., those with creatinine clearance of at least 50 mL/minute). However, patients with NSTE ACS who have a creatinine clearance of less than 50 mL/ minute (using Cockcroft-Gault equation) should receive a 180-mcg/kg IV loading dose of eptifibatide as soon as possible following diagnosis followed by IV infusion of 1 mcg/kg per minute.

In patients undergoing PCI who have a creatinine clearance of less than 50 mL/minute, an IV loading dose of 180 mcg/kg of eptifibatide should be given immediately prior to PCI followed by IV infusion of the drug at 1 mcg/kg per minute; a second IV loading dose of 180 mcg/kg should be given 10 minutes after the first loading dose.

Information on the pharmacokinetics or use of eptifibatide in patients with hepatic impairment is not available, and the manufacturer currently makes no specific dosage recommendations for such patients. Patients with hepatic disease severe enough to produce alterations in the synthesis of coagulation factors were excluded from clinical trials of eptifibatide, and use of the drug is contraindicated in such patients.

CAUTIONS

The incidence of adverse effects with eptifibatide therapy is based principally on data from 2 large, placebo-controlled studies, the PURSUIT study in patients with unstable angina or non-ST-segment-elevation myocardial infarction (NSTEMI) (i.e., non-ST-segment-elevation acute coronary syndromes [NSTE ACS]) and the IMPACT-II study in patients undergoing percutaneous coronary intervention (PCI). Patients in the PURSUIT study received 180 mcg/kg of eptifibatide as an IV loading dose followed by either 1.3 or 2 mcg/kg per minute by continuous IV infusion for up to 72–96 hours; patients in the IMPACT-II study received 135 mcg/kg of the drug as an IV loading dose immediately before PCI, followed by either 0.5 or 0.75 mcg/kg per minute by continuous IV infusion for 20–24 hours. (See Uses.) Almost all patients receiving eptifibatide in clinical studies received concomitant therapy with heparin and/or aspirin; therefore, the incidence of bleeding complications attributable solely to eptifibatide is difficult to determine. Because of the different eptifibatide dosage regimens used in the PURSUIT and IMPACT-II studies, data from these studies were not pooled.

The most frequent and severe adverse effect of eptifibatide therapy is bleeding. Bleeding complications, which usually are minor and develop at vascular access (e.g., femoral puncture) sites (e.g., in patients undergoing PCI), have been reported in 35–75% of patients receiving various dosages of eptifibatide in clinical studies. Bleeding is an extension of the pharmacologic action of eptifibatide and was classified in clinical trials principally according to criteria of the Thrombolysis in Myocardial Infarction (TIMI) study groups. Minor bleeding generally was defined as spontaneous gross hematuria or spontaneous hematemesis; observed blood loss with a decrease in hemoglobin concentration of 3–5 g/dL or a reduction in hematocrit of at least 10%; or a decrease of 4–5 g/dL or 12–15% in hemoglobin or hematocrit, respectively, with no identifiable bleeding site. Major bleeding was defined as intracranial hemorrhage or overt bleeding associated with a hemoglobin or hematocrit decrease of at least 5 g/dL or at least 15%, respectively.

In clinical trials, administration of eptifibatide was associated with an increase in major and minor bleeding complications compared with placebo. The overall incidence of major and minor bleeding according to TIMI criteria in the PURSUIT study was 23.5% compared with an incidence of 40–70% in smaller studies. Bleeding of any severity was reported in about 15–60% of patients receiving placebo (i.e., heparin and aspirin therapy alone). Bleeding episodes resulted in discontinuance of eptifibatide in 8, 4.6, or 3.5% of patients receiving the drug in the PURSUIT, ESPRIT, or IMPACT-II study, respectively.

● Hematologic Effects

Major bleeding events occurred in 4.4 or 4.7% of evaluable patients receiving eptifibatide 0.5 or 0.75 mcg/kg per minute, respectively, by IV infusion following an IV loading dose of 135 mcg/kg in the IMPACT-II study; major bleeding occurred in 10.5 or 10.8% of those receiving 1.3 or 2 mcg/kg per minute, respectively, of eptifibatide following an IV loading dose of 180 mcg/kg in the PURSUIT study. Major bleeding occurred in 1.3 or 0.4% of those receiving eptifibatide (2 IV loading doses of 180 mcg/kg each given 10 minutes apart followed by continuous infusion of 2 mcg/kg per minute initiated after the first loading dose) or placebo in the ESPRIT study, respectively. The incidence of bleeding increased as the activated clotting time (ACT) increased (mean ACT of 284 seconds) in those receiving eptifibatide. At the lower ACTs achieved in the ESPRIT trial, the incidence of bleeding was lower than that observed in the IMPACT-II and PURSUIT studies. The incidence of major bleeding with eptifibatide was similar to that with placebo in the IMPACT-II study and modestly increased compared with placebo in the PURSUIT study. The overall incidence of major bleeding was higher in the PURSUIT study than in the IMPACT-II study because coronary artery bypass grafting (CABG) was more commonly employed in the PURSUIT study (15.5% incidence within 30 days) than in the IMPACT-II study (4.3%); major bleeding was minimal (0.6%) in patients receiving medical management alone in the PURSUIT trial. However, bleeding episodes in patients who underwent CABG were not more frequent in patients receiving eptifibatide than in placebo recipients in either study.

In the PURSUIT and ESPRIT studies, the greatest increase in major bleeding with eptifibatide therapy compared with placebo was bleeding at the femoral vascular access site (2.8 and 1.3%, respectively, in the PURSUIT study and 0.8 and 0.1%, respectively, in the ESPRIT study) associated with PCI; oropharyngeal (principally gingival), genitourinary, GI, and retroperitoneal bleeding also were more common with eptifibatide therapy than with placebo. GI, pulmonary, and retroperitoneal hemorrhage, including fatalities, have been reported during postmarketing experience with eptifibatide given concomitantly with heparin and aspirin. Among patients experiencing major bleeding in the IMPACT-II study, an increase in bleeding with eptifibatide versus placebo was demonstrated only for bleeding at the femoral vascular access site (3.2 versus 2.8%, respectively). In the PURSUIT and ESPRIT studies, patient weight was inversely related to the number of major bleeding episodes in patients receiving eptifibatide; this relationship was not found in the IMPACT-II study.

Adverse hematologic effects with eptifibatide therapy have been severe enough to require blood or platelet transfusions. In the IMPACT-II study, the incidences of major bleeding events and transfusions (including whole blood, packed red blood cells, fresh frozen plasma, cryoprecipitate, platelets, and autotransfusion) were similar in patients receiving eptifibatide or placebo, while minor bleeding events were more common with eptifibatide therapy. Bleeding or thrombocytopenia requiring transfusions in the IMPACT-II study occurred in about 5.5 or 5.8% of patients receiving eptifibatide 0.5 or 0.75 mcg/kg per minute, respectively, following an IV loading dose of 135 mcg/kg, compared with about 5.1% of patients receiving placebo injection and infusion (based on treated-as-randomized analysis). In the PURSUIT study, transfusions were required in 12.8% of patients receiving eptifibatide and in 10.4% of patients receiving placebo. In the ESPRIT study, transfusions were required in 1.5% of patients receiving eptifibatide and in 1.1% of those receiving placebo.

Minor bleeding episodes occurred in about 11.7 or 14.2% of patients receiving 0.5 or 0.75 mcg/kg per minute, respectively, of eptifibatide following an IV loading dose of 135 mcg/kg in the IMPACT-II study, and in 10.5 or 13.1% of those receiving 1.3 or 2 mcg/kg per minute, respectively, following an IV loading dose of 180 mcg/kg in the PURSUIT study. Minor bleeding episodes occurred in 3 or 2% of patients receiving eptifibatide or placebo, respectively, in the ESPRIT study.

Decreases in platelet count or thrombocytopenia occur occasionally (2.3% overall) after therapy with GP IIb/IIIa-receptor inhibitors. Thrombocytopenia associated with administration of a GP IIb/IIIa-receptor inhibitor generally occurs within hours or days after administration of the drug. The incidence of thrombocytopenia (defined as a platelet count less than 100,000/mm^3 or a decrease of at least 50% in platelet count from baseline) and the need for platelet transfusions were similar in patients receiving eptifibatide in several clinical trials (IMPACT-II, PURSUIT, pilot studies) and in patients receiving placebo. In the ESPRIT study, the incidence of thrombocytopenia was 1.2 or 0.6% among patients receiving eptifibatide or placebo, respectively. A preliminary report based on pooled data from clinical trials indicates that the incidence of thrombocytopenia is not appreciably different among GP IIb/IIIa-receptor inhibitors (i.e., abciximab, eptifibatide, tirofiban), although the absolute risk of thrombocytopenia appears to increase (but not synergistically) with concomitant use of heparin. However, severe thrombocytopenia (i.e., platelet count less than 20,000 per mm^3) has been reported more frequently with abciximab than with eptifibatide. In the large PURSUIT study, the incidence of profound thrombocytopenia (defined as a platelet count less than 20,000/mm^3) was small (0.2%) in patients receiving eptifibatide, but greater than the incidence in those receiving placebo (less than 0.1%).

● Sensitivity Reactions

Anaphylaxis was reported in 7 patients (0.16%) receiving an eptifibatide infusion rate of 2 mcg/kg per minute, respectively, following an IV loading dose of 180 mcg/kg in the PURSUIT study and in 7 patients (0.15%) receiving placebo in this study; none of the patients receiving eptifibatide and one patient receiving placebo in the IMPACT-II study developed anaphylaxis. Allergic reactions were reported in 2 patients (0.19%) receiving eptifibatide and in one patient (0.1%) receiving placebo in the ESPRIT study. Of those who received eptifibatide in the PURSUIT study, the drug was discontinued in 3 patients (0.05%). In patients undergoing PCI and receiving the drug in the IMPACT-II study, eptifibatide therapy was discontinued in 2 patients (0.04%) because of allergic reactions.

While therapy with some platelet-aggregation inhibitors (e.g., abciximab) has been associated with development of antibodies to the drug, development of antibodies against eptifibatide has not been reported to date. No evidence of delayed-type hypersensitivity or antigenicity with eptifibatide was noted in studies in mice and guinea pigs. The low molecular weight of eptifibatide may account for its lack of antigenicity. Some clinicians suggest that the lack of antigenicity of eptifibatide and the rapidly reversible binding of the drug to platelets compared with abciximab may account for the relative lack of thrombocytopenia observed with eptifibatide.

● Cardiovascular Effects

Most adverse effects of eptifibatide other than bleeding in clinical trials were cardiovascular in nature and were typical of patients with unstable angina; the incidence of most of these effects, with the exception of hypotension, was similar in patients receiving eptifibatide or placebo.

Hypotension occurred in 7% of patients receiving eptifibatide and 6% of those receiving placebo in the PURSUIT study.

Stroke, including primary hemorrhagic stroke, cerebral infarction, or infarction with hemorrhagic conversion, occurred in 0.5% of patients receiving an eptifibatide infusion rate of 1.3 mcg/kg per minute following an IV loading dose of 180 mcg/kg in the PURSUIT study and in 0.5% of patients receiving an infusion rate of 0.5 mcg/kg per minute following an IV loading dose of 135 mcg/kg in the IMPACT-II study. The overall incidence of stroke was 0.7% in patients receiving an eptifibatide infusion rate of 2 mcg/kg per minute following an IV loading dose of 180 mcg/kg in the PURSUIT study and in 0.7% of patients receiving an infusion rate of 0.75 mcg/kg per minute following an IV loading dose of 135 mcg/kg in the IMPACT-II study. Hemorrhagic stroke occurred in 2 patients (0.19%) receiving eptifibatide and in one patient (0.1%) receiving placebo in the ESPRIT study.

Therapy with GP IIb/IIIa receptor inhibitors, including eptifibatide, has not been associated with an increased risk of intracranial hemorrhage. The incidence of stroke was similar among patients receiving eptifibatide or placebo in either the PURSUIT or IMPACT-II study. Most strokes occurring in these studies were nonhemorrhagic (thromboembolic) in nature (i.e., cerebral infarctions). Cerebral infarction occurred in one patient (0.1%) receiving eptifibatide in the ESPRIT study. The incidence of intracranial hemorrhage in the IMPACT-II study was low (0.1–0.2%) and also was similar in patients receiving eptifibatide or placebo. Cerebral hemorrhage, sometimes resulting in death, has been reported with eptifibatide, principally in combination with heparin and aspirin, during postmarketing experience. Adverse cardiovascular effects leading to discontinuance of eptifibatide therapy occurred in 0.3 or 1.4% of patients receiving the drug in the PURSUIT or IMPACT-II study, respectively.

● Other Adverse Effects

Serious adverse effects of eptifibatide other than bleeding occurred in 19% of patients receiving either eptifibatide or placebo, respectively, in the PURSUIT study and in 7 or 6% of patients receiving the drug or placebo, respectively, in the ESPRIT study. Other adverse effects in the PURSUIT study occurring in at least 0.1% of patients and leading to discontinuance of eptifibatide involved the digestive system (0.1%), hemic/lymphatic system (0.1%), nervous system (0.3%), urogenital system (0.1%), and whole body (0.2%); these adverse effects resulted in discontinuance of therapy in a similar percentage of placebo recipients. In patients undergoing PCI who received eptifibatide in the IMPACT-II study, adverse effects other than bleeding that resulted in discontinuance of drug therapy occurred in the following body systems: whole body (0.3% of patients), digestive system (0.2%), hemic/lymphatic system (0.2%), nervous system (0.3%), and respiratory system (0.1%).

● Precautions and Contraindications

The administration of eptifibatide in patients with NSTE ACS is associated with a small increase in the frequency of major bleeding compared with heparin and aspirin therapy alone. Bleeding with platelet glycoprotein (GP IIb/IIIa)-receptor inhibitors can be reduced by adherence to strict anticoagulation guidelines, the use of a short course of low-dose, weight-adjusted heparin, early arterial sheath removal, and careful patient and access site management. Prior to administration of eptifibatide, preexisting hemostatic and renal abnormalities should be identified by obtaining a prothrombin time (PT), serum creatinine, hematocrit or hemoglobin, and activated partial thromboplastin time (aPTT). In patients receiving heparin concomitantly with eptifibatide, the extent of heparin anticoagulation (as assessed by activated clotting time [ACT] or aPTT) should be monitored closely to minimize bleeding. The aPTT should be maintained at 50–70 seconds unless PCI is to be performed. In addition, the ACT should be measured in patients undergoing PCI. Current guidelines of the ACCP, ACC, and AHA and risk-benefit analyses in trials with GP IIb/IIIa-receptor inhibitors suggest that heparin sodium dosing should be adjusted to maintain the ACT at 200 seconds or greater during PCI in patients receiving GP IIb/IIIa-receptor inhibitors. (See Dosage and Administration: Dosage.) Routine use of postprocedural heparin is not recommended while GP IIb/IIIa-receptor inhibitor therapy is given. After PCI, the aPTT should be checked prior to arterial sheath removal, and the sheath should not be removed unless the aPTT is less than 45 seconds or the ACT is less than 150–180 seconds. The manufacturer recommends that concomitant thrombolytic therapy be used with caution.

Platelet counts should be determined prior to treatment with eptifibatide and periodically (e.g., daily) during concomitant eptifibatide and heparin therapy. The manufacturer states that there is no clinical experience with the use of eptifibatide in patients who have platelet counts less than 100,000/mm³ and that the drug should be used with caution in such patients. Abciximab, another GP IIb/IIIa-receptor inhibitor, has been associated with pseudothrombocytopenia caused by an in vitro anticoagulant (edetate disodium [EDTA]) interaction. Some clinicians suggest that a peripheral-blood smear be examined for the presence of platelet clumping or that blood for platelet counts be drawn into separate tubes containing EDTA, citrate, or heparin to exclude pseudothrombocytopenia in patients receiving eptifibatide. The possibility of heparin-induced thrombocytopenia also should be considered in the differential diagnosis of thrombocytopenia in patients receiving GP IIb/IIIa-receptor inhibitors concomitantly with heparin. If true thrombocytopenia (platelet count less than 100,000/mm³) is verified, eptifibatide should be discontinued and the condition appropriately monitored and treated. Thrombocytopenia is usually reversible following discontinuance of GP IIb/IIIa-receptor inhibitors and anticoagulant (heparin) therapy; however, platelet transfusions should be considered for the management of severe thrombocytopenia.

To minimize the possibility of bleeding associated with the use of eptifibatide, particularly at the site of femoral artery sheath placement, precautions in the placement, maintenance, and removal of the vascular access sheath should be observed. Placement of a femoral venous sheath should be avoided if possible. When inserting the femoral artery sheath, care should be taken so that only the anterior wall of the femoral artery is punctured; a Seldinger (through and through) technique for puncture of the artery should be avoided. Appropriate precautions should be observed while the vascular access sheath is in place (e.g., complete bed rest, elevation of the head of the bed not exceeding 30°, restraint of the limb in which the vascular access sheath is inserted, frequent monitoring of the vascular access site and the distal pulse in the involved limb). The femoral artery sheath may be removed during treatment with eptifibatide, provided that at least 3–4 hours have elapsed since heparin therapy was discontinued and its effects largely reversed (as indicated by an aPTT of less than 45 seconds or an ACT of less than 150–180 seconds). Early removal of femoral sheaths (4–6 hours after PCI) was encouraged in patients receiving PCI in both the PURSUIT and IMPACT-II studies while the study drug was being infused.

Both heparin and eptifibatide therapy should be discontinued and sheath hemostasis achieved with standard compressive techniques at least 4 hours before hospital discharge. Pressure (e.g., using manual compression or a mechanical hemostatic device) should be applied to the femoral artery for at least 20–30 minutes after sheath removal; after hemostasis, a pressure dressing should be applied. Any hematoma that forms should be measured and monitored for enlargement.

Careful monitoring of all potential bleeding sites should be undertaken during and following treatment with platelet aggregation inhibitors. Needle punctures (e.g., arterial, IM, IV, lumbar, subcutaneous, intradermal), cutdown sites, and use of nasotracheal intubation, nasogastric tubes, urinary catheterization, and automatic blood pressure cuffs should be minimized during and following treatment with eptifibatide. Establishment of IV access at noncompressible sites (e.g., in subclavian or jugular veins) should be avoided; an indwelling venipuncture device (e.g., heparin lock) should be considered for drawing blood; documentation and monitoring of vascular puncture sites should occur; and dressings should be removed gently and carefully. The manufacturer states that any occurrence of serious bleeding that cannot be controlled by pressure on the bleeding site should result in discontinuance of eptifibatide and concomitantly administered heparin therapy.

Because eptifibatide increases the risk of bleeding, the drug is contraindicated in patients with a history of bleeding diathesis or active abnormal bleeding (e.g., elevated hemostatic indices, recent noncompressible vascular punctures GI or genitourinary bleeding) within the previous 30 days. A low hematocrit value (less than 30%) at baseline could represent recent undetected bleeding, and patients with such values may not be able to tolerate additional bleeding episodes; eptifibatide should not be used in these patients. Eptifibatide also is contraindicated in patients with severe uncontrolled hypertension (systolic blood pressure exceeding 200 mm Hg or diastolic blood pressure exceeding 110 mm Hg with antihypertensive therapy); recent (within 6 weeks) major surgery; history of stroke within 30 days or any history of hemorrhagic stroke; current or planned therapy with another GP IIb/IIIa-receptor inhibitor; and patients receiving renal dialysis. No data are available on the use of eptifibatide in patients with serum creatinine concentrations of 4 mg/dL or greater; the dosage should be reduced in patients with serum creatinine concentrations between 2–4 mg/dL. (See Dosage in Renal and Hepatic Impairment under Dosage and Administration: Dosage.)

Eptifibatide also is contraindicated in patients with known hypersensitivity to any component of the commercially available preparation.

● Pediatric Precautions

Safety and efficacy of eptifibatide in pediatric patients have not been determined.

● Geriatric Precautions

Safety and efficacy of eptifibatide in geriatric patients have not been specifically studied to date; however, in clinical studies of eptifibatide involving over 14,000 patients up to 94 years of age, approximately 45% of the patients were 65 years of age or older, and 12% were 75 years of age or older. Clinical experience generally has not revealed age-related differences in efficacy with eptifibatide therapy. However, the incidence of bleeding complications in clinical trials was higher in geriatric than in younger patients receiving either placebo or eptifibatide in clinical trials. No dosage adjustment was made for geriatric patients in the principal clinical trials (PURSUIT, IMPACT II), but patients older than 75 years of age had to weigh at least 50 kg to be enrolled in the PURSUIT study because of a concern for an increased risk of bleeding in those weighing less than that. (See Cautions: Hematologic Effects.)

● Mutagenicity and Carcinogenicity

No evidence of mutagenicity was seen at the chromosomal or gene level when eptifibatide was evaluated in several in vitro and in vivo test systems. The drug was not genotoxic in the Ames microbial mutagen test, mouse micronucleus test, or mouse lymphoma cell forward mutation assay. Eptifibatide did not demonstrate any potential to induce chromosomal aberrations in human lymphocytes.

Since eptifibatide is designed to be used in acute-care settings, long-term studies in animals to evaluate the carcinogenic potential of eptifibatide have not been performed and are not planned.

● Pregnancy, Fertility, and Lactation
Pregnancy

Reproduction studies using continuous IV infusion of eptifibatide dosages at a total daily dosage of up to 72 mg/kg in pregnant rats and up to 36 mg/kg in pregnant rabbits (either dosage representing about 4 times the recommended maximum daily human dosage based on body surface area) have not revealed evidence of harm to the fetus. However, since animal reproduction studies are not always predictive of human response and there are no adequate or controlled studies to date using eptifibatide in pregnant women, eptifibatide should be used during pregnancy only when clearly needed.

Fertility

Reproduction studies in male and female rats using eptifibatide dosages up to 72 mg/kg daily (about 4 times the maximum recommended human daily dosage) by continuous IV infusion have not revealed evidence of impaired fertility.

Lactation

Since it is not known if eptifibatide is distributed into milk, the drug should be used with caution in nursing women.

DRUG INTERACTIONS

● Drugs Affecting Platelet Function

Limited data from preclinical and clinical studies in patients receiving eptifibatide (0.5 mcg/kg per minute by IV infusion) alone or concomitantly with aspirin, heparin, or both drugs suggest no substantial pharmacokinetic or pharmacodynamic interactions (e.g., additive effects on platelet-aggregation inhibition) between eptifibatide and aspirin. While coadministration of eptifibatide and aspirin resulted in up to a fivefold increase in bleeding time compared with baseline values, similar increases in bleeding time were observed with aspirin and placebo. Nevertheless, since eptifibatide inhibits platelet aggregation, caution should be observed when the drug is used with other drugs that affect hemostasis, including thrombolytic agents, oral anticoagulants, nonsteroidal anti-inflammatory agents (NSAIAs), or dipyridamole. (See Drug Interactions: Thrombolytic Therapy and also see Drug Interactions: Anticoagulants.) However, clopidogrel or ticlopidine was used routinely with eptifibatide in a large clinical, multicenter study (Enhanced Suppression of the Platelet IIb/IIIa Receptor with Integrilin Therapy [ESPRIT]) in patients undergoing coronary artery stent placement.

To minimize potentially additive pharmacologic effects, the manufacturer of eptifibatide states that concomitant therapy with other platelet glycoprotein (GP IIb/IIIa)-receptor inhibitors (e.g., abciximab, tirofiban) should be avoided.

● Thrombolytic Therapy

Eptifibatide has been administered concomitantly with thrombolytic agents (e.g., alteplase, streptokinase, tenecteplase) in a limited number of patients with acute myocardial infarction (MI) to reduce the risk of reocclusion of the infarct-related artery. (See Uses: Adjunctive Therapy During Thrombolysis to Prevent Reocclusion.) Some clinicians suggest that use of short-acting platelet-aggregation inhibitors such as eptifibatide concomitantly with thrombolytic therapy may provide optimal benefit while minimizing the risk of bleeding. However, use after thrombolysis of drugs that affect platelet function may increase the risk of bleeding complications, including those requiring blood transfusions, associated with thrombolytic therapy and has not been shown to be unequivocally effective to date; therefore, use of eptifibatide with thrombolytic therapy should be considered investigational and should be undertaken with caution.

In a small, placebo-controlled trial and dose-ranging study in patients with acute MI, combined therapy with eptifibatide (up to 180 mcg/kg as an IV loading dose followed by continuous infusion of 0.75 mcg/kg per minute for 24 hours) and alteplase (accelerated, weight-adjusted IV infusion up to 100 mg) was not associated with an increased incidence of major bleeding or transfusions compared with alteplase monotherapy. However, in another study in patients with acute MI receiving streptokinase (1.5 million units IV over 60 minutes) and eptifibatide (up to 180 mcg/kg as an IV loading dose followed by continuous infusion of 2 mcg/kg per minute for 72 hours), the higher infusion rates of eptifibatide (1.3 and 2 mcg/kg per minute) were associated with an increase in bleeding and the need for blood transfusion compared with streptokinase monotherapy. In the IMPACT-II study, 2 of 15 patients who received a thrombolytic agent concomitantly with eptifibatide (135 mcg/kg as an IV loading dose followed by 0.5 mcg/kg per minute by IV infusion) had a major bleeding episode, while 10 of 40 patients who received thrombolytic therapy and eptifibatide (180 mcg/kg as an IV loading dose followed by 2 mcg/kg per minute by IV infusion) in the PURSUIT study experienced major bleeding.

● Anticoagulants

Concomitant use of platelet-aggregation inhibitors and an anticoagulant (particularly in high dosages) may increase the risk of hemorrhage, and careful monitoring

for bleeding is necessary, especially at arterial puncture sites. Eptifibatide and concomitant heparin therapy should be discontinued immediately and appropriate therapy (e.g., protamine sulfate in patients receiving heparin) instituted as necessary if serious bleeding occurs (e.g., bleeding not controlled by pressure). In healthy individuals, enoxaparin sodium (1 mg/kg subcutaneously every 12 hours for 4 doses) did not alter the pharmacokinetics or pharmacodynamics (platelet aggregation) of eptifibatide. The manufacturer states that caution should be employed when using eptifibatide with oral anticoagulants.

In almost all patients receiving eptifibatide for non-ST-segment-elevation acute coronary syndromes or in patients undergoing percutaneous coronary intervention (PCI), heparin (generally combined with aspirin) has been administered before and during eptifibatide therapy to reduce the risk of coronary artery occlusion or new thrombi formation. When eptifibatide was given alone or in combination with heparin in a limited number of healthy individuals at eptifibatide infusion rates exceeding 0.5 mcg/kg per minute or for durations exceeding 6 hours, bleeding time was prolonged approximately twofold or greater; smaller dosages infused over 90 minutes had minimal effects on bleeding time.

LABORATORY TEST INTERFERENCES

In blood samples, binding of eptifibatide to the GP IIb/IIIa-receptor and the drug's subsequent inhibitory activity on platelet aggregation are dependent on the free calcium concentration, and therefore the type of anticoagulant used in the sample. In the IMPACT-II study, the assay used to determine inhibition of platelet aggregation involved anticoagulation with sodium citrate, which removes calcium bound to the GP IIb/IIIa receptor and results in enhanced binding of eptifibatide to the receptor. Therefore, the inhibitory activity of eptifibatide is overestimated in blood samples collected in citrate relative to that in samples anticoagulated with PPACK. (See Uses: Acute Ischemic Complications of Percutaneous Coronary Intervention.)

ACUTE TOXICITY

Limited information is available on the acute toxicity of eptifibatide. In general, overdosage of eptifibatide in humans may be expected to produce effects that are extensions of the pharmacologic and adverse effects of the drug, predominantly bleeding. (See Cautions: Hematologic Effects.) A small number of patients in each of the major clinical studies (IMPACT-II, PURSUIT) received doses of eptifibatide by IV injection and/or infusion that were more than twice those recommended or that were identified by study investigators as an overdose; none of these individuals had intracranial hemorrhage or other major bleeding.

In acute toxicity studies in animals (rats, rabbits, or monkeys) given 45 mg/kg of eptifibatide (about 2–5 times the maximum recommended daily human dose based on body surface area) over 90 minutes by continuous IV infusion, loss of righting reflex, dyspnea, ptosis, and decreased muscle tone were observed in rabbits, and petechial hemorrhages in the femoral and abdominal areas were observed in monkeys; no manifestations of toxicity were observed in rats given this dose of eptifibatide. In short-term toxicology studies (14–28 days) in monkeys, continuous IV infusion of eptifibatide in dosages exceeding 5 mcg/kg per minute produced contusions, hemorrhage, and petechial hemorrhages, resulting in anemia in some animals. At a dosage of 50 mcg/kg per minute, bleeding, decreased concentrations of plasma proteins, anemia, and death occurred. These effects were not observed in monkeys given eptifibatide 5 mcg/kg per minute (representing 1.1 times the mean steady-state plasma concentrations in patients undergoing PCI and receiving the recommended dosing regimen) in the IMPACT-II study.

PHARMACOLOGY

● Platelet Aggregation and Thrombosis

Eptifibatide is a selective, competitive, reversible inhibitor of platelet aggregation that is used to prevent acute ischemic complications associated with non-ST-segment-elevation acute coronary syndromes (NSTE ACS) and/or percutaneous coronary intervention (PCI). Because of its mechanism of action, eptifibatide, like abciximab and tirofiban, has been referred to as a platelet glycoprotein (GP) IIb/IIIa-receptor inhibitor. Platelet adhesion, activation, and aggregation are key processes leading to the formation of platelet-rich ("white") coronary artery thrombi and the development of ACS and ischemic complications associated with PCI. White thrombus formation is triggered by vascular injury (e.g., from PCI procedures), plaque rupture, or denudation of endothelium that exposes the subendothelial matrix of the vessel to circulating platelets. Upon exposure of the vessel subendothelium, potent thrombogenic stimuli (e.g., thrombin, collagen) present in both subendothelium and plaque, and/or high-shear stress, stimulate platelet adhesion and activation.

Activated platelets release intracellular granules consisting of vasoactive substances that are part of an autostimulatory loop for platelet aggregation; these vasoactive substances include thromboxane A_2, serotonin, and adenosine diphosphate (ADP); adhesive glycoproteins such as fibrinogen, fibronectin, and von Willebrand's factor; and plasminogen activator inhibitor-1 (PAI-1). Regardless of the initial stimulus for platelet activation, the final common pathway to platelet aggregation and thrombosis involves activation of the receptor function of the platelet glycoprotein (GP) IIb/IIIa complex (also known as $\alpha_{IIb}\beta_3$). GP IIb/IIIa receptors on the surface of activated platelets undergo a conformational change to accept soluble fibrinogen, von Willebrand's factor, and other ligands (e.g., fibronectin, vitronectin, thrombospondin). Some of these adhesive ligands form cross-links to GP IIb/IIIa receptors on the surface of adjacent activated platelets, causing aggregation and white thrombus formation. In addition, fibrinogen bound to the vessel wall or to other platelet aggregates can activate GP IIb/IIIa receptors on unstimulated platelets and recruit these platelets to growing white thrombi.

Progression of unstable angina or non-ST-segment-elevation myocardial infarction (NSTEMI) to ST-segment-elevation myocardial infarction (STEMI) or sudden death occurs when obstructive platelet-rich thrombi grow to become occlusive thrombi in the absence of perfusion beyond the obstruction through collateral blood vessels. Fibrin and erythrocytes comprise the outer layer of occlusive red thrombi that are formed on the surface of the platelet-rich inner core of the thrombus. While thrombolytic therapy effectively dissolves the occluding fibrin-rich portion of the thrombus, this process releases clot-bound thrombin and re-exposes the underlying disrupted plaque, which releases potent thrombogenic stimuli. This newly released thrombin then activates platelets, leading to platelet aggregation. In addition, activated platelets secrete a variety of factors associated with rethrombosis and thrombin production (e.g., PAI-1, fibrinogen, factor V) and bind factors Xa, VIIIa, and IXa, which are involved in further thrombin production. Platelet reactivity also may increase after thrombolysis. Use of platelet-aggregation inhibitors such as eptifibatide concomitantly with thrombolytic therapy may counter the thrombogenic activity of these agents and minimize the risk of reocclusion.

● Inhibition of Platelet Aggregation

Eptifibatide reversibly inhibits platelet aggregation by preventing the binding of fibrinogen, von Willebrand factor, and other adhesive ligands to resting and active GP IIb/IIIa receptors. Inhibition of platelet aggregation by eptifibatide occurs in a dose- and concentration-dependent manner via an increase in GP IIb/IIIa-receptor occupancy (as determined by ex vivo platelet aggregation assay with the direct thrombin inhibitor D-phenylalanyl-L-propyl-L-arginyl chloromethyl ketone [PPACK]). Some platelet-aggregation inhibitors such as aspirin, ticlopidine, and clopidogrel prevent platelet activation in response to one or more agonists (thromboxane A_2, adenosine diphosphate); agonists not affected by these drugs may continue to induce platelet aggregation. However, GP IIb/IIIa-receptor inhibitors such as abciximab, eptifibatide, and tirofiban prevent platelet aggregation regardless of the initial stimulus. In vitro studies indicate that eptifibatide is not effective in displacing fibrinogen cross-links from GP IIb/IIIa-receptors in platelet-rich thrombi when the bond between fibrinogen and GP IIb/IIIa becomes irreversible.

Following a single 180-mcg/kg IV dose of eptifibatide in healthy individuals or patients with NSTE ACS and/or those undergoing PCI, platelet aggregation was inhibited by greater than 90% within 15 minutes at physiologic calcium concentrations based on ex vivo platelet-aggregation assays using PPACK as the anticoagulant. Inhibition of platelet aggregation by eptifibatide also may depend on the degree of initial platelet activation, which may be influenced by concurrent disease states. In an ex vivo study, the concentration of eptifibatide needed to inhibit 50% of ADP-induced platelet aggregation was lowest in healthy men, higher in patients undergoing PCI, and highest in patients with NSTE ACS, perhaps reflecting differences in existing platelet activation. The pharmacodynamics of eptifibatide do not appear to be affected by age; differences in pharmacodynamic effects among ethnic groups have not been assessed.

● Hemostatic Effects

Since the effect of eptifibatide on platelet aggregation is rapidly reversible following cessation of the infusion, the drug has a modest effect on hemostatic indices (e.g., bleeding times) and platelet function. Normal hemostasis is restored more rapidly than with abciximab, a monoclonal antibody that dissociates very slowly from the GP IIb/IIIa-receptor.

When eptifibatide was administered alone or in combination with heparin in clinical trials, bleeding time was prolonged approximately twofold. At steady-state plasma eptifibatide concentrations in patients with NSTE ACS (who received a 180-mcg/kg IV loading dose followed by IV infusion of 2 mcg/kg per minute) or who were undergoing PCI (who received a 135-mcg/kg IV loading dose followed by IV infusion of 0.5 mcg/kg per minute) and also were receiving concomitant aspirin and heparin, bleeding time was prolonged up to 5 times the control value. Ex vivo ADP-induced platelet aggregation using PPACK in patients with NSTE ACS was restored toward baseline values (i.e., to less than 50% inhibition) within 4 hours after cessation of an eptifibatide infusion (180-mcg/kg IV loading dose followed by IV infusion of 2 mcg/kg per minute for 72–96 hours); 6 hours after discontinuance of the eptifibatide infusion, bleeding time averaged 1.4 times the control value. Data from an ex vivo platelet aggregation assay in these patients indicated a GP IIb/IIIa-receptor occupancy of less than 60% 8 hours after discontinuance of the eptifibatide infusion.

When administered alone, eptifibatide usually does not affect prothrombin time (PT) or activated partial thromboplastin time (aPTT).

● Effect of Calcium Concentration on Platelet-Aggregation Assays

The reported inhibitory effect of eptifibatide on platelet aggregation depends on the free calcium concentration (and therefore the type of anticoagulant used) in the samples to be assayed, which is negatively correlated with the inhibitory activity and can affect interpretation of results of platelet function tests. (See Laboratory Test Interferences.)

PHARMACOKINETICS

The pharmacokinetics of eptifibatide in healthy individuals are linear, and plasma concentrations are proportional to dose following IV loading doses of 90–250 mcg/kg and IV infusion rates of 0.5–3 mcg/kg per minute. Concomitant administration of aspirin or heparin does not appear to affect the pharmacokinetics of eptifibatide, nor does gender.

● Absorption

With recommended IV loading and maintenance infusions of eptifibatide, peak plasma drug concentrations occur within 5 minutes of IV injection and steady-state drug concentrations are attained within 4–6 hours. Following IV administration of an eptifibatide loading dose of 135 mcg/kg and an IV infusion of 0.5 mcg/kg per minute for 20–24 hours, plasma drug concentrations at steady state averaged 291 ng/mL in patients undergoing percutaneous coronary intervention (PCI). In geriatric patients with coronary artery disease, plasma concentrations are increased compared with those in younger adults. Following IV administration of an eptifibatide loading dose of 180 mcg/kg and IV infusion of 2 mcg/kg per minute for 24 or 72 hours, steady-state plasma drug concentrations (as determined using population pharmacokinetic methods) in patients with non-ST-segment-elevation acute coronary syndromes (NSTE ACS) or those undergoing PCI reportedly averaged 2.2 or 1.5 mcg/mL, respectively. In healthy individuals receiving eptifibatide infusion rates of 0.5–2 mcg/kg per minute for 24 hours, steady-state plasma drug concentrations reportedly average approximately 0.3–1.1 mcg/mL. In patients with moderate to severe renal impairment (estimated Cl_{cr} less than 50 mL/minute), steady-state plasma concentrations double.

Eptifibatide has a rapid onset and short duration of action; maximal inhibition of platelet aggregation occurs within 15 minutes after initiation of therapy and is rapidly reversible. Within 4 hours after cessation of drug infusion, platelet aggregation returned to greater than 50% of baseline in patients with NSTE ACS receiving recommended dosages of eptifibatide (180-mcg/kg IV loading dose followed by infusion of 2 mcg/kg per minute) and to less than 30% of peak values in patients undergoing PCI and receiving recommended dosages of the drug (135-mcg/kg IV loading dose followed by infusion of 0.5 mcg/kg per minute). Platelet aggregation usually returns toward normal within 4–8 hours after discontinuing eptifibatide in patients with NSTE ACS or ST-segment-elevation myocardial infarction (STEMI).

● Distribution

Eptifibatide is approximately 25% bound to plasma proteins, principally (9–16%) to albumin. The volume of distribution of eptifibatide in patients with coronary artery disease is about 185–260 mL/kg and is somewhat higher (220–270 mL/kg) in healthy individuals. It is not known whether eptifibatide is distributed into milk in humans.

● **Elimination**

Eptifibatide is eliminated by renal and nonrenal mechanisms. The drug appears to undergo rapid and nonmetabolic degradation in the urinary bladder after its elimination from plasma. Eptifibatide is metabolized principally through deamidation to a metabolite that has approximately 41% of the platelet-aggregation inhibitory activity of the parent compound, and through formation of other more polar metabolites. Approximately 27% of a dose of eptifibatide is broken down in plasma into naturally occurring amino acids; no major non-amino acid metabolites have been detected in plasma in humans. Following IV administration of a single, ^{14}C-radiolabeled dose of eptifibatide (135 mcg/kg) in healthy men, 34, 19, and 13% of the radioactivity was recovered in urine within the first 24 hours as parent compound, deamidated metabolite, and polar metabolites (as detected by radiochromatography), respectively. In healthy men receiving a single, radiolabeled IV dose of the drug (135 mcg/kg), 98, 1.5, and 0.8% of the dose was recovered in urine, feces, and breath carbon dioxide, respectively. In vitro studies indicate that eptifibatide is not extensively bound to plasma proteins; therefore, the drug may be removed from plasma by hemodialysis.

Plasma concentrations of eptifibatide decline in a biexponential manner following IV injection or infusion of the drug. The half-life of eptifibatide in patients with coronary artery disease averages 2.5–2.8 hours. In healthy individuals, half-life of the drug reportedly averages 0.83–2.4 hours. Clearance of eptifibatide in patients with coronary disease is 55–80 mL/kg per hour; clearance of the drug is twofold higher in healthy individuals. Plasma clearance of eptifibatide is proportional to body weight and estimated creatinine clearance and inversely proportional to age. Following a single IV dose of ^{14}C-radiolabeled eptifibatide (135 mcg/kg) in healthy men, renal clearance averaged approximately 40–50% of total body clearance. Clearance is reduced by 50% in patients with moderate to severe renal impairment (estimated Cl_{cr} less than 50 mL/minute). Total body clearance in geriatric patients with coronary artery disease is lower than that in younger adults.

CHEMISTRY AND STABILITY

● **Chemistry**

Eptifibatide, a synthetic cyclic heptapeptide, is a selective platelet-aggregation inhibitor. Eptifibatide, like abciximab and tirofiban, has been referred to as a platelet glycoprotein (GP) IIb/IIIa-receptor inhibitor. The drug is similar in structure to barbourin, a peptide constituent of the venom of the southeastern pigmy rattlesnake, *Sistrurus m. barbouri*.

Eptifibatide is composed of 6 amino acids and a mercaptopropionyl (desamino cysteinyl) residue with an interchain disulfide bridge between the cysteine amide and the mercaptopropionyl moieties. The active domain of eptifibatide contains a modified lysine-glycine-aspartate (KGD) amino acid sequence similar to the physiologic arginine-glycine-aspartate (RGD) sequence in von Willebrand's factor, vitronectin, fibrinogen, and fibronectin, adhesive ligands that bind to platelet glycoprotein (GP) IIb/IIIa receptors on activated platelets and cause platelet

aggregation. The substitution of lysine for arginine on the binding site in eptifibatide increases the selectivity of binding to the GP IIb/IIIa receptor.

Commercially available eptifibatide injection is a clear, colorless, sterile solution of the drug in sterile water for injection; sodium hydroxide and citric acid have been added to adjust the pH to 5.25. Eptifibatide is insoluble in nonpolar solvents such as hexane (0.02 mg/mL), but is freely soluble in polar aqueous solvents and in highly polar solvents such as dimethyl sulfoxide (exceeding 400 mg/mL). Eptifibatide has pK_as of 4 and exceeding 12.5.

● **Stability**

Eptifibatide should be refrigerated at between 2–8°C and protected from light until administration. Commercially available eptifibatide injection has an expiration date of 24 months following the date of manufacture when stored as directed. The injection may be transferred to room temperature storage (15–30°C) for a period not to exceed 2 months. When stored at room temperature, the injection container should be marked to indicate that any unused vials should be discarded after 2 months or by the manufacturer's labeled expiration date (whichever comes first). The manufacturer states that vials of the injection that have been left unrefrigerated only for a brief period (i.e., the vial is still cool to the touch) may be returned to refrigeration without the need to alter the expiration date.

The manufacturer states that eptifibatide is chemically and physically compatible (i.e., no evidence of precipitation, color or pH change, or loss of potency) with, and may be administered in the same IV line as alteplase, atropine, dobutamine, heparin, lidocaine, meperidine, metoprolol, midazolam, morphine, nitroglycerin, or verapamil. Eptifibatide is chemically/physically incompatible with furosemide (i.e., precipitate formation within 1 hour of mixing, exceeding 40% loss of furosemide potency at 24 hours, and decrease in pH from about 8.9 to 5.4), and these drugs should *not* be administered through the same IV line. Eptifibatide may be administered in the same IV line with 0.9% sodium chloride injection or 0.9% sodium chloride and 5% dextrose injection. With either vehicle, the infusion may contain up to 60 mEq/L of potassium chloride. No incompatibilities have been observed between eptifibatide and IV administration sets, and no data are available concerning the compatibility of eptifibatide with polyvinyl chloride (PVC) bags.

PREPARATIONS

Excipients in commercially available drug preparations may have clinically important effects in some individuals; consult specific product labeling for details.

Eptifibatide

Parenteral		
Injection, for IV Use	2 mg/mL (20 mg)	Integrilin®, Schering
	0.75 mg/mL (75 mg)	Integrilin®, Schering

† Use is not currently included in the labeling approved by the US Food and Drug Administration.

Selected Revisions September 18, 2017, © Copyright, November 1, 1999, American Society of Health-System Pharmacists, Inc.

Prasugrel Hydrochloride

20:12.18 • PLATELET-AGGREGATION INHIBITORS

■ Prasugrel hydrochloride, a thienopyridine P2Y12 platelet adenosine diphosphate (ADP)-receptor antagonist, is a platelet-activation and -aggregation inhibitor.

USES

● Acute Coronary Syndrome

Patients Managed with Percutaneous Coronary Intervention

Prasugrel is used in combination with aspirin for the reduction of thrombotic cardiovascular events (e.g., stent thrombosis, myocardial infarction [MI]) in patients with acute coronary syndrome (ACS) undergoing percutaneous coronary intervention (PCI). Prasugrel is used in patients with unstable angina or non-ST-segment-elevation MI (NSTEMI) undergoing PCI and in patients with ST-segment-elevation MI (STEMI) managed with primary or nonprimary/delayed (i.e., after medical treatment) PCI.

Dual antiplatelet therapy with a P2Y12 receptor inhibitor (e.g., clopidogrel, prasugrel, ticagrelor) and aspirin is part of the current standard of care in patients with ACS, including those undergoing PCI. The American College of Cardiology (ACC)/American Heart Association (AHA) has issued guidelines for treatment options and duration of dual antiplatelet therapy in patients with ACS. Recommendations are similar for patients with non-ST-segment-elevation ACS (NSTE-ACS) and those with ST-segment-elevation MI (STEMI) since both are part of the spectrum of ACS. Decisions about the duration of dual antiplatelet therapy should be individualized based on the risks of bleeding versus benefits of ischemic reduction, clinical judgment, and patient preference. Aspirin should almost always be continued indefinitely; therefore, recommendations are given for the duration of P2Y12 inhibitor therapy in patients treated with dual antiplatelet therapy. While the addition of a P2Y12 inhibitor to aspirin therapy reduces ischemic complications, this occurs at the expense of increased bleeding; a similar risk-benefit trade-off should be considered when determining whether to use a prolonged versus shorter duration of dual antiplatelet therapy. ACC/AHA generally recommends considering shorter duration dual antiplatelet therapy for patients at reduced ischemic, but high bleeding, risk and longer duration antiplatelet therapy for patients at high ischemic, but reduced bleeding, risk.

The current ACC/AHA guideline recommends that in patients with ACS who undergo PCI and stent implantation (bare-metal or drug-eluting), P2Y12 inhibitor therapy should be given for at least 12 months; in such patients who have tolerated dual antiplatelet therapy without bleeding complications and who do not have a high risk of bleeding, continuation of dual antiplatelet therapy for longer than 12 months may be reasonable. With regard to the specific P2Y12 inhibitor, evidence supports the use of clopidogrel, prasugrel, or ticagrelor in ACS patients treated with PCI. Patients with a history of stroke or transient ischemic attack (TIA) should not be administered prasugrel. In addition, prasugrel should not be initiated in patients who are likely to undergo urgent coronary artery bypass grafting (CABG) because of increased risk of bleeding. (See Bleeding under Cautions.) In patients treated with dual antiplatelet therapy after coronary stent implantation who subsequently undergo CABG, P2Y12 inhibitor therapy should be resumed after surgery to complete 12 months of therapy. Use of more potent P2Y12 inhibitors such as prasugrel or ticagrelor over clopidogrel results in a greater reduction in ischemic events and stent thrombosis, but increases the risk of bleeding. The ACC/AHA guideline states that it is reasonable to consider the use of prasugrel or ticagrelor over clopidogrel for maintenance P2Y12 inhibitor therapy in ACS patients treated with dual antiplatelet therapy after coronary stent implantation. The European Society of Cardiology (ESC) generally recommends dual antiplatelet therapy with prasugrel or ticagrelor over clopidogrel in patients with NSTE-ACS undergoing PCI; according to ESC, clopidogrel should be considered an alternative in such patients unable to receive prasugrel or ticagrelor therapy.

Unlike clopidogrel, genetic polymorphism of the cytochrome P-450 (CYP) 2C19 isoenzyme does not appear to affect the pharmacodynamic or clinical response to prasugrel. The Clinical Pharmacogenetics Implementation Consortium (CPIC) guidelines recommend the use of prasugrel as an alternative antiplatelet agent to clopidogrel when not contraindicated in patients who are poor or intermediate metabolizers of CYP2C19. Prasugrel inhibits platelet aggregation more potently and rapidly than standard or higher dosages of clopidogrel and is associated with less interpatient variability in antiplatelet effects. Such improved inhibition of platelet aggregation was associated with reduced ischemic events (e.g., reductions in stent thrombosis and MI) in a large prospective randomized study of patients with ACS undergoing PCI; however, these benefits were accompanied by an increased risk of bleeding. When considering the use of prasugrel over other P2Y12 inhibitors, clinicians should balance the anticipated greater benefits with prasugrel against the increased risk of bleeding, and also consider the patient populations in whom the drugs have been used. Some evidence suggests that certain patient populations (e.g., those with diabetes or previous MI) are more likely to benefit from prasugrel's greater inhibition of platelet aggregation, while others (e.g., geriatric patients, those with low body weight or history of stroke/TIA) may experience harm.

The indication for prasugrel in patients with ACS is based principally on results of a multicenter, randomized, double-blind parallel group study (Trial to Assess Improvement in Therapeutic Outcomes by Optimizing Platelet Inhibition with Prasugrel-Thrombolysis in Myocardial Infarction [TRITON-TIMI 38]) comparing efficacy and safety of prasugrel and clopidogrel in 13,608 high-risk ACS patients undergoing planned PCI. Patients with unstable angina or NSTEMI were eligible if they had ischemic manifestations lasting 10 minutes or more within 72 hours prior to randomization, a TIMI risk score of at least 3, and either ST-segment deviation of at least 1 mm or elevated levels of a cardiac biomarker of necrosis; patients with STEMI were enrolled within 12 hours of symptom onset if primary PCI was planned or within 14 days after receiving medical treatment for STEMI (delayed PCI). Patients received either clopidogrel (300-mg loading dose followed by 75 mg daily) or prasugrel (60-mg loading dose followed by 10 mg daily) for 6–15 months. The loading dose of the study drug was administered anytime between randomization and 1 hour after the patient was transferred from the cardiac catheterization laboratory; most patients (approximately 75%) received the study drug after the first coronary guidewire was placed or within 1 hour of PCI. Patients were required to receive concomitant treatment with aspirin 75–325 mg daily; other standard therapies (e.g., heparin, platelet glycoprotein [GP] IIb/IIIa-receptor inhibitors) were given at the discretion of the treating clinician. Most patients (94%) received at least one intracoronary stent.

Treatment with prasugrel resulted in a 19% relative reduction in the composite primary end point of cardiovascular death, nonfatal MI, or nonfatal stroke compared with clopidogrel; such benefits were apparent within 3 days and persisted throughout the duration of the study (median 14.5 months). The reduction in the primary end point was largely driven by a substantial reduction in MI (new or recurrent) with little or no difference in the incidence of stroke or cardiovascular death (other than from MI) between groups. Reductions in the rate of stent thrombosis and urgent target-vessel revascularization also favored prasugrel. Stent thrombosis was substantially reduced with prasugrel in patients who received at least one intracoronary stent irrespective of the stent type (bare-metal or drug-eluting).

The benefit of prasugrel in reducing ischemic events in the TRITON-TIMI 38 study was accompanied by an increased risk of bleeding. Major and minor bleeding complications, including life-threatening and fatal bleeding, occurred more frequently in patients receiving prasugrel compared with clopidogrel. (See Bleeding under Cautions.) When efficacy and bleeding end points were combined, the net clinical benefit (defined as death from any cause, nonfatal MI, nonfatal stroke, or non-CABG-related nonfatal TIMI major hemorrhage) favored prasugrel over clopidogrel in the overall study population, but not in all subgroups. In post hoc analyses, patients 75 years of age or older, those weighing less than 60 kg, and those with previous stroke or TIA were identified as subgroups experiencing no net clinical benefit and possibly harm with such therapy. In patients with diabetes mellitus, however, a trend towards greater efficacy of prasugrel compared with nondiabetics was noted without a relative increase in major bleeding. Results of such subgroup analyses should be considered exploratory and should be interpreted with caution.

The prasugrel dosage regimen used in the TRITON-TIMI 38 study (60-mg loading dose, 10 mg daily maintenance dosage) has been shown to produce substantially greater and more consistent inhibition of platelet aggregation than that produced by a clopidogrel loading dose of 600 mg and maintenance dosage of 150 mg daily, dosages higher than current FDA-labeled loading and maintenance dosages. In addition, while it is generally recommended that antiplatelet agents be administered promptly upon presentation or diagnosis in patients with ACS, administration of prasugrel and clopidogrel in the TRITON-TIMI 38 study was delayed until after coronary anatomy was determined to be appropriate for PCI. Therefore, this study does not provide information on the comparative efficacy and safety of clopidogrel and prasugrel in dosages that provide equivalent inhibition of platelet aggregation, nor does it directly address the potential effects on efficacy of routine pretreatment with clopidogrel or prasugrel before diagnostic cardiac catheterization.

In an open-label randomized study (Intracoronary Stenting and Antithrombotic Regimen: Rapid Early Action for Coronary Treatment [ISAR-REACT 5]), prasugrel (60 mg loading dose followed by 10 mg daily) was compared with ticagrelor (180 mg loading dosage followed by 90 mg twice daily) in approximately 4000 patients with ACS who were scheduled to undergo angiography. At 1 year, the primary end point (composite of death, MI, or stroke) occurred in substantially fewer patients treated with prasugrel (6.9%) compared with ticagrelor (9.3%). The incidence of major bleeding was not different between prasugrel and ticagrelor (5.4 and 4.8%, respectively). Limitations of the trial include its open-label design and limited data in patients who were treated medically or with CABG.

Although it is generally recommended that antiplatelet therapy be administered promptly in the management of ACS because many cardiovascular events occur within hours of initial presentation, results of a randomized, double-blind, event-driven study found no benefit with administering a loading dose of prasugrel prior to diagnostic coronary angiography compared with at the time of PCI. The ACCOAST (A Comparison of Prasugrel at the Time of Percutaneous Coronary Intervention Or as Pretreatment At the Time of Diagnosis in Patients with Non-ST-Elevation Myocardial Infarction) trial compared the effects of early administration of prasugrel prior to coronary angiography with a strategy of administration at the time of PCI in 4033 patients with NSTE-ACS. The pretreatment strategy did not reduce the rate of major ischemic events, but increased rates of major bleeding. Based on results of the ACCOAST study as well as other available evidence, routine pretreatment with prasugrel is not recommended in patients with NSTE-ACS; prasugrel should be initiated after coronary anatomy has been defined.

Patients Managed Medically without Revascularization

Prasugrel is currently not indicated for use in ACS patients undergoing conservative noninvasive (medical) management without revascularization†. Use of prasugrel in this setting was evaluated in the TRILOGY-ACS (The Targeted Platelet Inhibition to Clarify the Optimal Strategy to Medically Manage Acute Coronary Syndromes) study, which was a double-blind, randomized study that compared prolonged treatment with prasugrel compared with clopidogrel in more than 7000 patients with NSTE-ACS. Results showed that prasugrel was not superior to clopidogrel in reducing the primary end point of cardiovascular death, MI, or stroke despite signs of intensified platelet inhibition with prasugrel. However, there was a divergence in treatment effect after 12 months where prasugrel appeared to reduce the risk of ischemic events. An increased risk of bleeding was not observed with prasugrel compared with clopidogrel in this study. Additional study is needed to understand the differences in response to intensified platelet inhibition in patients undergoing medical management only (without revascularization) compared with those undergoing revascularization who receive prasugrel.

● Atrial Fibrillation and Acute Coronary Syndrome

Prasugrel also has been used in patients with atrial fibrillation and ACS. These patients have an indication for treatment with both antiplatelet and anticoagulant agents. Selecting the optimal antithrombotic regimen in such patients can be challenging.

Current guidelines from AHA/ACC/Heart Rhythm Society and other experts provide recommendations regarding the use of P2Y12 inhibitors in patients with atrial fibrillation who present with ACS and/or undergo PCI. Because of the high risk of bleeding associated with triple antithrombotic therapy (aspirin, a P2Y12 inhibitor, and an oral anticoagulant), experts generally recommend against this approach for most patients. Studies have shown similar or lower rates of bleeding and similar rates of thrombotic events with dual antithrombotic therapy compared with triple therapy. Therefore, the preferred strategy in patients with atrial fibrillation who have undergone recent PCI is to use dual antithrombotic therapy

(an oral anticoagulant and a P2Y12 inhibitor); if triple therapy is considered in patients with high thrombotic risk and low bleeding risk, such therapy should be given over the shortest possible duration. Clopidogrel is generally recommended over the more potent P2Y12 inhibitors (prasugrel, ticagrelor) when combination antithrombotic therapy is needed because of a lower risk of bleeding. Prasugrel is currently not recommended as a component of triple therapy because of limited data to support its use in this setting.

DOSAGE AND ADMINISTRATION

● Administration

Prasugrel is administered orally without regard to meals.

● Dosage

Dosage of prasugrel hydrochloride is expressed in terms of prasugrel.

Acute Coronary Syndromes

Patients Undergoing PCI

For the reduction of thrombotic cardiovascular events in patients with ACS undergoing PCI, the manufacturer recommends a loading dose of 60 mg of prasugrel, followed by 10 mg once daily. Aspirin (75–325 mg daily) should be given concomitantly. The majority of patients in the TRITON-TIMI 38 study received the loading dose of prasugrel after the first coronary guidewire was placed or within 1 hour of PCI.

In the TRITON-TIMI 38 study, the loading dose of prasugrel was administered after coronary anatomy was established in patients with NSTE-ACS and in patients with STEMI presenting more than 12 hours after symptom onset. The loading dose was administered at the time of diagnosis in STEMI patients presenting within 12 hours of symptom onset; however, most of these patients received prasugrel at the time of PCI. In patients who received urgent CABG after treatment with prasugrel, the risk of bleeding was substantially increased. (See Bleeding under Cautions.)

In the ACCOAST study that was conducted in patients with NSTEMI, administration of the prasugrel loading dose prior to diagnostic coronary angiography did not offer any clear benefit compared with administration at the time of PCI. The risk of bleeding was increased with early administration in patients undergoing PCI or early CABG.

The optimum duration of prasugrel therapy has not been determined. However, in patients undergoing PCI with stent implantation, premature discontinuance of any antiplatelet therapy (i.e., aspirin, a P2Y12-receptor antagonist) increases the risk of stent thrombosis, myocardial infarction, and death; therefore, long-term (e.g., at least 12 months) dual antiplatelet therapy is recommended in such patients unless the risk of bleeding outweighs the anticipated net benefit. (See Discontinuance of Therapy under Cautions.) Recommendations for duration of dual antiplatelet therapy can be found in ACC/AHA guidelines. (See Acute Coronary Syndrome under Uses.)

Discontinuance in Patients Undergoing Invasive Procedures

Prasugrel should be discontinued prior to elective surgery. In patients who require elective CABG, discontinuance of prasugrel therapy is recommended at least 7 days prior to surgery. Prasugrel should not be initiated in those who are likely to undergo emergent CABG. To minimize the risk of adverse cardiac events, thienopyridines, including prasugrel, and other antiplatelet therapy should be resumed as soon as possible after temporary discontinuance of therapy for adverse effects or invasive procedures. (See Discontinuance of Therapy under Cautions.)

● Special Populations

Renal Impairment

No dosage adjustment necessary in patients with renal impairment.

Hepatic Impairment

No dosage adjustment necessary in patients with mild to moderate hepatic impairment (Child-Pugh Class A and B). Not studied in patients with severe hepatic disease.

Patients Weighing <60 kg

A prasugrel maintenance dosage of 5 mg daily may be considered in patients weighing less than 60 kg, although safety and efficacy of this lower dosage has not been established. In patients with stable coronary artery disease, mean platelet inhibition was similar between patients weighing less than 60 kg receiving prasugrel 5 mg and patients weighing 60 kg or more receiving prasugrel 10 mg. However, the relationship between platelet inhibition and clinical activity has not been established. (See Bleeding under Cautions.)

Other Special Populations

Not known whether dosage adjustments based on age, weight or other patient characteristics will maintain effectiveness of prasugrel while decreasing risk of bleeding.

CAUTIONS

● Contraindications

● Presence of active pathological bleeding (e.g., peptic ulcer, intracranial hemorrhage).

● History of transient ischemic attack (TIA) or stroke.

● Hypersensitivity (e.g., anaphylaxis) to prasugrel or any component of the formulation.

● Warnings/Precautions

Warnings

Bleeding

Use of prasugrel is associated with a risk of serious, sometimes fatal bleeding. A black box warning about the risk of bleeding is included in the prescribing information for the drug. Major bleeding (defined as intracranial hemorrhage or clinically overt bleeding associated with a decline in hemoglobin concentration of at least 5 g/dL) and minor bleeding (defined as overt bleeding with a decrease in hemoglobin concentration of at least 3 g/dL but less than 5 g/dL) were more frequent in patients receiving prasugrel versus clopidogrel in the TRITON-TIMI 38 study. Major hemorrhage not related to CABG occurred in 2.4% of patients receiving prasugrel compared with 1.8% of those receiving clopidogrel; this included higher rates of life-threatening and fatal bleeding. Life-threatening bleeding occurred mostly at GI, intracranial, retroperitoneal, or puncture sites. CABG-related major bleeding occurred in 13.4% of patients receiving prasugrel versus 3.2% of those receiving clopidogrel. (See Bleeding Related to Coronary Artery Bypass Grafting under Cautions.) Subgroup analysis indicated that patients 75 years of age or older, those weighing less than 60 kg, and those with prior stroke or TIA had higher rates of bleeding than patients without these characteristics. Additional risk factors for bleeding include recent trauma, recent surgery (e.g., CABG), recent or recurrent GI bleeding, active peptic ulcer disease, severe hepatic impairment, and concurrent use of drugs that increase risk of bleeding (e.g., oral anticoagulants, sustained use of nonsteroidal anti-inflammatory agents, thrombolytic agents).

Prasugrel should not be used in patients who are actively bleeding and/or who have a history of stroke or TIA. The drug also should not be initiated in those who are likely to undergo emergent CABG. Bleeding should be suspected in any patient who is hypotensive and has recently undergone coronary angiography, PCI, CABG, or any other surgical procedure, even if there are no overt manifestations of bleeding. Risk of bleeding appears to be highest in the first several days of therapy. If possible, bleeding should be managed without discontinuing prasugrel; premature discontinuance is associated with an increased risk of subsequent cardiovascular events. (See Discontinuance of Therapy under Cautions.) If bleeding occurs, platelet transfusions may be given to restore homeostasis; however, such transfusions may be less effective within 6 hours of a loading dose or 4 hours of a maintenance dose. Withholding a dose of prasugrel is unlikely to resolve a bleeding episode or prevent bleeding associated with an invasive procedure because of the drug's prolonged inhibitory effects on platelet aggregation.

Patients with a History of TIA or Stroke

In the TRITON-TIMI 38 study, patients with a history of TIA or ischemic stroke had no evidence of a clinical benefit from prasugrel and a strong trend towards a higher rate of major bleeding compared with clopidogrel. In this subgroup, a higher incidence of stroke was observed during treatment with prasugrel compared with clopidogrel (6.5 or 1.2%, respectively). In patients without such a history, the incidence of stroke was similar (0.9 or 1%, respectively) between treatment groups. Strokes occurring in patients receiving prasugrel were both thrombotic and hemorrhagic, while those reported with clopidogrel were all thrombotic. Based on these findings, prasugrel should not be initiated in patients with a history of stroke or TIA and generally should be discontinued in those who experience an adverse cerebrovascular event during therapy.

Bleeding Related to Coronary Artery Bypass Grafting

Risk of bleeding is increased in patients receiving prasugrel who undergo CABG. (See Bleeding under Cautions.) CABG-related major and minor bleeding events occurred more frequently in patients receiving prasugrel than with clopidogrel in the TRITON-TIMI 38 study (14.1 versus 4.5%, respectively). Bleeding was reported in 26.7 or 5% of those who received prasugrel or clopidogrel, respectively, within 3 days prior to CABG. Although the bleeding risk decreased in both groups when the last dose of study drug was given 4–7 days prior to surgery, the incidence of bleeding remained comparatively higher in the prasugrel-treated group (11.3 versus 3.4%, respectively). Prasugrel should not be initiated in patients who are likely to undergo urgent CABG. In patients scheduled for CABG, prasugrel should be discontinued at least 7 days prior to surgery. CABG-related bleeding may be treated with blood product transfusions (e.g., packed red blood cells, platelets); however, platelet transfusions within 6 hours of a loading dose or 4 hours of a maintenance dose of prasugrel may be less effective in restoring homeostasis.

Other Warnings/Precautions

Discontinuance of Therapy

Prasugrel should be discontinued in patients who develop active bleeding, stroke, or TIA during therapy. (See Contraindications under Cautions.) The drug also should be discontinued prior to elective surgery to minimize risk of bleeding, but should be reinitiated postoperatively as soon as possible (e.g., once adequate hemostasis has been established).

In general, treatment with a thienopyridine derivative should not be discontinued prematurely, particularly in the first few weeks after ACS, because of the subsequent increased risk of cardiovascular events. Premature discontinuance of any antiplatelet therapy (e.g., thienopyridine derivative, aspirin) in patients undergoing PCI and coronary artery stent placement has been associated with an increased risk of stent thrombosis, MI, and/or death. (See Patients Managed with Percutaneous Coronary Intervention under Uses.)

Results of the DAPT (Dual Antiplatelet Therapy) study, a randomized, placebo-controlled, double-blind study, found that patients who received 30 months of dual antiplatelet therapy (aspirin plus clopidogrel or prasugrel) following placement of a drug-eluting stent had substantially reduced rates of stent thrombosis and major adverse cardiovascular and cerebrovascular events compared with those who received 12 months of dual antiplatelet therapy. However, the longer duration of therapy was associated with a higher incidence of moderate to severe bleeding and also an unexpected finding of an increased rate of noncardiovascular mortality (principally related to trauma or cancer). The increased risk of death with longer treatment was seen in the patients who received clopidogrel, but not in those who received prasugrel.

Patients should not discontinue prasugrel without first consulting their prescribing clinician, even if instructed by another health-care professional (e.g., dentist) to stop such therapy. Prior to scheduling an invasive procedure, patients should inform their clinicians (including dentists) that they currently are taking prasugrel, and clinicians performing the invasive procedure should consult with the prescribing clinician before discontinuing prasugrel therapy. If prasugrel must be temporarily discontinued because of an adverse event, therapy should be reinstituted as soon as possible.

Thrombotic Thrombocytopenic Purpura

Thrombotic thrombocytopenic purpura (TTP) has been reported rarely with use of thienopyridine derivatives, sometimes after brief exposure (less than 2 weeks). TTP is a potentially fatal condition that is characterized by thrombocytopenia, microangiopathic hemolytic anemia (schistocytes on peripheral blood smear), neurologic findings, renal dysfunction, and fever. Urgent treatment (e.g., plasmapheresis) is required in patients who develop TTP.

Specific Populations

Pregnancy

There are no adequate and well-controlled studies of prasugrel in pregnant women. In animal studies, no structural malformations were observed when rats and rabbits were administered prasugrel during organogenesis at dosages up to 30 times the recommended human dosage. The benefits and risks of prasugrel and possible risks to the fetus should be considered when prescribing prasugrel to a pregnant woman.

Lactation

Prasugrel metabolites are distributed into milk in rats; it is not known whether the drug is distributed into milk in humans. The drug should be used in nursing women only if the anticipated benefits to the mother outweigh potential risks to the infant.

Pediatric Use

Safety and efficacy of prasugrel have not been established in pediatric patients.

Geriatric Use

Geriatric patients, particularly those 75 years of age and older, appear to be at greater risk of bleeding (including fatal bleeding) with prasugrel therapy compared with younger patients. In the TRITON-TIMI 38 trial, about 39% of patients were 65 years of age or older and 13% were 75 years of age or older. Risk of bleeding increased with advancing age in both prasugrel and clopidogrel treatment groups. Among patients 75 years of age or older, fatal bleeding was more common with prasugrel than with clopidogrel (1 or 0.1%, respectively); symptomatic intracranial hemorrhage also was reported more frequently with prasugrel (0.8 or 0.3%, respectively). Mean exposure to the active metabolite of prasugrel is approximately 19% higher in patients 75 years or older compared with younger patients. Prasugrel generally should be avoided in patients 75 years of age or older because of a higher risk of bleeding and uncertain efficacy, but use may be considered in certain patients with high-risk conditions (e.g., diabetes, previous MI) in whom a greater net clinical benefit has been demonstrated.

Hepatic Impairment

Pharmacokinetics of prasugrel's active metabolite and its inhibition of platelet aggregation are similar in patients with mild to moderate hepatic impairment (Child-Pugh class A and B) and healthy individuals. The pharmacokinetics and pharmacodynamics of the drug have not been specifically studied in patients with severe hepatic impairment; however, such patients generally are at higher risk of bleeding.

Renal Impairment

Pharmacokinetics of prasugrel's active metabolite and its inhibition of platelet aggregation in patients with moderate renal impairment (creatinine clearance of 30–50 mL/minute) are similar to those observed in healthy individuals. In patients with end-stage renal impairment, exposure to the active metabolite was decreased to about half that of healthy individuals and those with moderate renal impairment; however, these patients are generally at higher risk of bleeding.

Low Body Weight

In the TRITON-TIMI 38 study, patients with low body weight (less than 60 kg) had an increased exposure to the active metabolite of prasugrel and an increased risk of bleeding. Clearance of prasugrel's active metabolite appears to increase exponentially with increasing body weight. (See Bleeding under Cautions.)

● Common Adverse Effects

Bleeding, including life-threatening and fatal bleeding, is the most commonly reported adverse reaction in patients receiving prasugrel.

DRUG INTERACTIONS

● Drugs Affecting or Metabolized by Hepatic Microsomal Enzymes

Prasugrel is metabolized by the cytochrome P-450 (CYP) microsomal enzyme system, principally by isoenzymes 3A4 and 2B6, and to a lesser extent by isoenzymes 2C9 and 2C19. In vitro studies indicate that prasugrel is not likely to inhibit CYP isoenzymes 1A2, 2C9, 2C19, 2D6, and 3A or induce CYP isoenzymes 1A2 or 3A. Prasugrel is a weak inhibitor of CYP2B6.

Clinically important drug interactions mediated by CYP isoenzymes are considered unlikely with prasugrel. Studies have shown that if one of the CYP isoenzymes involved in the metabolism of prasugrel is inhibited, others remain capable of forming the active metabolite. CYP3A4 inhibitors such as verapamil, diltiazem, indinavir, ciprofloxacin, clarithromycin, and grapefruit juice are not expected to have a substantial effect on the pharmacokinetics of prasugrel's active metabolite. In healthy individuals receiving prasugrel, concomitant administration of ketoconazole (a potent inhibitor of CYP3A4) decreased maximum concentrations of prasugrel's active metabolite by 34–46%, but did not alter systemic exposure or degree of inhibition of platelet aggregation. Similarly, CYP3A4 inducers (e.g., rifampin, carbamazepine) are not expected to substantially alter the pharmacokinetic or pharmacodynamic response to prasugrel; concomitant administration of rifampin, a potent inducer of CYP3A4 and CYP2B6, did not affect formation of the active prasugrel metabolite nor its ability to inhibit platelet aggregation. Concomitant administration of prasugrel and drugs principally metabolized by CYP2B6 (e.g., halothane, cyclophosphamide, propofol, nevirapine) may increase plasma concentrations and exposure of the concomitant drug; however, clinically important interactions are not expected because of weak inhibition of CYP2B6.

● Drugs Affecting Gastric Acidity

May be used concomitantly with proton pump inhibitors and histamine H_2-receptor antagonists. Maximum plasma concentrations of the active metabolite of prasugrel are decreased by 14 or 29% with ranitidine or lansoprazole, respectively, but systemic exposure of this metabolite is unaffected. In a pharmacokinetic study in healthy adults, concomitant daily administration of a single loading dose of prasugrel 60 mg with lansoprazole 30 mg decreased systemic exposure and peak plasma concentrations of prasugrel's active metabolite but did not affect inhibition of platelet aggregation.

● Digoxin

May be administered concomitantly. Prasugrel is not an inhibitor of the P-glycoprotein transport system and is not expected to affect clearance of digoxin.

● HMG-CoA Reductase Inhibitors (Statins)

May be used concomitantly without dosage adjustments. Coadministration of prasugrel and atorvastatin 80 mg daily had little effect on exposure to the active prasugrel metabolite and no effect on inhibition of platelet aggregation.

● Nonsteroidal Anti-inflammatory Agents

Increased risk of bleeding with concomitant long-term use of aspirin or other nonsteroidal anti-inflammatory agents (NSAIAs).

● Opiate Agonists

Concomitant use of opiate agonists may delay and reduce absorption of the active metabolite of prasugrel because of slowed gastric emptying. The use of a parenteral antiplatelet agent should be considered in patients with ACS who require coadministration of opiate agonists.

● Thrombolytic Agents

Increased risk of bleeding with concomitant use.

● Warfarin

Increased risk of bleeding in patients receiving concomitant therapy with warfarin. Bleeding time substantially prolonged with concomitant administration of a single 15-mg dose of warfarin.

● Other Antiplatelet or Antithrombotic Agents

The manufacturer states that prasugrel may be administered concomitantly with aspirin, heparin, and GP IIb/IIIa-receptor inhibitors. Concomitant use of prasugrel and aspirin 150 mg daily increased bleeding time compared with use of either drug alone, but inhibition of platelet aggregation was not altered. In a study in healthy individuals, concomitant use of prasugrel and aspirin 325 mg daily resulted in greater inhibition of platelet aggregation, but the combination was well tolerated; no clinically important bleeding events occurred. When a single IV dose of unfractionated heparin sodium 100 units/kg was given concomitantly with prasugrel, bleeding time was increased without any associated changes in coagulation or inhibition of platelet aggregation.

Although evidence from drug interaction studies generally is lacking, increased risk of bleeding is likely with concomitant use of prasugrel and other antiplatelet or antithrombotic agents; caution is advised.

DESCRIPTION

Prasugrel hydrochloride, a thienopyridine derivative structurally and pharmacologically related to clopidogrel, is a platelet-activation and aggregation inhibitor. Like clopidogrel, prasugrel is a prodrug that requires hepatic transformation to an active metabolite (R-138727) in order to exert its pharmacologic effect on the P2Y12 platelet adenosine diphosphate (ADP) receptor. Compared with clopidogrel, prasugrel inhibits ADP-mediated platelet aggregation more rapidly, more consistently, and to a greater extent; inhibition of platelet aggregation is at least 30% greater with prasugrel than with standard dosages of clopidogrel. The increased potency of prasugrel appears to be a result of more efficient conversion of the prodrug to its active metabolite. Genetic polymorphisms of cytochrome P-450 (CYP) isoenzymes (e.g., CYP2B6, CYP2C9, CYP2C19, CYP3A5) do not appear to affect the pharmacologic or clinical response to prasugrel.

Prasugrel is a P2Y12 platelet ADP-receptor antagonist; the active metabolite binds irreversibly to the P2Y12 class of ADP receptors on the surface of platelets, thereby inhibiting ADP-dependent platelet activation and aggregation for the life of the platelet (approximately 7–10 days). Following a 60-mg loading dose of prasugrel, at least 50% inhibition of platelet aggregation is achieved at 1 hour in approximately 90% of patients. Approximately 70% inhibition of platelet aggregation is achieved at steady state within 3–5 days with prasugrel 10 mg daily. The maximum inhibition of platelet aggregation attained with a 60-mg loading dose of prasugrel is about 80%. Platelet aggregation gradually returns to baseline values within 5–9 days following discontinuance of the drug. The relationship between inhibition of platelet aggregation and clinical activity of prasugrel has not been established.

Prasugrel is rapidly and completely (at least 79% of a dose) absorbed from the GI tract following oral administration. Once absorbed, the drug is rapidly hydrolyzed by esterases to an inactive thiolactone that is subsequently metabolized to the active metabolite (R-138727) by CYP enzymes (principally by 3A4 and 2B6, and to a lesser extent by 2C9 and 2C19). Compared with clopidogrel, which undergoes a 2-step oxidative process, prasugrel requires only a single step for metabolic activation; this may explain its faster onset of action. Peak plasma concentrations of the active metabolite of prasugrel are reached approximately 30 minutes after an oral dose, and there is no evidence of accumulation with repeated administration. The active metabolite of prasugrel is approximately 98% bound to human albumin. Administration of a high-fat or high-caloric meal to healthy individuals did not affect exposure to the active metabolite but decreased peak plasma concentrations by 49% and delayed time to peak concentration from 0.5 to 1.5 hours.

The manufacturer states that the elimination half-life of prasugrel's active metabolite (R-138727) averages about 7 hours (range: 2–15 hours), although a half-life of 3.7 hours has been reported in some studies. However, inhibition of platelet aggregation following prasugrel administration persists for about 96 hours. Prasugrel is eliminated principally in urine (68%) and to a lesser extent

in feces (27%) as inactive metabolites. Dialysis is not expected to remove the active metabolite.

● *Pharmacogenomics*

Genetic polymorphisms of the CYP2B6, CYP2C9, CYP2C19, or CYP3A5 enzyme do not appear to affect the pharmacokinetic or pharmacodynamic response of prasugrel.

ADVICE TO PATIENTS

- Importance of patients reading the FDA-approved patient labeling (medication guide).
- Importance of counseling patients about potential risks versus benefits of prasugrel.
- Importance of informing patients that they will bruise and/or bleed more easily and that a longer than usual time will be required to stop bleeding when taking prasugrel. Importance of informing clinicians about any unexpected, prolonged, or excessive bleeding, or blood in urine or stool.
- Importance of patients taking prasugrel exactly as prescribed and not discontinuing therapy without first consulting the prescribing clinician.
- Importance of informing clinicians (e.g., physicians, dentists) about prasugrel therapy before any invasive procedure or surgery is scheduled. Clinician performing invasive procedure should consult with prescribing clinician before discontinuing prasugrel.
- Importance of informing clinicians of changes in health status that may increase risk of bleeding, including recent trauma, GI bleeding, kidney or liver dysfunction, and decreases in weight.
- Risk of thrombotic thrombocytopenic purpura (TTP); importance of advising patients to immediately seek medical attention if they experience manifestations such as fever, weakness, extreme skin paleness, purple skin patches, yellowing of the skin or eyes, or otherwise unexplained neurologic changes.
- Importance of informing clinicians of existing or contemplated concomitant therapy, including prescription and OTC drugs, particularly drugs that affect bleeding (e.g., warfarin, NSAIAs).
- Importance of women informing clinicians if they are or plan to become pregnant or plan to breast-feed.
- Importance of informing patients of other important precautionary information. (See Cautions.)

PREPARATIONS

Excipients in commercially available drug preparations may have clinically important effects in some individuals; consult specific product labeling for details.

Prasugrel Hydrochloride

Oral

Tablets, film-coated	5 mg (of prasugrel)*	**Effient®**, Eli Lilly and Company (also promoted by Daiichi Sankyo Inc.)
	10 mg (of prasugrel)	**Effient®**, Eli Lilly and Company (also promoted by Daiichi Sankyo Inc.)

* available from one or more manufacturer, distributor, and/or repackager by generic (nonproprietary) name

Selected Revisions October 4, 2021, © Copyright, December 1, 2010, American Society of Health-System Pharmacists, Inc.

Ticagrelor

20:12.18 • PLATELET-AGGREGATION INHIBITORS

- Ticagrelor, a nonthienopyridine, reversible, P2Y12 platelet adenosine diphosphate (ADP)-receptor antagonist, is a platelet-activation and -aggregation inhibitor.

USES

● Acute Coronary Syndrome or History of Myocardial Infarction

Ticagrelor is used in combination with aspirin to reduce the risk of cardiovascular death, myocardial infarction (MI), and stroke in patients with acute coronary syndrome (ACS) or history of MI.

Patients with Acute Coronary Syndrome

Dual antiplatelet therapy with a P2Y12 receptor inhibitor (e.g., clopidogrel, prasugrel, ticagrelor) and aspirin is part of the current standard of care in patients with ACS. The American College of Cardiology (ACC)/American Heart Association (AHA) has issued guidelines for treatment options and duration of dual antiplatelet therapy in patients with ACS. Recommendations are similar for patients with non-ST-segment-elevation ACS (NSTE-ACS) and those with ST-segment-elevation MI (STEMI) since both are part of the spectrum of ACS. Decisions about the duration of dual antiplatelet therapy should be individualized based on the risks of bleeding versus benefits of ischemic reduction, clinical judgment, and patient preference. Aspirin should almost always be continued indefinitely; therefore, recommendations are given for the duration of P2Y12 inhibitor therapy in patients treated with dual antiplatelet therapy. While the addition of a P2Y12 inhibitor to aspirin therapy reduces ischemic complications, this occurs at the expense of increased bleeding; a similar risk-benefit trade-off should be considered when determining whether to use a prolonged versus shorter duration of dual antiplatelet therapy. ACC/AHA generally recommends considering shorter duration dual antiplatelet therapy for patients at reduced ischemic, but high bleeding, risk and longer duration dual antiplatelet therapy for patients at high ischemic, but reduced bleeding, risk.

The AHA/ACC guideline recommends that in patients with ACS who are managed medically (without revascularization or reperfusion therapy) or with percutaneous coronary intervention (PCI) and stent implantation (bare-metal or drug-eluting), P2Y12 inhibitor therapy should be given for at least 12 months; in such patients who have tolerated dual antiplatelet therapy without bleeding complications and who do not have a high risk of bleeding, continuation of dual antiplatelet therapy for longer than 12 months may be reasonable. With regard to the specific P2Y12 inhibitor, evidence supports the use of clopidogrel or ticagrelor in medically-managed ACS patients; clopidogrel, prasugrel, or ticagrelor may be used in ACS patients treated with PCI. In patients undergoing coronary artery bypass grafting (CABG), P2Y12 inhibitor therapy should be resumed after surgery to complete 12 months of therapy.

Use of more potent P2Y12 inhibitors such as ticagrelor or prasugrel over clopidogrel results in a greater reduction in ischemic events and stent thrombosis, but increases the risk of bleeding. In some clinical guidelines, ticagrelor or prasugrel is preferred or suggested for maintenance P2Y12 inhibitor therapy in ACS patients while clopidogrel is considered an alternative when these more potent P2Y12 inhibitors cannot be used. Other clinicians state that because of its reversibility and faster offset of action, ticagrelor may be preferred over the irreversible P2Y12-receptor antagonists (clopidogrel, prasugrel) in patients with ACS who are being managed with an early invasive strategy (e.g., those in whom coronary anatomy has not been determined and who are likely to undergo CABG). Ticagrelor also may be a reasonable alternative in patients who are nonresponsive to clopidogrel based on studies demonstrating that ticagrelor not only inhibits platelet aggregation in clopidogrel nonresponders, but also produces greater inhibition of platelet aggregation than clopidogrel in patients who remain nonresponsive to clopidogrel. Unlike clopidogrel, genetic polymorphism of the cytochrome P-450 (CYP) 2C19 isoenzyme does not appear to affect the pharmacodynamic or clinical response to ticagrelor. The Clinical Pharmacogenetics Implementation

Consortium (CPIC) guidelines recommend the use of ticagrelor as an alternative antiplatelet agent to clopidogrel in patients who are poor or intermediate metabolizers of CYP2C19. When selecting an appropriate antiplatelet regimen for the management of patients with ACS, clinicians should consider individual risks of ischemia and bleeding as well as the specific characteristics (e.g., adverse effects, drug interaction potential) of the drugs.

The indication for ticagrelor in patients with ACS is based principally on an international, randomized, double-blind study (PLATO). The study compared efficacy and safety of ticagrelor versus clopidogrel in reducing the rate of death from vascular causes, nonfatal MI (excluding silent MI), or nonfatal stroke in more than 18,000 patients hospitalized for ACS. Because the study was designed to evaluate patients at hospital presentation or diagnosis ("upstream"), patients across the spectrum of ACS were enrolled, including those in whom conservative or invasive management was planned. Approximately 50% of patients were pretreated with clopidogrel prior to randomization; PCI was performed in about 64% of the patients and approximately 10% underwent CABG. Within 24 hours of symptom onset and before PCI, patients received either ticagrelor (180-mg loading dose followed by 90 mg twice daily) or clopidogrel (300-mg loading dose followed by 75 mg daily) in addition to aspirin and other standard therapy; treatment was continued for at least 6 months up to a maximum of 12 months. Those undergoing PCI received an additional loading dose of study drug at the time of PCI (90 mg of ticagrelor if more than 24 hours had passed since the initial loading dose or 300 mg of clopidogrel at the investigator's discretion). Aspirin was administered to all patients in the study at a recommended loading dose of 160–500 mg and daily maintenance dosage of 75–100 mg; higher maintenance dosages (e.g., 325 mg daily for 6 months following stent placement) were permitted based on clinician judgment.

In the PLATO study, ticagrelor substantially reduced the rate of the primary composite end point of cardiovascular death, nonfatal MI, or nonfatal stroke compared with clopidogrel (Kaplan-Meier estimates of 9.8 versus 11.7%). The treatment difference was apparent by 30 days and maintained throughout the 12-month study period. The benefit associated with ticagrelor was based on a reduction in the incidence of cardiovascular death and MI, but not stroke. Although the overall rate of stroke was similar between the treatment groups, hemorrhagic strokes were more frequent in patients receiving ticagrelor. Among patients who received a coronary artery stent during the study, the rate of stent thrombosis was substantially lower with ticagrelor than with clopidogrel regardless of the type of stent (bare-metal or drug-eluting). In addition, death from any cause was reduced with ticagrelor (1.4% absolute reduction, 22% relative reduction). Some experts state, however, that additional study is needed to confirm this mortality benefit since all-cause mortality was not evaluated as a primary outcome in the PLATO study. The overall rate of major bleeding was similar for patients who received ticagrelor or clopidogrel; however, ticagrelor was associated with a higher incidence of non-CABG related major bleeding, including fatal intracranial bleeding. (See Bleeding under Cautions.)

In the PLATO study, clinical outcomes with ticagrelor generally were consistent across subgroups of patients with ACS regardless of whether a conservative or invasive management strategy was employed and regardless of the type of antiplatelet therapy received prior to the index ACS event. However, the benefits of ticagrelor appeared to be reduced in patients enrolled in North America compared with those enrolled in other regions. Results of additional statistical analyses of a variety of baseline and procedural differences between the US and non-US regions identified aspirin maintenance dosage as a possible factor accounting for this regional discrepancy. These analyses showed that ticagrelor was associated with a more favorable response than clopidogrel in patients receiving low (100 mg or less daily) maintenance dosages of aspirin. This was seen in both US and non-US patients; however, substantially more (about 54%) US patients were treated with aspirin dosages exceeding 300 mg daily, whereas patients in other countries rarely (only about 2% of patients) received such high aspirin dosages. Because of inherent limitations of subgroup analyses and the possibility that the effect of aspirin dosage on ticagrelor outcome could be due to chance, these findings should be interpreted with caution. Nevertheless, the manufacturer states that aspirin dosage should be limited to 75–100 mg daily in patients receiving ticagrelor; higher dosages do not have an established benefit in the management of ACS and may be associated with reduced efficacy of ticagrelor.

In an open-label randomized study (Intracoronary Stenting and Antithrombotic Regimen: Rapid Early Action for Coronary Treatment [ISAR-REACT 5]), prasugrel (60 mg loading dose followed by 10 mg daily) was compared with ticagrelor (180 mg loading dose followed by 90 mg twice daily) in approximately 4000 patients with ACS who were scheduled to undergo angiography. At 1 year, the primary end point (composite of death, MI, or stroke) occurred in substantially fewer patients treated with prasugrel (6.9%) compared with ticagrelor (9.3%). The incidence of major bleeding was not different between prasugrel and ticagrelor (4.8 and 5.4%, respectively). Limitations of the trial include its open-label design and limited data in patients who were treated medically or with CABG.

Patients with History of Myocardial Infarction

The initial indication for ticagrelor was expanded to include patients with a history of MI; in the clinical trial that established efficacy of ticagrelor for this indication (PEGASUS-TIMI 54), patients had a history of MI 1–3 years prior to study entry.

AHA/ACC states that in patients with stable ischemic heart disease (SIHD) being treated with dual antiplatelet therapy for an MI that occurred 1–3 years earlier, further continuation of such therapy may be reasonable if tolerated without any bleeding complications. Based on evidence from studies in post-MI patients, extended dual antiplatelet therapy for 18–36 months is associated with an absolute decrease in ischemic complications of approximately 1–3% and an absolute increase in bleeding complications of approximately 1%.

Use of ticagrelor for secondary prevention of MI is based on data from the randomized, double-blind, placebo-controlled, multicenter, multinational PEGASUS-TIMI 54 (Prevention of Cardiovascular Events in Patients with Prior Heart Attack Using Ticagrelor Compared to Placebo on a Background of Aspirin-Thrombolysis in Myocardial Infarction 54) trial. PEGASUS-TIMI 54 randomly assigned 21,162 patients (50 years of age or older) with a prior MI 1–3 years before enrollment and at least 1 additional high-risk feature (age 65 years or older, diabetes mellitus requiring drug therapy, creatinine clearance less than 60 mL/minute, evidence of multivessel coronary artery disease [CAD], or a second prior MI) to ticagrelor 90 mg twice daily, ticagrelor 60 mg twice daily, or placebo. All patients were also administered aspirin 75–150 mg daily. The primary efficacy end point was a composite of cardiovascular death, nonfatal MI, and nonfatal stroke; cardiovascular death and death from any cause were secondary end points. The primary safety end point was the occurrence of TIMI major bleeding. The median time from the qualifying MI to randomization was 1.7 years; 83% of patients had a history of PCI, and 59.4% had multivessel CAD. The median duration of follow-up was 33 months. Both ticagrelor dosages substantially reduced the rate of the primary composite end point compared with placebo, with Kaplan-Meier 3-year rates of 7.85% with ticagrelor 90 mg twice daily, 7.77% with ticagrelor 60 mg twice daily, and 9.04% with placebo. The occurrence of cardiovascular death and death from any cause was similar between the groups; however, there was a trend with ticagrelor toward a reduction in the rate of cardiovascular death alone. The treatment effect of ticagrelor appeared similar across major patient subgroups. The greatest reduction in ischemic events was seen in patients in whom P2Y12 inhibitor therapy either had not been discontinued or had been discontinued for no more than 30 days; there was no apparent benefit in patients who had stopped taking a P2Y12 inhibitor more than 1 year prior to study enrollment. The rates of TIMI major bleeding were increased in patients receiving ticagrelor compared with those receiving placebo. (See Bleeding under Cautions.)

• Coronary Artery Disease but No Prior Stroke or Myocardial Infarction

Ticagrelor is used in conjunction with aspirin to reduce the risk of an initial MI or stroke in patients with established CAD who are at high risk for these events. This indication is based on data from the randomized, double-blind, multicenter THEMIS (The Effect of Ticagrelor on Health Outcomes in Diabetes Mellitus Patients Intervention) study. In THEMIS, 19,220 patients (50 years of age or older) with stable CAD (defined as a history of PCI or CABG, or angiographic evidence of stenosis of at least 50% in at least 1 coronary artery) and type 2 diabetes mellitus were randomly assigned to ticagrelor plus aspirin or placebo plus aspirin. Ticagrelor was initially given at a dosage of 90 mg twice daily, but subsequently reduced to 60 mg twice daily after the PEGASUS-TIMI 54 results were known. Aspirin also was administered at a dosage of 75–150 mg daily. A composite of cardiovascular death, MI, or stroke was the primary efficacy end point, with TIMI major bleeding as the primary safety outcome. Enrolled patients had a median duration of diabetes of 10 years, and an estimated 25% reported having

diabetes-related complications. Over half (58%) of the patients had a history of PCI with or without stent placement; 21.8% had undergone CABG alone without PCI, and an additional 7% underwent both PCI and CABG. Patients with previous MI or stroke were excluded from the study. The median duration of follow-up was 39.9 months.

The primary composite efficacy end point occurred less frequently in the ticagrelor group compared to the placebo group (7.7 versus 8.5%, corresponding to Kaplan-Meier 3 year rates of 6.9 and 7.6%, respectively), with reduced incidences of MI and stroke driving the improved outcome with ticagrelor. There was no difference between treatment groups in cardiovascular death. Although the treatment effect was small, results of the THEMIS study support the use of ticagrelor in reducing the risk of a first MI and stroke in patients with CAD and type 2 diabetes mellitus. However, the reduced risk of ischemic events occurred at the expense of a higher risk of bleeding. The incidence of TIMI major bleeding occurred twice as often with ticagrelor than placebo. (See Bleeding under Cautions.)

Results of a predefined exploratory analysis of the THEMIS study showed no substantial difference between ticagrelor and placebo in irreversible harm (death from any cause, MI, stroke, fatal bleeding, or intracranial hemorrhage) suggesting that the drug does not have a favorable risk-benefit ratio among the patient population evaluated in the THEMIS study. In a substudy that was conducted in patients who had previous PCI (THEMIS-PCI), ticagrelor appeared to have a favorable net clinical benefit compared with patients without PCI, irrespective of time from the most recent PCI.

• Acute Ischemic Stroke or Transient Ischemic Attack

Ticagrelor is used in conjunction with aspirin to reduce the risk of stroke in patients with mild to moderate acute ischemic stroke (National Institutes of Health Stroke Scale [NIHSS] less than or equal to 5) or high-risk transient ischemic attack (TIA). This indication is based on results from the THALES (The Acute Stroke or Transient Ischemic Attack Treated with Ticagrelor and ASA for Prevention of Stroke and Death) trial. THALES was a randomized, placebo-controlled, double-blind, multicenter, multinational trial that enrolled 11,016 patients (40 years of age or older) with mild to moderate acute noncardioembolic ischemic stroke or high-risk TIA. Patients were randomly assigned to a 30-day regimen of either ticagrelor (180 mg as a loading dose, followed by 90 mg twice daily) plus aspirin or placebo plus aspirin within 24 hours after symptom onset. Aspirin was administered as a 300–325 mg loading dose on the first day of therapy followed by a maintenance dosage of 75–100 mg daily, with reduced loading doses recommended for patients who had already received aspirin after symptom onset but prior to randomization. The primary end point was a composite of stroke or death from randomization through 30 days of follow-up. Secondary end points included occurrence of the first subsequent ischemic stroke and overall disability. The first severe bleeding event was the primary safety outcome. Results from THALES revealed that the primary end point event occurred less frequently in the ticagrelor plus aspirin group compared to the aspirin only group (Kaplan-Meier event rate estimates of 5.4 versus 6.5%); the relative risk reduction was 17% and absolute risk reduction was 1.1%. The risk of a subsequent ischemic stroke was also reduced with ticagrelor plus aspirin compared with aspirin alone (5 versus 6.3%). Overall disability (defined as a score greater than 1 on the modified Rankin Scale [mRS]) was similar between the groups (incidence of about 24%). Severe bleeding occurred more frequently among patients who received ticagrelor and aspirin compared with those who received aspirin alone. (See Bleeding under Cautions.) The generalizability of these results is limited to the specific patient population studied and therefore excludes those with more severe stroke or cardioembolic stroke, those undergoing thrombectomy or thrombolysis, and those in whom treatment was administered more than 24 hours after symptom onset. An exploratory analysis of the THALES study evaluated time to occurrence of disabling stroke (progression of index event or new stroke) or death within 30 days, as measured by mRS; disabling stroke was defined as mRS greater than 1. Results of this analysis showed that ticagrelor plus aspirin substantially reduced the 30-day risk of disabling stroke or death compared with aspirin alone (4 versus 4.7%) and also produced a clinically meaningful reduction in disability burden following a recurrent ischemic stroke.

• Atrial Fibrillation and Acute Coronary Syndrome

Ticagrelor also has been used in patients with atrial fibrillation and ACS. These patients have an indication for treatment with both antiplatelet and anticoagulant agents. Selecting the optimal antithrombotic regimen in such patients can be challenging. Current guidelines from AHA/ACC/Heart Rhythm Society and other experts provide recommendations regarding the use of P2Y12 inhibitors in patients with atrial fibrillation who present with ACS and/or undergo PCI. Because of the high risk of bleeding associated with triple antithrombotic therapy (aspirin, a P2Y12 inhibitor, and an oral anticoagulant), experts generally recommend against this approach for most patients. Studies have shown similar or lower rates of bleeding and similar rates of thrombotic events with dual antithrombotic therapy compared with triple therapy. Therefore, the preferred strategy in patients with atrial fibrillation who have undergone recent PCI is to use dual antithrombotic therapy (an oral anticoagulant and a P2Y12 inhibitor); if triple therapy is considered in patients with high thrombotic risk and low bleeding risk, such therapy should be given over the shortest possible duration. Clopidogrel is generally recommended over the more potent P2Y12 inhibitors (prasugrel, ticagrelor) when combination antithrombotic therapy is needed because of a lower risk of bleeding; however, there is also some evidence to support the use of ticagrelor in this setting. The ACC Expert Consensus decision pathway states that ticagrelor may be used in place of clopidogrel in patients at high risk of stent thrombosis, although data are limited.

DOSAGE AND ADMINISTRATION

• Administration

Ticagrelor is administered orally without regard to meals.

If a dose is missed, the next dose should be taken at the regularly scheduled time.

Ticagrelor tablets may be crushed and mixed with water if a patient is unable to swallow the tablet whole. The mixture also may be administered via a nasogastric tube (CH8 or greater).

• Dosage

Acute Coronary Syndrome or History of Myocardial Infarction

For the reduction of thrombotic cardiovascular events (e.g., cardiovascular death, MI, and stroke) in patients with ACS or a history of MI, an initial ticagrelor loading dose of 180 mg is recommended, followed by a maintenance dosage of 90 mg twice daily during the first year. After the first year, the recommended maintenance dosage of ticagrelor is 60 mg twice daily.

Aspirin should be administered concomitantly at a maintenance dosage of 75–100 mg daily. The American College of Cardiology (ACC) states that the optimal maintenance dosage of aspirin in patients with CAD has not been established; recommendations for aspirin dosage vary across indications. However, since aspirin dosages exceeding 100 mg daily have been associated with reduced effectiveness of ticagrelor in patients with ACS, the manufacturer recommends that ticagrelor be administered with aspirin maintenance dosages of 75–100 mg daily. (See Reduced Response with Higher Aspirin Dosages in Patients with ACS under Cautions.)

The manufacturer makes no specific recommendations regarding duration of ticagrelor therapy; however, the drug was administered for up to 12 months in the PLATO study, and for this time period, ticagrelor was found to be superior to clopidogrel. Recommendations for duration of dual antiplatelet therapy can be found in the ACC/AHA guideline. (See Acute Coronary Syndrome or History of Myocardial Infarction under Uses.)

Transitioning from Clopidogrel to Ticagrelor Therapy

Patients may be transitioned directly from clopidogrel to ticagrelor therapy without interruption in antiplatelet effects. In clinical trials, patients who were switched from clopidogrel to ticagrelor received an initial loading dose of ticagrelor regardless of whether a previous loading dose of clopidogrel was given.

Coronary Artery Disease but no Prior Stroke or Myocardial Infarction

For reduction of the risk of initial MI or stroke in patients with CAD at high risk for these events, a dosage of ticagrelor 60 mg twice daily is recommended. Aspirin should be administered concomitantly at a maintenance dosage of 75–100 mg daily.

Acute Ischemic Stroke or Transient Ischemic Attack

For reduction of the risk of stroke in patients with acute ischemic stroke (NIHSS less than or equal to 5) or high-risk TIA, an initial ticagrelor loading dose of 180 mg is recommended, followed by a maintenance dosage of 90 mg twice daily for up to 30 days. Aspirin should be administered concomitantly, with a loading dose of 300–325 mg followed by a maintenance dosage of 75–100 mg daily.

Discontinuance of Therapy in Patients Undergoing Invasive Procedures

Antiplatelet agents generally should be discontinued prior to surgery or other invasive procedures to minimize the risk of perioperative bleeding. Whenever feasible, ticagrelor should be discontinued at least 5 days prior to surgery associated with a high risk of bleeding (e.g., CABG) and then resumed once hemostasis is achieved. If urgent CABG is required, the American College of Cardiology Foundation (ACCF) and AHA state that ticagrelor should be discontinued at least 24 hours before the procedure. In the PLATO study, ticagrelor was discontinued 24–72 hours prior to CABG surgery and was associated with bleeding rates comparable to those observed with clopidogrel when withheld for 5 days. (See Discontinuance of Therapy in Patients with Coronary Artery Disease under Cautions.)

• Special Populations

No dosage adjustments are necessary in patients with renal impairment or mild hepatic impairment (Child-Pugh class A).

CAUTIONS

• Contraindications

- History of intracranial hemorrhage.
- Active pathologic bleeding (e.g., peptic ulcer, intracranial hemorrhage).
- Hypersensitivity to the drug or any components.

• Warnings/Precautions

Warnings

Bleeding

Like other antiplatelet agents, ticagrelor increases the risk of bleeding, which may be serious and sometimes fatal. A black box warning about the risk of bleeding is included in the prescribing information for the drug. When all major and minor bleeding events were considered in the PLATO study, the overall risk of bleeding was somewhat greater with ticagrelor than with clopidogrel (7.7 versus 6.2%). There was a small but statistically significant increase in the rate of fatal intracranial bleeding with ticagrelor versus clopidogrel; fatal bleeding of other types was not increased. Many of the bleeding events occurred early, at the time of coronary angiography, percutaneous coronary intervention (PCI), CABG, or other procedures, but the risk persisted throughout therapy.

Major CABG-related bleeding occurred at a very high rate in the PLATO study (81.3% in patients treated with ticagrelor and 81.8% in patients treated with clopidogrel). There was no difference in major bleeding between the treatment groups when antiplatelet therapy was discontinued 5 days or less prior to CABG surgery, suggesting that the pharmacokinetic advantages of ticagrelor (i.e., faster offset of action, reversibility) do not translate into a lower risk of bleeding in patients undergoing CABG.

In the PEGASUS-TIMI 54 study, TIMI major bleeding was substantially increased in patients receiving ticagrelor compared with placebo (Kaplan-Meier 3-year rates of 2.6, 2.3, and 1.06% with ticagrelor 90 mg twice daily, ticagrelor 60 mg twice daily, and placebo, respectively). Although the incidence of fatal bleeding or nonfatal intracranial hemorrhage was less than 1% in all 3 groups over a treatment period of 3 years, the study excluded patients with recent bleeding, prior stroke, or need for oral anticoagulant therapy; therefore, findings from this study should not be generalized to other populations with increased risk of bleeding.

In the THEMIS study, TIMI major bleeding (2.2 versus 1%) and intracranial hemorrhage (0.7 versus 0.5%) occurred more frequently with ticagrelor than placebo. Discontinuance of therapy due to bleeding occurred more frequently among patients who received ticagrelor than those who received placebo (4.9 versus 1.3%).

Severe bleeding occurred more frequently among patients who received ticagrelor compared with those who received placebo in the THALES study (0.5 versus 0.1%). A composite of intracranial hemorrhage or fatal bleeding also was elevated with ticagrelor (0.4%) versus placebo (0.1%). Permanent discontinuance of treatment due to bleeding occurred more frequently among patients in the ticagrelor arm of the study (2.8 versus 0.6%).

Ticagrelor should not be used in patients who are actively bleeding or who have a history of intracranial hemorrhage. (See Contraindications under Cautions.) The drug also should not be initiated in patients undergoing urgent CABG. Risk factors for bleeding include advanced age, female gender, renal dysfunction, history of bleeding disorders, performance of PCI, and concurrent use of other drugs that increase risk of bleeding (e.g., anticoagulants, thrombolytic agents). If bleeding occurs, it should be managed without discontinuing ticagrelor if possible since premature discontinuance of such therapy increases the risk of subsequent cardiovascular events. (See Discontinuance of Therapy in Patients with Coronary Artery Disease under Cautions.)

In patients with acute ischemic stroke or TIA, ticagrelor is not recommended in those with NIHSS greater than 5 or in those receiving thrombolysis because of an increased risk of bleeding.

Reduced Response with Higher Aspirin Dosages in Patients with ACS

A black box warning about reduced response to ticagrelor with higher aspirin dosages in patients with ACS is included in the prescribing information for the drug. This finding was observed in patients receiving aspirin maintenance dosages exceeding 100 mg daily in the PLATO study. (See Acute Coronary Syndrome or History of Myocardial Infarction under Uses.) In patients with ACS, ticagrelor should be used in conjunction with an aspirin maintenance dosage of 75–100 mg daily; the manufacturer states that higher maintenance dosages may reduce the effectiveness of ticagrelor and should be avoided in patients with ACS.

Other Warnings and Precautions

Dyspnea

In clinical studies, dyspnea was commonly reported with ticagrelor (incidence of about 14% in PLATO and PEGASUS and 21% in THEMIS). In most cases, dyspnea was mild to moderate in severity and resolved with continued therapy. Discontinuance of ticagrelor therapy due to dyspnea occurred in 0.9, 1.0, 4.3, and 6.9% of patients in the PLATO, THALES, PEGASUS, and THEMIS trials, respectively. Although the mechanism of this adverse effect is unknown, it is thought to be an adenosine-mediated response. Ticagrelor does not appear to have adverse effects on cardiac or pulmonary function. Pulmonary function testing in a subset of patients from the PLATO study revealed no evidence of an adverse effect on pulmonary function after 1 month or after at least 6 months of chronic treatment with ticagrelor.

If new, prolonged, or worsening dyspnea related to ticagrelor occurs, the manufacturer states that no specific treatment is required and the drug may be continued without interruption if possible. If dyspnea is intolerable and results in discontinuance of ticagrelor therapy, another antiplatelet agent should be considered.

Discontinuance of Therapy in Patients with Coronary Artery Disease

In general, treatment with ticagrelor should not be discontinued prematurely in patients with CAD because this increases the risk of ischemic events. Premature discontinuance of antiplatelet therapy (e.g., P2Y12 inhibitors) in patients with coronary artery stents has been associated with an increased risk of ischemic cardiovascular events (e.g., stent thrombosis, MI, death). If temporary discontinuance of ticagrelor is necessary such as prior to elective surgery or for management of bleeding, the drug should be restarted as soon as possible.

Prior to scheduling surgery or a dental procedure, patients should inform clinicians and dentists that they are currently taking ticagrelor.

Bradyarrhythmias

Bradyarrhythmias, including ventricular pauses, have occurred in patients receiving ticagrelor. In the PLATO study, Holter monitor-detected ventricular pauses of at least 3 seconds were reported more frequently during the first week of therapy in patients receiving ticagrelor than in those receiving clopidogrel (5.8 versus 3.6%, respectively). There was no difference in the overall risk of clinically important bradycardic effects (e.g., syncope, need for pacemaker insertion) between the treatment groups. Ventricular pauses were mostly asymptomatic and attributed to sinoatrial nodal suppression.

Patients with a baseline increased risk of bradycardia (e.g., those with sick sinus syndrome, second- or third-degree AV block, syncope due to bradycardia without a pacemaker) were excluded from clinical studies and may be at elevated risk of bradyarrhythmia development with ticagrelor; therefore, some clinicians recommend that ticagrelor be used with caution in such patients.

• Laboratory Test Interference

Ticagrelor may cause false negative results in platelet function tests for patients with heparin-induced thrombocytopenia (e.g., heparin-induced platelet aggregation [HIPA] assay). Ticagrelor is not expected to affect PF4 antibody testing for heparin-induced thrombocytopenia.

Specific Populations

Pregnancy

Based on data from case reports in pregnant women, a drug-associated risk of major birth defects, miscarriage, or adverse maternal or fetal outcomes with ticagrelor therapy has not been identified.

Lactation

It is not known whether ticagrelor or its metabolites are distributed into human milk. The effects of the drug on breast-fed infants or on the production of milk are also unknown. Ticagrelor and its metabolites are distributed into milk in rats, indicating that the drug may be present in human milk. Breast-feeding is not recommended during ticagrelor therapy.

Pediatric Use

Safety and efficacy of ticagrelor have not been established in pediatric patients.

Geriatric Use

Of all enrolled patients in the PLATO, PEGASUS, THEMIS, and THALES trials, about 50% were 65 years of age or older and 15% were 75 years of age or older. No overall differences in effectiveness or safety were observed between geriatric and younger patients.

Age does not appear to substantially affect the pharmacokinetics of ticagrelor.

Hepatic Impairment

Because ticagrelor is metabolized by the liver, there is a potential for increased exposure and risk of bleeding in patients with impaired hepatic function. Ticagrelor use should be avoided in patients with severe hepatic impairment. Clinical experience with ticagrelor in patients with moderate hepatic impairment is limited; the risks and benefits of therapy should be considered in these patients.

Ticagrelor may be used in patients with mild hepatic impairment without the need for dosage adjustments. In a pharmacokinetic/pharmacodynamic study, systemic exposure to ticagrelor was slightly higher in individuals with mild (Child-Pugh class A) hepatic impairment compared with those with normal hepatic function; however, no clinically important effects of such impairment were observed.

Renal Impairment

No substantial differences in pharmacokinetics or clinical efficacy of ticagrelor have been observed in patients with renal impairment versus those with normal renal function.

Approximately 25% of patients enrolled in the PLATO study had chronic kidney disease (creatinine clearance less than 60 mL/minute); dosage reductions based on renal function were not required to prevent major bleeding. Patients with end-stage renal disease (ESRD) on dialysis were not enrolled in clinical studies of ticagrelor; however, clinically important differences in ticagrelor and metabolite concentrations, or in platelet inhibitory activity, are not expected in such patients receiving intermittent hemodialysis.

• Common Adverse Effects

The most common adverse reactions occurring at a rate greater than 5% in patients receiving ticagrelor include bleeding and dyspnea.

DRUG INTERACTIONS

● Drugs Affecting Hemostasis

Risk of bleeding may be increased when ticagrelor is used concomitantly with drugs that affect hemostasis (e.g., anticoagulants, thrombolytics, high doses of aspirin, chronic nonsteroidal anti-inflammatory agents [NSAIAs]). (See Bleeding under Cautions.)

Efficacy of ticagrelor may be affected by aspirin maintenance dosage. (See Aspirin under Drug Interactions.)

● Drugs Affecting or Metabolized by Hepatic Microsomal Enzymes

Ticagrelor is metabolized principally by the cytochrome P-450 (CYP) 3A4 isoenzyme. In vitro studies indicate that ticagrelor and its major active metabolite are weak inhibitors of CYP3A4 and potential activators of CYP3A5. Ticagrelor does not appear to inhibit CYP 1A2, 2C19, or 2E1.

Concomitant use of ticagrelor with potent CYP3A inhibitors (e.g., atazanavir, clarithromycin, itraconazole, ketoconazole, nefazodone, nelfinavir, ritonavir, saquinavir, voriconazole) may result in substantially increased exposure to ticagrelor and possible increased risk of bleeding, dyspnea, and other adverse events; such concomitant use should be avoided. Moderate CYP3A inhibitors (e.g., diltiazem) also may increase ticagrelor exposure, but to a lesser extent; therefore, these drugs may be used with ticagrelor without any dosage adjustments. Concomitant use of ticagrelor with potent inducers of CYP3A (e.g., carbamazepine, phenobarbital, phenytoin, rifampin) may result in substantially reduced plasma concentrations and possible reduced efficacy of ticagrelor; such concomitant use should be avoided.

Ticagrelor may increase serum concentrations of drugs metabolized by CYP3A4 (e.g., lovastatin, simvastatin). (See HMG-CoA Reductase Inhibitors [Statins] under Drug Interactions.)

● Drugs Affecting or Affected by P-glycoprotein Transport

Ticagrelor and its major active metabolite are substrates and weak inhibitors of the P-glycoprotein (P-gp) transport system. Increased serum concentrations of P-gp substrates (e.g., digoxin) are possible when these drugs are used concomitantly with ticagrelor; appropriate laboratory and/or clinical monitoring is recommended.

P-gp inhibitors (e.g., cyclosporine) can increase exposure to ticagrelor.

● Aspirin

When ticagrelor is used in conjunction with aspirin maintenance dosages exceeding 100 mg daily, efficacy of ticagrelor may be reduced. (See Reduced Response with Higher Aspirin Dosages in Patients with ACS under Cautions.)

Aspirin does not appear to substantially affect the pharmacokinetics of ticagrelor.

● Desmopressin

Desmopressin does not appear to affect peak concentrations of or systemic exposure to ticagrelor; no dosage adjustment is necessary when these drugs are used concomitantly.

● Digoxin

Concomitant administration of ticagrelor and digoxin did not substantially affect pharmacokinetics of digoxin; therefore, these drugs may be used concomitantly without dosage adjustments. However, because of the possibility of increased digoxin concentrations as a result of P-glycoprotein inhibition, serum digoxin concentrations should be monitored during initiation of and following any change in ticagrelor therapy.

● HMG-CoA Reductase Inhibitors (Statins)

Concomitant administration of ticagrelor and simvastatin (a CYP3A4 substrate) resulted in substantially increased exposure to simvastatin and its active metabolite. If ticagrelor is used concomitantly with simvastatin or lovastatin, the manufacturer states that dosage of the statin should not exceed 40 mg daily.

Concomitant administration of ticagrelor and atorvastatin did not substantially affect the pharmacokinetics of atorvastatin; therefore, these drugs may be used concomitantly without dosage adjustments.

● Ketoconazole

Concomitant use of ketoconazole 200 mg twice daily and ticagrelor substantially increased peak plasma concentrations of and systemic exposure to ticagrelor. Concomitant use of ticagrelor and ketoconazole should be avoided.

● Opiate Agonists

Concomitant use of opiate agonists may delay and reduce absorption of ticagrelor and its active metabolite because of slowed gastric emptying. Use of a parenteral antiplatelet agent should be considered in patients with ACS who require treatment with opiate agonists (e.g., morphine). Ticagrelor exposure was decreased and time to peak plasma concentration was delayed when the drug was coadministered with IV fentanyl or IV morphine in healthy adults and ACS patients undergoing PCI. Platelet inhibition was not delayed or decreased in healthy adults, but platelet aggregation was higher up to 3 hours after the loading dose was given in ACS patients who received these drugs concomitantly.

● Oral Contraceptives

In healthy women receiving stable dosages of an oral contraceptive containing ethinyl estradiol and levonorgestrel, administration of ticagrelor (90 mg twice daily) increased peak plasma concentrations of and systemic exposure to the estrogen component, but did not alter the pharmacokinetics of levonorgestrel. Ticagrelor is not expected to affect contraceptive efficacy; therefore, no dosage adjustment is necessary when the drug is administered with levonorgestrel or ethinyl estradiol.

● Proton-pump Inhibitors

Ticagrelor may be used concomitantly with proton-pump inhibitors. In a clinical study in patients with ACS, concomitant administration of ticagrelor with a proton-pump inhibitor did not affect the platelet response to ticagrelor.

● Rifampin

Concomitant administration of ticagrelor and rifampin 600 mg once daily substantially decreased peak plasma concentrations of and systemic exposure to ticagrelor. Concomitant use of ticagrelor and rifampin should therefore be avoided.

● Tolbutamide

Concomitant administration of ticagrelor and tolbutamide did not substantially affect pharmacokinetics of tolbutamide; therefore, the drugs may be used concomitantly without dosage adjustments.

● Other Concomitant Therapy

Concomitant administration of ticagrelor with heparin or enoxaparin did not affect peak plasma concentrations of or systemic exposure to ticagrelor; therefore, no dosage adjustments are required when these drugs are used concomitantly.

DESCRIPTION

Ticagrelor, a cyclopentyltriazolopyrimidine derivative, is a nonthienopyridine, P2Y12 ADP-receptor antagonist. In contrast to the thienopyridines (e.g., clopidogrel, prasugrel), ticagrelor binds reversibly to the P2Y12 ADP receptor and does not require hepatic transformation to exert its pharmacologic effect. Ticagrelor exhibits noncompetitive and reversible binding to the P2Y12 platelet ADP receptor, preventing signal transduction of the cyclic adenosine monophosphate (cAMP) pathway. This results in reduced exposure of fibrinogen binding sites to the platelet glycoprotein (GP) IIb/IIIa complex and subsequent inhibition of platelet activation and aggregation. In addition to platelet ADP-receptor blockade, ticagrelor inhibits reuptake of adenosine into erythrocytes, a mechanism that may account for some of the beneficial cardiovascular effects of the drug, while potentially contributing to some of its adverse effects (e.g., dyspnea, ventricular pauses).

Compared with clopidogrel, ticagrelor produces more rapid and effective inhibition of platelet aggregation and has a faster offset of action. In a 6-week randomized study comparing the antiplatelet effects of ticagrelor with clopidogrel in patients with stable coronary artery disease, higher and more consistent levels of platelet-aggregation inhibition as assessed by light transmission aggregometry were achieved with ticagrelor (180-mg loading dose followed by 90 mg twice daily) compared with clopidogrel (600-mg loading dose followed by 75 mg once daily). Following discontinuance of therapy, the offset of antiplatelet effect occurred at a faster rate with ticagrelor than with clopidogrel. The mean maximal inhibition of platelet aggregation following the last dose of study drug was higher with ticagrelor than clopidogrel initially, but approached equivalent levels after 24 hours. In patients receiving ticagrelor, inhibition of platelet aggregation returned to baseline levels 5 days after the last dose was administered. Maximum inhibition of platelet aggregation with ticagrelor is observed approximately 2 hours after a dose and is maintained for at least 8 hours. Patients who transition from clopidogrel to ticagrelor therapy appear to achieve additional inhibition of platelet aggregation (absolute increase of 26.4%). The relationship between inhibition of platelet aggregation and bleeding or thrombotic risk of either drug is not known.

Ticagrelor is rapidly absorbed following oral administration. The drug is metabolized principally by CYP isoenzyme 3A4 to an active metabolite that has similar antiplatelet activity as the parent drug. Plasma concentrations of ticagrelor and its active metabolite increase in a dose-dependent manner with peak concentrations achieved within approximately 1.5 and 2.5 hours, respectively. Ticagrelor is primarily eliminated in the feces and to a lesser extent in urine; less than 1% of a dose is recovered in urine as the parent drug and active metabolite. The mean terminal half-lives of ticagrelor and its active metabolite reportedly are about 7 and 9 hours, respectively. Both ticagrelor and its active metabolite are extensively (more than 99%) bound to human plasma proteins. Administration with a high-fat meal increases systemic exposure of ticagrelor by 21% and decreases peak plasma concentrations of the active metabolite by 22%, but has no effect on peak plasma concentrations of ticagrelor or on systemic exposure to the active metabolite.

● Pharmacogenomics

Genetic polymorphism of the CYP2C19 isoenzyme does not appear to affect the pharmacodynamic or clinical response to ticagrelor. In 2 genotype studies, ticagrelor demonstrated greater inhibition of platelet aggregation than clopidogrel regardless of CYP2C19 genotype or metabolizer status; in contrast, patients with a loss-of-function CYP2C19 variant had reduced antiplatelet effects during clopidogrel therapy. In addition, results of a genetic substudy of the PLATO trial showed that clinical outcomes with ticagrelor (reduction in the risk of

cardiovascular death, MI, or stroke) were superior to those with clopidogrel irrespective of CYP2C19 polymorphism.

ADVICE TO PATIENTS

- Importance of patients reading the FDA-approved patient labeling (medication guide).
- Importance of patients informing clinicians (e.g., physicians, dentists) about ticagrelor therapy before any surgery or dental procedure is performed.
- Importance of informing patients not to take aspirin dosages exceeding 100 mg daily; advise patients to not take any other aspirin-containing drugs.
- Importance of informing patients that they will bruise and/or bleed more easily and that a longer than usual time will be required to stop bleeding when taking ticagrelor. Importance of patients informing clinicians about any unexpected, prolonged, or excessive bleeding, or blood in urine or stool.
- Importance of informing patients that ticagrelor can cause dyspnea; advise patient to contact their clinician if they experience any unexpected shortness of breath.
- Importance of informing clinicians of existing or contemplated concomitant therapy, including prescription and OTC drugs, particularly drugs that affect bleeding risk (e.g., heparin, warfarin).
- Importance of women informing clinicians if they are or plan to become pregnant or plan to breast-feed.
- Importance of informing patients of other important precautionary information. (See Cautions.)

PREPARATIONS

Excipients in commercially available drug preparations may have clinically important effects in some individuals; consult specific product labeling for details.

Ticagrelor

Oral			
Tablets, film-coated	60 mg		Brilinta®, AstraZeneca
	90 mg*		Brilinta®, AstraZeneca
			Ticagrelor Tablets

* available from one or more manufacturer, distributor, and/or repackager by generic (nonproprietary) name

Selected Revisions October 4, 2021, © Copyright, November 27, 2012, American Society of Health-System Pharmacists, Inc.

Tirofiban

20:12.18 • PLATELET-AGGREGATION INHIBITORS

■ Tirofiban hydrochloride, a selective, competitive platelet-aggregation inhibitor, has been referred to as a platelet glycoprotein (GP) IIb/IIIa-receptor inhibitor.

USES

● Non-ST-Segment-Elevation Acute Coronary Syndromes

Tirofiban is used with anticoagulant therapy (e.g., heparin [referring throughout this monograph to unfractionated heparin], low molecular weight heparin), aspirin, and a P2Y12 platelet adenosine diphosphate (ADP)-receptor antagonist (e.g., clopidogrel, prasugrel, ticagrelor) to reduce the risk of acute cardiac ischemic events (death and/or myocardial infarction [MI]) in patients with unstable angina or non-ST-segment-elevation MI (NSTEMI) (i.e., non-ST-segment-elevation acute coronary syndromes [NSTE ACS]), both in patients who are to receive medical management and those undergoing percutaneous coronary intervention (PCI) (e.g., percutaneous transluminal coronary angioplasty [PTCA], stent placement, atherectomy). The goal of therapy in these patients is to maintain myocardial perfusion by inhibiting further platelet aggregation and thus preventing the progression of a nonocclusive thrombus to an occlusive thrombus. In clinical trials of tirofiban, NSTE ACS was defined by prolonged symptoms of cardiac ischemia (at least 10 minutes' duration within the previous 12–24 hours) occurring at rest or with minimal exertion that were associated with *transient* ST-segment changes (i.e., elevation or depression), T-wave inversion, or increased cardiac [MB] fraction of creatine kinase [CK, creatine phosphokinase, CPK]); patients who had MI associated with Q waves or *persistent* ST-segment elevation (exceeding 20 minutes) were not included in these studies. NSTEMI and unstable angina clinically may be indistinguishable at initial presentation and are managed similarly. Most of the patients in clinical trials of tirofiban received concomitant therapy with aspirin and IV heparin, and the efficacy and safety of tirofiban without adjunctive heparin and/or aspirin therapy have not been established.

Platelet glycoprotein (GP) IIb/IIIa-receptor inhibitors are used as an adjunct to standard therapeutic measures for managing NSTE ACS. These measures include therapy with aspirin and a P2Y12-receptor antagonist (e.g., clopidogrel, prasugrel, ticagrelor), nitrates (e.g., nitroglycerin), anticoagulant therapy (e.g., low molecular weight heparin, heparin), and β-blockers followed by either conservative medical management or early aggressive management, such as angiographic evaluation and revascularization procedures (e.g., PCI, coronary artery bypass grafting [CABG], coronary artery stent implantation) as required. Several meta-analyses of studies indicate that adjunctive therapy with a GP IIb/IIIa-receptor inhibitor can reduce the incidence of cardiac ischemic events, including subsequent MI and death, in patients with NSTE ACS. The benefits of GP IIb/IIIa-receptor inhibitors on mortality principally occur early during therapy (i.e., the first 48–96 hours).

The benefit of aspirin for secondary prevention of ischemic events in patients with NSTE ACS has been demonstrated in several studies and pooled analyses. Many clinicians recommend that all patients with NSTE ACS receive aspirin as soon as possible after hospital admission and then continued indefinitely unless they have documented hypersensitivity or other definite contraindications (e.g., active or recent major bleeding, peptic ulcer disease). (See Non-ST-Segment-Elevation Acute Coronary Syndromes under Thrombosis: Coronary Artery Disease and Myocardial Infarction, in Uses in Aspirin 28:08.04.24.) The American College of Cardiology Foundation (ACCF) and the American Heart Association (AHA) state that in patients with NSTE ACS in whom an initial invasive management strategy is planned, an additional antiplatelet agent (either clopidogrel or a GP IIb/IIIa-receptor inhibitor given IV) should be administered prior to diagnostic angiography ("upstream") as an adjunct to aspirin therapy. Eptifibatide or tirofiban is the preferred GP IIb/IIIa-receptor inhibitor for this use; abciximab is indicated only if there is no appreciable delay before angiography and PCI is likely to be performed.

Randomized controlled studies, including a meta-analysis of 16 randomized trials involving approximately 10,000 patients with ST-segment-elevation MI (STEMI) undergoing primary PCI, generally have failed to demonstrate benefits of GP IIb/IIIa-receptor blockade similar to those observed in patients with NSTE ACS. ACCF, AHA, the Society for Cardiovascular Angiography and Interventions (SCAI), and other experts currently do not recommend the *routine* use of GP IIb/IIIa-receptor inhibitors in patients with STEMI undergoing

PCI; however, selective use of these drugs as an adjunct to heparin may be reasonable in certain high-risk patients (e.g., those with large anterior MI and/or large thrombus). Studies evaluating the use of GP IIb/IIIa-receptor inhibitors in patients with NSTE ACS undergoing PCI have demonstrated reductions in ischemic outcomes, particularly in patients with high-risk features (e.g., elevated troponin); therefore, ACCF/AHA/SCAI states that it may be useful to administer a GP IIb/IIIa-receptor inhibitor at the time of PCI as an adjunct to heparin therapy in such high-risk patients who are not receiving bivalirudin and who are not adequately pretreated with clopidogrel. Regarding the choice of GP IIb/IIIa-receptor inhibitor in patients undergoing PCI, abciximab, "double-bolus" eptifibatide (i.e., two 180-mcg/kg direct IV injections given 10 minutes apart), and high-dose tirofiban (25 mcg/kg by direct IV injection) all have been shown to produce a high degree of platelet inhibition and reduce ischemic complications.

In patients with NSTE ACS with elevated troponin concentrations who were managed with conservative medical therapy, GP IIb/IIIa-receptor inhibitors were equally effective in men and women. However, in women with NSTE ACS who are not at high risk for acute cardiac ischemic events (e.g., no elevated troponin concentrations) and are managed with a conservative strategy, eptifibatide and tirofiban appear to show little benefit and may possibly have detrimental effects; these agents are not recommended by AHA in women at lower risk for adverse cardiac events.

The current labeled indication for tirofiban is based principally on the results of 3 large, randomized controlled studies evaluating the efficacy of tirofiban alone or in combination with heparin in patients with NSTE ACS, including those who subsequently underwent PCI. All patients in these studies also received aspirin (300–325 mg daily) for at least 48 hours after randomization (indefinitely in some patients) or within 12 hours prior to PCI unless the drug was contraindicated. In the Platelet Receptor Inhibition in Ischemic Syndrome Management in Patients Limited by Unstable Signs and Symptoms [PRISM-PLUS]) study, therapy with tirofiban (IV loading dose of 0.4 or 0.6 mcg/kg per minute given over 30 minutes followed by continuous IV infusion of 0.1 mcg/kg per minute for 48–108 hours) plus adjusted-dose heparin reduced the incidence of ischemic events compared with adjusted-dose heparin alone in patients with NSTE ACS. All patients received aspirin 325 mg daily unless the drug was contraindicated. Patients who received medical management alone (i.e., those not undergoing PCI) were given an IV loading dose of heparin sodium (5000 units) followed by an IV infusion (1000 units/hour) that was titrated to a target activated partial thromboplastin time (aPTT) of twice the control value. In patients undergoing PCI after at least 48 hours of medical management, the infusion of heparin sodium or heparin placebo was discontinued and an IV loading dose of heparin sodium (5000–7500 units) was administered, followed by an IV infusion (1000 units/hour) that was titrated with additional IV injections of heparin sodium as needed. Overall, patients in each group received the study drug(s) for an average of about 71 hours. Patients undergoing PCI received the study drug(s) for an average of 76 hours, of which an average of 15.4 hours was after PCI.

Beneficial effects of therapy with tirofiban and heparin were evident within 48 hours of initiating the tirofiban infusion and persisted for up to 6 months. The combined incidence of nonfatal MI or death at 48 hours in patients receiving tirofiban plus heparin was reduced by 66% (from 2.6 to 0.9%). The combined incidence of death, nonfatal MI, or refractory ischemia at 7 days (the primary composite end point) in patients receiving tirofiban plus heparin was reduced by 32% (from 17.9% to 12.9%); relative reductions of 47 and 30% occurred in the individual incidences of MI and refractory ischemia, respectively. The incidences of the composite end point at 30 days and 6 months, which also included hospital readmissions for unstable angina in patients receiving tirofiban and heparin, were reduced by 22% (from 22.3% to 18.5%) and 19% (from 32.1% to 27.7%), respectively, compared with heparin therapy alone. Data from a substudy of patients in PRISM-PLUS indicate that troponin I concentrations, a sensitive marker of myocardial injury or ischemia, were reduced to a greater extent in patients receiving tirofiban and heparin than in those receiving heparin alone. In another substudy of PRISM-PLUS, a reduction in angiographically evident thrombus formation was accompanied by an increase in blood flow to the affected coronary artery in patients receiving tirofiban and heparin. The incidence of major hemorrhage was similar in patients receiving tirofiban plus heparin (4%) or heparin alone (3%). Death occurred in 1.9% of each study group; no intracranial hemorrhages or hemorrhage-related deaths occurred in either group.

An initial third arm of the PRISM-PLUS study that included patients receiving tirofiban alone (without heparin) was discontinued prematurely because of unexpected excess mortality at 7 days (4.6%) compared with that in patients receiving heparin alone (1.1%); however, similar increases in the incidences of refractory ischemia, MI, or the composite end point did not occur. Also, another randomized study (Platelet Receptor Inhibition in Ischemic Syndrome Management [PRISM]) in which tirofiban therapy was compared with heparin therapy in patients with NSTE ACS demonstrated reductions in the composite end point of death, MI, or refractory ischemia at 48 hours and in mortality at 30 days. The PRISM-PLUS study included more high-risk patients than did the PRISM study (based on a higher percentage of patients with baseline ST-segment changes on ECG), and it has also been suggested that the large proportion (70%) of patients receiving IV heparin prior to randomization in the PRISM-PLUS study may have increased the likelihood of heparin rebound (i.e., ischemic events, including death, associated with recent or current heparin therapy in patients receiving concomitant aspirin). It has been suggested that the small number of events involved (16 of 345 patients receiving tirofiban alone versus 4 of 350 receiving heparin alone) also makes it possible that the higher incidence of death in PRISM-PLUS in patients receiving tirofiban alone compared with that in the PRISM study was attributable to chance. However, other variables potentially influencing the efficacy of tirofiban monotherapy (without heparin) include differences in the severity of NSTE ACS; the extent of use of PCI, angiography, or CABG; and the duration of the tirofiban infusion. Alternatively, concomitant thrombin inhibition (e.g., heparin, a low molecular weight heparin) may be needed for optimal efficacy of tirofiban, especially in high-risk patients with more severe NSTE ACS. Pooled analysis of data from the PRISM and PRISM-PLUS studies reportedly indicates that the effect of tirofiban therapy alone on mortality at 7 and 30 days was comparable to that of heparin therapy alone.

The efficacy of tirofiban in reducing composite clinical events associated with NSTE ACS in the PRISM-PLUS study was not affected by age or gender; the effect of race on efficacy could not be determined from the small number of non-white patients studied. Subgroup analyses indicated that beneficial effects of tirofiban and aspirin and heparin were particularly evident in patients receiving β-adrenergic blocking agents prior to study entry; benefit appeared to be consistent for all other factors studied (e.g., age, gender prior treatment with aspirin or heparin). While evaluation of patients who did or did not undergo PCI was not based on a randomized cohort, the incidence of the composite end point at 30 days in patients undergoing PCI was reduced from 15.3% in patients receiving heparin alone to 8.8% in patients receiving tirofiban and heparin (45% reduction).

In the Platelet Receptor Inhibition in Ischemic Syndrome Management [PRISM] study, therapy with tirofiban (IV loading dose of 0.6 mcg/kg per minute for 30 minutes followed by continuous IV infusion of 0.15 mcg/kg per minute for 48 hours) reduced the incidence of ischemic events compared with heparin sodium therapy (5000 units IV loading dose followed by 1000 units per hour for 48 hours, adjusted to achieve an aPTT of twice the control value). All patients received aspirin 300–325 mg before randomization and daily thereafter for at least 48 hours unless contraindicated. Approximately 25% of the patients in the PRISM study had evidence of NSTEMI, while 30% had no electrocardiographic evidence of cardiac ischemia (ST-segment depression).

Beneficial effects of tirofiban were apparent during infusion of the drug but diminished thereafter. The combined incidence of death, nonfatal MI, or refractory ischemia at 48 hours (the primary composite end point) was reduced by 33% in patients receiving tirofiban compared with those receiving heparin; reductions in the incidence of these end-point events at 7 and 30 days (10 and 8%, respectively) were no longer statistically significant. However, the effect of tirofiban on survival became more pronounced with time; death was less common at 30 days (risk reduction of 38%) in tirofiban-treated patients than in those who received heparin (2.3 versus 3.6% of patients, respectively). In patients treated with medical therapy alone (i.e., not undergoing PCI), the rate of death or MI at 30 days was reduced by 42% (from 6.2%, with heparin to 3.6% with tirofiban). The incidence of major bleeding was similar in both treatment groups.

In the Randomized Efficacy Study of Tirofiban for Outcome and Restenosis (RESTORE) study, therapy with tirofiban (IV loading dose of 10 mcg/kg followed by continuous IV infusion of 0.15 mcg/kg per minute for 36 hours, beginning immediately prior to coronary intervention) reduced the incidence of early ischemic events in patients at high risk for abrupt closure of the affected coronary artery who underwent urgent or emergency PCI, although this reduction was not sustained. Patients considered at high risk for abrupt closure of coronary blood vessels included those with NSTE ACS or acute STEMI. All patients were receiving adjunctive therapy with low-dose aspirin (325 mg within 12 hours before the procedure) and heparin sodium (IV loading dose of 10,000 units in patients weighing at least 70 kg or 150 units/kg in those weighing less than 70 kg) prior to PCI. Additional heparin sodium was administered during the procedure as required to maintain an activated clotting time (ACT) of 300–400 seconds; heparin generally was discontinued after completion of PCI.

Beneficial effects of tirofiban were most apparent during infusion of the drug and for several days after drug administration but declined thereafter. The relative risk reduction in the primary composite clinical end point of death, nonfatal MI, or additional surgical interventions (e.g., recurrent ischemia, complications, or procedural failure of initial PCI necessitating CABG, coronary artery stent implantation, or repeat PCI) at 48 hours was 38% (from 8.7% in placebo recipients to 5.4% in those receiving tirofiban); however, the reduction in these clinical events was no longer statistically significant at 30 days (16% relative risk reduction) or 6 months (11% relative risk reduction), principally because of nonemergency CABG and repeat PCI procedures. In an angiographic substudy of the RESTORE study, tirofiban had no effect on the angiographic measurements of restenosis at 6 months. The incidence of major bleeding complications or thrombocytopenia were similar in patients receiving tirofiban or placebo.

DOSAGE AND ADMINISTRATION

● Administration

Tirofiban hydrochloride is administered by IV infusion using either the diluted injection concentrate or the premixed injection in plastic (IntraVia™) containers. *Tirofiban hydrochloride injection concentrate for IV infusion must be diluted to the same concentration as the premixed injection (50 mcg/mL of tirofiban) before administration.* The injection concentrate is prepared for infusion by withdrawing and discarding 50 or 100 mL of solution from a 250- or 500-mL bag, respectively, of 0.9% sodium chloride or 5% dextrose injection and replacing this volume with 50 mL (12.5 mg of tirofiban) or 100 mL (25 mg of tirofiban) of tirofiban hydrochloride injection to achieve a final tirofiban concentration of 50 mcg/mL. The solution should be mixed well prior to infusion. Any unused drug solution should be discarded.

The plastic container of the premixed injection may be somewhat opaque because of moisture absorption during sterilization; this opacity will diminish gradually. The container of the premixed injection should be checked for minute leaks by firmly squeezing the bag. The premixed injection should be discarded if the seal is not intact, leaks are found, or the solution is cloudy or contains a precipitate. Additives should not be introduced into the injection container. The plastic IV containers should not be used in series connections with other plastic containers, since such use could result in air embolism from residual air being drawn from the primary container if the first container is empty.

In clinical trials, almost all patients receiving tirofiban also received concomitant aspirin and/or heparin. Tirofiban and heparin may be administered through the same IV line.

Parenteral tirofiban hydrochloride solutions should be inspected visually for particulate matter and discoloration prior to administration whenever solution and container permit.

● Dosage

Dosage of tirofiban hydrochloride is expressed in terms of tirofiban.

Non-ST-Segment-Elevation Acute Coronary Syndromes

For reducing the risk of death, nonfatal myocardial infarction (MI), and/or refractory ischemia/repeat revascularization procedures in patients with non-ST-segment-elevation acute coronary syndromes (NSTE ACS) who are receiving medical therapy alone, an IV loading dose consisting of 0.4 mcg/kg of tirofiban per minute for 30 minutes is given as soon as possible after diagnosis, followed by continuous IV infusion of tirofiban 0.1 mcg/kg per minute for at least 24–48 hours. Patients receiving tirofiban who undergo percutaneous coronary intervention (PCI) should receive the same IV loading dose of tirofiban (0.4 mcg/kg per minute for 30 minutes) followed by continuous IV infusion of 0.1 mcg/kg per minute given during angiography and for 12–24 hours after angioplasty or atherectomy. In the PRISM-PLUS study, the tirofiban infusion was continued in combination with heparin for 48–108 hours. In patients who require coronary artery bypass grafting (CABG), tirofiban should be discontinued at least 4–6 hours before the procedure. While females and geriatric patients had a higher incidence of adverse effects (both hemorrhagic and nonhemorrhagic) in clinical trials of tirofiban (see Cautions), the manufacturer does not recommend dosage adjustments for tirofiban in female or geriatric patients.

Adjunctive Antithrombotic Therapy

Adjunctive antithrombotic therapy with aspirin and heparin was used in most patients with NSTE ACS receiving tirofiban therapy in clinical trials. In the 3 large, randomized controlled studies evaluating the efficacy of tirofiban, patients received aspirin (300–325 mg daily) for at least 48 hours after randomization or within 12 hours prior to PCI, unless the drug was contraindicated; some patients received aspirin indefinitely. For additional details regarding aspirin dosage regimens in patients with ACS, see Non-ST-Segment-Elevation Acute Coronary Syndromes under Dosage: Thrombosis, in Dosage and Administration in Aspirin 28:08.04.24.

The American College of Cardiology Foundation (ACCF), American Heart Association (AHA), and Society of Cardiovascular Angiography and Interventions (SCAI) recommend that aspirin 325 mg be given prior to PCI in patients not already receiving maintenance therapy with aspirin. Patients already receiving maintenance therapy with aspirin should receive a dose of 81–325 mg of aspirin before the procedure. For additional details regarding aspirin dosage regimens in patients undergoing PCI, see Percutaneous Coronary Intervention and Revascularization Procedures under Dosage: Thrombosis, in Dosage and Administration in Aspirin 28:08.04.24.

In addition to aspirin, ACC/AHA/SCAI recommends administration of a loading dose of a P2Y12 platelet adenosine diphosphate (ADP)-receptor antagonist (clopidogrel, prasugrel, or ticagrelor) in patients undergoing PCI with stent placement.

In clinical trials with tirofiban in patients *not* undergoing PCI, an initial 5000-unit IV loading dose of heparin sodium was given, followed by IV infusion of 1000 units/hour and dosage titration to achieve a target activated partial thromboplastin time (aPTT) of twice the control value. In patients undergoing PCI after at least 48 hours of medical management with tirofiban and heparin in the PRISM-PLUS study, an IV loading dose of heparin sodium (5000–7500 units) was administered, followed by an IV infusion (1000 units/hour) that was titrated to an aPTT approximately 2 times the control value with additional IV injections of heparin sodium as needed. In the RESTORE trial, patients at high risk for abrupt closure of the affected coronary artery who underwent urgent or emergency PCI received heparin sodium as an IV loading dose (10,000 units in patients weighing at least 70 kg or 150 units/kg in those weighing less than 70 kg) prior to PCI. Additional heparin sodium was administered during the procedure as required to maintain an activated clotting time (ACT) of 300–400 seconds; heparin generally was discontinued after completion of PCI. Since tirofiban and other GP IIb/IIIa-receptor inhibitors may have additive effects on ACT in patients receiving one of these drugs concomitantly with heparin, the dosage of heparin required to maintain an appropriate ACT during such concomitant GP IIb/IIIa-receptor inhibitor therapy may be lower than with heparin monotherapy. Clinical experience from other studies with GP IIb/IIIa-receptor inhibitors (e.g., abciximab) and expert guidelines suggest that use of lower dosages of concomitant IV heparin sodium (e.g., 50–70 units/kg) given 6 hours prior to PCI and targeted to an ACT of at least 200 seconds may provide similar reductions in ischemic coronary events as dosages for higher target ACTs with less risk of major bleeding. In women and geriatric patients undergoing PCI and receiving adjunctive therapy with a GP IIb/IIIa-receptor inhibitor and heparin, a lower dosage of heparin should be considered to decrease the risk of minor bleeding that has been observed compared with that in men.

Postprocedural use of heparin generally is not recommended while GP IIb/IIIa-receptor inhibitor therapy is given.

● **Dosage in Renal and Hepatic Impairment**

Plasma clearance of tirofiban may be decreased substantially (more than 50%) in patients with severe renal impairment (i.e., creatinine clearance of 30 mL/minute or less), including patients requiring hemodialysis. These patients should receive half the usual rate of infusion of tirofiban.

In patients with mild to moderate hepatic impairment, plasma clearance of tirofiban is similar to that in healthy individuals; information on plasma clearance in patients with severe hepatic impairment is not available since these patients were excluded from participation in clinical trials of tirofiban. Metabolism of tirofiban appears to be limited, and the manufacturer does not make specific recommendations for dosage adjustment in patients with hepatic impairment.

CAUTIONS

The most frequent and severe adverse effect of tirofiban therapy is bleeding. Bleeding is an extension of the pharmacologic action of tirofiban and was classified in clinical trials principally according to criteria of the Thrombolysis in Myocardial Infarction (TIMI) study groups. Minor bleeding generally was defined as

spontaneous gross hematuria, hematemesis, hemoptysis, or observed blood loss with a decrease in hemoglobin concentration exceeding 3 but less than 5 g/dL; major bleeding was defined as intracranial bleeding, cardiac tamponade, or a hemoglobin decrease exceeding 5 g/dL with or without an observed bleeding site. Almost all patients receiving tirofiban in clinical trials received concomitant therapy with heparin and/or aspirin; therefore, the contribution of tirofiban to the incidence of bleeding complications in these trials is difficult to determine.

Approximately 30% of patients in clinical trials of tirofiban were female, and 43% were older than 65 years of age. Patients in these trials received tirofiban for up to 116 hours. Females (compared with males) and geriatric (compared with younger) patients receiving tirofiban plus heparin or heparin alone had a higher incidence of adverse effects (both hemorrhagic and nonhemorrhagic). However, the incremental risk of hemorrhage and the incidence of nonhemorrhagic adverse effects in patients treated with tirofiban and heparin versus heparin alone were comparable regardless of age or gender. The incidence of adverse effects was not affected by race or the presence of underlying hypertension, diabetes mellitus, or hypercholesterolemia.

● **Hematologic Effects**

Effects on Hemostasis

Administration of tirofiban is associated with a small increase in major and minor bleeding complications compared with heparin and/or aspirin therapy. Major bleeding events (as defined by TIMI criteria) occurred in about 1.4 or 0.8% of patients receiving tirofiban plus heparin or heparin monotherapy, respectively, in the PRISM-PLUS study, in about 2.4 or 2.1% of patients receiving tirofiban plus heparin or heparin monotherapy, respectively, in the RESTORE study, and in 0.4% of each respective treatment group in the PRISM study. Major bleeding episodes, including fatalities, have been reported during postmarketing experience. Bleeding complications resulted in discontinuance of tirofiban in 3.5 or 1.3% of patients receiving tirofiban plus heparin or heparin alone, respectively, in PRISM-PLUS. Spontaneous (i.e., unrelated to catheter or other puncture sites) bleeding occurred at retroperitoneal, genitourinary, or GI sites in 0, 0.1, or 0.1%, respectively, of patients during therapy with tirofiban plus heparin in the PRISM-PLUS study, and in 0.6%, 0%, or 0.2%, respectively, of patients receiving this drug combination in the RESTORE study. During postmarketing experience, pulmonary (alveolar) hemorrhage, spinal-epidural hematoma, and hemopericardium have been reported in patients receiving tirofiban. Blood transfusions were required in 4 versus 2.8% of patients receiving tirofiban and heparin or heparin alone, respectively, in the PRISM-PLUS study and in 4.3 versus 2.5% of patients receiving these respective therapies in the RESTORE study.

Most major bleeding in clinical trials of tirofiban occurred at the arterial access site for femoral sheath placement in patients undergoing revascularization procedures. In patients undergoing PCI (e.g., percutaneous transluminal coronary angioplasty [PTCA]) in the PRISM-PLUS study, the incidences of major bleeding prior to PCI, following angiography (performed in 89.8% of the patients), and following PCI were 0.3, 1.3, and 2.5%, respectively, in patients receiving tirofiban plus heparin and 0.1, 0.7, and 2.2%, respectively, in patients receiving heparin monotherapy. The incidence of major bleeding (in some instances possibly reflecting hemoglobin decreases related to hemodilution rather than actual bleeding) in patients receiving tirofiban plus heparin or heparin monotherapy and undergoing coronary artery bypass grafting (CABG) within 1 day of discontinuance of study drug was 17.2 or 35.4%, respectively, in the PRISM-PLUS study and 25 or 37.5%, respectively, in the RESTORE study.

Therapy with GP IIb/IIIa-receptor inhibitors, including tirofiban, has not been associated with an increased risk of intracranial hemorrhage. Intracranial hemorrhage occurred in 0.1 or 0.3% of patients receiving tirofiban and heparin or heparin alone, respectively, in the RESTORE study, and was not reported in patients receiving these therapies in the PRISM-PLUS study. The incidence of intracranial hemorrhage in patients receiving tirofiban or heparin in the PRISM study was 0.1% in each group. Retroperitoneal bleeding or hemopericardium has been reported during postmarketing experience in patients receiving tirofiban.

Minor bleeding episodes occurred in about 10.5 or 8% of patients receiving tirofiban plus heparin or heparin monotherapy, respectively, in the PRISM-PLUS study and in 12 or 6.3% of patients receiving tirofiban plus heparin or heparin alone, respectively, in the RESTORE study.

Other Hematologic Effects

Decreases in platelet count or thrombocytopenia occurs occasionally (2.3% overall) after therapy with GP IIb/IIIa-receptor inhibitors. Thrombocytopenia associated with administration of a GP IIb/IIIa-receptor inhibitor generally occurs within hours or days after administration of the drug. Decreases in platelet counts have been observed in patients with no prior history of thrombocytopenia following readministration of GP IIb/IIIa-receptor inhibitors. Severe thrombocytopenia (i.e., platelet count less than 20,000/mm³) has been reported more frequently with abciximab than with tirofiban. However, a preliminary report based on pooled data from clinical trials indicates that the incidence of thrombocytopenia is not appreciably different among GP IIb/IIIa-receptor inhibitors (i.e., abciximab, eptifibatide, tirofiban), although the absolute risk of thrombocytopenia appears to increase (but not synergistically) with concomitant use of heparin. In controlled clinical trials of tirofiban, the incidence of thrombocytopenia (defined as platelet counts less than 90,000/mm³) was increased in patients receiving tirofiban plus heparin (1.5%) compared with heparin monotherapy (0.6%), respectively; reductions in platelet count to less than 50,000/mm³ were observed in 0.3 or 0.1% of patients receiving tirofiban plus heparin or heparin alone, respectively, in clinical trials. In the PRISM study, the incidence of thrombocytopenia also was increased in patients receiving tirofiban versus those receiving heparin; platelet counts returned to normal several days after cessation of therapy without any other clinical sequelae. Decreased platelet counts associated with chills and a low-grade fever have been reported with tirofiban during postmarketing experience.

Reductions in hemoglobin or hematocrit were reported in 2.1 or 2.2%, respectively, of patients receiving tirofiban plus heparin and in 3.1 or 2.6%, respectively, of patients receiving heparin in controlled clinical trials. Microscopic hematuria or occult blood in the stool was noted in 10.7 or 18.3%, respectively, of patients receiving tirofiban plus heparin and in 7.8 or 12.2%, respectively, of those receiving heparin monotherapy in clinical trials.

Cardiovascular Effects

Adverse cardiovascular effects that occurred in greater than 1% of patients receiving tirofiban plus heparin in clinical trials were bradycardia (4%) or dissection of the coronary artery (5%). Edema/swelling or vasovagal reactions were reported in 2% of patients receiving tirofiban and heparin in these trials.

Dermatologic and Sensitivity Reactions

Sweating was reported in 2% of patients receiving tirofiban and heparin in controlled clinical trials. Anaphylaxis and/or urticaria requiring discontinuance of therapy was not reported in clinical trials of tirofiban, but anaphylaxis and other severe allergic reactions have been reported during postmarketing experience. Such reactions have occurred on the first day of tirofiban infusion, during initial treatment, and during readministration of the drug. Some severe allergic reactions have been associated with severe thrombocytopenia (platelet counts less than 10,000/mm³).

Therapy with some platelet-aggregation inhibitors (e.g., abciximab) has been associated with development of antibodies to the drug; limited information indicates that no antibodies to tirofiban have developed, but very few patients have received the drug on more than one occasion. However, as a nonpeptide GP IIb/IIIa-receptor inhibitor, tirofiban is expected to be less immunogenic than the monoclonal antibody abciximab.

Other Adverse Effects

Pelvic pain occurred in 6%, leg pain in 3%, and dizziness in 3% of patients receiving tirofiban plus heparin in clinical trials. Other adverse effects reported in greater than 1% of patients receiving tirofiban plus heparin in clinical trials include headache, nausea, and fever.

Precautions and Contraindications

The administration of tirofiban in patients with non-ST-segment-elevation acute coronary syndromes (NSTE ACS) has been associated with a small increase in the frequency of major bleeding compared with heparin and aspirin therapy alone. Bleeding with platelet glycoprotein (GP) IIb/IIIa-receptor inhibitors can be reduced by adherence to strict anticoagulation guidelines, the use of a short course of low-dose, weight-adjusted heparin, and in patients undergoing PCI, early arterial sheath removal and careful patient and access site management. Prior to administration of tirofiban, preexisting hemostatic abnormalities should be identified by obtaining determinations of hematocrit and hemoglobin; these parameters should then be monitored within 6 hours following the loading infusion and at least daily thereafter during therapy. In patients receiving heparin concomitantly with tirofiban, the extent of heparin anticoagulation (as assessed by

activated clotting time [ACT] or aPTT) should be monitored closely to minimize bleeding, which may be potentially life-threatening. The aPTT should be monitored 6 hours after the start of the heparin infusion and be maintained at 50–70 seconds or approximately 2 times the control value unless PCI is to be performed. In addition, the ACT should be measured in patients undergoing PCI.Current guidelines of the American College of Chest Physicians (ACCP) and other experts and risk-benefit analyses in trials with GP IIb/IIIa-receptor inhibitors suggest that heparin dosing should be adjusted to maintain the ACT at 200 seconds or greater during PCI in patients receiving GP IIb/IIIa-receptor inhibitors. (See Adjunctive Antithrombotic Therapy under Dosage: Non-ST-Segment-Elevation Acute Coronary Syndromes, in Dosage and Administration.) Routine use of postprocedural heparin generally is not recommended during GP IIb/IIIa-receptor inhibitor therapy. After PCI, the aPTT should be checked prior to arterial sheath removal, and the sheath should not be removed unless the aPTT is less than 45 seconds or the ACT is less than 180 seconds. Tirofiban should be used with caution in patients with hemorrhagic retinopathy, anemia (hemoglobin concentration less than 10–12 g/dL) and in those requiring chronic hemodialysis.

Platelet counts should be determined prior to treatment with tirofiban and periodically (e.g., within the first 6 hours of the loading infusion and daily thereafter) during concomitant tirofiban and heparin therapy. should be used with caution in patients with a platelet count less than 150,000/mm³. If a patient experiences a reduction in platelet count to less than 90,000/mm³, additional platelet counts should be performed to exclude the possibility of pseudothrombocytopenia. The possibility of heparin-induced thrombocytopenia also should be considered in the differential diagnosis of thrombocytopenia in patients receiving GP IIb/IIIa-receptor inhibitors concomitantly with heparin. If thrombocytopenia is confirmed, tirofiban should be discontinued and the condition appropriately monitored and treated. Thrombocytopenia is usually reversible following discontinuance of GP IIb/IIIa-receptor inhibitors and anticoagulant (heparin) therapy; however, platelet transfusions should be considered for the management of severe thrombocytopenia.

To minimize the possibility of bleeding associated with the use of tirofiban, particularly at the site of femoral artery sheath placement in patients undergoing PCI, precautions in the placement, maintenance, and removal of the vascular access sheath should be observed. Placement of a femoral venous sheath should be avoided if possible. When inserting the femoral artery sheath, care should be taken so that only the anterior wall of the femoral artery is punctured; a Seldinger (through and through) technique for puncture of the artery should be avoided. Appropriate precautions should be observed while the vascular access sheath is in place (e.g., complete bed rest, elevation of the head of the bed no more than 30°, restraint of the limb in which the vascular access sheath is inserted, frequent monitoring of the vascular access site and the distal pulse in the involved limb). The femoral artery sheath may be removed during treatment with tirofiban, provided at least 3–4 hours have elapsed since heparin therapy was discontinued and its effects largely have reversed (as indicated by an aPTT of less than 45 seconds or an ACT of less than 180 seconds).

Both heparin and tirofiban therapy should be discontinued and sheath hemostasis achieved with standard compressive techniques at least 4 hours before hospital discharge. Pressure (e.g., using manual compression or a mechanical hemostatic device) should be applied to the femoral artery for at least 20–30 minutes after sheath removal; after hemostasis, a pressure dressing should be applied. Any hematoma that forms should be measured and monitored for enlargement.

Careful monitoring of all potential bleeding sites should be undertaken during and following treatment with platelet aggregation inhibitors. Needle punctures (e.g., arterial, IM, IV, lumbar, subcutaneous, intradermal), cutdown sites, and use of nasotracheal intubation, nasogastric tubes, urinary catheterization, and automatic blood pressure cuffs should be minimized during and following treatment with tirofiban. Establishment of IV access at noncompressible sites (e.g., in subclavian or jugular veins) should be avoided; an indwelling venipuncture device (e.g., heparin lock) should be considered for drawing blood; documentation and monitoring of vascular puncture sites should occur; and dressings should gently and carefully be removed. The manufacturer states that any occurrence of serious bleeding that cannot be controlled by pressure on the bleeding site should result in discontinuance of tirofiban and concomitantly administered heparin therapy.

Because tirofiban increases the risk of bleeding, the drug is contraindicated in patients with active internal bleeding (including microscopic hematuria or a positive test for occult fecal blood) or a history of bleeding diathesis (e.g., GI or genitourinary bleeding, elevated hemostatic indices, recent noncompressible vascular punctures) within the previous 30 days; a history of intracranial hemorrhage, intracranial neoplasm, arteriovenous malformation, or aneurysm; a history of thrombocytopenia following prior exposure to tirofiban; history of stroke within 30 days or any history of hemorrhagic stroke; recent (within 1 month) major surgery or severe physical trauma; history, symptoms, or findings suggestive of aortic dissection; severe uncontrolled hypertension (systolic or diastolic blood pressure exceeding 180 or 110 mm Hg, respectively); concomitant therapy with another parenteral GP IIb/IIIa-receptor inhibitor; or acute pericarditis. Tirofiban also is contraindicated in patients with a known hypersensitivity to any component of the commercially available preparation.

● Pediatric Precautions

Safety and efficacy of tirofiban in pediatric patients younger than 18 years of age have not been determined.

● Geriatric Precautions

Safety and efficacy of tirofiban in geriatric patients have not been specifically studied to date; however, in large clinical trials, approximately 43% of patients were 65 years of age or older, while 11.7% were 75 years of age or older. Clinical experience generally has not revealed age-related differences in response to tirofiban therapy. Plasma clearance of tirofiban is about 19–26% lower in geriatric patients (exceeding 65 years of age) with coronary artery disease than in younger patients. While the incidence of bleeding complications was higher in geriatric patients receiving either heparin plus tirofiban or heparin monotherapy, the incremental risk of bleeding among patients receiving these 2 regimens was similar regardless of age. The overall incidence of nonhemorrhagic adverse effects was higher in older patients compared with younger patients receiving either treatment regimen (heparin or tirofiban plus heparin). In the RESTORE study, the loading dose of IV heparin was weight-adjusted in patients weighing less than 70 kg because of concern for an increased risk for bleeding in these patients. However, the manufacturer recommends no dosage adjustment for tirofiban in geriatric patients.

● Mutagenicity and Carcinogenicity

No evidence of mutagenicity was seen at the chromosomal or gene level when tirofiban was evaluated in several in vitro and in vivo test systems. The drug was not directly genotoxic in the in vitro alkaline elution or chromosomal aberration assay. Tirofiban did not induce chromosomal aberrations in bone marrow cells of male mice given the drug IV at dosages of up to 5 mg/kg daily (about 3 times the maximum recommended daily human dosage based on body surface area).

Studies have not been performed to date to evaluate the carcinogenic potential of tirofiban.

● Pregnancy, Fertility, and Lactation

Pregnancy

Reproduction studies using IV tirofiban dosages of up to 5 mg/kg daily in rats and rabbits (representing about 5 and 13 times, respectively, the recommended maximum daily human dosage based on body surface area) have not revealed evidence of harm to the fetus. However, animal reproduction studies are not always predictive of human response. There are no adequate or controlled studies to date using tirofiban in pregnant women, and the drug should be used during pregnancy only when clearly needed.

Fertility

Reproduction studies of tirofiban in male and female rats given up to 5 mg/kg daily IV (representing about 5 times the recommended maximum daily human dosage based on body surface area) have not revealed evidence of impaired fertility or reproductive performance.

Lactation

It is not known if tirofiban is distributed into milk in humans; however, the drug is distributed into milk in rats. Because of the potential for serious adverse effects in nursing infants, a decision should be made whether to discontinue nursing or tirofiban, taking into account the importance of the drug to the woman.

DRUG INTERACTIONS

● Drugs Affecting Hemostasis

Almost all patients receiving tirofiban in clinical trials have received concomitant therapy with heparin and/or aspirin, and such concomitant therapy has been associated with a small increase in bleeding complications compared with that in patients receiving aspirin and heparin alone. (See Effects on Hemostasis under Cautions: Hematologic Effects.) Caution should be observed when tirofiban is used with other drugs that affect hemostasis, including thrombolytic agents, oral anticoagulants (e.g., warfarin), nonsteroidal anti-inflammatory agents (NSAIAs), dipyridamole, ticlopidine, and clopidogrel; some clinicians also recommend against concomitant use of tirofiban and IV dextran.

In several studies evaluating pharmacokinetic and pharmacodynamic interactions with tirofiban in healthy individuals, the pharmacokinetics of tirofiban were not affected by pretreatment with aspirin (325 mg administered 1 and 24 hours prior to tirofiban) or ticlopidine (200 mg once daily for 4 days). However, aspirin or ticlopidine may enhance the inhibition of platelet aggregation produced by tirofiban. In healthy individuals and in patients with non-ST-segment-elevation acute coronary syndromes (NSTE ACS), bleeding time was prolonged by the combination of tirofiban and aspirin compared with tirofiban or aspirin therapy alone; aPTT was not affected (compared with baseline values). (See Pharmacology.)

No information is available concerning the use of tirofiban concomitantly with thrombolytic agents.

● Other Drugs

Data from a large clinical study (the PRISM study) indicate that concomitant administration of tirofiban and levothyroxine or omeprazole was associated with a higher clearance of tirofiban; the clinical importance of this effect is not known. Concomitant administration of the following drugs in the same study was not associated with clinically important effects on the plasma clearance of tirofiban: acebutolol, acetaminophen, alprazolam, amlodipine, aspirin preparations, atenolol, bromazepam, captopril, diazepam, digoxin, diltiazem, docusate sodium, enalapril, furosemide, glyburide, heparin, insulin, isosorbide, lorazepam, lovastatin, metoclopramide, metoprolol, morphine, nifedipine, nitrate preparations, oxazepam, potassium chloride, propranolol, ranitidine, simvastatin, sucralfate, or temazepam.

ACUTE TOXICITY

Limited information is available on the acute toxicity of tirofiban. In general, overdosage of tirofiban in humans may be expected to produce effects that are extensions of the pharmacologic and adverse effects of the drug, predominantly bleeding. (See Cautions: Hematologic Effects.) The most frequently reported manifestation of overdosage was bleeding, principally minor bleeding at mucocutaneous and cardiac catheterization sites. Inadvertent overdosage with tirofiban has occurred in doses of up to twice those recommended for an IV loading infusion and up to 9.8 times higher than the recommended maintenance infusion dosage of 0.15 mcg/kg per minute. In the event of overdosage, tirofiban therapy should be discontinued or the dosage adjusted and the patient's clinical status monitored as appropriate. Tirofiban is removed by hemodialysis.

PHARMACOLOGY

● Platelet Aggregation and Thrombosis

Tirofiban is a selective, competitive, reversible inhibitor of platelet aggregation that is used in combination with heparin to reduce the risk of acute ischemic events (death and/or myocardial infarction [MI]) associated with non-ST-segment-elevation acute coronary syndromes (NSTE ACS), including those undergoing percutaneous coronary intervention (PCI) (e.g., percutaneous transluminal coronary angioplasty [PTCA], atherectomy). Because of its mechanism of action, tirofiban, like abciximab and eptifibatide, has been referred to as a platelet glycoprotein (GP) IIb/IIIa-receptor inhibitor. Platelet adhesion, activation, and aggregation are key processes leading to the formation of platelet-rich ("white") coronary artery thrombi and the development of acute coronary artery syndromes and ischemic complications associated with PCI. White thrombus formation is triggered by vascular injury (e.g., from PCI procedures), plaque rupture, or denudation of endothelium that exposes the subendothelial matrix of the vessel to circulating platelets. Upon exposure of the vessel subendothelium, potent thrombogenic stimuli (e.g., thrombin, collagen) present in both subendothelium and plaque, and/or high-shear stress, stimulate platelet adhesion and activation.

Activated platelets release intracellular granules consisting of vasoactive substances that are part of an autostimulatory feedback loop for platelet aggregation; these substances include thromboxane A_2, serotonin, and adenosine diphosphate

(ADP); adhesive glycoproteins such as fibrinogen, fibronectin, and von Wille-brand's factor; and plasminogen activator inhibitor-1 (PAI-1). Regardless of the initial stimulus for platelet activation, the final common pathway to platelet aggregation and thrombosis involves activation of the receptor function of the GP IIb/IIIa complex (also known as $\alpha_{IIb}\beta_3$). Inactive GP IIb/IIIa receptors undergo a conformational change on the surface of activated platelets to accept soluble fibrinogen, von Willebrand's factor, and other ligands (e.g., fibronectin, vitronectin, thrombospondin). Some of these adhesive ligands form cross-links to other GP IIb/IIIa on surfaces of adjacent activated platelets, causing aggregation and white thrombus formation. In addition, fibrinogen bound to the vessel wall or to other platelet aggregates can activate GP IIb/IIIa receptors on unstimulated platelets and recruit these platelets to growing white thrombi.

Progression of NSTE ACS to ST-segment-elevation MI (STEMI) or sudden death occurs when obstructive platelet-rich thrombi grow to become occlusive thrombi in the absence of adequate perfusion beyond the obstruction through collateral blood vessels. Fibrin and erythrocytes comprise the outer layer of occlusive red thrombi that are formed on the surface of the platelet-rich inner core of the thrombus. While thrombolytic therapy effectively dissolves the occluding fibrin-rich portion of the thrombus, this process releases clot-bound thrombin and re-exposes the underlying disrupted plaque, which rereleases potent thrombogenic stimuli. These newly released thrombogenic stimuli then activate platelets, leading to platelet aggregation. In addition, activated platelets secrete a variety of factors (e.g., PAI-1, fibrinogen, factor V) associated with rethrombosis or thrombin production and bind factors Xa, VIIIa, and IXa, which are involved in further thrombin production. Platelet reactivity also may increase after thrombolysis. It has been suggested that use of platelet-aggregation inhibitors concomitantly with thrombolytic therapy may counter the thrombogenic activity of these agents and minimize the risk of reocclusion.

● Inhibition of Platelet Aggregation

Tirofiban reversibly inhibits platelet aggregation by preventing the binding of fibrinogen, von Willebrand's factor, and other adhesive ligands to resting and active GP IIb/IIIa receptors. Inhibition of platelet aggregation by tirofiban and other GP IIb/IIIa-receptor inhibitors occurs in a dose- and concentration-dependent manner via an increase in GP IIb/IIIa receptor occupancy (as determined by the ex vivo platelet aggregation assay for tirofiban using sodium citrate as the anticoagulant in blood samples); platelet aggregation is nearly completely abolished at receptor occupancy exceeding 80%. Sodium citrate reportedly does not affect binding of tirofiban to the GP IIb/IIIa receptor. Some platelet-aggregation inhibitors such as aspirin, ticlopidine, and clopidogrel prevent platelet aggregation by preventing platelet activation in response to one or more agonists (e.g., thromboxane A_2, adenosine diphosphate); agonists not affected by these drugs may continue to induce platelet aggregation. However, GP IIb/IIIa-receptor inhibitors such as abciximab, eptifibatide, and tirofiban prevent platelet aggregation regardless of the initial stimulus. Some in vitro data suggest that inhibition of platelet aggregation by tirofiban can be overcome by an increase in the concentration of fibrinogen, indicating reversible, competitive binding to the GP IIb/IIIa receptor. However, tirofiban or other GP IIb/IIIa-receptor inhibitors do not appear to be effective in displacing fibrinogen cross-links from GP IIb/IIIA receptors in established thrombi when the bond between fibrinogen and GP IIb/IIIa receptors becomes irreversible.

In vitro binding studies in platelets and human endothelial cells demonstrate that tirofiban is selective in binding to the platelet GP IIb/IIIa receptor; concentrations of the drug needed to inhibit the attachment of human endothelial cells to vitronectin or fibronectin receptors are approximately 1000-fold or greater than those required for inhibiting the attachment of platelets to fibrinogen.

Following the recommended IV loading infusion of tirofiban (0.4 mcg/kg per minute for 30 minutes) in patients with NSTE ACS receiving concomitant heparin and aspirin, inhibition of platelet aggregation exceeded 90% at the end of the infusion. Addition of heparin to tirofiban therapy (0.1 mcg/kg per minute by IV infusion) does not alter the percentage of individuals with platelet aggregation inhibition exceeding 70%.

● Hemostatic Effects

Since the effect of tirofiban on platelet aggregation is rapidly reversible following cessation of the infusion, the drug has a modest effect on hemostatic indices (e.g., bleeding times). Normal hemostasis is restored more rapidly than with abciximab, a monoclonal antibody that dissociates very slowly from the GP IIb/IIIa receptor.

In healthy individuals and patients with coronary artery disease, tirofiban prolongs bleeding time in a dose-dependent manner. Following administration of tirofiban as a loading infusion (0.4 mcg/kg per minute for 30 minutes)

concomitantly with heparin and aspirin in patients with NSTE ACS, bleeding time was prolonged to 2.9 times that of baseline values. During continuous infusion of tirofiban (0.1 mcg/kg per minute) with concomitant heparin and aspirin in patients with NSTE ACS, bleeding time exceeded 20–30 minutes. However, in patients with NSTE ACS receiving heparin titrated to an aPTT twice the control value, addition of tirofiban did not alter the aPTT. When administered without heparin in patients with NSTE ACS in several large clinical trials (the Platelet Receptor Inhibitor in Ischemic Syndrome Management in Patients Limited by Unstable Signs and Symptoms [PRISM-PLUS] study and the Platelet Receptor Inhibition in Ischemic Syndrome Management [PRISM] study), tirofiban and aspirin prolonged bleeding time to less than 20 minutes and aPTT was not affected (compared with baseline values). In patients with coronary artery disease receiving tirofiban, ex vivo adenosine diphosphate (ADP)-induced platelet aggregation using sodium citrate as an anticoagulant in blood samples was restored toward baseline values in approximately 90% of patients within 4–8 hours after discontinuance of the infusion.

PHARMACOKINETICS

The pharmacokinetics of tirofiban are linear, and plasma concentrations are proportional to dose following IV infusions of 0.05–0.4 mcg/kg per minute for 1 hour or 0.1–0.2 mcg/kg per minute for 4 hours in healthy individuals. Concomitant administration of aspirin or ticlopidine does not appear to affect the pharmacokinetics of tirofiban. (See Drug Interactions: Drugs Affecting Hemostasis.)

● Absorption

Information concerning plasma concentrations resulting from recommended loading and maintenance infusion dosages of tirofiban is not available. In a study in healthy individuals, plasma tirofiban concentrations of 10.9 and 20.7 ng/mL were reported after infusion of 0.1 mcg/kg per minute of tirofiban for 1 and 4 hours, respectively.

Tirofiban has a rapid onset and short duration of action. In patients with non-ST-segment-elevation acute coronary syndromes (NSTE ACS) receiving the recommended tirofiban regimen consisting of an IV loading infusion of 0.4 mcg/kg per minute for 30 minutes followed by 0.1 mcg/kg per minute for up to 48 hours, approximately 90% inhibition of ex vivo adenosine diphosphate (ADP)-induced platelet aggregation was achieved by the end of the loading infusion, with inhibition persisting for the duration of the maintenance infusion. Platelet function returned to near baseline levels in approximately 90% of these patients within 4–8 hours following discontinuance of the tirofiban infusion.

In a randomized study in a limited number of patients with NSTE ACS undergoing PCI, administration of the recommended regimen of tirofiban (0.4 mcg/kg per minute IV for 30 minutes followed by 0.1 mcg/kg per minute by IV infusion) for 20–24 hours was associated with a delayed onset and reduced intensity of platelet-aggregation inhibition (as measured by rapid platelet function assay [RPFA] or light transmission aggregometry using 20 μmol ADP) compared with that produced by recommended regimens of abciximab (0.25-mg/kg IV loading dose followed by 0.125 mcg/kg per minute, up to a maximum infusion rate of 10 mcg/minute, for 12 hours) or eptifibatide (180-mcg/kg IV loading dose followed by 2 mcg/kg per minute by IV infusion for 20–24 hours). The delayed onset of action of tirofiban was attributed to its comparatively long loading infusion duration (30 minutes) since in another study, maximal inhibition of platelet aggregation (96%) occurred within 5 minutes after infusion of a 10-mcg/kg IV loading dose over 3 minutes. The diminished intensity of platelet-aggregation inhibition was related in part to the strength of the agonist (20 μM) used in the platelet-aggregation assay, which is identical to that used in clinical trials of abciximab and eptifibatide but exceeds the concentration used in clinical trials of tirofiban (5 μM).

● Distribution

Tirofiban is approximately 65% bound to plasma proteins, and protein binding is independent of plasma drug concentration over the range of 0.01–25 mcg/mL. The steady-state volume of distribution of tirofiban ranges from 22–42 L. It is not known whether tirofiban is distributed into milk or crosses the placenta in humans; however, the drug is distributed into milk in rats and crosses the placenta in pregnant rats and rabbits.

● Elimination

Following administration in healthy individuals, plasma concentrations of tirofiban decline in a biphasic manner. The half-life of tirofiban averages approximately 1.2–2 hours. Tirofiban is cleared from the plasma mainly by renal excretion; metabolism of the drug appears to be limited.

About 65 and 25% of a single dose of tirofiban is excreted in urine and feces, respectively, principally as unchanged parent drug. Plasma clearance of tirofiban in healthy individuals ranges from 213–314 mL/minute, with renal clearance accounting for 39–69% of plasma clearance. In patients with coronary artery disease, the plasma clearance of tirofiban ranges from 152–267 mL/minute and does not appear to be influenced by gender or race; renal clearance in these patients accounts for 39% of plasma clearance. Plasma clearance is about 19–26% lower in geriatric patients (those exceeding 65 years of age) with coronary artery disease than in younger patients. Plasma clearance appears to be independent of dose in healthy individuals and is not appreciably affected by mild to moderate hepatic insufficiency. In patients with renal impairment (creatinine clearance less than 30 mL per minute), including those requiring hemodialysis, plasma clearance of tirofiban is decreased by greater than 50% compared with that in individuals with normal renal function. Tirofiban is removed by hemodialysis.

CHEMISTRY AND STABILITY

● Chemistry

Tirofiban hydrochloride, a synthetic nonpeptide tyrosine derivative, is a selective, competitive platelet-aggregation inhibitor. Tirofiban, like abciximab and eptifibatide, has been referred to as a platelet glycoprotein (GP) IIb/IIIa-receptor inhibitor.

Tirofiban is produced by the addition of an n-butylsulfonyl group to the C-terminus and a 4-(piperidin-4-yl)butyloxy group to the N-terminus of tyrosine; these modifications increase the potency of the drug's inhibitory effect on platelet aggregation.

The final step in platelet aggregation involves the binding of fibrinogen to the activated, membrane-bound platelet glycoprotein complex, GP IIb/IIIa, principally through a recognition site on the C-terminal peptide of the γ chain of fibrinogen that is structurally similar to the amino acid sequence arginine-glycine-aspartate (RGD). Other adhesive glycoproteins (e.g., von Willebrand's factor, fibronectin, vitronectin) appear to bind to activated GP IIb/IIIa through the RGD sequence. Unlike other GP IIb/IIIa-receptor inhibitors such as abciximab, which is an antibody to the GP IIb/IIIa receptor, and eptifibatide, which is a peptide mimetic of the GP IIb/IIIa receptor binding site, tirofiban is a nonpeptide amino acid derivative that mimics the geometric, stereotactic, and charge characteristics of the RGD binding site on the GP IIb/IIIa receptor. Molecular modeling studies suggest that the piperidine nitrogen of tirofiban replaces the basic guanidino moiety of arginine, the aromatic ring of tyrosine replaces the glycine residue, and the tyrosine carboxyl group substitutes for the carboxyl group of aspartic acid on the GP IIb/IIIa receptor binding site. In addition, the butylsulfonyl group of tirofiban appears to enhance potency of the drug by interacting with another site (exosite) on the GP IIb/IIIa receptor to which peptide mimetics (e.g., eptifibatide) do not bind.

Tirofiban is commercially available as the hydrochloride salt, which is monohydrated; potency of tirofiban hydrochloride is expressed in terms of tirofiban, calculated on the anhydrous basis.

Tirofiban hydrochloride monohydrate occurs as a white to off-white powder and is very slightly soluble in water and freely soluble (exceeding 100 mg/mL) in alcohol. The drug has pK$_a$ values of 3.6 and 11.1. Tirofiban hydrochloride is commercially available as a clear, colorless, sterile injection concentrate and as a clear, sterile premixed IV solution in water for injection that has been made iso-osmotic with sodium chloride. Tirofiban hydrochloride injections contain sodium citrate dihydrate and citric acid anhydrous as buffers; the injections contain no preservatives. Sodium hydroxide and/or hydrochloric acid may be added during manufacture to adjust the pH of the injections to 5.5–6.5. When tirofiban hydrochloride injection concentrate is diluted extemporaneously with 0.9% sodium chloride or 5% dextrose injection, the pH of the resulting IV solution is approximately 6. The osmolality of tirofiban hydrochloride injection concentrate after dilution or of the premixed IV solution is approximately 280 or 300 mOsm/kg, respectively.

Each mL of tirofiban hydrochloride injection concentrate contains 0.281 mg of tirofiban hydrochloride monohydrate equivalent to 0.25 mg of tirofiban base (250 mcg/mL of tirofiban). Each 500 mL of tirofiban hydrochloride injection premixed contains 28.09 mg of tirofiban hydrochloride monohydrate equivalent to 25 mg of tirofiban base (50 mcg/mL of tirofiban).

● Stability

Commercially available premixed tirofiban hydrochloride in 0.9% sodium chloride injection is provided in a flexible plastic (Intravia®) container fabricated from specially formulated, multilayered plastic (PL 2408). Premixed tirofiban hydrochloride injection or injection concentrate is stable for 18 or 24 months, respectively, following the date of manufacture when stored unopened as directed. Solutions in contact with the plastic container can leach out some of the container's chemical components in very small amounts within the expiration period of the injection; however, safety of the plastic container materials has been supported by USP biological tests.

Dopamine, lidocaine, potassium chloride, and famotidine injection may be administered in the same IV line with tirofiban hydrochloride injection; tirofiban should not be administered in the same IV line as diazepam.

Unused portions of tirofiban hydrochloride IV solutions should be discarded since these solutions contain no preservatives. Tirofiban hydrochloride injections should be stored at a temperature between 15 and 30°C and should be protected from light during storage; freezing should be avoided.

PREPARATIONS

Excipients in commercially available drug preparations may have clinically important effects in some individuals; consult specific product labeling for details.

Tirofiban Hydrochloride

Parenteral

For injection, concentrate, for IV infusion	250 mcg (of tirofiban) per mL (5 and 12.5 mg)	Aggrastat®, Medicure

Tirofiban Hydrochloride in Sodium Chloride

Parenteral

Injection, for IV infusion	50 mcg (of tirofiban) per mL (12.5 mg) in 0.9% Sodium Chloride	Aggrastat® Premixed in Iso-osmotic Sodium Chloride Injection (in IntraVia® flexible container), Medicure

Selected Revisions September 18, 2017, © Copyright, January 1, 2000, American Society of Health-System Pharmacists, Inc.

Alteplase

20:12.20 • THROMBOLYTIC AGENTS

■ Alteplase, a biosynthetic (recombinant DNA origin) form of the enzyme human tissue-type plasminogen activator (t-PA), is a thrombolytic agent.

USES

● Acute Myocardial Infarction

Alteplase, a recombinant tissue-type plasminogen activator, is used as a thrombolytic agent for reperfusion therapy in patients with acute myocardial infarction (MI) to reduce mortality and to reduce the incidence of heart failure. The term MI is used when there is evidence of myocardial necrosis in the setting of acute myocardial ischemia. MI is further distinguished based on the presence or absence of ST-segment elevation on ECG. Because patients with ST-segment-elevation MI (STEMI) typically have complete arterial occlusion, immediate reperfusion therapy is required. Reperfusion may be achieved with a pharmacologic (e.g., thrombolytic therapy) or mechanical (percutaneous coronary intervention [PCI]) strategy. The manufacturer states that the risk of stroke may outweigh the benefit of thrombolytic therapy in patients whose acute MI places them at low risk for death or heart failure.

Clinical Experience

Almost all clinical studies to date of tissue-type plasminogen activator (t-PA) in patients with acute MI have been conducted using either the predominantly two-chain (prepared by Genentech roller-bottle method but not currently available) form of recombinant t-PA (rt-PA) that was used in early clinical studies or the currently marketed, predominantly one-chain form of rt-PA (alteplase) (prepared by Genentech suspension-culture methods); the manufacturer states that all Genentech-sponsored studies of rt-PA initiated since August 1985 have used the predominantly one-chain form. Therefore, unless otherwise specified, the term rt-PA in the Uses section refers to studies in which either alteplase or predominantly two-chain rt-PA was evaluated.

Coronary Artery Patency

The overall rate of coronary artery reperfusion or patency after rt-PA administration exceeds that of placebo or IV streptokinase (no longer commercially available in the US). Reperfusion after thrombolytic therapy may be evident by appearance of arrhythmias, relief of chest pain, and/or early peaking of serum concentrations of AST (SGOT) and the cardiac fraction (MB fraction) of creatine kinase (CK, creatine phosphokinase, CPK); however, these are not definitive measures of recanalization. Creatine kinase concentrations usually return to baseline levels rapidly after reperfusion. Beneficial effects of rt-PA therapy on ventricular function or mortality generally have been limited to patients with infarct-related coronary arteries that became patent with therapy. Analyses of data from an angiographic substudy of patients in the Global Utilization of Streptokinase and Tissue Plasminogen Activator for Occluded Coronary Arteries (GUSTO-I) trial indicate that "normal" perfusion (TIMI grade 3 flow) in an infarct-related artery at 90 minutes post-thrombolysis was associated with a lower 30-day mortality rate regardless of the thrombolytic agent used; these data support the "open-artery" hypothesis regarding early restoration of coronary artery patency and subsequent mortality reduction beyond that expected from preservation of left ventricular function (myocardial salvage) alone. Some evidence suggests that while the early benefit of infarct-artery patency occurs as a result of myocardial salvage, the late mortality benefit occurs independent of improvements in ventricular function. This late benefit appears to result from a reduction of scar formation and attenuation of ventricular dilation and infarct remodeling, particularly in areas of the myocardium that depend on collateral circulation.

The extent of coronary recanalization after rt-PA therapy generally has been shown to be dose dependent. In studies employing pretreatment angiography to confirm coronary artery occlusion, rt-PA in dosages of 40–100 mg administered IV over 1–3 hours was associated with reperfusion after approximately 45–90 minutes in about 60–75% of infarct-related coronary arteries; at these dosages, coronary artery patency rates in studies not employing pretreatment angiography

have been similar or somewhat higher. However, patency rates may overestimate efficacy because of failure to exclude patients with patent infarct-related coronary arteries or early spontaneous recanalization. In dose-ranging studies conducted before the second phase of the Thrombolysis in Myocardial Infarction (TIMI) trial (TIMI-2), IV infusion of alteplase at a dose of 150 mg over 5–8 hours was associated with patency rates of 75% at 90 minutes. However, because an increased incidence of life-threatening intracranial bleeding was noted at this dose, the maximum recommended total dose was reduced to 100 mg. In phase 1 of the TIMI trial, a comparative trial of IV rt-PA and streptokinase in which *both* pre- and post-treatment angiography were used, the rate of reperfusion during the first 90 minutes after initiating therapy in patients with total or subtotal coronary artery occlusion was twice as high for rt-PA as for streptokinase (62 versus 31%, respectively). Although the average time from symptom onset until initiation of thrombolytic therapy was 4.75 hours in this study, the proportion of coronary arteries reperfused was greater for rt-PA than for streptokinase regardless of the time from symptom onset. An analysis of the combined results of the TIMI-1 trial and another randomized comparative trial also showed that the rate of coronary artery patency or reperfusion was greater with rt-PA than with streptokinase in patients treated both within 3 hours of symptom onset and 3–6 hours after onset of symptoms. These findings appear to confirm in vitro evidence indicating that the fibrinolytic efficacy of rt-PA is relatively unaffected by the age of a thrombus; however, delayed initiation of thrombolytic therapy is associated with a decreased likelihood of beneficial cardiac effects, regardless of the thrombolytic agent used.

Effects on Mortality Reduction

Several controlled studies have demonstrated a survival benefit in patients with acute MI receiving alteplase. In a large, placebo-controlled, multicenter study (Anglo-Scandinavian Study of Early Thrombolysis; ASSET), patients with acute MI who received alteplase 100 mg IV over a 3-hour period (an initial 10-mg loading dose followed by infusions of 50, 20, and 20 mg/hour during hours 1, 2, and 3, respectively) within 5 hours of onset of symptoms had a 26% reduction in mortality (death occurred in 9.8% of placebo-treated patients versus 7.2% of patients who received alteplase) at 1 month after discharge. The mortality reductions in patients treated within 3 hours or between 3–5 hours of symptom onset (e.g., chest pain) were similar, and the overall mortality reduction in the ASSET study was similar to that in patients receiving streptokinase within 6 hours of symptom onset in several large studies. In another study, the mortality rates in patients receiving alteplase 100 mg IV over 3 hours versus placebo were 2.8 versus 5.7% (51% mortality reduction) at 14 days and 5.1 versus 7.9% (36% mortality reduction) at 3 months; patients treated within 3 hours of onset of symptoms had 14-day and 3-month mortality reductions of 82% and 59%, respectively. All patients in this study received concomitant therapy for 10–22 days after admission with heparin by continuous IV infusion and low-dose aspirin every other day.

In 2 randomized, multicenter studies, >20,000 patients with acute evolving MI received either alteplase 100 mg IV over 3 hours or streptokinase 1.5 million units over 30–60 minutes, with or without subcutaneous heparin therapy (starting 12 hours after initiation of thrombolytic therapy). In-hospital mortality rates for the combined studies were low and similar in all 4 treatment groups: 9.2, 8.7, 7.9, or 9.2% in patients receiving either alteplase plus heparin, alteplase alone, streptokinase plus heparin, or streptokinase alone, respectively. Aspirin therapy (300–325 mg daily) and atenolol 5–10 mg IV were also administered to all study patients who had no specific contraindications to such therapy; aspirin and atenolol were given to approximately 96 and 23% of patients, respectively, in each treatment group. Although the overall incidence of complications and adverse effects was low, stroke was reported more often with alteplase than with streptokinase therapy (1.3 and 1% of patients, respectively), while major bleeding occurred more frequently in streptokinase-treated patients; streptokinase and heparin were both independently associated with an increased risk of bleeding. Adjunctive therapy with subcutaneous heparin (12,500 units twice daily during hospitalization) did not appear to provide additional benefit in patients receiving thrombolytic therapy since the incidences of stroke and reinfarction were similar whether or not concomitant heparin therapy was given.

Improved survival with a thrombolytic regimen containing alteplase compared with streptokinase-containing regimens has been demonstrated in a multicenter study in >41,000 patients with acute MI (GUSTO-1). In the GUSTO-1 study, patients were randomized to receive 1 of 4 thrombolytic regimens: alteplase (maximum dose: 100 mg) in an "accelerated-dose" schedule (i.e., total dose administered IV over 1.5 rather than the usual 3 hours, with two-thirds of the dose given in the first 30 minutes) in conjunction with *simultaneously initiated* IV heparin therapy; streptokinase (1.5 million units over 1 hour) with IV heparin;

streptokinase (1.5 million units over 1 hour) with subcutaneously administered heparin; or combined alteplase and streptokinase with IV heparin. Therapy with IV heparin (5000 units by rapid injection, then 1000–1200 units/hour) was initiated at the same time as thrombolytic therapy, while subcutaneously administered heparin (12,500 units twice daily) was begun 4 hours after initiation of thrombolytic therapy. In the combined alteplase-streptokinase regimen, streptokinase was given in a dosage of 1 million units over 1 hour; alteplase was administered in a dosage of 1 mg/kg (up to 90 mg) over 1 hour, with 10% of the dose given initially by rapid IV injection. The mortality rates at 30 days for the groups receiving streptokinase and subcutaneous heparin, streptokinase and IV heparin, accelerated-dose alteplase and IV heparin, and the combined alteplase-streptokinase regimen with IV heparin were 7.2, 7.4, 6.3, and 7%, respectively. The difference in these rates represent a 14% reduction in mortality with the accelerated-dose alteplase regimen compared with both streptokinase-only regimens and a 10% reduction compared with the combined alteplase-streptokinase regimen; there was no difference in 30 day-mortality between the 2 streptokinase-only regimens. Although hemorrhagic stroke occurred more frequently in patients receiving the accelerated-dose alteplase or combined alteplase-streptokinase regimens, the risk of the combined end point of death or disabling stroke was reduced with the accelerated-dose alteplase regimen compared with the streptokinase-only regimens, resulting in a net benefit of alteplase versus the other regimens.

Results of the GUSTO-1 study support previous data from smaller studies that demonstrated an association between early and complete coronary artery patency, improved left ventricular function, and increased survival after acute MI. In a subset of patients enrolled in the GUSTO-1 study who were randomly assigned to undergo coronary artery angiography at 90 minutes, 180 minutes, 24 hours, or 5–7 days after initiation of thrombolytic therapy, the rate of patency of the infarct-related artery and the percentage of patients with normal blood flow through that artery at 90 minutes was higher in the group given accelerated-dose alteplase with IV heparin than in those receiving other thrombolytic regimens; patency rates were similar for all groups at 180 minutes. Measures of left ventricular function paralleled the rate of patency at 90 minutes; ventricular function was best in the group given accelerated-dose alteplase with heparin and in patients with normal flow through the infarct-related artery regardless of treatment group. Likewise, mortality at 30 days was lowest (4.4%) among patients with normal blood flow in the infarct-related artery at 90-minute angiography and highest (8.9%) among those with no coronary blood flow in that artery. Failure of the combined alteplase-streptokinase regimen to produce an early patency rate similar to that of the accelerated-dose alteplase regimen has been attributed to the use of only a small initial rapid-injection dose of alteplase in the combined regimen.

Results from 2 large, comparative clinical trials (International Joint Efficacy Comparison of Thrombolytics [INJECT] trial, Global Utilization of Strategies to Open Occluded Coronary Arteries-III [GUSTO-III] trial) in patients with acute MI suggest similar effects of accelerated-dose alteplase (given as a 15-mg IV loading dose followed by 0.75 mg/kg [up to 50 mg] over 30 minutes, then 0.5 mg/kg [up to 35 mg] over 60 minutes), reteplase (2 doses of 10 units each given 30 minutes apart by direct IV injection), or streptokinase (1.5 million units IV over 60 minutes) on reduction of short-term (30 or 35 days) or long-term (6 months or 1 year) mortality. While previous studies had demonstrated improved coronary artery patency with reteplase compared with alteplase, analysis of >15,000 patients receiving the drugs in the GUSTO-III trial revealed very similar 30-day mortality rates (7.47 or 7.24% with reteplase or alteplase therapy, respectively); the incidences of other cardiovascular events, including stroke, bleeding, and intracranial hemorrhage, also were similar. The INJECT trial was not designed to demonstrate superiority of reteplase or streptokinase on reduction of mortality in patients with MI, only therapeutic equivalence; a trial in a larger number of patients would be required to demonstrate superiority of either agent. The occurrence of certain secondary clinical end points (i.e., stroke, reinfarction) was similar among patients with acute MI receiving any of the evaluated thrombolytic agents in these trials. The incidence of congestive heart failure also was lower in patients receiving reteplase than in those receiving streptokinase in the INJECT trial, and was similar among patients receiving reteplase or alteplase in the GUS-TO-III trial. All patients in these trials received adjunctive antithrombotic therapy with aspirin (160–350 mg initially followed by 75–350 mg daily) and unfractionated heparin (5000 units by direct IV injection prior to reteplase administration, followed by 1000 units hourly by continuous IV infusion for at least 24 hours). Overall clinical outcomes also were improved with alteplase compared with anistreplase (no longer commercially available in the US), although the difference in mortality rate at 6 weeks was not statistically significant.

Prevention of Reocclusion after Thrombolysis

Reocclusion of the infarct-related coronary artery following therapy with rt-PA generally has occurred in approximately 10–20% of patients, although higher reocclusion rates (up to 45%) have been reported. The reocclusion rate reported after rt-PA therapy for acute MI varies considerably but appears to be similar to or greater than that reported for streptokinase or urokinase (both no longer commercially available in the US). The rate of reocclusion is greater with a standard infusion of alteplase than with an accelerated infusion. Reocclusion usually occurs in the first 24 hours after thrombolysis, but may occur within 30 minutes after completion of the infusion and be clinically silent; late reocclusion (e.g., 4–10 days or longer after thrombolytic therapy) also can occur. The rate of reocclusion appears to depend principally on the degree of residual stenosis of the affected coronary artery, but also may be influenced by other factors, such as fluctuations in coronary blood flow during infusion of the thrombolytic agent, induction of a transient procoagulant state or possible platelet activation during thrombolytic therapy, the dosage and duration of the infusion of the thrombolytic agent, subsequent therapeutic measures (e.g., anticoagulant and/or platelet-aggregation inhibitor therapy), and the timing of angiography after thrombolytic therapy. In one study, all patients who developed reocclusion did so within 1 hour after discontinuance of the t-PA infusion when the plasma t-PA concentration had declined to less than 0.7 mcg/mL. However, in other studies, plasma rt-PA concentrations as low as 0.45 mcg/mL have been associated with prevention of reocclusion after thrombolytic therapy in patients with MI.

Several therapeutic measures (e.g., anticoagulation and/or antiplatelet therapy, prolonged infusion of the thrombolytic agent, or mechanical or surgical revascularization procedures) have been used to reduce the incidence of reocclusion after coronary artery thrombolysis with rt-PA. Anticoagulant therapy (e.g., heparin and/or oral anticoagulants) has been used concomitantly with and/or subsequent to rt-PA therapy in most patients treated for acute MI in clinical studies. Platelet-aggregation inhibitors (e.g., aspirin) and P2Y12-receptor antagonists (e.g., clopidogrel) also have been administered before, during, or after rt-PA therapy in many patients for secondary prevention of recurrent ischemic events. In addition, a vitamin K antagonist (i.e., warfarin) is recommended in patients who have other indications for anticoagulation, such as atrial fibrillation, mechanical heart valves, venous thromboembolism, or hypercoagulable disorders.

Since a substantial degree of coronary artery stenosis often remains even after successful thrombolysis and the presence of residual thrombus strongly predisposes to reocclusion, PCI also has been used after thrombolysis in an effort to maintain coronary artery patency and reduce the risk of reinfarction and recurrent ischemia.

Clinical Perspective

The principal goal of therapy in patients with STEMI is to reestablish coronary blood flow; therefore, the current standard of care in such patients is timely reperfusion (with primary PCI or thrombolytic therapy). Because of a demonstrated mortality benefit and lower rates of reinfarction with PCI compared with thrombolytic therapy, primary PCI is the preferred reperfusion strategy when it can be performed in a timely manner by experienced clinicians. Due to the limited number of PCI-capable facilities in the US, thrombolytic therapy is considered an acceptable alternative. Experts state that the appropriate and timely use of any form of reperfusion is likely more important than the choice of therapy.

The benefits of thrombolytic therapy in patients with STEMI are well established. When rt-PA is used by IV infusion in selected patients with acute MI, thrombolysis occurs usually within 1 hour after initiation of the IV infusion. The resulting reperfusion can limit infarct size, improve ventricular function (e.g., decrease ventricular arrhythmias), and reduce the incidence of congestive heart failure, cardiogenic shock, and death.

The American College of Cardiology Foundation (ACCF)/American Heart Association (AHA) guideline for the management of STEMI states that reperfusion therapy should be administered to all eligible patients with STEMI and onset of ischemic symptoms within the previous 12 hours. The appropriate reperfusion method (thrombolytic therapy or PCI) should be selected based on a risk-benefit analysis that incorporates the time from onset of MI symptoms, the clinical and hemodynamic status of the patient, presence of comorbidities (e.g., severe heart failure), bleeding risk, contraindications, and the availability (and timeliness) of PCI. Primary PCI is the preferred method of reperfusion when it can be performed in a timely manner. Thrombolytic therapy is recommended when it is anticipated that PCI cannot be performed within 120 minutes of first medical contact. Initial thrombolytic therapy is most appropriate for those patients with low bleeding risk who present early after symptom onset (less than 2–3 hours) to a non-PCI-capable hospital and who have longer delays to PCI. If therapy with rt-PA is selected, it should be instituted as soon as possible after acute MI since the potential clinical benefit diminishes as the time period from symptom onset to initiation of therapy increases. The greatest benefits of thrombolytic therapy in terms of reductions in mortality and morbidity have been observed when such therapy was initiated within the first 12 hours after symptom onset. Appreciable improvement of ventricular function (as assessed by left ventricular ejection fraction or regional wall motion), reduction in infarct size, and reduction in the incidence of congestive heart failure have been apparent when rt-PA was initiated within 6 hours of the onset of symptoms of MI, although the greatest clinical benefit has been observed when therapy was initiated earlier. ACCF and AHA recommend that thrombolytic therapy be administered within 30 minutes of hospital arrival.

Standard therapeutic measures for management of MI should be instituted concomitantly with rt-PA therapy. In all patients receiving rt-PA, the potential risk of serious hemorrhage must be weighed against the possible benefit of therapy with the drug.

The relative role of alteplase versus other thrombolytic agents in acute evolving MI remains to be fully elucidated. Many clinicians suggest that the particular thrombolytic agent used is less important for patient survival than reducing the delay in initiating treatment in patients with MI. Some clinicians state that tenecteplase may be preferred over alteplase due to its ease of IV administration as a single weight- and age-adjusted dose, lower risk of non-cerebral bleeds, and decreased necessity for blood transfusion. ACCF and AHA recommend the use of a fibrin-specific thrombolytic agent (e.g., alteplase, reteplase, tenecteplase).

• Pulmonary Embolism

Alteplase is used in adults for lysis of acute pulmonary emboli involving obstruction of blood flow to a lobe or multiple segments of the lungs, and for lysis of pulmonary emboli accompanied by unstable hemodynamics (i.e., when blood pressure cannot be maintained without supportive measures).

Clinical Experience

rt-PA, including alteplase, has been administered IV or via the pulmonary artery† in patients with acute pulmonary embolism. In a comparative study in adults with symptoms of pulmonary embolism of <2 weeks (usually <5 days) duration, 100 mg of alteplase infused over 2 hours produced moderate or marked lysis of pulmonary emboli (as documented by pulmonary angiography at 2 hours) in 59% of patients compared with 13% receiving urokinase. Improvement in lung perfusion scans 24 hours after alteplase therapy was similar to that produced by a 24-hour IV infusion of urokinase, although the biological activity of the alteplase dosage substantially exceeded that of the urokinase dosage.

The optimal therapeutic regimen for rt-PA in patients with pulmonary embolism has not been established. In IV dosages of 40–100 mg over 2–7 hours or via the pulmonary artery † in dosages of 30 or 50 mg over 1.5 or 2 hours, respectively, with or without concomitant heparin therapy, rt-PA produces clot lysis within 2–6 hours in more than 80% of patients with angiographically documented pulmonary emboli. However, substantial hemodynamic and angiographic improvement with such dosages of rt-PA has not been universally observed. Lysis of pulmonary emboli with rt-PA generally has been associated with early hemodynamic improvement and reversal of right ventricular dysfunction, and IV infusion appears to be as effective as administration via the pulmonary artery. Rapid IV injection† (e.g., over 2 minutes) of rt-PA also has been used effectively in a limited number of patients for the treatment of acute pulmonary embolism.

Clinical Perspective

Use of systemic thrombolytic therapy in the treatment of pulmonary embolism remains controversial, in part because it has not been definitely established in randomized controlled trials that thrombolytic therapy ultimately decreases mortality or prevents recurrent pulmonary embolism and because of the high risk of bleeding associated with such therapy. The American College of Chest Physicians (ACCP) generally recommends against the use of systemic thrombolytic therapy in most patients with acute pulmonary embolism; however, in such patients with associated hypotension (e.g., systolic blood pressure <90 mm Hg), thrombolytic therapy may provide some benefit in terms of a reduction in mortality, and is suggested by ACCP in patients without a high risk of bleeding. ACCP also

recommends systemic thrombolytic therapy in selected patients with acute pulmonary embolism who clinically deteriorate after starting anticoagulant therapy but have yet to develop hypotension and who have an acceptable bleeding risk. For additional information on treatment of pulmonary embolism, consult the most recent American College of Chest Physicians Evidence-based Clinical Practice Guidelines on Antithrombotic Therapy and Prevention of Thrombosis available at https://www.chestnet.org.

Further comparative studies are needed to establish the efficacy, safety, and optimum dosage of rt-PA compared with heparin, and to determine the effects of the therapies on morbidity and mortality, in the treatment of acute pulmonary embolism.

• Acute Ischemic Stroke

Alteplase is used in the management of acute ischemic stroke for improving neurologic recovery and reducing the incidence of disability. Current data from randomized, placebo-controlled studies and pooled analyses of such studies indicate that prompt initiation of alteplase treatment (within at least 3 hours but up to 4.5 hours following onset of stroke symptoms†) can result in long-term (e.g., 3-month) improvements in residual neurologic deficit, disability, and functional outcome following acute ischemic stroke with no net change in mortality. However, because benefit from thrombolytic therapy decreases substantially with time, such therapy should be administered as soon as possible following onset of stroke symptoms to obtain optimal benefit; experts recommend a "door-to-needle" time (i.e., from arrival at the treating facility until injection of alteplase) of ≤1 hour. Treatment with alteplase in these studies has been associated with an increased incidence of intracranial hemorrhage, and careful diagnosis and patient selection are necessary to minimize the risk of hemorrhage and maximize benefit in patients with acute ischemic stroke. Therapy with alteplase in acute ischemic stroke should be initiated only in patients carefully selected according to history and physical examination and in whom intracranial hemorrhage has been excluded by cranial computed tomography (CT) scan or other diagnostic imaging method sensitive for the presence of hemorrhage. Intracranial hemorrhage should be excluded as the primary cause of stroke signs and symptoms prior to initiation of treatment.

Clinical Experience

Reassurance regarding the safety and efficacy of alteplase in clinical practice is provided by the results of large phase 4 studies that included a variety of treatment centers, including academic and community hospitals with frequent and infrequent use of thrombolytic agents; a multicenter study (Safe Implementation of Thrombolysis in Stroke-Monitoring Study) in almost 6500 patients found incidences of symptomatic intracranial hemorrhage and 3-month mortality similar to or lower than those in placebo-controlled trials of alteplase given within 3 hours of symptom onset in acute stroke based on analyses of pooled data from those trials. Postmarketing surveillance and pooled analyses of data including a randomized trial in which alteplase was administered within 3–4.5 hours of symptom onset also indicate no increase in outcomes (risk of symptomatic intracranial hemorrhage, mortality, functional independence) compared with that in randomized trials in which the drug was given within 3 hours of symptom onset.

The importance of administering thrombolytic therapy as soon as possible after symptom onset is indicated by the results of a pooled analysis of data from 6 randomized, placebo-controlled trials of alteplase therapy in acute ischemic stroke, which found that such therapy was almost twice as effective when administered within 0–1.5 hours following onset of stroke symptoms (odds of a favorable outcome at 3 months: 2.81) as when administered 1.5–3 hours following onset of symptoms (odds of a favorable outcome at 3 months: 1.6). Based on a subsequent pooled analysis of data that also included a randomized study in which alteplase was administered up to 4.5 hours after symptom onset, it was estimated that substantial benefit was attained in 1 of 3 patients receiving the drug within 0–3 hours and in 1 of 6 patients receiving the drug within 3–4.5 hours after symptom onset. The safety of alteplase treatment administered >4.5 hours after symptom onset, in dosages >0.9 mg/kg and without careful blood-pressure management, has not been established; a pooled analysis of data from several randomized trials of alteplase in acute ischemic stroke suggests that administration of the drug >4.5 hours following onset of stroke symptoms may even be associated with an increased risk of mortality.

Several randomized, controlled trials in patients with acute ischemic stroke individually have failed to show statistically significant benefits of alteplase therapy in reducing disability from stroke; possible reasons for such findings include a lack of statistical power (e.g., small sample size), inclusion of patients who received the drug up to 6 hours after symptom onset or had less severe strokes, and/or choice of end points. Analyses of pooled data from these trials indicated that benefit from treatment decreased as time from stroke onset to start of treatment increased. In a subsequent 2-part, randomized, placebo-controlled study conducted by the National Institute of Neurological Disorders and Stroke (NINDS) rt-PA Stroke Study Group, treatment with alteplase (0.9 mg/kg IV to a maximum dose of 90 mg) was associated with improved functional outcome in adults with acute ischemic stroke who received the drug within 3 hours of symptom onset. All patients had CT scans at 24 hours and at 7–10 days after the onset of stroke and when clinical findings suggested intracranial hemorrhage. Blood pressure was carefully monitored and controlled (systolic and diastolic blood pressure maintained at 185 and 110 mm Hg, respectively, or less) in the study, and concomitant administration of aspirin or heparin was not allowed. In part 1 of the NINDS study, which evaluated neurologic improvement at 24 hours after stroke onset, the proportion of patients with an improvement of at least 4 points in the NIH Stroke Scale (NIHSS) or complete recovery (NIHSS score = 0) was not significantly different with alteplase or placebo treatment, although NIHSS scores suggested improvement in the condition of alteplase-treated patients at 3 months. This long-term (3-month) clinical benefit of alteplase treatment was confirmed in part 2 of the NINDS study; patients receiving alteplase were at least 30% more likely to have minimal or no disability at 3 months (as determined by median scores on the Barthel Index, Modified Rankin Scale, Glasgow Outcome Scale, and NIHSS) than those receiving placebo. In part 2, the favorable outcome of minimal or no disability occurred in at least 11% more patients treated with alteplase than in those receiving placebo. Alteplase treatment resulted in a more favorable outcome than placebo regardless of the type of stroke diagnosed at study entry or of prior aspirin use.

Combined analysis of the incidences of all-cause mortality, 90-day mortality, intracranial hemorrhage, and new ischemic stroke for patients in both parts of the NINDS study indicated a significant increase in intracranial hemorrhage, particularly symptomatic intracranial hemorrhage within 36 hours, with alteplase therapy compared with placebo. The total incidence of intracranial hemorrhage during the study follow-up period was 15.4 or 6.4% with alteplase or placebo, respectively. Symptomatic intracranial hemorrhage (defined as the occurrence of sudden clinical worsening followed by subsequent verification of intracranial hemorrhage on CT scan) occurred in 8 versus 1.3% of alteplase- or placebo-treated patients, respectively, while symptomatic intracranial hemorrhage within 36 hours after the onset of stroke was found in 6.4 versus 0.6% of these respective groups. The incidence of asymptomatic intracranial hemorrhage (defined as intracranial hemorrhage detected on a routine repeat CT scan without preceding clinical worsening) was similar among patients receiving alteplase (7.4%) or placebo (5.1%), as was the incidence of new ischemic stroke at 3 months (5.8 versus 4.5% with alteplase or placebo, respectively). Alteplase therapy was not associated with increases in the incidences of 90-day mortality or severe disability compared with placebo.

There was a trend toward increased risk of symptomatic intracranial hemorrhage within the first 36 hours in patients with severe neurologic deficit (e.g., NIHSS score >22) or those of advanced age (e.g., patients >77 years of age). Analyses of efficacy suggested a reduced but still favorable clinical outcome for alteplase-treated patients with severe neurologic deficit or advanced age on pretreatment evaluation.

In another randomized, placebo-controlled, phase 3 trial (ECASS-3), patients with acute ischemic stroke who received alteplase (0.9 mg/kg IV to a maximum dose of 90 mg) within up to 4.5 hours† following onset of stroke symptoms (median time: 3 hours 59 minutes following onset of symptoms) had more favorable clinical outcomes than those receiving placebo, and overall results with regard to efficacy and safety were consistent with those of an earlier trial (NINDS study) indicating efficacy of alteplase given within 3 hours of onset of stroke symptoms. The primary efficacy end point in the ECASS-3 trial, disability at day 90 (defined as a modified Rankin scale score of 0 or 1, indicating a favorable outcome of minimal or no disability) was achieved in 52.4 or 45.2% of those receiving alteplase or placebo, respectively. Alteplase recipients also had a 28% greater likelihood of attaining a favorable outcome in terms of a global composite secondary efficacy end point that assessed the patient's ability to return to an independent lifestyle. As in other trials of alteplase therapy for acute ischemic stroke, the incidence of symptomatic intracranial hemorrhage was higher with alteplase therapy (2.4%) than with placebo (0.2%); however, mortality was similar between the groups (7.7 or 8.4% with alteplase therapy or placebo, respectively). The incidence

of intracranial hemorrhage was not substantially increased despite allowing the use of subcutaneous heparin to prevent deep-vein thrombosis in the first 24 hours after alteplase treatment, an exclusion criterion in earlier trials. Patient selection criteria for the ECASS-3 trial were similar to those of earlier trials of alteplase in acute ischemic stroke (e.g., NINDS) except that patients >80 years of age, those with severe stroke (a baseline NIHSS score >25), and those with a history of both stroke and diabetes were excluded. Therefore, some clinicians recommend close adherence to the ECASS-3 inclusion and exclusion criteria when treating patients with onset of stroke symptoms between 3 and 4.5 hours.

Trials investigating alteplase treatment administered >4.5 hours after symptom onset† in patients with acute ischemic stroke using imaging biomarkers to determine eligibility for treatment have been conducted. The MRI-Guided Thrombolysis for Stroke with Unknown Time of Onset (WAKE-UP) trial was a multicenter, randomized, double-blind, placebo-controlled trial in patients with an unknown onset of stroke † and a time since last known to be well of ≥4.5 hours. Patients qualified if there was a mismatch between the presence of an abnormal signal on MRI diffusion-weighted imaging and no visible signal change on diffusion-positive fluid-attenuated inversion recovery (FLAIR) in the region of the acute stroke. Patients were excluded if MRI showed intracranial hemorrhage or regions larger than one-third of the territory of the middle cerebral artery (MCA); if thrombectomy was planned; or if they had severe stroke (NIHSS score >25). The incidence of a favorable outcome (a modified Rankin scale score of 0 or 1 at 90 days) was greater in patients who received alteplase (0.9 mg/kg IV up to a maximum dose of 90 mg) compared with patients receiving placebo (53.3 versus 41.8%). The median time from symptom recognition to administration of alteplase was 3.1 hours, and the median interval between the time the patient was last known to be well and treatment initiation was 10.3 hours. There was a trend toward a higher incidence of symptomatic intracranial hemorrhage (2 versus 0.4%) and mortality (4.1 versus 1.2%) with alteplase therapy compared with placebo.

In the Thrombolysis Guided by Perfusion Imaging up to 9 Hours after Onset of Stroke (EXTEND) clinical trial, CT-perfusion (CT-P) imaging was used to assess the eligibility for IV alteplase and suggested that the efficacy and safety of alteplase can extend to up to 9 hours† after stroke onset. The EXTEND trial was a multicenter, randomized, placebo-controlled trial in patients with NIHSS score of 4–26 and hypoperfused but salvageable regions of brain detected on automated perfusion imaging. Patients were randomly assigned to receive IV alteplase (0.9 mg/kg IV up to a maximum dose of 90 mg) or placebo between 4.5 and 9 hours after the onset of stroke or on awakening with stroke† (if within 9 hours from the midpoint of sleep). The incidence of a favorable outcome (a score of 0 or 1 on the modified Rankin scale at 90 days) was greater in patients who received alteplase compared with patients receiving placebo (35.4 versus 29.5%). As in other trials of alteplase therapy for acute ischemic stroke, the incidence of symptomatic intracranial hemorrhage was higher with alteplase therapy (6.2%) than with placebo (0.9%); however, mortality was similar between the groups (11.5 or 8.9% with alteplase therapy or placebo, respectively). Additional studies are needed to establish the safety and efficacy of IV alteplase in patients with acute ischemic stroke and unknown time of onset or time since onset of >4.5 hours.

Clinical Perspective

Current evidence from randomized studies and pooled analyses of data indicate that initiation of alteplase up to 4.5 hours following the onset of symptoms of stroke provides a net benefit in terms of reducing disability, and the American Heart Association/American Stroke Association (AHA/ASA) and other experts currently recommend administration of alteplase within up to 3–4.5 hours of the onset of symptoms in eligible patients. Therapy with alteplase in acute ischemic stroke should be initiated only in patients carefully selected according to history and physical examination and in whom intracranial hemorrhage has been excluded by cranial computed tomography (CT) scan or other diagnostic imaging method sensitive for the presence of hemorrhage.

According to the 2019 update to the 2018 guidelines for the early management of acute ischemic stroke from AHA/ASA, IV alteplase within 4.5 hours of stroke onset remains the standard of care for most patients with acute ischemic stroke. AHA/ASA state that patients who are eligible for IV alteplase should receive the drug even if mechanical thrombectomy is being considered. The benefits of both IV alteplase and mechanical thrombectomy are time-dependent, with greater benefits associated with treatment earlier in the time window; time from symptom onset to IV alteplase should be as short as possible, and generally never more than 4.5 hours.

AHA/ASA recommend IV alteplase within 3 hours of symptom onset in patients ≥18 years of age with severe stroke or mild but disabling stroke. IV alteplase is recommended within 3–4.5 hours of symptom onset in patients 18–80 years of age who meet the following criteria: absence of a history of both diabetes mellitus and prior stroke; NIHSS score ≤25; not taking any oral anticoagulants; and no imaging evidence of ischemic injury involving greater than one-third of the middle cerebral artery (MCA) territory. Additional eligibility criteria for treatment with IV alteplase include: ability to safely lower and maintain BP ≤185/110 mm Hg; blood glucose concentrations ≥50 mg/dL; mild to moderate early ischemic changes on noncontrast CT; and normal activated partial thromboplastin time (aPTT) in patients with end-stage renal disease. AHA/ASA state that IV alteplase is recommended for patients taking antiplatelet drug monotherapy or combination therapy (eg, aspirin and clopidogrel) before stroke on the basis of evidence that the benefit of alteplase outweighs a possible small increased risk of intracranial hemorrhage. IV alteplase is considered contraindicated in otherwise eligible patients with mild and nondisabling stroke (NIHSS ≤5).

According to AHA/ASA, individual assessment of the relative risks and benefits is required in patients with ischemic stroke presenting within 3–4.5 hours of symptom onset who: are >80 years of age; have a history of both prior stroke and diabetes mellitus; have a mild but disabling stroke; or who have NIHSS >25. Additional criteria which indicate a need for individual risk benefit assessment based on clinical characteristics, specifics of stroke presentation, medical history, and comorbid conditions are detailed in the guidelines and can be found at https://www.stroke.org/-/media/Stroke-Files/Ischemic-Stroke-Professional-Materials/AIS-Toolkit/Guidelines-for-Mangaging-Patients-with-AIS-2019-Update-to-2018-Guidelines.pdf.

AHA/ASA state that while IV alteplase remains the recommended thrombolytic agent, it may be reasonable to choose tenecteplase (single IV bolus of 0.25 mg/kg, maximum 25 mg) over IV alteplase in patients without contraindications for IV fibrinolysis who also are candidates to undergo mechanical thrombectomy. AHA/ASA also state that tenecteplase administered as a 0.4-mg/kg single IV bolus has not been proven to be superior or noninferior to alteplase but might be considered as an alternative to alteplase in patients with acute ischemic stroke who have minor neurological impairment and no major intracranial occlusion. However, in some studies, including a study in patients with moderate to severe stroke published after release of the AHA/ASA 2019 update, tenecteplase 0.4 mg/kg was associated with worse functional and safety outcomes compared to alteplase, and some clinicians recommend against use of this dosage of tenecteplase in patients with acute ischemic stroke. The administration of tenecteplase as a single IV bolus as opposed to the 1-hour infusion required for alteplase is mentioned by AHA/ASA as a potential advantage of tenecteplase.

Based on data from studies such as the WAKE-UP (Efficacy and Safety of MRI-based Thrombolysis in Wake-Up Stroke) trial, AHA/ASA state that in patients with acute ischemic stroke who awake with stroke symptoms † or have unclear time of onset >4.5 hours† from last known well or baseline state, MRI to identify diffusion-positive fluid-attenuated inversion recovery (FLAIR)-negative lesions can be useful for selecting those who can benefit from IV alteplase administration within 4.5 hours of stroke symptom recognition.

AHA/ASA state that use of intra-arterial infusion† of alteplase initiated within 6 hours of stroke onset† in carefully selected patients who have contraindications to the use of IV alteplase might be considered but that the clinical outcome of such treatment is uncertain. According to AHA/ASA, mechanical thrombectomy with stent retrievers is recommended over intra-arterial fibrinolysis as first-line therapy.

● *Arterial Thrombosis and Embolism*

rt-PA has been administered by selective intra-arterial injection in a limited number of adults for lysis of arterial occlusions† in peripheral vessels and bypass grafts. Angiographic and clinical improvement generally have occurred in more than 80% of patients treated with dosages of 0.05–0.1 mg/kg per hour, or even lower dosages (e.g., 0.02 mg/kg per hour) in a few patients, for 1–8 hours; however, most patients with acute arterial occlusion require further therapeutic intervention after thrombolysis. ACCP suggests the use of intra-arterial thrombolytic therapy in patients with acute limb ischemia due to arterial emboli or thrombosis; however, surgical reperfusion is preferred over thrombolytic therapy. If thrombolytic therapy is used in such patients, ACCP suggests that a recombinant tissue plasminogen activator (e.g., alteplase) or urokinase (no longer available in the U.S.) is preferred. In neonates and children with limb- or organ-threatening (via proximal extension) femoral artery thrombosis who fail to respond to initial treatment with unfractionated heparin, thrombolytic therapy is recommended unless such

therapy is contraindicated. Like other thrombolytic agents, rt-PA probably should be avoided in patients with arterial emboli originating from the left side of the heart (e.g., in patients with mitral stenosis accompanied by atrial fibrillation or those with left ventricular thrombi) because of the potential risk of new embolic episodes, including those involving cerebral vessels.

● *Occluded Catheters*

Alteplase is used to restore patency to central venous catheters obstructed by a thrombus (assessed by the ability to withdraw blood). Causes of catheter dysfunction other than thrombus formation, such as catheter malposition, mechanical failure, constriction by a suture, lipid deposits, or drug precipitates, should be considered before instillation of alteplase. Pooled results of a placebo-controlled study and a large open-label study indicate that about 68% of central venous catheters occluded for less than 14 days were cleared (as determined by the successful withdrawal of 3 mL of blood and infusion of 5 mL of saline through the catheter) with a single dose of alteplase (2 mg) and about 88% of occluded catheters were cleared after a second dose of alteplase, administered 120 minutes after the first dose. The incidence of recurrent catheter dysfunction within 30 days after treatment was 26%. Restoration of catheter function was similar among all catheter types studied (single, double, or triple lumen; implanted ports). Results of an open-label study evaluating the efficacy of the drug in restoring catheter function in pediatric patients (2 weeks to 17 years of age) indicated that 83% of the occluded catheters (defined by the inability to withdraw at least 3 mL of blood from the catheter in children weighing at least 10 kg or at least 1 mL in children weighing less than 10 kg) were cleared with up to 2 doses of alteplase (2 mg/2 mL in children weighing at least 30 kg or 110% of the estimated lumen volume not to exceed 2 mg/2 mL in children weighing less than 30 kg) in up to 120 minutes postdose.

Alteplase has been used for clearing totally or partially occluded hemodialysis access catheters†. Studies of alteplase in patients with occluded hemodialysis catheters have evaluated similar dosing regimens as those currently used for clearing central venous catheters.

DOSAGE AND ADMINISTRATION

● *General*

Pretreatment Screening

- In patients with acute ischemic stroke who have not received recent anticoagulation therapy (e.g., oral anticoagulants, heparin), therapy with alteplase may be initiated prior to coagulation study results. However, infusion of alteplase should be discontinued if pretreatment coagulation study results are abnormal (as indicated by an INR >1.7 or an elevated aPTT).

- In patients with acute ischemic stroke, obtain blood glucose concentrations prior to treatment with IV alteplase.

Patient Monitoring

- Frequently monitor and control blood pressure during and following IV infusion of alteplase in patients with acute ischemic stroke. AHA/ASA state that systolic/diastolic blood pressure should be maintained at <180/105 mm Hg for the first 24 hours after IV alteplase treatment.

- Carefully monitor all potential bleeding sites (e.g., sites of all venous cutdowns, arterial and venous punctures, needle punctures).

- Routine monitoring of hemostatic indices (e.g., fibrinogen concentrations or thrombin times) during therapy for acute MI is generally not recommended; however, monitoring hemostatic function has been suggested for patients who exhibit bleeding. Determination of plasma fibrinogen also may be useful after discontinuance of thrombolytic therapy for correcting potential hemostatic abnormalities before anticipated surgery or other invasive procedures; monitoring of other coagulation indices (e.g., activated partial thromboplastin time) may be indicated for adjusting subsequent anticoagulant therapy.

- Monitor patients for hypersensitivity reactions and treat appropriately.

Dispensing and Administration Precautions

- Based on the Institute for Safe Medication Practices (ISMP), alteplase is a high-alert medication that has a heightened risk of causing significant patient harm when used in error.

- The ISMP list of error-prone abbreviations, symbols, and dose designations states that the use of abbreviations for alteplase (e.g., t-PA) during the medication use process should be avoided as their use has been associated with serious medication errors.

Other General Considerations

- Institute therapy as soon as possible after acute MI.

- In patients with acute ischemic stroke, administer in facilities that can provide appropriate evaluation and management of intracranial hemorrhage.

- Initiate therapy for acute ischemic stroke within 3–4.5 hours of symptom onset. Prior to administration, exclude intracranial hemorrhage by cranial CT scan or other sensitive diagnostic imaging method.

● Administration

Alteplase is administered by IV infusion and by intracatheter instillation into occluded central venous catheters (Cathflo® Activase®), and the manufacturer states that the drug is intended for this method of administration only. When administered IV, the drug preferably should be administered via a controlled-infusion device using separate IV tubing. Do not add any other drugs to infusion solutions containing alteplase. Alteplase also has been administered by intracoronary† injection, selective intra-arterial† infusion, and intraocularly† via intracameral injection in a limited number of patients.

Extravasation during IV infusion of alteplase may cause ecchymosis and/or inflammation. If extravasation occurs, terminate the infusion at that IV site and apply local therapy.

IV Administration

Reconstitution and Dilution

Alteplase is reconstituted by adding 50 mL of sterile water for injection without preservatives to a vial labeled as containing 50 mg of drug using a large-bore (e.g., 18-gauge) needle and directing the stream of diluent into the lyophilized cake; do not use diluents other than sterile water for injection without preservatives for reconstitution. Do not use the vial if a vacuum is not present. The resultant solution contains approximately 1 mg of alteplase per mL. If foaming (usually slight) occurs during reconstitution, leave the vial undisturbed for several minutes after addition of the diluent to allow dissipation of any large bubbles. The reconstituted solution may be used as reconstituted (1 mg/mL) or may be further diluted just prior to administration to a concentration of approximately 0.5 mg/mL with 0.9% sodium chloride injection or 5% dextrose injection, using either polyvinyl chloride bags or glass vials; do not use more dilute solutions since precipitation of the drug may occur at concentrations <0.5 mg/mL. Other infusion solutions, including sterile water for injection without preservatives or preservative-containing solutions, should not be used for dilution of the reconstituted solution. During dilution of the reconstituted solution, mix the solution with gentle swirling and/or slow inversion of the infusion container; avoid excessive agitation.

Consult the manufacturer's labeling for information on the reconstitution and dilution of vials labeled as containing 100 mg of the drug and for detailed instructions on preparing doses of alteplase for IV infusion.

Visually inspect reconstituted solutions of alteplase for particulate matter and discoloration before further dilution or administration whenever solution and container permit. Because alteplase powder for injection and reconstituted and diluted solutions of the drug contain no preservatives, the solutions preferably should be prepared immediately before use, but may be used for up to 8 hours after reconstitution or dilution when stored at 2–30°C; discard any unused solution.

Standardize 4 Safety

Standardized concentrations for alteplase have been established through Standardize 4 Safety (S4S), a national patient safety initiative to reduce medication errors, especially during transitions of care. Multidisciplinary expert panels were convened to determine recommended standard concentrations. Because recommendations from the S4S panels may differ from the manufacturer's prescribing information, caution is advised when using concentrations that differ from labeling, particularly when using rate information from the label. For additional information on S4S (including updates that may be available), see https://www.ashp.org/pharmacy-practice/standardize-4-safety-initiative.

TABLE 1. Standardize 4 Safety Continuous Infusion Standards for Alteplase.

Patient Population	Concentration Standard	Dosing Units
Pediatric patients (<50 kg)	1 mg/mL	mg/kg per hour
Adults	1 mg/mL	mg/hour

Administration into Occluded Central Venous Catheters

Reconstitution

Alteplase powder for restoring patency of central venous catheters (Cathflo® Activase®) is reconstituted by adding 2.2 mL of sterile water for injection to a vial labeled as containing 2 mg of alteplase to provide a concentration of 1 mg/mL. Do not use bacteriostatic water for injection as a diluent. If foaming (usually slight) occurs during reconstitution, leave the vial undisturbed for several minutes after addition of the diluent to allow dissipation of any large bubbles.

Visually inspect reconstituted solutions of alteplase for particulate matter and discoloration before further dilution or administration whenever solution and container permit. Because alteplase powder intracatheter instillation and reconstituted solutions of the drug contain no preservatives, the drug preferably should be reconstituted immediately before use, but may be used for up to 8 hours after reconstitution when stored at 2–30°C; discard any unused solution.

● Dosage

Dosage of alteplase usually is expressed in mg of drug but also may be expressed in international units (IU, units); each mg is equivalent to 580,000 units.

Acute Myocardial Infarction

Alteplase therapy should be initiated as soon as possible after the onset of symptoms of myocardial infarction (MI) since potential clinical benefit diminishes as the time period to initiation of therapy increases. Some experts recommend that thrombolytic therapy be administered within 30 minutes of hospital arrival.

Various dosage regimens have been employed in patients treated with rt-PA for lysis of coronary artery thrombi. Alteplase may be administered by IV infusion over 3 hours or as an "accelerated" infusion over 1.5 hours. Controlled studies comparing clinical outcomes with these regimens have not been performed. However, pooled analyses of data from thrombolytic trials indicate that an accelerated infusion of alteplase is associated with greater rates of patency of the infarct-related artery than with a standard 3-hour infusion, and some experts consider the accelerated infusion regimen of alteplase to be the preferred method of administration. Although a dose of 150 mg of alteplase was used in early studies with the drug, this dose should not be used for the treatment of acute MI because of its association with an increased incidence of intracranial bleeding.

3-Hour Infusion

For lysis of coronary artery thrombi associated with acute MI, the usual adult dose (weight ≥65 kg) of alteplase currently recommended is 100 mg (58 million units) IV over a 3-hour period, given as an initial 60-mg (34.8 million units) lytic dose during the first hour (of which 6–10 mg is infused rapidly over 1–2 minutes) and a subsequent maintenance infusion at a rate of 20 mg (11.6 million units) per hour for the next 2 hours. For adults weighing <65 kg (lean or actual body weight, whichever is less), a dose of 1.25 mg/kg may be infused IV over 3 hours as an initial lytic dose of 0.75 mg/kg during the first hour (of which 0.075 mg/kg is infused rapidly over 1–2 minutes) and a subsequent maintenance infusion at a rate of 0.25 mg/kg per hour for the next 2 hours. The maximum recommended total dosage is 100 mg.

Accelerated Infusion

When administered as an accelerated infusion for lysis of coronary artery thrombi associated with MI, the dose of alteplase is based on patient weight but should not exceed 100 mg. In adults weighing >67 kg, the usual dose of alteplase is 100 mg given by IV infusion; an initial 15-mg dose is given by rapid IV injection (e.g., over 1–2 minutes) followed by 50 mg IV over the next 30 minutes then 35 mg IV over the next hour. In patients weighing ≤67 kg, an initial 15-mg dose of alteplase is given by rapid IV injection (e.g., over 1–2 minutes), followed by 0.75 mg/kg (not to exceed 50 mg) over the next 30 minutes then 0.5 mg/kg (not to exceed 35 mg) over the next hour. The manufacturer states that the safety and efficacy of alteplase given by accelerated infusion has only been evaluated with concomitant heparin and aspirin administration. Although a dose of 150 mg of alteplase was used in early studies with the drug, this dose is no longer recommended because of its association with an increased incidence of intracranial bleeding.

Pulmonary Embolism

Various dosage regimens of rt-PA, including alteplase, have been used in adults for the management of acute pulmonary embolism, and the optimal dosage regimen for rt-PA in patients with this condition has not been established. For lysis of acute pulmonary emboli involving obstruction of blood flow to a lobe or multiple segments of the lungs, the usual adult dose of alteplase currently recommended is 100 mg (58 million units) IV over a 2-hour period. The manufacturer states that parenteral anticoagulation should be instituted near the end of or immediately following the alteplase infusion when the activated partial thromboplastin time (aPTT) or thrombin time returns to twice the normal value or less. In the setting of cardiac arrest associated with pulmonary embolism, AHA guidelines suggest an alteplase dosage of 50 mg IV bolus with an option for a repeat bolus in 15 minutes; there is no consensus on the ideal dose of thrombolytic therapy in pulmonary embolism-associated cardiac arrest. Alteplase also has been infused via the pulmonary artery† in adults in dosages of 30 or 50 mg over 1.5 or 2 hours, respectively, with concomitant heparin therapy. Lysis of pulmonary emboli usually has occurred within 2–6 hours after initiation of the IV or intra-arterial infusion, and IV infusion of the drug appears to be as effective as administration via the pulmonary artery.

Acute Ischemic Stroke

For the treatment of acute ischemic stroke, the recommended dosage of alteplase is 0.9 mg/kg (up to a maximum dose of 90 mg). Initially, administer 10% of the dose by rapid IV infusion over 1 minute; infuse the remainder of the dose by IV infusion over 60 minutes. The dosage of alteplase for the treatment of acute ischemic stroke should not exceed 0.9 mg/kg (maximum 90 mg). For optimum benefit, alteplase should be administered as soon as possible, but must be given within 3–4.5 hours following onset of stroke symptoms. The manufacturer states that treatment should be initiated within 3 hours of onset of symptoms. Heparin anticoagulation that produces an elevated aPTT should not be used within 48 hours of the use of alteplase. Administration of aspirin within 24 hours of the use of a thrombolytic agent generally is not recommended by AHA and the American Stroke Association (ASA). In patients with acute ischemic stroke who have not received recent anticoagulation therapy (e.g., oral anticoagulants, heparin), therapy with alteplase may be initiated prior to coagulation study results. However, infusion of alteplase should be discontinued if pretreatment coagulation study results are abnormal (as indicated by an INR >1.7 or an elevated aPTT).

Arterial Thrombosis and Embolism

For lysis of arterial occlusion† in a peripheral vessel or bypass graft, alteplase usually has been infused intra-arterially in a dosage of 0.05–0.1 mg/kg per hour for 1–8 hours, although there is limited evidence that even lower dosages (e.g., 0.02 mg/kg per hour over 1–7 hours) may be effective. Regardless of the regimen used, however, some patients with acute arterial occlusion require further therapeutic intervention after thrombolysis.

Occluded Catheters

To clear an occluded central venous IV catheter, 2 mg of alteplase in 2 mL of sterile water for injection is administered into the occluded catheter in patients weighing ≥30 kg. In patients weighing <30 kg, a volume of the alteplase solution equal to 110% of the internal lumen volume of the catheter should be instilled, up to a maximum of 2 mg of alteplase in 2 mL of solution. After at least 30 minutes of dwell time, catheter function is assessed by attempting to aspirate blood. When patency is restored, 4–5 mL of blood in patients weighing ≥10 kg or 3 mL of blood in patients weighing <10 kg should be aspirated to remove all drug and residual clot. An aspiration attempt may be repeated at 120 minutes of dwell time, and a second injection of alteplase (up to 2 mg for a total of up to 4 mg) may be necessary in resistant cases. The American College of Chest Physicians (ACCP) suggests that a second dose of alteplase may be administered after 30 minutes of dwell time if the catheter remains occluded. The catheter should then be gently irrigated with 0.9% sodium chloride injection. If catheter patency is not successfully established after 2 doses of alteplase, ACCP suggests radiologic imaging to rule out a catheter-related thrombus.

When alteplase has been used to clear occluded hemodialysis access catheters,† several regimens have been employed. In a limited number of studies, 1–2 mg of alteplase were injected directly into the occluded catheter and allowed to remain for at least 30 minutes of dwell time. Catheter function was assessed by measurement of blood flow rate at the next hemodialysis session; blood flow rates of 200–300 mL/minute indicated successful restoration of patency of the hemodialysis access catheter. Some patients required additional intracatheter instillations of alteplase for reocclusion of hemodialysis access catheters after successful establishment of patency. Some clinicians have used 2 mg of alteplase in a total volume of 2 mL by direct injection into the catheter after a hemodialysis session and then aspirated the lumen contents before the next hemodialysis session in patients with indwelling catheters. Other clinicians have infused 2.5–5 mg of alteplase over 2–3 hours in each access port in patients with occluded hemodialysis catheters.

Special Populations

Geriatric Patients

Based on results of a trial with tenecteplase showing that an excess of intracranial hemorrhage in patients ≥75 years of age with acute MI was reduced after reducing the tenecteplase dosage by 50%, some clinicians suggest considering a 50% reduction in the dosage of alteplase in patients ≥75 years of age receiving the drug for acute MI.

CAUTIONS

● Contraindications

Acute MI or PE

- Active internal bleeding.
- History of recent stroke.
- Intracranial neoplasm.
- Aneurysm.
- Recent (within 3 months) intracranial or intraspinal surgery or serious head trauma.
- Bleeding diathesis.
- Arteriovenous malformation.
- Current severe uncontrolled hypertension.

Acute Ischemic Stroke

- Current intracranial hemorrhage, subarachnoid hemorrhage, history of intracranial hemorrhage, or active internal bleeding.
- Extensive regions of clear hypoattenuation on CT brain imaging.
- Bleeding diathesis.
- Recent (within 3 months) intracranial or intraspinal surgery, serious head trauma, or prior ischemic stroke.
- Current severe uncontrolled hypertension.
- Arteriovenous malformation or aneurysm.
- Symptoms consistent with infective endocarditis.
- Stroke known or suspected to be associated with aortic arch dissection.
- Intracranial neoplasm.
- Structural GI malignancy.
- Thrombocytopenia (platelets <100,000/mm³), INR >1.7, aPTT >40 seconds, or PT >15 seconds.
- Treatment dose of low molecular weight heparin within previous 24 hours.
- Current treatment with direct thrombin inhibitors or direct factor Xa inhibitors unless laboratory tests are normal or >48 hours since a dose of these agents was received (assuming normal renal metabolizing function).

● Warnings/Precautions

Effects on Hemostasis

Alteplase can cause serious, sometimes fatal, internal and external bleeding, especially at arterial and venous puncture sites. Bleeding and hemorrhagic complications, including intracranial hemorrhage and other major bleeding complications, are possible in patients receiving alteplase. Hemorrhage associated with alteplase may be more common in geriatric patients and those with a history of cerebrovascular accident or severe or poorly controlled hypertension.

Weigh increased risks of therapy against anticipated benefits in patients with recent major surgery (e.g., coronary artery bypass), cerebrovascular disease, obstetric delivery, organ biopsy, previous puncture of noncompressible vessels, hypertension (SBP >175 mm Hg and/or DBP >110 mm Hg), high likelihood of hemostatic defects (e.g., secondary to severe hepatic or renal disease), internal (e.g., GI or GU) bleeding, acute pericarditis, subacute bacterial endocarditis, pregnancy, septic thrombophlebitis or occluded arteriovenous cannula at seriously infected site, recent intracranial hemorrhage, or recent (within 2–4 weeks) trauma. Also, weigh risks against benefits of therapy in patients with diabetic hemorrhagic retinopathy or other hemorrhagic ophthalmic conditions. Weigh risks against benefits in patients receiving concurrent oral anticoagulant therapy (e.g., warfarin). Weigh risks against benefits in patients with any condition in which bleeding constitutes a substantial hazard or would be particularly difficult to manage because of its location.

Initiate therapy only after careful screening for contraindications (e.g., previous neurologic events, severe hypertension, and potential bleeding sites).

Minimize the risk of bleeding by carefully selecting patients and monitoring all potential bleeding sites (e.g., sites of all venous cutdowns, arterial and venous punctures, needle punctures). Avoid IM injections and nonessential handling of patient. Perform invasive venous procedures carefully and as infrequently as possible. Avoid arterial and venous invasive procedures in areas inaccessible to manual compression (e.g., internal jugular or subclavian punctures) before and during therapy. Use of an artery in an upper extremity (e.g., radial or brachial) is preferable if arterial puncture is essential. Apply pressure to the puncture site for ≥30 minutes, followed by a pressure dressing and frequent inspection of the puncture site for bleeding.

Severe spontaneous (i.e., unrelated to catheter or other puncture sites) bleeding, including cerebral, retroperitoneal, genitourinary, and GI bleeding, has occurred during rt-PA therapy and can be fatal (e.g., secondary to cerebral hemorrhage or other serious internal hemorrhage). Upper airway hemorrhage (sometimes fatal) at the site of traumatic intubation has been reported with alteplase therapy. Less severe spontaneous bleeding, such as superficial hematoma or ecchymoses, hematuria, hemoptysis, epistaxis, and gingival bleeding, also can occur in patients receiving rt-PA.

Aspirin and heparin have been administered concomitantly with and following infusions of alteplase in the management of acute MI and pulmonary embolism; however, the concomitant administration of heparin and aspirin with and following infusions of alteplase for the treatment of acute ischemic stroke during the first 24 hours after symptom onset has not been studied. Because heparin, aspirin, or alteplase may cause bleeding complications, carefully monitor for bleeding, especially at arterial puncture sites. Hemorrhage can occur one or more days after administration of alteplase, while patients are still receiving anticoagulant therapy.

If serious bleeding occurs, immediately discontinue alteplase therapy and initiate appropriate treatment. If serious bleeding at a critical location (e.g., intracranial, GI, retroperitoneal, pericardial) occurs with intracatheter instillation of alteplase, discontinue therapy immediately and withdraw the drug from the catheter.

Coagulation tests and measures of fibrinolytic activity may be unreliable during alteplase therapy, unless specific precautions are taken to prevent in vitro artifacts. When present in blood at pharmacologic concentrations, alteplase remains active under in vitro conditions, which can result in degradation of fibrinogen in blood samples removed for analysis.

Extravasation during IV infusion of alteplase may cause ecchymosis and/or inflammation. Terminate the infusion at that IV site and apply local therapy if extravasation occurs.

Cardiovascular Effects

Cardiovascular effects such as cardiogenic shock, heart failure, myocardial rupture, electromechanical dissociation, pericardial effusion, pericarditis, mitral regurgitation, or cardiac tamponade have occurred in patients with acute MI receiving alteplase. Pleural effusion has been reported in patients with pulmonary embolism receiving alteplase. Hypotension and pulmonary edema have been reported in patients with either acute MI or pulmonary embolism receiving alteplase. Potentially fatal adverse effects, such as thromboembolism or recurrent thromboembolic events (myocardial reinfarction, recurrent ischemia, or pulmonary

re-embolization) have occurred in patients with acute MI or pulmonary embolism receiving alteplase in clinical trials or during postmarketing surveillance.

Thromboembolic events may occur in patients receiving thrombolytic agents, including alteplase, who have a high likelihood of left heart thrombus, such as patients with mitral stenosis or atrial fibrillation. Alteplase has not been shown to adequately treat underlying deep vein thrombosis in patients with pulmonary embolism; consider the possible risk of re-embolization due to lysis of underlying deep vein thrombi in such patients. Weigh risks against anticipated benefits of therapy in patients with a high likelihood of left heart thrombus (e.g., mitral stenosis, atrial fibrillation, profound left ventricular dyskinesia), acute pericarditis, subacute bacterial endocarditis, septic thrombophlebitis, or an occluded arteriovenous cannula at a seriously infected site.

New embolic episodes, including those involving cerebral vessels, may occur in patients receiving alteplase. Like other thrombolytic agents, rt-PA probably should be avoided in patients with arterial emboli originating from the left side of the heart (e.g., in patients with mitral stenosis accompanied by atrial fibrillation or those with left ventricular thrombi) because of the potential risk of new embolic episodes, including those involving cerebral vessels.

Reocclusion of the infarct-related coronary artery following therapy with rt-PA generally has occurred in approximately 10–20% of patients, although higher reocclusion rates (up to 45%) have been reported. The rate of reocclusion is greater with a standard infusion of alteplase than with an accelerated infusion. Reocclusion usually occurs in the first 24 hours after thrombolysis, but may occur within 30 minutes after completion of the infusion and be clinically silent; late reocclusion (e.g., 4–10 days or longer after thrombolytic therapy) also can occur. Reduce incidence of reocclusion through concomitant anticoagulation (e.g., heparin and/or oral anticoagulants) and/or platelet-aggregation inhibitor (e.g., aspirin, dipyridamole) therapy, prolonged infusion of the thrombolytic agent, or mechanical or surgical revascularization procedures.

Cerebrovascular Effects

New ischemic stroke, which may be potentially fatal, has been reported in patients with an acute ischemic stroke receiving alteplase in clinical trials or during postmarketing surveillance. Therefore, it is important that the benefits versus risks of rt-PA therapy be carefully considered, particularly when the potential for acute intraventricular thrombus exists.

The manufacturer and other clinicians state that the risks of alteplase therapy for the treatment of acute ischemic stroke may be increased and should be weighed against anticipated benefits in patients with severe neurologic deficit (e.g., NIH Stroke Scale [NIHSS] score >22) on pretreatment evaluation (because of an increased risk of intracranial hemorrhage in such patients); clinicians state that this also applies to patients with major early infarct signs on CT scan (e.g., substantial edema, mass effect, midline shift). However, AHA and ASA state that thrombolytic therapy almost always should not be administered to patients with major early infarct signs (greater than one-third of the middle cerebral artery territory and clearly identifiable hypodensity on CT scan).

In patients with acute ischemic stroke, administer alteplase in facilities that can provide appropriate evaluation and management of intracranial hemorrhage. Frequently monitor and control blood pressure during and following administration. The safety of administering alteplase without careful blood pressure management has not been established.

Cholesterol Embolization

Cholesterol crystal embolization and associated serious complications in the absence of antecedent invasive vascular procedures have been reported rarely in patients receiving thrombolytic therapy, including alteplase. This serious condition, which can be fatal, also is associated with invasive vascular procedures (e.g., cardiac catheterization, angiography, vascular surgery) and/or anticoagulant therapy. Clinical features of cholesterol embolization may include livedo reticularis, "purple toe" syndrome, acute renal failure, gangrenous digits, hypertension, pancreatitis, MI, cerebral infarction, spinal cord infarction, retinal artery occlusion, bowel infarction, and rhabdomyolysis.

Arrhythmias

Rapid lysis of coronary artery thrombi by thrombolytic agents may be associated with reperfusion-related atrial and/or ventricular arrhythmias. Arrhythmias most commonly associated with reperfusion include accelerated idioventricular rhythm and ventricular premature complexes and, less frequently, ventricular fibrillation; atrial premature complexes, atrial fibrillation, junctional rhythm, ventricular tachycardia, and sinus bradycardia also have been observed. Reperfusion-related arrhythmias usually are transient, but immediate treatment occasionally may be required. Monitor patients receiving rt-PA, including alteplase, for acute MI carefully for possible arrhythmias during and immediately after administration of the drug; appropriate antiarrhythmic therapy for bradycardia and/or ventricular irritability should be available during administration of the drug.

AV block or cardiac arrest has been reported in patients with acute MI receiving alteplase in clinical trials and during postmarketing surveillance.

Hepatic Effects

Weigh the anticipated benefits of alteplase therapy against the increased risks in patients with substantial liver dysfunction.

Hypersensitivity Reactions

Hypersensitivity reactions (e.g., anaphylactoid reaction, laryngeal edema, angioedema, rash, urticaria), in rare cases fatal, have been reported with IV alteplase therapy. The onset of angioedema has occurred during and up to 2 hours after infusion of alteplase in patients with acute ischemic stroke or acute MI. In many instances, such patients were receiving concomitant angiotensin-converting enzyme (ACE) inhibitors.

Monitor patients during and several hours following alteplase infusion for signs of hypersensitivity reactions. If signs of hypersensitivity (e.g., anaphylactic reaction, angioedema) occur, discontinue alteplase and promptly administer appropriate therapy (e.g., antihistamines, epinephrine, IV corticosteroids).

Hypersensitivity reactions, including urticaria, angioedema, and anaphylaxis, also have been reported in patients receiving alteplase by intracatheter instillation. Monitor patients receiving alteplase by intracatheter instillation for hypersensitivity reactions and treat appropriately if necessary.

Specific Populations

Pregnancy

Although no adequate studies have been performed in pregnant women, animal reproduction studies indicate that IV alteplase was embryocidal in rabbits given the drug at a dosage of 3 mg/kg, approximately equal to the human dosage (based on AUC) used for the treatment of acute MI. No maternal or fetal toxicity was evident in rabbits or rats administered alteplase during organogenesis at doses approximately 0.3 or 0.6 times the human dose (based on body weight) for acute MI, respectively.

The risk of bleeding associated with thrombolytic therapy may be increased during pregnancy. Weigh the risk and benefits of alteplase prior to use during pregnancy.

The American Heart Association (AHA) and American Stroke Association (ASA) state that IV alteplase therapy for acute ischemic stroke may be considered in pregnancy when the anticipated benefits of treating moderate or severe stroke outweigh the anticipated increased risks of uterine bleeding. Therapy with rt-PA followed by IV heparin treatment has been used successfully for lysis of pulmonary emboli in a pregnant woman with congenital antithrombin III deficiency. Approximately 20 hours following discontinuance of rt-PA therapy, at week 35 of pregnancy, the patient delivered a male infant by cesarean section. No placental bleeding occurred and the infant showed no signs of bleeding, but he died later from complications related to respiratory distress syndrome. Another pregnant woman with massive pulmonary embolism and circulatory shock at week 31 of pregnancy who was treated successfully with rt-PA (10 mg/hour for 4 hours followed by 2 mg/hour for 1.5 hours) delivered an otherwise healthy premature infant 48 hours following thrombolytic therapy.

AHA and ASA state that the safety and efficacy of IV alteplase for the treatment of acute ischemic stroke in the early postpartum period (<14 days after delivery) have not been established.

Lactation

It is not known whether alteplase is distributed into human milk or whether the drug affects the breast-fed infant or affects milk production.

Females and Males of Reproductive Potential

It is not known whether alteplase can affect fertility.

Pediatric Use

Safety and efficacy of IV infusion of alteplase in pediatric patients have not been established. However, the drug has been used with some success in a few infants and children with thrombosis of the vena cava, aorta, or peripheral arteries; successful lysis of pulmonary emboli without bleeding complications also has been reported in at least one child with angiographically documented pulmonary emboli of undetermined duration who received 0.1 mg/kg of alteplase per hour for 11 hours via the pulmonary artery†. Thrombolytic therapy generally is not recommended for the treatment of venous thromboembolism in neonates and children unless vessel occlusion is life-threatening and/or causes organ dysfunction. If thrombolysis is required, ACCP states that alteplase is the drug of choice.

Use of thrombolytic therapy in children with arterial ischemic stroke is not recommended by ACCP outside of a research setting.

Safety and efficacy of intracatheter instillation of alteplase for the restoration of central venous catheters in pediatric patients (2 weeks to 17 years) is similar to that observed in adults.

Geriatric Use

Assess the risks against the anticipated benefits of therapy with alteplase in patients >75 years of age. Intracranial hemorrhage and other major bleeding complications are more common in patients >75 years compared with younger adults. Some clinicians suggest considering a 50% reduction in the dosage of alteplase in patients ≥75 years of age receiving the drug for acute MI.

The manufacturer states that efficacy results in patients with acute ischemic stroke suggest a reduced but still favorable clinical outcome for geriatric patients receiving alteplase.

In a large trial comparing 4 thrombolytic regimens, including accelerated-infusion alteplase, in patients with acute MI, 12% of patients were >75 years of age. The incidence of stroke in geriatric patients receiving accelerated-infusion alteplase was 4%, and the incidence of combined 30-day mortality or nonfatal stroke was 20.6%.

Hepatic Impairment

Limited data in animals suggests the possibility of a prolonged elimination half-life of t-PA in patients with severely impaired hepatic function and/or hepatic blood flow. Weigh the anticipated benefits of alteplase therapy against the risks of possible hemostatic defects associated with severe hepatic disease.

● Common Adverse Effects

Adverse effects reported in >5% of patients include hemorrhage.

DRUG INTERACTIONS

● Thrombolytic Agents

In vitro clot lysis studies have failed to show substantial synergistic effects with t-PA and an investigational plasminogen activator, single-chain urokinase plasminogen activator (scu-PA, prourokinase). However, in animals, simultaneous administration of t-PA and scu-PA in a molar ratio of 1:3 demonstrated synergistic thrombolytic effects without associated systemic fibrinogen breakdown. Synergistic thrombolysis also has been observed in preliminary studies in patients with acute MI who received predominantly two-chain rt-PA (no longer currently available in the US) and recombinant scu-PA in doses of each approximately one-fourth the usual doses. Concomitant administration of t-PA and urokinase (no longer commercially available in the US) has been associated with synergistic thrombolytic effects in animals. However, in a study in patients with acute MI, combined use of alteplase and urokinase was not associated with synergistic thrombolysis, although a substantial reduction in the rate of reocclusion after coronary thrombolysis did occur and was not accompanied by an increase in bleeding complications.

● Anticoagulants

In almost all patients receiving alteplase for the treatment of acute MI in clinical studies, heparin, followed by oral anticoagulants in some cases, has been administered before, during, and/or after alteplase therapy to reduce the risk of coronary artery reocclusion. However, concomitant use of alteplase and an anticoagulant may increase the risk of hemorrhage, and careful monitoring for bleeding is necessary, especially at arterial puncture sites. Anticoagulant therapy should be discontinued immediately and appropriate therapy (e.g., protamine sulfate in patients receiving heparin) instituted as necessary if serious bleeding occurs.

The American Heart Association (AHA) and the American Stroke Association (ASA) state that in patients with acute ischemic stroke, a follow-up CT or MRI scan should be performed at 24 hours after IV alteplase before starting treatment with anticoagulant agents.

• Drugs Affecting Platelet Function

Platelet-aggregation inhibitors (e.g., aspirin, clopidogrel) also have been administered after alteplase therapy for the treatment of acute MI to reduce the risk of reocclusion of the infarct-related artery. Drugs that affect platelet function (e.g., aspirin, dipyridamole, abciximab) may increase the risk of bleeding if administered prior to, during, or after alteplase therapy.

In patients with acute stroke, the American Heart Association (AHA) and the American Stroke Association (ASA) generally do not recommend administration of aspirin within 24 hours of the use of a thrombolytic agent, as such adjunctive use of aspirin may increase the risk of bleeding from thrombolytic agents. AHA/ASA state that concurrent administration of abciximab with IV alteplase, and administration of IV aspirin within 90 minutes of starting alteplase treatment, should be avoided. AHA/ASA also state that a follow-up CT or MRI scan should be performed at 24 hours after IV alteplase before starting antiplatelet agents.

• Angiotensin-Converting Enzyme Inhibitors

Angioedema has been reported in patients (primarily with acute ischemic stroke) receiving concomitant angiotensin-converting enzyme (ACE) inhibitors with alteplase.

DESCRIPTION

Alteplase, a recombinant DNA-derived form of human tissue-type plasminogen activator (t-PA), is a thrombolytic agent. The amino acid sequence and biological properties of human melanoma cell t-PA are similar or identical to those of endogenous human t-PA from uterine tissue, and the amino acid sequence of alteplase is identical to that of human melanoma cell t-PA; therefore, differences between alteplase and human uterine tissue or melanoma cell t-PA apparently relate to variability in the carbohydrate moieties of the molecules. In contrast to anticoagulants, which prevent propagation of thrombi, t-PA and other plasminogen activators such as streptokinase and urokinase (urinary-type plasminogen activator, u-PA) promote thrombolysis by hydrolyzing the arginine560-valine561 peptide bond in plasminogen to form the active proteolytic enzyme plasmin. Plasmin is a relatively nonspecific serine protease that is capable of degrading fibrin, fibrinogen, and other procoagulant proteins, such as factors V, VIII, and XII. Unlike streptokinase and urokinase (no longer commercially available in the US), t-PA is a relatively fibrin-selective plasminogen activator. Fibrinolytic activity is localized to the site of the thrombus due to formation of a ternary complex between t-PA, fibrin, and plasminogen. Alteplase induces thrombolysis without substantially activating circulating plasminogen or degrading fibrinogen. Thrombolytic therapy paradoxically may transiently activate the coagulation system, which may decrease the patency of successfully reperfused infarct-related arteries in patients with acute myocardial infarction (MI).

Alteplase is not absorbed after oral administration and must be administered parenterally. Thrombolysis of the infarct-related coronary artery usually occurs <1 hour after initiation of therapy. Lysis of pulmonary emboli usually occurs within 2–6 hours after initiation of therapy. The mechanisms involved in the elimination of t-PA from blood are poorly understood. t-PA appears to be cleared principally by the liver, which subsequently releases degradation products into the blood. In a study in patients with MI, the half-lives of alteplase in the initial distribution phase ($t\frac{1}{2}\alpha$) and in the terminal elimination phase ($t\frac{1}{2}\beta$) averaged 3.6–4.6 and 39–53 minutes, respectively; mean $t\frac{1}{2}\alpha$ and $t\frac{1}{2}\beta$ averaged 4.4 and 26.5 minutes, respectively, in patients with thrombo-occlusive disease. In healthy men receiving alteplase, $t\frac{1}{2}\alpha$ and $t\frac{1}{2}\beta$ averaged 3.3–4.2 and 26–36 minutes, respectively. Limited evidence in animals suggests that the elimination half-life of t-PA may be prolonged in patients with severely impaired hepatic function and/or hepatic blood flow. There is limited evidence from healthy adults receiving radiolabeled human melanoma cell t-PA that exogenously administered t-PA is excreted mainly in urine, with about 80% of total radioactivity being excreted within 18 hours.

ADVICE TO PATIENTS

- **Risk of bleeding.** Advise patients to contact clinicians if they experience symptoms or signs consistent with bleeding (e.g., unusual bruising, pink or brown urine, red or black or tarry stools, coughing up blood, vomiting blood or blood that looks like coffee grounds), headache, or stroke symptoms.

- Advise patients to inform clinicians of existing or contemplated concomitant therapy, including prescription and OTC drugs and dietary or herbal supplements, as well as any concomitant illnesses or recent surgery.

- Advise females of reproductive potential to inform clinicians if they are or plan to become pregnant or plan to breast-feed.

- Inform patients of other important precautionary information.

PREPARATIONS

Excipients in commercially available drug preparations may have clinically important effects in some individuals; consult specific product labeling for details.

Alteplase (Recombinant DNA Origin)

Parenteral

For injection, for IV infusion	50 mg	**Activase®** (with sterile water for injection diluent), Genentech
	100 mg	**Activase®** (with sterile water for injection diluent), Genentech
For solution, for IV catheter clearance	2 mg	**Cathflo® Activase®**, Genentech

† Use is not currently included in the labeling approved by the US Food and Drug Administration.

Table of Contents

24:00 CARDIOVASCULAR DRUGS

§ Omitted from the print version of *AHFS Drug Information®* because of space limitations. This monograph is available on the *AHFS Drug Information®* website, http://ahfsdruginformation.com.

Procainamide Hydrochloride

24:04.04.04 • CLASS Ia ANTIARRHYTHMICS

■ Procainamide hydrochloride is a class Ia antiarrhythmic agent.

USES

● Ventricular Arrhythmias

Procainamide hydrochloride is used for the treatment of ventricular arrhythmias (e.g., sustained ventricular tachycardia) that in the judgment of the physician are life-threatening, but the drug usually is not the antiarrhythmic of first choice. Because of the drug's arrhythmogenic potential, the lack of evidence for improved survival for class I antiarrhythmic agents, and the risk of serious (occurring in about 0.5% of patients), potentially fatal adverse hematologic effects (see Cautions: Hematologic Effects), particularly leukopenia or agranulocytosis, use of procainamide for less severe arrhythmias is not recommended by the manufacturer. Findings from the National Heart, Lung, and Blood Institute (NHLBI)'s Cardiac Arrhythmia Suppression Trial (CAST) study after an average of 10 months of follow-up have indicated that the rate of total mortality and nonfatal cardiac arrest in patients with recent myocardial infarction, mild-to-moderate left ventricular dysfunction, and asymptomatic or mildly symptomatic ventricular arrhythmias (principally frequent ventricular premature complexes [VPCs, PVCs]) who received encainide or flecainide increased substantially compared with placebo. (See Cautions in Flecainide 24:04.04.12.). Therefore, therapy with selected antiarrhythmic agents (e.g., procainamide) should be reserved for the suppression and prevention of documented life-threatening ventricular arrhythmias and treatment of patients with asymptomatic VPCs should be avoided. The manufacturers state that procainamide therapy should be initiated only in a hospital setting.

Procainamide has been used to suppress and prevent the recurrence of less severe but *symptomatic* ventricular arrhythmias†, including uniform, multiform, and/or coupled VPCs† and nonsustained ventricular tachycardia, and asymptomatic ventricular arrhythmias†; however, the arrhythmogenic potential of the drug and findings of the CAST study with other class I antiarrhythmic agents have called into question the safety of using such agents in arrhythmias that were not life-threatening. Therefore, procainamide therapy should be reserved for *life-threatening* ventricular arrhythmias in carefully selected patients in whom the benefits of procainamide therapy outweigh the possible risks.

Life-Threatening Ventricular Arrhythmias and Advanced Cardiovascular Life Support

Antiarrhythmic drugs are used during cardiac arrest to facilitate the restoration and maintenance of a spontaneous perfusing rhythm in patients with refractory (i.e., persisting or recurring after at least one shock) ventricular fibrillation or pulseless ventricular tachycardia; however, there is no evidence that these drugs increase survival to hospital discharge when given routinely during cardiac arrest. High-quality cardiopulmonary resuscitation (CPR) and defibrillation are integral components of advanced cardiovascular life support (ACLS) and the only proven interventions to increase survival to hospital discharge. Other resuscitative efforts, including drug therapy, are considered secondary and should be performed without compromising the quality and timely delivery of chest compressions and defibrillation. The principal goal of pharmacologic therapy during cardiac arrest is to facilitate return of spontaneous circulation (ROSC), and epinephrine is considered the drug of choice for this use. (See Uses: Advanced Cardiovascular Life Support and Cardiac Arrhythmias, in Epinephrine 12:12.12.) Antiarrhythmic drugs may be considered for the treatment of refractory ventricular fibrillation or pulseless ventricular tachycardia during cardiac resuscitation; however, experts generally recommend the use of amiodarone (or lidocaine). Procainamide may be used for the management of regular wide-complex tachycardias during the periarrest period and is included as a recommended antiarrhythmic agent in current ACLS guidelines for adult and pediatric tachycardia.

Monomorphic and Polymorphic Ventricular Tachycardia

Procainamide is one of several antiarrhythmic agents that may be used in the treatment of sustained, stable monomorphic ventricular tachycardia not associated with angina, pulmonary edema, or hypotension (blood pressure less than 90 mm Hg) in patients with preserved ventricular function. Drug regimens including amiodarone or procainamide may be used initially for the treatment of patients with episodes of sustained ventricular tachycardia that are somewhat better tolerated hemodynamically. If IV antiarrhythmic therapy is used for ventricular fibrillation or tachycardia, it probably should be discontinued (at least temporarily) after 6–24 hours so that the patient's ongoing need for antiarrhythmic drugs can be reassessed.

Although rare, episodes of drug-refractory sustained polymorphic ventricular tachycardia ("electrical storm") have been reported in cases of acute myocardial infarction. Some experts state that these episodes usually are treated with an IV β-adrenergic blocking agent, IV amiodarone, left stellate ganglion blockade, intra-aortic balloon counterpulsation (IABP), or emergency revascularization; IV magnesium also may be used. However, other experts recommend revascularization and β-blockade followed by IV antiarrhythmic drugs, such as procainamide or amiodarone, for patients with recurrent or incessant polymorphic ventricular tachycardia due to acute myocardial ischemia.

Ventricular Premature Complexes

Procainamide decreases the frequency of VPCs associated with acute myocardial infarction, but IV lidocaine is considered the drug of choice because normal doses of lidocaine do not decrease cardiac contractility or peripheral resistance or slow AV conduction to the degree produced by procainamide. Like other antiarrhythmic drugs, procainamide has not been shown to decrease mortality rate in patients with VPCs associated with acute myocardial infarction. The use of procainamide in the treatment of asymptomatic VPCs should be avoided. Procainamide generally is not used to treat cardiac glycoside-induced ventricular arrhythmias. (See Cautions: Precautions and Contraindications.)

● Supraventricular Tachyarrhythmias

Procainamide has been used for the treatment of various supraventricular tachycardias (SVTs)†; because of a higher risk of toxicity and proarrhythmic effects, antiarrhythmic agents generally should be reserved for patients who do not respond to or cannot be treated with AV nodal blocking agents (β-adrenergic blocking agents and nondihydropyridine calcium-channel blocking agents). Some experts state that procainamide may be useful for restoring sinus rhythm or slowing ventricular rate in patients with preexcited atrial fibrillation and rapid ventricular response associated with Wolff-Parkinson-White syndrome† since AV nodal blocking agents are contraindicated in such patients; however, direct-current cardioversion is the treatment of choice in hemodynamically compromised patients. Procainamide also has been used in the management of junctional tachycardia†, but the drug has a more limited role in this arrhythmia and is usually considered only when IV β-adrenergic blocking agents are ineffective.

● Other Uses

IV procainamide has been used effectively in the treatment of malignant hyperthermia†. Procainamide is also used parenterally (preferably IM) in the treatment of arrhythmias that occur during surgery and anesthesia.

DOSAGE AND ADMINISTRATION

● Administration

Procainamide hydrochloride may be administered by IM or IV injection or by IV infusion. ECG and blood pressure should be continuously monitored during IV administration of procainamide. IV administration may produce transient high plasma levels of the drug, which can cause severe hypotension.

Procainamide may be administered by intraosseous (IO) injection† in the setting of pediatric advanced cardiovascular life support (PALS); onset of action and systemic concentrations are comparable to those achieved with venous administration. The drug also has been administered orally; however, an oral dosage form no longer is commercially available in the US.

● Dosage

Dosage of procainamide must be carefully adjusted according to individual requirements and response, age, renal function, and the general condition and cardiovascular status of the patient. ECG monitoring of cardiac function and monitoring of renal function (i.e. creatinine clearance) is recommended during procainamide therapy, especially when the drug is given IV or when it is given in patients with increased risk of adverse reactions to procainamide, such as patients older than 50 years of age and patients with severe heart disease, hypotension, or hepatic or renal disease. Dosage should be reduced in patients with renal insufficiency and/or congestive heart failure and in critically ill patients; plasma concentrations of procainamide and its major metabolite N-acetyl procainamide (NAPA) should be determined and dosage should be adjusted to maintain desired concentrations.

Adult Dosage
Ventricular and Supraventricular Arrhythmias

The usual initial adult IM dosage of procainamide hydrochloride is 50 mg/kg given in divided doses (every 3–6 hours). For the treatment of arrhythmias that occur during surgery and anesthesia, 100–500 mg of procainamide hydrochloride may be administered parenterally (preferably IM) in adults.

To facilitate control of the rate of administration, it is recommended that commercially available injections of procainamide hydrochloride be diluted prior to direct IV injection. Administration of the drug by IV injection should be done slowly at a rate not exceeding 50 mg/minute. If procainamide hydrochloride is administered by IV infusion, the drug should be diluted with a suitable IV infusion fluid (usually 5% dextrose injection) to a concentration of 20 mg/mL (for initial loading infusion) or 2 or 4 mg/mL (for maintenance infusion). *Blood pressure and ECG should be monitored continuously and the rate of administration adjusted accordingly.* If a fall in blood pressure of more than 15 mm Hg occurs, or if excessive widening of the QRS complex (greater than 50%) or prolongation of the PR interval occurs, or if severe adverse effects appear, the drug should be temporarily discontinued.

For initial control of arrhythmias in adults, IV doses of 100 mg of procainamide hydrochloride may be given every 5 minutes until the arrhythmia is controlled, adverse effects occur, or until a total of 500 mg has been administered, after which it may be advisable to wait 10 minutes or longer to allow for distribution of the drug before additional doses are given. Alternatively, a loading-dose IV infusion of 500–600 mg may be administered at a constant rate over a period of 25–30 minutes. Although it is unusual to require more than 600 mg to initially control an arrhythmia, the maximum recommended total dose given by either method of IV administration is 1 g. To maintain therapeutic plasma concentrations subsequently, a continuous IV infusion of 2–6 mg/minute may be administered. Alternatively, some clinicians have recommended a maintenance IV infusion of 0.02–0.08 mg/kg per minute.

If used in adults with cardiac arrest, some experts recommend an IV infusion of 20 mg/minute up to a total maximum dose of 17 mg/kg.

Malignant Hyperthermia

Various dosages of procainamide hydrochloride have been given in the treatment of malignant hyperthermia†. The IV dosage has ranged from 200–900 mg and has generally been followed by a maintenance infusion.

Pediatric Dosage
Ventricular and Supraventricular Arrhythmias

The manufacturers have not established pediatric dosage recommendations for procainamide hydrochloride.

Pediatric parenteral dosage recommendations are variable, and clinicians should consult specialized references for specific information. Some clinicians recommend a pediatric IV dose of 2–6 mg/kg (not to exceed 100 mg) as a loading dose administered over 5 minutes, repeated as necessary at intervals of 5–10 minutes (not to exceed a total loading dose of 15 mg/kg or 500 mg in a 30-minute period). Also, some experts recommend a maintenance IV infusion dose of 0.02–0.08 mg (20–80 mcg)/kg per minute, up to a total maintenance infusion dose of 2 g in 24 hours. For pediatric resuscitation, some experts recommend an IV or IO† dose of 15 mg/kg given over 30–60 minutes with discontinuance of the drug if widening of the QRS complex (greater than 50%) from baseline occurs or hypotension develops. If the drug is administered IM, some clinicians recommend a pediatric dosage of 20–30 mg/kg daily (not to exceed 4 g in 24 hours), given in divided doses (every 4–6 hours).

CAUTIONS

Procainamide has numerous adverse effects which may necessitate cessation of therapy in many patients.

● Sensitivity Reactions

Prolonged use of procainamide often results in the development of positive antinuclear antibody (ANA) titers. ANA titers are found in at least

50% of patients receiving long-term procainamide therapy (usually within 2–18 months after starting therapy); the induction of ANA by the drug appears to be independent of the dosage. Patients with procainamide-induced increases in ANA titers may develop a syndrome resembling systemic lupus erythematosus (SLE), characterized by polyarthralgia, arthritis, pleurisy, pleural effusion, dyspnea, fever, chills, myalgia, skin lesions (including urticaria, erythema multiforme, and morbilliform eruptions), headache, fatigue, weakness, abdominal pain, nausea, vomiting, pericarditis, pericardial effusion, pericardial tamponade, acute hepatomegaly, splenomegaly, lymphadenopathy, acute pancreatitis, and the presence of LE cells in the blood. Patients with procainamide-induced SLE may have a positive direct antiglobulin (Coombs') test. Thrombocytopenia, Coombs' positive hemolytic anemia, increased serum concentrations of AST (SGOT), ALT (SGPT), and amylase rarely have been associated with procainamide-induced SLE. Procainamide-induced SLE syndrome probably represents a hypersensitivity reaction in which procainamide anti-DNA antibodies are formed.

If a positive ANA titer develops during procainamide therapy, the relative benefits and risks of continued therapy with the drug should be assessed. Procainamide should be discontinued in patients who develop symptoms of SLE and/or who have rising ANA titer, unless the benefit of antiarrhythmic therapy with the drug outweighs the potential risk. If procainamide-induced SLE develops in a patient with a life-threatening arrhythmia uncontrolled by other antiarrhythmic drugs, the manufacturers state that corticosteroid therapy may be used concomitantly with procainamide. Signs and symptoms of SLE usually regress when the drug is discontinued, but long-term treatment with corticosteroids may be necessary if symptoms do not regress. If arthralgia, fever, rash, malaise, or other unexplained symptoms occur, laboratory studies such as LE cell preparations and ANA titer determinations should be performed.

● Hematologic Effects

Serious adverse hematologic effects, including agranulocytosis, leukopenia, bone marrow depression, hypoplastic anemia, and thrombocytopenia, have been reported in 0.5% of patients receiving procainamide. Pure red cell aplasia also has been reported. In most reported cases, such effects occurred with usual recommended dosages of procainamide during the first 12 weeks of therapy. The drug should be discontinued if any of these adverse hematologic effects occurs. Although blood cell counts usually return to normal within 1 month after discontinuance of procainamide, adverse hematologic effects have been fatal in some cases (e.g., in about 20–25% of patients who developed agranulocytosis). Because of the risk of these effects, careful monitoring of hematologic status is necessary during procainamide therapy (see Cautions: Precautions and Contraindications), and use of the drug should be limited to patients in whom the potential benefits clearly outweigh the possible risks (see Uses).

Leukopenia, hemolytic anemia, and eosinophilia also have occurred rarely in patients receiving procainamide. In at least one case, pancytopenia with generalized ecchymoses has been reported. Adverse hematologic effects also have been associated with a procainamide-induced syndrome resembling systemic lupus erythematosus. (See Cautions: Sensitivity Reactions.)

● GI Effects

GI disturbances such as anorexia, bitter taste, abdominal pain, nausea, vomiting, and diarrhea may occur in patients receiving procainamide and are most common with dosages of 4 g or more daily.

● Nervous System Effects

Adverse nervous system effects of procainamide are rare and have included dizziness, giddiness, seizures, mental depression, confusion, and psychosis with hallucinations.

● Dermatologic Effects

Urticaria, pruritus, and maculopapular rash have occurred occasionally in patients receiving procainamide. An urticarial vasculitis also has occurred.

● Cardiovascular Effects

Paradoxically, an extremely rapid ventricular rate may occur when procainamide is used in the treatment of atrial fibrillation or flutter, because of a reduction in the degree of AV nodal block to a 1:1 ratio. Patients with atrial flutter or fibrillation should be cardioverted or digitalized prior to procainamide administration to avoid enhanced AV conduction, which may result in ventricular rate acceleration beyond tolerable limits. The anticholinergic action of the drug on the AV node may also increase the heart rate. Procainamide-induced ventricular tachycardia may be prevented by prior digitalization; however, in atrial flutter or fibrillation, adequate digitalization reduces but does not eliminate the possibility of sudden increase in ventricular rate as the atrial rate is slowed by procainamide. If cessation of atrial fibrillation is accompanied by depression of the normal pacemaker, an idioventricular rhythm (including ventricular tachycardia and fibrillation) may result. Procainamide-induced ventricular tachycardia is particularly hazardous in patients with extensive myocardial injury. Conversion of atrial fibrillation also may be associated with embolism. Therefore, anticoagulant therapy may be necessary before procainamide conversion of atrial fibrillation to normal sinus rhythm. (See Uses: Supraventricular Tachyarrhythmias.) The arrhythmogenic effect of procainamide may result in atypical ventricular tachycardia (torsades de pointes). (See Cautions: Precautions and Contraindications.)

Procainamide cardiotoxicity is evidenced by conduction defects (50% widening of the QRS complex), ventricular tachycardia, frequent ventricular premature complexes, and complete AV block. When these ECG signs appear, procainamide should be discontinued and the patient should be monitored closely. Less frequently, ECG signs of toxicity may include prolongation of the PR and QT intervals and decreases in voltage of the QRS complexes and T waves. Adverse cardiac effects occur most commonly when procainamide is administered IV. The hazard of ventricular fibrillation increases with increasing dosage of procainamide and may be accompanied by ECG signs of toxicity. Large IV doses of the drug may cause heart block and asystole, and death has occurred rarely.

The manufacturers state that phenylephrine or norepinephrine should be available to treat severe hypotension caused by IV procainamide.

● Other Adverse Effects

Other adverse effects of procainamide include fever, flushing, angioedema, hypergammaglobulinemia, and, rarely, generalized or digital vasculitis, proximal myopathy, and Sjögren's syndrome. Hepatomegaly with increased serum aminotransferase concentrations has been reported after a single oral dose of the drug. Liver aminotransferase concentrations have been elevated, with or without elevations in alkaline phosphatase and bilirubin concentrations, in patients receiving oral procainamide. Abnormal liver function test results in some patients were accompanied by malaise, right upper-quadrant pain, liver failure, and death secondary to liver failure.

● Precautions and Contraindications

Findings from the postmarketing Cardiac Arrhythmia Suppression Trial (CAST), a long-term, multicenter, randomized, double-blind study in patients with asymptomatic non-life-threatening ventricular arrhythmias who had had myocardial infarctions more than 6 days but less than 2 years previously, indicate that the rate of total mortality and nonfatal cardiac arrest was increased in patients treated with encainide or flecainide compared with that seen in patients who received placebo. The applicability of these results to other populations (e.g., those without recent myocardial infarction) is uncertain. The manufacturers state that because of the drug's arrhythmogenic potential, the lack of evidence for improved survival for class I antiarrhythmic agents, and the risk of serious (occurring in about 0.5% of patients), potentially fatal adverse hematologic effects (see Cautions: Hematologic Effects), use of procainamide hydrochloride in patients with ventricular arrhythmias should be limited to those with *life-threatening* arrhythmias in carefully selected patients in whom benefits of procainamide therapy outweigh the possible risks, taking into account possible alternative antiarrhythmic therapy. Use of procainamide in less severe arrhythmias currently is not recommended and treatment of asymptomatic VPCs should be avoided.

Since procainamide, like other antiarrhythmic agents, has been associated with the development or exacerbation of arrhythmias in some patients, clinical and ECG evaluations are essential prior to and during procainamide therapy to monitor for the appearance of arrhythmias and to determine the need for continued therapy. Procainamide should be used with extreme caution, if at all, in patients with marked disturbances of AV conduction, such as second- or third-degree heart block, bundle-branch block, or severe cardiac glycoside intoxication because procainamide may cause additional depression of conduction, resulting in ventricular asystole or fibrillation. The drug is contraindicated in patients with complete AV heart block and in patients with second- or third-degree AV nodal block unless an electrical pacemaker is operative. The dosage should be reduced in patients who exhibit or develop first-degree heart block with procainamide; if the block persists despite dosage reduction, risk versus benefit of continued therapy with increased heart block must be carefully evaluated. Procainamide should be administered with caution (especially parenterally) in the treatment of ventricular arrhythmias in patients with severe organic heart disease, since these patients may have undiagnosed complete heart block; if the ventricular rate is slowed by

procainamide and normal AV conduction does not occur, the drug should be discontinued and the patient reevaluated, since asystole may result. Procainamide also is contraindicated in patients with atypical ventricular tachycardia (torsades de pointes), since class IA antiarrhythmic agents may aggravate this ventricular arrhythmia. The possibility that potentially serious cardiac arrhythmias, including torsades de pointes, could occur if procainamide were used concomitantly with other drugs that prolong the QT_c interval also should be considered and such combined use should be avoided. Procainamide should be used with extreme caution in the treatment of ventricular tachycardia occurring during coronary occlusion. Hypokalemia, hypoxia, and disorders of acid-base balance must be eliminated as potentiating factors in patients who require large doses of antiarrhythmic agents to control ventricular arrhythmias. Procainamide should be used with caution in patients with congestive heart failure, acute ischemic heart disease, or cardiomyopathy, since even slight depression of contractility may further decrease cardiac output. Procainamide should be used with caution in patients with renal and hepatic disease, since accumulation of the drug may cause symptoms of overdosage, such as ventricular tachycardia and severe hypotension.

Commercially available formulations of procainamide hydrochloride injection may contain sulfites, which can cause allergic-type reactions, including anaphylaxis and life-threatening or less severe asthmatic episodes, in certain susceptible individuals. The overall prevalence of sulfite sensitivity in the general population is unknown but probably low; such sensitivity appears to occur more frequently in asthmatic than in nonasthmatic individuals.

Procainamide should be used with caution in patients with preexisting bone marrow depression or cytopenia of any type. Because of the risk of potentially severe, sometimes fatal adverse hematologic effects, the manufacturers recommend that complete blood cell counts, including differential leukocyte counts and platelet counts, optimally be performed at weekly intervals during the first 3 months of therapy and periodically thereafter. If a serious adverse hematologic effect is identified, the drug should be discontinued. Patients should be instructed to promptly report to their physician any sign of infection (e.g., sore mouth, throat, or gums; unexplained fever; chills), unusual bleeding or bruising, rash, arthralgia, myalgia, dark urine or icterus, wheezing, muscular weakness, chest or abdominal pain, palpitation, nausea, vomiting, anorexia, diarrhea, hallucinations, dizziness, or mental depression associated with procainamide therapy. If any of these signs and/or symptoms occur and granulocytopenia is present, the drug should be discontinued and appropriate treatment (e.g., measures to prevent infection) should be instituted immediately. Laboratory tests for detection of procainamide-induced SLE such as ANA titer determinations should be performed before and periodically during maintenance or prolonged procainamide therapy, even in asymptomatic patients. Procainamide is contraindicated in patients with an established diagnosis of SLE, since symptomatic aggravation is likely.

Procainamide is contraindicated in patients who are hypersensitive to the drug, and the possibility of cross-sensitivity to procaine and chemically related drugs (e.g., ester-type local anesthetics) must be considered, although cross-sensitivity is unlikely. Procainamide should not be used if it causes acute allergic dermatitis, asthma, or anaphylactic symptoms. Since procainamide has been reported to increase muscle weakness in patients with myasthenia gravis, the drug may be contraindicated in these patients. (See Drug Interactions: Anticholinesterase and Anticholinergic Agents.)

● Pediatric Precautions

Safety and efficacy of procainamide in pediatric patients have not been established. However, some experts state that procainamide may be considered in children with supraventricular tachycardia unresponsive to adenosine, vagal maneuvers, or electric cardioversion. Procainamide also has been used during pediatric resuscitation; expert consultation prior to use in a hemodynamically stable patient is strongly recommended. In addition, the drug should not be used in combination with another agent that prolongs the QT interval (e.g., amiodarone) without expert consultation.

● Geriatric Precautions

Clinical studies of procainamide did not include sufficient numbers of patients 65 years of age and older to determine whether geriatric patients respond differently than younger patients. Because the drug is known to be substantially excreted by the kidney, patients with renal impairment may be at increased risk of procainamide-induced toxicity. In general, dosage should be titrated carefully in geriatric patients, usually initiating therapy at the low end of the dosage range. (See Dosage and Administration: Dosage.) The greater frequency of decreased hepatic, renal, and/or cardiac function and of concomitant disease and drug therapy observed in the elderly also should be considered.

● **Mutagenicity and Carcinogenicity**

Studies to determine the mutagenic and carcinogenic potentials of procainamide have not been performed to date.

● **Pregnancy, Fertility, and Lactation**

Pregnancy

Animal reproduction studies have not been performed with procainamide. It is not known whether procainamide can cause fetal harm when administered to pregnant women or can affect reproduction capacity. Procainamide does cross the placenta, but the extent to which it does so has not been well characterized. Procainamide should be used during pregnancy only when clearly needed.

Lactation

Procainamide and NAPA are distributed into milk and can be absorbed by a nursing infant. Because of the potential for serious adverse reactions to procainamide in nursing infants, a decision should be made whether to discontinue nursing or the drug, taking into account the importance of the drug to the woman.

DRUG INTERACTIONS

● **Histamine H$_2$-Receptor Antagonists**

Concomitant administration of procainamide and cimetidine may result in increased plasma procainamide and NAPA concentrations and subsequent toxicity. This interaction may be more marked in geriatric patients and patients with renal impairment since such patients eliminate procainamide, NAPA, and cimetidine more slowly. Cimetidine decreases the renal clearance of procainamide and NAPA; however, additional mechanisms also may contribute to this interaction. Limited evidence suggests that ranitidine also may increase plasma concentrations of procainamide and NAPA, but to a lesser extent than cimetidine; the precise mechanisms for this interaction are complex and are not fully understood. Evidence to date suggests that famotidine does not substantially interact with procainamide. Caution should be exercised when either cimetidine or ranitidine is administered concomitantly with procainamide, particularly in geriatric patients and patients with renal impairment; the patient and plasma procainamide concentrations should be monitored closely and procainamide dosage adjusted accordingly.

● **Neuromuscular Blocking Agents**

Procainamide may enhance the effects of skeletal muscle relaxants. The drug may potentiate the effects of both nondepolarizing and depolarizing skeletal muscle relaxants, such as gallamine triethiodide (no longer commercially available in the US), metocurine iodide (no longer commercially available in the US), pancuronium bromide, succinylcholine chloride, and tubocurarine chloride. Although the clinical significance of this interaction has not been established, procainamide should be used with caution in conjunction with neuromuscular blocking agents.

● **Anticholinesterase and Anticholinergic Agents**

Procainamide should be used with caution, if at all, in patients with myasthenia gravis and the dose of anticholinesterase drugs such as neostigmine and pyridostigmine may have to be increased. Theoretically, the anticholinergic effect of procainamide may be additive with anticholinergic drugs or procainamide may enhance the effects of anticholinergic agents.

● **Cardiovascular Drugs**

Since procainamide may reduce blood pressure, patients receiving hypotensive drugs and procainamide parenterally or in high oral doses should be observed for possible additive hypotensive effects. β-adrenergic blocking agents may increase plasma procainamide concentrations.

Concomitant use of procainamide with drugs that prolong the QT interval may result in potentially serious cardiac arrhythmias, including torsades de pointes.

Concurrent use of procainamide with class IA antiarrhythmics (e.g., disopyramide, quinidine) may enhance conduction prolongation, contractility depression, and hypotension, especially in patients with cardiac decompensation; combined use should be reserved for serious arrhythmias unresponsive to monotherapy and only if close observation is possible. When procainamide is administered with other antiarrhythmic drugs such as lidocaine, phenytoin, propranolol, or quinidine, the cardiac effects may be additive or antagonistic and toxic effects may be additive.

Concomitant use of procainamide and amiodarone may result in increased plasma procainamide and N-acetylprocainamide (NAPA) concentrations and subsequent toxicity. In a limited number of patients receiving 2–6 g of procainamide hydrochloride daily, initiation of amiodarone hydrochloride (1200 mg daily for 5–7 days and then 600 mg daily) increased plasma procainamide and NAPA concentrations by about 55 and 33%, respectively, during the first week of amiodarone therapy. The exact mechanism(s) has not been elucidated, but it has been suggested that amiodarone may decrease the renal clearance of procainamide or NAPA and/or inhibit the hepatic metabolism of procainamide. In addition to a pharmacokinetic interaction, additive electrophysiologic effects, including increased QT and QRS intervals, occur during concomitant use; adverse electrophysiologic effects (e.g., acceleration of ventricular tachycardia) may also occur. Pending further accumulation of data, it is recommended that procainamide dosage be reduced by 20–33% when amiodarone therapy is initiated in patients currently receiving procainamide or that procainamide therapy be discontinued.

● **Other Drugs**

Concomitant administration of procainamide and trimethoprim may result in increased plasma procainamide and NAPA concentrations.

Because alcohol appears to enhance acetylation of procainamide to NAPA, alcohol consumption may reduce the half-life of procainamide.

Ofloxacin may decrease the renal clearance of procainamide, which may result in an increase in the area under the serum concentration-time curve (AUC) and peak concentration of procainamide by 20–25%.

Para-aminobenzoic acid may decrease the renal clearance of NAPA, which may result in an increase in the plasma concentration and half-life of NAPA.

ACUTE TOXICITY

● **Manifestations**

Overdosage of procainamide has produced hypotension, widening of the QRS complex, prolongation of PR and QT intervals, lowering of R and T waves, increasing AV block, ventricular extrasystole, ventricular tachycardia or fibrillation, junctional tachycardia, intraventricular conduction delay, oliguria, lethargy, confusion, nausea, and vomiting.

● **Treatment**

Management of procainamide overdosage generally involves symptomatic and supportive care with ECG and blood pressure monitoring. There is no known antidote to procainamide. If ingestion of the drug is recent, gastric lavage or emesis may reduce absorption. Procainamide toxicity can usually be treated, if necessary, by administering vasopressors after adequate fluid volume replacement. IV infusion of (1/6) M sodium lactate injection reportedly reduces the cardiotoxic effects of procainamide. If procainamide toxicity causes severe hypotension and renal insufficiency, urinary elimination of procainamide and NAPA is decreased and hemodialysis may be necessary. Peritoneal dialysis is not effective. One patient who ingested approximately 7 g of procainamide hydrochloride recovered after treatment consisting of IV norepinephrine, IV furosemide, attempted volume expansion with albumin, and hemodialysis. Another patient recovered after ingestion of 19 g of procainamide hydrochloride; this patient was treated with IV isoproterenol and IV epinephrine.

PHARMACOLOGY

● **Antiarrhythmic and Electrophysiologic Effects**

Procainamide is an antiarrhythmic agent whose cardiac actions appear to be similar to those of quinidine. Procainamide is regarded as a myocardial depressant because it decreases myocardial excitability and conduction velocity, and may depress myocardial contractility. Procainamide, like disopyramide and quinidine, also possesses anticholinergic properties which may modify the direct myocardial effects of the drug.

The exact mechanism of antiarrhythmic action of procainamide has not been established, but the drug is considered a class I (membrane-stabilizing) antiarrhythmic agent. Like other class I antiarrhythmic agents, procainamide is believed to combine with fast sodium channels in their inactive state and thereby inhibit recovery after repolarization in a time- and voltage-dependent manner which is associated with subsequent dissociation of the drug from the sodium channels. Procainamide exhibits electrophysiologic effects characteristic of class IA antiarrhythmic agents. The electrophysiologic characteristics of the subgroups of class

I antiarrhythmic agents may be related to quantitative differences in their rates of attachment to and dissociation from transmembrane sodium channels, with class IA agents exhibiting intermediate rates of attachment and dissociation. *N*-Acetylprocainamide (NAPA), a metabolite of procainamide, exhibits class III antiarrhythmic activity.

Like lidocaine and quinidine, procainamide suppresses automaticity in the His-Purkinje system. In usual doses, procainamide may decrease the automaticity of ectopic pacemakers, but the extent of this effect also depends upon the anticholinergic effect of the drug on the sinoatrial (SA) node, atria, and atrioventricular (AV) node. Extremely high concentrations of procainamide may increase myocardial automaticity. The drug decreases conduction velocity in the atria, ventricles, and His-Purkinje system, and may decrease or cause no change in conduction velocity through the AV node. Procainamide probably suppresses atrial fibrillation or flutter by prolonging the effective refractory period (ERP) and increasing the action potential duration in atrial and ventricular muscle and in the His-Purkinje system. Because prolongation of the ERP is greater than the increase in the duration of the action potential, the cardiac tissue remains refractory even after restoration of the resting membrane potential. Procainamide shortens the ERP of the AV node, and the anticholinergic action of the drug may also increase the conductivity of the AV node. The effects of procainamide on refractoriness and the action potential duration of atrial fibers may be modified by the anticholinergic effects of the drug. Procainamide decreases cardiac excitability both in diastole and in the relative refractory period by increasing the threshold potential for electrical excitation. In therapeutic plasma concentrations, procainamide causes prolongation of the PR and QT intervals, but the QRS complex is usually not prolonged beyond the normal range.

● Cardiovascular Effects

The effect of procainamide on heart rate is unpredictable, but generally the drug causes no change or slightly increases heart rate. Procainamide may have a direct negative inotropic effect, but therapeutic plasma concentrations of the drug do not usually depress contractility in the normal heart. Cardiac output is not usually decreased, except in the presence of myocardial damage. Procainamide may reduce peripheral resistance and blood pressure as a result of peripheral vasodilation. Decreased blood pressure is most likely to occur with high plasma concentrations of the drug. IV procainamide may decrease pulmonary arterial pressure. At high plasma concentrations, procainamide may produce sinus tachycardia because of reflex sympathetic response to its hypotensive effect.

● Other Effects

Procainamide has local anesthetic properties equal to but more sustained than those of procaine. Procainamide produces less CNS stimulation than does procaine.

PHARMACOKINETICS

● Absorption

Plasma procainamide concentrations of approximately 4–10 mcg/mL are required to suppress ventricular arrhythmias. Plasma procainamide concentrations exceeding 10 mcg/mL are increasingly associated with toxic findings, which are observed occasionally in the 10–12 mcg/mL range, more often in the 12–15 mcg/mL range, and commonly in patients with plasma concentrations greater than 15 mcg/mL; however, some clinicians state that plasma procainamide concentrations of 15–20 mcg/mL may be appropriate in selected patients with careful monitoring. With fixed dosage, there are large interindividual variations in the plasma concentrations of procainamide. Plasma concentrations of procainamide are approximately 25% higher than blood concentrations. *N*-Acetylprocainamide (NAPA), a metabolite of procainamide, has antiarrhythmic activity, and plasma concentrations of this metabolite may represent more than 50% of the total drug in the plasma. If renal excretion of procainamide is prolonged and conversion to NAPA is rapid, plasma concentrations of NAPA exceed procainamide concentrations at steady-state. The suggested therapeutic range for combined procainamide and NAPA concentrations is 5–30 mcg/mL.

Absorption of procainamide after IM administration is rapid, and the drug appears in the plasma in 2 minutes. Peak plasma procainamide concentrations after IM administration of the drug average 30% higher than after oral administration of the same dose. In one study in healthy individuals, peak plasma procainamide concentrations of 5–8.5 mcg/mL were attained in 15–60 minutes and plasma concentrations of 2–3 mcg/mL persisted for 6 hours after a single 1-g IM dose. The onset of action after IM administration of a single dose of the drug

occurs within 10–30 minutes. In one study in patients with atherosclerotic heart disease, plasma concentrations of the drug ranged from 5.8–16 mcg/mL at the end of an IV infusion of 500 mg of procainamide hydrochloride at a rate of 50 mg/minute.

● Distribution

Procainamide is rapidly distributed into the CSF, liver, spleen, kidneys, lungs, muscles, brain, and heart. The apparent volume of distribution of the drug at steady state is approximately 2 L/kg. The apparent volume of distribution of procainamide is decreased in patients with heart failure. Studies using radiolabeled procainamide indicate that 14–23% of the drug is bound to plasma proteins at therapeutic plasma concentrations. Procainamide crosses the placenta, but the extent to which it does has not been well characterized. Procainamide and NAPA are distributed into milk and can be absorbed by a nursing infant.

● Elimination

After IV administration, procainamide has an initial half-life of 4–5 minutes and a terminal half-life of 2.5–4.7 hours in individuals with normal renal function. The elimination half-life of procainamide may be increased in patients with renal impairment and in geriatric patients. The half-life of NAPA is 6–7 hours in patients with normal renal function. In patients with congestive heart failure and/or renal insufficiency, plasma concentrations of procainamide are higher and decrease more gradually.

Procainamide is acetylated, presumably in the liver, to form NAPA. Acetylation of procainamide is related to genetic acetylator phenotype. The rate of acetylation is genetically determined and varies among individuals; however, it is constant for each person.

The total amount of unchanged procainamide excreted in urine varies from 40–70% of a dose due to differences in acetylator phenotype and in renal excretion. NAPA and 2 unidentified metabolites are also excreted in urine. Less than 0.2% of the dose is excreted in urine as either *p*-acetamidobenzoic acid or aminobenzoic acid. Procainamide and NAPA are excreted by active tubular secretion and glomerular filtration. The rate of renal excretion of procainamide and NAPA is not affected by changes in urine pH nor by acetylator phenotype. Rapid and slow acetylators excrete approximately the same amount of procainamide as unchanged drug, but rapid acetylators excrete more of a dose as NAPA. In patients with renal insufficiency, excretion of procainamide and NAPA is decreased. Procainamide and NAPA are removed by hemodialysis but not by peritoneal dialysis. NAPA also is removed by arteriovenous hemofiltration and by arteriovenous hemodiafiltration.

CHEMISTRY AND STABILITY

● Chemistry

Procainamide hydrochloride is an antiarrhythmic agent. The drug differs structurally from procaine in the replacement of the ester group of procaine with an amide group. Procainamide hydrochloride occurs as a white to tan, hygroscopic, crystalline powder and is very soluble in water and soluble in alcohol. The drug has a pK_a of 9.23.

Procainamide hydrochloride injection is a sterile solution of the drug in water for injection and is colorless or has not more than a slight yellow color. Hydrochloric acid and/or sodium hydroxide is used to adjust the pH of the commercially available injection to 4–6. At the time of manufacture, the air in the vials of procainamide hydrochloride injection is replaced with nitrogen. Sodium metabisulfite is present in the injection principally to prevent discoloration caused by oxidation of *p*-aminobenzoic acid (a procainamide degradation product) rather than to maintain product potency. Sodium metabisulfite is present in the injection principally to prevent discoloration caused by oxidation of *p*-aminobenzoic acid (a procainamide degradation product) rather than to maintain product potency.

● Stability

Procainamide hydrochloride injections are colorless or may turn slightly yellow on standing; injection of air into vials of the drug causes darkening of the solution. Solutions of procainamide that are darker than light amber or are otherwise discolored should not be used. Although procainamide hydrochloride injection may be stored at room temperature (10–27°C), refrigeration retards oxidation and associated development of color.

When procainamide hydrochloride injection is diluted with 0.9% sodium chloride injection or sterile water for injection, solutions containing 2–4 mg/mL are stable for 24 hours at room temperature or for 7 days at 2–8°C. While solutions diluted in 5% dextrose have been described as being less stable than this secondary to possible formation of an association complex between the drug and dextrose,/ and such complexation may not be readily reversible, at least in vitro, this phenomenon has *only* been observed in vitro to date and its clinical importance, if any, remains unclear. There is in vitro evidence indicating that complexation is pH dependent and that its rate and extent can be minimized by adjusting the pH of procainamide hydrochloride in 5% dextrose solutions to 7.5 with sodium bicarbonate. However, because this complexation has not been observed in vivo and its clinical importance has not been established, the need for such precautions remains questionable. Therefore, the manufacturer currently states that procainamide hydrochloride that has been diluted to a final concentration of 2–4 mg/mL in 5% dextrose can be considered stable for at least 24 hours at room temperature or for 7 days when refrigerated. In addition, because use of IV procainamide hydrochloride generally is limited to clinical situations in which ECG and blood pressure are monitored continuously, any potential alterations in clinical bioavailability resulting from such dilutions probably would be readily apparent. Procainamide hydrochloride injection has been reported to be physically incompatible with some drugs, but the compatibility depends on several factors (e.g., concentrations of the drugs, specific diluents used, resulting pH, temperature). Specialized references should be consulted for specific compatibility information.

PREPARATIONS

Excipients in commercially available drug preparations may have clinically important effects in some individuals; consult specific product labeling for details.

Procainamide Hydrochloride

Parenteral

Injection	100 mg/mL*	Procainamide Hydrochloride Injection
	500 mg/mL*	Procainamide Hydrochloride Injection

* available from one or more manufacturer, distributor, and/or repackager by generic (nonproprietary) name

† Use is not currently included in the labeling approved by the US Food and Drug Administration.

Selected Revisions November 4, 2016, © Copyright, September 1, 1977, American Society of Health-System Pharmacists, Inc.

Lidocaine Hydrochloride (Systemic)

24:04.04.08 • CLASS Ib ANTIARRHYTHMICS

■ Lidocaine hydrochloride is an amide-type local anesthetic that is also used as a class Ib antiarrhythmic agent.

USES

● Ventricular Arrhythmias

Ventricular Arrhythmias Associated with Myocardial Infarction or Cardiac Manipulation

Lidocaine hydrochloride is used parenterally as an alternative to other antiarrhythmic drugs (e.g., amiodarone, procainamide, sotalol) for the acute treatment of life-threatening ventricular arrhythmias such as those that occur following myocardial infarction (MI) or during cardiac manipulative procedures such as cardiac surgery. Lidocaine previously was recommended for the prevention of ventricular arrhythmias associated with acute myocardial ischemia or infarction. Such use was supported largely by animal studies and extrapolation from historical use of the drug to suppress premature ventricular contractions (PVCs) and prevent ventricular fibrillation and potentially, sudden death, following acute MI. However, although pooled analysis of randomized controlled trials of prophylaxis with lidocaine demonstrated a reduction of approximately 33% in primary ventricular fibrillation following acute MI, this benefit was offset by a trend toward *increased* mortality, probably as a result of fatal episodes of bradycardia and asystole. Therefore, experts no longer recommend routine *prophylactic* use of lidocaine during acute MI, and such use has largely been abandoned.

Shock-Resistant Ventricular Fibrillation or Pulseless Ventricular Tachycardia

Lidocaine is used as adjunctive therapy for the management of ventricular fibrillation or pulseless ventricular tachycardia resistant to cardiopulmonary resuscitation (CPR), defibrillation, and a vasopressor (e.g., epinephrine).

Antiarrhythmic drugs are used during cardiac arrest to facilitate the restoration and maintenance of a spontaneous perfusing rhythm in patients with refractory (i.e., persisting or recurring after at least one shock) ventricular fibrillation or pulseless ventricular tachycardia; however, there is no evidence that these drugs increase survival to hospital discharge when given routinely during cardiac arrest. High-quality CPR and defibrillation are integral components of ACLS and the only proven interventions to increase survival to hospital discharge. Other resuscitative efforts, including drug therapy, are considered secondary and should be performed without compromising the quality and timely delivery of chest compressions and defibrillation. The principal goal of pharmacologic therapy during cardiac arrest is to facilitate return of spontaneous circulation (ROSC), and epinephrine is the drug of choice for this use. (See Uses: Advanced Cardiovascular Life Support and Cardiac Arrhythmias, in Epinephrine 12:12.12.) If an antiarrhythmic agent is needed for the treatment of refractory ventricular fibrillation or pulseless ventricular tachycardia during adult cardiac arrest, AHA recommends amiodarone as the first-line drug of choice because of its proven benefits in improving rates of ROSC and hospital admission; lidocaine may be used as an alternative. Results of several studies suggest that amiodarone is more effective than lidocaine in improving rates of ROSC and hospital admission in patients with shock-refractory ventricular fibrillation or pulseless ventricular tachycardia. In pediatric advanced life support (PALS), current evidence supports the use of either amiodarone or lidocaine for these arrhythmias.

In a randomized, double-blind, comparative study, approximately 23% of patients with out-of-hospital cardiac arrest due to defibrillation-refractory ventricular arrhythmias (i.e., ventricular fibrillation, pulseless ventricular tachycardia) who received IV amiodarone hydrochloride (5 mg/kg) or lidocaine-placebo survived to hospital admission compared with 12% of those who received IV lidocaine hydrochloride (1.5 mg/kg) or amiodarone-placebo following at least 3 precordial electrical shocks, IV epinephrine, and an additional precordial shock. Among patients for whom the time from dispatch of the ambulance to the administration of the drug was equal to or less than the median time (24 minutes), approximately 28% of those given amiodarone and 15% of those given lidocaine survived to hospital admission. Despite these results, only about 6 or 4% of patients receiving IV amiodarone or IV lidocaine, respectively, who survived to hospital admission lived to be discharged from the hospital. Evidence supporting the use of amiodarone and lidocaine in pediatric cardiac arrest is more limited and principally based on extrapolation of data from the adult population. In a retrospective cohort study that included data from 889 pediatric patients with in-hospital cardiac arrest, improved ROSC was observed with lidocaine compared with amiodarone. Neither drug was associated with improved survival to hospital discharge.

Monomorphic Ventricular Tachycardia

Lidocaine may be considered as an alternative to other antiarrhythmic agents or synchronized cardioversion for the treatment of hemodynamically stable monomorphic ventricular tachycardia; however, other agents are preferred. Available evidence suggests that lidocaine is less effective in treating ventricular tachycardia than either procainamide, sotalol, or amiodarone.

● Status Epilepticus

IV lidocaine has been used as a last resort for the treatment of status epilepticus†.

● Local Anesthesia

For the use of lidocaine hydrochloride as a local anesthetic, see Lidocaine 72:00.

DOSAGE AND ADMINISTRATION

● Administration

Parenteral Administration

Lidocaine hydrochloride is administered IV for the treatment of ventricular arrhythmias. The drug also has been administered by IM injection, but an IM formulation no longer is commercially available in the US. Lidocaine hydrochloride also has been administered by intraosseous (IO) injection† in the setting of advanced cardiovascular life support (ACLS) when IV administration is not possible; onset of action and systemic concentrations of the drug are comparable to those achieved with venous administration. *Lidocaine solutions that contain epinephrine must not be used to treat arrhythmias.*

Lidocaine hydrochloride also is available as solutions of the drug in 5% dextrose. Contents of lidocaine hydrochloride in dextrose injections should be inspected visually for discoloration and/or particulate matter prior to administration whenever solution and container permit. Additives should not be introduced into the solution container. Lidocaine hydrochloride in dextrose injection should not be used in series connections with other plastic containers, since such use could result in air embolism from residual air being drawn from the primary container before administration of fluid from the secondary container is complete. Commercially available solutions of the drug in 5% dextrose should not be administered unless the solution is clear and the container and seals are undamaged. When the commercially available IV infusion solution of lidocaine hydrochloride and 5% dextrose is used, the accompanying labeling should be consulted for proper methods of administration and other associated precautions.

Standardize 4 Safety

Standardized concentrations for lidocaine hydrochloride have been established through Standardize 4 Safety (S4S), a national patient safety initiative to reduce medication errors, especially during transitions of care. Multidisciplinary expert panels were convened to determine recommended standard concentrations. Because recommendations from the S4S panels may differ from the manufacturer's prescribing information, caution is advised when using concentrations that differ from labeling, particularly when using rate information from the label. For additional information on S4S (including updates that may be available), see https://www.ashp.org/pharmacy-practice/standardize-4-safety-initiative.

TABLE 1. Standardize 4 Safety Continuous IV Infusion Standard Concentrations for Lidocaine Hydrochloride

Patient Population	Concentration Standards	Dosing Units
Adults	8 mg/mL	mg/min
Pediatric patients (<50 kg)[a]	4 mg/mL	mcg/kg/min[b]
	8 mg/mL	

[a] The recommended concentrations are intended for cardiac indications only.

[b] dosing units differ from concentration units

Endotracheal Administration

Lidocaine hydrochloride may be administered via the endotracheal route† if vascular (IV or IO) access cannot be established during cardiac arrest; however, IV or IO administration is preferred whenever possible because of more predictable drug delivery and pharmacologic effect. (See Pharmacokinetics: Absorption.) For endotracheal administration in adults, the dose should be diluted in 5–10 mL of 0.9% sodium chloride or sterile water and administered directly into the endotracheal tube. In pediatric patients, the endotracheal dose should be followed with a flush of at least 5 mL of 0.9% sodium chloride injection. Absorption of lidocaine, when administered via an endotracheal tube, may be increased by diluting the drug in sterile water instead of 0.9% sodium chloride.

• Dosage

Dosage of lidocaine hydrochloride must be carefully adjusted according to individual requirements and response.

Ventricular Arrhythmias

Adult Dosage

For the initial treatment of ventricular arrhythmias, lidocaine hydrochloride usually is administered as a rapid (i.e., bolus) IV injection. The manufacturer states that the usual adult dose of lidocaine hydrochloride is 50–100 mg administered at a rate of approximately 25–50 mg/minute by direct IV injection. If the desired response is not achieved, a second dose may be administered 5 minutes after completion of the first injection. The manufacturer states that *no more than 200–300 mg should be administered during a 1-hour period.* Patients with congestive heart failure or cardiogenic shock may require smaller loading doses.

For the treatment of hemodynamically stable monomorphic ventricular tachycardia, the American Heart Association (AHA) recommends an initial adult dose of 1–1.5 mg/kg IV; additional doses of 0.5–0.75 mg/kg may be administered every 5–10 minutes as necessary, up to a maximum total dose of 3 mg/kg.

For the treatment of shock-resistant ventricular fibrillation or pulseless ventricular tachycardia during cardiac resuscitation, the initial adult loading dose of lidocaine hydrochloride is 1–1.5 mg/kg by IV or IO† injection, followed by 0.5–0.75 mg/kg repeated at 5- to 10-minute intervals as necessary, up to a maximum total dose of 3 mg/kg.

If IV or IO† access cannot be established during cardiac arrest, lidocaine may be administered via the endotracheal† route. Although the optimum endotracheal dose of lidocaine hydrochloride remains to be established, some experts state that typical doses should be 2–2.5 times those administered IV, and generally should be diluted in 5–10 mL of 0.9% sodium chloride or sterile water.

A maintenance infusion of lidocaine hydrochloride may be required to maintain normal sinus rhythm if oral antiarrhythmic therapy is not feasible. Following initial administration with direct IV injections, an IV infusion of lidocaine hydrochloride may be initiated at a rate of 1–4 mg/minute (14–57 mcg/kg per minute). Some clinicians recommend maintaining the infusion rate below 30 mcg/kg per minute in patients with congestive heart failure. In patients with liver disease, dosing must be carefully individualized.

Major differences in lidocaine pharmacokinetics may exist for different types of liver disease (e.g., cirrhosis, hepatitis) and no consistent correlation has been established between clearance of the drug and severity of liver disease (as determined by liver function tests). No dosing modification appears to be necessary in patients with renal failure.

When arrhythmias reappear during a constant infusion of lidocaine hydrochloride, a small bolus dose (e.g., 0.5 mg/kg) may be given to rapidly increase plasma concentrations of the drug; the infusion rate is maintained or increased simultaneously. If the infusion rate alone is increased, a plateau or peak concentration of lidocaine may not be reached for 3–4 half-lives (5–8 hours).

The infusion should be terminated as soon as the patient's basic cardiac rhythm appears to be stable or at the earliest sign of toxicity. If signs of excessive cardiac depression, such as prolongation of the PR interval and QRS complex or the appearance or aggravation of arrhythmias occur, the infusion should be stopped immediately. The manufacturers state that it should rarely be necessary to continue the infusion for longer than 24 hours. Clinical studies have reported continuation of lidocaine infusions for several days; however, there are data which indicate that the half-life of lidocaine may be increased to 3 hours or longer following infusions lasting longer than 24 hours, and dosage may need to be reduced accordingly (e.g., by 50%) to avoid accumulation of the drug and potential toxicity. If maintenance therapy is necessary, therapy should be changed to an oral antiarrhythmic agent.

Pediatric Dosage

Controlled clinical studies to establish pediatric dosing schedules of lidocaine hydrochloride have not been performed. Some clinicians have suggested that infants and children may be given an initial rapid IV injection (i.e., bolus) of 0.5–1 mg/kg; this dose may be repeated according to the response of the patient, but the total dose should not exceed 3–5 mg/kg. A maintenance IV infusion of 10–50 mcg/kg per minute may be given via an infusion pump.

For the treatment of shock-refractory ventricular fibrillation or pulseless ventricular tachycardia during pediatric resuscitation, the recommended dosage of lidocaine hydrochloride is an initial rapid IV or IO† injection (i.e., bolus) of 1 mg/kg, followed by a maintenance infusion of 20–50 mcg/kg per minute. A repeat IV injection should be given if there is more than a 15-minute delay from the time of the initial rapid IV injection dose to the onset of the infusion.

If IV or IO† access cannot be established, lidocaine may be administered via the endotracheal† route. Although the optimum endotracheal dose of lidocaine hydrochloride remains to be established, some experts state that typical doses should be 2–2.5 times those administered IV. If cardiopulmonary resuscitation (CPR) is in progress, chest compressions should be interrupted briefly to administer lidocaine. Following administration, the endotracheal tube should be flushed with 5 mL of 0.9% sodium chloride injection and followed by 5 consecutive positive-pressure ventilations.

Status Epilepticus

For the treatment of status epilepticus†, some clinicians have suggested an initial IV lidocaine hydrochloride bolus dose of 1 mg/kg. If the seizure is not terminated, 0.5 mg/kg may be given 2 minutes after completion of the first injection. A maintenance IV infusion of 30 mcg/kg per minute has been given to prevent recurrence of seizures.

CAUTIONS

Serious adverse reactions to lidocaine are uncommon. Adverse effects of the drug mainly involve the CNS, are usually of short duration, and are dose related.

If severe reactions occur, lidocaine administration should be discontinued; emergency resuscitative procedures and other supportive measures should be instituted. Maintenance of adequate ventilation and a patent airway are of primary importance. For the treatment of severe seizures, small IV doses of diazepam or an ultrashort-acting barbiturate (e.g., thiopental, thiamylal) may be given or, if these are not available, pentobarbital or secobarbital may be administered. If the patient is anesthetized, a short-acting neuromuscular blocking agent (e.g., succinylcholine) may be given IV. If circulatory depression occurs, IV fluids and vasopressors such as ephedrine or metaraminol may be used if necessary.

• Nervous System Effects

Adverse CNS reactions may be manifested by drowsiness; dizziness; disorientation; confusion; lightheadedness; tremulousness; psychosis; nervousness;

apprehension; agitation; euphoria; tinnitus; visual disturbances including blurred or double vision; nausea; vomiting; paresthesia; sensations of heat, cold, or numbness; difficulty swallowing; dyspnea; and slurred speech. Muscle twitching or tremors, seizures, unconsciousness or altered consciousness, coma, and respiratory depression and arrest may also occur.

● Dermatologic and Sensitivity Reactions

Hypersensitivity to lidocaine is rare and may be characterized by skin lesions, urticaria, edema, and anaphylactoid reactions.

● Cardiovascular Effects

Although usual doses of lidocaine generally produce no adverse cardiovascular effects, patients with high plasma concentrations of the drug or myocardial conduction defects may develop hypotension, arrhythmias, heart block, cardiovascular collapse, and bradycardia which may lead to cardiac arrest. However, cardiac arrest caused by lidocaine is usually secondary to respiratory arrest. In anesthetized patients, CNS toxicity and seizures may not occur; cardiovascular depression may be the first manifestation of toxicity in these patients.

● Administration Effects

Local thrombophlebitis may occur in patients receiving prolonged IV infusions of lidocaine.

● Precautions and Contraindications

Constant ECG monitoring is necessary during IV administration of lidocaine. ECG changes such as prolongation of the PR interval and QRS complex or the appearance or aggravation of arrhythmias necessitates prompt cessation of lidocaine infusion. Resuscitative equipment and drugs should be immediately available for the management of severe, adverse cardiovascular, respiratory, or CNS effects. If severe reactions occur, lidocaine should be discontinued and appropriate therapy instituted. Severe reactions are often preceded by somnolence and paresthesia, and these symptoms should *not* be ignored.

Although the manufacturers state that lidocaine should be used with caution in patients with severe renal disease, the drug has been used safely in these patients. Lidocaine should be administered with caution to patients with liver disease, congestive heart failure, marked hypoxia, severe respiratory depression, hypovolemia, or shock. Caution should be used when administering lidocaine to patients with sinus bradycardia or incomplete heart block for the treatment of ventricular premature contractions without prior acceleration of heart rate, since more frequent and serious ventricular arrhythmias or heart block may result. In addition, use of the drug in patients with symptomatic bradycardia may result in potentially life-threatening adverse effects (e.g., death), particularly if the bradycardia is a ventricular escape rhythm that is mistaken for preventricular contractions or slow ventricular tachycardia. Lidocaine may increase ventricular rate when it is administered to patients with atrial fibrillation. Hypokalemia, hypoxia, and disorders of acid-base balance must be eliminated as potentiating factors in patients who require large doses of antiarrhythmic agents to control ventricular irritability.

Lidocaine is contraindicated in patients with a known hypersensitivity to the amide-type local anesthetics. There have been no reports of cross-sensitivity reactions between lidocaine and procainamide or quinidine. Lidocaine should be used with caution in patients with any form of heart block and is contraindicated in patients with Adams-Stokes syndrome or with severe degrees of SA, AV, or intraventricular heart block in the absence of an artificial pacemaker. Although some manufacturers state that lidocaine is contraindicated in patients with Wolff-Parkinson-White syndrome, some clinicians have used the drug for the treatment of tachyarrhythmias in patients with this syndrome.

● Pediatric Precautions

Safety and efficacy of lidocaine in the management of ventricular arrhythmias in children have not been established by controlled clinical studies. However, lidocaine has been used for the treatment of ventricular arrhythmias in infants and children. Some experts state that use of the drug may be considered during pediatric resuscitation for the treatment of ventricular fibrillation or pulseless ventricular tachycardia that is resistant to cardiopulmonary resuscitation (CPR), cardioversion (i.e., defibrillation), and epinephrine.

● Pregnancy, Fertility, and Lactation

Pregnancy

Safe use of lidocaine during pregnancy (prior to labor) has not been established. The drug should be used during pregnancy only when clearly needed.

Lactation

Since lidocaine is distributed into milk, the drug should be used with caution in nursing women. Limited data suggest that the amount of drug that potentially would be ingested by a breast-fed infant is small.

DRUG INTERACTIONS

● Succinylcholine

In anesthetized individuals, the neuromuscular blocking effect of succinylcholine has been reported to be increased by IV administration of lidocaine prior to or following succinylcholine administration; however, this effect appears to be important only following administration of lidocaine in doses higher than those usually used clinically.

● Antiarrhythmic Agents

When lidocaine is administered with other antiarrhythmic drugs such as phenytoin, procainamide, propranolol, or quinidine, the cardiac effects may be additive or antagonistic and toxic effects may be additive. Phenytoin may stimulate the hepatic metabolism of lidocaine, but the clinical importance of this effect is not known.

● Other Drugs

Concurrent use of lidocaine with cimetidine or propranolol may result in increased serum concentrations of lidocaine with resultant toxicity. Cimetidine and propranolol substantially reduce the systemic clearance of lidocaine, apparently by reducing hepatic blood flow and hepatic extraction of the drug; other mechanisms (e.g., altered distribution or metabolism of lidocaine) may also be involved. If lidocaine and cimetidine or propranolol are used concurrently, the patient should be closely observed for signs of lidocaine toxicity, and serum lidocaine concentrations should be carefully monitored; reduction of lidocaine dosage may be necessary.

PHARMACOLOGY

Lidocaine hydrochloride is an amide-type local anesthetic that is also used as an antiarrhythmic agent. The cardiac actions of lidocaine appear to be similar to those of phenytoin. Lidocaine is considered a class I (membrane-stabilizing) antiarrhythmic agent. Like other class I antiarrhythmic agents, lidocaine is believed to combine with fast sodium channels in their inactive state and thereby inhibit recovery after repolarization in a time- and voltage-dependent manner which is associated with subsequent dissociation of the drug from the sodium channels. Lidocaine exhibits electrophysiologic effects characteristic of class IB antiarrhythmic agents. The electrophysiologic characteristics of the subgroups of class I antiarrhythmic agents may be related to quantitative differences in their rates of attachment to and dissociation from transmembrane sodium channels, with class IB agents exhibiting rapid rates of attachment and dissociation.

Lidocaine controls ventricular arrhythmias by suppressing automaticity in the His-Purkinje system and by suppressing spontaneous depolarization of the ventricles during diastole. These effects occur at lidocaine concentrations that do not suppress automaticity of the sinoatrial (SA) node. At therapeutic plasma concentrations, lidocaine has little effect on atrioventricular (AV) node conduction and His-Purkinje conduction in the normal heart. Specialized conducting tissues of the atria are less sensitive to the effects of lidocaine than are those of ventricular tissues. Lidocaine has a variable effect on the effective refractory period (ERP) of the AV node; the drug shortens the ERP and the action potential duration of the His-Purkinje system. Lidocaine does not appear to affect excitability of normal cardiac tissue.

Unlike quinidine and procainamide, lidocaine has little effect on autonomic tone and generally does not produce a substantial fall in blood pressure, decreased myocardial contractility, or diminished cardiac output in usual doses. Although lidocaine usually has little effect on heart rate, patients with a diseased or abnormal sinus node may be especially sensitive to the cardiac depressant effects of the drug. Lidocaine may increase coronary blood flow in patients with recent myocardial infarction.

Lidocaine is a CNS depressant and produces sedative, analgesic, and anticonvulsant effects. With high doses, seizures may result from depression of inhibitory influences on motor pathways; severe overdosage may cause respiratory arrest because of motor nerve paralysis and/or inadequate medullary blood flow. Lidocaine also suppresses the cough and gag reflexes.

PHARMACOKINETICS

● Absorption

Although lidocaine hydrochloride is absorbed from the GI tract, it passes into the hepatic portal circulation and only about 35% of an oral dose reaches systemic circulation unchanged. One study showed that therapeutic plasma concentrations are not achieved after oral administration of 250 or 500 mg of the drug, but toxic effects appear, perhaps because of high concentrations of toxic metabolites.

Plasma lidocaine concentrations of approximately 1–5 mcg/mL are required to suppress ventricular arrhythmias. Toxicity has been associated with plasma lidocaine concentrations greater than 5 mcg/mL. Following IV administration of a bolus dose of 50–100 mg of lidocaine hydrochloride, the drug has an onset of action within 45–90 seconds and a duration of action of 10–20 minutes. If an IV infusion is initiated without an initial bolus dose, the attainment of therapeutic plasma concentrations is relatively slow. For example, therapeutic plasma concentrations are achieved in 30–60 minutes after the start of a continuous infusion of 60–70 mcg/kg per minute when no loading dose is given. Plasma concentrations of 1.5–5.5 mcg/mL have been reported to be maintained with an initial IV bolus of 1.5 mg/kg followed by infusion of 50 mcg/kg per minute in patients with heart disease.

Lidocaine hydrochloride is absorbed in the trachea; when the drug is administered endotracheally, plasma concentrations generally are lower than those achieved with vascular administration. A biphasic pattern of absorption is observed following endotracheal administration of lidocaine (initial instantaneous absorption of a small fraction of the dose, followed by a late, delayed absorption phase). Absorption may be increased by diluting the drug in sterile water instead of 0.9% sodium chloride injection.

After intradeltoid injection (an IM formulation no longer is commercially available in the US) of lidocaine hydrochloride 4.5 mg/kg in one study in patients with ventricular premature contractions, peak blood concentrations of 2.9 mcg/mL were achieved in 10 minutes and blood concentrations of 2.2 mcg/mL persisted for 60 minutes. Intradeltoid injection produces higher blood concentrations and more rapid development of peak blood concentrations than do injections into the gluteus maximus or vastus lateralis.

● Distribution

Lidocaine is widely distributed into body tissues. After an IV bolus, there is an early, rapid decline in plasma concentrations of the drug, principally associated with distribution into highly perfused tissues such as the kidneys, lungs, liver, and heart, followed by a slower elimination phase in which metabolism and redistribution into skeletal muscle and adipose tissue occur. Lidocaine has a high affinity for fat and adipose tissue. As plasma concentrations of the drug fall, the diffusion gradient from tissue to blood increases and the lidocaine that initially entered the highly perfused tissues and fat diffuses back into the blood. The volume of distribution is decreased in patients with congestive heart failure and increased in patients with liver disease.

Binding of lidocaine to plasma proteins is variable and concentration dependent. At concentrations of 1–4 mcg/mL, the drug is approximately 60–80% bound to plasma proteins. Lidocaine is partially bound to α_1-acid glycoprotein (α_1-AGP), and the extent of binding to α_1-AGP depends on the plasma concentration of the protein. In patients with myocardial infarction, increases in plasma α_1-AGP concentration are associated with increased lidocaine binding and increased total plasma concentrations of the drug, but only small increases in plasma concentration of free drug; these changes in α_1-AGP concentration and lidocaine binding are believed to account in part for accumulation of the drug observed in patients with myocardial infarction receiving prolonged infusions.

Lidocaine readily crosses the blood-brain barrier and the placenta. Lidocaine also is distributed into milk; in one lactating woman, milk lidocaine concentration was approximately 40% of the serum concentration (from a sample obtained 2 hours earlier).

● Elimination

Lidocaine has an initial half-life of 7–30 minutes and a terminal half-life of 1.5–2 hours. In healthy individuals, the elimination half-lives of the active metabolites, monoethylglycinexylidide (MEGX) and glycinexylidide (GX) are 2 hours and 10 hours, respectively. In patients with myocardial infarction (with or without cardiac failure), the half-lives of lidocaine and MEGX have been reported to be prolonged; the half-life of GX is reportedly prolonged in patients with cardiac failure secondary to myocardial infarction. The half-life of lidocaine is reportedly also prolonged in patients with congestive heart failure or liver disease and may be prolonged following continuous IV infusions lasting longer than 24 hours. MEGX elimination may also be decreased in patients with congestive heart failure.

Approximately 90% of a parenteral dose of lidocaine is rapidly metabolized in the liver by de-ethylation to form MEGX and GX followed by cleavage of the amide bond to form xylidine and 4-hydroxyxylidine which are excreted in urine. Less than 10% of a dose is excreted unchanged in urine. MEGX and GX are pharmacologically active and may also cause CNS toxicity in some patients. The rate of metabolism of lidocaine appears to be limited by hepatic blood flow which may be reduced in patients after acute myocardial infarction and/or with congestive heart failure. Patients with congestive heart failure excrete more of a dose of lidocaine as unchanged drug and MEGX and less as GX and 4-hydroxyxylidine than do those without congestive heart failure. The rate of lidocaine metabolism may also be decreased in patients with liver disease, possibly because of altered perfusion in the liver or hepatic tissue necrosis. Distribution and elimination of lidocaine and MEGX appear to remain normal in patients with renal failure, but GX may accumulate in these patients when lidocaine is administered IV for several days.

CHEMISTRY AND STABILITY

● Chemistry

Lidocaine is an amide-type local anesthetic that is also used as an antiarrhythmic agent. The drug occurs as a white, crystalline powder having a slightly bitter taste and is very soluble in water and in alcohol. The pK_a of the drug is 7.86. Sodium hydroxide and/or hydrochloric acid are used to adjust the pH of the commercially available injections to 5–7. Commercially available lidocaine hydrochloride in 5% dextrose injections are sterile, nonpyrogenic solutions of the drug; sodium hydroxide may have been added to adjust pH to 4 (range: 3–7). Commercially available 0.4 or 0.8% solutions of lidocaine hydrochloride in 5% dextrose have osmolarities of 280–282, or 305–311 mOsm/L, respectively. Potency of lidocaine hydrochloride is calculated on the anhydrous basis.

● Stability

Lidocaine hydrochloride injections and commercially available solutions of the drug in 5% dextrose should be stored at 25°C but may be exposed to temperatures up to 40°C; the injection and solutions should not be frozen, and the solutions should be protected from excessive heat. Commercially available solutions of lidocaine hydrochloride in 5% dextrose usually are stable for 18 months after the date of manufacture. Commercially available solutions of lidocaine hydrochloride in 5% dextrose may be provided in plastic containers. The amount of water that can permeate from the container into the overwrap is insufficient to significantly affect the injection. Solutions in contact with the plastic can leach out some of the chemical components in very small amounts; however, safety of the plastic has been confirmed in tests in animals according to USP biological tests for plastic containers.

At concentrations of 1–4 mg/mL in 5% dextrose injection, extemporaneously prepared lidocaine hydrochloride solutions appear to be stable at room temperature for at least 24 hours.

Lidocaine hydrochloride injection is compatible with most commercially available IV infusion fluids, but the pH of the drug may adversely affect additives such as dopamine, epinephrine, norepinephrine, or isoproterenol that require low pH for stability. If such admixtures are prepared, they should be administered shortly after preparation. Specialized references should be consulted for specific compatibility information. The manufacturers state that the commercially available solutions of lidocaine hydrochloride in 5% dextrose should not be mixed with other drugs.

PREPARATIONS

Excipients in commercially available drug preparations may have clinically important effects in some individuals; consult specific product labeling for details.

Lidocaine Hydrochloride

Parenteral

| Injection, for direct IV injection | 10 mg/mL* | Lidocaine Hydrochloride Injection for Cardiac Arrhythmias |
| | 20 mg/mL* | Lidocaine Hydrochloride Injection for Cardiac Arrhythmias |

* available from one or more manufacturer, distributor, and/or repackager by generic (nonproprietary) name

Lidocaine Hydrochloride in Dextrose

Parenteral

| Injection, for IV infusion | 4 mg/mL (1 or 2 g) Lidocaine Hydrochloride in 5% Dextrose | 0.4% Lidocaine Hydrochloride and 5% Dextrose Injection |
| | 8 mg/mL (2 or 4 g) Lidocaine Hydrochloride in 5% Dextrose | 0.8% Lidocaine Hydrochloride and 5% Dextrose Injection |

† Use is not currently included in the labeling approved by the US Food and Drug Administration.

Selected Revisions September 10, 2024, © Copyright, September 1, 1977, American Society of Health-System Pharmacists, Inc.

Flecainide Acetate

24:04.04.12 • CLASS Ic ANTIARRHYTHMICS

■ Flecainide acetate is a local anesthetic-type class Ic antiarrhythmic agent.

USES

● Ventricular Arrhythmias

Flecainide acetate is used to suppress and prevent the recurrence of documented *life-threatening* ventricular arrhythmias (e.g., sustained ventricular tachycardia). Based on information from the National Heart, Lung, and Blood Institute (NHLBI) describing interim results of the Cardiac Arrhythmia Suppression Trial (CAST) (see the opening discussion in Cautions), flecainide therapy should be *reserved* for the suppression and prevention of documented ventricular arrhythmias that, in the clinician's judgment, are considered *life-threatening*.

Because of the drug's arrhythmogenic potential and associated risk of death identified in CAST, use of flecainide for less severe arrhythmias (e.g., nonsustained ventricular tachycardia†, frequent premature ventricular complexes† [PVCs]), even when the patient is symptomatic, is not recommended. The findings of CAST involved a select patient population with recent myocardial infarction (MI), mild-to-moderate left ventricular dysfunction (e.g., mean baseline ejection fraction of 0.4), and asymptomatic or mildly symptomatic ventricular arrhythmias† (mean baseline PVCs of 127/hour as evidenced via ambulatory ECG [Holter] monitoring during at least 18 hours of analyzable time, with about 20% of patients exhibiting at least one run of nonsustained ventricular tachycardia during such monitoring); such patients also had demonstrated drug-induced suppressibility of PVCs during the initial phase of the open trial. It currently is not known whether the findings of CAST can be extrapolated to other patient populations with non-life-threatening ventricular arrhythmias (e.g., patients with arrhythmias in the absence of ventricular dysfunction, myocardial ischemia, or recent MI). CAST principally involved suppression and prevention of PVCs, with only about 10% of patients exhibiting more than a single run of tachycardia at baseline. Some clinicians also question whether the results of CAST even can be extrapolated to patients with recurrent nonsustained ventricular tachycardia and ventricular dysfunction, since these patients are known to be at high risk of sudden death if untreated, and since CAST did not include sufficient numbers of such patients to clearly determine the benefit-to-risk ratio. However, despite the limitations of the CAST findings, the manufacturer, FDA, and other experts consider the potential risks of flecainide therapy substantial and currently do not recommend use of the drug in any patient with non-life-threatening ventricular arrhythmias in the absence of substantial evidence of safety and efficacy. The manufacturer states that it is prudent to consider the risks of class Ic antiarrhythmic agents and current lack of evidence of improved survival *unacceptable* in patients *without* life-threatening ventricular arrhythmias, even in patients experiencing unpleasant, but non-life-threatening signs and symptoms. However, some clinicians, while recognizing the strong evidence of risk in the patient population studied in CAST and the substantial limitations of current evidence on safety and efficacy in other patient populations, question such an extreme limitation of usage.

Life-threatening Ventricular Arrhythmias

The optimum role of flecainide in the suppression and prevention of ventricular arrhythmias remains to be clearly determined.

In addition, it remains to be determined whether antiarrhythmic agents, including flecainide, have a beneficial effect on mortality or sudden death. Although flecainide has been effective in suppressing and preventing ventricular arrhythmias in carefully selected patients, further studies are needed to evaluate the long-term efficacy and safety and the relative role of the drug. Therefore, it is recommended that flecainide generally be reserved for patients who have an insufficient therapeutic response to, or who do not tolerate, conventional orally administered antiarrhythmic agents (e.g., class Ia agents). In addition, because of flecainide's arrhythmogenic potential, some clinicians avoid use of the drug as a first-line agent in patients with life-threatening ventricular arrhythmias who also have congestive heart failure or substantial ventricular dysfunction. While it

currently is not known whether the findings of the CAST study apply to class Ic antiarrhythmic agents other than flecainide and encainide (no longer commercially available in the US), some experts state that, in the absence of specific evidence of safety and efficacy, other class Ic drugs should be considered to share these risks.

There is relatively limited experience with the use of flecainide for suppression and prevention of recurrent life-threatening ventricular arrhythmias. In the management of severe refractory arrhythmias, the efficacy of flecainide appears to be comparable to that of other first-line antiarrhythmic agents, with the drug being effective in up to about 40% of patients. Younger patients and patients without coronary heart disease and/or substantial ventricular dysfunction appear to have a greater likelihood of responding to flecainide. Further studies, including comparative studies with other antiarrhythmic agents, are needed to evaluate the use of flecainide in the management of life-threatening ventricular arrhythmias.

Limited information is available on the use of flecainide in conjunction with other antiarrhythmic agents for the management of severe refractory ventricular arrhythmias. (See Drug Interactions: Antiarrhythmic Agents.) In a limited number of patients, flecainide has been combined with amiodarone, with good results in selected patients; however, use of these two agents in combination requires extreme caution and is generally reserved for patients with life-threatening ventricular arrhythmias inadequately controlled by single-agent therapy with amiodarone or another antiarrhythmic agent. Combination antiarrhythmic therapy for severe refractory ventricular arrhythmias is generally empiric and must be individualized.

Other Ventricular Arrhythmias

Controlled and uncontrolled clinical studies in patients with chronic stable ventricular arrhythmias† have shown that flecainide is highly effective in suppressing and preventing nonsustained ventricular tachycardia and frequent PVCs, including complex PVCs. In short-term clinical studies, flecainide therapy produced at least 80–90% suppression of PVCs in about 80–90% of patients; in many patients, essentially complete suppression of uniform and multiform PVCs, complex PVCs, and/or nonsustained ventricular tachycardia may occur. However, despite such documented evidence of efficacy in suppressing and preventing these arrhythmias, there currently is no evidence of beneficial effect on mortality, and in at least one patient population (those with mild-to-moderate ventricular dysfunction and recent MI) with such arrhythmias, there was evidence of substantial risk (including mortality and nonfatal cardiac arrest) associated with flecainide or encainide therapy. (See the opening discussion of Cautions.) Therefore, use of flecainide in nonlife-threatening ventricular arrhythmias currently is *not* recommended by the manufacturer, FDA, and other experts.

● Supraventricular Tachyarrhythmias

Flecainide is used for the prevention of paroxysmal supraventricular tachycardia (PSVT), including atrioventricular (AV) nodal reentrant tachycardia and AV reentrant tachycardia (e.g., Wolff-Parkinson-White syndrome); other symptomatic, disabling supraventricular tachycardias of unspecified mechanisms; and symptomatic, disabling paroxysmal atrial fibrillation/flutter (PAF) in patients without structural heart disease. Controlled and uncontrolled clinical studies have shown that flecainide may prevent or delay recurrence of PSVT and PAF episodes or may increase the interval between episodes of PSVT and PAF in 31–81% of patients, depending on the type of arrhythmia; suppression of arrhythmias refractory to other antiarrhythmic agents also has occurred. In some patients with atrial fibrillation or flutter associated with ventricular preexcitation and Wolff-Parkinson-White syndrome, flecainide may slow the ventricular rate or possibly restore and maintain normal sinus rhythm. Because of the risk of proarrhythmia, flecainide should not be used in patients with structural heart disease or ischemic heart disease.

Based on findings from the CAST study demonstrating substantial flecainide-associated risk in certain patients with ventricular arrhythmias, some experts currently caution that use of flecainide in supraventricular arrhythmias be limited to the management of symptomatic, disabling supraventricular arrhythmias (PAF, AV junctional tachycardias) in patients *without* structural heart disease. However, some clinicians state that even these patients may be at risk of developing drug-induced arrhythmogenic effects (e.g., during exercise testing). The risks versus benefits of flecainide for the management of such arrhythmias in patients *with* structural heart defects remains to be elucidated, and assessment of the possible risks and potential benefits in such patients must be individualized.

Paroxysmal Supraventricular Tachycardia

For acute conversion of PSVT, vagal maneuvers, IV adenosine, AV nodal blocking agents (e.g., calcium-channel blocking agents, β-adrenergic blocking agents), and/or synchronized cardioversion are the treatments of choice. Flecainide is one of several drugs that may be used for the ongoing management of PSVT (to prevent recurrences of these arrhythmias) in patients without structural or ischemic heart disease; because of the risk of adverse effects, however, use of flecainide generally is reserved for patients in whom other therapies are ineffective or contraindicated. In a randomized, placebo-controlled, crossover study in 34 patients with symptomatic PSVT, episodes of PSVT occurred in 85% of patients receiving placebo but in only about 21% of patients receiving flecainide acetate in a median dosage of 300 mg daily (range: 100–400 mg daily in 2 divided doses) during the 16-week study period. The median time before initial recurrence of PSVT exceeded 55 days in patients receiving flecainide compared with 11 days in those receiving placebo, while median intervals between episodes of PSVT exceeded 55 days in patients receiving flecainide compared with 12 days in those receiving placebo.

Paroxysmal Atrial Fibrillation and Flutter

In another randomized, crossover placebo-controlled study in 48 patients with PAF, episodes of PAF occurred in 92% of patients receiving placebo versus 69% of patients who received flecainide acetate in a median dosage of 300 mg daily (range: 100–600 mg daily in 2 divided doses) during the 8-week study period. The median time before initial recurrence of PAF was approximately 15 days in patients receiving flecainide versus 3 days in those receiving placebo, while the median interval between episodes of PAF was 27 days in patients receiving flecainide and approximately 6 days in patients receiving placebo.

Self-administration for Conversion of Paroxysmal Atrial Fibrillation

Limited evidence suggests that out-of-hospital *self-administration* of a single oral loading dose† of flecainide or propafenone ("pill-in-the-pocket" approach) is safe and effective for terminating recent-onset PAF† and can reduce hospitalizations and emergency room visits in carefully selected patients who have mild or no heart disease. Experts state that an initial conversion trial in a monitored setting is recommended before this approach is undertaken in an unmonitored setting outside of the hospital. In-hospital administration of flecainide or propafenone (as immediate-release tablets) as a single oral dose for terminating acute atrial fibrillation† has been shown to be effective with a low incidence of adverse effects in several randomized, controlled studies; however, the safety of such treatment without initial evaluation in a hospital setting or in patients with substantial structural heart disease has not been established. In addition, additional study and experience are required to assess the possible need for concomitant antithrombotic (e.g., warfarin) therapy and potential for adverse drug interactions (e.g., with warfarin or digoxin) in patients self-administering antiarrhythmic agents for recent-onset paroxysmal atrial fibrillation on an out-of-hospital basis.

In a prospective, uncontrolled study, 268 patients (18–75 years of age) with mild or no heart disease who had hemodynamically well-tolerated atrial fibrillation of recent (less than 48 hours) onset were treated in-hospital (i.e., in the emergency room or cardiology ward) with a single oral dose of flecainide or immediate-release propafenone (according to clinician preference) to restore normal sinus rhythm. Patients weighing 70 kg or more received 300 mg of flecainide acetate or 600 mg of propafenone hydrochloride and those weighing less than 70 kg received 200 mg of flecainide acetate or 450 mg of propafenone hydrochloride. In-hospital treatment was considered effective if conversion of atrial fibrillation to sinus rhythm occurred within 6 hours of administration of the antiarrhythmic agent without clinically important adverse effects (i.e., symptomatic hypotension, symptomatic bradycardia after restoration of sinus rhythm, dyspnea, presyncope, syncope, conversion to atrial flutter or atrial tachycardia, or episodes of sustained or unsustained ventricular tachycardia). The time to conversion to sinus rhythm following in-hospital treatment with flecainide or propafenone in these patients averaged 135 minutes (median: 120 minutes). Patients in whom inpatient administration of these antiarrhythmics was effective and who were not excluded during subsequent examination were discharged and given flecainide or propafenone for treatment of subsequent episodes of palpitations (presumed recurrent atrial fibrillation) on an outpatient basis. These patients were instructed to take a single oral dose of the assigned antiarrhythmic drug 5 minutes after noting the onset of palpitations (self-assessed) and then to assume a resting state (e.g., a supine or sitting position) until resolution of the palpitations or for at least four hours.

Analysis of data from 2 of the study sites indicated that 12% of patients presenting to the emergency room for recent-onset atrial fibrillation were candidates for out-of-hospital treatment with propafenone or flecainide. During a mean follow-up period of 15 months (range: 7–19 months), 79% of patients included in the out-of-hospital phase of the study experienced episodes of palpitations (presumed atrial fibrillation); patients self-administered propafenone hydrochloride (mean dose: 555 mg) or flecainide acetate (mean dose: 263 mg) within a mean of 36 minutes (median: 10 minutes) after the onset of symptoms in 92% of such episodes. Each antiarrhythmic agent was effective in interrupting 94% of episodes of palpitations (a primary end point); time to resolution of symptoms after drug administration averaged 113 minutes (median: 98 minutes). In patients who had multiple recurrences of palpitations during the follow-up period, self-administration of flecainide or propafenone terminated all such episodes in 84% of patients. Self-administration of oral flecainide or propafenone also was associated with reductions in emergency room visits and hospital admissions (secondary end points); calls for emergency room intervention during the study averaged 4.9 per month compared with 45.6 per month during the year prior to the study, while the number of hospitalizations averaged 1.6 per month during the study compared with 15 per month during the prior year.

Atrial Fibrillation and Flutter

Flecainide is considered a drug of choice for pharmacologic cardioversion of atrial fibrillation or atrial flutter†. Conversion of atrial fibrillation or flutter to normal sinus rhythm may be associated with embolism, particularly when the arrhythmia has been present for more than 48 hours, unless the patient is adequately anticoagulated. (See Uses: Cardioversion of Atrial Fibrillation/Flutter, in Heparin 20:12.04.16.)

Limited data suggest that flecainide may also improve control of ventricular rate at rest and during exercise in digitalized patients with atrial fibrillation† in whom cardiac glycosides alone may not provide adequate control.

Some clinicians do not recommend the use of antiarrhythmic agents in patients with atrial fibrillation or flutter because increased mortality has been reported in patients receiving antiarrhythmic therapy after conversion of atrial fibrillation to normal sinus rhythm.

Other Supraventricular Tachycardias

Flecainide may be used for the ongoing management of focal atrial tachycardia† or junctional tachycardia† in patients without structural or ischemic heart disease. Limited data suggest that flecainide may be effective in suppressing and preventing recurrent atrial tachycardia†.

DOSAGE AND ADMINISTRATION

● *Administration*

Flecainide acetate is administered orally. Flecainide also has been administered IV†, but a parenteral dosage form of the drug is currently not commercially available in the US.

Flecainide acetate is administered orally, usually in 2 equally divided doses daily at 12-hour intervals; however, in patients in whom arrhythmias are not adequately controlled or the drug is not well tolerated with twice-daily dosing, the drug may be given in 3 divided doses daily at 8-hour intervals. The elimination half-life of flecainide suggests that once-daily oral dosing may be possible in some patients, but once-daily dosing regimens of the drug have not been evaluated to date.

Absorption of flecainide is not affected by food or antacids; however, milk may inhibit absorption in infants. Dosage reduction of flecainide acetate may be necessary when milk is removed from the diet in infants.

Because of the risk of proarrhythmia, initiation of therapy in a hospital setting is recommended in patients with sustained ventricular tachycardia, regardless of their cardiac status. Some clinicians recommend that withdrawal of therapy should also occur in a hospital setting under continuous ECG monitoring.

Extemporaneously Compounded Oral Solution

Extemporaneously compounded oral solutions of flecainide acetate have been prepared.

Standardize 4 Safety

Standardized concentrations for an extemporaneously compounded oral solution of flecainide have been established through Standardize 4 Safety (S4S), a national patient safety initiative to reduce medication errors, especially during transitions of care. Multidisciplinary expert panels were convened to determine recommended standard concentrations. Because recommendations from the S4S panels may differ from the manufacturer's prescribing information, caution is advised when using concentrations that differ from labeling, particularly when using rate information from the label. For additional information on S4S (including updates that may be available), see https://www.ashp.org/pharmacy-practice/standardize-4-safety-initiative.

TABLE 1. Standardize 4 Safety Compounded Oral Liquid Standards for Flecainide

Concentration Standards
10 mg/mL

● *Dosage*

Dosage of flecainide acetate should be carefully adjusted according to individual patient response and tolerance. Clinical and ECG monitoring of cardiac function is recommended during therapy with the drug. When feasible, plasma trough flecainide concentrations should be monitored; monitoring is required in patients with severe renal or hepatic impairment, and is recommended in other patients in whom elimination of the drug may be impaired (e.g., those with moderate renal impairment or congestive heart failure, or those receiving concomitant amiodarone therapy). Dosage should be adjusted to maintain trough plasma flecainide concentrations at less than 0.7–1 mcg/mL since concentrations above this range have been associated with a higher rate of adverse cardiac effects, especially when the trough concentration exceeds 1 mcg/mL. Since steady-state plasma concentrations of flecainide and the optimum therapeutic effect may not be attained for 3–5 days (or longer in some patients) at a given dosage in patients with normal renal and hepatic function, increases in flecainide dosage should be made at intervals of not less than 4 days. Once adequate control of arrhythmias has been attained, dosage reduction to minimize adverse effects or effects on cardiac conduction may be possible in some patients; however, efficacy of the drug at the lower dosage should be evaluated. If congestive heart failure, myocardial dysfunction, or renal or hepatic failure develops in patients receiving flecainide, dosage reduction may be necessary. Many clinicians recommend the use of low initial dosages in geriatric patients.

Any use of flecainide in children should be supervised directly by a cardiologist experienced in the treatment of arrhythmias in this age group. (See Cautions: Pediatric Precautions.) In pediatric patients, flecainide should be initiated in a hospital setting with facilities available for cardiac rhythm monitoring. Because of the evolving nature of flecainide use in children, specialized references should be consulted for the most recent information. The manufacturer states that the initial flecainide acetate dosage in infants younger than 6 months of age is approximately 50 mg/m^2 daily, divided into 2 or 3 equally spaced doses. For older children, an initial dosage of 100 mg/m^2 daily may be given. The maximum dosage recommended by the manufacturer for pediatric patients is 200 mg/m^2 daily, which should not be exceeded. Plasma trough flecainide concentrations (less than 1 hour before dosing) and ECGs should be obtained at presumed steady state (after at least 5 doses) after initiation of therapy or after any change in dosing, whether the dosage was increased for lack of effectiveness or for increased growth of the child. In some children receiving higher dosages, plasma drug concentrations are labile; while receiving the same dosage, plasma flecainide concentrations have increased rapidly to far above therapeutic concentrations, despite previously low plasma concentrations. Small changes in dosage also may lead to disproportionate increases in plasma drug concentrations. For the first year of flecainide treatment whenever the pediatric patient is seen for clinical follow-up, a 12-lead ECG and plasma trough flecainide concentrations are suggested. The usual therapeutic concentration of flecainide in children is 200–500 ng/mL, although concentrations up to 800 ng/mL may be required for adequate control in some children.

Since initial flecainide acetate dosages higher than those recommended and dosage adjustments at shorter intervals than recommended have resulted in an increased risk of arrhythmogenicity and congestive heart failure in patients with sustained ventricular tachycardia, especially during the first few days of flecainide

therapy, a loading dose of the drug is *not* recommended; however, single oral loading doses (e.g., 200–300 mg) have been used for conversion of recent-onset atrial fibrillation to normal sinus rhythm† in selected patients ("pill-in-the-pocket" approach). IV lidocaine has occasionally been used concomitantly and without any apparent adverse interaction until the therapeutic effect of oral flecainide therapy was attained; however, studies have not been performed to determine the value of this regimen.

Based on theoretical considerations, it is recommended that, when transferring patients from therapy with another antiarrhythmic agent to flecainide, at least 2–4 plasma half-lives of the agent being discontinued be allowed to elapse before therapy with flecainide is initiated at the usual dosage. When withdrawal of another antiarrhythmic agent is likely to result in life-threatening arrhythmias, initiation of flecainide therapy in a hospital setting should be considered.

Life-threatening Ventricular Arrhythmias

For the prevention of life-threatening ventricular arrhythmias (e.g., sustained ventricular tachycardia), the recommended initial adult dosage of flecainide acetate is 100 mg every 12 hours. Some clinicians suggest an initial dosage of 50 mg twice daily in these patients. Dosage may be increased in increments of 50 mg twice daily every 4 days until an effective response is attained. Most patients do not require dosages greater than 150 mg every 12 hours or 300 mg daily. The maximum recommended dosage of flecainide acetate in most patients with sustained ventricular tachycardia is 400 mg daily.

Supraventricular Tachyarrhythmias

For the prevention of paroxysmal supraventricular tachycardias (PSVT), including atrioventricular nodal reentrant tachycardia, atrioventricular reentrant tachycardia, and other disabling supraventricular tachycardias of unspecified mechanism, and disabling paroxysmal atrial fibrillation/flutter (PAF), the recommended initial adult dosage of flecainide acetate is 50 mg every 12 hours. Dosage may be increased in increments of 50 mg twice daily every 4 days until an effective response is attained. In patients with PAF who do not attain the desired response, the manufacturer states that increasing flecainide acetate dosage to 100 mg twice daily can increase effective response without increasing the incidence of adverse effects (which might lead to discontinuance of flecainide therapy). The maximum recommended dosage of flecainide in patients with paroxysmal supraventricular arrhythmias is 300 mg daily.

Self-administration for Conversion of Paroxysmal Atrial Fibrillation

For *self-administration*† on an outpatient basis for termination of atrial fibrillation of recent onset in carefully selected patients with mild or no heart disease ("pill-in-the-pocket" approach), flecainide acetate has been given as a single oral loading dose of 300 mg in patients weighing 70 kg or more or 200 mg in patients weighing less than 70 kg.

Some clinicians suggest that flecainide be taken 5 minutes after noting the onset of palpitations and that patients remain in a supine or sitting position until resolution of palpitations or for a period of at least 4 hours following the dose. Patients should seek medical advice if palpitations do not resolve within 6–8 hours, if previously unexperienced symptoms (e.g., dyspnea, presyncope, syncope) occur, or if a marked increase in heart rate occurs after taking the antiarrhythmic drug. Patients should not take more than a single oral dose of flecainide during a 24-hour period.

● *Dosage in Renal and Hepatic Impairment*

In patients with renal impairment, dosage of flecainide acetate must be carefully adjusted based on the degree of renal impairment. The recommended initial oral dosage of flecainide acetate in patients with severe renal impairment (creatinine clearance of 35 mL/minute per 1.73 m^2 or less) is 100 mg once daily (or 50 mg twice daily). In patients with less severe renal impairment, an initial dosage of 100 mg every 12 hours is recommended. Since the elimination half-life of the drug may be prolonged in patients with renal impairment, steady-state plasma concentrations with a given dosage may not be attained for longer than 4 days. Consequently, increases in dosage should be made with caution and at intervals of longer than 4 days, with the patient closely monitored for signs of adverse cardiac effects or other toxicity. Plasma trough flecainide concentrations should be monitored in patients with severe renal impairment and also may be useful in patients with moderate renal impairment.

Since flecainide is extensively metabolized, probably in the liver, elimination may be markedly prolonged in patients with substantial hepatic impairment, and therefore the drug should not be used in such patients unless the potential benefits are considered to clearly outweigh the risks. If flecainide is used in patients with hepatic impairment, plasma flecainide concentrations should be monitored closely to guide dosage, and dosage should be increased cautiously at intervals of longer than 4 days.

CAUTIONS

While clinical studies have indicated that adverse reactions to flecainide occur frequently but are usually mild to moderate in severity and transient, and the drug is generally well tolerated in most patients, concerns about the long-term safety and efficacy of the drug in patients with nonlife-threatening arrhythmias have been raised by findings of the Cardiac Arrhythmia Suppression Trial (CAST). Findings from the CAST study after an average of 10 months of follow-up indicate that the rate of total mortality and nonfatal cardiac arrest in patients with recent myocardial infarction (MI), mild-to-moderate left ventricular dysfunction, and asymptomatic or mildly symptomatic ventricular arrhythmias (principally frequent premature ventricular complexes [PVCs]) who received flecainide was increased substantially.

The CAST study, which began in 1987, was designed to evaluate the efficacy (in terms of reduced sudden cardiac death and total mortality) and safety of flecainide, encainide, and moricizine for the suppression and prevention of PVCs following recent MI (more than 6 days but less than 2 years previously) in patients with asymptomatic or mildly symptomatic ventricular arrhythmias. Findings from this large, multicenter, double-blind, placebo-controlled study, sponsored by the National Heart, Lung, and Blood Institute (NHLBI), indicate that the rates of total mortality (from arrhythmia, cardiac arrest, other cardiac causes, or noncardiac or unclassified causes) and nonfatal cardiac arrest combined in such patients receiving flecainide was increased substantially to 2.2 times that observed in patients receiving placebo. These findings were consistent across a variety of patient subgroups, and the degree of undesirable effects associated with flecainide or encainide was similar. When the effects of flecainide or encainide were considered together, the rate of total mortality and nonfatal cardiac arrest was 2.5 times that observed with placebo, and the rate of death secondary to arrhythmia or cardiac arrest for these drugs was 3.6 times that observed with placebo. Because there was evidence suggesting a potential harmful effect and no evidence of substantial benefit in the type of patient studied, flecainide and encainide were removed from the CAST study in early 1989. The relevance of the findings of the CAST study to patients with ventricular arrhythmias associated with a high risk of death currently is not known, and the manufacturers and FDA state that current evidence does *not* require discontinuance of flecainide in patients being treated for *life-threatening* arrhythmias.

The frequency of flecainide-induced adverse effects tends to decrease with time, and adverse effects tend to occur intermittently. Flecainide-induced adverse effects are often alleviated by dosage reduction, occasionally disappear despite continued treatment and without dosage reduction, and are usually reversible following discontinuance of the drug. The risk of adverse effects, particularly adverse cardiac effects, may increase when trough plasma flecainide concentrations increase above 0.7–1 mcg/mL, especially when the trough concentration exceeds 1 mcg/mL.

The most common adverse effects of flecainide are dizziness and visual disturbances, which are dose related, often occur concomitantly, and are also the most common adverse reactions requiring discontinuance of the drug. Adverse extracardiac effects requiring discontinuance of flecainide therapy occur in about 5–15% of patients. The need to discontinue flecainide results most often from multiple adverse effects rather than a single adverse effect, and adverse effects requiring discontinuance of the drug are most likely to occur during the first 2–4 weeks of therapy.

● *Nervous System Effects*

Dizziness (including dizziness, lightheadedness, faintness, unsteadiness, near syncope), which is dose related and often accompanied by visual disturbances, occurs in about 11–13% of patients receiving flecainide acetate dosages of 200–400 mg daily. Dizziness has required discontinuance of therapy in about 4–6% of patients. Flecainide-induced dizziness may also be associated with other adverse nervous

system effects (e.g., nervousness) and probably results from an effect of the drug on the CNS.

Headache, which appears to be dose related, occurs in about 5–9% of patients receiving flecainide acetate dosages of 200–400 mg daily. Headache has required discontinuance of therapy in less than 1% of patients.

Fatigue has occurred in about 3–8% of patients receiving flecainide and required discontinuance in about 1% of patients. Tremor or nervousness has occurred in about 3–5% of patients and required discontinuance in less than 1% of patients. Hypoesthesia and paresthesia, which tend to occur in the perioral region or the extremities, occur in about 1–3% of patients receiving flecainide. Other adverse nervous system effects occurring in about 1–3% of patients receiving the drug include paresis, ataxia, vertigo, syncope, somnolence, tinnitus, anxiety, insomnia, and depression. Twitching, weakness, change in taste perception, dry mouth, speech disorder, stupor, seizures, amnesia, confusion, neuropathy, hallucinations, depersonalization, euphoria, morbid dreams, and apathy have been reported in less than 1% of patients.

● *Ocular Effects*

Visual disturbances (including blurred vision, difficulty in focusing, spots before eyes), which are dose related and often associated with dizziness, occur in about 5–20% of patients receiving flecainide acetate dosages of 200–400 mg daily and about 18–30% of patients receiving 400–600 mg daily. Visual disturbances have required discontinuance of therapy in about 2–3% of patients. The most common visual disturbance is blurred vision on lateral gaze and/or turning the head to the side. Diplopia has occurred in about 1–3% of patients receiving flecainide, and photophobia, nystagmus, and ocular pain or irritation have occurred in less than 1% of patients.

Flecainide-induced visual disturbances tend to be mild to moderate in severity and transient; persistent disturbances often respond to dosage reduction. Visual disturbances occur intermittently, usually last only for a few seconds, and occur most often during the time of expected peak plasma concentrations following an individual dose. The mechanism(s) of flecainide-induced visual disturbances is not known, but blurred vision may result from difficulty in accommodation caused by a local anesthetic effect of the drug on the ciliary muscle, from an effect on vestibulo-ocular reflexes, or from an effect on the CNS.

● *Arrhythmogenic Effects*

Like other antiarrhythmic agents, flecainide can worsen existing arrhythmias or cause new arrhythmias, and the arrhythmogenic potential is the most serious risk associated with the drug. Arrhythmogenic effects associated with flecainide range from an increased frequency of PVCs to the development of new and/or more severe and potentially fatal ventricular tachyarrhythmias. About 75% of the arrhythmogenic effects associated with the drug have been new or worsened ventricular tachyarrhythmias (e.g., new occurrence of sustained or nonsustained ventricular tachycardia, including exercise-induced or spontaneous wide QRS complex tachycardia, or progression of ventricular tachycardia to ventricular fibrillation), with the remainder consisting of increased frequency of PVCs or new or worsened supraventricular arrhythmias. In some patients, principally those with factors predisposing them to the risk of arrhythmogenic effects, flecainide therapy has been associated with episodes of ventricular tachycardia or fibrillation that required prolonged or unusual resuscitative measures or that resulted in death despite resuscitative measures.

The risk of flecainide-induced arrhythmogenic effects appears to be directly related to dosage and underlying cardiac disease, including severity of the preexisting ventricular arrhythmia and myocardial dysfunction. Patients with atherosclerosis, cardiac disease, previous MI, congestive heart failure, or nonsustained ventricular tachycardia appear to have approximately twice the risk of arrhythmogenic effects during flecainide therapy as those without these conditions. Patients with a history of sustained ventricular tachycardia appear to have about a 10-fold overall increased risk, and patients with both a history of sustained ventricular tachycardia and structural heart disease appear to have about a 14-fold increased risk compared with those with structural heart disease and only PVCs. When flecainide is given according to currently recommended dosage regimens and precautions, the risk of arrhythmogenic effects appears to be comparable to that associated with other antiarrhythmic agents.

Because of difficulties in distinguishing spontaneous and drug-related variations in an underlying arrhythmia disorder in patients with complex arrhythmias, reported occurrence rates must be considered approximations. In clinical studies, new or worsened arrhythmias occurred with an overall frequency of about 1–7%. In patients with sustained ventricular tachycardia who also often had heart failure, a low left ventricular ejection fraction, a history of MI, and/or an episode of cardiac arrest, the incidence of arrhythmogenic effects during flecainide therapy was 13% when dosage was initiated at 200 mg daily, was titrated upward slowly, and did not exceed 300 mg daily in most patients. In early clinical studies in patients with sustained ventricular tachycardia who received an initial flecainide acetate dosage of 400 mg daily (twice the currently recommended initial dosage), the incidence of arrhythmogenic effects was 26%, and arrhythmogenic effects resulted in death in about 10% of patients receiving the drug despite immediate medical attention. With lower initial dosages in these patients, the incidence of arrhythmogenic effects resulting in death has decreased to about 0.5% of patients. In patients with less severe arrhythmias (chronic PVCs, nonsustained ventricular tachycardia) receiving flecainide, the overall incidence of arrhythmogenic effects appears to be approximately 3–4%. It is not known whether the incidence of arrhythmogenic effects is increased in patients with chronic atrial fibrillation, high ventricular rate, and/or exercise. Wide complex tachycardia and ventricular fibrillation have been reported in about 17% of patients with chronic atrial fibrillation who were undergoing maximal exercise tolerance testing.

In patients with supraventricular arrhythmias including paroxysmal atrial fibrillation (PAF), the incidence of arrhythmogenic effects during flecainide therapy was about 4%; proarrhythmic events resulted in one fatal case of ventricular tachycardia/ventricular fibrillation and one case of wide complex ventricular tachycardia.

Flecainide-induced arrhythmogenic effects appear to be directly related to dosage and the rate of dosage escalation, particularly in patients with sustained ventricular tachycardia. A relationship with plasma concentrations of the drug has not been established; however, some data suggest that arrhythmogenicity may be associated with plasma concentrations higher than 1 mcg/mL. Arrhythmogenic effects appear to be most likely to occur within 1–4 weeks of initiation of flecainide therapy and/or within 1 week of an increase in dosage. In patients with sustained ventricular tachycardia, 80% of the arrhythmogenic effects occur within 14 days of initiation of flecainide therapy. The exact role is not clear, but concomitant use of other antiarrhythmic agents may increase the risk of arrhythmogenic effects during flecainide therapy. When transferring patients from another antiarrhythmic drug to flecainide, a transition period is recommended to allow the effects of the previous antiarrhythmic to dissipate prior to initiating flecainide. (See Dosage and Administration: Dosage.) Because of the risk of arrhythmogenic effects, initiation of flecainide therapy in a hospital setting is recommended for patients with sustained ventricular tachycardia and should be considered for other patients in whom withdrawal of a previous antiarrhythmic agent is likely to produce life-threatening arrhythmia. (See Cautions: Precautions and Contraindications.)

● Cardiovascular Effects

Because of its mild to moderate negative inotropic effect, flecainide may cause or worsen congestive heart failure, particularly in patients with cardiomyopathy, preexisting severe heart failure (New York Heart Association [NYHA] class III or IV), or low left ventricular ejection fractions (less than 30%). New or worsened congestive heart failure associated with flecainide has occurred in about 6% of patients with PVCs, non-sustained or sustained ventricular tachycardia. Worsened congestive heart failure associated with flecainide therapy occurred with a frequency of about 26% in patients with a history of congestive heart failure and sustained ventricular tachycardia. New or worsened congestive heart failure occurred in about 0.4% of patients with supraventricular arrhythmias.

Exacerbation of preexisting congestive heart failure during flecainide therapy has occurred most frequently in patients with advanced stages of failure (i.e., NYHA class III or IV). When congestive heart failure has developed or worsened, the onset has occurred within hours to several months after initiation of therapy; the risk appears to be greatest during the first 1–4 weeks of treatment. Some patients who develop signs and/or symptoms of congestive heart failure during flecainide therapy can continue to receive the drug at the same dosage with adjustment of concomitant cardiac glycoside and/or diuretic therapy; however, others may require a reduction in flecainide dosage or discontinuance of the drug.

Palpitation has occurred in about 6%, chest pain in about 5%, and edema in about 3% of patients receiving flecainide. Tachycardia and flushing have occurred in about 1–3% of patients, and bradycardia, angina pectoris, hypertension, and hypotension have occurred in less than 1% of patients receiving the drug.

● Effects on Cardiac Conduction

Clinically important conduction disturbances occur infrequently during flecainide therapy in patients without preexisting conduction abnormalities; however, the risk of adverse cardiac effects appears to increase as plasma flecainide concentrations increase above 0.7–1 mcg/mL. Sinus bradycardia, pause, and arrest have occurred collectively in about 1.2% of patients. First-degree AV block occurs in about 30–40% of patients receiving flecainide. Second-degree AV block occurs in about 0.5% of patients and third-degree AV block in about 0.4% of patients. New bundle-branch block may develop rarely. Some patients with atrial flutter may develop 1:1 AV conduction with flecainide due to slowing of the atrial rate. Paradoxically, an increase in ventricular rate also may occur when flecainide is used in patients with atrial fibrillation. Discontinuance of the drug may be necessary in some patients unless a temporary or permanent artificial pacemaker is in place. (See Cautions: Precautions and Contraindications.) Syncope also has occurred rarely as a result of sinus node dysfunction. Torsades de pointes-type arrhythmia associated with flecainide therapy also has been reported rarely.

Flecainide-induced increases in PR and QRS intervals are usually not clinically important. The degree of lengthening of PR and QRS intervals does not allow prediction of therapeutic efficacy or the development of adverse cardiac effects, although some data suggest that absolute increases in PR and QRS intervals (at least 40 ms) may be associated with adverse cardiac effects. Although prolongation of PR and QRS intervals is to be expected during therapy with the drug and is usually not clinically important, substantial increases require caution and consideration of dosage reduction. (See Cautions: Precautions and Contraindications.) Rarely, substantial prolongation of QT_c may occur and also require caution and dosage reduction.

● GI Effects

Nausea occurs in about 9–10% of patients receiving flecainide and has required discontinuance of the drug in about 1% of patients. Dyspepsia, anorexia, vomiting, constipation, and diarrhea have occurred in about 1–4% of patients and flatulence in less than 1% of patients.

● Dermatologic Effects

Rash occurs in about 1–3% of patients receiving flecainide. Urticaria, pruritus, and exfoliative dermatitis have occurred in less than 1% of patients.

● Other Adverse Effects

Dyspnea has occurred in about 5–10% of patients receiving flecainide. Malaise, fever, and increased sweating have occurred in about 1–3% of patients receiving the drug. Decreased libido, impotence, polyuria, urinary retention, arthralgia, myalgia, bronchospasm, and swelling of the lips, tongue, and mouth have been reported in less than 1% of patients.

There have been rare reports of asymptomatic, isolated increases in serum alkaline phosphatase or aminotransferase concentrations in patients receiving long-term flecainide therapy; however, a causal relationship to the drug has not been established. There have also been rare reports of hepatic dysfunction, including cholestasis and hepatic failure, and extremely rare reports of blood dyscrasias (leukopenia, thrombocytopenia) in patients receiving flecainide, but these effects have not been directly attributed to the drug. (See Cautions: Precautions and Contraindications.) However, in one patient who developed granulocytopenia, there was evidence of a specific IgG antibody directed against a flecainide (hapten)-neutrophil complex.

● Precautions and Contraindications

Findings from the CAST study indicate that use of flecainide and other class I antiarrhythmic agents (e.g., disopyramide, quinidine, procainamide) may be associated with substantial risk in certain patients with ventricular arrhythmias. Therefore, the manufacturer, FDA, and some experts currently recommend that use of flecainide and other class I agents in patients with ventricular arrhythmias be limited to those with *life-threatening* arrhythmias. (See Uses.) Use in less severe ventricular arrhythmias, even when symptomatic, currently is not recommended. In addition, it has been recommended that use of these drugs in patients with supraventricular arrhythmias be limited to those with symptomatic disabling arrhythmias. It is essential that patients not alter their antiarrhythmic therapy without first consulting their physician. The decision to discontinue therapy with flecainide must be made by the physician, and physicians have been advised by

FDA and the manufacturers to contact their patients receiving the drug and determine whether alternative therapy is indicated, reserving therapy with flecainide only for arrhythmias considered *life-threatening*. Some experts state that discontinuance of therapy in patients with symptomatic sustained ventricular arrhythmias that have been treated effectively for prolonged periods seems unwarranted and is potentially dangerous. However, if withdrawal of therapy with flecainide is contemplated in these or other patients with sustained arrhythmias, it is recommended that it be performed in a hospital setting under continuous ECG monitoring. It also has been suggested that the need for hospitalization and ECG monitoring be considered when withdrawing therapy with these drugs in patients with nonsustained arrhythmias.

Since flecainide, like other antiarrhythmic agents, can worsen existing arrhythmias or cause new arrhythmias in some patients, clinical and ECG evaluations are essential prior to and during flecainide therapy to monitor for the appearance of arrhythmias and to determine the need for continued therapy. To minimize the risk of arrhythmogenic effects, the recommended flecainide dosage schedule should be closely followed, plasma drug concentrations should be monitored and concentrations higher than 1 mcg/mL avoided, ECG monitoring should be carefully evaluated before each dosage adjustment, and, if possible, concomitant use of other antiarrhythmic agents should be avoided. If flecainide is suspected or determined to be causing an increased frequency of PVCs despite adequate dosage or to be causing an increased frequency of complex PVCs or new and/or more serious arrhythmias, alternative therapy should be substituted. There is some evidence that exercise (e.g., treadmill) testing may be useful for detecting arrhythmogenic potential in some patients (e.g., those with preexisting sustained or nonsustained ventricular tachycardia and/or ventricular dysfunction), but additional study and experience are necessary.

Because of the relatively high incidence of arrhythmogenic effects in patients with sustained ventricular tachycardia and serious underlying heart disease and the need for careful dosage titration and monitoring, flecainide therapy should be initiated in a hospital setting with ECG monitoring in patients with sustained ventricular tachycardia, regardless of their cardiac status. Initiation of flecainide therapy in a hospital setting should also be considered for other patients with underlying structural heart disease, particularly those with serious disease, and for patients transferring from therapy with another antiarrhythmic agent in whom discontinuance of the current antiarrhythmic agent is likely to result in life-threatening arrhythmias. In patients with less severe and/or stable ventricular arrhythmias (frequent PVCs, nonsustained ventricular tachycardia), flecainide therapy may be initiated in an ambulatory setting with careful clinical and ECG monitoring.

Because of flecainide's mild to moderate negative inotropic effect, as well as an increased risk of arrhythmogenic effects, the drug should be used with caution in patients with a history of congestive heart failure or myocardial dysfunction, particularly those with advanced failure or dysfunction. Patients with a history of congestive heart failure or myocardial dysfunction who receive flecainide must be carefully monitored, and the recommended initial dosage in these patients should not be exceeded. When feasible, plasma flecainide concentrations should be monitored and dosage adjusted to maintain trough concentrations less than 0.7–1 mcg/mL. Particular attention should be given to maintenance of cardiac function, including optimum management with cardiac glycoside, diuretic, and/or other therapy. If myocardial dysfunction occurs, the patient may be managed with a reduction in flecainide dosage, discontinuance of therapy, or an adjustment in other drug therapy (e.g., diuretics, digoxin).

If the PR interval increases to 300 ms or greater, QRS duration increases to 180 ms or greater, or QT_c interval increases substantially during flecainide therapy, caution is necessary and dosage reduction should be considered. To minimize effects on cardiac conduction, an attempt should be made to manage patients on the lowest possible effective dosage. If second- or third-degree AV block or bifascicular block (right bundle-branch block associated with left hemiblock) occurs during flecainide therapy, the drug should be discontinued unless a temporary or implanted artificial ventricular pacemaker is in place to ensure an adequate ventricular rate.

Because its effects on sinus node function may be marked, flecainide should be used with particular caution in patients with preexisting sinus node dysfunction. Flecainide should be used only with extreme caution, if at all, in patients with sick sinus syndrome (including bradycardia-tachycardia syndrome), since the drug may cause sinus bradycardia, pause, or arrest in such patients.

Flecainide can increase acute and chronic endocardial pacing thresholds and may suppress ventricular escape rhythms; these effects are reversible following discontinuance of the drug. Flecainide should be used with particular caution in patients with permanent artificial pacemakers or temporary pacing electrodes and should not be administered to patients with existing poor thresholds or nonprogrammable artificial pacemakers unless suitable pacing rescue is available. In patients with pacemakers, the pacing threshold should be determined before and 1 week after initiating therapy with the drug and at regular intervals thereafter. Flecainide-induced changes in pacing threshold are generally within the range of multiprogrammable pacemakers and, when such changes occur, doubling of voltage or pulse width is usually sufficient to regain capture.

Since hypokalemia or hyperkalemia may alter the effects of class I antiarrhythmic agents, the possibility of a potassium imbalance should be evaluated and, if present, corrected before administration of flecainide.

Since elimination of flecainide may be impaired, the drug should be used with caution and dosage adjusted carefully in patients with renal impairment, particularly severe impairment. Because the urinary excretion of flecainide can be markedly affected by extremes of urinary pH, the potential effects of dietary regimens (e.g., very alkaline pH in strict vegetarians), disease states or conditions (e.g., renal tubular acidosis or metabolic alkalosis or acidosis), or concomitant drugs that may affect urinary pH should be kept in mind. Since flecainide is extensively metabolized, probably in the liver, elimination may be markedly prolonged in patients with substantial hepatic impairment, and therefore the drug should not be used in such patients unless the potential benefits are considered to clearly outweigh the risks. If flecainide is used in patients with severe renal or hepatic impairment, periodic monitoring of plasma concentrations of the drug is necessary.

Flecainide therapy should be discontinued in patients who develop unexplained jaundice, signs of hepatic dysfunction, or a blood dyscrasia to rule out the drug as a possible cause.

Use of flecainide in chronic atrial fibrillation is not recommended. Flecainide should not be used in patients with recent MI. In the absence of a pacemaker, flecainide is contraindicated in patients with preexisting second- or third-degree AV block or bifascicular block (right bundle-branch block associated with left hemiblock). Flecainide also is contraindicated in patients with cardiogenic shock or known hypersensitivity to the drug.

● *Pediatric Precautions*

The manufacturer states that safety and efficacy of flecainide in infants or children have not been established in randomized controlled studies. Limited data suggest that the drug may be useful in children for the management of refractory supraventricular tachycardias. The proarrhythmic effects of flecainide observed in adults also may occur in children. In pediatric patients with structural heart disease, flecainide has been associated with cardiac arrest and sudden death. Because of these risks, flecainide generally is not a preferred antiarrhythmic drug in pediatric patients; if use is necessary, therapy should be initiated in a hospital setting equipped with ECG monitoring and supervised directly by a cardiologist experienced in the treatment of arrhythmias in children.

● *Pregnancy, Fertility, and Lactation*

Pregnancy

Reproduction studies in rats and mice using oral flecainide acetate dosages up to 50 and 80 mg/kg daily, respectively, have not revealed evidence of fetal malformation; however, delayed sternebral and vertebral ossification were observed in rats receiving the highest dosages. Club paws, sternebral and vertebral abnormalities, pale hearts with contracted ventricular septum, and increased fetal resorptions were observed in one breed of rabbits (New Zealand white rabbits) receiving dosages of 30 and 35 mg/kg daily; reproduction studies in Dutch Belted rabbits using similar dosages did not reveal evidence of teratogenicity or embryotoxicity. There are no adequate and controlled studies to date using oral flecainide acetate in pregnant women, and the drug should be used during pregnancy only when the potential benefits justify the possible risks to the fetus. It is not known whether use of the drug during labor or delivery could have any immediate or delayed adverse effects on the mother or fetus, affect the duration of labor, or increase the likelihood of forceps delivery or other obstetrical intervention.

Fertility

The effect of flecainide on fertility in humans is not known. In vitro, the drug inhibits sperm motility. Reproduction studies in male and female rats using flecainide acetate dosages up to 50 mg/kg daily (7 times the usual human dosage) have not revealed evidence of impaired fertility.

Lactation

Limited data suggest that flecainide is distributed into milk in humans. In one study in postpartum women receiving multiple doses of flecainide, milk flecainide concentration averaged 2.5 times (sometimes as high as 4 times) that of maternal plasma concentrations. It is estimated that less than 3 mg of the drug would be ingested by a nursing infant (receiving about 700 mL of milk) over a 24-hour period assuming a maternal plasma flecainide concentration of 1 mcg/mL, which is considered at the top of the therapeutic range.

DRUG INTERACTIONS

● Drugs Affecting or Metabolized by Hepatic Microsomal Enzymes

Metabolism of flecainide is mediated by the cytochrome P-450 (CYP) isoenzyme 2D6, and concurrent use of flecainide with CYP2D6 inhibitors (e.g., quinidine) could result in increased plasma flecainide concentrations.

Limited data indicate that the rate of flecainide elimination is increased by 30% in patients receiving flecainide concurrently with enzyme inducers (e.g., carbamazepine, phenytoin, phenobarbital).

● Protein-bound Drugs

Flecainide is not extensively bound to plasma proteins. Concomitant use of flecainide with other drugs that are highly protein-bound (e.g., oral anticoagulants) is not expected to result in an interaction.

● Antiarrhythmic Agents

There is limited information on the use of flecainide in conjunction with other antiarrhythmic agents for the management of severe refractory ventricular or supraventricular† arrhythmias. Combination antiarrhythmic therapy for severe refractory arrhythmias is generally empiric and must be individualized. Since the cardiac effects of multiple antiarrhythmic agents may be additive, synergistic, or antagonistic and adverse effects may be additive, combination therapy must be used with particular caution and careful monitoring. Because concomitant administration may increase the risk of arrhythmogenic effects, it is generally recommended that concomitant use of flecainide with other antiarrhythmic agents be avoided, if possible; however, combination therapy may be useful in carefully selected and managed patients with severe refractory arrhythmias. When transitioning from another antiarrhythmic drug to flecainide, sufficient time should elapse (at least 2–4 half-lives of the discontinued antiarrhythmic agent) before initiating flecainide therapy. (See Dosage and Administration: Dosage.)

Flecainide has been used in combination with amiodarone, with good results in selected patients, for the management of severe refractory ventricular arrhythmias or refractory atrial fibrillation†. Combined therapy may allow the use of lower dosages of flecainide and/or amiodarone and thereby potentially reduce the risk of toxicity. Plasma flecainide concentrations adjusted for daily dosage increased by an average of 60% (range: 5–190%) when amiodarone therapy was initiated in a limited number of patients receiving flecainide. Although the mechanism(s) of this interaction is not known, it has been suggested that amiodarone may inhibit the hepatic metabolism and/or decrease the renal clearance of flecainide. Pending further accumulation of data, it is recommended that dosage of flecainide be reduced by 30–50% several days after initiation of amiodarone therapy; subsequently, the patient and plasma flecainide concentrations should be monitored closely and flecainide dosage adjusted as necessary.

The effects of concomitant administration of flecainide and disopyramide have not been evaluated and experience with combined use of the drugs is limited. Because both drugs have negative inotropic effects, there appears to be little rationale for their combined use and the manufacturer cautions that they not be used concomitantly unless the potential benefits are considered to outweigh the risks.

● Cardiac Glycosides

Studies in healthy individuals indicate that plasma digoxin concentrations may be increased by an average of about 13–25% when flecainide and digoxin are administered concomitantly. The increase in plasma digoxin concentration may occur within a few days of initiating flecainide therapy in patients receiving digoxin and may result from a decrease in the volume of distribution of digoxin. Although the

PR interval was substantially prolonged in most healthy individuals during concomitant administration of flecainide and digoxin, it was not determined whether this resulted from an additive effect of the drugs or mainly from flecainide. Flecainide has been administered concomitantly with cardiac glycosides without adverse effects. Additional studies to determine the potential importance of an interaction in patients with congestive heart failure are needed. Flecainide-induced increases in plasma digoxin concentration generally appear to be of a small magnitude and are unlikely to be clinically important in most cases; however, patients with AV nodal dysfunction, plasma digoxin concentrations in the upper end of the therapeutic range, and/or high plasma flecainide concentrations may be at increased risk of digoxin toxicity. Pending further accumulation of data, patients receiving flecainide and digoxin should be monitored for signs of digoxin toxicity.

● β-Adrenergic Blocking Agents

In healthy individuals, plasma flecainide concentrations are increased by about 20% and plasma propranolol concentrations are increased by about 30% when the drugs are administered concomitantly compared with administration of each drug alone. The mechanism(s) of this interaction is not known, but the elimination half-lives of both drugs are apparently unchanged. The negative inotropic effects of flecainide and propranolol are additive in healthy individuals, but the increases in PR interval produced by the drugs are less than additive. Flecainide has been administered concomitantly with β-adrenergic blocking agents in patients with ventricular arrhythmias without unusual adverse effects or an increased incidence of adverse effects; however, if flecainide and a β-adrenergic blocking agent are administered concomitantly, the possibility of additive negative inotropic effects should be considered.

● Calcium-Channel Blocking Agents

The effects of concomitant administration of flecainide and calcium-channel blocking agents have not been evaluated, and experience with combined use of the drugs is limited. Because verapamil also has a negative inotropic effect and decreases AV nodal conduction, the manufacturer cautions that flecainide and verapamil not be used concomitantly unless the potential benefits are considered to outweigh the risk. The manufacturer also cautions that there is insufficient experience with concomitant administration of flecainide and diltiazem or nifedipine to recommend such combined use.

● Acidifying and Alkalinizing Agents

The urinary excretion and systemic elimination of flecainide may be substantially affected by extremes of urinary pH, with urinary excretion of the drug decreased and elimination half-life increased in the presence of very alkaline urine and vice versa in the presence of very acidic urine. (See Pharmacokinetics: Elimination.) When drugs that can markedly affect urinary acidity (e.g., ammonium chloride) or alkalinity (e.g., high-dose antacids, carbonic anhydrase inhibitors, sodium bicarbonate) are administered concomitantly with flecainide, the potential effect on elimination of the antiarrhythmic agent and need for appropriate flecainide dosage adjustment should be kept in mind.

● Diuretics

Flecainide has been used concomitantly with diuretics in a large number of patients without any apparent drug interaction.

● Cimetidine

Plasma flecainide concentrations and half-life reportedly increased by approximately 30 and 10%, respectively, in a study in healthy individuals receiving flecainide in conjunction with cimetidine (1 g daily for 1 week). Further study of this potential interaction is needed, but these data suggest that reduction of flecainide dosage might be necessary in patients receiving cimetidine concomitantly.

ACUTE TOXICITY

Limited information is available on the acute toxicity of flecainide.

● Pathogenesis

The acute lethal dose of flecainide acetate in humans is not known. The oral and IV LD_{50}s of the drug in mice were 190 and 24 mg/kg, respectively. Following IV, intraperitoneal, or oral administration of single large doses of flecainide acetate (up to 500 mg/kg) in animals, vomiting, ataxia, dyspnea, seizures, and death were observed; death appeared to result from respiratory depression and arrest. Surviving animals recovered within several hours after administration of flecainide with no apparent residual effects.

● Manifestations

In general, overdosage of flecainide may be expected to produce effects that are extensions of pharmacologic effects, particularly those involving cardiac conduction and function. Animal studies and case reports in humans indicate that possible effects may include increases in PR, QRS, and QT intervals; conduction disturbances; hypotension; asystole; or cardiac arrest and death. In one adult who reportedly intentionally ingested 2.5 g of flecainide acetate, somnolence, tremor, and sweating resulted. Plasma flecainide concentrations 3 and 4.5 hours after ingestion of the drug were 1.9 and 3 mcg/mL, respectively, with an AV nodal escape rhythm and substantial prolongation of QRS and QT intervals occurring in association with the higher of these concentrations. The patient recovered following symptomatic and supportive treatment, as well as the use of charcoal hemoperfusion and forced diuresis to enhance elimination of the drug. Other ECG abnormalities associated with flecainide intoxication have included regular ventricular tachycardia with right bundle-branch block that progressed to polymorphous tachycardia (possibly torsades de pointes); substantial prolongation of the PR and JT intervals; broadened P waves; and inverted T waves. Regular or polymorphous ventricular tachycardia may progress to ventricular fibrillation and sudden death.

● Treatment

Treatment of flecainide overdosage generally involves symptomatic and supportive care, with ECG, blood pressure, and respiratory monitoring. There is no specific antidote for flecainide intoxication.

Supportive treatment may include IV administration of inotropic agents or cardiac stimulants (e.g., dopamine, dobutamine, isoproterenol), circulatory assistance (e.g., intra-aortic balloon counterpulsation), mechanically assisted respiration, and transvenous pacing. Because of the long elimination half-life of flecainide and the possibility of markedly nonlinear pharmacokinetics at very high doses, treatment for an extended period of time may be necessary. Hemodialysis is not an effective means for enhancing elimination of flecainide. Specific data are not available, but acidification of the urine may be potentially useful for enhancing elimination of flecainide, particularly if the urine is very alkaline; however, the potential effects of acidification on serum electrolyte concentrations (e.g., potassium) would have to be considered. The value of forced diuresis is not known.

PHARMACOLOGY

● Antiarrhythmic and Electrophysiologic Effects

Flecainide acetate is a local anesthetic-type antiarrhythmic agent. Studies in animals have shown that flecainide is at least as effective and more potent on a weight basis than most currently available antiarrhythmic agents in preventing and/or suppressing experimentally induced arrhythmias.

The exact mechanism of antiarrhythmic action of flecainide has not been conclusively determined, but the drug is considered a class I (membrane-stabilizing) antiarrhythmic agent. The principal effect of flecainide on cardiac tissue appears to be a concentration-dependent inhibition of the transmembrane influx of extracellular sodium ions via fast sodium channels, as indicated by a decrease in the maximal rate of depolarization of phase 0 of the action potential and a shift of the membrane-responsiveness curve in the hyperpolarizing direction. Like other class I antiarrhythmic agents, flecainide is believed to combine with fast sodium channels in their inactive state and thereby inhibit recovery after repolarization in a time- and voltage-dependent manner which is associated with subsequent dissociation of the drug from the sodium channels. Flecainide also appears to have a slight inhibitory effect on the transmembrane influx of extracellular calcium ions via slow calcium channels, but generally only at high drug concentrations. Flecainide has no vagomimetic, vagolytic, or β-adrenergic blocking activity and does not antagonize the positive inotropic effect of calcium on cardiac muscle.

Flecainide exhibits electrophysiologic effects characteristic of class Ic antiarrhythmic agents. The electrophysiologic characteristics of the subgroups of class I antiarrhythmic agents may be related to quantitative differences in their rates of attachment to and dissociation from transmembrane sodium channels,

with class Ic agents exhibiting slow rates of attachment and dissociation. Flecainide decreases the amplitude and maximal rate of rise of the action potential in a concentration-dependent manner and has little or no effect on resting potential. Like other class Ic antiarrhythmic agents, flecainide slows intracardiac conduction at low concentrations, has relatively small effects on refractoriness, and generally has little effect on repolarization and action potential duration (APD). The drug produces a slight increase in APD in atrial and ventricular muscle and a decrease in APD in Purkinje fibers. The electrophysiologic effects of flecainide generally appear to be comparable following multiple oral or single IV doses of the drug.

Effects on Cardiac Conduction and Refractoriness

Flecainide produces a dose-related decrease in intracardiac conduction throughout the heart, with the most marked effect on conduction within the His-Purkinje system. The effect of the drug on intra-atrial and atrioventricular (AV) conduction is less pronounced than its effect on intraventricular conduction. Flecainide may also prolong refractoriness in most parts of the heart, with the most marked effect on the ventricles; however, the effects of the drug on refractoriness are less pronounced than its effects on intracardiac conduction.

The effects of flecainide on intracardiac conduction are manifested by dose-related increases in PR, QRS, and, to a lesser degree, QT intervals. Increases in PR and QRS intervals average about 25% (40 and 20 ms, respectively) at dosages of 400 mg or more daily but may be as large as approximately 118 and 150%, respectively, in some patients. About 30–40% of patients may develop first-degree AV block during flecainide therapy, and many patients develop a QRS interval of 120 ms or longer; however, PR intervals usually do not increase to 300 ms or longer and QRS intervals usually do not increase to 180 ms or longer. Flecainide generally increases QT interval by about 8%, but about 60–90% of this increase is secondary to the increase in QRS interval. Consequently, the JT interval (QT minus QRS) increases by an average of about 4%. Substantial prolongation of the JT interval occurs in less than 2% of patients. The QT interval corrected for rate (QT$_c$) may be unchanged or slightly increased. AH and HV intervals are prolonged. The atrial effective refractory period (ERP) may be unchanged or slightly increased, and ventricular ERP may be increased by about 5–15%. The AV nodal ERP may be unchanged or slightly increased.

Effects on Sinus Node

Flecainide generally has minimal effects on normal sinus node function. Spontaneous sinus rate may be unchanged or decreased, and corrected sinus node recovery time following pacing and spontaneous cycle lengths is somewhat increased. Sinoatrial conduction time may be slightly increased. In contrast to its effects on normal sinus node function, flecainide may have a marked depressive effect on sinus node function in individuals with preexisting sinus node dysfunction; corrected sinus node recovery time and sinoatrial conduction time may be substantially increased in some individuals.

Effects on Dual AV Nodal and Anomalous AV Pathways

The relatively selective effects of flecainide on retrograde pathways of dual AV nodal and anomalous AV conduction are responsible for the drug's ability to effectively terminate paroxysmal reentrant supraventricular tachycardias in many patients. In patients with dual AV pathways, flecainide decreases conduction, markedly increases refractoriness of the retrograde fast pathway, and increases or has little effect on refractoriness of the anterograde fast pathway or the anterograde and retrograde slow pathways; complete block of the retrograde fast pathway and, rarely, the anterograde fast pathway may result. In patients with Wolff-Parkinson-White syndrome or concealed accessory AV pathways, flecainide decreases conduction and increases the refractoriness of anterograde and retrograde accessory pathways, with the effects more pronounced on the retrograde pathway. In addition, the effects of flecainide may be greater on accessory pathways that have a long pretreatment refractory period. Complete block of the retrograde pathway and, sometimes, the anterograde pathway may result.

Effects on Endocardial Pacing Threshold

Flecainide can increase acute and chronic endocardial pacing thresholds and may suppress ventricular escape rhythms; these effects are reversible following discontinuance of the drug. (See Cautions: Precautions and Contraindications.) Increases in endocardial pacing threshold as large as 200% have occurred. Flecainide-induced increases in endocardial pacing threshold appear to be correlated with plasma concentrations of the drug. Flecainide appears to have a greater effect on endocardial pacing threshold than most other class I antiarrhythmic agents.

● Arrhythmogenic Effects

Like other antiarrhythmic agents, flecainide can worsen existing arrhythmias or cause new arrhythmias. (See Cautions: Arrhythmogenic Effects.) The arrhythmogenic effects of the drug may range from an increased frequency of premature ventricular complexes (PVCs) to the development of more severe and potentially fatal ventricular tachyarrhythmias. The exact mechanism(s) by which various antiarrhythmic agents, including flecainide, produce arrhythmogenic effects has not been fully determined, but the arrhythmogenic potential of flecainide may be related to its effects on conduction and possibly myocardial contractility.

● Cardiovascular Effects

Flecainide generally exhibits minimal cardiovascular effects following oral or IV administration. The cardiovascular effects of the drug appear to be more pronounced following IV than oral administration, but evaluations have been more extensive following IV administration.

Flecainide exhibits a mild to moderate negative inotropic effect. The negative inotropic effect and other cardiovascular effects may be more pronounced and clinically important in patients with coronary heart disease, acute myocardial infarction (MI), congestive heart failure, or myocardial dysfunction. (See Cautions: Cardiovascular Effects.) The exact mechanism of flecainide's negative inotropic effect has not been determined, but it may be related in part to its effect on slow calcium channels. The myocardial depressant effect of flecainide appears to be less than that of disopyramide, but further evaluation is needed.

Heart rate is usually unchanged following oral or IV administration of flecainide, but slight increases may occur; occasionally, bradycardia or tachycardia has been reported. Similarly, blood pressure is usually unchanged following oral or IV administration of the drug, but small increases in mean systolic and/or diastolic blood pressure have been observed.

Following IV administration of flecainide in patients with coronary heart disease, acute MI, congestive heart failure, or myocardial dysfunction, cardiac output and left ventricular ejection fraction are generally decreased, pulmonary artery and/or wedge pressures are generally increased, and systemic vascular resistance may be unchanged or increased. The negative inotropic and other cardiovascular effects of IV flecainide are generally transient, being most marked during and immediately following administration of the drug, and are generally more pronounced in patients with preexisting ventricular dysfunction. Following chronic oral administration of flecainide, left ventricular ejection fraction generally appears to be unchanged or only slightly decreased, although both increases and decreases have been observed in patients receiving usual dosages of the drug. The drug can worsen or cause congestive heart failure, particularly in patients with a history of congestive heart failure and/or a preexisting ejection fraction of 30% or less. (See Cautions: Cardiovascular Effects.)

● Other Effects

Flecainide exhibits a local anesthetic action that is more potent and sustained than that of procaine (no longer commercially available in the US) in vitro. In animals, flecainide also exhibits anticonvulsant activity at doses higher than those required for antiarrhythmic action.

PHARMACOKINETICS

● Absorption

Flecainide acetate is rapidly and almost completely absorbed from the GI tract following oral administration. The absolute bioavailability of the commercially available flecainide acetate tablets averages approximately 85–90%. The rate of absorption may be slightly decreased by the presence of food, but the extent of absorption is not affected. The rate and extent of absorption are not affected by concomitant ingestion of an aluminum hydroxide antacid. Flecainide does not undergo any substantial first-pass metabolism.

Peak plasma flecainide concentrations usually occur within approximately 3 hours (range: 1–6 hours) after oral administration. Following oral administration of a single 200-mg dose of flecainide acetate in fasting, healthy adults, peak plasma flecainide concentrations of approximately 0.19–0.34 mcg/mL are attained. The pharmacokinetic profile of flecainide is apparently not substantially affected by dose or plasma concentrations at usual dosages, but does deviate somewhat from linearity. Within the usual dosage range, plasma concentrations

of the drug are approximately proportional to dosage, with average concentrations increasing from direct proportionality by about 10–15% per 100-mg increment in dosage. Although plasma flecainide concentrations are relatively linearly related and approximately proportional to dosage, there is considerable interindividual and intraindividual variation in plasma concentrations attained with a given dosage. Following single oral doses, total plasma concentrations of flecainide metabolites (free and conjugated) are generally 1–2 times higher than those of unchanged flecainide; however, free plasma concentrations of the 2 major metabolites, m-O-dealkylated flecainide and the m-O-dealkylated lactam derivative, are very low (less than 0.05 mcg/mL), even after multiple dosing. (See Pharmacokinetics: Elimination.)

In patients with premature ventricular complexes (PVCs), flecainide-induced decreases in single and multiple PVCs are related to dosage and plasma concentrations of the drug. The dose-related increases in PR, QRS, and, to a lesser degree, QT intervals also appear to be related to plasma concentrations of the drug. Based on greater than 90% suppression of PVCs, plasma flecainide concentrations of approximately 0.2–1 mcg/mL (mean of about 0.5–0.6 mcg/mL) appear to be necessary for optimum therapeutic effect, with minimum therapeutic concentrations ranging from about 0.2–0.4 mcg/mL. Plasma flecainide concentrations necessary to suppress serious ventricular arrhythmias are not clearly established, but trough plasma concentrations of the drug in patients effectively treated for recurrent ventricular tachycardia have also ranged from about 0.2–1 mcg/mL. The risk of adverse cardiac effects (e.g., conduction defects, bradycardia) increases as plasma flecainide concentrations increase above 0.7–1 mcg/mL, particularly when concentrations exceed 1 mcg/mL. A relationship between plasma flecainide concentrations and arrhythmogenic effects has not been established, but some data suggest that adverse cardiac effects may be associated with plasma concentrations higher than 1 mcg/mL. In clinical studies of patients with ventricular tachycardia, reduction of flecainide dosage (i.e., use of a lower initial dosage with slow upward titration) appeared to be associated with a decreased frequency and severity of arrhythmogenic effects.

● Distribution

Distribution of flecainide acetate into human body tissues and fluids has not been fully characterized. Following IV administration in rats, flecainide and/or its metabolites are distributed extensively into many tissues, including the heart, but only minimally into the CNS. Studies in animals also indicate that the drug and/or its metabolites are distributed into and may accumulate in pigmented ocular tissues; however, chronic toxicity studies in animals and clinical experience to date in humans have not revealed evidence of specific flecainide-induced ocular toxicity. Following IV administration in humans, flecainide is rapidly and apparently widely distributed. The apparent volume of distribution of the drug in healthy adults reportedly averages 5.5–8.7 L/kg (range: 5–13.4 L/kg) following a single IV dose and about 10 L/kg following a single oral dose.

In vitro, flecainide is approximately 40–50% bound to plasma proteins, mainly α_1-acid glycoprotein (α_1-AGP). At in vitro plasma flecainide concentrations of 0.015–10 mcg/mL, binding is independent of the plasma concentration of the drug. Following acute myocardial infarction, protein binding of flecainide may be increased to an average of approximately 60% for about 24 hours, but this effect is not likely to be clinically important in most circumstances.

It is not known whether flecainide crosses the placenta in humans, but the drug and/or its metabolites cross the placenta in rats. A multiple-dose study conducted in mothers soon after delivery indicated that flecainide is distributed into human milk in concentrations as high as 4 times (with average concentrations about 2.5 times) corresponding plasma concentrations; assuming a high maternal plasma concentration of 1 mcg/mL, the calculated daily dose to a nursing infant (assuming about 700 mL of breast milk over 24 hours) would be less than 3 mg.

● Elimination

Plasma concentrations of flecainide acetate appear to decline in a biphasic manner. Following a single IV dose in healthy adults, the half-life of flecainide in the initial distribution phase ($t_{1/2\alpha}$) is about 3–6 minutes and the half-life in the terminal elimination phase ($t_{1/2\beta}$) has been reported to average 11–14 hours (range: 7–19 hours). Following single or multiple oral doses in healthy adults, the elimination half-life has averaged 11.5–16 hours (range: 7–25 hours), but the half-life tends to be slightly more prolonged following multiple rather than single doses. The elimination half-life of flecainide following multiple oral doses in patients with PVCs is slightly longer than in healthy individuals, averaging 19–22 hours (range: 12–30 hours). The elimination half-life tends to increase with age in patients with PVCs. Although data are limited in infants younger than 1 year of age, currently available data suggest that half-life of flecainide at birth may be as long as 29 hours, decreasing to 11–12 hours by 3 months of age, and to 6 hours by 1 year of age. In children 1–12 years of age, the half-life of flecainide is approximately 8 hours. In adolescents 12–15 years of age, the plasma elimination half-life is approximately 11–12 hours. Following a single oral dose in patients with congestive heart failure, the elimination half-life is also slightly longer than in healthy individuals but similar to that in patients with PVCs, averaging 19 hours (range: 14–26 hours). Steady-state plasma concentrations are reached in 3–5 days; once at steady state, no additional accumulation of drug is expected during chronic therapy. Over the usual therapeutic range, plasma concentrations of flecainide increase in an approximately dose-proportional manner.

The elimination half-life of flecainide is prolonged in patients with renal impairment, particularly in those with severe renal impairment. Following a single oral dose, the elimination half-life reportedly averaged 17 hours (range: 12–26 hours) and 26 hours (range: 9–58 hours) in patients with creatinine clearances of 4–41 and 0–2 mL/minute per m², respectively. The elimination half-lives of flecainide metabolites have not been determined to date, but their elimination appears to occur somewhat more slowly than that of unchanged flecainide and free plasma concentrations of m-O-dealkylated flecainide appear to persist in some patients with severe renal impairment. Extremes of urinary pH can markedly affect the elimination half-life of flecainide, prolonging it when very alkaline (pH 7.2–8.3) and reducing it when very acidic (pH 4.4–5.8).

Flecainide is extensively metabolized, probably in the liver, to 2 major metabolites and to at least 3 unidentified minor metabolites. In vitro metabolic studies indicate that the cytochrome P-450 (CYP) isoenzyme 2D6 is involved in the drug's metabolism. The 2 major metabolites, m-O-dealkylated flecainide and the m-O-dealkylated lactam derivative, are formed by preferential O-dealkylation at the *meta* position of the benzamide ring and by subsequent oxidation of the piperidine ring of m-O-dealkylated flecainide, respectively. Both metabolites undergo extensive conjugation at the m-O-dealkylated position with glucuronic or sulfuric acid. Studies in animals indicate that, on a weight basis, m-O-dealkylated flecainide has up to 20–50% of the antiarrhythmic and electrophysiologic activity of flecainide and the m-O-dealkylated lactam derivative has less than 10% of the electrophysiologic activity of flecainide. Because free plasma concentrations of the major metabolites are so low following multiple oral doses, it is unlikely that these metabolites would contribute to the therapeutic or toxic effects of the parent drug under most clinical circumstances; however, further studies are needed to evaluate their potential contribution, if any, in the presence of conditions that might affect their formation and/or elimination (e.g., severe hepatic or renal impairment). The minor metabolites remain to be identified, but some data suggest that they may result from amide hydrolysis. Some data also suggest that cigarette smoking may induce metabolism of flecainide.

Following oral administration, flecainide and its metabolites are excreted almost completely in urine; only small amounts of the drug and/or its metabolites are excreted in feces. Flecainide appears to be excreted in urine mainly by glomerular filtration, but some tubular secretion may also occur. Following a single oral dose of flecainide in healthy individuals, about 80–90% of the dose is excreted in urine and about 5% in feces within 6 days; most excretion occurs within 24 hours, and excretion is almost complete within 72 hours. In healthy individuals, about 30% (range: 10–50%) of a single oral dose is excreted in urine as unchanged drug, 10–20% as m-O-dealkylated flecainide and its conjugates, 10–15% as the m-O-dealkylated lactam derivative and its conjugates, and 3% or less as 3 unidentified minor metabolites. The major metabolites of the drug are excreted in urine principally as conjugates.

The fraction of flecainide excreted in urine as unchanged drug decreases with decreasing renal function and is markedly reduced in patients with severe renal impairment. Following a single oral dose in patients with creatinine clearances of 4–41 and 0–2 mL/minute per m², the fraction excreted in urine within 72 hours as unchanged drug averaged approximately 15% (range: 5–30%) and 1% (range: 0–3%), respectively. The fraction of flecainide excreted in urine as unchanged drug is also inversely related to urinary pH, increasing with decreasing urinary pH and vice versa. Although usual variations in urinary pH would generally be expected to have minimal effects, extremes of urinary pH may substantially affect the fraction of unchanged flecainide excreted in urine, approximately

doubling it when very acidic (pH 4.4–5.8) and decreasing it by half when very alkaline (pH 7.2–8.3).

Following oral administration in healthy individuals, total apparent plasma clearance of flecainide averages approximately 10 mL/minute per kg (range: 4–20 mL/minute per kg); renal clearance of the drug is about 25–40% of the total plasma clearance. In healthy geriatric individuals, total apparent plasma clearance decreases following multiple oral doses, apparently as a result of decreased nonrenal clearance of the drug. Total apparent plasma clearance is decreased in patients with PVCs compared with healthy individuals, averaging 6.2 mL/minute per kg (range: 3.1–12.6 mL/minute per kg) in a small group of patients. Total apparent plasma clearance of flecainide is somewhat decreased in patients with congestive heart failure compared with healthy individuals, averaging 8.1 mL/minute per kg (range: 3.1–13.4 mL/minute per kg) in a small group of patients; renal clearance is also decreased in these patients, but still accounts for about 25% of total plasma clearance. It appears that an increase in nonrenal clearance can, to some extent, compensate for decreased renal clearance in some patients. Renal clearance of flecainide is inversely related to urinary pH, increasing with decreasing urinary pH and vice versa. Extremes of urinary pH may substantially affect renal clearance of the drug. The manufacturer states that elimination of flecainide from plasma may be markedly prolonged in patients with substantial hepatic impairment.

Only about 1% of an oral dose of flecainide is removed by hemodialysis as unchanged drug; however, about 10% of a dose is removed by hemodialysis as m-O-dealkylated flecainide and its conjugates. It is not known if flecainide and/or its metabolites are removed by peritoneal dialysis. There is some evidence that flecainide may be removed by charcoal hemoperfusion.

CHEMISTRY AND STABILITY

● *Chemistry*

Flecainide acetate is a local anesthetic-type antiarrhythmic agent. Flecainide is an amide-type local anesthetic and is structurally related to procainamide in that the drug is a benzamide derivative. The antiarrhythmic potency of flecainide is associated with the presence and positions of the trifluoroethoxy groups on the benzamide ring, which enhance lipophilicity, and with the presence of the nonsubstituted piperidylmethyl group in the amide side chain.

Flecainide acetate occurs as a white to slightly off-white crystalline powder and has a solubility of 48.4 mg/mL in water and 300 mg/mL in alcohol at 37°C. The drug has a pK$_a$ of 9.3.

● *Stability*

Flecainide acetate tablets should be stored in tight, light-resistant containers at 20–25°C. However, USP states that the tablets can be stored in well-closed containers.

PREPARATIONS

Excipients in commercially available drug preparations may have clinically important effects in some individuals; consult specific product labeling for details.

Flecainide Acetate

Oral		
Tablets	50 mg*	Flecainide Acetate Tablets
	100 mg*	Flecainide Acetate Tablets
	150 mg*	Flecainide Acetate Tablets

* available from one or more manufacturer, distributor, and/or repackager by generic (nonproprietary) name

† Use is not currently included in the labeling approved by the US Food and Drug Administration.

Propafenone Hydrochloride

24:04.04.12 • CLASS Ic ANTIARRHYTHMICS

■ Propafenone hydrochloride is a local anesthetic-type class Ic antiarrhythmic agent. The drug is commercially available as immediate-release tablets and extended-release capsules.

USES

● Supraventricular Tachyarrhythmias

When given as *immediate-release tablets*, propafenone hydrochloride is used to prolong the time to recurrence of symptomatic, disabling paroxysmal supraventricular tachycardia (PSVT) (e.g., atrioventricular [AV] nodal reentrant tachycardia or AV reentrant tachycardia [Wolff-Parkinson-White, WPW, syndrome]) and symptomatic, disabling paroxysmal atrial fibrillation/flutter (PAF) in patients without structural heart disease. While comparative studies are limited, propafenone appears to be comparable to other antiarrhythmic agents (e.g., quinidine, disopyramide, flecainide, procainamide, sotalol) in preventing recurrences of PAF and maintaining sinus rhythm following successful cardioversion of atrial fibrillation.

When given as *extended-release capsules*, propafenone is used to prolong the time to recurrence of symptomatic paroxysmal atrial fibrillation in patients without structural heart disease. The safety and efficacy of propafenone as extended-release capsules have not been established in patients with exclusively PSVT or atrial flutter.

Propafenone also has been used for termination of supraventricular tachycardias; analysis of combined data from controlled and uncontrolled clinical studies in patients receiving oral (immediate-release tablets) or IV (IV dosage form not commercially available in the US) propafenone therapy has demonstrated termination of PAF, PSVT, or tachycardia associated with WPW syndrome in 73, 57, or 45%, respectively, of patients. However, vagal maneuvers, IV adenosine, AV nodal blocking agents (e.g., calcium-channel blocking agents, β-adrenergic blocking agents) and/or synchronized cardioversion are the treatments of choice for acute conversion of PSVT.

The safety and efficacy of propafenone hydrochloride as immediate-release tablets or extended-release capsules have not been established in patients with chronic atrial fibrillation, and the manufacturer states that the drug should not be used to control ventricular rate in patients with atrial fibrillation.

Because of the risk of proarrhythmia, propafenone should not be used in patients with structural heart disease or ischemic heart disease.

Paroxysmal Atrial Fibrillation/Flutter and Paroxysmal Supraventricular Tachyarrhythmias

Immediate-release Propafenone Hydrochloride

Controlled and uncontrolled clinical studies have shown that propafenone (immediate-release tablets) may prevent or delay recurrence of PAF or increase the interval between recurrences of PAF in 39–64% of patients monitored for 6–18 months. Preliminary analysis of combined data from clinical studies indicates that propafenone prevented or delayed recurrence of PAF in 51 or 33% of patients monitored for 1 or 2 years, respectively, and prevented or delayed recurrence of PSVT or AV reentrant tachycardia (WPW syndrome) syndrome in 63 or 83%, respectively, of patients treated during a 10-month period. Long-term therapy with oral propafenone also has been effective in some patients for suppression and prevention of atrial fibrillation refractory to other antiarrhythmic agents. It has been suggested that propafenone may be more effective than flecainide in patients with adrenergically mediated atrial fibrillation or flutter, possibly because of its β-adrenergic blocking activity.

Control of ventricular rate should be the first therapeutic step in most patients with hemodynamically stable, acute atrial fibrillation. The goal of therapy should be a reduction of ventricular rate to less than 80–90 beats/minute and prevention of inappropriately high ventricular rates during activity. The use of propafenone in patients with chronic atrial fibrillation has not been adequately evaluated to date, and the manufacturer states that the drug should not be used to control ventricular rate in patients with atrial fibrillation. However, some experts and clinicians suggest that propafenone may be useful in controlling ventricular response rate

in patients with stable but rapid atrial fibrillation/flutter and ventricular preexcitation via an accessory pathway (e.g., WPW syndrome).

In a randomized, crossover clinical trial of approximately 2–3 months' duration, the median time to arrhythmia recurrence was greater than 98 days in patients with PAF or PSVT receiving propafenone and 8 or 12 days in patients with PAF or PSVT, respectively, receiving placebo. Recurrences of PAF or PSVT were completely prevented in 53 or 47%, respectively, of patients receiving propafenone and in 13 or 16%, respectively, of those receiving placebo. In another randomized, crossover clinical trial of 2–3 months' duration, the median time to arrhythmia recurrence in patients with PAF or PSVT was 62 or 31 days, respectively, with propafenone therapy and 5 or 8 days, respectively, with placebo. Recurrences of PAF or PSVT were completely prevented in 67 or 38%, respectively, of patients receiving propafenone and in 22 or 7%, respectively, of those receiving placebo. Patients enrolled in these 2 trials had a mean age of 57.3 years; 50% of patients were male, and 80% received a daily propafenone hydrochloride dosage of 600 mg. Patients with PSVT or PAF were equally represented in the 2 studies.

Propafenone has been used orally for the long-term management of AV nodal reentrant tachycardia; however, the drug is generally reserved for patients in whom other therapies (e.g., catheter ablation, β-adrenergic blocking agents, diltiazem, verapamil) are ineffective or contraindicated.

In a randomized crossover study, the rate of recurrence of tachycardia with propafenone therapy was approximately one-fifth that with placebo. Propafenone may be particularly effective and may be considered first-line therapy in patients with atrial fibrillation/flutter associated with ventricular preexcitation and WPW syndrome; in these patients, the drug may slow the ventricular rate and possibly restore and maintain normal sinus rhythm. However, in patients with WPW syndrome whose condition is unstable (e.g., those with hypotension or heart failure), immediate cardioversion may be required. In studies in patients with recurrent episodes of supraventricular tachyarrhythmia associated with WPW syndrome, administration of oral propafenone hydrochloride (300–1200 mg daily prevented arrhythmia recurrence in 38–100% of patients during 7–36 months of follow-up). Propafenone therapy also has been effective for arrhythmias associated with WPW syndrome and a short anterograde refractory period of the accessory pathway, although radiofrequency catheter ablation of the accessory pathway may be preferred for the long-term management of this condition.

Based on findings from the Cardiac Arrhythmia Suppression (CAST) study of substantial risk associated with flecainide or encainide therapy in certain patients with ventricular arrhythmias, some experts currently caution that use of class Ic antiarrhythmic agents in supraventricular arrhythmias be limited to the management of symptomatic, disabling supraventricular arrhythmias (paroxysmal atrial fibrillation, AV junctional tachycardias) in patients *without* structural heart disease. However, some clinicians state that even these patients may be at risk of developing drug-induced arrhythmogenic effects (e.g., during exercise testing). The risks versus benefits of propafenone for the management of such arrhythmias in patients *with* structural heart disease remain to be elucidated, and assessment of the possible risks and potential benefits in such patients must be individualized. Current evidence indicates that initiation of antiarrhythmic therapy in patients with atrial fibrillation is associated with a notable risk for adverse cardiac events, particularly in geriatric patients or those with structural heart disease (e.g., heart failure); initiation of antiarrhythmic therapy in such patients should be performed in a hospital setting with ECG monitoring for the initial 24–48 hours. Some clinicians do not recommend the use of antiarrhythmic agents in patients with atrial fibrillation or flutter because increased mortality has been reported in patients receiving antiarrhythmic therapy after conversion of atrial fibrillation to normal sinus rhythm.

Extended-release Propafenone Hydrochloride

The FDA-labeled indication for *extended-release* propafenone hydrochloride in prolonging the time to first recurrence of symptomatic paroxysmal atrial fibrillation is based principally on the results of 2 multicenter, randomized, double-blind, placebo-controlled trials in patients with a history of ECG-documented recurrent episodes of this arrhythmia. Patients had a median duration of paroxysmal atrial fibrillation of 13 months and ECG-documented symptomatic atrial fibrillation within 12 months in one trial, and a median duration of paroxysmal atrial fibrillation of 39.6 months and ECG-documented symptomatic atrial fibrillation within 28 days in the second trial. In the first trial, the median time to first recurrence of atrial fibrillation from day 1 of randomization (primary efficacy variable) was 112, 291, or 41 days in patients receiving extended-release propafenone hydrochloride 225 or 325 mg twice daily or placebo, respectively, for up to 39 weeks. Additional analysis indicated that extended-release propafenone hydrochloride 425 mg twice daily also increased the interval to first recurrence of symptomatic atrial fibrillation. A dose-response relationship was observed with respect to time to first recurrence of ECG-documented symptomatic atrial fibrillation. The time to first recurrence of atrial fibrillation from day 5 of randomization (primary efficacy variable) also was increased in patients receiving extended-release propafenone hydrochloride (325 or 425 mg twice daily) for 91 days in the second trial.

IV† Propafenone Hydrochloride

Propafenone has been administered IV† with some success in the acute treatment of supraventricular reentrant tachycardias. In a randomized, crossover, placebo-controlled study in patients with AV nodal reentrant tachycardia, intraatrial orthodromic reentrant tachycardia, or tachycardia associated with WPW syndrome, conversion to normal sinus rhythm occurred in 75% of patients receiving 1 or 2 rapid IV injections† of propafenone hydrochloride (2 mg/kg) and in no patients receiving placebo. However, an IV dosage form is not commercially available in the US and other therapies (e.g., vagal maneuvers, IV adenosine, calcium-channel blocking agents, β-adrenergic blocking agents, synchronized cardioversion) are recommended for acute conversion of PSVT.

Conversion of Atrial Fibrillation or Flutter to Normal Sinus Rhythm

Propafenone has been used for pharmacologic cardioversion of atrial fibrillation or flutter†. Both oral (immediate-release tablets) and IV propafenone (IV dosage form currently not commercially available in the US) have been effective for conversion of recent-onset atrial fibrillation, including atrial fibrillation occurring after open-heart surgery, to normal sinus rhythm†, and some clinicians suggest that propafenone may be considered first-line therapy for this use. Conversion rates are inversely related to both duration of atrial fibrillation, number of previous drug treatment failures, and degree of atrial enlargement. Some patients with atrial flutter receiving propafenone (immediate-release tablets) may develop 1:1 AV conduction and a rapid ventricular response; therefore, concomitant therapy with drugs that prolong the functional AV refractory period (e.g., cardiac glycoside, β-adrenergic blocking agent) is recommended in such patients.

In acute, hemodynamically stable atrial fibrillation of less than 48 hours' duration, antiarrhythmic drug therapy may result in conversion to sinus rhythm in about 60–90% of patients; however, such therapy is effective in only 15–30% or less of patients with atrial fibrillation of longer duration. Conversion of atrial fibrillation or flutter to normal sinus rhythm may be associated with embolism, particularly when the arrhythmia has been present for more than 48 hours, unless the patient is adequately anticoagulated. (See Uses: Cardioversion of Atrial Fibrillation/Flutter, in Heparin 20:12.04.16.)

Propafenone hydrochloride also has been administered orally (150–600 mg as immediate-release tablets) or IV (2 mg/kg over 10 minutes) as a single dose for restoration of sinus rhythm† in patients with infrequent episodes of paroxysmal atrial fibrillation when it is desirable to avoid potential adverse effects of long-term antiarrhythmic drug therapy. Limited data suggest that oral propafenone therapy (immediate-release tablets) initiated 48 hours prior to electrical cardioversion of patients with chronic atrial fibrillation† may decrease the recurrence rate of this arrhythmia without an untoward effect on defibrillation threshold or electrical cardioversion rates.

Self-administration for Conversion of Paroxysmal Atrial Fibrillation

Limited evidence suggests that out-of-hospital *self-administration*† ("pill-in-the-pocket" approach) of a single oral loading dose of propafenone hydrochloride (immediate-release tablets) or flecainide is safe and effective for terminating recent-onset paroxysmal atrial fibrillation† and can reduce hospitalizations and emergency room visits in carefully selected patients who have mild or no heart disease. *In-hospital administration* of propafenone hydrochloride (immediate-release tablets) or flecainide as a single oral dose for terminating acute atrial fibrillation† has been shown to be effective with a low incidence of adverse effects in several randomized, controlled studies; however, the safety of such treatment without initial evaluation in a hospital setting or in patients with substantial structural heart disease has not been established. In addition, additional study and experience are required to assess the possible need for concomitant antithrombotic (e.g., warfarin) therapy and potential for adverse drug interactions (e.g., with warfarin or digoxin) in patients self-administering antiarrhythmic agents for recent-onset paroxysmal atrial fibrillation on an out-of-hospital basis.

In a prospective, uncontrolled study, 268 patients (18–75 years of age) with mild or no heart disease who had hemodynamically well-tolerated atrial fibrillation of recent (less than 48 hours) onset were treated in-hospital (i.e., in the emergency room or cardiology ward) with a single oral dose of propafenone hydrochloride (immediate-release tablets) or flecainide (according to clinician preference) to restore normal sinus rhythm. Patients weighing 70 kg or more received 600 mg of propafenone hydrochloride (immediate-release tablets) or 300 mg of flecainide acetate and those weighing less than 70 kg received 450 mg of propafenone hydrochloride (immediate-release tablets) or 200 mg of flecainide acetate. In-hospital treatment was considered effective if conversion of atrial fibrillation to sinus rhythm occurred within 6 hours of administration of the antiarrhythmic agent without clinically important adverse effects (i.e., symptomatic hypotension, symptomatic bradycardia after restoration of sinus rhythm, dyspnea, presyncope, syncope, conversion to atrial flutter or atrial tachycardia, or episodes of sustained or unsustained ventricular tachycardia). The time to conversion to sinus rhythm following in-hospital treatment with propafenone hydrochloride (immediate-release tablets) or flecainide in these patients averaged 135 minutes (median: 120 minutes). Patients in whom inpatient administration of these antiarrhythmics was effective and who were not excluded during subsequent examination were discharged and given propafenone hydrochloride (immediate-release tablets) or flecainide for treatment of subsequent episodes of palpitations (presumed recurrent atrial fibrillation) on an outpatient basis. These patients were instructed to take a single oral dose of the assigned antiarrhythmic drug 5 minutes after noting the onset of palpitations (self-assessed) and then to assume a resting state (e.g., a supine or sitting position) until resolution of the palpitations or for a period of at least four hours.

Analysis of data from 2 of the study sites indicated that 12% of patients presenting to the emergency room for recent-onset atrial fibrillation were candidates for out-of-hospital treatment with propafenone hydrochloride or flecainide. During a mean follow-up period of 15 months (range: 7–19 months), 79% of patients included in the out-of-hospital phase of the study experienced episodes of palpitations (presumed atrial fibrillation); patients self-administered propafenone hydrochloride (immediate-release tablets) (mean dose: 555 mg) or flecainide acetate (mean dose: 263 mg) within a mean of 36 minutes (median: 10 minutes) after the onset of symptoms in 92% of such episodes. Each antiarrhythmic agent was effective in interrupting 94% of episodes of palpitations (a primary end point); time to resolution of symptoms after drug administration averaged 113 minutes (median: 98 minutes). In patients who had multiple recurrences of palpitations during the follow-up period, self-administration of propafenone or flecainide hydrochloride terminated all such episodes in 84% of patients. Self-administration of oral propafenone (immediate-release tablets) or flecainide also was associated with reductions in emergency room visits and hospital admissions (secondary end points); calls for emergency room intervention during the study averaged 4.9 per month compared with 45.6 per month during the year prior to the study, while the number of hospitalizations averaged 1.6 per month during the study compared with 15 per month during the prior year.

Other Atrial Tachycardias

Propafenone is one of several drugs that may be used for the ongoing management of focal atrial tachycardia† or junctional tachycardia† in patients without structural or ischemic heart disease.

Supraventricular Tachyarrhythmias in Children

Although controlled studies generally are lacking, oral (immediate-release tablets) or IV propafenone (IV dosage form currently not commercially available in the US) has been used successfully for the management of supraventricular tachyarrhythmias (e.g., PSVT, postoperative or congenital junctional ectopic tachycardia, atrial ectopic tachycardia, chaotic atrial tachycardia, atrial fibrillation or flutter) in children†. Oral propafenone (immediate-release tablets) reportedly has been effective in treating refractory atrial flutter in children†; however, experience is limited and the drug cannot currently be recommended as first-line therapy for this use.

● Ventricular Arrhythmias

Propafenone hydrochloride (immediate-release tablets) is used orally to suppress and prevent the recurrence of documented *life-threatening* ventricular arrhythmias (e.g., sustained ventricular tachycardia, ventricular fibrillation). Based on the results of the Cardiac Arrhythmia Suppression Trial (CAST) (see the opening discussion in Cautions in Flecainide Acetate 24:04.04.12), FDA, the manufacturer, and many clinicians recommend that therapy with antiarrhythmic agents, including propafenone, be *reserved* for the suppression and prevention of documented ventricular tachyarrhythmias that, in the clinician's judgment, are considered *life-threatening*.

Because of propafenone's arrhythmogenic potential and the associated risk of death identified with other class Ic antiarrhythmic drugs (encainide, flecainide) in CAST, use of propafenone for less severe ventricular arrhythmias (e.g., asymptomatic ventricular premature complexes† [VPCs]), is *not* recommended. The findings of CAST involved a select patient population with recent myocardial infarction, mild to moderate left ventricular dysfunction (e.g., mean baseline ejection fraction of 40%), and asymptomatic or mildly symptomatic ventricular arrhythmias (mean baseline VPCs of 127/hour as evidenced by ambulatory ECG [Holter] monitoring during at least 18 hours of analyzable time, with about 20% of patients exhibiting at least one run of nonsustained ventricular tachycardia during such monitoring); such patients also had demonstrated drug-induced suppressibility of VPCs during the initial phase of the open trial.

It currently is not known whether the findings of CAST can be extrapolated to other patient populations with non-life-threatening ventricular arrhythmias (e.g., patients with arrhythmias in the absence of ventricular dysfunction, myocardial ischemia, or recent myocardial infarction) or to other antiarrhythmic drugs (e.g., propafenone). CAST principally involved suppression and prevention of VPCs, with only about 10% of patients exhibiting more than a single run of tachycardia at baseline. Some clinicians also question whether the results of CAST even can be extrapolated to patients with recurrent nonsustained ventricular tachycardia and ventricular dysfunction, since these patients are known to be at high risk of sudden death if untreated, and since CAST did not include sufficient numbers of such patients to clearly determine the benefit-to-risk ratio. However, despite the limitations of the CAST findings, the manufacturer, FDA, and other experts consider the potential risks of antiarrhythmic therapy substantial and currently do not recommend use of propafenone in any patient with non-life-threatening ventricular arrhythmias in the absence of substantial evidence of safety and efficacy. They state that it is prudent to consider the risks of class Ic antiarrhythmic agents and current lack of evidence of improved survival *unacceptable* in patients *without* life-threatening ventricular arrhythmias, even in patients experiencing unpleasant but non-life-threatening manifestations. However, some clinicians, while recognizing the strong evidence of risk in the patient population studied in CAST and the substantial limitations of current evidence on safety and efficacy in other patient populations, question such an extreme limitation of usage.

Life-threatening Ventricular Arrhythmias
Monotherapy

The optimum role of propafenone (immediate-release tablets) in the suppression and prevention of ventricular arrhythmias remains to be clearly determined. In addition, it remains to be determined whether antiarrhythmic agents, including propafenone, have a beneficial effect on mortality or sudden death. Although propafenone (immediate-release tablets) has been used for chronic suppression and prevention of ventricular arrhythmias in carefully selected patients, further study is needed to evaluate the long-term efficacy and safety and the relative role of the drug in such patients. Therefore, it is recommended that propafenone (immediate-release tablets) generally be reserved for patients who have an insufficient therapeutic response to, or who do not tolerate, conventional orally administered antiarrhythmic agents (e.g., class IA agents). In addition, because of propafenone's negative inotropic potential, some clinicians would avoid use of the drug as a first-line agent in patients with life-threatening ventricular arrhythmias who also have congestive heart failure and/or substantial ventricular dysfunction (e.g., left ventricular ejection fraction less than 30%). While it currently is not known whether the findings of the CAST study apply to class Ic antiarrhythmic agents other than flecainide and encainide, some experts state that, in the absence of specific evidence of safety and efficacy, other class Ic drugs should be considered to share the risks of flecainide and encainide.

Available data suggest that the efficacy of propafenone (immediate-release tablets) for suppression and prevention of recurrent, life-threatening ventricular arrhythmias is comparable to that of other antiarrhythmic agents (e.g., quinidine, procainamide, disopyramide), with propafenone considered effective in approximately 22–50% of patients. The decision to use propafenone therapy (immediate-release tablets) should be based on an analysis of each patient's risk profile, including consideration of the type and prognosis of the specific arrhythmia, presence of underlying heart disease, degree of ventricular dysfunction, and any other serious comorbidities (e.g., hepatic or renal impairment, conduction abnormalities). Additional studies, including comparative studies with other antiarrhythmic agents, are needed to evaluate the use of propafenone (immediate-release tablets) in the management of life-threatening ventricular arrhythmias.

In a cohort study, oral propafenone hydrochloride (750–900 mg daily) (immediate-release tablets) was effective in rendering arrhythmias noninducible in 26%

of patients with documented sustained ventricular arrhythmias and/or ventricular fibrillation as determined by programmed ventricular stimulation. An analysis of 27 studies in a combined total of 684 patients with malignant ventricular arrhythmias receiving propafenone yielded overall efficacy rates of 61 and 71% as determined by invasive and noninvasive testing methods, respectively. In the invasive method efficacy studies, propafenone therapy (immediate-release tablets) was considered effective in 25% of patients whose arrhythmias became noninducible, 32% of patients whose arrhythmias remained inducible but who developed improved hemodynamic tolerance and prolongation of ventricular tachycardia cycle length (100 msec or greater), and 4% of patients whose inducible sustained ventricular tachycardia was improved to inducible nonsustained ventricular tachycardia. In the noninvasive method efficacy studies, short-term propafenone therapy (1–5 days) (immediate-release tablets) was considered effective in 53–92% (mean: 71%) of patients as determined by the complete elimination of ventricular tachycardia, greater than 90% reduction in frequency of ventricular coupled beats, or greater than 50% reduction in the total number of VPCs compared with baseline arrhythmia frequency. Overall long-term efficacy, defined as the absence of symptomatic recurrence of the baseline arrhythmia, was determined by evaluation of the 90% of patients who had a positive initial response to therapy (measured by invasive or noninvasive efficacy criteria) and who continued propafenone therapy (immediate-release tablets) after hospital discharge. Long-term propafenone therapy (immediate-release tablets) (mean duration of follow-up: 14 months; range: 1–57 months) was considered effective in 67% of patients discharged on the drug and in 36% of the combined total of patients enrolled in the studies.

Combination Therapy

Limited information is available on the use of propafenone (immediate-release tablets) in conjunction with other antiarrhythmic agents for the management of severe, refractory ventricular arrhythmias. In a limited number of patients, propafenone (immediate-release tablets) has been combined with procainamide, quinidine, or mexiletine with good results in selected patients. (See Drug Interactions: Antiarrhythmic Agents.)

Concomitant use of 2 or more antiarrhythmic drugs requires extreme caution and generally is reserved for patients with life-threatening ventricular arrhythmias inadequately controlled by single-agent therapy with propafenone (immediate-release tablets) or another antiarrhythmic agent. Combination antiarrhythmic therapy for severe refractory ventricular arrhythmias generally is empiric and must be individualized.

Other Ventricular Arrhythmias

Controlled and uncontrolled clinical studies in patients with chronic stable ventricular arrhythmias† have shown that propafenone (immediate-release tablets) is highly effective in suppressing and preventing nonsustained ventricular tachycardia and frequent VPCs, including complex VPCs. In short-term clinical studies, propafenone therapy (immediate-release tablets) produced approximately 66–98% suppression of VPCs in about 90% of patients; in approximately 75% of patients, ventricular tachycardia was abolished and ventricular couplets suppressed. However, despite such documented evidence of efficacy in suppressing and preventing these arrhythmias, there currently is no evidence of a beneficial effect on mortality, and in at least one patient population (those with mild-to-moderate ventricular dysfunction and recent myocardial infarction) with such arrhythmias treated with other class Ic antiarrhythmic drugs (i.e., flecainide, encainide), there was evidence of substantial risk (including mortality and nonfatal cardiac arrest) associated with therapy. (For additional information, see the opening discussion of Cautions in Flecainide Acetate 24:04.04.12.) Therefore, use of propafenone in non-life-threatening ventricular arrhythmias currently is *not* recommended by the manufacturer, FDA, and other experts.

Although controlled studies generally are lacking, both oral (immediate-release tablets) and IV propafenone (IV dosage form currently not commercially available in the US) have been used successfully in the management of ventricular arrhythmias (e.g., VPCs, coupled VPCs, nonsustained ventricular tachycardia) in children†.

DOSAGE AND ADMINISTRATION

● *Administration*

Propafenone hydrochloride is administered orally. Propafenone hydrochloride is commercially available as conventional (immediate-release) tablets and extended-release capsules. The drug also has been administered IV†, but a parenteral dosage form of propafenone hydrochloride currently is not commercially available in the US.

Propafenone hydrochloride (immediate-release tablets) usually is administered orally in 3 equally divided doses daily at 8-hour intervals. Administration of single doses of propafenone hydrochloride (immediate-release tablets) with food has increased the rate and extent of drug absorption in healthy individuals with the extensive-metabolizer phenotype, and limited data indicate that this effect also may occur in those with the poor-metabolizer phenotype. Therefore, while appreciable alterations in propafenone bioavailability have not been documented during multiple-dose administrations of immediate-release tablets with food, patients should be advised of the importance of taking propafenone hydrochloride (immediate-release tablets) in a consistent manner relative to food intake to ensure consistent bioavailability and clinical effect.

Extended-release capsules of propafenone hydrochloride usually are administered orally in equally divided doses every 12 hours. The extended-release capsules should be swallowed intact and should *not* be crushed; extended-release capsules of the drug may be taken without regard to food.

Concomitant oral administration of grapefruit juice with drugs that undergo hepatic oxidation by cytochrome P-450 isoenzymes (e.g., cyclosporine, midazolam, felodipine, nifedipine) has been reported to increase bioavailability of these drugs, resulting in increased plasma concentrations of the unchanged drugs and potential adverse effects. The possibility that a similar interaction could occur between grapefruit juice and propafenone should be considered since the reported increase in bioavailability appears to result from inhibition, probably prehepatic, of the cytochrome P-450 enzyme system. Therefore, pending further accumulation of data, clinicians should be aware of this potential interaction and should discourage patients from ingesting grapefruit juice concomitantly with propafenone. For additional information on drug interactions with grapefruit juice, see Grapefruit Juice, under Drug Interactions: Drugs and Foods Affecting Hepatic Microsomal Enzymes, in the Antihistamines General Statement 4:00.

● Dosage

Dosage of propafenone hydrochloride must be adjusted carefully according to individual requirements and response, patient tolerance, and the general condition and cardiovascular status of the patient. The manufacturer recommends that propafenone therapy (immediate-release tablets) for life-threatening ventricular arrhythmias be initiated in a hospital setting. Clinical and ECG monitoring of cardiac function, including appropriate ambulatory ECG monitoring (e.g., Holter monitoring), is recommended during therapy with the drug. However, ECG determination of propafenone's effect on the QT interval may be confounded by drug-induced prolongation of the QRS interval. (See Effects on Cardiac Conduction under Cautions.) Because of considerable interindividual variation in plasma concentrations of propafenone and its metabolites with a given dosage and their variable contribution to clinical response, the value of monitoring plasma concentrations of the drug and its metabolites has not been established.

At a given dosage, the relative proportion of propafenone in plasma is substantially higher in poor metabolizers than in extensive metabolizers. (See Pharmacokinetics: Absorption.) However, these differences in plasma propafenone concentrations are smaller at higher dosages of the drug and the pharmacologic effects of the drug in poor metabolizers are attenuated by the lack of the active 5-OHP metabolite; in addition, steady state is achieved after 4–5 days of dosing in all patients. Therefore, based on pharmacokinetic considerations and clinical experience, the recommended oral dosage regimens for propafenone are appropriate for initial dosing regardless of the patient's genetically determined ability to metabolize the drug. Reduction of the initial dosage of immediate-release tablets should be considered in patients weighing less than 70 kg.

The manufacturer and some clinicians state that oral loading doses of propafenone hydrochloride (immediate-release tablets) may lead to acute toxicity and are not recommended; however, oral loading doses (e.g., 450–750 mg as immediate-release tablets have been used with apparent safety for conversion of recent-onset atrial fibrillation to normal sinus rhythm† in individuals without heart failure. (See Conversion of Atrial Fibrillation or Flutter to Normal Sinus Rhythm, under Uses: Supraventricular Tachyarrhythmias.)

Since steady-state plasma concentrations of propafenone and the optimum therapeutic effect may not be attained for 1–3 days at a given dosage (immediate-release tablets) in patients with normal renal and hepatic function, increases in propafenone hydrochloride (immediate-release tablets) dosage should be made at intervals of not less than 3–4 days. More gradual dosage escalation should be performed in geriatric patients and patients with marked previous myocardial

damage during initiation of propafenone therapy (immediate-release tablets). Increases in propafenone hydrochloride dosage as (extended-release capsules) should be made at intervals of not less than 5 days. Dosage reduction also should be considered in patients who develop excessive prolongation of the PR interval, excessive QRS widening, or second- or third-degree AV block during propafenone therapy. While it has been suggested that a reduction in propafenone hydrochloride dosage (immediate-release tablets) from initial levels may be needed because of a decrease in propafenone metabolism with long-term therapy, other limited data suggest that a partial tolerance to the antiarrhythmic effects of the drug may develop with continued therapy. (See Pharmacokinetics: Absorption.)

Supraventricular Arrhythmias

For the prevention of paroxysmal supraventricular tachycardia (PSVT) associated with disabling symptoms and for disabling paroxysmal atrial fibrillation/flutter (PAF), the recommended initial adult dosage of propafenone hydrochloride (immediate-release tablets) is 150 mg every 8 hours. Dosage (immediate-release tablets) may be increased after 3–4 days to 225 mg 3 times daily if necessary. If the desired therapeutic response is not attained after an additional 3–4 days, dosage (immediate-release tablets) may be increased again to 300 mg 3 times daily. The safety and efficacy of propafenone hydrochloride dosages (immediate-release tablets) exceeding 900 mg daily have not been established.

Some clinicians suggest a maximum daily propafenone hydrochloride dosage (immediate-release tablets) of 600 mg/m^2 in children.

When propafenone hydrochloride is given as *extended-release capsules* for the prevention of symptomatic atrial fibrillation, the recommended initial adult dosage is 225 mg every 12 hours. Dosage may be increased after at least 5 days to 325 mg every 12 hours if necessary. If the desired therapeutic response is not attained after an additional 5 days, dosage may be increased again to 425 mg every 12 hours. If a dose of propafenone hydrochloride as extended-release capsules is missed, the patient should take only the next scheduled dose (i.e., the next dose should *not* be doubled to make up for the missed dose).

During relative bioavailability studies, a higher daily dosage of propafenone hydrochloride as extended-release capsules was required to obtain similar exposure to propafenone compared with that following immediate-release tablets. Because of decreased saturation of hepatic metabolic pathways and increased first-pass hepatic metabolism associated with the extended-release formulation compared with the immediate-release formulation, the bioavailability of propafenone hydrochloride 325 mg given every 12 hours as extended-release capsules is similar to that following 150 mg of the drug given every 8 hours as immediate-release tablets. Therefore, when switching therapy in a patient who currently is receiving the immediate-release dosage form to the extended-release dosage form, the dosage conversion ratio is *not* a 1:1 substitution (e.g., a patient who currently is receiving 150 mg every 8 hours of propafenone hydrochloride immediate-release tablets may be switched to 325 mg of extended-release capsules every 12 hours).

Self-administration for Conversion of Paroxysmal Atrial Fibrillation

For *self-administration* on an outpatient basis for termination of atrial fibrillation of recent onset in carefully selected patients with mild or no heart disease†, propafenone hydrochloride (immediate-release tablets) has been given as a single oral loading dose of 600 mg in patients weighing 70 kg or more and 450 mg in patients weighing less than 70 kg. Some clinicians suggest that propafenone hydrochloride (immediate-release tablets) be taken 5 minutes after noting the onset of palpitations and that patients remain in a supine or sitting position until resolution of palpitations or for a period of at least four hours following the dose. Patients should seek medical advice if palpitations do not resolve within 6–8 hours, if previously unexperienced symptoms (e.g., dyspnea, presyncope, syncope) occur, or if a marked increase in heart rate occurs after taking the antiarrhythmic drug. Patients should not take more than a single oral dose of propafenone hydrochloride (immediate-release tablets) during a 24-hour period.

Life-threatening Ventricular Arrhythmias

For the suppression and prevention of life-threatening ventricular arrhythmias (e.g., sustained ventricular tachycardia), the recommended initial adult dosage of propafenone hydrochloride (immediate-release tablets) is 150 mg every 8 hours. Dosage (immediate-release tablets) may be increased after 3–4 days to 225 mg 3 times daily if necessary. If the desired therapeutic response is not attained after an additional 3–4 days, dosage (immediate-release tablets) may be increased again to 300 mg 3 times daily. The safety and efficacy of propafenone hydrochloride dosages (immediate-release tablets) exceeding 900 mg daily have not been established.

Some clinicians suggest a maximum daily propafenone hydrochloride dosage (immediate-release tablets) of 600 mg/m² in children.

● Dosage in Renal and Hepatic Impairment

Propafenone should be used with caution in patients with renal impairment since a considerable proportion of the dose (approximately 20–40%) administered as the immediate-release formulation is excreted in urine as active metabolites over a 48-hour period. The amount of the extended-release formulation excreted in urine has not been determined. The manufacturer states that data currently are insufficient to recommend a propafenone hydrochloride dosage for patients with renal impairment; however, such patients should be monitored closely for manifestations of toxicity, including hypotension, somnolence, bradycardia, conduction disturbances (intra-atrial and intraventricular), seizures, and serious ventricular arrhythmias.

Elimination of propafenone may be decreased in patients with hepatic impairment, including cirrhosis and alcoholic liver disease; the terminal elimination half-life of propafenone (immediate-release tablets) of the drug is increased to approximately 9 hours in such patients. (See Pharmacokinetics: Elimination.) In addition, the bioavailability of propafenone (immediate-release tablets) is increased to approximately 70% in patients with substantial hepatic impairment compared with a range of 3–40% in patients with normal hepatic function; absolute bioavailability of propafenone as the extended-release formulation has not been determined. When propafenone (immediate-release tablets) is used in patients with hepatic impairment, the initial dosage of the drug should be approximately 20–30% of the dosage given to patients with normal hepatic function (i.e., a 70–80% reduction in dosage), and these patients should be monitored for signs of toxicity, including hypotension, somnolence, bradycardia, conduction disturbances (intra-atrial and intraventricular), seizures, and/or ventricular arrhythmias.

CAUTIONS

The most common adverse effects of propafenone involve the GI, cardiovascular, and central nervous systems and generally are dose related. Discontinuance of propafenone therapy was required in about 20% of patients receiving the drug in clinical trials. Drug discontinuance in patients treated for ventricular arrhythmias was required most frequently (i.e., in greater than 1% of patients) for proarrhythmia (4.7%), nausea and/or vomiting (3.4%), dizziness (2.4%), dyspnea (1.6%), congestive heart failure (1.4%), and ventricular tachycardia (1.2%). In patients treated for supraventricular arrhythmias in clinical trials, discontinuance of therapy was required most frequently (i.e., in greater than 1% of patients) for nausea and/or vomiting (2.9%), wide-complex tachycardia (1.9%), dizziness (1.7%), fatigue (1.5%), unusual taste (1.3%), and weakness (1.3%).

Propafenone-induced adverse effects tend to decrease with time and may be attenuated by dosage reduction and/or adjustment of dosage interval. Patients with the poor-metabolizer phenotype (see Pharmacokinetics: Elimination) and geriatric patients may be at increased risk of adverse effects because of increased plasma propafenone concentrations. In a multicenter, randomized study in patients with paroxysmal atrial fibrillation or paroxysmal supraventricular tachycardia (PSVT) who had no evidence of ischemic heart disease, the safety and tolerability (i.e., the incidence of adverse effects, including proarrhythmic events) of propafenone hydrochloride (450–900 mg daily, mean daily dosage: 569 mg) was comparable to that of flecainide acetate (100–300 mg daily, mean daily dosage: 167 mg) during a 12-month period of follow-up. In another multicenter, randomized study in patients with paroxysmal atrial fibrillation (more than 90% who were New York Heart Association [NYHA] functional class I) receiving extended-release capsules of propafenone hydrochloride (225 mg, 325 mg, or 425 mg twice daily) for up to 39 weeks, the most common adverse events included dizziness, chest pain, palpitations, taste disturbance, dyspnea, nausea, constipation, anxiety, fatigue, upper respiratory tract infection, influenza, first-degree heart block, and vomiting. The incidence of adverse effects in patients treated with extended-release propafenone hydrochloride capsules in this study was similar regardless of age or gender.

● Nervous System Effects

Adverse nervous system effects reported in US clinical trials in patients receiving propafenone for the treatment of ventricular arrhythmias included dizziness and/or lightheadedness in 13% of patients, fatigue/lethargy in 6%, and headache in 5%. Weakness, ataxia, insomnia, or anxiety was reported in 2%, and tremor or drowsiness in 1% of patients receiving propafenone for ventricular arrhythmias. Pain or

loss of balance also has been reported with propafenone therapy in patients with ventricular arrhythmias.

In US clinical trials in patients with supraventricular arrhythmias, adverse nervous system effects reported with propafenone therapy included dizziness in 9% of patients, headache or fatigue in 6%, weakness in 3%, and tremor or ataxia in 2%. Abnormal dreams, abnormal speech, agitation, delusions, disorientation, coma, confusion, decreased libido, depression, memory loss, paranoia, paresthesia/numbness, psychosis/mania, seizures, unusual smell sensation, or vertigo has been reported in less than 1% of patients receiving propafenone in clinical trials or during postmarketing experience.

Transient global amnesia, which resolved within hours after drug discontinuance, has been reported in at least one patient receiving propafenone. Peripheral neuropathy, which was characterized by episodic jabbing and crushing pain in the hands and feet and hyperesthesia of the extremities and resolved following discontinuance of the drug, has been reported rarely with propafenone therapy.

● GI Effects

The most common adverse GI effect of propafenone therapy is nausea and/or vomiting, which was reported in 11% of patients receiving the drug for ventricular arrhythmias in US clinical trials. Propafenone is secreted by the salivary glands, and unusual (e.g., metallic or salty) taste (dysgeusia) was reported in 9% of patients treated for ventricular arrhythmias. Constipation occurred in 7%; dyspepsia and/or diarrhea in 3%; dry mouth, anorexia, and/or abdominal pain/cramps in 2%; and flatulence in 1% of patients receiving the drug for ventricular arrhythmias. Esophagitis and gastroenteritis also have been reported in clinical trials or during postmarketing experience in patients treated with propafenone for ventricular arrhythmias.

Unusual taste or nausea and/or vomiting was reported in 14 or 11%, respectively, of patients receiving propafenone for supraventricular arrhythmias in US clinical trials. Constipation occurred in 8% and anorexia or diarrhea in 2% of patients with supraventricular arrhythmias.

● Arrhythmogenic Effects

Like other antiarrhythmic agents, propafenone can worsen existing arrhythmias or cause new arrhythmias; the arrhythmogenic potential is the most serious risk associated with the drug. Arrhythmogenic effects associated with propafenone range from an increased frequency of ventricular premature complexes (VPCs) to the development of new and/or more severe and potentially fatal ventricular tachyarrhythmias. Because of difficulties in distinguishing between spontaneous and drug-related variations in an underlying arrhythmia disorder in patients with complex arrhythmias, reported occurrence rates must be considered approximations.

Arrhythmogenic events associated with propafenone therapy in clinical trials reportedly have occurred with an overall frequency of about 5%. In patients with malignant ventricular arrhythmias monitored by invasive and noninvasive methods, the incidence of arrhythmogenic effects during propafenone therapy was 8–19%. About 82–85% of the arrhythmogenic effects associated with the drug have been new or worsened ventricular tachyarrhythmias (e.g., new occurrence of sustained or nonsustained ventricular tachycardia, including spontaneous wide-QRS complex tachycardia, torsades de pointes, progression of ventricular tachycardia to ventricular fibrillation), with the remainder consisting of increased frequency of VPCs. VPCs were reported in 2% of patients receiving propafenone for treatment of ventricular arrhythmias in US clinical trials.

An increased incidence of arrhythmogenic events also has been reported during propafenone therapy in patients with supraventricular tachyarrhythmias. Wide-QRS complex tachycardia was reported in 2% of patients receiving propafenone for supraventricular arrhythmias in overall US clinical trials. In a long-term multicenter trial in patients with symptomatic supraventricular tachycardia, ventricular tachycardia or ventricular fibrillation developed in 9 of 474 patients (1.9 %) receiving propafenone therapy. Ventricular tachycardia or ventricular fibrillation developed within the first 14 days of therapy in 6 of 9 patients; ventricular tachycardia appeared to be of atrial origin in 4 of these 9 patients. Approximately 2.3% of patients in this trial may have experienced an arrhythmogenic event manifested as a recurrence of supraventricular tachycardia. Increased VPCs, ventricular tachycardia, ventricular fibrillation, and death have been reported in patients with atrial fibrillation/flutter receiving propafenone therapy. The overall annual mortality rate based on data from 8 clinical studies was 2.5 or 4% per year in patients receiving propafenone (extended-release or immediate-release formulation) or placebo, respectively.

Although the occurrence of propafenone-induced arrhythmias generally is unpredictable, the risk of arrhythmogenic effects generally appears to be related to dosage and underlying cardiac disease, including severity of the preexisting ventricular arrhythmia and myocardial dysfunction (e.g., low left ventricular ejection fraction, congestive heart failure (New York Heart Association [NYHA] functional class III or IV), myocardial ischemia). Of patients in clinical trials who had worsening of ventricular tachycardia while receiving propafenone, 92% had a history of ventricular tachycardia and/or ventricular fibrillation, 71% had coronary artery disease, and 68% had a history of myocardial infarction. During long-term (mean: 14.4 months) therapy in patients with symptomatic atrial fibrillation, atrial flutter, or supraventricular tachycardia, propafenone therapy was associated with a 20% incidence of adverse cardiovascular effects (e.g., arrhythmogenicity, congestive heart failure, conduction disturbance) in patients with structural heart disease compared with a 13% incidence in those without structural heart disease. While the overall incidence of adverse reactions was similar for patients with or without structural heart disease, the incidence was directly related to dosage and age. The incidence of proarrhythmia in patients receiving propafenone for less serious or benign arrhythmias, including an increased frequency of VPCs, was 1.6%.

Although most proarrhythmic events occurred during the first week of therapy in clinical trials with propafenone, such events also occurred later in therapy, and results of the CAST study suggest that an increased risk of proarrhythmic events is present throughout treatment with antiarrhythmic agents. When propafenone is administered according to currently recommended dosage regimens and precautions, the risk of arrhythmogenic effects appears to be comparable to or less than that associated with other antiarrhythmic agents (e.g., encainide, flecainide).

● *Effects on Cardiac Conduction*

Clinically important conduction disturbances may occur during propafenone therapy in patients without preexisting conduction abnormalities; however, the risk of adverse cardiac effects probably increases progressively as plasma propafenone concentrations increase. There is a correlation between propafenone dosage, plasma concentration, and the degree of lengthening of PR and QRS intervals.

First-, second-, or third-degree AV block occurred in about 2.5, 0.6, or 0.2%, respectively, of patients with ventricular arrhythmias receiving propafenone (immediate-release tablets) in clinical trials. First-degree AV block occurred in approximately 2–3% of patients with symptomatic paroxysmal atrial fibrillation receiving the extended-release formulation of propafenone hydrochloride in a clinical trial. There were no cases of sinus rhythm with Mobitz type I (Wenckenbach) second-degree AV block, sinus rhythm with Mobitz Type II second-degree AV block, third-degree AV block, or increased sinus bradycardia in a clinical trial of patients with symptomatic paroxysmal atrial fibrillation receiving the extended-release formulation of the drug. Dosage reduction or discontinuance of the drug may be necessary in patients who develop second- or third-degree AV block. (See Cautions: Precautions and Contraindications.) Bundle branch block, intraventricular conduction delay/increased QRS duration, or bradycardia occurred in about 1–2% of patients with ventricular arrhythmias in clinical trials. Bradycardia was reported in 2% of patients receiving propafenone therapy for supraventricular arrhythmias in clinical trials. A paradoxical increase in ventricular rate also has occurred with propafenone therapy in patients with atrial flutter or fibrillation because of a reduction in the degree of AV nodal block or enhanced conduction through an accessory bypass tract (e.g., in patients with Wolff-Parkinson-White [WPW] syndrome). (See Cautions: Precautions and Contraindications.)

● *Cardiovascular Effects*

The manufacturer states that clinically important decreases in left ventricular ejection fraction with oral propafenone therapy did not occur in clinical trials in patients with depressed baseline ejection fraction (mean ejection fraction: 33.5%). However, because of propafenone's dose-related β-adrenergic blocking and negative inotropic effects, the drug may cause or worsen congestive heart failure, particularly in patients with preexisting heart failure or decreased left ventricular ejection fraction (less than 30%). New or worsened congestive heart failure occurred in about 1–4% of patients treated for ventricular arrhythmias in clinical trials. In patients in whom these adverse effects were considered probably or definitely related to propafenone therapy (about 1%), 80% had preexisting heart failure and 85% had coronary artery disease. Patients with no prior history of congestive heart failure receiving propafenone rarely (less than 0.2%) developed congestive heart failure. Congestive heart failure or palpitations occurred in about 2% of patients receiving propafenone therapy for supraventricular arrhythmias (PAF or PSVT) in clinical trials.

Chest pain or angina, palpitations, or syncope/near syncope occurred in about 2–5% of patients receiving propafenone in clinical trials for treatment of ventricular arrhythmias. Atrial fibrillation or edema has occurred in about 1% of

patients receiving propafenone therapy for ventricular arrhythmias. Atrial flutter, AV dissociation, cardiac arrest, flushing, hot flashes, sick sinus syndrome, sinus pause, sinus arrest, or supraventricular tachycardia has been reported in less than 1% of patients receiving propafenone.

● *Hepatic Effects*

Propafenone is extensively metabolized in the liver and should be administered with caution to patients with impaired hepatic function. (See Cautions: Precautions and Contraindications.) There have been postmarketing reports of hepatic dysfunction, including hepatocellular, cholestatic, and mixed hepatotoxicity in patients receiving the drug. In at least one case, hepatotoxicity recurred upon rechallenge with propafenone. Cholestasis, hepatitis, and increases in serum aminotransferase (AST [SGOT], ALT [SGPT]) and alkaline phosphatase concentrations have been reported in patients receiving the drug. In toxicology studies, fatty degenerative liver changes were observed in rats following long-term (6 months) administration of oral propafenone hydrochloride at a dosage of 270 mg/kg daily (about 3 times the maximum recommended human daily dosage based on body surface area) but not at 90 mg/kg daily (equivalent to the maximum recommended human daily dosage based on body surface area).

● *Dermatologic and Sensitivity Reactions*

Rash has been reported in 3% of patients with ventricular arrhythmias receiving propafenone in clinical trials, and diaphoresis has been reported in 1% of such patients. Pruritus also have been reported in patients receiving the drug. Possible propafenone-associated drug fever has been reported in at least one patient receiving oral propafenone therapy for sustained ventricular tachycardia. Fever and an erythematous, papular rash developed 10 days after initiation of propafenone therapy and resolved following drug discontinuance; fever recurred upon rechallenge with the drug but resolved completely upon termination of therapy.

Alopecia also has been reported with propafenone therapy.

● *Hematologic Effects*

Granulocytopenia, leukopenia, lymphopenia, leukocytosis, thrombocytosis, thrombocytopenia, purpura, anemia, bruising, and increased bleeding time have been reported in less than 1% of patients receiving propafenone. Agranulocytosis (fever, chills, weakness, and neutropenia) also has been reported with propafenone therapy, generally within 8 weeks after initiation of therapy. The leukocyte count generally returned to normal within 14 days after discontinuance of therapy. The possibility of agranulocytosis should be considered in any patient receiving propafenone who develops unexplained fever and/or decreases in leukocyte count, particularly during the 3 months following initiation of therapy. (See Cautions: Precautions and Contraindications.)

● *Musculoskeletal Effects*

Joint pain occurred in about 1% of patients receiving propafenone for ventricular arrhythmias in clinical trials. Arthritis, arthralgia, gout, muscle pain, muscle weakness, or muscle cramps were reported in less than 1% of such patients. Lupus erythematosus has been reported in less than 1% of patients receiving propafenone therapy in clinical trials or during postmarketing experience; in at least one patient, propafenone-induced lupus erythematosus recurred following rechallenge with the drug but resolved completely upon discontinuance of therapy. Positive antinuclear antibody (ANA) titers have been reported with propafenone therapy; these abnormalities generally were not associated with clinical manifestations and resolved upon discontinuance of the drug or even with continued therapy. In a randomized, controlled trial, positive ANA titers were found in about 24% of patients who had negative ANA titers before initiation of propafenone therapy.

Exacerbation of myasthenia gravis, which was evident within a few hours after initiation of propafenone hydrochloride (450 mg daily) in a patient with ocular myasthenia gravis and resolved upon drug discontinuance, has been reported with propafenone therapy.

● *Other Adverse Effects*

Blurred vision occurred in 4% of patients receiving propafenone therapy for ventricular arrhythmias in clinical trials; abnormal vision also has been reported. Asthma, increased serum glucose concentration, diabetes mellitus, hypochloremia, hyponatremia, syndrome of inappropriate antidiuretic hormone (SIADH) secretion, nephrotic syndrome, renal failure, nasal congestion, ocular irritation, tinnitus, pneumonia, respiratory failure, pain, increased urinary frequency or urgency, impotence, or prostatitis occurred in less than 1% of patients receiving propafenone for treatment of ventricular arrhythmias in clinical trials.

Blurred vision was reported in 3% and dyspnea in 2% of patients receiving propafenone therapy for supraventricular arrhythmias in clinical trials.

Both inflammatory and noninflammatory lesions in the renal tubules, with accompanying interstitial nephritis, have been observed in rats following administration of oral propafenone hydrochloride for 6 months at dosages of 180 and 360 mg/kg daily (2 or 4 times the maximum recommended human daily dosage based on body surface area) but not at 90 mg/kg daily (equivalent to the maximum recommended human daily dosage based on body surface area). However, these lesions appeared reversible as they were not found 6 weeks after discontinuance of the drug.

● Precautions and Contraindications

Findings from the postmarketing Cardiac Arrhythmia Suppression Trial (CAST), a long-term, multicenter, randomized, double-blind study in patients with asymptomatic, non-life-threatening ventricular arrhythmias who had had a myocardial infarction more than 6 days but less than 2 years previously, indicate that the rate of total mortality and nonfatal cardiac arrest in patients treated with encainide or flecainide (7.7%) was increased compared with that seen in patients who received placebo (3%). The applicability of these results to other populations (e.g., those without recent myocardial infarction) or to other antiarrhythmic drugs is uncertain; however, the manufacturer of propafenone states that use of any class Ic antiarrhythmic drug in patients with structural heart disease may be associated with substantial risk. In addition, the manufacturer, FDA, and some experts currently recommend that use of propafenone or other class I agents in patients with ventricular arrhythmias be limited to those with *life-threatening* arrhythmias. (See Uses.) Use in less severe ventricular arrhythmias, including even those with unpleasant manifestations, currently is not recommended, and treatment of asymptomatic VPCs should be avoided. In addition, current evidence indicates that initiation of antiarrhythmic therapy in patients with atrial fibrillation is associated with a notable risk for adverse cardiac events, particularly in geriatric patients or those with structural heart disease.

Since propafenone, like other antiarrhythmic agents, can worsen existing arrhythmias or cause new arrhythmias in some patients, clinical and ECG evaluations are essential prior to and during propafenone therapy to monitor for the appearance of arrhythmias and to determine the need for continued therapy. Use of propafenone in patients with atrial flutter has resulted in an increase in AV conduction (1:1 ratio) and the development of very rapid ventricular rates. (See Cautions: Effects on Cardiac Conduction.) Risk of this tachycardia may be reduced by concomitant administration of a cardiac glycoside or a β-adrenergic blocking agent. Patients with permanent artificial pacemakers should be monitored and, if necessary, have their pacemakers reprogrammed since propafenone may affect endocardial pacing and sensing thresholds (e.g., increased stimulation threshold) of these devices.

The patient's medication history should be carefully screened prior to and during propafenone therapy, including obtaining information on all OTC, prescription, and herbal/natural preparations with emphasis on those that may affect the pharmacodynamics or pharmacokinetics of propafenone. (See Drug Interactions.) Patients should be advised to inform their health-care providers of any change in the use of medications (OTC, prescription) and supplements. Patients should be advised to inform their health-care providers that they are receiving propafenone when hospitalized or prescribed a new medication for any condition. Patients should be advised to immediately inform their health care providers if they experience symptoms associated with electrolyte imbalance (e.g., excessive or prolonged diarrhea, sweating, vomiting, loss of appetite or thirst).

Because of propafenone's mild to moderate negative inotropic and β-adrenergic blocking effects, as well as an increased risk of arrhythmogenic effects, the immediate-release formulation of the drug should be used with caution in patients with a history of congestive heart failure or myocardial dysfunction; the manufacturer of the extended-release formulation of propafenone states that the drug should not be used in patients with congestive heart failure. Congestive heart failure should be fully compensated before propafenone therapy with the immediate-release formulation is initiated. If cardiovascular manifestations increase, therapy should be discontinued (unless congestive heart failure is caused by the cardiac arrhythmia) and adequate cardiac compensation reestablished before resuming propafenone therapy, if indicated, at a lower dosage of the immediate-release formulation.

Propafenone slows AV conduction and may cause AV block. A correlation exists between dosage and plasma concentrations of propafenone hydrochloride and the degree of lengthening of PR and QRS intervals. Some clinicians have suggested limiting QRS interval increases to 25% or less in patients receiving propafenone. If second- or third-degree AV block occurs during propafenone therapy, the dosage should be reduced or the drug discontinued.

Because reversible granulocytopenia and agranulocytosis have occurred rarely with propafenone therapy, patients receiving the drug should be advised to promptly report fever, sore throat, chills, or any other manifestations of infection.

Positive antinuclear antibody (ANA) titers have been reported in patients receiving propafenone therapy. (See Cautions: Musculoskeletal Effects.) Patients who develop an abnormal ANA test following initiation of propafenone therapy should be monitored carefully and, if titers remain elevated or increase further, drug discontinuance should be considered.

Propafenone is extensively metabolized in the liver, and dosage should be reduced substantially in patients with impaired hepatic function. The drug also should be used with caution in patients with renal dysfunction since a considerable portion of the dose is excreted in urine as active metabolites. (See Dosage and Administration: Dosage in Renal and Hepatic Impairment.)

Reversible disorders of spermatogenesis have been demonstrated in animals following high-dose IV administration of propafenone. Transient, reversible decreases (within the normal range) in sperm count have been reported in healthy men receiving short-term propafenone therapy but subsequent evaluations in patients receiving long-term therapy have suggested no effect of the drug on sperm count. (See Cautions: Pregnancy, Fertility, and Lactation.)

Pending further accumulation of data, patients should be discouraged from ingesting grapefruit juice concomitantly with propafenone because of the potential for increased propafenone bioavailability and possible adverse effects associated with such concomitant administration. (See Dosage and Administration: Administration.)

Propafenone, like other agents with nonselective β-adrenergic blocking activity, generally should *not* be used in patients with asthma/bronchospastic disease or nonallergic bronchospastic disease (e.g., chronic bronchitis, emphysema) since the drugs may inhibit bronchodilation produced by endogenous catecholamines.

Propafenone has been reported to exacerbate myasthenia gravis, and it has been suggested that use of the drug be avoided in patients with this condition.

Propafenone (immediate-release formulation) is contraindicated in patients with uncontrolled congestive heart failure; the extended-release formulation of the drug is contraindicated in patients with congestive heart failure. Propafenone is contraindicated in patients with cardiogenic shock, atrioventricular or intraventricular disorders of impulse generation and/or conduction (e.g., sick sinus node syndrome, atrioventricular block) unless an artificial pacemaker is present, bradycardia, severe hypotension, marked electrolyte imbalance, or known hypersensitivity to the drug.

The manufacturer of ritonavir states that concomitant use of ritonavir with propafenone is contraindicated because such use is likely to produce substantially increased plasma concentrations of propafenone and associated serious toxicity. (See Drug Interactions: Ritonavir.)

● Pediatric Precautions

Safety and efficacy of propafenone in patients younger than 18 years of age have not been established. However, the drug has been used successfully and without unusual adverse effects in a limited number of infants and children for the management of various refractory supraventricular (e.g., PSVT, junctional ectopic tachycardia, atrial fibrillation or flutter) and ventricular (e.g., VPCs, ventricular tachycardia) arrhythmias. (See Uses.)

● Geriatric Precautions

Data from clinical studies with propafenone (immediate-release tablets) in patients 65 years of age or older is insufficient to determine whether geriatric patients respond differently than younger adults. Dosage of propafenone (immediate-release tablets) should be selected with caution and generally initiated at the lower end of the recommended range since geriatric patients are more likely to have impaired renal, hepatic, and/or cardiac function and concomitant disease and drug therapy. Data from clinical studies indicate that safety and efficacy of propafenone as extended-release capsules are similar in geriatric patients and younger adults. Nevertheless, the manufacturer states that the possibility that some older patients may exhibit increased sensitivity to the drug as extended-release capsules cannot be ruled out.

● Mutagenicity and Carcinogenicity

No evidence of propafenone-induced mutagenicity was seen with in vitro microbial (Ames test), dominant lethal tests in mice, mammalian mutagenicity assays using Chinese hamster spermatogonoia and bone marrow cells, rat bone marrow, and Chinese hamster micronucleus test.

No evidence of carcinogenesis was seen in mice and rats receiving oral propafenone hydrochloride dosages up to 360 mg/kg (about 2 times the maximum recommended human daily dosage based on body surface area) and 270 mg/kg daily (about 3 times the maximum recommended human daily dosage based on body surface area), respectively.

● Pregnancy, Fertility, and Lactation

Pregnancy

Propafenone has been shown to be embryotoxic, but not teratogenic, in rabbits and rats when given at a dosage 3 (150 mg/kg daily) and 6 times (600 mg/kg daily), respectively, the maximum recommended human daily dose based on body surface area. Embryotoxic effects were not observed in rats given propafenone hydrochloride dosages up to 270 mg/kg daily (about 3 times the maximum recommended human daily dose based on body surface area); however, dose-dependent increases in post-implantation loss were observed in rabbits given propafenone hydrochloride dosages as low as 15 mg/kg daily (about 33% of the maximum recommended human daily dose based on body surface area). Increased maternal death was observed in rats receiving oral propafenone hydrochloride dosages as low as 90 mg/kg daily (equivalent to the maximum recommended human daily dosage) from mid-gestation through weaning. Decreases in neonatal survival, weight gain, and physiologic development were observed in rats receiving oral propafenone hydrochloride dosages of 360 mg/kg or more daily (4 or more times the maximum recommended human daily dosage) from mid-gestation through weaning. Unchanged propafenone and its metabolite, 5-hydroxy-propafenone (5-OHP), have been reported to cross the placenta in humans. However, there are no adequate and controlled studies to date using propafenone in pregnant women, and the drug should be used during pregnancy only when the potential benefits justify the possible risks to the fetus. It is not known whether use of the drug during labor or delivery could have any immediate or delayed adverse effects on the mother or fetus, affect the duration of labor, or increase the likelihood of forceps delivery or other obstetrical intervention.

Fertility

The effect of propafenone on fertility in humans is not known. Temporary decreases in sperm count have been observed in healthy men receiving short-term, oral propafenone therapy; this effect was reversible following discontinuance of the drug and did not persist during long-term propafenone therapy. Administration of large IV doses of propafenone in monkeys, dogs, and rabbits has caused transient, reversible decreases in spermatogenesis; this effect was observed only at lethal or sublethal dosages and was not seen in rats receiving oral or IV propafenone. Reproduction studies in male rabbits using an oral propafenone hydrochloride dosage of 120 mg/kg daily (about 2.4 times the maximum recommended human daily dosage based on body surface area) or an IV dosage of 3.5 mg/kg daily (a dosage associated with impairment of spermatogenesis) have not revealed evidence of impaired fertility. In addition, reproduction studies in male and female rats using oral propafenone hydrochloride dosages up to 270 mg/kg daily (about 3 times the maximum recommended human daily dosage based on body surface area) have not revealed evidence of impaired fertility.

Lactation

Since propafenone is distributed in milk, caution is advised if the drug is administered in nursing women. (See Pharmacokinetics: Distribution.) Because of the potential for serious adverse reactions to propafenone in nursing infants, a decision should be made whether to discontinue nursing or the drug, taking into account the importance of the drug to the woman.

DRUG INTERACTIONS

● Drugs Affecting or Metabolized by Hepatic Microsomal Enzymes

Metabolism of propafenone is mediated by the cytochrome P-450 (CYP) isoenzyme system, including CYP2D6 (major metabolic pathway), CYP1A2 and CYP3A4; patients should be monitored and dosage of propafenone hydrochloride should be reduced accordingly when the drug is used concurrently with inhibitors of CYP2D6 (e.g., desipramine, paroxetine, quinidine, ritonavir, sertraline), CYP1A2 (e.g., amiodarone), or CYP3A4 (e.g., erythromycin, ketoconazole, ritonavir, saquinavir), because plasma propafenone concentrations may increase.

In addition, propafenone inhibits CYP2D6 and caution is advised if the drug is used concurrently with substrates of CYP2D6 (e.g., desipramine, haloperidol, imipramine, metoprolol, propranolol, venlafaxine) since increased plasma concentrations of these drugs may occur, and consideration should be given to reduction of dosage for drugs that are substrates of CYP2D6 when such drugs are used concurrently with propafenone.

● Drugs Metabolized by P-glycoprotein Transporter

The effect, if any, of propafenone on the p-glycoprotein transport system has not been systematically evaluated.

● Digoxin

Concomitant administration of propafenone and oral or IV digoxin has resulted in increased serum or plasma digoxin concentrations, associated in some cases with enhanced effects of digoxin (e.g., decreased heart rate, shortened QT interval) and at least one case of digoxin toxicity.In some studies, increases in serum digoxin concentrations with propafenone hydrochloride dosages of 450 or 900 mg daily averaged about 35 or 85%, respectively; such increases in digoxin concentrations have been maintained over a period of up to 16 months of concomitant therapy with the drugs. Changes in digoxin concentrations in patients receiving concomitant propafenone therapy have exhibited wide interindividual and intra-individual variation, with a relationship to propafenone and/or digoxin dosage or plasma propafenone concentration being reported in some studies.

Although the exact mechanism of this interaction has not been established, some evidence suggests that propafenone may reduce the renal clearance of digoxin by inhibiting renal tubular transport of the drug. Other data suggest no alterations in digoxin renal clearance, but decreases in total body and/or nonrenal clearance or volume of distribution of digoxin have been reported.

Digoxin dosage generally should be reduced in patients in whom propafenone therapy is initiated, especially in those who have relatively high digoxin dosages or serum concentrations. Careful monitoring of serum digoxin concentrations and appropriate adjustments in digoxin dosage should be performed in patients receiving concomitant propafenone and digoxin therapy.

● β-Adrenergic Blocking Agents

In healthy individuals, concomitant administration of propafenone and propranolol or metoprolol has resulted in substantial increases in plasma concentrations and terminal elimination half-lives of the β-adrenergic blocking agents; plasma propafenone concentrations were unchanged. These increases in plasma concentration and half-life apparently are the result of propafenone's inhibition of the hydroxylation pathway responsible for metabolism of the β-adrenergic blocking agents. Increases in plasma metoprolol concentrations may result in loss of the drug's relative cardioselectivity and an increase in adverse effects. Although pharmacokinetics of propafenone were not affected and concomitant use of β-adrenergic blocking agents was not associated with an increased incidence of adverse effects in clinical trials of propafenone, an increase in the manifestations of acute metoprolol-induced brain syndrome (e.g., delirium, fatigue, lassitude) has been reported in a patient receiving concomitant metoprolol and propafenone. Patients receiving propafenone and β-adrenergic blocking agents concomitantly may require a reduction in the dosage of the β-adrenergic blocking agent.

● Antiarrhythmic Agents

There is limited information on the use of propafenone in conjunction with other antiarrhythmic agents for the management of severe, refractory ventricular or supraventricular arrhythmias. (See Combination Therapy under Ventricular Arrhythmias: Life-threatening Ventricular Arrhythmias, in Uses.) Combination antiarrhythmic therapy for severe refractory arrhythmias generally is empiric and must be individualized. Since the cardiac effects of multiple antiarrhythmic agents may be additive, synergistic, or antagonistic and adverse effects may be additive, combination therapy must be used only when the increased risk is justified and with careful monitoring.

The manufacturer of propafenone states that the extended-release formulation of the drug should *not* be used concomitantly with class Ia or III antiarrhythmic agents (including quinidine or amiodarone) and that class Ia or III antiarrhythmic agents should be withheld for at least 5 half-lives prior to administration of extended-release propafenone. Experience is limited with the concomitant use of propafenone and class Ib or other class Ic antiarrhythmic agents.

Quinidine

Quinidine, even at small doses, completely inhibits the CYP2D6 hydroxylation pathway responsible for propafenone's metabolism; therefore, patients receiving concomitant quinidine and propafenone effectively are rendered poor metabolizers. Propafenone clearance decreased by 60%, plasma steady-state propafenone concentrations increased twofold, and 5-hydroxypropafenone (5-OHP) concentrations were reduced by approximately 50%, in patients with the extensive-metabolizer phenotype who received concomitant quinidine (50 mg 3 times daily) and propafenone as the immediate-release formulation (150 mg every 8 hours); steady-state plasma propafenone concentrations increased threefold in such patients who received concomitant quinidine at a dosage of 100 mg every 8 hours. Poor metabolizers receiving the 2 drugs concomitantly did not exhibit changes in plasma concentrations of propafenone or 5-OHP.

In a limited number of patients with ventricular arrhythmias refractory to procainamide or quinidine monotherapy, combined therapy with propafenone and quinidine or procainamide resulted in a substantial reduction in the frequency of ventricular premature complexes (VPCs) compared with drug-free baseline VPC frequencies. VPC frequency was reduced from a baseline geometric mean of 406/hour before treatment to 33/hour in patients receiving concomitant propafenone/quinidine therapy and from a baseline geometric mean of 211/hour to 27/hour in patients receiving concomitant propafenone/procainamide.

The manufacturer states that the concomitant use of propafenone and quinidine is not recommended; however, some clinicians have suggested that such combined therapy may be useful in selected patients.

Mexiletine

Combined therapy with propafenone and mexiletine was effective in preventing the induction of ventricular tachycardia by programmed electrical stimulation in 3 of 16 patients with refractory sustained ventricular tachycardia; however, ventricular tachycardia with hemodynamic deterioration requiring defibrillation occurred in 5 patients (31%) receiving propafenone alone and 2 patients (13%) receiving propafenone and mexiletine. Additional data are needed to determine whether the observed benefit from combined therapy is attributable to potential synergism of the electrophysiologic effects of the 2 drugs or to alterations in hepatic metabolism of the drug(s), resulting in increased plasma concentrations of one or both drugs and decreased plasma concentrations of drug metabolites.

Lidocaine

In patients with ventricular arrhythmias who received propafenone and lidocaine concomitantly by IV infusion, the negative inotropic effect of propafenone was increased and the effect of propafenone in prolonging atrial and ventricular refractoriness was attenuated. Although propafenone and lidocaine have been used concomitantly without notable effect on the pharmacokinetics of either drug, an increased risk of lidocaine-related adverse effects involving the central nervous system has been reported in patients receiving such concomitant therapy.

Other Antiarrhythmic Agents

Sotalol or amiodarone reportedly may enhance the antiarrhythmic effect of propafenone. However, prolongation of the QT interval and atypical ventricular tachycardia (torsades de pointes) have been reported rarely in patients receiving concomitant propafenone and amiodarone therapy. Concomitant use of propafenone and amiodarone may affect cardiac conduction and repolarization. The manufacturer of propafenone states that concomitant use of propafenone and amiodarone is not recommended.

● Other Drugs That Prolong QT Interval

Although specific pharmacokinetic drug interaction studies are not available, the manufacturer of propafenone states that the drug should *not* be used concomitantly with other drugs that prolong the QT interval, including certain phenothiazines, cisapride, bepridil (not currently commercially available in the US), tricyclic antidepressant agents, or macrolides.

● Ritonavir

Although specific pharmacokinetic drug interaction studies are not available, the manufacturer of ritonavir states that ritonavir should *not* be used concomitantly with certain cardiovascular agents, including propafenone, because of the potential for substantially increased plasma concentrations of these cardiovascular drugs and potentially serious and/or life-threatening adverse effects. (See Cautions: Precautions and Contraindications, in Ritonavir 8:18.08.08.) This pharmacokinetic interaction may occur because ritonavir has high affinity for several cytochrome P-450 (CYP) isoenzymes (e.g., CYP3A, CYP2D6, CYP1A2) involved in propafenone metabolism. (See Drug Interactions in Ritonavir 8:18.08.08.)

● Local Anesthetic Agents

The manufacturer states that concomitant use of propafenone and local anesthetic agents (i.e., during pacemaker implantation, surgery, or dental procedures) may increase the risk of adverse nervous system effects.

● Warfarin

Concomitant administration of propafenone and warfarin results in increased plasma warfarin concentrations and corresponding increases in prothrombin times (PTs), possibly because of competition for a common metabolic pathway. Steady-state plasma warfarin concentrations and PTs increased an average of 39 and 25%, respectively, in a limited number of healthy individuals receiving concomitant propafenone and warfarin therapy. PTs or international normalized ratios (INRs) should be monitored closely and, if required, adjustments in warfarin dosage should be made in patients receiving concurrent propafenone and warfarin therapy.

● Cimetidine

In a limited number of healthy individuals receiving concomitant propafenone and cimetidine therapy, steady-state plasma propafenone concentrations averaged 20% higher than those with propafenone therapy alone.

● Theophylline

Increased serum theophylline concentrations have been reported in patients receiving theophylline concomitantly with propafenone and some clinicians suggest that serum theophylline concentrations and ECGs be monitored closely in patients receiving such combined therapy.

● Rifampin

Rifampin may increase the metabolism of concomitant propafenone; reductions in plasma propafenone concentrations and decreased antiarrhythmic efficacy have been reported in patients receiving these drugs concomitantly. Plasma propafenone concentrations decreased 67%, 5-OHP concentrations were reduced by 65%, and N-depropylpropafenone (NDPP) concentrations were increased by 35% in patients with the extensive-metabolizer phenotype who received concomitant propafenone and rifampin. Plasma propafenone concentrations decreased 50%, NDPP exposure and peak plasma concentration increased by 74 and 20%, respectively, and urinary excretion of propafenone, 5-OHP, and NDPP was reduced in patients with the poor-metabolizer phenotype who received such concomitant therapy. Propafenone exposure and peak plasma concentration both decreased by 84% and 5-OHP exposure and peak plasma concentration decreased by 69 and 57% in elderly patients with the poor-metabolizer phenotype who received concomitant propafenone and rifampin.

● Phenobarbital

Concomitant therapy with phenobarbital and propafenone reportedly may increase the clearance of propafenone, resulting in decreased plasma propafenone concentrations.

● Fluoxetine

Concomitant therapy with fluoxetine and propafenone in patients with the extensive-metabolizer phenotype increased the peak plasma concentrations and area under the plasma concentration-time curve (AUC) of the S-enantiomer by 39 and 59%, respectively, and the peak plasma concentrations and AUC of the R-enantiomer by 71 and 50%, respectively.

● Orlistat

Orlistat may limit absorption of propafenone during concomitant therapy with the drugs. There have been postmarketing reports of severe adverse effects, including seizures, atrioventricular block, and acute circulatory failure that occurred following abrupt discontinuance of orlistat in patients receiving chronic propafenone therapy.

● Other Drugs

Increases in blood cyclosporine or serum desipramine concentrations have been reported during concomitant administration of propafenone.

The manufacturer states that clinical experience in patients receiving propafenone concomitantly with calcium-channel blocking agents or diuretics has not revealed evidence of clinically important adverse interactions.

ACUTE TOXICITY

Limited information is available on the acute toxicity of propafenone.

● Manifestations

In general, overdosage of propafenone may be expected to produce effects that are extensions of the drug's pharmacologic effects, particularly those involving cardiac conduction and function and the CNS. Overdosage of propafenone may result in nausea and/or vomiting, hypotension, somnolence, intra-atrial and intraventricular conduction disturbances, and high-grade ventricular arrhythmias; fatalities also have occurred. Cardiac manifestations may occur within 30–120 minutes after ingestion. Manifestations of overdosage generally are most severe during the 3 hours following the overdose. Nausea generally is the first manifestation of toxicity and may occur within 30 minutes of ingestion of the drug.

● Treatment

Effective management of propafenone overdosage requires early diagnosis and prompt detoxification, since no specific antidote is available and resuscitative measures (e.g., external cardiac massage, assisted mechanical ventilation) and supportive measures (e.g., pacemaker placement, cardiopulmonary bypass) may be of limited benefit. Some clinicians state that any adult or pediatric patient who has ingested a propafenone hydrochloride dose exceeding 1 g or exceeding 600 mg/m², respectively, should be admitted to intensive care and monitored closely for 24 hours. If ingestion of the drug is recent, emesis or gastric lavage with at least 30 g of activated charcoal may reduce absorption. Some experts recommend insertion of a transvenous pacemaker prior to gastric lavage, since vagal stimulation associated with such lavage may induce bradycardia. Defibrillation and IV infusion of dopamine and isoproterenol have been used successfully to restore normal cardiac rhythm and blood pressure, while IV diazepam has been used to control seizures. Limited data suggest that alkalinization with IV sodium lactate and potassium chloride may be of benefit in propafenone overdosage. IV infusion of small amounts of a concentrated (20%) sodium chloride injection reportedly has been used successfully in a patient with propafenone overdosage unresponsive to hemoperfusion.

Hemodialysis is probably of no value in enhancing elimination of propafenone hydrochloride since the drug is highly bound to plasma proteins and has a large volume of distribution.

PHARMACOLOGY

● Antiarrhythmic and Electrophysiologic Effects

Propafenone hydrochloride is a local anesthetic-type antiarrhythmic agent. Studies in animals have demonstrated the effectiveness of propafenone in preventing and/or suppressing experimentally induced arrhythmias.

Propafenone is considered a class I (membrane stabilizing) antiarrhythmic agent, although the antiarrhythmic and electrophysiologic actions of the drug are complex in that it also has demonstrated some β-adrenergic blocking and calcium-channel blocking activity. Like encainide and flecainide, the principal effect of propafenone on cardiac tissue appears to be a concentration-dependent inhibition of the transmembrane influx of extracellular sodium ions via fast sodium channels, as indicated by a decrease in the maximal rate of depolarization of phase 0 of the action potential and a shift of the membrane-responsiveness curve in the hyperpolarizing direction. Since this effect is greater at higher stimulation frequencies and less negative membrane potentials, the drug's sodium blockade is enhanced in ischemic cardiac tissue. Studies in cardiac tissue in animals indicate that propafenone binds to fast sodium channels in both their active and inactive states; the drug thereby inhibits recovery after repolarization in a time- and voltage-dependent manner, which is associated with subsequent dissociation of the drug from the sodium channels. Propafenone induces phasic (frequency-dependent) sodium channel blockade faster than encainide or flecainide, while recovery is similar to flecainide and faster than encainide. Propafenone also appears to have a slight inhibitory effect (approximately 1/75 the potency of verapamil) on the transmembrane influx of extracellular calcium ions via slow calcium channels (calcium-channel blocking effect), but this effect generally occurs only at high drug concentrations and probably does not contribute to antiarrhythmic efficacy. Propafenone has no vagomimetic or vagolytic effect on cardiac muscle.

Propafenone exhibits electrophysiologic effects characteristic of class Ic antiarrhythmic agents, with local anesthetic effects and a direct stabilizing action on myocardial membranes. The electrophysiologic characteristics of the subgroups of class

I antiarrhythmic agents may be related to quantitative differences in their rates of attachment to and dissociation from transmembrane sodium channels, with class Ic agents exhibiting slow rates of attachment and dissociation. Propafenone decreases the amplitude and maximal rate of rise (phase 0) of the action potential in a concentration-dependent manner and has little or no effect on resting potential. Like other class Ic antiarrhythmic agents, propafenone slows intracardiac conduction at low concentrations, has relatively minimal effects on refractoriness, and generally has little effect on repolarization. The drug increases action potential duration (APD) in the sinus node and ventricular myocytes and decreases APD in Purkinje fibers. Propafenone decreases cardiac excitability in diastole by increasing the threshold potential for electrical excitation and prolonging the effective refractory period in the atria, AV node, and, to a lesser extent, the ventricles. The effective refractory period in accessory pathways also is prolonged, and both anterograde and retrograde conduction are decreased by the drug. The electrophysiologic effects of propafenone in ischemic cardiac tissue are qualitatively similar to those in healthy cardiac tissue but are more marked; increases in action potential amplitude and refractoriness and decreases in conduction velocity have been attributed to the voltage-dependent sodium channel blockade produced by the drug. This differential activity in ischemic versus healthy cardiac tissue may contribute to propafenone's antiarrhythmic action in ischemic heart disease.

The antiarrhythmic and electrophysiologic effects of propafenone result from the parent drug and its 2 major metabolites, 5-hydroxypropafenone (5-OHP) and N-depropylpropafenone (NDPP). (See Pharmacokinetics.) Concentrations and relative proportions of propafenone and its metabolites attained in plasma vary considerably depending on the patient's genetically determined ability to metabolize the drug, dosage, and duration of drug administration. Consequently, the observed effects of propafenone are a somewhat complex aggregate that depends on the relative proportions and serum concentrations of parent drug and metabolites. Following acute IV administration (IV dosage form currently not commercially available in the US), antiarrhythmic and electrophysiologic effects appear to result principally from propafenone regardless of the patient's metabolizer phenotype; however, following long-term oral administration, these effects appear to result principally from propafenone and 5-OHP in patients with the extensive-metabolizer phenotype and principally from propafenone in patients with the poor-metabolizer phenotype.

Effects on Cardiac Conduction and Refractoriness

Propafenone and its metabolites produce a dose-related decrease in intracardiac conduction within the His-Purkinje system, atrioventricular (AV) node, and intraventricular pathways. The effects of the drug on conduction are manifested by dose-related increases in PR, QRS, AH, and HV intervals; at higher workload and heart rates, dose-related increases in QT interval also occur. PR interval increased about 11–28% with oral propafenone hydrochloride dosages of 450–1200 mg daily (immediate-release tablets), while QRS duration was prolonged from 8–32% after 1 or 2 IV doses of 1–2 mg/kg or oral dosages of 450–1200 mg daily (immediate-release tablets). Increases in mean PR interval of 9–21 msec, mean QRS duration of 4–6 msec, and the mean QT interval corrected for rate (QT_c) of 2–6 msec were observed with oral propafenone hydrochloride dosages of 500–850 mg daily as extended-release capsules. The range of maximum increases in the QT_c observed were greater than 20, 10–20, or 10% or less compared to baseline in 1–5, 16–26, or 72–83%, respectively, of patients receiving oral propafenone hydrochloride dosages of 500–850 mg daily as extended-release capsules. Effects on PR and QRS intervals (prolongation) were maintained for up to 2 years in patients receiving propafenone hydrochloride 600–900 mg daily (immediate-release tablets). Increases in AH and HV intervals of about 16–32% and up to 67% or less, respectively, were observed with dosages of 900–1200 mg daily (immediate-release tablets). Conduction slowing was greatest in patients with prolonged baseline HV intervals. 5-OHP further prolongs QRS duration and, to a lesser degree, PR interval.

Propafenone also prolongs atrial and ventricular refractoriness. Increases of approximately 17% in ventricular effective refractory period (ERP) during ventricular pacing have been reported with a propafenone hydrochloride dosage of 900 mg daily. In patients with recurrent ventricular tachycardia receiving 2 mg/kg of propafenone hydrochloride IV, atrial and AV nodal ERP were prolonged. Ventricular repolarization as determined by the QT interval corrected for rate (QT_c) has been reported to be increased by 7–15% or unaffected. The JT_c interval (QT_c-QRS interval) does not appear to be affected by propafenone.

Effects on Sinus Node

Propafenone appears to have minimal effects on normal sinus node function, although some depression of function may occur. Sinus node recovery time, sinus cycle length, sinus node automaticity, and sinoatrial conduction time may increase or remain unaffected. Sinus cycle length generally is unchanged by propafenone; however, an 8% decrease in sinus cycle length was observed in children with recurrent paroxysmal supraventricular tachycardia (PSVT) receiving propafenone hydrochloride 1.5 mg/kg IV over 3 minutes. In patients with ventricular tachycardia, propafenone may have a depressant effect on sinus node function; sinus node recovery time increased by approximately 0.2 seconds in such patients receiving usual dosages of the drug.

Effects on Dual AV Nodal and Anomalous AV Pathways

In patients with Wolff-Parkinson-White (WPW) syndrome or dual AV nodal pathways, propafenone decreases conduction and increases the refractoriness of anterograde and retrograde accessory pathways; complete block of the anterograde accessory pathway may result.

● *Arrhythmogenic Effects*

Like other antiarrhythmic agents, propafenone can worsen existing arrhythmias or cause new arrhythmias. (See Cautions: Arrhythmogenic Effects.) The arrhythmogenic effects of the drug may range from an increased frequency of ventricular premature complexes (VPCs) to the development of more severe and potentially fatal ventricular tachyarrhythmias. The exact mechanism(s) by which various antiarrhythmic agents, including propafenone, produce arrhythmogenic effects has not been fully determined, but the arrhythmogenic potential of propafenone may be related to its effects on conduction. The risk of arrhythmogenesis during propafenone therapy appears to correlate directly with the severity of the presenting arrhythmia and the degree of ventricular dysfunction, if present.

● *Cardiovascular Effects*
Inotropic Effects

Propafenone exhibits a dose-dependent negative inotropic effect. The exact mechanism of the drug's negative inotropic effect has not been determined but may involve blockade of sodium channels as well as β-adrenergic receptors and/or, at high concentrations, calcium-channel blockade. Both propafenone and 5-OHP exhibit negative inotropic effects at high concentrations in vitro and, in large doses, have depressed left ventricular function in animals. The negative inotropic effect and other cardiovascular effects of propafenone may be more pronounced and clinically important in patients with coronary artery disease, acute myocardial infarction, congestive heart failure, or myocardial dysfunction. (See Cautions: Cardiovascular Effects.) However, conflicting data have been reported regarding the depressant effects of propafenone on left ventricular function, and reductions in left ventricular ejection fraction (LVEF) with oral propafenone therapy may be less than that with flecainide or disopyramide. No appreciable effects of propafenone on LVEF were observed in a study in patients with ventricular arrhythmias who had baseline LVEFs less than 40%. However, in another study, patients with baseline LVEFs less than 50% had reductions of 20–26% in LVEF with propafenone therapy compared with reductions of only 4–8% in patients who had no preexisting impairment in LVEF. Reductions in left ventricular function as measured by peak flow velocity have been observed in patients with ventricular arrhythmias receiving propafenone, but left ventricular ejection time was not affected. Increases in left ventricular end-systolic and end-diastolic diameter have been reported in patients with impaired left ventricular function receiving the drug. Increases in intracardiac pressure (assessed by measurement of right atrial, pulmonary artery, and pulmonary capillary wedge pressure) manifested as a depression of cardiac index have been reported in some patients receiving IV propafenone but not in others.

β-Adrenergic Blocking Effects

Propafenone has β-adrenergic blocking activity in humans about 1–5% that of propranolol on a molar basis. While the clinical importance of propafenone's β-adrenergic blocking activity has not been fully elucidated, clinically important β-adrenergic blocking effects potentially could occur at usual dosages of the drug since long-term therapy may result in steady-state plasma propafenone concentrations 10–50 times greater than those of propranolol. Because plasma propafenone concentrations are high relative to those of propranolol, the functional relative β-adrenergic blocking activity of propafenone may be up to one-fourth the potency of propranolol.

β-Adrenergic blockade associated with propafenone is evidenced by inhibition of the positive inotropic effects of isoproterenol and attenuation of isoproterenol-induced increases in left ventricular pressure, contractile index, heart rate, and carotid arterial pressure. In addition, up-regulation of β2-adrenergic

receptors similar to that observed with nonselective β-adrenergic blocking agents has been reported in patients with symptomatic VPCs receiving 450–900 mg of propafenone hydrochloride daily. The extent of propafenone's β-adrenergic blocking activity may vary with a patient's genetically determined metabolizer phenotype and the differing ratios of parent drug to metabolites. The 2 principal metabolites of propafenone, 5-hydroxypropafenone (5-OHP) and N-depropylpropafenone (NDPP), have no clinically relevant β-adrenergic blocking effects at concentrations achieved with usual therapeutic dosages of propafenone. Therefore, in patients whose ability to metabolize the drug into 5-OHP is impaired (i.e., poor metabolizers), plasma concentrations of propafenone are increased, and β-adrenergic blocking effects are more evident, than those in whom the drug is rapidly and extensively metabolized (i.e., extensive metabolizers). Patients with poor-metabolizer phenotypes receiving 450–900 mg of propafenone hydrochloride daily had increased plasma propafenone concentrations and greater attenuation of exercise- and isoproterenol-induced tachycardia than patients with the extensive-metabolizer phenotype.

The β-adrenergic blocking effect of propafenone appears to be stereoselective. The S-enantiomer of propafenone possesses 50–100 times greater affinity for β-adrenergic receptors than the R-enantiomer and has a dissociation constant (Ki value) for these receptors about 140 times less than that of the R-enantiomer. Although conflicting data exist regarding the effects of propafenone on heart rate and blood pressure, decreases of 4–5% in systolic blood pressure consistent with a negative inotropic or a peripheral vasodilatory effect have been reported in healthy individuals after oral or IV administration of S-propafenone or a racemic mixture of the drug, but not with the R-enantiomer.

Chronotropic Effects

Following oral or IV administration of propafenone, heart rate may be reduced or unchanged. Propafenone's effect on heart rate varies at least in part according to evaluative conditions; sinus rate generally is unaffected at usual dosages in patients with arrhythmias, but decreases in heart rate have been reported in patients receiving such dosages during exercise. Propafenone-induced decreases in diurnal and nocturnal heart rate of 14–31 and 6.3–8.3%, respectively, have been reported; however, the normal circadian variation in heart rate was not affected. Propafenone-induced bradycardia is associated with high plasma drug concentrations and may be related to the patient's metabolizer phenotype; patients with the poor-metabolizer phenotype develop bradycardia more frequently than those with the extensive-metabolizer phenotype. The bradycardic effect appears to be attributable only to the parent drug.

● *Local Anesthetic Effects*

Propafenone exhibits a local anesthetic action approximately equal to that of procaine (no longer commercially available in the US).

PHARMACOKINETICS

● *Absorption*

Propafenone hydrochloride (immediate-release tablets) is rapidly and almost completely absorbed from the GI tract following oral administration. The absolute bioavailability averages approximately 5–50% for propafenone immediate-release tablets and has not been determined for extended-release capsules. The absolute bioavailability of propafenone depends principally on a patient's genetically determined ability to metabolize the drug. (See Pharmacokinetics: Elimination.) In most patients (those with the extensive-metabolizer phenotype), propafenone is metabolized extensively and undergoes first-pass metabolism in the liver, producing the 2 major, active metabolites 5-hydroxypropafenone (5-OHP) and N-depropylpropafenone (NDPP). In these patients, the absolute bioavailability of propafenone is dependent on dosage and dosage form; 150- and 300-mg immediate-release tablets of propafenone hydrochloride had absolute bioavailabilities of 3.4 and 10.6%, respectively, while a more rapidly absorbed solution of propafenone hydrochloride 3.5 mg/mL had an absolute bioavailability of 21.4%. In patients with the extensive-metabolizer phenotype, the drug exhibits nonlinear pharmacokinetics: a threefold increase in propafenone hydrochloride dosage (300 versus 900 mg as immediate-release tablets) results in a 10-fold increase in steady-state plasma concentration, while in a small fraction of patients (those with the poor-metabolizer phenotype or those receiving concurrent quinidine) (see Antiarrhythmic Agents: Quinidine, in Drug Interactions) propafenone exhibits linear pharmacokinetics, and 5-OHP is not formed or only minimally formed because the drug undergoes little or no first-pass metabolism. The nonlinear pharmacokinetics observed in patients with the extensive-metabolizer phenotype has been attributed to the saturation of the hydroxylation pathway.

Although the rate and extent of propafenone absorption were increased (bioavailability was increased by an average of 147%) when the drug was administered with food in a single-dose study in healthy individuals, the manufacturer states that bioavailability of the drug is not appreciably affected by food during multiple-dose administration of immediate-release tablets. Propafenone exposure was increased 4-fold when a single 425-mg extended-release capsule was administered with food in healthy individuals; however, the bioavailability of the drug is not appreciably affected by food during multiple-dose administration (425-mg extended-release capsules twice daily).

Bioavailability of propafenone is increased in patients with hepatic impairment (e.g., cirrhosis) and is inversely proportional to indocyanine green clearance. Bioavailability of immediate-release propafenone averages approximately 60–70% in patients with marked hepatic impairment (indocyanine green clearance of 7 mL/minute or less) and 3–40% in patients with normal hepatic function; the relative bioavailability of the extended-release formulation has not been determined.

Peak plasma propafenone concentrations generally occur approximately 2–3.5 hours after oral administration of immediate-release tablets in most individuals. Peak plasma concentration of propafenone after a single 300-mg oral dose of propafenone hydrochloride immediate-release tablets in patients with ventricular arrhythmias averaged 416 ng/mL; peak drug concentrations were 1198 and 1213 ng/mL with a dosage of 900 mg (immediate-release tablets) daily for 1 and 3 months, respectively. Increases in area under the plasma concentration-time curve (AUC) in these patients were similar following single- or multiple-dose drug administration of immediate-release tablets. Following single-dose administration of propafenone immediate-release tablets, the ratio of the AUCs of parent drug to 5-OHP was 0.43; with multiple dosing for 1 or 3 months, the ratio was 0.24 or 0.25, respectively. Peak plasma propafenone concentrations generally occur approximately 3–8 hours after oral administration of extended-release capsules in most individuals.

In healthy individuals, administration of propafenone hydrochloride as a single oral (300- or 450-mg immediate-release tablet) or IV (35–50 mg) dose produced similar peak plasma concentrations of the parent drug (278 versus 295 ng/mL, respectively). However, neither 5-OHP nor NDPP was detectable in plasma after IV administration in these individuals. Since 5-OHP and NDPP has clinically important antiarrhythmic activity, propafenone's effect may differ with oral versus IV administration. Considerable interindividual variation exists in plasma concentrations of propafenone and its metabolites with a given dosage. Peak plasma concentrations of 5-OHP and NDPP average 101–288 and 8–40 ng/mL, respectively, in healthy individuals after administration of a single oral dose (300–450 mg) of propafenone hydrochloride immediate-release tablets. Propafenone, 5-OHP, and NDPP exhibit nonlinear pharmacokinetics in patients with the extensive-metabolizer phenotype, although the pharmacokinetics of 5-OHP and NDPP deviate from linearity only to a small extent. The pharmacokinetic profiles of propafenone, 5-OHP, and NDPP apparently are not affected substantially by age or gender.

The considerable degree of interindividual variability observed in the pharmacokinetics of propafenone in individuals with the extensive-metabolizer phenotype is principally attributable to first-pass hepatic metabolism and non-linear pharmacokinetics. The degree of interindividual variability in propafenone pharmacokinetic parameters is increased following single and multiple dose administration of propafenone hydrochloride extended-release capsules. The fact that interindividual variability in the pharmacokinetics of propafenone appears to be substantially less in individuals with the poor-metabolizer phenotype than in those with the extensive-metabolizer phenotype suggests that such variability may be due to CYP2D6 polymorphism rather than to the formulation.

The pattern of plasma concentrations of propafenone and its metabolites observed in an individual patient with long-term oral propafenone therapy depends principally on the genetically determined metabolizer phenotype and, to a lesser extent, on hepatic blood flow and enzyme function. (See Pharmacokinetics: Elimination.) Following oral administration of propafenone (immediate-release tablets), steady-state plasma concentrations of the parent drug and its metabolites are attained within 4–5 days in individuals with normal hepatic and renal function. Plasma concentrations of 5-OHP and NDPP generally average less than 20% those of propafenone. Poor metabolizers achieve plasma propafenone concentrations 1.5–2 times higher than those of extensive metabolizers at propafenone hydrochloride dosages of 675–900 mg (immediate-release tablets) daily; at lower dosages, poor metabolizers may attain plasma propafenone concentrations more than fivefold higher than those of extensive metabolizers.

In patients with ventricular arrhythmias and the extensive-metabolizer phenotype receiving 337.5, 450, 675, or 900 mg of propafenone hydrochloride daily (immediate-release tablets), the proportions of 5-OHP to propafenone in plasma were 45, 40, 24, or 19%, respectively, while a subset of patients with the poor-metabolizer phenotype had higher relative plasma concentrations of the parent drug at each dosage and no detectable 5-OHP. Ratios of NDPP to propafenone are similar in extensive and poor metabolizers (approximately 10 and 6%, respectively). In poor metabolizers, NDPP is the principal metabolite and 5-OHP may not be detectable. Following oral administration of propafenone hydrochloride 300 mg (immediate-release tablets) every 8 hours for 14 days, plasma propafenone, 5-OHP, and NDPP concentrations averaged 1010, 174, and 179 ng/mL, respectively, in healthy individuals with the extensive-metabolizer phenotype. In an individual presumed to have the poor-metabolizer phenotype, plasma concentrations of propafenone, 5-OHP, and NDPP concentrations were 1048, undetectable, and 219 ng/mL, respectively, following oral administration of immediate-release tablets. Following administration of extended-release capsules of propafenone hydrochloride, plasma concentrations of 5-OHP and NDPP are generally less than 40 and 10% of plasma propafenone concentrations, respectively.

In extensive metabolizers, propafenone bioavailability following administration of extended-release capsules is less than that following administration of the immediate-release tablets; the more gradual release of propafenone from the extended-release formulation results in an increase in the extent of first-pass hepatic metabolism. During relative bioavailability studies, higher daily dosages of propafenone administered as extended-release capsules compared with immediate-release tablets were required to obtain similar exposure to propafenone. The bioavailability of propafenone following 325-mg extended-release capsules given twice daily is similar to 150-mg immediate-release tablets given 3 times daily. Following administration of extended-release capsules, the mean exposure to 5-OHP was approximately 20-25% higher compared with such exposure following immediate-release tablets.

Because propafenone, 5-OHP, and NDPP are pharmacologically active and plasma concentrations of the parent drug and these metabolites vary considerably depending on the patient's metabolizer phenotype, duration of drug administration, and dosage formulation relationships between plasma concentrations of propafenone and/or its metabolites and antiarrhythmic and electrophysiologic effects are complex. (See Pharmacology: Antiarrhythmic and Electrophysiologic Effects.) Limited data suggest that in patients with the extensive-metabolizer phenotype, the antiarrhythmic and electrophysiologic effects are correlated principally with plasma concentrations of unchanged propafenone and 5-OHP. In patients with the poor-metabolizer phenotype, the antiarrhythmic and electrophysiologic effects appear to be correlated with plasma concentrations of unchanged propafenone. In a study in patients with chronic ventricular arrhythmias, plasma propafenone concentrations of 250–490 ng/mL were associated with at least 90% suppression of ventricular premature complexes (VPCs), ventricular coupled beats, and nonsustained ventricular tachycardia in 47, 70, and 78% of patients, respectively; propafenone concentrations of 1500 ng/mL or higher produced at least 90% suppression of VPCs, ventricular coupled beats, and nonsustained ventricular tachycardia in 67, 83, and 100% of patients, respectively.

Following long-term administration of 850 mg of propafenone hydrochloride daily as extended-release capsules, plasma concentrations of propafenone in individuals with the poor-metabolizer phenotype was approximately twice that observed in individuals with the extensive-metabolizer phenotype. Following lower daily dosages of propafenone hydrochloride as extended-release capsules, the difference in plasma concentrations of propafenone is larger between the metabolizer phenotypes; plasma concentrations of propafenone in individuals with the poor-metabolizer phenotype are approximately 3–4 times higher than those observed in individuals with the extensive-metabolizer phenotype. Following saturation of the hydroxylation pathway (CYP2D6) in individuals with the extensive-metabolizer phenotypes, plasma propafenone concentrations increase at a greater-than-linear rate after administration of extended-release capsules of propafenone hydrochloride. In individuals with the poor-metabolizer phenotype, propafenone exhibits linear pharmacokinetics.

Despite the complex nature of the contribution of propafenone and its metabolites to clinical response in individual patients, clinical response generally is related to dosage and the usually effective dosages in patients with the poor- or extensive-metabolizer phenotype are comparable. (See Dosage and Administration: Dosage.) This recommendation is based on consideration of propafenone pharmacokinetics including the fact that differences in pharmacokinetics between metabolizer phenotypes decrease as dosage is increased, mitigation by the lack of the active 5-OHP metabolite in individuals with the poor-metabolizer phenotype, and the fact that steady-state occurs following 4–5 days of therapy in all patients. However, plasma concentrations of the drug may increase disproportionately during dosage titration in patients with the poor-metabolizer phenotype, resulting in an increased occurrence of adverse effects, especially CNS effects (e.g., dizziness, blurred vision, taste disturbances).

Limited data suggest that a partial tolerance to the antiarrhythmic effects of propafenone may develop during long-term therapy so that higher plasma concentrations are required to produce equivalent effects.

A relationship between plasma concentrations of propafenone or its metabolites and arrhythmogenic effects has not been established. (See Cautions: Arrhythmogenic Effects.)

● Distribution

Distribution of propafenone and its metabolites into human body tissues and fluids has not been fully characterized. Propafenone is highly lipophilic and rapidly distributed into lung, liver, and heart tissue. The apparent volume of distribution of propafenone averages 3 L/kg (range: 2.5–4 L/kg). In patients receiving propafenone who underwent heart surgery, 5-OHP was detected in higher concentrations in right atrial tissue than in plasma, and ratios of parent drug to metabolites were lower in plasma than in atrial tissue (1.7 versus 3.9, respectively).

The degree of protein binding of propafenone is concentration dependent. In healthy individuals, 81–97% of propafenone is bound in vitro to plasma proteins at plasma propafenone concentrations of 0.25–100 mcg/mL, while protein binding averages 96% at plasma propafenone concentrations of 0.5–2 mcg/mL. Most propafenone in plasma is bound to α_1-acid glycoprotein and a lesser extent to albumin.

In patients with severe hepatic dysfunction, approximately 88% of propafenone is bound in vitro to plasma proteins.

Propafenone and 5-OHP cross the placenta and are distributed into milk. (See Cautions: Pregnancy, Fertility, and Lactation.)

● Elimination

There are two principal patterns of propafenone metabolism. These patterns are genetically determined by an individual's ability to metabolize the drug via a hepatic oxidation pathway. The ability to oxidatively metabolize propafenone is dependent on an individual's ability to metabolize debrisoquin (debrisoquin phenotype). The debrisoquin phenotype or the observed pattern of propafenone metabolites may be used to determine an individual's metabolic phenotype for propafenone. Individuals who extensively metabolize propafenone via the oxidation pathway exhibit the extensive-metabolizer phenotype, while those who have an impaired ability to metabolize the drug by this pathway exhibit the poor-metabolizer phenotype. Approximately 90–95% of Caucasians exhibit the extensive-metabolizer phenotype, with the remainder being poor metabolizers. Propafenone metabolism in patients with the poor-metabolizer phenotype is characterized by a linear dose-concentration relationship and a relatively long terminal elimination half-life; these individuals have increased plasma propafenone concentrations relative to individuals with the extensive-metabolizer phenotype and are more likely to experience β-adrenergic blocking and adverse effects of the drug.

Following single or multiple oral doses of immediate-release tablets in adults with the extensive-metabolizer phenotype and normal renal and hepatic function, the elimination half-life of propafenone averages about 1–3 hours (range: 2–10 hours). The half-life of propafenone averages approximately 8–13 hours (range: 6–36 hours) in adults with the poor-metabolizer phenotype. Following a single oral dose of 300 mg of propafenone hydrochloride as immediate-release tablets, a half-life of 3.5 hours was reported; after administration of 300 mg of propafenone hydrochloride daily for 1 and 3 months, the reported half-lives were 6.7 and 5.8 hours, respectively. Steady-state plasma elimination half-life of propafenone is prolonged in poor metabolizers, averaging 17.2 hours (range: 10–32 hours) compared with 5.5 hours (range: 2–10 hours) in extensive metabolizers.

In individuals with the extensive-metabolizer phenotype, propafenone is metabolized in the liver to 2 active metabolites and at least 9 additional metabolites. The 2 active metabolites, 5-hydroxypropafenone (5-OHP) and N-depropylpropafenone (NDPP), are formed through hydroxylation and dealkylation of the parent drug. Propafenone hydroxylation via cytochrome CYP2D6, a cytochrome P-450 isoenzyme under genetic control, produces 5-OHP. Formation of NDPP is catalyzed by different isoenzymes, cytochrome CYP1A2 and CYP3A4. Differences in metabolism between R- and S-propafenone related to stereoselective interaction with the CYP2D6 isoenzyme have been observed in animals and humans receiving single enantiomers of the drug. Following a 250-mg oral

dose of R- or S-propafenone hydrochloride administered to adults with the extensive-metabolizer phenotype, the mean values for elimination half-life, clearance, and volume of distribution for R-propafenone were smaller than those for S-propafenone, while AUC was larger; however, these stereospecific effects were not observed in an adult with the poor-metabolizer phenotype who received the separate drug enantiomers. In vitro and in vivo studies indicate that the R-enantiomer is cleared faster than the S-enantiomer via the 5-hydroxylation pathway (CYP2D6). This results in a higher ratio of the S-enantiomer to R-enantiomer at steady state. Although the enantiomers have equivalent sodium-channel blocking potency, the S-enantiomer is a more potent β-adrenergic antagonist than the R-enantiomer. Following administration of propafenone hydrochloride (immediate-release tablets or extended-release capsules), the observed ratio of S-enantiomer to R-enantiomer (S/R ratio) for AUC was approximately 1.7. The S/R ratios after administration of 225-, 325-, or 425-mg extended-release capsules were independent of dose. In addition, similar S/R ratios were observed among metabolizer genotypes and following long-term administration.

When racemic propafenone is administered, some data indicate that metabolic inhibition between the enantiomers appears to result in reversal of these enantiomer-dependent pharmacokinetic differences. In patients with extensive or poor metabolizer phenotypes receiving propafenone hydrochloride 450 mg daily (immediate-release tablets), the clearance of R-propafenone was approximately 1.7 times that of the S-enantiomer, and the AUC was smaller for R-propafenone regardless of metabolizer phenotype. In adults with the poor-metabolizer phenotype, the clearance of both enantiomers is reduced; however, the clearance of the R-enantiomer still exceeds that of the S-enantiomer.

Although conflicting data exist, clearance of propafenone appears to be reduced during long-term administration, presumably as a result of reduced hepatic metabolism. Increases in steady-state bioavailability, elimination half-life, and peak plasma concentration have been reported following oral administration of propafenone hydrochloride (150–300 mg as immediate-release tablets 3 times daily) for 5–30 days compared with these values after single-dose administration, suggesting a reduction in propafenone clearance during chronic dosing. However, the minimum plasma propafenone concentration required for antiarrhythmic efficacy also has been reported to increase with long-term therapy, suggesting the development of partial tolerance to the drug. (See Pharmacokinetics: Absorption.)

Propafenone clearance directly correlates with hepatic function as indicated by indocyanine green clearance, prothrombin time, and serum concentrations of albumin, total bilirubin, and AST (SGOT). The drug's terminal elimination half-life is increased to approximately 9 hours in patients with moderate to severe hepatic impairment (e.g., cirrhosis).

The volume of distribution, clearance, and elimination half-life of propafenone were similar in healthy individuals, patients undergoing hemodialysis, and those with moderate renal impairment (mean creatinine clearance: about 40 mL/minute per 1.73 m²) receiving a single IV dose of the drug. Propafenone is not removed by hemodialysis.

Limited data indicate that mean interdose plasma propafenone concentrations in patients with the extensive-metabolizer phenotype and renal impairment receiving maintenance therapy with oral propafenone hydrochloride 450 mg daily (immediate-release tablets) may be decreased slightly compared with those in healthy individuals with normal renal function. However, steady-state concentrations of 5-OHP were decreased, and those of NDDP were increased, in patients with the extensive-metabolizer phenotype and renal impairment compared with those concentrations in healthy individuals with normal renal function. In another study, impaired renal function did not alter plasma concentrations of propafenone or 5-OHP at steady state in patients receiving 600 mg of propafenone hydrochloride (immediate-release tablets) daily for 4 days. The disposition of propafenone hydrochloride after administration of a single IV dose (70 mg) was similar in a limited number of patients with renal impairment (mean creatinine clearance: 0.66 mL/minute per 1.73 m²) or renal failure compared with those with normal renal function (mean creatinine clearance: 1.43 mL/minute per 1.73 m²). More data from long-term studies are needed to determine the effect of decreased renal function on the pharmacokinetics of propafenone.

Less than 1% of a dose of propafenone is excreted unchanged in urine or feces following oral administration of the drug; metabolites are mainly excreted in feces via biliary elimination. Urinary excretion of propafenone and its metabolites in patients with the extensive-metabolizer phenotype and cirrhosis generally is similar to that in healthy individuals with the same metabolizer phenotype, although the fraction of the dose excreted as unchanged drug is increased substantially and some NDDP also is excreted.

CHEMISTRY AND STABILITY

● *Chemistry*

Propafenone hydrochloride is a local anesthetic-type antiarrhythmic agent. Propafenone is structurally related to other class Ic antiarrhythmic drugs and also to β-adrenergic blocking agents (e.g., propranolol); both propafenone and β-adrenergic blocking agents contain an aromatic ring joined by a methylenenoxy bridge to the asymmetric carbon atom of *N*-substituted hydroxyethylamine.

Propafenone hydrochloride is commercially available as a racemic mixture. While limited data suggest that the *R*- and *S*-enantiomers of the drug have similar antiarrhythmic activity, only the *S*-isomer exerts a β-adrenergic blocking effect. (See Pharmacology.)

Propafenone hydrochloride occurs as a white crystalline powder or as colorless crystals and is slightly soluble in water and alcohol, having solubilities of 5 mg/mL in water and 11 mg/mL in alcohol. The drug has a pK$_a$ of 9.

● *Stability*

Commercially available propafenone hydrochloride immediate-release tablets and extended-release capsules should be stored in tight containers at a controlled room temperature of 25°C, but may be exposed to temperatures ranging from 15–30°C. Propafenone hydrochloride immediate-release tablets should be stored in light-resistant containers. When stored under such conditions, the commercially available immediate-release tablets have an expiration date of 3 years following the date of manufacture.

PREPARATIONS

Excipients in commercially available drug preparations may have clinically important effects in some individuals; consult specific product labeling for details.

Propafenone Hydrochloride

Oral		
Capsules, extended-release	225 mg	**Rythmol®SR**, Reliant
	325 mg	**Rythmol®SR**, Reliant
	425 mg	**Rythmol®SR**, Reliant
Tablets, film-coated	150 mg*	**Propafenone Hydrochloride Tablets**
		Rythmol® (scored), Reliant
	225 mg*	**Propafenone Hydrochloride Tablets**
		Rythmol® (scored), Reliant
	300 mg*	**Propafenone Hydrochloride Tablets**
		Rythmol® (scored), Reliant

* available from one or more manufacturer, distributor, and/or repackager by generic (nonproprietary) name

† Use is not currently included in the labeling approved by the US Food and Drug Administration.

Selected Revisions November 14, 2016, © Copyright, November 1, 1998, American Society of Health-System Pharmacists, Inc.

Amiodarone Hydrochloride

24:04.04.20 • CLASS III ANTIARRHYTHMICS

■ Amiodarone hydrochloride is considered to be predominantly a class III antiarrhythmic agent, but the drug also appears to exhibit activity in each of the 4 Vaughn-Williams antiarrhythmic classes, including some class I (membrane-stabilizing) antiarrhythmic action.

USES

Amiodarone appears to be effective in the management of a wide variety of ventricular as well as supraventricular arrhythmias†. Because of amiodarone's potentially life-threatening adverse effects and the management difficulties associated with its use, the drug previously was not considered a first-line antiarrhythmic but generally was reserved for use in life-threatening ventricular arrhythmias. The drug also was used infrequently for the suppression or prevention of any type of arrhythmia and only when conventional antiarrhythmic therapy was considered ineffective or was not tolerated. However, amiodarone generally appears to exhibit greater efficacy and a lower incidence of proarrhythmic effects than class I or other class III antiarrhythmic drugs and therefore has become a mainstay in the management of various tachyarrhythmias, including expert recommendations for advanced cardiovascular life support (ACLS), despite labeling that continues to recommend more limited use. In addition, although no antiarrhythmic agent given routinely during cardiac arrest has been shown to increase survival to hospital discharge, amiodarone has been shown to increase short-term survival to hospital admission relative to lidocaine or placebo. Amiodarone should be used only by clinicians who are familiar with and have access to, either directly or through referral, the use of all currently available modalities for the management of recurrent life-threatening ventricular arrhythmias and who have access to appropriate evaluative and monitoring procedures, including continuous ECG monitoring and electrophysiologic techniques for evaluating the patient in both ambulatory and hospital settings.

● Ventricular Arrhythmias

Amiodarone is used orally or IV to suppress and prevent the recurrence of documented life-threatening ventricular arrhythmias (recurrent ventricular fibrillation and recurrent, hemodynamically unstable ventricular tachycardia) that do not respond to documented adequate dosages of other currently available antiarrhythmic agents or when alternative antiarrhythmic agents are not tolerated. Amiodarone is designated an orphan drug by the FDA for use in this condition. Amiodarone may be used IV to treat patients with ventricular tachycardia or fibrillation in whom oral amiodarone therapy is indicated, but who are unable to take oral medication.

It is difficult to assess the overall efficacy of amiodarone since response to the drug depends on many factors, including the specific cardiac arrhythmia being treated, the criteria used to evaluate efficacy, the presence of underlying cardiac disease in the patient, the number of antiarrhythmic agents used prior to amiodarone, the duration of follow-up, and the concomitant use of other antiarrhythmic agents. In addition, overall arrhythmia recurrence rates (fatal and nonfatal) appear to be highly variable and depend on many factors, including response to programmed electrical stimulation (PES) or other measures, and whether patients who do not appear to respond initially are included. When considering only those patients who responded well enough to amiodarone to be placed on long-term treatment, ventricular arrhythmia recurrence rates have ranged from 20–40% in most studies having an average follow-up period of 1 year or longer.

Life-Threatening Ventricular Arrhythmias and Advanced Cardiovascular Life Support

There is relatively limited experience from controlled studies with the use of amiodarone for suppression and prevention of recurrent life-threatening ventricular arrhythmias. Although comparative data are lacking, the efficacy of amiodarone in the management of severe refractory arrhythmias generally is considered to be at least comparable to and probably better than that of other

antiarrhythmic agents (e.g., quinidine, procainamide). Data from most clinical studies indicate that the drug is effective in approximately 50–80% of patients with life-threatening ventricular arrhythmias, including those refractory to other antiarrhythmic agents. Previously, the potential severity of the drug's adverse effects generally had precluded amiodarone from being considered a first-line† agent in the management of life-threatening ventricular arrhythmias, and use of the drug generally was reserved for patients in whom other antiarrhythmic agents were ineffective or not tolerated. Currently, however, amiodarone is considered a preferred† or alternative agent for the management of various life-threatening ventricular arrhythmias, in part because of comparable or better efficacy and its apparent reduced risk of proarrhythmic activity.

Shock-Resistant Ventricular Fibrillation or Pulseless Ventricular Tachycardia

Amiodarone is used as adjunctive therapy for the treatment of ventricular fibrillation or pulseless ventricular tachycardia resistant to cardiopulmonary resuscitation (CPR), defibrillation, and a vasopressor (e.g., epinephrine).

Antiarrhythmic drugs are used during cardiac arrest to facilitate the restoration and maintenance of a spontaneous perfusing rhythm in patients with refractory (i.e., persisting or recurring after at least one shock) ventricular fibrillation or pulseless ventricular tachycardia; however, there is no evidence that these drugs increase survival to hospital discharge when given routinely during cardiac arrest. High-quality CPR and defibrillation are integral components of ACLS and the only proven interventions to increase survival to hospital discharge. Other resuscitative efforts, including drug therapy, are considered secondary and should be performed without compromising the quality and timely delivery of chest compressions and defibrillation. The principal goal of pharmacologic therapy during cardiac arrest is to facilitate return of spontaneous circulation (ROSC), and epinephrine is the drug of choice for this use. (See Uses: Advanced Cardiovascular Life Support and Cardiac Arrhythmias, in Epinephrine 12:12.12.) If an antiarrhythmic agent is needed for the treatment of refractory ventricular fibrillation or pulseless ventricular tachycardia during adult cardiac arrest, the American Heart Association (AHA) recommends amiodarone as the first-line drug of choice because of its proven benefits in improving rates of ROSC and hospital admission; lidocaine may be used as an alternative. Results of several studies suggest that amiodarone is more effective than lidocaine in improving rates of ROSC and hospital admission in patients with shock-refractory ventricular fibrillation or pulseless ventricular tachycardia. In pediatric advanced life support (PALS), current evidence supports the use of either amiodarone or lidocaine for these arrhythmias.

Results of a randomized, double-blind, placebo-controlled study in patients with out-of-hospital cardiac arrest due to defibrillation-refractory ventricular arrhythmias (i.e., ventricular fibrillation, pulseless ventricular tachycardia) who received a single 300-mg dose of IV amiodarone hydrochloride (after at least 3 precordial electrical shocks were administered) indicate that the drug improved the rate of survival to hospital admission by 29%. In a randomized, double-blind, comparative study with lidocaine, approximately 23% of patients with out-of-hospital cardiac arrest due to defibrillation-refractory ventricular arrhythmias who received IV amiodarone hydrochloride (5 mg/kg) or its matching placebo survived to hospital admission compared with 12% of those who received IV lidocaine (1.5 mg/kg) or its matching placebo following at least 3 precordial electrical shocks, IV epinephrine, and an additional precordial electrical shock. Among patients for whom the time from dispatch of the ambulance to the administration of the drug was equal to or less than the median time (24 minutes), approximately 28% of those given amiodarone and 15% of those given lidocaine survived to hospital admission. Despite these results, only about 5% of patients receiving IV amiodarone who survived to hospital admission lived to be discharged from the hospital compared with about 3% of those receiving IV lidocaine. Evidence supporting the use of amiodarone and lidocaine in pediatric cardiac arrest is more limited and principally based on extrapolation of data from the adult population. In a retrospective cohort study that included data from 889 pediatric patients with in-hospital cardiac arrest, improved ROSC was observed with lidocaine compared with amiodarone. Neither drug was associated with improved survival to hospital discharge.

IV amiodarone also may be used for the treatment of regular wide-complex tachycardias during the periarrest period and is included as a recommended antiarrhythmic agent in current ACLS guidelines for both adult and pediatric tachycardia.

Monomorphic and Polymorphic Ventricular Tachycardia

Some experts recommend that sustained monomorphic ventricular tachycardia not associated with angina, pulmonary edema, or hypotension (blood pressure less than 90 mm Hg)† be treated with amiodarone or synchronized electrical cardioversion. Other experts recommend amiodarone for control of hemodynamically stable monomorphic ventricular tachycardia†. Drug regimens including amiodarone or procainamide may be used initially† for the treatment of patients with episodes of sustained ventricular tachycardia that are associated with myocardial infarction and somewhat better tolerated hemodynamically. If IV antiarrhythmic therapy is used for ventricular fibrillation or tachycardia, it probably should be discontinued (at least temporarily) after 6–24 hours so that the patient's ongoing need for antiarrhythmic drugs can be reassessed.

Amiodarone also may be used for the treatment of polymorphic (irregular) ventricular tachycardia† associated with myocardial ischemia in the absence of QT interval prolongation. Although rare, episodes of drug-refractory sustained polymorphic ventricular tachycardia (electrical storm) have been reported in cases of acute myocardial infarction. Some experts state that these episodes should be managed by aggressive attempts at reducing myocardial ischemia†, including therapies such as an IV β-adrenergic blocking agent, IV amiodarone, left stellate ganglion blockade, intra-aortic balloon counterpulsation (IABP), or emergency revascularization (percutaneous transluminal coronary angioplasty [PTCA], coronary artery bypass graft [CABG] surgery); IV magnesium also may be used. Polymorphic ventricular tachycardia associated with QT interval prolongation usually is treated with IV magnesium sulfate.

Prevention of Ventricular Arrhythmias and Death Associated with Cardiac Arrest

Primary Prevention

Oral amiodarone has been used for primary prevention† of sustained ventricular tachycardia (i.e., ventricular tachycardia lasting greater than 30 seconds and/or associated with hemodynamic compromise), ventricular fibrillation, or sudden cardiac death in patients with nonsustained ventricular arrhythmia following myocardial infarction. Such use of the drug was once thought to prevent sudden cardiac death because ventricular premature complexes (VPCs) were believed to be harbingers of more serious ventricular arrhythmias (e.g. ventricular fibrillation or tachycardia). However, conflicting results have been reported in studies evaluating the efficacy of antiarrhythmic agents on the risk of sudden death from cardiac causes in post-myocardial infarction patients.

Results of 2 multicenter, randomized, placebo-controlled studies in patients with frequent or repetitive ventricular premature complexes (Canadian Amiodarone Myocardial Infarction Arrhythmia Trial [CAMIAT]) or with left ventricular dysfunction (European Myocardial Infarct Amiodarone Trial [EMIAT]) indicate that therapy with oral amiodarone in patients who had survived a recent myocardial infarction appeared to reduce resuscitated cardiac arrest or ventricular fibrillation or arrhythmic death but was *not* associated with reduction of total mortality after 1–2 years of follow-up. These data are consistent with results of pooled analysis of small controlled trials in patients with structural heart disease, including post-myocardial infarction patients. However, in a smaller study (Basel Antiarrhythmic Study of Infarct Survival [BASIS]) comparing amiodarone with usual care in patients with persisting asymptomatic complex arrhythmias (multiform or repetitive ventricular arrhythmias [Lown class 3 or 4b]) after acute myocardial infarction, long-term therapy with amiodarone was associated with a reduction in mortality at 1 year compared with no antiarrhythmic therapy, possibly as a result of a decreased incidence of sudden death from ventricular tachycardia and fibrillation. In addition, analysis of pooled data from several other randomized studies in patients at risk of sudden cardiac death (e.g., those with congestive heart failure or left ventricular dysfunction, recent myocardial infarction, prior cardiac arrest) suggested that amiodarone therapy may reduce total mortality by 10–19%, and such risk reduction associated with the drug may be similar in the mentioned patient populations.

Findings from the National Heart, Lung, and Blood Institute (NHLBI)'s Cardiac Arrhythmia Suppression Trial (CAST) study indicated a substantially increased rate of total mortality and nonfatal cardiac arrest in patients with recent myocardial infarction, mild to moderate left ventricular dysfunction, and asymptomatic or mildly symptomatic ventricular arrhythmias (principally frequent VPC) who received encainide or flecainide (class I antiarrhythmic drugs) compared with placebo after an average of 10 months of follow-up, which resulted in considerably modified clinicians' use of not only class IC antiarrhythmics,

but also class I antiarrhythmic agents in general, in post-myocardial infarction patients. Although it has been suggested that the applicability of the CAST results to other populations (e.g., those without recent myocardial infarction) or to predominantly class III antiarrhythmic agents such as amiodarone (a drug that has some characteristics of class IA and IC antiarrhythmic agents) is uncertain, the American College of Cardiology (ACC) and AHA state that β-adrenergic blocking agents are preferred over amiodarone for general prophylaxis. In addition, results of prospective, randomized clinical studies indicate improved survival following use of implantable cardioverter defibrillator (ICD) therapy compared with conventional drug therapy, including amiodarone, in patients with nonsustained ventricular tachycardia, reduced ejection fraction (less than 40%), and/or a history of myocardial infarction. However, preliminary reports suggest that only a small proportion of patients with a previous myocardial infarction would benefit from ICD therapy and it remains unclear whether routinely screening patients with impaired left ventricular function for prophylactic ICD therapy is clinically feasible and cost-effective.

Secondary Prevention

Amiodarone hydrochloride is used orally or IV to suppress or prevent the recurrence of documented life-threatening ventricular arrhythmias (e.g., recurrent ventricular fibrillation and recurrent, hemodynamically unstable ventricular tachycardia) that do not respond to documented adequate dosages of other currently available antiarrhythmic agents or when alternative antiarrhythmic agents cannot be tolerated. The effectiveness of IV amiodarone in suppressing recurrent ventricular fibrillation or hemodynamically unstable (destabilizing) ventricular tachycardia is supported by 2 randomized, parallel, dose-response studies of approximately 300 patients each. In patients with recurrent ventricular fibrillation or destabilizing ventricular tachycardia that was refractory to first-line (e.g., lidocaine) therapy, amiodarone produced a dose-dependent decrease in arrhythmia recurrence, although not in mortality. Patients with at least 2 episodes of ventricular fibrillation or hemodynamically unstable ventricular tachycardia within the preceding 24 hours were randomly assigned to receive IV amiodarone hydrochloride doses of 125 mg or 1 g over 24 hours; one study also evaluated a dose of 500 mg. After 48 hours, patients were eligible to receive open access to any treatment deemed necessary (including IV amiodarone) to control their arrhythmias. Amiodarone was administered in a 3-phase sequence, with an initial rapid loading infusion, followed by a slower 6-hour loading infusion, and a subsequent 18-hour maintenance infusion. Maintenance infusion was continued up through hour 48. Additional supplemental 10-minute infusions of 150 mg were administered for breakthrough arrhythmias; these occurred more frequently in patients receiving the 125-mg dosage regimen. Fewer patients receiving the 1-g IV amiodarone hydrochloride regimen required supplemental infusions. During treatment with IV amiodarone, median episodes of ventricular tachycardia or ventricular fibrillation were 0.02/hour in the group receiving the 1-g dosage regimen and 0.07/hour in the group receiving the 125-mg dosage regimen, or approximately 0.5 versus 1.7 episodes daily in patients receiving the 1-g versus 125-mg dosage regimen, respectively. In one study, the time to first episode of ventricular tachycardia or ventricular fibrillation was approximately 10 or 14 hours in patients receiving the 125- or 1000-mg amiodarone hydrochloride dosage regimens, respectively. Mortality rate was not affected by treatment in either of these studies.

Because there has been no evidence of improved survival with use of antiarrhythmic agents, including amiodarone and β-adrenergic blocking agents, whereas such evidence does exist for ICD therapy, ICDs have increasingly been used in the secondary prevention of life-threatening ventricular arrhythmias. In comparative studies, ICD therapy has been shown to be superior to antiarrhythmic drugs, principally amiodarone, for increasing overall survival of patients who had been resuscitated from near-fatal ventricular fibrillation or sustained ventricular tachycardia. Analysis of pooled data indicates that ICD therapy prolongs life by 2.1 or 4.4 months compared with amiodarone after a follow-up period of 3 or 6 years, respectively. Subgroup analysis of patients enrolled in the Antiarrhythmics Versus Implantable Defibrillators (AVID) study indicates that patients with an isolated episode of ventricular fibrillation in the absence of cerebrovascular disease or history of prior arrhythmia who have undergone revascularization or who have moderately preserved left ventricular function (i.e., left ventricular ejection fraction greater than 27%) are not likely to benefit from ICD therapy compared with amiodarone therapy. However, results of this analysis must be considered speculative because the specific criteria used in defining the subgroups were not planned prior to collection of data, and additional studies are needed to verify these findings.

Prediction of the efficacy of any antiarrhythmic agent in the long-term prevention of recurrent ventricular tachycardia and ventricular fibrillation is difficult and controversial. Many authorities currently recommend the use of ambulatory ECG monitoring, programmed electrical stimulation (PES), or a combination of both to assess patient response to amiodarone. There is no consensus on many aspects of how best to assess patient response to the drug; however, there is reasonable agreement on some aspects. If a patient with a prior history of cardiac arrest does not manifest a hemodynamically unstable arrhythmia during ECG monitoring prior to treatment, some provocative approach such as exercise or PES is required to assess the efficacy of amiodarone. The need for provocation in patients who do manifest life-threatening arrhythmias spontaneously remains to be established, although there are reasons to consider PES or other means of provocation in such patients. In patients whose PES-induced arrhythmia is made noninducible by amiodarone, the prognosis is almost uniformly excellent, with very low rates of arrhythmia recurrence or sudden death. The meaning of continued inducibility during therapy with the drug is controversial. Although not clearly established, increased difficulty of arrhythmia induction by PES and/or the ability to tolerate the induced ventricular tachycardia without severe symptoms may be useful criteria for identifying patients who may benefit from amiodarone therapy despite continued inducibility of the arrhythmia during therapy with the drug. Generally, easier inducibility or poorer tolerance of the induced arrhythmia should suggest consideration of the need to revise treatment. Other criteria for predicting the efficacy of amiodarone therapy, including complete suppression of nonsustained ventricular tachycardia determined by ambulatory ECG monitoring and the documentation of very low rates of VPCs, also have been suggested. These issues remain unsettled for amiodarone as well as for other antiarrhythmic agents. Specialized references should be consulted for additional information.

Combination Antiarrhythmic Regimens

Amiodarone has been used in combination with numerous other antiarrhythmic agents for the management of severe refractory ventricular arrhythmias; however, such combination therapy has not been evaluated in well-controlled studies and is associated with an increased risk of adverse cardiovascular effects.

Other Ventricular Arrhythmias

Amiodarone has been used with good results in a limited number of patients experiencing life-threatening ventricular arrhythmias associated with postinfarction aneurysm† or with chronic myocarditis induced by Chagas' disease.† IV amiodarone has been used with some success in a limited number of patients for the management of ventricular tachycardia and ventricular fibrillation associated with cardiac glycoside intoxication†.

● Supraventricular Tachyarrhythmias

Amiodarone appears to be effective in the suppression and prevention of various supraventricular tachycardias (SVTs)†; because of a higher risk of toxicity and proarrhythmic effects, antiarrhythmic agents generally should be reserved for patients who do not respond to or cannot be treated with AV nodal blocking agents (β-adrenergic blocking agents and nondihydropyridine calcium-channel blocking agents). Some experts state that amiodarone may be useful in situations where ventricular rate control is needed but AV nodal blocking agents are contraindicated, such as in patients with preexcited atrial arrhythmias associated with an accessory pathway†. However, IV amiodarone is potentially harmful when used for the acute treatment of patients with preexcited atrial fibrillation since it has the potential to accelerate the ventricular response and precipitate fatal arrhythmias.

Atrial Fibrillation and Flutter

Amiodarone has been used orally and IV in the management of atrial fibrillation† or flutter†.

Amiodarone is one of several antiarrhythmic agents that may be used to maintain sinus rhythm in patients with atrial fibrillation or flutter. Long-term therapy with oral amiodarone alone or in combination with other antiarrhythmic agents has been effective for suppression and prevention of refractory atrial fibrillation†. Limited data indicate that long-term amiodarone therapy may be effective in about 70% (range: 35–95%) of patients with atrial fibrillation†, including those whose arrhythmia is refractory to conventional therapy. Although not clearly established, the efficacy of amiodarone in the suppression of atrial fibrillation†

may result from the drug's ability to maintain normal sinus rhythm (probably by increasing atrial refractoriness), suppress atrial premature complexes (which may precipitate atrial fibrillation), and control ventricular rate. There is some evidence that amiodarone may be substantially more effective than sotalol or propafenone for long-term prevention of recurrent atrial fibrillation. Whether maintaining sinus rhythm in patients with recurrent atrial fibrillation will result in improved survival or a reduction in the risk of thromboembolic complications remains to be established.

Oral or IV† amiodarone may be effective for conversion of atrial fibrillation† to normal sinus rhythm (i.e., rhythm control). In current expert guidelines, amiodarone is considered a reasonable option for pharmacological conversion of atrial fibrillation; however, other antiarrhythmic agents (e.g., flecainide, dofetilide, propafenone, ibutilide) are preferred. IV amiodarone may be harmful, and therefore should not be used, in patients with Wolff-Parkinson-White (WPW) syndrome who have preexcited atrial fibrillation because the drug can accelerate ventricular rate and potentially cause life-threatening ventricular arrhythmias. Conversion of atrial fibrillation to normal sinus rhythm may be associated with embolism, particularly when atrial fibrillation has been present for more than 48 hours, unless the patient is adequately anticoagulated. (See Uses: Cardioversion of Atrial Fibrillation/Flutter, in Heparin 20:12.04.16.)

Further studies are needed to evaluate the comparative efficacy and safety of oral amiodarone, other antiarrhythmic agents, and cardioversion (direct-current countershock). Although cardioversion has been used safely and effectively following oral or IV amiodarone administration, decreased efficacy of cardioversion in patients receiving the drug has also been reported. Further studies are needed to evaluate the effect of amiodarone therapy on the efficacy of cardioversion.

Paroxysmal Supraventricular Tachycardia

Limited data suggest that IV amiodarone is effective in terminating paroxysmal supraventricular tachycardia (PSVT)†, including atrioventricular nodal reentrant tachycardia (AVNRT) and atrioventricular reentrant tachycardia (AVRT) (e.g., WPW syndrome). Some experts state that IV amiodarone may be considered for the acute treatment of hemodynamically stable patients with AVNRT when other therapies are ineffective or contraindicated. However, IV use of amiodarone can be potentially harmful in patients with preexcited atrial fibrillation because the drug may accelerate ventricular rate and cause life-threatening ventricular arrhythmias.

Long-term oral amiodarone therapy appears to be particularly effective in the suppression and prevention of paroxysmal reentrant supraventricular tachycardias† (AVNRT and AVRT [e.g., WPW syndrome]) including those refractory to other antiarrhythmic agents. Some experts state that oral amiodarone may be reasonable for ongoing management of AVNRT or AVRT in patients who are not candidates for, or prefer not to undergo, catheter ablation and in whom first-line drugs (e.g., β-adrenergic blocking agents, diltiazem, verapamil) are not effective or contraindicated. Oral amiodarone also has been effective in some patients for the suppression and prevention of atrial fibrillation or flutter associated with WPW syndrome†. Although amiodarone also has been used IV in such patients, IV use of the drug has resulted in acceleration of ventricular rate.

Atrial Tachycardia

IV amiodarone may be used for the acute treatment of patients with hemodynamically stable focal atrial tachycardia† (i.e., regular SVT arising from a localized atrial site), and oral amiodarone may be reasonable for the ongoing management of such patients.

While evidence is more limited, amiodarone also has been used in patients with multifocal atrial tachycardia† (i.e., rapid, irregular rhythm with at least 3 distinct P-wave morphologies). However, such arrhythmia is commonly associated with an underlying condition (e.g., pulmonary, coronary, or valvular heart disease) and is generally not responsive to antiarrhythmic therapy. Antiarrhythmic drug therapy usually is reserved for patients who do not respond to initial attempts at correcting or managing potential precipitating factors (e.g., exacerbation of chronic obstructive pulmonary disease or congestive heart failure, electrolyte and/or ventilatory disturbances, infection, theophylline toxicity).

Junctional Tachycardia

Amiodarone may be used for the treatment of junctional tachycardia† (i.e., nonreentrant SVT originating from the AV junction), a rapid, occasionally irregular, narrow-complex tachycardia; however, efficacy data is available only for pediatric patients. β-Adrenergic blocking agents generally are considered the drugs of choice for terminating and/or reducing the incidence of junctional tachycardia.

Bradycardia-Tachycardia Syndrome

Amiodarone has been effective in the prevention of supraventricular arrhythmias associated with bradycardia-tachycardia syndrome† in a limited number of patients; however, the drug should be used with caution in such patients, since it may depress sinoatrial node function, possibly resulting in marked bradycardia. Some clinicians recommend insertion of a temporary or permanent artificial pacemaker prior to initiation of amiodarone therapy in patients with bradycardia-tachycardia syndrome†.

● Angina

Amiodarone has been used in a limited number of patients for the management of chronic stable angina pectoris†. Limited data suggest that amiodarone is as effective as diltiazem and more effective than sublingual nitroglycerin in increasing exercise tolerance and decreasing ST-segment depression in patients with chronic stable angina pectoris†. Amiodarone also has been used with good results in some patients with Prinzmetal variant angina†. Because of the potential toxicity associated with amiodarone, the drug generally is not considered a first-line agent for the management of chronic stable angina pectoris† or Prinzmetal variant angina† but may have a beneficial antianginal effect in patients receiving the drug for the management of arrhythmias.

● Hypertrophic Cardiomyopathy

Amiodarone has been used with good results in some patients for the management of ventricular and supraventricular arrhythmias associated with hypertrophic cardiomyopathy†. In addition to its antiarrhythmic effects, the drug may also relieve symptoms and increase exercise capacity in some patients, including those whose arrhythmias are refractory to conventional treatment. Pending further accumulation of data, some clinicians recommend that treatment with amiodarone be considered only in patients with refractory hypertrophic cardiomyopathy†.

DOSAGE AND ADMINISTRATION

● Reconstitution and Administration

Amiodarone hydrochloride is administered orally or by IV infusion. Amiodarone also has been administered by intraosseous (IO) injection† in the setting of advanced cardiovascular life support (ACLS); however, there is limited experience with the drug given by this route.

Oral Administration

For the management of life-threatening ventricular arrhythmias, oral amiodarone hydrochloride usually is administered once daily. When dosages of 1 g or more daily are administered (e.g., during the loading-dose phase of therapy) or when intolerable adverse GI effects occur with once-daily dosing, it is recommended that the drug be given in divided doses (e.g., twice daily) with meals. Because food can increase the rate and extent of absorption of amiodarone, the drug should be administered in a consistent manner relative to food intake.

Patients should be advised not to stop taking amiodarone without their clinician's knowledge, even if they feel better, as their condition may worsen. If a patient misses an oral dose of amiodarone, a double dose should not be taken to make up for the missed dose; instead, the next dose should be taken at the regularly scheduled time. If additional oral doses of amiodarone are ingested, patients should seek medical attention urgently by contacting their clinician or immediately proceeding to the nearest hospital emergency department.

Extemporaneous Oral Suspension

Extemporaneous oral suspensions of amiodarone have been prepared using the tablets and a commercially available vehicle.

Standardize 4 Safety

Standardized concentrations for an extemporaneously prepared oral suspension of amiodarone have been established through Standardize 4 Safety (S4S), a national

patient safety initiative to reduce medication errors, especially during transitions of care. Multidisciplinary expert panels were convened to determine recommended standard concentrations. Because recommendations from the S4S panels may differ from the manufacturer's prescribing information, caution is advised when using concentrations that differ from labeling, particularly when using rate information from the label. For additional information on S4S (including updates that may be available), see https://www.ashp.org/pharmacy-practice/standardize-4-safety-initiative

---

TABLE 1. Standardize 4 Safety Compounded Oral Liquid Standards for Amiodarone[a]

Concentration Standards
5 mg/mL
20 mg/mL for doses of 75 mg or greater

[a] Amiodarone needs to have a pH very close to 8 to assure particle consistency.

IV Infusion

Commercially available amiodarone hydrochloride concentrate for injection containing 50 mg of the drug per mL *must* be diluted prior to administration. To produce the solution required for the first rapid loading infusion or for supplemental amiodarone infusions, 3 mL of amiodarone hydrochloride concentrate should be added to 100 mL of 5% dextrose, resulting in a final concentration of 1.5 mg/mL. To produce the solution for slow infusion and the maintenance infusion, 18 mL of amiodarone hydrochloride concentrate should be added to 500 mL of 5% dextrose, resulting in a final amiodarone concentration of 1.8 mg/mL. For subsequent maintenance infusions, solutions containing a final amiodarone hydrochloride concentration of 1–6 mg/mL may be used. Parenteral amiodarone hydrochloride solutions should be inspected visually for particulate matter whenever solution and container permit.

For IV infusion, the recommended dose of the diluted amiodarone hydrochloride solution is administered in a 3-phase sequence: a rapid loading phase, a slow loading phase, and a maintenance infusion phase. Parenteral amiodarone therapy should be used for acute antiarrhythmic therapy until the patient's cardiac rhythm is stabilized and oral therapy can be initiated. The manufacturer states that most patients will require IV therapy for 48–96 hours, but that parenteral therapy may be administered safely for longer periods of time.

Solutions containing an amiodarone hydrochloride concentration of 2 mg/mL or more should be administered via a central venous catheter, although the manufacturer states that parenteral amiodarone solutions should be administered via a central venous catheter dedicated to administration of the drug whenever possible. An in-line filter also should be used for administration of IV amiodarone hydrochloride solutions. Amiodarone hydrochloride infusions that will exceed 2 hours must be administered in glass or polyolefin bottles. (See Chemistry and Stability: Stability.) Although amiodarone hydrochloride adsorbs to polyvinyl chloride (PVC), the drug dosages used in clinical trials were designed to take this factor into account; therefore, the manufacturer recommends that solutions containing amiodarone hydrochloride injection be administered through PVC tubing. Polysorbate (Tween®) 80, a component of IV amiodarone, can cause leaching of diethylhexylphthalate (DEHP) from IV tubing, including PVC tubing. Leaching of DEHP increases at lower than recommended flow rates and at higher than recommended infusion concentrations. Therefore, the manufacturer's dosage recommendations should be followed closely.

The surface properties of solutions containing amiodarone hydrochloride injection are altered such that the drop size may be reduced. This reduction may lead to underdosage of the patient by up to 30% if drop counter infusion sets are used. Therefore, the manufacturer states that solutions containing amiodarone hydrochloride injection must be administered by a volumetric infusion pump.

Standardize 4 Safety

Standardized concentrations for IV amiodarone have been established through Standardize 4 Safety (S4S), a national patient safety initiative to reduce medication errors, especially during transitions of care. Multidisciplinary expert panels were convened to determine recommended standard concentrations. Because recommendations from the S4S panels may differ from the manufacturer's prescribing information, caution is advised when using concentrations that differ from labeling, particularly when using rate information from the label. For additional information on S4S (including updates that may be available), see https://www.ashp.org/pharmacy-practice/standardize-4-safety-initiative.

TABLE 2. Standardize 4 Safety Continuous IV Infusion Standard Concentrations for Amiodarone

Patient Population	Concentration Standards	Dosing Units
Adults	1.8 mg/mL	mg/min
Pediatric patients (<50 kg)	1.8 mg/mL	mcg/kg/min[a]
	3.6 mg/mL	

[a] Dosing units differ from concentration units

● Dosage

A uniform and optimal dosage schedule for amiodarone hydrochloride has not been established. *Amiodarone is a highly toxic drug, and the lowest effective dosage should be used to minimize the risk and occurrence of adverse effects.* Dosage of amiodarone hydrochloride must be carefully adjusted according to individual requirements and response, patient tolerance, and the general condition and cardiovascular status of the patient. Clinical and ECG monitoring of cardiac function, including appropriate ambulatory ECG monitoring (e.g., Holter monitoring) and/or programmed electrical stimulation (PES), as appropriate, is recommended during therapy with the drug. When dosage adjustment is necessary, the patient should be monitored closely for an extended period of time because of the long and variable elimination half-life of amiodarone and the difficulty in predicting the length of time required to attain a new steady-state plasma concentration of the drug. When feasible, monitoring of plasma amiodarone concentrations may be helpful in evaluating patients who are not responding to the drug or who experience unexpectedly severe toxicity. Monitoring of plasma amiodarone concentrations may also be useful in identifying patients whose concentrations are unusually low and who might benefit from an increase in dosage or those whose concentrations are unusually high in whom dosage reduction might minimize the risk of adverse effects.

Patients should be advised not to double the next dose if a dose is missed.

Although amiodarone dosage requirements generally appear to be similar in geriatric and younger adults, relatively high dosages should be used with caution in geriatric patients since they may be more susceptible to bradycardia and conduction disturbances induced by the drug. In addition, some manufacturers state that dosage in general for geriatric patients should be selected carefully, usually starting at the low end of the dosage range, because these individuals frequently have decreased hepatic, renal, and/or cardiac function and concomitant disease and drug therapy.

Life-threatening Ventricular Arrhythmias in Adults
Oral Dosage

For the management of life-threatening ventricular arrhythmias, loading doses of amiodarone hydrochloride are required to ensure an antiarrhythmic effect without waiting several months. The loading-dose phase of therapy should be performed in a hospital setting. Close monitoring of patients is necessary, especially until the risk of recurrent ventricular tachycardia or fibrillation has abated. Upon initiating amiodarone therapy in patients receiving other antiarrhythmic agents, an attempt should be made to gradually discontinue the other antiarrhythmic agents.

In adults, oral amiodarone hydrochloride loading dosages of 800–1600 mg daily generally are required for 1–3 weeks (and occasionally for longer periods of time) until an initial therapeutic response occurs. Some clinicians have used oral loading dosages exceeding 1600 mg daily or IV† loading-dose regimens. Clinicians should consult published protocols for specific information on oral loading-dose regimens using dosages greater than 1600 mg daily or on IV loading-dose regimens. If an IV loading-dose regimen is used, oral therapy should be initiated as soon as possible after an adequate response is obtained and IV amiodarone therapy gradually eliminated. If adverse effects become excessive during the

loading-dose phase of therapy, a reduction in dosage is recommended. Elimination of recurrent ventricular tachycardia and recurrent ventricular fibrillation as well as reduction in VPCs and total ventricular ectopic beats usually occur within about 1–3 weeks.

When adequate control of ventricular arrhythmias is achieved or adverse effects become prominent, the dosage of amiodarone hydrochloride should be reduced to 600–800 mg daily for about 1 month and then reduced again to the lowest effective maintenance dosage, usually 400 mg daily. Further cautious reductions in maintenance dosage (e.g., to 200 mg daily) may be possible in some patients. Adequate maintenance dosages generally range from less than 400 mg daily up to 600 mg daily. Because absorption and elimination of amiodarone are variable, adjustment of maintenance dosage is difficult, and it is not unusual to require dosage reductions or temporary withdrawal or discontinuance of the drug.

Parenteral Dosage

For the management of life-threatening ventricular arrhythmias, the recommended starting dose of IV amiodarone hydrochloride over the first 24 hours is approximately 1000 mg. The amiodarone hydrochloride dose for the first rapid loading infusion is 150 mg administered at a rate of 15 mg/minute (i.e., over 10 minutes); the initial infusion rate should not exceed 30 mg/minute. The slow loading phase of the infusion is 360 mg of amiodarone hydrochloride administered at a rate of 1 mg/minute (i.e., over 6 hours). The first maintenance phase of the infusion is 540 mg of amiodarone hydrochloride administered at a rate of 0.5 mg/minute (i.e., over 18 hours). The first 24-hour dose of amiodarone hydrochloride may be individualized for each patient; however, in controlled clinical trials, mean daily dosages exceeding 2.1 g were associated with an increased risk of hypotension.

After the first 24 hours, the maintenance infusion rate of 0.5 mg/minute (i.e., 720 mg over 24 hours) should be continued; however, the rate of the maintenance infusion may be increased to achieve effective arrhythmia suppression. In the event of breakthrough episodes of ventricular fibrillation or hemodynamically unstable ventricular tachycardia, supplemental amiodarone hydrochloride infusions of 150 mg administered at a rate of 15 mg/minute (i.e., over 10 minutes) may be given. Based on experience from clinical trials of IV amiodarone hydrochloride, a maintenance infusion of up to 0.5 mg/minute can be administered with caution for 2–3 weeks, regardless of the patient's age, renal function, or left ventricular function. The manufacturer states that there is limited experience in patients receiving parenteral amiodarone hydrochloride for longer than 3 weeks.

For cardiac arrest secondary to pulseless ventricular tachycardia or ventricular fibrillation, experts recommend an initial adult loading dose of amiodarone hydrochloride of 300 mg, given by rapid IV or IO† injection; an additional dose of 150 mg may be considered.

Supraventricular Arrhythmias in Adults

For acute treatment of supraventricular tachycardia (SVT) in adults, an IV amiodarone hydrochloride loading dose of 150 mg over 10 minutes is recommended. The drug should then be administered at a rate of 1 mg/minute for 6 hours, then 0.5 mg/minute for the remaining 18 hours or until oral dosing is initiated. For ongoing management of SVT, some experts recommend an oral amiodarone hydrochloride loading dosage of 400–600 mg daily (in divided doses) in adults for approximately 2–4 weeks, followed by a maintenance dosage of 100–200 mg daily. Clinicians should consult published protocols for specific information on oral loading-dose regimens using higher dosages.

When used for rate control of atrial fibrillation, some experts recommend an initial IV amiodarone hydrochloride dose of 300 mg over 1 hour, followed by 10–50 mg/hr over 24 hours; the usual oral maintenance dose is 100–200 mg daily.

For the long-term management of recurrent atrial fibrillation† in adults, an oral dosage regimen that includes an initial amiodarone hydrochloride loading dose of 10 mg/kg daily for 14 days, followed by 300 mg daily for 4 weeks, and then by a maintenance dosage of 200 mg daily has been used effectively to prevent recurrences.

Pediatric Dosage
Oral Dosage

Pediatric dosage of oral amiodarone hydrochloride has not been established, and dosage may vary considerably. For the management of ventricular and supraventricular arrhythmias in children†, some clinicians have recommended oral amiodarone hydrochloride loading dosages of 10–15 mg/kg daily or 600–800 mg/1.73 m² daily for approximately 4–14 days and/or until adequate control of cardiac arrhythmias is achieved or adverse effects become prominent. Dosage of the drug is then reduced to 5 mg/kg daily or 200–400 mg/1.73 m² for several weeks. If possible, dosage is then reduced gradually to the lowest effective level. Children younger than 1 year of age appear to require higher loading and maintenance dosages of amiodarone hydrochloride than older children when dosage of the drug is calculated on the basis of body weight, but not on the basis of body surface area.

Parenteral Dosage

The manufacturer states that pediatric dosage of IV amiodarone hydrochloride has not been established. For the management of refractory ventricular fibrillation or pulseless ventricular tachycardia† during pediatric resuscitation, the recommended amiodarone hydrochloride IV or IO† dose is 5 mg/kg as a rapid bolus injection. Some experts recommend that if adequate control of cardiac arrhythmia is not achieved, the dose may be repeated twice (maximum single dose of 300 mg) up to a total dosage of 15 mg/kg. If used for the management of wide-complex tachycardias or SVT in pediatric patients who are not in cardiac arrest, an IV amiodarone hydrochloride dose of 5 mg/kg is recommended (infused slowly over 20–60 minutes depending on the urgency). Alternative methods of dosing IV amiodarone hydrochloride (e.g., loading dose of 5 mg/kg given in 5 divided doses of 1 mg/kg, with each incremental dose infused over 5–10 minutes) may be considered in order to minimize pediatric exposure to the plasticizer DEHP.

Conversion from IV to Oral Dosage

Patients whose arrhythmias have been controlled successfully with IV amiodarone hydrochloride may be switched to oral therapy. The manufacturer states that since there are some differences in the safety and efficacy profiles of the oral and IV preparations of amiodarone, clinicians should review the prescribing information for oral amiodarone when switching from IV to oral therapy. The optimal dose of oral amiodarone hydrochloride will depend on the dose and duration of IV therapy, as well as the bioavailability of the oral drug. The manufacturer suggests that for patients receiving a daily dose of 720 mg of amiodarone hydrochloride IV (assuming an infusion rate of 0.5 mg/minute) for less than 1 week, 1–3 weeks, or longer than 3 weeks, the initial daily oral amiodarone hydrochloride dose should be 800–1600, 600–800, or 400 mg of the drug, respectively. These recommendations are made on the basis of a comparable total body amount of amiodarone hydrochloride delivered by IV and oral routes, taking into consideration the drug's oral bioavailability of 50%. When switching from IV to oral amiodarone hydrochloride therapy, clinical monitoring is recommended, particularly for geriatric patients.

● Dosage in Renal and Hepatic Impairment

Routine reduction of amiodarone hydrochloride dosage in patients with renal impairment does not appear to be necessary, although the risk of excessive accumulation of iodine and possible resultant thyroid effects should be considered.

The effects of hepatic impairment on the elimination of amiodarone have not been evaluated. Because the drug is extensively metabolized, probably in the liver, some clinicians caution that dosage reduction is probably warranted in patients with substantial hepatic impairment. Dosage reduction or discontinuance of amiodarone may be necessary in patients who develop evidence of hepatotoxicity during therapy with the drug.

CAUTIONS

Amiodarone is a highly toxic drug and exhibits several potentially fatal toxicities, notably pulmonary toxicity. Adverse reactions to amiodarone are common in nearly all patients receiving the drug for the treatment of ventricular arrhythmias. With relatively large dosages of amiodarone hydrochloride (400 mg or more daily), adverse reactions occur in about 75% of patients and require discontinuance of the drug in about 5–20% of patients.

The most severe reactions to oral amiodarone are pulmonary toxicity, arrhythmogenic effects, and rare, but potentially serious, liver injury; however, numerous other adverse reactions to the drug also may be clinically important.

Amiodarone-induced adverse effects are often reversible following dosage reduction and nearly always reversible following discontinuance of the drug, although adverse effects may persist for weeks or months after discontinuance of therapy because of the drug's prolonged elimination. The most common adverse reactions requiring discontinuance of oral amiodarone are pulmonary infiltrates or fibrosis, paroxysmal ventricular tachycardia, congestive heart failure, and elevations of serum hepatic enzyme concentrations. The likelihood of most adverse reactions appears to increase after the first 6 months of therapy with the drug and then remains relatively constant beyond 1 year of therapy. The most common adverse effect observed with IV amiodarone therapy in clinical trials was hypotension, which resulted in discontinuation of therapy in less than 2% of patients. Additional experience with amiodarone is needed to more fully characterize the adverse effect profile of the drug, particularly in relation to duration of therapy and dosage.

● Pulmonary Effects

Pulmonary toxicity, which is potentially fatal, is the most severe adverse effect associated with oral amiodarone therapy with or without initial IV therapy. Acute-onset (days to weeks) pulmonary toxicity has been reported during postmarketing experience; manifestations include radiographic evidence of pulmonary infiltrates and/or mass, pulmonary alveolar hemorrhage, pleural effusion, bronchospasm, wheezing, fever, dyspnea, cough, hemoptysis, hypoxia, or adult respiratory distress syndrome (ARDS), sometimes leading to respiratory failure and/or death.

Amiodarone-induced pulmonary toxicity may result from pulmonary interstitial pneumonitis (or alveolitis) or from hypersensitivity pneumonitis (e.g., eosinophilic pneumonia). Clinically apparent interstitial pneumonitis (or alveolitis), hypersensitivity pneumonitis, and pulmonary fibrosis have occurred in up to 10–17% of patients with ventricular arrhythmias receiving amiodarone hydrochloride therapy at oral dosages of about 400 mg daily, and an abnormal diffusion capacity without symptoms occurs in a much higher percentage of patients. Only one patient in clinical trials of IV amiodarone therapy developed pulmonary fibrosis; in this patient, the condition was diagnosed 3 months after IV therapy, during which time the patient had begun treatment with oral amiodarone. Amiodarone-induced pulmonary toxicity has been fatal in about 10% of cases. Rarely, amiodarone has been associated with exacerbation of bronchial asthma, possibly because of its antiadrenergic effects. Hemoptysis has been reported during postmarketing experience.

Amiodarone pneumonitis is a clinical syndrome consisting of progressive dyspnea and cough accompanied by functional, radiographic, scintigraphic, and pathological data consistent with pulmonary toxicity. The clinical course of pulmonary toxicity appears to be quite variable. Although a slow, progressive course is often described, an abrupt onset of febrile illness resembling infectious illness (e.g., pneumonia) also may occur. Early symptoms may include dyspnea (particularly with exertion), cough (generally without sputum production), fever or chills, chest pain (generally pleuritic), malaise, weakness, fatigue, myalgia, myopathy, nausea, anorexia, and/or weight loss. Bronchiolitis obliterans organizing pneumonia (that may be fatal) and pleuritis have been reported during postmarketing experience.

The overall incidence of amiodarone-induced pulmonary toxicity has generally been reported to range from about 2–7%, but some studies indicate that pulmonary toxicity may occur in about 10–17% of patients receiving the drug orally. Adult respiratory distress syndrome (ARDS) and lung edema were reported in 2% and less than 2%, respectively, of patients receiving IV amiodarone therapy. Limited evidence suggests that the incidence may increase with duration of therapy, total daily dose, age of the patient, and cumulative dose. However, pulmonary toxicity has been reported during postmarketing experience in patients receiving low dosages. Although not clearly established, limited data suggest that patients with evidence of pulmonary disease prior to amiodarone therapy may have an increased risk of amiodarone-induced pulmonary toxicity, although there may be a bias toward detection in such patients. Some clinicians state, however, that preexisting pulmonary disease does not appear to increase the risk of amiodarone-induced pulmonary toxicity; however, these patients have a poorer prognosis than patients without preexisting pulmonary disease if toxicity develops. The syndrome is usually reversible following discontinuance of the drug (with or without corticosteroid therapy), but pulmonary toxicity may be fatal in some patients.

Hypersensitivity pneumonitis has been reported in about one-third of patients with amiodarone-induced pulmonary toxicity, and may occur earlier during amiodarone therapy than interstitial pneumonitis. Hypersensitivity pneumonitis does not appear to be dose related and may be characterized by acute onset of symptoms (e.g., fever). Alveolar infiltrates appear to be the most common radiographic findings in patients with amiodarone-induced hypersensitivity pneumonitis; increased suppressor/cytotoxic ($CD8^+$, $T8^+$) T cells and neutrophils often are found in the bronchoalveolar lavage of these patients. It is not known whether fatalities secondary to amiodarone-induced hypersensitivity pneumonitis occur more frequently than fatalities secondary to other pulmonary toxicity induced the drug. The precise mechanism of amiodarone-induced hypersensitivity pneumonitis, including the possible role of immunoglobulins, complement deposition, and cytokines in the development of pulmonary toxicity, remains to be more fully elucidated.

Physical findings in patients with amiodarone interstitial pneumonitis (alveolitis) may include rales, decreased breath sounds, and/or a pleuritic friction rub. Laboratory abnormalities may include hypoxemia, hypercarbia, leukocytosis, and elevated erythrocyte sedimentation rate. Diffuse interstitial infiltrates appear to be the most common radiographic finding in patients with amiodarone-induced pulmonary toxicity; however, airspace opacities (particularly patchy, peripheral alveolar infiltrates), well-localized infiltrates, and mixed interstitial and airspace disease patterns have also been reported.

Microscopic tissue changes in patients with amiodarone pneumonitis appear to be nonspecific but generally are consistent. Pathologic changes may include accumulation of foamy macrophages in alveolar spaces (the presence of lamellated cytoplasmic inclusions probably causes their foamy appearance), hyperplasia of type II pneumocytes, and thickening of the alveolar septal membrane by connective tissue. Although lamellated cytoplasmic inclusions appear to occur predominantly in macrophages, they may also occur in epithelial cells of respiratory bronchioles, type II pneumocytes, endothelial cells, and interstitial cells. Interstitial thickening secondary to an infiltrate of lymphocytes, histiocytes, and occasional plasma cells may also occur. Because foamy alveolar macrophages and lamellated cytoplasmic inclusions have been reported in approximately 50% of patients receiving amiodarone without clinical evidence of pulmonary toxicity, these pathologic changes alone should not be relied on in the diagnosis of amiodarone pneumonitis.

Pulmonary function tests most commonly reveal impairment of diffusion capacity, but reductions of total lung capacity (TLC) and forced vital capacity (FVC) may also occur. Limited data suggest that pulmonary function testing is neither sensitive nor specific enough to be the only method employed in monitoring for amiodarone-induced pulmonary toxicity.

Patients receiving amiodarone should be carefully monitored for the development of pulmonary toxicity. If hypersensitivity pneumonitis occurs, corticosteroid therapy should be initiated and amiodarone discontinued. Rechallenge with the drug in patients with hypersensitivity pneumonitis results in more rapid and more severe adverse effects. If interstitial pneumonitis (alveolitis) occurs, dosage reduction and preferably discontinuance of the drug is necessary, especially in patients in whom other acceptable antiarrhythmic therapies are available. Following dosage reduction or discontinuance of amiodarone in patients with interstitial pneumonitis, clinical improvement usually is evident within the first week and is maximal after 2 or 3 weeks; radiographic abnormalities usually resolve within 2–4 months. In some patients with interstitial pneumonitis, rechallenge with a lower dosage of amiodarone has not resulted in recurrence of pulmonary toxicity; however, in some patients (e.g., those with severe alveolar damage), pulmonary lesions have been irreversible. Treatment of amiodarone pneumonitis is mainly supportive and may include mechanical ventilation, if necessary. Although data from uncontrolled studies suggest that corticosteroid therapy is of some benefit, controlled studies are needed to fully evaluate the safety and efficacy of corticosteroids in the management of amiodarone-induced pulmonary toxicity. Some patients have received prednisone dosages of 40–60 mg daily, which were tapered in small decrements during several weeks, depending on the patient's condition.

Adult respiratory distress syndrome (ARDS) has occurred occasionally following cardiothoracic or other surgery in patients with or without preexisting amiodarone-induced pulmonary toxicity. A causal relationship between ARDS and amiodarone has not been clearly established, and other factors (e.g., prolonged pump-oxygenator time, oxygen toxicity, anesthetic agents) may have contributed to the development of the syndrome. Although patients usually have responded to vigorous respiratory therapy, fatalities have occurred rarely. Some manufacturers state that forced inspiratory oxygen (FiO_2) and determinants of tissue oxygenation (e.g., arterial oxygen saturation [SaO_2], arterial oxygen pressure [PaO_2]) should be monitored closely.

● Hepatic Effects

Abnormalities of liver function test results have generally been reported in about 3–20% of patients receiving amiodarone, although the incidence has been as high as 40–55% in some studies. Nonspecific hepatic disorders have occurred in about 1–3% of patients.

Amiodarone-induced elevations in serum AST (SGOT), ALT (SGPT), γ-glutamyltransferase (GGT, γ-glutamyltranspeptidase, GGTP), and alkaline phosphatase concentrations usually are minor, not accompanied by clinical symptoms, and generally return to normal following dosage reduction or discontinuance of the drug. Rarely, severe hepatic injury (i.e., clinical hepatitis, cholestatic hepatitis, hepatocellular necrosis, cirrhosis), which has been fatal in some patients (including at least one child), has occurred. Signs and symptoms of amiodarone-induced hepatotoxicity may include hepatomegaly, ascites, abdominal pain, nausea, vomiting, anorexia, and weight loss. Hypoalbuminemia, hyperbilirubinemia, and hyperammonemia have also been reported.

Liver biopsies performed in a limited number of patients with amiodarone-induced hepatic dysfunction have revealed histologic changes resembling alcoholic hepatitis or cirrhosis. Microscopic tissue changes may include Mallory bodies within hepatocytes, mixed inflammatory infiltrates, collagen deposits and/or fibrosis, steatosis, hepatocyte destruction, and/or cholangitis. Electron microscopic studies have revealed the presence of phospholipid-laden lysosomal inclusions within hepatocytes, bile duct epithelium, Kupffer cells, and endothelial cells, even in the absence of clinically apparent hepatic disease. Although the exact mechanism of amiodarone-induced hepatic injury has not been determined, limited evidence suggests that the drug may form amiodarone-phospholipid complexes within lysosomes, resulting in phospholipidosis. Acute centrolobular confluent hepatocellular necrosis, leading to hepatic coma, acute renal failure, and death, has been associated with administration of IV amiodarone at a much higher loading dose concentration and more rapid infusion rate than recommended.

Serum hepatic enzyme concentrations should be monitored in patients receiving amiodarone. Persistent elevations in enzyme concentrations or the development of hepatomegaly may necessitate dosage reduction or discontinuance of the drug.

● Arrhythmogenic Effects

Like other antiarrhythmic agents, amiodarone can worsen existing arrhythmias or cause new arrhythmias. Arrhythmogenic effects associated with amiodarone have occurred in approximately 2–5% of patients and have included progression of ventricular tachycardia to ventricular fibrillation, sustained ventricular tachycardia, increased resistance to cardioversion, atrial fibrillation, nodal arrhythmia, and atypical ventricular tachycardia (torsades de pointes). Transient exacerbation of preexisting cardiac arrhythmias with subsequent control during continued therapy has also been reported. Prolongation of the QT interval was reported in less than 2% of patients receiving IV amiodarone. Acceleration of ventricular rate was reported in a patient receiving IV amiodarone for the treatment of atrial fibrillation associated with Wolff-Parkinson-White syndrome. In most cases, amiodarone-induced arrhythmogenic effects should be manageable in the proper clinical setting.

Arrhythmogenic effects do not appear to occur more frequently with amiodarone than with other antiarrhythmic agents; however, such effects may be prolonged if they occur. Concomitant use of cardiac glycosides and/or other antiarrhythmic agents may increase the risk of arrhythmogenic effects during amiodarone therapy. Limited data suggest that hypokalemia may increase the risk of amiodarone-induced atypical ventricular tachycardia.

Chronic administration of antiarrhythmic drugs (e.g., amiodarone) in patients with an implanted cardiac device (e.g., defibrillator, pacemaker) may affect pacing and/or defibrillating thresholds. Therefore, the manufacturer recommends that pacing and defibrillation thresholds should be assessed at the inception of and during amiodarone therapy.

● Nervous System Effects

Adverse nervous system effects occur in approximately 20–40% of patients receiving oral amiodarone. Amiodarone-induced nervous system effects may be alleviated by dosage reduction and rarely require discontinuance of the drug.

Malaise and fatigue, tremor and/or involuntary movements, lack of coordination, abnormal gait and/or ataxia, dizziness, and paresthesia occur in about

4–9% of patients. Other adverse nervous system effects occurring in about 1–3% of patients receiving the drug include abnormal smell, insomnia, sleep disturbances, headache, and decreased libido. Adverse nervous system effects occurring less frequently include difficulty in handwriting, postural instability, dyskinetic movements, decreased ability to concentrate, confusion, memory loss, and mood lability. Delirium, hallucination, confusional state, disorientation, and parkinsonian symptoms (e.g., akinesia, bradykinesia) have been reported during postmarketing experience.

Peripheral neuropathy, demyelinating polyneuropathy, and proximal myopathy have been reported rarely in patients receiving amiodarone. Although not fully established, these adverse effects may be dose related. Amiodarone-induced peripheral neuropathy, which occurs rarely during chronic oral administration of the drug, is usually symmetrical and involves all four limbs; the neurologic deficit is usually more marked in the lower limbs than in the upper limbs. Signs and symptoms may include distal sensory loss, sensory ataxia, loss of vibratory sensation, paresthesia, and/or decreased tendon reflexes. Proximal muscle weakness also may be present. Nerve biopsies in patients with amiodarone-induced peripheral neuropathy have demonstrated complete loss of large myelinated fibers, marked reduction of small myelinated and unmyelinated axons, and evidence of lysosomal inclusion bodies within Schwann cells. Nerve conduction studies have demonstrated normal or reduced nerve conduction velocities. Although the mechanism(s) of amiodarone-induced peripheral neuropathy has not been fully determined, the mechanism may involve formation of drug-phospholipid complexes within neurons. Peripheral neuropathy and proximal myopathy generally are slowly reversible following dosage reduction or discontinuance of the drug, although resolution of peripheral neuropathy has been incomplete.

Amiodarone-induced tremor generally presents as a fine hand tremor that is clinically indistinguishable from essential tremor; the tremor may be more prominent on one side of the body than the other. Amiodarone has also reportedly exacerbated preexisting tremor or parkinsonian tremor in some patients. Although limited data suggest that cautious use of propranolol may be of some benefit in the management of amiodarone-induced tremor, further study is needed.

Pseudotumor cerebri (with papilledema) has been reported rarely during postmarketing experience in patients receiving amiodarone. Although a causal relationship has not been established, chronic anxiety reactions have also occurred during therapy with the drug.

● Thyroid Effects

Thyroid nodules or thyroid cancer, sometimes accompanied by hyperthyroidism, has been reported during postmarketing experience.

Amiodarone alters thyroid function test results in many patients and thyroid function in some patients. Because amiodarone appears to partially inhibit the peripheral conversion of thyroxine (T_4) to triiodothyronine (T_3), serum T_4 and reverse triiodothyronine (reverse T_3, rT_3) concentrations may be increased and serum T_3 concentrations may be decreased. Most patients remain clinically euthyroid despite these changes in serum thyroid hormone concentrations; however, clinical hypothyroidism or hyperthyroidism may occur, and thyroid function should therefore be monitored in patients receiving amiodarone. Geriatric patients and/or patients with a history of thyroid dysfunction (e.g., goiter, hypothyroidism, hyperthyroidism, thyroid nodules) may be more likely to develop adverse thyroid effects while receiving the drug. Because of the slow elimination of amiodarone and its metabolites from the body, increased plasma iodide concentration, alterations in thyroid function, and/or abnormal thyroid function test results may persist for several weeks or months following discontinuance of the drug.

Amiodarone-induced increases in serum T_4 and rT_3 concentrations with normal or decreased serum T_3 concentrations often occur in patients receiving amiodarone and generally are not accompanied by clinical evidence of thyroid dysfunction. Such changes may be referred to as "euthyroid hyperthyroxinemia" and generally do not require specific treatment. Periodic monitoring of thyroid function tests, including serum T_3, T_4, and thyrotropin (thyroid-stimulating hormone, TSH) concentrations, is recommended in these patients.

Amiodarone-induced hypothyroidism has been reported in about 2–4% of patients receiving oral drug therapy in most clinical studies, although this effect has occurred more frequently (8–10%) in some patient series. Although not clearly established, limited data suggest that hypothyroidism may be more likely to occur in females and in patients with a prior history of thyroid dysfunction. The clinical manifestations of hypothyroidism associated with amiodarone appear to be the same as those occurring in primary idiopathic hypothyroidism.

Amiodarone-induced hypothyroidism is probably best detected by monitoring for the signs and symptoms of hypothyroidism and for an elevation in serum thyrotropin concentration, a decrease in serum T_3 concentration, and/or a decrease or no change in free serum T_4 concentration compared with baseline values.

Hypothyroidism induced by amiodarone may be managed by reduction in amiodarone dosage and/or careful supplementation with thyroid agents (e.g., levothyroxine sodium) if necessary. Some clinicians have recommended cautious titration of levothyroxine sodium until serum T_4 concentrations, but not serum thyrotropin concentrations, are within the normal range. Thyroid agents must be administered with extreme caution, however, in patients with angina pectoris or cardiovascular disease; if chest pain or aggravation of cardiovascular disease occurs, dosage of the thyroid agent should be reduced or the thyroid agent discontinued. Amiodarone-induced hypothyroidism may require discontinuance of the drug in some patients and appears to regress slowly once the drug is discontinued, usually over a period of 2–3 months.

Amiodarone-induced hyperthyroidism occurs in approximately 2% of patients receiving the drug orally and may require dosage reduction or discontinuance of amiodarone therapy. Hyperthyroidism may occur more frequently in geographic areas where iodine intake is relatively low. Hyperthyroidism may occur 3 or more months following discontinuance of amiodarone therapy. Hyperthyroidism associated with amiodarone therapy generally is more difficult to diagnose and manage and more poorly tolerated than hypothyroidism. Amiodarone-associated hyperthyroidism can be fatal. The clinical manifestations of amiodarone-induced hyperthyroidism may include weight loss, anxiety, tremor, heat intolerance, thyrotoxicosis, and breakthrough arrhythmias or exacerbation of cardiac arrhythmias. Patients receiving the drug should contact their physician if exacerbation of angina or recurrence of cardiac arrhythmias occurs after an initial apparent response to therapy, even several months after discontinuing the drug, since these signs may suggest the presence of amiodarone-induced hyperthyroidism. Hyperthyroidism is probably best detected by monitoring for signs and symptoms associated with hyperthyroidism and by monitoring for elevations in serum T_3 concentrations, elevations in serum T_4 concentrations, or subnormal serum thyrotropin concentrations. A thyrotropin-releasing hormone (protirelin) stimulation test may be performed in patients with suspected hyperthyroidism to confirm diagnosis in equivocal cases, although the availability of sensitive assays for serum thyrotropin concentrations has virtually eliminated the need for such a test. Secretion of thyrotropin, induced by exogenous administration of synthetic thyrotropin-releasing hormone (protirelin), is flat or blunted in such patients.

Because clinical manifestations of hyperthyroidism (i.e., cardiac arrhythmias) may be potentially serious in patients receiving amiodarone, aggressive therapy is indicated including dosage reduction or discontinuance of amiodarone, if necessary. Conventional antithyroid agents (e.g., methimazole, propylthiouracil) have been recommended for the management of amiodarone-induced hyperthyroidism; however, these agents appear to be of limited benefit when used alone, since the intrathyroidal thyroglobulin stores generally are fully iodinated in patients receiving long-term amiodarone therapy. High intrathyroidal iodine stores antagonize the inhibitory effects of antithyroid drugs on thyroidal iodine utilization. Combination therapy with methimazole and potassium perchlorate has been used with good results in a limited number of patients with hyperthyroidism and evidence of goiter. The use of β-adrenergic blocking agents (e.g., propranolol) and/or corticosteroids may be of some benefit in the management of hyperthyroidism associated with amiodarone therapy. Radioactive iodine therapy is contraindicated in patients with amiodarone-associated hyperthyroidism because of the low radioiodine uptake due to the high concentrations of circulating iodine from amiodarone therapy and the large intrathyroidal iodine load. In patients in whom aggressive treatment of thyrotoxicosis has failed or amiodarone cannot be discontinued because it is the only drug effective against the resistant arrhythmia, surgical management may be an option. Experience with thyroidectomy as a treatment for amiodarone-induced thyrotoxicosis is limited and could induce thyroid storm. Therefore, careful surgical and anesthetic management is required. Transient hypothyroidism occasionally may occur following resolution of amiodarone-induced hyperthyroidism. Further studies are needed to determine the optimum management of hyperthyroidism in patients receiving amiodarone.

● GI Effects

Adverse GI effects, principally nausea, vomiting, constipation, and anorexia, occur in about 25% of patients receiving amiodarone orally but only rarely necessitate discontinuance of the drug. Amiodarone-induced GI disturbances occur most commonly during administration of relatively large oral dosages of the drug (e.g., loading doses) and usually are alleviated by dosage reduction or administration in divided doses with meals.

Nausea and vomiting occur in about 10–33% of patients receiving oral amiodarone; nausea and vomiting occur in approximately 4% and less than 2% of patients receiving IV amiodarone, respectively. Constipation and anorexia have occurred in about 4–9% of patients, and abdominal pain, abnormal salivation, and abnormal taste have occurred in about 1–3% of patients. Epigastric burning or fullness and diarrhea have been reported rarely in patients receiving oral amiodarone; however, a causal relationship to the drug has not been established. Diarrhea has been reported in less than 2% of patients receiving the drug IV. Pancreatitis has been reported during postmarketing experience.

● **Ocular Effects**

Asymptomatic corneal microdeposits are present in practically all adults who receive oral amiodarone for longer than 6 months. These corneal deposits generally are detectable only by slit-lamp ophthalmologic examination and usually are not associated with visual disturbances; however, subjective visual disturbances including halo vision (particularly at night and/or while looking at bright objects), blurred vision, photophobia, and dry eyes may occur in up to 10% of patients receiving the drug.

The development of amiodarone-induced corneal deposits appears to be related to both dosage and duration of therapy. Limited data suggest that more extensive deposits occur in patients receiving amiodarone hydrochloride dosages of 400–1400 mg daily than in patients receiving dosages of 100–200 mg daily. The corneal deposits generally develop within 1–4 months but have occurred as soon as a few weeks after beginning therapy with the drug. Amiodarone keratopathy appears to occur rarely in pediatric patients, possibly because of greater lacrimal secretion and more rapid lacrimal circulation in children than in adults.

Corneal microdeposits generally occur bilaterally and symmetrically. Slit-lamp examination during the early stage of amiodarone keratopathy usually demonstrates fine, punctate, gray to golden brown opacities in a horizontal, linear pattern in the inferior cornea; these deposits then progress gradually into a characteristic, whorl-like pattern with continued therapy. Although the mechanism of amiodarone-induced keratopathy is not known, the presence of complex lipid deposits within lysosome-like intracytoplasmic inclusions suggests possible deposition of amiodarone-phospholipid complexes or lipofuscin within corneal epithelium as well as other epithelial structures of the eye. Corneal microdeposits and visual disturbances are reversible following dosage reduction or discontinuance of amiodarone, usually within about 3 months (range: 2–7 months). Methylcellulose ophthalmic solutions have been used in patients receiving amiodarone in an attempt to decrease the severity of existing microdeposits and progression of the keratopathy, but the efficacy of such therapy has not been established. The presence of asymptomatic corneal microdeposits does *not* necessitate dosage reduction or withdrawal of amiodarone. If severe and/or persistent visual disturbances occur, they may subside with dosage reduction if continued amiodarone therapy is considered necessary.

Optic neuropathy and/or optic neuritis, which may occur at any time following initiation of amiodarone therapy and usually results in visual impairment, has been reported in patients receiving amiodarone. In some patients, such visual impairment has progressed to permanent blindness. Diplopia, nystagmus, and itching of the eyes have been reported rarely. In addition, papilledema, corneal degeneration, scotoma, lens opacities, ocular discomfort, and macular degeneration have been reported in patients receiving amiodarone therapy. Visual disturbances infrequently impair visual acuity to a substantial degree and rarely require discontinuance of the drug.

● **Local, Dermatologic, and Sensitivity Reactions**

Local injection-site reactions (i.e., pain, erythema, edema, pigment changes, phlebitis, cellulitis, necrosis, skin sloughing) have been reported during postmarketing experience in patients receiving IV injection of amiodarone in recommended dosages.

Adverse dermatologic reactions occur in about 15% of patients receiving oral amiodarone. The most common adverse dermatologic effect associated with amiodarone is photosensitivity, which occurs in about 10% of patients but usually does not require discontinuance of the drug. When photosensitivity occurs, it generally begins within 2 hours of exposure to sunlight, and symptoms may consist of a burning or tingling sensation followed by erythema; blistering

occurs infrequently. Swelling of sunlight-exposed areas has been reported rarely. Amiodarone-induced photosensitivity reactions generally last for 1–3 days, but may last as long as a week in severe cases. Photosensitivity reactions may occur up to 4 months following discontinuance of the drug. Enhanced tanning ability has also been reported in some patients receiving the drug.

Since exposure to visible light (wavelengths longer than 400 nm) and/or ultraviolet (UV) wavelengths near the visible spectrum (longer than 320 nm) has resulted in photosensitivity reactions in patients receiving amiodarone, both sunlight and light transmitted through window glass may potentially induce photosensitivity reactions in patients receiving the drug. Sunscreen agents may help to at least partially prevent amiodarone-induced photosensitivity reactions, particularly opaque physical sunscreens (i.e., agents containing zinc oxide, titanium dioxide) and chemical sunscreens that absorb longer UV light wavelengths (i.e., dioxybenzone, oxybenzone). Protective clothing and avoidance of exposure to sunlight are also recommended to at least partially prevent photosensitivity reactions. Although administration of pyridoxine hydrochloride has been recommended for the prevention of photosensitivity in patients receiving amiodarone, in vitro data and data from clinical use suggest that pyridoxine does not prevent and possibly may worsen amiodarone-induced photosensitivity reactions. Reduction in amiodarone dosage may partially alleviate photosensitivity reactions in some patients.

Long-term administration of amiodarone is associated with pigment deposition resulting in a blue-gray discoloration of the skin. The manufacturer states that blue-gray skin pigmentation occurred in less than 1% of patients who had received the drug for an average of about 440 days (range: 2–1515 days); however, in clinical studies, blue-gray skin pigmentation was reported in approximately 2–5% of patients. The incidence appears to be related to both the cumulative dosage and duration of therapy. Pigmentary changes of the skin generally are restricted to exposed areas of the body, particularly the face and hands, and may be mistaken for cyanosis. Exposure to sunlight or visible light and fairness of complexion appear to be risk factors. Although not clearly established, limited data suggest that photosensitivity reactions may predispose to the development of blue-gray pigmentation. The mechanism(s) of amiodarone-induced blue-gray discoloration is not known; however, histologic examination in a limited number of patients has revealed lysosomal, membrane-bound bodies containing amiodarone, *N*-desethylamiodarone, lipids, and possibly lipofuscin. Blue-gray pigmentation is of cosmetic importance only. The pigmentation usually is slowly reversible following discontinuance of the drug, although this may require up to a year in some cases. Occasionally, the pigmentation may not be completely reversible. Skin cancer has been reported during postmarketing experience with amiodarone.

Rash and hair loss have been reported in less than 1% of patients receiving oral amiodarone. Toxic epidermal necrolysis (sometimes fatal) and generalized pustular psoriasis also have been reported in patients receiving amiodarone. Exfoliative dermatitis and erythema multiforme also have been reported. Stevens-Johnson syndrome has been reported in less than 2% of patients receiving the drug IV and also has been reported during postmarketing experience with amiodarone. Pruritus has been reported during postmarketing experience with amiodarone.

Angioedema, urticaria, eczema, or bronchospasm has been reported during postmarketing experience with amiodarone therapy; anaphylactic/anaphylactoid reactions, including shock, also have been reported during postmarketing experience in patients receiving amiodarone.

Granuloma has been reported through postmarketing experience in patients receiving amiodarone.

● **Cardiovascular Effects**

New or worsened heart failure reportedly occurs in about 3% or about 2% of patients receiving oral or IV amiodarone therapy, respectively; however, it is often difficult to distinguish between spontaneous and amiodarone-induced depression of left ventricular function. Congestive heart failure rarely requires discontinuance of the drug.

Hypotension was the most frequent adverse effect observed in clinical trials of IV amiodarone, occurring in approximately 16% of patients. Hypotension has occurred in less than 1% of patients receiving oral amiodarone. Hypotension refractory to treatment and resulting in death has been reported during postmarketing experience with IV amiodarone. The relationship to amiodarone is not known, but hypotension (probably resulting from decreased cardiac output and/or decreased peripheral vascular resistance) has occurred rarely during open-heart surgery (during and/or following cardiopulmonary bypass) in patients receiving the drug. An interaction between amiodarone and various anesthetic agents has been suggested but not clearly established. Some manufacturers and clinicians state that close perioperative monitoring is recommended in amiodarone-treated patients undergoing general anesthesia, since amiodarone may sensitize patients to the myocardial depressant and conduction effects of halogenated hydrocarbon general anesthetics.

Flushing and edema have occurred in about 1–3% of patients receiving oral amiodarone. In patients receiving IV amiodarone, cardiac arrest and shock have been reported in 2.9% and less than 2% of patients, respectively; asystole also has been reported. Venous thrombosis and thrombophlebitis have been reported with IV amiodarone during postmarketing experience.

● Effects on Cardiac Conduction and Sinus Node Function

Clinically important conduction disturbances, mainly AV and intraventricular block, occur infrequently in patients receiving amiodarone and are reversible following discontinuance of the drug. Sinoatrial block has also been reported. Rarely, amiodarone-induced QT prolongation has been associated with arrhythmogenicity.

Amiodarone generally depresses sinus node function. SA node dysfunction, including symptomatic sinus bradycardia or sinus arrest with suppression of escape foci, has occurred in approximately 1–5% of patients. Concomitant administration of a cardiac glycoside, β-adrenergic blocking agent, and/or calcium-channel blocking agent may increase the risk of sinus bradyarrhythmias. The relationship to amiodarone is not known, but atropine-resistant sinus bradycardia, sinus arrest, and/or AV block have also occurred in some amiodarone-treated patients undergoing general anesthesia, mainly for open-heart surgery. Patients with preexisting sinus bradycardia or sinus node disease may have an increased risk of amiodarone-induced sinus bradyarrhythmias. Sinus bradycardia induced by amiodarone generally is not fully responsive to atropine.Bradycardia usually responds to dosage reduction, but administration of a β-adrenergic agonist (e.g., isoproterenol) and/or insertion of an artificial ventricular pacemaker may be necessary in patients with severe amiodarone-induced sinus bradyarrhythmias; amiodarone has been discontinued in several patients because of bradycardia.

● Hematologic Effects

Coagulation abnormalities have occurred in about 1–3% of patients receiving oral amiodarone, and spontaneous ecchymosis has occurred in less than 1% of patients receiving the drug. Severe thrombocytopenia, resulting in ecchymoses and petechiae, has occurred in a few patients receiving the drug. Following discontinuance of amiodarone and initiation of corticosteroid therapy, platelet counts gradually increased to normal values over a period of 12–16 days; subsequent administration of the drug resulted in recurrence of thrombocytopenia. Thrombocytopenia has been reported in less than 2% of patients receiving IV amiodarone. Although not clearly established, positive lymphocyte stimulation test results suggest that a delayed hypersensitivity reaction may be responsible for the thrombocytopenia. Hemolytic anemia, aplastic anemia, pancytopenia, agranulocytosis, and neutropenia have been reported during postmarketing experience in patients receiving amiodarone.

● Other Adverse Effects

Noninfectious epididymitis or epididymo-orchitis and/or scrotal pain have occurred in some patients receiving high oral dosages of amiodarone and/or long-term therapy with the drug. In patients who developed epididymitis, epididymal enlargement initially occurred unilaterally but later progressed bilaterally. Epididymitis subsided in some patients with reduction of amiodarone dosage but resolved in other patients despite continued therapy without dosage adjustment. Abnormal kidney function has been reported in less than 2% of patients receiving the drug IV. Renal insufficiency/impairment or acute renal failure has been reported with IV amiodarone during postmarketing experience. Impotence also has been reported during postmarketing experience with amiodarone therapy.

Gynecomastia, which was reversible following withdrawal of amiodarone but recurred upon rechallenge, has been reported. Hyperglycemia, symptomatic hypoglycemia, and vasculitis have been reported rarely. Myopathy, rhabdomyolysis, and muscle weakness have been reported during postmarketing experience in patients receiving amiodarone. Syndrome of inappropriate antidiuretic hormone secretion (SIADH) has been reported during postmarketing experience in patients receiving amiodarone therapy.

Symptomatic bradycardia, sometimes requiring pacemaker intervention, has been reported in patients receiving amiodarone concomitantly with a hepatitis C virus (HCV) treatment regimen containing sofosbuvir in conjunction with another HCV direct-acting antiviral (DAA), including ledipasvir, simeprevir, or daclatasvir. Fatal cardiac arrest was reported in a patient receiving amiodarone concomitantly with the fixed combination containing ledipasvir and sofosbuvir (ledipasvir/sofosbuvir). In most reported cases, bradycardia occurred within hours to days after HCV treatment containing sofosbuvir with another DAA was initiated in patients receiving amiodarone, but has been observed up to 2 weeks after initiation of such HCV treatment regimens in patients receiving amiodarone. Bradycardia generally resolved after the HCV treatment regimen was discontinued. The mechanism for this adverse cardiovascular effect is unknown. Patients who may be at increased risk for symptomatic bradycardia if amiodarone is used concomitantly with an HCV treatment regimen containing sofosbuvir and another DAA include those also receiving a β-adrenergic blocking agent, those with underlying cardiac comorbidities, and/or those with advanced liver disease. Because of these reports of symptomatic bradycardia, concomitant use of amiodarone with an HCV treatment regimen containing sofosbuvir with another DAA (e.g., ledipasvir, simeprevir, daclatasvir) is not recommended.

● Precautions and Contraindications

Patients should be instructed to read the medication guide provided by the manufacturer before initiating therapy with amiodarone and each time the prescription is refilled, since new information may be available.

Amiodarone is a highly toxic drug and exhibits several potentially fatal toxicities, notably pulmonary toxicity. Because of its pharmacokinetic properties, difficult dosing schedule, and severity of adverse effects in patients who are improperly monitored, amiodarone should be administered only by clinicians who are experienced in the management of life-threatening arrhythmias, who are thoroughly familiar with the risks and benefits associated with amiodarone therapy, and who have access to laboratory facilities necessary to adequately monitor the efficacy and adverse effects of the drug, including continuous ECG monitoring and electrophysiologic techniques for evaluating the patient in both ambulatory and hospital settings. Because of the risks of substantial toxicity, amiodarone therapy currently is reserved principally for the management of documented life-threatening ventricular arrhythmias. Even in patients at high risk of death from arrhythmia, in whom the risks of toxicity are acceptable, use of amiodarone poses major management difficulties that could be life-threatening in a patient population at risk of sudden death, and maximum efforts should be made to utilize alternative antiarrhythmic agents initially.

Because of the life-threatening nature of the arrhythmias treated, lack of a predictable time course of antiarrhythmic effect, and the risks of arrhythmogenic effects and potential interactions with previous drug therapy, the loading-dose phase of oral amiodarone therapy should be performed in a hospital setting. Close monitoring of patients during the loading-dose phase of therapy is necessary, especially until the risk of recurrent ventricular tachycardia or fibrillation has abated. The difficulties associated with using amiodarone effectively and safely pose substantial risks to the patient. Even with an oral loading-dose regimen, a response to orally administered drug generally requires at least 1 week and usually 2 or more weeks of therapy. Because absorption and elimination of amiodarone are variable, adjustment of maintenance dosage is difficult, it is not unusual to require dosage reduction or temporary withdrawal or discontinuance of the drug. Patients who experience serious adverse effects during therapy with amiodarone should immediately contact their clinician or seek medical attention; in addition, patients should contact their clinician before discontinuance of the drug.

The time at which a previously controlled life-threatening arrhythmia will recur after reduction of amiodarone dosage or discontinuance of the drug is unpredictable, ranging from weeks to months. During this period, the patient is at great risk and may need prolonged hospitalization or intensive ambulatory monitoring (e.g., via telemetric ECG), possibly with periodic determination of plasma concentrations of the drug. Attempts to substitute other antiarrhythmic agents when amiodarone must be discontinued because of inefficacy or intolerance are difficult because of the gradually, but unpredictably, changing body burden of the drug, the drug's residual effects, and its potential interactions with subsequent treatment.

Because amiodarone may cause pulmonary toxicity that is potentially fatal, baseline pulmonary function tests, including diffusion capacity, should be performed prior to initiation of oral amiodarone therapy, and periodic chest radiographs and clinical evaluation should be performed every 3–6 months during therapy with the drug. Periodic pulmonary function testing also should be considered. Preoperative pulmonary function tests are recommended for patients undergoing cardiothoracic surgery since ARDS may develop postoperatively in patients receiving the drug. Until further studies have been performed, some manufacturers recommend that FiO_2 and tissue oxygenation (as determined by SaO_2 or PaO_2) be closely monitored in patients receiving amiodarone. Amiodarone should be used with caution, if at all, in patients with preexisting pulmonary disease, including chronic obstructive disease, or reduced pulmonary diffusion capacity. Patients should inform their clinician of preexisting lung or breathing disorders prior to initiation of amiodarone therapy. The possibility of amiodarone-induced pulmonary toxicity should be considered in any patient developing a new respiratory symptom during therapy with the drug. Patients should contact their clinician if dyspnea, wheezing, coughing, chest pain, hemoptysis, or any other breathing disorders occur during therapy with amiodarone. Clinical and radiographic evaluation, as well as scintigraphic and pulmonary function testing (including diffusion capacity), if necessary, are recommended in such patients. Respiratory symptoms should be carefully assessed and other causes of respiratory impairment (e.g., congestive heart failure, pulmonary embolism, malignancy) should be ruled out before discontinuance of the drug. Measurement of pulmonary capillary wedge pressure may help exclude congestive heart failure as a cause of symptoms or radiographic findings. Since amiodarone-induced pulmonary toxicity may mimic infection, possible infectious causes should be excluded; bronchoalveolar lavage, transbronchial lung biopsy, and/or open lung biopsy may aid in the diagnosis, especially in patients in whom alternative antiarrhythmic therapy is not available. The manufacturer states that the presence of suppressor/cytotoxic (CD8[+], T8[+]) T-cell lymphocytosis in bronchoalveolar lavage specimens should be considered confirmatory of hypersensitivity pneumonitis. If hypersensitivity pneumonitis occurs, corticosteroid therapy should be initiated and amiodarone should be discontinued. If evidence of interstitial pneumonitis (alveolitis) is present, dosage of amiodarone should be reduced and, preferably, therapy with the drug withdrawn in an attempt to determine whether the toxicity is reversible; however, amiodarone should be discontinued with caution in patients with life-threatening arrhythmias, since sudden cardiac death is common in these patients.

Because amiodarone can alter results of thyroid function tests and/or cause clinical hypothyroidism or hyperthyroidism, thyroid function tests should be performed prior to initiating amiodarone therapy and at periodic intervals (approximately every 3–6 months) thereafter, particularly in geriatric patients and/or in patients with a prior history of thyroid nodules, goiter, or other thyroid dysfunction. Patients should inform their clinician if they have thyroid dysfunction or a history of such dysfunction prior to initiation of therapy. In addition, patients receiving amiodarone should be instructed to report episodes of chest pain, weight loss or gain, weakness, heat or cold intolerance, hair thinning, diaphoresis, menstrual cycle changes, swelling in the neck (e.g., goiter), nervousness, irritability, restlessness, decreased concentration, depression in geriatric patients, tremor, or aggravation of cardiovascular disease to their clinician, since such manifestations may indicate amiodarone-induced thyroid dysfunction. If any new signs of cardiac arrhythmias appear, the possibility of hyperthyroidism should be considered. The risks and benefits of amiodarone therapy in patients with thyroid dysfunction should be carefully considered because of the potential for arrhythmia breakthrough or exacerbation of arrhythmias, which may result in death, in such patients.

Because amiodarone may cause elevations in serum hepatic enzyme concentrations and may rarely cause severe, potentially fatal, hepatic injury, serum hepatic enzyme concentrations should be monitored at regular intervals in patients receiving the drug, particularly those receiving relatively high maintenance dosages. Patients should inform their clinician of preexisting liver dysfunction prior to initiation of amiodarone therapy. Patients should contact their clinician if nausea or vomiting, dark urine, fatigue, jaundice, or stomach pain occurs during amiodarone therapy. In patients with life-threatening arrhythmias, the potential risk of hepatic injury should be weighed against the potential benefit of IV amiodarone therapy. If serum hepatic enzyme concentrations increase to more than 3 times normal values in patients with normal pretreatment values or twice baseline pretreatment values in patients with elevated values prior to amiodarone therapy, or if hepatomegaly or progressive hepatic injury occurs, a reduction in oral amiodarone dosage, a decrease in the infusion rate during parenteral amiodarone therapy, or discontinuance of the drug should be considered. Because the risk of hepatic necrosis during IV amiodarone therapy may be related to the use of rapid infusion rates and excessive drug concentrations in the initial loading dose, the initial amiodarone concentration and IV infusion rate should be monitored closely and should not exceed those recommended by the manufacturer. Liver biopsy with ultrastructural study by electron microscopy may aid in the diagnosis of amiodarone-induced hepatic toxicity.

Because amiodarone causes corneal microdeposits in almost all patients and optic neuropathy occasionally may result in visual disturbances, the manufacturer and some clinicians recommend that a baseline ophthalmologic examination (e.g., a slit-lamp evaluation) be performed before initiating therapy with the drug and then possibly at periodic intervals during long-term therapy (e.g., after the first 6 months and then annually and/or as necessary). Patients experiencing visual disturbances or those receiving long-term therapy should be monitored carefully. Patients experiencing visual disturbances (e.g., blurred vision, visual halos, ocular photosensitivity) should contact their clinician. The presence of nonprogressive, asymptomatic corneal microdeposits does *not* necessitate dosage reduction or discontinuance of amiodarone. In addition, optic neuropathy and/or optic neuritis (usually resulting in visual impairment, which sometimes may progress to permanent blindness) has been reported in patients receiving amiodarone and although a causal relationship to the drug has not been clearly established, some manufacturers state that if visual impairment occurs (e.g., changes in visual acuity, decreases in peripheral vision), a prompt ophthalmologic examination should be performed. If optic neuropathy and/or optic neuritis has developed, amiodarone therapy should be reevaluated and the described risks and complications should be weighed against the possible benefits of antiarrhythmic therapy. Routine ophthalmologic examinations, including slit-lamp and funduscopic tests, should be performed in patients receiving amiodarone therapy. Most manufacturers of corneal refractive laser surgery devices consider the procedure to be contraindicated in patients receiving amiodarone.

The use of sunscreen agents and protective clothing and avoidance of excessive exposure to sunlight are recommended to help prevent photosensitivity reactions associated with amiodarone therapy. Patients with fair complexions or excessive exposure to sunlight or those who have received prolonged amiodarone therapy and/or relatively large cumulative doses appear to be more susceptible to amiodarone-induced blue-gray skin discoloration.

Hypotension has been reported during open-heart surgery (during and/or following cardiopulmonary bypass) in amiodarone-treated patients. Patients should inform their clinician of blood pressure abnormalities prior to initiating amiodarone therapy. Atropine-resistant sinus bradycardia, sinus arrest, and/or AV block also have occurred in some amiodarone-treated patients undergoing general anesthesia for major surgery. The relationship of these effects to amiodarone is not known. An interaction between the antiarrhythmic agent and various anesthetic agents has been suggested but not clearly established. The hypotension may be severe in some patients and require larger than usual dosages of sympathomimetic agents and/or intra-aortic balloon counterpulsation. Sinus bradyarrhythmias and/or AV block may require insertion of an artificial pacemaker. Pending further evaluation, the anesthesiologist should be aware of potential complications in patients undergoing general anesthesia who are currently receiving amiodarone or who have previously received the drug within the past 1–2 months. In addition, close perioperative monitoring is recommended in patients undergoing general anesthesia while receiving amiodarone, since amiodarone may sensitize patients to the myocardial depressant and conduction effects of halogenated hydrocarbon general anesthetics.

Because IV amiodarone therapy is associated with bradycardia, patients with a known predisposition to bradycardia or AV block should be treated with IV amiodarone in a setting where a temporary pacemaker is available. Patients should contact their clinician if they experience heart pounding, irregular heart beat, very fast or slow heartbeat, lightheadedness, or faintness during amiodarone therapy. Also, because of the risk of proarrhythmia during parenteral amiodarone therapy, patients should be monitored for QT_c prolongation during infusion of amiodarone. The need to coadminister amiodarone with other drugs that are known to prolong the QT_c interval must be based on a careful assessment of the potential risks and benefits in individual patients.

Since antiarrhythmic agents, including amiodarone, may be less effective and/or more arrhythmogenic in patients with hypokalemia or hypomagnesemia, the possibility of a potassium or magnesium deficiency should be evaluated and, if present, corrected prior to initiation of amiodarone therapy. Special attention should be given to electrolyte and acid-base balance in patients experiencing severe or prolonged diarrhea or in patients receiving concomitant diuretics.

Because of the possibility of clinically important interactions when amiodarone is used concomitantly with other drugs, patients should inform their clinicians of their use of other drugs, including prescription and nonprescription drugs, or of dietary and herbal supplements such as St. John's wort. Grapefruit juice is known to inhibit cytochrome P-450 (CYP) 3A4-mediated metabolism of oral amiodarone, resulting in increased plasma concentrations of the drug; therefore, patients should be instructed not to consume grapefruit juice during treatment with oral amiodarone.

Amiodarone is contraindicated in patients with cardiogenic shock, in patients with severe sinus node dysfunction resulting in marked sinus bradycardia, in patients with second- or third-degree AV block, and in patients with episodes of bradycardia that have caused syncope, except when used concomitantly with an artificial pacemaker. Amiodarone also is contraindicated in patients with known hypersensitivity to the drug or any ingredient in the formulation, including iodine; IV amiodarone is contraindicated in patients with known hypersensitivity to any components of the parenteral formulation, including iodine.

● Pediatric Precautions

Safety and efficacy of amiodarone in children† have not been established. In a clinical trial in pediatric patients 30 days to 15 years of age, hypotension (36%), bradycardia (20%), and atrioventricular block (15%) were common dose-related adverse effects, and in some cases were severe or life-threatening. In this trial, injection-site reactions were observed in 5 of 20 patients receiving IV amiodarone through a peripheral vein. Limited data suggest that the drug may be useful in carefully selected cases for the management of refractory supraventricular or ventricular tachycardias in children, and current guidelines for pediatric advanced life support (PALS) recommend the use of amiodarone or lidocaine for the treatment of shock-refractory ventricular fibrillation or pulseless ventricular tachycardia. This recommendation is based principally on extrapolation of data from adult studies as well as an observational study in pediatric patients suggesting improved return of spontaneous circulation (ROSC) with lidocaine compared with amiodarone.

Each mL of the commercially available amiodarone hydrochloride IV injection contains 20.2 mg of benzyl alcohol as a preservative. Although a causal relationship has not been established, administration of injections preserved with benzyl alcohol has been associated with toxicity in neonates. Toxicity appears to have resulted from administration of large amounts (i.e., 100–400 mg/kg daily) of benzyl alcohol in these neonates. Although use of drugs preserved with benzyl alcohol should be avoided in neonates whenever possible, the American Academy of Pediatrics states that the presence of small amounts of the preservative in a commercially available injection should not proscribe its use when indicated in neonates.

In addition, the commercially available amiodarone hydrochloride IV injection has been found to leach diethylhexyl phthalate (DEHP) plasticizer from IV tubing (e.g., PVC tubing). Leaching of DEHP is increased when IV amiodarone hydrochloride is infused at higher concentrations and slower infusion rates than those recommended by the manufacturer. After reviewing data from animal studies and limited experience in humans, an expert panel of the National Toxicology Program Center for the Evaluation of Risks to Human Reproduction (NTP-CERHR) concluded that exposure to DEHP may adversely affect male reproductive tract development during fetal, infant, and toddler stages of development if the exposure at these stages is severalfold higher than that in adults, a situation that might be associated with intensive medical procedures such as those performed in critically ill infants. In studies in sexually mature rats, an oral amiodarone hydrochloride dosage of 3.7–14 mg/kg daily was associated with no observable adverse effects; however, in rats at the postnatal stage, a dosage level associated with no observable adverse effects was not identified. The maximum anticipated exposure to DEHP following IV administration of amiodarone hydrochloride in pediatric patients has been calculated to be about 1.9 mg/kg daily for a 3-kg infant, which provides about a 2- to 7-fold margin of safety. In pediatric patients requiring therapy with IV amiodarone hydrochloride, dosing methods that may reduce potential exposure to DEHP (e.g., IV loading dose of 5 mg/kg given in 5 divided doses of 1 mg/kg, with each incremental dose infused over 5–10 minutes) may be considered.

● Geriatric Precautions

While clinical experience to date has not revealed age-related differences in response to amiodarone, clinical studies evaluating the drug have not included sufficient numbers of adults 65 years of age and older to determine whether geriatric patients respond differently than younger adults. The manufacturers state that dosage in general for geriatric patients should be selected carefully, usually starting at the low end of the dosage range, because these individuals frequently have decreased hepatic, renal, and/or cardiac function and concomitant disease and drug therapy. In addition, geriatric patients may be more susceptible to bradycardia and conduction disturbances induced by the drug.

● Pregnancy, Fertility, and Lactation

Pregnancy

Reproduction studies in pregnant rats or rabbits receiving oral amiodarone hydrochloride dosages of 25 mg/kg daily (approximately 0.4 and 0.9 times, respectively, the maximum recommended human maintenance dosage of 600 mg for a 50-kg patient [calculated on the basis of body surface area]) revealed no evidence of harm to the fetus. However, in pregnant rabbits receiving oral amiodarone hydrochloride dosages of 75 mg/kg daily (approximately 2.7 times the maximum recommended human maintenance dosage of 600 mg for a 50-kg patient [calculated on the basis of body surface area]), abortions occurred in more than 90% of these rabbits. Slight displacement of the testes and an increased incidence of incomplete ossification of some skull and digital bones were reported in pregnant rats receiving oral amiodarone hydrochloride dosages of 50 mg/kg daily (approximately 0.8 times the maximum recommended human maintenance dosage of 600 mg for a 50-kg patient [calculated on the basis of body surface area]) or more. In addition, in rats receiving oral amiodarone hydrochloride dosages of 100 mg/kg daily (approximately 1.6 times the maximum recommended human maintenance dosage of 600 mg for a 50-kg patient [calculated on the basis of body surface area] or more, or 200 mg/kg daily (approximately 1.6 or 3.2 times the maximum recommended human maintenance dosage of 600 mg for a 50-kg patient [calculated on the basis of body surface area]), reduced fetal body weight or increased incidence of fetal resorptions, respectively, were observed. Adverse effects on fetal growth and survival also were reported in 1 of 2 strains of mice receiving oral amiodarone hydrochloride dosages of 5 mg/kg daily (approximately 0.04 times the maximum recommended human maintenance dosage of 600 mg for a 50-kg patient [calculated on the basis of body surface area]).

In a reproductive study in which amiodarone was administered IV to rabbits at dosages of 5, 10, or 25 mg/kg daily (approximately 0.1, 0.3, or 0.7 times the recommended maximum human dose on the basis of body surface area, respectively), maternal deaths occurred in all groups, including controls. Embryotoxicity, as manifested by fewer full-term fetuses and increased resorptions with concomitantly lower litter weights, occurred at dosages of 10 mg/kg and greater. No evidence of embryotoxicity was observed at the 5 mg/kg dosage and no teratogenicity was observed at any dosage level tested. In a teratology study in which amiodarone was administered by continuous IV infusion to rats at dosages of 25, 50, or 100 mg/kg daily (approximately 0.4, 0.7, or 1.4 times the recommended maximum human dose on the basis of body surface area, respectively), maternal toxicity (as evidenced by reduced weight gain and food consumption) and embryotoxicity (as evidenced by increased resorptions, decreased live litter size, reduced body weights, and retarded sternum and metacarpal ossification) were observed in the group receiving 100 mg/kg daily.

Amiodarone and N-desethylamiodarone cross the placenta to a limited extent. QT prolongation and transient sinus bradycardia have been observed in neonates of a limited number of pregnant women who received the drug during the second and/or third trimester. Specific data are not available, but there are concerns that amiodarone potentially could adversely affect fetal thyroid function and overall development. Congenital goiter/hypothyroidism and hyperthyroidism have been observed in a limited number of neonates born to women who received amiodarone during pregnancy. Amiodarone should be used during pregnancy only when the potential benefits justify the possible risks to the fetus. Women should inform their clinicians if they are or plan to become pregnant or plan to breast-feed. If amiodarone is used during pregnancy or if the patient becomes pregnant while receiving the drug, the patient should be apprised of the potential hazard to the fetus. Women of childbearing potential should avoid becoming pregnant during amiodarone therapy. The prolonged elimination of amiodarone from the body after discontinuance of the drug should be considered when a woman of childbearing potential receiving amiodarone plans to become pregnant. It is not known whether use of amiodarone during labor and delivery could have any immediate or delayed adverse effects on the mother or fetus. Studies in rodents have not shown any effect of the drug on duration of gestation or on parturition.

Fertility

Reproduction studies in male and female rats using oral amiodarone hydrochloride dosages of 90 mg/kg daily (approximately 1.4 times the maximum recommended human maintenance dosage of 600 mg for a 50-kg patient [calculated on the basis of body surface area]) and initiated 9 weeks prior to mating, have revealed evidence of reduced fertility. Amiodarone and N-desethylamiodarone are distributed in high concentrations into human testes and semen. No fertility studies were conducted with IV amiodarone.

Lactation

Amiodarone and, to a lesser extent, N-desethylamiodarone are distributed into milk in concentrations substantially higher than concurrent maternal plasma concentrations. Nursing offspring of lactating rats receiving amiodarone have been shown to be less viable and to have reduced bodyweight gains. Because nursing may expose the infant to a substantial dose of amiodarone and its metabolite, it is recommended that nursing be discontinued during amiodarone therapy. The slow elimination of amiodarone from the body after discontinuance of the drug should also be considered.

DRUG INTERACTIONS

While only a limited number of drug interactions with amiodarone have been investigated, most drugs studied to date have been shown to interact with amiodarone. Few data are available on drug interactions with parenteral amiodarone therapy; most of the information on drug interactions with amiodarone comes from experience with *oral* administration of the drug. The possibility of interactions with any concomitantly administered drug and amiodarone should be anticipated, particularly for drugs with potentially serious toxic effects such as other antiarrhythmic agents. If such drugs are needed, their dosage should be carefully reassessed and adjusted as necessary, and plasma concentrations of such drugs should be measured, if appropriate.

Because of the long and variable elimination half-life of amiodarone, the potential for interactions exists not only with concomitantly administered drugs but also with drugs administered after discontinuance of amiodarone therapy.

● *Drugs Affecting the QT Interval*

Amiodarone prolongs the QT_c interval, and clinicians should consider the possibility that potentially serious cardiac arrhythmias, including torsades de pointes, could occur if amiodarone were used concomitantly with other drugs that prolong the QT_c interval (e.g., cisapride [no longer commercially available in the US], halofantrine [no longer commercially available in the US], dolasetron, pimozide, disopyramide, fluoroquinolones, loratadine, macrolide antibiotics, trazodone, ziprasidone, azole antifungal agents). Use of amiodarone with any other agent known to prolong the QT_c interval must be based on a careful assessment of the potential risks and benefits of such combination therapy. Some manufacturers state that such combined use should be avoided or is contraindicated. If dolasetron and amiodarone are used concomitantly, caution should be exercised and cardiac function should be monitored.

● *Drugs with P-Glycoprotein-mediated Clearance*

Amiodarone inhibits the P-glycoprotein transport system, which may result in unexpectedly high plasma concentrations of drugs that are substrates for this transport system.

● *Drugs, Foods, and Dietary or Herbal Supplements Affecting Hepatic Microsomal Enzymes*

Amiodarone is metabolized by the cytochrome P-450 (CYP) microsomal enzyme system, principally the isoenzymes CYP3A4 and CYP2C8. Therefore, amiodarone has the potential for interactions with drugs or substances that may be substrates, inhibitors, or inducers of CYP3A4 and CYP2C8. Amiodarone also inhibits CYP2D6, CYP1A2, CYP2C9, and CYP3A4 isoenzymes. Inhibition of these isoenzymes by amiodarone may result in unexpectedly high plasma concentrations of other drugs which are metabolized by these isoenzymes.

Antiarrhythmic Agents

The use of amiodarone in conjunction with other antiarrhythmic agents generally should be reserved for patients with life-threatening arrhythmias who do not respond completely to either a single antiarrhythmic agent or amiodarone alone. When combination therapy with amiodarone is employed, it is generally recommended that dosage of the currently administered antiarrhythmic agent(s) be reduced by 30–50% several days after initiation of amiodarone therapy, since the onset of amiodarone's antiarrhythmic effect may be delayed. The necessity of continuing the other antiarrhythmic agent(s) should be assessed after the antiarrhythmic effect of amiodarone has been established, and discontinuance of the other antiarrhythmic agent(s) usually should be attempted. If combination therapy with the other antiarrhythmic agent(s) is continued, patients should be monitored with particular care for possible adverse effects, especially conduction disturbances and exacerbation of tachyarrhythmias. In patients already receiving amiodarone, the initial dosage of other antiarrhythmic agents should be reduced to approximately 50% of their usual recommended initial dosages.

Atypical ventricular tachycardia (torsades de pointes) has been reported rarely when amiodarone was administered concomitantly with various antiarrhythmic agents, including disopyramide, mexiletine, propafenone, and quinidine. Pending further accumulation of data, amiodarone should be used with caution when administered concomitantly with other antiarrhythmic agents, particularly class IA antiarrhythmic agents.

Flecainide

Plasma flecainide concentrations adjusted for daily dosage increased by an average of about 60% (range: 5–190%) when amiodarone therapy was initiated in a limited number of patients receiving flecainide. Although the mechanism(s) of this interaction is not known, it has been suggested that amiodarone may inhibit the hepatic metabolism and/or decrease the renal clearance of flecainide. Pending further accumulation of data, it is recommended that the dosage of flecainide be reduced by 30–50% several days after initiation of amiodarone therapy; subsequently, the patient and plasma flecainide concentrations should be monitored closely and flecainide dosage adjusted as necessary.

Procainamide

Concomitant use of amiodarone and procainamide may result in increased plasma procainamide and N-acetylprocainamide (NAPA) concentrations and subsequent toxicity. In a limited number of patients receiving 2–6 g of procainamide hydrochloride daily, initiation of amiodarone hydrochloride (1200 mg daily for 5–7 days and then 600 mg daily) increased plasma procainamide and NAPA concentrations by about 55 and 33%, respectively, during the first week of amiodarone therapy. The exact mechanism(s) has not been elucidated, but it has been suggested that amiodarone may decrease the renal clearance of procainamide or NAPA and/or inhibit the hepatic metabolism of procainamide. In addition to a pharmacokinetic interaction, additive electrophysiologic effects, including increased QT_c and QRS intervals, occur during concomitant use; adverse electrophysiologic effects (e.g., acceleration of ventricular tachycardia) may also occur. Pending further accumulation of data, it is recommended that procainamide dosage be reduced by 20–33% when amiodarone therapy is initiated in patients currently receiving procainamide or that procainamide therapy be discontinued.

Quinidine

Serum quinidine concentrations may increase following initiation of amiodarone therapy in patients currently receiving quinidine, with subsequent toxicity occurring in some patients. Administration of amiodarone hydrochloride (1200 mg daily for 5–7 days then reduced to 600 mg daily) to a limited number of patients receiving quinidine gluconate or sulfate (average dose of about 3 g daily) resulted in an increase in serum quinidine concentrations of about 33%. Serum quinidine concentrations may begin to increase within a couple days after initiation of amiodarone therapy. The mechanism of the interaction is not fully established, but it has been suggested that amiodarone may inhibit hepatic clearance or decrease renal clearance of quinidine and/or displace quinidine from tissue- and/or protein-binding sites. Although not clearly established, combination therapy with amiodarone and quinidine may also cause marked QT prolongation, predisposing patients to atypical ventricular tachycardia (torsades de pointes). It is generally recommended that quinidine dosage be reduced by 33–50% when amiodarone therapy is initiated in patients currently receiving quinidine or that quinidine therapy be discontinued. Serum quinidine concentrations should be monitored carefully and quinidine dosage reduced as necessary in patients receiving concomitant amiodarone and quinidine therapy; patients should be observed closely for signs of toxicity, including QT prolongation.

Lidocaine

Sinus bradycardia was observed in a patient receiving oral amiodarone who was given lidocaine for local anesthesia. Seizures associated with increased lidocaine concentrations were observed in one patient receiving concomitant IV amiodarone therapy.

HIV Protease Inhibitors

HIV protease inhibitors inhibit CYP3A4 to varying degrees, which may result in a decrease in the metabolism of amiodarone. Concomitant use of amiodarone and an HIV protease inhibitor used with low-dose ritonavir (*ritonavir-boosted*) or without low-dose ritonavir (unboosted) may result in increased plasma concentrations of amiodarone and the HIV protease inhibitor.

Concomitant use of amiodarone and *ritonavir-boosted* saquinavir or *ritonavir-boosted* tipranavir is not recommended. If amiodarone is used concomitantly with other *ritonavir-boosted* HIV protease inhibitors or with unboosted HIV protease inhibitors, some experts recommend caution and state that the patient should be monitored for amiodarone toxicity and consideration given to monitoring ECG and amiodarone plasma concentrations.

Histamine H$_2$-Receptor Antagonists

Cimetidine inhibits CYP3A4 and can increase plasma amiodarone concentrations.

Histamine H$_1$-Receptor Antagonists

Use of amiodarone with loratadine may result in a decrease in the metabolism of loratadine, a substrate of CYP3A4. QT-interval prolongation and torsades de pointes have been reported with concomitant use of amiodarone and loratadine.

Cyclosporine

Amiodarone inhibits CYP3A4, which may result in a decrease in the metabolism of cyclosporine, a substrate of CYP3A4. Concomitant use of amiodarone and cyclosporine has been reported to produce persistently elevated plasma concentrations of cyclosporine, resulting in elevated serum creatinine concentrations despite reduction in the dose of cyclosporine.

HMG-CoA Reductase Inhibitors (Statins)

Potent inhibitors of CYP3A4 can increase plasma concentrations of HMG-CoA reductase inhibitory activity and increase the risk of myopathy. Because the risk of myopathy/rhabdomyolysis is increased following concomitant use of amiodarone with higher dosages of certain HMG-CoA reductase inhibitors (e.g., simvastatin dosages exceeding 20 mg daily), the daily dosage of lovastatin or simvastatin should not exceed 40 or 20 mg, respectively, during concomitant therapy with amiodarone.

Rifampin

Concomitant administration of amiodarone and rifampin has been associated with decreases in plasma concentrations of amiodarone and desethylamiodarone because of induction of CYP3A4 by rifampin.

St. John's Wort (Hypericum perforatum)

St. John's wort is an extract of hypericum and contains at least 7 different components that may contribute to its pharmacologic effects, including hypericin, pseudohypericin, and hyperforin. There is evidence that hypericum extracts can induce several different CYP isoenzymes, including CYP3A4 and CYP1A2. Since amiodarone is a substrate for CYP3A4, concomitant use of amiodarone and St. John's wort has the potential to result in decreased plasma concentrations of amiodarone.

Other Drugs Affecting Hepatic Microsomal Enzymes

Concomitant administration of fentanyl and amiodarone may result in hypotension, bradycardia, and decreased cardiac output. Prolonged (exceeding 2 weeks) administration of oral amiodarone impairs the metabolism of dextromethorphan, phenytoin, and methotrexate.

Use of amiodarone concurrently with trazodone may result in a decrease in the metabolism of trazodone, a substrate of CYP3A4. QT-interval prolongation and torsades de pointes have been reported with concomitant use of amiodarone and trazodone.

Clopidogrel undergoes biotransformation through the CYP3A4 isoenzyme, and concomitant use with amiodarone may decrease the biotransformation of clopidogrel to the active form. Ineffective inhibition of platelet aggregation has been reported during concomitant use of clopidogrel and amiodarone.

Grapefruit Juice

Grapefruit juice inhibits CYP3A4-mediated metabolism of oral amiodarone in intestinal mucosa, resulting in increased plasma concentrations of amiodarone. In healthy individuals receiving grapefruit juice and oral amiodarone concurrently, the area under the plasma concentration-time curve (AUC) and peak plasma concentration of amiodarone increased by 50 and 84%, respectively, and desethylamiodarone plasma concentrations decreased to below the detection limits of the assay. Therefore, grapefruit juice should not be consumed during treatment with oral amiodarone. This interaction should be considered when switching from IV to oral amiodarone therapy.

Phenytoin

Concomitant use of amiodarone and phenytoin has resulted in a twofold to threefold increase in steady-state serum concentrations of phenytoin and subsequent signs of phenytoin toxicity (e.g., nystagmus, ataxia, lethargy) in a limited number of patients. The increase in serum phenytoin concentrations occurred within 3–4 weeks of initiating amiodarone therapy. Although the exact mechanism(s) has not been clearly established, amiodarone may inhibit hepatic metabolism of phenytoin. Patients receiving phenytoin should be monitored closely for signs of phenytoin toxicity when amiodarone is administered concomitantly; serum phenytoin concentrations also should be monitored and dosage of phenytoin reduced as necessary.

Phenytoin has been reported to decrease plasma amiodarone concentrations.

● Anticoagulants

An increase in prothrombin time (PT) appears to occur in almost all patients treated with amiodarone and a coumarin or indandione anticoagulant concomitantly and can result in serious or fatal hemorrhage. The increase in PT usually begins within 3–4 days, although onset of the effect may be delayed for 1–3 weeks in some patients. Bleeding episodes generally have been reported to occur 1–4 weeks following initiation of amiodarone therapy. The magnitude of the increase in PT appears to average 100%. Because of amiodarone's long elimination half-life, the PT may not return to normal for 1–4 months following discontinuance of the antiarrhythmic agent. The exact mechanism is not fully established, but amiodarone appears to decrease the hepatic clearance of warfarin. If amiodarone therapy is initiated in patients receiving warfarin or another coumarin or indandione anticoagulant, a reduction in anticoagulant dosage of 33–50% is recommended. In patients receiving amiodarone and an oral anticoagulant concomitantly, the PT should be determined frequently and patients should be observed closely for adverse effects; dosage of the anticoagulant should be adjusted as necessary.

● Cardiac Glycosides

Concomitant use of amiodarone and digoxin regularly results in increased serum digoxin concentrations, which may reach toxic levels with subsequent digoxin toxicity. Serum digoxin concentrations generally increase by an average of 70–100% in adults, but substantial variability exists in the magnitude of the increase. Limited data suggest that the magnitude of the increase may be much greater in children than in adults (i.e., 70–800%).

The amiodarone-induced increase in serum digoxin concentrations usually begins within 1–7 days and progresses gradually over a period of several weeks or even months. The exact mechanism(s) of this interaction appears to be complex and remains to be fully established, but data indicate that amiodarone may decrease the renal and/or nonrenal clearance of digoxin. It has also been suggested that amiodarone may increase the oral bioavailability of digoxin or displace digoxin from tissue binding sites. When initiating amiodarone therapy in patients receiving digoxin, the need for continued cardiac glycoside therapy should be reassessed, and digoxin discontinued if appropriate; if concomitant therapy is considered necessary in patients receiving digoxin, a 50% reduction in digoxin dosage is recommended when amiodarone therapy is begun. Serum digoxin concentrations should be monitored carefully and digoxin dosage reduced as necessary in patients receiving amiodarone and digoxin concomitantly; patients should be observed closely for signs of cardiac glycoside toxicity. In addition, thyroid function should be monitored carefully in patients receiving concurrent amiodarone and digoxin therapy, since amiodarone-induced changes in thyroid function may increase or decrease serum digoxin concentrations or alter sensitivity to the therapeutic and toxic effects of the cardiac glycoside.

● Other Cardiovascular Drugs

Amiodarone should be used with caution in patients receiving calcium-channel blocking agents (e.g., diltiazem, verapamil) and/or β-adrenergic blocking agents (e.g. propranolol), since possible potentiation of sinus bradycardia, sinus arrest, and AV block may occur. If amiodarone therapy is considered necessary, the drug may continue to be used in patients with severe sinus bradycardia or sinus arrest following insertion of an artificial pacemaker and institution of cardiac monitoring.

● General Anesthetics

The effects of concomitant administration of amiodarone and anesthetic agents have not been fully evaluated. However, potentially serious adverse cardiovascular and cardiac effects have occurred in some amiodarone-treated patients undergoing general anesthesia, suggesting the possibility of an interaction between the antiarrhythmic agent and various anesthetic agents. In addition, close perioperative monitoring is recommended in patients undergoing general anesthesia while receiving amiodarone, since amiodarone may sensitize patients to the myocardial depressant and conduction effects of halogenated hydrocarbon general anesthetics.

● HCV Antivirals

Concomitant use of amiodarone and a hepatitis C virus (HCV) treatment regimen containing sofosbuvir with another HCV direct-acting antiviral (DAA), including ledipasvir, simeprevir, or daclatasvir, may result in serious symptomatic bradycardia and is not recommended. The mechanism for this adverse cardiovascular effect is unknown; the effect of concomitant use of amiodarone with these HCV treatment regimens on plasma concentrations of the drugs is unknown. If there are no alternative HCV treatment options and a regimen of sofosbuvir with another DAA (e.g., ledipasvir, simeprevir, daclatasvir) must be used in a patient receiving amiodarone, the patient should be advised about the risk of serious symptomatic bradycardia before HCV treatment is initiated. Cardiac monitoring should be performed in an inpatient setting during the first 48 hours of concomitant use of amiodarone and a regimen containing sofosbuvir with another DAA; heart rate monitoring should then be performed daily (outpatient or self-monitoring) through at least the first 2 weeks of concomitant use. Similar cardiac monitoring is recommended in patients who discontinued amiodarone just prior to initiation of a regimen that includes sofosbuvir with another DAA or if an alternative antiarrhythmic agent cannot be used and amiodarone must be initiated in a patient already receiving such sofosbuvir regimens. Patients receiving amiodarone concomitantly with a regimen containing sofosbuvir with another DAA should be advised about the risk of serious symptomatic bradycardia and the importance of immediately contacting a clinician if signs or symptoms of bradycardia (e.g., near-fainting or fainting, dizziness, lightheadedness, malaise, weakness, excessive tiredness, shortness of breath, chest pain, confusion, memory problems) occur.

Concomitant use of oral amiodarone and simeprevir is expected to result in modestly increased amiodarone concentrations due to intestinal CYP3A4 inhibition by simeprevir. If amiodarone is used concomitantly with a simeprevir-containing HCV treatment regimen that does *not* include sofosbuvir, caution is warranted and therapeutic drug monitoring of the antiarrhythmic agent, if available, is recommended.

Concomitant use of amiodarone and the fixed combination of ombitasvir, paritaprevir, and ritonavir (ombitasvir/paritaprevir/ritonavir) with dasabuvir is expected to increase plasma concentrations of amiodarone. If amiodarone is used concomitantly with ombitasvir/paritaprevir/ritonavir with dasabuvir, caution is warranted and therapeutic drug monitoring of the antiarrhythmic agent, if available, is recommended.

● Cholestyramine Resin

Limited data indicate that administration of cholestyramine resin following a single oral dose of amiodarone may decrease the elimination half-life and plasma concentrations of amiodarone, possibly by interfering with enterohepatic circulation of the antiarrhythmic agent. Further evaluation of this potential interaction is needed.

● Agalsidase Beta

Some clinicians state that because of a theoretical risk of inhibited intracellular α-galactosidase activity with amiodarone, it should not be administered concurrently with agalsidase beta, a biosynthetic form of α-galactosidase.

ACUTE TOXICITY

Limited information is available on the acute toxicity of amiodarone. However, cases of amiodarone overdosage, sometimes fatal, have been reported. If an overdosage occurs, patients should contact their clinician or proceed immediately to a hospital emergency room.

● Pathogenesis

The acute lethal dose of amiodarone hydrochloride in humans is not known. The oral LD_{50} of the drug in rats, mice, and dogs is greater than 3 g/kg. Following oral administration of single large doses of amiodarone hydrochloride (up to 3 g/kg) in dogs, emesis, tremors, and hindlimb paresis were observed.

● Manifestations

In general, overdosage of amiodarone may be expected to produce effects that are extensions of pharmacologic effects, including sinus bradycardia and/or heart block, hypotension, and QT prolongation. The most likely effects of an inadvertent overdosage of IV amiodarone are hypotension, cardiogenic shock, bradycardia, AV block, and hepatotoxicity. Nausea is likely to occur with ingestions of greater than 1 g of the drug. Slight, asymptomatic bradycardia and QT prolongation occurred about 1–3 days following acute ingestion of 2.6–8 g of amiodarone hydrochloride in 3 patients. In an adult who reportedly intentionally ingested 8 g of amiodarone hydrochloride and an unknown amount of diazepam and lorazepam, profuse perspiration occurred within 12 hours and slight bradycardia and QT prolongation (to about 500 ms) occurred 2–3 days after ingestion. In another adult who had received 200 mg of amiodarone hydrochloride daily for 1 week and then intentionally ingested 2.6 g of the drug, no ECG changes were apparent 6 hours after ingestion, but QT prolongation, T-wave inversion, and transient disappearance of precordial R waves occurred the day following ingestion. No symptoms were reported, and the patient's heart rate remained normal; repolarization returned to baseline about 10 days after ingestion. No deaths or permanent sequelae occurred in these patients.

● Treatment

Management of amiodarone overdosage generally involves symptomatic and supportive care, with ECG and blood pressure monitoring. In case of hypotension or cardiogenic shock in patients receiving amiodarone IV, the infusion rate should be decreased. There is no specific antidote for amiodarone intoxication.

Following recent acute ingestion of amiodarone, the stomach should be emptied immediately by inducing emesis or by gastric lavage. If the patient is comatose, having seizures, or lacks the gag reflex, gastric lavage may be performed if an endotracheal tube with cuff inflated is in place to prevent aspiration of gastric contents. Administration of activated charcoal after emesis or gastric lavage may be useful in minimizing absorption of amiodarone, although specific data are not available. Because the onset of toxicity may be delayed, ECG monitoring may be necessary for several days following acute ingestion of the drug. For bradycardia, IV administration of a β-adrenergic agonist (e.g., isoproterenol) or use of a transvenous cardiac pacemaker is recommended; amiodarone-induced bradycardia generally is not fully responsive to atropine. For AV block, the use of a transvenous cardiac pacemaker may be necessary. Administration of IV fluids and placement of the patient in Trendelenburg's position is recommended for the initial treatment of hypotension. An inotropic agent or vasopressor (e.g., dopamine, norepinephrine) should be given for hypotension accompanied by signs of inadequate tissue perfusion. Hepatic enzymes also should be monitored closely in the case of IV amiodarone overdosage. Hemodialysis or peritoneal dialysis is not useful for enhancing elimination of amiodarone or N-desethylamiodarone in acute overdosage.

PHARMACOLOGY

● Antiarrhythmic and Electrophysiologic Effects

The antiarrhythmic and electrophysiologic actions of amiodarone hydrochloride are complex and differ from those of other currently available antiarrhythmic agents. Studies in animals have shown that amiodarone is effective in preventing and/or suppressing experimentally induced arrhythmias.

The exact mechanism(s) of antiarrhythmic action of amiodarone has not been conclusively determined. Amiodarone is considered to be predominantly a class III antiarrhythmic agent, but the drug also appears to exhibit activity in each of the four Vaughn-Williams antiarrhythmic classes, including some class I (membrane-stabilizing) antiarrhythmic action. The principal effect of amiodarone on cardiac tissue is to delay repolarization by prolonging the action potential duration (APD) and effective refractory period (ERP). The drug also appears to inhibit transmembrane influx of extracellular sodium ions via fast sodium channels, as indicated by a decrease in the maximal rate of depolarization of phase 0 of the action potential. Like class I antiarrhythmic agents, amiodarone is believed to combine with fast sodium channels in their inactive state and thereby inhibit recovery after repolarization in a time- and voltage-dependent manner, which is associated with subsequent dissociation of the drug from the sodium channels. Amiodarone appears to have little affinity for activated fast sodium channels. Amiodarone also produces a noncompetitive inhibition of α- and β-adrenergic activity that may contribute to the drug's antiarrhythmic activity. Limited data suggest that the drug may possess some vagolytic and/or calcium-channel blocking activity, and that recovery from calcium-channel blockade may be substantially more rapid than that with diltiazem or verapamil, but additional study is needed. Amiodarone does not appear to have vagomimetic or local anesthetic activity.

Amiodarone predominantly exhibits electrophysiologic effects characteristic of class III antiarrhythmic agents (i.e., prolonged repolarization and refractoriness), but the drug also appears to exhibit activity in each of the four Vaughn-Williams antiarrhythmic classes, including some electrophysiologic effects characteristic of class I (particularly class IA or IC) antiarrhythmic agents. The drug prolongs APD in atrial and ventricular muscle, the sinus node, the atrioventricular (AV) node, and the His-Purkinje system without substantially altering resting membrane potential or action potential height, except in automatic cells (e.g., those in the sinus node or His-Purkinje system) in which it reduces the slope of diastolic depolarization and thereby generally reduces automaticity. Although several investigators have suggested that the myocardial effects observed during chronic amiodarone therapy are comparable to those associated with hypothyroidism and may be related to competitive inhibition of sodium-potassium-activated adenosine triphosphatase (Na$^+$-K$^+$-ATPase) activity, other data suggest that amiodarone's effects on thyroid function contribute minimally, if at all, to the overall electrophysiologic effects of the drug.

Effects on Cardiac Conduction and Refractoriness

Amiodarone appears to prolong refractoriness throughout the myocardium including the atria, ventricles, His-Purkinje system, sinus node, and AV node, as well as in accessory pathways, if present. The effect of amiodarone on cardiac conduction is less well defined, but the drug appears to decrease AV conduction following a single IV dose or chronic oral administration; the decrease appears to be heart-rate dependent, with substantially larger reductions in AV conduction at high rates. Amiodarone may also partially impair conduction within the His-Purkinje system. When administered IV, amiodarone prolongs intranodal conduction and AV node refractoriness, but has little to no effect on sinus cycle length, refractoriness of the right atrium or right ventricle, repolarization, intraventricular conduction, or intranodal conduction. At higher than usual IV doses (e.g., greater than 10 mg/kg), amiodarone prolongation of right ventricular refractoriness and modest prolongation of the QRS complex have been observed. Differences in the effect between parenterally versus orally administered amiodarone are seen predominantly in effects on AV nodal conduction; IV amiodarone causes an intranodal conduction delay and increased nodal refractoriness secondary to slow-channel blockade (class IV activity) and noncompetitive adrenergic antagonism (class II activity). The effects of amiodarone on intracardiac conduction may result from its class I antiarrhythmic activity; the drug's effects on slow calcium channels also may be involved. Further studies are needed to fully determine the effects of the drug on intracardiac conduction.

The effects of amiodarone on refractoriness and intracardiac conduction are manifested by increases in PR and QT intervals. Following chronic oral administration of the drug, increases in PR interval and QT interval corrected for rate (QT$_c$) average about 10–17% and 10–23%, respectively. Limited data suggest that amiodarone-induced QT prolongation may constitute an antiarrhythmic mechanism, although additional study is necessary. Rarely, QT prolongation induced by the drug is associated with arrhythmogenicity. QRS intervals may be unchanged or increased. Amiodarone generally increases the AH interval but has a variable effect on the HV interval, which may be unchanged or prolonged following chronic oral administration of the drug. Changes in T-wave contour, such as widening, bifurcation, or reduction in amplitude, and the development of prominent U waves may also occur during amiodarone therapy.

The antiarrhythmic and electrophysiologic effects of amiodarone following single IV doses appear to differ substantially from those observed during chronic oral administration of the drug. Following a single IV dose, the major effect of the drug is on the AV node with lengthening of ERP and prolongation of intranodal conduction time, whereas during chronic oral therapy, prolongation of APD and ERP in the atria, ventricles, and AV nodal tissue occurs. At a constant oral dosage, the electrophysiologic effects of amiodarone, including increases in APD and refractoriness, appear to develop as a function of time.

Effects on Sinus Node

Amiodarone generally depresses sinus node function. Following chronic oral administration of amiodarone, sinus rate is reduced by about 10–20%; however, changes in sinus rate following single IV doses of the drug do not appear to be substantial. Marked sinus bradycardia or sinus arrest and heart block may occur in some patients. Amiodarone appears to depress sinus node automaticity. Data are conflicting, but amiodarone may in part reduce automaticity by increasing the APD and depressing the slope of diastolic depolarization in the sinus node. Administration of propranolol or atropine does not appear to substantially influence these changes, but a low calcium concentration enhances the drug's negative chronotropic effect. Following chronic administration of amiodarone, spontaneous cycle lengths are increased. The effects of amiodarone on sinus node recovery time (SNRT) and sinoatrial conduction time (SACT) have not been fully established; however, prolongation of both SNRT and SACT has occurred in some patients receiving long-term therapy with the drug.

Effects on His-Purkinje System

In addition to prolonging repolarization and refractoriness, amiodarone reduces the maximum rate of phase 0 depolarization in Purkinje fibers in a use-dependent manner (i.e., the magnitude of depression of the maximum rate of phase 0 depolarization increases at faster stimulation rates). Clinical experience indicates that chronic oral therapy with the drug may result in prolongation of intraventricular conduction as manifested by lengthening of the HV interval. However, amiodarone's effect on the HV interval appears to be variable; data from clinical studies indicate that the HV interval may either be unchanged or prolonged by up to about 15–30% during chronic administration of the drug. In addition, amiodarone therapy reportedly has exacerbated preexisting His-Purkinje delay in some patients.

Effects on Accessory AV Pathways and Reentry Mechanisms

The electrophysiologic effects of amiodarone on accessory pathways, the AV node, the His-Purkinje system, and/or atrial and ventricular myocardium may contribute to the drug's efficacy in terminating and preventing paroxysmal reentrant supraventricular tachycardias. In patients with Wolff-Parkinson-White syndrome or concealed accessory AV pathways, amiodarone generally increases refractoriness of the anterograde and retrograde accessory pathways, but the effect on refractoriness of the retrograde accessory pathway appears to be somewhat more variable and less pronounced. Limited data indicate that the effects of amiodarone may be greater on anterograde accessory pathways that have relatively long pretreatment refractory periods. In addition to its effects on accessory pathways, amiodarone may increase refractoriness in atrial and ventricular tissue, the AV node, and the His-Purkinje system, resulting in possible prevention or interruption of reentrant tachyarrhythmias. Amiodarone may also decrease the occurrence of atrial premature complexes (APCs) and ventricular premature complexes (VPCs) responsible for initiation of reentrant tachyarrhythmias.

● Antiadrenergic Effects

Amiodarone noncompetitively inhibits α- and β-adrenergic responses to sympathetic stimulation and catecholamine administration. In vitro and in vivo data indicate that the drug noncompetitively antagonizes cardiovascular effects (e.g., tachycardia, hypertension, increase in myocardial oxygen consumption) induced by epinephrine, norepinephrine, and/or isoproterenol. The precise mechanism of adrenergic inhibition is unclear. Some data suggest that amiodarone does not bind directly to the catecholamine-recognition site on β-adrenergic receptors but instead may reduce β-adrenergic activity by decreasing the number of β-adrenergic receptors. Although conflicting results have been reported, limited data suggest that amiodarone may also inhibit the release of neurotransmitter from presynaptic adrenergic neurons. Although not clearly established, the antiadrenergic activity of amiodarone may contribute to its antiarrhythmic and antianginal efficacy.

● Arrhythmogenic Effects

Like other antiarrhythmic agents, amiodarone can worsen existing arrhythmias or cause new arrhythmias. The arrhythmogenic effects of the drug have included ventricular fibrillation, sustained ventricular tachycardia, increased resistance to cardioversion, and atypical ventricular tachycardia (torsades de pointes).

● Cardiovascular Effects

Amiodarone generally exhibits minimal cardiovascular effects following oral administration. The cardiovascular effects of the drug appear to be more pronounced following IV than oral administration, but evaluations have been more extensive following IV administration. In addition, some cardiovascular effects observed following IV administration may be related to the solvent, polysorbate (Tween®) 80, used in the parenteral dosage form of the drug.

Long-term oral administration of amiodarone generally depresses sinus node function, and heart rate is reduced by an average of about 10–20%. Following a single IV dose of amiodarone, heart rate may be increased, decreased, or unchanged; however, changes in heart rate after IV administration, if present, generally are minimal and transient. Amiodarone generally does not appear to have a substantial negative inotropic effect following long-term oral administration, even in patients with depressed left ventricular ejection fraction (LVEF); however, a mild negative inotropic effect (possibly related to the rate of injection) may occur following IV administration of the drug.

Amiodarone generally relaxes cardiac and vascular smooth muscle, thereby dilating both systemic and coronary arteries. Following IV administration of 5 mg/kg of amiodarone hydrochloride, systemic blood pressure, systemic vascular resistance, coronary vascular resistance, and left ventricular end-diastolic pressure (LVEDP) are generally decreased, while coronary sinus flow may increase transiently and cardiac index may increase slightly. Studies in humans and animals indicate that IV amiodarone may produce a transient, dose-related increase in coronary artery blood flow, mainly as a result of a direct relaxant effect on coronary arteries, but reductions in contractility and LVEF may also be involved. Although not clearly established, limited data suggest that the transient reduction in coronary and systemic vascular resistance observed following IV administration may at least partially result from the vasodilatory effects of polysorbate 80 present as a solvent in the injection. Studies in humans and animals also suggest that amiodarone reduces myocardial oxygen consumption, resulting in a protective effect on ischemic myocardium. Although not clearly established, decreased myocardial oxygen consumption appears to result from a reduction in heart rate, systemic vascular resistance, and possibly myocardial contractility.

Long-term oral administration of amiodarone generally does not appear to produce substantial changes in LVEF, even in patients with left ventricular dysfunction. The drug, however, has been associated with new or worsened heart failure in some patients receiving chronic oral therapy. (See Cautions: Cardiovascular Effects.) IV administration of amiodarone may transiently depress left ventricular function, probably as a result of the drug's negative inotropic effect, particularly in patients with preexisting left ventricular dysfunction or at high doses. Although decreases in left ventricular function following IV administration of the drug are generally transient and well tolerated, severe hypotension has occurred rarely in patients with severe heart failure.

● Thyroid Effects

Amiodarone has variable and complex effects on thyroid function. The drug's principal effect appears to be inhibition of extrathyroidal deiodinases, resulting in decreased peripheral conversion of thyroxine (T_4) to triiodothyronine (T_3) and a subsequent increase in serum T_4 and inactive reverse triiodothyronine (reverse T_3, rT_3) concentrations and decrease in serum T_3 concentrations. Serum concentrations of thyrotropin (thyroid-stimulating hormone, TSH) usually increase initially but return to baseline or slightly below baseline values within a few months to a year despite continued therapy. In addition, the thyrotropin response to protirelin initially may be accentuated in patients receiving amiodarone; normal or depressed responses may occur during long-term therapy.

Despite the changes in serum thyroid hormone concentrations, most patients receiving amiodarone remain clinically euthyroid; however, clinical hypothyroidism or hyperthyroidism may occur. The mechanism(s) of amiodarone-induced hypothyroidism or hyperthyroidism has not been fully elucidated, but may be related to the iodine content of amiodarone and/or involve a direct effect of the drug or its major metabolite on thyroid function. It has also been proposed that amiodarone may alter the sensitivity of the pituitary gland and peripheral organs to the actions of thyroid hormones; however, additional study is needed.

● Other Effects

Amiodarone inhibits phospholipase (including phospholipase A_1, A_2, and C) activity in vitro. In patients receiving the drug, histologic examination has revealed the presence of phospholipid-laden lysosomal inclusions within pulmonary cells, liver cells, Schwann cells, leukocytes, epithelial cells in skin, and possibly within epithelial cells in the eye. The exact mechanism(s) of amiodarone-induced injury to various body organs remains to be clearly established; however, the production of amiodarone-phospholipid complexes within certain organs may play a role in the development of many of the adverse effects associated with the drug. It also has been suggested that accumulation of phospholipids within pulmonary cells also may result from increased phospholipid synthesis. In addition, amiodarone-induced pulmonary toxicity may be related to surfactant ingestion by macrophages, release of free oxygen radicals, increased iodide content, and/or altered cellular function secondary to the amphophilic nature of the drug. Although pulmonary toxicity appears to result from a hypersensitivity reaction in some patients, and there was evidence of an IgG-mediated immune response initiated against an amiodarone/native pulmonary protein complex (hapten-protein complex) in at least one patient, the mechanism of amiodarone-induced hypersensitivity, including the possible role of immunoglobulins, complement deposition, and cytokines in this reaction remains to be more fully elucidated. In patients developing amiodarone-induced hypersensitivity pneumonitis, suppressor/cytotoxic ($CD8^+$, $T8^+$) T-cell lymphocytosis often is present in bronchoalveolar lavage specimens.

Amiodarone theoretically can inhibit intracellular α-galactosidase activity. (See Drug Interactions: Agalsidase Beta.)

The effects of amiodarone on serum lipid concentrations have not been clearly established. Serum cholesterol and triglyceride concentrations in patients receiving the drug have variably been reported to be increased or decreased.

PHARMACOKINETICS

● Absorption

Amiodarone hydrochloride is slowly and variably absorbed from the GI tract following oral administration. The absolute bioavailability of commercially available amiodarone hydrochloride tablets averages approximately 50%, but varies considerably, ranging from 22–86%. The sometimes low and often variable bioavailability of amiodarone may possibly result from N-dealkylation or other metabolism in the intestinal lumen and/or GI mucosa, from first-pass metabolism in the liver, and/or from poor dissolution characteristics of the drug. Food increases the rate and extent of absorption of amiodarone. Results of a study in healthy adults indicate that administration of a single 600-mg oral dose of amiodarone hydrochloride after a high-fat meal increases the area under the plasma concentration-time curve (AUC) and the peak plasma concentration of amiodarone by 2.3 (range: 1.7–3.6) and 3.8 (range: 2.7–4.4) times, respectively, compared with administration in the fasting state. Food also increases the rate of absorption of amiodarone; when administered with food, the time to achieve peak plasma concentration of unchanged drug is decreased by about 37% to 4.5 hours. The mean AUC and mean peak plasma concentrations of N-desethylamiodarone (the major metabolite) increase by about 55 and 32%, respectively; however, the time to peak plasma concentration of this metabolite remains unchanged in the presence of food. Limited data suggest that the drug may undergo enterohepatic circulation.

Following oral administration, peak plasma amiodarone concentrations usually occur within 3–7 hours (range: 2–12 hours). Following oral administration of a single 400-mg dose of amiodarone hydrochloride in fasting, healthy adults, peak plasma amiodarone concentrations of approximately 0.15–0.7 mcg/mL are attained. Within the oral dosage range of 100–600 mg daily, steady-state plasma concentrations of the drug are approximately proportional to dosage, increasing by an average of 0.5 mcg/mL per 100-mg increment in dosage; however, there is considerable interindividual variation in plasma concentrations attained with a given dosage. Following continuous oral administration of the drug in the absence of an initial loading-dose regimen, steady-state plasma amiodarone concentrations would not be attained for at least 1 month and generally not for up to 5 months or longer. Following chronic oral administration of amiodarone, plasma concentrations of N-desethylamiodarone, the major metabolite of the drug, are approximately 0.5–2 times those of unchanged drug.

In a study of single-dose IV amiodarone hydrochloride (5 mg/kg over 15 minutes) in healthy individuals, peak drug concentration ranged from 5–41mcg/mL. Following 10-minute IV infusions of amiodarone hydrochloride at a dose of 150 mg in patients with ventricular fibrillation or hemodynamically unstable ventricular tachycardia, peak drug concentration ranged from 7–26 mcg/mL. Because of a rapid distribution phase, the concentration of amiodarone declines to 10% of peak values within 30–45 minutes after the end of the infusion. In clinical trials after 48 hours of continuous IV infusions (125, 500, or 1000 mg daily) plus supplemental infusions (150 mg) as needed for recurrent arrhythmias, mean plasma concentrations of amiodarone ranged from 0.7–1.4 mcg/mL.Following administration of a single IV dose of amiodarone in patients with cirrhosis, lower peak and mean plasma concentrations of N-desethylamiodarone are observed; mean amiodarone concentration remains unchanged.

Following oral administration of amiodarone, the onset of antiarrhythmic activity is highly variable. A therapeutic response may begin within 2–3 days in some patients but generally is not evident until 1–3 weeks after beginning therapy with the drug, even when loading doses are administered. Limited data suggest that the onset of action occurs earlier in patients receiving loading doses of the drug and in pediatric patients. Although not clearly established, the time of maximal antiarrhythmic effect usually occurs within 1–5 months after initiating oral amiodarone therapy. Antiarrhythmic effects generally persist for 10–150 days following withdrawal of long-term amiodarone therapy; however, duration of antiarrhythmic activity is variable and unpredictable and appears to depend on the length of therapy as well as the type of cardiac arrhythmia being treated. In general, when amiodarone therapy is resumed after prior discontinuance of the drug and subsequent recurrence of the arrhythmia, control of the arrhythmia occurs relatively rapidly compared to the initial response, presumably because tissues are not fully depleted of the drug at the time therapy is resumed.

There is considerable interindividual variation in the relationship between plasma amiodarone concentrations and antiarrhythmic effects. Limited data suggest that prolongation of the QT$_c$ interval is correlated with plasma amiodarone concentrations. Based on suppression of arrhythmias, plasma amiodarone concentrations of approximately 1–2.5 mcg/mL are usually necessary for optimum therapeutic effect, although therapeutic response may be apparent at lower concentrations in some patients; plasma concentrations higher than 2.5 mcg/mL are generally not necessary. There is no established relationship between drug concentration and therapeutic response for short-term IV amiodarone therapy. Although considerable overlap exists between therapeutic and toxic plasma concentrations, certain adverse reactions including adverse hepatic, ocular, and neuromuscular effects appear to occur more frequently when plasma amiodarone concentrations exceed 2.5 mcg/mL.

● **Distribution**

Distribution of amiodarone into human body tissues and fluids has not been fully characterized. Following IV administration in rats, amiodarone is distributed extensively into many tissues, including adipose tissue, liver, kidneys, heart, and, to a lesser extent, the CNS. Following chronic oral administration of the drug in humans, amiodarone and N-desethylamiodarone are distributed extensively into many body tissues and fluids, including adipose tissue, liver, lung, spleen, skeletal muscle, bone marrow, adrenal glands, kidneys, pancreas, testes, semen, saliva, lymph nodes, myocardium, thyroid gland, skin, and brain. Amiodarone is also distributed into bile. Limited data indicate that peak biliary concentrations

of the drug may be approximately 50 times greater than peak plasma concentrations. Tissue concentrations of amiodarone generally exceed concurrent plasma concentrations of the drug. N-Desethylamiodarone appears to accumulate in the same body tissues as amiodarone; however, after long-term therapy, concentrations of the metabolite are usually substantially higher than concentrations of unchanged drug in almost all tissues, except adipose tissue, which mainly contains amiodarone. N-Desethylamiodarone and, to a lesser extent, amiodarone also distribute into erythrocytes. Ratios of erythrocyte-to-plasma concentrations of amiodarone and N-desethylamiodarone were 0.33 and 0.67, respectively, after a single oral dose of amiodarone and 0.38–0.48 and 1.3–1.76, respectively, after long-term oral therapy with the drug. Following a single IV dose, the mean blood-to-plasma ratio for amiodarone is 0.73.

Following IV administration, amiodarone is rapidly and widely distributed. The apparent volume of distribution of the drug or its major metabolite, N-desethylamiodarone, in healthy adults reportedly averages 65.8 L/kg (range: 18.3–147.7 L/kg) or ranges from 68–168 L/kg, respectively, following a single IV dose.

In vitro, amiodarone is approximately 96% bound to plasma proteins, mainly to albumin and, to a lesser extent, a high-density lipoprotein that is probably β-lipoprotein.

Amiodarone and N-desethylamiodarone cross the placenta to a limited extent. In pregnant women receiving amiodarone, ratios of umbilical venous to maternal venous plasma concentrations of amiodarone and N-desethylamiodarone were 0.1–0.28 and 0.25–0.55, respectively. Amiodarone and its major metabolite are distributed into milk in concentrations substantially higher than concurrent maternal plasma concentrations. Limited data in a lactating woman indicate amiodarone and N-desethylamiodarone milk-to-plasma ratios ranging from 2.3–9.1 and 0.8–3.8, respectively.

● **Elimination**

Plasma concentrations of amiodarone appear to decline in at least a biphasic manner, although more complex, multicompartment pharmacokinetics have been described. Following a single IV dose in healthy adults, the half-life of the drug in the terminal elimination phase (t$_{½β}$) has been reported to average 25 days (range: 9–47 days). The elimination half-life of the major metabolite, N-desethylamiodarone, is equal to or longer than that of the parent drug. Following single-dose administration of amiodarone in a limited number of healthy individuals, amiodarone exhibits multicompartmental pharmacokinetics; the mean apparent terminal plasma elimination half-life of amiodarone and N-desethylamiodarone were 58 (range: 15–142) and 36 (range: 14–75) days, respectively. The half-life of amiodarone appears to be substantially more prolonged following multiple rather than single doses. It has been suggested that differences in reported elimination half-lives may result in part from misinterpretation of slow distribution phases as elimination phases following IV administration of the drug. Following chronic oral administration of amiodarone hydrochloride in patients with cardiac arrhythmias (200–600 mg daily for 2–52 months), the drug appears to be eliminated in a biphasic manner with an initial elimination half-life of about 2.5–10 days, which is followed by a terminal elimination half-life averaging 53 days (range: 26–107 days), with most patients exhibiting a terminal elimination half-life in the range of 40–55 days. The elimination half-life of the major metabolite, N-desethylamiodarone, averages 57–61 days (range: 20–118 days) following long-term oral administration of amiodarone. The elimination profile of amiodarone probably reflects an initial elimination of the drug from well-perfused tissues followed by prolonged elimination from poorly perfused tissues such as adipose tissue.

In a study of single-dose amiodarone hydrochloride (5 mg/kg over 15 minutes) in healthy individuals, clearance of the drug and its major active metabolite, N-desethylamiodarone, ranged from 90–158 and 197–290 mL/hour per kg, respectively. In clinical studies lasting 2–7 days, clearance of IV amiodarone in patients with ventricular fibrillation or ventricular tachycardia ranged from 220–440 mL/hour per kg. Clearance of the drug in healthy geriatric individuals (i.e., older than 65 years of age) was decreased to approximately 100 mL/hour per kg, as compared with clearance of approximately 150 mL/hour per kg in younger individuals; in addition, the elimination half-life of the drug was increased in these geriatric individuals to 47 days, as compared with 20 days in younger individuals.

The exact metabolic fate of amiodarone has not been fully elucidated, but the drug appears to be extensively metabolized, probably in the liver and possibly in the intestinal lumen and/or GI mucosa, to at least one major metabolite.

The major metabolite, *N*-desethylamiodarone, is formed by *N*-deethylation. Although not clearly established, limited data in animals indicate that the desethyl metabolite possesses substantial electrophysiologic and antiarrhythmic activity similar to amiodarone's. Following IV administration of a single dose of *N*-desethylamiodarone in animals, the metabolite prolonged atrial and ventricular refractoriness and decreased conduction within the AV node; however, further studies are needed to determine the effects of the desethyl metabolite following chronic administration. The precise role of *N*-desethylamiodarone in the antiarrhythmic activity of amiodarone has not been clearly established. The development of maximal ventricular class III antiarrhythmic effects after oral amiodarone administration in humans correlates more closely with *N*-desethylamiodarone accumulation over time than with amiodarone accumulation. A minor metabolite of amiodarone, di-*N*-desethylamiodarone, has been identified in animals following chronic administration of the drug. Amiodarone and *N*-desethylamiodarone may undergo deiodination to form deiodoamiodarone and deiodo-*N*-desethylamiodarone, respectively; iodine (in the form of iodide); and possibly other iodine-containing metabolites. It is not known whether deiodinated metabolites are pharmacologically active.

The excretory patterns of amiodarone and its metabolite have not been well characterized. Following oral or IV administration, amiodarone appears to be excreted almost completely in feces as unchanged drug and *N*-desethylamiodarone, presumably via biliary elimination. Although not clearly established, limited data suggest that amiodarone may undergo enterohepatic circulation. Renal excretion of amiodarone and *N*-desethylamiodarone appears to be negligible.

Following IV administration of amiodarone in healthy individuals, total plasma clearance of the drug averages approximately 1.9 mL/minute per kg (range: 1.4–2.5 mL/minute per kg). Although not clearly established, total apparent plasma clearance of the drug appears to decrease with time. Clinical experience suggests that clearance of amiodarone may be more rapid in pediatric patients; however, further studies are needed to fully determine the effects of age on clearance of the drug. Factors of age, gender, or renal or hepatic disease appear to have no effect on the disposition of amiodarone or its major metabolite, *N*-desethylamiodarone.

In patients with severe left ventricular dysfunction, the pharmacokinetics of amiodarone are not significantly altered; however, the terminal elimination half-life of *N*-desethylamiodarone is prolonged in these patients.

Amiodarone and *N*-desethylamiodarone are not appreciably removed by hemodialysis or peritoneal dialysis.

CHEMISTRY AND STABILITY

● Chemistry

Amiodarone hydrochloride is an iodinated benzofuran-derivative antiarrhythmic agent. The drug differs structurally and pharmacologically from other currently available antiarrhythmic agents.

Amiodarone hydrochloride occurs as a white to cream-colored, crystalline powder and has solubilities of approximately 0.72 mg/mL in water and 12.8 mg/mL in alcohol at 25°C. The drug is highly lipophilic. Amiodarone hydrochloride contains 37.3% iodine; each 200-mg tablet of the drug or each mL of the commercially available injection contains approximately 75 or 18.7 mg of iodine, respectively. The commercially available injection contains benzyl alcohol as a preservative. Amiodarone has a pK_a of approximately 6.6.

● Stability

Amiodarone hydrochloride tablets should be protected from light and stored in tight containers at 20–25°C. The manufacturer of one commercially available amiodarone hydrochloride tablet preparation (Pacerone®) states that the tablets may be exposed to temperatures ranging from 15–30°C. Commercially available amiodarone tablets have an expiration date of 3 years following the date of manufacture.

Commercially available amiodarone hydrochloride injection concentrate should be stored at 20–25°C and protected from light and excessive heat. Ampuls containing the injection concentrate should be stored in the carton to protect the solution from light until used. Diluted solutions of amiodarone hydrochloride injection do not need to be protected from light during administration.

Although amiodarone hydrochloride adsorbs to polyvinyl chloride (PVC) tubing, the parenteral drug doses and administration schedule studied in clinical trials were designed to take this fact into account. Therefore, the manufacturer recommends using PVC tubing and closely following the suggested infusion regimen when administering amiodarone hydrochloride by IV infusion. Leaching of diethylhexyl phthalate (DEHP) from IV tubing may occur.

Following dilution of amiodarone hydrochloride injection concentrate to a concentration of 1–6 mg/mL in 5% dextrose in a PVC container, there is physical compatibility, with a loss of less than 10% of drug at 2 hours at room temperature. Following dilution of amiodarone hydrochloride injection concentrate to a concentration of 1–6 mg/mL in 5% dextrose in a glass or polyolefin container, there is physical compatibility, with no loss of drug at 24 hours at room temperature. Therefore, the manufacturer states that amiodarone hydrochloride infusions exceeding 2 hours should be administered in 5% dextrose in a glass or polyolefin containers. However, evacuated glass containers should not be used since incompatibility with a buffer in the container may cause precipitation.

When admixed in 5% dextrose, amiodarone hydrochloride injection is incompatible with aminophylline, cefamandole nafate, cefazolin sodium, mezlocillin sodium, heparin sodium, or sodium bicarbonate. Specialized references should be consulted for specific compatibility information.

Clinicians should provide information to patients regarding proper techniques for storage and disposal of out-of-date amiodarone tablets.

PREPARATIONS

Excipients in commercially available drug preparations may have clinically important effects in some individuals; consult specific product labeling for details.

Amiodarone Hydrochloride

Oral			
Tablets		100 mg	Pacerone®, Upsher-Smith
		200 mg*	**Amiodarone Hydrochloride Tablets**
			Cordarone® (scored), Wyeth
			Pacerone® (scored), Upsher-Smith
		400 mg*	**Amiodarone Hydrochloride Tablets**
			Pacerone® (scored), Upsher-Smith
Parenteral			
Concentrate for injection, for IV infusion	50 mg/mL*		**Amiodarone Hydrochloride Injection**

* available from one or more manufacturer, distributor, and/or repackager by generic (nonproprietary) name

† Use is not currently included in the labeling approved by the US Food and Drug Administration.

Selected Revisions June 10, 2024, © Copyright, September 1, 1987, American Society of Health-System Pharmacists, Inc.

Dofetilide

24:04.04.20 • CLASS III ANTIARRHYTHMICS

■ Dofetilide is a class III antiarrhythmic agent.

REMS

FDA approved a REMS for dofetilide to ensure that the benefits outweigh the risks. However, FDA later rescinded REMS requirements. See the FDA REMS page (https://www.accessdata.fda.gov/scripts/cder/rems/index.cfm).

USES

● Supraventricular Tachyarrhythmias

Dofetilide is used for the maintenance of normal sinus rhythm in patients with atrial fibrillation/ atrial flutter of more than 1 week duration who have been converted to normal sinus rhythm. Because dofetilide can cause life-threatening ventricular arrhythmias, it should be reserved for patients in whom atrial fibrillation/ atrial flutter is highly symptomatic. Dofetilide also is used for the conversion of atrial fibrillation and atrial flutter to normal sinus rhythm. Dofetilide has not been shown to be effective in patients with paroxysmal atrial fibrillation.

In 2 randomized, double-blind, dose-response studies, about 30% of patients with atrial fibrillation/ atrial flutter who received 500 mcg of dofetilide twice daily were successfully converted to normal sinus rhythm compared with about 10 or 6% of those receiving 250 or 125 mcg twice daily and 1% of those who received placebo. Approximately 70% of the patients who successfully achieved normal sinus rhythm did so within 24–36 hours of beginning dofetilide therapy. After 12 months of therapy, the probabilities of remaining in normal sinus rhythm were 58–66 or 25–21% in patients who had converted to normal sinus rhythm and were still receiving dofetilide (500 mcg twice daily) or placebo, respectively. In one of these studies, dofetilide also was more effective than sotalol (80 mg orally twice daily) in converting atrial fibrillation to normal sinus rhythm or maintaining normal sinus rhythm for up to 12 months. In a third study, dofetilide was effective in converting and preventing the recurrence of atrial fibrillation without affecting mortality in patients with congestive heart failure and reduced left ventricular function.

DOSAGE AND ADMINISTRATION

● Administration

Dofetilide is administered orally twice daily without regard to meals.

Restricted Distribution Program

Commercially available dofetilide must be obtained through a restricted distribution program. Clinicians and pharmacies in institutions must confirm their participation in a designated Tikosyn® educational program before prescribing or ordering the drug; the drug is not available through community pharmacies. The status of clinicians who have participated in these programs may be verified on the internet (www.tikosynlist.com); for information regarding such educational programs, contact the manufacturer at 877-845-6796.

● Dosage

The recommended adult dosage of dofetilide is 500 mcg twice daily, which is modified according to creatinine clearance and QT$_c$ interval. The risk of torsades de pointes is related to the dosage of dofetilide, and clinicians may elect to initiate therapy with lower dosages. Dosages exceeding 500 mcg twice daily have been associated with an increased incidence of torsades de pointes.

Because of the arrhythmogenic potential of dofetilide, the manufacturer recommends that both initiation of therapy with the drug and any subsequent increases in dosage be performed in a hospital setting where creatinine clearance calculations, continuous ECG monitoring, and cardiac resuscitation can be performed and where the patient can be monitored by personnel trained in the management of serious ventricular arrhythmias. Prior to initiation of dofetilide, the creatinine clearance must be calculated and QT$_c$ interval (or QT interval if

the heart rate is less than 60 beats/minute) must be determined using an average of 5–10 beats. If the QT$_c$ interval exceeds 440 msec (500 msec in patients with ventricular conduction abnormalities), dofetilide is contraindicated. If creatinine clearance is less than 60 mL/minute, the initial dosage of dofetilide must be reduced. (See Dosage and Administration: Special Populations.) Serum potassium should be within the normal range (above 3.6–4 mEq/L) before initiation of dofetilide therapy and maintained in that range during therapy. Within 2–3 hours of administering the first dose of dofetilide, determine the QT$_c$ interval. If QT$_c$ interval has increased by more than 15% or exceeds 500 msec (550 msec in patients with ventricular conduction abnormalities), adjust subsequent dosages as indicated in Table 1.

TABLE 1.

Initial Dosage (Based on Creatinine Clearance)	Adjusted Dosage (for QT$_c$ Prolongation)
500 mcg twice daily	250 mcg twice daily
250 mcg twice daily	125 mcg twice daily
125 mcg twice daily	125 mcg once daily

Within 2–3 hours after each subsequent dose of dofetilide (for in-hospital doses 2–5), determine the QT$_c$ interval. No further downward titration of dofetilide based on QT$_c$ is recommended. However, if at any time after the second dose of dofetilide is given the QT$_c$ exceeds 500 msec (550 msec in patients with ventricular conduction abnormalities), discontinue dofetilide. Continuous ECG monitoring should be performed for a minimum of 3 days or for a minimum of 12 hours after electrical or pharmacologic conversion to normal sinus rhythm, whichever is greater.

Reevaluate renal function and QT$_c$ interval every 3 months or as medically warranted. If QT$_c$ exceeds 500 msec (550 msec in patients with ventricular conduction abnormalities), discontinue dofetilide and carefully monitor the patient until QT$_c$ returns to baseline levels. If renal function deteriorates, adjust dosage as described in Dosage and Administration: Special Populations.

The manufacturer recommends that patients be hospitalized and closely monitored for 3 days (until steady-state plasma concentrations are obtained) whenever treatment is initiated or reinitiated or when dofetilide dosage is increased. Previously successful use of such dosages of dofetilide does not eliminate the need for rehospitalization when the dosage is increased.

● Special Populations

In patients with impaired renal function, dosage of dofetilide must be modified according to the degree of impairment. *Because increase in QT interval and the risk of ventricular arrhythmias are directly related to plasma dofetilide concentrations, dosage adjustment based on calculated creatinine clearance is essential.* The patient's creatinine clearance (Ccr) can be estimated by using the following formulas:

$$Ccr\ male = \frac{(140 - age) \times weight}{72 \times serum\ creatinine}$$
$$Ccr\ female = 0.85 \times Ccr\ male$$

where age is in years, weight is in kg, and serum creatinine is in mg/dL.

The manufacturer recommends that patients receive the following dosage based on calculated creatinine clearance (see Table 2).

TABLE 2.

Calculated Creatinine Clearance (mL/minute)	Dosage
>60	500 mcg twice daily
40–60	250 mcg twice daily
20 to <40	125 mcg twice daily
<20	Dofetilide is contraindicated

No dosage adjustment is required in patients with mild to moderate hepatic impairment (Child-Pugh class A or B). The pharmacokinetics of the drug have not been studied in patients with severe hepatic insufficiency (Child-Pugh class C) and such patients should be treated cautiously.

CAUTIONS

● Contraindications

Congenital or acquired long QT syndromes; baseline QT or QT_c interval exceeding 440 msec (500 msec in patients with ventricular conduction abnormalities). Severe renal impairment (calculated creatinine clearance below 20 mL/minute). Concomitant use of verapamil or cation transport system inhibitors (e.g., cimetidine, ketoconazole, megestrol, prochlorperazine, trimethoprim [alone or in combination with sulfamethoxazole]). Concomitant use of hydrochlorothiazide (alone or in combination with triamterene). (See Drug Interactions.) Known hypersensitivity to dofetilide.

● Warnings/Precautions

Warnings

Arrhythmogenic Effects

Dofetilide may cause serious ventricular arrhythmias, principally polymorphic ventricular tachycardia associated with QT interval prolongation (i.e., torsades de pointes). The risk of torsades de pointes can be reduced by controlling the plasma concentration (e.g., adjustment of initial dofetilide dosage according to creatinine clearance, avoiding certain drug interactions) and monitoring the ECG for excessive increases in the QT interval. In clinical trials, the overall incidence of torsades de pointes was 0.8% and was dose-related in patients with supraventricular arrhythmias. Most episodes of torsades de pointes occurred within the first 3 days of dofetilide therapy, and the risk was threefold greater in women than in men.

Drug Interactions

Because there is a linear relationship between plasma dofetilide concentration and QT_c, drug interactions that increase plasma dofetilide concentrations either through decreased renal excretion (e.g., inhibitors of cationic renal secretion) or decreased metabolism (e.g., inhibitors of cytochrome P-450 [CYP] isoenzyme 3A4) may increase the risk of torsades de pointes. Use of dofetilide with other drugs that prolong the QT interval has not been studied, and concomitant use of dofetilide with such drugs is not recommended. Carefully screen patients' medication history, including all over-the-counter, prescription, and herbal/natural preparations with emphasis on those that may affect dofetilide pharmacokinetics. If dofetilide must be discontinued to permit administration of potentially interacting drug(s), allow a washout period of at least 2 days. (See Drug Interactions.)

General Precautions

Effects on Cardiac Conduction

Animal and human studies have not shown any adverse effects of dofetilide on conduction velocity. No effect on AV nodal conduction following dofetilide treatment was noted in normal volunteers or in patients with first degree heart block. Dofetilide has been used safely in conjunction with pacemakers.

Drug Transfer

The manufacturer recommends a transition period for patients being transferred from another antiarrhythmic agent to dofetilide. Class I and class III antiarrhythmic agents should be withheld for at least 3 half-lives prior to initiating dofetilide. Amiodarone should be withheld for at least 3 months or until serum amiodarone concentration is less than 0.3 mcg/mL prior to administering dofetilide. (See Drug Interactions.)

Anticoagulants

Patients with atrial fibrillation should receive appropriate anticoagulant therapy. (See Uses: Embolism Associated with Mitral Valve Disease and/or Atrial Fibrillation in Warfarin 20:12.04.08.)

Electrolyte Imbalance

Hypokalemia or hypomagnesemia may increase the risk of torsades de pointes in patients receiving dofetilide. Patients experiencing prolonged or excessive

diarrhea, sweating, vomiting, loss of appetite, or thirst or receiving concomitant therapy with drugs that may increase the risk of such electrolyte imbalance (e.g., diuretics) should be closely monitored. Hypokalemia should be corrected before initiation of dofetilide. (See Drug Interactions.)

Specific Populations

Pregnancy

Category C. (See Users' Guide.)

Lactation

Not known whether dofetilide is distributed in milk. Patients should not breast-feed while receiving dofetilide.

Pediatric Use

Safety and efficacy not established in children younger than 18 years of age.

Geriatric Use

No substantial differences in safety and efficacy relative to younger adults. Because geriatric patients may have decreased renal function, cautious dosage selection is advised.

Renal Impairment

Safety and efficacy not established in patients with creatinine clearance less than 20 mL/minute. (See Dosage and Administration: Special Populations.)

Hepatic Impairment

No dosage adjustment necessary in mild to moderate hepatic impairment. Use with caution in patients with severe hepatic impairment. (See Dosage and Administration: Special Populations.)

● Common Adverse Effects

Adverse effects occurring in 2% or more of patients receiving dofetilide and more frequently than placebo include headache, chest pain, dizziness, respiratory tract infection, dyspnea, nausea, flu syndrome, insomnia, accidental injury, back pain, medical, surgical, or other health service procedure, diarrhea, rash, and abdominal pain.

DRUG INTERACTIONS

● Drugs Inhibiting Renal Tubular Cationic Transport

Pharmacokinetic interaction (decreased dofetilide excretion) when dofetilide is used with drugs inhibiting renal tubular cationic transport (e.g., cimetidine, ketoconazole, megestrol, prochlorperazine, trimethoprim [with or without sulfamethoxazole]). (See Cautions: Contraindications.)

● Drugs Secreted by Renal Tubular Cationic Transport

Potential pharmacokinetic interaction (decreased dofetilide excretion and increased plasma concentration) when dofetilide is used with drugs secreted by renal tubular cationic transport (e.g., amiloride, metformin, triamterene). (See Cautions: Contraindications.)

● Verapamil

Pharmacokinetic interaction (increased dofetilide concentrations). (See Cautions: Contraindications.)

● Drugs Affecting Hepatic Microsomal Enzymes

Potential pharmacokinetic interaction (decreased dofetilide metabolism and possible increased systemic exposure to dofetilide) with inhibitors of cytochrome P-450 (CYP) 3A4 isoenzyme (e.g., macrolide antibiotics, azole antifungal agents, protease inhibitors, serotonin reuptake inhibitors, amiodarone, cannabinoids, diltiazem, grapefruit juice, nefazodone, norfloxacin, quinine, zafirlukast).

● Drugs that Prolong QT Interval

Potential pharmacodynamic interaction (increased toxicity) when dofetilide is used with drugs that prolong QT interval (e.g., class I or III antiarrhythmic agents, bepridil, cisapride, phenothiazines, tricyclic antidepressants, certain oral macrolides, hydrochlorothiazide-containing preparations).

● **Warfarin**

Pharmacodynamic or pharmacokinetic interaction unlikely.

● **Potassium-depleting Diuretics**

Potential pharmacodynamic interaction (increased dofetilide toxicity). Concomitant use with hydrochlorothiazide alone or in combination (e.g., with triamterene) is contraindicated.

DESCRIPTION

Dofetilide, a class III antiarrhythmic agent, is a methanesulfonamide derivative that is structurally related to sotalol. Dofetilide exhibits electrophysiologic effects characteristic of class III antiarrhythmic agents (e.g., prolongs repolarization and refractoriness without affecting cardiac conduction velocity and sinus node function). However, unlike ibutilide and sotalol, dofetilide has no effect on sodium channels (associated with class I antiarrhythmic agents) or β-adrenergic receptors at clinically relevant concentrations.

Dofetilide prolongs the action potential duration and effective refractory period in both atrial and ventricular cardiac tissue, principally due to delayed repolarization. The antiarrhythmic action of dofetilide results from selective inhibition of the rapidly activating component of the potassium channel involved in repolarization of cardiac cells (i.e., the rapidly activated component of the delayed rectifier potassium current I_{Kr}). Like other class III antiarrhythmics, effects on cardiac repolarization induced by the drug can result in proarrhythmic effects (principally torsades de pointes).

Dofetilide, like ibutilide, appears to be more selective in its cellular actions than some other currently available class III antiarrhythmic agents (e.g., amiodarone, sotalol) and therefore has been referred to as a "pure" class III antiarrhythmic. Dofetilide has negligible effects on heart rate or blood pressure and may slightly improve cardiac contractility.

ADVICE TO PATIENTS

Importance of reading the manufacturer's patient information prior to beginning therapy and rereading it each time the prescription is refilled in case status has changed. (See REMS.)

Importance of informing clinician immediately if new rapid heartbeats, light-headedness, or fainting occur; if clinician cannot be contacted, go to nearest hospital emergency room.

Importance of adherence to dosage and medical appointment schedule. Take drug at same time each day and omit any missed doses.

Importance of informing clinicians of existing or contemplated concomitant therapy, including prescription and OTC drugs, as well as concomitant illnesses. Importance of women informing clinicians if they are or plan to become pregnant or breast-feed.

PREPARATIONS

Distribution of dofetilide is restricted. (See Restricted Distribution under Dosage and Administration: Administration.)

Excipients in commercially available drug preparations may have clinically important effects in some individuals; consult specific product labeling for details.

Dofetilide

Oral			
Capsules	0.125 mg		Tikosyn®, Pfizer
	0.25 mg		Tikosyn®, Pfizer
	0.5 mg		Tikosyn®, Pfizer

Selected Revisions June 2, 2016, © Copyright, January 1, 2002, American Society of Health-System Pharmacists, Inc.

Dronedarone Hydrochloride

24:04.04.20 • CLASS III ANTIARRHYTHMICS

■ Dronedarone hydrochloride is considered to be predominantly a class III antiarrhythmic agent, but the drug appears to exhibit activity in each of the 4 Vaughan-Williams antiarrhythmic classes.

REMS

FDA approved a REMS for dronedarone hydrochloride to ensure that the benefits outweigh the risks. However, FDA later rescinded REMS requirements. See the FDA REMS page (https://www.accessdata.fda.gov/scripts/cder/rems/index.cfm).

USES

● *Supraventricular Tachyarrhythmias*

Dronedarone hydrochloride is used to reduce the risk of hospitalization for atrial fibrillation in patients in sinus rhythm who have a history of paroxysmal or persistent atrial fibrillation. Current evidence from a comparative trial suggests that dronedarone is less effective than amiodarone in preventing recurrence of atrial fibrillation but has an improved safety profile (based on short-term follow-up) with regard to certain serious adverse effects (e.g., thyroid, neurologic) and potential for drug interactions (e.g., with warfarin). However, long-term data and experience are needed to fully elucidate the relative safety and tolerability of dronedarone versus amiodarone because some adverse effects of amiodarone (e.g., pulmonary toxicity) have been reported to occur up to 2–3 years after initiation of therapy.

Dronedarone should *not* be used in patients with *permanent* atrial fibrillation (i.e., patients in whom normal sinus rhythm will not or cannot be restored); results of a clinical trial indicate an increased risk of cardiovascular events and death in such patients. (See Cardiovascular Death and Heart Failure in Patients with Permanent Atrial Fibrillation under Warnings/Precautions: Warnings, in Cautions.)

The efficacy of retreatment with dronedarone in patients who relapse after initial successful treatment or in those who fail therapy with amiodarone remains to be determined. Some clinicians suggest that based on current data, dronedarone should be considered alternative (e.g., second- or third-line) therapy in selected patients in whom control of ventricular rate alone is not feasible or successful and who do not have advanced (i.e., New York Heart Association [NYHA] class IV or recently decompensated class II or III) heart failure and are not receiving drugs that prolong QT interval or strongly inhibit cytochrome P-450 (CYP) isoenzyme 3A4 (CYP3A4). (See Cautions: Contraindications.) Treatment of atrial fibrillation/flutter should be individualized, with consideration given to the relative benefits and risks of various therapies (e.g., rhythm versus rate control, nondrug therapies such as ablation and pacemaker implantation), patient age, as well as patient preference and tolerance of the arrhythmia.

In a multicenter, placebo-controlled, double-blind, parallel-arm trial to assess the efficacy of dronedarone for the prevention of hospitalization for cardiovascular events or death from any cause in patients with atrial fibrillation/flutter (ATHENA study), the incidence of the combined primary outcome (first hospitalization due to cardiovascular events or death from any cause) was reduced with dronedarone compared with placebo. In this study, 4628 patients with a recent history of paroxysmal or persistent atrial fibrillation/flutter were randomized to receive dronedarone (400 mg twice daily) or placebo in addition to conventional therapy for cardiovascular diseases (i.e., β-adrenergic blocking agents, angiotensin-converting enzyme [ACE] inhibitors, angiotensin II receptor antagonists, digoxin, calcium-channel blocking agents, HMG-CoA reductase inhibitors, oral anticoagulants, aspirin, other maintenance antiplatelet therapy, and diuretics). Eligible patients included those who were at least 75 years of age or those at least 70 years of age who had one or more risk factors (i.e., hypertension, diabetes, prior cerebrovascular accident, left atrial diameter of 50 mm or greater, left ventricular ejection fraction of 40% or less) and who were in sinus rhythm or were to undergo cardioversion to sinus rhythm. Patients ineligible for participation in the study included, but were not limited to, patients with NYHA class IV heart failure. The median duration of follow-up was 22 months (range: 12–30 months).

In the ATHENA study, the combined primary outcome of first hospitalization due to cardiovascular events or death from any cause occurred in 31.9% of patients who received dronedarone (individual event rates of 29.3 and 2.6% were reported for cardiovascular hospitalization and death from any cause, respectively) compared with 39.4% of patients who received placebo (individual event rates of 36.9 and 2.5% were reported for cardiovascular hospitalizations and death from any cause, respectively). The reduction in the rate of the combined primary outcome with dronedarone was mainly attributable to a reduction in the rate of first hospitalization due to cardiovascular events, principally hospitalization related to atrial fibrillation; the incidence of death from any cause was not substantially reduced. The numbers of first hospitalizations for congestive heart failure (CHF), ventricular arrhythmia, nonfatal cardiac arrest, or syncope were similar for patients who received dronedarone or placebo; however, there were fewer first hospitalizations for acute coronary syndromes in the dronedarone group.

In 2 other multicenter, double-blind, placebo-controlled trials in outpatients with atrial fibrillation/flutter receiving dronedarone for the maintenance of sinus rhythm (the EURIDIS study in 12 European countries and the ADONIS study in the US, Canada, Australia, South Africa, and Argentina), patients who received dronedarone had a longer median time to first recurrence of atrial fibrillation/flutter (116 versus 53 days) and a lower rate of recurrence at 12 months (64.1 versus 75.2%) than those who received placebo. In these studies, a total of 1237 patients 21 years of age or older who had at least one episode of atrial fibrillation/flutter (as documented by electrocardiogram [ECG]) during the previous 3 months and were in sinus rhythm for at least 1 hour were randomized to receive dronedarone (400 mg twice daily) or placebo, in addition to conventional therapy, for 12 months. Patients ineligible for participation in the studies included, but were not limited to, patients with NYHA class III or IV congestive heart failure. The primary outcome was time from randomization to first documented recurrence of atrial fibrillation/flutter, which was defined as an episode lasting for at least 10 minutes and confirmed by 2 consecutive ECG or transtelephonic recordings taken 10 minutes apart.

In another double-blind, placebo-controlled trial of dronedarone therapy in patients with moderate to severe CHF (ANDROMEDA study), the study was terminated prematurely (after enrollment of 627 of 1000 planned patients and a median follow-up of 63 days) because of excess mortality, mainly as a result of worsening heart failure, in the dronedarone group (8.1%) compared with the placebo group (3.8%). However, at study termination, the combined primary end point of death from any cause or hospitalization for worsening heart failure was not significantly different between patients who received dronedarone or placebo (crude estimate: 17.1 versus 12.6%). After an additional 6 months of follow-up without study treatment, the rate of mortality and the percentage of patients who had reached the combined primary end point were not significantly different between the 2 groups.

In the ANDROMEDA study, patients 18 years of age or older who were hospitalized with new or worsening heart failure and who had at least one episode of shortness of breath on minimal exertion or at rest (NYHA class III or IV heart failure) or paroxysmal nocturnal dyspnea within the previous month and a wall-motion index of 1.2 or less (ejection fraction of about 35% or less) were randomized to receive dronedarone (400 mg twice daily) or placebo. Outcomes were assessed up to the day active treatment was discontinued, 1 month after the date of cessation of the active-treatment phase, and at the end of a 6-month follow-up phase following completion of the study. The study was originally scheduled to last for 2 years and each patient was to be treated for a minimum of 12 months; however, 7 months after the first patient was assigned to a study group, enrollment and treatment were discontinued for safety reasons on the recommendation of the data and safety monitoring board. Dronedarone is contraindicated in patients with NYHA class IV heart failure or heart failure with recent decompensation requiring hospitalization. (See Cautions: Contraindications and also see Cardiovascular Death in Decompensated Heart Failure under Warnings/Precautions: Warnings, in Cautions.)

Dronedarone appears to be less effective than amiodarone in preventing recurrence of atrial fibrillation but may be less likely to cause serious adverse effects, at least in the short term. In a randomized, double-blind study (DIONYSOS) in 504 amiodarone-naive patients (mean age: 64 years) with persistent atrial fibrillation, the primary composite (efficacy/safety) end point (time to first ECG-documented recurrence of atrial fibrillation or premature discontinuance of the study drug due to lack of efficacy or intolerance) was reached in 75.1% of patients receiving dronedarone (400 mg twice daily) compared with 58.8% of those receiving amiodarone (600 mg daily for 28 days, then 200 mg daily) at 12 months; the median duration of treatment was 7 months (maximum treatment duration of 13.8 months in both groups).

Patients enrolled in the DIONYSOS study had documented atrial fibrillation of more than 72 hours' duration, and almost all (95.6%) were receiving concomitant oral anticoagulant therapy. Recurrence of atrial fibrillation (including documented atrial fibrillation after successful conversion, unsuccessful electrical cardioversion, and no spontaneous conversion and no electrical cardioversion on days 10–28) accounted for the largest component of the composite primary end point (63.5 or 42% for dronedarone or amiodarone, respectively) compared with the premature drug discontinuance component (10.4 or 13.3% for dronedarone or amiodarone, respectively). Recurrence of atrial fibrillation after successful conversion was more frequent with dronedarone than with amiodarone (36.5 versus 24.3%, respectively). The incidence of the predefined main safety end point, which included thyroid, hepatic, pulmonary, neurologic, skin, ocular, and GI adverse effects as well as premature drug discontinuance, was similar for dronedarone and amiodarone at 12 months. Bradycardia and QT_c (QT interval corrected for rate, Bazett's formula) prolongation, thyroid and neurologic events, and premature drug discontinuance due to adverse effects were less frequent with dronedarone; however, GI events, none of which were serious (mainly diarrhea), occurred at a higher incidence in the dronedarone group. However, when GI events were excluded, the relative risk of the main safety end point was reduced by 39% with dronedarone. In addition, the proportion of patients with supratherapeutic INR levels (exceeding 4.5) was smaller and the incidence of hemorrhagic events was reduced with dronedarone compared with amiodarone therapy.

In the PALLAS study, patients with permanent atrial fibrillation (defined as the presence of atrial fibrillation or atrial flutter for at least 6 months prior to randomization and patient and clinician decision not to make further efforts to restore sinus rhythm) and additional cardiovascular risk factors who received dronedarone had a higher incidence of heart failure, stroke, and cardiovascular death than those receiving placebo, and the study was terminated early for safety reasons. In this study, patients received dronedarone (400 mg twice daily) or placebo in addition to standard therapy (e.g., drugs to control heart rate, digoxin, anticoagulation with a vitamin K antagonist [e.g., warfarin]). Patients were at least 65 years of age and considered at high risk for vascular events because of the presence of at least one of the following risk factors: coronary artery disease, previous stroke or transient ischemic attack (TIA); symptomatic heart failure, left ventricular ejection fraction of 40% or less; peripheral arterial disease; or the combination of age exceeding 75 years, hypertension, and diabetes. Dronedarone therapy was associated with a more-than-twofold increase in the rate of the first coprimary outcome (stroke, myocardial infarction, systemic embolism, or cardiovascular death) and a near-doubling of the second coprimary outcome (unplanned hospitalization for cardiovascular causes or death). Dronedarone is contraindicated in patients with *permanent* atrial fibrillation. (See Cautions: Contraindications and see Cardiovascular Death and Heart Failure in Patients with Permanent Atrial Fibrillation under Warnings/Precautions: Warnings, in Cautions.)

DOSAGE AND ADMINISTRATION

● Administration

Dronedarone hydrochloride is administered orally twice daily with the morning and evening meals (to enhance bioavailability). (See Description.)

● Dosage

Dosage of dronedarone hydrochloride is expressed in terms of dronedarone.

Supraventricular Tachyarrhythmias

The recommended dosage of dronedarone to reduce the risk of hospitalization for atrial fibrillation in selected patients in sinus rhythm who have a history of paroxysmal or persistent atrial fibrillation (See Uses: Supraventricular Tachyarrhythmias) is 400 mg twice daily with the morning and evening meals.

In a small dose-response study, patients with recurrent atrial fibrillation received dronedarone dosages of 400, 600, or 800 mg twice a day; dosages above 400 mg twice daily were not more effective and were less well tolerated.

Treatment with class I or III antiarrhythmic agents or drugs that are potent inhibitors of the cytochrome P-450 (CYP) 3A isoenzyme must be discontinued prior to initiating dronedarone therapy. (See Cautions: Contraindications and also see Drug Interactions.)

● Special Populations

No dosage adjustment is required in patients with moderate hepatic impairment. However, dronedarone is contraindicated in patients with severe hepatic impairment. (See Hepatic Impairment under Warnings/Precautions: Specific Populations, in Cautions.)

No dosage adjustment is required in patients with renal impairment. (See Renal Impairment under Warnings/Precautions: Specific Populations, in Cautions.)

The manufacturer states that no dosage of dronedarone other than 400 mg twice daily is recommended for any population at this time.

CAUTIONS

● Contraindications

Permanent atrial fibrillation (patients in whom normal sinus rhythm will not or cannot be restored).

Symptomatic heart failure with NYHA Class IV symptoms or recent decompensation requiring hospitalization.

Second- or third-degree atrioventricular (AV) block or sick sinus syndrome (except in patients with a functioning pacemaker).

Bradycardia (less than 50 beats/minute).

QT interval corrected for rate (Bazett's formula, QT_c) of 500 milliseconds or greater or PR interval exceeding 280 milliseconds. (See Other Warnings and Precautions: Prolongation of QT Interval, under Cautions: Warnings/Precautions.)

Concomitant use of potent inhibitors of the cytochrome P-450 (CYP) 3A isoenzyme (e.g., clarithromycin, cyclosporine, itraconazole, ketoconazole, nefazodone, ritonavir, telithromycin, voriconazole). (See Drug Interactions: Drugs Affecting Hepatic Microsomal Enzymes and also see Drug Interactions: Drugs Metabolized by Hepatic Microsomal Enzymes.)

Concomitant use with drugs or herbal supplements that prolong the QT interval and may increase the risk of torsades de pointes (e.g., class I or III antiarrhythmic agents, phenothiazine antipsychotics, tricyclic antidepressants, certain oral macrolides [e.g., erythromycin]). (See Drug Interactions: Drugs that Prolong the QT Interval.)

Liver toxicity related to previous use of amiodarone. (See Other Warnings and Precautions: Severe Hepatic Injury, under Warnings/Precautions, in Cautions.)

Severe hepatic impairment. (See Hepatic Impairment under Warnings/Precautions: Specific Populations.)

Women who are or may become pregnant. (See Other Warnings and Precautions: Fetal/Neonatal Morbidity and Mortality under Cautions: Warnings/Precautions.)

Nursing women.

● Warnings/Precautions

Warnings

Cardiovascular Death in Decompensated Heart Failure

Dronedarone should not be used in patients with NYHA Class IV heart failure or symptomatic heart failure and recent decompensation requiring hospitalization because of a twofold increase in cardiovascular death in such patients receiving the drug. (See Cautions: Contraindications.)

Cardiovascular Death and Heart Failure in Patients with Permanent Atrial Fibrillation

Dronedarone doubles the risk of cardiovascular death (principally due to arrhythmia) and heart failure in patients with *permanent* atrial fibrillation (i.e., those who cannot or will not be converted to normal sinus rhythm); the drug offers no benefit and is contraindicated in such patients.

Patients receiving dronedarone should have heart rate monitored by electrocardiogram (ECG) at least every 3 months. Patients who have atrial fibrillation should have dronedarone therapy discontinued or, if clinically indicated, should undergo cardioversion.

Increased Risk of Stroke in Patients with Permanent Atrial Fibrillation

Dronedarone should only be initiated in patients in sinus rhythm who are receiving appropriate antithrombotic therapy. In a placebo-controlled study in patients with permanent atrial fibrillation, dronedarone therapy was associated with an increased risk of stroke, particularly during the first 2 weeks of therapy.

Other Warnings and Precautions

New-Onset or Worsening Heart Failure

New-onset or worsening heart failure has been reported in patients receiving dronedarone during postmarketing experience. In a placebo-controlled study in patients with permanent atrial fibrillation, increased rates of heart failure were observed in patients with normal left ventricular function and no history of symptomatic heart failure, and also in those with a history of heart failure or left ventricular dysfunction. If heart failure develops or worsens, dronedarone therapy should be discontinued. In addition, the manufacturer states that dronedarone is contraindicated in patients with NYHA class IV heart failure or heart failure with recent decompensation requiring hospitalization. (See Cautions: Contraindications.)

Severe Hepatic Injury

Severe hepatocellular injury, including acute hepatic failure requiring liver transplantation, has been reported during postmarketing experience in patients receiving dronedarone. Hepatic failure requiring transplantation was reported in 2 women 4.5 and 6 months, respectively, after initiation of dronedarone therapy. No alternative etiologies for hepatic failure were identified in either case; in both cases, the explanted liver showed evidence of extensive hepatocellular necrosis. A causal relationship between dronedarone exposure and hepatic failure has not been established because these events were reported voluntarily from a population of unknown size.

Patients should be advised to contact a clinician immediately if they experience manifestations of hepatic injury (e.g., anorexia, nausea, vomiting, fever, malaise, fatigue, right upper quadrant pain, jaundice, dark urine, itching) while taking dronedarone. Clinicians should consider periodic monitoring of serum hepatic enzymes in patients receiving dronedarone, especially during the first 6 months of therapy; it is not known whether routine periodic monitoring of hepatic enzymes will prevent development of severe hepatic injury. If hepatic injury is suspected, dronedarone therapy should be discontinued promptly and serum hepatic enzymes (AST, ALT, and alkaline phosphatase) and bilirubin assessed. Appropriate therapy should be initiated if hepatic injury is found, and the probable cause of such injury should be investigated. Dronedarone should not be reinitiated in patients who experience hepatic injury without another explanation for such injury.

Hypokalemia and Hypomagnesemia

Hypokalemia or hypomagnesemia may occur in patients receiving dronedarone concomitantly with potassium-depleting diuretics. Serum potassium and magnesium concentrations should be within the normal range prior to initiation of dronedarone therapy and maintained within the normal range during dronedarone therapy.

Prolongation of QT Interval

Dronedarone prolongs the QT_c interval by an average of about 10 milliseconds; however, much greater prolongation of the QT_c interval has been observed. If the QT_c interval is 500 milliseconds or greater, dronedarone should be discontinued. (See Cautions: Contraindications.)

Increased Serum Creatinine Concentrations

Small increases in serum creatinine concentrations (about 0.1 mg/dL) following initiation of dronedarone therapy have been reported to result from inhibition of the tubular secretion of creatinine by dronedarone.

Larger increases in serum creatinine after dronedarone initiation have been reported during postmarketing experience. In clinical studies, a 10–15% increase in serum creatinine concentration has been observed in healthy individuals and patients receiving dronedarone without any clinical or laboratory evidence of structural renal damage. The increase in serum creatinine concentration associated with dronedarone has a rapid onset, reaches a plateau after 7 days, and is reversible following discontinuance of the drug. In some cases, increases in BUN were also reported. These effects generally appear to be reversible upon drug discontinuance. Renal function should be monitored periodically in patients receiving dronedarone.

Fetal/Neonatal Morbidity and Mortality

Dronedarone may cause fetal harm; teratogenicity has been demonstrated in animals at dosages equivalent to human dosages. Pregnancy should be avoided during therapy. Women of childbearing potential (i.e., premenopausal women who have not undergone hysterectomy or oophorectomy) should be counseled regarding appropriate contraceptive choices and must use effective contraception while receiving dronedarone. If dronedarone is used during pregnancy or if the patient becomes pregnant while receiving the drug, the patient should be apprised of the potential hazard to the fetus. (See Advice to Patients.) Dronedarone is contraindicated in women who are or may become pregnant.

Specific Populations

Pregnancy

Category X. (See Cautions: Contraindications and also see Fetal/Neonatal Morbidity and Mortality under Cautions: Warnings/Precautions.)

Lactation

Dronedarone and its metabolites are distributed into milk in rats. It is not known whether dronedarone is distributed into human milk. Because of the potential for serious adverse reactions to dronedarone in nursing infants, a decision should be made whether to discontinue nursing or the drug, taking into account the importance of the drug to the woman. Dronedarone is contraindicated in nursing women.

Pediatric Use

Safety and efficacy have not been established in children or adolescents younger than 18 years of age.

Geriatric Use

No substantial differences in safety and efficacy have been observed in geriatric patients compared with younger adults. In clinical studies, exposure to dronedarone was increased by 23% in patients 65 years of age or older compared with younger adults.

Hepatic Impairment

Dronedarone has not been studied in patients with severe hepatic impairment and limited clinical experience is available in patients with moderate hepatic impairment. Dronedarone is contraindicated in patients with severe hepatic impairment.

Severe liver injury has been reported rarely with dronedarone therapy. (See Severe Hepatic Injury under Warnings/Precautions, in Cautions.)

In patients with moderate hepatic impairment, the mean exposure to dronedarone increased by 1.3-fold compared with that in individuals with normal hepatic function, and the mean exposure to the N-debutyl metabolite decreased by about 50%. The pharmacokinetics of dronedarone have not been studied in patients with severe hepatic impairment.

Renal Impairment

Because dronedarone undergoes minimal renal excretion, the manufacturer states that dosage adjustment in patients with renal impairment is not necessary.

No apparent differences in the pharmacokinetics of dronedarone have been observed in individuals with mild or moderate renal impairment versus those with normal renal function or in patients with atrial fibrillation with mild to severe renal impairment versus those with normal renal function. (See Dosage and Administration: Special Populations.)

● Common Adverse Effects

Adverse effects reported in at least 1% of patients receiving dronedarone and more frequently than with placebo include early increases in serum creatinine (at least 10% increase), prolonged QT interval corrected for rate (QT_c, Bazett's formula), diarrhea, asthenic conditions, nausea, skin reactions (e.g., rash [generalized, macular, maculopapular, erythematous], pruritus, eczema, dermatitis, allergic dermatitis), abdominal pain, bradycardia, vomiting, and dyspeptic manifestations. (See Cautions: Contraindications and also see Other Warnings and Precautions: Prolongation of QT Interval and Other Warnings and Precautions: Increased Serum Creatinine Concentrations under Cautions: Warnings/Precautions.)

DRUG INTERACTIONS

Dronedarone is metabolized mainly by the cytochrome P-450 (CYP) 3A isoenzyme.

Dronedarone is a moderate inhibitor of CYP 3A and 2D6; however, the drug does not appear to substantially inhibit CYP 1A2, 2C9, 2C19, 2C8, or 2B6. Dronedarone may potentially inhibit the P-glycoprotein transport system. Dronedarone or its metabolites are weak inhibitors of organic cation transporter (OCT1), organic anion transporting polypeptide (OATP1B1, OATP1B3), and organic anion transporter (OAT3) in vitro.

● Drugs Affecting Hepatic Microsomal Enzymes

Potent inhibitors of CYP3A (e.g., clarithromycin, cyclosporine, itraconazole, ketoconazole, nefazodone, ritonavir, telithromycin, voriconazole): Pharmacokinetic interaction (increased peak plasma concentrations of and exposure to drone-darone). Concomitant use is contraindicated.

Moderate inhibitors of CYP3A (e.g., diltiazem, verapamil): Potential pharmacokinetic interaction (increased exposure to dronedarone). Initiate calcium-channel blocking agents at a low dosage and increase dosage only after ECG verification of good tolerability.

Inducers of CYP3A (e.g., carbamazepine, phenobarbital, phenytoin, rifampin, St. John's wort [*Hypericum perforatum*]): Potential pharmacokinetic interaction (substantially decreased exposure to dronedarone). Concomitant use should be avoided.

● Drugs Metabolized by Hepatic Microsomal Enzymes

Substrates of CYP3A: Potential pharmacokinetic interaction (possible increased plasma concentrations of the CYP3A substrate). Initiation of dronedarone therapy in one patient receiving sirolimus following kidney transplantation resulted in a threefold increase in trough sirolimus concentrations compared with the patient's baseline trough concentration. The manufacturer states that plasma concentrations of sirolimus, tacrolimus, and other CYP3A substrates with a narrow therapeutic index when administered orally should be monitored and dosage of these drugs should be adjusted appropriately when used concomitantly with dronedarone. Some clinicians state that dronedarone should be used with caution in patients receiving drugs with a narrow therapeutic index that are metabolized by CYP3A4. Due to the potential for sirolimus toxicity and excessive immunosuppression, some clinicians recommend that concurrent use of sirolimus and dronedarone be avoided when possible. However, if concurrent administration cannot be avoided, these clinicians suggest a 50–75% reduction in sirolimus dosage prior to dronedarone initiation and regular monitoring (possibly even daily) of trough sirolimus concentrations during the titration phase.

Substrates of CYP2D6 (e.g., β-adrenergic blocking agents, selective serotonin-reuptake inhibitors [SSRIs], tricyclic antidepressants): Potential pharmacokinetic interaction (possible increased exposure to the CYP2D6 substrate).

● Drugs that Prolong the QT Interval

Pharmacologic interaction (potential risk of torsades de pointes-type ventricular tachycardia). Concomitant use of dronedarone with drugs that prolong the QT interval (e.g., class I or III antiarrhythmic agents such as amiodarone, disopyramide, dofetilide, flecainide, propafenone, quinidine, sotalol; tricyclic antidepressants; certain phenothiazines; certain oral macrolides) is contraindicated.

● Drugs Affected by the P-glycoprotein Transport System

Potential pharmacokinetic interaction; increased exposure to substrates of the P-glycoprotein transport system (e.g., dabigatran, digoxin) is expected when such drugs are used concomitantly with dronedarone. Some clinicians state that dronedarone should be used with caution in patients receiving drugs with a narrow therapeutic index that are metabolized by the P-glycoprotein transport system.

● β-Adrenergic Blocking Agents

Potential pharmacologic and pharmacokinetic interactions. In clinical studies, bradycardia was observed more frequently when dronedarone was given concomitantly with β-adrenergic blocking agents. Dronedarone increases exposure to propranolol and metoprolol.

If dronedarone is used concomitantly with a β-adrenergic blocking agent, a lower initial dosage of the β-adrenergic blocking agent is recommended and the dosage should be increased only if well tolerated as documented by electrocardiogram (ECG). (Also see Drug Interactions: Drugs Metabolized by Hepatic Microsomal Enzymes.)

● Calcium-channel Blocking Agents

Potential pharmacologic and pharmacokinetic interactions. Calcium-channel blocking agents associated with depressant effects on the sinus and AV nodes may potentiate the myocardial conduction effects of dronedarone. In addition, dronedarone may increase exposure to calcium-channel blocking agents (diltiazem, nifedipine, verapamil). Initiate calcium-channel blocking agents at a low dosage and increase dosage only after ECG verification of good tolerability.

In addition, verapamil and diltiazem (moderate CYP3A inhibitors) may increase exposure to dronedarone. (See Drug Interactions: Drugs Affecting Hepatic Microsomal Enzymes.)

● Clopidogrel

Concomitant administration of dronedarone does not require dosage adjustment of clopidogrel.

● Dabigatran

Potential pharmacokinetic interaction. Concomitant administration of dronedarone may increase systemic exposure to dabigatran. (See Drug Interactions: Drugs Affected by the P-glycoprotein Transport System.)

● Digoxin

Potential pharmacologic and pharmacokinetic interactions. Digoxin may potentiate the electrophysiologic effects of dronedarone (e.g., decreased AV node conduction). In clinical studies, increased serum digoxin concentrations and an increased incidence of GI disorders were reported with concomitant use of dronedarone and digoxin. When dronedarone therapy is initiated in patients receiving digoxin, the need for continued digoxin therapy should be reassessed and digoxin discontinued if appropriate; if digoxin therapy is continued, a 50% reduction in digoxin dosage is recommended when dronedarone therapy is initiated. In addition, serum digoxin concentrations should be monitored carefully and patients should be observed closely for signs of digoxin toxicity if dronedarone and digoxin are used concomitantly. (See Drug Interactions: Drugs Affected by the P-glycoprotein Transport System.)

● Grapefruit Juice

Potential pharmacokinetic interaction (grapefruit juice increases exposure to dronedarone by threefold); use of grapefruit juice during dronedarone therapy should be avoided.

● HMG-CoA Reductase Inhibitors (Statins)

Simvastatin: Potential pharmacokinetic interaction; dronedarone increases exposure to simvastatin and simvastatin acid by fourfold and twofold, respectively. Simvastatin dosages exceeding 10 mg once daily should be avoided.

Other statins (e.g., atorvastatin, rosuvastatin): The manufacturer's labeling for the respective statin should be consulted for specific recommendations regarding concomitant use with CYP3A or P-glycoprotein transport system inhibitors, such as dronedarone. Concomitant administration of dronedarone does not require adjustment of atorvastatin or rosuvastatin dosage.

● Ketoconazole

Pharmacokinetic interaction; concomitant administration of ketoconazole, a potent CYP3A inhibitor, results in substantially increased exposure to dronedarone. Concomitant use of ketoconazole and dronedarone is contraindicated.

● Losartan

No losartan dosage adjustment required with concomitant administration of dronedarone and losartan.

● Metformin

No dosage adjustment to metformin hydrochloride required with concomitant dronedarone.

● Oral Contraceptives

No dosage adjustments to ethinyl estradiol or levonorgestrel required with concomitant dronedarone.

● Omeprazole

No dosage adjustment to omeprazole required with concomitant dronedarone.

● Pantoprazole

Pantoprazole does not necessitate dosage adjustment of concomitant dronedarone.

● Potassium-depleting Diuretics

Potential pharmacologic interaction (possible risk of hypokalemia or hypomagnesemia) with concomitant use of dronedarone and potassium-depleting diuretics. (See Other Warnings and Precautions: Hypokalemia and Hypomagnesemia under Cautions: Warnings/Precautions.)

● *Rifampin*

Potential pharmacokinetic interaction (rifampin substantially decreases exposure to dronedarone); concomitant use of dronedarone and rifampin should be avoided.

● *Theophylline*

No adjustment of theophylline dosage is required with concomitant dronedarone.

● *Warfarin*

Concomitant administration of dronedarone and warfarin resulted in slightly increased exposure to S-warfarin; however, there was no clinically important increase in the international normalized ratio (INR). In the ATHENA study, more patients experienced clinically important increases in INR (INR ≥5) usually within 1 week after adding dronedarone to warfarin therapy compared with placebo, but an excess risk of bleeding was not observed in such patients. However, cases of increased INR with or without bleeding events have been reported during postmarketing experience in warfarin-treated patients who received dronedarone. The INR should be monitored after initiation of dronedarone therapy in patients taking warfarin.

DESCRIPTION

Dronedarone hydrochloride is considered to be predominantly a class III anti-arrhythmic agent, but the drug also appears to exhibit activity in each of the 4 Vaughan-Williams antiarrhythmic classes. The exact mechanism of antiarrhythmic action has not been fully elucidated, and the exact contribution of each of these activities to the clinical effect of dronedarone is unknown. Dronedarone is a benzofuran derivative that is structurally related to amiodarone, but with structural modifications that include removal of the iodine moiety and addition of a methane-sulfonyl group. The removal of the iodine group was intended to reduce the risk of non-target organ (e.g., thyroid, pulmonary) adverse effects associated with amiodarone, while the addition of the methane-sulfonyl group was aimed at reducing lipophilicity and thus decreasing the risk of neurotoxic adverse effects and shortening the half-life of dronedarone. Dronedarone also has an electro-physiologic profile similar to that of amiodarone, but with different relative effects on individual ion channels. Dronedarone prolongs the action potential duration (APD), principally due to inhibition of potassium channels including transmembrane delayed rectifier, ultrarapid delayed rectifier, inward rectifier, and transient outward potassium currents. Dronedarone also appears to inhibit sodium currents (at rapid pacing rates), calcium channels and slow L-type calcium currents, and demonstrates noncompetitive, antiadrenergic (α- and β-blocking) activity. Dronedarone prolongs the PR interval and slows the sinus rate by prolonging the atrial and ventricular refractory periods. Similar to amiodarone, dronedarone produces a dose-dependent increase in the PR interval, as well as moderate prolongation of the QT interval corrected for rate (QT$_c$, Bazett's formula). The drug also prolongs the RR and QT intervals.

Because dronedarone undergoes first-pass metabolism, the drug has low systemic bioavailability; the absolute bioavailability is about 4% when administered without food. Bioavailability is increased when the drug is given with meals and is approximately 15% when administered with a high-fat meal. Peak plasma concentrations of dronedarone and its main circulating N-debu-tyl metabolite are reached within 3–6 hours following oral administration with food. Steady-state concentrations are achieved within 4–8 days following repeated oral administration of dronedarone 400 mg twice daily. Dronedarone and its N-debutyl metabolite are greater than 98% bound to plasma proteins, mainly albumin; plasma protein binding does not appear to be saturable. Dronedarone is extensively metabolized, mainly by the cytochrome P-450 (CYP) 3A isoenzyme. The initial metabolic pathway includes N-debu-tylation to form the active N-debutyl metabolite, oxidative deamination to form the inactive propanoic acid metabolite, and direct oxidation. Monoamine oxidases contribute partially to the metabolism of the active metabolite of dronedarone. The metabolites undergo further metabolism to yield over 30 uncharacterized metabolites. The N-debutyl metabolite exhibits pharmacodynamic activity, but is only up to one-third as potent as dronedarone. Approximately 6 and 84% of an oral dose is excreted in urine and feces, respectively, mainly as metabolites; no unchanged drug is excreted in urine. The elimination half-life of dronedarone ranges from 13–19 hours following IV administration.

ADVICE TO PATIENTS

Importance of instructing patients to carefully read the manufacturer's patient information (medication guide) before initiating therapy and each time the prescription is refilled. (See REMS.)

Importance of patients not taking dronedarone if they have signs and symptoms of heart failure that recently worsened or required hospitalization, or if they have severe heart failure, because of an increased risk of dying. Importance of informing clinicians if signs or symptoms of heart failure (e.g., weight gain, dependent edema, increasing shortness of breath) occur during dronedarone treatment.

May cause hepatic injury, including life-threatening hepatic failure. Importance of patients not taking dronedarone if they have severe hepatic injury or had hepatic injury after using amiodarone. Importance of advising patients receiving dronedarone to immediately report symptoms suggesting hepatic injury (e.g., anorexia, nausea, vomiting, fever, malaise, fatigue, right upper quadrant pain or discomfort, jaundice, dark urine, itching).

Importance of patients not taking dronedarone if they have permanent atrial fibrillation. Importance of patients informing clinicians immediately if they notice an irregular pulse (a sign of atrial fibrillation) during treatment with dronedarone.

Importance of advising patients to avoid grapefruit juice while taking dronedarone. (See Drug Interactions: Grapefruit Juice.)

Importance of women informing clinicians immediately if they are or plan to become pregnant or plan to breast-feed; necessity of clinicians advising women to avoid pregnancy and breast-feeding during dronedarone therapy. Necessity of advising women of childbearing potential to use an effective method of contraception while receiving therapy and importance of advising these patients regarding appropriate contraceptive choices (taking into consideration their underlying medical conditions and lifestyle preferences). If pregnancy occurs, advise patient of risk to the fetus.

Importance of informing clinicians of existing or contemplated concomitant therapy, including prescription and OTC drugs and herbal supplements (e.g., St. John's wort) (see Drug Interactions), as well as any concomitant illnesses (e.g., heart failure, rhythm disturbance other than atrial fibrillation/flutter, uncorrected hypokalemia).

Importance of taking dronedarone exactly as prescribed (e.g., with meals). Importance of advising patients that if a dose of dronedarone is missed, the next dose should be taken at the regularly scheduled time; the dose should not be doubled.

Importance of informing patients of other important precautionary information. (See Cautions.)

PREPARATIONS

Excipients in commercially available drug preparations may have clinically important effects in some individuals; consult specific product labeling for details.

Dronedarone Hydrochloride

Oral

Tablets, film-coated	400 mg (of dronedarone)	**Multaq®**, Sanofi-Aventis

Selected Revisions June 2, 2016, © Copyright, January 1, 2011, American Society of Health-System Pharmacists, Inc.

Ibutilide Fumarate

24:04.04.20 • CLASS III ANTIARRHYTHMICS

■ Ibutilide fumarate is a class III antiarrhythmic agent.

USES

● *Supraventricular Tachyarrhythmias*

Ibutilide fumarate is used IV for the rapid conversion of recent-onset atrial fibrillation or atrial flutter to sinus rhythm. Ibutilide is considered a drug of choice for pharmacologic cardioversion of atrial fibrillation or flutter. Some experts also state that ibutilide may be useful for restoring sinus rhythm or slowing ventricular rate in hemodynamically stable patients with preexcited atrial fibrillation and rapid ventricular response (e.g., Wolff-Parkinson-White syndrome)†, although direct-current (DC) cardioversion is the intervention of choice for this indication when the patient is hemodynamically compromised. In addition, IV ibutilide may be considered for the treatment of focal atrial tachycardia†, usually after failure of other preferred therapies (e.g., diltiazem, verapamil, β-adrenergic blocking agents). Atrial arrhythmias that are not of recent onset are less likely to respond to the drug, and ibutilide's effectiveness has not been determined in atrial arrhythmias of more than 90 days' duration.

Ibutilide may cause potentially fatal arrhythmias, particularly sustained polymorphic ventricular tachycardia, usually associated with QT prolongation (i.e., torsades de pointes), but occasionally without documented QT interval prolongation; such ventricular arrhythmias that were severe enough to require treatment with DC cardioversion occurred during or within a few hours of ibutilide fumarate administration in 1.7% of patients in clinical trials. The risk of torsades de pointes may be increased in patients with bradycardia, varying heart rate, or hypokalemia. In addition, patients with a history of congestive heart failure or low ventricular ejection fraction appear to have a higher incidence of sustained polymorphic ventricular tachycardia. Therefore, it is essential that the drug be administered in a setting of continuous ECG monitoring and by personnel trained in the identification and treatment of acute ventricular arrhythmias, especially polymorphic ventricular tachycardia. In addition, the manufacturer states that patients with atrial fibrillation of more than 2 to 3 days' duration must be adequately anticoagulated, generally for at least 2 weeks before administration of ibutilide. Conversion of atrial fibrillation or flutter to normal sinus rhythm may be associated with embolism, particularly when the arrhythmia has been present for more than 48 hours, unless the patient is adequately anticoagulated. (See Uses: Cardioversion of Atrial Fibrillation/Flutter, in Heparin 20:12.04.16.) Ibutilide is *not* recommended for use in patients with a history of polymorphic ventricular tachycardia (e.g., torsades de pointes).

Chronic atrial fibrillation that has been converted by treatment such as ibutilide to sinus rhythm has a strong tendency to revert, and therapy required to maintain sinus rhythm is associated with risks. Therefore, patients for whom parenteral ibutilide therapy is considered should be selected carefully such that the expected benefits of conversion to sinus rhythm and continuous treatment to maintain it outweigh the immediate risks associated with use of ibutilide and the risks of maintenance therapy, and that they are likely to offer an advantage compared with alternative management methods for atrial flutter or fibrillation.

Because of their potential to prolong refractoriness, class Ia (e.g., disopyramide, quinidine, procainamide) or III (e.g., amiodarone, sotalol) antiarrhythmic agents should *not* be administered concomitantly with, or within 4 hours after completion of, ibutilide administration. In clinical trials, class I or III agents were withheld for at least 5 half-lives prior to, and 4 hours after completion of, ibutilide infusion, but thereafter were permitted at the clinician's discretion. The possibility that drugs that prolong the QT interval (e.g., certain antihistamines such as terfenadine [no longer commercially available in the US] and astemizole [no longer commercially available in the US], phenothiazines, tricyclic or tetracyclic antidepressants) may potentiate the proarrhythmic effects of ibutilide should be considered.

Current evidence of safety and efficacy of ibutilide in the acute termination of recent-onset atrial arrhythmias is based on several placebo-controlled studies that included hundreds of patients with atrial flutter and/or fibrillation of 3 hours'

to 90 days' duration and in one active treatment (i.e., sotalol)-controlled study that included 319 patients with such arrhythmias of 3 hours' to 45 days' duration. In one study comparing single doses of ibutilide and sotalol, conversion to sinus rhythm reportedly occurred in 53 or 70% of patients with atrial flutter, and in 22 or 43% of patients with atrial fibrillation receiving a 1 or 2 mg of ibutilide fumarate IV, respectively; conversion to sinus rhythm occurred in 18% of those with atrial flutter, and 10% of patients with atrial fibrillation receiving 1.5 mg/kg of sotalol hydrochloride, respectively. In another placebo-controlled study, 14, 30, 58, or 55 % of patients with atrial flutter, and 10, 35, 32, or 40% of those with atrial fibrillation reportedly experienced conversion to sinus rhythm after receiving a single IV ibutilide fumarate dose of 0.005, 0.01, 0.015, or 0.025 mg/kg, respectively. In the other placebo-controlled study in which patients received up to 2 doses of ibutilide (i.e., an initial IV ibutilide fumarate dose of 1 mg followed by a second IV dose of either 0.5 or 1 mg), 48 or 63% of eligible patients with atrial flutter and 38 or 25% of those with atrial fibrillation receiving a total dose of 1.5 or 2 mg, respectively, converted to sinus rhythm.

In a double-blind, placebo-controlled, dose-ranging study in patients with atrial flutter or fibrillation of 1 hour's to 3 days' duration that developed 1–7 days after coronary bypass graft or valvular surgery, 56, 61, or 78% of patients with atrial flutter and 28, 42, or 44% of those with atrial fibrillation treated with two 10-minute IV ibutilide fumarate infusions (10 minutes apart) of 0.25, 0.5, or 1 mg (each), respectively, reportedly experienced conversion to sinus rhythm at 90 minutes. Four or 20% of patients with atrial flutter or atrial fibrillation, respectively, reportedly experienced conversion to sinus rhythm after receiving two 10-minute infusions of placebo. The mean time to conversion to sinus rhythm decreased as the dose of ibutilide fumarate was increased. In addition, 53 or 72% of patients who experienced conversion to sinus rhythm after receiving 10-minute IV ibutilide fumarate infusions of 0.5 or 1 mg (each), respectively, remained in sinus rhythm for 24 hours without the use of additional antiarrhythmic agents.

Direct-current (DC) cardioversion often is the treatment of choice for patients with atrial flutter and/or fibrillation, and up to 70–95% of such arrhythmias may initially be converted to sinus rhythm by DC cardioversion. However, while ibutilide also can effectively convert such arrhythmias in many patients, the role of the drug, particularly in light of its proarrhythmic potential, relative to DC cardioversion for acute conversion of atrial flutter or fibrillation to sinus rhythm remains to be established.

DOSAGE AND ADMINISTRATION

● *Administration*

Ibutilide fumarate is administered by IV infusion. The commercially available injection containing 0.1 mg (100 mcg) of the drug per mL may be administered undiluted. Alternatively, ibutilide fumarate injection may be diluted prior to administration by adding the contents of a 10-mL vial of the drug to 50 mL of 0.9% sodium chloride or 5% dextrose injection, resulting in a final ibutilide fumarate concentration of about 0.017 mg/mL (17 mcg/mL). Undiluted or diluted infusion solutions of ibutilide should be administered IV over 10 minutes.

● *Dosage*

Dosage of ibutilide fumarate is expressed in terms of the hemifumarate salt. Safety and efficacy of the drug in children younger than 18 years of age have not been established.

Proarrhythmic effects of ibutilide must be anticipated, and the drug should be administered only by skilled personnel in a setting in which proper equipment (e.g., cardiac monitors, intracardiac pacing, cardioverter/defibrillator) and therapy for sustained ventricular tachycardia such as polymorphic ventricular tachycardia are available during and after administration of ibutilide. In clinical trials, many initial episodes of such proarrhythmic effects were observed after completion of the ibutilide infusion but no later than 40 minutes after initiation of the infusion. However, instances of recurrent polymorphic ventricular tachycardia occurring about 3 hours after the initial infusion also were observed in these trials. Therefore, patients should be observed with continuous ECG monitoring for at least 4–6 hours after completion of ibutilide administration or until the corrected QT interval (QT$_c$) has returned to baseline. Longer monitoring may be required if any arrhythmic activity is noted. Most cases of ventricular tachycardia observed in clinical trials responded to cardiac pacing and magnesium sulfate infusions, although degeneration to ventricular fibrillation requiring immediate defibrillation also can occur. If polymorphic ventricular tachycardia occurs in patients receiving ibutilide, the manufacturer recommends that the drug be discontinued and that electrolyte abnormalities (especially potassium and magnesium) be corrected and overdrive cardiac pacing, electrical cardioversion, and/or defibrillation be undertaken as necessary. Treatment with antiarrhythmic drugs generally should be avoided, although pharmacologic intervention with magnesium sulfate infusions may prove beneficial.

Supraventricular Tachyarrhythmias

For the acute management of recent-onset atrial flutter or fibrillation in adults weighing 60 kg or more, 1 mg of ibutilide fumarate should be given initially; for adults weighing less than 60 kg, an initial dose of 0.01 mg/kg (10 mcg/kg) is recommended. If the arrhythmia does not terminate within 10 minutes after completion of the initial infusion, the initial dose may be repeated 10 minutes after completion of such infusion. In a clinical study comparing ibutilide with sotalol, 2 mg of ibutilide fumarate administered as a single infusion to patients weighing more than 60 kg also was effective in terminating atrial flutter or fibrillation. Results of a clinical study in patients who developed atrial flutter and/or fibrillation after undergoing coronary bypass graft or valvular surgery indicate that lower doses (i.e., 1 or 2 infusions of 0.5 mg each [0.005 mg/kg per dose for patients weighing less than 60 kg]) was effective in producing conversion to sinus rhythm in these patients. The value and patient tolerance of additional doses of the drug have not been established and currently are not recommended by the manufacturer.

Clinical studies of ibutilide did not include sufficient numbers of patients younger than 65 years of age to determine whether they respond differently than older patients. While other clinical experience has not revealed age-related differences in response, dosage of ibutilide should be selected with caution for geriatric patients, usually initiating therapy at the low end of the dosing range. The greater frequency of decreased hepatic, renal, and/or cardiac function and of concomitant disease or other drug therapy observed in geriatric patients also should be considered.

● Dosage in Renal and Hepatic Impairment

The safety, efficacy, and pharmacokinetics of ibutilide fumarate in patients with renal and/or hepatic impairment have not been established. The manufacturer states that it is unlikely that dosing adjustments based on renal or hepatic function are necessary. Nonetheless, because the drug undergoes substantial hepatic clearance, the manufacturer recommends that patients with abnormal liver function undergo continuous ECG monitoring that extends beyond the usual 4-hour period recommended for other patients.

DESCRIPTION

Ibutilide fumarate is a class III antiarrhythmic agent. Like sotalol, ibutilide is a methanesulfonanilide derivative, and exhibits electrophysiologic effects characteristic of class III antiarrhythmic agents (e.g., prolongs repolarization and refractoriness without affecting conduction). However, unlike sotalol, ibutilide lacks β-adrenergic blocking activity.

Ibutilide fumarate prolongs repolarization of cardiac tissue by prolonging the action potential duration (APD) and effective refractory period (ERP) in both atrial and ventricular cardiac tissue. In vitro studies of its electrophysiologic effects suggest that the antiarrhythmic action of ibutilide may result at least in part from activation of a slow, predominantly sodium, inward current at very low (i.e., less than nanomolar) concentrations, and/or from inhibition of the rapidly activating component of the potassium channel involved in repolarization of cardiac cells (i.e., the rapidly activated component of the delayed rectifier potassium current I_{Kr}) at higher (100-fold) concentrations. However, the exact mechanism of action of the drug remains to be more fully elucidated. Like other class III antiarrhythmics, effects on cardiac repolarization induced by the drug can result in proarrhythmic effects (principally torsades de pointes). (See Uses.)

Ibutilide appears to be more selective in its cellular actions than some other currently available class III antiarrhythmic agents (e.g., amiodarone, sotalol), and therefore has been referred to as a "pure" class III antiarrhythmic. Ibutilide has negligible effects on heart rate, cardiac contractility, or blood pressure.

PREPARATIONS

Excipients in commercially available drug preparations may have clinically important effects in some individuals; consult specific product labeling for details.

Ibutilide Fumarate

Parenteral

Injection, for IV infusion	1 mg (0.1 mg/mL)*	Corvert®, Pfizer
		Ibutilide Fumarate Injection

* available from one or more manufacturer, distributor, and/or repackager by generic (nonproprietary) name

† Use is not currently included in the labeling approved by the US Food and Drug Administration.

Selected Revisions November 15, 2016, © Copyright, June 1, 1996, American Society of Health-System Pharmacists, Inc.

Adenosine

24:04.04.24 • CLASS IV ANTIARRHYTHMICS

■ Adenosine, an endogenous nucleoside present in all cells of the body, is an antiarrhythmic and pharmacologic stress test agent.

USES

● Treatment of Supraventricular Tachyarrhythmias

Adenosine is used as initial drug therapy for termination of paroxysmal supraventricular tachycardia (PSVT), including that associated with accessory bypass tracts (e.g., Wolff-Parkinson-White [WPW] syndrome). Adenosine is considered a drug of choice for terminating stable, regular narrow-complex tachycardias, the most common of which are reentry supraventricular tachycardias (SVTs) such as PSVT due to AV nodal reentrant tachycardia (AVNRT) and AV reentrant tachycardia (AVRT). In addition, the American Heart Association (AHA) states that a trial of adenosine may be considered in selected patients with unstable, narrow-complex tachycardia before cardioversion†. There also is evidence suggesting that adenosine may be useful for both diagnosis and treatment of stable, regular monomorphic wide-complex tachycardias† if the etiology of the rhythm cannot be determined. Appropriate vagal maneuvers (e.g., Valsalva maneuver, carotid sinus massage) should be attempted prior to adenosine administration when clinically indicated.

In controlled clinical studies, the cumulative percentage of patients with PSVT that converted to sinus rhythm within 1 minute after administration of 6 or 12 mg of adenosine by rapid IV injection was 60 or 92%, respectively; the conversion rate following 1–4 injections of placebo was 7–16%. Response to adenosine was not influenced by factors such as concomitant digoxin therapy, presence of WPW syndrome, gender, or race (black, white, Hispanic).

Adenosine is not effective in terminating arrhythmias that are not due to reentry involving the AV or sinus node; these arrhythmias include atrial flutter, atrial fibrillation, and ventricular tachycardia. Although a transient AV block with modest slowing of ventricular response may occur immediately following administration of adenosine in patients with atrial fibrillation or flutter, which may help clarify the type of arrhythmia present, serious arrhythmias and/or hypotension has occurred in some patients with preexcited arrhythmias who received the drug. (See Cardiovascular and Cerebrovascular Effects under Cautions: Warnings/Precautions.) Some clinicians state that adenosine is contraindicated in patients with atrial fibrillation or atrial flutter associated with WPW syndrome because of the risk of dramatically accelerating ventricular rate.

In pediatric patients, adenosine is considered the drug of choice for conversion of supraventricular tachycardia (SVT) when pharmacologic therapy is indicated. If IV or intraosseous (IO) access is readily available, adenosine should be administered; synchronized cardioversion is recommended if IV/IO access is not available, the patient is hemodynamically unstable, or adenosine is not effective. Some experts also state that adenosine may be useful for diagnosis and treatment of wide-complex tachycardias of supraventricular origin in pediatric patients if the rhythm is regular and monomorphic. Synchronized cardioversion is the treatment of choice in hemodynamically unstable patients. (See Cardiovascular and Cerebrovascular Effects under Cautions: Warnings/Precautions.)

● Adjunct to Thallium Stress Test

Adenosine is used as an adjunct to thallous (thallium) chloride TI 201 myocardial perfusion scintigraphy (thallium stress test) in patients unable to exercise adequately.

Adenosine substantially increases blood flow in normal coronary arteries while producing little or no increase in blood flow in stenotic arteries. Because myocardial uptake of thallous chloride TI 201 is directly proportional to coronary blood flow, relatively less thallous chloride TI 201 uptake as well as slower washout occurs in myocardium perfused by stenotic versus normal coronary arteries and the differences in blood flow between areas served by stenotic versus normal arteries are enhanced during thallium testing with adenosine infusion. Intracoronary Doppler flow catheter studies showed maximum coronary artery hyperemia (relative to intracoronary papaverine) in about 95% of cases within 2–3 minutes following initiation of an adenosine infusion at 140 mcg/kg per minute. Coronary artery blood flow velocity returns to baseline within 1–2 minutes after discontinuing the infusion.

In crossover, comparative studies in 319 individuals who could exercise, including 213 patients known or suspected to have coronary artery disease and 106 healthy individuals, thallium images obtained after IV infusion of adenosine or after a treadmill exercise test yielded comparable findings by blind assessment. Agreement regarding the presence of perfusion defects between thallium images obtained after adenosine and after exercise was 85.5% by global analysis and up to 93% when considered by coronary vascular territory. The sensitivity and specificity of thallium imaging using adenosine versus exercise in the detection of angiographically significant coronary artery disease (i.e., more than 50% reduction in the luminal diameter of at least one coronary artery) were determined by comparing results of thallium imaging with those of recent coronary arteriography in 193 patients. The sensitivity (true positive thallium stress tests divided by number of patients with positive [abnormal] angiograms) was 64% with use of either adenosine or exercise, while the specificity (true negative thallium stress tests divided by the number of patients with negative angiograms) was 54 or 65% with use of adenosine or exercise, respectively. The 95% confidence intervals for the sensitivity and specificity of adenosine were 56–78% and 37–71%, respectively.

● Diagnosis of Supraventricular Tachycardias

Adenosine has been used to aid diagnosis of stable, regular narrow-complex SVTs†. A transient AV block may occur following administration of the drug, which can unmask atrial activity in certain arrhythmias such as atrial tachycardia and atrial flutter. Adenosine also has been used diagnostically in patients with stable, regular wide-complex tachycardias; if the tachycardia is a result of SVT with aberrancy, adenosine will likely be effective in slowing or converting the arrhythmia to normal sinus rhythm. Some clinicians discourage overuse of adenosine for diagnostic purposes and recommend that the drug be used only when an arrhythmia of supraventricular origin is strongly suspected. (See Cardiovascular and Cerebrovascular Effects under Cautions: Warnings/Precautions.) Appropriate resuscitative equipment should be readily available during use of the drug.

DOSAGE AND ADMINISTRATION

● Administration

Supraventricular Tachyarrhythmias

For termination of paroxysmal supraventricular tachycardia (PSVT), adenosine is administered by rapid (over 1–2 seconds) IV ("bolus") injection into a peripheral vein. The drug also has been administered via a central vein† or by intraosseous (IO) injection† in pediatric patients without reliable/immediate IV access.

To ensure that the drug reaches the systemic circulation, the solution should be administered either directly into a vein or an IV line at a site as close to the patient as possible, followed by a rapid flush of 0.9% sodium chloride injection (e.g., flush with 5 mL or more for pediatric patients and 20 mL for adults).

Adjunct to Thallium Stress Testing

For use as an adjunct to thallium stress testing, adenosine is administered by continuous IV infusion into a peripheral vein; the drug should be infused over a period of 6 minutes.

Safety and efficacy of intracoronary administration of adenosine as an adjunct to thallium stress testing has not been established.

● Dosage

Supraventricular Tachyarrhythmias

When used for the treatment of PSVT in children weighing less than 50 kg, the manufacturer recommends an initial adenosine dose of 0.05–0.1 mg/kg by rapid IV (bolus) injection. If conversion does not occur within 1–2 minutes, subsequent doses should be increased by 0.05–0.1 mg/kg until sinus rhythm is established or a maximum single dose of 0.3 mg/kg (not exceeding 12 mg) has been given. When used for the treatment of PSVT in children weighing 50 kg or more, the manufacturer recommends an initial dose of 6 mg by rapid IV (bolus) injection. If conversion does not occur within 1–2 minutes, a 12-mg dose should be administered and repeated once, if necessary. The manufacturer states that doses greater than 12 mg are not recommended. Some experts recommend a maximum single dose of 6 mg for the initial injection in pediatric patients.

When used for the treatment of PSVT in adults, an initial adenosine dose of 6 mg by rapid IV (bolus) injection (over 1–3 seconds) is recommended. If conversion does not occur within 1–2 minutes, a 12-mg dose should be administered and repeated once, if necessary. Patients receiving methylxanthines (e.g., theophylline) may require higher adenosine doses because of decreased sensitivity to the effects of adenosine, but experience with such doses is limited and the manufacturer does not recommend doses exceeding 12 mg. (See Drug Interactions: Methylxanthines.) Some experts state that recurrences of PSVT may be treated with additional doses of adenosine or a longer-acting AV nodal blocking agent (e.g., diltiazem, β-adrenergic blocking agent). If adenosine fails to convert PSVT, rate control may be attempted with a nondihydropyridine calcium-channel blocking agent (e.g., diltiazem, verapamil) or a β-adrenergic blocking agent.

The manufacturer-recommended dosage regimen for adenosine in the treatment of PSVT is based on clinical studies of the drug administered by peripheral IV injection. However, the manufacturer and some clinicians suggest that a lower initial dose of adenosine (3 mg for adults or 50% of the usual recommended initial dose for children) may be effective if the drug is given via a central vein because the rhythm effects of adenosine are concentration dependent. In addition, the drug is metabolized by an enzyme on the surface of erythrocytes and more of the dose will be metabolized before reaching the heart when given by peripheral versus central IV injection.

Adjunct to Thallium Stress Testing

When used as an adjunct to thallium stress testing, adenosine is administered by continuous IV infusion at a rate of 0.14 mg/kg per minute for 6 minutes (total dose of 0.84 mg/kg). The appropriate rate of infusion corrected for total body weight may be determined using the following formula:

$$\text{infusion rate (mL/minute)} = \frac{0.14 \text{ mg/kg per minute} \times \text{total body weight (kg)}}{\text{adenosine concentration (3 mg/mL)}}$$

The required dose of thallous (thallium) chloride TI 201 should be administered at the midpoint (i.e., after the first 3 minutes) of the adenosine infusion.

Adenosine and thallous chloride TI 201 are physically compatible, allowing direct injection of thallous chloride TI 201 into the infusion set containing adenosine. Thallous chloride TI 201 should be injected as close as possible to the venous access site to prevent an inadvertent increase in the dose of adenosine (the contents of the IV tubing) being administered.

● Special Populations

Adenosine should be administered with caution to cardiac transplant recipients because of cardiac denervation-related hypersensitivity to the drug. (See Cardiovascular and Cerebrovascular Effects under Cautions: Warnings/Precautions.)

CAUTIONS

● Contraindications

Known hypersensitivity to adenosine.

Second- or third-degree AV block (except in patients with a functioning artificial pacemaker).

Sinus node disease, such as sick sinus syndrome or symptomatic bradycardia (except in patients with a functioning artificial pacemaker).

Known or suspected bronchoconstrictive or bronchospastic lung disease (e.g., asthma).

● Warnings/Precautions

Cardiovascular and Cerebrovascular Effects

Serious cardiovascular and cerebrovascular events, including myocardial ischemic events, rhythm and conduction abnormalities, hypotension, hypertension, and stroke, have been reported rarely in patients receiving adenosine. Cardiac resuscitation equipment and trained staff should be available prior to administration of the drug.

Myocardial Ischemic Events

Fatal or nonfatal cardiac arrest, sustained ventricular arrhythmias (e.g., ventricular tachycardia), and myocardial infarction, have occurred in patients receiving adenosine as a cardiac stress test agent during myocardial perfusion imaging. At least 6 cases of myocardial infarction and 27 deaths associated with the use of adenosine (as Adenoscan®) have been reported to the FDA Adverse Event Reporting System since the date of initial marketing of the drug. A similar risk has been observed with regadenoson, another pharmacologic stress test agent used in myocardial perfusion

imaging. (See Myocardial Ischemic Events under Warnings/Precautions: Cardiovascular and Cerebrovascular Effects, in Cautions in Regadenoson 36:18.) Available data indicate that these adverse cardiovascular events tended to occur within 6 hours following administration of adenosine (as Adenoscan®). Fatal outcomes with adenosine (as Adenoscan®) were most often associated with cardiorespiratory arrest, dyspnea, cardiac arrest, respiratory arrest, and ventricular tachycardia. A few cases of myocardial infarction also have been reported in the medical literature in patients receiving adenosine or regadenoson as a pharmacologic stress test agent. Published studies generally do not suggest a difference in the incidence of cardiovascular events between adenosine and regadenoson. However, many factors, including differences in patient exposure, underlying cardiac risk factors that may influence choice of drug, and longer time on the market for adenosine, may complicate analysis of the true incidence of such adverse events with these drugs.

Prior to performing a cardiac stress test with adenosine, clinicians should assess the suitability of patients to receive the drug. Because patients with signs or symptoms of acute myocardial ischemia (e.g., unstable angina, cardiovascular instability) may be at increased risk of serious cardiovascular events with adenosine, the drug should not be used in such patients.

Rhythm and Conduction Abnormalities

When adenosine is used for termination of paroxysmal supraventricular tachycardia (PSVT), new arrhythmias (ventricular premature complexes [VPCs], atrial premature complexes, atrial fibrillation, sinus bradycardia, sinus tachycardia, skipped beats, and varying degrees of AV nodal block) may appear at the time of conversion to normal sinus rhythm. These arrhythmias generally last only a few seconds and resolve without intervention. However, transient or prolonged episodes of asystole, sometimes fatal, have been reported with IV injection of adenosine. Ventricular fibrillation has been reported rarely with IV injection of the drug, including both resuscitated and fatal events. In most cases, these adverse effects occurred in patients receiving concomitant therapy with digoxin or, less frequently, digoxin and verapamil, although a causal relationship has not been established. (See Drug Interactions: Digoxin or Digoxin/Verapamil.) Atrial fibrillation also has been reported in patients receiving continuous IV infusion of adenosine (as Adenoscan®) as a pharmacologic stress test agent; the abnormal rhythm generally occurred shortly (1.5–3 minutes) after administration, was not persistent (lasting only 15 seconds to 6 hours), and converted to normal sinus rhythm spontaneously. Some clinicians state that adenosine should not be used in patients with wide-complex tachycardias of unknown origin because of the risk of inducing potentially serious arrhythmias, including atrial fibrillation with a rapid ventricular rate or prolonged asystole with severe hypotension in preexcited tachycardias (e.g., atrial flutter); the drug also may induce ventricular fibrillation in patients with severe coronary artery disease.

Because of adenosine's depressant effects on the SA and AV nodes, sinus bradycardia, varying degrees of AV block (asymptomatic and transient), and (rarely) sinus pauses may occur following IV administration of the drug; however, these effects generally are transient due to the short half-life of the drug. Cardiac denervation in patients who have undergone cardiac transplantation reportedly may enhance sensitivity to the bradycardic effects of adenosine. Adenosine should not be used in patients with sinus node dysfunction or high-grade AV block unless the patient has a functioning artificial pacemaker (see Cautions: Contraindications); caution is advised if the drug is used in patients with preexisting first-degree AV block or bundle branch block. If persistent or symptomatic high-grade AV block occurs during therapy, adenosine should be discontinued.

Hemodynamic and Associated Effects

Adenosine may decrease or increase blood pressure. Marked hypotension is possible due to the potent peripheral vasodilating effects of adenosine, and the risk of serious hypotension may be increased in patients with autonomic dysfunction, stenotic valvular heart disease, pericarditis or pericardial effusions, stenotic carotid artery disease with cerebrovascular insufficiency, or hypovolemia. Adenosine should be discontinued in any patient who develops persistent or symptomatic hypotension. Clinically important *increases* in systolic and diastolic blood pressure also have occurred in patients receiving adenosine; these effects generally are transient but reportedly have lasted for several hours in some cases.

Cerebrovascular events, including hemorrhagic and ischemic stroke, have occurred in patients receiving adenosine, and may be associated with the drug's effects on blood pressure.

Respiratory Effects

Adenosine is a respiratory stimulant and adverse respiratory effects, including dyspnea, bronchospasm, bronchoconstriction, and respiratory compromise, have occurred in patients receiving the drug. Dyspnea was reported in approximately 28 or 12% of patients receiving adenosine for pharmacologic stress testing or conversion of PSVT, respectively, in clinical trials. In addition, respiratory compromise has occurred during adenosine infusion in patients with obstructive pulmonary disease. Other respiratory effects reported during postmarketing experience with the drug include bronchospasm, respiratory arrest, and throat tightness.

Adenosine should not be used in patients with bronchoconstriction or bronchospasm (e.g., asthma) since the drug may exacerbate respiratory symptoms in such patients; caution is advised if adenosine is used in patients with obstructive pulmonary disease not associated with bronchoconstriction (e.g., emphysema, bronchitis). (See Cautions: Contraindications.) Appropriate resuscitative measures should be available prior to administration of the drug. Adenosine should be discontinued in any patient who develops severe respiratory difficulties.

CNS Effects

New-onset or recurrent seizures, including tonic-clonic (grand mal) seizures, have been reported following administration of adenosine. In some cases, seizure activity was prolonged and required emergency management. Concomitant use of aminophylline may increase the risk of seizures. (See Drug Interactions: Methylxanthines.)

Sensitivity Reactions
Hypersensitivity

Hypersensitivity reactions may occur following administration of adenosine, possibly requiring resuscitative measures; reported manifestations have included dyspnea, throat tightness, flushing, erythema, and chest discomfort. Prior to administration of adenosine, clinicians should ensure that appropriate personnel and resuscitative equipment are available. (See Cautions: Contraindications.)

Specific Populations
Pregnancy

Category C. Some clinicians suggest that because of its rapid onset and brief duration of action, adenosine may have advantages over other antiarrhythmic agents (e.g., verapamil, digoxin) in the acute treatment of PSVT in pregnant women in whom vagal maneuvers have failed. However, caution is advised because hypotension may compromise placental (fetal) blood flow.

Lactation

It is not known whether adenosine is distributed into human milk. Because of the potential for serious adverse reactions from adenosine in nursing infants, a decision should be made whether to discontinue nursing or the drug, taking into account the importance of the drug to the woman. Some clinicians suggest that use of adenosine during lactation may be possible because of the drug's short half-life.

Pediatric Use

Although the manufacturer states that controlled studies establishing the safety and efficacy of adenosine for treatment of PSVT in pediatric patients are lacking, the drug has been used for the treatment of PSVT in neonates, infants, children, and adolescents, and some clinicians consider it a drug of choice for SVT in pediatric patients.

Safety and efficacy as an adjunct to thallium stress testing not established in children 18 years of age or younger.

Geriatric Use

Insufficient experience in patients 65 years of age or older to determine whether geriatric patients respond differently than younger adults. However, use with caution because increased sensitivity cannot be ruled out; some geriatric patients may have diminished cardiac function, nodal dysfunction, or concomitant disease or drug therapy that may alter hemodynamic function and result in severe bradycardia or AV block.

Hepatic Impairment

Adenosine does not require hepatic function for therapeutic effect or inactivation; therefore, hepatic dysfunction would not be expected to alter the drug's effectiveness or tolerability.

Renal Impairment

Adenosine does not require renal function for therapeutic effect or inactivation; therefore, renal dysfunction would not be expected to alter the drug's effectiveness or tolerability.

● Common Adverse Effects

Adverse effects reported in at least 1% of patients receiving adenosine for the treatment of PSVT in controlled clinical trials include facial flushing, shortness of breath/dyspnea, chest pressure, nausea, headache, lightheadedness, dizziness, numbness, and tingling in the arms.

Adverse effects reported in at least 1% of patients receiving adenosine as an adjunct to thallium stress testing in controlled and uncontrolled clinical trials include facial flushing; chest discomfort; dyspnea or urge to breathe deeply; headache; discomfort in the throat, neck, or jaw; GI discomfort; lightheadedness/dizziness; upper extremity discomfort; ST-segment depression; first-degree AV block; second-degree AV block; paresthesia; hypotension; nervousness; and arrhythmias.

DRUG INTERACTIONS

When possible, drugs that may augment or inhibit adenosine effects should be withheld for 5 half-lives prior to adenosine administration.

● ACE Inhibitors

Potential pharmacodynamic interaction (additive or synergistic depressant effects on SA and AV nodes); the drugs should be used concomitantly with caution.

● β-Adrenergic Blocking Agents

Potential pharmacodynamic interaction (additive or synergistic depressant effects on SA and AV nodes); the drugs should be used concomitantly with caution.

● Calcium-channel Blocking Agents

Potential pharmacodynamic interaction (additive or synergistic depressant effects on SA and AV nodes); the drugs should be used concomitantly with caution.

● Carbamazepine

Potential pharmacodynamic interaction (higher degrees of heart block).

● Digoxin or Digoxin/Verapamil

Potential pharmacodynamic interaction (additive or synergistic depressant effects on SA and AV nodes); serious and/or life-threatening effects (asystole, ventricular fibrillation) have been reported rarely. (See Cardiovascular and Cerebrovascular Effects under Cautions: Warnings/Precautions.) The drugs should be used concomitantly with caution and with appropriate resuscitative measures available.

● Dipyridamole

Potential pharmacodynamic interaction (potentiation of vasoactive effects of adenosine). caution should be exercised.

The manufacturer of adenosine (Adenoscan®) states that safety and efficacy of the drug in the presence of dipyridamole have not been established. In general, administration of drugs that may inhibit or augment the pharmacologic effects of adenosine should be withheld for at least 5 half-lives prior to administration of adenosine.

● Methylxanthines

Potential pharmacodynamic interaction (inhibition of vasoactive effects of adenosine) with methylxanthines such as caffeine, aminophylline, or theophylline; larger doses of adenosine may be required or the drug may not be effective during such concomitant therapy. (See Advice to Patients.) The manufacturer of adenosine (Adenoscan®) states that safety and efficacy of the drug in the presence of methylxanthines have not been established. In general, administration of drugs that may inhibit or augment the pharmacologic effects of adenosine should be withheld for at least 5 half-lives prior to administration of adenosine.

Methylxanthines are competitive adenosine receptor antagonists, and theophylline has been used effectively to terminate persistent adverse effects of adenosine. However, the manufacturer states that aminophylline may increase the risk of seizures associated with adenosine and that methylxanthines should not be used in patients who experience adenosine-induced seizures. (See CNS Effects under Cautions: Warnings/Precautions.)

● Quinidine

Potential pharmacodynamic interaction (additive or synergistic depressant effects on SA and AV nodes); the drugs should be used concomitantly with caution.

DESCRIPTION

Adenosine is an endogenous nucleoside present in all cells of the body. Adenosine may exert its pharmacologic effects by activation of purine (cell-surface A_1 and A_2 adenosine) receptors; relaxation of vascular smooth muscle may be mediated by reduction in calcium uptake through inhibition of slow inward calcium current and activation of adenylate cyclase in smooth muscle cells. Adenosine may reduce vascular tone by modulation of sympathetic neurotransmission.

Adenosine has negative chronotropic, dromotropic, and inotropic effects on the heart. The drug slows conduction time through the AV node and can interrupt AV nodal reentry pathways, leading to restoration of normal sinus rhythm in patients with paroxysmal supraventricular tachycardia (PSVT), including that associated with Wolff-Parkinson-White syndrome.

Adenosine is a potent vasodilator in most vascular beds; however, vasoconstriction is produced in renal afferent arterioles and hepatic veins. The drug typically produces a net mild to moderate reduction in systolic, diastolic, and mean arterial blood pressure and a reflex increase in heart rate. Adenosine increases blood flow in normal coronary arteries with little or no increase in stenotic arteries, resulting in a relative difference in thallous (thallium) chloride TI 201 uptake in myocardium supplied by normal versus stenotic coronary arteries.

Adenosine is a respiratory stimulant, probably because of activation of carotid body chemoreceptors; IV administration produces an increase in minute ventilation and a reduction in arterial PCO_2, resulting in respiratory alkalosis.

Adenosine is rapidly metabolized intracellularly to the inactive metabolites adenosine monophosphate and inosine; the plasma half-life of adenosine is less than 10 seconds. The drug is cleared by cellular uptake, principally by erythrocytes and vascular endothelial cells, via a specific transmembrane nucleoside transport system.

ADVICE TO PATIENTS

Importance of informing patients about serious adverse effects associated with adenosine, such as myocardial infarction, arrhythmias, cardiac arrest, heart block, substantial changes in blood pressure, bronchoconstriction, hypersensitivity reactions, seizures, and stroke.

Importance of patient informing clinicians of existing or contemplated concomitant therapy, including prescription and OTC drugs (e.g., aminophylline, theophylline), caffeine-containing foods or beverages, as well as any concomitant illnesses (e.g., asthma, chronic obstructive pulmonary disease [COPD]).

Importance of women informing clinicians if they are or plan to become pregnant or plan to breast-feed.

Importance of informing patients of other important precautionary information. (See Cautions.)

PREPARATIONS

Excipients in commercially available drug preparations may have clinically important effects in some individuals; consult specific product labeling for details.

Adenosine

Parenteral		
Injection, for rapid IV injection only	3 mg/mL*	Adenocard®, Astellas Adenosine Injection
Injection, for IV infusion only	3 mg/mL	Adenoscan®, Astellas

* available from one or more manufacturer, distributor, and/or repackager by generic (nonproprietary) name

† Use is not currently included in the labeling approved by the US Food and Drug Administration.

Selected Revisions November 15, 2016, © Copyright, January 1, 2006, American Society of Health-System Pharmacists, Inc.

dilTIAZem Hydrochloride

24:04.04.24 • CLASS IV ANTIARRHYTHMICS

■ Diltiazem is a nondihydropyridine calcium-channel blocking agent (calcium-channel blocker).

USES

Diltiazem is used in the management of Prinzmetal variant angina, chronic stable angina pectoris, supraventricular tachycardias, and hypertension.

● Angina

Diltiazem is used in the management of angina, including chronic stable angina, Prinzmetal variant angina, and unstable angina†. Calcium-channel blockers (used alone or in combination with nitrates) are considered the drugs of choice for the management of Prinzmetal variant angina. β-Adrenergic blocking agents (β-blockers) are recommended as the anti-ischemic drugs of choice in most patients with chronic stable angina; however, calcium-channel blockers may be substituted or added in patients who do not tolerate or respond adequately to β-blockers. In short-term, controlled clinical studies in patients with chronic stable angina, oral diltiazem reduced the frequency of attacks, allowed a decrease in sublingual nitroglycerin dosage, and increased exercise tolerance. All classes of calcium-channel blockers appear to be equally effective in reducing anginal episodes; however, choice of a specific agent should be individualized since the pharmacologic properties of these drugs differ.

Diltiazem also may be beneficial in patients with unstable angina†; experts recommend the use of a nondihydropyridine calcium-channel blocker (e.g., diltiazem, verapamil) for the relief of ongoing or recurrent ischemia when β-blocker therapy is inadequate, not tolerated, or contraindicated in patients with unstable angina who do not have clinically important left ventricular dysfunction, increased risk of cardiogenic shock, or AV block.

Although concurrent use of some calcium-channel blockers and a β-blocker may have beneficial effects in some patients (e.g., reduction of dihydropyridine-induced tachycardia through β-blockade), combined use of diltiazem with a β-blocker generally should be avoided because of the potential adverse effects on AV nodal conduction, heart rate, and cardiac contractility. (See β-Adrenergic Blocking Agents under Drug Interactions: Drugs Known to Impair Cardiac Contractility and Conduction.)

● Hypertension

Oral diltiazem is used alone or in combination with other classes of antihypertensive agents in the management of hypertension. Only extended-release formulations of diltiazem are recommended for the management of hypertension.

Calcium-channel blockers (e.g., diltiazem) are considered one of several preferred antihypertensive drug classes for the initial management of hypertension according to current evidence-based hypertension guidelines; other preferred options include angiotensin-converting enzyme (ACE) inhibitors, angiotensin II receptor antagonists, and thiazide diuretics. While there may be individual differences with respect to recommendations for initial drug selection and use in specific patient populations, current evidence indicates that these antihypertensive drug classes all generally produce comparable effects on overall mortality and cardiovascular, cerebrovascular, and renal outcomes. (See Uses: Hypertension, in Amlodipine 24:28.08.)

Calcium-channel blockers may be particularly useful in the management of hypertension in patients with certain coexisting conditions such as ischemic heart disease (e.g., angina) and in geriatric patients, including those with isolated systolic hypertension. (See Uses: Hypertension, in Amlodipine 24:28.08.) In addition, nondihydropyridine calcium-channel blockers may be beneficial in hypertensive patients with coexisting atrial fibrillation and a rapid ventricular rate. However, some experts recommend against the use of nondihydropyridine calcium-channel blockers in patients who have heart failure with reduced ejection fraction because of the drugs' myocardial depressant activity and unfavorable outcomes in some clinical trials in patients with heart failure receiving the drugs.

In the Antihypertensive and Lipid-lowering Treatment to Prevent Heart Attack Trial (ALLHAT), the long-term cardiovascular morbidity and mortality benefit of a long-acting dihydropyridine calcium-channel blocker (amlodipine), a thiazide-like diuretic (chlorthalidone), and an ACE inhibitor (lisinopril) were compared in a broad population of patients with hypertension at risk for coronary heart disease. Although these antihypertensive agents were comparably effective in providing important cardiovascular benefit, apparent differences in certain secondary outcomes were observed. Patients receiving the ACE inhibitor experienced higher risks of stroke, combined cardiovascular disease, GI bleeding, and angioedema, while those receiving the calcium-channel blocker were at higher risk of developing heart failure. The ALLHAT investigators suggested that the observed differences in cardiovascular outcome may be attributable, at least in part, to the greater antihypertensive effect of the calcium-channel blocker compared with that of the ACE inhibitor, especially in women and black patients. (See Clinical Benefits of Thiazides in Hypertension under Hypertension in Adults: Treatment Benefits, in Uses in the Thiazides General Statement 40:28.20.)

Most patients with hypertension, especially black patients, will require at least 2 antihypertensive drugs to achieve adequate blood pressure control. Calcium-channel blockers may be particularly useful in the management of hypertension in black patients; these patients tend to have greater blood pressure response to calcium-channel blockers and thiazide diuretics than to other antihypertensive drug classes (e.g., ACE inhibitors, angiotensin II receptor antagonists). However, the combination of an ACE inhibitor or an angiotensin II receptor antagonist with a calcium-channel blocker or thiazide diuretic produces similar blood pressure lowering in black patients as in other racial groups. (See Race under Hypertension: Other Special Considerations for Antihypertensive Therapy, in Uses in Amlodipine 24:28.08.)

For additional information on the role of calcium-channel blockers in the management of hypertension, see Uses: Hypertension, in Amlodipine 24:28.08. For information on overall principles and expert recommendations for treatment of hypertension, see Uses: Hypertension in Adults, and also see Uses: Hypertension in Pediatric Patients, in the Thiazides General Statement 40:28.20.

● Supraventricular Arrhythmias

Diltiazem is used in the management of supraventricular tachycardias (SVTs), including rapid conversion to sinus rhythm of paroxysmal supraventricular tachycardia (PSVT) (e.g., tachycardia associated with Wolff-Parkinson-White or Lown-Ganong-Levine syndrome), and control of rapid ventricular rate in atrial flutter or fibrillation. The American College of Cardiology/American Heart Association/Heart Rhythm Society (ACC/AHA/HRS) guideline for the management of adults with supraventricular tachycardia recommends the use of diltiazem in the treatment of various SVTs (e.g., atrial flutter, junctional tachycardia, focal atrial tachycardia, atrioventricular nodal reentrant tachycardia [AVNRT]); in general, IV diltiazem is recommended for acute treatment while oral diltiazem is recommended for ongoing management of these arrhythmias. Vagal maneuvers and/or IV adenosine are considered first-line interventions for the acute treatment of patients with SVT and should be attempted prior to other therapies when clinically indicated; if such measures are ineffective or not feasible, a nondihydropyridine calcium-channel blocker (i.e., diltiazem or verapamil) may be considered. Diltiazem should only be used in hemodynamically stable patients who do not have impaired ventricular function.

Paroxysmal Supraventricular Tachycardia

IV diltiazem is used for rapid conversion of PSVT that is uncontrolled or unconverted by vagal maneuvers and adenosine, including atrioventricular nodal reentrant tachycardias and PSVT associated with extranodal accessory pathways (e.g., Wolff-Parkinson-White or Lown-Ganong-Levine syndrome). In about 86–88% of patients with PSVT, IV diltiazem produces rapid conversion (usually within 2–3 minutes of the first or second dose) to sinus rhythm; conversion to sinus rhythm appears to be dose related. Limited data indicate that conversion to sinus rhythm may occur spontaneously in 25% of placebo-treated patients with PSVT. Transient ventricular premature complexes may be present following conversion of PSVT to sinus rhythm but appear to be benign and of little clinical importance. While comparative trials have not been performed with IV diltiazem and other calcium-channel blockers, the efficacy rate of IV diltiazem in converting PSVT to sinus rhythm appears to be similar to that of verapamil.

Oral diltiazem also has been used to prevent PSVT, but efficacy of the drug for this condition has not been established.

Atrial Fibrillation and Flutter

Nondihydropyridine calcium-channel blockers (e.g., diltiazem, verapamil) are recommended as one of several drug therapy options for ventricular rate control in patients with nonpreexcited atrial fibrillation or flutter. Management of atrial fibrillation or flutter depends on the clinical situation and the patient's condition. For acute treatment of atrial fibrillation, IV diltiazem may be used. Cardioversion is indicated, however, in hemodynamically unstable patients. IV diltiazem should *not* be used when atrial flutter or fibrillation is associated with an accessory pathway that has a short refractory period (e.g., Wolff-Parkinson-White or Lown-Ganong-Levine syndrome) or with preexcited ventricular complexes or wide QRS complexes, since ventricular tachyarrhythmias, including ventricular fibrillation and cardiac arrest, may be precipitated. Although approximately 95% of patients with atrial flutter or fibrillation respond to direct IV injection of 1 or 2 doses with at least a 20% reduction in ventricular rate and this reduction in heart rate is maintained in at least 83% of patients with continuous IV infusion of the drug, IV diltiazem alone rarely (i.e., less than 10% of patients) converts atrial flutter or fibrillation to normal sinus rhythm; limited data indicate that conversion to sinus rhythm may be dose-related and is not usually seen with recommended doses. Conversion to sinus rhythm after drug therapy is more likely to occur in atrial flutter or atrial fibrillation that is of recent onset (i.e., within 24–48 hours) in patients without structural heart disease.

While comparative trials have not been performed with IV diltiazem and IV digoxin, pharmacokinetic data indicate that diltiazem has a faster onset of action than digoxin and may be more useful for slowing ventricular response in patients with atrial flutter or fibrillation. Calcium-channel blockers (i.e., diltiazem or verapamil) may be used for the management of atrial fibrillation associated with an acute myocardial infarction (MI) in patients with a β-blocker intolerance. (See Uses: Acute Myocardial Infarction.)

Oral diltiazem also has been used to reduce heart rate in patients with atrial fibrillation†, but efficacy of the drug for this condition has not been established.

Atrial Tachycardia

IV diltiazem may be used for the acute treatment of patients with hemodynamically stable focal atrial tachycardia† (i.e., regular SVT arising from a localized atrial site), and oral diltiazem may be used for ongoing management.

IV diltiazem also may be used in patients with multifocal atrial tachycardia† (i.e., rapid, irregular rhythm with at least 3 distinct P-wave morphologies), although such arrhythmia is commonly associated with an underlying condition (e.g., pulmonary, coronary, or valvular heart disease) and is generally not responsive to antiarrhythmic drugs. Antiarrhythmic drug therapy usually is reserved for patients who do not respond to initial attempts at correcting or managing potential precipitating factors (e.g., exacerbation of chronic obstructive pulmonary disease or congestive heart failure, electrolyte and/or ventilatory disturbances, infection, theophylline toxicity) or in whom a precipitating factor cannot be identified. While specific studies have not been performed with IV diltiazem in patients with multifocal atrial tachycardia, the effects of the drug are expected to be similar to that of IV verapamil, which has been shown to have some efficacy in the acute treatment of this arrhythmia. Orally administered diltiazem may be a reasonable choice for chronic suppression of recurrent symptomatic multifocal atrial tachycardia.

Junctional Tachycardia

Diltiazem may be used for the treatment of junctional tachycardia† (i.e., nonreentrant SVT originating from the AV junction), a rapid, occasionally irregular, narrow-complex tachycardia. β-Adrenergic blocking agents generally are used for acute termination and/or ongoing management of junctional tachycardia; limited evidence suggests there may be a role for diltiazem when β-blocking agents (particularly propranolol) are ineffective.

Acute Myocardial Infarction

Calcium-channel blockers have been used in the early treatment and secondary prevention of acute MI†; although these drugs are effective anti-ischemic agents, they have not demonstrated mortality benefits and therefore are generally used as an alternative to β-blockers. A review of 28 randomized controlled studies involving 19,000 patients found no benefit with regard to infarct size, rate of reinfarction, or death when calcium-channel blockers were used during the acute or convalescent phase of ST-segment-elevation MI (STEMI). Although some studies demonstrated a reduced risk of reinfarction when verapamil or diltiazem was administered after MI in patients without left ventricular dysfunction, other studies have not confirmed this finding. Calcium-channel blockers generally are used for their anti-ischemic and blood pressure-reducing properties in the MI setting, and only when β-blockers (which have been shown to reduce mortality after MI) are ineffective, not tolerated, or contraindicated; because the nondihydropyridine calcium-channel blockers (verapamil and diltiazem) can cause substantial negative inotropic effects, their use should be limited to patients without left ventricular dysfunction.

Current expert guidelines state that a calcium-channel blocker may be used to relieve ischemic symptoms, lower blood pressure, or control rapid ventricular response associated with atrial fibrillation in patients with STEMI who are intolerant to β-blockers. A nondihydropyridine calcium-channel blocker (e.g., verapamil or diltiazem) may be used as an alternative to β-blockers for relief of ongoing or recurring ischemia when β-blocker therapy is inadequate, not tolerated, or contraindicated in patients with non-ST-segment-elevation MI (NSTEMI) who do not have clinically important left ventricular dysfunction, increased risk of cardiogenic shock, or AV block. The use of immediate-release nifedipine is generally contraindicated because of the potential for hypotension and reflex sympathetic activation.

● Other Uses

Diltiazem has been used with good results as an alternative to β-adrenergic blocking agents (e.g., propranolol) for short-term adjunctive therapy in the treatment of tachycardia and tachyarrhythmias in a limited number of patients with hyperthyroidism and/or thyrotoxicosis†. Diltiazem hydrochloride (160–480 mg daily in divided doses) has reduced heart rate, blood pressure, and ventricular and supraventricular premature complexes in patients with these conditions. Diltiazem does not affect the underlying disease, which must be treated with antithyroid therapy. While additional study and experience are necessary, diltiazem may be a useful alternative to β-adrenergic blocking agents in patients in whom therapy with these agents is contraindicated or not tolerated.

DOSAGE AND ADMINISTRATION

● Administration

Diltiazem hydrochloride is administered by direct IV injection, continuous IV infusion, or orally.

Oral Administration

Diltiazem hydrochloride is administered orally as conventional tablets, extended-release capsules, and extended-release tablets. Diltiazem also has been available as diltiazem malate alone or in combination with enalapril, but these preparations no longer are commercially available in the US.

Directions for administration (e.g., dosing frequency, whether to administer with or without food, potential for opening capsules and mixing with food) may vary by manufacturer and formulation; the manufacturer's information for a specific preparation should be consulted for detailed information.

IV Administration

Diltiazem hydrochloride is administered by direct IV injection or continuous IV infusion in the management of supraventricular tachyarrhythmias.

For direct IV injection or continuous IV infusion, diltiazem is given slowly under continuous ECG and blood pressure monitoring during the administration period. Solutions of the drug should be inspected visually for particulate matter or discoloration prior to IV administration whenever solution and container permit.

IV injection: When administered by direct IV injection, diltiazem hydrochloride injection containing 5 mg/mL requires no further dilution.

IV Infusion: When administered as a continuous IV infusion, 25, 50, or 50 mL of diltiazem hydrochloride injection containing 5 mg/mL should be added to 100, 250, or 500 mL of a compatible infusion solution (i.e., 0.9% sodium chloride, 5% dextrose, or 5% dextrose and 0.45% sodium chloride) to produce a final diltiazem hydrochloride concentration of 1, 0.83, or 0.45 mg/mL, respectively. Alternatively, IV infusions with a final concentration of 1 mg/mL can be prepared using the single-dose 100-mg ADD-Vantage® vials of diltiazem hydrochloride.

Standardize 4 Safety

Standardized concentrations for IV diltiazem have been established through Standardize 4 Safety (S4S), a national patient safety initiative to reduce medication errors, especially during transitions of care. Multidisciplinary expert panels were convened to determine recommended standard concentrations. Because recommendations from the S4S panels may differ from the manufacturer's prescribing information, caution is advised when using concentrations that differ from labeling, particularly when using rate information from the label. For additional information on S4S (including updates that may be available), see https://www.ashp.org/pharmacy-practice/standardize-4-safety-initiative.

TABLE 1. Standardize 4 Safety Continuous IV Infusion Standard Concentrations for Diltiazem Hydrochloride

Patient Population	Concentration Standards	Dosing Units
Adults	1 mg/mL	mg/hour

• Dosage

Potency of diltiazem hydrochloride preparations is expressed in terms of the hydrochloride.(See Chemistry and Stability: Chemistry.)

Dosage of diltiazem hydrochloride must be carefully adjusted according to individual requirements, tolerance, and response. The manufacturers state that dosage of diltiazem for geriatric patients should be selected carefully because these individuals frequently have decreased hepatic, renal, and/or cardiac function and concomitant disease and drug therapy.

Angina

For the management of Prinzmetal variant angina or chronic stable angina pectoris, the usual initial adult dosage of diltiazem hydrochloride as conventional tablets is 30 mg 4 times daily. Generally, dosage is gradually increased at 1- to 2-day intervals until optimum control of angina is obtained. The average optimum adult dosage range for diltiazem hydrochloride tablets appears to be 180–360 mg daily given in 3 or 4 divided doses. Geriatric patients may respond to lower dosages. After anginal symptoms are controlled, dosage should be gradually reduced to the lowest level that will maintain relief of symptoms.

When diltiazem hydrochloride is administered as extended-release capsules (Tiazac®, Dilt-XR®, Taztia XT®) or extended-release tablets (Cardizem® LA, Matzim® LA) for the management of chronic stable angina, the usual initial adult dosage is 120 mg (Dilt-XR®), 120–180 mg (Tiazac®, Taztia XT®) or 180 mg (Cardizem® LA, Matzim® LA) once daily. When diltiazem hydrochloride is administered as Cardizem® CD or Cartia XT® extended-release capsules for the management of chronic stable angina and angina secondary to coronary artery spasm, the usual initial adult dosage is 120–180 mg once daily.

Dosage should be individualized based on response; when dosage increases are necessary, they should be titrated over 7–14 days. Some patients may respond to higher dosages of up to 360 mg (Cardizem® LA, Matzim® LA), 480 mg (Dilt-XR®, Cardizem CD®, Cartia XT®), or 540 mg (Tiazac®, Taztia XT®) once daily.

Hypertension

Usual Dosage

For the management of hypertension in adults receiving diltiazem hydrochloride as monotherapy, the usual initial dosage as the extended-release capsules (Cardizem® CD, Cartia XT®, Dilt-XR®) or extended-release tablets (Cardizem® LA, Matzim® LA) is 180–240 mg once daily. When the extended-release capsules of diltiazem hydrochloride (Tiazac®, Taztia XT®) are used, the usual initial dosage is 120–240 mg once daily. Dosage of the drug should be adjusted according to the patient's blood pressure response. Some patients may respond to lower initial dosages; the manufacturer of Dilt-XR® states that patients 60 years of age or older may respond to an initial dosage of 120 mg daily. The maximum hypotensive effect associated with a given dosage level usually is observed within 14 days. Some manufacturers state that maintenance dosages usually range from 240–360 mg daily, although diltiazem hydrochloride extended-release capsules (Dilt-XR®) have been administered during clinical trials in dosages of 180–480 mg once daily, and the diltiazem hydrochloride extended-release capsules (Tiazac®, Taztia

XT®, Dilt-XR®) and the extended-release tablets (Cardizem® LA, Matzim® LA) may be administered at dosages of 120–540 mg once daily. Some experts state that the usual maintenance dosage of extended-release diltiazem hydrochloride for the management of hypertension is 120–360 mg once daily.

The manufacturers of Cardizem® CD or Cartia XT® extended-release capsules or Cardizem® LA or Matzim® LA extended-release tablets state that patients whose blood pressure is adequately controlled with diltiazem therapy alone or in combination with another antihypertensive agent may be safely switched to Cardizem® CD, Cartia XT®, Cardizem® LA, or Matzim® LA at the nearest equivalent daily dosage. Subsequent titration of dosage may be necessary depending on the clinical response of the patient. The manufacturers of Cardizem® CD or Cartia XT® extended-release capsules and Cardizem® LA extended-release tablets also state that there is limited clinical experience with diltiazem doses exceeding 360 mg, but doses up to 540 mg have been used during clinical trials; the incidence of adverse effects (especially first-degree AV block, dizziness, sinus bradycardia) increases with increasing dosage. The manufacturer of Dilt-XR® states that although clinical experience is limited, Dilt-XR® extended-release capsules have been administered in 540-mg doses with little or no increased risk of adverse effects.

Blood Pressure Monitoring and Treatment Goals

Blood pressure should be monitored regularly (i.e., monthly) during therapy and dosage of the antihypertensive drug adjusted until blood pressure is controlled. If an adequate blood pressure response is not achieved with diltiazem monotherapy, another antihypertensive agent with demonstrated benefit and preferably with a complementary mechanism of action (e.g., angiotensin-converting enzyme [ACE] inhibitor, angiotensin II receptor antagonist, thiazide diuretic) may be added; if goal blood pressure is still not achieved with the use of 2 antihypertensive agents, a third drug may be added.(See Uses: Hypertension in Adults, in the Thiazides General Statement 40:28.20.) In patients who develop unacceptable adverse effects with diltiazem, the drug should be discontinued and another antihypertensive agent from a different pharmacologic class should be initiated.

The goal of hypertension management and prevention is to achieve and maintain optimal control of blood pressure. However, the optimum blood pressure threshold for initiating antihypertensive drug therapy and specific treatment goals remain controversial. While other hypertension guidelines have based target blood pressure goals on age and comorbidities, the 2017 American College of Cardiology (ACC)/ American Heart Association (AHA) hypertension guideline incorporates underlying cardiovascular risk into decision making regarding treatment and generally recommends the same target blood pressure (i.e., less than 130/80 mm Hg) in all adults. Many patients will require at least 2 drugs from different pharmacologic classes to achieve this blood pressure goal; the potential benefits of hypertension management and drug cost, adverse effects, and risks associated with the use of multiple antihypertensive drugs also should be considered when deciding a patient's blood pressure treatment goal.

For additional information on target levels of blood pressure and on monitoring therapy in the management of hypertension, see Blood Pressure Monitoring and Treatment Goals under Dosage: Hypertension, in Dosage and Administration in the Thiazides General Statement 40:28.20.

Supraventricular Arrhythmias

Paroxysmal Supraventricular Tachycardia

For rapid conversion to normal sinus rhythm in patients with paroxysmal supraventricular tachycardia (PSVT) or for stable, narrow-complex, reentry mechanism tachycardias (reentry SVT), if the rhythm is unresponsive to (i.e., not controlled or converted by) vagal maneuvers or adenosine, the usual initial IV dose of diltiazem hydrochloride is 0.25 mg/kg based on actual body weight (20 mg is reasonable for the average adult) given by direct IV injection over 2 minutes; some patients may respond to an initial dose of 0.15 mg/kg, but duration of action may be shorter and clinical experience with this dose is limited. If the patient tolerates the dose but response is inadequate (i.e., conversion to normal sinus rhythm does not occur) and no hypotension is observed, a second dose of 0.35 mg/kg based on actual body weight (25 mg is reasonable for the average adult) may be given 15 minutes after the initial dose. Subsequent doses should be individualized for each patient. Some clinicians suggest that additional doses of diltiazem should be given at intervals of no less than 15 minutes to allow for the full effect of the drug on AV conduction to be observed. Greater than recommended dosages (e.g., 0.45 mg/

kg)† do not appear to be more effective in terminating PSVT. Patients with low body weights should be dosed on a mg/kg basis. The usual adult IV maintenance infusion dose of diltiazem hydrochloride is 5–15 mg/hour.

Atrial Fibrillation and Flutter

For temporary control of rapid ventricular rates in adults with atrial flutter or atrial fibrillation, an IV diltiazem hydrochloride loading dose of 0.25 mg/kg based on actual body weight (20 mg is reasonable for the average adult) is administered by direct IV injection over 2 minutes; some patients may respond to an initial dose of 0.15 mg/kg, but clinical experience with this dose is limited. If the patient tolerates but does not respond adequately to the initial dose (i.e., does not experience the desired reduction in ventricular rate), a second dose of 0.35 mg/kg based on actual body weight (25 mg is reasonable for the average adult) may be given 15 minutes after the initial dose. Subsequent doses should be individualized for each patient. Some clinicians suggest that additional doses of diltiazem should be given at intervals of not less than 15 minutes to allow for the full effect of the drug on AV conduction to be observed. For continued reduction of ventricular rate in patients with atrial flutter or fibrillation who have responded to initial therapy with diltiazem, the rate and duration of the diltiazem maintenance infusion should be adjusted carefully according to the patient's tolerance (e.g., reduction in blood pressure) and response (i.e., reduction in heart rate); infusions may be maintained for up to 24 hours. An initial maintenance infusion at the rate of 10 mg/hour (range: 5–15 mg/hour) is recommended. The maintenance infusion rate may be increased in increments of 5 mg/hour up to, but not exceeding, 15 mg/hour, as needed, if further reduction in heart rate is required. Optimal response usually is achieved with diltiazem hydrochloride maintenance dosages of 10–15 mg/hour, but some patients (e.g., those with small body frame) may achieve adequate heart rate control with infusion rates as low as 5 mg/hour; maintenance dosage requirements may be lower in patients with liver disease or in geriatric patients. The safety and efficacy of maintenance infusion rates exceeding 15 mg/hour for longer than 24 hours have not been established, and use of such dosages is not recommended by the manufacturers.

Once adequate control of heart rate or conversion to normal sinus rhythm has been achieved with diltiazem therapy, therapy with antiarrhythmic agents may be necessary to maintain reduced heart rate in patients with atrial fibrillation or atrial flutter or to prevent the further occurrence of paroxysmal supraventricular tachycardia. Attempts to transfer the patient to alternative antiarrhythmic therapy (e.g., IV or oral digoxin, quinidine, procainamide, oral calcium-channel blockers, oral β-adrenergic blockers) should be made. In controlled clinical trials, transference of therapy occurred within 3–24 hours of administration of direct IV injection of diltiazem. Clinical experience with transferring therapy following maintenance infusion of diltiazem hydrochloride is limited. In determining the appropriateness of transferring therapy, characteristics and dosing guidelines for the alternative drug must be considered.

After an acute reduction of heart rate in patients with atrial fibrillation or flutter is obtained with diltiazem therapy, clinicians may consider cardioversion, anticoagulant therapy (e.g., warfarin) to decrease the risk of peripheral embolization, or oral long-term antiarrhythmic agents, depending on the duration of atrial fibrillation and presence of concurrent cardiac disease.

Other Supraventricular Arrhythmias

For the treatment of other supraventricular tachycardias (e.g., junctional tachycardia†, atrial tachycardia†) in adults, an initial diltiazem hydrochloride dose of 0.25 mg/kg has been administered by direct IV injection over 2 minutes, followed by a maintenance IV infusion of 5–10 mg/hour (up to 15 mg/hour).

● Dosage in Renal and Hepatic Impairment

Diltiazem is metabolized extensively by the liver and excreted in urine and bile. Although specific dosage recommendations for patients with impaired renal function are not available, dosage of diltiazem hydrochloride should be titrated cautiously in these patients. However, some evidence suggests that the pharmacokinetics and bioavailability of the oral drug and its major active metabolite deacetyldiltiazem may not be altered substantially in patients with renal failure.

Diltiazem should be used with caution in patients with hepatic impairment, since acute hepatic injury has been reported rarely.(See Cautions: Hepatic Effects.) In addition, systemic clearance and half-life of the drug are increased in patients with liver cirrhosis receiving oral diltiazem; however, the manufacturers make no specific recommendations for dosage adjustment in patients with impaired hepatic function.

CAUTIONS

In therapeutic dosage, diltiazem usually is well tolerated. Serious adverse reactions requiring discontinuance of diltiazem therapy or dosage adjustment are rare; however, GI tract disturbances, skin eruptions, and bradycardia may result in discontinuance of the drug in about 1% of patients.

● Cardiovascular Effects

The most common adverse cardiovascular effect noted with IV diltiazem is symptomatic or asymptomatic hypotension, which occurred in 3.2 or 4.3%, respectively, of patients receiving the drug in clinical trials. Hypotension or postural hypotension also was noted in approximately 1% or less of patients receiving oral diltiazem. If symptomatic hypotension occurs, appropriate therapy (e.g., placement of the patients in the Trendelenburg's position, plasma volume expansion) should be initiated. Hypotension occurred secondary to the vasodilating action of diltiazem on vascular smooth muscle. Vasodilation or flushing occurred in 1.7% of patients receiving IV diltiazem and in approximately 1% or less of patients receiving oral diltiazem in clinical trials.

Adverse cardiovascular effects of diltiazem generally occurring in approximately 1% or less of patients include angina; arrhythmia (e.g., junctional rhythm or isorhythmic dissociation); bradycardia; atrial fibrillation or flutter; chest pain; heart murmur; tachycardia; pallor; phlebitis; asymptomatic asystole; bigeminal extrasystole, ventricular extrasystole; sinus pause; sinus node dysfunction; congestive heart failure; worsening of congestive heart failure (in patients with impaired ventricular function); first-, second-, or third-degree AV block; bundle-branch block; ECG abnor   malities; ST elevation; ventricular premature complexes; ventricular tachycardia; ventricular fibrillation; syncope; and palpitation. Some of these effects (e.g., first-degree AV block, bradycardia, ECG abnormalities, flushing) have been reported more frequently (but less than 10%) in patients receiving the drug in placebo-controlled studies for the treatment of angina or hypertension. Swelling and/or edema have been reported in about 2.5–9% or less than 1% of patients receiving the drug orally or IV, respectively. Myocardial infarction (MI) or ischemia also has been reported rarely in patients receiving diltiazem; however, this adverse effect is not readily distinguishable from the natural history of the disease in these patients.

● GI Effects

Nausea occurs in up to 3% of patients receiving diltiazem. Anorexia, vomiting, diarrhea, abdominal pain, paralytic ileus, dyspepsia, dysgeusia, tooth disorder, eructation, colitis, flatulence, GI hemorrhage, gastric ulcers, thirst, and weight gain have occurred in less than 2% of patients receiving the drug. Constipation or dry mouth has been reported in less than 2% of patients receiving the drug orally and in less than 1% of patients receiving the drug IV.

● Nervous System Effects

Adverse nervous system effects of diltiazem generally occurring in about 1–5% of patients include headache, somnolence, insomnia, and abnormal dreams. Dizziness or asthenia occurs in 1–5% of patients receiving the drug orally and in less than 1% of patients receiving the drug IV. However, headache, dizziness, and asthenia reportedly occurred in 8–12, 6–7, and 3–5%, respectively, of patients receiving the drug for hypertension. Other adverse nervous system effects including amnesia, depression, gait abnormality, neuropathy, sweating,paresthesia, personality change, malaise, fever, tinnitus, tremor, vertigo, hypertonia, nervousness, abnormal thinking, and hallucinationshave been reported in less than 1% of patients receiving the drug. Extrapyramidal reactions have been reported rarely in patients receiving diltiazem.

● Hepatic Effects

Mild to marked elevations in liver function test results (e.g., serum AST [SGOT], ALT [SGPT], LDH, creatine kinase [CK, creatine phosphokinase, CPK], alkaline phosphatase, bilirubin) and hepatocellular injury have been reported rarely in patients receiving oral diltiazem, usually early in therapy (e.g., 1–8 weeks after initiation); although a causal relationship to the drug is uncertain in most cases, it is likely in some cases. Mild elevations usually were transient and frequently resolved despite continued oral diltiazem therapy. Elevations in some indices of liver function (i.e., AST [SGOT], alkaline phosphatase) also have been reported in less than 1% of patients receiving IV diltiazem. Adverse hepatic effects of oral diltiazem have been reversible following discontinuance of the drug.

High dosages of diltiazem hydrochloride have been associated with hepatic damage in dogs and rats during subacute and chronic toxicity studies. Histologic liver changes occurred in rats receiving oral doses of 125 mg/kg or greater, but the changes were reversible following discontinuance of the drug. Doses of 20 mg/kg have also been associated with hepatic effects in dogs; however, the effects were reversible despite continued administration of the drug.

● Local and Dermatologic Effects and Sensitivity Reactions

Pruritus or burning at the injection site was reported in 3.9% of patients receiving IV diltiazem in clinical trials.

Rash has been reported in about 1% of patients receiving diltiazem. A generalized rash characterized by leukocytoclastic vasculitis also has been reported, but a causal relationship to the drug has not been established. Photosensitivity reactions, petechiae, urticaria, contact dermatitis, and skin hypertrophy (nevus) have occurred in less than 1% of patients receiving the drug orally; other allergic reactions also have been reported. Pruritus has been reported in less than 1% of patients receiving the drug orally or IV in clinical trials. Diaphoresis was reported in less than 1% of patients receiving IV diltiazem in clinical trials. Alopecia has occurred infrequently, but a causal relationship to the drug has not been established. Adverse dermatologic effects (e.g., rash) associated with diltiazem may be transient and resolve despite continued therapy with the drug; however, skin eruptions infrequently have progressed to erythema multiforme, toxic epidermal neurolysis, Stevens-Johnson syndrome, and/or exfoliative dermatitis. Recurrence of exfoliative dermatitis with rechallenge also has been reported.(See Cautions: Precautions and Contraindications.) Angioedema (including facial or periorbital edema) has been reported infrequently in patients receiving diltiazem. In at least one patient, a diffuse pruritic erythematous rash was associated with generalized lymphadenopathy and appeared to be a hypersensitivity reaction, which resolved following discontinuance of the drug.

● Other Adverse Effects

Hyperuricemia was reported in less than 1% of patients receiving IV diltiazem in clinical trials. Other adverse effects of diltiazem include amblyopia, dyspnea, respiratory distress, epistaxis, rhinitis, pharyngitis, pharyngeal edema,sinusitis or sinus disorder, bronchitis, ocular irritation, ophthalmitis, ocular hemorrhage, otic pain, otitis media, hyperglycemia, nasal congestion, sinus congestion, cough increase, flu syndrome, infection, pain, ecchymosis, osteoarticular pain, respiratory disorder, nocturia, polyuria, albuminuria, crystalluria, cystitis, kidney stones, renal failure, pyelonephritis, urinary tract infection, dysmenorrhea, vaginitis, prostate disease, gout, bone pain, neck pain, neck rigidity, blurred vision, muscle cramps, myalgia, back pain, arthrosis, arthralgia, bursitis, fatigue, accidental injury, gynecomastia, and sexual difficulties (e.g., impotence). Gingival hyperplasia, leukopenia, hemolytic anemia, increased bleeding time, purpura, myopathy, retinopathy, thrombocytopenia, and lymphadenopathy also have been reported rarely; however, a definite causal relationship to the drug has not been established.

● Precautions and Contraindications

Some findings concerning possible risks of calcium-channel blockers raised concerns about the safety and efficacy of these agents (mainly conventional [short-acting] preparations of nifedipine).(See Cautions, in Nifedipine 24:28.08.) Findings of the Antihypertensive and Lipid-Lowering Treatment to Prevent Heart Attack Trial (ALLHAT), which compared long-term therapy with a dihydropyridine-derivative calcium-channel blocker, a thiazide-like diuretic, or an angiotensin-converting enzyme (ACE) inhibitor, however, have failed to support these findings.(See Clinical Benefits of Thiazides in Hypertension under Hypertension in Adults: Treatment Benefits, in Uses in the Thiazides General Statement 40:28.20.)

Diltiazem shares the toxic potentials of other nondihydropyridine calcium-channel blockers, and the usual precautions of these agents should be observed.

IV diltiazem initially should be used only in a setting where ECG and hemodynamic monitoring can be performed and where resuscitative therapy and

equipment (e.g., direct-current cardioconverter) are readily available. Once a clinician becomes familiar with an individual patient's response to diltiazem, IV administration of the drug in an office setting may be acceptable. All patients receiving IV diltiazem should be monitored electocardiographically. Because diltiazem decreases peripheral vascular resistance and occasionally causes symptomatic hypotension, blood pressure should be monitored carefully, especially during initiation of therapy or upward adjustment of dosage. In addition, the frequency, duration, and severity of angina may rarely increase during initiation of therapy or upward adjustment of dosage.

Diltiazem should be used with caution in patients with congestive heart failure, especially in those receiving concomitant β-adrenergic blocking agents or digoxin, since diltiazem may precipitate or worsen heart failure in these patients secondary to possible negative inotropic effects. Although negative inotropic effects have been noted in vitro with diltiazem, hemodynamic studies in humans with normal ventricular function and in patients with a compromised myocardium, (e.g., severe congestive heart failure, acute MI, hypertrophic cardiomyopathy) have not shown a reduction in cardiac index nor consistent negative effects on contractility. While IV diltiazem has been used successfully in patients with atrial flutter or fibrillation and concurrent moderate to severe congestive heart failure, clinical experience with IV diltiazem in patients with impaired ventricular function is limited, and the manufacturers state that the drug should be used with caution in such patients. Peripheral edema occurring during the course of diltiazem therapy should always be investigated as it may indicate deterioration in left ventricular function induced by the drug.

The manufacturers warn that diltiazem rarely may cause second- or third-degree AV block. If high-degree AV block occurs in patients with sinus rhythm, IV diltiazem should be discontinued and appropriate supportive measures instituted. Diltiazem has been administered IV to patients receiving chronic oral β-adrenergic blocking therapy and the combination generally is well tolerated. However, the possibility of detrimental effects on myocardial contractility, heart rate, or AV conduction with such concomitant therapy should be considered. (See β-Adrenergic Blocking Agents under Drug Interactions: Drugs Known to Impair Cardiac Contractility and Conduction.)

The possibility that diltiazem-induced skin eruptions may progress to severe dermatologic reactions (e.g., erythema multiforme, exfoliative dermatitis) should be considered. While these dermatologic effects have not yet been reported with IV diltiazem, they potentially could occur with such administration. If an adverse dermatologic effect persists during diltiazem therapy, the drug should be discontinued.

The manufacturer of diltiazem hydrochloride extended-release capsules (Dilt-XR®) states that although the drug is contained in a slowly disintegrating matrix instead of nondeformable material, such capsules should be used with caution in patients with preexisting GI narrowing. While obstructive symptoms have not been reported in patients receiving diltiazem extended-release preparations, there have been reports of obstructive symptoms in patients with known GI strictures who were receiving other preparations containing nondeformable materials.

Diltiazem is contraindicated in patients with known hypersensitivity to the drug, sick sinus syndrome (unless a functioning ventricular pacemaker is in place), second- or third-degree AV block (unless a functioning ventricular pacemaker is in place), or severe hypotension (systolic blood pressure less than 90 mm Hg) or cardiogenic shock. Oral diltiazem is contraindicated in patients with acute MI with radiographically documented pulmonary congestion. Diltiazem should not be administered IV concomitantly with or within a few hours of IV β-adrenergic blocking agents. Prompt cardioversion to normal sinus rhythm is usually necessary in those patients with supraventricular tachycardias and hemodynamic compromise. Diltiazem also should not be used in patients with ventricular tachycardia, since administration of the drug in patients with wide-complex ventricular tachycardia (i.e., QRS of 0.12 seconds or longer) can result in marked hemodynamic deterioration and ventricular fibrillation; proper diagnosis and differentiation from wide-complex supraventricular tachycardia is imperative when administration of diltiazem is considered. The drug should not be used for the management of atrial flutter or fibrillation in patients with an accessory pathway (e.g., those with Wolff-Parkinson-White or Lown-Ganong-Levine syndrome) since life-threatening adverse effects (e.g., ventricular fibrillation, cardiac arrest) may be precipitated secondary to accelerated AV conduction across aberrant pathways that bypass the AV node.

● **Pediatric Precautions**

Safety and efficacy of diltiazem in children have not been established. For information on overall principles and expert recommendations for treatment of hypertension in pediatric patients, see Uses: Hypertension in Pediatric Patients, in the Thiazides General Statement 40:28.20.

● **Geriatric Precautions**

Diltiazem should be used with caution in geriatric patients, since the plasma half-life of the drug may be prolonged in these patients. Since diltiazem is extensively metabolized in the liver and is excreted by the kidneys, renal and hepatic function should be monitored periodically and the drug should be used cautiously in patients with renal or hepatic impairment. Pending further accumulation of data regarding the long-term safety of diltiazem, the manufacturers recommend that laboratory determinations be made at regular intervals when the drug is used for prolonged periods. While clinical experience to date has not revealed age-related differences in response to diltiazem, clinical studies evaluating diltiazem have not included sufficient numbers of adults 65 years of age or older to determine whether geriatric patients respond differently than younger adults. The manufacturers of diltiazem state that dosage for geriatric patients should be selected carefully because these individuals frequently have decreased hepatic, renal, and/or cardiac function and concomitant disease and drug therapy.

● **Mutagenicity and Carcinogenicity**

In vitro bacterial studies using diltiazem have not shown evidence of mutagenicity. No evidence of carcinogenicity was observed in rats or mice receiving diltiazem dosages up to 100 or 30 mg/kg daily for 24 or 21 months, respectively.

● **Pregnancy, Fertility, and Lactation**

Pregnancy

Diltiazem has produced embryocidal and fetocidal effects, skeletal abnormalities, and reductions in early individual pup weights and survival rates during reproduction studies in mice, rats, and rabbits when given in dosages 5–10 times the usual human daily dosage, and an increased incidence of stillbirths at dosages 20 times or more the usual human dosage. There are no adequate and controlled studies to date with diltiazem in pregnant women, and the drug should be used during pregnancy only when the potential benefits justify the possible risks to the fetus.

Fertility

Reproduction studies in male and female rats using diltiazem dosages of up to 100 mg/kg daily have not revealed evidence of impaired fertility.

Lactation

Because diltiazem is distributed into milk, the manufacturers state that women receiving the drug should not breastfeed their infants; an alternative method of infant feeding should be used if diltiazem therapy is considered necessary in nursing women.

DRUG INTERACTIONS

In all drug interactions described in the Drug Interactions section, diltiazem hydrochloride was used.

Because of the potential for additive cardiovascular effects, the manufacturers recommend caution when diltiazem is administered concomitantly with other drugs that may decrease peripheral resistance or myocardial filling, contractility, or impulse conduction.

● **Cardiac Glycosides**

There are conflicting reports on whether diltiazem substantially affects the pharmacokinetics of digoxin when the drugs are administered concomitantly. In some studies, diltiazem reportedly increased average steady-state serum digoxin concentrations by about 20–50%, possibly by decreasing the renal and nonrenal clearance of the glycoside; however, in other studies, diltiazem did not substantially alter serum digoxin concentrations. Despite conflicting reports, serum digoxin concentrations should be carefully monitored and the patient observed closely

for signs of digoxin toxicity when diltiazem and digoxin are administered concomitantly, especially in geriatric patients, patients with unstable renal function, or those with serum digoxin concentrations in the upper therapeutic range before diltiazem is administered; digoxin dosage should be reduced if necessary. Digoxin does not appear to affect the pharmacokinetics of diltiazem. Concomitant use of diltiazem and a cardiac glycoside may result in an additive effect on AV nodal conduction. Although concomitant therapy with the drugs generally has been well tolerated, patients should be monitored for excessive slowing of the heart rate and/or AV block.

● **Drugs Affecting Hepatic Microsomal Enzymes**

Metabolism of diltiazem is mediated principally by the cytochrome P-450 (CYP) isoenzyme 3A4. The possibility exists that drugs that induce, inhibit, or compete for this isoenzyme may alter metabolism of diltiazem and therefore, may alter the efficacy and adverse effect profile of diltiazem.

Diltiazem may competitively inhibit CYP3A4-dependent metabolism of other drugs, potentially altering oral bioavailability and/or clearance of these drugs. Diltiazem has been shown to inhibit metabolism of aminopyrine in vitro, and the drug has substantially reduced antipyrine clearance via apparent inhibition of oxidative metabolism in healthy adults.

Dosage of drugs metabolized via CYP3A4 may require adjustment when concomitant diltiazem therapy is initiated or discontinued in order to maintain optimum therapeutic concentrations of such drugs, particularly drugs with a low therapeutic index or in patients with renal and/or hepatic impairment.

H₂-Receptor Antagonists

Concomitant administration of diltiazem and cimetidine may result in increased plasma diltiazem concentrations. Peak plasma diltiazem concentrations were increased by approximately 58% and area under the plasma concentration-time curve by approximately 50% in several healthy adults who received a single, 60-mg oral dose of diltiazem after 1 week of oral cimetidine therapy (1.2 g daily). Concomitant administration of ranitidine produced some but not substantial alterations in these pharmacokinetic parameters of diltiazem. Cimetidine and ranitidine increased peak plasma deacetyldiltiazem concentrations by about 65 and 60%, respectively. Although the precise mechanism of this interaction is not known, cimetidine-induced inhibition of the cytochrome P-450 system may play a role; other mechanisms for the decreased clearance of diltiazem and its deacetyl metabolite also may be involved. Although the clinical importance of this potential interaction has not been elucidated, the effects of diltiazem should be monitored carefully when cimetidine therapy is initiated or discontinued in patients receiving cimetidine; dosage adjustment of diltiazem may be necessary.

Cyclosporine

Concomitant use of diltiazem and cyclosporine has resulted in increased blood cyclosporine concentrations and consequent cyclosporine-induced nephrotoxicity. Although further study is needed, it has been suggested that diltiazem may interfere with metabolism of cyclosporine via CYP3A4 inhibition. The possibility that diltiazem may increase serum cyclosporine concentrations and thereby increase its nephrotoxic potential should be considered if the drugs are used concomitantly. Concomitant administration of cyclosporine with diltiazem (especially when diltiazem therapy is initiated, adjusted, or discontinued) requires monitoring of the concentration of cyclosporine in biologic fluid with appropriate adjustment of cyclosporine dosage.

Carbamazepine

Concomitant use of oral diltiazem and carbamazepine can result in increased serum or plasma carbamazepine concentrations and subsequent neurologic and sensory manifestations of carbamazepine toxicity (e.g., dizziness, diplopia, nausea, anorexia, ataxia, fatigue, listlessness, lethargy, nystagmus, dysmetria, headache, paresthesia, depression, speech disturbances, visual hallucinations, hyperacusis); carbamazepine concentrations may increase by 40–72%. Limited experience indicates that a similar interaction also may occur when verapamil, but not nifedipine, is administered concomitantly with carbamazepine. Although further study is needed, it has been suggested that diltiazem may inhibit hepatic metabolism of carbamazepine via CYP3A4. Because of the risk of carbamazepine toxicity and the possibility of reduced diltiazem effect, concurrent use of diltiazem and carbamazepine should be avoided, if possible. If the combination is used, patients should be monitored closely for manifestations of carbamazepine toxicity and alterations in the pharmacokinetics of the drug during concomitant therapy, adjusting carbamazepine dosage accordingly.

Benzodiazepines

Concomitant use of diltiazem and certain benzodiazepines (e.g., midazolam, triazolam) may result in increased plasma concentrations and decreased plasma clearance of those benzodiazepines. Although the exact mechanism has not been elucidated, diltiazem appears to inhibit the CYP3A4 isoenzyme responsible for metabolism of midazolam and triazolam. Results of clinical studies indicate that concomitant use of diltiazem with midazolam or triazolam increases area under the plasma concentration-time curve (AUC), peak plasma concentrations, and elimination half-lives of these benzodiazepines by about 300–400, 200, and 150–250%, respectively (compared with placebo). This interaction may result in increased adverse effects (e.g., prolonged sedation, respiratory depression) associated with the benzodiazepines.

Buspirone

Concomitant use of diltiazem with buspirone may result in increased mean AUC and peak plasma concentrations of buspirone. Results of a placebo-controlled clinical study indicate that concomitant use of diltiazem with buspirone increases the AUC and peak plasma concentration of buspirone by about 550 and 410%, respectively. The elimination half-life and time to peak plasma concentration of buspirone were not affected by diltiazem. This interaction may result in enhanced effects and increased adverse reactions associated with buspirone. In patients receiving buspirone concomitantly with diltiazem, dosage adjustment of buspirone may be necessary.

Lovastatin

Concomitant use of diltiazem with lovastatin may result in increased mean AUCs and peak plasma concentrations of lovastatin and an increased risk of myopathy/rhabdomyolysis. This drug interaction was not observed when diltiazem was used concomitantly with pravastatin. Results of a study in a limited number of individuals indicate that administration of diltiazem dosages of 120 mg twice daily for 2 weeks increases the mean AUC and peak plasma concentration of lovastatin (single dose of 20 mg) by 3- to 4-fold. When concomitant use is required, lovastatin therapy should be initiated at a dosage of 10 mg once daily and may be increased up to a maximum of 20 mg once daily. When a statin is required in a patient receiving diltiazem, a non-CYP3A4-metabolized statin should be used if possible. Patients receiving concomitant lovastatin concomitantly with diltiazem should be monitored for evidence of lovastatin toxicity (e.g., rhabdomyolysis, myositis).

Quinidine

Concomitant use of diltiazem with quinidine may result in increases in mean AUC and elimination half-life quinidine and a decrease in oral clearance of quinidine. Results of clinical studies indicate that concomitant use of diltiazem with quinidine increases the AUC and elimination half-life of quinidine by about 51 and 36%, respectively, and decreases quinidine oral clearance by about 33%. Patients receiving quinidine concomitantly with diltiazem should be monitored for evidence of quinidine toxicity and quinidine dosage should be adjusted as necessary.

Rifampin

Rifampin reduces the bioavailability and increases the clearance of diltiazem after oral administration via induction of CYP3A enzymes responsible for the metabolism of diltiazem. In a clinical study, concomitant use of rifampin with diltiazem lowered the plasma diltiazem concentrations to undetectable levels. Concomitant use of diltiazem with rifampin (or any other known inducer of CYP3A4) should be avoided when possible and alternative therapy should be considered.

Simvastatin

Concomitant use of simvastatin with diltiazem may result in increased systemic exposure to simvastatin and possible increased risk of myopathy and rhabdomyolysis. In a limited number of healthy individuals, administration of a single 20-mg dose of simvastatin in patients who had been receiving extended-release diltiazem 120 mg twice daily for 2 weeks resulted in a fivefold increase in mean simvastatin AUC. Based on computer simulations using these data, administration of diltiazem 480 mg once daily may be expected to result in an eightfold to

ninefold increase in mean simvastatin AUC. When a statin is required in a patient receiving diltiazem, a non-CYP3A4-metabolized statin should be used if possible. When concomitant use is required, daily dosages of diltiazem and simvastatin should not exceed 240 and 10 mg, respectively. Patients receiving simvastatin concomitantly with diltiazem should be monitored for evidence of simvastatin toxicity (e.g., rhabdomyolysis, myositis).

Atazanavir

Concomitant use of diltiazem and atazanavir sulfate may result in increased plasma concentrations and AUC of diltiazem and an additive effect on PR interval prolongation. Caution is advised if diltiazem and atazanavir are used concomitantly; a 50% reduction in diltiazem dosage and ECG monitoring also are recommended.

● Drugs Known to Impair Cardiac Contractility and Conduction

Concomitant use of diltiazem with drugs known to affect cardiac conduction or contractility may increase the risk of bradycardia, AV block, and heart failure.

β-Adrenergic Blocking Agents

Concomitant use of diltiazem or other nondihydropyridine calcium-channel blockers with β-adrenergic blocking agents (β-blockers) can have additive negative effects on myocardial contractility, heart rate, and AV conduction. Although controlled studies indicate that concomitant use of diltiazem and a β-blocker in patients with chronic stable angina may reduce the frequency of angina attacks and increase exercise tolerance and usually is well tolerated, the risk of excessive bradycardia, cardiac conduction abnormalities (AV block), and congestive heart failure may be increased compared with diltiazem alone. Reflex enhancement in autonomic tone secondary to peripheral hypotensive effects has been noted with diltiazem alone, and concomitant use of β-blockers may increase the sensitivity of the AV node to the direct depressant effects of diltiazem or other nondihydropyridine calcium-channel blocker. Slowing or complete suppression of SA node activity with development of slow ventricular rates (e.g., 30–40 bpm), often misdiagnosed as complete AV block, has been reported in patients receiving the nondihydropyridine calcium-channel blocker mibefradil (no longer commercially available in the US), principally in geriatric patients and in association with concomitant β-blocker therapy.

Diltiazem has been administered IV to patients maintained on oral β-blockers therapy, and the combination generally is well tolerated. However, the possibility of detrimental effects on myocardial contractility, heart rate, or AV conduction with such concomitant therapy should be considered. When IV propranolol is used concomitantly with IV diltiazem in patients with coronary artery disease, heart rate and cardiac output are decreased and the PR interval is prolonged. Because of the depressive effects of the drugs on myocardial contractility and AV conduction, IV diltiazem and IV β-blockers should not be administered within a few hours of each other.

Oral bioavailability of propranolol has been increased by approximately 50% when diltiazem was administered concomitantly in several healthy individuals. Diltiazem has been shown to increase the mean plasma concentrations, elimination half-lives, AUC, and maximum plasma concentrations of propranolol or metoprolol. However, the mean plasma concentration and the pharmacokinetics of atenolol were not affected by concomitant use with diltiazem. In vitro, propranolol appears to be displaced from its binding sites by diltiazem. Dosage adjustment of propranolol may be necessary when concomitant diltiazem therapy is initiated or discontinued.

General Anesthetics

Depression of cardiac contractility, conductivity, and automaticity as well as vascular dilation associated with the use of general anesthetics may be potentiated by concomitant use of a calcium-channel blocker, including diltiazem. When used concomitantly, anesthetics and calcium-channel blockers should be titrated carefully.

Ivabradine

Concomitant use of diltiazem and ivabradine increases the systemic exposure of ivabradine and may exacerbate bradycardia and conduction disturbances. Concomitant use of ivabradine and diltiazem should be avoided.

● Nitrates

The manufacturers of diltiazem state that sublingual nitroglycerin may be administered as required during diltiazem therapy for relief of acute angina pectoris. The manufacturers also state that concomitant prophylactic therapy with short- or long-acting nitrates may be administered safely during diltiazem therapy, but that controlled studies to evaluate concomitant use of the drugs have not been performed.

● Other Drugs

Sinus bradycardia resulting in hospitalization and pacemaker insertion has been reported in patients receiving diltiazem and clonidine concomitantly. Patients receiving such concomitant therapy should have their heart rate monitored.

ACUTE TOXICITY

Limited information is available on the acute toxicity of diltiazem. Because of the extensive metabolism of diltiazem, blood concentrations of the drug may vary tenfold. Therefore, the usefulness of such concentrations as a guide in the management of acute overdosages of diltiazem is limited.

Acute overdosages of diltiazem (up to 18 g) have been reported. Fatalities as a result of these overdosages usually occurred in individuals who ingested diltiazem in combination with other drugs. Most patients with a known outcome recovered.

● Pathogenesis

The acute lethal dose of diltiazem in humans is not known, but blood concentrations greater than 800 ng/mL have not been associated with toxicity. The oral LD_{50} of diltiazem hydrochloride is 415–740 and 560–810 mg/kg in mice and rats, respectively, and the IV LD_{50} in these animals is 60 and 38 mg/kg, respectively. The oral LD_{50} of diltiazem is greater than 50 mg/kg in dogs, and doses of 360 mg/kg are lethal in monkeys.

● Manifestations

Overdosage of diltiazem may be expected to produce signs and symptoms that are mainly extensions of common adverse reactions. Adverse effects observed following overdosage of diltiazem included bradycardia, hypotension, heart block, and heart failure.

● Treatment

If diltiazem overdosage or an exaggerated response to the drug occurs, general supportive and symptomatic treatment should be initiated in addition to gastric lavage and administration of activated charcoal. If bradycardia or second- or third-degree AV block occurs, IV atropine sulfate (0.6–1 mg) should be administered. If bradycardia and AV block do not respond to vagal blockade, isoproterenol hydrochloride may be administered with caution. Fixed second- or third-degree AV block should be treated with cardiac pacing. Sympathomimetic agents (e.g., isoproterenol, dopamine, dobutamine) and diuretics may be administered to treat cardiac failure. Ventilatory support also may be needed in some patients. Hypotension may be treated with fluids and a vasopressor agent (e.g., dopamine, levarterenol bitartrate, norepinephrine). IV calcium salts also may be useful for the management of hypotension, and possibly some other cardiovascular disturbances; however, use of IV calcium salts in the treatment of diltiazem overdosage has yielded conflicting results. In a few reported cases of calcium-channel blocker overdosage, hypotension and bradycardia that initially were refractory to atropine became more responsive to atropine following IV administration of calcium. In some cases, IV calcium (1 g calcium chloride or 3 g calcium gluconate) has been administered over 5 minutes and repeated every 10–20 minutes as needed. In addition, calcium gluconate has been administered by continuous IV infusion, at a rate of 2 g/hour for 10 hours; calcium infusions lasting 24 hours or more may be required. Patients receiving IV calcium should be monitored for signs of hypercalcemia. It appears that diltiazem is not eliminated by hemodialysis or peritoneal dialysis. Charcoal hemoperfusion has been used effectively, as adjunctive therapy, in eliminating diltiazem. Limited data suggest that plasmapheresis may hasten diltiazem elimination following overdosage.

PHARMACOLOGY

Diltiazem has pharmacologic actions similar to those of other calcium-channel blockers (e.g., nifedipine, verapamil). The principal physiologic action of diltiazem is to inhibit the transmembrane influx of extracellular calcium ions across the membranes of myocardial cells and vascular smooth muscle cells, without changing serum calcium concentrations.

Calcium plays important roles in the excitation-contraction coupling processes of the heart and vascular smooth muscle cells and in the electrical discharge of the specialized conduction cells of the heart. The membranes of these cells contain numerous channels that carry a slow inward current and that are selective for calcium. Activation of these slow calcium channels contributes to the plateau phase (phase 2) of the action potential of cardiac and vascular smooth muscle cells.

The exact mechanism whereby diltiazem inhibits calcium ion influx across the slow calcium channels is not known, but the drug is thought to inhibit ion-control gating mechanisms of the channel, deform the slow channel, and/or interfere with the release of calcium from the sarcoplasmic reticulum.

By inhibiting calcium influx, diltiazem inhibits the contractile processes of cardiac and vascular smooth muscle, thereby dilating the main coronary and systemic arteries and decreasing myocardial contractility. In patients with Prinzmetal variant angina (vasospastic angina), inhibition of spontaneous and ergonovine-induced coronary artery spasm by diltiazem results in increased myocardial oxygen delivery. Dilation of systemic arteries by diltiazem results in a decrease in total peripheral resistance, a decrease in systemic blood pressure, a decrease in the afterload of the heart, and, at high doses (e.g., 210 mg), an increase in the cardiac index. Decreases in peripheral vascular resistance usually occur without orthostatic decreases in blood pressure or tachycardia; however, orthostatic hypotension has occurred occasionally when the upright position was assumed suddenly. The reduction in afterload, seen at rest and with exercise, and its resultant decrease in myocardial oxygen consumption, are thought to be responsible for the effects of diltiazem in patients with chronic stable angina pectoris. Diltiazem also appears to reduce left ventricular mass and wall thickness that are associated with hypertension.

In contrast to nifedipine, diltiazem has substantial inhibitory effects on the cardiac conduction system, acting principally at the atrioventricular (AV) node, with some effects at the sinus node. When administered IV, diltiazem prolongs intranodal AV conduction and refractoriness, thereby prolonging the atria-His bundle (AH) interval; the drug usually has little or no effect on the His-Purkinje conduction system or intra-atrial or intraventricular conduction. Diltiazem increases AV nodal refractoriness by binding to calcium channels; binding is enhanced during depolarization, and the drug tends to unbind in a time-dependent manner during repolarization. Therefore, when heart rate is increased (e.g., tachycardia), calcium channel-bound diltiazem reportedly increases as a result of a greater number of depolarizations (allowing drug binding) and shorter diastolic periods (limiting drug unbinding). This frequency-dependent effect of diltiazem on AV nodal conduction allows it to selectively decrease heart rate during tachyarrhythmias involving the AV node while having little or no effect on normal AV nodal conduction at normal heart rates. Although diltiazem rarely produces clinically important changes in the rate of sinoatrial (SA) node discharge or recovery time, in patients without SA node dysfunction, the drug may decrease heart rate and prolong sinus cycle length, and may produce sinus arrest or sinus block in patients with SA node disease (e.g., sick sinus syndrome). Diltiazem has little effect on the QT interval and does not affect the His-Purkinje conduction system. In patients with paroxysmal supraventricular tachycardia (PSVT), including AV nodal reentrant tachycardias and reciprocating tachycardias associated with extranodal accessory pathways (e.g., Wolff-Parkinson-White [WPW] syndrome, short PR syndrome), the drug's effect at the AV node results in an interruption of conduction along the reentrant pathway and restoration of normal sinus rhythm. Similarly, diltiazem's effect on the AV node reduces rapid ventricular response rate (generally 150 bpm) caused by atrial flutter or atrial fibrillation. However, the drug does not prolong the refractoriness of the accessory pathway in patients with atrial flutter or fibrillation associated with an accessory pathway (e.g., WPW syndrome, short PR syndrome); these patients may experience a potentially life-threatening increase in heart rate accompanied by hypotension.

Although negative inotropic effects have been noted in vitro and in animal studies with diltiazem, they are rarely seen clinically. Major increases in left ventricular end-diastolic pressure (LVEDP) or volume (LVEDV) or decreases in cardiac ejection fraction usually are not seen following diltiazem administration in patients with normal ventricular function. However, worsening of congestive heart failure has been reported in patients with impaired ventricular function.

Diltiazem does not appear to affect blood glucose, serum insulin, and plasma renin or aldosterone concentrations. Following oral administration of diltiazem in hypertensive patients, serum total cholesterol, high- (HDL) and low-density lipoprotein (LDL)-cholesterol, and triglyceride concentrations have generally been unchanged. In patients with hypertension, diltiazem generally does not change renal plasma flow or glomerular filtration rate while it decreases renal vascular resistance; the drug does not cause sodium or water retention.

PHARMACOKINETICS

Unless otherwise specified, in all studies described in the Pharmacokinetics section, diltiazem was administered as the hydrochloride salt. The pharmacokinetics of diltiazem are subject to considerable interindividual variation.

● Absorption

Approximately 80% of an oral dose of diltiazem hydrochloride is rapidly absorbed from the GI tract following oral administration of conventional tablets of the drug. Only about 40% of an oral dose reaches systemic circulation as unchanged drug since diltiazem undergoes extensive metabolism on first pass through the liver. Oral bioavailability and average plasma concentrations at steady state reportedly are equivalent following oral administration of diltiazem hydrochloride dosages of 120 mg twice daily as extended-release capsules or 60 mg 4 times daily as conventional tablets; however, peak plasma concentration at steady state is lower and the time to peak concentrations is longer with extended-release capsules. The oral bioavailability of diltiazem from Cardizem® CD extended-release capsules at steady state is about 95% when compared with that of conventional diltiazem hydrochloride tablets. Oral bioavailability of diltiazem hydrochloride increases disproportionately with increasing doses; as the dosage of extended-release capsules increases from 120 to 240 mg daily (60 to 120 mg twice daily), oral bioavailability of the drug approximately triples, as the dosage of conventional tablets or extended-release capsules increases from 240 to 360 mg daily, the oral bioavailability approximately doubles, and as the dosage of extended-release capsules increases from 120 to 540 mg daily, the oral bioavailability of the drug approximately increases sevenfold. As the dose of diltiazem extended-release tablets (Cardizem® LA) increases from 120 to 240 mg, the area under the plasma concentration-time curve (AUC) increases by 250%.

Food does not appear to affect the extent of absorption of the (Cardizem® CD, Cartia XT®) extended-release diltiazem hydrochloride capsules or the (Cardizem® LA) extended-release diltiazem hydrochloride tablets; however, rate of absorption may be increased if the extended-release capsules (Tiazac®, Taztia XT®) are taken with a high-fat meal. Food may affect extent of absorption of some extended-release diltiazem hydrochloride capsules (Dilt-XR®); AUC was increased by 13 or 19%, while peak plasma concentrations increased by 37 or 51%, when Dilt-XR® extended-release capsules were administered with a high-fat meal. In healthy geriatric individuals 65–77 years of age who received oral or IV diltiazem, mean AUC of the drug was increased by approximately 50% relative to that in younger adults; these increases were attributed to slower elimination in the geriatric individuals.

Peak serum concentrations usually are reached within 2–3 or 4–11 hours after oral administration of conventional tablets or extended-release capsules, respectively; peak serum concentrations usually are reached within 10–14 hours after oral administration of Cardizem® CD extended-release capsules. Peak serum concentrations usually are reached within 11–18 hours following oral administration of diltiazem extended-release tablets (Cardizem® LA). In healthy adults, direct IV injection over 3 minutes of a single 10- or 15-mg dose of diltiazem hydrochloride results in median plasma diltiazem concentrations of 104 or 492 ng/mL, respectively. Following continuous infusion of 10 or 15 mg/hour of diltiazem, peak plasma concentrations average 242 or 470 ng/mL, respectively, in patients with atrial flutter/fibrillation and 170 or 270 ng/mL in healthy adults, respectively. After continuous IV infusion at a rate of 10 mg/hour in healthy adults, steady-state plasma diltiazem concentrations average approximately 160 ng/mL.

Plasma concentrations of 50–200 ng/mL appear to be required for antianginal effect. The manufacturer of diltiazem extended-release capsules (Cardizem® CD) states that administration of the capsules once daily provides 24-hour blood pressure control. When diltiazem is administered as a continuous IV infusion, plasma diltiazem concentrations of approximately 80–300 ng/mL are required to lower heart rate by 20–40% in patients with atrial flutter or atrial fibrillation; reductions in heart rate tend to correlate with plasma concentrations in these patients but not in healthy adults. Following administration of 1 or 2 direct IV injections of diltiazem hydrochloride, reductions in heart rate usually occur within 3 minutes; maximal heart rate reduction generally occurs within 2–7 minutes and persists for 1–3 hours. Following direct IV injection of diltiazem hydrochloride over a 2-minute period, hemodynamic effects (e.g., decrease in blood pressure) generally occur by the end of the 2-minute period and reach a maximum within 2–11 minutes. Blood pressure reductions following direct IV injection of diltiazem, if they occur, generally are short-lived but may last 1–3 hours. Plasma diltiazem concentrations required to prolong the AH interval in patients with paroxysmal supraventricular tachycardia (PSVT) vary considerably, ranging from 65–260 ng/mL following initial direct IV injection; conversion to normal sinus rhythm usually occurs within a mean of 0.4–8 minutes. Increases in plasma diltiazem concentrations or dosage roughly correlate with prolongation of AV nodal conduction in healthy individuals and patients with PSVT; individual differences in the extent of protein binding, tissue distribution, and autonomic tone may account for variability in the dose-response relationship. After initiation of a continuous IV infusion of diltiazem, effects on the AV node generally occur within minutes and may persist for 0.5–10 hours postinfusion. No consistent relationship has been established between plasma diltiazem concentrations or dosage and overall blood pressure reduction in healthy adults.

● Distribution

Diltiazem has a large volume of distribution because of its lipophilicity and is rapidly and extensively distributed into body tissues. The extensive distribution also may be secondary to the relatively high unbound fraction in plasma. The mean apparent volume of distribution of diltiazem at steady state ranges from 360–391 L in healthy adults receiving an IV infusion of 4.8–13.2 mg/hour for 24 hours. About 70–85% of diltiazem is bound to plasma proteins, but only 30–40% is bound to albumin.

Diltiazem is distributed into milk, apparently in concentrations approximately equal to maternal serum concentrations.

● Elimination

Following oral administration in healthy individuals, diltiazem has a plasma half-life of 2–11 hours; however, plasma half-life of unidentified metabolites may be increased to about 20 hours. Half-life may be slightly prolonged after multiple oral dosing. Following a single IV injection of diltiazem in healthy adults, pharmacokinetics are dose proportional over a dosage range of 10.5–21 mg with a half-life of approximately 3.4 hours and a systemic clearance of approximately 65 L/hour. In patients with atrial flutter or fibrillation receiving a single IV injection of diltiazem hydrochloride 2.5–38.5 mg, the systemic clearance averages 36 L/hour. After continuous IV infusion (10 and 15 mg/hour) in healthy adults, the plasma elimination half-life increases to 4.1–5 hours and the systemic clearance decreases to 52–68 or 48 L/hour, respectively; pharmacokinetics are nonlinear after continuous IV infusion. In patients with atrial fibrillation or atrial flutter receiving 10 or 15 mg/hour of diltiazem via continuous IV infusion, the half-life increases to 6.8 or 6.9 hours and the systemic clearance decreases to 42 or 31 L/hour, respectively. Plasma half-life of the drug may be increased in geriatric patients, but is unchanged or only slightly increased in patients with renal impairment. Liver cirrhosis has been shown to reduce diltiazem's apparent oral clearance and to prolong its half-life.

Diltiazem is rapidly and almost completely metabolized in the liver via deacetylation, N-demethylation, and O-demethylation to several active and at least 5 inactive metabolites principally via the cytochrome P-450 (CYP) microsomal enzyme system and mainly by the isoenzyme 3A4 (CYP3A4); the drug and its metabolites also undergo glucuronide and/or sulfate conjugation. Plasma diltiazem concentrations are higher following multiple oral doses of the drug than after single oral doses, indicating saturation of hepatic microsomal enzyme systems. Following single diltiazem doses administered via direct IV injection, plasma concentrations of the principal metabolites, deacetyldiltiazem and N-monodesmethyldiltiazem, are low or undetectable; plasma concentrations of active metabolites are detectable generally within 30 minutes of initiation of continuous IV infusion and peak at 0.25–5 hours after infusion. About 10–35% of diltiazem is metabolized to deacetyldiltiazem, which exhibits 25–50% of the coronary vasodilating activity of diltiazem.

The contribution of deacetyldiltiazem and N-monodesmethyldiltiazem to the observed efficacy of diltiazem is unclear. In one study, the plasma concentrations of the active metabolites were low in patients with atrial flutter or fibrillation receiving diltiazem hydrochloride by a continuous IV infusion; the metabolites are thought to contribute little to clinical response. However, data from a study in healthy individuals indicate the presence of appreciable concentrations of active metabolites following continuous IV infusion of the drug. Other unidentified metabolites were noted in the plasma after short-term IV administration in healthy adults and appeared in higher concentrations than unchanged diltiazem; these metabolites were more slowly eliminated than the parent drug.

Approximately 2–4% of a dose of the drug is excreted in urine unchanged. The remainder of the drug is eliminated in urine and via bile, mainly as metabolites.

CHEMISTRY AND STABILITY

● Chemistry

Diltiazem is a benzothiazepine-derivative calcium-channel blocker. Because most currently available calcium-channel blockers are dihydropyridines, diltiazem, like verapamil and mibefradil (no longer commercially available in the US), has been referred to as a nondihydropyridine calcium-channel blocker. Diltiazem is commercially available as diltiazem hydrochloride oral extended-release capsules, extended-release tablets, conventional tablets, and parenteral injections and powder for injection. Diltiazem also has been commercially available as diltiazem malate extended-release tablets and diltiazem malate extended-release tablets in fixed combination with enalapril; however, these preparations are no longer commercially available in the US. Diltiazem hydrochloride occurs as a bitter-tasting, white to off-white crystalline powder that is soluble in water and alcohol. Diltiazem malate occurs as a white to off-white crystalline powder that is soluble in water and slightly soluble in alcohol.

USP temporarily stated that potency of diltiazem hydrochloride preparations should be expressed both in terms of the salt and the base ("active moiety"). However, USP recently reverted to its previous standard that potency be expressed *only* in terms of diltiazem hydrochloride. Dosage of diltiazem hydrochloride currently is expressed in terms of diltiazem hydrochloride. Therefore, care should be taken to avoid confusion between potencies that during a transitional period may be labeled as the salt and/or base and dosage of diltiazem hydrochloride.

Diltiazem hydrochloride injection is a clear, colorless, nonpyrogenic, sterile solution of the drug in sorbitol and water for injection. Hydrochloric acid or sodium hydroxide may be added to the solution during manufacture to adjust the pH to 3.7–4.1. Diltiazem hydrochloride powder for IV infusion in ADD-Vantage® vials contains mannitol.

Each extended-release diltiazem hydrochloride capsule (Dilt-XR®) consists of multiple 60-mg tablets contained in a swellable matrix core that slowly releases the drug over approximately 24 hours. The commercially available Cardizem® CD extended-release diltiazem capsules contain 2 types of beads of diltiazem hydrochloride; the beads differ in the thickness of their copolymer membranes that surround the beads. In Cardizem® CD extended-release capsules 40% of the beads (surrounded by the thinner copolymer membrane) release the drug within 12 hours of oral administration of the extended-release diltiazem hydrochloride capsules and 60% of the beads (surrounded by the thicker copolymer membrane) release the drug throughout the last 12 hours of a 24-hour period following oral administration of these extended-release capsules. The manufacturer states that Cardizem® CD extended-release capsules and Cardizem® LA extended-release tablets provide continuous therapeutic plasma concentrations of diltiazem over a 24-hour period.

● Stability

Unless otherwise specified by the manufacturer, diltiazem hydrochloride conventional tablets, extended-release capsules, and extended-release tablets should be stored in tight, light-resistant, containers at a controlled room temperature of 25°C but may be exposed to temperatures ranging from 15–30°C; excessive humidity should be avoided.

Diltiazem hydrochloride injection in vials should be refrigerated at 2–8°C; freezing of the injection should be avoided. Diltiazem hydrochloride injection may be stored at room temperature for up to 1 month; after that time, the injection should be discarded. Diltiazem hydrochloride powder for IV infusion in ADD-Vantage® vials should be stored at a room temperature of 20–25°C; freezing of the powder for IV infusion should be avoided.

In concentrations up to 1 mg/mL, diltiazem hydrochloride-containing solutions are stable for at least 24 hours at controlled room temperature (15–30°C) or under refrigeration at 2–8°C, when stored in glass or polyvinyl chloride (PVC) bags in the following IV infusions: 0.9% sodium chloride, 5% dextrose, or 5% dextrose and 0.45% sodium chloride injection. The manufacturers state that, for IV infusion, diltiazem hydrochloride injection should be diluted to a final concentration of 0.45, 0.83, or 1 mg/mL by adding 250, 250, or 125 mg of diltiazem hydrochloride to 500, 250, or 100 mL, respectively, of a compatible IV infusion solution; these IV infusion solutions should be stored at room temperature or under refrigeration until administration and used within 24 hours.

After the ADD-Vantage® vials containing diltiazem hydrochloride 100 mg have been connected to an appropriate diluent container (containing 100 mL of 0.9% sodium chloride or 5% dextrose injection) and activated for dilution, the resultant 1-mg/mL solution is stable for 24 hours at controlled room temperature (15–30°C) or under refrigeration at 2–8°C; these IV infusion solutions should be stored at room temperature or under refrigeration until administration and used within 24 hours.

Diltiazem hydrochloride is potentially physically incompatible with many drugs, including acetazolamide, acyclovir, aminophylline, ampicillin, ampicillin sodium in fixed combination with sulbactam sodium, cefamandole, cefoperazone, diazepam, furosemide, heparin, hydrocortisone sodium succinate, insulin (regular; 100 units/mL), methylprednisolone sodium succinate, mezlocillin, nafcillin, phenytoin, rifampin, and sodium bicarbonate. Specialized references should be consulted for specific compatibility information.

PREPARATIONS

Excipients in commercially available drug preparations may have clinically important effects in some individuals; consult specific product labeling for details.

dilTIAZem Hydrochloride

Oral

Capsules, extended-release	60 mg*	Diltiazem Hydrochloride Capsules Extended-release (12 hours)
	90 mg*	Diltiazem Hydrochloride Capsules Extended-release (12 hours)
	120 mg*	Cardizem® CD (24 hours), Valeant
		Cartia XT® (24 hours), Actavis
		Dilt-XR® (24 hours), Apotex
		Diltiazem Hydrochloride Capsules Extended-release (12 hours)
		Diltiazem Hydrochloride Capsules Extended-release (24 hours)
		Taztia® XT (24 hours), Actavis
		Tiazac® (24 hours), Valeant
	180 mg*	Cardizem® CD (24 hours), Valeant
		Cartia XT® (24 hours), Actavis
		Dilt-XR® (24 hours), Apotex
		Diltiazem Hydrochloride Capsules Extended-release (24 hours)
		Taztia® XT (24 hours), Actavis
		Tiazac® (24 hours), Valeant

240 mg*	Cardizem® CD (24 hours), Valeant
	Cartia XT® (24 hours), Actavis
	Dilt-XR® (24 hours), Apotex
	Diltiazem Hydrochloride Capsules Extended-release (24 hours)
	Taztia® XT (24 hours), Actavis
	Tiazac® (24 hours), Valeant
300 mg*	Cardizem® CD (24 hours), Valeant
	Cartia XT® (24 hours), Actavis
	Dilt XR® (24 hours), Apotex
	Diltiazem Hydrochloride Capsules Extended-release (24 hours)
	Taztia® XT (24 hours), Actavis
	Tiazac® (24 hours), Valeant
360 mg*	Cardizem®CD (24 hours), Valeant
	Diltiazem Hydrochloride Capsules Extended-release (24 hours)
	Taztia® XT (24 hours), Actavis
	Tiazac® (24 hours), Valeant
420 mg	Tiazac® (24 hours), Valeant
Tablets 30 mg*	Cardizem®, Valeant
	Diltiazem Hydrochloride Tablets
60 mg*	Cardizem® (scored), Valeant
	Diltiazem Hydrochloride Tablets
90 mg*	Cardizem® (scored), Valeant
	Diltiazem Hydrochloride Tablets
120 mg*	Cardizem® (scored), Valeant
	Diltiazem Hydrochloride Tablets

Tablets, extended-release	120 mg*	Cardizem® LA (24 hours), Valeant
		Diltiazem Hydrochloride Tablets Extended-release (24 hours)
	180 mg*	Cardizem® LA (24 hours), Valeant
		Diltiazem Hydrochloride Tablets Extended-release (24 hours)
		Matzim® LA (24 hours), Actavis
	240 mg*	Cardizem® LA (24 hours), Valeant
		Diltiazem Hydrochloride Tablets Extended-release (24 hours)
		Matzim® LA (24 hours), Actavis
	300 mg*	Cardizem® LA (24 hours), Valeant
		Diltiazem Hydrochloride Tablets Extended-release (24 hours)
		Matzim® LA (24 hours), Actavis
	360 mg*	Cardizem® LA (24 hours), Valeant
		Diltiazem Hydrochloride Tablets Extended-release (24 hours)
		Matzim® LA (24 hours), Actavis
	420 mg*	Cardizem® LA (24 hours), Valeant
		Diltiazem Hydrochloride Tablets Extended-release (24 hours)
		Matzim® LA (24 hours), Actavis

Parenteral		
For injection, for IV infusion only	100 mg*	Diltiazem Hydrochloride for Injection ADD-Vantage®, Hospira
Injection	5 mg/mL (25, 50, and 125 mg)*	Diltiazem Hydrochloride Injection

* available from one or more manufacturer, distributor, and/or repackager by generic (nonproprietary) name

† Use is not currently included in the labeling approved by the US Food and Drug Administration.

Selected Revisions June 10, 2024, © Copyright, January 1, 1984, American Society of Health-System Pharmacists, Inc.

Verapamil Hydrochloride

24:04.04.24 • CLASS IV ANTIARRHYTHMICS

■ Verapamil hydrochloride is a nondihydropyridine calcium-channel blocking agent (calcium-channel blocker).

USES

Verapamil is used in the management of supraventricular tachycardias (SVTs). The drug also is used for the management of Prinzmetal variant angina and unstable and chronic stable angina pectoris, and for the management of hypertension.

● Supraventricular Arrhythmias

Verapamil is used for rapid conversion to sinus rhythm of paroxysmal supraventricular tachycardia (PSVT), including tachycardia associated with Wolff-Parkinson-White or Lown-Ganong-Levine syndrome; the drug also is used for control of rapid ventricular rate in nonpreexcited atrial flutter or fibrillation. The American College of Cardiology/American Heart Association/Heart Rhythm Society (ACC/AHA/HRS) guideline for the management of adult patients with supraventricular tachycardia recommends the use of verapamil in the treatment of various SVTs (e.g., atrial flutter, junctional tachycardia, focal atrial tachycardia, atrioventricular nodal reentrant tachycardia [AVNRT]); in general, IV verapamil is recommended for acute treatment, while oral verapamil is recommended for ongoing management of these arrhythmias. Vagal maneuvers and/or IV adenosine are considered first-line interventions for the acute treatment of patients with SVT and should be attempted prior to other therapies when clinically indicated; if such measures are ineffective or not feasible, a nondihydropyridine calcium-channel blocker (i.e., verapamil or diltiazem) may be considered. Verapamil should only be used in hemodynamically stable patients who do not have impaired ventricular function.

Paroxysmal Supraventricular Tachycardia

IV verapamil is used for rapid conversion of PSVT that is uncontrolled or unconverted by vagal maneuvers and adenosine, including atrioventricular nodal reentrant tachycardias and PSVT associated with accessory bypass tracts (e.g., Wolff-Parkinson-White or Lown-Ganong-Levine syndrome). In 60–100% of patients with PSVT, rapid (usually within 10 minutes after administration) conversion to sinus rhythm is achieved with IV verapamil.

Verapamil is used orally to prevent recurrent PSVT and is considered a drug of choice for this arrhythmia. The drug appears to be more effective in preventing PSVT associated with AV nodal reentry than that associated with a concealed accessory pathway.

Atrial Fibrillation and Flutter

Nondihydropyridine calcium-channel blockers (e.g., diltiazem, verapamil) are recommended as one of several drug therapy options for ventricular rate control in patients with nonpreexcited atrial fibrillation or flutter. Management of atrial fibrillation or flutter depends on the clinical situation and the patient's condition. For acute treatment of atrial fibrillation, IV verapamil may be used to temporarily control rapid ventricular rate, usually decreasing heart rate by at least 20%. Cardioversion is indicated, however, in hemodynamically unstable patients. Verapamil should not be used when atrial flutter or fibrillation (especially when preexcited ventricular complexes are present) is associated with an accessory bypass tract (e.g., Wolff-Parkinson-White or Lown-Ganong-Levine syndrome), since ventricular tachyarrythmias, including ventricular fibrillation, and cardiac arrest may be precipitated. (See Cautions: Cardiovascular Effects.) Although approximately 70% of patients with atrial flutter and/or fibrillation respond to IV verapamil with a reduction in ventricular rate, the drug alone rarely converts atrial flutter or fibrillation to normal sinus rhythm. Conversion is more likely to occur in atrial flutter or fibrillation that is of recent onset and/or associated with only mild or moderate left-atrial enlargement.

Calcium-channel blockers (i.e., verapamil or diltiazem) may be used for the management of atrial fibrillation associated with acute myocardial infarction (MI) in patients with a β-blocker intolerance. (See Uses: Acute Myocardial Infarction.)

Oral verapamil is used in conjunction with a cardiac glycoside (e.g., digoxin) to control ventricular rate at rest and during stress in patients with chronic atrial fibrillation and/or flutter. Verapamil has also been used alone† and in combination with quinidine† to control ventricular rate in these patients. The drug should not be used when these arrhythmias are associated with an accessory bypass tract. Unlike cardiac glycosides, verapamil may be particularly useful in controlling tachycardia induced by exercise and stress. Verapamil reduces heart rate at rest (e.g., by 15–30%) and increases exercise capacity in patients with chronic atrial fibrillation and/or flutter, and has been effective in patients who did not respond adequately to a cardiac glycoside alone. Improvement in maximal exercise capacity occurs with a concomitant decrease in heart rate, blood pressure, and double product (heart rate times systolic blood pressure) at maximal exertion during verapamil therapy. Combined therapy with verapamil and a cardiac glycoside appears to be somewhat more effective than verapamil or a cardiac glycoside alone. Cardioversion has been used safely and effectively following IV or oral verapamil administration.

Although controlled studies have not been conducted to date, IV verapamil also has been used successfully in the management of PSVT and atrial fibrillation or flutter in neonates and children. However, most experts state that verapamil should *not* be used in infants because it may cause refractory hypotension and cardiac arrest and should be used with caution in children because it may cause hypotension and myocardial depression. (see Cautions: Pediatric Precautions.)

Atrial Tachycardia

IV verapamil may be used for the acute treatment of patients with hemodynamically stable focal atrial tachycardia† (i.e., regular SVT arising from a localized atrial site), and oral verapamil may be used for ongoing management.

While evidence is more limited, IV verapamil also has been used in patients with multifocal atrial tachycardia† (i.e., rapid, irregular rhythm with at least 3 distinct P-wave morphologies) to control ventricular rate and convert to normal sinus rhythm. However, such arrhythmia is commonly associated with an underlying condition (e.g., pulmonary, coronary, or valvular heart disease) and is generally not responsive to antiarrhythmic therapy. Antiarrhythmic drug therapy usually is reserved for patients who do not respond to initial attempts at correcting or managing potential precipitating factors (e.g., exacerbation of chronic obstructive pulmonary disease or congestive heart failure, electrolyte and/or ventilatory disturbances, infection, theophylline toxicity). Therapy with verapamil has been associated with slowing of atrial and ventricular rates and conversion to sinus rhythm in some patients with this arrhythmia. Therefore, some clinicians suggest that IV verapamil may be useful for the acute treatment of patients with multifocal atrial tachycardia who do not have ventricular dysfunction, sinus node dysfunction, or AV block. Verapamil also may be useful orally for chronic suppression of recurrent symptomatic multifocal atrial tachycardia.

Junctional Tachycardia

Verapamil may be used for the treatment of junctional tachycardia† (i.e., nonreentrant SVT originating from the AV junction), a rapid, occasionally irregular, narrow-complex tachycardia. β-Adrenergic blocking agents generally are used for acute termination and/or ongoing management of junctional tachycardia; limited evidence suggest there may be a role for verapamil when β-blocking agents (particularly propranolol) are ineffective.

● Angina

Verapamil is used in the management of angina, including chronic stable angina, unstable angina, and Prinzmetal variant angina. Calcium-channel blockers (used alone or in combination with nitrates) are considered the drugs of choice for the management of Prinzmetal variant angina. β-Blockers are recommended as the anti-ischemic drugs of choice in most patients with chronic stable angina; however, calcium-channel blockers may be substituted or added in patients who do not tolerate or respond adequately to β-blockers. In patients with chronic stable angina, verapamil may reduce the frequency of attacks, allow a decrease in sublingual nitroglycerin dosage, and increase exercise tolerance. All classes of calcium-channel blockers appear to be equally effective in reducing anginal episodes; however, choice of a specific agent should be individualized since the pharmacologic properties of these drugs differ. Verapamil also may be beneficial in patients with unstable angina; experts recommend the use of a nondihydropyridine calcium-channel blocker (e.g., diltiazem, verapamil) for the relief of ongoing or recurring ischemia when β-blocker therapy is inadequate, not tolerated, or contraindicated in patients with unstable angina who do not have clinically important left ventricular dysfunction, increased risk of cardiogenic shock, or AV block.

Although concurrent use of some calcium-channel blockers and a β-blocker may have beneficial effects in some patients (e.g., reduction of dihydropyridine-induced tachycardia through β-blockade), combined use of verapamil with a β-blocker generally should be avoided because of the potential adverse effects on AV nodal conduction, heart rate, and cardiac contractility. (See Drug Interactions: β-Adrenergic Blocking Agents.)

● Hypertension

Verapamil is used alone or in combination with other classes of antihypertensive agents in the management of hypertension.

Calcium-channel blockers (e.g., verapamil) are considered one of several preferred antihypertensive drugs for the initial management of hypertension according to current evidence-based hypertension guidelines; other preferred options include angiotensin-converting enzyme (ACE) inhibitors, angiotensin II receptor antagonists, and thiazide diuretics. While there may be individual differences with respect to recommendations for initial drug selection and use in specific patient populations, current evidence indicates that these antihypertensive drug classes all generally produce comparable effects on overall mortality and cardiovascular, cerebrovascular, and renal outcomes. (See Uses: Hypertension, in Amlodipine 24:28.08.)

Calcium-channel blockers may be particularly useful in the management of hypertension in patients with certain coexisting conditions such as ischemic heart disease (e.g., angina) and in geriatric patients, including those with isolated systolic hypertension. (See Uses: Hypertension, in Amlodipine 24:28.08.) In addition, nondihydropyridine calcium-channel blockers (e.g., diltiazem, verapamil) may be beneficial in hypertensive patients with coexisting atrial fibrillation and a rapid ventricular rate. However, some experts recommend against the use of nondihydropyridine calcium-channel blockers in patients who have heart failure with reduced ejection fraction because of the drugs' myocardial depressant activity and unfavorable outcomes in some clinical trials in patients with heart failure receiving the drugs.

In the Antihypertensive and Lipid-lowering Treatment to Prevent Heart Attack Trial (ALLHAT), the long-term cardiovascular morbidity and mortality benefit of a long-acting dihydropyridine calcium-channel blocker (amlodipine), a thiazide-like diuretic (chlorthalidone), and an ACE inhibitor (lisinopril) were compared in a broad population of patients with hypertension at risk for coronary heart disease. Although these antihypertensive agents were comparably effective in providing important cardiovascular benefit, apparent differences in certain secondary outcomes were observed. Patients receiving the ACE inhibitor experienced higher risks of stroke, combined cardiovascular disease, GI bleeding, and angioedema, while those receiving the calcium-channel blocker were at higher risk of developing heart failure. The ALLHAT investigators suggested that the observed differences in cardiovascular outcome may be attributable, at least in part, to the greater antihypertensive effect of the calcium-channel blocker compared with that of the ACE inhibitor, especially in women and black patients. (See Clinical Benefits of Thiazides in Hypertension under Hypertension in Adults: Treatment Benefits, in Uses in the Thiazides General Statement 40:28.20.)

Most patients with hypertension, especially black patients, will require at least 2 antihypertensive drugs to achieve adequate blood pressure control. Calcium-channel blockers may be particularly useful in the management of hypertension in black patients; these patients tend to have greater blood pressure response to calcium-channel blockers and thiazide diuretics than to other antihypertensive drug classes (e.g., ACE inhibitors, angiotensin II receptor antagonists). However, the combination of an ACE inhibitor or an angiotensin II receptor antagonist with a calcium-channel blocker or thiazide diuretic produces similar blood pressure lowering in black patients as in other racial groups. (See Race under Hypertension: Other Special Considerations for Antihypertensive Therapy, in Uses in Amlodipine 24:28.08.)

For additional information on the role of calcium-channel blockers in the management of hypertension, see Uses: Hypertension, in Amlodipine 24:28.08. For information on overall principles and expert recommendations for treatment of hypertension, see Uses: Hypertension in Adults, in the Thiazides General Statement 40:28.20.

● Hypertrophic Cardiomyopathy

Verapamil has been used as adjunctive therapy in the management of hypertrophic cardiomyopathy†. The drug is used to relieve cardiac manifestations

(e.g., angina, dyspnea) and improve exercise capacity and quality of life associated with cardiomyopathy-induced outflow tract obstruction and also may alleviate and suppress concomitant supraventricular tachyarrhythmias. Verapamil therapy also has produced clinical improvement in patients without evidence of outflow obstruction. The drug can reduce the outflow tract gradient in patients with obstruction and enhance left ventricular diastolic filling (e.g., rate) and relaxation; the drug also appears to reduce regional systolic and diastolic asynchrony. In addition, limited evidence suggests that verapamil may limit the extent of ischemic myocardial changes in some patients with hypertrophic cardiomyopathy; however, the drug may not alter the underlying hypertrophic process, which apparently can progress slowly despite clinical and cardiac functional improvements induced by the drug and evidence of an increase in the number of calcium-channel blocker receptors (1,4-dihydropyridine receptors) in the myocardium of patients with this condition.

While clinical improvement frequently occurs in patients with hypertrophic cardiomyopathy treated with verapamil, improvement in the extent of hypertrophy as evidenced by changes in intraventricular septum (IVS) and left ventricular posterior wall (LVPW) thickness and in left ventricular diameters appears to occur only occasionally. In one study, there was no change in these parameters overall in patients receiving verapamil, although 13% of these patients exhibited decreases in IVS and/or LVPW thickness. The clinical importance of such changes is not known, but some evidence suggests that decreases in LVPW thickness in patients with hypertrophic cardiomyopathy actually may result in left ventricular systolic dysfunction.

Despite evidence of a lack of substantial effect on the underlying hypertrophic process, functional cardiac changes induced by verapamil, particularly those involving left ventricular diastolic filling, relaxation, and asynchrony, can result in decreased ischemic manifestations, including symptomatic improvement and increased exercise tolerance. While the role of chronic drug therapy in *asymptomatic* patients with hypertrophic cardiomyopathy remains controversial, verapamil has improved reversible perfusion defects and exercise capacity in such patients, and some clinicians suggest that such therapy can be considered for relatively young patients with a family history of premature sudden death and those with marked ventricular hypertrophy or marked subaortic stenosis.

Verapamil appears to be more effective than propranolol as adjunctive therapy in the management of hypertrophic cardiomyopathy† and often is effective and can delay the need for surgery in patients who fail to respond to β-adrenergic blocker therapy. In one study, most such patients improved clinically following discontinuance of propranolol and initiation of verapamil, and in many of those in whom symptoms were considered severe enough to warrant surgery, improvement was sufficient to delay the need for surgery. In another comparative study, clinical and hemodynamic improvement was greater with verapamil than with propranolol. However, because response to drug therapy in patients with hypertrophic cardiomyopathy is variable, probably secondary to the complexity and relative contribution of various underlying pathophysiologic mechanisms in this condition, such therapy should be individualized.

Additional study and experience are necessary to determine whether the beneficial effects of verapamil in hypertrophic cardiomyopathy† persist during long-term therapy. Some evidence suggests that potential benefits may diminish with time. In addition, verapamil should be used for hypertrophic cardiomyopathy with extreme caution and only when other alternatives are not considered suitable in patients with elevated pulmonary venous pressures (particularly when combined with a baseline outflow obstruction), paroxysmal nocturnal dyspnea or orthopnea, or clinically important SA nodal or AV junctional conduction abnormalities (unless a functional artificial ventricular pacemaker is in place).

● Acute Myocardial Infarction

Calcium-channel blockers have been used in the early treatment and secondary prevention of acute MI†; although these drugs are effective anti-ischemic agents, they have not demonstrated mortality benefits and therefore are generally used as an alternative to β-blockers. A review of 28 randomized controlled studies involving 19,000 patients found no benefit with regard to infarct size, rate of reinfarction, or death when calcium-channel blockers were used during the acute or convalescent phase of ST-segment-elevation MI (STEMI). Although some studies demonstrated a reduced risk of reinfarction when verapamil or diltiazem was administered after MI in patients without left ventricular dysfunction, other studies have not confirmed this finding. Calcium-channel blockers generally are used for their anti-ischemic and blood pressure-reducing properties in the MI setting, and only when β-blockers (which have been shown to reduce mortality after MI) are ineffective, not tolerated, or contraindicated; because the nondihydropyridine calcium-channel blockers (verapamil and diltiazem) can cause substantial negative inotropic effects, their use should be limited to patients without left ventricular dysfunction.

Current expert guidelines state that a calcium-channel blocker may be used to relieve ischemic symptoms, lower blood pressure, or control rapid ventricular response associated with atrial fibrillation in patients with STEMI who are intolerant to β-blockers. A nondihydropyridine calcium-channel blocker (e.g., verapamil or diltiazem) may be used as an alternative to β-blockers for relief of ongoing or recurring ischemia when β-blocker therapy is inadequate, not tolerated, or contraindicated in patients with non-ST-segment-elevation MI (NSTEMI) who do not have clinically important left ventricular dysfunction, increased risk of cardiogenic shock, or AV block. The use of immediate-release nifedipine is generally contraindicated because of the potential for hypotension and reflex sympathetic activation.

● **Other Uses**

Verapamil has been used orally with some success in a limited number of patients for the management of manic manifestations of bipolar disorder†, but additional study is needed.

DOSAGE AND ADMINISTRATION

● **Administration**

Verapamil hydrochloride is administered by direct IV injection or orally. The drug has also been administered by IV infusion†, but safety and efficacy of this method of administration have not been established.

For IV administration, verapamil hydrochloride is given *slowly* under continuous ECG and blood pressure monitoring as a direct injection over a period of not less than 2 minutes or, in geriatric patients, of not less than 3 minutes. Solutions of the drug should be inspected visually for particulate matter prior to IV administration whenever solution and container permit.

The manufacturers recommend that extended-release tablets of the drug be administered with food, since smaller differences between peak and trough serum verapamil concentrations occur with such administration. Oral bioavailability of the extended-release tablets is not affected by halving the tablets. Conventional tablets, extended-release capsules, and controlled extended-release capsules can be administered without regard to food.

The commercially available extended-release capsules containing pellets of verapamil hydrochloride (Verelan®) may be swallowed intact and should not be chewed. Alternatively, the entire contents of a capsule may be sprinkled on a small amount of applesauce immediately prior to administration; patients should drink a glass of cool water to ensure complete swallowing the pellets. In addition, the applesauce should not be hot, and should be soft enough to be swallowed without chewing. The mixture of applesauce and pellets should not be stored for future use; subdividing the contents of a capsule is not recommended. Studies to establish bioequivalence of controlled extended-release pellets (Verelan PM®) sprinkled on applesauce have not been conducted to date.

● **Dosage**

Potency of verapamil hydrochloride preparations is expressed in terms of the hydrochloride salt. (See Chemistry and Stability: Chemistry.)

Dosage of verapamil hydrochloride must be carefully titrated according to individual requirements and response. Safety and efficacy of adult oral verapamil hydrochloride dosages exceeding 480 mg daily have not been established.

Supraventricular Arrhythmias

Parenteral Dosage

For the management of supraventricular tachycardia (SVT) in adults, the usual initial IV dose of verapamil hydrochloride recommended by the manufacturer is 5–10 mg (0.075–0.15 mg/kg). Slower infusion rates (over at least 3 minutes) should be used in geriatric patients in order to minimize the risk of adverse effects. If the patient tolerates but does not respond adequately to the initial IV dose, a second IV dose of 10 mg (0.15 mg/kg) may be given 30 minutes after the initial dose.

For the management of SVT in children younger than 1 year of age, the usual initial IV dose of verapamil hydrochloride recommended by the manufacturer is 0.75–2 mg (0.1–0.2 mg/kg) administered over at least 2 minutes under continuous ECG monitoring. In children 1–15 years of age, the usual initial IV dose is 2–5 mg (0.1–0.3 mg/kg), but should not exceed 5 mg. The initial pediatric dose may be repeated once after 30 minutes if an adequate response is not achieved. In children 1–15 years of age, the repeat dose should not exceed 10 mg.

Because severe adverse cardiovascular effects have been associated with IV administration of verapamil, most experts state that IV verapamil should *not* be used in infants and should be used with caution in children. (See Cautions: Pediatric Precautions.)

Oral Dosage

The usual oral dosage of verapamil hydrochloride for the prevention of recurrent paroxysmal supraventricular tachycardia (PSVT) in adults is 240–480 mg daily given in 3 or 4 divided doses as conventional tablets. To control ventricular rate in digitalized adults with chronic atrial flutter and/or fibrillation, the usual adult oral dosage of verapamil hydrochloride is 240–320 mg daily given in 3 or 4 divided doses as conventional tablets. Maximum antiarrhythmic effects are generally apparent within 48 hours after initiating a given verapamil dosage.

Angina

For the management of Prinzmetal variant angina or unstable or chronic stable angina pectoris, the usual initial adult oral dosage of verapamil hydrochloride is 80 mg every 6–8 hours. Dosage of the drug may be gradually increased by 80-mg increments at weekly intervals or, in patients with unstable angina, at daily intervals until optimum control of angina is obtained. Lower dosages (e.g., 40 mg every 8 hours) may be necessary in geriatric or other patients who may have an increased response to the drug. Although maximum pharmacologic effects may occur 24–48 hours after dosage adjustment, maximum pharmacologic and therapeutic response may be delayed since the half-life of the drug increases during this period of time after dosage adjustment. The adult oral maintenance dosage ranges from 240–480 mg daily but usually is 320–480 mg daily, given in 3 or 4 divided doses.

Hypertension

For the management of hypertension in adults, verapamil hydrochloride extended-release capsules, extended-release tablets, or controlled extended-release capsules may be preferred because of less frequent dosing and potentially smoother blood pressure control.

The hypotensive effect of verapamil is usually evident within the first week of therapy. The need for upward titration of dosage with the extended-release capsules or tablets should be based on efficacy and safety and blood pressure determinations evaluated weekly at approximately 24 hours after a dose. When verapamil hydrochloride is administered at bedtime as controlled extended-release capsules, blood pressure determinations the following morning or early afternoon are necessary to determine maximum effect.

Verapamil Therapy

For the management of hypertension in adults, the usual dosage of verapamil as extended-release capsules (e.g., Verelan®) is 240 mg once daily in the morning; when given as extended-release tablets (e.g., Calan® SR), the usual initial dosage is 180 mg once daily in the morning. In patients who may have an increased response to the drug, such as geriatric patients and those of small stature, it may be preferable to initially administer 120 mg once daily in the morning as extended-release capsules or tablets.

If an adequate response is not obtained with an initial dosage of 120 mg once daily in the morning (as extended-release capsules [e.g., Verelan®]), the dosage may be adjusted upward as follows according to the patient's blood pressure response:

Extended-release capsules (e.g., Verelan®)

- 180 mg once daily in the morning;
- 240 mg once daily in the morning;
- 360 mg once daily in the morning;
- 480 mg once daily in the morning.

If an adequate response is not obtained with an initial dosage of 180 mg once daily in the morning (as extended-release tablets [e.g., Calan® SR]), the dosage may be adjusted upward as follows according to the patient's blood pressure response:

Extended-release tablets (e.g., Calan® SR)

* 240 mg each morning;
* 180 mg each morning plus 180 mg each evening, OR 240 mg each morning plus 120 mg each evening;
* 240 mg every 12 hours.

Some experts recommend a usual dosage range of 120–360 mg given as a single dose or in 2 divided doses daily as the extended-release capsules or tablets.

The usual manufacturer-recommended initial adult dosage of verapamil hydrochloride controlled extended-release capsules (Verelan® PM) is 200 mg daily at bedtime. Dosage may be increased to 300 mg daily at bedtime; if an adequate response is not achieved, dosage of the controlled extended-release capsules may be further increased to 400 mg (two 200-mg capsules) daily at bedtime. In patients who may have an increased response to the drug (e.g., elderly, low weight, those with impaired renal or hepatic function), an initial dosage of 100 mg daily may be warranted in rare instances.

Some experts recommend a usual dosage range of 100–300 mg once daily administered in the evening for verapamil delayed-onset extended-release capsules.

Conventional Tablets (e.g., Calan®)

If a conventional (immediate-release) preparation is used for the management of hypertension in adults, the usual initial oral dosage of verapamil hydrochloride as monotherapy is 40 or 80 mg 3 times daily. Initiation of therapy with dosages at the lower end of this range should be considered in patients who might respond to low dosages, such as geriatric patients and those of small stature. Oral dosages up to 480 mg daily have been used in some adults, but there is no evidence that dosages exceeding 360 mg daily as conventional tablets provide any additional benefit in the management of hypertension. Some experts recommend a usual dosage range of 120–360 mg daily (given in 3 divided doses) as conventional tablets.

When switching from conventional verapamil hydrochloride tablets to extended-release capsules or tablets, the total daily dose may remain the same.

Verapamil/Trandolapril Fixed-combination Therapy

When combination therapy is required for the management of hypertension, the commercially available preparations containing verapamil in fixed combination with trandolapril should not be used for initial therapy. Instead, dosage should first be adjusted by administering each drug separately. If it is determined that the optimum maintenance dosage corresponds to the ratio in a commercial combination preparation, the fixed combination may be used. For patients receiving verapamil hydrochloride (up to 240 mg) and trandolapril (up to 8 mg) in separate tablets once daily, replacement with the fixed combination can be attempted using tablets containing the same component doses. Clinical trials with the verapamil and trandolapril fixed combination have investigated only once-daily dosing.

The fixed-combination tablets contain verapamil hydrochloride in an extended-release component and trandolapril in an immediate-release component. The antihypertensive effect or the adverse effects of adding 4 mg once daily of trandolapril to extended-release verapamil hydrochloride (120 mg twice daily) have not been studied, nor have the effects of adding 180 mg of verapamil hydrochloride extended-release tablets daily to 1 mg of trandolapril twice daily been evaluated. Over the dosage range of extended-release verapamil hydrochloride of 120–240 mg once daily and trandolapril 0.5–8 mg once daily, the effects of the fixed combination increase with increasing doses of either component.

Blood Pressure Monitoring and Treatment Goals

Blood pressure should be monitored regularly (i.e., monthly) during therapy and dosage of the antihypertensive drug adjusted until blood pressure is controlled. If an adequate blood pressure response is not achieved with verapamil monotherapy, another antihypertensive agent with demonstrated benefit and preferably with a complementary mechanism of action (e.g., angiotensin-converting enzyme [ACE] inhibitor, angiotensin II receptor antagonist, thiazide diuretic) may be added; if goal blood pressure is still not achieved with the use of 2 antihypertensive

agents, a third drug may be added. (See Uses: Hypertension in Adults, in the Thiazides General Statement 40:28.20.) In patients who develop unacceptable adverse effects with verapamil, the drug should be discontinued and another antihypertensive agent from a different pharmacologic class should be initiated.

The goal of hypertension management and prevention is to achieve and maintain optimal control of blood pressure. However, the optimum blood pressure threshold for initiating antihypertensive drug therapy and specific treatment goals remain controversial. While other hypertension guidelines have based target blood pressure goals on age and comorbidities, the 2017 ACC/AHA hypertension guideline incorporates underlying cardiovascular risk into decision making regarding treatment and generally recommends the same target blood pressure (i.e., less than 130/80 mm Hg) in all adults. Many patients will require at least 2 drugs from different pharmacologic classes to achieve this blood pressure goal; the potential benefits of hypertension management and drug cost, adverse effects, and risks associated with the use of multiple antihypertensive drugs also should be considered when deciding a patient's blood pressure treatment goal.

For additional information on target levels of blood pressure and on monitoring therapy in the management of hypertension, see Blood Pressure Monitoring and Treatment Goals under Dosage: Hypertension, in Dosage and Administration in the Thiazides General Statement 40:28.20.

● Dosage in Hepatic and Renal Impairment

Patients with impaired hepatic and/or renal function should be monitored for prolongation of the PR interval on ECG, blood pressure changes, or other signs of overdosage during therapy with verapamil hydrochloride. Neither verapamil nor norverapamil appear to be removed appreciably by hemodialysis; therefore, supplemental doses in patients undergoing hemodialysis are not necessary.

Because approximately 70% of a dose of verapamil is excreted renally as metabolites (norverapamil, the principal metabolite, is pharmacologically active) in patients with normal renal function, the manufacturers recommend that the drug be used cautiously and with close monitoring in patients with impaired renal function pending further accumulation of data. Some evidence suggests that the pharmacokinetics of the drug may not be altered substantially in patients with impaired renal function; however, the manufacturer of the controlled extended-release capsules (Verelan®PM) states that an initial dosage of 100 mg daily at bedtime rarely may be necessary in patients with impaired renal function.

In adults with severe hepatic impairment, dose and/or frequency of administration of verapamil hydrochloride must be modified according to the degree of impairment and the tolerance and therapeutic response of the patient. Usual oral daily doses for adults may need to be reduced by up to 60–70% in adults with severe hepatic dysfunction. The manufacturer of the controlled extended-release capsules (Verelan®PM) states that an initial dosage of 100 mg daily at bedtime rarely may be necessary in patients with impaired hepatic function.

CAUTIONS

Verapamil shares the toxic potentials of the calcium-channel blockers, and the usual precautions of these agents should be observed. In therapeutic dosage, verapamil usually is well tolerated. Serious adverse effects requiring dosage reduction occur in 6.3% of patients receiving the drug orally; adverse effects requiring discontinuance of oral verapamil occur in approximately 5.5% of patients. The incidence and severity of adverse effects are increased in patients receiving the drug IV; in patients with hypertrophic cardiomyopathy, moderate to severe congestive heart failure, or sick sinus syndrome; and in patients receiving β-adrenergic blocking agents or digoxin concurrently with verapamil.

● Cardiovascular Effects

Serious adverse effects attributed to verapamil's action on the cardiac conduction system occurring in less than 2% of patients include bradycardia; first-, second-, and third-degree AV block; AV dissociation; and bundle-branch block. First-degree AV block may be asymptomatic. Prolongation of the PR interval is correlated with plasma verapamil concentrations, especially during initial titration of therapy with the drug, but this correlation may disappear during chronic therapy. When first-degree AV block and transient bradycardia, sometimes accompanied by nodal escape rhythms, occur with oral verapamil, they usually are associated with peaks in serum concentrations of the drug. In patients with hypertrophic cardiomyopathy receiving the drug orally, the incidence of these adverse effects may be increased; in one study, 11% of these patients had bradycardia, 4% had second-degree AV block, and 2% had sinus arrest. Cardiovascular collapse, which may be fatal, has occurred rarely in patients receiving verapamil for hypertrophic cardiomyopathy and may be related to electrophysiologic and/or hemodynamic effects of the drug. Asystole has occurred with IV verapamil but AV nodal or normal sinus rhythm usually has returned within a few seconds. Conduction disturbances, including marked first-degree block or progression to second- or third-degree block, generally respond to discontinuance of IV verapamil, reduction of oral verapamil dosage, or, in the case of increased ventricular response rate, to cardioversion; severe AV block may rarely require discontinuance of the drug and initiation of appropriate treatment (e.g., IV atropine, isoproterenol, calcium), depending on the clinical situation. During clinical trials, ventricular rates less than 50 bpm and asymptomatic hypotension occurred in 15 and 5%, respectively, of patients with atrial fibrillation or flutter receiving verapamil and cardiac glycoside therapy to control ventricular response.

In patients with atrial fibrillation and/or flutter and an accessory AV pathway (e.g., Wolff-Parkinson-White or Lown-Ganong-Levine syndrome), increased anterograde conduction across aberrant pathways that bypass the AV node may result in a verapamil-induced increase in ventricular response rate. Ventricular fibrillation with loss of consciousness and atrial fibrillation with markedly increased ventricular response rate and resultant profound hypotension and syncope have occurred within minutes after IV administration of verapamil in patients with an accessory AV pathway. The risk of these effects occurring when the drug is used orally in patients with atrial fibrillation and/or flutter and an accessory AV pathway has not been established, but a similar risk may be associated with oral use of the drug. Because of the risk of potentially fatal adverse effects, verapamil should not be used (parenterally or orally) in these patients. (See Cautions: Precautions and Contraindications.)

Congestive heart failure or pulmonary edema, resulting from verapamil's negative inotropic action, occurs in less than 2% of patients receiving the drug orally. Most patients who develop congestive heart failure or pulmonary edema require reduction of verapamil dosage or discontinuance of the drug.

Adverse effects attributed to the vasodilating action of verapamil on vascular smooth muscle include dizziness or symptomatic hypotension, which occur in less than 4% of patients receiving the drug. Systolic and diastolic blood pressures less than 90 and 60 mm Hg, respectively, occur in 5–10% of patients receiving IV verapamil. Hypotension rarely may require treatment with an IV calcium salt (e.g., 7–14 mEq of calcium in adults) or vasopressor (e.g., dopamine, isoproterenol, metaraminol, methoxamine, norepinephrine, phenylephrine). Pretreatment with IV calcium chloride may prevent the hemodynamic changes associated with IV verapamil. Decreases in blood pressure to lower than normal are unusual in hypertensive patients receiving the drug.

Peripheral edema occurs in about 2% of patients receiving the drug orally and flushing occurs occasionally. Myocardial infarction (MI) has occurred in 1% or less of patients receiving oral verapamil, principally in those being treated for unstable angina; however, it is difficult to conclude whether this effect is drug related or associated with the natural history of the underlying disease. Angina, chest pain, palpitation, syncope, and claudication have also been reported in 1% or less of patients receiving oral verapamil but has not been directly attributed to the drug.

● GI Effects

The most common adverse effect of oral verapamil is constipation, occurring in less than 9% of patients. Nausea, dyspepsia, and abdominal discomfort occur in less than 3% of patients receiving the drug orally and in less than 1% receiving the drug IV. Dry mouth, gingival hyperplasia, GI distress, and diarrhea have been reported in 1% or less of patients receiving the drug orally but have not been directly attributed to the drug. Paralytic ileus, which was reversible following discontinuance of the drug, has been reported rarely in patients receiving verapamil.

● Nervous System Effects

Dizziness occurs in about 4% of patients receiving verapamil orally and in less than 2% of patients receiving the drug IV. Headache, lethargy, and fatigue occur in about 5, 3, and less than 2% of patients receiving oral verapamil, respectively; headache has occurred in less than 2% of patients receiving the drug IV. Seizures have occurred occasionally following IV administration of the drug.

Confusion, sleep disturbances (e.g., insomnia), sleepiness, equilibrium disorders, muscle cramps, paresthesia, shakiness, cerebrovascular accident, and psychotic symptoms have been reported in patients receiving oral verapamil but many of these have not been directly attributed to the drug. Similarly, mental depression, sleepiness, muscle fatigue, and vertigo have been reported with, but not directly attributed to, IV verapamil. Vivid, disturbing dreams, which recurred with rechallenge, have been reported in several patients receiving the drug for migraine headache prophylaxis. Morbid dreams (paroniria) also have been reported in several other patients receiving the drug.

● Hepatic Effects

Transient increases in serum concentrations of AST (SGOT) and ALT (SGPT), with or without concomitant increases in alkaline phosphatase and bilirubin, have been reported rarely with oral verapamil. These increases are occasionally transient and may resolve despite continued verapamil therapy. However, hepatocellular injury, which recurred during rechallenge, has occurred in several patients and may be accompanied by clinical symptoms of hepatotoxicity, including malaise, fever, and/or right upper quadrant pain. Periodic monitoring of liver function is recommended during chronic verapamil therapy.

● Other Adverse Effects

Blurred vision, tinnitus, dyspnea, hair loss, rash and arthralgia, Stevens-Johnson syndrome, erythema multiforme, macular eruptions, ecchymosis, bruising, purpura (vasculitis), exanthema, urticaria, hyperkeratosis, gynecomastia, urinary frequency, impotence, and spotty menstruation have been reported in approximately 1% of patients receiving oral verapamil, but some of these have not been directly attributed to the drug; myalgia also have been reported. Diaphoresis has been reported occasionally in patients receiving the drug IV or orally, and rotary nystagmus has been reported in a few patients receiving the drug IV. Rarely, hypersensitivity to verapamil has been manifested as bronchospasm and/or laryngospasm accompanied by pruritus and urticaria. Hyperprolactinemia, with or without galactorrhea, has occurred occasionally in females receiving verapamil; these effects were not associated with amenorrhea and subsided following discontinuance of the drug.

● Precautions and Contraindications

Some findings concerning possible risks of calcium-channel blockers have raised concerns about the safety and efficacy of these agents (mainly conventional [short-acting] preparations of nifedipine). (See Cautions, in Nifedipine 24:28.08.) Findings of the Antihypertensive and Lipid-Lowering Treatment to Prevent Heart Attack Trial (ALLHAT), which compared long-term therapy with a dihydropyridine-derivative calcium-channel blocker, a thiazide-like diuretic, or an angiotensin-converting enzyme (ACE) inhibitor, however, have failed to support these findings. (See Clinical Benefits of Thiazides in Hypertension under Hypertension in Adults: Treatment Benefits, in Uses in the Thiazides General Statement 40:28.20.)

Verapamil shares the toxic potentials of other nondihydropyridine calcium-channel blockers, and the usual precautions of these agents should be observed.

IV verapamil initially should only be used in a hospital setting using ECG and hemodynamic monitoring and where resuscitative therapy and equipment (e.g., direct-current cardioverter) are readily available. Once the physician becomes familiar with an individual patient's response to verapamil, the drug may be administered IV in an office setting. All patients receiving IV verapamil should be monitored electrocardiographically.

Because verapamil decreases peripheral vascular resistance and occasionally causes symptomatic hypotension, blood pressure should be monitored carefully.

Verapamil should be used with caution or not at all in patients with moderately severe to severe ventricular dysfunction or heart failure since the drug may precipitate or worsen heart failure. Signs and symptoms of heart failure in these patients should be controlled with a cardiac glycoside (e.g., digoxin) (see Drug Interactions: Digoxin) and/or diuretics before initiating verapamil therapy. The drug should also be used with caution in patients with hypertrophic cardiomyopathy since serious and sometimes fatal adverse cardiovascular effects (e.g., pulmonary edema, hypotension, second-degree AV block, sinus arrest) have occurred in such patients during verapamil therapy.

Dosage should be reduced, verapamil discontinued, and/or appropriate therapy or resuscitative measures instituted if congestive heart failure or conduction disturbances occur. (See Cautions: Cardiovascular Effects.)

Verapamil should be used with caution in patients with hepatic or renal impairment. Some clinicians state that extended-release preparations of verapamil hydrochloride should be used with caution in patients with renal impairment, since serious adverse (e.g., cardiovascular, metabolic, hepatic) effects secondary to accumulation of the drug and/or its metabolites have been reported in some of these patients. When the drug is administered orally or when multiple IV doses are given to these patients, the usual dosage should generally be reduced and the patient should be carefully monitored for signs (e.g., prolongation of the PR interval) and symptoms of overdosage. Because of the apparent potential for verapamil-induced hepatocellular toxicity, liver function should be determined periodically during chronic verapamil therapy.

Although verapamil has been used in a limited number of patients with pseudohypertrophic (Duchenne type) muscular dystrophy†, only minimal ergometric benefit was apparent during therapy with the drug, and the manufacturers state that verapamil should be used with caution in patients with this condition since the drug can precipitate respiratory paralysis. Caution should also be exercised and appropriate monitoring performed when verapamil is used in patients with supratentorial tumors who are undergoing anesthesia induction, since increased intracranial pressure can occur.

Patients with sick sinus syndrome and patients with atrial flutter and/or fibrillation with an accessory bypass tract are at increased risk of developing conduction disturbances during verapamil therapy. The drug should not be used for the management of atrial flutter or fibrillation in patients with an accessory bypass tract (e.g., those with Wolff-Parkinson-White or Lown-Ganong-Levine syndrome) since life-threatening adverse effects (e.g., ventricular fibrillation, cardiac arrest) may be precipitated secondary to accelerated AV conduction. Verapamil also should not be used in patients with ventricular tachycardia, since administration of the drug in patients with wide-complex ventricular tachycardia (QRS of 0.12 seconds or longer) can result in marked hemodynamic deterioration and ventricular fibrillation; proper diagnosis and differentiation of wide-complex ventricular tachycardia from wide-complex supraventricular tachycardia is imperative when administration of verapamil is considered.

Verapamil generally should not be used in patients with severe left ventricular dysfunction (i.e., pulmonary wedge pressure greater than 20 mm Hg, left ventricular ejection fraction less than 20–30%), unless the heart failure is caused by a supraventricular tachycardia amenable to verapamil, nor should the drug be used in patients with moderate to severe symptoms of cardiac failure. The drug also should generally not be used in patients with ventricular dysfunction or AV conduction abnormalities if they are receiving a β-adrenergic blocking agent. Verapamil is contraindicated in patients with severe hypotension (systolic blood pressure less than 90 mm Hg) or cardiogenic shock and, unless a functioning artificial ventricular pacemaker is in place, in patients with second- or third-degree AV block or with sick sinus syndrome. Verapamil also is contraindicated in patients with known hypersensitivity to the drug. Some experts state that verapamil is contraindicated in patients with borderline hypotension associated with drug-induced hemodynamically significant tachycardia, because the drug may further lower blood pressure.

● Pediatric Precautions

Controlled studies with verapamil in children have not been performed to date, but experience using IV verapamil in more than 250 children (about 50% were younger than 12 months of age and 25% were neonates) indicates that the drug produces effects similar to those in adults. However, severe adverse cardiovascular effects (e.g., refractory hypotension, cardiac arrest) have occurred rarely following IV administration of verapamil in neonates and infants. Therefore, the manufacturer states that IV verapamil should be used with caution in neonates and infants. However, some experts state that IV verapamil should *not* be used in infants. These experts also state that IV verapamil should be used with caution in children because such use also may result in adverse cardiovascular effects (e.g., hypotension, myocardial depression). Safety and efficacy of oral verapamil in children younger than 18 years of age have not been established. For information on overall principles and expert recommendations for treatment of hypertension in pediatric patients, see Uses: Hypertension in Pediatric Patients, in the Thiazides General Statement 40:28.20.

● Mutagenicity and Carcinogenicity

At a concentration of 3 mg/plate, verapamil was not mutagenic in the Ames microbial mutagen test with or without metabolic activation.

Studies in rats using verapamil dosages of 6 times the recommended maximum human dosage for 18 months did not reveal evidence of carcinogenicity.

There was also no evidence of carcinogenic potential in rats receiving oral verapamil hydrochloride dosages approximately 1, 3.5, and 12 times the recommended maximum human dosage for 2 years.

● Pregnancy, Fertility, and Lactation

Pregnancy

Reproduction studies in rabbits and rats using oral verapamil dosages up to 1.5 (15 mg/kg daily) and 6 (60 mg/kg daily) times the usual human oral dosage, respectively, have not revealed evidence of teratogenicity. However, in rats, this dosage has been shown to be embryocidal and was associated with retarded fetal growth and development, probably as a result of adverse maternal effects as evidenced by reduced maternal weight gain; this dosage has been shown to cause hypotension in rats. There are no adequate and controlled studies to date using verapamil in pregnant women, and the drug should be used during pregnancy only when clearly needed. Although the effects of verapamil on the mother and fetus during labor and delivery have not been fully determined, the drug has been used short-term without prolonging the duration of labor or increasing the need for forceps delivery or other obstetric intervention and without apparent adverse fetal effect in women who received verapamil as therapy for adverse cardiac effects induced by β-adrenergic agonists that were used in the management of premature labor.

Fertility

Reproduction studies in female rats using oral verapamil hydrochloride dosages up to 5.5 times the recommended maximum human dosage have not revealed evidence of impaired fertility. The effects of verapamil on male fertility have not been determined, but the drug has increased human sperm motility in vitro.

Lactation

Verapamil is distributed into milk. Because of the potential for serious adverse effects of verapamil in nursing infants, the manufacturers recommend that nursing be discontinued during therapy with the drug.

DRUG INTERACTIONS

● Protein-bound Drugs

Because verapamil is highly protein bound, it theoretically could be displaced from binding sites by, or could displace from binding sites, other protein-bound drugs such as oral anticoagulants, hydantoins, salicylates, sulfonamides, and sulfonylureas. Verapamil should be used with caution in patients receiving any highly protein-bound drug.

● β-Adrenergic Blocking Agents

Concomitant use of nondihydropyridine calcium-channel blockers (e.g., verapamil, diltiazem, mibefradil [no longer commercially available in the US]) and β-adrenergic blocking agents can have additive negative effects on myocardial contractility, heart rate, and AV conduction. The incidence of congestive heart failure (CHF), arrhythmia, and severe hypotension may be increased when verapamil is administered concurrently with a β-adrenergic blocking agent (e.g., propranolol), especially if high doses of the latter agent are used, if the drugs are administered IV, or if the patient has moderately severe or severe CHF (e.g., left ventricular ejection fraction less than 20–30%), severe cardiomyopathy, or recent myocardial infarction (MI). In several studies in patients with chronic stable angina whose symptoms were inadequately controlled by conventional therapy, concomitant administration of verapamil and a β-adrenergic blocking agent (i.e., propranolol) resulted in greater antianginal effect than either drug alone; patients studied were usually refractory to propranolol or intolerant of its adverse effects. When low or moderate dosages of propranolol (i.e., 320 mg or less daily) were used concomitantly with verapamil, substantial negative inotropic, chronotropic, or dromotropic effects generally were not produced by combined therapy in patients with preserved left ventricular function; however, such effects have occurred in some patients.

Slowing or complete suppression of SA node activity with development of slow ventricular rates (e.g., 30–40 bpm), often misdiagnosed as complete AV block, has been reported in patients receiving the nondihydropyridine calcium-channel blocker mibefradil, principally in geriatric patients and in association with concomitant β-adrenergic blocker therapy. The hypotensive effects of concomitant therapy with verapamil and a β-adrenergic blocking agent are usually additive; this effect has been used to therapeutic advantage in some hypertensive patients, but careful adjustment of dosage is necessary. However, excessive bradycardia and AV block, including complete heart block, occasionally have occurred in hypertensive patients receiving combined therapy with the drugs, and the risks of such combined hypotensive therapy may outweigh the benefits. Verapamil should be used cautiously with a β-adrenergic blocking agent for the management of hypertension and only with close monitoring.

Patients considered for combined therapy with verapamil and a β-adrenergic blocking agent must be carefully selected and monitored. Pending further accumulation of data, concomitant therapy with the drugs should generally be avoided or used with extreme caution after conventional therapy has failed in patients with any degree of left ventricular dysfunction, patients with AV conduction abnormalities, and patients receiving drugs with a negative inotropic effect. If verapamil is used with a β-adrenergic blocking agent, the possibility of detrimental interactions on myocardial contractility or AV conduction should be considered, dosage of both drugs may need to be reduced, the clinical status of the patient should be carefully monitored, and the need for concomitant therapy should be reassessed periodically. Because of the depressant effects of the drugs on myocardial contractility and AV conduction, IV verapamil and an IV β-adrenergic blocking agent should not be administered within a few hours of each other.

Severe bradycardia (e.g., 36 bpm), which was associated with a wandering atrial pacemaker in one patient, and transient asystole have been reported when oral verapamil and ophthalmic timolol were used concomitantly. A single IV dose of atropine was effective in managing serious bradycardia in at least one patient. Verapamil should be used with extreme caution in patients receiving ophthalmic timolol; when therapy with a calcium-channel blocker is indicated (e.g., for angina) in such patients, an agent with minimal effects on the sinoatrial node and cardiac conduction (e.g., nifedipine) should be used if possible.

Verapamil may substantially increase the oral bioavailability of metoprolol, a lipophilic drug. Area under the plasma metoprolol concentration-time curve has increased up to 300% following initiation of verapamil therapy. Verapamil appears to increase oral bioavailability of metoprolol by decreasing its hepatic clearance, although the exact mechanism(s) has not been elucidated. A similar pharmacokinetic interaction does not appear to occur when atenolol (a hydrophilic drug) and verapamil are used concomitantly, although long-term administration of verapamil may increase steady-state plasma concentrations of atenolol. Concomitant use of verapamil and metoprolol should be avoided if possible and another β-adrenergic blocker with which verapamil does not interact pharmacokinetically (e.g., atenolol) preferably used when combined therapy is required. If verapamil and metoprolol are used concomitantly, dosage of metoprolol should be adjusted carefully and the patient monitored closely. Verapamil also may decrease oral clearance of propranolol; minimal increases in plasma propranolol concentrations have been reported in some individuals receiving verapamil concomitantly.

● **Digoxin**

Oral verapamil may increase serum digoxin concentrations by 50–75% during the first week of verapamil therapy. This effect may be more substantial in patients with underlying hepatic disease (e.g., cirrhosis). When verapamil is administered to a patient receiving digoxin, dosage of the glycoside generally should be reduced and the patient monitored closely for clinical response and cardiac glycoside toxicity. Combined therapy with the drugs is usually well tolerated if dosages of digoxin are properly adjusted. Whenever cardiac glycoside toxicity is suspected, dosage of digoxin should be further reduced and/or temporarily withheld. If verapamil is discontinued in a patient stabilized on digoxin, the patient should be monitored closely and dosage of the glycoside increased as necessary to avoid underdigitalization. Because of the possibility of additive effects of verapamil and digoxin on AV nodal conduction, patients receiving the drugs concomitantly should undergo periodic ECG monitoring for AV block or severe bradycardia during chronic therapy.

● **Hypotensive Agents**

Verapamil may be additive with or potentiate the hypotensive actions of hypotensive agents (e.g., diuretics, angiotensin-converting enzyme inhibitors, vasodilators). This effect is usually used to therapeutic advantage in hypertensive patients, but careful adjustment of dosage is necessary when these drugs are used concomitantly. An excessive reduction in blood pressure may occur in patients receiving verapamil concomitantly with drugs that attenuate α-adrenergic response (e.g., methyldopa, prazosin). In healthy normotensive individuals, 160 mg of oral verapamil hydrochloride substantially enhanced the

hypotensive effect of 1 mg of oral prazosin. Patients receiving verapamil for the management of hypertension concomitantly with a hypotensive agent that inhibits α-adrenergic activity should be monitored closely for an exaggerated hypotensive effect.

● **Antiarrhythmic Agents**

A substantial hypotensive effect has occurred in some patients with hypertrophic cardiomyopathy when verapamil was used concurrently with quinidine; pending further accumulation of data on the safety of combined therapy, concomitant use of verapamil and quinidine in such patients should probably be avoided. Excessive hypotension has also been reported following an IV dose of verapamil in several other patients who were receiving quinidine therapy concomitantly but did not have hypertrophic cardiomyopathy. There is in vitro evidence that verapamil and quinidine have additive adrenergic-blocking activity at α₁- and α₂-receptors. Verapamil and quinidine have reportedly been used effectively in combination in a limited number of patients for the treatment of atrial fibrillation; verapamil has counteracted the effects of quinidine on AV conduction. The drugs have been used concomitantly in these patients without serious adverse effects; however, controlled studies to determine the safety and efficacy of this combination have not been conducted to date and the drugs should be used concomitantly with caution. There is also evidence that verapamil may substantially increase plasma quinidine concentrations during concomitant use. In one patient, the elimination half-life and peak and steady-state plasma concentrations of quinidine increased and clearance and volume of distribution decreased during verapamil therapy, requiring a reduction in quinidine dosage; an increase in quinidine dosage was subsequently necessary when verapamil was discontinued after 5 months of combined therapy.

Disopyramide should not be administered concomitantly with IV or oral verapamil because of the possibility of additive effects and impairment of left ventricular function. Pending further accumulation of data on the safety of combined therapy, disopyramide should be discontinued 48 hours prior to initiating verapamil therapy and should not be reinstituted until 24 hours after verapamil has been discontinued.

● **Carbamazepine**

Concomitant use of verapamil and carbamazepine may result in increased plasma carbamazepine concentrations and subsequent toxicity. In several patients receiving 1–2 g of carbamazepine daily, initiation of 360 mg of verapamil hydrochloride daily resulted in development of neurologic manifestations (e.g., diplopia, dizziness, ataxia, nystagmus) of carbamazepine toxicity within 36–96 hours. Plasma total and unbound carbamazepine concentrations increased by a mean of 46 and 33%, respectively, but returned to baseline values within 1 week after discontinuance of verapamil; manifestations of toxicity also resolved during this period. The ratio of plasma carbamazepine 10,11-epoxide to unchanged drug decreased during verapamil therapy but returned toward pretreatment levels following discontinuance of verapamil. Limited experience suggests that a similar interaction may also occur when diltiazem, but not nifedipine, is administered concomitantly with carbamazepine. It appears that verapamil and possibly diltiazem inhibit hepatic metabolism of carbamazepine via the cytochrome P-450 microsomal enzyme system.

If verapamil is initiated in patients receiving carbamazepine, a 40–50% reduction in carbamazepine dosage may be necessary during concomitant therapy. Patients should be monitored closely for manifestations of carbamazepine toxicity and for alterations in the pharmacokinetics of carbamazepine during concomitant therapy, adjusting carbamazepine dosage accordingly. If verapamil is discontinued, dosage of carbamazepine should be increased to avoid loss of seizure control.

● **Rifampin**

Rifampin may substantially reduce the oral bioavailability of verapamil. In a patient receiving 600 mg of rifampin daily, the patient's arrhythmias were resistant to oral verapamil therapy, requiring a verapamil hydrochloride dosage of 1920 mg daily. Steady-state trough serum concentrations of verapamil were 123 ng/mL at this dosage during rifampin use; 9 days after discontinuance of rifampin, trough serum verapamil concentrations increased almost fourfold. Arrhythmias were subsequently controlled at a lower verapamil dosage. It appears that rifampin may decrease oral bioavailability of verapamil by increasing first-pass metabolism via induction of hepatic microsomal enzymes. Patients receiving verapamil should be monitored closely for reduced clinical efficacy or for toxicity whenever rifampin is initiated or discontinued, respectively, and dosage of verapamil should be adjusted accordingly; the effects of this interaction may persist for several days or longer following discontinuance of rifampin.

● Cimetidine

Several manufacturers state that the pharmacokinetics of IV verapamil are not affected by concomitant use of cimetidine. However, conflicting data regarding the effects of cimetidine on clearance of IV or oral verapamil and on bioavailability of oral verapamil have been reported. Studies to date have determined the effects of cimetidine on single IV or oral doses of verapamil and may not reflect the effects during multiple-dose verapamil therapy. Pending further accumulation of data from well-designed studies performed under steady-state conditions for verapamil, some clinicians recommend that patients receiving verapamil should be monitored closely for alterations in the drug's pharmacokinetics and therapeutic and toxic effects whenever cimetidine is added to or deleted from the drug regimen and that verapamil dosage should be reduced if necessary (e.g., if oral bioavailability is increased and/or clearance is decreased).

● Lithium

Serum lithium concentrations may decrease, increase, or remain unchanged during concomitant use of verapamil. In a patient with bipolar disorder whose lithium dosage had been stabilized for several years, manic symptoms emerged and serum lithium concentrations decreased to subtherapeutic levels within 1 month after initiating 320 mg of verapamil hydrochloride daily, requiring an increase in lithium carbonate dosage from 900–1200 mg daily to 1800–2100 mg daily. Serum lithium concentrations also decreased in another patient and urinary excretion of the cation increased. Although the mechanism of this interaction currently is not known, serum lithium concentrations and the patient should be monitored closely and lithium dosage adjusted accordingly when verapamil is initiated or discontinued in patients receiving lithium therapy.

There is also some evidence that verapamil may potentiate the neurotoxic effects of lithium. When 240 mg of verapamil hydrochloride daily was initiated as investigational antimanic therapy in a patient whose bipolar disorder was inadequately controlled with a therapeutic dosage of lithium, bipolar disorder was controlled within 1 week after initiating combined therapy, but manifestations of neurotoxicity occurred 2 days later despite therapeutic serum lithium concentrations. Neurotoxicity subsided within 2 days following discontinuance of verapamil but recurred when the patient was rechallenged with verapamil in an attempt to regain control of the bipolar disorder. Verapamil did not appear to affect the pharmacokinetics of lithium in this patient. The mechanism of this interaction is not known, but a similar interaction has been described in a patient receiving lithium and diltiazem concomitantly. Calcium-channel blockers appear to share some of the neuropharmacologic effects of lithium, and combined therapy with the drugs may potentiate neurotoxicity. Pending further accumulation of data, verapamil and possibly other calcium-channel blockers should be used concomitantly with lithium cautiously.

● Flecainide

Experience with combined use of verapamil and flecainide is limited. In a small number of healthy individuals, concomitant administration of verapamil and flecainide showed possible additive effects on myocardial contractility. Because flecainide also has a negative inotropic effect and decreases AV nodal conduction, the manufacturer of flecainide cautions that flecainide and verapamil not be used concomitantly unless the potential benefits are considered to outweigh the risk.

● Theophylline

Concomitant use of verapamil in individuals receiving theophylline has resulted in decreased clearance of theophylline, elevated serum theophylline concentrations, and a prolonged serum half-life of the bronchodilator. Patients receiving theophylline should be closely monitored for signs of theophylline toxicity when verapamil is administered concomitantly; serum theophylline concentrations should be monitored and dosage of the bronchodilator reduced if indicated.

● Alcohol

Verapamil may increase blood alcohol concentrations and prolong its effects. Following oral administration of a single oral dose of alcohol (e.g., 0.8 g/kg of body weight) to healthy men receiving verapamil (80 mg 3 times daily for 5 days) or placebo, mean peak blood alcohol concentrations increased by 17% and the area under the blood alcohol concentration-time curve (AUC_{0-12}) increased by 30%.

● Other Drugs

Verapamil can produce marked increases in blood cyclosporine concentrations. Therefore, the drugs should be used concomitantly with caution; patients should be monitored closely for possible cyclosporine toxicity, and dosage of the drug should be adjusted accordingly.

Verapamil and a neuromuscular blocking agent should be used concomitantly with caution since there is some evidence that verapamil may potentiate the neuromuscular blockade of these agents. Careful monitoring of neuromuscular function is necessary, and dosage of verapamil and/or the neuromuscular blocking agent should be decreased as necessary.

The manufacturers state that dosages of each agent should be titrated carefully when a calcium slow-channel blocker such as verapamil is used concomitantly with inhalation anesthetics that depress cardiovascular activity since potentiation of this depression may occur.

Phenobarbital can increase the clearance of total and unbound verapamil, possibly via induction of hepatic cytochrome P-450 microsomal metabolism. Combined therapy with the drugs may decrease oral bioavailability of verapamil secondary to increased first-pass metabolism in the liver. The possibility that verapamil dosage may need to be adjusted following initiation or discontinuance of barbiturate therapy should be considered.

The clinical relevance to humans is not known, but animal studies suggest that concomitant use of IV verapamil and IV dantrolene may result in cardiovascular collapse.

ACUTE TOXICITY

● Manifestations

Overdosage of oral or IV verapamil produces symptoms that are mainly extensions of common adverse reactions. Hypotension, bradycardia, and conduction abnormalities (junctional rhythm with AV dissociation and high degree AV block [including asystole]) have been reported in patients with verapamil overdosage. Other symptoms secondary to hypoperfusion (e.g., metabolic acidosis, hyperglycemia, hyperkalemia, renal dysfunction, seizures) also may occur.

● Treatment

All overdosages of verapamil should be considered serious; patients should be observed for at least 48 hours (especially those who ingested extended-release preparations) and preferably in a hospital setting. Delayed pharmacologic effects may occur following ingestion of the delayed-release preparations. Verapamil may decrease GI transit time. Ingestion of an overdose of verapamil extended-release tablets has been associated occasionally with intestinal or stomach concretions that were not detected by abdominal radiograph. GI evacuation techniques have not proven effective in removing such concretions; endoscopy may be considered in cases of large overdoses when symptoms last for an unusually long time.

In verapamil overdosage, supportive and symptomatic treatment, including administration of IV fluids and placement of the patient in Trendelenburg's position, should be initiated. Except in patients with hypertrophic cardiomyopathy, β-adrenergic agonists and IV calcium salts may be useful since they may increase the flux of calcium ions across the slow calcium channel. Clinically important hypotension should be treated with an IV calcium salt or vasopressor agent (e.g., isoproterenol, norepinephrine); in patients with hypertrophic cardiomyopathy, α-adrenergic agents (e.g., metaraminol, methoxamine, phenylephrine) should be used to treat hypotension, and isoproterenol and norepinephrine should be avoided. Bradycardia or a fixed second- or third-degree AV block should be treated with IV atropine, isoproterenol, calcium salt, or norepinephrine or a temporary cardiac pacemaker. In patients with bradycardia initially refractory to atropine, response was enhanced after the addition of large doses of calcium chloride (about 1 g/hour IV for more than 24 hours).

In calcium-channel blocker toxicity, an IV dose of 20 mg/kg (0.2 mL/kg) of 10% calcium chloride over 5–10 minutes has been administered; if a beneficial effect was observed from this dose, an IV infusion of 20–50 mg/kg per hour has been administered. Asystole should be treated using the appropriate resuscitative measures (e.g., isoproterenol, other vasopressor agents, cardiopulmonary resuscitation).

Rapid ventricular response rate secondary to anterograde conduction (e.g., in patients with Wolff-Parkinson-White or Lown-Ganong-Levine syndrome) can be managed with direct-current cardioversion, possibly requiring high energy, or with IV lidocaine or procainamide. Verapamil is not removed by hemodialysis.

IV glucagon, sodium bicarbonate, and/or an infusion of insulin and glucose also has been used in calcium-channel blocker toxicity. Some experts state that isoproterenol should be used with caution, if at all, for the treatment of shock or hypotension associated with calcium-channel blocker toxicity. Also, atropine and prophylactic transvenous pacing should be used with caution, if at all, for brady-cardia associated with calcium-channel blocker toxicity; atropine is seldom help-ful for drug-induced bradycardia except for cholinesterase inhibitor poisoning. The effectiveness of IV calcium salt administration in calcium-channel blocker toxicity is variable. Ionized calcium concentrations should be monitored to pre-vent hypercalcemia in patients receiving calcium salts.

PHARMACOLOGY

Verapamil has pharmacologic actions similar to those of other calcium-channel blockers (e.g., diltiazem, nifedipine). The principal physiologic action of ver-apamil is to inhibit the transmembrane influx of extracellular calcium ions across the membranes of myocardial cells and vascular smooth muscle cells, without changing serum calcium concentrations.

Calcium plays important roles in the excitation-contraction coupling process of the heart and vascular smooth muscle cells and in the electrical discharge of the specialized conduction cells of the heart. The membranes of these cells contain numerous channels that carry a slow inward current and that are selective for cal-cium. Activation of these slow calcium channels contributes to the plateau phase (phase 2) of the action potential of cardiac and vascular smooth muscle cells.

The exact mechanism whereby verapamil inhibits calcium ion influx across the slow calcium channels is not known, but the drug is thought to inhibit ion-control gating mechanisms of the channel, deform the slow channel, and/or inter-fere with the release of calcium from the sarcoplasmic reticulum.

By inhibiting calcium influx, verapamil inhibits the contractile processes of cardiac and vascular smooth muscle, thereby dilating the main coronary and sys-temic arteries. In patients with Prinzmetal variant angina (vasospastic angina), inhibition of spontaneous and ergonovine-induced coronary artery spasm by verapamil results in increased myocardial oxygen delivery. Dilation of systemic arteries by verapamil results in a decrease in total peripheral resistance, systemic blood pressure, and the afterload of the heart. Decreases in peripheral vascular resistance usually occur without orthostatic decreases in blood pressure or reflex tachycardia. The reduction in afterload, seen at rest and with exercise, and its resultant decrease in oxygen consumption are thought to be responsible for the effects of verapamil in patients with unstable and chronic stable angina pectoris.

In contrast to nifedipine, verapamil has substantial inhibitory effects on the cardiac conduction system and is considered a class IV antiarrhythmic agent. Although verapamil rarely produces clinically important changes in the rate of sinoatrial (SA) node discharge or recovery time, the drug may reduce the resting heart rate and produce sinus arrest or SA block in patients with SA node disease (e.g., sick sinus syndrome). Verapamil also slows conduction and prolongs refrac-toriness in the atrioventricular (AV) node, thereby prolonging the AH (atria-His bundle) interval. This usually also results in PR-interval prolongation on ECG, which is correlated with plasma verapamil concentrations (especially during ini-tial titration of verapamil therapy), and may rarely cause second- or third-degree AV block (even in patients without preexisting conduction defects). The correla-tion between plasma drug concentrations and PR-interval prolongation may dis-appear during chronic therapy. Verapamil has little effect on the QT interval. In patients with paroxysmal supraventricular tachycardia, including that associated with accessory pathways, verapamil's effects at the AV node result in an interrup-tion of the reentrant pathway and restoration of normal sinus rhythm. Similarly, the drug's effects on the AV node reduce rapid ventricular rate caused by atrial flutter and/or fibrillation. Verapamil has minimal or no effects on anterograde or retrograde conduction of accessory bypass pathways. The drug may depress velocity of depolarization and amplitude and prolong intra-atrial conduction times in diseased or depressed but not normal atrial tissue. The drug does not alter normal intraventricular conduction, but acceleration of ventricular rate and/ or ventricular fibrillation can occur in patients with atrial flutter or fibrillation and a coexisting accessory AV pathway.

Verapamil reduces afterload and myocardial contractility. Although nega-tive inotropic effects have been noted in vitro and in animal studies of verapamil, they are seldom seen clinically in patients with normal left ventricular function. Even in patients with cardiac disease, the negative inotropic effect of verapamil is offset by reduced afterload, and cardiac index usually is not reduced; how-ever, in patients with moderately severe or severe heart failure (i.e., pulmonary wedge pressure greater than 20 mm Hg, left ventricular ejection fraction less than 20–30%), substantial increases in left ventricular end-diastolic pressure (LVEDP) or volume (LVEDV) and decreases in cardiac ejection fraction may occur.

Verapamil also exhibits local anesthetic action (about 1.6 times that of pro-caine), but the clinical importance of this effect has not been determined.

PHARMACOKINETICS

In all studies described in the Pharmacokinetics section, verapamil was adminis-tered as the hydrochloride salt.

● *Absorption*

Approximately 90% of an oral dose of verapamil hydrochloride is rapidly absorbed from the GI tract following oral administration of conventional tablets of the drug. Only about 20–35% of an oral dose reaches systemic circulation as unchanged drug following administration of conventional tablets since verapamil is metabolized on first pass through the liver. The manufacturers state that oral bioavailability of extended-release capsules or tablets of the drug is similar to that of the conventional tablets when the drug is administered under fasting condi-tions. Oral bioavailability of the drug may be substantially increased in patients with hepatic dysfunction (e.g., in those with hepatic cirrhosis).

Considerable interindividual and intraindividual variations in plasma con-centrations attained with a specific oral dose of verapamil have been reported. In healthy adults, peak plasma concentrations are reached within 1–2 hours after oral administration of conventional tablets of the drug, within 7–9 or 4–8 hours after extended-release capsules or tablets, respectively, and within about 11 hours after extended-release core tablets or controlled extended-release cap-sules. Following oral administration of a single 240-mg extended-release capsule or tablet under fasting conditions, mean peak plasma verapamil concentrations of about 77 or 150–165 ng/mL, respectively, were achieved, but there was consid-erable interindividual variation. Food decreases the rate and extent of absorption of extended-release verapamil tablets but produces smaller differences between peak and trough plasma concentrations of the drug; food does not appear to sub-stantially affect the absorption of conventional tablets, extended-release capsules, or controlled extended-release capsules. of the drug. Mean steady-state plasma concentrations of verapamil range from 125–400 ng/mL following long-term oral administration of 120 mg every 6 hours as conventional tablets in healthy adults. Peak plasma concentrations after a 10-mg IV dose of verapamil range from 10–1500 ng/mL. In a limited number of infants receiving 1–3 mg/kg of the drug orally every 8 hours, peak plasma verapamil concentrations were attained within 1–4 hours after a dose but varied considerably, ranging from about 30–150 ng/mL.

Plasma concentrations greater than 100 ng/mL usually are required for acute antiarrhythmic effect, and PR-interval prolongation linearly correlates with plasma verapamil concentrations ranging from 10–250 ng/mL during initial dose titration, but this correlation may disappear during chronic therapy. Hemody-namic effects of verapamil usually peak at about 2 hours and persist for 6–8 hours after a single oral dose of the drug as conventional tablets. After a single IV injec-tion of verapamil, hemodynamic effects peak within 5 minutes and persist for 10–20 minutes; effects on the AV node occur within 1–2 minutes, peak at 10–15 minutes, and usually persist for 30–60 minutes, but may persist for as long as 6 hours. No relationship has been established between plasma verapamil concen-trations and blood pressure reduction.

● *Distribution*

The steady-state volume of distribution of verapamil ranges from 4.5–7 L/kg in healthy adults. An apparent volume of distribution of 12 L/kg has been reported in patients with hepatic cirrhosis. Approximately 90% of verapamil is bound to plasma proteins. Verapamil and norverapamil distribute into the CNS. Following oral administration of 120 mg of the drug 4 times daily in several schizophrenic patients, mean CSF concentrations of verapamil and norverapamil were 6 and 4%, respectively, of mean plasma concentrations.

Verapamil crosses the placenta and is present in umbilical vein blood at delivery. The drug is distributed into milk, reaching concentrations in breast milk similar to those in maternal plasma in some women.

● Elimination

Plasma concentrations of verapamil appear to decline in a biphasic or triphasic manner following IV administration of the drug. After IV infusion or administration of a single oral dose, verapamil has a plasma half-life of 2–8 hours. After 1–2 days of oral administration of the drug, plasma half-life may increase to 4.5–12 hours, presumably because of saturation of hepatic enzymes. Plasma half-life of the drug also is increased to 14–16 hours in patients with hepatic cirrhosis. Plasma elimination half-life also appears to be increased and clearance is decreased in geriatric patients. An elimination half-life of 4.4–6.9 hours has been reported in several infants.

Verapamil is rapidly and almost completely metabolized in the liver to at least 12 dealkylated or demethylated metabolites; only norverapamil is present in plasma in more than trace amounts. The drug appears to undergo stereoselective first-pass metabolism, with the *l*-isomer being preferentially metabolized. Norverapamil, an active (approximately 20% of the cardiovascular activity of verapamil) metabolite, achieves plasma concentrations approximately equal to those of verapamil within 4–6 hours of administration. Food decreases the rate and extent of drug reaching systemic circulation as norverapamil following oral administration of extended-release verapamil tablets. Approximately 70 and 16% of an oral or IV dose are excreted as metabolites in urine and feces, respectively, within 5 days. Only 3–4% of a dose is excreted in urine as unchanged drug. Metabolism of verapamil may differ in infants; in several infants receiving the drug orally, plasma concentrations of norverapamil were only 50% those of unchanged drug, and concentrations of 2 inactive metabolites were similar to or exceeded those of unchanged drug. Neither verapamil nor norverapamil appear to be removed appreciably by hemodialysis.

CHEMISTRY AND STABILITY

● Chemistry

Verapamil hydrochloride is a phenylalkylamine-derivative calcium-channel blocker. Because most currently available calcium-channel blockers are dihydropyridines, verapamil, like diltiazem and mibefradil (no longer commercially available in the US), has been referred to as a nondihydropyridine calcium-channel blocker. Verapamil hydrochloride is commercially available as a racemic mixture. The *l*-isomer of verapamil has been shown to inhibit the adenosine triphosphate (ATP)-dependent calcium-transport properties of the sarcolemma and intrinsic calcium-sensitive adenosine triphosphatase (ATPase). The *l*-isomer appears to be principally responsible for the negative dromotropic effects of the drug on atrioventricular nodal conduction.

Verapamil hydrochloride occurs as a white or practically white, crystalline powder with a bitter taste and is soluble in water and sparingly soluble in alcohol. Verapamil hydrochloride injection is a sterile solution of the drug in water for injection. The injection has a pH of 4–6.5.

The commercially available controlled extended-release capsules of verapamil hydrochloride (Verelan® PM) contain the drug in an oral diffusion delivery system formulation that also is designed to initiate delivery of the drug 4–5 hours after ingestion. The diffusion delivery system consists of controlled-release coated pellets enclosed in a hard gelatin capsule. The nonenteric controlled-release coat contains water-soluble and water-insoluble polymers. When exposed to water in the GI tract, the soluble polymer on individual pellets slowly dissolves, allowing the drug to diffuse through the resultant pores, while the insoluble polymer continues to act as a barrier maintaining controlled release of the drug into the GI tract. The rate of verapamil delivery in the GI tract is independent of posture, pH, GI motility, and presence of food in the GI tract.

● Stability

Verapamil hydrochloride injection should be stored at 15–30°C and protected from light; freezing of the injection should be avoided. Verapamil hydrochloride conventional tablets usually should be stored in tight, light-resistant containers at 15–25°C. Verapamil hydrochloride extended-release tablets should be stored in tight, light-resistant containers at 15–25°C. Verapamil hydrochloride extended-release capsules (Verelan®) should be stored in tight, light-resistant

containers at 20–25°C. Verapamil hydrochloride controlled extended-release capsules (Verelan® PM) should be stored in tight, light-resistant containers at a controlled room temperature of 25°C, but may be exposed to temperatures ranging from 15–30°C.

Verapamil hydrochloride injection is reportedly physically compatible with parenteral solutions having a pH of 3–6. The drug is physically and chemically stable for at least 24 hours at 25°C in most common infusion solutions when protected from light. Dilution of the drug in (1/6) *M* sodium lactate injection in PVC containers is not recommended. In solutions with a pH greater than 6, the drug will precipitate. Admixing the drug with albumin human, amphotericin B, hydralazine hydrochloride, or co-trimoxazole should be avoided.

PREPARATIONS

Excipients in commercially available drug preparations may have clinically important effects in some individuals; consult specific product labeling for details.

Verapamil Hydrochloride

Oral

Capsules, controlled- and extended-release (containing pellets)	100 mg	Verelan® PM, Schwarz
	200 mg	Verelan® PM, Schwarz
	300 mg	Verelan® PM, Schwarz
Capsules, extended-release (containing pellets)	120 mg*	Verapamil Hydrochloride Extended-Release Capsules Verelan®, Schwarz
	180 mg	Verapamil Hydrochloride Extended-Release Capsules Verelan®, Schwarz
	240 mg	Verapamil Hydrochloride Extended-Release Capsules Verelan®, Schwarz
	360 mg	Verelan®, Schwarz
Tablets, extended-release, film-coated	120 mg*	Calan® SR Caplets®, Pfizer
	180 mg*	Calan® SR Caplets® (scored), Pfizer
	240 mg*	Calan® SR Caplets® (scored), Pfizer
Tablets, film-coated	40 mg*	Calan®, Pfizer
	80 mg*	Calan® (scored), Pfizer
	120 mg*	Calan® (scored), Pfizer

Parenteral

Injection, for IV use	2.5 mg/mL*	Verapamil Hydrochloride Injection

* available from one or more manufacturer, distributor, and/or repackager by generic (nonproprietary) name

Verapamil Hydrochloride Combinations

Oral

Tablets, extended-release core (containing verapamil hydrochloride 180 mg), film-coated	180 mg with Trandolapril 2 mg	Tarka®, Abbott
Tablets, extended-release core (containing verapamil hydrochloride 240 mg), film-coated	240 mg with Trandolapril 1 mg	Tarka®, Abbott
Tablets, extended-release core (containing verapamil hydrochloride 240 mg), film-coated	240 mg with Trandolapril 2 mg	Tarka®, Abbott
Tablets, extended-release core (containing verapamil hydrochloride 240 mg), film-coated	240 mg with Trandolapril 4 mg	Tarka®, Abbott

† Use is not currently included in the labeling approved by the US Food and Drug Administration.

Digoxin

24:04.08 • CARDIOTONIC AGENTS

■ Digoxin is a cardiac glycoside with positive inotropic and antiarrhythmic effects.

USES

Digoxin is a cardiac glycoside that is used principally in the management of heart failure and atrial fibrillation. Cardiac glycosides are a class of drugs that increase force and velocity of myocardial systolic contraction (positive inotropic action) and also decrease conduction velocity through the atrioventricular (AV) node. Although several cardiac glycoside preparations were previously available for medicinal use (see Chemistry and Stability: Chemistry), digoxin is currently the only commercially available cardiac glycoside in the US.

● Heart Failure

Digoxin is used in conjunction with other agents in the management of mild to moderate (New York Heart Association [NYHA] class II-III) heart failure associated with left ventricular systolic dysfunction. Although digoxin has been used extensively in the management of heart failure, current use is generally limited because of the lack of demonstrated survival benefit, potential for serious adverse effects, and availability of other drugs that have been shown to substantially reduce morbidity and mortality.

Current guidelines for the management of heart failure in adults generally recommend inhibition of the renin-angiotensin-aldosterone system with a combination of drug therapies, including neurohormonal antagonists (e.g., angiotensin-converting enzyme [ACE] inhibitors, angiotensin II receptor antagonists, angiotensin receptor-neprilysin inhibitors [ARNIs], β-adrenergic blocking agents [β-blockers], aldosterone receptor antagonists) to inhibit the detrimental compensatory mechanisms in heart failure and reduce morbidity and mortality. (See Uses: Heart Failure, in Enalaprilat/Enalapril 24:32.04 and in Sacubitril and Valsartan 24:32.92.) Additional agents (e.g., digoxin, diuretics, sinoatrial modulators [i.e., ivabradine]) added to a heart failure treatment regimen in selected patients have been associated with symptomatic improvement of heart failure and/or reduction in heart failure-related hospitalizations. Experts state that digoxin therapy may be initiated in severely symptomatic patients with heart failure and reduced left ventricular ejection fraction who have started, but not yet responded to, an ACE inhibitor or a β-blocker. Alternatively, digoxin may be withheld until the patient's symptomatic response to the ACE inhibitor or β-blocker has been defined and then used only in those patients who remain symptomatic while receiving ACE inhibitor or β-blocker therapy. In patients with heart failure who are receiving digoxin without an ACE inhibitor or β-blocker, digoxin should not be withdrawn, but appropriate therapy with an ACE inhibitor and/or a β-blocker should be added. The beneficial effects of digoxin have been shown to be additive with those of ACE inhibitors and/or diuretics; symptomatic and functional deterioration can occur when digoxin is withdrawn from patients whose heart failure was stabilized on a regimen of combined therapy.

In patients with heart failure, digoxin may alleviate symptoms and decrease heart failure-related hospitalizations. Although data demonstrating an overall survival benefit of digoxin are lacking, a large, controlled study (the Digitalis Investigation Group [DIG] study) showed reductions in hospitalization rates, both overall and for worsening heart failure, as well as a reduction in the combined incidence of death from worsening heart failure and hospitalization for such worsening, when digoxin was added to a regimen of ACE inhibitors and/or diuretics in patients with normal sinus rhythm and chronic left ventricular heart failure (principally mild to moderate). The decision to use digoxin in patients with symptomatic heart failure caused by systolic left ventricular dysfunction should be based not on an anticipated improvement in survival but on potential benefits of less deterioration of the condition and associated improvement in hospitalization rates as well as of improved symptomatic and functional status.

Digoxin increases left ventricular ejection fraction and improves symptoms of heart failure (as evidenced by exercise capacity, heart failure-related hospitalizations and emergency care), while having no apparent effect on overall mortality. The acute and sustained hemodynamic efficacy of digoxin is well established, at least in patients with symptomatic heart failure caused by predominant systolic ventricular dysfunction. Digoxin is less effective in the management of high-output heart failure caused by bronchopulmonary insufficiency, infection, hyperthyroidism, anemia, fever, arteriovenous fistula, thiamine deficiency, Paget's disease, cor pulmonale, acute glomerulonephritis, or toxic or infectious myocarditis (e.g., diphtheria, acute rheumatic fever). Heart failure resulting from hypermetabolic or hyperdynamic states (e.g., hyperthyroidism, hypoxia, AV shunt) is best treated by addressing the underlying condition rather than by using digoxin. In addition, digoxin is of limited value in the management of heart failure caused by mechanical disturbances such as constrictive pericarditis, pericardial tamponade, mitral stenosis with normal sinus rhythm, and pure valvular aortic stenosis. Patients with idiopathic hypertrophic subaortic stenosis receiving digoxin may have a worsening of outflow obstruction as a result of the inotropic effects of the drug.

● Supraventricular Tachyarrhythmias

Atrial Fibrillation

Digoxin is used for controlling rapid ventricular rate in patients with chronic atrial fibrillation; however, the drug is not considered first-line therapy for this use, in part because of its slow onset of action. In addition, concerns have been raised regarding possible increased mortality in patients with atrial fibrillation receiving digoxin, particularly when used for long-term therapy. In the AFFIRM (AF Follow-up Investigation of Rhythm Management) study, use of digoxin was associated with a 41% increase in mortality in patients with atrial fibrillation; however, additional post-hoc analyses have reported conflicting results.

Experts recommend the use of β-blockers or nondihydropyridine calcium-channel blocking agents (e.g., diltiazem, verapamil) as the preferred drugs for ventricular rate control in patients with atrial fibrillation. Digoxin may be used in combination with one of these agents to improve heart rate control during exercise and also may be useful in patients with concomitant heart failure. (See Uses: Heart Failure.) Choice of therapy should be individualized based on the clinical situation and patient-related factors. Digoxin should not be used in patients with preexcited atrial fibrillation because the drug may increase ventricular response and result in ventricular fibrillation.

Other Supraventricular Tachycardias

Digoxin also is used in the management of paroxysmal supraventricular tachycardia (PSVT) due to AV nodal reentry tachycardia (AVNRT) or AV reentry tachycardia (AVRT)†. Some experts state that oral digoxin may be reasonable for ongoing management of PSVT in patients who are not candidates for, or prefer not to undergo, catheter ablation. Because of the potential for adverse effects, digoxin generally is reserved as a third-line agent for patients who are not responsive to, or are not candidates for, the preferred therapies (e.g., β-blockers, nondihydropyridine calcium-channel blocking agents, flecainide, propafenone). If acute treatment of PSVT is necessary, however, measures to increase vagal tone (such as carotid sinus massage and Valsalva maneuver) or administration of adenosine are the treatments of choice.

Digoxin has been used in the management of regular supraventricular (reciprocating) tachycardia associated with Wolff-Parkinson-White (WPW) syndrome†, but the drug may be potentially harmful if used in patients with WPW syndrome and preexcited atrial fibrillation because acceleration of the ventricular rate may occur. Digoxin should therefore not be administered to patients with WPW syndrome and preexcited atrial fibrillation. The preferred treatment of choice in hemodynamically compromised patients with WPW syndrome usually is prompt direct-current cardioversion.

● Myocardial Infarction

Use of digoxin in acute myocardial infarction (MI) is controversial. (See Cautions: Precautions and Contraindications.) Because the drug can increase myocardial oxygen demand and exacerbate ongoing ischemia, it is generally not recommended during acute MI. However, digoxin may be used in selected patients with left ventricular systolic dysfunction after acute MI. (See Uses: Heart Failure.)

DOSAGE AND ADMINISTRATION

● *Administration*

Digoxin usually is administered orally. When oral therapy is not feasible or when rapid therapeutic effect is necessary, the drug may be administered parenterally. Although digoxin may be given IM or IV, the IV route of administration is preferred because IM injection can cause severe local irritation and pain at the site of injection. If the drug must be administered by the IM route, injections should be made deep into the muscle followed by massage of the injection site, and no more than 2 mL of the drug should be injected at a single site.

Oral Administration

Digoxin is administered orally as tablets or oral solution. The manufacturers recommend once-daily dosing in adults and children older than 10 years of age; divided daily dosing is recommended in infants and children younger than 10 years of age.

The manufacturer recommends that the oral solution be used to obtain the appropriate dose in infants, young children, or patients with very low body weights. The calibrated dosing syringe supplied by the manufacturer should be used to measure doses of the oral digoxin solution; a separate measuring device should be used to accurately measure doses less than 0.1 mL.

IV Administration

For IV administration, digoxin injection may be given undiluted or may be diluted with a fourfold or greater volume of sterile water for injection, 5% dextrose injection, or 0.9% sodium chloride injection; use of less than a fourfold volume of diluent may cause precipitation of the drug. Diluted IV solutions of digoxin should be used immediately.

Digoxin should be administered by slow IV infusion (over at least 5 minutes); rapid IV (i.e., bolus) administration may cause systemic and coronary vasoconstriction and should be avoided.

Mixing of digoxin injection with other drugs in the same container or simultaneous administration in the same IV line is not recommended.

● *Dosage*

General Considerations

Digoxin has a narrow therapeutic index; therefore, cautious dosage determination is essential and dosage must be carefully individualized based on clinical assessment and therapeutic drug monitoring. Dosage guidelines provided are based upon average patient response and substantial patient variation can be expected. When selecting an appropriate dosage, the patient's renal function, body weight, age, concomitant disease states, concurrent drugs, and other factors likely to alter serum concentrations of digoxin should be considered. Because the drug is largely distributed into tissues, lean body weight should be used for dosage calculations. Serum digoxin concentrations can be used to guide dosing, but should always be interpreted in the overall clinical context.

Digoxin dosage may be initiated with or without a loading dose depending on whether rapid titration or a more gradual titration is desired; the different approaches vary in dosage and frequency of administration but achieve the same total amount of digoxin accumulated in the body. Loading doses may be used to reach adequate and effective drug concentrations for control of ventricular response in patients with atrial fibrillation. However, in patients with heart failure, experts state there is no reason to use loading doses and maintenance dosing can be initiated immediately.

Loading doses of digoxin are administered in divided doses, with about 50% of the total dose given as the first (i.e., initial) dose and additional fractions (usually 25%) usually administered every 6–8 hours with careful assessment of the patient's clinical response (including possible toxicity) before each additional dose. If a change from the calculated loading dose is required, then the maintenance dosage should be calculated based upon the amount (i.e., total loading dose) actually administered.

More gradual attainment of digoxin concentrations can be achieved by initiating therapy with a maintenance dosage without a loading dose. Steady-state serum digoxin concentrations will be achieved in about 5 half-lives of the drug for the individual patient; depending on the patient's renal function, this may take approximately 1–3 weeks.

Differences in the bioavailability of parenteral and oral preparations of digoxin should be considered when patients are switched from one dosage form to another. Because the absolute bioavailability of digoxin tablets and solution are similar, equivalent dosages may be used. (See Pharmacokinetics: Absorption.) When switching from oral to IV therapy, dosage of digoxin should be reduced by about 20–25%.

Since daily maintenance digoxin dosage is a replacement of daily digoxin loss from the body, an alternative dosing method has been used where the maintenance dosage for a particular patient is *estimated* by multiplying the daily percentage loss (see Pharmacokinetics: Elimination) by the peak body stores (i.e., loading dose) that produced a satisfactory response. The percentage of digoxin eliminated from the body daily can be *estimated* by the following equation: daily % loss = 14 + (creatinine clearance [in mL/minute] / 5)

Heart Failure in Adults

Loading doses are generally not required in patients with heart failure. If a loading dose is to be given, the manufacturers recommend an oral loading dose of 10–15 mcg/kg or an IV loading dose of 8–12 mcg/kg in adults, administered in divided doses. (See General Considerations under Dosage and Administration: Dosage.)

Experts state that digoxin is commonly initiated and maintained at a dosage of 125–250 mcg (0.125–0.25 mg) daily for the management of heart failure in adults. The manufacturers recommend an initial oral digoxin maintenance dosage of 3.4–5.1 mcg/kg once daily as tablets or 3–4.5 mcg/kg once daily as the oral solution in adults with normal renal function; dosage may be increased every 2 weeks according to clinical response, serum digoxin concentrations, and toxicity. If IV administration is necessary, the manufacturer recommends an initial IV maintenance dosage of 2.4–3.6 mcg/kg once daily in adults with normal renal function; dosage may be increased every 2 weeks according to clinical response, serum digoxin concentrations, and toxicity. The manufacturer's prescribing information should be consulted for recommended maintenance oral and IV dosages based on renal function.

Atrial Fibrillation in Adults

If a loading dose is to be given for rate control in patients with atrial fibrillation, the manufacturers recommend an oral loading dose of 10–15 mcg/kg or an IV loading dose of 8–12 mcg/kg in adults, administered in divided doses. (See General Considerations under Dosage and Administration: Dosage.) Some experts recommend an initial IV dose of 250 mcg (0.25 mg) with repeat dosing to a maximum of 1500 mcg (1.5 mg) over 24 hours. These experts state that the usual oral maintenance dosage of digoxin for ventricular rate control in adults with atrial fibrillation is 125–250 mcg (0.125–0.25 mg) daily.

Heart Failure in Pediatric Patients

Dosage should be carefully titrated in neonates, especially in premature infants, because renal clearance of digoxin is reduced in such patients. Infants and young children (up to 10 years of age) generally require proportionally larger doses than children older than 10 years of age and adults when calculated on the basis of lean body weight or body surface area. Children older than 10 years of age require adult dosages in proportion to the child's body weight.

Loading doses and maintenance dosages recommended by the manufacturers for the treatment of heart failure in pediatric patients are given in the tables that follow based on the dosage form administered. (See General Considerations under Dosage and Administration: Dosage.)

TABLE 1. Usual Pediatric Loading Doses and Maintenance Dosages for Digoxin Tablets (normal renal function, based on lean body weight)

Age	Oral Loading Dose[a]	Initial Oral Maintenance Dosage
5–10 years	20–45 mcg/kg	3.2–6.4 mcg/kg twice daily
>10 years	10–15 mcg/kg	3.4–5.1 mcg/kg once daily

[a] Loading doses are administered in divided doses, with about 50% of the total dose given as the first (i.e., initial) dose; additional 25% fractions are administered every 6–8 hours

TABLE 2. Usual Pediatric Loading Doses and Maintenance Dosages for Digoxin Solution (normal renal function, based on lean body weight)

Age	Oral Loading Dose[a]	Initial Oral Maintenance Dosage
Premature neonates	20–30 mcg/kg	2.3–3.9 mcg/kg twice daily
Full-term neonates	25–35 mcg/kg	3.8–5.6 mcg/kg twice daily
1–24 months	35–60 mcg/kg	5.6–9.4 mcg/kg twice daily
2–5 years	30–45 mcg/kg	4.7–6.6 mcg/kg twice daily
5–10 years	20–35 mcg/kg	2.8–5.6 mcg/kg twice daily
>10 years	10–15 mcg/kg	3–4.5 mcg/kg once daily

[a] Loading doses are administered in divided doses, with about 50% of the total dose given as the first (i.e., initial) dose; additional fractions may be administered every 4–8 hours

TABLE 3. Usual Pediatric Loading Doses and Maintenance Dosages for IV Digoxin (normal renal function, based on lean body weight)

Age	IV Loading Dose[a]	Initial IV Maintenance Dosage
Premature neonates	15–25 mcg/kg	1.9–3.1 mcg/kg twice daily
Full-term neonates	20–30 mcg/kg	3–4.5 mcg/kg twice daily
1–24 months	30–50 mcg/kg	4.5–7.5 mcg/kg twice daily
2–5 years	25–35 mcg/kg	3.8–5.3 mcg/kg twice daily
5–10 years	15–30 mcg/kg	2.3–4.5 mcg/kg twice daily
>10 years	8–12 mcg/kg	2.4–3.6 mcg/kg once daily

[a] Loading doses are administered in divided doses, with 50% of the total dose given as the first (i.e., initial) dose; additional 25% fractions are administered every 6–8 hours

Geriatric Dosage

Dosage of digoxin should be selected carefully in geriatric patients since they are more likely to have impaired renal function. (See Dosage in Renal Impairment under Dosage and Administration: Dosage.) Lower dosages (125 mcg [0.125 mg] daily or every other day) are recommended for the management of heart failure in geriatric patients older than 70 years of age.

Dosage in Hepatic Impairment

No dosage adjustment is necessary in patients with hepatic impairment; however, serum digoxin concentrations may be used to guide dosing in such patients.

Dosage in Renal Impairment

Renal function should be considered during dosage selection. Digoxin is principally excreted by the kidneys and impaired renal function may predispose patients to digoxin toxicity. Dosage should be reduced and titrated carefully in patients with renal impairment based on clinical response and serum digoxin concentrations as appropriate.

CAUTIONS

In addition to toxicity (see Acute Toxicity and also see Chronic Toxicity), other adverse effects may occur in patients receiving digoxin.

● Adverse Effects

GI effects, including nausea, vomiting, abdominal pain, and intestinal ischemia and hemorrhagic necrosis, have occurred in patients receiving digoxin.

CNS effects associated with digoxin include headache, weakness, dizziness, apathy, confusion, and mental disturbances (e.g., anxiety, depression, delirium, hallucinations).

Estrogen-like effects may occur with chronic administration of cardiac glycosides, especially in geriatric men and women whose endogenous concentrations of sex hormones are low. Cardiac glycosides increase plasma estrogen and decrease serum luteinizing hormone in men and postmenopausal women and decrease plasma testosterone in men. Gynecomastia and enlargement of the mammary glands in women have been reported after chronic therapy with digoxin and were reversible when the drug was withdrawn. Digoxin also may produce vaginal cornification in postmenopausal women and result in the incorrect diagnosis of endometrial carcinoma. The estrogen-like effects of cardiac glycosides also cause reduced excretion of pituitary gonadotropin in postmenopausal women. Digoxin may cause an increase in urinary 17-hydroxycorticosteroids.

Hypersensitivity reactions to cardiac glycosides are rare but may occur, usually within 6–10 days after initiating therapy. Skin reactions may be erythematous, scarlatiniform, papular, vesicular, or bullous. Rashes usually are accompanied by eosinophilia; eosinophilia also may occur without skin reactions. Urticaria; fever; pruritus; facial, angioneurotic, or laryngeal edema; alopecia of the scalp; shedding of finger and toe nails; and desquamation have been reported. Rarely, thrombocytopenic purpura has been reported to occur during administration of cardiac glycosides.

● Precautions and Contraindications

The possibility that use of digoxin in patients with acute myocardial infarction (MI) may increase oxygen demand and associated ischemia should be considered. Patients with idiopathic hypertrophic subaortic stenosis may experience worsening of their condition because of the inotropic effects of digoxin. Patients with certain disorders involving heart failure associated with preserved left ventricular ejection fraction (e.g., restrictive cardiomyopathy, constrictive pericarditis, amyloid heart disease, acute cor pulmonale) may experience decreased cardiac output with digoxin. Digoxin should not be administered to patients with substantial sinus or atrioventricular (AV) block, unless the conduction block has been addressed with a permanent pacemaker. Digoxin should be used cautiously with other drugs that can depress sinus or AV nodal function.

Digoxin should be used with caution in patients with Wolff-Parkinson-White (WPW) syndrome and atrial fibrillation since the drug may enhance conduction via the accessory pathway and result in extremely rapid ventricular rates and ventricular fibrillation. (See Other Supraventricular Tachycardias under Uses: Supraventricular Tachyarrhythmias.) Carotid sinus massage has caused ventricular fibrillation in patients receiving cardiac glycosides.

Since digoxin can induce ventricular arrhythmias, it is recommended that dosage of the drug be reduced or therapy discontinued for 1–2 days before elective cardioversion in patients with atrial fibrillation; however, clinicians should consider the consequences of increasing the ventricular response if digoxin is decreased or withdrawn. Elective cardioversion should be postponed in patients with signs and symptoms of cardiac glycoside toxicity. If it is not possible to delay cardioversion, the lowest possible energy level should be used to avoid provoking ventricular arrhythmias.

Digoxin is contraindicated in patients with ventricular fibrillation.

Digoxin is contraindicated in patients who have demonstrated hypersensitivity to the drug or to other forms of digitalis.

● Pediatric Precautions

Safety and efficacy of digoxin in controlling ventricular rate have not been established in pediatric patients with atrial fibrillation.

The manufacturer states that safety and efficacy of digoxin in pediatric patients with heart failure have not been established in adequate and well-controlled studies; however, improvements in hemodynamics and clinical manifestations have been reported in pediatric patients with heart failure of various etiologies in the published literature.

Neonates exhibit considerable variability in their tolerance to digoxin. Premature and immature infants are particularly sensitive to the drug, and dosage must be reduced and individualized according to maturity. The adverse effect profile of digoxin differs in infants and children, particularly in regard to initial signs of toxicity. Cardiac arrhythmias, including sinus bradycardia, usually occur earliest and most frequently. In children, any arrhythmia can occur. Therefore, any arrhythmia or alteration in cardiac conduction in a child should be considered a sign of toxicity.

Pregnancy, Fertility, and Lactation

Pregnancy

Available data from retrospective clinical studies and case reports have not identified a drug-associated risk of major birth defects, miscarriage, or adverse maternal and fetal effects with digoxin. However, the underlying maternal condition (e.g., heart failure, atrial fibrillation) may increase the risk of adverse pregnancy outcomes during digoxin therapy. Animal reproduction studies have not been conducted with the drug.

Dosage requirements for digoxin may increase during pregnancy and decrease during the postpartum period; serum digoxin concentrations should be monitored.

Because digoxin crosses the placenta and is found in amniotic fluid, neonates should be monitored for signs and symptoms of digoxin toxicity (e.g., vomiting, cardiac arrhythmias).

Lactation

Although digoxin is distributed into milk, the quantities present are unlikely to be clinically important. The effects of digoxin on the breast-fed infant or on milk production are not known.

DRUG INTERACTIONS

Because digoxin has a narrow therapeutic window, increased monitoring of serum digoxin concentrations and for possible clinical manifestations of digoxin toxicity is necessary when initiating, adjusting, or discontinuing therapy with any drugs that may interact with digoxin. Clinicians should also consult the prescribing information for any drugs that are concurrently administered with digoxin for potential drug interaction information.

Concomitant use of certain drugs may increase serum concentrations of digoxin by interfering with absorption of the cardiac glycoside via P-glycoprotein (P-gp) interaction or other mechanisms. Drugs that have been shown to increase serum digoxin concentrations by more than 50% include amiodarone, captopril, clarithromycin, dronedarone, gentamicin, erythromycin, itraconazole, lapatinib, propafenone, quinidine, ranolazine, ritonavir, tetracycline, and verapamil. Serum digoxin concentrations should be measured prior to initiating these drugs and dosage of digoxin should be adjusted by either decreasing the dose by approximately 30–50% or modifying the dosing frequency and continuing monitoring.

Drugs that have been shown to increase digoxin concentrations by less than 50% include atorvastatin, carvedilol, conivaptan, diltiazem, indomethacin, mirabegron, nefazodone, nifedipine, propantheline, quinine, rabeprazole, saquinavir, spironolactone, telmisartan, ticagrelor, tolvaptan, and trimethoprim. Serum digoxin concentrations should be measured prior to initiating these drugs and dosage of digoxin should be adjusted by either decreasing the dose by approximately 15–30% or modifying the dosing frequency and continuing monitoring.

Drugs that have been shown to increase serum digoxin concentrations with unclear magnitude include alprazolam, azithromycin, cyclosporine, diclofenac, diphenoxylate, epoprostenol, esomeprazole, ibuprofen, ketoconazole, lansoprazole, metformin, and omeprazole. Serum digoxin concentrations should be measured prior to initiating these drugs; monitoring should be continued and dosage of digoxin should be reduced as necessary.

Drugs or therapies that have been shown to decrease serum digoxin concentrations include acarbose, albuterol, antacids, certain cancer chemotherapy or radiation therapy, cholestyramine, colestipol, exenatide, kaolin-pectin, metoclopramide, miglitol, neomycin, penicillamine, phenytoin, rifampin, St. John's wort (*Hypericum perforatum*), sucralfate, and sulfasalazine. Serum digoxin concentrations should be measured prior to initiating these drugs or therapies; monitoring should be continued and dosage of digoxin should be increased by approximately 20–40% as necessary.

Drugs Affecting P-glycoprotein Transport

Digoxin is a substrate of the P-gp transport protein at the level of intestinal absorption, renal tubular secretion, and biliary-intestinal secretion. Clinically important interactions may occur when digoxin is used concomitantly with drugs that induce (e.g., rifampin, neomycin, penicillamine) or inhibit (e.g., amiodarone, dronedarone, verapamil, propafenone, quinidine, cyclosporine, atorvastatin, simvastatin, darunavir, saquinavir, ritonavir) P-gp.

Drugs Affecting GI Absorption of Digoxin

A number of drugs are capable of binding digoxin and/or inhibiting the absorption of the cardiac glycoside from the GI tract, which may result in low serum concentrations of the glycoside.

Single-dose studies indicate that aluminum hydroxide, magnesium hydroxide, magnesium trisilicate, kaolin-pectin, aminosalicylic acid, metoclopramide, and sulfasalazine reduce GI absorption of digoxin (resulting in low serum digoxin concentrations), especially when these drugs are administered at the same time as digoxin; therefore, doses of these drugs should be spaced as far apart as possible from doses of digoxin.

Orally administered neomycin may cause malabsorption of digoxin, which may result in low serum digoxin concentrations, but administration of neomycin to digitalized patients apparently does not affect the terminal half-life of digoxin.

Macrolide antibiotics (e.g., clarithromycin, erythromycin) may increase oral bioavailability of digoxin by altering the GI flora that metabolize digoxin, possibly resulting in increased serum concentrations of digoxin and risk of digoxin toxicity. (See Drug Interactions: Anti-infective Agents.)

GI absorption of oral digoxin tablets may be substantially reduced in patients receiving radiation therapy, certain antineoplastic agents, or various combination chemotherapy regimens, possibly as a result of temporary damage to intestinal mucosa caused by the radiation or cytotoxic agents. Colestipol and cholestyramine may bind digoxin in the GI tract and impair its absorption (resulting in low serum digoxin concentrations), particularly if the glycoside and colestipol or cholestyramine are administered simultaneously or close together. Digoxin should be given at least 1.5–2 hours before cholestyramine or colestipol. Drugs that alter GI transit time and/or motility of the GI tract, such as antimuscarinics and diphenoxylate, may alter the rate of absorption of digoxin. Patients receiving an antimuscarinic and digoxin should be closely observed for signs of digitalis toxicity.

Drugs Affecting Electrolyte Balance

In patients receiving digoxin, electrolyte disturbances produced by diuretics such as ethacrynic acid, furosemide, and thiazides (primarily hypokalemia but also hypomagnesemia and, with the thiazides, hypercalcemia) predispose the patient to digoxin toxicity. Fatal cardiac arrhythmias may result. Periodic electrolyte determinations must be performed in patients concurrently receiving digoxin and a diuretic, and corrective measures undertaken if warranted. Other drugs that deplete body potassium (e.g., amphotericin B, corticosteroids, corticotropin, edetate disodium, laxatives, sodium polystyrene sulfonate) or that reduce extracellular potassium (e.g., glucagon, large doses of dextrose, dextrose-insulin infusions) also may predispose digitalized patients to toxicity.

Drugs Affecting Renal Function

Drugs that affect renal function (e.g., angiotensin-converting enzyme [ACE] inhibitors, angiotensin II receptor antagonists, nonsteroidal anti-inflammatory agents [NSAIAs]) may impair elimination of digoxin, and thus predispose patients to digoxin toxicity.

Calcium Salts

The inotropic and toxic effects of digoxin and calcium are synergistic and arrhythmias may occur if these drugs are given together (particularly when calcium is administered rapidly IV). IV administration of calcium should be avoided in patients receiving digoxin; if necessary, calcium should be given slowly in small amounts.

Antiarrhythmic Agents

Although quinidine, procainamide, disopyramide, phenytoin, propranolol, and lidocaine have been used effectively in conjunction with digoxin to treat arrhythmias and also alone to treat cardiac glycoside-induced arrhythmias, these antiarrhythmic agents may have negative inotropic effects with larger than usual doses, especially in patients with cardiac glycoside toxicity (propranolol has negative inotropic effects with usual doses).

Amiodarone

Concomitant administration of digoxin and amiodarone may result in increased serum digoxin concentrations and subsequent digoxin toxicity. Serum digoxin concentrations generally increase by an average of 70–100% in adults, but substantial variability exists in the magnitude of the increase. Limited data suggest that the magnitude of the increase may be much greater in children than in adults (i.e., 70–800%).

The amiodarone-induced increase in serum digoxin concentrations usually begins within 1–7 days and progresses gradually over a period of several weeks or even months. The exact mechanism(s) of this interaction appears to be complex and remains to be fully established, but data indicate that amiodarone may decrease the renal and/or nonrenal clearance of digoxin. It also has been suggested that amiodarone may increase the oral bioavailability of digoxin or displace digoxin from tissue binding sites. When initiating amiodarone therapy in patients receiving digoxin, the need for continued digoxin therapy should be reassessed, and digoxin discontinued if appropriate; if concomitant therapy is considered necessary, serum digoxin concentrations should be measured prior to initiating amiodarone and dosage of digoxin adjusted by either decreasing the dose by approximately 30–50% or modifying the dosing frequency. Patients should be observed closely for signs of cardiac glycoside toxicity. In addition, thyroid function should be monitored carefully in patients receiving concurrent amiodarone and digoxin therapy, since amiodarone-induced changes in thyroid function may increase or decrease serum digoxin concentrations or alter sensitivity to the therapeutic and toxic effects of the cardiac glycoside.

Dofetilide

Concomitant use of dofetilide and digoxin was associated with an increased risk of torsades de pointes. Dosage of digoxin should be individualized when used concomitantly with dofetilide.

Dronedarone

Concomitant use of digoxin and dronedarone (a P-gp inhibitor) may result in a substantial increase (150%) in systemic exposure to digoxin; possible digoxin toxicity may occur. In clinical studies, baseline use of digoxin was associated with an increased risk of arrhythmic or sudden death in patients receiving dronedarone. Because digoxin can potentiate the electrophysiologic effects of dronedarone and dronedarone can increase exposure to digoxin, concomitant use of these drugs is not recommended. If concomitant use of dronedarone is necessary in a patient receiving digoxin, serum digoxin concentrations should be determined prior to initiating dronedarone and dosage of digoxin should be reduced by decreasing the dose by approximately 30–50% or modifying the dosing frequency.

Flecainide

Studies in healthy individuals indicate that serum digoxin concentrations may be increased by an average of about 15–25% when flecainide and digoxin are administered concomitantly. The increase in serum digoxin concentration may occur within a few days of initiating flecainide therapy in patients receiving digoxin and may result from a decrease in the volume of distribution of digoxin. Although the PR interval was substantially prolonged in most healthy individuals during concomitant administration of flecainide and digoxin, it was not determined whether this resulted from an additive effect of the drugs or mainly from flecainide. Flecainide has been administered concomitantly with cardiac glycosides in patients with ventricular arrhythmias without unusual adverse effects. Additional studies to determine the potential importance of an interaction in patients with heart failure are needed. Flecainide-induced increases in serum digoxin concentration generally appear to be of a small magnitude and are unlikely to be clinically important in most cases; however, patients with AV nodal dysfunction, serum digoxin concentrations in the upper end of the therapeutic range, and/or high plasma flecainide concentrations may be at increased risk of digoxin toxicity. Pending further accumulation of data, patients receiving flecainide and digoxin should be monitored for signs of digoxin toxicity.

Quinidine

Concomitant administration of quinidine and digoxin increases serum concentrations of digoxin (in 90% or more of patients), which may result in digoxin toxicity. Although variability exists in the magnitude of the increase, serum digoxin concentrations usually increase twofold to threefold when quinidine therapy is

initiated in patients digitalized with digoxin. Serum digoxin concentrations may begin to increase within a few hours after initiating quinidine therapy, but at least 5–7 days are usually required to achieve a new steady-state serum digoxin concentration. The magnitude of the increase appears to depend on the serum quinidine concentration. Both the clearance (principally renal clearance) and volume of distribution of digoxin generally are decreased, but serum half-life of the drug may be unaffected.

When quinidine therapy is initiated in a patient receiving digoxin, serum digoxin concentrations should be carefully monitored and digoxin dosage reduced (by decreasing dose by approximately 30–50% or modifying dosing frequency) as needed; the patient should be observed closely for signs of toxicity. Because of the variability in magnitude of the interaction, additional dosage adjustments are likely to be necessary. If digoxin therapy is initiated in a patient receiving quinidine, lower than usual dosages of digoxin may be sufficient to produce desired serum concentrations of the cardiac glycoside. If quinidine is discontinued in a patient stabilized on therapy with both drugs, the patient should be observed for signs of decreased response to digoxin and dosage of the cardiac glycoside adjusted as necessary.

Sotalol

In clinical studies, proarrhythmic events were more common in patients receiving sotalol and digoxin concomitantly than when either drug was used alone. It is not known if this represents an adverse drug interaction or is related to the presence of heart failure, which is a known risk factor for proarrhythmia, in patients receiving digoxin. Dosage of digoxin should be individualized when used concomitantly with sotalol.

• β-Adrenergic Blocking Agents

Concomitant use of digoxin and β-adrenergic blocking agents (β-blockers) can have additive negative effects on AV conduction, which can result in complete heart block. Although such combined therapy may be useful in controlling ventricular rate in patient with atrial fibrillation and/or flutter, digoxin dosage in patients receiving such therapy should be carefully individualized given the considerable variability of these interactions.

• Calcium-channel Blocking Agents

Although combination therapy with digoxin and calcium-channel blocking agents may be useful in controlling atrial fibrillation, such concomitant use can have negative effects on AV conduction, which can result in complete heart block. Digoxin dosage should be carefully individualized when used in conjunction with calcium-channel blocking agents because of the considerable variability of these interactions.

Diltiazem

There are conflicting reports on whether diltiazem substantially affects the pharmacokinetics of digoxin when the drugs are administered concomitantly. In some studies, diltiazem reportedly increased average steady-state serum digoxin concentrations by about 20–50%, possibly by decreasing the renal and nonrenal clearance of the glycoside; however, in other studies, diltiazem did not substantially alter serum digoxin concentrations. Despite conflicting reports, serum digoxin concentrations should be carefully monitored and the patient observed closely for signs of digoxin toxicity when diltiazem and digoxin are administered concomitantly, especially in geriatric patients, patients with unstable renal function, or those with serum digoxin concentrations in the upper therapeutic range before diltiazem is administered. Dosage of digoxin should be reduced by either decreasing the dose by approximately 15–30% or modifying the dosing frequency. Digoxin does not appear to affect the pharmacokinetics of diltiazem.

Nifedipine

Most evidence indicates that nifedipine does not substantially affect the pharmacokinetics of digoxin when the drugs are administered concomitantly; however, some data suggest that serum digoxin concentrations may increase by about 15–45% during concomitant therapy. Further evaluation of this potential interaction is needed. Patients receiving the drugs concomitantly should be monitored for signs and symptoms of digoxin toxicity. Serum digoxin concentrations should be determined prior to initiating nifedipine and dosage of digoxin should be reduced by either decreasing the dose by approximately 15–30% or modifying the dosing frequency.

Verapamil

Verapamil, a potent P-gp inhibitor, may increase serum digoxin concentrations by 50–75% during the first week of verapamil therapy. This effect may be more substantial in patients with underlying hepatic disease (e.g., cirrhosis). When verapamil is administered to a patient receiving digoxin, serum digoxin concentrations should be measured and dosage of digoxin adjusted by either decreasing the dose by approximately 30–50% or modifying the dosing frequency. The patient should be monitored closely for clinical response and digoxin toxicity. Combined therapy with the drugs (e.g., for control of ventricular rate in patients with atrial fibrillation and/or flutter) usually is well tolerated if dosage of digoxin is properly adjusted.

● Other Cardiovascular Drugs

Sympathomimetics (e.g., dopamine, epinephrine, norepinephrine) should be used with caution in patients receiving digoxin, since the risk of arrhythmias may be increased in patients receiving these drugs concomitantly.

Altered responses to digoxin therapy have occurred in patients receiving digoxin and amiloride concomitantly. In healthy individuals in one study, amiloride increased the renal clearance but decreased the extrarenal clearance of digoxin, resulting in slight increases in serum digoxin concentration. Inhibition of the positive inotropic effect of digoxin has also been observed in healthy individuals receiving amiloride. Patients receiving amiloride and digoxin concurrently should be carefully observed for altered responses to digoxin therapy. Further studies are needed to determine the clinical importance of the potential drug interaction between amiloride and digoxin.

Concomitant use of captopril and digoxin has been reported to increase serum concentrations and systemic exposure to digoxin by about 58 and 39%, respectively. Such increases may result from decreased renal clearance (probably both glomerular filtration and tubular secretion) of digoxin and, possibly, displacement of the glycoside from tissue-binding sites by captopril-induced increases in serum potassium. Captopril has been administered concomitantly with digoxin in patients with congestive heart failure *without* unusual adverse effects or apparent increased risk of cardiac glycoside toxicity. It has been postulated that captopril-induced increases in serum potassium may offset the potential toxic effects of increased serum digoxin concentrations. If captopril is initiated in a patient receiving digoxin, serum digoxin concentrations should be measured prior to initiating captopril and dosage of digoxin should be adjusted by either decreasing the dose by approximately 30–50% or modifying the dosing frequency.

● Anti-infective Agents

Data suggest that, in about 10% of patients receiving digoxin, substantial amounts of the drug are metabolized by bacteria within the lumen of the large intestine to cardioinactive compounds (reduced metabolites) following oral and possibly parenteral administration. The extent of such metabolism following oral administration appears to vary inversely with the bioavailability of the preparation. In patients who form substantial amounts of reduced metabolites, alteration of enteric bacterial flora by some anti-infective agents (e.g., oral erythromycin or tetracycline hydrochloride) may result in an increase in the bioavailability of active drug and as much as a twofold increase in serum digoxin concentrations. When concomitant therapy with a systemic anti-infective agent is administered in patients receiving digoxin, the possibility that serum digoxin concentrations may increase should be considered and dosage of the cardiac glycoside should be reduced if necessary.

Concomitant administration of digoxin and itraconazole may result in increased serum digoxin concentrations (by 80%); digoxin toxicity may occur. If itraconazole is initiated in a patient receiving digoxin, serum digoxin concentrations should be measured prior to initiating itraconazole and dosage of digoxin should be adjusted by either decreasing the dose by approximately 30–50% or modifying the dosing frequency. Such patients should be observed for clinical manifestations of digoxin toxicity.

● Other Drugs

Succinylcholine appears to potentiate the effects of digoxin on conduction and ventricular irritability. Cardiac arrhythmias have occurred in patients receiving these drugs concomitantly and, therefore, succinylcholine should be administered with caution in patients receiving digoxin. Dosage of digoxin should be individualized when used concomitantly with neuromuscular blocking agents such as succinylcholine.

Teriparatide can transiently increase serum calcium concentrations, which may predispose patients to digoxin toxicity.

Thyroid supplements may increase dosage requirements of digoxin.

Indomethacin may prolong the elimination half-life and increase serum concentrations of digoxin; the mechanism of this interaction requires further elucidation. (See Drug Interactions: Digoxin, in Indomethacin 28:08.04.92.) Serum digoxin concentrations should be monitored carefully in patients receiving the drugs concomitantly. The manufacturer states that dosage of digoxin should be reduced by either decreasing the dose by approximately 15–30% or modifying the dosing frequency.

LABORATORY TEST INTERFERENCES

Digoxin may cause false-positive ST-T changes during exercise testing.

ACUTE TOXICITY

The widespread use of digoxin and the very narrow margin between effective therapeutic and toxic dosages contribute to the high incidence of toxicity and the relatively high associated mortality rate.

Toxic effects of digoxin are mainly GI, CNS, biochemical, and cardiac in origin. The minimum toxic and lethal doses of digoxin are not well established. Based on both accidental and suicidal ingestions, the single oral lethal dose in otherwise healthy individuals is approximately 20–50 times the usual daily maintenance dose. However, patients with predisposing factors (e.g., preexisting heart disease) and patients receiving chronic digoxin therapy may tolerate lesser amounts. Infants and children appear to be more tolerant to the therapeutic and toxic actions of digoxin; children without underlying cardiac problems can usually tolerate an acute dose of several milligrams of the drug without potentially life-threatening cardiac toxicity.

Serum digoxin concentrations are useful in confirming the diagnosis of intoxication; however, clinical diagnosis and management should not be based on serum concentrations alone but should always be interpreted in the overall clinical context with all other relevant information. At least 6–10 hours usually are necessary for digoxin to equilibrate between plasma and tissue; plasma specimens drawn prior to this time may show digoxin concentrations greater than those present after equilibration. Many factors, including adequacy of tissue oxygenation, electrolyte and acid-base balance, thyroid function, autonomic nervous system tone, age of the patient, renal function, other concurrently administered drugs, and the nature and severity of the underlying cardiac disease, influence whether a patient manifests toxicity with a given dosage or serum concentration. There is some concern that therapeutic serum concentrations of digoxin (e.g., less than 2 ng/mL) may exert deleterious cardiovascular effects in the long term, although such concentrations appear to be well tolerated in the short term.

● Manifestations

Overdosage of digoxin is manifested by a wide variety of signs and symptoms that are difficult to distinguish from effects associated with cardiac disease (e.g., adverse GI effects, arrhythmias). Before additional doses of the drug are administered, attempts should be made to determine whether the patient's manifestations are glycoside induced. However, this may be difficult since signs of intoxication do not occur in regular sequence, and subjective signs of toxicity are frequently less easily recognized in infants and children than in adults.

Extracardiac Effects

The extracardiac manifestations of digoxin intoxication are similar in both acute and chronic intoxication. However, GI effects and, to a lesser extent, CNS and visual disturbances may be more pronounced following acute overdosage. Acute toxicity may cause hyperkalemia, whereas patients with chronic toxicity may be hypokalemic or normokalemic. In addition, patients receiving chronic digoxin therapy may be hyperkalemic, normokalemic, or hypokalemic if acute intoxication occurs. In pediatric patients, drowsiness and vomiting are often the most prominent extracardiac effects. However, life-threatening cardiac arrhythmias have developed suddenly in children without evidence of any extracardiac signs of intoxication.

Anorexia, nausea, and vomiting are common early signs of toxicity and may precede or follow evidence of cardiotoxicity. Clinical evaluation of the cause of these symptoms should be attempted before further administration of digoxin; determination of serum digoxin concentrations may aid in deciding whether or not toxicity is present. GI effects probably are at least partially mediated by the area postrema of the medulla since they occur following administration by all routes. Large doses of cardiac glycosides may also produce emesis by direct GI irritation. Episodes of nausea and vomiting may start and stop abruptly. Other GI effects include salivation, epigastric or abdominal pain, abdominal distention, diarrhea, constipation, and weight loss. Acute hemorrhage and intestinal, esophageal, and gastric necrosis have occurred rarely in patients receiving cardiac glycosides.

Headache, fatigue, malaise, drowsiness, and generalized muscle weakness are common nervous system signs of cardiac glycoside toxicity. Dizziness, vertigo, syncope, apathy, lethargy, excitement, euphoria, insomnia, irritability, agitation, hiccups, restlessness, nervousness, seizures, opisthotonos, stupor, and coma also have occurred.

Severe facial pain, simulating trigeminal neuralgia and usually involving the lower third of the face, has occurred in some patients. The pain usually is characterized by aching of the teeth and lower jaw and sharp stabbing pain throughout the mandible and maxilla. Neuralgic pain also has occurred in the upper extremities and lumbar area; paresthesias and tremors have accompanied the pain.

Visual disturbances induced by toxic doses of digoxin probably result from a direct effect on the retina (cones are affected more than rods). Transient retrobulbar neuritis has been reported to cause visual changes in digoxin intoxication; however, it is likely that most visual disturbances result from functional changes of the retina in the presence of high concentrations of the drug. Color vision is commonly affected and objects may appear yellow or green or, less commonly, brown, red, blue, or white. Blurred vision, flashes or flickering of light, photophobia, halos or borders on objects (often are white and appear on dark objects), diplopia, macropsia, and micropsia may occur. Transient or permanent amblyopia and scotoma, including teichopsia, also have occurred. Visual disorders generally are reversible after withdrawal of digoxin therapy; transient or total blindness is rare.

Patients with digoxin toxicity are often hypokalemic or normokalemic. However, severe intoxication may cause hyperkalemia, presumably secondary to inhibition of the Na^+-K^+-ATPase pump. Hyperkalemia may develop rapidly and can result in life-threatening cardiac manifestations, such as AV block and asystole. Presence of hyperkalemia during the early stages of intoxication appears to be a poor prognostic indicator; data from clinical studies indicate that mortality correlates better with the severity of initial hyperkalemia than with the dosage of digoxin ingested, initial serum glycoside concentration, or initial ECG changes in patients treated with conventional supportive and symptomatic measures that do not include digoxin immune Fab therapy.

Cardiac Effects

The most well defined and most dangerous toxic actions of digoxin are those affecting the heart. Cardiac signs of glycoside toxicity may occur with or without other signs of toxicity and often precede other toxic effects. Digoxin has caused almost every kind of cardiac arrhythmia, and various combinations of arrhythmias may occur in the same patient. In addition, arrhythmias associated with digoxin intoxication may result in worsening of heart failure.

Since most of the toxic cardiac effects of digoxin also can occur as manifestations of heart disease, it is often difficult to determine whether toxic cardiac effects are caused by an underlying heart disease or the glycoside. The type of arrhythmia, presence or absence of other manifestations of toxicity, serum concentrations of the drug, and the patient's age, disease state, renal function, and serum potassium concentration should be considered.

Cardiac effects occurring in acute overdosage in otherwise healthy individuals often differ from those in patients with underlying heart disease who are receiving chronic digoxin therapy. Otherwise healthy individuals with acute toxicity frequently present with atrioventricular (AV) conduction disturbances and supraventricular arrhythmias, such as sinus bradycardia. Ventricular arrhythmias are uncommon in these individuals; however, when present, they are associated with severe toxicity and high mortality.

Pediatric patients with healthy hearts often present with sinus bradycardia and conduction disturbances; ventricular arrhythmias also occur but are less common than in adults. In neonates, premonitory signs of toxicity may include sinus bradycardia, sinoatrial (SA) arrest, or prolongation of the PR interval. Multifocal premature ventricular complexes (PVCs), including bigeminy and trigeminy, and, less commonly, unifocal PVCs are common arrhythmias in adults with digoxin toxicity, especially in the presence of heart disease. Patients with glycoside-induced ventricular tachycardia have a high mortality rate, since ventricular fibrillation or asystole may result. Bidirectional ventricular tachycardia may occur in severe digoxin toxicity.

First-degree AV block is common in patients receiving digoxin and generally indicates a therapeutic rather than a toxic effect. However, AV block may progressively increase in patients with toxicity. Mobitz type I (Wenckebach) second-degree AV block and AV junctional exit block are relatively common AV conduction disorders associated with digoxin toxicity; complete (third-degree) AV block may occur in advanced intoxication.

Paroxysmal and nonparoxysmal AV junctional rhythms, especially nonparoxysmal AV junctional tachycardia, AV dissociation (with or without some degree of AV block), and paroxysmal atrial tachycardia with variable AV block, are common in both adults and children and somewhat characteristic of digoxin toxicity.

Digoxin toxicity also may cause various atrial and SA nodal arrhythmias and conduction disorders, including atrial tachycardia, atrial fibrillation, atrial flutter, atrial premature complexes, wandering atrial pacemaker, sinus bradycardia, SA arrest, SA exit block, and sinus tachycardia. Junctional premature complexes also may occur. Sinus bradycardia may be a sign of impending digoxin intoxication, especially in infants and children.

Electrolyte imbalances, especially hypokalemia and, to a lesser extent, hypomagnesemia or hypercalcemia, may predispose patients to the cardiotoxic effects of digoxin. Potassium depletion sensitizes the myocardium to digoxin, and calcium has effects similar to digoxin on contractility and excitability of the heart. Conversely, hypocalcemia may cause resistance to the effects of digoxin on the AV node, and digoxin may be ineffective until serum calcium is restored to normal.

● Treatment

If signs of toxicity appear, digoxin should be discontinued immediately and serum digoxin concentrations obtained; the patient should be placed on a cardiac monitor while possible contributing factors (e.g., electrolyte and thyroid abnormalities, concomitant drugs) are addressed.

Measures to Reduce Absorption or Enhance Elimination of Digoxin

Activated charcoal may be administered if acute ingestion (intentionally or accidently) of a potentially toxic amount of digoxin occurs. Administration of activated charcoal appears to be useful in preventing further absorption of the glycoside. Although activated charcoal is most effective when administered soon after ingestion, doses given later also appear to be effective, presumably because of the prolonged absorption and/or enterohepatic circulation of the drug. Multiple oral doses of activated charcoal have been used to enhance the elimination of digoxin, especially in patients with substantial renal impairment, since the drug undergoes enterohepatic circulation. Adults have been given 20–60 g of activated charcoal every 4–12 hours until objective evidence and clinical observations indicated that serum glycoside concentration had declined to the subtoxic range.

An anion-exchange resin such as cholestyramine or colestipol administered soon after ingestion of digoxin may reduce initial absorption of the glycoside. When administered after onset of toxicity, these resins also may reduce the duration of toxicity by binding digoxin in the GI tract during enterohepatic circulation. These agents probably do not have substantial value in the treatment of advanced digoxin toxicity.

Although these measures may be used to reduce the absorption or enhance elimination of digoxin, severe digoxin toxicity generally should be treated with digoxin-specific antibody fragments (digoxin immune Fab).

Therapeutic Measures

Supportive and symptomatic treatment should be initiated depending on the type of cardiotoxicity; continuous ECG monitoring is recommended to monitor for signs of arrhythmias and hyperkalemia. Serum electrolytes, especially potassium, and serum digoxin concentrations should be monitored carefully. Hypoxia and acid-base and fluid and electrolyte imbalances should be corrected, when necessary.

Milder forms of cardiotoxicity, such as occasional PVCs, AV junctional rhythm with a slow rate, and possibly atrial fibrillation with a slow ventricular rate, usually are treated by temporary withdrawal of digoxin and, if necessary, careful correction of hypokalemia and subsequent adjustment of dosage to prevent recurrence. However, cardiac irregularities that impair cardiac output because of substantial bradycardia or tachycardia should be treated. Ventricular tachycardia, bidirectional ventricular tachycardia, nonparoxysmal AV junctional rhythm with rapid rate or with exit block, and frequent multifocal PVCs generally should be treated since these arrhythmias may be forerunners of ventricular fibrillation. In hypokalemic patients, some clinicians believe these ventricular arrhythmias should be treated initially with potassium supplements and/or IV phenytoin. In patients with ventricular arrhythmias who are normokalemic or hyperkalemic or in whom potassium is ineffective or contraindicated, phenytoin and/or lidocaine may be used. Phenytoin appears to be particularly useful in the treatment of ventricular arrhythmias, especially in the presence of AV block, because the drug improves conduction through the AV node. Limited data suggest that phenytoin is also occasionally useful in the treatment of supraventricular arrhythmias.

Although propranolol is effective in the treatment of cardiac glycoside-induced ventricular and supraventricular arrhythmias, the drug should be used with caution because it may compromise conduction through the AV node and also may cause bradycardia. Refractory ventricular or junctional tachycardia has been treated with ventricular overdrive pacing, but temporary ventricular pacing has been associated with decreased fibrillatory threshold of the ventricle and with mechanical damage to the heart in rare instances. Therefore, use of digoxin immune Fab, if available, generally is preferable in the management of ventricular or junctional tachyarrhythmias unresponsive to conventional therapy.

In adults with severe sinus bradycardia, SA arrest, or second- or third-degree AV block, 0.6–2 mg of atropine sulfate administered IV or IM may be effective, especially in those without heart disease. In pediatric patients, recommended dosages of atropine sulfate range from 0.01–0.03 mg/kg per dose. If atropine is ineffective, administration of digoxin immune Fab, if available, may reverse severe sinus bradycardia and advanced AV block. Insertion of a transvenous bipolar electrode catheter may be necessary if sinus bradyarrhythmias and/or AV block result in hemodynamic compromise.

Cardioversion is used only as a last resort for refractory supraventricular or ventricular tachycardia or for ventricular fibrillation caused by cardiac glycosides. Cardioversion is potentially hazardous in the treatment of ectopic rhythms induced by glycoside toxicity because it may cause ventricular tachycardia or fibrillation that is resistant to further cardioversion. If cardioversion is mandatory, initial shocks should be at low energy levels (e.g., 5, 20, then 40 watt-seconds) and gradually increased in successive shocks until the arrhythmia is terminated or evidence of worsened electrophysiologic instability emerges. Many clinicians recommend administration of phenytoin or lidocaine prophylactically before cardioversion and to suppress PVCs if they occur after cardioversion.

In patients with hypokalemia, potassium supplementation should be given to maintain serum concentrations between 4 and 5.5 mEq/L. Potassium generally should not be administered to patients with second- or third-degree AV block caused by cardiac glycosides since excess potassium may further impair AV conduction. Caution should be exercised when using potassium in acute digoxin intoxication since potentially life-threatening hyperkalemia may develop rapidly in advanced toxicity. Close ECG monitoring for evidence of hyperkalemia (e.g., tall peaked T-waves) is recommended.

Hypomagnesemia also should be corrected. Rarely, magnesium sulfate has been used slowly IV as an antiarrhythmic (e.g., to control ventricular arrhythmias unresponsive to other antiarrhythmics) and to correct demonstrated magnesium deficiency in patients with cardiac glycoside toxicity.

Digoxin immune Fab (ovine) is a specific antidote that can be used in the treatment of life-threatening or potentially life-threatening acute or chronic digoxin toxicity. Specific antigen-binding fragments present in the immune Fab bind to free (unbound) digoxin intravascularly and in extracellular fluid, thereby preventing and reversing the pharmacologic and toxic effects of the glycoside and enhancing its elimination as the bound, inactivated glycoside-Fab fragment complex. In cases of potentially life-threatening cardiotoxicity or hyperkalemia, digoxin immune Fab should be administered. Clinical trials with the immune Fab

have been promising, with complete reversal of toxicity occurring in most cases. Massive glycoside overdosage may cause hyperkalemia, which can be refractory to conventional therapy. Prognosis appears to correlate with serum potassium concentration (i.e., the greater the serum potassium concentration, the worse the prognosis) in patients treated by conventional symptomatic and supportive measures that do not include digoxin immune Fab. Severe hyperkalemia refractory to standard measures is an indication for digoxin immune Fab. For further information on the immune Fab, see Digoxin Immune Fab 80:04. If digoxin immune Fab is not readily available, emergency measures for the treatment of hyperkalemia have included IV administration of glucose and insulin, sodium bicarbonate, peritoneal dialysis or hemodialysis, and/or use of exchange resins; however, these treatments have not been shown to reduce mortality. Use of calcium infusions in the treatment of hyperkalemia traditionally has been avoided because calcium may worsen cardiac irregularities.

Forced diuresis does not accelerate the renal elimination of cardiac glycosides and may worsen electrolyte imbalances. Because of the large volume of distribution and extensive protein binding of digoxin, hemodialysis and peritoneal dialysis are ineffective in removing the glycoside from the body and potentially may worsen toxicity because of a reduction in body potassium. Hemoperfusion using charcoal or extracorporeal resins or hemofiltration may result in limited removal of digoxin from the body. However, because of the risks involved in these procedures, their use cannot be routinely recommended.

CHRONIC TOXICITY

Most cases of digoxin toxicity occur following multiple doses and result, at least in part, from the cumulative effects of the drug. Administration of digoxin in conjunction with diuretics (see Drug Interactions: Drugs Affecting Electrolyte Balance) is a frequent cause of chronic digoxin toxicity. Failure to individualize dosage is another contributing factor in many cases of toxicity.

Patients with chronic digoxin toxicity commonly present with ventricular arrhythmias, such as PVCs or ventricular tachycardia. AV conduction disturbances also are frequent in chronic toxicity. The extracardiac manifestations of digoxin intoxication are similar in both acute and chronic intoxication. Neuropsychiatric disturbances are especially likely to develop in geriatric patients with atherosclerotic disease and are easily overlooked in patients receiving chronic digoxin therapy. These effects include disorientation, confusion, depression, memory impairment, amnesia, aphasia, bad dreams, delirium, delusions, illusions, and hallucinations.

The initial treatment of chronic overdosage is the same as in an acute overdosage situation. (See Acute Toxicity.) If signs of toxicity appear, digoxin should be discontinued immediately and serum digoxin concentrations obtained; the patient should be placed on a cardiac monitor while possible contributing factors (e.g., electrolyte and thyroid abnormalities, concomitant drugs) are addressed. In patients with hypokalemia, potassium supplementation should be given to maintain serum concentrations between 4 and 5.5 mEq/L.

PHARMACOLOGY

The main pharmacologic property of cardiac glycosides is their ability to increase the force and velocity of myocardial systolic contraction (positive inotropic action) by a direct action on the myocardium both in patients with nonfailing hearts and in those with failing hearts. When the force of contraction is increased in patients with failing hearts, cardiac output is increased, systolic emptying is more complete, and diastolic heart size is decreased. Elevated ventricular end-diastolic pressure also is reduced and, consequently, pulmonary and systemic venous pressures are decreased. However, in normal subjects, cardiac output is unchanged or slightly decreased, and total peripheral resistance is increased by direct constriction of vascular smooth muscle and by CNS-mediated increase in sympathetic tone. In patients with heart failure, cardiac glycosides cause reflex reduction in peripheral resistance by increasing myocardial contractility; this compensates for the direct vasoconstrictor action of the drugs and, therefore, total peripheral resistance usually is reduced.

Digoxin inhibits the activity of sodium-potassium-activated adenosine triphosphatase (Na^+-K^+-ATPase), an enzyme required for active transport of sodium across myocardial cell membranes. Inhibition of this enzyme in cardiac cells results in an increase in the contractile state of the heart. Toxic doses of digoxin cause efflux of potassium from the myocardium and concurrent influx of sodium. Toxicity results in part from loss of intracellular potassium associated with inhibition of Na^+-K^+-ATPase. With therapeutic doses, augmentation of calcium influx to the contractile proteins with resultant enhancement of excitation-contraction coupling is involved in the positive inotropic action of cardiac glycosides; the role of Na^+-K^+-ATPase in this effect is controversial.

In patients with heart failure, increased myocardial contractility and cardiac output reflexly reduce sympathetic tone, thus slowing increased heart rate and causing diuresis in edematous patients. In patients without heart failure, increased myocardial contractility produced by cardiac glycosides is accompanied by increased myocardial oxygen consumption. In patients with heart failure, reduced ventricular end-diastolic pressure and increased myocardial contractility produce a net decrease or no change in myocardial oxygen consumption. Cardiac glycosides do not decrease coronary blood flow, and in patients with heart failure the restoration of efficient heart action may improve coronary circulation. Cardiac glycosides have a minor inotropic effect on skeletal muscle.

Digoxin decreases conduction velocity through the atrioventricular (AV) node and prolongs the effective refractory period (ERP) of the AV node by increasing vagal activity, by a direct effect on the AV node, and by a sympatholytic effect. The effects of the drug on the AV node are not apparent clinically when the atrial rate is slow enough to allow time for the AV node to recover between each beat, but in patients with supraventricular tachyarrhythmias such as atrial flutter or atrial fibrillation, the number of waves of depolarization reaching the ventricles is decreased. With usual doses, conduction velocity and refractoriness of the His-Purkinje system are not directly affected. Digoxin shortens the ERP of the atria and increases conduction velocity by a reflex increase in vagal tone and by a direct effect on the atria. With therapeutic doses, digoxin may cause prolongation of the PR interval and ST segment depression, but these ECG effects are not indicative of toxicity.

Digoxin-induced slowing of heart rate in patients without heart failure is negligible and is primarily due to vagal (cholinergic) and sympatholytic effects on the sinoatrial (SA) node, but with toxic doses is due to direct depression of SA node automaticity. Therapeutic doses of digoxin apparently have minimal direct effects and do not have cholinergic or sympatholytic effects on the ventricles. Low concentrations of digoxin produce little effect on the action potential, but toxic concentrations cause progressive loss of resting membrane potential, decreased rate of rise of the action potential, and increased rate of spontaneous diastolic depolarization producing increased automaticity and ectopic impulse activity, especially in the ventricles. Therefore, toxic doses of digoxin increase the automaticity (increased spontaneous diastolic depolarization) of all areas of the heart except the SA node.

Anorexia, nausea, and vomiting caused by cardiac glycosides are probably mediated by chemoreceptors located in the area postrema of the medulla.

PHARMACOKINETICS

● Absorption

Absorption of digoxin is mainly from the small intestine, presumably by a passive, nonsaturable process. The presence of food in the GI tract may slow the rate, but not extent, of absorption of orally administered digoxin from the tablet formulation. Decreased absorption may occur if the drug is administered with a high fiber meal. Gastric pH apparently does not affect the degree of digoxin absorption. Intestinal absorption of the drug may be impaired in patients with certain malabsorption states (e.g., short bowel syndrome, celiac sprue, jejunoileal bypass). Digoxin is a substrate of P-glycoprotein (P-gp), a transport protein involved in absorption of the drug.

There are interindividual variations in plasma concentrations of digoxin with a specific dose and in plasma concentrations of the drug that produce therapeutic and toxic effects. A specific plasma concentration may be therapeutic or toxic in an individual patient depending on factors other than dosage (e.g., serum electrolytes, acid-base balance, concurrently administered drugs, thyroid status, underlying disease states). Plasma concentrations of digoxin are the same as its serum concentrations. If plasma concentrations of digoxin are to be determined, blood samples should be obtained at least 6–8 hours after the daily dose and preferably

just prior to the next scheduled daily dose. Therapeutic plasma concentrations of digoxin in adults generally are 0.5–2 ng/mL. Some experts suggest that plasma concentrations of 0.5–0.9 ng/mL are sufficient for the treatment of heart failure in adults; however, limited data are available. In adults, toxicity is usually, but not always, associated with steady-state plasma digoxin concentrations exceeding 2 ng/mL. Toxicity may also occur with lower digoxin levels, especially if hypokalemia, hypomagnesemia, or hypothyroidism coexists. Although neonates and infants appear to tolerate higher plasma concentrations of digoxin than do adults, evidence suggests that plasma concentrations greater than those in the generally accepted therapeutic ranges for adults are associated with little, if any, additional therapeutic benefit in these patients. *Serum concentrations of digoxin should be interpreted in the overall clinical context; thus, an isolated serum concentration measurement should not be used alone as the basis for adjusting dosage.*

Following oral administration of a single dose of digoxin, onset of action occurs in 0.5–2 hours and maximal effects occur in 2–6 hours. After IV administration of a single dose of digoxin, the onset of action occurs in 5–30 minutes depending on the rate of infusion and maximal effects occur in 1–4 hours.

The absolute bioavailability of digoxin tablets is 60–80% and the absolute bioavailability of the oral solution is 70–85%; when switching from IV to oral dosage forms, the differences in bioavailability should be considered.

● Distribution

Cardiac glycosides are widely distributed in body tissues; highest concentrations are found in the heart, kidneys, intestine, stomach, liver, and skeletal muscle. Lowest concentrations are in the plasma and brain. In the myocardium, cardiac glycosides are found in the sarcolemma-T system bound to a receptor (probably Na^+-K^+-ATPase). Only small amounts of digoxin are distributed into fat. Digoxin crosses the placenta and, in pregnant women receiving digoxin, fetal and maternal plasma concentrations are equal. Maternal concentrations of digoxin in plasma and milk are similar.

With therapeutic plasma concentrations, about 20–30% of digoxin in the blood is bound to plasma proteins.

● Elimination

In patients with normal renal function, the elimination half-life ($t_{\frac{1}{2}}$) of digoxin is 36 hours. The elimination $t_{\frac{1}{2}}$ of digoxin is increased in patients with impaired renal function. In undigitalized patients, institution of fixed daily maintenance doses of digoxin without an initial loading dose results in steady-state plasma concentrations after 4–5 elimination $t_{\frac{1}{2}}$s.

Digoxin is not metabolized appreciably (only about 13%) prior to excretion. Metabolism includes stepwise cleavage of the sugar molecules, hydroxylation, epimerization, and formation of glucuronide and sulfate conjugates. The cytochrome P-450 (CYP) system is not involved in the metabolism of digoxin. Digoxin is also apparently metabolized by bacteria within the lumen of the large intestine following oral administration and possibly after biliary elimination following parenteral administration.

Digoxin is excreted primarily by the kidneys mainly as unchanged drug. In healthy individuals, about 50–70% of an IV dose of digoxin is excreted unchanged in urine. Digoxin is eliminated from the body by first-order kinetics, with a fixed proportion of the residual drug in the body being eliminated each day. Renal excretion of digoxin is proportional to creatinine clearance and is largely independent of urine flow. Orally administered activated charcoal has been shown to enhance total body clearance and elimination of digoxin, probably by adsorbing the cardiac glycoside in the GI tract with subsequent excretion in feces. Digoxin is not appreciably removed by hemodialysis or peritoneal dialysis. Similarly, only minor amounts of the drug are removed during cardiopulmonary bypass or exchange transfusion.

CHEMISTRY AND STABILITY

● Chemistry

Digoxin is a cardiac glycoside, a class of drugs with common specific effects on the myocardium. Glycosides with positive inotropic actions on the diseased heart occur widely in nature and/or can be prepared synthetically. Cardiac glycosides of medicinal importance have been obtained from *Digitalis purpurea* Linné

(Fam. *Scrophulariaceae*) (digitoxin, digitalis, gitalin), *Digitalis lanata* Ehrhart (Fam. *Scrophulariaceae*) (digoxin, digitoxin, lanatoside C, deslanoside, acetyldigitoxin), *Strophanthus gratus* (ouabain), and *Acokanthera schimperi* (ouabain). The term "digitalis" is sometimes used to designate the entire class of cardiac glycosides. Currently, digoxin is the only cardiac glycoside commercially available in the US.

Cardiac glycosides have a characteristic ring structure known as an aglycone (or genin) coupled with one or more types of sugars. The aglycone portion of the glycoside consists of a steroid nucleus (cyclopentanoperhydrophenanthrene nucleus) and an α,β-unsaturated 5- or 6-membered lactone ring at the C 17 position of the steroid nucleus. A β-oriented hydroxyl substitution usually is present at the C 3 and C 14 positions. Increasing the number of hydroxyl groups on the aglycone increases polarity and decreases lipid solubility; additional sugars also may increase polarity. The sugar portion of the glycoside is attached to the steroid nucleus, usually through a hydroxyl group at the C 3 position. The sugar moiety affects in part the activity of the cardiac glycoside by influencing solubility, absorption, distribution, and toxicity.

Digoxin has an hydroxyl group at the C 12 position and a tridigitoxose at the C 3 position.

Digoxin occurs as clear to white crystals or as a white, crystalline powder and has a bitter taste. Digoxin is practically insoluble in water, slightly soluble in diluted alcohol, and very slightly soluble in 40% propylene glycol. The pH of commercially available digoxin injection is 6.8–7.2.

● **Stability**

Digoxin preparations should be protected from light and stored at 20–25°C.

Digoxin injection is compatible with most commercially available IV infusion fluids. Before IV administration, digoxin injection may be diluted with a fourfold or greater volume of sterile water for injection, 5% dextrose injection, or 0.9% sodium chloride injection; use of less than a fourfold volume of diluent may cause precipitation of digoxin. Diluted solutions of digoxin should be used immediately.

Solutions of digoxin have been reported to be physically incompatible with other drugs, but the compatibility depends on several factors (e.g., concentrations of the drugs, specific diluents used, resulting pH, temperature). Specialized references should be consulted for specific compatibility information.

PREPARATIONS

Excipients in commercially available drug preparations may have clinically important effects in some individuals; consult specific product labeling for details.

Digoxin

Oral		
Solution	50 mcg/mL*	Digoxin Oral Solution
Tablets	62.5 mcg	Lanoxin®, Concordia
	125 mcg*	Digitek®, Mylan
		Digoxin Tablets
		Lanoxin® (scored), Concordia
	187.5 mcg	Lanoxin®, Concordia
	250 mcg*	Digitek®, Mylan
		Digoxin Tablets
		Lanoxin® (scored), Concordia
Parenteral		
Injection	100 mcg/mL	Lanoxin® Injection Pediatric, Covis
	250 mcg/mL*	Digoxin Injection
		Lanoxin®, Covis

* available from one or more manufacturer, distributor, and/or repackager by generic (nonproprietary) name

† Use is not currently included in the labeling approved by the US Food and Drug Administration.

Selected Revisions April 10, 2024, © Copyright, July 1, 1978, American Society of Health-System Pharmacists, Inc.

Ivabradine Hydrochloride

24:04.08 • CARDIOTONIC AGENTS

■ Ivabradine hydrochloride, a hyperpolarization activated cyclic nucleotide-gated (HCN) channel (funny-channel [f-channel]) blocking agent, is a sinoatrial modulator.

USES

● Heart Failure

Ivabradine is used to reduce the risk of hospitalization for worsening heart failure in patients with stable, symptomatic, mild to severe chronic heart failure (New York Heart Association [NYHA] class II–IV) with reduced ejection fraction (left ventricular ejection fraction [LVEF] of 35% or less), who are in sinus rhythm with a resting heart rate of 70 beats/minute or more and are either on maximally tolerated dosages of a β-adrenergic blocking agent (β-blocker) or have a contraindication to β-blocker use.

Current guidelines for the management of heart failure in adults generally recommend a combination of drug therapies to reduce morbidity and mortality, including neurohormonal antagonists (e.g., angiotensin-converting enzyme [ACE] inhibitors, angiotensin II receptor antagonists, angiotensin receptor-neprilysin inhibitors [ARNIs], β-blockers, aldosterone receptor antagonists) that inhibit the detrimental compensatory mechanisms in heart failure. (See Uses: Heart Failure, in Enalapril 24:32.04 and in Sacubitril and Valsartan 24:32.92.) Additional agents (e.g., cardiac glycosides, diuretics, sinoatrial modulators [i.e., ivabradine]) added to a heart failure treatment regimen in selected patients have been associated with symptomatic improvement and/or reduction in heart-failure related hospitalizations. Experts recommend that all *asymptomatic* patients with reduced LVEF (i.e., American College of Cardiology Foundation [ACCF]/American Heart Association [AHA] stage B heart failure) receive therapy with an ACE inhibitor and a β-blocker to prevent symptomatic heart failure and to reduce morbidity and mortality. In patients *with prior or current symptoms* of chronic heart failure with reduced LVEF (ACCF/AHA stage C heart failure), ACCF, AHA, and the Heart Failure Society of America (HFSA) recommend inhibition of the renin-angiotensin-aldosterone (RAA) system with an ACE inhibitor, angiotensin II receptor antagonist, or ARNI in conjunction with a β-blocker, and an aldosterone antagonist in selected patients, to reduce morbidity and mortality. If a patient cannot tolerate a β-blocker or if increasing the dosage of the β-blocker is ineffective, experts suggest that ivabradine be considered in symptomatic patients as an alternative or additional treatment option to reduce heart failure-related hospitalizations. Unlike β-blockers, ivabradine selectively reduces heart rate without any adverse effects on myocardial contractility, left ventricular relaxation, and coronary tone. Ivabradine also has a use-dependent mechanism of action, in which the reduction in heart rate is greater at higher heart rates than at lower heart rates, minimizing the risk of severe bradycardia. (See Description.) Unlike β-blockers, ivabradine has not been shown to reduce cardiovascular mortality. Given the well-established mortality benefits of β-blocker therapy, it remains important to initiate and titrate the dosage of β-blockers upwards to optimal level, as tolerated, before assessing the resting heart rate for consideration of ivabradine therapy.

Efficacy and safety of ivabradine as an adjunct to or a substitute for therapy with a β-blocker in the management of chronic heart failure has been established principally by the results of a randomized, double-blind, placebo-controlled trial (SHIFT) in patients with chronic heart failure receiving standard-of-care therapy at baseline, which included a β-blocker if tolerated. In this trial, ivabradine reduced the risk of the combined end point of hospitalization for worsening heart failure or cardiovascular death by 18% when added to guideline- and evidence-based treatment within 3 months. The trial was conducted in 6558 adults with stable NYHA class II–IV chronic heart failure with an LVEF of 35% or less, who were in sinus rhythm with a resting heart rate of 70 beats/minute or more and had been admitted to the hospital for worsening of heart failure within the previous 12 months. Patients received ivabradine or placebo in addition to standard-of-care therapy that included maximally tolerated dosages of β-blockers. Approximately 89% of enrolled patients received a β-blocker; 26% of patients were receiving

guideline-defined target daily dosages of these drugs. The predominant reasons for patients not achieving target dosages of β-blockers were hypotension, fatigue, dyspnea, dizziness, cardiac decompensation, and excessive bradycardia. Approximately 11% of patients did not receive a β-blocker, principally because of chronic obstructive pulmonary disease (COPD), asthma, or hypotension. Most patients' baseline treatment regimens included an ACE inhibitor or angiotensin II receptor antagonist (91% of patients), diuretic (83%), and aldosterone antagonist (60%). The initial dosage of ivabradine was 5 mg twice daily. After a 14-day titration period, the dosage was increased to 7.5 mg twice daily unless the resting heart rate was 60 beats/minute or less. The dosage of ivabradine was adjusted throughout the trial (range: 2.5–7.5 mg twice daily) as tolerated to maintain a resting heart rate of 50–60 beats/minute. The primary end point of the trial was the composite of cardiovascular death or hospital admission for worsening heart failure.

The benefit of ivabradine in the SHIFT trial was attributable mainly to a reduction in the risk of hospitalization for worsening heart failure with ivabradine compared with placebo (15.6 versus 20.2%, respectively). Ivabradine did not have a favorable effect on the mortality component of the primary end point and did not substantially reduce cardiovascular death in the overall treatment population. The beneficial effect of ivabradine on the primary end point appeared to diminish as the dosage of β-blockers increased, with negligible benefit seen in patients taking guideline-defined target dosages of β-blockers. The composite end point of hospitalization for worsening heart failure or cardiovascular death was not substantially reduced by ivabradine in the subgroup of patients receiving at least 50% of the evidence-based target daily dosage of a β-blocker. Ivabradine therapy was associated with an average reduction in heart rate of 15 beats/minute (baseline value 80 beats/minute), which was generally maintained throughout the course of the trial. Patients with heart rates higher than the median were at increased risk of an end point event and exhibited greater event-reducing benefit from ivabradine than those with lower heart rates. A diminishing benefit of ivabradine was also seen in patients with lower baseline heart rates (less than 77 beats/minute). It has been suggested that this diminished benefit may be due to the lower risk of all end points in patients with lower heart rates and/or ivabradine's use-dependent mechanism of action, which may limit the heart rate reduction in patients with lower baseline heart rates. Whether ivabradine can improve patient outcomes when added to optimally managed heart failure therapies has not been established.

● Angina

Ivabradine also has been used for the treatment of chronic stable angina pectoris† in patients with normal sinus rhythm as an adjunct to, or a substitute for, β-blockers in patients whose symptoms are inadequately controlled by β-blockers or in those who have a contraindication or intolerance to the drugs. In some clinical trials in patients with chronic stable angina, ivabradine has reduced heart rate, improved exercise capacity, and decreased the number of anginal attacks. Evidence from randomized controlled trials using standard stress testing indicates that ivabradine may be as effective as atenolol or amlodipine in patients with stable coronary artery disease and that adding ivabradine to atenolol therapy may provide better control of heart rate and anginal symptoms. However, clinical trials (e.g., BEAUTIFUL, SIGNIFY) have not demonstrated any benefit of ivabradine in terms of cardiovascular outcomes (e.g., myocardial infarction [MI], cardiovascular death) among patients who have stable coronary artery disease with or without stable heart failure and are receiving guideline-based therapy for angina (e.g., including aspirin, statins, ACE inhibitors, β-blockers). Some clinical trial data suggest that ivabradine should be used with caution in patients with more severe forms of angina due to the possibility of an increased risk of death due to cardiovascular causes or nonfatal MI; however, further study and experience are needed to confirm these findings. Since ivabradine therapy has not been associated with a reduction in cardiovascular mortality, it is important to ensure that dosages of β-blockers (which do reduce cardiovascular mortality) are adjusted to clinically optimal levels before initiating ivabradine therapy.

The BEAUTIFUL trial was a randomized, double-blind placebo-controlled trial evaluating the use of ivabradine in approximately 11,000 patients with coronary artery disease, LVEF less than 40%, and a heart rate of at least 60 beats/minute. Eligible patients had heart failure and/or angina with stable symptoms for at least 3 months and were receiving conventional drug therapy for these conditions at stable dosages for at least 1 month. Patients who received ivabradine were given an initial dosage of 5 mg twice daily, which was increased to 7.5 mg twice daily depending on resting heart rate and tolerability. The primary end point was the composite of time to cardiovascular death, hospitalization for acute MI, or hospitalization for new-onset or worsening heart failure. After a median follow-up of 19 months, the primary composite end point was not reduced with ivabradine therapy. However, in a post hoc analysis of a subgroup of patients with activity-limiting anginal symptoms (e.g., pain, fatigue, palpitations, dyspnea) and a heart rate of at least 70 beats/minute at the time of randomization, ivabradine therapy was associated with reductions in the primary composite end point of cardiovascular death or hospitalization for fatal and nonfatal MI or heart failure and in coronary revascularization; these reductions were observed despite almost all patients in the subgroup receiving concomitant β-blocker therapy.

The findings of the post hoc subgroup analysis in the BEAUTIFUL trial, which were generally considered hypothesis generating, were further evaluated in the SIGNIFY trial in which approximately 19,000 patients with stable coronary artery disease, no clinical heart failure (NYHA class I), and a heart rate of at least 70 beats/minute received ivabradine or placebo in addition to standard therapy. After a median follow-up of 24.1 months, ivabradine did not substantially affect the primary end point (first occurrence of either cardiovascular death or MI). However, in the prespecified subgroup of patients with angina of Canadian Cardiovascular Society (CCS) class II or higher in the SIGNIFY trial, ivabradine increased the absolute risk of the primary composite end point of death from cardiovascular causes or nonfatal MI (7.6 versus 6.5%) compared with placebo, despite improving angina symptoms. The use of β-blockers was not required for inclusion in the SIGNIFY trial, but approximately 83% of patients in the ivabradine and placebo groups received a β-blocker as a part of their therapy. Approximately 12,000 patients in the trial had activity-limiting (CSS Class II or greater) angina. Ivabradine was initiated at a dosage of 7.5 mg twice daily, which could be increased to 10 mg twice daily or decreased to 5 mg twice daily to achieve a target heart rate of 55–60 beats/minute. Further study is needed to evaluate the adverse effects seen in the subgroup analysis of SIGNIFY as these effects may be attributable to the high dosages of ivabradine (10 mg twice daily) used in the trial and potentially exacerbated by concurrent use of drugs that increase ivabradine plasma concentrations and have negative chronotropic actions (e.g., verapamil, diltiazem). However, some experts currently suggest that ivabradine not be used in patients with activity-limiting angina who do not have clinical heart failure.

DOSAGE AND ADMINISTRATION

● General

Dosage of ivabradine should be individualized according to the patient's heart rate response and tolerance to a target resting heart rate of 50–60 beats/minute.

● Administration

Ivabradine is administered orally twice daily with meals. If a dose is missed, the next dose should be taken at the usual time; the dose should not be doubled to make up for the missed dose. (See Advice to Patients.)

● Dosage

Dosage of ivabradine hydrochloride is expressed in terms of ivabradine.

Heart Failure

For the management of chronic symptomatic heart failure, the initial dosage of ivabradine is 5 mg twice daily. In patients with a history of conduction defects, or other patients in whom bradycardia could lead to hemodynamic compromise, therapy should be initiated at a dosage of 2.5 mg twice daily. Patients should be assessed 2 weeks after initiation of therapy and the dosage adjusted to achieve a resting heart rate of 50–60 beats/minute. After the initial adjustment period, the dosage may be adjusted as needed based on resting heart rate and tolerability. If the heart rate exceeds 60 beats/minute, the dosage should be increased by 2.5 mg (given twice daily) up to a maximum of 7.5 mg twice daily. If the heart rate is less than 50 beats/minute or if the patient is experiencing signs and symptoms of bradycardia, the dosage should be decreased by 2.5 mg (given twice daily). If a patient is receiving ivabradine 2.5 mg twice daily and their heart rate is less than 50 beats/minute or they are experiencing signs and symptoms of bradycardia, ivabradine therapy should be discontinued.

Angina

For the treatment of chronic stable angina†, ivabradine dosages of 2.5–10 mg twice daily have been used. In 2 large clinical trials in patients with stable angina with or without heart failure, ivabradine was initiated at dosages of 5 or 7.5 mg twice daily and titrated after 2–4 weeks to a target heart rate of 50–60 beats/minute. In the BEAUTIFUL trial, if the patient's resting heart rate was less than 50 beats/minute or if signs or symptoms of bradycardia were present, the dosage was titrated downward. In clinical trials, ivabradine was discontinued if the resting heart rate was less than 50 beats/minute or if signs or symptoms related to bradycardia were present despite reduction of ivabradine dosage.

Specific Populations

Hepatic Impairment

No dosage adjustment is required in patients with mild or moderate hepatic impairment. Ivabradine is contraindicated in patients with severe hepatic impairment (Child-Pugh class C) as safety and efficacy have not been established in this population and an increase in systemic exposure is expected. (See Cautions: Contraindications.)

Renal Impairment

No dosage adjustment is required in patients with creatinine clearance 15–60 mL/minute. Data are lacking on use of ivabradine in patients with creatinine clearance less than 15 mL/minute.

CAUTIONS

● Contraindications

- Acute decompensated heart failure.
- Blood pressure less than 90/50 mm Hg.
- Heart rate less than 60 beats/minute prior to treatment.
- Severe hepatic impairment. (See Hepatic Impairment under Warnings/Precautions: Specific Populations, in Cautions.)
- Pacemaker dependence (heart rate maintained exclusively by the pacemaker).
- Concomitant use of potent cytochrome P-450 (CYP) isoenzyme 3A4 inhibitors. (See Drug Interactions: Drugs and Foods Affecting Hepatic Microsomal Enzymes.)
- Sick sinus syndrome, sinoatrial (SA) block, or third-degree atrioventricular (AV) block (unless a functioning demand pacemaker is present).

● Warnings/Precautions

Fetal Toxicity

Based on findings in animal studies, ivabradine may cause fetal toxicity and teratogenicity when administered to pregnant women. Embryofetal toxicity and cardiac teratogenic effects (abnormal shape of the heart, interventricular septal defect, complex anomalies of primary arteries) were observed in fetuses of pregnant rats treated with ivabradine during organogenesis at exposures 1–3 times the human exposures at the maximum recommended human dose. Reduced fetal and placental weights and teratogenic effects (ectrodactylia) were observed in pregnant rabbits treated with ivabradine during organogenesis at exposures 15 times the human exposures at the maximum recommended human dose.

Women of childbearing potential should be advised to use effective contraception while taking ivabradine. (See Advice to Patients.)

Atrial Fibrillation

Ivabradine increases the risk of atrial fibrillation. In the SHIFT trial, the rate of atrial fibrillation was 5 versus 3.9% per patient-year in patients treated with ivabradine or placebo, respectively. Results of a meta-analysis evaluating clinical trial data from 11 studies indicated a 15% increase in the relative risk of atrial fibrillation with ivabradine therapy. Patients receiving ivabradine should receive regular cardiac rhythm monitoring and the drug should be discontinued if atrial fibrillation occurs.

Bradycardia and Conduction Disturbances

Bradycardia, sinus arrest, and heart block have occurred with ivabradine therapy. The rate of bradycardia was 6% per patient-year with ivabradine (2.7%

symptomatic; 3.4% asymptomatic) and 1.3% per patient-year with placebo. Risk factors for bradycardia include sinus node dysfunction, conduction defects (e.g., first or second degree AV block, bundle branch block), ventricular dyssynchrony, and the use of other negative chronotropes (e.g., digoxin, diltiazem, verapamil, amiodarone). Concurrent use of verapamil or diltiazem can increase ivabradine exposure, may contribute to heart rate lowering, and should be avoided. (See Drug Interactions: Calcium-channel Blocking Agents.)

Ivabradine should be avoided in patients with second degree AV block, unless a functioning demand pacemaker is present. (See Cautions: Contraindications.) Patients with demand pacemakers set to a rate of 60 beats/minute or more cannot achieve a target heart rate less than 60 beats/minute, and these patients were excluded from clinical trials. The use of ivabradine is not recommended in patients with demand pacemakers set to rates of 60 beats/minute or higher.

Sensitivity Reactions

Hypersensitivity

Hypersensitivity reactions (e.g., angioedema, erythema, rash, pruritus, urticaria) have been reported during postmarketing experience in patients receiving ivabradine.

Specific Populations

Pregnancy

There are no adequate and well-controlled studies of ivabradine in pregnant women. Studies in rats and rabbits indicate that ivabradine can cause fetal harm when administered to pregnant women. (See Fetal Toxicity under Cautions: Warnings/Precautions.) Increased postnatal mortality was associated with the teratogenic effects seen in rats. In pregnant rabbits, increased postimplantation loss was observed at an exposure 5 times the human exposure at the maximum recommended human dose. Pregnant women receiving ivabradine should be informed of the potential risk to the fetus.

Stroke volume and heart rate increase during pregnancy, which increases cardiac output, especially during the first trimester. Pregnant patients with left ventricular ejection fraction (LVEF) less than 35% on maximally tolerated dosages of β-adrenergic blocking agents (β-blockers) may be particularly dependent on increases in heart rate for augmentation of cardiac output. Therefore, pregnant patients taking ivabradine, especially during the first trimester, should be closely monitored for destabilization of their heart failure that could result from heart rate slowing. Pregnant women with chronic heart failure in their third trimester of pregnancy should be monitored for preterm birth.

Lactation

Ivabradine is distributed into milk in rats; it is not known whether ivabradine is distributed into human milk. Because of the potential risk to breast-fed infants from exposure to ivabradine, breast-feeding is not recommended.

Pediatric Use

Safety and efficacy have not been established in patients younger than 18 years of age.

Geriatric Use

No pharmacokinetic differences with ivabradine have been observed in patients 65 years of age or older compared with the overall population. However, there is limited experience with ivabradine in patients 75 years of age or older.

Renal Impairment

Renal impairment (creatinine clearance 15–60 mL/minute) has minimal effect on the pharmacokinetics of ivabradine. Data are lacking on use of ivabradine in patients with creatinine clearance less than 15 mL/minute.

Hepatic Impairment

In patients with mild or moderate hepatic impairment, the pharmacokinetics of ivabradine were similar to that in patients with normal hepatic function. Safety and efficacy have not been established in patients with severe hepatic impairment (Child-Pugh class C); use is contraindicated in these patients as increased systemic exposure is anticipated. (See Cautions: Contraindications.)

● Common Adverse Effects

Adverse effects reported in more than 1% of patients receiving ivabradine in the SHIFT trial and occurring at least 1% more frequently with ivabradine than with placebo include bradycardia, hypertension, atrial fibrillation, and phosphenes/visual brightness. Phosphenes are described as a transiently enhanced brightness in a limited area of the visual field, or as halos, image decomposition (stroboscopic or kaleidoscopic effects), colored bright lights, or multiple images (retinal persistency). Phosphenes generally are triggered by sudden changes in light intensity. Phosphenes generally become apparent within the first 2 months of treatment, after which they may occur repeatedly. This phenomenon generally has been of mild to moderate intensity and usually has resolved during or after ivabradine treatment.

DRUG INTERACTIONS

● Drugs and Foods Affecting Hepatic Microsomal Enzymes

Ivabradine is metabolized principally by cytochrome P-450 (CYP) isoenzyme 3A4. The major metabolite of ivabradine is the N-desmethylated derivative (S 18982), which is also metabolized by CYP3A4. Drugs that inhibit or induce CYP3A4 can increase or decrease, respectively, ivabradine plasma concentrations; increased concentrations may exacerbate bradycardia and conduction disturbances. Concomitant use of potent CYP3A4 inhibitors such as azole antifungal agents, macrolide antibiotics, HIV protease inhibitors, and nefazodone is contraindicated. (See Cautions: Contraindications.) The concomitant use of moderate CYP3A4 inhibitors such as diltiazem, verapamil, and grapefruit juice should be avoided. Inducers of CYP3A4 such as St. John's wort (Hypericum perforatum), rifampin, barbiturates, and phenytoin also should be avoided during ivabradine therapy.

● Azole Antifungal Agents

Concomitant use of ivabradine and potent CYP3A4 inhibitors such as azole antifungal agents (e.g., itraconazole, ketoconazole) increases the plasma concentrations of ivabradine and is contraindicated. (See Cautions: Contraindications.)

● Calcium-channel Blocking Agents

Concomitant use of ivabradine and moderate CYP3A4 inhibitors such as diltiazem and verapamil increases plasma ivabradine concentrations and should be avoided. Calcium-channel blocking agents such as diltiazem and verapamil that act as negative chronotropes also may increase the risk of bradycardia. Heart rate should be monitored in patients taking ivabradine with other negative chronotropes.

● HIV Protease Inhibitors

Concomitant use of ivabradine and potent CYP3A4 inhibitors such as HIV protease inhibitors (e.g., nelfinavir) increases plasma concentrations of ivabradine and is contraindicated. (See Cautions: Contraindications.)

● Macrolide Antibiotics

Concomitant use of ivabradine and potent CYP3A4 inhibitors such as macrolide antibiotics (e.g., clarithromycin, telithromycin) increases plasma concentrations of ivabradine and is contraindicated. (See Cautions: Contraindications.)

● Metformin

Ivabradine (10 mg twice daily dosed to steady state) did not affect the pharmacokinetics of concomitantly administered metformin, an organic cation transporter (OCT2) sensitive substrate. No dosage adjustment is required for metformin when administered with ivabradine.

● Nefazodone

Concomitant use of ivabradine and potent CYP3A4 inhibitors such as nefazodone increases plasma concentrations of ivabradine and is contraindicated. (See Cautions: Contraindications.)

● **Negative Chronotropes**

The risk of bradycardia increases with concomitant administration of drugs that slow heart rate (e.g., digoxin, amiodarone, β-adrenergic blocking agents [β-blockers]). Heart rate should be monitored in patients taking ivabradine with other negative chronotropes. Digoxin exposure did not change when used concomitantly with ivabradine.

● **Proton-pump Inhibitors**

Concomitant administration of lansoprazole (60 mg daily) or omeprazole (40 mg daily) did not have a clinically important effect on the pharmacokinetics of ivabradine; no dosage adjustment is required.

● **Sildenafil**

Sildenafil (100 mg) did not have a clinically important effect on the pharmacokinetics of ivabradine; no dosage adjustment is required.

● **Simvastatin**

Simvastatin (20 mg daily) did not have a clinically important effect on the pharmacokinetics of ivabradine; no dosage adjustment is required.

● **Warfarin**

Warfarin (1–5 mg daily) did not have a clinically important effect on the pharmacokinetics of ivabradine; no dosage adjustment is required.

DESCRIPTION

Ivabradine is a hyperpolarization-activated cyclic nucleotide-gated (HCN) channel (funny-channel [f-channel]) blocking agent that reduces the spontaneous pacemaker activity of the sinoatrial (SA) node by selectively inhibiting the funny-current (I_f) in pacemaker cells, resulting in heart rate reduction with no effect on ventricular repolarization or myocardial contractility.

The f-channels are part of the HCN channel family, which is comprised of many distinct isoforms (HCN 1–4), and are expressed in the heart and nervous system. The HCN4 channel is found in the heart and is active in the pacemaker cells of the SA node. The f-channels, unlike other voltage-gated ion channels, open with hyperpolarization rather than depolarization and have a mixed permeability to sodium and potassium ions. These channels open and close in response to ambient voltage and local intracellular cyclic adenosine monophosphate (cAMP) concentrations. Adrenergic agonists activate adenylate cyclase, which causes an increase in intracellular cAMP, whereas cholinergic transmitters decrease local cAMP by inhibiting adenylate cyclase. Intracellular cAMP acts as a second messenger and favors f-channel opening by direct binding to the c-terminus of the channel, which induces a depolarizing shift of the activation curve, leading to an increase in the number of open f-channels. The I_f current, which is a mixed sodium-potassium current, is able to move across open f-channels; this causes a deeper slope of diastolic depolarization and a reduction in diastolic duration, leading to an elevation in heart rate.

Ivabradine has a unique mechanism of action in that it displays state-dependent, use-dependent, and current-dependent properties. Ivabradine enters cardiac pacemaker cells and blocks the f-channel from the cytoplasmic side of the membrane preferentially when the channel is in an open state (state-dependence) and is more efficient at depolarized than hyperpolarized voltages. Therefore, the interaction between ivabradine and the f-channel binding site is dependent upon the rate of opening and closing of the channels in response to repolarization and depolarization (i.e., related to heart rate). As a result of this use-dependent inhibition, the reduction in pacemaker activity by ivabradine is more pronounced at higher firing rates in the SA node. Ivabradine also displays a current-dependence property by which ivabradine is drawn to the binding site of the f-channel by the electrostatic forces generated by the depolarization process and dissociates from the binding site in response to the inward current generated from the repolarization process. The blockade of f-channels by ivabradine inhibits the I_f current, which leads to a reduction in the slow diastolic depolarization phase of the SA node action potential, thereby reducing heart rate. The selective binding of ivabradine to f-channels makes it a pure

heart-rate-reducing agent. Reduction in heart rate with ivabradine decreases myocardial oxygen consumption and increases oxygen supply due to prolongation of diastolic perfusion time.

The adverse effects of ivabradine on vision are due to interaction of ivabradine with retinal ion channels (I_h current), which closely resemble the I_f channels in the SA node. The I_h current is involved in curtailing retinal responses to bright light stimuli. Under circumstances that trigger these I_h channels (e.g., rapid changes in luminosity), partial inhibition of the I_h current by ivabradine may cause the luminous phenomena experienced by some patients. (See Cautions: Common Adverse Effects.)

Following oral administration, peak plasma concentrations of ivabradine are reached in approximately 1 hour under fasting conditions. Food delays absorption by approximately 1 hour and increases plasma ivabradine exposure by 20–40%; therefore, it is recommended that the drug be taken with meals to reduce individual variability in systemic exposure. (See Dosage and Administration: Administration.) The absolute oral bioavailability of ivabradine is approximately 40% due to first-pass elimination in gut and liver via cytochrome P-450 (CYP) isoenzyme 3A4-mediated oxidation. The major metabolite of ivabradine is the N-desmethylated derivative (S 18982), which is equipotent to ivabradine and circulates at concentrations approximately 40% that of ivabradine and is also metabolized by CYP3A4. Ivabradine has a low affinity for CYP3A4 and does not modify CYP3A4 substrate metabolism or plasma concentrations. Conversely, potent inhibitors and inducers may substantially affect ivabradine's bioavailability and plasma concentrations. (See Drug Interactions: Drugs and Foods Affecting Hepatic Microsomal Enzymes.) Ivabradine is approximately 70% bound to plasma proteins. Ivabradine plasma concentrations decline with a distribution half-life of 2 hours and an effective half-life of approximately 6 hours.

ADVICE TO PATIENTS

Importance of advising patients to read the FDA-approved patient labeling (medication guide).

Importance of women informing clinicians if they are or plan to become pregnant or plan to breast-feed. Importance of advising females of reproductive potential to use effective contraception and to notify their healthcare provider about a known or suspected pregnancy. Importance of informing pregnant women about the potential risks to the fetus.

Importance of advising patients to report substantial decreases in heart rate or symptoms such as dizziness, fatigue, or hypotension.

Importance of advising patients to report symptoms of atrial fibrillation, such as heart palpitations or racing pulse, chest pressure, or worsened shortness of breath. Importance of patients receiving regular cardiac rhythm monitoring.

Importance of advising patients about the possible occurrence of luminous phenomena (phosphenes) in the field of vision. Importance of advising patients to use caution if they are driving or using machines in situations where sudden changes in light intensity could occur, especially when driving at night. Importance of informing patients that phosphenes may subside spontaneously during continued treatment with ivabradine.

Importance of informing clinician of existing or contemplated concomitant therapy, including prescription and OTC drugs, as well as any concomitant diseases. Importance of advising patients to avoid ingestion of grapefruit juice or St. John's wort.

Importance of advising patients to take ivabradine twice daily with meals. If a dose is missed, the next dose should be taken at the usual time; the dose should not be doubled to make up for the missed dose.

Importance of informing patients of other important precautionary information. (See Cautions.)

PREPARATIONS

Excipients in commercially available drug preparations may have clinically important effects in some individuals; consult specific product labeling for details.

Ivabradine Hydrochloride

Oral

| Tablets (film-coated) | 5 mg (of ivabradine) | Corlanor®, Amgen |
| | 7.5 mg (of ivabradine) | Corlanor®, Amgen |

† Use is not currently included in the labeling approved by the US Food and Drug Administration.

Selected Revisions April 10, 2024, © Copyright, January 31, 2017, American Society of Health-System Pharmacists, Inc.

Ezetimibe

24:06.05 • CHOLESTEROL ABSORPTION INHIBITORS

■ Ezetimibe, a cholesterol absorption inhibitor, is an antilipemic agent.

USES

● *Dyslipidemias*

Ezetimibe is used alone or in combination with other antilipemic agents (e.g., a hydroxymethylglutaryl-coenzyme A [HMG-CoA] reductase inhibitor [statin], fenofibrate) as an adjunct to dietary therapy in the treatment of primary hyperlipidemia and mixed dyslipidemia, homozygous familial hypercholesterolemia, and/or homozygous familial sitosterolemia. The effects of ezetimibe on cardiovascular morbidity and mortality have not been established. The fixed-combination preparation containing ezetimibe and simvastatin (e.g., Vytorin®) is indicated for use in patients with primary hyperlipidemia, mixed dyslipidemia, or homozygous familial hypercholesterolemia; the manufacturer states that no incremental benefit of the fixed combination on cardiovascular morbidity and mortality over and above that demonstrated for simvastatin has been established. Efficacy of ezetimibe, alone or in fixed combination with simvastatin, in patients with Fredrickson type I, III, IV, or V dyslipidemias has not been established.

The fixed-combination preparation containing bempedoic acid and ezetimibe (Nexlizet®) is used as an adjunct to diet and maximally tolerated statin therapy in patients with heterozygous familial hypercholesterolemia or established atherosclerotic cardiovascular disease (ASCVD) who require additional reduction in low-density lipoprotein (LDL)-cholesterol concentrations; the effects of the combination preparation on cardiovascular morbidity and mortality have not been established.

The 2018 American Heart Association (AHA)/American College of Cardiology (ACC) cholesterol management guideline emphasizes lifestyle modification as the foundation of ASCVD risk reduction. Patients with clinical ASCVD (defined as those with acute coronary syndromes [ACS], history of myocardial infarction [MI], stable or unstable angina or coronary or other arterial revascularization, stroke, transient ischemic attack [TIA], or peripheral artery disease [PAD]) also should be treated with a statin in conjunction with lifestyle modification to reduce LDL cholesterol, the lipoprotein fraction found to be a major cause of ASCVD. Nonstatin drugs may be considered as adjunctive therapy in certain high-risk patients who do not achieve adequate reductions in LDL-cholesterol concentrations with maximally tolerated statin therapy. An expert consensus panel was convened by ACC to provide further guidance on the role of nonstatin drugs in the management of ASCVD, specifically in regard to the patient populations and clinical situations in which these drugs may be considered. According to these experts, patients who may benefit from the addition of a nonstatin drug include those with clinical ASCVD with or without comorbidities (including severe elevations of baseline LDL-cholesterol concentrations greater than 190 mg/dL) who have not met certain thresholds of LDL-cholesterol reduction (e.g., at least 50% reduction in LDL cholesterol, or an absolute LDL-cholesterol concentration of less than 70 mg/dL or non-high-density lipoprotein [non-HDL]-cholesterol concentration of less than 100 mg/dL) while receiving maximally tolerated statin therapy; nonstatin drugs that may be considered include ezetimibe or a proprotein convertase subtilisin kexin type 9 (PCSK9) inhibitor (or possibly both) depending on the specific situation. Selection of a nonstatin drug should be based on a favorable benefit-risk ratio (i.e., demonstrated benefit of ASCVD risk reduction outweighs risks of adverse effects and drug interactions) and patient preferences. Prior to initiation of nonstatin antilipemic drugs, it is critical that patients are treated first with maximally tolerated statin therapy and that lifestyle modifications are intensified/optimized. Because true statin intolerance is uncommon, patients should be systematically and rigorously evaluated for this condition to encourage adherence to evidence-based statin therapy. For additional details on prevention of ASCVD, see the HMG-CoA Reductase Inhibitors General Statement 24:06.08.

Primary Hyperlipidemia and Mixed Dyslipidemia

Efficacy and safety of ezetimibe monotherapy in the management of primary hyperlipidemia were established in 2 multicenter, randomized, double-blind, placebo-controlled studies of 12 weeks' duration in approximately 1700 patients with primary hyperlipidemia. In these studies, patients who received ezetimibe (10 mg daily) had mean reductions of approximately 12–13% in total cholesterol, 18% in LDL-cholesterol, 15–16% in apo B, 16% in non-HDL-cholesterol, and 7–9% in triglyceride concentrations; increases in high-density lipoprotein (HDL)-cholesterol concentrations in patients receiving ezetimibe were negligible (1%). In most patients with primary hyperlipidemia, maximal or near-maximal reductions in serum lipoprotein and apolipoprotein concentrations are achieved within 2 weeks and maintained during continued therapy. Reductions in LDL-cholesterol concentrations appear to be consistent across age, gender, and baseline LDL-cholesterol concentrations.

The manufacturer states that ezetimibe may be used in combination with a statin or fenofibrate for incremental antilipemic effect. Data from several multicenter, randomized, double-blind, placebo-controlled studies indicate that concomitant therapy with ezetimibe and a statin may produce additive antilipemic effects. In a study in patients with primary hyperlipidemia and either multiple cardiovascular risk factors or documented coronary heart disease (CHD) who had not achieved their target LDL-cholesterol goal with diet and statin monotherapy, addition of ezetimibe (10 mg daily) to existing statin therapy reduced total cholesterol, LDL-cholesterol, apo B, non-HDL-cholesterol, and triglyceride concentrations by an additional 17, 25, 19, 23, and 14%, respectively, at 8 weeks and increased HDL-cholesterol concentrations by an additional 3% compared with statin monotherapy. For patients whose LDL-cholesterol levels were above the target levels recommended by the Second Report of the National Cholesterol Education Program (NCEP) (Adult Treatment Panel [ATP] II), approximately 72% of patients receiving combination therapy achieved their target LDL-cholesterol goal compared with 19% of those receiving statin monotherapy. In 4 multicenter, randomized, double-blind, placebo-controlled studies in hyperlipidemic patients, combination therapy with ezetimibe (10 mg daily) and a statin (i.e., atorvastatin 10–80 mg daily, lovastatin 10–40 mg daily, pravastatin 10–40 mg daily, or simvastatin 10–80 mg daily) for 12 weeks reduced total cholesterol, LDL-cholesterol, apo B, non-HDL-cholesterol, and triglyceride concentrations and, except for the combination of ezetimibe and pravastatin, increased HDL-cholesterol concentrations compared with monotherapy with the corresponding statin. The addition of ezetimibe to statin therapy has been shown to increase the magnitude of LDL-cholesterol lowering by approximately 13–20%.

Similar additive antilipemic effects have been observed following therapy with the fixed-combination preparation containing ezetimibe and simvastatin. Data from several randomized, double-blind studies in patients with primary hyperlipidemia indicated that reductions in LDL-cholesterol concentrations achieved with pooled doses of the fixed-combination preparation were greater than those achieved with pooled doses of atorvastatin, rosuvastatin, or simvastatin monotherapy. In one study, LDL-cholesterol concentrations were reduced by 47–59% following therapy with the fixed-combination preparation containing ezetimibe (10 mg) and simvastatin (10–80 mg) and by 36–53% following monotherapy with atorvastatin (10–80 mg daily). In another study, LDL-cholesterol concentrations were reduced by 52–61% following therapy with the fixed-combination preparation containing ezetimibe (10 mg) and simvastatin (20–80 mg) and by 46–57% following monotherapy with rosuvastatin (10–40 mg daily). In the third study, LDL-cholesterol concentrations were reduced by 45–60% following therapy with the fixed-combination preparation containing ezetimibe (10 mg) and simvastatin (10–80 mg) and by 33–49% following monotherapy with simvastatin (10–80 mg daily).

Despite its additive effects on LDL-cholesterol reduction, early findings from a randomized, double-blind, active-controlled study (Ezetimibe and Simvastatin in Hypercholesterolemia Enhances Atherosclerosis Regression [ENHANCE]) in patients with heterozygous familial hypercholesterolemia indicated that the fixed-combination preparation containing ezetimibe and simvastatin (10 and 80 mg daily, respectively) was *not* superior to simvastatin monotherapy (80 mg daily) in reducing carotid intimal-medial wall thickness (cIMT). In this study, treatment with the fixed-combination preparation for 2 years resulted in a change in cIMT (increase of 0.011 mm) that was not statistically different from the change in cIMT observed with simvastatin monotherapy (increase of 0.006 mm). However, reductions in LDL-cholesterol concentrations achieved with the fixed-combination preparation (56%) were substantially greater than those achieved with simvastatin monotherapy (39%). Although the greater reductions in LDL-cholesterol concentrations did not translate into substantial improvement in cIMT in the ENHANCE study, the cardiovascular benefits of reducing LDL-cholesterol concentrations are well established and have been demonstrated in other studies.

The addition of ezetimibe to simvastatin therapy resulted in further LDL-cholesterol lowering and improved cardiovascular outcomes in the Improved Reduction of Outcomes: Vytorin® Efficacy International (IMPROVE-IT) study. IMPROVE-IT was a large randomized, double-blind study in 18,144 patients who had been hospitalized for ACS in the preceding 10 days and had baseline LDL-cholesterol concentrations of 50–125 mg/dL (or 50–100 mg/dL if they were receiving lipid-lowering therapy). Patients were randomized to receive the fixed-combination preparation containing ezetimibe and simvastatin (10 and 40 mg daily, respectively) or simvastatin monotherapy (40 mg daily). After a median duration of follow-up of 6 years, the fixed-combination preparation produced a 24% further reduction in mean LDL-cholesterol concentration and also reduced the rate of the primary end point (composite of cardiovascular death, nonfatal myocardial infarction [MI], unstable angina requiring hospitalization, coronary revascularization, or nonfatal stroke) compared with simvastatin monotherapy; the absolute risk reduction for the primary composite outcome was 2% over 7 years. The treatment benefit of combined simvastatin/ezetimibe therapy began to emerge after 1 year and appeared to be particularly pronounced in patients with diabetes mellitus and geriatric patients (75 years of age or older).

The combination of ezetimibe and fenofibrate has been shown to reduce total and LDL-cholesterol, apo B, and non-HDL-cholesterol concentrations in patients with mixed dyslipidemia. In a randomized, double-blind, placebo-controlled study in patients with mixed dyslipidemia, combination therapy with ezetimibe and fenofibrate (160 mg daily) was superior to fenofibrate monotherapy in reducing total cholesterol (22 versus 11%), LDL-cholesterol (20 versus 6%), apo B (26 versus 15%), and non-HDL-cholesterol (30 versus 16%) concentrations at 12 weeks. Effects on triglyceride and HDL-cholesterol concentrations in patients receiving combination therapy were comparable to those in patients receiving fenofibrate monotherapy. Following an additional 48 weeks of combination therapy or monotherapy, changes in lipoprotein concentrations were consistent with those observed at 12 weeks of therapy. The manufacturer states that efficacy and safety of ezetimibe in combination with a fibric acid derivative other than fenofibrate have not been studied and currently is not recommended. (See Fibric Acid Derivatives under Drug Interactions: Antilipemic Agents.)

Results of a systematic meta-analysis of 26 randomized controlled studies comparing ezetimibe plus other lipid-modifying therapies with other lipid-modifying therapies alone in patients with or without cardiovascular disease found that the addition of ezetimibe to statin therapy had a modest benefit in reducing the risk of nonfatal MI and nonfatal stroke, but that the addition of ezetimibe to statin or fenofibrate therapy had little to no effect on death from any cause. The results from this analysis were driven largely by the IMPROVE-IT study (in patients with established ASCVD, predominately with ACS) and by studies of ezetimibe in combination with statins; only one study compared the combination of ezetimibe and fenofibrate. Therefore, the observed cardiovascular benefits may not apply to combination therapy with ezetimibe and fenofibrate. Additional studies are needed to evaluate the role of ezetimibe in primary prevention of cardiovascular disease and the effects of ezetimibe monotherapy in the prevention of cardiovascular disease also need to be further investigated.

Patients with Chronic Kidney Disease

Chronic kidney disease is a risk-enhancing factor for ASCVD. The 2018 AHA/ACC cholesterol management guideline states that initiation of a moderate-intensity statin or moderate-intensity statin combined with ezetimibe may be useful in adults 40–75 years of age with chronic kidney disease (not treated with dialysis or kidney transplantation) who have LDL-cholesterol concentrations of 70–189 mg/dL and a 10-year ASCVD risk of 7.5% or higher. For additional details, see the HMG-CoA Reductase Inhibitors General Statement 24:06.08.

In the Study of Heart and Renal Protection (SHARP), the fixed-combination preparation containing ezetimibe and simvastatin was shown to reduce the risk of major vascular and atherosclerotic events in patients with chronic kidney disease. More than 9000 patients with moderate to severe chronic kidney disease (33% receiving dialysis) and no known history of MI or coronary revascularization were initially randomized in a 4:4:1 ratio to receive the fixed-combination preparation containing ezetimibe and simvastatin (10 and 20 mg daily, respectively), placebo, or simvastatin alone (20 mg daily) for 1 year to assess the safety of adding ezetimibe to simvastatin; patients in the simvastatin monotherapy group were then re-randomized to the fixed-combination preparation or placebo. After a median duration of follow up of 4.9 years, the risk of a major vascular event (nonfatal MI or cardiac death, stroke, or revascularization excluding dialysis

access procedures) was reduced by 16% (based on the primary intent-to-treat analysis in patients initially randomized to the fixed-combination preparation or placebo groups) and the risk of a major atherosclerotic event (nonfatal MI or cardiac death, nonhemorrhagic stroke, or arterial revascularization excluding dialysis access procedures) was reduced by 17% (based on the total number of patients randomized at any time to the fixed-combination preparation or placebo groups) with the fixed-combination preparation compared with placebo. The treatment effect was largely driven by a substantial reduction in ischemic strokes and arterial revascularization procedures. The subgroup of patients receiving dialysis at baseline experienced a smaller risk reduction benefit compared with those not receiving dialysis. In addition, therapy with the fixed-combination preparation did not appear to slow the progression to end-stage renal disease.

Homozygous Familial Hypercholesterolemia

Ezetimibe may be used in combination with atorvastatin or simvastatin to decrease elevated serum total and LDL-cholesterol concentrations in patients with homozygous familial hypercholesterolemia as an adjunct to other lipid-lowering therapies (e.g., plasma LDL apheresis) or when such therapies are not available. Ezetimibe in fixed combination with simvastatin (Vytorin®) is used to decrease elevated serum total cholesterol and LDL cholesterol in patients with homozygous familial hypercholesterolemia as an adjunct to other lipid-lowering therapies (e.g., plasma LDL apheresis) or if such treatments are unavailable.

Efficacy and safety of ezetimibe combined with atorvastatin or simvastatin for the management of homozygous familial hypercholesterolemia were established in a randomized, double-blind study of 12 weeks' duration in a limited number of patients with a clinical and/or genotypic diagnosis of homozygous familial hypercholesterolemia who were already receiving atorvastatin (40 mg daily) or simvastatin (40 mg daily), with or without concomitant LDL apheresis. In this study, patients were randomized to receive 1 of 3 regimens: atorvastatin (80 mg daily) or simvastatin (80 mg daily) monotherapy; ezetimibe (10 mg daily) with either atorvastatin (40 mg daily) or simvastatin (40 mg daily); or ezetimibe (10 mg daily) with either atorvastatin (80 mg daily) or simvastatin (80 mg daily). The addition of ezetimibe (10 mg daily) to therapy with atorvastatin (40 or 80 mg daily) or simvastatin (40 or 80 mg daily) was more effective in reducing LDL-cholesterol concentrations (21% additional reduction based on pooled data from 40-mg and 80-mg groups) than increasing the dosage of atorvastatin or simvastatin monotherapy from 40 to 80 mg daily (7% additional reduction based on pooled data from 40-mg and 80-mg groups).

In the entire group of patients receiving higher dosages (80 mg daily) of either atorvastatin or simvastatin in combination with ezetimibe (10 mg daily), LDL-cholesterol concentrations were reduced by approximately 27% compared with a 7% reduction with statin monotherapy. Comparable reductions in LDL-cholesterol concentrations were observed in the subgroup of patients with genotype-confirmed homozygous familial hypercholesterolemia.

Beneficial effects of ezetimibe combined with atorvastatin or simvastatin in patients with homozygous familial hypercholesterolemia who currently are undergoing LDL apheresis compared with effects in patients not undergoing the procedure have not been established. Effects on clinical outcome and modification of other disease parameters (e.g., xanthoma formation, regression of atherosclerosis) also have not been established.

Homozygous Familial Sitosterolemia (Phytosterolemia)

Ezetimibe is used as an adjunct to dietary therapy to decrease elevated serum sitosterol and campesterol concentrations in patients with homozygous familial sitosterolemia.

Efficacy and safety of ezetimibe in the management of homozygous sitosterolemia were established in a randomized, double-blind study of 8 weeks' duration in a limited number of patients with homozygous sitosterolemia who had plasma sitosterol concentrations exceeding 5 mg/dL and were already receiving standard antilipemic therapy (dietary therapy, bile acid sequestrants, statins, ileal bypass surgery, and/or LDL apheresis). In this study, treatment with ezetimibe (10 mg daily) reduced plasma sitosterol and campesterol concentrations by 21 and 24%, respectively, compared with increases of 4 and 3% in placebo-treated patients. Reductions in sitosterol and campesterol concentrations were consistent between patients receiving ezetimibe with or without bile acid sequestrants. The effect of reducing plasma concentrations of sitosterol and campesterol on cardiovascular morbidity and mortality has not been established.

For additional information on the role of antilipemic therapy in the treatment of lipoprotein disorders, prevention of cardiovascular events, and other conditions, see General Principles of Antilipemic Therapy in the HMG-CoA Reductase Inhibitors General Statement 24:06.08.

DOSAGE AND ADMINISTRATION

● *Administration*

Ezetimibe is administered orally without regard to meals. Ezetimibe in fixed combination with simvastatin (e.g., Vytorin®) is administered orally in the evening without regard to meals. Patients should be placed on a standard cholesterol-lowering diet before initiation of ezetimibe therapy and should remain on this diet during treatment with the drug.

When used in combination with a hydroxymethylglutaryl-coenzyme A [HMG-CoA] reductase inhibitor (statin) or fenofibrate for additive antilipemic effects, ezetimibe may be administered at the same time as the statin or fenofibrate, in accordance with the recommended dosing schedule for these drugs. When used in combination with a bile acid sequestrant, ezetimibe should be administered at least 2 hours before or at least 4 hours after administration of the bile acid sequestrant. The manufacturer states that pending further accumulation of data, use of ezetimibe in combination with a fibric acid derivative other than fenofibrate is not recommended. (See Drug Interactions: Antilipemic Agents.)

Antilipemic therapy is an adjunct to, not a substitute for, lifestyle modification therapies that reduce the risk of atherosclerotic cardiovascular disease (ASCVD). Adherence to lifestyle modifications for ASCVD risk reduction in addition to statin therapy should be reinforced periodically.

● *Dosage*

Ezetimibe

For the management of primary hyperlipidemia, mixed dyslipidemia, homozygous familial hypercholesterolemia, or homozygous familial sitosterolemia in adults and children 10 years of age and older, the recommended dosage of ezetimibe (alone or in combination with a statin or fenofibrate) is 10 mg once daily without regard to meals.

Ezetimibe/Simvastatin Combination Therapy

The recommended initial dosage of the commercially available fixed-combination preparation (Vytorin®) for the management of primary hyperlipidemia or mixed dyslipidemia in adults is 10 mg of ezetimibe and 10 or 20 mg of simvastatin once daily in the evening. Patients requiring reductions in LDL-cholesterol concentration of more than 55% to achieve their goal may receive an initial dosage of 10 mg of ezetimibe and 40 mg of simvastatin once daily in the absence of moderate to severe renal impairment (estimated glomerular filtration rate [eGFR] less than 60 mL/minute per 1.73 m²). Serum lipoprotein concentrations should be determined 2 or more weeks after initiation or titration of therapy, and dosage adjusted as needed. The usual maintenance dosage of ezetimibe in fixed combination with simvastatin is 10 mg of ezetimibe and 10–40 mg of simvastatin once daily. Because higher simvastatin dosages (e.g., 80 mg daily) have been associated with a greater risk of myopathy, including rhabdomyolysis, particularly during the first year of treatment, the manufacturer states that patients who are unable to achieve their LDL-cholesterol target goal with the fixed-combination preparation containing 10 mg of ezetimibe and 40 mg of simvastatin should *not* be titrated to the dosage containing 10 mg of ezetimibe and 80 mg of simvastatin but should be switched to alternative antilipemic agents that provide greater LDL-cholesterol reduction. The manufacturer also states that use of the fixed-combination preparation containing 10 mg of ezetimibe and 80 mg of simvastatin should be restricted to patients who have been receiving long-term therapy (e.g., 12 months or longer) at this dosage without evidence of muscle toxicity. (See Cautions.) Patients currently tolerating the fixed-combination preparation containing 10 mg of ezetimibe and 80 mg of simvastatin who require therapy with an interacting drug (i.e., a drug with which concomitant use is contraindicated or is associated with a dose limit for simvastatin) should be switched to an alternative statin or statin-based regimen with less drug interaction potential.

The recommended dosage of ezetimibe in fixed combination with simvastatin for the management of homozygous familial hypercholesterolemia in adults is 10 mg of ezetimibe and 40 mg of simvastatin once daily in the evening. Ezetimibe in fixed combination with simvastatin should be used as an adjunct to other lipid-lowering treatments (e.g., LDL apheresis) in these patients or as an alternative if such therapy is unavailable.

Bempedoic Acid/Ezetimibe Combination Therapy

The recommended dosage of the fixed-combination preparation containing bempedoic acid and ezetimibe (Nexlizet®) as an adjunct to maximally tolerated statin therapy in adults with heterozygous familial hypercholesterolemia or established ASCVD is 180 mg of bempedoic acid and 10 mg of ezetimibe once daily. Lipoprotein concentrations should be monitored within 8–12 weeks after initiation of therapy.

● *Special Populations*

Ezetimibe

No dosage adjustment of ezetimibe is necessary in geriatric patients (65 years of age or older), in patients with mild hepatic impairment, or in patients with renal impairment. However, the manufacturer states that ezetimibe should not be used in patients with moderate or severe hepatic impairment. (See Specific Populations under Cautions: Warnings/Precautions.)

Ezetimibe/Simvastatin Fixed Combination

In patients receiving ezetimibe in fixed combination with simvastatin, the manufacturer states that no dosage adjustment is necessary in geriatric patients or in patients with mild renal impairment (eGFR of 60 mL/minute per 1.73 m² or greater). However, in patients with chronic kidney disease and an eGFR of less than 60 mL/minute per 1.73 m², the dosage of the fixed-combination preparation is 10 mg of ezetimibe and 20 mg of simvastatin once daily in the evening; in such patients, higher dosages should be used with caution and close monitoring.

Bempedoic Acid/Ezetimibe Fixed Combination

In patients receiving ezetimibe in fixed combination with bempedoic acid, the manufacturer states that no dosage adjustment of the fixed-combination preparation is necessary in patients with mild or moderate renal impairment; there is limited to no experience with bempedoic acid in patients with severe renal impairment (eGFR less than 30 mL/minute per 1.73 m²) or end-stage renal disease requiring dialysis.

CAUTIONS

● *Contraindications*

Known hypersensitivity to ezetimibe or any ingredient in the formulation.

Ezetimibe, in combination with a hydroxymethylglutaryl-coenzyme A (HMG-CoA) reductase inhibitor (statin), is contraindicated in patients with active liver disease or unexplained, persistent increases in serum aminotransferase (transaminase) concentrations.

All statins are contraindicated in pregnant or nursing women. If ezetimibe is used in combination with a statin in a woman of childbearing age, the prescribing information for the statin should be consulted for detailed information on contraindications of the drug.

Concomitant use of the fixed combination of ezetimibe and simvastatin with potent inhibitors of cytochrome P-450 (CYP) isoenzyme 3A4, cyclosporine, danazol, or gemfibrozil is contraindicated.

● *Warnings/Precautions*

Sensitivity Reactions

Anaphylaxis, angioedema, rash, and urticaria have been reported.

Hepatic Effects

Consecutive elevations in serum aminotransferase (transaminase) concentrations (i.e., AST, ALT) exceeding 3 times the upper limit of normal were reported in approximately 0.5% of patients receiving ezetimibe and in 0.3% of those receiving placebo in clinical studies. In studies in which ezetimibe was initiated concurrently with a statin, these elevations were reported in 1.3% of patients receiving combination therapy and in 0.4% of those receiving statin monotherapy. Consecutive elevations in serum transaminase concentrations exceeding 3 times the upper limit of normal were reported in approximately 1.7–1.8% of patients receiving the fixed-combination preparation containing ezetimibe and simvastatin; these elevations appeared to be dose related and occurred in 2.6–3.6% of patients receiving the fixed combination containing 10 mg of ezetimibe and 80 mg of simvastatin. In a study in which ezetimibe was used in combination with fenofibrate, consecutive elevations in serum transaminase concentrations exceeding 3 times the upper limit of normal were reported in 2.7% of patients receiving combination therapy and in 4.5% of those receiving fenofibrate monotherapy. Increases in transaminase concentrations generally were asymptomatic and not associated with cholestasis; transaminase concentrations usually returned to pretreatment values during continued therapy or following discontinuance of ezetimibe. Hepatitis has been reported during postmarketing surveillance; however, a causal relationship to the drug has not been established.

When ezetimibe is used in combination with a statin, liver function tests should be performed at initiation of therapy and in accordance with the recommended monitoring schedule for the specific statin and as clinically indicated. If ALT or AST concentrations increase to 3 or more times the upper limit of normal (ULN) and are persistent, discontinuance of ezetimibe and/or the statin should be considered.

Musculoskeletal Effects

Marked (exceeding 10 times the upper limit of normal) elevations of serum creatine kinase (CK, creatine phosphokinase, CPK) were reported in 0.2% of patients receiving ezetimibe and in 0.1% of patients receiving placebo in clinical studies. In clinical studies evaluating safety and efficacy of ezetimibe in combination with a statin, these elevations were reported in 0.1% of patients receiving combination therapy and in 0.4% of those receiving statin monotherapy.

In clinical studies, the incidence of myopathy (manifested as unexplained muscle pain, tenderness, or weakness and increases in serum CK concentration exceeding 10 times the upper limit of normal) or rhabdomyolysis appears to be similar among patients receiving ezetimibe, statin monotherapy, or placebo. Myalgia, myopathy, and/or rhabdomyolysis have been reported during postmarketing surveillance in patients receiving ezetimibe alone or in combination with other antilipemic agents. Most reported cases of rhabdomyolysis have occurred in patients who were receiving statin therapy prior to initiating ezetimibe. However, rhabdomyolysis also has been reported following ezetimibe monotherapy or following addition of ezetimibe to therapy with agents known to be associated with increased risk of rhabdomyolysis (e.g., fibric acid derivatives).

Predisposing factors for the development of myopathy and/or rhabdomyolysis include increased dosages of statins, age exceeding 65 years, uncontrolled hypothyroidism, renal impairment, and potential statin-drug interactions. Patients initiating therapy with ezetimibe should be advised of the risk of myopathy and instructed to promptly report any unexplained muscle pain, tenderness, or weakness, particularly if accompanied by malaise or fever or if such manifestations persist after discontinuance of therapy. If myopathy is diagnosed or suspected, ezetimibe and other concomitant antilipemic agents (e.g., statin, fibric acid derivative) should be discontinued immediately.

General Precautions

Combination Therapy

When ezetimibe is used in combination with other drugs (e.g., statins, fenofibrate, bempedoic acid), the usual cautions, precautions, and contraindications associated with the other drug should be considered.

Risk of Cancer

The fixed combination of ezetimibe and simvastatin was reported in the Simvastatin and Ezetimibe in Aortic Stenosis (SEAS) study to be possibly associated with an increased risk of cancer; these findings prompted the FDA to issue an early communication in 2008 about this potential safety risk. Results of this study in 1873 patients with mild to moderate asymptomatic aortic stenosis revealed a higher incidence of cancer and cancer-related deaths (11.1 and 4.1%, respectively) in patients receiving the fixed-combination preparation compared with those receiving placebo (7.5 and 2.5%, respectively). However, results of 2 subsequent large randomized studies (the Study of Heart and Renal Protection [SHARP] and the Improved Reduction of Outcomes: Vytorin® Efficacy International Trial [IMPROVE-IT]) involving a combined study population of 27,414 patients with chronic kidney disease or acute coronary syndrome found no consistent pattern of increased cancer

risk among patients receiving the fixed-combination preparation of ezetimibe and simvastatin. In the SHARP study, cancer or cancer-related mortality occurred in 9.4 or 2.8%, respectively, of patients receiving the fixed-combination preparation, and these rates were similar to those reported in placebo recipients. In the IMPROVE-IT study, cancer or cancer-related mortality occurred in 10.2 or 3.8%, respectively, of patients receiving the fixed combination of ezetimibe and simvastatin and these rates were similar to those reported in patients who received simvastatin monotherapy. Based on the currently available evidence, FDA has concluded that neither ezetimibe nor the fixed-combination preparation of ezetimibe and simvastatin is likely to increase the risk of cancer or cancer-related deaths.

Specific Populations

Pregnancy

Category C. (See Users Guide.)

Category X for fixed combination of ezetimibe and simvastatin (due to simvastatin component). (See Users Guide.)

Lactation

Ezetimibe is distributed into milk in rats. It is not known whether ezetimibe is distributed into milk in humans. Because many drugs are distributed into human milk, caution should be used if ezetimibe is used in nursing women; the drug should not be used in nursing women unless the potential benefits justify the possible risks to the infant.

Pediatric Use

There are no differences in the pharmacokinetics of ezetimibe between adolescents and adults. Pharmacokinetic data are not available for pediatric patients younger than 10 years of age.

Use of ezetimibe in combination with simvastatin has been evaluated in a limited number of adolescent boys and girls with heterozygous familial hypercholesterolemia. In a randomized, double-blind, controlled study in boys and postmenarchal girls 10–17 years of age with heterozygous familial hypercholesterolemia, discontinuance of therapy because of adverse effects occurred in more patients receiving ezetimibe in combination with simvastatin (10–40 mg daily) (6%) than in those receiving simvastatin monotherapy (2%); in addition, increases in aminotransferase or CK concentrations also occurred more frequently in patients receiving combination therapy (3 or 2%, respectively) than in those receiving simvastatin monotherapy (2 or 0%, respectively). There were no detectable adverse effects on growth or sexual maturation in adolescent boys or girls or on duration of menstrual cycle in girls. Use of ezetimibe in combination with simvastatin dosages exceeding 40 mg daily has not been evaluated in adolescents; safety and efficacy of ezetimibe, alone or in fixed combination with simvastatin, have not been evaluated in prepubertal girls or in children younger than 10 years of age.

Safety and efficacy of ezetimibe in fixed combination with bempedoic acid have not been established in pediatric patients.

Geriatric Use

In clinical studies in patients receiving ezetimibe, 28% of patients were 65 years of age or older, and 5% of patients were 75 years of age or older. Following administration of ezetimibe (10 mg daily for 10 days), plasma concentrations of the drug were approximately twofold higher in geriatric individuals (65 years of age or older) than in younger adults; however, no overall differences in safety and efficacy of ezetimibe have been observed in geriatric patients relative to younger adults. Nevertheless, the manufacturer states that the possibility that some older patients may exhibit increased sensitivity to the drug cannot be ruled out.

In clinical studies in patients receiving ezetimibe in fixed combination with simvastatin, 32% of patients were 65 years of age or older, and 8% of patients were 75 years of age or older. No substantial differences in safety or efficacy of the fixed-combination preparation were observed in geriatric patients relative to younger patients; however, greater sensitivity in some older patients cannot be ruled out. Because advanced age (65 years of age or older) is a risk factor for myopathy, including rhabdomyolysis, ezetimibe in fixed combination with simvastatin should be used with caution in geriatric patients.

Hepatic Impairment

Following a single 10-mg dose of ezetimibe, the mean area under the plasma concentration-time curve (AUC) of total ezetimibe was increased by approximately 1.7 fold in individuals with mild hepatic impairment (Child-Pugh score 5–6). In individuals with moderate (Child-Pugh score 7–9) or severe (Child-Pugh score 10–15) hepatic impairment, the mean AUC of total ezetimibe was increased by approximately threefold to fourfold and that of ezetimibe was increased by approximately fivefold to sixfold. In a multiple-dose study, administration of ezetimibe (10 mg daily) for 14 days resulted in fourfold increases in the AUCs of total ezetimibe and ezetimibe on days 1 and 14 in patients with moderate hepatic impairment compared with healthy individuals. Because the effects of increased exposure to ezetimibe in patients with moderate or severe hepatic impairment currently are not known, the manufacturer states that the drug is not recommended in such patients.

Renal Impairment

Following a single 10-mg dose of ezetimibe, the mean AUC of ezetimibe was increased by approximately 1.5-fold in individuals with severe renal impairment (mean creatinine clearance of 30 mL/minute per 1.73 m^2 or less) compared with healthy individuals. When ezetimibe is used as monotherapy, no dosage adjustment is necessary in patients with renal impairment. (See Dosage and Administration: Special Populations.)

In the SHARP study in patients with moderate to severe renal impairment, the incidence of serious adverse effects, adverse effects leading to discontinuance of therapy, or adverse effects of special interest (adverse musculoskeletal effects, liver enzyme abnormalities, incident cancer) was similar in patients receiving the fixed combination of ezetimibe 10 mg and simvastatin 20 mg compared with those receiving placebo following a median of 4.9 years. However, because renal impairment is a risk factor for statin-associated myopathy, dosages of the fixed-combination preparation exceeding ezetimibe 10 mg and simvastatin 20 mg daily should be used with caution and close monitoring in patients with moderate to severe renal impairment. (See Dosage and Administration: Special Populations.)

● Common Adverse Effects

Adverse effects occurring in 2% or more of patients receiving ezetimibe and more frequently with the drug than with placebo include upper respiratory tract infection, diarrhea, arthralgia, sinusitis, pain in extremity, fatigue, and influenza.

Adverse effects occurring in patients receiving ezetimibe in combination with statins generally were similar to those reported in patients receiving statin therapy alone. However, the incidence of increased transaminase concentrations was higher in patients receiving combination therapy (1.3%) than in those who received statin monotherapy (0.4%). (See Hepatic Effects under Warnings/Precautions: Major Toxicities, in Cautions.) Adverse effects occurring in 2% or more of patients receiving ezetimibe in fixed combination with simvastatin include headache, increased ALT, myalgia, upper respiratory tract infection, and diarrhea.

Adverse effects occurring in 2% or more of patients receiving ezetimibe in fixed combination with bempedoic acid include upper respiratory tract infection, muscle spasms, hyperuricemia, back pain, abdominal pain or discomfort, bronchitis, extremity pain, anemia, increased hepatic enzymes, diarrhea, arthralgia, sinusitis, fatigue, and influenza.

DRUG INTERACTIONS

When using the fixed-combination preparation containing ezetimibe and simvastatin, the drug interactions associated with simvastatin should be considered. No formal drug interaction studies have been performed to date with the fixed-combination preparation other than that with extended-release niacin. (See Niacin under Drug Interactions: Antilipemic Agents.)

When using the fixed-combination preparation containing ezetimibe and bempedoic acid, the drug interactions associated with bempedoic acid should be considered.

● Drugs Affecting Hepatic Microsomal Enzymes

Based on results of a study evaluating possible interactions with caffeine, dextromethorphan, tolbutamide, and IV midazolam in a limited number of healthy men, the potential for drug interactions mediated by hepatic cytochrome P-450 (CYP) isoenzymes with ezetimibe is low.

● Antacids

Concomitant use of ezetimibe (10 mg) and an aluminum and magnesium hydroxides-containing antacid decreased AUC and peak plasma concentration of total ezetimibe by 4 and 30%, respectively.

● Antilipemic Agents

Bile Acid Sequestrants

Concomitant administration of cholestyramine (4 g twice daily for 14 days) and ezetimibe (10 mg) decreased the AUC and peak plasma concentration of total ezetimibe by 55 and 4%, respectively. Reduced LDL-cholesterol lowering effect may occur as a result of this interaction. Ezetimibe should be administered at least 2 hours before or at least 4 hours after administration of the bile acid sequestrant.

Fibric Acid Derivatives

Concomitant use of fenofibrate (200 mg daily for 14 days) and ezetimibe (10 mg) increased AUC and peak plasma concentration of total ezetimibe by 48 and 64%, respectively. Concomitant use of fenofibrate (200 mg daily for 14 days) and ezetimibe (10 mg daily for 14 days) increased AUC and peak plasma concentration of fenofibrate by 11 and 7%, respectively.

Concomitant use of gemfibrozil (600 mg twice daily for 7 days) and ezetimibe (10 mg) increased AUC and peak plasma concentration of total ezetimibe by 64 and 91%, respectively. Concomitant use of gemfibrozil (600 mg twice daily for 7 days) and ezetimibe (10 mg daily for 7 days) decreased AUC and peak plasma concentration of gemfibrozil by 1 and 11%, respectively.

Fibric acid derivatives may increase cholesterol excretion into bile, leading to cholelithiasis, and ezetimibe has been shown to increase cholesterol in the gall bladder bile in animals. In clinical studies, cholecystectomy has been reported in 1.7% of patients receiving ezetimibe concomitantly with fenofibrate and in 0.6% of those receiving fenofibrate monotherapy.

The efficacy and safety of concomitant use of ezetimibe with a fibric acid derivative other than fenofibrate have not been established. Such concomitant use currently is *not* recommended pending further accumulation of data from adequate study in humans. Concomitant use of the fixed combination of ezetimibe and simvastatin with gemfibrozil is contraindicated. (See Ezetimibe/Simvastatin Combination Therapy under Dosage and Administration: Dosage.) If cholelithiasis is suspected in a patient receiving ezetimibe with fenofibrate, gallbladder studies should be performed, and alternative antilipemic therapy should be considered.

Hydroxymethylglutaryl-Coenzyme A (HMG-CoA) Reductase Inhibitors (Statins)

Concomitant use of atorvastatin (10 mg daily for 14 days) and ezetimibe (10 mg) decreased AUC of total ezetimibe by 2% and increased peak plasma concentration of total ezetimibe by 12%. Concomitant use of atorvastatin (10 mg daily for 14 days) and ezetimibe (10 mg daily for 14 days) decreased AUC of atorvastatin by 4% and increased peak plasma concentration of atorvastatin by 7%.

Concomitant use of fluvastatin (20 mg daily for 14 days) and ezetimibe (10 mg) decreased AUC of total ezetimibe by 19% and increased peak plasma concentration of total ezetimibe by 7%. Concomitant use of fluvastatin (20 mg daily for 14 days) and ezetimibe (10 mg daily for 14 days) decreased AUC and peak plasma concentration of fluvastatin by 39 and 27%, respectively.

Concomitant use of lovastatin (20 mg daily for 7 days) and ezetimibe (10 mg) increased AUC and peak plasma concentration of total ezetimibe by 9 and 3%, respectively. Concomitant use of lovastatin (20 mg daily for 7 days) and ezetimibe (10 mg daily for 7 days) increased AUC and peak plasma concentration of lovastatin by 19 and 3%, respectively.

Concomitant use of pravastatin (20 mg daily for 14 days) and ezetimibe (10 mg) increased AUC and peak plasma concentration of total ezetimibe by 7 and 23%, respectively. Concomitant use of pravastatin (20 mg daily for 14 days) and ezetimibe (10 mg daily for 14 days) decreased AUC and peak plasma concentration of pravastatin by 20 and 24%, respectively.

Concomitant use of rosuvastatin (10 mg daily for 14 days) and ezetimibe (10 mg) increased AUC and peak plasma concentration of total ezetimibe by 13 and 18%, respectively. Concomitant use of rosuvastatin (10 mg daily for 14 days) and ezetimibe (10 mg daily for 14 days) increased AUC and peak plasma concentration of rosuvastatin by 19 and 17%, respectively.

Mipomersen

No clinically relevant pharmacokinetic interactions were observed when ezetimibe was used concomitantly with mipomersen. Therefore, dosage adjustment of ezetimibe and mipomersen is not necessary during such concomitant use.

Niacin

When using the fixed-combination ezetimibe/simvastatin preparation, it should be considered that cases of myopathy and rhabdomyolysis have been reported with concomitant use of simvastatin and niacin dosages of 1 g daily or greater; the risk is increased in Chinese patients. Concomitant use of simvastatin and niacin dosages of 1 g or more daily is therefore not recommended in Chinese patients.

• Cimetidine

Concomitant use of cimetidine (400 mg twice daily for 7 days) and ezetimibe (10 mg) increased AUC and peak plasma concentration of total ezetimibe by 6 and 22%, respectively.

• Cyclosporine

Concomitant use of cyclosporine (75–150 mg twice daily) and ezetimibe (10 mg) in renal transplant recipients with normal renal function or mild renal impairment increased AUC and peak plasma concentration of total ezetimibe by 3.4- and 3.9-fold, respectively. Exposure to ezetimibe may be greater in patients with severe renal insufficiency. In a renal transplant patient with severe renal impairment (creatinine clearance 13.2 mL/minute per 1.73 m^2) receiving multiple medications in addition to cyclosporine and ezetimibe, a 12-fold increase in total ezetimibe exposure occurred.

Concomitant use of cyclosporine (single 100-dose on day 7) and ezetimibe (20 mg daily for 8 days) increased AUC and peak plasma concentration of cyclosporine by 15 and 10%, respectively.

Because of increased exposure to ezetimibe and cyclosporine, caution should be exercised with concomitant use and cyclosporine concentrations should be monitored. The potential benefits versus risks of such concomitant therapy should be considered.

• Digoxin

Concomitant use of digoxin (single 0.5-mg dose) and ezetimibe (10 mg daily for 8 days) increased AUC of digoxin by 2% and decreased peak plasma concentration of digoxin by 7%.

• Fat-soluble Vitamins

Pharmacokinetic interactions with vitamins A, D, and E are unlikely.

• Glipizide

Concomitant use of glipizide (single 10-mg dose) and ezetimibe (10 mg) increased AUC of total ezetimibe by 4% and decreased peak plasma concentration of total ezetimibe by 8%. Concomitant use of glipizide (10 mg on days 1 and 9) and ezetimibe (10 mg daily on days 2–9) decreased AUC and peak plasma concentration of glipizide by 3 and 5%, respectively.

• Oral Contraceptives

Concomitant use of an oral contraceptive containing ethinyl estradiol and levonorgestrel (daily for 21 days) and ezetimibe (10 mg daily on days 8–14) decreased the peak plasma concentrations of ethinyl estradiol and levonorgestrel by 9 and 5%, respectively; AUCs of both components remained unchanged.

• Warfarin

Pharmacokinetic or pharmacodynamic interaction with ezetimibe is unlikely based on one small study. Concomitant use of warfarin (single 25-mg dose on day 7) and ezetimibe (10 mg daily for 11 days) decreased the AUCs of R- and S-warfarin by 2 and 4%, respectively, and increased peak plasma concentrations of R- and S-warfarin by 3 and 1%, respectively.

Increased international normalized ratio (INR) with concomitant use of ezetimibe and warfarin has been reported during postmarketing experience; however, most patients also were receiving other drugs. If ezetimibe is initiated in a patient receiving warfarin, the INR should be monitored.

DESCRIPTION

Ezetimibe, a cholesterol absorption inhibitor, is an antilipemic agent that differs chemically and pharmacologically from other currently available antilipemic agents. Following absorption, the drug localizes at the brush border of the small intestine and inhibits absorption of cholesterol through the sterol transporter, Niemann-Pick C1-Like 1 (NPC1L1), resulting in decreased delivery of intestinal cholesterol to the liver. This causes a reduction in hepatic cholesterol stores, a compensatory increase in hepatic uptake of cholesterol from systemic circulation, and consequently, an increase in systemic clearance of cholesterol. Ezetimibe does not appear to inhibit hepatic cholesterol synthesis or increase bile acid excretion.

Intestinal absorption of cholesterol reportedly was reduced by approximately 54% in a limited number of patients with hypercholesterolemia who received ezetimibe (10 mg daily) for 2 weeks. The cholesterol-lowering effects of ezetimibe and hydroxymethylglutaryl-coenzyme A (HMG-CoA) reductase inhibitors (statins) or of ezetimibe and fenofibrate are additive. In addition to reducing lipoprotein concentrations, ezetimibe also has been shown to reduce concentrations of noncholesterol sterols, including sitosterol and campesterol.

Ezetimibe does not appear to inhibit the absorption of triglycerides, fatty acids, bile acids, progesterone, or ethinyl estradiol. In 2 separate studies in more than 100 patients each, ezetimibe exhibited no clinically relevant effects on plasma concentrations of fat-soluble vitamins A, D, or E and did not appear to impair adrenocortical steroid production.

Following oral administration, approximately 93% of a radiolabeled dose of ezetimibe is absorbed systemically (as ezetimibe and ezetimibe glucuronide). Food does not appear to affect the extent of absorption of ezetimibe; however, concomitant administration of the drug with a high-fat meal resulted in a 38% increase in peak plasma concentrations of the drug. Following absorption, ezetimibe is rapidly and extensively metabolized in the small intestine and liver to a pharmacologically active phenolic glucuronide metabolite, ezetimibe glucuronide; the drug or its glucuronide metabolite constitutes 10–20 or 80–90%, respectively, of the total absorbed drug in plasma. Ezetimibe and ezetimibe glucuronide are more than 90% bound to human plasma proteins. The preparation containing ezetimibe in fixed combination with simvastatin is bioequivalent to corresponding dosages of the individual components.

Ezetimibe and ezetimibe glucuronide are each slowly eliminated from plasma with a half-life of approximately 22 hours. Plasma concentration-time profiles of ezetimibe exhibit multiple peaks, suggesting that the drug and its active metabolite may undergo enterohepatic recycling. Following oral administration of 20 mg of ^{14}C-ezetimibe, approximately 78 or 11% of the radioactivity was excreted in feces or urine, respectively, in 10 days; ezetimibe was the major component in feces, while ezetimibe glucuronide was the major component in urine.

Based on a meta-analysis of multiple-dose pharmacokinetic studies, there were no differences in pharmacokinetic parameters between blacks and Caucasians. Studies in Asian individuals indicated that the pharmacokinetics of ezetimibe were similar to those seen in Caucasian individuals.

ADVICE TO PATIENTS

Importance of adherence to prescribed directions for use, particularly when used concomitantly with other antilipemic agents.

Importance of adherence to a standard cholesterol-lowering diet.

Risk of myopathy and/or rhabdomyolysis; risk is increased when used concomitantly with certain other drugs or grapefruit juice. Importance of promptly informing clinicians of any unexplained muscle pain, tenderness, or weakness, particularly if accompanied by malaise or fever or if such manifestations persist after discontinuance of therapy.

Risk of adverse hepatic effects. Importance of monitoring liver function tests at initiation of ezetimibe if used in combination with a statin and thereafter in accordance with the recommendation of the statin. Importance of promptly reporting any symptoms suggestive of liver injury (e.g., fatigue, anorexia, right upper abdominal discomfort, dark urine, jaundice) when ezetimibe is used in combination with simvastatin.

Importance of women informing clinicians if they are or plan to become pregnant. Importance of advising women and adolescent girls to avoid pregnancy (i.e., using effective and appropriate contraceptive methods) and informing pregnant women of the risk to the fetus when using ezetimibe in combination with statin therapy.

Importance of avoiding breast-feeding when using ezetimibe in combination with statin therapy. If the patient has a lipid disorder and is breast-feeding, importance of contacting a clinician to discuss other antilipemic treatment options.

Importance of informing clinicians of existing or contemplated concomitant therapy, including prescription and OTC drugs, as well as concomitant illnesses.

Importance of informing patients of other important precautionary information. (See Cautions.)

PREPARATIONS

Excipients in commercially available drug preparations may have clinically important effects in some individuals; consult specific product labeling for details.

Ezetimibe

Oral		
Tablets	10 mg*	**Ezetimibe Tablets**
		Zetia®, Merck

* available from one or more manufacturer, distributor, and/or repackager by generic (nonproprietary) name

Ezetimibe Combinations

Oral		
Tablets	10 mg with Simvastatin 10 mg*	**Ezetimibe and Simvastatin Tablets Vytorin®**, Merck
	10 mg with Simvastatin 20 mg*	**Ezetimibe and Simvastatin Tablets Vytorin®**, Merck
	10 mg with Simvastatin 40 mg*	**Ezetimibe and Simvastatin Tablets Vytorin®**, Merck
	10 mg with Simvastatin 80 mg*	**Ezetimibe and Simvastatin Tablets Vytorin®**, Merck
Tablets, film-coated	10 mg with Bempedoic Acid 180 mg	**Nexlizet®**, Esperion

* available from one or more manufacturer, distributor, and/or repackager by generic (nonproprietary) name

Selected Revisions May 10, 2021, © Copyright, March 1, 2003, American Society of Health-System Pharmacists, Inc.

Isosorbide Dinitrate, Isosorbide Mononitrate

24:08.08 · NITRATES AND NITRITES

■ Isosorbide dinitrate and isosorbide mononitrate, organic nitrates, are vasodilating agents.

USES

Angina

Isosorbide dinitrate and isosorbide mononitrate share the actions of the other nitrates and nitrites. The drugs are used for the acute relief of angina pectoris, for prophylactic management in situations likely to provoke angina attacks, and for long-term prophylactic management of angina pectoris. (For further information on the use of isosorbide dinitrate and isosorbide mononitrate in the management of stable and unstable angina, see Uses: Angina in the Nitrates and Nitrites General Statement 24:12.08.)

Heart Failure

Isosorbide dinitrate is used in fixed combination with hydralazine (BiDil®) as an adjunct to standard therapy for the treatment of heart failure in self-identified black patients to improve survival, decrease rate of hospitalization for worsened heart failure, and improve patient-reported functional status. Current guidelines for the management of heart failure in adults generally recommend a combination of drug therapies to reduce morbidity and mortality, including neurohormonal antagonists (e.g., angiotensin-converting enzyme [ACE] inhibitors, angiotensin II receptor antagonists, angiotensin receptor-neprilysin inhibitors [ARNIs], β-adrenergic blocking agents [β-blockers], aldosterone receptor antagonists) that inhibit the detrimental compensatory mechanisms in heart failure. (See Uses: Heart Failure in Carvedilol 24:24 and in Sacubitril and Valsartan 24:32.92.) The combination of isosorbide dinitrate and hydralazine is recommended by the American College of Cardiology Foundation (ACCF) and American Heart Association (AHA) for self-identified black patients with New York Heart Association (NYHA) functional class III or IV heart failure and reduced ejection fraction who are receiving optimal therapy with ACE inhibitors and β-blockers (unless contraindicated). ACCF and AHA also state that combined therapy with isosorbide dinitrate and hydralazine may be considered in patients with current or prior symptomatic heart failure and reduced ejection fraction who cannot receive an ACE inhibitor or angiotensin II receptor antagonist† because of drug intolerance, hypotension, or renal insufficiency. For further information on the use of isosorbide dinitrate in the management of heart failure, see Uses: Heart Failure and Low-output Syndromes in the Nitrates and Nitrites General Statement 24:12.08.

Diffuse Esophageal Spasm

In a limited number of patients with diffuse esophageal spasm without gastroesophageal reflux†, isosorbide dinitrate has been used effectively to relieve pain, dysphagia, and spasm.

DOSAGE AND ADMINISTRATION

Administration

Isosorbide Dinitrate

Isosorbide dinitrate is administered sublingually, intrabuccally, or orally. The possibility that sublingual or intrabuccal nitrates may be inadequately absorbed, with resultant decreased efficacy, in patients with dry oral mucous membranes (e.g., xerostomia) should be considered. Chewable tablets (no longer commercially available in the US) should be chewed thoroughly before swallowing. Extended-release preparations should *not* be chewed. The patient should be sitting immediately after administration of isosorbide dinitrate sublingually or as a chewable tablet.

Isosorbide Mononitrate

Isosorbide mononitrate is administered orally. Isosorbide mononitrate extended-release tablets can be administered as whole or halved tablets, but these should be swallowed intact and not chewed or crushed. In addition, isosorbide extended-release tablets should be administered with adequate amounts of fluid (e.g., 120 mL) on arising in the morning.

Dosage

Dosage of isosorbide dinitrate and isosorbide mononitrate must be carefully adjusted according to the patient's requirements and response and the smallest effective dosage should be used.

When isosorbide dinitrate is used in fixed combination with hydralazine, the cautions, precautions, and contraindications associated with hydralazine must be considered in addition to those associated with isosorbide dinitrate (see Cautions and Precautions and Contraindications in the Nitrates and Nitrites General Statement 24:12.08).

Clinical studies of isosorbide dinitrate alone or in fixed combination with hydralazine did not include sufficient numbers of patients 65 years of age and older to determine whether geriatric patients respond differently than younger patients. Although other clinical experience has not revealed age-related differences in response or tolerance, drug dosage generally should be titrated carefully in geriatric patients, usually initiating therapy at the low end of the dosage range. The greater frequency of decreased hepatic, renal, and/or cardiac function and of concomitant disease and drug therapy observed in the elderly also should be considered. Elimination of isosorbide dinitrate and its metabolites may occur more slowly in geriatric patients than in younger adults.

Clinical studies of isosorbide mononitrate did not include sufficient numbers of patients 65 years of age and older to determine whether geriatric patients respond differently than younger patients. Other clinical experience has not identified any differences in responses between geriatric and younger patients. One manufacturer of isosorbide mononitrate states that if isosorbide mononitrate is used in geriatric patients, dosage of the drug should be selected with caution, usually initiating therapy at the low end of the dosage range, although age, renal, hepatic, and cardiovascular dysfunction do not appear to have a significant effect on the clearance of the drug.

Angina

Acute Symptomatic Relief and Prophylactic Management

For the acute relief of angina pectoris or for prophylactic management in situations likely to provoke angina attacks in patients who fail to respond to nitroglycerin lingual or sublingual preparations, 2.5–5 mg of isosorbide dinitrate is administered sublingually, intrabuccally, or as a chewable tablet (no longer commercially available in the US). If relief is not attained after a single dose during an acute attack, additional doses may be given at 5- to 10-minute intervals; no more than 3 doses should be given in a 15- to 30- minute period.

For the prophylactic management in situations likely to provoke angina attacks in patients who fail to respond to sublingual nitroglycerin, 2.5–5 mg of isosorbide dinitrate should be placed under the tongue approximately 15 minutes prior to engaging in such activities.

Since the onset of action of extended-release preparations containing isosorbide dinitrate or any preparation containing isosorbide mononitrate is not sufficiently rapid to be efficacious in aborting an acute anginal episode, such preparations are not indicated for use in the management of acute relief of angina or in the prophylactic management in situations likely to provoke angina attacks.

Long-term Prophylactic Management

For long-term prophylactic management of angina pectoris, the usual initial dosage of oral isosorbide dinitrate conventional tablets (e. g., Isordil® Titradose®) is 5–20 mg administered 2 or 3 times daily. The usual recommended maintenance dosage is 10–40 mg 2 or 3 times daily, although some patients may require higher dosages. Some clinicians recommend that such dosages be administered at 7 a.m., 12 p.m., and 5 p.m. in most patients with chronic stable angina or at 7 a.m. and 12 p.m. in patients with less severe symptoms of angina in order to allow for a nitrate-free interval of 10–14 hours. Patients who arise earlier than 7 a.m. may need to adjust this schedule since early morning angina is common. There is some evidence that less frequent administration of isosorbide dinitrate in patients with angina pectoris may reduce the development of tolerance to the drug's antianginal effects (see Cautions: Tolerance and Dependence, in the Nitrates and Nitrites General Statement). In addition, the manufacturer of isosorbide dinitrate extended-release capsules (Dilatrate®-SR) states that results of the only multiple-dose study performed using an extended-release preparation of isosorbide dinitrate indicate that when these extended-release capsules were given twice daily (6 hours apart), the antianginal efficacy of the drug after 4 weeks of therapy was comparable to that of placebo. This manufacturer also states that an interdosing interval sufficient to avoid tolerance with these extended-release capsules is not known, but it must exceed 18 hours. The maximum daily dosages of Dilatrate® should not exceed 160 mg (4 capsules).

Alternatively, conventional or extended-release tablets of isosorbide mononitrate may be used for long-term prophylactic management of angina. The usual initial dosage of conventional isosorbide mononitrate tablets (e.g., Ismo®, Monoket®) is 20 mg twice daily, with the 2 doses administered 7 hours apart. Patients of particularly small stature may receive initial dosages of 5 mg (administered as one-half of a 10-mg tablet) twice daily, but since such a lower dosage is only effective (as determined by exercise tolerance) on the first day of therapy, the dosage should be increased to at least 10 mg twice daily by the second or third day of therapy. The recommended initial dosage of the extended-release isosorbide mononitrate tablets (e.g., Imdur®) is 30 (administered as a single 30-mg tablet or as one-half of a 60-mg tablet) or 60 mg (administered as a single 60-mg tablet) once daily. Dosage may be increased to 120 mg (administered as a single 120-mg tablet or as two 60-mg tablets) once daily after several days of therapy; dosages of 240 mg of these extended-release tablets are rarely needed.

Heart Failure

For the adjunctive treatment of heart failure in self-identified black patients, the recommended initial dosage of the fixed-combination preparation is 20 mg of isosorbide dinitrate and 37.5 mg of hydralazine hydrochloride (1 tablet of BiDil®) 3 times daily. The dosage may be titrated to a maximum tolerated dosage, not to exceed 2 tablets (a total of 40 mg of isosorbide dinitrate and 75 mg of hydralazine hydrochloride) 3 times daily. Although rapid titration (over 3–5 days) of dosage can be undertaken, slower titration may be needed in some patients who experience adverse effects. In patients who experience intolerable adverse effects, the dosage may be decreased to as little as one-half of the fixed-combination tablet 3 times daily; however, an attempt should be made to titrate the dosage up once the adverse effects subside.

If the drugs are administered separately in the treatment of heart failure†, an initial dosage of isosorbide dinitrate 20–30 mg 3 or 4 times daily, given concomitantly with hydralazine hydrochloride 25–50 mg 3 or 4 times daily, is recommended by the American College of Cardiology Foundation (ACCF) and American Heart Association (AHA). Dosages of the drugs should be titrated to levels similar to those recommended for the fixed-combination preparation and administered at least 3 times daily. The maximum recommended dosages are isosorbide dinitrate 120 mg daily and hydralazine hydrochloride 300 mg daily.

Diffuse Esophageal Spasm

In a limited number of patients with diffuse esophageal spasm without gastroesophageal reflux†, 10–30 mg of isosorbide dinitrate has been given orally 4 times daily.

PHARMACOKINETICS

● Absorption

Isosorbide dinitrate is readily (and almost completely) absorbed from the GI tract and oral mucosa, but considerable variations in the bioavailability of the drug (10–90%) have been reported as a result of extensive first-pass metabolism in the liver. The bioavailability of isosorbide dinitrate, as unchanged drug, following oral administration of conventional tablets (25%) generally appears to be about half that following sublingual administration (40–50%); however, in one study,

systemic bioavailability of the drug was similar (about 29%) for both oral conventional tablets and sublingual tablets. It has been suggested that the reduced bioavailability of sublingual tablets of isosorbide dinitrate may result from swallowing a portion of the drug dissolved from such tablets, possibly because absorption of the drug is slow relative to the time that a sublingual dose might reasonably be retained in the mouth. Although multiple-dose studies of isosorbide dinitrate sublingual tablets have not been conducted, multiple-dose studies of isosorbide dinitrate oral conventional tablets indicate that progressive increases in bioavailability may occur during chronic therapy.

Although some evidence suggests that systemic bioavailability of isosorbide dinitrate from extended-release oral tablets is similar but slightly less than that from conventional oral tablets, other evidence suggests that considerable variability exists for various extended-release preparations and that some preparations may be substantially less bioavailable than conventional tablets. Because pharmacologic effects of the drug also depend on serum concentrations of active metabolites (e.g., isosorbide-5-mononitrate, isosorbide-2-mononitrate), comparisons should extend beyond systemic bioavailability of unchanged drug alone. Unfortunately, many studies do not specify or provide incomplete data on these metabolites. In addition, although most studies have employed single doses, the pharmacokinetics and/or bioavailability of the drug may be affected substantially during multiple dosing because the metabolites may decrease the metabolic clearance of isosorbide dinitrate; therefore, predictions based on single-dose studies are uncertain.

Although food may decrease substantially mean peak plasma concentrations of isosorbide dinitrate, total bioavailability of the drug does not seem to be affected.

Considerable interindividual variations (approximately 5- to 11-fold) in peak plasma concentrations attained have been reported with a specific oral dose of isosorbide dinitrate. Following administration of isosorbide dinitrate as sublingual or conventional oral tablets, peak plasma isosorbide dinitrate concentrations are reached in 10–15 or 60 minutes, respectively. Elevated blood concentrations of isosorbide dinitrate have been observed in patients with cirrhosis.

Isosorbide mononitrate also is readily absorbed from the GI tract. Because isosorbide mononitrate, unlike isosorbide dinitrate, does not undergo first-pass hepatic metabolism, the bioavailability of isosorbide mononitrate conventional or extended-release tablets is approximately 100 or 77–80%, respectively.

In general, food was found to delay the rate but not the extent of absorption (less than 10%) of conventional or extended-release isosorbide mononitrate tablets. Following oral administration of conventional or extended-release isosorbide mononitrate tablets, peak plasma concentrations of isosorbide mononitrate are achieved within 0.5–1 or about 3–4.5 hours, respectively. In one study, following oral administration of a 40-mg conventional isosorbide mononitrate tablet in fasted healthy individuals, mean peak plasma concentrations of about 930 ng/mL were achieved within about 1 hour. In addition, in another study, following oral administration of a 60- or 120-mg extended-release tablet of isosorbide mononitrate in healthy individuals, peak plasma concentrations of about 557 or 1151 ng/mL were achieved within about 3 hours, respectively.

Following oral administration of a single 40-mg dose of isosorbide dinitrate given in fixed combination with 75 mg of hydralazine hydrochloride (2 tablets of BiDil®) in a limited number of healthy adults, peak plasma isosorbide concentrations of 76 ng/mL per 65 kg were reached in 1 hour. The effect of food on the bioavailability of isosorbide dinitrate when administered in fixed combination with hydralazine hydrochloride is not known.

Although optimal therapeutic plasma concentrations have not been determined, it has been suggested that the therapeutic plasma concentration of isosorbide mononitrate (both for the management of angina and heart failure) is 100 ng/mL. In addition, evidence from clinical studies of isosorbide dinitrate and isosorbide mononitrate have shown that dosing regimens that result in plasma isosorbide mononitrate concentrations that fall below 100 ng/L prior to the administration of the next dose may be associated with a lower risk of developing tolerance.

The approximate onset and duration of action of various dosage forms of isosorbide dinitrate (ISDN) and isosorbide mononitrate (ISMN) are shown in Table 1 and Table 2.

TABLE 1. Antianginal Effects

Dosage Form	Onset	Duration
sublingual ISDN	within 3 min	2 h
chewable ISDN	within 3 min	2–2.5 h
oral ISDN	1 h	up to 8 h
oral ISMN	1 h	5–7 h
extended-release ISDN	1 h	8 h
extended-release ISMN	1 h	12 h

TABLE 2. Hemodynamic Effects

Dosage Form	Onset	Duration
sublingual ISDN	within 15–30 min	1.5–4 h
chewable ISDN	5 min	2–3 h
oral ISDN	within 20–60 min	4–6 h
oral ISMN	10–30 min	at least 6 h
extended-release ISDN	within 2 h	up to 12 h
extended-release ISMN	20–30 min	at least 6 h

The onset and duration of action following intrabuccal administration are probably similar to those after sublingual administration of isosorbide dinitrate; however, no studies are available.

● Distribution

Distribution of isosorbide dinitrate or isosorbide mononitrate into human body tissues and fluids has not been fully characterized. Once absorbed, isosorbide dinitrate is widely distributed into body tissues and fluids including smooth muscle cells of blood vessels with the apparent volume of distribution reported to be 2–4 L/kg in adults. Under steady-state conditions, substantial accumulation (relative to simultaneous plasma concentrations) of isosorbide dinitrate may occur in the pectoral muscle and saphenous vein walls. Following IV administration, isosorbide mononitrate is distributed into total body water in about 9 minutes with an apparent volume of distribution of approximately 0.6–0.7 L/kg in adults. Isosorbide mononitrate also is distributed into blood cells and saliva.

Isosorbide dinitrate and isosorbide mononitrate are approximately 28 and 4–5% bound to plasma proteins, respectively.

Although isosorbide dinitrate reportedly was detected in milk, it currently is not known if isosorbide dinitrate and isosorbide mononitrate are distributed into milk in humans.

● Elimination

The elimination half-life of isosorbide dinitrate is approximately 1 hour (although a longer half-life [about 2 hours] has been reported when administered in fixed combination with hydralazine hydrochloride). Isosorbide mononitrate has an elimination half-life of about 5 hours.

Isosorbide dinitrate is metabolized (denitrated) extensively; about 15–25 and 75–85% of a dose is metabolized to isosorbide-2-mononitrate and isosorbide-5-mononitrate (referred to simply as isosorbide mononitrate), respectively. Both metabolites are pharmacologically active, especially the isosorbide mononitrate.

Isosorbide mononitrate is metabolized principally in the liver, but unlike isosorbide dinitrate, it does not undergo first-pass metabolism. About 50% of a dose of isosorbide mononitrate undergoes denitration to form isosorbide, followed by partial dehydration to form sorbitol. Isosorbide mononitrate also appears to undergo glucuronidation to form the 5-mononitrate glucuronide. These metabolites apparently do not have pharmacologic activity.

After a single oral dose of isosorbide dinitrate, 80–100% of the amount is excreted in urine within 24 hours, chiefly as metabolites. Isosorbide mononitrate also is excreted mainly in the urine; compounds recovered in urine after isosorbide mononitrate administration have included isosorbide, sorbitol, and conjugates; only 2% of a dose is excreted as unchanged drug. About 96% of an administered dose of isosorbide mononitrate is excreted in urine and about 1% in feces within 5 days; most excretion (about 93%) occurs within 48 hours.

The plasma clearance of isosorbide dinitrate reportedly is 2–4 L/minute. Since plasma clearance exceeds hepatic blood flow, it appears that the drug also is metabolized at extrahepatic sites.

Renal clearance of isosorbide mononitrate accounts only for about 4% of total body clearance. Plasma clearance of isosorbide mononitrate does not appear to be affected by age, cardiac disease, or renal or hepatic impairment. Isosorbide mononitrate is substantially removed by hemodialysis.

CHEMISTRY AND STABILITY

● Chemistry

Isosorbide is commercially available as dinitrate and mononitrate organic salts. Organic nitrates (e.g., isosorbide dinitrate, isosorbide mononitrate) are powerful explosives that are rendered nonexplosive by the addition of an inert excipient such as lactose.

● Isosorbide Dinitrate

Isosorbide dinitrate occurs as a white to off-white, crystalline powder. Isosorbide dinitrate is sparingly soluble in water and freely soluble in alcohol. The drug is diluted with lactose, mannitol, or other suitable inert excipients to permit safe handling. Diluted isosorbide dinitrate occurs as an ivory-white, odorless powder.

Isosorbide dinitrate is commercially available as conventional tablets (e.g., Sorbitrate® and Isordil® Titradose®), extended-release capsules (e.g., Dilatrate®-SR), extended-release tablets, and sublingual-intrabuccal (e.g., Isordil®) tablets. The commercially available extended-release capsules of isosorbide dinitrate (Dilatrate-SR®) contain the drug in a microdialysis membrane delivery system that slowly releases the drug.

● Isosorbide Mononitrate

Isosorbide mononitrate is the major active metabolite of isosorbide dinitrate. Isosorbide mononitrate occurs as a white, crystalline, odorless powder, and is freely soluble in water and alcohol.

The drug is commercially available as conventional (e.g., Monoket®, Ismo®) or extended-release (e.g., Imdur®) tablets. The commercially available extended-release isosorbide mononitrate tablets contain the drug in an insoluble matrix designed for extended release. Isosorbide mononitrate also may be available as extended-release capsules (not commercially available in the US) that contain 30% of the drug in an immediate-release layer and the remaining 70% in controlled-release coated pellets.

● Stability

Isosorbide Dinitrate

Isosorbide dinitrate tablets should be stored in tight, light-resistant containers at room temperature (25°C) and should not be exposed to extremes in temperature. Commercially available fixed-combination tablets of isosorbide dinitrate and hydralazine hydrochloride should be stored in tight, light-resistant containers at a controlled room temperature of 25°C but may be exposed to temperatures ranging from 15–30°C.

Isosorbide Mononitrate

Some isosorbide mononitrate extended-release (Imdur®) and conventional tablets (Ismo®) should be stored in tight, light-resistant containers at 20–25°C; however, other conventional tablets of isosorbide mononitrate (e.g., Monoket®) should be stored in tight, light-resistant containers at 15–30°C.

PREPARATIONS

Excipients in commercially available drug preparations may have clinically important effects in some individuals; consult specific product labeling for details.

Isosorbide Dinitrate

Oral

Capsules, extended-release	40 mg	**Dilatrate®-SR, Schwarz**
Tablets	5 mg*	**Isordil® Titradose® (scored), Biovail**
		Isosorbide Dinitrate Tablets
	10 mg*	**Isosorbide Dinitrate Tablets**
	20 mg*	**Isosorbide Dinitrate Tablets**
	30 mg*	**Isosorbide Dinitrate Tablets**
	40 mg*	**Isordil® Titradose® (scored), Biovail**
Tablets, extended-release	40 mg*	**Isosorbide Dinitrate Tablets ER**

Sublingual-intrabuccal

Tablets	2.5 mg*	**Isosorbide Dinitrate Tablets**
	5 mg*	**Isosorbide Dinitrate Tablets**

* available from one or more manufacturer, distributor, and/or repackager by generic (nonproprietary) name

Isosorbide Mononitrate

Oral

Tablets	10 mg*	**Isosorbide Mononitrate Tablets**
		Monoket® (scored), Schwarz
	20 mg*	**Isosorbide Mononitrate Tablets**
		Monoket® (scored), Schwarz
Tablets, extended-release	30 mg*	**Imdur® (scored), Schering-Plough**
		Isosorbide Mononitrate Tablets ER
	60 mg*	**Imdur® (scored), Schering-Plough**
		Isosorbide Mononitrate Tablets ER
	120 mg*	**Imdur®, Schering-Plough**
		Isosorbide Mononitrate Tablets ER
Tablets, extended-release, film-coated	20 mg	**Ismo®, ESP Pharma**

* available from one or more manufacturer, distributor, and/or repackager by generic (nonproprietary) name

Isosorbide Dinitrate Combinations

Oral

Tablets, film-coated	20 mg with Hydralazine Hydrochloride 37.5 mg	**BiDil® (scored), NitroMed**

† Use is not currently included in the labeling approved by the US Food and Drug Administration.

Selected Revisions April 10, 2024, © Copyright, June 1, 1979, American Society of Health-System Pharmacists, Inc.

Nitroglycerin

24:08.08 · NITRATES AND NITRITES

- Nitroglycerin, an organic nitrate, is a vasodilating agent.

USES

● Angina

Nitroglycerin is used for the acute relief of angina pectoris secondary to coronary artery disease, for prophylactic management in situations likely to provoke angina attacks, and for long-term prophylactic management of chronic stable angina. The drug is commercially available in various dosage forms and preparations. Short-acting preparations (e.g., sublingual tablets, lingual aerosol) are used for acute relief of angina, but also may be used for prophylactic management in situations likely to provoke an angina attack. The ointment and transdermal preparations are indicated for the prevention of angina due to coronary artery disease; the onset of action of these dosage forms is not sufficiently rapid enough to abort an acute anginal episode.

Chronic Coronary Disease

Guidelines for the management of patients with chronic coronary disease have been published by the American Heart Association (AHA), American College of Cardiology (ACC), and other experts. The guidelines recommend antianginal therapy with either a β-blocker, a calcium channel blocker, or a long-acting nitrate for relief of angina in patients with chronic coronary disease. Sublingual nitroglycerin or nitroglycerin spray is recommended for immediate short-term relief of angina. Studies comparing nitroglycerin spray with the sublingual formulation have shown the spray to be more effective and efficient at relieving angina with less headache.

Non-ST-Segment-Elevation Acute Coronary Syndromes

Nitroglycerin is used for relief of angina in patients with non-ST-segment-elevation acute coronary syndromes (NSTE ACS). Patients with NSTE ACS have either unstable angina or non-ST-segment-elevation MI (NSTEMI); because these conditions are part of a continuum of acute myocardial ischemia and have indistinguishable clinical features upon presentation, the same initial treatment strategies are recommended. The American Heart Association/American College of Cardiology (AHA/ACC) guideline for the management of patients with NSTE ACS recommends sublingual nitroglycerin (0.3–0.4 mg every 5 minutes for up to 3 doses) for the relief of ongoing ischemic pain in patients with NSTE ACS; IV nitroglycerin may be used in patients with persistent ischemia who do not respond to sublingual therapy and administration of a β-blocker or those with heart failure or hypertension. Topical nitrates may be used as an alternative to IV nitroglycerin for patients who do not have refractory or recurrent ischemia. Nitrates should not be administered to patients with hypotension or those who have received a phosphodiesterase inhibitor, and should be used with caution in patients with right ventricular infarction.

ST-Segment Elevation Myocardial Infarction (STEMI)

Nitroglycerin is used for the management of ongoing chest pain in patients with STEMI. Nitroglycerin injection is specifally indicated for control of congestive heart failure (CHF) in the setting of acute MI. The American College of Cardiology Foundation/American Heart Association (ACCF/AHA) guideline for the management of STEMI states that IV nitroglycerin may be beneficial in patients with STEMI and heart failure or hypertension. The manufacturer of some other formulations of nitroglycerin state that the benefits of these formulations in patients with acute MI or CHF have not been established; if the drug is used in this setting, careful hemodynamic and clinical monitoring is essential because of the possibility of hypotension and tachycardia. In addition to potentially alleviating ischemic myocardial pain, beneficial hemodynamic effects of nitroglycerin include vasodilation of the coronary arteries (especially at or near the site of recent plaque disruption), peripheral arteries, and venous capacitance vessels; however, the drug generally does not reduce myocardial injury associated with epicardial coronary artery occlusion unless there is substantial vasospasm. Although studies conducted prior to the routine use of reperfusion therapy suggested a mortality benefit with nitrates in patients with acute MI, this benefit was not confirmed in 2 large randomized controlled studies.

● Hypertension

IV nitroglycerin is used for the treatment of perioperative hypertension and for induction of intraoperative hypotension.

IV nitroglycerin also has been used to control blood pressure in perioperative hypertension, especially hypertension associated with cardiovascular procedures; to control blood pressure in patients with severe hypertension† or in hypertensive crises† for the immediate reduction of blood pressure in patients in whom such reduction is considered an emergency (hypertensive emergencies), especially those associated with coronary complications (e.g., coronary ischemia, acute coronary insufficiency, acute left ventricular failure, postoperative hypertension [especially following coronary bypass surgery]) and/or acute pulmonary edema; and to produce controlled hypotension during surgical procedures.

Hypertensive emergencies are those rare situations requiring immediate blood pressure reduction, although not necessarily to normal ranges, in order to prevent or limit target organ damage. Examples of such emergency situations include hypertensive encephalopathy, intracerebral hemorrhage, unstable angina pectoris, acute myocardial infarction (MI), acute left ventricular failure with pulmonary edema, dissecting aortic aneurysm, and eclampsia. Elevated blood pressure alone, in the absence of symptoms or new or progressive target organ damage, rarely is a hypertensive crisis requiring emergency therapy.

● Heart Failure and Low-output Syndromes

IV nitroglycerin has been used effectively for the treatment of acutely decompensated (e.g., congestive) heart failure† or other low cardiac output states†, including those associated with acute MI. (See ST-Segment Elevation Myocardial Infarction [STEMI] undr Uses.) The precipitating cause of acute heart failure decompensation should be carefully assessed to inform appropriate treatment, optimize outcomes, and prevent future acute events in patients with heart failure. Current guidelines for the management of heart failure in adults generally recommend inhibition of the renin-angiotensin-aldosterone system with a combination of drug therapies, including neurohormonal antagonists (e.g., angiotensin-converting enzyme [ACE] inhibitors, angiotensin II receptor antagonists, angiotensin receptor-neprilysin inhibitors [ARNIs], β-adrenergic blocking agents [β-blockers], aldosterone receptor antagonists), to inhibit the detrimental compensatory mechanisms in heart failure and reduce morbidity and mortality. IV vasodilators have not been shown to improve outcomes in patients hospitalized for heart failure; however, in the absence of symptomatic hypotension, IV nitroglycerin may be considered as an adjunct to diuretic therapy for relief of dyspnea in patients hospitalized for acutely decompensated heart failure. IV nitroglycerin causes venodilation, which lowers preload and may help to rapidly reduce pulmonary congestion. Patients with heart failure and hypertension, coronary ischemia, or substantial mitral regurgitation are often considered ideal candidates for the use of IV nitroglycerin. However, tachyphylaxis to nitroglycerin may develop within 24 hours, and up to 20% of those with heart failure may have inadequate response to even high doses.

DOSAGE AND ADMINISTRATION

● Administration

Nitroglycerin is administered lingually, sublingually, topically, or by IV infusion.

Sublingual and Lingual Administration

Nitroglycerin tablets for sublingual administration are dissolved under the tongue and should not be swallowed.

Nitroglycerin lingual preparations (aerosol or solution in a spray pump) are administered using a metered-dose spray pump; the aerosol or solution should be administered onto or under the tongue and not inhaled. Do not expectorate the drug or rinse the mouth for 5–10 minutes following administration. The possibility that lingual or sublingual nitroglycerin may be inadequately absorbed, with resultant decreased efficacy, in patients with dry oral mucous membranes (e.g., xerostomia) should be considered.

Transdermal Administration (Transdermal System)

Nitroglycerin transdermal system is preferably applied at the same time each day to areas of clean, dry, hairless skin of the upper arm or body; the system should not be applied to the extremities below the knee or elbow. Skin areas with irritation, extensive scarring, or calluses should be avoided, and application sites should be rotated to avoid causing skin irritation. Nitroglycerin transdermal systems should be removed from the site(s) of application prior to attempting defibrillation or cardioversion since altered electrical conductivity and enhanced potential for electrical arcing may occur.

Topical Administration (Ointment)

When applied topically as an ointment, the appropriate amount of nitroglycerin ointment should be squeezed onto the manufacturer-supplied applicator and placed ointment side down on the desired non-hairy area of skin (usually on the chest or back). The ointment is then spread on the skin area in a thin, uniform layer without massaging or rubbing and using the applicator to prevent absorption of the ointment through the fingers. Using the size of the applicator to measure the coverage area allows the ointment to be absorbed through a smaller area of skin than that used in clinical trials; the clinical importance of this difference is not known. The applicator should be taped into place after application. To protect clothing, plastic wrap held in place by an elastic bandage, hosiery, or tape may be used to cover the ointment applicator. Application of the ointment over the chest may provide an additional psychological effect. As with transdermal nitroglycerin systems, nitroglycerin ointment has been reported to alter electrical conductivity, and some clinicians suggest that areas of the chest where defibrillation paddles typically are placed not be used for application of the ointment if possible.

IV Administration

The commercially available injection concentrate must be diluted in 5% dextrose or 0.9% sodium chloride injection before administration. The drug should be diluted and stored only in glass bottles; avoid using filters since some filters absorb nitroglycerin. Nitroglycerin also is commercially available as a premixed solution in 5% dextrose injection for IV administration. *Because nitroglycerin readily migrates into many plastics, the manufacturers' specific instructions for dilution, dosage, and administration must be carefully followed.*

Nitroglycerin injection should not be admixed with other drugs.

Standardize 4 Safety

Standardized concentrations for IV nitroglycerin have been established through Standardize 4 Safety (S4S), a national patient safety initiative to reduce medication errors, especially during transitions of care. Multidisciplinary expert panels were convened to determine recommended standard concentrations. Because recommendations from the S4S panels may differ from the manufacturer's prescribing information, caution is advised when using concentrations that differ from labeling, particularly when using rate information from the label. For additional information on S4S (including updates that may be available), see https://www.ashp.org/pharmacy-practice/standardize-4-safety-initiative.

TABLE 1. Standardize 4 Safety Continuous IV Infusion Standard Concentrations for Nitroglycerin

Patient Population	Concentration Standards	Dosing Units
Adults	200 mcg/mL	mcg/min
Pediatric patients (<50 kg)	200 mcg/mL	mcg/kg/min
	400 mcg/mL	

● Dosage

Dosage of nitroglycerin must be carefully adjusted according to the patient's requirements and response and the smallest effective dosage should be used. When nitroglycerin is administered IV, the type of IV administration set used, polyvinyl chloride (PVC) or non-PVC, must be considered in dosage estimations. *It should be noted that dosages commonly used in early published studies were based on the use of PVC administration sets and are too high when non-PVC administration sets are used.*

Continuous monitoring of blood pressure and heart rate, as well as other appropriate parameters (e.g., pulmonary capillary wedge pressure), must be performed in all patients. Adequate systemic blood pressure and coronary perfusion pressure must be maintained. Some patients with normal or low left ventricular filling pressures or pulmonary capillary wedge pressure may be extremely sensitive to the effects of IV nitroglycerin and may respond fully to dosages as low as 5 mcg/minute; these patients require particularly careful monitoring and dosage titration.

Angina

Lingual Dosage

For the acute relief of angina pectoris, 1 or 2 sprays (0.4 or 0.8 mg, respectively) of nitroglycerin as a lingual solution or aerosol may be administered. If relief is not attained after the initial spray(s), additional single sprays may be given at 5-minute intervals as necessary; no more than 3 sprays should be given in a 15-minute period. If pain persists after a total of 3 doses within a 15-minute period, prompt medical attention is recommended. Nitroglycerin lingual solution or aerosol also may be used prophylactically 5–10 minutes before situations likely to provoke angina attacks.

Sublingual Dosage

For the acute relief of angina pectoris, the manufacturer recommends 0.3–0.6 mg of nitroglycerin as sublingual tablets, placed under the tongue and allowed to dissolve at the first sign of an acute attack. Most patients respond within 5 minutes of taking 1 or 2 doses. If relief is not attained after a single dose during an acute attack, additional doses may be given at 5-minute intervals. If chest pain persists after a total of 3 doses within a 15-minute period, or if the pain is different from the pain that is typically experienced, patients should be advised to seek prompt medical attention. For prophylactic management in situations likely to provoke angina attacks, nitroglycerin sublingual tablets may be administered 5–10 minutes prior to engaging in such activities.

Transdermal and Topical Dosage

When a nitroglycerin transdermal system is used for the long-term prophylactic management of angina pectoris, the usual initial adult dosage is one transdermal dosage system, delivering the smallest available dose of nitroglycerin in its dosage series, applied every 24 hours. To minimize the occurrence of tolerance to the effects of nitroglycerin, a nitrate-free interval of 10–14 hours has been recommended; however, the minimum nitrate-free interval necessary for restoration of full first-dose effects of nitrate therapy has not been determined. Dosage may be adjusted by changing to the next larger dosage system in the series or by a combination of dosage systems in the series. The transdermal systems should *not* be used to treat acute attacks of angina.

When nitroglycerin is applied topically as an ointment, a suggested initial dosage is 0.5 inch (as squeezed from the tube) of the 2% ointment (i.e., approximately 7.5 mg) applied twice daily (once upon arising in the morning and repeated 6 hours later). When the dose to be applied is in multiples of whole inches, unit-dose preparations that provide the equivalent of 1 inch of the 2% ointment also may be used. The initial dose may be doubled (i.e., increased to 1 inch or approximately 15 mg) and subsequently doubled again (i.e., increased to 2 inches or approximately 30 mg) if tolerated in patients failing to respond adequately. Doses used in clinical trials have ranged from 0.5–2 inches (approximately 7.5–30 mg). Dosage should be titrated upward until angina is effectively controlled or adverse effects preclude further dosage increases.

The amount of nitroglycerin reaching the circulation varies directly with the size of the area of application and the amount of ointment applied. Coverage of an area approximately the size of the applicator (3.5 by 2.25 inches) should be sufficient to obtain the desired clinical effects, however, a larger area may be used. In clinical trials, the ointment generally has been spread over an area of 6 by 6 inches.

As with other nitroglycerin formulations, all regimens of nitroglycerin ointment should include a daily nitrate-free interval to avoid development of tolerance. It is not known whether nitroglycerin ointment is effective in preventing exertional angina for longer than 7 hours after application of a dose.

The onset of action of topical nitroglycerin ointment is not sufficiently rapid to treat acute attacks of angina; therefore, the ointment should *not* be used for this purpose.

IV Dosage

The recommended initial adult IV dosage when non-PVC administration sets are used is 5 mcg/minute, with increases of 5 mcg/minute every 3–5 minutes until a blood pressure response is obtained or until the infusion rate is 20 mcg/minute. If no effect is obtained with 20 mcg/minute, dosage may be increased by increments of 10 mcg/minute and if later necessary, by increments of 20 mcg/minute. When PVC administration sets are used, higher dosages generally are required; the usual initial adult dosage when these sets are used is 25 mcg/minute. Dosage is then titrated according to the response and tolerance of the patient.

Non-ST-Segment-Elevation Acute Coronary Syndromes

Sublingual Dosage

For the treatment of continuing ischemic pain in patients with non-ST-segment-elevation acute coronary syndromes (NSTE ACS), sublingual nitroglycerin 0.3–0.4 mg every 5 minutes for up to 3 doses is recommended.

IV Dosage

Following use of sublingual nitroglycerin, the need for IV nitroglycerin should be assessed, if not contraindicated; experts state that IV nitroglycerin may be useful in patients with heart failure, hypertension, or persistent ischemia not relieved with sublingual nitroglycerin and administration of a β-blocker.

The recommended initial adult IV dosage of nitroglycerin when a nonadsorptive (e.g., non-PVC) administration set is used is 5 mcg/minute, with increases of 5 mcg/minute every 3–5 minutes until a blood pressure response is obtained or until the infusion rate is 20 mcg/minute. If no effect is obtained with 20 mcg/minute, dosage may be increased by increments of 10 mcg/minute and, if necessary, by increments of 20 mcg/minute. When a PVC administration set is used, higher dosages generally are required; the usual initial adult dosage when these sets are used is 25 mcg/minute. Dosage should be titrated according to the patient's response. Blood pressure and heart rate should be continuously monitored during IV administration.

ST-Segment Elevation Myocardial Infarction (STEMI)

IV Dosage

When IV nitroglycerin is used after acute MI, some experts recommend an initial continuous IV infusion rate of 10 mcg/minute, increasing the dosage as necessary according to hemodynamic and clinical response. Dosage will vary considerably among patients and should be adjusted based on individual requirements, blood pressure response, and adverse effects. The manufacturer states that the usual initial adult dosage of nitroglycerin when a nonadsorptive (e.g., non-PVC) administration set is used is 5 mcg/minute; the rate may be increased by 5 mcg/minute every 3–5 minutes until blood pressure response is obtained or the infusion rate is 20 mcg/minute. If no effect is obtained with 20 mcg/minute, dosage may be further increased by increments of 10 mcg/minute and, if necessary, by increments of 20 mcg/minute. When a PVC administration set is used, higher dosages generally are required; the usual initial adult dosage when these sets are used is 25 mcg/minute. Dosage should then be titrated according to the patient's response. Blood pressure and heart rate should be continuously monitored during IV administration.

Continuous IV infusions of nitroglycerin have been given for 12 hours with no attenuation of effect.

Hypertension

IV Dosage

When nitroglycerin is used to control perioperative hypertension or for the induction of intraoperative hypotension, the manufacturer recommends an initial adult IV dosage (using a nonadsorptive [e.g., non-PVC] administration set) of 5 mcg/minute, with increases of 5 mcg/minute every 3–5 minutes until a blood pressure response is obtained or an infusion rate of 20 mcg/minute is reached. If no effect is obtained with 20 mcg/minute, dosage may be increased by increments of 10 mcg/minute and, if necessary, by increments of 20 mcg/minute. When a PVC administration set is used, higher dosages generally are required; an initial infusion rate of 25 mcg/minute or greater has been used in studies employing PVC tubing. Dosage should be titrated according to the patient's response and possible adverse effects. Blood pressure and heart rate should be continuously monitored during IV administration; in many cases, invasive monitoring of pulmonary capillary wedge pressure is indicated.

When nitroglycerin is used IV in hypertensive emergencies†, some experts recommend an initial adult dosage of 5 mcg/minute, with increases of 5 mcg/minute every 3–5 minutes up to a maximum of 20 mcg/minute. Adults with a hypertensive emergency with a compelling indication (e.g., eclampsia or severe preeclampsia or pheochromocytoma crisis) should have their systolic blood pressure reduced to less than 140 mm Hg during the first hour and, in patients with acute aortic dissection, to less than 120 mm Hg within the first 20 minutes.

The risks of overly aggressive therapy in any hypertensive crisis must always be considered. The initial goal of IV nitroglycerin therapy for a hypertensive emergency in adults without a compelling indication is to reduce systolic blood pressure by no more than 25% within the first hour, followed by further blood pressure reduction if stable to 160/110 or 160/100 mm Hg within the next 2–6 hours, avoiding excessive declines in pressure that could precipitate renal, cerebral, or coronary ischemia.

PHARMACOKINETICS

● Absorption

The approximate onset and duration of action of various dosage forms of nitroglycerin are as follows:

TABLE 2. Antianginal Effects

Dosage Form	Onset	Duration
sublingual	within 2 min	up to 30 min
ointment	30 min	3 h
oral extended-release	1 h	up to 12 h

TABLE 3. Hemodynamic Effects

Dosage Form	Onset	Duration
sublingual	2 min	up to 30 min
ointment	within 1 h	3–6 h

The onset of action of transdermal systems of nitroglycerin is delayed and the duration prolonged compared with other currently available dosage forms of the drug. Transdermal systems of the drug are designed to provide continuous, controlled release of nitroglycerin to the skin from which the drug undergoes percutaneous absorption. The rates of delivery and absorption of the drug vary depending on the specific preparation, and the individual manufacturers' information should be consulted for specific descriptions of these rates and other characteristics of the preparation. The rate of delivery is linearly dependent on the active surface area of the applied system. In general, each transdermal system contains a reservoir of excess nitroglycerin, which establishes a concentration gradient to promote delivery of the drug out of the system and into the skin, and not all of the drug is delivered from the system during normal use. The preparations currently are labeled in terms of the approximate rate of drug delivery per hour; previously, they were labeled in terms of the approximate rate of drug delivery per 24 hours.

Several studies suggest that percutaneous absorption of nitroglycerin ointment varies with the site of application, with application to the chest resulting in higher blood concentrations of the drug and greater hemodynamic effects than application to the extremities; however, there are conflicting data, and further studies are needed to more fully evaluate the effect of the application site on absorption and hemodynamic effects.

● Distribution

Nitroglycerin is widely distributed in the body. It is not known if nitroglycerin is distributed into milk.

At plasma concentrations of 50–500 ng/mL, nitroglycerin is about 60% bound to plasma proteins while its metabolites, 1,3-glyceryl dinitrate and 1,2-glyceryl dinitrate, are approximately 60 and 30% bound, respectively.

Elimination

The plasma half-life of nitroglycerin is about 1–4 minutes. Clearance of nitroglycerin occurs at a rate of about 1 L/kg per minute.

Nitroglycerin is metabolized to 1,3-glyceryl dinitrate, 1,2-glyceryl dinitrate, and glyceryl mononitrate. In animals, the vasodilator effects of nitroglycerin are 10–14 times greater than those of the dinitrate metabolites. Glyceryl mononitrate, which is inactive, is the principal metabolite. The dinitrate metabolites are metabolized further to inactive mononitrates and are metabolized ultimately to glycerol and carbon dioxide. Clearance of nitroglycerin exceeds hepatic blood flow. Extrahepatic sites of metabolism include red blood cells and vascular walls.

CHEMISTRY AND STABILITY

Chemistry

Nitroglycerin an organic nitrate, is a vasodilator with peripheral and coronary vascular effects.

Stability

Nitroglycerin sublingual tablets should be stored in the original glass container at 20–25°C and tightly capped after each use to prevent loss of tablet potency.

Nitroglycerin lingual spray pump and lingual aerosol should be stored at 25°C but may be exposed to temperatures ranging from 15–30°C. Because the contents of nitroglycerin lingual spray or lingual aerosol contain 20% alcohol or a highly flammable propellant (butane), respectively, the containers should *not* be forcefully opened, sprayed toward a flame, or placed into a fire or incinerator for disposal. Nitroglycerin ointment should be stored in tight containers at 20–25°C. Nitroglycerin transdermal systems should be stored at 15–30°C; do not store in the refrigerator.

Since nitroglycerin readily migrates into many plastics, nitroglycerin IV solutions should be diluted and stored only in glass bottles; since some filters also absorb nitroglycerin, use of filters with IV solutions should be avoided. Nitroglycerin IV solutions should not be admixed with other drugs. Specialized references and the manufacturers' labeling should be consulted for specific stability and compatibility information.

PREPARATIONS

Excipients in commercially available drug preparations may have clinically important effects in some individuals; consult specific product labeling for details.

Nitroglycerin

Lingual		
Aerosol	0.4 mg/spray*	**Nitroglycerin Lingual Spray**
		NitroMist®, Evus
Solution	0.4 mg/spray*	**Nitroglycerin Lingual Spray**

Parenteral		
For injection concentrate, for IV infusion	5 mg/mL (50 mg)	**Nitroglycerin Injection**

Sublingual		
Tablets	0.3 mg*	**Nitroglycerin Sublingual Tablets**
		Nitrostat®, Pfizer
	0.4 mg*	**Nitroglycerin Sublingual Tablets**
		Nitrostat®, Pfizer
	0.6 mg*	**Nitroglycerin Sublingual Tablets**
		Nitrostat®, Pfizer

Topical		
Ointment	2%	**Nitro-Bid®**, Fougera
Transdermal System	0.1 mg/hour (total nitroglycerin content and transdermal system size may vary by manufacturer)*	**Nitro-Dur®**, Merck **Nitroglycerin Transdermal System**
	0.2 mg/hour (total nitroglycerin content and transdermal system size may vary by manufacturer)*	**Nitro-Dur®**, Ingenus **Nitroglycerin Transdermal System**
	0.3 mg/hour (60 mg/15 cm2)	**Nitro-Dur®**, Ingenus
	0.4 mg/hour (total nitroglycerin content and transdermal system size may vary by manufacturer)*	**Nitro-Dur®**, Ingenus **Nitroglycerin Transdermal System**
	0.6 mg/hour (total nitroglycerin content and transdermal system size may vary by manufacturer)*	**Nitro-Dur®**, Ingenus **Nitroglycerin Transdermal System**
	0.8 mg/hour (160 mg/40 cm2)	**Nitro-Dur®**, Ingenus

* available from one or more manufacturer, distributor, and/or repackager by generic (nonproprietary) name

Nitroglycerin in Dextrose

Parenteral		
Injection, for IV use only	100 mcg/mL (25 or 50 mg) Nitroglycerin in 5% Dextrose*	**Nitroglycerin in 5% Dextrose Injection**
	200 mcg/mL (50 mg) Nitroglycerin in 5% Dextrose*	**Nitroglycerin in 5% Dextrose Injection**
	400 mcg/mL (100 or 200 mg) Nitroglycerin in 5% Dextrose*	**Nitroglycerin in 5% Dextrose Injection**

* available from one or more manufacturer, distributor, and/or repackager by generic (nonproprietary) name

† Use is not currently included in the labeling approved by the US Food and Drug Administration.

Selected Revisions October 10, 2024, © Copyright, June 1, 1979, American Society of Health-System Pharmacists, Inc.

Vericiguat

24:08.10 • cGMP SYNTHESIS AGENTS

- Vericiguat, a soluble guanylate cyclase (sGC) stimulator, is a vasodilator.

USES

● Heart Failure

Vericiguat is used to reduce the risk of cardiovascular death and heart failure (HF) hospitalization following a hospitalization for heart failure or need for outpatient IV diuretics, in adults with symptomatic chronic HF and left ejection fraction (LVEF) less than 45%.

Clinical Experience

Efficacy and safety of vericiguat for this use have been established principally by the results of a randomized, double-blind, placebo-controlled trial (VICTORIA) in patients with chronic heart failure (New York Heart Association [NYHA] class II–IV) following a worsening heart failure event and receiving guideline-based medical therapy at baseline. The trial was conducted in 5050 adults with NYHA class II–IV chronic heart failure, LVEF less than 45%, an elevated natriuretic peptide level within 30 days of randomization, and evidence of worsening heart failure defined as hospitalization in the prior 6 months or use of IV diuretics for heart failure in the prior 3 months of randomization. Patients with concurrent or anticipated use of long-acting nitrates, soluble guanylate cyclase stimulators, or phosphodiesterase type 5 inhibitors or systolic blood pressure of less than 100 mm Hg were excluded. Vericiguat was initiated at a dosage of 2.5 mg once daily and then increased at approximately 2 week intervals to 5 mg once daily and then to the target dosage of 10 mg once daily, in a blinded manner, as guided by evaluation of blood pressure and clinical symptoms; placebo doses were similarly adjusted.

The mean age of patients was 67 years; 76% were male, 64% were white, 22% were Asian, and 5% were Black. At randomization, 59% of patients were NYHA class II, 40% were NYHA class III, and 1% were NYHA class IV. The mean LVEF was 29%; approximately half of all patients had an LVEF <30%, 85.7% had an LVEF <40%, and 14% had an LVEF between 40 and 45%. The median N-terminal pro b-type natriuretic peptide (NT-proBNP) level was 2800 pg/mL at randomization; 67% of the patients were enrolled within 3 months of a HF-hospitalization index event. At baseline, 91% of patients were treated with 2 or more HF medications which included a beta-adrenergic blocking agent, any renin-angiotensin system inhibitor, or mineralocorticoid receptor antagonist, and 60% of patients were treated with all 3 drug classes. The 10 mg vericiguat target dose was reached by 90% of patients in both treatment groups after approximately 1 year.

The primary outcome, a composite of death from cardiovascular causes or first hospitalization for heart failure, occurred in 35.5 and 38.5% of vericiguat and placebo patients, respectively; the difference was statistically significant. The individual components of the composite primary outcome did not differ, however the secondary outcome of total events of HF-hospitalization occurred less frequently in the vericiguat group (38.3 versus 42.4 events per 100 patient-years at risk).

Clinical Perspective

Current American Heart Association/American College of Cardiology/Heart Failure Society of America (AHA/ACC/HFSA) guidelines for the management of heart failure (HF) with reduced ejection fraction (HFrEF) in adults generally recommend a combination of drug therapies (e.g., angiotensin-converting enzyme [ACE] inhibitors, angiotensin II receptor antagonists, angiotensin receptor-neprilysin inhibitors [ARNIs], beta-adrenergic blocking agents, aldosterone receptor antagonists, sodium-glucose cotransporter 2 [SGLT2] inhibitors), also known as guideline-directed medical therapy (GDMT), to reduce morbidity and mortality. Additional agents (e.g., cardiac glycosides, diuretics, sinoatrial modulators [i.e., ivabradine], oral soluble guanylate cyclase stimulators [i.e., vericiguat]) in selected patients already on GDMT have been associated with symptomatic improvement and/or reduction in heart failure-related hospitalizations.

Experts (ACC/AHA/HFSA) recommend that all asymptomatic patients with reduced LVEF ≤40% (i.e., ACC/AHA stage B pre-heart failure) receive therapy with an ACE inhibitor and a beta-adrenergic blocking agent to prevent symptomatic heart failure and to reduce morbidity and mortality. In patients with prior or current symptoms of HFrEF (LVEF ≤40%, ACC/AHA stage C symptomatic HF), experts recommend inhibition of the renin-angiotensin-aldosterone (RAA) system with an ACE inhibitor, angiotensin II receptor antagonist, or ARNI in conjunction with a beta-adrenergic blocking agent, SGLT2 inhibitor, and an aldosterone receptor antagonist.

Experts state an oral soluble guanylate cyclase stimulator (i.e., vericiguat) may be considered in selected high-risk patients with HFrEF (stage C, New York Heart Association [NYHA] class II-IV) and recent worsening of HF (recent HF-hospitalization, IV diuretics) already on GDMT, to reduce HF-hospitalization and cardiovascular death.

DOSAGE AND ADMINISTRATION

● General

Pretreatment Screening

- Obtain a pregnancy test in females of reproductive potential prior to start of treatment with vericiguat.

● Administration

Oral Administration

Vericiguat is administered orally once daily with food. If a dose of vericiguat is missed, the missed dose may be administered as soon as possible on the same day of the missed dose. Do not administer 2 doses on the same day to make up for a missed dose.

For patients who are unable to swallow whole tablets, vericiguat may be crushed and mixed with water immediately before administration.

Store vericiguat tablets at 20–25°C (excursions permitted between 15–30°C).

● Dosage

Adult Dosage

Heart Failure

The recommended initial dosage of vericiguat for the treatment of heart failure in adults is 2.5 mg once daily. Double the dose of vericiguat approximately every 2 weeks to reach the target maintenance dosage of 10 mg once daily, as tolerated by the patient.

● Special Populations

Hepatic Impairment

The manufacturer makes no specific dosage recommendations for patients with mild or moderate hepatic impairment (Child-Pugh class A or B). Vericiguat has not been studied in patients with severe hepatic impairment (Child-Pugh class C).

Renal Impairment

The manufacturer makes no specific dosage recommendations for patients with estimated glomerular filtration rate (eGFR) ≥15 mL/minute per 1.73 m^2 who are not on dialysis. Vericiguat has not been studied in patients with eGFR <15 mL/minute per 1.73 m^2 or on dialysis.

Geriatric Patients

No dosage adjustment is required in geriatric patients; however, greater sensitivity of some older patients cannot be ruled out.

CAUTIONS

● Contraindications

- Pregnancy.
- Concomitant therapy with other soluble guanylate cyclase stimulators.

● Warnings/Precautions

Warnings

Embryo-fetal Toxicity

A boxed warning about the risk of embryo-fetal toxicity is included in the prescribing information for vericiguat. Based on data from animal reproduction studies, vericiguat may cause fetal harm when administered to a pregnant woman. Obtain a pregnancy test before initiating vericiguat.

Advise females of reproductive potential of the potential risk to a fetus and to use effective contraception during treatment with vericiguat and for at least one month after the final dose.

Specific Populations

Pregnancy

Based on data from animal reproduction studies, vericiguat may cause embryo-fetal toxicity when administered to a pregnant woman and is contraindicated during pregnancy. There are no available data with vericiguat use in pregnant women.

In animal reproduction studies, oral administration of vericiguat to pregnant rabbits during organogenesis, at ≥4 times the human exposure (total AUC) with the maximum recommended human dose (MRHD) of 10 mg, resulted in malformations of the heart and major vessels, as well as an increased number of abortions and resorptions. In a pre/postnatal toxicity study, vericiguat administered orally to rats during gestation through lactation caused maternal toxicity, which resulted in decreased pup body weight gain (dosage ≥10 times the MRHD) and increased pup mortality (dosage 24 times the MRHD) during the preweaning period. [^{14}C]-vericiguat was administered orally to pregnant rats at a dose of 3 mg/kg and vericiguat-related material was transferred across the placenta, with fetal plasma concentrations of approximately 67% maternal concentrations on gestation day 19.

There is a Pregnancy Surveillance Program that monitors pregnancy outcomes in women exposed to vericiguat during pregnancy. Healthcare providers should report any prenatal exposure to vericiguat by calling 1-877-888-4231 or at https://pregnancyreporting.verquvo-us.com.

Lactation

There are no data on the presence of vericiguat in human milk, the effects on the breastfed infant, or the effects on milk production. Vericiguat is present in the milk of lactating rats and it is likely that vericiguat or its metabolites are present in human milk. Because of the potential for serious adverse reactions in breastfed infants from vericiguat, advise women not to breastfeed during treatment with vericiguat.

Females and Males of Reproductive Potential

Verify the pregnancy status in females of reproductive potential prior to initiating vericiguat. Vericiguat may cause fetal harm when administered to a pregnant woman. Advise females of reproductive potential to use effective contraception during treatment and for at least one month after the final dose.

Pediatric Use

Safety and effectiveness of vericiguat have not been established in pediatric patients.

Geriatric Use

No dosage adjustment of vericiguat is required in geriatric patients. In the VICTORIA study, a total of 1,596 (63%) patients treated with vericiguat were 65 years of age and older, and 783 (31%) patients treated with vericiguat were 75 years of age and older. No overall differences in safety or efficacy of vericiguat were observed between patients 65 years of age and older compared to younger patients, but greater sensitivity of some older individuals cannot be ruled out.

Hepatic Impairment

No dosage adjustment of vericiguat is recommended in patients with mild or moderate hepatic impairment (Child-Pugh class A or B). Vericiguat has not been studied in patients with severe hepatic impairment (Child-Pugh class C).

Mean vericiguat exposures were 21 and 47% higher in individuals with mild and moderate hepatic impairment (Child Pugh class A and B), respectively, compared to healthy controls. The manufacturer states increased vericiguat AUC, normalized for body weight, is not clinically relevant.

Renal Impairment

No dosage adjustment of vericiguat is recommended in patients with estimated glomerular filtration rate (eGFR) ≥15 mL/minute per 1.73 m^2 who are not on dialysis. Vericiguat has not been studied in patients with eGFR <15 mL/minute per 1.73 m^2 at treatment initiation or on dialysis.

In patients with heart failure with mild, moderate, and severe renal impairment not requiring dialysis, the mean exposure (AUC) to vericiguat was increased 5, 13, and 20%, respectively, compared to those with normal renal function. These differences in exposure are not considered clinically relevant.

● Common Adverse Effects

The most common adverse reactions reported in ≥5% of patients receiving vericiguat are hypotension and anemia.

DRUG INTERACTIONS

Vericiguat primarily undergoes glucuronidation by uridine diphosphate-glucuronosyltransferase (UGT) enzymes 1A9 and, to a lesser extent, by UGT1A1 to form an inactive N-glucuronide metabolite. Vericiguat is not an inhibitor of UGT1A1, 1A4, 1A6, 1A9, 2B4, or 2B7 in vitro.

In vitro studies suggest that vericiguat is not an inhibitor of cytochrome P-450 (CYP) isoenzymes 1A2, 2B6, 2C8, 2C9, 2C19, 2D6, 3A4 and is not an inducer of CYP1A2, 2B6, or 3A4.

Vericiguat is a substrate of P-glycoprotein (P-gp) and breast cancer resistance protein (BCRP) transporters in vitro. In vitro studies suggest vericiguat is not a substrate of organic cation transporter (OCT) 1 or organic anion transporting (OAT) polypeptides OATP1B1 and OATP1B3 and not an inhibitor of P-gp, BCRP, bile salt export pump (BSEP), OATP1B1/1B3, OAT1, OAT3, OCT1, OCT2, multidrug and toxin extrusion (MATE) 1, or MATE2K.

● Drugs Affecting Uridine Diphosphate Glucuronosyltransferase Enzymes

No clinically significant differences on vericiguat pharmacokinetics were observed with coadministration of mefenamic acid (UGT1A9 inhibitor); no clinically significant differences on vericiguat pharmacokinetics were predicted with coadministration of atazanavir (UGT1A1 inhibitor).

● Drugs Affecting or Metabolized by Hepatic Microsomal Enzymes

No clinically significant differences on the pharmacokinetics of midazolam (CYP3A substrate) were observed when coadministered with vericiguat in healthy subjects. No clinically significant differences on vericiguat pharmacokinetics were observed with coadministration of ketoconazole (multi-pathway CYP and transporter inhibitor).

● Drugs Affecting Gastric Acidity

Vericiguat is less soluble at neutral than at acidic pH. Pre- and coadministration with drugs that increase gastric pH, omeprazole or aluminum hydroxide/magnesium hydroxide combination, decreased vericiguat exposure (AUC) by about 32.2 and 27.1%, respectively, following fasted administration. However, no clinically significant differences were observed with coadministration of drugs that increase gastric pH (e.g., proton pump inhibitors, H$_2$-receptor antagonists, antacids) in patients with heart failure when vericiguat was taken with food based on population pharmacokinetic analysis.

● Drugs Affecting or Affected by Transport Systems

No clinically significant differences on vericiguat pharmacokinetics were observed with coadministration of ketoconazole (multi-pathway CYP and transporter inhibitor) or digoxin (P-gp substrate).

● *Phosphodiesterase Type 5 Inhibitors*

Co-administration of vericiguat with phosphodiesterase (PDE) type 5 inhibitors is not recommended because of the potential for hypotension. No clinically significant differences on sildenafil pharmacokinetics were observed with coadministration in healthy subjects. Concomitant use of vericiguat 10 mg with single doses of sildenafil (25, 50, or 100 mg) was associated with additional seated blood pressure reduction of up to 5.4 mm Hg, compared to administration of vericiguat alone with no evidence of a sildenafil dose-related effect. Standing blood pressure and standing and seated heart rate were similar between treatment groups. There is limited experience with concomitant use of vericiguat and PDE type 5 inhibitors in patients with heart failure.

● *Soluble Guanylate Cyclase Stimulators*

Co-administration of vericiguat is contraindicated in patients receiving other soluble guanylate cyclase stimulators.

DESCRIPTION

Vericiguat is a stimulator of soluble guanylate cyclase (sGC), an important enzyme in the nitric oxide (NO) signaling pathway. When NO binds to sGC, the enzyme catalyzes the synthesis of intracellular cyclic guanosine monophosphate (cGMP), a second messenger that plays a role in the regulation of vascular tone, cardiac contractility, and cardiac remodeling. Heart failure is associated with impaired synthesis of NO and decreased activity of sGC, which may contribute to myocardial and vascular dysfunction. By directly stimulating sGC, independently of and synergistically with NO, vericiguat augments levels of intracellular cGMP, leading to smooth muscle relaxation and vasodilation. Mean systolic blood pressure was 1–2 mm Hg lower in patients who received vericiguat compared to those who received placebo. Dose-dependant reductions in N-terminal pro b-type natriuretic peptide (NT-proBNP), a biomarker for heart failure, were observed in heart failure patients receiving vericiguat compared to placebo. There was no evidence of proarrhythmic risk in an in vitro assessment of vericiguat or its major N-glucuronide metabolite, no inhibition of cardiac ion channels were observed at the recommended target dose of 10 mg, and risk assessment of nonclinical and clinical data supports that administration of vericiguat 10 mg is not associated with clinically meaningful QT_c interval prolongation.

Vericiguat has an absolute bioavailability of 93% when taken with food; results were comparable when vericiguat was administered orally as a whole tablet or as a crushed tablet in water. Administration of vericiguat 10 mg with a high-fat, high-calorie meal increases time to peak concentration from about 1 hour (fasted) to about 4 hours (fed), reduces pharmacokinetic variability, and increases AUC by 44% and peak concentration by 41% compared with administration in the fasted state. Results were similar when vericiguat was administered with a low-fat, low-calorie meal when compared to administration with a high-fat, high-calorie meal. Vericiguat is about 98% protein bound, primarily to serum albumin. Half-life is 30 hours in patients with heart failure; steady-state is achieved in approximately 6 days. Vericiguat primarily undergoes glucuronidation by uridine diphosphate glucuronosyltransferase (UGT) enzymes 1A9 and, to a lesser extent, by UGT1A1 to form an inactive N-glucuronide metabolite. Cytochrome P-450 isoenzyme-mediated metabolism is a minor clearance pathway (<5%). Following oral administration of radiolabeled vericiguat to healthy subjects, approximately 53% of the dose was excreted in urine (primarily as inactive metabolite) and 45% in feces (primarily as unchanged drug).

Mean vericiguat exposures were 21 and 47% higher in individuals with mild and moderate hepatic impairment (Child-Pugh class A and B), respectively, compared to healthy controls. Vericiguat has not been studied in patients with severe hepatic impairment (e.g., Child-Pugh class C). In patients with heart failure with mild, moderate, and severe renal impairment not requiring dialysis, the mean exposure (AUC) to vericiguat was increased 5, 13, and 20%, respectively, compared to those with normal renal function. Vericiguat has not been studied in patients with an estimated glomerular filtration rate (eGFR) <15 mL/minute per 1.73 m² at treatment initiation or on dialysis. No clinically significant differences in the pharmacokinetics of vericiguat were observed based on age, sex, race/ethnicity (Black, white, Asian, Hispanic, Latino), body weight, or baseline NT-proBNP.

ADVICE TO PATIENTS

- Advise patients to read the FDA-approved patient labeling (Medication Guide).

- If a dose is missed, advise patients to take it as soon as it is remembered on the same day of the missed dose. Patients should not take two doses of vericiguat on the same day.

- Advise pregnant women and females of reproductive potential of the potential risk to a fetus and to inform their healthcare provider of a known or suspected pregnancy. Advise females of reproductive potential to use effective contraception during treatment with vericiguat and for at least one month after the final dose.

- Advise women who are exposed to vericiguat during pregnancy to report the pregnancy to their healthcare provider. Health care providers should report any prenatal exposure to vericiguat by calling 1-877-888-4231 or at https://pregnancyreporting.verquvo-us.com.

- Advise women not to breastfeed during treatment with vericiguat.

- Advise patients that vericiguat tablets should be administered with food and swallowed whole.

- Advise patients unable to swallow a whole vericiguat tablet that they may crush the tablet(s) and mix with water right before taking the dose.

- Advise patients to inform their clinician of existing or contemplated concomitant therapy, including prescription and OTC drugs and dietary or herbal supplements, as well as any concomitant illnesses.

- Inform patients of other important precautionary information.

PREPARATIONS

Excipients in commercially available drug preparations may have clinically important effects in some individuals; consult specific product labeling for details.

Vericiguat

Oral

Tablets, film-coated	2.5 mg	Verquvo®, Merck
	5 mg	Verquvo®, Merck
	10 mg	Verquvo®, Merck

† Use is not currently included in the labeling approved by the US Food and Drug Administration.

Sodium Nitroprusside

24:08.16 • DIRECT VASODILATORS

■ Sodium nitroprusside is a vasodilating and hypotensive agent.

USES

● Hypertensive Crises

IV sodium nitroprusside is used in hypertensive crises for immediate reduction of blood pressure in patients in whom such reduction is considered an emergency (hypertensive emergencies). The drug is consistently effective in the management of hypertensive emergencies, irrespective of etiology; however, sodium nitroprusside is contraindicated in compensatory hypertension (e.g., arteriovenous shunt or coarctation of the aorta). Because of the potential for serious toxicity (see Cautions), sodium nitroprusside should be used for treatment of hypertensive emergencies in carefully selected patients.

Hypertensive emergencies are those rare situations requiring immediate blood pressure reduction (not necessarily to normal ranges) to prevent or limit target organ damage. Such emergencies may be associated with hypertensive encephalopathy, acute myocardial infarction (MI), unstable angina pectoris, acute left ventricular failure with pulmonary edema, acute renal failure, acute ischemic stroke, eclampsia, or aortic dissection. Some experts state that the use of sodium nitroprusside is contraindicated for the treatment of eclampsia or preeclampsia. (For additional information on the use of antihypertensive drugs in women with preeclampsia, see Uses: Hypertension, Severe Hypertension during Pregnancy, in Hydralazine 24:08.20.) Patients with hypertensive emergencies require hospitalization and are treated initially with an appropriate parenteral agent. Several antihypertensive drugs from various pharmacologic classes are available for the treatment of hypertensive emergencies; because of the lack of evidence to support the use of one antihypertensive drug over another, experts state that selection of an appropriate agent should be individualized based on the underlying cause of hypertension, degree of target organ damage, desired rate of blood pressure reduction, specific drug characteristics, and patient comorbidities. Excessive falls in blood pressure should be avoided in any hypertensive crisis since they may precipitate renal, cerebral, or coronary ischemia. Hypertensive urgencies (i.e., situations in which there is severe elevation in blood pressure without acute or impending target organ damage) generally can be managed with intensification or reinstitution (e.g., following noncompliance) of the current antihypertensive regimen; there is no indication that hospitalization and immediate reduction of blood pressure is required in these situations.

Almost any desired blood pressure can be maintained by varying the rate of IV sodium nitroprusside infusion. Blood pressure reduction by sodium nitroprusside is a temporary measure. Administration of other longer-acting hypotensive agents should be started as soon as possible while the blood pressure is being controlled by sodium nitroprusside to minimize the duration of sodium nitroprusside therapy. The IV infusion should be slowed or stopped as the other medication takes effect.

● Congestive Heart Failure

Sodium nitroprusside is used in the management of acute decompensated (e.g., congestive) heart failure. The precipitating cause of acute heart failure decompensation should be carefully assessed to inform appropriate treatment, optimize outcomes, and prevent future acute events in patients with heart failure. Current guidelines for the management of heart failure in adults generally recommend inhibition of the renin-angiotensin-aldosterone system with a combination of drug therapies, including neurohormonal antagonists (e.g., angiotensin-converting enzyme [ACE] inhibitors, angiotensin II receptor antagonists, angiotensin receptor-neprilysin inhibitors [ARNIs], β-adrenergic blocking agents [β-blockers], aldosterone receptor antagonists), to inhibit the detrimental compensatory mechanisms in heart failure and reduce morbidity and mortality. (See Uses: Heart Failure in Carvedilol 24:24 and in Sacubitril and Valsartan 24:32.92.) IV vasodilators have not been shown to improve outcomes in patients hospitalized for heart failure; however, in the absence of symptomatic hypotension, sodium nitroprusside may be considered as an adjunct to diuretic therapy

for relief of dyspnea in patients hospitalized for acutely decompensated heart failure. Administration of the drug produces rapid hemodynamic and clinical improvement by inducing arteriolar dilatation with subsequent reduction in systemic vascular resistance, thereby increasing cardiac output; by producing vasodilation and thus decreasing left ventricular filling, ventricular filling pressures are reduced. In addition, sodium nitroprusside has been reported to be particularly useful in the management of severe heart failure caused by the regurgitant valvular lesions of aortic insufficiency and mitral regurgitation. Some experts state that sodium nitroprusside may also be potentially useful in the management of heart failure in patients with severe pulmonary congestion and hypertension.

● Controlled Hypotension during Surgery

Sodium nitroprusside also is used to produce controlled hypotension during anesthesia in order to reduce bleeding during surgical procedures when appropriate. Use of the drug is contraindicated in patients with inadequate cerebral circulation or in patients requiring emergency surgery who are near death.

● Acute Myocardial Infarction

Vasodilators such as sodium nitroprusside also have been used to improve cardiac output in patients with left ventricular failure and low cardiac output after acute MI†. An inotropic agent (e.g., dobutamine) should be used initially to improve myocardial contractility and cardiac output; if blood pressure permits, afterload-reducing agents may be added to decrease cardiac work and pulmonary congestion. Use of sodium nitroprusside may be limited by coronary steal, a phenomenon whereby altered myocardial blood flow distribution causes diversion of blood away from ischemic areas. Nitroglycerin is the preferred vasodilator in patients with acute MI because of its ability to relieve ischemia by reducing left ventricular preload and increasing coronary blood flow.

DOSAGE AND ADMINISTRATION

● Administration

Sodium nitroprusside is administered by IV infusion only using a controlled-infusion device (i.e., infusion pump); *IV infusion devices regulated only by gravity or mechanical clamps should not be used*. The rate of administration should be adjusted to maintain the desired hypotensive effect, as determined by continuous monitoring of blood pressure, using either a continually reinflated sphygmomanometer or, preferably, an intra-arterial pressure sensor. Because of the potential for toxicity, the drug should be administered for the shortest possible duration. Prolonged infusions should not exceed a rate of 3 mcg/kg per minute to prevent thiocyanate (byproduct of sodium nitroprusside metabolism) concentrations from reaching neurotoxic levels; thiocyanate concentrations should be monitored daily if this rate is exceeded.

Commercially available sodium nitroprusside injection concentrate (25 mg/mL) *must be further diluted* prior to IV infusion. The contents of one vial containing 50 mg of the drug should be diluted in 250–1000 mL of 5% dextrose injection. Vials of the drug are for single use only. Nitroprusside solutions should be protected from light by promptly wrapping the containers in the supplied opaque sleeve, aluminum foil, or other opaque material; it is not necessary to cover the infusion drip chamber or IV tubing. If properly protected from light, diluted solutions of the drug are stable for 24 hours. (See Chemistry and Stability: Stability.) Parenteral solutions of the drug should be inspected visually for particulate matter and discoloration prior to administration. The freshly prepared infusion solution has a very faint brownish tint; if it is highly colored (e.g., blue, green, red) or contains particulate matter, it should be discarded. No other drug should be added to the infusion fluid for simultaneous administration with sodium nitroprusside.

Standardize 4 Safety

Standardized concentrations for sodium nitroprusside have been established through Standardize 4 Safety (S4S), a national patient safety initiative to reduce medication errors, especially during transitions of care. Multidisciplinary expert panels were convened to determine recommended standard concentrations. Because recommendations from the S4S panels may differ from the manufacturer's prescribing information, caution is advised when using concentrations that differ from labeling, particularly when using rate information from the label. For additional information on S4S (including updates that may be available), see https://www.ashp.org/pharmacy-practice/standardize-4-safety-initiative.

TABLE 1. Standardize 4 Safety Continuous IV Infusion Standard Concentrations for Sodium Nitroprusside

Patient Population	Concentration Standards	Dosing Units
Adults	200 mcg/mL	mcg/kg/min
	500 mcg/mL	
Pediatric patients (<50 kg)	200 mcg/mL	mcg/kg/min
	500 mcg/mL	

● Dosage

Hypertensive Crises or Controlled Hypotension during Surgery

In adults and pediatric patients receiving sodium nitroprusside for hypertensive crises or for controlled hypotension during surgery, the manufacturer states that the average effective IV dosage is about 3 mcg/kg per minute, with a range of 0.5–10 mcg/kg per minute; however, some patients will experience profound hypotension when receiving the drug at this rate. Therefore, the infusion should be started at a very low rate (e.g., 0.3 mcg/kg per minute) and gradually titrated upward every few minutes until adequate blood pressure control is achieved or the maximum recommended infusion rate of 10 mcg/kg per minute has been reached. Some experts state that for management of severe hypertension with life-threatening symptoms in children and adolescents, an initial infusion rate of 0–3 mcg/kg per minute should be used. These experts suggest that blood pressure be reduced by no more than 25% of the planned reduction over the first 8 hours, with the remainder of the planned reduction over the next 12–24 hours. For the management of a hypertensive emergency in adults, some experts recommend an initial dosage of 0.3–0.5 mcg/kg per minute, with increases in increments of 0.5 mcg/kg per minute, up to a maximum rate of 10 mcg/kg per minute, to achieve desired blood pressure control. The infusion duration should be as short as possible; if an adequate reduction in blood pressure is not obtained within 10 minutes at this maximum infusion rate, the infusion should be immediately discontinued. Because of the rapidity of sodium nitroprusside's hypotensive onset and dissipation of effect, small changes in infusion rate can lead to large, undesirable fluctuations in blood pressure. The manufacturer states that prior to increasing dosage, the drug's effects should be confirmed by measuring blood pressure 5 minutes after any change in infusion rate to achieve the desired blood pressure response.

Diastolic blood pressure usually is decreased and maintained about 30–40% below pretreatment levels with sodium nitroprusside dosages of 3 mcg/kg per minute. Smaller dosages of sodium nitroprusside are adequate in patients receiving other hypotensive agents and in geriatric patients.

In adults who have a hypertensive emergency *with* a compelling indication (i.e., aortic dissection, pheochromocytoma crisis), some experts recommend that systolic blood pressure be reduced to less than 140 mm Hg during the first hour and, in patients with acute aortic dissection, to less than 120 mm Hg within the first 20 minutes. In adults who have a hypertensive emergency *without* a compelling indication, systolic blood pressure should be reduced by no more than 25% over the first hour, followed by further blood pressure reduction *if stable* to 160/110 or 160/100 mm Hg within the next 2–6 hours; excessive declines in pressure that could precipitate renal, cerebral, or coronary ischemia should be avoided. If this blood pressure is well tolerated and the patient is clinically stable, further gradual reductions toward normal can be implemented in the next 24–48 hours.

Longer-acting hypotensive agents should be administered concomitantly with sodium nitroprusside to minimize the duration of sodium nitroprusside therapy.

Congestive Heart Failure

When sodium nitroprusside is used in adults and pediatric patients with acute congestive heart failure, the manufacturer recommends that the infusion be initiated at a rate of 0.3 mcg/kg per minute. Dosage should be gradually titrated upward every few minutes until the desired effect is achieved or the maximum recommended infusion rate of 10 mcg/kg per minute has been reached. The

manufacturer states that the average effective dosage is about 3 mcg/kg (range: 0.5–10 mcg/kg) per minute. Adjustment of the infusion rate must be guided by the results of invasive hemodynamic monitoring and monitoring of urine output. Titration of sodium nitroprusside dosage can be accomplished by increasing the infusion rate until cardiac output is no longer increasing, systemic blood pressure cannot be further reduced without compromising vital organ perfusion, or the maximum recommended infusion rate is reached, whichever occurs first. While specific hemodynamic goals must be tailored to the clinical situation, improvements in cardiac output and left ventricular filling pressure must not be achieved at the expense of undue hypotension and consequent hypoperfusion.

CAUTIONS

The most clinically important adverse effects of sodium nitroprusside are profound hypotension and cyanide toxicity. Other adverse effects are less common and develop less rapidly.

● Hypotension

Sodium nitroprusside can produce precipitous decreases in blood pressure and profound hypotension when administered at transient, slightly excessive infusion rates; the subsequent hemodynamic changes can result in a variety of associated symptoms, or blood pressure may decrease to the point where perfusion of vital organs may be compromised. The hypotensive effect of the drug occurs rapidly and the possible sequelae of hypotension (e.g., irreversible ischemic injury, death) are serious.

● Cyanogenic Effects

Manifestations

Sodium nitroprusside infusions at rates exceeding 2 mcg/kg per minute generate cyanogen (cyanide radical) in amounts greater than can be effectively buffered by the methemoglobin normally present in the body; cyanide toxicity can result when this buffering system is exhausted. The capacity of this system is exceeded when more than 500 mcg/kg of sodium nitroprusside is given; this amount is produced in less than 1 hour when the drug is administered at a rate of 10 mcg/kg per minute. Most cases of cyanide toxicity have occurred when sodium nitroprusside is used for prolonged periods or at high dosages; however, elevated cyanide levels, metabolic acidosis, and marked clinical deterioration have been reported occasionally in patients receiving the drug at recommended rates of infusion for only a few hours, and in one case, for only 35 minutes. Infusions of sodium nitroprusside at the maximum recommended rate of 10 mcg/kg per minute should never last longer than 10 minutes; if blood pressure is not adequately controlled after 10 minutes, the infusion should be discontinued immediately.

The toxic effects of cyanide may be rapid, serious, and possibly fatal and may manifest as venous hyperoxemia (secondary to the inability of tissues to extract oxygen from erythrocytes, with resultant bright red venous blood), lactic acidosis, air hunger, confusion, and death. While acid-base balance and venous oxygen concentrations should be monitored and may indicate cyanide toxicity, these tests alone should not be relied upon to guide therapy. Cyanide toxicity resulting from causes other than sodium nitroprusside has been associated with angina and myocardial infarction, ataxia, seizures, stroke, and other diffuse ischemic damage.

Treatment

Sodium thiosulfate has been administered concomitantly with sodium nitroprusside at infusion rates 5–10 times that of the sodium nitroprusside infusion to accelerate the metabolism of cyanide; however, coadministration of these agents has not been extensively researched and further study is necessary. Caution must be exercised to avoid prolonged or excessive dosages of sodium nitroprusside with sodium thiosulfate, since thiocyanate toxicity and/or hypovolemia may result. The same precautions and contraindications apply to this method of administration as to the administration of sodium nitroprusside alone.

● Methemoglobinemia

Infusions of sodium nitroprusside can result in the sequestration of hemoglobin as methemoglobin; cyanide combines with methemoglobin to form cyanmethemoglobin. Although the conversion of methemoglobin back to hemoglobin is normally rapid, clinically important methemoglobinemia (greater than 10%)

rarely may occur. Even patients who are congenitally incapable of converting methemoglobin back to hemoglobin should demonstrate 10% methemoglobinemia only following a total sodium nitroprusside dose of 10 mg/kg (i.e., infusion at the maximum recommended rate of 10 mcg/kg per minute for greater than 16 hours). Methemoglobinemia should be suspected in patients who have received greater than 10 mg/kg of sodium nitroprusside and who exhibit signs of impaired oxygen delivery despite adequate cardiac output and arterial PaO$_2$.

● Thiocyanate Accumulation

Thiocyanate may accumulate in the blood of patients receiving sodium nitroprusside therapy, especially in those with impaired renal function, or in patients receiving prolonged infusions of sodium nitroprusside at infusion rates exceeding 3 mcg/kg per minute or receiving sodium thiosulfate concomitantly with sodium nitroprusside to accelerate the metabolism of cyanide. (See Cautions: Precautions and Contraindications, and Chronic Toxicity.) Thiocyanate is mildly neurotoxic (e.g., tinnitus, miosis, hyperreflexia) at serum concentrations of 60 mcg/mL and may be life-threatening at concentrations of 200 mcg/mL. (See Cautions: Precautions and Contraindications

Since thiocyanate inhibits both uptake and binding of iodine, symptoms of hypothyroidism may occur. Thiocyanate retention and hypothyroidism have been reported in one patient with severe hypertension and uremia who had received 3.9 g of sodium nitroprusside IV over a period of 21 days. Elevated plasma thiocyanate concentrations and signs of hypothyroidism diminished after peritoneal dialysis.

● Other Metabolic Effects

Cyanogen (cyanide radical) as well as thiocyanate may interfere with vitamin B$_{12}$ distribution and metabolism. A fall in total plasma cobalamins has been reported during administration of sodium nitroprusside; however, a rise in plasma cyanocobalamin has been noted in patients receiving the drug for prolonged periods.

● Renal Effects

Increases in serum creatinine concentrations, which returned to normal after the infusion was stopped, have also occurred during sodium nitroprusside use.

● Other Adverse Effects

Other adverse effects resulting from IV administration of sodium nitroprusside are uncommon and are usually associated with a too-rapid reduction in blood pressure. Nausea, retching, diaphoresis, apprehension, headache, restlessness, muscle twitching, retrosternal discomfort, palpitation, dizziness, and abdominal pain or cramps have been reported during use of the drug. These symptoms may be relieved by slowing the rate of infusion or temporarily discontinuing the drug, or minimized by keeping the patient supine. In addition, bradycardia, tachycardia, ECG changes, rash, decreased platelet aggregation, ileus, increased intracranial pressure, flushing, venous streaking, and irritation at the site of injection have been reported.

● Precautions and Contraindications

Sodium nitroprusside injection concentrate is *not* suitable for direct injection; the drug *must* be further diluted in 5% dextrose injection before IV infusion. (See Dosage and Administration: Administration.)

Because sodium nitroprusside can produce precipitous decreases in blood pressure, the drug should be administered only when adequate facilities, equipment, and personnel are available for close monitoring of blood pressure. Hypotension generally is self-limiting within 1–10 minutes following the discontinuance of the infusion; during this time, patients may benefit from being placed in Trendelenburg's position to maximize venous return. If blood pressure does not normalize within a few minutes, sodium nitroprusside may not be the principal cause of the hypotension and another cause should be sought.

Except when used for short periods of time or at low infusion rates (e.g., 2 mcg/kg per minute or slower), therapy with sodium nitroprusside can result in the production of clinically important levels of cyanide, which can reach toxic or potentially lethal concentrations. If excessive dosages of sodium nitroprusside are used and/or sulfur (usually thiosulfate) stores become depleted, cyanogen toxicity may occur. (See Cautions: Cyanogenic Effects and see Chronic Toxicity.) Sodium

nitroprusside infusions at the maximum recommended infusion rate of 10 mcg/kg per minute should never last longer than 10 minutes; if after 10 minutes the blood pressure has not been adequately controlled, the infusion should be immediately discontinued.

Sodium nitroprusside should be used with caution in patients with hepatic insufficiency, hypothyroidism, or hyponatremia. Thiocyanate may accumulate in patients with renal impairment or in patients receiving prolonged infusions of sodium nitroprusside at rates exceeding 3 mcg/kg per minute. To maintain the steady-state concentration of thiocyanate below 60 mcg/mL (the level at which mild neurotoxic effects have been observed), infusion rates of sodium nitroprusside should be maintained below 3 mcg/kg per minute in patients with normal renal function or 1 mcg/kg per minute in anuric patients. When prolonged infusions are more rapid than these, serum thiocyanate concentrations should be monitored daily. Some clinicians recommend that plasma cyanogen concentrations be monitored daily after 1 or 2 days in patients with impaired hepatic function. Peritoneal dialysis or hemodialysis may be required to remove excess thiocyanate and relieve the symptoms. (See Chronic Toxicity: Treatment.)

Because sodium nitroprusside may interfere with vitamin B$_{12}$ distribution and metabolism, the drug should be used with caution in patients with low plasma vitamin B$_{12}$ concentrations. Because hydroxocobalamin is an antidote for cyanogen (combining to form cyanocobalamin), its use may be advisable before and during sodium nitroprusside administration in these patients.

Frequent monitoring of acid-base balance is necessary in all patients, particularly if tolerance to the pharmacologic effects of sodium nitroprusside develops during therapy (manifested as the need for higher infusion rates to control blood pressure), since metabolic acidosis is one of the earliest and most reliable signs of cyanogen toxicity; however, laboratory tests alone should not be relied upon to guide therapy since acidosis may not be evident until more than 1 hour after the development of toxic cyanogen concentrations. If signs of metabolic acidosis or increased tolerance to the hypotensive effect of the drug occurs during sodium nitroprusside therapy, the drug should be discontinued and alternative treatment should be administered.

In patients with symptomatic methemoglobinemia (i.e., 10% or greater), 1–2 mg/kg of methylene blue should be administered IV slowly over several minutes. However, treatment of methemoglobinemia should be undertaken with extreme caution in patients who are likely to have substantial amounts of cyanide bound to methemoglobin as cyanmethemoglobin.

Young, healthy males may require higher than recommended dosages of sodium nitroprusside for hypotensive anesthetic procedures; however, the maximum infusion rate of 10 mcg/kg per minute should not be exceeded. (See Dosage and Administration: Dosage.) Deepening of anesthesia in these patients may produce adequate hypotension with administration of sodium nitroprusside in the recommended dosage range.

Sodium nitroprusside, like other vasodilating agents, can produce increases in intracranial pressure; therefore, the drug should be used only with extreme caution in patients with preexisting increased intracranial pressure.

When IV sodium nitroprusside is used for controlled hypotension during anesthesia, tolerance to loss of blood, anemia, and hypovolemia may be decreased. If possible, preexisting anemia and hypovolemia should be corrected prior to use of the drug. Hypotensive anesthetic techniques also may affect pulmonary ventilation perfusion ratio. In patients who cannot tolerate additional dead air space at normal oxygen partial pressure, higher oxygen partial pressure may be beneficial. Sodium nitroprusside IV infusion should be used with extreme caution in patients who are especially poor surgical risks.

The use of sodium nitroprusside to produce controlled hypotension during surgery is contraindicated in patients with inadequate cerebral circulation and is not intended for use during emergency surgery in patients near death. Sodium nitroprusside should not be used in the treatment of compensatory hypertension (e.g., arteriovenous shunt or coarctation of the aorta). Use of the drug also should be avoided in patients with congenital (Leber's) optic atrophy or tobacco amblyopia; these conditions, although rare, are associated with absent or deficient thiosulfate sulfurtransferase (rhodanase), and these patients have unusually high cyanogen to thiocyanate ratios. The manufacturer states that sodium nitroprusside should not be used in patients with acute heart failure associated with reduced peripheral vascular resistance, such as high-output heart failure that may accompany endotoxic sepsis. Concomitant use of sodium nitroprusside and phosphodiesterase (PDE) type 5 inhibitors (e.g., sildenafil) or soluble guanylate cyclase stimulators (e.g., riociguat) is contraindicated because of the potential for additive hypotensive effects.

• Pediatric Precautions

Sodium nitroprusside has been used to induce hypotension in a limited number of patients younger than 17 years of age; at least 50% of such patients were prepubertal, and about 50% of prepubertal patients were younger than 2 years of age, including 4 neonates. Efficacy of the drug in pediatric patients has been established in a parallel, dose-ranging study and a long-term infusion study in which sodium nitroprusside dosage was titrated according to blood pressure; the primary efficacy variable in these studies was mean arterial pressure (MAP). Both studies demonstrated the blood pressure-lowering effect of sodium nitroprusside. In the latter study, sodium nitroprusside reduced MAP below that of placebo control for at least 12 hours. Similar effects on MAP were observed in all age groups in these studies, and no novel safety issues were noted.

• Pregnancy, Fertility, and Lactation

Pregnancy

Animal reproduction studies have not been performed with sodium nitroprusside. It is also not known whether the drug can cause fetal harm when administered to pregnant women. The manufacturer states that sodium nitroprusside should be used during pregnancy only when clearly needed; some experts state that the drug is contraindicated in women with preeclampsia or eclampsia.

The effects of sodium thiosulfate administration during pregnancy, either alone or in conjunction with sodium nitroprusside, are unknown.

Fertility

It is not known whether sodium nitroprusside affects fertility in humans.

Lactation

It is not known if sodium nitroprusside and its metabolites are distributed into human milk. Because many drugs are distributed into milk and because of the potential for serious adverse effects in nursing infants, a decision should be made whether to discontinue nursing or the drug, taking into account the importance of the drug to the woman.

DRUG INTERACTIONS

• Hypotensive Agents

The hypotensive effects of sodium nitroprusside are additive when used concomitantly with ganglionic blocking agents, negative inotropic agents, general anesthetics (e.g., enflurane), and most other circulatory depressants.

• Phosphodiesterase Inhibitors

Additive hypotensive effects can occur if sodium nitroprusside is used concomitantly with phosphodiesterase (PDE) type 5 inhibitors (e.g., sildenafil). Concomitant use of these drugs is contraindicated.

• Soluble Guanylate Cyclase Stimulators

Additive hypotensive effects can occur if sodium nitroprusside is used concomitantly with soluble guanylate cyclase stimulators (e.g., riociguat). Concomitant use of these drugs is contraindicated.

CHRONIC TOXICITY

• Pathogenesis

Following IV administration, sodium nitroprusside is rapidly metabolized to cyanogen (cyanide radical) and subsequently converted to thiocyanate by the enzyme rhodanase. The rate of conversion from cyanogen to thiocyanate depends on the availability of sulfur, usually thiosulfate; however, cyanide toxicity can occur if excessive dosages of sodium nitroprusside are used and/or sulfur stores become depleted.

The toxicity of sodium nitroprusside has been attributed to cyanogen; however, the role of cyanogen in sodium nitroprusside poisoning has been questioned and it has been postulated that some toxic effects may be caused by profound hypotension.

The first signs of overdosage with sodium nitroprusside are those related to severe hypotension. Increasing tolerance to the hypotensive effects of the drug and metabolic acidosis are also early indications of overdosage with sodium nitroprusside and may be associated with or followed by dyspnea, headache, vomiting, dizziness, ataxia, or loss of consciousness. Frequent monitoring of acid-base balance is necessary in all patients receiving sodium nitroprusside, particularly in patients who develop tolerance to the drug's pharmacologic effects, since metabolic acidosis is the most reliable sign of cyanogen toxicity; however, laboratory tests alone should not be relied upon to guide therapy since acidosis may not be evident until more than 1 hour after the development of toxic cyanogen concentrations. Reasonable suspicion of cyanogen toxicity is adequate basis for initiation of treatment. If signs of metabolic acidosis or tolerance to the hypotensive effect of the drug occurs during sodium nitroprusside therapy, the drug should be discontinued and alternative treatment should be administered. Signs or symptoms of cyanogen toxicity may include coma, imperceptible pulse, absent reflexes, dilated pupils, pink coloration of the skin, distant heart sounds, or shallow breathing.

Deaths clearly caused by sodium nitroprusside are limited to cases in which large oral doses were taken in suicides. Autopsy showed all organs to be congested and some evidence of cyanogen poisoning was observed.

In the event of overdosage with sodium nitroprusside, nitrites should be administered to induce methemoglobin formation. Oxygen administration alone will not provide relief. Methemoglobin combines with cyanogen bound to cytochrome-c oxidase to yield cytochrome-c oxidase and cyanmethemoglobin, a nontoxic complex. Cyanogen gradually dissociates from cyanmethemoglobin and is converted to sodium thiocyanate by administration of thiosulfate in the presence of thiosulfate sulfurtransferase (rhodanase).

When overdosage with sodium nitroprusside occurs with signs of cyanogen toxicity, sodium nitroprusside should be discontinued; amyl nitrite inhalations may be administered until IV access can be established for sodium nitrite administration. A 3% sodium nitrite solution should then be administered IV at a dosage of 4–6 mg/kg (approximately 0.2 mL/kg of the 3% solution) injected over 2–4 minutes. This dose can be expected to convert about 10% of the patient's hemoglobin to methemoglobin; however, this degree of methemoglobinemia alone is not associated with any important hazard. Blood pressure should be carefully monitored during sodium nitrite administration since vasodilation and hypotension may occur; hypotension should be managed routinely. Following these steps, a 10 or 25% solution of sodium thiosulfate is administered IV in a dose of 150–200 mg/kg; a typical adult dose is 50 mL of the 25% solution. Injections of sodium nitrite and sodium thiosulfate may be repeated at one-half the initial recommended doses after 2 hours.

Thiosulfate treatment of acute cyanide toxicity will increase the serum concentration of thiocyanate; however, the increase should not pose any risk to the patient. Physiologic methods (e.g., altering urinary pH) have not been demonstrated to increase the elimination of thiocyanate. Although hemodialysis is ineffective for the removal of cyanide from circulation, most thiocyanate will be removed by this procedure; the clearance rate of thiocyanate can approach the blood flow rate of the dialyzer.

PHARMACOLOGY

Sodium nitroprusside is a potent direct arterial and venous dilator. When sodium nitroprusside is administered by IV infusion to hypertensive or normotensive patients, a marked lowering of arterial blood pressure is produced. Venous pressure is also lowered and a moderate reduction in total peripheral resistance occurs. The effects of the drug on blood pressure are more pronounced in hypertensive than in normotensive patients.

The hypotensive action of sodium nitroprusside results from peripheral vasodilation caused by a direct action on vascular smooth muscle. Animal tests performed *in situ* have demonstrated no relaxation of other smooth muscle tissue, such as the uterus or duodenum, by sodium nitroprusside. The drug has no direct effect on vasomotor centers, sympathetic nerves, or adrenergic receptors. The hypotensive effect of sodium nitroprusside is augmented by concomitant use of other hypotensive agents and is not blocked by adrenergic blocking agents or vagotomy. Pressor agents such as epinephrine which stimulate the myocardium directly are the only drugs that cause an increase in blood pressure during sodium nitroprusside therapy. Resistance to the drug's hypotensive effects is very rare.

The effects of sodium nitroprusside on cardiac performance appear to depend on preexisting performance. Changes in cardiac performance are attributed mainly to a reduction in left ventricular afterload resulting from vasodilation but may also be related to reduction in venous return to the heart resulting from peripheral vascular pooling of blood, decreased arteriolar resistance, and increased diastolic compliance. The drug may exert a direct coronary vasodilator effect. When sodium nitroprusside is administered to hypertensive patients, a slight increase in heart rate usually occurs and cardiac output is usually decreased slightly. Decreases in cardiac index and stroke index are common; however, these decreases do not occur consistently and increases have occurred in some patients. When sodium nitroprusside is administered to patients with refractory heart failure and/or acute myocardial infarction, substantial improvement in left ventricular performance results with cardiac output, cardiac index, and stroke volume being increased and left ventricular filling pressure being decreased. In patients with congestive heart failure, a slight but clinically important slowing of the heart rate results, as well as reduction or cessation of arrhythmias. A reduction in myocardial oxygen consumption during sodium nitroprusside use has been noted which could prove beneficial when infarcted areas of the heart are already short of oxygen. In patients with congestive heart failure, improvement in cardiac performance is accompanied by prompt diuresis, with urine volume and sodium excretion both being increased.

Moderate doses of sodium nitroprusside in hypertensive patients produce renal vasodilation without an appreciable increase in renal blood flow or a decrease in glomerular filtration. Mean renal arterial pressure and renal vascular resistance are slightly decreased. The acute reduction in mean arterial pressure is accompanied by an increase in renin activity of renal venous plasma.

PHARMACOKINETICS

● Absorption

IV infusion of sodium nitroprusside produces an almost immediate reduction in blood pressure. Blood pressure begins to rise immediately when the infusion is slowed or stopped and returns to pretreatment levels within 1–10 minutes.

● Distribution

Distribution of nitroprusside in the body as well as passage across the placenta, into milk, or across the blood-brain barrier has not been studied.

● Elimination

Sodium nitroprusside is rapidly metabolized, probably by interaction with sulfhydryl groups in the erythrocytes and tissues. Cyanogen (cyanide radical) is produced which is converted to thiocyanate in the liver by the enzyme thiosulfate sulfurtransferase (rhodanase). This mitochondrial enzyme normally is present in excess quantities such that the rate-limiting step in the conversion of cyanogen to thiocyanate usually is the availability of sulfur donors (e.g., thiosulfate, cystine, cysteine). A thiocyanate oxidase present in the erythrocytes may oxidize small quantities of thiocyanate back to cyanogen. Toxic symptoms begin to appear at plasma thiocyanate concentrations of 50–100 mcg/mL; fatalities have been reported at concentrations of 200 mcg/mL.

Sodium nitroprusside is excreted entirely as metabolites, principally thiocyanate. In animals, sodium nitroprusside metabolites are excreted mainly in urine, exhaled air, and probably in feces. The elimination half-life of thiocyanate is 2.7–7 days when renal function is normal but is longer in patients with impaired renal function or hyponatremia.

CHEMISTRY AND STABILITY

● Chemistry

Sodium nitroprusside is a hypotensive agent which is structurally unrelated to other available hypotensive agents. Sodium nitroprusside is commercially available as the dihydrate, and potency is expressed in terms of the hydrated drug. The drug occurs as reddish-brown, practically odorless, crystals or powder and is freely soluble in water and slightly soluble in alcohol.

● Stability

Sodium nitroprusside is sensitive to, and must be protected from, light, heat, and moisture. Sodium nitroprusside injection concentrate should be protected from light and stored at 20–25°C.

Exposure of sodium nitroprusside solutions to light causes deterioration which may be evidenced by a change from a brown to a blue color caused by reduction of the ferric ion to the ferrous ion. It has been reported that approximately 20% of sodium nitroprusside in solution in glass bottles undergoes degradation within 4 hours when exposed to fluorescent light. Solutions in Viaflex® bags exposed to fluorescent light are degraded even more rapidly. Specialized references should be consulted for specific stability information. Sodium nitroprusside solutions should be protected from light by wrapping the container with aluminum foil or other opaque material. If properly protected from light, diluted solutions of the drug are stable for 24 hours. Sodium nitroprusside solution is rapidly degraded by trace contaminants often forming highly colored products, usually blue, green, or red. If this occurs, the solution should be discarded. No other drug or preservative should be added to sodium nitroprusside infusions.

PREPARATIONS

Excipients in commercially available drug preparations may have clinically important effects in some individuals; consult specific product labeling for details.

Sodium Nitroprusside

Parenteral

Injection concentrate, for IV infusion only	25 mg/mL*	**Nitropress®**, Hospira
		Sodium Nitroprusside Injection

* available from one or more manufacturer, distributor, and/or repackager by generic (nonproprietary) name

† Use is not currently included in the labeling approved by the US Food and Drug Administration.

Doxazosin Mesylate

24:16 • α-ADRENERGIC BLOCKING AGENTS

■ Doxazosin mesylate is a quinazoline-derivative postsynaptic α₁-adrenergic blocking agent.

USES

● Hypertension

Doxazosin mesylate is used alone or in combination with other classes of antihypertensive agents for the management of hypertension. However, because of established clinical benefits (e.g., reductions in overall mortality and in adverse cardiovascular, cerebrovascular, and renal outcomes), current evidence-based practice guidelines for the management of hypertension in adults generally recommend the use of drugs from 4 classes of antihypertensive agents (angiotensin-converting enzyme [ACE] inhibitors, angiotensin II receptor antagonists, calcium-channel blockers, and thiazide diuretics).

In a randomized, double-blind clinical study (the Antihypertensive and Lipid-Lowering Treatment to Prevent Heart Attack Trial [ALLHAT]), doxazosin, an α₁-blocker, was less effective in lowering mean systolic blood pressure (by about 2–3 mm Hg) than chlorthalidone, a thiazide-like diuretic. In order to achieve target blood pressure in hypertensive patients, use of doxazosin required additional hypotensive therapy more frequently than chlorthalidone. In addition, interim analysis (median follow-up: 3.3 years) of this study indicated that use of doxazosin in high-risk (at least 2 risk factors for coronary heart disease) hypertensive patients 55 years of age and older was associated with a higher risk of stroke and a higher incidence of combined cardiovascular disease events (including twice the risk of congestive heart failure) than use of chlorthalidone. Study investigators concluded that such increased risk of congestive heart failure could not have been caused by the relatively small difference in the mean target systolic blood pressure observed in patients receiving doxazosin compared with those receiving chlorthalidone. Therefore, based on these findings, the trial's Data Safety and Monitoring Board recommended that the doxazosin treatment arm be terminated prematurely. The remaining antihypertensive arms (e.g., calcium-channel blockers, ACE enzyme inhibitors, diuretics) and lipid-lowering (pravastatin vs usual care) components of the study subsequently were completed and reported.

Current antihypertensive and urology guidelines no longer recommend α₁-blockers as preferred *first-line* therapy for any patients with hypertension, principally because of negative findings observed in ALLHAT. However, α₁-blockers are effective antihypertensive drugs and many experts still consider their use appropriate for the management of resistant hypertension as a component of combination therapy. Therapy with an α₁-blocker is most effective when used in combination with a diuretic. Some experts state that an α₁-blocker may be a second-line agent in antihypertensive treatment regimens in men with coexisting benign prostatic hyperplasia (BPH); the American Urology Association (AUA) states that monotherapy with these drugs is not optimal in hypertensive patients with lower urinary tract symptoms (LUTS) or BPH and that such conditions should be managed separately.

The beneficial effects of α₁-blockers on blood glucose and lipid concentrations may mitigate some of the adverse metabolic effects of diuretics, and α₁-blockers may offer some advantage in patients with underlying lipoprotein disorders (e.g., hypercholesterolemia) or in those with lipoprotein abnormalities induced by other antihypertensive agents (e.g., thiazide diuretics). The possibility that geriatric patients may be more susceptible than younger patients to the postural hypotensive effects of α₁-blockers should be considered in the selection of therapy. Blood pressure response to α₁-blockers appears to be comparable in white and black patients.

For further information on overall principles and expert recommendations for treatment of hypertension, see Uses: Hypertension in Adults and also see Uses: Hypertension in Pediatric Patients, in the Thiazides General Statement 40:28.20.

● Benign Prostatic Hyperplasia

Doxazosin is used to reduce urinary obstruction and relieve associated manifestations in hypertensive or normotensive patients with symptomatic benign prostatic hyperplasia (BPH, benign prostatic hypertrophy). For patients who can tolerate the potential cardiovascular and other effects of α₁-adrenergic blockade, doxazosin can effectively relieve mild to moderate obstructive manifestations (e.g., hesitancy, terminal dribbling of urine, interrupted or weak stream, impaired size and force of stream, sensation of incomplete bladder emptying or straining) and improve urinary flow rates in a substantial proportion of patients and may be a useful alternative to surgery, particularly in those who are awaiting or are unwilling to undergo surgical correction of the hyperplasia (e.g., via transurethral resection of the prostate [TURP]) or who are not candidates for such surgery.

Therapy with α₁-blockers appears to be less effective in relieving irritative (e.g., nocturia, daytime frequency, urgency, dysuria) than obstructive symptomatology. In addition, therapy with the drugs generally can be expected to produce less subjective and objective improvement than prostatectomy, and periodic monitoring (e.g., performance of digital rectal examinations, serum creatinine determinations, serum prostate specific antigen [PSA] assays) is indicated in these patients to detect and manage other potential complications of or conditions associated with BPH (e.g., obstructive uropathy, prostatic carcinoma). While symptomatic improvement has been maintained for at least up to 2 years of doxazosin therapy in some patients, the long-term effects of α-blockers on the need for surgery and on the frequency of developing BPH-associated complications such as acute urinary obstruction remain to be established.

Although the etiology of benign prostatic hyperplasia currently is unclear, age-associated changes in circulating hormones (e.g., androgens, estrogens) appear to be involved; approximately 40% of men have been reported to have clinical evidence of BPH by age 70. Hyperplasia of the prostatic tissue encircling the urethra produces narrowing of the bladder neck and prostatic urethra, leading to both obstructive (e.g., urinary hesitancy, slow/weak stream, straining, incomplete voiding) and irritative (e.g., urinary frequency, urgency, nocturia) manifestations; progressive obstruction of urinary flow eventually may lead to urinary retention and subsequent complications (e.g., urinary tract infection, bladder calculi, hydronephrosis).

In addition to the mechanical component of urethral obstruction caused by the enlarged gland, a dynamic component of obstruction may be prominent in some patients; current evidence suggests that approximately 50% of prostate outflow obstruction is caused by reversible α-adrenergic (principally α₁) receptor-mediated contractions of smooth muscle in the prostatic capsule, prostatic adenoma, and bladder neck. While nonselective α-adrenergic blockers such as phenoxybenzamine have been used successfully to treat BPH, such nonselective blockade has been associated with adverse effects such as postural hypotension, dizziness, and tachycardia because blockade of α₂-adrenergic receptors interferes with the negative feedback mechanism controlling norepinephrine release from presynaptic nerve terminals. As a result, nonselective α-blocker therapy currently is not recommended for BPH; instead, therapy with selective α₁-blockers, which can relieve α₁-adrenergic-mediated bladder outflow obstruction, is recommended.

Patients with mildly symptomatic BPH and those with moderate to severe symptoms that are not bothersome (i.e., that do not interfere with daily activities of living) generally should simply be followed rather than actively treated. Active therapy (e.g., drug therapy; minimally invasive therapies such as transurethral microwave heat; surgery such as TURP) should be considered for patients with moderate to severe BPH that is bothersome; the potential benefits and possible risks of various therapeutic options, including watchful waiting, should be discussed with the patient. Although drug therapy usually is not as effective as surgical therapy, it may provide adequate symptomatic relief with fewer and less serious adverse effects compared with surgery. Most experts currently consider therapy with an α₁-adrenergic blocker such as doxazosin to be an appropriate option for symptomatic treatment of bothersome lower urinary tract symptoms in patients with BPH. With the exception of prazosin (for which there are insufficient data to compare), currently available α₁-adrenergic blockers are considered comparably effective. Therapy with an α₁-adrenergic blocker generally is more effective in relieving lower urinary tract symptoms than that with a 5α-reductase inhibitor (e.g., finasteride), and 5α-reductase inhibitors are ineffective in patients without prostatic enlargement.

Combination Therapy

Although studies of up to 1 year in duration generally have found combination therapy with an α₁-blocker and 5α-reductase inhibitor (e.g., finasteride) to be no more effective than α₁-adrenergic blocker monotherapy in providing symptomatic relief of BPH, a long-term (mean follow-up: 4.5 years), double-blind study (Medical Therapy of Prostatic Symptoms [MTOPS]) found that combined therapy with doxazosin (4–8 mg daily) and finasteride (5 mg daily) was more effective than therapy with either drug alone in preventing symptom progression (defined as an increase from baseline of at least 4 points in the American Urological Association [AUA] symptom score, acute urinary retention, urinary incontinence, renal insufficiency, or recurrent urinary tract infection). The percent reduction in the risk of symptom progression (generally manifested as an increase in AUA symptom score) relative to placebo was 34% with finasteride, 39% with doxazosin, and 67% with combination therapy. The risks of long-term acute urinary retention and the need for invasive therapy were reduced by combination therapy and by finasteride monotherapy but not by doxazosin monotherapy. Combination therapy or doxazosin or finasteride monotherapy each were effective in providing improvement in symptom scores, with combination therapy providing greater improvement than either drug alone.

Most experts state that combined therapy with an α₁-adrenergic blocker and 5α-reductase inhibitor can be considered for men with bothersome moderate to severe BPH and demonstrable prostatic enlargement, weighing the benefit of preventing progression of BPH with the risks and cost of the combination. Men at risk for BPH progression are most likely to benefit from combination therapy. Although the benefit of combination therapy was not as substantial in men with low baseline prostate-specific antigen (PSA) levels compared with those with high baseline values in the MTOPS study, the potential benefit appears to be greatest in those in whom baseline risk of progression generally is high rather than specifically in those with larger prostates or higher PSA levels at baseline.

Adverse effects associated with combined α₁-adrenergic blocker and 5α-reductase inhibitor therapy generally reflect the combined toxicity profile of each drug alone, although certain adverse effects (e.g., effects on sexual function and libido, postural hypotension, peripheral edema, dizziness, asthenia, rhinitis) may be more common with combined therapy. For further information on adverse effects associated with combined doxazosin and finasteride therapy, see Cautions in Finasteride 92:08.

DOSAGE AND ADMINISTRATION

● Administration

Doxazosin mesylate is administered orally.

The pharmacokinetics and safety were similar with morning or evening dosing of doxazosin conventional (immediate-release) tablets in a limited number of normotensive patients in one study; however, the area under the plasma concentration-time curve (AUC) was 11% less with morning dosing, and the time to peak concentration occurred later with evening dosing (5.6 versus 3.5 hours).

Peak plasma concentrations and oral bioavailability are increased by approximately 32 and 18%, respectively, when doxazosin mesylate extended-release tablets (Cardura® XL) are administered with food. Therefore, to provide more consistent systemic exposure to the drug, extended-release tablets should be administered with breakfast.

Doxazosin mesylate extended-release tablets should be swallowed intact and should *not* be chewed, crushed, or broken. Patients should be advised *not* to become alarmed if they notice a tablet-like substance in their stools; this is normal since the tablet is designed to release the drug slowly from a nonabsorbable shell during passage through the GI tract.

● Dosage

Dosage of doxazosin mesylate is expressed in terms of doxazosin and must be adjusted according to the patient's blood pressure response and tolerance.

Hypertension
Usual Dosage

For the management of hypertension in adults, the usual initial dosage of doxazosin conventional (immediate-release) tablets is 1 mg once daily. Because of the risk of postural effects (see Cautions: Postural Effects), it is essential that therapy with the drug *not* be initiated with higher dosages. Patient response (standing blood pressure) should be assessed 2–6 and 24 hours after the initial dose and any subsequent dosage adjustments. Because postural effects are most likely to occur 2–6 hours after a dose, it is particularly important that the standing blood pressure response be assessed during this period after the first dose and any increases.

If blood pressure is not adequately controlled at a doxazosin dosage of 1 mg daily as conventional tablets, the dosage may be increased to 2 mg once daily in adults; subsequent dosage adjustments can be made by doubling the dose until the desired blood pressure control is achieved, the drug is not tolerated, or a maximum dosage of 16 mg once daily is reached. Some experts state that the usual adult dosage ranges from 1–16 mg once daily. The manufacturer recommends that dosage increases be made no more frequently than every 2 weeks. Doxazosin dosages exceeding 4 mg daily as conventional tablets are associated with an increased likelihood of excessive postural effects including syncope, dizziness, vertigo, and hypotension, and those exceeding 16 mg daily are *not* recommended because of the substantial risk of postural effects.

If doxazosin is used for the management of hypertension in children†, some experts have recommended an initial dosage of 1 mg once daily as conventional tablets; dosage may be increased as necessary to a maximum of 4 mg once daily. (See Cautions: Pediatric Precautions.) For information on overall principles and expert recommendations for treatment of hypertension in pediatric patients, see Uses: Hypertension in Pediatric Patients, in the Thiazides General Statement 40:28.20.

Extended-release doxazosin tablets (Cardura® XL) currently are not FDA-labeled for use in the management of hypertension.

Blood Pressure Monitoring and Treatment Goals

Blood pressure should be monitored regularly (i.e., monthly) during therapy and dosage adjusted until blood pressure is controlled. If an adequate blood pressure response is not achieved, the dosage may be increased or another antihypertensive agent with demonstrated benefit and preferably with a complementary mechanism of action (e.g., angiotensin-converting enzyme [ACE] inhibitor, angiotensin II receptor antagonist, calcium-channel blocker, thiazide diuretic) may be added; if target blood pressure is still not achieved with the use of 2 antihypertensive agents, a third drug may be added. (See Uses: Hypertension.) In patients who develop unacceptable adverse effects with doxazosin, the drug should be discontinued and another antihypertensive agent from a different pharmacologic class should be initiated.

The goal of hypertension management and prevention is to achieve and maintain optimal control of blood pressure. However, the optimum blood pressure threshold for initiating antihypertensive drug therapy and specific treatment goals remain controversial. A 2017 multidisciplinary hypertension guideline from the American College of Cardiology (ACC), American Heart Association (AHA), and a number of other professional organizations generally recommends a blood pressure goal of less than 130/80 mm Hg in all adults, regardless of comorbidities or level of atherosclerotic cardiovascular disease (ASCVD) risk. Many patients will require at least 2 drugs from different pharmacologic classes to achieve this blood pressure goal; the potential benefits of hypertension management and drug cost, adverse effects, and risks associated with the use of multiple antihypertensive drugs also should be considered when deciding a patient's blood pressure treatment goal.

For additional information on target levels of blood pressure and on monitoring therapy in the management of hypertension, see Blood Pressure Monitoring and Treatment Goals under Dosage: Hypertension, in Dosage and Administration in the Thiazides General Statement 40:28.20.

Benign Prostatic Hyperplasia

For the management of benign prostatic hyperplasia (BPH), the usual initial adult dosage of doxazosin as conventional (immediate-release) tablets is 1 mg daily, given in the morning or in the evening. Some clinicians state that it is preferable to administer the drug at bedtime to minimize postural effects. Because of the risk of postural effects (see Cautions: Postural Effects), it is essential that therapy with the drug *not* be initiated with higher dosages.

To achieve the desired improvement in symptoms and urodynamics, subsequent doxazosin dosage as conventional tablets may be increased in a stepwise manner to 2, 4, and 8 mg daily as necessary; it is recommended that each doubling of dosage occur at intervals of not less than 1–2 weeks. Although higher dosages (e.g., 16 mg daily) have been used, maximally tolerable and effective dosages have not been established and the manufacturer and most experts recommend that the dosage for BPH not exceed 8 mg daily as conventional tablets. Blood pressure should be evaluated routinely in patients receiving doxazosin therapy, particularly with initiation of therapy and subsequent dosage adjustment (see Dosage: Hypertension).

In a study demonstrating the combined efficacy of an α₁-adrenergic blocker and 5α-reductase inhibitor, doxazosin therapy as conventional tablets was initiated at a dosage of 1 mg daily at bedtime for the first week and then doubled at 1-week intervals until a dosage of 8 mg daily was achieved. In patients who could not tolerate the 8-mg dose, dosage was reduced to 4 mg daily as conventional tablets; those unable to tolerate the 4-mg dose were counted as having discontinued the drug. Finasteride was administered concomitantly at a dosage of 5 mg daily at bedtime.

Alternatively, when extended-release tablets are used for the management of BPH, the usual initial dosage is 4 mg once daily with breakfast. This dosage also should be used initially in patients being switched from conventional tablets. Depending on patient response and tolerability, extended-release dosage may be increased to a maximum of 8 mg once daily with breakfast. If extended-release therapy is interrupted, it should be reinitiated at 4 mg once daily.

● Dosage in Renal and Hepatic Impairment

Clinically important alterations in the pharmacokinetics of doxazosin in patients with impaired renal function have not been observed to date, and the manufacturer makes no specific recommendations for modification of dosage in such patients.

The effect of hepatic impairment on the disposition of doxazosin has not been established in controlled clinical studies. However, administration of a single 2-mg dose of doxazosin as conventional tablets to patients with cirrhosis (Child-Pugh class A) resulted in a 40% increase in systemic exposure to the drug. Because doxazosin is eliminated almost entirely by metabolism in the liver, the manufacturer states that the drug should be administered cautiously in patients with hepatic impairment.

● Dosage in Geriatric Patients

While the manufacturer makes no specific recommendations for titration of doxazosin dosage in geriatric patients, patients in this age group generally are less tolerant of the postural hypotensive effects of α₁-adrenergic blocking agents because of impaired cardiovascular reflexes, and caution should be exercised. Therefore, dosage escalation in elderly hypertensive patients generally should be slower than in younger adults. Clinically important alterations in the pharmacokinetics of the drug in geriatric patients have not been observed to date.

CAUTIONS

Adverse effects occurring most frequently during doxazosin mesylate therapy for hypertension include dizziness, headache, drowsiness, lack of energy (e.g, lethargy, fatigue), nausea, edema, and rhinitis. In patients receiving the drug for benign prostatic hyperplasia (BPH), the most frequent adverse effects are dizziness, headache, fatigue, edema, dyspnea, abdominal pain, and diarrhea. The frequency of adverse effects in controlled clinical trials generally has been lower in patients receiving doxazosin for BPH than in those receiving the drug for hypertension; however, dosages employed for this condition also generally have been lower than those for hypertension.

While adverse effects occur frequently in patients receiving the drug, most are mild to moderate in severity, and discontinuance of doxazosin secondary to adverse effects was required in only 7% of patients with hypertension during clinical trials. The principal reasons for discontinuance in patients with hypertension were postural effects in 2% of patients and edema, malaise/fatigue, and heart rate disturbance each in about 0.7% of patients. In controlled clinical trials in patients with hypertension, only dizziness (including postural effects), weight gain, somnolence, and malaise/fatigue occurred at rates significantly greater than those for placebo; postural effects and edema appeared to be dose related. Only dizziness, fatigue, hypotension, edema, and dyspnea occurred significantly more frequently with the drug than placebo in controlled clinical trials for BPH; dizziness and dyspnea appeared to be dose-related.

● Postural Effects

Doxazosin, like other α₁-adrenergic blocking agents, can cause marked hypotension, which may be accompanied by syncope and other postural effects. While syncope is the most severe orthostatic effect of the drug, other less severe symptoms, such as dizziness, lightheadedness, and vertigo, also can be associated with doxazosin-induced reductions in blood pressure. Syncope is uncommon when doxazosin dosage is initiated at low levels and titrated slowly, but dizziness and/or lightheadedness are frequent, occurring in about 20 or 16% of patients receiving the drug for hypertension or BPH, respectively, in controlled trials. Vertigo has been reported in 2%, syncope in 0.7%, and postural hypotension in 0.3% of hypertensive patients in controlled trials. In patients receiving the drug for BPH in controlled clinical trials, postural hypotension was reported in 0.3% and syncope in 0.5–0.7% of patients.

Doxazosin-induced postural effects are dose related, particularly likely in the upright position following an initial dose, and most likely to develop between 2–6 hours after administration. With continued therapy after careful dosage titration, adaptation of reflex mechanisms to α₁-blockade develop and the risk of postural effects generally subsides. However, marked hypotension also can occur with subsequent dosage increases or after therapy is interrupted for more than a few days. In clinical trials in patients with hypertension, postural effects occurred in 23% of patients receiving the drug and required discontinuance in 2% of patients. In clinical trials in patients with BPH receiving doxazosin dosages up to 8 mg daily, discontinuance of the drug for postural effects was required in 3.3% of patients. While the adverse effect profiles of doxazosin and prazosin generally appear to be similar, it has been suggested that postural effects may be less likely with doxazosin in part because of the drug's slower onset of action and reduced affinity for α₁-receptors; however, additional study and experience are needed to elucidate the relative risks of postural effects.

The risk of first-dose syncope with α₁-adrenergic blocking agents generally can be minimized by initiating therapy at low doses (i.e., 1 mg of doxazosin daily) and lessening the level of salt restriction and avoiding diuretics just prior to initiation of α₁-blocker therapy. It is essential that doxazosin therapy *not* be initiated at dosages exceeding 1 mg daily and that dosage escalation be slow with patient evaluations. In addition, it is important that standing blood pressure be evaluated 2 minutes after standing. If syncope develops, the patient should be placed in the recumbent position and treated supportively as necessary. Patients should be advised to lie or sit down if they develop any postural symptom (e.g., dizziness, vertigo) and to exercise caution upon standing from a sitting or supine position. Patients also should be cautioned to avoid situations, both during the day and through the night, that could result in injury if syncope were to occur. Other antihypertensive therapy should added cautiously in patients receiving doxazosin.

In an early dose-ranging study of the safety and tolerance of doxazosin in several normotensive individuals, two-thirds of these individuals could not tolerate dosages exceeding 2 mg daily because of symptomatic postural hypotension. In other studies in normotensive individuals, approximately 30% of individuals receiving initial doxazosin dosages of 2 mg daily experienced symptomatic hypotension 0.5–6 hours after the dose, and in subsequent trials in hypertensive patients in which doxazosin therapy was initiated at 1 mg daily, postural effects were observed following the initial dose in 4% of patients but were not associated with syncope. In multiple-dose clinical trials in hypertensive patients involving dosage initiation at 1 mg daily and titration every 1–2 weeks, syncope was reported in less than 1% of patients, occurring in no patients at a dosage of 1 mg daily but in 1.2% of those titrated to 16 mg daily. In dose titration trials, the frequency of orthostatic effects could be minimized by initiating therapy at 1 mg daily and titrating dosage no more frequently than every 2 weeks to a maximum of 2.4–8 mg daily. The frequency of orthostatic effects in these titration trials in hypertensive patients was about 12% in those receiving 16 mg of doxazosin once daily, 10% in those receiving 8 mg or more once daily, and 5% in those receiving 1–4 mg once daily. In controlled trials in patients with BPH, the frequency of orthostatic hypotension was not dose related at dosages up to 8 mg daily, titrated at intervals of 1–2 weeks.

● Nervous System Effects

Besides dizziness (see Cautions: Postural Effects), headache is the most common adverse nervous system effect associated with doxazosin therapy, occurring in about 14 or 10% of patients receiving the drug for hypertension or BPH, respectively. Somnolence occurs in 5 or 3% of such patients, respectively, and pain in 2% of patients. Nervousness occurs in about 2% of patients receiving doxazosin for hypertension, and insomnia and anxiety occur in 1.2 and 1.1%, respectively, of those receiving the drug for BPH; insomnia occurs in 1% of hypertensive patients. Adverse nervous system effects occurring in 0.5–1% of patients include paresthesia, kinetic disorders, ataxia, hypertonia, hypoesthesia, agitation, depression, and decreased libido. Paresis, tremor, twitching, confusion, migraine, paroniria, amnesia, emotional lability, impaired concentration, abnormal thinking, and depersonalization have been reported in less than 0.5% of patients, but a causal relationship to the drug has not been established.

● GI Effects

Nausea, diarrhea, and dry mouth are the most common adverse GI effects of doxazosin in hypertensive patients, occurring in 3, 2, and 2% of such patients, respectively, and abdominal pain, diarrhea, dyspepsia, nausea, and dry mouth are the most common in those with BPH, occurring in 2.4, 2.3, 1.7, 1.5, and 1.4% of such patients, respectively; dyspepsia occurs in 1% of hypertensive patients. Constipation and flatulence occur in 1% of patients receiving the drug for hypertension. Increased appetite, anorexia, fecal incontinence, and gastroenteritis have been reported in less than 0.5% of hypertensive patients but not directly attributed to the drug. Vomiting has been reported during postmarketing experience with doxazosin.

● Cardiovascular Effects

Besides postural effects of the drug (see Cautions: Postural Effects), other cardiovascular effects reported in patients receiving doxazosin for hypertension or BPH include edema in 4 or 2.7%, respectively, and palpitation and chest pain in 2 or 1.2% of such patients, respectively. Arrhythmia occurs in 1% of hypertensive patients, and tachycardia and angina pectoris occur in 0.9 and 0.6%, respectively, of patients with BPH. Tachycardia and peripheral ischemia have been reported in 0.3% of hypertensive patients. Hot flushes, ischemia, angina pectoris, myocardial infarction, and cerebral vascular accident have been reported in less that 0.5% of hypertensive patients, but a causal relationship has not been established. In addition, bradycardia has been reported with doxazosin during postmarketing experience.

An increased incidence of myocardial necrosis and fibrosis has been observed in Sprague-Dawley rats after 6 months of oral doxazosin dosages of 80 mg/kg daily, and after 12 months of oral dosages of 40 mg/kg daily (AUC exposure in rats was 8 times the human AUC exposure associated with a 12 mg daily dosage). Myocardial fibrosis also was observed in both rats and mice receiving an oral dosage of 40 mg/kg daily for 18 months (AUC exposure in rats was 8 times the human exposure and in mice was somewhat equivalent to the human exposure). No cardiotoxicity was associated with lower dosages (e.g., 10 or 20 mg/kg daily, depending on the study) in either species, and such effects also were not observed following 12 months of administration in dogs receiving maximum oral doxazosin dosages of 20 mg/kg daily nor in Wistar rats receiving maximum oral dosages of 100 mg/kg daily. While the clinical relevance of these findings to human is not known, the manufacturer states that there currently is no evidence that similar lesions occur in humans.

● Dermatologic Effects

Adverse dermatologic effects associated with doxazosin include rash, pruritus, and facial edema. In controlled clinical trials, these effects were reported in 1% of hypertensive patients. Pallor, alopecia, dry skin, and eczema have been reported in less than 0.5% of hypertensive patients receiving doxazosin, but a causal relationship to the drug has not been established.

● Musculoskeletal Effects

Arthralgia/arthritis, muscle weakness, myalgia, and muscle cramps have been reported in 1% of hypertensive patients receiving doxazosin. Back pain was reported in 1.8% or less than 0.5% of patients receiving the drug for BPH or hypertension, respectively.

● Respiratory Effects

Rhinitis occurs in 3% of hypertensive patients receiving doxazosin. Dyspnea occurs in 2.6 or 1% of patients with BPH or hypertension, respectively, and respiratory disorder occurs in 1.1% of those with BPH. Bronchospasm, sinusitis, cough, and pharyngitis have been reported in less than 0.5% of hypertensive patients but not directly attributed to the drug. In addition, aggravated bronchospasm has been reported with doxazosin during postmarketing experience.

● Genitourinary Effects

Polyuria occurs in 2% of hypertensive patients receiving doxazosin and urinary incontinence occurs in 1% of such patients. Sexual dysfunction occurred in 2% of hypertensive patients and impotence occurred in 1.1% of those with BPH receiving the drug. Urinary tract infection and dysuria were reported in 1.4 and 0.5%, respectively, of patients with BPH receiving doxazosin, but they occurred less frequently than with placebo. Renal calculus has been reported in less than 0.5% of hypertensive patients, but a causal relationship has not been established. Priapism (painful penile erection sustained for hours and unrelieved by sexual intercourse or masturbation) has been reported rarely (probably less frequently than 1 in several thousand patients) in patients receiving an α₁-adrenergic antagonist (e.g., doxazosin). Urinary frequency, nocturia, hematuria, and unspecified micturition disorder have been reported with doxazosin during postmarketing experience.

● Ocular and Otic Effects

Visual abnormalities occur in 2 or 1.4% of patients receiving doxazosin for hypertension of BPH, respectively, and conjunctivitis/ocular pain occurs in 1% of hypertensive patients. Tinnitus also occurs in 1% of patients receiving the drug. Photophobia, abnormal lacrimation, and earache have been reported in less than 0.5% of hypertensive patients, but these effects have not been directly attributed to the drug.

● Hematologic Effects

Adverse hematologic effects reported with doxazosin include decreased leukocyte and neutrophil counts. Mean reductions in these counts relative to placebo were 2.4 and 1%, respectively, in clinical trials in hypertensive patients. In clinical trials in patients with BPH, clinically important leukocyte abnormalities occurred in 0.4% of patients receiving doxazosin and in 0% of those receiving placebo, but the difference in incidence between these groups was not statistically different. Leukopenia and thrombocytopenia have been reported with doxazosin during postmarketing experience.

A search by the manufacturer of a database that included information on 2400 hypertensive patients and 665 with BPH revealed 4 cases in the hypertensive group and one case in the BPH group in which doxazosin-related neutropenia could not be ruled out. In 2 hypertensive patients, stable, nonprogressive neutropenia of about 1000/mm³ was observed over periods of 20–40 weeks. In a patient with BPH, the leukocyte count decreased from 4800 to 2700/mm³ at the end of the study, but there was no evidence of clinical impairment. In cases where follow-up was possible, leukocyte and neutrophil counts returned to normal after discontinuance of doxazosin; no cases of symptomatic reductions have been reported to date. Similar reductions in leukocyte and neutrophil counts have been observed with other α₁-adrenergic blocking agents.

● Other Adverse Effects

Sweating has been reported in 1.1 or 0.5–1% of patients receiving doxazosin for BPH or hypertension, respectively, and flu-like symptoms have been reported in 1.1 or less than 0.5% of such patients, respectively. Weight gain has been reported in 0.5–1% of hypertensive patients receiving the drug and thirst, gout, hypokalemia, lymphadenopathy, purpura, breast pain, taste perversion, parosmia, infection, fever/rigors, and weight loss have been reported in less than 0.5% of patients. In addition, gynecomastia, hepatitis, and cholestatic hepatitis have been reported with doxazosin during postmarketing experience.

● Precautions and Contraindications

Patients should be warned of the possibility of doxazosin-induced postural dizziness and measures to take if it develops (e.g., sitting, lying down). (See Cautions: Postural Effects.) During initiation of doxazosin therapy, the patient should be cautioned to avoid situations, both day and night, where injury could result if syncope occurs. If syncope occurs, the patient should be placed in the recumbent position and treated supportively as necessary. Patients who engage in potentially hazardous activities such as operating machinery or driving motor vehicles should be warned about possible drowsiness, dizziness, or lightheadedness.

Patients also should be advised that priapism has been reported rarely in patients receiving an α₁-adrenergic antagonist (e.g., doxazosin). Priapism is a medical emergency that could result in penile tissue damage and permanent loss of potency if not treated immediately; therefore, patients should be advised to report promptly to their clinician or, if their clinician is unavailable, to seek alternative immediate medical attention if an erection occurs that persists longer than several (e.g., 4–6) hours or is painful.

Experience to date with doxazosin under controlled conditions is limited to patients with normal liver function. However, because the drug is almost completely metabolized in the liver, particular caution should be exercised when using doxazosin in patients with impaired liver function or who are receiving other agents (e.g., cimetidine) that could influence hepatic clearance of the drug.

The possibility of carcinoma of the prostate and other conditions associated with manifestations that mimic those of BPH should be excluded in any patient for whom doxazosin therapy for presumed BPH is being considered. No evidence of an effect on plasma concentrations of prostate specific antigen (PSA) has been observed in patients treated with doxazosin for up to 3 years.

Doxazosin is contraindicated in patients with known sensitivity to the drug or any other quinazoline derivative (e.g., prazosin, terazosin).

● Pediatric Precautions

The manufacturer states that safety and efficacy of doxazosin in children and adolescents younger than 18 years of age have not been established. Some experts state that use of centrally acting antihypertensive agents (e.g., doxazosin) should be reserved for children who are not responsive to 2 or more of the preferred classes of antihypertensive agents (angiotensin-converting enzyme [ACE] inhibitors, angiotensin II receptor antagonists, long-acting calcium-channel blockers, or thiazide diuretics). For information on overall principles and expert recommendations for treatment of hypertension in pediatric patients, see Uses: Hypertension in Pediatric Patients, in the Thiazides General Statement 40:28.20.

● Geriatric Precautions

Geriatric patients may be particularly susceptible to postural effects of α₁-adrenergic blocking agents such as doxazosin. (See Dosage and Administration: Dosage.) The manufacturer states that certain pharmacokinetic parameters (i.e., plasma half-life, oral clearance) were similar for geriatric individuals 65 years of age or older compared with younger adults. In addition, safety and efficacy of the drug in patients with BPH were similar in those 65 years of age or older compared with younger patients. Clinical studies of doxazosin in patients with hypertension did not include sufficient numbers of patients 65 years of age and older to determine whether geriatric patients respond differently than younger patients. While other clinical experience has not revealed age-related differences in response, drug dosage generally should be titrated carefully in geriatric patients, usually initiating therapy at the low end of the dosage range. The greater frequency of decreased hepatic, renal, and/or cardiac function and of concomitant disease and drug therapy observed in the elderly also should be considered.

● Mutagenicity and Carcinogenicity

The manufacturer states that there was no evidence of mutagenicity associated with doxazosin or its metabolites at the chromosomal or subchromosomal level in mutagenicity studies.

No evidence of carcinogenicity was seen in rats receiving the maximally tolerated oral doxazosin dosage of 40 mg/kg daily (8 times the human AUC exposure) for up to 24 months. There also was no evidence of carcinogenicity in a similarly conducted study in mice receiving oral doxazosin for up to 18 months; however, the relevance, if any, of the findings of this study in mice is unclear since the maximally tolerated dosage was not employed.

● Pregnancy, Fertility, and Lactation

Pregnancy

Reproduction studies in rabbits and rats using doxazosin dosages up to 41 and 20 mg/kg daily (plasma concentrations 10 and 4 times the peak plasma concentration and AUC exposures of humans receiving a dosage of 12 mg daily) have not revealed evidence of harm to the fetus. Postnatal development (weight gain, anatomical features, reflexes) was delayed in some offspring of rats given maternal oral doxazosin dosages of 40–50 mg/kg daily, and decreased fetal survival was associated with dosages of 82 mg/kg daily (in rabbits). There are no adequate and controlled studies to date using doxazosin in pregnant women, and the drug should be used during pregnancy only when clearly needed.

Fertility

Reproduction studies in male rats using oral doxazosin dosages of 20 mg/kg daily demonstrated a reversible decrease in fertility; however, oral dosages of 10 mg/kg or less daily were not associated with impaired fertility. There have been no reports of adverse effects of the drug on fertility in men.

Lactation

Since it is not known whether doxazosin is distributed into human milk, the drug should be used with caution in nursing women. Accumulation of the drug has been observed in the milk of lactating rats given a single 1-mg/kg oral dose; in these rats, concentrations of radiolabeled doxazosin in milk were about 20 times greater than those in maternal plasma.

DESCRIPTION

Doxazosin mesylate is a quinazoline-derivative postsynaptic α₁-adrenergic blocking agent. The drug is chemically and pharmacologically related to prazosin and

terazosin. On a weight basis, the postsynaptic α₁-adrenergic blocking potency of doxazosin is half that of prazosin, and the α₁-receptor selectivity is one-fourth that of terazosin when tested in human prostate adenoma.

Doxazosin reduces peripheral vascular resistance and blood pressure as a result of its vasodilating effects; the drug produces both arterial and venous dilation. Doxazosin reduces blood pressure in both supine and standing patients; the effect is most pronounced on standing blood pressure, and postural hypotension can occur. Doxazosin generally causes no change in heart rate or cardiac output in the supine position. Cardiovascular responses to exercise (e.g., increased heart rate and cardiac output) are maintained during doxazosin therapy.

Effects of doxazosin on the cardiovascular system are mediated by the drug's activity at α₁-receptor sites on vascular smooth muscle. α₁-Adrenergic receptors also are located in nonvascular smooth muscle (e.g., bladder trigone and sphincters, GI tract and sphincters, prostate adenoma and capsule, ureters, uterus) and in nonmuscular tissues (e.g., CNS, liver, kidneys). Because of the prevalence of α-receptors on the prostate capsule, prostate adenoma, and the bladder trigone and the relative absence of these receptors on the bladder body, α-blockers decrease urinary outflow resistance in men.

Doxazosin may improve to a limited extent the serum lipid profile (e.g., small increases in high-density lipoprotein cholesterol concentrations [HDL] and HDL/total cholesterol ratio, small decreases in low-density lipoprotein cholesterol [LDL], total cholesterol, and triglyceride concentrations), and can reduce blood glucose and serum insulin concentrations. The drug does not appear to affect plasma renin activity appreciably.

Commercially available extended-release tablets of doxazosin mesylate (Cardura® XL) contain the drug in an oral osmotic delivery system formulation (elementary osmotic pump, GI therapeutic system [GITS]). The osmotic delivery system consists of an osmotically active core (comprised of a layer containing the drug and a layer containing osmotically active but pharmacologically inert components) that is surrounded by a semipermeable membrane with a laser-drilled delivery orifice and is designed to deliver the drug at an approximately constant rate over a 24-hour period (approximately zero-order delivery). The inert tablet ingredients remain intact and are eliminated in feces. Oral bioavailability from extended-release tablets at steady state with 4- or 8-mg doses is 54 or 59%, respectively, of that achieved with conventional (immediate-release) tablets. Food increases peak plasma concentrations and bioavailability achieved with extended-release tablets.

PREPARATIONS

Excipients in commercially available drug preparations may have clinically important effects in some individuals; consult specific product labeling for details.

Doxazosin Mesylate

Oral

Tablets	1 mg (of doxazosin)*	Cardura® (scored), Pfizer
		Doxazosin Mesylate Tablets
	2 mg (of doxazosin)*	Cardura® (scored), Pfizer
		Doxazosin Mesylate Tablets
	4 mg (of doxazosin)*	Cardura® (scored), Pfizer
		Doxazosin Mesylate Tablets
	8 mg (of doxazosin)*	Cardura® (scored), Pfizer
		Doxazosin Mesylate Tablets
Tablets, extended-release	4 mg (of doxazosin)	Cardura® XL, Pfizer
	8 mg (of doxazosin)	Cardura® XL, Pfizer

* available from one or more manufacturer, distributor, and/or repackager by generic (nonproprietary) name

† Use is not currently included in the labeling approved by the US Food and Drug Administration.

Prazosin Hydrochloride

24:16 • α-ADRENERGIC BLOCKING AGENTS

■ Prazosin hydrochloride is an α₁-adrenergic blocking agent.

USES

● Hypertension

Prazosin hydrochloride is used alone or in combination with other classes of antihypertensive agents in the management of hypertension. However, because of established clinical benefits (e.g., reductions in overall mortality and in adverse cardiovascular, cerebrovascular, and renal outcomes), current evidence-based practice guidelines for the management of hypertension in adults generally recommend the use of drugs from 4 classes of antihypertensive agents (angiotensin-converting enzyme [ACE] inhibitors, angiotensin II receptor antagonists, calcium-channel blockers, and thiazide diuretics).

In a randomized, double-blind clinical study (the Antihypertensive and Lipid-Lowering Treatment to Prevent Heart Attack Trial [ALLHAT]), doxazosin, an α₁-blocker, was less effective in lowering mean systolic blood pressure (by about 2–3 mm Hg) than chlorthalidone, a thiazide-like diuretic. In order to achieve target blood pressure in hypertensive patients, use of doxazosin required additional hypotensive therapy more frequently than chlorthalidone. In addition, interim analysis (median follow-up: 3.3 years) of this study indicated that use of doxazosin in high-risk (at least 2 risk factors for coronary heart disease) hypertensive patients 55 years of age and older was associated with a higher risk of stroke and a higher incidence of combined cardiovascular disease events (including twice the risk of congestive heart failure than use of chlorthalidone. Study investigators concluded that such increased risk of congestive heart failure could not have been caused by the relatively small difference in the mean target systolic blood pressure observed in patients receiving doxazosin compared with those receiving chlorthalidone. Therefore, based on these findings, the trial's Data Safety and Monitoring Board recommended that the α-blocker treatment arm be terminated prematurely. The remaining antihypertensive arms (e.g., calcium-channel blocking agents, angiotensin-converting enzyme [ACE] inhibitors, diuretics) and lipid-lowering (pravastatin vs usual care) components of the study subsequently were completed and reported.

Current antihypertensive and urology guidelines no longer recommend α₁-blockers as preferred *first-line* therapy for any patients with hypertension, principally because of negative findings observed in ALLHAT. However, α₁-blockers are effective antihypertensive drugs and many experts still consider their use appropriate for the management of resistant hypertension as a component of combination therapy. Therapy with an α₁-blocker is most effective when used in combination with a diuretic. Some experts state that an α₁-blocker may be a second-line agent in antihypertensive treatment regimens in men with coexisting benign prostatic hyperplasia (BPH); the American Urology Association (AUA) states that monotherapy with these drugs is not optimal in hypertensive patients with lower urinary tract symptoms (LUTS) or BPH and that such conditions should be managed separately.

The beneficial effects of α₁-blockers on blood glucose and lipid concentrations may mitigate some of the adverse metabolic effects of diuretics, and α₁-blockers may offer some advantage in patients with underlying lipoprotein disorders (e.g., hypercholesterolemia) or in those with lipoprotein abnormalities induced by other antihypertensive agents (e.g., thiazide diuretics). The possibility that geriatric patients may be more susceptible than younger patients to the postural hypotensive effects of α₁-blockers should be considered in the selection of therapy. Blood pressure response to α₁-blockers appears to be comparable in white and black patients.

Prazosin generally is most effective when used with a diuretic. The use of a diuretic may permit reduction of prazosin dosage. Prazosin has also been used with other hypotensive drugs, permitting a reduction in the dosage of each drug and, in some patients, minimizing adverse effects while maintaining blood pressure control. (See Drug Interactions: Diuretics and Hypotensive Agents.)

For further information on overall principles and expert recommendations for treatment of hypertension, see Uses: Hypertension in Adults, in the Thiazides General Statement 40:28.20.

● Benign Prostatic Hyperplasia

Prazosin has been used to reduce urinary obstruction and relieve associated manifestations (e.g., urinary hesitancy and/or urgency, nocturia) in patients with symptomatic benign prostatic hyperplasia† (BPH, benign prostatic hypertrophy) but efficacy relative to other α₁-blockers remains to be established. For patients who can tolerate the potential cardiovascular and other effects of α₁-adrenergic blockade, the drug can effectively relieve mild to moderate obstructive manifestations in a substantial proportion of patients, at least in the short term, and may be a useful alternative to surgery, particularly in those who are awaiting or are unwilling to undergo surgical correction of the hyperplasia (e.g., via transurethral resection of the prostate [TURP]) or who are not candidates for such surgery.

Therapy with α₁-blockers appears to be less effective in relieving irritative than obstructive symptomatology. In addition, therapy with the drugs generally can be expected to produce less subjective and objective improvement than prostatectomy, and periodic monitoring (e.g., performance of digital rectal examination, serum creatinine determinations, serum prostate specific antigen [PSA] assays) is indicated in these patients to detect and manage other potential complications of or conditions associated with BPH (e.g., obstructive uropathy, prostatic carcinoma). While symptomatic improvement has been observed in the short term in some patients receiving prazosin therapy, the long-term effects of α₁-blockers on the need for surgery and on the frequency of developing BPH-associated complications such as acute urinary obstruction remain to be established. Currently available α₁-adrenergic blockers (with the exception of prazosin, for which there are insufficient data to compare) are considered comparably effective.

Current evidence from principally uncontrolled, short-term studies suggests that the α₁-selective adrenergic blocker prazosin produces beneficial effects in approximately 60–70% of treated patients without the degree of adverse effects associated with nonselective adrenergic blockers; alleviation of both obstructive and irritative manifestations of the hyperplasia has been reported in some patients with prazosin therapy. In a few placebo-controlled or comparative studies, therapy with prazosin in dosages of 1–9 mg daily (generally 2 mg twice daily) has improved urinary flow rates and reduced urinary frequency and nocturia in patients with BPH.

Combination therapy with an α₁-blocker and 5α-reductase inhibitor (e.g., finasteride) has been more effective than therapy with either drug alone in preventing long-term BPH symptom progression; combined therapy also can reduce the risks of long-term acute urinary retention and the need for invasive therapy compared with α₁-blocker monotherapy.

For additional information on the use of α₁-blockers in the management of BPH, see Uses: Benign Prostatic Hyperplasia, in Doxazosin 24:20.

● Posttraumatic Stress Disorder

Prazosin has been used in the management of posttraumatic stress disorder (PTSD)†, particularly in combat veterans and in patients experiencing nighttime PTSD symptoms (e.g., nightmares, sleep disturbances). Nightmares and other sleep disturbances reportedly occur in about 70–87% of patients with PTSD; such patients often have decreased sleep efficiency because of more frequent nocturnal awakenings, as well as a higher incidence of other parasomnias and sleep-related breathing disorders compared with patients who have idiopathic nightmares.

Although selective serotonin-reuptake inhibitors (SSRIs; e.g., paroxetine, sertraline) generally have been considered the drugs of choice for the pharmacologic treatment of PTSD, they usually have not been effective in treating nighttime PTSD symptoms, which can be very disturbing and substantially interfere with the patient's quality of life. Atypical antipsychotic agents also have been studied in the treatment of PTSD and have been shown to reduce nighttime PTSD symptoms and may help reduce accompanying psychotic and other symptoms (e.g., agitation, irritability) in some patients; however, routine and long-term use of these drugs is discouraged by some clinicians because of the risk of clinically important adverse effects, such as weight gain and diabetes mellitus.

Clinical experience with prazosin in PTSD to date, which is mainly from small case series, case reports, retrospective or open-label studies, and several small randomized placebo-controlled studies, indicates that the drug is effective in suppressing or eliminating the nighttime sleep-related symptoms associated with PTSD. In several open-label and retrospective studies, prazosin therapy substantially improved trauma-related nightmares and reduced the severity of PTSD (as assessed by the recurrent distressing dreams item of the Clinician-Administered PTSD Scale [CAPS] and/or the Clinical Global Impression of Change [CGI-C] Scale, a 7-point clinician-rated assessment measuring overall PTSD severity and function).

In 2 randomized, double-blind, placebo-controlled trials conducted in combat veterans with PTSD, prazosin was found to be superior to placebo in reducing trauma-related nightmares and sleep disturbances. In the first study, 10 Vietnam combat veterans (mean age: 53 years) with chronic PTSD and severe trauma-related nightmares were randomized to receive prazosin or placebo with crossover to the opposite treatment arm occurring midway through the 20-week study. Prazosin was found to be more effective than placebo in reducing nightmares and sleep disturbances (assessed by CAPS) as well as improving overall PTSD severity and functional status (assessed by the CGI-C Scale). The second study, which was 8 weeks in duration, was conducted in a larger group of patients (40 US combat veterans; mean age: 56 years) with chronic PTSD, distressing trauma nightmares, and sleep disturbances. Compared with placebo, patients receiving prazosin in this study experienced substantially greater improvements in each of the 3 primary outcome measures addressing frequency and intensity of trauma-related nightmares and sleep quality used in this study (the CAPS recurrent distressing dreams item, the Pittsburgh Sleep Quality Index, and the CGI-C).

In a double-blind, placebo-controlled study in 13 patients with civilian trauma-related PTSD, prazosin reduced trauma-related nightmares, distressed awakenings, and total PTSD Checklist-Civilian scores; improved Clinical Global Impression of Improvement scores; and changed the PTSD Dream Rating Scale toward normal dreaming compared with placebo; the drug also improved objective measures of sleep (total sleep time, total REM sleep time, mean REM period duration) without changing sleep onset latency. In a historical prospective cohort study using retrospective chart review, the short-term effectiveness of prazosin (62 patients) and quetiapine (175 patients) in treating nighttime PTSD symptoms in combat veterans was found to be similar. However, long-term effectiveness (3–6 years) of prazosin was better compared with quetiapine; the quetiapine-treated patients were found to be more likely to discontinue therapy because of adverse effects than the prazosin-treated patients (approximately 35 and 18%, respectively). Prazosin therapy was generally found to be well tolerated when used in the treatment of PTSD-associated nightmares and other symptoms.

Some clinicians recommend prazosin as either first-line or alternative therapy when treating PTSD patients with prominent nighttime symptoms (e.g., nightmares, insomnia, sleep disturbances), particularly in combat veterans. Prazosin therapy could potentially be beneficial in some older PTSD patients who have hypertension and/or benign prostatic hyperplasia, since these conditions also may respond to therapy with the drug. Although preliminary findings have been very encouraging, larger, well controlled studies are needed to more fully define the role and optimum dosing of prazosin in the pharmacologic management of PTSD. In addition, further studies are needed to determine the safety and efficacy of prazosin in civilians with noncombat trauma-related PTSD and in the treatment of daytime symptoms associated with PTSD. Several controlled studies, including comparative and augmentation trials, are planned or currently underway to further evaluate prazosin in patients with this disorder.

For additional information on management of PTSD, see Uses: Posttraumatic Stress Disorder, in Paroxetine 28:16.04.20.

● **Other Uses**

Prazosin has been effective in conjunction with cardiac glycosides and diuretics for the management of severe congestive heart failure† , often producing improvements in cardiac function indexes and exercise tolerance. Although partial or complete tolerance to the hemodynamic effects of prazosin has reportedly developed rapidly in some patients, the attenuated response may be transient and/or corrected by dosage adjustment, by temporarily withdrawing the drug, and/or by the addition of an aldosterone antagonist (e.g., spironolactone) to the treatment regimen; acute hemodynamic attenuation does not preclude a beneficial hemodynamic response, especially during exercise. Most studies evaluating the long-term effects of prazosin have suggested that beneficial clinical and hemodynamic effects are sustained; however, conflicting results have been reported. Further studies are needed to determine the efficacy and role of prazosin for the long-term treatment of severe congestive heart failure.

Prazosin has been used with good results alone or in combination with a β-blocker for the preoperative management of the signs and symptoms of pheochromocytoma† in a limited number of patients; however, these patients may be particularly susceptible to a marked hypotensive response to the initial dose of prazosin. Limited data also suggest that prazosin may be useful for the treatment of Raynaud's disease† or phenomenon† and ergotamine-induced peripheral ischemia† .

DOSAGE AND ADMINISTRATION

● **Administration**

Prazosin hydrochloride is administered orally.

● **Dosage**

Dosage of prazosin hydrochloride is expressed in terms of prazosin and must be adjusted according to the patient's blood pressure response and tolerance.

Hypertension

Usual Dosage

For the management of hypertension in adults, the usual initial dosage of prazosin is 1 mg given 2 or 3 times daily; higher doses should not be used for initial therapy, since initiation of therapy with doses in excess of 1 mg may cause syncope. (See Cautions: Postural Effects.) It has been suggested that syncopal episodes can be minimized by limiting the initial dose of the drug to 1 mg, by subsequently increasing dosage gradually, and by introducing other hypotensive agents into the patient's regimen cautiously. Dosage of prazosin may be gradually increased if necessary to a total dosage of 20 mg daily administered in divided doses. Higher dosages usually do not increase efficacy, but a few patients may benefit from up to 40 mg of prazosin daily in divided doses. The manufacturer states that the usual maintenance dosage is 6–15 mg daily given in divided doses. For maintenance therapy, prazosin may be administered twice daily in some patients. Some experts state that the usual dosage range is 2–20 mg daily, administered in 2 or 3 divided doses.

When other hypotensive agents or diuretics are added to existing prazosin therapy, the dosage of prazosin in adults should be reduced to 1 or 2 mg given 3 times daily and gradually increased according to the response and tolerance of the patient.

If prazosin is used for the management of hypertension in children† , some experts have recommended an initial dosage of 0.05–0.1 mg/kg daily given in 3 divided doses; dosage may be increased as necessary to a maximum of 0.5 mg/kg daily given in 3 divided doses. (See Cautions: Pediatric Precautions.) For information on overall principles and expert recommendations for treatment of hypertension in pediatric patients, see Uses: Hypertension in Pediatric Patients, in the Thiazides General Statement 40:28.20.

Blood Pressure Monitoring and Treatment Goals

Blood pressure should be monitored regularly (i.e., monthly) during therapy and dosage of the antihypertensive drug adjusted until blood pressure is controlled. If an adequate blood pressure response is not achieved, the dosage may be increased or another antihypertensive agent with demonstrated benefit and preferably with a complementary mechanism of action (e.g., angiotensin-converting enzyme [ACE] inhibitor, angiotensin II receptor antagonist, calcium-channel blocker, thiazide diuretic) may be added; if target blood pressure is still not achieved with the use of 2 antihypertensive agents, a third drug may be added. (See Uses: Hypertension.) In patients who develop unacceptable adverse effects with prazosin, the drug should be discontinued and another antihypertensive agent from a different pharmacologic class should be initiated.

The goal of hypertension management and prevention is to achieve and maintain optimal control of blood pressure. However, the optimum blood pressure threshold for initiating antihypertensive drug therapy and specific treatment goals remain controversial. A 2017 multidisciplinary hypertension guideline from the American College of Cardiology (ACC), American Heart Association (AHA), and a number of other professional organizations generally recommends a blood pressure goal of less than 130/80 mm Hg in all adults, regardless of comorbidities or level of atherosclerotic cardiovascular disease (ASCVD) risk. Many patients will require at least 2 drugs from different pharmacologic classes to achieve this blood pressure goal; the potential benefits of hypertension management and drug cost, adverse effects, and risks associated with the use of multiple antihypertensive drugs also should be considered when deciding a patient's blood pressure treatment goal.

For additional information on target levels of blood pressure and on monitoring therapy in the management of hypertension, see Blood Pressure Monitoring and Treatment Goals under Dosage: Hypertension, in Dosage and Administration in the Thiazides General Statement 40:28.20.

Benign Prostatic Hyperplasia

In the treatment of benign prostatic hyperplasia†, prazosin generally has been used in a dosage of 2 mg twice daily; however, dosages ranging from 1–9 mg daily also have been used.

Posttraumatic Stress Disorder

The optimum dosage regimen of prazosin for the management of posttraumatic stress disorder (PTSD)† in adults has not been fully established. However, in clinical studies, prazosin usually was initiated at a dosage of 1 mg given at bedtime; the dosage was gradually increased (i.e., in 1- or 2-mg increments every few days or week) until an effective (i.e., nighttime symptoms associated with PTSD, such as nightmares and sleep disturbances, were substantially reduced) and well tolerated dosage was reached. Some clinicians recommend monitoring patients receiving prazosin for PTSD for first-dose syncope and orthostatic hypotension, particularly early in therapy. (See Cautions: Postural Effects and also see Cautions: Precautions and Contraindications.) In the available clinical studies, maintenance dosages ranging from 1 to 25 mg daily have been used. Some experts recommend a target maintenance dosage of 1–10 mg daily, while others recommend a higher target maintenance dosage of 2–20 mg daily. Although prazosin usually has been given once daily at bedtime, particularly when lower daily dosages have been used, some clinicians recommend a twice-daily regimen to help control daytime PTSD symptoms; further trials are needed to determine the optimal timing of doses for symptom control. Symptom relief appears to occur within several days to 2 weeks after beginning therapy with the drug.

Although the optimal duration of therapy has not been established, PTSD is often a chronic disorder and requires long-term therapy (i.e., for at least 1 to 2 years). Some PTSD patients have received the drug for up to 6 years. Because a rapid return of symptoms following prazosin discontinuance has been reported, some patients may require therapy indefinitely.

● Dosage in Renal Impairment

For the management of hypertension in adults with renal failure, therapy with prazosin should be initiated with 1 mg twice daily. Patients with chronic renal failure may require only small doses of the drug.

CAUTIONS

Adverse effects occurring most frequently during prazosin hydrochloride therapy include dizziness, lightheadedness, headache, drowsiness, lack of energy, weakness, palpitation, and nausea. These effects may diminish with continued therapy or may be relieved by a reduction in dosage.

● Postural Effects

Prazosin may cause syncope with sudden loss of consciousness. (See Cautions: Precautions and Contraindications.) Syncopal episodes occur unpredictably and have no relationship to plasma prazosin concentrations. The incidence of syncope is greatest in patients given an initial dose of 2 mg or more (approximately 1%) and may be minimized by administering 1 mg of the drug initially with subsequent gradual increases in dosage. Results of one study suggest that administration of prazosin with food may reduce the frequency of hypotension and dizziness in some patients. Syncope, which is self-limiting, may result from an excessive postural hypotensive effect; syncopal episodes occasionally have been preceded by tachycardia with heart rates of 120–160 beats/minute. Syncopal episodes usually have occurred within 30–90 minutes after the initial dose of prazosin and occasionally have been associated with rapid dosage increases or the introduction of another hypotensive drug to the regimen of patients taking high dosages of prazosin.

● Intraoperative Floppy Iris Syndrome

A condition named intraoperative floppy iris syndrome (IFIS) has been observed during cataract surgery in some patients treated with α₁-adrenergic blocking agents. IFIS is a variant of small pupil syndrome and is characterized by the combination of a flaccid iris that billows in response to intraoperative irrigation currents, progressive intraoperative miosis despite preoperative dilation with mydriatics, and potential prolapse of the iris toward the phacoemulsification incisions. Most reported cases of IFIS occurred in patients who continued α₁-blocker therapy at the time of cataract surgery. Some cases were reported in patients who had discontinued such therapy prior to surgery, generally 2 to 14 days prior to surgery, but occasionally 5 weeks to 9 months prior to surgery. (See Cautions: Precautions and Contraindications.)

● GI Effects

Nausea is the most common adverse GI effect of prazosin, occurring in about 5% of patients. Other adverse GI effects such as vomiting, diarrhea, constipation, and abdominal discomfort and/or pain have also been reported.

● Cardiovascular Effects

Palpitation is the most common adverse cardiovascular effect of prazosin, occurring in about 5% of patients. In addition to syncope, other adverse cardiovascular effects of the drug include edema, dyspnea, orthostatic hypotension, tachycardia, and angina. (See Cautions: Postural Effects.) Nonspecific chest pain also has been reported in a patient receiving prazosin for posttraumatic stress disorder.

● Nervous System Effects

Dizziness is the most common adverse effect of prazosin, occurring in about 10% of patients. Headache or drowsiness occur in about 8% of patients, and lack of energy or weakness occur in about 7% of patients. Other adverse nervous system effects of prazosin which occur rarely include nervousness, vertigo, depression, paresthesia, hallucinations, and insomnia.

Worsening of narcolepsy (e.g., exacerbation of associated cataplexy) has been associated with prazosin therapy in patients with a history of this disorder. Although the manufacturers state that a causal relationship to prazosin has not been established to date, the frequency of cataplectic attacks decreased when the drug was withdrawn and increased when it was resumed in at least 2 patients. In addition, prazosin has been shown to exacerbate canine narcolepsy-cataplexy, probably secondary to inhibition of a subtype of α₁-adrenergic receptor (e.g., α₁ᵦ) in the CNS. Therefore, some clinicians recommend that prazosin not be used in patients with a history of narcolepsy.

● Dermatologic Effects

Adverse dermatologic effects associated with prazosin include rash, pruritus, alopecia, and lichen planus.

● Other Adverse Effects

Other adverse effects reported to occur with prazosin include urinary frequency, incontinence, impotence, priapism, blurred vision, epistaxis, tinnitus, reddened sclera, dry mouth, nasal congestion, liver function test result abnormalities, pancreatitis, diaphoresis, fever, positive ANA titer, and arthralgia. A transient fall in leukocyte count and increased serum uric acid and BUN concentrations have also been reported during prazosin therapy. Single reports of pigmentary mottling and serous retinopathy, and a few cases of cataract development or disappearance have been reported, but these have not been directly attributable to the drug. In slit-lamp and funduscopic studies, no drug-related abnormal ophthalmologic findings have been reported.

● Precautions and Contraindications

Because syncope and orthostatic hypotension may occur in patients receiving prazosin, careful monitoring of blood pressure during initial titration or subsequent upward adjustment in dosage is recommended in patients receiving prazosin; patients also should be monitored for possible symptoms of orthostatic hypotension. Patients receiving prazosin should be warned of the possibility of prazosin-induced postural dizziness and advised of measures to take if it develops (e.g., lying down). During initiation of prazosin therapy, the patient should be cautioned to avoid situations where injury could result if syncope occurs.

If syncope occurs, the patient should be placed in the recumbent position and treated supportively as necessary. Patients who engage in potentially hazardous activities such as operating machinery or driving motor vehicles should be warned about possible drowsiness, dizziness, or lightheadedness. (See Cautions: Postural Effects.)

Intraoperative floppy iris syndrome (IFIS) has been observed during cataract surgery in some patients treated with α₁-adrenergic blocking agents (see Cautions: Intraoperative Floppy Iris Syndrome). If a patient scheduled for cataract surgery has received such agents, the ophthalmologist should be prepared to modify the surgical technique (e.g., through use of iris hooks, iris dilator rings, or viscoelastic substances) to minimize complications of IFIS. There does not appear to be a benefit from discontinuing α₁-blocker therapy prior to cataract surgery.

The possibility of carcinoma of the prostate and other conditions associated with manifestations that mimic those of benign prostatic hyperplasia (BPH) should be excluded in any patient for whom prazosin therapy for presumed BPH is being considered.

Patients receiving prazosin for posttraumatic stress disorder (PTSD)† should be informed that prazosin may help reduce nightmares and improve their sleep and other symptoms, but that the drug does not cure PTSD and that their nightmares, anxiety, and other PTSD-related symptoms may return if the drug is stopped.

Caution should be used when adding prazosin to a preexisting antihypertensive regimen or when adding other hypotensive agents to a prazosin regimen in order to avoid a possible rapid fall in blood pressure. (See Drug Interactions: Diuretics and Hypotensive Agents.) Caution also should be used when administering prazosin to patients with chronic renal failure as they may require only small doses of the drug.

Prazosin is contraindicated in patients with known hypersensitivity to the drug, any other quinazoline derivative (e.g., alfuzosin, doxazosin, terazosin), or any ingredient in the commercially available formulation.

● Pediatric Precautions

The manufacturers state that safety and efficacy of prazosin in children have not been established. (See Dosage and Administration: Dosage.) Some experts state that use of centrally acting antihypertensive agents (e.g., prazosin) should be reserved for children who are not responsive to 2 or more of the preferred classes of antihypertensive agents (angiotensin-converting enzyme [ACE] inhibitors, angiotensin II receptor antagonists, calcium-channel blockers, or thiazide diuretics).

For information on overall principles and expert recommendations for treatment of hypertension in pediatric patients, see Uses: Hypertension in Pediatric Patients, in the Thiazides General Statement 40:28.20.

● Mutagenicity and Carcinogenicity

No evidence of prazosin-induced mutagenicity was seen with in vivo tests.

No evidence of carcinogenesis was seen in rats receiving prazosin hydrochloride dosages more than 225 times the usual maximum recommended human dosage for 18 months.

● Pregnancy, Fertility, and Lactation

Pregnancy

Prazosin hydrochloride has been associated with decreased litter size at birth and at 1, 4, and 21 days of age in rats receiving more than 225 times the usual maximum recommended human dosage; no evidence of drug-related external, visceral, or skeletal fetal abnormalities was observed. No prazosin-related external, visceral, or skeletal abnormalities were observed in the offspring of pregnant rabbits and monkeys receiving dosages more than 225 and 12 times the usual maximum recommended human dosage, respectively. Prazosin has been used alone or in combination with other hypotensive agents for the management of severe hypertension in a limited number of pregnant women without apparent adverse effect on the fetus. There are no adequate and well-controlled studies to date using prazosin in pregnant women, however, and the drug should be used during pregnancy only when the potential benefits justify the possible risks to the fetus.

Fertility

Decreased fertility has occurred in male and female rats receiving prazosin dosages of 75 mg/kg (225 times the usual maximum recommended human dosage) but did not occur in those receiving 25 mg/kg (75 times the usual maximum recommended human dosage). Testicular changes consisting of atrophy and necrosis have occurred in rats and dogs receiving prazosin dosages of 25 mg/kg daily for a year or longer but no such changes occurred in those receiving 10 mg/kg daily (30 times the usual maximum recommended human dosage). Because of the testicular changes observed in animals, a group of patients receiving long-term prazosin therapy was monitored for 17-ketosteroid excretion, but no changes indicating a drug effect were observed. In addition, a group of males receiving prazosin for up to 51 months did not exhibit changes in sperm morphology suggestive of a drug effect.

Lactation

Since prazosin is distributed into milk in small amounts, the drug should be used with caution in nursing women.

DRUG INTERACTIONS

● Analgesics and Antipyretics

Although clinical experience is limited, prazosin has been administered concomitantly with aspirin, indomethacin, phenylbutazone (no longer commercially available in the US), or propoxyphene (no longer commercially available in the US) without any apparent adverse interaction.

● Antiarrhythmic Agents

Although clinical experience to date is limited, prazosin has been administered concomitantly with procainamide, propranolol (see Drug Interactions: Diuretics and Hypotensive Agents), or quinidine without any apparent adverse drug interaction.

● Antidiabetic Agents

Although clinical experience to date is limited, prazosin has been administered concomitantly with insulin, chlorpropamide, phenformin (no longer commercially available in the US), tolazamide, and tolbutamide without any apparent adverse drug interaction.

● Antigout Agents

Although clinical experience is limited, prazosin has been administered concurrently with allopurinol, colchicine, or probenecid without any apparent adverse interaction.

● CNS Depressants

Although clinical experience is limited, prazosin has been administered concurrently with chlordiazepoxide, diazepam, or phenobarbital without any apparent adverse interaction.

● Digoxin

Although clinical experience is limited, prazosin has been administered concomitantly with digoxin without any apparent adverse interaction.

● Diuretics and Hypotensive Agents

When prazosin is administered with diuretics or other hypotensive agents, particularly β-adrenergic blocking agents (e.g., propranolol), the hypotensive effect of prazosin may be increased. This effect is usually used to therapeutic advantage, but careful adjustment of dosage is necessary when these drugs are used concomitantly. (See Dosage and Administration: Dosage.)

● Phosphodiesterase Type 5 Inhibitors

Concomitant administration of prazosin and a phosphodiesterase type 5 (PDE5) inhibitor (e.g., sildenafil, tadalafil, vardenafil) may result in additive hypotensive effects and symptomatic hypotension. Therefore, PDE5 inhibitor therapy should be initiated at the lowest possible dosage in patients receiving prazosin. (See Dosage and Administration: Dosage.)

For further information on this potential drug interaction, see Drug Interactions: Antihypertensive and Hypotensive Agents, in Sildenafil 24:12.12.

● Protein-bound Drugs

Since prazosin is highly bound to plasma proteins, the possibility that it may interact with other highly protein-bound drugs should be considered.

ACUTE TOXICITY

● Manifestations

The manufacturers state that ingestion of at least 50 mg of prazosin by a 2-year-old child produced profound drowsiness and depressed reflexes. There was no decrease in blood pressure and recovery was uneventful. A 19-year-old man who ingested approximately 200 mg of prazosin had normal CNS responses and slightly decreased blood pressure. Treatment of overdosage consisted of induction of emesis and maintaining the patient in a supine position with the head of the bed lowered; recovery was uneventful.

● Treatment

If overdosage of prazosin causes hypotension, supportive therapy should be initiated. The patient should be kept in the supine position; if necessary, shock may be treated with plasma volume expanders and vasopressor drugs. Renal function should be monitored. The manufacturers state that laboratory data indicate prazosin is not dialyzable because it is highly protein bound.

PHARMACOLOGY

Prazosin reduces peripheral vascular resistance and blood pressure as a result of its vasodilating effects; the drug produces both arterial and venous dilation. Prazosin's effects appear to result principally from its selective, competitive inhibition of α_1-adrenergic receptors. Prazosin's effects were initially attributed to a direct effect on vascular smooth muscle, inhibition of phosphodiesterase, and/or inhibition of dopamine β-hydroxylase with a resultant reduction in neurotransmitter synthesis; however, it is unlikely that concentrations of the drug necessary for these effects are achieved when prazosin is administered in therapeutic doses. Animal studies indicate that prazosin does not have its antihypertensive effect in the CNS. Prazosin does not interfere with nerve impulse transmission across sympathetic ganglia nor does it cause adrenergic neuronal blockade.

Prazosin reduces blood pressure in both supine and standing patients; the effect is most pronounced on diastolic blood pressure. The drug may cause postural hypotension. (See Cautions: Postural Effects.) Tolerance to the hypotensive effect has not been observed during long-term prazosin therapy in hypertensive patients. Prazosin generally causes no change in heart rate or cardiac output in the supine position. Cardiovascular responses to exercise (e.g., increased heart rate and cardiac output) are maintained during prazosin therapy. Reports on the effect of the drug on glomerular filtration rate and renal plasma flow indicate that these parameters may increase or show no marked change. In patients with chronic renal failure, prazosin produces no clinically important change in renal function. In a limited number of patients treated with prazosin, plasma renin activity (PRA) decreased; however, no appreciable effect on PRA was demonstrated in other patients.

In patients with congestive heart failure, prazosin markedly decreases systemic and pulmonary venous pressures and right atrial pressure, and increases cardiac output. Systemic blood pressure and systemic vascular resistance are moderately decreased in these patients; pulmonary vascular resistance is decreased and heart rate may be slightly decreased or unchanged. In patients with congestive heart failure precipitated or exacerbated by mitral or aortic regurgitation, prazosin may increase cardiac output and decrease regurgitant volume.

The precise mechanism of action of prazosin in posttraumatic stress disorder (PTSD) has not been fully elucidated; however, preliminary studies suggest that norepinephrine and α_1-adrenergic receptors play an important role in the pathophysiology of PTSD-associated nightmares, arousal, selective attention, and vigilance. Norepinephrine concentrations in the cerebrospinal fluid appear to correlate with PTSD symptom severity. Hyperresponsiveness of postsynaptic α_1-adrenergic receptors occurs primarily at night and can disrupt certain stages of the sleep cycle (stage 1, stage 2, rapid eye movement [REM]) in which PTSD-associated nightmares are known to occur. In preclinical and clinical studies, prazosin has been shown to reduce the effects of α_1-adrenergic receptor hyperstimulation and to help normalize the sleep cycle. In a placebo-controlled trial of prazosin in civilian trauma-related PTSD, prazosin increased total sleep time, REM sleep time, and mean REM period duration compared with placebo without producing a sedative-like effect on sleep onset latency.

PHARMACOKINETICS

● Absorption

There is intraindividual and interindividual variation in the rate of absorption and plasma concentrations of prazosin. The absolute oral bioavailability of prazosin is also variable but is reported to average about 60% (range: 43–82%). Results of one study indicate that the presence of food may delay absorption of the drug in some patients, but does not affect the extent of absorption.

Following oral administration of prazosin hydrochloride, plasma concentrations of the drug reach a peak in 2–3 hours in most fasting patients. Plasma concentrations of prazosin generally do not correlate with therapeutic effect. One manufacturer reports that plasma concentrations of the drug after a single 5-mg dose range from 0.01–0.075 mcg/mL. Blood pressure begins to decrease within 2 hours after an oral dose; the maximum decrease occurs in 2–4 hours. The hypotensive effect of prazosin lasts less than 24 hours. At fixed dosage levels, 4–6 weeks of therapy are required before the full antihypertensive effect of the drug is achieved.

● Distribution

Animal studies indicate that prazosin is widely distributed in body tissues. After IV administration in dogs, highest concentrations of the drug are found in the lungs, coronary arteries, aorta, paw arteries and heart; the lowest concentrations are in the brain. During prazosin therapy, approximately 97% of the drug in plasma is bound to proteins. Prazosin crosses the blood-brain barrier. It is not known whether the drug crosses the placenta. Prazosin is distributed into milk in small amounts.

● Elimination

The plasma half-life of prazosin after oral administration has been reported to be 2–4 hours.

Animal studies show that prazosin hydrochloride is metabolized extensively in the liver, principally by demethylation and conjugation, and excreted as unchanged drug (5–11%) and metabolites. Four of the metabolites have been shown to possess 10–25% of the hypotensive activity of prazosin and they may contribute to the antihypertensive effect of the drug. Approximately 6–10% of a dose is excreted in urine and the remainder in feces via bile.

CHEMISTRY AND STABILITY

● Chemistry

Prazosin hydrochloride is a quinazoline-derivative postsynaptic α_1-adrenergic blocking agent. The drug is chemically and pharmacologically related to alfuzosin, doxazosin, and terazosin. Prazosin hydrochloride occurs as a white to tan powder, is slightly soluble in water and very slightly soluble in alcohol, and has a pK_a of 6.5 in 1:1 water and ethanol solution.

● Stability

Prazosin hydrochloride capsules should be stored in well-closed, light-resistant containers at 20-25°C.

PREPARATIONS

Excipients in commercially available drug preparations may have clinically important effects in some individuals; consult specific product labeling for details.

Prazosin Hydrochloride

Oral

Capsules	1 mg (of prazosin)*	**Minipress**®, Pfizer
		Prazosin Hydrochloride Capsules
	2 mg (of prazosin)*	**Minipress**®, Pfizer
		Prazosin Hydrochloride Capsules,
	5 mg (of prazosin)*	**Minipress**®, Pfizer
		Prazosin Hydrochloride Capsules,

* available from one or more manufacturer, distributor, and/or repackager by generic (nonproprietary) name

† Use is not currently included in the labeling approved by the US Food and Drug Administration.

Selected Revisions April 10, 2024, © Copyright, May 1, 1977, American Society of Health-System Pharmacists, Inc.

Terazosin Hydrochloride

24:16 • α-ADRENERGIC BLOCKING AGENTS

■ Terazosin hydrochloride is a α₁-adrenergic blocking agent.

USES

● Hypertension

Terazosin hydrochloride is used alone or in combination with other classes of antihypertensive agents for the management of hypertension. However, because of established clinical benefits (e.g., reductions in overall mortality and in adverse cardiovascular, cerebrovascular, and renal outcomes), current evidence-based practice guidelines for the management of hypertension in adults generally recommend the use of drugs from 4 classes of antihypertensive agents (angiotensin-converting enzyme [ACE] inhibitors, angiotensin II receptor antagonists, calcium-channel blockers, and thiazide diuretics).

In a randomized, double-blind clinical study (the Antihypertensive and Lipid-Lowering Treatment to Prevent Heart Attack Trial; [ALLHAT]), doxazosin, an α₁-blocker, was less effective in lowering mean systolic blood pressure (by about 2–3 mm Hg) than chlorthalidone, a thiazide-like diuretic. In order to achieve target blood pressure in hypertensive patients, use of doxazosin required additional hypotensive therapy more frequently than chlorthalidone. In addition, interim analysis (median follow-up: 3.3 years) of this study indicated that use of doxazosin in high-risk (at least 2 risk factors for coronary heart disease) hypertensive patients 55 years of age and older was associated with a higher risk of stroke and a higher incidence of combined cardiovascular disease events (including twice the risk of congestive heart failure) than use of chlorthalidone. Study investigators concluded that such increased risk of congestive heart failure could not have been caused by the relatively small difference in the mean target systolic blood pressure observed in patients receiving doxazosin compared with those receiving chlorthalidone. Therefore, based on these findings, the trial's Data Safety and Monitoring Board recommended that the α-blocker treatment arm be terminated prematurely. The remaining antihypertensive arms (e.g., calcium-channel blockers, ACE inhibitors, diuretics) and lipid-lowering (pravastatin vs usual care) components of the study subsequently were completed and reported.

Current antihypertensive and urology guidelines no longer recommend α₁-blockers as preferred *first-line* therapy for any patients with hypertension, principally because of negative findings observed in ALLHAT. However, α₁-blockers are effective antihypertensive drugs and many experts still consider their use appropriate for the management of resistant hypertension as a component of combination therapy. Therapy with an α₁-blocker is most effective when used in combination with a diuretic. Some experts state that an α₁-blocker may be a second-line agent in antihypertensive treatment regimens in men with coexisting benign prostatic hyperplasia (BPH); the American Urology Association (AUA) states that monotherapy with these drugs is not optimal in hypertensive patients with lower urinary tract symptoms (LUTS) or BPH and that such conditions should be managed separately.

The beneficial effects of α₁-blockers on blood glucose and lipid concentrations may mitigate some of the adverse metabolic effects of diuretics, and α₁-blockers may offer some advantage in patients with underlying lipoprotein disorders (e.g., hypercholesterolemia) or in those with lipoprotein abnormalities induced by other antihypertensive agents (e.g., thiazide diuretics). The possibility that geriatric patients may be more susceptible than younger patients to the postural hypotensive effects of α₁-blockers should be considered in the selection of therapy. Blood pressure response to α₁-blockers appears to be comparable in white and black patients.

For further information on overall principles and expert recommendations for treatment of hypertension, see Uses: Hypertension in Adults and also see Uses: Hypertension in Pediatric Patients, in the Thiazides General Statement 40:28.20.

● Benign Prostatic Hyperplasia

Terazosin hydrochloride is used to reduce urinary obstruction and relieve associated manifestations in patients with symptomatic benign prostatic hyperplasia (BPH, benign prostatic hypertrophy). For patients who can tolerate the potential cardiovascular and other effects of α₁-adrenergic blockade, the drug can effectively relieve mild to moderate obstructive manifestations (e.g., hesitancy, terminal dribbling of urine, interrupted stream, impaired size and force of stream, sensation of incomplete bladder emptying or straining) and urinary flow rates in a substantial proportion of patients and may be a useful alternative to surgery, particularly in those who are awaiting or are unwilling to undergo surgical correction of the hyperplasia (e.g., via transurethral resection of the prostate [TURP]) or who are not candidates for such surgery.

Therapy with α₁-blockers appears to be less effective in relieving irritative (e.g., nocturia, daytime frequency, urgency, dysuria) than obstructive symptomatology. In addition, therapy with the drugs generally can be expected to produce less subjective and objective improvement than prostatectomy, and periodic monitoring (e.g., performance of digital rectal examinations, serum creatinine determinations, serum prostate specific antigen [PSA] assays) is indicated in these patients to detect and manage other potential complications of or conditions associated with BPH (e.g., obstructive uropathy, prostatic carcinoma). While symptomatic improvement has been maintained for at least up to 2 years of terazosin therapy in some patients, the long-term effects of the drug on the need for surgery and on the frequency of developing BPH-associated complications such as acute urinary obstruction remain to be established.

Combination therapy with an α₁-blocker and 5α-reductase inhibitor (e.g., finasteride) has been more effective than therapy with either drug alone in preventing long-term BPH symptom progression; combined therapy also can reduce the risks of long-term acute urinary retention and the need for invasive therapy compared with α-blocker monotherapy.

For additional information on the use of α₁-blockers in the management of BPH, see Uses: Benign Prostatic Hyperplasia, in Doxazosin 24:20.

Because many of the signs and symptoms of BPH can occur with carcinoma of the prostate and with certain genitourinary conditions, including prostatitis and neurologic disorders, the possibility of such conditions, particularly this carcinoma, should be ruled out in any patient for whom terazosin therapy for presumed hyperplasia is being considered.

DOSAGE AND ADMINISTRATION

● Administration

Terazosin hydrochloride is administered orally. Food has little, if any, effect on the extent of absorption of terazosin but may delay achievement of peak plasma concentrations by about 1 hour.

● Dosage

Dosage of terazosin hydrochloride is expressed in terms of terazosin and must be individualized according to the patient's response and tolerance.

Hypertension

Usual Dosage

For the management of hypertension, terazosin dosage should be adjusted according to blood pressure response and tolerance. The usual initial adult dosage of the drug is 1 mg once daily at bedtime. Because of the risk of postural effects (see Cautions: Postural Effects), it is essential that therapy with the drug *not* be initiated with higher dosages.

If blood pressure is not adequately controlled at a terazosin dosage of 1 mg daily, the dosage may be increased gradually up to 5 mg once daily in adults, but each incremental increase should be delayed until blood pressure has stabilized at a given dosage; some patients may benefit from further titration up to 20 mg daily. Maintenance doses of the drug can be administered in the morning rather than at bedtime. Blood pressure should be monitored at the end of the dosing interval to ensure maintenance of control, and additional measurements 2–3 hours after dosing may be helpful in determining whether peak and trough responses are similar and in assessing potential manifestations (e.g., dizziness, palpitation) of an excessive response. If blood pressure response is diminished substantially 24 hours after a dose, an increased dose may provide adequate control. If necessary for optimal blood pressure control, the daily dose can be divided and administered every 12 hours.

Some experts state the usual adult dosage of terazosin for the management of hypertension ranges from 1–20 mg daily administered as a single dose or in

2 divided doses daily. While higher dosages have been employed, those exceeding 20 mg daily do not appear to be associated with improved hypertensive control and those exceeding 40 mg daily have not been studied systematically. If terazosin is discontinued for several days or longer, therapy with drug should be reinstituted at 1 mg daily at bedtime and titrated as usual.

If terazosin is used for the management of hypertension in children†, some experts have recommended an initial dosage of 1 mg once daily; dosage may be increased as necessary to a maximum dosage of 20 mg once daily. (See Cautions: Pediatric Precautions.) For information on overall principles and expert recommendations for treatment of hypertension in pediatric patients, see Uses: Hypertension in Pediatric Patients, in the Thiazides General Statement 40:28.20.

Blood Pressure Monitoring and Treatment Goals

Blood pressure should be monitored regularly (i.e., monthly) during therapy and dosage of the antihypertensive drug adjusted until blood pressure is controlled. If an adequate blood pressure response is not achieved, the dosage may be increased or another antihypertensive agent with demonstrated benefit and preferably with a complementary mechanism of action (e.g., angiotensin-converting enzyme [ACE] inhibitor, angiotensin II receptor antagonist, calcium-channel blocker, thiazide diuretic) may be added; if target blood pressure is still not achieved with the use of 2 antihypertensive agents, a third drug may be added. (See Uses: Hypertension.) In patients who develop unacceptable adverse effects with terazosin, the drug should be discontinued and another antihypertensive agent from a different pharmacologic class should be initiated.

The goal of hypertension management and prevention is to achieve and maintain optimal control of blood pressure. However, the optimum blood pressure threshold for initiating antihypertensive drug therapy and specific treatment goals remain controversial. A 2017 multidisciplinary hypertension guideline from the American College of Cardiology (ACC), American Heart Association (AHA), and a number of other professional organizations generally recommends a blood pressure goal of less than 130/80 mm Hg in all adults, regardless of comorbidities or level of atherosclerotic cardiovascular disease (ASCVD) risk. Many patients will require at least 2 drugs from different pharmacologic classes to achieve this blood pressure goal; the potential benefits of hypertension management and drug cost, adverse effects, and risks associated with the use of multiple antihypertensive drugs also should be considered when deciding a patient's blood pressure treatment goal.

For additional information on target levels of blood pressure and on monitoring therapy in the management of hypertension, see Blood Pressure Monitoring and Treatment Goals under Dosage: Hypertension, in Dosage and Administration in the Thiazides General Statement 40:28.20.

Benign Prostatic Hyperplasia

For the management of benign prostatic hyperplasia (BPH), the usual initial adult dosage of terazosin is 1 mg once daily at bedtime. Because of the risk of postural effects (see Cautions: Postural Effects), it is essential that therapy with the drug *not* be initiated with higher dosages. To achieve the desired improvement in symptoms and/or urinary flow rates, subsequent dosage may be increased in a stepwise manner to 2, 5, and 10 mg daily as necessary. Titration to a dosage of 10 mg once daily generally is required for adequate clinical response. A minimum of 4–6 weeks may be needed to adequately assess the response at this dosage, but some patients may not respond despite appropriate titration. While additional benefit occasionally may be observed by increasing the dosage to 20 mg daily, maximally tolerable and effective dosages have not been established and there currently is insufficient experience with this dosage in the management of BPH to draw definitive conclusions. In addition, there currently are insufficient data to support the use of dosages exceeding 20 mg daily in patients with an inadequate or no response at lower dosages. If terazosin therapy is discontinued for several days or longer, therapy should be restarted using the recommended initial dosage.

● Dosage in Renal and Hepatic Impairment

Clinically important alterations in the pharmacokinetics of terazosin in patients with impaired renal function have not been observed to date, and modification of dosage in such patients generally does not appear to be necessary. In addition, administration of supplemental doses of the drug following hemodialysis does not appear to be necessary.

The effects, if any, of hepatic impairment on the pharmacokinetics of terazosin have not been elucidated, and the manufacturer makes no specific recommendations for modification of terazosin dosage in patients with hepatic impairment.

● Dosage in Geriatric Patients

While the manufacturer makes no specific recommendations for titration of terazosin dosage in geriatric patients, patients in this age group generally are less tolerant of the postural hypotensive effects of α₁-adrenergic blocking agents because of impaired cardiovascular reflexes, and caution should be exercised. Therefore, dosage escalation in elderly patients generally should be slower than in younger adults. In addition, the elimination half-life may be prolonged and plasma clearance of the drug decreased in patients 70 years of age and older.

CAUTIONS

Adverse effects occurring most frequently during terazosin hydrochloride therapy for hypertension include dizziness, headache, asthenia (weakness, tiredness, lassitude, fatigue), nasal congestion, peripheral edema, somnolence, nausea, and palpitation. In patients receiving the drug for benign prostatic hyperplasia (BPH), the most frequent adverse effects are dizziness, asthenia, headache, postural hypotension, and somnolence. The frequency of adverse effects in controlled clinical trials generally has been lower in patients receiving terazosin for BPH than in those receiving the drug for hypertension; however, dosages employed for this condition also generally have been lower than those for hypertension.

While adverse effects occur frequently in patients receiving terazosin, most are mild to moderate in severity, and discontinuance of the drug secondary to adverse effects was required in only 9% of patients with BPH and in only 13–21% of patients with hypertension during clinical trials. The principal reasons for discontinuance in patients with hypertension were postural effects (e.g., dizziness in about 3% of patients) and asthenia, palpitation, headache, and dyspnea each in about 1–2% of patients. In patients with BPH, the principal reasons for discontinuance were dizziness, headache, and blurred vision/amblyopia in 2, 1.1, and 0.6%, respectively, of patients and postural hypotension, syncope, vertigo, dyspnea, fever, nausea, and urinary tract infection each in 0.5% of patients. In controlled clinical trials in patients with hypertension, only dizziness (including postural effects), asthenia, blurred vision, nasal congestion, nausea, peripheral edema, palpitation, and somnolence occurred at rates significantly greater than those for placebo. Only asthenia, postural hypotension, dizziness, somnolence, nasal congestion/rhinitis, and impotence occurred significantly more frequently with the drug than with placebo in controlled clinical trials for BPH. The risk of postural hypotension and syncope appears to be higher in geriatric patients (i.e., those 65 years of age and older) than in younger patients. Asthenia and postural effects, including dizziness, appear to be dose related.

● Postural Effects

Terazosin, like other α₁-adrenergic blocking agents, can cause marked hypotension, which may be accompanied by syncope and other postural effects. While syncope is the most severe orthostatic effect of the drug, other less severe symptoms, such as dizziness, lightheadedness, tachycardia, palpitation, and vertigo, also can be associated with terazosin-induced reductions in blood pressure. Syncope is uncommon when terazosin dosage is initiated at low levels and titrated slowly, but dizziness is frequent, occurring in about 20 or 10% of patients receiving the drug for hypertension or BPH, respectively, in controlled trials. Palpitation has been reported in 4.3% of hypertensive patients receiving terazosin, and tachycardia (especially in the standing position) and postural hypotension have been reported in 1–2% of such patients. Postural hypotension, vertigo, and syncope have been reported in about 4, 1.4, and 0.6% of patients, respectively, receiving the drug for BPH; however, in several clinical trials in such patients, the frequency of postural hypotension ranged from 3.7–5.2%.

Terazosin-induced postural hypotension is dose related, particularly likely in the upright position following an initial dose, and most likely to develop shortly after dosing (e.g., within 90 minutes), particularly during the initial week of therapy. With continued therapy after careful dosage titration, adaptation of reflex mechanisms to α₁-blockade develops and the risk of postural effects generally subsides. However, marked hypotension also can occur with subsequent dosage increases or after therapy is interrupted for more than a few days. Occasionally, syncopal episodes have been preceded by episodes of severe supraventricular tachycardia with heart rates of 120–160 bpm. In addition, the possibility exists that hemodilution induced by the drug may contribute to postural hypotension. While the adverse effect profiles of terazosin and prazosin generally appear to be similar, it has been suggested that postural effects may be less likely with terazosin in part because of the drug's slower onset of action and reduced affinity for α₁-receptors; however, additional study and experience are needed to elucidate the relative risks of postural effects.

The risk of first-dose syncope with α₁-adrenergic blocking agents generally can be minimized by initiating therapy at low doses (i.e., 1 mg of terazosin daily), lessening the level of salt restriction and avoiding diuretics just prior to initiation of α₁-blocker therapy, and administering initial doses at bedtime. It is essential that terazosin therapy *not* be initiated at dosages exceeding 1 mg daily and that dosage escalation be slow. If syncope develops, the patient should be placed in the recumbent position and treated supportively as necessary. Patients should be advised to lie or sit down if they develop any postural symptom (e.g., dizziness, vertigo) and to exercise caution upon standing from a sitting or supine position. Patients also should be advised to contact their physician if dizziness, lightheadedness, or palpitations become bothersome since dosage adjustment may be necessary. Other antihypertensive therapy, especially verapamil (see Precautions and Contraindications), should be added cautiously in patients receiving terazosin.

In early trials in which increasing single terazosin doses up to 7.5 mg were administered at 3-day intervals, tolerance to the first-dose phenomenon did not necessarily develop, and first-dose postural effects were observed at all doses. In addition, syncope occurred in about 20% of patients at single-dose levels of 2.5, 5, or 7.5 mg, and a few patients developed severe orthostatic hypotension (blood pressure declining to 50/0 mm Hg) at these dosing levels. These effects occurred within 90 minutes of dosing in all cases.

● Nervous System Effects

Besides dizziness (see Cautions: Postural Effects), headache is the most common adverse nervous system effect associated with terazosin therapy, occurring in about 16 or 5% of patients receiving the drug for hypertension or BPH, respectively. Asthenia (weakness, tiredness, lassitude, fatigue) occurs in 11.3 or 7.4% of such patients, respectively, and somnolence occurs in 5.4 or 3.6%, respectively. Paresthesia and nervousness occur in 2–3% of patients receiving the drug for hypertension, and depression occurs in 0.3%. Anxiety and insomnia have been reported occasionally, but a causal relationship to the drug has not been established.

● GI Effects

Nausea is the most common adverse GI effect of terazosin, occurring in 4.4 or 1.7% of patients receiving the drug for hypertension or BPH, respectively. Constipation, diarrhea, dry mouth, dyspepsia, flatulence, abdominal pain, and vomiting have been reported occasionally, but these effects have not been directly attributed to the drug.

● Cardiovascular Effects

Besides postural effects of the drug (see Cautions: Postural Effects), other cardiovascular effects reported with terazosin include peripheral edema in about 6 or 1% of patients receiving the drug for hypertension or BPH, respectively, and tachycardia and nonperipheral edema in about 1–2% of those receiving the drug for hypertension. Arrhythmia, chest pain, and vasodilation have been reported occasionally, but a causal relationship has not been established. While clinically important nonpostural decreases in blood pressure generally are not observed in normotensive patients receiving the drug for BPH, some reduction may occur, and hypotension develops in less than 1% of patients. Atrial fibrillation has been reported during postmarketing surveillance in patients receiving terazosin.

● Dermatologic and Sensitivity Reactions

Adverse dermatologic effects have been reported occasionally in patients receiving terazosin, but a causal relationship to the drug has not been established. Such effects include facial edema, pruritus, and rash.

Allergic reactions, including anaphylaxis, have been reported rarely in patients receiving terazosin.

● Musculoskeletal Effects

Back pain or flu-like syndrome occurs in 2.4% of patients receiving terazosin for hypertension or BPH, respectively. These effects also have been reported in hypertensive patients, but a causal relationship to the drug could not be established. Other musculoskeletal effects for which a causal relationship has not been established include neck or shoulder pain, arthralgia, arthritis, joint disorder, and myalgia. Pain in the extremities also has been reported.

● Respiratory Effects

Nasal congestion/rhinitis occurs in about 6 or 2% of patients receiving terazosin for hypertension or BPH, respectively, and dyspnea occurs in about 3.1 and 1.7%, respectively. Sinusitis occurs in 2.6% of hypertensive patients receiving the drug. Occasionally, cold symptoms, bronchitis, epistaxis, cough, and pharyngitis have been reported, but these effects have not been directly attributed to the drug.

● Genitourinary Effects

Impotence is the most common adverse genitourinary effect of terazosin, occurring in 1.2 or 1.6% of patients receiving the drug for hypertension or BPH, respectively. Priapism (painful penile erection sustained for hours and unrelieved by sexual intercourse or masturbation) has been reported rarely (probably less frequently than 1 per several thousand patients) in patients receiving an α₁-adrenergic antagonist (e.g., terazosin). Urinary tract infection was reported in 1.3% of patients with BPH receiving the drug, but this frequency was less than that reported with placebo. Urinary tract infection also has been reported in hypertensive patients receiving terazosin but could not be directly attributed to the drug. Other adverse genitourinary effects for which a causal relationship has not been established include urinary frequency and urinary incontinence (principally in postmenopausal women).

● Ocular and Otic Effects

Blurred vision/amblyopia occurs in 1.6 or 1.3% of patients receiving terazosin for hypertension or BPH, respectively. Visual abnormalities, conjunctivitis, and tinnitus have been reported occasionally but have not been directly attributed to the drug.

● Hematologic Effects

Small decreases in hemoglobin concentration, hematocrit, leukocyte count, and total protein and albumin concentrations have been observed following administration of terazosin and were suggestive of hemodilution. Similar changes have been observed with other α₁-adrenergic blocking agents and attributed to hemodilution. Thrombocytopenia has been reported during postmarketing surveillance in patients receiving terazosin.

● Other Adverse Effects

Weight gain (in both males and females) occurs in 0.5% of patients receiving terazosin for hypertension or BPH, and decreased libido occurs in 0.6% of those receiving the drug for hypertension. Some evidence suggests that the likelihood of weight gain may increase with increasing dosage and/or duration of therapy in some patients. Other adverse effects have been reported occasionally with terazosin but have not been directly attributed to the drug. Such effects include fever, gout, and sweating.

● Precautions and Contraindications

Patients should be warned of the possibility of terazosin-induced postural dizziness and measures to take if it develops (e.g., sitting, lying down). (See Cautions: Postural Effects.) During initiation of terazosin therapy, the patient should be cautioned to avoid, for 12 hours after the first dose, subsequent dosage increases, and resumption of therapy, situations where injury could result (e.g., driving, hazardous tasks) if syncope were to occur. If syncope occurs, the patient should be placed in the recumbent position and treated supportively as necessary. Patients who engage in potentially hazardous activities such as operating machinery or driving motor vehicles should be warned about possible somnolence, drowsiness, or dizziness.

While the manufacturer questions the need for caution, some clinicians state that α₁-adrenergic blocking agents should be avoided in patients with micturition-associated syncope because of the risk of exaggerated postural effects.

Patients also should be advised that priapism has been reported rarely in patients receiving an α₁-adrenergic antagonist (e.g., terazosin). Priapism is a medical emergency that could result in penile tissue damage and permanent loss of potency if not treated immediately; therefore, patients should be advised to report promptly to their clinician or, if their clinician is unavailable, to seek alternative immediate medical attention if an erection occurs that persists longer than several (e.g., 4–6) hours or is painful.

The possibility of carcinoma of the prostate and other conditions associated with manifestations that mimic those of BPH should be excluded in any patient for whom terazosin therapy for presumed BPH is being considered.

Caution should be exercised when adding terazosin to a preexisting antihypertensive regimen or when adding other hypotensive agents to a terazosin regimen in order to avoid a possible rapid fall in blood pressure and exacerbation of postural effects. Dosage reduction and/or retitration of therapy may be necessary. Particular caution may be necessary when terazosin and verapamil are used concomitantly because of an added potential pharmacokinetic interaction (i.e., verapamil-induced increases in plasma terazosin concentrations).

Terazosin is contraindicated in patients with known sensitivity to the drug or any other quinazoline derivative (e.g., doxazosin, prazosin).

● Pediatric Precautions

The manufacturer states that safety and efficacy of terazosin in patients younger than 21 years of age have not been established. Some experts state that use of centrally acting antihypertensive agents (e.g., terazosin) should be reserved for children who are not responsive to 2 or more of the preferred classes of antihypertensive agents (angiotensin-converting enzyme [ACE] inhibitors, angiotensin II receptor antagonists, long-acting calcium-channel blockers, or thiazide diuretics). For information on overall principles and expert recommendations for treatment of hypertension in pediatric patients, see Uses: Hypertension in Pediatric Patients, in the Thiazides General Statement 40:28.20.

● Geriatric Precautions

Geriatric patients (e.g., those 65 years of age and older) may be particularly susceptible to postural as well as certain other adverse effects of terazosin. (See Dosage and Administration: Dosage.)

● Mutagenicity and Carcinogenicity

There was no evidence of terazosin-induced mutagenicity in in vitro and in vivo test systems (Ames test, in vivo cytogenetics, dominant lethal test in mice, in vivo Chinese hamster chromosome aberration test, V79 forward mutation assay).

Oral terazosin dosages of 250 mg/kg daily (695 times the maximum recommended human dosage of 20 mg daily adjusted for a 55-kg man) for 2 years were associated with an increase in benign adrenal medullary tumors in male rats; females were unaffected. The drug was not oncogenic in mice receiving oral dosages of 32 mg/kg daily for 2 years. The absence of mutagenicity in a battery of in vivo and in vitro tests, of tumorigenicity of any cell type in the mouse carcinogenicity assay, of increased total tumor incidence in rats or mice, and of proliferative adrenal lesions in female rats suggests that the observed increase in benign medullary tumors is a male-rat species-specific effect. In addition, numerous other drugs and chemicals have been associated with increased benign adrenal medullary tumors in male rats without evidence of carcinogenic effects in humans.

● Pregnancy, Fertility, and Lactation

Pregnancy

Terazosin was not teratogenic in rats or rabbits at oral dosages up to 1330 or 165 times the maximum recommended human dosage, respectively. Fetal resorptions occurred in rats at an oral dosage of 480 mg/kg daily, which is approximately 1330 times the maximum recommended human dosage. Increased fetal resorptions, decreased fetal weight, and increased supernumerary ribs were observed in offspring of rabbits that received 165 times the maximum recommended human dosage. These fetal findings were most likely secondary to maternal toxicity. There are no adequate and controlled studies in pregnant women, and safety of terazosin during pregnancy has not been established. The drug should be used during pregnancy only when potential benefits justify the possible risks to the mother and fetus.

In a perinatal and postnatal development study in rats, there was an increased frequency of deaths in the offspring during the first 3 weeks postpartum at a maternal oral terazosin dosage of 120 mg/kg daily (more than 300 times the maximum recommended human dosage).

Fertility

In reproduction studies in rats receiving oral terazosin dosages of 8, 30, or 120 mg/kg daily, failure to sire litters was observed in males receiving the latter 2 dosages, but testicular weight and morphology were unaffected. However, vaginal smears

at these latter dosages appeared to contain less sperm than smears from control matings, and a positive correlation between sperm count and subsequent pregnancy was observed. An increase in testicular atrophy has been observed in rats receiving terazosin dosages of 40 or 250 mg/kg daily but not in those receiving 8 mg/kg daily (more than 20 times the maximum recommended human dosage). Testicular atrophy also was observed in dogs receiving 300 mg/kg daily (more than 800 times the maximum recommended human dosage) for 3 months but not with 1 year of administration at 20 mg/kg daily. Such atrophy also has been observed with prazosin.

Lactation

Since it is not known whether terazosin is distributed into milk, the drug should be used with caution in nursing women.

DESCRIPTION

Terazosin hydrochloride is a quinazoline-derivative postsynaptic α_1-adrenergic blocking agent. The drug is chemically and pharmacologically related to prazosin and doxazosin. On a molar basis, the postsynaptic α_1-adrenergic receptor affinity of terazosin is one-third that of prazosin when tested in rat liver, and the α_1-receptor selectivity is 4 times that of doxazosin when tested in human prostate adenoma.

Terazosin reduces peripheral vascular resistance and blood pressure as a result of its vasodilating effects; the drug produces both arterial and venous dilation. Terazosin reduces blood pressure in both supine and standing patients; the effect is most pronounced on standing blood pressure, and postural hypotension can occur. Terazosin generally causes no change in heart rate or cardiac output in the supine position. Cardiovascular responses to exercise (e.g., increased heart rate and cardiac output) are maintained during terazosin therapy.

Effects of terazosin on the cardiovascular system are mediated by the drug's activity at α_1-receptor sites in vascular smooth muscle. α_1-Adrenergic receptors also are located in nonvascular smooth muscle (e.g., bladder trigone and sphincters, GI tract and sphincters, prostate adenoma and capsule, ureters, uterus) and in nonmuscular tissues (e.g., CNS, liver, kidneys). Because of the prevalence of α-receptors in the prostate capsule, prostate adenoma, and the bladder trigone and the relative absence of these receptors on the bladder body, α-blockers decrease urinary outflow resistance in men.

Terazosin may improve to a limited extent the serum lipid profile (e.g., small increases in high-density lipoprotein cholesterol concentrations [HDL]/total cholesterol ratio, small decreases in low-density lipoprotein [LDL] cholesterol, total cholesterol, and triglyceride concentrations). In addition, such potential effects of terazosin may counteract the negative effects of thiazide diuretics on serum lipoprotein concentrations.

PREPARATIONS

Excipients in commercially available drug preparations may have clinically important effects in some individuals; consult specific product labeling for details.

Terazosin Hydrochloride

Oral		
Capsules	1 mg (of terazosin)*	**Terazosin Hydrochloride Capsules**
	2 mg (of terazosin)*	**Terazosin Hydrochloride Capsules**
	5 mg (of terazosin)*	**Terazosin Hydrochloride Capsules**
	10 mg (of terazosin)*	**Terazosin Hydrochloride Capsules**

* available from one or more manufacturer, distributor, and/or repackager by generic (nonproprietary) name

† Use is not currently included in the labeling approved by the US Food and Drug Administration.

Selected Revisions April 10, 2024, © Copyright, January 1, 1994, American Society of Health-System Pharmacists, Inc.

Atenolol

24:20 • β-ADRENERGIC BLOCKING AGENTS

■ Atenolol is a β₁-selective adrenergic blocking agent (β-blocker).

USES

Atenolol is used for the management of hypertension, angina, and acute myocardial infarction (MI). The drug also has been used for the management of supraventricular and ventricular tachyarrhythmias†, management of acute alcohol withdrawal (in conjunction with a benzodiazepine)†, and prophylaxis of migraine headache†.

The choice of a β-adrenergic blocking agent (β-blocker) depends on numerous factors, including pharmacologic properties (e.g., relative β-selectivity, intrinsic sympathomimetic activity, membrane-stabilizing activity, lipophilicity), pharmacokinetics, intended use, and adverse effect profile, as well as the patient's coexisting disease states or conditions, response, and tolerance. While specific pharmacologic properties and other factors may appropriately influence the choice of a β-blocker in individual patients, evidence of clinically important differences among the agents in terms of overall efficacy and/or safety is limited. Patients who do not respond to or cannot tolerate one β-blocker may be successfully treated with a different agent.

In the management of hypertension or chronic stable angina pectoris in patients with chronic obstructive pulmonary disease (COPD) or type 1 diabetes mellitus, many clinicians prefer to use low dosages of a β₁-selective adrenergic blocking agent (e.g., atenolol, metoprolol), rather than a nonselective agent (e.g., nadolol, pindolol, propranolol, timolol). However, selectivity of these agents is relative and dose dependent. Some clinicians also will recommend using a β₁-selective agent or an agent with intrinsic sympathomimetic activity (ISA) (e.g., pindolol), rather than a nonselective agent, for the management of hypertension or angina pectoris in patients with peripheral vascular disease, but there is no evidence that the choice of β-blocker substantially affects efficacy.

● Hypertension

Atenolol is used alone or in combination with other classes of antihypertensive agents in the management of hypertension. β-Blockers often are used concurrently with a diuretic because of their additive effects. β-Blockers also have been combined with vasodilators (e.g., hydralazine, minoxidil) to counteract the reflex tachycardia that occurs with vasodilators.

Current evidence-based practice guidelines for the management of hypertension in adults generally recommend the use of drugs from 4 classes of antihypertensive agents (angiotensin-converting enzyme [ACE] inhibitors, angiotensin II receptor antagonists, calcium-channel blockers, and thiazide diuretics). Most guidelines no longer recommend β-blockers as first-line therapy for hypertension because of the lack of established superiority over other recommended drug classes and evidence from at least one study (with atenolol) demonstrating that β-blockers may be less effective than angiotensin II receptor antagonists in preventing cardiovascular death, MI, or stroke. (See Uses: Hypertension in Adults, in the Thiazides General Statement 40:28.20.) However, therapy with a β-blocker may still be considered in hypertensive patients who have a compelling indication (e.g., prior MI, ischemic heart disease, heart failure) for their use or as add-on therapy in those who do not respond adequately to the preferred drug classes. (See Considerations for Drug Therapy in Patients with Underlying Cardiovascular and Other Risk Factors, under Uses: Hypertension.) Ultimately, choice of antihypertensive therapy should be individualized, considering the clinical characteristics of the patient (e.g., age, ethnicity/race, comorbid conditions, cardiovascular risk factors) as well as drug-related factors (e.g., ease of administration, availability, adverse effects, costs).

General Considerations for Initial and Maintenance Antihypertensive Therapy

Nonpharmacologic Therapy

Nonpharmacologic measures (i.e., lifestyle/behavioral modifications) that are effective in lowering blood pressure include weight reduction (for those who are overweight or obese), dietary changes to include foods such as fruits, vegetables, whole grains, and low-fat dairy products that are rich in potassium, calcium, magnesium, and fiber (i.e., adoption of the Dietary Approaches to Stop Hypertension [DASH] eating plan), sodium reduction, increased physical activity, and moderation of alcohol intake. Such lifestyle/behavioral modifications, including smoking cessation, enhance antihypertensive drug efficacy and decrease cardiovascular risk and remain an indispensable part of the management of hypertension. Lifestyle/behavioral modifications without antihypertensive drug therapy are recommended for individuals classified by a 2017 multidisciplinary hypertension guideline of the American College of Cardiology (ACC), American Heart Association (AHA), and a number of other professional organizations as having elevated blood pressure (systolic blood pressure 120–129 mm Hg and diastolic blood pressure less than 80 mm Hg) and in those with stage 1 hypertension (systolic blood pressure 130–139 mm Hg or diastolic blood pressure 80–89 mm Hg) who do *not* have preexisting cardiovascular disease or an estimated 10-year atherosclerotic cardiovascular disease (ASCVD) risk of 10% or greater.

Initiation of Drug Therapy

Drug therapy in the management of hypertension must be individualized and adjusted based on the degree of blood pressure elevation while also considering cardiovascular risk factors. Drug therapy generally is reserved for patients who respond inadequately to nondrug therapy (i.e., lifestyle modifications such as diet [including sodium restriction and adequate potassium and calcium intake], regular aerobic physical activity, moderation of alcohol consumption, and weight reduction) or in whom the degree of blood pressure elevation or coexisting risk factors, especially increased cardiovascular risk, requires more prompt or aggressive therapy; however, the optimum blood pressure threshold for initiating antihypertensive drug therapy and specific treatment goals remain controversial.

The 2017 ACC/AHA hypertension guideline and many experts currently state that the treatment of hypertension should be based not only on blood pressure values but also on patients' cardiovascular risk factors. For *secondary prevention* of recurrent cardiovascular disease events in adults with clinical cardiovascular disease or for *primary prevention* in adults with an estimated 10-year ASCVD risk of 10% or higher, the 2017 ACC/AHA hypertension guideline recommends initiation of antihypertensive drug therapy in conjunction with lifestyle/behavioral modifications at an average systolic blood pressure of 130 mm Hg or an average diastolic blood pressure of 80 mm Hg or higher. For *primary prevention* of cardiovascular disease events in adults with a low (less than 10%) estimated 10-year risk of ASCVD, the 2017 ACC/AHA hypertension guideline recommends initiation of antihypertensive drug therapy in conjunction with lifestyle/behavioral modifications at a systolic blood pressure of 140 mm Hg or higher or a diastolic blood pressure of 90 mm Hg or higher. After initiation of antihypertensive drug therapy, regardless of the ASCVD risk, the 2017 ACC/AHA hypertension guideline generally recommends a blood pressure goal of less than 130/80 mm Hg in all adults. In addition, a systolic blood pressure goal of less than 130 mm Hg also is recommended for noninstitutionalized ambulatory patients 65 years of age or older. While these blood pressure goals are lower than those recommended for most patients in previous guidelines, they are based upon clinical studies demonstrating continuing reduction of cardiovascular risk at progressively lower levels of systolic blood pressure.

Most data indicate that patients with a higher cardiovascular risk will benefit the most from tighter blood pressure control; however, some experts state this treatment goal also may be beneficial in those at lower cardiovascular risk. Other clinicians believe that the benefits of such blood pressure lowering do not outweigh the risks in those patients considered to be at lower risk of cardiovascular disease and that reclassifying individuals formerly considered to have prehypertension as having hypertension may potentially lead to use of drug therapy in such patients without consideration of cardiovascular risk. Previous hypertension guidelines, such as those from the JNC 8 expert panel, generally have recommended initiation of antihypertensive treatment in patients with a systolic blood pressure of at least 140 mm Hg or diastolic blood pressure of at least 90 mm Hg, targeted a blood pressure goal of less than 140/90 mm Hg regardless of cardiovascular risk, and used higher systolic blood pressure thresholds and targets in geriatric patients. Some clinicians continue to support the target blood pressures recommended by the JNC 8 expert panel because of concerns that such recommendations in the 2017 ACC/AHA hypertension guideline are based on extrapolation of data from the high-risk population in the SPRINT study to a lower-risk population. Also, because more than 90% of patients in SPRINT were already receiving antihypertensive drugs at baseline, data are lacking on the effects of *initiating* drug therapy at a lower blood pressure threshold (130/80 mm Hg) in patients at high risk of cardiovascular disease. The potential benefits of hypertension management and drug cost, adverse effects, and risks associated with the use of multiple antihypertensive drugs should be considered when deciding a patient's treatment goal.

The 2017 ACC/AHA hypertension guideline recommends an ASCVD risk assessment for all adults with hypertension; however, experts state that it can be assumed that patients with hypertension and diabetes mellitus or chronic kidney disease (CKD) are at high risk for cardiovascular disease and that antihypertensive drug therapy should be initiated in these patients at a blood pressure of 130/80 mm Hg or higher. ACC/AHA also recommends a blood pressure goal of less than 130/80 mm Hg in patients with hypertension and diabetes mellitus or CKD. These recommendations are based on a systematic review of high-quality evidence from randomized controlled trials, meta-analyses, and post hoc analyses that have demonstrated substantial reductions in the risk of important clinical outcomes (e.g., cardiovascular events) regardless of comorbid conditions or age when systolic blood pressure is lowered to less than 130 mm Hg. However, some clinicians have questioned the generalizability of findings from some of the trials (e.g., SPRINT) used to support the 2017 ACC/AHA hypertension guideline. For example, SPRINT included adults (mean age: 68 years) *without* diabetes mellitus who were at high risk of cardiovascular disease. While benefits of intensive blood pressure control were observed in this patient population, some clinicians have questioned whether these findings apply to younger patients who have a low risk of cardiovascular disease. In patients with CKD in the SPRINT trial, intensive blood pressure management (achieving a mean systolic blood pressure of approximately 122 mm Hg compared with 136 mm Hg with standard treatment) provided a similar beneficial reduction in the composite cardiovascular disease primary outcome and all-cause mortality as in the full patient cohort. Because most patients with CKD die from cardiovascular complications, the findings of this study further support a lower blood pressure target of less than 130/80 mm Hg. Data are lacking to determine the ideal blood pressure goal in patients with hypertension and diabetes mellitus; also, studies evaluating the benefits of intensive blood pressure control in patients with diabetes mellitus have provided conflicting results.

Clinical studies reviewed for the 2017 ACC/AHA hypertension guideline have shown similar quantitative benefits from blood pressure lowering in hypertensive patients with or without diabetes mellitus. In a randomized, controlled study (ACCORD-BP) that compared a higher (systolic blood pressure less than 140 mm Hg) versus lower (systolic blood pressure less than 120 mm Hg) blood pressure goal in patients with diabetes mellitus, there was no difference in the incidence of cardiovascular outcomes (e.g., composite outcome of cardiovascular death, nonfatal MI, and nonfatal stroke). However, some experts state that this study was underpowered to detect a difference between the 2 treatment groups and that the factorial design of the study complicated interpretation of the results. Although SPRINT did not include patients with diabetes mellitus, patients in this study with prediabetes demonstrated a similar cardiovascular benefit from intensive treatment of blood pressure as normoglycemic patients. A meta-analysis of data from ACCORD and SPRINT suggests that the findings of both studies are consistent and that patients with diabetes mellitus benefit from more intensive blood pressure control. These data support the 2017 ACC/AHA hypertension guideline recommendation of a blood pressure treatment goal of less than 130/80 mm Hg in patients with hypertension and diabetes mellitus. Alternatively, the American Diabetes Association (ADA) recommends a blood pressure goal of less than 140/90 mm Hg in patients with diabetes mellitus. The ADA states that a lower blood pressure goal (e.g., less than 130/80 mm Hg) may be appropriate for patients with a high risk of cardiovascular disease and diabetes mellitus if it can be achieved without undue treatment burden.

Further study is needed to more clearly define optimum blood pressure goals in patients with hypertension, particularly in high-risk groups (e.g., patients with diabetes mellitus, cardiovascular disease, or cerebrovascular disease; black patients); when determining appropriate blood pressure goals, individual risks and benefits should be considered in addition to the evidence from clinical studies.

Experts state that in patients with stage 1 hypertension (especially the elderly, those with a history of hypotension, or those who have experienced adverse drug effects), it is reasonable to initiate drug therapy using the stepped-care approach in which one drug is initiated and titrated and other drugs are added sequentially to achieve the target blood pressure. However, although some patients can begin treatment with a single antihypertensive agent, the 2017 ACC/AHA hypertension guideline recommends initiation of antihypertensive therapy with 2 drugs from different pharmacologic classes (either as separate agents or in a fixed-dose combination) in patients with stage 2 hypertension and an average blood pressure more than 20/10 mm Hg above their target blood pressure. Such combined therapy may increase the likelihood of achieving goal blood pressure in a more timely fashion, but also may increase the risk of adverse effects (e.g., orthostatic hypotension) in some patients (e.g., elderly). Drug regimens with complementary activity, where a second antihypertensive agent is used to block compensatory responses to the first agent or affect a different pressor mechanism, can result in additive blood pressure lowering and are preferred. Drug combinations that have similar mechanisms of action or clinical effects (e.g., the combination of an ACE inhibitor and an angiotensin II receptor antagonist) generally should be avoided. Many patients who begin therapy with a single antihypertensive agent will subsequently require at least 2 drugs from different pharmacologic classes to achieve their blood pressure goal. Experts state that other patient-specific factors, such as age, concurrent medications, drug adherence, drug interactions, the overall treatment regimen, cost, and comorbidities, also should be considered when deciding on an antihypertensive drug regimen. For any stage of hypertension, antihypertensive drug dosages should be adjusted and/or other agents substituted or added until goal blood pressure is achieved. (See Follow-up and Maintenance Drug Therapy under Hypertension: General Considerations for Initial and Maintenance Antihypertensive Therapy, in Uses.)

Follow-up and Maintenance Drug Therapy

Several strategies are used for the titration and combination of antihypertensive drugs; these strategies, which are generally based on those used in randomized controlled studies, include maximizing the dosage of the first drug before adding a second drug, adding a second drug before achieving maximum dosage of the initial drug, or initiating therapy with 2 drugs simultaneously (either as separate preparations or as a fixed-dose combination). Combined use of an ACE inhibitor and angiotensin II receptor antagonist should be avoided because of the potential risk of adverse renal effects. After initiating a new or adjusted antihypertensive drug regimen, patients should have their blood pressure reevaluated monthly until adequate blood pressure control is achieved. Effective blood pressure control can be achieved in most hypertensive patients, but many will ultimately require therapy with 2 or more antihypertensive drugs. In addition to measuring blood pressure, clinicians should evaluate patients for orthostatic hypotension, adverse drug effects, adherence to drug therapy and lifestyle modifications, and the need for drug dosage adjustments. Laboratory testing such as electrolytes and renal function status and other assessments of target organ damage also should be performed.

Considerations for Drug Therapy in Patients with Underlying Cardiovascular and Other Risk Factors

Drug therapy in patients with hypertension and underlying cardiovascular or other risk factors should be carefully individualized based on the underlying disease(s), concomitant drugs, tolerance to drug-induced adverse effects, and blood pressure goal. (See Table 2 on Compelling Indications for Drug Classes based on Comorbid Conditions, under Uses: Hypertension in Adults, in the Thiazides General Statement 40:28.20.)

Ischemic Heart Disease

The selection of an appropriate antihypertensive agent in patients with ischemic heart disease should be based on individual patient characteristics and may include a β-blocker, with the addition of other drugs (e.g., ACE inhibitors, thiazide diuretics, calcium-channel blockers) as necessary to achieve blood pressure goals. Because of the demonstrated mortality benefit of β-blockers following MI, these drugs should be administered in all patients who have survived an MI. The 2017 ACC/AHA hypertension guideline states that β-blockers used for ischemic heart disease/angina that are also effective in lowering blood pressure include bisoprolol, carvedilol, metoprolol succinate, metoprolol tartrate, nadolol, propranolol, and timolol. However, ACC/AHA state that the use of atenolol for the management of hypertension in patients with stable ischemic heart disease should be *avoided* because the drug has been shown to be less effective than placebo in reducing cardiovascular events and is not as effective in treating hypertension as other antihypertensive agents.

Heart Failure

While β-blockers as single therapies are not superior to other antihypertensive agents in the reduction of all cardiovascular outcomes, certain β-blockers (bisoprolol, carvedilol, extended-release metoprolol succinate) have been shown to be effective in reducing the incidence of heart failure† and associated morbidity and mortality. (See Uses: Heart Failure, in Carvedilol 24:24.)

Other Special Considerations for Antihypertensive Drug Therapy

Race

Most patients with hypertension, especially black patients, will require at least 2 antihypertensive drugs to achieve adequate blood pressure control. In general, black hypertensive patients tend to respond better to monotherapy with thiazide diuretics or calcium-channel blocking agents than to monotherapy with β-blockers, ACE inhibitors, or angiotensin II receptor antagonists. However, such diminished response to a β-blocker is largely eliminated when the drug is administered concomitantly with a thiazide diuretic. In addition, some experts state that when use of β-blockers is indicated in hypertensive patients with underlying cardiovascular or other risk factors, these indications should be applied equally to black hypertensive patients.

For information on overall principles and expert recommendations for treatment of hypertension, see Uses: Hypertension in Adults, in the Thiazides General Statement 40:28.20.

● Chronic Stable Angina

Atenolol is used for the management of chronic stable angina pectoris. β-Blockers are recommended as the anti-ischemic drugs of choice in most patients with chronic stable angina; despite differences in cardioselectivity, intrinsic sympathomimetic activity, and other clinical factors, all β-blockers appear to be equally effective for this indication. Long-term use of β-blockers in patients with chronic stable angina pectoris has been shown to reduce the frequency of anginal attacks, allow a reduction in nitroglycerin dosage, and increase exercise tolerance.

Combination therapy with a β-blocker and a nitrate appears to be more effective than either drug alone because β-blockers attenuate the increased sympathetic tone and reflex tachycardia associated with nitrate therapy while nitrate therapy (e.g., nitroglycerin) counteracts the potential increase in left-ventricular wall tension associated with a decrease in heart rate. Combined therapy with a β-blocker and a dihydropyridine calcium-channel blocker also may be useful because the tendency to develop tachycardia with the calcium-channel blocker is counteracted by the β-blocker. However, caution should be exercised in the concomitant use of β-blockers and the nondihydropyridine calcium-channel blockers verapamil or diltiazem because of the potential for excessive fatigue, bradycardia, or atrioventricular (AV) block. (See Drug Interactions: Cardiovascular Drugs.)

● Non-ST-Segment-Elevation Acute Coronary Syndromes

β-Blockers are used as part of the standard therapeutic measures for managing non-ST-segment-elevation acute coronary syndromes (NSTE ACS). Patients with NSTE ACS have either unstable angina or non-ST-segment-elevation MI (NSTEMI); because these conditions are part of a continuum of acute myocardial ischemia and have indistinguishable clinical features upon presentation, the same initial treatment strategies are recommended. The American Heart Association/American College of Cardiology (AHA/ACC) guideline for the management of patients with NSTE ACS recommends an early invasive strategy (angiographic evaluation with the intent to perform revascularization procedures such as percutaneous coronary intervention [PCI] with coronary artery stent implantation or coronary artery bypass grafting [CABG]) or an ischemia-guided strategy (initial medical management followed by cardiac catheterization and revascularization if indicated) in patients with definite or likely NSTE ACS; standard medical therapies for all patients should include a β-blocker, antiplatelet agents (aspirin and/or a P2Y12-receptor antagonist), anticoagulant agents (e.g., low molecular weight or unfractionated heparin), nitrates (e.g., nitroglycerin), and analgesic agents regardless of the initial management approach. The guideline states that oral β-blocker therapy should be initiated within the first 24 hours in patients who do not have manifestations of heart failure, evidence of a low-output state, increased risk of cardiogenic shock, or any other contraindications to β-blocker therapy; use of IV β-blockers is potentially harmful in patients with risk factors for cardiogenic shock. Continued therapy with a β-blocker proven to reduce mortality (bisoprolol, carvedilol, or metoprolol succinate) is recommended in patients

with stabilized heart failure and reduced systolic function. (See Uses: Heart Failure, in Carvedilol 24:24.)

● Acute Myocardial Infarction

Atenolol is used to reduce the risk of cardiovascular mortality in hemodynamically stable patients with definite or suspected acute MI. The term MI is used when there is evidence of myocardial necrosis in the setting of acute myocardial ischemia. ST-segment-elevation MI (STEMI) is distinguished from NSTEMI based on the presence or absence of ST-segment elevation on ECG. Patients with STEMI typically have complete arterial occlusion; therefore, immediate reperfusion therapy (with primary PCI or thrombolytic agents) is the current standard of care for such patients. Because the clinical presentation of NSTEMI is similar to that of unstable angina, these conditions are considered together in current expert guidelines. (See Uses: Non-ST-Segment-Elevation Acute Coronary Syndromes.) During the early stage of a definite or suspected MI, atenolol has been initiated with IV doses (no longer commercially available in the US), followed by continued oral dosing; however, experts currently recommend that early IV use of β-blockers be limited to selected patients.

Because β-blockers can reduce myocardial oxygen demand during the first few hours of an acute MI by reducing heart rate, arterial blood pressure, and myocardial contractility, and also have been shown to reduce mortality, early IV therapy with these drugs was routinely recommended following acute MI. Evidence supporting this recommendation was generally based on studies conducted prior to the reperfusion era demonstrating a reduction in mortality and other clinical benefits (i.e., reduced infarct size, incidence of ventricular arrhythmias, chest pain, and cardiac enzyme elevations) with early use of β-blockers during MI. In one such study (the First International Study of Infarct Survival; ISIS-1), therapy with atenolol (initiated IV within the first 12 hours of symptom onset and continued orally for 7 days) was shown to reduce cardiovascular mortality by approximately 15% during the first few days of therapy, but did not substantially reduce cardiovascular mortality beyond this initial period. The difference in vascular mortality rate between those receiving atenolol or placebo was evident almost entirely during the first 2 days of therapy. Analysis of data from a subset of patients who died during early treatment in ISIS-1 suggested that the principal mechanism of early mortality reduction associated with atenolol therapy was prevention of cardiac rupture and of cardiac electromechanical dissociation. However, the relevance of these study findings to current clinical practice has been questioned since patients did not receive reperfusion therapy and only 5% received an antiplatelet agent.

Studies conducted after the widespread use of reperfusion therapy generally have demonstrated more attenuated benefits with early β-blocker therapy in patients with acute MI; while β-blockers may still confer benefits (e.g., reduction in the risk of reinfarction and ventricular arrhythmias), there is less certainty regarding the drugs' effects on mortality in patients receiving contemporary revascularization and pharmacologic therapies (antiplatelet agents, ACE inhibitors, and lipid-lowering therapies). In addition, early use of β-blockers (particularly when administered IV) has been associated with an increased risk of cardiogenic shock. (See Uses: Acute Myocardial Infarction in Metoprolol 24:24.) Based on the currently available evidence, the American College of Cardiology Foundation/American Heart Association (ACCF/AHA) guideline for the management of STEMI recommends oral β-blocker therapy in all patients who do not have manifestations of heart failure, evidence of a low-output state, increased risk of cardiogenic shock, or any other contraindications to β-blocker therapy. Such therapy should be initiated within the first 24 hours following acute MI and continued during and after hospitalization. Because of conflicting evidence of benefit and the potential for harm, the guidelines recommend limiting use of IV β-blockers to patients with refractory hypertension or ongoing ischemia.

Although the efficacy of atenolol in reducing cardiovascular mortality has been established only during the first 7 days after an acute MI, the benefits of long-term β-blocker therapy for secondary prevention have been well established in numerous clinical studies. Patients with MI complicated by heart failure, left ventricular dysfunction, or ventricular arrhythmias appear to derive the most benefit from long-term β-blocker therapy. Data from studies using other β-blockers suggest that optimum benefit may be achieved if treatment with these agents is continued for at least 1–3 years if not indefinitely after infarction unless contraindicated. Several large, randomized studies have demonstrated that prolonged oral therapy with a β-blocker can reduce the rates of reinfarction and mortality (e.g., sudden and nonsudden cardiac death) following acute MI. It is estimated that such therapy could result in a relative reduction in mortality of about 25% annually for years 1–3 after infarction, with high-risk patients exhibiting the greatest potential benefit; the benefit of continued therapy may persist for at least several years beyond this period, although less substantially. Therefore, atenolol, like other β-blockers, can be used for secondary prevention following acute MI to reduce the risk of reinfarction and mortality. The AHA/ACCF secondary prevention guideline recommends β-blocker therapy in all patients with left ventricular systolic dysfunction (ejection fraction of 40% or less) and a prior MI; use of a β-blocker with proven mortality benefit (bisoprolol, carvedilol, or metoprolol succinate) is recommended. (See Uses: Heart Failure, in Carvedilol 24:24.) Although the benefits of long-term β-blockade in post-MI patients with normal left ventricular function are less well established, the guideline recommends continued β-blocker therapy for at least 3 years in such patients. Further studies are needed to establish the optimal duration of β-blocker therapy for secondary prevention of MI.

● **Supraventricular Arrhythmias**

β-Blockers, including atenolol, have been used to slow ventricular rate in patients with supraventricular tachycardia (SVT)†. The American College of Cardiology/American Heart Association/Heart Rhythm Society (ACC/AHA/HRS) guideline for the management of adult patients with supraventricular tachycardia recommends the use of β-adrenergic blocking agents in the treatment of various SVTs (e.g., atrial flutter, junctional tachycardia, focal atrial tachycardia, atrioventricular nodal reentrant tachycardia [AVNRT]); in general, an IV β-blocker is recommended for acute treatment, while an oral preparation is recommended for ongoing management of these arrhythmias. Vagal maneuvers and/or IV adenosine are considered first-line interventions for the acute treatment of patients with SVT and should be attempted prior to other therapies when clinically indicated; if such measures are ineffective or not feasible, an IV β-blocker may be considered in hemodynamically stable patients. Although evidence of efficacy is limited, experts state that the overall safety of β-adrenergic blockers warrants their use in patients with SVT. Patients should be closely monitored for hypotension and bradycardia during administration of these drugs.

Atrial Fibrillation and Flutter

β-Blockers are recommended as one of several drug therapy options for ventricular rate control in patients with nonpreexcited atrial fibrillation or flutter†. For acute treatment of atrial fibrillation or flutter, an IV β-adrenergic blocking agent (e.g., esmolol, propranolol, metoprolol) may be used for ventricular rate control in patients without preexcitation; an oral β-blocker such as atenolol may be used for ongoing rate control in such patients. Choice of a specific β-blocker should be individualized based on the patient's clinical condition.

Atrial Tachycardia

IV β-blockers may be used for the treatment of patients with hemodynamically stable focal atrial tachycardia† (i.e., regular SVT arising from a localized atrial site), and an oral β-blocker may be used for ongoing management. Multifocal atrial tachycardia, characterized by a rapid, irregular rhythm with at least 3 distinct P-wave morphologies, is commonly associated with an underlying condition (e.g., pulmonary, coronary, or valvular heart disease) and is generally not responsive to antiarrhythmic drug therapy. Antiarrhythmic drug therapy usually is reserved for patients who do not respond to initial attempts at correcting or managing potential precipitating factors (e.g., exacerbation of chronic obstructive pulmonary disease or congestive heart failure, hypoxemia, anemia) or in whom a precipitating factor cannot be identified.

Paroxysmal Supraventricular Tachycardia

IV β-blockers may be used for the acute treatment of hemodynamically stable patients with paroxysmal supraventricular tachycardia (PSVT), including AVNRT†, that is uncontrolled or unconverted by vagal maneuvers and adenosine; an oral β-blocker may be used for the ongoing management of such patients who are not candidates for, or prefer not to undergo, catheter ablation.

Junctional Tachycardia

β-Blockers are considered one of several drug therapy options that may be used for the treatment of junctional tachycardia† (i.e., nonreentrant SVT originating from the AV junction), a rapid, occasionally irregular, narrow-complex tachycardia. While evidence is limited, there is some data indicating that β-blockers (specifically propranolol) are modestly effective in terminating and/or reducing the incidence of junctional tachycardia.

● **Ventricular Arrhythmias**

β-Blockers also have been used in patients with cardiac arrest precipitated by ventricular fibrillation or pulseless ventricular tachycardia†. However, AHA states that routine administration of β-blockers after cardiac arrest is potentially harmful (e.g., may worsen hemodynamic instability, exacerbate heart failure, or cause bradyarrhythmias) and is therefore not recommended.

β-Blockers may be useful in the management of certain forms of polymorphic ventricular tachycardia† (e.g., associated with acute ischemia).

● **Vascular Headache**

Migraine

Atenolol has been used for the prophylaxis of migraine headache†. When used prophylactically, atenolol can prevent migraine or reduce the number of attacks in some patients. However, the US Headache Consortium states that the quality of evidence for atenolol is not as compelling as it is for propranolol for this indication. Atenolol is not recommended for the treatment of a migraine attack that has already started. For further information on management and classification of migraine headache, see Vascular Headaches: General Principles in Migraine Therapy, under Uses in Sumatriptan 28:32.28.

● **Alcohol Withdrawal**

Atenolol has been used in conjunction with a benzodiazepine in the management of acute alcohol withdrawal†. β-Blockers such as atenolol appear to be effective in reducing manifestations of the hyperadrenergic state associated with alcohol withdrawal, including elevated blood pressure, increased heart rate, and anxiety. However, β-blockers have not been shown to prevent delirium or seizures, and such drugs should be used only as adjuncts to benzodiazepines (not as monotherapy) for the treatment of alcohol withdrawal. (See Uses: Alcohol Withdrawal, in the Benzodiazepines General Statement 28:24.08.) Some clinicians state that the use of β-blockers may be particularly helpful in patients with certain coexisting conditions (e.g., coronary artery disease).

DOSAGE AND ADMINISTRATION

● **Administration**

Atenolol is administered orally; the drug also has been administered by IV injection, however a parenteral preparation no longer is commercially available in the US.

Oral administration of atenolol more frequently than once daily for the management of hypertension usually is not necessary. If atenolol is used in patients with bronchospastic disorders, therapy should be initiated cautiously; concomitant administration of a β_2-adrenergic agonist and twice-daily dosing of atenolol may minimize the risk of bronchospasm in some patients.

Extemporaneous Liquid Formulation

An oral liquid formulation containing 2 mg/mL of atenolol has been extemporaneously prepared using the commercially available tablets and various vehicles (e.g., simple syrup, Ora-Sweet, Ora-Plus, Ora-Sweet SF, methylcellulose-based vehicle).

Standardize 4 Safety

Standardized concentrations for an extemporaneously prepared oral liquid formulation of atenolol have been established through Standardize 4 Safety (S4S), a national patient safety initiative to reduce medication errors, especially during transitions of care. Multidisciplinary expert panels were convened to determine recommended standard concentrations. Because recommendations from the S4S panels may differ from the manufacturer's prescribing information, caution is advised when using concentrations that differ from labeling, particularly when using rate information from the label. For additional information on S4S (including updates that may be available), see https://www.ashp.org/pharmacy-practice/standardize-4-safety-initiative.

TABLE 1. Standardize 4 Safety Compounded Oral Liquid Standards for Atenolol

Concentration Standards
2 mg/mL

● *Dosage*

Dosage of atenolol must be individualized and adjusted according to the patient's response and tolerance. If atenolol therapy is to be discontinued, dosage of the drug should be reduced gradually over a period of about 2 weeks. (See Cautions: Precautions and Contraindications.)

Hypertension

Atenolol Therapy

The manufacturer recommends an initial adult atenolol dosage of 50 mg once daily, either alone or in combination with diuretic therapy; the full antihypertensive effect may not be evident for 1–2 weeks. If response is inadequate after a sufficient trial at the initial dosage, the manufacturer states that dosage should be increased to 100 mg once daily. Some experts state that the usual adult dosage range for treatment of hypertension is 25–100 mg daily administered in 2 divided doses. Dosages exceeding 100 mg daily usually do not result in further improvement in blood pressure control.

If atenolol is used for the management of hypertension in children†, some experts have recommended an initial oral dosage of 0.5–1 mg/kg daily given as a single dose or in 2 divided doses. Such experts have suggested that dosage may be increased as necessary to a maximum dosage of 2 mg/kg (up to 100 mg) daily given as a single dose or in 2 divided doses. For information on overall principles and expert recommendations for treatment of hypertension in pediatric patients, see Uses: Hypertension in Pediatric Patients, in the Thiazides General Statement 40:28.20.

Atenolol/Chlorthalidone Fixed-combination Therapy

When combination therapy is required, commercially available preparations containing atenolol in combination with chlorthalidone should not be used initially. Dosage should first be adjusted by administering each drug separately. If it is determined that the optimum maintenance dosage corresponds to the ratio in the commercial combination preparation, such a preparation may be used. If the fixed-combination preparation is used, the manufacturer recommends an initial dosage of 50 mg of atenolol and 25 mg of chlorthalidone once daily. If an optimal response is not achieved, the fixed-combination preparation containing 100 mg of atenolol and 25 mg of chlorthalidone may be used once daily.

Blood Pressure Monitoring and Treatment Goals

Blood pressure should be monitored regularly (i.e., monthly) during therapy and dosage of the antihypertensive drug adjusted until blood pressure is controlled. If an adequate blood pressure response is not achieved, the dosage may be increased or another antihypertensive agent with demonstrated benefit and preferably with a complementary mechanism of action (e.g., angiotensin-converting enzyme [ACE] inhibitor, angiotensin II receptor antagonist, calcium-channel blocker, thiazide diuretic) may be added; if target blood pressure is still not achieved with the use of 2 antihypertensive agents, a third drug may be added. (See Uses: Hypertension.) In patients who develop unacceptable adverse effects with atenolol, the drug should be discontinued and another antihypertensive agent from a different pharmacologic class should be initiated.

The goal of hypertension management and prevention is to achieve and maintain optimal control of blood pressure. However, the optimum blood pressure threshold for initiating antihypertensive drug therapy and specific treatment goals remain controversial. While other hypertension guidelines have based target blood pressure goals on age and comorbidities, the 2017 American College of Cardiology/American Heart Association (ACC/AHA) hypertension guideline incorporates underlying cardiovascular risk into decision making regarding treatment and generally recommends the same target blood pressure (i.e., less than 130/80 mm Hg) for all adults. Many patients will require at least 2 drugs from different pharmacologic classes to achieve this blood pressure goal; the potential benefits of hypertension management and drug cost, adverse effects, and risks associated with the use of multiple antihypertensive drugs also should be considered when deciding a patient's blood pressure treatment goal. (See General Considerations for Initial and Maintenance Antihypertensive Therapy under Uses: Hypertension.)

For additional information on target levels of blood pressure and on monitoring therapy in the management of hypertension, see Blood Pressure Monitoring and Treatment Goals under Dosage: Hypertension, in Dosage and Administration in the Thiazides General Statement 40:28.20.

Chronic Stable Angina

For the management of chronic stable angina pectoris, the initial adult oral dosage of atenolol is 50 mg once daily. If an optimum response is not achieved within one week, oral dosage should be increased to 100 mg once daily. Some patients may require an oral atenolol dosage of 200 mg once daily for optimum effect. Dosage of β-blockers in angina pectoris usually is adjusted according to clinical response and to maintain a resting heart rate of 55–60 beats/minute. Control of angina pectoris over a 24-hour period with once-daily dosing of atenolol is achieved by the use of doses larger than those necessary to achieve an immediate maximum effect. The maximum early effect on exercise tolerance occurs with oral atenolol doses of 50–100 mg, but the effect at 24 hours is attenuated at these doses, averaging about 50–75% of that observed with once-daily oral doses of 200 mg.

Acute Myocardial Infarction

Early Treatment

Atenolol therapy may be initiated as soon as possible after an acute myocardial infarction (MI) when the patient's hemodynamic condition has stabilized. During the early stage of a definite or suspected MI, atenolol has been initiated with IV doses, followed by continued oral dosing; however, a parenteral preparation of atenolol is no longer commercially available in the US. When IV dosing is excluded, atenolol can be administered orally at a dosage of 50 mg twice daily or 100 mg once daily for at least 7 days.

The American College of Cardiology Foundation (ACCF)/AHA guideline for the management of ST-segment-elevation MI (STEMI) recommends initiation of oral β-blocker therapy within the first 24 hours of an acute MI in all patients who do not have manifestations of heart failure, evidence of a low-output state, increased risk of cardiogenic shock, or any other contraindications to β-blocker therapy.

Long-term Secondary Prevention

The optimal duration of β-blocker therapy following MI remains to be clearly established. Experts generally recommend that such therapy be continued long-term in post-MI patients with left ventricular systolic dysfunction, and for at least 3 years in those with normal left ventricular function.

Supraventricular Arrhythmias

For the ongoing treatment of various supraventricular tachycardias (SVTs)† (e.g., atrial flutter†, atrial tachycardia†, junctional tachycardia†) or atrial fibrillation† after initial IV therapy in adults, some experts recommend an initial oral atenolol dose of 25–50 mg daily and usual maintenance dosage of 25–100 mg daily.

Vascular Headaches

Migraine

Although oral dosage of atenolol for the prophylaxis of migraine† in adults has not been established, the usual effective dosage of the drug in clinical studies was 100 mg daily.

● *Dosage in Renal Impairment*

In patients with impaired renal function, doses and/or frequency of administration of atenolol must be modified in response to the degree of renal impairment. Because decreased renal function is a physiologic consequence of aging, the possibility that modification of atenolol dosage may be necessary in geriatric patients should be considered. Initiation of oral atenolol therapy at 25 mg daily may be necessary in some renally impaired or geriatric patients being treated for hypertension; if this dosage is employed, measurement of blood pressure just prior to a dose is recommended to ensure persistence of adequate blood pressure reduction. Although similar, low-dose initial therapy may be warranted for other conditions, data currently are not available.

A maximum oral atenolol dosage of 50 mg daily is recommended for patients with creatinine clearances of 15–35 mL/minute per 1.73 m^2; 25 mg daily or 50 mg every other day is recommended when creatinine clearance is less than 15 mL/minute per 1.73 m^2. In patients undergoing hemodialysis, a 25- or 50-mg oral dose of atenolol may be administered after each dialysis; since marked reductions in blood pressure may occur, it is recommended that the supplemental dose be given under careful supervision.

CAUTIONS

Atenolol shares the toxic potentials of β-adrenergic blocking agents (β-blockers). In therapeutic dosage, atenolol usually is well tolerated and has a low incidence of adverse effects. The incidence and severity of adverse reactions may occasionally be obviated by a reduction in dosage. Abrupt withdrawal of the drug should be avoided, especially in patients with coronary artery disease, since it may exacerbate angina or precipitate myocardial infarction (MI).

● Cardiovascular Effects

Potentially serious adverse cardiovascular effects of atenolol include bradycardia, which occurs in 3% of patients; profound hypotension; second- or third-degree atrioventricular (AV) block; and precipitation of severe heart failure, which is more likely to occur in patients with preexisting left ventricular dysfunction. Sick sinus syndrome has been reported during postmarketing experience in patients receiving atenolol-containing therapy. Atenolol-containing therapy is not recommended for use in patients with untreated pheochromocytoma. Bradycardia and hypotension usually can be reversed with an antimuscarinic agent like IV atropine. Isoproterenol or a transvenous cardiac pacemaker may be required for AV block. Other adverse cardiovascular effects include coldness of the extremities, reportedly occurring in 0–12% of patients; postural hypotension (which may be associated with syncope), in 2–4% of patients; and leg pain, in 0–3% of patients. When IV and oral atenolol were used in the early post-MI infarction period (for up to 10 days after onset of symptoms) in clinical trials, the principal adverse effects were bradycardia and hypotension, which occurred in up to 25% of patients receiving the drug (often combined with other therapy) and required reduction in dosage or discontinuance of atenolol in many patients. In addition, analysis of data from a subset of patients who died during early treatment in the First International Study of Infarct Survival (ISIS-1) revealed evidence of a small but not statistically significant increase in early death secondary to bradycardia and shock associated with atenolol therapy, but this potential adverse effect was outweighed substantially by beneficial effects of the drug on reduction of mortality from other causes. Atenolol may aggravate peripheral arterial circulatory disorders.

● CNS Effects

Adverse CNS effects of atenolol include dizziness, fatigue, and mental depression. Lethargy, drowsiness, unusual dreams, lightheadedness, and vertigo usually occur in less than 3% of patients. Headache and hallucinations also have been reported in patients receiving atenolol. Adverse CNS effects seen with other β-blockers that may occur with atenolol include visual disturbances, disorientation, short-term memory impairment, emotional lability, psychoses, catatonia, and impaired performance on neuropsychometric tests.

● GI Effects

Adverse GI reactions include diarrhea and nausea, which reportedly occur in 2–4% of patients receiving atenolol. A few cases of mesenteric arterial thrombosis and ischemic colitis have been reported in patients receiving other β-blockers. Dry mouth also has been reported in patients receiving atenolol.

● Endocrine Effects

Results of a large prospective cohort study of nondiabetic adults 45–64 years of age indicate that use of β-blockers in hypertensive patients is associated with increased risk (about 28%) of developing type 2 diabetes mellitus compared with hypertensive patients who were not receiving hypotensive therapy. In this study, the number of new cases of diabetes per 1000 person-years was 33.6 or 26.3 in patients receiving a β-blocker or no drug therapy, respectively. The association between the risk of developing diabetes mellitus and use of β-blockers reportedly was not confounded by weight gain, hyperinsulinemia, or differences in heart rate. It is not known if the risk of developing type 2 diabetes is affected by β-receptor selectivity. Further studies are needed to determine whether concomitant use of ACE inhibitors (which may improve insulin sensitivity) would abrogate β-blocker-induced adverse effects related to glucose intolerance. Therefore, until results of such studies are available, the proven benefits of β-blockers in reducing cardiovascular events in hypertensive patients must be weighed carefully against the possible risks of developing type 2 diabetes mellitus.

Hypoglycemia, which may result in loss of consciousness, also may occur in nondiabetic patients receiving β-blockers. Patients most at risk for the development of β-blocker-induced hypoglycemia are those undergoing dialysis, prolonged fasting, or severe exercise regimens.

β-Blockers may mask signs and symptoms of hypoglycemia (e.g., palpitation, tachycardia, tremor) and potentiate insulin-induced hypoglycemia. Although it has been suggested that nonselective β-blockers are more likely to induce hypoglycemia than selective β-blockers, such an adverse effect also has been reported with selective β-blocking agents (e.g., atenolol). In addition, selective β-blockers are less likely to mask symptoms of hypoglycemia or delay recovery from insulin-induced hypoglycemia than nonselective β-blockers because of their vascular sparing effects; however, selective β-blockers can decrease insulin sensitivity by approximately 15–30%, which may result in increased insulin requirements.

● Other Adverse Effects

Wheezing and dyspnea have occurred in patients receiving atenolol and are more likely to occur when dosage of the drug exceeds 100 mg daily. Rashes (which may be psoriasiform), exacerbation of psoriasis, lupus syndrome, drying of the eyes, visual disturbances, reversible alopecia, Peyronie's disease, antinuclear antibodies (ANA), impotence, elevated serum concentrations of hepatic enzymes and bilirubin, purpura, and thrombocytopenia also have been reported with atenolol.

The possibility that other adverse effects associated with other β-blockers may occur during atenolol therapy should be considered. These include hematologic reactions (e.g., agranulocytosis, nonthrombocytopenic or thrombocytopenic purpura); allergic reactions characterized by fever, sore throat, laryngospasm, and respiratory distress; Raynaud's phenomenon; conjunctivitis sicca; otitis; sclerosing serositis; and erythematous rash.

● Precautions and Contraindications

Atenolol shares the toxic potentials of β-blockers, and the usual precautions of these agents should be observed. When atenolol is used as a fixed-combination preparation that includes chlorthalidone, the cautions, precautions, and contraindications associated with thiazide diuretics must be considered in addition to those associated with atenolol.

In patients with heart failure, sympathetic stimulation is vital for the support of circulatory function. Atenolol should be used with caution in patients with inadequate cardiac function, since heart failure may be precipitated by blockade of β-adrenergic stimulation when atenolol therapy is administered. In addition, in patients with latent cardiac insufficiency, prolonged β-adrenergic blockade may lead to cardiac failure. Although β-blockers should be avoided in patients with overt heart failure, atenolol may be administered cautiously, if necessary, to patients with well-compensated heart failure (e.g., those controlled with cardiac glycosides and/or diuretics). Patients receiving atenolol therapy should be instructed to consult their physician at the first sign or symptom of impending cardiac failure and should be adequately treated (e.g., with a cardiac glycoside and/or diuretic) and observed closely; if cardiac failure continues, atenolol should be discontinued, gradually if possible. In patients with acute MI, use of atenolol is contraindicated in those whose congestive heart failure cannot be controlled promptly and effectively with a parenteral loop diuretic or comparable therapy. In addition, good clinical judgment suggests that patients whose cardiac output and/or blood pressure depends on sympathetic stimulation are not good candidates for β-adrenergic blocker therapy for acute MI, and such use is not recommended for patients whose systolic blood pressure or heart rate persistently is less than 100 mm Hg or 50–60 beats/minute, respectively.

Since β-blockers may inhibit bronchodilation produced by endogenous catecholamines, the drugs generally should not be used in patients with bronchospastic disease; however, because of its relative β₁-selective adrenergic blocking activity, atenolol may be used with caution in patients with bronchospastic disease who do not respond to or cannot tolerate other hypotensive agents. If atenolol is used in such patients, the initial dosage should be 50 mg daily and the smallest effective dosage should be used. In patients who develop symptoms of bronchospasm, atenolol dosage should be reduced or the drug discontinued (gradually if possible), and supportive treatment administered. In patients with bronchospastic disease, concomitant administration of a β₂-adrenergic agonist and/or twice-daily dosing of the drug may minimize the risk of bronchospasm.

Abrupt withdrawal of atenolol may exacerbate angina symptoms and/or precipitate MI and ventricular arrhythmias in patients with coronary artery disease, or may precipitate thyroid storm in patients with thyrotoxicosis. Therefore, patients receiving atenolol (especially those with ischemic heart disease) should be warned not to interrupt or discontinue therapy without consulting their physician. Because coronary artery disease is common and may be undiagnosed, abrupt withdrawal also should be avoided in patients receiving atenolol for other conditions (e.g., hypertension). When atenolol is discontinued in patients with coronary artery disease or suspected thyrotoxicosis, the patients should be observed carefully; patients with coronary artery disease should be advised to temporarily limit their physical activity. If exacerbation of angina occurs or acute coronary insufficiency develops after atenolol therapy is interrupted or discontinued, treatment with the drug should be reinstituted, at least temporarily.

Patients who have a history of anaphylactic reactions to a variety of allergens reportedly may be more reactive to repeated accidental, diagnostic, or therapeutic challenges with such allergens while taking β-blockers. These patients may be unresponsive to usual doses of epinephrine or may develop a paradoxical response to epinephrine when used to treat anaphylactic reactions.

Atenolol should be used with caution in patients undergoing major surgery involving general anesthesia. The necessity of withdrawing β-adrenergic blocking therapy prior to major surgery is controversial. Severe, protracted hypotension and difficulty in restarting or maintaining a heart beat have occurred during surgery in some patients who have received β-blockers. As with other β-blockers, the effects of atenolol can be reversed by administration of β-agonists (e.g., dobutamine, isoproterenol). If atenolol is discontinued, this should be done 2 days before surgery. If patients continue to receive atenolol prior to or during surgery in which anesthetics with negative inotropic activity are used, the patients should be observed for signs and symptoms of heart failure; if vagal stimulation occurs, atropine may be administered.

Atenolol should be used with caution in patients with hyperthyroidism since the drug may mask the tachycardia associated with hyperthyroidism. In addition, it is recommended that atenolol be used with caution in patients with diabetes mellitus since β-blockers may mask the tachycardia associated with hypoglycemia (a few cases have been reported in patients with type 2 diabetes mellitus), and β-blockers, especially nonselective ones, may potentially precipitate severe, acute hyperglycemia. (See Cautions: Endocrine Effects.) However, many clinicians state that patients with diabetes mellitus may be particularly likely to experience a reduction in morbidity and mortality with the use of these drugs. β-Blockers usually will not mask dizziness and sweating seen with hypoglycemia.

Atenolol should be used with caution and in reduced dosage in patients with impaired renal function, especially when creatinine clearance is less than 35 mL/minute per 1.73 m². The manufacturers recommend that patients receiving atenolol after hemodialysis be administered the drug under close supervision in a hospital setting, since marked hypotension may occur.

Atenolol is contraindicated in patients with sinus bradycardia, AV block greater than first degree, cardiogenic shock, known hypersensitivity to any component of the drug formulations, and overt or decompensated cardiac failure. Atenolol-containing therapy is not recommended for use in patients with untreated pheochromocytoma.

● Pediatric Precautions

Safety and efficacy of atenolol in pediatric patients have not been established; however, some experts have suggested dosages for hypertension based on clinical experience.

● Geriatric Precautions

Clinical studies of atenolol (used for angina pectoris associated with coronary atherosclerosis or hypertension) and of atenolol in fixed combination with chlorthalidone (used for hypertension) did not include sufficient numbers of patients 65 years of age and older to determine whether geriatric patients respond differently than younger adults. In addition, in a large clinical study (ISIS-1) evaluating atenolol in 8037 patients for the management of suspected acute MI, 2644 patients (about 33%) were 65 years of age or older, and there were no overall differences in safety or efficacy observed between geriatric individuals and younger adults; however, geriatric patients with systolic blood pressure below 120 mmHg seemed less likely to benefit from atenolol therapy. Although other clinical experience has not revealed age-related differences in response to the drug, care should be taken in dosage selection of atenolol. Because of greater frequency of decreased hepatic, renal, and/or cardiac function and of concomitant disease and drug therapy in geriatric patients, the manufacturers suggest that patients in this age group receive initial dosages of the drug in the low end of the usual range.

The manufacturers state that evaluation of geriatric patients with hypertension or MI always should include assessment of renal function.

● Pregnancy, Fertility, and Lactation

Pregnancy

Atenolol has been shown to cause a dose-related increase in embryonal and fetal resorptions in rats when given at dosages 25 or more times the maximum human antihypertensive dosage; similar effects were not observed in rabbits receiving atenolol dosages up to 12.5 times the maximum human antihypertensive dosage. Atenolol crosses the placenta and has been detected in cord blood. Atenolol can cause fetal harm when administered to pregnant women. There are no studies on use of the drug during the first trimester of pregnancy and the possibility of fetal injury cannot be excluded. Atenolol therapy initiated in the second trimester of pregnancy has been associated with birth of infants who were small for gestational age. Atenolol has been used effectively under close supervision for the management of hypertension during the third trimester in a limited number of women and was well tolerated, and apparently did not adversely affect the fetus. However, use of the drug for longer periods of time for the management of mild to moderate hypertension in pregnant women has been associated with intrauterine growth retardation. Neonates born to mothers who receive atenolol at parturition may be at risk for developing hypoglycemia and bradycardia. Caution is recommended when atenolol is administered during pregnancy. If atenolol is administered during pregnancy or if the patient becomes pregnant while receiving the drug, the patient should be informed of the potential hazard to the fetus.

Fertility

Reproduction studies in male and female rats using atenolol dosages up to 200 mg/kg daily (100 times the maximum recommended human antihypertensive dosage) have not revealed evidence of impaired fertility.

Lactation

Atenolol is distributed into milk. The drug distributes into milk in concentrations 1.5–6.8 times those in maternal serum. In at least one infant, potentially toxic serum atenolol concentrations (2 mcg/mL) have been reported 48 hours after discontinuance of breast-feeding. Neonates of mothers who receive atenolol during breast-feeding may be at risk of developing hypoglycemia and adverse β-adrenergic effects (e.g., bradycardia). Therefore, the manufacturers state that atenolol should be used cautiously in nursing women. Because clearance of the drug may be substantially impaired, premature neonates, and infants with impaired renal function, may be at increased risk of developing adverse effects from ingested atenolol during breast-feeding. If a woman receiving atenolol breast-feeds, the infant should be monitored closely for potential systemic effects of the drug. Alternatively, β-blockers that distribute less extensively into milk (e.g., propranolol) can be considered, although caution still must be exercised.

DRUG INTERACTIONS

● Cardiovascular Drugs

Concomitant administration of atenolol with reserpine may increase the incidence of hypotension and bradycardia as compared with atenolol alone, because of reserpine's catecholamine-depleting activity. Atenolol also is additive with and may potentiate the hypotensive actions of other hypotensive agents (e.g., calcium-channel blockers, hydralazine, methyldopa). This effect usually is used to therapeutic advantage, but dosage should be carefully adjusted when these drugs are used concurrently. Because β-blockers may exacerbate rebound hypertension that may occur following discontinuance of clonidine therapy, atenolol should be discontinued several days before clonidine when clonidine therapy is to be discontinued in patients receiving atenolol and clonidine concurrently.

Patients currently receiving another β-blocker must be evaluated carefully prior to initiating atenolol therapy. Depending on clinical findings (e.g., blood pressure, pulse), initial and subsequent atenolol dosage can be adjusted downward.

Slowing or complete suppression of SA node activity with development of slow ventricular rates (e.g., 30–40 bpm), often misdiagnosed as complete AV block, has been reported in patients receiving the nondihydropyridine calcium-channel blocking agent mibefradil (no longer commercially available in the US), principally in geriatric patients and in association with concomitant β-adrenergic blocker therapy.

Parenteral atenolol should be used with caution in patients who recently have received another drug that also may have a negative inotropic effect on the myocardium. Concomitant therapy with a β-blocker and verapamil can result in potentially serious adverse reactions, particularly in patients with severe cardiomyopathy, heart failure, or recent myocardial infarction (MI). (See Drug Interactions: β-Adrenergic Blocking Agents, in Verapamil Hydrochloride 24:28.92.)

● Nonsteroidal Anti-inflammatory Agents

Concurrent use of cyclooxygenase (prostaglandin synthase) inhibitors (e.g., indomethacin) may decrease the hypotensive effects of β-blockers. However, information on concomitant use of atenolol and aspirin is limited. Evidence from several studies (e.g., Thrombolysis in Myocardial Infarction Phase II [TIMI-II], Second International Study of Infarct Survival [ISIS-2]) suggests a lack of any clinically important adverse interaction and that the drugs can be used safely and effectively together in patients with MI.

ACUTE TOXICITY

● Manifestations

Limited information is available on atenolol overdosage. In one woman who reportedly ingested 1.2 g of the drug, no unusual effects occurred and the patient's recovery was uncomplicated, and adults have survived acute doses up to 5 g; however, in a woman 15 years of age who reportedly ingested a single 500-mg dose of atenolol, severe sinus bradycardia, hypotension, and marked hypoglycemia occurred, and death occurred in a man who may have ingested up to 10 g acutely. In general, overdosage of atenolol may be expected to produce effects that are mainly extensions of pharmacologic effects, including symptomatic bradycardia, hypotension, bronchospasm, and acute cardiac failure; hypoglycemia, impaired conduction, decreased cardiac contractility, heart block, shock, and cardiac arrest may also occur.

● Treatment

In acute atenolol overdose, the stomach should be emptied immediately by gastric lavage. Supportive and symptomatic treatment should be initiated. For symptomatic bradycardia, IV atropine sulfate may be given and for second- or third-degree AV block, IV isoproterenol hydrochloride or a transvenous cardiac pacemaker may be used. A vasopressor (e.g., dobutamine, dopamine, epinephrine, norepinephrine) may be given for severe hypotension; IV glucagon may be useful if hypotension is refractory to vasopressors. For heart failure, a cardiac glycoside, diuretic, and oxygen should be used; IV glucagon also may be useful. Hypoglycemia should be treated with IV dextrose. Hemodialysis may be useful in enhancing elimination of atenolol in patients with severe overdosage.

PHARMACOLOGY

Atenolol has pharmacologic actions similar to those of other β-blockers. The principal physiologic action of atenolol is to competitively block adrenergic stimulation of β-adrenergic receptors within the myocardium and within vascular smooth muscle. Like metoprolol, low doses of atenolol selectively inhibit cardiac and lipolytic β_1-adrenergic receptors while having little effect on the β_2-adrenergic receptors of bronchial and vascular smooth muscle. At high doses (e.g., greater than 100 mg daily), this selectivity of atenolol for β_1-adrenergic receptors usually diminishes, and the drug will competitively block β_1- and β_2-adrenergic receptors. Atenolol does not exhibit the intrinsic sympathomimetic activity seen with pindolol or the membrane-stabilizing activity possessed by propranolol or pindolol.

By inhibiting myocardial β_1-adrenergic receptors, atenolol produces negative chronotropic and inotropic activity. The negative chronotropic action of atenolol on the sinoatrial (SA) node results in a decrease in the rate of SA node discharge and an increase in recovery time, thereby decreasing resting and exercise-stimulated heart rate and reflex orthostatic tachycardia by about 25–35%. High doses of the drug may produce sinus arrest, especially in patients with SA node disease (e.g., sick sinus syndrome). Atenolol also slows conduction in the atrioventricular (AV) node. Although stroke index may be increased moderately by

about 10%, atenolol usually reduces cardiac output by about 20%, probably secondary to its effect on heart rate. The decrease in myocardial contractility and heart rate, as well as the reduction in blood pressure, produced by atenolol generally lead to a reduction in myocardial oxygen consumption which accounts for the effectiveness of the drug in chronic stable angina pectoris; however, atenolol can increase oxygen requirements by increasing left ventricular fiber length and end-diastolic pressure, particularly in patients with cardiac failure.

Atenolol suppresses plasma renin activity and suppresses the renin-aldosterone-angiotensin system. The renin-lowering effect of β-blockers may lead to a minimal reduction in glomerular filtration rate and occasionally may reduce renal blood flow; however, other mechanisms (e.g., decreased cardiac output, unopposed α-mediated renal vasoconstriction) also probably contribute to these effects. Because of the suppression of aldosterone production, β-blockers usually produce no measurable increases in plasma volume or sodium and water retention.

The precise mechanism of atenolol's hypotensive effect has not been determined. Single doses of atenolol may increase peripheral vascular resistance at rest and with exercise. It has been postulated that β-blockers reduce blood pressure by blocking peripheral (especially cardiac) adrenergic receptors (decreasing cardiac output), by decreasing sympathetic outflow from the CNS, and/or by suppressing renal renin release.

Because of its β_1-receptor selectivity, low doses (100 mg or less) of atenolol usually have little effect on bronchial airway resistance. Higher doses of atenolol may result in an increase in airway resistance (as measured by decreasing forced expiratory volume in 1 second), especially in patients with asthma and/or chronic obstructive pulmonary disease (COPD).

Low doses of atenolol produce no changes in serum insulin concentrations or in time to recover from insulin-induced hypoglycemia, and little change in free fatty acid response to hypoglycemia. The drug reduces serum free fatty acid concentrations and slightly increases serum triglyceride concentrations.

PHARMACOKINETICS

● Absorption

Atenolol is rapidly but incompletely absorbed from the GI tract. Only about 50–60% of an oral dose of atenolol is absorbed. In healthy adults, peak plasma concentrations of 1–2 mcg/mL are achieved 2–4 hours after oral administration of a single 200-mg dose of atenolol. An approximately fourfold interindividual variation in plasma concentrations attained has been reported with a specific oral dose of atenolol. In geriatric patients, plasma concentrations are increased. Peak plasma atenolol concentrations are achieved within 5 minutes following direct IV injection of the drug, and decline rapidly during an initial distribution phase; after the first 7 hours, plasma concentrations reportedly decline with an elimination half-life similar to that of orally administered drug.

The effect of atenolol on heart rate usually has an onset of 1 hour, peaks at 2–4 hours, and persists for 24 hours following oral administration of the drug. Following IV administration of a single 10-mg dose, the effect on heart rate usually peaks within 5 minutes and generally is negligible by 12 hours after the dose. The antihypertensive and β-adrenergic blocking effect of a single 50- to 100-mg oral dose usually persists for 24 hours. Atenolol's effect on heart rate, but not on blood pressure, correlates linearly with plasma atenolol concentrations of 0.02–200 mcg/mL.

● Distribution

In animals, atenolol is well distributed into most tissues and fluids except brain and CSF. Unlike propranolol, only a small portion of atenolol is apparently distributed into the CNS.

Approximately 6–16% of atenolol is bound to plasma protein.

Atenolol readily crosses the placenta and has been detected in cord blood. During continuous administration, fetal serum concentrations of the drug are probably equivalent to those in maternal serum. Atenolol is distributed into milk; peak milk concentrations of the drug are higher than peak serum concentrations after an individual dose, and the area under the milk concentration-time curve (AUC) is substantially greater than that of the serum AUC in lactating women receiving the drug continuously. (See Cautions: Pregnancy, Fertility, and Lactation.)

• *Elimination*

In patients with normal renal function, atenolol has a plasma half-life ($t_{1/2}$) of 6–7 hours. Children with normal renal function may exhibit a shorter elimination half-life. In one study in children 5–16 (mean: 8.9) years of age with arrhythmias and normal renal and hepatic function, the terminal elimination half-life averaged 4.6 hours. The plasma half-life($t_{1/2}$) of atenolol is markedly prolonged in geriatric patients compared with that in younger patients. Plasma $t_{1/2}$ of the drug increases to 16–27 hours in patients with creatinine clearances of 15–35 mL/minute per 1.73 m^2 and exceeds 27 hours with progressive renal impairment. Little or no metabolism of atenolol occurs in the liver. Approximately 40–50% of an oral dose of the drug is excreted in urine unchanged. The remainder is excreted unchanged in feces, principally as unabsorbed drug. About 1–12% of atenolol is reportedly removed by hemodialysis.

In geriatric patients, total plasma clearance of atenolol is reduced by about 50% compared with that in younger patients, resulting in higher plasma concentrations of the drug. The decreased clearance in geriatric adults may be related to decreased renal function in this age group.

CHEMISTRY AND STABILITY

• *Chemistry*

Atenolol is a β$_1$-selective adrenergic blocking agent. The drug occurs as a white, crystalline powder and has a solubility of 26.5 mg/mL in water at 37°C.

• *Stability*

Atenolol tablets alone or in fixed combination with chlorthalidone should be protected from heat, light, and moisture and stored in well-closed, light-resistant containers at 20–25°C.

PREPARATIONS

Excipients in commercially available drug preparations may have clinically important effects in some individuals; consult specific product labeling for details.

Atenolol

Oral		
Tablets	25 mg*	**Atenolol Tablets**
		Tenormin®, AstraZeneca
	50 mg*	**Atenolol Tablets**
		Tenormin® (scored), AstraZeneca
	100 mg*	**Atenolol Tablets**
		Tenormin®, AstraZeneca

* available from one or more manufacturer, distributor, and/or repackager by generic (nonproprietary) name

Atenolol Combinations

Oral		
Tablets	50 mg with Chlorthalidone 25 mg*	**Atenolol and Chlorthalidone Tablets**
		Tenoretic® (scored), AstraZeneca
	100 mg with Chlorthalidone 25 mg*	**Atenolol and Chlorthalidone Tablets**
		Tenoretic® (scored), AstraZeneca

* available from one or more manufacturer, distributor, and/or repackager by generic (nonproprietary) name

† Use is not currently included in the labeling approved by the US Food and Drug Administration.

Selected Revisions June 10, 2024, © Copyright, January 1, 1984, American Society of Health-System Pharmacists, Inc.

Carvedilol

24:20 · β-ADRENERGIC BLOCKING AGENTS

■ Carvedilol is a nonselective β-adrenergic blocking agent (β-blocker) with selective α₁-adrenergic blocking activity.

USES

Carvedilol is used for the management of hypertension and heart failure. Carvedilol also is used to reduce the risk of cardiovascular mortality in clinically stable patients with left ventricular dysfunction (manifested as a left ventricular ejection fraction [LVEF] of 40% or less) with or without symptomatic heart failure following an acute myocardial infarction (MI).

The choice of a β-adrenergic blocking agent (β-blocker) depends on numerous factors, including intended use, pharmacologic properties (e.g., relative β-selectivity, intrinsic sympathomimetic activity, membrane-stabilizing activity, lipophilicity), pharmacokinetics, and adverse effect profile, as well as the patient's coexisting disease states or conditions, response, and tolerance. While specific pharmacologic properties and other factors may appropriately influence the choice of a β-blocker in individual patients, evidence of clinically important differences among the agents in terms of overall efficacy and/or safety is limited. Patients who do not respond to or cannot tolerate a given β-blocker may be successfully treated with a different one.

● Hypertension

Carvedilol is used alone or in combination with other classes of antihypertensive agents in the management of hypertension.

Current evidence-based practice guidelines for the management of hypertension in adults generally recommend the use of drugs from 4 classes of antihypertensive agents (angiotensin-converting enzyme [ACE] inhibitors, angiotensin II receptor antagonists, calcium-channel blockers, and thiazide diuretics). Most guidelines no longer recommend β-blockers as first-line therapy for hypertension because of the lack of established superiority over other recommended drug classes and evidence from at least one study demonstrating that β-blockers may be less effective than angiotensin II receptor antagonists in preventing cardiovascular death, MI, or stroke. However, therapy with a β-blocker may still be considered in hypertensive patients who have a compelling indication (e.g., prior MI, ischemic heart disease, heart failure) for their use or as add-on therapy in those who do not respond adequately to the preferred drug classes. (See Considerations for Drug Therapy in Patients with Underlying Cardiovascular and Other Risk Factors under Uses: Hypertension, in Atenolol 24:24 and in Metoprolol 24:24.) Ultimately, choice of antihypertensive therapy should be individualized, considering the clinical characteristics of the patient (e.g., age, ethnicity/race, comorbid conditions, cardiovascular risk factors) as well as drug-related factors (e.g., ease of administration, availability, adverse effects, costs).

A 2017 multidisciplinary hypertension guideline of the American College of Cardiology (ACC), American Heart Association (AHA), and a number of other professional organizations generally recommends a target blood pressure goal (i.e., blood pressure to achieve with drug therapy and/or nonpharmacologic intervention) of less than 130/80 mm Hg in all adults regardless of comorbidities or level of atherosclerotic cardiovascular disease (ASCVD) risk. In addition, a systolic blood pressure goal of less than 130 mm Hg generally is recommended for noninstitutionalized ambulatory patients 65 years of age or older with an average systolic blood pressure of at least 130 mm Hg. These blood pressure goals are based upon clinical studies demonstrating continuing reduction of cardiovascular risk at progressively lower levels of systolic blood pressure. Previous hypertension guidelines, such as those from an expert panel of the Eighth Joint National Committee on the Prevention, Detection, Evaluation, and Treatment of High Blood Pressure (JNC 8), generally have recommended initiation of antihypertensive treatment in patients with a systolic blood pressure of at least 140 mm Hg or diastolic blood pressure of at least 90 mm Hg, targeted a blood pressure goal of less than 140/90 mm Hg regardless of cardiovascular risk, and used higher systolic blood pressure thresholds and targets in geriatric patients compared with those recommended by the 2017 ACC/AHA hypertension guideline. The blood

pressure thresholds used to define hypertension, the optimum blood pressure threshold at which to initiate antihypertensive drug therapy, and the ideal target blood pressure values remain controversial.

Most patients with hypertension, especially black patients, will require at least 2 antihypertensive drugs to achieve adequate blood pressure control. In general, black hypertensive patients tend to respond better to monotherapy with thiazide diuretics or calcium-channel blocking agents than to monotherapy with β-blockers. Although β-blockers have lowered blood pressure in all races studied, monotherapy with these agents has produced a smaller reduction in blood pressure in black hypertensive patients; however, this population difference in response does not appear to occur during combined therapy with a β-blocker and a thiazide diuretic. (See Race under Hypertension: Other Special Considerations for Antihypertensive Therapy, in Uses in Atenolol 24:24 and in Metoprolol 24:24.)

For additional information on the role of β-blockers in the management of hypertension, see Uses: Hypertension, in Atenolol 24:24 and in Metoprolol 24:24. For information on overall principles and expert recommendations for treatment of hypertension, see Uses: Hypertension in Adults, in the Thiazides General Statement 40:28.20. For information on overall principles and expert recommendations for treatment of hypertension in pediatric patients, see Uses: Hypertension in Pediatric Patients, in the Thiazides General Statement 40:28.20.

● Heart Failure

Carvedilol is used (usually in conjunction with other heart failure therapies) in the management of mild to severe (New York Heart Association [NYHA] class II–IV) heart failure of ischemic or cardiomyopathic origin to increase survival and to reduce the risk of hospitalization. Current guidelines for the management of heart failure in adults generally recommend a combination of drug therapies to reduce morbidity and mortality, including neurohormonal antagonists (e.g., ACE inhibitors, angiotensin II receptor antagonists, angiotensin receptor-neprilysin inhibitors [ARNIs], β-blockers, aldosterone receptor antagonists), that inhibit the detrimental compensatory mechanisms in heart failure. Additional agents (e.g., cardiac glycosides, diuretics, sinoatrial modulators [i.e., ivabradine]) added to a heart failure treatment regimen in selected patients have been associated with symptomatic improvement of heart failure and/or reduction in heart failure-related hospitalizations. Experts recommend that all asymptomatic patients with reduced LVEF (American College of Cardiology Foundation [ACCF]/American Heart Association [AHA] stage B heart failure) receive therapy with an ACE inhibitor and a β-blocker to prevent symptomatic heart failure and reduce morbidity and mortality. In patients with prior or current symptoms of chronic heart failure and reduced LVEF (ACCF/AHA stage C heart failure), ACCF, AHA, and the Heart Failure Society of America (HFSA) recommend inhibition of the renin-angiotensin-aldosterone (RAA) system with an ACE inhibitor, angiotensin II receptor antagonist, or ARNI in conjunction with a β-blocker, and an aldosterone antagonist in selected patients, to reduce morbidity and mortality. While ACE inhibitors have been the preferred drugs for inhibition of the RAA system because of their established benefits in patients with heart failure and reduced ejection fraction, some evidence indicates that therapy with an ARNI (sacubitril/valsartan) may be more effective than ACE inhibitor therapy (enalapril) in reducing cardiovascular death and heart failure-related hospitalization in such patients. ACCF, AHA, and HFSA recommend that patients with chronic symptomatic heart failure and reduced LVEF (NYHA class II or III) who are able to tolerate an ACE inhibitor or angiotensin II receptor antagonist be switched to therapy containing an ARNI to further reduce morbidity and mortality.

Because of favorable effects on survival and disease progression, therapy with a clinical trial-proven β-blocker (bisoprolol, carvedilol, extended-release metoprolol succinate) should be initiated as soon as the patient is diagnosed with heart failure and reduced LVEF. While bisoprolol, carvedilol, and extended-release metoprolol have been effective in reducing the risk of death in patients with chronic heart failure, these positive findings should not be considered indicative of a β-blocker class effect. Even when symptoms are mild or improve with other therapies, β-blocker therapy should not be delayed until symptoms return or the disease progresses. Despite concerns about β-blockade potentially masking some signs of hypoglycemia, patients with diabetes mellitus may be particularly likely to experience a reduction in morbidity and mortality with the use of β-blockers. If a patient cannot tolerate a β-blocker or if increasing the β-blocker dosage to optimal levels is ineffective, ivabradine should be considered as an alternative or additional treatment option. Some evidence suggests that ivabradine is effective in reducing hospitalizations related to heart failure, but unlike β-blockers, ivabradine has not been shown to reduce cardiovascular mortality. (See Uses: Heart Failure, in Ivabradine 24:04.92.)

In individualizing the decision to use a β-blocker, clinicians should consider that clinical studies establishing the effects of these drugs on morbidity and mortality excluded patients who were hospitalized or had unstable symptoms and enrolled few patients with current or recent NYHA class IV symptoms. The efficacy of β-blockers in such patients is not known, and they may be at particular risk of deterioration following initiation of therapy with β-blockers. In the Carvedilol Prospective Randomized Cumulative Survival Trial (COPERNICUS) evaluating such patients with severe but stable heart failure (patients with marked fluid retention or severe pulmonary disease or requiring intensive care, IV vasodilators, or positive inotropic agents were excluded), carvedilol decreased the rate of death and the combined risk of death and hospitalization for any reason compared with placebo.

The beneficial effects of β-blockers in the management of heart failure are thought to result principally from inhibition of the effects of the sympathetic nervous system. (See Description.) Although the specific effects on the heart and circulation that are responsible for progression of heart failure remain to be established, sympathetic activity can increase ventricular volumes and pressure secondary to peripheral vasoconstriction and by impairing sodium excretion by the kidneys. Other sympathetic effects (e.g., induction of cardiac hypertrophy, arrhythmogenic activity) also may be involved. The beneficial effect of carvedilol in patients with severe heart failure may be the result of other effects (α-adrenergic blockade, antioxidant activity, antiendothelin effects) in addition to β-adrenergic blockade. Collective experience indicates that long-term therapy with β-blockers, like that with ACE inhibitors, can reduce heart failure symptoms and improve clinical status in patients with chronic heart failure and also can decrease the risk of death as well as the combined risk of death and hospitalization. These beneficial effects were demonstrated in patients already receiving an ACE inhibitor, suggesting that combined inhibition of the renin-angiotensin system and sympathetic nervous system can produce additive effects.

β-Blockers should not be used in patients with acutely decompensated heart failure requiring IV inotropic therapy and those with substantial fluid retention requiring intensive diuresis. In the absence of hemodynamic instability or contraindications, it has been recommended that patients with heart failure and a reduced ejection fraction who are hospitalized for a symptomatic exacerbation continue to receive maintenance treatment with standard oral therapy for heart failure (e.g., β-blocker, ACE inhibitor). Withholding of or reduction in β-blocker therapy should be considered only in patients hospitalized after recent initiation or increase in β-blocker therapy or in those with marked volume overload or low/marginal cardiac output. Initiation of β-blocker therapy in hospitalized patients is recommended once the patient's condition is stabilized (i.e., after optimization of volume status and successful discontinuance of IV diuretics, vasodilators, and inotropic agents). Caution should be used when initiating β-blockers in patients who have required inotrope therapy during hospitalization.

Carvedilol has been shown in controlled studies to improve left ventricular function, symptoms, and submaximal exercise tolerance (although not in all studies) in patients with wide-ranging severity of manifestations. Change in NYHA classification was a secondary endpoint in all of the studies, and a trend toward improvement in NYHA class was reported in all studies. Subjective quality-of-life determined by a standard questionnaire was not improved in patients receiving carvedilol compared with those receiving placebo; however, global assessments by patients and clinicians supported an improvement in such assessments in patients receiving carvedilol.

● Left Ventricular Dysfunction After Acute Myocardial Infarction

Carvedilol is used to reduce the risk of cardiovascular mortality following the acute phase of MI in clinically stable patients with left ventricular dysfunction (manifested as an ejection fraction of 40% or less) with or without symptomatic heart failure. In these patients, when compared with those receiving placebo, carvedilol therapy initiated within 21 days after an acute MI reduced mortality from any cause by about 23%; all-cause mortality or cardiovascular hospitalization was reduced by 8%, which was not statistically significant. In addition, a 40% reduction in fatal and nonfatal MI was observed in patients receiving carvedilol. This evidence of efficacy was obtained from a large, double-blind, placebo-controlled, multicenter long-term (about 16 months) study (Carvedilol Post-Infarct Survival Control in Left Ventricular Dysfunction Study; CAPRICORN). For information on the use of β-blockers during the acute phase of MI, see Uses in Metoprolol 24:24.

The benefits of long-term β-blocker therapy for secondary prevention of MI have been well established in numerous clinical studies. Patients with MI complicated by heart failure, left ventricular dysfunction, or ventricular arrhythmias appear to derive the most benefit from long-term β-blocker therapy. AHA/ACCF secondary prevention guideline recommends β-blocker therapy in all patients with left ventricular systolic dysfunction (ejection fraction of 40% or less) and a prior MI; use of a β-blocker with proven mortality benefit (bisoprolol, carvedilol, or metoprolol succinate) is recommended. (See Uses: Heart Failure.)

For additional information on the use of β-blockers in the management of MI, see Uses in Metoprolol 24:24.

DOSAGE AND ADMINISTRATION

● Administration

Carvedilol and carvedilol phosphate are administered orally. Food has little, if any, effect on the oral bioavailability of carvedilol immediate-release tablets but may decrease the rate of absorption, resulting in reduced and delayed peak plasma concentrations. Therefore, to potentially decrease the risk of orthostatic hypotension, it is recommended that carvedilol be administered with food. In addition, the manufacturer suggests that manifestations of vasodilation in patients receiving concomitant therapy with an angiotensin-converting enzyme (ACE) inhibitor may be reduced by administering carvedilol 2 hours prior to the latter drug.

Food increases the bioavailability of carvedilol phosphate extended-release capsules and the manufacturer states that the extended-release capsules should be taken with food. Carvedilol extended-release capsules should be taken once daily in the morning and should be swallowed whole; the capsule and/or its contents should not be crushed, chewed, or taken in divided doses. However, carvedilol extended-release capsules may be opened carefully and the entire contents sprinkled over a spoonful of applesauce, immediately prior to administration. The applesauce should not be warm, and the drug and applesauce mixture should be consumed in entirety. The drug and applesauce mixture should not be stored for future use. The absorption of the beads sprinkled on foods other than applesauce has not been studied.

● Dosage

Patients whose conditions are controlled with immediate-release carvedilol tablets alone or in combination with other drugs may be switched to carvedilol phosphate extended-release capsules. Patients who are receiving a daily carvedilol dosage of 6.25 (3.125 mg twice daily), 12.5 (6.25 mg twice daily), 25 (12.5 mg twice daily), or 50 mg (25 mg twice daily) as immediate-release tablets may be switched to a dosage of 10, 20, 40, or 80 mg once daily, respectively, as carvedilol phosphate extended-release capsules. Subsequent titration to higher or lower dosages may be necessary and should be guided by the patient's clinical response.

Hypertension

Dosage of carvedilol must be individualized and adjusted according to the patient's blood pressure response and tolerance.

In hypertensive patients with left ventricular dysfunction, including those with heart failure who already are receiving a cardiac glycoside, diuretic, and/or an ACE inhibitor, the manufacturer states that the usual carvedilol dosages and instructions recommended for the treatment of heart failure should be followed instead of those for hypertension, since such patients generally depend, at least in part, on β-adrenergic stimulation for maintaining cardiovascular compensation. (See Heart Failure under Dosage and Administration: Dosage.)

Usual Dosage

For the management of hypertension in adults, the usual initial dosage of carvedilol (as immediate-release tablets) is 6.25 mg twice daily. The manufacturer recommends that patient response and tolerance to the initial dosage and subsequent dosage adjustments be evaluated by measurement of standing systolic blood pressure 1 hour after administration of carvedilol (trough blood pressure). In patients whose blood pressure is not controlled adequately with the initial carvedilol dosage, dosage can be increased gradually (usually increasing dosage every 7–14 days), as tolerated up to a maximum of 50 mg daily. For patients who received an initial dosage of 6.25 mg twice daily, the dosage may be increased to 12.5 mg twice daily and, if needed, to 25 mg twice daily. Some experts state the usual dosage range is 12.5–50 mg daily, administered in 2 divided doses.

For the management of hypertension in adults, the usual initial dosage of carvedilol phosphate extended-release capsules is 20 mg once daily. The manufacturer recommends that patient tolerance to the initial dosage and subsequent dosage adjustments be evaluated by measurement of standing systolic blood pressure 1 hour after administration of carvedilol phosphate extended-release capsules. In patients whose blood pressure is not controlled adequately with the initial carvedilol phosphate dosage (given as extended-release capsules), dosage can be increased gradually (usually increasing dosage every 7–14 days) up to a maximum of 80 mg once daily (given as carvedilol phosphate extended-release capsules). Some experts state the usual dosage range is 20–80 mg once daily administered as extended-release capsules.

Addition of a diuretic to carvedilol therapy or of carvedilol to diuretic therapy can be expected to produce additive effects. When carvedilol and a thiazide diuretic are used concomitantly, an additive hypotensive response, including an increased risk of orthostatic hypotension, can be expected.

Blood Pressure Monitoring and Treatment Goals

Blood pressure should be monitored regularly (i.e., monthly) during therapy and dosage of the antihypertensive drug adjusted until blood pressure is controlled. If an adequate blood pressure response is not achieved, the dosage may be increased or another antihypertensive agent with demonstrated benefit and preferably with a complementary mechanism of action (e.g., ACE inhibitor, angiotensin II receptor antagonist, calcium-channel blocker, thiazide diuretic) may be added; if target blood pressure is still not achieved with the use of 2 antihypertensive agents, a third drug may be added. (See Uses: Hypertension.) In patients who develop unacceptable adverse effects with carvedilol, the drug should be discontinued and another antihypertensive agent from a different pharmacologic class should be initiated.

The goal of hypertension management and prevention is to achieve and maintain optimal control of blood pressure. However, the optimum blood pressure threshold for initiating antihypertensive drug therapy and specific treatment goals remain controversial. While previous hypertension guidelines have based target blood pressure goals on age and comorbidities, the 2017 American College of Cardiology/American Heart Association (ACC/AHA) hypertension guideline incorporates underlying cardiovascular risk into decision making regarding treatment and generally recommends the same target blood pressure (i.e., less than 130/80 mm Hg) for all adults. Many patients will require at least 2 drugs from different pharmacologic classes to achieve this blood pressure goal; the potential benefits of hypertension management and drug cost, adverse effects, and risks associated with the use of multiple antihypertensive drugs also should be considered when deciding a patient's blood pressure treatment goal.

For additional information on target levels of blood pressure and on monitoring therapy in the management of hypertension, see Blood Pressure Monitoring and Treatment Goals under Dosage: Hypertension, in Dosage and Administration in the Thiazides General Statement 40:28.20.

Heart Failure

Prior to initiation of carvedilol therapy for heart failure, fluid retention should be minimized, and patients who are receiving treatment that includes a cardiac glycoside, diuretic, and/or ACE inhibitor should be stabilized with respect to the dosage of these drugs. Initiation of carvedilol therapy for heart failure and subsequent dosage adjustments should occur under very close medical supervision, since the risk of cardiac decompensation and/or severe hypotension is highest during the initial 30 days of therapy.

For the management of mild to severe (NYHA class II–IV) heart failure, carvedilol often is administered in conjunction with other agents such as a cardiac glycoside, ACE inhibitor, and/or diuretic. Treatment with carvedilol should be initiated at a very low dosage. The usual initial carvedilol dosage as immediate-release tablets for the management of heart failure in adults is 3.125 mg twice daily for 2 weeks. The usual initial dosage of carvedilol phosphate extended-release capsules for the management of heart failure in adults is 10 mg once daily for 2 weeks. Prior to dosage increases, the patient's response and tolerance to carvedilol therapy should be determined in a clinical setting and should include an assessment of manifestations of declining cardiovascular status, vasodilation (e.g., dizziness, lightheadedness, symptomatic hypotension), and bradycardia.

If the patient experiences increases in manifestations of heart failure such as edema during the initiation and titration phases of carvedilol therapy, further increases in carvedilol dosage should be delayed until the patient regains clinical stability; such manifestations may require an increase in diuretic dosage. If increased manifestations of heart failure do not resolve in response to an increase in diuretic dosage, consideration should be given to decreasing the carvedilol dosage or temporarily discontinuing the drug. The occurrence of increased manifestations of heart failure during initiation of carvedilol therapy or dosage titration that require dosage decreases or discontinuance of the drug should not prevent future consideration of resuming therapy with or increasing dosage of carvedilol. If the patient develops manifestations of vasodilation, consideration should be given to decreasing the patient's dosage of diuretic or ACE inhibitor; however, if these dosage reductions do not result in improved circulatory status, carvedilol dosage may be decreased. Separating the time of dosing of carvedilol from that of the ACE inhibitor also may reduce vasodilatory symptoms. If the patient becomes bradycardic (heart rate less than 55 beats/minute), carvedilol dosage should be reduced. If the patient develops manifestations of worsening heart failure or vasodilation, carvedilol dosage should not be increased until the patient's cardiovascular status is stable.

If the patient tolerates the initial dosage, carvedilol dosage may be increased to 6.25 mg twice daily as the immediate-release tablets or to 20 mg once daily as carvedilol phosphate extended-release capsules for 2 weeks. When increases in dosage are considered, the patient should be observed in a clinical setting for manifestations of hypotension (e.g., dizziness, light-headedness) for 1 hour after administration of the initial dose at the increased dosage. Dosage of carvedilol as the immediate-release tablets and carvedilol phosphate as extended-release capsules can be doubled every 2 weeks if necessary (with strict adherence to the monitoring regimen described above) to the highest tolerated dosage that does not exceed the maximum recommended dosage of 50 mg daily (in patients weighing less than 85 kg) and 100 mg daily (in those weighing more than 85 kg) as carvedilol immediate-release tablets and of 80 mg once daily as carvedilol phosphate extended-release capsules.

Left Ventricular Dysfunction After Acute Myocardial Infarction

Prior to initiation of carvedilol therapy for left ventricular dysfunction following acute myocardial infarction (MI), fluid retention should be minimized, and patients should be hemodynamically stable. Initiation of carvedilol therapy and subsequent dosage adjustments should occur under very close medical supervision, since the risk of cardiac decompensation and/or severe hypotension is highest during the initial 30 days of therapy. Therapy may be initiated on an inpatient or outpatient basis after the patient is hemodynamically stable and fluid retention is minimized.

To decrease the likelihood of syncope or excessive hypotension, treatment with carvedilol should be initiated at a low dosage of 6.25 mg twice daily as the immediate-release tablets or 20 mg of carvedilol phosphate once daily as the extended-release capsules. If the patient tolerates the initial dosage, carvedilol dosage may be increased after 3–10 days to 12.5 mg twice daily as the immediate-release tablets or 40 mg once daily as carvedilol phosphate extended-release capsules, and then to the target dosage of 25 mg twice daily as the immediate-release tablets or 80 mg of carvedilol phosphate once daily as the extended-release capsules. A lower initial dosage of 3.125 mg twice daily as the immediate-release tablets or 10 mg of carvedilol phosphate once daily as the extended-release capsules and/or a slower rate of dosage titration may be used when clinically indicated (e.g., low blood pressure or heart rate, fluid retention). Alteration of the recommended dosage regimen is not necessary in patients who received IV or oral treatment with a β-blocker during the acute phase of MI.

Although the optimal duration of β-blocker therapy following MI remains to be clearly established, experts generally recommend that such therapy be continued long-term in post-MI patients with left ventricular systolic dysfunction.

● Special Populations

Use of carvedilol is not recommended in patients with clinical manifestations of hepatic impairment or with otherwise severe impairment. (See Contraindications.)

Although the manufacturer makes no specific recommendations for dosage adjustments in patients with renal impairment, plasma concentrations of carvedilol based on comparison of mean plasma concentration-time curves (AUC) reportedly are 40–50% higher in patients with hypertension and moderate to severe renal impairment compared with patients with hypertension and normal renal function receiving carvedilol therapy as the immediate-release tablets. Although the ranges of AUC values were similar for both groups, mean peak plasma concentrations were approximately 12–26% higher in patients with impaired renal function compared with those in patients with no such impairment. Carvedilol does not appear to be removed by hemodialysis.

If a deterioration in renal function is detected in patients with heart failure, dosage of carvedilol should be decreased or the drug should be discontinued.

Some clinicians suggest using a reduced initial carvedilol dosage in geriatric patients, since such patients are at increased risk of developing orthostatic hypotension and experience is limited regarding the use of the drug in patients 75 years of age or older.

CAUTIONS

● *Contraindications*

- Bronchial asthma or related bronchospastic conditions.
- Second or third degree AV block.
- Sick sinus syndrome or severe bradycardia (unless permanent pacemaker is in place).
- Cardiogenic shock or decompensated heart failure requiring IV inotropic therapy; initiate carvedilol only after the patient is weaned from IV therapy.
- Clinically apparent or otherwise severe hepatic impairment.
- History of serious hypersensitivity reaction (e.g., Stevens-Johnson syndrome, anaphylactic reaction, angioedema) to carvedilol or any ingredient in the formulation.

● *Warnings/Precautions*

Warnings

Abrupt Withdrawal of Therapy

Abrupt withdrawal of carvedilol may exacerbate angina symptoms and/or precipitate myocardial infarction (MI) and ventricular arrhythmias in patients with coronary artery disease or may precipitate thyroid storm in patients with thyrotoxicosis. Therefore, patients receiving carvedilol (especially those with ischemic heart disease) should be warned not to interrupt or discontinue therapy without consulting their clinician. Because coronary artery disease is common and may be undiagnosed, abrupt withdrawal also should be avoided in patients receiving carvedilol for other conditions (e.g., hypertension). When carvedilol is discontinued in patients with coronary artery disease or suspected thyrotoxicosis, the patient should be observed carefully; patients with coronary artery disease should be advised to temporarily limit their physical activity. If exacerbation of angina occurs or acute coronary insufficiency develops after carvedilol therapy is interrupted or discontinued, treatment with the drug should be reinstituted, at least temporarily.

If carvedilol therapy, alone or combined with another antihypertensive agent (e.g., a thiazide diuretic), is to be discontinued, dosage should be reduced gradually in a deliberate and progressive manner, if possible. When such cessation of therapy is planned, the manufacturer recommends that therapy with the drug be withdrawn gradually over approximately 1–2 weeks. Patients should be monitored closely during this period and, if manifestations of withdrawal (e.g., angina, exacerbation of hypertension) develop, dosage should be increased or the drug reinstituted, at least temporarily.

Peripheral Vascular Disease

Possible precipitation or aggravation of arterial insufficiency in patients with peripheral vascular disease. Use with caution.

Anesthesia and Major Surgery

If carvedilol therapy is continued perioperatively, use particular caution when anesthetic agents that depress myocardial function (e.g., ether, cyclopropane, trichloroethylene) are used. (See Drug Interactions.)

Diabetes and Hypoglycemia

β-Adrenergic blocking agents (β-blockers) may mask some of the manifestations of hypoglycemia (e.g., tachycardia). Non-selective β-blockers (e.g., carvedilol) are more likely to potentiate insulin-induced hypoglycemia and delay recovery of serum glucose concentrations.

In patients with heart failure and diabetes mellitus, blood glucose should be monitored when carvedilol therapy is initiated or discontinued or the dosage adjusted, since carvedilol therapy may worsen hyperglycemia.

Thyrotoxicosis

β-Adrenergic blockade may mask clinical signs of hyperthyroidism (e.g., tachycardia). Abrupt withdrawal of β-blockade may be followed by an exacerbation of symptoms of hyperthyroidism or may precipitate thyroid storm.

General Precautions

Carvedilol shares the toxic potentials of β-adrenergic and α₁-adrenergic blocking agents; observe the usual precautions recommended with these agents.

Bradycardia

May cause bradycardia; dosage should be reduced if heart rate is less than 55 beats/minute.

Hypotension

May cause hypotension, postural hypotension, or syncope. Risk is highest in first 30 days of therapy in patients with heart failure. To decrease risk of orthostatic hypotension, administer with food and strictly adhere to the usual starting dose and titration recommendations. (See Dosage and Administration.)

Pheochromocytoma

In patients with pheochromocytoma, an α-adrenergic blocking agent should be administered before using a β-blocker. Although carvedilol has both α- and β-blocking pharmacologic activities, there has been no experience with its use in this condition; use with caution.

Prinzmetal's Variant Angina

Nonselective β-blockers may provoke chest pain in patients with Prinzmetal's variant angina; use with caution.

History of Anaphylactic Reactions

Possible increased reactivity to a variety of allergens; patients may be unresponsive to usual doses of epinephrine used to treat anaphylactic reactions.

Bronchospastic Disease

Bronchospasm reported rarely; deaths secondary to status asthmaticus have been reported following single doses of carvedilol. Patients with bronchospastic disease (e.g., chronic bronchitis, emphysema) generally should not receive β-blockers. Carvedilol should be used in patients with bronchospastic disease only when they are nonresponsive or intolerant of other antihypertensive agents; if used in such patients, the drug should be administered with caution and at the lowest dosage that achieves the desired clinical effect to minimize the drug's inhibition of endogenous or exogenous β-adrenergic agonists. (See Contraindications under Cautions.) If bronchospasm occurs, dosage should be reduced.

The manufacturer recommends that carvedilol be used with caution and strict adherence to recommendations regarding dosage titration in patients with heart failure and bronchospastic disease. If any evidence of bronchospasm occurs during initiation and/or titration of carvedilol, the dosage should be reduced.

Specific Populations

Pregnancy

Category C. (See Users Guide.)

Crosses the placenta in rats. Perinatal and neonatal distress have been reported with other α- and β-blockers.

Lactation

Distributed into milk in rats; not known whether distributed into human milk. Because of the risk of adverse effects in the infant, discontinue nursing or the drug, taking into account the importance of the drug to the woman.

Pediatric Use

Safety and efficacy not established in children younger than 18 years of age.

In a clinical trial in pediatric patients (mean age 6 years, range 2 months to 17 years) with chronic heart failure (NYHA class II–IV), carvedilol resulted in β-blockade activity as demonstrated by a placebo-corrected heart rate reduction of 4–6 beats/minute; however, no clinically important effect on treatment outcome was observed after 8 months of follow-up. Common adverse effects included chest pain, dizziness, and dyspnea.

Geriatric Use

No substantial differences in safety or efficacy relative to younger adults, but possibility exists of increased sensitivity to carvedilol in some individuals. Some clinicians suggest using a reduced initial carvedilol dosage in geriatric patients, since such patients are at increased risk of developing orthostatic hypotension and experience is limited regarding the use of the drug in patients 75 years of age or older. Plasma concentrations of carvedilol are about 50% higher in geriatric individuals than in younger individuals.

Hepatic Impairment

Not recommended for use in patients with manifestations of hepatic impairment or severe hepatic impairment. (See Contraindications under Cautions.)

Patients with hepatic cirrhosis developed plasma drug concentrations approximately 4–7 times higher than those in healthy individuals after a single dose of immediate-release carvedilol tablets.

Renal Impairment

Deterioration of renal function has been reported in patients receiving carvedilol.

Patients at risk appear to be those with low blood pressure (systolic blood pressure less than 100 mm Hg), ischemic heart disease and diffuse vascular disease, and/or underlying renal insufficiency. Renal function should be monitored in these patients during the dosage titration period; the drug should be discontinued or dosage reduced if worsening of renal function occurs.

• Common Adverse Effects

Adverse effects reported in 5% or more of patients with heart failure receiving immediate-release carvedilol tablets include dizziness, headache, fatigue, asthenia, arthralgia, hypotension, bradycardia, generalized edema, diarrhea, nausea, vomiting, hyperglycemia, weight gain, increased BUN, increased nonprotein nitrogen (NPN), increased cough, and abnormal vision.

Adverse effects reported in patients with left ventricular dysfunction following MI receiving immediate-release carvedilol tablets generally were similar to those in patients receiving the drug for the treatment of heart failure. Additional adverse effects reported in 3% or more of such patients include anemia, dyspnea, and pulmonary edema.

Adverse effects reported in 2% or more of patients receiving immediate-release carvedilol tablets for the treatment of hypertension include dizziness, bradycardia, diarrhea, insomnia, and postural hypotension.

Adverse effects reported in 2% or more of patients receiving extended-release carvedilol phosphate capsules for the treatment of hypertension include nasopharyngitis, dizziness, nausea, and peripheral edema.

DRUG INTERACTIONS

Metabolized by cytochrome P-450 (CYP) isoenzymes, principally CYP2D6 and CYP2C9; also metabolized to a lesser extent by CYP3A4, CYP2C19, CYP1A2, CYP2E1.

• Drugs Affecting Hepatic Microsomal Enzymes

Potent inhibitors of CYP2D6 (e.g., fluoxetine, paroxetine, propafenone, quinidine): potential pharmacokinetic interaction (increased plasma concentrations of R(+)-carvedilol); however interactions with carvedilol have not been studied.

• Antidiabetic Agents (Oral and Parenteral [Insulin])

Possible increased hypoglycemic effect. Blood glucose concentrations should be monitored regularly.

• Calcium-channel Blocking Agents

Possible conduction disturbance, rarely with hemodynamic compromise. Blood pressure and ECG should be monitored during concomitant use with diltiazem or verapamil.

• Cardiac Glycosides

Potential pharmacokinetic and pharmacodynamic interaction. Digoxin concentrations are increased by about 15% in patients receiving concomitant therapy with digoxin and carvedilol. Both cardiac glycosides and carvedilol slow AV conduction and decrease heart rate; concomitant use may increase risk of bradycardia. Digoxin therapy should be carefully monitored when carvedilol dosage is initiated, adjusted, or discontinued.

• Catecholamine-depleting Agents (e.g., reserpine, MAO inhibitors)

Potential additive effects (e.g., hypotension, bradycardia). Patients should be monitored closely for symptoms (e.g., vertigo, syncope, postural hypotension).

• Cimetidine

Potential decreased carvedilol metabolism and increased (by 30%) bioavailability (area under the plasma concentration-time curve [AUC]) of carvedilol. No apparent change in peak plasma concentration of carvedilol.

• Clonidine

Potential additive effects (e.g., hypotension, bradycardia). If carvedilol is used concomitantly with clonidine, caution should be exercised, particularly when discontinuing therapy; carvedilol generally should be discontinued first, and clonidine continued for several days thereafter with gradual downward dosage titration.

• Cyclosporine

Possible increased cyclosporine concentrations. Cyclosporine concentrations should be closely monitored during carvedilol dosage titration; adjust cyclosporine dosage as necessary.

• Fluoxetine

Potential pharmacokinetic and pharmacodynamic interaction; potential for increased plasma concentrations of R(+)-carvedilol that may result in increased α-adrenergic blockade effects (vasodilation).

• Glyburide

Pharmacokinetic interaction unlikely.

• Hydrochlorothiazide

Pharmacokinetic interaction unlikely.

• Myocardial Depressant General Anesthetics (ether, cyclopropane, trichloroethylene)

Potential for increased risk of hypotension and heart failure. Use with caution.

• Pantoprazole

No clinically important increases in AUC and peak plasma concentrations of carvedilol reported with concomitant administration of carvedilol and pantoprazole.

• Paroxetine

Potential pharmacokinetic and pharmacodynamic interaction; potential for increased plasma concentrations of R(+)-carvedilol that may result in increased α-adrenergic blockade effects (vasodilation).

• Propafenone

Potential pharmacokinetic interaction; potential for increased plasma concentrations of R(+)-carvedilol that may result in increased α-adrenergic blockade effects (vasodilation).

• Quinidine

Potential pharmacokinetic interaction; potential for increased plasma concentrations of R(+)-carvedilol that may result in increased α-adrenergic blockade effects (vasodilation).

• Rifampin

In a pharmacokinetic study, rifampin decreased peak plasma concentration (by 70%) and AUC (by 70%) of carvedilol.

● **Torsemide**

Pharmacokinetic interaction unlikely.

● **Warfarin**

No effect on steady-state prothrombin times or warfarin pharmacokinetics.

DESCRIPTION

Carvedilol is a nonselective β-adrenergic blocking agent (β-blocker) with selective α_1-adrenergic blocking activity. The principal physiologic action of carvedilol is to competitively block adrenergic stimulation of β-receptors within the myocardium (β_1-receptors) and within bronchial and vascular smooth muscle (β_2-receptors), and to a lesser extent α_1-receptors within vascular smooth muscle. The β_1-antagonist activity of carvedilol is similar to that of propranolol and greater than that of labetalol, and the duration of carvedilol's effect is longer than those of labetalol and propranolol. Studies in animals indicate that the drug may exert an antioxidant effect on the myocardium and an antiproliferative effect on intimal tissue. The commercially available drug is a racemic mixture of the 2 enantiomers, $(R)[+]$ and $(S)[-]$, and both enantiomers have equal α_1-adrenergic blocking activity; however, only the S(-)-enantiomer of carvedilol has β-adrenergic blocking activity. Carvedilol does not exhibit intrinsic sympathomimetic (β_1-agonist) activity and possesses only weak membrane-stabilizing (local anesthetic) activity.

Vasodilation resulting in reduced total peripheral resistance mediated through carvedilol's α_1-adrenergic blockade and reduced sympathetic tone appear to play a major role in the drug's hypotensive effect. Carvedilol causes reductions in cardiac output, exercise-induced tachycardia, isoproterenol-induced tachycardia, and reflex orthostatic tachycardia. Clinically important β-adrenergic blocking activity of carvedilol usually is evident within 1 hour of oral administration, and the drug's hypotensive effect is similar to that of metoprolol. Carvedilol's α_1-adrenergic blocking effects, which contribute to the drug's hypotensive effects, generally are evident within 30 minutes of oral administration and include reductions in phenylephrine-induced pressor effects, vasodilation, and decreased peripheral vascular resistance. The dose-dependent hypotensive effect of carvedilol results in blood pressure (systolic and diastolic) reductions of 5–46% with little, if any, reflex tachycardia. This hypotensive effect occurs approximately 30 minutes after oral administration and has a maximum effect 1.5–7 hours after oral administration.

Carvedilol reduces peripheral vascular resistance and blood pressure as a result of its vasodilating effects; the drug produces both arterial and venous dilation. Carvedilol reduces blood pressure in both supine and standing patients; as a result of α_1-blockade, the effect is most pronounced on standing blood pressure, and orthostatic hypotension can occur. The manufacturer states that the frequency and severity of orthostatic hypotension may be decreased by administering the drug with food and by strictly adhering to the usual starting dose and titration recommendations. (See Dosage and Administration.)

The precise mechanism of the beneficial effects of carvedilol in the treatment of heart failure has not been fully elucidated. β-Adrenergic blockade and vasodilation generally are associated with reflex tachycardia and peripheral vasoconstriction in therapeutic agents in which one of these pharmacologic effects predominates, but the combined effects of carvedilol appear to attenuate these two major untoward responses by balancing the potential adverse effects associated with adrenergic blockade and vasodilation. The drug's vasodilatory action appears to enable the patient to tolerate the negative inotropic effect of carvedilol during the initiation and titration of therapy in the treatment of compensated heart failure. Chronic adrenergic stimulation and resultant activation of the renin-angiotensin system associated with compensated chronic heart failure result in sodium retention and vasoconstriction that, in turn, can induce further increases in preload and afterload that decrease cardiac output and stimulate additional sympathetic output. Some evidence suggests that the combined adrenergic effects of carvedilol, especially vasodilation, may ameliorate the negative inotropic effects that could otherwise lead to myocardial dysfunction in the compensating heart failure patient.

In patients with chronic heart failure and left ventricular dysfunction, carvedilol is associated with improvements in myocardial function through reduction in afterload as evidenced by improved left ventricular ejection fraction, reduced left ventricular volumes, and prevention of progression of left ventricular dilatation. Reductions in systemic blood pressure, pulmonary artery pressure, pulmonary capillary wedge pressure, and heart rate were observed in patients with heart failure (New York Heart Association [NYHA] functional class II–IV) receiving angiotensin-converting enzyme (ACE) inhibitors, cardiac glycosides, and/or diuretics after initiating concurrent carvedilol therapy. During initial therapy with carvedilol, small and variable responses in cardiac output, stroke volume index, and systemic vascular resistance occur. Chronic carvedilol therapy (12–14 weeks) is associated with reductions in systemic blood pressure, pulmonary artery pressure, right atrial pressure, systemic vascular resistance, and heart rate, and increased stroke volume index. Increases (7%) in left ventricular ejection fraction (LVEF) were observed in patients with heart failure (NYHA class II-III) receiving carvedilol at a target dosage of 25–50 mg twice daily for 26–52 weeks. The effect of carvedilol on LVEF was dose-related, with increases of 5, 6, and 8% reported with twice-daily doses of 6.25 mg, 12.5 mg, and 25 mg, respectively.

The precise mechanism of the beneficial effects of carvedilol in the treatment of left ventricular dysfunction following myocardial infarction (MI) has not been fully elucidated.

Carvedilol is rapidly and extensively absorbed following oral administration. Food decreases the rate of the drug's absorption (i.e., increases time to peak plasma concentration), but not the extent (i.e., no effect on bioavailability) of absorption. Administration with food may decrease the risk of orthostatic hypotension. Carvedilol is substantially distributed into extravascular tissues. The half-life of carvedilol is 7–10 hours; 5–9 hours for $R(+)$-carvedilol, and 7–11 hours for $S(-)$-carvedilol. The drug is more than 98% bound to plasma proteins. Carvedilol is extensively metabolized; phenol ring demethylation and hydroxylation produce 3 metabolites with β-adrenergic blocking activity and (weak) vasodilating activity. Plasma concentrations of active metabolites are about 10% those of carvedilol. The 4'-hydroxyphenyl metabolite is 13 times more potent than carvedilol in β-adrenergic blocking activity. Carvedilol is excreted principally in feces as metabolites; less than 2% is excreted in urine unchanged.

ADVICE TO PATIENTS

Importance of taking carvedilol exactly as prescribed. Importance of taking with food.

Importance of advising patients receiving carvedilol phosphate extended-release capsules not to crush or chew the capsules.

Importance of not interrupting or discontinuing therapy without consulting clinician. When discontinuing therapy, importance of advising patients to temporarily limit physical activity.

Importance of advising patients to sit or lie down and avoid hazardous tasks (e.g., driving) if dizziness or fatigue occur. Importance of informing clinician if dizziness or faintness from decreased blood pressure occurs; dosage adjustment may be necessary.

Importance of diabetic patients informing clinician if changes in blood glucose concentrations occur. Importance of warning patients receiving insulin or oral hypoglycemic agents or those subject to spontaneous hypoglycemia about these potential effects.

Importance of immediately informing clinician at the first sign or symptom (e.g., weight gain, shortness of breath) of heart failure.

Importance of informing contact lens wearers that they may experience decreased lacrimation.

Importance of advising patients undergoing major surgery to inform anesthesiologist or dentist that they are receiving the drug.

Importance of informing clinicians of existing or contemplated therapy, including prescription and OTC drugs.

Importance of women informing clinicians if they are or plan to become pregnant or plan to breast-feed.

Importance of informing patient of other important precautionary information. (See Cautions.)

PREPARATIONS

Excipients in commercially available drug preparations may have clinically important effects in some individuals; consult specific product labeling for details.

Carvedilol

Oral

Tablets, film-coated	3.125 mg*	**Carvedilol Tablets**
		Coreg®, GlaxoSmithKline
	6.25 mg*	**Carvedilol Tablets**
		Coreg® Tiltabs®, GlaxoSmithKline
	12.5 mg*	**Carvedilol Tablets**
		Coreg® Tiltabs®, GlaxoSmithKline
	25 mg*	**Carvedilol Tablets**
		Coreg® Tiltabs®, GlaxoSmithKline

* available from one or more manufacturer, distributor, and/or repackager by generic (nonproprietary) name

Carvedilol Phosphate

Oral

Capsules, extended-release	10 mg (with 12.5% immediate-release and 87.5% extended-release)	**Coreg CR®,** GlaxoSmithKline
	20 mg (with 12.5% immediate-release and 87.5% extended-release)	**Coreg CR®,** GlaxoSmithKline
	40 mg (with 12.5% immediate-release and 87.5% extended-release)	**Coreg CR®,** GlaxoSmithKline
	80 mg (with 12.5% immediate-release and 87.5% extended-release)	**Coreg CR®,** GlaxoSmithKline

† Use is not currently included in the labeling approved by the US Food and Drug Administration.

Selected Revisions April 10, 2024, © Copyright, January 1, 1998, American Society of Health-System Pharmacists, Inc.

Labetalol Hydrochloride

24:20 • β-ADRENERGIC BLOCKING AGENTS

■ Labetalol hydrochloride is an α- and β-adrenergic blocking agent.

USES

Labetalol is used for the management of hypertension. The drug is used for hypertension associated with angina or pheochromocytoma and during pregnancy. IV labetalol is used for hypertension associated with myocardial infarction (MI) and to control blood pressure in patients with severe hypertension or in hypertensive crises.

In addition, IV labetalol has been used to produce controlled hypotension during anesthesia† and to control blood pressure in eclampsia† or preeclampsia†. The drug also has been used in the management of sympathetic overactivity syndrome with severe tetanus† and in angina†.

The choice of a β-adrenergic blocking agent (β-blocker) depends on numerous factors, including pharmacologic properties (e.g., relative β-selectivity, intrinsic sympathomimetic activity, membrane-stabilizing activity, lipophilicity), pharmacokinetics, intended use, and adverse effect profile, as well as the patient's coexisting disease states or conditions, response, and tolerance. While specific pharmacologic properties and other factors may appropriately influence the choice of a β-blocker in individual patients, evidence of clinically important differences among the agents in terms of overall efficacy and/or safety is limited. Patients who do not respond to or cannot tolerate one β-blocker may be successfully treated with a different agent.

● Hypertension

Labetalol hydrochloride is used alone or in combination with other classes of antihypertensive agents in the management of hypertension.

Current evidence-based practice guidelines for the management of hypertension in adults generally recommend the use of drugs from 4 classes of antihypertensive agents (angiotensin-converting enzyme [ACE] inhibitors, angiotensin II receptor antagonists, calcium-channel blockers, and thiazide diuretics). Most guidelines no longer recommend β-blockers as first-line therapy for hypertension because of the lack of established superiority over other recommended drug classes and evidence from at least one study demonstrating that β-blockers may be less effective than angiotensin II receptor antagonists in preventing cardiovascular death, MI, or stroke. However, therapy with a β-blocker may still be considered in hypertensive patients who have a compelling indication (e.g., prior MI, ischemic heart disease, heart failure) for their use or as add-on therapy in those who do not respond adequately to the preferred drug classes. (See Considerations for Drug Therapy in Patients with Underlying Cardiovascular and Other Risk Factors under Uses: Hypertension, in Atenolol 24:24 and in Metoprolol 24:24.) Ultimately, choice of antihypertensive therapy should be individualized, considering the clinical characteristics of the patient (e.g., age, ethnicity/race, comorbid conditions, cardiovascular risk factors) as well as drug-related factors (e.g., ease of administration, availability, adverse effects, costs).

A 2017 multidisciplinary hypertension guideline of the American College of Cardiology (ACC), American Heart Association (AHA), and a number of other professional organizations generally recommends a target blood pressure goal (i.e., blood pressure to achieve with drug therapy and/or nonpharmacologic intervention) of less than 130/80 mm Hg in all adults regardless of comorbidities or level of atherosclerotic cardiovascular disease (ASCVD) risk. In addition, a systolic blood pressure goal of less than 130 mm Hg generally is recommended for noninstitutionalized ambulatory patients 65 years of age or older. These blood pressure goals are based upon clinical studies demonstrating continuing reduction of cardiovascular risk at progressively lower levels of systolic blood pressure. Previous hypertension guidelines, such as those from an expert panel of the Eighth Joint National Committee on the Prevention, Detection, Evaluation, and Treatment of High Blood Pressure (JNC 8), generally have recommended initiation of antihypertensive treatment in patients with a systolic blood pressure of at least 140 mm Hg or diastolic blood pressure of at least 90 mm Hg, targeted a

blood pressure goal of less than 140/90 mm Hg regardless of cardiovascular risk, and used higher systolic blood pressure thresholds and targets in geriatric patients compared with those recommended by the 2017 ACC/AHA hypertension guideline. The blood pressure thresholds used to define hypertension, the optimum blood pressure threshold at which to initiate antihypertensive drug therapy, and the ideal target blood pressure values remain controversial.

Most patients with hypertension, especially black patients, will require at least 2 antihypertensive drugs to achieve adequate blood pressure control. In general, black hypertensive patients tend to respond better to monotherapy with thiazide diuretics or calcium-channel blocking agents than to monotherapy with β-blockers. Although β-blockers have lowered blood pressure in all races studied, monotherapy with these agents has produced a smaller reduction in blood pressure in black hypertensive patients; however, this population difference in response does not appear to occur during combined therapy with a β-blocker and a thiazide diuretic. (See Race under Hypertension: Other Special Considerations for Antihypertensive Drug Therapy, in Uses in Atenolol 24:24 and in Metoprolol 24:24.)

For additional information on the role of β-blockers in the management of hypertension, see Uses: Hypertension, in Atenolol 24:24 and in Metoprolol 24:24. For information on overall principles and expert recommendations for treatment of hypertension, see Uses: Hypertension, in Adults, in the Thiazides General Statement 40:28.20.

Hypertension Associated with Angina or Myocardial Infarction

Oral labetalol has been used effectively for the management of hypertension in patients with coexisting angina pectoris, and IV labetalol has been used effectively for the management of hypertension associated with acute myocardial infarction. In patients with hypertension and ischemic heart disease, oral labetalol therapy reduced blood pressure and heart rate and was associated with elimination or reduction of anginal pain, improvement in exercise tolerance, and decreased consumption of nitroglycerin. In the management of hypertension associated with acute myocardial infarction, IV infusions of labetalol decreased blood pressure and heart rate and generally decreased cardiac index and pulmonary artery wedge pressure, without producing adverse hemodynamic effects.

Hypertension during Pregnancy

Labetalol has been used for the management of hypertension in pregnant women. The drug has been effective in controlling blood pressure in pregnant women with moderate to severe hypertension, in those with severe pregnancy-induced hypertension, and in those with hypertension and superimposed pregnancy-induced hypertension. In addition, in hypertensive pregnant women with proteinuria, labetalol therapy has resulted in substantially less proteinuria.

The goal of antihypertensive treatment in pregnant women with hypertension is to minimize the acute complications of maternal hypertension while avoiding therapy that would compromise fetal well-being. Antihypertensive therapy is recommended in pregnant women with chronic hypertension who have persistent, severely elevated blood pressure (e.g., systolic blood pressure of 160 mm Hg or higher or diastolic blood pressure of 105 mm Hg or higher); it is less clear whether antihypertensive therapy should be initiated in women with mild to moderate chronic hypertension. If initiation of antihypertensive therapy is considered necessary in a pregnant woman, use of labetalol, nifedipine, or methyldopa is recommended by the American College of Obstetricians and Gynecologists (ACOG) and other experts. In women who are already receiving antihypertensive therapy prior to pregnancy, ACOG states that data are insufficient to make recommendations regarding the continuance or discontinuance of such therapy; treatment decisions should be individualized in these situations. Some other experts state that women with hypertension who become pregnant or who are planning to become pregnant should have their antihypertensive therapy transitioned to methyldopa, nifedipine, and/or labetalol during pregnancy. Antihypertensive therapy can reduce the risk of severe hypertension but has not been shown to prevent the development of preeclampsia. Use of labetalol in association with careful prenatal management during pregnancy does not appear to adversely affect the fetus. (See Cautions: Pregnancy, Fertility, and Lactation.)

Labetalol also has been used parenterally in the hospital setting for urgent lowering of blood pressure in severely hypertensive pregnant women, including those with preeclampsia† or eclampsia†. Recommendations for the management of such patients are based principally on experience in women with preeclampsia or gestational hypertension in the third trimester. Delivery is the preferred method of management for women with severe preeclampsia; however, use of antihypertensive drugs is recommended in such women who have severely elevated blood pressures (sustained systolic blood pressure of at least 160 mm Hg or diastolic blood pressure of at least 110 mm Hg) to prevent potentially life-threatening cardiovascular, renal, and cerebrovascular complications. Results of several randomized clinical trials evaluating antihypertensive therapy in women with severe hypertension during pregnancy suggest that IV labetalol, IV hydralazine, or oral nifedipine are appropriate antihypertensives for urgently lowering blood pressure in such patients; choice of therapy should be based on clinician experience and preference as well as patient-specific factors (e.g., concomitant medical conditions or therapies) and drug-related factors (e.g., route of administration, adverse effects, contraindications, local availability, cost). Although hydralazine historically has been considered the agent of choice for management of hypertensive emergencies associated with pregnancy, some clinicians now prefer IV labetalol for its more rapid onset and shorter duration of action and its more predictable hypotensive effect.

Hypertension Associated with Pheochromocytoma

Because of labetalol's α- and β-adrenergic blocking activity, the drug has been used alone to control hypertension and symptoms resulting from excessive β-receptor stimulation in patients with pheochromocytoma. Labetalol generally appears to be effective in these patients; some evidence suggests that the drug may be more effective in patients whose tumors predominantly secrete epinephrine rather than norepinephrine and in patients with sustained rather than paroxysmal hypertension. Since there have been reports that oral labetalol may induce a paradoxical hypertensive crisis in some patients with pheochromocytoma (possibly because the drug's predominant β-adrenergic blockade leaves α-adrenergic stimulation relatively unopposed), the manufacturers recommend that the drug be used with caution in patients with this tumor. Although labetalol has some α-adrenergic blocking activity, some clinicians caution that the drug, like other β-adrenergic blocking agents, should not be used in patients with pheochromocytoma unless they have received pretreatment with an α-adrenergic blocking agent (e.g., IV phentolamine). If labetalol is used in patients with known or suspected pheochromocytoma, appropriate methods for determining urinary catecholamines should be employed. (See Laboratory Test Interferences: Urinary Catecholamines.)

Severe Hypertension and Hypertensive Crises

IV labetalol hydrochloride is used to control blood pressure in patients with severe hypertension or in hypertensive crises for the immediate reduction in blood pressure in patients in whom such reduction is considered an emergency (hypertensive emergencies). Hypertensive emergencies are those rare situations requiring immediate blood pressure reduction (not necessarily to normal ranges) to prevent or limit target organ damage. Such emergency situations include hypertensive encephalopathy, acute MI, intracerebral hemorrhage, acute left ventricular failure with pulmonary edema, eclampsia, dissecting aortic aneurysm, unstable angina pectoris, acute ischemic stroke, and acute renal failure, and labetalol generally is suitable for most hypertensive emergencies (e.g., acute aortic dissection, acute coronary syndromes) except when acute cardiac failure is present. Patients with hypertensive emergencies require hospitalization and are treated with an appropriate parenteral agent. Elevated blood pressure alone, in the absence of manifestations or other evidence of target organ damage, rarely requires emergency therapy. The risks of overly aggressive therapy in any hypertensive crisis must always be considered. Excessive falls in blood pressure should be avoided in any hypertensive crisis since they may precipitate renal, cerebral, or coronary ischemia.

Labetalol usually produces a prompt, but gradual reduction of blood pressure without substantial changes in heart rate or cardiac output. IV labetalol appears to adequately reduce blood pressure in about 80–90% of patients with severe hypertension or hypertensive emergencies, irrespective of etiology, and may be useful even when other drugs have failed. The exact effects of previous antihypertensive therapy on the efficacy of IV labetalol have not been fully determined. IV labetalol generally appears to be effective regardless of whether patients have received other hypotensive drugs, including β-blockers; however, in some studies, the drug was reported to be ineffective, usually in patients who received a single IV injection and who were receiving other hypotensive drugs, including β-blockers. The possibility of a diminished response to IV labetalol should be considered in patients receiving α- or β-blockers.

The comparative efficacy and safety of IV labetalol and other currently available parenteral hypotensive agents in the management of severe hypertension and hypertensive emergencies have not been fully evaluated, but IV labetalol

is considered one of several parenteral drugs of choice for the management of these forms of hypertension. IV labetalol appears to be as effective as IV diazoxide (parenteral formulation no longer commercially available in the US), but may be less likely to induce excessive hypotension and adverse neurologic or cardiovascular sequelae. Because of its usual lack of substantial changes in heart rate or cardiac output, IV labetalol may be particularly useful in severely hypertensive patients with ischemic heart disease. In addition, IV labetalol has an advantage over most other parenteral hypotensive agents in that oral therapy with the drug may be continued after parenteral therapy when long-term control of blood pressure is necessary. IV labetalol also has been used effectively to control blood pressure and the rate of left ventricular pressure rise (dp/dt) in a few patients with acute dissection of the aorta; the drug produced a gradual reduction in blood pressure without a concomitant increase in heart rate.

Hypertensive urgencies are those situations in which there is a severe elevation in blood pressure without progressive target organ damage. Hypertensive urgencies generally can be managed by intensification or reinstitution (e.g., following noncompliance) of the current antihypertensive regimen and treatment of anxiety if needed. Experts state that there is no need for rapid reduction of blood pressure in the emergency department in such patients and hospitalization also is unnecessary.

IV labetalol has been used effectively in a small number of patients for the management of hypertensive crises following discontinuance of clonidine†, and oral labetalol has been used effectively in a small number of patients to prevent such crises during withdrawal from clonidine therapy†. However, since severe rebound hypertension reportedly has occurred in at least one patient during gradual withdrawal of clonidine and concurrent oral administration of labetalol, some clinicians caution that labetalol not be used in such patients unless they have received pretreatment with an α-blocker (e.g., IV phentolamine).

● Controlled Hypotension during Anesthesia

IV labetalol hydrochloride has been used effectively to produce controlled hypotension during anesthesia† in order to reduce bleeding resulting from surgical procedures. When labetalol and halothane are used concomitantly, a synergistic hypotensive effect results, which may be used to therapeutic advantage. (See Drug Interactions: Halothane.) Labetalol has also been effective in the management of uncontrolled hypertension before anesthesia and during surgery†, and for the management and/or prevention of acute hypertensive responses during laryngoscopy†.

● Chronic Stable Angina

Labetalol has been used in a limited number of patients for the long-term management of chronic stable angina pectoris†. Use of the drug has been associated with a reduction in the frequency and severity of anginal attacks, a decrease in nitrate dosage, and an increase in exercise tolerance. β-Blockers are recommended as the anti-ischemic drugs of choice in most patients with chronic stable angina; despite differences in cardioselectivity, intrinsic sympathomimetic activity, and other clinical factors, all β-blockers appear to be equally effective for this indication. For additional information on the role of β-blockers in the management of chronic stable angina, see Uses: Chronic Stable Angina, in Metoprolol 24:24.

● Tetanus

Labetalol has been used with good results for the management of the sympathetic overactivity syndrome associated with severe tetanus†. The drug generally has been effective in stabilizing the cardiovascular disturbances, including hypertension, tachycardia, and increased systemic arteriolar resistance, that occur in patients with severe tetanus.

DOSAGE AND ADMINISTRATION

● Administration

Labetalol hydrochloride is usually administered orally, but may be administered by slow, direct IV injection or by slow, continuous IV infusion.

Oral Administration

Labetalol hydrochloride is usually administered orally in 2 divided doses daily; however, if adverse effects (e.g., nausea, dizziness) occur and are intolerable (particularly with dosages of 1.2 g daily or higher), administration of the drug in 3 divided doses daily may improve patient tolerance and/or facilitate dosage titration.

Labetalol also has been administered as an extemporaneously compounded oral suspension using the commercially available tablets.

Standardize 4 Safety

Standardized concentrations for an oral compounded liquid formulation of labetalol have been established through Standardize 4 Safety (S4S), a national patient safety initiative to reduce medication errors, especially during transitions of care. Because recommendations from the S4S panels may differ from the manufacturer's prescribing information, caution is advised when using concentrations that differ from labeling, particularly when using rate information from the label. For additional information on S4S (including updates that may be available), see http://www.ashp.org/pharmacy-practice/standardize-4-safety-initiative.

TABLE 1. Standardize 4 Safety Standards for Labetalol Hydrochloride Compounded Oral Liquid

Concentration Standard
40 mg/mL

IV Administration

To control blood pressure in patients with severe hypertension or hypertensive emergencies, repeated doses of labetalol hydrochloride may be given by slow, direct IV injection over a 2-minute period at intervals of 10 minutes, or a diluted solution of the drug may be administered by slow, continuous IV infusion. For IV infusion, labetalol hydrochloride solutions are prepared by diluting the injection to an appropriate concentration in a compatible IV infusion solution. (See Chemistry and Stability: Stability.) For example, 200 mg of the drug may be added to 160 mL of 5% dextrose injection to provide a solution containing 1 mg/mL. To facilitate a desired rate of infusion, diluted solutions of the drug can be administered via a controlled-infusion device. Labetalol hydrochloride injection and diluted solutions of the drug should be inspected visually for particulate matter and discoloration prior to administration whenever solution and container permit. Prefilled syringes of the drug should be destroyed and discarded if damaged in any manner; if the cannula is bent, no attempt should be made to straighten it.

Patients receiving IV labetalol must be kept in a supine position during administration of the drug; a substantial fall in blood pressure on standing should be expected in these patients. Since symptomatic orthostatic hypotension is likely to occur if these patients are tilted upward or allowed to assume an upright position within 3 hours after administration of the drug, they should remain in a supine position during this time period. The patient's ability to tolerate an upright position must be established before any ambulation is permitted. (See Cautions: Precautions and Contraindications.) Blood pressure must be closely monitored during and after completion of IV administration of labetalol. Rapid or excessive reductions in systolic or diastolic blood pressure during IV therapy with the drug should be avoided. In patients with excessive systolic hypertension, the decrease in systolic pressure, as well as the decrease in diastolic pressure, should be used to assess response to the drug. When labetalol is administered by direct IV injection, blood pressure should be monitored before and at 5-minute intervals after each injection; the maximum hypotensive effect usually occurs within 5–15 minutes after each injection. When the drug is administered by continuous IV infusion, the rate of infusion may be adjusted according to the supine blood pressure response. After the desired supine blood pressure is attained or the maximum recommended cumulative dose has been given, IV administration of labetalol should be discontinued. Following discontinuance of IV labetalol, blood pressure is usually monitored at 5-minute intervals for 30 minutes, then at 30-minute intervals for 2 hours, then hourly for about 6 hours, and as necessary thereafter. Oral therapy with the drug may be initiated when it has been established that the supine diastolic blood pressure has begun to increase (usually determined by an increase of 10 mm Hg).

Standardize 4 Safety

Standardized concentrations for IV labetalol have been established through Standardize 4 Safety (S4S), a national patient safety initiative to reduce medication

errors, especially during transitions of care. Multidisciplinary expert panels were convened to determine recommended standard concentrations. Because recommendations from the S4S panels may differ from the manufacturer's prescribing information, caution is advised when using concentrations that differ from labeling, particularly when using rate information from the label. For additional information on S4S (including updates that may be available), see https://www.ashp.org/pharmacy-practice/standardize-4-safety-initiative.

TABLE 2. Standardize 4 Safety Continuous IV Infusion Standard Concentrations for Labetalol Hydrochloride

Patient Population	Concentration Standards	Dosing Units
Adults	1 mg/mL	mg/min
	5 mg/mL	
Pediatric patients (<50 kg)	1 mg/mL	mg/kg/hour
	5 mg/mL	

• Dosage

Hypertension

Dosage of oral labetalol hydrochloride should be adjusted according to standing blood pressure. Some adverse effects (e.g., nausea, dizziness) of the drug may be minimized or avoided and patient tolerance improved if dosage is adjusted more gradually (e.g., every 2–4 weeks) over a period of 4–12 weeks. The maximum, steady-state blood pressure response with twice-daily dosing occurs within 1–3 days and, with continued dosing, blood pressure can be measured approximately 12 hours after a dose to determine if further dosage titration is necessary. Since the maximum hypotensive effect of the drug is usually evident within 1–4 hours, lack of an excessive hypotensive response to the initial dose or a dose increment can usually be established in an ambulatory clinical setting.

If long-term labetalol therapy is to be discontinued, dosage of the drug should be reduced gradually over a period of 1–2 weeks. (See Cautions: Precautions and Contraindications.)

Usual Dosage

For the management of hypertension in adults, the recommended initial oral dosage of labetalol hydrochloride is 100 mg twice daily, given alone or in combination with a diuretic. Dosage may be adjusted in increments of 100 mg twice daily every 2 or 3 days until the optimum blood pressure response is achieved.

The usual oral maintenance dosage of labetalol hydrochloride recommended by the manufacturers for adults is 200–400 mg twice daily. Some experts recommend a lower usual dosage range of 100–400 mg twice daily; the rationale for this reduced dosage is that it usually is preferable to add another antihypertensive agent to the regimen than to continue increasing labetalol hydrochloride dosage since the patient may not tolerate such continued increases. Because some geriatric individuals eliminate labetalol more slowly than younger adults, a lower maintenance dosage than that recommended for the general population may be adequate to control blood pressure in these older patients. Some manufacturers suggest that a maintenance dosage of 100–200 mg twice daily may be adequate for most geriatric patients. The manufacturers state that some adults with severe hypertension may require labetalol hydrochloride dosages of up to 2.4 g daily given in 2 divided doses, administered alone or in combination with a diuretic; in these patients, dosage titration increments should not exceed 200 mg twice daily.

When diuretic therapy is initiated in a patient already receiving labetalol hydrochloride, adjustment of labetalol dosage may be necessary. Optimum maintenance dosage of oral labetalol hydrochloride is usually lower in patients also receiving a diuretic.

When patients are transferred from therapy with other antihypertensive agents, oral therapy with labetalol hydrochloride should be initiated in the usual initial dosage and dosage of the existing regimen gradually decreased.

If labetalol hydrochloride is used for the management of hypertension in children†, some experts have recommended an initial oral dosage of 1–3 mg/kg daily given in 2 divided doses. Such experts have suggested that dosage may be increased as necessary to a maximum dosage of 10–12 mg/kg (up to 1.2 g) daily given in 2 divided doses.For information on overall principles and expert recommendations for treatment of hypertension in pediatric patients, see Uses: Hypertension in Pediatric Patients, in the Thiazides General Statement 40:28.20.

Blood Pressure Monitoring and Treatment Goals

Blood pressure should be monitored regularly (i.e., monthly) during therapy and dosage of the antihypertensive drug adjusted until blood pressure is controlled. If an adequate blood pressure response is not achieved, the dosage may be increased or another antihypertensive agent with demonstrated benefit and preferably with a complementary mechanism of action (e.g., angiotensin-converting enzyme [ACE] inhibitor, angiotensin II receptor antagonist, calcium-channel blocker, thiazide diuretic) may be added; if target blood pressure is still not achieved with the use of 2 antihypertensive agents, a third drug may be added. (See Uses: Hypertension.) In patients who develop unacceptable adverse effects with labetalol, the drug should be discontinued and another antihypertensive agent from a different pharmacologic class should be initiated.

The goal of hypertension management and prevention is to achieve and maintain optimal control of blood pressure. However, the optimum blood pressure threshold for initiating antihypertensive drug therapy and specific treatment goals remain controversial. While previous hypertension guidelines have based target blood pressure goals on age and comorbidities, the 2017 American College of Cardiology/American Heart Association (ACC/AHA) hypertension guideline incorporates underlying cardiovascular risk into decision making regarding treatment and generally recommends the same target blood pressure (i.e., less than 130/80 mm Hg) for all adults. Many patients will require at least 2 drugs from different pharmacologic classes to achieve this blood pressure goal; the potential benefits of hypertension management and drug cost, adverse effects, and risks associated with the use of multiple antihypertensive drugs also should be considered when deciding a patient's blood pressure treatment goal.

For additional information on target levels of blood pressure and on monitoring therapy in the management of hypertension, see Blood Pressure Monitoring and Treatment Goals under Dosage: Hypertension, in Dosage and Administration in the Thiazides General Statement 40:28.20.

Severe Hypertension and Hypertensive Crises

Dosage of labetalol hydrochloride must be adjusted according to the severity of hypertension and the patient's blood pressure response and tolerance. IV dosage of labetalol hydrochloride should be adjusted according to supine blood pressure. When IV labetalol hydrochloride is used in the management of a hypertensive emergency in adults *without* a compelling indication, the initial goal of such therapy is to reduce systolic blood pressure by no more than 25% within the first hour, followed by further blood pressure reduction *if stable* to 160/110 or 160/100 mm Hg within the next 2–6 hours, avoiding excessive declines in pressure that could precipitate renal, cerebral, or coronary ischemia. If this blood pressure is well tolerated and the patient is clinically stable, further gradual reductions toward normal can be implemented in the next 24–48 hours. Adults who have hypertensive crisis *with* a compelling indication (e.g., aortic dissection, severe preeclampsia or eclampsia, pheochromocytoma crisis) should have their systolic blood pressure reduced to less than 140 mm Hg during the first hour, and, in patients with aortic dissection, to less than 120 mm Hg within the first 20 minutes.

To control blood pressure in adults with severe hypertension or hypertensive emergencies, the manufacturer recommends that IV labetalol hydrochloride be given in an initial dose of 20 mg by slow (over 2 minutes), direct IV injection. Alternatively, some experts recommend an initial IV labetalol dosage of 0.3–1 mg/kg (maximum 20 mg) administered by slow, direct IV injection every 10 minutes. Higher initial doses (e.g., 1–2 mg/kg) have been administered by direct IV injection, but the 20-mg dose is recommended to minimize adverse effects (e.g., nausea, excessive hypotension) and the risks associated with too rapid reduction in blood pressure. Additional labetalol doses of 40 or 80 mg may be given at 10-minute intervals until the desired supine blood pressure is achieved or a total cumulative dose of 300 mg has been administered; IV labetalol should then be discontinued and oral therapy with the drug (administered as tablets) may be initiated when the supine diastolic blood pressure begins to increase.

As an alternative to direct IV injections, the manufacturer states that labetalol hydrochloride may be given by continuous IV infusion at an initial rate of 2 mg/minute, with the rate of infusion adjusted according to the blood pressure

response. Some experts recommend an initial IV infusion rate of 0.4–1 mg/kg per hour and increasing the rate as needed up to 3 mg/kg per hour. The usual effective cumulative dose administered by IV infusion is 50–200 mg, although up to 300 mg may be required in some patients. A total cumulative dose of 300 mg has been recommended by some experts. Because of the elimination half-life of labetalol, steady-state plasma concentrations of the drug are not attained during the usual infusion period. The infusion should be continued until an adequate response is obtained (or the maximum recommended cumulative dose has been given) and then discontinued, and oral therapy with the drug initiated when the supine diastolic blood pressure begins to increase. Some clinicians have used a progressive, incremental IV infusion regimen† (i.e., infusing 20, 40, 80, and 160 mg/hour for 1 hour at each dose level, or until the desired blood pressure is achieved) and believe this method may result in a more gradual reduction of blood pressure and minimize adverse effects compared with repeated IV injections of the drug; however, controlled comparisons of the various methods of IV administration are not available. Some clinicians have also used oral regimens† for urgent reduction of blood pressure in severely hypertensive patients.

For rapid reduction of blood pressure in children and adolescents with acute severe hypertension† and life-threatening symptoms, some experts recommend administration of labetalol hydrochloride as a direct IV injection of 0.2–1 mg/kg per dose, up to 40 mg per dose. As an alternative to direct IV injections, labetalol hydrochloride may be given by continuous IV infusion at a rate of 0.25–3 mg/kg per hour. These experts suggest that blood pressure should be reduced by no more than 25% of the planned reduction over the first 8 hours.For information on overall principles and expert recommendations for treatment of hypertension in pediatric patients, see Uses: Hypertension in Pediatric Patients, in the Thiazides General Statement 40:28.20.

When oral labetalol therapy is initiated following IV therapy with the drug, the recommended initial oral dose in adults is 200 mg, followed in 6–12 hours by an additional oral dose of 200 or 400 mg, depending on the blood pressure response. Thereafter, while the patient is hospitalized, oral dosage may be increased in usual increments at 1-day intervals (dosage range: 400–2400 mg daily administered in 2 or 3 divided doses), if necessary, to achieve the desired blood pressure control; for subsequent outpatient dosage titration or maintenance dosing, the usual oral dosage recommendations should be followed.

Severe Hypertension During Pregnancy

To control acute severe hypertension in pregnant women, including preeclampsia†, some experts recommend an initial IV labetalol hydrochloride dose of 10–20 mg administered by direct IV injection, followed by 20–80 mg every 20–30 minutes as needed up to a maximum cumulative dose of 300 mg. Alternatively, the drug may be administered by continuous IV infusion at a rate of 1–2 mg/minute. Antihypertensive therapy is recommended for women with preeclampsia who have persistent systolic blood pressures of 160 mm Hg or higher or diastolic blood pressures of 110 mm Hg or higher.

Controlled Hypotension during Anesthesia

To produce controlled hypotension during halothane anesthesia† in adults, IV labetalol hydrochloride has been given in an initial dose of 20 mg (range: 10–25 mg) following induction of anesthesia; if necessary, additional doses of 5–10 mg (range: 2.5–15 mg) were given. When IV labetalol hydrochloride and halothane anesthesia are used concomitantly, the degree and duration of the synergistic hypotensive response can be controlled by adjusting the inspired halothane concentration. (See Drug Interactions: Halothane.) To produce controlled hypotension during anesthesia with other anesthetic agents† in adults, IV labetalol hydrochloride has been given in an initial dose of 30 mg, with additional doses of 5–10 mg given if necessary.

● Dosage in Renal and Hepatic Impairment

Modification of labetalol hydrochloride dosage does not appear to be necessary in patients with mild to moderate renal impairment. In patients with severe renal impairment (i.e., creatinine clearance less than 10 mL/minute) undergoing dialysis, adequate blood pressure control may be possible with once-daily dosing of the drug.

Although specific data are currently not available, dosage reduction may be necessary in patients with impaired hepatic function since metabolism of the drug may be decreased in these patients.

CAUTIONS

Labetalol hydrochloride shares the toxic potentials of β-adrenergic and postsynaptic α_1-adrenergic blocking agents. Most adverse reactions to labetalol are mild, transient, and occur early in the course of treatment. Adverse effects of labetalol can generally be divided into 3 groups (in decreasing order of frequency): nonspecific effects, effects related to the α-adrenergic blocking activity of the drug, and effects related to its β-adrenergic blocking activity. During controlled clinical studies in patients receiving oral labetalol for 3–4 months, adverse reactions requiring discontinuance of the drug occurred in about 7% of patients; in these same comparative studies, adverse reactions requiring discontinuance of therapy occurred in 8–10% of patients receiving pure β-adrenergic blocking agents (i.e., metoprolol, propranolol) and in 30% of patients receiving a centrally acting adrenergic inhibitor (i.e., methyldopa). Evidence from clinical studies in patients receiving oral labetalol hydrochloride dosages of 200 mg to 2.4 g daily suggests that some adverse effects, including dizziness, fatigue, nausea, vomiting, dyspepsia, paresthesia, nasal congestion, failure to ejaculate, impotence, and edema, are dose related. The incidence and/or severity of some labetalol-induced adverse reactions may occasionally be obviated by slow, upward titration of dosage over 4–12 weeks.

● Cardiovascular Effects

The most frequent adverse cardiovascular effect of labetalol is symptomatic orthostatic hypotension, which occurs in about 1–5% or 60% of patients following oral or IV administration of the drug, respectively. Orthostatic hypotension has been associated with loss of consciousness occasionally following IV administration and rarely following oral administration. Symptomatic orthostatic hypotension is likely to occur if supine patients are tilted upward or allowed to assume the upright position within 3 hours following IV administration of labetalol. (See Cautions: Precautions and Contraindications.) Moderate hypotension occurs in about 1% of patients in the supine position who are receiving the drug IV. Following oral administration, orthostatic hypotension appears to occur more frequently during initiation of therapy, in patients receiving concomitant administration of a diuretic, and in those receiving higher dosages of the drug.

Development or exacerbation of heart failure has occurred in some patients receiving labetalol, although the drug appears to be less likely to precipitate heart failure than pure β-adrenergic blocking agents. At the first sign or symptom of impending cardiac failure during labetalol therapy, patients should receive adequate treatment (e.g., cardiac glycoside, diuretic) and should be observed closely; if cardiac failure continues, labetalol should be discontinued, gradually if possible.

Ventricular arrhythmia (including ventricular premature contractions), edema or fluid retention, bradycardia, hypotension, syncope, chest pain, atrioventricular (AV) conduction delay, and AV block have occurred during therapy with labetalol.

● Nervous System Effects

Adverse nervous system effects occur with variable frequency with labetalol and most of these effects appear to be dose related. At the usual labetalol hydrochloride dosage of 200–400 mg twice daily, most adverse nervous system effects occur in 5% or less of patients. Adverse nervous system effects of the drug include drowsiness or tiredness, dizziness or lightheadedness (often posture related), headache, fatigue, lethargy, and nightmares or vivid dreams. Paresthesia, usually mild, transient tingling of the scalp or skin, may also occur following oral or IV administration of the drug, usually at the beginning of therapy. Hypoesthesia or numbness and circumoral paresthesia have also occurred. Mental depression, paroniria, vertigo, somnolence, yawning, tremor, asthenia, and insomnia have also been reported. Some adverse nervous system effects such as fatigue, mental depression, and sleep disorders may occur less frequently with labetalol than with pure β-adrenergic blocking agents. Adverse nervous system effects of labetalol may be obviated by a reduction in dosage or alteration of dosage schedule.

● GI Effects

The most frequent adverse GI effects associated with labetalol therapy are nausea, dyspepsia, and vomiting. Alteration or distortion in taste, abdominal pain, constipation, diarrhea, and flatulence have also been reported.

● Hepatic Effects

Elevated liver function test results, including reversible increases in serum aminotransferase concentrations; jaundice (including cholestatic jaundice); and

hepatitis have been reported in patients receiving labetalol. Severe hepatocellular injury, which has recurred during rechallenge, has occurred rarely during labetalol therapy; hepatocellular injury may be accompanied by clinical symptoms of hepatotoxicity, including pruritus, dark urine, persistent anorexia, jaundice, flu-like syndrome, and/or right upper quadrant tenderness. Hepatocellular injury is usually reversible; however, hepatic necrosis and death have been reported. Hepatic injury may occur after short- or long-term labetalol therapy. Similar severe adverse hepatic effects, including at least 2 fatalities, have been reported with dilevalol hydrochloride; dilevalol is one of the 4 stereoisomers that make up the racemic mixture labetalol. (See Chemistry and Stability: Chemistry.)

● Respiratory Effects

Adverse respiratory effects of labetalol, including dyspnea, wheezing, bronchospasm, and nasal congestion, occur occasionally. Rhinorrhea and rhinitis also have been reported.

● Genitourinary Effects

Ejaculatory failure, impotence, difficult or painful micturition, and acute urinary retention have occurred occasionally in patients receiving labetalol alone or in fixed combination with hydrochlorothiazide. Peyronie's disease and priapism have been reported rarely. Urinary frequency, nocturia, and polyuria have been reported when the drug was used in fixed combination with hydrochlorothiazide.

● Dermatologic and Sensitivity Reactions

Rashes, including maculopapular, lichenoid, urticarial, and psoriasiform lesions, have developed in some patients during labetalol therapy (alone or in fixed combination with hydrochlorothiazide). Pruritus, bullous lichen planus, facial erythema, and reversible alopecia have also occurred. Hypersensitivity (e.g., rash, urticaria, pruritus, angioedema, dyspnea) and anaphylactoid reactions have been reported rarely in patients receiving labetalol.

● Endocrine Effects

Results of a large prospective cohort study of nondiabetic adults 45–64 years of age indicate that use of β-adrenergic blocking agents in hypertensive patients is associated with increased risk (about 28%) of developing type 2 diabetes mellitus compared with hypertensive patients who were not receiving hypotensive therapy. In this study, the number of new cases of diabetes per 1000 person-years was 33.6 or 26.3 in patients receiving a β-adrenergic blocking agents or no drug therapy, respectively. The association between the risk of developing type 2 diabetes mellitus and use of β-adrenergic blocking agents reportedly was not confounded by weight gain, hyperinsulinemia, or differences in heart rate. It is not known if the risk of developing diabetes is affected by β-receptor selectivity. Further studies are needed to determine whether concomitant use of ACE inhibitors (which may improve insulin sensitivity) would abrogate β-blocker-induced adverse effects related to glucose intolerance. Therefore, until results of such studies are available, the proven benefits of β-adrenergic blocking agents in reducing cardiovascular events in hypertensive patients must be weighed carefully against the possible risks of developing type 2 diabetes mellitus.

Hypoglycemia, which may result in loss of consciousness, also may occur in nondiabetic patients receiving β-adrenergic blocking agents. Patients most at risk for the development of β-blocker-induced hypoglycemia are those undergoing dialysis, prolonged fasting, or severe exercise regimens.

β-Adrenergic blocking agents may mask signs and symptoms of hypoglycemia (e.g., palpitation, tachycardia, tremor) and potentiate insulin-induced hypoglycemia. Although it has been suggested that nonselective β-adrenergic blocking agents are more likely to induce hypoglycemia than selective β-blockers agents, such an adverse effect also has been reported with selective β-blocking agents (e.g., atenolol). In addition, selective β-adrenergic blocking agents are less likely to mask symptoms of hypoglycemia or delay recovery from insulin-induced hypoglycemia than nonselective β-adrenergic blocking agents because of their vascular sparing effects; however, selective β-blockers can decrease insulin sensitivity by approximately 15–30%, which may result in increased insulin requirements.

● Other Adverse Effects

Lupus erythematosus-like illness, positive antinuclear antibody (ANA) titer, mild hyperglycemia, leukopenia, and development of positive antimitochondrial antibodies have occurred in patients receiving labetalol. Transient increases in BUN and serum creatinine concentrations associated with decreases in blood pressure have also occurred, usually in patients with renal insufficiency. Flushing or a feeling of warmth, fever, rigors, increased sweating, dry mouth or eyes, blurred vision, visual disturbances, pallor, shivering, decreased libido, muscle cramps, toxic myopathy, claudication, Raynaud's phenomenon, burning sensation of the groin, and pain at the injection site have been reported. In addition, leg cramps, pain, gout, increased appetite, hypokalemia, and increased serum creatine kinase (CK, creatine phosphokinase, CPK) concentrations have been reported when the drug was used in fixed combination with hydrochlorothiazide.

The possibility that other adverse effects associated with other β-adrenergic blocking agents may occur during labetalol therapy should be considered. These include, but may not be limited to, hematologic reactions (e.g., agranulocytosis, nonthrombocytopenic or thrombocytopenic purpura); allergic reactions characterized by fever, sore throat, laryngospasm, and respiratory distress; GI reactions including mesenteric thrombosis or ischemic colitis; and CNS reactions including reversible mental depression progressing to catatonia, short-term memory loss, decreased performance on neuropsychometric tests, and oculomucocutaneous syndrome.

● *Precautions and Contraindications*

Labetalol shares the toxic potentials of β-adrenergic and postsynaptic α₁-adrenergic blocking agents, and the usual precautions of these agents should be observed.

In patients with heart failure, sympathetic stimulation is vital for the support of circulatory function. Labetalol should be used with caution in patients with inadequate cardiac function, since heart failure may be precipitated by blockade of β-adrenergic stimulation when labetalol therapy is administered. In addition, in patients with latent cardiac insufficiency, prolonged β-adrenergic blockade may lead to cardiac failure. Although β-adrenergic blocking agents should be avoided in patients with overt heart failure, labetalol may be administered cautiously, if necessary, to patients with well-compensated heart failure (e.g., those controlled with cardiac glycosides and/or diuretics). Patients receiving labetalol therapy should be instructed to consult their clinician at the first sign or symptom of impending cardiac failure and should be adequately treated (e.g., with a cardiac glycoside and/or diuretic) and observed closely; if cardiac failure continues, labetalol should be discontinued, gradually if possible.

Further experience is necessary, but labetalol may be less likely than pure β-adrenergic blocking agents to produce adverse cardiovascular withdrawal reactions (e.g., angina, rebound hypertension) following abrupt withdrawal. Although angina pectoris has *not* been reported to date following discontinuance of labetalol therapy, exacerbation of angina pectoris and precipitation of myocardial infarction have occurred following abrupt cessation of therapy with some β-adrenergic blocking agents in patients with coronary artery disease. Therefore, patients receiving labetalol (especially those with ischemic heart disease) should be warned not to interrupt or discontinue therapy without consulting their clinician. When discontinuance of long-term labetalol therapy is planned, particularly in patients with ischemic heart disease, dosage of the drug should be gradually reduced over a period of 1–2 weeks. When labetalol therapy is discontinued, patients should be carefully monitored and advised to temporarily limit their physical activity. If exacerbation of angina occurs or acute coronary insufficiency develops after labetalol therapy is interrupted or discontinued, treatment with the drug should be reinstituted promptly, at least temporarily, and appropriate measures for the management of unstable angina pectoris should be initiated. Because coronary artery disease is common and may be unrecognized, the manufacturers caution that it may be prudent not to discontinue labetalol therapy abruptly, even in patients being treated only for hypertension.

Since β-adrenergic blocking agents may inhibit bronchodilation produced by endogenous catecholamines, the drugs generally should not be used in patients with bronchospastic disease; however, oral labetalol may be used with caution in patients with nonallergic bronchospasm (e.g., chronic bronchitis, emphysema) who do not respond to or cannot tolerate other hypotensive agents. (See Pharmacology: Respiratory Effects.) If oral labetalol is administered to such patients, the smallest effective dose should be used so that inhibition of endogenous or exogenous β-adrenergic agonist activity is minimized. Because IV labetalol at the usual therapeutic doses has not been studied in patients with nonallergic bronchospasm, the manufacturers state that it should not be used in these patients.

Although labetalol has been used effectively in the management of hypertension and relief of symptoms associated with pheochromocytoma, the drug should be used with caution in patients with this tumor since paradoxical hypertensive responses have been reported in a few patients. (See Hypertension Associated with Pheochromocytoma under Uses: Hypertension.)

It is recommended that labetalol be used with caution in patients with diabetes mellitus receiving hypoglycemic agents, especially those with labile disease or those prone to hypoglycemia since the drug may mask the signs and symptoms associated with acute hypoglycemia (e.g., tachycardia and blood pressure changes but not sweating). β-Adrenergic blocking agents also may impair glucose tolerance; delay the rate of recovery of blood glucose concentration following drug-induced hypoglycemia; alter the hemodynamic response to hypoglycemia, possibly resulting in an exaggerated hypertensive response; and possibly impair peripheral circulation. (See Cautions: Endocrine Effects.) However, many clinicians state that patients with diabetes mellitus may be particularly likely to experience a reduction in morbidity and mortality with the use of β-adrenergic blocking agents. (See Uses: Heart Failure, in Metoprolol 24:24.) If labetalol is used in diabetic patients receiving hypoglycemic agents, it may be necessary to adjust the dosage of the hypoglycemic agent.

The necessity of withdrawing β-adrenergic blocking therapy prior to major surgery is controversial. Severe, protracted hypotension and difficulty in restarting or maintaining a heart beat have occurred during surgery in some patients who have received β-adrenergic blocking agents. The effect of labetalol's α-adrenergic activity in patients undergoing major surgery has not been evaluated. However, several deaths have been reported in patients in whom labetalol hydrochloride injection was used during surgery, including those receiving the drug to control bleeding. In addition, a synergistic hypotensive response occurs in patients receiving IV labetalol and halothane anesthesia concomitantly. (See Drug Interactions: Halothane.) If labetalol therapy is continued in a patient undergoing major surgery, the anesthesiologist should be informed that the patient is receiving the drug.

Caution must be employed when reducing severely elevated blood pressure. The manufacturers state that IV labetalol is intended for use in hospitalized patients. When IV labetalol is used in patients with severely elevated blood pressure, the desired blood pressure reduction should be achieved over as long a period of time as is compatible with the patient's clinical status. Serious adverse effects, including cerebral infarction, optic nerve infarction, angina, and ischemic changes in the ECG, have been reported with other hypotensive agents when severely elevated blood pressure was reduced over periods ranging from several hours to as long as 1 or 2 days. Rapid or excessive reductions in systolic or diastolic blood pressure should be avoided; while these effects are unlikely with the recommended dosage schedules of IV labetalol, they can occasionally occur. Transient hypotension occurring with IV labetalol is usually readily managed by placing the patient in Trendelenburg's position, administering IV fluids, and/or temporarily discontinuing administration of the drug. Patients should remain supine during and for up to 3 hours after IV administration of the drug, since symptomatic orthostatic hypotension is likely to occur if they are tilted upward or allowed to assume an upright position during this period. The patient's ability to tolerate an upright position should be established before any ambulation (e.g., use of toilet facilities) is permitted; the patient should be advised on how to proceed gradually to become ambulatory and should be observed at the time of initial ambulation.

Labetalol should be used with caution in patients with impaired hepatic function, since metabolism of the drug may be decreased in such patients. Since labetalol has been rarely associated with the development of jaundice, hepatitis, severe hepatocellular injury, and elevated liver function test results, the manufacturers recommend that the drug be discontinued immediately if jaundice or laboratory evidence of hepatic injury occurs. Jaundice and hepatic dysfunction usually are reversible following discontinuance of the drug. Liver function tests should be performed at the first signs or symptoms of liver dysfunction (e.g., pruritus, dark urine, persistent anorexia, jaundice, right upper quadrant tenderness, flu-like syndrome).

Routine laboratory tests are usually not required before or after IV administration of labetalol, but the manufacturers recommend that laboratory parameters be monitored at regular intervals in patients receiving long-term oral therapy with the drug. In patients with concomitant illnesses (e.g., impaired renal function), appropriate tests should be performed to monitor these conditions.

Patients should be advised that transient scalp tingling may occur, usually during initiation of labetalol therapy.

Patients with a history of atopy or severe anaphylactic reactions to a variety of allergens may be more reactive to repeated, accidental, diagnostic, or therapeutic challenge with such allergens while receiving a β-adrenergic blocking agent. These patients may be less responsive than other patients to usual dosages of epinephrine or may develop a paradoxical response to epinephrine when that drug is used to treat anaphylactic reactions.

Labetalol is contraindicated in patients with a history of obstructive airway disease (e.g., bronchial asthma), overt cardiac failure, heart block of severity greater than first degree, cardiogenic shock, severe bradycardia, and/or other conditions associated with severe and prolonged hypotension. The drug also is contraindicated in patients with a history of hypersensitivity to any component of the formulation.

Because of similarity in spelling between labetalol hydrochloride and Lamictal® (the trade name for lamotrigine, an anticonvulsant agent), several dispensing errors have been reported to the manufacturer of Lamictal® (GlaxoSmithKline). These medication errors may be associated with serious adverse events either due to lack of appropriate therapy for seizures (e.g., in patients not receiving the prescribed anticonvulsant, lamotrigine, which may lead to status epilepticus) or, alternatively, to the risk of developing adverse effects (e.g., serious rash) associated with the use of lamotrigine in patients for whom the drug was not prescribed and consequently was not properly titrated. Therefore, the manufacturer of Lamictal® cautions that extra care should be exercised in ensuring the accuracy of both oral and written prescriptions for Lamictal® and labetalol. The manufacturer also recommends that when appropriate, clinicians might consider including the intended use of the particular drug on the prescription in addition to alerting patients to carefully check the drug they receive and promptly bring any question or concern to the attention of the dispensing pharmacist. The manufacturer also recommends that pharmacists assess the measures of avoiding dispensing errors and implement them as appropriate (e.g., placing drugs with similar names apart from one another in product storage areas, patient counseling).

● Pediatric Precautions

Although safety and efficacy remain to be fully established in children, some experts have recommended pediatric dosages for hypertension based on clinical experience.For information on overall principles and expert recommendations for treatment of hypertension in pediatric patients, see Uses: Hypertension in Pediatric Patients, in the Thiazides General Statement 40:28.20.

● Geriatric Precautions

Orthostatic hypotension, dizziness, or lightheadedness, similar to that reported in younger adults, have been reported in geriatric patients (i.e., those 60 years of age or older) receiving labetalol. Geriatric individuals are generally more likely than younger adults to experience orthostatic symptoms and these individuals should be cautioned about the possibility of these adverse effects during therapy with the drug. Because elimination of labetalol may be decreased in some geriatric patients, usual maintenance dosage of the drug is slightly lower in geriatric individuals than in younger adults. (See Dosage and Administration: Dosage.)

● Mutagenicity and Carcinogenicity

It is not known if labetalol is mutagenic or carcinogenic in humans. No evidence of labetalol-induced mutagenesis was seen with the modified Ames test or in studies in mice and rats using dominant lethal assays.

No evidence of carcinogenesis was seen in mice receiving oral labetalol hydrochloride dosages up to 200 mg/kg daily for 18 months or in rats receiving oral dosages up to 225 mg/kg daily for up to 113 weeks in females and up to 116 weeks in males.

● Pregnancy, Fertility, and Lactation

Pregnancy

Reproduction studies in rats and rabbits using oral labetalol hydrochloride dosages up to about 6 and 4 times the maximum recommended human dosage, respectively, have not revealed reproducible evidence of fetal malformation; however, oral dosages approximating the maximum recommended human dosage were associated with an increased incidence of fetal resorption in both species. There was no evidence of drug-related fetotoxicity in rabbits receiving IV dosages of the drug up to 1.7 times the maximum recommended human dosage.In rats, oral administration of labetalol hydrochloride at dosages 2–4 times the maximum recommended human dosage during the period of late gestation through weaning was associated with decreased neonatal survival. Reproduction studies in rats or rabbits using combined oral labetalol hydrochloride and hydrochlorothiazide dosages up to about 15 and 80 times the maximum recommended human dosage,

respectively, have not revealed evidence of teratogenicity, although combined oral dosages 3.5 and 20 times the maximum recommended human dosage, respectively, were maternotoxic with resultant fetotoxicity in rabbits. The combination appeared to be more toxic than either drug alone in rabbits.

Labetalol has been used orally for the management of hypertension in pregnant women and IV to control blood pressure in severely hypertensive pregnant women requiring urgent blood pressure reduction. (See Hypertension during Pregnancy under Uses: Hypertension.) Labetalol has been effective for the management of hypertension associated with pregnancy, and is one of several preferred agents for such use. Infants of mothers who received labetalol for the management of hypertension during pregnancy have not appeared to be adversely affected by the drug; however, transient hypotension (including slight decreases in systolic blood pressure during the first 24 hours after delivery), bradycardia, respiratory depression, and hypoglycemia have been reported rarely in neonates. Maternal labetalol therapy reportedly has been associated with a beneficial effect on development of fetal pulmonary maturity. Use of labetalol in pregnant women with hypertension does not appear to affect the usual course of labor and delivery, and the drug has been used IV to treat severe hypertension during labor. Following a single IV dose of the drug in pregnant women with preeclampsia, maternal blood pressure was reduced but placental and fetal blood flow were not affected. The manufacturers state that there are no adequate and controlled studies to date using labetalol in pregnant women, and the drug should be used during pregnancy only when the potential benefits justify the possible risks to the fetus.

Fertility

The effects of labetalol on fertility in humans have not been fully determined. Ejaculatory failure and impotence in males and decreased libido have been reported in patients receiving labetalol.

Lactation

Since small amounts (about 0.004% of the maternal dose) of labetalol are distributed into milk, the drug should be used with caution in nursing women.

DRUG INTERACTIONS

Since IV labetalol hydrochloride may be administered to patients receiving other drugs, including other hypotensive agents, careful monitoring of these patients is necessary to detect and promptly treat any adverse effect resulting from concomitant administration.

● Diuretics and Cardiovascular Drugs

When labetalol is administered with diuretics or other hypotensive drugs, the hypotensive effect may be increased. This effect is usually used to therapeutic advantage, but careful adjustment of dosage is necessary to avoid excessive hypotension when these drugs are used concomitantly. When β-adrenergic blocking agents are administered with calcium-channel blocking agents, therapeutic as well as adverse effects may be additive. Slowing or complete suppression of SA node activity with development of slow ventricular rates (e.g., 30–40 bpm), often misdiagnosed as complete AV block, has been reported in patients receiving the nondihydropyridine calcium-channel blocking agent mibefradil (no longer commercially available in the US), principally in geriatric patients and in association with concomitant β-adrenergic blocker therapy. The manufacturers of labetalol and some clinicians state that labetalol and a calcium-channel blocking agent (e.g., verapamil, diltiazem) should be used concomitantly with caution.

● Halothane

Concomitant administration of IV labetalol and halothane anesthesia results in a synergistic hypotensive effect, the degree and duration of which may be controlled by adjusting the halothane concentration; however, excessive hypotension can result in a large reduction in cardiac output and an increase in central venous pressure. To minimize the risk of excessive hypotension during controlled hypotensive anesthesia with IV labetalol and halothane, inspired halothane concentrations of 3% or higher should *not* be used. If labetalol therapy is continued in a patient undergoing major surgery, the anesthesiologist should be informed that the patient is receiving the drug.

● *Cimetidine*

Concomitant administration of oral cimetidine has been shown to substantially increase the absolute bioavailability of oral labetalol, possibly via enhanced absorption or decreased first-pass hepatic metabolism of labetalol. If labetalol and cimetidine are administered concomitantly, dosage of labetalol required for optimal control of blood pressure should be carefully adjusted.

● *Glutethimide*

Concomitant administration of oral glutethimide (no longer commercially available in the US) has been shown to substantially decrease the absolute bioavailability of oral labetalol, possibly by increasing first-pass hepatic metabolism (glucuronidation) of labetalol. If labetalol and glutethimide are administered concomitantly, dosage of labetalol required for optimal control of blood pressure should be carefully adjusted.

● *Other Drugs*

Labetalol, like other drugs with β-adrenergic blocking activity, can antagonize the bronchodilation produced by β-adrenergic agonists in patients with bronchospasm, and greater than usual dosages of β-adrenergic agonist bronchodilators may be required in patients receiving labetalol.

Labetalol antagonizes the reflex tachycardia produced by nitroglycerin without preventing the hypotensive effect of the nitrate. If labetalol is used concurrently with nitroglycerin, an additive hypotensive effect may occur.

An increased incidence of tremor has been reported in patients receiving labetalol and tricyclic antidepressants concomitantly compared with those receiving labetalol alone. Although the contribution of each drug to this adverse reaction is not known, the possibility of a drug interaction cannot be excluded.

LABORATORY TEST INTERFERENCES

● *Urinary Catecholamines*

The presence of labetalol metabolites in urine may result in false-positive elevations of urinary free and total catecholamines, metanephrine, normetanephrine, and 3-methoxy-4-hydroxymandelic acid (vanillylmandelic acid, VMA) measured by fluorometric or photometric methods. When screening labetalol-treated patients suspected of having pheochromocytoma or when evaluating labetalol-treated patients with the tumor, specific assay methods such as high-performance liquid chromatography (HPLC) with solid phase extraction should be used to determine concentrations of catecholamines or their metabolites.

ACUTE TOXICITY

● *Pathogenesis*

The acute lethal dose of labetalol in humans is not known. The oral LD_{50} of labetalol hydrochloride is approximately 0.6, greater than 2, and greater than 1 g/kg in mice, rats, and dogs, respectively; the IV LD_{50} in these species is about 50–60 mg/kg.

● *Manifestations*

In general, overdosage of labetalol may be expected to produce effects that are extensions of pharmacologic effects, particularly those involving the cardiovascular system; hypotension (which is posture dependent and may be severe), bradycardia (which may be severe), cardiac failure, and bronchospasm may occur. Common, dose-related adverse effects (e.g., nausea, vomiting, headache) might also occur. In one adult who was reported to have intentionally ingested labetalol hydrochloride 7.2 g, acebutolol hydrochloride 9.6 g, and trimipramine 625 mg, loss of consciousness, bradycardia, and profound hypotension resulted.

● *Treatment*

Treatment of labetalol overdosage generally involves symptomatic and supportive care. Following acute ingestion of the drug, the stomach should be emptied immediately by inducing emesis or by gastric lavage. If the patient is comatose, having seizures, or lacks the gag reflex, gastric lavage may be performed if an endotracheal tube with cuff inflated is in place to prevent aspiration of gastric contents.

Administration of activated charcoal after emesis or gastric lavage may be useful in preventing absorption of labetalol, although specific data are not available. Patients should be placed in a supine position and their legs elevated if necessary to improve blood supply to the brain. For symptomatic bradycardia, atropine or epinephrine may be given. A vasopressor (e.g., norepinephrine, dopamine) may be given for severe hypotension. For heart failure, a cardiac glycoside and diuretic may be used; dopamine or dobutamine may also be useful. Glucagon may also be useful for the management of myocardial depression and hypotension. A β₂-adrenergic agonist and/or a theophylline derivative may be used for bronchospasm. For seizures, diazepam may be used. Labetalol is not appreciably removed (less than 1% of a dose) by hemodialysis or peritoneal dialysis.

PHARMACOLOGY

Labetalol is a nonselective β-adrenergic blocking agent and a selective α₁-adrenergic blocking agent. The pharmacology of labetalol is complex and in some ways resembles that of other β-adrenergic blocking agents and that of postsynaptic α₁-adrenergic blocking agents such as prazosin; however, the overall pharmacologic profile of labetalol differs from that of these other drugs. The β-adrenergic blocking activity of labetalol is approximately 3 or 7 times greater than the α-adrenergic blocking activity following oral or IV administration, respectively; it has not been clearly established whether the ratio changes with dosage of the drug or following long-term administration.

The principal physiologic action of labetalol is to competitively block adrenergic stimulation of β-receptors within the myocardium (β₁-receptors) and within bronchial and vascular smooth muscle (β₂-receptors) and α₁-receptors within vascular smooth muscle. In addition to inhibiting access of endogenous or exogenous catecholamines to β-adrenergic receptors, labetalol has been shown to exhibit some intrinsic β₂-agonist activity in animals; however, the drug exerts little, if any, intrinsic β₁-agonist activity. Labetalol does not exhibit intrinsic α-adrenergic agonist activity. There is some evidence from animal studies suggesting that the drug may have a vasodilating effect, possibly resulting from a direct or β₂-agonist action. In animals, at doses greater than those required for α- or β-adrenergic blockade, labetalol also has a membrane-stabilizing effect on the heart which is similar to that of quinidine; however, this effect is unlikely to be clinically important since it occurs only at doses higher than those required for α- or β-adrenergic blockade.

● *Cardiovascular Effects*

The hemodynamic effects of labetalol are variable following oral or IV administration. Labetalol, unlike pure β-adrenergic blocking agents, produces a dose-dependent (at usual doses) decrease in systemic arterial blood pressure and systemic vascular resistance without a substantial reduction in resting heart rate, cardiac output, or stroke volume, apparently because of its combined α- and β-adrenergic blocking activity. Labetalol effectively reduces blood pressure in the standing or supine position, but because of the drug's α₁-adrenergic blocking activity, the effect on blood pressure is position dependent; labetalol-induced decreases in blood pressure are greater in the standing than in the supine position, and orthostatic hypotension can occur. (See Cautions: Cardiovascular Effects.) The blunting of exercise-induced increases in blood pressure by oral or IV labetalol is generally greater than that produced by pure β-adrenergic blocking agents (e.g., propranolol), but the blunting of exercise-induced tachycardia produced by labetalol is generally less than that produced by pure β-adrenergic blocking agents.

Following oral administration of labetalol hydrochloride dosages of 200 mg to 2.4 g daily for 1 week to 20 months in clinical studies in patients with hypertension, blood pressure and heart rate were reduced at rest or during exercise and in the supine or standing position. During oral labetalol therapy, cardiac output is generally decreased or unchanged and stroke volume is generally increased or unchanged; however, unlike most pure β-adrenergic blocking agents, oral labetalol usually decreases systemic vascular resistance. Following IV administration of single labetalol doses in patients with hypertension, the drug decreases blood pressure and systemic vascular resistance in the supine position without substantially reducing cardiac output or stroke volume. Although substantial changes in heart rate usually do not occur in the supine position following IV administration, heart rate and cardiac output generally are reduced in an upright or tilted upright position or during exercise. In one study in patients with severe hypertension, an initial 0.25-mg/kg IV dose of the drug decreased supine blood pressure by an average of 11/7 mm Hg; additional 0.5-mg/kg IV doses administered at 15-minute intervals up to a total cumulative dose of 1.75 mg/kg caused further dose-related decreases in blood pressure in these patients. Similar results in patients with severe hypertension have also been produced with an initial 20-mg IV dose followed by IV doses of 40 or 80 mg at 10-minute intervals until blood pressure was adequately controlled or a total cumulative dose of 300 mg was administered. Following continuous IV infusion of a mean labetalol hydrochloride dose of 136 mg (range: 27–300 mg) over 2–3 hours in patients with severe hypertension, blood pressure was reportedly decreased by an average of 60/35 mm Hg. IV administration of a single labetalol dose does not appear to produce a clinically important reduction in cerebral blood flow following rapid reduction of blood pressure in severely hypertensive patients, and long-term oral administration of the drug also does not appear to affect cerebral blood flow.

Following IV administration of labetalol in normotensive patients with coronary artery disease, blood pressure, heart rate, systemic vascular resistance, and coronary vascular resistance are generally decreased; cardiac index, left ventricular end-diastolic pressure (LVEDP), and pulmonary artery wedge pressure are generally unchanged; and coronary sinus blood flow may be increased. In patients with hypertension associated with acute myocardial infarction, IV labetalol decreases blood pressure and heart rate and generally decreases cardiac index and pulmonary artery wedge pressure. In normotensive patients with acute myocardial infarction, IV labetalol may decrease blood pressure, heart rate, and cardiac index without affecting systemic vascular resistance.

The electrophysiologic effects of labetalol are variable and appear to be mediated via the drug's myocardial β_1-adrenergic blocking activity. Labetalol may decrease conduction velocity through the atrioventricular (AV) node and increase the atrial effective refractory period (ERP), but the drug appears to have inconsistent effects on sinoatrial (SA) conduction time and the AV nodal refractory period; the decrease in AV nodal conduction velocity produced by labetalol is less than that produced by pure β-adrenergic blocking agents. In healthy individuals and in patients with cardiac disease (e.g., coronary artery disease), labetalol generally has little effect on sinus rate, intraventricular conduction, the His-Purkinje system, or duration of the QRS complex. In one study in hypertensive patients, oral labetalol therapy was associated with a substantial reduction in ventricular premature contractions, and in another study in hypertensive patients, IV labetalol rapidly restored sinus rhythm in some patients with supraventricular or ventricular arrhythmias. Further studies are needed to adequately evaluate the drug's antiarrhythmic activity.

● Renal Effects

Unlike therapy with some pure β-adrenergic blocking agents (e.g., propranolol), labetalol therapy does not appear to be associated with a reduction in glomerular filtration rate or renal plasma flow following short- or long-term administration in patients with hypertension and normal renal function. Labetalol's apparent lack of effect on renal hemodynamics may be related to the drug's α-adrenergic blocking action on renal vasculature or its minimal effect on cardiac output. Use of the drug in patients with hypertension and chronic renal failure has generally not been associated with any deterioration in renal function. Although not consistently found, increases in plasma volume have been reported in some patients with hypertension receiving oral labetalol alone, and edema and/or fluid retention have been reported in some patients during therapy with the drug.

In several studies in patients with hypertension and elevated plasma renin activity (PRA), long-term oral administration of labetalol hydrochloride (150 mg to 2.4 g daily) has been reported to suppress PRA at rest and during exercise, and in the supine and standing positions; in most of the studies, the net suppressive effect on renin was generally proportional to basal PRA. In other studies, labetalol has been reported to have an inconsistent overall effect on resting PRA, but there was considerable interindividual variation in PRA in these studies. Following acute IV administration, labetalol has been reported to produce substantial reductions in plasma angiotensin II concentration, particularly in patients with high basal values. Although labetalol has been reported to have little, if any, effect on plasma aldosterone concentration following long-term oral administration in several studies, there is some evidence that the drug may decrease plasma aldosterone concentration following oral or IV administration. Labetalol has also been reported to decrease urinary aldosterone excretion following oral administration in patients with hypertension.

● Endocrine and Metabolic Effects

The exact mechanism is unknown and the effect has not been clinically important, but labetalol may increase plasma glucose concentration. Serum cholesterol

and triglyceride concentrations have generally been unchanged or very slightly decreased during labetalol therapy; although data currently are limited, long-term administration of the drug does not appear to be associated with any clinically important adverse effects on plasma lipid concentrations. Labetalol does not appear to substantially alter serum concentrations of insulin, C-peptide, free fatty acids, growth hormone, or prolactin; however, following IV administration in one preliminary study, labetalol caused a substantial increase in serum prolactin concentration which was more marked in females than in males. Although subsequent studies have not demonstrated an effect on serum prolactin concentration following oral administration of the drug, IV administration appears to be associated with hyperprolactinemia, apparently resulting from a drug-induced CNS effect; the clinical importance of this finding is not known.

● Respiratory Effects

Through its β_2-adrenergic blocking action in the respiratory tract, labetalol may increase airway resistance, especially in patients with asthma or chronic obstructive pulmonary disease; however, since α-adrenergic receptors in the respiratory tract may be involved in the pathogenesis of bronchoconstriction, it is possible that the α-adrenergic blocking action of labetalol may attenuate some of the potential adverse respiratory effects resulting from the drug's β-adrenergic blocking action. In addition, labetalol's apparent β_2-adrenergic agonist activity may contribute to attenuation of the drug's potential adverse respiratory effects. Although an increase in airway resistance as measured by forced expiratory volume in 1 second (FEV_1) or by resting and post-exercise peak expiratory flow rates was not observed in many studies in healthy individuals or patients with asthma or chronic obstructive pulmonary disease (COPD) who received labetalol, evidence of increased airway resistance has occurred in some studies in healthy individuals or in patients with or without COPD who received the drug. Labetalol's effect on airway resistance generally appears to be less than that of nonselective β-adrenergic blocking agents (e.g., propranolol), but generally comparable to that of β_1-selective agents (e.g., atenolol). Labetalol has been used without evidence of a substantial increase in airway resistance in a limited number of hypertensive patients with bronchial asthma in whom propranolol had increased airway resistance.

PHARMACOKINETICS

● Absorption

Labetalol hydrochloride is rapidly and approximately 90–100% absorbed from the GI tract following oral administration, but the drug undergoes extensive first-pass metabolism in the liver and/or GI mucosa. Only about 25% of an oral dose reaches systemic circulation unchanged in fasted adults. Although absolute bioavailability in one study reportedly ranged from 11–86% (mean: 33%) following oral administration of a single 100-mg dose in fasted adults, the considerable interindividual variability in this study may have resulted from use of a relatively insensitive spectrofluorometric assay. Food delays GI absorption of labetalol hydrochloride but increases absolute bioavailability of the drug, possibly by decreasing first-pass metabolism and/or hepatic blood flow. Following oral administration of a single 200-mg dose in healthy adults in one study, absolute bioavailability of the drug averaged 26 and 36% in the fasted and nonfasted state, respectively. First-pass metabolism may also be reduced and bioavailability substantially increased in geriatric patients and in patients with hepatic dysfunction. However, in one study in patients with hepatosplenic schistosomiasis, mean absolute bioavailability of the drug was reportedly decreased when compared with healthy individuals. Oral cimetidine increases, and glutethimide decreases, the bioavailability of labetalol. (See Drug Interactions.) Concomitant oral administration of labetalol hydrochloride and hydrochlorothiazide does not affect the bioavailability of either drug.

Following multiple-dose oral administration of labetalol hydrochloride, peak plasma concentrations are generally achieved within 40 minutes to 2 hours. Peak plasma concentrations reportedly increase proportionately with oral dosage at dosages ranging from 100 mg to 3 g daily. In one study in hypertensive patients, peak plasma labetalol concentration following oral administration of 200 mg 3 times daily or 300 mg twice daily averaged 323 or 430 ng/mL, respectively, and the steady-state plasma drug concentration averaged 149 or 145 ng/mL, respectively; based on pharmacokinetic and pharmacodynamic (i.e., blood pressure response) evaluation, these dosage regimens were considered equivalent.

Following IV injection over 1 minute of a 1.5-mg/kg dose of labetalol hydrochloride in one study, a mean peak plasma concentration of about 5.7 mcg/mL occurred 2 minutes after injection and plasma concentration had declined to an average of 575 ng/mL at 10.5 minutes after injection.

The relationship between plasma labetalol concentration and pharmacologic effects of the drug has not been clearly established. Relationships between pharmacologic effects (e.g., blood pressure response, response of exercise-induced tachycardia) and dose, logarithm of plasma labetalol concentration, and/or area under the plasma concentration-time curve (AUC) have been reported in some studies, but such relationships were not found in other studies. In general, there appears to be a correlation between plasma labetalol concentration and blood pressure reduction, particularly in the upright position, but there is wide interindividual variation.

Following oral administration of labetalol hydrochloride, the hypotensive effect of the drug is generally apparent within 20 minutes to 2 hours, maximal within 1–4 hours, and persists in a dose-dependent manner for about 8–12 or 12–24 hours after a single 200- or 300-mg dose, respectively. The maximum, steady-state blood pressure response with twice-daily dosing occurs within 1–3 days. Following slow, direct IV injection of the drug, the hypotensive effect is apparent within 2–5 minutes, is usually maximal within 5–15 minutes, and generally persists for about 2–4 hours, although a longer duration of effect (i.e., up to 24 hours) has been reported in some patients.

● Distribution

Following IV administration, labetalol is rapidly and widely distributed into the extravascular space. The drug has an apparent volume of distribution of 3.2–15.7 L/kg. In one study in healthy adults, the volume of distribution in the central compartment (V_c) and at steady state (V_{ss}) averaged 1.1 and 9.4 L/kg, respectively. The apparent volume of distribution is reportedly decreased in patients with impaired hepatic function but is similar to that of healthy individuals in patients with impaired renal function or in pregnant women. In animals, the drug distributes in highest concentrations into the lungs, liver, and kidneys; only minimal amounts cross the blood-brain barrier.

In vitro, labetalol is approximately 50% bound to plasma proteins at plasma labetalol concentrations of 0.1–50 mcg/mL.

Labetalol crosses the placenta. In one study in several pregnant women receiving the drug orally (200 mg 3 times daily) for about 7 days, the median ratio of fetal cord to maternal plasma concentration at parturition was 0.5. Small amounts of unchanged labetalol have been shown to distribute into the fetal uveal tract following administration of radiolabeled drug in pregnant animals; the drug bound reversibly to melanin in the uveal tract but was not oculotoxic. Small amounts of labetalol and its metabolites are distributed into milk, principally as unbound labetalol.

● Elimination

Plasma concentrations of labetalol appear to decline in a biphasic or possibly triphasic manner. In healthy adults and adults with hypertension, the half-life in the distribution phase ($t_{1/2\alpha}$) has been reported to average 6–44 minutes and the half-life in the terminal elimination phase ($t_{1/2\beta}$) has been reported to average 2.5–8 hours. The variability in reported mean half-lives for the drug may have resulted in part from use of a relatively insensitive spectrofluorometric assay in some studies. The manufacturers state that the drug has a plasma elimination half-life of 5.5 or 6–8 hours following IV or oral administration, respectively. The elimination half-life of the drug appears to be unchanged in individuals with renal or hepatic impairment, but may be increased in patients with severe renal impairment (i.e., creatinine clearance less than 10 mL/minute) undergoing dialysis. Results of some studies indicate that elimination of labetalol may be reduced in geriatric individuals; elimination half-life of the drug reportedly may be slightly increased (but within the reported range) in some geriatric individuals. Total body clearance of labetalol from plasma has been reported to average 19–33 mL/minute per kg in individuals with normal renal and hepatic function. Plasma clearance appears to be unaffected by renal impairment but may be decreased in patients with hepatic impairment.

Labetalol is extensively metabolized in the liver and possibly in the GI mucosa following oral administration, principally by conjugation with glucuronic acid. The major metabolite is the O-alkylglucuronide, with smaller amounts of the O-phenylglucuronide and N-glucuronide being formed. Following oral administration, labetalol undergoes extensive first-pass metabolism in the liver and/or GI mucosa. (See Pharmacokinetics: Absorption.)

Labetalol and its metabolites are excreted in feces via biliary elimination and in urine. About 55–60% of a dose is excreted in urine, mainly as glucuronide conjugates, within 24 hours, and about 30% is excreted in feces within 4 days. Less than 5% of a dose is excreted unchanged in urine. Labetalol is not appreciably removed (less than 1% of a dose) by hemodialysis or peritoneal dialysis.

CHEMISTRY AND STABILITY

● Chemistry

Labetalol hydrochloride is an α- and β-adrenergic blocking agent. The drug is commercially available as a racemic mixture of its 4 stereoisomers. The RR-isomer, dilevalol, makes up 25% of the racemic mixture. Dilevalol has about 2–4 times the β-adrenergic blocking activity of the racemic mixture but has only minimal α_1-adrenergic blocking activity; dilevalol also appears to possess some β_2-agonist activity. Most of the α_1-adrenergic blocking activity of labetalol hydrochloride is attributable to the SR-isomer.

Labetalol hydrochloride occurs as a white or off-white crystalline powder and is sparingly soluble in water (approximately 20 mg/mL) and freely soluble to soluble in alcohol (at least 100 mg/mL). Labetalol is less lipophilic than propranolol but more lipophilic than most other currently available β-adrenergic blocking agents. The drug has a pK_a of 9.3. Labetalol hydrochloride injection is a sterile, isotonic solution of the drug in water for injection. The injection occurs as a clear, colorless to light yellow solution and has a pH of 3–4. The injection also contains parabens as preservatives, dextrose, and edetate sodium; citric acid and sodium hydroxide may be added during manufacture of the injection to adjust pH.

● Stability

Labetalol hydrochloride tablets should be stored in well-closed containers at 2–30°C; tablets in unit-dose packages should be protected from excessive moisture. Labetalol hydrochloride injection should be stored at 2–30°C and protected from light and freezing. Labetalol hydrochloride tablets and injection have an expiration date of 3 and 2 years, respectively, after the date of manufacture.

Labetalol hydrochloride is most stable in solutions having a pH of 2–4. The drug is physically and chemically compatible with the following IV solutions: 5% dextrose; 0.9% sodium chloride; 2.5% dextrose and 0.45% sodium chloride; 5% dextrose and 0.2, 0.33, or 0.9% sodium chloride; 5% dextrose and lactated Ringer's or Ringer's; lactated Ringer's; or Ringer's. Following dilution of labetalol hydrochloride injection with one of these IV solutions, solutions containing 1.25–3.75 mg/mL are stable for at least 24 hours when refrigerated or stored at room temperature. In one study, these solutions were stable for at least 72 hours at 4 or 25°C. Appreciable changes in pH or osmolarity of these IV solutions did not occur following admixture of labetalol hydrochloride injection. The drug is physically and/or chemically incompatible with 5% sodium bicarbonate injection; labetalol hydrochloride solutions containing 1.25–3.75 mg/mL in 5% sodium bicarbonate have a pH of 7.6–8 and form a white precipitate, probably the free base, within 6 hours after admixture. A white precipitate also has been observed following concomitant infusion of other alkaline drugs (e.g., furosemide) and labetalol hydrochloride injection; therefore, labetalol hydrochloride injection should not be given in the same infusion line with other alkaline solutions.

PREPARATIONS

Excipients in commercially available drug preparations may have clinically important effects in some individuals; consult specific product labeling for details.

Labetalol Hydrochloride

Oral

Tablets, film-coated	100 mg*	Labetalol Hydrochloride Tablets
	200 mg*	Labetalol Hydrochloride Tablets
	300 mg*	Labetalol Hydrochloride Tablets

Parenteral

Injection, for IV use	5 mg/mL*	Labetalol Hydrochloride Injection

* available from one or more manufacturer, distributor, and/or repackager by generic (nonproprietary) name

† Use is not currently included in the labeling approved by the US Food and Drug Administration.

Selected Revisions June 10, 2024, © Copyright, August 1, 1985, American Society of Health-System Pharmacists, Inc.

Metoprolol Succinate, Metoprolol Tartrate

24:20 • β-ADRENERGIC BLOCKING AGENTS

■ Metoprolol is a β_1-selective adrenergic blocking agent (β-blocker).

USES

Metoprolol is used for the management of hypertension, angina, acute myocardial infarction (MI), and heart failure. The drug also has been used for supraventricular and ventricular tachyarrhythmias† and prophylaxis of migraine headache†.

The choice of a β-adrenergic blocking agent (β-blocker) depends on numerous factors, including pharmacologic properties (e.g., relative β-selectivity, intrinsic sympathomimetic activity, membrane-stabilizing activity, lipophilicity), pharmacokinetics, intended use, and adverse effect profile, as well as the patient's coexisting disease states or conditions, response, and tolerance. While specific pharmacologic properties and other factors may appropriately influence the choice of a β-blocker in individual patients, evidence of clinically important differences among the agents in terms of overall efficacy and/or safety is limited. Patients who do not respond to or cannot tolerate one β-blocker may be successfully treated with a different agent.

In the management of hypertension or chronic stable angina pectoris in patients with chronic obstructive pulmonary disease (COPD) or type 1 diabetes mellitus, many clinicians prefer to use low dosages of a β_1-selective adrenergic blocking agent (e.g., atenolol, metoprolol), rather than a nonselective agent (e.g., nadolol, pindolol, propranolol, timolol). However, selectivity of these agents is relative and dose dependent. Some clinicians also will recommend using a β_1-selective agent or an agent with intrinsic sympathomimetic activity (ISA) (e.g., pindolol), rather than a nonselective agent, for the management of hypertension or angina pectoris in patients with peripheral vascular disease, but there is no evidence that the choice of β-blocker substantially affects efficacy.

● Hypertension

Metoprolol is used alone or in combination with other classes of antihypertensive agents in the management of hypertension. β-Blockers often are used concurrently with a diuretic because of their additive effects. β-Blockers also have been combined with vasodilators (e.g., hydralazine, minoxidil) to counteract the reflex tachycardia that occurs with vasodilators.

Metoprolol's efficacy in the management of hypertension is similar to that of other β-blockers; however, metoprolol may be preferred over a nonselective β-blocker, like propranolol, in hypertensive patients with certain concomitant disease states. Metoprolol may be associated with less risk of bronchospasm than propranolol in patients with bronchitis. Metoprolol's relative cardioselectivity may be advantageous in hypertensive patients with concomitant heart failure controlled by diuretics and cardiac glycosides; however, it remains to be established whether metoprolol is less likely to cause heart failure in these patients than is propranolol. In patients with catecholamine excess (e.g., pheochromocytoma, drug-induced hypoglycemia, or acute withdrawal of adrenergic blocking agents), metoprolol reportedly is less likely to produce impairment of peripheral circulation, heart failure, and hypertensive reactions than is propranolol. Because metoprolol may cause less inhibition of glycogenolysis than does propranolol, metoprolol may be preferred in patients with diabetes mellitus who are receiving insulin or oral antidiabetic agents (e.g., sulfonylurea drugs); however, additional study is required.

In contrast to many other antihypertensive agents, metoprolol lowers blood pressure equally well in the upright or supine position. The drug appears to be safe and effective in the management of hypertension in patients with renal damage. Although metoprolol is apparently more effective in reducing blood pressure in patients with normal or elevated plasma renin concentrations, the drug also lowers blood pressure in patients with low renin hypertension. Tolerance to the antihypertensive effect of metoprolol apparently does not occur during long-term administration.

Current evidence-based practice guidelines for the management of hypertension in adults generally recommend the use of drugs from 4 classes of antihypertensive agents (angiotensin-converting enzyme [ACE] inhibitors, angiotensin II receptor antagonists, calcium-channel blockers, and thiazide diuretics). Most guidelines no longer recommend β-blockers as first-line therapy for hypertension because of the lack of established superiority over other recommended drug classes and evidence from at least one study demonstrating that β-blockers may be less effective than angiotensin II receptor antagonists in preventing cardiovascular death, MI, or stroke. However, therapy with a β-blocker may still be considered in hypertensive patients who have a compelling indication (e.g., prior MI, ischemic heart disease, heart failure) for their use or as add-on therapy in those who do not respond adequately to the preferred drug classes. (See Considerations for Drug Therapy in Patients with Underlying Cardiovascular and Other Risk Factors, under Uses: Hypertension.) Ultimately, choice of antihypertensive therapy should be individualized, considering the clinical characteristics of the patient (e.g., age, ethnicity/race, comorbid conditions, cardiovascular risk factors) as well as drug-related factors (e.g., ease of administration, availability, adverse effects, costs).

General Considerations for Initial and Maintenance Antihypertensive Therapy

Nonpharmacologic Therapy

Nonpharmacologic measures (i.e., lifestyle/behavioral modifications) that are effective in lowering blood pressure include weight reduction (for those who are overweight or obese), dietary changes to include foods such as fruits, vegetables, whole grains, and low-fat dairy products that are rich in potassium, calcium, magnesium, and fiber (i.e., adoption of the Dietary Approaches to Stop Hypertension [DASH] eating plan), sodium reduction, increased physical activity, and moderation of alcohol intake. Such lifestyle/behavioral modifications, including smoking cessation, enhance antihypertensive drug efficacy and decrease cardiovascular risk and remain an indispensable part of the management of hypertension. Lifestyle/behavioral modifications without antihypertensive drug therapy are recommended for individuals classified by a 2017 multidisciplinary hypertension guideline of the American College of Cardiology (ACC), American Heart Association (AHA), and a number of other professional organizations as having elevated blood pressure (systolic blood pressure 120–129 mm Hg and diastolic blood pressure less than 80 mm Hg) and in those with stage 1 hypertension (systolic blood pressure 130–139 mm Hg or diastolic blood pressure 80–89 mm Hg) who do *not* have preexisting cardiovascular disease or an estimated 10-year atherosclerotic cardiovascular disease (ASCVD) risk of 10% or greater.

Initiation of Drug Therapy

Drug therapy in the management of hypertension must be individualized and adjusted based on the degree of blood pressure elevation while also considering cardiovascular risk factors. Drug therapy generally is reserved for patients who respond inadequately to nondrug therapy (i.e., lifestyle modifications such as diet [including sodium restriction and adequate potassium and calcium intake], regular aerobic physical activity, moderation of alcohol consumption, and weight reduction) or in whom the degree of blood pressure elevation or coexisting risk factors requires more prompt or aggressive therapy; however, the optimum blood pressure threshold for initiating antihypertensive drug therapy and specific treatment goals remain controversial.

The 2017 ACC/AHA hypertension guideline and many experts currently state that the treatment of hypertension should be based not only on blood pressure values but also on patients' cardiovascular risk factors. For *secondary prevention* of recurrent cardiovascular disease events in adults with clinical cardiovascular disease or for *primary prevention* in adults with an estimated 10-year ASCVD risk of 10% or higher, the 2017 ACC/AHA hypertension guideline recommends initiation of antihypertensive drug therapy in conjunction with lifestyle/behavioral modifications at an average systolic blood pressure of 130 mm Hg or an average diastolic blood pressure of 80 mm Hg or higher. For *primary prevention* of cardiovascular disease events in adults with a low (less than 10%) estimated 10-year risk of ASCVD, the 2017 ACC/AHA hypertension guideline recommends initiation of antihypertensive drug therapy in conjunction with lifestyle/behavioral modifications at a systolic blood pressure of 140 mm Hg or higher or a diastolic blood pressure of 90 mm Hg or higher. After initiation of antihypertensive drug therapy, regardless of the ASCVD risk, the 2017 ACC/AHA hypertension guideline generally recommends a blood pressure goal of less than 130/80 mm Hg in all adults. In addition, a systolic blood pressure goal of less than 130 mm Hg also is recommended for noninstitutionalized ambulatory patients 65 years of age or older with an average systolic blood pressure of at least 130 mm Hg. While these blood pressure goals are lower than those recommended for most patients in previous guidelines, they are based upon clinical studies demonstrating continuing reduction of cardiovascular risk at progressively lower levels of systolic blood pressure.

Most data indicate that patients with a higher cardiovascular risk will benefit the most from tighter blood pressure control; however, some experts state this treatment goal also may be beneficial in those at lower cardiovascular risk. Other clinicians believe that the benefits of such blood pressure lowering do not outweigh the risks in those patients considered to be at lower risk of cardiovascular disease and that reclassifying individuals formerly considered to have prehypertension as having hypertension may potentially lead to use of drug therapy in such patients without consideration of cardiovascular risk. Previous hypertension guidelines, such as those from the JNC 8 expert panel, generally have recommended initiation of antihypertensive treatment in patients with a systolic blood pressure of at least 140 mm Hg or a diastolic blood pressure of at least 90 mm Hg, targeted a blood pressure goal of less than 140/90 mm Hg regardless of cardiovascular risk, and used higher systolic blood pressure thresholds and targets in geriatric patients. Some clinicians continue to support the target blood pressures recommended by the JNC 8 expert panel because of concerns that such recommendations in the 2017 ACC/AHA hypertension guideline are based on extrapolation of data from the high-risk population in the SPRINT study to a lower-risk population. Also, because more than 90% of patients in SPRINT were already receiving antihypertensive drugs at baseline, data are lacking on the effects of *initiating* drug therapy at a lower blood pressure threshold (130/80 mm Hg) in patients at high risk of cardiovascular disease. The potential benefits of hypertension management and drug cost, adverse effects, and risks associated with the use of multiple antihypertensive drugs should be considered when deciding a patient's treatment goal.

The 2017 ACC/AHA hypertension guideline recommends an ASCVD risk assessment for all adults with hypertension; however, experts state that it can be assumed that patients with hypertension and diabetes mellitus or chronic kidney disease (CKD) are at high risk for cardiovascular disease and that antihypertensive drug therapy should be initiated in these patients at a blood pressure of 130/80 mm Hg or higher. ACC/AHA also recommends a blood pressure goal of less than 130/80 mm Hg in patients with hypertension and diabetes mellitus or CKD. These recommendations are based on a systematic review of high-quality evidence from randomized controlled trials, meta-analyses, and post hoc analyses that have demonstrated substantial reductions in the risk of important clinical outcomes (e.g., cardiovascular events) regardless of comorbid conditions or age when systolic blood pressure is lowered to less than 130 mm Hg. However, some clinicians have questioned the generalizability of findings from some of the trials (e.g., SPRINT) used to support the 2017 ACC/AHA hypertension guideline. For example, SPRINT included adults (mean age: 68 years) *without* diabetes mellitus who were at high risk of cardiovascular disease. While benefits of intensive blood pressure control were observed in this patient population, some clinicians have questioned whether these findings apply to younger patients who have a low risk of cardiovascular disease. In patients with CKD in the SPRINT trial, intensive blood pressure management (achieving a mean systolic blood pressure of approximately 122 mm Hg compared with 136 mm Hg with standard treatment) provided a similar beneficial reduction in the composite cardiovascular disease primary outcome and all-cause mortality as in the full patient cohort. Because most patients with CKD die from cardiovascular complications, the findings of this study further support a lower blood pressure target of less than 130/80 mm Hg. Data are lacking to determine the ideal blood pressure goal in patients with hypertension and diabetes mellitus; also, studies evaluating the benefits of intensive blood pressure control in patients with diabetes mellitus have provided conflicting results.

Clinical studies reviewed for the 2017 ACC/AHA hypertension guideline have shown similar quantitative benefits from blood pressure lowering in hypertensive patients with or without diabetes mellitus. In a randomized, controlled study (ACCORD-BP) that compared a higher (systolic blood pressure less than 140 mm Hg) versus lower (systolic blood pressure less than 120 mm Hg) blood pressure goal in patients with diabetes mellitus, there was no difference in the incidence of cardiovascular outcomes (e.g., composite outcome of cardiovascular death, nonfatal MI, and nonfatal stroke). However, some experts state that this study was underpowered to detect a difference between the 2 treatment groups and that the factorial design of the study complicated interpretation of the results. Although SPRINT did not include patients with diabetes mellitus, patients in this study with prediabetes demonstrated a similar cardiovascular benefit from intensive treatment of blood pressure as normoglycemic patients. A meta-analysis of data from ACCORD and SPRINT suggests that the findings of both studies are consistent and that patients with diabetes mellitus benefit from more intensive blood pressure control. These data support the 2017 ACC/AHA hypertension guideline recommendation of a blood pressure treatment goal of less than 130/80 mm Hg in patients with hypertension and diabetes mellitus. Alternatively, the American Diabetes Association (ADA) recommends a blood pressure goal of less than 140/90 mm Hg in patients with diabetes mellitus. The ADA states that a lower blood pressure goal (e.g., less than 130/80 mm Hg) may be appropriate for patients with a high risk of cardiovascular disease and diabetes mellitus if it can be achieved without undue treatment burden.

Further study is needed to more clearly define optimum blood pressure goals in patients with hypertension, particularly in high-risk groups (e.g., patients with diabetes mellitus, cardiovascular disease, or cerebrovascular disease; black patients); when determining appropriate blood pressure goals, individual risks and benefits should be considered in addition to the evidence from clinical studies.

Experts state that in patients with stage 1 hypertension (especially the elderly, those with a history of hypotension, or those who have experienced adverse drug effects), it is reasonable to initiate drug therapy using the stepped-care approach in which one drug is initiated and titrated and other drugs are added sequentially to achieve the target blood pressure. However, although some patients can begin treatment with a single antihypertensive agent, the 2017 ACC/AHA hypertension guideline recommends initiation of antihypertensive therapy with 2 drugs from different pharmacologic classes (either as separate agents or in a fixed-dose combination) in patients with stage 2 hypertension and an average blood pressure more than 20/10 mm Hg above their target blood pressure. Such combined therapy may increase the likelihood of achieving goal blood pressure in a more timely fashion, but also may increase the risk of adverse effects (e.g., orthostatic hypotension) in some patients (e.g., elderly). Drug regimens with complementary activity, where a second antihypertensive agent is used to block compensatory responses to the first agent or affect a different pressor mechanism, can result in additive blood pressure lowering and are preferred. Drug combinations that have similar mechanisms of action or clinical effects (e.g., the combination of an ACE inhibitor and an angiotensin II receptor antagonist) generally should be avoided. Many patients who begin therapy with a single antihypertensive agent will subsequently require at least 2 drugs from different pharmacologic classes to achieve their blood pressure goal. Experts state that other patient-specific factors, such as age, concurrent medications, drug adherence, drug interactions, the overall treatment regimen, cost, and comorbidities, also should be considered when deciding on an antihypertensive drug regimen. For any stage of hypertension, antihypertensive drug dosages should be adjusted and/or other agents substituted or added until goal blood pressure is achieved. (See Follow-up and Maintenance Drug Therapy under Hypertension: General Considerations for Initial and Maintenance Antihypertensive Therapy, in Uses.)

Follow-up and Maintenance Drug Therapy

Several strategies are used for the titration and combination of antihypertensive drugs; these strategies, which are generally based on those used in randomized controlled studies, include maximizing the dosage of the first drug before adding a second drug, adding a second drug before achieving maximum dosage of the initial drug, or initiating therapy with 2 drugs simultaneously (either as separate preparations or as a fixed-dose combination). Combined use of an ACE inhibitor and angiotensin II receptor antagonist should be avoided because of the potential risk of adverse renal effects. After initiating a new or adjusted antihypertensive drug regimen, patients should have their blood pressure reevaluated monthly until adequate blood pressure control is achieved. Effective blood pressure control can be achieved in most hypertensive patients, but many will ultimately require therapy with 2 or more antihypertensive drugs. In addition to measuring blood pressure, clinicians should evaluate patients for orthostatic hypotension, adverse drug effects, adherence to drug therapy and lifestyle modifications, and the need for drug dosage adjustments. Laboratory testing such as electrolytes and renal function status and other assessments of target organ damage also should be performed.

Considerations for Drug Therapy in Patients with Underlying Cardiovascular and Other Risk Factors

Drug therapy in patients with hypertension and underlying cardiovascular or other risk factors should be carefully individualized based on the underlying disease(s), concomitant drugs, tolerance to drug-induced adverse effects, and blood pressure goal. (See Table 2 on Compelling Indications for Drug Classes based on Comorbid Conditions, under Uses: Hypertension in Adults, in the Thiazides General Statement 40:28.20.)

Ischemic Heart Disease

The selection of an appropriate antihypertensive agent in patients with ischemic heart disease should be based on individual patient characteristics, and may include a β-blocker, with the addition of other drugs (e.g., ACE inhibitors, thiazide diuretics, calcium-channel blockers) as necessary to achieve blood pressure goals. Because of the demonstrated mortality benefit of β-blockers following MI, these drugs should be administered in all patients who have survived an MI. The 2017 ACC/AHA hypertension guideline states that β-blockers used for ischemic heart disease/angina that are also effective in lowering blood pressure include bisoprolol, carvedilol, metoprolol succinate, metoprolol tartrate, nadolol, propranolol, and timolol.

Heart Failure

While β-blockers as single therapies are not superior to other antihypertensive agents in the reduction of all cardiovascular outcomes, certain β-blockers (bisoprolol, carvedilol, extended-release metoprolol succinate) have been shown to be effective in reducing the incidence of heart failure and associated morbidity and mortality. (See Uses: Heart Failure.)

Other Special Considerations for Antihypertensive Drug Therapy
Race

Most patients with hypertension, especially black patients, will require at least 2 antihypertensive drugs to achieve adequate blood pressure control. In general, black hypertensive patients tend to respond better to monotherapy with thiazide diuretics or calcium-channel blockers than to monotherapy with β-blockers, ACE inhibitors, or angiotensin II receptor antagonists. However, such diminished response to a β-blocker is largely eliminated when the drug is administered concomitantly with a thiazide diuretic. In addition, some experts state that when use of β-blockers is indicated in hypertensive patients with underlying cardiovascular or other risk factors, these indications should be applied equally to black hypertensive patients.

For information on overall principles and expert recommendations for treatment of hypertension, see Uses: Hypertension in Adults, in the Thiazides General Statement 40:28.20.

• Chronic Stable Angina

Metoprolol is used for the management of chronic stable angina pectoris. β-Blockers are recommended as the anti-ischemic drugs of choice in most patients with chronic stable angina; despite differences in cardioselectivity, intrinsic sympathomimetic activity, and other clinical factors, all β-blockers appear to be equally effective for this indication. In placebo-controlled studies, metoprolol reduced the frequency of anginal attacks, reduced nitroglycerin consumption, and increased exercise tolerance.

Combination therapy with a β-blocker and a nitrate appears to be more effective than either drug alone because β-blockers attenuate the increased sympathetic tone and reflex tachycardia associated with nitrate therapy while nitrate therapy (e.g., nitroglycerin) counteracts the potential increase in left-ventricular wall tension associated with a decrease in heart rate. Combined therapy with a β-blocker and a dihydropyridine calcium-channel blocker also may be useful because the tendency to develop tachycardia with the calcium-channel blocker is counteracted by the β-blocker. However, caution should be exercised in the concomitant use of β-blockers and the nondihydropyridine calcium-channel blockers verapamil or diltiazem because of the potential for excessive fatigue, bradycardia, or atrioventricular (AV) block. Concomitant use of metoprolol with cardiac glycosides may be beneficial in patients with angina pectoris, especially in those with cardiomegaly, because both drugs reduce myocardial oxygen consumption; however, the potential effect of combined therapy on AV conduction should be considered. (See Drug Interactions: Cardiovascular Drugs.)

• Non-ST-Segment-Elevation Acute Coronary Syndromes

β-Blockers are used as part of the standard therapeutic measures for managing non-ST-segment-elevation acute coronary syndromes (NSTE ACS). Patients with NSTE ACS have either unstable angina or non-ST-segment-elevation MI (NSTEMI); because these conditions are part of a continuum of acute myocardial ischemia and have indistinguishable clinical features upon presentation, the same initial treatment strategies are recommended. The American Heart Association/American College of Cardiology (AHA/ACC) guideline for the management of patients with NSTE ACS recommends an early invasive strategy (angiographic evaluation with the intent to perform revascularization procedures such as percutaneous coronary intervention [PCI] with coronary artery stent implantation or coronary artery bypass grafting [CABG]) or an ischemia-guided strategy (initial medical management followed by cardiac catheterization and revascularization if indicated) in patients with definite or likely NSTE ACS; standard medical therapies for all patients should include a β-blocker, antiplatelet agents (aspirin and/or a P2Y12-receptor antagonist), anticoagulant agents (e.g., low-molecular weight or unfractionated heparin), nitrates (e.g., nitroglycerin), and analgesic agents regardless of the initial management approach. The guideline states that oral β-blocker therapy should be initiated within the first 24 hours in patients who do not have manifestations of heart failure, evidence of a low-output state, increased risk of cardiogenic shock, or any other contraindications to β-blocker therapy; use of IV β-blockers is potentially harmful in patients with risk factors for cardiogenic shock. Continued therapy with a β-blocker proven to reduce mortality (bisoprolol, carvedilol, or metoprolol succinate) is recommended in patients with stabilized heart failure and reduced systolic function. (See Uses: Heart Failure, in Carvedilol 24:24.)

• Acute Myocardial Infarction

Metoprolol tartrate is used orally and IV to reduce the risk of cardiovascular mortality in hemodynamically stable patients with definite or suspected acute MI. The term MI is used when there is evidence of myocardial necrosis in the setting of acute myocardial ischemia. ST-segment-elevation MI (STEMI) is distinguished from NSTEMI based on the presence or absence of ST-segment elevation on ECG. Patients with STEMI typically have complete arterial occlusion; therefore, immediate reperfusion therapy (with primary PCI or thrombolytic agents) is the current standard of care for such patients. Because the clinical presentation of NSTEMI is similar to that of unstable angina, these conditions are considered together in current expert guidelines. (See Uses: Non-ST-Segment Elevation Acute Coronary Syndromes.) During the early stage of a definite or suspected MI, metoprolol has been initiated with IV doses, followed by continued oral dosing; however, experts currently recommend that early IV use of β-blockers be limited to selected patients.

Because β-blockers can reduce myocardial oxygen demand during the first few hours of an acute MI by reducing heart rate, arterial blood pressure, and/or myocardial contractility, and also have been shown to reduce mortality, early IV therapy with these drugs was routinely recommended following acute MI. Evidence supporting this recommendation was generally based on studies conducted prior to the reperfusion era demonstrating a reduction in mortality and other clinical benefits (i.e., reduced infarct size, incidence of ventricular arrhythmias, chest pain, and cardiac enzyme elevations) with early use of β-blockers during MI. In one double-blind, placebo-controlled study in patients with definite or suspected acute MI, therapy with metoprolol tartrate (initiated IV as soon as possible after arrival to the hospital and continued orally for 3 months) was associated with a 36% reduction in mortality. The mortality benefit of metoprolol was similar between patients who were treated early (no more than 8 hours from the onset of symptoms) and those who initiated treatment at a later time. Patients receiving metoprolol also had substantial reductions in ventricular fibrillation and chest pain. (See Uses: Acute Myocardial Infarction, in Atenolol 24:24.)

Studies conducted after the widespread use of reperfusion therapy generally have demonstrated more attenuated benefits with early β-blocker therapy in patients with acute MI; while β-blockers may still confer benefits (e.g., reduction in the risk of reinfarction and ventricular arrhythmias), there is less certainty regarding the drugs' effects on mortality in patients receiving contemporary revascularization and pharmacologic therapies (antiplatelet agents, ACE inhibitors, and lipid-lowering therapies). In addition, early use of β-blockers (particularly when administered IV) has been associated with an increased risk of cardiogenic shock. In the Clopidogrel and Metoprolol in Myocardial

Infarction Trial (COMMIT), there was no difference in mortality or the combined end point of death, reinfarction, or cardiac arrest between patients receiving early metoprolol therapy (initiated IV for up to 3 doses and continued orally) and those receiving placebo. Although patients who received metoprolol had a lower risk of reinfarction and ventricular fibrillation, these benefits were accompanied by a substantially higher risk of cardiogenic shock, particularly within the first day of treatment. Based on the currently available evidence, the American College of Cardiology Foundation/American Heart Association (ACCF/AHA) guideline for the management of STEMI recommends oral β-blocker therapy in all patients who do not have manifestations of heart failure, evidence of a low-output state, increased risk of cardiogenic shock, or any other contraindications to β-blocker therapy. Such therapy should be initiated within the first 24 hours following acute MI and continued during and after hospitalization. Because of conflicting evidence of benefit and the potential for harm, the guidelines recommend limiting use of IV β-blockers to patients with refractory hypertension or ongoing ischemia.

Although the efficacy of metoprolol tartrate following administration of the drug for longer than 3 months has not been conclusively established, the benefits of long-term β-blocker therapy for secondary prevention have been well established in numerous clinical studies. Patients with MI complicated by heart failure, left ventricular dysfunction, or ventricular arrhythmias appear to derive the most benefit from long-term β-blocker therapy. Data from studies using other β-blockers suggest that treatment should be continued for at least 1–3 years if not indefinitely after infarction unless contraindicated. Several large, randomized studies have demonstrated that long-term therapy with a β-blocker can reduce the rates of reinfarction and mortality (e.g., sudden or nonsudden cardiac death) following acute MI. It is estimated that such therapy could result in a relative reduction in mortality of about 25% annually for years 1–3 after infarction, with high-risk patients exhibiting the greatest potential benefit; the benefit of continued therapy may persist for at least several years beyond this period, although less substantially. Therefore, metoprolol, like other β-blockers, can be used for secondary prevention following acute MI to reduce the risk of reinfarction and mortality. The AHA/ACCF secondary prevention guideline recommends β-blocker therapy in all patients with left ventricular systolic dysfunction (ejection fraction of 40% or less) and a prior MI; use of a β-blocker with proven mortality benefit (bisoprolol, carvedilol, or metoprolol succinate) is recommended. (See Uses: Heart Failure, in Carvedilol 24:24.) Although the benefits of long-term β-blockade in post-MI patients with normal left ventricular function are less well established, the guideline recommends continued β-blocker therapy for at least 3 years in such patients. Further studies are needed to establish the optimal duration of β-blocker therapy for secondary prevention of MI.

● Supraventricular Arrhythmias

β-Blockers, including metoprolol, have been used to slow ventricular rate in patients with supraventricular tachycardia† (SVT). The American College of Cardiology/American Heart Association/Heart Rhythm Society (ACC/AHA/HRS) guideline for the management of adult patients with supraventricular tachycardia recommends the use of β-blockers in the treatment of various SVTs (e.g., atrial flutter, junctional tachycardia, focal atrial tachycardia, AV nodal reentrant tachycardia [AVNRT]); in general, an IV β-blocker is recommended for acute treatment, while an oral β-blocker is recommended for ongoing management of these arrhythmias. Vagal maneuvers and/or IV adenosine are considered first-line interventions for the acute treatment of SVT and should be attempted prior to other therapies when clinically indicated; if such measures are ineffective or not feasible, an IV β-blocker may be considered in hemodynamically stable patients. Although evidence of efficacy is limited, experts state that the overall safety of β-adrenergic blockers warrants their use in patients with SVT. Patients should be closely monitored for hypotension and bradycardia during administration of these drugs.

Atrial Fibrillation and Flutter

β-Blockers, including metoprolol, have been used to slow rapid ventricular response in patients with atrial fibrillation† or atrial flutter†. IV β-blockers (e.g., esmolol, propranolol, metoprolol) are recommended as one of several drug therapy options for ventricular rate control in patients with nonpreexcited atrial fibrillation or flutter; an oral β-blocker may be used for ongoing rate control in such patients. Choice of a specific β-blocker should be individualized based on the patient's clinical condition.

Atrial Tachycardia

IV β-blockers may be used for the acute treatment of patients with hemodynamically stable focal atrial tachycardia† (i.e., regular SVT arising from a localized atrial site), and an oral β-blocker may be used for ongoing management.

While evidence is more limited, IV metoprolol also has been used in patients with multifocal atrial tachycardia† (rapid, irregular rhythm with at least 3 distinct P-wave morphologies) to control ventricular rate and convert to normal sinus rhythm. Multifocal atrial tachycardia is commonly associated with an underlying condition (e.g., pulmonary, coronary, or valvular heart disease) and is generally not responsive to antiarrhythmic drug therapy. Antiarrhythmic drug therapy usually is reserved for patients who do not respond to initial attempts at correcting or managing potential precipitating factors (e.g., exacerbation of COPD or congestive heart failure, electrolyte and/or ventilatory disturbances, infection, theophylline toxicity) or in whom a precipitating factor cannot be identified. Therapy with IV metoprolol has been associated with slowing of atrial and ventricular rates and conversion to sinus rhythm in many patients with this arrhythmia; therefore, some experts state that IV metoprolol may be useful for the acute treatment of patients with multifocal atrial tachycardia who do not have respiratory decompensation, sinus node dysfunction, or AV block. Metoprolol also may be useful orally for chronic suppression of symptomatic multifocal atrial tachycardia.

Paroxysmal Supraventricular Tachycardia

IV β-blockers may be used for the acute treatment of hemodynamically stable patients with paroxysmal supraventricular tachycardia (PSVT), including AVNRT†, that is uncontrolled or unconverted by vagal maneuvers and adenosine; an oral β-blocker may be used for the ongoing management of such patients who are not candidates for, or prefer not to undergo, catheter ablation.

Junctional Tachycardia

β-Blockers are considered one of several drug therapy options for the treatment of junctional tachycardia† (i.e., nonreentrant SVT originating from the AV junction), a rapid, occasionally irregular, narrow-complex tachycardia. While evidence is limited, there is some data indicating that β-blocking agents (specifically propranolol) are modestly effective in terminating and/or reducing the incidence of junctional tachycardia.

● Ventricular Arrhythmias

Ventricular Fibrillation

β-Blockers have been used in patients with cardiac arrest precipitated by ventricular fibrillation or pulseless ventricular tachycardia†. However, AHA states that routine administration of β-adrenergic blocking agents after cardiac arrest is potentially harmful (e.g., may worsen hemodynamic instability, exacerbate heart failure, or cause bradyarrhythmias) and is therefore not recommended.

Polymorphic Ventricular Tachycardia

β-Blockers may be useful in the management of certain forms of polymorphic ventricular tachycardia† (e.g., associated with acute ischemia).

● Heart Failure

Metoprolol is used (usually in conjunction with other heart failure therapies) in the management of mild to moderately severe (New York Heart Association [NYHA] class II or III) heart failure of ischemic, hypertensive, or cardiomyopathic origin. In clinical studies, metoprolol (as extended-release metoprolol succinate) increased survival and reduced the risk of hospitalization in patients with chronic heart failure. Current guidelines for the management of heart failure in adults generally recommend a combination of drug therapies to reduce morbidity and mortality, including neurohormonal antagonists (e.g., ACE inhibitors, angiotensin II receptor antagonists, angiotensin receptor-neprilysin inhibitors [ARNIs], β-blockers, aldosterone receptor antagonists) that inhibit the detrimental compensatory mechanisms in heart failure. Additional agents (e.g., cardiac glycosides, diuretics, sinoatrial modulators [i.e., ivabradine]) added to a heart failure treatment regimen in selected patients have been associated with symptomatic improvement and/or reduction in heart-failure related hospitalizations. Experts recommend that all asymptomatic patients with reduced left ventricular ejection fraction (LVEF) (ACCF/AHA stage B heart failure) receive therapy with an ACE inhibitor and a β-blocker to prevent symptomatic heart failure and to reduce morbidity and mortality. In patients with prior or current symptoms of heart failure and reduced LVEF (ACCF/AHA stage C heart failure), ACCF, AHA, and the Heart Failure Society of America (HFSA) recommend inhibition of the renin-angiotensin-aldosterone (RAA) system with an ACE inhibitor, angiotensin II receptor antagonist, or ARNI in conjunction with a β-blocker, and an aldosterone antagonist in selected patients, to reduce morbidity and mortality. While ACE inhibitors have been the preferred drugs for inhibition of the RAA system because of their established benefits in patients with heart failure and reduced ejection fraction, some evidence indicates that therapy with an ARNI may be more effective than ACE inhibitor therapy in reducing cardiovascular death and heart failure-related hospitalization in such patients. ACCF, AHA, and HFSA recommend that patients with chronic symptomatic heart failure with reduced LVEF (NYHA class II or III) who are able to tolerate an ACE inhibitor or angiotensin II receptor antagonist be switched to therapy containing an ARNI to further reduce morbidity and mortality.

Because of favorable effects on survival and disease progression, therapy with a clinical trial-proven β-blocker (bisoprolol, carvedilol, extended-release metoprolol succinate) should be initiated as soon as the patient is diagnosed with heart failure and reduced LVEF. While bisoprolol, carvedilol, and extended-release metoprolol have been effective in reducing the risk of death in patients with chronic heart failure, these positive findings should not be considered indicative of a β-blocker class effect. Even when symptoms are mild or improve with other therapies, β-blocker therapy should not be delayed until symptoms return or the disease progresses. Despite concerns about β-blockade potentially masking some signs of hypoglycemia, patients with diabetes mellitus may be particularly likely to experience a reduction in morbidity and mortality with the use of β-blockers. If a patient cannot tolerate a β-blocker or if increasing the β-blocker dosage is ineffective, ivabradine should be considered an alternative or additional treatment option. Some evidence suggests that ivabradine is effective in reducing hospitalizations related to heart failure, but unlike β-blockers, ivabradine has not been shown to reduce cardiovascular mortality.(See Uses: Heart Failure, in Ivabradine 24:04.92.)

In individualizing the decision to use a β-blocker, clinicians should consider that clinical studies establishing the effects of these drugs on morbidity and mortality excluded patients who were hospitalized or had unstable symptoms and enrolled few patients with current or recent NYHA class IV symptoms. The efficacy of β-blockers in such patients is not known, and they may be at particular risk of deterioration following initiation of therapy with β-blockers.

In a large, randomized, double-blind, placebo-controlled study (Metoprolol CR/XL Randomized Intervention Trial in Congestive Heart Failure [MERIT-HF]) in patients with mild to severe (NYHA class II–IV) heart failure and a left ventricular ejection fraction of 0.4 or less, therapy with metoprolol succinate (as extended-release tablets) 12.5–25 mg daily as the tartrate (initial dosage depending on NYHA class, with dosage increased over 8 weeks to a target daily dosage of 200 mg daily) in addition to optimal standard therapy (principally ACE inhibitors and diuretics) was associated with a reduction in all-cause mortality of 34% (mortality rates of 7.2 and 11% with metoprolol and placebo, respectively). The MERIT-HF trial was terminated early because of the favorable effects of metoprolol on overall mortality; the mean follow-up period was 1 year. Sudden deaths and deaths from worsening heart failure also were reduced with metoprolol therapy. In addition to improved survival, metoprolol therapy improved NYHA class, reduced hospitalizations due to worsening heart failure, and resulted in beneficial effects on patient well-being (as determined by quality-of-life measurements); the composite end point of overall mortality and hospitalization for any cause was reduced by 19%. Metoprolol therapy appeared to be well tolerated, with 64% of patients achieving the target dosage of 200 mg daily and 87% tolerating a daily dosage of 100 mg; the mean daily dosage of metoprolol as the tartrate was 159 mg.

The beneficial effects of β-blockers in the management of heart failure are thought to result principally from inhibition of the effects of the sympathetic nervous system. Although the specific effects on the heart and circulation that are responsible for progression of heart failure remain to be established, sympathetic activity can increase ventricular volumes and pressure secondary to peripheral vasoconstriction and by impairing sodium excretion by the kidneys. Other sympathetic effects (e.g., induction of cardiac hypertrophy, arrhythmogenic activity) also may be involved. Collective experience indicates that long-term therapy with β-blockers, like that with ACE inhibitors, can reduce heart failure symptoms and improve clinical status in patients with chronic heart failure and also can decrease

the risk of death as well as the combined risk of death and hospitalization. These beneficial effects were demonstrated in patients already receiving an ACE inhibitor, suggesting that combined inhibition of the renin-angiotensin system and sympathetic nervous system can produce additive effects.

β-Blockers should not be used in patients with acutely decompensated heart failure requiring IV inotropic therapy (see Cautions: Precautions and Contraindications) and those with substantial fluid retention requiring intensive diuresis. In the absence of hemodynamic instability or contraindications, it has been recommended that patients with heart failure and a reduced ejection fraction who are hospitalized for a symptomatic exacerbation continue to receive maintenance treatment with standard oral therapy (e.g., β-blocker, ACE inhibitor). Withholding of, or reduction in, β-blocker therapy may be considered in patients hospitalized after recent initiation or increase in β-blocker therapy. Initiation of β-blocker therapy in hospitalized patients is recommended once the patient's condition is stabilized (i.e., after optimization of volume status and successful discontinuance of IV diuretics, vasodilators, and inotropic agents). Caution should be used when initiating β-blockers in patients who have required inotrope therapy during their hospitalization.

● Vascular Headache

Migraine

Metoprolol has been used for the prophylaxis of migraine headache†. When used prophylactically, metoprolol can prevent migraine or reduce the number of attacks in some patients. Results of comparative studies suggest that metoprolol may be comparable to propranolol for this indication. However, the US Headache Consortium states that the quality of evidence for metoprolol is not as compelling as it is for propranolol for this indication. Metoprolol is not recommended for the treatment of a migraine attack that has already started. For further information on management and classification of migraine headache, see Vascular Headaches: General Principles in Migraine Therapy, under Uses in Sumatriptan 28:32.28.

DOSAGE AND ADMINISTRATION

● Administration

Metoprolol tartrate and metoprolol succinate are administered orally. Metoprolol tartrate also may be administered IV.

Absorption of metoprolol tartrate may be enhanced by administration with food. The manufacturer recommends that metoprolol tartrate be administered with or immediately following meals. Although administration with meals is not required, metoprolol tartrate should be given in a standardized relation to meals to minimize variance in effect. Food does not appear to affect the bioavailability of metoprolol succinate extended-release tablets.

Metoprolol tartrate may be administered daily as a single dose or in divided doses; metoprolol succinate extended-release tablets should be administered daily as a single dose. If a dose is missed, the patient should take only the next scheduled dose (i.e., the next dose should not be doubled). Metoprolol succinate extended-release tablets are scored and can be divided; however, the tablet or half tablet should be swallowed whole and should not be chewed or crushed.

Dispensing and Administration Precautions

Because of similarity in spelling between Toprol-XL® (a trade name for metoprolol succinate) and Topamax® (the trade name for topiramate, an anticonvulsant and antimigraine agent), the potential exists for dispensing or prescribing errors involving these drugs. In addition, there is a potential for dispensing errors involving confusion between Toprol-XL® and Tegretol® or Tegretol®-XR (trade names for carbamazepine, an anticonvulsant that also is used for relief of pain associated with trigeminal neuralgia, as well as for various psychiatric disorders). According to medication error reports, the overlapping tablet strengths between Toprol-XL® and Topamax® (25, 50, 100, and 200 mg) and between Toprol-XL® and Tegretol® or Tegretol®-XR (100 and 200 mg) and the fact that these drugs were stored closely together in pharmacies also may have been contributing factors in causing these errors. Another contributing factor to dispensing errors associated with Toprol-XL® and Topamax® may be the use of mnemonic abbreviations in computerized listings incorporating the first 3 letters and dose strength (e.g., "TOP25"). Extra care should be exercised to ensure the accuracy of both oral and written prescriptions for these drugs. The manufacturers of Toprol-XL® and Topamax® also recommend that pharmacists assess various measures of avoiding dispensing errors and implement them as appropriate (e.g., by verifying all orders for these drugs by citing both the trade and generic names to prescribers, attaching reminders to pharmacy shelves, separating the drugs on pharmacy shelves, counseling patients).(See Cautions: Precautions and Contraindications.)

Extemporaneously Compounded Oral Liquid

An extemporaneously compounded oral liquid formulation of metoprolol tartrate containing 10 mg/mL has been prepared using the commercially available tablets and sweetened vehicles.

Standardize 4 Safety

Standardized concentrations for an extemporaneously prepared oral liquid formulation of metoprolol have been established through Standardize 4 Safety (S4S), a national patient safety initiative to reduce medication errors, especially during transitions of care. Multidisciplinary expert panels were convened to determine recommended standard concentrations. Because recommendations from the S4S panels may differ from the manufacturer's prescribing information, caution is advised when using concentrations that differ from labeling, particularly when using rate information from the label. For additional information on S4S (including updates that may be available), see https://www.ashp.org/pharmacy-practice/standardize-4-safety-initiative.

TABLE 1. Standardize 4 Safety Compounded Oral Liquid Standards for Metoprolol

Concentration Standards
10 mg/mL

● Dosage

Dosages of metoprolol tartrate and metoprolol succinate are expressed in terms of the tartrate. Since there is no consistent interpatient correlation between the dosage of metoprolol and therapeutic response, dosage must be individualized according to the response of the patient. Blood pressure should be measured near the end of a dosing interval to determine whether satisfactory control is being maintained throughout the day. When patients receiving metoprolol tartrate conventional tablets are switched to metoprolol succinate extended-release tablets, the same daily dosage should be used. If long-term metoprolol therapy is to be discontinued, dosage of the drug should be gradually reduced over a period of 1–2 weeks. (See Cautions: Precautions and Contraindications.)

Hypertension

Metoprolol Therapy

The manufacturers state that the usual initial adult oral dosage of metoprolol tartrate conventional tablets, given alone or in combination with a diuretic, is 100 mg daily given in single or divided doses. When administered as metoprolol succinate extended-release tablets, the manufacturers state that the recommended initial dosage in terms of metoprolol tartrate is 25–100 mg administered once daily. Some clinicians recommend an initial dosage of at least 50 mg 3 times daily as metoprolol tartrate conventional tablets, for better control. Dosage may be increased at weekly (or longer) intervals until optimum hypotensive effect is achieved. In general, the maximum effect of any given dosage will be apparent within 1 week. The manufacturers state that oral dosages in terms of metoprolol tartrate should not exceed 450 mg daily as conventional tablets or 400 mg daily as extended-release tablets; dosages of the respective formulations exceeding these have not been studied.

Some experts state the usual dosage range is 100–200 mg daily, given in 2 divided doses daily as conventional tablets or 50–200 mg once daily given as extended-release tablets.

The fact that β₁-adrenergic blocking selectivity of metoprolol diminishes as dosage is increased should be considered.

Patients with severe hypertension may require more uniform plasma concentrations for adequate control and in some hypertensive patients, especially when lower dosages (e.g., 100 mg daily) are used, blood pressure increases slightly toward the end of the dosing interval with once- or twice-daily administration. If a satisfactory response is not maintained throughout the day, larger doses, more frequent administration, or use of extended-release tablets may achieve better control.

If metoprolol tartrate is used for the management of hypertension in children 1–17 years of age†, some experts have recommended an initial oral dosage of 1–2 mg/kg daily given in 2 divided doses. Such experts have suggested that dosage may be increased as necessary to a maximum dosage of 6 mg/kg (up to 200 mg) daily given in 2 divided doses. The manufacturer states that if extended-release metoprolol succinate is used for hypertension in children 6 years of age or older, an initial oral dosage of 1 mg/kg (up to 50 mg) daily in terms of metoprolol tartrate is recommended. The dosage should be adjusted according to blood pressure response. The safety and efficacy of dosages exceeding 2 mg/kg (or 200 mg) once daily have not been established in pediatric patients. For information on overall principles and expert recommendations for treatment of hypertension in pediatric patients, see Uses: Hypertension in Pediatric Patients, in the Thiazides General Statement 40:28.20.

Metoprolol/Hydrochlorothiazide Fixed-combination Therapy

When combination therapy is required, the manufacturer recommends that commercially available preparations containing metoprolol tartrate in fixed combination with a thiazide diuretic should not be used initially. Dosage should first be adjusted by administering each drug separately. If it is determined that the optimum maintenance dosage corresponds to the ratio in the commercial combination preparation, the fixed combination may be used. Dosage regimens using fixed-combination preparations that exceed 50 mg of hydrochlorothiazide daily are not recommended.

Blood Pressure Monitoring and Treatment Goals

Blood pressure should be monitored regularly (i.e., monthly) during therapy and dosage of the antihypertensive drug adjusted until blood pressure is controlled. If an adequate blood pressure response is not achieved, the dosage may be increased or another antihypertensive agent with demonstrated benefit and preferably with a complementary mechanism of action (e.g., angiotensin-converting enzyme [ACE] inhibitor, angiotensin II receptor antagonist, calcium-channel blocker, thiazide diuretic) may be added; if target blood pressure is still not achieved with the use of 2 antihypertensive agents, a third drug may be added.(See Uses: Hypertension.) In patients who develop unacceptable adverse effects with metoprolol, the drug should be discontinued and another antihypertensive agent from a different pharmacologic class should be initiated.

The goal of hypertension management and prevention is to achieve and maintain optimal control of blood pressure. However, the optimum blood pressure threshold for initiating antihypertensive drug therapy and specific treatment goals remain controversial. While previous hypertension guidelines have based target blood pressure goals on age and comorbidities, the 2017 American College of Cardiology/American Heart Association (ACC/AHA) hypertension guideline incorporates underlying cardiovascular risk into decision making regarding treatment and generally recommends the same target blood pressure (i.e., less than 130/80 mm Hg) for all adults. Many patients will require at least 2 drugs from different pharmacologic classes to achieve this blood pressure goal; the potential benefits of hypertension management and drug cost, adverse effects, and risks associated with the use of multiple antihypertensive drugs also should be considered when deciding a patient's blood pressure treatment goal.

For additional information on target levels of blood pressure and on monitoring therapy in the management of hypertension, see Blood Pressure Monitoring and Treatment Goals under Dosage: Hypertension, in Dosage and Administration in the Thiazides General Statement 40:28.20.

Chronic Stable Angina

For the long-term management of angina pectoris, the initial adult dosage of metoprolol tartrate (conventional tablets) or metoprolol succinate (extended-release tablets) is 100 mg as the tartrate daily given in 2 divided doses or in a single dose, respectively. Dosage may be increased at weekly intervals until optimum control of angina is obtained or there is pronounced slowing of the heart rate. The usual maintenance dosage of metoprolol tartrate (conventional tablets) or metoprolol succinate (extended-release tablets) is 100–400 mg (expressed in terms of metoprolol tartrate) daily. Oral dosages exceeding 400 mg daily (given as metoprolol tartrate conventional tablets or as metoprolol succinate extended-release tablets) have not been studied. When discontinuance of metoprolol therapy is planned, dosage of the drug should be gradually reduced over a period of about 1–2 weeks. (See Cautions: Precautions and Contraindications.)

Acute Myocardial Infarction

Early Treatment

The manufacturer states that metoprolol therapy may be initiated as soon as possible after an acute myocardial infarction (MI) when the patient's hemodynamic condition has stabilized. During the early stage of a definite or suspected MI, the manufacturer recommends that treatment with metoprolol tartrate be initiated with the administration of three 5-mg rapid IV injections given at approximately 2-minute intervals as tolerated. Heart rate, blood pressure, and ECG should be monitored during IV administration, and the drug should be titrated to response. In patients who tolerate the full IV dose (15 mg), the manufacturer states that oral administration of metoprolol tartrate should be initiated 15 minutes after the last IV dose at a dosage of 50 mg every 6 hours for 48 hours. Thereafter, an oral maintenance dosage of 100 mg twice daily should be used. Patients who appear not to tolerate the usual total IV dose should initially receive an oral metoprolol tartrate dosage of 25 or 50 mg (depending on the degree of intolerance) every 6 hours beginning 15 minutes after the last IV dose or as soon as their clinical condition allows. In patients with severe intolerance, metoprolol should be discontinued.

The American College of Cardiology Foundation/American Heart Association (ACCF/AHA) guideline for the management of ST-segment-elevation MI (STEMI) recommends initiation of oral β-blocker therapy within the first 24 hours in patients who do not have manifestations of heart failure, evidence of a low-output state, increased risk of cardiogenic shock, or any other contraindications to β-blocker therapy. The recommended oral dosage of metoprolol tartrate is 25–50 mg every 6–12 hours; patients should be transitioned over the following 2–3 days to twice-daily dosing (using metoprolol tartrate) or daily dosing (using metoprolol succinate). Dosage should be titrated up to a total daily dose of 200 mg as tolerated. Because IV β-blockers can be potentially harmful in patients with risk factors for cardiogenic shock, these experts recommend that IV use be limited to patients who have refractory hypertension or have ongoing ischemia at the time of presentation. If IV therapy is employed, the recommended IV dosage of metoprolol tartrate is 5 mg every 5 minutes as tolerated up to 3 doses.

Late Treatment and Long-term Secondary Prevention

In patients who have contraindications to metoprolol therapy during the early phase of definite or suspected acute MI, in patients who appear not to tolerate the full early treatment, or in patients in whom therapy is delayed for any other reason, the manufacturer recommends initiation of metoprolol therapy with an oral dosage of 100 mg twice daily as soon as their clinical condition allows. The manufacturer states that oral metoprolol therapy should be continued for at least 3 months; however, the optimal duration of β-blocker therapy following MI remains to be clearly established. Experts generally recommend that such therapy be continued long-term in post-MI patients with left ventricular systolic dysfunction, and for at least 3 years in those with normal left ventricular function.

Atrial Fibrillation

To slow rapid ventricular response in adults with atrial fibrillation†, metoprolol tartrate has been administered IV in doses of 2.5–5 mg administered over 2 minutes, up to a total of 3 doses. Once adequate control of heart rate or conversion to normal sinus rhythm has been achieved with parenteral metoprolol therapy, some experts suggest an oral metoprolol tartrate dosage of 25–100 mg twice daily or extended-release metoprolol succinate at a dosage of 50–400 mg once daily for long-term rate control in patients with atrial fibrillation.

Other Supraventricular Arrhythmias

For the acute treatment of supraventricular tachycardia (SVT) (e.g., atrial flutter†, junctional tachycardia†, paroxysmal supraventricular tachycardia [PSVT]†, atrial tachycardia†) in adults, some experts recommend an initial IV metoprolol tartrate dose of 2.5–5 mg administered over 2 minutes; additional doses may be given every 10 minutes up to a maximum of 3 doses. The usual oral maintenance dosage for ongoing treatment of SVT is 200 mg twice daily (as metoprolol tartrate tablets) or 400 mg once daily (as metoprolol succinate extended-release tablets).

Heart Failure

Prior to initiation of therapy with a β-blocker in patients with heart failure, the dosage of any concomitant heart failure therapy should be stabilized. Because of the potential for severe adverse effects (e.g., hypotension, bradycardia, fluid retention, worsening of heart failure), initiation of β-blocker therapy for heart failure and subsequent dosage adjustments should occur under close medical supervision.

For the management of symptomatic heart failure, the manufacturer recommends an initial metoprolol succinate (extended-release tablets) dosage of 25 mg (expressed as the tartrate) once daily in adults with New York Heart Association (NYHA) class II heart failure; adults with more severe heart failure should receive an initial dosage of 12.5 mg once daily. The manufacturer recommends that the dosage be doubled every 2 weeks until a dosage of 200 mg once daily or the highest tolerated dosage is reached. Some experts recommend initiation of β-blocker therapy at a very low dosage (e.g., a metoprolol succinate dosage of 12.5–25 mg once daily [expressed as metoprolol tartrate] using the extended-release tablets) in patients with heart failure, with the dosage gradually titrated upward as tolerated (maximum dosage 200 mg once daily). If deterioration of heart failure (usually transient) becomes evident during titration of metoprolol therapy, the dosage of the concurrent diuretic should be increased and the dosage of metoprolol not escalated until symptoms of worsening heart failure (e.g., fluid retention) have stabilized; it may be necessary to decrease the dosage of metoprolol or temporarily discontinue the drug. Should patients with heart failure experience symptomatic bradycardia (e.g., dizziness) or second- or third-degree heart block, the dosage of metoprolol should be reduced. Initial difficulty in titrating metoprolol dosage should not preclude subsequent attempts to successfully titrate the dosage.

It should be recognized that symptomatic improvement may not be evident for 2–3 months after initiating therapy with β-blockers. However, β-blocker therapy may reduce the risk of disease progression even if symptomatic improvement is not evident. In clinical trials, metoprolol dosages were *not* adjusted according to response but instead were increased as tolerated to a prespecified target dose. Once titrated to the target or highest tolerated dosage, therapy generally can be maintained at this level long term. In clinical trials, dosages usually were titrated up to 150–200 mg daily.

Vascular Headaches

Migraine

Although dosages of metoprolol tartrate or metoprolol succinate for the prophylaxis of migraine† in adults have not been established, oral dosages of 50–300 mg daily have been used in clinical studies. The usual effective dosage of the drug in these studies was 200 mg daily.

CAUTIONS

Metoprolol shares the toxic potentials of β-adrenergic blocking agents (β-blockers). Most adverse effects of metoprolol are mild and transient and occur more frequently at the onset of therapy than during prolonged treatment. The most frequent adverse effects are dizziness, tiredness, insomnia, and gastric upset.

● Cardiovascular and Cerebrovascular Effects

The most common adverse cardiovascular effects of metoprolol are shortness of breath and bradycardia, occurring in about 3% of patients with hypertension or angina receiving metoprolol tartrate in clinical trials. Severe bradycardia should be treated with IM or IV administration of atropine sulfate. If there is an inadequate response to atropine, IV isoproterenol may be administered with caution. Cold extremities, arterial insufficiency (e.g., Raynaud's phenomenon), palpitations, congestive heart failure, peripheral edema, syncope, chest pain, or hypotension has been reported in about 1% of patients with hypertension or angina receiving metoprolol tartrate. Gangrene has been reported very rarely in patients with preexisting severe peripheral circulatory disorders receiving metoprolol tartrate. Claudication has been reported in patients with myocardial infarction (MI) receiving metoprolol tartrate, although a relationship to the drug is unclear. Raynaud's phenomenon may be treated by keeping the patient warm, stopping the drug, and, if necessary, administering a vasodilator. Adverse cardiovascular events occurring in greater than 1% of patients with heart failure receiving metoprolol succinate extended-release tablets but with a similar incidence (within 0.5%) in patients receiving placebo include MI, coronary artery disorder, cerebrovascular disorder, ventricular tachycardia, or aggravation of arrhythmia.

If hypotension (systolic blood pressure of 90 mm Hg or less) occurs in patients with MI, metoprolol should be discontinued and appropriate cardiovascular monitoring and therapy instituted as necessary. (See Cautions: Precautions and Contraindications.) In patients without a prior history of heart failure, prolonged depression of the myocardium by metoprolol occasionally has resulted in heart failure. Intensification of AV block has occurred with other β-blockers and is a potential adverse effect of metoprolol. AV dissociation, AV conduction delays, complete heart block or cardiac arrest also may occur, especially in patients with preexisting heart block caused by digitalis or other factors.

During surgery, some patients who have received β-blockers may experience severe, protracted hypotension and, occasionally, difficulty in restarting and maintaining heart beat. The untoward effects of metoprolol may be reversed during surgery by IV administration of β-adrenergic agonists (e.g., isoproterenol, dopamine, dobutamine).

Nervous System Effects

Tiredness or dizziness has occurred in about 10% of patients with hypertension or angina receiving metoprolol tartrate in clinical trials; tiredness has been reported in about 1% of patients with MI receiving the drug. In addition, vertigo, sleep disturbances/insomnia, hallucinations, nightmares, headache, dizziness, visual disturbances, and confusion have been reported in patients with MI receiving the drug, although a causal relationship is unclear. Somnolence or increased dreaming also has been reported with metoprolol therapy; these effects may be alleviated by avoiding late-evening dosage. Rarely, impotence, nervousness, and general weakness have occurred. Depression has been reported in about 5% of patients receiving metoprolol tartrate for hypertension or angina. Reversible mental depression occurs less frequently with metoprolol than with propranolol but is a reason for withdrawal of the drugs, as it may progress to catatonia. An acute reversible syndrome characterized by disorientation to time and place, short-term memory loss, emotional lability, slightly clouded sensorium, and decreased performance on neuropsychometric tests has been reported with other β-blockers and should be considered a potential adverse effect of metoprolol. Lethargy and, rarely, fullheadedness have occurred.

GI Effects

Diarrhea has occurred in about 5% of patients receiving metoprolol tartrate in clinical trials. Other GI symptoms such as nausea, gastric pain, constipation, flatulence, digestive tract disorders, heartburn, xerostomia, and hiccups also have been reported with oral metoprolol therapy. Nausea and abdominal pain have occurred in less than 1% of patients with MI receiving IV or oral metoprolol.

Endocrine Effects

Unstable diabetes mellitus has been reported in patients with MI receiving metoprolol tartrate, although a relationship to the drug is unclear. Results of a large prospective cohort study of adults 45–64 years of age indicate that use of β-blockers in hypertensive patients is associated with increased risk (about 28%) of developing diabetes mellitus. In this study, the number of new cases of diabetes per 1000 person-years was 33.6 or 26.3 in patients receiving a β-blocker or no drug therapy, respectively. The association between the risk of developing diabetes mellitus and use of β-blockers reportedly was not confounded by weight gain, hyperinsulinemia, or differences in heart rate. It is not known if the risk of developing diabetes is affected by β-receptor selectivity. Further studies are needed to determine whether concomitant use of ACE inhibitors (which may improve insulin sensitivity) would abrogate β-blocker-induced adverse effects related to glucose intolerance. Therefore, until results of such studies are available, the proven benefits of β-blockers in reducing cardiovascular events in hypertensive patients must be weighed carefully against the possible risks of developing diabetes mellitus.

Hypoglycemia, which may result in loss of consciousness, also may occur in nondiabetic patients receiving β-adrenergic blocking agents. Patients most at risk for the development of β-blocker-induced hypoglycemia are those undergoing dialysis, prolonged fasting, or severe exercise regimens.

β-Blockers may mask signs and symptoms of hypoglycemia (e.g., palpitation, tachycardia, tremor) and potentiate insulin-induced hypoglycemia. Although it has been suggested that nonselective β-blockers are more likely to induce hypoglycemia than selective β-blockers, such an adverse effect also has been reported with selective β-blockers (e.g., atenolol). Selective β-blockers are less likely to mask symptoms of hypoglycemia or delay recovery from insulin-induced hypoglycemia than nonselective β-blockers; however, selective β-blockers can decrease insulin sensitivity by approximately 15–30%, which may result in increased insulin requirements.

Other Adverse Effects

In spite of its relative β_1-blocking selectivity, β_2-adrenergic blockade leading to bronchoconstriction, dyspnea, and wheezing may occur with metoprolol dosages greater than 100 mg daily, particularly in patients with a history of asthma. Wheezing or dyspnea has been reported in about 1% of patients with hypertension or angina receiving metoprolol, and dyspnea of pulmonary origin has been reported in less than 1% of patients with MI receiving the drug. Rhinitis also has been reported in patients receiving metoprolol tartrate. In a large clinical trial, pneumonia was reported in greater than 1% of patients with heart failure receiving metoprolol succinate extended-release tablets but with a similar incidence (within 0.5%) in patients receiving placebo.

Peyronie's disease, tinnitus, restless legs, a polymyalgia-like syndrome, musculoskeletal pain, decreased libido, blurred vision, dry mucous membranes, and sweating have occurred rarely in patients receiving metoprolol. Fatigue was reported in greater than 1% of patients with heart failure receiving metoprolol succinate extended-release tablets in a large clinical trial but with a similar incidence (within 0.5%) in patients receiving placebo.

Pruritus, dry skin, worsening of psoriasis, and psoriasiform, maculopapular, and urticarial rash have occurred in some patients receiving metoprolol. Allergic reactions reported in patients receiving other β-blockers include erythematous rash, fever combined with aching and sore throat, laryngospasm, and respiratory distress. Reversible alopecia, agranulocytosis, thrombocytopenia, weight gain, arthritis, retroperitoneal fibrosis, and dry eyes have been reported rarely with metoprolol therapy. Discontinuance of the drug should be considered if any such reaction is not otherwise explicable. There have been some reported cases of increased antinuclear factor (ANF) levels during metoprolol therapy; however, other reports indicate decreased ANF levels, and no positive ANF findings have been associated with adverse effects of metoprolol involving the skin and eyes.

Potential hematologic effects of β-blockers include eosinophilia, agranulocytosis, and nonthrombocytopenic and thrombocytopenic purpura.

Other β-blockers may cause elevated BUN and serum creatinine concentrations in patients with severe heart disease, presumably because of decreased renal blood flow. Hepatitis, jaundice, or nonspecific hepatic dysfunction has been reported during postmarketing experience in patients receiving metoprolol. Subclinical hepatitis of unknown etiology occurred in one patient receiving metoprolol therapy for 6 months. Isolated instances of elevated serum transaminase, alkaline phosphatase, and lactate dehydrogenase concentrations also have been reported during postmarketing experience with metoprolol therapy. Metoprolol may increase serum uric acid concentration.

Precautions and Contraindications

Metoprolol shares the toxic potentials of β-blockers, and the usual precautions of these agents should be observed. When metoprolol is used as a fixed-combination preparation that includes hydrochlorothiazide, the cautions, precautions, and contraindications associated with thiazide diuretics must be considered in addition to those associated with metoprolol.

In patients with heart failure, sympathetic stimulation is vital for the support of circulatory function. Metoprolol should be used with caution in patients with inadequate myocardial function, since heart failure may be precipitated by blockade of β-adrenergic stimulation when metoprolol therapy is administered. Exercise tolerance may decrease in patients with left ventricular dysfunction. In addition, in patients with latent cardiac insufficiency, prolonged β-adrenergic blockade may lead to cardiac failure. Although β-blockers should be avoided in patients with overt or decompensated heart failure, metoprolol may be administered cautiously to patients with well-compensated heart failure (e.g., those controlled with ACE inhibitors, diuretics, and/or cardiac glycosides). Patients receiving metoprolol therapy should be instructed to consult their physician at the first sign or symptom of impending cardiac failure (e.g., weight gain, increasing shortness of breath) and should be adequately treated (e.g., with a cardiac glycoside and/or diuretic) and observed closely; if cardiac failure continues, metoprolol should be discontinued, gradually if possible. Metoprolol should be administered with caution in patients with sinus node dysfunction, since the drug can depress SA node automaticity.

Abrupt withdrawal of β-blocker therapy may exacerbate angina symptoms or precipitate MI in patients with coronary artery disease. Therefore, patients receiving metoprolol (especially those with ischemic heart disease) should be warned not to interrupt or discontinue therapy without consulting their physician. When discontinuance of metoprolol therapy is planned, particularly in patients with ischemic heart disease, dosage of the drug should be gradually reduced over a period of about 1–2 weeks. When metoprolol therapy is discontinued, patients should be monitored carefully and advised to temporarily limit their physical activity. If exacerbation of angina occurs or acute coronary insufficiency develops after metoprolol therapy is interrupted, metoprolol therapy should be reinstituted promptly, at least temporarily, and appropriate measures for the management of unstable angina pectoris should be initiated. Because coronary artery disease is common and may be unrecognized, it may be prudent not to discontinue metoprolol therapy abruptly, even in patients receiving the drug for conditions other than angina.

In patients with MI, hemodynamic status should be carefully monitored during metoprolol therapy. If heart rate decreases to less than 40 beats/minute in patients receiving the drug, particularly if associated with evidence of decreased cardiac output, the manufacturer recommends that IV atropine be administered; if the bradycardia is refractory to atropine, the manufacturer recommends that metoprolol be discontinued and that cautious administration of isoproterenol or use of a cardiac pacemaker be considered. If heart block occurs in patients with MI during metoprolol therapy, the manufacturer recommends that the drug be discontinued and IV atropine be administered; if the heart block is refractory to atropine, the manufacturer recommends that cautious administration of isoproterenol or use of a cardiac pacemaker be considered. If hypotension (systolic blood pressure of 90 mm Hg or less) occurs in patients with MI, the manufacturer recommends that metoprolol be discontinued and the hemodynamic status of the patient and the extent of myocardial damage be carefully assessed. Invasive monitoring of central venous, pulmonary capillary wedge, and arterial pressures may be necessary; appropriate therapy with IV fluids and other treatment modalities should be instituted. If hypotension is associated with severe bradycardia or heart block, treatment should be directed at reversing these effects.

Metoprolol should be used with caution in patients undergoing major surgery involving general anesthesia, and the anesthetic used should be one that does not cause myocardial depression. (See Drug Interactions: Other Drugs.) The necessity of withdrawing β-adrenergic blocking therapy prior to major surgery is controversial. Metoprolol may impair the ability of the heart to respond to reflex β-adrenergic stimuli and may increase the risks associated with general anesthesia such as severe hypotension and maintenance of heart beat. As with other β-blockers, the effects of metoprolol can be reversed by administration of β-agonists (e.g., dobutamine, isoproterenol). If metoprolol is continued during major or dental surgery, the anesthesiologist or dentist should be informed that the patient is receiving the drug.

Since β-blockers may inhibit bronchodilation produced by endogenous catecholamines, the drugs generally should not be used in patients with bronchospastic disease; however, because of its relative β_1-selective adrenergic blocking activity, metoprolol may be used with caution in patients with bronchospastic disease who do not respond to or cannot tolerate other hypotensive agents. In such patients, the lowest effective dosage of metoprolol should be used in addition to maximal therapy with a β_2-adrenergic agonist (e.g., terbutaline); in addition, it would be prudent to initially administer metoprolol in lower dosage given in 3 divided doses daily to avoid the higher plasma concentrations of the drug associated with twice-daily dosing. Patients receiving metoprolol should contact their physician if any difficulty in breathing occurs. Bronchoconstriction is readily reversed with β_2-adrenergic agonists.

Although the oculomucocutaneous syndrome associated with practolol use has not occurred with metoprolol, some patients have experienced dry eyes and decreased tear production, minimal injection of conjunctivae and/or eyelids, punctate keratitis, keratoconjunctivitis or corneal ulceration; therefore, patients receiving metoprolol should be observed carefully for potential ocular adverse effects.

Signs of hyperthyroidism (e.g., tachycardia) may be masked by metoprolol, and patients having or suspected of developing thyrotoxicosis should be monitored carefully because abrupt withdrawal of β-adrenergic blockade might precipitate thyroid storm. In addition, it is recommended that metoprolol be used with caution in patients with diabetes mellitus (especially those with labile diabetes) since the drug also may mask signs and symptoms of hypoglycemia (e.g., tachycardia, palpitation, blood pressure changes, tremor, feelings of anxiety, but not sweating) and may potentiate insulin-induced hypoglycemia.(see Cautions: Endocrine Effects.) However, many clinicians state that patients with diabetes mellitus may be particularly likely to experience a reduction in morbidity and mortality with the use of β-blockers.

The manufacturer states that metoprolol should be used with caution in patients with impaired hepatic function.

Because of similarity in spelling between Toprol-XL® (metoprolol succinate) and Topamax® (the trade name for topiramate, an anticonvulsant and antimigraine agent), the potential exists for dispensing or prescribing errors involving these drugs. In addition, there is a potential for dispensing errors involving confusion between Toprol-XL® and Tegretol® or Tegretol®-XR (trade names for carbamazepine, an anticonvulsant that also is used for relief of pain associated with trigeminal neuralgia, as well as for various psychiatric disorders). These medication errors have been associated with serious adverse events sometimes requiring hospitalization as a result of either lack of the intended medication (e.g., seizure recurrence, return of hallucinations, suicide attempt, hypertension recurrence) or exposure to the wrong drug (e.g., bradycardia in a patient erroneously receiving metoprolol). Therefore, extra care should be exercised to ensure the accuracy of both oral and written prescriptions for these drugs. (See Dispensing and Administration Precautions, in Dosage and Administration: Administration.) Patients should be advised to carefully check their medications and to bring any questions or concerns to the attention of the dispensing pharmacist. Dispensing errors involving Toprol-XL® (metoprolol succinate) and Topamax® (topiramate) or Tegretol® or Tegretol®–XR (carbamazepine) should be reported to the manufacturers, the USP/ISMP (Institute for Safe Medication Practices) Medication Errors Reporting Program by phone (800-233-7767), or directly to the FDA MedWatch program by phone (800-FDA-1088), fax (800-FDA-0178), or internet (http://www.fda.gov/Safety/MedWatch).

Metoprolol should be used with caution, if at all, in patients with AV conduction defects. The drug should be used with extreme caution in patients with substantial cardiomegaly. Metoprolol is contraindicated in patients with hypertension or angina who have sinus bradycardia, heart block greater than first degree, cardiogenic shock, overt or decompensated cardiac failure, severe peripheral, arterial circulatory disorders, pheochromocytoma (unless administered after initiating treatment with an alpha-adrenergic blocking agent), or sick sinus syndrome (unless a permanent pacemaker is in place). The drug is contraindicated in patients with acute MI who have a heart rate less than 45–60 beats/minute, heart block greater than first degree, systolic blood pressure less than 100 mm Hg, or moderate to severe cardiac failure. Metoprolol also is contraindicated in patients with a known history of hypersensitivity to metoprolol or any component of the formulations and in patients with a known history of hypersensitivity to other β-blockers.

● Pediatric Precautions

Although safety and efficacy of metoprolol tartrate remain to be fully established in children, some experts have recommended pediatric dosages for hypertension based on currently limited clinical experience.

The safety and efficacy of extended-release metoprolol succinate in pediatric patients has been evaluated in a placebo-controlled study in hypertensive patients 6–16 years of age. In this study, patients received extended-release metoprolol succinate 0.2, 1, or 2 mg/kg orally once daily (dosage expressed in terms of metoprolol tartrate) or placebo and were followed for 4 weeks. Although the primary efficacy end point (dose response for reduction in systolic blood pressure) was not met, several prespecified secondary end points were achieved. Compared with placebo, extended-release metoprolol succinate substantially reduced systolic blood pressure at the 1- and 2-mg/kg once-daily dosages, reduced diastolic blood pressure at the 2-mg/kg once-daily dosage, and demonstrated a dose-response relationship for reductions in diastolic blood pressure. No substantial differences in safety relative to adults were observed. Safety and efficacy of metoprolol succinate has not been established in children younger than 6 years of age.

For information on overall principles and expert recommendations for treatment of hypertension in pediatric patients, see Uses: Hypertension in Pediatric Patients, in the Thiazides General Statement 40:28.20.

● Geriatric Precautions

Clinical trials of conventional metoprolol tartrate or extended-release metoprolol succinate tablets for hypertension did not include sufficient numbers of patients 65 years and older to determine whether they respond differently than younger adults. While clinical experience generally has not revealed age-related differences in response to the drug, care should be taken in dosage selection of metoprolol. Safety and efficacy of conventional metoprolol tartrate tablets are similar in geriatric adults with MI and younger adults. However, since the possibility of greater sensitivity of some older patients cannot be ruled out, initial dosage should be selected carefully in these patients. Safety and efficacy of extended-release metoprolol succinate are similar in geriatric adults with heart failure and in younger adults. Because of the greater frequency of decreased hepatic, renal, and/or cardiac function and of concomitant disease and drug therapy in geriatric patients, the manufacturer suggests that patients in this age group receive initial dosages of the drug in the lower end of the usual range.

● Mutagenicity and Carcinogenicity

There has been no evidence of mutagenic potential in tests performed to date with metoprolol. No evidence of metoprolol tartrate-induced mutagenicity was observed in dominant lethal tests in mice, chromosome tests in somatic cells, *Salmonella* mammalian microsome tests, or nucleus anomaly tests in somatic interphase nuclei. No evidence of mutagenicity was observed in the *Salmonella* mammalian microsome test using metoprolol succinate. In chronic toxicity studies, benign lung tumors (small adenomas) occurred more frequently in female Swiss albino mice receiving oral dosages of metoprolol tartrate up to 750 mg/kg daily (representing 18 times the daily dosage of 200 mg in a 60-kg patient on a mg/m^2 basis) for 21 months than in untreated control animals, although there was no increase in malignant lung tumors or total (benign plus malignant) lung tumors. In CD-1 mice, however, no differences were observed between treated and control mice of either gender for any tumor. In a 2-year study in rats, there was no evidence of increased development of spontaneously occurring benign or malignant neoplasms at dosages of metoprolol tartrate up to 800 mg/kg daily. However, in these rats, histologic changes included an increased incidence of mild focal accumulation of foamy macrophages in alveolar spaces and slight increases of biliary hyperplasia.

● Pregnancy, Fertility, and Lactation

Pregnancy

Distribution studies in mice have shown that the fetus is exposed to metoprolol when the drug is administered during pregnancy. Although there are no adequate and controlled studies to date in humans, metoprolol has been shown to increase postimplantation loss and to decrease neonatal survival in rats when given at metoprolol succinate dosages (expressed as the tartrate) up to 22 times a daily dosage of 200 mg in a 60-kg patient (on a mg/m^2 basis) or metoprolol tartrate dosages up to 55.5 times the maximum recommended human dosage of 450 mg daily. Metoprolol should be used during pregnancy only when clearly needed.

Fertility

Reproduction studies in rats using metoprolol succinate dosages (expressed as the tartrate) up to 22 times a daily dosage of 200 mg in a 60-kg patient (on a mg/m^2 basis) or metoprolol tartrate dosages up to 55.5 times the maximum recommended human dosage of 450 mg have not revealed evidence of impaired fertility. Metoprolol has rarely caused Peyronie's disease in human males.

Lactation

Since metoprolol is distributed into milk, the drug should be used with caution in nursing women. The extent to which metoprolol distributes into milk has not been clearly established, but the amount of drug a nursing infant would ingest (less than 1 mg/L of milk consumed daily) is believed to be too small to be clinically important; however, if a woman receiving metoprolol breastfeeds, the infant should be monitored for potential systemic effects of the drug.

DRUG INTERACTIONS

● Cardiovascular Drugs

When metoprolol is administered with diuretics or other hypotensive drugs, the hypotensive effect of metoprolol may be increased. This effect is usually used to therapeutic advantage, but careful adjustment of dosage is necessary when these drugs are used concomitantly. An additive effect may be obtained when metoprolol is given to patients receiving catecholamine-depleting drugs, such as reserpine and monoamine oxidase inhibitors, resulting in hypotension and/or bradycardia. The β$_1$-adrenergic stimulating effects of sympathomimetic agents are antagonized by usual doses of metoprolol.

Concomitant use of β-adrenergic blocking agents (β-blockers) and certain other cardiovascular drugs (e.g., cardiac glycosides, nondihydropyridine calcium-channel blocking agents) can have additive negative effects on SA or AV nodal conduction. Caution should be exercised in the concomitant administration of β-blockers and other cardiovascular drugs (e.g., nondihydropyridine calcium-channel blocking agents). Slowing or complete suppression of SA node activity with development of slow ventricular rates (e.g., 30–40 bpm), often misdiagnosed as complete AV block, has been reported in patients receiving the nondihydropyridine calcium-channel blocking agent mibefradil (no longer commercially available in the US), principally in geriatric patients and in association with concomitant β-blocker therapy.

Because β-blockers may exacerbate rebound hypertension that may occur following discontinuance of clonidine therapy, β-blockers should be discontinued several days before gradual withdrawal of clonidine when clonidine therapy is to be discontinued in patients receiving a β-blocker and clonidine concurrently. If clonidine therapy is to be replaced by a β-blocker, administration of the β-blocker should be delayed for several days after clonidine therapy has been discontinued.

Verapamil may substantially increase the oral bioavailability of metoprolol, a lipophilic drug. Area under the plasma metoprolol concentration-time curve has increased up to 300% following initiation of verapamil therapy. Verapamil appears to increase oral bioavailability of metoprolol by decreasing its hepatic clearance, although the exact mechanism(s) has not been elucidated. A similar pharmacokinetic interaction does not appear to occur when atenolol, a hydrophilic drug, and verapamil are used concomitantly. Concomitant use of verapamil and metoprolol should be avoided if possible and another β-blocker with which verapamil does not interact pharmacokinetically (e.g., atenolol) preferably used when combined therapy is required. If verapamil and metoprolol are used concomitantly, dosage of metoprolol should be adjusted carefully and the patient monitored closely.

● Drugs Affecting Hepatic Microsomal Enzymes

Metabolism of certain β-blockers (e.g., metoprolol, timolol) is mediated by the cytochrome (CYP) P-450 isoenzyme 2D6 (CYP2D6), and concurrent use of metoprolol with drugs that inhibit CYP2D6 (e.g., bupropion, cimetidine, diphenhydramine, fluoxetine, hydroxychloroquine, paroxetine, propafenone, quinidine, ritonavir, terbinafine, thioridazine) may increase plasma metoprolol concentrations, resulting in decreased cardioselectivity of the drug. Pending further experience with combination therapy with paroxetine and metoprolol, caution should be exercised when paroxetine and metoprolol are used concomitantly. In healthy individuals with an extensive metabolizer phenotype, coadministration of quinidine (100 mg) and metoprolol conventional tablets (200 mg) doubled the half life of metoprolol and tripled the plasma concentration of the S-enantiomer. In a limited number of patients with cardiovascular disease, concurrent administration of propafenone (150 mg 3 times daily) with metoprolol conventional tablets (50 mg 3 times daily) resulted in a twofold to fivefold increase in the steady-state plasma concentration of metoprolol.

● Other Drugs

Use of myocardial depressant general anesthetics (e.g., diethyl ether) in patients receiving a β-blocker, such as metoprolol, leads to a risk of hypotension and heart failure.

Administration of a β-blocker with a vasodilator, such as hydralazine, in patients with uremia could cause pulmonary hypertension secondary to β-adrenergic blockade of the pulmonary vasculature and to the increased cardiac output caused by the vasodilator.

ACUTE TOXICITY

● Pathogenesis

The acute lethal dose of metoprolol in humans is not known. The oral LD$_{50}$ of the drug is 1158–2460 and 3090–4670 mg/kg in mice and rats, respectively.

● Manifestations

Limited information is available on acute metoprolol toxicity; several cases of overdosage with metoprolol tartrate or metoprolol succinate have been reported, some resulting in death. A 19-year-old man who ingested 10 g of metoprolol tartrate (160 mg/kg) was conscious with peripheral cyanosis, weak heart sounds, and no measurable blood pressure. Treatment consisted of gastric lavage, IV infusion of Ringer's injection, IV administration of sodium bicarbonate to correct acidosis, furosemide to relieve fluid retention, and glucagon and metaraminol to restore blood pressure. Within 12 hours after admission to the hospital, the patient exhibited no signs of cardiac depression. In general, overdosage of metoprolol may be expected to produce effects that are mainly extensions of pharmacologic effects, including symptomatic bradycardia, hypotension, bronchospasm, and acute cardiac failure; impaired conduction, decreased cardiac contractility, heart block, shock, and cardiac arrest also may occur. Other manifestations associated with overdosage of metoprolol succinate as extended-release tablets include atrioventricular block, cardiogenic shock, cardiac arrest, impairment of consciousness, nausea, vomiting, and cyanosis.

● Treatment

In acute metoprolol overdose, the stomach should be emptied immediately by gastric lavage. Supportive and symptomatic treatment should be initiated. For symptomatic bradycardia, IV atropine sulfate may be given; if bradycardia persists, IV isoproterenol hydrochloride may be administered cautiously. A vasopressor (e.g., dopamine, norepinephrine) may be given for severe hypotension; IV glucagon may be useful if hypotension is refractory to vasopressors. A β-adrenergic agonist (e.g., isoproterenol) and/or a theophylline derivative may be given for bronchospasm. For heart failure, a cardiac glycoside, diuretic, and oxygen should be used; IV glucagon also may be useful.

PHARMACOLOGY

At low doses, metoprolol is a selective inhibitor of β_1-adrenergic receptors. Like propranolol, metoprolol inhibits response to adrenergic stimuli by competitively blocking β_1-adrenergic receptors within the myocardium. Unlike propranolol, however, metoprolol blocks β_2-adrenergic receptors within bronchial and vascular smooth muscle only in high doses.

Through its myocardial β_1-adrenergic blocking action, metoprolol decreases resting heart rate and reflex orthostatic tachycardia, inhibits exercise-induced increases in heart rate, decreases myocardial contractility, and decreases cardiac output at rest and during exercise without a compensatory increase in peripheral resistance. The drug increases systolic ejection time and cardiac output; stroke volume is unchanged. Metoprolol also decreases conduction velocity through the sinoatrial (SA) and atrioventricular (AV) nodes and decreases myocardial automaticity via β_1-adrenergic blockade. The drug has no intrinsic sympathomimetic activity and little or no membrane-stabilizing effect on the heart; membrane-stabilizing effects occur only at plasma concentrations much higher than those required for β-adrenergic blocking action.

The precise mechanism of metoprolol's hypotensive action has not been determined. It has been postulated that β-adrenergic blocking agents (β-blockers) reduce blood pressure by blocking peripheral (especially cardiac) adrenergic receptors (decreasing cardiac output), by decreasing sympathetic outflow from the CNS, and/or by suppressing renin release. Results of several studies suggest a reduction in peripheral resistance by inhibition of release of norepinephrine as a basis for metoprolol's hypotensive effect, but this requires further study. Like propranolol, metoprolol decreases blood pressure in both supine and standing positions.

In patients with normal or high concentrations of circulating renin, low doses of metoprolol are associated with a fall in plasma renin concentrations, possibly due, at least partly, to acute peripheral β_1-adrenergic blockade. Metoprolol also substantially reduces furosemide-induced renin release. Metoprolol and propranolol produce similar decreases in plasma renin activity (PRA) in patients with high PRA. The importance of these effects in decreasing blood pressure in hypertensive patients requires further investigation.

A small increase in serum potassium has been observed during metoprolol therapy and may be related to β_2-adrenergic blockade and reduced PRA and plasma aldosterone concentration.

The exact mechanism of action of metoprolol in patients with suspected or definite myocardial infarction (MI) has not been determined. In patients with MI, metoprolol reduces heart rate, systolic blood pressure, and cardiac output, but stroke volume, diastolic blood pressure, and pulmonary artery end diastolic pressure remain unchanged; the drug also appears to decrease the occurrence of ventricular fibrillation in these patients.

In the management of angina pectoris, the mechanism of action of metoprolol is thought to be blockade of catecholamine-induced increases in heart rate, velocity and extent of myocardial contraction, and blood pressure, which results in a net decrease in myocardial oxygen consumption. In some studies, metoprolol (given as extended-release tablets) has improved left ventricular ejection fraction and has been shown to delay increases in left ventricular end-systolic and end-diastolic volumes after 6 months of therapy.

Usual doses of metoprolol increase airway resistance and decrease ventilatory capacity in asthmatic patients but, because of its relatively selective β_1-adrenergic blocking activity, to a lesser degree than does an equivalent β_1-adrenergic receptor blocking dose of propranolol. Unlike propranolol, low dosages (up to 100 mg daily) of metoprolol tartrate do not appreciably inhibit isoproterenol-induced bronchodilation. Because of its relative β_1-adrenergic blocking selectivity, metoprolol causes little inhibition of glycogenolysis in skeletal and cardiac muscles. Metoprolol inhibits the increase in plasma glycerol caused by exercise. Metoprolol may cause less inhibition of insulin release than does propranolol and may therefore result in better glucose tolerance than does propranolol in patients with diabetes mellitus; however, results of studies of this effect are conflicting. Metoprolol does not appear to reduce free fatty acid concentrations in healthy individuals. Fasting triglyceride concentrations have been increased in some patients, while in others no consistent changes have occurred. Metoprolol may increase the peripheral platelet count by interfering with β-adrenergic receptors involved in platelet level regulation in the spleen.

PHARMACOKINETICS

● Absorption

Metoprolol tartrate is rapidly and almost completely absorbed from the GI tract; absorption of a single oral dose of 20–100 mg is complete in 2.5–3 hours. After an oral dose, about 50% of the drug administered as conventional tablets appears to undergo first-pass metabolism in the liver. Bioavailability of orally administered metoprolol tartrate increases with increased doses, indicating a possible saturable disposition process of low capacity such as tissue binding in the liver. Steady-state oral bioavailability of extended-release tablets of metoprolol succinate given once daily at dosages equivalent to 50–400 mg of metoprolol tartrate is about 77% of that of conventional tablets at corresponding dosages given once daily or in divided doses. Food does not appear to affect bioavailability of metoprolol succinate extended-release tablets. Following a single oral dose as conventional tablets, metoprolol appears in the plasma within 10 minutes and peak plasma concentrations are reached in about 90 minutes. When metoprolol tartrate conventional tablets are administered with food rather than on an empty stomach, peak plasma concentrations are higher and the extent of absorption of the drug is increased. Following oral administration of metoprolol succinate as extended-release tablets, peak plasma metoprolol concentrations are about 25–50% of those attained after administration of metoprolol tartrate conventional tablets given once daily or in divided doses. However, in patients with heart failure, peak plasma concentrations attained after administration of metoprolol succinate as extended-release tablets (200 mg [expressed as the tartrate] once daily) are similar to those attained with conventional metoprolol tartrate tablets (50 mg 3 times daily). Time to peak concentration is longer with extended-release tablets, with peak plasma concentrations being reached in about 7 hours following administration of such tablets.

Plasma concentrations attained 1 hour after an oral dose are linearly related to metoprolol tartrate doses ranging from 50–400 mg as conventional tablets. After an oral dose of metoprolol tartrate, plasma concentrations attained are quite variable among individuals (particularly in geriatric patients) and apparently do not correlate with hypotensive effects. However, oral doses ranging from 50–400 mg appear to cause dose-dependent reductions in systolic blood pressure and exercise-induced heart rate. In addition, a linear relationship between plasma concentration of the drug and reduction in exercise-induced heart rate appears to exist. In healthy adults, plasma metoprolol concentrations of 8–144 ng/mL are associated with an 8–23% reduction in exercised-induced tachycardia;

plasma concentration-effect curves reach a plateau at about 53.5–80 ng/mL, and higher metoprolol plasma concentrations produce little additional β_1-adrenergic blocking effects. The relative β_1 selectivity of the drug diminishes at higher plasma metoprolol concentrations while β_2-blocking effects increase at higher plasma metoprolol concentrations. Such effects diminish at higher plasma metoprolol concentrations while β_2-adrenergic blocking effects increase at higher plasma metoprolol concentrations.

Following oral administration of dosages equivalent to 100–400 mg of metoprolol tartrate given once daily as metoprolol succinate extended-release tablets in healthy individuals, steady-state β-adrenergic blocking effects (as measured by blockade of exercise-induced increases in heart rate) over a 24-hour period were similar to those following administration of metoprolol tartrate conventional tablets given 1–4 times daily. However, β-adrenergic blocking effects over a 24-hour period were higher following oral administration of metoprolol succinate extended-release tablets given once daily in a dosage equivalent to 50 mg of metoprolol tartrate compared with those following administration of the same dosage given as metoprolol tartrate conventional tablets. Following oral administration of metoprolol succinate as extended-release tablets, reduction in exercise-induced heart rate is stable throughout the entire dosing interval, and oral doses (equivalent to the tartrate) ranging from 50–400 mg appear to cause dose-dependent reductions in exercise-induced heart rate while a larger peak effect on exercise-induced tachycardia occurs following administration of 50–100 mg once daily as conventional tablets; this effect is not observed 24 hours after dosing. To achieve a similar effect to that attained with metoprolol succinate extended-release tablets, a total daily dosage of 200–400 mg is given in 3 or 4 divided doses if administered as conventional metoprolol tartrate tablets. In a randomized, crossover trial in patients with heart failure who had prior chronic therapy with metoprolol, the reduction in the average or exercise-induced heart rate over 24 hours was greater during short-term therapy with metoprolol succinate 200 mg (expressed as the tartrate) daily as extended-release tablets than with metoprolol tartrate 50 mg 3 times daily as conventional tablets. The manufacturer of Toprol XL® states that the relationship between plasma metoprolol concentrations and reduction in exercise-induced heart rate is independent of the pharmaceutical formulation. In patients with angina pectoris, a relationship between metoprolol tartrate dose and exercise capacity and reductions in left ventricular ischemia appears to exist for oral doses ranging from 50–400 mg. Following oral administration of multiple doses of metoprolol tartrate (50–80 mg 3 times daily), peak plasma concentrations range from 20–340 ng/mL.

In hypertensive patients, a reduction in systolic blood pressure during exercise has been reported within 15 minutes after a single oral dose of 50–80 mg of metoprolol tartrate and the effect persisted for 6 hours. Dosages of 150–450 mg daily cause a dose-dependent decrease in systolic blood pressure which averages 20 mm Hg; the effect is usually maximal within 1 week in healthy or hypertensive patients at rest and during exercise. The same dosage causes a less rapid but appreciable reduction in diastolic blood pressure which averages 10–15 mm Hg. Metoprolol succinate extended-release tablets given once daily at dosages equivalent to 100–400 mg of metoprolol tartrate produce similar hypotensive effects as conventional metoprolol tartrate tablets at similar dosages given 2–4 times daily; the hypotensive effect of extended-release tablets may persist for 24 hours. Duration of the β-adrenergic blocking effect (as measured by blockade of exercise-induced increases in heart rate) is dose related, increasing with increasing doses. With chronic therapy, hypotensive effects may persist for up to 4 weeks after withdrawal of the drug, possibly as a result of tissue-bound drug.

Plasma metoprolol concentrations attained after IV administration of the drug are approximately 2 times those attained following oral administration. Following IV infusion of metoprolol over 10 minutes in healthy individuals, maximum β-adrenergic blocking activity occurred at 20 minutes. In healthy individuals, a maximum reduction in exercise-induced heart rate of approximately 10 and 15% occurs following IV administration of a single 5- and 15-mg metoprolol dose, respectively; the effect on exercise-induced heart rate decreased linearly with time at the same rate for both doses and persisted for approximately 5 and 8 hours for the 5- and 15-mg doses, respectively.

● Distribution

Metoprolol is widely distributed into body tissues. The concentration of the drug is greater in the heart, liver, lungs, and saliva than in the plasma. Metoprolol is 11–12% bound to serum proteins, apparently only to albumin. Following therapeutic doses, metoprolol concentrations in erythrocytes are about 20% greater than those in plasma, but the drug is available for elimination from these two sites

at the same rate. Metoprolol crosses the placenta, and maternal and fetal blood concentrations are about equal. The drug crosses the blood-brain barrier; the concentration of metoprolol in CSF is about 78% of the simultaneous concentration in plasma. Metoprolol is distributed into milk in a concentration about 3–4 times that of maternal plasma concentrations, but the actual amount distributed into milk appears to be very small.

● Elimination

Elimination of metoprolol appears to follow first-order kinetics and occurs mainly in the liver; the time required for the process apparently is independent of dose and duration of therapy. In healthy individuals and hypertensive patients, the elimination half-life of both unchanged drug and metabolites is about 3–4 hours. In poor hydroxylators of the drug, the elimination half-life is prolonged to about 7.6 hours. There is more interindividual variation in elimination half-lives in geriatric patients than in young healthy individuals. The half-life of metoprolol does not increase appreciably with impaired renal function.

Metoprolol is metabolized by the cytochrome P-450 (CYP) microsomal enzyme system, predominantly by the 2D6 isoenzyme (CYP2D6). When administered orally, metoprolol exhibits stereoselective metabolism that is dependent on oxidation phenotype. The CYP2D6 isoenzyme is absent in about 8% of Caucasians (poor metabolizers) and about 2% of most other populations. Since CYP2D6 can be inhibited by other drugs, concomitant use of such drugs with metoprolol in poor metabolizers will lead to increases in plasma metoprolol concentrations and a decrease in the β_1-selectivity of the drug. Metoprolol does not inhibit or enhance its own metabolism. Three main metabolites of the drug are formed by oxidative deamination, O-dealkylation with subsequent oxidation, and aliphatic hydroxylation; these metabolites account for 85% of the total urinary excretion of metabolites. The metabolites apparently do not have appreciable pharmacologic activity. The rate of hydroxylation, resulting in α-hydroxymetoprolol, is genetically determined and is subject to considerable interindividual variation. Poor hydroxylators of metoprolol have increased areas under the plasma concentration-time curves (AUCs), prolonged elimination half-lives (about 7.6 hours), higher urinary concentrations of unchanged drug, and negligible urinary concentrations of α-hydroxymetoprolol compared with extensive hydroxylators. β-Adrenergic blockade of exercise-induced tachycardia persists for at least 24 hours after administration of a single 200-mg oral dose of metoprolol tartrate in poor hydroxylators.

Metoprolol and its metabolites are excreted in urine mainly via glomerular filtration, although tubular secretion and reabsorption may be involved. About 95% of a single oral dose is excreted in urine within 72 hours. Less than 5% and approximately 10% of a metoprolol dose is excreted unchanged in urine following oral and IV administration of the drug, respectively.

CHEMISTRY AND STABILITY

● Chemistry

Metoprolol is a β_1-selective adrenergic blocking agent. Metoprolol is commercially available as the tartrate salt in oral tablets and parenteral injection and as the succinate salt in oral extended-release tablets containing controlled-release coated pellets. Metoprolol tartrate is commercially available as a racemic mixture. Metoprolol tartrate occurs as a white, crystalline powder with a bitter taste and is very soluble in water and freely soluble in alcohol. The drug has a pK_a of 9.68. Metoprolol succinate occurs as a white, crystalline powder and is freely soluble in water and sparingly soluble in alcohol.

● Stability

Commercially available preparations of metoprolol tartrate should be protected from light. Metoprolol tartrate tablets should be protected from moisture and stored in tight, light-resistant containers at 25°C but may be exposed to temperatures ranging from 15–30°C. Metoprolol tartrate injection should be stored at a temperature of 25°C but may be exposed to temperatures ranging from 15–30°C; freezing of the injection should be avoided.

PREPARATIONS

Excipients in commercially available drug preparations may have clinically important effects in some individuals; consult specific product labeling for details.

Metoprolol Succinate

Oral

Tablets, extended-release, film-coated	23.75 mg (equivalent to 25 mg of metoprolol tartrate)*	**Metoprolol Succinate Extended-release Tablets** Toprol XL® (scored), AstraZeneca
	47.5 mg (equivalent to 50 mg of metoprolol tartrate)*	**Metoprolol Succinate Extended-release Tablets** Toprol XL® (scored), AstraZeneca
	95 mg (equivalent to 100 mg of metoprolol tartrate)*	**Metoprolol Succinate Extended-release Tablets** Toprol XL® (scored), AstraZeneca
	190 mg (equivalent to 200 mg of metoprolol tartrate)*	**Metoprolol Succinate Extended-release Tablets** Toprol XL® (scored), AstraZeneca

* available from one or more manufacturer, distributor, and/or repackager by generic (nonproprietary) name

Metoprolol Tartrate

Oral

Tablets	50 mg*	**Lopressor®** (scored), Validus **Metoprolol Tartrate Tablets**
	100 mg*	**Lopressor®** (scored), Validus **Metoprolol Tartrate Tablets**

Parenteral

Injection	1 mg/mL*	**Lopressor®**, Novartis **Metoprolol Tartrate Injection**

* available from one or more manufacturer, distributor, and/or repackager by generic (nonproprietary) name

Metoprolol Tartrate and Hydrochlorothiazide

Oral

Tablets	50 mg Metoprolol Tartrate and Hydrochlorothiazide 25 mg*	**Lopressor® HCT** (scored), Validus **Metoprolol Tartrate and Hydrochlorothiazide Tablets**
	100 mg Metoprolol Tartrate and Hydrochlorothiazide 25 mg*	**Lopressor® HCT** (scored), Validus **Metoprolol Tartrate and Hydrochlorothiazide Tablets**
	100 mg Metoprolol Tartrate and Hydrochlorothiazide 50 mg*	**Lopressor® HCT** (scored), Validus **Metoprolol Tartrate and Hydrochlorothiazide Tablets**

* available from one or more manufacturer, distributor, and/or repackager by generic (nonproprietary) name

† Use is not currently included in the labeling approved by the US Food and Drug Administration.

Selected Revisions June 10, 2024, © Copyright, June 1, 1979, American Society of Health-System Pharmacists, Inc.

Propranolol Hydrochloride

24:20 • β-ADRENERGIC BLOCKING AGENTS

■ Propranolol hydrochloride is a nonselective β-adrenergic blocking agent (β-blocker).

USES

Propranolol is used for the management of hypertension, angina, supraventricular and ventricular arrhythmias, acute myocardial infarction (MI), and essential tremor. Propranolol also is used for prophylaxis of migraine headache, management of hypertrophic subaortic stenosis, and as an adjunct in the management of pheochromocytoma. The drug also has been used in the management of thyrotoxicosis†.

The choice of a β-adrenergic blocking agent (β-blocker) depends on numerous factors, including pharmacologic properties (e.g., relative β-selectivity, intrinsic sympathomimetic activity, membrane-stabilizing activity, lipophilicity), pharmacokinetics, intended use, and adverse effect profile, as well as the patient's coexisting disease states or conditions, response, and tolerance. While specific pharmacologic properties and other factors may appropriately influence the choice of a β-blocker in individual patients, evidence of clinically important differences among the agents in terms of overall efficacy and/or safety is limited. Patients who do not respond to or cannot tolerate one β-blocker may be successfully treated with a different agent.

In the management of hypertension or chronic stable angina pectoris in patients with chronic obstructive pulmonary disease (COPD) or type 1 diabetes mellitus, many clinicians prefer to use low dosages of a β_1-selective adrenergic blocking agent (e.g., atenolol, metoprolol), rather than a nonselective agent (e.g., nadolol, pindolol, propranolol, timolol). However, selectivity of these agents is relative and dose dependent. Some clinicians also will recommend using a β_1-selective agent or an agent with intrinsic sympathomimetic activity (e.g., pindolol), rather than a nonselective agent, for the management of hypertension or angina pectoris in patients with peripheral vascular disease, but there is no evidence that the choice of β-blocker substantially affects efficacy. Nonselective β-blockers are preferred for the management of hypertension or angina pectoris in patients with coexisting essential tremor or vascular (e.g., migraine) headache. For further information on management and classification of migraine headache, see Vascular Headaches: General Principles in Migraine Therapy, under Uses in Sumatriptan 28:32.28.

● Hypertension

Propranolol is used alone or in combination with other classes of antihypertensive agents in the management of hypertension.

Current evidence-based practice guidelines for the management of hypertension in adults generally recommend the use of drugs from 4 classes of antihypertensive agents (angiotensin-converting enzyme [ACE] inhibitors, angiotensin II receptor antagonists, calcium-channel blockers, and thiazide diuretics). Most guidelines no longer recommend β-blockers as first-line therapy for hypertension because of the lack of established superiority over other recommended drug classes and evidence from at least one study demonstrating that β-blockers may be less effective than angiotensin II receptor antagonists in preventing cardiovascular death, MI, or stroke. However, therapy with a β-blocker may still be considered in hypertensive patients who have a compelling indication (e.g., prior MI, ischemic heart disease, heart failure) for their use or as add-on therapy in those who do not respond adequately to the preferred drug classes. (See Considerations for Drug Therapy in Patients with Underlying Cardiovascular and Other Risk Factors under Uses: Hypertension, in Atenolol 24:24 and in Metoprolol 24:24.) Ultimately, choice of antihypertensive therapy should be individualized, considering the clinical characteristics of the patient (e.g., age, ethnicity/race, comorbid conditions, cardiovascular risk factors) as well as drug-related factors (e.g., ease of administration, availability, adverse effects, costs).

A 2017 multidisciplinary hypertension guideline of the American College of Cardiology (ACC), American Heart Association (AHA), and a number of other professional organizations generally recommends a target blood pressure goal (i.e., blood pressure to achieve with drug therapy and/or nonpharmacologic intervention) of less than 130/80 mm Hg in all adults regardless of comorbidities or level of atherosclerotic cardiovascular disease (ASCVD) risk. In addition, a systolic blood pressure goal of less than 130 mm Hg generally is recommended for noninstitutionalized ambulatory patients 65 years of age or older with an average systolic blood pressure of at least 130 mm Hg. These blood pressure goals are based upon clinical studies demonstrating continuing reduction of cardiovascular risk at progressively lower levels of systolic blood pressure. Previous hypertension guidelines, such as those from an expert panel of the Eighth Joint National Committee on the Prevention, Detection, Evaluation, and Treatment of High Blood Pressure (JNC 8), generally have recommended initiation of antihypertensive treatment in patients with a systolic blood pressure of at least 140 mm Hg or diastolic blood pressure of at least 90 mm Hg, targeted a blood pressure goal of less than 140/90 mm Hg regardless of cardiovascular risk, and used higher systolic blood pressure thresholds and targets in geriatric patients compared with those recommended by the 2017 ACC/AHA hypertension guideline. The blood pressure thresholds used to define hypertension, the optimum blood pressure threshold at which to initiate antihypertensive drug therapy, and the ideal target blood pressure values remain controversial.

Most patients with hypertension, especially black patients, will require at least 2 antihypertensive drugs to achieve adequate blood pressure control. In general, black hypertensive patients tend to respond better to monotherapy with thiazide diuretics or calcium-channel blocking agents than to monotherapy with β-blockers. Although β-blockers have lowered blood pressure in all races studied, monotherapy with these agents has produced a smaller reduction in blood pressure in black hypertensive patients; however, this population difference in response does not appear to occur during combined therapy with a β-blocker and a thiazide diuretic. (See Race under Hypertension: Other Special Considerations for Antihypertensive Drug Therapy, in Uses in Atenolol 24:24 and in Metoprolol 24:24.)

Propranolol is *not* indicated for the treatment of hypertensive emergencies.

In contrast to many other antihypertensive agents, propranolol lowers blood pressure equally well in the upright or supine position. The drug appears to be safe and effective for the treatment of hypertension in patients with renal damage. Although it apparently is more effective in patients with normal or elevated plasma renin concentrations than in those with low plasma renin concentrations, propranolol does lower blood pressure in patients with low-renin hypertension.

For additional information on the role of β-blockers in the management of hypertension, see Uses: Hypertension, in Atenolol 24:24 and in Metoprolol 24:24. For information on overall principles and expert recommendations for treatment of hypertension, see Uses: Hypertension in Adults and also see Uses: Hypertension in Pediatric Patients, in the Thiazides General Statement 40:28.20.

● Chronic Stable Angina

Propranolol is used for the long-term management of chronic stable angina pectoris. β-Blockers are recommended as the anti-ischemic drugs of choice in most patients with chronic stable angina; despite differences in cardioselectivity, intrinsic sympathomimetic activity, and other clinical factors, all β-blockers appear to be equally effective for this indication. In a double-blind study in patients with stable angina, propranolol reduced the frequency of anginal attacks and increased exercise tolerance compared with placebo.

Combination therapy with a β-blocker and a nitrate appears to be more effective than either drug alone because β-blockers attenuate the increased sympathetic tone and reflex tachycardia associated with nitrate therapy while nitrate therapy (e.g., nitroglycerin) counteracts the potential increase in left-ventricular wall tension associated with a decrease in heart rate. Combined therapy with a β-blocker and a dihydropyridine calcium-channel blocker also may be useful because the tendency to develop tachycardia with the calcium-channel blocker is counteracted by the β-blocker. However, caution should be exercised in the concomitant use of β-blockers and the nondihydropyridine calcium-channel blockers verapamil or diltiazem because of the potential for excessive fatigue, bradycardia, or atrioventricular (AV) block. (See Drug Interactions: Diuretics and Cardiovascular Drugs.)

● Cardiac Arrhythmias

Supraventricular Arrhythmias

β-Blockers, including propranolol, are used to slow ventricular rate in patients with supraventricular tachycardia (SVT). The American College of Cardiology/American Heart Association/Heart Rhythm Society (ACC/AHA/HRS) guideline for the management of adult patients with supraventricular tachycardia recommends the use of β-blockers in the treatment of various SVTs (e.g., atrial flutter, junctional tachycardia, focal atrial tachycardia, atrioventricular nodal reentrant tachycardia [AVNRT]); in general, an IV β-blocker is recommended for acute treatment, while an oral β-blocker is recommended for ongoing management of these arrhythmias. Vagal maneuvers and/or IV adenosine generally are considered first-line interventions for the acute treatment of SVT and should be attempted prior to other therapies when clinically indicated; if such measures are ineffective or not feasible, an IV β-blocker may be considered in hemodynamically stable patients. Although evidence of efficacy is limited, experts state that the overall safety of β-blockers warrants their use in patients with SVT. Patients should be closely monitored for hypotension and bradycardia during administration of these drugs.

IV β-blockers may be used for the acute treatment of patients with hemodynamically stable focal atrial tachycardia (i.e., regular SVT arising from a localized atrial site), and an oral β-blocker may be used for ongoing management. Multifocal atrial tachycardia, characterized by a rapid, irregular rhythm with at least 3 distinct P-wave morphologies, is commonly associated with an underlying condition (e.g., pulmonary, coronary, or valvular heart disease) and is generally not responsive to antiarrhythmic drug therapy.

Propranolol is used to slow ventricular rate in patients with atrial fibrillation or atrial flutter when ventricular rate cannot be controlled with standard measures. For acute treatment of atrial fibrillation or flutter, an IV β-blocker (e.g., esmolol, propranolol, metoprolol) may be used for ventricular rate control in patients without preexcitation; an oral β-blocker may be used for ongoing rate control in such patients. Choice of a specific β-blocker should be individualized based on the patient's clinical condition.

IV β-blockers may be used for the acute treatment of hemodynamically stable patients with paroxysmal supraventricular tachycardia (PSVT), including AVNRT, that is uncontrolled or unconverted by vagal maneuvers and adenosine; an oral β-blocker may be used for the ongoing management of such patients who are not candidates for, or prefer not to undergo, catheter ablation. Propranolol may be useful in the prophylactic management of refractory PSVT, especially when caused by catecholamines or cardiac glycosides or associated with Wolff-Parkinson-White syndrome.

β-Blockers are considered one of several drug therapy options for the treatment of junctional tachycardia (i.e., nonreentrant SVT originating from the AV junction), a rapid, occasionally irregular, narrow-complex tachycardia. While evidence is limited, there is some data indicating that β-blockers (specifically propranolol) are modestly effective in terminating and/or reducing the incidence of junctional tachycardia.

Ventricular Arrhythmias

Although propranolol generally is less effective in the management of ventricular arrhythmias than supraventricular arrhythmias and is usually not the first drug of choice for ventricular arrhythmias, it may be considered when cardioversion or other drugs are not effective. Propranolol also may be used in the treatment of persistent premature ventricular complexes that impair the well-being of the patient and do not respond to conventional therapy.

β-Blockers may be useful in the management of certain forms of polymorphic ventricular tachycardia (e.g., associated with acute ischemia).

β-Blockers also have been used in patients with cardiac arrest precipitated by ventricular fibrillation† or pulseless ventricular tachycardia†. However, AHA states that routine administration of β-blockers after cardiac arrest is potentially harmful (e.g., may worsen hemodynamic instability, exacerbate heart failure, or cause bradyarrhythmias) and is therefore not recommended.

Tachyarrhythmias Associated with Cardiac Glycoside Intoxication

When AV block is not present, propranolol may be useful in the management of supraventricular or ventricular tachyarrhythmias associated with cardiac glycoside toxicity; however, because of the risk of adverse cardiovascular effects, the drug has a limited role in the management of these arrhythmias and other drugs are usually preferred. Propranolol can compromise conduction through the SA and AV nodes (possibly resulting in sinus bradycardia or asystole) and decrease myocardial automaticity; in addition, β-adrenergic blockade may result in deterioration of hemodynamic status in patients whose myocardial contractility depends on increased sympathetic nervous system activity. Oral propranolol may be useful in some patients for the management of cardiac glycoside-induced tachyarrhythmias that persist following discontinuance of the glycoside and correction of electrolyte abnormalities. IV propranolol should be used only if arrhythmias caused by cardiac glycoside intoxication are life-threatening and other therapy is ineffective. Use of digoxin immune Fab, if available, may be preferable and should be considered for the management of life-threatening cardiac glycoside-induced tachyarrhythmias that are unresponsive to conventional therapy.

Resistant Tachyarrhythmias Associated with Catecholamine Excess During Anesthesia

Propranolol may be used with extreme caution and constant ECG and central venous pressure monitoring in the management of resistant tachyarrhythmias associated with catecholamine excess during anesthesia; however, more effective and less hazardous therapy such as lessening the depth of anesthesia or improving ventilation is preferred. (See Cautions: Precautions and Contraindications.)

● Hypertrophic Subaortic Stenosis

Propranolol may be of benefit in the management of exertional or other stress-induced angina, vertigo, syncope, and palpitation in some patients with hypertrophic subaortic stenosis; however, clinical improvement may be only temporary.

● Pheochromocytoma

An α-adrenergic blocking agent (e.g., phenoxybenzamine or phentolamine) alone is usually sufficient for management of the signs and symptoms of pheochromocytoma. Propranolol, however, may be used as an adjunct to α-adrenergic blocking agents to control symptoms resulting from excessive β-receptor stimulation in patients with inoperable or metastatic pheochromocytoma, or to control tachycardia prior to or during surgery in patients with pheochromocytoma. To prevent severe hypertension caused by unopposed α-adrenergic stimulation, treatment with an α-adrenergic blocking agent must always be instituted prior to the use of propranolol and continued during propranolol therapy in patients with pheochromocytoma.

● Thyrotoxicosis

Propranolol, which will not alter thyroid function tests, may be used orally as short-term (2–4 weeks) adjunctive therapy in the treatment of tachycardia and supraventricular arrhythmias in patients with thyrotoxicosis when these symptoms are distressful or hazardous, or when immediate therapy is necessary. Propranolol has been used IV and orally to treat symptomatic hypercalcemia secondary to thyrotoxicosis†, but this use requires further study. Propranolol has also been used for the management of thyrotoxicosis in neonates†. Safety of long-term administration of the drug in patients with thyrotoxicosis has not been established. The drug does not affect the underlying disease, which must be treated with an antithyroid agent.

● Vascular Headache

Migraine

Propranolol may be used for the prophylaxis of common migraine headache. When used prophylactically, the drug can prevent common migraine or reduce the number of attacks in some patients. The US Headache Consortium states that there is good evidence from multiple well-designed clinical trials that propranolol has medium to high efficacy for the prophylaxis of migraine headache. Propranolol is not recommended for the treatment of a migraine attack that has already started nor for the prevention or treatment of cluster headaches. For further information on management and classification of migraine headache, see Vascular Headaches: General Principles in Migraine Therapy, under Uses in Sumatriptan 28:32.28.

● Myocardial Infarction

Propranolol is used to reduce the risk of cardiovascular mortality in patients who have survived the acute phase of MI and are clinically stable. In these patients, long-term (up to 39 months) administration of propranolol (begun within 5–21 days following MI) reduced overall mortality, cardiovascular mortality, arteriosclerotic heart disease (ASHD) mortality, and sudden death mortality within the ASHD category. Evidence of efficacy was obtained from a double-blind, placebo-controlled, multicenter study (Beta-Blocker Heart Attack Trial; BHAT). The effect of propranolol on reinfarction remains to be fully evaluated. For information on the use of β-blockers during the acute phase of MI, see Uses in Metoprolol 24:24.

The benefits of long-term β-blocker therapy for secondary prevention of MI have been well established in numerous clinical studies. Patients with MI complicated by heart failure, left ventricular dysfunction, or ventricular arrhythmias appear to derive the most benefit from long-term β-blocker therapy. Several large, randomized studies have demonstrated that prolonged oral therapy with a β-blocker can reduce the long-term rates of reinfarction and mortality (e.g., sudden or nonsudden cardiac death) following acute MI. It is estimated that such therapy could result in a relative reduction in mortality of about 25% annually for years 1–3 after infarction, with high-risk patients exhibiting the greatest potential benefit; the benefit of continued therapy may persist for at least several years beyond this period, although less substantially. Therefore, propranolol, like other β-blockers, can be used for secondary prevention following acute MI to reduce the risk of reinfarction and mortality. The American Heart Association/American College of Cardiology Foundation (AHA/ACCF) secondary prevention guideline recommends β-blocker therapy in all patients with left ventricular systolic dysfunction (ejection fraction of 40% or less) and prior MI; use of a β-blocker with proven mortality benefit (e.g., bisoprolol, carvedilol, or metoprolol succinate) is recommended. (See Uses: Heart Failure, in Carvedilol 24:24.) Although the benefits of long-term β-blockade in post-MI patients with normal left ventricular function are less well established, the guideline recommends continued β-blocker therapy for at least 3 years in such patients.

Essential Tremor

Propranolol is used for the management of essential (familial, hereditary) tremor. The tremor is a postural and action tremor manifested as involuntary, rhythmic, oscillatory movements, principally of the upper limbs and, less frequently, the head; other areas, including the voice, legs, jaw, eyelids, and mouth, also may be involved. Essential tremor occurs during active movement and when the limb is held in a fixed posture or position against gravity; the tremor usually is absent at rest, although, when it is of large amplitude, tremor occasionally may be evident at rest, particularly in geriatric patients.

Propranolol decreases the amplitude but not the frequency of essential tremor; complete suppression of the tremor rarely is achieved with treatment. Response to propranolol therapy is variable, but the drug appears to be most effective in the management of high-amplitude, low-frequency tremor. Clinical benefit often is most evident for tremor affecting the upper extremities, although benefit also has been observed for head and other tremors; voice tremor may be less responsive to therapy with the drug. Propranolol hydrochloride doses of 120–320 mg generally produce tremor amplitude reductions averaging about 4–50%; however, reductions averaging 25–75% have been reported. Therapy with the drug may improve functional ability (e.g., handwriting, eating, drinking, dressing) and provide some subjective improvement (e.g., reduced anxiety and embarrassment), but patients should be advised that complete relief rarely is achieved so that their expectations about potential therapeutic benefit are realistic. Although propranolol often is used for chronic suppressive therapy in essential tremor, single oral doses may be useful in some patients to prevent or minimize tremor that is considered bothersome during specific, planned activity or to manage an exacerbation of tremor during periods of stress (e.g., business meetings, examinations).

Other Uses

Propranolol has been used in the management of cyanotic spells of Fallot's tetralogy†, acute exacerbations of schizophrenic disorder† and anxiety states†, recurrent GI bleeding in patients with cirrhosis†, and many other conditions. In addition to essential tremor (see Uses: Essential Tremor), propranolol also has been used in the management of other action tremors†, including those associated with lithium therapy (see Cautions: Nervous System and Neuromuscular Effects, in Lithium Salts 28:28), anxiety, and thyrotoxicosis.

DOSAGE AND ADMINISTRATION

Administration

Propranolol hydrochloride is usually administered orally. When administered orally in divided doses, the drug should be given before meals and at bedtime. When propranolol hydrochloride extended-release capsules are administered, the entire daily dose is given once daily. When propranolol hydrochloride oral concentrate solution is used, the dose should be diluted (e.g., with water, juice, carbonated beverages) or mixed with semisolid foods (e.g., applesauce, puddings) just prior to administration.

For the treatment of cardiac arrhythmias, propranolol has been given IV. Oral therapy should replace IV therapy as soon as possible.

Dosage

Since there is no consistent interpatient correlation between the dosage of propranolol hydrochloride and therapeutic response, especially after oral administration, dosage must be carefully individualized according to the response of the patient. If patients are switched from the conventional tablets to the extended-release capsules, care should be taken to ensure that the desired therapeutic effect is maintained. The extended-release capsules should not be considered a simple substitute for the conventional tablets on a mg-for-mg basis, since the capsules produce lower blood concentrations. If patients are switched to the extended-release capsules, the need for dosage retitration should be considered, especially to maintain effectiveness at the end of the dosing interval.

The manufacturers of propranolol hydrochloride injection state that a reduction in the dosage of propranolol hydrochloride may be necessary in geriatric patients.

Hypertension

Propranolol Therapy

For the management of hypertension in adults, the initial oral dosage of propranolol hydrochloride, administered either alone or in combination with a diuretic, is 40 mg twice daily as conventional tablets or oral solution or 80 mg once daily as extended-release capsules. The usual effective oral dosage is 120–240 mg daily as conventional tablets or oral solution or 120–160 mg once daily as extended-release capsules; some manufacturers state that some patients may require dosages up to 640 mg daily. However, the manufacturer of Innopran XL® states that dosage of the extended-release capsules may be increased, if needed, up to 120 mg once daily, since dosages exceeding 120 mg once daily did not provide additional hypotensive effects. Some experts state the usual dosage range is 80–160 mg daily given in 2 divided doses as conventional tablets or oral solution or 80–160 mg once daily as extended-release capsules. It usually is preferable to add another antihypertensive agent to the regimen than to continue increasing propranolol hydrochloride dosage since the patient may not tolerate such continued increases. The full hypotensive effect of the drug usually is evident within 2–3 weeks, but the timing is variable. While twice-daily dosing using the conventional tablets or oral solution is usually effective, some patients may require larger doses or 3 divided doses daily to maintain effective blood pressure control throughout the day.

Propranolol/Hydrochlorothiazide Fixed-combination Therapy

When combination therapy is required, the manufacturers recommend that commercially available preparations containing propranolol hydrochloride in fixed combination with a thiazide diuretic should not be used initially. Dosage should first be adjusted by administering each drug separately. If it is determined that the optimum maintenance dosage corresponds to the ratio in the commercial combination preparation, the fixed combination may be used. Therapy with propranolol hydrochloride in fixed combination with hydrochlorothiazide is administered twice daily for a total daily dosage of up to 160 mg of propranolol hydrochloride and 50 mg of hydrochlorothiazide; use of this combination formulation is not appropriate for propranolol hydrochloride dosages exceeding 160 mg daily since it would provide an excessive dosage of the thiazide component. When necessary, another antihypertensive agent may be added gradually using half of the usual initial dosage to avoid an excessive decrease in blood pressure.

Blood Pressure Monitoring and Treatment Goals

Blood pressure should be monitored regularly (i.e., monthly) during therapy and dosage of the antihypertensive drug adjusted until blood pressure is controlled. If an adequate blood pressure response is not achieved, the dosage may be increased or another antihypertensive agent with demonstrated benefit and preferably with a complementary mechanism of action (e.g., angiotensin-converting enzyme [ACE] inhibitor, angiotensin II receptor antagonist, calcium-channel blocker, thiazide diuretic) may be added; if target blood pressure is still not achieved with the use of 2 antihypertensive agents, a third drug may be added. (See Uses: Hypertension.) In patients who develop unacceptable adverse effects with propranolol, the drug should be discontinued and another antihypertensive agent from a different pharmacologic class should be initiated.

The goal of hypertension management and prevention is to achieve and maintain optimal control of blood pressure. However, the optimum blood pressure threshold for initiating antihypertensive drug therapy and specific treatment goals remain controversial. While previous hypertension guidelines have based target blood pressure goals on age and comorbidities, the 2017 American College of Cardiology/American Heart Association (ACC/AHA) hypertension guideline incorporates underlying cardiovascular risk into decision making regarding treatment and generally recommends the same target blood pressure (i.e., less than 130/80 mm Hg) for all adults. Many patients will require at least 2 drugs from different pharmacologic classes to achieve this blood pressure goal; the potential benefits of hypertension management and drug cost, adverse effects, and risks associated with the use of multiple antihypertensive drugs also should be considered when deciding a patient's blood pressure treatment goal.

For additional information on target levels of blood pressure and on monitoring therapy in the management of hypertension, see Blood Pressure Monitoring and Treatment Goals under Dosage: Hypertension, in Dosage and Administration in the Thiazides General Statement 40:28.20.

Chronic Stable Angina

For the management of angina pectoris, the initial oral dosage of propranolol hydrochloride as extended-release capsules is 80 mg daily; dosage is gradually increased as needed to control symptoms, usually at 3- to 7-day intervals. Although optimum response usually occurs at a dosage of 160 mg daily, there is a wide variation in individual requirements.

When using conventional tablets or oral solutions, the usual dosage of propranolol hydrochloride is 80–320 mg daily (given in 2–4 divided doses). The value and safety of dosages greater than 320 mg daily have not been established, but some clinicians have stated that dosage may be increased further if there is only a partial response to usual dosage.

During long-term therapy, the patient should be periodically reevaluated to determine the need for dosage alteration or continued therapy. When propranolol hydrochloride is to be discontinued, dosage should be reduced slowly over a period of at least a few weeks (about 2). (See Cautions: Precautions and Contraindications.)

Cardiac Arrhythmias

The usual adult oral dosage of propranolol hydrochloride for the treatment of arrhythmias is 10–30 mg 3 or 4 times daily as conventional tablets or oral solution. For arrhythmias in adults which are life-threatening or occur during anesthesia, the manufacturer states that 1–3 mg may be administered IV under careful monitoring (e.g., ECG, central venous pressure). If necessary, a second IV dose may be administered after 2 minutes. Additional IV doses may be administered at intervals of no less than 4 hours until the desired response is obtained.

For the acute treatment of supraventricular tachycardia (SVT) (e.g., atrial flutter, junctional tachycardia, paroxysmal supraventricular tachycardia [PSVT], atrial tachycardia) in adults, some experts recommend an initial IV propranolol hydrochloride dose of 1 mg administered over 1 minute; additional doses may be given every 2 minutes up to a total of 3 doses. The usual oral maintenance dosage for ongoing treatment of SVT is 40–160 mg daily in divided doses or single doses (with long-acting preparations). To slow ventricular response in adults with acute atrial fibrillation, experts recommend an initial IV propranolol hydrochloride dose of 1 mg administered over 1 minute; additional doses may be given at 2-minute intervals up to a total of 3 doses. The usual oral maintenance dosage for ongoing treatment of atrial fibrillation is 40–160 mg daily in divided doses.

Hypertrophic Subaortic Stenosis

Hypertrophic subaortic stenosis in adults is usually treated with 20–40 mg of propranolol hydrochloride orally 3 or 4 times daily as conventional tablets or oral solution or 80–160 mg once daily as extended-release capsules.

Pheochromocytoma

In adults with pheochromocytoma, 60 mg of oral propranolol hydrochloride may be administered daily in divided doses as conventional tablets or oral solution in conjunction with an α-adrenergic blocking agent for 3 days prior to surgery. As an adjunct to prolonged treatment of inoperable pheochromocytoma, 30 mg of propranolol hydrochloride daily in divided doses with an α-adrenergic blocker is usually sufficient.

Vascular Headaches

Migraine

For prophylaxis of migraine in adults, the initial oral dosage of propranolol hydrochloride is 80 mg daily, given in divided doses as the conventional tablets or oral solution or once daily as the extended-release capsules. Dosage may be increased gradually to achieve optimum migraine prophylaxis. The usual effective dosage is 80–240 mg daily. If an adequate response is not obtained within 4–6 weeks after reaching the maximum dose, propranolol therapy should be discontinued; it may be advisable to withdraw the drug gradually over several weeks.

Myocardial Infarction

When used for secondary prevention after the acute phase of myocardial infarction (MI), the recommended oral dosage of propranolol hydrochloride is 180–240 mg daily (in divided doses) as conventional tablets or oral solution. In the study demonstrating mortality benefit with propranolol, the drug was initiated 5–21 days following infarction. Although the drug was given in 3 or 4 divided doses daily in clinical studies, there are considerable clinical, pharmacologic, and pharmacokinetic data suggesting that a twice-daily dosing regimen would also be adequate. Safety and efficacy of propranolol hydrochloride dosages exceeding 240 mg daily for the prevention of cardiac mortality have not been established; however, higher dosages may be required for the treatment of coexisting conditions such as angina or hypertension. Although the optimal duration of β-blocker therapy following MI remains to be clearly established, experts generally recommend that such therapy be continued long-term in post-MI patients with left ventricular systolic dysfunction, and for at least 3 years in those with normal left ventricular function.

Essential Tremor

The initial oral dosage of propranolol hydrochloride for the management of essential tremor in adults is 40 mg twice daily as conventional tablets. Response to the drug is variable and dosage must be individualized; optimum suppression of tremor usually is achieved with a dosage of 120–320 mg daily (administered in 3 divided doses when conventional tablets are used). In adjusting propranolol hydrochloride dosage, it should be remembered that complete suppression of essential tremor rarely is achieved. Some evidence suggests that dosages exceeding 320 mg daily do not provide substantial added benefit but are associated with an increased risk of adverse effects. Although currently not recommended by the manufacturer, usual dosages administered once daily each morning as extended-release capsules appear to be at least as effective as equivalent dosages administered in divided doses daily as conventional tablets. Some patients may benefit from intermittent rather than maintenance therapy; single 80- to 120-mg doses as conventional tablets have been administered 1–3 hours before planned activity or anticipated stress associated with tremor.

Pediatric Dosage

Hypertension

For the management of hypertension in children†, some experts have recommended an initial oral propranolol hydrochloride dosage of 1–2 mg/kg daily given in 2 or 3 divided doses as an immediate-release formulation. Dosage may be increased as necessary to a maximum dosage of 4 mg/kg (up to 640 mg) daily given in 2 or 3 divided doses. The extended-release formulation may be administered once daily.

Cardiac Arrhythmias

Although parenteral propranolol hydrochloride currently is not recommended by the manufacturer for use in children†, an initial IV dose of 10–20 mcg/kg infused over 10 minutes has been recommended by some clinicians for the treatment of cardiac arrhythmias in children. Some clinicians state that pediatric oral dosages exceeding 4 mg/kg daily may be necessary for the management of supraventricular tachyarrhythmias. Oral propranolol hydrochloride therapy has been initiated at 1.5–2 mg/kg daily and titrated upward as necessary to control the arrhythmia, up to a maximum dosage of 16 mg/kg daily given in 4 divided doses.

Thyrotoxicosis

For the treatment of tachyarrhythmias in neonates with thyrotoxicosis†, an oral propranolol hydrochloride dosage of 2 mg/kg daily given in 2–4 divided doses has been used, although higher dosages occasionally may be needed.

● Dosage in Hepatic Impairment

The manufacturers of propranolol hydrochloride injection state that a reduction in the dosage of propranolol hydrochloride may be necessary in patients with hepatic impairment.

CAUTIONS

The most common, serious adverse effects of propranolol hydrochloride are related to its β-adrenergic blocking activity. Adverse reactions are more frequent and may be more severe after IV administration than after oral administration. In one large study of hospitalized patients receiving propranolol, reactions were most common in azotemic patients and in those older than 60 years of age. The incidence of adverse reactions to oral propranolol was unrelated to the dose, and adverse reactions usually occurred soon after the initiation of therapy. The investigators concluded that many severe adverse reactions result from the inability of severely ill patients to withstand a decrease in normal β-adrenergic stimulation.

● Cardiovascular Effects

The most common adverse cardiovascular effect of propranolol is bradycardia, especially in patients with digitalis intoxication. Bradycardia is occasionally severe and may be accompanied by hypotension, syncope, shock, or angina pectoris. Severe bradycardia should be treated with IM or IV administration of atropine sulfate. (See Drug Interactions: Sympathomimetic Agents.) In patients with Wolff-Parkinson-White syndrome, propranolol has produced severe bradycardia requiring a demand pacemaker.

In patients with heart failure, sympathetic stimulation is vital for the support of circulatory function. In patients with inadequate cardiac function, heart failure may be precipitated as a result of removal of β-adrenergic stimulation when propranolol therapy is initiated. A decrease in exercise tolerance may be experienced by patients with left ventricular dysfunction. In patients without a prior history of heart failure, prolonged depression of the myocardium by propranolol has resulted in heart failure in rare instances. (See Cautions: Precautions and Contraindications.) Intensification of AV block, AV dissociation, AV conduction delays, complete heart block, or cardiac arrest may occur, especially in patients with preexisting partial heart block caused by a cardiac glycoside or other factors. Ventricular fibrillation has been reported in a patient with hypertrophic subaortic stenosis.

After sudden cessation of propranolol therapy in some patients treated for angina, increased frequency, duration, and severity of angina episodes have occurred, often within 24 hours. These episodes are unstable and are not relieved by nitroglycerin. Acute and sometimes fatal myocardial infarction and sudden death have also occurred after abrupt withdrawal of propranolol therapy in some patients treated for angina. In hypertensive patients, sudden cessation of propranolol has produced a syndrome similar to florid thyrotoxicosis, characterized by tenseness, anxiety, tachycardia, and excessive perspiration; these symptoms occurred within one week of cessation of the drug and were relieved by reinstituting propranolol therapy.

During surgery, some patients who have been receiving propranolol may experience severe, protracted hypotension and, occasionally, difficulty in restarting and maintaining heart beat. These adverse cardiovascular effects of propranolol may be reversed during surgery by IV administration of β-adrenergic agonists such as isoproterenol or norepinephrine.

Severe hypertension has been reported in a few patients with schizophrenic disorder who received only propranolol orally in rapidly increasing doses; the hypertension responded to treatment with IV phentolamine followed by oral phenoxybenzamine.

Fluid retention, pulmonary edema, and peripheral arterial insufficiency, usually of the Raynaud's type, may occur in patients receiving propranolol. When the drug is used alone, dietary sodium restriction may be necessary. Intermittent claudication has occurred in patients with previously asymptomatic peripheral arterial disease who received propranolol, although one study which used the drug for the treatment of intermittent claudication did not note any deterioration of occlusive peripheral arterial disease.

● Nervous System Effects

A number of adverse CNS effects, which are usually reversible after withdrawal of the drug, have been reported with propranolol. Adverse CNS effects usually occur after long-term treatment with high dosages of propranolol hydrochloride and range from lightheadedness, giddiness, ataxia, dizziness, irritability, sleepiness, hearing loss, and visual disturbances to vivid dreams, hallucinations, and confusion. Insomnia, lassitude, weakness, fatigue, and mental depression progressing to catatonia have been reported. Dosages exceeding 160 mg daily, when administered in divided doses exceeding 80 mg each, may be associated with an increased incidence of fatigue, lethargy, and vivid dreams. Organic brain syndrome, characterized by disorientation to time and place, short-term memory loss, emotional lability, slightly clouded sensorium, and decreased performance on neuropsychometric tests, has been reported rarely. Paresthesia of the hands, peripheral neuropathy, and precipitation of myotonia have been reported. Impotence has been reported rarely. Ptosis has been reported in at least 2 patients. A few patients receiving propranolol for hypertrophic obstructive cardiomyopathy have developed migraine in some cases associated with sensory disturbances and teichopsia.

● GI Effects

Adverse GI effects such as nausea, vomiting, diarrhea, epigastric distress, abdominal cramping, constipation, and flatulence may occur in patients receiving propranolol and occasionally necessitate reduction of dosage or withdrawal of the drug. Mesenteric arterial thrombosis and ischemic colitis have also occurred.

● Dermatologic and Sensitivity Reactions

Rarely, rashes have been reported during propranolol usage. Rashes are most commonly erythematous (maculopapular or acneiform), dry, scaly, pruritic, psoriasiform lesions which occur on the trunk, extremities, and scalp. Hyperkeratosis of the scalp, palms, and soles of the feet have been reported during treatment with propranolol; nail changes such as thickening, pitting, and discoloration have occurred. At least one case of exfoliative dermatitis has been reported. Dermatologic reactions disappear after the drug is withdrawn. Other allergic manifestations reported during propranolol therapy include fever accompanied by aching and sore throat, rhinitis, dry mouth, laryngospasm, respiratory distress, and pharyngitis. A lupus-like syndrome characterized by fever, pruritus, severe myalgia, and positive lupus erythematosus cell tests has been reported. Reversible alopecia, which recurred following readministration of the drug, also has been reported.

● Hematologic Effects

Adverse hematologic effects of propranolol include transient eosinophilia (a pharmacologic effect of β-adrenergic blockade) and idiosyncratic reactions including thrombocytopenic and nonthrombocytopenic purpura and, rarely, agranulocytosis.

● Endocrine Effects

Results of a large prospective cohort study of adults 45–64 years of age indicate that use of β-adrenergic blocking agents (β-blockers) in hypertensive patients is associated with increased risk (about 28%) of developing type 2 diabetes mellitus compared with hypertensive patients who were not receiving hypotensive therapy. In this study, the number of new cases of diabetes per 1000 person-years was 33.6 or 26.3 in patients receiving a β-blocker or no drug therapy, respectively. The association between the risk of developing diabetes mellitus and use of β-blockers reportedly was not confounded by weight gain, hyperinsulinemia, or differences in heart rate. It is not known if the risk of developing diabetes is affected by β-receptor selectivity. Further studies are needed to determine whether concomitant use of ACE inhibitors (which may improve insulin sensitivity) would abrogate β-blocker-induced adverse effects related to glucose intolerance. Therefore, until results of such studies are available, the proven benefits of β-blockers in reducing cardiovascular events in hypertensive patients must be weighed carefully against the possible risks of developing diabetes mellitus.

Hypoglycemia, which may result in loss of consciousness, also may occur in nondiabetic patients receiving β-blockers. Patients most at risk for the development of β-blocker-induced hypoglycemia are those undergoing dialysis, prolonged fasting, or severe exercise regimens.

β-Blockers may mask signs and symptoms of hypoglycemia (e.g., palpitation, tachycardia, tremor) and potentiate insulin-induced hypoglycemia. Acute increases in blood pressure have occurred after insulin-induced hypoglycemia in patients receiving propranolol. Although it has been suggested that nonselective β-blockers are more likely to induce hypoglycemia than selective β-blockers, such an adverse effect also has been reported with selective β-blockers (e.g., atenolol). In addition, selective β-blockers are less likely to mask symptoms of hypoglycemia or delay recovery from insulin-induced hypoglycemia than nonselective β-blockers because of their vascular sparing effects; however, selective β-blockers can decrease insulin sensitivity by approximately 15–30%, which may result in increased insulin requirements.

● *Other Adverse Effects*

Propranolol may cause elevated BUN in patients with severe heart disease, elevated serum creatinine, aminotransferase, alkaline phosphatase, or lactic dehydrogenase concentrations. In hypertensive patients, propranolol may cause small increases in serum potassium concentration. Peyronie's disease has been reported rarely. Generalized hyperemia of the conjunctivae with decreased tear production and a prickling sensation of the eyes, eye dryness, eye pain, discoloration of the tongue, and bad taste have been reported rarely.

● *Precautions and Contraindications*

Propranolol shares the toxic potentials of β-blockers, and the usual precautions of these agents should be observed. When propranolol is used as a fixed-combination preparation that includes hydrochlorothiazide, the cautions, precautions, and contraindications associated with thiazide diuretics must be considered in addition to those associated with propranolol.

In patients with heart failure, sympathetic stimulation is vital for the support of circulatory function. Propranolol should be used with caution in patients with inadequate cardiac function, since heart failure may be precipitated by blockade of β-adrenergic stimulation when propranolol therapy is administered. In addition, in patients with latent cardiac insufficiency, prolonged β-adrenergic blockade may lead to cardiac failure. Although β-blockers should be avoided in patients with overt heart failure, propranolol may be administered cautiously, if necessary, to patients with well-compensated heart failure (e.g., those controlled with cardiac glycosides and/or diuretics). Patients receiving propranolol therapy should be instructed to consult their physician at the first sign or symptom of impending cardiac failure and should be adequately treated (e.g., with a cardiac glycoside and/or diuretic) and observed closely; if cardiac failure continues, propranolol should be discontinued, gradually if possible.

Abrupt withdrawal of propranolol may exacerbate angina symptoms or precipitate myocardial infarction in patients with coronary artery disease. Abrupt withdrawal of the drug in patients treated for hypertension has also been associated with adverse effects. (See Cautions: Cardiovascular Effects.) Therefore, patients receiving propranolol (especially those with ischemic heart disease) should be warned not to interrupt or discontinue therapy without consulting their clinician. When discontinuance of propranolol therapy is planned, particularly in patients with ischemic heart disease, dosage of the drug should be gradually reduced over a period of at least a few (about 2) weeks. When propranolol therapy is discontinued, patients should be carefully monitored and their activity restricted. If exacerbation of angina occurs after propranolol therapy is interrupted, treatment with the drug should generally be reinstituted and appropriate measures taken for the management of unstable angina pectoris. Because coronary artery disease is common and may be unrecognized, the manufacturers caution that it may be prudent not to discontinue propranolol therapy abruptly, even in patients receiving the drug for conditions other than angina.

The necessity of withdrawing β-adrenergic blocking therapy prior to major surgery is controversial. Severe, protracted hypotension and difficulty in restarting or maintaining a heart beat have occurred during surgery in some patients who have received β-blockers. As with other β-blockers, the effects of propranolol can be reversed by administration of β-agonists (e.g., dobutamine, isoproterenol). If propranolol therapy is discontinued prior to major surgery, oral therapy with the drug may be restarted as soon after surgery as possible; patients who are unable to take oral drugs after surgery may be treated with IV propranolol if necessary.

Caution should be used when administering propranolol to patients with sinus node dysfunction, since the drug can cause marked depression of SA node automaticity. Propranolol should be used with extreme caution for the management of arrhythmias occurring during anesthesia with myocardial depressant anesthetics, since excessive myocardial depression, bradycardia, and hypotension may occur.

Signs of hyperthyroidism may be masked by propranolol, and patients with thyrotoxicosis who receive the drug should be monitored closely. In addition, the drug may alter thyroid function test results, increasing thyroxine (T_4) and reverse triiodothyronine (rT_3) and decreasing triiodothyronine (T_3) determinations.

It is recommended that propranolol be used with caution in patients with diabetes mellitus (especially those with labile diabetes or those prone to hypoglycemia) since the drug also may block the signs and symptoms of hypoglycemia (e.g., tachycardia and blood pressure changes but not sweating). However, many clinicians state that patients with diabetes mellitus may be particularly likely to experience a reduction in morbidity and mortality with the use of β-blockers. In addition, the drug occasionally causes hypoglycemia, even in nondiabetic patients, presumably by interfering with catecholamine-induced glycogenolysis. Propranolol may also inhibit the insulin-releasing mechanism of the pancreas and has been implicated in hyperglycemic reactions. Propranolol-induced alterations in glucose tolerance appear to occur only rarely. (See Cautions: Endocrine Effects.) Some sources state that hypertensive patients who are prone to hypoglycemia should not receive propranolol because the drug may cause a sharp rise in blood pressure.

Since β-blockers may inhibit bronchodilation produced by endogenous catecholamines, the drugs generally should not be used in patients with bronchospastic disease. Propranolol should be used with caution in patients with a history of nonallergic bronchospasm (e.g., chronic bronchitis, emphysema). β-adrenergic blockade may lead to an increase in airway resistance and bronchospasm, particularly in patients with a history of asthma. Bronchospasm may be treated with IV administration of aminophylline; isoproterenol may also be administered. (See Drug Interactions: Sympathomimetic Agents.) IV administration of atropine has been suggested if the patient fails to respond to the above or if bradycardia is present.

Since treatment with β-blockers (e.g., propranolol) may reduce intraocular pressure, patients should be advised that such therapy may interfere with glaucoma screening tests. Withdrawal of propranolol may lead to an increase in intraocular pressure.

Propranolol should be used with caution in patients with renal or hepatic impairment. Laboratory parameters should be monitored in patients receiving prolonged therapy with the drug.

Patients with a history of severe anaphylactic reactions to a variety of allergens may be more reactive to repeated, accidental, diagnostic, or therapeutic challenge with such allergens while receiving a β-blocker. These patients may be unresponsive to usual doses of epinephrine or may develop a paradoxical response to epinephrine when it is used to treat anaphylactic reactions.

Propranolol is contraindicated in patients with Raynaud's syndrome, bronchial asthma, sinus bradycardia and heart block greater than first degree, and overt and decompensated heart failure (unless the failure is secondary to a tachyarrhythmia treatable with propranolol). The drug is not indicated in the management of hypertensive emergencies. Although the manufacturers state that propranolol is contraindicated in patients with cardiogenic shock, results of some studies indicate that the drug may have a beneficial effect in patients with myocardial infarction with or without cardiogenic shock. (See Uses: Acute Myocardial Infarction.) Because propranolol has produced a myasthenic condition characterized by ptosis, weakness of limbs, and double vision in 2 patients, the drug may be contraindicated in patients with myasthenia gravis. In addition, since propranolol appears to impair metabolism of thioridazine which may result in increased plasma concentrations of thioridazine that may be associated with prolongation of the QT interval, the manufacturer of thioridazine states that concomitant use of thioridazine and propranolol is contraindicated. (See Drug Interactions: Phenothiazines and Other Psychotherapeutic Agents.)

● Pediatric Precautions

Although safety and efficacy of propranolol have not been as extensively or systematically studied in children as in adults, current information from the medical literature allows fair estimates, and specific dosing information has been reasonably studied. Cardiovascular diseases that are common to adults and children generally are as responsive to propranolol therapy in children as in adults, and adverse reactions also are similar. For information on overall principles and expert recommendations for treatment of hypertension in pediatric patients, see Uses: Hypertension in Pediatric Patients, in the Thiazides General Statement 40:28.20. One manufacturer states that the possibility that oral bioavailability of propranolol hydrochloride may be increased in children with Down's syndrome should be considered. Safety and efficacy of propranolol hydrochloride extended-release capsules, oral solution, and injection have not been established in children.

● Geriatric Precautions

Clinical studies of propranolol tablets, injections, and extended-release capsules did not include sufficient numbers of patients 65 years of age and older to determine whether geriatric patients respond differently than younger patients. If propranolol is used in geriatric patients, dosage of the drug should be selected with caution, usually initiating therapy at the low end of the dosage range since decreased hepatic, renal, or cardiac function and concomitant disease or other drug therapy are more common in this age group than in younger patients.

Decreased propranolol clearance and a prolonged elimination half-life have been reported in geriatric patients receiving propranolol hydrochloride injection, and the manufacturers recommend that dosage reduction be considered in these patients.

● Mutagenicity and Carcinogenicity

In long-term studies in animals, no evidence of propranolol-related tumorigenic effects was observed.

● Pregnancy, Fertility, and Lactation

Pregnancy

There are no adequate and well-controlled studies to date using propranolol in pregnant women. Safe use of propranolol during pregnancy has not been established. Low birthweight infants with respiratory distress and hypoglycemia have been born to women who received propranolol throughout pregnancy. Bradycardia, hypoglycemia, and respiratory depression also have been reported in neonates whose mothers received propranolol at parturition; adequate facilities for monitoring such infants at birth should be available. The manufacturers state that the drug should be used during pregnancy only when the possible benefits outweigh the potential risks to the fetus.

Embryotoxicity (reduced litter size, increased resorption rates) and neonatal toxicity (deaths) have been reported in reproductive studies in rats receiving propranolol hydrochloride 150 mg/kg daily by gavage or in the diet throughout pregnancy and lactation; however, such effects were not observed in rats receiving 80 mg/kg daily (equivalent to the maximum recommended human dosage on a mg/m² basis). No evidence of embryotoxicity or neonatal toxicity was observed in rabbits receiving oral doses of propranolol hydrochloride of up to 150 mg/kg daily (about 5 times the maximum recommended oral human daily dose) throughout pregnancy and lactation.

Fertility

Reproduction studies in animals using propranolol have not revealed evidence of impaired fertility.

Lactation

Since propranolol is distributed into milk, the drug should be used with caution in nursing women.

DRUG INTERACTIONS

● Drugs Affecting or Metabolized by Hepatic Microsomal Enzymes

Because metabolism of propranolol is mediated by cytochrome P-450 (CYP) isoenzymes 2D6, 1A2, and 2C19, drugs that induce or inhibit these isoenzymes may alter the metabolism of propranolol, which may result in clinically important drug interactions. Inhibitors or substrates of the isoenzymes 2D6 (e.g., amiodarone, cimetidine, delavirdine, fluoxetine, paroxetine, quinidine, ritonavir), 1A2 (e.g., cimetidine, ciprofloxacin, fluvoxamine, imipramine, isoniazid, ritonavir, rizatriptan, theophylline, zileuton, zolmitriptan), or 2C19 (e.g., cimetidine, fluconazole, fluoxetine, fluvoxamine, teniposide, tolbutamide) could decrease the metabolism and increase plasma concentrations of propranolol. Drugs that induce cytochrome P-450 activity (e.g., alcohol, rifampin) may increase the metabolism of propranolol and decrease its plasma concentrations; in current smokers, plasma propranolol concentrations also may be decreased because cigarette smoking may induce hepatic metabolism of the drug, increasing propranolol clearance up to 100%.

● Phenothiazines and Other Psychotherapeutic Agents

Phenothiazines and propranolol may have additive hypotensive activity, especially when phenothiazines are administered in large doses. Chlorpromazine has been shown to reduce the clearance of propranolol and increase plasma propranolol concentrations. Increased plasma concentrations of chlorpromazine also have been reported in patients receiving the drug concomitantly with propranolol. Hypotension and cardiac arrest have occurred during concomitant therapy with propranolol and haloperidol.

In addition, since propranolol may inhibit metabolism of thioridazine, concomitant use of propranolol hydrochloride (100–800 mg daily) and thioridazine, reportedly resulted in increased plasma concentrations of thioridazine and its metabolites by about 50–400 and 80–300%, respectively. Because such increased concentrations of thioridazine may enhance thioridazine-induced prolongation of the QT_c interval, and increase the risk of serious, potentially fatal cardiac arrhythmias (e.g., torsades de pointes), the manufacturer of thioridazine states that concomitant use of thioridazine and propranolol is contraindicated.

Complete heart block has been reported in a patient receiving fluoxetine concomitantly with propranolol. The mechanism of this interaction is not known; however, it has been postulated that fluoxetine may inhibit metabolism of lipophilic β-adrenergic blocking agents (β-blockers) (e.g., propranolol, metoprolol), increase their bioavailability, and increase their β-adrenergic blocking effects. Therefore, some clinicians recommend that fluoxetine be administered with caution in patients receiving β-blockers and in those with impaired cardiac conduction.

The hypotensive effects of monoamine oxidase (MAO) inhibitors or tricyclic antidepressants may be exacerbated in patients receiving β-blockers.

Decreased metabolism and increased plasma concentrations of diazepam and its metabolites have been reported in patients receiving the drug concomitantly with propranolol; propranolol does not appear to alter pharmacokinetics of other benzodiazepines (e.g., alprazolam, lorazepam, oxazepam, triazolam). Diazepam does not alter pharmacokinetics of propranolol.

● Sympathomimetic Agents

The β-adrenergic stimulating effects of sympathomimetic agents are antagonized by propranolol. This interaction is especially pronounced with isoproterenol, and very large doses of isoproterenol may be needed to overcome the β-adrenergic blocking effects of propranolol. The effects of propranolol also can be reversed by administration of dobutamine. In addition, propranolol may reduce sensitivity to dobutamine stress echocardiography in patients undergoing evaluation for myocardial ischemia. Patients receiving long-term propranolol therapy may experience uncontrolled hypertension upon administration of epinephrine as a result of unopposed α-receptor stimulation. In patients receiving propranolol, epinephrine should be administered with caution since a decrease in pulse rate with first- and second-degree heart block may occur.

● Antimuscarinic Agents and Drugs with Anticholinergic Effects

Antimuscarinic agents, such as atropine, may counteract the bradycardia caused by propranolol by reestablishing the balance between sympathetic and parasympathetic actions on the heart. Tricyclic antidepressants (e.g., amitriptyline) also have anticholinergic activity and may similarly antagonize the cardiac β-adrenergic blocking effects of propranolol, although not as intensely as do the antimuscarinics.

● Catecholamine-depleting Drugs

When propranolol and a catecholamine-depleting drug (e.g., reserpine) are administered concomitantly, the effects of the drugs may be additive. Excessive reduction of resting sympathetic nervous system activity, which may lead to hypotension, severe bradycardia, vertigo, syncope, or orthostatic hypotension, has been reported in patients receiving both drugs concurrently. Concomitant use of reserpine and propranolol also may potentiate depression.

● Selective Serotonin Agonists

Increased concentrations of zolmitriptan and rizatriptan have been reported in patients receiving concomitant propranolol therapy.

● Diuretics and Cardiovascular Drugs

When propranolol is administered with diuretics or other antihypertensive drugs, the hypotensive effect of propranolol may be increased. This effect is usually used to therapeutic advantage, but careful adjustment of dosage is necessary when these drugs are used concomitantly. In addition to its potentially additive hypotensive effect, reserpine theoretically may add to the β-adrenergic blocking activity of propranolol through its catecholamine-depleting activity. (See Drug Interactions: Catecholamine-depleting Drugs.)

Clonidine

The antihypertensive effects of clonidine may be antagonized by β-blockers, including propranolol. Because β-blockers (e.g., propranolol) may exacerbate rebound hypertension that may occur following discontinuance of clonidine therapy, β-blockers should be discontinued several days before gradual withdrawal of clonidine when clonidine therapy is to be discontinued in patients receiving a β-blocker and clonidine concurrently.

Angiotensin-converting Enzyme Inhibitors

Concomitant therapy with angiotensin-converting enzyme (ACE) inhibitors and β-blockers (e.g., propranolol) may result in hypotension, particularly in patients with acute myocardial infarction. Increased bronchial hyperreactivity has been reported in patients receiving ACE inhibitors concomitantly with propranolol.

α-Adrenergic Blocking Agents

Prolonged hypotension associated with administration of a first prazosin dose has been reported in patients receiving β-blockers. In addition, postural hypotension has been reported in patients receiving β-blockers concomitantly with terazosin or doxazosin.

Other Cardiovascular Agents

When propranolol is administered with antiarrhythmic drugs such as lidocaine, phenytoin, procainamide, quinidine, or verapamil (see Drug Interactions: β-Adrenergic Blocking Agents, in Verapamil 24:28.92), cardiac effects may be additive or antagonistic and toxic effects may be additive.

Concomitant use of β-blockers (e.g., propranolol) and certain other cardiovascular drugs (e.g., cardiac glycosides, lidocaine, nondihydropyridine calcium-channel blocking agents) can have additive negative effects on SA or AV nodal conduction. Slowing or complete suppression of SA node activity with development of slow ventricular rates (e.g., 30–40 bpm), often misdiagnosed as complete AV block, has been reported in patients receiving the nondihydropyridine calcium-channel blocking agent mibefradil (no longer commercially available in the US), principally in geriatric patients and in association with concomitant β-adrenergic blocker therapy. Concomitant therapy with an IV β-blocker and IV verapamil has resulted rarely in serious adverse

reactions, especially in patients with severe cardiomyopathy, heart failure, or recent myocardial infarction. Severe bradycardia, heart failure, and cardiovascular collapse have been reported in patients receiving verapamil concomitantly with β-blockers.

Caution should be used in patients receiving propranolol concomitantly with a calcium-channel blocking agent with negative inotropic and/or chronotropic effects, since both drugs may depress myocardial contractility and AV conduction. Severe bradycardia, asystole, heart failure, and cardiovascular collapse have been reported in patients receiving propranolol concomitantly with disopyramide or verapamil. In addition, bradycardia, hypotension, high-degree heart block, and heart failure have been reported in patients with cardiac disease receiving concomitant therapy with propranolol and diltiazem. Concomitant use of propranolol with amiodarone also may result in additive negative chronotropic effects, while additive negative inotropic and β-adrenergic blocking effects may occur when propafenone and propranolol are used concomitantly. In patients currently receiving a cardiac glycoside, concomitant propranolol therapy may reduce the positive inotropic effect of the glycoside. (See Cautions: Precautions and Contraindications.)

Increased propafenone exposure has been reported in patients receiving the drug concomitantly with propranolol. Verapamil does not appear to affect pharmacokinetics of propranolol and propranolol does not affect pharmacokinetics of verapamil or norverapamil. Increased propranolol concentrations have been reported in patients receiving concomitant therapy with nisoldipine or nicardipine with propranolol; increased concentrations of nifedipine may occur in patients receiving the drug concomitantly with propranolol.

Administration of quinidine has been reported to cause decreased propranolol metabolism, resulting in increased propranolol plasma concentrations and increased β-blocking effects (and possible postural hypotension). Reduced lidocaine metabolism and clearance resulting in lidocaine toxicity have been reported in patients receiving the drug concomitantly with propranolol.

● Antilipemic Agents

Decreased propranolol plasma concentrations have been reported in patients receiving the drug concomitantly with cholestyramine or colestipol. Decreased plasma concentrations of lovastatin and pravastatin have been reported in patients receiving the drugs concomitantly with propranolol; however, the pharmacodynamics of the antilipemics were not altered.

● Warfarin

Increases in warfarin bioavailability and prothrombin time have been reported in patients receiving warfarin concomitantly with propranolol. Prothrombin time should be monitored in patients receiving warfarin concomitantly with propranolol.

● Neuromuscular Blocking Agents

High doses of propranolol may potentiate the effects of neuromuscular blocking agents such as tubocurarine chloride, possibly because of propranolol's interference with ionic permeability of the postjunctional membrane. Propranolol should be administered with caution to patients who are receiving neuromuscular blocking agents or who are recovering from their effects.

● Antidiabetic Agents

β-Blockers may impair glucose tolerance; increase the frequency or severity of hypoglycemia; block hypoglycemia-induced tachycardia but not hypoglycemic sweating, which may actually be increased; delay the rate of recovery of blood glucose concentration following drug-induced hypoglycemia; alter the hemodynamic response to hypoglycemia, possibly resulting in an exaggerated hypertensive response; and possibly impair peripheral circulation. Nonselective β-blockers (e.g., propranolol, nadolol) without intrinsic sympathomimetic activity are more likely to affect glucose metabolism than more selective β-blockers (e.g., metoprolol, atenolol) or those with intrinsic sympathomimetic activity (e.g., acebutolol, pindolol). Signs of hypoglycemia (e.g., tachycardia, blood pressure changes, tremor, feelings of anxiety) mediated by catecholamines may be masked by either nonselective or selective β-blockers. When an oral antidiabetic agent or insulin and a β-blocker are used concomitantly, the patient should be advised about and monitored closely for altered antidiabetic response.

● **Ergot Alkaloids**

One case of severe peripheral vasoconstriction with pain and cyanosis has been reported in a patient who received propranolol orally and high doses of ergotamine in a rectal suppository concurrently for the treatment of migraine; however, several patients have received these drugs concomitantly without adverse effects. Caution should be used during simultaneous administration of propranolol and high doses of ergot alkaloids because of the possibility of additive peripheral vasoconstriction.

● **Cimetidine**

Cimetidine can substantially reduce the clearance of propranolol (apparently by inhibiting the hepatic metabolism of propranolol), which results in increased propranolol concentrations. If propranolol and cimetidine are administered concomitantly, the patient should be monitored for signs and symptoms of increased β-adrenergic blocking activity.

● **Antacids**

Concomitant oral administration of an aluminum hydroxide antacid with propranolol may reduce the GI absorption of propranolol. In a study in healthy adults, oral administration of 30 mL of an aluminum hydroxide (1.2 g) suspension with a single, 80-mg dose of propranolol hydrochloride reduced the peak plasma propranolol concentration and bioavailability of the drug by about 60%. The mechanism of this potential interaction has not been elucidated, but propranolol adsorption to or complexation with aluminum hydroxide does not appear to be involved. In another study in healthy adults, however, concomitant oral administration of 30 mL of an aluminum hydroxide suspension with a single, 40-mg dose of propranolol hydrochloride did *not* substantially affect bioavailability of propranolol. The need to avoid concomitant use or stagger dosing of an aluminum hydroxide antacid and propranolol has not been fully elucidated, but increasing propranolol dosage may be considered if an interaction is suspected.

● **Levodopa**

Propranolol may antagonize the hypotensive and positive inotropic effects of levodopa. This interaction is not well documented; however, the possibility of its occurrence should be kept in mind.

● **Nonsteroidal Anti-inflammatory Agents**

The possibility that nonsteroidal anti-inflammatory agents (NSAIAs; e.g., indomethacin) may reduce the hypotensive effect of β-blockers such as propranolol should be considered. (See Drug Interactions, in Indomethacin 28:08.04.92.)

● **Theophylline**

Propranolol decreases the clearance of theophylline in a dose-dependent manner by inhibiting hepatic microsomal metabolism (principally demethylation). In addition, propranolol can antagonize theophylline-induced bronchodilation.

ACUTE TOXICITY

● **Manifestations**

Limited information is available on the acute toxicity of propranolol hydrochloride. In adults who intentionally ingested the drug, estimates of the ingested doses have ranged from 0.8–6 g. The principal manifestations of overdosage were bradycardia and severe hypotension (which may result in peripheral cyanosis); loss of consciousness and seizures have also occurred. In most cases of acute propranolol overdosage, the patient recovered; however, in a few cases, toxicity was severe enough to result in death. Two small children who ingested a total of 150 mg of propranolol hydrochloride became drowsy, perspired, and experienced periods of SA node block; they were treated with IV and oral dextrose. Severe paradoxical rise in blood pressure has been reported in 8 patients with schizophrenic disorder who received propranolol hydrochloride in rapidly increasing doses (600 mg in the first 24 hours); these patients responded to IV phentolamine.

● **Treatment**

Treatment of propranolol hydrochloride overdosage generally involves symptomatic and supportive care. Following acute ingestion of the drug, the stomach should be emptied immediately by inducing emesis or by gastric lavage. If the patient is comatose, having seizures, or lacks the gag reflex, gastric lavage may be performed if an endotracheal tube with cuff inflated is in place to prevent aspiration of gastric contents. For symptomatic bradycardia, IV atropine may be given; if bradycardia persists, IV isoproterenol hydrochloride may be administered cautiously (large doses may be required), and in refractory cases, use of a transvenous cardiac pacemaker should be considered. A vasopressor (e.g., norepinephrine, dopamine) may be given for severe hypotension. For heart failure, a cardiac glycoside and diuretic may be used. Because of the possibility of uncontrolled hypertension secondary to unopposed α-receptor stimulation in patients receiving long-term propranolol therapy, epinephrine is not indicated for the treatment of propranolol overdosage. Glucagon also may be useful for the management of myocardial depression and hypotension. Phosphodiesterase inhibitors also may be useful in the management of propranolol overdosage. A β_2-adrenergic agonist and/or a theophylline derivative may be used for bronchospasm. IV diazepam may be useful for controlling seizures. Hemodialysis is probably not useful for enhancing elimination of propranolol in acute overdosage.

PHARMACOLOGY

Propranolol hydrochloride is a nonselective β-adrenergic blocking agent (β-blocker). Propranolol inhibits response to adrenergic stimuli by competitively blocking β-adrenergic receptors within the myocardium and within bronchial and vascular smooth muscle. Only the *l*-isomer of propranolol has substantial β-adrenergic blocking activity. Propranolol has no intrinsic sympathomimetic activity.

Through its myocardial β-adrenergic blocking action, propranolol decreases heart rate and prevents exercise-induced increases in heart rate, decreases myocardial contractility, decreases cardiac output, increases systolic ejection time, and increases cardiac volume. The drug also decreases conduction velocity through the sinoatrial (SA) and atrioventricular (AV) nodes and decreases myocardial automaticity via β-adrenergic blockade. At blood concentrations greater than those required for β-adrenergic blockade, propranolol has a membrane-stabilizing effect on the heart which is similar to that of quinidine. The clinical importance of this effect is not clear, but it appears to be less important than its β-adrenergic blocking activity.

β-Adrenergic blockade may also increase peripheral resistance initially, but peripheral resistance tends to decrease after chronic administration of the drug as a result of unopposed α-adrenergic vasoconstriction. The cardiac effects of β-adrenergic blockade cause an increase in sodium reabsorption because of alterations in renal hemodynamics; renal blood flow and glomerular filtration rate generally decrease during chronic therapy. Plasma volume may increase if dietary sodium is not restricted. Hepatic blood flow is decreased.

The precise mechanism of propranolol's hypotensive effect has not been determined. It has been postulated that β-blockers reduce blood pressure by blocking peripheral (especially cardiac) adrenergic receptors (decreasing cardiac output), by decreasing sympathetic outflow from the CNS, and/or by suppressing renin release. In patients with high concentrations of circulating renin, low doses of the drug are associated with a fall in both blood pressure and in plasma renin concentrations, probably because of acute peripheral β-adrenergic blockade. With higher doses of propranolol, the hypotensive effect is probably unrelated to plasma renin activity and may be caused by a delayed centrally mediated reduction of adrenergic outflow. However, there appears to be some overlap between these mechanisms, and both mechanisms seem to be operative with usual therapeutic doses. Propranolol decreases blood pressure in both the supine and standing positions.

Several effects of propranolol may contribute to its usefulness in the management of angina pectoris. The drug usually causes decreased myocardial oxygen consumption and, secondarily, a decrease in coronary blood flow. The drug may reduce the oxygen requirements of the heart because of its β-adrenergic blockade. Propranolol also appears to cause redistribution of 2,3-diphosphoglyceric acid in erythrocytes which results in a decrease in the affinity of hemoglobin for oxygen, enhancing oxygen delivery to the tissues. This action is unrelated to β-adrenergic blockade. Propranolol may also affect platelet aggregation through a nonspecific platelet membrane effect unrelated to β-adrenergic blockade and possibly because of interference with calcium flux. In one study of patients with angina, the drug restored previously elevated platelet aggregability to normal. Abrupt withdrawal of the drug in patients with angina may cause rebound platelet hyperaggregability.

When used prophylactically, propranolol can prevent common migraine or reduce the number of attacks in some patients. β-Adrenergic receptors have been shown to be present in the pial vessels of the brain; however, the exact mechanism of the antimigraine effect of propranolol is not known. Some evidence suggests that propranolol may prevent migraines through diminishing central catecholaminergic hyperactivity, possibly by inhibiting norepinephrine release, reducing neuronal activity and excitability, exerting membrane-stabilizing effects, and inhibiting nitric oxide production.

Through its β-adrenergic blocking action in other body systems, propranolol increases airway resistance (especially in asthmatic patients), inhibits glycogenolysis in the skeletal and cardiac muscles, blocks the release of free fatty acids and insulin by adrenergic stimulation, and increases the number of circulating eosinophils. Propranolol increases uterine activity, more in the nonpregnant than in the pregnant uterus.

PHARMACOKINETICS

● Absorption

Propranolol is almost completely absorbed from the GI tract; however, plasma concentrations attained are quite variable among individuals. There is no difference in the rate of absorption of the 2 isomers of propranolol. Propranolol appears in the plasma within 30 minutes, and peak plasma concentrations are reached about 60–90 minutes after oral administration of the conventional tablets. The time when peak plasma concentrations are reached may be delayed, but concentrations are not necessarily lowered, when the drug is administered with food. One manufacturer states that oral bioavailability of the drug may be increased in children with Down's syndrome; higher than expected plasma propranolol concentrations have been observed in such children. Bioavailability of a single 40-mg oral dose of propranolol hydrochloride as a conventional tablet or oral solution reportedly is equivalent in adults. Propranolol is slowly absorbed following administration of the drug as extended-release capsules, and peak blood concentrations are reached about 6 hours after administration. When measured at steady-state over a 24-hour period, the area under the plasma concentration-time curve (AUC) for the extended-release capsules is about 60–65% of the AUC for a comparable divided daily dose of the conventional tablets. The lower AUC is probably caused by the slower rate of absorption of the drug from the extended-release capsules with resultant greater hepatic metabolism. After administration of a single dose of propranolol hydrochloride as the extended-release capsules, blood concentrations of propranolol are fairly constant for about 12 hours and then decline exponentially during the following 12 hours.

Plasma propranolol concentrations attained after IV administration of the drug are relatively consistent among individuals. After administration of a 0.5-mg IV bolus of propranolol hydrochloride, peak plasma propranolol concentrations of 40 ng/mL are produced in 1 minute and the drug is undetectable in the plasma in 5 minutes. Following IV administration of propranolol, the onset of action is almost immediate. Animal studies indicate that propranolol is rapidly absorbed after IM administration.

After absorption from the GI tract, propranolol is bound by the liver through nonspecific tissue binding. There are large individual differences in hepatic extraction, probably because of differences in hepatic blood flow. Following oral administration, the drug does not reach the general circulation until hepatic binding sites are saturated. Once saturation occurs, hepatic binding no longer affects the passage of the drug into the blood. The amount of drug that reaches the circulation after oral administration also depends on the amount of drug metabolized on the first pass through the liver. Propranolol decreases its own rate of metabolism by decreasing hepatic blood flow. Studies indicate that hepatic extraction and possibly metabolism of propranolol are reduced following oral administration of the drug in patients with chronic renal disease, resulting in higher peak plasma concentrations of the drug after the first dose than are attained in patients with normal renal function.

There is considerable interpatient variation in the relationship of plasma propranolol concentrations and therapeutic effect, but therapeutic plasma concentrations of propranolol are usually 50–100 ng/mL. Concentrations of 100 ng/mL generally represent a high degree of β-adrenergic blockade. There are several possible metabolic explanations for the discrepancies between plasma concentrations and therapeutic effect. (See Pharmacokinetics: Elimination.) Individual differences in sympathetic tone may also contribute to interpatient differences in response.

● Distribution

Propranolol is widely distributed into body tissues including lungs, liver, kidneys, and heart. Propranolol readily crosses the blood-brain barrier and the placenta. The drug is distributed into milk.

The apparent volume of distribution of propranolol at steady-state varies widely in proportion to the fraction of unbound drug in whole blood. Propranolol is more than 90% bound to plasma proteins over a wide range of blood concentrations. Both free and protein-bound propranolol are metabolized. Increased plasma protein binding of the drug increases its metabolism and decreases its volume of distribution, resulting in a shorter terminal half-life.

● Elimination

Elimination of propranolol appears to follow first-order kinetics and seems to be independent of plasma concentration or the dose administered, at least with oral doses of 160–320 mg/day. The reported elimination half-life varies considerably among different studies. After IV administration of 10 mg of propranolol hydrochloride at a rate of 1.03 mg/minute in one study, plasma concentrations declined in a biphasic manner; the half-life during the initial phase ($t_{1/2}\alpha$) was 10 minutes and that during the terminal phase ($t_{1/2}\beta$) was 2.3 hours. Results from one study indicate that the half-life of the l-isomer is about 50% longer than that of the d-isomer. When usual therapeutic doses of propranolol hydrochloride are administered chronically, the half-life of propranolol ranges from 3.4–6 hours. Single-dose studies generally have shown a shorter half-life of 2–3 hours. This difference in half-life between chronic and single-dose studies may be the result of initial removal of the drug into a large extravascular space (especially hepatic binding sites) and also a saturation of systemic clearance (including drug metabolizing enzymes and excretion). The half-life of propranolol may decrease with decreasing renal function; however, there is insufficient evidence to indicate that any alteration in maintenance dosage is necessary in patients with impaired renal function.

During initial oral therapy (but not during IV or chronic oral therapy), an active metabolite, 4-hydroxypropranolol, is formed. 4-Hydroxypropranolol has about the same β-adrenergic blocking potency as does propranolol and may be present in plasma in amounts about equal to propranolol. This metabolite is eliminated more rapidly than propranolol and is virtually absent from the plasma 6 hours after oral administration of the drug. Results of one study indicate that after IV administration or chronic oral administration of propranolol, 4-hydroxypropranolol is not formed to a substantial extent, and β-adrenergic blocking activity is more closely reflected by propranolol concentrations. Individual variations in ability to hydroxylate propranolol to the active metabolite may also exist. In addition, some other metabolites of propranolol may possess antiarrhythmic activity without β-adrenergic blocking activity.

Propranolol is almost completely metabolized in the liver and at least 8 metabolites have been identified in urine. Only 1–4% of an oral or IV dose of the drug appears in feces as unchanged drug and metabolites. In patients with severely impaired renal function, a compensatory increase in fecal excretion of propranolol occurs. Reduced propranolol plasma clearance and increased peak plasma concentrations have been reported in patients with chronic renal failure compared with healthy individuals and patients receiving dialysis. Chronic renal failure may be associated with reduced drug metabolism secondary to downregulation of hepatic cytochrome P-450 (CYP) enzyme system activity. Propranolol is apparently not substantially removed by hemodialysis.

Decreased propranolol clearance and prolonged elimination half-life have been reported in geriatric patients compared with younger patients. In addition, reduced clearance, increased volume of distribution, decreased protein binding, and considerable variation in elimination half-life of propranolol have been reported in patients with chronic liver disease compared with individuals with normal liver function. Increased propranolol exposure and decreased clearance also have been reported in obese individuals compared with nonobese individuals.

CHEMISTRY AND STABILITY

● Chemistry

Propranolol hydrochloride is a nonselective β-adrenergic blocking agent (β-blocker). Propranolol hydrochloride occurs as a white or off-white, crystalline powder with a bitter taste and is soluble in water and in alcohol. The commercially available drug is a racemic mixture of the 2 optical isomers. Solutions of propranolol hydrochloride fluoresce at pH 4–5. The injection is adjusted to pH 2.8–3.5 with citric acid.

● Stability

Propranolol hydrochloride preparations should be protected from light and stored at room temperature (20–25°C). The manufacturer recommends that propranolol hydrochloride extended-release capsules be stored in tight, light-resistant containers and be protected from moisture, freezing, and excessive heat. Propranolol hydrochloride injection also should be protected from freezing and excessive heat. USP recommends that propranolol hydrochloride preparations be stored in well-closed containers. Solutions of the drug have maximum stability at pH 3 and decompose rapidly at alkaline pH. Decomposition in aqueous solution is accompanied by a lowered pH and discoloration. Propranolol hydrochloride injection is reportedly compatible with 0.9% sodium chloride injection; however, specialized references should be consulted for specific compatibility information.

PREPARATIONS

Excipients in commercially available drug preparations may have clinically important effects in some individuals; consult specific product labeling for details.

Propranolol Hydrochloride

Oral

Capsules, extended-release	60 mg	Inderal® LA, Ani Pharms
	80 mg	Inderal® LA, Ani Pharms
		Innopran® XL, Ani Pharms
	120 mg	Inderal® LA, Ani Pharms
		Innopran® XL, Ani Pharms
	160 mg	Inderal® LA, Ani Pharms

Solution	20 mg/5 mL*	Propranolol Hydrochloride Solution
	40 mg/5 mL*	Propranolol Hydrochloride Solution
Tablets	10 mg*	Propranolol Hydrochloride Tablets
	20 mg*	Propranolol Hydrochloride Tablets
	40 mg*	Propranolol Hydrochloride Tablets
	60 mg*	Propranolol Hydrochloride Tablets
	80 mg*	Propranolol Hydrochloride Tablets

Parenteral

| Injection | 1 mg/mL* | Propranolol Hydrochloride Injection |

* available from one or more manufacturer, distributor, and/or repackager by generic (nonproprietary) name

Propranolol Hydrochloride and Hydrochlorothiazide

Oral

| Tablets | 40 mg Propranolol Hydrochloride and Hydrochlorothiazide 25 mg* | Propranolol Hydrochloride and hydroCHLOROthiazide Tablets |
| | 80 mg Propranolol Hydrochloride and Hydrochlorothiazide 25 mg* | Propranolol Hydrochloride and hydroCHLOROthiazide Tablets |

* available from one or more manufacturer, distributor, and/or repackager by generic (nonproprietary) name

† Use is not currently included in the labeling approved by the US Food and Drug Administration.

Selected Revisions April 10, 2024, © Copyright, July 1, 1977, American Society of Health-System Pharmacists, Inc.

Sotalol Hydrochloride

24:20 • β-ADRENERGIC BLOCKING AGENTS

■ Sotalol hydrochloride is a nonselective β-adrenergic blocking agent that exhibits antiarrhythmic activity characteristic of class II and class III antiarrhythmic agents.

USES

Sotalol is used to suppress and prevent the recurrence of documented life-threatening ventricular arrhythmias (e.g., sustained ventricular tachycardia). The drug also is used to maintain normal sinus rhythm in patients with symptomatic atrial fibrillation or flutter who are currently in sinus rhythm. Sotalol also has been used in the management of other supraventricular arrhythmias such as paroxysmal supraventricular tachycardia (PSVT)†.

The choice of a β-adrenergic blocking agent depends on numerous factors, including pharmacologic properties (e.g., relative β-selectivity, intrinsic sympathomimetic activity, membrane-stabilizing activity, lipophilicity), pharmacokinetics, intended use, and adverse effect profile, as well as the patient's coexisting disease states or conditions, response, and tolerance. While specific pharmacologic properties and other factors may appropriately influence the choice of a β-blocker in individual patients, evidence of clinically important differences among the agents in terms of overall efficacy and/or safety is limited. Patients who do not respond to or cannot tolerate one β-blocker may be successfully treated with a different agent.

● Ventricular Arrhythmias

Sotalol is used to suppress and prevent the recurrence of documented life-threatening ventricular arrhythmias (e.g., sustained ventricular tachycardia) and has been designated an orphan drug by the FDA for such use.

Although antiarrhythmic agents, including sotalol, may suppress the recurrence of arrhythmias and improve symptoms, there is no evidence from randomized controlled studies indicating that these drugs have a beneficial effect on mortality or sudden death. Findings from the National Heart, Lung, and Blood Institute (NHLBI)'s Cardiac Arrhythmia Suppression Trial (CAST) after an average of 10 months of follow-up have indicated that the rate of total mortality and nonfatal cardiac arrest in patients with recent myocardial infarction (MI), mild to moderate left ventricular dysfunction, and asymptomatic or mildly symptomatic ventricular arrhythmias (principally frequent premature ventricular complexes [PVCs]) who received encainide or flecainide (class I antiarrhythmic drugs) increased substantially compared with placebo. (See Cautions in Flecainide 24:04.04.12.) Like other antiarrhythmic agents, sotalol can worsen existing arrhythmias or cause new arrhythmias, including torsades de pointes. Because of the drug's arrhythmogenic potential, use of sotalol for less severe arrhythmias, even if symptomatic, is not recommended by the manufacturer, and treatment of asymptomatic PVCs should be avoided. (See Cautions: Arrhythmogenic Effects.)

Although comparative data are limited, sotalol generally is considered to be as effective as some other antiarrhythmic agents (e.g., procainamide, quinidine) for the management of severe refractory arrhythmias. Data from clinical studies indicate that the drug is effective in approximately 55–85% of patients with life-threatening ventricular arrhythmias, including those refractory to other antiarrhythmic agents, and also is effective in patients with less severe arrhythmias. Sotalol can reduce PVCs, paired PVCs, and nonsustained ventricular tachycardia in patients with frequent PVCs, and can also suppress the recurrence of ventricular tachyarrhythmias in patients with ventricular tachycardia and/or fibrillation. The drug also has suppressed Holter monitor evidence of sustained ventricular tachycardia and ventricular tachycardia induced by programmed electrical stimulation (PES). Although some studies have shown that sotalol may reduce the risk of death from any cause and from cardiac causes compared with several class I antiarrhythmics (e.g., mexiletine, procainamide, propafenone, quinidine) in patients with ventricular tachyarrhythmias, the effect of the drug on survival (e.g., relative to placebo) remains to be established.

Life-threatening Ventricular Arrhythmias During Cardiac Arrest

Antiarrhythmic drugs are used during cardiac arrest to facilitate and maintain a spontaneous perfusing rhythm in patients with refractory (i.e., persisting or recurring after at least one shock) ventricular fibrillation or pulseless ventricular tachycardia; however, there is no evidence that these drugs increase survival to hospital discharge when given routinely during cardiac arrest. High-quality cardiopulmonary resuscitation (CPR) and defibrillation are integral components of advanced cardiovascular life support (ACLS) and the only proven interventions to increase survival to hospital discharge. Other resuscitative efforts, including drug therapy, are considered secondary and should be performed without compromising the quality and timely delivery of chest compressions and defibrillation. The principal goal of pharmacologic therapy during cardiac arrest is to facilitate return of spontaneous circulation (ROSC), and epinephrine is considered the drug of choice for this use. (See Uses: Advanced Cardiovascular Life Support and Cardiac Arrhythmias, in Epinephrine 12:12.12.) Antiarrhythmic drugs may be considered for the treatment of refractory ventricular fibrillation or pulseless ventricular tachycardia during cardiac resuscitation; however, experts generally recommend the use of amiodarone (or lidocaine). IV sotalol may be used for the management of hemodynamically stable sustained monomorphic ventricular tachycardia during the periarrest period and is included as a recommended antiarrhythmic agent in current ACLS guidelines for adult tachycardia.

● Supraventricular Arrhythmias

Sotalol appears to be effective in the suppression and prevention of various supraventricular tachycardias (SVTs), including atrial fibrillation or flutter and PSVT†. Because of a higher risk of toxicity and proarrhythmic effects, antiarrhythmic agents such as sotalol generally should be reserved for patients who are not candidates for catheter ablation and who do not respond to or cannot be treated with AV nodal blocking agents (i.e., β-adrenergic blocking agents, nondihydropyridine calcium-channel blocking agents).

Atrial Fibrillation and Flutter

Sotalol is used to maintain normal sinus rhythm in patients with symptomatic atrial fibrillation or flutter who are currently in sinus rhythm. Because of the potential to cause life-threatening ventricular arrhythmias, the manufacturer states that sotalol should be reserved for the treatment of highly symptomatic atrial fibrillation/flutter. (See Cautions: Arrhythmogenic Effects.) In addition, patients with paroxysmal atrial fibrillation that is easily reversed (e.g., by the Valsalva maneuver) should *not* receive sotalol.

Available data suggest that the efficacy of oral sotalol for prevention of recurrences of atrial fibrillation or flutter is comparable to that of quinidine or propafenone and less than that of amiodarone. Maintenance of sinus rhythm with oral sotalol does not appear to be related to either duration of previous episodes of atrial fibrillation (e.g., paroxysmal or persistent atrial fibrillation) or the degree of atrial enlargement.

Other Supraventricular Tachycardias

Sotalol also has been used in patients with other SVTs, including PSVT due to AV nodal reentry tachycardia (AVNRT) or AV reentry tachycardia (AVRT).† However, vagal maneuvers and IV adenosine generally are preferred for initial treatment of PSVT in patients without contraindications. Sotalol may be a reasonable choice of therapy for the ongoing management of symptomatic SVT in patients who are not candidates for, or prefer not to undergo, catheter ablation and in whom first-line drugs (e.g., β-adrenergic blocking agents, diltiazem, verapamil) are not effective or are contraindicated.

DOSAGE AND ADMINISTRATION

● Administration

Sotalol hydrochloride is administered orally or by IV infusion when oral administration is not feasible.

Because of the arrhythmogenic potential of sotalol, initiation or reinitiation of therapy, or conversion from IV to oral therapy should be performed in a facility capable of providing cardiac resuscitation, continuous electrocardiogram (ECG) monitoring, and calculation of creatinine clearance; treatment should be initiated in the presence of personnel trained in the management of serious arrhythmias. Patients should be closely monitored for at least 3 days (or until steady-state plasma concentrations are achieved) whenever treatment is initiated or dosage is increased. Prior to initiating therapy, the patient's baseline QT interval and creatinine clearance should be determined; therapy should not be initiated if the QT interval corrected for rate (QT_c) exceeds 450 msec or creatinine clearance is less than 40 mL/minute. Because the potential for arrhythmogenic events increases with increasing dosage, patients should be monitored closely during the dose titration phase until steady-state concentrations are reached. When titrating dosage, QT interval should be determined 2–4 hours after each dose increase (if the drug is given orally) or after completion of each IV infusion; dose should be reduced, dosing interval increased, or therapy discontinued if prolongation of the QT interval to 500 msec or greater occurs.

Patients should be advised not to discontinue or interrupt sotalol therapy without consulting their clinician. Patients should be given an adequate supply of the drug upon hospital discharge to allow uninterrupted therapy until their outpatient prescription can be filled.

Patients with atrial fibrillation should be anticoagulated according to usual medical practice. (See Uses: Embolism Associated with Atrial Fibrillation in Warfarin 20:12.04.08.)

Oral Administration

Sotalol hydrochloride is administered orally as tablets or oral solution.

If the drug is administered as an oral solution, the commercially available oral solution containing 25 mg/5 mL may be used or an oral solution may be extemporaneously prepared by adding five 120-mg tablets to a 180-mL polyethylene terephthalate (PET) prescription bottle containing 120 mL of simple syrup with 0.1% sodium benzoate (syrup NF); alternatively, the syrup may be added to the tablets. An oversized bottle is used to allow more effective shaking of the mixture. The tablets may be added intact to the syrup or crushed; if crushed, care should be taken to transfer the entire quantity of tablet powder to the syrup. The mixture should be shaken to wet the tablets and the tablets allowed to hydrate for at least 2 hours. The bottle should then be shaken intermittently over another 2 hours until dispersion of fine particles is obtained; alternatively, the tablets may be allowed to hydrate overnight to simplify the disintegration process. An appropriate measuring device (e.g., oral dosing syringe) should be used to administer oral solutions of sotalol; use of a teaspoon or tablespoon may result in dosing errors and is not recommended.

Administration of oral sotalol within 2 hours of administration of an aluminum oxide and magnesium hydroxide-containing antacid resulted in decreased absorption of sotalol as evidenced by 26 and 20% reductions in peak plasma concentrations and area under the plasma concentration-time curve (AUC), respectively, of the drug. Since such decreased absorption was associated with a 25% reduction in bradycardic effect, the manufacturer states that antacids should not be administered within 2 hours of administration of sotalol; however, when the antacid was administered 2 hours after sotalol, no effects on the pharmacokinetics or pharmacodynamics of sotalol were observed.

IV Administration

Sotalol hydrochloride is administered by IV infusion over 5 hours using a volumetric pump to ensure that the drug is delivered at a constant rate.

The commercially available 15-mg/mL injection concentrate must be diluted with a suitable diluent (i.e., 0.9% sodium chloride injection, 5% dextrose injection, lactated Ringer's injection) prior to administration. The manufacturer recommends that the volume of injection concentrate used to prepare the infusion solution and the final infusion solution volume exceed those required for the intended dose to account for the volume loss in the dead space of the infusion set. Preparation of a final volume of 120 or 300 mL is recommended; however, the actual volume that should be infused is 100 or 250 mL, respectively. For a dose of 75 mg, the manufacturer recommends that 6 mL of the injection concentrate be diluted with 114 or 294 mL of diluent to prepare a final volume of 120 or 300 mL, respectively. For a dose of 112.5 mg, the manufacturer recommends that 9 mL of the injection concentrate be diluted with 111 or 291 mL of diluent to prepare a final volume of 120 or 300 mL, respectively. For a dose of 150 mg, the manufacturer recommends that 12 mL of injection concentrate be diluted with 108 or 288 mL of diluent to prepare a final volume of 120 or 300 mL, respectively.

● Dosage

Dosage of sotalol hydrochloride must be adjusted carefully according to individual requirements and response, patient tolerance, renal function, and QT interval.

Appropriate dosage adjustments should be made for patients with impaired renal function to minimize the risk of drug accumulation and arrhythmogenic events. (See Dosage and Administration: Dosage in Renal and Hepatic Impairment.) If a dose is missed, patients should be advised to take the next dose at the regularly scheduled time and to not take a double dose or increase the dosing frequency to compensate for the missed dose.

Adult Oral Dosage

Life-threatening Ventricular Arrhythmias

For the management of life-threatening ventricular arrhythmias in adults with normal renal function (creatinine clearance exceeding 60 mL/minute), an initial oral sotalol hydrochloride dosage of 80 mg twice daily is recommended. Dosage may be increased every 3 days in increments of 80 mg daily provided QT_c does not exceed 500 msec. The usual oral maintenance dosage in adults is 160–320 mg daily, given in 2 or 3 divided doses; because of the long elimination half-life of the drug, dosing more than 2 times a day usually is not necessary. In patients with life-threatening refractory ventricular arrhythmias, oral sotalol hydrochloride dosages as high as 480–640 mg daily have been used; however, the risk of serious arrhythmias increases with higher dosages.

Atrial Fibrillation/Flutter

For maintenance of normal sinus rhythm in adults with atrial fibrillation or flutter who have normal renal function (creatinine clearance exceeding 60 mL/minute), an initial oral sotalol hydrochloride dosage of 80 mg twice daily is recommended. Dosage may be increased every 3 days in increments of 80 mg daily provided QT_c does not exceed 500 msec. In a dose-response study, the most effective dosage in preventing recurrence of atrial fibrillation or flutter was 120 mg once or twice daily. Some clinicians state that dosage may be increased up to a maximum of 160 mg twice daily (provided the drug is well tolerated without excessive QT interval prolongation) if patients continue to experience recurrences of symptomatic atrial fibrillation or flutter.

Adult Parenteral Dosage

When oral therapy is not feasible, sotalol may be administered as an IV infusion. Because oral bioavailability of sotalol is 90–100%, equivalent IV doses are lower than oral doses. The manufacturer recommends the following dose equivalencies when converting between oral and IV dosing: 75 mg IV for an oral dose of 80 mg, 112.5 mg IV for an oral dose of 120 mg, and 150 mg IV for an oral dose of 160 mg.

Life-threatening Ventricular Arrhythmias

The recommended initial IV dosage of sotalol hydrochloride for the management of life-threatening ventricular arrhythmias in adults is 75 mg once or twice daily (depending on creatinine clearance) by IV infusion over 5 hours. (See Dosage and Administration: Dosage in Renal and Hepatic Impairment.) If the desired response has not been achieved and the drug is well tolerated without excessive QT interval prolongation, dosage may be increased to 112.5 mg once or twice daily (depending on creatinine clearance); the manufacturer recommends that dosage be increased in increments of 75 mg daily every 3 days. Based on experience with oral sotalol hydrochloride, the usual therapeutic effect should be observed with IV dosages of 75–150 mg once or twice daily; however, patients with life-threatening refractory ventricular arrhythmias have received higher dosages (e.g., oral dosages of 240–320 mg once or twice daily corresponding to IV dosages of 225–300 mg once or twice daily).

Atrial Fibrillation/Flutter

The recommended initial IV dosage of sotalol hydrochloride for the maintenance of normal sinus rhythm in adults with atrial fibrillation or flutter is 75 mg once or twice daily (depending on creatinine clearance) by IV infusion over 5 hours. (See Dosage and Administration: Dosage in Renal and Hepatic Impairment.) If the desired response has not been achieved and the drug is well tolerated without excessive QT interval prolongation, dosage may be increased after at least 3 days to 112.5 mg once or twice daily (depending on creatinine clearance). Based on experience with oral sotalol hydrochloride, the usual therapeutic effect should be observed with an IV dosage of 112.5 mg once or twice daily; however, the manufacturer states that IV dosage may be increased up to 150 mg once or twice daily if necessary provided the drug is well tolerated.

Pediatric Dosage

Dosage of sotalol hydrochloride in pediatric patients is based on pharmacokinetic data. (See Cautions: Pediatric Precautions.) The usual precautions observed in adults should also be taken when initiating or reinitiating therapy in pediatric patients. Dosage increases should preferably be performed in an inpatient setting where patients can be closely monitored. Because sotalol has similar potency in children and adults, dosages used in pediatric patients should achieve plasma concentrations similar to those within the adult dosage range; however, dosage should be individualized based on clinical response, heart rate, and QT_c. There are no studies of IV sotalol hydrochloride in pediatric patients.

The recommended initial oral dosage of sotalol hydrochloride for the management of ventricular arrhythmias or atrial fibrillation/flutter in children about 2 years of age or older with normal renal function is 30 mg/m^2 3 times daily (total daily dose of 90 mg/m^2); dosage may be increased up to a maximum of 60 mg/m^2 3 times daily, allowing at least 36 hours to elapse between dosage escalations to achieve steady-state concentrations.

Dosage of sotalol hydrochloride in children about 2 years of age or younger should be reduced from the usual oral dosage for older children (i.e., 30 mg/m^2 3 times daily) by an age-dependent factor obtained from the manufacturer's prescribing information. The age-dependent factor is approximately 0.3 in neonates about 1 week old, 0.68 in infants 1 month of age, and 0.97 in infants 20 months of age. The calculated dose after multiplying the age-dependent factor by 30 mg/m^2 is 9 mg/m^2 in neonates about 1 week old, 20 mg/m^2 in infants 1 month of age, and 29.1 mg/m^2 in infants 20 months of age, administered 3 times daily.

Use of sotalol in pediatric patients with renal impairment has not been evaluated; in general, lower doses should be used or the dosing interval should be increased.

Conversion from other Antiarrhythmic Agents

The manufacturer recommends a transition period when converting patients from another antiarrhythmic agent to sotalol therapy. In general, initiation of sotalol therapy should be delayed for a period of at least 2–3 elimination half-lives of the previously administered antiarrhythmic; the patient should be monitored carefully during the transition. Class I or Class III antiarrhythmic agents should be withheld for at least 3 half-lives prior to dosing with sotalol hydrochloride.

● Dosage in Renal and Hepatic Impairment

In patients with renal impairment, the dose or dosing frequency of sotalol hydrochloride should be reduced to minimize the risk of proarrhythmia; as in patients with normal renal function, QT interval and heart rate should be closely monitored. (See Cautions: Arrhythmogenic Effects.) Dosing interval should be modified according to the patient's estimated creatinine clearance. In general, the initial oral adult sotalol hydrochloride dose of 80 mg and subsequent doses should be administered twice daily in patients with a creatinine clearance greater than 60 mL/minute and once daily in patients with a creatinine clearance of 40–60 mL/minute. The drug is generally contraindicated in patients with creatinine clearance less than 40 mL/minute. In patients with ventricular arrhythmias, some manufacturers recommend a dosing interval of 36–48 hours in adults with creatinine clearance of 10–29 mL/minute and individualized dosing in those with creatinine clearance less than 10 mL/minute. Since terminal elimination half-life of the drug is prolonged in patients with renal impairment, dosage increases generally should be made after administration of at least 5 doses at appropriate intervals. Sotalol is partially removed by dialysis; however, the manufacturers make no dosing recommendations for patients undergoing dialysis. Dosage of sotalol hydrochloride in children with renal impairment has not been established; however, reduced doses and increased dosing intervals are recommended in patients of all age groups with renal impairment.

The manufacturer states that clearance of sotalol is not altered by impaired hepatic function.

CAUTIONS

Sotalol shares the toxic potentials of nonselective β-adrenergic blocking agents and, in therapeutic dosage, generally is well tolerated during long-term therapy. However, as a class III antiarrhythmic agent (see Description), sotalol, unlike conventional β-blockers, can prolong the QT interval and precipitate torsades de pointes. Adverse effects associated with sotalol are generally dose related and typically result from the drug's class II (beta-blocking) and class III (cardiac action potential duration prolongation) effects.

The most serious adverse effect of sotalol is torsades de pointes, which occurred in almost 4 or 1% of patients with a history of sustained ventricular tachycardia or other less serious ventricular arrhythmias, respectively, who received the drug orally in clinical studies. The most frequent adverse effects of sotalol involve the cardiovascular and nervous systems and GI tract, and occasionally they may be severe enough to require discontinuance of the drug. The most common adverse effects resulting in discontinuance of the drug include effects usually associated with β-blockade. Fatigue caused discontinuance of sotalol in 4–5% of patients, bradycardia (heart rate less than 50 bpm) in 2–3%, dyspnea in 2–3%, arrhythmogenic effects in 1.5–3%, asthenia in 2%, and dizziness in 2% of patients receiving the drug in clinical trials. Overall, discontinuance of sotalol as a result of adverse effects occurred in 17% of patients receiving the drug in clinical trials and in 10% of those treated for at least 2 weeks. Abrupt withdrawal of sotalol should be avoided, especially in patients with coronary artery disease, since it may exacerbate angina or precipitate myocardial infarction (MI).

● Arrhythmogenic Effects

Like other antiarrhythmic agents, sotalol can worsen existing arrhythmias or cause new arrhythmias, including sustained ventricular tachycardia or ventricular fibrillation which potentially may be fatal; the arrhythmogenic potential is the most serious risk associated with the drug. Because sotalol prolongs the QT interval corrected for rate (QT_c), torsades de pointes, a polymorphic ventricular tachycardia with prolongation of the QT interval and a shifting electrical axis, is the most common arrhythmogenic effect of the drug, occurring in about 0.6 or 4% of patients with a history of supraventricular arrhythmias (i.e., atrial fibrillation or flutter) or ventricular arrhythmias (i.e., sustained ventricular tachycardia or ventricular fibrillation), respectively. The risk of torsades de pointes increases progressively with prolongation of the QT interval and is worsened by a reduction in heart rate and serum potassium concentration. (See Cautions: Precautions and Contraindications.)

In patients with a history of sustained ventricular tachycardia, the frequency of torsades de pointes was 4% and the frequency of worsened ventricular tachycardia was about 1%; in patients with other, less serious ventricular arrhythmias, the frequency of torsades de pointes was 1% and the frequency of new or worsened ventricular tachycardia was 0.7%.

In clinical trials of sotalol, the incidence of cardiac mortality was 3.8% overall and 5.9% in patients with sustained ventricular tachycardia or ventricular fibrillation. Overall, cardiac death was associated with low left ventricular ejection fraction, history of congestive heart failure and/or cardiomegaly, and increasing age; the risk of death in patients with a history of both cardiomegaly and congestive heart failure was more than 3 times that in patients with no history of either condition. In patients with sustained ventricular tachycardia or ventricular fibrillation, the risk of cardiac death was most strongly associated with a history of cardiomegaly and then with a history of congestive heart failure and low ventricular ejection fraction. A clear relationship between sotalol dosage and the frequency of death has not been demonstrated to date.

Prolongation of the QT_c interval and the occurrence of torsades de pointes are dose related. In patients with sustained ventricular tachycardia or ventricular fibrillation, the incidence of torsades de pointes ranged from 0.5% at 160 mg daily to 1.6% at 320 mg daily but increased more abruptly at higher dosages, to about 4% at 480–640 mg daily and to almost 6% at higher dosages. The frequency of torsades de pointes in patients with ventricular arrhythmias was 1.6% when the change in QT_c interval was less than 65 msec but increased by about 1% with each additional increase of about 20–30 msec in the QT_c interval, with a frequency of 7.1% at QT_c interval increases exceeding 130 msec. In addition, the risk of sotalol-induced torsades de pointes was increased with female gender, reduced renal function, large doses of the drug, and a history of cardiomegaly or heart failure. Patients with sustained ventricular tachycardia and a history of heart failure appeared to be at greatest risk of a serious arrhythmogenic event, with an occurrence rate of 7%. Approximately two-thirds of patients experiencing sotalol-induced torsades de pointes reverted spontaneously to their baseline rhythm. The remaining patients required either cardioversion or overdrive pacing or treatment with other drugs. Although it is not possible to determine whether some sudden deaths resulted from episodes of torsades de pointes, some instances of sudden death did follow documented episodes. Most cases of torsades de pointes required discontinuance of sotalol therapy, but 17% of patients continued the drug at a lower dosage. Sotalol should be used with particular caution if the QT_c interval exceeds 500 msec during treatment, and dosage reduction or discontinuance of the drug should be seriously considered when the QT_c interval exceeds 500 msec. Regardless of the QT_c interval, caution should be exercised because of the multiple risk factors associated with torsades de pointes.

Sotalol-induced arrhythmogenic events can occur not only when initiating therapy, but with every upward dosage adjustment. About 75% of such serious events (e.g., torsades de pointes, worsened ventricular tachycardia) occur within 7 days of initiating therapy with the drug, and about 60% occur within 3 days of initiation of the drug or dosage adjustment. Initiation of sotalol therapy at low dosages with gradual upward titration and appropriate monitoring should reduce the risk of arrhythmogenic events. Because of the arrhythmogenic potential of the drug and the life-threatening nature of the arrhythmias against which the drug is being employed, the manufacturer recommends that both initiation and reinitiation of sotalol therapy and any subsequent upward dosage adjustments be performed in an institutional setting.

Cardiovascular Effects

Sympathetic stimulation is necessary for supporting circulatory function in heart failure. Therefore, because of its β-adrenergic blocking effects, sotalol may cause or worsen heart failure, particularly in patients with preexisting heart failure (New York Heart Association [NYHA] class II–IV) or sustained ventricular tachycardia or ventricular fibrillation, and/or a history of cardiomegaly, cardiomyopathy, coronary artery disease, or myocardial infarction. The effect of these risk factors appears to be cumulative, with patients exhibiting more risk factors being at greater risk for precipitated or worsened heart failure during therapy with the drug.

New or worsened heart failure occurred in 3% of patients receiving sotalol in premarketing studies and required discontinuance of the drug in about 1% of patients. The frequency of new or worsened heart failure was 5% in patients with sustained ventricular tachycardia or ventricular fibrillation and 7% in patients with a history of heart failure. In patients with sustained ventricular tachycardia or ventricular fibrillation, the most reliable predictive risk factors were a history of congestive heart failure or cardiomegaly. The 1-year frequency of new or worsened heart failure was 3% in patients without a previous history and 10% in those with a previous history of heart failure. The risk of new or worsened heart failure was closely related to NYHA classification. The occurrence of heart failure was not related to dosage of sotalol, regardless of heart failure history. New or worsened heart failure occurred in 2.7% of patients with nonsustained ventricular tachycardia or premature ventricular complexes (PVCs) and in 2.3% of patients with supraventricular arrhythmias.

Chest pain and palpitation occurred in 16 and 14%, respectively, of patients with sustained ventricular tachycardia or ventricular fibrillation receiving sotalol in clinical trials, but each of these adverse effects required discontinuance of the drug in less than 1% of patients. In pooled data from several clinical trials in a limited number of patients with atrial fibrillation or flutter, angina pectoris occurred in 1.6–2% of patients receiving sotalol hydrochloride 160–320 mg daily. Nonanginal chest pain occurred in 2.5–4.6% of these patients. Edema was reported in 8%, abnormal ECG in 7%, and syncope in 5% of patients with a history of ventricular arrhythmias receiving sotalol, and each of these adverse effects required discontinuance of the drug in 1% of patients. Hypotension was reported in 6% of patients with a history of ventricular arrhythmias and required discontinuance in 2% of patients. Presyncope was reported in 4%; peripheral vascular disorder, cardiovascular disorder, vasodilation, or AICD discharge in 3%; and hypertension in 2% of patients with a history of ventricular arrhythmias receiving sotalol, and each of these adverse effects required discontinuance of the drug in less than 1% of patients.

Effects on Cardiac Conduction

Sinus bradycardia (heart rate less than 50 bpm), which increases the risk of torsades de pointes, occurred in 13% of patients with sustained ventricular tachycardia or ventricular fibrillation receiving sotalol in clinical trials and required discontinuance of the drug in about 2.4% of patients. Pooled data from several clinical trials in patients with atrial fibrillation or flutter indicate that bradycardia occurred in 12–13% of patients receiving oral sotalol; discontinuance of therapy was required in 2.4% of these patients. Sinus pause, arrest, and nodal dysfunction occurred in less than 1% of patients, and second- or third-degree AV block occurred in about 1% of patients receiving sotalol.

QRS intervals are affected minimally by sotalol; however, at dosages of 160–640 mg daily, sotalol causes dose-related mean increases of 40–100 msec in the QT interval and 10–40 msec in the QT_c interval. Excessive prolongation of the QT interval (to greater than 550 msec) can promote serious arrhythmias and should be avoided during sotalol therapy. (See Cautions: Arrhythmogenic Effects.)

Nervous System Effects

Fatigue, dizziness, and asthenia, which appear to be dose related, are the most common adverse nervous system effects of sotalol, occurring in 20% of patients with sustained ventricular tachycardia or ventricular fibrillation receiving the drug in clinical trials. Fatigue and dizziness also are the most common adverse nervous system effects of sotalol in patients with a history of atrial fibrillation or flutter, occurring in 18.9–19.6 or 13.1–16.3% of these patients, respectively. Fatigue resulted in discontinuance of sotalol in 4.6% of patients with a history of these supraventricular arrhythmias. Lightheadedness, dizziness, and syncope also are symptoms of torsades de pointes. Asthenia and lightheadedness were reported in 13 and 12%, respectively, of patients with a history of ventricular arrhythmias receiving sotalol in clinical trials. Weakness was reported in about 5% of patients with a history of atrial fibrillation or flutter receiving sotalol in clinical trials. Headache and sleep disturbances were reported in 8% of patients with ventricular arrhythmias receiving sotalol and required discontinuance in less than 1% of patients. Insomnia was reported in 2.6–4.1% of patients with a history of atrial fibrillation or flutter receiving sotalol in clinical trials. Perspiration was reported in 6% of patients; altered consciousness, depression, paresthesia, or anxiety in 4% of patients; and localized pain, mood change, or appetite disorder in 3% of patients with a history of ventricular arrhythmias receiving sotalol in clinical trials; each of these adverse effects required discontinuance of the drug in less than 1% of patients. Cold sensation was reported in 2–2.5% of patients with a history of atrial fibrillation or flutter receiving sotalol in clinical trials. Rarely, emotional lability, slightly clouded sensorium, incoordination, vertigo, and paralysis have been reported during postmarketing experience. One case of peripheral neuropathy, which resolved on discontinuance of sotalol therapy and recurred when the patient was rechallenged with the drug, also has been reported.

Respiratory Effects

Dyspnea was reported in 21% of patients with sustained ventricular tachycardia or ventricular fibrillation receiving the drug in clinical trials but required discontinuance of therapy in only 2% of patients. Dyspnea also has been reported in 9.2–9.8% of patients with a history of atrial fibrillation or flutter receiving sotalol in clinical trials, requiring discontinuance of therapy in 2% of these patients. Pulmonary problems were reported in 8%, upper respiratory tract problems in 5%, and asthma in 2% of patients with ventricular arrhythmias receiving sotalol; each of these adverse effects required discontinuance of therapy in less than 1% of patients. Influenza or upper respiratory tract infection has been reported in 0.8–2 or 2.6–3.3%, respectively, of patients with a history of atrial fibrillation or flutter receiving sotalol in clinical trials. Cough or tracheobronchitis has been reported in 2.5–3.3 or 0.7–3.3%, respectively, of patients with a history of these supraventricular arrhythmias receiving sotalol in clinical trials. Rarely, pulmonary edema has been reported during postmarketing experience with the drug. As with other nonselective β-adrenergic blocking agents, sotalol can increase airway resistance by inhibiting bronchodilation mediated by endogenous or exogenous catecholamine stimulation of $β_2$-adrenergic receptors; such changes may be clinically important in patients with underlying airway disease. (See Cautions: Precautions and Contraindications.)

GI Effects

Nausea and vomiting are the most frequent adverse GI effects of sotalol, occurring in 5.7–7.8 or 10% of patients with supraventricular (i.e., atrial fibrillation or flutter) or ventricular (i.e., sustained ventricular tachycardia or ventricular fibrillation) arrhythmias, respectively, receiving the drug in clinical trials and requiring discontinuance in up to 1% of patients. Other adverse GI effects each required discontinuance of sotalol in less than 1% of patients with ventricular arrhythmias. Diarrhea and dyspepsia were reported in 7 and 6%, respectively, of patients with ventricular arrhythmias receiving sotalol in clinical trials. Diarrhea or dyspepsia was reported in 5.2–5.7 or 2–2.5% of patients, respectively, with a history of atrial fibrillation or flutter receiving sotalol in controlled clinical trials. Abdominal pain and colon problems occurred in 3% of patients, and flatulence occurred in 2% of patients with ventricular arrhythmias. Abdominal pain or abdominal distension was reported in 2.5–3.9% or 0.7–2.5%, respectively, of patients with a history of atrial fibrillation or flutter receiving sotalol in controlled clinical trials.

● Hepatic Effects

Increased serum concentrations of hepatic enzymes have occurred occasionally with sotalol therapy, but a causal relationship to the drug has not been established.

● Genitourinary Effects

Genitourinary disorders and sexual dysfunction were reported in 3 and 2%, respectively, of patients with ventricular arrhythmias receiving sotalol in clinical trials and each required discontinuance of the drug in less than 1% of patients.

● Musculoskeletal Effects

Extremity pain and back pain were reported in 7 and 3%, respectively, of patients with ventricular arrhythmias receiving sotalol in clinical trials and each required discontinuance of the drug in less than 1% of patients. Rarely, myalgia has been reported during postmarketing experience with the drug. Musculoskeletal pain or musculoskeletal chest pain has been reported in 2.6–4.1 or 2–2.5%, respectively, of patients with a history of atrial fibrillation or flutter receiving sotalol in clinical trials.

● Dermatologic Effects

Rash was reported in 5% of patients with ventricular arrhythmias receiving sotalol in clinical trials and required discontinuance of the drug in less than 1% of patients. Rarely, photosensitivity reactions, pruritus, and alopecia have been reported during postmarketing experience with the drug. Hyperhidrosis has been reported in 4.9–5.2% of patients with a history of atrial fibrillation or flutter receiving sotalol in clinical trials.

● Hematologic Effects

Bleeding was reported in 2% of patients with ventricular arrhythmias receiving sotalol in clinical trials and required discontinuance of the drug in less than 1% of patients. Rarely, thrombocytopenia, leukopenia, and eosinophilia have been reported during postmarketing experience with the drug.

● Ocular Effects

Visual disorders were reported in 5% of patients with ventricular arrhythmias receiving sotalol in clinical trials and required discontinuance of the drug in less than 1% of patients. Visual disturbances were reported in 0.8–2.6% of patients with a history of atrial fibrillation or flutter receiving sotalol in clinical trials.

● Other Adverse Effects

Fever, infection, and abnormal laboratory test results were each reported in 4% of patients and weight change in 2% of patients with sustained ventricular tachycardia or ventricular fibrillation receiving sotalol in clinical trials, and each of these adverse effects required discontinuance of the drug in less than 1% of patients. Pooled data from several clinical trials in patients with a history of atrial fibrillation or flutter indicate that fever was reported in 0.7–3.3% of patients receiving sotalol. Increases in blood glucose concentration and insulin requirements can occur in patients with diabetes mellitus receiving sotalol. Rarely, hyperlipidemia has been reported during postmarketing experience with the drug.

● Precautions and Contraindications

Sotalol shares the toxic potentials of other nonselective β-adrenergic blocking agents, and the usual precautions of these agents should be observed. In addition, as a class III antiarrhythmic agent, sotalol, unlike conventional β-blockers, can precipitate torsades de pointes.

Sotalol, like other antiarrhythmics, has been associated with the development or exacerbation of arrhythmias in some patients. (See Cautions: Arrhythmogenic Effects.) Concerns about the long-term safety and efficacy of several antiarrhythmic agents (e.g., encainide, flecainide, moricizine) in patients with nonlife-threatening arrhythmias have been raised by the postmarketing Cardiac Arrhythmia Suppression Trial (CAST). Findings from the CAST study after an average of 10 months of follow-up indicated that the rate of total mortality and nonfatal cardiac arrest in patients with recent MI, mild-to-moderate left ventricular dysfunction, and asymptomatic or mildly symptomatic ventricular

arrhythmias (principally frequent PVCs) who received encainide or flecainide was increased substantially. (For additional information on the CAST study, see Cautions, in Flecainide 24:04.04.12.)

While sotalol can be used safely and effectively in the chronic management of life-threatening ventricular arrhythmias following MI, experience with the drug in the management of arrhythmias during the early phase of recovery from an acute MI is limited and at least at high initial doses (i.e., nontitrated initial dosage of 320 mg daily or 320 mg twice daily) has not been reassuring. Sotalol is devoid of class I antiarrhythmic activity, and there was no evidence of excess mortality associated with sotalol hydrochloride dosages up to 320 mg daily in a large (1456 patients), double-blind, placebo-controlled secondary prevention trial in patients with recent MI (but not necessarily concurrent ventricular arrhythmias). However, in patients who received an initial (i.e., not titrated) dosage of 320 mg daily in the study and in high-risk postinfarction patients who received high dosages (320 mg twice daily) in another smaller study, there was some evidence of a possible excess in early (within 2 weeks) sudden deaths. Therefore, sotalol should be used cautiously and with careful titration of dosage if the drug is used during the first 2 weeks following an acute MI, particularly in patients with markedly impaired ventricular function. Although specific studies of sotalol in treating supraventricular arrhythmias after a recent MI have not been performed to date, the usual precautions regarding heart failure, avoidance of hypokalemia, bradycardia, or prolonged QT interval apply.

Since sotalol, like other antiarrhythmic agents, can worsen existing arrhythmias or cause new arrhythmias in some patients, clinical and ECG evaluations are essential prior to and during sotalol therapy to monitor for the appearance of arrhythmias and to determine the need for continued therapy or dosage adjustment. (See Cautions: Arrhythmogenic Effects.) Arrhythmogenic events must be anticipated not only when sotalol therapy is initiated, but also with each upward dosage titration. To minimize the risk of arrhythmogenic effects, the recommendations for initiation of sotalol therapy and dosage adjustments should be closely followed. (See Dosage and Administration.) In addition, excessive accumulation of the drug in patients with diminished renal function should be avoided with appropriate dosage adjustment. Because of the arrhythmogenic potential, the manufacturer recommends that patients be hospitalized for a minimum of 3 days (or until steady-state concentrations are achieved) for initiation or reinitiation of sotalol therapy in a facility capable of providing cardiac resuscitation and continuous ECG monitoring.

Sotalol increases QT_c interval in a dose-related fashion and thereby increases the risk of torsades de pointes. Therefore, the QT interval should be monitored during therapy and dosage adjusted accordingly. (See Dosage and Administration: Administration.) Sotalol should not be *initiated* in patients with a QT interval exceeding 450 msec. If the QT interval exceeds 500 msec, the dose should be reduced, the dosing interval increased, or the drug should be discontinued. Excessive prolongation of the QT interval (to greater than 500 msec) can promote serious arrhythmias and should be avoided during sotalol therapy. The possibility that the development of syncope and/or dizziness may be signs of undetected torsades de pointes should be considered. Because of the multiple risk factors associated with torsades de pointes, however, caution should be exercised regardless of the QT_c interval.

Sotalol should not be used in patients with hypokalemia or hypomagnesemia until these imbalances are corrected, since such electrolyte abnormalities can exaggerate the degree of QT prolongation and increase the risk of torsades de pointes. Special attention should be given to electrolyte and acid-base balance in patients with severe or prolonged diarrhea and in patients receiving diuretics concomitantly. Patients should be advised to report immediately to their clinician conditions, concomitant therapy (e.g., diuretics), and/or manifestations associated with altered electrolyte balance such as severe or prolonged diarrhea, unusual sweating, vomiting, loss of appetite, or thirst. Sotalol generally should not be used concomitantly with other drugs known to prolong the QT interval (e.g., class I or other class III antiarrhythmic agents, certain oral macrolides [e.g., azithromycin, clarithromycin], phenothiazines, tricyclic antidepressants, certain quinolones [e.g., ciprofloxacin, levofloxacin]). The manufacturers state that class Ia antiarrhythmic agents such as disopyramide, quinidine, and procainamide and class III antiarrhythmic agents such as amiodarone should not be used concomitantly with sotalol and should be discontinued for at least 3 half-lives prior to dosing with sotalol. In clinical trials in patients with a history of atrial fibrillation or flutter, sotalol was not administered in patients previously treated with oral amiodarone for longer than 1 month in the previous 3 months. There is only limited experience with concomitant use of class Ib or Ic antiarrhythmics and sotalol. The manufacturers state that additive class II effects should be anticipated with the use of other β-blocking agents concomitantly with sotalol.

Sotalol is contraindicated in patients with sinus bradycardia, second- or third-degree AV block, or sick sinus syndrome, unless a functioning pacemaker is present. The risk of torsades de pointes in patients with atrial fibrillation and sinus node dysfunction is increased, especially after cardioversion. Because sotalol has a greater effect in prolonging the QT interval and the action potential duration at lower heart rates (reverse rate dependence), bradycardia following cardioversion in such patients is associated with greater QT_c prolongation than observed at higher heart rates.

Sotalol should be used with caution in patients with inadequate cardiac function. Because sympathetic stimulation is necessary to support circulatory function in patients with heart failure, β-blockade with sotalol carries the potential risk of depressing myocardial contractility and precipitating more severe heart failure. However, the fact that sotalol and cardiac glycosides both slow AV conduction also should be considered.

Since β-adrenergic blocking agents may inhibit bronchodilation produced by endogenous catecholamines, the drugs generally should not be used in patients with bronchospastic diseases. Use of sotalol is not recommended in patients with nonallergic bronchospasm (e.g., chronic bronchitis, emphysema). If sotalol is administered, it is prudent to use the lowest effective dosage to minimize inhibition of bronchodilation produced by endogenous or exogenous catecholamine stimulation of β_2-adrenergic receptors.

It is recommended that sotalol be used with caution in patients with diabetes mellitus (especially those with labile diabetes or those prone to hypoglycemia) since the drug may mask certain signs and symptoms associated with acute hypoglycemia (e.g., tachycardia). Sotalol may increase blood glucose concentrations and insulin requirements in diabetic patients. The drug also should be used with caution in patients with a history of episodic spontaneous hypoglycemia. However, many clinicians state that patients with diabetes mellitus may be particularly likely to experience a reduction in morbidity and mortality with the use of β-adrenergic blocking agents.

There is some controversy regarding the perioperative use of β-adrenergic blocking agents. Severe, protracted hypotension, bradycardia, and stroke have occurred during surgery in some patients who have received β-adrenergic blocking agents; in addition, it is unclear whether such use confers any mortality benefit or risk. It is generally recommended that β-blockers be continued during surgery in patients who are already receiving these drugs for a chronic condition. However, the risks versus benefits should be carefully considered in individual patients.

While receiving β-blockers such as sotalol, patients with a history of anaphylactic reaction to a variety of allergens may have a more severe reaction on repeated accidental, diagnostic, or therapeutic challenge. These patients may be unresponsive to the usual doses of epinephrine used to treat the reaction.

Abrupt withdrawal of sotalol may exacerbate angina symptoms and/or precipitate MI in patients with ischemic heart disease, or may precipitate thyroid storm (since signs of hyperthyroidism such as tachycardia may be masked by the drug) in patients with thyroid disease. Therefore, patients receiving sotalol (especially those with ischemic heart disease) should be warned not to interrupt or discontinue therapy without consulting their clinician. If possible, sotalol hydrochloride dosage should be reduced gradually and with close monitoring over 1–2 weeks, especially in patients with ischemic heart disease. If exacerbation of angina occurs or acute coronary insufficiency develops after sotalol therapy is interrupted or discontinued, appropriate treatment (e.g., temporary use of another β-blocker) should be instituted.

Sotalol reduces systolic and diastolic blood pressures and may result in hypotension. Hemodynamic monitoring is recommended in patients with marginal cardiac compensation.

Sotalol is contraindicated in patients with bronchial asthma or related bronchospastic conditions, sinus bradycardia (less than 50 beats per minute during waking hours), second- or third-degree AV block (unless a functioning pacemaker is present), congenital or acquired long-QT syndromes, cardiogenic shock, decompensated heart failure, hypokalemia (serum potassium concentrations less than 4 mEq/L), or hypersensitivity to the drug. In addition, sotalol is contraindicated for the treatment of atrial fibrillation or flutter in patients with baseline QT interval exceeding 450 msec and in patients with creatinine clearance less than 40 mL/minute.

● Pediatric Precautions

Safety and efficacy of sotalol in children younger than 18 years of age have not been established. Sotalol has been used in a limited number of infants younger than 3 months of age and children younger than 18 years of age and was effective for the treatment of supraventricular arrhythmias and to a lesser degree for the treatment of ventricular arrhythmias. Mild sinus bradycardia occurred in most of the infants, and fatigue, which required discontinuance in a few patients, occurred in several of the children receiving the drug. The physiologic effects and pharmacokinetics of sotalol have been evaluated in infants and children 3 days to 12 years of age. Dosage recommendations in pediatric patients are based on pharmacokinetic data. Similar to adults, serious adverse events including death, torsades de pointes, other proarrhythmias, AV block, and bradycardia have been reported in infants and children; therefore, the usual precautions in adults should also be observed when sotalol is used in pediatric patients.

● Geriatric Precautions

Safety and efficacy of sotalol in geriatric patients have not been studied specifically to date; however, life-threatening ventricular arrhythmias such as sustained ventricular tachycardia, for which safety and efficacy have been established, occur in many patients older than 50 years of age and clinical trials of sotalol included many such patients. In sotalol clinical trials, the overall risk of cardiac death was associated with increasing age. Because geriatric patients may have decreased renal function and because patients with renal impairment may be at increased risk of sotalol-induced toxicity, patients in this age group should be monitored closely and dosage adjusted accordingly.

● Mutagenicity and Carcinogenicity

Specific assays to determine the mutagenic or clastogenic potential of sotalol have not been performed to date.

There was no evidence of carcinogenic potential in a 24-month study in rats receiving sotalol hydrochloride dosages of 137–275 mg/kg daily (approximately 30 times the maximum recommended human oral dosage on a mg/kg basis or 5 times the maximum recommended human oral dosage on a mg/m² basis). There also was no evidence of carcinogenic potential in a study in mice receiving sotalol hydrochloride dosages of 4141–7122 mg/kg daily (approximately 450–750 times the maximum recommended human oral dosage on a mg/kg basis or 36–63 times the maximum recommended human oral dosage on a mg/m² basis).

● Pregnancy, Fertility, and Lactation

Pregnancy

Reproduction studies in rats and rabbits during organogenesis did not reveal any teratogenic potential at sotalol hydrochloride doses that were 100 and 22 times the maximum recommended human oral dose on a mg/kg basis (9 and 7 times the maximum recommended human oral dose on a mg/m² basis), respectively. However, higher sotalol hydrochloride dosages of 160 mg/kg daily (16 times the maximum recommended human oral dosage on a mg/kg basis or 6 times the maximum recommended human oral dosage on a mg/m² basis) in rabbits were associated with a slight increase in fetal death likely resulting from maternal toxicity. A sotalol hydrochloride dosage of 80 mg/kg daily (8 times the maximum recommended human oral dosage on a mg/kg basis or 3 times the maximum recommended human oral dosage on a mg/m² basis) did not produce this effect. An increase in the number of early resorptions was associated with a sotalol hydrochloride dosage of 1000 mg/kg daily in rats (100 times the maximum recommended human oral dosage on a mg/kg basis or 18 times the maximum recommended human oral dosage on a mg/m² basis), while no increase was observed at 14 times the maximum recommended human oral dosage on mg/kg basis (2.5 times the maximum recommended human oral dosage on a mg/m² basis). Animal data are not always indicative of human response. There are no adequate and well-controlled studies using sotalol in pregnant women, but the drug has been shown to cross the placenta and is found in amniotic fluid.

Lactation

Sotalol is distributed into milk, apparently in concentrations approximately 2.5–5.5 times concurrent maternal serum concentrations. Because of the potential for adverse reactions to sotalol in nursing infants, a decision should be made whether to discontinue nursing or the drug, taking into account the importance of the drug to the woman.

DESCRIPTION

Sotalol hydrochloride (MJ 1999) is a nonselective β-adrenergic blocking agent. Like propranolol, sotalol inhibits response to adrenergic stimuli by competitively blocking $β_1$-adrenergic receptors within the myocardium and $β_2$-adrenergic receptors within bronchial and vascular smooth muscle. In addition, sotalol, like propranolol, exhibits antiarrhythmic activity characteristic of class II antiarrhythmic agents. However, unlike propranolol, sotalol does not exhibit membrane-stabilizing activity but, as a methanesulfonanilide derivative, does exhibit electrophysiologic effects characteristic of class III antiarrhythmic agents (e.g., prolongs repolarization and refractoriness without affecting conduction). Sotalol does not exhibit intrinsic sympathomimetic activity.

The electrophysiologic effects of sotalol, like other methanesulfonanilide derivatives, also differ from those of many other commonly used antiarrhythmics (e.g., class I agents). In vitro studies suggest that sotalol selectively inhibits the rapidly activating component of the potassium channel involved in repolarization of cardiac cells (i.e., the rapidly activated inward component of the delayed rectifier potassium current I_{Kr}). In addition, sotalol does not appear to block sodium channels at usual doses (although it may at relatively high doses), and pharmacologic differences of the drug at potassium and sodium channels compared with class I antiarrhythmic agents (e.g., mexiletine, procainamide, propafenone, quinidine) have been proposed as possibly contributing to potential clinical superiority of sotalol in the management of ventricular tachyarrhythmias. However, other factors also may be involved.

Commercially available sotalol is a racemic mixture of the 2 optical isomers. Both isomers exhibit class III antiarrhythmic activity, but only the *l*-isomer exhibits its β-blocking activity.

PREPARATIONS

Excipients in commercially available drug preparations may have clinically important effects in some individuals; consult specific product labeling for details.

Sotalol Hydrochloride

Oral		
Solution	25 mg/5 mL	Sotylize®, Arbor
Tablets	80 mg*	Betapace® (scored), Covis
		Betapace AF® (scored), Covis
		Sorine® (scored), Upsher-Smith
		Sotalol Hydrochloride Tablets (scored)
	120 mg*	Betapace® (scored), Covis
		Betapace AF® (scored), Covis
		Sorine® (scored), Upsher-Smith
		Sotalol Hydrochloride Tablets (scored),
	160 mg*	Betapace® (scored), Covis
		Betapace AF® (scored), Covis
		Sorine® (scored), Upsher-Smith
		Sotalol Hydrochloride Tablets (scored),
	240 mg*	Sorine® (scored), Upsher-Smith
		Sotalol Hydrochloride Tablets (scored),
Parenteral		
Injection concentrate, for IV infusion	15 mg/mL*	Sotalol Hydrochloride Injection

* available from one or more manufacturer, distributor, and/or repackager by generic (nonproprietary) name

† Use is not currently included in the labeling approved by the US Food and Drug Administration.

Selected Revisions April 10, 2024, © Copyright, September 1, 1993, American Society of Health-System Pharmacists, Inc.

amLODIPine Besylate

24:28.08 • DIHYDROPYRIDINES

■ Amlodipine is a 1,4-dihydropyridine-derivative calcium-channel blocking agent with an intrinsically long duration of action.

USES

● Hypertension

Amlodipine is used alone or in combination with other classes of antihypertensive agents in the management of hypertension. Amlodipine in fixed combination with atorvastatin (Caduet®) is used in patients for whom treatment with both amlodipine and atorvastatin is appropriate.

Current evidence-based practice guidelines for the management of hypertension in adults generally recommend the use of drugs from 4 classes of antihypertensive agents (angiotensin-converting enzyme [ACE] inhibitors, angiotensin II receptor antagonists, calcium-channel blockers, and thiazide diuretics); data from clinical outcome trials indicate that lowering blood pressure with any of these drug classes can reduce the complications of hypertension and provide similar cardiovascular protection. However, recommendations for initial drug selection and use in specific patient populations may vary across these expert guidelines. This variability is due, in part, to differences in the guideline development process and the types of studies (e.g., randomized controlled studies only versus a range of studies with different study designs) included in the evidence reviews. Ultimately, choice of antihypertensive therapy should be individualized, considering the clinical characteristics of the patient (e.g., age, ethnicity/race, comorbid conditions, cardiovascular risk factors) as well as drug-related factors (e.g., ease of administration, availability, adverse effects, costs). Because many patients eventually will need drugs from 2 or more antihypertensive classes, experts generally state that the emphasis should be placed on achieving appropriate blood pressure control rather than on identifying a preferred drug to achieve that control.

Disease Overview

Worldwide, hypertension is the most common modifiable risk factor for cardiovascular events and mortality. The lifetime risk of developing hypertension in the US exceeds 80%, with higher rates observed among African Americans and Hispanics compared with whites or Asians. The systolic blood pressure and diastolic blood pressure values defined as hypertension in adults (see Blood Pressure Classification under Uses: Hypertension) in a 2017 multidisciplinary guideline of the American College of Cardiology (ACC), American Heart Association (AHA), and a number of other professional organizations (subsequently referred to as the 2017 ACC/AHA hypertension guideline in this monograph) are lower than those defined in the Seventh Report of the Joint National Committee on Prevention, Detection, Evaluation, and Treatment of High Blood Pressure (JNC 7) guidelines, which results in an increase of approximately 14% in the prevalence of hypertension in the US. However, this change in definition results in only a 2% increase in the percentage of patients requiring antihypertensive drug therapy because non-pharmacologic treatment is recommended for most adults now classified by the 2017 ACC/AHA hypertension guideline as hypertensive who would *not* meet the JNC 7 definition of hypertension. Among US adults receiving antihypertensive drugs, approximately 53% have inadequately controlled blood pressure according to current ACC/AHA treatment goals.

Cardiovascular and Renal Sequelae

The principal goal of preventing and treating hypertension is to reduce the risk of cardiovascular and renal morbidity and mortality, including target organ damage. The relationship between blood pressure and cardiovascular disease is continuous, consistent, and independent of other risk factors. It is important that very high blood pressure be managed promptly to reduce the risk of target organ damage. The higher the blood pressure, the more likely the development of myocardial infarction (MI), heart failure, stroke, and renal disease. For adults 40–70 years of age, each 20-mm Hg increment in systolic blood pressure or 10-mm Hg increment in diastolic blood pressure doubles the risk of developing cardiovascular disease across the entire blood pressure range of 115/75 to 185/115 mm Hg. For those older than 50 years of age, systolic blood pressure is a much more important risk factor for developing cardiovascular disease than is diastolic blood pressure.

The rapidity with which treatment is required depends on the patient's clinical presentation (presence of new or worsening target organ damage) and the presence or absence of cardiovascular complications; the 2017 ACC/AHA hypertension guideline states that treatment of very high blood pressure should be initiated within at least 1 week.

Blood Pressure Classification

Accurate blood pressure measurement is essential for the proper diagnosis and management of hypertension. Error in measuring blood pressure is a major cause of inadequate blood pressure control and may lead to overtreatment. Because a patient's blood pressure may vary in an unpredictable fashion, a single blood pressure measurement is not sufficient for clinical decision-making. An average of 2 or 3 blood pressure measurements obtained on 2–3 separate occasions using proper technique should be used to minimize random error and provide a more accurate blood pressure reading. Out-of-office blood pressure measurements may be useful for confirming and managing hypertension. The 2017 ACC/AHA hypertension guideline document (available on the ACC and AHA websites) should be consulted for key steps on properly measuring blood pressure.

According to the 2017 ACC/AHA hypertension guideline, blood pressure in adults is classified into 4 categories: normal, elevated, stage 1 hypertension, and stage 2 hypertension. (See Table 1.) The 2017 ACC/AHA hypertension guideline lowers the blood pressure threshold used to define hypertension in the US; previous hypertension guidelines (JNC 7) considered adults with systolic blood pressure of 120–139 mm Hg or diastolic blood pressure of 80–89 mm Hg to have prehypertension, those with systolic blood pressure of 140–159 mm Hg or diastolic blood pressure of 90–99 mm Hg to have stage 1 hypertension, and those with systolic blood pressure of 160 mm Hg or higher or diastolic blood pressure of 100 mm Hg or higher to have stage 2 hypertension. The blood pressure definitions in the 2017 ACC/AHA hypertension guideline are based upon data from studies evaluating the association between systolic blood pressure/diastolic blood pressure and cardiovascular risk and the benefits of blood pressure reduction. Individuals with systolic blood pressure and diastolic blood pressure in 2 different categories should be designated as being in the higher blood pressure category.

TABLE 1. ACC/AHA Blood Pressure Classification in Adults [ab]

Category	SBP [c] (mm Hg)		DBP [d] (mm Hg)
Normal	<120	and	<80
Elevated	120–129	and	<80
Hypertension, Stage 1	130–139	or	80–89
Hypertension, Stage 2	≥140	or	≥90

[a] Source: Whelton PK, Carey RM, Aronow WS et al. 2017 ACC/AHA/AAPA/ABC/ACPM/AGS/APhA/ASH/ASPC/NMA/PCNA guideline for the prevention, detection, evaluation, and management of high blood pressure in adults: a report of the American College of Cardiology/American Heart Association Task Force on Clinical Practice Guidelines. Hypertension. 2018;71:e13-115.

[b] Individuals with SBP and DBP in 2 different categories (e.g., elevated SBP and normal DBP) should be designated as being in the higher blood pressure category (i.e., elevated BP).

[c] Systolic blood pressure

[d] Diastolic blood pressure

The blood pressure thresholds used to define hypertension, when to initiate drug therapy, and the ideal target blood pressure values remain controversial. The 2017 ACC/AHA hypertension guideline recommends a blood pressure goal of less than 130/80 mm Hg in all adults who have confirmed hypertension and known cardiovascular disease or a 10-year atherosclerotic cardiovascular disease (ASCVD) event risk of 10% or higher; the ACC/AHA guideline also states that this blood pressure goal is reasonable to attempt to achieve in adults with confirmed hypertension who do *not* have increased cardiovascular risk. The lower blood pressure values used to define hypertension and the lower target blood pressure goals outlined in the 2017 ACC/AHA hypertension guideline are based on clinical studies demonstrating a substantial reduction in the composite end point of major cardiovascular disease events and the combination of fatal and nonfatal stroke when a lower systolic blood pressure/diastolic blood pressure value (i.e., 130/80 mm Hg) was used to define hypertension. These lower target blood pressure goals also are based upon clinical studies demonstrating continuing reduction of cardiovascular risk at progressively lower levels of systolic blood pressure. A linear relationship has been demonstrated between cardiovascular risk and blood pressure even at low systolic blood pressures (e.g., 120–124 mm Hg). The 2017 ACC/AHA hypertension guideline recommends estimating a patient's ASCVD risk using the ACC/AHA Pooled Cohort equations (available online at http://tools.acc.org/ASCVD-Risk-Estimator), which are based on a variety of factors including age, race, gender, cholesterol levels, statin use, blood pressure, treatment for hypertension, history of diabetes mellitus, smoking status, and aspirin use. While the 2017 ACC/AHA hypertension guideline has lowered the threshold for *diagnosing* hypertension in adults, the threshold for *initiating drug therapy* has only been lowered for those patients who are at high risk of cardiovascular disease. Clinicians who support the 2017 ACC/AHA hypertension guideline believe that these recommendations have the potential to increase hypertension awareness, encourage lifestyle modification, and focus antihypertensive drug initiation and intensification in those adults at high risk for cardiovascular disease.

The lower blood pressure goals advocated in the 2017 ACC/AHA hypertension guideline have been questioned by some clinicians who have concerns regarding the guideline's use of extrapolated observational data, the lack of generalizability of some of the randomized trials (e.g., SPRINT) used to support the guideline, the difficulty of establishing accurate representative blood pressure values in typical clinical practice settings, and the accuracy of the cardiovascular risk calculator used in the guideline. Some clinicians state the lower blood pressure threshold used to define hypertension in the 2017 ACC/AHA hypertension guideline is not fully supported by clinical data, and these clinicians have expressed concerns about the possible harms (e.g., adverse effects of antihypertensive therapy) associated with classifying more patients as being hypertensive. Some clinicians also state that using this guideline, a large number of young, low-risk patients would need to be treated in order to observe a clinical benefit, while other clinicians state that the estimated gains in life-expectancy attributable to long-term use of blood pressure-lowering drugs are correspondingly greater in this patient population.

Treatment Benefits

In clinical trials, antihypertensive therapy has been found to reduce the risk of developing stroke by about 34–40%, MI by about 20–25%, and heart failure by more than 50%. In a randomized, controlled study (SPRINT) that included hypertensive patients without diabetes mellitus who had a high risk of cardiovascular disease, intensive systolic blood pressure lowering of approximately 15 mm Hg was associated with a 25% reduction in cardiovascular disease events and a 27% reduction in all-cause mortality. However, the exclusion of patients with diabetes mellitus, prior stroke, and those younger than 50 years of age may decrease the generalizability of these findings. Some experts estimate that if the systolic blood pressure goals of the 2017 ACC/AHA hypertension guideline are achieved, major cardiovascular disease events may be reduced by an additional 340,000 and total deaths by an additional 156,000 compared with implementation of the JNC 8 expert panel guideline goals but these benefits may be accompanied by an increase in the frequency of adverse events. While there was no overall difference in the occurrence of serious adverse events in patients receiving intensive therapy for blood pressure control (systolic blood pressure target of less than 120 mm Hg) compared with those receiving less intense control (systolic blood pressure target of less than 140 mm Hg) in the SPRINT study, hypotension, syncope, electrolyte abnormalities, and acute kidney injury or acute renal failure occurred in substantially more patients receiving intensive therapy.

In the Antihypertensive and Lipid-lowering Treatment to Prevent Heart Attack Trial (ALLHAT), the long-term cardiovascular morbidity and mortality benefit of a long-acting dihydropyridine calcium-channel blocker (amlodipine), a thiazide-like diuretic (chlorthalidone), and an ACE inhibitor (lisinopril) were compared in a broad population of patients with hypertension at risk for coronary heart disease. Although these antihypertensive agents were comparably effective in providing important cardiovascular benefit, apparent differences in certain secondary outcomes were observed. Patients receiving the ACE inhibitor experienced higher risks of stroke, combined cardiovascular disease, GI bleeding, and angioedema, while those receiving the calcium-channel blocker were at higher risk of developing heart failure. The ALLHAT investigators suggested that the observed differences in cardiovascular outcome may be attributable, at least in part, to the greater antihypertensive effect of the calcium-channel blocker compared with that of the ACE inhibitor, especially in women and black patients. (See Clinical Benefits of Thiazides in Hypertension under Hypertension in Adults: Treatment Benefits in Uses in the Thiazides General Statement 40:28.20.)

General Considerations for Initial and Maintenance Antihypertensive Therapy
Nonpharmacologic Therapy

Nonpharmacologic measures (i.e., lifestyle/behavioral modifications) that are effective in lowering blood pressure include weight reduction (for those who are overweight or obese), dietary changes to include foods such as fruits, vegetables, whole grains, and low-fat dairy products that are rich in potassium, calcium, magnesium, and fiber (i.e., adoption of the Dietary Approaches to Stop Hypertension [DASH] eating plan), sodium reduction, increased physical activity, and moderation of alcohol intake. Such lifestyle/behavioral modifications, including smoking cessation, enhance antihypertensive drug efficacy and decrease cardiovascular risk and remain an indispensable part of the management of hypertension. Lifestyle/behavioral modifications without antihypertensive drug therapy are recommended for adults classified by the 2017 ACC/AHA hypertension guideline as having elevated blood pressure (systolic blood pressure 120–129 mm Hg and diastolic blood pressure less than 80 mm Hg) and in those with stage 1 hypertension (systolic blood pressure 130–139 mm Hg or diastolic blood pressure 80–89 mm Hg) who do *not* have preexisting cardiovascular disease or an estimated 10-year ASCVD risk of 10% or greater.

Initiation of Drug Therapy

Drug therapy in the management of hypertension must be individualized and adjusted based on the degree of blood pressure elevation while also considering cardiovascular risk factors. Drug therapy generally is reserved for patients who respond inadequately to nondrug therapy (i.e., lifestyle modifications such as diet [including sodium restriction and adequate potassium and calcium intake], regular aerobic physical activity, moderation of alcohol consumption, and weight reduction) or in whom the degree of blood pressure elevation or coexisting risk factors, especially increased cardiovascular risk, require more prompt or aggressive therapy; however, the optimum blood pressure threshold for initiating antihypertensive drug therapy and specific treatment goals remain controversial.

The 2017 ACC/AHA hypertension guideline and many experts currently state that the treatment of hypertension should be based not only on blood pressure values but also on patients' cardiovascular risk factors. For *secondary prevention* of recurrent cardiovascular disease events in adults with clinical cardiovascular disease or for *primary prevention* in adults with an estimated 10-year ASCVD risk of 10% or higher, the 2017 ACC/AHA hypertension guideline recommends initiation of antihypertensive drug therapy in conjunction with lifestyle/behavioral modifications at an average systolic blood pressure of 130 mm Hg or an average diastolic blood pressure of 80 mm Hg or higher. For *primary prevention* of cardiovascular disease events in adults with a low (less than 10%) estimated 10-year risk of ASCVD, the 2017 ACC/AHA hypertension guideline recommends initiation of antihypertensive drug therapy in conjunction with lifestyle/behavioral modifications at a systolic blood pressure of 140 mm Hg or higher or a diastolic blood pressure of 90 mm Hg or higher. After initiation of antihypertensive drug therapy, regardless of the ASCVD risk, the 2017 ACC/AHA hypertension guideline generally recommends a blood pressure goal of less than 130/80 mm Hg in all patients. In addition, a systolic blood pressure goal of less than 130 mm Hg also is recommended for noninstitutionalized ambulatory patients 65 years of age or older. While these blood pressure goals are lower than those recommended for most patients in previous guidelines, they are based upon clinical studies demonstrating continuing reduction of cardiovascular risk at progressively lower levels of systolic blood pressure.

Most data indicate that patients with a higher cardiovascular risk will benefit the most from tighter blood pressure control; however, some experts state this treatment goal also may be beneficial in those at lower cardiovascular risk. Other clinicians believe that the benefits of such blood pressure lowering do not outweigh the risks in those patients considered to be at lower risk of cardiovascular disease and that reclassifying individuals formerly considered to have prehypertension as having hypertension may potentially lead to use of drug therapy in such patients without consideration of cardiovascular risk. Previous hypertension guidelines, such as those from the JNC 8 expert panel, generally recommended initiation of antihypertensive treatment in patients with a systolic blood pressure of at least 140 mm Hg or diastolic blood pressure of at least 90 mm Hg, targeted a blood pressure goal of less than 140/90 mm Hg regardless of cardiovascular risk, and used higher systolic blood pressure thresholds and targets in geriatric patients. Some clinicians continue to support the target blood pressures recommended by the JNC 8 expert panel because of concerns that such recommendations in the 2017 ACC/AHA hypertension guideline are based on extrapolation of data from the high-risk population in the SPRINT study to a lower-risk population. Also, because more than 90% of patients in SPRINT were already receiving antihypertensive drugs at baseline, data are lacking on the effects of *initiating* drug therapy at a lower blood pressure threshold (130/80 mm Hg) in patients at high risk of cardiovascular disease. The potential benefits of hypertension management and drug cost, adverse effects, and risks associated with the use of multiple antihypertensive drugs should be considered when deciding a patient's blood pressure treatment goal.

The 2017 ACC/AHA hypertension guideline recommends an ASCVD risk assessment for all adults with hypertension; however, experts state that it can be assumed that patients with hypertension and diabetes mellitus or chronic kidney disease (CKD) are at high risk for cardiovascular disease and that antihypertensive drug therapy should be initiated in these patients at a blood pressure of 130/80 mm Hg or higher. The 2017 ACC/AHA hypertension guideline also recommends a blood pressure goal of less than 130/80 mm Hg in patients with hypertension and diabetes mellitus or CKD. These recommendations are based on a systematic review of high-quality evidence from randomized controlled trials, meta-analyses, and post hoc analyses that have demonstrated substantial reductions in the risk of important clinical outcomes (e.g., cardiovascular events) regardless of comorbid conditions or age when systolic blood pressure is lowered to less than 130 mm Hg. However, some clinicians have questioned the generalizability of findings from some of the trials (e.g., SPRINT) used to support the 2017 ACC/AHA hypertension guideline. For example, SPRINT included adults (mean age: 68 years) *without* diabetes mellitus who were at high risk of cardiovascular disease. While benefits of intensive blood pressure control were observed in this patient population, some clinicians have questioned whether these findings apply to younger patients who have a low risk of cardiovascular disease. In patients with CKD in the SPRINT trial, intensive blood pressure management (achieving a mean systolic blood pressure of approximately 122 mm Hg compared with 136 mm Hg with standard treatment) provided a similar beneficial reduction in the composite cardiovascular disease primary outcome and all-cause mortality as in the full patient cohort. Because most patients with CKD die from cardiovascular complications, the findings of this study further support a lower blood pressure target of less than 130/80 mm Hg.

Data are lacking to determine the ideal blood pressure goal in adult patients with hypertension and diabetes mellitus; also, studies evaluating the benefits of intensive blood pressure control in patients with diabetes mellitus have provided conflicting results. Clinical studies reviewed for the 2017 ACC/AHA hypertension guideline have shown similar quantitative benefits from blood pressure lowering in hypertensive patients with or without diabetes mellitus. In a randomized, controlled study (ACCORD-BP) that compared a higher (systolic blood pressure less than 140 mm Hg) versus lower (systolic blood pressure less than 120 mm Hg) blood pressure goal in patients with diabetes mellitus, there was no difference in the incidence of cardiovascular outcomes (e.g., composite outcome of cardiovascular death, nonfatal MI, and nonfatal stroke). However, some experts state that this study was underpowered to detect a difference between the 2 treatment groups and that the factorial design of the study complicated interpretation of the results. Although SPRINT did not include patients with diabetes mellitus, patients in this study with prediabetes demonstrated a similar cardiovascular benefit from intensive treatment of blood pressure as normoglycemic patients. A meta-analysis of data from the ACCORD and SPRINT studies suggests that the findings of both studies are consistent and that patients with diabetes mellitus benefit from more intensive blood pressure control. These data support the 2017 ACC/AHA hypertension guideline recommendation of a blood pressure treatment goal of less than 130/80 mm Hg in adult patients with hypertension and diabetes mellitus. Alternatively, the American Diabetes Association (ADA) recommends a blood pressure goal of less than 140/90 mm Hg in patients with diabetes mellitus. The ADA states that a lower blood pressure goal (e.g., less than 130/80 mm Hg) may be appropriate for patients with a high risk of cardiovascular disease and diabetes mellitus if it can be achieved without undue treatment burden.

Further study is needed to more clearly define optimum blood pressure goals in patients with hypertension, particularly in high-risk groups (e.g., patients with diabetes mellitus, cardiovascular disease, or cerebrovascular disease; black patients); when determining appropriate blood pressure goals, individual risks and benefits should be considered in addition to the evidence from clinical studies.

Choice of Initial Drug Therapy

In current hypertension management guidelines, calcium-channel blockers are recommended as one of several preferred drugs for the initial treatment of hypertension; other preferred options include ACE inhibitors, angiotensin II receptor antagonists, and thiazide diuretics. (See Hypertension: Treatment Benefits, in Uses.) The 2017 ACC/AHA adult hypertension guideline states that a calcium-channel blocker, ACE inhibitor, angiotensin II receptor antagonist, or thiazide or thiazide-like diuretic (preferably chlorthalidone) are all acceptable choices for initial antihypertensive drug therapy in the general population of nonblack patients, including those with diabetes mellitus; drugs from any of these classes generally produce similar benefits in terms of overall mortality and cardiovascular, cerebrovascular, and renal outcomes. Calcium-channel blockers may be particularly useful in the management of hypertension in black patients; these patients tend to have a greater blood pressure response to calcium-channel blockers and thiazide diuretics than to other antihypertensive drug classes (e.g., ACE inhibitors, angiotensin II receptor antagonists). (See Race under Hypertension: Other Special Considerations for Antihypertensive Therapy, in Uses.) In black patients, including those with diabetes mellitus, the initial drug choice should include a thiazide diuretic or calcium-channel blocker. Use of a calcium-channel blocker also may be beneficial in patients with certain coexisting conditions such as ischemic heart disease (e.g., angina) and in geriatric patients, including those with isolated systolic hypertension. (See Considerations for Drug Therapy in Patients with Underlying Cardiovascular and Other Risk Factors and also see Other Special Considerations for Antihypertensive Drug Therapy, under Uses: Hypertension in Adults, in the Thiazides General Statement 40:28.20.) Because many patients eventually will need more than one antihypertensive drug to achieve blood pressure control, any of the recommended drug classes may be considered for add-on therapy.

Experts state that in patients with stage 1 hypertension (especially the elderly, those with a history of hypotension, or those who have experienced adverse drug effects), it is reasonable to initiate drug therapy using the stepped-care approach in which one drug is initiated and titrated and other drugs are added sequentially to achieve the target blood pressure. Although some patients can begin treatment with a single antihypertensive agent, starting with 2 first-line drugs in different pharmacologic classes (either as separate agents or in a fixed-dose combination) is recommended in patients with stage 2 hypertension and an average blood pressure more than 20/10 mm Hg above their target blood pressure. Such combined therapy may increase the likelihood of achieving goal blood pressure in a more timely fashion, but also may increase the risk of adverse effects (e.g., orthostatic hypotension) in some patients (e.g., elderly). Drug regimens with complementary activity, where a second antihypertensive agent is used to block compensatory responses to the first agent or affect a different pressor mechanism, can result in additive blood pressure lowering and are preferred. Drug combinations that have similar mechanisms of action or clinical effects (e.g., the combination of an ACE inhibitor and an angiotensin II receptor antagonist) generally should be avoided. Many patients who begin therapy with a single antihypertensive agent will subsequently require at least 2 drugs from different pharmacologic classes to achieve their blood pressure goal. Experts state that other patient-specific factors, such as age, concurrent medications, drug adherence, drug interactions, the overall treatment regimen, cost, and comorbidities, also should be considered when deciding on an antihypertensive drug regimen. For any stage of hypertension, antihypertensive drug dosages should be adjusted and/or other agents substituted or added until goal blood pressure is achieved. (See Follow-up and Maintenance Drug Therapy under Hypertension: General Considerations for Initial and Maintenance Antihypertensive Therapy, in Uses.)

Follow-up and Maintenance Drug Therapy

Several strategies are used for the titration and combination of antihypertensive drugs; these strategies, which are generally based on those used in randomized controlled studies, include maximizing the dosage of the first drug before adding a second drug, adding a second drug before achieving maximum dosage of the initial drug, or initiating therapy with 2 drugs simultaneously (either as separate preparations or as a fixed-dose combination). Combined use of an ACE inhibitor and angiotensin II receptor antagonist should be avoided because of the potential risk of adverse renal effects. After initiating a new or adjusted antihypertensive drug regimen, patients should have their blood pressure reevaluated monthly until adequate blood pressure control is achieved. Effective blood pressure control can be achieved in most hypertensive patients, but many will ultimately require therapy with 2 or more antihypertensive drugs. In addition to measuring blood pressure, clinicians should evaluate patients for orthostatic hypotension, adverse drug effects, adherence to drug therapy and lifestyle modifications, and the need for drug dosage adjustments. Laboratory testing such as electrolytes and renal function status and other assessments of target organ damage also should be performed.

Considerations for Drug Therapy in Patients with Underlying Cardiovascular and Other Risk Factors

Drug therapy in patients with hypertension and underlying cardiovascular or other risk factors should be carefully individualized based on the underlying disease(s), concomitant drugs, tolerance to drug-induced adverse effects, and blood pressure goal. (See Table 2: Compelling Indications for Drug Classes based on Comorbid Conditions, in Considerations for Drug Therapy in Patients with Underlying Cardiovascular and Other Risk Factors under Uses: Hypertension in Adults, in the Thiazides General Statement 40:28.20.)

Other Special Considerations for Antihypertensive Therapy
Race

Most patients with hypertension, especially black patients, will require at least 2 antihypertensive drugs to achieve adequate blood pressure control. Blood pressure response to calcium-channel blockers appears to be comparable in white and black patients. In general, black hypertensive patients tend to respond better to monotherapy with calcium-channel blockers or thiazide diuretics than to monotherapy with other drug classes (e.g., ACE inhibitors, angiotensin II receptor antagonists, β-blockers). In a prespecified subgroup analysis of the ALLHAT study, a calcium-channel blocker was more effective than an ACE inhibitor in lowering blood pressure and was associated with a substantially reduced rate of stroke in black patients. When compared with a thiazide diuretic, the calcium-channel blocker appeared to be less effective in preventing heart failure, but comparable with respect to other outcomes (e.g., cerebrovascular, cardiovascular, renal, mortality). (See Clinical Benefits of Thiazides in Hypertension under Hypertension in Adults: Treatment Benefits, in Uses in the Thiazides General Statement 40:28.20.) However, the combination of an ACE inhibitor or an angiotensin II receptor antagonist with a calcium-channel blocker or thiazide diuretic produces similar blood pressure lowering in black patients as in other racial groups. In addition, some experts state that when use of ACE inhibitors, angiotensin II receptor antagonists, or β-blockers is indicated in hypertensive patients with underlying cardiovascular or other risk factors, these indications should be applied equally to black hypertensive patients. (See Considerations for Drug Therapy in Patients with Underlying Cardiovascular and Other Risk Factors under Uses: Hypertension in Adults, in the Thiazides General Statement 40:28.20.)

Advanced Age

Antihypertensive drugs recommended for initial therapy in geriatric patients, including those with isolated systolic hypertension, generally are the same as those recommended for younger patients. Antihypertensive therapy initiated with a calcium-channel blocking agent has been shown to reduce cardiovascular morbidity and mortality in older patients with isolated systolic hypertension.

Although some experts state that calcium-channel blocking agents or diuretics may be preferred in geriatric patients, ACE inhibitors and angiotensin II receptor antagonists also have shown beneficial effects and may be considered in this population.

For further information on overall principles and expert recommendations for treatment of hypertension, see Uses: Hypertension in Adults, and also see Uses: Hypertension in Pediatric Patients, in the Thiazides General Statement 40:28.20.

Hypertensive Crises

Because of the slow onset of hypotensive effect with amlodipine, this drug is *not* suitable for use as acute therapy in rapidly reducing blood pressure in patients with severe hypertension in whom reduction of blood pressure is considered urgent (i.e., hypertensive urgencies) nor in hypertensive emergencies.

For additional information on the role of dihydropyridine calcium-channel blocking agents in the management of hypertension and angina, see Uses in Nifedipine 24:28.08.

● Coronary Artery Disease

Amlodipine in fixed combination with atorvastatin (Caduet®) is used in patients for whom treatment with both amlodipine and atorvastatin is appropriate.

Angina

Amlodipine is used for the management of Prinzmetal variant angina and chronic stable angina pectoris. The drug has been used alone or in combination with other antianginal agents.

Angiographically Documented Coronary Artery Disease

Amlodipine is used in patients with recently documented coronary artery disease by angiography (without heart failure or an ejection fraction less than 40%), to reduce the risk of coronary revascularization procedure and hospitalization due to angina.

DOSAGE AND ADMINISTRATION

● Administration

Amlodipine besylate is administered orally. Amlodipine generally can be given without regard to meals.

● Dosage

Dosage of amlodipine besylate is expressed in terms of amlodipine.

Hypertension
Amlodipine Therapy

The manufacturers state that the usual initial adult dosage of amlodipine is 2.5–5 mg once daily as monotherapy. In geriatric patients and small or frail individuals, an initial dosage of 2.5 mg once daily is recommended. This reduced initial dosage also can be used in adults when amlodipine is added to an existing antihypertensive drug regimen. Subsequent dosage of amlodipine should be adjusted according to the patient's blood pressure response and tolerance and usually should not exceed 10 mg once daily. Generally, dosage is increased gradually at 7- to 14-day intervals until optimum control of blood pressure is maintained. However, more rapid titration of dosage can be undertaken when clinically warranted, provided response and tolerance are assessed frequently. The usual maintenance dosage of amlodipine for the management of hypertension in adults is 2.5–10 mg once daily.

The manufacturer states that the safety and efficacy of amlodipine have not been established in pediatric patients younger than 6 years of age; however, for the management of hypertension in children 1–5 years of age†, an initial dosage of 0.1 mg/kg once daily and a maximum dosage of 0.6 mg/kg daily (up to 5 mg daily) has been recommended by some experts. In children 6 years of age and older, some experts recommend an initial dosage of 2.5 mg once daily and a maximum dosage of 10 mg once daily. However, the manufacturer states that the safety and efficacy of dosages exceeding 5 mg daily have not been established in pediatric patients. The manufacturer states that the usual effective dosage of amlodipine in children 6 years of age and older is 2.5–5 mg once daily. Experts state that the drug should be initiated at the low end of the dosage range; the dosage may be increased every 2–4 weeks until blood pressure is controlled, the maximum dosage is reached, or adverse effects occur. For information on overall principles and expert recommendations for treatment of hypertension in pediatric patients, see Uses: Hypertension in Pediatric Patients, in the Thiazides General Statement 40:28.20.

Amlodipine/Benazepril Fixed-combination Therapy

Therapy with the commercially available preparations containing amlodipine in fixed combination with benazepril hydrochloride usually should be initiated only after an adequate response is not achieved with amlodipine (or another dihydropyridine-derivative calcium-channel blocker) or benazepril (or another ACE inhibitor) alone. Alternatively, such fixed combinations may be used if amlodipine dosages necessary for adequate response have been associated with development of edema. The fixed combination containing amlodipine and benazepril also may be used as a substitute for the individually titrated drugs. The recommended initial dosage is amlodipine 2.5 mg in fixed combination with benazepril hydrochloride 10 mg once daily. Dosage of the fixed combination containing amlodipine and benazepril should be adjusted according to the patient's response. The antihypertensive effect of a given dosage is largely attained with 2 weeks; if necessary, dosage of the fixed combination may be increased up to a maximum dosage of 10 mg of amlodipine in fixed combination with 40 mg of benazepril hydrochloride once daily.

The addition of benazepril to amlodipine therapy usually does not provide additional antihypertensive effects in black patients; however, benazepril appears to reduce the development of amlodipine-associated edema regardless of race. The manufacturers state that when the fixed combinations containing 2.5–10 mg of amlodipine with 10–40 mg of benazepril hydrochloride have been used, the antihypertensive effects of these combinations have increased with increasing dosages of amlodipine in all patients; in addition, antihypertensive effects increased with increasing dosages of benazepril in nonblack patients.

Amlodipine/Olmesartan Fixed-combination Therapy

In patients who do not respond adequately to monotherapy with amlodipine (or another dihydropyridine-derivative calcium-channel blocker) or, alternatively, with olmesartan medoxomil (or another angiotensin II receptor antagonist), combined therapy with the drugs can be used to provide additional antihypertensive effects. The fixed-combination preparation containing amlodipine and olmesartan medoxomil also can be used as a substitute for the individually titrated drugs. The patient can be switched to the fixed-combination preparation containing the corresponding individual doses of amlodipine and olmesartan medoxomil; alternatively, the dosage of one or both components can be increased for additional antihypertensive effects. If needed, dosage of the fixed combination may be increased after 2 weeks. Dosage adjustments generally should involve one drug at a time, although dosages of both drugs can be increased to achieve more rapid blood pressure control. Daily dosages exceeding 10 mg of amlodipine given in fixed combination with 40 mg of olmesartan medoxomil are not recommended by the manufacturer.

Commercially available preparations containing amlodipine in fixed combination with olmesartan medoxomil may be used for initial treatment of hypertension in patients likely to require combined therapy with multiple antihypertensive drugs to achieve blood pressure control. In such patients, therapy with the fixed-combination preparation usually should be initiated at a dosage of 5 mg of amlodipine and 20 mg of olmesartan medoxomil once daily. If necessary, dosage of the fixed combination may be increased after 1–2 weeks for additional blood pressure control (but should not exceed a maximum dosage of 10 mg of amlodipine and 40 mg of olmesartan medoxomil once daily). In patients whose baseline blood pressure is 160/100 mm Hg, the estimated probability of achieving control of systolic blood pressure (defined as systolic blood pressure of less than 140 mm Hg) is 48, 46, or 68% and of achieving control of diastolic blood pressure (defined as diastolic blood pressure of less than 90 mm Hg) is 51, 60, or 85% with olmesartan medoxomil (40 mg daily) alone, amlodipine (10 mg daily) alone, or amlodipine combined with olmesartan medoxomil (at the same dosages), respectively.

Amlodipine/Olmesartan/Hydrochlorothiazide Fixed-combination Therapy

The fixed-combination preparation containing amlodipine, olmesartan, and hydrochlorothiazide may be used to provide additional blood pressure control in patients who do not respond adequately to combination therapy with any 2 of the following classes of antihypertensive agents given at maximally tolerated, labeled, or usual dosages: calcium-channel blockers, angiotensin II receptor antagonists, or diuretics. Patients who experience dose-limiting adverse effects of amlodipine, olmesartan, or hydrochlorothiazide while receiving any dual combination of these drugs may be switched to a lower dosage of that drug, given as a fixed-combination preparation containing all 3 of these drugs, to achieve similar blood pressure reductions. The fixed-combination preparation containing amlodipine, olmesartan, and hydrochlorothiazide also can be used as a substitute for the individually titrated drugs. If necessary, dosage of the fixed-combination preparation may be increased after 2 weeks for additional blood pressure control (but should not exceed a maximum dosage of 10 mg of amlodipine, 40 mg of olmesartan medoxomil, and 25 mg of hydrochlorothiazide once daily). The commercially available preparation containing amlodipine in fixed combination with olmesartan and hydrochlorothiazide should not be used for the initial management of hypertension.

Amlodipine/Perindopril Fixed-combination Therapy

The commercially available preparation containing amlodipine in fixed combination with perindopril arginine may be used in patients receiving amlodipine monotherapy when amlodipine dosages necessary for adequate response have been associated with development of edema. In addition, patients who do not respond adequately to monotherapy may be switched to therapy with the fixed combination of amlodipine and perindopril arginine. Dosage of the fixed-combination preparation should be adjusted according to the patient's response at intervals of 7–14 days.

Commercially available preparations containing amlodipine in fixed combination with perindopril may be used for initial treatment of hypertension in patients likely to require combined therapy with multiple antihypertensive drugs to achieve blood pressure control. In such patients, therapy with the fixed-combination preparation usually should be initiated at a dosage of 2.5 mg of amlodipine and 3.5 mg of perindopril arginine once daily. The decision to use the fixed combination of amlodipine and perindopril for initial management of hypertension should be based on assessment of potential benefits and risks of such therapy, including consideration of whether the patient is likely to tolerate the lowest available dosage of the combined drugs. Dosage may be adjusted as needed at intervals

of 7–14 days to a maximum dosage of amlodipine 10 mg and perindopril arginine 14 mg once daily.

In patients whose baseline blood pressure is 170/105 mm Hg, the estimated probability of achieving control of systolic blood pressure (defined as systolic blood pressure of less than 140 mm Hg) is 26, 40, or 50% and of achieving control of diastolic blood pressure (defined as diastolic blood pressure of less than 90 mm Hg) is 31, 46, or 65% with perindopril erbumine (16 mg daily) alone, amlodipine (10 mg daily) alone, or amlodipine (10 mg daily) combined with perindopril arginine (14 mg daily), respectively.

In black patients and patients with diabetes mellitus, the addition of perindopril arginine (14 mg daily) to amlodipine (10 mg daily) did not provide additional antihypertensive effects beyond those achieved with amlodipine monotherapy.

Amlodipine/Telmisartan Fixed-combination Therapy

The fixed-combination preparation containing amlodipine and telmisartan can be used as a substitute for the individually administered drugs; patients may be switched to the fixed-combination preparation containing the corresponding individual doses of amlodipine and telmisartan or, alternatively, the dosage of one or both components can be increased for additional antihypertensive effects. In addition, the manufacturers state that patients who do not respond adequately to monotherapy with amlodipine (or another dihydropyridine-derivative calcium-channel blocker) or, alternatively, with telmisartan (or another angiotensin II receptor antagonist) may be switched to therapy with the fixed-combination preparation containing amlodipine and telmisartan. Patients who experience dose-limiting adverse effects (e.g., edema) during monotherapy with amlodipine 10 mg may be switched to the fixed combination containing amlodipine 5 mg and telmisartan 40 mg to achieve similar blood pressure control. If needed, dosage of the fixed-combination preparation may be increased to a maximum dosage of 10 mg of amlodipine and 80 mg of telmisartan given once daily; because most of the antihypertensive effect of a given dosage is achieved within 2 weeks, dosage may be adjusted after at least 2 weeks, if needed, to attain blood pressure control.

Commercially available preparations containing amlodipine in fixed combination with telmisartan may be used for initial treatment of hypertension in patients likely to require combined therapy with multiple antihypertensive drugs to achieve blood pressure control. In such patients, therapy with the fixed-combination preparation usually should be initiated at a dosage of 5 mg of amlodipine and 40 mg of telmisartan once daily. An initial dosage of 5 mg of amlodipine and 80 mg of telmisartan once daily may be used in patients requiring larger blood pressure reductions. The decision to use the fixed combination of amlodipine and telmisartan for initial management of hypertension should be based on assessment of potential benefits and risks of such therapy, including consideration of whether the patient is likely to tolerate the lowest available dosage of the combined drugs. In patients whose baseline blood pressure is 160/110 mm Hg, the estimated probability of achieving control of systolic blood pressure (defined as systolic blood pressure of less than 140 mm Hg) is 46, 69, or 79% and of achieving control of diastolic blood pressure (defined as diastolic blood pressure of less than 90 mm Hg) is 26, 22, or 55% with telmisartan (80 mg daily) alone, amlodipine (10 mg daily) alone, or amlodipine combined with telmisartan (at the same dosages), respectively.

Amlodipine/Valsartan Fixed-combination Therapy

Patients whose hypertension is adequately controlled with amlodipine and valsartan administered separately may be switched to the fixed-combination preparation containing the corresponding individual doses. Alternatively, the manufacturers state that patients who do not respond adequately to monotherapy with amlodipine (or another dihydropyridine-derivative calcium-channel blocker) or, alternatively, with valsartan (or another angiotensin II receptor antagonist) may be switched to therapy with the fixed-combination preparation containing amlodipine and valsartan. In addition, patients who experience dose-limiting adverse effects during monotherapy with amlodipine or valsartan can be switched to a lower dosage of that drug, given as a fixed-combination preparation containing amlodipine and valsartan, to achieve similar blood pressure control; dosage should be adjusted according to the patient's response after 3–4 weeks of therapy. If needed, dosage of the fixed-combination preparation may be increased to a maximum of 10 mg of amlodipine and 320 mg of valsartan given once daily; because most of the antihypertensive effect of a given dosage is achieved within 2 weeks, dosage may be adjusted after 1–2 weeks, if needed, to attain blood pressure control.

Commercially available preparations containing amlodipine in fixed combination with valsartan may be used for initial treatment of hypertension in patients likely to require combined therapy with multiple antihypertensive drugs to achieve blood pressure control. In such patients, therapy with the fixed-combination preparation should be initiated at a dosage of 5 mg of amlodipine and 160 mg of valsartan once daily in individuals without depletion of intravascular volume. The decision to use the fixed combination of amlodipine and valsartan for initial management of hypertension should be based on assessment of potential benefits and risks of such therapy, including consideration of whether the patient is likely to tolerate the lowest available dosage of the combined drugs. In patients whose baseline blood pressure is 160/100 mm Hg, the estimated probability of achieving control of systolic blood pressure (defined as systolic blood pressure of less than 140 mm Hg) is 47, 67, or 80% and of achieving control of diastolic blood pressure (defined as diastolic blood pressure of less than 90 mm Hg) is 62, 80, or 85% with valsartan (320 mg daily) alone, amlodipine (10 mg daily) alone, or amlodipine combined with valsartan (at the same dosages), respectively.

Amlodipine/Valsartan/Hydrochlorothiazide Fixed-combination Therapy

The fixed-combination preparation containing amlodipine, valsartan, and hydrochlorothiazide may be used to provide additional blood pressure control in patients who do not respond adequately to combination therapy with any 2 of the following classes of antihypertensive agents: calcium-channel blockers, angiotensin II receptor antagonists, or diuretics. Patients who experience dose-limiting adverse effects of amlodipine, valsartan, or hydrochlorothiazide while receiving any dual combination of these drugs may be switched to a lower dosage of that drug, given as a fixed-combination preparation containing all 3 of these drugs, to achieve similar blood pressure reductions. The fixed-combination preparation containing amlodipine, valsartan, and hydrochlorothiazide also can be used as a substitute for the individually titrated drugs. If necessary, dosage of the fixed-combination preparation may be increased after 2 weeks for additional blood pressure control (but should not exceed a maximum dosage of 10 mg of amlodipine, 320 mg of valsartan, and 25 mg of hydrochlorothiazide given once daily). The commercially available preparation containing amlodipine in fixed combination with valsartan and hydrochlorothiazide should not be used for the initial management of hypertension.

Amlodipine/Atorvastatin Fixed-combination Therapy

The fixed-combination preparation containing amlodipine and atorvastatin may be used as a substitute for individually titrated drugs. In patients currently receiving amlodipine and atorvastatin, the initial dosage of the fixed-combination preparation is the equivalent of titrated dosages of amlodipine and atorvastatin. Increased amounts of amlodipine, atorvastatin, or both components may be added for additional antihypertensive or antilipemic effects.

The fixed-combination preparation may be used to provide additional therapy for patients currently receiving one component of the preparation. The initial dosage of the fixed-combination preparation should be selected based on the dosage of the current component being used and the recommended initial dosage for the added monotherapy.

The fixed-combination preparation may be used to initiate treatment in patients with hypertension and dyslipidemias. The initial dosage of the fixed-combination preparation should be selected based on the recommended initial dosages of the individual components. For dosage recommendations for atorvastatin, see Dosage and Administration: Dosage, in Atorvastatin 24:06.08. The maximum dosage of amlodipine or atorvastatin in the fixed-combination preparation is 10 or 80 mg daily, respectively.

Blood Pressure Monitoring and Treatment Goals

Blood pressure monitoring using an out-of-office (home [self-monitored]) or ambulatory method (using a device that measures blood pressure over a 24-hour period) as an adjunct to in-office monitoring generally is recommended to provide a more reliable assessment of blood pressure; studies suggest that out-of-office blood pressure may be a better predictor of hypertension-induced organ damage and cardiovascular risk than office blood pressure. Periodic determination of blood pressure in both the morning and evening (before taking the morning or evening dose) is useful in monitoring daytime control and ensuring that the surge in blood pressure that occurs with arising has been modulated adequately. Occasionally, particularly in geriatric patients and those with orthostatic symptoms, monitoring should include blood pressure determinations in both the seated position and, to recognize possible postural hypotension, after standing quietly for 2–5 minutes.

Once antihypertensive drug therapy has been initiated, dosage generally is adjusted at approximately monthly intervals if blood pressure control is inadequate at a given dosage; additional drugs may need to be added to an antihypertensive drug regimen to achieve adequate blood pressure control. Once blood pressure has been stabilized, follow-up visits generally can be scheduled at 3- to 6-month intervals, depending on patient status.

Blood pressure should be monitored regularly (i.e., monthly) during therapy and dosage of the antihypertensive drug adjusted until blood pressure is controlled. In patients who develop unacceptable adverse effects with amlodipine, the drug should be discontinued and another antihypertensive agent from a different pharmacologic class should be initiated. If an adequate blood pressure response is not achieved with amlodipine monotherapy, another antihypertensive agent with demonstrated benefit and preferably a complementary mechanism of action (e.g., angiotensin-converting enzyme [ACE] inhibitor, angiotensin II receptor antagonist, thiazide diuretic) may be added; if goal blood pressure is still not achieved with the use of 2 antihypertensive agents, a third drug may be added. (See Uses: Hypertension.)

The goal of hypertension management and prevention is to achieve and maintain optimal control of blood pressure. However, the optimum blood pressure threshold for initiating antihypertensive drug therapy and specific treatment goals remain controversial. While other hypertension guidelines have based target blood pressure goals on age and comorbidities, the 2017 American College of Cardiology (ACC)/American Heart Association (AHA) hypertension guideline incorporates underlying cardiovascular risk into decision making regarding treatment and generally recommends the same target blood pressure (i.e., less than 130/80 mm Hg) for all adults. Many patients will require at least 2 drugs from different pharmacologic classes to achieve this blood pressure goal; the potential benefits of hypertension management and drug cost, adverse effects, and risks associated with the use of multiple antihypertensive drugs also should be considered when deciding a patient's blood pressure treatment goal. (See General Considerations for Initial and Maintenance Antihypertensive Therapy under Uses: Hypertension.)

For additional information on target levels of blood pressure and on monitoring therapy in the management of hypertension, see Blood Pressure Monitoring and Treatment Goals under Dosage: Hypertension, in Dosage and Administration in the Thiazides General Statement 40:28.20.

In children with hypertension with or without diabetes mellitus, blood pressure should be reduced to less than the corresponding age-adjusted 90th percentile value and to less than 130/80 mm Hg in adolescents at least 13 years of age. In children and adolescents with hypertension and chronic kidney disease (CKD), the 24-hour mean arterial pressure (MAP) as determined by ambulatory blood pressure monitoring should be decreased to a value less than the 50th percentile.

Coronary Artery Disease
Angina

For the management of Prinzmetal variant angina or chronic stable angina, the usual adult dosage of amlodipine is 5–10 mg once daily. The manufacturers state that adequate control of angina usually requires a maintenance dosage of 10 mg daily.

Amlodipine has been used concomitantly with other antihypertensive and antianginal drugs, including thiazide diuretics, angiotensin-converting enzyme inhibitors, β-adrenergic blocking agents, long-acting nitrates, and/or sublingual nitroglycerin.

Angiographically Documented Coronary Artery Disease

For the management of coronary artery disease, the recommended adult dosage of amlodipine is 5–10 mg once daily. In clinical studies the majority of patients required a dosage of 10 mg daily.

Amlodipine/Atorvastatin Combination Therapy in Coronary Artery Disease

The fixed-combination preparation containing amlodipine and atorvastatin may be used as a substitute for individually titrated drugs. In patients currently receiving amlodipine and atorvastatin, the initial dosage of the fixed-combination preparation is the equivalent of titrated dosages of amlodipine and atorvastatin. Increased amounts of amlodipine, atorvastatin, or both components may be added for additional antianginal or antilipemic effects.

The fixed-combination preparation may be used to provide additional therapy for patients currently receiving one component of the preparation. The initial dosage of the fixed-combination preparation should be selected based on the dosage of the current component being used and the recommended initial dosage for the added monotherapy.

The fixed-combination preparation may be used to *initiate treatment* in patients with angina *and* dyslipidemias. The initial dosage of the fixed-combination preparation should be selected based on the recommended initial dosages of the individual components. For dosage recommendations for atorvastatin, see Dosage and Administration: Dosage, in Atorvastatin 24:06.08. The maximum dosage of amlodipine or atorvastatin in the fixed-combination preparation is 10 or 80 mg daily, respectively.

● *Special Populations*

Hepatic Impairment

Since the elimination of amlodipine may be impaired substantially in patients with hepatic impairment, resulting in increased exposure to the drug (area under the plasma concentration-time curve [AUC] increases of 40–60%), a reduced initial amlodipine dosage may be required and subsequent dosage should be titrated slowly in such patients.

For the management of hypertension in adults with hepatic insufficiency, an initial amlodipine dosage of 2.5 mg once daily generally is recommended. Subsequent dosage should be adjusted according to patient response and tolerance but usually should not exceed 10 mg once daily. Commercially available preparations containing amlodipine in fixed combination with olmesartan medoxomil (with or without hydrochlorothiazide), telmisartan, or valsartan (with or without hydrochlorothiazide) exceed the recommended initial dosage of amlodipine (2.5 mg daily) for patients with hepatic insufficiency. The manufacturer states that preparations containing amlodipine in fixed combination with perindopril are not recommended in patients with hepatic impairment, as insufficient data are available to support dosage recommendations.

For the management of Prinzmetal variant angina or chronic stable angina in patients with hepatic insufficiency, an amlodipine dosage of 5 mg daily is recommended. The manufacturers state that adequate control of angina usually requires a maintenance dosage of 10 mg daily.

Renal Impairment

Adjustment of amlodipine dosage generally is not necessary in patients with renal impairment since elimination of the drug is not altered substantially by such impairment. However, use of the commercially available preparation containing benazepril in fixed combination with amlodipine is not recommended for patients with severe renal impairment (creatinine clearance of 30 mL/minute or less). In addition, use of preparations containing amlodipine in fixed combination with olmesartan medoxomil and hydrochlorothiazide are not recommended in patients with severe renal impairment; a loop diuretic generally is preferred over a thiazide diuretic in such patients. The safety and efficacy of preparations containing amlodipine in fixed combination with valsartan (with or without hydrochlorothiazide) in patients with creatinine clearances less than 30 mL/minute have not been established. The manufacturer states that preparations containing amlodipine in fixed combination with perindopril are not recommended in patients with creatinine clearances of less than 60 mL/minute, as insufficient data are available to support dosage recommendations. Dosage of the fixed combination of amlodipine and telmisartan should be titrated slowly in patients with severe renal impairment.

Geriatric Patients

Since the elimination of amlodipine may be impaired substantially in geriatric patients, resulting in increased exposure to the drug (AUC increases of 40–60%), a reduced initial amlodipine dosage should be considered in such patients. For management of hypertension, some manufacturers recommend an initial amlodipine dosage of 2.5 mg once daily for geriatric patients; other manufacturers recommend this reduced dosage for geriatric patients 75 years of age or older. For management of Prinzmetal variant angina or chronic stable angina in geriatric patients, an amlodipine dosage of 5 mg daily is recommended; the manufacturers state that adequate control of angina usually requires a maintenance dosage of 10 mg once daily. Commercially available preparations containing amlodipine in fixed combination with olmesartan medoxomil (with or without hydrochlorothiazide), telmisartan, or valsartan (with or without hydrochlorothiazide) exceed the recommended initial dosage of amlodipine (2.5 mg daily) for geriatric patients. The manufacturer states that preparations containing amlodipine in fixed combination with perindopril are not recommended in geriatric patients, as insufficient data are available to support dosage recommendations.

Heart Failure

Patients with moderate to severe heart failure have an increased AUC for amlodipine similar to that of geriatric patients and those with hepatic impairment, but the manufacturers currently make no specific recommendations for dosage adjustment in patients with congestive heart failure. The manufacturer states that

preparations containing amlodipine in fixed combination with perindopril are not recommended in patients with heart failure, as insufficient data are available to support dosage recommendations.

CAUTIONS

● *Contraindications*

Amlodipine is contraindicated in patients with known hypersensitivity to the drug.

● *Warnings/Precautions*

Hypotension

Symptomatic hypotension may occur in patients receiving amlodipine, particularly in individuals with severe aortic stenosis; however, acute hypotension is unlikely because of the gradual onset of action of the drug.

Increased Angina or Acute Myocardial Infarction

Worsening of angina or acute myocardial infarction can occur, particularly in patients with severe obstructive coronary artery disease, upon initiation of amlodipine therapy or an increase in amlodipine dosage.

Use of Fixed Combinations

When amlodipine is used in fixed combination with other drugs (e.g., other antihypertensive agents, atorvastatin), cautions, precautions, contraindications, and interactions associated with the concomitant agent(s) should be considered in addition to those associated with amlodipine. Cautionary information applicable to specific populations (e.g., pregnant or nursing women, individuals with hepatic or renal impairment, geriatric patients) also should be considered for each drug in the fixed combination.

Heart Failure

Although some calcium-channel blockers have been shown to worsen the clinical status of patients with heart failure, no evidence of worsening heart failure (based on exercise tolerance, New York Heart Association [NYHA] class, symptoms, or left ventricular ejection fraction) and no adverse effects on overall survival and cardiac morbidity were observed in controlled studies of amlodipine in patients with heart failure. Cardiac morbidity and overall mortality rates in these studies were similar in patients receiving amlodipine and those receiving placebo.

In patients with moderate to severe heart failure, amlodipine clearance is decreased and area under the concentration-time curve (AUC) is increased by about 40–60%.

Specific Populations

Pregnancy

Category C. (See Users Guide.)

Lactation

It is not known whether amlodipine is distributed into milk; the manufacturer recommends discontinuance of nursing if amlodipine is used.

Pediatric Use

Safety and efficacy of amlodipine in children younger than 6 years of age have not been established. Efficacy of amlodipine (2.5–5 mg daily) for the treatment of hypertension has been established in pediatric patients 6–17 years of age.

Safety and efficacy of amlodipine in fixed combination with atorvastatin, benazepril, olmesartan (with or without hydrochlorothiazide), perindopril, telmisartan, or valsartan (with or without hydrochlorothiazide) have not been established in children.

Geriatric Use

In geriatric patients, amlodipine clearance is decreased and AUC is increased by about 40–60%. Therefore, amlodipine dosage should be selected carefully, usually initiating therapy with dosages at the lower end of the recommended range. The greater frequency of decreased hepatic, renal, and/or cardiac function and of concomitant disease and drug therapy observed in the elderly also should be considered. (See Geriatric Patients under Dosage and Administration: Special Populations.)

Clinical studies of amlodipine did not include sufficient numbers of patients 65 years of age and older to determine whether geriatric patients respond differently than younger patients; however, other clinical experience has not revealed age-related differences in response or tolerance. No substantial differences in safety and efficacy relative to younger adults have been observed in geriatric patients receiving amlodipine in fixed combination with benazepril, olmesartan (with or without hydrochlorothiazide), telmisartan, or valsartan (with or without hydrochlorothiazide), but increased sensitivity cannot be ruled out.

The manufacturer states that use of amlodipine in fixed combination with perindopril in geriatric patients is not recommended, as insufficient data are available to support dosage recommendations.

The manufacturers state that safety and efficacy of amlodipine in fixed combination with atorvastatin have not been established in geriatric patients.

Hepatic Impairment

In patients with hepatic impairment, amlodipine clearance is decreased and AUC is increased by about 40–60%. A reduced initial dosage of the drug is recommended, and subsequent dosage should be titrated slowly. (See Hepatic Impairment under Dosage and Administration: Special Populations.)

● Common Adverse Effects

Adverse effects reported in 1% or more of patients receiving amlodipine include edema, dizziness, flushing, palpitations, fatigue, nausea, abdominal pain, and somnolence. Edema, flushing, palpitations, and somnolence may occur more commonly in women than in men. Edema is dose related and may be less frequent with concomitant use of an angiotensin-converting enzyme (ACE) inhibitor or angiotensin II receptor antagonist.

DRUG INTERACTIONS

When amlodipine is used in fixed combination with other drugs, interactions associated with the concomitant agent(s) must be considered in addition to those associated with amlodipine.

● Drugs Affecting Hepatic Microsomal Enzymes

Concomitant use of amlodipine with moderate (e.g., diltiazem) or potent (e.g., clarithromycin, itraconazole) inhibitors of cytochrome P-450 (CYP) 3A isoenzymes (CYP3A) results in increased systemic exposure to amlodipine. Reduction of amlodipine dosage may be necessary; patients receiving concomitant therapy with CYP3A inhibitors should be monitored for symptoms of hypotension or edema, which may indicate a need for dosage adjustment.

Data on the effects of CYP3A inducers on amlodipine exposure are lacking; blood pressure should be closely monitored in patients receiving such concomitant therapy.

● Alcohol

Concomitant administration of alcohol with amlodipine did not alter systemic exposure to alcohol.

● Antacids

Concomitant administration of a magnesium- and aluminum hydroxide-containing antacid with amlodipine did not alter systemic exposure to amlodipine.

● Cimetidine

Concomitant administration of cimetidine with amlodipine did not alter systemic exposure to amlodipine.

● Digoxin

Concomitant administration of amlodipine with digoxin did not alter systemic exposure to digoxin.

● Diltiazem

Concomitant use of diltiazem hydrochloride (180 mg daily) with amlodipine (5 mg) in geriatric patients with hypertension resulted in a 60% increase in amlodipine exposure.

● Erythromycin

Concomitant administration of erythromycin with amlodipine did not substantially alter systemic exposure to amlodipine in healthy individuals.

● Grapefruit Juice

The manufacturer states that concomitant administration of grapefruit juice with amlodipine did not alter systemic exposure to amlodipine. Although there is some evidence from healthy individuals that concomitant administration with grapefruit juice may increase oral bioavailability of the drug compared with concomitant administration with water, there currently is no evidence of altered amlodipine pharmacodynamics by concurrent ingestion of grapefruit juice in healthy individuals. Concomitant oral administration of other 1,4-dihydropyridine-derivative calcium-channel blocking agents (e.g., felodipine, nifedipine, nisoldipine) with grapefruit juice has resulted in potentially clinically important increases in the hemodynamic effects of these drugs. (See Drug Interactions: Grapefruit Juice, in Nifedipine 24:28.08.)

● HMG-CoA Reductase Inhibitors

Atorvastatin

Concomitant administration of amlodipine with atorvastatin did not alter systemic exposure to atorvastatin.

Simvastatin

Concomitant administration of amlodipine (multiple 10-mg doses) with simvastatin (80 mg) resulted in a 77% increase in simvastatin exposure compared with simvastatin alone. In patients receiving amlodipine, simvastatin dosage should not exceed 20 mg daily.

● Immunosuppressants

Cyclosporine

Concomitant use of cyclosporine and amlodipine may result in increased systemic exposure to cyclosporine. Concomitant use of amlodipine with cyclosporine in renal allograft recipients resulted in a 40% increase in trough concentrations of the immunosuppressant. If concomitant use is required, cyclosporine concentrations should be monitored frequently and cyclosporine dosage adjusted as needed.

Tacrolimus

Concomitant use of tacrolimus and amlodipine may result in increased systemic exposure to tacrolimus. If concomitant use is required, tacrolimus concentrations should be monitored frequently and tacrolimus dosage adjusted as needed.

In healthy Chinese individuals who expressed the CYP3A5 isoenzyme, concomitant administration of amlodipine with tacrolimus resulted in a 2.5- to 4-fold increase in tacrolimus exposure compared with tacrolimus alone; this finding was not observed in individuals who did not express CYP3A5. However, in a renal transplant patient who did not express CYP3A5, a threefold increase in systemic exposure to tacrolimus was observed following initiation of amlodipine therapy for posttransplantation hypertension; reduction in tacrolimus dosage was required. Irrespective of CYP3A5 genotype, the possibility of an interaction between tacrolimus and amlodipine cannot be excluded.

● Protein-bound Drugs

In vitro data indicate that amlodipine does not alter plasma protein binding of digoxin, indomethacin, phenytoin, or warfarin.

● Sildenafil

Concomitant administration of sildenafil with amlodipine did not alter systemic exposure to amlodipine; however, additional reductions in blood pressure are possible with such concomitant use. Patients receiving sildenafil concomitantly with amlodipine should be monitored for hypotension.

● Warfarin

Concomitant administration of amlodipine with warfarin did not alter prothrombin time.

DESCRIPTION

Amlodipine is a 1,4-dihydropyridine-derivative calcium-channel blocking agent that is structurally related to felodipine, nifedipine, and nimodipine. Unlike other currently available agents in the dihydropyridine class, amlodipine has an intrinsically long duration of action.

Following oral administration of amlodipine besylate, peak plasma concentrations of the drug are attained within 6–12 hours. Absolute bioavailability ranges from 64–90%; food does not affect bioavailability of amlodipine. Amlodipine is approximately 93% bound to plasma proteins. The drug is extensively (approximately 90%) metabolized to inactive metabolites in the liver. Amlodipine is excreted in urine as metabolites (60%) and unchanged drug (10%). The terminal elimination half-life of amlodipine is 30–50 hours.

ADVICE TO PATIENTS

When amlodipine is used in fixed combination with other drugs, importance of informing patients of important cautionary information about the concomitant agent(s).

Importance of instructing patients not to remove tablets containing amlodipine in fixed combination with telmisartan from the blister package until immediately before administration.

Importance of informing clinicians of existing or contemplated concomitant therapy, including prescription and OTC drugs, as well as any concomitant illnesses.

Importance of women informing clinicians if they are or plan to become pregnant or plan to breast-feed.

Importance of advising patients of other important precautionary information. (See Cautions.)

PREPARATIONS

Excipients in commercially available drug preparations may have clinically important effects in some individuals; consult specific product labeling for details.

amLODIPine Besylate

Oral

Tablets	2.5 mg (of amlodipine)*	**Amlodipine Besylate Tablets**
		Norvasc®, Pfizer
	5 mg (of amlodipine)*	**Amlodipine Besylate Tablets**
		Norvasc®, Pfizer
	10 mg (of amlodipine)*	**Amlodipine Besylate Tablets**
		Norvasc®, Pfizer

* available from one or more manufacturer, distributor, and/or repackager by generic (nonproprietary) name

amLODIPine Besylate Combinations

Oral

Capsules	2.5 mg (of amlodipine) with Benazepril Hydrochloride 10 mg*	**Amlodipine Besylate and Benazepril Hydrochloride Capsules**
		Lotrel®, Novartis
	5 mg (of amlodipine) with Benazepril Hydrochloride 10 mg*	**Amlodipine Besylate and Benazepril Hydrochloride Capsules**
		Lotrel®, Novartis
	5 mg (of amlodipine) with Benazepril Hydrochloride 20 mg*	**Amlodipine Besylate and Benazepril Hydrochloride Capsules**
		Lotrel®, Novartis
	5 mg (of amlodipine) with Benazepril Hydrochloride 40 mg*	**Amlodipine Besylate and Benazepril Hydrochloride Capsules**
		Lotrel®, Novartis
	10 mg (of amlodipine) with Benazepril Hydrochloride 20 mg*	**Amlodipine Besylate and Benazepril Hydrochloride Capsules**
		Lotrel®, Novartis
	10 mg (of amlodipine) with Benazepril Hydrochloride 40 mg*	**Amlodipine Besylate and Benazepril Hydrochloride Capsules**
		Lotrel®, Novartis

Tablets	2.5 mg (of amlodipine) with Perindopril Arginine 3.5 mg	**Prestalia®**, Symplmed
	5 mg (of amlodipine) with Olmesartan Medoxomil 20 mg	**Azor®**, Daiichi-Sankyo
	5 mg (of amlodipine) with Olmesartan Medoxomil 40 mg	**Azor®**, Daiichi-Sankyo
	5 mg (of amlodipine) with Perindopril Arginine 7 mg	**Prestalia®**, Symplmed
	10 mg (of amlodipine) with Olmesartan Medoxomil 20 mg	**Azor®**, Daiichi-Sankyo
	10 mg (of amlodipine) with Olmesartan Medoxomil 40 mg	**Azor®**, Daiichi-Sankyo
	10 mg (of amlodipine) with Perindopril Arginine 14 mg	**Prestalia®**, Symplmed
Tablets, film-coated	2.5 mg (of amlodipine) with Atorvastatin Calcium 10 mg (of atorvastatin)*	**Amlodipine Besylate and Atorvastatin Calcium Tablets**
		Caduet®, Pfizer
	2.5 mg (of amlodipine) with Atorvastatin Calcium 20 mg (of atorvastatin)*	**Amlodipine Besylate and Atorvastatin Calcium Tablets**
		Caduet®, Pfizer
	2.5 mg (of amlodipine) with Atorvastatin Calcium 40 mg (of atorvastatin)*	**Amlodipine Besylate and Atorvastatin Calcium Tablets**
		Caduet®, Pfizer
	5 mg (of amlodipine) with Atorvastatin Calcium 10 mg (of atorvastatin)*	**Amlodipine Besylate and Atorvastatin Calcium Tablets**
		Caduet®, Pfizer
	5 mg (of amlodipine) with Atorvastatin Calcium 20 mg (of atorvastatin)*	**Amlodipine Besylate and Atorvastatin Calcium Tablets**
		Caduet®, Pfizer
	5 mg (of amlodipine) with Atorvastatin Calcium 40 mg (of atorvastatin)*	**Amlodipine Besylate and Atorvastatin Calcium Tablets**
		Caduet®, Pfizer
	5 mg (of amlodipine) with Atorvastatin Calcium 80 mg (of atorvastatin)*	**Amlodipine Besylate and Atorvastatin Calcium Tablets**
		Caduet®, Pfizer
	5 mg (of amlodipine) with Hydrochlorothiazide 12.5 mg and Olmesartan Medoxomil 20 mg	**Tribenzor®**, Daiichi Sankyo
	5 mg (of amlodipine) with Hydrochlorothiazide 12.5 mg and Olmesartan Medoxomil 40 mg	**Tribenzor®**, Daiichi Sankyo
	5 mg (of amlodipine) with Hydrochlorothiazide 12.5 mg and Valsartan 160 mg*	**Amlodipine Besylate, Valsartan, and Hydrochlorothiazide Tablets**
		Exforge HCT®, Novartis
	5 mg (of amlodipine) with Hydrochlorothiazide 25 mg and Olmesartan Medoxomil 40 mg	**Tribenzor®**, Daiichi Sankyo
	5 mg (of amlodipine) with Hydrochlorothiazide 25 mg and Valsartan 160 mg*	**Amlodipine Besylate, Valsartan, and Hydrochlorothiazide Tablets**
		Exforge HCT®, Novartis
	5 mg (of amlodipine) with Valsartan 160 mg*	**Amlodipine Besylate and Valsartan Tablets**
		Exforge®, Novartis
	5 mg (of amlodipine) with Valsartan 320 mg*	**Amlodipine Besylate and Valsartan Tablets**
		Exforge®, Novartis
	10 mg (of amlodipine) with Atorvastatin Calcium 10 mg (of atorvastatin)*	**Amlodipine Besylate and Atorvastatin Calcium Tablets**
		Caduet®, Pfizer

10 mg (of amlodipine) with Atorvastatin Calcium 20 mg (of atorvastatin)*	**Amlodipine Besylate and Atorvastatin Calcium Tablets** **Caduet®**, Pfizer
10 mg (of amlodipine) with Atorvastatin Calcium 40 mg (of atorvastatin)*	**Amlodipine Besylate and Atorvastatin Calcium Tablets** **Caduet®**, Pfizer
10 mg (of amlodipine) with Atorvastatin Calcium 80 mg (of atorvastatin)*	**Amlodipine Besylate and Atorvastatin Calcium Tablets** **Caduet®**, Pfizer
10 mg (of amlodipine) with Hydrochlorothiazide 12.5 mg and Olmesartan Medoxomil 40 mg	**Tribenzor®**, Daiichi Sankyo
10 mg (of amlodipine) with Hydrochlorothiazide 12.5 mg and Valsartan 160 mg*	**Amlodipine Besylate, Valsartan, and Hydrochlorothiazide Tablets** **Exforge HCT®**, Novartis
10 mg (of amlodipine) with Hydrochlorothiazide 25 mg and Olmesartan Medoxomil 40 mg	**Tribenzor®**, Daiichi Sankyo
10 mg (of amlodipine) with Hydrochlorothiazide 25 mg and Valsartan 160 mg*	**Amlodipine Besylate, Valsartan, and Hydrochlorothiazide Tablets** **Exforge HCT®**, Novartis
10 mg (of amlodipine) with Hydrochlorothiazide 25 mg and Valsartan 320 mg*	**Amlodipine Besylate, Valsartan, and Hydrochlorothiazide Tablets** **Exforge HCT®**, Novartis

	10 mg (of amlodipine) with Valsartan 160 mg*	**Amlodipine Besylate and Valsartan Tablets** **Exforge®**, Novartis
	10 mg (of amlodipine) with Valsartan 320 mg*	**Amlodipine Besylate and Valsartan Tablets** **Exforge®**, Novartis
Tablets, multilayer	5 mg (of amlodipine) with Telmisartan 40 mg*	**Telmisartan and Amlodipine Besylate Tablets** **Twynsta®**, Boehringer Ingelheim
	5 mg (of amlodipine) with Telmisartan 80 mg*	**Telmisartan and Amlodipine Besylate Tablets** **Twynsta®**, Boehringer Ingelheim
	10 mg (of amlodipine) with Telmisartan 40 mg*	**Telmisartan and Amlodipine Besylate Tablets** **Twynsta®**, Boehringer Ingelheim
	10 mg (of amlodipine) with Telmisartan 80 mg*	**Telmisartan and Amlodipine Besylate Tablets** **Twynsta®**, Boehringer Ingelheim

* available from one or more manufacturer, distributor, and/or repackager by generic (nonproprietary) name

† Use is not currently included in the labeling approved by the US Food and Drug Administration.

Selected Revisions October 21, 2019, © Copyright, October 1, 1992, American Society of Health-System Pharmacists, Inc.

NIFEdipine

24:28.08 • DIHYDROPYRIDINES

■ Nifedipine is a 1,4-dihydropyridine-derivative calcium-channel blocking agent.

USES

● Angina

Nifedipine is used in the management of Prinzmetal variant angina and chronic stable angina pectoris. Calcium-channel blocking agents (used alone or in combination with nitrates) are considered the drugs of choice for the management of Prinzmetal variant angina. β-Adrenergic blocking agents (β-blockers) are recommended as the anti-ischemic drugs of choice in most patients with chronic stable angina; however, calcium-channel blockers may be substituted or added in patients who do not tolerate or respond adequately to β-blockers. In controlled clinical studies of up to 8 weeks' duration in patients with chronic stable angina, nifedipine reduced the frequency of attacks, allowed a decrease in sublingual nitroglycerin dosage, and increased exercise tolerance. All classes of calcium-channel blockers appear to be equally effective in reducing anginal episodes; however, choice of a specific agent should be individualized since the pharmacologic properties of these drugs differ. The potential risks of *short-acting* (conventional, immediate-release) nifedipine should be considered. (See Cautions.)

Calcium-channel blockers also have been used for the relief of ongoing or recurrent ischemia in patients with unstable angina†; however, a nondihydropyridine calcium-channel blocker (e.g., diltiazem, verapamil) generally is recommended.

Concurrent use of nifedipine and a β-blocker may have beneficial effects in some patients with chronic stable angina (e.g., reduction of dihydropyridine-induced tachycardia through β-blockade).

● Hypertension

Nifedipine is used alone or in combination with other classes of antihypertensive agents in the management of hypertension. Because of concerns about potentially serious adverse cardiovascular effects and increased mortality associated with short-acting (conventional, immediate-release) nifedipine (see Cautions), only extended-release formulations of the drug are recommended for the management of hypertension.

Calcium-channel blockers (e.g., nifedipine) are considered one of several preferred antihypertensive drugs for the initial management of hypertension according to current evidence-based hypertension guidelines; other preferred options include angiotensin-converting enzyme (ACE) inhibitors, angiotensin II receptor antagonists, and thiazide diuretics. While there may be individual differences with respect to recommendations for initial drug selection and use in specific patient populations, current evidence indicates that these antihypertensive drug classes all generally produce comparable effects on overall mortality and cardiovascular, cerebrovascular, and renal outcomes. (See Uses: Hypertension, in Amlodipine 24:28.08.)

Most patients with hypertension, especially black patients, will require at least 2 antihypertensive drugs to achieve adequate blood pressure control. Calcium-channel blockers may be particularly useful in the management of hypertension in black patients; these patients tend to have greater blood pressure response to calcium-channel blockers and thiazide diuretics than to other antihypertensive drug classes (e.g., ACE inhibitors, angiotensin II receptor antagonists). However, the combination of an ACE inhibitor or an angiotensin II receptor antagonist with a calcium-channel blocker or thiazide diuretic produces similar blood pressure lowering in black patients as in other racial groups. (See Race under Hypertension: Other Special Considerations for Antihypertensive Therapy, in Uses in Amlodipine 24:28.08.) Use of a calcium-channel blocker also may be beneficial in patients with certain coexisting conditions such as ischemic heart disease (e.g., angina) and in geriatric patients, including those with isolated systolic hypertension. (See Uses: Hypertension, in Amlodipine 24:28.08.)

In the Antihypertensive and Lipid-lowering Treatment to Prevent Heart Attack Trial (ALLHAT), the long-term cardiovascular morbidity and mortality benefit of a long-acting dihydropyridine calcium-channel blocker (amlodipine), a thiazide-like diuretic (chlorthalidone), and an ACE inhibitor (lisinopril) were compared in a broad population of patients with hypertension at risk of coronary heart disease. Although these antihypertensive agents were comparably effective in providing important cardiovascular benefit, apparent differences in certain secondary outcomes were observed. Patients receiving the ACE inhibitor experienced higher risks of stroke, combined cardiovascular disease, GI bleeding, and angioedema, while those receiving the calcium-channel blocker were at higher risk of developing heart failure. The ALLHAT investigators suggested that the observed differences in cardiovascular outcome may be attributable, at least in part, to the greater antihypertensive effect of the calcium-channel blocker compared with that of the ACE inhibitor, especially in women and black patients. (See Clinical Benefits of Thiazides in Hypertension under Hypertension in Adults: Treatment Benefits, in Uses in the Thiazides General Statement 40:28.20.)

For more detailed information on the role of calcium-channel blockers in the management of hypertension, see Uses: Hypertension, in Amlodipine 24:28.08. For information on overall principles and expert recommendations for treatment of hypertension, see Uses: Hypertension in Adults, in the Thiazides General Statement 40:28.20.

Hypertensive Crises

In the past, when oral therapy was considered preferable to parenteral therapy in selected patients, short-acting (conventional, immediate-release capsules) nifedipine had been used for rapidly reducing blood pressure in patients with hypertensive crises† in whom reduction of blood pressure was considered urgent (hypertensive urgencies) or an emergency (hypertensive emergencies); however, most clinicians and the manufacturers now question the safety of short-acting nifedipine for this use because of occasional reports of poorly tolerated severe hypotension and the potential adverse cardiovascular consequences (e.g., cerebrovascular ischemia, stroke, myocardial ischemia and infarction, death). As a result of these and other (see Cautions) concerns and absence of substantial evidence clearly establishing superiority (both in terms of safety and efficacy) of nifedipine for this use, it is recommended that short-acting nifedipine no longer be used for the management of any form of hypertension, including hypertensive crises.

Patients with hypertensive emergencies (i.e., those rare situations requiring immediate blood pressure reduction, although not necessarily to normal ranges, in order to prevent or limit target organ damage) require hospitalization and are treated with an appropriate parenteral antihypertensive agent (e.g., labetalol, esmolol, fenoldopam, nicardipine, sodium nitroprusside). Hypertensive urgencies (i.e., situations in which there is severe elevation in blood pressure without progressive target organ damage) generally can be managed by intensification or reinstitution (e.g., following noncompliance) of the current antihypertensive regimen and treatment of anxiety if needed. Experts state that there is no need for rapid reduction of blood pressure in such patients and hospitalization or referral to the emergency department also is unnecessary. Excessive falls in blood pressure should be avoided in any hypertensive crisis since they may precipitate renal, cerebral, or coronary ischemia.

Hypertension During Pregnancy

Antihypertensive therapy is recommended in pregnant women with chronic hypertension who have persistent, severely elevated blood pressure (e.g., systolic blood pressure of 160 mm Hg or higher or diastolic blood pressure of 105 mm Hg or higher); it is less clear whether antihypertensive therapy should be initiated in women with mild to moderate chronic hypertension. If initiation of antihypertensive therapy is necessary in a pregnant woman, use of labetalol, nifedipine, or methyldopa is recommended by the American College of Obstetricians and Gynecologists (ACOG) and other experts. In women who are already receiving antihypertensive therapy prior to pregnancy, ACOG states there are insufficient data to make recommendations regarding the continuance or discontinuance of such therapy; treatment decisions should be individualized in these situations. Alternatively, other experts state that women with hypertension who became pregnant, or are planning to become pregnant, should have their antihypertensive therapy transitioned to methyldopa, nifedipine, and/or labetalol during pregnancy.

Nifedipine also has been used orally in the hospital setting for urgent lowering of blood pressure in severely hypertensive pregnant women, including those with preeclampsia†. However, short-acting (conventional) formulations of nifedipine are not labeled by the US Food and Drug Administration (FDA) for acute reduction of blood pressure; cases of profound hypotension and other serious adverse cardiovascular consequences have been reported with the use of these preparations. (For additional information on the use of antihypertensive drugs in women with preeclampsia, see Uses: Hypertension, in Hydralazine 24:08.20.)

• Raynaud's Phenomenon

Nifedipine has been used effectively in the management of Raynaud's phenomenon† and is considered a drug of choice for the management of this condition. The drug has reduced the frequency, duration, and severity of attacks in patients with this condition. However, not all patients with this condition respond to nifedipine, and intolerable adverse effects (e.g., headache, flushing, orthostatic hypotension) may limit the usefulness of the drug in some other patients. Although most experience with nifedipine in the management of Raynaud's phenomenon had been with short-acting (conventional, immediate-release) formulations of the drug, recent concerns (e.g., risks of serious hypotension and associated cardiovascular consequences) about the safety of short-acting (conventional) nifedipine have prompted the manufacturers to warn against use of this preparation in conditions for which safety and efficacy have not been fully established. (See Cautions.) Therefore, while not studied as extensively as short-acting nifedipine, extended-release nifedipine (e.g., 30–60 mg daily) preferably should be used when the drug is indicated for the management of Raynaud's phenomenon. The extended-release preparation of nifedipine appears to be tolerated better than the short-acting preparation in patients with this condition. The principal troublesome adverse effect during long-term therapy in these patients appears to be peripheral (ankle) edema.

• Preterm Labor

Nifedipine has been used in selected patients to inhibit uterine contractions in preterm labor† (tocolysis) and thus prolong gestation when such prolongation of intrauterine life was expected to benefit pregnancy outcome. Current ACOG guidelines for management of preterm labor state that there is no clear first-line tocolytic agent because of conflicting results regarding efficacy in comparative trials. In addition, concerns about the safety of short-acting (conventional) nifedipine (e.g., risks of serious hypotension and associated cardiovascular consequences) have prompted the manufacturers to warn against use of this preparation in conditions for which safety and efficacy have not been fully established. (See Cautions.) However, an analysis of pooled data from a number of randomized, controlled studies suggests that calcium-channel blockers (principally nifedipine) may be more effective than, and preferable to, other agents (e.g., magnesium sulfate, β-adrenergic agonists) when tocolysis is deemed necessary. Results of this pooled analysis suggest that calcium-channel blockers are more effective in reducing births within 7 days of initiation of tocolytic treatment and before 34 weeks' gestation and are associated with improved neonatal outcomes (e.g., less neonatal respiratory distress syndrome, intraventricular hemorrhage, necrotizing enterocolitis, jaundice) and a reduced frequency of maternal adverse effects leading to treatment discontinuance compared with other tocolytic agents. A number of different dosages and dosage forms of nifedipine were used in these studies, and an optimal dosage regimen for the drug as a tocolytic has not been determined.

The main benefit currently derived from tocolytic therapy may be to forestall labor and provide time for patients to receive corticosteroids to increase fetal lung maturation and/or to be transferred to other (e.g., tertiary-care) facilities; any other potential benefits of prolonging pregnancy are unclear. For additional information, see Uses: Preterm Labor in Magnesium Sulfate 28:12.92.

• Acute Myocardial Infarction

Calcium-channel blocking agents have been used in the early treatment and secondary prevention of acute myocardial infarction (MI)†; although these drugs are effective anti-ischemic agents, they have not demonstrated mortality benefits and therefore are generally used as an alternative to β-blockers. A review of 28 randomized controlled studies involving 19,000 patients found no benefit with regard to infarct size, rate of reinfarction, or death when calcium-channel blockers were used during the acute or convalescent phase of ST-segment-elevation MI (STEMI). Calcium-channel blockers generally are used for their anti-ischemic and blood pressure-reducing properties in the MI setting, and only when β-blockers (which have been shown to reduce mortality after MI) are ineffective, not tolerated, or contraindicated.

Current expert guidelines state that a calcium-channel blocker may be used to relieve ischemic symptoms, lower blood pressure, or control rapid ventricular response associated with atrial fibrillation in patients with STEMI who are intolerant to β-blockers. A nondihydropyridine calcium-channel blocker (e.g., verapamil or diltiazem) may be used as an alternative to β-blockers for the relief of ongoing or recurring ischemia when β-blocker therapy is inadequate, not tolerated, or contraindicated in patients with non-ST-segment-elevation MI (NSTEMI) who do not have clinically important left ventricular dysfunction, increased risk of cardiogenic shock, or AV block.

The use of short-acting (conventional, immediate-release) nifedipine is generally contraindicated in patients with MI because of its negative inotropic effects and the reflex sympathetic activation, tachycardia, and hypotension associated with its use. Short-acting nifedipine may be particularly detrimental in patients with hypotension and/or tachycardia since the drug may induce a reduction in coronary perfusion pressure, disproportionate dilatation of coronary arteries adjacent to ischemic areas ("steal" phenomenon), and/or reflex activation of the sympathetic nervous system, resulting in an increase in myocardial oxygen demands. These findings are based on numerous clinical trials, including the Nifedipine Angina Myocardial Infarction Trial (NAMIS), the Trial of Early Nifedipine Treatment in Acute Myocardial Infarction (TRENT), the Norwegian Nifedipine Multicenter Trial, and the Secondary Prevention Reinfarction Israeli Nifedipine Trial (SPRINT).

DOSAGE AND ADMINISTRATION

• Administration

Nifedipine is administered orally. The drug also has been administered sublingually† or intrabuccally† (e.g., for rapid reduction of blood pressure). When nifedipine is administered sublingually or intrabuccally, the conventional liquid-filled capsule must be punctured, chewed, and/or squeezed to express the liquid into the mouth. However, based on pharmacokinetic considerations (see Pharmacokinetics: Absorption), some clinicians recommend that when a relatively rapid response is desired the drug preferably be administered as conventional liquid-filled capsules that are bitten and then swallowed.

Nifedipine extended-release tablets should be swallowed intact and should *not* be chewed, crushed, or broken. The manufacturer of Adalat® CC states that the extended-release nifedipine tablets should be taken on an empty stomach. Patients should be advised *not* to become alarmed if they notice a tablet-like substance in their stools; this is normal since the tablet containing the drug is designed to remain intact and slowly release the drug from a nonabsorbable shell during passage through the GI tract.

Whenever extended-release tablets of nifedipine are dispensed or administered, care should be taken to ensure that the extended-release dosage form actually was prescribed. The manufacturers recommend that dosage of extended-release nifedipine tablets should be decreased gradually with close clinical supervision when discontinuance of the drug is required.

The manufacturer of Adalat® CC states that two 30-mg Adalat® CC extended-release tablets may be interchanged with one 60-mg Adalat® CC extended-release tablet; however, three 30-mg Adalat® CC extended-release tablets should *not* be considered interchangeable with one 90-mg Adalat® CC extended-release tablet (see Pharmacokinetics: Absorption).

Concomitant oral administration of 1,4-dihydropyridine-derivative calcium-channel blocking agents (e.g., nifedipine) with grapefruit juice usually should be avoided since potentially clinically important increases in hemodynamic effects may result. (See Grapefruit Juice under Drug Interactions: Drugs and Foods Affecting Hepatic Microsomal Enzymes.)

Extemporaneously Compounded Oral Liquid

Extemporaneously compounded oral liquid formulations of nifedipine have been prepared.

Standardize 4 Safety

Standardized concentrations for an extemporaneously prepared oral liquid formulation of nifedipine have been established through Standardize 4 Safety (S4S), a national patient safety initiative to reduce medication errors, especially during transitions of care. Multidisciplinary expert panels were convened to determine recommended standard concentrations. Because recommendations from the S4S panels may differ from the manufacturer's prescribing information, caution is advised when using concentrations that differ from labeling, particularly when using rate information from the label. For additional information on S4S (including updates that may be available), see https://www.ashp.org/pharmacy-practice/standardize-4-safety-initiative.

TABLE 1. Standardize 4 Safety Compounded Oral Liquid Standards for NIFEdipine

Concentration Standards
4 mg/mL

● Dosage
Angina

The National Heart, Lung, and Blood Institute (NHLBI) states that, pending further accumulation of data, it seems prudent that conventional liquid-filled (short-acting) capsules of nifedipine, especially at high doses, be used in the management of angina with great caution, if at all. (See Cautions.)

If short-acting nifedipine is used for the management of Prinzmetal variant angina or chronic stable angina pectoris, the usual initial adult dosage of the drug as conventional liquid-filled capsules that are swallowed intact is 10 mg 3 times daily. Alternatively, nifedipine antianginal therapy can be initiated with extended-release tablets at a dosage of 30 or 60 mg once daily. Generally, dosage is gradually increased at 7- to 14-day intervals until optimum control of angina is obtained. If symptoms so warrant and the patient's tolerance and response to therapy are assessed frequently, dosage may be increased more rapidly to 90 mg daily in increments of 30 mg/day over a 3-day period using conventional liquid-filled capsules or after steady state is achieved (usually achieved on the second day of therapy with a given dose) using extended-release tablets. In hospitalized patients who are closely monitored, nifedipine dosage may be increased in 10-mg increments using conventional liquid-filled capsules at 4- to 6-hour intervals, as necessary to control pain and arrhythmias caused by ischemia. Single doses usually should not exceed 30 mg.

The usual adult maintenance dosage of nifedipine as conventional liquid-filled capsules is 10–20 mg 3 times daily. In some patients, especially those with evidence of coronary artery spasm, higher dosages (using conventional liquid-filled capsules or extended-release tablets) and/or more frequent administration (using conventional liquid-filled capsules *only*) are necessary. In such patients, the usual maintenance dosage is 20–30 mg 3 or 4 times daily using conventional liquid-filled capsules; rarely, more than 120 mg daily is necessary. Experience with antianginal dosages exceeding 90 mg once daily using the extended-release tablets is limited; therefore, higher dosages using this dosage form should be employed with caution and only when clinically necessary.

Dosage generally should not exceed 180 mg daily as conventional liquid-filled capsules or 120 mg daily as extended-release tablets, since the safety and efficacy of higher dosages have not been established. After anginal symptoms are controlled, dosage should be gradually reduced to the lowest level that will maintain relief of symptoms.

In patients whose angina is controlled with conventional liquid-filled capsules of nifedipine alone or in combination with other antianginal agents, extended-release tablets of nifedipine can be substituted for the conventional capsules at the nearest equivalent total daily dose. Thus, patients who are receiving a nifedipine dosage of 30 mg 3 times daily as conventional liquid-filled capsules can be switched to a dosage of 90 mg once daily as extended-release tablets. When the total daily dose as conventional liquid-filled capsules does not correspond exactly to the strength of a commercially available extended-release tablet, the nearest equivalent daily dose can be substituted; the extended-release tablets should *not* be divided in an attempt to exactly match total daily doses of conventional capsules. Subsequent titration to higher or lower dosages may be necessary and should be guided by the patient's clinical response and tolerance.

Hypertension

Dosage of nifedipine should be adjusted according to the patient's blood pressure response and tolerance.

Usual Dosage

For the management of hypertension in adults, the usual initial dosage of nifedipine as extended-release tablets is 30 or 60 mg once daily. Generally, dosage is increased gradually at 7- to 14-day intervals until optimum control of blood pressure is obtained. If symptoms so warrant and the patient's tolerance and response to therapy are assessed frequently, dosage may be increased more rapidly. Steady state usually is achieved during the second day of therapy with a given dose as extended-release tablets. The manufacturers state that dosages exceeding 90 mg once daily (Adalat® CC) or 120 mg once daily (Procardia XL®) as extended-release tablets are not recommended. Some experts recommend a usual dosage range of 30–90 mg once daily.

If nifedipine is used for the management of hypertension in children†, some experts recommend a usual initial dosage of 0.2–0.5 mg/kg daily, administered as extended-release tablets once daily or in 2 divided doses daily. Dosage may be increased as necessary to a maximum dosage of 3 mg/kg (up to 120 mg), given once daily or in 2 divided doses. Experts state that the drug should be initiated at the low end of the dosage range and the dosage may be increased every 2–4 weeks until blood pressure is controlled, the maximum dosage is reached, or adverse effects occur. For information on overall principles and expert recommendations for treatment of hypertension in pediatric patients, see Uses: Hypertension in Pediatric Patients, in the Thiazides General Statement 40:28.20.

Because of concerns about potential cardiovascular risks associated with conventional liquid-filled (short-acting) capsules of the drug, short-acting preparations of nifedipine are no longer recommended for use in the management of hypertension.

Blood Pressure Monitoring and Treatment Goals

Blood pressure should be monitored regularly (i.e., monthly) during therapy and dosage of the antihypertensive drug adjusted until blood pressure is controlled. If an adequate blood pressure response is not achieved with nifedipine monotherapy, another antihypertensive agent with demonstrated benefit and preferably a complementary mechanism of action (e.g., angiotensin-converting enzyme [ACE] inhibitor, angiotensin II receptor antagonist, thiazide diuretic) may be added; if goal blood pressure is still not achieved with the use of 2 antihypertensive agents, a third drug may be added. (See Uses: Hypertension in Adults, in the Thiazides General Statement 40:28.20.) In patients who develop unacceptable adverse effects with nifedipine, the drug should be discontinued and another antihypertensive agent from a different pharmacologic class should be initiated.

The goal of hypertension management and prevention is to achieve and maintain optimal control of blood pressure. However, the optimum blood pressure threshold for initiating antihypertensive drug therapy and specific treatment goals remain controversial. While other hypertension guidelines have based target blood pressure goals on age and comorbidities, the 2017 American College of Cardiology (ACC)/American Heart Association (AHA) hypertension guideline incorporates underlying cardiovascular risk into decision making regarding treatment and generally recommends the same target blood pressure (i.e., less than 130/80 mm Hg) in all adults. Many patients will require at least 2 drugs from different pharmacologic classes to achieve this blood pressure goal; the potential benefits of hypertension management and drug cost, adverse effects, and risks associated with the use of multiple antihypertensive drugs also should be considered when deciding a patient's blood pressure treatment goal.

For additional information on target levels of blood pressure and on monitoring therapy in the management of hypertension, see Blood Pressure Monitoring and Treatment Goals under Dosage: Hypertension, in Dosage and Administration in the Thiazides General Statement 40:28.20.

CAUTIONS

While serious adverse reactions requiring discontinuance of nifedipine therapy or dosage adjustments are uncommon, concerns about safety and efficacy of calcium-channel blocking agents (mainly conventional [short-acting] preparations of dihydropyridine derivatives) have been raised by findings of several studies. Results of a case-control study indicate dose-dependent increases in the risk of myocardial infarction (MI) (by about 60%) in hypertensive patients (with or without diagnosed cardiovascular disease, but excluding MI or heart failure) receiving a short-acting calcium-channel blocking agent (e.g., nifedipine, diltiazem, verapamil) compared with those receiving a diuretic or a β-adrenergic blocking agent (β-blocker). In addition, findings of several pooled analyses of studies indicate an increased risk of mortality (by about 16%) and reinfarction (by about 19%) in patients who have had an MI or in those with stable or unstable angina who were receiving dihydropyridine-derivative calcium-channel blocking agents (mainly conventional [short-acting] preparations of nifedipine) compared with those receiving placebo. Results of a pooled analysis of 16 studies indicate that the nifedipine-associated mortality may be dose dependent, especially in patients receiving short-acting nifedipine dosages of 80 mg or more daily when compared with those receiving placebo.

The National Heart, Lung, and Blood Institute (NHLBI) concluded from the apparent concordance of findings from observational studies in hypertensive patients and from randomized studies principally in acute MI and unstable angina patients that it seems prudent and consistent with current evidence to recommend that *short-acting* nifedipine, especially at high doses, be used in the management of hypertension, angina, or MI with great caution, if at all. In arriving at this conclusion, the NHLBI recognized the potential biases of observational studies. The NHLBI and some clinicians also state that while other calcium-channel blocking agents (e.g., diltiazem, verapamil) also were associated with increased risk of MI in the described case-control study, results of previous well-designed clinical studies indicate that the use of calcium-channel blocking agents was not associated with an increased risk of death; therefore, the adverse effects associated with short-acting nifedipine may not necessarily apply to other calcium-channel blocking agents, including other short-acting dihydropyridines (e.g., isradipine), or to long-acting preparations of nifedipine. Findings from the Antihypertensive and Lipid-Lowering Treatment to Prevent Heart Attack Trial (ALL-HAT), which compared long-term therapy with an ACE inhibitor (lisinopril) or dihydropyridine-derivative calcium-channel blocker (amlodipine) revealed no difference in the primary outcome of combined fatal coronary heart disease or nonfatal MI among these therapies.

The increased risk of MI and death in patients receiving short-acting calcium-channel blocking agents may be associated with the arrhythmogenic, proischemic, negative inotropic, and/or prohemorrhagic effects of these agents; proischemic effects may result from reflex increases in sympathetic activity or from a reduction of coronary perfusion pressure induced by short-acting calcium-channel blocking agents. However, some clinicians state that while current evidence indicates an increased relative risk of MI associated with calcium-channel blocking agents, the actual increased risk for an individual patient may be low. Therefore, patients should not discontinue such therapy independently, but instead should consult their clinician about possible alternatives based on full evaluation of their medical condition, since the known risks of uncontrolled hypertension may be far greater than the postulated but unproven hazards associated with calcium-channel blocking agents.

● *Cardiovascular Effects*

Serious adverse reactions requiring discontinuance of nifedipine therapy or dosage adjustment are relatively rare. An increase in the frequency, intensity, and duration of angina, possibly resulting from hypotension, has occurred rarely during initiation of nifedipine therapy. Additional serious adverse effects including MI, congestive heart failure or pulmonary edema, and ventricular arrhythmia or conduction defects have reportedly occurred in 4%, 2%, and less than 0.5% of patients receiving conventional nifedipine capsules, respectively, but these have not been directly attributed to the drug. For additional information on potential serious cardiovascular effects associated with nifedipine, see the introductory discussion in Cautions and see also Cautions: Precautions and Contraindications.

Chest pain (nonspecific) has been reported in less than 3% of patients receiving extended-release nifedipine tablets in clinical trials. Adverse cardiovascular effects reported in up to 1% of patients receiving extended-release nifedipine tablets include substernal chest pain, arrhythmia, atrial fibrillation, bradycardia, tachycardia, cardiac arrest, extrasystole, hypotension, postural hypotension, syncope, increased angina, phlebitis, and cutaneous angiectases.

Most of the common adverse reactions to nifedipine result from its vasodilating action on vascular smooth muscle and include dizziness, lightheadedness, giddiness, flushing or heat sensation, and headache, reportedly occurring in up to 25% of patients, and less frequently, hypotension (usually mild to moderate and well tolerated), weakness, peripheral edema, and palpitation. The incidence and severity of syncope, peripheral (ankle) edema, and hypotension generally are dose related and occasionally may be obviated by a reduction in dosage. In patients receiving conventional liquid-filled (short-acting) nifedipine capsules, transient

hypotension occurred in about 2% of patients receiving less than 60 mg daily and in about 5% of patients receiving 120 mg or more daily. Nifedipine-induced peripheral edema of the lower extremities usually responds to diuretic therapy. The relatively common adverse effects reported with conventional liquid-filled (short-acting) nifedipine capsules are similar in nature to those reported with extended-release tablets of the drug. However, some evidence indicates that the risk of certain adverse effects may be increased with short-acting preparations of the drug, particularly at high doses. (See the introductory discussion in Cautions.)

Although the hypotensive effect of nifedipine is modest and well tolerated in most patients receiving the drug for angina, excessive and poorly tolerated hypotension occurs occasionally in such patients. Such excessive hypotension usually occurs during initial dosage titration or subsequent upward titration of dosage, and may be more likely in patients receiving a β-blocker concomitantly. Severe hypotension and/or increased fluid requirements also have been reported in patients who were receiving these drugs concomitantly and underwent coronary artery bypass surgery involving high-dose fentanyl anesthesia. (See Drug Interactions: Fentanyl.) Several cases of profound hypotension, cerebrovascular ischemia or stroke, myocardial ischemia or infarction, and/or death have been reported when conventional short-acting preparations of nifedipine were used for the management of hypertensive crises, and therefore, the manufacturers currently warn that short-acting preparations should not be used for acute reduction in blood pressure. (See Hypertensive Crises under Uses: Hypertension.) However, profound hypotension, myocardial ischemia or infarction, and/or death also have been reported occasionally in patients receiving conventional short-acting preparations of the drug for other uses (e.g., angina, pulmonary hypertension). The manufacturers also warn that short-acting preparations of nifedipine should not be used for the chronic management of hypertension.

The frequency of nifedipine-induced peripheral edema appears to be dose related and reportedly occurs in 10–30% of patients receiving the drug. The edema is localized and probably occurs secondary to vasodilation of dependent arterioles and small blood vessels rather than to left ventricular dysfunction or generalized fluid retention. Intolerable adverse effects associated with nifedipine-induced vasodilation (e.g., headache, flushing, orthostatic hypotension) may limit the usefulness of nifedipine in some patients receiving the drug for Raynaud's phenomenon. The extended-release preparations of nifedipine appear to be tolerated better than the short-acting preparation in patients with this condition. The principal troublesome adverse effect during long-term therapy in these patients appears to be peripheral (ankle) edema.

Erythromelalgia has been reported in about 0.5% of patients receiving nifedipine. Characteristic manifestations of erythromelalgia include burning pain, increased skin temperature, and erythema of the extremities, usually the feet and lower legs, and less commonly, the hands. Manifestations resolve following discontinuance of the drug.

● *Nervous System Effects*

In patients receiving conventional liquid-filled (short-acting) nifedipine capsules, weakness was reported in 12% of patients, while tremor, nervousness, and mood changes occurred in about 7–8% of patients; fever and chills were reported in up to 2% of patients, and shakiness, jitteriness, disturbed sleep, and difficulty with postural balance occurred occasionally; mental depression and paranoid syndrome were reported rarely. In patients receiving extended-release nifedipine tablets, fatigue and asthenia were reported in about 4–6% of patients, pain occurred in less than 3% of patients, and paresthesia, vertigo, asthenia, insomnia, nervousness, and somnolence were reported in up to 3% of patients, while migraine, anxiety, confusion, ataxia, depression, hypertonia, hypoesthesia, paroniria, fever, and tremor were reported in up to 1% of patients. Chills occurred in less than 1% of patients. For nervous system effects associated with the vasodilating effect of nifedipine, see Cautions: Cardiovascular Effects.

● *GI Effects*

In patients receiving conventional liquid-filled (short-acting) nifedipine capsules, nausea and heartburn occurred in 11% of patients, while diarrhea, constipation, cramps, and flatulence were reported occasionally, and gingival hyperplasia occurred rarely. In patients receiving extended-release nifedipine tablets, nausea and constipation were reported in about 2–3 and about 1–3%, respectively, while abdominal pain, diarrhea, dry mouth, dyspepsia, and flatulence occurred in less than 3% of patients, and dysphagia, eructation, gastroesophageal reflux, esophagitis, vomiting, melena, GI hemorrhage, gum hemorrhage, gum hyperplasia, gum disorder, unspecified GI disorder, and taste perversion were reported in up to 1% of patients. GI irritation and GI bleeding have been reported in less than 1% of patients receiving Procardia XL® extended-release nifedipine tablets in open-label trials and during post-marketing experience, although a causal relationship to the drug has not been established.

Symptoms of GI obstruction have occurred in several patients with a history of GI strictures who were receiving extended-release tablets of the drug. (See Cautions: Precautions and Contraindications.) GI obstruction also has occurred in at least one patient with no preexisting abnormality who was receiving conventional capsules of the drug concomitantly with diltiazem; it was suggested that obstruction in this patient may have resulted from a pharmacologic effect on intestinal smooth muscle.

● Dermatologic and Sensitivity Reactions

In patients receiving conventional liquid-filled (short-acting) nifedipine capsules, dermatitis, pruritus, urticaria, and sweating have been reported occasionally, while angioedema (principally oropharyngeal edema and occasionally breathing difficulty) occurred in less than 0.5% of patients. Exfoliative dermatitis, exfoliative or bullous skin reactions (including erythema multiforme, Stevens-Johnson syndrome, and toxic epidermal necrolysis), and photosensitivity reactions have been reported rarely.

In patients receiving extended-release nifedipine tablets, rash and pruritus have been reported in up to 3% of patients, while angioedema, allergic reaction, cellulitis, facial edema, periorbital edema, alopecia, sweating, urticaria, photosensitivity reactions, and petechial rash were reported in up to 1% of patients.

Anaphylactic reactions have been reported rarely in patients receiving nifedipine.

● Respiratory Effects

In patients receiving conventional liquid-filled (short-acting) nifedipine capsules, dyspnea, cough, wheezing, nasal congestion, and sore throat occurred in 6% of patients, while chest congestion and shortness of breath have been reported in up to 2% of patients.

In patients receiving extended-release nifedipine tablets, dyspnea, epistaxis, and rhinitis were reported in up to 3% of patients, while cough, pharyngitis, sinusitis, upper respiratory tract infection, respiratory disorder, rales, and stridor were reported in up to 1% of patients.

● Musculoskeletal Effects

In patients receiving conventional liquid-filled (short-acting) nifedipine capsules, muscle cramps occurred in 8% of patients, while musculoskeletal complaints of inflammation and joint stiffness have been reported occasionally, and myalgia and arthritis with increased antinuclear antibodies (ANA) have been reported rarely.

In patients receiving extended-release nifedipine tablets, arthralgia, leg pain, and leg cramps occurred in up to 3% of patients, while myalgia, arthritis, joint disorder, myasthenia, back pain, neck pain, and gout occurred in up to 1% of patients.

● Genitourinary Effects

In patients receiving conventional liquid-filled (short-acting) nifedipine capsules, sexual difficulty has been reported occasionally, while gynecomastia, nocturia, and polyuria have been reported rarely.

In patients receiving extended-release nifedipine tablets, impotence, polyuria, and urinary frequency have been reported in up to 3% of patients, while decreased libido, breast pain, pelvic pain, dysuria, hematuria, and nocturia occurred in up to 1% of patients, and renal calculi, urogenital disorder, and breast engorgement were reported in less than 1% of patients. Gynecomastia has been reported in less than 1% of patients receiving Procardia XL® extended-release nifedipine tablets in open-label trials and during postmarketing experience, although a causal relationship to the drug has not been established.

● Hepatic Effects

Abnormal laboratory test results including mild to moderately increased serum concentrations of alkaline phosphatase, LDH, creatine kinase (CK, creatine phosphokinase, CPK), AST (SGOT), and ALT (SGPT) have been reported rarely in

patients receiving nifedipine. Although a definite causal relationship of these laboratory test results to the drug has not been established, the relationship has been considered probable in several cases. In most cases, the laboratory test abnormalities were not associated with clinical symptoms; however, cholestasis (with or without jaundice) has been reported. Small increases (about 5%) in mean alkaline phosphatase concentrations have been reported in patients receiving extended-release nifedipine tablets; however, these increases were clinically asymptomatic, isolated incidents that rarely resulted in values outside the normal range. Increased γ-glutamyltransferase (GGT, γ-glutamyltranspeptidase, GGTP) concentrations have been reported in less than 1% of patients receiving Adalat® CC extended-release nifedipine tablets. Allergic hepatitis has occurred rarely.

● Renal Effects

In patients with preexisting chronic renal insufficiency receiving nifedipine, reversible increases in blood urea nitrogen (BUN) and serum creatinine concentrations have been reported rarely. Although a definite causal relationship of these laboratory test results to the drug has not been established, the relationship has been considered probable in several cases.

● Ocular and Otic Effects

In patients receiving conventional liquid-filled (short-acting) nifedipine capsules, blurred vision has been reported occasionally, while transient blindness at peak serum nifedipine concentrations and transient unilateral loss of vision have been reported rarely.

In patients receiving extended-release nifedipine tablets, abnormal lacrimation and vision abnormalities have been reported in up to 1% of patients, while amblyopia, conjunctivitis, diplopia, eye disorder, and ocular hemorrhage have been reported in less than 1% of patients.

Tinnitus has been reported in up to 1% of patients receiving nifedipine.

● Hematologic Effects

In patients receiving conventional liquid-filled (short-acting) nifedipine capsules, thrombocytopenia, anemia, leukopenia, and purpura have been reported rarely. In patients receiving extended-release nifedipine tablets, purpura occurred in up to 1% of patients, and eosinophilia and lymphadenopathy occurred in less than 1% of patients. Positive antiglobulin (Coombs') test results, with or without hemolytic anemia, have been reported in patients receiving nifedipine, but a causal relationship to the drug has not been established.

Like other calcium-channel blocking agents, nifedipine decreases platelet aggregation in vitro. A moderate decrease in platelet aggregation and increases in bleeding time, believed to be related to inhibition of calcium transport across the platelet membrane, have been reported in patients receiving nifedipine in a limited number of clinical studies; however, these findings were not considered to be clinically important.

● Metabolic Effects

Weight gain has been reported in up to 1% of patients receiving Procardia XL® extended-release nifedipine tablets, while weight loss has been reported in less than 1% of patients receiving Adalat® CC extended-release nifedipine tablets.

● Other Adverse Effects

In patients receiving extended-release nifedipine tablets, hot flushes (flashes), rigors, and malaise were reported in up to 1% of patients in clinical trials.

● Precautions and Contraindications

Some findings concerning possible risks of calcium-channel blocking agents have raised concerns about the safety and efficacy of these agents (mainly conventional [short-acting] preparations of nifedipine). However, findings with amlodipine in the ALLHAT study have shown a beneficial effect of dihydropyridine-derivative calcium-channel blockers on fatal coronary heart disease and nonfatal MI in patients treated with the drug for hypertension.

Nifedipine shares the toxic potentials of the calcium-channel blocking agents, and the usual precautions of these agents should be observed.

Because nifedipine decreases peripheral vascular resistance and occasionally causes excessive and poorly tolerated hypotension, blood pressure should be monitored carefully, especially during initiation of therapy and titration or upward adjustment of dosage. In addition, the manufacturers warn that the frequency, duration, and severity of angina may increase during initiation of therapy or upward adjustment of dosage.

Nifedipine should be used with caution in patients with congestive heart failure or aortic stenosis, especially in those receiving concomitant β-blockers, because nifedipine may precipitate or worsen heart failure in these patients. Peripheral edema occurring during the course of nifedipine therapy should be investigated, especially in patients with congestive heart failure, since it may indicate deterioration in left ventricular function induced by the drug.

Patients with acute stroke or acute MI may be at particular risk for the negative cardiovascular effects (both direct and reflex) of rapid blood pressure reduction, and the manufacturers warn that short-acting nifedipine should not be used during the first 1–2 weeks after acute MI. Preexisting hypovolemia or recent antihypertensive therapy may increase the risk of severe hypotension as may repeated doses of nifedipine. In patients with coronary artery disease and/or myocardial ischemia, reflex sympathetic activity with resultant increases in myocardial contractility, heart rate, and workload may aggravate preexisting myocardial ischemia. The manufacturers warn that short-acting nifedipine should be avoided in patients with acute coronary syndrome when MI may be imminent. When nifedipine therapy is initiated in patients with angina, they should be warned that the drug may cause increased angina, especially if β-blocker therapy is withdrawn abruptly when nifedipine therapy is being initiated. (See Drug Interactions: β-Adrenergic Blocking Agents.)

As with other nondeformable material, extended-release nifedipine tablets should be used with caution in patients with underlying severe GI narrowing (pathologic or iatrogenic) since obstruction may occur.

Nifedipine is contraindicated in patients with known hypersensitivity to the drug.

● **Pediatric Precautions**

Although safety and efficacy remain to be fully established in children younger than 18 years of age, some experts have recommended pediatric dosages for hypertension based on clinical experience. For information on overall principles and expert recommendations for treatment of hypertension in pediatric patients, see Uses: Hypertension in Pediatric Patients, in the Thiazides General Statement 40:28.20.

● **Geriatric Precautions**

Although a prolonged elimination half-life and an increase in peak plasma concentration and area under the plasma concentration-time curve (AUC) have been observed in pharmacokinetic studies in small numbers of patients (see Pharmacokinetics: Elimination), clinical studies of nifedipine did not include sufficient numbers of patients 65 years of age and older to determine whether geriatric patients respond differently than younger adults. While other clinical experience generally has not revealed age-related differences in response or tolerance, drug dosage generally should be titrated carefully in geriatric patients, usually initiating therapy at the low end of the dosage range and adjusting dosage as necessary based on patient response. The greater frequency of decreased hepatic, renal, and/or cardiac function and of concomitant disease and drug therapy observed in the elderly also should be considered.

● **Mutagenicity and Carcinogenicity**

In vivo studies using nifedipine have not revealed evidence of mutagenicity. No evidence of carcinogenicity was observed in rats receiving oral nifedipine for 2 years.

● **Pregnancy, Fertility, and Lactation**
Pregnancy

Nifedipine has been shown to be teratogenic in rats and rabbits. Digital anomalies similar to those reported with phenytoin also have been reported in the offspring of animals receiving nifedipine or other dihydropyridines; these anomalies may occur secondary to compromised uterine blood flow. Nifedipine administration in rats, mice, rabbits, and monkeys also has been associated with a variety of other embryotoxic, placentotoxic, and fetotoxic effects, including stunted fetuses (rats, mice, and rabbits), rib deformities (mice), cleft palate (mice), small

placentas and underdeveloped chorionic villi (monkeys), embryonic and fetal deaths (rats, mice, and rabbits), and prolonged pregnancy/decreased neonatal survival (rats; not evaluated in other species). The dosages (on a mg/kg basis) of nifedipine associated with teratogenic, embryotoxic, or fetotoxic effects in animals were higher (3.5–42 times) than the maximum recommended human dosage (120 mg daily); however, such dosages were within one order of magnitude of the maximum recommended human dosage. The dosages of nifedipine associated with placentotoxic effects in monkeys were equivalent to or lower than the maximum recommended human dosage on a mg/m² basis. There are no adequate and well-controlled studies using nifedipine in pregnant women, and the drug should be used during pregnancy only when the potential benefits justify the possible risks to the fetus.

Fertility

Nifedipine caused decreased fertility when given to rats prior to mating at a dosage approximately 30 times the maximum recommended human dosage. A reversible reduction in the ability of human sperm to bind to and fertilize an ovum in vitro has been reported in a limited number of infertile men who were receiving usual dosages of nifedipine when the sperm was obtained.

Lactation

Nifedipine is distributed into milk. In one lactating woman who received 10, 20, and 30 mg of the drug every 8 hours as conventional capsules, peak milk concentrations of nifedipine occurred within 1 hour after a dose and ranged from about 13–53 ng/mL; the drug generally was not detectable during the hour prior to a dose. Because of the potential for serious adverse reactions to nifedipine in nursing infants, a decision should be made whether to discontinue nursing or the drug, taking into account the importance of the drug to the woman.

DRUG INTERACTIONS

● **Drugs and Foods Affecting Hepatic Microsomal Enzymes**

Metabolism of nifedipine is mediated by the cytochrome P-450 (CYP) microsomal enzyme system (principally the 3A isoenzyme) and concomitant use of nifedipine with inhibitors or inducers of CYP3A4 may be associated with altered nifedipine exposure resulting in favorable or adverse effects. In addition, in vitro and in vivo data indicate that nifedipine may inhibit metabolism of drugs that are substrates of CYP3A, thereby increasing exposure of other drugs. Nifedipine does not appear to affect the metabolism of CYP2D6 substrates.

Quinidine

Quinidine appears to be a substrate of the CYP isoenzyme system and has been shown to inhibit CYP3A in vitro. In a multiple-dose study in healthy individuals, concomitant use of quinidine sulfate (200 mg 3 times daily) and nifedipine (20 mg 3 times daily) increased the area under the plasma concentration-time curve (AUC) and peak plasma concentration values of nifedipine 2.3 and 1.37 times, respectively. Heart rate during the initial interval following drug administration increased by up to 17.9 beats per minute. Heart rate should be monitored and nifedipine dosage adjusted as needed in patients receiving concomitant therapy with quinidine and nifedipine.

Although exposure to quinidine was not substantially affected by nifedipine in the previous study, nifedipine may decrease serum quinidine concentrations in some patients. Reductions or increases in serum quinidine concentrations occasionally have been observed following initiation or discontinuance, respectively, of nifedipine. Such changes can be substantial and may manifest as therapeutic resistance to usual quinidine dosages during concomitant therapy and/or altered ECGs (e.g., prolongation in corrected QT interval following discontinuance of nifedipine). While it had been postulated that alterations in quinidine pharmacokinetics during concomitant nifedipine therapy may have resulted from changes in hemodynamics induced by the latter drug (e.g., reduced peripheral vascular resistance with resultantly increased quinidine volume of distribution) in some patients (e.g., those with left ventricular dysfunction), subsequent study failed to confirm left ventricular dysfunction as a predictor of this interaction. Therefore, the mechanism of this interaction remains to be established, and possible identification of patients at risk requires further study. The possibility of this interaction should be considered in any patient exhibiting unpredictably low serum quinidine concentrations during concomitant nifedipine therapy. Serum quinidine concentrations should be monitored whenever nifedipine is initiated or discontinued in patients maintained on the antiarrhythmic, and quinidine dosage adjusted accordingly.

Verapamil

Verapamil, an inhibitor of the isoenzyme CYP3A, may inhibit the metabolism of nifedipine. In patients receiving concomitant therapy with verapamil and nifedipine, blood pressure should be monitored, and nifedipine dosage reduction should be considered.

Diltiazem

Since metabolism of diltiazem also is mediated principally by the CYP3A isoenzyme, diltiazem may competitively inhibit CYP3A4-dependent metabolism of other drugs (e.g., nifedipine). Administration of diltiazem 30- or 90-mg doses 3 times daily followed by a single 20-mg dose of nifedipine in healthy individuals increased nifedipine AUC values by 2.2 or 3.1 times, respectively, and peak plasma nifedipine concentrations by 2 or 1.7 times, respectively.

Angiotensin II Receptor Antagonists

Nifedipine has been shown to inhibit the formation of oxidized metabolites of irbesartan in vitro; however, concomitant nifedipine therapy had no effect on irbesartan pharmacokinetics in clinical studies.

In addition, since candesartan is not substantially metabolized by the CYP isoenzyme system, no substantial drug interaction has been reported in individuals receiving nifedipine concomitantly with candesartan.

Antifungal Agents

Concomitant use of nifedipine with ketoconazole, itraconazole, or fluconazole may affect the pharmacokinetics of nifedipine, possibly secondary to the inhibition of the CYP3A isoenzyme, and increased exposure of nifedipine may occur. Blood pressure should be monitored, and a decrease in nifedipine dosage should be considered.

Antiretroviral Agents

Concomitant use of nifedipine with antiretroviral agents (HIV protease inhibitors [e.g., amprenavir, atazanavir, fosamprenavir, indinavir, nelfinavir, ritonavir] and nonnucleoside reverse transcriptase inhibitors [e.g., delavirdine]) may affect the pharmacokinetics of nifedipine, possibly secondary to the inhibition of the CYP3A isoenzyme, and may result in decreased nifedipine metabolism and increased nifedipine exposure. Caution is advised if nifedipine is administered concomitantly with these antiretroviral agents; patients should be monitored carefully.

Antituberculosis Agents

Rifamycin derivatives (e.g., rifampin, rifabutin) can induce certain cytochrome P-450 liver enzymes (e.g., CYP3A isoenzyme) responsible for the metabolism of nifedipine. Concomitant use of these rifamycin derivatives and nifedipine may result in decreased plasma concentrations of nifedipine. In healthy individuals, concomitant use of oral rifampin (600 mg daily) and oral nifedipine (20 mcg/kg) or IV nifedipine resulted in an 87 or 30% decrease in nifedipine exposure, respectively. Adjustment of nifedipine dosage may be needed in patients receiving nifedipine concomitantly with rifamycin derivatives.

Quinupristin and Dalfopristin

Concomitant use of nifedipine with quinupristin and dalfopristin may affect the pharmacokinetics of nifedipine, possibly secondary to the inhibition of the isoenzyme CYP3A. In healthy individuals, concomitant administration of repeated oral doses of nifedipine with IV quinupristin and dalfopristin increased the median peak plasma concentration and the AUC of nifedipine by 18 and 44%, respectively. In patients receiving nifedipine concomitantly with quinupristin and dalfopristin, blood pressure should be monitored and nifedipine dosage reduced if needed.

Erythromycin

Concomitant use of erythromycin (an inhibitor of the CYP3A4 isoenzyme) and nifedipine may result in inhibition of the metabolism of nifedipine and increased nifedipine exposure. Blood pressure should be monitored and nifedipine dosage reduced if necessary in patients in whom erythromycin is used concomitantly with nifedipine.

Histamine H₂-Receptor Antagonists

Concomitant use of nifedipine (single 10-mg doses and 40–60 mg daily) with cimetidine (up to 1 g daily) in healthy individuals increased peak plasma nifedipine concentrations by approximately 60–102% and AUC of nifedipine by approximately 52–101%; plasma clearance of nifedipine was decreased by approximately 40%. Increases in the effect of nifedipine on blood pressure also have been observed in hypertensive patients receiving concomitant therapy with cimetidine (1 g daily) and nifedipine (10 mg daily). Peak plasma concentrations and AUCs of nifedipine also have increased with concomitant nifedipine and ranitidine therapy, but to a lesser degree than with cimetidine. Although the precise mechanism of these interactions is not known, cimetidine-induced inhibition of the cytochrome P-450 mixed-function oxidase system (the enzyme system that is probably responsible for the first-pass metabolism of nifedipine) may play a role. Pending further accumulation of data, cautious dosage titration of nifedipine is recommended in patients receiving cimetidine; a reduction in nifedipine dosage may be necessary in some patients previously stabilized on the drug when cimetidine therapy is initiated.

Since ranitidine interacts with the hepatic cytochrome P-450 (microsomal) enzyme system differently than does cimetidine, ranitidine appears to only minimally inhibit hepatic metabolism of some drugs. Results of several studies indicate that concomitant use of ranitidine with nifedipine did not affect exposure of nifedipine and no effects on blood pressure or heart rate have been observed when these drugs were used concomitantly in healthy individuals or hypertensive patients.

Anticonvulsant Agents

Concomitant use of phenytoin with nifedipine may affect the pharmacokinetics of nifedipine. Phenytoin is an inducer of the CYP3A4 isoenzyme and may cause decreased nifedipine exposure. Concomitant use of nifedipine (as a 10-mg capsule or a 60-mg extended-release tablet) with phenytoin decreased (by about 70%) the AUC and peak plasma concentrations of nifedipine. Phenytoin toxicity has occurred within 4 weeks after initiating nifedipine in a patient stabilized on phenytoin. Manifestations of phenytoin toxicity (e.g., headaches, nystagmus, tremors, slurred speech, ataxia, mental depression) resolved and plasma concentrations of the drug decreased within 2 weeks after discontinuance of nifedipine. While the mechanism of this interaction has not been elucidated, it was suggested that nifedipine may have reduced the metabolism of phenytoin.

Phenytoin toxicity also reportedly has occurred in at least one patient with subarachnoid hemorrhage receiving nimodipine, another 1,4-dihydropyridine calcium-channel blocker. Whether this effect represented an actual drug interaction between phenytoin and nimodipine has not been determined to date. However, most patients with subarachnoid hemorrhage receiving nimodipine also received concomitant therapy with phenytoin or barbiturates reportedly with no apparent evidence of drug interactions.

Pending further accumulation of data, patients and plasma phenytoin concentrations should be monitored carefully whenever therapy with a 1,4-dihydropyridine calcium-channel blocker is initiated or withdrawn from a patient receiving phenytoin. Blood pressure should be monitored and nifedipine dosage adjusted as needed in patients receiving concomitant nifedipine and phenytoin therapy.

Phenobarbital and carbamazepine also may decrease exposure to nifedipine by inducing the CYP3A isoenzyme. In patients receiving nifedipine concomitantly with phenobarbital or carbamazepine, adjustment of nifedipine dosage may be needed. Conversely, nifedipine exposure may be increased in patients receiving valproic acid concomitantly with nifedipine; blood pressure should be monitored, and a reduction in nifedipine dosage should be considered in these patients.

Immunosuppressive Agents

Because nifedipine may inhibit metabolism of tacrolimus, a substrate of CYP3A4, concomitant use of nifedipine and tacrolimus may result in increased tacrolimus exposure. In patients who underwent transplantation and received such concomitant therapy, tacrolimus dosage reductions of 26–38% were required; tacrolimus blood concentrations should be monitored, and a reduction in tacrolimus dosage should be considered in these patients.

Although sirolimus is a substrate for the isoenzyme 3A4, no clinically important pharmacokinetic interactions were observed in patients receiving nifedipine (a single 60-mg dose) concomitantly with oral sirolimus (a single 10-mg dose).

Dolasetron

Although hydrodolasetron (the main active metabolite of dolasetron) is extensively metabolized, principally via the CYP system, including the 2D6 and 3A4 isoenzymes, concomitant use of IV or oral dolasetron with nifedipine did not alter the clearance of the metabolite.

Other Drugs Affecting Hepatic Microsomal Enzymes

Ethanol can increase the oral bioavailability of nifedipine, possibly via inhibition of hepatic cytochrome P-450 microsomal metabolism. In one study in healthy adults, concomitant administration of ethanol with a single 20-mg oral dose of nifedipine capsules resulted in a 54% increase in the AUC of nifedipine.

Nefazodone, an inhibitor of the CYP3A isoenzyme, may inhibit the metabolism of nifedipine and increase nifedipine exposure; blood pressure should be monitored, and a reduction of nifedipine dosage should be considered in patients receiving nefazodone concomitantly with nifedipine.

St. John's wort may decrease nifedipine exposure by inducing the CYP3A4 isoenzyme. Adjustment of nifedipine dosage may be necessary in patients receiving nifedipine concomitantly with St. John's wort.

Grapefruit Juice

Concomitant oral administration of grapefruit juice with nifedipine has been reported to increase bioavailability of the drug. Peak plasma concentrations and AUC values of nifedipine have been reported to increase by approximately twofold (with no change in elimination half-life) when the drug is administered with grapefruit juice. The interaction between grapefruit juice and the oral bioavailability of some 1,4-dihydropyridine-derivative calcium-channel blocking agents appears to result from inhibition, probably prehepatic, of the cytochrome P-450 enzyme system by some constituent(s) in the juice. Following oral administration of nifedipine, such prehepatic inhibition of drug metabolism by grapefruit juice appears mainly to involve the CYP3A4 isoenzyme, principally within the wall of the small intestine (e.g., in the jejunum), thus increasing systemic availability of the drug. (See Grapefruit Juice under Drug Interactions: Drugs and Foods Affecting Hepatic Microsomal Enzymes, in Cyclosporine 92:44.) Concomitant oral administration of grapefruit juice and nifedipine should be avoided. Consumption of grapefruit juice should be discontinued at least 3 days prior to initiating nifedipine therapy.

● β-Adrenergic Blocking Agents

Although concomitant therapy usually is well tolerated, the risk of severe hypotension, exacerbation of angina, congestive heart failure, and arrhythmia may be increased when nifedipine is used concomitantly with a β-adrenergic blocking agent (β-blocker) (e.g., propranolol, timolol), as compared with nifedipine alone. One manufacturer states that clinical monitoring is recommended in patients receiving nifedipine concomitantly with a β-blocker, and adjustment of nifedipine dosage should be considered. Exacerbation of anginal pain also has been observed when β-blocker therapy was being withdrawn concurrently with initiation of nifedipine therapy; gradual reduction of β-blocker dosage instead of abrupt withdrawal may minimize the risk of this effect.

● Fentanyl

Severe hypotension has occurred during surgery in patients receiving nifedipine, a β-blocker, and fentanyl concomitantly. The manufacturers recommend temporarily withholding nifedipine for at least 36 hours before surgery in which use of high-dose fentanyl is contemplated, if the patient's condition permits.

● Digoxin

Most evidence indicates that nifedipine does not substantially affect the pharmacokinetics of digoxin when the drugs are administered concomitantly; however, some data suggest that serum digoxin concentrations may increase by about 15–45% during concomitant therapy. Further evaluation of this potential interaction is needed. Since there have been isolated reports of increased serum digoxin concentrations during concomitant administration, serum digoxin concentrations should be monitored when nifedipine therapy is initiated or discontinued

or dosage of nifedipine is adjusted in patients receiving digoxin. Patients receiving the drugs concomitantly should be monitored for signs and symptoms of digoxin toxicity and dosage of the cardiac glycoside reduced if necessary.

● Antidiabetic Agents

Since nifedipine may produce hyperglycemia which may lead to loss of glycemic control, glucose concentrations should be carefully monitored and adjustment of nifedipine dosage should be considered in patients receiving concomitant therapy with nifedipine and acarbose.

Nifedipine appears to enhance absorption of metformin. In healthy individuals, concomitant use of nifedipine with metformin was associated with 20 and 9% increases in peak plasma concentrations and AUC of metformin, respectively.

● Omeprazole

Administration of omeprazole 20 mg daily for 8 days followed by a single 10-mg dose of nifedipine in healthy individuals increased AUC of nifedipine by 26% and decreased peak plasma concentrations of nifedipine by 13% when compared with placebo followed by a single 10-mg dose of nifedipine. Concomitant use of omeprazole and nifedipine did not alter the effects of nifedipine on blood pressure or heart rate. The effect of omeprazole on nifedipine pharmacokinetics is unlikely to be clinically important.

● Hypotensive Agents

Concomitant administration of nifedipine with hypotensive agents (e.g., methyldopa, hydralazine, captopril, doxazosin) may increase the incidence of severe hypotension. When nifedipine is added to an existing antihypertensive therapy regimen, the patient should be observed closely for severe hypotension, especially during initial titration or upward adjustment of nifedipine dosage.

Attenuation of the tachycardic effect of nifedipine has been observed in patients receiving concomitant benazepril.

● Anticoagulants

Increased prothrombin time has been reported rarely in patients receiving concomitant therapy with nifedipine and coumarin anticoagulants; however, a causal relationship to nifedipine has not been established.

● Platelet-aggregation Inhibitors

No clinically important interactions have been reported in patients receiving nifedipine concomitantly with clopidogrel or tirofiban.

● Other Drugs

The manufacturer of Adalat® CC extended-release nifedipine tablets states that clinical experience is insufficient to recommend concomitant use of nifedipine with flecainide.

ACUTE TOXICITY

Experience with acute overdosage of nifedipine is limited. Generally, overdosage with the drug would be expected to produce toxic effects that are extensions of the usual adverse effects of the drug, including pronounced hypotension. If pronounced hypotension occurs, symptomatic and supportive care should be initiated, including active cardiovascular support that includes monitoring of cardiovascular and respiratory function, elevation of the extremities, and judicious use of parenteral calcium salts, vasopressors, and fluids. Other symptoms associated with severe nifedipine overdosage include loss of consciousness, heart rhythm disturbances, metabolic acidosis, hypoxia, and cardiogenic shock with pulmonary edema. Clearance of nifedipine would be expected to be prolonged in patients with impaired hepatic function, since the drug is metabolized in the liver. Because nifedipine is highly protein bound, hemodialysis is unlikely to promote elimination of the drug; however, plasmapheresis may prove beneficial.

In a young man who intentionally ingested 4.8 g of extended-release nifedipine tablets, the principal manifestations of overdosage initially were dizziness, palpitations, flushing, and nervousness. Nausea, vomiting, and generalized edema developed within several hours following ingestion of the drug; however, no substantial hypotension developed approximately 18 hours after ingestion. Mild, transient elevation of serum creatinine and modest elevations in serum LDH and creatine kinase (CK, creatine phosphokinase, CPK) were observed, but serum AST was normal. The patient's vital signs remained stable, no ECG abnormalities were observed, and renal function returned to normal within 24–48 hours with routine supportive measures only. No prolonged sequelae were observed.

In a patient with angina and a history of bundle branch block who was receiving tricyclic antidepressants and ingested a single 900-mg dose of nifedipine capsules, loss of consciousness (within 30 minutes of nifedipine ingestion) and profound hypotension (which responded to calcium infusion, pressor agents, and fluid replacement) were observed. Because ECG abnormalities (e.g., sinus bradycardia, varying degrees of AV block) developed, a temporary ventricular pacemaker was required; thereafter, ECG abnormalities resolved spontaneously. Substantial hyperglycemia also was observed but resolved rapidly without treatment.

Ingestion of a single 280-mg dose of nifedipine capsules in a young patient with hypertension and advanced renal failure resulted in marked hypotension which responded to calcium infusion and fluids. No AV conduction abnormalities, arrhythmias, pronounced change in heart rate, or further deterioration in renal function were observed.

PHARMACOLOGY

Nifedipine has pharmacologic actions similar to those of other dihydropyridine calcium-channel blocking agents (e.g., felodipine, nisoldipine). The principal physiologic action of nifedipine is to inhibit the transmembrane influx of extracellular calcium ions across the membranes of myocardial cells and vascular smooth muscle cells, without changing serum calcium concentrations.

Calcium plays important roles in the excitation-contraction coupling processes of the heart and vascular smooth muscle cells and in the electrical discharge of the specialized conduction cells of the heart. The membranes of these cells contain numerous channels that carry a slow inward current and that are selective for calcium. Activation of these slow calcium channels contributes to the plateau phase (phase 2) of the action potential of cardiac and vascular smooth muscle cells.

The exact mechanism whereby nifedipine inhibits calcium ion influx across the slow calcium channels is not known, but the drug is thought to inhibit ion-control gating mechanisms of the channel, deform the slow channel, and/or interfere with release of calcium from the sarcoplasmic reticulum.

By inhibiting calcium influx, nifedipine inhibits the contractile processes of cardiac and vascular smooth muscle, thereby dilating the main coronary and systemic arteries. In patients with Prinzmetal variant angina (vasospastic angina), inhibition of spontaneous and ergonovine-induced coronary artery spasm by nifedipine results in increased myocardial oxygen delivery. Dilation of systemic arteries by nifedipine results in a decrease in total peripheral resistance, a usually modest decrease in systemic blood pressure (e.g., a decrease of 5–10 mm Hg), a decrease in the afterload of the heart, a small reflex increase in heart rate, and an increase in the cardiac index. The reduction in afterload, seen at rest and with exercise, and its resultant decrease in myocardial oxygen consumption are thought to be responsible for the effects of nifedipine in patients with chronic stable angina pectoris.

In contrast to verapamil and diltiazem, nifedipine has little or no effect on sinoatrial (SA) and atrioventricular (AV) nodal conduction at therapeutic doses.

Although negative inotropic effects have been noted in vitro and in animal studies with nifedipine, they are rarely, if ever, seen clinically, probably because of reflex responses to the drug's vasodilating actions including a small increase in heart rate. Major increases in left ventricular end-diastolic pressure (LVEDP) or volume (LVEDV) or decreases in cardiac ejection fraction usually are not seen following nifedipine administration in patients with normal ventricular function. In patients with impaired ventricular function, some increase in ejection fraction and reduction in left ventricular filling pressure may be seen acutely.

PHARMACOKINETICS

● *Absorption*

Approximately 90% of an oral dose of nifedipine is rapidly absorbed from the GI tract following oral administration of the drug as conventional capsules. Only about 45–75% of an oral dose as conventional capsules reaches systemic circulation

as unchanged drug since nifedipine is metabolized on first pass through the liver. Peak serum concentrations usually are reached within 0.5–2 hours after oral administration as conventional capsules. Food appears to decrease the rate but not the extent of absorption of nifedipine as conventional capsules.

The manufacturer states that relative oral bioavailability differs little if conventional nifedipine capsules are swallowed intact, bitten and swallowed, or bitten and held sublingually. However, some data indicate that the rate and extent of absorption of nifedipine following sublingual administration may be decreased substantially. In several studies, peak plasma concentrations of nifedipine appeared to be delayed and decreased following sublingual administration. In one crossover study in healthy adults in which a 10-mg conventional capsule of the drug was bitten and held sublingually for 20 minutes or bitten and swallowed, the bioavailability following sublingual administration was 17% (range: 7–28%) of that following oral administration of a bitten capsule; on average, 86% of the dose remained in the mouth at the end of the 20-minute sublingual retention period. In this study, peak serum nifedipine concentrations following sublingual or oral administration of a bitten capsule occurred within 50 (range: 20–99) or 30 (range: 15–49) minutes, respectively, and averaged 10 (range: 5–17) or 82 (range: 44–146) ng/mL, respectively. Oral bioavailability of nifedipine may be increased up to twofold in patients with liver cirrhosis.

The commercially available extended-release tablets of nifedipine (Procardia XL®) contain the drug in an oral osmotic delivery system formulation (elementary osmotic pump, gastrointestinal therapeutic system [GITS]). The osmotic delivery system consists of an osmotically active core (comprised of a layer containing the drug and a layer containing osmotically active but pharmacologically inert components) that is surrounded by a semipermeable membrane with a laser-drilled delivery orifice and is designed to deliver the drug at an approximately constant rate over a 24-hour period (approximately zero-order delivery). When exposed to water in the GI tract, water is drawn osmotically into the core at a controlled rate that is determined by the permeability of the outer membrane and the osmotic pressure of the core formulation; as water enters the formulation, a resulting suspension of the drug is pushed out the delivery orifice of the membrane into the GI tract. Delivery of nifedipine from the formulation depends on the existence of an osmotic gradient between the fluid in the GI tract and the osmotically active core of the tablet, with drug delivery remaining approximately constant as long as the gradient is maintained and then declining parabolically to zero as the concentration inside the tablet falls below saturation. The rate of nifedipine delivery in the GI tract is independent of pH over the range of 1.2–7.5 and probably GI motility. The inert tablet ingredients remain intact and are eliminated in feces.

Extended-release tablets (Procardia XL®) labeled as containing 30, 60, or 90 mg of nifedipine reportedly deliver the drug into the GI tract at an approximately constant rate of 1.7, 3.4, and 5.1 mg/hour, respectively, throughout the 24-hour dosing period. Following oral administration of a single dose of the drug as extended-release tablets, plasma nifedipine concentrations increase gradually, reaching a peak at approximately 6 hours, and bioavailability is approximately 55–65% of that achieved with the same doses administered orally as conventional capsules. Following multiple doses, oral bioavailability from the extended-release tablets increases to approximately 75–86% of that achieved with the same doses administered as conventional capsules. Administration of Procardia XL® nifedipine extended-release tablets with food can increase the early rate of GI absorption but reportedly does not affect overall bioavailability.

The commercially available extended-release tablets of nifedipine (Adalat® CC) are composed of a slow-release outer coat and an immediate-release core. The bioavailability of nifedipine as Adalat® CC extended-release tablets relative to conventional nifedipine capsules is about 84–89%. Following oral administration of Adalat® CC in fasting individuals, peak plasma concentrations occur within 2.5–5 hours, with a small second peak (or "shoulder") occurring within 6–12 hours. Following oral administration of Adalat® CC extended-release nifedipine 30-mg tablets over a dosage range of 30–90 mg, the area under the plasma-concentration time curve (AUC) was proportional to the dose administered; however, peak plasma concentrations of the 90-mg dose (three 30-mg tablets) were 29% greater than that predicted from the 30- and 60-mg doses. Once-daily dosing of Adalat® CC extended-release tablets, under fasting conditions, resulted in less fluctuation in plasma nifedipine concentrations when compared with 3-times-daily dosing with conventional nifedipine capsules. Following administration of a single Adalat® CC 90-mg extended-release tablet under fasting conditions, mean peak plasma nifedipine concentration of about 115 ng/mL were reported. Administration of Adalat® CC extended-release tablets immediately after a high-fat meal increases peak plasma nifedipine concentrations by 60% and delays the time to peak plasma concentrations; however, no substantial changes in AUC occur. Peak plasma concentrations of nifedipine following administration of Adalat® CC extended-release tablets after a high-fat meal are slightly lower compared with those occurring after administration of the same daily dosage given in 3 divided doses as the conventional nifedipine capsules; this difference may be attributed to the lower bioavailability of Adalat® CC extended-release tablets compared with that of conventional nifedipine capsules.

Following oral administration of Adalat® CC extended-release nifedipine tablets in healthy geriatric individuals (older than 60 years of age), the mean peak plasma concentrations and average plasma concentrations of nifedipine increased by 36 and 70%, respectively, compared with those observed in younger adults.

With another extended-release tablet formulation (Adalat L®, not commercially available in the US), both the rate and extent (over 12 hours) of absorption of a single dose of nifedipine were increased by administration with food. Because orally administered nifedipine undergoes extensive metabolism on first pass through the liver, bioavailability of the drug from extended-release tablets is increased substantially in patients with liver cirrhosis and may be particularly increased in those with portacaval shunts. Substantial reductions in GI retention time for prolonged periods (e.g., in patients with short-bowel syndrome) can result in decreased absorption of nifedipine from extended-release tablets.

● **Distribution**

Binding of nifedipine to plasma proteins is concentration dependent and ranges from 92–98%. Protein binding may be reduced in patients with renal or hepatic (e.g., liver cirrhosis) impairment.

● **Elimination**

In patients with normal renal and hepatic function, the plasma half-life of nifedipine is about 2 hours when administered as conventional capsules, and about 7 hours when administered as extended-release tablets (Adalat® CC). The drug is extensively metabolized in the liver (to highly water-soluble, inactive metabolites) by the cytochrome P-450 microsomal enzyme system, including CYP3A. Approximately 60–80% of an oral dose of nifedipine is excreted as metabolites in the urine, with only traces (less than 0.1%) of an oral dose being excreted in urine as unchanged drug. The remainder of a dose is excreted in the feces as metabolites, possibly via biliary elimination. Nifedipine appears to be negligibly removed by hemodialysis or hemoperfusion.

Adalat® CC extended-release tablets should be used with caution in patients with renal impairment because absorption of the drug may be altered in such patients. In patients with hepatic impairment, elimination of the drug may be altered. The elimination half-life of nifedipine has been reported to increase to 7 hours in patients with liver cirrhosis; oral bioavailability of the drug also is increased in such patients.

Following IV administration of nifedipine, body clearance of the drug is 519 and 348 mL/minute in young adults and geriatric individuals, respectively.

CHEMISTRY AND STABILITY

● **Chemistry**

Nifedipine is a 1,4-dihydropyridine-derivative calcium-channel blocking agent. The drug occurs as a yellow, crystalline powder and is practically insoluble in water and soluble in alcohol.

● **Stability**

Nifedipine liquid-filled capsules should be protected from light and moisture and stored in tight, light-resistant containers at a temperature of 15–25°C, and extended-release tablets of the drug should be protected from light and moisture and stored in tight, light-resistant containers at a temperature less than 30°C.

PREPARATIONS

Excipients in commercially available drug preparations may have clinically important effects in some individuals; consult specific product labeling for details.

NIFEdipine

Oral

Capsules, liquid-filled	10 mg*	**NIFEdipine Capsules**
		Procardia®, Pfizer
	20 mg*	**NIFEdipine Capsules**
Tablets, extended-release, film-coated	30 mg*	**Adalat® CC**, Bayer
		Afeditab® CR, Watson
		Nifedical® XL, Teva
		NIFEdipine ER
		Procardia XL®, Pfizer
	60 mg*	**Adalat® CC**, Bayer
		Afeditab® CR, Watson
		Nifedical® XL, Teva
		NIFEdipine ER
		Procardia XL®, Pfizer
	90 mg*	**Adalat® CC**, Bayer
		NIFEdipine ER,
		Procardia XL®, Pfizer

* available from one or more manufacturer, distributor, and/or repackager by generic (nonproprietary) name

† Use is not currently included in the labeling approved by the US Food and Drug Administration.

Benazepril Hydrochloride

24:32.04 • ANGIOTENSIN-CONVERTING ENZYME INHIBITORS

■ Benazepril is an angiotensin-converting enzyme (ACE) inhibitor.

USES

Benazepril hydrochloride is used alone or in combination with other classes of antihypertensive agents (e.g., thiazide diuretics) in the management of hypertension.

● Hypertension

Benazepril is used alone or in combination with other classes of antihypertensive agents in the management of hypertension.

ACE inhibitors are considered one of several preferred antihypertensive drugs for the initial management of hypertension according to current evidence-based hypertension guidelines; other preferred options include angiotensin II receptor antagonists, calcium-channel blockers, and thiazide diuretics. While there may be individual differences with respect to recommendations for initial drug selection and use in specific patient populations, current evidence indicates that these antihypertensive drug classes all generally produce comparable effects on overall mortality and cardiovascular, cerebrovascular, and renal outcomes. (See Uses: Hypertension, in Captopril 24:32.04.)

ACE inhibitors may be particularly useful in the management of hypertension in patients with certain coexisting conditions such as heart failure, ischemic heart disease, diabetes mellitus, chronic kidney disease (CKD), or cerebrovascular disease or following myocardial infarction (MI). (See Uses: Hypertension in Captopril 24:32.04 and in Enalaprilat/Enalapril 24:32.04.)

In patients with hypertension and compelling indications (e.g., CKD with albuminuria [urine albumin 300 mg/day or greater, or urine albumin:creatinine ratio of 300 mg/g or equivalent in the first morning void]), angiotensin II receptor antagonists are usually considered an alternative for ACE inhibitor-intolerant patients. However, data indicate no difference in efficacy between ACE inhibitors and angiotensin II receptor antagonists with regard to blood pressure lowering and clinical outcomes (i.e., all-cause mortality, cardiovascular mortality, MI, heart failure, stroke, and end-stage renal disease). Adverse events (e.g., cough, angioedema) leading to drug discontinuance occur more frequently with ACE inhibitor therapy than with angiotensin II receptor antagonist therapy. Because of similar efficacy and a lower frequency of adverse effects, some experts believe that an angiotensin II receptor antagonist should be used instead of an ACE inhibitor for the treatment of hypertension or hypertension with certain compelling indications.

Most patients with hypertension, especially black patients, will require at least 2 antihypertensive drugs to achieve adequate blood pressure control. In general, black hypertensive patients tend to respond better to monotherapy with thiazide diuretics or calcium-channel blockers than to monotherapy with ACE inhibitors. Although ACE inhibitors have lowered blood pressure in all races studied, monotherapy with these agents has produced a smaller reduction in blood pressure in black hypertensive patients, a population associated with low renin hypertension. However, the combination of an ACE inhibitor or an angiotensin II receptor antagonist with a calcium-channel blocker or thiazide diuretic produces similar blood pressure lowering in black patients as in other racial groups. In addition, ACE inhibitors appear to produce a higher incidence of angioedema in black patients than in other races. (See Race under Hypertension: Other Special Considerations for Antihypertensive Drug Therapy, in Uses in Captopril 24:32.04 and in Enalaprilat/Enalapril 24:32.04.)

For additional information on the role of ACE inhibitors in the management of hypertension, see Uses in Captopril 24:32.04 and in Enalaprilat/Enalapril 24:32.04. For information on overall principles and expert recommendations for treatment of hypertension, see Uses: Hypertension in Adults and also see Uses: Hypertension in Pediatric Patients, in the Thiazides General Statement 40:28.20.

● Heart Failure

ACE inhibitors have been used in the management of heart failure†, usually in conjunction with other agents such as cardiac glycosides, diuretics, and β-adrenergic blocking agents (β-blockers).

Current guidelines for the management of heart failure in adults generally recommend a combination of drug therapies to reduce morbidity and mortality, including neurohormonal antagonists (e.g., ACE inhibitors, angiotensin II receptor antagonists, angiotensin receptor-neprilysin inhibitors [ARNIs], β-blockers, aldosterone receptor antagonists) that inhibit the detrimental compensatory mechanisms in heart failure. Additional agents (e.g., cardiac glycosides, diuretics, sinoatrial modulators [i.e., ivabradine]) added to a heart failure treatment regimen in selected patients have been associated with symptomatic improvement and/or reduction in heart failure-related hospitalizations. Experts recommend that all asymptomatic patients with reduced left ventricular ejection fraction (LVEF) (American College of Cardiology Foundation [ACCF]/American Heart Association [AHA] stage B heart failure) receive therapy with an ACE inhibitor and β-blocker to prevent symptomatic heart failure and to reduce morbidity and mortality. If ACE inhibitors are not tolerated, then an angiotensin II receptor antagonist is recommended as alternative therapy. In patients with prior or current symptoms of chronic heart failure with reduced LVEF (ACCF/AHA stage C heart failure), ACCF, AHA, and the Heart Failure Society of America (HFSA) recommend inhibition of the renin-angiotensin-aldosterone (RAA) system with an ACE inhibitor, angiotensin II receptor antagonist, or ARNI in conjunction with a β-blocker, and an aldosterone antagonist in selected patients, to reduce morbidity and mortality. While ACE inhibitors have been the preferred drugs for inhibition of the RAA system because of their established benefits in patients with heart failure and reduced ejection fraction, some evidence indicates that therapy with sacubitril/valsartan, an ARNI, may be more effective than ACE inhibitor therapy (enalapril) in reducing cardiovascular death and heart failure-related hospitalization in such patients. ACCF, AHA, and HFSA recommend that patients with chronic symptomatic heart failure and reduced LVEF (New York Heart Association [NYHA] class II or III) who are able to tolerate an ACE inhibitor or angiotensin II receptor antagonist be switched to therapy containing an ARNI to further reduce morbidity and mortality. However, in patients in whom an ARNI is not appropriate, continued use of an ACE inhibitor for all classes of heart failure with reduced ejection fraction remains strongly advised. In patients in whom an ARNI or ACE inhibitor is not appropriate, an angiotensin II receptor antagonist may be used. For additional information on the use of ACE inhibitors in the management of heart failure, see Uses: Heart Failure, in Captopril 24:32.04 and in Enalaprilat/Enalapril 24:32.04. For further information on the use of ARNIs in patients with heart failure, see Uses: Heart Failure, in Sacubitril and Valsartan 24:32.92.

● Diabetic Nephropathy

Both ACE inhibitors and angiotensin II receptor antagonists have been shown to slow the rate of progression of renal disease in patients with diabetes mellitus and persistent albuminuria†, and use of a drug from either class is recommended in such patients with modestly elevated (30–300 mg/24 hours) or higher (exceeding 300 mg/24 hours) levels of urinary albumin excretion. The usual precautions of ACE inhibitor or angiotensin II receptor antagonist therapy in patients with substantial renal impairment should be observed. For additional information on the use of ACE inhibitors in the treatment of diabetic nephropathy, see Diabetic Nephropathy under Uses: Nephropathy, in Captopril 24:32.04.

DOSAGE AND ADMINISTRATION

● Administration

Benazepril hydrochloride is administered orally.

For adult or pediatric patients unable to swallow tablets or those children for whom the daily dose does not correspond exactly to the strength of commercially available tablets, benazepril hydrochloride may be administered orally as an extemporaneously prepared suspension.

An extemporaneous suspension containing benazepril hydrochloride 2 mg/mL can be prepared in the following manner. First, 75 mL of suspending vehicle (Ora-Plus®) is added to an amber polyethylene terephthalate (PET) bottle containing fifteen 20-mg tablets of benazepril hydrochloride, and the contents are shaken for at least 2 minutes. The concentrated suspension should be allowed to stand for at least 60 minutes following reconstitution, and then should be shaken for an additional minute. The concentrated suspension of benazepril hydrochloride should be diluted with 75 mL of syrup (Ora-Sweet®), and the container then shaken to disperse the ingredients. The suspension should be shaken before dispensing each dose. The extemporaneous suspension is stable for 30 days when stored at 2–8°C.

● Dosage

Dosage of benazepril hydrochloride must be adjusted according to patient tolerance and response. Because of the risk of inducing hypotension, initiation of benazepril therapy requires consideration of recent and current antihypertensive therapy, the extent of blood pressure elevation, sodium intake, fluid status, and other clinical circumstances. If blood pressure is not controlled adequately with the ACE inhibitor alone, a low dosage of a diuretic may be added.

Hypertension

Benazepril Therapy

For the management of hypertension in adults *not* receiving a diuretic, the usual initial dosage of benazepril hydrochloride is 10 mg once daily. In patients currently receiving a diuretic, an initial benazepril hydrochloride dosage of 5 mg daily is recommended. The divided-dose regimen has been more effective in controlling trough (pre-dose) blood pressure than the same dose given once daily.

The manufacturer states that the usual maintenance dosage in adults is 20–40 mg daily, given as a single dose or in 2 divided doses daily. Some experts state that the usual dosage range is 10–40 mg daily, given as a single dose or in 2 divided doses. Higher dosages (i.e., 80 mg daily) reportedly have resulted in increased response; however, there is limited experience with such dosages. The safety and efficacy of dosages exceeding 80 mg daily have not been established. If blood pressure is not controlled with benazepril alone, a second antihypertensive agent (e.g., diuretic) may be added.

For the management of hypertension in children 6 years of age or older, the usual initial dosage of benazepril hydrochloride is 0.2 mg/kg (up to 10 mg) once daily. Dosage may be adjusted until the desired blood pressure goal is achieved. Experts state that the dosage should be increased every 2–4 weeks until blood pressure is controlled, the maximum dosage is reached, or adverse effects occur. The safety and efficacy of dosages exceeding 0.6 mg/kg or in excess of 40 mg daily have not been established in pediatric patients. For information on overall principles and expert recommendations for treatment of hypertension in pediatric patients, see Uses: Hypertension in Pediatric Patients, in the Thiazides General Statement 40:28.20.

Benazepril/Hydrochlorothiazide Fixed-combination Therapy

The manufacturers state that therapy with the commercially available preparations containing benazepril hydrochloride in fixed combination with hydrochlorothiazide should only be initiated in adults after an adequate response is not achieved with benazepril or hydrochlorothiazide monotherapy. Alternatively, the fixed combination containing benazepril with hydrochlorothiazide may be used in patients who had been receiving the drugs separately and in whom dosage of the individual drugs has been adjusted. Patients whose blood pressure is not adequately controlled with benazepril or hydrochlorothiazide monotherapy may receive the fixed combination containing 10 mg of benazepril hydrochloride and 12.5 mg of hydrochlorothiazide initially. The maximum recommended dosage of the fixed combination preparation is 20 mg of benazepril hydrochloride and 25 mg of hydrochlorothiazide once daily.

Benazepril/Amlodipine Fixed-combination Therapy

The manufacturer states that therapy with the commercially available preparations containing benazepril hydrochloride in fixed combination with amlodipine should only be initiated in adults in whom an adequate response has not been achieved with benazepril or amlodipine monotherapy. Alternatively, such fixed combinations may be used if amlodipine dosages necessary for adequate response have been associated with development of edema. The fixed combination containing benazepril hydrochloride with amlodipine also may be used in patients who have been receiving the drugs separately, provided that the optimum dosage corresponds to the ratio in the commercial fixed-combination preparation. Dosage of the fixed combination containing benazepril hydrochloride and amlodipine should be adjusted according to the patient's response. The manufacturer states that when the fixed combinations containing 10–40 mg of benazepril hydrochloride and 2.5–10 mg of amlodipine have been used, the antihypertensive effects of these combinations have increased with increasing dosages of amlodipine regardless of race; in addition, antihypertensive effects increased with increasing dosages of benazepril in nonblack patients. The addition of benazepril to amlodipine therapy usually does not provide additional antihypertensive effects in black patients. The maximum recommended dosage of the fixed combination of benazepril hydrochloride and amlodipine is 40 mg of benazepril hydrochloride and 10 mg of amlodipine daily.

Blood Pressure Monitoring and Treatment Goals

Blood pressure should be monitored regularly (i.e., monthly) during therapy and dosage of the antihypertensive drug adjusted until blood pressure is controlled. If an adequate blood pressure response is not achieved with ACE inhibitor monotherapy, the dosage may be increased or another antihypertensive agent with demonstrated

benefit and preferably with a complementary mechanism of action (e.g., calcium-channel blocker, thiazide diuretic) may be added; if target blood pressure is still not achieved, a third drug may be added. (See Uses: Hypertension.) In patients who develop unacceptable adverse effects with benazepril, the drug should be discontinued and another antihypertensive agent from a different pharmacologic class should be initiated.

The goal of hypertension management and prevention is to achieve and maintain optimal control of blood pressure. However, the optimum blood pressure threshold for initiating antihypertensive drug therapy and specific treatment goals remain controversial. While other hypertension guidelines have based target blood pressure goals on age and comorbidities, a 2017 multidisciplinary hypertension guideline from the American College of Cardiology (ACC), American Heart Association (AHA), and a number of other professional organizations incorporates underlying cardiovascular risk into decision making regarding treatment and generally recommends the same target blood pressure (i.e., less than 130/80 mm Hg) in all adults. Many patients will require at least 2 drugs from different pharmacologic classes to achieve this blood pressure goal; the potential benefits of hypertension management and drug cost, adverse effects, and risks associated with the use of multiple antihypertensive drugs also should be considered when deciding a patient's blood pressure treatment goal.

For additional information on target levels of blood pressure and on monitoring therapy in the management of hypertension, see Blood Pressure Monitoring and Treatment Goals under Dosage: Hypertension, in Dosage and Administration in the Thiazides General Statement 40:28.20.

● Special Populations

If benazepril is used in patients with impaired renal function, dosage must be modified in response to the degree of renal impairment, and, as with other ACE inhibitors, the theoretical risk of neutropenia must be considered. In adults with creatinine clearances less than 30 mL/minute per 1.73 m^2 or serum creatinine concentrations exceeding 3 mg/dL, the recommended initial dosage of benazepril hydrochloride is 5 mg once daily. If an adequate response is not achieved, dosage may be increased gradually until blood pressure is controlled or a maximum benazepril hydrochloride dosage of 40 mg daily is reached. There are insufficient data to date to make recommendations regarding dosage of benazepril hydrochloride in children with creatinine clearances less than 30 mL/minute per 1.73 m^2, and the manufacturer recommends that benazepril therapy not be used in such patients. Safety and efficacy of the fixed combination containing benazepril and hydrochlorothiazide have not been established in patients with severe renal impairment. Use of the commercially available preparation containing benazepril in combination with amlodipine is not recommended for patients with severe renal impairment.

Because of the greater frequency of decreased renal function in geriatric patients, the manufacturer states that dosage selection should be made with care and that it may be useful to monitor renal function in such patients receiving benazepril.

Preparations containing benazepril hydrochloride in fixed combination with 5 or 10 mg of amlodipine exceed the recommended initial dosage of amlodipine (2.5 mg daily) in geriatric patients and patients with hepatic impairment.

CAUTIONS

● Contraindications

Benazepril is contraindicated in patients with known hypersensitivity to benazepril, other angiotensin-converting enzyme (ACE) inhibitors, or any ingredient in the formulation; those with a history of angioedema with or without prior ACE inhibitor therapy; and in patients with diabetes mellitus who are receiving aliskiren therapy. Benazepril also is contraindicated in combination with a neprilysin inhibitor (e.g., sacubitril) and should not be administered within 36 hours of switching to or from sacubitril/valsartan.

● Warnings/Precautions

Warnings

Fetal/Neonatal Morbidity and Mortality

Drugs that act directly on the renin-angiotensin system (e.g., ACE inhibitors, angiotensin II receptor antagonists) reduce fetal renal function and can cause fetal and neonatal morbidity and mortality when used during pregnancy. Such potential risks of these drugs occur throughout pregnancy, especially during the second and third trimesters. ACE inhibitors also have been reported to increase the risk of major congenital malformations when administered during the first trimester of pregnancy. Potential neonatal effects include skull hypoplasia, anuria, hypotension, renal failure, and death. Resulting oligohydramnios can be associated with fetal lung hypoplasia and skeletal deformations. ACE inhibitors (e.g., benazepril) should be discontinued as soon as possible when pregnancy is detected, unless continued use is considered lifesaving. Nearly all women can be transferred successfully to alternative therapy for the remainder of pregnancy. For additional information on the risk of ACE inhibitors during pregnancy, see Cautions: Pregnancy, Fertility, and Lactation, in Captopril 24:32.04 and in Enalaprilat/Enalapril 24:32.04.

Sensitivity Reactions

Sensitivity reactions, including anaphylactoid reactions and angioedema (including laryngeal angioedema and tongue edema), are potentially fatal. Head and neck angioedema have occurred in patients receiving an ACE inhibitor and have been reported at a higher rate in black patients compared with patients of other races. Patients with a history of angioedema unrelated to ACE inhibitor therapy may be at increased risk of angioedema while receiving an ACE inhibitor. In addition, concomitant use of an ACE inhibitor and a mammalian target of rapamycin (mTOR) inhibitor (e.g., everolimus, sirolimus, temsirolimus) or a neprilysin inhibitor (e.g., sacubitril) may increase the risk of angioedema; patients should be monitored for signs of angioedema during such concomitant therapy. Head and neck angioedema involving the tongue, glottis, or larynx may cause airway obstruction, especially in those with a history of airway surgery. If laryngeal stridor or angioedema of the face, tongue, or glottis occurs, ACE inhibitors (e.g., benazepril) should be discontinued promptly and appropriate therapy (e.g., epinephrine) and monitoring initiated until complete and sustained resolution of manifestations of angioedema has occurred.

Intestinal angioedema (occasionally without a prior history of facial angioedema or elevated serum levels of complement 1 [C1] esterase inhibitor) also has been reported in patients receiving ACE inhibitors. Intestinal angioedema, which frequently presents as abdominal pain (with or without nausea or vomiting), usually is diagnosed by abdominal CT scan, ultrasound, or surgery; symptoms usually have resolved after discontinuance of the ACE inhibitor. Intestinal angioedema should be considered in the differential diagnosis of patients who develop abdominal pain during therapy with an ACE inhibitor.

Life-threatening anaphylactoid reactions have been reported in at least 2 patients receiving ACE inhibitors while undergoing desensitization treatment with hymenoptera venom. When ACE inhibitors were temporarily discontinued before desensitization with the venom, anaphylactoid reactions did not recur; however, such reactions recurred after inadvertent rechallenge. Anaphylactoid reactions also have been reported following initiation of hemodialysis that used a high-flux membrane in patients receiving an ACE inhibitor. In addition, anaphylactoid reactions have been reported in patients undergoing low-density lipoprotein (LDL) apheresis with dextran sulfate absorption. In such patients, dialysis must be stopped immediately, and aggressive treatment for anaphylactoid reactions must be initiated. Antihistamine treatment has been ineffective in the alleviation of symptoms in these situations. In these patients, consideration should be given to using a different type of dialysis membrane or a different class of antihypertensive drug.

Other Warnings and Precautions
Renal Effects

Deterioration of renal function, including acute renal failure, may occur in patients receiving ACE inhibitor therapy. Patients whose renal function depends on the activity of the renin-angiotensin system, particularly those with unilateral or bilateral renal artery stenosis, chronic kidney disease (CKD), severe congestive heart failure, myocardial infarction (MI), or volume depletion, may be at particular risk of developing acute renal failure while receiving benazepril. Increases in BUN and serum creatinine concentrations have occurred in patients with unilateral or bilateral renal artery stenosis; such increases generally are reversible following discontinuance of benazepril and/or diuretic therapy. Renal function should be monitored periodically in patients receiving benazepril. Withholding or discontinuance of therapy should be considered in patients who develop clinically important decreases in renal function while receiving benazepril.

Cardiovascular Effects

Symptomatic hypotension may occur; patients at particular risk include those with heart failure with systolic blood pressure less than 100 mm Hg, ischemic heart disease, cerebrovascular disease, hyponatremia, high-dose diuretic therapy, renal dialysis, or severe volume and/or salt depletion of any etiology. Symptomatic hypotension also may occur in patients with severe aortic stenosis. Volume and/or salt depletion should be corrected before starting benazepril therapy.

Excessive hypotension may occur in patients with heart failure (with or without associated renal impairment), which may be associated with oliguria and/or progressive azotemia and, rarely, acute renal failure and/or death. In patients with heart failure, benazepril therapy should be started under close medical supervision and patients should be followed closely for at least 2 weeks after initiation of benazepril or diuretic therapy or dosage adjustment of either drug. (See Dosage and Administration: Dosage.) Benazepril therapy should be avoided in patients who have hemodynamic instability following MI.

If hypotension occurs, the patient should be placed in the supine position, and if necessary, an IV infusion of 0.9% sodium chloride injection to expand fluid volume may be administered. Benazepril therapy usually may be continued following restoration of blood pressure and volume.

Hypotension may occur in patients undergoing major surgery or during anesthesia with agents that produce hypotension due to ACE inhibitor blockade of angiotensin II formation secondary to compensatory renin release. Hypotension in such patients may be corrected by volume expansion.

Effects on Potassium

Hyperkalemia can develop in patients receiving drugs that inhibit the renin-angiotensin system, especially in those with renal impairment or diabetes mellitus and those receiving other drugs that can increase serum potassium concentration (e.g., potassium-sparing diuretics, potassium supplements, potassium-containing salt substitutes). Serum potassium concentrations should be monitored periodically in patients receiving benazepril.

Hepatic Effects

An ACE inhibitor-associated clinical syndrome manifested initially by cholestatic jaundice has occurred; the syndrome may progress to fulminant hepatic necrosis and is potentially fatal. Patients receiving an ACE inhibitor, including benazepril, who develop jaundice or marked elevations of hepatic enzymes should discontinue the drug and receive appropriate monitoring and medical follow-up.

Hematologic Effects

Neutropenia/agranulocytosis, particularly in patients with renal impairment (especially those with concomitant collagen vascular disease), have been reported with another ACE inhibitor (captopril). Data are insufficient to rule out a similar incidence of agranulocytosis with benazepril in patients without prior reactions to other ACE inhibitors. Monitoring of leukocyte counts in patients with collagen vascular disease, especially if renal impairment exists, should be considered.

Respiratory Effects

Persistent, nonproductive cough has been reported with all ACE inhibitors; this effect resolves after drug discontinuance. ACE inhibitor-induced cough should be considered in the differential diagnosis of patients who develop cough during benazepril therapy.

Use of Fixed Combinations

When hydrochlorothiazide, amlodipine, or other drugs are used in fixed combination with benazepril, the usual cautions, precautions, and contraindications associated with these other drugs must be considered in addition to those associated with benazepril. (See Cautions, in the Thiazides General Statement 40:28.20 and in Amlodipine Besylate 24:28.08.)

Specific Populations
Pregnancy

Category D. (See Users Guide.) Benazepril can cause fetal and neonatal morbidity and mortality when administered to a pregnant woman. Benazepril should be discontinued as soon as possible when pregnancy is detected. (See Fetal/Neonatal Morbidity and Mortality under Warnings/Precautions: Warnings, in Cautions.)

Lactation

Benazepril and benazeprilat are distributed into human milk in minimal amounts. Because of the unknown effects of benazepril or benazeprilat in nursing infants, a decision should be made whether to discontinue nursing or benazepril, taking into account the importance of the drug(s) to the woman.

Pediatric Use

If oliguria or hypotension occurs in neonates with a history of in utero exposure to benazepril, blood pressure and renal function should be supported; exchange transfusions or dialysis may be required. (See Fetal/Neonatal Morbidity and

Mortality under Warnings/Precautions: Warnings, in Cautions.) Benazepril, which crosses the placenta, can theoretically be removed from the neonatal circulation by these means. There are occasional reports of benefit from these maneuvers with another ACE inhibitor; however, experience is limited.

Safety and efficacy of benazepril have not been established in children younger than 6 years of age and in pediatric patients with creatinine clearances of less than 30 mL/minute. Safety and efficacy of benazepril in fixed combination with amlodipine or hydrochlorothiazide have not been established in children. The long-term effects of benazepril on growth and development in children have not been studied. Although the safety profile of benazepril in pediatric patients is similar to that in adults, because of the potential for adverse effects on kidney development, ACE inhibitors should not be administered to pediatric patients younger than 1 year of age. For information on overall principles and expert recommendations for treatment of hypertension in pediatric patients, see Uses: Hypertension in Pediatric Patients, in the Thiazides General Statement 40:28.20.

Geriatric Use

No substantial differences in safety and efficacy have been observed in geriatric patients relative to younger adults, but increased sensitivity cannot be ruled out.

Because geriatric patients are more likely to have decreased renal function, dosage should be selected cautiously; it may be useful to monitor renal function in such patients.

Renal Impairment

Renal function may decrease with ACE inhibitor therapy in susceptible patients. Benazepril should be used with caution in those with renal impairment.

Benazepril in fixed combination with amlodipine is not recommended in patients with severe renal impairment; the recommended daily dosage of benazepril hydrochloride in such patients is 5 mg, which is not available in this combination preparation. (See Dosage and Administration: Special Populations and also Renal Effects under Warnings/Precautions: Other Warnings and Precautions, in Cautions.)

Black Patients

ACE inhibitors are not as effective and are associated with a higher incidence of angioedema in black patients compared with patients of other races. (See Uses: Hypertension.)

● Common Adverse Effects

Adverse effects reported in at least 2% of patients receiving benazepril and at an incidence more than 1% greater than that with placebo include headache, dizziness, somnolence, and postural dizziness. Adverse effects reported in greater than 1% of patients receiving benazepril in fixed combination with hydrochlorothiazide and possibly or probably study drug-related include dizziness, fatigue, postural dizziness, headache, cough, hypertonia, vertigo, nausea, impotence, and somnolence. Adverse effects reported in greater than 1% of patients receiving benazepril in fixed combination with amlodipine and possibly or probably drug-related include cough, headache, dizziness, and edema.

DRUG INTERACTIONS

● Antidiabetic Agents

Concomitant administration of benazepril and insulin or oral antidiabetic agents may increase the risk of hypoglycemia. Patients receiving these drugs concomitantly should be informed of the possibility of hypoglycemia and monitored appropriately; dosage of the antidiabetic drug may need to be altered.

● Antihypertensive Agents and Drugs that Block the Renin-Angiotensin System

Benazepril potentiates the antihypertensive effect of other antihypertensive agents and drugs that block the renin-angiotensin system (e.g., curare derivatives, guanethidine, methyldopa, β-adrenergic blocking agents, vasodilators, calcium-channel blocking agents, ACE inhibitors, angiotensin II receptor antagonists, direct renin inhibitors [DRIs]).

Dual blockade of the renin-angiotensin system with angiotensin II receptor antagonists, ACE inhibitors, or aliskiren is associated with increased risks of

hypotension, hyperkalemia, and changes in renal function (including acute renal failure) compared with monotherapy. Most patients receiving the combination of 2 renin-angiotensin system blocking agents do not obtain additional benefit compared with monotherapy. Concomitant use of 2 renin-angiotensin system blocking agents generally should be avoided. Blood pressure, renal function, and electrolytes should be closely monitored in patients receiving benazepril with other agents that affect the renin-angiotensin system.

● Diuretics

Potential pharmacokinetic and pharmacologic interaction (hypotensive effect).

● Drugs Increasing Serum Potassium Concentration

Potential pharmacologic interaction (additive hyperkalemic effect). Includes potassium-sparing diuretics, potassium supplements, and other drugs that can cause hyperkalemia. (See Effects on Potassium under Warnings/Precautions: Cautions: Other Warnings and Precautions, in Cautions.)

● Gold

Nitritoid reactions (e.g., facial flushing, nausea, vomiting, hypotension) have been reported rarely in patients receiving concomitant therapy with injectable gold (sodium aurothiomalate) and an ACE inhibitor.

● Lithium

Potential pharmacokinetic interaction (increased lithium concentrations and clinical toxicity). Lithium toxicity usually is reversible following discontinuance of lithium or benazepril. Serum lithium concentrations should be monitored during such concomitant use.

● Mammalian Target of Rapamycin Inhibitors

Concomitant use of an ACE inhibitor and a mammalian target of rapamycin (mTOR) inhibitor (e.g., everolimus, sirolimus, temsirolimus) may increase the risk of angioedema. (See Sensitivity Reactions under Cautions: Warnings/Precautions.)

● Neprilysin Inhibitors

Concomitant use of benazepril and a neprilysin inhibitor (e.g., sacubitril) may increase the risk for angioedema. (See Sensitivity Reactions under Cautions: Warnings/Precautions.)

● Nonsteroidal Anti-inflammatory Agents

In geriatric patients, patients who are volume depleted (including those who are receiving diuretic therapy), or in patients with compromised renal function, concomitant use of nonsteroidal anti-inflammatory agents (NSAIAs), including cyclooxygenase-2 (COX-2) inhibitors, with ACE inhibitors may result in the deterioration of renal function, including possible renal failure. These effects are usually reversible. Renal function should be monitored periodically in patients receiving concomitant benazepril and NSAIA therapy.

DESCRIPTION

Benazepril is an angiotensin-converting enzyme (ACE, bradykininase, kininase II) inhibitor. Benazepril, the ethylester of benazeprilat, is a prodrug and has little pharmacologic activity until hydrolyzed in the liver to benazeprilat. Like enalapril, fosinopril, lisinopril, quinapril, and ramipril, but unlike captopril, benazepril does not contain a sulfhydryl group.

ADVICE TO PATIENTS

When benazepril is used in fixed combination with hydrochlorothiazide, amlodipine, or other drugs, importance of advising patients about important precautionary information regarding the concomitant agent.

Risk of angioedema (including laryngeal edema), anaphylactoid, and other sensitivity reactions. Importance of discontinuing drug and reporting manifestations suggestive of angioedema (e.g., edema of face, eyes, lips, or tongue; swallowing or breathing with difficulty) to a clinician.

Risk of symptomatic hypotension (e.g., lightheadedness, syncope), especially during initial therapy or with volume depletion secondary to excessive perspiration, vomiting, or diarrhea; importance of reporting such symptoms to clinician. Importance of discontinuing drug and contacting clinician if syncope occurs.

Importance of informing clinicians of existing or contemplated concomitant therapy, including prescription and OTC drugs. Risk of hyperkalemia and hypoglycemia. Importance of avoiding the use of potassium supplements or salt substitutes containing potassium without consulting a clinician. Importance of monitoring closely for hypoglycemia in patients receiving oral antidiabetic agents or insulin, especially during first month of combined use with benazepril.

Risks of use during pregnancy. Importance of women informing clinicians immediately if they are or plan to become pregnant or plan to breast-feed; importance of discussing other options for hypertension treatment if pregnancy occurs.

Importance of informing patients of other important precautionary information. (See Cautions.)

PREPARATIONS

Excipients in commercially available drug preparations may have clinically important effects in some individuals; consult specific product labeling for details.

Benazepril Hydrochloride

Oral

Tablets, film-coated	5 mg*	**Benazepril Hydrochloride Tablets** Lotensin®, Validus
	10 mg*	**Benazepril Hydrochloride Tablets** Lotensin®, Validus
	20 mg*	**Benazepril Hydrochloride Tablets** Lotensin®, Validus
	40 mg*	**Benazepril Hydrochloride Tablets** Lotensin®, Validus

* available from one or more manufacturer, distributor, and/or repackager by generic (nonproprietary) name

Benazepril Hydrochloride Combinations

Oral

Capsules	10 mg with Amlodipine Besylate 2.5 mg (of amlodipine)*	**Amlodipine Besylate and Benazepril Hydrochloride Capsules** Lotrel®, Novartis
	10 mg with Amlodipine Besylate 5 mg (of amlodipine)*	**Amlodipine Besylate and Benazepril Hydrochloride Capsules** Lotrel®, Novartis
	20 mg with Amlodipine Besylate 5 mg (of amlodipine)*	**Amlodipine Besylate and Benazepril Hydrochloride Capsules** Lotrel®, Novartis
	20 mg with Amlodipine Besylate 10 mg (of amlodipine)*	**Amlodipine Besylate and Benazepril Hydrochloride Capsules** Lotrel®, Novartis
	40 mg with Amlodipine Besylate 5 mg (of amlodipine)*	**Amlodipine Besylate and Benazepril Hydrochloride Capsules** Lotrel®, Novartis
	40 mg with Amlodipine Besylate 10 mg (of amlodipine)*	**Amlodipine Besylate and Benazepril Hydrochloride Capsules** Lotrel®, Novartis
Tablets, film-coated	5 mg with Hydrochlorothiazide 6.25 mg*	**Benazepril with Hydrochlorothiazide Tablets** Lotensin® HCT (scored), Validus
	10 mg with Hydrochlorothiazide 12.5 mg*	**Benazepril with Hydrochlorothiazide Tablets** Lotensin® HCT (scored), Validus
	20 mg with Hydrochlorothiazide 12.5 mg*	**Benazepril with Hydrochlorothiazide Tablets** Lotensin® HCT (scored), Validus
	20 mg with Hydrochlorothiazide 25 mg*	**Benazepril with Hydrochlorothiazide Tablets** Lotensin® HCT (scored), Validus

* available from one or more manufacturer, distributor, and/or repackager by generic (nonproprietary) name

† Use is not currently included in the labeling approved by the US Food and Drug Administration.

Selected Revisions November 5, 2018, © Copyright, May 1, 1992, American Society of Health-System Pharmacists, Inc.

Captopril, Captopril and Hydrochlorothiazide

24:32.04 • ANGIOTENSIN CONVERTING ENZYME INHIBITORS

■ Captopril is an angiotensin-converting enzyme (ACE) inhibitor.

USES

● Hypertension

Captopril is used alone or in combination with other classes of antihypertensive agents in the management of hypertension. Because captopril can cause serious adverse effects (e.g., neutropenia, agranulocytosis), particularly in patients with renal impairment (especially those with collagen vascular disease) or in patients receiving immunosuppressive therapy, the drug was previously reserved for hypertension (usually severe) that was not manageable with maximal therapeutic dosages of other hypotensive agents in combination regimens (e.g., usually a diuretic, a β-adrenergic blocking agent [β-blocker], and a vasodilator) or when such regimens produced intolerable adverse effects. However, clinical experience with low dosages (up to 150 mg daily) has shown captopril to have a favorable benefit-to-risk ratio in the management of mild to moderate hypertension and the drug may currently be used as initial therapy in patients with normal renal function, in whom the risk of adverse hematologic effects is relatively low. In patients with impaired renal function, especially those with collagen vascular disease, captopril should be reserved for patients in whom other antihypertensive agents produce intolerable adverse effects or who do not have an adequate response to combination regimens of antihypertensive agents.

Current evidence-based practice guidelines for the management of hypertension in adults generally recommend the use of drugs from 4 classes of antihypertensive agents (angiotensin-converting enzyme [ACE] inhibitors, angiotensin II receptor antagonists, calcium-channel blockers, and thiazide diuretics); data from clinical outcome trials indicate that lowering blood pressure with any of these drug classes can reduce the complications of hypertension and provide similar cardiovascular protection. However, recommendations for initial drug selection and use in specific patient populations may vary across these expert guidelines. This variability is due, in part, to differences in the guideline development process and the types of studies (e.g., randomized controlled studies only versus a range of studies with different study designs) included in the evidence reviews. Ultimately, choice of antihypertensive therapy should be individualized, considering the clinical characteristics of the patient (e.g., age, ethnicity/race, comorbid conditions, cardiovascular risk factors) as well as drug-related factors (e.g., ease of administration, availability, adverse effects, costs). Because many patients eventually will need drugs from 2 or more antihypertensive classes, experts generally state that the emphasis should be placed on achieving appropriate blood pressure control rather than on identifying a preferred drug to achieve that control.

Disease Overview

Worldwide, hypertension is the most common modifiable risk factor for cardiovascular events and mortality. The lifetime risk of developing hypertension in the US exceeds 80%, with higher rates observed among African Americans and Hispanics compared with whites or Asians. The systolic blood pressure and diastolic blood pressure values defined as hypertension (see Blood Pressure Classification under Uses: Hypertension) in a 2017 multidisciplinary guideline of the American College of Cardiology (ACC), American Heart Association (AHA), and a number of other professional organizations (subsequently referred to as the 2017 ACC/AHA hypertension guideline in this monograph) are lower than those defined in the Seventh Report of the Joint National Committee on Prevention, Detection, Evaluation, and Treatment of High Blood Pressure (JNC 7) guidelines, which results in an increase of approximately 14% in the prevalence of hypertension in the US. However, this change in definition results in only a 2% increase in the percentage of patients requiring antihypertensive drug therapy because nonpharmacologic treatment is recommended for most adults now classified by the 2017 ACC/AHA hypertension guideline as hypertensive who would *not* meet the JNC 7 definition of hypertension. Among US adults receiving antihypertensive drugs,

approximately 53% have inadequately controlled blood pressure according to current ACC/AHA treatment goals.

Cardiovascular and Renal Sequelae

The principal goal of preventing and treating hypertension is to reduce the risk of cardiovascular and renal morbidity and mortality, including target organ damage. The relationship between blood pressure and cardiovascular disease is continuous, consistent, and independent of other risk factors. It is important that very high blood pressure be managed promptly to reduce the risk of target organ damage. The higher the blood pressure, the more likely the development of myocardial infarction (MI), heart failure, stroke, and renal disease. For adults 40–70 years of age, each 20-mm Hg increment in systolic blood pressure or 10-mm Hg increment in diastolic blood pressure doubles the risk of developing cardiovascular disease across the entire blood pressure range of 115/75 to 185/115 mm Hg. For those older than 50 years of age, systolic blood pressure is a much more important risk factor for developing cardiovascular disease than is diastolic blood pressure. The rapidity with which treatment is required depends on the patient's clinical presentation (presence of new or worsening target organ damage) and the presence or absence of cardiovascular complications; the 2017 ACC/AHA hypertension guideline states that treatment of very high blood pressure should be initiated within 1 week.

Blood Pressure Classification

Accurate blood pressure measurement is essential for the proper diagnosis and management of hypertension. Error in measuring blood pressure is a major cause of inadequate blood pressure control and may lead to overtreatment. Because a patient's blood pressure may vary in an unpredictable fashion, a single blood pressure measurement is not sufficient for clinical decision-making. An average of 2 or 3 blood pressure measurements obtained on 2–3 separate occasions using proper technique should be used to minimize random error and provide a more accurate blood pressure reading. Out-of-office blood pressure measurements may be useful for confirming and managing hypertension. The 2017 ACC/AHA hypertension guideline document (available on the ACC and AHA websites) should be consulted for key steps on properly measuring blood pressure.

According to the 2017 ACC/AHA hypertension guideline, blood pressure in adults is classified into 4 categories: normal, elevated, stage 1 hypertension, and stage 2 hypertension.(See Table 1.) The 2017 ACC/AHA hypertension guideline lowers the blood pressure threshold used to define hypertension in the US; previous hypertension guidelines (JNC 7) considered adults with systolic blood pressure of 120–139 mm Hg or diastolic blood pressure of 80–89 mm Hg to have prehypertension, those with systolic blood pressure of 140–159 mm Hg or diastolic blood pressure of 90–99 mm Hg to have stage 1 hypertension, and those with systolic blood pressure of 160 mm Hg or higher or diastolic blood pressure of 100 mm Hg or higher to have stage 2 hypertension. The blood pressure definitions in the 2017 ACC/AHA hypertension guideline are based upon data from studies evaluating the association between systolic blood pressure/diastolic blood pressure and cardiovascular risk and the benefits of blood pressure reduction. Individuals with systolic blood pressure and diastolic blood pressure in 2 different categories should be designated as being in the higher blood pressure category.

TABLE 1. ACC/AHA Blood Pressure Classification in Adults[ab]

Category	SBP[c] (mm Hg)		DBP[d] (mm Hg)
Normal	<120	and	<80
Elevated	120–129	and	<80
Hypertension, Stage 1	130–139	or	80–89
Hypertension, Stage 2	≥140	or	≥90

[a] Source: Whelton PK, Carey RM, Aronow WS et al. 2017 ACC/AHA/AAPA/ABC/ACPM/AGS/APhA/ASH/ASPC/NMA/PCNA guideline for the prevention, detection, evaluation, and management of high blood pressure in adults: a report of the American College of Cardiology/American Heart Association Task Force on Clinical Practice Guidelines. *Hypertension*. 2018;71:e13-115.

[b] Individuals with SBP and DBP in 2 different categories (e.g., elevated SBP and normal DBP) should be designated as being in the higher blood pressure category (i.e., elevated BP).

[c] Systolic blood pressure

[d] Diastolic blood pressure

The blood pressure thresholds used to define hypertension, when to initiate drug therapy, and the ideal target blood pressure values remain controversial. The 2017 ACC/AHA hypertension guideline recommends a blood pressure goal of less than 130/80 mm Hg in all adults who have confirmed hypertension and known cardiovascular disease or a 10-year atherosclerotic cardiovascular disease (ASCVD) event risk of 10% or higher; the ACC/AHA guideline also states that this blood pressure goal is reasonable to attempt to achieve in adults with confirmed hypertension who do *not* have increased cardiovascular risk. The lower blood pressure values used to define hypertension and the lower target blood pressure goals outlined in the 2017 ACC/AHA hypertension guideline are based on clinical studies demonstrating a substantial reduction in the composite end point of major cardiovascular disease events and the combination of fatal and nonfatal stroke when a lower systolic blood pressure/diastolic blood pressure value (i.e., 130/80 mm Hg) was used to define hypertension. These lower target blood pressure goals also are based upon clinical studies demonstrating continuing reduction of cardiovascular risk at progressively lower levels of systolic blood pressure. A linear relationship has been demonstrated between cardiovascular risk and blood pressure even at low systolic blood pressures (e.g., 120–124 mm Hg). The 2017 ACC/AHA hypertension guideline recommends estimating a patient's ASCVD risk using the ACC/AHA Pooled Cohort equations (available online at http://tools.acc.org/ASCVD-Risk-Estimator), which are based on a variety of factors including age, race, gender, cholesterol levels, statin use, blood pressure, treatment for hypertension, history of diabetes mellitus, smoking status, and aspirin use. While the 2017 ACC/AHA hypertension guideline has lowered the threshold for *diagnosing* hypertension in adults, the threshold for *initiating drug therapy* has only been lowered for those patients who are at high risk of cardiovascular disease. Clinicians who support the 2017 ACC/AHA hypertension guideline believe that these recommendations have the potential to increase hypertension awareness, encourage lifestyle modification, and focus antihypertensive drug initiation and intensification in those adults at high risk for cardiovascular disease.

The lower blood pressure goals advocated in the 2017 ACC/AHA hypertension guideline have been questioned by some clinicians who have concerns regarding the guideline's use of extrapolated observational data, the lack of generalizability of some of the randomized trials (e.g., SPRINT) used to support the guideline, the difficulty of establishing accurate representative blood pressure values in typical clinical practice settings, and the accuracy of the cardiovascular risk calculator used in the guideline. Some clinicians state the lower blood pressure threshold used to define hypertension in the 2017 ACC/AHA hypertension guideline is not fully supported by clinical data, and these clinicians have expressed concerns about the possible harms (e.g., adverse effects of antihypertensive therapy) associated with classifying more patients as being hypertensive. Some clinicians also state that using this guideline, a large number of young, low-risk patients would need to be treated in order to observe a clinical benefit, while other clinicians state that the estimated gains in life expectancy attributable to long-term use of blood pressure-lowering drugs are correspondingly greater in this patient population.

Treatment Benefits

In clinical trials, antihypertensive therapy has been found to reduce the risk of developing stroke by about 34–40%, MI by about 20–25%, and heart failure by more than 50%. In a randomized, controlled study (SPRINT) that included hypertensive patients without diabetes mellitus who had a high risk of cardiovascular disease, intensive systolic blood pressure lowering of approximately 15 mm Hg was associated with a 25% reduction in cardiovascular disease events and a 27% reduction in all-cause mortality. However, the exclusion of patients with diabetes mellitus, prior stroke, and those younger than 50 years of age may decrease the generalizability of these findings. Some experts estimate that if the systolic blood pressure goals of the 2017 ACC/AHA hypertension guideline are achieved, major cardiovascular disease events may be reduced by an additional 340,000 and total deaths by an additional 156,000 compared with implementation of the JNC 8 expert panel guideline goals but these benefits may be accompanied by an increase in the frequency of adverse events. While there was no overall difference in the occurrence of serious adverse events in patients receiving intensive therapy for blood pressure control (systolic blood pressure target of less than 120 mm Hg) compared with those receiving less intense control (systolic blood pressure target of less than 140 mm Hg) in the SPRINT study, hypotension, syncope, electrolyte abnormalities, and acute kidney injury or acute renal failure occurred in substantially more patients receiving intensive therapy.

In the Antihypertensive and Lipid-lowering Treatment to Prevent Heart Attack Trial (ALLHAT), the long-term cardiovascular morbidity and mortality benefit of a long-acting dihydropyridine calcium-channel blocker (amlodipine), a thiazide-like diuretic (chlorthalidone), and an ACE inhibitor (lisinopril) were compared in a broad population of patients with hypertension at risk for coronary heart disease. Although these antihypertensive agents were comparably effective in providing important cardiovascular benefit, apparent differences in certain secondary outcomes were observed. Patients receiving the ACE inhibitor experienced higher risks of stroke, combined cardiovascular disease, GI bleeding, and angioedema, while those receiving the calcium-channel blocker were at higher risk of developing heart failure. The ALLHAT investigators suggested that the favorable cardiovascular outcome may be attributable, at least in part, to the greater antihypertensive effect of the calcium-channel blocker compared with that of the ACE inhibitor, especially in women and black patients. See Clinical Benefit of Thiazides in Hypertension under Hypertension in Adults: Treatment Benefits, in Uses in the Thiazides General Statement 40:28.20.

General Considerations for Initial and Maintenance Antihypertensive Therapy

Nonpharmacologic Therapy

Nonpharmacologic measures (i.e., lifestyle/behavioral modifications) that are effective in lowering blood pressure include weight reduction (for those who are overweight or obese), dietary changes to include foods such as fruits, vegetables, whole grains, and low-fat dairy products that are rich in potassium, calcium, magnesium, and fiber (i.e., adoption of the Dietary Approaches to Stop Hypertension [DASH] eating plan), sodium reduction, increased physical activity, and moderation of alcohol intake. Such lifestyle/behavioral modifications, including smoking cessation, enhance antihypertensive drug efficacy and decrease cardiovascular risk and remain an indispensable part of the management of hypertension. Lifestyle/behavioral modifications without antihypertensive drug therapy are recommended for individuals classified by the 2017 ACC/AHA hypertension guideline as having elevated blood pressure (systolic blood pressure 120–129 mm Hg and diastolic blood pressure less than 80 mm Hg) and in those with stage 1 hypertension (systolic blood pressure 130–139 mm Hg or diastolic blood pressure 80–89 mm Hg) who do *not* have preexisting cardiovascular disease or an estimated 10-year ASCVD risk of 10% or greater.

Initiation of Drug Therapy

Drug therapy in the management of hypertension must be individualized and adjusted based on the degree of blood pressure elevation while also considering cardiovascular risk factors. Drug therapy generally is reserved for patients who respond inadequately to nondrug therapies or in whom the degree of blood pressure elevation or coexisting risk factors, especially increased cardiovascular risk, require more prompt or aggressive therapy; however, the optimum blood pressure threshold for initiating antihypertensive drug therapy and specific treatment goals remain controversial. Recommendations generally are based on specific blood pressure levels shown in clinical studies to produce clinical benefits and can therefore vary depending on the studies selected for review.

The 2017 ACC/AHA hypertension guideline and many experts currently state that the treatment of hypertension should be based not only on blood pressure values but also on patients' cardiovascular risk factors. For *secondary prevention* of recurrent cardiovascular disease events in adults with clinical cardiovascular disease or for *primary prevention* in adults with an estimated 10-year ASCVD risk of 10% or higher, the 2017 ACC/AHA hypertension guideline recommends initiation of antihypertensive drug therapy in conjunction with lifestyle/behavioral modifications at an average systolic blood pressure of 130 mm Hg or an average diastolic blood pressure of 80 mm Hg or higher. For *primary prevention* of cardiovascular disease events in adults with a low (less than 10%) estimated 10-year risk of ASCVD, the 2017 ACC/AHA hypertension guideline recommends initiation of antihypertensive drug therapy in conjunction with lifestyle/behavioral modifications at a systolic blood pressure of 140 mm Hg or higher or a diastolic blood pressure of 90 mm Hg or higher. After initiation of antihypertensive drug therapy, regardless of the ASCVD risk, the 2017 ACC/AHA hypertension guideline generally recommends a blood pressure goal of less than 130/80 mm Hg in all adults. In addition, a systolic blood pressure goal of less than 130 mm Hg is also recommended for noninstitutionalized ambulatory patients 65 years of age or older. While these blood pressure goals are lower than those recommended for most patients in previous guidelines, they are based upon clinical studies demonstrating continuing reduction of cardiovascular risk at progressively lower levels of systolic blood pressure.

Most data indicate that patients with a higher cardiovascular risk will benefit the most from tighter blood pressure control; however, some experts state this treatment goal also may be beneficial in those at lower cardiovascular risk. Other clinicians believe that the benefits of such blood pressure lowering do not outweigh the risks in those patients considered to be at lower risk of cardiovascular disease and that reclassifying individuals formerly considered to have prehypertension as having hypertension may potentially lead to use of drug therapy in such patients without consideration of cardiovascular risk. Previous hypertension guidelines, such as those from the JNC 8 expert panel, generally recommended initiation of antihypertensive treatment in patients with a systolic blood pressure of at least 140 mm Hg or diastolic blood pressure of at least 90 mm Hg, targeted a blood pressure goal of less than 140/90 mm Hg regardless of cardiovascular risk, and used higher systolic blood pressure thresholds and targets in geriatric patients. Some clinicians continue to support the target blood pressures recommended by the JNC 8 expert panel because of concerns that such recommendations in the 2017 ACC/AHA hypertension guideline are based on extrapolation of data from the high-risk population in the SPRINT study to a lower-risk population. Also, because more than 90% of patients in SPRINT were already receiving antihypertensive drugs at baseline, data are lacking on the effects of *initiating* drug therapy at a lower blood pressure threshold (130/80 mm Hg) in patients at high risk of cardiovascular disease. The potential benefits of hypertension management and drug cost, adverse effects, and risks associated with the use of multiple antihypertensive drugs should be considered when deciding a patient's blood pressure treatment goal.

The 2017 ACC/AHA hypertension guideline recommends an ASCVD risk assessment for all adults with hypertension; however, experts state that it can be assumed that patients with hypertension and diabetes mellitus or chronic kidney disease (CKD) are at high risk for cardiovascular disease and that antihypertensive drug therapy should be initiated in these patients at a blood pressure of 130/80 mm Hg or higher. The 2017 ACC/AHA guideline also recommends a blood pressure goal of less than 130/80 mm Hg in patients with hypertension and diabetes mellitus or CKD. These recommendations are based on a systematic review of high-quality evidence from randomized controlled trials, meta-analyses, and post-hoc analyses that have demonstrated substantial reductions in the risk of important clinical outcomes (e.g., cardiovascular events) regardless of comorbid conditions or age when systolic blood pressure is lowered to less than 130 mm Hg. However, some clinicians have questioned the generalizability of findings from some of the trials (e.g., SPRINT) used to support the 2017 ACC/AHA hypertension guideline. For example, SPRINT included adults (mean age: 68 years) *without* diabetes mellitus who were at high risk of cardiovascular disease. While benefits of intensive blood pressure control were observed in this patient population, some clinicians have questioned whether these findings apply to younger patients who have a low risk of cardiovascular disease. In patients with CKD in the SPRINT trial, intensive blood pressure management (achieving a mean systolic blood pressure of approximately 122 mm Hg compared with 136 mm Hg with standard treatment) provided a similar beneficial reduction in the composite cardiovascular disease primary outcome and all-cause mortality as in the full patient cohort. Because most patients with CKD die from cardiovascular complications, the findings of this study further support a lower blood pressure target of less than 130/80 mm Hg.

Data are lacking to determine the ideal blood pressure goal in patients with hypertension and diabetes mellitus; also, studies evaluating the benefits of intensive blood pressure control in patients with diabetes mellitus have provided conflicting results. Clinical studies reviewed for the 2017 ACC/AHA hypertension guideline have shown similar quantitative benefits from blood pressure lowering in hypertensive patients with or without diabetes mellitus. In a randomized, controlled study (ACCORD-BP) that compared a higher (systolic blood pressure less than 140 mm Hg) versus lower (systolic blood pressure less than 120 mm Hg) blood pressure goal in patients with diabetes mellitus, there was no difference in the incidence of cardiovascular outcomes (e.g., composite outcome of cardiovascular death, nonfatal MI, and nonfatal stroke). However, some experts state that this study was underpowered to detect a difference between the 2 treatment groups and that the factorial design of the study complicated interpretation of the results. Although SPRINT did not include patients with diabetes mellitus, patients in this study with prediabetes demonstrated a similar cardiovascular benefit from intensive treatment of blood pressure as normoglycemic patients. A meta-analysis

of data from ACCORD and SPRINT suggests that the findings of both studies are consistent and that patients with diabetes mellitus benefit from more intensive blood pressure control. These data support the 2017 ACC/AHA hypertension guideline recommendation of a blood pressure treatment goal of less than 130/80 mm Hg in patients with hypertension and diabetes mellitus. Alternatively, the American Diabetes Association (ADA) recommends a blood pressure goal of less than 140/90 mm Hg in patients with diabetes mellitus. The ADA states that a lower blood pressure goal (e.g., less than 130/80 mm Hg) may be appropriate for patients with a high risk of cardiovascular disease and diabetes mellitus if it can be achieved without undue treatment burden.

Further study is needed to more clearly define optimum blood pressure goals in patients with hypertension, particularly in high-risk groups (e.g., patients with diabetes mellitus, cardiovascular disease, or cerebrovascular disease; black patients); when determining appropriate blood pressure goals, individual risks and benefits should be considered in addition to the evidence from clinical studies.

Choice of Initial Drug Therapy

In current hypertension management guidelines, ACE inhibitors are recommended as one of several preferred drugs for the initial treatment of hypertension; other options include angiotensin II receptor antagonists, calcium-channel blockers, and thiazide diuretics. The 2017 ACC/AHA hypertension guideline states that an ACE inhibitor, angiotensin II receptor antagonist, calcium-channel blocker, or thiazide diuretic (preferably chlorthalidone) are all acceptable choices for initial antihypertensive drug therapy in the general population of nonblack patients, including those with diabetes mellitus; drugs from any of these classes generally produce similar benefits in terms of overall mortality and cardiovascular, cerebrovascular, and renal outcomes. ACE inhibitors may be particularly useful in the management of hypertension in patients with certain coexisting conditions such as heart failure, ischemic heart disease, diabetes mellitus, CKD, or cerebrovascular disease or following myocardial infarction (MI). (See Considerations for Drug Therapy in Patients with Underlying Cardiovascular and Other Risk Factors under Uses: Hypertension.)

In patients with hypertension and compelling indications (e.g., CKD with albuminuria [urine albumin 300 mg/day or greater, or urine albumin:creatinine ratio of 300 mg/g or equivalent in the first morning void]), angiotensin II receptor antagonists are usually considered an alternative for ACE inhibitor-intolerant patients. (See Chronic Kidney Disease under Hypertension: Considerations for Drug Therapy in Patients with Underlying Cardiovascular and Other Risk Factors, in Uses.) However, data indicate no difference in efficacy between ACE inhibitors and angiotensin II receptor antagonists with regard to blood pressure lowering and clinical outcomes (i.e., all-cause mortality, cardiovascular mortality, MI, heart failure, stroke, and end-stage renal disease). Adverse events (e.g., cough, angioedema) leading to drug discontinuance occur more frequently with ACE inhibitor therapy than with angiotensin II receptor antagonist therapy. Because of similar efficacy and a lower frequency of adverse effects, some experts believe that angiotensin II receptor antagonists should be used instead of an ACE inhibitor for the treatment of hypertension or hypertension with certain compelling indications.

Experts state that in patients with stage 1 hypertension (especially the elderly, those with a history of hypotension, or those who have experienced adverse drug effects), it is reasonable to initiate drug therapy using the stepped-care approach in which one drug is initiated and titrated and other drugs are added sequentially to achieve the target blood pressure. Although some patients can begin treatment with a single antihypertensive agent, starting with 2 drugs in different pharmacologic classes (either as separate agents or in a fixed-dose combination) is recommended in patients with stage 2 hypertension and an average blood pressure more than 20/10 mm Hg above their target blood pressure. Such combined therapy may increase the likelihood of achieving goal blood pressure in a more timely fashion, but also may increase the risk of adverse effects (e.g., orthostatic hypotension) in some patients (e.g., elderly). Drug regimens with complementary activity, where a second antihypertensive agent is used to block compensatory responses to the first agent or affect a different pressor mechanism, can result in additive blood pressure lowering and are preferred. Drug combinations that have similar mechanisms of action or clinical effects (e.g., the combination of an ACE inhibitor and an angiotensin II receptor antagonist) generally should be avoided. Many patients who begin therapy with a single antihypertensive agent will subsequently require at least 2 drugs from different pharmacologic classes to achieve their blood pressure goal. Experts state that other patient-specific factors, such as age, concurrent medications, drug adherence, drug interactions, the overall treatment regimen, cost, and comorbidities, also should be considered when deciding on an antihypertensive drug regimen. For any stage of hypertension, antihypertensive drug dosages should be adjusted and/or other agents substituted or added until goal blood pressure is achieved. (See Follow-up and Maintenance Drug Therapy under Hypertension: General Considerations for Initial and Maintenance Antihypertensive Therapy, in Uses.)

Follow-up and Maintenance Drug Therapy

Several strategies are used for the titration and combination of antihypertensive drugs; these strategies, which are generally based on those used in randomized controlled studies, include maximizing the dosage of the first drug before adding a second drug, adding a second drug before achieving maximum dosage of the initial drug, or initiating therapy with 2 drugs simultaneously (either as separate preparations or as a fixed-dose combination). Combined use of an ACE inhibitor and angiotensin II receptor antagonist should be avoided because of the potential risk of adverse renal effects. After initiating a new or adjusted antihypertensive drug regimen, patients should have their blood pressure reevaluated monthly until adequate blood pressure control is achieved. Effective blood pressure control can be achieved in most hypertensive patients, but many will ultimately require therapy with 2 or more antihypertensive drugs. In addition to measuring blood pressure, clinicians should evaluate patients for orthostatic hypotension, adverse drug effects, adherence to drug therapy and lifestyle modifications, and the need for drug dosage adjustments. Laboratory testing such as electrolytes and renal function status and other assessments of target organ damage also should be performed.

Captopril can be used for the management of hypertension as initial monotherapy or as a component of a multiple-drug regimen. When captopril is used alone but the patient's hypertension does not respond adequately, addition of a thiazide diuretic often adequately controls blood pressure. Such combined therapy generally produces additive reduction in blood pressure and may permit dosage reduction of either or both drugs and minimize adverse effects while maintaining blood pressure control.

Captopril may be effective in the management of hypertension resistant to other drugs. Although captopril occasionally may be effective alone in patients with severe hypertension, it is usually necessary to use it in conjunction with a diuretic. (See Drug Interactions: Hypotensive Agents and Diuretics.)

Tolerance to the hypotensive effect of captopril apparently does not occur during long-term administration, particularly if the drug is used with a diuretic. Abrupt withdrawal of captopril therapy results in a gradual return of hypertension; rapid increases in blood pressure have not been reported to date.

Considerations for Drug Therapy in Patients with Underlying Cardiovascular and Other Risk Factors

Drug therapy in patients with hypertension and underlying cardiovascular or other risk factors should be carefully individualized based on the underlying disease(s), concomitant drugs, tolerance to drug-induced adverse effects, and blood pressure goal. See Table 2 on Compelling Indications for Drug Classes based on Comorbid Conditions, under Uses: Hypertension in Adults, in the Thiazides General Statement 40:28.20.

Ischemic Heart Disease

The selection of an appropriate antihypertensive agent in patients with ischemic heart disease should be based on individual patient characteristics and may include ACE inhibitors and/or β-blockers, with the addition of other drugs such as thiazide diuretics or calcium-channel blockers as necessary to achieve blood pressure goals. Many experts recommend the use of an ACE inhibitor (or an angiotensin II receptor antagonist) and/or a β-blocker in hypertensive patients with stable ischemic heart disease because of the cardioprotective benefits of these drugs; in addition, all patients who have survived an MI should be treated with a β-blocker because of the demonstrated mortality benefit of these agents.

Heart Failure

While ACE inhibitors as single therapies are not superior to other antihypertensive agents in the reduction of cardiovascular outcomes, ACE inhibitors, usually in conjunction with other agents such as cardiac glycosides, diuretics, and β-blockers, have been shown to reduce morbidity and mortality in patients with existing heart failure. (See Uses: Heart Failure.) ACE inhibitors also have been shown to prevent subsequent heart failure and reduce morbidity and mortality in patients with systolic dysfunction following an acute MI. (See Uses: Left Ventricular Dysfunction after Acute Myocardial Infarction.)

Diabetes Mellitus

Experts state that initial treatment of hypertension in adults with diabetes mellitus and hypertension should include any of the usual first-line agents (ACE inhibitors, angiotensin II receptor antagonist, calcium-channel blockers, thiazide diuretics). In adults with diabetes mellitus, hypertension, and albuminuria, treatment with an ACE inhibitor or angiotensin II receptor antagonist may be considered to reduce the progression of kidney disease. While there is evidence demonstrating the benefits of ACE inhibitors in reducing the development or progression of microvascular or macrovascular complications in hypertensive patients with type 1 or type 2 diabetes mellitus, in the absence of albuminuria, the risk of progressive kidney disease is low, and ACE inhibitors and angiotensin II receptor antagonists have not demonstrated superior cardioprotection when compared with other first-line agents. Results of several studies indicate that adequate control of blood pressure in patients with type 2 diabetes mellitus reduces the development or progression of complications of diabetes (e.g., death related to diabetes, stroke, heart failure, microvascular disease). Most patients with diabetes mellitus will require 2 or more antihypertensive agents to achieve blood pressure control.

Chronic Kidney Disease

Hypertensive patients with CKD (glomerular filtration rate [GFR] less than 60 mL/minute per 1.73 m² or kidney damage for 3 or more months) usually will require more than one antihypertensive agent to reach target blood pressure. Use of ACE inhibitors or angiotensin II receptor antagonists may be reasonable in patients with diabetic or nondiabetic CKD (stage 1 or 2 with albuminuria or stage 3 or higher); these drugs have been shown to slow the progression of kidney disease. Evidence of a renoprotective benefit is strongest in those with higher levels of albuminuria. Increases in serum creatinine (up to 30%) may be observed as a result of a decrease in intraglomerular pressure and concurrent reduction in GFR. The 2017 ACC/AHA hypertension guideline states that in patients with less severe kidney disease (i.e., stage 1 or 2 CKD without albuminuria), any of the first-line antihypertensive agents (e.g., ACE inhibitors, angiotensin II receptor antagonists, calcium-channel blockers, thiazide diuretics) can be used for the initial treatment of hypertension. Diuretics also may be useful in the management of CKD, and may potentiate the effects of ACE inhibitors, angiotensin II receptor antagonists, and other antihypertensive agents when used in combination.

Cerebrovascular Disease

Some experts recommend a blood pressure goal of less than 140/90 mm Hg in patients with ischemic stroke or transient ischemic attack (TIA), while others state that a blood pressure goal of less than 130/80 mm Hg may be reasonable. The 2017 ACC/AHA hypertension guideline states that adults not previously treated for hypertension who experience a stroke or TIA and who have an established blood pressure of 140/90 mm Hg or higher should receive antihypertensive therapy within a few days after the event to reduce the risk of recurrent stroke or other vascular events. In patients with a recent lacunar stroke, experts suggest that a systolic blood pressure goal of 130 mm Hg may be reasonable based on results of a randomized open-label study (the Secondary Prevention of Small Subcortical Strokes [SPS3] trial). Although experts state that the optimal choice of drug for the management of hypertension in patients with a previous TIA or ischemic stroke is uncertain, available data indicate that an ACE inhibitor, angiotensin II receptor antagonist, thiazide diuretic, or the combination of a thiazide diuretic and an ACE inhibitor may be effective. Administration of an ACE inhibitor in combination with a thiazide diuretic has been shown to lower rates of recurrent stroke.

Other Special Considerations for Antihypertensive Drug Therapy
Race

Most patients with hypertension, especially black patients, will require at least 2 antihypertensive drugs to achieve adequate blood pressure control. In general, black hypertensive patients tend to respond better to monotherapy with thiazide diuretics or calcium-channel blockers than to monotherapy with ACE inhibitors. In a prespecified subgroup analysis of the ALLHAT study, a thiazide-type diuretic was more effective than an ACE inhibitor in improving cerebrovascular and cardiovascular outcomes in black patients; when compared with a calcium-channel blocker, the ACE inhibitor was less effective in reducing blood pressure and was associated with a 51% higher rate of stroke. (See Clinical Benefit of Thiazides in Hypertension under Hypertension in Adults: Treatment Benefits, in Uses in the Thiazides General Statement 40:28.20.) However, the combination of an ACE inhibitor or an angiotensin II receptor antagonist with a calcium-channel blocker or thiazide diuretic produces similar blood pressure lowering in black patients as in other racial groups. In addition, some experts state that when use of ACE inhibitors is indicated in hypertensive patients with underlying cardiovascular or other risk factors, these indications should be applied equally to black hypertensive patients.

Although captopril has lowered blood pressure in all races studied, monotherapy with this agent has produced a smaller reduction in blood pressure in black hypertensive patients, a population associated with low renin hypertension; however, this population difference in response does not appear to occur during combined therapy with captopril and a thiazide diuretic. In addition, ACE inhibitors appear to produce a higher incidence of angioedema in black patients than in other races studied.

For further information on overall principles and expert recommendations for treatment of hypertension, see Uses: Hypertension in Adults and also see Uses: Hypertension in Pediatric Patients, in the Thiazides General Statement 40:28.20.

Renovascular or Malignant Hypertension

Captopril also has been effective in the management of renovascular or malignant hypertension and, in some patients, in the management of hypertension associated with chronic renal failure.

Hypertensive Crises

Captopril has been used orally for rapidly reducing blood pressure in patients with hypertensive crises† in whom reduction of blood pressure was considered urgent (hypertensive urgencies) or emergent (hypertensive emergencies). Because even oral therapy for hypertensive crises can result in profound hypotension and associated adverse cardiovascular effects (e.g., myocardial ischemia or infarction, cerebrovascular hypoperfusion or stroke), captopril should not be used indiscriminately, and the benefits versus risks of rapidly reducing blood pressure with the drug must be weighed carefully.

Hypertensive urgencies are those situations in which there is a severe elevation in blood pressure without progressive target organ damage. Hypertensive urgencies generally can be managed by intensification or reinstitution (e.g., following noncompliance) of the current antihypertensive regimen and treatment of anxiety if needed. Experts state that there is no need for rapid reduction of blood pressure in such patients and hospitalization or referral to the emergency department also is unnecessary.

Hypertensive emergencies are those rare situations requiring immediate blood pressure reduction (not necessarily to normal ranges) to prevent or limit target organ damage. Such emergencies include hypertensive encephalopathy, acute MI, intracerebral hemorrhage, acute left ventricular failure with pulmonary edema, eclampsia, dissecting aortic aneurysm, unstable angina pectoris, acute ischemic stroke, and acute renal failure. Although oral therapy with captopril has been used to rapidly reduce blood pressure in such emergencies, patients with hypertensive emergencies should be hospitalized and treated initially with appropriate parenteral antihypertensive therapy (e.g., labetalol, esmolol, fenoldopam, nicardipine, sodium nitroprusside).

● Nephropathy

Captopril may be used in patients with nephropathy, including diabetic nephropathy. Use of ACE inhibitors or angiotensin II receptor antagonists is recommended in the management of diabetic or nondiabetic† CKD to slow progression of the disease. ACE inhibitors have stabilized or improved effective renal blood flow and glomerular filtration rate and decreased proteinuria in hypertensive or normotensive patients with moderately impaired renal function, moderate to severe renal disease, or diabetic nephropathy. Short-term administration of captopril improved blood flow and glomerular filtration rate in some hypertensive patients with moderately impaired renal function; however, long-term captopril therapy has not maintained sustained improvement in renal blood flow and glomerular filtration rate. In general, captopril should be used with caution in

patients with impaired renal function, especially those with bilateral renal-artery stenosis or renal-artery stenosis in a solitary kidney. (See Cautions: Renal Effects and see Cautions: Hematologic Effects, and also see Precautions and Contraindications.) Captopril appears to be ineffective in the management of hypertension in anephric patients. (See Pharmacology: Renal and Electrolyte Effects.)

Diabetic Nephropathy

Captopril is used in the management of diabetic nephropathy manifested by proteinuria (urinary protein excretion exceeding 500 mg per 24 hours) in patients with type 1 diabetes mellitus and diabetic retinopathy.

Both ACE inhibitors and angiotensin II receptor antagonists have been shown to slow the rate of progression of renal disease in patients with diabetes mellitus and persistent albuminuria, and use of a drug from either class is recommended in such patients with modestly elevated (30–300 mg per 24 hours) or higher (exceeding 300 mg per 24 hours) levels of urinary albumin excretion. Comparative trials evaluating the efficacy of ACE inhibitors and angiotensin II receptor antagonists for improving renal outcomes in diabetic patients are lacking. Evidence supporting use of ACE inhibitors generally is based on studies in patients with type 1 diabetes mellitus, while evidence supporting use of angiotensin II receptor antagonists generally is based on studies in patients with type 2 diabetes mellitus. Findings from these studies indicate that both drug classes delay progression of increased urinary albumin excretion in patients with diabetes mellitus and also may slow the decline in renal function. Because the available data are consistent, some experts suggest that the effects of both drug classes in improving renal outcomes in patients with diabetes mellitus and proteinuria are likely to be similar. Drugs that inhibit the renin-angiotensin system (i.e., ACE inhibitors, angiotensin II receptor antagonists) have been shown to delay the onset of albuminuria in patients with type 2 diabetes mellitus and hypertension who have normal levels of urinary albumin excretion†; however, experts state that in the absence of albuminuria, the risk of progressive kidney disease is low. Combined therapy with ACE inhibitors and angiotensin II receptor antagonists provides no additional cardiovascular benefit and increases the risk of adverse effects (e.g., impaired renal function, hyperkalemia). The American Diabetes Association (ADA) states that the use of an ACE inhibitor or angiotensin II receptor antagonist is not recommended for the primary prevention of diabetic nephropathy in patients with diabetes mellitus who are normotensive, have normal levels of urinary protein excretion, and have a normal glomerular filtration rate.

In a multicenter, controlled study in hypertensive and normotensive individuals who had type 1 diabetes mellitus for at least 7 years, diabetic retinopathy, proteinuria, and a serum creatinine concentration of 2.5 mg/dL or less, deterioration in renal function was substantially less pronounced in patients receiving long-term captopril therapy (median: 3 years [range: 1.8–4.8 years]) than in those receiving placebo. Patients with hypertension received hypotensive agents (e.g., diuretics, β-blockers, α-adrenergic blocking agents, vasodilators) as needed. Overall, patients receiving captopril had a 48% reduction in the risk of doubling of serum creatinine concentration. Captopril therapy was especially useful in patients with more advanced renal disease (i.e., baseline serum creatinine exceeding 1.5 mg/dL). Captopril therapy was associated with a 30% reduction in urinary protein excretion within 3 months and was evident throughout the study. In addition, patients receiving captopril had a 50% reduction in the risk of death and need for dialysis or renal transplantation, particularly in those with more advanced renal disease. It has been suggested that captopril and other ACE inhibitors may slow the progression of renal nephropathy by a mechanism independent of its antihypertensive properties.

Captopril also has been shown to delay the onset of diabetic nephropathy in normotensive patients with diabetes mellitus and microalbuminuria†. In multicenter controlled studies in normotensive patients with type 1 diabetes mellitus, retinopathy, and microalbuminuria (20–200 mcg/minute), treatment with captopril (50 mg twice daily) for 2 years was associated with a substantial reduction in the risk of developing diabetic nephropathy (based on progression of microalbuminuria to proteinuria). In one study, albumin excretion rate increased from a mean baseline value of 52 to 76 mcg/minute at 2 years in patients receiving placebo, while rates determined at the same time points in patients receiving captopril decreased from 52 to 41 mcg/minute. While clinical studies indicate that treatment with captopril can postpone the development of diabetic nephropathy in normotensive type 1 diabetic patients with microalbuminuria, the long-term clinical benefit of reducing the progression of microalbuminuria to proteinuria has not been determined.

● **Heart Failure**

Captopril is used in the management of heart failure, usually in conjunction with other agents such as cardiac glycosides, diuretics, and β-blockers.

Current guidelines for the management of heart failure in adults generally recommend a combination of drug therapies to reduce morbidity and mortality, including neurohormonal antagonists (e.g., ACE inhibitors, angiotensin II receptor antagonists, angiotensin receptor-neprilysin inhibitors [ARNIs], β-blockers, aldosterone receptor antagonists) that inhibit the detrimental compensatory mechanisms in heart failure. Additional agents (e.g., cardiac glycosides, diuretics, sinoatrial modulators [i.e., ivabradine]) added to a heart failure treatment regimen in selected patients have been associated with symptomatic improvement and/or reduction in heart failure-related hospitalizations. Experts recommend that all asymptomatic patients with reduced left ventricular ejection fraction (LVEF) (American College of Cardiology Foundation [ACCF]/American Heart Association [AHA] stage B heart failure) receive therapy with an ACE inhibitor and β-blocker to prevent symptomatic heart failure and to reduce morbidity and mortality. In patients with prior or current symptoms of chronic heart failure with reduced LVEF, ACCF, AHA, and the Heart Failure Society of America (HFSA) recommend inhibition of the renin-angiotensin-aldosterone (RAA) system with an ACE inhibitor, angiotensin II receptor antagonist, or ARNI in conjunction with a β-blocker, and an aldosterone antagonist in selected patients, to reduce morbidity and mortality. While ACE inhibitors have been the preferred drugs for inhibition of the RAA system because of their established benefits in patients with heart failure and reduced ejection fraction, some evidence indicates that therapy with sacubitril/valsartan, an ARNI, may be more effective than ACE inhibitor therapy (enalapril) in reducing cardiovascular death and heart failure-related hospitalization in such patients. ACCF, AHA, and HFSA recommend that patients with chronic symptomatic heart failure and reduced LVEF (New York Heart Association [NYHA] class II or III) who are able to tolerate an ACE inhibitor or angiotensin II receptor antagonist be switched to therapy containing an ARNI to further reduce morbidity and mortality. However, in patients in whom an ARNI is not appropriate, continued use of an ACE inhibitor for all classes of heart failure with reduced ejection fraction remains strongly advised. In patients in whom an ARNI or ACE inhibitor is not appropriate, an angiotensin II receptor antagonist may be used. For further information on the use of ARNIs in patients with heart failure, see Uses: Heart Failure, in Sacubitril and Valsartan 24:32.92.

Some clinicians state that ACE inhibitors usually are prescribed in clinical practice at dosages lower than those determined as target dosages in clinical trials, although results of several studies suggest that high dosages are associated with greater hemodynamic, neurohormonal, symptomatic, and prognostic benefits than lower dosages. Results of a large, randomized, double-blind study (Assessment of Treatment with Lisinopril and Survival [ATLAS] study) in patients with heart failure (NYHA class II–IV) indicate that high lisinopril dosages (32.5–35 mg daily) were associated with a 12% lower risk of death or hospitalization for any cause and 24% fewer hospitalizations for heart failure than low dosages (2.5–5 mg) of the drug.

Once ACE inhibitor therapy is initiated for heart failure, it generally is continued indefinitely, if tolerated, since withdrawal of an ACE inhibitor may lead to clinical deterioration. Patients with NYHA class II or III heart failure who are tolerating therapy with an ACE inhibitor may be switched to therapy containing an ARNI to further reduce morbidity and mortality; however, the ARNI should not be administered concomitantly with an ACE inhibitor or within 36 hours of the last dose of an ACE inhibitor.

Diuretics are recommended in all patients with heart failure and reduced ejection fraction who have evidence of fluid retention, unless contraindicated, to improve symptoms. Digoxin may be beneficial to patients with heart failure with reduced ejection fraction to decrease hospitalization for heart failure, especially in those with persistent symptoms despite treatment with guideline-directed medical therapy. The manufacturer states that most experience from controlled studies has been with combined captopril, cardiac glycoside, and diuretic therapy; however, the manufacturer also states that the beneficial effect of captopril does not require concomitant cardiac glycoside therapy. The addition of a sinoatrial modulator (i.e., ivabradine) is recommended in selected patients with chronic heart failure and reduced LVEF who are already receiving guideline-directed medical therapy, to reduce heart failure-related hospitalizations. (See Uses: Heart Failure, in Ivabradine 24:04.92.)

Results of a randomized, multicenter, double-blind, placebo-controlled study (Randomized Aldactone Evaluation Study [RALES]) indicate that addition of low-dosage spironolactone (25–50 mg daily) to standard therapy (e.g., an ACE inhibitor and a loop diuretic with or without a cardiac glycoside) in patients with severe (NYHA class IV within 6 months before enrollment and NYHA class III or IV at the time of enrollment) heart failure and LVEF of 35% or less was associated with decreases in overall mortality and hospitalization (for worsening heart failure) rates of approximately 30 and 35%, respectively, compared with standard therapy and placebo. Based on results of RALES and other studies, ACCF and AHA recommend the addition of an aldosterone antagonist (i.e., spironolactone or eplerenone) in selected patients with heart failure (NYHA class II–IV) and reduced LVEF (35% or less) who are already receiving standard therapy to reduce morbidity and mortality. (See Uses: Heart Failure, in Spironolactone 24:32.20.)

Many patients with heart failure respond to captopril with improvement in cardiac function indexes, symptomatic relief, improved functional capacity, and increased exercise tolerance. In some studies, improvement in cardiac function indexes and exercise tolerance were sustained for up to 6 months. In some patients, beneficial effects have been sustained for up to 1 year or longer. Captopril also has been effective in conjunction with cardiac glycosides and diuretics in the management of heart failure resistant to or inadequately controlled by cardiac glycosides, diuretics, and vasodilators.

ACE inhibitors also are used to prevent symptomatic heart failure in patients with ACCF/AHA stage B heart failure (see Uses: Asymptomatic Left Ventricular Dysfunction) and have been shown to reduce mortality after MI or acute coronary syndrome. (See Uses: Left Ventricular Dysfunction after Acute Myocardial Infarction.)

In patients with heart failure in whom renal perfusion is severely compromised, the renin-angiotensin system appears to substantially contribute to preservation of glomerular filtration; therefore, therapy with an ACE inhibitor may adversely affect renal function in such patients. (See Cautions: Renal Effects.)

● **Left Ventricular Dysfunction After Acute Myocardial Infarction**

Captopril is used to improve survival following acute MI in clinically stable patients with left ventricular dysfunction (manifested as an ejection fraction of 40% or less) and to reduce the incidence of overt heart failure and subsequent hospitalizations for heart failure in these patients.

Studies with various ACE inhibitors have shown that these drugs reduce fatal and nonfatal cardiovascular events in patients with recent MI. The magnitude of benefit appears to be greatest in certain high-risk patients (e.g., those with an anterior infarct, ejection fraction of 40% or less, heart failure, prior infarction, or tachycardia). In addition to their effects on mortality, ACE inhibitors also are used to minimize or prevent the development of left ventricular dilatation and dysfunction (ventricular "remodeling") following acute MI. Evidence regarding the efficacy of such therapy has been somewhat conflicting, particularly when parenteral therapy was initiated early (within 24–48 hours) and included patients with no evidence of baseline dysfunction. (See Uses: Left Ventricular Dysfunction After Acute Myocardial Infarction, in Enalaprilat/Enalapril 24:32.04.) However, the preponderance of evidence has shown a benefit of early oral therapy with ACE inhibitors, even in patients with no baseline dysfunction. In a multicenter, controlled study involving captopril in which initiation of therapy with the drug was delayed until 3–16 days after acute MI and limited to patients with low ejection fractions (40% or less), long-term (mean: 42 months; range: 24–60 months) therapy with the drug was associated with a reduction in overall mortality as well as a reduction in morbidity and mortality secondary to cardiovascular causes. In several other studies in which captopril was initiated within 24 hours to 4 weeks after acute MI, a beneficial effect also was observed, at least in terms of effects on left ventricular volume and/or infarct expansion.

Current expert guidelines recommend the use of an oral ACE inhibitor within the first 24 hours of acute MI in patients with an anterior infarction, heart failure, or ejection fraction of 40% or less who do not have any contraindications (e.g., hypotension, shock, renal dysfunction). While early treatment within the first 24 hours of MI has been shown to be beneficial, ACE inhibitors should be used with caution (and with gradual upward titration) during the initial postinfarction period because of the possibility of hypotension or renal dysfunction. ACE inhibitor therapy generally should be continued indefinitely in all patients with left ventricular dysfunction or other compelling indications for use (e.g., hypertension, diabetes mellitus, CKD). The benefits of long-term ACE inhibitor therapy are less certain in low-risk patients who have undergone revascularization and are receiving aggressive antilipemic therapy.

● Asymptomatic Left Ventricular Dysfunction

ACE inhibitors have been used to attenuate left ventricular enlargement and prevent progression to symptomatic dysfunction in asymptomatic patients with heart failure† (ACCF/AHA stage B heart failure). Captopril has reduced the development of symptomatic heart failure and associated morbidity and mortality in such patients. The drug's beneficial effect in preventing the development of symptomatic heart failure in these patients may result either from relieving symptoms that otherwise would have become apparent or from slowing the progression of asymptomatic ventricular dysfunction to overt, symptomatic disease. (See Uses: Asymptomatic Left Ventricular Dysfunction, in Enalaprilat/Enalapril 24:32.04.) If an ACE inhibitor is not tolerated, then an angiotensin II receptor antagonist is recommended as alternative therapy.

● Other Uses

Captopril has been shown to increase digital circulation in one patient with Raynaud's phenomenon† and decrease the orthostatic sodium and water retention in several women with idiopathic edema†. Therefore, it has been suggested that the drug may be useful in the treatment of these conditions; however, additional evaluation is necessary.

ACE inhibitors have been used to reduce the risk of cardiovascular events in patients 55 years of age or older who are at high risk for cardiovascular events† (e.g., diabetes mellitus, history of cardiovascular disease, stroke, peripheral vascular disease, dyslipidemia, smoking, microalbuminuria, hypertension). (See Uses: Prevention of Cardiovascular Events, in Ramipril 24:32.04.)

DOSAGE AND ADMINISTRATION

● Administration

Captopril is administered orally. The manufacturer recommends that the drug be taken 1 hour before meals to ensure maximum absorption.

Extemporaneously Compounded Oral Liquid

An extemporaneously compounded oral liquid formulation of captopril has been prepared.

Standardize 4 Safety

Standardized concentrations for an extemporaneously prepared oral liquid formulation of captopril have been established through Standardize 4 Safety (S4S), a national patient safety initiative to reduce medication errors, especially during transitions of care. Multidisciplinary expert panels were convened to determine recommended standard concentrations. Because recommendations from the S4S panels may differ from the manufacturer's prescribing information, caution is advised when using concentrations that differ from labeling, particularly when using rate information from the label. For additional information on S4S (including updates that may be available), see https://www.ashp.org/pharmacy-practice/standardize-4-safety-initiative.

TABLE 2. Standardize 4 Safety Compounded Oral Liquid Standards for Captopril

Concentration Standards
1 mg/mL

● Dosage

Dosage of captopril must be adjusted according to the patient's tolerance and response.

Hypertension

Because of the risk of inducing hypotension, initiation of captopril therapy requires consideration of recent antihypertensive therapy, the extent of blood pressure elevation, sodium intake, fluid status, and other clinical circumstances. Except in patients with severe hypertension, it is recommended that other antihypertensive therapy be discontinued, if possible, 1 week before initiating captopril to minimize the possibility of severe hypotension. If captopril therapy is initiated in patients already receiving a diuretic, treatment with the drug should be initiated under close supervision, following the usual dosage and titration recommendations.

Concomitant sodium restriction may be helpful when captopril is used alone.

Captopril Therapy

The manufacturer states that the usual initial adult dosage of captopril for the management of hypertension in adults with normal renal function is 25 mg 2 or 3 times daily. However, lower initial dosages (e.g., 6.25 mg twice daily to 12.5 mg 3 times daily) may be effective in some patients, particularly in those already receiving a diuretic. Because the reduction in blood pressure may be gradual, most clinicians do not increase dosage during the first 1–2 weeks of captopril therapy. If blood pressure is not adequately controlled after 1–2 weeks, dosage may be increased to 50 mg 2 or 3 times daily. Similar dosages generally have been used in the management of hypertension in geriatric patients, although dosages of 6.25–12.5 mg 1–4 times daily have occasionally been used. The manufacturer states that it usually is not necessary to exceed a captopril dosage of 150 mg daily; if blood pressure is not adequately controlled after 1–2 weeks at a dosage of 50 mg 3 times daily, a thiazide diuretic should also be administered in a low dosage (e.g., 15 mg of hydrochlorothiazide daily). Because the full effect of a combined dose of therapy with captopril and a diuretic may not be attained for 6–8 weeks, dosage of either drug in a combined regimen generally should be increased no more frequently than every 6 weeks, unless the clinical situation requires more rapid adjustment. Diuretic dosage may be increased until its maximum usual antihypertensive dose is reached. If further reduction of blood pressure is necessary, dosage of captopril may be increased to 100 mg 2 or 3 times daily and, if necessary, to 150 mg 2 or 3 times daily, while continuing diuretic therapy. Although a β-adrenergic blocking agent (β-blocker) may be used with captopril, the hypotensive effects are less than additive and this combination is rarely employed. (See Uses: Hypertension.) For further information on dosage of captopril used in combination therapy, see Captopril/Hydrochlorothiazide Fixed-combination Therapy under Dosage: Hypertension. The usual adult maintenance dosage of captopril recommended by the manufacturers is 25–150 mg 2 or 3 times daily, and the maximum dosage is 450 mg daily.

The need for divided (2 or 3 doses) daily dosing of captopril may deter patient compliance and adequate blood pressure control throughout the day; optimally, the antihypertensive drug or dosage form should provide 24-hour efficacy with once-daily dosing, with at least 50% of the peak antihypertensive effect remaining at the end of the dosing interval.

Clinical experience with captopril in pediatric patients is limited (see Cautions: Pediatric Precautions), and dosage must be carefully titrated. In general, dosage for children has been reduced in proportion to body weight. Some experts have recommended an initial captopril dosage in infants of 0.05 mg/kg 1–4 times daily and an initial dosage of 0.5 mg/kg 3 times daily in children. Some experts state that the drug should be initiated at the low end of the dosage range and the dosage may be increased every 2–4 weeks until blood pressure is controlled, the maximum dosage (6 mg/kg per day) is reached, or adverse effects occur. For information on overall principles and expert recommendations for treatment of hypertension in pediatric patients, see Uses: Hypertension in Pediatric Patients, in the Thiazides General Statement 40:28.20.

Captopril/Hydrochlorothiazide Fixed-combination Therapy

When combination therapy is required for the management of hypertension, dosage first can be adjusted by administering each drug separately. If it is determined that the optimum maintenance dosage corresponds to the ratio in a commercial combination preparation, the fixed combination may be used. Alternatively, certain fixed-combination preparations containing low doses of captopril and hydrochlorothiazide can be used initially, thereby potentiating the antihypertensive effect of either drug alone while minimizing the likelihood of dose-related adverse effects. If combination therapy is initiated with the fixed-combination preparation, the initial adult dosage is 25 mg of captopril and 15 mg of hydrochlorothiazide once daily. Subsequent dosage can be adjusted by administering each drug separately or by advancing the once-daily administered fixed-combination preparation to that containing captopril and hydrochlorothiazide 50 and 15 mg, respectively; 25 and 25 mg, respectively; or 50 and 25 mg, respectively. The manufacturer states that dosage adjustments generally should be made at 6-week intervals. It may be necessary to administer captopril separately in divided doses in order to maintain adequate trough (prior to a dose) blood pressure control. Generally, combined dosage of captopril and hydrochlorothiazide in adults should not exceed 150 and 50 mg daily, respectively.

Blood Pressure Monitoring and Treatment Goals

Blood pressure should be monitored regularly (i.e., monthly) during therapy and dosage of the antihypertensive drug adjusted until blood pressure is controlled. If an adequate blood pressure response is not achieved with ACE inhibitor monotherapy, the dosage may be increased or another antihypertensive agent with demonstrated benefit and preferably with a complementary mechanism of action (e.g., calcium-channel blocking agent, thiazide diuretic) may be added; if target blood pressure is still not achieved, a third drug may be added. (See Uses: Hypertension.) In patients who develop unacceptable adverse effects with captopril, the drug should be discontinued and another antihypertensive agent from a different pharmacologic class should be initiated.

The goal of hypertension management and prevention is to achieve and maintain optimal control of blood pressure. However, the optimum blood pressure threshold for initiating antihypertensive drug therapy and specific treatment goals remain controversial. While other hypertension guidelines have based target blood pressure goals on age and comorbidities, the 2017 American College of Cardiology/American Heart Association (ACC/AHA) hypertension guideline incorporates underlying cardiovascular risk into decision making regarding treatment and generally recommends the same target blood pressure (i.e., less than 130/80 mm Hg) in all adults. Many patients will require at least 2 drugs from different pharmacologic classes to achieve this blood pressure goal; the potential benefits of hypertension management and drug cost, adverse effects, and risks associated with the use of multiple antihypertensive drugs also should be considered when deciding a patient's blood pressure treatment goal. (See General Considerations for Initial and Maintenance Antihypertensive Therapy under Uses: Hypertension.)

For additional information on target levels of blood pressure and on monitoring therapy in the management of hypertension, see Blood Pressure Monitoring and Treatment Goals under Dosage: Hypertension, in Dosage and Administration in the Thiazides General Statement 40:28.20.

Hypertensive Crises

In adults with severe hypertension (e.g., accelerated or malignant hypertension) in whom prompt blood pressure reduction is indicated or in whom temporary discontinuance of current antihypertensive therapy is not practical or desirable, diuretic therapy should be continued, other hypotensive agents should be discontinued, and captopril should be initiated promptly at a dosage of 25 mg 2 or 3 times daily, under close supervision with frequent monitoring of the patient's blood pressure.

When necessary, dosage of captopril may be increased at intervals of 24 hours or less under continuous supervision until the optimum blood pressure response is attained or 450 mg daily is given; in this regimen, a diuretic such as furosemide may also be necessary. If adequate control of blood pressure is not attained initially with captopril alone or in combination with a diuretic, some clinicians believe that temporary, adjunctive therapy with other hypotensive agents may be necessary.

Although acute captopril therapy (e.g., 12.5–25 mg, repeated once or twice if necessary at intervals of 30–60 minutes or longer) has been used orally in adults with hypertensive crises†, including those with severe hypertension in whom reduction of blood pressure was considered urgent† (hypertensive urgencies) or an emergency† (hypertensive emergencies), other management methods generally are preferred for patients with these conditions. (See Hypertensive Crises under Uses: Hypertension.)

Diabetic Nephropathy

The recommended dosage of captopril for the long-term treatment of diabetic nephropathy is 25 mg 3 times daily. If adequate control of blood pressure is not attained with captopril alone, additional hypotensive agents (e.g., diuretics, β-blockers, calcium-channel blocking agents) may be administered concomitantly.

Heart Failure

For the management of symptomatic heart failure, captopril usually is administered in conjunction with other agents such as a cardiac glycoside, a diuretic, and a β-blocker. Captopril therapy must be initiated under very close medical supervision with consideration given to recent diuretic therapy and the possibility of severe sodium and/or fluid depletion. ACE inhibitor therapy should be initiated with caution in patients with very low systemic blood pressure (systolic blood pressure less than 80 mm Hg), markedly increased serum concentrations of creatinine (greater than 3 mg/dL), bilateral renal artery stenosis, or elevated concentrations of serum potassium (greater than 5 mEq/L). Experts recommend that renal function and serum potassium should be assessed within 1–2 weeks of initiation of therapy and periodically thereafter, especially in patients with preexisting hypotension, hyponatremia, diabetes mellitus, or azotemia, or in those taking potassium supplements.

It should be recognized that although symptoms of heart failure may improve within 48 hours after initiating ACE inhibitor therapy in some patients, such improvement usually is not evident for several weeks or months after initiating ACE inhibitor therapy. In addition, it should be considered that such therapy may reduce the risk of disease progression even if symptomatic improvement is not evident. Therefore, dosages generally should be titrated to a prespecified target (i.e., 150 mg of captopril daily) or highest tolerated dosage rather than according to response.

The usual initial adult dosage of captopril recommended by the manufacturer for the management of heart failure in patients with normal renal function is 25 mg 3 times daily. In patients with normal or low blood pressure who have been vigorously treated with diuretics and who may be hyponatremic and/or hypovolemic, an initial dosage of 6.25 or 12.5 mg 3 times daily may minimize the magnitude or duration of the hypotensive effect; titration to the usual daily dosage can then be made within the next several days. Dosage is increased gradually according to the patient's tolerance and response. After a dosage of 50 mg 3 times daily is reached, further increases in dosage should be delayed when possible for at least 2 weeks to determine if an adequate response occurs.

Alternatively, the American College of Cardiology (ACC) and American Heart Association (AHA) recommend that captopril be initiated at low dosage (i.e., 6.25 mg 3 times daily) and titrated gradually upward as tolerated to a maximum dosage of 50 mg 3 times daily. It has been recommended that therapy with ACE inhibitors be titrated upwards to dosages that have been shown to reduce the risk of cardiovascular events in clinical trials rather than titrating based on a patient's therapeutic response. Most patients have an adequate response with 50 or 100 mg 3 times daily. The manufacturer states that a maximum dosage of 450 mg daily should not be exceeded. Some experts suggest a maximum dosage of 50 mg 3 times daily in patients with chronic heart failure.

Alternatively, for the management of heart failure in geriatric patients, some clinicians have initiated captopril therapy at a dosage of 6.25 mg twice daily; if necessary, dosage was increased to 25 mg twice daily after 2 weeks and was subsequently increased if heart failure was not adequately controlled after 4 weeks of therapy at this dosage. The median dosage after 12 weeks of therapy in these geriatric patients was 75 mg daily in 2 divided doses.

Left Ventricular Dysfunction After Acute Myocardial Infarction

When used following acute myocardial infarction (MI) in adults with left ventricular dysfunction, the manufacturer states that captopril therapy may be initiated as early as 3 days following MI. When this approach is followed, an initial 6.25-mg dose of captopril should be given, followed by 12.5 mg 3 times daily. During the next several days, dosage should be increased to 25 mg 3 times daily and then, during the next several weeks as tolerated, dosage should be increased to 50 mg 3 times daily. Some clinicians recommend initiation of therapy within the first 24 hours following MI. The recommended maintenance dosage for long-term use following MI is 50 mg 3 times daily.

● Dosage in Renal Impairment

If captopril is used in patients with impaired renal function, doses and/or frequency of administration must be modified in response to the degree of renal impairment and the risk of neutropenia must be considered. (See Cautions: Precautions and Contraindications.) The initial dosage of captopril should be reduced in these patients (i.e., less than 75 mg daily), and dosage should be slowly increased in small increments at 1- to 2-week intervals. After the desired therapeutic effect has been attained, dosage should be slowly decreased to the minimum effective level. It has been suggested that, after the minimum effective daily dosage has been determined in patients with impaired renal function, the dosing interval may be increased with appropriate dose modification; however, criteria for dosage adjustment have not been clearly established. Some clinicians suggest that patients with creatinine clearances of 10–50 mL/minute can receive 75% of the usual captopril dosage or the usual dose can be administered every 12–18 hours, and that those with creatinine clearances less than 10 mL/minute can receive 50% of the usual dosage or the usual dose can be administered every 24 hours. Patients undergoing hemodialysis may require a supplemental dose after dialysis.

When combination therapy with captopril and hydrochlorothiazide is required for the management of hypertension in patients with impaired renal function, the risk of precipitating hypotension during initiation of combined therapy should be considered. (See Cautions: Cardiovascular Effects and see Precautions and Contraindications.) Dosages of the drugs should be titrated carefully by slowly increasing the dosage of each drug separately in small increments. After the desired therapeutic effect has been attained, the manufacturer recommends that the dosing interval be increased and/or the doses decreased until the minimal effective daily dosage has been achieved. If after careful titration of each drug separately it is determined that the optimum maintenance dosage corresponds to the ratio in commercial combination preparation, the fixed combination may be substituted but should be replaced with the individual drugs if subsequent dosage adjustment is necessary. If concomitant diuretic therapy is required in patients with severe renal impairment, a loop diuretic such as furosemide is preferred to a thiazide diuretic. Therefore, use of commercially available preparations containing captopril in fixed combination with hydrochlorothiazide is usually not recommended for patients with severe renal impairment.

CAUTIONS

Captopril is generally well tolerated in most patients; however, serious adverse effects (e.g., neutropenia, agranulocytosis, proteinuria, aplastic anemia) have been reported rarely, mainly in patients with renal impairment (especially those with collagen vascular disease). Captopril-induced adverse effects are often alleviated by dosage reduction, occasionally disappear despite continued treatment and without dosage reduction, and are usually reversible following discontinuance of the drug. The most common adverse effects of captopril are rash and loss of taste perception. Adverse effects requiring discontinuance of captopril therapy occur in about 4–12% of patients.

● Hematologic Effects

Neutropenia (less than 1000 neutrophils/mm^3) and agranulocytosis, both associated with myeloid hypoplasia, have occurred rarely in patients receiving captopril. In addition to myeloid hypoplasia, erythroid hypoplasia and decreased numbers of megakaryocytes (e.g., hypoplastic bone marrow and pancytopenia) were frequently observed in patients with captopril-induced neutropenia; anemia and thrombocytopenia also occurred occasionally in these patients. Systemic or oral cavity infections or other effects associated with agranulocytosis occurred in about half of the patients who developed neutropenia.

Neutropenia has occurred within 3–12 weeks after beginning treatment with captopril. The risk of captopril-induced neutropenia appears to depend principally on the degree of renal impairment and the presence of collagen vascular disease (e.g., systemic lupus erythematosus, scleroderma). In clinical studies in patients with some degree of renal impairment (serum creatinine concentration of at least 1.6 mg/dL), neutropenia occurred in about 0.2% of patients, a frequency greater than 15 times that in patients with uncomplicated hypertension who have normal renal function. Most of the patients with renal impairment received relatively high dosages, particularly in relation to their renal function; in some reports, the neutropenia was associated with concomitant administration of allopurinol while in other reports this association was not apparent. In clinical studies, neutropenia has occurred in about 3.7% of patients with collagen vascular disease and renal impairment. Neutropenia has also occurred in some patients receiving captopril for the management of heart failure and the risk factors appear to be similar; about 50% of the patients developing neutropenia had impaired renal function and about 75% were receiving procainamide concomitantly.

Following discontinuance of captopril and other drugs, the neutrophil count generally returned to normal in about 2 weeks. Serious infections have been limited to patients with complex clinical conditions. Death has occurred in about 13% of patients who developed neutropenia, but almost all deaths occurred in patients with serious illness who had collagen vascular disease, renal failure, and/or heart failure and/or who were receiving immunosuppressive therapy. Although a few patients have been rechallenged with captopril (usually with lower dosages) without recurrence, others have reportedly experienced recurrence, even with lower dosages. Although a causal relationship to captopril has not been established, anemia (e.g., aplastic, hemolytic) has been reported in some patients receiving the drug.

● Renal Effects

Proteinuria (total urinary proteins exceeding 1 g/day) has occurred in about 0.7% of patients receiving captopril, and nephrotic syndrome occurred in about one-fifth of these patients. About 90% of patients who have developed proteinuria during captopril therapy had evidence of prior renal disease and/or received relatively high dosages of the drug (greater than 150 mg daily). If proteinuria develops, it usually occurs by the eighth month of treatment with captopril, consists mainly of albumin, and is rarely accompanied by increases in BUN or serum creatinine concentrations. Renal biopsies in some patients who developed proteinuria showed that membranous glomerulopathy was present; however, it was not definitely established that this effect was caused by the drug since these patients did not have pretreatment renal biopsies, and membranous glomerulopathy has occurred in hypertensive patients who did not receive the drug. Proteinuria usually subsides or clears within 6 months whether or not captopril therapy is continued; however, in some patients, it may persist.

Deterioration in renal function, manifested as transient increases in BUN and serum creatinine concentrations may occur following administration of captopril, especially in patients with impaired renal function, sodium depletion, or hypovolemia; patients with renovascular hypertension, particularly those with bilateral renal-artery stenosis or those with renal-artery stenosis in a solitary kidney; or patients with chronic or severe hypertension in whom the glomerular filtration rate may decrease transiently. This effect was usually reversible following discontinuance of captopril and/or diuretic therapy. Acute reversible renal failure also may occur. Renal function should be monitored closely during the first few weeks of therapy and periodically thereafter in patients with bilateral renal-artery stenosis or those with renal-artery stenosis in a solitary kidney. (See Cautions: Precautions and Contraindications.) About 5–15% or 15–30% of patients with mild to moderate or severe heart failure, respectively, treated with an angiotensin-converting enzyme (ACE) inhibitor develop substantial elevations of serum creatinine concentrations (e.g., exceeding 5 mg/dL) and BUN. Some patients with heart failure, including those with severe preexisting renal disease, may require discontinuance of ACE inhibitor therapy, including captopril, because of progressively increasing serum creatinine concentration. The rapidity of onset and magnitude of captopril-induced renal insufficiency in patients with heart failure may depend in part on the degree of sodium depletion.

Because the renin-angiotensin system appears to contribute substantially to maintenance of glomerular filtration in patients with heart failure in whom renal perfusion is severely compromised, renal function may deteriorate markedly during therapy with an ACE inhibitor in these patients. Such drug-induced deterioration is generally well tolerated, and does not usually necessitate discontinuance of effective therapy with the drug when symptomatic improvement of the heart failure occurs. In addition, the magnitude of deterioration in renal function can usually be ameliorated by reducing the dosage of concomitantly administered diuretics and/or by liberalizing dietary sodium intake, since concomitant diuretic therapy and/or sodium restriction potentially increase the role of angiotensin II in maintaining glomerular filtration in these patients. In patients in whom renal perfusion pressure is very low and is further reduced by ACE inhibitor therapy, however, deterioration in renal function may be clinically important. Patients with concomitant underlying diabetes mellitus may be at risk for developing renal insufficiency during ACE inhibitor therapy; however, ACE inhibitors, including captopril, have been beneficial in the management of diabetic nephropathy.

Although a definite causal relationship to captopril has not been established, renal insufficiency, polyuria, oliguria, and urinary frequency have been reported in about 0.1–0.2% of patients.

● Dermatologic and Sensitivity Reactions

The most common adverse effect of captopril is rash, which occurs in about 4–7% of patients (depending on renal function and dosage) and is usually maculopapular and rarely urticarial. Rash is often accompanied by pruritus and erythema and sometimes by fever, arthralgia, eosinophilia, and/or positive antinuclear antibody (ANA) titers. Eosinophilia and/or positive ANA titers have been reported in 7–10% of patients with captopril-induced rash. The rash occurs most frequently on the upper extremities and trunk but may occur at other sites. It generally occurs during the first 4 weeks of therapy and has occurred rarely within 30 minutes after the initial dose of the drug. The rash is usually mild and disappears within a few days after dosage reduction, short-term treatment with an oral antihistamine, and/or discontinuance of the drug. In some patients, the rash may disappear despite continued treatment and without dosage adjustment. Although the cause has not been clearly determined, it has been suggested that the rash may be a reaction mediated by kinins. Pruritus without rash occurs in about 2% of patients receiving captopril.

Photosensitivity has occurred, and captopril has been associated with reversible, pemphigoid lesions. Bullous pemphigoid also has been reported; however, a causal relationship to the drug has not been established.

Angioedema of the face, mucous membranes, lips, tongue, larynx, glottis, or extremities has occurred in about 0.1% of patients and may be reversible following discontinuance of therapy. (See Cautions: Precautions and Contraindications.) Intestinal angioedema (occasionally without a prior history of facial angioedema or elevated serum levels of complement 1 [C1] esterase inhibitor) also has been reported in patients receiving ACE inhibitors. Intestinal angioedema, which frequently presents as abdominal pain (with or without nausea or vomiting), usually is diagnosed by abdominal CT scan, ultrasound, or surgery; manifestations usually have resolved after discontinuance of the ACE inhibitor. Intestinal angioedema should be considered in the differential diagnosis of patients who develop abdominal pain during therapy with an ACE inhibitor.

Other hypersensitivity reactions have included vasculitis and hypersensitivity pneumonitis, which was associated with eosinophilia and pulmonary infiltrates. Rarely, a serum sickness type of reaction with rash or other dermatologic manifestations, fever, myalgia, arthralgia, interstitial nephritis, increased erythrocyte sedimentation rate (ESR), and/or difficulty in breathing has been reported in patients receiving captopril. Alopecia has occurred, but a causal relationship to the drug has not been established.

Severe, sudden anaphylactoid reactions, which can be fatal, have been reported following initiation of hemodialysis that utilized a high-flux polyacrylonitrile [PAN] membrane (e.g., AN 69®) in patients receiving an ACE inhibitor. Manifestations of these reactions included nausea, abdominal cramps, burning, angioedema, and shortness of breath; progression to severe hypotension can develop rapidly. Dialysis should be stopped immediately and aggressive supportive and symptomatic therapy should be initiated as indicated. Antihistamines do *not* appear to be effective in providing symptomatic relief. While it currently does not seem to be necessary to exclude the use of ACE inhibitors in patients undergoing hemodialysis that involves PAN membranes, caution should be exercised during concomitant use. The mechanism of this interaction has not been established, and the incidence and risk of its occurrence remain to be elucidated. In these patients, consideration should be given to using a different type of dialysis membrane or a drug other than an ACE inhibitor. In addition, anaphylactoid reactions also have been reported in patients undergoing low-density lipoprotein (LDL) apheresis with dextran sulfate absorption, a procedure utilizing devices not approved in the US. Manifestations of these reactions included flushing, dyspnea, bradycardia, and hypotension. It has been postulated that these reactions may be associated with accumulation of polypeptides (e.g., bradykinin) since endogenous concentration of such polypeptides may be increased by LDL-apheresis with dextran sulfate and their metabolism may be decreased by ACE inhibitors. To avoid these anaphylactoid reactions, some clinicians recommend withdrawal of ACE inhibitors 12–30 hours before apheresis, while others state that ACE inhibitors should not be used in patients treated with LDL apheresis.

Life-threatening anaphylactoid reactions have been reported in at least 2 patients receiving ACE inhibitors while undergoing desensitization treatment with hymenoptera venom. When ACE inhibitors were temporarily discontinued 24 hours before desensitization with the venom, anaphylactoid reactions did not recur; however, such reactions recurred after inadvertent rechallenge.

Onycholysis and dystrophic changes in the fingernails have occurred rarely in patients receiving captopril. In at least one patient, these changes were associated with other manifestations of zinc deficiency (e.g., alopecia, asteatosis, dysgeusia, cutaneous eruptions). Although serum zinc concentrations were within the normal range in this patient, manifestations of zinc deficiency showed some

improvement when captopril dosage was reduced and then gradually resolved when supplemental zinc therapy was initiated. However, other manifestations of zinc deficiency have been absent and serum zinc concentrations normal in other patients with nail changes, and the relationship, if any, of these effects to captopril-induced zinc deficiency has not been established.

● *Effects on Taste*

Decrease in taste acuity, or alteration (persistent metallic or salty taste) or loss of taste perception is another common adverse effect of captopril, occurring in about 2–4% of patients (depending on renal function and dosage). Taste impairment usually occurs during the first 3 months of therapy; it is usually reversible within 2–3 months even when captopril therapy is continued. In some patients, taste impairment has been associated with subsequent weight loss. The mechanism of taste impairment has not been established. In patients not receiving captopril, alterations in taste perception have been associated with decreased plasma zinc concentrations, but normal plasma zinc concentrations have been reported in a few patients with captopril-induced taste impairment and these patients did not respond to oral zinc supplements.

● *Cardiovascular Effects*

Excessive hypotension occurs rarely in hypertensive patients receiving captopril. Transient decreases in mean blood pressure greater than 20% may occur in about half of patients with heart failure treated with captopril. Hypotension has required discontinuance of therapy in about 3–5% of patients with heart failure receiving captopril.

Captopril-induced hypotension may occasionally be alleviated by initial dosage reduction (i.e., 6.25 or 12.5 mg 3 times daily), but hypotension has also occurred after low doses (i.e., a single 6.25-mg dose) of the drug. Orthostatic hypotension appears to occur more frequently during initiation of therapy and in patients with sodium depletion, hypovolemia, markedly elevated plasma renin or angiotensin II concentration, or overdosage. Transient hypotension in patients with heart failure or with hypertension may occur after any of the first several doses and usually is well tolerated, producing no symptoms or occasionally associated with brief, mild lightheadedness or dizziness, blurred vision, syncope, and, rarely, bradycardia or conduction defects. One patient with congestive heart failure who had markedly elevated PRA developed fatal refractory ventricular fibrillation, associated with hypotension, following two 6.25-mg doses of captopril. Patients who are volume and/or sodium depleted such as those receiving diuretics, especially those in whom diuretic therapy was recently initiated (e.g., patients with severe congestive heart failure), those whose sodium intake is severely restricted, and those who are undergoing dialysis, may occasionally experience a precipitous reduction of blood pressure within the first 3 hours after the initial dose of captopril. Symptomatic hypotension that occurs later in a course of captopril therapy (e.g., after the first 48 hours) may indicate the presence of sodium depletion (e.g., secondary to restriction of sodium intake or increased diuretic dosage).

Enalapril, another ACE inhibitor, has produced severe hypotension in patients with severe heart failure with or without renal insufficiency, which was occasionally associated with oliguria and/or progressive azotemia and, rarely, with acute renal failure, myocardial ischemia, and/or death. Captopril, which has a shorter duration of action than enalapril, may have a decreased risk associated with these adverse effects. Because of the risk of developing severe hypotension and potential compromise of the patient's hemodynamic status, patients with heart failure should be monitored closely for 2 weeks after initiation of captopril therapy and whenever dosage of captopril and/or a concomitantly administered diuretic is increased.

The possibility of severe hypotension may be minimized by withholding diuretic therapy and/or increasing sodium intake approximately 3–7 days prior to initiating captopril therapy. If hypotension occurs in patients receiving captopril, the patient should be placed in the supine or Trendelenburg's position; if hypotension is severe, IV infusion of 0.9% sodium chloride injection to expand fluid volume should be considered. Transient hypotension is not a contraindication to additional doses of captopril, and therapy with the drug can be cautiously reinstated after blood pressure has been stabilized (e.g., with volume expansion). Asymptomatic hypotension often does not require specific therapy and may be well tolerated with continued captopril therapy; however, severe hypotension occasionally may require discontinuance of captopril therapy. In patients with heart failure, the reduction in blood pressure stabilizes within 1–2 weeks after starting captopril therapy, and blood pressure generally returns to pretreatment levels within 2 months without a decrease in therapeutic efficacy. Hypotension may also occur in captopril-treated patients during major surgery or during anesthesia with agents that produce hypotension. This hypotensive effect results from inhibition by captopril of the angiotensin II formation that occurs subsequent to compensatory renin release, and, if it is thought to be caused by captopril, can generally be corrected with fluid volume expansion.

Tachycardia, chest pain, and palpitations have each occurred in about 1% of patients receiving captopril. Flushing, pallor, angina pectoris, myocardial infarction (MI), Raynaud's phenomenon, and heart failure have been reported rarely. Captopril has also produced hyperkinetic circulation (tachycardia, greatly increased cardiac output, and decreased mean blood transit time) in at least one patient with congestive heart failure. Although a causal relationship has not been established, other adverse cardiovascular effects that have been reported in patients receiving captopril include cardiac arrest, cerebrovascular accident and/or insufficiency, rhythm disturbances, and syncope.

● Effects on Potassium

Although small increases in serum potassium concentration occur frequently in patients receiving captopril without a thiazide diuretic, hyperkalemia has occurred rarely. Patients with impaired renal function or heart failure and patients concomitantly receiving drugs that can increase serum potassium concentration (e.g., potassium-sparing diuretics, potassium supplements, potassium-containing salt substitutes) may be at increased risk of developing hyperkalemia during captopril therapy, especially those with diabetes mellitus; serum potassium concentration should be monitored carefully in these patients, and potassium intake should be controlled and therapy with drugs that can increase serum potassium modified or discontinued as necessary. In a clinical trial in patients with type 1 diabetes mellitus who were receiving captopril for proteinuria, the drug was discontinued in about 2% of patients secondary to hyperkalemia. However, hyperkalemia was not reported in another trial in normotensive patients with type 1 diabetes mellitus who were receiving captopril for microalbuminuria.

● Respiratory Effects

Cough has been reported in about 0.5–2% of patients receiving captopril. However, cough often is overlooked as a potential adverse effect of ACE inhibitors and may occur more frequently (in about 5–15% of patients). The cough generally is persistent and nonproductive and reversible following discontinuance of the drug. It has been suggested that accumulation of kinins in the respiratory tract secondary to ACE inhibition may in part be responsible for this cough. Concomitant therapy with a nonsteroidal anti-inflammatory agent (i.e., sulindac) appeared to minimize cough in a few patients, but additional study of the safety (e.g., effects on renal function) of such combined therapy is necessary. Dyspnea and bronchospasm have been reported rarely during captopril therapy. Angioedema has occurred in 0.1% of patients receiving captopril, and, if associated with laryngeal edema or angioedema of the tongue or glottis, airway obstruction may occur, and angioedema may be fatal. (See Cautions: Precautions and Contraindications.)

● Hepatic Effects

Hepatitis (including rare cases of hepatic necrosis), cholestasis, jaundice, and elevations in serum concentrations of hepatic enzymes, alkaline phosphatase, and bilirubin have been reported occasionally but have not been directly attributed to the drug, and rare cases of cholestatic jaundice and of hepatocellular injury (with or without secondary cholestasis) have been associated with captopril therapy.

A clinical syndrome that usually is manifested initially by cholestatic jaundice and may progress to fulminant hepatic necrosis (which occasionally may be fatal) has been reported rarely in patients receiving ACE inhibitors. The mechanism of this reaction is not known.

● Other Adverse Effects

Hyponatremia (which may be symptomatic) has been reported occasionally in patients receiving captopril; some of these patients had heart failure or were receiving a low-sodium diet or concomitant diuretics. In at least one patient, gynecomastia occurred while receiving captopril, which was reversible following discontinuance of the drug.

Although a causal relationship has not been established, other adverse effects that have occurred rarely in patients receiving captopril include dry mouth,

aphthous ulcers, ulceration of the tongue, reversible lymphadenopathy, abdominal pain, nausea, vomiting, diarrhea, anorexia, constipation, dyspepsia, gastric irritation, peptic ulcer, pancreatitis, glossitis, headache, dizziness, paresthesia, malaise, asthenia, myalgia, myasthenia, ataxia, confusion, depression, nervousness, somnolence, blurred vision, impotence, and insomnia.

● Precautions and Contraindications

Captopril may cause serious adverse effects (e.g., neutropenia) and must be used under close supervision, particularly in patients with renal impairment (especially those with collagen vascular disease). When the drug is used, the risk of neutropenia and agranulocytosis must be considered. When captopril is used as a fixed combination that includes hydrochlorothiazide, the cautions, precautions, and contraindications associated with thiazide diuretics must be considered in addition to those associated with captopril.

Because cough has been associated with the use of many ACE inhibitors, including captopril, it should be considered in the differential diagnosis of patients who develop cough during captopril therapy.

The possibility that proteinuria can develop and may progress to nephrotic syndrome in patients receiving captopril should be considered, particularly in those with preexisting renal disease or receiving captopril dosages exceeding 150 mg daily. (See Cautions: Renal Effects.)

Renal function should be evaluated prior to initiation of captopril therapy, and the drug should be used with caution in patients with renal impairment, particularly those with known or suspected renovascular disease. Reduction of captopril dosage, reduction in dosage or discontinuance of diuretic therapy, and/or adequate sodium repletion may be necessary in some patients who develop impaired renal function during captopril therapy; it may be impossible to reduce blood pressure to normal levels and maintain adequate renal perfusion. Because of an increased risk of reducing renal perfusion to a critically low level, captopril should be used with caution and renal function monitored closely for the first few weeks of therapy in patients with bilateral renal-artery stenosis and in those with renal-artery stenosis in a solitary kidney. Serum creatinine and electrolyte concentrations should be evaluated prior to and 1 week following initiation of therapy with ACE inhibitors in patients with heart failure. In patients with heart failure who have some degree of renal impairment (baseline serum creatinine concentrations less than 2 mg/dL) or more severe renal impairment (baseline serum creatinine concentrations exceeding 2 mg/dL), an increase in serum creatinine concentration exceeding 0.5 or 1 mg/dL, respectively, should prompt consideration of discontinuing ACE inhibitor therapy while additional renal evaluation and corrective action is undertaken. The possibility that ACE inhibitors might precipitate severe, sudden, potentially life-threatening anaphylactoid reactions in patients undergoing hemodialysis involving a high-flux membrane should be considered. (See Cautions: Dermatologic and Hypersensitivity Reactions.)

In patients with collagen vascular disease (e.g., systemic lupus erythematosus, scleroderma) or in those receiving other drugs known to affect leukocytes or immune response, particularly those with coexisting impaired renal function, captopril should be used only after an assessment of the benefits and risks, and then with caution. If captopril is administered to patients with any of these conditions and/or with impaired renal function, complete and differential leukocyte counts should be performed prior to initiation of therapy, at approximately 2-week intervals for the first 3 months of therapy, and periodically thereafter. In other patients receiving captopril, complete leukocyte counts may be performed at approximately 2-week intervals for the first 3 months of therapy and periodically thereafter; differential leukocyte counts should be performed if the complete leukocyte count is less than 4000/mm³ or half of the pretreatment count. If the neutrophil count is less than 1000/mm³, captopril should be discontinued and the patient closely monitored. Patients should be instructed to notify their clinician if any signs or symptoms of infection such as fever or sore throat occur. If infection is suspected, blood cell counts should be performed immediately.

Because rare cases of cholestatic jaundice and fulminant hepatic necrosis (sometimes fatal) have occurred in patients receiving ACE inhibitors, including captopril, the drug should be discontinued and patients monitored appropriately if jaundice or marked elevations in hepatic enzymes occur during therapy. (See Cautions: Hepatic Effects.)

Captopril should be used with caution in patients with sodium depletion or hypovolemia, those receiving diuretics, and those undergoing dialysis since severe hypotension may occur. The drug should also be used with caution in patients in whom excessive hypotension may have serious consequences (e.g., patients with coronary or cerebrovascular insufficiency). ACE inhibitor therapy should be initiated with caution in patients with very low systemic blood pressure (systolic blood pressure less than 80 mm Hg), markedly increased serum concentrations of creatinine (greater than 3 mg/dL), bilateral renal artery stenosis, or elevated concentrations of serum potassium (greater than 5 mEq/L). Experts recommend that treatment with an ACE inhibitor be initiated at low doses and gradually titrated upward as tolerated. Patients with heart failure should be closely monitored for the first 2 weeks of therapy and whenever the dosage of captopril and/or the diuretic is increased. Patients receiving captopril therapy should be informed that vomiting, diarrhea, excessive perspiration, and dehydration may lead to an exaggerated decrease in blood pressure because of fluid volume reduction; patients should notify their clinician if any of these conditions occurs. The possibility that patients with aortic stenosis might be at risk of decreased coronary perfusion when treated with captopril should be considered.

Patients receiving captopril should be warned not to interrupt or discontinue therapy unless instructed by their clinician. Patients with heart failure receiving captopril should be cautioned against rapid increases in physical activity.

Although captopril and penicillamine are not pharmacologically related, many adverse effects (e.g., rash, taste impairment, proteinuria) of these drugs are similar. Because captopril and penicillamine contain sulfhydryl groups and are structurally related, it has been suggested that the common toxicities may in part result from the chemical and structural characteristics of the drugs; however, such a relationship has not been clearly determined. Since therapy with ACE inhibitors has been associated with development of a rare syndrome that usually is manifested initially by cholestatic jaundice that may progress to fulminant hepatic necrosis and occasionally may be fatal, patients receiving an ACE inhibitor, including captopril, who develop jaundice or marked elevations of hepatic enzymes should discontinue the drug and receive appropriate medical follow-up. (See Cautions: Hepatic Effects.)

Angioedema may occur in patients receiving an ACE inhibitor (e.g., captopril), and, if associated with laryngeal edema, may be fatal. If swelling is confined to the extremities, face, lips, and mucous membranes of the mouth, the condition usually responds without treatment. Swelling of the tongue, glottis, or larynx may cause airway obstruction, and appropriate therapy (e.g., epinephrine) should be initiated immediately. Patients should be informed that swelling of the face, eyes, lips, tongue, larynx, or extremities or difficulty in breathing or in swallowing may be signs and symptoms of angioedema, and that they should discontinue captopril and notify their clinician immediately if any of these conditions occurs. The possibility that patients with a history of angioedema unrelated to ACE inhibitors may be at increased risk of developing angioedema while receiving the drugs should be considered.

Captopril is contraindicated in patients with known hypersensitivity to the drug or to another ACE inhibitor (e.g., those who experienced angioedema during therapy with another ACE inhibitor).

● *Pediatric Precautions*

Although there is limited clinical experience with captopril in children, safety and efficacy of the drug in children have not been established; however, pediatric dosage was reported to be comparable or less than dosage used in adults when calculated on the basis of body weight. Infants, especially neonates, may have increased susceptibility to captopril-induced adverse hemodynamic effects. Excessive, prolonged, and unpredictable decreases in blood pressure and associated complications (e.g., oliguria, seizures) have been reported in children receiving the drug. The manufacturer states that captopril should be used in children only when other measures for controlling blood pressure have not been effective. For information on overall principles and expert recommendations for treatment of hypertension in pediatric patients, see Uses: Hypertension in Pediatric Patients, in the Thiazides General Statement 40:28.20.

● *Pregnancy, Fertility, and Lactation*
Pregnancy

Fetal and neonatal morbidity and mortality have been reported in at least 50 women who were receiving ACE inhibitors during pregnancy. Very limited epidemiologic data indicate that the rate of fetal and neonatal morbidity resulting from exposure to ACE inhibitors during the second and third trimesters may be as high as 10–20%. Hypotension, reversible or irreversible renal failure, anuria, skull hypoplasia, and/or death were reported in neonates whose mothers had received ACE inhibitors during the second and third trimesters of pregnancy. Other adverse effects associated with such use included oligohydramnios, presumably due to decreased renal function in the fetus, prematurity, fetal death, and patent ductus arteriosus; however, it is not known if these effects were associated with ACE inhibition or underlying maternal disease. Oligohydramnios has been associated with contractures of the limbs, craniofacial deformities, hypoplasia of the lungs, and intrauterine growth retardation.

Although fetal exposure limited to the first trimester previously was considered not to be associated with substantial risk, data from an epidemiologic study have shown that infants whose mothers had taken an ACE inhibitor during the first trimester of pregnancy have an increased risk of major congenital malformations compared with infants who had not undergone first trimester exposure to ACE inhibitors. The risk of major congenital malformations, primarily affecting the cardiovascular and central nervous systems, was increased by about 2.7 times in infants whose mothers had taken an ACE inhibitor during the first trimester of pregnancy compared with infants who had not undergone such exposure. Every effort should be made to discontinue captopril therapy as soon as possible in any woman who becomes pregnant while receiving the drug, regardless of the period of gestation. In addition, all women of childbearing potential who are receiving an ACE inhibitor should be advised to report pregnancy to their clinician as soon as possible. Women of childbearing potential who are receiving an ACE inhibitor also should be advised to inform their clinician if they are planning to become pregnant or think they might be pregnant. Nearly all women can be transferred successfully to alternative therapy for the remainder of their pregnancy. Rarely (probably less frequently than once in every 1000 pregnancies), no adequate alternative can be identified; in such rare cases, the woman should be informed of the potential hazard to the fetus and serial ultrasound examinations should be performed to assess the intra-amniotic environment. If oligohydramnios is present, captopril therapy should be discontinued, unless use of the drug is considered life-saving for the woman. Contraction stress testing (CST), a nonstress test (NST), or biophysical profiling may be performed, if appropriate, depending on the period of gestation. However, both clinicians and patients should realize that oligohydramnios may not become apparent until after irreversible fetal injury already has occurred.

Infants exposed in utero to ACE inhibitors should be observed closely for hypotension, oliguria, and hyperkalemia. If oliguria occurs, supportive measures (e.g., administration of fluids and pressor agents) to correct hypotension and renal perfusion should be considered. Exchange transfusion or dialysis may be required to reverse hypotension and/or substitute for impaired renal function. Although captopril may be removed by hemodialysis in adults, it is not known if the drug is removed from circulation of neonates or older children by hemodialysis. Peritoneal dialysis is not effective in enhancing the elimination of captopril, and it is not known whether the drug may be removed by exchange transfusion.

Reproduction studies in hamsters and rats using 150 and 625 times the maximum human dosage, respectively, of captopril have not revealed evidence of teratogenic effects. However, the drug was associated with a low incidence of craniofacial malformations in rabbits when given at dosages 0.8–70 times the maximum human dosage. Reduction in neonatal survival occurred in the offspring of rats receiving captopril dosages 400 times the usual human dosage continuously during gestation and lactation, and an increased incidence of stillbirths has reportedly occurred in ewes.

Fertility

Reproduction studies in rats using captopril have not revealed evidence of impaired fertility.

Lactation

Captopril is distributed into milk in concentrations about 1% of those in maternal blood. Because of the potential for serious adverse reactions to captopril in nursing infants, a decision should be made whether to discontinue nursing or the drug, taking into account the importance of the drug to the woman.

DRUG INTERACTIONS

• Hypotensive Agents and Diuretics

When captopril is administered with diuretics or other hypotensive drugs, the hypotensive effect of captopril is increased. The effect is usually used to therapeutic advantage, but careful adjustment of dosage is necessary when these drugs are used concomitantly.

Captopril and diuretics appear to have additive hypotensive effects; however, severe hypotension and reversible renal insufficiency may occasionally occur, especially in volume- and/or sodium-depleted patients. (See Cautions: Cardiovascular Effects.) In addition, the duration of hypotensive effect is extended by concomitant diuretic therapy. The hypotensive effects of captopril and β-adrenergic blocking agents (β-blockers) (e.g., propranolol) are less than additive. Hypotensive drugs that cause release of renin (e.g., diuretics) will increase the hypotensive effect of captopril. Reduction of captopril dosage and/or dosage reduction or discontinuance of diuretic therapy may be necessary. Patients should be monitored closely during initiation and dosage adjustment of concomitant therapy with captopril and a diuretic; in patients already receiving diuretics, the risk of these effects may be minimized by withholding diuretic therapy and/or increasing sodium intake for 3–7 days prior to initiating captopril therapy.

While captopril may have pharmacodynamic interactions in patients receiving diuretics, use of furosemide concurrently with captopril in patients with renal impairment and hypertension does not alter the pharmacokinetics of captopril.

Hypotensive drugs that affect sympathetic nervous system activity such as ganglionic blocking agents (e.g., trimethaphan camsylate [no longer commercially available in the US]) or adrenergic neuron blocking agents (e.g., guanethidine sulfate) should be used with caution in patients receiving captopril, since the sympathetic nervous system may be especially important in maintaining blood pressure in patients treated with captopril.

• Vasodilating Agents

Data on the effect of concomitant use of captopril and other vasodilators in the management of heart failure are not currently available. Pending accumulation of clinical data on such concomitant use, nitroglycerin or other nitrates or other drugs with vasodilating activity (e.g., hydralazine, prazosin) should be discontinued if possible before starting captopril; if such agents are resumed during captopril therapy, they should be administered with caution and possibly at lower dosage.

• Drugs Increasing Serum Potassium Concentration

Since captopril decreases aldosterone secretion, small increases in serum potassium concentration frequently occur, especially in patients with impaired renal function; hyperkalemia has occurred rarely. Potassium-sparing diuretics (e.g., amiloride, spironolactone, triamterene), potassium supplements, or potassium-containing salt substitutes should be used with caution in patients receiving captopril and only if hypokalemia is documented, since hyperkalemia may occur; serum potassium should be monitored carefully. Dosage of the potassium-sparing diuretic and/or potassium supplement should be reduced or the diuretic and/or supplement discontinued as necessary. Patients with renal impairment may be at increased risk of hyperkalemia. If the patient has received spironolactone at any time up to several months before captopril is administered, serum potassium concentration should be determined frequently when captopril is administered since the potassium-sparing effect of spironolactone may persist. However, angiotensin-converting enzyme (ACE) inhibitors have been administered with low-dosage spironolactone therapy and hyperkalemia was reported rarely. (See Uses: Heart Failure.)

• Cardiac Glycosides

A study in healthy men revealed no evidence of a pharmacokinetic interaction between captopril and digoxin. However, studies in patients with heart failure indicate that serum digoxin concentrations may increase by about 15–30% when captopril and digoxin are used concomitantly. Such increases may result from decreased renal clearance (probably both glomerular filtration and tubular secretion) of digoxin and, possibly, displacement of the glycoside from tissue-binding sites by captopril-induced increases in serum potassium. Captopril has been administered concomitantly with digoxin in patients with heart failure *without*

unusual adverse effects or apparent increased risk of cardiac glycoside toxicity. It has been postulated that captopril-induced increases in serum potassium may offset the potential toxic effects of increased serum digoxin concentrations. Reduction in digoxin dosage does not appear to be necessary when captopril is initiated; however, serum digoxin concentrations should be monitored and the patient observed for signs of glycoside toxicity when the drugs are used concomitantly. Further studies are needed to determine the clinical importance of this potential interaction.

• Nonsteroidal Anti-inflammatory Agents

Because ACE inhibitors may promote kinin-mediated prostaglandin synthesis and/or release, concomitant administration of drugs that inhibit prostaglandin synthesis (e.g., aspirin, ibuprofen) may reduce the blood pressure response to ACE inhibitors, including captopril. Limited data indicate that concomitant administration of ACE inhibitors with nonsteroidal anti-inflammatory agents (NSAIAs) occasionally may result in acute reduction of renal function; however, the possibility cannot be ruled out that one drug alone may cause such an effect. Blood pressure should be monitored carefully when an NSAIA is initiated in patients receiving ACE inhibitor therapy; in addition, clinicians should be alert for evidence of impaired renal function. Some clinicians suggest that if a drug interaction between an ACE inhibitor and an NSAIA is suspected, the NSAIA should be discontinued, or a different hypotensive agent used or, alternatively, the dosage of the hypotensive agent should be modified.

Aspirin and other NSAIAs also can attenuate the hemodynamic actions of ACE inhibitors in patients with heart failure. Because ACE inhibitors share and enhance the effects of the compensatory hemodynamic mechanisms of heart failure, with aspirin and other NSAIAs interacting with the compensatory mechanisms rather than with a given ACE inhibitor per se, these desirable mechanisms are particularly susceptible to the interaction and a subsequent potential loss of clinical benefits. As a result, the more severe the heart failure and the more prominent the compensatory mechanisms, the more appreciable the interaction between NSAIAs and ACE inhibitors. Even if optimal dosage of an ACE inhibitor is used in the treatment of heart failure, the potential cardiovascular and survival benefit may not be seen if the patient is receiving an NSAIA concomitantly. In several multicenter studies, concomitant administration of a single 350-mg dose of aspirin in patients with heart failure inhibited favorable hemodynamic effects associated with ACE inhibitors, attenuating the favorable effects of these drugs on survival and cardiovascular morbidity. However, these findings have not been confirmed by other studies. In one retrospective analysis of pooled data, patients who received an ACE inhibitor concomitantly with aspirin (160–325 mg daily) during the acute phase following myocardial infarction (MI) had proportional reductions in 7- and 30-day mortality rates comparable to patients who received an ACE inhibitor alone. Some clinicians have questioned the results of this study because of methodologic concerns (e.g., unsubstantiated assumptions about aspirin therapy [dosage, time of initiation, duration]; disparate distribution of patients). Although it has been suggested that patients requiring long-term management of heart failure avoid the concomitant use of ACE inhibitors and aspirin (and perhaps substitute another platelet-aggregation inhibitor for aspirin [e.g., clopidogrel, ticlopidine]), many clinicians state that existing data are insufficient to recommend a change in the current prescribing practices of clinicians concerning the use of aspirin in patients receiving therapy with an ACE inhibitor.

• Antacids

Concomitant oral administration of captopril and antacids may decrease the rate and extent of GI absorption of captopril. Oral administration of a single, 50-mg dose of captopril 15 minutes after an oral dose of an antacid containing magnesium carbonate and aluminum and magnesium hydroxides resulted in a 40–45% decrease in captopril bioavailability, and a delay and decrease in peak serum concentrations of the drug. However, there is some evidence that this potential interaction may not be clinically important, but additional study is necessary.

• Probenecid

Concomitant administration of probenecid may increase blood concentrations of captopril and its metabolites, probably through decreased tubular secretion of captopril and subsequently increased metabolism of the drug (the latter effect probably occurring indirectly as a result of decreased renal clearance of the drug). Prolongation of ACE inhibition by captopril and possible subsequent potentiation of clinical and toxic effects of the drug may occur during concomitant therapy, but the potential for such interaction has not been fully elucidated.

● Other Drugs

Neuropathy reportedly developed in 2 patients receiving captopril and cimetidine; however, further documentation of this potential interaction is necessary.

Initiation of captopril therapy has been associated with unexplained hypoglycemia in several diabetic patients whose diabetes had been controlled with insulin or oral antidiabetic agents. Testing in these patients indicated that captopril may increase insulin sensitivity; the mechanism of this effect is not known. The risk of precipitating hypoglycemia should be considered when captopril therapy is initiated in diabetic patients.

Lithium and an ACE inhibitor (e.g., captopril) should be used concomitantly with caution and serum lithium concentrations should be monitored frequently since elevated serum lithium concentrations and lithium toxicity have occurred following concomitant therapy with the drugs. The risk of lithium toxicity in patients receiving captopril may be increased in patients who are also receiving diuretic therapy.

LABORATORY TEST INTERFERENCES

Captopril may cause false-positive results in urine acetone determinations using sodium nitroprusside reagent.

PHARMACOLOGY

The mechanism(s) of action of captopril has not been fully elucidated. The drug appears to reduce blood pressure in hypertensive patients and produce beneficial hemodynamic effects in patients with heart failure mainly by suppressing the renin-angiotensin-aldosterone system.

● Effects on Renin-Angiotensin-Aldosterone System

Captopril prevents the conversion of angiotensin I to angiotensin II (a potent vasoconstrictor) by competing with the physiologic substrate (angiotensin I) for the active site of angiotensin-converting enzyme (ACE); the affinity of the drug for ACE is approximately 30,000 times greater than that of angiotensin I.

Inhibition of ACE results in decreased plasma angiotensin II concentrations and, consequently, blood pressure may be reduced in part through decreased vasoconstriction. Plasma renin activity (PRA) increases, possibly as a result of loss of feedback inhibition (mediated by angiotensin II) on the release of renin from the kidneys and/or stimulation of reflex mechanisms via baroreceptors (as a result of the decrease in blood pressure). It has been suggested that the hypotensive effect of ACE inhibitors may in part result from a local effect (e.g., in vascular wall). By decreasing local angiotensin II production, ACE inhibitors may decrease vascular tone by reducing direct angiotensin II-induced vasoconstriction and/or angiotensin II-induced increases in sympathetic activity. The hypotensive effect of captopril persists longer than inhibition of ACE in blood; it is not known whether ACE is inhibited longer in vascular endothelium than in blood.

Captopril alone is apparently more effective in reducing blood pressure in patients with high or normal renin hypertension. The drug also may lower blood pressure in patients with low renin hypertension, but these patients are unlikely to respond unless a diuretic is given in conjunction with captopril. A positive correlation between pretreatment PRA and short-term reduction in blood pressure with captopril has been reported and is particularly evident when data from a large number of patients are combined; the magnitude of the initial decrease in blood pressure appears to be proportional to the pretreatment PRA. Although some clinicians have reported a positive correlation between pretreatment PRA and long-term response to captopril, such a correlation has not been consistently found and remains to be clearly established. Some clinicians believe that an individual pretreatment PRA is not useful in predicting a response to captopril because of the wide interpatient variation in PRA values. Since captopril increases PRA, renin profiling should not be performed during captopril therapy.

Decreases in plasma angiotensin II concentrations lead to decreased aldosterone secretion from the adrenal cortex and, therefore, decreased plasma aldosterone concentrations and decreased urinary aldosterone excretion. However, there is increasing evidence to suggest that plasma aldosterone concentrations may not decrease during therapy with usual dosages of ACE inhibitors in some patients and may return to pretreatment levels in others during prolonged therapy. It has been suggested that the addition of spironolactone, a drug that competitively inhibits the physiologic effects of aldosterone, appears to augment the suppressive effect of ACE inhibitors on aldosterone. The hypotensive effect of captopril may result in part from decreased sodium and water retention as a result of the reduction in aldosterone secretion.

● Effects on Catecholamines and Autacoids

Circulating plasma norepinephrine concentration is not affected by captopril, and the drug does not inhibit the increase in plasma norepinephrine concentration that results from orthostatic reflexes. However, by inhibiting angiotensin II formation, ACE inhibitors may affect catecholamine release and reuptake by noradrenergic nerve endings and/or may decrease vascular sensitivity to vasopressors. There is some evidence that high doses of ACE inhibitors may inhibit presynaptic norepinephrine release and postsynaptic α_2-adrenoceptor activity, thereby interfering with sympathetic reflexes, but the clinical importance of this finding is not known since dosages tested in animals substantially exceed usual human hypotensive dosages.

Because ACE also degrades the vasodilator bradykinin, it has been suggested that inhibition of ACE by captopril may cause accumulation of bradykinin in plasma or tissues with resultant vasodilation. However, the effects of captopril on plasma bradykinin concentration have varied, possibly because of the difficulties in measuring bradykinin; the contribution of bradykinin-mediated effects to the hypotensive action of captopril remains to be clearly established. It has been suggested that prostaglandins also may mediate some of the pharmacologic effects of captopril, since there is some evidence that the drug may increase prostaglandin production or release; prostaglandin release may in part result from increased concentrations of bradykinin. Some clinicians have reported that captopril may control blood pressure in patients with renovascular hypertension without affecting urinary excretion of prostaglandin E_2. However, the effects of captopril on prostaglandins have been inconsistent, and further evaluation is necessary to determine the importance of any prostaglandin-mediated effects. (See Drug Interactions: Nonsteroidal Anti-Inflammatory Agents.)

● Cardiovascular Effects

In hypertensive patients, captopril reduces blood pressure by decreasing total peripheral resistance with no change or an increase in heart rate, stroke volume, or cardiac output; these effects are independent of pretreatment blood pressure or cardiac output. The drug causes arterial and possibly venous dilation. Captopril generally decreases systolic and diastolic blood pressure by 15–25%; blood pressure is decreased to about the same extent in both the supine and standing positions. Orthostatic hypotension and tachycardia occur infrequently but are more common in sodium-depleted or hypovolemic patients. (See Cautions: Cardiovascular Effects.) Plasma volume has been reported to be unchanged or slightly increased. Animal studies indicate that captopril does not have a direct effect on vascular smooth muscle. The drug appears to have no direct effect on baroreceptor sensitivity although reflex stimulation may occur during captopril therapy.

In patients with heart failure, captopril decreases total peripheral resistance, pulmonary vascular resistance, pulmonary capillary wedge pressure, and mean arterial and right atrial pressures. Cardiac index, cardiac output, stroke volume, and exercise tolerance are increased in these patients; heart rate decreases or is unchanged. The drug may also cause regional redistribution of blood flow, principally increasing renal blood flow with slight or no increase in flow in the forearm or hepatic vasculature, respectively.

● Renal and Electrolyte Effects

Renal blood flow may increase but glomerular filtration rate is usually unchanged during captopril therapy. In some patients, however, both BUN and serum creatinine concentrations have occasionally increased. Increased BUN and serum creatinine occur more frequently in patients with preexisting renal impairment, in those receiving concomitant therapy with a diuretic, and in those with heart failure. In patients with heart failure and renal perfusion pressures less than 70 mm Hg, changes in creatinine clearance induced by 1–3 months of captopril therapy have varied linearly and inversely with pretreatment PRA; however, creatinine clearance was not substantially affected by the drug in patients with renal perfusion pressures of 70 mm Hg or greater. Transient increases in BUN and serum creatinine concentrations are more frequent in patients with renovascular hypotension than in hypertensive patients with normal renal function. In addition, renal function can markedly deteriorate during therapy with an ACE inhibitor in patients with preexisting, severely compromised renal function. (See Cautions: Renal Effects.) Although anephric patients may respond to captopril immediately following hemodialysis (i.e., when hypovolemia exists), they apparently do not respond to the drug when fluid repleted.

Small increases in serum potassium concentration may occur secondary to captopril-induced decreases in aldosterone secretion, especially in patients with impaired renal function. Concomitant administration of thiazide diuretics generally offsets this increase. Captopril apparently does not cause sodium retention. Urinary sodium excretion may be increased during the first 2-3 days of captopril therapy.

● Other Effects

Serum prolactin concentration has been reported to increase during captopril therapy.

PHARMACOKINETICS

● Absorption

Approximately 60-75% of an oral dose of captopril is rapidly absorbed from the GI tract in fasting healthy individuals or hypertensive patients. Food may decrease absorption of captopril by up to 25-40%, although there is some evidence that this effect is not clinically important. Following oral administration of a single 100-mg dose of captopril in fasting healthy individuals in one study, average peak blood drug concentrations of 800 ng/mL were attained in 1 hour.

The hypotensive effect of a single dose of orally administered captopril may be apparent within 15 minutes and is usually maximal in 1-2 hours. The duration of action is generally 2-6 hours but appears to increase with increasing doses and has been prolonged up to 12 hours in some patients receiving high doses. The reduction in blood pressure may be gradual, and several weeks of therapy may be required before the full effect of the drug is achieved. The reduction in blood pressure observed with the initial dose of captopril has been reported by some clinicians to be positively correlated with the reduction in blood pressure achieved by long-term therapy with the drug. Some clinicians have observed a triphasic hypotensive effect during the first 1-2 weeks of therapy: the initial blood pressure reduction in the first few days is followed by a period lasting 3-9 days during which blood pressure increases toward pretreatment levels or remains stable, and then, a further reduction in blood pressure occurs. Because of the apparent resistance that may occur, increases in captopril dosage are usually avoided in the first 1-2 weeks of therapy since the eventual reduction in blood pressure does not reflect the response observed during this period. After withdrawal of the drug, blood pressure gradually returns to pretreatment levels within 1-7 days; rebound hypertension has not been reported to date.

● Distribution

Animal studies indicate that captopril is rapidly distributed into most body tissues, except the CNS. Captopril crosses the placenta in humans and is distributed into milk in concentrations about 1% of maternal blood concentrations.

Captopril is approximately 25-30% bound to plasma proteins, mainly albumin.

● Elimination

The elimination half-life of unchanged captopril appears to be less than 2 hours in patients with normal renal function. The elimination half-life of captopril and its metabolites is correlated with creatinine clearance and increases to about 20-40 hours in patients with creatinine clearances less than 20 mL/minute and as long as 6.5 days in anuric patients.

About half the absorbed dose of captopril is rapidly metabolized, mainly to captopril-cysteine disulfide and the disulfide dimer of captopril. In vitro studies suggest that captopril and its metabolites may undergo reversible interconversions. It has been suggested that the drug may be more extensively metabolized in patients with renal impairment than in patients with normal renal function.

Captopril and its metabolites are excreted in urine. Renal excretion of unchanged captopril occurs principally via tubular secretion. In patients with normal renal function, more than 95% of an absorbed dose is excreted in urine in 24 hours; about 40-50% of the drug excreted in urine is unchanged captopril and the remainder is mainly the disulfide dimer of captopril and captopril-cysteine disulfide. In one study in healthy individuals, about 20% of a single dose of captopril was recovered in feces in 5 days, apparently representing unabsorbed drug. Captopril is removed by hemodialysis.

PREPARATIONS

Excipients in commercially available drug preparations may have clinically important effects in some individuals; consult specific product labeling for details.

Captopril

Oral Tablets		
	12.5 mg*	Captopril Tablets
	25 mg*	Captopril Tablets
	50 mg*	Captopril Tablets
	100 mg*	Captopril Tablets

* available from one or more manufacturer, distributor, and/or repackager by generic (nonproprietary) name

Captopril and Hydrochlorothiazide

Oral Tablets		
	25 mg Captopril and Hydrochlorothiazide 15 mg*	Captopril and Hydrochlorothiazide Tablets
	25 mg Captopril and Hydrochlorothiazide 25 mg*	Captopril and Hydrochlorothiazide Tablets
	50 mg Captopril and Hydrochlorothiazide 15 mg*	Captopril and Hydrochlorothiazide Tablets
	50 mg Captopril and Hydrochlorothiazide 25 mg*	Captopril and Hydrochlorothiazide Tablets

* available from one or more manufacturer, distributor, and/or repackager by generic (nonproprietary) name

† Use is not currently included in the labeling approved by the US Food and Drug Administration.

Selected Revisions June 10, 2024, © Copyright, March 1, 1982, American Society of Health-System Pharmacists, Inc.

Enalaprilat
Enalapril Maleate

24:32.04 • ANGIOTENSIN-CONVERTING ENZYME INHIBITORS

■ Enalaprilat and enalapril are angiotensin-converting enzyme (ACE) inhibitors; enalapril, the ethylester of enalaprilat, is a prodrug and has little pharmacologic activity until hydrolyzed in the liver to enalaprilat.

USES

● Hypertension

Enalapril is used alone or in combination with other classes of antihypertensive agents in the management of hypertension. Enalaprilat is used in the management of hypertension when oral therapy is not practical. Because captopril, another angiotensin-converting enzyme (ACE) inhibitor, may cause serious adverse effects (e.g., neutropenia, agranulocytosis), particularly in patients with renal impairment (especially those with collagen vascular disease) or in patients receiving immunosuppressive therapy, the possibility that similar adverse effects may occur with enalapril or enalaprilat should be considered since current experience is insufficient to rule out such risk. Enalapril has occasionally been used without recurrence of adverse effect in patients who developed intolerable adverse effects (i.e., rash, taste disturbances) during captopril therapy. Further studies are needed to evaluate the possible risks associated with the long-term use of enalapril. The hypotensive efficacy of enalapril in hypertensive patients is similar to that of captopril or β-adrenergic blocking agents (β-blockers). Enalapril may have a greater effect on systolic blood pressure at rest (but not with exercise) than do β-blockers, but additional study is necessary to establish the comparative efficacy of enalapril and β-blockers.

Current evidence-based practice guidelines for the management of hypertension in adults generally recommend the use of drugs from 4 classes of antihypertensive agents (ACE inhibitors, angiotensin II receptor antagonists, calcium-channel blockers, and thiazide diuretics); data from clinical outcome trials indicate that lowering blood pressure with any of these drug classes can reduce the complications of hypertension and provide similar cardiovascular protection. However, recommendations for initial drug selection and use in specific patient populations may vary across these expert guidelines. This variability is due, in part, to differences in the guideline development process and the types of studies (e.g., randomized controlled studies only versus a range of studies with different study designs) included in the evidence reviews. Ultimately, choice of antihypertensive therapy should be individualized, considering the clinical characteristics of the patient (e.g., age, ethnicity/race, comorbid conditions, cardiovascular risk factors) as well as drug-related factors (e.g., ease of administration, availability, adverse effects, costs). Because many patients eventually will need drugs from 2 or more antihypertensive classes, experts generally state that the emphasis should be placed on achieving appropriate blood pressure control rather than on identifying a preferred drug to achieve that control.

Disease Overview

Worldwide, hypertension is the most common modifiable risk factor for cardiovascular events and mortality. The lifetime risk of developing hypertension in the US exceeds 80%, with higher rates observed among African Americans and Hispanics compared with whites or Asians. The systolic blood pressure and diastolic blood pressure values defined as hypertension (see Blood Pressure Classification under Uses: Hypertension) in a 2017 multidisciplinary guideline of the American College of Cardiology (ACC), American Heart Association (AHA), and a number of other professional organizations (subsequently referred to as the 2017 ACC/AHA hypertension guidelines in this monograph) are lower than those defined in the Seventh Report of the Joint National Committee on Prevention, Detection, Evaluation, and Treatment of High Blood Pressure (JNC 7) guidelines, which results in an increase of approximately 14% in the prevalence of hypertension in the US. However, this change in definition results in only a 2% increase in the percentage of patients requiring antihypertensive drug therapy because nonpharmacologic treatment is recommended for most adults now classified by the 2017 ACC/AHA hypertension guideline as hypertensive who would *not* meet the JNC 7 definition of hypertension. Among US adults receiving antihypertensive drugs,

approximately 53% have inadequately controlled blood pressure according to current ACC/AHA treatment goals.

Cardiovascular and Renal Sequelae

The principal goal of preventing and treating hypertension is to reduce the risk of cardiovascular and renal morbidity and mortality, including target organ damage. The relationship between blood pressure and cardiovascular disease is continuous, consistent, and independent of other risk factors. It is important that very high blood pressure be managed promptly to reduce the risk of target organ damage. The higher the blood pressure, the more likely the development of myocardial infarction (MI), heart failure, stroke, and renal disease. For adults 40–70 years of age, each 20-mm Hg increment in systolic blood pressure or 10-mm Hg increment in diastolic blood pressure doubles the risk of developing cardiovascular disease across the entire blood pressure range of 115/75 to 185/115 mm Hg. For those older than 50 years of age, systolic blood pressure is a much more important risk factor for developing cardiovascular disease than is diastolic blood pressure. The rapidity with which treatment is required depends on the patient's clinical presentation (presence of new or worsening target organ damage) and the presence or absence of cardiovascular complications; the 2017 ACC/AHA hypertension guideline states that treatment of very high blood pressure should be initiated within 1 week.

Blood Pressure Classification

Accurate blood pressure measurement is essential for the proper diagnosis and management of hypertension. Error in measuring blood pressure is a major cause of inadequate blood pressure control and may lead to overtreatment. Because a patient's blood pressure may vary in an unpredictable fashion, a single blood pressure measurement is not sufficient for clinical decision-making. An average of 2 or 3 blood pressure measurements obtained on 2–3 separate occasions using proper technique should be used to minimize random error and provide a more accurate blood pressure reading. Out-of-office blood pressure measurements may be useful for confirming and managing hypertension. The 2017 ACC/AHA hypertension guideline document (available on the ACC and AHA websites) should be consulted for key steps on properly measuring blood pressure.

According to the 2017 ACC/AHA hypertension guideline, blood pressure in adults is classified into 4 categories: normal, elevated, stage 1 hypertension, and stage 2 hypertension. (See Table 1.) The 2017 ACC/AHA hypertension guideline lowers the blood pressure threshold used to define hypertension in the US; previous hypertension guidelines (JNC 7) considered adults with systolic blood pressure of 120–139 mm Hg or diastolic blood pressure of 80–89 mm Hg to have prehypertension, those with systolic blood pressure of 140–159 mm Hg or diastolic blood pressure of 90–99 mm Hg to have stage 1 hypertension, and those with systolic blood pressure of 160 mm Hg or higher or diastolic blood pressure of 100 mm Hg or higher to have stage 2 hypertension. The blood pressure definitions in the 2017 ACC/AHA hypertension guideline are based upon data from studies evaluating the association between systolic blood pressure/diastolic blood pressure and cardiovascular risk and the benefits of blood pressure reduction. Individuals with systolic blood pressure and diastolic blood pressure in 2 different categories should be designated as being in the higher blood pressure category.

TABLE 1. ACC/AHA Blood Pressure Classification in Adults [a,b]

Category	SBP [c] (mm Hg)		DBP [d] (mm Hg)
Normal	<120	and	<80
Elevated	120–129	and	<80
Hypertension, Stage 1	130–139	or	80–89
Hypertension, Stage 2	≥140	or	≥90

[a] Source: Whelton PK, Carey RM, Aronow WS et al. 2017 ACC/AHA/AAPA/ABC/ACPM/AGS/APhA/ASH/ASPC/NMA/PCNA guideline for the prevention, detection, evaluation, and management of high blood pressure in adults: a report of the American College of Cardiology/American Heart Association Task Force on Clinical Practice Guidelines. Hypertension. 2018;71:e13-115.

[b] Individuals with SBP and DBP in 2 different categories (e.g., elevated SBP and normal DBP) should be designated as being in the higher blood pressure category (i.e., elevated BP).

[c] Systolic blood pressure

[d] Diastolic blood pressure

The blood pressure thresholds used to define hypertension, when to initiate drug therapy, and the ideal target blood pressure values remain controversial. The 2017 ACC/AHA hypertension guideline recommends a blood pressure goal of less than 130/80 mm Hg in all adults who have confirmed hypertension and known cardiovascular disease or a 10-year atherosclerotic cardiovascular disease (ASCVD) event risk of 10% or higher; the ACC/AHA guideline also states that this blood pressure goal is reasonable to attempt to achieve in adults with confirmed hypertension who do *not* have increased cardiovascular risk. The lower blood pressure values used to define hypertension and the lower target blood pressure goals outlined in the 2017 ACC/AHA hypertension guideline are based on clinical studies demonstrating a substantial reduction in the composite end point of major cardiovascular disease events and the combination of fatal and nonfatal stroke when a lower systolic blood pressure/diastolic blood pressure value (i.e., 130/80 mm Hg) was used to define hypertension. These lower target blood pressure goals also are based upon clinical studies demonstrating continuing reduction of cardiovascular risk at progressively lower levels of systolic blood pressure. A linear relationship has been demonstrated between cardiovascular risk and blood pressure even at low systolic blood pressures (e.g, 120–124 mm Hg). The 2017 ACC/AHA hypertension guideline recommends estimating a patient's ASCVD risk using the ACC/AHA Pooled Cohort equations (available online at http://tools.acc.org/ASCVD-Risk-Estimator), which are based on a variety of factors including age, race, gender, cholesterol levels, statin use, blood pressure, treatment for hypertension, history of diabetes mellitus, smoking status, and aspirin use. While the 2017 ACC/AHA hypertension guideline has lowered the threshold for *diagnosing* hypertension in adults, the threshold for *initiating drug therapy* has only been lowered for those patients who are at high risk of cardiovascular disease. Clinicians who support the 2017 ACC/AHA hypertension guideline believe that these recommendations have the potential to increase hypertension awareness, encourage lifestyle modification, and focus antihypertensive drug initiation and intensification in those adults at high risk for cardiovascular disease.

The lower blood pressure goals advocated in the 2017 ACC/AHA hypertension guideline have been questioned by some clinicians who have concerns regarding the guideline's use of extrapolated observational data, the lack of generalizability of some of the randomized trials (e.g., SPRINT) used to support the guideline, the difficulty of establishing accurate representative blood pressure values in typical clinical practice settings, and the accuracy of the cardiovascular risk calculator used in the guideline. Some clinicians state the lower blood pressure threshold used to define hypertension in the 2017 ACC/AHA hypertension guideline is not fully supported by clinical data, and these clinicians have expressed concerns about the possible harms (e.g., adverse effects of antihypertensive therapy) associated with classifying more patients as being hypertensive. Some clinicians also state that using this guideline, a large number of young, low-risk patients would need to be treated in order to observe a clinical benefit, while other clinicians state that the estimated gains in life expectancy attributable to long-term use of blood pressure-lowering drugs are correspondingly greater in this patient population.

Treatment Benefits

In clinical trials, antihypertensive therapy has been found to reduce the risk of developing stroke by about 34–40%, MI by about 20–25%, and heart failure by more than 50%. In a randomized, controlled study (SPRINT) that included hypertensive patients without diabetes mellitus who had a high risk of cardiovascular disease, intensive systolic blood pressure lowering of approximately 15 mm Hg was associated with a 25% reduction in cardiovascular disease events and a 27% reduction in all-cause mortality. However, the exclusion of patients with diabetes mellitus, prior stroke, and those younger than 50 years of age may decrease the generalizability of these findings. Some experts estimate that if the systolic blood pressure goals of the 2017 ACC/AHA hypertension guideline are achieved, major cardiovascular disease events may be reduced by an additional 340,000 and total deaths by an additional 156,000 compared with implementation of the JNC 8 expert panel guideline goals but these benefits may be accompanied by an increase in the frequency of adverse events. While there was no overall difference in the occurrence of serious adverse events in patients receiving intensive therapy for blood pressure control (systolic blood pressure target of less than 120 mm Hg) compared with those receiving less intense control (systolic blood pressure target of less than 140 mm Hg) in the SPRINT study, hypotension, syncope, electrolyte abnormalities, and acute kidney injury or acute renal failure occurred in substantially more patients receiving intensive therapy.

In the Antihypertensive and Lipid-lowering Treatment to Prevent Heart Attack Trial (ALLHAT), the long-term cardiovascular morbidity and mortality benefit of a long-acting dihydropyridine calcium-channel blocker (amlodipine),

a thiazide-like diuretic (chlorthalidone), and an ACE inhibitor (lisinopril) were compared in a broad population of patients with hypertension at risk for coronary heart disease. Although these antihypertensive agents were comparably effective in providing important cardiovascular benefit, apparent differences in certain secondary outcomes were observed. Patients receiving the ACE inhibitor experienced higher risks of stroke, combined cardiovascular disease, GI bleeding, and angioedema, while those receiving the calcium-channel blocker were at higher risk of developing heart failure. The ALLHAT investigators suggested that the favorable cardiovascular outcome may be attributable, at least in part, to the greater antihypertensive effect of the calcium-channel blocker compared with that of the ACE inhibitor, especially in women and black patients. (See Clinical Benefit of Thiazides in Hypertension under Hypertension in Adults: Treatment Benefits, in Uses in the Thiazides General Statement 40:28.20.)

General Considerations for Initial and Maintenance Antihypertensive Therapy

Nonpharmacologic Therapy

Nonpharmacologic measures (i.e., lifestyle/behavioral modifications) that are effective in lowering blood pressure include weight reduction (for those who are overweight or obese), dietary changes to include foods such as fruits, vegetables, whole grains, and low-fat dairy products that are rich in potassium, calcium, magnesium, and fiber (i.e., adoption of the Dietary Approaches to Stop Hypertension [DASH] eating plan), sodium reduction, increased physical activity, and moderation of alcohol intake. Such lifestyle/behavioral modifications, including smoking cessation, enhance antihypertensive drug efficacy and decrease cardiovascular risk and remain an indispensable part of the management of hypertension. Lifestyle/behavioral modifications without antihypertensive drug therapy are recommended for individuals classified by the 2017 ACC/AHA hypertension guideline as having elevated blood pressure (systolic blood pressure 120–129 mm Hg and diastolic blood pressure less than 80 mm Hg) and in those with stage 1 hypertension (systolic blood pressure 130–139 mm Hg or diastolic blood pressure 80–89 mm Hg) who do *not* have preexisting cardiovascular disease or an estimated 10-year ASCVD risk of 10% or greater.

Initiation of Drug Therapy

Drug therapy in the management of hypertension must be individualized and adjusted based on the degree of blood pressure elevation while also considering cardiovascular risk factors. Drug therapy generally is reserved for patients who respond inadequately to nondrug therapy (i.e., life-style modifications such as diet [including sodium restriction and adequate potassium and calcium intake], regular aerobic physical activity, moderation of alcohol consumption, and weight reduction) or in whom the degree of blood pressure elevation or coexisting risk factors, especially cardiovascular risk, require more prompt or aggressive therapy; however, the optimum blood pressure threshold for initiating antihypertensive drug therapy and specific treatment goals remain controversial. Recommendations generally are based on specific blood pressure levels shown in clinical studies to produce clinical benefits and can therefore vary depending on the studies selected for review.

The 2017 ACC/AHA hypertension guideline and many experts currently state that the treatment of hypertension should be based not only on blood pressure values but also on patients' cardiovascular risk factors. For *secondary prevention* of recurrent cardiovascular disease events in adults with clinical cardiovascular disease or for *primary prevention* in adults with an estimated 10-year ASCVD risk of 10% or higher, the 2017 ACC/AHA hypertension guideline recommends initiation of antihypertensive drug therapy in conjunction with lifestyle/behavioral modifications at an average systolic blood pressure of 130 mm Hg or an average diastolic blood pressure of 80 mm Hg or higher. For *primary prevention* of cardiovascular disease events in adults with a low (less than 10%) estimated 10-year risk of ASCVD, the 2017 ACC/AHA hypertension guideline recommends initiation of antihypertensive drug therapy in conjunction with lifestyle/behavioral modifications at a systolic blood pressure of 140 mm Hg or higher or a diastolic blood pressure of 90 mm Hg or higher. After initiation of antihypertensive drug therapy, regardless of the ASCVD risk, the 2017 ACC/AHA hypertension guideline generally recommends a blood pressure goal of less than 130/80 mm Hg in all adults. In addition, a systolic blood pressure goal of less than 130 mm Hg is also recommended for noninstitutionalized ambulatory patients 65 years of age or older. While these blood pressure goals are lower than those recommended for most patients in previous guidelines, they are based upon clinical studies demonstrating continuing reduction of cardiovascular risk at progressively lower levels of systolic blood pressure.

Most data indicate that patients with a higher cardiovascular risk will benefit the most from tighter blood pressure control; however, some experts state this treatment goal also may be beneficial in those at lower cardiovascular risk. Other clinicians believe that the benefits of such blood pressure lowering do not outweigh the risks in those patients considered to be at lower risk of cardiovascular disease and that reclassifying individuals formerly considered to have prehypertension as having hypertension may potentially lead to use of drug therapy in such patients without consideration of cardiovascular risk. Previous hypertension guidelines, such as those from the JNC 8 expert panel, generally recommended initiation of antihypertensive treatment in patients with a systolic blood pressure of at least 140 mm Hg or diastolic blood pressure of at least 90 mm Hg, targeted a blood pressure goal of less than 140/90 mm Hg regardless of cardiovascular risk, and used higher systolic blood pressure thresholds and targets in geriatric patients. Some clinicians continue to support the target blood pressures recommended by the JNC 8 expert panel because of concerns that such recommendations in the 2017 ACC/AHA hypertension guideline are based on extrapolation of data from the high-risk population in the SPRINT study to a lower-risk population. Also, because more than 90% of patients in SPRINT were already receiving antihypertensive drugs at baseline, data are lacking on the effects of *initiating* drug therapy at a lower blood pressure threshold (130/80 mm Hg) in patients at high risk of cardiovascular disease. The potential benefits of hypertension management and drug cost, adverse effects, and risks associated with the use of multiple antihypertensive drugs should be considered when deciding a patient's blood pressure treatment goal.

The 2017 ACC/AHA hypertension guideline recommends an ASCVD risk assessment for all adults with hypertension; however, experts state that it can be assumed that patients with hypertension and diabetes mellitus or chronic kidney disease (CKD) are at high risk for cardiovascular disease and that antihypertensive drug therapy should be initiated in these patients at a blood pressure of 130/80 mm Hg or higher. The 2017 ACC/AHA hypertension guideline also recommends a blood pressure goal of less than 130/80 mm Hg in patients with hypertension and diabetes mellitus or CKD. These recommendations are based on a systematic review of high-quality evidence from randomized controlled trials, meta-analyses, and post-hoc analyses that have demonstrated substantial reductions in the risk of important clinical outcomes (e.g., cardiovascular events) regardless of comorbid conditions or age when systolic blood pressure is lowered to less than 130 mm Hg. However, some clinicians have questioned the generalizability of findings from some of the trials (e.g., SPRINT) used to support the 2017 ACC/AHA hypertension guideline. For example, SPRINT included adults (mean age: 68 years) *without* diabetes mellitus who were at high risk of cardiovascular disease. While benefits of intensive blood pressure control were observed in this patient population, some clinicians have questioned whether these findings apply to younger patients who have a low risk of cardiovascular disease. In patients with CKD in the SPRINT trial, intensive blood pressure management (achieving a mean systolic blood pressure of approximately 122 mm Hg compared with 136 mm Hg with standard treatment) provided a similar beneficial reduction in the composite cardiovascular disease primary outcome and all-cause mortality as in the full patient cohort. Because most patients with CKD die from cardiovascular complications, the findings of this study further support a lower blood pressure target of less than 130/80 mm Hg.

Data are lacking to determine the ideal blood pressure goal in patients with hypertension and diabetes mellitus; also, studies evaluating the benefits of intensive blood pressure control in patients with diabetes mellitus have provided conflicting results. Clinical studies reviewed for the 2017 ACC/AHA hypertension guideline have shown similar quantitative benefits from blood pressure lowering in hypertensive patients with or without diabetes mellitus. In a randomized, controlled study (ACCORD-BP) that compared a higher (systolic blood pressure less than 140 mm Hg) versus lower (systolic blood pressure less than 120 mm Hg) blood pressure goal in patients with diabetes mellitus, there was no difference in the incidence of cardiovascular outcomes (e.g., composite outcome of cardiovascular death, nonfatal MI, and nonfatal stroke). However, some experts state that this study was underpowered to detect a difference between the 2 treatment groups and that the factorial design of the study complicated interpretation of the results. Although SPRINT did not include patients with diabetes mellitus, patients in this study with prediabetes demonstrated a similar cardiovascular benefit from intensive treatment of blood pressure as normoglycemic patients. A meta-analysis of data from ACCORD and SPRINT suggests that the findings of both studies are consistent and that patients with diabetes mellitus benefit from more intensive blood pressure control. These data support the 2017 ACC/AHA hypertension guideline recommendation of a blood pressure treatment goal of less than 130/80 mm Hg in patients with hypertension and diabetes mellitus. Alternatively, the American Diabetes Association (ADA) recommends a blood pressure goal of less than 140/90 mm Hg in patients with diabetes mellitus. The ADA states that a lower blood pressure goal (e.g., less than 130/80 mm Hg) may be appropriate for patients with a high risk of cardiovascular disease and diabetes mellitus if it can be achieved without undue treatment burden.

Further study is needed to more clearly define optimum blood pressure goals in patients with hypertension, particularly in high-risk groups (e.g., patients with diabetes mellitus, cardiovascular disease, or cerebrovascular disease; black patients); when determining appropriate blood pressure goals, individual risks and benefits should be considered in addition to the evidence from clinical studies.

Choice of Initial Drug Therapy

In current hypertension management guidelines, ACE inhibitors are recommended as one of several preferred drugs for the initial treatment of hypertension; other options include angiotensin II receptor antagonists, calcium-channel blockers, and thiazide diuretics. The 2017 ACC/AHA hypertension guideline states that an ACE inhibitor, angiotensin II receptor antagonist, calcium-channel blocker, or thiazide diuretic (preferably chlorthalidone) are all acceptable choices for initial antihypertensive drug therapy in the general population of nonblack patients, including those with diabetes mellitus; drugs from any of these classes generally produce similar benefits in terms of overall mortality and cardiovascular, cerebrovascular, and renal outcomes. ACE inhibitors may be particularly useful in the management of hypertension in patients with certain coexisting conditions such as heart failure, ischemic heart disease, diabetes mellitus, CKD, or cerebrovascular disease or following myocardial infarction (MI). (See Considerations for Drug Therapy in Patients with Underlying Cardiovascular and Other Risk Factors under Uses: Hypertension.)

In patients with hypertension and compelling indications (e.g., CKD with albuminuria [urine albumin 300 mg/day or greater, or urine albumin:creatinine ratio of 300 mg/g or equivalent in the first morning void]), angiotensin II receptor antagonists are usually considered an alternative for ACE inhibitor-intolerant patients. (See Chronic Kidney Disease under Hypertension: Considerations for Drug Therapy in Patients with Underlying Cardiovascular and Other Risk Factors, in Uses.) However, data indicate no difference in efficacy between ACE inhibitors and angiotensin II receptor antagonists with regard to blood pressure lowering and clinical outcomes (i.e., all-cause mortality, cardiovascular mortality, MI, heart failure, stroke, and end-stage renal disease). Adverse events (e.g., cough, angioedema) leading to drug discontinuance occur more frequently with ACE inhibitor therapy than with angiotensin II receptor antagonist therapy. Because of similar efficacy and a lower frequency of adverse effects, some experts believe that angiotensin II receptor antagonists should be used instead of an ACE inhibitor for the treatment of hypertension or hypertension with certain compelling indications.

Experts state that in patients with stage 1 hypertension (especially the elderly, those with a history of hypotension, or those who have experienced adverse drug effects), it is reasonable to initiate drug therapy using the stepped-care approach in which one drug is initiated and titrated and other drugs are added sequentially to achieve the target blood pressure. Although some patients can begin treatment with a single antihypertensive agent, starting with 2 drugs in different pharmacologic classes (either as separate agents or in a fixed-dose combination) is recommended in patients with stage 2 hypertension and an average blood pressure more than 20/10 mm Hg above their target blood pressure. Such combined therapy may increase the likelihood of achieving goal blood pressure in a more timely fashion, but also may increase the risk of adverse effects (e.g., orthostatic hypotension) in some patients (e.g., elderly). Drug regimens with complementary activity, where a second antihypertensive agent is used to block compensatory responses to the first agent or affect a different pressor mechanism, can result in additive blood pressure lowering and are preferred. Drug combinations that have similar mechanisms of action or clinical effects (e.g., the combination of an ACE inhibitor and an angiotensin II receptor antagonist) generally should be avoided. Many patients who begin therapy with a single antihypertensive agent will subsequently require at least 2 drugs from different pharmacologic classes to achieve their blood pressure goal. Experts state that other patient-specific factors, such as age, concurrent medications, drug adherence, drug interactions, the overall treatment regimen, cost, and comorbidities, also should be considered when deciding on an antihypertensive drug regimen. For any stage of hypertension, antihypertensive drug dosages should be adjusted and/or other agents substituted or added until goal blood pressure is achieved. (See Follow-up and Maintenance Drug Therapy under Hypertension: General Considerations for Initial and Maintenance Antihypertensive Therapy, in Uses.)

Follow-up and Maintenance Drug Therapy

Several strategies are used for the titration and combination of antihypertensive drugs; these strategies, which are generally based on those used in randomized controlled studies, include maximizing the dosage of the first drug before adding a second drug, adding a second drug before achieving maximum dosage of the initial drug, or initiating therapy with 2 drugs simultaneously (either as separate preparations or as a fixed-dose combination). Combined use of an ACE inhibitor and angiotensin II receptor antagonist should be avoided because of the potential risk of adverse renal effects. After initiating a new or adjusted antihypertensive drug regimen, patients should have their blood pressure reevaluated monthly until adequate blood pressure control is achieved. Effective blood pressure control can be achieved in most hypertensive patients, but many will ultimately require therapy with 2 or more antihypertensive drugs. In addition to measuring blood pressure, clinicians should evaluate patients for orthostatic hypotension, adverse drug effects, adherence to drug therapy and lifestyle modifications, and the need for drug dosage adjustments. Laboratory testing such as electrolytes and renal function status and other assessments of target organ damage also should be performed.

Enalapril can be used for the management of hypertension as initial monotherapy or as a component of a multiple-drug regimen. When enalapril alone is used but the patient's hypertension does not respond adequately, addition of a thiazide diuretic often adequately controls blood pressure. Such combined therapy generally produces additive reduction in blood pressure and may permit dosage reduction of either or both drugs and minimize adverse effects while maintaining blood pressure control.

Enalapril may be effective in the management of hypertension resistant to other drugs. Although enalapril occasionally may be effective alone in patients with severe hypertension, it is usually necessary to use the drug in conjunction with a diuretic. (See Drug Interactions: Hypotensive Agents and Diuretics.) Enalapril has been used in some diabetic hypertensive patients with no adverse effect on control or therapy of diabetes; however, hypoglycemia has occasionally occurred when the drug was used in patients whose diabetes had been controlled with insulin or oral hypoglycemic agents. (See Drug Interactions: Other Drugs.)

Tolerance to the hypotensive effect of enalapril apparently does not occur during long-term administration, particularly if the drug is used with a diuretic. Abrupt withdrawal of enalapril or enalaprilat therapy results in a gradual return of hypertension; rapid increases in blood pressure have not been reported to date.

IV enalaprilat may be used in the management of hypertension when oral therapy is not practical. Enalaprilat generally produces a prompt reduction in blood pressure, usually without an orthostatic response, and with a slight reduction in heart rate. Occasional hypotension, or symptomatic postural hypotension in volume-depleted patients, might be anticipated. Enalaprilat also has been used effectively to control blood pressure in adults with severe hypertension or hypertensive emergencies† (see Hypertensive Crises under Uses: Hypertension) and in a small number of neonates with severe hypertension†.

Considerations for Drug Therapy in Patients with Underlying Cardiovascular and Other Risk Factors

Drug therapy in patients with hypertension and underlying cardiovascular or other risk factors should be carefully individualized based on the underlying disease(s), concomitant drugs, tolerance to drug-induced adverse effects, and blood pressure goal. See Table 2 on Compelling Indications for Drug Classes based on Comorbid Conditions under Uses: Hypertension in Adults, in the Thiazides General Statement 40:28.20.

Ischemic Heart Disease

The selection of an appropriate antihypertensive agent in patients with ischemic heart disease should be based on individual patient characteristics and may include ACE inhibitors and/or β-blockers, with the addition of other drugs such as thiazide diuretics or calcium-channel blockers as necessary to achieve blood pressure goals. Many experts recommend the use of an ACE inhibitor (or an angiotensin II receptor antagonist) and/or a β-blocker in hypertensive patients with stable ischemic heart disease because of the cardioprotective benefits of these drugs; all patients who have survived an MI should be treated with a β-blocker because of the demonstrated mortality benefit of these agents.

Heart Failure

While ACE inhibitors as single therapies are not superior to other antihypertensive agents in the reduction of cardiovascular outcomes, ACE inhibitors, usually in conjunction with other agents such as cardiac glycosides, diuretics, and β-blockers, have been shown to reduce morbidity and mortality in patients with existing heart failure. (See Uses: Heart Failure.) ACE inhibitors also have been used to prevent subsequent heart failure and reduce morbidity and mortality in patients with systolic dysfunction following acute MI†. (See Uses: Left Ventricular Dysfunction After Acute Myocardial Infarction.)

Diabetes Mellitus

Experts state that initial treatment of hypertension in adults with diabetes mellitus and hypertension should include any of the usual first-line agents (ACE inhibitors, angiotensin II receptor antagonists, calcium-channel blockers, thiazide diuretics). In adults with diabetes mellitus, hypertension, and albuminuria, treatment with an ACE inhibitor or angiotensin II receptor antagonist may be considered to reduce the progression of kidney disease. While there is evidence demonstrating the benefits of ACE inhibitors in reducing the development or progression of microvascular or macrovascular complications in hypertensive patients with type 1 or type 2 diabetes mellitus, in the absence of albuminuria, the risk of progressive kidney disease is low, and ACE inhibitors and angiotensin II receptor antagonists have not demonstrated superior cardioprotection when compared with other first-line agents. Results of several studies indicate that adequate control of blood pressure in patients with type 2 diabetes mellitus reduces the development or progression of complications of diabetes (e.g., death related to diabetes, stroke, heart failure, microvascular disease). Most patients with diabetes mellitus will require 2 or more antihypertensive agents to achieve blood pressure control.

Chronic Kidney Disease

Hypertensive patients with CKD (glomerular filtration rate [GFR] less than 60 mL/minute per 1.73 m² or kidney damage for 3 or more months) usually will require more than one antihypertensive agent to reach target blood pressure. Use of ACE inhibitors or angiotensin II receptor antagonists may be reasonable in patients with diabetic or nondiabetic CKD (stage 1 or 2 with albuminuria or stage 3 or higher); these drugs have been shown to slow the progression of kidney disease. Evidence of a renoprotective benefit is strongest in those with higher levels of albuminuria. Increases in serum creatinine (up to 30%) may be observed as a result of a decrease in intraglomerular pressure and concurrent reduction in GFR. The 2017 ACC/AHA hypertension guideline states that in patients with less severe kidney disease (i.e., stage 1 or 2 CKD without albuminuria), any of the first-line antihypertensive agents (e.g., ACE inhibitors, angiotensin II receptor antagonists, calcium-channel blockers, thiazide diuretics) can be used for the initial treatment of hypertension. Diuretics also may be useful in the management of CKD, and may potentiate the effects of ACE inhibitors, angiotensin II receptor antagonists, and other antihypertensive agents when used in combination. (See Diabetic Nephropathy under Uses: Nephropathy, in Captopril 24:32.04.)

Cerebrovascular Disease

Some experts recommend a blood pressure goal of less than 140/90 mm Hg in patients with ischemic stroke or transient ischemic attack (TIA), while others state that a blood pressure goal of less than 130/80 mm Hg may be reasonable. The 2017 ACC/AHA hypertension guideline states that adults not previously treated for hypertension who experience a stroke or TIA and who have an established blood pressure of 140/90 mm Hg should receive antihypertensive therapy within a few days after the event to reduce the risk of recurrent stroke or other vascular events. In patients with a recent lacunar stroke, experts suggest that a systolic blood pressure goal of 130 mm Hg may be reasonable based on results of a randomized open-label study (the Secondary Prevention of Small Subcortical Strokes [SPS3] trial). Although experts state that the optimal choice of drug for the management of hypertension in patients with a previous TIA or ischemic stroke is uncertain, available data indicate that an ACE inhibitor, angiotensin II receptor antagonist, thiazide diuretic, or the combination of a thiazide diuretic and an ACE inhibitor may be effective. Administration of an ACE inhibitor in combination with a thiazide diuretic has been shown to lower rates of recurrent stroke.

Hypertension Associated with Scleroderma Renal Crisis

Enalapril has been effective for the management of hypertension associated with scleroderma renal crisis† in a limited number of patients who were unable to tolerate captopril because of adverse effects. Maintenance therapy with enalapril (5–30 mg daily) controlled blood pressure in these patients and was accompanied by improvement in renal function. Some clinicians consider ACE inhibitors the drugs of choice for this condition.

Other Special Considerations for Antihypertensive Drug Therapy
Race

Most patients with hypertension, especially black patients, will require at least 2 antihypertensive drugs to achieve adequate blood pressure control. In general, black hypertensive patients tend to respond better to monotherapy with thiazide diuretics or calcium-channel blockers than to monotherapy with ACE inhibitors. In a prespecified subgroup analysis of the ALLHAT study, a thiazide-type diuretic was more effective than an ACE inhibitor in improving cerebrovascular and cardiovascular outcomes in black patients; when compared with a calcium-channel blocker, the ACE inhibitor was less effective in reducing blood pressure and was associated with a 51% higher rate of stroke. (See Clinical Benefit of Thiazides in Hypertension under Hypertension in Adults: Treatment Benefits, in Uses in the Thiazides General Statement 40:28.20.) However, the combination of an ACE inhibitor or an angiotensin II receptor antagonist with a calcium-channel blocker or thiazide diuretic produces similar blood pressure lowering in black patients as in other racial groups. In addition, some experts state that when use of ACE inhibitors is indicated in hypertensive patients with underlying cardiovascular or other risk factors, these indications should be applied equally to black hypertensive patients.

Although enalapril has lowered blood pressure in all races studied, monotherapy with enalapril has produced a smaller reduction in blood pressure in black hypertensive patients, a population associated with low renin hypertension; however, this population difference in response does not appear to occur during combined therapy with enalapril and a thiazide diuretic. In addition, ACE inhibitors appear to produce a higher incidence of angioedema in black patients than in other races studied.

For further information on overall principles and expert recommendations for treatment of hypertension, see Uses: Hypertension in Adults and also see Uses: Hypertension in Pediatric Patients, in the Thiazides General Statement 40:28.20.)

Renovascular or Malignant Hypertension

Enalapril also has been effective in the management of renovascular or malignant hypertension, renal hypertension secondary to renal-artery stenosis, and, in some patients, hypertension associated with chronic renal failure. In addition to the drugs' hypotensive effect, ACE inhibitors also have stabilized or improved effective renal blood flow and glomerular filtration rate and decreased proteinuria in some hypertensive patients with moderately impaired renal function, moderate to severe renal disease, or diabetic nephropathy. However, enalapril should be used with caution in patients with impaired renal function, especially those with bilateral renal-artery stenosis or with renal-artery stenosis in a solitary kidney. (See Cautions: Renal Effects and see Hematologic Effects and see Precautions and Contraindications.)

Hypertensive Crises

Enalaprilat has been used effectively to reduce blood pressure in adults with severe hypertension or hypertensive emergencies†.

Hypertensive emergencies are those rare situations requiring immediate blood pressure reduction (not necessarily to normal ranges) to prevent or limit target organ damage. Such emergencies include hypertensive encephalopathy, acute MI, intracerebral hemorrhage, acute left ventricular failure with pulmonary edema, eclampsia, dissecting aortic aneurysm, unstable angina pectoris, acute ischemic stroke, and acute renal failure. Patients with hypertensive emergencies require hospitalization and are treated initially with an appropriate parenteral agent. Elevated blood pressure alone, in the absence of manifestations or other evidence of target organ damage, rarely requires emergency therapy.

Acute enalaprilat therapy (e.g., 1.25–5 mg IV, repeated every 6 hours as necessary) is one of several parenteral regimens currently recommended for rapidly reducing blood pressure in patients with hypertensive crises in whom reduction of blood pressure is considered an emergency. However, reduction of blood pressure in a prompt but controlled manner may be more easily achieved with short-acting antihypertensive agents administered by continuous IV infusion (e.g., labetalol, esmolol, fenoldopam, nicardipine, sodium nitroprusside), and some clinicians state that such agents generally are preferred.

The risks of overly aggressive therapy in any hypertensive crisis must always be considered, as excessive falls in blood pressure may precipitate renal, cerebral, or coronary ischemia.

● Heart Failure

Enalapril is used in the management of symptomatic heart failure, usually in conjunction with other agents such as cardiac glycosides, diuretics, and β-blockers.

Current guidelines for the management of heart failure in adults generally recommend a combination of drug therapies to reduce morbidity and mortality, including neurohormonal antagonists (e.g., ACE inhibitors, angiotensin II receptor antagonists, angiotensin receptor-neprilysin inhibitors [ARNIs], β-blockers, aldosterone receptor antagonists) that inhibit the detrimental compensatory mechanisms in heart failure. Additional agents (e.g., cardiac glycosides, diuretics,

sinoatrial modulators [i.e., ivabradine]) added to a heart failure treatment regimen in selected patients have been associated with symptomatic improvement and/or reduction in heart failure-related hospitalizations. In patients with prior or current symptoms of chronic heart failure with reduced left ventricular ejection fraction (LVEF) (American College of Cardiology Foundation [ACCF]/AHA stage C heart failure), ACCF, AHA, and the Heart Failure Society of America (HFSA) recommend inhibition of the renin-angiotensin-aldosterone (RAA) system with an ACE inhibitor, angiotensin II receptor antagonist, or ARNI (e.g., sacubitril/valsartan) in conjunction with a β-blocker, and an aldosterone antagonist in selected patients, to reduce morbidity and mortality. While ACE inhibitors have been the preferred drugs for inhibition of the RAA system because of their established benefits in patients with heart failure and reduced ejection fraction, some evidence indicates that therapy with an ARNI (sacubitril/valsartan) may be more effective than ACE inhibitor therapy (enalapril) in reducing cardiovascular death and heart failure-related hospitalization in such patients. ACCF, AHA, and HFSA recommend that patients with chronic symptomatic heart failure with reduced LVEF (New York Heart Association [NYHA] class II or III) who are able to tolerate an ACE inhibitor or angiotensin II receptor antagonist be switched to therapy containing an ARNI to further reduce morbidity and mortality. However, in patients in whom an ARNI is not appropriate, continued use of an ACE inhibitor for all classes of heart failure with reduced ejection fraction remains strongly advised. In patients in whom an ARNI or ACE inhibitor is not appropriate, an angiotensin II receptor antagonist may be used. For further information on the use of ARNIs in patients with heart failure, see Uses: Heart Failure, in Sacubitril and Valsartan 24:32.92.

Some clinicians state that ACE inhibitors usually are prescribed in clinical practice at dosages lower than those determined as target dosages in clinical trials, although results of several studies suggest that high dosages are associated with greater hemodynamic, neurohormonal, symptomatic, and prognostic benefits than lower dosages. Results of a large, randomized, double-blind study (Assessment of Treatment with Lisinopril and Survival [ATLAS] study) in patients with heart failure (NYHA class II–IV) indicate that high lisinopril dosages (32.5–35 mg daily) were associated with a 12% lower risk of death or hospitalization for any cause and 24% fewer hospitalizations for heart failure than low dosages (2.5–5 mg) of the drug.

Once ACE inhibitor therapy is initiated for heart failure, it generally is continued indefinitely, if tolerated, since withdrawal of an ACE inhibitor may lead to clinical deterioration. Patients with NYHA class II or III heart failure who are tolerating therapy with an ACE inhibitor may be switched to therapy containing an ARNI to further reduce morbidity and mortality; however, the ARNI should not be administered concomitantly with an ACE inhibitor or within 36 hours of the last dose of an ACE inhibitor.

Current evidence supports the use of ACE inhibitors and β-blocker therapy to prevent development of left ventricular dilatation and dysfunction ("ventricular remodeling") in patients with heart failure. (See Uses: Asymptomatic Left Ventricular Dysfunction.) The addition of other agents such as diuretics, cardiac glycosides, aldosterone antagonists, and/or sinoatrial modulators in the management of heart failure should be individualized. Unless contraindicated, diuretics are recommended in all patients with heart failure and reduced ejection fraction who have evidence of fluid retention to improve symptoms. Digoxin may be beneficial to patients with heart failure with reduced ejection fraction to decrease hospitalization for heart failure, especially in those with persistent symptoms despite treatment with guideline-directed medical therapy. The addition of a sinoatrial modulator (i.e., ivabradine) is recommended in selected patients with chronic heart failure and reduced LVEF who are already receiving guideline-directed medical therapy, to reduce heart failure-related hospitalizations. (See Uses: Heart Failure, in Ivabradine 24:04.92.)

Results of a randomized, multicenter, double-blind, placebo-controlled study (Randomized Aldactone Evaluation Study [RALES]) indicate that addition of low-dosage spironolactone (25–50 mg daily) to standard therapy (e.g., an ACE inhibitor and a loop diuretic with or without a cardiac glycoside) in patients with severe (NYHA class IV within 6 months before enrollment and NYHA class III or IV at the time of enrollment) heart failure and an LVEF of 35% or less, was associated with decreases in overall mortality and hospitalization (for worsening heart failure) rates of approximately 30 and 35%, respectively, compared with standard therapy and placebo. Based on the results of RALES and other studies, ACCF and AHA recommend the addition of an aldosterone antagonist (i.e., spironolactone or eplerenone) in selected patients with heart failure (NYHA class II–IV) and reduced LVEF (35% or less) who are already receiving standard therapy to reduce morbidity and mortality. (See Uses: Heart Failure, in Spironolactone 24:32.20.)

Many patients with heart failure respond to enalapril with improvement in cardiac function indexes, symptomatic (e.g., dyspnea, fatigue) relief, improved functional capacity, and increased exercise tolerance. In some studies, improvement in cardiac function indexes and exercise tolerance were sustained for up to 4 months. In some patients, beneficial effects have been sustained for up to 2–21 months. Enalapril also has been effective in conjunction with cardiac glycosides and diuretics for the management of heart failure resistant to or inadequately controlled by cardiac glycosides, diuretics, and vasodilators. In a multicenter, placebo-controlled study in patients with severe heart failure (NYHA class IV), the addition of enalapril to the therapeutic regimen (which included cardiac glycosides, diuretics, and/or vasodilators) was associated with a 40% reduction in overall mortality at 6 months and a 31% reduction at 12 months compared with patients who did not receive an ACE inhibitor, although the incidence of sudden cardiac death did not differ. In addition, there was a substantial improvement in NYHA functional class for patients receiving enalapril in this study. Follow-up of surviving patients 2 years after completion of the blinded, placebo-controlled phase showed a carry-over effect of enalapril on mortality reduction despite the availability of enalapril therapy for all surviving patients (whether treated initially with the drug or not) and the poorer clinical condition of the initial enalapril-treated group at the outset of follow-up; during follow-up, the carry-over effect on mortality reduction of initial enalapril therapy persisted for 15 months.

In 2 multicenter, controlled studies, enalapril substantially reduced mortality in patients with mild to moderate heart failure (NYHA class I–III) when added to a conventional therapeutic regimen (most commonly cardiac glycosides and diuretics); in these patients, enalapril therapy also may substantially reduce the rate of hospitalization. In one of these studies, the reduction in mortality was substantially greater with enalapril than with combined hydralazine and isosorbide dinitrate, although the latter regimen produced substantially greater improvement in exercise performance and left ventricular function. The beneficial effects of enalapril on reduction in mortality may result from a delay in worsening of heart failure, although other mechanisms (e.g., on causes of sudden death) may be involved. Analysis of the results of these studies according to racial subgroup indicates that white patients had substantially greater reductions in blood pressure and the risk of hospitalization for heart failure than black patients receiving similar dosages of enalapril. (See Race under Hypertension: Other Special Considerations for Antihypertensive Therapy, in Uses.) However, the risk of death in either racial subgroup was not altered by enalapril therapy.

It has not been determined whether addition of a vasodilator (e.g., hydralazine) to an ACE inhibitor is more effective than an ACE inhibitor alone. The efficacy of enalapril appears to be similar to that of captopril. However, because of enalapril's relatively long duration of action compared with captopril, enalapril may produce more prolonged hypotensive effects, particularly at high dosages, which potentially could result in adverse cerebral and renal effects. In addition, because the renin-angiotensin system appears to substantially contribute to preservation of glomerular filtration in patients with heart failure in whom renal perfusion is severely compromised, therapy with an ACE inhibitor in such patients may adversely affect renal function. (See Cautions: Renal Effects.)

ACE inhibitors also are used in patients with ACCF/AHA stage B heart failure (see Uses: Asymptomatic Left Ventricular Dysfunction) to prevent symptomatic heart failure and have been shown to reduce mortality after MI or acute coronary syndrome (ACS). (See Uses: Left Ventricular Dysfunction After Acute Myocardial Infarction.)

● **Asymptomatic Left Ventricular Dysfunction**

Enalapril is used in clinically stable asymptomatic patients with left ventricular dysfunction (manifested as an ejection fraction of 35% or less) in an effort to decrease the rate of development of overt heart failure and subsequent hospitalizations for heart failure in these patients. Experts recommend that all asymptomatic patients with reduced LVEF (ACCF/AHA stage B heart failure) receive therapy with an ACE inhibitor and β-blocker to prevent symptomatic heart failure and to reduce morbidity and mortality. If ACE inhibitors are not tolerated, then an angiotensin II receptor antagonist is recommended as an alternative.

Enalapril's beneficial effect in preventing the development of symptomatic heart failure in patients with asymptomatic left ventricular dysfunction may result either from relieving symptoms that otherwise would have become apparent or from slowing the progression of asymptomatic ventricular dysfunction to overt, symptomatic disease. In a multicenter, placebo-controlled study in patients with left ventricular dysfunction who did not have symptomatic heart failure (NYHA class I and II) and were not being treated for such at initiation of ACE inhibitor therapy, enalapril reduced the incidence of heart failure and rate of related hospitalizations relative to those receiving placebo during an average of 37.4 months

of follow-up. Patients with higher ejection fractions and black patients appeared to benefit less from enalapril therapy than those with lower fractions and white patients, respectively. The effect of enalapril in preventing the development of heart failure was evident within 3 months after initiation of the drug and continued to increase for the remaining study period (approximately 3 years). Mortality rates increased substantially in patients who developed overt heart failure, suggesting the possibility of a secondary benefit on prognosis from prevention of symptomatic progression. In a follow-up study, treatment with enalapril for 3–4 years led to a sustained improvement in survival (11–12 years) in patients with reduced LVEF, including those who were asymptomatic at baseline.

● **Left Ventricular Dysfunction After Acute Myocardial Infarction**

ACE inhibitors, including enalapril and enalaprilat, have been used to reduce mortality and prevent the development of left ventricular dilatation and dysfunction following acute MI†. Studies with various ACE inhibitors have shown that these drugs reduce fatal and nonfatal cardiovascular events in patients with recent MI. The magnitude of benefit appears to be greatest in certain high-risk patients (e.g., those with an anterior infarct, ejection fraction of 40% or less, heart failure, prior infarction, or tachycardia). Evidence regarding the efficacy of such therapy has been somewhat conflicting, particularly when parenteral therapy was initiated early (within 24–48 hours) and included patients with no evidence of baseline dysfunction. While the preponderance of evidence (including a large, multinational, multicenter study) has shown a benefit of early oral therapy involving other ACE inhibitors, even in patients with no baseline dysfunction, one large study involving parenteral and oral enalapril found little if any early (within several months) benefit, particularly in terms of survival, from such therapy. In this multicenter, controlled study, IV enalaprilat (followed by oral enalapril) was initiated within 24 hours of the onset of chest pain associated with acute MI and continued for up to approximately 6 months; there was no evidence of improved survival from enalapril therapy during the 6-month period after MI and, in some patients, an actual worsening of heart failure was observed. In addition, enalapril therapy was associated with a substantial risk of hypotensive episodes, and long-term mortality was higher among patients who experienced hypotension with the first dose of enalapril than among other patients receiving the drug or among those who experienced hypotension with placebo. The lack of survival benefit observed in this study applied overall as well as to subgroups of patients (e.g., those with Q-wave infarction, anterior infarction, previous infarction, or current infarction complicated by pulmonary edema or heart failure). The results of this study are in contrast to other studies involving other ACE inhibitors initiated within 24 hours to 4 weeks after acute MI in which a beneficial effect was observed, in terms of effects on left ventricular volume, infarct expansion, and/or survival.

The reason for the differences in potential benefit observed between studies involving enalapril and those involving other ACE inhibitors (e.g., captopril, lisinopril, ramipril) is unclear, but the lack of benefit in the enalapril study may have resulted in part from an early adverse effect of ACE inhibition (e.g., inhibition of angiotensin II-stimulated protein synthesis involved in healing) combined with a rapid decrease in blood pressure associated with the initial administration of enalaprilat and with an inadequate period of follow-up to detect a delayed beneficial effect. Current expert guidelines recommend the use of an oral ACE inhibitor within the first 24 hours of acute MI in patients with an anterior infarction, heart failure, or ejection fraction of 40% or less who do not have any contraindications (e.g., hypotension, shock, renal dysfunction). While early treatment within the first 24 hours of MI has been shown to be beneficial, ACE inhibitors should be used with caution (and with gradual upward titration) during the initial postinfarction period because of the possibility of hypotension or renal dysfunction. ACE inhibitor therapy generally should be continued indefinitely in patients with left ventricular dysfunction or other compelling indications for use (e.g., hypertension, diabetes mellitus, CKD). The benefits of long-term ACE inhibitor therapy are less certain in low-risk patients who have undergone revascularization and are receiving aggressive antilipemic therapy.

● **Diabetic Nephropathy**

Both ACE inhibitors and angiotensin II receptor antagonists have been shown to slow the rate of progression of renal disease in patients with diabetes mellitus and persistent albuminuria†, and use of a drug from either class is recommended in such patients with modestly elevated (30–300 mg/24 hours) or higher (exceeding 300 mg/24 hours) levels of urinary albumin excretion. The usual precautions of ACE inhibitor or angiotensin II receptor antagonist therapy in patients with substantial renal impairment should be observed. For additional information on the use of ACE inhibitors in the treatment of diabetic nephropathy, see Diabetic Nephropathy under Uses: Nephropathy, in Captopril 24:32.04.

DOSAGE AND ADMINISTRATION

● Administration

Oral Administration

Enalapril maleate alone or in fixed combination with hydrochlorothiazide is administered orally. For patients unable to swallow tablets, enalapril maleate may be administered orally as an extemporaneously prepared suspension. The drug can be given before, during, or after meals since food does not appear to substantially affect the rate or extent of absorption of enalapril.

An extemporaneous suspension containing enalapril maleate 1 mg/mL can be prepared in the following manner. First, 50 mL of sodium citrate dihydrate (Bicitra®) is added to a polyethylene terephthalate (PET) bottle containing ten 20-mg tablets of enalapril maleate, and the contents are shaken for at least 2 minutes. The concentrated suspension should be allowed to stand for 60 minutes following reconstitution, and then should be shaken for an additional minute. The concentrated suspension of enalapril maleate should be diluted with 150 mL of syrup (Ora-Sweet SF®), and the container then shaken to disperse the ingredients. The suspension should be shaken before dispensing of each dose.

IV Administration

Enalaprilat is administered by slow IV infusion over a period of at least 5 minutes. The drug should not be administered by other parenteral routes of administration. Enalaprilat may be administered by slow, direct IV infusion, or the injection can be diluted in up to 50 mL of compatible IV infusion solution for administration. (See Chemistry and Stability: Stability.) Enalaprilat injection and diluted solutions of the drug should be inspected visually for particulate matter and discoloration prior to administration whenever solution and container permit.

● Dosage

Dosage of enalapril maleate and enalaprilat must be adjusted according to the patient's tolerance and response. *Since enalapril maleate is a prodrug of enalaprilat and is well absorbed following oral administration, dosage of the two drugs is not identical and clinicians must give careful attention to dosage when converting from oral to IV therapy or vice versa.*

Because of the risk of inducing hypotension, initiation of enalapril maleate or enalaprilat therapy requires consideration of recent antihypertensive therapy, the extent of blood pressure elevation, sodium intake, fluid status, and other clinical circumstances. If therapy is initiated in patients already receiving a diuretic, symptomatic hypotension may occur following the initial dose of the angiotensin-converting enzyme (ACE) inhibitor. The possibility of hypotension may be minimized by discontinuing the diuretic, reducing the diuretic dosage, or cautiously increasing salt intake prior to initiation of oral enalapril maleate or IV enalaprilat therapy. (See Cautions: Cardiovascular Effects.) For information on initiating oral enalapril maleate or IV enalaprilat therapy when diuretic therapy is not being withheld, see the disease-specific dosage sections in Dosage and Administration: Dosage.

Hypertension
Oral Dosage

The manufacturer states that the usual initial adult dosage of enalapril maleate for the management of hypertension in patients *not* receiving a diuretic is 5 mg once daily. In patients who are receiving a diuretic, it is recommended that diuretic therapy be discontinued, if possible, 2–3 days before initiating therapy. (See Cautions: Precautions and Contraindications.) If blood pressure is not adequately controlled with the ACE inhibitor alone, diuretic therapy may be resumed cautiously. If diuretic therapy cannot be discontinued, an initial enalapril maleate dose of 2.5 mg should be administered under medical supervision for at least 2 hours and until blood pressure has stabilized for at least an additional hour.

The usual initial pediatric (1 month to 16 years of age) dosage of enalapril maleate is 0.08 mg/kg once daily, up to 5 mg. Some experts state that the dose may be administered as a single dose or in 2 divided doses daily. Such experts also state that the dosage may be increased every 2–4 weeks until blood pressure is controlled, the maximum dosage is reached, or adverse effects occur. The manufacturer states that dosages of enalapril maleate exceeding 0.58 mg/kg or in excess of 40 mg daily have not been studied in pediatric patients. (For information on overall principles and expert recommendations for treatment of hypertension in pediatric patients, see Uses: Hypertension in Pediatric Patients, in the Thiazides General Statement 40:28.20.)

Dosage of enalapril maleate should be adjusted according to the patient's blood pressure response. If the blood pressure response diminishes toward the end of the dosing interval during once-daily administration, increasing the dosage or giving the drug in 2 divided doses daily should be considered. Because the reduction in blood pressure may be gradual, some clinicians suggest that enalapril maleate dosage generally be titrated at 2- to 4-week intervals if necessary. The manufacturer states that the usual maintenance dosage of enalapril maleate in adults is 10–40 mg daily, given as a single dose or in 2 divided doses daily, although most patients can be maintained on once-daily dosing. Some experts state that the usual adult dosage is 5–40 mg daily, given as a single dose or in 2 divided doses daily. Optimum blood pressure reduction may require several weeks of therapy in some patients. If blood pressure is not adequately controlled with enalapril alone, a second antihypertensive agent (e.g., a diuretic) may be added.

When oral therapy is initiated following IV enalaprilat therapy in adults *not* receiving a diuretic, the recommended initial dosage of enalapril maleate is 5 mg once daily with subsequent dosage adjustment as necessary. When oral therapy is initiated following IV enalaprilat therapy in adults receiving a diuretic, the recommended initial dosage of enalapril maleate in those who responded to enalaprilat 0.625 mg every 6 hours is 2.5 mg once daily with subsequent dosage adjustment as necessary.

Enalapril/Hydrochlorothiazide Fixed-combination Oral Therapy

To minimize the likelihood of adverse effects, therapy with the commercially available preparations containing enalapril in fixed combination with hydrochlorothiazide should only be initiated in adults after an adequate response is not achieved with enalapril or hydrochlorothiazide monotherapy. Alternatively, the fixed combination containing enalapril with hydrochlorothiazide may be used in adults who had been receiving the drugs separately and in whom dosage of the individual drugs has been adjusted. The recommended initial adult dosage of the commercially available fixed-combination tablets is 5 mg of enalapril maleate and 12.5 mg of hydrochlorothiazide or 10 mg of enalapril maleate and 25 mg of hydrochlorothiazide once daily. Further increases of either or both drugs depend on clinical response; however, generally, dosage of hydrochlorothiazide should not be increased for about 2–3 weeks after initiation of therapy. Because the suggested maximum adult dosage of enalapril maleate and hydrochlorothiazide during combined antihypertensive therapy is 20 or 50 mg daily, respectively, the combined dosage of enalapril maleate and hydrochlorothiazide in the fixed combination should not exceed these respective levels.

Blood Pressure Monitoring and Treatment Goals

Blood pressure should be monitored regularly (i.e., monthly) during therapy and dosage of the antihypertensive drug adjusted until blood pressure is controlled. If an adequate blood pressure response is not achieved with ACE inhibitor monotherapy, the dosage may be increased or another antihypertensive agent with demonstrated benefit and preferably with a complementary mechanism of action (e.g., calcium-channel blocking agent, thiazide diuretic) may be added; if target blood pressure is still not achieved, a third drug may be added. (See Uses: Hypertension.) In patients who develop unacceptable adverse effects with enalapril, the drug should be discontinued and another antihypertensive agent from a different pharmacologic class should be initiated.

The goal of hypertension management and prevention is to achieve and maintain optimal control of blood pressure. However, the optimum blood pressure threshold for initiating antihypertensive drug therapy and specific treatment goals remain controversial. While other hypertension guidelines have based target blood pressure goals on age and comorbidities, the 2017 American College of Cardiology/American Heart Association (ACC/AHA) hypertension guideline incorporates underlying cardiovascular risk into decision making regarding treatment and generally recommends the same target blood pressure (i.e., less than 130/80 mm Hg) in all adults. Many patients will require at least 2 drugs from different pharmacologic classes to achieve this blood pressure goal; the potential benefits of hypertension management and drug cost, adverse effects, and risks associated with the use of multiple antihypertensive drugs also should be considered when deciding a patient's blood pressure treatment goal. (See General Considerations for Initial and Maintenance Antihypertensive Therapy under Uses: Hypertension.)

For additional information on target levels of blood pressure and on monitoring therapy in the management of hypertension, see Blood Pressure Monitoring and Treatment Goals under Dosage: Hypertension, in Dosage and Administration in the Thiazides General Statement 40:28.20.

IV Dosage

When oral therapy is not feasible, the recommended initial IV enalaprilat dosage in adults *not* receiving a diuretic or in those converting from enalapril maleate therapy (without concomitant diuretic therapy) is 1.25 mg every 6 hours. Reduction in blood pressure usually occurs within 15 minutes, but the maximal hypotensive response after the first dose may not occur for up to 4 hours after administration. The maximum effects of the second and subsequent doses may exceed those of the first dose. Although no regimen has been shown to be more effective than 1.25 mg every 6 hours, dosages as high as 5 mg every 6 hours were well tolerated for up to 36 hours in controlled clinical studies. Experience with dosages greater than 20 mg daily is insufficient. In studies of patients with hypertension, enalaprilat was not administered for longer than 48 hours, but in other studies it has been administered for as long as 7 days.

When oral therapy is not feasible in adults receiving a diuretic, the recommended initial IV enalaprilat dose is 0.625 mg. A reduction in blood pressure usually occurs within 15 minutes. Although most of the effect is usually apparent within the first hour, the maximal hypotensive response may not occur for up to 4 hours after the initial dose. If the blood pressure response after 1 hour is inadequate, another dose of 0.625 mg may be given. Additional doses of 1.25 mg may be administered at 6-hour intervals.

To reduce blood pressure rapidly in adults with a hypertensive emergency†, an IV enalaprilat dosage of 1.25–5 mg, repeated every 6 hours as necessary, has been recommended. If IV enalaprilat is used in the management of a hypertensive emergency in adults without a compelling condition, the initial goal of such therapy is to reduce systolic blood pressure by no more than 25% within 1 hour, followed by further reduction *if stable* toward 160/100 to 110 mm Hg within the next 2–6 hours, avoiding excessive declines in pressure that could precipitate renal, cerebral, or coronary ischemia. If this blood pressure is well tolerated and the patient is clinically stable, further gradual reductions toward normal can be implemented in the next 24–48 hours. Enalaprilat is most useful in hypertensive emergencies associated with high plasma renin activity.

For information on converting patients from IV to oral therapy, see Oral Dosage under Dosage: Hypertension, in Dosage and Administration.

Heart Failure

Because of the risk of severe hypotension, enalapril maleate therapy for heart failure should be initiated under very close medical supervision (e.g., in a hospital setting) with consideration given to recent diuretic therapy and the possibility of severe sodium and/or fluid depletion. ACE inhibitor therapy should be initiated with caution in patients with very low systemic blood pressure (systolic blood pressure less than 80 mm Hg), markedly increased serum concentrations of creatinine (greater than 3 mg/dL), bilateral renal artery stenosis, or elevated concentrations of serum potassium (greater than 5 mEq/L). Experts recommend that renal function and serum potassium be assessed within 1–2 weeks of initiation of therapy and periodically thereafter in patients receiving an ACE inhibitor, especially in those with preexisting hypotension, hyponatremia, diabetes mellitus, or azotemia, or in those taking potassium supplements. Use of low initial enalapril maleate dosages and reduction of the dosage of concomitantly administered diuretics may decrease the initial risk of hypotension. However, the long-term hemodynamic benefit of low enalapril maleate dosages (e.g., 10–20 mg daily) in this condition has not been established.

It should be recognized that although symptoms of heart failure may improve within 48 hours after initiating ACE inhibitor therapy in some patients, such improvement usually is not evident for several weeks or months after initiating ACE inhibitor therapy. In addition, it should be considered that such therapy may reduce the risk of disease progression even if symptomatic improvement is not evident. Therefore, dosages generally should be titrated to a prespecified target (i.e., at least 20 mg of enalapril daily) or highest tolerated dosage rather than according to response.

For the management of symptomatic heart failure, enalapril maleate often is administered in conjunction with other agents such as a cardiac glycoside, a

diuretic, and a β-blocker. Enalapril maleate dosage for heart failure should be initiated at low doses and titrated gradually upward if lower doses have been well tolerated. The usual initial enalapril maleate dosage for the management of heart failure in adults with normal renal function and serum sodium concentration is 2.5 mg twice daily. After the initial dose, the patient should be monitored closely for at least 2 hours and for at least one additional hour after blood pressure has stabilized. Hypotension occurring after the initial dose does not preclude the administration of subsequent doses of the drug, provided due caution is exercised and the hypotension has been managed effectively. To minimize the likelihood of hypotension, the dosage of any diuretic given concomitantly with enalapril should be reduced, if possible. The usual maintenance dosage of enalapril maleate for heart failure is 2.5–20 mg twice daily. The maximum recommended daily dosage of the drug is 40 mg, given in 2 divided doses.

Asymptomatic Left Ventricular Dysfunction

When used in adults with asymptomatic left ventricular dysfunction, enalapril maleate therapy has been initiated using a dosage of 2.5 mg twice daily. Therapy is then titrated as tolerated to a target daily dosage of 20 mg given in divided doses. After the initial dose of enalapril, the patient should be closely observed for at least 2 hours and for at least one additional hour after blood pressure has stabilized. To minimize the likelihood of hypotension, the dosage of any concomitant diuretic should be reduced, if possible. The appearance of hypotension after the initial dose of enalapril does not preclude subsequent carefully titrated doses of the drug after the hypotension has been effectively managed.

● *Dosage in Renal or Hepatic Impairment, Hyponatremia, Pediatric Patients, and Geriatric Patients*

If enalapril maleate or enalaprilat is used in patients with impaired renal function, dosage must be modified in response to the degree of renal impairment, and the theoretical risk of neutropenia must be considered. (See Cautions: Hematologic Effects.)

The manufacturer states that hypertensive adults with moderate renal impairment (i.e., creatinine clearances greater than 30 mL/minute) may receive the usual dosage of enalapril maleate. In adults with severe renal impairment (i.e., creatinine clearances of 30 mL/minute or less), dosage of enalapril maleate should be initiated at 2.5 mg daily. If an adequate response is not achieved, dosage may then be gradually increased until blood pressure is controlled or a maximum dosage of 40 mg daily is reached. Alternatively, some clinicians suggest that patients with creatinine clearances of 10–50 mL/minute can receive 75–100% of the usual dosage and those with creatinine clearances less than 10 mL/minute can receive 50% of the usual dosage. Patients undergoing hemodialysis should receive a supplemental dose of the drug after dialysis. The manufacturer recommends that hemodialysis patients be given a dose of 2.5 mg on dialysis days; on days between dialysis periods, enalapril maleate dosage should be adjusted according to the patient's blood pressure response.

For hypertensive adults with moderate renal impairment (i.e., creatinine clearances greater than 30 mL/minute) in whom oral therapy is not feasible, the recommended dosage of IV enalaprilat is 1.25 mg every 6 hours. In adults with severe renal impairment (i.e., creatinine clearances of 30 mL/minute or less), the initial dose of IV enalaprilat should be 0.625 mg; if the blood pressure response is inadequate after 1 hour, another dose of 0.625 mg may be given. Additional doses of 1.25 mg may be administered at 6-hour intervals. For patients undergoing dialysis, the initial dosage of IV enalaprilat should be 0.625 mg every 6 hours. When oral therapy is initiated following IV enalaprilat therapy, the recommended initial dosage of enalapril maleate is 5 mg once daily in patients with creatinine clearances greater than 30 mL/minute and 2.5 mg once daily in patients with creatinine clearances of 30 mL/minute or less. Dosage is subsequently adjusted according to the patient's blood pressure response.

The manufacturer states that adults with heart failure and hyponatremia (serum sodium concentration less than 130 mEq/L) or serum creatinine concentration greater than 1.6 mg/dL should receive an initial enalapril maleate dosage of 2.5 mg daily under close monitoring (see Heart Failure under Dosage and Administration: Dosage). Subsequent dosage may be increased gradually as necessary, usually at intervals of 4 or more days, to 2.5 mg twice daily, then 5 mg twice daily, and then higher, provided excessive hypotension or deterioration of renal function is not present at the time of intended dosage adjustment; dosage should not exceed 40 mg daily.

If concomitant diuretic therapy is required in patients with severe renal impairment, a loop diuretic is preferred to a thiazide diuretic. Therefore, use of commercially available preparations containing enalapril maleate in fixed combination with hydrochlorothiazide is not recommended for patients with severe renal impairment. The manufacturers state that dosage adjustment of commercially available preparations containing enalapril maleate in fixed combination with hydrochlorothiazide is not needed in patients with renal impairment whose creatinine clearance exceeds 30 mL/minute per 1.73 m². (For information on dosage of hydrochlorothiazide in other special populations, see Dosage and Administration, in Hydrochlorothiazide 40:28.20.)

Enalapril maleate is *not* recommended for neonates or for pediatric patients who have a glomerular filtration rate of less than 30 mL/minute per 1.73 m², since no data are available in such patients.

Since it is not known whether geriatric patients 65 years of age or older respond the same to enalapril in fixed combination with hydrochlorothiazide as younger adults, the manufacturer suggests that patients in this age group receive initial dosages of the fixed combination in the lower end of the usual range.

CAUTIONS

Adverse reactions to enalapril usually are mild and transient but have required discontinuance of therapy in about 3 or 6% of patients receiving the drug for the management of hypertension or heart failure, respectively. Enalaprilat usually is well tolerated. Since enalapril is metabolized to enalaprilat, administration of enalaprilat can be expected to produce adverse effects associated with enalapril therapy. Overall, the frequency of many adverse effects produced by enalapril appears to be similar to or less than that produced by captopril. However, unlike captopril, enalapril lacks the sulfhydryl group which has been associated with certain captopril-induced adverse effects (e.g., cutaneous reactions, taste disturbances, proteinuria), and the risk of these effects may be decreased during enalapril therapy. Additional experience to determine the relative safety of enalapril is necessary, and the possibility that the risk may be similar should be considered. Because of enalapril's long duration of action, the risk of some adverse effects (e.g., hypotension, deterioration in renal function) may be increased compared with short-acting ACE inhibitors, particularly in patients whose cardiovascular and renal systems have increased dependency on the renin-angiotensin system (e.g., those with severe heart failure).

Adverse nervous system effects (e.g., headache, dizziness, fatigue) occur most frequently during enalapril therapy for hypertension. Although adverse effects of enalapril generally are mild, discontinuance of the drug has been necessary in about 6% of patients, principally because of dizziness, headache, hypotension, or rash. The manufacturer states that the incidence of the most frequently reported adverse effects was similar in patients receiving enalapril or placebo in clinical trials. In patients with heart failure, symptomatic hypotension, deterioration in renal function, and increased serum potassium concentration appear to occur most frequently, particularly during initiation of enalapril therapy in volume- and/or sodium-depleted patients (e.g., those receiving concomitant diuretic therapy).

The frequency of some adverse reactions may be increased during therapy with enalapril in fixed combination with hydrochlorothiazide compared with either drug alone, but the manufacturer states that adverse reactions reported to date with the combination have been reported previously with the individual drugs. No reactions peculiar to the combination have been reported.

● Nervous System Effects

Headache and dizziness occur in about 5% of patients receiving enalapril alone for hypertension, requiring discontinuance in 0.4 and 0.3% of patients, respectively, and occur in about 6 and 9%, respectively, of hypertensive patients receiving the drug in fixed combination with hydrochlorothiazide. In patients receiving enalapril for heart failure, dizziness and headache occurred in approximately 8 and 2% of patients, respectively, and required discontinuance of the drug in 0.6 and 0.1%, respectively. Headache has been reported in about 3% of patients receiving enalaprilat. Fatigue has occurred in about 3% of patients receiving the drug alone for hypertension, requiring discontinuance in less than 0.1%, and has occurred in about 4% of hypertensive patients receiving the drug in fixed combination with hydrochlorothiazide. Fatigue, fever, and dizziness have been reported in 0.5–1% of patients receiving enalaprilat. Vertigo has occurred in about 2% of patients receiving enalapril for heart failure and required discontinuance in about 0.1% of patients. Insomnia, nervousness, peripheral neuropathy (e.g., paresthesia, dysesthesia, asthenia, and somnolence occur in about 0.5–2% of patients receiving enalapril alone or in fixed combination with hydrochlorothiazide. Hyperesthesia

of the oral mucosa, CNS depression, malaise, nightmares, confusion, ataxia, and coldness of the extremities have been reported rarely.

● GI Effects

Diarrhea and nausea occur in about 1–2% of patients with hypertension receiving enalapril alone or in fixed combination with hydrochlorothiazide and in patients with heart failure receiving the drug, and have required discontinuance of the drug in 0.2% or less of patients. Nausea has been reported in about 1% of patients receiving enalaprilat. Abdominal pain, vomiting, stomatitis, and dyspepsia occur in 0.5–2% of patients receiving enalapril, and ulceration of the oral mucosa, ileus, melena, anorexia, glossitis, dry mouth, and flatulence have been reported rarely. Constipation has been reported in 0.5–1% of patients receiving enalaprilat.

● Hepatic Effects

A clinical syndrome that usually is manifested initially by cholestatic jaundice and may progress to fulminant hepatic necrosis (which occasionally may be fatal), has been reported rarely in patients receiving ACE inhibitors. The mechanism of this reaction is not known.

● Cardiovascular Effects

The most frequent adverse cardiovascular effect of enalapril or enalaprilat is hypotension (including postural hypotension and other orthostatic effects), which occurs in about 1–2% of patients with hypertension and in about 5–7% of those with heart failure, following an initial dose or during extended therapy. Syncope occurred in approximately 0.5 or 2% of patients with hypertension or heart failure, respectively. Hypotension or syncope has required discontinuance of therapy in about 0.1 or 2% of patients with hypertension or heart failure, respectively, receiving enalapril.

Hypotensive effects, including excessive and/or symptomatic hypotension, appear to occur more frequently in patients receiving enalapril for heart failure rather than for uncomplicated hypertension. Some reduction in blood pressure occurs in most patients receiving the drug for heart failure and generally is beneficial when secondary to afterload reduction; however, pronounced hypotension can occur and may adversely affect renal and myocardial perfusion (see later discussion in this section). Enalapril-induced hypotension may occasionally be alleviated by dosage reduction, but severe hypotension has also occurred after low doses (i.e., a single 2.5- or 5-mg dose) of the drug.

The value of initiating enalapril therapy at low doses to decrease the risk of hypotension has not been fully elucidated, but such dosing has been suggested, particularly for patients at risk (e.g., those with heart failure). Orthostatic hypotension appears to occur more frequently during initiation of therapy and in patients with sodium depletion or hypovolemia. Transient hypotension in patients with heart failure or with hypertension may occur after any of the first several doses (i.e., with the first 24–48 hours), and sometimes is associated with dizziness, blurred vision, nausea, syncope, and, rarely, bradycardia. Patients who are volume and/or sodium depleted such as those receiving diuretics, especially those in whom diuretic therapy was recently initiated (e.g., patients with severe congestive heart failure), those whose sodium intake is severely restricted, and those who are undergoing dialysis, may occasionally experience a precipitous reduction in blood pressure within the first 3–4 hours after a dose of enalapril. The risk of orthostatic hypotension associated with concomitant use of enalapril and a diuretic may be affected by the sequence of initiation of therapy with each drug; the risk may be higher when enalapril is added to diuretic therapy than when a diuretic is added to enalapril therapy. Symptomatic hypotension that occurs later in a course of enalapril therapy (e.g., after the first 48 hours) may indicate the presence of sodium depletion (e.g., secondary to restriction of sodium intake or increased diuretic dosage).

When enalapril was used in fixed combination with hydrochlorothiazide in clinical trials in hypertensive patients, hypotension, orthostatic hypotension, and other orthostatic effects occurred in 0.9, 1.5, and 2.3% of patients, respectively. Syncope occurred in 1.3% of patients receiving the fixed combination, but the frequency of this effect can be minimized by proper titration of each drug separately and substitution with the combination preparation only when the optimum dosages correspond to the fixed ratio in the preparation.

Severe enalapril-induced hypotension may be associated with oliguria and/or progressive azotemia and, rarely, with acute renal failure, myocardial ischemia, and/or death in patients with heart failure, hyponatremia, or severe sodium or volume depletion of any etiology; patients undergoing dialysis; and those receiving high-dose or recent intensive diuretic therapy or in whom the diuretic dosage was recently increased. In such patients, it may be advisable to discontinue diuretic therapy (except in patients with heart failure), reduce the diuretic dosage, or cautiously increase salt intake, if possible, prior to initiating therapy with enalapril. Patients at risk for excessive hypotension should be closely monitored after an initial dose of the drug, and should be followed closely for 2 weeks after initiation of enalapril therapy and whenever dosage of enalapril and/or a concomitantly administered diuretic is increased. Some experts state that patients with heart failure should be under very close medical supervision (e.g., in a hospital setting) when enalapril therapy is initiated, since severe hypotension could potentially compromise the patient's hemodynamic status. The risk of hypotension and potential detrimental hemodynamic and clinical effects in patients with severe heart failure appears to be higher during therapy with a long-acting ACE inhibitor such as enalapril than with a short-acting inhibitor.

If hypotension occurs in patients receiving enalapril, the patient should be placed in the supine or Trendelenburg's position; if hypotension is severe or prolonged, IV infusion of 0.9% sodium chloride injection to expand fluid volume should be considered. Transient hypotension is not a contraindication to additional doses of enalapril, and therapy with the drug can usually be cautiously reinitiated after blood pressure has been stabilized (e.g., with volume expansion); enalapril dosage reduction and/or dosage reduction or discontinuance of concomitantly administered diuretics may be necessary. Some clinicians state that asymptomatic hypotension often does not require specific therapy and may be well tolerated with continued enalapril therapy. However, severe hypotension occasionally may require discontinuance of enalapril therapy, and the possibility should be considered that hypotension may persist for prolonged periods (e.g., for a week or longer) after discontinuance of the drug because of the drug's long duration of action. Patients with heart failure or those undergoing dialysis may be at particular risk of prolonged hypotension. The possibility of severe hypotension may be minimized by withholding diuretic therapy and/or increasing sodium intake for 2–3 days prior to initiating enalapril therapy.

Hypotension also may occur in enalapril-treated patients during major surgery or during anesthesia with agents that produce hypotension. This hypotensive effect results from inhibition by enalapril of the angiotensin II formation that occurs subsequent to compensatory renin release, and, if it is thought to be caused by enalapril, can generally be corrected with fluid volume expansion.

Palpitation and chest pain occur in about 0.5–2% of patients with hypertension receiving enalapril alone or in fixed combination with hydrochlorothiazide. Tachycardia, bradycardia, and development or worsening of Raynaud's phenomenon have been reported rarely in patients receiving the drug. Cardiac arrest or cerebrovascular accident, possibly secondary to excessive hypotension in high-risk patients, pulmonary embolism and infarction, pulmonary edema, rhythm disturbances (including atrial tachycardia and bradycardia), flushing, and atrial fibrillation have been reported in about 0.5–1% of patients with hypertension or heart failure. Angina or myocardial infarction (MI) was reported in about 1–1.5% of patients receiving enalapril for heart failure in controlled and uncontrolled studies, and required discontinuance in about 0.1–0.3% of patients, but a similar incidence for these effects was reported in patients receiving placebo in controlled studies. MI was reported in 0.5–1% of patients receiving enalaprilat.

● Renal Effects

Deterioration in renal function, manifested as transient increases in BUN and serum creatinine concentrations, has occurred in about 20% of patients with renovascular hypertension, especially those with bilateral renal-artery stenosis or those with renal-artery stenosis in a solitary kidney. This effect was usually reversible following discontinuance of enalapril and/or diuretic therapy. Renal function should be monitored closely during the first few weeks of therapy in these patients. (See Cautions: Precautions and Contraindications.) Transient increases in BUN and serum creatinine concentrations have also occurred in about 0.2% of patients with hypertension, but without preexisting renal vascular disease, who were receiving enalapril alone. These effects occur more frequently in patients receiving concomitant diuretic therapy, in patients with heart failure, and in patients with some degree of preexisting renal dysfunction. Dosage reduction of enalapril and/or dosage reduction or discontinuance of diuretic therapy may be necessary. The rapidity of onset and magnitude of enalapril-induced renal insufficiency in patients with heart failure may depend in part on the degree of sodium depletion. About 5–15 or 15–30% of patients with mild to moderate or severe heart failure, respectively, treated with an ACE inhibitor develop substantial elevations of serum creatinine concentrations (e.g., greater than 5 mg/dL). Acute reversible renal failure, flank pain, oliguria, uremia, glycosuria, and proteinuria have been reported rarely in patients receiving enalapril. Urinary tract infection has been reported in about 1% of patients receiving enalapril for heart failure in controlled and uncontrolled studies, but this effect occurred in about 2% of patients receiving placebo in controlled studies.

Because the renin-angiotensin system appears to contribute substantially to maintenance of glomerular filtration in patients with heart failure in whom renal perfusion is severely compromised, renal function may deteriorate markedly during therapy with an ACE inhibitor in these patients. Such drug-induced deterioration is generally well tolerated, and does not usually necessitate discontinuance of effective therapy with the drug when symptomatic improvement of the heart failure occurs. In addition, the magnitude of deterioration in renal function can usually be ameliorated by reducing the dosage of concomitantly administered diuretics and/or by liberalizing dietary sodium intake, since concomitant diuretic therapy and/or sodium restriction potentially increase the role of angiotensin II in maintaining glomerular filtration in these patients. In patients in whom renal perfusion pressure is very low and is further reduced by ACE-inhibitor therapy, however, deterioration in renal function may be clinically important. Patients with concomitant underlying diabetes mellitus may be at particular risk for developing renal insufficiency during ACE-inhibitor therapy. In some patients with severe heart failure, with or without associated renal insufficiency, treatment with an ACE inhibitor, including enalapril, may be associated with oliguria and/or progressive azotemia, and rarely with acute renal failure and/or death. The risk of developing functional renal insufficiency appears to be higher during therapy with a long-acting ACE inhibitor such as enalapril than with a short-acting inhibitor.

● Dermatologic and Sensitivity Reactions

The most frequent adverse dermatologic effect of enalapril is rash, which occurs in about 1.5% of patients and is usually maculopapular and rarely urticarial. Rash may sometimes be accompanied by pruritus, erythema, or eosinophilia, and has required discontinuance of the drug in approximately 0.3% of patients. A patient who developed enalapril-induced rash was subsequently treated with captopril without recurrence. However, the frequency of enalapril-induced rash appears to be less than that of captopril, possibly because enalapril lacks the sulfhydryl group, and several patients who developed captopril-induced rash have subsequently been treated with enalapril without recurrence of rash. Rash has been reported in 0.5–1% of patients receiving enalaprilat.

Pruritus, without rash, and excessive sweating have been reported in 0.5–2% of patients receiving enalapril alone or in fixed combination with hydrochlorothiazide. Alopecia has been reported in 0.5–1% of patients receiving enalapril. A symptom complex, consisting of positive ANA titer, increased erythrocyte sedimentation rate (ESR), arthralgias and/or arthritis, myalgias, fever, serositis, vasculitis, leukocytosis, eosinophilia, photosensitivity, rash, and other dermatologic reactions has been reported in 0.5–1% of patients receiving enalapril therapy. Exfoliative dermatitis, toxic epidermal necrolysis, Stevens-Johnson syndrome, pemphigus, herpes zoster, and erythema multiforme have been reported rarely in patients receiving enalapril therapy.

Severe, sudden anaphylactoid reactions, which can be fatal, have been reported following initiation of hemodialysis that utilized a high-flux polyacrylonitrile [PAN] membrane (e.g., AN 69®) in patients receiving an ACE inhibitor. Manifestations of these reactions included nausea, abdominal cramps, burning, angioedema, and shortness of breath; progression to severe hypotension can develop rapidly. Dialysis should be stopped immediately and aggressive supportive and symptomatic therapy should be initiated as indicated. Antihistamines do *not* appear to be effective in providing symptomatic relief. While it currently does not seem to be necessary to exclude the use of ACE inhibitors in patients undergoing hemodialysis that involves PAN membranes, caution should be exercised during concomitant use. The mechanism of this interaction has not been established, and the incidence and risk of its occurrence remain to be elucidated. The possibility that ACE inhibitors may precipitate similar reactions in patients undergoing hemodialysis involving other membrane types (new or reprocessed) should be considered. In addition, anaphylactoid reactions also have been reported in patients undergoing low-density lipoprotein (LDL) apheresis with dextran sulfate absorption. Manifestations of these reactions included flushing, dyspnea, bradycardia, and hypotension. It has been postulated that these reactions may be associated with accumulation of polypeptides (e.g., bradykinin) since endogenous concentration of such polypeptides may be increased by LDL-apheresis with dextran sulfate and their metabolism may be decreased by ACE inhibitors. To avoid these anaphylactoid reactions, some clinicians recommend withdrawal of ACE inhibitors 12–30 hours before apheresis, while others state that ACE inhibitors should not be used in patients treated with LDL apheresis.

Life-threatening anaphylactoid reactions have been reported in at least 2 patients receiving ACE inhibitors while undergoing desensitization treatment with hymenoptera venom. When ACE inhibitors were temporarily discontinued 24 hours before desensitization with the venom, anaphylactoid reactions did not recur; however, such reactions recurred after inadvertent rechallenge.

Angioedema of the face, lips, tongue, larynx, glottis, or extremities has occurred in patients receiving ACE inhibitor therapy, including enalapril. (See Cautions: Precautions and Contraindications.) In addition, intestinal angioedema (occasionally without a prior history of facial angioedema or elevated serum levels of complement 1 [C1] esterase inhibitor) has been reported in patients receiving ACE inhibitors. Intestinal angioedema, which frequently presents as abdominal pain (with or without nausea or vomiting), usually is diagnosed by abdominal CT scan, ultrasound, or surgery; manifestations usually have resolved after discontinuance of the ACE inhibitor. Intestinal angioedema should be considered in the differential diagnosis of patients who develop abdominal pain during therapy with an ACE inhibitor.

● Hematologic Effects

Decreases in hemoglobin and hematocrit averaging approximately 0.3 g/dL and 1%, respectively, occur frequently in hypertensive patients receiving enalapril alone or in fixed combination with hydrochlorothiazide, but rarely are clinically important unless another cause of anemia also exists. Enalapril-induced anemia has required discontinuance of therapy in less than 0.1% of patients. Hemolytic anemia, including cases of hemolysis in a few patients with glucose-6-phosphate-dehydrogenase (G-6-PD) deficiency, has been reported in patients receiving enalapril maleate therapy; a causal relationship has not been established.

Neutropenia (less than 1000 neutrophils/mm³) and agranulocytosis, both associated with myeloid hypoplasia, have occurred rarely in patients receiving captopril. (See Cautions: Hematologic Effects, in Captopril 24:32.04.) Several cases of neutropenia, agranulocytosis, or thrombocytopenia have been reported, and a causal relationship to enalapril cannot be excluded. Because of pharmacologic and structural similarities between captopril and enalapril and the current lack of sufficient data to establish the relative risk of these adverse hematologic effects in patients receiving enalapril, the possibility that bone marrow depression, neutropenia, and agranulocytosis could occur in patients receiving enalapril should be considered. Experience with captopril indicates that patients with renal impairment, especially those with collagen vascular disease, appear to be at increased risk of these adverse hematologic effects, and complete and differential leukocyte counts should be performed periodically during enalapril therapy in these patients. Enalapril lacks a sulfhydryl group, the structural feature suggested as being associated with this toxicity in patients receiving captopril; however, this structural relationship has not been established and the lack of this group in enalapril may not exclude the possibility of these effects in patients receiving the drug.

● Effects on Taste

Loss of taste perception and decrease in taste acuity have been reported infrequently during enalapril therapy. Hyperesthesia of the oral mucosa has occurred in at least one patient receiving enalapril but was reversible following discontinuance of the drug. Patients with intolerable captopril-induced taste disturbances may tolerate enalapril better.

● Effects on Potassium

Although small increases (i.e., by an average of 0.2 mEq/L) in serum potassium concentrations frequently occur in patients receiving enalapril without a thiazide diuretic, hyperkalemia (i.e., increases to greater than 5.7 mEq/L) occurs in approximately 1 or 4% of patients with hypertension or heart failure, respectively, receiving the drug. In most cases, these were isolated increases that resolved despite continued therapy with the drug; however, hyperkalemia required discontinuance of enalapril therapy in about 0.3% of patients receiving the drug for hypertension. Hyperkalemia is less frequent in patients receiving enalapril and hydrochlorothiazide concomitantly, occurring in about 0.1% of patients. Patients with diabetes mellitus, impaired renal function, or heart failure and patients concomitantly receiving drugs that can increase serum potassium concentration (e.g., potassium-sparing diuretics, potassium supplements, potassium-containing salt substitutes) may be at increased risk of developing hyperkalemia during enalapril therapy; serum potassium concentration should be monitored frequently in these patients, and potassium intake should be controlled and therapy with drugs that can increase serum potassium modified or discontinued as necessary. The manufacturer recommends that potassium-sparing diuretics generally *not* be used in patients receiving enalapril for heart failure.

● Respiratory Effects

Cough has been reported in 1.3 or 3.5% of patients receiving enalapril alone or in fixed combination with hydrochlorothiazide for hypertension, respectively, and in about 2% of those receiving the drug for heart failure; discontinuance of the drug was required in less than 0.5% of patients. Nonproductive cough, particularly at night, may occur more frequently, especially in patients with chronic obstructive pulmonary disease. Some clinicians state that cough often is overlooked as a potential adverse effect of ACE inhibitors and may occur more frequently (in about 5–15% of patients). The cough generally is persistent and nonproductive, is not associated with other respiratory symptoms, and is reversible following discontinuance of the drug. Nasal congestion also has been reported. It has been suggested that accumulation of kinins in the respiratory tract secondary to ACE inhibition may in part be responsible for cough and nasal congestion. Concomitant therapy with a nonsteroidal anti-inflammatory agent (i.e., sulindac) appeared to minimize cough in a few patients, but additional study of the safety (e.g., effects on renal function) of such combined therapy is necessary. If cough develops in a patient receiving enalapril, ACE inhibitor-induced cough should be considered as part of the differential diagnosis.

Dyspnea and wheezing, which may persist if therapy with the drug is continued, have been reported in about 1% or less of patients receiving enalapril. Pneumonia or bronchitis has been reported in about 1% of patients receiving enalapril for heart failure. Asthma, upper respiratory infection, bronchospasm, pulmonary infiltrates, eosinophilic pneumonitis, and rhinorrhea also have been reported in patients receiving enalapril maleate therapy. Angioedema has occurred in 0.2 or 0.6% of patients receiving enalapril alone or in fixed combination with hydrochlorothiazide, respectively, and, if associated with laryngeal edema, may be fatal. ACE inhibitors appear to produce a higher incidence of angioedema in black patients than in other races studied. (See Cautions: Precautions and Contraindications.)

● Other Adverse Effects

Muscle cramps, and impotence have been reported in 0.5–1% of patients receiving enalapril alone, and decreased libido has been reported rarely. These effects have occurred more frequently when the drug was administered in fixed combination with hydrochlorothiazide. Hearing loss, which was reversible following discontinuance of the drug, has been reported rarely; however, the mechanism of this adverse effect is not known. Pancreatitis, hepatitis or cholestatic jaundice, hepatic failure, sore throat, hoarseness, anosmia, conjunctivitis, dry eyes, tearing eyes, gynecomastia, and myalgia have been reported in patients receiving enalapril. Vulvovaginal pruritus, burning urination, and dysuria were reported in at least one patient receiving enalapril.

Although a definite causal relationship to enalapril has not been established, elevations of serum hepatic enzymes and/or bilirubin concentrations have been reported rarely when enalapril was administered alone or in fixed combination with hydrochlorothiazide.

● Precautions and Contraindications

Since enalapril is metabolized to enalaprilat, both drugs share the same cautions, precautions, and contraindications. Because captopril, another ACE inhibitor, can cause serious adverse effects (e.g., neutropenia, agranulocytosis), particularly in patients with renal impairment (especially those with collagen vascular disease), the possibility that similar adverse effects may occur with enalapril should be considered. Periodic monitoring of leukocyte counts should be considered in these patients. (See Cautions: Hematologic Effects.) Patients should be instructed to notify their clinician if any sign or symptom of infection such as fever or sore throat occurs. When enalapril is used in fixed combination with hydrochlorothiazide, the cautions, precautions, and contraindications associated with thiazide diuretics must be considered in addition to those associated with enalapril. To minimize dose-independent adverse effects, it is recommended that therapy with enalapril in fixed combination with hydrochlorothiazide only be initiated in patients in whom an adequate response is not achieved with enalapril or hydrochlorothiazide monotherapy.

Renal function should be evaluated prior to initiation of enalapril therapy, and the drug should be used with caution in patients with renal impairment, particularly those with known or suspected renovascular disease. Reduction of enalapril dosage, reduction in dosage or discontinuance of diuretic therapy, and/or adequate sodium repletion may be necessary in some patients who develop impaired renal function during enalapril therapy. Because of an increased risk of reducing renal perfusion to a critically low level, enalapril should be used with caution and renal function monitored closely for the first few weeks of therapy in patients with bilateral renal-artery stenosis and those with renal-artery stenosis in a solitary kidney. Serum creatinine and electrolyte concentrations should be evaluated prior to and 1 week following initiation of therapy with ACE inhibitors in patients with heart failure. In patients with heart failure who have some degree of renal impairment (baseline serum creatinine concentrations less than 2 mg/dL) or more severe renal impairment (baseline serum creatinine concentrations exceeding 2 mg/dL), an increase in serum creatinine concentration exceeding 0.5 or 1 mg/dL, respectively, should prompt consideration of discontinuing ACE inhibitor therapy while additional renal evaluation and corrective action is undertaken. The possibility that ACE inhibitors might precipitate severe, sudden, potentially life-threatening anaphylactoid reactions in patients undergoing hemodialysis involving a high-flux membrane should be considered. (See Cautions: Dermatologic and Sensitivity Reactions.)

Enalapril should be used with caution in patients with sodium depletion or hypovolemia, those receiving diuretics, and those undergoing dialysis since severe hypotension may occur. The drug should also be used with caution in patients in whom excessive hypotension may have serious consequences (e.g., patients with coronary or cerebrovascular insufficiency). Because of the potential decrease in blood pressure in patients with heart failure, enalapril therapy should be initiated under very close medical supervision in these patients. (See Cautions: Cardiovascular Effects.) Like all vasodilators, enalapril should be administered with caution in patients with obstruction in the outflow tract of the left ventricle (e.g., aortic stenosis, hypertrophic cardiomyopathy). Patients at risk for excessive hypotension should be monitored closely for the first 2 weeks of therapy and whenever the dosage of enalapril and/or a concomitantly administered diuretic is increased. Patients receiving enalapril therapy should be informed that vomiting, diarrhea, excessive perspiration, and dehydration may lead to an exaggerated decrease in blood pressure because of fluid volume reduction; patients should notify their clinician if any of these conditions occurs. Patients should also be warned to report light headedness, especially during the first few days of therapy; if actual syncope occurs, they should discontinue enalapril therapy and contact their clinician. Since therapy with ACE inhibitors has been associated with development of a rare syndrome that usually is manifested initially by cholestatic jaundice, which may progress to fulminant hepatic necrosis and occasionally may be fatal, patients receiving an ACE inhibitor, including enalapril, who develop jaundice or marked elevations of hepatic enzymes should discontinue the drug and receive appropriate medical follow-up. (See Cautions: Hepatic Effects.)

Angioedema may occur, especially following the first dose of enalapril, and, if associated with laryngeal edema, may be fatal. If laryngeal stridor or angioedema of the face, extremities, lips, tongue, or glottis occurs, enalapril should be discontinued and the patient carefully observed until swelling disappears. If swelling is confined to the face and lips, the condition generally responds without treatment; however, antihistamines may provide symptomatic relief. Swelling of the tongue, glottis, or larynx may cause airway obstruction, and appropriate therapy (e.g., epinephrine, maintenance of patent airway) should be initiated immediately. Patients should be informed that swelling of the face, eyes, lips, or tongue or difficulty in breathing may be signs and symptoms of angioedema, and that they should discontinue enalapril and notify their clinician immediately if any of these conditions occurs. The possibility that patients with a history of angioedema unrelated to ACE inhibitors may be at increased risk of developing angioedema while receiving the drugs should be considered. Enalapril is contraindicated in patients with a history of angioedema related to ACE inhibitor therapy and those with hereditary or idiopathic angioedema. Enalapril also is contraindicated in patients with known hypersensitivity to the drug or any ingredient in the formulation.

Pediatric Precautions

Antihypertensive effects of enalapril maleate have been established in hypertensive pediatric patients 1 month to 16 years of age. Enalapril maleate is not recommended for neonates or for pediatric patients with a glomerular filtration rate of less than 30 mL/minute per 1.73 m², since no data are available. The adverse effect profile of enalapril maleate in pediatric patients is similar to that in adults. Safety and efficacy of enalaprilat injection or of enalapril in fixed combination with hydrochlorothiazide in children have not been established. For information on overall principles and expert recommendations for treatment of hypertension in pediatric patients, see Uses: Hypertension in Pediatric Patients, in the Thiazides General Statement 40:28.20.

Geriatric Precautions

Clinical studies of enalapril in fixed combination with hydrochlorothiazide did not include sufficient numbers of patients 65 years of age and older to determine whether geriatric patients respond differently than younger patients. While other clinical experience has not revealed age-related differences in response, drug dosage generally should be titrated carefully in geriatric patients, usually initiating therapy at the low end of the dosage range. The greater frequency of decreased hepatic, renal, and/or cardiac function and of concomitant disease and drug therapy observed in the elderly also should be considered. Enalapril is substantially eliminated by the kidneys; because geriatric patients may have decreased renal function and because patients with renal impairment may be at increased risk of toxicity, renal function should be monitored and dosage should be selected carefully.

Mutagenicity and Carcinogenicity

No evidence of enalapril- or enalaprilat-induced mutagenicity or of mutagenicity induced by concomitant testing of enalapril and hydrochlorothiazide was seen with an in vitro microbial test system (Ames test) with or without metabolic activation. Enalapril alone or combined with hydrochlorothiazide also was not mutagenic in several other in vitro test systems, including mammalian systems, and in in vivo cytogenetic tests using mouse bone marrow.

No evidence of carcinogenesis was seen in rats or in male and female mice receiving enalapril maleate dosages up to 90 or 90 and 180 mg/kg daily, respectively (about 26 or 13 times the maximum daily human dosage on a mg/m² basis, respectively), for 106 or 94 weeks, respectively. Carcinogenicity studies have not been performed with enalaprilat.

While an excess rate of GI cancer relative to placebo has been observed in several large trials in patients receiving prolonged ACE-inhibitor therapy, a causal relationship to the drugs has not been established. Some evidence suggests that such a relationship is unlikely since the observed risk did not increase with increasing exposure to the drugs and because of the heterogeneity of the reported cancers (involving the rectum, cecum, colon, esophagus, stomach, gallbladder, pancreas, or liver). However, the possibility of a causal relationship cannot be excluded, and additional study to further elucidate any possible relationship between use of ACE inhibitors and these cancers is necessary.

Pregnancy, Fertility, and Lactation
Pregnancy

Fetal and neonatal morbidity and mortality have been reported in at least 50 pregnant women who were receiving ACE inhibitors during pregnancy. Very limited epidemiologic data indicate that the rate of fetal and neonatal morbidity resulting from exposure to ACE inhibitors during the second and third trimesters may be as high as 10–20%. Hypotension, reversible or irreversible renal failure, anuria, skull hypoplasia (defective skull ossification in some cases), and/or death were reported in neonates whose mothers had received ACE inhibitors during the second and third trimesters of pregnancy. In one premature neonate (35 weeks' gestation) born with acute, reversible renal failure following exposure to enalapril for several weeks prior to delivery, plasma ACE activity was completely suppressed at birth, and plasma active and total renin concentrations and renin activity were substantially increased in the neonate; the renal failure was managed with peritoneal dialysis, which was discontinued after 10 days. Other adverse effects associated with such use included oligohydramnios, presumably due to decreased renal function in the fetus, prematurity, fetal death, and patent ductus arteriosus; however, it is not known whether these effects were associated with ACE inhibition or underlying maternal disease. Oligohydramnios has been associated with contractures of the limbs, craniofacial deformities, hypoplasia of the lungs, and intrauterine growth retardation.

Although fetal exposure limited to the first trimester previously was considered not to be associated with substantial risk, data from an epidemiologic study have shown that infants whose mothers had taken an ACE inhibitor during the first trimester of pregnancy have an increased risk of major congenital malformations compared with infants who had not undergone first trimester exposure to ACE inhibitors. The risk of major congenital malformations, primarily affecting the cardiovascular and central nervous systems, was increased by about 2.7 times in infants whose mothers had taken an ACE inhibitor during the first trimester of pregnancy compared with infants who had not undergone such exposure. Every effort should be made to discontinue enalapril or enalaprilat therapy as soon as possible in any woman who becomes pregnant while receiving either of the drugs, regardless of the period of gestation. In addition, all women of childbearing potential who are receiving an ACE inhibitor should be advised to report pregnancy to their clinician as soon as possible. Women of childbearing potential who are receiving an ACE inhibitor also should be advised to inform their clinician if they are planning to become pregnant or think they might be pregnant. Nearly all women can be transferred successfully to alternative therapy for the remainder of their pregnancy. Rarely (probably less frequently than once in every 1000 pregnancies), no adequate alternative can be identified; in such rare cases, the woman should be informed of the potential hazard to the fetus and serial ultrasound examinations should be performed to assess the intra-amniotic environment. If oligohydramnios is present, enalapril therapy should be discontinued, unless use of the drug is considered life-saving for the woman.Contraction stress testing (CST), a nonstress test (NST), or biophysical profiling may be performed, if appropriate depending on the period of gestation. However, both clinicians and patients should realize that oligohydramnios may not become apparent until after irreversible fetal injury already has occurred.

Infants exposed in utero to ACE inhibitors should be observed closely for hypotension, oliguria, and hyperkalemia. If oliguria occurs, supportive measures (e.g., administration of fluids and pressor agents) to correct hypotension and renal perfusion should be considered. Exchange transfusion or dialysis may be required to reverse hypotension and/or substitute for impaired renal function. Enalapril, which crosses the placenta, has been removed from neonatal circulation by peritoneal dialysis with some clinical benefit. The manufacturer states that the drug theoretically may be removed by exchange transfusion; however, this latter procedure has not been used to date.

Reproduction studies in rats using enalapril maleate dosages up to 200 mg/kg daily (about 333 times the maximum daily human dosage) have not revealed evidence of teratogenicity or fetotoxicity. Decreases in average fetal weight occurred in rats receiving enalapril maleate dosages of 1200 mg/kg daily, but fetotoxicity did not occur when rats received a diet supplemented with sodium chloride. Fetotoxicity (decreased fetal weight) has been observed in rats receiving oral dosages up to 90 mg/kg of enalapril maleate combined with 10 mg/kg of hydrochlorothiazide daily (representing 26 and 1.6 times the maximum recommended human daily dosage of enalapril maleate and hydrochlorothiazide, respectively, on a mg/m^2 basis) and in mice receiving combined oral therapy with up to 30 and 10 mg/kg daily of enalapril maleate and hydrochlorothiazide, respectively (representing 4.3 and 0.8 times the maximum recommended human daily dosage of enalapril maleate and hydrochlorothiazide, respectively, on a mg/m^2 basis), but did not occur when lower dosages of enalapril maleate (30 and 10 mg/kg daily, respectively) were combined with 10 mg/kg of hydrochlorothiazide daily in these animals. Reproduction studies in rabbits receiving enalapril maleate dosages up to 30 mg/kg daily during days 6–18 of gestation did not reveal evidence of teratogenicity, but maternotoxicity and fetotoxicity occurred in rabbits at dosages of 1 mg/kg daily. Fetotoxicity and maternotoxicity did not occur in rabbits receiving enalapril maleate dosages of 3–10 mg/kg daily when their diet was supplemented with sodium chloride, but did occur at dosages of 30 mg/kg daily even when the diet was supplemented.

Fertility

Reproduction studies in male and female rats using enalapril maleate dosages of 10–90 mg/kg daily (representing up to 4.3 and 0.8 times the maximum recommended human daily dosage of enalapril maleate and hydrochlorothiazide, respectively, on a mg/m^2 basis) have not revealed adverse effects on reproductive performance. Impotence and decreased libido have been reported occasionally in patients receiving enalapril alone or in fixed combination with hydrochlorothiazide.

Lactation

Because enalapril alone or thiazide diuretics alone are distributed into human milk and potentially may cause serious adverse reactions in nursing infants, a decision should be made whether to discontinue nursing or enalapril (either alone or in fixed combination with hydrochlorothiazide), taking into account the importance of the drug(s) to the woman.

DRUG INTERACTIONS

In addition to the drug interactions described, the possibility that other drug interactions reported with other angiotensin-converting enzyme (ACE) inhibitors (e.g., captopril) might occur with enalapril should be considered.

● Hypotensive Agents and Diuretics

When enalapril is administered with diuretics or other hypotensive drugs, the hypotensive effect of enalapril is increased. The effect is usually used to therapeutic advantage, but careful adjustment of dosage is necessary when these drugs are used concomitantly.

Enalapril and diuretics appear to have additive hypotensive effects; however, severe hypotension and reversible renal insufficiency may occasionally occur, especially in volume- and/or sodium-depleted patients. (See Cautions: Cardiovascular Effects; and Renal Effects.) Hypotensive drugs that cause release of renin (e.g., diuretics) will increase the hypotensive effect of enalapril. Reduction of enalapril dosage and/or dosage reduction or discontinuance of diuretic therapy may be necessary. Patients should be monitored closely during initiation and dosage adjustment of concomitant therapy with enalapril and a diuretic; in patients already receiving diuretics, the risk of these effects may be minimized by withholding diuretic therapy and/or increasing sodium intake for 2–3 days prior to initiating enalapril therapy. If diuretic therapy cannot be withheld, the patient should be under medical supervision for at least 2 hours after the initial dose of enalapril and until blood pressure has stabilized for at least an additional hour.

● Drugs Increasing Serum Potassium Concentration

Potassium-sparing diuretics (e.g., amiloride, spironolactone, triamterene), potassium supplements, or potassium-containing salt substitutes should be used with caution and serum potassium should be determined frequently in patients receiving enalapril, since hyperkalemia may occur. Dosage of the potassium-sparing diuretic and/or potassium supplement should be reduced or the diuretic and/or supplement discontinued as necessary. The manufacturer recommends that potassium-sparing diuretics generally not be used in patients receiving enalapril for heart failure. However, ACE inhibitors have been administered with low-dosage spironolactone therapy and hyperkalemia was reported rarely. (See Uses: Heart Failure.) Patients should be advised to not use potassium-containing salt substitutes unless otherwise instructed by their clinician. Patients with renal impairment may be at increased risk of hyperkalemia.

● Nonsteroidal Anti-inflammatory Agents

Because ACE inhibitors may promote kinin-mediated prostaglandin synthesis and/or release, concomitant administration of drugs that inhibit prostaglandin synthesis (e.g., aspirin, ibuprofen) may reduce the blood pressure response to ACE inhibitors, including enalapril. Limited data indicate that concomitant administration of ACE inhibitors with nonsteroidal anti-inflammatory agents (NSAIAs) occasionally may result in acute reduction of renal function; however, the possibility cannot be ruled out that one drug alone may cause such an effect. Blood pressure should be monitored carefully when an NSAIA is initiated in patients receiving ACE inhibitor therapy; in addition, clinicians should be alert for evidence of impaired renal function. Some clinicians suggest that if a drug interaction between an ACE inhibitor and an NSAIA is suspected, the NSAIA should be discontinued, or a different hypotensive agent used or, alternatively, the dosage of the hypotensive agent should be modified.

Aspirin and other NSAIAs also can attenuate the hemodynamic actions of ACE inhibitors in patients with heart failure. Because ACE inhibitors share and enhance the effects of the compensatory hemodynamic mechanisms of heart failure, with aspirin and other NSAIAs interacting with the compensatory mechanisms rather than with a given ACE inhibitor per se, these desirable mechanisms are particularly susceptible to the interaction and a subsequent potential loss of clinical benefits. As a result, the more severe the heart failure and the more prominent the compensatory mechanisms, the more appreciable the interaction between NSAIAs and ACE inhibitors. Even if optimal dosage of an ACE inhibitor is used in the treatment of heart failure, the potential cardiovascular and survival benefit may not be seen if the patient is receiving an NSAIA concomitantly. In several multicenter studies, concomitant administration of a NSAIA (i.e., a single 350-mg dose of aspirin) in patients with heart failure inhibited favorable hemodynamic effects associated with ACE inhibitors, attenuating the favorable effects of these drugs on survival and cardiovascular morbidity. However, these findings have not been confirmed by other studies. In one retrospective analysis of pooled data, patients who received an ACE inhibitor concomitantly with aspirin (160– 325 mg daily) during the acute phase following myocardial infarction (MI) had proportional reductions in 7- and 30-day mortality rates comparable to patients who received an ACE inhibitor alone. Some clinicians have questioned the results of this study because of methodologic concerns (e.g., unsubstantiated assumptions about aspirin therapy [dosage, time of initiation, duration]; disparate distribution of patients). Although it has been suggested that patients requiring long-term management of heart failure avoid the concomitant use of ACE inhibitors and aspirin (and perhaps substitute another platelet-aggregation inhibitor for aspirin [e.g., clopidogrel, ticlopidine]), some clinicians state that existing data are insufficient to recommend a change in the current prescribing practices of clinicians concerning the use of aspirin in patients receiving therapy with an ACE inhibitor.

● Lithium

Lithium toxicity has occurred following concomitant administration of enalapril and lithium carbonate and was reversible following discontinuance of both drugs. In one patient, the toxicity was associated with elevated plasma lithium concentration and was manifested as ataxia, dysarthria, tremor, confusion, and altered EEG; bradycardia and T-wave depression also occurred. Moderate renal insufficiency (serum creatinine of 2.2 mg/dL) or acute renal failure has also occurred in these patients. The exact mechanism of this interaction remains to be established, but it has been suggested that enalapril may decrease renal elimination of lithium, possibly by increasing sodium excretion secondary to decreased aldosterone secretion or by altering renal function secondary to ACE inhibition. Renal function has returned to baseline within 2–4 days after discontinuing enalapril, and plasma lithium concentrations have returned to within normal limits following discontinuance of enalapril and temporary withdrawal of lithium therapy. The manufacturer of enalapril recommends that serum lithium concentrations be monitored frequently when enalapril and lithium are administered concomitantly.

● Other Drugs

Enalapril may reduce fasting blood glucose concentrations in nondiabetic individuals and may produce hypoglycemia in diabetic patients whose diabetes has been controlled with insulin or oral antidiabetic agents. Further studies are needed to evaluate the hypoglycemic effect of enalapril; however, similar effects have been reported in patients receiving captopril, and the risk of precipitating hypoglycemia should be considered when therapy with an ACE inhibitor is initiated in diabetic patients.

Concomitant use of enalapril and some vasodilating agents (e.g., nitrates) or anesthetic agents may cause an exaggerated hypotensive response. Patients receiving enalapril concomitantly with nitrates or with anesthetic agents that produce hypotension should be observed for possible additive hypotensive effects. Fluid volume expansion can correct hypotension during surgery or anesthesia if it is thought to result from an enalapril-induced inhibition of the angiotensin II formation that occurs secondary to compensatory renin release.

ACUTE TOXICITY

Limited information is available on the acute toxicity of enalapril in humans. Specific information on overdosage with the fixed combination of enalapril and hydrochlorothiazide currently is not available.

● Pathogenesis

The oral LD_{50} of enalapril maleate ranged from 2000–3500 mg/kg in mice and male rats and 2000–3000 mg/kg in female rats. The IV LD_{50} ranged from 700–950 mg/kg in female mice and male rats, and the subcutaneous LD_{50} was 1150, 1400, 1500, and 1750 mg/kg in male mice, female rats, female mice, and male rats, respectively. The IV LD_{50} of enalaprilat was 3740–5890 mg/kg in female mice. In clinical studies, some hypertensive patients received a maximum IV enalaprilat dose of 80 mg over a 15-minute period, but no adverse effects other than those associated with the recommended dosages were observed. In animals, sublethal doses of enalapril produced ptosis, decreased activity, and bradypnea. In dogs, a single 200-mg/kg dose was lethal, but a single 100-mg/kg dose was not toxic. In mice and rats, single oral doses exceeding 1000 mg/kg or at least 1775 mg/kg, respectively, were lethal.

● Manifestations

Overdosage of enalapril produces effects that are mainly extensions of the drug's pharmacologic effects as an ACE inhibitor. Plasma ACE activity was completely suppressed within 10–15 hours after acute ingestion of 300–440 mg of enalapril maleate in 2 patients. The most likely manifestation of enalapril overdosage is hypotension, which may be profound. Onset and duration of the hypotensive effect may be prolonged following acute overdosage.Hypotension may be accompanied by stupor. Renal dysfunction, including acute renal failure; hyperkalemia; and hyponatremia may also occur.

● Treatment

Management of enalapril overdosage is mainly supportive and symptomatic. Hypotension can be corrected with fluid volume expansion (e.g., IV infusion of 0.9% sodium chloride injection). Renal function also improves during supportive

therapy with sodium chloride infusion. Because of the long ACE-inhibitory effect of enalapril, prolonged observation (e.g., for several weeks) and supportive treatment may be necessary following overdosage with the drug. Treatment of acute oral overdosage may also include gastric lavage and administration of activated charcoal to prevent further GI absorption of the drug. The active metabolite enalaprilat may be removed by hemodialysis. Management of overdosage with the fixed combination of enalapril and hydrochlorothiazide should also include measures for the management of thiazide overdosage.

PHARMACOLOGY

Enalapril maleate is a prodrug of enalaprilat and has little pharmacologic activity until hydrolyzed in vivo to enalaprilat. Pharmacologic effects described for enalapril generally apply to enalaprilat, although the latter drug is substantially more potent on a weight basis. The mechanism(s) of action of enalaprilat and enalapril have not been fully elucidated. The drugs appear to reduce blood pressure in normotensive individuals and hypertensive patients and to produce beneficial hemodynamic effects in patients with heart failure mainly by suppressing the renin-angiotensin-aldosterone system.

● Effects on Renin-Angiotensin-Aldosterone System

Enalapril prevents the conversion of angiotensin I to angiotensin II (a potent vasoconstrictor) through inhibition of angiotensin-converting enzyme (ACE). The drug competes with physiologic substrate (angiotensin I) for the active site of ACE; the affinity of enalaprilat for ACE is approximately 200,000 times greater than that of angiotensin I. In vitro on a molar basis, the affinity of enalaprilat for ACE is 300–1000 or 2–17 times that of enalapril or captopril, respectively. However, in vitro on a molar basis, the ACE-inhibitory effect of enalapril was shown to be similar to that of enalaprilat in rat plasma and kidneys, because these tissues extensively hydrolyze enalapril to form enalaprilat. The drug apparently does not inhibit brain ACE in animals.

Inhibition of ACE initially results in decreased plasma angiotensin II concentrations and, consequently, blood pressure may be reduced in part through decreased vasoconstriction. Plasma renin activity (PRA) increases, possibly as a result of loss of feedback inhibition (mediated by angiotensin II) on the release of renin from the kidneys and/or stimulation of reflex mechanisms via baroreceptors (as a result of the decrease in blood pressure). Enalapril-induced increases in PRA are greater in the upright than in the supine position, and the effects of the drug on PRA and plasma angiotensin II concentrations may be potentiated by restriction of sodium intake. The initial hypotensive effect of enalapril appears to be proportional to inhibition of ACE in blood, but the hypotensive effect of the drug appears to persist longer than decreased angiotensin II concentrations. It has been suggested that the hypotensive effect of ACE inhibitors may in part also result from a local effect (e.g., in vascular wall). By decreasing local angiotensin II production, ACE inhibitors may decrease vascular tone by reducing direct angiotensin II-induced vasoconstriction and/or angiotensin II-induced increases in sympathetic activity. During prolonged enalapril use, plasma angiotensin II concentrations may return toward pretreatment levels, and inhibition of the renin-angiotensin system in various tissues (e.g., arterial wall, kidneys) rather than in blood may be more important determinants of the hypotensive effect of the drug, particularly long term.

Enalapril alone may be more effective in reducing blood pressure in patients with high or normal renin hypertension, but the drug may also lower blood pressure in patients with low renin hypertension. Although enalapril has lowered blood pressure in all races studied, the drug was less effective in black hypertensive patients, a population associated with low renin hypertension. Correlation between pretreatment PRA and short-term reduction in blood pressure has varied. Some clinicians have reported no correlation between pretreatment PRA and short-term reduction in blood pressure, while others have reported initial decreases in blood pressure to be proportional to pretreatment PRA. Correlation between pretreatment PRA and long-term response to the drug has not been consistently found.

Initial decreases in plasma angiotensin II concentrations lead to decreased aldosterone secretion from the adrenal cortex and, therefore, to decreased plasma concentrations and urinary excretion of aldosterone. However, there is increasing evidence to suggest that plasma aldosterone concentrations may not decrease with usual dosages of ACE inhibitors in some patients and may return to pretreatment levels in others during prolonged therapy. In addition, plasma aldosterone concentrations may not accurately reflect changes in aldosterone secretion, and reductions in these concentrations are usually greater when measured during ambulation than during rest in the supine position. It has been suggested that the addition of spironolactone, a drug that competitively inhibits the physiologic effects of aldosterone, appears to augment the suppressive effect of ACE inhibitors on aldosterone. Enalapril has blunted secondary hyperaldosteronism in healthy individuals receiving diuretics; the drug corrected hypokalemia associated with thiazides and increased sodium excretion. The drug has also improved potassium balance, increased PRA, decreased aldosterone secretion, and reduced blood pressure in a limited number of patients with idiopathic hyperaldosteronism.

● Effects on Catecholamines and Autacoids

Circulating plasma norepinephrine concentration generally is not affected by enalapril, but the drug has reduced these concentrations in some patients with hypertension or heart failure. In addition, the drug has attenuated the increase in plasma norepinephrine concentration that results from orthostatic reflexes. By inhibiting angiotensin II formation, ACE inhibitors may affect catecholamine release and reuptake by noradrenergic nerve endings and/or may decrease vascular sensitivity to vasopressors. There is some evidence that high doses of ACE inhibitors may inhibit presynaptic norepinephrine release and postsynaptic α_2-adrenoceptor activity, thereby interfering with sympathetic reflexes, but the clinical importance of this finding is not known since dosages tested in animals substantially exceed usual human hypotensive dosages.

Because ACE also degrades the vasodilator bradykinin, it has been suggested that inhibition of ACE may cause accumulation of bradykinin in plasma or tissues with resultant vasodilation; however, plasma and/or urinary concentrations of bradykinin and/or its metabolites have been unchanged in enalapril-responsive patients. Plasma and urinary concentrations of bradykinin may not indicate tissue activity of the peptide, and its role, if any, in the therapeutic effects of enalapril remains to be elucidated. It has been suggested that prostaglandins also may mediate some of the pharmacologic effects of enalapril since there is some evidence that the drug may increase prostaglandin production or release; however, most available evidence currently indicates that enalapril does not substantially affect prostaglandins, and further evaluation is necessary to determine the importance of any prostaglandin-mediated effects. (See Drug Interactions: Nonsteroidal Anti-inflammatory Agents.) Urinary concentration of thromboxane and prostacyclin metabolites have been unchanged during enalapril therapy.

● Cardiovascular Effects

In hypertensive patients, enalapril reduces blood pressure by decreasing total peripheral resistance with a slight increase or no change in heart rate, stroke volume, or cardiac output. The drug causes arterial and possibly venous dilation. Enalapril generally decreases systolic and diastolic blood pressures by approximately 10–15%; blood pressure is decreased to about the same extent in both the supine and standing positions.Orthostatic hypotension and tachycardia occur infrequently but are more common in sodium-depleted or hypovolemic patients. (See Cautions: Cardiovascular Effects.) Plasma volume has been reported to be unchanged or slightly increased; erythrocyte volume, extracellular fluid volume, and total body water have been unchanged. The drug appears to have no direct effect on baroreceptor sensitivity in normotensive or hypertensive individuals on a normal sodium diet. However, slight potentiation of baroreceptor sensitivity has been reported in mildly sodium-depleted individuals.

In patients with heart failure, enalapril, usually in conjunction with cardiac glycosides and diuretics, decreases total peripheral resistance, pulmonary capillary wedge pressure, heart size, and mean arterial and right atrial pressures. Cardiac index, cardiac output, stroke volume, and exercise tolerance increase in these patients; mean ejection fraction increases or remains unchanged; and heart rate decreases slightly or is unchanged. The drug may also cause a regional redistribution of blood flow, principally increasing renal blood flow with slight or no increase in flow in the forearm or hepatic vasculature, respectively.

● Renal and Electrolyte Effects

Renal blood flow may increase, but glomerular filtration rate is usually unchanged during enalapril therapy. In some patients, however, both renal blood flow and glomerular filtration rate have increased. BUN and serum creatinine concentrations have occasionally increased during long-term enalapril therapy. Increased BUN and serum creatinine occur more frequently in patients with preexisting renal impairment, in those receiving concomitant therapy with a diuretic, and in those with heart failure. However, in some hypertensive patients with preexisting renal impairment, renal blood flow and glomerular filtration rate have increased, presumably secondary to enalapril-induced intrarenal effects. In patients with heart failure and renal perfusion pressures less than 70 mm Hg, changes in creatinine clearance induced by 1–3 months of enalapril therapy have varied linearly and inversely with pretreatment PRA; however, creatinine clearance was not substantially affected by the drug in patients with renal perfusion pressures of 70 mm Hg or greater. Enalapril's effects on renal blood flow and glomerular filtration in patients with renovascular hypertension appear to be similar to those in hypertensive patients with normal renal function; however, transient increases in BUN and serum creatinine concentrations are more frequent in patients with renovascular hypertension than in hypertensive patients with normal renal function. In addition, renal function can markedly deteriorate during therapy with an ACE inhibitor in patients with preexisting, severely compromised renal perfusion. (See Cautions: Renal Effects.)

Increases in serum potassium concentration may occur secondary to enalapril-induced decreases in aldosterone secretion, especially in patients with impaired renal function. Concomitant administration of thiazide diuretics generally offsets this increase. Urinary sodium excretion may be increased during the first 2–3 days of enalapril therapy and may persist for longer periods in some patients with normal sodium intake, probably secondary to reduced tubular reabsorption of the ion. The hypotensive effect of enalapril may also result in part from decreased sodium and water retention secondary to reduced aldosterone secretion; however, decreases in aldosterone secretion during enalapril therapy are generally small.

PHARMACOKINETICS

● Absorption

Enalapril maleate, unlike enalaprilat, is well absorbed following oral administration. Although enalaprilat is a more potent angiotensin-converting enzyme (ACE) inhibitor than enalapril, it is poorly absorbed from the GI tract because of its high polarity, with only about 3–12% of an orally administered dose being absorbed. Approximately 55–75% of an oral dose of enalapril maleate is rapidly absorbed from the GI tract in healthy individuals and hypertensive patients. Food does not appear to substantially affect the rate or extent of absorption of enalapril maleate. Following oral administration, enalapril maleate appears to undergo first-pass metabolism principally in the liver, being hydrolyzed to enalaprilat. Concomitant oral administration of enalapril maleate and hydrochlorothiazide has little, if any, effect on the bioavailability of either drug. Oral administration of the commercially available fixed combination containing the drugs reportedly is bioequivalent to concurrent administration of the drugs as individual preparations. (See Pharmacokinetics: Elimination.)

Peak serum enalapril concentrations of 40–80 ng/mL occur within about 0.5–1.5 hours following oral administration of a single 10-mg dose of enalapril maleate in healthy individuals or hypertensive patients. Peak serum enalaprilat concentrations reportedly increase proportionally with oral doses of enalapril maleate ranging from 2.5–40 mg. Following oral administration of a single 2.5-, 5-, 10-, 20-, or 40-mg dose of enalapril maleate in these patients, average peak serum enalaprilat concentrations of 6–8, 15–28, 37–50, 70–80, or 123–150 ng/mL, respectively, occur within about 3–4.5 hours. Steady-state serum concentrations of enalaprilat were reached within 30–60 hours in patients with normal renal function receiving oral enalapril maleate dosages of 10 mg daily for 8 days; appreciable accumulation of the metabolite did not occur.

The hypotensive effect of a single oral dose of enalapril maleate is usually apparent within 1 hour and maximal in 4–8 hours. The hypotensive effect of usual doses of the drug generally persists for 12–24 hours but may diminish toward the end of the dosing interval in some patients. The reduction in blood pressure may be gradual, and several weeks of therapy may be required before the full effect is achieved. Following IV administration of enalaprilat, the hypotensive effect is usually apparent within 5–15 minutes with maximal effect occurring within 1–4 hours; the duration of hypotensive effect appears to be dose related, but with the recommended doses, the duration of action in most patients is approximately 6 hours. Plasma ACE inhibition and reduction in blood pressure appear to be correlated to a plasma enalaprilat concentration of 10 ng/mL, a concentration at which maximal blockade of plasma ACE is achieved. After withdrawal of enalapril or enalaprilat, blood pressure gradually returns to pretreatment levels; rebound hypertension following abrupt withdrawal of the drug has not been reported to date.

The onset and duration of hemodynamic effects of enalapril maleate appear to be slower and more prolonged than those of captopril. In patients with heart failure, the hemodynamic effects of enalapril maleate are generally apparent within 2–4 hours and may persist for up to 24 hours after an oral dose.

● **Distribution**

Distribution of enalapril into human body tissues and fluids has not been fully characterized.

Approximately 50–60% of enalaprilat is bound to plasma proteins. Two binding sites have been identified, a low-affinity, high-capacity site and a high-affinity, low-capacity site. Drug bound to the latter site may represent enalaprilat bound to circulating serum ACE, possibly accounting for the prolonged terminal elimination of the drug.

Information on distribution into the CNS is limited, but enalapril appears to cross the blood-brain barrier poorly, if at all, and enalaprilat does not appear to distribute into the CNS. The drug did not accumulate in any tissue following multiple-dose administration in animals. The drug crosses the placenta. In a premature neonate (35 weeks' gestation) whose mother received 20 mg of enalapril maleate daily for 17 days prior to delivery, plasma enalaprilat concentration soon after birth in the neonate was 28 ng/mL. Enalapril and enalaprilat are distributed into milk in trace amounts.

● **Elimination**

Following oral administration, the half-life of unchanged enalapril appears to be less than 2 hours in healthy individuals and in patients with normal hepatic and renal functions, but may be increased in patients with heart failure. Following oral administration of a single 5- or 10-mg dose of enalapril maleate in patients with heart failure, the half-life of enalapril was 3.4 or 5.8 hours, respectively. Serum concentrations of enalaprilat, the active metabolite of enalapril, appear to decline in a multiphasic manner. Elimination of enalaprilat may also be prolonged in patients with heart failure or impaired hepatic function compared with healthy individuals and patients with hypertension. Observations of serum concentrations of enalaprilat over long periods following oral or IV administration suggest that enalaprilat has an average terminal half-life of about 35–38 hours (range: 30–87 hours). The observed prolonged terminal phase may actually reflect enalaprilat binding to the high-affinity, low-capacity binding site of circulating serum ACE. The effective half-life for accumulation of enalaprilat (determined from urinary recovery) has been reported to average about 11 or 14 hours in healthy adults with normal renal function or in hypertensive pediatric patients, respectively.

Peak and trough enalaprilat concentrations and areas under the serum concentration-time curves (AUCs) may increase, time to peak and steady-state serum concentration may be delayed, and the effective half-life for accumulation may be prolonged in patients with impaired renal function. In patients with creatinine clearances less than 30 mL/minute, the effective half-life for accumulation of enalaprilat following multiple doses of enalapril maleate is prolonged. In patients with moderate renal impairment (i.e., creatinine clearances of 30–60 mL/minute), this half-life is not substantially prolonged, and there appears to be a lack of correlation between AUCs and creatinine clearance. Decreased urinary excretion of enalapril may increase the extent of hydrolysis of enalapril to enalaprilat or may increase extrarenal elimination of the drug (e.g., via biliary excretion).

About 60% of an absorbed dose of enalapril is extensively hydrolyzed to enalaprilat, principally in the liver via esterases. About 20% appears to be hydrolyzed on first pass through the liver; this hydrolysis does not appear to occur in plasma in humans. Enalaprilat is a more potent ACE inhibitor than enalapril. There is no evidence of other metabolites of enalapril in humans, rats, or dogs. However, a despropyl metabolite of enalaprilat was identified in urine in rhesus monkeys, accounting for 13% of an oral dose of enalapril maleate. Hydrolysis of enalapril to enalaprilat may be delayed and/or impaired in patients with severe hepatic impairment, but the pharmacodynamic effects of the drug do not appear to be significantly altered.

Following oral administration, enalapril and enalaprilat are excreted in urine and feces. In healthy individuals, a mean of 60–78% (a mean of 43–56% as enalaprilat and the remainder as unchanged drug) of a 10-mg oral dose of enalapril maleate is excreted in urine within 24–48 hours after administration and approximately 33% (about 27% as enalaprilat and 6% as unchanged drug) is excreted in feces within 24–48 hours. In a multiple-dose study (10 mg daily) in healthy individuals with normal renal function, urinary excretion of enalaprilat and total drug increased during the first 4 days of therapy and then stabilized; urinary excretion of the metabolite

averaged 45% of the cumulative dose and that of total drug averaged 62%. In a multiple-dose study (0.07–0.14 mg/kg of enalapril maleate daily) in hypertensive pediatric patients (2 months to 16 years), 67% (64–76% as enalaprilat and the remainder as unchanged drug) of the administered dose is recovered in urine within 24 hours. It is not known whether enalapril and enalaprilat excreted in feces represent unabsorbed drug or that excreted via biliary elimination. Biliary excretion of enalapril and enalaprilat occurs in animals; however, this route of elimination has not been demonstrated in humans.

Renal clearance of enalaprilat and enalapril are reported to be approximately 100–158 and 300 mL/minute, respectively, in adults with normal renal function. The higher renal clearance of enalapril compared with that of the metabolite may indicate some degree of active tubular secretion of unchanged drug. Renal clearance may be decreased in hypertensive patients. In geriatric individuals, renal clearance and/or volume of distribution may decrease.

Enalaprilat is removed by hemodialysis. The amount of drug removed during hemodialysis depends on several factors (e.g., type of coil used, dialysis flow rate); however, the hemodialysis clearance of enalaprilat is reportedly 62 mL/minute. Enalaprilat also appears to be removed by peritoneal dialysis.

CHEMISTRY AND STABILITY

● **Chemistry**

Enalaprilat and enalapril are angiotensin-converting enzyme (ACE, bradykininase, kininase II) inhibitors. Enalapril, the ethylester of enalaprilat, is a prodrug and has little pharmacologic activity until hydrolyzed in the liver to enalaprilat. Enalapril is commercially available as the maleate salt and differs structurally from enalaprilat by the presence of an ethoxycarbonyl group rather than a carboxy group at position 1 of l-alanyl-l-proline and by the presence of the maleate salt. These structural modifications result in increased GI absorption of enalapril compared with enalaprilat, which is poorly absorbed from the GI tract. Enalapril is structurally and pharmacologically similar to captopril but contains a disubstituted nitrogen rather than a sulfhydryl group at position 3 of 2-methyl-1-oxopropyl-l-proline. The lack of the sulfhydryl group in enalapril may result in decreased risk of certain adverse effects (e.g., cutaneous reactions, taste disturbances, proteinuria).

Enalaprilat occurs as a white to off-white crystalline powder and is slightly soluble in water and sparingly soluble in methanol. Commercially available enalaprilat injection is a sterile, clear, colorless solution of the drug. Sodium chloride is added during manufacture of the injection to adjust tonicity, and sodium hydroxide is added to adjust pH; the injection also contains 0.9% benzyl alcohol as a preservative. Enalapril maleate occurs as a white to off-white, crystalline powder and has solubilities of 25 mg/mL in water and 80 mg/mL in alcohol at room temperature. The apparent pK_as of enalapril are 3 and 5.4 at 25°C.

● **Stability**

Commercially available enalaprilat injection should be stored at a temperature less than 30°C. Following dilution of enalaprilat injection in 5% dextrose, 0.9% sodium chloride, 5% dextrose and 0.9% sodium chloride, 5% dextrose in lactated Ringer's, or Isolyte® E, solutions of the drug are stable for 24 hours at room temperature. Enalaprilat is physically incompatible with amphotericin B and phenytoin sodium. Specialized references should be consulted for specific compatibility information.

The manufacturer recommends that enalapril maleate tablets be stored in tight containers at a temperature less than 30°C and that transient exposure to temperatures warmer than 50°C be avoided. The tablets should be protected from moisture. The tablets have an expiration date of 30 months following the date of manufacture when stored at less than 30°C. The manufacturer states that extemporaneous preparation of oral solutions of enalapril maleate should be avoided since the drug is not sufficiently stable in solution.

An extemporaneous preparation of enalapril maleate tablets in syrup (Ora-Sweet SF®) and sodium citrate dihydrate (Bicitra®) containing enalapril maleate 1 mg/mL is stable for 30 days when stored at 2–8°C.

PREPARATIONS

Excipients in commercially available drug preparations may have clinically important effects in some individuals; consult specific product labeling for details.

Enalaprilat

Parenteral

Injection, for IV use only	equivalent to 1.25 mg of anhydrous enalaprilat per mL*	**Enalaprilat Injection**

* available from one or more manufacturer, distributor, and/or repackager by generic (nonproprietary) name

Enalapril Maleate

Oral

Tablets	2.5 mg*	**Enalapril Maleate Tablets**
		Vasotec® (scored), Valeant
	5 mg*	**Enalapril Maleate Tablets**
		Vasotec® (scored), Valeant
	10 mg*	**Enalapril Maleate Tablets**
		Vasotec® (scored), Valeant
	20 mg*	**Enalapril Maleate Tablets**
		Vasotec® (scored), Valeant

* available from one or more manufacturer, distributor, and/or repackager by generic (nonproprietary) name

Enalapril Maleate and Hydrochlorothiazide

Oral

Tablets	5 mg Enalapril Maleate and Hydrochlorothiazide 12.5 mg*	**Enalapril Maleate and Hydrochlorothiazide Tablets**
	10 mg Enalapril Maleate and Hydrochlorothiazide 25 mg*	**Enalapril Maleate and Hydrochlorothiazide Tablets**
		Vaseretic®, Valeant

* available from one or more manufacturer, distributor, and/or repackager by generic (nonproprietary) name

† Use is not currently included in the labeling approved by the US Food and Drug Administration.

Selected Revisions November 5, 2018, © Copyright, November 1, 1986, American Society of Health-System Pharmacists, Inc.

Lisinopril

24:32.04 • ANGIOTENSIN-CONVERTING ENZYME INHIBITORS

■ Lisinopril is an angiotensin-converting enzyme (ACE) inhibitor.

USES

Lisinopril is used alone or in combination with other classes of antihypertensive agents (e.g., thiazide diuretics) in the management of hypertension. Lisinopril also is used in conjunction with other agents such as β-adrenergic blocking agents (β-blockers), cardiac glycosides, and diuretics in the management of heart failure. In addition, lisinopril may be used in conjunction with thrombolytic agents, aspirin, and/or β-blockers to improve survival in patients with acute myocardial infarction (MI) who are hemodynamically stable.

Because captopril, another angiotensin-converting enzyme (ACE) inhibitor, may cause serious adverse effects, (e.g., neutropenia, agranulocytosis), particularly in patients with renal impairment (especially those with collagen vascular disease) or in patients receiving immunosuppressive therapy, the possibility that similar adverse effects may occur with lisinopril should be considered since current evidence is insufficient to rule out such risk. (See Cautions: Hematologic Effects, in Captopril 24:32.04.)

● Hypertension

Lisinopril is used alone or in combination with other classes of antihypertensive agents in the management of hypertension. ACE inhibitors are considered one of several preferred antihypertensive drugs for the initial management of hypertension according to current evidence-based hypertension guidelines; other preferred options include angiotensin II receptor antagonists, calcium-channel blockers, and thiazide diuretics. While there may be individual differences with respect to recommendations for initial drug selection and use in specific patient populations, current evidence indicates that these antihypertensive drug classes all generally produce comparable effects on overall mortality and cardiovascular, cerebrovascular, and renal outcomes. (See Uses: Hypertension, in Captopril 24:32.04.)

ACE inhibitors may be particularly useful in the management of hypertension in patients with certain coexisting conditions such as heart failure, ischemic heart disease, diabetes mellitus, chronic kidney disease (CKD), or cerebrovascular disease or following MI. (See Uses: Hypertension in Captopril 24:32.04 and in Enalaprilat/Enalapril 24:32.04.)

In patients with hypertension and compelling indications (e.g., CKD with albuminuria [urine albumin 300 mg/day or greater, or urine albumin:creatinine ratio of 300 mg/g or equivalent in the first morning void]), angiotensin II receptor antagonists are usually considered an alternative for ACE inhibitor-intolerant patients. However, data indicate no difference in efficacy between ACE inhibitors and angiotensin II receptor antagonists with regard to blood pressure lowering and clinical outcomes (i.e., all-cause mortality, cardiovascular mortality, MI, heart failure, stroke, and end-stage renal disease). Adverse events (e.g., cough, angioedema) leading to drug discontinuance occur more frequently with ACE inhibitor therapy than with angiotensin II receptor antagonist therapy. Because of similar efficacy and a lower frequency of adverse effects, some experts believe that an angiotensin II receptor antagonist should be used instead of an ACE inhibitor for the treatment of hypertension or hypertension with certain compelling indications.

Most patients with hypertension, especially black patients, will require at least 2 antihypertensive drugs to achieve adequate blood pressure control. In general, black hypertensive patients tend to respond better to monotherapy with thiazide diuretics or calcium-channel blockers than to monotherapy with ACE inhibitors. Although ACE inhibitors have lowered blood pressure in all races studied, monotherapy with an ACE inhibitor has produced a smaller reduction in blood pressure in black hypertensive patients, a population associated with low renin hypertension. However, the combination of an ACE inhibitor or an angiotensin II receptor antagonist with a calcium-channel blocker or thiazide diuretic produces similar blood pressure lowering in black patients as in other racial groups. In addition, ACE inhibitors appear to produce a higher incidence of angioedema in black patients than in other races studied. (See ALLHAT study below and also see Race under Hypertension: Other Special Considerations for Antihypertensive Drug Therapy, in Uses in Captopril 24:32.04 and in Enalaprilat/Enalapril 24:32.04.)

The ALLHAT study, a large (33,357 patients), multicenter, randomized, active-control study in hypertensive patients 55 years of age or older with at least one other coronary heart disease risk factor, compared the cardiovascular benefit of therapy with an ACE inhibitor (lisinopril 10–40 mg daily) or a dihydropyridine-derivative calcium-channel blocker (amlodipine 2.5–10 mg daily) relative to therapy with a thiazide diuretic (chlorthalidone 12.5–25 mg daily). After a mean follow-up of 4.9 years, an intent-to-treat analysis revealed no difference in the primary outcome of combined fatal coronary heart disease or nonfatal MI among the treatments.

Compared with chlorthalidone, the relative risks for the primary outcome were 0.99 for lisinopril and 0.98 for amlodipine. In addition, all-cause mortality, a secondary outcome, did not differ among the treatments. Although each drug decreased blood pressure substantially, the extent of reduction was not equivalent. Five-year systolic blood pressures were significantly higher in the lisinopril (2 mm Hg) and amlodipine (0.8 mm Hg) groups relative to that achieved with chlorthalidone, and 5-year diastolic blood pressure was significantly lower with amlodipine (0.8 mm Hg) relative to the thiazide. Control of hypertension (systolic and diastolic blood pressures less than 140 and 90 mm Hg, respectively) was achieved in approximately two-thirds of patients by 5 years of follow-up (61, 66, or 68% of patients treated with lisinopril, amlodipine, lisinopril, or chlorthalidone, respectively).

Subgroup analysis of the ALLHAT study for race-related effects revealed no difference in the primary outcome of combined fatal coronary heart disease or nonfatal MI among the treatments in both black and nonblack patients. However, substantial race-related effects were observed in the incidence of secondary outcomes (e.g., stroke, combined cardiovascular disease events, heart failure). Compared with chlorthalidone, the relative risk for lisinopril was 1.4 or 1 (in black or nonblack patients, respectively) for stroke and 1.19 or 1.06 (in black or nonblack patients, respectively) for combined cardiovascular disease events. When amlodipine was compared with chlorthalidone, the only race-related difference observed was in the incidence of heart failure; the relative risk was 1.46 or 1.32 (in black or nonblack patients, respectively). The relative risk for heart failure in black versus nonblack patients receiving lisinopril was not considered to be statistically significant, and the overall relative risk for both groups was 1.19. In addition, after 4 years, in each treatment group, blood pressure reductions were greater in nonblack than in black patients; about 68 or 60% of nonblack or black patients, respectively, achieved a systolic/diastolic blood pressure of less than 140/90 mmHg. In nonblack patients receiving chlorthalidone, amlodipine, or lisinopril 69, 69, or 67% achieved the mentioned blood pressure, respectively, while in black patients receiving chlorthalidone, amlodipine, or lisinopril 63, 60, or 54% achieved such blood pressure, respectively.

Although the ALLHAT study provides strong evidence that these classes of antihypertensive agents (ACE inhibitors, dihydropyridine-derivative calcium-channel blockers, thiazide diuretics) are comparably effective in providing important cardiovascular benefit, apparent differences in certain secondary outcomes were observed. Thiazide diuretic therapy was superior to ACE inhibitor therapy in preventing aggregate cardiovascular events, principally stroke, heart failure, angina, and the need for coronary revascularization. Thiazide therapy also was better tolerated than ACE inhibitor therapy (e.g., angioedema, which was more likely in blacks than nonblacks).

Post hoc analysis of the ALLHAT study directly comparing cardiovascular and other outcomes in patients receiving amlodipine or lisinopril revealed no difference in the primary outcome of combined fatal coronary heart disease or nonfatal MI between patients receiving the ACE inhibitor and those receiving the calcium-channel blocking agent. However, patients receiving lisinopril were at higher risk for stroke, combined cardiovascular disease, GI bleeding, and angioedema, while those receiving amlodipine were at higher risk of developing heart failure. ALLHAT investigators suggested that the observed differences in cardiovascular outcome may be attributable, at least in part, to the greater antihypertensive effect of amlodipine compared with that of lisinopril, especially in women and black patients.

For additional information on the role of ACE inhibitors in the management of hypertension, see Uses in Captopril 24:32.04 and in Enalaprilat/Enalapril 24:32.04. For information on overall principles and expert recommendations for treatment of hypertension, see Uses: Hypertension in Adults and also see Uses: Hypertension in Pediatric Patients, in the Thiazides General Statement 40:28.20.

● Heart Failure

Lisinopril is used as adjunctive therapy in the management of heart failure in patients who do not respond adequately to diuretics and a cardiac glycoside.

Current guidelines for the management of heart failure in adults generally recommend a combination of drug therapies to reduce morbidity and mortality, including neurohormonal antagonists (e.g., ACE inhibitors, angiotensin II receptor antagonists, angiotensin receptor-neprilysin inhibitors [ARNIs], β-blockers, aldosterone receptor antagonists) that inhibit the detrimental compensatory mechanisms in heart failure. Additional agents (e.g., cardiac glycosides, diuretics, sinoatrial modulators [i.e., ivabradine]) added to a heart failure treatment regimen in selected patients have been associated with symptomatic improvement and/or reduction in heart failure-related hospitalizations. Experts recommend that all asymptomatic patients with reduced left ventricular ejection fraction (LVEF) (American College of Cardiology Foundation [ACCF]/American Heart Association [AHA] stage B heart failure) receive therapy with an ACE inhibitor and β-blocker to prevent symptomatic heart failure and to reduce morbidity and mortality. If ACE inhibitors are not tolerated, then an angiotensin II receptor antagonist is recommended as alternative therapy. In patients with prior or current symptoms of chronic heart failure and reduced LVEF (ACCF/AHA stage C heart failure), ACCF, AHA, and the Heart Failure Society of America (HFSA) recommend inhibition of the renin-angiotensin-aldosterone (RAA) system with an ACE inhibitor, angiotensin II receptor antagonist, or ARNI in conjunction with a β-blocker, and an aldosterone antagonist in selected patients, to reduce morbidity and mortality. While ACE inhibitors have been the preferred drugs for inhibition of the RAA system because of their established benefits in patients with heart failure and reduced ejection fraction, some evidence indicates that therapy with sacubitril/valsartan, an ARNI, may be more effective than ACE inhibitor therapy (enalapril) in reducing cardiovascular death and heart failure-related hospitalization in such patients. ACCF, AHA, and HFSA recommend that patients with chronic symptomatic heart failure and reduced LVEF (New York Heart Association [NYHA] class II or III) who are able to tolerate an ACE inhibitor or angiotensin II receptor antagonist be switched to therapy containing an ARNI to further reduce morbidity and mortality. However, in patients in whom an ARNI is not appropriate, continued use of an ACE inhibitor for all classes of heart failure with reduced ejection fraction remains strongly advised. In patients in whom an ARNI or ACE inhibitor is not appropriate, an angiotensin II receptor antagonist may be used. For additional information on the use of ACE inhibitors in the management of heart failure, see Uses: Heart Failure, in Captopril 24:32.04 and in Enalaprilat/Enalapril 24:32.04 For further information on the use of ARNIs in patients with heart failure, see Uses: Heart Failure, in Sacubitril and Valsartan 24:32.92.

Some clinicians state that ACE inhibitors usually are prescribed in clinical practice at dosages lower than those determined as target dosages in clinical trials, although results of several studies suggest that high dosages are associated with greater hemodynamic, neurohormonal, symptomatic, and prognostic benefits than lower dosages. Results of a large, randomized, double blind study (Assessment of Treatment with Lisinopril and Survival [ATLAS] study) in patients with heart failure (NYHA class II–IV) indicate that high lisinopril dosages (32.5–35 mg daily) were associated with a 12% lower risk of death or hospitalization for any cause and 24% fewer hospitalizations for heart failure than low dosages (2.5–5 mg) of the drug.

Many patients with heart failure respond to lisinopril with improvement in cardiac function indexes, symptomatic (e.g., dyspnea, fatigue) relief, improved functional capacity, and increased exercise tolerance. In some studies, improvement in cardiac function indexes and exercise tolerance were sustained for up to 3 months. Although additional studies are needed to determine the specific role of lisinopril in the management of heart failure and its long-term efficacy, the efficacy of the drug appears to be similar to that of captopril and enalapril. However, like enalapril, lisinopril has a relatively long duration of action compared with captopril; therefore, the drug may produce more prolonged hypotensive effects, particularly at high doses, which potentially could result in adverse cerebral and renal effects. In addition, because the renin-angiotensin system appears to contribute substantially to preservation of glomerular filtration in patients with heart failure in whom renal function is severely compromised, therapy with an ACE inhibitor may adversely affect renal function. (See Cautions: Renal Effects in Captopril 24:32.04 and in Enalaprilat/Enalapril 24:32.04.)

● Mortality Reduction After Acute Myocardial Infarction

Lisinopril is used in conjunction with standard therapies (e.g., thrombolytic agents, aspirin, β-blockers) to improve survival in hemodynamically stable patients with acute MI. Results of a multicenter, controlled, randomized, clinical study indicate that patients who received lisinopril or lisinopril concomitantly with nitrates within 24 hours of MI in addition to conventional therapy (thrombolytic agents, aspirin, β-blockers) had an 11% lower risk of death (6 weeks after infarction) compared with patients receiving conventional therapy only; mortality rates were 6.4 or 7.2% in patients receiving lisinopril and conventional therapy or conventional therapy alone, respectively.

Studies with various ACE inhibitors have shown that these drugs reduce fatal and nonfatal cardiovascular events in patients with recent MI. The magnitude of benefit appears to be greatest in certain high-risk patients (e.g., those with an anterior infarct, ejection fraction of 40% or less, heart failure, prior infarction, or tachycardia). In addition to their effects on mortality, ACE inhibitors also are used to minimize or prevent the development of left ventricular dilatation and dysfunction (ventricular "remodeling") following acute MI. Evidence regarding the efficacy of such therapy has been somewhat conflicting, particularly when parenteral therapy was initiated early (within 24–48 hours) and included patients with no evidence of baseline dysfunction. (See Uses: Left Ventricular Dysfunction After Acute Myocardial Infarction, in Enalaprilat/Enalapril 24:32.04.) However, the preponderance of evidence has shown a benefit of early oral therapy with ACE inhibitors, even in patients with no baseline dysfunction.

Current expert guidelines recommend the use of an ACE inhibitor within the first 24 hours of acute MI in patients with an anterior infarction, heart failure, or ejection fraction of 40% or less who do not have any contraindications (e.g., hypotension, shock, renal dysfunction). While early treatment within the first 24 hours of MI has been shown to be beneficial, ACE inhibitors should be used with caution (and with gradual upward titration) during the initial postinfarction period because of the possibility of hypotension or renal dysfunction. ACE inhibitor therapy generally should be continued indefinitely in all patients with left ventricular dysfunction or other compelling indications for use (e.g., hypertension, diabetes mellitus, CKD). The benefits of long-term ACE inhibitor therapy are less certain in low-risk patients who have undergone revascularization and are receiving aggressive antilipemic therapy.

● Diabetic Nephropathy

Both ACE inhibitors and angiotensin II receptor antagonists have been shown to slow the rate of progression of renal disease in patients with diabetes mellitus and persistent albuminuria†, and use of a drug from either class is recommended in such patients with modestly elevated (30–300 mg/24 hours) or higher (exceeding 300 mg/24 hours) levels of urinary albumin excretion. The usual precautions of ACE inhibitor or angiotensin II receptor antagonist therapy in patients with substantial renal impairment should be observed. For additional information on the use of ACE inhibitors in the treatment of diabetic nephropathy, see Diabetic Nephropathy under Uses: Nephropathy, in Captopril 24:32.04.

DOSAGE AND ADMINISTRATION

● Administration

Lisinopril is administered orally. The manufacturers state that the absorption of lisinopril is not affected by the presence of food in the GI tract.

For pediatric patients and patients unable to swallow tablets, lisinopril may be administered orally as an extemporaneously prepared suspension. An extemporaneous suspension containing lisinopril 1 mg/mL can be prepared in the following manner. First, 10 mL of purified water is added to a polyethylene terephthalate (PET) bottle containing ten 20-mg tablets of lisinopril, and the contents are shaken for at least 1 minute. The concentrated suspension of lisinopril should be diluted with 30 mL of sodium citrate dihydrate (Bicitra®) and 160 mL of syrup (Ora-Sweet®), and the container then shaken gently for several seconds to disperse the ingredients. The suspension should be shaken before dispensing of each dose. The extemporaneous suspension is stable for 4 weeks when stored at or below 25°C.

● Dosage

Dosage of lisinopril must be adjusted according to patient tolerance and response. Because of the risk of inducing hypotension, initiation of lisinopril therapy requires consideration of recent antihypertensive therapy, the extent of blood pressure elevation, sodium intake, fluid status, and other clinical circumstances. If therapy is initiated in a patient already receiving a diuretic, symptomatic hypotension may occur following the initial dose of the angiotensin-converting enzyme (ACE) inhibitor. The possibility of hypotension may be minimized by discontinuing the diuretic, reducing the diuretic dosage, or cautiously increasing salt intake prior to initiation of lisinopril therapy. If diuretic therapy cannot be discontinued, lisinopril should be initiated in adults at a dosage of 5 mg daily under close medical supervision until blood pressure has stabilized. (See Cardiovascular Effects under Warnings/Precautions: Warnings, in Cautions.) For additional information on initiating lisinopril in patients receiving diuretic therapy, see the disease-specific dosage sections in Dosage and Administration.

Hypertension

Lisinopril Therapy

For the management of uncomplicated hypertension in adults *not* receiving a diuretic, the usual initial dosage of lisinopril is 10 mg once daily. In patients currently receiving diuretic therapy, it is recommended that the diuretic be discontinued, if possible, 2–3 days before initiating lisinopril. If blood pressure is not adequately controlled with the ACE inhibitor alone, diuretic therapy may be resumed cautiously. If diuretic therapy cannot be discontinued, lisinopril should be initiated in adults at a reduced dosage of 5 mg daily under close medical supervision for at least 2 hours and until blood pressure has stabilized for at least an additional hour.

Dosage of lisinopril should be adjusted according to blood pressure response. If the blood pressure response diminishes toward the end of the dosing interval during once-daily administration, which may be particularly likely with a dosage of 10 mg or less daily, consideration should be given to increasing the dosage. The manufacturer states that the usual maintenance dosage of lisinopril in adults is 20–40 mg daily, given as a single dose. Some experts state that the usual dosage range is 10–40 mg daily, given as a single dose. Dosages up to 80 mg daily have been used, but do not appear to give a greater effect.

For the management of hypertension in children 6 years of age and older, the usual initial dosage of lisinopril is 0.07 mg/kg (up to 5 mg) once daily. Some experts state that the dosage may be increased every 2–4 weeks until blood pressure is controlled, the maximum dosage is reached, or adverse effects occur. The safety and efficacy of doses exceeding 0.61 mg/kg or in excess of 40 mg have not been established. For information on overall principles and expert recommendations for treatment of hypertension in pediatric patients, see Uses: Hypertension in Pediatric Patients, in the Thiazides General Statement 40:28.20.

Lisinopril/Hydrochlorothiazide Fixed-combination Therapy

The manufacturer states that therapy with the commercially available preparations containing lisinopril in fixed combination with hydrochlorothiazide should only be initiated in adults after an adequate response is not achieved with lisinopril or hydrochlorothiazide monotherapy. Alternatively, the fixed combination containing lisinopril with hydrochlorothiazide may be used in patients who have been receiving the drugs separately and in whom dosage of the individual drugs has been adjusted to the ratio in a commercial combination preparation. Such fixed combinations also may be used to prevent hydrochlorothiazide-induced potassium loss. Volume and/or salt depletion should be corrected before initiating therapy with lisinopril in fixed combination with hydrochlorothiazide. Patients whose blood pressure is not adequately controlled with lisinopril or hydrochlorothiazide monotherapy may receive the fixed combination containing 10 mg of lisinopril and 12.5 mg of hydrochlorothiazide or, alternatively, the preparation containing 20 mg of lisinopril and 12.5 mg of hydrochlorothiazide. Further increases of either or both drugs depend on clinical response; however, dosage of hydrochlorothiazide generally should not be increased for about 2–3 weeks after initiation of therapy. Patients whose blood pressure has been adequately controlled with a hydrochlorothiazide dosage of 25 mg daily, but who experienced potassium loss, may achieve a similar response if they are switched to therapy with the fixed-combination preparation containing 10 mg of lisinopril and 12.5 mg of hydrochlorothiazide. The dosages of lisinopril and hydrochlorothiazide should not exceed 80 and 50 mg daily, respectively.

Blood Pressure Monitoring and Treatment Goals

Blood pressure should be monitored regularly (i.e., monthly) and dosage of the antihypertensive drug adjusted until blood pressure is controlled. If an adequate blood pressure response is not achieved with ACE inhibitor monotherapy, the dosage may be increased or another antihypertensive agent with demonstrated benefit and preferably with a complementary mechanism of action (e.g., calcium-channel blocker, thiazide diuretic) may be added; if target blood pressure is still not achieved, a third drug may be added. (See Uses: Hypertension.) In patients who develop unacceptable adverse effects with lisinopril, the drug should be discontinued and another antihypertensive agent from a different pharmacologic class should be initiated.

The goal of hypertension management and prevention is to achieve and maintain optimal control of blood pressure. However, the optimum blood pressure threshold for initiating antihypertensive drug therapy and specific treatment goals remain controversial. While other hypertension guidelines have based target blood pressure goals on age and comorbidities, a 2017 multidisciplinary hypertension guideline from the American College of Cardiology (ACC), American Heart Association (AHA), and a number of professional organizations incorporates underlying cardiovascular risk into decision making regarding treatment and generally recommends the same target blood pressure (i.e., less than 130/80 mm Hg) in all adults. Many patients will require at least 2 drugs from different pharmacologic classes to achieve this blood pressure goal; the potential benefits of hypertension management and drug cost, adverse effects, and risks associated with the use of multiple antihypertensive drugs also should be considered when deciding a patient's blood pressure treatment goal.

For additional information on target levels of blood pressure and on monitoring therapy in the management of hypertension, see Blood Pressure Monitoring and Treatment Goals under Dosage: Hypertension, in Dosage and Administration in the Thiazides General Statement 40:28.20.

Heart Failure

Because of the risk of severe hypotension, lisinopril therapy for heart failure should be initiated under very close medical supervision (e.g., in a hospital setting), especially in patients with low blood pressure (i.e., systolic blood pressure less than 80–100 mm Hg), with consideration given to recent diuretic therapy and the possibility of severe sodium and/or fluid depletion. Experts suggest that ACE inhibitor therapy also be initiated with caution in patients with markedly increased serum concentrations of creatinine (exceeding 3 mg/dL), bilateral renal artery stenosis, or elevated concentrations of serum potassium (exceeding 5 mEq/L).

For the management of heart failure, the usual initial dosage of lisinopril in adults with normal renal function and serum sodium concentration is 2.5–5 mg once daily. The usual effective dosage of lisinopril in adults with heart failure is 5–40 mg once daily.

Lisinopril often is administered in conjunction with other agents such as a cardiac glycoside, a diuretic, and a β-adrenergic blocking agent (β-blocker). After the initial dose, the patient should be monitored closely (especially those with systolic blood pressure less than 100 mg Hg) until blood pressure has stabilized. The mean peak blood pressure lowering usually occurs 6–8 hours after administration of a dose. Hypotension occurring after the initial dose does not preclude the administration of subsequent doses of the drug, provided due caution is exercised and the hypotension has been managed effectively. Evidence from a large clinical trial in patients with heart failure suggests that hypotension with lisinopril is dose-related. To minimize the likelihood of hypotension, the dosage of any diuretic given concomitantly with lisinopril should be reduced, if possible.

It should be recognized that although symptoms of heart failure may improve within 48 hours after initiating ACE inhibitor therapy in some patients, such improvement usually is not evident for several weeks or months after initiating ACE inhibitor therapy. In addition, it should be considered that such therapy may reduce the risk of disease progression even if symptomatic improvement is not evident. Therefore, some experts recommend that dosages generally be titrated to a prespecified target (i.e., 20–40 mg of lisinopril daily) or highest tolerated dosage rather than according to response. However, one manufacturer states that dosage adjustment of lisinopril should be based on the clinical response of individual patients. Patients with severe heart failure, with or without renal impairment, should be monitored closely for the first 2 weeks of lisinopril therapy and periodically thereafter (e.g., whenever dosage of the drug and/or concomitantly administered diuretic is increased), especially those taking potassium supplements or those with preexisting hypotension, hyponatremia, diabetes mellitus, or azotemia.

Mortality Reduction After Acute Myocardial Infarction

Because of the risk of persistent hypotension (i.e., systolic blood pressure of less than 90 mm Hg lasting for more that 1 hour), lisinopril therapy should *not* be initiated in patients with myocardial infarction (MI) who are at risk of further severe hemodynamic deterioration (i.e., systolic blood pressure of 100 mm Hg or less after receiving therapy with a vasodilator) or who are in cardiogenic shock. In addition, because severe hypotension in patients with MI may result in MI or cerebrovascular accident, lisinopril therapy should be initiated under very close medical supervision in such patients, with close monitoring for the first 2 weeks of therapy and whenever dosage of the drug and/or concomitantly administered diuretic is increased. (See Hypotension under Warnings/Precautions: Warnings, in Cautions.)

To improve survival after acute MI in hemodynamically stable patients, the manufacturers state a 5-mg dose of lisinopril should be given within 24 hours of onset of symptoms of MI followed by a 5- and 10-mg dose 24 and 48 hours later, respectively; the drug should be administered in conjunction with standard therapies such as thrombolytic agents, aspirin, and/or β-blockers as appropriate. Thereafter, a maintenance dosage of 10 mg daily of lisinopril should be used and continued for 6 weeks. Patients who have low blood pressure (i.e., systolic pressure of 120 mm Hg or less) when lisinopril therapy is initiated or during the first 3 days after MI should be given a lower dose (i.e., 2.5 mg) of lisinopril; in addition, if hypotension (i.e., systolic pressure less than 100 mm Hg) occurs, the maintenance dosage should be reduced to 5 mg daily, which may be temporarily reduced further to 2.5 mg daily if needed. If prolonged hypotension occurs (i.e., systolic pressure less than 90 mm Hg lasting for more than 1 hour), lisinopril should be discontinued. Alternatively, experts recommend an initial lisinopril dosage of 2.5–5 mg daily (initiated within 24 hours of MI) titrated upward to 10 mg daily or higher as tolerated in patients with MI. For patients who develop symptoms of heart failure, the dosage indicated for heart failure should be administered. (See Dosage and Administration: Heart Failure).

● Special Populations

The manufacturers state that modification of the usual initial dosage (10 mg once daily) of lisinopril is not necessary in hypertensive adults with creatinine clearances exceeding 30 mL/minute per 1.73 m². If the drug is used in hypertensive adults with more than mildly impaired renal function, dosage must be modified in response to the degree of renal impairment, and as with other ACE inhibitors, the theoretical risk of neutropenia must be considered. Hypertensive adults with creatinine clearances of 10–30 mL/minute can receive an initial lisinopril dosage of 5 mg once daily and those with creatinine clearances less than 10 mL/minute (usually on hemodialysis) can receive an initial dosage of 2.5 mg once daily. Subsequent dosage should be titrated according to individual tolerance and blood pressure response up to a maximum of 40 mg once daily. The manufacturers state that use of lisinopril in hypertensive pediatric patients with creatinine clearances less than 30 mL/minute per 1.73 m² is not recommended.

The manufacturers state that adults with heart failure and hyponatremia (serum sodium concentration less than 130 mEq/L) or moderate to severe renal impairment (i.e., creatinine clearance of 30 mL/minute or less or serum creatinine exceeding 3 mg/dL) should receive an initial lisinopril dosage of 2.5 mg daily under close monitoring. (See Dosage and Administration: Dosage.)

The manufacturers state that lisinopril should be initiated with caution in patients with MI and renal impairment (serum creatinine concentrations exceeding 2 mg/dL). The manufacturers also state that dosage adjustments in patients with MI and severe renal impairment have not been evaluated. If renal impairment (serum creatinine concentrations exceeding 3 mg/dL) develops or if baseline serum creatinine concentrations are increased by 100% during lisinopril therapy, discontinuance of the drug should be considered.

When combination therapy with lisinopril and hydrochlorothiazide is required for the management of hypertension in patients with impaired renal function, the risk of precipitating hypotension during initiation of combined therapy should be considered. Dosages of the drugs should be titrated carefully by increasing slowly the dosage of each drug separately in small increments and the patient should be monitored closely. After careful titration of each drug separately, a fixed combination preparation can be substituted. If concomitant diuretic therapy is required in patients with severe renal impairment, a loop diuretic such as furosemide is preferred to a thiazide diuretic. Therefore, use of commercially available preparations containing lisinopril in fixed combination with hydrochlorothiazide is not recommended for patients with severe renal impairment.

CAUTIONS

● Contraindications

History of angioedema related to previous angiotensin-converting enzyme (ACE) inhibitor treatment or of hereditary or idiopathic angioedema.

Known hypersensitivity to lisinopril, other ACE inhibitors, or any ingredient in the formulation.

Concomitant use of lisinopril and aliskiren in patients with diabetes mellitus. (See Drug Interactions: Drugs that Block the Renin-Angiotensin System.)

● Warnings/Precautions

Warnings

When hydrochlorothiazide is used in fixed combination with lisinopril, the usual cautions, precautions, and contraindications associated with hydrochlorothiazide must be considered in addition to those associated with lisinopril. (See Cautions, in the Thiazides General Statement 40:28.20.)

Hypotension

Symptomatic hypotension may occur, sometimes associated with oliguria and/or progressive azotemia and, rarely, acute renal failure and/or death. Patients at particular risk include those with heart failure with systolic blood pressure less than 100 mm Hg, hyponatremia, high-dose or recent intensive diuretic therapy, recent increase in diuretic dose, dialysis, or severe volume and/or salt depletion of any etiology. In such patients, it may be advisable to discontinue the diuretic (except in patients with heart failure), reduce the diuretic dosage, or cautiously increase salt intake, if possible, prior to initiating lisinopril therapy. Treatment with lisinopril must not be initiated in patients with acute myocardial infarction (MI) at risk of further serious hemodynamic deterioration following treatment with a vasodilator (e.g., systolic blood pressure of 100 mm Hg or lower) or in those with cardiogenic shock. Marked hypotension may result in MI or stroke in those with acute MI or ischemic cardiovascular or cerebrovascular disease.

Hematologic Effects

Neutropenia/agranulocytosis, particularly in patients with renal impairment (especially those with concomitant collagen vascular disease), reported with captopril. Data insufficient to rule out similar incidence of agranulocytosis with lisinopril in patients without prior reactions with other ACE inhibitors. Hemolytic anemia reported rarely; causal relationship to lisinopril cannot be ruled out. Myelosuppression, leukopenia/neutropenia, and thrombocytopenia reported rarely.

Hepatic Effects

Rare ACE inhibitor-associated clinical syndrome manifested initially by cholestatic jaundice or hepatitis; may progress to fulminant hepatic necrosis and is potentially fatal. Patients receiving an ACE inhibitor, including lisinopril, who develop jaundice or marked elevations in hepatic enzymes should discontinue the drug and receive appropriate monitoring.

Fetal/Neonatal Morbidity and Mortality

ACE inhibitors can cause fetal and neonatal morbidity and mortality when used in pregnancy during the second and third trimesters. ACE inhibitors also increase the risk of major congenital malformations when administered during the first trimester of pregnancy. Discontinue as soon as possible when pregnancy is detected, unless continued use is considered lifesaving. Nearly all women can be transferred successfully to alternative therapy for the remainder of their pregnancy. For additional information on the risk of ACE inhibitors during pregnancy, see Cautions: Pregnancy, Fertility, and Lactation, in Captopril 24:32.04 and Enalaprilat/Enalapril 24:32.04.

Sensitivity Reactions

Sensitivity reactions, including anaphylactoid reactions and angioedema (including laryngeal edema, tongue edema), are potentially fatal. Patients with head and neck angioedema involving the tongue, glottis, or larynx are likely to experience airway obstruction, especially in those with a history of airway surgery. If laryngeal stridor or angioedema of the face, lips, tongue, or glottis occurs, lisinopril should be discontinued and appropriate therapy (e.g., epinephrine) should be initiated immediately. Antihistamines and corticosteroids may not provide sufficient relief of symptoms even in patients experiencing only swelling of the tongue; prolonged observation may be necessary. Caution in patients with history of angioedema unrelated to ACE inhibitor therapy.

Intestinal angioedema (occasionally without a prior history of facial angioedema or elevated serum levels of complement 1 [C1] esterase inhibitor) also has been reported in patients receiving ACE inhibitors. Intestinal angioedema, which frequently presents as abdominal pain (with or without nausea or vomiting), usually is diagnosed by abdominal CT scan, ultrasound, or surgery; manifestations usually have resolved after discontinuance of the ACE inhibitor. Intestinal angioedema should be considered in the differential diagnosis of patients who develop abdominal pain during therapy with an ACE inhibitor.

Life-threatening anaphylactoid reactions reported in at least 2 patients receiving ACE inhibitors while undergoing desensitization with hymenoptera venom. Such reactions did not occur when ACE inhibitors were temporarily discontinued before desensitization but did recur following inadvertent rechallenge. Sudden and potentially life-threatening anaphylactoid reactions also have been reported in patients receiving ACE inhibitors while undergoing hemodialysis using high-flux membranes. In such patients, dialysis should be discontinued immediately, and aggressive therapy for anaphylactic reactions should be initiated.

Antihistamines have not been effective for relieving symptoms in these patients; use of a different type of dialysis membrane or a different class of antihypertensive agent should be considered. In addition, anaphylactoid reactions have been reported in patients undergoing low-density lipoprotein (LDL) apheresis with dextran sulfate absorption.

General Precautions
Aortic Stenosis/Hypertrophic Cardiomyopathy

Like other vasodilators, lisinopril should be administered with caution in patients with obstruction in the outflow tract of the left ventricle (e.g., aortic stenosis, hypertrophic cardiomyopathy).

Renal Effects

Inhibition of the renin-angiotensin-aldosterone (RAA) system may cause renal impairment and rarely renal failure and/or death in susceptible patients (e.g., those whose renal function depends on the activity of the RAA system such as patients with severe heart failure).

Deterioration of renal function, usually reversible upon discontinuance of the drug, manifested as minor and transient increases in BUN and serum creatinine concentrations, may occur following administration of ACE inhibitor therapy, particularly in hypertensive patients with unilateral or bilateral renal artery stenosis, preexisting renal impairment, or concomitant diuretic therapy. Renal function should be monitored during the first few weeks of therapy in such patients; dosage reduction and/or discontinuance of lisinopril and/or the diuretic may be required.

Renal artery stenosis, preexisting renal impairment, and concomitant diuretic therapy also are risk factors for renal impairment during ACE inhibitor therapy. In patients with acute MI who have evidence of renal dysfunction (i.e., serum creatinine concentration exceeding 2 mg/dL), consider discontinuance of lisinopril if serum creatinine exceeds 3 mg/dL or doubles from pretreatment value.

Hyperkalemia

Hyperkalemia can develop, especially in those with renal impairment or diabetes mellitus and those receiving drugs that can increase serum potassium concentration (e.g., potassium-sparing diuretics, potassium supplements, potassium-containing salt substitutes). Hyperkalemia can result in serious, potentially fatal, cardiac arrhythmias.

Cough

Persistent and nonproductive cough reported with all ACE inhibitors; resolves after drug discontinuance.

Surgery/Anesthesia

Hypotension may occur in patients undergoing surgery or during anesthesia with agents that produce hypotension.

Specific Populations
Pregnancy

Category C (first trimester); Category D (second and third trimesters). (See Users Guide.) (See: Fetal/Neonatal Morbidity and Mortality under Warnings/Precautions: Warnings, in Cautions.)

Lactation

Lisinopril is distributed into milk (as determined by presence of radioactivity following administration of radiolabeled drug) in rats; not known whether the drug is distributed into milk in humans. Hydrochlorothiazide is distributed into human milk. Because of the potential for serious adverse reactions to ACE inhibitors (e.g., lisinopril) in nursing infants, a decision should be made whether to discontinue nursing or lisinopril (either alone or in fixed combination with hydrochlorothiazide), taking into account the importance of the drug(s) to the woman.

Pediatric Use

Safety and efficacy not established in children less than 6 years of age and in pediatric patients with creatinine clearances less than 30 mL/minute per 1.73 m². For information on overall principles and expert recommendations for treatment of hypertension in pediatric patients, see Uses: Hypertension in Pediatric Patients, in the Thiazides General Statement 40:28.20.

Geriatric Use

Clinical studies of lisinopril alone or in fixed combination with hydrochlorothiazide did not include sufficient numbers of patients (with hypertension and heart failure) 65 years of age and older to determine whether geriatric patients respond differently than younger patients, but other clinical experience has not revealed age-related differences. In pharmacokinetic studies, peak plasma concentrations and area under the plasma concentration-time curve (AUC) of lisinopril were increased in geriatric individuals compared with younger individuals. Drug dosage generally should be titrated carefully in geriatric patients, usually initiating therapy at the low end of the dosage range. The greater frequency of decreased hepatic, renal, and/or cardiac function and of concomitant disease and drug therapy observed in the elderly also should be considered.

Renal Impairment

Renal function may decrease with ACE inhibitor therapy in susceptible patients. Use with caution in those with renal impairment. (See Dosage and Administration: Special Populations and also Renal Effects under Warnings/Precautions: General Precautions, in Cautions.)

Black Patients

ACE inhibitors not as effective for decreasing blood pressure. Increased incidence of angioedema. (See Uses: Hypertension.)

● Common Adverse Effects

Adverse effects reported in greater than 1% of patients receiving lisinopril or lisinopril in fixed combination with hydrochlorothiazide for the management of hypertension and more frequently than with placebo include headache, dizziness, cough, fatigue, diarrhea, upper respiratory tract infection, nausea, asthenia, rash, orthostatic effects, hypotension, vomiting, hyperkalemia, or minor increases in BUN and serum creatinine concentrations. Additional adverse effects reported in 1% or more of patients receiving lisinopril in fixed combination with hydrochlorothiazide include dyspepsia, muscle cramps, paresthesia, decreased libido, vertigo, nasal congestion, influenza, or impotence.

Adverse effects reported in greater than 1% of patients receiving lisinopril for the management of heart failure and more frequently than with placebo include dizziness, hypotension, headache, diarrhea, chest pain, nausea, abdominal pain, rash, and upper respiratory tract infection.

In a large trial in patients with acute MI, hypotension and renal dysfunction occurred more frequently in patients receiving lisinopril than in those not receiving the drug.

DRUG INTERACTIONS

● Drugs that Block the Renin-Angiotensin System

Increased risk of hypotension, syncope, hyperkalemia, and changes in renal function (e.g., acute renal failure) with concomitant use of other drugs that block the renin-angiotensin system (e.g., aliskiren, angiotensin II receptor antagonists); when lisinopril is used concomitantly with such drugs, blood pressure, renal function, and serum electrolyte concentrations should be monitored closely. Concomitant use of lisinopril and aliskiren is contraindicated in patients with diabetes mellitus; in addition, such concomitant use should be avoided in patients with renal impairment (glomerular filtration rate [GFR] less than 60 mL/minute per 1.73 m²). (See Cautions in Aliskiren Hemifumarate 24:32.40.)

● Drugs Increasing Serum Potassium Concentration

Potential pharmacologic interaction (additive hyperkalemic effect). Includes potassium-sparing diuretics, potassium supplements, and other drugs that can increase serum potassium. The manufacturer states that lisinopril should be used cautiously (with frequent monitoring of serum potassium), if at all, with potassium supplements or salt substitutes containing potassium.

● Antidiabetic Agents

Potential pharmacologic interaction (increased hypoglycemic effect), especially during initial weeks of combined treatment and in patients with renal impairment.

● Digoxin

Clinically important adverse interaction not observed.

● **Diuretics**

Potential pharmacokinetic and pharmacologic interaction (hypotensive effect).

● **Gold Compounds**

Rare reports of nitritoid reactions (manifested by facial flushing, nausea, vomiting, and hypotension) in patients receiving parenteral aurothioglucose and gold sodium thiomalate concomitantly with ACE inhibitors, including lisinopril.

● **Lithium**

Potential pharmacokinetic interaction (increased lithium concentrations and clinical toxicity).

● **Nonsteroidal Anti-inflammatory Agents**

Potential pharmacologic interaction (decreased antihypertensive effect) when lisinopril is used concomitantly concurrently with nonsteroidal anti-inflammatory agents (NSAIAs). Potential pharmacologic interaction (decreased renal function) when lisinopril is used concomitantly with NSAIAs in patients with impaired renal function. (See Drug Interactions in Captopril 24:32.04.)

● **Propranolol**

Clinically important pharmacokinetic interaction not observed.

DESCRIPTION

Lisinopril is an angiotensin-converting enzyme (ACE, bradykinase, kininase II) inhibitor. Like benazepril, enalapril, fosinopril, quinapril, and ramipril but unlike captopril, lisinopril does not contain a sulfhydryl group.

Unlike enalapril, quinapril, fosinopril, and ramipril but like captopril, lisinopril is *not* a prodrug but instead is active unchanged.

ADVICE TO PATIENTS

Risk of angioedema, anaphylactoid, and other sensitivity reactions and importance of discontinuing the drug and reporting suggestive manifestations (e.g., edema of face, eyes, lips, or tongue; swallowing or breathing with difficulty) to a clinician.

Risk of hypotension (e.g., lightheadedness, syncope), especially during initial therapy and with volume depletion secondary to excessive perspiration or dehydration, vomiting, or diarrhea. Importance of adequate fluid intake. Importance of discontinuing drug and contacting clinician if symptoms of syncope occur.

Importance of contacting a clinician promptly if manifestations of infection or neutropenia (e.g., sore throat, fever) develop.

Importance of informing clinicians of existing or contemplated concomitant therapy, including prescription and OTC drugs. Risk of hyperkalemia; importance of avoiding use of potassium supplements or salt substitutes containing potassium without consultation with a clinician.

Risk of hypoglycemia in patients receiving concomitant therapy with insulin or oral antidiabetic agents. Importance of closely monitoring blood glucose concentrations, especially during the first month of combined use.

Importance of women informing clinicians immediately if they are or plan to become pregnant or plan to breast-feed. Risk of use during first, second, and third trimesters of pregnancy.

Importance of informing patients of other important precautionary information. (See Cautions.)

PREPARATIONS

Excipients in commercially available drug preparations may have clinically important effects in some individuals; consult specific product labeling for details.

Lisinopril

Oral

Tablets	2.5 mg*	**Zestril®**, AstraZeneca
	5 mg*	**Prinivil®**, Merck
		Zestril®, AstraZeneca
	10 mg*	**Prinivil®**, Merck
		Zestril®, AstraZeneca
	20 mg*	**Prinivil®**, Merck
		Zestril®, AstraZeneca
	30 mg*	**Zestril®**, AstraZeneca
	40 mg*	**Zestril®**, AstraZeneca

* available from one or more manufacturer, distributor, and/or repackager by generic (nonproprietary) name

Lisinopril Combinations

Oral

Tablets	10 mg with Hydrochlorothiazide 12.5 mg*	**Prinzide®**, Merck **Zestoretic®**, AstraZeneca
	20 mg with Hydrochlorothiazide 12.5 mg*	**Prinzide®**, Merck **Zestoretic®**, AstraZeneca
	20 mg with Hydrochlorothiazide 25 mg*	**Prinzide®**, Merck **Zestoretic®**, AstraZeneca

* available from one or more manufacturer, distributor, and/or repackager by generic (nonproprietary) name

† Use is not currently included in the labeling approved by the US Food and Drug Administration.

Selected Revisions November 5, 2018, © Copyright, January 1, 1995, American Society of Health-System Pharmacists, Inc.

Ramipril

24:32.04 • ANGIOTENSIN CONVERTING ENZYME INHIBITORS

■ Ramipril is an angiotensin-converting enzyme (ACE) inhibitor.

USES

Ramipril is used alone or in combination with other classes of antihypertensive agents (e.g., thiazide diuretics) in the management of hypertension. Ramipril also is used to reduce the risk of mortality (mainly cardiovascular mortality) following myocardial infarction (MI) in hemodynamically stable patients who have demonstrated clinical signs of heart failure within a few days following acute MI; ramipril therapy also may reduce rate of heart failure-associated hospitalization and progression to severe and/or resistant heart failure. In addition, ramipril has been shown to reduce the rate of death, MI, and stroke in patients at high risk for cardiovascular events†.

Because captopril, another angiotensin-converting enzyme (ACE) inhibitor, may cause serious adverse effects (e.g., neutropenia, agranulocytosis), particularly in patients with renal impairment (especially those with collagen vascular disease) or in patients receiving immunosuppressive therapy, the possibility that similar adverse effects may occur with ramipril should be considered since current evidence is insufficient to rule out such risk. (See Cautions: Hematologic Effects, in Captopril 24:32.04.)

● Hypertension

Ramipril is used alone or in combination with other classes of antihypertensive agents in the management of hypertension. ACE inhibitors are considered one of several preferred antihypertensive drugs for the initial management of hypertension according to current evidence-based hypertension guidelines; other preferred options include angiotensin II receptor antagonists, calcium-channel blockers, and thiazide diuretics. While there may be individual differences with respect to recommendations for initial drug selection and use in specific patient populations, current evidence indicates that these antihypertensive drug classes all generally produce comparable effects on overall mortality and cardiovascular, cerebrovascular, and renal outcomes. (See Uses: Hypertension, in Captopril 24:32.04.)

ACE inhibitors may be particularly useful in the management of hypertension in patients with certain coexisting conditions such as heart failure, ischemic heart disease, diabetes mellitus, chronic kidney disease (CKD), or cerebrovascular disease or following MI. (See Uses: Hypertension in Captopril 24:32.04 and in Enalaprilat/Enalapril 24:32.04.)

In patients with hypertension and compelling indications (e.g., CKD with albuminuria [urine albumin 300 mg/day or greater, or urine albumin:creatinine ratio of 300 mg/g or equivalent in the first morning void]), angiotensin II receptor antagonists are usually considered an alternative for ACE inhibitor-intolerant patients. However, data indicate no difference in efficacy between ACE inhibitors and angiotensin II receptor antagonists with regard to blood pressure lowering and clinical outcomes (i.e., all-cause mortality, cardiovascular mortality, MI, heart failure, stroke, and end-stage renal disease). Adverse events (e.g., cough, angioedema) leading to drug discontinuance occur more frequently with ACE inhibitor therapy than with angiotensin II receptor antagonist therapy. Because of similar efficacy and a lower frequency of adverse effects, some experts believe that an angiotensin II receptor antagonist should be used instead of an ACE inhibitor for the treatment of hypertension or hypertension with certain compelling indications.

Most patients with hypertension, especially black patients, will require at least 2 antihypertensive drugs to achieve adequate blood pressure control. In general, black hypertensive patients tend to respond better to monotherapy with diuretics or calcium-channel blockers than to monotherapy with ACE inhibitors. Although ACE inhibitors have lowered blood pressure in all races studied, monotherapy with these agents has produced a smaller reduction in blood pressure in black hypertensive patients, a population associated with low renin hypertension. However, the combination of an ACE inhibitor or an angiotensin II receptor antagonist with a calcium-channel blocker or thiazide diuretic produces similar blood pressure lowering in black patients as in other racial groups. In addition, ACE inhibitors appear to produce a higher incidence of angioedema in black patients than in other races studied. (See Race under Hypertension: Other Special Considerations for Antihypertensive Drug Therapy, in Uses in Captopril 24:32.04 and in Enalaprilat/Enalapril 24:32.04.)

For additional information on the role of ACE inhibitors in the management of hypertension, see Uses in Captopril 24:32.04 and in Enalaprilat/Enalapril 24:32.04. For information on overall principles and expert recommendations for treatment of hypertension, see Uses: Hypertension in Adults and also see Uses: Hypertension in Pediatric Patients, in the Thiazides General Statement 40:28.20.

● Heart Failure After Acute Myocardial Infarction

Ramipril is used to reduce the risk of mortality (mainly cardiovascular mortality) following MI in hemodynamically stable patients who have demonstrated clinical signs of heart failure within a few days following acute MI; ramipril therapy also may reduce the rate of heart failure-associated hospitalization and progression to severe and/or resistant heart failure. In these patients, when compared with those receiving placebo, ramipril therapy initiated on average 5 (range: 2–9) days after acute MI reduced risk of mortality from any cause by approximately 27% (90% of mortality was cardiovascular, mainly sudden death); risk of progression to severe heart failure and heart failure-associated hospitalization were reduced by 23 and 26%, respectively. In addition, ramipril reduced risk of mortality combined with other events (e.g., reinfarction, stroke, development of severe heart failure) by 19%. This evidence of efficacy was obtained from a large, controlled, long-term (average: 15 months; range: 6–46 months) study (the Acute Infarction Ramipril Efficacy; AIRE). Benefits of ramipril were observed by day 30 of drug therapy and were not affected by gender, exact timing of initiation of drug therapy, or by concomitant drugs (e.g., aspirin, nitrates, β-adrenergic blocking agents [β-blockers], thrombolytic agents, calcium-channel blocking agents, cardiac glycosides); however, such benefits appeared to be increased in patients 65 years and older and in those receiving diuretics. Ramipril did not appear to reduce the rates of reinfarction, although there was a trend to fewer such events when compared with placebo.

Studies with various ACE inhibitors have shown that these drugs reduce fatal and nonfatal cardiovascular events in patients with recent MI. The magnitude of benefit appears to be greatest in certain high-risk patients (e.g., those with an anterior infarct, ejection fraction of 40% or less, heart failure, prior infarction, or tachycardia). In addition to their effects on mortality, ACE inhibitors also are used to minimize or prevent the development of left ventricular dilatation and dysfunction (ventricular "remodeling") following acute MI. Evidence regarding the efficacy of such therapy has been somewhat conflicting, particularly when parenteral therapy was initiated early (within 24–48 hours) and included patients with no evidence of baseline left ventricular dysfunction. (See Uses: Left Ventricular Dysfunction After Acute Myocardial Infarction in Enalaprilat/Enalapril 24:32.04.) However, the preponderance of evidence has shown a benefit of early oral therapy with ACE inhibitors, even in patients with no baseline dysfunction.

Current expert guidelines recommend the use of an oral ACE inhibitor within the first 24 hours of acute MI in patients with an anterior infarction, heart failure, or ejection fraction of 40% or less who do not have any contraindications (e.g., hypotension, shock, renal dysfunction). While early treatment within the first 24 hours of MI has been shown to be beneficial, ACE inhibitors should be used with caution (and with gradual upward titration) during the initial postinfarction period because of the possibility of hypotension or renal dysfunction. ACE inhibitor therapy generally should be continued indefinitely in all patients with left ventricular dysfunction or other compelling indications for use (e.g., hypertension, diabetes mellitus, CKD). The benefits of long-term ACE inhibitor therapy are less certain in low-risk patients who have undergone revascularization and are receiving aggressive antilipemic therapy.

● Prevention of Major Cardiovascular Events

Ramipril may reduce the rate of death, MI, and stroke in patients 55 years of age and older who are at high risk for cardiovascular events (e.g., those with a history of coronary artery disease, stroke, peripheral vascular disease, or diabetes mellitus, in addition to at least one other cardiovascular risk factor, including hypertension, elevated serum total cholesterol and/or decreased high-density lipoprotein [HDL]-cholesterol concentrations, smoking, or documented microalbuminuria) and who are not known to have low left ventricular ejection fraction (LVEF) or heart failure. Ramipril may be used concomitantly with antihypertensive, antiplatelet, or antilipemic drugs. Results of a randomized, multicenter, double-blind, placebo-controlled study (Heart Outcomes Prevention Evaluation [HOPE]) of approximately 5 years' duration in more than 9000 patients 55 years of age or older with a history of coronary artery disease, stroke, peripheral vascular disease, and at least one other cardiovascular risk factor (see above) indicate that ramipril (10 mg daily after an initial dosage of 2.5 mg daily for 1 week followed by 5 mg daily for 3 weeks) reduced the risk of cardiovascular death, stroke, and MI by about 25, 32, and 20%, respectively, compared with placebo. When compared with placebo, the drug also reduced the risk of cardiac arrest and heart failure by approximately 34 and 21%, respectively, and the need for coronary revascularization procedures by 15%. The exact mechanism of the beneficial effects of ramipril in high-risk patients for cardiovascular events has not been fully elucidated, but it appears that ACE inhibitors may antagonize the direct effects of angiotensin II thereby preventing the proliferation of vascular smooth muscle cells and rupture of fibrous plaques. ACE inhibitors also may improve vascular endothelial function, reduce left ventricular hypertrophy, and enhance fibrinolysis.

In addition to these beneficial cardiovascular effects, a reduction in the incidence of diabetic complications was reported in 6.2% of patients receiving ramipril compared with 7.4% of those receiving placebo. New diagnosis of diabetes was reported in fewer patients receiving ramipril compared with those receiving placebo. Although the exact mechanism of the endocrine effects of ramipril is not known, it has been suggested that ACE inhibitors may prevent diabetic complications and new diagnosis of diabetes by improving insulin sensitivity and blood flow to the pancreas and by decreasing hepatic clearance of insulin. In addition, results of other studies indicate that in patients with type 2 diabetes mellitus, intensive control of blood pressure (e.g., an approximate target systolic pressure of less than 150 mm Hg and diastolic pressure of less than 85 mm Hg) using an ACE inhibitor (e.g., captopril) or a β-blocker (e.g., atenolol) resulted in a reduction of development or progression of complications of diabetes (e.g., death related to diabetes, stroke, heart failure, microvascular disease).

In the HOPE study, reduction of cardiovascular risk factors was observed within 1 year of initiation of ramipril therapy and continued throughout the study (approximately 5 years). Because interim analysis of this study after about 5 years revealed a clear evidence of a beneficial effect of ramipril, the study was discontinued.

Heart Failure

ACE inhibitors have been used in the management of heart failure†, usually in conjunction with other agents such as cardiac glycosides, diuretics, and β-blockers.

Current guidelines for the management of heart failure in adults generally recommend a combination of drug therapies to reduce morbidity and mortality, including neurohormonal antagonists (e.g., ACE inhibitors, angiotensin II receptor antagonists, angiotensin receptor-neprilysin inhibitors [ARNIs], β-blockers, aldosterone receptor antagonists) that inhibit the detrimental compensatory mechanisms in heart failure. Additional agents (e.g., cardiac glycosides, diuretics, sinoatrial modulators [i.e., ivabradine]) added to a heart failure treatment regimen in selected patients have been associated with symptomatic improvement and/or reduction in heart failure-related hospitalizations. Experts recommend that all asymptomatic patients with reduced LVEF (American College of Cardiology Foundation [ACCF]/American Heart Association [AHA] stage B heart failure) receive therapy with an ACE inhibitor and β-blocker to prevent symptomatic heart failure and to reduce morbidity and mortality. In patients with prior or current symptoms of chronic heart failure and reduced LVEF (ACCF/AHA stage C heart failure), ACCF, AHA, and the Heart Failure Society of America (HFSA) recommend inhibition of the renin-angiotensin-aldosterone (RAA) system with an ACE inhibitor, angiotensin II receptor antagonist, or ARNI in conjunction with a β-blocker, and an aldosterone antagonist in selected patients, to reduce morbidity and mortality. While ACE inhibitors have been the preferred drugs for inhibition of the RAA system because of their established benefits in patients with heart failure and reduced ejection fraction, some evidence indicates that therapy with sacubitril/valsartan, an ARNI, may be more effective than ACE inhibitor therapy (enalapril) in reducing cardiovascular death and heart failure-related hospitalization in such patients. ACCF, AHA, and HFSA recommend that patients with chronic symptomatic heart failure and reduced LVEF (New York Heart Association [NYHA] class II or III) who are able to tolerate an ACE inhibitor or angiotensin II receptor antagonist be switched to therapy containing an ARNI to further reduce morbidity and mortality. However, in patients in whom an ARNI is not appropriate, continued use of an ACE inhibitor for all classes of heart failure with reduced ejection fraction remains strongly advised. In patients in whom an ARNI

or ACE inhibitor is not appropriate, an angiotensin II receptor antagonist may be used. For additional information on the use of ACE inhibitors in the management of heart failure, see Uses: Heart Failure, in Captopril 24:32.04 and in Enalaprilat/Enalapril 24:32.04. For further information on the use of ARNIs in patients with heart failure, see Uses: Heart Failure, in Sacubitril and Valsartan 24:32.92.

● Diabetic Nephropathy

Both ACE inhibitors and angiotensin II receptor antagonists have been shown to slow the rate of progression of renal disease in patients with diabetes mellitus and persistent albuminuria†, and use of a drug from either class is recommended in such patients with modestly elevated (30–300 mg/24 hours) or higher (exceeding 300 mg/24 hours) levels of urinary albumin excretion. The usual precautions of ACE inhibitor or angiotensin II receptor antagonist therapy in patients with substantial renal impairment should be observed. For additional information on the use of ACE inhibitors in the treatment of diabetic nephropathy, see Diabetic Nephropathy under Uses: Nephropathy, in Captopril 24:32.04.

DOSAGE AND ADMINISTRATION

● Administration

Ramipril is administered orally. The rate but not the extent of GI absorption of the drug may be reduced by administration with food. Ramipril capsules usually are swallowed whole. However, if needed such capsules also may be opened and contents sprinkled in a small amount (about 120 mL) of applesauce or mixed in 120 mL of water or apple juice. To ensure that no drug is lost, the entire mixture should be consumed. These mixtures are stable for 24 hours at room temperature and 48 hours when refrigerated. The manufacturers state that serum ramiprilat concentrations are not affected when contents of ramipril capsules are mixed in applesauce or dissolved in water or apple juice.

● Dosage

Dosage of ramipril must be adjusted according to patient tolerance and response. Because of the risk of inducing hypotension, initiation of ramipril therapy requires consideration of recent antihypertensive therapy, the extent of blood pressure elevation, sodium intake, fluid status, and other clinical circumstances. If therapy is initiated in a patient already receiving a diuretic, symptomatic hypotension may occur following the initial dose of the angiotensin-converting enzyme (ACE) inhibitor. To minimize the possibility of hypotension, especially in patients in whom diuretic therapy was recently initiated, it is recommended that diuretic therapy be discontinued, the diuretic dosage decreased, or salt intake increased, if possible, before initiating ramipril. If such changes are not possible, ramipril therapy should be initiated at a reduced dosage of 1.25 mg once daily. (See Cardiovascular Effects under Warnings/Precautions: Warnings, in Cautions.) For additional information on initiating ramipril in patients receiving diuretic therapy, see the disease-specific dosage sections in Dosage and Administration. Hypotension does not preclude the administration of subsequent doses of the drug, provided the hypotension has been managed effectively.

Hypertension
Usual Dosage

For the management of hypertension in adults *not* receiving a diuretic, the manufacturer states that the usual initial dosage of ramipril is 2.5 mg once daily. In patients currently receiving a diuretic, an initial ramipril dosage of 1.25 mg once daily is recommended; however, discontinuance or dosage reduction of the diuretic or an increase in salt intake is preferred. (See the introductory discussion under Dosage and Administration: Dosage.) Subsequent dosage of ramipril should be adjusted according to the patient's blood pressure response. If the blood pressure response diminishes toward the end of the dosing interval during once-daily administration, increasing the dosage or giving the drug in 2 divided doses daily should be considered. The usual maintenance dosage recommended by the manufacturer and some experts in adults is 2.5–20 mg daily, given as a single dose or in 2 divided doses.

Blood Pressure Monitoring and Treatment Goals

Blood pressure should be monitored regularly (i.e., monthly) during therapy and dosage of the antihypertensive drug adjusted until blood pressure is controlled. If an adequate blood pressure response is not achieved with ACE inhibitor monotherapy, the dosage may be increased or another antihypertensive agent with demonstrated benefit and preferably with a complementary mechanism of action (e.g., calcium-channel blocker, thiazide diuretic) may be added; if target blood pressure is still not achieved, a third drug may be added. (See Uses: Hypertension.) In patients who develop unacceptable adverse effects with ramipril, the drug should be discontinued and another antihypertensive agent from a different pharmacologic class should be initiated.

The goal of hypertension management and prevention is to achieve and maintain optimal control of blood pressure. However, the optimum blood pressure threshold for initiating antihypertensive drug therapy and specific treatment goals remain controversial. While other hypertension guidelines have based target blood pressure goals on age and comorbidities, a 2017 multidisciplinary hypertension guideline from the American College of Cardiology (ACC), American Heart Association (AHA), and a number of other professional organizations incorporates underlying cardiovascular risk into decision making regarding treatment and generally recommends the same target blood pressure (i.e., less than 130/80 mm Hg) in all adults. Many patients will require at least 2 drugs from different pharmacologic classes to achieve this blood pressure goal; the potential benefits of hypertension management and drug cost, adverse effects, and risks associated with the use of multiple antihypertensive drugs also should be considered when deciding a patient's blood pressure treatment goal.

For additional information on target levels of blood pressure and on monitoring therapy in the management of hypertension, see Blood Pressure Monitoring and Treatment Goals under Dosage: Hypertension, in Dosage and Administration in the Thiazides General Statement 40:28.20.

Heart Failure After Acute Myocardial Infarction

When used after myocardial infarction (MI) in adults with clinical signs of heart failure, the manufacturer recommends an initial ramipril dosage of 2.5 mg twice daily, but if hypotension occurs, dosage should be reduced to 1.25 mg twice daily. Some clinicians recommend initiation of therapy within the first 24 hours following MI. After one week at the initial dosage, therapy is then titrated as tolerated, at intervals of about 3 weeks, to a target daily dosage of 5 mg twice daily. After the initial dose of ramipril, the patient should be observed closely for at least 2 hours and for at least 1 additional hour after blood pressure has stabilized. To minimize the likelihood of hypotension, the dosage of any concomitant diuretic should be reduced, if possible. The appearance of hypotension after the initial dose of ramipril does not preclude subsequent carefully titrated doses of the drug after the hypotension has been effectively managed. Dosage should be adjusted carefully under close medical supervision in patients with heart failure because of the risk of hypotension; such patients should be followed closely for at least 2 weeks after initiation of ramipril therapy or any increase in ramipril or diuretic dosage.

Prevention of Major Cardiovascular Events

For reduction in the risk of MI, stroke, and death from cardiovascular causes, the manufacturers recommend that patients receive 2.5 mg once daily for the first week of therapy and 5 mg once daily for the following 3 weeks; dosage then may be increased, as tolerated, to a maintenance dosage of 10 mg once daily. In patients with hypertension or those with recent MI, dosage of ramipril may be given in divided doses.

Heart Failure

In patients with prior or current symptoms of chronic heart failure and reduced LVEF (American College of Cardiology Foundation [ACCF]/American Heart Association [AHA] stage C heart failure†), ACCF and AHA recommend an initial ramipril dosage of 1.25–2.5 mg once daily. The dosage should be slowly titrated upward as tolerated to dosages that have been shown to reduce the risk of cardiovascular events in clinical trials; if such target dosages cannot be achieved or are poorly tolerated, ACCF and AHA state that intermediate doses should be used. ACCF and AHA recommend a maximum ramipril dosage of 10 mg once daily for patients with ACCF/AHA stage C heart failure.

● Special Populations

If ramipril is used in patients with impaired renal function, dosage must be modified in response to the degree of renal impairment, and as with other ACE inhibitors, the theoretical risk of neutropenia must be considered. In adults with creatinine clearances less than 40 mL/minute, 25% of the usual doses are expected to induce full therapeutic concentrations of ramiprilat. For the management of

hypertension in these patients, the usual initial dosage of ramipril is 1.25 mg once daily. Subsequent dosage should be titrated according to individual tolerance and blood pressure response, up to a maximum of 5 mg daily. In patients with heart failure following acute MI and who have creatinine clearances less than 40 mL/minute, the usual initial dosage of ramipril is 1.25 mg once daily; dosage may be increased to 1.25 mg twice daily. Subsequent dosage should be titrated according to individual clinical response and tolerance up to a maximum dosage of 2.5 mg twice daily.

Patients with known or suspected renal artery stenosis should receive an initial ramipril dosage of 1.25 mg once daily; subsequent dosage should be adjusted based on blood pressure response.

Since ramipril is primarily metabolized by hepatic esterases to ramiprilat (its active moiety), hepatic impairment may result in increased ramipril plasma concentrations. In addition, the renin-angiotensin-aldosterone (RAA) system (see Renal Effects under Warnings/Precautions: General Precautions, in Cautions) may be activated in hypertensive patients with severe hepatic impairment (e.g., severe liver cirrhosis and/or ascites). However, the manufacturers make no specific recommendations regarding dosage adjustment in patients with hepatic impairment.

For additional information on initiating and adjusting ramipril dosage in the management of hypertension, including recommendations for blood pressure monitoring, see Dosage: Hypertension, under Dosage and Administration, in Captopril 24:32.04 and in Enalaprilat/Enalapril 24:32.04.

CAUTIONS

● Contraindications

History of angioedema related to previous angiotensin-converting enzyme (ACE) inhibitor treatment.

Known hypersensitivity to ramipril, other ACE inhibitors, or any ingredient in the formulation.

Concomitant use of ramipril and aliskiren in patients with diabetes mellitus. (See Drug Interactions: Drugs that Block the Renin-Angiotensin System.)

● Warnings/Precautions

Warnings

Hypotension

Like other ACE inhibitors, ramipril rarely is associated with hypotension in patients with uncomplicated hypertension. Symptomatic hypotension may occur; patients at particular risk include those with severe volume and/or salt depletion secondary to prolonged diuretic therapy, dietary salt restriction, dialysis, diarrhea, or vomiting. Volume and/or salt depletion should be corrected before starting ramipril therapy.

Marked hypotension may occur in patients with heart failure (with or without associated renal impairment), which may be associated with oliguria and/or progressive azotemia and, rarely, acute renal failure and/or death. In patients with heart failure, ramipril therapy should be started under close medical supervision, and patients should be followed closely for at least 2 weeks after initiation of ramipril or diuretic therapy or dosage adjustment of either drug. (See Dosage and Administration: Dosage.)

If hypotension occurs, the patient should be placed in the supine position, and if necessary, an IV infusion of 0.9% sodium chloride injection to expand fluid volume should be administered. Ramipril therapy usually may be continued following restoration of blood pressure and volume.

Hematologic Effects

Neutropenia/agranulocytosis, anemia, leukopenia, thrombocytopenia, pancytopenia may occur in patients receiving ACE inhibitors, particularly in patients with renal impairment (especially those with concomitant collagen vascular disease [e.g., systemic lupus erythematosus, scleroderma]). Monitoring of leukocytes in patients with collagen vascular disease, especially if renal impairment exists, should be considered.

Fetal/Neonatal Morbidity and Mortality

ACE inhibitors can cause fetal and neonatal morbidity and mortality when used in pregnancy during the second and third trimesters. ACE inhibitors also increase the risk of major congenital malformations when administered during the first trimester of pregnancy. Discontinue as soon as possible when pregnancy is detected, unless continued use is considered lifesaving. Nearly all women can be transferred successfully to alternative therapy for the remainder of their pregnancy. For additional information on the risk of ACE inhibitors during pregnancy, see Cautions: Pregnancy, Fertility, and Lactation, in Captopril 24:32.04.

Hepatic Effects

Rare ACE inhibitor-associated clinical syndrome manifested initially by cholestatic jaundice may occur; may progress to fulminant hepatic necrosis and is potentially fatal. Patients receiving an ACE inhibitor, including ramipril, who develop jaundice or marked elevations in hepatic enzymes should discontinue the drug and receive appropriate monitoring.

Sensitivity Reactions

Sensitivity reactions, including anaphylactic reactions and angioedema (including laryngeal or tongue edema) are potentially fatal. Head and neck angioedema involving the tongue, glottis, or larynx may cause airway obstruction. If laryngeal stridor or angioedema of the face, tongue, or glottis occurs, ramipril should be discontinued and appropriate therapy (e.g., epinephrine) should be initiated immediately.

Intestinal angioedema (occasionally without a prior history of facial angioedema or elevated serum levels of complement 1 [C1] esterase inhibitor) also has been reported in patients receiving ACE inhibitors. Intestinal angioedema, which frequently presents as abdominal pain (with or without nausea or vomiting), usually is diagnosed by abdominal CT scan, ultrasound, or surgery; symptoms usually have resolved after discontinuance of the ACE inhibitor. Intestinal angioedema should be considered in the differential diagnosis of patients who develop abdominal pain during therapy with an ACE inhibitor.

Patients receiving concomitant mammalian target of rapamycin (mTOR) inhibitors (e.g., temsirolimus) may be at increased risk for angioedema.

Life-threatening anaphylactoid reactions have been reported in at least 2 patients receiving ACE inhibitors while undergoing desensitization treatment with hymenoptera venom. When ACE inhibitors were temporarily discontinued before desensitization with the venom, anaphylactoid reactions did not recur; however, such reactions recurred after inadvertent rechallenge. Anaphylactoid reactions have been reported following initiation of hemodialysis that used a high-flux membrane in patients receiving an ACE inhibitor. In addition, anaphylactoid reactions have been reported in patients undergoing low-density lipoprotein (LDL) apheresis with dextran sulfate absorption.

General Precautions

Renal Effects

Inhibition of the renin-angiotensin-aldosterone (RAA) system may cause renal impairment and rarely renal failure and/or death in susceptible patients (e.g., those whose renal function depends on the activity of the RAA system such as patients with severe heart failure).

Deterioration in renal function, manifested as transient increases in BUN and serum creatinine concentrations may occur following administration of ACE inhibitor therapy, particularly in hypertensive patients with unilateral or bilateral renal-artery stenosis, preexisting renal impairment, or concomitant diuretic therapy. This effect was usually reversible following discontinuance of ACE inhibitor and/or diuretic therapy. Renal function should be monitored closely during the first few weeks of therapy and periodically thereafter in such patients.

Effects on Potassium

Hyperkalemia can develop, especially in those with renal impairment or diabetes mellitus and those receiving drugs that can increase serum potassium concentration (e.g., potassium-sparing diuretics, potassium supplements, potassium-containing salt substitutes).

Cough

Persistent and nonproductive; resolves after drug discontinuance.

Surgery/Anesthesia

Hypotension may occur in patients undergoing surgery or during anesthesia with agents that produce hypotension. Hypotension in such patients may be corrected by volume expansion.

Specific Populations

Pregnancy

Category C (first trimester); Category D (second and third trimesters). (See Users Guide.) (See Fetal/Neonatal Morbidity and Mortality under Warnings/Precautions: Warnings, in Cautions.)

Lactation

Ramipril and its metabolites were undetectable in breast milk following a single 10-mg oral dose of the drug in nursing women; however, milk concentrations resulting from multiple doses of the drug have not been determined. Because of the potential for serious adverse reactions from ramipril in nursing infants, the manufacturers state that women receiving the drug should not breast-feed.

Pediatric Use

The manufacturers state that safety and efficacy of ramipril in children younger than 18 years of age have not been established. For information on overall principles and expert recommendations for treatment of hypertension in pediatric patients, see Uses: Hypertension in Pediatric Patients, in the Thiazides General Statement 40:28.20.

Geriatric Use

No substantial differences in safety and efficacy relative to younger adults, but increased sensitivity cannot be ruled out. Increased ramiprilat plasma concentrations and area under the concentration-time curve (AUC) have been reported in some geriatric patients.

Renal Impairment

Renal function may decrease with ACE inhibitor therapy in susceptible patients. Use with caution in those with renal impairment. (See Dosage and Administration: Special Populations and also under Warnings/Precautions: General Precautions, Renal Effects, in Cautions.)

Hepatic Impairment

Use with caution. (See Dosage and Administration: Special Populations.)

Black Patients

ACE inhibitors not as effective. (See Uses: Hypertension.)

● Common Adverse Effects

Adverse effects reported in 1% or more of patients receiving ramipril and considered possibly or probably related to treatment include asthenia/fatigue, hypotension, postural hypotension, increased cough, dizziness, headache, angina pectoris, nausea, syncope, vomiting, vertigo, abnormal kidney function, and diarrhea.

DRUG INTERACTIONS

● Drugs that Block the Renin-Angiotensin System

Increased risk of renal impairment, hyperkalemia, and hypotension with concomitant use of other drugs that block the renin-angiotensin system (e.g., aliskiren, angiotensin II receptor antagonists); when ramipril is used concomitantly with such drugs, blood pressure, renal function, and serum concentrations of electrolytes should be monitored closely. Concomitant use of ramipril and aliskiren is contraindicated in patients with diabetes mellitus; in addition, such concomitant use should be avoided in patients with renal impairment (glomerular filtration rate [GFR] less than 60 mL/minute per 1.73 m²). (See Cautions in Aliskiren Hemifumarate 24:32.40.)

● Drugs Increasing Serum Potassium Concentration

Potential pharmacologic interaction (additive hyperkalemic effect). Includes potassium-sparing diuretics, potassium supplements, and other drugs that can cause hyperkalemia.

● Diuretics

Potential pharmacokinetic and pharmacologic interaction (hypotensive effect).

● **Lithium**

Potential pharmacokinetic interaction (increased lithium concentrations and clinical toxicity).

● **mTOR Inhibitors**

Patients receiving concomitant mammalian target of rapamycin (mTOR) inhibitors (e.g., temsirolimus) may be at increased risk for angioedema.

● **Nonsteroidal Anti-inflammatory Agents**

Potential pharmacologic interaction (decreased renal function and increased serum potassium concentrations). (See Drug Interactions in Captopril 24:32.04.)

DESCRIPTION

Ramipril is an angiotensin-converting enzyme (ACE, bradykininase, kininase II) inhibitor. Unlike captopril or lisinopril but similar to benazepril, enalapril, fosinopril, moexipril, perindopril, quinapril, and trandolapril, ramipril is a prodrug and has little pharmacologic activity until hydrolyzed in the liver to ramiprilat. Like benazepril, enalapril, fosinopril, lisinopril, moexipril, and quinapril but unlike captopril, ramipril does not contain a sulfhydryl group.

ADVICE TO PATIENTS

Risk of angioedema, anaphylactoid, and other sensitivity reactions; importance of discontinuing the drug and immediately reporting suggestive manifestation (e.g., edema of face, eyes, lips, or tongue; swallowing or breathing with difficulty) to a clinician.

Risk of hypotension (e.g., lightheadedness, syncope), especially during initial therapy or with volume depletion secondary to excessive perspiration, vomiting, or diarrhea. Importance of adequate fluid intake. Importance of discontinuing drug and contacting clinician if symptoms of syncope occur.

Importance of contacting a clinician promptly if manifestations of infection or neutropenia (e.g., sore throat, fever) develop.

Importance of informing clinicians of existing or contemplated concomitant therapy, including prescription and OTC drugs. Risk of hyperkalemia. Importance of avoiding the use of potassium supplements or salt substitutes containing potassium without consultation with a clinician.

Importance of women informing clinicians immediately if they are or plan to become pregnant or plan to breast-feed. Risk of use during first, second, and third trimesters of pregnancy.

Importance of informing patients of other important precautionary information. (See Cautions.)

PREPARATIONS

Excipients in commercially available drug preparations may have clinically important effects in some individuals; consult specific product labeling for details.

Ramipril

Oral			
Capsules	1.25 mg*		Altace®, Pfizer
			Ramipril Capsules
	2.5 mg*		Altace®, Pfizer
			Ramipril Capsules
	5 mg*		Altace®, Pfizer
			Ramipril Capsules
	10 mg*		Altace®, Pfizer
			Ramipril Capsules

* available from one or more manufacturer, distributor, and/or repackager by generic (nonproprietary) name

† Use is not currently included in the labeling approved by the US Food and Drug Administration.

Irbesartan

24:32.08 • ANGIOTENSIN II RECEPTOR ANTAGONISTS

■ Irbesartan, a nonpeptide tetrazole derivative, is an angiotensin II type 1 (AT$_1$) receptor antagonist (also referred to as an angiotensin II receptor blocker [ARB]).

USES

● Hypertension

Irbesartan is used alone or in combination with other classes of antihypertensive agents in the management of hypertension. Angiotensin II receptor antagonists, such as irbesartan, are considered one of several preferred antihypertensive drugs for the initial management of hypertension according to current evidence-based hypertension guidelines; other preferred options include angiotensin-converting enzyme (ACE) inhibitors, calcium-channel blockers, and thiazide diuretics. While there may be individual differences with respect to recommendations for initial drug selection and use in specific patient populations, current evidence indicates that these antihypertensive drug classes all generally produce comparable effects on overall mortality and cardiovascular, cerebrovascular, and renal outcomes. (See Uses: Hypertension, in Valsartan 24:32.08.)

Angiotensin II receptor antagonists or ACE inhibitors may be particularly useful in the management of hypertension in patients with certain coexisting conditions such as diabetes mellitus or chronic kidney disease (CKD); angiotensin II receptor antagonists also may be preferred, generally as an alternative to ACE inhibitors, in hypertensive patients with heart failure or ischemic heart disease and/or following myocardial infarction (MI). (See Uses: Hypertension, in Valsartan 24:32.08.)

In patients with hypertension and compelling indications (e.g., CKD with albuminuria [urine albumin 300 mg/day or greater, or urine albumin:creatinine ratio of 300 mg/g or equivalent in the first morning void]), angiotensin II receptor antagonists are usually considered an alternative for ACE inhibitor-intolerant patients. However, data indicate no difference in efficacy between ACE inhibitors and angiotensin II receptor antagonists with regard to blood pressure lowering and clinical outcomes (i.e., all-cause mortality, cardiovascular mortality, MI, heart failure, stroke, and end-stage renal disease). Adverse events (e.g., cough, angioedema) leading to drug discontinuance occur more frequently with ACE inhibitor therapy than with angiotensin II receptor antagonist therapy. Because of similar efficacy and a lower frequency of adverse effects, some experts believe that angiotensin II receptor antagonists should be used instead of an ACE inhibitor for the treatment of hypertension or hypertension with certain compelling indications.

Efficacy of irbesartan for the management of hypertension has been established by controlled studies of 8–12 weeks' duration in patients with hypertension of mild to moderate severity in outpatient settings. Clinical studies have shown that the hypotensive effect of usual dosages of irbesartan in patients with mild to moderate hypertension is greater than that of placebo and comparable to that of usual dosages of losartan, enalapril, or atenolol.

Most patients with hypertension, especially black patients, will require at least 2 antihypertensive drugs to achieve adequate blood pressure control. Like ACE inhibitors, angiotensin II receptor antagonists such as irbesartan may produce a smaller blood pressure response in hypertensive black patients compared with nonblack patients. (See Race under Hypertension: Other Special Considerations for Antihypertensive Drug Therapy, in Uses in Valsartan 24:32.08.)

For additional information on the management of hypertension, see Uses: Hypertension, in Valsartan 24:32.08. For information on overall principles and expert recommendations for treatment of hypertension, see Uses: Hypertension in Adults and also see Uses: Hypertension in Pediatric Patients, in the Thiazides General Statement 40:28.20.

● Diabetic Nephropathy

Irbesartan is used in the management of diabetic nephropathy manifested by elevated serum creatinine and proteinuria (urinary protein excretion exceeding 300 mg daily) in patients with type 2 diabetes mellitus and hypertension.

Both angiotensin II receptor antagonists and ACE inhibitors have been shown to slow the rate of progression of renal disease in patients with diabetes mellitus and persistent albuminuria, and use of a drug from either class is recommended in such patients with modestly elevated (30–300 mg/24 hours) or higher (exceeding 300 mg/24 hours) levels of urinary albumin excretion. Some evidence suggests that these drugs may slow the progression of nephropathy by a mechanism independent of their antihypertensive effects.

Comparative trials evaluating the efficacy of angiotensin II receptor antagonists and ACE inhibitors for improving renal outcomes in diabetic patients are lacking. Evidence supporting use of ACE inhibitors generally is based on studies in patients with type 1 diabetes mellitus, while evidence supporting use of angiotensin II receptor antagonists generally is based on studies in patients with type 2 diabetes mellitus. Findings from these studies indicate that both drug classes delay progression of increased urinary albumin excretion in patients with diabetes mellitus and may also slow the decline in renal function. Because the available data are consistent, some experts suggest that the effects of both drug classes in improving renal outcomes in patients with diabetes mellitus and proteinuria are likely to be similar.

Drugs that inhibit the renin-angiotensin system (i.e., angiotensin II receptor antagonists, ACE inhibitors) also have been shown to delay the onset of albuminuria in patients with type 2 diabetes mellitus and hypertension who have normal levels of urinary albumin excretion†; however, some experts state that in the absence of albuminuria, the risk of progressive kidney disease is low. The American Diabetes Association (ADA) states that the use of an ACE inhibitor or angiotensin II receptor antagonist is not recommended for the primary prevention of diabetic nephropathy in patients with diabetes mellitus who are normotensive, have normal levels of urinary protein excretion, and have a normal glomerular filtration rate (GFR).

Combined therapy with ACE inhibitors and angiotensin II receptor antagonists provides no additional cardiovascular benefit and increases the risk of adverse effects (e.g., impaired renal function, hyperkalemia). The usual precautions of angiotensin II receptor antagonist therapy in patients with substantial renal impairment should be observed.

The current labeled indication for irbesartan in hypertensive patients with type 2 diabetes mellitus and nephropathy (indicated by an elevated serum creatinine and proteinuria exceeding 300 mg/day) is based principally on the results of a long-term (mean duration of follow-up: 2.6 years), multicenter, comparative controlled trial, the Irbesartan Diabetic Nephropathy Trial (IDNT). In the IDNT, therapy with irbesartan (dosage titrated from 75 to 300 mg daily) reduced the risk of the primary composite end point, which was defined as a doubling of the baseline serum creatinine concentration, end-stage renal disease (i.e., initiation of dialysis, renal transplantation, or a serum creatinine concentration of at least 6 mg/dL), or death, by 23% compared with amlodipine therapy (dosage titrated from 2.5 to 10 mg daily) and by 20% compared with placebo. Additional antihypertensive agents (diuretics, β-adrenergic blocking agents [β-blockers], peripheral α-adrenergic blocking agents, or central α$_2$-adrenergic agonists) were used as needed in all treatment groups to achieve a trough blood pressure of 135/85 mm Hg or less in the sitting position or 10 mm Hg reduction in systolic blood pressure if higher than 160 mm Hg; ACE inhibitors, other angiotensin II receptor antagonists, and calcium-channel blocking agents could not be used. Most of the delay in time to occurrence of composite clinical events seen with irbesartan-containing therapy was the result of a reduction in the risk of doubling of serum creatinine concentration; irbesartan-containing therapy had no appreciable effect on overall mortality, onset of end-stage renal disease, or secondary composite cardiovascular end point (death from cardiovascular causes, nonfatal myocardial infarction, hospitalization for heart failure, stroke with permanent neurologic deficit, amputation) compared with other treatments. Mean blood pressure achieved with either irbesartan- or amlodipine-containing therapies was similar (142/77 or 142/76 mm Hg, respectively) and lower than that achieved with placebo plus other antihypertensive agents (145/79 mm Hg). Despite therapy with an average of 3 other nonstudy antihypertensive agents per patient in all treatment groups, none of the treatment groups achieved the target blood pressure goal.

● Heart Failure

Angiotensin II receptor antagonists have been used in the management of heart failure†.

Current guidelines for the management of heart failure in adults generally recommend a combination of drug therapies to reduce morbidity and mortality, including neurohormonal antagonists (e.g., ACE inhibitors, angiotensin II receptor antagonists, angiotensin receptor-neprilysin inhibitors [ARNIs], β-blockers, aldosterone receptor antagonists) that inhibit the detrimental compensatory mechanisms in heart failure. Additional agents (e.g., cardiac glycosides, diuretics, sinoatrial modulators [i.e., ivabradine]) added to a heart failure treatment regimen in selected patients have been associated with symptomatic improvement and/or reduction in heart failure-related hospitalizations. Experts recommend that all asymptomatic patients with reduced left ventricular ejection fraction (LVEF) (American College of Cardiology Foundation [ACCF]/American Heart Association [AHA] stage B heart failure) receive therapy with an ACE inhibitor and β-blocker to prevent symptomatic heart failure and reduce morbidity and mortality. In patients with prior or current symptoms of chronic heart failure with reduced LVEF (ACCF/AHA stage C heart failure), ACCF, AHA, and the Heart Failure Society of America (HFSA) recommend inhibition of the renin-angiotensin-aldosterone (RAA) system with an ACE inhibitor, angiotensin II receptor antagonist, or ARNI in conjunction with a β-blocker, and an aldosterone antagonist in selected patients, to reduce morbidity and mortality. While ACE inhibitors have been the preferred drugs for inhibition of the RAA system because of their established benefits in patients with heart failure and reduced ejection fraction, some evidence indicates that therapy with sacubitril/valsartan, an ARNI, may be more effective than ACE inhibitor therapy (enalapril) in reducing cardiovascular death and heart failure-related hospitalization. ACCF, AHA, and HFSA recommend that patients with chronic symptomatic heart failure and reduced LVEF (New York Heart Association [NYHA] functional class II or III) who are able to tolerate an ACE inhibitor or angiotensin II receptor antagonist be switched to therapy containing an ARNI to further reduce morbidity and mortality. However, in patients in whom an ARNI is not appropriate, continued use of an ACE inhibitor for all classes of heart failure with reduced ejection fraction remains strongly advised. In patients in whom an ARNI or ACE inhibitor is not appropriate, an angiotensin II receptor antagonist may be used. For additional information on the use of angiotensin II receptor antagonists in the management of heart failure, see Uses: Heart Failure, in Valsartan 24:32.08 and in Candesartan 24:32.08. For further information on the use of ARNIs in patients with heart failure, see Uses: Heart Failure, in Sacubitril and Valsartan 24:32.92.

Several clinical trials in patients with heart failure have evaluated the use of angiotensin II receptor antagonists as add-on therapy to conventional regimens compared with an ACE inhibitor, as add-on therapy to conventional regimens including an ACE inhibitor, as combination therapy with an ACE inhibitor compared with therapy with either type of agent alone, or as an alternative therapy in patients intolerant of ACE inhibitors. Data from these and other long-term placebo-controlled clinical trials indicate that angiotensin II receptor antagonists produce hemodynamic and neurohormonal effects associated with their suppression of the renin-angiotensin system; reduced hospitalizations and mortality also have been demonstrated. However, in some studies, these drugs did not show consistent effects on cardiac symptoms or exercise tolerance.

While angiotensin II receptor antagonists are considered reasonable alternatives in patients who are unable to tolerate ACE inhibitors (e.g., because of cough or angioedema), urticaria and angioedema (e.g., swelling of the face, lips, pharynx, and/or tongue) have been reported rarely during postmarketing experience in patients receiving irbesartan. (See Sensitivity Reactions under Cautions: Warnings/Precautions.)

DOSAGE AND ADMINISTRATION

● Administration

Irbesartan is administered orally. Since food does not affect the oral bioavailability of irbesartan, the manufacturer states that the drug can be taken without regard to meals.

● Dosage

Hypertension

Dosage of irbesartan must be individualized and adjusted according to blood pressure response.

Irbesartan Therapy

The manufacturer states that the usual initial dosage of irbesartan in adults is 150 mg once daily in patients without depletion of intravascular volume; in adults with depletion of intravascular volume, the usual initial dosage is 75 mg once daily. If blood pressure response is inadequate with the initial dosage, dosage may be increased as tolerated to 300 mg daily or a diuretic may be added. Increasing irbesartan dosages beyond 300 mg daily or dividing the total daily dosage into 2 doses usually does not result in additional therapeutic effect. Some experts state

that the usual dosage range is 150–300 mg once daily. Addition of a diuretic generally has a greater effect on blood pressure reduction than dosage increases of irbesartan beyond 300 mg daily. Irbesartan also can be used concomitantly with other antihypertensive agents.

The manufacturer states that some of the irbesartan dosages used in a clinical study did not effectively lower blood pressure in pediatric patients 6–16 years of age. (See Pediatric Use under Cautions: Specific Populations.) In children 6–12 years of age, experts recommend an initial irbesartan dosage of 75 mg once daily and a maximum dosage of 150 mg once daily. In children at least 13 years of age, experts recommend an initial irbesartan dosage of 150 mg once daily and a maximum dosage of 300 mg once daily. These experts state the dosage may be increased every 2–4 weeks until blood pressure is controlled, the maximum dosage is reached, or adverse effects occur. For information on overall principles and expert recommendations for treatment of hypertension in pediatric patients, see Uses: Hypertension in Pediatric Patients, in the Thiazides General Statement 40:28.20.

Irbesartan/Hydrochlorothiazide Fixed-combination Therapy

In patients who do not respond adequately to monotherapy with irbesartan or, alternatively, with hydrochlorothiazide, combined therapy with the drugs can be used. The manufacturer states that combined therapy with the commercially available fixed-combination preparation containing 150 mg of irbesartan and 12.5 mg of hydrochlorothiazide, 300 mg of irbesartan and 12.5 mg of hydrochlorothiazide, or 300 mg of irbesartan and 25 mg of hydrochlorothiazide (in order of increasing mean effect) can be used in patients whose blood pressure is not adequately controlled by monotherapy with irbesartan or hydrochlorothiazide. The maximum antihypertensive effect is attained about 2–4 weeks after a change in dosage. Dosage of the fixed-combination preparation should not exceed 300 mg of irbesartan and 25 mg of hydrochlorothiazide once daily.

Irbesartan in fixed combination with hydrochlorothiazide also can be used for initial treatment of hypertension in patients who are likely to need multiple drugs to achieve their blood pressure goals. The decision to use irbesartan in fixed combination with hydrochlorothiazide as initial therapy should be based on an assessment of potential benefits and risks. Patients with moderate to severe hypertension are at relatively high risk for cardiovascular events (e.g., stroke, myocardial infarction, heart failure), kidney failure, and vision problems; therefore, prompt treatment is clinically important. The decision to use combination therapy as initial treatment should be individualized taking into account baseline blood pressure, target goal, and incremental likelihood of achieving blood pressure goal with combination therapy compared with monotherapy. In patients receiving fixed-combination tablets as initial therapy, the usual starting dosage is irbesartan 150 mg and hydrochlorothiazide 12.5 mg once daily. Dosage may be increased after 1–2 weeks of therapy to a maximum of irbesartan 300 mg and hydrochlorothiazide 25 mg once daily.

Blood Pressure Monitoring and Treatment Goals

Blood pressure should be monitored regularly (i.e., monthly) during therapy and dosage of the antihypertensive drug adjusted until blood pressure is controlled. If an adequate blood pressure response is not achieved with angiotensin II receptor antagonist monotherapy, the dosage may be increased or another antihypertensive agent with demonstrated benefit and preferably with a complementary mechanism of action (e.g., calcium-channel blocker, thiazide diuretic) may be added; if target blood pressure is still not achieved, a third drug may be added. (See Uses: Hypertension.) In patients who develop unacceptable adverse effects with irbesartan, the drug should be discontinued and another antihypertensive agent from a different pharmacologic class should be initiated.

The goal of hypertension management and prevention is to achieve and maintain optimal control of blood pressure. However, the optimum blood pressure threshold for initiating antihypertensive drug therapy and specific treatment goals remain controversial. While previous hypertension guidelines have based target blood pressure goals on age and comorbidities, the 2017 ACC/AHA hypertension guideline incorporates underlying cardiovascular risk into decision making regarding treatment and generally recommends the same target blood pressure (i.e., less than 130/80 mm Hg) in all adults. Many patients will require at least 2 drugs from different pharmacologic classes to achieve their blood pressure goal; the potential benefits of hypertension management and drug cost, adverse effects, and risks associated with the use of multiple antihypertensive drugs also should be considered when deciding a patient's blood pressure treatment goal.

For additional information on target levels of blood pressure and on monitoring therapy in the management of hypertension, see Blood Pressure Monitoring and Treatment Goals under Dosage: Hypertension, in Dosage and Administration in the Thiazides General Statement 40:28.20.

Diabetic Nephropathy

For the management of diabetic nephropathy in patients with type 2 diabetes mellitus, the recommended target maintenance dosage of irbesartan is 300 mg once daily. No data are available on the effects of lower dosages of irbesartan on diabetic nephropathy. In a large clinical trial, approximately 83% of patients had dosage titrated from 75 mg daily initially up to 300 mg daily and maintained that dosage for more than 50% of the study period.

● Special Populations

Volume and/or salt depletion should be corrected prior to initiation of therapy or, alternatively, therapy should be initiated using a lower initial dosage (75 mg once daily). Fixed-combination tablets containing irbesartan and hydrochlorothiazide are *not* recommended as initial therapy in patients with intravascular volume depletion.

The manufacturer states that dosage modification of irbesartan is not necessary for adults with renal impairment; however, irbesartan should be used with caution in patients with renal impairment and depletion of intravascular volume. If concomitant diuretic therapy is required in patients with severe renal impairment (i.e., creatinine clearance less than 30 mL/minute), a loop diuretic is preferred to a thiazide diuretic. Therefore, commercially available preparations containing irbesartan in fixed combination with hydrochlorothiazide usually are *not* recommended for patients with severe renal impairment. Irbesartan is not removed by hemodialysis.

The manufacturer states that dosage adjustment is not necessary in patients with hepatic impairment.

The manufacturer states that dosage modification of irbesartan because of age in geriatric adults is not necessary. Because of the greater frequency of decreased hepatic, renal, and/or cardiac function and of concomitant disease and/or drug therapy in geriatric patients, dosage of irbesartan in fixed combination with hydrochlorothiazide should be carefully selected in such patients. The manufacturer recommends that dosage of the fixed combination be initiated at the lower end of the usual range in geriatric patients.

CAUTIONS

● Contraindications

Known hypersensitivity to irbesartan or any ingredient in the formulation.

Concomitant use of irbesartan and aliskiren in patients with diabetes mellitus. (See Drug Interactions: Drugs that Block the Renin-Angiotensin System.)

● Warnings/Precautions

Warnings

Fetal/Neonatal Morbidity and Mortality

Drugs that act on the renin-angiotensin system (e.g., angiotensin-converting enzyme [ACE] inhibitors, angiotensin II receptor antagonists) reduce fetal renal function and increase fetal and neonatal morbidity and mortality when used in pregnancy during the second and third trimesters. Resulting oligohydramnios can be associated with fetal lung hypoplasia and skeletal deformations. Potential neonatal effects include skull hypoplasia, anuria, hypotension, renal failure, and death. Irbesartan should be discontinued as soon as possible when pregnancy is detected, unless continued use is considered life-saving. Nearly all women can be transferred successfully to alternative therapy for the remainder of their pregnancy. For additional information on the risk of such drugs during pregnancy, see Cautions: Pregnancy, Fertility, and Lactation, in Captopril 24:32.04 and Enalaprilat/Enalapril 24:32.04.

Sensitivity Reactions

Sensitivity reactions, including various anaphylactoid reactions and/or angioedema, have been reported with use of angiotensin II receptor antagonists, including irbesartan. Irbesartan is not recommended in patients with a history of angioedema associated with or unrelated to ACE inhibitor or angiotensin II receptor antagonist therapy.

Other Warnings and Precautions

Hypotension

Symptomatic hypotension has been reported in patients receiving irbesartan, especially in volume- and/or salt-depleted patients (e.g., those treated with

diuretics or undergoing dialysis). Volume and/or salt depletion should be corrected before initiation of irbesartan therapy or a lower initial dosage should be used. (See Dosage and Administration: Special Populations.)

Transient hypotension is not a contraindication to additional doses; therapy may be reinstated cautiously after blood pressure is stabilized (e.g., with volume expansion).

Malignancies

In July 2010, the US Food and Drug Administration (FDA) initiated a safety review of angiotensin II receptor antagonists after a published meta-analysis suggested a possible association between the use of these agents and an increased risk of cancer. The meta-analysis, which combined cancer-related findings from 5 randomized, controlled trials in over 60,000 patients, found a modest but significant increase in the risk of new cancer occurrence in patients receiving an angiotensin II receptor antagonist (mostly telmisartan) compared with those in control groups (7.2 versus 6%, respectively; risk ratio 1.08). However, because of several limitations of the study (e.g., trials included in the meta-analysis were not specifically designed to evaluate cancer outcomes, lack of individual patient data), the validity of these findings has been questioned.

Subsequent studies, including a larger, more comprehensive meta-analysis conducted by FDA, have not shown an increased risk of cancer in patients receiving angiotensin II receptor antagonists. FDA's meta-analysis, which included trial-level data from 31 randomized studies (total of approximately 156,000 patients), found no evidence of an increased risk of cancer in patients who received an angiotensin II receptor antagonist compared with those who received other treatments (placebo or active control). The overall rate of new cancer occurrence was essentially the same in both groups of patients (1.82 and 1.84 cases per 100 patient-years, respectively). In addition, there was no difference in the risk of cancer-related death, breast cancer, lung cancer, or prostate cancer between the groups. Based on these results and a review of all currently available data related to this potential safety concern, FDA has concluded that use of angiotensin II receptor antagonists is not associated with an increased risk of cancer.

Renal Effects

Because the renin-angiotensin-aldosterone (RAA) system appears to contribute substantially to maintenance of glomerular filtration in patients with heart failure in whom renal perfusion is severely compromised, renal function may deteriorate markedly (e.g., oliguria, progressive azotemia, renal failure, death) in these patients during therapy with an ACE inhibitor or an angiotensin II receptor antagonist (e.g., irbesartan). Increases in BUN and serum creatinine also may occur in patients with renal artery stenosis, chronic kidney disease (CKD), or volume depletion. Renal function should be monitored periodically in these patients. The clinician should consider withholding or discontinuing irbesartan in patients who develop a clinically important reduction in renal function while receiving irbesartan. (See Cautions: Renal Effects, in Enalapril 24:32.04.)

Fixed-combination Preparations

When hydrochlorothiazide is used in fixed combination with irbesartan, the usual cautions, precautions, and contraindications associated with hydrochlorothiazide must be considered in addition to those associated with irbesartan. (See Cautions, in the Thiazides General Statement 40:28.20.)

Specific Populations

Pregnancy

Category D. (See Users Guide)

Irbesartan can cause fetal and neonatal morbidity and mortality when administered to a pregnant woman. Irbesartan should be discontinued as soon as possible when pregnancy is detected. (See Fetal/Neonatal Morbidity and Mortality under Warnings/Precautions: Warnings, in Cautions.)

Lactation

Irbesartan is distributed into milk in rats; it is not known whether the drug is distributed into human milk. Because of the potential risk in nursing infants, a decision should be made whether to discontinue nursing or the drug.

Pediatric Use

If oliguria or hypotension occurs in neonates with a history of in utero exposure to irbesartan, blood pressure and renal function should be supported; exchange transfusions or dialysis may be required. (See Fetal/Neonatal Morbidity and Mortality under Warnings/Precautions: Warnings, in Cautions.)

Administration of irbesartan in dosages of up to 4.5 mg/kg once daily did not appear to effectively lower blood pressure in pediatric patients 6–16 years of age. Safety and efficacy of irbesartan in children younger than 6 years of age have not been established.

Safety and efficacy of the fixed-combination preparation containing irbesartan and hydrochlorothiazide in pediatric patients have not been established.

For information on overall principles and expert recommendations for treatment of hypertension in pediatric patients, see Uses: Hypertension in Pediatric Patients, in the Thiazides General Statement 40:28.20.

Geriatric Use

No substantial differences in safety or efficacy of irbesartan monotherapy or fixed-combination irbesartan/hydrochlorothiazide tablets have been observed in geriatric patients relative to younger adults, but increased sensitivity cannot be ruled out.

Renal Impairment

Irbesartan should be used with caution in patients with renal impairment.

Deterioration of renal function may occur in patients receiving irbesartan.

Use of irbesartan in fixed combination with hydrochlorothiazide is *not* recommended in patients with severe renal impairment.

Black Patients

Blood pressure reduction may be smaller in black patients compared with nonblack patients; clinicians should consider using irbesartan in combination with a diuretic or calcium-channel blocker.

● Common Adverse Effects

Adverse effects occurring in at least 1% of patients with hypertension receiving irbesartan and at a higher incidence than with placebo in clinical trials include diarrhea, dyspepsia/heartburn, and fatigue. In patients receiving irbesartan for the treatment of diabetic nephropathy, dizziness, orthostatic dizziness, and orthostatic hypotension occurred with an incidence of at least 5% and were reported more frequently than in those receiving placebo.

DRUG INTERACTIONS

● Agents that Increase Serum Potassium

Concomitant administration of irbesartan with potassium-sparing diuretics, potassium supplements, potassium-containing salt substitutes, or other drugs that increase serum potassium concentrations may result in hyperkalemia. Serum potassium concentrations should be monitored in such patients.

● Drugs Affecting Hepatic Microsomal Enzymes

Metabolized principally by cytochrome P-450 (CYP) 2C9 isoenzyme. Does not substantially induce or inhibit CYP1A1, 1A2, 2A6, 2B6, 2D6, 2E1, or 3A4. Potential pharmacokinetic interaction (decreased irbesartan metabolism) with CYP2C9 inhibitors.

● Drugs that Block the Renin-Angiotensin System

Increased risk of hypotension, hyperkalemia, and changes in renal function (e.g., renal impairment) with concomitant use of other drugs that block the renin-angiotensin system (e.g., angiotensin-converting enzyme [ACE] inhibitors, angiotensin II receptor antagonists, aliskiren); when irbesartan is used concomitantly with such drugs, blood pressure, renal function, and serum electrolyte concentrations should be monitored closely. The manufacturer states that most patients do not derive additional benefit from combination therapy with 2 renin-angiotensin system inhibitors compared with monotherapy. Concomitant use of irbesartan and aliskiren is contraindicated in patients with diabetes mellitus; in addition, such concomitant use should be avoided in patients with renal impairment (glomerular filtration rate [GFR] less than 60 mL/minute). (See Use in Combination with Angiotensin-converting Enzyme Inhibitors or Angiotensin II Receptor Antagonists under Warnings/Precautions: Other Warnings and Precautions, in Cautions in Aliskiren Hemifumarate 24:32.40.)

● Digoxin

Pharmacologic and/or pharmacokinetic interactions unlikely when irbesartan is used concomitantly with digoxin.

● Hydrochlorothiazide

Pharmacokinetic interactions unlikely when irbesartan is used concomitantly with hydrochlorothiazide.

Additive hypotensive effects expected when irbesartan is used concomitantly with hydrochlorothiazide.

● Lithium

Elevations in lithium concentrations and lithium toxicity have been reported when irbesartan is used concomitantly with lithium. Serum lithium concentrations should be carefully monitored.

● Nifedipine

Decreased irbesartan metabolism in vitro observed with nifedipine; alteration of irbesartan pharmacokinetics not observed in vivo when irbesartan is used concomitantly with nifedipine.

● Nonsteroidal Anti-inflammatory Agents

Possible deterioration of renal function in geriatric, volume-depleted (including those receiving concomitant diuretic therapy), or renally impaired patients; renal function should be monitored periodically in patients receiving concomitant therapy with irbesartan and a nonsteroidal anti-inflammatory agent (NSAIA), including selective cyclooxygenase-2 (COX-2) inhibitors.

Potential pharmacologic interaction (attenuated hypotensive effects) when angiotensin II receptor antagonists are used concomitantly with NSAIAs, including selective COX-29 inhibitors.

● Tolbutamide

Possible decreased irbesartan metabolism when irbesartan is used concomitantly with tolbutamide.

● Warfarin

Pharmacologic and/or pharmacokinetic interaction unlikely when irbesartan is used concomitantly with warfarin.

DESCRIPTION

Irbesartan, a nonpeptide tetrazole derivative, is an angiotensin II type 1 (AT_1) receptor antagonist. Irbesartan has pharmacologic actions similar to those of losartan; however, unlike losartan, irbesartan is not a prodrug and its pharmacologic activity does not depend on hydrolysis in the liver.

Irbesartan blocks the physiologic actions of angiotensin II, including vasoconstrictor and aldosterone-secreting effects, by selectively inhibiting access of angiotensin II to AT_1 receptors within many tissues, including vascular smooth muscle and the adrenal gland. By comparison, angiotensin-converting enzyme (ACE, kininase II) inhibitors block the conversion of angiotensin I to angiotensin II; however, the blockade of angiotensin II production by ACE inhibitors is not complete since the vasopressor hormone can be formed via other enzymes that are not blocked by ACE inhibitors. Because irbesartan, unlike ACE inhibitors, does not inhibit ACE, the drug does not interfere with response to bradykinins and substance P; a beneficial consequence is the absence of certain ACE inhibitor-induced adverse effects (e.g., cough), but possible renal and/or cardioprotective effects may be sacrificed.

ADVICE TO PATIENTS

Importance of informing women of risks of use during pregnancy. Importance of women informing clinicians if they plan to become pregnant or plan to breastfeed. All women of childbearing potential should be advised to report pregnancy to their clinician as soon as possible. See Fetal/Neonatal Morbidity and Mortality under Warnings/Precautions: Warnings, in Cautions.

Importance of informing clinicians of existing or contemplated concomitant therapy, including prescription and OTC drugs.

Importance of informing patients of other important precautionary information. (See Cautions.)

PREPARATIONS

Excipients in commercially available drug preparations may have clinically important effects in some individuals; consult specific product labeling for details.

Irbesartan

Oral

Tablets	75 mg	**Avapro®**, Sanofi-Aventis
	150 mg	**Avapro®**, Sanofi-Aventis
	300 mg	**Avapro®**, Sanofi-Aventis

Irbesartan Combinations

Oral

Tablets	150 mg with Hydrochlorothiazide 12.5 mg	**Avalide®**, Sanofi-Aventis
	300 mg with Hydrochlorothiazide 12.5 mg	**Avalide®**, Sanofi-Aventis

† Use is not currently included in the labeling approved by the US Food and Drug Administration.

Selected Revisions November 5, 2018, © Copyright, June 1, 1998, American Society of Health-System Pharmacists, Inc.

Losartan Potassium

24:32.08 • ANGIOTENSIN II RECEPTOR ANTAGONISTS

■ Losartan potassium, a nonpeptide tetrazole derivative, is an angiotensin II type 1 (AT_1) receptor antagonist (also referred to as an angiotensin II receptor blocker [ARB]).

USES

● Hypertension

Losartan is used alone or in combination with other classes of antihypertensive agents, including diuretics, in the management of hypertension.

Angiotensin II receptor antagonists, such as losartan, are considered one of several preferred antihypertensive drugs for the initial management of hypertension according to current evidence-based hypertension guidelines; other preferred options include angiotensin-converting enzyme (ACE) inhibitors, calcium-channel blockers, and thiazide diuretics. While there may be individual differences with respect to recommendations for initial drug selection and use in specific patient populations, current evidence indicates that these antihypertensive drug classes all generally produce comparable effects on overall mortality and cardiovascular, cerebrovascular, and renal outcomes. (See Uses: Hypertension, in Valsartan 24:32.08.)

Angiotensin II receptor antagonists or ACE inhibitors may be particularly useful in the management of hypertension in patients with certain coexisting conditions such as diabetes mellitus or chronic kidney disease (CKD); angiotensin II receptor antagonists also may be preferred, generally as an alternative to ACE inhibitors, in hypertensive patients with heart failure or ischemic heart disease and/or following myocardial infarction (MI). (See Uses: Hypertension, in Valsartan 24:32.08.)

In patients with hypertension and compelling indications (e.g., CKD with albuminuria [urine albumin 300 mg/day or greater, or urine albumin:creatinine ratio of 300 mg/g or equivalent in the first morning void]), angiotensin II receptor antagonists are usually considered an alternative for ACE inhibitor-intolerant patients. However, data indicate no difference in efficacy between ACE inhibitors and angiotensin II receptor antagonists with regard to blood pressure lowering and clinical outcomes (i.e., all-cause mortality, cardiovascular mortality, MI, heart failure, stroke, and end-stage renal disease). Adverse events (e.g., cough, angioedema) leading to drug discontinuance occur more frequently with ACE inhibitor therapy than with angiotensin II receptor antagonist therapy. Because of similar efficacy and a lower frequency of adverse effects, some experts believe that angiotensin II receptor antagonists should be used instead of an ACE inhibitor for the treatment of hypertension or hypertension with certain compelling indications.

Efficacy of losartan in the treatment of hypertension was established in placebo-controlled studies of 6–12 weeks' duration in patients with hypertension (baseline diastolic blood pressure: 95–115 mm Hg). In these patients, losartan potassium dosages of 50–150 mg once daily were associated with mean decreases in systolic blood pressure of 5.5–10.5 mm Hg and diastolic blood pressure of 3.5–7.5 mm Hg. Daily dosages of 150 mg did not result in greater decreases in blood pressure compared with daily dosages of 50–100 mg. Larger decreases in trough blood pressures were observed with twice-daily dosing compared with once daily dosing in patients receiving daily dosages of 50–100 mg. Rebound hypertension following abrupt withdrawal of the drug has not been reported.

Most patients with hypertension, especially black patients, will require at least 2 antihypertensive drugs to achieve adequate blood pressure control. Like ACE inhibitors, angiotensin II receptor antagonists such as losartan may produce a smaller blood pressure response in hypertensive black patients compared with nonblack patients. However, the combination of an ACE inhibitor or an angiotensin II receptor antagonist with a calcium-channel blocker or thiazide diuretic produces similar blood pressure lowering in black patients as in other racial groups. (See Race under Hypertension: Other Special Considerations for Antihypertensive Drug Therapy, in Uses in Valsartan 24:32.08.)

For additional information on the management of hypertension, see Uses: Hypertension, in Valsartan 24:32.08. For information on overall principles and expert recommendations for treatment of hypertension, see Uses: Hypertension in Adults and also see Uses: Hypertension in Pediatric Patients, in the Thiazides General Statement 40:28.20.

● Prevention of Cardiovascular Morbidity and Mortality

Losartan is used alone or in combination with other antihypertensive agents (e.g., hydrochlorothiazide) to reduce the risk of stroke in patients with hypertension and left ventricular hypertrophy; however, there is evidence that the benefit associated with such losartan-based antihypertensive therapy does not apply to black patients. In a randomized, double-blind, comparative study (Losartan Intervention for Endpoint [LIFE] reduction in hypertension) of approximately 4 years' duration in more than 9000 patients, losartan-based antihypertensive therapy (e.g., losartan 50–100 mg with hydrochlorothiazide 12.5–25 mg daily) reduced the risk of the primary outcome of combined cardiovascular death, stroke, and myocardial infarction (relative risk reduction of about 13%, adjusted for Framingham risk score and baseline left ventricular hypertrophy) compared with atenolol-containing therapy (e.g., atenolol 50–100 mg with hydrochlorothiazide 12.5–25 mg daily) despite similar control of blood pressure with each regimen. In addition, the rate of drug-related adverse events and the incidence of new-onset diabetes mellitus was less in patients receiving losartan-based therapy. The study population consisted primarily of white patients 55–80 years of age with ECG evidence of left ventricular hypertrophy but who did not have low left-ventricular ejection fraction (40% or less) or heart failure. The results of the study provided no evidence that the benefits of losartan in reducing the risk of cardiovascular events in patients with hypertension and left ventricular hypertrophy apply to black patients. Among black patients in the study, the risk of experiencing the primary outcome of combined cardiovascular death, stroke, and myocardial infarction was lower in patients receiving atenolol (11%) than in patients receiving losartan (17%).

Subgroup analysis of the LIFE study (mean follow-up 4.7 years) suggests that aspirin therapy at baseline in patients receiving losartan reduced the risk of the primary outcome of combined cardiovascular death, stroke, and myocardial infarction (relative risk reduction of about 32%, adjusted for Framingham risk score and baseline left ventricular hypertrophy) compared with aspirin therapy at baseline in patients receiving atenolol, despite similar control of blood pressure with each regimen. Further studies are needed to determine whether these differences are associated with a pharmacologic interaction or a selection by aspirin use of patients more likely to respond to losartan therapy.

● Diabetic Nephropathy

Losartan is used in the management of diabetic nephropathy manifested by elevated serum creatinine and proteinuria (urinary albumin to creatinine ratio of 300 mg/g or greater) in patients with type 2 diabetes mellitus and hypertension.

Both angiotensin II receptor antagonists and ACE inhibitors have been shown to slow the rate of progression of renal disease in patients with diabetes mellitus and persistent albuminuria, and use of a drug from either class is recommended in such patients with modestly elevated (30–300 mg/24 hours) or higher (exceeding 300 mg/24 hours) levels of urinary albumin excretion. Some evidence suggests that these drugs may slow the progression of nephropathy by a mechanism independent of their antihypertensive effects.

Comparative trials evaluating the efficacy of angiotensin II receptor antagonists and ACE inhibitors for improving renal outcomes in diabetic patients are lacking. Evidence supporting use of ACE inhibitors generally is based on studies in patients with type 1 diabetes mellitus, while evidence supporting use of angiotensin II receptor antagonists generally is based on studies in patients with type 2 diabetes mellitus. Findings from these studies indicate that both drug classes delay progression of increased urinary albumin excretion in patients with diabetes mellitus and also may slow the decline in renal function. Because the available data are consistent, some experts suggest that the effects of both drug classes in improving renal outcomes in patients with diabetes mellitus and proteinuria are likely to be similar.

Drugs that inhibit the renin-angiotensin system (i.e., ACE inhibitors, angiotensin II receptor antagonists) also have been shown to delay the onset of albuminuria in patients with type 2 diabetes mellitus and hypertension who have normal levels of urinary albumin excretion†; however, some experts state that in the absence of albuminuria, the risk of progressive kidney disease is low. The American Diabetes Association (ADA) states that the use of an ACE inhibitor or angiotensin II receptor antagonist is not recommended for the primary prevention of diabetic nephropathy in patients with diabetes mellitus who are normotensive, have normal levels of urinary protein excretion, and have a normal glomerular filtration rate (GFR).

Combined therapy with ACE inhibitors and angiotensin II receptor antagonists provides no additional cardiovascular benefit and increases the risk of adverse effects (e.g., impaired renal function, hyperkalemia). The usual precautions of angiotensin II receptor antagonist therapy in patients with substantial renal impairment should be observed.

The current labeled indication for losartan in hypertensive patients with type 2 diabetes mellitus and nephropathy (indicated by an elevated serum creatinine and urinary albumin to creatinine ratio of 300 mg/g or greater) is based principally on the results of a long-term (mean duration of follow-up: 3.4 years), multicenter, placebo-controlled trial, the Reduction of Endpoints in NIDDM with the Angiotensin II Receptor Antagonist Losartan (RENAAL) study. In the RENAAL trial, therapy with losartan potassium (50 mg daily initially and titrated to 100 mg daily) reduced the risk of the primary composite clinical end point, which was defined as a doubling of the baseline serum creatinine concentration, end-stage renal disease (i.e., need for dialysis or renal transplantation), or death, by 16% compared with placebo. Additional antihypertensive agents (diuretics, calcium-channel blocking agents, α- or β-adrenergic blocking agents (β-blockers), and/or centrally acting agents) were used as needed in all treatment groups to achieve a trough blood pressure of less than 140/90 mm Hg in the sitting position; ACE inhibitors and other angiotensin II receptor antagonists could not be used. Most of the delay in time to occurrence of composite clinical events seen with losartan-containing therapy was the result of a reduction in the risk of doubling serum creatinine concentration and end-stage renal disease (25 and 28% reductions, respectively); losartan-containing therapy had no appreciable effect on overall mortality. Similar mean blood pressures were achieved with losartan or placebo plus conventional antihypertensive therapy.

● Heart Failure

Angiotensin II receptor antagonists have been used in the management of heart failure†.

Current guidelines for the management of heart failure in adults generally recommend a combination of drug therapies to reduce morbidity and mortality, including neurohormonal antagonists (e.g., ACE inhibitors, angiotensin II receptor antagonists, angiotensin receptor-neprilysin inhibitors [ARNIs], β-blockers, aldosterone receptor antagonists) that inhibit the detrimental compensatory mechanisms in heart failure. Additional agents (e.g., cardiac glycosides, diuretics, sinoatrial modulators [i.e., ivabradine]) added to a heart failure treatment regimen in selected patients have been associated with symptomatic improvement and/or reduction in heart failure-related hospitalizations. Experts recommend that all asymptomatic patients with reduced left ventricular ejection fraction (LVEF) (American College of Cardiology Foundation [ACCF]/American Heart Association [AHA] stage B heart failure) receive therapy with an ACE inhibitor and β-blocker to prevent symptomatic heart failure and reduce morbidity and mortality. In patients with prior or current symptoms of chronic heart failure with reduced LVEF (ACCF/AHA stage C heart failure), ACCF, AHA, and the Heart Failure Society of America (HFSA) recommend inhibition of the renin-angiotensin-aldosterone (RAA) system with an ACE inhibitor, angiotensin II receptor antagonist, or ARNI in conjunction with a β-blocker, and an aldosterone antagonist in selected patients, to reduce morbidity and mortality. While ACE inhibitors have been the preferred drugs for inhibition of the RAA system because of their established benefits in patients with heart failure and reduced ejection fraction, some evidence indicates that therapy with sacubitril/valsartan, an ARNI, may be more effective than ACE inhibitor therapy (enalapril) in reducing cardiovascular death and heart failure-related hospitalization. ACCF, AHA, and HFSA recommend that patients with chronic symptomatic heart failure and reduced LVEF (New York Heart Association [NYHA] functional class II or III) who are able to tolerate an ACE inhibitor or angiotensin II receptor antagonist be switched to therapy containing an ARNI to further reduce morbidity and mortality. However, in patients in whom an ARNI is not appropriate, continued use of an ACE inhibitor for all classes of heart failure with reduced ejection fraction remains strongly advised. In patients in whom an ARNI or ACE inhibitor is not appropriate, an angiotensin II receptor antagonist may be used. For additional information on the use of angiotensin II receptor antagonists in the management of heart failure, see Uses: Heart Failure, in Valsartan 24:32.08 and in Candesartan 24:32.08. For further information on the use of ARNIs in patients with heart failure, see Uses: Heart Failure, in Sacubitril and Valsartan 24:32.92.

Several clinical trials have evaluated the use of angiotensin II receptor antagonists as add-on therapy to conventional regimens including an ACE inhibitor, as add-on therapy to conventional regimens compared with an ACE inhibitor, as combination therapy with an ACE inhibitor compared with therapy with either type of agent alone, or as an alternative therapy in patients intolerant of ACE inhibitors. Data from these and other long-term placebo-controlled clinical trials indicate that angiotensin II receptor antagonists produce hemodynamic and neurohormonal effects associated with their suppression of the renin-angiotensin system; reduced hospitalizations and mortality also have been demonstrated. However, in some studies, these drugs did not show consistent effects on cardiac symptoms or exercise tolerance.

In one comparative study (Evaluation of Losartan in the Elderly [ELITE]) in geriatric patients 65 years of age and older who received losartan (up to 50 mg daily) or captopril (up to 150 mg daily) in addition to conventional therapy for 48 weeks, patients receiving losartan had a 46% lower risk of death and also experienced a lower incidence of adverse effects than those receiving captopril. However, after interim analysis of data, the difference in survival was no longer significant and no difference in morbidity and mortality or frequency in hospitalizations for heart failure was found between the 2 therapies. Results of a follow-up study (ELITE II), failed to confirm a survival benefit for losartan therapy compared with captopril. In this study, losartan did not provide a statistically significant difference in reduction of overall death, sudden cardiac death, and/or resuscitated cardiac arrest compared with captopril, although ELITE II was not designed to demonstrate equivalence between the 2 therapies. For additional details on the use of angiotensin II receptor antagonists in the management of heart failure, see Uses: Heart Failure, in Valsartan 24:32.08 and in Candesartan 24:32.08.

While angiotensin II receptor antagonists are considered reasonable alternatives in patients who are unable to tolerate ACE inhibitors (e.g., because of cough or angioedema), angioedema, including swelling of the larynx and glottis (causing airway obstruction) and/or swelling of the face, lips, pharynx, and/or tongue, has been reported rarely during postmarketing experience in patients receiving losartan. The manufacturer states that some of these patients had a history of angioedema associated with other drugs (e.g., ACE inhibitors). (See Sensitivity Reactions under Cautions: Warnings/Precautions.)

DOSAGE AND ADMINISTRATION

● Administration

Losartan is administered orally. Although food may decrease the rate of absorption of losartan and peak concentrations achieved, the magnitude of effect is not clinically important; the manufacturer states that the drug can be given without regard to meals.

For pediatric patients or patients unable to swallow tablets, losartan may be administered orally as an extemporaneously prepared suspension. An extemporaneous suspension containing losartan potassium 2.5 mg/mL can be prepared in the following manner. First, 10 mL of purified water is added to a 240-mL amber polyethylene terephthalate (PET) bottle containing ten 50-mg tablets of losartan potassium, and the contents are shaken for at least 2 minutes. The concentrated suspension should be allowed to stand for 60 minutes following reconstitution, and then should be shaken for an additional minute. A mixture containing equal parts (by volume) of syrup (Ora-Sweet SF®) and suspending vehicle (Ora-Plus®) should be prepared separately. The concentrated suspension of losartan should be diluted with 190 mL of the Ora-Sweet SF® and Ora-Plus® mixture, and the container then shaken an additional minute to disperse the ingredients. The suspension should be shaken before dispensing of each dose. The extemporaneous suspension is stable for up to 4 weeks when stored at 2–8°C.

● Dosage

Available as losartan potassium; dosage expressed in terms of the salt.

Hypertension

Dosage of losartan potassium must be individualized and adjusted according to blood pressure response. Substantial therapeutic response to losartan generally occurs within 1 week of treatment initiation, but in some studies the maximum therapeutic response occurred in 3–6 weeks.

Losartan Therapy

The manufacturer states that the usual initial dosage of losartan potassium in adults is 50 mg daily; lower initial dosages (e.g., 25 mg daily) may be used in patients with possible depletion of intravascular volume, including those receiving a diuretic, or with hepatic impairment. (See Dosage and Administration: Special Populations.) The manufacturer states that the usual maintenance dosage is

25–100 mg daily given in 1 dose or 2 divided doses. Some experts state that the usual dosage range is 50–100 mg daily, given in 1 dose or 2 divided doses.

The usual initial dosage of losartan potassium in children 6 years of age and older is 0.7 mg/kg (up to 50 mg) once daily. Some experts state that the dosage may be increased every 2–4 weeks until blood pressure is controlled, the maximum dosage is reached, or adverse effects occur. The safety and efficacy of dosages exceeding 1.4 mg/kg or in excess of 100 mg daily have not been established. For information on overall principles and expert recommendations for treatment of hypertension in pediatric patients, see Uses: Hypertension in Pediatric Patients, in the Thiazides General Statement 40:28.20.

Losartan/Hydrochlorothiazide Fixed-combination Therapy

In patients who do not respond adequately to monotherapy with losartan or, alternatively, with hydrochlorothiazide, combined therapy with the drugs can be used. When combination therapy is necessary, the commercially available preparation containing losartan in fixed combination with hydrochlorothiazide generally should not be used initially. Dosage preferably should first be adjusted by titrating the dosage of each drug separately; if it is determined that the optimum maintenance dosage corresponds to the ratio in the commercial combination preparation, this product may be used. Alternatively, the manufacturer states that combined therapy can be initiated with the commercially available preparation in patients whose blood pressure is not adequately controlled with losartan monotherapy or with 25 mg daily of hydrochlorothiazide alone, in those in whom control is maintained but hypokalemia is problematic at this hydrochlorothiazide dosage, or in those with severe hypertension in whom the potential benefit of achieving prompt blood pressure control outweighs the potential risk of initiating therapy with the commercially available fixed combination. In such patients, the manufacturer states that combination therapy can be initiated with 50 mg of losartan potassium and 12.5 mg of hydrochlorothiazide daily as the fixed combination. In patients whose blood pressure is not adequately controlled with losartan 100 mg monotherapy, combination therapy can be initiated with 100 mg of losartan potassium and 12.5 mg of hydrochlorothiazide once daily as the fixed combination. If blood pressure is not controlled after about 3 weeks (or after 2–4 weeks of therapy in those with severe hypertension), dosage may be increased to 100 mg of losartan potassium and 25 mg of hydrochlorothiazide daily (administered as 2 tablets of the fixed combination containing 50 mg of losartan potassium and 12.5 mg of hydrochlorothiazide, or, alternatively, as 1 tablet of the fixed combination containing 100 mg of losartan potassium and 25 mg of hydrochlorothiazide). Additional increases using the fixed combination are not recommended. The fixed combination is *not* recommended for use in patients with creatinine clearances of 30 mL/minute or less, those with hepatic impairment, or those with intravascular volume depletion (e.g., patients receiving diuretics). (See Dosage and Administration: Special Populations.)

Blood Pressure Monitoring and Treatment Goals

Blood pressure should be monitored regularly (i.e., monthly) during therapy and dosage of the antihypertensive drug adjusted until blood pressure is controlled. If an adequate blood pressure response is not achieved with angiotensin II receptor antagonist monotherapy, the dosage may be increased or another antihypertensive agent with demonstrated benefit and preferably with a complementary mechanism of action (e.g., calcium-channel blocker, thiazide diuretic) may be added; if target blood pressure is still not achieved, a third drug may be added. (See Uses: Hypertension.) In patients who develop unacceptable adverse effects with losartan, the drug should be discontinued and another antihypertensive agent from a different pharmacologic class should be initiated.

The goal of hypertension management and prevention is to achieve and maintain optimal control of blood pressure. However, the optimum blood pressure threshold for initiating antihypertensive drug therapy and specific treatment goals remain controversial. While previous hypertension guidelines have based target blood pressure goals on age and comorbidities, the 2017 ACC/AHA hypertension guideline incorporates underlying cardiovascular risk into decision making regarding treatment and generally recommends the same target blood pressure (i.e., less than 130/80 mm Hg) in all adults. Many patients will require at least 2 drugs from different pharmacologic classes to achieve their blood pressure goal; the potential benefits of hypertension management and drug cost, adverse effects, and risks associated with the use of multiple antihypertensive drugs also should be considered when deciding a patient's blood pressure treatment goal.

For additional information on target levels of blood pressure and on monitoring therapy in the management of hypertension, see Blood Pressure Monitoring and Treatment Goals under Dosage: Hypertension, in Dosage and Administration in the Thiazides General Statement 40:28.20.

Diabetic Nephropathy

For the management of diabetic nephropathy in patients with type 2 diabetes mellitus, the usual initial adult dosage of losartan potassium is 50 mg once daily. Dosage of losartan potassium may be increased to 100 mg once daily based on blood pressure response. In a large clinical trial, approximately 72% of patients had dosage titrated from 50 mg daily initially up to 100 mg daily and maintained that dosage for more than 50% of the study period.

Prevention of Cardiovascular Morbidity and Mortality

When losartan potassium is used to reduce the risk of stroke in high-risk patients with hypertension and left ventricular hypertrophy, the usual starting dose is 50 mg once daily. Treatment should be adjusted based on blood pressure response. Adjustment of therapy, when indicated, should include the addition of hydrochlorothiazide 12.5 mg daily and/or an increase in losartan potassium dosage to 100 mg daily; subsequently, the hydrochlorothiazide dosage may be increased to 25 mg once daily. Alternatively, the fixed combination containing losartan potassium and hydrochlorothiazide may be used at the appropriate dosage.

Heart Failure

In patients with prior or current symptoms of heart failure† and reduced left ventricular ejection fraction (LVEF) (American College of Cardiology Foundation [ACCF]/American Heart Association [AHA] stage C heart failure), ACCF and AHA recommend an initial losartan potassium dosage of 25–50 mg once daily. Blood pressure (including postural blood pressure changes), renal function, and serum potassium concentrations should be reevaluated within 1–2 weeks after initiation of therapy, and these parameters should be monitored closely after changes in dosage. ACCF and AHA recommend a maximum losartan potassium dosage of 50–150 mg once daily for patients with ACCF/AHA stage C heart failure.

● Special Populations

The manufacturer recommends that patients with depletion of intravascular volume (e.g., patients receiving treatment with a diuretic) should have this condition corrected prior to initiation of losartan potassium therapy, or alternatively, therapy should be initiated using a lower initial dosage (25 mg once daily). The manufacturer states that modification of losartan potassium dosage is not necessary for geriatric patients nor for other adults with renal impairment, including those undergoing hemodialysis. In patients with hepatic impairment, the manufacturer recommends that therapy be initiated with a lower dosage of losartan potassium (25 mg once daily).

The commercially available preparation containing losartan in fixed combination with hydrochlorothiazide is not recommended for patients with renal impairment whose creatinine clearance is less than 30 mL/minute, and such preparations should be used with caution in patients with hepatic impairment. The commercially available preparation containing losartan potassium in fixed combination with hydrochlorothiazide is not recommended for initial titration in patients with hepatic impairment, because the appropriate starting dose of losartan potassium (25 mg once daily) is not available as a fixed-ratio preparation.

CAUTIONS

● Contraindications

Known hypersensitivity to losartan or any ingredient in the formulation.

Concomitant therapy with aliskiren in patients with diabetes mellitus. (See Drug Interactions: Drugs that Block the Renin-Angiotensin System.)

● Warnings/Precautions

Warnings

Fetal/Neonatal Morbidity and Mortality

Drugs that act on the renin-angiotensin system (e.g., angiotensin-converting enzyme [ACE] inhibitors, angiotensin II receptor antagonists, aliskiren) reduce fetal renal function and increase fetal and neonatal morbidity and mortality when administered during pregnancy during the second and third trimesters. Resulting oligohydramnios can be associated with fetal lung hypoplasia and skeletal deformations. Potential neonatal effects include skull hypoplasia, anuria, hypotension, renal failure, and death. Losartan should be discontinued as soon as possible when pregnancy is detected, unless continued use is considered life-saving. Nearly all women can be transferred successfully to alternative therapy for the remainder of their pregnancy. For additional information on the risk of such drugs (i.e., angiotensin II antagonists and ACE inhibitors) during pregnancy, see Cautions: Pregnancy, Fertility, and Lactation, in Captopril 24:32.04 and in Enalaprilat/Enalapril 24:32.04.

Sensitivity Reactions

Sensitivity reactions, including anaphylactoid reactions and/or angioedema, have been reported with use of angiotensin II receptor antagonists, including losartan. Losartan is not recommended in patients with a history of angioedema associated with or unrelated to ACE inhibitor or angiotensin II receptor antagonist therapy.

Other Warnings and Precautions
Hypotension

Symptomatic hypotension has been reported in patients receiving losartan, especially in volume- and/or salt-depleted patients (e.g., those receiving diuretics). (See Dosage and Administration: Special Populations.)

Malignancies

In July 2010, the US Food and Drug Administration (FDA) initiated a safety review of angiotensin II receptor antagonists after a published meta-analysis suggested a possible association between the use of these agents and an increased risk of cancer. The meta-analysis, which combined cancer-related findings from 5 randomized, controlled trials in over 60,000 patients, found a modest but significant increase in the risk of new cancer occurrence in patients receiving an angiotensin II receptor antagonist (mostly telmisartan) compared with those in control groups (7.2 versus 6%, respectively; risk ratio 1.08). However, because of several limitations of the study (e.g., trials included in the meta-analysis were not specifically designed to evaluate cancer outcomes, lack of individual patient data), the validity of these findings has been questioned.

Subsequent studies, including a larger, more comprehensive meta-analysis conducted by FDA, have not shown an increased risk of cancer in patients receiving angiotensin II receptor antagonists. FDA's meta-analysis, which included trial-level data from 31 randomized studies (total of approximately 156,000 patients), found no evidence of an increased risk of cancer in patients who received an angiotensin II receptor antagonist compared with those who received other treatments (placebo or active control). The overall rate of new cancer occurrence was essentially the same in both groups of patients (1.82 and 1.84 cases per 100 patient-years, respectively). In addition, there was no difference in the risk of cancer-related death, breast cancer, lung cancer, or prostate cancer between the groups. Based on these results and a review of all currently available data related to this potential safety concern, FDA has concluded that use of angiotensin II receptor antagonists is not associated with an increased risk of cancer.

Renal Effects

Because the renin-angiotensin-aldosterone (RAA) system appears to contribute substantially to maintenance of glomerular filtration in patients with heart failure in whom renal perfusion is severely compromised, renal function may deteriorate markedly (e.g., oliguria, progressive azotemia, renal failure, death) in these patients during therapy with an ACE inhibitor or an angiotensin II receptor antagonist (e.g., losartan). Increases in BUN and serum creatinine may occur in patients with unilateral or bilateral renal artery stenosis, chronic kidney disease (CKD), or volume depletion. The clinician should consider withholding or discontinuing losartan in patients who develop a clinically important reduction in renal function while receiving losartan. (See Cautions: Renal Effects, in Enalapril 24:32.04.)

Effects on Potassium

Hyperkalemia can develop, especially in patients receiving agents that can increase serum potassium concentration (e.g., potassium-sparing diuretics, potassium supplements, potassium-containing salt substitutes). (See Drug Interactions: Agents that Increase Serum Potassium.)

Fixed-combination Preparations

When losartan is used in fixed combination with hydrochlorothiazide, the cautions, precautions, and contraindications associated with thiazide diuretics must be considered in addition to those associated with losartan.

Specific Populations
Pregnancy

Category D. (See Users Guide.)

Losartan can cause fetal and neonatal morbidity and mortality when administered to a pregnant woman. Losartan should be discontinued as soon as possible when pregnancy is detected. (See Fetal/Neonatal Morbidity and Mortality under Warnings/Precautions: Warnings, in Cautions.)

Lactation

Losartan is distributed into milk in rats; it is not known whether the drug is distributed into human breast milk. A decision should be made whether to discontinue nursing or the drug because of the potential risk in nursing infants.

Pediatric Use

If oliguria or hypotension occurs in neonates with a history of in utero exposure to losartan, blood pressure and renal function should be supported; exchange transfusions or dialysis may be required. (See Fetal/Neonatal Morbidity and Mortality under Warnings/Precautions: Warnings, in Cautions.)

Safety and efficacy of losartan in pediatric patients younger than 6 years of age and in pediatric patients with glomerular filtration rate less than 30 mL/minute per 1.73 m² have not been established. For information on overall principles and expert recommendations for treatment of hypertension in pediatric patients, see Uses: Hypertension in Pediatric Patients, in the Thiazides General Statement 40:28.20.

Geriatric Use

No overall differences in safety and efficacy of losartan for the treatment of hypertension have been observed in geriatric patients relative to younger adults, but increased sensitivity cannot be ruled out.

No overall differences in efficacy with the fixed combination preparation containing losartan and hydrochlorothiazide have been observed in patients 65 years of age or older compared with younger adults. Geriatric patients had a somewhat higher incidence of adverse effects than younger patients; dosage should be selected with caution.

Hepatic Impairment

Systemic exposure to losartan and its active metabolite may be increased in patients with hepatic impairment. Initial dosage adjustment is recommended. (See Losartan Therapy under Dosage: Hypertension, in Dosage and Administration.)

Use of losartan in fixed combination with hydrochlorothiazide is not recommended in patients with hepatic impairment because the dosage of losartan potassium in the fixed-combination tablets exceeds the recommended initial dosage.

Renal Impairment

Deterioration of renal function may occur in patients with renal impairment receiving losartan. (See Renal Effects under Warnings/Precautions: Other Warnings and Precautions, in Cautions.)

Use of losartan in fixed combination with hydrochlorothiazide is not recommended in patients with creatinine clearances of 30 mL/minute or less.

Black Patients

Blood pressure reduction may be smaller in black patients compared with non-black patients; losartan should be used in combination with a diuretic or calcium-channel blocker in such patients.

There is no evidence that the benefits of therapy in reducing the risk of cardiovascular events in hypertensive patients with left ventricular hypertrophy apply to black patients.

● Common Adverse Effects

Adverse effects occurring in at least 1% of patients with hypertension receiving losartan and at a higher incidence than with placebo include upper respiratory infection, dizziness, nasal congestion, back pain, leg pain, muscle cramp, and sinusitis. The incidence of adverse effects was not affected by age, gender, or race. In patients receiving losartan for the treatment of diabetic nephropathy, urinary tract infection, diarrhea, anemia, asthenia/fatigue, hypoglycemia, back pain, chest pain, cough, bronchitis, diabetic vascular disease, influenza-like disease, cataracts, cellulitis, hyperkalemia, hypotension, muscular weakness, sinusitis, gastritis, hypoesthesia, infection, knee pain, and leg pain occurred with an incidence of at least 5% and were reported more frequently than in those receiving placebo.

DRUG INTERACTIONS

● Agents that Increase Serum Potassium

Hyperkalemia may occur with concomitant administration of losartan and potassium-sparing diuretics, potassium supplements, potassium-containing salt substitutes, or other drugs that increase serum potassium concentrations. Serum potassium concentrations should be monitored in patients receiving such concomitant therapy.

● Drugs Affecting Hepatic Microsomal Enzymes

Formation of active metabolite appears to be mediated by cytochrome P-450 (CYP) 2C9 isoenzyme. CYP3A4 apparently contributes to formation of inactive metabolites.

Potential pharmacokinetic interaction (inhibition of the formation of losartan's active metabolite) with CYP2C9 inhibitors. Clinically important interactions unlikely with CYP3A4 inhibitors (possible increased concentration of losartan, but no effects on formation of active metabolite observed).

● Drugs that Block the Renin-Angiotensin System

Increased risk of hypotension, hyperkalemia, and changes in renal function (e.g., renal impairment) with concomitant use of other drugs that block the renin-angiotensin system (e.g., angiotensin-converting enzyme [ACE] inhibitors, angiotensin II receptor antagonists, aliskiren); when losartan is used concomitantly with such drugs, blood pressure, renal function, and serum concentrations of electrolytes should be monitored closely. The manufacturer states that most patients do not derive additional benefit from combination therapy with 2 renin-angiotensin system inhibitors compared with monotherapy. Concomitant use of losartan and aliskiren is contraindicated in patients with diabetes mellitus; in addition, such concomitant use should be avoided in patients with renal impairment (glomerular filtration rate [GFR] less than 60 mL/minute). (See Use in Combination with Angiotensin-converting Enzyme Inhibitors or Angiotensin II Receptor Antagonists under Warnings/Precautions: Other Warnings and Precautions, in Cautions in Aliskiren Hemifumarate 24:32.40.)

● Cimetidine

Pharmacokinetic interactions unlikely when losartan is used concomitantly with cimetidine.

● Digoxin

Pharmacokinetic interactions unlikely when losartan is used concomitantly with digoxin.

● Erythromycin

Clinically important pharmacokinetic interactions unlikely when losartan is used concomitantly with erythromycin.

● Fluconazole

Decreased plasma concentrations of losartan's active metabolite and increased plasma losartan concentrations have been reported when losartan is used concomitantly with fluconazole.

● Hydrochlorothiazide

Pharmacokinetic interactions unlikely when losartan is used concomitantly with hydrochlorothiazide.

Additive hypotensive effects observed when losartan is used concomitantly with hydrochlorothiazide, which is used for therapeutic advantage. (See Uses and see Dosage and Administration: Dosage.)

● Ketoconazole

Conversion of losartan to its active metabolite unaffected when losartan is used concomitantly with ketoconazole.

● Lithium

Lithium excretion may be reduced. Serum lithium concentrations should be carefully monitored.

● Nonsteroidal Anti-inflammatory Agents

Potential pharmacologic interaction (attenuated hypotensive effects) when angiotensin II receptor antagonists are used concomitantly with nonsteroidal anti-inflammatory agents (NSAIAs), including selective cyclooxygenase-2 (COX-2) inhibitors.

Possible deterioration of renal function in geriatric, volume-depleted (including those receiving concomitant diuretic therapy), or renally impaired patients; renal function should be monitored periodically in patients receiving concomitant therapy with losartan and an NSAIA, including selective COX-2 inhibitors.

● Phenobarbital

Pharmacokinetic interactions unlikely when losartan is used concomitantly with phenobarbital.

● Rifampin

Decreased plasma concentrations of losartan and its active metabolite observed when losartan is used concomitantly with rifampin.

● Warfarin

Pharmacokinetic interactions unlikely when losartan is used concomitantly with warfarin.

DESCRIPTION

Losartan, a nonpeptide tetrazole derivative, is an angiotensin II receptor (type AT_1) antagonist. Losartan is a prodrug and requires activation in the liver to exert its pharmacologic activity. Losartan's active carboxylic acid metabolite is 10 to 40 times more potent by weight than losartan and appears to be a reversible, noncompetitive inhibitor of the AT_1 receptor.

Losartan blocks the physiologic actions of angiotensin II, including vasoconstrictor and aldosterone-secreting effects. Losartan does not interfere with response to bradykinins and does not share the angiotensin-converting enzyme (ACE) inhibitor common adverse effect of dry cough. For additional information on the pharmacology of angiotensin II receptor antagonists, see Description in Irbesartan 24:32.08.

ADVICE TO PATIENTS

Importance of advising patients not to use potassium supplements or salt substitutes containing potassium without consulting their clinician.

Importance of informing women of risks of use during pregnancy. Importance of women informing clinicians if they are or plan to become pregnant or to breast-feed. All women of childbearing potential should be advised to report pregnancy to their clinician as soon as possible. (See Fetal/Neonatal Morbidity and Mortality under Warnings/Precautions: Warnings, in Cautions.)

Importance of informing clinicians of existing or contemplated concomitant therapy, including prescription and OTC drugs (including salt substitutes containing potassium).

Importance of informing patients of other important precautionary information. (See Cautions.)

PREPARATIONS

Excipients in commercially available drug preparations may have clinically important effects in some individuals; consult specific product labeling for details.

Losartan Potassium

Oral

Tablets, film-coated	25 mg	Cozaar®, Merck
	50 mg	Cozaar®, Merck
	100 mg	Cozaar®, Merck

Losartan Potassium Combinations

Oral

Tablets, film-coated	50 mg with Hydrochlorothiazide 12.5 mg	Hyzaar®, Merck
	100 mg with Hydrochlorothiazide 12.5 mg	Hyzaar®, Merck
	100 mg with Hydrochlorothiazide 25 mg	Hyzaar®, Merck

† Use is not currently included in the labeling approved by the US Food and Drug Administration.

Olmesartan Medoxomil

24:32.08 • ANGIOTENSIN II RECEPTOR ANTAGONISTS

■ Olmesartan medoxomil is a nonpeptide, benzimidazole derivative angiotensin II type 1 (AT$_1$) receptor antagonist (also referred to as an angiotensin II receptor blocker [ARB]).

USES

● Hypertension

Olmesartan medoxomil is used alone or in combination with other classes of antihypertensive agents in the management of hypertension.

Angiotensin II receptor antagonists, such as olmesartan medoxomil, are considered one of several preferred antihypertensive drugs for the initial management of hypertension according to current evidence-based hypertension guidelines; other preferred options include angiotensin-converting enzyme (ACE) inhibitors, calcium-channel blockers, and thiazide diuretics. While there may be individual differences with respect to recommendations for initial drug selection and use in specific patient populations, current evidence indicates that these antihypertensive drug classes all generally produce comparable effects on overall mortality and cardiovascular, cerebrovascular, and renal outcomes. (See Uses: Hypertension, in Valsartan 24:32.08.)

Angiotensin II receptor antagonists or ACE inhibitors may be particularly useful in the management of hypertension in patients with certain coexisting conditions such as diabetes mellitus or chronic kidney disease (CKD); angiotensin II receptor antagonists also may be preferred, generally as an alternative to ACE inhibitors, in hypertensive patients with heart failure or ischemic heart disease, and/or following myocardial infarction (MI). (See Uses: Hypertension, in Valsartan 24:32.08.)

In patients with hypertension and compelling indications (e.g., CKD with albuminuria [urine albumin 300 mg/day or greater, or urine albumin:creatinine ratio of 300 mg/g or equivalent in the first morning void]), angiotensin II receptor antagonists are usually considered an alternative for ACE inhibitor-intolerant patients. However, data indicate no difference in efficacy between ACE inhibitors and angiotensin II receptor antagonists with regard to blood pressure lowering and clinical outcomes (i.e., all-cause mortality, cardiovascular mortality, MI, heart failure, stroke, and end-stage renal disease). Adverse events (e.g., cough, angioedema) leading to drug discontinuance occur more frequently with ACE inhibitor therapy than with angiotensin II receptor antagonist therapy. Because of similar efficacy and a lower frequency of adverse effects, some experts believe that angiotensin II receptor antagonists should be used instead of an ACE inhibitor for the treatment of hypertension or hypertension with certain compelling indications.

Efficacy of olmesartan medoxomil in the treatment of hypertension has been established in several placebo-controlled studies of 6–12 weeks' duration in patients with mild to moderate hypertension. In these patients, usual dosages of olmesartan medoxomil (20–40 mg administered once daily) decreased placebo-corrected systolic blood pressure by about 10–12 mm Hg and diastolic blood pressure by about 6–7 mm Hg 24 hours after dosing. There was no evidence of tachyphylaxis during long-term (e.g., 1 year) olmesartan therapy, and rebound hypertension following abrupt withdrawal of the drug has not been reported. Clinical studies have shown that the hypotensive effect of olmesartan in patients with mild to moderate hypertension is greater than that of placebo and comparable to or greater than that of captopril, irbesartan, losartan, and valsartan. In addition, olmesartan appears to be as effective as atenolol when used in conjunction with hydrochlorothiazide in the treatment of patients with moderate to severe hypertension.

Most patients with hypertension, especially black patients, will require at least 2 antihypertensive drugs to achieve adequate blood pressure control. Like ACE inhibitors, angiotensin II receptor antagonists such as olmesartan may produce a smaller blood pressure response in hypertensive black patients compared with nonblack patients. (See Race under Hypertension: Other Special Considerations for Antihypertensive Drug Therapy, in Uses in Valsartan 24:32.08.)

For additional information on the management of hypertension, see Uses: Hypertension, in Valsartan 24:32.08. For information on overall principles and expert recommendations for treatment of hypertension, see Uses: Hypertension in Adults and also see Uses: Hypertension in Pediatric Patients, in the Thiazides General Statement 40:28.20.

● Diabetic Nephropathy

Both angiotensin II receptor antagonists and ACE inhibitors have been shown to slow the rate of progression of renal disease in patients with diabetes mellitus and persistent albuminuria†, and use of a drug from either class is recommended in such patients with modestly elevated (30–300 mg/24 hours) or higher (exceeding 300 mg/24 hours) levels of urinary albumin excretion. The usual precautions of angiotensin II receptor antagonist or ACE inhibitor therapy in patients with substantial renal impairment should be observed. (See Renal Effects under Warnings/Precautions: Other Warnings and Precautions, in Cautions.) For additional information on the use of angiotensin II receptor antagonists in the treatment of diabetic nephropathy, see Uses: Diabetic Nephropathy, in Losartan 24:32.08 and in Irbesartan 24:32.08.

● Heart Failure

Angiotensin II receptor antagonists have been used in the management of heart failure†.

Current guidelines for the management of heart failure in adults generally recommend a combination of drug therapies to reduce morbidity and mortality, including neurohormonal antagonists (e.g., ACE inhibitors, angiotensin II receptor antagonists, angiotensin receptor-neprilysin inhibitors [ARNIs], β-adrenergic blocking agents [β-blockers], aldosterone receptor antagonists) that inhibit the detrimental compensatory mechanisms in heart failure. Additional agents (e.g., cardiac glycosides, diuretics, sinoatrial modulators [i.e., ivabradine]) added to a heart failure treatment regimen in selected patients have been associated with symptomatic improvement and/or reduction in heart failure-related hospitalizations. Experts recommend that all asymptomatic patients with reduced left ventricular ejection fraction (LVEF) (American College of Cardiology Foundation [ACCF]/American Heart Association [AHA] stage B heart failure) receive therapy with an ACE inhibitor and β-blocker to prevent symptomatic heart failure and reduce morbidity and mortality. In patients with prior or current symptoms of chronic heart failure with reduced LVEF (ACCF/AHA stage C heart failure), ACCF, AHA, and the Heart Failure Society of America (HFSA) recommend inhibition of the renin-angiotensin-aldosterone (RAA) system with an ACE inhibitor, angiotensin II receptor antagonist, or ARNI in conjunction with a β-blocker, and an aldosterone antagonist in selected patients, to reduce morbidity and mortality. While ACE inhibitors have been the preferred drugs for inhibition of the RAA system because of their established benefits in patients with heart failure and reduced ejection fraction, some evidence indicates that therapy with sacubitril/valsartan, an ARNI, may be more effective than ACE inhibitor therapy (enalapril) in reducing cardiovascular death and heart failure-related hospitalization. ACCF, AHA, and HFSA recommend that patients with chronic symptomatic heart failure and reduced LVEF (New York Heart Association [NYHA] class II or III) who are able to tolerate an ACE inhibitor or angiotensin II receptor antagonist be switched to therapy containing an ARNI to further reduce morbidity and mortality. However, in patients in whom an ARNI is not appropriate, continued use of an ACE inhibitor for all classes of heart failure with reduced ejection fraction remains strongly advised. In patients in whom an ARNI or ACE inhibitor is not appropriate, an angiotensin II receptor antagonist may be used. For additional information on the use of angiotensin II receptor antagonists in the management of heart failure, see Uses: Heart Failure, in Valsartan 24:32.08 and in Candesartan 24:32.08. For further information on the use of ARNIs in patients with heart failure, see Uses: Heart Failure, in Sacubitril and Valsartan 24:32.92.

While angiotensin II receptor antagonists are considered reasonable alternatives in patients who are unable to tolerate ACE inhibitors (e.g., because of cough or angioedema), angioedema and anaphylactic reactions have been reported rarely during postmarketing experience in patients receiving olmesartan. (See Sensitivity Reactions under Cautions: Warnings/Precautions.)

DOSAGE AND ADMINISTRATION

● Administration

Olmesartan medoxomil is administered orally without regard to meals. Twice-daily dosing offers no therapeutic advantage over the same total dose given once daily.

For pediatric patients unable to swallow tablets, olmesartan may be administered orally as an extemporaneously prepared suspension. An extemporaneous suspension containing olmesartan medoxomil 2 mg/mL can be prepared in the following manner. First, 50 mL of purified water is added to an amber polyethylene terephthalate (PET) bottle containing twenty 20-mg tablets of olmesartan medoxomil, and the contents allowed to stand for a minimum of 5 minutes. The container should then be shaken for at least 1 minute and allowed to stand for at least 1 minute; this step of alternating shaking and standing should be repeated 4 additional times. The concentrated suspension should then be diluted with 100 mL of syrup (Ora-Sweet®) and 50 mL of a suspending vehicle (Ora-Plus®) and the container shaken well for at least 1 minute to disperse the ingredients. The suspension should be shaken well before dispensing each dose. The extemporaneous suspension is stable for up to 4 weeks when stored at 2–8°C. Olmesartan medoxomil tablets and the extemporaneously prepared oral suspension of the drug are bioequivalent.

● Dosage

Hypertension

Dosage of olmesartan medoxomil must be individualized and adjusted according to blood pressure response.

Olmesartan Therapy

The usual initial dosage of olmesartan medoxomil as monotherapy is 20 mg once daily in adults without depletion of intravascular volume. If blood pressure response is inadequate with the initial dosage, dosage may be increased as tolerated to 40 mg daily or a diuretic may be added. Some experts state that the usual dosage of olmesartan medoxomil in adults is 20–40 mg once daily. Olmesartan medoxomil dosages exceeding 40 mg daily do not appear to provide additional therapeutic benefit. The antihypertensive effect of olmesartan medoxomil generally is evident within 2 weeks, with a maximum reduction observed after 4 weeks.

Dosage of olmesartan medoxomil in pediatric patients is based on weight. For pediatric patients 6–16 years of age weighing 20 to less than 35 kg, the usual initial dosage of olmesartan medoxomil is 10 mg once daily; dosage may be increased to a maximum of 20 mg once daily after 2 weeks if further reduction in blood pressure is needed. For pediatric patients 6–16 years of age weighing 35 kg or more, the recommended initial dosage of olmesartan medoxomil is 20 mg once daily; if necessary, dosage may be increased to a maximum of 40 mg once daily after 2 weeks.

Olmesartan/Amlodipine Fixed-combination Therapy

In patients who do not respond adequately to monotherapy with olmesartan medoxomil (or another angiotensin II receptor antagonist) or, alternatively, with amlodipine (or another dihydropyridine-derivative calcium-channel blocker), combined therapy with the drugs can be used to provide additional antihypertensive effects. The fixed-combination preparation containing olmesartan medoxomil and amlodipine also can be used as a substitute for the individually titrated drugs. The patient can be switched to the fixed-combination preparation containing the corresponding individual doses of olmesartan medoxomil and amlodipine; alternatively, the dosage of one or both components can be increased for additional antihypertensive effects. If needed, dosage of the fixed combination may be increased after 2 weeks. Dosage adjustments generally should involve one drug at a time, although dosages of both drugs can be increased to achieve more rapid blood pressure control. Daily dosages exceeding 40 mg of olmesartan medoxomil given in fixed combination with 10 mg of amlodipine are not recommended by the manufacturer.

Commercially available preparations containing olmesartan medoxomil in fixed combination with amlodipine may be used for initial treatment of hypertension in patients likely to require combined therapy with multiple antihypertensive drugs to achieve blood pressure control. In such patients, therapy with the fixed-combination preparation usually should be initiated at a dosage of 20 mg of olmesartan medoxomil and 5 mg of amlodipine once daily. If necessary, dosage of the fixed combination may be increased after 1–2 weeks for additional blood pressure control (but should not exceed a maximum dosage of 40 mg of olmesartan medoxomil and 10 mg of amlodipine once daily). In patients whose baseline blood pressure is 160/100 mm Hg, the estimated probability of achieving control of systolic blood pressure (defined as systolic blood pressure of less than 140 mm Hg) is 48, 46, or 68% and of achieving control of diastolic blood pressure (defined as diastolic blood pressure of less than 90 mm Hg) is 51, 60, or 85% with olmesartan medoxomil (40 mg daily) alone, amlodipine (10 mg daily) alone, or amlodipine combined with olmesartan medoxomil (at the same dosages), respectively.

Olmesartan/Hydrochlorothiazide Fixed-combination Therapy

In patients who do not respond adequately to monotherapy with olmesartan medoxomil or, alternatively, with hydrochlorothiazide, combined therapy with the drugs can be used. When combination therapy is necessary, the commercially available preparation containing olmesartan medoxomil in fixed combination with hydrochlorothiazide generally should not be used initially. Dosage preferably should first be adjusted by titrating the dosage of each drug separately; if it is determined that the optimum maintenance dosage corresponds to the ratio in the commercial combination preparation, this product may be used. The manufacturer states that combined therapy with the commercially available fixed-combination preparation containing 20 mg of olmesartan medoxomil and 12.5 mg of hydrochlorothiazide can be used in patients whose blood pressure is not adequately controlled by monotherapy with olmesartan medoxomil or 25 mg daily of hydrochlorothiazide. If needed, dosage of the fixed combination may be increased up to a maximum of 40 mg of olmesartan medoxomil and 25 mg of hydrochlorothiazide daily after 2–4 weeks. Daily dosages exceeding 40 mg of olmesartan medoxomil and 25 mg of hydrochlorothiazide given in combination are not recommended by the manufacturer.

Olmesartan/Amlodipine/Hydrochlorothiazide Fixed-combination Therapy

The fixed-combination preparation containing olmesartan medoxomil, amlodipine, and hydrochlorothiazide may be used to provide additional blood pressure control in patients who do not respond adequately to combination therapy with any 2 of the following classes of antihypertensive agents given at maximally tolerated, labeled, or usual dosages: angiotensin II receptor antagonists, calcium-channel blockers, or diuretics. Patients who experience dose-limiting adverse effects of olmesartan medoxomil, amlodipine, or hydrochlorothiazide while receiving any dual combination of these drugs may be switched to a lower dosage of that drug, given as a fixed-combination preparation containing all 3 of these drugs, to achieve similar blood pressure reductions. The fixed-combination preparation containing olmesartan medoxomil, amlodipine, and hydrochlorothiazide also can be used as a substitute for the individually titrated drugs. If necessary, dosage of the fixed combination preparation may be increased after 2 weeks for additional blood pressure control (but should not exceed a maximum dosage of 40 mg of olmesartan medoxomil, 10 mg of amlodipine, and 25 mg of hydrochlorothiazide daily). The commercially available preparation containing olmesartan medoxomil in fixed combination with amlodipine and hydrochlorothiazide should not be used for the initial management of hypertension.

Blood Pressure Monitoring and Treatment Goals

Blood pressure should be monitored regularly (i.e., monthly) during therapy and dosage of the antihypertensive drug adjusted until blood pressure is controlled. If an adequate blood pressure response is not achieved with angiotensin II receptor antagonist monotherapy, the dosage may be increased or another antihypertensive agent with demonstrated benefit and preferably with a complementary mechanism of action (e.g., calcium-channel blocker, thiazide diuretic) may be added; if target blood pressure is still not achieved, a third drug may be added. (See Uses: Hypertension.) In patients who develop unacceptable adverse effects with olmesartan, the drug should be discontinued and another antihypertensive agent from a different pharmacologic class should be initiated.

The goal of hypertension management and prevention is to achieve and maintain optimal control of blood pressure. However, the optimum blood pressure threshold for initiating antihypertensive drug therapy and specific treatment goals remain controversial. While previous hypertension guidelines have based target blood pressure goals on age and comorbidities, the 2017 ACC/AHA hypertension guideline incorporates underlying cardiovascular risk into decision making regarding treatment and generally recommends the same target blood pressure (i.e., less than 130/80 mm Hg) in all adults. Many patients will require at least 2 drugs from different pharmacologic classes to achieve their blood pressure goal; the potential benefits of hypertension management and drug cost, adverse effects, and risks associated with the use of multiple antihypertensive drugs also should be considered when deciding a patient's blood pressure treatment goal.

For additional information on target levels of blood pressure and on monitoring therapy in the management of hypertension, see Blood Pressure Monitoring and Treatment Goals under Dosage: Hypertension, in Dosage and Administration in the Thiazides General Statement 40:28.20.

● Special Populations

The manufacturer recommends that patients with depletion of intravascular volume be monitored closely and consideration be given to administering a lower initial dose of the drug. The manufacturer states that no adjustment in initial olmesartan medoxomil dosage is necessary in geriatric patients or in those with moderate-to-severe hepatic or renal impairment (creatinine clearance less than 40 mL/minute). However, some clinicians state that consideration should be given to administering a lower initial dose of the drug in patients with severe renal impairment (creatinine clearance less than 20 mL/minute) and recommend a maximum dosage of 20 mg once daily in such patients. The appropriate dosage in patients with end-stage renal disease has not been determined.

If concomitant diuretic therapy is required in patients with severe renal impairment (i.e., creatinine clearance of 30 mL/minute or less), a loop diuretic is preferred to a thiazide diuretic. Therefore, commercially available preparations containing olmesartan medoxomil in fixed combination with hydrochlorothiazide usually are not recommended for patients with severe renal impairment.

The amount of amlodipine in fixed-combination preparations containing olmesartan medoxomil and amlodipine exceeds the recommended initial dosage of amlodipine (2.5 mg daily) in patients 75 years of age or older and in those with hepatic impairment.

CAUTIONS

● Contraindications

Concomitant therapy with aliskiren in patients with diabetes mellitus. (See Drug Interactions: Drugs that Block the Renin-Angiotensin System.)

● Warnings/Precautions

Warnings

Fetal/Neonatal Morbidity and Mortality

Drugs that act on the renin-angiotensin system (e.g., angiotensin-converting enzyme [ACE] inhibitors, angiotensin II receptor antagonists, aliskiren) can reduce fetal renal function and increase fetal and neonatal morbidity and mortality when used in pregnancy during the second and third trimesters. ACE inhibitors also may increase the risk of major congenital malformations when administered during the first trimester of pregnancy. Resulting oligohydramnios can be associated with fetal lung hypoplasia and skeletal deformations. Potential neonatal effects include skull hypoplasia, anuria, hypotension, renal failure, and death. Olmesartan should be discontinued as soon as possible when pregnancy is detected, unless continued use is considered life-saving. Nearly all women can be transferred successfully to alternative therapy for the remainder of their pregnancy. For additional information on the risk during pregnancy of drugs that act on the renin-angiotensin system, see Cautions: Pregnancy, Fertility, and Lactation, in Captopril 24:32.04 and in Enalaprilat/Enalapril 24:32.04.

Sensitivity Reactions

Facial edema has occurred in patients receiving olmesartan. Sensitivity reactions, including various anaphylactoid reactions and/or angioedema have been reported in patients receiving angiotensin II receptor antagonists.

Extreme caution is advised in patients with history of angioedema associated with or unrelated to ACE inhibitor or angiotensin II receptor antagonist therapy.

Other Warnings and Precautions

Infant Morbidity

Olmesartan must not be used for the treatment of hypertension in infants younger than 1 year of age because drugs that act on the renin-angiotensin-aldosterone (RAA) system can affect the development of immature kidneys. (See Pediatric Use under Warnings/Precautions: Specific Populations, in Cautions.)

Hypotension

Because symptomatic hypotension may occur in patients with an activated RAA system (e.g., patients with volume or salt depletion secondary to salt restriction or prolonged diuretic therapy), olmesartan should be initiated in such patients under close medical supervision and consideration should be given to administering a lower initial dose of the drug.

If hypotension occurs in patients receiving olmesartan, the patient should be placed in the supine position; if hypotension is severe, IV infusion of 0.9% sodium chloride injection to expand fluid volume should be considered. Transient hypotension is not a contraindication to additional doses of olmesartan, and therapy with the drug can be cautiously reinstated after blood pressure has been stabilized (e.g., with volume expansion).

Malignancies

In July 2010, FDA initiated a safety review of angiotensin II receptor antagonists after a published meta-analysis suggested a possible association between the use of these agents and an increased risk of cancer. The meta-analysis,

which combined cancer-related findings from 5 randomized, controlled trials in over 60,000 patients, found a modest but significant increase in the risk of new cancer occurrence in patients receiving an angiotensin II receptor antagonist (mostly telmisartan) compared with those in control groups (7.2 versus 6%, respectively; risk ratio 1.08). However, because of several limitations of the study (e.g., trials included in the meta-analysis were not specifically designed to evaluate cancer outcomes, lack of individual patient data), the validity of these findings has been questioned.

Subsequent studies, including a larger, more comprehensive meta-analysis conducted by FDA, have not shown an increased risk of cancer in patients receiving angiotensin II receptor antagonists. FDA's meta-analysis, which included trial-level data from 31 randomized studies (total of approximately 156,000 patients), found no evidence of an increased risk of cancer in patients who received an angiotensin II receptor antagonist compared with those who received other treatments (placebo or active control). The overall rate of new cancer occurrence was essentially the same in both groups of patients (1.82 and 1.84 cases per 100 patient-years, respectively). In addition, there was no difference in the risk of cancer-related death, breast cancer, lung cancer, or prostate cancer between the groups. Based on these results and a review of all currently available data related to this potential safety concern, FDA has concluded that use of angiotensin II receptor antagonists is not associated with an increased risk of cancer.

Renal Effects

Because the RAA system appears to contribute substantially to maintenance of glomerular filtration in patients with heart failure in whom renal perfusion is severely compromised, renal function may deteriorate markedly (e.g., oliguria, progressive azotemia, renal failure, death) in these patients during therapy with an ACE inhibitor or an angiotensin II receptor antagonist (e.g., olmesartan). Renal artery stenosis also is a risk factor for renal impairment during therapy with drugs that inhibit the RAA system. Although reports received to date have involved patients treated with ACE inhibitors, this adverse effect also would be expected to occur when drugs with similar pharmacologic activity (e.g., angiotensin II receptor antagonists) are used in a similar manner. (See Cautions: Renal Effects, in Enalaprilat/Enalapril 24:32.04.)

Sprue-like Enteropathy

Sprue-like enteropathy, an intestinal condition characterized by severe chronic diarrhea with substantial weight loss, has been reported during postmarketing experience in patients receiving olmesartan; in some cases, intestinal biopsy revealed villous atrophy. At least 23 cases of sprue-like enteropathy were identified through the FDA Adverse Event Reporting System, and an additional 22 patients were described as having a similar condition in a published case series. Clinical manifestations developed months to years after initiation of olmesartan therapy and sometimes resulted in hospitalization. In all of the reported cases, clinical improvement occurred after the drug was discontinued, and a positive rechallenge was observed in some of the patients. Although the exact mechanism of this adverse effect is not known, certain findings suggest that it may be associated with a localized delayed hypersensitivity or cell-mediated immune response to the prodrug olmesartan medoxomil.

If symptoms of sprue-like enteropathy develop during olmesartan therapy, the possibility of other etiologies (e.g., celiac disease) should be excluded; if no other causative factor can be identified, discontinuance of the drug should be considered. Sprue-like enteropathy has not been associated with other angiotensin II receptor antagonists to date and is not considered to be a class effect of the drugs.

Increased Cardiovascular Risk in Patients with Diabetes

Findings from 2 long-term, randomized, double-blind, placebo-controlled trials (the Randomized Olmesartan and Diabetes Microalbuminuria Prevention Study [ROADMAP] and the Olmesartan Reducing Incidence of End-stage Renal Disease in Diabetic Nephropathy Trial [ORIENT]) prompted concerns that high-dose olmesartan may be associated with an increased risk of cardiovascular death in patients with diabetes mellitus. The trials were designed to evaluate the renoprotective effects of olmesartan in patients with type 2 diabetes mellitus over a period of about 4–5 years, but unexpectedly found an increased risk of cardiovascular deaths (e.g., fatal myocardial infarction, sudden cardiac death) associated with olmesartan therapy. However, in the ROADMAP trial, there was a trend toward a lower incidence of nonfatal myocardial infarction in the olmesartan group. The US Food and Drug Administration (FDA) has reviewed the results of these studies in addition to several other studies to further evaluate this safety concern; although some studies appeared to support the initial findings of the ROADMAP trial, results were inconsistent and, in some cases, not statistically significant. In one such study (an observational study conducted in a large [more than 300,000 patient-years of exposure] cohort of patients 65 years of age or older), an increased risk of death was observed in patients receiving olmesartan as compared with other angiotensin II receptor antagonists, but only in the subgroup of patients with diabetes mellitus who received the highest dosage of the drug (40 mg daily) for longer than 6 months; in nondiabetic patients, high-dose olmesartan was associated with a lower incidence of death as compared with other angiotensin II receptor antagonists. FDA has concluded after considering all of the available data that the collective evidence to date is insufficient to clearly demonstrate an association between olmesartan and increased cardiovascular risk in diabetic patients. FDA states that the benefits of olmesartan in hypertensive patients continue to outweigh its potential risks when used according to the manufacturer's labeling.

Fixed-combination Preparations

When olmesartan is used in fixed combination with hydrochlorothiazide and/or amlodipine, the cautions, precautions, and contraindications associated with the concomitant agent(s) must be considered in addition to those associated with olmesartan.

Specific Populations

Pregnancy

Category D. (See Users Guide.)

Olmesartan may cause fetal and neonatal morbidity and mortality when administered to a pregnant woman. Olmesartan should be discontinued as soon as possible when pregnancy is detected. (See Fetal/Neonatal Morbidity and Mortality under Warnings/Precautions: Warnings, in Cautions.)

Lactation

Olmesartan is distributed into milk in rats; it is not known whether the drug is distributed into milk in humans. Because of the potential for serious adverse reactions to olmesartan in nursing infants, a decision should be made whether to discontinue nursing or the drug, taking into account the importance of the drug to the woman.

Pediatric Use

If oliguria or hypotension occurs in neonates with a history of in utero exposure to olmesartan, blood pressure and renal function should be supported; exchange transfusions or dialysis may be required. (See Fetal/Neonatal Morbidity and Mortality under Warnings/Precautions: Warnings, in Cautions.)

Safety and efficacy of olmesartan have been established in a randomized, double-blind, placebo-controlled trial in pediatric patients 6–16 years of age with hypertension. Patients in the study were enrolled into 1 of 2 cohorts (an all-black or mixed racial cohort, 18% of whom were black). In both groups, olmesartan (given in a weight-adjusted dosage) substantially reduced systolic and diastolic blood pressures from baseline in a dose-dependent manner; systolic and diastolic blood pressures were, on average, 3.2 and 2.8 mm Hg lower, respectively, in patients receiving olmesartan than in those receiving placebo. Similar to that observed in the adult population, smaller blood pressure reductions were observed in the black compared with the predominantly nonblack pediatric patient cohort. The same pediatric study also included 59 patients who were 1–5 years of age; treatment with olmesartan medoxomil (0.3 mg/kg once daily) in this age group did not result in a statistically significant reduction in blood pressure compared with placebo. Adverse effects reported in the pediatric patients evaluated in this study generally were similar to those observed in adults.

Pharmacokinetics of olmesartan have been evaluated in pediatric patients 1–16 years of age; clearance of the drug (adjusted for body weight) in these pediatric patients was similar to that observed in adults.

The manufacturer states that olmesartan has not been shown to be effective for hypertension in patients younger than 6 years of age.

Olmesartan has not been evaluated in infants younger than 1 year of age; because of the possibility of abnormal kidney development, the drug *must* not be used in this age group.

Safety and efficacy of olmesartan in fixed combination with hydrochlorothiazide and/or amlodipine in pediatric patients have not been established.

For information on overall principles and expert recommendations for treatment of hypertension in pediatric patients, see Uses: Hypertension in Pediatric Patients, in the Thiazides General Statement 40:28.20.

Geriatric Use

No overall differences in safety and efficacy of olmesartan have been observed in geriatric patients 65 years of age or older relative to younger adults, but increased sensitivity to the drug cannot be ruled out. In general, dosage should be selected with caution because of age-related decreases in hepatic, renal, and/or cardiac function and concomitant disease and drug therapy.

Hepatic Impairment

Systemic exposure to olmesartan may be increased in patients with moderate hepatic impairment compared with those with normal hepatic function; however, no initial dosage adjustment is required in patients with moderate or severe hepatic impairment.

Renal Impairment

Serum concentrations of olmesartan may be increased in patients with renal impairment compared with those with normal renal function; however, the manufacturer states that no initial dosage adjustment is required. (See Dosage and Administration: Special Populations.)

Deterioration of renal function may occur during therapy. (See Renal Effects under Warnings/Precautions: Other Warnings and Precautions, in Cautions.)

Black Patients

Blood pressure reduction with olmesartan may be smaller in black patients than in patients of other races.

● Common Adverse Effects

Adverse effects occurring in 1% or more of patients receiving olmesartan, but also occurring at about the same or greater incidence in patients receiving placebo, include back pain, bronchitis, diarrhea, headache, hematuria, hyperglycemia, hypertriglyceridemia, influenza-like symptoms, pharyngitis, rhinitis, sinusitis, and upper respiratory tract infection. In placebo-controlled studies, the only adverse effect that occurred in more than 1% of patients receiving olmesartan and at an incidence greater than with placebo was dizziness. The incidence of adverse effects was not affected by age, gender, or race.

DRUG INTERACTIONS

● Drugs Affecting or Metabolized by Hepatic Microsomal Enzymes

Olmesartan is not metabolized by the cytochrome P-450 (CYP) isoenzyme system and does not alter activity of CYP isoenzymes; pharmacokinetic interactions are unlikely with inhibitors or inducers of CYP isoenzymes or with drugs that are metabolized by these isoenzymes.

● Drugs that Block the Renin-Angiotensin System

Increased risk of renal impairment, hyperkalemia, and hypotension with concomitant use of other drugs that block the renin-angiotensin system (e.g., angiotensin-converting enzyme [ACE] inhibitors, angiotensin II receptor antagonists, aliskiren); when olmesartan is used concomitantly with such drugs, blood pressure, renal function, and serum concentrations of electrolytes should be monitored closely. The manufacturer states that most patients do not derive additional benefit from combination therapy with 2 renin-angiotensin system inhibitors compared with monotherapy. Concomitant use of olmesartan and aliskiren is contraindicated in patients with diabetes mellitus; in addition, such concomitant use should be avoided in patients with renal impairment (glomerular filtration rate [GFR] less than 60 mL/minute). (See Use in Combination with Angiotensin-converting Enzyme Inhibitors or Angiotensin II Receptor Antagonists under Warnings/Precautions: Other Warnings and Precautions, in Cautions in Aliskiren Hemifumarate 24:32.40.)

● **Antacids**

Pharmacokinetic interactions unlikely.

● **Colesevelam Hydrochloride**

Pharmacokinetic interaction (decreased systemic exposure and peak plasma concentrations of olmesartan). Administration of olmesartan at least 4 hours prior to colesevelam decreases the extent of this interaction and should be considered.

● **Digoxin**

Pharmacokinetic interactions unlikely.

● **Lithium**

Increased serum lithium concentrations resulting in lithium toxicity have been reported when angiotensin II receptor antagonists are used concomitantly with lithium. Serum lithium concentrations should be carefully monitored.

● **Nonsteroidal Anti-inflammatory Agents**

Potential pharmacologic interaction (attenuated hypotensive effects) when angiotensin II receptor antagonists are used concomitantly with nonsteroidal anti-inflammatory agents (NSAIAs), including selective cyclooxygenase-2 (COX-2) inhibitors. Possible deterioration of renal function, including possible acute renal failure, in geriatric, volume-depleted (including those receiving concomitant diuretic therapy), or renally impaired patients; renal function should be monitored periodically in patients receiving concomitant therapy with olmesartan and an NSAIA, including selective COX-2 inhibitors.

● **Warfarin**

Pharmacokinetic and pharmacologic interactions unlikely.

DESCRIPTION

Olmesartan medoxomil is a nonpeptide, benzimidazole-derivative angiotensin II type 1 (AT$_1$) receptor antagonist. For additional information on the pharmacology of angiotensin II receptor antagonists, see Description in Irbesartan 24:32.08 and Valsartan 24:32.08.

Olmesartan medoxomil is a prodrug that has little, if any, pharmacologic activity until hydrolyzed during absorption in the GI tract to olmesartan. Following rapid and complete ester hydrolysis of olmesartan medoxomil to olmesartan, there is virtually no further metabolism of olmesartan. Approximately 35–50% of an absorbed dose is recovered in urine while the remainder is excreted in feces via the bile. Olmesartan is not metabolized by the cytochrome P-450 (CYP) microsomal enzyme system.

ADVICE TO PATIENTS

When olmesartan is used in fixed combination with amlodipine and/or hydrochlorothiazide, importance of advising patients of important precautionary information about the concomitant agent(s).

Importance of informing clinicians of existing or contemplated concomitant therapy, including prescription and OTC drugs.

Importance of women informing clinicians if they are or plan to become pregnant or plan to breast-feed. Importance of advising women of childbearing age about the potential risks to the fetus if the drug is used during pregnancy. All women of childbearing potential should be advised to report pregnancy to their clinician as soon as possible. (See Fetal/Neonatal Morbidity and Mortality under Warnings/Precautions: Warnings, in Cautions.)

Importance of informing patients of other important precautionary information. (See Cautions.)

PREPARATIONS

Excipients in commercially available drug preparations may have clinically important effects in some individuals; consult specific product labeling for details.

Olmesartan Medoxomil

Oral

Tablets, film-coated	5 mg	**Benicar®**, Daiichi Sankyo
	20 mg	**Benicar®**, Daiichi Sankyo
	40 mg	**Benicar®**, Daiichi Sankyo

Olmesartan Medoxomil Combinations

Oral

Tablets	20 mg with Amlodipine Besylate 5 mg (of amlodipine)	**Azor®**, Daiichi Sankyo
	20 mg with Amlodipine Besylate 10 mg (of amlodipine)	**Azor®**, Daiichi Sankyo
	40 mg with Amlodipine Besylate 5 mg (of amlodipine)	**Azor®**, Daiichi Sankyo
	40 mg with Amlodipine Besylate 10 mg (of amlodipine)	**Azor®**, Daiichi Sankyo
Tablets, film-coated	20 mg with Amlodipine Besylate 5 mg (of amlodipine) and Hydrochlorothiazide 12.5 mg	**Tribenzor®**, Daiichi Sankyo
	20 mg with Hydrochlorothiazide 12.5 mg	**Benicar® HCT**, Daiichi Sankyo
	40 mg with Amlodipine Besylate 5 mg (of amlodipine) and Hydrochlorothiazide 12.5 mg	**Tribenzor®**, Daiichi Sankyo
	40 mg with Amlodipine Besylate 5 mg (of amlodipine) and Hydrochlorothiazide 25 mg	**Tribenzor®**, Daiichi Sankyo
	40 mg with Amlodipine Besylate 10 mg (of amlodipine) and Hydrochlorothiazide 12.5 mg	**Tribenzor®**, Daiichi Sankyo
	40 mg with Amlodipine Besylate 10 mg (of amlodipine) and Hydrochlorothiazide 25 mg	**Tribenzor®**, Daiichi Sankyo
	40 mg with Hydrochlorothiazide 12.5 mg	**Benicar® HCT**, Daiichi Sankyo
	40 mg with Hydrochlorothiazide 25 mg	**Benicar® HCT**, Daiichi Sankyo

† Use is not currently included in the labeling approved by the US Food and Drug Administration.

Selected Revisions November 5, 2018, © Copyright, October 1, 2002, American Society of Health-System Pharmacists, Inc.

Valsartan

24:32.08 • ANGIOTENSIN II RECEPTOR ANTAGONISTS

■ Valsartan is an angiotensin II type 1 (AT₁) receptor antagonist (also referred to as an angiotensin II receptor blocker [ARB]). Valsartan also is commercially available in fixed combination with sacubitril, a neprilysin inhibitor. (See the monograph on Sacubitril and Valsartan in 24:32.92.)

USES

● *Hypertension*

Valsartan is used alone or in combination with other classes of antihypertensive agents (e.g., thiazide diuretics) in the management of hypertension. Efficacy of valsartan for the management of hypertension has been established by controlled studies of 8–12 weeks' duration in patients with hypertension of mild to moderate severity in outpatient settings. The efficacy of valsartan for long-term use (i.e., exceeding 12 weeks) has been established in noncontrolled, follow-up studies in which the drug was used for up to 2 years without apparent loss of clinical effect. Clinical studies have shown that the hypotensive effect of usual dosages of valsartan in patients with mild to moderate hypertension is greater than that of placebo and comparable to that of usual dosages of amlodipine, enalapril, lisinopril, or hydrochlorothiazide.

Current evidence-based practice guidelines for the management of hypertension in adults generally recommend the use of drugs from 4 classes of antihypertensive agents (angiotensin-converting enzyme [ACE] inhibitors, angiotensin II receptor antagonists, calcium-channel blockers, and thiazide diuretics); data from clinical outcome trials indicate that lowering blood pressure with any of these drug classes can reduce the complications of hypertension and provide similar cardiovascular protection. However, recommendations for initial drug selection and use in specific patient populations may vary across these expert guidelines. This variability is due, in part, to differences in the guideline development process and the types of studies (e.g., randomized controlled studies only versus a range of studies with different study designs) included in the evidence reviews. Ultimately, choice of antihypertensive therapy should be individualized, considering the clinical characteristics of the patient (e.g., age, ethnicity/race, comorbid conditions, cardiovascular risk factors) as well as drug-related factors (e.g., ease of administration, availability, adverse effects, costs). Because many patients eventually will need drugs from 2 or more antihypertensive classes, experts generally state that the emphasis should be placed on achieving appropriate blood pressure control rather than on identifying a preferred drug to achieve that control.

Disease Overview

Worldwide, hypertension is the most common modifiable risk factor for cardiovascular events and mortality. The lifetime risk of developing hypertension in the US exceeds 80%, with higher rates observed among African Americans and Hispanics compared with whites or Asians. The systolic blood pressure and diastolic blood pressure values defined as hypertension in adults (see Blood Pressure Classification under Uses: Hypertension) in a 2017 multidisciplinary guideline of the American College of Cardiology (ACC), American Heart Association (AHA), and a number of other professional organizations (subsequently referred to as the 2017 ACC/AHA hypertension guideline in this monograph) are lower than those defined in the Seventh Report of the Joint National Committee on Prevention, Detection, Evaluation, and Treatment of High Blood Pressure (JNC 7) guidelines, which results in an increase of approximately 14% in the prevalence of hypertension in the US. However, this change in definition results in only a 2% increase in the percentage of patients requiring antihypertensive drug therapy because non-pharmacologic treatment is recommended for most adults now classified by the 2017 ACC/AHA hypertension guideline as hypertensive who would *not* meet the JNC 7 definition of hypertension. Among US adults receiving antihypertensive drugs, approximately 53% have inadequately controlled blood pressure according to current ACC/AHA treatment goals.

Cardiovascular and Renal Sequelae

The principal goal of preventing and treating hypertension is to reduce the risk of cardiovascular and renal morbidity and mortality, including target organ damage.

The relationship between blood pressure and cardiovascular disease is continuous, consistent, and independent of other risk factors. It is important that very high blood pressure be managed promptly to reduce the risk of target organ damage. The higher the blood pressure, the more likely the development of myocardial infarction (MI), heart failure, stroke, and renal disease. For adults 40–70 years of age, each 20-mm Hg increment in systolic blood pressure or 10-mm Hg increment in diastolic blood pressure doubles the risk of developing cardiovascular disease across the entire blood pressure range of 115/75 to 185/115 mm Hg. For those older than 50 years of age, systolic blood pressure is a much more important risk factor for developing cardiovascular disease than is diastolic blood pressure. The rapidity with which treatment is required depends on the patient's clinical presentation (presence of new or worsening target organ damage) and the presence or absence of cardiovascular complications; the 2017 ACC/AHA hypertension guideline states that treatment of very high blood pressure should be initiated within 1 week.

Blood Pressure Classification

Accurate blood pressure measurement is essential for the proper diagnosis and management of hypertension. Error in measuring blood pressure is a major cause of inadequate blood pressure control and may lead to overtreatment. Because a patient's blood pressure may vary in an unpredictable fashion, a single blood pressure measurement is not sufficient for clinical decision-making. An average of 2 or 3 blood pressure measurements obtained on 2–3 separate occasions using proper technique should be used to minimize random error and provide a more accurate blood pressure reading. Out-of-office blood pressure measurements may be useful for confirming and managing hypertension. The 2017 ACC/AHA hypertension guideline document (available on the ACC and AHA websites) should be consulted for key steps on properly measuring blood pressure.

According to the 2017 ACC/AHA hypertension guideline, blood pressure in adults is classified into 4 categories: normal, elevated, stage 1 hypertension, and stage 2 hypertension. (See Table 1.) The 2017 ACC/AHA hypertension guideline lowers the blood pressure threshold used to define hypertension in the US; previous hypertension guidelines (JNC 7) considered adults with systolic blood pressure of 120–139 mm Hg or diastolic blood pressure of 80–89 mm Hg to have prehypertension, those with systolic blood pressure of 140–159 mm Hg or diastolic blood pressure of 90–99 mm Hg to have stage 1 hypertension, and those with systolic blood pressure of 160 mm Hg or higher or diastolic blood pressure of 100 mm Hg or higher to have stage 2 hypertension. The blood pressure definitions in the 2017 ACC/AHA hypertension guideline are based upon data from studies evaluating the association between systolic blood pressure/diastolic blood pressure and cardiovascular risk and the benefits of blood pressure reduction. Individuals with systolic blood pressure and diastolic blood pressure in 2 different categories should be designated as being in the higher blood pressure category.

TABLE 1. ACC/AHA Blood Pressure Classification in Adults [a][b]

Category	SBP [c] (mm Hg)		DBP [d] (mm Hg)
Normal	<120	and	<80
Elevated	120–129	and	<80
Hypertension, Stage 1	130–139	or	80–89
Hypertension, Stage 2	≥140	or	≥90

[a] Source: Whelton PK, Carey RM, Aronow WS et al. 2017 ACC/AHA/AAPA/ABC/ACPM/AGS/APhA/ASH/ASPC/NMA/PCNA guideline for the prevention, detection, evaluation, and management of high blood pressure in adults: a report of the American College of Cardiology/American Heart Association Task Force on Clinical Practice Guidelines. Hypertension. 2018;71:e13-115.

[b] Individuals with SBP and DBP in 2 different categories (e.g., elevated SBP and normal DBP) should be designated as being in the higher blood pressure category (i.e., elevated BP).

[c] Systolic blood pressure

[d] Diastolic blood pressure

The blood pressure thresholds used to define hypertension, when to initiate drug therapy, and the ideal target blood pressure values remain controversial.

The 2017 ACC/AHA hypertension guideline recommends a blood pressure goal of less than 130/80 mm Hg in all adults who have confirmed hypertension and known cardiovascular disease or a 10-year atherosclerotic cardiovascular disease (ASCVD) event risk of 10% or higher; the ACC/AHA guideline also states that this blood pressure goal is reasonable to attempt to achieve in adults with confirmed hypertension who do *not* have increased cardiovascular risk. The lower blood pressure values used to define hypertension and the lower target blood pressure goals outlined in the 2017 ACC/AHA hypertension guideline are based on clinical studies demonstrating a substantial reduction in the composite end point of major cardiovascular disease events and the combination of fatal and nonfatal stroke when a lower systolic blood pressure/diastolic blood pressure value (i.e., 130/80 mm Hg) was used to define hypertension. These lower target blood pressure goals also are based upon clinical studies demonstrating continuing reduction of cardiovascular risk at progressively lower levels of systolic blood pressure. A linear relationship has been demonstrated between cardiovascular risk and blood pressure even at low systolic blood pressures (e.g., 120–124 mm Hg). The 2017 ACC/AHA hypertension guideline recommends estimating a patient's ASCVD risk using the ACC/AHA Pooled Cohort equations (available online at http://tools.acc.org/ASCVD-Risk-Estimator), which are based on a variety of factors including age, race, gender, cholesterol levels, statin use, blood pressure, treatment for hypertension, history of diabetes mellitus, smoking status, and aspirin use. While the 2017 ACC/AHA hypertension guideline has lowered the threshold for *diagnosing* hypertension in adults, the threshold for *initiating drug therapy* has only been lowered for those patients who are at high risk of cardiovascular disease. Clinicians who support the 2017 ACC/AHA hypertension guideline believe that these recommendations have the potential to increase hypertension awareness, encourage lifestyle modification, and focus antihypertensive drug initiation and intensification in those adults at high risk for cardiovascular disease.

The lower blood pressure goals advocated in the 2017 ACC/AHA hypertension guideline have been questioned by some clinicians who have concerns regarding the guideline's use of extrapolated observational data, the lack of generalizability of some of the randomized trials (e.g., SPRINT) used to support the guideline, the difficulty of establishing accurate representative blood pressure values in typical clinical practice settings, and the accuracy of the cardiovascular risk calculator used in the guideline. Some clinicians state the lower blood pressure threshold used to define hypertension in the 2017 ACC/AHA hypertension guideline is not fully supported by clinical data, and these clinicians have expressed concerns about the possible harms (e.g., adverse effects of antihypertensive therapy) associated with classifying more patients as being hypertensive. Some clinicians also state that using this guideline, a large number of young, low-risk patients would need to be treated in order to observe a clinical benefit, while other clinicians state that the estimated gains in life-expectancy attributable to long-term use of blood pressure-lowering drugs are correspondingly greater in this patient population.

Treatment Benefits

In clinical trials, antihypertensive therapy has been found to reduce the risk of developing stroke by about 34–40%, MI by about 20–25%, and heart failure by more than 50%. In a randomized, controlled study (SPRINT) that included hypertensive patients without diabetes mellitus who had a high risk of cardiovascular disease, intensive systolic blood pressure lowering of approximately 15 mm Hg was associated with a 25% reduction in cardiovascular disease events and a 27% reduction in all-cause mortality. However, the exclusion of patients with diabetes mellitus, prior stroke, and those younger than 50 years of age may decrease the generalizability of these findings. Some experts estimate that if the systolic blood pressure goals of the 2017 ACC/AHA hypertension guideline are achieved, major cardiovascular disease events may be reduced by an additional 340,000 and total deaths by an additional 156,000 compared with implementation of the JNC 8 expert panel guideline goals but these benefits may be accompanied by an increase in the frequency of adverse events. While there was no overall difference in the occurrence of serious adverse events in patients receiving intensive therapy for blood pressure control (systolic blood pressure target of less than 120 mm Hg) compared with those receiving less intense control (systolic blood pressure target of less than 140 mm Hg) in the SPRINT study, hypotension, syncope, electrolyte abnormalities, and acute kidney injury or acute renal failure occurred in substantially more patients receiving intensive therapy.

In the Antihypertensive and Lipid-lowering Treatment to Prevent Heart Attack Trial (ALLHAT), the long-term cardiovascular morbidity and mortality benefit of a long-acting dihydropyridine calcium-channel blocker (amlodipine), a thiazide-like diuretic (chlorthalidone), and an ACE inhibitor (lisinopril) were compared in a broad population of patients with hypertension at risk for coronary heart disease. Although these antihypertensive agents were comparably effective in providing important cardiovascular benefit, apparent differences in certain secondary outcomes were observed. Patients receiving the ACE inhibitor experienced higher risks of stroke, combined cardiovascular disease, GI bleeding, and angioedema, while those receiving the calcium-channel blocker were at higher risk of developing heart failure. The ALLHAT investigators suggested that the observed differences in cardiovascular outcome may be attributable, at least in part, to the greater antihypertensive effect of the calcium-channel blocker compared with that of the ACE inhibitor, especially in women and black patients. (See Clinical Benefits of Thiazides in Hypertension under Hypertension in Adults: Treatment Benefits, in Uses in the Thiazides General Statement 40:28.20.)

General Considerations for Initial and Maintenance Antihypertensive Therapy

Nonpharmacologic Therapy

Nonpharmacologic measures (i.e., lifestyle/behavioral modifications) that are effective in lowering blood pressure include weight reduction (for those who are overweight or obese), dietary changes to include foods such as fruits, vegetables, whole grains, and low-fat dairy products that are rich in potassium, calcium, magnesium, and fiber (i.e., adoption of the Dietary Approaches to Stop Hypertension [DASH] eating plan), sodium reduction, increased physical activity, and moderation of alcohol intake. Such lifestyle/behavioral modifications, including smoking cessation, enhance antihypertensive drug efficacy and decrease cardiovascular risk and remain an indispensable part of the management of hypertension. Lifestyle/behavioral modifications without antihypertensive drug therapy are recommended for individuals classified by the 2017 ACC/AHA hypertension guideline as having elevated blood pressure (systolic blood pressure 120–129 mm Hg and diastolic blood pressure less than 80 mm Hg) and in those with stage 1 hypertension (systolic blood pressure 130–139 mm Hg or diastolic blood pressure 80–89 mm Hg) who do *not* have preexisting cardiovascular disease or an estimated 10-year ASCVD risk of 10% or greater.

Initiation of Drug Therapy

Drug therapy in the management of hypertension must be individualized and adjusted based on the degree of blood pressure elevation while also considering cardiovascular risk factors. Drug therapy generally is reserved for patients who respond inadequately to nondrug therapy (i.e., lifestyle modifications such as diet [including sodium restriction and adequate potassium and calcium intake], regular aerobic physical activity, moderation of alcohol consumption, and weight reduction) or in whom the degree of blood pressure elevation or coexisting risk factors, especially increased cardiovascular risk, requires more prompt or aggressive therapy; however, the optimum blood pressure threshold for initiating antihypertensive drug therapy and specific treatment goals remain controversial. Recommendations generally are based on specific blood pressure levels shown in clinical studies to produce clinical benefits and can therefore vary depending on the studies selected for review.

The 2017 ACC/AHA hypertension guideline and many experts currently state that the treatment of hypertension should be based not only on blood pressure values but also on patients' cardiovascular risk factors. For *secondary prevention* of recurrent cardiovascular disease events in adults with clinical cardiovascular disease or for *primary prevention* in adults with an estimated 10-year ASCVD risk of 10% or higher, the 2017 ACC/AHA hypertension guideline recommends initiation of antihypertensive drug therapy in conjunction with lifestyle/behavioral modifications at an average systolic blood pressure of 130 mm Hg or an average diastolic blood pressure of 80 mm Hg or higher. For *primary prevention* of cardiovascular disease events in adults with a low (less than 10%) estimated 10-year risk of ASCVD, the 2017 ACC/AHA hypertension guideline recommends initiation of antihypertensive drug therapy in conjunction with lifestyle/behavioral modifications at a systolic blood pressure of 140 mm Hg or higher or a diastolic blood pressure of 90 mm Hg or higher. After initiation of antihypertensive drug therapy, regardless of the ASCVD risk, the 2017 ACC/AHA hypertension guideline generally recommends a blood pressure goal of less than 130/80 mm Hg in all patients. In addition, a systolic blood pressure goal of less than 130 mm Hg also is recommended for noninstitutionalized ambulatory patients 65 years of age or older. While these blood pressure goals are lower than those recommended for most patients in previous guidelines, they are based upon clinical studies demonstrating continuing reduction of cardiovascular risk at progressively lower levels of systolic blood pressure.

Most data indicate that patients with a higher cardiovascular risk will benefit the most from tighter blood pressure control; however, some experts state this treatment goal also may be beneficial in those at lower cardiovascular risk. Other clinicians believe that the benefits of such blood pressure lowering do not outweigh the risks in those patients considered to be at lower risk of cardiovascular disease and that reclassifying individuals formerly considered to have prehypertension as having hypertension may potentially lead to use of drug therapy in such patients without consideration of cardiovascular risk. Previous hypertension guidelines, such as those from the JNC 8 expert panel, generally recommended initiation of antihypertensive treatment in patients with a systolic blood pressure of at least 140 mm Hg or diastolic blood pressure of at least 90 mm Hg, targeted a blood pressure goal of less than 140/90 mm Hg regardless of cardiovascular risk, and used higher systolic blood pressure thresholds and targets in geriatric patients. Some clinicians continue to support the target blood pressures recommended by the JNC 8 expert panel because of concerns that such recommendations in the 2017 ACC/AHA hypertension guideline are based on extrapolation of data from the high-risk population in the SPRINT study to a lower-risk population. Also, because more than 90% of patients in SPRINT were already receiving antihypertensive drugs at baseline, data are lacking on the effects of *initiating* drug therapy at a lower blood pressure threshold (130/80 mm Hg) in patients at high risk of cardiovascular disease. The potential benefits of hypertension management and drug cost, adverse effects, and risks associated with the use of multiple antihypertensive drugs should be considered when deciding a patient's blood pressure treatment goal.

The 2017 ACC/AHA hypertension guideline recommends an ASCVD risk assessment for all adults with hypertension; however, experts state that it can be assumed that patients with hypertension and diabetes mellitus or chronic kidney disease (CKD) are at high risk for cardiovascular disease and that antihypertensive drug therapy should be initiated in these patients at a blood pressure of 130/80 mm Hg or higher. The 2017 ACC/AHA hypertension guideline also recommends a blood pressure goal of less than 130/80 mm Hg in patients with hypertension and diabetes mellitus or CKD. These recommendations are based on a systematic review of high-quality evidence from randomized controlled trials, meta-analyses, and post-hoc analyses that have demonstrated substantial reductions in the risk of important clinical outcomes (e.g., cardiovascular events) regardless of comorbid conditions or age when systolic blood pressure is lowered to less than 130 mm Hg. However, some clinicians have questioned the generalizability of findings from some of the trials (e.g., SPRINT) used to support the 2017 ACC/AHA hypertension guideline. For example, SPRINT included adults (mean age: 68 years) *without* diabetes mellitus who were at high risk of cardiovascular disease. While benefits of intensive blood pressure control were observed in this patient population, some clinicians have questioned whether these findings apply to younger patients who have a low risk of cardiovascular disease. In patients with CKD in the SPRINT trial, intensive blood pressure management (achieving a mean systolic blood pressure of approximately 122 mm Hg compared with 136 mm Hg with standard treatment) provided a similar beneficial reduction in the composite cardiovascular disease primary outcome and all-cause mortality as in the full patient cohort. Because most patients with CKD die from cardiovascular complications, the findings of this study further support a lower blood pressure target of less than 130/80 mm Hg.

Data are lacking to determine the ideal blood pressure goal in adult patients with hypertension and diabetes mellitus; also, studies evaluating the benefits of intensive blood pressure control in patients with diabetes mellitus have provided conflicting results. Clinical studies reviewed for the 2017 ACC/AHA hypertension guideline have shown similar quantitative benefits from blood pressure lowering in hypertensive patients with or without diabetes mellitus. In a randomized, controlled study (ACCORD-BP) that compared a higher (systolic blood pressure less than 140 mm Hg) versus lower (systolic blood pressure less than 120 mm Hg) blood pressure goal in patients with diabetes mellitus, there was no difference in the incidence of cardiovascular outcomes (e.g., composite outcome of cardiovascular death, nonfatal MI, and nonfatal stroke). However, some experts state that this study was underpowered to detect a difference between the 2 treatment groups and that the factorial design of the study complicated interpretation of the results. Although SPRINT did not include patients with diabetes mellitus, patients in this study with prediabetes demonstrated a similar cardiovascular benefit from intensive treatment of blood pressure as normoglycemic patients. A meta-analysis of data from the ACCORD and SPRINT studies suggests that the findings of both studies are consistent and that patients with diabetes mellitus benefit from more intensive blood pressure control. These data support the 2017 ACC/AHA hypertension guideline recommendation of a blood pressure treatment goal of less than 130/80 mm Hg in adult patients with hypertension and diabetes mellitus. Alternatively, the American Diabetes Association (ADA) recommends a blood pressure goal of less than 140/90 mm Hg in patients with diabetes mellitus. The ADA states that a lower blood pressure goal (e.g., less than 130/80 mm Hg) may be appropriate for patients with a high risk of cardiovascular disease and diabetes mellitus if it can be achieved without undue treatment burden.

Further study is needed to more clearly define optimum blood pressure goals in patients with hypertension, particularly in high-risk groups (e.g., patients with diabetes mellitus, cardiovascular disease, or cerebrovascular disease; black patients); when determining appropriate blood pressure goals, individual risks and benefits should be considered in addition to the evidence from clinical studies.

Choice of Initial Drug Therapy

In current hypertension management guidelines, angiotensin II receptor antagonists are recommended as one of several preferred drugs for the initial treatment of hypertension; other preferred options include ACE inhibitors, calcium-channel blockers, and thiazide diuretics. The 2017 ACC/AHA adult hypertension guideline states that an ACE inhibitor, angiotensin II receptor antagonist, calcium-channel blocker, or thiazide or thiazide-like diuretic (preferably chlorthalidone) are all acceptable choices for initial antihypertensive drug therapy in the general population of nonblack patients, including those with diabetes mellitus; drugs from any of these classes generally produce similar benefits in terms of overall mortality and cardiovascular, cerebrovascular, and renal outcomes. Angiotensin II receptor antagonists or ACE inhibitors may be particularly useful in the management of hypertension in patients with certain coexisting conditions such as diabetes mellitus or CKD; angiotensin II receptor antagonists also may be preferred, generally as an alternative to ACE inhibitors, in hypertensive patients with heart failure or ischemic heart disease and/or following MI. (See Considerations for Drug Therapy in Patients with Underlying Cardiovascular and Other Risk Factors under Uses: Hypertension.)

In patients with hypertension and compelling indications (e.g., CKD with albuminuria [urine albumin 300 mg/day or greater, or urine albumin:creatinine ratio of 300 mg/g or equivalent in the first morning void]), angiotensin II receptor antagonists are usually considered an alternative for ACE inhibitor-intolerant patients. (See Chronic Kidney Disease under Hypertension: Considerations for Drug Therapy in Patients with Underlying Cardiovascular and Other Risk Factors, in Uses.) However, data indicate no difference in efficacy between ACE inhibitors and angiotensin II receptor antagonists with regard to blood pressure lowering and clinical outcomes (i.e., all-cause mortality, cardiovascular mortality, MI, heart failure, stroke, and end-stage renal disease). Adverse events (e.g., cough, angioedema) leading to drug discontinuance occur more frequently with ACE inhibitor therapy than with angiotensin II receptor antagonist therapy. Because of similar efficacy and a lower frequency of adverse effects, some experts believe that angiotensin II receptor antagonists should be used instead of an ACE inhibitor for the treatment of hypertension or hypertension with certain compelling indications.

Experts state that in patients with stage 1 hypertension (especially the elderly, those with a history of hypotension, or those who have experienced adverse drug effects), it is reasonable to initiate drug therapy using the stepped-care approach in which one drug is initiated and titrated and other drugs are added sequentially to achieve the target blood pressure. Although some patients can begin treatment with a single antihypertensive agent, starting with 2 first-line drugs in different pharmacologic classes (either as separate agents or in a fixed-dose combination) is recommended in patients with stage 2 hypertension and an average blood pressure more than 20/10 mm Hg above their target blood pressure. Such combined therapy may increase the likelihood of achieving goal blood pressure in a more timely fashion, but also may increase the risk of adverse effects (e.g., orthostatic hypotension) in some patients (e.g., elderly). Drug regimens with complementary activity, where a second antihypertensive agent is used to block compensatory responses to the first agent or affect a different pressor mechanism, can result in additive blood pressure lowering and are preferred. Drug combinations that have similar mechanisms of action or clinical effects (e.g., the combination of an ACE inhibitor and an angiotensin II receptor antagonist) generally should be avoided. Many patients who begin therapy with a single antihypertensive agent will subsequently require at least 2 drugs from different pharmacologic classes to achieve their blood pressure goal. Experts state that other patient-specific factors, such as age, concurrent medications, drug adherence, drug interactions, the overall treatment regimen, cost, and comorbidities, also should be considered when deciding on an antihypertensive drug regimen. For any stage of hypertension, antihypertensive drug dosages should be adjusted and/or other agents substituted or added until goal blood pressure is achieved. (See Follow-up and Maintenance Drug Therapy under Hypertension: General Considerations for Initial and Maintenance Antihypertensive Therapy, in Uses.)

Follow-up and Maintenance Drug Therapy

Several strategies are used for the titration and combination of antihypertensive drugs; these strategies, which are generally based on those used in randomized controlled studies, include maximizing the dosage of the first drug before adding a second drug, adding a second drug before achieving maximum dosage of the initial drug, or initiating therapy with 2 drugs simultaneously (either as separate preparations or as a fixed-dose combination). Combined use of an ACE inhibitor and angiotensin II receptor antagonist should be avoided because of the potential risk of adverse renal effects. After initiating a new or adjusted antihypertensive drug regimen, patients should have their blood pressure reevaluated monthly until adequate blood pressure control is achieved. Effective blood pressure control can be achieved in most hypertensive patients, but many will ultimately require therapy with 2 or more antihypertensive drugs. In addition to measuring blood pressure, clinicians should evaluate patients for orthostatic hypotension, adverse drug effects, adherence to drug therapy and lifestyle modifications, and the need for drug dosage adjustments. Laboratory testing such as electrolytes and renal function status and other assessments of target organ damage also should be performed.

Considerations for Drug Therapy in Patients with Underlying Cardiovascular and Other Risk Factors

Drug therapy in patients with hypertension and underlying cardiovascular or other risk factors should be carefully individualized based on the underlying disease(s), concomitant drugs, tolerance to drug-induced adverse effects, and blood pressure goal. (See Table 2 on Compelling Indications for Drug Classes based on Comorbid Conditions, in Considerations for Drug Therapy in Patients with Underlying Cardiovascular and Other Risk Factors under Uses: Hypertension in Adults, in the Thiazides General Statement 40:28.20.)

Ischemic Heart Disease

The selection of an appropriate antihypertensive agent in patients with ischemic heart disease should be based on individual patient characteristics but may include ACE inhibitors and/or β-blockers, with the addition of other drugs such as thiazide diuretics or calcium-channel blockers as necessary to achieve blood pressure goals. Many experts recommend the use of an ACE inhibitor (or an angiotensin II receptor antagonist if ACE inhibitors are not tolerated) and/or a β-blocker in hypertensive patients with stable ischemic heart disease because of the cardioprotective benefits of these drugs; all patients who have survived an MI should be treated with a β-blocker because of the demonstrated mortality benefit of these agents.

Heart Failure

While available evidence suggests that angiotensin II receptor antagonists as single therapies are not superior to other antihypertensive agents in the reduction of cardiovascular outcomes, angiotensin II receptor antagonists, usually in conjunction with other agents such as cardiac glycosides, diuretics, and β-blockers, have been shown to reduce morbidity and mortality in patients with existing heart failure. Because of the established benefits of ACE inhibitors in patients with heart failure, the American College of Cardiology Foundation (ACCF), AHA, and Heart Failure Society of America (HFSA) recommend the use of these drugs in all patients with symptomatic or asymptomatic (i.e., structural heart disease but no signs or symptoms) heart failure with reduced left ventricular ejection fraction (LVEF). Experts recommend an angiotensin II receptor antagonist as an alternative to therapy with an ACE inhibitor in patients with symptomatic or asymptomatic (i.e., structural heart disease but no signs or symptoms) heart failure with reduced LVEF. (See Uses: Heart Failure.)

Diabetes Mellitus

Experts state that initial treatment of hypertension in adults with diabetes mellitus and hypertension should include any of the usual first-line agents (ACE inhibitors, angiotensin II receptor antagonists, calcium-channel blockers, thiazide diuretics). In adults with diabetes mellitus, hypertension, and albuminuria, treatment with an ACE inhibitor or angiotensin II receptor antagonist may be considered to reduce the progression of kidney disease. While there is evidence demonstrating the benefits of angiotensin II receptor antagonists in reducing the development or progression of microvascular or macrovascular complications in hypertensive patients with type 1 or type 2 diabetes mellitus, in the absence of albuminuria, the risk of progressive kidney disease is low, and ACE inhibitors and angiotensin II receptor antagonists have not demonstrated superior cardioprotection when compared with other first-line agents. Results of several studies indicate that adequate control of blood pressure in patients with type 2 diabetes mellitus reduces the development or progression of complications of diabetes (e.g., death related to diabetes, stroke, heart failure, microvascular disease). Most patients with diabetes mellitus will require 2 or more antihypertensive agents to achieve blood pressure control.

Chronic Kidney Disease

Hypertensive patients with CKD (glomerular filtration rate [GFR] less than 60 mL/minute per 1.73 m^2 or kidney damage for 3 or more months) usually will require more than one antihypertensive agent to reach target blood pressure. Use of angiotensin II receptor antagonists or ACE inhibitors may be reasonable in patients with diabetic or nondiabetic CKD (Stage 1 or 2 with albuminuria or Stage 3 or higher); these drugs have been shown to slow the progression of kidney disease. Evidence of a renoprotective benefit is strongest in those with higher levels of albuminuria. Increases in serum creatinine (up to 30%) may be observed as a result of a decrease in intraglomerular pressure and concurrent reduction in GFR. The 2017 ACC/AHA hypertension guideline states that in patients with less severe kidney disease (i.e., stage 1 or 2 CKD without albuminuria), any of the first-line antihypertensive agents (e.g., ACE inhibitors, angiotensin II receptor antagonists, calcium-channel blockers, thiazide diuretics) can be used for the initial treatment of hypertension. Diuretics also may be useful in the management of CKD, and may potentiate the effects of angiotensin II receptor antagonists, ACE inhibitors, and other antihypertensive agents when used in combination.

Cerebrovascular Disease

Some experts recommend a blood pressure goal of less than 140/90 mm Hg in patients with ischemic stroke or transient ischemic attack (TIA), while others state that a blood pressure goal of less than 130/80 mm Hg may be reasonable. The 2017 ACC/AHA hypertension guideline states that adults not previously treated for hypertension who experience a stroke or TIA and who have an established blood pressure of 140/90 mm Hg or higher should receive antihypertensive therapy a few days after the event to reduce the risk of recurrent stroke or other vascular events. In patients with a recent lacunar stroke, experts suggest that a systolic blood pressure goal of 130 mm Hg may be reasonable based on results of a randomized open-label study (the Secondary Prevention of Small Subcortical Strokes [SPS3] trial). Although experts state that the optimal choice of drug for the management of hypertension in patients with a previous TIA or ischemic stroke is uncertain, available data indicate that an ACE inhibitor, angiotensin II receptor antagonist, thiazide diuretic, or the combination of a thiazide diuretic and an ACE inhibitor may be effective. Administration of an ACE inhibitor in combination with a thiazide diuretic has been shown to lower rates of recurrent stroke.

Other Special Considerations for Antihypertensive Drug Therapy
Race

Most patients with hypertension, especially black patients, will require at least 2 antihypertensive drugs to achieve adequate blood pressure control. Like ACE inhibitors, angiotensin II receptor antagonists may produce a smaller blood pressure response in hypertensive black patients compared with nonblack patients. In general, black patients tend to respond better to thiazide diuretics or calcium-channel blocking agents than to angiotensin II receptor antagonists. However, the combination of an ACE inhibitor or an angiotensin II receptor antagonist with a calcium-channel blocker or thiazide diuretic produces similar blood pressure lowering in black patients as in other racial groups. In addition, some experts state that when use of angiotensin II receptor antagonists is indicated in hypertensive patients with underlying cardiovascular or other risk factors, these indications should be applied equally to black hypertensive patients.

For further information on overall principles and expert recommendations for treatment of hypertension, see Uses: Hypertension in Adults and also see Uses: Hypertension in Pediatric Patients, in the Thiazides General Statement 40:28.20.

• Diabetic Nephropathy

Both angiotensin II receptor antagonists (e.g., valsartan) and ACE inhibitors have been shown to slow the rate of progression of renal disease in patients with diabetes mellitus and persistent albuminuria†, and use of a drug from either class is recommended in such patients with modestly elevated (30–300 mg/24 hours) or higher (exceeding 300 mg/24 hours) levels of urinary albumin excretion. The ADA states that the use of an ACE inhibitor or angiotensin II receptor antagonist is not recommended for the primary prevention of diabetic nephropathy in patients with diabetes mellitus who are normotensive, have normal levels of urinary protein excretion, and have a normal GFR. The usual precautions of angiotensin II receptor antagonist or ACE inhibitor therapy in patients with substantial renal impairment should be observed. (See Renal Effects under Warnings/Precautions: Other Warnings/Precautions, in Cautions.) For additional information on the use of angiotensin II receptor antagonists in the treatment of diabetic nephropathy, see Uses: Diabetic Nephropathy, in Losartan 24:32.08 and in Irbesartan 24:32.08.

● Heart Failure

Valsartan is used in the management of heart failure.

Current guidelines for the management of heart failure in adults generally recommend a combination of drug therapies to reduce morbidity and mortality, including neurohormonal antagonists (e.g., ACE inhibitors, angiotensin II receptor antagonists, angiotensin receptor-neprilysin inhibitors [ARNIs], β-blockers, aldosterone receptor antagonists) that inhibit the detrimental compensatory mechanisms in heart failure. Additional agents (e.g., cardiac glycosides, diuretics, sinoatrial modulators [i.e., ivabradine]) added to a heart failure treatment regimen in selected patients have been associated with symptomatic improvement and/or reduction in heart failure-related hospitalizations. Experts recommend that all asymptomatic patients with reduced LVEF (ACCF/AHA stage B heart failure) receive therapy with an ACE inhibitor and β-blocker to prevent symptomatic heart failure and to reduce morbidity and mortality. In patients with prior or current symptoms of chronic heart failure with reduced LVEF (ACCF/AHA stage C heart failure), ACCF, AHA, and HFSA recommend inhibition of the renin-angiotensin-aldosterone (RAA) system with an ACE inhibitor, angiotensin II receptor antagonist, or ARNI in conjunction with a β-blocker, and an aldosterone antagonist in selected patients, to reduce morbidity and mortality. While ACE inhibitors have been the preferred drugs for inhibition of the RAA system because of their established benefits in patients with heart failure and reduced ejection fraction, some evidence indicates that therapy with sacubitril/valsartan, an ARNI, may be more effective than ACE inhibitor therapy (enalapril) in reducing cardiovascular death and heart failure-related hospitalization in such patients. ACCF, AHA, and HFSA recommend that patients with chronic symptomatic heart failure and reduced LVEF (New York Heart Association [NYHA] class II or III) who are able to tolerate an ACE inhibitor or angiotensin II receptor antagonist be switched to therapy containing an ARNI to further reduce morbidity and mortality. However, in patients in whom an ARNI is not appropriate, continued use of an ACE inhibitor for all classes of heart failure with reduced ejection fraction remains strongly advised. In patients in whom an ARNI or ACE inhibitor is not appropriate, an angiotensin II receptor antagonist may be used. For further information on the use of ARNIs in patients with heart failure, see Uses: Heart Failure, in Sacubitril and Valsartan 24:32.92.

While angiotensin II receptor antagonists are considered reasonable alternatives in patients who are unable to tolerate ACE inhibitors (e.g., because of cough or angioedema), angioedema has been reported rarely with the use of valsartan during postmarketing experience. (See Sensitivity Reactions under Cautions: Warnings/Precautions.)

Several clinical trials have evaluated the use of angiotensin II receptor antagonists in patients with heart failure as add-on therapy to conventional regimens compared with an ACE inhibitor, as add-on therapy to conventional regimens including an ACE inhibitor, as combination therapy with an ACE inhibitor compared with therapy with either type of agent alone, or as an alternative therapy in patients intolerant of ACE inhibitors. In a large, double-blind, placebo-controlled study (Valsartan Heart Failure Trial [Val-HeFT]) in patients with mild to severe (NYHA class II–IV) heart failure and LVEF less than 40%, addition of valsartan 40 mg twice daily (initial dosage, with dosage doubled every 2 weeks to a target dosage of 160 mg twice daily) to standard therapy (principally ACE inhibitors, diuretics, digoxin, and β-blockers) was associated with a reduction in the composite end point of heart failure-related morbidity and mortality (defined as cardiac arrest with resuscitation, hospitalization for worsening heart failure, or administration of IV inotropic or vasodilator drugs for 4 or more hours without hospitalization) after an average of approximately 23 months. Valsartan therapy also improved secondary cardiovascular outcomes such as NYHA class, ejection fraction, and symptoms of heart failure (dyspnea, fatigue, edema, rales), and prevented deterioration of the patients' well-being (as determined by quality of life measurements). However, improvement in heart failure morbidity occurred principally in patients not receiving adjunctive therapy with an ACE inhibitor, and overall mortality was not affected by valsartan therapy. For additional details of studies on the use of angiotensin II receptor antagonists in the management of heart failure, see Uses: Heart Failure, in Losartan 24:32.08 and and Candesartan 24:32.08.

Data from other long-term placebo-controlled clinical trials indicate that angiotensin II receptor antagonists produce hemodynamic and neurohormonal effects associated with their suppression of the renin-angiotensin system; reduced hospitalizations and mortality also have been demonstrated. However, these drugs did not show consistent effects on cardiac symptoms or exercise tolerance in some studies. In one comparative (Evaluation of Losartan in the Elderly [ELITE]) study in geriatric patients 65 years of age and older who received losartan (up to 50 mg daily) or captopril (up to 150 mg daily) in addition to conventional therapy for 48 weeks, patients receiving losartan had a 46% lower risk of death and also experienced a lower incidence of adverse effects than those receiving captopril. However, after interim analysis of data, the difference in survival was no longer statistically significant and no difference in morbidity and mortality or frequency in hospitalizations for heart failure was found between the 2 therapies. Results of a follow-up study (ELITE II) failed to confirm a survival benefit for losartan therapy compared with captopril. In this study, losartan did not provide a statistically significant difference in reduction of overall death, sudden cardiac death, and/or resuscitated cardiac arrest compared with captopril, although ELITE II was not designed to demonstrate equivalence between the 2 therapies. In addition, results of another study (Randomized Evaluation of Strategies for Left Ventricular Dysfunction [RESOLVD]) in patients with ischemic or nonischemic dilated cardiomyopathy and mild to moderate heart failure showed no differences in exercise capacity or risk of cardiac events in patients receiving candesartan (up to 16 mg daily), enalapril (up to 20 mg daily), or a combination of candesartan and enalapril, in addition to conventional therapy.

● Heart Failure or Left Ventricular Dysfunction After Acute Myocardial Infarction

Valsartan is used to reduce the risk of cardiovascular mortality following acute MI in clinically stable patients with demonstrated clinical evidence of heart failure (signs, symptoms, radiologic evidence) or left ventricular systolic dysfunction (i.e., LVEF 40% or less). While ACE inhibitors generally are the preferred agents for this use because of their established benefits, angiotensin II receptor antagonists may be substituted in patients who are intolerant to ACE inhibitor therapy.

Efficacy of valsartan for reducing risk of mortality from any cause has been evaluated in a large, double-blind, randomized, long-term (median follow-up: 24.7 months) study (VALsartan In Acute myocardial iNfarcTion trial [VALIANT]) involving 14,703 patients with acute MI complicated by heart failure or left ventricular systolic dysfunction. The primary end point of this study was death from any cause, while secondary end points included time to cardiovascular mortality and time to the first occurrence of cardiovascular reinfarction or hospitalization for heart failure. A prespecified analysis was designed to demonstrate the noninferiority or equivalence of valsartan to captopril in the event that valsartan would not clearly be shown to be superior to the ACE inhibitor. Such analysis also was based on results from previous placebo-controlled studies, in which administration of ACE inhibitors has been associated with reduction in mortality.

Results of VALIANT indicate that when compared with those receiving captopril (titrated to 50 mg 3 times daily) or the combination of valsartan (titrated to 80 mg twice daily) and captopril (titrated to 50 mg 3 times daily), valsartan therapy (titrated to 160 mg twice daily) initiated 0.5–10 days after an acute MI was associated with a reduction of all-cause mortality similar to the reduction observed among those receiving captopril or the combination of valsartan and captopril. Nine hundred and seventy-nine (19.9%) patients receiving valsartan died (hazard ratio of 1; 97.5% confidence interval: 0.9–1.11) compared with 958 (19.5%) of those receiving captopril. In addition, 941 (19.3%) patients receiving valsartan in combination with captopril died (compared with 19.5% of those receiving captopril) (hazard ratio of 0.98; 97.5% confidence interval: 0.89–1.09). Valsartan therapy also was comparable to ACE inhibitor therapy in terms of the composite end point of fatal and nonfatal cardiovascular events (hospitalization for heart failure and recurrent nonfatal MI). Benefits associated with valsartan were not affected by age, gender, race, or baseline therapies. In this study, combined therapy with valsartan and captopril increased the rate of adverse effects without providing further benefit on survival. Although findings of this study provide evidence of comparable benefit, at least in high-risk patients, most experts continue to recommend that angiotensin II receptor antagonists be reserved for patients who do not tolerate ACE inhibitors since experience with ACE inhibitors is more extensive.

DOSAGE AND ADMINISTRATION

● Administration

Valsartan is administered orally. Although food may decrease the rate and extent (e.g., by about 40%) of valsartan absorption, the manufacturers state that the drug can be administered without regard to meals.

Valsartan may be administered as an extemporaneously prepared oral suspension in pediatric patients who are unable to swallow tablets or in those for whom the calculated daily dosage does not correspond to the available tablet strengths. An extemporaneous suspension containing valsartan 4 mg/mL can be prepared in the following manner. First, 80 mL of suspending vehicle (e.g., Ora-Plus®) is added to an amber glass bottle containing eight 80-mg tablets of valsartan, and the contents are shaken for at least 2 minutes. The concentrated suspension should be allowed to stand for at least 1 hour following reconstitution and then should be shaken for at least an additional minute. The concentrated suspension of valsartan should be diluted with 80 mL of sweetening vehicle (e.g., Ora-Sweet SE®), and the container then shaken for at least 10 seconds to disperse the contents. The suspension should be shaken for at least 10 seconds before each dose is dispensed. When stored in an amber glass bottle with child-resistant screw-cap closure at a temperature of less than 30°C or at 2–8°C, the extemporaneous suspension is stable for up to 30 or up to 75 days, respectively.

● Dosage

Hypertension

Dosage of valsartan must be individualized and adjusted according to blood pressure response.

Valsartan Therapy

The manufacturers state the usual initial dosage of valsartan as monotherapy in adults is 80 or 160 mg once daily in patients without depletion of intravascular volume; patients requiring greater reductions in blood pressure initially may be started at the higher dosage. If blood pressure response is inadequate with the initial dosage, dosage may be increased as tolerated up to a maximum of 320 mg daily or a diuretic may be added. The usual maintenance dosage of valsartan is 80–320 mg given once daily. However, addition of a diuretic generally has a greater effect on blood pressure reduction than dosage increases of valsartan as dosage exceeds 80 mg daily. Valsartan also can be used concomitantly with other antihypertensive agents.

The usual initial dosage of valsartan in children and adolescents 6–16 years of age with hypertension is 1.3 mg/kg (up to 40 mg) once daily. Dosage should be adjusted according to blood pressure response. Some experts state that the dosage may be increased every 2–4 weeks until blood pressure is controlled, the maximum dosage is reached, or adverse effects occur. Dosages exceeding 2.7 mg/kg (up to 160 mg) once daily have not been evaluated in pediatric patients. Because systemic exposure to valsartan is 1.6 times greater when the drug is administered as an extemporaneously prepared suspension compared with administration as the commercially available tablets, children being switched from the suspension to the oral tablets may require an increase in dosage of the drug. For information on overall principles and expert recommendations for treatment of hypertension in pediatric patients, see Uses: Hypertension in Pediatric Patients, in the Thiazides General Statement 40:28.20.

Valsartan/Hydrochlorothiazide Fixed-combination Therapy

Commercially available preparations containing valsartan in fixed combination with hydrochlorothiazide can be used as a substitute for the individually titrated drugs. Alternatively, in patients who do not respond adequately to monotherapy with valsartan (or another angiotensin II receptor antagonist) or, alternatively, with hydrochlorothiazide, combined therapy with the drugs can be used. The manufacturers state that patients who do not respond adequately to monotherapy with valsartan (or another angiotensin II receptor antagonist) or hydrochlorothiazide may be switched to therapy with the fixed-combination preparation at an initial dosage of valsartan 160 mg and hydrochlorothiazide 12.5 mg once daily. In addition, patients who experience dose-limiting adverse effects during monotherapy with valsartan or hydrochlorothiazide can be switched to a lower dosage of that drug, given as a fixed-combination preparation containing valsartan and hydrochlorothiazide, to achieve similar blood pressure control. If needed, dosage of the fixed combination may be increased up to a maximum of 320 mg of valsartan and 25 mg of hydrochlorothiazide (given once daily) after 3–4 weeks. The maximum antihypertensive effect is attained within 2–4 weeks after initiation of therapy or a change in dosage.

Commercially available preparations containing valsartan in fixed combination with hydrochlorothiazide may be used for initial treatment of hypertension in patients likely to require combined therapy with multiple antihypertensive drugs to achieve blood pressure control. In such patients, therapy with the fixed-combination preparation should be initiated at a dosage of 160 mg of valsartan and 12.5 mg of hydrochlorothiazide once daily. Dosage should be adjusted according to the patient's response after 1–2 weeks of therapy. The decision to use the fixed combination of valsartan and hydrochlorothiazide for initial treatment of hypertension

should be based on assessment of potential benefits and risks of such therapy. The fixed combination of valsartan and hydrochlorothiazide is not recommended as initial therapy in patients with depletion of intravascular volume. In patients whose baseline blood pressure is 160/100 mm Hg, the estimated probability of achieving control of systolic blood pressure (defined as systolic blood pressure of less than 140 mm Hg) is 41, 50, or 84% and of achieving control of diastolic blood pressure (defined as diastolic blood pressure of less than 90 mm Hg) is 60, 57, or 80% with valsartan (320 mg daily) alone, hydrochlorothiazide (25 mg daily) alone, or valsartan combined with hydrochlorothiazide (at the same dosages), respectively.

Valsartan/Amlodipine Fixed-combination Therapy

Patients whose hypertension is adequately controlled with valsartan and amlodipine administered separately may be switched to the fixed-combination preparation containing the corresponding individual doses. Alternatively, the manufacturers state that patients who do not respond adequately to monotherapy with valsartan (or another angiotensin II receptor antagonist) or, alternatively, with amlodipine (or another dihydropyridine-derivative calcium-channel blocker) may be switched to therapy with the fixed-combination preparation containing valsartan and amlodipine. In addition, patients who experience dose-limiting adverse effects during monotherapy with valsartan or amlodipine can be switched to a lower dosage of that drug, given as a fixed-combination preparation containing valsartan and amlodipine, to achieve similar blood pressure control; dosage should be adjusted according to the patient's response after 3–4 weeks of therapy. If needed, dosage of the fixed-combination preparation may be increased up to a maximum of 320 mg of valsartan and 10 mg of amlodipine given once daily; because most of the antihypertensive effect of a given dosage is achieved within 2 weeks, dosage may be adjusted after 1–2 weeks, if needed, to attain blood pressure control.

Commercially available preparations containing valsartan in fixed combination with amlodipine may be used for initial treatment of hypertension in patients likely to require combined therapy with multiple antihypertensive drugs to achieve blood pressure control. In such patients, therapy with the fixed-combination preparation should be initiated at a dosage of 160 mg of valsartan and 5 mg of amlodipine once daily in individuals without depletion of intravascular volume. The decision to use the fixed combination of valsartan and amlodipine for initial management of hypertension should be based on assessment of potential benefits and risks of such therapy, including consideration of whether the patient is likely to tolerate the lowest available dosage of the combined drugs. In patients whose baseline blood pressure is 160/100 mm Hg, the estimated probability of achieving control of systolic blood pressure (defined as systolic blood pressure of less than 140 mm Hg) is 47, 67, or 80% and of achieving control of diastolic blood pressure (defined as diastolic blood pressure of less than 90 mm Hg) is 62, 80, or 85% with valsartan (320 mg daily) alone, amlodipine (10 mg daily) alone, or valsartan combined with amlodipine (at the same dosages), respectively.

Valsartan/Amlodipine/Hydrochlorothiazide Fixed-combination Therapy

The fixed-combination preparation containing valsartan, amlodipine, and hydrochlorothiazide may be used to provide additional blood pressure control in patients who do not respond adequately to combination therapy with any 2 of the following classes of antihypertensive agents: angiotensin II receptor antagonists, calcium-channel blockers, or diuretics. Patients who experience dose-limiting adverse effects of valsartan, amlodipine, or hydrochlorothiazide while receiving any dual combination of these drugs may be switched to a lower dosage of that drug, given as a fixed-combination preparation containing all 3 of these drugs, to achieve similar blood pressure reductions. The fixed-combination preparation containing valsartan, amlodipine, and hydrochlorothiazide also can be used as a substitute for the individually titrated drugs. If necessary, dosage of the fixed-combination preparation may be increased after 2 weeks for additional blood pressure control (but should not exceed a maximum dosage of 320 mg of valsartan, 10 mg of amlodipine, and 25 mg of hydrochlorothiazide once daily). The commercially available preparation containing valsartan in fixed combination with amlodipine and hydrochlorothiazide should not be used for the initial management of hypertension.

Blood Pressure Monitoring and Treatment Goals

Blood pressure should be monitored regularly (i.e., monthly) during therapy and dosage of the antihypertensive drug adjusted until blood pressure is controlled. If an adequate blood pressure response is not achieved with angiotensin II receptor antagonist monotherapy, the dosage may be increased or another antihypertensive agent with demonstrated benefit and preferably with a complementary mechanism of action (e.g., calcium-channel blocker, thiazide diuretic) may be added; if target blood pressure is still not achieved, a third drug may be added. (See Uses: Hypertension.) In patients who develop unacceptable adverse effects with valsartan, the drug should be discontinued and another antihypertensive agent from a different pharmacologic class should be initiated.

The goal of hypertension management and prevention is to achieve and maintain optimal control of blood pressure. However, the optimum blood pressure threshold for initiating antihypertensive drug therapy and specific treatment goals remain controversial. While previous hypertension guidelines have based target blood pressure goals on age and comorbidities, the 2017 ACC/AHA hypertension guideline incorporates underlying cardiovascular risk into decision making regarding treatment and generally recommends the same target blood pressure (i.e., less than 130/80 mm Hg) in all adults. Many patients will require at least 2 drugs from different pharmacologic classes to achieve their blood pressure goal; the potential benefits of hypertension management and drug cost, adverse effects, and risks associated with the use of multiple antihypertensive drugs also should be considered when deciding a patient's blood pressure treatment goal. (See General Considerations for Initial and Maintenance Antihypertensive Therapy under Uses: Hypertension.)

For additional information on target levels of blood pressure and on monitoring therapy in the management of hypertension, see Blood Pressure Monitoring and Treatment Goals under Dosage: Hypertension, in Dosage and Administration in the Thiazides General Statement 40:28.20.

Heart Failure

For the management of heart failure (New York Heart Association [NYHA] class II–IV) in patients unable to tolerate therapy with angiotensin-converting enzyme (ACE) inhibitors, the manufacturers recommend an initial valsartan dosage of 40 mg twice daily; some experts recommend an initial dosage of 20–40 mg twice daily in patients with chronic heart failure and reduced left ventricular ejection fraction (LVEF) (American College of Cardiology Foundation [ACCF]/American Heart Association [AHA] stage C heart failure). Dosage of valsartan should be increased until a dosage of 160 mg twice daily (the maximum dosage used in clinical trials) or the highest tolerated dosage is reached. While patients with heart failure generally have some reduction in blood pressure with valsartan therapy, discontinuance of therapy usually is not necessary when dosage recommendations are followed. Consideration should be given to reducing the dosage of concurrent diuretic therapy.

Heart Failure or Left Ventricular Dysfunction after Acute Myocardial Infarction

When used after myocardial infarction (MI) in adults with clinical signs of heart failure or left ventricular systolic dysfunction, valsartan therapy may be initiated as early as 12 hours after the MI. An initial dosage of 20 mg twice daily is recommended. Dosage may be increased within 7 days to 40 mg twice daily with subsequent titrations to a target maintenance dosage of 160 mg twice daily, as tolerated. If hypotension or renal dysfunction occurs, dosage reduction should be considered. While post-MI patients generally have some reduction in blood pressure with valsartan therapy, discontinuance of therapy usually is not necessary when dosage recommendations are followed. Valsartan may be given with other standard post-MI therapy (e.g., thrombolytics, aspirin, β-adrenergic blocking agents [β-blockers], hydroxymethylglutaryl-CoA [HMG-CoA] reductase inhibitors [statins]).

• Special Populations

The manufacturers state that modification of valsartan dosage is not necessary for patients with mild to moderate renal impairment; however, valsartan has not been studied in patients with creatinine clearances of less than 10 mL/minute and should be used with caution in adults with severe renal impairment. Valsartan is not removed by hemodialysis. Use of valsartan in pediatric patients with glomerular filtration rates of less than 30 mL/minute per 1.73 m² has not been studied. Safety and efficacy of commercially available preparations containing valsartan in fixed combination with hydrochlorothiazide have not been established in patients with severe renal impairment.

The manufacturers state that valsartan should be used with caution in patients with hepatic impairment. Although systemic exposure to valsartan (as measured by area under the serum concentration-time curve [AUC]) is increased approximately twofold in patients with mild to moderate chronic liver disease, the manufacturers state that modification of valsartan dosage is not necessary for these

patients. The amount of amlodipine in fixed-combination preparations containing valsartan and amlodipine exceeds the recommended initial dosage of amlodipine (2.5 mg daily) for patients with hepatic impairment.

The manufacturers state that modification of valsartan dosage is not necessary for geriatric patients. However, the amount of amlodipine in fixed-combination preparations containing valsartan and amlodipine exceeds the recommended initial dosage of amlodipine (2.5 mg daily) for geriatric patients.

CAUTIONS

• Contraindications

Known hypersensitivity to valsartan or any ingredient in the formulation.

Concomitant use of valsartan and aliskiren in patients with diabetes mellitus. (See Drug Interactions: Drugs that Block the Renin-Angiotensin System.)

• Warnings/Precautions

Warnings

Fetal/Neonatal Morbidity and Mortality

Drugs that act directly on the renin-angiotensin system (e.g., angiotensin-converting enzyme [ACE] inhibitors, angiotensin II receptor antagonists) can cause fetal and neonatal morbidity and mortality when used in pregnancy during the second and third trimesters. Valsartan should be discontinued as soon as possible when pregnancy is detected, unless continued use is considered life-saving. Nearly all women can be transferred successfully to alternative therapy for the remainder of their pregnancy. For additional information on the risk of such drugs (i.e., angiotensin II antagonists and ACE inhibitors) during pregnancy, see Cautions: Pregnancy, Fertility, and Lactation, in Captopril 24:32.04 and in Enalaprilat/Enalapril 24:32.04.

Sensitivity Reactions

Sensitivity reactions, including various anaphylactoid reactions and/or angioedema, have been reported in patients receiving angiotensin II receptor antagonists, including valsartan. These drugs should be used with extreme caution in patients with a history of angioedema associated with or unrelated to ACE inhibitor or angiotensin II receptor antagonist therapy. The manufacturer states that valsartan should not be readministered to patients with a history of angioedema.

Other Warnings/Precautions

Cardiovascular Effects

Valsartan rarely is associated with severe hypotension in patients with uncomplicated hypertension. Symptomatic hypotension may occur in patients with an activated renin-angiotensin system (e.g., patients with volume or salt depletion secondary to salt restriction or high-dose diuretic therapy). Volume and/or salt depletion should be corrected before starting valsartan therapy, or therapy should be initiated under close medical supervision.

Patients with heart failure and those with clinical signs of left ventricular systolic dysfunction following acute myocardial infarction (MI) generally have some reduction in blood pressure with valsartan therapy, but drug discontinuance generally is not necessary when recommended dosages are used. Caution should be observed when initiating valsartan therapy in these patients.

If symptomatic hypotension occurs, the patient should be placed in the supine position; if hypotension is severe, IV infusion of 0.9% sodium chloride injection to expand fluid volume should be considered. Transient hypotension is not a contraindication to additional doses of valsartan, and therapy with the drug can be reinstated cautiously after blood pressure has been stabilized (e.g., with volume expansion).

Malignancies

In July 2010, the US Food and Drug Administration (FDA) initiated a safety review of angiotensin II receptor antagonists after a published meta-analysis suggested a possible association between the use of these agents and an increased risk of cancer. The meta-analysis, which combined cancer-related findings from 5 randomized, controlled trials in over 60,000 patients, found a modest but significant increase in the risk of new cancer occurrence in patients receiving an angiotensin II receptor antagonist (mostly telmisartan) compared with those in control groups (7.2 versus 6%, respectively; risk ratio 1.08). However, because of several limitations of the study (e.g., trials included in the meta-analysis were not specifically designed to evaluate cancer outcomes, lack of individual patient data), the validity of these findings has been questioned.

Subsequent studies, including a larger, more comprehensive meta-analysis conducted by FDA, have not shown an increased risk of cancer in patients receiving angiotensin II receptor antagonists. FDA's meta-analysis, which included trial-level data from 31 randomized studies (total of approximately 156,000 patients), found no evidence of an increased risk of cancer in patients who received an angiotensin II receptor antagonist compared with those who received other treatments (placebo or active control). The overall rate of new cancer occurrence was essentially the same in both groups of patients (1.82 and 1.84 cases per 100 patient-years, respectively). In addition, there was no difference in the risk of cancer-related death, breast cancer, lung cancer, or prostate cancer between the groups. Based on these results and a review of all currently available data related to this potential safety concern, FDA has concluded that use of angiotensin II receptor antagonists is not associated with an increased risk of cancer.

Renal Effects

Because the renin-angiotensin-aldosterone (RAA) system appears to contribute substantially to maintenance of glomerular filtration in patients with heart failure in whom renal perfusion is severely compromised, renal function may deteriorate markedly (e.g., renal failure) in these patients during therapy with an ACE inhibitor or an angiotensin II receptor antagonist (e.g., valsartan). Dosage reduction or discontinuance of valsartan or diuretic therapy may be required. Renal artery stenosis, preexisting renal impairment, and concomitant diuretic therapy also are risk factors for renal impairment during therapy with drugs that inhibit the RAA system. Although reports received to date have involved patients treated with ACE inhibitors, this adverse effect also would be expected to occur when drugs with similar pharmacologic activity (e.g., angiotensin II receptor antagonists) are used in a similar manner. (See Cautions: Renal Effects, in Enalapril 24:32.04.)

Hyperkalemia

Hyperkalemia may occur in patients receiving valsartan, especially in those with heart failure and preexisting renal impairment. Dosage reduction or discontinuance of valsartan therapy may be required.

Fixed-combination Preparations

When valsartan is used as a fixed combination that includes amlodipine and/or hydrochlorothiazide, the cautions, precautions, and contraindications associated with the concomitant agent(s) must be considered in addition to those associated with valsartan.

Specific Populations

Pregnancy

Category D. (See Users Guide.)

Valsartan can cause fetal and neonatal morbidity and mortality when administered to a pregnant woman. Valsartan should be discontinued as soon as possible when pregnancy is detected. (See Fetal/Neonatal Morbidity and Mortality under Warnings/Precautions: Warnings, in Cautions.)

Lactation

Valsartan is distributed into milk in rats. It is not known whether valsartan is distributed into human milk. A decision should be made whether to discontinue nursing or the drug because of the potential risk in nursing infants.

Pediatric Use

Safety and efficacy of valsartan have been established in a randomized, double-blind clinical trial in pediatric patients 6–16 years of age with hypertension; adverse effects of the drug in this age group were similar to those observed in adults. Although there was some evidence of efficacy in randomized, double-blind clinical trials in pediatric patients 6 months to 5 years of age with hypertension, 2 deaths and 3 cases of transaminase elevations were observed in a one-year open-label extension study in patients 1–5 years of age. A causal relationship to the drug has not been established; however, use of valsartan in pediatric patients younger than 6 years of age is not recommended. In pediatric patients with hypertension in whom underlying renal abnormalities may be more common, renal function and serum potassium should be carefully monitored. Pharmacokinetics of the drug have been studied in pediatric patients 1–16 years of age.

Safety and efficacy of valsartan in fixed combination with hydrochlorothiazide and/or amlodipine in pediatric patients have not been established.

Safety and efficacy of valsartan in pediatric patients with glomerular filtration rates of less than 30 mL/minute per 1.73 m² have not been established.

For information on overall principles and expert recommendations for treatment of hypertension in pediatric patients, see Uses: Hypertension in Pediatric Patients, in the Thiazides General Statement 40:28.20.

Geriatric Use

No substantial differences in safety and efficacy of valsartan in geriatric patients relative to younger adults have been observed, but increased sensitivity cannot be ruled out.

Hepatic Impairment

Valsartan should be used with caution in patients with obstructive biliary disease or hepatic impairment since the drug is eliminated primarily by biliary excretion and clearance of the drug may be reduced.

Renal Impairment

Valsartan should be used with caution in patients with severe renal impairment. (See Renal Effects and also see Hyperkalemia under Warning/Precautions: Other Warnings/Precautions, in Cautions.)

● Common Adverse Effects

Adverse effects occurring in 1% or more of adults with hypertension receiving valsartan and more frequently than with placebo include viral infection, fatigue, and abdominal pain; adverse effects in pediatric patients 6–16 years of age generally are similar to those in adults.

Adverse effects occurring in 2% or more of patients with heart failure receiving valsartan and more frequently than with placebo include dizziness, hypotension, diarrhea, arthralgia, fatigue, back pain, postural dizziness, hyperkalemia, and postural hypotension. In patients receiving valsartan following acute MI, the most common adverse effects resulting in discontinuation of the drug included hypotension, cough, and increased serum creatinine concentration.

DRUG INTERACTIONS

● Drugs Affecting or Metabolized by Hepatic Microsomal Enzymes

In vitro studies suggest valsartan is minimally metabolized by cytochrome P-450 (CYP) microsomal isoenzyme 2C9 and does not inhibit CYP enzymes at therapeutic concentrations. Therefore, drug interactions mediated by CYP enzymes are considered unlikely with valsartan.

● Drugs That Inhibit Hepatic Transport Systems

In vitro data suggest that valsartan is a substrate of organic anion transporter protein (OATP) 1B1 (hepatic uptake transporter) and multidrug resistance protein MRP2 (hepatic efflux transporter). Use of valsartan concomitantly with inhibitors of OATP 1B1 (e.g., cyclosporine, rifampin) or MRP2 (e.g., ritonavir) may result in increased systemic exposure to valsartan.

● Drugs that Block the Renin-Angiotensin System

Concomitant use of valsartan with other drugs that block the renin-angiotensin system (e.g., angiotensin-converting enzyme [ACE] inhibitors, aliskiren) may increase the risk of renal impairment, hyperkalemia, and hypotension; when valsartan is used concomitantly with such drugs, blood pressure, renal function, and serum concentrations of electrolytes should be monitored closely. Concomitant use of valsartan with aliskiren is contraindicated in patients with diabetes mellitus; in addition, such concomitant use should be avoided in patients with renal impairment (glomerular filtration rate [GFR] less than 60 mL/minute per 1.73 m²). (See Cautions in Aliskiren Hemifumarate 24:32.40.)

● Drugs or Foods That Increase Serum Potassium Concentration

Concomitant use of potassium-sparing diuretics (e.g., amiloride, spironolactone, triamterene), potassium supplements, potassium-containing salt substitutes, or other drugs that may increase serum potassium concentrations (e.g., heparin) with valsartan may result in increased hyperkalemic effects and, in patients with heart failure, increases in serum creatinine concentration. Monitoring of serum potassium concentrations is recommended during concomitant use.

● Atenolol

Antihypertensive effect of combined atenolol and valsartan therapy exceeds that of either drug alone, but the reduction in heart rate with the drugs in combination does not exceed that observed with atenolol alone. Pharmacokinetic interaction is unlikely.

● Hydrochlorothiazide

Hypotensive effects of valsartan and hydrochlorothiazide are additive; pharmacokinetic interaction is unlikely.

● Lithium

Increased lithium concentrations and clinical toxicity have been reported in patients receiving valsartan concomitantly with lithium. Monitoring of serum lithium concentrations is recommended during concomitant use.

● Nonsteroidal Anti-inflammatory Agents

Hypotensive effects of angiotensin II receptor antagonists may be attenuated when these agents are used concomitantly with nonsteroidal anti-inflammatory agents (NSAIAs), including selective cyclooxygenase-2 (COX-2) inhibitors.

Deterioration of renal function may occur when angiotensin II receptor antagonists are used concomitantly with NSAIAs, including selective COX-2 inhibitors, in geriatric patients, patients with volume depletion (including those receiving concomitant diuretic therapy), or patients with renal impairment; renal function should be monitored periodically in patients receiving concomitant therapy with valsartan and an NSAIA.

● Warfarin

Concurrent use of valsartan and warfarin did not affect the pharmacokinetics of valsartan or the anticoagulant effect of warfarin.

● Other Drugs

Pharmacokinetic interactions with amlodipine, cimetidine, digoxin, furosemide, glyburide, and indomethacin are unlikely.

DESCRIPTION

Valsartan, a nonpeptide tetrazole derivative, is an angiotensin II type 1 (AT$_1$) receptor antagonist. Valsartan has pharmacologic actions similar to those of losartan; however, unlike losartan, valsartan is not a prodrug and its pharmacologic activity does not depend on hydrolysis in the liver.

Valsartan blocks the physiologic actions of angiotensin II, including vasoconstrictor and aldosterone-secreting effects, by selectively inhibiting access of angiotensin II to AT$_1$ receptors within many tissues, including vascular smooth muscle and the adrenal gland. By comparison, angiotensin-converting enzyme (ACE, kininase II) inhibitors block the conversion of angiotensin I to angiotensin II; however, the blockade of angiotensin II production by ACE inhibitors is not complete since the vasopressor hormone can be formed via other enzymes that are not blocked by ACE inhibitors. Because valsartan, unlike ACE inhibitors, does not inhibit ACE, the drug does not interfere with response to bradykinins and substance P; a beneficial consequence is the absence of certain ACE inhibitor-induced adverse effects (e.g., cough), but possible renal and/or cardioprotective effects may be sacrificed. Valsartan also does not interfere with angiotensin II synthesis.

Valsartan is eliminated mainly by biliary excretion; following oral administration, about 83% of the administered dose is recovered in feces and 13% in urine. The drug is eliminated mainly as unchanged drug, with only about 20% of a dose recovered as metabolites. In vitro studies indicate that valsartan is minimally metabolized by cytochrome P-450 (CYP) microsomal isoenzyme 2C9.

ADVICE TO PATIENTS

When valsartan is used in fixed combination with hydrochlorothiazide and/or amlodipine, importance of advising patients of important precautionary information about the concomitant agent(s).

Importance of informing women of childbearing potential about the risks of use during pregnancy.

Importance of women informing clinicians if they are or plan to become pregnant or plan to breast-feed. All women of childbearing potential should be advised to report pregnancy to their clinician as soon as possible. (See Fetal/Neonatal Morbidity and Mortality under Warnings/Precautions: Warnings, in Cautions.)

Importance of contacting clinician if dizziness or faintness develops or if unexplained weight gain or swelling of the feet, ankles, or hands occurs.

Importance of informing clinicians of existing or contemplated concomitant therapy, including prescription and OTC drugs.

Importance of informing patients of other important precautionary information. (See Cautions.)

PREPARATIONS

Excipients in commercially available drug preparations may have clinically important effects in some individuals; consult specific product labeling for details.

Valsartan

Oral		
Tablets	40 mg*	**Diovan®** (scored), Novartis
		Valsartan Tablets
	80 mg*	**Diovan®**, Novartis
		Valsartan Tablets
	160 mg*	**Diovan®**, Novartis
		Valsartan Tablets
	320 mg*	**Diovan®**, Novartis
		Valsartan Tablets

* available from one or more manufacturer, distributor, and/or repackager by generic (nonproprietary) name

Valsartan Combinations

Oral		
Tablets, film-coated	80 mg with Hydrochlorothiazide 12.5 mg*	**Diovan® HCT**, Novartis
		Valsartan and Hydrochlorothiazide Tablets
	160 mg with Amlodipine Besylate 5 mg (of amlodipine)*	**Amlodipine Besylate and Valsartan Tablets**
		Exforge®, Novartis
	160 mg with Amlodipine Besylate 5 mg (of amlodipine) and Hydrochlorothiazide 12.5 mg*	**Amlodipine Besylate, Valsartan, and Hydrochlorothiazide Tablets**
		Exforge HCT®, Novartis
	160 mg with Amlodipine Besylate 5 mg (of amlodipine) and Hydrochlorothiazide 25 mg*	**Amlodipine Besylate, Valsartan, and Hydrochlorothiazide Tablets**
		Exforge HCT®, Novartis
	160 mg with Amlodipine Besylate 10 mg (of amlodipine)*	**Amlodipine Besylate and Valsartan Tablets**
		Exforge®, Novartis
	160 mg with Amlodipine Besylate 10 mg (of amlodipine) and Hydrochlorothiazide 12.5 mg*	**Amlodipine Besylate, Valsartan, and Hydrochlorothiazide Tablets**
		Exforge HCT®, Novartis
	160 mg with Amlodipine Besylate 10 mg (of amlodipine) and Hydrochlorothiazide 25 mg*	**Amlodipine Besylate, Valsartan, and Hydrochlorothiazide Tablets**
		Exforge HCT®, Novartis

160 mg with Hydrochlorothiazide 12.5 mg*	**Diovan® HCT**, Novartis **Valsartan and Hydrochloro-thiazide Tablets**
160 mg with Hydrochlorothiazide 25 mg*	**Diovan® HCT**, Novartis **Valsartan and Hydrochloro-thiazide Tablets**
320 mg with Amlodipine Besylate 5 mg (of amlodipine)*	**Amlodipine Besylate and Valsartan Tablets** **Exforge®**, Novartis
320 mg with Amlodipine Besylate 10 mg (of amlodipine)*	**Amlodipine Besylate and Valsartan Tablets** **Exforge®**, Novartis
320 mg with Amlodipine Besylate 10 mg (of amlodipine) and Hydrochlorothiazide 25 mg*	**Amlodipine Besylate, Valsartan, and Hydrochloro-thiazide Tablets** **Exforge HCT®**, Novartis

320 mg with Hydrochlorothiazide 12.5 mg*	**Diovan® HCT**, Novartis **Valsartan and Hydrochloro-thiazide Tablets**
320 mg with Hydrochlorothiazide 25 mg*	**Diovan® HCT**, Novartis **Valsartan and Hydrochloro-thiazide Tablets**

* available from one or more manufacturer, distributor, and/or repackager by generic (nonproprietary) name

† Use is not currently included in the labeling approved by the US Food and Drug Administration.

Selected Revisions November 5, 2018, © Copyright, June 1, 1997, American Society of Health-System Pharmacists, Inc.

Sacubitril and Valsartan

24:32.12 • ANGIOTENSIN II RECEPTOR ANTAGONISTS/
NEPROLYSIN INHIBITORS

■ Sacubitril and valsartan (sacubitril/valsartan) is a fixed combination of sacubitril (a neprilysin [neutral endopeptidase] inhibitor) and valsartan (an angiotensin II type 1 [AT₁] receptor antagonist [i.e., angiotensin II receptor blocker, ARB]); such drug combinations have been referred to as angiotensin receptor-neprilysin inhibitors (ARNIs).

USES

● Heart Failure

Sacubitril and valsartan in fixed combination (sacubitril/valsartan) is used to reduce the risk of cardiovascular death and hospitalization for patients with chronic heart failure (New York Heart Association [NYHA] class II–IV) and reduced ejection fraction. Sacubitril/valsartan is usually administered in conjunction with other heart failure therapies (e.g., β-adrenergic blocking agent [β-blocker], aldosterone antagonist, diuretic) as a substitute for therapy with an angiotensin-converting enzyme (ACE) inhibitor or other angiotensin II receptor antagonist. Current evidence indicates that sacubitril/valsartan results in improved outcomes compared with enalapril based on reductions in cardiovascular death and heart failure hospitalization in patients with chronic heart failure and reduced ejection fraction receiving optimal heart failure therapy.

Current guidelines for the management of heart failure in adults generally recommend a combination of drug therapies to reduce morbidity and mortality, including neurohormonal antagonists (e.g., ACE inhibitors, angiotensin II receptor antagonists, angiotensin receptor-neprilysin inhibitors [ARNIs], β-blockers, aldosterone receptor antagonists) that inhibit the detrimental compensatory mechanisms in heart failure. Sacubitril/valsartan achieves dual neurohormonal modulation of the renin-angiotensin-aldosterone (RAA) system and neprilysin enzyme; the beneficial effects of RAA inhibition by valsartan are augmented by enhanced natriuretic peptide activity due to sacubitril. Additional agents (e.g., cardiac glycosides, diuretics, sinoatrial modulators [i.e., ivabradine]) added to a heart failure treatment regimen in selected patients have been associated with symptomatic improvement and/or reduction in heart failure-related hospitalizations.

Experts recommend that all asymptomatic patients with reduced left ventricular ejection fraction (LVEF) (i.e., American College of Cardiology Foundation [ACCF]/American Heart Association [AHA] stage B heart failure) receive therapy with an ACE inhibitor and β-blocker to prevent symptomatic heart failure and to reduce morbidity and mortality. In patients with prior or current symptoms of chronic heart failure with reduced LVEF (ACCF/AHA stage C), ACCF, AHA, and the Heart Failure Society of America (HFSA) recommend inhibition of the RAA system with an ACE inhibitor, angiotensin II receptor antagonist, or ARNI in conjunction with a β-blocker, and an aldosterone antagonist in selected patients, to reduce morbidity and mortality. While ACE inhibitors have been the preferred drugs for inhibition of the RAA system because of their established benefits in patients with heart failure and reduced ejection fraction, some evidence indicates that therapy with an ARNI (sacubitril/valsartan) may be more effective than ACE inhibitor therapy (enalapril) in reducing cardiovascular death and heart failure-related hospitalization and that such ARNI therapy is cost-effective. ACCF, AHA, and HFSA recommend that patients with NYHA class II or III chronic symptomatic heart failure with reduced LVEF who are able to tolerate an ACE inhibitor or angiotensin II receptor antagonist be switched to therapy containing an ARNI to further reduce morbidity and mortality. However, in patients in whom an ARNI is not appropriate, ACCF, AHA, and HFSA strongly advise continued use of an ACE inhibitor for all classes of heart failure with reduced ejection fraction. In patients in whom therapy with an ARNI or ACE inhibitor is not appropriate, an angiotensin II receptor antagonist may be used. For additional information on the use of angiotensin II receptor antagonists in the management of heart failure, see Uses: Heart Failure, in Valsartan 24:32.08 and in Candesartan 24:32.08.

Efficacy and safety of sacubitril/valsartan in the management of heart failure have been established principally by the results of a randomized, double-blind trial (PARADIGM-HF) comparing the long-term efficacy and safety of sacubitril/valsartan with that of enalapril in addition to standard-of-care therapy in 8442 patients with symptomatic (NYHA class II–IV) chronic heart failure and reduced ejection fraction (LVEF of 40% or less). In this trial, sacubitril/valsartan was superior to enalapril in reducing the risk of death and hospitalization for heart failure in patients who were receiving these drugs in addition to the best available medical therapy; the benefit of sacubitril/valsartan was similar for both death and hospitalization and was consistent across subgroups. Benefits of sacubitril/valsartan were observed in comparison with optimal therapy with enalapril; the mean dosage of enalapril was similar to the well-established target dosages shown to reduce mortality in patients with chronic heart failure and reduced ejection fraction.

Patients enrolled in the PARADIGM-HF trial were receiving an ACE inhibitor or angiotensin II receptor antagonist at a dosage equivalent to at least 10 mg of enalapril daily for at least 4 weeks prior to trial screening in addition to maximally tolerated dosages of β-blockers. Most patients also received diuretics and mineralocorticoid receptor antagonists and had mild to moderate heart failure symptoms. Patients with a systolic blood pressure of less than 100 mm Hg at the time of screening were excluded from the trial. All enrolled patients discontinued their existing ACE inhibitor or angiotensin II receptor antagonist therapy and entered sequential single-blind run-in periods during which they received enalapril 10 mg twice daily (a dosage that has previously been shown to reduce mortality), followed by sacubitril 49 mg/valsartan 51 mg twice daily, increasing to a target maintenance dosage of sacubitril 97 mg/valsartan 103 mg twice daily. To minimize the potential for angioedema caused by overlapping ACE and neprilysin inhibition, enalapril was withheld a day before initiating sacubitril/valsartan, and sacubitril/valsartan was withheld a day before initiating randomized therapy. The most common reason for patients failing to successfully complete the enalapril and sacubitril/valsartan run-in period was an adverse event, often related to renal dysfunction, hyperkalemia, or hypotension. Patients who successfully completed the sequential run-in periods were randomized to receive either sacubitril 97 mg/valsartan 103 mg twice daily or enalapril 10 mg twice daily in addition to standard-of-care therapy. The primary end point was a composite of death from cardiovascular causes or first hospitalization for heart failure.

The PARADIGM-HF trial was terminated prematurely following the revelation of a substantially lower rate of the primary composite outcome of cardiovascular death or heart failure hospitalization in the sacubitril/valsartan treatment group at a prespecified interim analysis. After a median follow-up duration of 27 months, sacubitril/valsartan reduced the primary end point by approximately 20% compared with enalapril. The treatment effect of sacubitril/valsartan compared with that of enalapril reflected a reduction in both cardiovascular death (20% reduction; event rate 13.3 or 16.5%, respectively) and first hospitalization for worsening heart failure (21% reduction; event rate 12.8 or 15.6%, respectively). Therapy with sacubitril/valsartan reduced the likelihood of a first hospitalization as well as of multiple hospitalizations. Sacubitril/valsartan therapy also improved measures of nonfatal clinical deterioration, including the need for intensification of outpatient treatment, frequency of emergency department visits for worsening heart failure, the requirement for intensive care or IV inotropic support during hospitalization, and the incidence of progression to heart failure mechanical device implantation or cardiac transplantation. Sacubitril/valsartan also substantially improved overall survival evidenced by a 16% reduction in all-cause mortality, which was attributable principally to a lower incidence of cardiovascular mortality. Symptomatic hypotension occurred more frequently with sacubitril/valsartan therapy than with enalapril (14 or 9.2%, respectively) but was not associated with an increased rate of discontinuance of therapy due to hypotension-related adverse effects. There were numerically more cases of angioedema with sacubitril/valsartan than with enalapril therapy but the difference was not statistically significant. While it has been stated that the final adverse event rate for sacubitril/valsartan may not reflect clinical practice because of exclusion of patients with intolerance to the drug during the initial run-in period, the overall number of patients who were excluded during this period was small and was higher in the enalapril treatment group; therefore, it is considered unlikely that the implementation of a run-in period in this trial substantially affected the observed safety profile of sacubitril/valsartan.

DOSAGE AND ADMINISTRATION

● General

Each fixed-combination tablet of sacubitril and valsartan (sacubitril/valsartan [Entresto®]) contains sacubitril 24 mg/valsartan 26 mg, sacubitril 49 mg/valsartan 51 mg, or sacubitril 97 mg/valsartan 103 mg.

Bioavailability of the valsartan component of sacubitril/valsartan tablets is 40–60% higher than that of valsartan in other commercially available tablet formulations; the valsartan dose of 26, 51, or 103 mg in the fixed combination of sacubitril/valsartan is equivalent to valsartan doses of 40, 80, or 160 mg, respectively, in other commercially available valsartan tablets.

When switching from an angiotensin-converting enzyme (ACE) inhibitor to sacubitril/valsartan, ACE inhibitor treatment should be stopped 36 hours prior to initiation of sacubitril/valsartan therapy. (See Contraindications under Cautions.) Therapy with an angiotensin II receptor antagonist also should be discontinued before initiation of sacubitril/valsartan therapy. (See Drug Interactions: Drugs that Block the Renin-Angiotensin System.)

● Administration

Sacubitril/valsartan is administered orally twice daily without regard to food.

● Dosage

Heart Failure

Dosage of sacubitril/valsartan in fixed combination is expressed in terms of both sacubitril and valsartan components.

Initial Dosage

The recommended initial dosage of sacubitril/valsartan in patients with chronic heart failure switching from therapy with an ACE inhibitor or angiotensin II receptor antagonist is sacubitril 49 mg/valsartan 51 mg twice daily; sacubitril/valsartan therapy should begin *after discontinuance* of the angiotensin II receptor antagonist or *36 hours after discontinuance* of the ACE inhibitor. (See Cautions: Contraindications.)

The recommended initial dosage of sacubitril/valsartan in patients switching from low dosages of an ACE inhibitor (i.e., in a clinical trial, "low dosage" was considered to be enalapril 10 mg daily or less or an equivalent dosage of another ACE inhibitor) or angiotensin II receptor antagonist (i.e., in a clinical trial, "low dosage" was considered to be valsartan 160 mg daily or less or an equivalent dosage of another angiotensin II receptor antagonist) is sacubitril 24 mg/valsartan 26 mg twice daily. Sacubitril/valsartan therapy in such patients should begin *after discontinuance* of the angiotensin II receptor antagonist or *36 hours after discontinuance* of the ACE inhibitor. (See Cautions: Contraindications.)

The recommended initial dosage of sacubitril/valsartan in patients *not* currently taking an ACE inhibitor or an angiotensin II receptor antagonist is sacubitril 24 mg/valsartan 26 mg twice daily.

Maintenance Dosage

The dosage of sacubitril/valsartan should be doubled every 2–4 weeks, as tolerated, to a target maintenance dosage of sacubitril 97 mg/valsartan 103 mg twice daily.

● Special Populations

Hepatic Impairment

No adjustment of sacubitril/valsartan dosage is necessary in patients with mild hepatic impairment (Child-Pugh class A). An initial dosage of sacubitril 24 mg/valsartan 26 mg twice daily is recommended for patients with moderate hepatic impairment (Child-Pugh class B). The dosage of sacubitril/valsartan should be doubled every 2–4 weeks, as tolerated, to a target maintenance dosage of sacubitril 97 mg/valsartan 103 mg twice daily. Sacubitril/valsartan is not recommended in patients with severe hepatic impairment (Child-Pugh class C). (See Hepatic Impairment under Warnings/Precautions: Specific Populations, in Cautions.)

Renal Impairment

No adjustment of sacubitril/valsartan dosage is necessary in patients with mild or moderate renal impairment. An initial dosage of sacubitril 24 mg/valsartan 26 mg twice daily is recommended for patients with severe renal impairment (estimated glomerular filtration rate [GFR] less than 30 mL/minute per 1.73 m²). The dosage of sacubitril/valsartan should be doubled every 2–4 weeks, as tolerated, to a target maintenance dosage of sacubitril 97 mg/valsartan 103 mg twice daily. Safety and efficacy have not been established in patients undergoing dialysis. (See Renal Impairment under Warnings/Precautions: Specific Populations, in Cautions.)

Volume- and/or Salt-Depleted Patients

Patients with volume and/or salt depletion should have these imbalances corrected prior to the initiation of sacubitril/valsartan therapy; alternatively, sacubitril/valsartan may be initiated at a lower dosage.

CAUTIONS

● Contraindications

- Known hypersensitivity to sacubitril, valsartan, or any ingredient in the formulation.

- History of angioedema related to prior treatment with an angiotensin-converting enzyme (ACE) inhibitor or angiotensin II receptor antagonist.

- Concomitant use of ACE inhibitors. Sacubitril/valsartan should *not* be administered within 36 hours of switching from or to an ACE inhibitor.

- Concomitant use of aliskiren in patients with diabetes mellitus.

● Warnings/Precautions

Warnings

Fetal/Neonatal Morbidity and Mortality

Drugs that act directly on the renin-angiotensin system (e.g., angiotensin-converting enzyme [ACE] inhibitors, angiotensin II receptor antagonists) can cause fetal and neonatal morbidity and mortality when used in pregnancy during the second and third trimesters. The fixed combination of sacubitril and valsartan (sacubitril/valsartan) should be discontinued as soon as possible when pregnancy is detected, unless continued use is considered life-saving. For additional information on the risk of such drugs (i.e., angiotensin II antagonists and ACE inhibitors) during pregnancy, see Cautions: Pregnancy, Fertility, and Lactation, in Captopril 24:32.04 and in Enalaprilat/Enalapril 24:32.04.

Sensitivity Reactions

Angioedema may occur with sacubitril/valsartan therapy, and if associated with laryngeal edema, may be fatal. In cases of confirmed angioedema where swelling has been confined to the face and lips, the condition generally resolves without treatment; however, antihistamines may provide symptomatic relief. Swelling of the tongue, glottis, or larynx may cause airway obstruction, and appropriate therapy (e.g., epinephrine, maintenance of patent airway) should be initiated. Sacubitril/valsartan should *not* be used in patients with a known history of angioedema related to previous ACE inhibitor or angiotensin II receptor antagonist therapy (see Cautions: Contraindications); black patients and those with a prior history of angioedema may be at an increased risk of angioedema with sacubitril/valsartan therapy.

Other Warnings/Precautions

Precautions Related to Use of Fixed Combinations

When the fixed combination of sacubitril/valsartan is used, the cautions, precautions, contraindications, and drug interactions associated with sacubitril and valsartan must be considered. Cautionary information applicable to specific populations (e.g., pregnant or nursing women, individuals with hepatic or renal impairment, geriatric patients) should be considered for each drug. (For cautionary information specific to valsartan, see Cautions in Valsartan 24:32.08.)

Cardiovascular Effects

Sacubitril/valsartan lowers blood pressure and may cause symptomatic hypotension. Symptomatic hypotension may occur in patients with an activated renin-angiotensin-aldosterone (RAA) system (e.g., patients with volume or salt depletion secondary to salt restriction or high-dose diuretic therapy). (See Volume- and/or Salt-Depleted Patients under Dosage and Administration: Special Populations.)

If hypotension occurs, dosage adjustments of diuretics or concomitant antihypertensive drugs, and treatment of other causes of hypotension (e.g., hypovolemia) should be considered. If hypotension persists despite such measures, the dosage of sacubitril/valsartan should be reduced or the drug temporarily discontinued. Permanent discontinuance of therapy is usually not required.

Renal Effects

Because the RAA system appears to contribute substantially to maintenance of glomerular filtration in patients with heart failure in whom renal perfusion is severely compromised, renal function may deteriorate markedly (e.g., leading to oliguria, progressive azotemia, and rarely acute renal failure and death) in these patients during therapy with an ACE inhibitor or an angiotensin II receptor antagonist (e.g., valsartan). Dosage reduction or interruption of sacubitril/valsartan therapy may be required in patients who develop a clinically important decrease in renal function. As with all drugs that affect the RAA system, sacubitril/valsartan may increase blood urea and serum creatinine concentrations in patients with bilateral or unilateral renal artery stenosis; renal function should be monitored. (See Cautions: Renal Effects, in Enalaprilat/Enalapril 24:32.04.)

Hyperkalemia

Hyperkalemia may occur in patients receiving sacubitril/valsartan, especially in those with severe renal impairment, diabetes mellitus, hypoaldosteronism, or a potassium-rich diet. Serum potassium should be monitored periodically and elevated values treated appropriately. Dosage reduction or interruption of sacubitril/valsartan therapy may be required in some instances of hyperkalemia.

Specific Populations

Pregnancy

Sacubitril/valsartan can cause fetal and neonatal morbidity and mortality when administered to a pregnant woman. Sacubitril/valsartan should be discontinued as soon as possible when pregnancy is detected, unless continued use is considered life-saving; in such cases, the woman should be advised of the risk to the fetus. (See Advice to Patients.) Reproduction studies in rats and rabbits using sacubitril/valsartan during organogenesis have demonstrated increased embryofetal death and teratogenic effects. (See Fetal/Neonatal Morbidity and Mortality under Warnings/Precautions: Warnings, in Cautions.)

Lactation

Sacubitril/valsartan is distributed into milk in rats. It is not known whether sacubitril/valsartan is distributed into human milk. Because of the potential for serious adverse reactions to sacubitril/valsartan in nursing infants, a decision should be made whether to discontinue nursing or the drug, taking into account the importance of the drug to the woman.

Pediatric Use

Safety and efficacy of sacubitril/valsartan in pediatric patients have not been established.

Geriatric Use

No clinically relevant pharmacokinetic differences have been observed in patients 65 years of age and older compared with the overall population.

Hepatic Impairment

Results of a pharmacokinetic study indicate that sacubitril/valsartan exposure is increased in patients with mild or moderate hepatic impairment (Child-Pugh class A or B). Dosage adjustments are not necessary for patients with mild hepatic impairment; a lower initial dosage is recommended in patients with moderate hepatic impairment. (See Hepatic Impairment under Dosage and Administration: Special Populations.)

Sacubitril/valsartan is not recommended in patients with severe hepatic impairment (Child-Pugh class C); safety and efficacy have not been established in this population.

Renal Impairment

Results of a pharmacokinetic study indicate that exposure to LBQ657 (the active metabolite of sacubitril) is increased by approximately twofold in patients with mild or moderate renal impairment (creatinine clearance 30–80 mL/minute) and 2.7-fold in patients with severe renal impairment (creatinine clearance less than 30 mL/minute). Exposure to sacubitril and valsartan was not substantially altered in patients with renal impairment.

In the PARADIGM-HF trial, there was no increase in adverse events associated with the increased exposure to LBQ657 in patients with mild or moderate renal impairment; dosage adjustments are not necessary in these patients.

Sacubitril/valsartan should be used with caution in patients with severe renal impairment. (See Renal Effects and also see Hyperkalemia under Warnings/Precautions: Other Warnings/Precautions, in Cautions.) In patients with severe renal impairment, no change to the target maintenance dosage is recommended; however, a lower initial dosage of sacubitril/valsartan should be used in these patients. (See Renal Impairment under Dosage and Administration: Special Populations.) A lower initial dosage and slower titration to the target maintenance dosage may reduce potential tolerability issues.

Safety and efficacy have not been established in patients undergoing dialysis. Sacubitril/valsartan is unlikely to be removed by hemodialysis due to high protein binding.

● Common Adverse Effects

Adverse effects occurring in at least 5% of patients with heart failure receiving sacubitril/valsartan in the double-blind phase of the PARADIGM-HF trial included hypotension, cough, dizziness, and renal failure or acute renal failure. Laboratory abnormalities occurring in at least 5% of patients receiving sacubitril/valsartan in the double-blind phase of the PARADIGM-HF trial included decreases in hemoglobin and hematocrit exceeding 20%, increases in serum creatinine concentration exceeding 50%, and serum potassium concentrations exceeding 5.5 mEq/L.

DRUG INTERACTIONS

● Drugs Affecting Hepatic Microsomal Enzymes

Cytochrome P-450 (CYP) enzyme-mediated metabolism of sacubitril and valsartan (sacubitril/valsartan) is minimal; therefore, drugs that affect activity of CYP enzymes are not expected to affect the pharmacokinetics of sacubitril/valsartan.

● Drugs Affected by Hepatic Transport Systems

In vitro data suggest that sacubitril inhibits organic anion transporter protein (OATP) 1B1 and OATP1B3 (hepatic uptake transporters). Sacubitril may increase systemic exposure of OATP1B1 and OATP1B3 substrates (e.g., atorvastatin).

● Drugs that Block the Renin-Angiotensin System

Concomitant therapy with sacubitril/valsartan and an angiotensin-converting enzyme (ACE) inhibitor is contraindicated because of the increased risk of angioedema. Concomitant therapy with sacubitril/valsartan and an angiotensin II receptor antagonist should be avoided because the valsartan component of sacubitril/valsartan is an angiotensin II receptor antagonist. Concomitant therapy with sacubitril/valsartan and aliskiren, a direct renin inhibitor, is contraindicated in patients with diabetes mellitus; in addition, such concomitant therapy should be avoided in patients with renal impairment (glomerular filtration rate [GFR] less than 60 mL/minute per 1.73 m²). (See Cautions in Aliskiren Hemifumarate 24:32.40.)

● Drugs or Foods that Increase Serum Potassium Concentration

Concomitant use of potassium-sparing diuretics (e.g., amiloride, spironolactone, triamterene), potassium supplements, or potassium-containing salt substitutes with valsartan may result in an increased risk of hyperkalemia. Serum potassium concentrations should be monitored periodically during such concomitant use.

● Amlodipine

No clinically relevant pharmacokinetic interaction was observed with coadministration of sacubitril/valsartan and amlodipine.

● Atorvastatin

Concomitant administration of sacubitril/valsartan and atorvastatin did not alter systemic exposure to sacubitril/valsartan to a clinically important degree; however, the area under the concentration-time curve (AUC) and peak plasma concentration of atorvastatin were increased.

● Cardiac Drugs

No clinically relevant pharmacokinetic interactions were observed when sacubitril/valsartan was coadministered with carvedilol or digoxin.

● Diuretics

Volume depletion may potentiate symptomatic hypotension in patients receiving concomitant therapy with diuretics and sacubitril/valsartan. No clinically relevant pharmacokinetic interactions were observed when sacubitril/valsartan was coadministered with hydrochlorothiazide or furosemide.

● Lithium

Increased serum lithium concentrations and lithium toxicity have been reported with concomitant use of angiotensin II receptor antagonists and lithium. Monitoring of serum lithium concentrations is recommended during such concomitant use.

● Metformin

No clinically relevant pharmacokinetic interaction was observed with coadministration of sacubitril/valsartan and metformin.

● Nonsteroidal Anti-inflammatory Agents

Deterioration of renal function, including possible acute renal failure, may occur when sacubitril/valsartan is used concomitantly with nonsteroidal anti-inflammatory agents (NSAIAs), including selective cyclooxygenase-2 (COX-2) inhibitors, in geriatric patients, patients with volume depletion (including those receiving concomitant diuretic therapy), or patients with renal impairment. These effects are usually reversible; renal function should be monitored periodically in such patients receiving concomitant therapy with sacubitril/valsartan and an NSAIA.

● Omeprazole

No clinically relevant pharmacokinetic interaction was observed with concomitant administration of sacubitril/valsartan and omeprazole.

● Oral Contraceptives

No clinically relevant pharmacokinetic interaction was observed with concomitant administration of sacubitril/valsartan and an oral contraceptive containing ethinyl estradiol and levonorgestrel.

● Sildenafil

No clinically relevant pharmacokinetic interaction was observed with concomitant administration of sacubitril/valsartan and sildenafil. Coadministration of a 50-mg single dose of sildenafil with sacubitril/valsartan at steady state (sacubitril 194 mg/valsartan 206 mg once daily for 5 days) in patients with hypertension was associated with additive reductions in blood pressure (approximately 5 or 4 mm Hg for systolic or diastolic blood pressure, respectively) compared with administration of sacubitril/valsartan alone. Patients should be advised about potential adverse effects due to blood pressure-lowering effects with concomitant use of sacubitril/valsartan and sildenafil.

● Warfarin

No clinically relevant pharmacokinetic interaction was observed with concomitant administration of sacubitril/valsartan and warfarin.

DESCRIPTION

Sacubitril and valsartan (sacubitril/valsartan) is a combination of a neprilysin inhibitor (sacubitril) and an angiotensin II type 1 (AT$_1$) receptor antagonist (valsartan). The dual mechanism of sacubitril/valsartan suppresses harmful compensatory mechanisms of heart failure that are mediated by the renin-angiotensin-aldosterone (RAA) system, while simultaneously enhancing the beneficial adaptive mechanisms of natriuretic peptides by inhibiting their degradation.

The natriuretic peptide system consists of 3 major peptides (atrial natriuretic peptide [ANP], B-type natriuretic peptide [BNP], and C-type natriuretic peptide [CNP]), which are involved in maintaining normal hemodynamics and plasma volume. Natriuretic peptides stimulate natriuresis and diuresis, promote vasodilation, and oppose acute effects of volume overload by inhibiting the RAA system and the sympathetic nervous system. Natriuretic peptides also have been shown to attenuate the development of cardiac hypertrophy and fibrosis and enhance endothelial function. The effects of natriuretic peptides are mediated through guanylyl cyclase receptors. Activation of these receptors increases intracellular cyclic guanosine monophosphate (cGMP), which is ultimately responsible for the physiologic effects of natriuretic peptides.

Natriuretic peptides are predominantly catabolized via enzymatic cleavage by the membrane-bound, zinc-dependent enzyme neprilysin (also known as neutral endopeptidase or membrane-metallo-endopeptidase). Other substrates of neprilysin include enkephalins, oxytocin, gastrin, angiotensin I and II, endothelin-1, substance P, and bradykinin. Degradation of these substrates is inhibited by sacubitril, which results in increased concentrations of natriuretic peptides and enhances their beneficial counterregulatory effects in heart failure patients. Sole inhibition of neprilysin results in increased ANP, BNP, and cGMP concentrations but at the expense of increased potent vasoconstrictors (angiotensin II and endothelin-1), which partly counteracts the benefits of increased natriuretic peptides. Augmentation of natriuretic peptide effects through neprilysin inhibition requires concomitant suppression of angiotensin II to yield a beneficial effect. Valsartan blocks the physiologic actions of angiotensin II, including vasoconstrictor and aldosterone-secreting effects, by selectively inhibiting access of angiotensin II to AT$_1$ receptors within many tissues, including vascular smooth muscle and the adrenal gland. For additional information on the pharmacology of angiotensin II receptor antagonists, see Description in Irbesartan 24:32.08 and Valsartan 24:32.08

Following oral administration, sacubitril/valsartan dissociates into sacubitril and valsartan. The absolute oral bioavailability of sacubitril is at least 60%, and the bioavailability of valsartan from sacubitril/valsartan is 40–60% higher than that of valsartan administered as a single agent. Sacubitril is a prodrug; its neprilysin-inhibitory activity is dependent upon conversion to the active metabolite (LBQ657) by deethylation via plasma esterases. LBQ657 is not further metabolized to a substantial extent and valsartan is minimally metabolized; approximately 20% of the dose of valsartan is recovered as metabolites. The primary metabolite of valsartan, accounting for less than 10% of the dose, is a hydroxyl metabolite formed by metabolism via the cytochrome P-450 (CYP) isoenzyme 2C9. Administration of sacubitril/valsartan with food has no clinically important effect on the systemic exposure of sacubitril, LBQ657, or valsartan. The peak plasma concentrations of sacubitril, LBQ657, and valsartan are reached in 0.5, 2 , and 1.5 hours, respectively. Sacubitril, LBQ657, and valsartan are 94–97% bound to plasma proteins. The average elimination half-lives of sacubitril, LBQ657, and valsartan are 1.4, 11.5, and 9.9 hours, respectively. Sacubitril (mainly as LBQ657) is excreted in urine (52–68%) and feces (37–48%). Valsartan and its metabolites are excreted in urine (approximately 13%) and feces (86%).

ADVICE TO PATIENTS

Importance of advising patients to read the manufacturer's patient information.

Importance of women informing clinicians if they are or plan to become pregnant or plan to breast-feed. Importance of advising women of childbearing age about the potential risks to the fetus if sacubitril/valsartan is used during pregnancy. All women of childbearing potential should be advised to report pregnancy to their clinician as soon as possible. (See Fetal/Neonatal Morbidity and Mortality under Warnings/Precautions: Warnings, in Cautions.)

Risk of angioedema. Importance of advising patients to discontinue use of any angiotensin-converting enzyme (ACE) inhibitor or angiotensin II receptor antagonist before taking sacubitril/valsartan. Importance of advising patients to allow a 36-hour wash-out period if switching from or to an ACE inhibitor. (See Cautions: Contraindications and also see Sensitivity Reactions under Cautions: Warnings/Precautions.)

Importance of informing clinicians of existing or contemplated concomitant therapy, including prescription and OTC drugs (including salt substitutes containing potassium), as well as any concomitant diseases.

Importance of informing patients of other important precautionary information. (See Cautions.)

PREPARATIONS

Excipients in commercially available drug preparations may have clinically important effects in some individuals; consult specific product labeling for details.

Sacubitril and Valsartan

Oral		
Tablets, film-coated	Sacubitril 24 mg and Valsartan 26 mg	**Entresto®**, Novartis
	Sacubitril 49 mg and Valsartan 51 mg	**Entresto®**, Novartis
	Sacubitril 97 mg and Valsartan 103 mg	**Entresto®**, Novartis

† Use is not currently included in the labeling approved by the US Food and Drug Administration.

Selected Revisions April 10, 2024, © Copyright, November 17, 2016, American Society of Health-System Pharmacists, Inc.

Spironolactone

24:32.20.08 · STEROIDAL MINERALOCORTICOID (ALDO-STERONE) RECEPTOR ANTAGONISTS

■ Spironolactone is a mineralocorticoid (aldosterone) receptor antagonist (aldosterone antagonist) and a potassium-sparing diuretic.

USES

● Edema

Spironolactone is used in the management of edema associated with excessive aldosterone excretion such as idiopathic edema and edema accompanying cirrhosis of the liver, nephrotic syndrome, and heart failure, usually in conjunction with other diuretics. Careful etiologic diagnosis should precede the use of any diuretic. Although thiazides and chlorthalidone are more rapidly acting and more effective diuretics, spironolactone does not cause potassium depletion as may result from thiazide or chlorthalidone therapy. In addition, spironolactone is a useful adjunct to thiazide therapy when diuresis is inadequate or reduction of potassium excretion is necessary. When used in conjunction with a thiazide diuretic in the treatment of edema associated with cirrhosis of the liver, spironolactone should be given for 2–3 days prior to administration of the thiazide diuretic in order to prevent potassium depletion and precipitation of hepatic coma.

● Hypertension

Spironolactone is used in the management of hypertension, usually in conjunction with other diuretics or hypotensive agents. Used alone, spironolactone produces a modest lowering of blood pressure in most patients with hypertension, and blood pressure returns to within normal limits in about 20% of patients.

Because of established clinical benefits (e.g., reductions in overall mortality and in adverse cardiovascular, cerebrovascular, and renal outcomes), current evidence-based practice guidelines for the management of hypertension in adults generally recommend the use of drugs from 4 classes of antihypertensive agents (angiotensin-converting enzyme [ACE] inhibitors, angiotensin II receptor antagonists, calcium-channel blockers, and thiazide diuretics). However, aldosterone antagonists (e.g., spironolactone, eplerenone) may be considered as add-on therapy if goal blood pressure cannot be achieved with the recommended drugs, and are considered preferred add-on therapy by some experts for resistant hypertension and for hypertension associated with primary aldosteronism. Some experts also state that aldosterone antagonists such as spironolactone may be useful for the management of resistant hypertension in patients with type 2 diabetes mellitus when added to an existing treatment regimen consisting of a renin-angiotensin system inhibitor (e.g., ACE inhibitor, angiotensin II receptor antagonist), diuretic, and calcium-channel blocker. However, therapy with an ACE inhibitor or angiotensin II receptor antagonist in conjunction with an aldosterone antagonist may increase the risk of hyperkalemia. Additionally, aldosterone antagonists may be particularly useful in selected patients with heart failure or following myocardial infarction (MI). For information on antihypertensive therapy for patients with heart failure or following MI, see Heart Failure and also see Ischemic Heart Disease under Hypertension in Adults: Considerations for Drug Therapy in Patients with Underlying Cardiovascular and Other Risk Factors, in Uses in the Thiazides General Statement 40:28.20.

Spironolactone may be useful to decrease the potassium loss caused by other diuretics and potentiate the hypotensive effects of those agents or other more potent hypotensive agents. In addition, the drug may be useful in hypertensive patients with gout or diabetes mellitus that may be aggravated by thiazide diuretics. Spironolactone should be avoided in patients with renal insufficiency and in those receiving potassium supplements or other potassium-sparing diuretics.

For additional information on the role of aldosterone antagonists in the management of hypertension in patients with underlying cardiovascular risk factors and information on overall principles and expert recommendations for treatment of hypertension, see Uses: Hypertension in Adults, in the Thiazides General Statement 40:28.20.

● Heart Failure

Spironolactone is used in the management of severe heart failure (New York Heart Association [NYHA] functional class III-IV) in conjunction with standard therapy for heart failure to increase survival and reduce heart failure-related hospitalizations.

Current guidelines for the management of heart failure in adults generally recommend a combination of drug therapies to reduce morbidity and mortality, including neurohormonal antagonists (e.g., ACE inhibitors, angiotensin II receptor antagonists, angiotensin receptor-neprilysin inhibitors [ARNIs], β-blockers, aldosterone receptor antagonists) that inhibit the detrimental compensatory mechanisms in heart failure. Additional agents (e.g., cardiac glycosides, diuretics, sinoatrial modulators [i.e., ivabradine]) added to a heart failure treatment regimen in selected patients have been associated with symptomatic improvement and/or reduction in heart failure-related hospitalizations. For additional information on the management of heart failure, see Uses: Heart Failure, in Carvedilol 24:24, Enalaprilat/Enalapril 24:32.04, and Sacubitril and Valsartan 24:32.92. The American College of Cardiology Foundation (ACCF) and American Heart Association (AHA) recommend the addition of an aldosterone antagonist (i.e., spironolactone or eplerenone) in selected patients with heart failure and reduced LVEF who are already receiving a β-blocker and an agent to inhibit the renin-angiotensin-aldosterone (RAA) system (e.g., ACE inhibitor, angiotensin II receptor antagonist, ARNI); careful patient selection is required to minimize the risk of hyperkalemia and renal insufficiency. (See Cautions: Electrolyte and Metabolic Effects.)

Aldosterone receptor antagonists are also recommended, unless contraindicated, in conjunction with other heart failure therapy to reduce morbidity and mortality following acute MI in patients with reduced LVEF who develop symptoms of heart failure or who have a history of diabetes mellitus†. ACCF and AHA state that there are limited data to support or refute whether spironolactone and eplerenone are interchangeable. The perceived difference between eplerenone and spironolactone is attributed to the selectivity of aldosterone receptor antagonism and not the effectiveness of mineralocorticoid-blocking activity. (See Pharmacology.)

The concomitant use of spironolactone and an ACE inhibitor had been considered relatively contraindicated because of the potential for developing severe hyperkalemia. In addition, it was believed that ACE inhibitors would inhibit formation of aldosterone, a hormone associated with the pathophysiology of heart failure, by suppressing the RAA system. However, results of several studies have indicated that ACE inhibitors only transiently inhibit the production of aldosterone, and the addition of spironolactone to ACE inhibitor therapy may augment the suppressive effect of ACE inhibitors on aldosterone. (See Pharmacology: Cardiovascular Effects.)

Results of a randomized, multicenter, controlled study (Randomized Aldactone Evaluation Study [RALES]) in 1663 patients with moderate or severe heart failure (NYHA functional class III or IV) and LVEF of 35% or less indicate that addition of low-dose (25–50 mg daily) spironolactone to standard therapy (e.g., an ACE inhibitor and a loop diuretic with or without a cardiac glycoside) was associated with decreases in overall mortality and hospitalization (for worsening heart failure) rates of approximately 30 and 35%, respectively, compared with standard therapy and placebo. The reduction in mortality and hospitalization rates was observed within 2–3 months of initiation of combined therapy and continued throughout the study (mean follow-up: 24 months). The combined therapy also was associated with an improvement in NYHA functional class in about 41% of patients. Because interim analysis of this study after a mean follow-up of 24 months revealed that morbidity and death were reduced significantly in patients receiving spironolactone concomitantly with standard therapy compared with those receiving standard therapy and placebo, the study was discontinued.

Spironolactone also is used for the management of edema and sodium retention in patients with heart failure who do not respond adequately to or are intolerant of other therapeutic measures. (See Uses: Edema.)

● Primary Hyperaldosteronism

Spironolactone is used for the short-term preoperative treatment of primary hyperaldosteronism and for long-term maintenance therapy in patients with discrete aldosterone-producing adrenal adenomas who are not candidates for surgery (e.g., adrenalectomy). The drug also is used for long-term maintenance therapy for patients with bilateral micronodular or macronodular adrenal hyperplasia (idiopathic hyperaldosteronism).

● Precocious Puberty

Spironolactone is used for its antiandrogenic effects in combination with testolactone in the management of certain forms of gonadotropin releasing hormone (GnRH)-independent (peripheral) precocious puberty† (e.g., familial male precocious puberty [testotoxicosis]). Such therapy has effectively controlled acne, spontaneous erections, and aggressive behavior and slowed accelerated growth and skeletal maturation, at least in the short term (e.g., 2 years), in boys with familial precocious puberty†. Neither drug alone effectively controls pubertal characteristics nor the rate of growth and skeletal maturation in boys with this condition, although some benefit (e.g., on height velocity) with testolactone alone may be apparent. Testolactone generally prevents the gynecomastia that may be associated with spironolactone. Testolactone also has been used in combination with other antiandrogens (e.g., flutamide) in the management of this condition, but experience is less extensive. While spironolactone currently is the most widely used antiandrogenic drug in familial male precocious puberty, alternative antiandrogenic drugs (e.g., flutamide) that avoid some of the potentially serious adverse effects of spironolactone therapy (e.g., mineralocorticoid-antagonist effects) are being studied for this condition and congenital adrenal hyperplasia. However, concerns about potential hepatotoxic effects of flutamide may limit the use of this drug in such precocious puberty. A gradual escape from the beneficial effects of combined therapy with spironolactone and testolactone may occur during long-term therapy because of the development of secondary GnRH-dependent precocity or pubertal increases in gonadotropins. In such cases, a GnRH analog has been added to the regimen to restore effective control of puberty progression. Additional study and experience are needed to elucidate further the optimum regimens for the management of these forms of precocious puberty and the long-term effects of such therapy, and such patients should be managed in consultation with experts in the diagnosis and treatment of these conditions. Combinations of testolactone with flutamide or with spironolactone also have been studied as a component in the complex regimen of therapy for boys and girls with congenital adrenal hyperplasia caused by steroid 21-hydroxylase or 11-hydroxylase deficiency†; the rationale for the addition of such therapy to the therapeutic regimen was similar to that for familial male precocious puberty (i.e., to control androgenic effects and accelerated growth and skeletal maturation).

● Other Uses

Spironolactone has been used effectively in the treatment of hirsutism† in women with polycystic ovary syndrome or idiopathic hirsutism. In the treatment of hirsutism, spironolactone appears to exert its therapeutic effects by interfering with ovarian androgen secretion and peripheral androgen activity.

Spironolactone has also been used as an adjunct in the treatment of myasthenia gravis† and familial periodic paralysis†.

DOSAGE AND ADMINISTRATION

● Administration

Spironolactone is administered orally.

Administration of spironolactone with food increases the bioavailability of the drug by approximately 90–100%. The manufacturers state that patients should establish a routine time for taking the drug with regard to meals.

Spironolactone tablets should be stored in tight, light-resistant containers at a temperature less than 25°C.

The commercially available oral suspension (CaroSpir®) is *not therapeutically equivalent* to spironolactone oral tablets (e.g., Aldactone®). In patients who require a dose exceeding 100 mg, tablets should be used; doses of CaroSpir® suspension exceeding 100 mg may result in higher than expected serum spironolactone concentrations. The oral suspension (CaroSpir®) should be stored at a controlled room temperature of 20–25°C but may be exposed to temperatures ranging from 15–30°C.

Although it has frequently been recommended that spironolactone tablets be administered in 3 or 4 doses daily, more recent information suggests that 1 or 2 doses daily may be adequate.

Extemporaneously Compounded Oral Suspension

Spironolactone tablets may be pulverized and administered as an oral suspension in cherry syrup.

Standardize 4 Safety

Standardized concentrations for an extemporaneously prepared oral suspension of spironolactone have been established through Standardize 4 Safety (S4S), a national patient safety initiative to reduce medication errors, especially during transitions of care. Multidisciplinary expert panels were convened to determine recommended standard concentrations. Because recommendations from the S4S panels may differ from the manufacturer's prescribing information, caution is advised when using concentrations that differ from labeling, particularly when using rate information from the label. For additional information on S4S (including updates that may be available), see https://www.ashp.org/pharmacy-practice/standardize-4-safety-initiative.

TABLE 1. Standardize 4 Safety Compounded Oral Liquid Standards for Spironolactone

Concentration Standards
5 mg/mL

● Dosage

Edema

Spironolactone Therapy

For the management of edema associated with hepatic cirrhosis or nephrotic syndrome in adults, the recommended initial adult dosage of spironolactone (as oral tablets) is 100 mg daily administered as a single dose or in divided doses, but initial dosage may range from 25–200 mg daily.

When the commercially available oral suspension (CaroSpir®) is used for the treatment of edema associated with hepatic cirrhosis, the recommended initial adult dosage is 75 mg daily administered in a single dose or divided doses.

The manufacturers state that spironolactone should be initiated in patients with cirrhosis in a hospital setting and dosage titrated slowly.

Experts state that diuretics should be administered at a dosage sufficient to achieve optimal volume status and relieve congestion without inducing an excessively rapid reduction in intravascular volume, which could result in hypotension, renal dysfunction, or both.

For the management of edema in children, a spironolactone dosage of 3.3 mg/kg daily (as oral tablets) administered as a single dose or in divided doses has been suggested. Alternatively, an initial pediatric dosage of 60 mg/m² daily (as oral tablets) administered in divided doses has been suggested.

When used alone for the management of edema, spironolactone should be administered in the usual initial dosage for at least 5 days. If a satisfactory response is obtained, dosage may be adjusted to the optimal therapeutic or maintenance dosage.

Spironolactone/Hydrochlorothiazide Fixed-combination Therapy

The manufacturer of the fixed combination of spironolactone and hydrochlorothiazide states that the optimal dosage should be established by individual titration of the drug components.

For the management of edema in adults, the usual maintenance dosage of the fixed combination of spironolactone and hydrochlorothiazide is 100 mg each of spironolactone and hydrochlorothiazide daily administered as a single dose or in divided doses. The effective dosage may range from 25–200 mg of each component daily depending on the response to the initial titration. In some instances, it may be beneficial to administer separate tablets of either spironolactone or hydrochlorothiazide in addition to the fixed combination of spironolactone and hydrochlorothiazide in order to provide optimal individual therapy.

Hypertension

Spironolactone Therapy

For the management of hypertension in adults, the usual initial dosage of spironolactone (as oral tablets) is 25–100 mg daily administered as a single dose or in divided doses. The dosage may be titrated at 2-week intervals. Dosages exceeding 100 mg daily generally do not provide additional reductions in blood pressure.

When the commercially available oral suspension (CaroSpir®) is used for the treatment of hypertension in adults, the recommended initial dosage is 20–75 mg daily administered in a single dose or divided doses. The dosage may be titrated at 2-week intervals. Dosages exceeding 75 mg daily generally do not provide additional reductions in blood pressure.

For the management of hypertension in children†, some experts have recommended an initial spironolactone dosage of 1 mg/kg daily (as tablets) administered as a single dose or in 2 divided doses. Such experts have suggested that dosage may be increased as necessary to a maximum dosage of 3.3 mg/kg (up to 100 mg) daily (as tablets) given as a single dose or in 2 divided doses. For information on overall principles and expert recommendations for treatment of hypertension in pediatric patients, see Uses: Hypertension in Pediatric Patients, in the Thiazides General Statement 40:28.20.

Spironolactone should be administered for a minimum of 2 weeks in order to assess its effectiveness in the management of hypertension in a specific patient. Subsequent dosage should be determined by the response of the patient.

Spironolactone/Hydrochlorothiazide Fixed-combination Therapy

The manufacturer of the fixed combination of spironolactone and hydrochlorothiazide states that the optimal dosage should be established by individual titration of the drug components. When the fixed combination is used for the management of hypertension, the dosage will vary depending on the results of the titration of the individual drug components. Most patients will have an optimal response to 50–100 mg each of spironolactone and hydrochlorothiazide daily administered as a single dose or in divided doses.

Monitoring and Blood Pressure Treatment Goals

The patient's renal function and electrolytes should be assessed 2–4 weeks after initiation of diuretic therapy. Blood pressure should be monitored regularly (i.e., monthly) during therapy and dosage of the antihypertensive drug adjusted until blood pressure is controlled. If an adequate blood pressure response is not achieved, the dosage may be increased or another antihypertensive agent with demonstrated benefit and preferably with a complementary mechanism of action (e.g., angiotensin-converting enzyme [ACE] inhibitor, angiotensin II receptor antagonist, calcium-channel blocker, thiazide diuretic) may be added. (See Uses: Hypertension.) In patients who develop unacceptable adverse effects with spironolactone, the drug should be discontinued and another antihypertensive agent from a different pharmacologic class should be initiated.

The goal of hypertension management and prevention is to achieve and maintain optimal control of blood pressure. However, the optimum blood pressure threshold for initiating antihypertensive drug therapy and specific treatment goals remain controversial. A 2017 multidisciplinary hypertension guideline from the American College of Cardiology (ACC), American Heart Association (AHA), and a number of other professional organizations generally recommends a blood pressure goal of less than 130/80 mm Hg in all adults, regardless of comorbidities or level of atherosclerotic cardiovascular disease (ASCVD) risk. Many patients will require at least 2 drugs from different pharmacologic classes to achieve this blood pressure goal; the potential benefits of hypertension management and drug cost, adverse effects, and risks associated with the use of multiple antihypertensive drugs also should be considered when deciding a patient's blood pressure treatment goal.

For additional information on target levels of blood pressure and on monitoring therapy in the management of hypertension, see Blood Pressure Monitoring and Treatment Goals under Dosage: Hypertension, in the Thiazides General Statement 40:28.20.

Heart Failure

For the management of severe heart failure, the manufacturer recommends an initial spironolactone dosage of 25 mg once daily (as oral tablets) in adults who have a serum potassium concentration of 5 mEq/L or less and an estimated glomerular filtration rate (eGFR) exceeding 50 mL/minute per 1.73 m². In patients who tolerate this initial dosage, dosage may be increased to 50 mg once daily as clinically indicated; those who do not tolerate the initial dosage (i.e., develop hyperkalemia) may receive 25 mg once every *other* day. Alternatively, the American College of Cardiology Foundation (ACCF) and the American Heart Association

(AHA) recommend an initial spironolactone dosage of 12.5–25 mg once daily and a maintenance dosage (after 4 weeks of therapy) of 25 mg once or twice daily (as tablets) in patients who have a serum potassium concentration of 5 mEq/L or less and adequate renal function (eGFR at least 50 mL/minute per 1.73 m²).

For the management of edema associated with heart failure in adults, some experts recommend initiating spironolactone (oral tablets) at a low dosage (e.g., 12.5–25 mg once daily) and increasing the dosage (maximum of 50 mg daily; higher dosages may be used with close monitoring) until urine output increases and weight decreases, generally by 0.5–1 kg daily.

The manufacturer recommends that serum potassium and renal function be monitored 1 week after initiation and then regularly thereafter; more frequent monitoring may be necessary when spironolactone is given with other drugs that cause hyperkalemia or in patients with impaired renal function. ACCF and AHA recommend that serum potassium and renal function be checked within 2–3 days and again 7 days after initiation of an aldosterone antagonist. Subsequent monitoring should be performed as needed based upon the stability of renal function and fluid status but should occur at least monthly for the first 3 months and then every 3 months thereafter. If hyperkalemia occurs, the dosage of spironolactone should be decreased or the drug discontinued and hyperkalemia should be treated. ACCF and AHA recommend withholding therapy with an aldosterone receptor antagonist if the patient's serum potassium concentration exceeds 5.5 mEq/L or if renal function worsens; therapy may be resumed at a reduced dosage after confirming resolution (for at least 72 hours) of hyperkalemia (i.e., serum potassium concentration decreases to less than 5 mEq/L) and of renal insufficiency. ACCF and AHA state that patients should also be specifically instructed to stop taking an aldosterone receptor antagonist if they have diarrhea or are dehydrated or if therapy with a concomitant loop diuretic is interrupted.

When the commercially available oral suspension (CaroSpir®) is used for the management of heart failure, the manufacturer recommends an initial dosage of 20 mg once daily in adults who have a serum potassium concentration of 5 mEq/L or less and an eGFR exceeding 50 mL/minute per 1.73 m². In patients who tolerate this initial dosage, dosage may be increased to 37.5 mg once daily as clinically indicated; those who develop hyperkalemia on the initial dosage may have their dosage reduced to 20 mg once every *other* day.

Primary Hyperaldosteronism

After the diagnosis of hyperaldosteronism has been established, 100–400 mg of spironolactone (as oral tablets) may be administered daily for short-term preoperative therapy. When spironolactone is used for the treatment of primary hyperaldosteronism in patients unable or unwilling to undergo surgery, spironolactone may be used as long-term maintenance therapy at the lowest effective dosage determined for the individual patient.

Other Uses

For the treatment of hirsutism† in women with polycystic ovary syndrome or idiopathic hirsutism, the usual dosage of spironolactone is 50–200 mg daily (as oral tablets). Regression of hirsutism is generally evident within 2 months, maximal within 6 months, and has been maintained up to at least 16 months with continued treatment.

● Dosage in Hepatic Impairment

In patients with cirrhosis, spironolactone should be initiated with the lowest dose and titrated slowly; patients with cirrhosis and ascites should have therapy initiated in the hospital. (See Cautions: Precautions and Contraindications.)

● Dosage in Renal Impairment

The manufacturer states, for the treatment of heart failure in patients with an eGFR of 30–50 mL/minute per 1.73 m², initiation of spironolactone at a dosage of 25 mg every *other* day (as oral tablets) should be considered because of the risk of hyperkalemia. Alternatively, ACCF and AHA state that the dosage of spironolactone should be reduced in heart failure patients with marginal renal function (eGFR 30–49 mL/minute per 1.73 m²); an initial dosage of 12.5 mg once daily or every *other* day and a maintenance dosage of 12.5–25 mg once daily as tablets (after 4 weeks of therapy and if serum potassium is 5 mEq/L or less) has been recommended. The manufacturer of the commercially available spironolactone oral suspension (CaroSpir®) states in patients with heart failure and an eGFR of 30–50 mL/minute per 1.73 m², a reduced initial dosage of 10 mg once daily (as the oral suspension) should be considered because of the risk of hyperkalemia. The use of an aldosterone antagonist may be harmful in patients with an eGFR less than 30 mL/minute per 1.73 m² because of potentially life-threatening hyperkalemia or renal insufficiency. (See Cautions: Electrolyte and Metabolic Effects.)

CAUTIONS

In general, adverse effects with recommended dosage of spironolactone are mild and respond to withdrawal of the drug.

● Electrolyte and Metabolic Effects

Patients receiving spironolactone may develop hyperkalemia. The risk of developing hyperkalemia is increased by impaired renal function or concomitant potassium supplementation, potassium-containing salt substitutes, or drugs that increase serum potassium (e.g., angiotensin-converting enzyme [ACE] inhibitors, angiotensin II receptor antagonists). (See Drug Interactions.) Hyperkalemia can cause cardiac irregularities that may be fatal.

Reversible hyperchloremic metabolic acidosis, usually in association with hyperkalemia, has occurred in some patients with decompensated hepatic cirrhosis, even in the presence of normal renal function. Mild acidosis also has occurred during spironolactone therapy. Spironolactone also may cause hypochloremic alkalosis.

Dehydration and hyponatremia manifested by a low serum sodium concentration, dry mouth, thirst, drowsiness, and lethargy may occur during spironolactone therapy, especially when spironolactone is used concomitantly with other diuretics. In patients with severe cirrhosis, dehydration and hyponatremia may be followed by further hepatic decompensation and asterixis. Hyponatremia occurs most frequently in patients with advanced cirrhosis and may be prevented by restriction of water intake, administration of corticosteroids, or administration of mannitol.

Spironolactone may cause hypomagnesemia, hypocalcemia, and hyperglycemia. Asymptomatic hyperuricemia also may occur and gout may rarely be precipitated.

Sudden alterations of fluid and electrolyte balance may precipitate impaired neurologic function, worsening hepatic encephalopathy, and coma in patients with hepatic disease with cirrhosis and ascites.

● GI Effects

Anorexia, nausea, vomiting, diarrhea, abdominal cramping, gastritis, gastric bleeding, and ulceration have occurred during spironolactone therapy.

● Nervous System Effects

Headache, drowsiness, lethargy, ataxia, mental confusion, and fever have occurred during spironolactone therapy. In addition, severe fatigue and lassitude have been associated with the rapid and profound weight loss that occurs at the start of high-dose spironolactone therapy in patients with primary hyperaldosteronism.

● Dermatologic and Sensitivity Reactions

Maculopapular and erythematous rashes (sometimes accompanied by eosinophilia), anaphylactic reaction, vasculitis, and urticaria have been reported rarely in patients receiving spironolactone. Stevens-Johnson Syndrome (SJS), toxic epidermal necrolysis (TEN), drug rash with eosinophilia and systemic symptoms (DRESS), alopecia, pruritus, and chloasma have also been reported in patients receiving spironolactone therapy.

● Endocrine Effects

Adverse effects related to the steroid-like structure of spironolactone include painful gynecomastia, decreased libido, and relative impotence in males, and menstrual irregularities, amenorrhea, postmenopausal bleeding, and breast soreness in females. Gynecomastia appears to be related to both dosage and duration of therapy (onset varies from 1–2 months to more than a year) and is usually reversible following discontinuance of spironolactone; however, some breast enlargement may rarely persist. Spironolactone may be associated with a greater risk of gynecomastia than eplerenone. In the RALES study, approximately 9% of the male patients who received spironolactone (mean dosage: 26 mg once daily) developed gynecomastia. Carcinoma of the breast has been reported in patients receiving spironolactone; however, a causal relationship to the drug has not been established. Androgen-like adverse effects such as hirsutism and deepening of the voice have also been reported.

● Renal Effects and Hypotension

Excessive diuresis may cause symptomatic dehydration, hypotension, and worsening renal function, especially in patients who are salt-depleted or those taking an ACE inhibitor or angiotensin II receptor antagonist. Worsening of renal function also may occur when spironolactone is used in conjunction with nephrotoxic drugs (e.g., aminoglycosides, cisplatin, nonsteroidal anti-inflammatory agents [NSAIAs]).

● Other Adverse Effects

Leg cramps, leukopenia (including agranulocytosis), and thrombocytopenia have been reported during spironolactone therapy. Mixed cholestatic/hepatocellular toxicity, with at least one fatality, has been reported rarely with spironolactone administration.

● Precautions and Contraindications

When spironolactone is used as a fixed-combination preparation that includes hydrochlorothiazide, the cautions, precautions, and contraindications associated with thiazide diuretics must be considered in addition to those associated with spironolactone.

Unless spironolactone is given concomitantly with another diuretic and a corticosteroid, the concurrent use of potassium supplements should generally be avoided. Serum electrolyte, uric acid, and blood glucose concentrations should be monitored periodically in patients receiving spironolactone. The manufacturer states that serum potassium concentrations should be monitored within 1 week of initiating or titrating spironolactone therapy and regularly thereafter. More frequent monitoring may be necessary when spironolactone is administered with other drugs that cause hyperkalemia or in patients with renal impairment. Serum potassium concentrations should be checked when concomitant ACE inhibitor or angiotensin II receptor antagonist therapy is altered. The patient's volume status and renal function also should be monitored periodically while on spironolactone therapy. Patients should be warned to avoid excessive ingestion of potassium-rich foods or salt substitutes. If hyperkalemia, occurs, the dosage of spironolactone should be decreased or the drug discontinued and hyperkalemia should be treated.

Spironolactone should be used with caution in patients with impaired renal function or hepatic disease. Spironolactone is contraindicated in patients with hyperkalemia. Some clinicians consider spironolactone to be contraindicated in patients whose serum creatinine or BUN concentration is more than twice normal. Spironolactone is also contraindicated in patients with Addison's disease or with concomitant use of eplerenone.

● Pediatric Precautions

The manufacturer states that safety and efficacy of spironolactone have not been established in pediatric patients.

● Pregnancy, Fertility, and Lactation

Pregnancy

The use of spironolactone during pregnancy may affect the sex differentiation of a male fetus during embryogenesis. Studies in rats indicate that spironolactone may cause feminization of male fetuses and endocrine dysfunction in female fetuses exposed to the drug in utero. Data from published case reports and case series have not demonstrated an association of major malformations or other adverse pregnancy outcomes with spironolactone use. Because of the potential risk to the male fetus due to the antiandrogenic properties of spironolactone, the drug should be avoided during pregnancy; pregnant women who receive spironolactone should be advised of the potential risk to a male fetus.

Lactation

Spironolactone is not distributed into milk; however, the active metabolite, canrenone, is distributed into milk in low amounts that are expected to be clinically inconsequential. The developmental and health benefits of breastfeeding along with the mother's clinical need for spironolactone and any potential adverse effects on the breastfed child from spironolactone or from the underlying maternal condition should be considered.

DRUG INTERACTIONS

● Drugs that Block the Renin-Angiotensin System

Concomitant administration of spironolactone and an angiotensin-converting enzyme (ACE) inhibitor or angiotensin II receptor antagonist may cause severe hyperkalemia. Serum potassium concentrations should be monitored closely in patients receiving concomitant therapy with an ACE inhibitor or angiotensin II receptor antagonist and spironolactone.

● Drugs or Foods that Increase Serum Potassium Concentration

Concomitant use of spironolactone, potassium supplements or other substances containing potassium (e.g., salt substitutes), or potassium-rich diets may increase the risk of severe hyperkalemia as compared with spironolactone therapy alone. In general, potassium supplementation should be discontinued in patients with heart failure who are initiating spironolactone.

Spironolactone should not be used concurrently with another potassium-sparing agent or aldosterone receptor antagonist (e.g., eplerenone) since concomitant therapy with these drugs may increase the risk of severe hyperkalemia as compared with spironolactone alone; concomitant use of spironolactone and eplerenone is contraindicated. Concomitant use of spironolactone and other drugs that are known to cause hyperkalemia, such as ACE inhibitors, angiotensin II receptor antagonists, nonsteroidal anti-inflammatory agents (NSAIAs), heparin or low molecular weight heparin, or trimethoprim, may cause severe hyperkalemia.

● Aminoglycosides

Worsening of renal function may occur with concomitant use; the patient's renal function and volume status should be monitored periodically.

● Antihypertensive and Hypotensive Agents

When used in conjunction with other diuretics or hypotensive agents, spironolactone may be additive with or may potentiate the action of these drugs. Therefore, dosage of these drugs, particularly ganglionic blocking agents, may need to be reduced by at least 50% when concomitant spironolactone therapy is instituted.

● Cholestyramine

Hyperkalemic metabolic acidosis has been reported in patients who received spironolactone concurrently with cholestyramine.

● Cisplatin

Worsening of renal function may occur with concomitant use; the patient's renal function and volume status should be monitored periodically.

● CNS Depressants

Concomitant use of spironolactone and CNS depressants, including alcohol, barbiturates, and opiate agonists, may potentiate orthostatic hypotension.

● Corticosteroids

Concomitant use of spironolactone and corticosteroids may intensify electrolyte depletion, particularly hypokalemia.

● Digoxin

Spironolactone and its metabolites interfere with radioimmunoassays for digoxin and increase the apparent exposure to digoxin. The extent, if any, to which spironolactone actually increases digoxin exposure is unknown. In patients receiving concomitant therapy with spironolactone and digoxin, an assay that does not interact with spironolactone should be used to measure serum digoxin concentrations.

● Lithium

Renal clearance of lithium is decreased in patients receiving diuretics, and lithium toxicity may result. Serum lithium concentrations should be monitored periodically during concomitant spironolactone and lithium use.

● Nondepolarizing Neuromuscular Blocking Agents

Concomitant use of spironolactone and nondepolarizing neuromuscular blocking agents may potentially increase the neuromuscular blockade.

● Nonsteroidal Anti-inflammatory Agents

Concomitant use of spironolactone and NSAIAs (e.g., indomethacin) may cause severe hyperkalemia. NSAIAs, including aspirin, can reduce the diuretic, natriuretic, and antihypertensive effect of diuretics. When these drugs are used concomitantly, the maintenance dosage of spironolactone may need to be increased and the patient should be monitored closely to determine if the desired therapeutic effect of spironolactone is being achieved. Worsening of renal function also may occur with concomitant use; the patient's renal function and volume status should be monitored periodically.

● Vasopressors

Spironolactone reportedly reduces vascular responsiveness to norepinephrine, and regional or general anesthesia should be used with caution in patients receiving spironolactone.

LABORATORY TEST INTERFERENCES

● Tests for Plasma and Urinary Steroids

Because spironolactone metabolites produce fluorescence, the drug may interfere with fluorometric determinations of plasma and urinary 17-hydroxycorticosteroids (cortisol). Spurious plasma and urine fluorescence may persist for several days after termination of spironolactone therapy. It has been reported that spironolactone administration may also interfere with determinations of urinary 17-hydroxycorticosteroids by the Porter-Silber technique, urinary 17-ketosteroids by the Klendshoj, Feldstein and Sprague technique, and possibly urinary 17-ketogenic steroids.

● Tests for Urinary Aldosterone

Most methods of determining urinary aldosterone appear to be unaffected by spironolactone metabolites, but one report indicates that the metabolites may interfere with aldosterone radioimmunoassay procedures.

● Tests for Serum Digoxin

Spironolactone may cause false elevations in measurements of serum digoxin concentrations when radioimmunoassay procedures are used.

PHARMACOLOGY

Spironolactone is a synthetic steroid mineralocorticoid (aldosterone) receptor antagonist (aldosterone antagonist) that exhibits potassium-sparing diuretic and probably cardioprotective effects.

Spironolactone is a nonselective mineralocorticoid receptor antagonist, as well as an androgen and progesterone receptor antagonist. Spironolactone exhibits magnesium- and potassium-sparing, natriuretic, diuretic, and hypotensive effects by competitively inhibiting the physiologic effects of the adrenocortical hormone aldosterone on the distal renal tubules, myocardium, and vasculature.

● Renal Effects

Spironolactone competitively inhibits the physiologic effects of the adrenocortical hormone aldosterone on the distal renal tubules, thereby producing increased excretion of sodium chloride and water, and decreased excretion of potassium, magnesium, ammonium, titratable acid, and phosphate. Spironolactone is a potassium-sparing diuretic that has diuretic activity only in the presence of aldosterone, and its effects are most pronounced in patients with hyperaldosteronism.

Spironolactone does not interfere with renal tubular transport mechanisms and does not inhibit carbonic anhydrase. Renal plasma flow and glomerular filtration rate usually are unaffected, but free water clearance may increase. Prolonged administration of spironolactone may cause increased aldosterone secretion; however, reports are conflicting. Because most sodium is reabsorbed in the proximal renal tubules, spironolactone is relatively ineffective when administered alone, and concomitant administration of a diuretic which blocks reabsorption of sodium proximal to the distal portion of the nephron, such as a thiazide or loop diuretic, is required for maximum diuretic effects. When administered with other diuretics, spironolactone produces an additive or synergistic diuretic response and decreases potassium excretion caused by the other diuretic.

Cardiovascular Effects

Spironolactone reportedly has hypotensive activity when given to hypertensive patients. The precise mechanism of hypotensive action has not been determined, but it has been suggested that the drug may act by blocking the effect of aldosterone on arteriolar smooth muscle or by altering the extracellular-intracellular sodium gradient.

Spironolactone appears to have cardioprotective effects when given to patients with severe heart failure. The exact mechanism of the cardioprotective action of spironolactone in patients with heart failure has not been fully elucidated, but it appears to be related more to the drug's ability to competitively inhibit the physiologic effects of aldosterone on the myocardium than to its diuretic effect. In addition to promoting retention of sodium and excretion of magnesium and potassium, aldosterone causes sympathetic activation, parasympathetic inhibition, myocardial and vascular fibrosis, direct vascular damage, and baroreceptor dysfunction; aldosterone also impairs arterial compliance and apparently prevents uptake of norepinephrine by the myocardium. Spironolactone appears to benefit patients with heart failure by increasing myocardial norepinephrine uptake and preventing myocardial fibrosis, sodium retention, and potassium and/or magnesium excretion. In addition, preliminary studies in animals and humans suggest that spironolactone may restore baroreceptor sensitivity and modulate baroreflex function in patients with heart failure.

It generally has been believed that angiotensin-converting enzyme (ACE) inhibitors would inhibit formation of aldosterone by suppressing the renin-angiotensin-aldosterone system. However, there is increasing evidence to suggest that plasma aldosterone concentrations may not decrease during therapy with usual dosages of ACE inhibitors in some patients and may return to pretreatment levels in others during prolonged therapy. Results of several studies indicate that the addition of spironolactone to ACE inhibitor therapy appears to augment the suppressive effect of the ACE inhibitors on aldosterone. In addition, although it has been suggested that concomitant administration of an ACE inhibitor and spironolactone was relatively contraindicated because of the potential for developing severe hyperkalemia, a low incidence of severe hyperkalemia has been reported in clinical studies in patients with heart failure receiving such combined therapy.

Antiandrogenic Effects

Spironolactone exhibits antiandrogenic effects in males and females. The mechanism of antiandrogenic activity of spironolactone is complex and appears to involve several effects of the drug. Spironolactone decreases testosterone biosynthesis by inhibiting steroid 17α-monooxygenase (17α-hydroxylase) activity, possibly secondary to destruction of microsomal cytochrome P-450 in tissues with high steroid 17α-monooxygenase activity (e.g., testes, adrenals). The drug also appears to competitively inhibit binding of dihydrotestosterone to its cytoplasmic receptor protein, thus decreasing androgenic actions at target tissues. Spironolactone-induced increases in serum estradiol concentration also may contribute to its antiandrogenic activity, although such increases may not occur consistently; such increases appear to result from increased conversion of testosterone to estradiol. Spironolactone may have variable effects on serum 17-hydroxyprogesterone concentrations, possibly decreasing its production by inhibiting steroid 17α-monooxygenase activity or decreasing its conversion (with resultant accumulation) to androstenedione by inhibiting cytochrome P450-dependent 17α-hydroxyprogesterone aldolase (17,20-desmolase) activity. Serum progesterone concentrations may increase with the drug secondary to decreased hydroxylation (via steroid 17α-monooxygenase) to 17-hydroxyprogesterone. In children, compensatory increases in lutropin (luteinizing hormone, LH) and follicle-stimulating hormone (FSH) secretion can occur, probably secondary to the drug's antiandrogenic effects (i.e., a feedback response to decreasing serum testosterone concentrations and/or peripheral androgenic activity).

PHARMACOKINETICS

Absorption

Absorption of spironolactone from the GI tract depends on the formulation in which it is administered. When spironolactone is administered as oral tablets, peak plasma concentrations of spironolactone and its active metabolite canrenone are achieved 2.6 and 4.3 hours, respectively, after dosing in healthy individuals.

When spironolactone is administered as the oral suspension (CaroSpir®), peak plasma concentrations of spironolactone are achieved 0.5–1.5 hours after dosing in healthy individuals; peak plasma concentrations of the active metabolite canrenone are reached 2.5–5 hours after dosing. When spironolactone (tablets or oral suspension) is administered concomitantly with food, peak serum concentrations and areas under the serum concentration-time curves (AUCs) of the drug and, to a lesser degree, its principal metabolites are increased substantially compared with the fasting state. (See Dosage and Administration: Administration.) At equivalent doses, serum concentrations of spironolactone are 15–37% higher following administration of the oral suspension (CaroSpir®) than with the oral tablets (Aldactone®)

When administered alone, spironolactone has a gradual onset of diuretic action with the maximum effect being reached on the third day of therapy. The delay in onset may result from the time required for adequate concentrations of the drug or metabolites to accumulate. After withdrawal of spironolactone, diuresis persists for 2 or 3 days. When a thiazide diuretic is used concomitantly with spironolactone, diuresis usually occurs on the first day of therapy.

Distribution

Spironolactone and canrenone, a major metabolite of the drug, are both more than 90% bound to plasma proteins.

Spironolactone or its metabolites may cross the placenta. Canrenone, a major metabolite of spironolactone, is distributed into milk.

Elimination

Spironolactone is rapidly and extensively metabolized. Spironolactone undergoes deacetylation at its sulfur group to form 7α-thiospironolactone

The half-life of spironolactone averages 1–2 hours,

PREPARATIONS

Excipients in commercially available drug preparations may have clinically important effects in some individuals; consult specific product labeling for details.

Spironolactone

Oral		
Suspension	25 mg/5 mL	**CaroSpir®**, CMP
Tablets, film-coated	25 mg*	**Aldactone®**, Pfizer **Spironolactone Tablets**
	50 mg*	**Aldactone®** (scored), Pfizer **Spironolactone Tablets**
	100 mg*	**Aldactone®** (scored), Pfizer **Spironolactone Tablets**

* available from one or more manufacturer, distributor, and/or repackager by generic (nonproprietary) name

Spironolactone and Hydrochlorothiazide

Oral		
Tablets, film-coated	25 mg Spironolactone and Hydrochlorothiazide 25 mg*	**Aldactazide®**, Pfizer **Spironolactone and Hydrochlorothiazide Tablets**
	50 mg Spironolactone and Hydrochlorothiazide 50 mg	**Aldactazide®** (scored), Pfizer

* available from one or more manufacturer, distributor, and/or repackager by generic (nonproprietary) name

† Use is not currently included in the labeling approved by the US Food and Drug Administration.

Selected Revisions June 10, 2024, © Copyright, March 1, 1974, American Society of Health-System Pharmacists, Inc.

Colchicine

24:44 · CARDIOVASCULAR DRUGS, NONSTEROIDAL ANTI-INFLAMMATORY

■ Colchicine is an antigout and antimitotic agent.

USES

● Gout Flare

Colchicine is used to relieve acute gout flares (acute attacks of gouty arthritis). Nonsteroidal anti-inflammatory agents (NSAIAs) (e.g., indomethacin, ibuprofen, naproxen, sulindac, piroxicam, ketoprofen) are as effective as, and better tolerated than, usual dosages of colchicine for short-term use in relieving acute attacks of gouty arthritis. (See Indomethacin 28:08.04.24.) Corticosteroids also are used to relieve acute attacks of gouty arthritis. Colchicine is considered a second-line agent; colchicine may be used for the treatment of acute gouty arthritis in patients who have not responded to or who cannot tolerate recommended therapies (i.e., NSAIAs, corticosteroids).

Colchicine should be initiated at the first sign of an acute gout flare. When colchicine is administered orally within 12 hours of the onset of an acute gout flare, 38% of patients receiving the drug in the currently recommended dosage have a favorable response.

Colchicine also is used in the prophylactic treatment of recurrent gout flares. Colchicine has no effect on plasma concentrations or urinary excretion of uric acid; therefore, concomitant administration of allopurinol or a uricosuric agent (e.g., febuxostat, probenecid, sulfinpyrazone) is necessary to decrease serum urate concentrations. Prophylactic doses of colchicine should be administered *before* the initiation of allopurinol or uricosuric therapy because sudden changes in serum urate concentrations may precipitate acute gout attacks. After the serum urate concentration has been reduced to the desired level and acute gout attacks have not occurred for 3–6 months (some clinicians suggest 1–12 months), colchicine may be discontinued and the patient may be treated with urate-lowering agents alone. Colchicine is frequently used in combination with probenecid to facilitate prophylactic therapy in patients with chronic gouty arthritis. The usefulness of the commercially available fixed-dosage preparation is limited, however, because the colchicine present exceeds the amount required by most patients.

● Familial Mediterranean Fever

Colchicine is used in the management of familial Mediterranean fever. The drug has been used effectively for chronic prophylactic therapy to reduce the frequency and severity of the episodic attacks of painful serositis in patients with familial Mediterranean fever. Chronic prophylactic therapy reportedly is associated with marked amelioration of attacks (both frequency and severity) or remission in about 90% of patients with this condition, but therapy with the drug is not curative and manifestations of this condition return to pretreatment levels following discontinuance of colchicine. Chronic prophylactic therapy also appears to prevent amyloidosis, manifested by nephropathy, in patients with familial Mediterranean fever who lack evidence of amyloidosis when therapy is initiated. Colchicine appears to be effective in preventing amyloidosis regardless of whether patients continue to experience episodic attacks of serositis during chronic prophylactic therapy with the drug. Colchicine may prevent deterioration in patients in the proteinuric phase of the disease when amyloid involvement is minimal. The drug generally appears to be of limited value in altering the effects of amyloid deposits when clinical amyloidosis is evident, particularly when proteinuria has progressed to nephrosis, although a beneficial effect (e.g., restoration of serum albumin concentrations toward normal, slight improvement in renal function) may be evident in some patients.

● Regulatory Actions Affecting Colchicine

Colchicine injection became available in the US in the 1950s and has been used for the treatment of acute attacks of gout. Colchicine injection preparations that have been commercially available have *not* been approved by the US Food and Drug Administration (FDA). Serious adverse events, some fatal, have been reported in patients receiving colchicine injection. (See Cautions: Adverse Effects.) Because of the potentially serious health risks associated with unapproved colchicine injection, FDA announced on February 8, 2008, that it would take enforcement action (e.g., seizure, injunction, other judicial proceeding) against all firms, including compounding pharmacies, attempting to manufacture, ship, or deliver colchicine injection.

Although commercially available, single-entity, oral preparations of colchicine also lacked FDA approval, FDA did not take action against colchicine tablets in February 2008; risks associated with use of the tablets are believed to be lower than those associated with use of the injection. In July 2009, FDA approved a single-ingredient oral colchicine preparation. During the review process, FDA identified 2 safety concerns associated with use of colchicine. Reports suggested that drug interactions play an important role in the development of colchicine toxicity. There also was evidence that the dosage of colchicine previously used for treatment of acute gout flares could be reduced without reducing the drug's efficacy. The labeling now includes extensive information on drug interactions and a new (lower) dosage for acute gout flare. Colchicine in fixed combination with probenecid is approved by the FDA for the management of recurrent gouty arthritis.

DOSAGE AND ADMINISTRATION

● Administration

Colchicine is administered orally without regard to meals. Colchicine has been administered by IV injection; however, IV preparations of colchicine have been withdrawn from the US market because of safety concerns. (See Uses: Regulatory Actions Affecting Colchicine and see Cautions.)

Patients receiving colchicine should be instructed on how to resume therapy in the event of a missed dose. Patients with gout who are receiving colchicine for treatment of an acute flare but not for prophylaxis of recurrent flares should be instructed to take the missed dose as soon as possible. Those receiving the drug to treat an acute gout flare during colchicine prophylaxis should be instructed to take the missed dose immediately and then wait 12 hours before resuming the previous dosing schedule. Patients receiving colchicine for treatment of familial Mediterranean fever or for prophylaxis of recurrent gout flares (without treatment for an acute gout flare) should be instructed to take the missed dose as soon as possible and then resume their usual dosing schedule, but not to take a double dose to make up for the missed dose.

● Dosage

Dosage of colchicine depends on the patient's age, renal and hepatic function, and whether the drug is administered concomitantly with or within 14 days following therapy with drugs that affect hepatic metabolism or the P-glycoprotein transport system.

Treatment of Acute Gout Flare

The recommended oral dosage of colchicine for relief of an acute gout flare in patients who are *not* receiving concomitant therapy with a moderate or potent inhibitor of cytochrome P-450 (CYP) isoenzyme 3A4 or an inhibitor of the P-glycoprotein transport system, and who have not received such therapy during the prior 14 days, is 1.2 mg given at the first sign of flare followed by 0.6 mg one hour later. The maximum recommended dosage for treatment of acute gout flare is 1.8 mg administered over a one-hour period. Higher dosages of colchicine have not been shown to be more effective in relieving acute gout flares. Additional courses of colchicine therapy for treatment of an acute gout flare should not be repeated until 3 days have elapsed. Patients receiving colchicine for prevention of gout flares who are not receiving a CYP3A4 inhibitor also may receive colchicine (1.2 mg initially followed by 0.6 mg 1 hour later) to relieve an acute gout flare; following the 2-dose treatment course, 12 hours should elapse before prophylactic doses of the drug are resumed.

In patients receiving concomitant therapy with a *potent inhibitor* of CYP3A4, such as atazanavir, boceprevir, clarithromycin, darunavir with low-dose ritonavir (*ritonavir-boosted* darunavir), *ritonavir-boosted* fosamprenavir, indinavir, itraconazole, ketoconazole, nefazodone, nelfinavir, ritonavir, saquinavir, telaprevir, telithromycin, *ritonavir-boosted* tipranavir, the fixed combination of lopinavir and ritonavir (lopinavir/ritonavir), or the fixed combination of elvitegravir, cobicistat, emtricitabine, and tenofovir, and those who have received such therapy during the prior 14 days, the recommended oral dosage of colchicine for relief of an acute gout flare is 0.6 mg given at the first sign of flare followed by 0.3 mg 1 hour later. Additional courses of colchicine therapy for treatment of an acute gout flare should not be repeated until 3 days have elapsed. Use of colchicine for the treatment of acute gout flares is not recommended in individuals receiving the drug for prevention of gout flares who also are receiving therapy with a CYP3A4 inhibitor.

In patients receiving concomitant therapy with a *moderate inhibitor* of CYP3A4, such as aprepitant, diltiazem, erythromycin, fluconazole, fosamprenavir (without ritonavir), grapefruit juice, or verapamil, and those who have received such therapy during the prior 14 days, the recommended oral dosage of colchicine for relief of an acute gout flare is a single 1.2-mg dose given at the first sign of flare. Additional courses of colchicine therapy for treatment of an acute gout flare should not be repeated until 3 days have elapsed. Use of colchicine for the treatment of acute gout flare is not recommended in individuals receiving the drug for prevention of gout flares who also are receiving therapy with a CYP3A4 inhibitor.

In patients receiving concomitant therapy with a drug that inhibits the P-glycoprotein transport system, such as cyclosporine or ranolazine, and those who have received such therapy during the prior 14 days, the recommended oral dosage of colchicine for relief of an acute gout flare is a single 0.6-mg dose given at the first sign of flare. Additional courses of colchicine therapy for treatment of an acute gout flare should not be repeated until 3 days have elapsed.

The safety and efficacy of repeat courses of colchicine for treatment of acute gout flare have not been evaluated.

Prophylactic Treatment of Recurrent Gout Flare

The recommended oral dosage of colchicine for prophylaxis of recurrent gout flares in adults and adolescents older than 16 years of age who are not receiving concomitant therapy with a moderate or potent inhibitor of CYP3A4 or an inhibitor of the P-glycoprotein transport system, and who have not received such therapy during the prior 14 days, is 0.6 mg once or twice daily. The maximum recommended dosage is 1.2 mg daily.

In patients receiving concomitant therapy with a *potent inhibitor* of CYP3A4, such as atazanavir, boceprevir, clarithromycin, *ritonavir-boosted* darunavir, *ritonavir-boosted* fosamprenavir, indinavir, itraconazole, ketoconazole, nefazodone, nelfinavir, ritonavir, saquinavir, telaprevir, telithromycin, *ritonavir-boosted* tipranavir, lopinavir/ritonavir, or the fixed combination of elvitegravir, cobicistat, emtricitabine, and tenofovir, and those who have received such therapy during the prior 14 days, the recommended oral dosage of colchicine for prophylaxis of recurrent gout flares is 0.3 mg daily or every other day.

In patients receiving concomitant therapy with a *moderate inhibitor* of CYP3A4, such as aprepitant, diltiazem, erythromycin, fluconazole, fosamprenavir (without ritonavir), grapefruit juice, or verapamil, and those who have received such therapy during the prior 14 days, the recommended oral dosage of colchicine for prophylaxis of recurrent gout flares is 0.3 mg twice daily, 0.6 mg once daily, or 0.3 mg once daily.

In patients receiving concomitant therapy with a drug that inhibits the P-glycoprotein transport system, such as cyclosporine or ranolazine, and those who have received such therapy during the prior 14 days, the recommended oral dosage of colchicine for prophylaxis of recurrent gout flares is 0.3 mg once daily or every other day.

Familial Mediterranean Fever

For management of familial Mediterranean fever in patients who are *not* receiving concomitant therapy with a moderate or potent inhibitor of CYP3A4 or an inhibitor of the P-glycoprotein transport system, and who have not received such therapy during the prior 14 days, colchicine may be given in a dosage of 1.2–2.4 mg daily in adults and adolescents older than 12 years of age, a dosage of 0.9–1.8 mg daily in children 6–12 years of age, and a dosage of 0.3–1.8 mg daily in children 4–6 years of age. The daily dosage may be given once daily or in 2 divided doses. Dosage of the drug may be increased in increments of 0.3 mg daily to the maximum recommended dosage. Alternatively, in patients experiencing intolerable adverse effects, dosage may be decreased in increments of 0.3 mg daily.

In adults and adolescents receiving concomitant therapy with a *potent inhibitor* of CYP3A4, such as atazanavir, boceprevir, clarithromycin, *ritonavir-boosted* darunavir, *ritonavir-boosted* fosamprenavir, indinavir, itraconazole, ketoconazole, nefazodone, nelfinavir, ritonavir, saquinavir, telaprevir, telithromycin, *ritonavir-boosted* tipranavir, lopinavir/ritonavir, or the fixed combination of elvitegravir,

cobicistat, emtricitabine, and tenofovir, and those who have received such therapy during the prior 14 days, the maximum recommended dosage of colchicine for the management of familial Mediterranean fever is 0.6 mg daily; the daily dosage may be given as 0.3 mg twice daily.

In adults and adolescents receiving concomitant therapy with a *moderate inhibitor* of CYP3A4, such as aprepitant, diltiazem, erythromycin, fluconazole, fosamprenavir (without ritonavir), grapefruit juice, or verapamil, and those who have received such therapy during the prior 14 days, the maximum recommended dosage of colchicine for the management of familial Mediterranean fever is 1.2 mg daily; the daily dosage may be given as 0.6 mg twice daily.

In adults and adolescents receiving concomitant therapy with a drug that inhibits the P-glycoprotein transport system, such as cyclosporine or ranolazine, and those who have received such therapy during the prior 14 days, the maximum recommended dosage of colchicine for the management of familial Mediterranean fever is 0.6 mg daily; the daily dosage may be given as 0.3 mg twice daily.

These maximum recommended dosages for patients with familial Mediterranean fever who are receiving CYP3A4 or P-glycoprotein inhibitors are intended for individuals for whom a dosage range of 1.2–2.4 mg daily would be appropriate in the absence of interacting drugs (i.e., adults and adolescents older than 12 years of age). The manufacturer currently makes no specific recommendations regarding maximum colchicine dosage in children 4–12 years of age who are receiving CYP3A4 or P-glycoprotein inhibitors.

• **Dosage in Renal and Hepatic Impairment**

Dosage in Renal Impairment

Use of colchicine in combination with a potent CYP3A4 inhibitor, such as atazanavir, boceprevir, clarithromycin, *ritonavir-boosted* darunavir, *ritonavir-boosted* fosamprenavir, indinavir, itraconazole, ketoconazole, nefazodone, nelfinavir, ritonavir, saquinavir, telaprevir, telithromycin, *ritonavir-boosted* tipranavir, lopinavir/ritonavir, or the fixed combination of elvitegravir, cobicistat, emtricitabine, and tenofovir, or with a P-glycoprotein inhibitor, such as cyclosporine or ranolazine, in patients with renal impairment is contraindicated.

Gout Flare

Use of colchicine for the treatment of an acute gout flare is not recommended in patients with renal impairment who are receiving the drug for prevention of gout flares.

Colchicine dosage adjustment is not needed in patients with mild (creatinine clearance 50–80 mL/minute) to moderate (creatinine clearance 30–50 mL/minute) renal impairment who are receiving the drug for treatment of an acute gout flare or for prophylaxis of recurrent gout flares; however, such patients should be monitored for adverse effects.

In patients with severe renal impairment, the recommended initial dosage of colchicine for prophylaxis of recurrent gout flares is 0.3 mg daily; close monitoring is needed if the dosage is increased. When colchicine is used for the treatment of an acute gout flare in patients with severe renal impairment, dosage adjustment is not needed, but additional courses of colchicine therapy for acute gout flares should not be repeated until 2 weeks have elapsed. Alternative therapy should be considered for patients with severe renal impairment requiring repeat courses of therapy.

In patients who are undergoing dialysis, the recommended dosage of colchicine for prophylaxis of recurrent gout flares is 0.3 mg twice weekly; close monitoring is advised. When colchicine is used for the treatment of an acute gout flare in patients who are undergoing dialysis, the recommended dosage of colchicine is 0.6 mg at the first sign of flare. Additional courses of colchicine therapy for acute gout flares should not be repeated until 2 weeks have elapsed.

Familial Mediterranean Fever

Patients with mild (creatinine clearance 50–80 mL/minute) to moderate (creatinine clearance 30–50 mL/minute) renal impairment who are receiving colchicine for management of familial Mediterranean fever should be monitored for adverse effects. Dosage adjustment may be needed.

In patients with severe (creatinine clearance less than 30 mL/minute) renal impairment or undergoing dialysis, the recommended initial dosage of colchicine for management of familial Mediterranean fever is 0.3 mg daily. Dosage can be increased with careful monitoring.

Dosage in Hepatic Impairment

Use of colchicine in combination with a potent CYP3A4 inhibitor, such as atazanavir, boceprevir, clarithromycin, *ritonavir-boosted* darunavir, *ritonavir-boosted* fosamprenavir, indinavir, itraconazole, ketoconazole, nefazodone, nelfinavir, ritonavir, saquinavir, telaprevir, telithromycin, *ritonavir-boosted* tipranavir, lopinavir/ritonavir, the fixed combination of elvitegravir, cobicistat, emtricitabine, and tenofovir, or with a P-glycoprotein inhibitor, such as cyclosporine or ranolazine, in patients with hepatic impairment is contraindicated.

Gout Flare

Colchicine dosage adjustment is not needed in patients with mild to moderate hepatic impairment who are receiving the drug for treatment of an acute gout flare or for prophylaxis of recurrent gout flares; however, such patients should be monitored for adverse effects.

Dosage reduction should be considered in patients with severe hepatic impairment who are receiving colchicine for prophylaxis of recurrent gout flares. When colchicine is used for the treatment of an acute gout flare in patients with severe hepatic impairment, dosage adjustment is not needed, but additional courses of colchicine therapy for acute gout flares should not be repeated until 2 weeks have elapsed. Alternative therapy should be considered for patients with severe hepatic impairment requiring repeat courses of therapy.

Familial Mediterranean Fever

Patients with mild to moderate hepatic impairment who are receiving colchicine for management of familial Mediterranean fever should be monitored for adverse effects.

Dosage adjustment should be considered for patients with severe hepatic impairment who are receiving colchicine for management of familial Mediterranean fever.

CAUTIONS

● Adverse Effects

The most common adverse effects of oral colchicine therapy are nausea, abdominal discomfort, vomiting, and diarrhea. Pharyngolaryngeal pain has been reported.

Bladder spasm, paralytic ileus, stomatitis, hypothyroidism, nonthrombocytopenic purpura, and prostration have also been reported with colchicine therapy.

Myelosuppression, disseminated intravascular coagulation, and renal, hepatic, circulatory, and CNS cellular injury have been reported in patients receiving colchicine, generally in those receiving excessive dosages of the drug. Leukopenia, granulocytopenia, thrombocytopenia, pancytopenia, and aplastic anemia have been reported. Death has occurred in one patient with normal renal and hepatic function who developed pancytopenia and bone marrow aplasia following IV administration of 10 mg of colchicine (IV preparations are no longer commercially available in the US) over a 5-day period.

Neuromuscular toxicity and rhabdomyolysis have been reported in patients receiving long-term colchicine therapy. Patients with renal dysfunction and geriatric patients, including those with normal renal and hepatic function, are at increased risk. Concomitant therapy with an HMG-CoA reductase inhibitor (statin), fibric acid derivative, or cyclosporine also may increase the risk for development of myopathy. Following discontinuance of colchicine, symptoms generally resolve within one week to several months.

Loss of body and scalp hair, rash, vesicular dermatitis, peripheral neuritis or neuropathy, myopathy, rhabdomyolysis, anuria, renal damage, hematuria, and one case of purpura have been reported with prolonged administration of colchicine. Colchicine may also cause increased serum concentrations of alkaline phosphatase, aminotransferases (AST, ALT), and creatine kinase (CK, creatine phosphokinase, CPK). Other reported adverse effects include sensory motor neuropathy, maculopapular rash, abdominal pain or cramping, lactose intolerance, myotonia, muscle weakness or pain, azoospermia, and oligospermia.

Serious adverse events have been reported in patients receiving IV colchicine. Many of these adverse effects were the result of colchicine toxicity. As of June 2007, the US Food and Drug Administration (FDA) was aware of 50 reports of adverse effects associated with use of IV colchicine; 23 of these events were fatal. Reported adverse effects included neutropenia, acute renal failure, thrombocytopenia, congestive heart failure, and pancytopenia. Three deaths were associated with use of compounded IV colchicine. Tests of vials from the same lot used to treat these 3 patients indicated that the concentration of colchicine was 4 mg/mL; labeling on the vial indicated that the concentration of colchicine was 0.5 mg/mL. Because of the potentially serious health risks associated with colchicine injection, FDA announced on February 8, 2008, that it would take enforcement action against all firms, including compounding pharmacies, attempting to manufacture, ship, or deliver colchicine injection.

Oral preparations containing colchicine remain on the market; risks associated with use of the tablets are believed to be lower than those associated with use of the injection.

● Precautions and Contraindications

Concomitant use of colchicine with certain drugs is contraindicated or requires particular caution. (See Drug Interactions and also see Dosage and Administration: Dosage.)

Colchicine is contraindicated in patients with renal or hepatic impairment who are receiving a drug that inhibits the P-glycoprotein transport system or is a potent CYP3A4 inhibitor (see Dosage and Administration: Dosage in Renal and Hepatic Impairment); fatal or life-threatening colchicine toxicity has occurred in such patients following therapeutic doses of colchicine.

● Pediatric Precautions

Safety and efficacy of colchicine for treatment of gout in children have not been established.

Safety and efficacy of colchicine for management of familial Mediterranean fever in children have been evaluated in uncontrolled studies. Long-term use of colchicine did not appear to affect growth in children with familial Mediterranean fever.

● Geriatric Precautions

Clinical studies of colchicine for treatment of acute gout flares, prophylactic treatment of recurrent gout flares, or management of familial Mediterranean fever did not include sufficient numbers of patients 65 years of age and older to determine whether geriatric patients respond differently than younger patients. Drug dosage generally should be titrated carefully in geriatric patients with gout; the greater frequency of decreased renal function and of concomitant disease and drug therapy observed in geriatric patients also should be considered.

● Pregnancy, Fertility, and Lactation

Pregnancy

Chromosomal aberrations have been reported in a limited number of patients receiving prolonged colchicine therapy. Colchicine crosses the placenta in humans and has been shown in animal reproduction and development studies to cause embryofetal toxicity, teratogenic effects, and altered postnatal development at exposure levels within or above the therapeutic range. Although there are no adequate and controlled studies to date in humans, results of one study suggest that patients receiving prolonged colchicine therapy may have a greater risk of producing trisomic offspring if conception occurs during therapy with the drug. Other clinicians, however, contend that this study is inconclusive and at most merely suggestive of a probable increased risk to the offspring. Data from a limited number of published studies indicate that use of colchicine for the treatment of familial Mediterranean fever in pregnant women was not associated with increased risk of miscarriage, stillbirth, or teratogenic effects. Colchicine should be used during pregnancy only if the potential benefits outweigh the risks.

The effect of colchicine on labor and delivery is not known.

Fertility

Colchicine has adversely affected spermatogenesis in humans and animals. Reversible azoospermia has been reported in a 36-year-old man who received 0.6 mg of colchicine twice daily for several months.

Lactation

Colchicine is distributed into milk. (See Pharmacokinetics: Distribution.) Limited information suggests that exclusively breast-fed infants receive less than 10% of the maternal weight-adjusted dose. Although the drug can affect GI cell renewal and permeability, some experts state that the actual amounts of the drug distributed into breast milk are not high enough to warrant cessation of nursing. No adverse effects have been reported to date in breast-fed infants of women receiving colchicine therapy who were observed over periods of up to 10 months. The American Academy of Pediatrics (AAP) states that the drug usually is compatible with breast-feeding. Some clinicians have suggested that exposure of the infant to the drug could be minimized by waiting 8–12 hours after a dose to breast-feed the infant. The manufacturer states that caution is advised; the infant should be observed for adverse effects.

DRUG INTERACTIONS

● *Drugs Affecting Hepatic Microsomal Enzymes*

Colchicine is metabolized by cytochrome P-450 (CYP) isoenzyme 3A4. In vitro studies indicate that colchicine does not inhibit or induce CYP isoenzymes 1A2, 2A6, 2B6, 2C8, 2C9, 2C19, 2D6, 2E1, or 3A4.

Concomitant use of colchicine with potent CYP3A4 inhibitors, such as atazanavir, boceprevir, clarithromycin, *ritonavir-boosted* darunavir, *ritonavir-boosted* fosamprenavir, indinavir, itraconazole, ketoconazole, nefazodone, nelfinavir, ritonavir, saquinavir, telaprevir, telithromycin, *ritonavir-boosted* tipranavir, lopinavir/ritonavir, or the fixed combination of elvitegravir, cobicistat, emtricitabine, and tenofovir, or with moderate CYP3A4 inhibitors, such as aprepitant, diltiazem, erythromycin, fluconazole, fosamprenavir (without ritonavir), grapefruit juice, or verapamil, may result in substantially increased plasma concentrations of colchicine. If concomitant therapy is required, the dosage of colchicine must be reduced or treatment with colchicine may need to be interrupted. (See Dosage and Administration: Dosage.) Use of colchicine in combination with a potent CYP3A4 inhibitor in patients with renal or hepatic impairment is contraindicated.

Clarithromycin

An increase in plasma colchicine concentrations (227% increase in peak plasma concentration, 281% increase in area under the plasma concentration-time curve [AUC]) was observed when a single 0.6-mg dose of colchicine was administered concomitantly with clarithromycin (250 mg twice daily for 7 days). Severe or fatal colchicine toxicity has been reported with concomitant clarithromycin and colchicine therapy.

Ketoconazole

An increase in plasma colchicine concentrations (102% increase in peak plasma concentration, 212% increase in AUC) was observed when a single 0.6-mg dose of colchicine was administered concomitantly with ketoconazole (200 mg twice daily for 5 days).

Ritonavir

An increase in plasma colchicine concentrations (184% increase in peak plasma concentration, 296% increase in AUC) was observed when a single 0.6-mg dose of colchicine was administered concomitantly with ritonavir (100 mg twice daily for 5 days).

Verapamil

An increase in plasma colchicine concentrations (40% increase in peak plasma concentration, 103% increase in AUC) was observed when a single 0.6-mg dose of colchicine was administered concomitantly with verapamil (240 mg daily for 5 days). Neuromuscular toxicity has been reported with concomitant verapamil and colchicine therapy.

Diltiazem

An increase in plasma colchicine concentrations (44% increase in peak plasma concentration, 93% increase in AUC) was observed when a single 0.6-mg dose of colchicine was administered concomitantly with diltiazem (240 mg daily for 7 days). Neuromuscular toxicity has been reported with concomitant diltiazem and colchicine therapy.

Grapefruit Juice

No substantial change in plasma concentrations of colchicine was observed when a single 0.6-mg dose of colchicine was administered concomitantly with grapefruit juice (240 mL twice daily for 4 days). However, when colchicine was given concomitantly with other moderate CYP3A4 inhibitors (e.g., diltiazem, verapamil), substantial increases in plasma colchicine concentrations were reported. The manufacturer states that patients receiving colchicine should be advised not to consume grapefruit or grapefruit juice. If a moderate CYP3A4 inhibitor (including grapefruit juice) is given concomitantly with colchicine, the manufacturer recommends adjustment of colchicine dosage (see Dosage and Administration: Dosage).

● *Drugs Affecting the P-glycoprotein Transport System*

Concomitant use of colchicine with drugs that inhibit the P-glycoprotein transport system, such as cyclosporine or ranolazine, results in substantially increased plasma concentrations of colchicine. If use of a P-glycoprotein inhibitor is required, the dosage of colchicine must be reduced or treatment with colchicine may need to be interrupted. (See Dosage and Administration: Dosage.) Use of colchicine in combination with a P-glycoprotein inhibitor in patients with renal or hepatic impairment is contraindicated.

Cyclosporine

Administration of a single 100-mg dose of cyclosporine, a P-glycoprotein inhibitor, concomitantly with a single 0.6-mg dose of colchicine resulted in increases in plasma colchicine concentrations (270% increase in peak plasma concentration, 259% increase in AUC). Fatal colchicine toxicity has been reported with concomitant cyclosporine and colchicine therapy. Concomitant use of cyclosporine and colchicine also may result in increased cyclosporine concentrations and additive nephrotoxic effects; therefore, renal function and blood concentrations of cyclosporine should be monitored and cyclosporine dosage should be adjusted accordingly if colchicine is initiated or discontinued or the colchicine dosage is altered in patients receiving cyclosporine.

● *Antilipemic Agents*

Addition of an HMG-CoA reductase inhibitor (statin) or other lipid-lowering agents (e.g., fibric acid derivatives) to long-term therapy with colchicine or addition of colchicine to long-term therapy with these antilipemic agents has resulted in myopathy and rhabdomyolysis; death has been reported. Potential benefits and risks of such concomitant therapy should be weighed. Patients should be monitored for muscle pain, tenderness, and weakness, especially during the initial phase of such concomitant therapy.

● *Azithromycin*

An increase in plasma colchicine concentrations (22% increase in peak plasma concentration, 57% increase in AUC) was observed when a single 0.6-mg dose of colchicine was administered concomitantly with azithromycin (500 mg initially, followed by 250 mg daily for 4 days).

● *Digoxin*

Digoxin is a P-glycoprotein transport system substrate. Rhabdomyolysis has been reported in an individual receiving colchicine and digoxin concomitantly. Potential benefits and risks of concomitant therapy with colchicine and digoxin should be weighed. Patients should be monitored for muscle pain, tenderness, and weakness, especially during the initial phase of such concomitant therapy.

● *Estrogens or Progestins*

Administration of an oral contraceptive (ethinyl estradiol 35 mcg with norethindrone 1 mg) concomitantly with colchicine (0.6 mg twice daily for 14 days) in healthy women did not alter the plasma concentrations of either the estrogen or the progestin.

● *Theophylline*

No change in plasma concentrations of theophylline was observed when theophylline was administered concomitantly with colchicine (0.6 mg twice daily for 14 days) in healthy individuals.

LABORATORY TEST INTERFERENCES

Colchicine has been reported to interfere with urinary determinations of 17-hydroxycorticosteroids using the Reddy, Jenkins, and Thorn procedure. Colchicine may cause false-positive results in urine tests for erythrocytes or hemoglobin.

ACUTE TOXICITY

● Manifestations

Poisoning may occur from repeated administration of large doses or from a single toxic dose of colchicine. Death has occurred following ingestion of as little as 7 mg of colchicine, although individuals have survived larger doses. The lethal dose in humans has been estimated to be 65 mg. In individuals receiving IV colchicine, death has occurred following cumulative doses as low as 5.5 mg. The median IV lethal dose in rats is 1.7 mg/kg. There is usually a delay of a few hours between ingestion of the toxic dose of colchicine and the appearance of the first toxic symptoms, regardless of the route of administration.

The first stage of acute colchicine toxicity typically begins within 24 hours of ingestion and includes adverse GI effects resulting in fluid loss and volume depletion; peripheral leukocytosis also may occur. Life-threatening complications occur during the second stage, which occurs 24–72 hours after administration, and result from multiorgan failure.

The first symptoms of acute colchicine toxicity involve the GI tract and include nausea, anorexia, abdominal pain, vomiting, paralytic ileus, and diarrhea which may be severe and bloody due to hemorrhagic gastroenteritis. Stomatitis, arthralgia, malaise, hypocalcemia, fever, and rashes including scarlatiniform rash may also occur. Dehydration may occur resulting in oliguria. Renal damage as evidenced by hematuria and oliguria has been reported. Hepatomegaly and liver tenderness with elevated serum concentrations of AST (SGOT) and alkaline phosphatase may occur. Extreme vascular damage may result in shock and cardiovascular collapse. Leukopenia may occur and may persist for several days followed by leukocytosis with numerous metamyelocytes and myelocytes. Other hematologic manifestations of colchicine toxicity include bone marrow depression, thrombocytopenia, granulocytopenia, immature leukocytes, pancytopenia, anemia with anisocytosis, polychromasia, and basophilic stippling. Muscular weakness is marked and an ascending paralysis of the CNS may develop, although the patient usually remains conscious. Mental confusion, delirium, and seizures may occur. There may be a loss of deep tendon and Achilles tendon reflexes, and Babinski's reflex may be elicited. Death usually occurs as a result of respiratory depression or cardiovascular collapse.

● Treatment

There is no specific antidote for colchicine poisoning. Gastric lavage should be performed initially and measures initiated to prevent shock. Other treatment is symptomatic and supportive. Colchicine is not removed by dialysis.

PHARMACOLOGY

● Gout

Colchicine possesses antigout activity. The drug also has weak anti-inflammatory activity but has no analgesic activity. The drug has no effect on urinary excretion of uric acid or on serum urate concentration, solubility, or binding to serum proteins. Although the mechanism of the antigout effect of colchicine is not completely known, the drug appears to disrupt cytoskeletal functions through inhibition of β-tubulin polymerization into microtubules, thus preventing activation, degranulation, and migration of neutrophils believed to mediate some gout symptoms.

● Familial Mediterranean Fever

The mechanism of colchicine's beneficial effects in familial Mediterranean fever has not been fully elucidated. Colchicine may interfere with intracellular assembly of the inflammasome complex in neutrophils and monocytes that mediates activation of interleukin-1β.

PHARMACOKINETICS

● Absorption

Following oral administration, colchicine is absorbed from the GI tract and is partially metabolized in the liver. The drug and its metabolites re-enter the intestinal tract via biliary secretions and the unchanged drug may be reabsorbed from the intestine. Following oral administration of colchicine 1.8 mg over 1 hour under fasting conditions, peak plasma concentrations of 6.2 ng/mL were reached in 1.8 hours. Following oral administration of 0.6 mg twice daily for 10 days, a mean peak plasma concentration of 3.6 ng/mL was reached at 1.3 hours after a dose. Administration of colchicine with food did not affect rate of absorption but decreased the extent of absorption by 15%. Absolute bioavailability is reported to be approximately 45%.

The presence of a secondary peak in colchicine concentrations, ranging from 39–155% of the height of the initial peak concentration, has been reported in some individuals 3–36 hours after oral administration and has been attributed to intestinal secretion and reabsorption and/or biliary circulation.

● Distribution

Colchicine is about 39% bound to serum proteins, mainly albumin.

Colchicine crosses the placenta. Fetal plasma concentrations of the drug are reported to be approximately 15% of the maternal concentration.

Colchicine is distributed into milk. In a limited number of nursing women receiving long-term colchicine therapy at dosages of 1–1.5 mg daily, peak concentrations of the drug in milk were similar to serum concentrations and ranged from 1.9–8.6 ng/mL. Higher concentrations of the drug in milk (31, 24–27, or 10 ng/mL at 2, 4, or 7 hours, respectively, after a dose) have been reported in the absence of concurrent serum concentration data in a nursing woman receiving colchicine 1 mg daily.

● Elimination

Following IV administration of a single therapeutic dose (IV preparations are no longer commercially available in the US), colchicine is rapidly removed from the plasma; plasma half-life is about 20 minutes. The drug has a half-life of about 60 hours in leukocytes.

Colchicine is demethylated in the liver by cytochrome P-450 (CYP) isoenzyme 3A4. In healthy individuals, 40–65% of an orally administered 1-mg dose of the drug is excreted unchanged in urine. Enterohepatic circulation and biliary excretion may occur. A half-life of 26.6–31.2 hours has been reported in healthy young adults receiving colchicine 0.6 mg orally twice daily. Colchicine is a substrate of the P-glycoprotein transport system. Colchicine is not removed by hemodialysis.

Clearance of colchicine is decreased in patients with renal impairment. In one study, patients with severe renal disease eliminated little or no colchicine or its metabolites in the urine, resulting in a prolonged plasma half-life. Total body clearance of colchicine was reduced by 75% in patients with end-stage renal disease requiring dialysis.

In patients with hepatic impairment, substantial interpatient variability in colchicine pharmacokinetics has been observed. In some patients with mild to moderate cirrhosis, clearance of colchicine was decreased substantially and plasma half-life was prolonged compared with healthy individuals; however, no consistent trends were observed in patients with primary biliary cirrhosis.

CHEMISTRY AND STABILITY

● Chemistry

Colchicine, a phenanthrene derivative, is an antigout drug obtained from species of *Colchicum*. Colchicine occurs as pale yellow, amorphous scales or powder and is soluble in water and freely soluble in alcohol.

● Stability

Colchicine darkens on exposure to light and should be stored in tight, light-resistant containers.

PREPARATIONS

Excipients in commercially available drug preparations may have clinically important effects in some individuals; consult specific product labeling for details.

Colchicine

Oral		
Tablets	0.6 mg	**Colcrys®** (scored), Takeda

Probenecid and Colchicine

Oral		
Tablets	500 mg Probenecid and Colchicine 0.5 mg*	**Probenecid and Colchicine Tablets**

* available from one or more manufacturer, distributor, and/or repackager by generic (nonproprietary) name

† Use is not currently included in the labeling approved by the US Food and Drug Administration.

Selected Revisions April 10, 2024, © Copyright, April 1, 1973, American Society of Health-System Pharmacists, Inc.

Table of Contents

§ Omitted from the print version of *AHFS Drug Information*® because of space limitations. This monograph is available on the *AHFS Drug Information*® website, http://ahfsdruginformation.com.

Etomidate

28:04.08 · NON-BARBITURATES

■ Etomidate is a sedative and hypnotic agent used for general anesthesia.

USES

● Induction and Maintenance of Anesthesia

Etomidate is used IV for induction of general anesthesia. Etomidate may be particularly useful in patients with compromised cardiopulmonary function because of its minimal hemodynamic effects and decreased respiratory depressant effects relative to other IV anesthetics (e.g., barbiturates, propofol). However, the manufacturers state that the potential benefits of the drug's hemodynamic effects must be weighed carefully against the possible risk of involuntary skeletal muscle movements (e.g., myoclonus). (See Cautions: Common Adverse Effects.)

Etomidate also is used during maintenance of anesthesia to supplement subpotent anesthetic agents (e.g., nitrous oxide and oxygen) during short surgical procedures (e.g., dilatation and curettage, cervical conization). Use of the drug for longer procedures is not recommended due to an increased risk of prolonged adrenal suppression. (See Adrenal Suppression under Cautions: Warnings/Precautions.)

When used for induction of anesthesia, etomidate is administered IV by rapid (over 30–60 seconds) injection. Induction with IV etomidate is rapid and results in dose-related hypnotic effects (progressing from light sleep to unconsciousness); the drug also has some amnestic effects, but lacks analgesic properties. Following administration of a standard induction dose of 0.3 mg/kg, hypnosis occurs in less than 1 minute and is maintained for about 3–10 minutes.

For further information on induction and maintenance of anesthesia, see Uses: Induction and Maintenance of Anesthesia, in Propofol 28:04.92.

● Rapid Sequence Intubation

Because of its rapid onset and favorable hemodynamic profile, etomidate is commonly used (and often the preferred induction agent) for rapid sequence intubation. Rapid sequence intubation involves the administration of a potent sedative (induction agent) and a neuromuscular blocking agent virtually simultaneously to facilitate rapid tracheal intubation. However, the potential for etomidate to cause adrenal suppression may limit its use in critically ill patients (particularly those with sepsis). (See Adrenal Suppression under Cautions: Warnings/Precautions.)

● Procedural Sedation

Etomidate has been used for procedural sedation† in the emergency department and other outpatient settings (e.g., clinic). Because of its relatively short duration of action, the drug is best suited for procedures of short duration. Etomidate does not exhibit analgesic properties and generally is used concomitantly with an opiate agonist (e.g., fentanyl).

Procedural sedation is a technique in which sedative or dissociative agents are administered with or without analgesics to allow patients to tolerate painful or unpleasant medical procedures; a depressed state of consciousness is intentionally induced while cardiorespiratory function is maintained. Because sedation is a continuum ranging from minimal sedation to general anesthesia, airway reflexes and cardiorespiratory function may be impaired if a deeper than intended level of sedation is produced. The appropriate level of sedation should be individualized according to the specific procedure and needs of the patient.

In clinical studies conducted in both adults and pediatric patients, etomidate (in doses less than those used for anesthesia) produced adequate sedation and facilitated the successful completion of a short painful procedure (e.g., fracture reduction, laceration repair, shoulder relocation). Time to onset of sedation and recovery with etomidate are comparable to those achieved with propofol, but considerably shorter than with midazolam. Adverse effects that occur more frequently with etomidate than with other sedative agents include myoclonus and pain at the injection site. Although respiratory depression or apnea also has been reported to occur in some patients receiving etomidate, the incidence is generally the same or less than that with other sedative agents.

DOSAGE AND ADMINISTRATION

● General

Etomidate should be administered only by clinicians experienced in the use of general anesthetic drugs and in the management of possible complications associated with their use (e.g., airway or respiratory compromise).

Common premedications such as benzodiazepines (to relieve anxiety and produce anterograde amnesia) and opiate agonists (to relieve pain) may be administered as appropriate.

● Administration

Etomidate is administered by IV injection over 30–60 seconds. The drug should be injected undiluted by direct IV injection. Some clinicians state that etomidate may be administered by intraosseous (IO) injection† in the setting of pediatric rapid sequence intubation. Although the drug has been administered as a continuous IV infusion†, this method of delivery is currently not recommended because of the risk of adrenal toxicity. (See Adrenal Suppression under Cautions: Warnings/Precautions.)

Etomidate injection should be inspected visually for particulate matter and discoloration prior to administration whenever solution and container permit. The injection should not be administered unless the solution is clear and the container is undamaged; unused portions should be discarded.

Limited data from clinical and animal studies indicate that inadvertent intra-arterial administration of etomidate injection does not appear to be associated with tissue necrosis distant from the injection site; however, intra-arterial use of the drug is not recommended. Pain at the injection site, which occurs frequently and usually is mild to moderate in severity (although occasionally may be severe), can be minimized if the larger, more proximal veins of the forearm, rather than the smaller, distal hand or wrist veins are used. To prevent needlestick injuries, needles should not be recapped, bent, or broken by hand.

Etomidate injection is compatible with commonly used premedicants administered prior to induction of anesthesia.

● Dosage

Dosage of etomidate should be adjusted according to individual requirements and response, age, physical and clinical status, underlying pathologic conditions (e.g., shock, intestinal obstruction, malnutrition, anemia, burns, advanced malignancy, ulcerative colitis, uremia, alcoholism), and the type and amount of premedication or concomitant medication(s). In addition, dosage of the drug should be titrated to clinical effect.

Induction and Maintenance of Anesthesia

The usual dose of etomidate for induction of anesthesia in adults and children older than 10 years of age is 0.3 mg/kg (0.2–0.6 mg/kg), administered by IV injection over 30–60 seconds.

When etomidate is used during maintenance of anesthesia to supplement subpotent anesthetic agents during short surgical procedures, smaller increments of etomidate may be administered.

Rapid Sequence Intubation

For rapid sequence intubation, etomidate is usually administered in a dose of 0.3 mg/kg IV. The manufacturers state that there are inadequate data to make dosage recommendations for pediatric patients younger than 10 years of age; however, in published reports, etomidate was used in pediatric patients as young as 18 days of age at an average dose of 0.3 mg/kg. Some clinicians recommend an etomidate dose of 0.3 mg/kg by IV or IO† injection for pediatric rapid sequence intubation.

Procedural Sedation

Doses of etomidate used for procedural sedation† are usually less than those used for induction of anesthesia; in clinical studies, an initial IV etomidate dose of 0.1–0.2 mg/kg was usually administered, followed by additional doses of 0.05–0.1 mg/kg given as needed for adequate sedation (average total dose of up to 0.26 mg/kg per procedure) in adults and pediatric patients. Some studies have found that a dose of 0.2 mg/kg was the most effective initial dose for short pediatric procedures in the emergency department.

● **Special Populations**

Since clinical studies have revealed pharmacokinetic differences (decreased initial distribution volumes and total clearance, decreased serum protein binding to albumin) between geriatric and younger patients, geriatric patients may require lower dosages of etomidate than younger patients.

CAUTIONS

● **Contraindications**

Known hypersensitivity to etomidate.

● **Warnings/Precautions**

Administration Precautions

To minimize the risk of adverse effects, recommendations for administration and monitoring of etomidate therapy should be followed. (See Dosage and Administration.)

Adrenal Suppression

Etomidate is known to cause adrenal suppression by inhibiting 11-β-hydroxylase activity, the enzyme responsible for production of cortisol and aldosterone. Decreased plasma concentrations of cortisol, which usually persist for 6–8 hours and are unresponsive to stimulation by corticotropin (ACTH), have been reported following IV administration of a single induction dose of etomidate (0.3 mg/kg). Because of the risk of prolonged suppression of endogenous cortisol and aldosterone secretion from the adrenal cortex, administration of etomidate as a continuous IV infusion is not recommended.

Although it is well established that etomidate can cause adrenal suppression, there is controversy regarding the clinical importance of this observed effect. Some evidence from a randomized controlled study suggested a possible link between the use of etomidate and increased mortality in critically ill patients (particularly those with sepsis); however, other studies have not found such an association. Studies comparing etomidate to other induction agents (e.g., midazolam, ketamine) for endotracheal intubation have not shown any strong evidence that etomidate increases mortality when compared with these other agents.

Specific Populations

Pregnancy

There are no adequate and well controlled studies of etomidate in pregnant women; in animal reproduction studies, reduced pup survival and maternal toxicity have been observed.

Based on animal data, repeated or prolonged use of general anesthetics and sedation drugs, including etomidate, during the third trimester of pregnancy may result in adverse neurodevelopmental effects in the fetus. The clinical relevance of these animal findings to humans is not known; the potential risk of adverse neurodevelopmental effects should be considered and discussed with pregnant women undergoing procedures requiring general anesthetics and sedation drugs. (See Pediatric Use under Warnings/Precautions: Specific Populations, in Cautions.)

There are insufficient data to support the use of etomidate during labor and delivery; use is therefore not recommended in the obstetric setting, including in patients undergoing cesarean section.

Lactation

It is not known whether etomidate is distributed into milk in humans. Because many drugs are distributed into human milk, caution is advised if etomidate is used in nursing women.

Pediatric Use

The manufacturers state that safety and efficacy of etomidate for induction or maintenance of anesthesia have not been established in children younger than 10 years of age. However, the drug has been used for rapid sequence intubation in pediatric patients as young as 18 days of age. Etomidate also has been used in children of all ages for procedural sedation† in the emergency department.

FDA warns that repeated or prolonged use of general anesthetics and sedation drugs, including etomidate, in children younger than 3 years of age or during the third trimester of pregnancy may affect brain development. Animal studies in multiple species, including nonhuman primates, have demonstrated that use for longer than 3 hours of anesthetic and sedation drugs that block N-methyl-D-aspartic acid (NMDA) receptors and/or potentiate γ-aminobutyric acid (GABA) activity leads to widespread neuronal and oligodendrocyte cell loss and alterations in synaptic morphology and neurogenesis in the brain, resulting in long-term deficits in cognition and behavior. Across animal species, vulnerability to these neurodevelopmental changes occurs during the period of rapid brain growth or synaptogenesis; this period is thought to correlate with the third trimester of pregnancy through the first year of life in humans, but may extend to approximately 3 years of age. The clinical relevance of these animal findings to humans is not known.

While some published evidence suggests that similar deficits in cognition and behavior may occur in children following repeated or prolonged exposure to anesthesia early in life, other studies have found no association between pediatric anesthesia exposure and long-term adverse neurodevelopmental outcomes. Most studies to date have had substantial limitations, and it is not clear whether the adverse neurodevelopmental outcomes observed in children were related to the drug or to other factors (e.g., surgery, underlying illness). There is some clinical evidence that a single, relatively brief exposure to general anesthesia in generally healthy children is unlikely to cause clinically detectable deficits in global cognitive function or serious behavioral disorders; however, further research is needed to fully characterize the effects of exposure to general anesthetics in early life, particularly for prolonged or repeated exposures and in more vulnerable populations (e.g., less healthy children). For further information, see Cautions: Pediatric Precautions, in Propofol 28:04.92.

Anesthetic and sedation drugs are an essential component of care for children and pregnant women who require surgery or other procedures that cannot be delayed; no specific general anesthetic or sedation drug has been shown to be less likely to cause neurocognitive deficits than any other such drug. Pending further accumulation of data in humans from well-designed studies, decisions regarding the timing of elective procedures requiring anesthesia should take into consideration both the benefits of the procedure and the potential risks. When procedures requiring the use of general anesthetics or sedation drugs are considered for young children or pregnant women, clinicians should discuss with the patient, parent, or caregiver the benefits, risks (including potential risk of adverse neurodevelopmental effects), and appropriate timing and duration of the procedure. FDA states that procedures that are considered medically necessary should not be delayed or avoided.

Geriatric Use

Clinical data indicate that etomidate may be associated with cardiac depression (decreased heart rate and cardiac index) and decreased mean arterial blood pressure in geriatric patients, especially those with hypertension. Etomidate is substantially excreted by the kidneys and the risk of severe adverse reactions to the drug may be increased in patients with impaired renal function. Because geriatric patients may have decreased renal function, it may be useful to monitor renal function, and dosage should be selected with caution in such patients. (See Dosage and Administration: Special Populations.)

Hepatic Impairment

Etomidate is metabolized by the liver; patients with hepatic insufficiency may be at higher risk of adverse effects (e.g., adrenal insufficiency). In patients with cirrhosis, elimination half-life of etomidate is approximately double that seen in healthy individuals.

Renal Impairment

Because etomidate is substantially excreted renally, the risk of serious adverse effects is increased in patients with renal impairment.

● **Common Adverse Effects**

The most frequent adverse effects associated with IV use of etomidate are transient venous pain at the injection site and transient skeletal muscle movements (i.e., myoclonus), which occur in about 20% (range: 1–42%) and 32% (range: 23–63%) of patients, respectively. Although generally mild to moderate in severity, such adverse effects can occasionally be severe.

Most (74%) cases of transient skeletal muscle movements have been classified as myoclonic, but tonic movements (10%), ocular movements (9%), and averting movements (7%) also have been noted. Such movements are usually bilateral (of the arms, legs, shoulders, neck, chest wall, trunk, and/or all 4 extremities, with one or more muscle groups predominating), with an electroencephalogram (EEG) suggesting that they are manifestations of cortical disinhibition in the absence of evidence of seizure activity. Alternatively, muscle movements may be unilateral or predominate on one side (e.g., predominance of movement of the arm in which the IV was started), or a mixture of bilateral and unilateral types may occur. The incidence of skeletal muscle movements, particularly those considered disturbing, has been minimized with IV administration of fentanyl immediately before induction of anesthesia with etomidate.

Other adverse effects reported in patients receiving etomidate include hyperventilation, hypoventilation, apnea (duration: 5–90 seconds), laryngospasm, hiccups and snoring (may be associated with partial upper airway obstruction), hypertension, hypotension, arrhythmias (e.g., tachycardia, bradycardia), and postoperative nausea and vomiting.

DRUG INTERACTIONS

● Neuromuscular Blocking Agents

Etomidate does not appear to alter usual dosage requirements of neuromuscular blocking agents used for endotracheal intubation or any other purpose.

● Opiate Agonists

Because of a potential additive pharmacologic effect when etomidate is used with an opiate agonist (e.g., fentanyl), dosage adjustments (i.e., decrease in etomidate dosage) may be necessary.

DESCRIPTION

Etomidate, a carboxylated imidazole, is a sedative and hypnotic agent used for general anesthesia. The drug is structurally unrelated to other currently available IV anesthetics.

Following IV injection, etomidate has a rapid onset of action and will produce loss of consciousness within 1 arm-brain circulation time (i.e., usually within about 60 seconds). Etomidate produces its anesthetic activity by enhancing the activity of γ-aminobutyric acid (GABA), the principal inhibitory neurotransmitter in the CNS, through modulation and direct activation of the GABA$_A$ receptor complex.

Etomidate is capable of producing all levels of CNS depression—from light sleep to deep coma—depending on the dosage; however, the drug has no analgesic activity. The degree of depression and duration of action depend on dosage, rate and route of administration, and pharmacokinetics of the drug. Substantial changes on the EEG appear to occur following induction doses of etomidate. The EEG changes are indicative of the various stages of anesthesia and appear to be similar to those occurring following induction of anesthesia with barbiturates. Etomidate may decrease cerebral blood flow and intracranial

pressure, while cerebral perfusion pressure is increased or maintained during induction of anesthesia.

Etomidate causes minimal hemodynamic changes and is associated with a decreased incidence and severity of cardiovascular effects compared with other IV anesthetic agents. Minor increases in cardiac index and slight decreases in heart rate, systemic vascular resistance, and arterial blood pressure have been reported with use of etomidate. In addition, equivalent induction doses of etomidate cause less respiratory depression than propofol or barbiturates. Increases in carbon dioxide tension (PCO_2) have been reported with administration of etomidate.

Some data suggest that etomidate usually reduces intraocular pressure (IOP).

The pharmacokinetic profile of etomidate is characterized by a rapid distribution from blood into CNS, rapid clearance from the brain, and substantial tissue uptake. Following the usual induction dose (0.3 mg/kg) of etomidate, duration of hypnosis is short (about 3–10 minutes) and dose dependent. The elimination half-life of etomidate is about 1.25–5 hours. The drug is rapidly metabolized in the liver, principally by hydrolysis, to form etomidate carboxylic acid, which appears to be pharmacologically inactive. About 75% of an administered dose is excreted in urine within 24 hours, mainly (about 80%) as the carboxylic acid metabolite, while 13 and 10% of a dose are excreted in feces and bile, respectively.

ADVICE TO PATIENTS

When procedures requiring general anesthetics or sedation drugs, including etomidate, are considered for young children or pregnant women, importance of discussing with the patient, parent, or caregiver the benefits, risks (including potential risk of adverse neurodevelopmental effects), and appropriate timing and duration of the procedure.

Importance of informing clinicians of existing or contemplated concomitant therapy, including prescription and OTC drugs.

Importance of women informing clinicians if they are or plan to become pregnant or are breast-feeding.

Importance of informing patients of other important precautionary information. (See Cautions.)

PREPARATIONS

Excipients in commercially available drug preparations may have clinically important effects in some individuals; consult specific product labeling for details.

Etomidate

Parenteral

| Injection, for IV use | 2 mg/mL (20 and 40 mg)* | Amidate®, Hospira |
| | | Etomidate Injection |

* available from one or more manufacturer, distributor, and/or repackager by generic (nonproprietary) name

† Use is not currently included in the labeling approved by the US Food and Drug Administration.

Selected Revisions June 10, 2024, © Copyright, January 1, 2004, American Society of Health-System Pharmacists, Inc.

Ketamine Hydrochloride

28:04.08 • NON-BARBITURATES

Notice: On October 10, 2023, FDA issued a warning to patients and health care providers about potential risks associated with compounded ketamine products, including oral formulations, for the treatment of psychiatric disorders. Ketamine is *not* FDA approved for the treatment of any psychiatric disorder. In addition, compounded drugs, including compounded ketamine products, are *not* FDA approved and have not been evaluated for safety, effectiveness, or quality prior to marketing. Home use of compounded ketamine products presents additional risk because onsite monitoring by a health care provider is *not* available. FDA has identified potential safety concerns associated with the use of compounded ketamine products from compounders and telemedicine platforms, including abuse and misuse, psychiatric events, increases in blood pressure, respiratory depression, and lower urinary tract and bladder symptoms. For additional information see https://www.fda .gov/drugs/human-drug-compounding/fda-warns-patients-and-health-care -providers-about-potential-risks-associated-compounded-ketamine.

■ Ketamine hydrochloride, an *N*-methyl-D-aspartate (NMDA) receptor antagonist, is a nonbarbiturate general anesthetic that also has analgesic and antidepressant properties.

USES

Ketamine hydrochloride was initially developed as an anesthetic agent; however, the drug can also produce profound analgesia and other pharmacologic effects, and is therefore used for a variety of other indications such as procedural sedation, pain management†, sedation and analgesia in the intensive care setting†, and some psychiatric indications, including treatment-resistant depression and suicidality†.

● Induction and Maintenance of Anesthesia

Ketamine is used IV or IM for induction of anesthesia prior to administration of other general anesthetic agents. Ketamine also may be used as the sole anesthetic agent for diagnostic and surgical procedures that do not require skeletal muscle relaxation or as a supplement to other general anesthetic agents. While the manufacturer states that safety and effectiveness of ketamine in patients younger than 16 years of age have not been established, the drug has been used widely in pediatric patients†.

Induction of anesthesia with ketamine is rapid and results in a trance-like cataleptic state characterized by profound analgesia and amnesia, with retention of protective airway reflexes, spontaneous respirations, and cardiopulmonary stability. The anesthetic state produced by ketamine is distinct from that of other general anesthetic drugs (e.g., barbiturates, propofol, benzodiazepines, inhalation anesthetics). Dissociated patients are nonresponsive and unable to respond to external stimuli (including pain). Unlike other anesthetic or sedative drugs, increasing the dose of ketamine beyond the dissociative threshold does not enhance or deepen sedation.

Efficacy of ketamine as an anesthetic agent has been evaluated in over 12,000 operative and diagnostic procedures involving over 10,000 patients from 105 studies. Procedures for which ketamine has been used include debridement, dressing changes, and skin grafting in burn patients; neurodiagnostic procedures (e.g., myelograms, lumbar punctures); diagnostic and operative procedures of the eye, ear, nose, and mouth, including dental extractions; sigmoidoscopy and minor surgery of the anus and rectum; circumcision; short gynecologic procedures (e.g., dilatation and curettage); orthopedic procedures (e.g., closed reductions, manipulations, femoral pinning, amputations, biopsies); and cardiac catheterization.

Due to the risk of emergence reactions and the availability of other anesthetic agents, current use of ketamine is generally limited to certain patient populations (e.g., those with hemodynamic instability) or settings (e.g., prehospital environments that lack appropriate monitoring and respiratory support) where the drug's unique pharmacologic properties may be advantageous. Because ketamine produces sympathomimetic effects, the drug may be particularly useful for induction of anesthesia in hemodynamically unstable patients (e.g., those with traumatic injury or septic shock). Because of its bronchodilating effects, ketamine is generally considered the induction agent of choice in patients with reactive airway disease (e.g., asthma) or active bronchospasm.

Ketamine is commonly used as an induction agent for rapid sequence intubation, particularly in patients with reactive airway disease or hemodynamic compromise; studies have shown that ketamine may produce similar outcomes to etomidate and may be used as an alternative.

● Procedural Sedation

Ketamine is used as a procedural sedation agent to facilitate short painful or emotionally disturbing procedures (e.g., fracture reduction, laceration repair, abscess drainage, emergency cardioversion, chest tube insertion, central line placement) in the emergency department and other clinical settings (e.g., radiology suite, dental office, cardiac catheterization laboratories).

Procedural sedation is a technique in which sedative or dissociative agents are administered with or without analgesics to allow patients to tolerate painful or unpleasant medical procedures; a depressed state of consciousness is intentionally induced while cardiorespiratory function is maintained. In contrast to other procedural sedation agents, ketamine produces dissociative sedation and does not follow the usual sedation continuum where the more drug that is given, the deeper the patient will progress in their level of sedation; once the dissociative threshold has been reached, additional administration of ketamine will not enhance or deepen sedation. Administration of a single IV or IM dose of ketamine can effectively produce a dissociative state for approximately 5–10 or 20–30 minutes, respectively, while maintaining cardiovascular stability, spontaneous respiration, and protective airway reflexes.

Ketamine is widely used for procedural sedation in pediatric patients† and is particularly useful for facilitating painful procedures as well as procedures requiring immobilization of uncooperative patients. A benefit of the drug is that it can be administered via the IM route in patients in whom IV administration may be difficult (e.g., severely agitated or combative patients, young children, patients with extensive burns). Although ketamine is used less frequently in adults due to an increased risk of emergence delirium, the current evidence also suggests that the drug can be used safely and effectively in the adult population. Ketamine has a well-established role in the care of burn patients undergoing painful procedures (e.g., dressing changes, debridement, grafts).

Ketamine is commonly administered in combination with propofol to provide deep sedation for painful procedures; the combination regimen is given to potentiate the advantages of each drug while decreasing the risks (e.g., propofol-associated hypotension and respiratory depression; ketamine-associated vomiting and recovery agitation).

Studies comparing the use of ketamine with other sedative/analgesic agents (e.g., propofol, benzodiazepines, etomidate, opiate analgesics) have reported various findings, and outcomes have differed based on whether the drug was used alone or in combination with other agents.

● Pain

Ketamine exhibits potent analgesic properties in low (i.e., subanesthetic or subdissociative) doses and has been used for a variety of acute and chronic pain conditions†. Such conditions include acute pain† in the emergency department and prehospital settings, postoperative pain†, and chronic pain† of various etiologies. In addition to its analgesic effects, ketamine also can prevent the development of central sensitization, hyperalgesia, and opiate tolerance, which may be particularly useful in patients who are opiate tolerant or opiate dependent.

Postoperative Pain

Ketamine in low (i.e., subanesthetic or subdissociative) doses has been used for the management of postoperative pain† following a variety of surgical procedures in both adults and pediatric patients. The drug should be used as part of a multimodal regimen consisting of a combination of pharmacologic and nonpharmacologic methods targeting different pain mechanisms in the peripheral and central nervous systems.

Efficacy of low-dose ketamine in the postoperative setting is well established and supported by numerous studies demonstrating reduced opiate requirements and, in some cases, additional reductions in postoperative pain when the drug was used as a component of multimodal analgesia; although some studies reported discrepant results, the inconsistency may be due to differences in patient populations, dosage regimens, and concomitant analgesics used. Because ketamine appears to be most beneficial for procedures associated with severe pain, some experts state that subanesthetic ketamine infusions should be reserved for patients undergoing surgeries in which the postoperative pain is expected to be severe; such procedures include thoracic, abdominal (upper, lower, and intra-abdominal), and orthopedic (limb and spinal) surgeries. These experts state that patients undergoing procedures associated with only mild postoperative pain (e.g., tonsillectomy, head and neck surgery) have not been shown to benefit from perioperative ketamine. For these procedures, standard analgesia with low dosages of opiates, nonsteroidal anti-inflammatory agents (NSAIAs), and local anesthetics usually can provide adequate pain relief. However, management of post-tonsillectomy pain in children can be difficult and several studies have demonstrated that administration of a single IV dose of ketamine 0.5 mg/kg (alone or in combination with other analgesics) can provide effective postoperative pain control.

Ketamine may be particularly useful in the management of opiate-tolerant or opiate-dependent patients undergoing surgery. In a randomized controlled study in opiate-dependent patients undergoing spinal surgery, intraoperative use of ketamine was associated with reduced opiate consumption at 48 hours and reduced opiate usage at 6 weeks. Ketamine also may be considered as an adjunct to reduce postoperative opiate consumption in patients who have an increased risk of opiate-related respiratory depression (e.g., those with obstructive sleep apnea).

Acute Pain

Ketamine (in subanesthetic doses) has been used alone or as an adjunct to other analgesics (e.g., opiates) for relief of acute pain† in the emergency department and prehospital settings (e.g., ambulance). Studies evaluating subanesthetic ketamine for analgesia in these settings have been conducted principally in the adult population. However, low or subanesthetic doses of ketamine also have been used for analgesia in pediatric patients 3 months of age or older presenting to the emergency department. When used as an adjunct to opiate analgesics in the emergency department or prehospital setting, ketamine has resulted in greater reduction in pain scores compared with opiate therapy alone, and/or decreased opiate requirements. When given as a single agent for acute pain in the emergency department, IV ketamine has been reported to provide comparable reductions in pain scores to IV morphine.

Although evidence is limited, ketamine may be useful in opiate-dependent patients with acute exacerbations of chronic pain conditions (e.g., sickle cell disease)†.

Chronic Pain

Ketamine has been used as an adjunct analgesic for the management of chronic pain of various etiologies, including complex regional pain syndrome (CRPS)†, neuropathic pain associated with spinal cord injury†, phantom limb pain†, fibromyalgia†, ischemic pain†, cancer pain†, and migraine pain†, in adults and pediatric patients. Evidence of efficacy varies depending on the specific pain condition treated and generally is limited to small randomized controlled studies, observational studies, and case reports demonstrating short-term benefits of ketamine infusions during and for a short time following the infusion; however, ketamine dosages and administration protocols varied widely in these studies.

Ketamine has been evaluated most extensively in chronic pain conditions associated with a neuropathic component. With regard to specific conditions, some experts state that there is weak to moderate evidence that ketamine infusions are effective for reducing pain related to CRPS in adults and pediatric patients; the evidence to date includes mostly systematic reviews, case reports, and observational studies with only a few small randomized controlled studies. In one study in 19 patients with CRPS, reductions in pain were reported for up to 12 weeks with continuous IV infusion of ketamine (maximum rate of 0.35 mg/kg per hour over 4 hours daily for 10 days). There also is weak evidence supporting ketamine infusions for short-term improvements in neuropathic pain associated with spinal cord injury. Other chronic pain syndromes that have been investigated generally have not responded to or only minimally responded to ketamine therapy; experts state that the available evidence remains inconclusive

for the efficacy of ketamine infusions for mixed neuropathic pain, phantom limb pain, postherpetic neuralgia, fibromyalgia, ischemic pain, migraine, and low-back pain.

Although data are limited regarding the use of ketamine as an adjuvant treatment of cancer pain, some experts state that oral or IV ketamine may be considered for the management of refractory cancer pain in adults. Evidence to date remains inconclusive for the efficacy of ketamine in chronic cancer pain and is mostly based on case reports and uncontrolled studies. While a few randomized controlled studies indicate that the drug may have some benefit as an adjunct analgesic in cancer-related pain, these studies generally were small and had short durations of follow-up relative to the chronic nature of the pain being treated. In a larger controlled clinical trial in 214 adults with cancer-related neuropathic pain inadequately treated with adjuvant analgesics, the addition of oral ketamine (up to 400 mg daily for 16 days) was no more effective than placebo in improving pain scores. In another controlled clinical trial in 185 adults in palliative care settings who had refractory cancer-related pain, adjunctive therapy with ketamine (administered as a subcutaneous infusion in escalating doses up to 500 mg every 24 hours over 5 days) also was no more effective than placebo in improving pain scores. Studies of IV and oral ketamine have been conducted in children with cancer pain; although these studies were mostly retrospective, there is some evidence suggesting that pain control can be achieved with ketamine in these patients.

Additional study is needed to establish the role of ketamine in patients with chronic pain and to determine optimum dosages, durability of response, and long-term benefits and risks of the drug. Some clinicians recommend that use of ketamine be restricted to patients with refractory pain who have failed to obtain adequate relief from standard analgesics and nonpharmacologic treatments.

● Treatment-resistant Depression and Suicidality

Ketamine has been used in low (i.e., subanesthetic) doses for the treatment of severe and treatment-resistant depression associated with major depressive disorder or bipolar disorder†. Although there are various definitions for treatment-resistant depression, the condition often has been defined as the failure of at least 2 trials of first-line antidepressants given in an adequate dosage for an adequate duration of therapy. In patients with refractory forms of depression, ketamine usually has been given in subanesthetic doses as an IV infusion.

Ketamine has demonstrated rapid and potent antidepressant effects when administered to depressed patients in controlled studies and case series, with improvement in depression reported within several hours to a day following a single IV infusion of the drug. In controlled studies, single, low-dose IV infusions of the drug have resulted in response rates of approximately 37–71% in patients with treatment-resistant depression.

Most depressed patients who respond to a single IV infusion of ketamine experience a relapse of depression within several days to a week or two following the initial infusion. Therefore, multiple-infusion regimens of ketamine (i.e., weekly, biweekly, 3 times weekly) have been studied in depressed patients in open-label as well as blinded studies with encouraging results suggesting that repeated infusions are more effective than a single infusion and can extend the duration of depressive symptom remission. However, the long-term efficacy and safety of repeated infusions of ketamine have not been fully determined to date and further studies are needed to evaluate relapse prevention therapy with the drug. There is some concern that multiple-infusion regimens of ketamine may cause long-term cognitive impairment or neurotoxicity, although no evidence of such impairment has been seen in preliminary studies. Some clinicians have suggested that the optimal use of ketamine infusions may be short-term to produce rapid antidepressant and antisuicidal effects until a less invasive relapse prevention strategy for a patient can be implemented.

In addition to its antidepressant effects, randomized controlled studies suggest that ketamine may be helpful in the short-term treatment of suicidal ideation†. In a systematic review and individual participant data meta-analysis, suicidal ideation rapidly decreased (within 1 day) following a single IV infusion of ketamine and the effect lasted for up to 1 week even among patients whose depression did not fully respond to ketamine therapy, suggesting that the drug may have a partially independent antisuicidal effect.

Despite the increasingly widespread use of IV ketamine to treat patients with treatment-resistant depression and suicidality, including in outpatient ketamine infusion centers and psychiatric clinics, some clinicians currently recommend that the drug's use for these psychiatric indications be limited to controlled settings under the care of skilled clinicians. Clinicians and patients should consider enrollment in clinical studies evaluating ketamine's efficacy and safety so that further data can be collected and analyzed to improve clinical practice.

When considering the use of ketamine for treating mood disorders, the American Psychiatric Association's (APA's) Council of Research Task Force on Novel Biomarkers and Treatments recommends balancing the potential benefits of ketamine infusion therapy with the potential risks of long-term exposure to the drug, including neurotoxicity, cystitis, and abuse potential. A thorough pretreatment evaluation process to determine the appropriateness of ketamine therapy is recommended in such cases. If ketamine is prescribed outside of a controlled setting, careful screening, monitoring during treatment, and follow-up of patients are necessary.

Since conventional oral antidepressants generally require several weeks or months to be effective, the addition of ketamine to oral antidepressant therapy has been suggested as one possible method to produce a more rapid antidepressant response in patients with depression. In a randomized, double-blind, placebo-controlled study, the efficacy and safety of single-infusion ketamine augmentation of oral escitalopram therapy (10 mg daily) were evaluated in 30 outpatients with severe major depressive disorder. Ketamine was given as a single IV infusion (0.5 mg/kg over 40 minutes) on day 1 of escitalopram therapy. At 4 weeks, response occurred in significantly more escitalopram plus ketamine-treated patients than in the escitalopram plus placebo-treated patients (approximately 92 and 57% of patients, respectively). In addition, the escitalopram plus ketamine-treated patients had a shorter mean time to response than the escitalopram plus placebo-treated patients (6 days compared with 27 days).

Some clinicians state that electroconvulsive therapy (ECT) should still be considered as a first-line therapy for patients with refractory depression, and have expressed concern that a trial of single- or multiple-dose ketamine therapy might delay patients from being referred for an ECT consultation. Preliminary experience with the adjunctive use of ketamine in the course of ECT for depression does not suggest improved efficacy or tolerability.

Preliminary evidence suggests that intranasal† ketamine given in 50-mg doses is effective in rapidly improving depressive symptoms in patients with major depressive disorder and generally is well tolerated; however, further study is needed to more clearly determine the efficacy, tolerability, and optimal dosing of this alternative route of administration. The APA's Council of Research Task Force on Novel Biomarkers and Treatments currently advises against the prescription of self-administration of ketamine at home and recommends medical supervision whenever the drug is used pending further accumulation of safety data from controlled settings.

For information on the intranasal use of esketamine hydrochloride, the *S*-enantiomer of racemic ketamine, for treatment-resistant depression, see Esketamine Hydrochloride 28:16.04.92.

● Sedation and Analgesia in Critical Care Settings

Ketamine has been used by continuous IV infusion to provide sedation in critically ill patients† in the intensive care unit (ICU) setting. Sedative agents are administered in ICU patients to reduce pain, agitation, and anxiety, and increase tolerance to invasive procedures (e.g., mechanical ventilation). The provision of adequate analgesia and other measures to ensure patient comfort is recommended before sedatives are administered. Common drugs used for ICU sedation include benzodiazepines (e.g., midazolam, lorazepam), propofol, and dexmedetomidine. Although ketamine also has been used for this indication, there is limited, but increasing, experience describing such use; available data evaluating ketamine in the ICU from randomized controlled trials and observational studies are heterogenous in terms of therapeutic indications, dosages used, concomitant drugs, and target levels of sedation.

Ketamine also has been used for pain management in critically ill patients†. Although opiate analgesics generally are considered the first-line drugs for management of non-neuropathic pain in this setting, some experts suggest the use of low-dose ketamine (e.g., 0.5 mg/kg by IV injection followed by 0.06–0.12 mg/kg per hour as an IV infusion) as an adjunct to opiates when attempting to reduce opiate requirements in postsurgical ICU patients. This recommendation

is based principally on indirect evidence from non-ICU patients and limited data from a randomized controlled study in postsurgical patients in the ICU.

DOSAGE AND ADMINISTRATION

● General

Pretreatment Screening

● Obtain baseline liver function tests, including alkaline phosphatase and gamma glutamyl transferase, in patients receiving ketamine as part of a treatment plan that utilizes recurrent dosing.

Patient Monitoring

● Continuously monitor vital signs and cardiac function during administration of ketamine. Maintain adequate oxygenation and ventilation.

Dispensing and Administration Precautions

● When used for general anesthesia, administer by or under supervision of clinicians experienced in the use and complications of general anesthetics. When used in anesthetic doses, administer in a monitored setting in the presence of personnel trained in advanced airway management and cardiovascular life support; resuscitative equipment should be readily available.

● When used in subanesthetic doses in the emergency department, adverse effects generally are mild and self-limiting; therefore, some experts state that ketamine administration may follow the same procedures and policies used for other analgesics in this setting. Consult local protocols since expectations may differ.

● When used for procedural sedation in the emergency department, administer by appropriately trained individuals who can safely administer and manage complications of the drug. Experts recommend the presence of 2 individuals during procedure (one to perform procedure and one to monitor patient). Patients should be continuously observed by a dedicated healthcare professional until recovery is well established.

● When used by IV infusion for mood disorders (e.g., treatment-resistant depression, suicidality)†, administer by experienced clinicians in a facility where adequate monitoring for and management of possible adverse reactions (e.g., altered cardiovascular and respiratory function, acute dissociative and psychotomimetic effects) are possible.

Other General Considerations

● May administer benzodiazepines (e.g., diazepam, midazolam) concomitantly to reduce risk of psychotomimetic effects during emergence in adults receiving ketamine anesthesia. Routine benzodiazepine prophylaxis is not recommended in pediatric patients because of uncertain benefit.

● Administer anticholinergic agents (e.g., atropine, glycopyrrolate) prior to or concomitantly with ketamine to reduce hypersalivation and risk of laryngospasm. Because of uncertain benefit, some experts state that such prophylaxis should be reserved for patients with clinically important hypersalivation or impaired ability to mobilize secretions.

● Consider the risk of aspiration and vomiting; the manufacturer states that ketamine is not recommended in patients who have not followed "nothing by mouth (NPO)" guidelines. Although protective laryngeal and pharyngeal reflexes generally are preserved with ketamine, coadministered anesthetics and muscle relaxants may impair such reflexes.

● Because nausea and vomiting may occur following ketamine administration, prophylactic use of antiemetics (e.g., ondansetron) may be beneficial, particularly in patients at higher risk (e.g., early adolescents receiving ketamine for procedural sedation).

● Administration

Ketamine hydrochloride usually is administered by slow (e.g., over 60 seconds) IV injection, IV infusion, or IM injection. Ketamine also has been used in IV patient-controlled analgesia (PCA), either as the sole analgesic or in combination with opioids to improve pain control and reduce opioid-related adverse effects. Ketamine also has been administered by oral†, intranasal†, rectal†, subcutaneous†, and intraosseous (IO)† routes. Because of extensive first-pass metabolism, the bioavailability of ketamine following oral or rectal administration is limited (approximately 20–30%). Although ketamine has been administered epidurally† or intrathecally†, there have been concerns about potential neurotoxicity with these routes, and some experts state it may be prudent to avoid neuraxial administration of the drug.

Some experts state that IV administration of ketamine is preferred to IM administration when access can be obtained readily. IM administration is associated with a higher rate of vomiting and longer recovery times compared with IV administration. In addition, IV access can permit convenient administration of additional doses for longer procedures and allow for rapid treatment of adverse effects (e.g., IV benzodiazepines for emergence reactions). In certain patients (e.g., severely agitated or uncooperative patients, young children), IM administration may be preferred.

Store ketamine hydrochloride injection at controlled room temperature between 20–25°C (excursions permitted between 15–30°C) and protect from light.

Ketamine has been reported to be compatible with several drugs when administered as additives, simultaneously in the same syringe, or when a Y-type administration set is used; specialized references should be consulted for more specific information.

Dilution

Ketamine hydrochloride is commercially available as an injection containing 10, 50, or 100 mg/mL of ketamine for IV or IM use. The 100-mg/mL concentration should *not* be administered IV without proper dilution; the commercially available injection concentrate must be diluted with an equal volume of sterile water for injection, 0.9% sodium chloride injection, or 5% dextrose injection prior to IV injection.

For IV infusion, a diluted solution containing 1 mg of ketamine per mL (1 mg/mL) may be prepared by adding 500 mg of ketamine (10 mL from a vial labeled as containing 50 mg/mL of ketamine or 5 mL from a vial labeled as containing 100 mg/mL of ketamine) to an infusion bag containing 500 mL of 0.9% sodium chloride injection or 5% dextrose injection. In patients requiring fluid restriction, a 2-mg/mL solution may be prepared by adding 500 mg of ketamine (10 mL from a vial labeled as containing 50 mg/mL of ketamine or 5 mL from a vial labeled as containing 100 mg/mL of ketamine) to an infusion bag containing 250 mL of 0.9% sodium chloride injection or 5% dextrose injection. The manufacturer states that the 10-mg/mL vial of ketamine hydrochloride is not recommended for dilution; however, some stability studies have used ketamine hydrochloride solutions prepared by diluting a 10-mg/mL solution of the drug with 0.9% sodium chloride injection.

Use immediately after dilution.

Rate of Administration

For induction of anesthesia, administer ketamine slowly (e.g., over 60 seconds); rapid IV administration can cause respiratory depression and enhanced vasopressor response. Induction dose may be administered by IV infusion at rate of 0.5 mg/kg per minute.

For maintenance of anesthesia, repeat one-half to full induction dosages as needed; may be given by slow microdrip infusion technique at a dosage of 0.1–0.5 mg/minute.

For dissociative sedation in emergency department settings, IV administration over 30–60 seconds has been recommended.

When ketamine is used in subanesthetic doses for acute pain†, some clinicians have recommended that the drug be administered as a short IV infusion over 15 minutes.

When ketamine is administered in subanesthetic doses for the treatment of severe and treatment-resistant depression and/or suicidality†, the drug is usually given as an IV infusion over 40 minutes. Although shorter and longer infusion rates have been used in some patients, clinical experience is too limited to recommend an alternative infusion rate at this time.

Standardize 4 Safety

Standardized concentrations for ketamine have been established through Standardize 4 Safety (S4S), a national patient safety initiative to reduce medication errors, *especially during transitions of care. Multidisciplinary expert panels were convened to determine recommended standard concentrations. Because recommendations from the S4S panels may differ from the manufacturer's prescribing information, caution is advised when using concentrations that differ from labeling, particularly when using rate information from the label. For additional information on S4S (including updates that may be available), see* https://www.ashp.org/pharmacy-practice/standardize-4-safety-initiative.

TABLE 1. Standardize 4 Safety Continuous Infusion Standards for Ketamine[a]

Patient Population	Concentration standard	Dosing units
Pediatric patients (<50 kg)	2 mg/mL	mg/kg/hr
	10 mg/mL	

[a] Ketamine is not included in the adult continuous infusion standards

TABLE 2. Standardize 4 Safety PCA Standard Concentrations for Ketamine

Patient Population	Concentration standard	Dosing units
Pediatric patients (<50 kg)	2 mg/mL	mg/kg/hr
	10 mg/mL	
Adults	5 mg/mL	mg/kg/hr
	10 mg/mL	

● Dosage

Dosage of ketamine hydrochloride is expressed in terms of ketamine.

Dose-dependency of Effects

Dosage of ketamine depends on the intended use and desired pharmacologic effect. At low doses, ketamine produces analgesia and sedation, and at higher doses, the drug produces a state of dissociative anesthesia. Ketamine has a dosing threshold at which dissociation occurs; doses at or above the threshold are referred to as "dissociative" or "anesthetic," and doses below this threshold are referred to as "subdissociative" or "subanesthetic." Although specific dosing ranges have not been established, dissociation generally appears at an IV dose of approximately 1–1.5 mg/kg or an IM dose of approximately 3–5 mg/kg. Once the dissociative threshold has been reached, additional administration of ketamine will not enhance or deepen sedation.

Induction and Maintenance of Anesthesia

As with other general anesthetics, individual response to ketamine is variable and can depend on factors such as dosage, route of administration, patient age, or concomitant drugs. Dosage should be individualized based on therapeutic response and the patient's anesthetic needs. In general, higher doses of ketamine correspond with longer times to complete recovery from anesthesia.

Adult Dosage

For induction of anesthesia in adults, the manufacturer recommends an initial IV ketamine dose of 1–4.5 mg/kg or an initial IM dose of 6.5–13 mg/kg. Administer IV ketamine doses by slow IV injection over 60 seconds or as an IV infusion at a rate of 0.5 mg/kg per minute. On average, an IV dose of 2 mg/kg will produce surgical anesthesia for 5–10 minutes within 30 seconds of administration, and an IM dose of 9–13 mg/kg will produce surgical anesthesia for 12–25 minutes within 3–4 minutes following administration.

For maintenance of anesthesia in adults, additional IV doses of 0.5–4.5 mg/kg or IM doses of 3.25–13 mg/kg may be administered as needed. The manufacturer additionally states that a slow microdrip IV infusion, using a dosage of 0.1–0.5 mg/minute will maintain general anesthesia after induction with ketamine. A continuous IV infusion of 1–6 mg/kg per hour also has been recommended for maintenance of anesthesia. The maintenance dosage should be adjusted based on the patient's anesthetic requirements and concomitant use of other anesthetic agents.

The manufacturer states that the incidence of psychologic manifestations during emergence, particularly dream-like observations and emergence delirium, may be reduced by using lower recommended dosages of ketamine in conjunction with an IV benzodiazepine during induction and maintenance of anesthesia.

Pediatric Dosage

In general, pediatric patients require higher doses of ketamine compared with adults, although there is considerable interpatient variability in dosing requirements.

Some experts recommend an initial IV ketamine dose of 1-3 mg/kg for induction of anesthesia in pediatric patients†; supplemental IV doses of 0.5-1 mg/kg may be given if clinically indicated. The recommended IM dose of ketamine for induction of anesthesia in pediatric patients is 5-10 mg/kg. Because of possible airway complications, some experts state that ketamine is contraindicated in infants younger than 3 months of age.

Procedural Sedation

Adult Dosage

For dissociative sedation in adults undergoing short painful or emotionally disturbing procedures in the emergency department, the usual IV dose of ketamine is 1 mg/kg administered by IV injection over 30-60 seconds. Dissociative sedation is usually achieved with a single IV loading dose; however, if sedation is inadequate or a prolonged period of sedation is needed for longer procedures, additional IV doses of 0.5-1 mg/kg may be administered every 5-15 minutes as needed. Lower IV doses of ketamine (e.g., 0.2-0.75 mg/kg) also have been used to produce analgesia, particularly if a dissociative effect is not required for the procedure.

Although the IM route is not preferred in adults, some experts state that an IM dose of 4-5 mg/kg may be administered; additional doses of 2-5 mg/kg may be given after 5-10 minutes if initial sedation is inadequate or additional doses are needed for longer procedures. Lower IM doses of ketamine (e.g., 0.4-2 mg/kg) also have been used, particularly if a dissociative effect is not required for the procedure.

Pediatric Dosage

For dissociative sedation in pediatric patients† 3 months of age or older undergoing short painful or emotionally disturbing procedures in the emergency department, some experts state that the usual IV dose of ketamine is 1.5-2 mg/kg administered by IV injection over 30-60 seconds. Dissociative sedation is usually achieved with a single IV loading dose; however, if initial sedation is inadequate or prolonged sedation is necessary for longer procedures, additional incremental IV doses of 0.5-1 mg/kg may be administered every 5-15 minutes as needed. These experts state that the minimum IV dose that will reliably elicit the dissociative state in children is 1.5 mg/kg; however, lower IV doses (e.g., 0.25-1 mg/kg) also have been used successfully to provide adequate procedural sedation in pediatric patients, particularly if a dissociative effect is not required for the procedure.

The recommended IM dose of ketamine for dissociative sedation in pediatric patients† 3 months of age or older undergoing short painful or emotionally disturbing procedures in the emergency department is 4-5 mg/kg. Although dissociative sedation is usually achieved with a single IM dose, additional doses of 2-5 mg/kg may be administered after 5-10 minutes if initial sedation is inadequate or additional doses are needed for longer procedures. Although some experts state that the minimum IM dose that will reliably elicit the dissociative state in children is 4-5 mg/kg, lower IM doses (e.g., 1-2 mg/kg) also have been used successfully, particularly if a dissociative effect is not required for the procedure.

Sedation and Analgesia in Critical Care Settings

There is increasing experience with the use of ketamine for ICU sedation, but dosages described in the literature are highly variable. Available data evaluating ketamine in the ICU from randomized controlled trials and observational studies are heterogenous in terms of therapeutic indications, dosages used, concomitant drugs, and target levels of sedation. Although adult and pediatric dosages of continuous IV ketamine have varied in these published studies, they generally fall within the broad range associated with analgosedative effects; the desired target level of sedation and concomitant use of other sedative/analgesic agents

are some factors that may influence dose variability. Continuous infusion dosages have ranged between 0.02-3 mg/kg per hour; lower dosages have been more commonly used when ketamine is used as part of patient-controlled analgesia. Use of initial bolus IV injections (range 0.3-0.5 mg/kg) and continuous infusion titration based on sedation or pain scores have also been reported.

For pain management in postsurgical patients in the ICU, some experts have suggested the use of low-dose ketamine (e.g., 0.5 mg/kg by IV injection followed by IV infusion of 0.06-0.12 mg/kg per hour as an adjunct to opioid therapy); other dosage regimens also have been used.

Pain

Ketamine is used in low (i.e., subanesthetic or subdissociative) dosages for the management of pain; however, a dosage range that is considered subanesthetic has not been consistently defined. Most acute pain studies used IV bolus doses less than 0.5 mg/kg and infusion rates of 0.5 mg/kg per hour or less; however, there is wide variability in the dosage ranges and routes of administration used.

Postoperative Pain

For the management of postoperative pain† in pediatric patients and adults, IV ketamine bolus doses ranging from 0.1-0.5 mg/kg with or without continuous IV infusion (at rates usually ranging from 0.1-0.6 mg/kg per hour) have been commonly used in clinical studies; however, dosages and timing of administration in relation to the surgical procedure varied widely in these studies and the optimum dosage regimen is not known. Some experts state that there is moderate evidence supporting the use of IV ketamine bolus doses up to 0.35 mg/kg and IV infusions up to 1 mg/kg per hour as an adjunct to opiates for perioperative analgesia. In several studies, administration of a single IV ketamine dose of 0.5 mg/kg (alone or in combination with other analgesics) was effective in achieving postoperative pain control in children undergoing tonsillectomy. Because of possible airway complications, some experts state that ketamine is contraindicated in infants younger than 3 months of age.

IM administration of analgesic agents for postoperative pain is not recommended because of unreliable absorption and substantial pain at the site of injection.

Acute Pain

For the management of acute pain† in the emergency department and prehospital settings, the usual IV dose of ketamine is 0.1-0.3 mg/kg administered as a slow IV injection or short IV infusion over 10-15 minutes based on studies conducted principally in adults; although longer infusions of ketamine are rare in this setting, continuous IV infusions of 0.1-0.3 mg/kg per hour have been used. Non-weight-based IV ketamine doses ranging from 10-20 mg also have been used in clinical studies of ketamine for the treatment of acute pain in adults. When ketamine is used for acute pain in settings without intensive monitoring, some experts state that IV bolus doses should not exceed 0.35 mg/kg and infusion rates generally should not exceed 1 mg/kg per hour, but also acknowledge that higher or lower doses may be necessary due to interindividual differences in response.

Because of possible airway complications, some experts state that ketamine is contraindicated in infants younger than 3 months of age.

Ketamine may be administered IM for acute pain in the emergency department or prehospital settings; however, experts state that a dosage range has not been definitively established and analgesic effects are less predictable when the drug is administered by IM injection.

Chronic Pain

Although there is no consensus on dosages or administration protocols for ketamine in patients with chronic pain†, the drug generally is administered in subanesthetic doses by IV infusion. There is some evidence suggesting that administration of higher dosages over longer periods and more frequent infusions may provide more benefit. Some experts state that it is reasonable to initiate a single outpatient infusion of ketamine at a minimum dose of 80 mg for at least 2 hours and then reassess before initiating further treatments. In a study in children and adolescents 12-17 years of age with chronic pain conditions (e.g., chronic headache, fibromyalgia, complex regional pain syndrome), ketamine was administered by continuous IV infusion at a rate of 0.1-0.3 mg/kg per hour for 4-8 hours each day up to a maximum of 16 hours (in total, up to a maximum of 3 consecutive days). Children with severe cancer-related pain have been treated with IV infusions of ketamine at 0.1-1 mg/kg per hour. Based on limited evidence,

IV ketamine bolus doses up to 0.35 mg/kg followed by IV infusions of 0.5–2 mg/kg per hour have been recommended by some experts for the management of chronic pain; however, higher (e.g., up to 7 mg/kg per hour for the treatment of refractory pain) or lower (e.g., 0.1–0.5 mg/kg per hour) infusion rates also have been used.

Treatment-resistant Depression and Suicidality

For severe and treatment-resistant depression and suicidality† in adults, ketamine usually is given as a low-dose (i.e., subanesthetic dose) IV infusion of 0.5 mg/kg over 40 minutes. Obese patients (i.e., body mass index [BMI] of 30 or higher) appear to be at increased risk for ketamine-associated hypertension and other adverse hemodynamic effects and potentially may benefit from adjusting the ketamine dosage to their calculated ideal body weight rather than actual body weight; further clinical experience to determine optimal dosing in such patients is needed. There is limited evidence that higher ketamine infusion dosages (e.g., 0.75 mg/kg) may be necessary in certain chronically ill and/or severely treatment-resistant patients, but further study is needed to determine the efficacy and safety of such higher-dosage regimens.

There currently is limited clinical experience with longer-term (multiple-dose) ketamine infusion therapy for treatment-resistant depression and suicidality; however, IV infusions of ketamine have been given once, twice, or 3 times weekly for the first 2 weeks during the acute treatment phase in some patients and sometimes have been continued once or twice weekly for another 2–4 weeks during the continuation phase for a total of 4–6 weeks of therapy or gradually tapered. Patients who do not initially respond to several infusions of ketamine appear unlikely to respond to subsequent infusions. Discontinuance of ketamine therapy is recommended by some experts if the interval between infusions cannot be extended to one week or longer by the second month of treatment; these experts state that the goal should be to eventually taper and discontinue ketamine treatment until additional long-term safety data with the drug become available.

● Special Populations

Hepatic Impairment

The manufacturer makes no specific dosage recommendations for patients with hepatic impairment.

Renal Impairment

The manufacturer makes no specific dosage recommendations for patients with renal impairment.

Geriatric Patients

The manufacturer recommends that dosages in geriatric patients should generally be started on the lower end of the dosing range to accommodate any underlying hepatic, renal, or cardiac dysfunction and any comorbidities or other drug therapy.

CAUTIONS

● Contraindications

- Patients in whom substantial blood pressure elevation would constitute a serious hazard.

- Known hypersensitivity to ketamine or any ingredient in the formulation.

- Some experts state that relative contraindications may include history of airway instability, tracheal surgery, or tracheal stenosis; active pulmonary infection or disease; known or suspected cardiovascular disease (e.g., angina, congestive heart failure [CHF], hypertension); CNS masses, abnormalities, or hydrocephalus; elevated intraocular pressure (IOP) (e.g., glaucoma, acute globe injury); and porphyria, hyperthyroidism, or concomitant thyroid replacement therapy.

● Warnings/Precautions

Cardiovascular Effects

Ketamine inhibits the reuptake of catecholamines and has other direct and indirect sympathomimetic effects at subanesthetic and anesthetic doses. Typical cardiovascular effects include increases in heart rate, blood pressure, cardiac output, and myocardial oxygen consumption; hypotension, bradycardia, arrhythmias, and cardiac decompensation also have been observed. Ketamine also causes direct relaxation of vascular smooth muscle; however, systemic vascular resistance usually is unaffected. The sympathomimetic effects of ketamine often are used to therapeutic advantage (e.g., in patients with severe hypotension, sepsis, or other hemodynamically compromised states).

Transient increases in blood pressure, heart rate, and cardiac output can occur following administration of ketamine at anesthetic or subanesthetic doses. When ketamine is administered IV in anesthetic doses, increased blood pressure usually occurs shortly after the IV injection, reaches a maximum within a few minutes, and returns to preanesthetic levels within 15 minutes. Systolic and diastolic blood pressure usually peaks at 10–50% over baseline values, but increases can be higher or last longer in some individuals. In healthy individuals receiving subanesthetic doses of ketamine (0.5 mg/kg by IV infusion over 40 minutes), increases in blood pressure were observed 10 minutes after the start of infusion; mean maximum increases in systolic and diastolic blood pressure of 13.38 and 12.65 mm Hg, respectively, occurred approximately 28 minutes after initiation of the infusion and returned to baseline levels within 2 hours. The mean maximum increase in heart rate in these individuals was 10.69 beats per minute.

Elevated blood pressure and/or heart rate may occur during IV infusions of ketamine for treatment-resistant depression and suicidality; these hemodynamic effects usually are transient and subside following completion of the IV infusion. Transient but significantly elevated blood pressure occurred in nearly one-third of ketamine-treated patients in one study. Short-term antihypertensive therapy sometimes has been used to treat ketamine infusion-associated blood pressure elevations in this and other studies.

Monitor vital signs and cardiac function during ketamine administration. Ketamine should be used with caution or avoided in patients with known or suspected cardiac conditions that may be exacerbated by the sympathomimetic effects of the drug (e.g., unstable angina, coronary artery disease, myocardial infarction [MI], congestive heart failure, hypertension). The manufacturer states that ketamine is contraindicated in patients in whom a substantial elevation of blood pressure would constitute a serious hazard.

Emergence Reactions

Emergence reactions have been reported during the recovery period in patients receiving ketamine; the manufacturer reports an incidence of approximately 12% in patients receiving ketamine for anesthesia, although higher rates have been reported in the published literature. The duration of such reactions is generally a few hours. Emergence reactions occur more frequently in adults (approximately 30–50%) than in pediatric patients (approximately 5–15%).

Emergence manifestations vary in severity from pleasant to unpleasant dream-like states, vivid imagery, hallucinations, alterations in mood and body image, floating sensations, extracorporeal (out-of-body) experiences, and emergence delirium; in some cases, these states have been accompanied by confusion, excitement, and irrational behavior, which some patients recall as an unpleasant experience. The manufacturer states that no residual psychologic effects have been reported from ketamine use during induction and maintenance of anesthesia.

Emergence reactions may be less frequent when ketamine is given IM. The incidence of emergence reactions may be reduced if verbal, tactile, and visual stimulation of the patient is minimized during the recovery period; however, this should not preclude appropriate monitoring of vital signs. Prophylactic administration of benzodiazepines (e.g., diazepam, midazolam) may reduce the incidence of ketamine-induced psychological manifestations during emergence, and the manufacturer suggests a regimen using a decreased dosage of ketamine in conjunction with an IV benzodiazepine during induction and maintenance of anesthesia. Benzodiazepines also may be used to terminate severe or unpleasant emergence reactions.

Respiratory Effects

Adverse respiratory effects are rare with ketamine; however, respiratory depression may occur following rapid IV administration or overdosage of the drug. When given in anesthetic doses, clinically important respiratory depression usually does not occur. Respiration is frequently stimulated, but ketamine may occasionally cause a transient and minimal respiratory depression

When used in subanesthetic doses for the treatment of depression in otherwise healthy individuals, ketamine usually does not cause clinically important adverse respiratory effects.

Ketamine also produces bronchodilation, likely through vagolytic and other centrally mediated mechanisms.

Airway or respiratory complications have been reported in about 3.9% of pediatric patients receiving ketamine for dissociative sedation in the emergency department; transient apnea and respiratory depression have been reported in about 0.8% and transient laryngospasm has been reported in about 0.3% of pediatric patients in this setting.

Maintain adequate oxygenation and ventilation during administration of ketamine. IV injections of ketamine should be administered slowly (e.g., over 60 seconds).

Risks with Pharynx, Larynx, or Bronchial Tree Procedures

Ketamine does not suppress pharyngeal or laryngeal reflexes. Therefore, ketamine as a sole anesthetic should be avoided during procedures of the pharynx, larynx, or bronchial tree, including mechanical stimulation of the pharynx. Muscle relaxants may be required for successful completion of these procedures.

Pediatric Neurotoxicity

Prolonged use of general anesthetics and sedation drugs, including ketamine, in children younger than 3 years of age or during the third trimester of pregnancy may affect brain development. Animal studies in multiple species, including nonhuman primates, have demonstrated that use for longer than 3 hours of anesthetic and sedation drugs that block N-methyl-D-aspartic acid (NMDA) receptors and/or potentiate γ-aminobutyric acid (GABA) activity leads to widespread neuronal and oligodendrocyte cell loss and alterations in synaptic morphology and neurogenesis in the developing brain, resulting in long-term deficits in cognition and behavior. Across animal species, vulnerability to these neurodevelopmental changes occurs during the period of rapid brain growth or synaptogenesis; this period is thought to correlate with the third trimester of pregnancy through the first year of life in humans, but may extend to approximately 3 years of age. The clinical relevance of these animal findings to humans is not known.

While some published evidence suggests that similar deficits in cognition and behavior may occur in children following repeated or prolonged exposure to anesthesia early in life, other studies have found no association between pediatric anesthesia exposure and long-term adverse neurodevelopmental outcomes. Most studies to date have had substantial limitations, and it is not clear whether the adverse neurodevelopmental outcomes observed in children were related to the drug or to other factors (e.g., surgery, underlying illness). There is some clinical evidence that a single, relatively brief exposure to general anesthesia in generally healthy children is unlikely to cause clinically detectable deficits in global cognitive function or serious behavioral disorders; however, further research is needed to fully characterize the effects of exposure to general anesthetics in early life, particularly for prolonged or repeated exposures and in more vulnerable populations (e.g., less healthy children).

Results from an observational study (the Pediatric Anesthesia Neurodevelopment Assessment [PANDA] study) and from a multicenter, randomized trial (the General Anesthesia Compared to Spinal Anesthesia [GAS] trial) provide some evidence that a single, relatively brief exposure to general anesthesia in generally healthy children is unlikely to cause clinically detectable deficits in global cognitive function or serious behavioral disorders. The PANDA study compared global cognitive function (as measured by intelligence quotient [IQ] score) of children 8–15 years of age who had a single anesthesia exposure for elective inguinal hernia surgery before the age of 3 years with that of a biologically related sibling who had no anesthesia exposure before the age of 3 years. All of the children had a gestational age at birth of at least 36 weeks, and sibling pairs were within 3 years of being the same age. Children who underwent the elective procedure were mostly males (90%) and generally healthy. The mean duration of anesthesia was 84 minutes; 16% of those receiving anesthesia had exposures exceeding 2 hours. The study found no substantial difference in IQ score between children who had a single anesthesia exposure before the age of 3 years and their siblings who had not. The GAS trial was designed to compare neurodevelopmental outcomes in children who received general anesthesia in infancy with those in children who received awake regional (caudal and/or spinal) anesthesia in infancy for inguinal

herniorrhaphy before they reached a postmenstrual age of 60 weeks (with a gestational age at birth of more than 26 weeks); the primary outcome was the Wechsler Preschool and Primary Scale of Intelligence Third Edition (WPPSI-III) Full Scale IQ at 5 years of age. In an interim analysis at the age of 2 years, no difference in composite cognitive score (as measured by the Bayley Scales of Infant and Toddler Development III) was detected between children who had received sevoflurane anesthesia of less than 1 hour's duration (median duration: 54 minutes) compared with those who had received awake regional anesthesia. This result was confirmed in a subsequent analysis of the GAS trial of neurodevelopmental outcomes at 5 years of age.

Anesthetic and sedation drugs are an essential component of care for children and pregnant women who require surgery or other procedures that cannot be delayed; no specific general anesthetic or sedation drug has been shown to be less likely to cause neurocognitive deficits than any other such drug. Pending further accumulation of data in humans from well-designed studies, decisions regarding the timing of elective procedures requiring anesthesia should take into consideration both the benefits of the procedure and the potential risks. When procedures requiring the use of general anesthetics or sedation drugs are considered for young children or pregnant women, clinicians should discuss with the patient, parent, or caregiver the benefits, risks (including potential risk of adverse neurodevelopmental effects), and appropriate timing and duration of the procedure. FDA states that procedures that are considered medically necessary should not be delayed or avoided.

Hepatic Injury

Recurrent use of ketamine (e.g., misuse/abuse or medically supervised unapproved indications) is associated with hepatobiliary dysfunction, most often a cholestatic pattern. For patients who receive recurrent doses of ketamine as part of a treatment plan, obtain baseline liver function tests, including alkaline phosphatase and gamma glutamyl transferase. Monitor patients receiving recurrent therapy at periodic intervals during treatment.

Elevated hepatic enzyme concentrations may occur with anesthetic and subanesthetic doses of ketamine, particularly following prolonged infusion and/or repeated doses within a short time frame. Hepatotoxicity has been reported following longer-term use (e.g., more than 3–4 days). Increased hepatic enzyme concentrations have been reported in approximately 10% of patients receiving repetitive low doses or continuous high doses of ketamine infusions clinically. In a small study in patients receiving IV infusions of S-ketamine for chronic pain, hepatic enzyme elevations up to 3 times the upper limit of normal occurred following a second exposure to the drug. Hepatic enzyme concentrations generally return to baseline over several months.

Increased Intracranial Pressure

Ketamine increases cerebral metabolism and cerebral blood flow, and can also potentially increase intracranial pressure. Monitor patients with elevated intracranial pressure with frequent neurologic assessments.

Some experts state that the drug should be avoided in patients with elevated intracranial pressure. However, there is some controversy regarding the use of ketamine in patients with head trauma. Despite concerns of increased intracranial pressure, cerebral perfusion is maintained and there is evidence that ketamine can be safely and effectively used in patients with head injuries or risk of intracranial hypertension.

Studies suggest that intracranial pressure increases are minimal in patients with normal ventilation and are associated with concomitant elevations in cerebral perfusion. In a systematic review of data from studies using ketamine in mechanically ventilated patients with traumatic brain injury, ketamine was not associated with increased intracranial pressure; in some cases, intracranial pressure was decreased.

Because of concerns about increased intracranial pressure, some experts state that ketamine should be used with caution or avoided in patients with CNS masses, abnormalities, or hydrocephalus.

Other Warnings and Precautions

Laryngospasm

Laryngospasm and airway obstruction may occur during ketamine administration. Although the risk of laryngospasm is low with minor oropharyngeal procedures typically performed in the emergency department, efforts should be made to avoid vigorous stimulation of the posterior pharynx and accumulation of secretions or blood during these procedures.

Ocular Effects

Elevation of intraocular pressure (IOP) may occur. Blurred vision and pupillary dilation have been reported with subanesthetic doses of ketamine. Transient blindness also has been reported.

Use with caution or avoid use in patients with elevated IOP (e.g., glaucoma, acute globe injury).

Genitourinary Effects

Urinary tract complications, including dysuria, urinary frequency, urgency, urge incontinence, cystitis, hematuria, postmicturition pain, and secondary renal failure, reported, generally in association with chronic ketamine use or abuse.

In patients experiencing urinary symptoms without evidence of infection, consider interruption of ketamine therapy and evaluation by a specialist. The manufacturer states to consider discontinuance of ketamine if genitourinary pain continues in the setting of other genitourinary symptoms. Some experts advise that patients receiving long-term ketamine therapy for mood disorders be assessed for urinary symptoms (e.g., discomfort) during therapy.

Schizophrenia/Psychosis

Ketamine can exacerbate schizophrenia, and generally should be avoided in patients with schizophrenia or active psychosis. Although data are limited, caution is advised when ketamine is used for procedural sedation or acute pain in patients with other psychiatric disorders, including substance abuse-induced psychosis.

Long-term use of ketamine can cause persistent neuropsychiatric symptoms, cognitive impairment, and psychologic abnormalities.

When used for treatment-resistant depression and suicidality, acute dissociative and psychotomimetic effects (e.g., psychotic symptoms) have been reported with IV infusions of ketamine. Such effects generally occur only during and immediately following ketamine infusion and resolve within 2–4 hours following the end of the infusion, are generally mild in severity, and are well tolerated. Clinical experience to date suggests that dissociative symptoms occur more commonly than psychotomimetic effects when ketamine is used in patients with treatment-resistant depression.

Overdosage

Changes in heart rate and blood pressure, respiratory depression, and apnea may occur with overdosage or by a rapid rate of administration of ketamine. Monitor patients for clinically relevant changes in heart rate and blood pressure. Assisted ventilation, including mechanical ventilation, may be required.

Several cases of accidental ketamine overdosage (with doses up to 10 or 100 times the intended dose in adults or children, respectively) resulted in prolonged sedation, but no other clinically important adverse effects or complications; ventilator support was required rarely. Death secondary to acute ketamine overdosage in the absence of multidrug intoxication is rare, although accidental deaths have been reported. A lethal dose of ketamine in humans has not been identified.

Abuse, Tolerance, and Dependence

Ketamine is a known drug of abuse and is subject to control under the Federal Controlled Substances Act of 1970 as a schedule III drug. Although cases of abuse and dependence have been reported with ketamine, the abuse potential with the drug has not been clearly defined. The pharmacologic and behavioral effects of ketamine are similar to, but somewhat less intense and shorter in duration than those of phencyclidine (PCP). Ketamine is most commonly abused by nasal insufflation (i.e., snorting) of the powder (evaporated from the injectable liquid), although IV, IM, and oral routes also have been used. Reported desired effects of ketamine include feelings of dissociation and unreality, altered state of consciousness, enhanced sensory perception, hallucinations, intoxication, mild euphoria, and a sensation of floating. Most cases of ketamine abuse have been reported in the context of multidrug or polysubstance abuse. Surveys and studies examining the use pattern of ketamine indicate that abuse of the drug may be more prevalent in certain geographic regions (e.g., Hong Kong). The annual

prevalence rate for ketamine use in adolescents (17–18 years of age) in the US was 1.5% in 2012.

Although brief exposure to ketamine in a hospital setting is not likely to cause addiction, the possibility of addiction exists and patients should be individually assessed for their risk. Abuse of ketamine can result in adverse urinary, CNS, and hepatobiliary effects. The manufacturer states that ketamine should be prescribed and administered with caution because of the risk of abuse.

Tolerance to the drug's effects may develop following prolonged administration of ketamine. A sevenfold increase in the dose required for a desired "high" has been reported after 2 months of continuous use in recreational users of ketamine.

Although reported rarely, dependence on ketamine is possible. Cases of ketamine abuse resulting in physical or psychologic dependence have been reported. Withdrawal symptoms have been reported following discontinuation of frequent (more than weekly) use of large doses of ketamine for long periods of time. Reported symptoms of withdrawal associated with daily administration of large doses of ketamine include craving, fatigue, poor appetite, and anxiety.

Chronic Toxicity

Long-term abuse of ketamine has been associated with urinary tract complications, hepatobiliary toxicity, neuropsychiatric effects (e.g., hallucinatory flashbacks, inability to concentrate, memory impairment), and MRI abnormalities.

Urinary tract complications have been reported in association with long-term ketamine use, generally in the setting of chronic drug abuse, but also with clinical use of the drug. Reported lower urinary tract and bladder symptoms include cystitis, hematuria, dysuria, increased urinary frequency, urgency, incontinence, and postmicturition pain; secondary renal damage also can occur in severe cases. The exact mechanism of urinary tract damage is not clear, but ketamine and/or its metabolites are thought to have a direct irritant effect on the urothelium or interstitial cells of the bladder. Decreased bladder capacity and compliance, bladder wall thickening, transmural inflammation, detrusor muscle dysfunction, vesicoureteric reflux, hydronephrosis, and papillary necrosis have been observed.

Hepatobiliary toxicity also has been associated with long-term use of ketamine for therapeutic purposes or in the setting of chronic drug abuse. Epigastric pain, bile duct dilatation, and abnormal liver function tests consistent with posthepatic obstruction have been observed in chronic ketamine abusers.

Long-term use of ketamine has been reported to cause neuropsychiatric effects including hallucinatory flashbacks, inability to concentrate, and other cognitive deficits, possibly resulting from long-term effects of N-methyl-D-aspartic acid (NMDA)-receptor blockade. Both short-term and long-term memory impairment have been reported in chronic ketamine users.

MRI studies in chronic ketamine abusers have found areas of degeneration in the superficial white matter as early as 1 year of ketamine abuse; cortical atrophy and substantially decreased thalamocortical connectivity in the brain also have been observed.

Specific Populations

Pregnancy

There are no adequate and well-controlled studies of ketamine in pregnant women. Although ketamine has been used for induction of anesthesia during vaginal delivery and caesarean sections, the manufacturer states that the drug is not recommended for use during pregnancy or delivery because safety has not been established. Some neonates exposed to ketamine at maternal IV doses of 1.5 mg/kg or higher during delivery have experienced respiratory depression and low Apgar scores requiring resuscitation. Marked increases in maternal blood pressure and uterine tone have been observed following administration of IV ketamine doses greater than 2 mg/kg.

In animal reproduction studies using IM ketamine doses approximately 0.3–0.6 times the usual human IM dose of 10 mg/kg (based on body surface area), developmental delays, skeletal hypoplasia, and increased fetal resorptions were observed.

Based on animal data, repeated or prolonged use of general anesthetics and sedation drugs, including ketamine, during the third trimester of pregnancy may result in adverse neurodevelopmental effects in the fetus. The clinical relevance of these animal findings to humans is not known; the potential risk of adverse neurodevelopmental effects should be considered and discussed with pregnant women undergoing procedures requiring general anesthetics and sedation drugs.

Lactation

It is not known whether ketamine is distributed into milk. Because the drug should be undetectable in plasma approximately 11 hours after administration, nursing after this time period should not expose the infant to clinically relevant amounts of ketamine.

Pediatric Use

Although the manufacturer states that safety and efficacy of ketamine have not been established in patients younger than 16 years of age, the drug has been used widely in pediatric patients† in a variety of clinical settings for anesthesia, procedural sedation and analgesia, postoperative analgesia, and chronic pain management. Ketamine frequently is used in children to facilitate painful procedures in the emergency department and is considered a drug of choice for this use. Ketamine may be particularly useful in pediatric patients because the drug may be administered IM.

Repeated or prolonged use of general anesthetics and sedation drugs, including ketamine, in children <3 years of age or during the third trimester of pregnancy may adversely affect neurodevelopment. In animals, use of anesthetic and sedation drugs that block NMDA receptors and/or potentiate GABA activity leads to widespread neuronal apoptosis in the brain and long-term deficits in cognition and behavior when used for longer than 3 hours; however, the clinical relevance to humans is unknown.

Ketamine may be preferred for induction of anesthesia in children with congenital heart disease with right-to-left shunt† because of its sympathomimetic effects and hemodynamic stability.

Ketamine generally should *not* be used in infants younger than 3 months of age because of the potential increased risk of airway complications (e.g., airway obstruction, laryngospasm, apnea) thought to be due to age-specific differences in airway reactivity and anatomy.

Geriatric Use

While reported clinical experience to date has not revealed age-related differences in response to ketamine when used as an anesthetic agent, clinical studies have not included sufficient numbers of patients ≥65 years of age to determine whether geriatric patients respond differently than younger adults. When ketamine is used as an anesthetic agent in geriatric patients, the dosage should be selected carefully, usually starting at the low end of the dosing range, because of the greater frequency of age-related decreases in hepatic, renal, and/or cardiac function, and of concomitant disease or other drug therapy.

Hepatic Impairment

Prolonged effects of ketamine may occur in patients with hepatic impairment. Some experts recommend that use of ketamine be avoided or limited in patients with severe hepatic disease or cirrhosis, and that the drug be used with caution (e.g., with monitoring of liver function tests) in patients with moderate hepatic disease. Discontinuance of ketamine therapy is recommended if hepatotoxicity occurs.

Renal Impairment

Ketamine concentrations have been reported to be 20% higher in individuals with acute renal failure than in those with normal renal function.

● Common Adverse Effects

The most common adverse reactions with ketamine are emergence reactions and elevated blood pressure and pulse.

DRUG INTERACTIONS

Ketamine principally undergoes *N*-demethylation to the active metabolite norketamine. *N*-Demethylation of ketamine to norketamine is mediated principally by cytochrome P-450 (CYP) isoenzyme 2B6 and 3A4 and, to a lesser extent, by other CYP enzymes.

Ketamine, and its active norketamine metabolite, are principally metabolized by CYP3A4 with lesser involvement by CYP2B6 and CYP2C9.

● Drugs and Foods Affecting Hepatic Microsomal Enzymes

Drugs that inhibit or induce CYP3A4 and CYP2B6 may increase or decrease, respectively, the systemic exposure of ketamine or norketamine.

Grapefruit Juice

In healthy individuals, concomitant administration of the CYP3A4 inhibitor grapefruit juice (200 mL 3 times daily for 5 days) and *S*-ketamine (single oral dose of 0.2 mg/kg) increased peak plasma concentrations and AUC of ketamine by twofold and threefold, respectively. This interaction may be clinically important if ketamine is taken orally.

Itraconazole

Concomitant administration of the CYP3A inhibitor itraconazole (200 mg orally once daily) and *S*-ketamine (single oral dose of 0.2 mg/kg) in healthy individuals had no effect on the AUC of ketamine.

Macrolide Antibiotics

Concomitant administration of the CYP3A4 inhibitor clarithromycin and *S*-ketamine (single oral dose of 0.2 mg/kg) in healthy individuals increased peak plasma concentration and AUC of ketamine by 3.6- and 2.6-fold, respectively, and decreased the ratio of norketamine to ketamine by 54%. In addition, self-reported pharmacologic effects of ketamine were increased when *S*-ketamine was administered following pretreatment with clarithromycin. Erythromycin, but not azithromycin, is expected to have similar effects on the pharmacokinetics of *S*-ketamine.

Rifampin

Concomitant use of the potent CYP3A4 and CYP2B6 inducer rifampin (600 mg orally daily for 5 days) and *S*-ketamine (0.57–1.14 mg/kg by IV infusion over 2 hours) in healthy individuals decreased the AUC of *S*-ketamine and *S*-norketamine by 10 and 50%, respectively.

St. John's Wort

In healthy individuals, concomitant administration of the CYP3A4 inducer St. John's wort (*Hypericum perforatum*) and *S*-ketamine (single oral dose of 0.3 mg/kg) decreased peak plasma concentration and AUC of *S*-ketamine by 66 and 58%, respectively, and of *S*-norketamine by 18 and 23%, respectively.

Ticlopidine

Concomitant use of the CYP2B6 inhibitor ticlopidine (250 mg orally twice daily) and *S*-ketamine (single oral dose of 0.2 mg/kg) in healthy individuals increased the AUC of *S*-ketamine by 2.4-fold and decreased the ratio of norketamine to ketamine.

● CNS Depressants

Concomitant use of ketamine with CNS depressants (e.g., alcohol, benzodiazepines, opiate agonists, skeletal muscle relaxants) may result in additive CNS depression and increased risk of profound sedation, respiratory depression, coma, or death. Concomitant use of opiate agonists with ketamine during anesthesia may prolong recovery time.

Closely monitor the patient's neurological status and respiratory parameters, including respiratory rate and pulse oximetry; consider dosage adjustment based on the individual clinical situation.

Barbiturates

Decreased half-life and plasma concentrations of ketamine have been observed in patients receiving long-term therapy with barbiturates, likely due to hepatic enzyme induction.

Benzodiazepines

Increased half-life of ketamine has been reported in patients who were premedicated with diazepam rectally (as a single dose) prior to anesthesia; these patients required lower doses of ketamine. *Decreased* ketamine half-life was observed in patients who had been receiving long-term therapy with oral diazepam.

Ketamine metabolism was not substantially altered in patients who received IV clorazepate prior to anesthesia.

Administration of lorazepam has been reported to diminish the antidepressant response to repeated ketamine infusions in a patient with severe depression associated with bipolar disorder. Based on limited clinical evidence and theoretic concerns based on proposed mechanisms of action that benzodiazepines may diminish the antidepressant effects of ketamine, some clinicians recommend avoiding benzodiazepine administration for 8–12 hours prior to ketamine infusions.

● Ergonovine

Concomitant use of ketamine and ergonovine may result in increased blood pressure.

● Lamotrigine

Limited data suggest that lamotrigine, which inhibits the release of glutamate, may antagonize some of the effects of ketamine. Attenuated effects of ketamine, including perceptual abnormalities, schizophrenia-like symptoms, and learning and memory impairment, have been observed in healthy individuals who were pretreated with lamotrigine (300 mg) prior to receiving ketamine (0.26 mg/kg by IV injection or 0.65 mg/kg per hour by IV infusion). Failure of ketamine anesthesia following administration of IV doses totaling approximately 3.125 mg/kg has been reported in a patient with lamotrigine overdosage.

Lamotrigine has been reported to reduce ketamine cravings in a patient with ketamine abuse disorder.

● Neuromuscular Blocking Agents

Ketamine may potentiate the neuromuscular blocking effects of atracurium, resulting in respiratory depression and apnea. It is not known whether ketamine affects the duration of neuromuscular blockade of other neuromuscular blocking agents.

● Sympathomimetics and Vasopressin

Concomitant use with sympathomimetics or vasopressin may result in an enhanced sympathomimetic effect of ketamine. If these drugs are used concomitantly, closely monitor vital signs and consider dosage adjustments based on the individual clinical situation.

● Theophyllines

Concomitant use of ketamine and aminophylline or theophylline may result in a clinically important reduction in the seizure threshold. Tonic seizures have been reported during ketamine anesthesia in patients receiving aminophylline or theophylline. Consider use of an alternative to ketamine in patients receiving theophylline or aminophylline.

● Thyroid Agents

Patients receiving thyroid replacement therapy may have an increased risk of ketamine-induced hypertension and tachycardia.

DESCRIPTION

Ketamine is a nonbarbiturate general anesthetic that also has analgesic, amnestic, anti-inflammatory, and antidepressant properties. The drug is an arylcycloalkylamine derived from phencyclidine (PCP). Ketamine is commercially available in the US as a racemic mixture containing equal amounts of the R- and S-enantiomers. S-Ketamine, which is commercially available as esketamine in the US and some other countries, has a higher binding affinity for N-methyl-D-aspartate (NMDA) receptors and has approximately 3–4 times greater anesthetic potency than R-ketamine. S-Ketamine also appears to be associated with more frequent psychotomimetic adverse effects compared with R-ketamine.

The pharmacologic effects of ketamine are dose dependent and mediated principally by its actions on the N-methyl-D-aspartate (NMDA) receptor, with contributory effects from other receptor interactions. The anesthetic, amnestic, analgesic, and psychotomimetic effects of ketamine have been attributed to the drug's noncompetitive antagonism of the NMDA receptor. The NMDA receptor is a ligand-gated channel complex that plays an important role in excitatory glutamate-mediated neurotransmission, which can affect cognition, chronic pain, opiate tolerance, and mood regulation. The receptor is blocked at resting state by extracellular magnesium. Upon neuronal depolarization, magnesium is released, resulting in ligand-induced channel opening and calcium influx. Ketamine binds to the phencyclidine (PCP) site of the NMDA receptor channel, decreasing the frequency of channel opening and duration of time in the open active state, thereby inhibiting receptor activation and excitatory glutamatergic neurotransmission.

The NMDA receptor is closely involved in the development of opiate tolerance, opiate-induced hyperalgesia, and central sensitization (a condition closely related to the development of chronic pain). Activation of the NMDA receptor enhances neuronal excitability that can lead to hyperalgesia and allodynia. In the development of opiate tolerance and opiate-induced hyperalgesia, repeated activation of opiate receptors causes phosphorylation and opening of the NMDA receptor channel, leading to downregulation of opiate receptors and a reduction in opiate responsiveness. In chronic pain states, prolonged nociceptive stimulation causes activation and upregulation of NMDA receptors at dorsal horn synapses, resulting in enhanced and amplified trafficking of pain signals to the brain (central sensitization). Therefore, antagonism of NMDA receptors by ketamine decreases amplification of the response to repeated opiate receptor stimulation and can also prevent or reduce central sensitization.

In addition to its effects on the NMDA receptor, ketamine also acts on a wide range of other targets, including opiate, α-amino-3-hydroxy-5-methyl-4-isoxazolepropionic acid (AMPA), γ-aminobutyric acid A (GABA$_A$), cholinergic, nicotinic, and muscarinic receptors; L-type voltage-dependent calcium channels, hyperpolarization-activated cyclic nucleotide (HCN) channels, voltage-gated sodium channels, and large-conductance potassium (BK) channels; and the monoaminergic system.

Ketamine produces dissociative anesthesia as a result of a functional and electrophysiologic dissociation between the thalamocortical and limbic systems. The drug appears to selectively depress sensory association areas in the cortex, limbic systems, and thalamus without substantially obtunding the more primitive pathways (reticular-activating and limbic systems). At anesthetic doses, ketamine disrupts frontal-to-posterior corticocortical connectivity while maintaining thalamocortical somatosensory pathways. Thus, sensory input may reach cortical receiving areas but fail to be observed in some of the association areas, effectively dissociating the CNS from outside stimuli. At subanesthetic doses, ketamine has been shown to alter functional connectivity between the subgenual anterior cingulate cortex and a network cluster involving the thalamus, hippocampus, and the retrosplenial cortex, without reported loss of consciousness.

At anesthetic doses, ketamine produces a dissociative, cataleptic state characterized by profound analgesia, sedation, and amnesia. Although there is some variability, ketamine dissociation usually occurs at a dosing threshold of approximately 1–1.5 mg/kg when given IV or 3–4 mg/kg when given IM. Plasma ketamine concentrations associated with dissociative anesthesia have been reported to range from approximately 1.2–3 mcg/mL; concentrations associated with hypnosis and amnesia during surgery range from 0.8–4 mcg/mL and awakening usually occurs at plasma concentrations of 0.5–1.1 mcg/mL.

At doses and plasma concentrations lower than those used for anesthesia, ketamine produces analgesia and sedation. Although there is some variability, doses less than 1 mg/kg generally have been considered subanesthetic. Following IV or IM administration, analgesic effects are associated with plasma ketamine concentrations ranging from 0.07–0.2 mcg/mL. Analgesic effects following oral administration occur at plasma ketamine concentrations of 0.04 mcg/mL, possibly due to a higher ratio of norketamine.

The precise mechanism(s) of ketamine's antidepressant activity has not been clearly established. Considerable preclinical research suggests that the NMDA class of glutamate receptors plays a role in the pathophysiology of depression as well as in the mechanism of action of antidepressant treatments. In addition, NMDA receptor antagonists, including ketamine, have been shown to be effective in animal models of depression and in models that predict antidepressant activity in many studies. Preclinical and clinical data suggest that the antidepressant effects of ketamine may be mediated by an increase in glutamate, which leads to a cascade of events that results in synaptogenesis and reversal of the negative effects of chronic stress and depression, particularly in the prefrontal cortex. Following IV infusion of 0.5 mg/kg of ketamine over 40 minutes in patients with treatment-resistant major depressive disorder, peak plasma ketamine concentrations of 0.07–0.2 mcg/mL are achieved. These concentrations usually are associated with antidepressant effects but not general anesthetic effects.

Like PCP, ketamine may cause psychotomimetic effects as a result of NMDA-receptor antagonism; such effects can occur following anesthetic or subanesthetic doses. At higher ketamine doses used for anesthesia, psychotomimetic effects appear to be dose related; however, a dose-related effect has not been clearly established at subanesthetic doses. The analgesic properties of ketamine are closely related to its psychotomimetic effects. Psychotomimetic effects of ketamine may occur at IV doses in the range of 0.1–1 mg/kg or IM doses in the range of 25–200 mg.

Ketamine has a rapid onset of anesthetic action when given IV or IM. Following IV administration of the usual induction dose of 2 mg/kg, onset of surgical anesthesia occurs within 30 seconds and the duration of anesthetic effect is 5–10 minutes. Following IM administration of doses ranging from 9–13 mg/kg, onset of surgical anesthesia occurs within 3–4 minutes and the duration of anesthetic effect is usually 12–25 minutes. Following IV administration of a 2.5-mg/kg dose, ketamine has an initial distribution phase (α) lasting about 45 minutes and a half-life of 10–15 minutes, which is associated with the duration of anesthetic effect (about 20 minutes). Norketamine, the main active metabolite of ketamine, appears in the blood 2–3 minutes following IV administration of the drug and reaches peak plasma concentration in approximately 30 minutes.

Peak plasma concentrations following oral administration of ketamine occur within 20–120 minutes. Bioavailability of ketamine following IM administration is 93% in adults; lower IM bioavailability has been reported in children. Due to extensive first-pass metabolism, bioavailability following oral or rectal administration is low (16–30 or 11–30%, respectively), with relatively higher concentrations of norketamine. Bioavailability of ketamine following intranasal administration has been reported to be up to 45–50%, but can vary substantially. In children 4–10 years of age, plasma ketamine concentrations are similar to those observed in adults. Plasma concentrations of norketamine are higher in children than adults following equivalent weight-adjusted doses.

Ketamine is rapidly and widely distributed into highly perfused tissues, including the CNS, with a distribution half-life of 10–15 minutes. Animal studies have shown ketamine to be highly concentrated in body fat, liver, and lung. Because ketamine is lipophilic, it has a large volume of distribution. Termination of the anesthetic effect of ketamine occurs partly via redistribution from the CNS to peripheral tissues and partly by hepatic biotransformation.

Ketamine crosses the placenta. Following an IM dose of 250 mg (approximately 4.2 mg/kg) in parturient patients, placental transfer rate of ketamine from maternal artery to umbilical vein was 47% at the time of delivery (average of 12 minutes from the time of injection to vaginal delivery). It is not known whether ketamine is distributed into milk. Ketamine is less than 50% bound to plasma proteins (α₁-acid glycoprotein or albumin). Ketamine is metabolized extensively in the liver, principally undergoing N-demethylation to the active metabolite norketamine, which has approximately one-third the anesthetic activity of the parent drug. N-demethylation of ketamine to norketamine is mediated principally by cytochrome P-450 (CYP) isoenzyme 2B6 and 3A4 and, to a lesser extent, by other CYP enzymes. Norketamine is further metabolized to hydroxynorketamines and dehydronorketamine. Other biotransformation pathways of ketamine include hydroxylation of the cyclohexone ring, conjugation with glucuronic acid, and dehydration of the hydroxylated metabolites to form a cyclohexene derivative. About 90% of a parenteral dose of ketamine is excreted in the urine, mostly as conjugates of hydroxylated metabolites. Less than 5% of a dose is excreted unchanged in feces and urine. Because ketamine is extensively metabolized prior to excretion, the effect of renal function on the pharmacokinetics of ketamine and norketamine is minimal. Plasma concentrations of ketamine have been reported to be 20% higher in individuals with acute renal failure than in those with normal renal function.

Ketamine is not appreciably removed by hemodialysis or hemofiltration (10 or 4%, respectively). The elimination half-life of ketamine is approximately 2–4 hours and is shorter in children (approximately 100 minutes) than in adults. The half-life of norketamine is 12 hours.

ADVICE TO PATIENTS

- May cause residual anesthetic effects and drowsiness. Importance of advising patients not to operate hazardous machinery, including driving a motor vehicle, or engage in hazardous activities within 24 hours of receiving ketamine.

- When procedures requiring general anesthetics or sedation drugs, including ketamine, are considered for young children or pregnant women, importance of discussing with the patient, parent, or caregiver the benefits, risks (including potential risk of adverse neurodevelopmental effects), and appropriate timing and duration of the procedure.

- Advise patients to inform their clinician of existing or contemplated concomitant therapy, including prescription and OTC drugs and dietary and herbal supplements, as well as any concomitant illnesses.

- Advise women to inform their clinician if they are or plan to become pregnant or plan to breast-feed.

- Advise patients of other important precautionary information. (See Cautions.)

PREPARATIONS

Ketamine is subject to control under the Federal Controlled Substances Act of 1970 as a schedule III (C-III) drug.

Excipients in commercially available drug preparations may have clinically important effects in some individuals; consult specific product labeling for details.

Ketamine Hydrochloride

Parenteral

Injection	10 mg (of ketamine) per mL*		Ketalar® (C-III), Par
			Ketamine Hydrochloride Injection (C-III)
	50 mg (of ketamine) per mL*		Ketalar® (C-III), Par
			Ketamine Hydrochloride Injection (C-III)
	100 mg (of ketamine) per mL*		Ketalar® (C-III), Par
			Ketamine Hydrochloride Injection (C-III)

* available from one or more manufacturer, distributor, and/or repackager by generic (nonproprietary) name

† Use is not currently included in the labeling approved by the US Food and Drug Administration.

Selected Revisions June 10, 2024, © Copyright, June 24, 2019, American Society of Health-System Pharmacists, Inc.

Propofol

28:04.08 · NON-BARBITURATES

■ Propofol is a sedative and hypnotic agent.

USES

Propofol is used for IV induction and maintenance of sedation and general anesthesia. Although propofol was initially developed as a general anesthetic agent, use of the drug has expanded to include procedural sedation in nonsurgical or ambulatory settings, monitored anesthesia care (MAC) sedation, and sedation in patients undergoing local or regional anesthesia. In addition, propofol is used for sedation in intubated and mechanically ventilated patients in a critical care setting (e.g., intensive care unit [ICU]).

● Induction and Maintenance of General Anesthesia

Propofol is used for IV induction and maintenance of general anesthesia. The drug is FDA-labeled for use as an IV induction agent for general anesthesia in adults and pediatric patients ≥3 years of age and for maintenance anesthesia in adults and pediatric patients ≥2 months of age.

General anesthesia is defined as a drug-induced depression of the CNS that results in loss of response to and perception of all external stimuli; patients enter a state of unconsciousness where they are not arousable, even to painful stimuli. The ability to maintain ventilatory function is often impaired, requiring assistance to maintain a patent airway; cardiovascular function also may be impaired. During general anesthesia, hypnosis, amnesia, analgesia, and muscle relaxation are provided using a combination of drugs. General anesthesia consists of 3 phases: induction, maintenance, and emergence. Induction of general anesthesia is generally achieved with an IV agent such as propofol; alternatively, an inhalation agent (e.g., sevoflurane) may be used, but will result in a slower onset of effect. Once unconsciousness is induced, anesthesia is maintained with either an inhalation agent (e.g., sevoflurane, desflurane, isoflurane) or IV anesthetic agent in addition to a combination of other drugs to provide attenuation of autonomic responses to surgery (e.g., cardiovascular, respiratory, GI), immobility, anterograde amnesia, analgesia, and muscle relaxation. The use of an IV anesthetic agent for both induction and maintenance of anesthesia (total IV anesthesia) may offer some advantages over inhalation anesthesia such as more rapid recovery and reduced risk of postoperative nausea and vomiting. Ideally, recovery from general anesthesia should be rapid without residual adverse effects.

Propofol is a preferred agent for IV induction and maintenance of anesthesia because of its favorable characteristics. Following IV administration, induction with propofol is rapid and results in dose-related hypnotic effects (progressing from light sleep to unconsciousness) and anterograde amnesia; however, the analgesic properties of the drug have not been conclusively demonstrated. A propofol dose of 2–2.5 mg/kg generally produces loss of consciousness in less than 1 minute (time required for one arm-brain circulation). Following induction, anesthesia can be maintained by continuous IV infusion or intermittent IV injections. Emergence from propofol anesthesia is rapid because of fast redistribution and metabolic clearance of the drug.

Compared with other IV anesthetic agents (e.g., etomidate, methohexital), propofol usually is associated with a similar or faster time to recovery from anesthesia, more rapid recovery of psychomotor performance and time to discharge, and a lower incidence of adverse effects (e.g., nausea, vomiting, cough, hiccups). When compared with other IV induction agents, propofol usually produces a more substantial decrease in blood pressure (especially when the drug is used concomitantly with opiates). Results of several comparative studies indicate that hemodynamic parameters (e.g., heart rate, systemic blood pressure, systemic vascular resistance) associated with use of propofol for maintenance anesthesia are similar to those associated with other IV anesthetics. Compared with the inhalation anesthetics (e.g., sevoflurane, desflurane, isoflurane), propofol is associated with a consistent and clinically relevant lower incidence of postoperative nausea and vomiting. However, comparative findings with respect to other outcomes have differed based on the specific comparisons. While early recovery usually is faster with the use of desflurane compared with propofol, time to intermediate recovery (return of cognitive and psychomotor functions) and time to discharge appear to be similar. Time to emergence after discontinuance of anesthesia appears to be comparable with propofol and sevoflurane, but may be faster with propofol compared with isoflurane.

Use of propofol as a general anesthetic agent is supported by numerous studies. The drug has produced adequate anesthesia in patients undergoing various types of surgery, including neurosurgery (e.g., craniotomy, intracranial aneurysm repair) and cardiovascular (e.g., coronary artery bypass graft [CABG]); abdominal; ocular; ear, nose and throat (ENT); orthopedic; and general surgery. Because propofol decreases cerebral blood flow, intracranial pressure, and cerebral metabolic requirements and is associated with fast recovery from anesthesia, which can facilitate rapid postoperative neurologic assessment, the drug may be particularly useful in patients undergoing neurosurgery. Propofol can substantially decrease intraocular pressure (IOP), which may be advantageous in patients undergoing ocular surgery. Although propofol has been studied extensively in patients with coronary artery disease, experience in patients with hemodynamically significant valvular or congenital heart disease is limited. When propofol is used for induction of anesthesia, substantial decreases in arterial pressure (by about 30%; 30–40 mm Hg) may occur in patients with normal or impaired ventricular or cardiac function.

Propofol has been used safely in patients who are susceptible to malignant hyperthermia and patients with porphyria; however, further studies are needed.

● Procedural Sedation

Propofol is used for sedation in patients undergoing diagnostic or therapeutic procedures across various clinical settings (e.g., emergency department, cardiac catheterization laboratories, radiology suites, endoscopy suites, dental offices). Propofol is a preferred sedative agent for this use because of its rapid onset of effect, short duration, and rapid time to recovery. The current evidence indicates that the drug can be used safely and effectively for procedures outside the operating room, provided it is administered and monitored appropriately by trained individuals. Although propofol is not FDA-labeled for use as a sedative agent in children undergoing procedures, the drug has been used widely for pediatric procedural sedation†.

Procedural sedation is a technique in which sedative or dissociative agents are administered with or without analgesics to allow patients to tolerate painful or unpleasant medical procedures; a depressed state of consciousness is intentionally induced while cardiorespiratory function is maintained. Because sedation is a continuum ranging from minimal sedation to general anesthesia, it is not always possible to predict how a patient will respond. If a deeper than intended level of sedation occurs, airway reflexes and cardiorespiratory function may be impaired; therefore, propofol should only be administered by clinicians who have the requisite training and skills to manage complications and rescue patients if an unintended level of deep sedation is achieved.

Propofol is generally used to provide moderate or deep sedation depending on the procedure, clinical setting, and patient requirements. Propofol may be used under monitored anesthesia care (MAC) or in conjunction with local or regional anesthesia. (See Monitored Anesthesia Care under Uses.) Because propofol can produce rapid and profound changes in the depth of sedation and lacks a reversal agent, the American Society of Anesthesiologists (ASA) states that even if moderate sedation is intended, patients should receive the same level of care required for deep sedation. Patients should be continuously monitored during propofol administration to assess their level of consciousness and identify early signs of hypotension, bradycardia, apnea, airway obstruction, and oxygen desaturation.

Propofol may be used alone or in combination with opiate analgesics and/or benzodiazepines to achieve the appropriate level of sedation; combination therapy may allow for reduced dosage requirements of the individual drugs and minimize the potential for adverse effects. Propofol is commonly administered with ketamine; the combination regimen is given to potentiate the advantages of each drug while decreasing the risks (e.g., propofol-associated hypotension and respiratory depression; ketamine-associated vomiting and recovery agitation).

Studies comparing the use of propofol with other sedative agents (e.g., benzodiazepines, ketamine, etomidate, opiate analgesics) have reported various findings, and outcomes have differed based on whether the drug was used alone or in combination with other agents; however, these studies generally demonstrate a faster recovery and similar adverse effect profile with propofol compared with these other sedative agents.

● Monitored Anesthesia Care

Propofol is used for initiation and maintenance of monitored anesthesia care (MAC) sedation in adults. When used for MAC sedation, propofol may be used alone, but is often used in combination with other sedative, analgesic, and hypnotic agents (e.g., opiate analgesics, benzodiazepines).

MAC is a specific anesthesia service performed by a qualified anesthesia provider and does not refer to a specific level of sedation. The service involves all aspects of anesthesia care, including an assessment of the patient's comorbidities and risk factors; administration of sedatives, analgesics, anesthetic agents, and hypnotics as needed; support of vital functions (e.g., hemodynamic stability, airway management); and other provisions to ensure patient comfort and safety during the procedure. The MAC provider is focused exclusively on the patient's anesthetic needs and is prepared to manage any complications, including conversion to general anesthesia if necessary. Factors to consider when determining whether MAC sedation is indicated include the nature of the procedure, the patient's clinical condition, risk factors, and/or need for deeper levels of analgesia and sedation than can be provided by moderate sedation (including the need to convert to general or regional anesthesia). MAC sedation is distinguished from moderate sedation, which is a drug-induced depression of consciousness during which patients respond purposefully to verbal commands. (For additional information on the use of propofol for procedural sedation, see Procedural Sedation under Uses.)

● Sedation in Critical Care Settings

Propofol is used as a continuous IV infusion for sedation in intubated and mechanically ventilated adults in a critical care setting (e.g., ICU). Efficacy and safety of propofol for this indication are based principally on the results of several comparative (with benzodiazepines and/or opiates) clinical trials in adults. Propofol, alone or in combination with an opiate analgesic (e.g., morphine, fentanyl), has been effective in achieving a desired level of sedation using the standardized Ramsay or modified Glasgow sedation scale and providing adequate sedation in intubated and mechanically ventilated patients.

Sedative agents are administered in critically ill patients to reduce agitation and anxiety, and increase tolerance to invasive procedures (e.g., mechanical ventilation). The provision of adequate analgesia and other measures to ensure patient comfort is recommended before sedatives are administered. Common sedative agents used in the ICU include benzodiazepines (e.g., midazolam, lorazepam), propofol, and dexmedetomidine. These agents appear to be similarly effective in providing adequate sedation in critically ill, mechanically ventilated adults. However, modest benefits with respect to other clinical outcomes (e.g., reduced duration of mechanical ventilation, shorter time to extubation, reduced risk of delirium) have been observed with the nonbenzodiazepine sedatives (dexmedetomidine and propofol) compared with benzodiazepines. Because of the apparent advantages and an overall favorable benefit-to-risk profile, nonbenzodiazepine sedatives (propofol or dexmedetomidine) are generally preferred to benzodiazepines (midazolam or lorazepam) in mechanically ventilated, critically ill adults. This recommendation should be considered in the context of the specific clinical situation since benzodiazepines may still be preferred in certain situations (e.g., patients with anxiety, seizures, or alcohol or benzodiazepine withdrawal). When selecting an appropriate sedative agent, the patient's individual sedation goals should be considered in addition to specific drug-related (e.g., pharmacology, pharmacokinetics, adverse effects, availability, cost) and patient-related (e.g., comorbid conditions) factors.

Comparative studies have shown that propofol may have a less variable effect on recovery of consciousness and time to recovery of function after cessation of therapy than midazolam. However, propofol may be associated with less frequent amnestic effects and more frequent hypotension than midazolam. When receiving short-term (less than 24 hours), intermediate-term (1–3 days), or long-term (more than 3 days) sedation, time to spontaneous breathing (ability to wean from mechanical ventilation), recovery (awakening or response to voice command), or extubation is often shorter in patients (especially those awakening from deep sedation) receiving propofol than in those receiving midazolam. However, certain clinical outcomes (e.g., discharge from an ICU) may be similar when the drugs are used for short- or intermediate-term sedation. Because of its short duration of sedative effect, some experts state that propofol may be particularly useful in patients requiring frequent awakenings (e.g., for neurologic assessments) or undergoing daily sedation interruption protocols. Results of several studies suggest that when used for long-term sedation, propofol is associated with more

reliable and rapid awakening than use of midazolam. However, long-term administration of propofol can lead to prolonged emergence. Prolonged use of propofol also may be associated with increased serum lipid concentrations (e.g., hypertriglyceridemia) secondary to the injectable emulsion formulation. Studies comparing propofol and dexmedetomidine for ICU sedation generally have not found any important differences in clinical outcomes between the drugs.

● Other Uses

Propofol also has been used in the management of refractory status epilepticus†, postoperative or cancer chemotherapy-induced nausea and vomiting†, and spinal opiate- or cholestasis-induced pruritus†.

Although propofol has been associated rarely with development of seizures or seizure-like activity, the drug has been used in patients with refractory status epilepticus†, usually administered IV by rapid injection followed by continuous infusion. In some patients with status epilepticus refractory to conventional anticonvulsants, termination of seizure activity and/or EEG burst suppression occurred within seconds after administration of propofol by rapid IV ("bolus") injection and was sustained during propofol infusion (lasting 2 hours to 12 days). In at least one patient, propofol also has been used in the management of refractory complex-partial seizures†.

Because propofol appears to possess direct antiemetic activity, the drug has been administered in subhypnotic doses (10–15 mg IV) for the management of postoperative nausea and vomiting†. In addition, propofol (usually administered with conventional antiemetics) has been used effectively for the prevention of nausea and vomiting associated with emetogenic cancer chemotherapy†.

Subhypnotic doses of propofol have been used effectively for relief of pruritus† associated with use of spinal opiates or cholestasis.

DOSAGE AND ADMINISTRATION

● General

Patient Monitoring

- During administration of propofol, closely monitor patient's cardiorespiratory function.
- In elderly, debilitated, or American Society of Anesthesiologists-Physical Status (ASA-PS) III or IV patients, continuously monitor for early signs of hypotension and/or bradycardia during administration of propofol.

Dispensing and Administration Precautions

- Strict aseptic technique must be used when preparing and administering propofol to avoid microbial contamination and transmission of infections. (See Guidelines for Aseptic Technique under Dosage and Administration.)
- Due to the potential for rapid and profound changes in the depth of anesthesia and sedation, special precautions are required when administering propofol. The ASA states that even if moderate sedation is intended, patients receiving propofol should receive care consistent with that required for deep sedation.
- There are different considerations when propofol is used for sedation of intubated, ventilated patients in a critical care setting. Administration of propofol is regulated at the state, regional, and local levels; guidance from these areas should be consulted.
- When used for general anesthesia or monitored anesthesia care (MAC) sedation, propofol should be administered by individuals experienced in the use of general anesthesia who are not involved in the conduct of the surgical and/or diagnostic procedure. Sedated patients should be constantly monitored and equipment necessary for intubation, assisted respiration, administration of oxygen, and cardiopulmonary resuscitation must be readily available.
- When used for sedation in intubated, mechanically ventilated patients in the ICU, propofol should be administered only by individuals qualified in the management of critically ill patients and trained in cardiovascular resuscitation and airway management. Since excessively high blood concentrations of propofol may occur in patients receiving the drug for prolonged periods, the infusion rate should be reduced and titrated according to individual clinical response and sedation levels should be evaluated at least daily when

the drug is used for long durations. Opioids and paralytic agents should be discontinued and respiratory function optimized prior to weaning patients from mechanical ventilation. Abrupt discontinuance of propofol should be avoided since this may result in rapid awakening accompanied by anxiety, agitation, and resistance to mechanical ventilation. Therefore, the manufacturers recommend that administration of propofol be continued to maintain a light level of sedation throughout the weaning process until about 10–15 minutes prior to extubation.

- Based on the Institute for Safe Medication Practices (ISMP), propofol is a high-alert medication that has a heightened risk of causing significant patient harm when used in error.

● Administration

Propofol injectable emulsion is administered by IV infusion or IV injection. When the drug is administered by IV infusion, use of a controlled infusion device (e.g., syringe or volumetric pump) is recommended. In patients undergoing magnetic resonance imaging (MRI) who are receiving IV infusion of propofol, metered controlled devices may be used when mechanical pumps are not suitable. Rarely, the drug also has been administered by continuous IV infusion using a patient-controlled infusion device† in individuals receiving monitored anesthesia care (MAC) sedation while undergoing diagnostic or surgical procedures.

Propofol injectable emulsion should be shaken well prior to administration. The drug should not be used if there is evidence of excessive creaming or aggregation, if large droplets are visible, or if there are other forms of phase separation indicating that the stability of the product has been compromised. Slight creaming, which may be visible upon prolonged standing, should disappear after shaking.

Clinical experience with use of inline filters for propofol administration during general anesthesia, MAC, or critical care sedation is limited. An inline membrane filter may be used during administration of the drug; however, the mean pore diameter of the filter should not be less than 5 μm, unless it has been demonstrated that the filter does not restrict the flow and/or cause the breakdown of the emulsion. Filters should be used with caution and only when clinically appropriate. Continuous monitoring for restricted flow and breakdown of the emulsion is required.

Commercially available propofol injectable emulsions should be stored at 4–25°C depending on the preparation and should be protected from freezing. Since propofol undergoes oxidative degradation in the presence of oxygen, the commercially available injectable emulsions are packaged under nitrogen to prevent such degradation.

The commercially available 1% (10 mg/mL) propofol injectable emulsion is a ready-to-use formulation that does not require dilution but may be diluted (see Dilution under Dosage and Administration). When the emulsion is administered directly from the original container, administration should be completed within 12 hours and unused portions should be discarded. If propofol injectable emulsion is transferred to another container, administration should begin promptly and be completed within 12 hours; unused portions also should be discarded. If dilution of propofol injectable emulsion is necessary, the drug may be diluted with 5% dextrose injection to a concentration of not less than 0.2% (2 mg/mL). It appears that stability of the diluted solutions is greater in glass than in plastic containers; potency of the diluted emulsions may decrease by about 5–8% after continuous IV infusion of propofol through a plastic (PVC) tubing for 2 hours. Potency may decrease even further (up to 35%) when the diluted solution is left stationary in a PVC tubing. It has been suggested that propofol injectable emulsion may adsorb to plastic IV tubing and such adsorption may be decreased by maintaining a constant flow of the solution.

The manufacturers state that propofol is compatible with several IV fluids (e.g., 5% dextrose, 5% dextrose and lactated Ringer's, lactated Ringer's, 5% dextrose and 0.2% or 0.45% sodium chloride) when a Y-type administration set is used. Propofol should *not* be administered through the same catheter as blood, serum, or plasma because compatibility has not been established. In vitro tests have shown that aggregates of the globular component of the vehicle containing propofol may form when the drug is in contact with blood, serum, or plasma. The clinical importance of these effects is not known.

Addition of lidocaine to propofol in quantities greater than 20 mg of lidocaine per 200 mg of propofol may cause instability of the propofol emulsion, resulting in increases in globule sizes over time; reduction of anesthetic potency has been reported in rats. The manufacturers recommend that lidocaine be given prior to administration of propofol or, alternatively, that lidocaine be added to propofol immediately before administration, in quantities not exceeding 20 mg lidocaine/200 mg propofol.

Propofol should *not* be mixed with other therapeutic agents prior to administration. Propofol has been reported to be physically and/or chemically incompatible with several drugs, but the compatibility depends on several factors (e.g., concentration of the drugs, specific diluents used, resulting pH, temperature). Specialized references should be consulted for more specific information.

Dilution

Commercially available 1% (10 mg/mL) propofol injectable emulsion may be used without dilution. If dilution is necessary, the drug should only be diluted with 5% dextrose injection and should not be diluted to a concentration less than 0.2% (2 mg/mL) in order to maintain the emulsion. The drug should not be used if there is evidence of separation of the emulsion. When diluted with 5% dextrose injection, propofol has been shown to be more stable in glass rather than in plastic containers. Propofol injectable emulsion and dilutions of the drug should be inspected visually for particulate matter and discoloration prior to administration whenever the emulsion and container permit.

Standardize 4 Safety

Standardized concentrations for propofol have been established through Standardize 4 Safety (S4S), a national patient safety initiative to reduce medication errors, especially during transitions of care. Multidisciplinary expert panels were convened to determine recommended standard concentrations. Because recommendations from the S4S panels may differ from the manufacturer's prescribing information, caution is advised when using concentrations that differ from labeling, particularly when using rate information from the label. For additional information on S4S (including updates that may be available), see https://www.ashp.org/pharmacy-practice/standardize-4-safety-initiative.

TABLE 1. Standardize 4 Safety Continuous Infusion Standards for Propofol

Patient Population	Concentration standard	Dosing units
Adults	10 mg/mL	mcg/kg/min[a]
Pediatric patients (<50 kg)	10 mg/mL	mcg/kg/min[a]

[a] Dosing units differ from concentration units

Guidelines for Aseptic Technique

Strict aseptic technique must be used when preparing and administering propofol. Although commercially available preparations of propofol injectable emulsion contain ingredients that inhibit the rate of growth of microorganisms (e.g., edetate disodium, sodium metabisulfite, sodium benzoate, benzyl alcohol), the emulsion may still support growth of microorganisms. Vials are intended for single-patient use and single access only. Any unused drug should be discarded within the specified time limits. Failure to observe strict aseptic technique has resulted in microbial contamination and transmission of infections. Propofol should not be used if contamination is suspected.

To administer propofol, contents of a vial may be transferred into a sterile, single-use syringe immediately after the vial is opened and after cleaning the rubber stopper with 70% isopropyl alcohol; when withdrawing the drug from vials, a sterile vented spike should be used. Syringes should be labeled with appropriate information, including the date and time the vial was opened.

When used for general anesthesia or MAC sedation, the manufacturers state that administration of propofol should be started promptly and completed within 12 hours after vials have been opened. Propofol injectable emulsion should be prepared for use just prior to initiation of each individual anesthetic/sedative procedure. The manufacturers also state that any unused portion, reservoirs, dedicated administration tubing, and/or solutions containing propofol injectable emulsion should be discarded at the end of the anesthetic procedure or after 12 hours, whichever occurs sooner. Following reports of acute febrile reactions associated with the administration of propofol, FDA recommended that administration be completed within 6 hours of opening of a single vial when used for general anesthesia or procedural sedation. The IV line should be flushed every 12 hours and at the end of the procedure to remove residual propofol emulsion.

When propofol is used for sedation in critical care settings, manipulations of IV lines should be minimized and administration should be started promptly and completed within 12 hours after the vial has been spiked. A sterile vent spike and sterile tubing must be used for administration of propofol injectable emulsion. When used for sedation in critical care settings, any unused portion and IV tubing should be discarded at the end of the procedure or after 12 hours.

Injection-site Pain

Injection-site pain occurs frequently with propofol. Pain can be minimized by administering the drug into larger veins of the forearm or antecubital fossa rather than hand veins, and by administering IV lidocaine (either as a pretreatment or admixed with propofol). Because of the possibility that lidocaine may cause instability of the propofol emulsion, the manufacturers recommend that lidocaine be administered prior to propofol administration or that lidocaine be added to propofol immediately before administration in a quantity not exceeding 20 mg of lidocaine per 200 mg of propofol.

Rate of Administration

Propofol should be administered slowly to minimize adverse effects (e.g., hypotension, respiratory depression). Cardiorespiratory depression is more likely to occur at higher blood propofol concentrations resulting from rapid IV ("bolus") injection or rapid increases in the rate of infusion. The drug should not be administered by rapid IV ("bolus") injection (single or repeated doses) in geriatric, debilitated, or American Society of Anesthesiologists (ASA) physical status III or IV patients since such administration may result in cardiorespiratory depression (e.g., hypotension, oxyhemoglobin desaturation, apnea, airway obstruction) during general anesthesia or MAC sedation.

When propofol is administered as a continuous IV infusion, depth of anesthesia is controlled by the rate of infusion. In the absence of clinical signs indicating light anesthesia and until a mild response to surgical stimulation develops, propofol IV infusion rates always should be titrated downward to avoid drug administration at rates higher than clinically necessary. To optimize recovery times, adults usually should receive propofol at a rate of about 50–100 mcg/kg per minute.

● Dosage

Because individual response to propofol is variable, dosage (including the infusion rate or amount and frequency of incremental doses) of the drug should always be adjusted to clinical effect and account for individual requirements, response, age, weight, clinical status (e.g., ASA physical status, degree of debilitation), blood lipid profile, underlying pathologic conditions (e.g., shock, intestinal obstruction, malnutrition, anemia, burns, advanced malignancy, ulcerative colitis, uremia, alcoholism), and the type and amount of premedication or concomitant medication(s) used. To provide adequate anesthesia in patients undergoing minor surgical procedures (e.g., on the body surface), propofol may be administered concomitantly with 60–70% nitrous oxide, while for major (e.g., intra-abdominal) surgical procedures or if nitrous oxide is not available or appropriate, administration rates of propofol and/or opiates may be increased. Similar to other sedatives, there appears to be wide interpatient variation in propofol dosage requirements that may increase or decrease with time. In general, the smallest effective dosage should be used.

Induction and Maintenance of General Anesthesia

Healthy Adults (Younger Than 65 Years of Age)

For induction of anesthesia, the manufacturers recommend that the majority of patients with ASA Physical Status I or II receive 2–2.5 mg/kg of propofol. Titrate the dosage against patient response and until there are clinical signs consistent with the onset of anesthesia.

For maintenance of anesthesia in patients undergoing general surgery, the usual initial IV infusion rate of propofol is 100–200 mcg/kg per minute (6–12 mg/kg per hour), administered concomitantly with inhaled 60–70% nitrous oxide and oxygen. Immediately following induction, higher IV infusion rates of 150–200 mcg/kg per minute generally may be required for the first 10–15 minutes, and

then decreased by 30–50% during the first 30 minutes of maintenance anesthesia. The manufacturers state that IV infusion rates of 50–100 mcg/kg per minute usually are used to optimize recovery times.

Alternatively, for maintenance anesthesia, healthy adults may receive propofol doses of 25–50 mg by intermittent IV injection in combination with inhaled nitrous oxide. These incremental boluses may be given if necessary, as determined by changes in vital signs (increases in pulse rate, blood pressure, sweating and/or lacrimation) indicating a stress response to surgical stimulation or emergence from anesthesia.

Geriatric (65 Years of Age and Older) or Debilitated Patients

Geriatric, debilitated, or ASA III or IV physical status patients usually require lower induction dosages of propofol because of possible reduced clearance and higher blood drug concentrations. For induction of anesthesia, such patients usually receive 1–1.5 mg/kg of propofol. Titrate the dosage against patient response and until there are clinical signs consistent with the onset of anesthesia. A rapid propofol bolus during induction may increase the likelihood of undesirable cardiorespiratory depression in these patients.

For maintenance of anesthesia, the usual IV infusion rate is 50–100 mcg/kg per minute (3–6 mg/kg per hour), administered concomitantly with inhaled 60–70% nitrous oxide and oxygen.

Pediatric Patients

In healthy (ASA I or II physical status) pediatric patients 3–16 years of age, the usual suggested IV induction dosage of propofol is 2.5–3.5 mg/kg until induction onset, as determined by the clinical response of the patient. Within this dosage range, younger pediatric patients may require higher induction dosages than older pediatric patients. However, a lower dosage for induction of anesthesia is recommended for pediatric patients with ASA physical status of III or IV.

For maintenance of anesthesia in healthy (ASA I or II physical status) pediatric patients 2 months to 16 years of age, propofol can be administered by infusion or intermittent IV bolus injection. The usual IV infusion rate is 125–300 mcg/kg per minute (7.5–18 mg/kg per hour) administered concomitantly with inhaled 60–70% nitrous oxide and oxygen. Immediately following induction, higher IV infusion rates of 200–300 mcg/kg per minute generally may be required for the first 30 minutes, which may be decreased to 125–150 mcg/kg per minute (unless clinical signs of light anesthesia develop) by titration, according to the patient's response. Younger pediatric patients may require higher maintenance infusion rates than older pediatric patients.

For intermittent IV bolus administration, an initial bolus of 1–4 mg/kg, followed by administration of 0.5–2 mg/kg injections based on patient response, may be sufficient for anesthesia maintenance.

Patients Undergoing Cardiac Anesthesia

For induction of anesthesia, adults undergoing cardiac surgery usually receive 0.5–1.5 mg/kg of propofol until the onset of induction, as determined by clinical response of the patient.

The maintenance dose of propofol in adult cardiac patients should be administered as 25–100 mcg/kg/min, adjusted according to the patient's sedation level and clinical response.

Patients Undergoing Neurosurgery

For induction of anesthesia, adults undergoing neurosurgery usually receive 1–2 mg/kg of propofol until the onset of induction, as determined by clinical response of the patient. For maintenance of anesthesia, the usual IV infusion rate is 100–200 mcg/kg per minute (6–12 mg/kg per hour).

Procedural Sedation

Various dosage regimens of propofol have been used for procedural sedation. Propofol is usually given as an initial IV bolus injection followed by intermittent injections or continuous IV infusion to maintain the desired level of sedation, but the drug also has been given by IV infusion throughout the procedure. Administration by IV infusion may allow for more precise control of the level of sedation compared with a repeated bolus technique. The appropriate dose and depth of sedation should be individualized based on the procedure and needs of the patient.

In clinical studies, an IV propofol dose of 1 mg/kg was commonly used to achieve initial sedation in adults undergoing a diagnostic or therapeutic procedure; however, lower (e.g., 0.5 mg/kg) or higher (e.g, 1.5 mg/kg) initial doses also have been used. To maintain the desired level of sedation, additional doses (e.g., 0.25-0.5 mg/kg by intermittent IV injection) usually are administered as needed.

In pediatric patients undergoing procedural sedation†, an initial IV propofol dose of 1 mg/kg has been used. In one study, children 3–18 years of age undergoing an emergency orthopedic procedure received an initial IV propofol dose of 1 mg/kg, followed by smaller intermittent doses based on patient response. In another study in children 2 years of age or older who received propofol sedation for closed orthopedic reductions, the drug was given as an initial 1-mg/kg bolus dose over 2 minutes, followed by an IV infusion of 67–100 mcg/kg per minute until cast completion. To maintain the desired level of sedation, additional bolus doses of 1 mg/kg were administered and/or the infusion rate was adjusted.

For dosages recommended by the manufacturer for MAC sedation, see Monitored Anesthesia Care Sedation under Dosage and Administration.

Monitored Anesthesia Care Sedation

Healthy Adults (Younger Than 65 Years of Age)

For initiation of MAC sedation in healthy adults younger than 65 years of age, a slow rate of IV infusion or slow IV injection is recommended to reduce the risk of apnea and hypotension. These patients usually require an initial propofol infusion of 100–150 mcg/kg per minute (6–9 mg/kg per hour) for 3–5 minutes or a slow injection of 0.5 mg/kg over 3–5 minutes immediately followed by a maintenance IV infusion. Initial propofol dosages of 100–150 mcg/kg per minute (administered over 3–5 minutes) usually are associated with a rapid onset of action (within 1–3 minutes) and recovery. If a procedure is longer than expected and a deeper level of anesthesia is required, an increase in the rate of infusion or administration of incremental rapid IV ("bolus") doses of the drug (titrated to effect) will result in an easy transition to general anesthesia.

The manufacturers state that a variable infusion rate is preferred to intermittent bolus administration for maintenance of MAC sedation in healthy adults to minimize undesirable cardiorespiratory effects. The usual initial IV maintenance dosage of propofol in this patient population is 25–75 mcg/kg per minute (1.5–4.5 mg/kg per hour) for the first 10–15 minutes and then it is decreased over time to a dosage of 25–50 mcg/kg per minute and adjusted to clinical response. When dosage is adjusted according to clinical effect, approximately 2 minutes should be allowed for onset of peak drug response. Alternatively, intermittent IV propofol injections of 10 or 20 mg may be administered; however, the possibility of developing respiratory depression or transient increases in sedation depth and/or prolongation of recovery should be considered.

Geriatric and Debilitated Patients

For initiation of MAC sedation in geriatric (65 years of age and older), debilitated, or ASA III or IV physical status patients, the manufacturers state that most patients require dosages similar to healthy adults Rapid boluses of propofol are to be avoided..

However, for maintenance of MAC sedation, the manufacturers recommend that the usual adult dosage of propofol be reduced by approximately 20% in geriatric, debilitated, ASA III or IV physical status, or neurosurgical patients according to the patient's condition, response, and vital signs. Rapid IV injection is *not* recommended in this patient population because of an increased risk of developing adverse cardiorespiratory effects.

Sedation in Critical Care Settings

Dosage of sedative agents should be titrated to the desired level of sedation; in most cases, a light rather than deep level of sedation is recommended in critically ill, mechanically ventilated adults because of improved clinical outcomes that have been demonstrated (e.g., shortened duration of mechanical ventilation, reduced ICU length of stay). The depth and quality of sedation should be assessed frequently using a validated and reliable assessment tool (e.g., Richmond Agitation-Sedation Scale [RASS], Sedation-Agitation Scale [SAS]).

For sedation in intubated and mechanically ventilated adults in the ICU, propofol should be initiated slowly with a continuous IV infusion to minimize

the risk of hypotension. Because most patients will have residual effects from previous anesthetic or sedative agents, the manufacturers recommend an initial infusion rate of 5 mcg/kg per minute (0.3 mg/kg per hour) for at least 5 minutes. The rate of infusion may be increased slowly in increments of 5–10 mcg/kg per minute (0.3–0.6 mg/kg per hour) until the desired level of sedation is achieved; a minimum period of 5 minutes should be allowed between dosage adjustments to assess clinical effects. Factors such as patient comorbidities, concomitant medications, age, ASA-physical status classification, and level of debilitation should be considered when determining an appropriate dosage of propofol for ICU sedation. In addition, the patient's clinical response, vital signs, and blood lipid profiles should be monitored and dosage should be adjusted accordingly. The usual maintenance infusion rate of propofol in adults is 5–50 mcg/kg per minute (0.3–3 mg/kg per hour); higher maintenance infusion rates occasionally may be required in some patients (e.g., patients who have recovered from general anesthesia or deep sedation), but the manufacturers state that the infusion rate should not exceed 4 mg/kg per hour unless the benefits outweigh the risks. Infusion rates greater than 4 mg/kg per hour have been associated with propofol infusion syndrome. (See Propofol Infusion Syndrome under Cautions.) Rapid IV ("bolus") administration of 10- or 20-mg doses of propofol may be used to rapidly increase depth of sedation in patients in whom development of hypotension is unlikely. Patients with impaired myocardial function, intravascular volume depletion, or abnormally low vascular tone (sepsis) may be more susceptible to hypotension. Assessment of the level of sedation and CNS function should be performed at regular intervals (at least daily during maintenance sedation) and the IV infusion rate should be adjusted accordingly. Abrupt discontinuation of propofol prior to weaning or for daily evaluation of sedation levels should be avoided.

Because certain propofol injectable emulsion formulations (i.e., Diprivan®) contain edetate disodium, a heavy metal antagonist, patients receiving continuous IV infusions for sedation in critical care settings should not receive this formulation for longer than 5 days without a drug-free interval, to allow replacement of estimated or measured urinary zinc losses.

During long-term therapy (exceeding 7 days), some tolerance to the sedative effects of the drug may occur requiring an increase in the infusion rate. It has been suggested, however, that such effects may be associated with changes in drug elimination or an improved health status of the patient.

Other Uses

For the management of patients with refractory status epilepticus†, 1- to 2-mg/kg doses of propofol have been administered initially by IV injection, over 5 minutes, which were repeated when seizure activity was no longer adequately controlled. In these patients, the rate of the IV maintenance infusion was adjusted to 2–10 mg/kg per hour until the lowest rate of infusion needed to suppress epileptiform activity was achieved; dosage was then decreased gradually to prevent withdrawal seizures.

Propofol has been administered in subhypnotic (10- to 15-mg) doses for the management of postoperative nausea and vomiting†. In addition, propofol, administered as a continuous IV infusion at a rate of 1 mg/kg per hour, also has been used for the prevention of nausea and vomiting associated with emetogenic cancer chemotherapy†.

For relief of pruritus associated with use of spinal opiates or cholestasis†, subhypnotic propofol doses given by direct IV injection (10 or 15 mg, respectively) or by IV infusion (at a rate of 0.5–1 or 1–1.5 mg/kg per hour, respectively) have been used.

● Special Populations

Hepatic Impairment

The manufacturer makes no specific dosage recommendations for patients with hepatic impairment.

Renal Impairment

The manufacturer makes no specific dosage recommendations for patients with renal impairment.

Geriatric Patients

Lower doses are recommended for initiation and maintenance of sedation and anesthesia in geriatric patients.

CAUTIONS

● *Contraindications*

● Known hypersensitivity to propofol or any ingredient in the formulation.

● Known hypersensitivity to eggs, egg products, soybeans, or soy products.

● *Warnings/Precautions*

Anaphylactic and Anaphylactoid Reactions

Propofol has been associated with fatal and life-threatening anaphylactic and anaphylactoid reactions.

Sulfite Sensitivity

Some commercially available formulations of propofol contain a sulfite that may cause allergic-type reactions, including anaphylaxis and life-threatening or less severe asthmatic episodes, in certain susceptible individuals. The overall prevalence of sulfite sensitivity in the general population is unknown but probably low; such sensitivity appears to occur more frequently in asthmatic than in nonasthmatic individuals.

Potential for Microbial Contamination

Propofol is commercially available in a lipid-based formulation that has been found to support rapid microbial growth at room temperature. Although currently available formulations contain an agent to retard the growth of microorganisms, they are not considered antimicrobially preserved products by USP standards. Contamination of propofol even with very small numbers of microorganisms may result in clinical disease. Therefore, strict aseptic technique and strict adherence to the manufacturer's preparation and handling instructions are required. When proper aseptic technique has not been used in handling propofol injectable emulsion, microbial contamination of the injection and consequent development of fever, infection, sepsis, other life-threatening illness, or death has occurred; in addition, transmission of bloodborne pathogens (e.g., hepatitis B, hepatitis C, human immunodeficiency virus [HIV]) has been reported as a result of unsafe injection practices and use of single-use propofol vials on multiple patients.

Several propofol-related infectious disease outbreaks have been reported worldwide following initial marketing of the drug. The outbreaks were associated with the use of propofol for a diverse range of procedures in various settings and determined to be caused mainly by extrinsic microbial contamination secondary to improper handling and use. Several practices were identified that were thought to contribute to this contamination: preparation of multiple syringes of propofol at one time for use throughout the day; reuse of vials, syringes, and/or infusion-pump lines on different patients; use of propofol syringes that had been prepared up to 24 hours in advance; failure to wear sterile gloves during handling of propofol; failure to disinfect the rubber stopper of propofol vials prior to use; use of opened vials for longer than recommended by the manufacturer; and transfer of prepared syringes of propofol between operating rooms or facilities.

The frequency of reports of infection declined substantially after an agent to retard microbial growth was added to propofol vials and after the prescribing information was revised to include warnings to use strict aseptic technique, adhere to requirements to use a vial or syringe for a single patient only, begin administration immediately after opening the vial or syringe, and discard unused product within specified time limits. Propofol formulations containing 0.005% disodium edetate, 1.5 mg/mL benzyl alcohol and 0.7 mg/mL sodium benzoate, or 0.25 mg/mL sodium metabisulfite can inhibit microbial growth for up to 12 hours as demonstrated by test data for representative USP organisms; however, strict aseptic technique and adherence to handling guidelines still are necessary to avoid the risk of infection.

Propofol injectable emulsion should not be used if contamination is suspected, and unused portions should be discarded within the required time limits as recommended by the manufacturers. Failure to follow proper aseptic technique has resulted in microbial contamination of the propofol injection and consequent development of fever, infection, sepsis, other life-threatening illness, or death.

Respiratory and Cardiovascular Effects

Propofol is a respiratory depressant; apnea and airway obstruction can occur, especially following rapid bolus injection and/or administration of larger doses such as those used for induction of anesthesia. In clinical trials in adults receiving propofol for induction of anesthesia, duration of apnea was less than 30, 30–60, and more than 60 seconds in 7, 24, and 12% of patients, respectively. In clinical trials in pediatric patients (neonates and children 16 years of age and younger) receiving 1- to 3.6-mg/kg doses of rapid IV propofol injections for induction of anesthesia, duration of apnea was less than 30, 30–60, and more than 60 seconds in 12, 10, and 5% of patients, respectively. The respiratory depressant effects of propofol appear to be similar to those of other IV induction anesthetics; however, the incidence and duration of apnea associated with propofol may be greater. During maintenance of general anesthesia, propofol causes a decrease in spontaneous minute ventilation, usually associated with increased carbon dioxide tension ($PaCO_2$), the likelihood of which depends on the rate of administration of propofol and other concomitantly used drugs (e.g., opiates, sedatives). Although the respiratory depressant effects of propofol are not clinically important during mechanical ventilation, such effects may be important during the weaning process.

Propofol is a cardiovascular depressant with effects similar to or greater than those associated with other IV anesthetic induction agents. The main adverse cardiovascular effect of propofol is hypotension, with decreases of 30% or more in both systolic and diastolic blood pressure observed following an induction dose. This effect is principally a result of arterial vasodilation due to reduced vascular sympathetic tone. Propofol-induced hypotension is more pronounced at higher plasma concentrations of the drug such as those achieved during induction of anesthesia. Concomitant use of propofol with other drugs such as opiate agonists, benzodiazepines, antihypertensives, and beta-adrenergic blocking agents also may increase the risk of severe hypotension. Administration of additional fluids and a cautious rate of IV infusion may help to prevent propofol-induced hypotension. Severe hypotensive effects may be alleviated by medical intervention.

Although propofol has no vagolytic activity, cases of bradycardia, asystole, and rarely, cardiac arrest have been reported, especially in pediatric patients who received concomitant administration with fentanyl. Administration of IV anticholinergic agents (e.g., atropine, glycopyrrolate) should be considered to modify potential increases in vagal tone associated with surgical stimuli or concomitant use of certain drugs, including succinylcholine. Apnea, which may persist for more than 60 seconds, occurs frequently during induction of anesthesia and ventilatory support should be considered.

Because propofol may produce cardiovascular depression, patients receiving the drug should be monitored for early signs of hypotension and bradycardia. Patients also should be monitored for adverse respiratory effects (e.g., apnea, airway obstruction, and/or oxygen desaturation), especially those undergoing MAC sedation. These cardiorespiratory effects are more likely to occur following administration of rapid IV ("bolus") injections, especially in patients with American Society of Anesthesiologists (ASA) physical status III or IV, and in geriatric or debilitated patients. Therefore, such patients should receive lower induction doses and slower maintenance infusion rates than other patients.

Seizures

Propofol appears to be associated with both anticonvulsant activity and excitatory effects on the nervous system. Propofol has been used effectively in patients with refractory status epilepticus, and the drug may substantially decrease seizures associated with electroconvulsive therapy (ECT). However, propofol also has been associated with a variety of excitatory effects (e.g., seizures, myoclonus, opisthotonos) on the nervous system, possibly resulting from glycine antagonism at subcortical sites.

Patients with a history of seizure disorders who are receiving propofol are at increased risk of developing seizures during the recovery phase of anesthesia.

Neurosurgical Anesthesia

When propofol is used for anesthesia in patients with increased intracranial pressure or impaired cerebral circulation who are undergoing neurosurgery, substantial decreases in mean arterial pressure should be avoided because of the resultant decreases in cerebral perfusion pressure. To avoid substantial hypotension and decreases in cerebral perfusion pressure, propofol should be administered IV by an infusion or a slow injection.

If increased intracranial pressure is suspected, administer in combination with hyperventilation and hypocarbia.

Cardiac Anesthesia

Slower rates of IV administration should be used during cardiac anesthesia in patients undergoing cardiac surgery who received premedication, geriatric patients, and those with recent fluid imbalance or hemodynamic instability. Correct fluid depletion prior to administration of propofol.

If additional fluid therapy is contraindicated, management of hypotension may include discontinuance of propofol, elevation of the lower extremities, and/or use of vasopressors.

Propofol has been studied extensively in patients with coronary artery disease and in patients with hemodynamically significant valvular or congenital heart disease. No significant safety issues or changes to the induction of anesthesia is generally required for these patients; dosing should be titrated based on depth of anesthesia.

Critical Care Sedation

Failure to reduce the infusion rate in patients receiving propofol for extended periods may result in excessively high blood concentrations of the drug; therefore, titration to clinical response and daily evaluation of sedation levels are important when propofol is used for ICU sedation, especially for long durations. Evaluate sedation levels at least daily.

Prior to weaning patients from mechanical ventilator assistance, discontinue neuromuscular blocking agents or reverse neuromuscular blockade and discontinue opiate therapy or adjust the dosage to optimize respiratory function and/or to maintain a light level of sedation. If respiratory depression does not develop, maintain this level of sedation during the weaning process since abrupt withdrawal has been associated with rapid awakening accompanied by anxiety, agitation, and resistance to mechanical ventilation, thus making the weaning process difficult. Therefore, the manufacturers recommend that administration of propofol be continued to produce a light level of sedation until about 10–15 minutes prior to extubation.

Propofol Infusion Syndrome

Propofol infusion syndrome, a potentially life-threatening constellation of metabolic derangements and organ system failures, has been reported in adult and pediatric patients receiving propofol for ICU sedation. The syndrome, characterized by severe metabolic acidosis, hyperkalemia, lipidemia, rhabdomyolysis, hepatomegaly, and cardiac, renal, or circulatory failure, has occurred most frequently in patients receiving prolonged, high-dose infusions of propofol (greater than 5 mg/kg per hour for more than 48 hours) or high dosages of vasoconstrictors, corticosteroids, or inotropes; however, the syndrome also has occurred following short-term, high-dose infusions during surgical anesthesia. Other risk factors include decreased oxygen delivery to tissues, serious neurological injury, and sepsis.

Patients should be closely monitored for development of unexplained acidosis, rhabdomyolysis, and cardiac and/or renal failure. The manufacturers state that alternate means of sedation should be considered in the setting of prolonged need for sedation, increasing propofol dosage requirements to maintain a constant level of sedation, or onset of metabolic acidosis during propofol infusion.

Effects on Lipids

Because commercially available propofol preparations are oil-in-water emulsions, the drug should be used with caution in patients with disorders of lipid metabolism (e.g., primary hyperlipoproteinemia, diabetic hyperlipemia, pancreatitis). Since prolonged administration of the drug may result in increased serum lipid concentrations (e.g., hypertriglyceridemia), patients undergoing sedation in a critical care setting (e.g., an ICU) who are at risk of developing hyperlipidemia should be monitored for increases in serum triglyceride concentrations or serum turbidity. The manufacturers state that the quantity of concurrently administered lipids (e.g., fat emulsions for parenteral nutrition) in these patients should be reduced in order to compensate for the amount of lipids contained in the propofol emulsion formulation (1 mL of propofol injectable emulsion contains 0.1 g of fat [1.1 kcal]).

Zinc Loss

Certain formulations of propofol injectable emulsion (Diprivan®) contain edetate disodium, which is a strong chelator of trace metals, including zinc. IV infusions of propofol should not be administered for longer than 5 days without a drug-free interval to replace urine zinc losses. This drug-free interval is intended to allow replacement of estimated or measured urinary zinc losses. In patients who are predisposed to zinc deficiency (e.g., those with burns, diarrhea, major sepsis), the need for supplemental zinc should be considered during prolonged therapy with edetate disodium-containing formulations of propofol. Although renal toxicity has been reported rarely in patients receiving high (2–3 g daily) dosages of edetate disodium, decreased renal function has not been observed in clinical studies conducted to date in patients with normal or impaired renal function receiving propofol (Diprivan®) injectable emulsion. However, the manufacturer of Diprivan® recommends that urinalysis and urine sediment should be checked prior to initiation of sedation and during (every other day) propofol therapy in patients at risk for developing renal impairment.

Use in Debilitated, Elderly, or ASA-PS III or IV Patients

A lower induction dose and a slower maintenance rate of administration should be used in elderly, debilitated, or ASA-PS III or IV patients. Patients should be continuously monitored for early signs of hypotension and/or bradycardia. Apnea requiring ventilatory support often occurs during induction and may persist for more than 60 seconds.

Local Effects

Pain at the injection site occurs frequently (in up to 70% of patients) following peripheral IV administration of propofol. Pain on injection occurred frequently in pediatric patients (45%) when a small vein of the hand was utilized without lidocaine pretreatment. Pain at the injection site can be minimized by using the larger veins of the forearm or antecubital fossa rather than hand veins and by administering lidocaine (either as a pretreatment or admixed with propofol). Because of the possibility that lidocaine may cause instability of the propofol emulsion, the manufacturers recommend that lidocaine be administered prior to propofol administration or that lidocaine be added to propofol immediately before administration in a quantity not exceeding 20 mg of lidocaine per 200 mg of propofol. For prevention of pain at the propofol injection site, other methods, including pretreatment with opiates or other analgesic agents and venous occlusion with a tourniquet may be beneficial.

Phlebitis or venous thrombosis has been reported. In addition, accidental intra-arterial injection has occurred; other than pain, there were no major sequelae. Local pain, swelling, blisters and/or tissue necrosis has been reported rarely following inadvertent extravasation in postmarketing surveillance of propofol. The manufacturers state that in clinical trials, burning, stinging, or pain at the injection site was reported in 17.6% of adults undergoing anesthesia or MAC sedation and in 10% of pediatric patients.

Aggregation if Administered through the Same IV Catheter with Blood or Plasma

Propofol should *not* be administered through the same catheter as blood or plasma because compatibility has not been established. In vitro tests have shown that aggregates of the globular component of the vehicle containing propofol may form when the drug is in contact with blood, serum, or plasma. The clinical importance of these effects is not known.

Postoperative Effects

Propofol has been associated rarely with a period of postoperative unconsciousness (sometimes preceded by a brief period of wakefulness), which may be accompanied by increased muscle tone; recovery has been spontaneous.

Perioperative Myoclonia

Perioperative myoclonia, rarely including convulsions and opisthotonos, has occurred in association with propofol administration.

Pulmonary Edema

Pulmonary edema has been reported rarely in temporal relationship to the administration of propofol, although a causal relationship has not been established.

Pancreatitis

Pancreatitis (sometimes requiring hospitalization) has been reported in patients undergoing induction of anesthesia or prolonged sedation with propofol in a critical care setting. A causal relationship with propofol has not been established.

Dependence, Tolerance, and Abuse

Cases of propofol abuse and dependence, in some cases resulting in death (following repeated *self-administration* of propofol by healthcare providers), have been reported. While most reported cases have involved healthcare professionals (primarily anesthesiology personnel), cases of propofol abuse among lay persons also have been reported.

Propofol currently is not subject to control under the Federal Controlled Substances Act of 1970; however, some clinicians have suggested that the drug should be subject to such control (or some other means of ensuring greater accountability).

Data regarding regulation of propofol by pharmacy departments in academic anesthesia programs indicate a greater prevalence of abuse and related deaths at locations where there was no established system to control or monitor propofol use. The manufacturers and some clinicians recommend that restriction of access and accounting procedures appropriate to the particular practice setting should be used to prevent diversion of propofol. Some clinicians also suggest routine testing of drug screenings for propofol in individuals considered to be at risk for abuse.

Specific Populations

Pregnancy

There are no adequate and controlled studies to date using propofol in pregnant women. Reproduction studies in rats and rabbits using IV propofol dosages of 15 mg/kg daily (approximately equivalent to the human propofol induction dose on a mg/m^2 basis) did not reveal any evidence of harm to the fetus, but decreased pup survival and increased postimplantation loss were observed.

Propofol readily crosses the placenta and similar to other general anesthetics, administration of propofol may be associated with neonatal depression. Limited data indicate that the ratio of umbilical vein to maternal vein concentration at parturition is about 0.7 after rapid IV ("bolus") administration of 2.5 mg/kg of propofol to women undergoing cesarean section. In one study, mean propofol concentrations of 0.078 mcg/mL were detected 2 hours after delivery in neonates whose mothers had received an IV propofol infusion of 5 mg/kg per hour for about 26 minutes while undergoing cesarean section. The manufacturers state that propofol is not recommended for obstetric surgery (e.g., cesarean section).

Based on animal data, repeated or prolonged use of general anesthetics and sedation drugs, including propofol, during the third trimester of pregnancy may result in adverse neurodevelopmental effects in the fetus. The clinical relevance of these animal findings to humans is not known; the potential risk of adverse neurodevelopmental effects should be considered and discussed with pregnant women undergoing procedures requiring general anesthetics and sedation drugs.

Lactation

Propofol reportedly is distributed into human milk. The manufacturers state that the drug should not be used in nursing women because the effects of oral absorption of small amounts of propofol are not known. Some clinicians state that nursing women undergoing surgery may receive usual anesthetic induction doses of propofol; however, since trace amounts of the drug may be present in milk, drowsiness of the infants may occur on the day of the procedure. It should be considered that in reproduction studies in rats and rabbits, IV propofol dosages (15 mg/kg daily) administered to dams during lactating periods have been shown to cause maternal deaths and decreased pup survival. It has been suggested that the pharmacologic effect (anesthesia) of propofol on the dams probably is responsible for the adverse effects observed in the offspring.

Females and Males of Reproductive Potential

Reproduction studies in female rats receiving IV propofol dosages up to 15 mg/kg daily (approximately equivalent to the human propofol induction dose on a mg/m^2 basis) for 2 weeks before pregnancy up to day 7 of gestation did not reveal evidence of impaired fertility. Impairment of male fertility was not observed in a dominant lethal study in rats receiving propofol dosages up to 15 mg/kg daily for 5 days.

Pediatric Use

The manufacturers state that the safety and efficacy of propofol for the induction of general anesthesia have not been established in pediatric patients younger than 3 years of age. For maintenance of general anesthesia, the manufacturers state that safety and efficacy of the drug have not been established in pediatric patients younger than 2 months of age. In addition, the manufacturers state that propofol is not recommended for ICU sedation, for use in combination with regional anesthesia, or for MAC sedation in pediatric patients younger than 16 years of age, because safety for these procedures in this patient population has not been established.

Propofol has been used in pediatric patients undergoing ICU sedation. Although a causal relationship to propofol has not been definitely established, case reports describe a severe, progressive metabolic (e.g., lactic) acidosis syndrome (that may progress to death) in several ventilated pediatric patients (mainly with respiratory infections) receiving propofol for ICU sedation. In some of these children, increasing metabolic acidosis was accompanied or followed by hypocalcemia, hypoglycemia, high serum lipid concentrations (hypertriglyceridemia), elevated serum liver enzyme concentrations, enlarged liver, oliguria, myoglobinuria, fever, multisystem organ failure, cardiac failure, bradycardia, hypotension, AV block of varying degrees, bundle branch block, asystole, and death. The mechanism of this syndrome is not known and the possibility that causes other than administration of propofol may be involved has been suggested.

Results of a multicenter, comparative, clinical trial in pediatric patients undergoing ICU sedation (excluding those with upper respiratory infection) indicate that the incidence of mortality was increased in those receiving propofol (9%) compared with those receiving standard sedative agents (4%). Although a causal relationship of such incidence of mortality to propofol has not been established, the manufacturer and FDA state that there may be important safety concerns associated with the use of propofol injectable emulsion in pediatric patients undergoing sedation in critical care settings. Therefore, propofol is *not* labeled and should not be employed for such use in children 16 years of age or younger.

Propofol also has been used in pediatric patients undergoing MAC sedation for surgical, diagnostic, and other procedures (e.g., lumbar puncture with intrathecal chemotherapy, bone marrow aspiration and biopsy, central venous catheter placement, transesophageal echocardiogram, cardiac catheterization, radiologic examinations, orthopedic manipulations). However, the manufacturers state that propofol should not be used for MAC sedation in pediatric patients, because safety and efficacy for such use have not been established.

In pediatric patients receiving prolonged IV infusions of propofol, abrupt discontinuance of the drug may result in flushing of the hands and feet, agitation, tremulousness, hyperirritability, increased incidence of bradycardia, agitation, or jitteriness.

FDA warns that repeated or prolonged use of general anesthetics and sedation drugs, including propofol, in children younger than 3 years of age or during the third trimester of pregnancy may affect brain development. Animal studies in multiple species, including nonhuman primates, have demonstrated that use for longer than 3 hours of anesthetic and sedation drugs that block N-methyl-D-aspartic acid (NMDA) receptors and/or potentiate γ-aminobutyric acid (GABA) activity leads to widespread neuronal and oligodendrocyte cell loss and alterations in synaptic morphology and neurogenesis in the brain, resulting in long-term deficits in cognition and behavior. Across animal species, vulnerability to these neurodevelopmental changes occurs during the period of rapid brain growth or synaptogenesis; this period is thought to correlate with the third trimester of pregnancy through the first year of life in humans, but may extend to approximately 3 years of age. The clinical relevance of these animal findings to humans is not known.

While some published evidence suggests that similar deficits in cognition and behavior may occur in children following repeated or prolonged exposure to anesthesia early in life, other studies have found no association between pediatric anesthesia exposure and long-term adverse neurodevelopmental outcomes. Most studies to date have had substantial limitations, and it is not clear whether the adverse neurodevelopmental outcomes observed in children were related to the drug or to other factors (e.g., surgery, underlying illness). There is some clinical evidence that a single, relatively brief exposure to general anesthesia in generally healthy children is unlikely to cause clinically detectable deficits in global cognitive function or serious behavioral disorders; however, further research is needed to fully characterize the effects of exposure to general anesthetics in early life, particularly for prolonged or repeated exposures and in more vulnerable populations (e.g., less healthy children).

Results from an observational study (the Pediatric Anesthesia Neurodevelopment Assessment [PANDA] study) and preliminary results from an ongoing multicenter, randomized trial (the General Anesthesia Compared to Spinal Anesthesia [GAS] trial) provide some evidence that a single, relatively brief exposure to general anesthesia in generally healthy children is unlikely to cause clinically detectable deficits in global cognitive function or serious behavioral disorders. The PANDA study compared global cognitive function (as measured by intelligence quotient [IQ] score) of children 8–15 years of age who had a single anesthesia exposure for elective inguinal hernia surgery before the age of 3 years with that of a biologically related sibling who had no anesthesia exposure before the age of 3 years. All of the children had a gestational age at birth of at least 36 weeks, and sibling pairs were within 3 years of being the same age. Children who underwent the elective procedure were mostly males (90%) and generally healthy. The mean duration of anesthesia was 84 minutes; 16% of those receiving anesthesia had exposures exceeding 2 hours. The study found no substantial difference in IQ score between children who had a single anesthesia exposure before the age of 3 years and their siblings who had not. The GAS trial was designed to compare neurodevelopmental outcomes in children who received general anesthesia with those in children who received awake regional (caudal and/or spinal) anesthesia for inguinal herniorrhaphy before they reached a postmenstrual age of 60 weeks (with a gestational age at birth of more than 26 weeks); the primary outcome was the Wechsler Preschool and Primary Scale of Intelligence Third Edition (WPPSI-III) Full Scale IQ at 5 years of age. In an interim analysis at the age of 2 years, no difference in composite cognitive score (as measured by the Bayley Scales of Infant and Toddler Development III) was detected between children who had received sevoflurane anesthesia of less than 1 hour's duration (median duration: 54 minutes) compared with those who had received awake regional anesthesia.

Anesthetic and sedation drugs are an essential component of care for children and pregnant women who require surgery or other procedures that cannot be delayed; no specific general anesthetic or sedation drug has been shown to be less likely to cause neurocognitive deficits than any other such drug. Pending further accumulation of data in humans from well-designed studies, decisions regarding the timing of elective procedures requiring anesthesia should take into consideration both the benefits of the procedure and the potential risks. When procedures requiring the use of general anesthetics or sedation drugs are considered for young children or pregnant women, clinicians should discuss with the patient, parent, or caregiver the benefits, risks (including potential risk of adverse neurodevelopmental effects), and appropriate timing and duration of the procedure. FDA states that procedures that are considered medically necessary should not be delayed or avoided.

Geriatric Use

Studies in geriatric patients have shown that these patients may require lower dosages of propofol for anesthesia and other indications. The manufacturers state that lower induction doses and a slower rate of maintenance IV infusion should be used in patients 55 years of age and older. In addition, to minimize the risk of adverse effects, including cardiorespiratory depression (e.g., hypotension), apnea, airway obstruction, and/or arterial oxygen desaturation, rapid (single or repeated) IV ("bolus") administration of propofol should not be used in geriatric patients during general anesthesia or MAC sedation.

Hepatic Impairment

Long-term propofol therapy in patients with hepatic insufficiency has not been evaluated to date. The pharmacokinetics of propofol do not appear to be altered in patients with chronic hepatic impairment; the effects of acute hepatic failure on the pharmacokinetics of the drug have not been studied.

Renal Impairment

Long-term propofol therapy in patients with renal failure has not been evaluated to date. The pharmacokinetics of propofol do not appear to be altered in patients with chronic renal impairment; the effects of acute renal failure on the pharmacokinetics of the drug have not been studied.

● Common Adverse Effects

The most common adverse reactions (>1%) reported with propofol were bradycardia, arrhythmia, tachycardia, hypotension, hypertension, decreased cardiac output, movement, apnea, respiratory acidosis during weaning, rash, pruritus, burning/stinging or pain at injection site, and hyperlipemia.

In adults, the adverse effect profile in patients undergoing monitored anesthesia care (MAC) sedation was similar to that of patients undergoing anesthesia, although more severe adverse respiratory effects (e.g., cough, upper airway obstruction, apnea, hypoventilation, dyspnea) were reported in those undergoing MAC sedation. In addition, the adverse effect profile in pediatric patients 6 days to 16 years of age undergoing anesthesia was similar to that of adults receiving propofol for anesthesia, although apnea may occur more frequently in children than in adults.

DRUG INTERACTIONS

● Drugs Affecting Hepatic Microsomal Enzymes

In vitro data indicate that propofol is metabolized mainly by cytochrome P-450 (CYP) isoenzyme 2B6 and to a lesser extent by 2C9. In addition, results of in vitro studies indicate that propofol is an inhibitor of the CYP isoenzymes 1A1, 1A2, 2B1, 2C9, 2D6, 2E1, and 3A4, and the possibility exists that propofol may alter the pharmacokinetics of drugs metabolized by these isoenzymes. However, it has been suggested that because of the increased value for hepatic extraction (50 μM) of propofol, there have been relatively few clinically important drug interactions mediated by the cytochrome P-450 system.

Concomitant use of propofol with alfentanil in healthy young men reportedly has resulted in increased (up to 22%) blood concentrations of propofol. Limited data indicate that concomitant use of propofol with opiate agonists (e.g., alfentanil, fentanyl, sufentanil) may result in increased (10–20%) blood concentrations of the opiates. These effects presumably occur via inhibition of CYP isoenzymes involved in the metabolism of propofol and the opiates. However, alfentanil also may reduce both distribution and clearance of propofol. Although these variations in blood concentrations of propofol and opiates are unlikely to be clinically important, concomitant use of propofol with opiates has resulted in greater sedation and analgesia than those associated with administration of each drug alone.

● CNS Depressants

Concomitant use of propofol with other CNS depressants including sedatives (e.g., benzodiazepines), hypnotics (e.g., opiates), and inhalation anesthetics (e.g., nitrous oxide, isoflurane) may increase the sedative, anesthetic, and cardiorespiratory depressant effects of propofol. Increased serum concentrations of propofol have been reported with concomitant use of propofol and inhalation anesthetics possibly associated with decreased hepatic blood flow that may result in decreased clearance of propofol. Therefore, the manufacturers state that the induction dose requirements of propofol may need to be reduced in patients receiving premedication with IV or IM opiates (e.g., meperidine, morphine, fentanyl) or in those receiving a combination of opiates with sedatives (e.g., benzodiazepines, barbiturates, chloral hydrate, droperidol). In addition, during maintenance of anesthesia or sedation, IV infusion rates of propofol may need to be reduced with concomitant use of CNS depressants.

Limited data suggest that IV propofol may act synergistically with IV midazolam to produce induction of anesthesia and sedation (e.g., in an ICU). It has been postulated that the synergism observed between propofol and midazolam is the result of a pharmacodynamic interaction occurring at the $GABA_A$ receptors in the brain. In addition, concomitant use of propofol and midazolam resulted in increased (by about 20%) mean free plasma concentration of midazolam, although mean free concentrations of propofol did not appear to be affected.

In pediatric patients, concomitant use of propofol with fentanyl may result in severe bradycardia.

● Neuromuscular Blocking Agents

Propofol does not appear to cause clinically important changes in the onset, intensity, or duration of action of commonly used neuromuscular blocking agents (e.g., succinylcholine, nondepolarizing skeletal muscle relaxants).

● Anticoagulants

Limited data indicate that IV administration of lipids (e.g., those contained in the propofol injectable emulsion) may decrease patient response to warfarin in patients with malabsorptive states secondary to disease (e.g., those with Crohn's disease). The mechanism of such an interaction has not been elucidated, but lipid emulsions may interfere pharmacodynamically with warfarin activity by increasing synthesis of functional blood coagulation factors, increasing platelet aggregation, or supplying vitamin K. It is recommended that until further studies are available to evaluate this interaction, heparin therapy should be administered for initial anticoagulation in patients with malabsorptive states receiving high-dose lipid emulsions who require reliable anticoagulation. If warfarin is given, international normalized ratio (INR) should be monitored daily in these patients.

● Other Drugs

In one study, concomitant use of droperidol with propofol was found to increase twofold the frequency of postoperative incidence of nausea and vomiting associated with administration of propofol alone, suggesting a potential interaction between the drugs.

DESCRIPTION

Propofol is an IV anesthetic agent that is structurally unrelated to other currently available IV anesthetics.

The exact mechanism(s) by which propofol exerts its effect on the CNS has not been fully elucidated. However, it is believed that such effects are related, at least partially, to the drug's ability to enhance the activity of γ-aminobutyric acid (GABA), the principal inhibitory neurotransmitter in the CNS, by interacting with the $GABA_A$ receptor complex both at spinal and supraspinal synapses. There is evidence that the drug enhances GABA-mediated transmission at a site distinct from benzodiazepine receptors and such activity may vary depending on plasma propofol concentrations. Propofol also may interact with other neurotransmitter sites (e.g., nicotinic, glutamate, G-protein coupled receptors) and inhibit sodium channels.

Propofol is capable of producing all levels of CNS depression—from light sleep to deep coma—depending on the dosage. The degree of depression and duration of action depend on dosage, rate of administration, and pharmacokinetics of the drug. In addition, the patient's age, weight, medical condition, type of surgical procedure, and/or concurrent use of other drugs may alter the response. Following IV injection, propofol has a rapid onset of action and will produce a loss of consciousness within 1 arm-brain circulation time (the time required for the drug to travel from the site of injection to the site of action in the brain) (i.e., usually within 40–60 seconds).

The analgesic effects of propofol have not been conclusively determined. Limited data indicate that hypnotic doses of propofol may be associated with analgesic effects, while responses to subhypnotic doses of the drug may vary from analgesia to hyperalgesia. Propofol also may be associated with some level of amnesia; however, the drug has lesser amnesic effects than the benzodiazepines. Limited data indicate that subhypnotic doses of propofol may be associated with anxiolytic effects comparable to those of midazolam or methohexital.

The pharmacokinetics of propofol after IV administration are best described by a 3-compartment model and appear to be linear. The drug's pharmacokinetic profile is characterized by rapid distribution from blood into tissues, rapid metabolic clearance from blood, and slow redistribution from the peripheral compartment. The pharmacokinetics of propofol have been studied in adults and in pediatric patients 3–12 years of age. Distribution and clearance of propofol in pediatric patients are similar to those reported in adults. There is no evidence of gender-related differences in the pharmacokinetics of the drug.

Following a single (e.g., 2.5 mg/kg) IV injection, propofol has a rapid onset because the drug is distributed rapidly from plasma to the CNS. The onset of action of propofol as determined by time to unconsciousness (i.e., loss of response to voice command) usually ranges from 15–30 seconds, and depends on the rate of administration. Following a single rapid IV injection, propofol blood concentrations decline so rapidly that peak plasma concentrations cannot be readily measured; duration of action of the drug usually is about 5–10 minutes. Following initiation of a continuous IV infusion of propofol, there is an initial rapid increase in blood concentrations of the drug, followed by a slower rate of increase, probably associated with a rapid distribution from the blood to tissues. Since propofol is rapidly distributed from CNS to inactive storage sites, recovery from anesthesia is rapid. Following daily titration of propofol to achieve only the minimum effective therapeutic concentration, rapid awakening within 10–15 minutes may occur even after long-term administration. However, if higher than necessary infusion rates have been maintained for a long time, redistribution of propofol from fat and muscle to the plasma may be substantial resulting in slow recovery. Recovery from anesthesia may be more rapid following administration of propofol than barbiturates (e.g., thiopental [no longer commercially available in the US], methohexital) or possibly, etomidate.

Propofol is highly lipophilic and is rapidly distributed from plasma into human body tissues, including the CNS. Following IV administration, the drug is widely distributed, initially to highly perfused tissues (e.g., brain), then to lean muscle tissue, and finally to fat tissue. In humans, equilibration of propofol between blood and CSF occurs within about 2–3 minutes. F Volume of distribution of propofol may be reduced in geriatric patients when compared with younger individuals, perhaps because of a reduction in the volume of highly perfused tissues relative to body mass or a reduction in perfusion of these tissues associated with decreased cardiac output. Propofol is approximately 95–99% bound to plasma proteins, mainly albumin and hemoglobin. Protein binding appears to be independent of the plasma concentration of the drug. Propofol readily crosses the placenta and is distributed into human milk in low concentrations.

Plasma concentrations of propofol decline in a triphasic manner, with a very rapid initial distribution. In adults receiving IV propofol either as a single rapid injection or a continuous infusion, in the initial (distribution) phase ($t_{\frac{1}{2}\alpha}$) reportedly averages 1.8–9.5 minutes, in the second (redistribution) phase ($t_{\frac{1}{2}\beta}$) averages 21–70 minutes, and in the terminal (elimination) phase ($t_{\frac{1}{2}\gamma}$) averages 1.5–31 hours. The terminal plasma half-life may not affect clinical outcome as substantially as the distribution half-life, because once blood propofol concentrations decrease below the range required for hypnosis, rapid awakening from anesthesia will occur. Propofol is rapidly and extensively metabolized in the liver. The drug mainly undergoes glucuronidation, but hydroxylation also may occur to form 4-hydroxypropofol which is subsequently conjugated with sulfuric and/or glucuronic acid. Hydroxypropofol has been reported to have approximately (1/3) of the hypnotic activity of propofol. Hydroxylation of propofol is mediated by the cytochrome P-450 (CYP) isoenzyme 2B6 and to a lesser extent by the 2C9 isoenzyme. Propofol is excreted mainly in the urine principally as sulfate and/or glucuronide conjugates; less than 0.3% of the drug is eliminated unchanged in the urine. Limited data indicate that less than 2% of a dose of propofol is eliminated in feces. Total body clearance of propofol may be substantially lower in geriatric patients compared with younger adults, possibly because of decreased hepatic metabolism resulting from decreased hepatic blood flow. The drug also appears to be metabolized at extrahepatic sites. Mean total body clearance of propofol appears to be proportional to body weight; obese patients have a substantially higher body clearance than leaner individuals.

ADVICE TO PATIENTS

- Inform patients that their ability to perform activities requiring mental alertness (e.g., driving, operating machinery, signing legal documents) may be impaired for some time after undergoing general anesthesia or sedation.

- When procedures requiring general anesthetics or sedation drugs, including propofol, are considered for young children or pregnant women, importance of discussing with the patient, parent, or caregiver the benefits, risks (including potential risk of adverse neurodevelopmental effects), and appropriate timing and duration of the procedure.

- Advise patients to inform their clinicians of existing or contemplated concomitant therapy, including prescription and OTC drugs, as well as any concomitant illnesses.

- Advise women to inform their clinicians if they are or plan to become pregnant or plan to breast-feed.

- Inform patients of other important precautionary information.

PREPARATIONS

Excipients in commercially available drug preparations may have clinically important effects in some individuals; consult specific product labeling for details.

Propofol

Parenteral

Injectable emulsion, **for IV use**	10 mg/mL*	**Diprivan® Emulsion** (available as ready-to-use single patient vials), Fresenius Kabi **Propofol Injectable Emulsion**

* available from one or more manufacturer, distributor, and/or repackager by generic (nonproprietary) name

† Use is not currently included in the labeling approved by the US Food and Drug Administration.

Selected Revisions June 10, 2024, © Copyright, January 1, 2003, American Society of Health-System Pharmacists, Inc.

Diclofenac Sodium, Diclofenac Potassium, Diclofenac Epolamine

28:08.04.04 • REVERSIBLE COX-1/COX-2 INHIBITORS

■ Diclofenac is a prototypical nonsteroidal anti-inflammatory agent (NSAIA) that also exhibits analgesic and antipyretic activity.

USES

● *Inflammatory Diseases*

Diclofenac sodium and diclofenac potassium are used orally for anti-inflammatory and analgesic effects in the symptomatic treatment of rheumatoid arthritis, osteoarthritis, ankylosing spondylitis, and other inflammatory conditions.

Diclofenac sodium in fixed combination with misoprostol is used orally for anti-inflammatory activity and analgesic effects in the symptomatic treatment of rheumatoid arthritis and osteoarthritis in patients at high risk of developing NSAIA-induced gastric or duodenal ulcers and in patients at high risk of developing complications from these ulcers.

Diclofenac sodium 1% gel and diclofenac sodium 1.5 or 2% topical solution are used topically for the symptomatic treatment of osteoarthritis-related joint pain. The gel is used for joints amenable to topical therapy (e.g., hands, wrists, elbows, knees, ankles, feet); the gel has not been evaluated for use on joints of the spine, hip, or shoulder. The topical solution is used for symptoms (e.g., pain) affecting the knees.

The potential benefits and risks of diclofenac therapy as well as alternative therapies should be considered prior to initiating diclofenac therapy. The lowest possible effective dosage and shortest duration of therapy consistent with treatment goals of the patient should be employed.

Rheumatoid Arthritis and Osteoarthritis

When used in the symptomatic treatment of rheumatoid arthritis, oral diclofenac has relieved pain and stiffness; reduced swelling, tenderness, and the number of joints involved; and improved mobility and grip strength. In the symptomatic treatment of osteoarthritis, diclofenac has relieved pain and stiffness, improved knee joint function, and increased range of motion and functional activity. Diclofenac appears to be only palliative in these conditions and has not been shown to permanently arrest or reverse the underlying disease process.

Most clinical studies have shown that the anti-inflammatory and analgesic effects of usual oral dosages of diclofenac sodium in the management of rheumatoid arthritis or osteoarthritis are greater than those of placebo and about equal to those of usual dosages of salicylates, diflunisal, ibuprofen, indomethacin, ketoprofen, mefenamic acid, naproxen, phenylbutazone (no longer commercially available in the US), piroxicam, or sulindac. In controlled clinical studies of 3 months' duration in patients with rheumatoid arthritis or osteoarthritis, diclofenac sodium dosages of 100–200 mg daily, given as delayed-release (enteric-coated) tablets, were as effective as 2.4–4.8 g of aspirin daily, 500 mg of naproxen daily, or 2.4 g of ibuprofen daily. Patient response to oral NSAIAs is variable; patients who do not respond to or cannot tolerate one NSAIA might be successfully treated with a different agent. However, NSAIAs are generally contraindicated in patients in whom sensitivity reactions (e.g., urticaria, bronchospasm, severe rhinitis) are precipitated by aspirin or other NSAIAs. (See Contraindications under Cautions.)

In the management of rheumatoid arthritis in adults, NSAIAs may be useful for initial symptomatic treatment; however, NSAIAs do not alter the course of the disease or prevent joint destruction. Disease-modifying antirheumatic drugs (DMARDs) (e.g., abatacept, hydroxychloroquine, leflunomide, methotrexate, rituximab, sulfasalazine, tocilizumab, tofacitinib, tumor necrosis factor [TNF; TNF-α] blocking agents) have the potential to reduce or prevent joint damage and to preserve joint integrity and function. DMARD therapy should be initiated early in the disease course to prevent irreversible joint damage. (For further information on the treatment of rheumatoid arthritis, including considerations in selecting a DMARD regimen, see Uses: Rheumatoid Arthritis, in Methotrexate 10:00.)

Medical management of osteoarthritis of the hip, knee, and/or hand includes both pharmacologic therapy and nonpharmacologic (e.g., educational, behavioral, psychosocial, physical) interventions to reduce pain, maintain and/or improve joint mobility, limit functional impairment, and enhance overall well-being. The American College of Rheumatology (ACR) strongly recommends exercise, weight loss when necessary in patients with osteoarthritis of the knee and/or hip, self-efficacy and self-management programs, tai chi, cane use, hand orthoses, knee bracing, topical NSAIAs for osteoarthritis of the knee, oral NSAIAs, and intra-articular glucocorticoid injections for osteoarthritis of the knee or hip. Other pharmacologic or nonpharmacologic interventions may be recommended conditionally. Interventions and the order of their selection are patient specific. Factors to consider when making decisions regarding therapy for osteoarthritis include patients' values and preferences, the presence of risk factors for serious adverse GI effects, existing comorbidities (e.g., hypertension, heart failure, other cardiovascular disease, chronic kidney disease), injuries, disease severity, surgical history, and access to and availability of the interventions. Pharmacologic therapy should be initiated with treatments resulting in the least systemic exposure or toxicity. For some patients with limited disease, topical NSAIAs may be an appropriate initial choice for pharmacologic therapy; for other patients, particularly those with osteoarthritis of the hip or with polyarticular involvement, oral NSAIAs may be more appropriate.

When used for the symptomatic treatment of osteoarthritis of the hand or knee, diclofenac sodium 1% gel has been more effective than vehicle (placebo) in relieving pain; however, results of clinical trials evaluating the formulation suggest that its analgesic effects may be modest.

When used for the symptomatic treatment of osteoarthritis of the knee, diclofenac sodium 1.5% topical solution (formulated with dimethyl sulfoxide [DMSO] 45.5%) has been more effective than placebo (containing DMSO 2.3%) and/or vehicle (containing DMSO 45.5%) in relieving pain, improving physical function, and resulting in clinical improvement as measured by a patient global or overall health assessment tool. When used for the symptomatic treatment of pain associated with osteoarthritis of the knee, diclofenac sodium 2% topical solution has been more effective than vehicle (placebo) in relieving pain.

Ankylosing Spondylitis

In the symptomatic treatment of ankylosing spondylitis, oral diclofenac appears to provide relief of spinal pain, tenderness and/or spasm, morning stiffness, and pain at rest (including night pain) and to improve motion, posture, chest expansion, and spinal mobility. The anti-inflammatory and analgesic effects of usual dosages of diclofenac in the management of ankylosing spondylitis are about equal to those of usual dosages of indomethacin or sulindac. In a controlled clinical study in patients with ankylosing spondylitis, diclofenac sodium dosages of 75–125 mg daily, given as delayed-release (enteric-coated) tablets, were as effective as indomethacin 75–125 mg daily.

Juvenile Arthritis

Diclofenac has been used orally with good results in a number of children for the management of juvenile rheumatoid arthritis†. Results of these studies suggest that usual dosages of the drug are more effective than placebo and at least as effective as usual dosages of salicylates, naproxen, or tolmetin in decreasing the number of painful, swollen, and tender joints. Further studies are needed to evaluate the efficacy and safety of diclofenac in the management of juvenile rheumatoid arthritis. (See Pediatric Precautions under Cautions.)

Other Inflammatory Conditions

Oral diclofenac has been effective in a limited number of patients for the symptomatic relief of acute gouty arthritis†. The drug does not appear to correct hyperuricemia but has been used instead for its anti-inflammatory and analgesic effects to relieve pain, joint tenderness, and swelling associated with this condition.

Oral diclofenac also has been used for the symptomatic treatment of acute painful shoulder† (bursitis and/or tendinitis), sciatic pain†, backache†, myositis†, and radiohumeral bursitis† (radiohumeral epicondylitis, tennis elbow). The drug has been injected locally† (a parenteral dosage form currently is not commercially available in the US) for the relief of myofascial pain† in a limited number of patients with fibrositis, but additional study is necessary.

Oral or topical diclofenac has been used for the symptomatic treatment of infusion-related superficial thrombophlebitis†. In a controlled clinical trial in a limited number of patients, symptoms of thrombophlebitis improved in 60% of patients receiving diclofenac either orally (75 mg every 12 hours) or topically (as a gel applied to affected area every 8 hours) for 48 hours compared with 20% of those receiving placebo.

● *Pain*

Diclofenac potassium is used orally for symptomatic relief of mild to moderate acute pain, postoperative pain (including that associated with orthopedic, gynecologic, and oral surgery), and orthopedic pain (including musculoskeletal sprains and traumatic joint distortions). Diclofenac epolamine transdermal system is used for symptomatic relief of acute pain due to minor strains, sprains, and contusions.

The potential benefits and risks of diclofenac therapy as well as alternative therapies should be considered prior to initiating diclofenac therapy. The lowest possible effective dosage and shortest duration of therapy consistent with treatment goals of the patient should be employed.

In patients with dental extraction or gynecologic surgery pain, single oral 50- and 100-mg doses of diclofenac potassium have been reported to be as effective as single 650-mg doses of aspirin; the duration of diclofenac potassium's analgesic effect appears to be longer than that of aspirin. When used to relieve postoperative orthopedic surgery pain, 50- or 100-mg doses of diclofenac potassium followed by 50 mg every 8 hours were as effective as 550 mg of naproxen sodium followed by 275 mg every 8 hours. When used to relieve orthopedic pain, 150 mg of diclofenac potassium daily was more effective than placebo and at least as effective as 1.2 g of ibuprofen daily or 20 mg of piroxicam daily.

In patients with pain following bunionectomy with osteotomy, therapy with diclofenac potassium liquid-filled capsules (25 mg every 6 hours for 4 days; the initial 25-mg dose could be repeated upon patient request) was more effective than placebo in reducing pain intensity over 48 hours of inpatient treatment. The median time to onset of pain relief was less than 1 hour in patients receiving the liquid-filled capsules.

Diclofenac sodium also has been used orally for symptomatic relief of postoperative (including that associated with dental surgery), postpartum, and orthopedic (including musculoskeletal strains or sprains) pain†, and visceral pain associated with cancer†. Because of the relatively slow onset of action of delayed-release (enteric-coated) or extended-release tablets of diclofenac sodium, other more rapid-acting NSAIAs (e.g., diclofenac potassium) may be preferred when prompt relief of acute pain is required. Diclofenac also has been used parenterally† (a parenteral dosage form is currently not commercially available in the US) for the relief of acute biliary or renal colic†, and for relief of postoperative pain† (including that associated with gynecologic and orthopedic surgery).

When used to relieve mild to moderate acute pain†, single oral diclofenac sodium doses of 50–150 mg have been more effective than placebo and at least as effective as usual analgesic doses of other NSAIAs or mild opiate analgesics. Diclofenac sodium dosages of 75–150 mg daily have been as effective as aspirin dosages of 0.9–2.7 g daily or ibuprofen dosages of 1.2 g daily. In patients with oral surgery pain†, 50-mg doses of diclofenac sodium have been reported to be as effective as 100-mg doses of pentazocine.

Efficacy of diclofenac epolamine transdermal system (Flector®) for the management of pain in patients with minor strains, sprains, and contusions has been demonstrated in 2 of 4 clinical studies. In one of these studies, diclofenac epolamine transdermal system (applied *twice* daily for 2 weeks) was more effective than a placebo transdermal system in relieving pain due to an acute minor sports injury. In a 7-day clinical study in patients with ankle sprain and a 14-day study in patients with muscle contusion, diclofenac epolamine transdermal system (Licart®, applied *once* daily) was more effective that placebo in reducing pain upon movement on day 3 of treatment.

● *Migraine*

Diclofenac potassium is used as an oral solution for the acute treatment of attacks of migraine with or without aura; diclofenac should *not* be used for the prophylaxis of migraine. Safety and efficacy have *not* been established for the treatment of cluster headache, which occurs in an older, predominantly male population.

In 2 randomized, double-blind, placebo-controlled trials, efficacy of diclofenac potassium (50-mg dose given as an oral solution) for the acute treatment of migraine attacks was evaluated in a total of 1212 adults (85% female, 86% White, mean age of 40 years) experiencing a migraine attack causing moderate to severe pain. Greater proportions of patients receiving diclofenac compared with those receiving placebo reported freedom from headache pain at 2 hours after the dose (24–25 versus 10–13%) and reported sustained freedom from headache pain from 2–24 hours after the dose (19–22 versus 7–10%). The incidence of associated symptoms (i.e., nausea, photophobia, phonophobia) also was reduced in patients receiving diclofenac compared with those receiving placebo.

● *Dysmenorrhea*

Diclofenac potassium is used orally in the management of primary dysmenorrhea. In patients with primary dysmenorrhea, NSAIAs may relieve pain and reduce the frequency and severity of uterine contractions, possibly as a result of inhibition of prostaglandin synthesis.

The potential benefits and risks of diclofenac therapy as well as alternative therapies should be considered prior to initiating diclofenac therapy. The lowest possible effective dosage and shortest duration of therapy consistent with treatment goals of the patient should be employed.

When used to relieve primary dysmenorrhea, 50- or 100-mg doses of diclofenac potassium followed by 50 mg every 8 hours were as effective as 550 mg of naproxen sodium followed by 275 mg every 8 hours.

Diclofenac sodium as delayed-release (enteric-coated) tablets also has been used for the symptomatic relief of dysmenorrhea†. When used to relieve dysmenorrhea, diclofenac sodium (delayed-release [enteric-coated]) dosages of 50–150 mg daily were more effective than placebo and as effective as naproxen dosages of 250–1250 mg daily.

● *Other Uses*

Oral diclofenac sodium has been used for its antipyretic effect in the management of fever†, usually associated with infection. In one study, the antipyretic effect of usual dosages of diclofenac sodium as delayed-release (enteric-coated) tablets was about equal to that of usual dosages of aspirin. The drug, however, should not be used routinely as an antipyretic because of its potential adverse effects.

Results from a large, prospective, population-based cohort study in geriatric individuals indicate a lower prevalence of Alzheimer's disease† among patients who received an NSAIA for 2 years or longer. Similar findings have been reported from some other, but not all, observational studies.

Diclofenac sodium also is used topically as an ophthalmic solution for the treatment of postoperative ocular inflammation in patients undergoing cataract extraction.

For use of diclofenac sodium in the topical treatment of actinic keratoses, see Diclofenac Sodium 84:06.20.

DOSAGE AND ADMINISTRATION

● *Administration*

The potential benefits and risks of diclofenac therapy as well as alternative therapies should be considered prior to initiating diclofenac therapy.

Diclofenac sodium, diclofenac sodium in fixed combination with misoprostol, and diclofenac potassium are administered orally. Diclofenac sodium also is administered topically as a solution or gel. The drug also has been administered rectally† and parenterally† (by IM injection), but commercially available dosage forms for the rectal and parenteral routes of administration currently are not available in the US. Diclofenac epolamine is administered topically as a transdermal system.

Oral Administration

When diclofenac potassium powder for oral solution is used, the contents of one packet containing 50 mg of buffered diclofenac potassium for oral solution should be emptied into a cup containing 30–60 mL of water, mixed well, and swallowed immediately. Liquids other than water should not be used. Administration of the oral solution with food may decrease peak plasma concentrations of the drug and result in reduced efficacy compared with administration on an empty stomach.

Topical Administration

Diclofenac sodium is administered topically as a 1% gel or as a 1.5 or 2% solution, and diclofenac epolamine is administered topically as a transdermal system.

Patients receiving diclofenac sodium 1% topical gel should be instructed in the use of the gel and given a copy of the patient instructions provided by the manufacturer. Diclofenac sodium 1% gel should be applied 4 times daily to the affected joint(s). To measure the appropriate dose using the dosing card provided by the manufacturer, gel is applied within the oblong area of the dosing card up to the appropriate line (i.e., 2.25- or 4.5-inch line, corresponding to 2 or 4 g of gel, respectively); the dosing card can be used to apply the gel. The gel should be massaged gently into the skin, ensuring application to the entire joint (e.g., foot [including sole, top of foot, and toes], knee, ankle, hand [including palm, back of hand, and fingers], elbow, wrist). The patient should be advised to wait 10 minutes before covering the treated area with clothing and at least 60 minutes before bathing or showering. Hands should be washed after application of the gel unless the treated joint is in the hand. Diclofenac sodium gel should not be applied to open wounds or areas of skin afflicted with cuts, infections, or rashes; contact with eyes and mucous membranes should be avoided. The treated joint should not be exposed to external heat or to natural or artificial sunlight; use of occlusive dressings has not been evaluated and should be avoided. Other topical preparations (e.g., sunscreens, cosmetics, lotions, moisturizers, insect repellents, other topical medications) should not be applied to the treated joint; such use has not been evaluated.

Diclofenac sodium 1.5% topical solution is administered as drops dispensed directly onto the affected knee(s) or into the palm of the hand and then applied to the affected knee(s). To avoid spillage, the drops should be applied in 4 increments of 10 drops each per joint; following each incremental application, the topical solution should be spread evenly around the front, back, and sides of the knee. Diclofenac sodium 2% topical solution is administered via pump dispenser (2 pump actuations per affected joint) into the palm of the hand and then the entire volume of solution is applied evenly around the front, back, and sides of the knee. The pump must be primed before first use by fully depressing the pump mechanism 4 times while holding the bottle in an upright position. Patients receiving therapy with diclofenac sodium 1.5 or 2% topical solution should be advised to wait until the treated area is dry before covering the area with clothing and to wait at least 30 minutes before bathing or showering. Hands should be washed after application of the topical solution. In addition, other individuals should avoid skin-to-skin contact with the treated area until the area is completely dry. Diclofenac sodium topical solution should not be applied to open wounds, infected or inflamed areas of skin, or areas affected with exfoliative dermatitis; contact with eyes and mucous membranes should be avoided. The treated knee should not be exposed to external heat, and exposure to natural or artificial sunlight should be avoided; use of occlusive dressings also should be avoided. The treated knee should be allowed to dry completely before other topical preparations (e.g., sunscreen, insect repellant, lotions, moisturizers, cosmetics, other topical medications) are applied to the same area.

Diclofenac epolamine is administered by topical application of a transdermal system. Patients receiving diclofenac epolamine transdermal system should be instructed in the use of the system. The manufacturer states that the transdermal system should be applied to the most painful area once daily (Licart®) or twice daily (Flector®). The system should be applied to intact skin only; application to damaged skin (e.g., wounds, burns, infected areas of skin, areas affected with eczema or exudative dermatitis) should be avoided. Hands should be washed after handling the system. Contact with the eyes and mucous membranes should be avoided. The transdermal system should not be worn while bathing or showering. If a system should begin to peel off during the period of use, the edges of the system may be taped to the skin. If problems with adhesion persist, a nonocclusive mesh netting sleeve (e.g., Curad® Hold Tite®, Surgilast® Tubular Elastic Dressing) may be used when appropriate (e.g., over ankles, knees, or elbows) to secure the system. In one study in which diclofenac epolamine transdermal system (Licart®) was applied to the lower leg above the ankle, evaluations performed every 4 hours during the 24-hour application period indicated 90% or greater adhesion at each evaluation.

● Dosage

The lowest possible effective dosage and shortest duration of therapy consistent with treatment goals of the patient should be employed. Dosage of diclofenac must be carefully adjusted according to individual requirements and response, using the lowest possible effective dosage.

Based on safety reviews conducted to evaluate available data on cardiovascular risk of diclofenac, some authorities (e.g., Health Canada) recommend that the dosage of systemically administered diclofenac not exceed 100 mg daily (except on the first day of treatment for dysmenorrhea when a total dose of 200 mg may be administered). (See Cardiovascular Effects under Cautions.)

Different strengths and formulations of oral diclofenac are not interchangeable. Commercially available diclofenac sodium enteric-coated tablets, diclofenac sodium extended-release tablets, and diclofenac potassium conventional tablets are not necessarily bioequivalent on a mg per mg basis. In addition, diclofenac potassium liquid-filled capsules and conventional tablets are not equivalent.

Each actuation of the pump dispenser of diclofenac sodium 2% topical solution delivers 20 mg of diclofenac sodium in 1 g of solution. The 1.5% topical solution contains diclofenac sodium 16.05 mg/mL. The 1% gel contains 10 mg of diclofenac sodium per 1 g of gel.

Inflammatory Diseases

Based on safety reviews conducted to evaluate cardiovascular risk of diclofenac, some authorities (e.g., Health Canada) recommend that systemic diclofenac dosage for inflammatory diseases not exceed 100 mg daily. (See Cardiovascular Effects under Cautions.)

Rheumatoid Arthritis and Osteoarthritis

For the symptomatic treatment of acute or chronic rheumatoid arthritis, the usual initial adult dosage of diclofenac sodium delayed-release (enteric-coated) tablets or diclofenac potassium conventional tablets is 150–200 mg daily, administered in divided doses of 75 mg (diclofenac sodium delayed-release [enteric-coated] tablets only) twice daily or 50 mg (diclofenac sodium delayed-release [enteric-coated] tablets or diclofenac potassium conventional tablets) 3 or 4 times daily. For the management of rheumatoid arthritis, the usual initial adult dosage of diclofenac sodium extended-release tablets is 100 mg daily. If dosage increase is necessary in patients receiving diclofenac sodium 100 mg daily as extended-release tablets, dosage can be increased to 100 mg twice daily.

When diclofenac is used in fixed combination with misoprostol for the symptomatic treatment of chronic rheumatoid arthritis, the usual dosage is 50 mg of diclofenac sodium 3 or 4 times daily. Dosage may be changed to 50 or 75 mg of diclofenac sodium twice daily in patients who do not tolerate the usual dosage; however, these dosages may be less effective in preventing NSAIA-induced ulcers. When therapy with diclofenac and misoprostol is required for the treatment of chronic rheumatoid arthritis, the commercially available combination of diclofenac in fixed combination with misoprostol should not be used for initial therapy. Instead, dosage should first be adjusted by administering each drug separately. If it is determined that the optimum maintenance dosage corresponds to the ratio in the commercial combination preparation, the fixed combination may be used. If clinically indicated, supplemental doses of misoprostol or diclofenac as the individual component can be administered with the fixed combination.

For the symptomatic treatment of osteoarthritis, the usual adult dosage of diclofenac sodium delayed-release (enteric-coated) tablets or diclofenac potassium conventional tablets is 100–150 mg daily, administered in divided doses of 75 mg (diclofenac sodium delayed-release [enteric-coated] tablets only) twice daily or 50 mg (diclofenac sodium delayed-release [enteric-coated] tablets or diclofenac potassium conventional tablets) 2 or 3 times daily. For the management of osteoarthritis, the recommended adult dosage of diclofenac sodium extended-release tablets is 100 mg daily.

When diclofenac is used in fixed combination with misoprostol for the symptomatic treatment of osteoarthritis, the usual dosage is 50 mg of diclofenac sodium 3 times daily. Dosage may be changed to 50 or 75 mg of diclofenac sodium twice daily in patients who do not tolerate the usual dosage; however, these dosages may be less effective in preventing NSAIA-induced ulcers. When therapy with diclofenac and misoprostol is required for the treatment of osteoarthritis, the commercially available combination of diclofenac in fixed combination with misoprostol should not be used for initial therapy. Instead, dosage should first be adjusted by administering each drug separately. If it is determined that the optimum maintenance dosage corresponds to the ratio in the commercial combination preparation, the fixed combination may be used. If clinically indicated, supplemental doses of misoprostol or diclofenac as the individual component can be administered with the fixed combination.

When diclofenac sodium 1% gel is used for the management of lower extremity (i.e., knees, ankles, feet) joint pain due to osteoarthritis, 4 g of gel is massaged into the affected joint 4 times daily. When the gel is used for the management of upper extremity (i.e., elbows, wrists, hands) joint pain, 2 g of gel is massaged into the affected joint 4 times daily. The total daily dose applied to all affected joints should *not* exceed 32 g of gel, with no more than 16 g of gel applied daily to any single lower extremity joint and no more than 8 g of gel applied daily to any single upper extremity joint. When diclofenac sodium 1% gel is used for *self-medication* for the temporary relief of arthritis pain, no more than 2 body areas should be treated at the same time, with no more than 16 g of gel applied daily to any single lower extremity (i.e., knees, ankles, feet) joint and no more than 8 g of gel applied daily to any single upper extremity (i.e., elbows, wrists, hands) joint. For *self-medication*, diclofenac sodium 1% gel may be used for up to 21 days unless otherwise directed by a clinician, and should be discontinued if no pain relief is obtained in 7 days.

When diclofenac sodium 1.5% topical solution is used for the symptomatic treatment of osteoarthritis of the knee, the recommended dosage is 40 drops (approximately 1.2 mL of a 16.05-mg/mL solution) applied to each affected knee 4 times daily. When diclofenac sodium 2% topical solution is used for the management of knee pain due to osteoarthritis, the recommended dosage is 40 mg of diclofenac sodium (2 pump actuations) applied to each affected knee twice daily.

Ankylosing Spondylitis

For the symptomatic treatment of ankylosing spondylitis, the usual adult dosage of diclofenac sodium delayed-release (enteric-coated) tablets is 100–125 mg daily, administered in divided doses of 25 mg 4 or 5 times daily. When diclofenac potassium is used for the management of ankylosing spondylitis, a dosage of 50 mg twice daily has been suggested by the manufacturers.

Pain and Dysmenorrhea

When diclofenac potassium conventional tablets are used for relief of pain or primary dysmenorrhea, an initial dose of 50 mg is recommended, followed by 50 mg every 8 hours as needed; some patients may benefit from an initial dose of 100 mg, followed by 50 mg every 8 hours as needed. Based on safety reviews conducted to evaluate available data on cardiovascular risk of diclofenac, some authorities (e.g., Health Canada) now recommend that the dosage of systemically administered diclofenac not exceed 100 mg daily (except on the first day of treatment for dysmenorrhea when a total dose of 200 mg may be administered). (See Cardiovascular Effects under Cautions.)

When diclofenac potassium liquid-filled capsules are used for relief of mild to moderate acute pain, the recommended dosage is 25 mg 4 times daily.

When diclofenac epolamine transdermal system is used for relief of acute pain due to strains, sprains, and contusions, the manufacturers state that one system should be applied to the most painful area once daily (Licart®) or twice daily (Flector®).

Migraine

For the acute treatment of migraine with or without aura, the usual adult dosage of diclofenac potassium is a single 50-mg dose (contents of one packet containing diclofenac potassium for oral solution mixed with water). The safety and efficacy of administering a second dose have not been established.

● Dosage in Renal or Hepatic Impairment

Diclofenac dosage reductions do not appear to be necessary in patients with renal impairment. However, use of diclofenac should be avoided in patients with advanced renal disease unless the benefits are expected to outweigh the risk of worsening renal function. If diclofenac is used, such patients should be monitored for signs of worsening renal function. (See Renal, Electrolyte, and Genitourinary Effects under Cautions.)

Reduction of oral diclofenac dosage may be necessary in patients with hepatic impairment. The manufacturer of diclofenac potassium liquid-filled capsules states that treatment should be initiated at the lowest dosage in such patients;

if efficacy is not achieved at that dosage, diclofenac should be discontinued and alternative treatment considered.

CAUTIONS

Adverse reactions to oral diclofenac are usually mild and transient and mainly involve the upper GI tract; however, adverse effects may be severe enough to require discontinuance of the drug in about 1.5–2% of patients. Most diclofenac-induced adverse effects occur during the first 3–6 months of treatment. The relationship of the frequency of adverse effects to dosage remains to be established. Overall, the frequency and nature of adverse effects produced by diclofenac sodium delayed-release (enteric-coated) tablets, diclofenac potassium conventional tablets, and ibuprofen appear to be similar. When diclofenac potassium was administered short-term (2 weeks or less), the incidence of adverse effects was about 10–50% of that associated with long-term administration of the drug.

● Cardiovascular Effects

Fluid retention manifested principally as edema has occurred in up to 10% of patients receiving oral diclofenac. Edema also has been reported in 3% of patients receiving diclofenac sodium topical solution. Adverse cardiovascular effects reported occasionally in diclofenac-treated patients include congestive heart failure, hypertension, tachycardia, and syncope. Arrhythmia, myocardial infarction, chest pain, palpitations, vasculitis, thrombophlebitis, hypotension, angina-like attack, and circulatory shock or distress have occurred rarely.

Nonsteroidal anti-inflammatory agents (NSAIAs), including selective cyclooxygenase-2 (COX-2) inhibitors and prototypical NSAIAs, increase the risk of serious adverse cardiovascular thrombotic events, including myocardial infarction and stroke (which can be fatal), in patients with or without cardiovascular disease or risk factors for cardiovascular disease. Use of NSAIAs also is associated with an increased risk of heart failure.

The association between cardiovascular complications and use of NSAIAs is an area of ongoing concern and study. Findings of an FDA review of published observational studies of NSAIAs, a meta-analysis of published and unpublished data from randomized controlled trials of these drugs, and other published information indicate that NSAIAs may increase the risk of serious adverse cardiovascular thrombotic events by 10–50% or more, depending on the drugs and dosages studied. Available data suggest that the increase in risk may occur early (within the first weeks) following initiation of therapy and may increase with higher dosages and longer durations of use. Although the relative increase in cardiovascular risk appears to be similar in patients with or without known underlying cardiovascular disease or risk factors for cardiovascular disease, the absolute incidence of serious NSAIA-associated cardiovascular thrombotic events is higher in those with cardiovascular disease or risk factors for cardiovascular disease because of their elevated baseline risk. (See Cautions: Cardiovascular Effects, in Celecoxib 28:08.04.08.)

Results from observational studies utilizing Danish national registry data indicated that patients receiving NSAIAs following a myocardial infarction were at increased risk of reinfarction, cardiovascular-related death, and all-cause mortality beginning in the first week of treatment. Patients who received NSAIAs following myocardial infarction had a higher 1-year mortality rate compared with those who did not receive NSAIAs (20 versus 12 deaths per 100 person-years). Although the absolute mortality rate declined somewhat after the first year following the myocardial infarction, the increased relative risk of death in patients who received NSAIAs persisted over at least the next 4 years of follow-up.

In 2 large controlled clinical trials of a selective COX-2 inhibitor for the management of pain in the first 10–14 days following coronary artery bypass graft (CABG) surgery, the incidence of myocardial infarction and stroke was increased. Therefore, NSAIAs are contraindicated in the setting of CABG surgery.

Findings from some systematic reviews of controlled observational studies and meta-analyses of data from randomized studies of NSAIAs suggest that naproxen may be associated with a lower risk of cardiovascular thrombotic events compared with other NSAIAs. However, limitations of these observational studies and the indirect comparisons used to assess cardiovascular risk of the prototypical NSAIAs (e.g., variability in patients' risk factors, comorbid conditions, concomitant drug therapy, drug interactions, dosage, and duration of therapy) affect the validity of the comparisons; in addition, these studies were not designed to demonstrate superior safety of one NSAIA compared with another. Therefore, FDA states that definitive conclusions regarding relative risks of NSAIAs are not possible at this time. (See Cautions: Cardiovascular Effects, in Celecoxib 28:08.04.08.)

Findings from some of these meta-analyses and systematic reviews also suggest that the cardiovascular risk associated with diclofenac, particularly at higher dosages (e.g., 150 mg or more daily), is similar to that observed with selective COX-2 inhibitors. (See Experience with Prototypical NSAIAs under Cautions: Cardiovascular Effects, in Celecoxib 28:08.04.08.) Some authorities (e.g., Health Canada) now recommend that the dosage of systemically administered diclofenac not exceed 100 mg daily (except for the first day of treatment for dysmenorrhea). (See Dosage and Administration: Dosage.)

Data from observational studies also indicate that use of NSAIAs in patients with heart failure is associated with increased morbidity and mortality. Results from a retrospective study utilizing Danish national registry data indicated that use of selective COX-2 inhibitors or prototypical NSAIAs in patients with chronic heart failure was associated with a dose-dependent increase in the risk of death and an increased risk of hospitalization for myocardial infarction or heart failure. In addition, findings from a meta-analysis of published and unpublished data from randomized controlled trials of NSAIAs indicated that use of selective COX-2 inhibitors or prototypical NSAIAs was associated with an approximate twofold increase in the risk of hospitalization for heart failure. Fluid retention and edema also have been observed in some patients receiving NSAIAs.

There is no consistent evidence that use of low-dose aspirin mitigates the increased risk of serious cardiovascular events associated with NSAIAs.

● GI Effects

Adverse GI effects, which mainly involve the upper GI tract, occur in up to 10% of patients receiving oral diclofenac. Adverse GI effects require discontinuance of the drug in about 3% of patients. Peptic ulcer, GI bleeding, and/or perforation have been reported in up to 10% of patients receiving oral diclofenac in controlled clinical studies. There is some evidence that the incidence of diclofenac-induced peptic ulcers and gastric lesions may be reduced with concomitant use of an appropriate ulcer preventive regimen. Nausea, diarrhea, constipation, abdominal pain or cramps, flatulence, vomiting, and dyspepsia occur in up to 10% of patients receiving oral diclofenac. Esophagitis, gastritis, glossitis, stomatitis, aphthous stomatitis, changes in appetite, dry mouth and mucous membranes, pancreatitis (with or without hepatitis), thirst, colitis, ulceration of the colon, and distress have occurred during diclofenac therapy. The incidence of abdominal pain, diarrhea, and other GI symptoms may be higher in patients receiving diclofenac in fixed combination with misoprostol than in patients receiving diclofenac without misoprostol. Dyspepsia, abdominal pain, flatulence, diarrhea, nausea, and constipation have occurred in 3–8% of patients receiving diclofenac sodium topical solution. Nausea, altered taste, dyspepsia, or other adverse GI effects (including gastritis, vomiting, diarrhea, constipation, upper abdominal pain, and dry mouth) have occurred in 1–3% of patients receiving diclofenac epolamine transdermal system (Flector®). Nausea has been reported in 3% of patients receiving diclofenac potassium oral solution for acute treatment of migraine attacks compared with 2% of those receiving placebo.

Usual oral dosages of diclofenac sodium reportedly produce fewer adverse GI effects than usual anti-inflammatory dosages of aspirin or naproxen. In healthy individuals, GI bleeding as determined by fecal blood loss was less in individuals receiving 150 mg of diclofenac sodium daily than in those receiving 3000, 750, or 150 mg of aspirin, naproxen, or indomethacin daily, respectively, for 3 weeks. In healthy adults, the frequency of GI mucosal lesions observed with endoscopic examination was lower with diclofenac than with naproxen. However, the clinical importance of these findings is not known since currently there is no evidence to indicate that diclofenac is less likely to produce serious GI lesions during chronic therapy than other prototypical NSAIAs.

Serious, sometimes fatal, adverse GI effects (e.g., bleeding, ulceration, or perforation of the esophagus, stomach, or small or large intestine) can occur at any time in patients receiving NSAIA therapy, and such effects may *not* be preceded by warning signs or symptoms. Only 1 in 5 patients who develop a serious upper GI adverse event while receiving NSAIA therapy is symptomatic. Therefore, clinicians should remain alert to the possible development of serious GI effects (e.g., bleeding, ulceration) in any patient receiving NSAIA therapy, and such patients

should be followed chronically for the development of manifestations of such effects and advised of the importance of this follow-up. Patients receiving concomitant low-dose aspirin therapy for cardiac prophylaxis should be monitored even more closely for evidence of GI bleeding. In addition, patients should be advised about the signs and symptoms of serious NSAIA-induced GI toxicity and what action to take if they occur. If signs and symptoms of a serious GI event develop, additional evaluation and treatment should be initiated promptly; the NSAIA should be discontinued until appropriate diagnostic studies have ruled out a serious GI event.

Results of studies to date are inconclusive concerning the relative risk of various prototypical NSAIAs in causing serious GI effects. In patients receiving NSAIAs and observed in clinical studies of several months' to 2 years' duration, upper GI ulcers, gross bleeding, or perforation appeared to occur in approximately 1% of patients treated for 3–6 months and in about 2–4% of those treated for 1 year. Longer duration of therapy with an NSAIA increases the likelihood of a serious GI event. However, short-term therapy is not without risk. High dosages of any NSAIA probably are associated with increased risk of such effects, although controlled studies documenting this probable association are lacking for most NSAIAs. Therefore, whenever use of relatively high dosages (within the recommended dosage range) is considered, sufficient benefit to offset the potential increased risk of GI toxicity should be anticipated.

Studies have shown that patients with a history of peptic ulcer disease and/or GI bleeding who are receiving NSAIAs have a greater than tenfold increased risk of developing GI bleeding than patients without these risk factors. In addition to a history of ulcer disease, pharmacoepidemiologic studies have identified several comorbid conditions and concomitant therapies that may increase the risk for GI bleeding, including concomitant use of oral corticosteroids, anticoagulants, aspirin, or selective serotonin-reuptake inhibitors (SSRIs); longer duration of NSAIA therapy; smoking; alcohol use; older age; and poor general health status. Risk of GI bleeding also is increased in patients with advanced liver disease and/or coagulopathy. Patients with rheumatoid arthritis are more likely to experience serious GI complications from NSAIA therapy than are patients with osteoarthritis. In addition, geriatric or debilitated patients appear to tolerate GI ulceration and bleeding less well than other individuals, and most spontaneous reports of fatal GI effects have been in such patients.

For patients at high risk for complications from NSAIA-induced GI ulceration (e.g., bleeding, perforation), concomitant use of misoprostol can be considered for preventive therapy. (See Misoprostol 56:28.28.) Alternatively, some clinicians suggest that a proton-pump inhibitor (e.g., omeprazole) may be used concomitantly to decrease the incidence of serious GI toxicity associated with NSAIA therapy. In one study, therapy with high dosages of famotidine (40 mg twice daily) was more effective than placebo in preventing peptic ulcers in NSAIA-treated patients; however, the effect of the drug was modest. In addition, efficacy of usual dosages of H_2-receptor antagonists for the prevention of NSAIA-induced gastric and duodenal ulcers has not been established. Therefore, most clinicians do not recommend use of H_2-receptor antagonists for the prevention of NSAIA-associated ulcers. Another approach in high-risk patients who would benefit from NSAIA therapy is use of an NSAIA that is a selective inhibitor of COX-2 (e.g., celecoxib), since these agents are associated with a lower incidence of serious GI bleeding than prototypical NSAIAs. However, while celecoxib (200 mg twice daily) was comparably effective to diclofenac sodium (75 mg twice daily) plus omeprazole (20 mg daily) in preventing recurrent ulcer bleeding (recurrent ulcer bleeding probabilities of 4.9 versus 6.4%, respectively, during the 6-month study) in *H. pylori*-negative arthritis (principally osteoarthritis) patients with a recent history of ulcer bleeding, the protective efficacy was unexpectedly low for both regimens and it appeared that neither could completely protect patients at high risk. Additional study is necessary to elucidate optimal therapy for preventing GI complications associated with NSAIA therapy in high-risk patients.

● Nervous System Effects

Headache or dizziness has been reported in up to 10% of patients receiving oral diclofenac. Anxiety, asthenia, confusion, depression, abnormal dreams, drowsiness, insomnia, malaise, nervousness, paresthesia, somnolence, tremors, irritability, and vertigo have occurred occasionally in patients receiving the drug. Tingling sensation, dreams, myoclonus, and migraine have occurred rarely. Headache, paresthesia, somnolence, or other adverse nervous system effects (including hypoesthesia, dizziness, and hyperkinesias) have occurred in 1% of patients receiving diclofenac epolamine transdermal system (Flector®). Paresthesia also has occurred in 2% of patients receiving diclofenac sodium topical solution. Dizziness has been reported in 1% of patients receiving diclofenac potassium oral solution for acute treatment of migraine attacks compared with 0.5% of those receiving placebo. Although a causal relationship to diclofenac has not been established, seizures, coma, hallucinations, and meningitis have been reported during therapy with the drug.

● Renal, Electrolyte, and Genitourinary Effects

Diclofenac has caused impairment of renal function, resulting in acute renal failure, interstitial nephritis, nephrotic syndrome, increased BUN and serum creatinine concentrations, and renal papillary necrosis in patients receiving the drug. In at least one patient receiving oral diclofenac, acute renal failure became chronic. Cystitis, dysuria, hematuria, oliguria/polyuria, and proteinuria have been reported occasionally in patients receiving diclofenac. Urinary tract infection, renal calculi, and hyponatremia have occurred rarely. Hyperkalemia also has been reported in patients receiving NSAIAs, including in individuals without renal impairment; in those with normal renal function, this effect has been attributed to a hyporenin-hypoaldosterone state.

● Hepatic Effects

Severe hepatic reactions (sometimes fatal or requiring liver transplantation), including jaundice and fulminant hepatitis, liver necrosis, cholestasis, hepatic failure, asymptomatic hepatitis, acute hepatitis, and chronic active hepatitis, have been reported rarely in patients receiving diclofenac. Meaningful (more than 3 times the upper limit of normal) elevations of serum AST concentration have occurred in approximately 2% of patients at some time during therapy with diclofenac. Increased serum concentrations of bilirubin have been reported rarely in patients receiving diclofenac therapy.

In one large, open-label, controlled study, meaningful or marked (more than 8 times the upper limit of normal) elevations of serum AST and/or ALT concentrations occurred in 4 or 1% of patients, respectively, receiving diclofenac for 2–6 months. In that open-label study, borderline, moderate, and marked elevations of ALT or AST were observed more frequently with diclofenac than with other NSAIAs. In addition, aminotransferase elevations were observed more frequently in patients with osteoarthritis than in those with rheumatoid arthritis. Almost all meaningful elevations of aminotransferase concentrations were detected before patients became symptomatic. During clinical trials, test results were abnormal during the first 2 months of diclofenac therapy in 82% of patients who developed marked aminotransferase elevations. During postmarketing experience, cases of drug-induced hepatotoxicity have been reported during the first month of diclofenac therapy and, in some cases, during the first 2 months of therapy, but can occur at any time during treatment with the drug.

In a retrospective population-based, case-control study of drug-induced liver injury, which included 10 cases of diclofenac-associated liver injury, current use of diclofenac was associated with an increased risk of liver injury (adjusted odds ratio of 4.1) compared with nonuse of the drug; the study findings suggested an increased risk in women compared with men and with use of higher doses (150 mg or more) and longer durations of therapy (more than 90 days).

Misoprostol does not appear to exacerbate hepatic effects (e.g., increases in liver function test values) associated with diclofenac therapy.

Diclofenac should be discontinued immediately if abnormal liver function test results persist or worsen, if clinical signs and symptoms consistent with liver disease develop, or if systemic manifestations occur. (See Hepatic Precautions under Cautions.)

● Dermatologic and Sensitivity Reactions

Rash or pruritus occurs in up to 10% of patients receiving oral diclofenac. Other adverse dermatologic reactions, including alopecia, photosensitivity, and excessive perspiration, have occurred occasionally. Bullous eruption, Stevens-Johnson syndrome, erythema multiforme, exfoliative dermatitis, toxic epidermal necrolysis, urticaria, and angioedema, have occurred rarely.

Sensitivity reactions, including anaphylaxis; swelling of the eyelids, tongue, lips, pharynx, or larynx; urticaria; asthma; bronchospasm; laryngeal edema; dyspnea; chest tightness; wheezing; anaphylactoid reactions; eosinophilic

pneumonitis and angioedema, sometimes with concomitant, potentially severe hypotension, have been reported in patients receiving diclofenac. Anaphylactic reactions have been reported in patients with or without known hypersensitivity to the drug, as well as in patients with aspirin-sensitivity asthma.

In clinical studies that evaluated diclofenac sodium 1% gel, the most common adverse effect reported was dermatitis at the application site; this adverse effect has been reported in 4–11% of patients receiving the gel. Application site pruritus, erythema, paresthesia, dryness, vesicles, irritation, or papules also have occurred in patients receiving diclofenac gel.

In clinical studies that evaluated diclofenac sodium 2% topical solution, dryness at the application site has been reported in 22% of patients receiving the topical solution, while application site exfoliation, erythema, pruritus, pain, induration, and rash have been reported in 2–7% of patients, and scabbing has been reported in less than 1% of patients. In clinical studies that evaluated diclofenac sodium 1.5% topical solution, dryness at the application site has been reported in 32% of patients receiving the topical solution, while contact dermatitis characterized by skin erythema and induration, contact dermatitis with vesicles, and pruritus have been reported in 2–9% of patients. Other application site reactions (e.g., paresthesia, vasodilation, acne, urticaria) have occurred in patients receiving diclofenac sodium topical solution. Rash, pruritus, and dry skin that are not localized to the application site also have occurred in 2–3% of patients receiving diclofenac sodium topical solution.

Application site reactions (i.e., pruritus, dermatitis, burning, dryness, irritation, erythema, atrophy, discoloration, hyperhidrosis, vesicles) have been reported in 11% of patients receiving therapy with diclofenac epolamine transdermal system (Flector®) in clinical studies. Rash also has been reported in patients receiving diclofenac epolamine transdermal system. Skin infection developed in one individual after the diclofenac system that had been applied to the foot was subjected to prolonged exposure to wetness. Edema and abnormal sensation at the treated site and allergic skin reactions also have been reported. Pruritus or other reactions (i.e., irritation, erythema, rash, inflammation, blister) at the application site have occurred in approximately 1% of patients receiving therapy with diclofenac epolamine transdermal system (Licart®) in clinical studies.

● Otic and Ocular Effects

Tinnitus has occurred in up to 10% of patients receiving oral diclofenac.

Adverse ocular effects (including blurred vision and conjunctivitis) and hearing impairment have occurred in diclofenac-treated patients.

● Hematologic Effects

Anemia has been reported in up to 10% of patients receiving oral diclofenac and may be due to occult or gross blood loss, fluid retention, or an incompletely described effect on erythropoiesis. Leukopenia, thrombocytopenia, purpura, ecchymosis, eosinophilia, melena, and rectal bleeding have occurred occasionally in patients receiving diclofenac. Ecchymosis has been reported in 2% of patients receiving diclofenac sodium topical solution. Agranulocytosis, lymphadenopathy, hemolytic anemia, aplastic anemia, and pancytopenia have been reported rarely in diclofenac-treated patients. Bruising in the extremities and abdomen, spontaneous bleeding, and hematoma formation also have been reported rarely in patients receiving the drug. Diclofenac may inhibit platelet aggregation and prolong bleeding time. However, administration of diclofenac sodium 1.5% topical solution at the maximum recommended dosage for 7 days in healthy individuals resulted in no substantial change in platelet aggregation. Diclofenac usually does not affect platelet count, prothrombin time, partial thromboplastin time, or thrombin time.

● Respiratory Effects

Asthma or dyspnea has been reported occasionally in patients receiving diclofenac. Respiratory tract infection (e.g., pneumonia, pharyngitis, bronchitis) or respiratory depression has been reported rarely.

● Other Adverse Effects

Fever, infection, and sepsis have occurred in patients receiving diclofenac. Back, leg, or joint pain and hyperglycemia have occurred rarely. Although a causal relationship to diclofenac has not been established, weight changes have occurred in patients receiving the drug.

● *Precautions and Contraindications*

Multiple diclofenac-containing preparations should not be used concomitantly. Concomitant use of topical formulations of diclofenac with oral NSAIAs may result in increased adverse effects.

When diclofenac sodium is used in fixed combination with misoprostol, the cautions, precautions, and contraindications associated with misoprostol must be considered in addition to those associated with diclofenac.

Patients should be advised that diclofenac, like other NSAIAs, is not free of potential adverse effects, including some that can cause discomfort, and that more serious effects (e.g., myocardial infarction, stroke, GI bleeding), which may require hospitalization and may even be fatal, also can occur.

Patients should be advised to read the medication guide for NSAIAs that is provided to the patient each time the drug is dispensed.

Cardiovascular Precautions

NSAIAs increase the risk of serious adverse cardiovascular thrombotic events. (See Cardiovascular Effects under Cautions.) To minimize the potential risk of adverse cardiovascular events, the lowest effective dosage and shortest possible duration of therapy should be employed. Some clinicians suggest that it may be prudent to avoid use of NSAIAs whenever possible in patients with cardiovascular disease. Patients receiving NSAIAs (including those without previous symptoms of cardiovascular disease) should be monitored for the possible development of cardiovascular events throughout therapy. Patients should be informed about the signs and symptoms of serious cardiovascular toxicity (chest pain, dyspnea, weakness, slurring of speech) and instructed to seek immediate medical attention if such toxicity occurs. Diclofenac should be avoided in patients with recent myocardial infarction unless the benefits of therapy are expected to outweigh the risk of recurrent cardiovascular thrombotic events; if diclofenac is used in such patients, the patient should be monitored for cardiac ischemia.

There is no consistent evidence that concomitant use of low-dose aspirin mitigates the increased risk of serious cardiovascular events associated with NSAIAs. Concomitant use of aspirin and an NSAIA increases the risk for serious GI events. (See Nonsteroidal Anti-inflammatory Agents under Drug Interactions.)

Use of NSAIAs can result in the onset of hypertension or worsening of preexisting hypertension; either of these occurrences may contribute to the increased incidence of cardiovascular events. Patients receiving NSAIAs may have an impaired response to diuretics (i.e., thiazide or loop diuretics), angiotensin-converting enzyme (ACE) inhibitors, angiotensin II receptor antagonists, or β-adrenergic blocking agents. Blood pressure should be monitored closely during initiation of NSAIA therapy and throughout therapy.

Because NSAIAs increase morbidity and mortality in patients with heart failure, the manufacturer states that diclofenac should be avoided in patients with severe heart failure unless the benefits of therapy are expected to outweigh the risk of worsening heart failure; if diclofenac is used in such patients, the patient should be monitored for worsening heart failure. Some experts state that use of NSAIAs should be avoided whenever possible in patients with reduced left ventricular ejection fraction and current or prior symptoms of heart failure. Patients receiving NSAIAs should be advised to inform their clinician if they experience symptoms of heart failure, including dyspnea, unexplained weight gain, and edema. Use of NSAIAs may diminish the cardiovascular effects of certain drugs used to treat heart failure and edema (e.g., diuretics, ACE inhibitors, angiotensin II receptor antagonists). (See Drug Interactions.)

GI Precautions

The risk of potentially serious adverse GI effects should be considered in patients receiving diclofenac, particularly in patients receiving chronic therapy with the drug. (See GI Effects under Cautions.) Because peptic ulceration and/or GI bleeding have been reported in patients receiving the drug, patients should be advised to promptly report signs or symptoms of GI ulceration or bleeding to their clinician.

To minimize the potential risk of adverse GI effects, the lowest effective dosage and shortest possible duration of therapy should be employed, and use of more than one NSAIA at a time should be avoided. (See Nonsteroidal Anti-inflammatory Agents under Drug Interactions.) In addition, use of NSAIAs should be avoided in patients at higher risk (see GI Effects under Cautions) unless the benefits of therapy are expected to outweigh the increased risk of bleeding; for patients who are at high risk, as well as for those with active GI bleeding, alternative therapy other than an NSAIA should be considered.

Concomitant use of corticosteroids during NSAIA therapy may increase the risk of GI ulceration; therefore, NSAIAs should be used with caution when used concomitantly with corticosteroids.

Hepatic Precautions

Because severe hepatotoxic effects may develop without symptoms of liver dysfunction, serum aminotransferase concentrations should be measured at baseline and monitored periodically during long-term therapy with diclofenac. While the optimum timing of aminotransferase determinations during diclofenac therapy has not been determined, serum aminotransferase values should be obtained 4–8 weeks after therapy with the drug is initiated. Diclofenac should be discontinued immediately if abnormal liver function test results persist or worsen, if clinical signs and symptoms consistent with liver disease develop, or if systemic manifestations (e.g., eosinophilia, rash) occur. (See Hepatic Effects under Cautions.) Patients receiving diclofenac should be informed of the warning signs and symptoms of hepatotoxicity (e.g., nausea, anorexia, fatigue, lethargy, pruritus, jaundice, right upper quadrant tenderness, flu-like syndrome) and the appropriate actions to take if any of these manifestations develop.

To minimize the potential risk of adverse hepatic effects, the lowest effective dosage and shortest possible duration of therapy should be employed, and diclofenac should be used with caution in patients receiving concomitant therapy with other potentially hepatotoxic drugs (e.g., acetaminophen, certain antibiotics, anticonvulsant agents).

Because diclofenac is almost completely metabolized in the liver, patients with hepatic impairment may require reduced oral dosages of the drug.

Renal Precautions

Renal toxicity has been observed in patients in whom renal prostaglandins have a compensatory role in maintaining renal perfusion. Administration of an NSAIA to such patients may cause a dose-dependent reduction in prostaglandin formation and thereby precipitate overt renal decompensation. Patients at greatest risk of this reaction are those with impaired renal function, heart failure, or hepatic dysfunction; those with extracellular fluid depletion (e.g., patients receiving diuretics); those taking an ACE inhibitor or angiotensin II receptor antagonist concomitantly; and geriatric patients. Fluid depletion should be corrected prior to initiation of diclofenac therapy, and renal function should be monitored during diclofenac therapy in patients with renal or hepatic impairment, heart failure, dehydration, or hypovolemia. Patients should be advised to consult their clinician promptly if unexplained weight gain or edema occurs. Recovery of renal function to pretreatment levels usually occurs following discontinuance of NSAIA therapy.

The renal effects of diclofenac may hasten the progression of renal dysfunction in patients with preexisting renal disease. Patients with preexisting renal disease should be monitored for worsening renal function.

Diclofenac has not been evaluated in patients with severe renal impairment, and the manufacturers state that use of the drug should be avoided in patients with advanced renal disease unless the benefits of therapy are expected to outweigh the risk of worsening renal function. If diclofenac is used in patients with advanced renal disease, close monitoring of renal function is recommended.

Precautions Related to Dermatologic or Hypersensitivity Reactions

Anaphylactic reactions have been reported in patients receiving diclofenac. Patients receiving diclofenac should be informed of the signs and symptoms of an anaphylactoid reaction (e.g., difficulty breathing, swelling of the face or throat) and advised to seek immediate medical attention if an anaphylactoid reaction develops.

Serious skin reactions (e.g., exfoliative dermatitis, Stevens-Johnson syndrome, toxic epidermal necrolysis) can occur in patients receiving diclofenac. These serious skin reactions may occur without warning; patients should be advised to consult their clinician if skin rash and blisters, fever, or other signs of hypersensitivity reaction (e.g., pruritus) occur. Diclofenac should be discontinued at the first appearance of rash or any other sign of hypersensitivity.

Multi-organ hypersensitivity (also known as drug reaction with eosinophilia and systemic symptoms [DRESS]), a potentially fatal or life-threatening syndrome, has been reported in patients receiving NSAIAs. The clinical presentation is variable, but typically includes eosinophilia, fever, rash, lymphadenopathy, and/or facial swelling, possibly associated with other organ system involvement such as hepatitis, nephritis, hematologic abnormalities, myocarditis, or myositis. Symptoms may resemble those of an acute viral infection. Early manifestations of hypersensitivity, such as fever or lymphadenopathy, may be present in the absence of rash. If such signs or symptoms develop, diclofenac should be discontinued and the patient evaluated immediately.

Precautions Related to Transdermal or Other Topical Use

When topical diclofenac preparations (e.g., diclofenac sodium topical gel or topical solution, diclofenac epolamine transdermal system) are used, patients should be advised to avoid contact with the eyes or mucous membranes. If the topical preparation does come in contact with the eyes, the eyes should be thoroughly rinsed with water or saline. Patients should be advised to consult a clinician if ocular irritation persists for longer than one hour.

Patients receiving diclofenac sodium 1% gel for *self-administration* should be advised that the gel should not be used in larger dosages or for longer periods of time than recommended and should not be used for symptomatic relief of strains, sprains, bruises, or sports injuries. Up to 7 days of use may be required for relief of osteoarthritis joint pain; if no relief is obtained within 7 days, *self-administration* of the 1% gel should be discontinued.

Topical application of diclofenac gel formulations has resulted in early onset of ultraviolet (UV) light-related skin tumors in animal studies. Patients receiving therapy with diclofenac sodium gel or topical solution should be advised to avoid exposure of treated areas to natural or artificial sunlight. The potential effects of topical diclofenac sodium gel or solution on skin response to UV damage in humans are not known.

Patients receiving therapy with diclofenac epolamine transdermal system should be advised to bathe or shower after removing one system but before applying a new system; patients should not wear the system while bathing or showering.

Patients should be advised to store and discard diclofenac epolamine transdermal systems in a manner that avoids accidental exposure or ingestion by children or pets.

Hematologic Precautions

Diclofenac should be used with caution in patients who may be adversely affected by a prolongation of bleeding time (e.g., patients receiving anticoagulant therapy), since the drug may inhibit platelet function.

NSAIAs, including diclofenac, may increase the risk of bleeding. Patients with certain coexisting conditions such as coagulation disorders and those receiving concomitant therapy with anticoagulants, antiplatelet agents, or serotonin-reuptake inhibitors may be at increased risk and should be monitored for signs of bleeding. (See Drug Interactions.)

If signs and/or symptoms of anemia occur during therapy with diclofenac, hemoglobin concentration and hematocrit should be determined.

Other Precautions

Patients receiving long-term NSAIA therapy should have a complete blood cell count and chemistry profile performed periodically.

Some clinicians state that NSAIAs should be used with caution in patients with systemic lupus erythematosus (SLE) since serious adverse CNS effects (e.g., aseptic meningitis) and possible activation of SLE occasionally have been observed in patients with SLE receiving NSAIAs.

Because NSAIAs have caused adverse ocular effects, patients who experience visual disturbances during diclofenac therapy should have an ophthalmologic examination.

The possibility that the antipyretic and anti-inflammatory effects of diclofenac may mask the usual signs and symptoms of infection or other diseases should be considered.

Diclofenac is not a substitute for corticosteroid therapy, and the drug is not effective in the management of adrenal insufficiency. Abrupt withdrawal of corticosteroids may exacerbate corticosteroid-responsive conditions. If corticosteroid therapy is to be discontinued after prolonged therapy, the dosage should be tapered gradually.

Excessive use of drugs indicated for the management of acute migraine attacks (e.g., use of NSAIAs, serotonin type 1 [5-HT$_1$] receptor agonists, ergotamine, or opiate analgesics on a regular basis for 10 or more days per month) may result in migraine-like daily headaches or a marked increase in the frequency of migraine attacks. Detoxification, including withdrawal of the overused drugs and treatment of withdrawal symptoms (which often include transient worsening of headaches), may be necessary. Patients should be encouraged to record the frequency of migraine headaches and medication use and to contact their clinician if the frequency of migraine attacks increases.

Contraindications

The manufacturers state that diclofenac is contraindicated in patients with known hypersensitivity (e.g., anaphylaxis, serious dermatologic reactions) to the drug or any ingredient in the formulation. In addition, NSAIAs, including diclofenac, generally are contraindicated in patients in whom asthma, urticaria, or other sensitivity reactions are precipitated by aspirin or other NSAIAs, since there is potential for cross-sensitivity between NSAIAs and aspirin, and severe, often fatal, anaphylactic reactions may occur in such patients. Although NSAIAs generally are contraindicated in these patients, the drugs have occasionally been used in NSAIA-sensitive patients who have undergone desensitization. Because patients with asthma may have aspirin-sensitivity asthma, patients with asthma but without known aspirin sensitivity who are receiving diclofenac should be monitored for changes in manifestations of asthma. In patients with asthma, aspirin sensitivity is manifested principally as bronchospasm and usually is associated with nasal polyps; the association of aspirin sensitivity, asthma, and nasal polyps is known as the aspirin triad. For a further discussion of cross-sensitivity of NSAIAs, see Cautions: Sensitivity Reactions, in the Salicylates General Statement 28:08.04.24.

NSAIAs are contraindicated in the setting of CABG surgery.

Use of diclofenac epolamine transdermal system on nonintact or damaged skin, regardless of the etiology (e.g., exudative dermatitis, eczema, infected lesions, burns, wounds), is contraindicated.

● *Pediatric Precautions*

The manufacturers state that safety and efficacy of diclofenac in children have not been established. However, oral diclofenac has been used with good results for the management of juvenile rheumatoid arthritis† in a limited number of children 3–16 years of age. Further studies are needed to establish the optimum dosages and indications for use in children.

● *Geriatric Precautions*

Geriatric patients are at increased risk for NSAIA-associated serious adverse cardiovascular, GI, and renal effects. Many of the spontaneous reports of fatal adverse GI effects in patients receiving NSAIAs involve geriatric individuals. If the anticipated benefits of diclofenac therapy outweigh the potential risks, diclofenac should be initiated at the lower end of the dosing range and patients should be monitored for adverse effects.

Of the total number of patients studied in clinical trials of diclofenac sodium 1% topical gel, 498 were 65 years of age or older. Although no overall differences in safety or efficacy were observed between geriatric individuals and younger adults in these studies, the possibility that some older patients may exhibit increased sensitivity to the drug cannot be ruled out.

In phase 3 clinical trials of diclofenac sodium 1.5% topical solution, 49% of patients receiving the drug were 65 years of age or older. In an open-label, long-term safety study, 42% of patients receiving diclofenac sodium 1.5% topical solution were 65 years of age or older, while 13% were 75 years of age or older. No age-related differences in the incidence of adverse effects were observed in these studies.

Clinical trials of diclofenac epolamine transdermal system or diclofenac potassium oral solution did not include sufficient numbers of patients 65 years of age and older to determine whether they respond differently than younger adults. Other clinical experience has not identified differences in response between geriatric and younger patients.

Diclofenac is substantially excreted by the kidneys, and the risk of toxicity may be greater in patients with renal impairment. Because geriatric patients are more likely to have decreased renal function, diclofenac should be used with caution; it may be useful to monitor renal function in such patients.

● Mutagenicity and Carcinogenicity

No evidence of diclofenac sodium-induced mutagenicity was seen with several in vitro test systems, including the microbial (Ames test) and mammalian (mouse lymphoma) test systems. Also, there was no evidence of mutagenicity when diclofenac sodium was tested with in vitro and in vivo mammalian tests, including dominant lethal and male germinal epithelial chromosomal tests in mice and nucleus anomaly and chromosome aberration tests in Chinese hamsters.

No evidence of carcinogenic potential was seen in rats receiving oral diclofenac sodium dosages up to 2 mg/kg daily (12 mg/m^2 daily; about the maximum recommended human dosage) for 2 years. In addition, no evidence of oncogenic potential was seen in male and female mice receiving diclofenac sodium dosages up to 0.3 (0.9 mg/m^2) and 1 mg/kg (3 mg/m^2) daily, respectively, for 2 years. There was an increase, however, in benign mammary fibroadenomas in female rats receiving oral diclofenac sodium dosages of 0.25–2 mg/kg for 2 years.

Animal photocarcinogenicity studies indicate a shortened time to skin tumor formation following application of diclofenac sodium gel in a concentration up to 0.035%.

● Pregnancy, Fertility, and Lactation

Pregnancy

Use of NSAIAs during pregnancy at about 30 weeks of gestation or later can cause premature closure of the fetal ductus arteriosus, and use at about 20 weeks of gestation or later has been associated with fetal renal dysfunction resulting in oligohydramnios and, in some cases, neonatal renal impairment. Because of these risks, use of NSAIAs should be avoided in pregnant women at about 30 weeks of gestation or later; if NSAIA therapy is necessary between about 20 and 30 weeks of gestation, the lowest effective dosage and shortest possible duration of treatment should be used. Monitoring of amniotic fluid volume via ultrasound examination should be considered if the duration of NSAIA treatment exceeds 48 hours; if oligohydramnios occurs, the drug should be discontinued and follow-up instituted according to clinical practice. Pregnant women should be advised to avoid use of NSAIAs beginning at 20 weeks' gestation unless otherwise advised by a clinician; they should be informed that NSAIAs should be avoided beginning at 30 weeks' gestation because of the risk of premature closure of the fetal ductus arteriosus and that monitoring for oligohydramnios may be necessary if NSAIA therapy is required for longer than 48 hours' duration between about 20 and 30 weeks of gestation.

Known effects of NSAIAs on the human fetus during the third trimester of pregnancy include prenatal constriction of the ductus arteriosus, tricuspid incompetence, and pulmonary hypertension; nonclosure of the ductus arteriosus during the postnatal period (which may be resistant to medical management); and myocardial degenerative changes, platelet dysfunction with resultant bleeding, intracranial bleeding, renal dysfunction or renal failure, renal injury or dysgenesis potentially resulting in prolonged or permanent renal failure, oligohydramnios, GI bleeding or perforation, and increased risk of necrotizing enterocolitis.

Fetal renal dysfunction resulting in oligohydramnios and, in some cases, neonatal renal impairment has been observed, on average, following days to weeks of maternal NSAIA use, although oligohydramnios has been observed infrequently as early as 48 hours after initiation of NSAIA therapy. Oligohydramnios is often, but not always, reversible (generally within 3–6 days) following discontinuance of NSAIA therapy. Complications of prolonged oligohydramnios may include limb contracture and delayed lung maturation. A limited number of case reports have described maternal NSAIA use and neonatal renal dysfunction, in some cases irreversible, without oligohydramnios. Some cases of neonatal renal dysfunction have required treatment with invasive procedures such as exchange transfusion or dialysis. Deaths associated with neonatal renal failure have been reported. Methodologic limitations of these postmarketing studies and case reports include lack of a control group; limited information regarding dosage, duration, and timing of drug exposure; and concomitant use of other drugs. These limitations preclude establishing a reliable estimate of the risk of adverse fetal and neonatal outcomes with maternal NSAIA use. Available data on neonatal outcomes generally involved preterm infants, and the extent to which certain reported risks can be generalized to full-term infants is uncertain.

Diclofenac crosses the placenta in mice, rats, and humans. Reproduction studies in rabbits, rats, and mice receiving oral diclofenac sodium dosages up to 10, 10, and 20 mg/kg daily, respectively, have not revealed evidence of teratogenicity; however, these dosages produced maternal (e.g., dystocia, prolonged gestation) and fetal (e.g., reduced weight, growth, and survival) toxicity.

Animal data indicate that prostaglandins have an important role in endometrial vascular permeability, blastocyst implantation, and decidualization. In animal studies, inhibitors of prostaglandin synthesis, such as diclofenac, were associated with increased pre- and post-implantation losses. Prostaglandins also have an important role in fetal kidney development. In animal studies, inhibitors of prostaglandin synthesis impaired kidney development at clinically relevant doses.

The effects of diclofenac on labor and delivery in humans currently are not known. In animal studies, NSAIAs, including diclofenac, inhibit prostaglandin synthesis, delay parturition, and increase the incidence of stillbirth.

Diclofenac sodium in fixed combination with misoprostol is contraindicated in women who are pregnant because misoprostol exhibits abortifacient activity and can cause serious fetal harm. In addition, it is recommended that diclofenac in fixed combination with misoprostol be used in women of childbearing potential *only* if they require NSAIA therapy and are considered at high risk of complications resulting from NSAIA-induced gastric or duodenal ulceration or at high risk of developing gastric or duodenal ulceration. (See Cautions: Pregnancy, Fertility, and Lactation, in Misoprostol 56:28.28.)

Fertility

Use of NSAIAs, including diclofenac, may delay or prevent ovarian follicular rupture, which has been associated with reversible infertility in some women. Reversible delays in ovulation have been observed in limited studies in women receiving NSAIAs, and animal studies indicate that inhibitors of prostaglandin synthesis can disrupt prostaglandin-mediated follicular rupture required for ovulation. Therefore, withdrawal of diclofenac should be considered in women who are experiencing difficulty conceiving or are undergoing evaluation of infertility.

Reproduction studies in male and female rats using diclofenac sodium dosages up to 4 mg/kg (24 mg/m^2) daily have not revealed evidence of impaired fertility.

Lactation

Diclofenac may be distributed into milk. While diclofenac was not detectable in breast milk in 12 women who received diclofenac 100 mg orally daily for 7 days or a single 50-mg IM dose administered in the immediate postpartum period, the drug was detected in breast milk at a concentration of 100 mcg/L (equivalent to an infant dose of about 0.03 mg/kg daily) in one woman receiving a diclofenac salt at a dosage of 150 mg daily.

The developmental and health benefits of breast-feeding should be considered along with the mother's clinical need for diclofenac and any potential adverse effects on the breast-fed infant from the drug or from the underlying maternal condition.

DRUG INTERACTIONS

● Drugs Affecting Hepatic Microsomal Enzymes

Diclofenac is metabolized by cytochrome P-450 (CYP) isoenzymes, mainly by CYP2C9. Concomitant use of CYP2C9 inhibitors (e.g., voriconazole) may increase systemic exposure to diclofenac and the risk of adverse effects; conversely, concomitant use of CYP2C9 inducers (e.g., rifampin) may reduce efficacy of diclofenac. Concomitant administration of voriconazole (inhibitor of CYP isoenzymes 2C9, 2C19, and 3A4) increased the peak concentration and area under the concentration-time curve (AUC) of diclofenac by 114 and 78%, respectively. Dosage adjustment may be required when diclofenac is used concomitantly with CYP2C9 inhibitors or inducers.

● Protein-bound Drugs

Because diclofenac is highly protein bound, it could be displaced from binding sites by, or it theoretically could displace from binding sites, other protein-bound drugs. In vitro studies suggest that diclofenac only minimally displaces from protein binding sites other highly protein-bound drugs (e.g., prednisolone, salicylates, tolbutamide, warfarin), although diclofenac may be displaced from binding sites by high doses of ionized protein-bound drugs (e.g., salicylates).

When NSAIAs were administered with aspirin, protein binding of the NSAIAs was reduced, although clearance of the free (unbound) NSAIAs was not altered; the clinical relevance of this interaction has not been established.

● **Antacids**

Concomitant administration of diclofenac and an aluminum and magnesium hydroxides antacid may result in delayed diclofenac absorption; however, extent of absorption is not affected.

Because magnesium-containing antacids may increase the incidence of misoprostol-induced diarrhea, concomitant administration of diclofenac in fixed combination with misoprostol with a magnesium-containing antacid is not recommended. Antacids and food appear to decrease the oral bioavailability of misoprostol. (See Drug Interactions: Food and Antacids, in Misoprostol 56:28.28.)

● **Antihypertensive Agents**

Concomitant use of NSAIAs with angiotensin-converting enzyme (ACE) inhibitors, angiotensin II receptor antagonists, or β-adrenergic blocking agents may reduce the blood pressure response to the antihypertensive agent. Therefore, blood pressure should be monitored to ensure that target blood pressure is achieved.

Concomitant use of diclofenac with ACE inhibitors or angiotensin II receptor antagonists in geriatric patients or patients with volume depletion or renal impairment may result in reversible deterioration of renal function, including possible acute renal failure; such patients should be monitored for signs of worsening renal function. Patients receiving concomitant therapy with diclofenac and ACE inhibitors or angiotensin II receptor antagonists should be adequately hydrated, and renal function should be assessed when concomitant therapy is initiated and periodically thereafter.

● **Anticoagulants**

The effects of warfarin and NSAIAs on GI bleeding are synergistic. Concomitant use of diclofenac and warfarin is associated with a higher risk of GI bleeding compared with use of either agent alone.

In short-term controlled studies in patients receiving maintenance doses of coumarin derivatives, diclofenac did not substantially alter the hypothrombinemic effect of these anticoagulants when the drugs were administered concomitantly. However, because diclofenac may cause GI bleeding, inhibit platelet aggregation, and prolong bleeding time, the drug should be used with caution and with careful monitoring for signs of bleeding in patients receiving any anticoagulant (e.g., warfarin).

● **Cyclosporine**

Concomitant administration of diclofenac and cyclosporine may increase the nephrotoxic effects of cyclosporine; this interaction may be related to inhibition of renal prostaglandin (e.g., prostacyclin) synthesis. Patients should be monitored for signs of worsening renal function.

● **Digoxin**

Concomitant use of diclofenac and digoxin has been reported to result in increased serum concentrations and prolonged half-life of digoxin. Serum digoxin concentrations should be monitored.

● **Diuretics**

Patients receiving diuretics may have an increased risk of developing renal failure secondary to decreased renal blood flow resulting from prostaglandin inhibition by NSAIAs, including diclofenac. (See Renal Precautions under Cautions.) In addition, NSAIAs may interfere with the natriuretic response to diuretics with activity that depends in part on prostaglandin-mediated alterations in renal blood flow (e.g., furosemide, thiazides). In patients with hypertension, the antihypertensive effect of hydrochlorothiazide was attenuated by diclofenac. Patients receiving concomitant NSAIA and diuretic therapy should be monitored for worsening renal function and for adequacy of diuretic and antihypertensive effects.

Concomitant use of diclofenac and potassium-sparing diuretics may be associated with increased serum potassium concentrations.

Concomitant administration of diclofenac and triamterene has resulted in reversible impairment of renal function. Similar adverse renal effects have been reported with concomitant use of triamterene and other NSAIAs (e.g.,

indomethacin), progressing to acute renal failure in some patients. Therefore, diclofenac and triamterene should be used concomitantly with caution. The mechanism of this interaction has not been determined, but it has been postulated that NSAIAs may inhibit triamterene-mediated renal vasoconstriction.

● **Lithium**

Diclofenac increases plasma lithium concentrations and reduces renal lithium clearance. The mechanism involved in the reduction of lithium clearance by NSAIAs (including diclofenac) is not known, but has been attributed to inhibition of prostaglandin synthesis, which may interfere with the renal elimination of lithium. With concomitant NSAIA use, the mean increase in trough lithium concentrations is 15% and renal clearance is decreased by approximately 20%. In one study in healthy women, plasma lithium concentration was increased by 26% and renal clearance was reduced by 23%. In a patient receiving 1 g of lithium daily together with diclofenac sodium dosages of 75 mg daily, plasma lithium concentrations increased about fivefold; manifestations of lithium intoxication developed but resolved following discontinuance of both diclofenac and lithium. If diclofenac and lithium are administered concurrently, the patient should be closely observed for signs of lithium toxicity and plasma lithium concentrations should be monitored carefully during the initial stages of combined therapy or subsequent dosage adjustment. In addition, appropriate adjustment of lithium dosage may be required when therapy with diclofenac is discontinued.

● **Methotrexate**

Concomitant use of NSAIAs and methotrexate may increase the risk for methotrexate toxicity (e.g., neutropenia, thrombocytopenia, renal dysfunction). Severe, sometimes fatal, toxicity has occurred following concomitant administration of diclofenac and methotrexate. The toxicity was associated with elevated serum concentrations of methotrexate. Patients at greatest risk of this reaction are those with renal impairment and those receiving relatively high (e.g., antineoplastic) dosages of methotrexate. Patients receiving concomitant diclofenac and methotrexate therapy should be monitored for methotrexate toxicity. (See Drug Interactions: Nonsteroidal Anti-inflammatory Agents, in Methotrexate 10:00.)

● **Nonsteroidal Anti-inflammatory Agents**

In controlled clinical trials, concomitant use of NSAIAs and analgesic dosages of aspirin did not produce any greater therapeutic effect than use of NSAIAs alone. However, concomitant use of aspirin and an NSAIA increases the risk for bleeding and serious GI events. Because of the potential for increased adverse effects, concomitant use of diclofenac with other NSAIAs or with analgesic dosages of aspirin generally is not recommended.

Concomitant use of oral and topical NSAIAs may result in a higher incidence of hemorrhage and abnormal values for creatinine, urea, and hemoglobin. Incidences of rectal hemorrhage and abnormal creatinine, urea, and hemoglobin concentrations were greater in patients receiving concomitant therapy with diclofenac sodium 1.5% topical solution and oral diclofenac (3, 12, 20, and 13%, respectively) compared with those receiving oral diclofenac alone (less than 1, 7, 12, and 9%, respectively); however, no difference in the incidence of aminotransferase elevations was observed. Topical diclofenac formulations (e.g., gels, solutions, transdermal systems) should not be used concomitantly with oral NSAIAs unless expected benefits outweigh risks and periodic laboratory evaluations are performed.

Patients receiving diclofenac should be advised not to take low-dose aspirin without consulting their clinician. Diclofenac is not a substitute for low-dose aspirin therapy for prophylaxis of cardiovascular events, and patients receiving antiplatelet agents such as aspirin concomitantly with diclofenac should be monitored closely for bleeding. There is no consistent evidence that use of low-dose aspirin mitigates the increased risk of serious cardiovascular events associated with NSAIAs.

While multiple-dose administration of ibuprofen may inhibit the cardioprotective effects of aspirin, limited data indicate that administration of diclofenac sodium delayed-release tablets (75 mg twice daily) does not inhibit the antiplatelet effect of aspirin (81 mg daily).

Following concomitant administration of diclofenac and aspirin in healthy individuals, protein binding of diclofenac is decreased, biliary excretion of diclofenac may be increased, and peak plasma concentrations and AUC of diclofenac are reduced. Pretreatment with diclofenac for 14 days before administration of aspirin appeared to enhance renal elimination of salicylate. The clinical importance of these pharmacokinetic interactions remains to be determined.

● Pemetrexed

Concomitant use of diclofenac and pemetrexed may increase the risk of pemetrexed-associated myelosuppression, renal toxicity, and GI toxicity. Administration of NSAIAs with short elimination half-lives (e.g., diclofenac, indomethacin) should be avoided beginning 2 days before and continuing through 2 days after pemetrexed administration. In the absence of data regarding potential interactions between pemetrexed and NSAIAs with longer half-lives (e.g., meloxicam, nabumetone), administration of NSAIAs with longer half-lives should be interrupted beginning at least 5 days before and continuing through 2 days after pemetrexed administration. Patients with renal impairment with a creatinine clearance of 45–79 mL/minute should be monitored for myelosuppression, renal toxicity, and GI toxicity if they receive concomitant diclofenac and pemetrexed therapy.

● Quinolones

It has been suggested that concomitant use of ciprofloxacin and an NSAIA (e.g., diclofenac) could increase the risk of CNS stimulation (e.g., seizures), but additional study and experience are necessary.

● Serotonin-reuptake Inhibitors

Serotonin release by platelets plays an important role in hemostasis. Results of case-control and epidemiologic cohort studies indicate that concomitant use of NSAIAs and drugs that interfere with serotonin reuptake may potentiate the risk of bleeding beyond that associated with an NSAIA alone. Patients receiving concomitant therapy with diclofenac and selective serotonin-reuptake inhibitors (SSRIs) or selective serotonin- and norepinephrine-reuptake inhibitors (SNRIs) should be monitored for signs of bleeding.

● Other Drugs

Concomitant use of ulcerogenic drugs such as corticosteroids during NSAIA therapy may increase the risk of GI ulceration. Concomitant administration of more than one diclofenac-containing product should be avoided.

ACUTE TOXICITY

Limited information is available on the acute toxicity of diclofenac.

● Pathogenesis

The acute lethal dose of diclofenac sodium in humans is not known. Individuals have survived reported ingestions of up to 4 g of the drug. The oral LD_{50} of diclofenac sodium is 55–240, 500, and 3200 mg/kg in rats, dogs, and monkeys, respectively. Hydroxylated metabolites of the drug have exhibited less toxic potential than did the unchanged drug in LD_{50} studies in rats.

Acute diclofenac overdosage produces manifestations that are mainly extensions of adverse effects of the drug. Loss of consciousness, increased intracranial pressure, and aspiration pneumonitis were reported in a 17-year-old male, who died 2 days after ingesting 5 g of diclofenac. No signs or symptoms of toxicity were observed in a few patients who ingested 3.75–4 g of diclofenac. However, vomiting and drowsiness occurred in an adolescent who ingested 2.37 g of the drug. Several other adults who ingested overdosages of diclofenac along with other drugs, including CNS depressants, developed confusion, hypotonia, and loss of consciousness (requiring intubation and ventilation). In one of these patients, plasma diclofenac concentrations were 60.1 and 0.19 mcg/mL 7 and 15 hours after ingestion, respectively.

In acute diclofenac overdosage, general measures should include immediately emptying the stomach by inducing emesis or by gastric lavage, followed by initiation of symptomatic and supportive treatment. Administration of activated charcoal after emesis or gastric lavage may be useful in minimizing absorption of diclofenac and reabsorption of enterohepatically recirculated drug. Forced diuresis, alkalinization of urine, hemodialysis, or hemoperfusion may not be beneficial in enhancing elimination of diclofenac, because the drug is highly protein bound. If forced diuresis is used in an attempt to enhance urinary excretion of the drug,

fluid and electrolyte balance should be monitored carefully, since potentially serious electrolyte disturbances and fluid retention may occur.

PHARMACOLOGY

Diclofenac has pharmacologic actions similar to those of other prototypical NSAIAs. The drug exhibits anti-inflammatory, analgesic, and antipyretic activity. The exact mechanisms have not been clearly established, but many of the actions appear to be associated principally with the inhibition of prostaglandin synthesis. Diclofenac inhibits the synthesis of prostaglandins in body tissues by inhibiting cyclooxygenase; at least 2 isoenzymes, cyclooxygenase-1 (COX-1) and -2 (COX-2) (also referred to as prostaglandin G/H synthase-1 [PGHS-1] and -2 [PGHS-2], respectively), have been identified that catalyze the formation of prostaglandins in the arachidonic acid pathway. Diclofenac, like other prototypical NSAIAs, inhibits both COX-1 and COX-2. Although the exact mechanisms have not been clearly established, NSAIAs appear to exert anti-inflammatory, analgesic, and antipyretic activity principally through inhibition of the COX-2 isoenzyme; COX-1 inhibition presumably is responsible for the drugs' unwanted effects on GI mucosa and platelet aggregation.

● Anti-inflammatory, Analgesic, and Antipyretic Effects

The anti-inflammatory, analgesic, and antipyretic effects of diclofenac and other NSAIAs, including selective inhibitors of COX-2 (e.g., celecoxib), appear to result from inhibition of prostaglandin synthesis. While the precise mechanism of the anti-inflammatory and analgesic effects of NSAIAs continues to be investigated, these effects appear to be mediated principally through inhibition of the COX-2 isoenzyme at sites of inflammation with subsequent reduction in the synthesis of certain prostaglandins from their arachidonic acid precursors.

High concentrations of diclofenac have been reported to inhibit formation of other arachidonic acid metabolites, including leukotrienes and 5- hydroxyeicosatetraenoic acid (5-HETE). Diclofenac may inhibit the migration of leukocytes, including polymorphonuclear leukocytes, into inflammatory sites. However, inhibition of leukotriene formation and migration of leukocytes do not appear to result from direct diclofenac-induced inhibition of lipoxygenase. Diclofenac also inhibits lysosomal enzyme release from polymorphonuclear leukocytes and may inhibit superoxide production and chemotaxis of polymorphonuclear leukocytes.

On a weight basis, the anti-inflammatory potency of diclofenac has been shown to be less than that of piroxicam, and to be about 2.5, 10, 24, 80, or 430 times that of indomethacin, naproxen, phenylbutazone, ibuprofen, or aspirin, respectively, as determined by inhibition of carrageenan-induced paw edema in rats. In adjuvant-induced arthritis in rats, the anti-inflammatory activity of diclofenac is similar to that of indomethacin, and about 30, 95, or 380 times that of naproxen, phenylbutazone, or ibuprofen, respectively. The anti-inflammatory activity of topically applied 4% diclofenac sodium is similar to that of topically applied 2–4% ibuprofen or indomethacin and 10% meclofenamic acid, mefenamic acid, or phenylbutazone, as determined by inhibition of UV light-induced erythema in animals.

On a weight basis, as determined by antagonism of phenylbenzoquinone-induced writhing in mice, the analgesic potency of diclofenac was similar to that of indomethacin and about 5, 10, 22, or 38 times that of naproxen, ibuprofen, phenylbutazone, or aspirin, respectively. On a weight basis in human studies, the analgesic effect of diclofenac was similar to that of codeine and about 3–8, 8–16, and 12–18 times that of naproxen, ibuprofen, and aspirin, respectively.

Tolerance to the analgesic effect of diclofenac apparently does not occur during long-term administration.

Diclofenac lowers body temperature in animals with antigen-induced fever. Although the mechanism of antipyretic effect of NSAIAs is not known, it has been suggested that suppression of prostaglandin synthesis in the CNS (probably in the hypothalamus) may be involved. In rats, the antipyretic activity of diclofenac 0.5 mg/kg was similar to that of 1.2, 24, 35, 55, or 185 mg/kg of indomethacin, ibuprofen, phenylbutazone, naproxen, or aspirin, respectively.

● Genitourinary and Renal Effects

Diclofenac has relieved symptoms associated with primary dysmenorrhea, probably by inhibiting the synthesis and/or actions of prostaglandins. Whether the increased production of prostaglandins associated with primary dysmenorrhea is mediated by COX-1 or COX-2 remains to be determined.

Diclofenac has been reported to adversely affect renal function. (See Renal, Electrolyte, and Genitourinary Effects under Cautions.) Although the exact mechanism of adverse renal effects of NSAIAs has not been determined, the effects may be related to inhibition of renal prostaglandin synthesis.

Diclofenac exhibited an antiproteinuric effect in a limited number of patients with glomerulonephritis and normal renal function. The mechanism(s) of this decreased proteinuria remains to be established.

Diclofenac does not appear to have uricosuric activity when administered in usual dosages.

● GI Effects

Diclofenac can cause gastric mucosal damage, which may result in ulceration and/or bleeding. These gastric effects have been attributed to inhibition of the synthesis of prostaglandins produced by COX-1. Other factors possibly involved in NSAIA-induced gastropathy include local irritation, promotion of acid back-diffusion into gastric mucosa, uncoupling of oxidative phosphorylation, and enterohepatic recirculation of the drugs.

Misoprostol, a synthetic prostaglandin E_1 analog, inhibits gastric acid secretion and protects the mucosa from irritant and/or other (e.g., pharmacologic) effects of certain drugs (e.g., nonsteroidal anti-inflammatory agents [NSAIAs]). (See Pharmacology, in Misoprostol 56:28.28.)

Epidemiologic and laboratory studies suggest that NSAIAs may reduce the risk of colon cancer. Although the exact mechanism by which NSAIAs may inhibit colon carcinogenesis remains to be determined, it has been suggested that inhibition of prostaglandin synthesis may be involved.

● Hematologic Effects

Diclofenac can inhibit platelet aggregation and may prolong bleeding time. Like other prototypical NSAIAs, these effects of diclofenac appear to be associated with inhibition of the synthesis of prostaglandins produced by COX-1. In a study in healthy individuals, the drug did not substantially affect collagen-induced platelet aggregation, platelet count, prothrombin time, or bleeding time. Administration of diclofenac sodium 1.5% topical solution at the maximum recommended dosage for 7 days in healthy individuals resulted in no substantial change in platelet aggregation. Reports of the effect of parenterally administered diclofenac on bleeding time have been equivocal. However, parenterally administered diclofenac has produced a dose-dependent increase in bleeding time in healthy adults when administered by IV infusion.

● Other Effects

Diclofenac may increase free fatty acid concentrations and plasma post-heparin lipoprotein lipase activity. In healthy men, diclofenac does not appear to alter substantially plasma concentrations of follicle-stimulating hormone, luteinizing hormone, or thyrotropin (thyroid-stimulating hormone, TSH) but has decreased plasma prolactin concentrations.

Like some other NSAIAs, diclofenac inhibits prostaglandin synthesis in the conjunctiva and uvea following topical application to the eye and thereby may prevent and/or decrease disruption of the blood-aqueous humor barrier.

PHARMACOKINETICS

● Absorption

Diclofenac sodium and diclofenac potassium are almost completely absorbed from the GI tract; however, the drugs undergo extensive first-pass metabolism in the liver, with only about 50–60% of a dose of diclofenac sodium or diclofenac potassium reaching systemic circulation as unchanged drug. Diclofenac also is absorbed into systemic circulation following rectal administration and percutaneously following topical application to the skin as a gel, solution, or transdermal system.

Measurable plasma concentrations of diclofenac have been observed in some fasting individuals within 10 minutes of receiving diclofenac potassium conventional tablets and within 5 minutes of receiving diclofenac potassium oral

solution. Onset of absorption is delayed when diclofenac sodium is administered orally as delayed-release (enteric-coated) tablets, but the extent of absorption does not appear to be affected. Peak plasma concentrations of diclofenac generally occur within 1 hour (range: 0.33–2 hours) or 2–3 hours (range: 1–4 hours) after oral administration of diclofenac potassium conventional tablets or delayed-release (enteric-coated) diclofenac sodium tablets, respectively. Peak plasma concentrations occur within 10–30 minutes after administration of an oral solution of diclofenac sodium and in approximately 15 minutes in fasting individuals receiving diclofenac potassium oral solution. Following oral administration of a single 25-mg dose as diclofenac potassium liquid-filled capsules under fasting conditions, peak diclofenac concentrations of approximately 1.1 mcg/mL occur at a mean of 0.47 hours. Following oral administration of a single 25-, 50-, 75-, or 150-mg dose as delayed-release (enteric-coated) diclofenac sodium tablets in healthy adults, average peak plasma diclofenac concentrations of 0.5–1, 1–1.5, 2, and 2.5 mcg/mL, respectively, occur within about 1.5–3 hours. The area under the plasma concentration-time curve (AUC) increases linearly with single diclofenac sodium doses of 25–150 mg. There is considerable interindividual and intraindividual variation in plasma concentrations attained with a given dosage, and onset of absorption is variable secondary to differing dissolution of the enteric coating of diclofenac sodium delayed-release tablets. Following oral administration of a single 100-mg dose of diclofenac sodium as an extended-release tablet, mean peak plasma concentrations of 417 ng/mL generally occur within 5–6 hours. Following rectal administration of a single 25-, 50-, or 100-mg diclofenac sodium suppository in healthy adults, peak plasma diclofenac concentrations of approximately 0.6, 0.7, or 1.8 mcg/mL, respectively, occur within about 1 hour. The relationship between plasma diclofenac concentrations and therapeutic effect has not been established.

Food decreases the rate of absorption of conventional tablets of diclofenac potassium and of delayed-release (enteric-coated) tablets of diclofenac sodium, resulting in delayed and decreased peak plasma concentrations; however, the extent of absorption is not affected substantially. When diclofenac potassium conventional tablets are administered with food, time to achieve peak plasma concentrations of the drug is increased and peak plasma concentrations of the drug are decreased by approximately 30%. Administration of diclofenac potassium oral solution after a high-fat meal did not substantially alter the extent of diclofenac absorption, but reduced peak plasma concentrations by approximately 70%. Food decreases the rate of absorption of diclofenac potassium liquid-filled capsules, resulting in a 47% decrease in peak concentration and a twofold increase in the time to peak concentration; the extent of absorption is not affected substantially. When single doses of diclofenac sodium delayed-release (enteric-coated) tablets are taken with food, the onset of absorption usually is delayed by 1–4.5 hours but may be delayed up to 12 hours in some patients. These food-induced alterations in GI absorption of the drug result from delayed transit of the delayed-release (enteric-coated) tablets to the small intestine, the site of dissolution. When diclofenac sodium extended-release tablets are taken with food, onset of absorption is delayed 1–2 hours and peak plasma concentrations are increased twofold; however, extent of absorption is not substantially affected. Absorption of diclofenac does not appear to be affected substantially by the presence of food following continuous dosing of the drug. Antacids also may decrease the rate but not the extent of absorption of diclofenac.

Peak plasma diclofenac concentrations attained following administration of the drug may be reduced in patients with rheumatoid arthritis compared with those in healthy adults; however, AUCs appear to be similar. Peak plasma concentrations and AUCs of the drug in geriatric individuals may be increased up to about fourfold and twofold those, respectively, observed in younger individuals, although a lack of substantial age-related alterations also has been reported. No differences in pharmacokinetic values for diclofenac have been detected in patients with renal impairment relative to healthy adults.

Diclofenac is absorbed into systemic circulation following topical application, but plasma concentrations generally are very low compared with oral administration. Following application of a single diclofenac epolamine transdermal system (Flector®) to intact skin on the upper arm, peak plasma diclofenac concentrations of 0.7–6 ng/mL occur in 10–20 hours. Following application of the system twice daily for 5 days, plasma diclofenac concentrations of 1.3–8.8 ng/mL have been reported. No difference in systemic absorption was observed between healthy individuals at rest and those engaging in moderate exercise.

Following application of diclofenac epolamine transdermal system (Licart®) to the anterior thigh once daily for 4 days, peak plasma diclofenac concentrations of 0.4–2.9 ng/mL occur in 4–20 hours; the mean plasma diclofenac concentration during the 24-hour application period is 0.5–0.9 ng/mL. On average, when the system is applied to the medial aspect of the upper arm for 24 hours, about 7 mg of diclofenac is released from the system. Moderate exercise, application of an occlusion dressing over the system, or moderate heat increases peak plasma concentrations and systemic exposure by approximately 20%.

Following topical application of 4 g of diclofenac sodium 1% gel 4 times daily to one knee, mean peak plasma diclofenac concentrations of 15 ng/mL occur in about 14 hours. Following application of the gel to both knees and both hands 4 times daily (48 g of gel), mean peak plasma diclofenac concentrations of 53.8 ng/mL occur in about 10 hours. Systemic exposure to the drug at these dosage levels (16 or 48 g of gel daily) is about 6 or 20%, respectively, of the systemic exposure attained when diclofenac sodium is administered orally at a dosage of 50 mg 3 times daily. Application of a heat patch for 15 minutes before application of the gel did not affect systemic absorption. It has not been established whether application of a heat patch following gel application affects systemic absorption of the drug. Moderate exercise did not affect systemic absorption of the drug.

Following topical application of the maximum recommended dosage of diclofenac sodium 1.5% solution to both knees (40 drops per knee) 4 times daily for 7 days, mean peak plasma diclofenac concentrations of 19.4 ng/mL were achieved about 4 hours after a dose. Following topical application of diclofenac sodium 2% solution (40 mg per knee) twice daily for 7.5 days, mean peak plasma diclofenac concentrations at steady state on day 8 were 25.3 ng/mL; studies have not established whether application of heat, occlusive dressings, or exercise following application of the topical solution affects systemic absorption of the drug.

● Distribution

Distribution of diclofenac into human body tissues and fluids has not been fully characterized. Following IV administration of diclofenac in rats, the drug is widely distributed, achieving highest concentrations in bile, liver, blood, heart, lungs, and kidneys and lower concentrations in adrenals, thyroid glands, salivary glands, pancreas, spleen, muscles, brain, and spinal cord.

Like other NSAIAs, diclofenac is distributed into synovial fluid, achieving peak synovial fluid concentrations about 60–70% of those attained in plasma following oral administration; however, synovial fluid concentrations of the drug and its metabolites substantially exceed those in plasma after 3–6 hours. Following oral administration of a single 75-mg dose of diclofenac sodium, peak synovial fluid concentrations of approximately 225 ng/mL occur within about 4 hours, but there is considerable interindividual variation in synovial concentrations attained with a given dosage of the drug. Diclofenac appears to be eliminated from synovial fluid less rapidly than from plasma.

The apparent total volume of distribution of diclofenac reportedly averages about 1.3–1.4 L/kg.

Diclofenac is extensively but reversibly bound to plasma proteins, mainly albumin. At plasma diclofenac concentrations of 0.15–105 mcg/mL, the drug is 99–99.8% protein bound in vitro. Two binding sites have been identified, a high-affinity, low capacity site and a low-affinity, high capacity site. In patients with rheumatoid arthritis, protein binding of diclofenac in synovial fluid appears to be lower than in plasma.

Diclofenac and its metabolites cross the placenta in mice and rats. While substantial distribution of the drug into the milk of lactating women does not appear to occur with oral diclofenac sodium dosages of 100 mg daily, milk diclofenac concentrations of approximately 100 ng/mL were achieved in at least one woman receiving 150 mg of the drug daily.

● Elimination

Plasma concentrations of diclofenac appear to decline in a triphasic manner. Following IV administration of diclofenac sodium in healthy adults, the half-life of diclofenac reportedly averages about 3 minutes in the initial distribution phase, about 16 minutes in the intermediate (redistribution) phase, and about 1–2 hours in the terminal (elimination) phase. Following oral administration of delayed-release (enteric-coated) diclofenac sodium tablets in healthy individuals or in patients with rheumatoid arthritis, the elimination half-life of the drug was approximately 1.2–2 hours. Following application of diclofenac epolamine transdermal system, the elimination half-life of diclofenac is approximately 12 hours. The elimination half-life of diclofenac in patients with moderate renal impairment

appears to be similar to that in patients with normal renal function; however, half-life may be prolonged with severe renal impairment.

The exact metabolic fate of diclofenac has not been fully elucidated, but the drug is rapidly and extensively metabolized in the liver. Diclofenac undergoes extensive hydroxylation and subsequent conjugation with glucuronic acid, taurine amide, sulfuric acid, and other biogenic ligands. Conjugation of unchanged drug also may occur. Hydroxylation of the dichlorophenyl aromatic ring results in formation of 4'-hydroxydiclofenac (the principal metabolite of diclofenac) and 3'-hydroxydiclofenac, both of which subsequently undergo conjugation. Diclofenac also may undergo hydroxylation of the phenylacetic acid ring and subsequent conjugation to form conjugates of 5-hydroxydiclofenac and 4',5-dihydroxydiclofenac. Formation of 4'-hydroxydiclofenac is mediated mainly by cytochrome P-450 (CYP) isoenzyme 2C9, while formation of the minor metabolites 5-hydroxydiclofenac and 3'-hydroxydiclofenac is mediated by CYP3A4. Uridine diphosphate-glucuronosyltransferase (UGT) 2B7 and CYP2C8 may mediate acyl glucuronidation and oxidation reactions, respectively. Conjugation with glucuronic acid and taurine usually occurs at the carboxyl group of the phenylacetic ring, while conjugation with sulfuric acid mainly occurs at the 4' hydroxyl group of the dichlorophenyl aromatic ring; 3'- and/or 4'-hydroxydiclofenac may undergo further 4'-O-methylation to form 3'-hydroxy-4'-methoxydiclofenac.

Studies in animals indicate that on a weight basis, 4'-hydroxydiclofenac has about 3% of the anti-inflammatory potency of diclofenac and about 6 times the anti-inflammatory potency of aspirin. 3'-Hydroxydiclofenac also may have some anti-inflammatory activity, but other metabolites of the drug appear to be pharmacologically inactive.

Following oral or IV administration, diclofenac is excreted in urine and feces, with only minimal amounts being excreted unchanged. Fecal excretion of the drug occurs mainly via biliary elimination. Conjugates of unchanged diclofenac are excreted principally in bile, while hydroxylated metabolites are excreted in urine. Although there is evidence from animal studies that diclofenac undergoes enterohepatic circulation, such recirculation is minimal in humans.

Following oral or IV administration of diclofenac in healthy adults, about 50–70% of a dose is excreted in urine and about 30–35% is excreted in feces within 96 hours. About 20–30% of a dose is excreted in urine as conjugates of 4'-hydroxydiclofenac, 10–20% as conjugates of 5-, 3'-, and 4',5-dihydroxydiclofenac, 5–10% as conjugates of unchanged diclofenac, 2% as unconjugated metabolites, 1.4% as an unidentified metabolite (with an elimination half-life of 80 hours), and less than 1% as unchanged drug. Approximately 10–20% of a dose is excreted in bile as conjugates of 4'-hydroxydiclofenac, 1–5% as conjugates of unchanged diclofenac, and about 5–6% total as conjugates of the other 3 major metabolites.

Following IV administration of diclofenac in healthy individuals, plasma clearance of the drug averages about 263–350 mL/minute. Plasma clearance of diclofenac does not appear to be affected by renal impairment, although clearance of metabolites may be decreased.

The degree of accumulation of metabolites of diclofenac in patients with renal failure has not been systematically evaluated. Metabolites of diclofenac may accumulate in patients with severe renal impairment. In these patients, steady-state plasma metabolite concentrations may be up to four times higher than those observed in healthy individuals.

It is not known whether diclofenac is removed from systemic circulation by hemodialysis, hemoperfusion, or peritoneal dialysis.

CHEMISTRY AND STABILITY

● Chemistry

Diclofenac, a phenylacetic acid derivative, is a prototypical nonsteroidal anti-inflammatory agent (NSAIA). The drug is structurally related to meclofenamate sodium and mefenamic acid, but unlike these anthranilic acid (2-aminobenzoic) acid derivatives, diclofenac is a 2-aminobenzeneacetic acid derivative.

Diclofenac is commercially available as diclofenac sodium delayed-release (enteric-coated) tablets, diclofenac sodium extended-release tablets, diclofenac potassium conventional tablets, diclofenac potassium liquid-filled capsules, and diclofenac potassium powder for oral solution. Diclofenac also is commercially available as a fixed combination of diclofenac sodium in an enteric-coated core and misoprostol in an outer shell. Diclofenac sodium also is commercially available as a topical gel or topical solution. Diclofenac epolamine is commercially available as a transdermal system. The transdermal system consists of an adhesive material containing diclofenac epolamine (13 mg of drug per g of adhesive) that is applied to a polyester felt backing and is covered with a polypropylene liner; the liner is removed prior to application to the skin. Each transdermal system measures 10×14 cm and contains 180 mg (Flector®) or 182 mg (Licart®) of diclofenac epolamine in an aqueous base.

Diclofenac sodium and diclofenac potassium occur as faintly yellowish white to light beige, practically odorless, slightly hygroscopic crystalline powders and, at 25°C, have a pK_a of approximately 4.

● Stability

Diclofenac sodium delayed-release (enteric-coated) tablets, diclofenac sodium extended-release tablets, diclofenac potassium tablets, and diclofenac potassium liquid-filled capsules should be protected from moisture and stored in tight containers at room temperature; the manufacturer's labeling should be consulted for specific storage temperatures. Diclofenac potassium powder for oral solution should be stored at 25°C, but may be exposed to temperatures ranging from 15–30°C. Diclofenac sodium and misoprostol tablets should be stored at 20–25°C but may be exposed to temperatures ranging from 15–30°C. Diclofenac sodium delayed-release (enteric-coated) tablets have an expiration date of 2 years following the date of manufacture.

Diclofenac sodium 1% gel should be stored at 20–25°C and should not be frozen. Diclofenac sodium 1.5% topical solution should be stored in an upright position at 20–25°C. Diclofenac sodium 2% topical solution should be stored at 25°C but may be exposed to temperatures ranging from 15–30°C. Diclofenac epolamine transdermal system should be stored at 20–25°C but may be exposed to temperatures ranging from 15–30°C; once an envelope containing diclofenac epolamine transdermal systems (Licart®) has been opened, the systems are stable for up to 6 months if stored at room temperature in the resealed envelope.

PREPARATIONS

Excipients in commercially available drug preparations may have clinically important effects in some individuals; consult specific product labeling for details.

Diclofenac Epolamine

Topical		
Transdermal System	1.3%*	Diclofenac Epolamine Transdermal System
		Flector®, Pfizer
		Licart®, IBSA

* available from one or more manufacturer, distributor, and/or repackager by generic (nonproprietary) name

Diclofenac Potassium

Oral		
Capsules, liquid-filled	25 mg	Zipsor®, Depomed
For oral solution	50 mg*	Cambia®, Assertio
		Diclofenac Potassium for Oral Solution
Tablets	50 mg*	Diclofenac Potassium Tablets

* available from one or more manufacturer, distributor, and/or repackager by generic (nonproprietary) name

Diclofenac Sodium

Oral		
Tablets, delayed-release (enteric-coated)	25 mg*	Diclofenac Sodium Delayed-release Tablets
	50 mg*	Diclofenac Sodium Delayed-release Tablets
	75 mg*	Diclofenac Sodium Delayed-release Tablets
Tablets, extended-release	100 mg*	Diclofenac Sodium Extended-release Tablets
Topical		
Gel	1%*	Diclofenac Sodium Gel
		Voltaren®, Endo
		Voltaren® Arthritis Pain, GlaxoSmithKline
Solution	1.5%*	Diclofenac Sodium Topical Solution
	2%	Pennsaid®, Horizon

* available from one or more manufacturer, distributor, and/or repackager by generic (nonproprietary) name

Diclofenac Sodium Combinations

Oral		
Tablets, delayed-release (enteric-coated core), film-coated	50 mg diclofenac sodium enteric-coated core, with 200 mcg of misoprostol outer layer*	Arthrotec®, Pfizer
		Diclofenac Sodium and Misoprostol Delayed-release Tablets
	75 mg diclofenac sodium enteric-coated core, with 200 mcg of misoprostol outer layer*	Arthrotec®, Pfizer
		Diclofenac Sodium and Misoprostol Delayed-release Tablets

* available from one or more manufacturer, distributor, and/or repackager by generic (nonproprietary) name

† Use is not currently included in the labeling approved by the US Food and Drug Administration.

Ibuprofen, Ibuprofen Lysine

28:08.04.04 · REVERSIBLE COX-1/COX-2 INHIBITORS

■ Ibuprofen is a prototypical nonsteroidal anti-inflammatory agent (NSAIA) that also exhibits analgesic and antipyretic activity.

USES

Ibuprofen is used orally for anti-inflammatory and analgesic effects in the symptomatic treatment of rheumatoid arthritis, juvenile rheumatoid arthritis, and osteoarthritis. Ibuprofen also is used orally to relieve mild to moderate pain and for the management of primary dysmenorrhea.

Ibuprofen has been used orally in the management of pericarditis†.

Ibuprofen also may be used orally for *self-medication* for analgesic effects to provide temporary relief of *minor* aches and pains, including those of arthritis and of dysmenorrhea, for relief of migraine headaches, and for its antipyretic effect to reduce fever.

Ibuprofen is used IV to relieve mild to moderate pain, to relieve moderate to severe pain (in conjunction with opiates), and to reduce fever.

Ibuprofen lysine is used IV in the treatment of patent ductus arteriosus (PDA) in premature neonates.

The potential benefits and risks of ibuprofen therapy as well as alternative therapies should be considered prior to initiating ibuprofen therapy. The lowest possible effective dosage and shortest duration of therapy consistent with treatment goals of the patient should be employed.

● Inflammatory Diseases

Rheumatoid Arthritis, Juvenile Arthritis, and Osteoarthritis

Ibuprofen is used orally for anti-inflammatory and analgesic effects in the symptomatic treatment of acute and chronic rheumatoid arthritis and osteoarthritis. A fixed-combination preparation containing ibuprofen and famotidine may be used for the symptomatic treatment of rheumatoid arthritis and osteoarthritis when use of famotidine to reduce the risk of upper GI ulcers is appropriate. Efficacy of the fixed combination in reducing the risk of gastric and/or duodenal ulcers was demonstrated in studies of 6 months' duration in patients without a history of GI ulcer who were generally younger than 65 years of age. Ibuprofen is also used orally for anti-inflammatory and analgesic effects in the symptomatic treatment of nonarticular (e.g., muscular) inflammation.

When used in the treatment of rheumatoid arthritis, ibuprofen has relieved pain and stiffness, reduced swelling, and improved grip strength and joint flexion. The drug does not, however, alter the basic rheumatoid process. Most clinical studies have shown that the analgesic and anti-inflammatory effects of ibuprofen in the treatment of rheumatoid arthritis and/or osteoarthritis are greater than those of placebo, about equal to those of salicylates or indomethacin, and less than those of phenylbutazone or prednisolone. Patient response to oral NSAIAs is variable; patients who do not respond to or cannot tolerate one NSAIA might be successfully treated with a different agent. However, NSAIAs generally are contraindicated in patients in whom sensitivity reactions (e.g., urticaria, bronchospasm, severe rhinitis) are precipitated by aspirin or other NSAIAs. (See Contraindications under Cautions.)

In the management of rheumatoid arthritis in adults, NSAIAs may be useful for initial symptomatic treatment; however, NSAIAs do not alter the course of the disease or prevent joint destruction. Disease-modifying antirheumatic drugs (DMARDs) (e.g., abatacept, hydroxychloroquine, leflunomide, methotrexate, rituximab, sulfasalazine, tocilizumab, tofacitinib, tumor necrosis factor [TNF; TNF-α] blocking agents) have the potential to reduce or prevent joint damage and to preserve joint integrity and function. DMARDs are used in conjunction with anti-inflammatory agents (i.e., NSAIAs, intra-articular and oral glucocorticoids) and physical and occupational therapies for the management of rheumatoid arthritis. DMARD therapy should be initiated early in the disease course to prevent irreversible joint damage. For further information on the treatment of rheumatoid

arthritis, including considerations in selecting a DMARD regimen, see Uses: Rheumatoid Arthritis, in Methotrexate 10:00.

Ibuprofen is used orally in the symptomatic management of juvenile rheumatoid arthritis. In a very limited number of patients with juvenile rheumatoid arthritis receiving alternate-day corticosteroid therapy, ibuprofen relieved joint stiffness when administered on the corticosteroid "off" day.

Other Inflammatory Conditions

Ibuprofen has been used with some success in other inflammatory diseases including ankylosing spondylitis†, gout†, and psoriatic arthritis†.

● Pericarditis

Ibuprofen has been used to reduce the pain, fever, and inflammation of pericarditis†; however, in the treatment of post-myocardial infarction pericarditis, NSAIAs are potentially harmful and aspirin is considered the treatment of choice. (See Cardiovascular Effects and also see Cardiovascular Precautions under Cautions.)

● Pain

Ibuprofen is used orally or IV for the relief of mild to moderate pain. Ibuprofen also may be used orally for *self-medication* for the temporary relief of minor aches and pains associated with the common cold, influenza, or sore throat; headache (including migraine); toothache; muscular aches; backache; and minor pain of arthritis.

Some experts state that an NSAIA (e.g., ibuprofen) is a reasonable first-line therapy for mild to moderate migraine attacks or for severe attacks that have responded in the past to similar NSAIAs or non-opiate analgesics. For further information on management and classification of migraine headache, see Vascular Headaches: General Principles in Migraine Therapy, under Uses in Sumatriptan 28:32.28.

Ibuprofen has been used to relieve postoperative pain (including that associated with dental or orthopedic surgery or episiotomy). In the relief of postoperative pain, ibuprofen has been shown to be more effective than placebo or propoxyphene and at least as effective as aspirin.

Ibuprofen has been used IV in conjunction with opiates to relieve pain following abdominal hysterectomy, other abdominal surgical procedures, or orthopedic surgery.

The fixed-combination preparation containing ibuprofen and hydrocodone bitartrate is used in the short-term treatment of acute pain that is severe enough to require an opiate analgesic and for which alternative treatments are inadequate.

● Dysmenorrhea

Ibuprofen is used orally for the relief of primary dysmenorrhea. Ibuprofen also may be used for *self-medication* for the relief of pain of menstrual cramps (dysmenorrhea). Ibuprofen has been used to relieve dysmenorrhea associated with insertion of an intrauterine contraceptive device†.

When used to relieve dysmenorrhea, ibuprofen has been reported to be as effective as mefenamic acid and more effective than placebo, aspirin, or propoxyphene. In patients with primary dysmenorrhea, ibuprofen has reduced resting and active intrauterine pressure and the frequency of uterine contractions, probably as a result of inhibition of prostaglandin synthesis.

● Fever

Ibuprofen is used orally or IV to reduce fever. Ibuprofen also may be used orally for *self-medication* to reduce fever.

When used to lower body temperature in febrile children (6 months–12 years of age) with viral infections and temperatures of 39°C or less, single oral ibuprofen doses of 10 mg/kg have been as effective as single ibuprofen doses of 5 mg/kg or single acetaminophen doses of 10–15 mg/kg; however, in children with temperatures exceeding 39°C, single oral 10-mg/kg doses of ibuprofen were most effective.

● Patent Ductus Arteriosus

Ibuprofen lysine is used IV in the treatment of patent ductus arteriosus (PDA) in premature neonates and is designated an orphan drug by the US Food and Drug

Administration (FDA) for use in this condition. The drug is used IV to promote closure of a clinically important PDA in premature neonates weighing 500–1500 g who are no more than 32 weeks' gestational age when usual medical management (e.g., fluid restriction, diuretics, respiratory support) is ineffective. Ibuprofen lysine has been evaluated in premature neonates with echocardiographic evidence of PDA who were asymptomatic from their PDA at the time of study enrollment. Efficacy was determined by the need for rescue therapy (indomethacin, open-label ibuprofen, or surgery) for a hemodynamically important PDA through study day 14. Rescue therapy was indicated if the neonate developed a hemodynamically important PDA that was confirmed by echocardiography. Rescue therapy was required by 25% of neonates receiving ibuprofen compared with 48% of those receiving placebo. Neonates enrolled in this study were followed for a short period of time (up to 8 weeks) following treatment; long-term consequences of such therapy have not been determined. Use of the drug should be reserved for neonates with clinically important PDA.

● Other Uses

Results from a large, prospective, population-based cohort study in geriatric individuals indicate a lower prevalence of Alzheimer's disease† among patients who received an NSAIA for 2 years or longer. Similar findings have been reported from some other, but not all, observational studies.

DOSAGE AND ADMINISTRATION

● Administration

The potential benefits and risks of ibuprofen therapy as well as alternative therapies should be considered prior to initiating ibuprofen therapy.

Ibuprofen is administered orally or IV. Ibuprofen lysine is administered IV.

Ibuprofen is administered by IV infusion over a period of at least 30 minutes in adults and at least 10 minutes in pediatric patients 6 months to 17 years of age. All patients receiving IV ibuprofen should be well hydrated.

For *self-medication* in pediatric patients, ibuprofen is commercially available as oral drops, an oral suspension, chewable tablets, and film-coated tablets. The calibrated dosing device provided by the manufacturer should be used by parents or caregivers for measurement of the dose of oral drops; the calibrated dosage cup provided by the manufacturer should be used by parents or caregivers for measurement of the dose of pediatric oral suspension. Ibuprofen oral drops generally are used in infants 6–23 months of age, the oral suspension and the 100-mg chewable tablets commonly are used in children 2–11 years of age, and the 100-mg film-coated tablets may be used in children 6–11 years of age.

If GI disturbances occur, ibuprofen should be administered with meals or with milk or dosage should be reduced.

Tablets containing ibuprofen in fixed combination with famotidine should be swallowed whole, and should not be chewed, divided, crushed, or cut to provide a lower dose.

For IV administration, ibuprofen injection concentrate containing 100 mg/mL must be diluted with a compatible IV solution (e.g., 0.9% sodium chloride injection, 5% dextrose injection, lactated Ringer's injection) to provide a solution containing 4 mg/mL (less-concentrated solutions are acceptable). IV administration of the undiluted concentrate can result in hemolysis. The commercially available ibuprofen 4-mg/mL (800 mg in 200 mL) premixed injection should be used for administration of 800-mg doses only. Parenteral solutions of ibuprofen should be inspected visually for particulate matter and/or discoloration prior to administration whenever solution and container permit. The solution should not be used if opaque particles, discoloration, or other foreign particulate matter is present.

For IV administration, ibuprofen lysine injection should be diluted with an appropriate volume of dextrose injection or sodium chloride injection and administered within 30 minutes of preparation. The drug should be administered using the IV port that is nearest to the IV insertion site. The dose should be infused over a period of 15 minutes. Care should be taken to avoid extravasation of the drug since it may be irritating to extravascular tissues. Ibuprofen lysine should not be infused simultaneously through the same IV line as parenteral nutrition solutions; if the same IV line must be used, infusion of the nutrition solution should be interrupted for 15 minutes before and after ibuprofen lysine administration, and patency of the IV line maintained by infusion of dextrose injection or sodium

chloride injection. Parenteral solutions of ibuprofen lysine should be inspected visually for particulate matter and/or discoloration prior to administration whenever solution and container permit. The solution should be discarded if particulate matter is observed. Ibuprofen lysine injection contains no preservatives and is intended for single use only; any unused portion should be discarded.

● Dosage

The lowest possible effective dosage and shortest duration of therapy consistent with treatment goals of the patient should be employed. Dosage of ibuprofen must be carefully adjusted according to individual requirements and response, using the lowest possible effective dosage.

Patients receiving ibuprofen for *self-medication* should be advised to use the lowest effective dosage and not to exceed the recommended dosage or duration of therapy.

Dosage of ibuprofen lysine is expressed in terms of ibuprofen.

Patients should be warned that the risk of GI bleeding is increased when recommended durations of *self-medication* are exceeded and when more than one NSAIA are used concomitantly.

Inflammatory Diseases
Rheumatoid Arthritis, Juvenile Arthritis, and Osteoarthritis

The usual adult oral dosage of ibuprofen in the symptomatic treatment of rheumatoid arthritis and osteoarthritis is 400–800 mg 3 or 4 times daily. Dosage should be adjusted according to the response and tolerance of the patient and should not exceed 3.2 g daily. Although well-controlled clinical studies did not show that the average response was greater with 3.2 g daily than with 2.4 g daily, some patients may have a better response with 3.2 g daily; in patients receiving 3.2 g daily, an adequate increase in clinical benefit should be evident to justify potential increased risks associated with this dosage. Optimum therapeutic response may occur within a few days to 1 week but usually occurs within 2 weeks after beginning ibuprofen therapy if the dosage is adequate. The manufacturers state that patients with rheumatoid arthritis usually require a higher dosage of ibuprofen than do patients with osteoarthritis. When a satisfactory response to ibuprofen therapy occurs, dosage of the drug should be reviewed and adjusted as required.

When ibuprofen is used in fixed combination with famotidine (to reduce the risk of upper GI ulcers), the recommended ibuprofen dosage for symptomatic treatment of rheumatoid arthritis or osteoarthritis is 800 mg orally 3 times daily.

For the management of juvenile rheumatoid arthritis, the recommended ibuprofen oral dosage is 30–40 mg/kg daily divided into 3 or 4 doses. An ibuprofen dosage of 20 mg/kg daily in divided doses may be adequate for children with mild disease. Dosages exceeding 50 mg/kg daily are not recommended in children with juvenile arthritis, since such dosages have not been studied. In addition, dosages exceeding 40 mg/kg daily may increase the risk of drug-induced adverse effects. Optimum therapeutic response occurs from a few days to several weeks in children with juvenile rheumatoid arthritis. Once a clinical effect is obtained, the dosage should be reduced to the lowest dosage needed to maintain adequate control of symptoms. Children receiving ibuprofen dosages exceeding 30 mg/kg daily and those who have had abnormal liver function test results associated with prior NSAIA therapy should be carefully monitored for signs and symptoms of early liver dysfunction.

Pain

For relief of mild to moderate pain, the usual adult oral dosage of ibuprofen is 400 mg every 4–6 hours as necessary. Alternatively, for *self-medication* of minor aches and pain, the usual adult dosage is 200 mg every 4–6 hours; dosage may be increased to 400 mg every 4–6 hours if pain does not respond to the lower dosage but should not exceed 1.2 g daily unless directed by a clinician. For *self-medication* of migraine pain, the usual adult dosage of ibuprofen liquid-filled capsules is 400 mg; unless directed by a clinician, dosage should not exceed 400 mg in a 24-hour period. *Self-medication* of pain should not exceed 10 days unless otherwise directed by a clinician. Doses greater than 400 mg have *not* provided a greater analgesic effect than the 400-mg dose.

For *self-medication* of minor aches and pain in adolescents 12 years of age and older, the usual dosage of ibuprofen is 200 mg every 4–6 hours; dosage may be increased to 400 mg every 4–6 hours if pain does not respond to the lower dosage but should not exceed 1.2 g daily unless directed by a clinician. *Self-medication* of pain should not exceed 10 days unless otherwise directed by a clinician.

When ibuprofen is used in fixed combination with acetaminophen for *self-medication* of minor aches and pain in adults and adolescents 12 years of age and older, the usual and maximum dosage (unless otherwise directed by a clinician) of ibuprofen is 250 mg every 8 hours while pain persists. *Self-medication* of pain should not exceed 10 days unless otherwise directed by a clinician.

For relief of mild to moderate pain in children 6 months up to 2 years of age, the recommended ibuprofen oral dosage is 10 mg/kg every 6–8 hours, administered in a manner that does not disrupt the child's sleep pattern; the maximum dosage of ibuprofen is 40 mg/kg daily. For *self-medication* of minor aches and pain in pediatric patients, ibuprofen dosages should be calculated based on body weight rather than age whenever possible. (See Pediatric Precautions under Cautions.) Infants 6–11 months of age or those weighing 12–17 pounds (approximately 5–8 kg) may receive 50 mg of ibuprofen, infants 12–23 months of age or those weighing 18–23 pounds (approximately 8–10 kg) may receive 75 mg, children 2–3 years of age or those weighing 24–35 pounds (approximately 11–16 kg) may receive 100 mg, children 4–5 years of age or those weighing 36–47 pounds (approximately 16–21 kg) may receive 150 mg, children 6–8 years of age or those weighing 48–59 pounds (approximately 22–27 kg) may receive 200 mg, children 9–10 years of age or those weighing 60–71 pounds (approximately 27–32 kg) may receive 200–250 mg, and children 11 years of age or those weighing 72–95 pounds (approximately 33–43 kg) may receive 300 mg; these doses may be administered every 6–8 hours and no more than 4 times daily. Parents and caregivers should be instructed to discontinue use of ibuprofen and contact the child's clinician if minor aches and pain do not improve within 24 hours or if pain increases or lasts longer than 3 days.

For relief of pain, adults may receive ibuprofen in a dosage of 400–800 mg infused IV over at least 30 minutes every 6 hours as needed; ibuprofen dosage should not exceed 3.2 g in a 24-hour period. Adolescents 12–17 years of age may receive a dosage of 400 mg infused IV over at least 10 minutes every 4–6 hours as needed; ibuprofen dosage should not exceed 2.4 g in a 24-hour period. Children 6 months to younger than 12 years of age may receive a dosage of 10 mg/kg (up to 400 mg) infused IV over at least 10 minutes every 4–6 hours as needed; ibuprofen dosage should not exceed 40 mg/kg or 2.4 g, whichever is less, in a 24-hour period.

When ibuprofen is used in fixed combination with hydrocodone bitartrate for short-term management of acute pain, the usual oral dosage is 200 mg of ibuprofen every 4–6 hours, as needed; ibuprofen dosage should not exceed 1 g in a 24-hour period.

Dysmenorrhea

For the relief of primary dysmenorrhea, ibuprofen therapy should be started with the earliest onset of pain; the usual adult oral dosage in these patients is 400 mg every 4 hours as necessary for relief of pain. Alternatively, for *self-medication* of dysmenorrhea in adults and adolescents 12 years of age and older, the usual dosage is 200 mg every 4–6 hours; dosage may be increased to 400 mg every 4–6 hours if necessary but should not exceed 1.2 g daily unless otherwise directed by a clinician.

Fever

For antipyresis in children 6 months up to 2 years of age, the usual oral dosage of ibuprofen is 5 mg/kg for temperatures below 39°C and 10 mg/kg for temperatures of 39°C or higher. The maximum daily dosage of ibuprofen in febrile children is 40 mg/kg.

For *self-medication* of fever in pediatric patients, ibuprofen dosages should be calculated based on body weight rather than age whenever possible. (See Pediatric Precautions under Cautions.) Infants 6–11 months of age or those weighing 12–17 pounds (approximately 5–8 kg) may receive 50 mg of ibuprofen, infants 12–23 months of age or those weighing 18–23 pounds (approximately 8–10 kg) may receive 75 mg, children 2–3 years of age or those weighing 24–35 pounds (approximately 11–16 kg) may receive 100 mg, children 4–5 years of age or those weighing 36–47 pounds (approximately 16–21 kg) may receive 150 mg, children 6–8 years of age or those weighing 48–59 pounds (approximately 22–27 kg) may receive 200 mg, children 9–10 years of age or those weighing 60–71 pounds (approximately 27–32 kg) may receive 200–250 mg, and children 11 years of age or those weighing 72–95 pounds (approximately 33–43 kg) may receive 300 mg; these doses may be administered every 6–8 hours and no more than 4 times

daily. Parents and caregivers should be instructed to contact the child's clinician if fever does not improve within 24 hours or if fever increases or lasts longer than 3 days.

For *self-medication* of fever in adults and adolescents 12 years of age and older, the usual dosage of ibuprofen is 200 mg every 4–6 hours; dosage may be increased to 400 mg every 4–6 hours if fever is not adequately reduced at the lower dosage but should not exceed 1.2 g daily unless otherwise directed by a clinician. In addition, limited data indicate that adequate antipyresis may be maintained in some patients in whom initial doses of ibuprofen were followed with lower doses of the drug. *Self-medication* of fever should not exceed 3 days unless otherwise directed by a clinician.

For reduction of fever, adults may receive an initial dose of ibuprofen 400 mg IV followed by 400 mg IV every 4–6 hours or 100–200 mg IV every 4 hours; doses should be infused over at least 30 minutes. Ibuprofen dosage in adults should not exceed 3.2 g in a 24-hour period. Adolescents 12–17 years of age may receive a dosage of 400 mg infused IV over at least 10 minutes every 4–6 hours as needed; ibuprofen dosage should not exceed 2.4 g in a 24-hour period. Children 6 months to younger than 12 years of age may receive a dosage of 10 mg/kg (up to 400 mg) infused IV over at least 10 minutes every 4–6 hours as needed; ibuprofen dosage should not exceed 40 mg/kg or 2.4 g, whichever is less, in a 24-hour period.

Patent Ductus Arteriosus

For the treatment of patent ductus arteriosus (PDA) in premature neonates, ibuprofen lysine is administered by IV infusion over 15 minutes. A course of therapy consists of 3 doses of ibuprofen lysine administered at 24-hour intervals. All doses are based on the neonate's birth weight. The first IV dose of ibuprofen in the course is 10 mg/kg; the second and third doses are 5 mg/kg each, administered 24 and 48 hours after the first dose. If anuria or oliguria (i.e., urine output less than 0.6 mL/kg per hour) is present at the time of the second or third dose, the dose should be withheld until laboratory determinations indicate that renal function has returned to normal. Subsequent doses are not necessary if the ductus arteriosus closes or is substantially constricted after completion of the first course of ibuprofen therapy. If the ductus fails to close or reopens, a second course of ibuprofen, alternative pharmacologic therapy, or surgery may be needed.

● *Pharmacogenomic Dosage Considerations*

Clinical Pharmacogenetics Implementation Consortium (CPIC) guidelines state that, in patients who are CYP2C9 poor metabolizers, ibuprofen should be initiated at a dosage that is 25–50% of the lowest recommended initial dosage and cautiously titrated to a clinically effective dosage, up to a dosage that is 25–50% of the maximum recommended dosage. Dosage should not be increased until steady-state concentrations are attained (at least 5 days following the initial dose in poor metabolizers). Alternatively, a drug that is not metabolized by CYP2C9 or is not substantially affected by CYP2C9 genetic variants in vivo should be considered. In addition, CPIC guidelines state that, in patients who are CYP2C9 intermediate metabolizers with a diplotype functional activity score (AS) of 1, ibuprofen may be initiated at the lowest recommended initial dosage and cautiously titrated to a clinically effective dosage, up to the maximum recommended dosage. Intermediate metabolizers with an AS of 1.5 may receive dosages recommended for normal metabolizers. These dosage recommendations apply to both nonprescription (over-the-counter, OTC) and prescription use of the drug. (See Pharmacogenomic Precautions under Cautions.)

CAUTIONS

● *Cardiovascular Effects*

Peripheral edema and fluid retention have been reported during ibuprofen therapy. Congestive heart failure has occurred in patients with marginal cardiac function. Increased blood pressure, hypotension, cerebrovascular accident, and palpitations also have been reported. Although a causal relationship has not been established, arrhythmias, including sinus tachycardia or bradycardia, have been reported during therapy with the drug.

Tachycardia, cardiac failure, hypotension, and pulmonary hypertension have occurred in premature neonates receiving ibuprofen for treatment of patent ductus arteriosus (PDA), although a causal relationship to the drug has not been established.

Nonsteroidal anti-inflammatory agents (NSAIAs), including selective cyclo-oxygenase-2 (COX-2) inhibitors and prototypical NSAIAs, increase the risk of serious adverse cardiovascular thrombotic events, including myocardial infarction and stroke (which can be fatal), in patients with or without cardiovascular disease or risk factors for cardiovascular disease. Use of NSAIAs also is associated with an increased risk of heart failure.

The association between cardiovascular complications and use of NSAIAs is an area of ongoing concern and study. Findings of an FDA review of published observational studies of NSAIAs, a meta-analysis of published and unpublished data from randomized controlled trials of these drugs, and other published information indicate that NSAIAs may increase the risk of serious adverse cardiovascular thrombotic events by 10–50% or more, depending on the drugs and dosages studied. Available data suggest that the increase in risk may occur early (within the first weeks) following initiation of therapy and may increase with higher dosages and longer durations of use. Although the relative increase in cardiovascular risk appears to be similar in patients with or without known underlying cardiovascular disease or risk factors for cardiovascular disease, the absolute incidence of serious NSAIA-associated cardiovascular thrombotic events is higher in those with cardiovascular disease or risk factors for cardiovascular disease because of their elevated baseline risk.

Results from observational studies utilizing Danish national registry data indicated that patients receiving NSAIAs following a myocardial infarction were at increased risk of reinfarction, cardiovascular-related death, and all-cause mortality beginning in the first week of treatment. Patients who received NSAIAs following myocardial infarction had a higher 1-year mortality rate compared with those who did not receive NSAIAs (20 versus 12 deaths per 100 person-years). Although the absolute mortality rate declined somewhat after the first year following the myocardial infarction, the increased relative risk of death in patients who received NSAIAs persisted over at least the next 4 years of follow-up.

In 2 large controlled clinical trials of a selective COX-2 inhibitor for the management of pain in the first 10–14 days following coronary artery bypass graft (CABG) surgery, the incidence of myocardial infarction and stroke was increased. Therefore, NSAIAs are contraindicated in the setting of CABG surgery.

Findings from some systematic reviews of controlled observational studies and meta-analyses of data from randomized studies of NSAIAs suggest that naproxen may be associated with a lower risk of cardiovascular thrombotic events compared with other NSAIAs. However, limitations of these observational studies and the indirect comparisons used to assess cardiovascular risk of the prototypical NSAIAs (e.g., variability in patients' risk factors, comorbid conditions, concomitant drug therapy, drug interactions, dosage, and duration of therapy) affect the validity of the comparisons; in addition, these studies were not designed to demonstrate superior safety of one NSAIA compared with another. Therefore, FDA states that definitive conclusions regarding relative risks of NSAIAs are not possible at this time. (See Cautions: Cardiovascular Effects, in Celecoxib 28:08.04.08.)

Data from observational studies also indicate that use of NSAIAs in patients with heart failure is associated with increased morbidity and mortality. Results from a retrospective study utilizing Danish national registry data indicated that use of selective COX-2 inhibitors or prototypical NSAIAs in patients with chronic heart failure was associated with a dose-dependent increase in the risk of death and an increased risk of hospitalization for myocardial infarction or heart failure. In addition, findings from a meta-analysis of published and unpublished data from randomized controlled trials of NSAIAs indicated that use of selective COX-2 inhibitors or prototypical NSAIAs was associated with an approximate twofold increase in the risk of hospitalization for heart failure. Fluid retention and edema also have been observed in some patients receiving NSAIAs.

There is no consistent evidence that use of low-dose aspirin mitigates the increased risk of serious cardiovascular events associated with NSAIAs.

● GI Effects

The most frequent adverse effects of ibuprofen involve the GI tract and have included dyspepsia, heartburn, nausea, vomiting, anorexia, diarrhea, constipation, stomatitis, flatulence, bloating, epigastric pain, and abdominal pain. Peptic ulcer and GI bleeding (including evidence of occult blood in stools), sometimes severe, have also been reported. Although a causal relationship has not been established, a few cases of GI ulceration with perforation and bleeding resulting in death have occurred.

Nonnecrotizing enterocolitis has occurred in premature neonates receiving ibuprofen for treatment of PDA. Gastroesophageal reflux, gastritis, ileus, GI perforation, and necrotizing enterocolitis also have occurred, although a causal relationship to the drug has not been established.

The frequency of mild adverse GI effects with usual dosages of ibuprofen is reported to be less than that with usual dosages of oral aspirin or indomethacin. It is not known whether ibuprofen causes less peptic ulceration than does aspirin. Usual dosages of ibuprofen generally have been associated with only minimal GI blood loss, and limited data indicate that the risk of GI bleeding and/or perforation with ibuprofen appears to be less than that with other prototypical NSAIAs (e.g., piroxicam, indomethacin, ketoprofen, naproxen, diclofenac).

Adverse GI effects of orally administered ibuprofen may be minimized by administering the drug with meals or milk. Close supervision of ibuprofen therapy is necessary, particularly in patients with a history of upper GI disease.

Serious, sometimes fatal, adverse GI effects (e.g., bleeding, ulceration, or perforation of the esophagus, stomach, or small or large intestine) can occur at any time in patients receiving NSAIA therapy, and such effects may *not* be preceded by warning signs or symptoms. Only 1 in 5 patients who develop a serious upper GI adverse event while receiving NSAIA therapy is symptomatic. Therefore, clinicians should remain alert to the possible development of serious GI effects (e.g., bleeding, ulceration) in any patient receiving NSAIA therapy, and such patients should be followed chronically for the development of manifestations of such effects and advised of the importance of this follow-up. Patients receiving concomitant low-dose aspirin therapy for cardiac prophylaxis should be monitored even more closely for evidence of GI bleeding. In addition, patients should be advised about the signs and symptoms of serious NSAIA-induced GI toxicity and what action to take if they occur. If signs and symptoms of a serious GI event develop, additional evaluation and treatment should be initiated promptly; the NSAIA should be discontinued until appropriate diagnostic studies have ruled out a serious GI event.

Results of studies to date are inconclusive concerning the relative risk of various prototypical NSAIAs in causing serious GI effects. In patients receiving NSAIAs and observed in clinical studies of several months' to 2 years' duration, upper GI ulcers, gross bleeding, or perforation appeared to occur in approximately 1% of patients treated for 3–6 months and in about 2–4% of those treated for 1 year. Longer duration of therapy with an NSAIA increases the likelihood of a serious GI event. However, short-term therapy is not without risk. High dosages of any NSAIA probably are associated with increased risk of such effects, although controlled studies documenting this probable association are lacking for most NSAIAs. Therefore, whenever use of relatively high dosages (within the recommended dosage range) is considered, sufficient benefit to offset the potential increased risk of GI toxicity should be anticipated.

Studies have shown that patients with a history of peptic ulcer disease and/or GI bleeding who are receiving NSAIAs have a greater than tenfold increased risk of developing GI bleeding than patients without these risk factors. In addition to a history of ulcer disease, pharmacoepidemiologic studies have identified several comorbid conditions and concomitant therapies that may increase the risk for GI bleeding, including concomitant use of oral corticosteroids, anticoagulants, aspirin, or selective serotonin-reuptake inhibitors (SSRIs); longer duration of NSAIA therapy; smoking; alcohol use; older age; and poor general health status. Risk of GI bleeding also is increased in patients with advanced liver disease and/or coagulopathy. Patients with rheumatoid arthritis are more likely to experience serious GI complications from NSAIA therapy than are patients with osteoarthritis. In addition, geriatric or debilitated patients appear to tolerate GI ulceration and bleeding less well than other individuals, and most spontaneous reports of fatal GI effects have been in such patients.

For patients at high risk for complications from NSAIA-induced GI ulceration (e.g., bleeding, perforation), concomitant use of misoprostol can be considered for preventive therapy. (See Misoprostol 56:28.28.) Alternatively, some clinicians suggest that a proton-pump inhibitor (e.g., omeprazole) may be used concomitantly to decrease the incidence of serious GI toxicity associated with NSAIA therapy. In one study, therapy with high dosages of famotidine (40 mg twice daily) was more effective than placebo in preventing peptic ulcers in NSAIA-treated patients; however, the effect of the drug was modest. In addition, efficacy of usual dosages of H_2-receptor antagonists for the prevention of NSAIA-induced gastric and duodenal ulcers has not been established. Therefore, most clinicians do not recommend use of H_2-receptor antagonists for the prevention of NSAIA-associated ulcers.

Another approach in high-risk patients who would benefit from NSAIA therapy is use of a NSAIA that is a selective inhibitor of COX-2 (e.g., celecoxib), since these agents are associated with a lower incidence of serious GI bleeding than are prototypical NSAIAs. However, while celecoxib (200 mg twice daily) was comparably effective to diclofenac sodium (75 mg twice daily) plus omeprazole (20 mg daily) in preventing recurrent ulcer bleeding (recurrent ulcer bleeding probabilities of 4.9 versus 6.4%, respectively, during the 6-month study) in *H. pylori*-negative arthritis (principally osteoarthritis) patients with a recent history of ulcer bleeding, the protective efficacy was unexpectedly low for both regimens and it appeared that neither could completely protect patients at high risk. Additional study is necessary to elucidate optimal therapy for preventing GI complications associated with NSAIA therapy in high-risk patients.

Nervous System Effects

Adverse CNS effects of ibuprofen include dizziness, headache, and nervousness. Fatigue, drowsiness, malaise, lightheadedness, anxiety, confusion, mental depression, and emotional lability have also been reported. Although a causal relationship has not been established, paresthesia, hallucinations, dream abnormalities, and pseudotumor cerebri also have been reported.

Aseptic meningitis with fever and coma has occurred rarely in patients receiving ibuprofen, and has recurred upon rechallenge with the drug. Although meningitis probably is more likely to occur in patients with systemic lupus erythematosus or related connective tissue diseases, it has been reported in some patients without evidence of any underlying chronic disease. Other associated manifestations have included GI symptoms (e.g., nausea, vomiting, abdominal pain), transient conjunctivitis, CNS signs (e.g., confusion, combativeness, lethargy, headache), and hypotension. If signs and/or symptoms of meningitis develop in a patient receiving ibuprofen, the possibility that these effects may be associated with the drug should be considered.

Intraventricular (intracranial) hemorrhage has occurred in premature neonates receiving ibuprofen for treatment of PDA. Seizures also have occurred, although a causal relationship to the drug has not been established.

Otic and Ocular Effects

Patients receiving ibuprofen have experienced tinnitus. Decreased hearing and amblyopia (blurred and/or decreased visual acuity, scotomata and/or changes in color vision) have also been reported. Vision generally has gradually improved when the drug was discontinued in patients with visual disturbances. Although a causal relationship has not been established, conjunctivitis, diplopia, optic neuritis, and cataracts have also been reported in patients receiving the drug. Ibuprofen should be discontinued and an ophthalmologic examination performed in patients who experience visual disturbances during therapy with the drug.

Hepatic Effects

Severe (sometimes fatal) reactions including jaundice, fulminant hepatitis, liver necrosis, and hepatic failure have been reported rarely in patients receiving NSAIAs, including ibuprofen. A transitory rise in serum AST, ALT, and serum alkaline phosphatase also has occurred in patients receiving ibuprofen therapy.

Borderline elevations of one or more liver function test results may occur in up to 15% of patients treated with NSAIAs; meaningful (3 times the upper limit of normal) elevations of serum ALT or AST concentration have occurred in approximately 1% of patients receiving NSAIAs in controlled clinical studies. Ibuprofen should be discontinued immediately if signs or symptoms consistent with liver disease develop or if systemic manifestations (e.g., eosinophilia, rash) occur, and clinical evaluation of the patient should be performed. (See Hepatic Precautions under Cautions.)

Although a causal relationship to the drug has not been established, jaundice and cholestasis have occurred in premature neonates receiving ibuprofen for treatment of PDA.

Dermatologic and Sensitivity Reactions

Urticarial, vesiculobullous, and erythematous macular rashes, erythema multiforme, exfoliative dermatitis, toxic epidermal necrolysis (Lyell's syndrome), and photosensitivity reactions have occurred occasionally during ibuprofen therapy. Pruritus without evidence of a rash has occurred in a few patients. Stevens-Johnson syndrome, flushes, alopecia, rectal itching, and acne have also been reported.

Hypersensitivity reactions manifested as a syndrome of abdominal pain, fever, chills, nausea, and vomiting have occasionally occurred during ibuprofen therapy. Anaphylaxis, anaphylactoid reactions, and bronchospasm have also occurred. Anaphylactic reactions have been reported in patients with or without known hypersensitivity to the drug, as well as in patients with aspirin-sensitivity asthma. Although a causal relationship has not been established, serum sickness, lupus erythematosus syndrome, Henoch-Schönlein vasculitis, and angioedema have also been reported during therapy with the drug.

Skin lesion/irritation has occurred in premature neonates receiving ibuprofen for treatment of PDA.

Hematologic Effects

Adverse hematologic effects of ibuprofen include neutropenia, agranulocytosis, aplastic anemia, hemolytic anemia (with or without positive direct antiglobulin test results), and thrombocytopenia (with or without purpura). Anemia may be due to occult or gross blood loss, fluid retention, or an incompletely described effect on erythropoiesis. Slight, dose-dependent reductions in serum hemoglobin concentrations and hematocrit have occurred in patients receiving ibuprofen dosages of 1.2–3.2 g daily, and the total decrease in hemoglobin may exceed 1 g in patients receiving 3.2 g or more of the drug. Data from clinical use indicate that a decrease in hemoglobin concentration of 1 g or more occurs in about 17% of patients receiving 1.6 g of ibuprofen daily and in about 23% of patients receiving 2.4 g of the drug daily. In the absence of clinical signs of bleeding, the decrease in hemoglobin probably is not clinically important. Although a causal relationship has not been established, bleeding episodes (e.g., epistaxis, menorrhagia, occult blood in the stool) have been reported during therapy with the drug. Ibuprofen can inhibit platelet aggregation and may prolong bleeding time. It appears that ibuprofen's inhibitory effect on platelet aggregation is of shorter duration and less pronounced than that of aspirin. Patients who may be adversely affected by a prolongation of bleeding time should be carefully observed during ibuprofen therapy.

Anemia and bleeding have occurred in premature neonates receiving ibuprofen for treatment of PDA. Neutropenia and thrombocytopenia also have occurred, although a causal relationship to the drug has not been established.

Renal and Electrolyte Effects

Acute renal failure has been reported in patients receiving ibuprofen and may be accompanied by acute tubular necrosis. Such acute deterioration in renal function may be evident soon (e.g., within several days) after initiation of ibuprofen therapy in certain patients at risk (e.g., those with preexisting renal impairment) (see Renal Precautions under Cautions) and may be accompanied by hyperkalemia. Polyuria, azotemia, cystitis, hematuria, and decreased creatinine clearance also have been reported in patients receiving the drug. Elevations in serum creatinine concentrations and increases in BUN without other manifestation of renal failure also have occurred occasionally. In addition, acute interstitial nephritis accompanied by hematuria, proteinuria, and occasionally nephrotic syndrome has occurred. Recurrence of nephrotic syndrome has occurred in at least one patient during ibuprofen therapy. Increases in serum uric acid concentration, tubular necrosis, glomerulitis, and renal papillary necrosis also have been reported. Long-term studies in rats and monkeys have shown histologic evidence of ibuprofen-induced mild renal toxicity manifested as papillary edema and necrosis in some animals. An association between prolonged (e.g., daily for 1 year or longer) NSAIA use, including ibuprofen, and chronic renal failure also has been described in certain high-risk patients, but current evidence suggests that the potential risk, if any, is low overall in patients receiving the drug, and additional study and experience are necessary to confirm and elucidate these findings.

Renal insufficiency (including oliguria), increases in BUN (sometimes accompanied by hematuria), increases in serum creatinine concentration, and renal failure have been reported in ibuprofen-treated premature neonates. Reversible decreases in urine output have occurred in premature neonates receiving ibuprofen therapy for PDA. Urine output usually decreases during the first 2–6 days of life; this is followed by a compensatory increase in output by day 9.

Hyperkalemia has been reported in patients receiving NSAIAs, including in individuals without renal impairment; in those with normal renal function, this effect has been attributed to a hyporenin-hypoaldosterone state.

● Other Adverse Effects

Other adverse effects of ibuprofen include dry mouth, gingival ulceration, and rhinitis. Although a causal relationship has not been established, gynecomastia, hypoglycemic reactions, and acidosis have also been reported during therapy with the drug.

Infections (e.g., sepsis, respiratory infection, urinary tract infection), apnea, respiratory failure, atelectasis, edema, adrenal insufficiency, hypoglycemia, hypocalcemia, and hypernatremia have occurred in premature neonates receiving ibuprofen for treatment of PDA. Hyperglycemia, abdominal distension, feeding problems, inguinal hernia, and injection site reactions also have occurred, although a causal relationship to the drug has not been established.

● Precautions and Contraindications

Patients should be advised that ibuprofen, like other NSAIAs, is not free of potential adverse effects, including some that can cause discomfort, and that more serious effects (e.g., myocardial infarction, stroke, GI bleeding), which may require hospitalization and may even be fatal, also can occur. When preparations containing ibuprofen in combination with other drugs are used, the precautions and contraindications associated with each ingredient also must be considered.

Patients should be advised to read the medication guide for NSAIAs that is provided to the patient each time the drug is dispensed.

Cardiovascular Precautions

NSAIAs increase the risk of serious adverse cardiovascular thrombotic events. (See Cardiovascular Effects under Cautions.) To minimize the potential risk of adverse cardiovascular events, the lowest effective dosage and shortest possible duration of therapy should be employed. Some clinicians suggest that it may be prudent to avoid use of NSAIAs whenever possible in patients with cardiovascular disease. Patients receiving NSAIAs (including those without previous symptoms of cardiovascular disease) should be monitored for the possible development of cardiovascular events throughout therapy. Patients should be informed about the signs and symptoms of serious cardiovascular toxicity (chest pain, dyspnea, weakness, slurring of speech) and instructed to seek immediate medical attention if such toxicity occurs. Ibuprofen should be avoided in patients with recent myocardial infarction unless the benefits of therapy are expected to outweigh the risk of recurrent cardiovascular thrombotic events; if ibuprofen is used in such patients, the patient should be monitored for cardiac ischemia.

There is no consistent evidence that concomitant use of low-dose aspirin mitigates the increased risk of serious cardiovascular events associated with NSAIAs. Concomitant use of aspirin and an NSAIA increases the risk for serious GI events. (See Nonsteroidal Anti-inflammatory Agents under Drug Interactions.)

Use of NSAIAs can result in the onset of hypertension or worsening of preexisting hypertension; either of these occurrences may contribute to the increased incidence of cardiovascular events. Patients receiving NSAIAs may have an impaired response to diuretics (i.e., thiazide or loop diuretics), angiotensin-converting enzyme (ACE) inhibitors, angiotensin II receptor antagonists, or β-adrenergic blocking agents. Blood pressure should be monitored closely during initiation of NSAIA therapy and throughout therapy.

Because NSAIAs increase morbidity and mortality in patients with heart failure, the manufacturer states that ibuprofen should be avoided in patients with severe heart failure unless the benefits of therapy are expected to outweigh the risk of worsening heart failure; if ibuprofen is used in such patients, the patient should be monitored for worsening heart failure. Some experts state that use of NSAIAs should be avoided whenever possible in patients with reduced left ventricular ejection fraction and current or prior symptoms of heart failure. Patients receiving NSAIAs should be advised to inform their clinician if they experience symptoms of heart failure, including dyspnea, unexplained weight gain, and edema. Use of NSAIAs may diminish the cardiovascular effects of certain drugs used to treat heart failure and edema (e.g., diuretics, ACE inhibitors, angiotensin II receptor antagonists). (See Antihypertensive Agents and also Diuretics under Drug Interactions.)

GI Precautions

The risk of potentially serious adverse GI effects should be considered in patients receiving ibuprofen, particularly in patients receiving chronic therapy with the drug. Since peptic ulceration and/or GI bleeding have been reported in patients receiving the drug, patients should be advised to promptly report signs or symptoms of GI ulceration or bleeding to their clinician.

To minimize the potential risk of adverse GI effects, the lowest effective dosage and shortest possible duration of therapy should be employed, and use of more than one NSAIA at a time should be avoided. (See Nonsteroidal Anti-inflammatory Agents under Drug Interactions.) In addition, use of NSAIAs should be avoided in patients at higher risk (see GI Effects under Cautions) unless the benefits of therapy are expected to outweigh the increased risk of bleeding; for patients who are at high risk, as well as for those with active GI bleeding, alternative therapy other than an NSAIA should be considered.

Use of corticosteroids during NSAIA therapy may increase the risk of GI ulceration, and the drugs should be used concomitantly with caution.

Hepatic Precautions

Liver function should be monitored periodically during long-term ibuprofen therapy. Elevations in serum ALT may be the most sensitive indicator of NSAIA-induced liver dysfunction. Patients who experience signs and/or symptoms suggestive of liver dysfunction or an abnormal liver function test result while receiving ibuprofen should be evaluated for evidence of the development of a more severe hepatic reaction. Severe reactions, including jaundice and fatal fulminant hepatitis, liver necrosis, and hepatic failure (sometimes fatal), have been reported in patients receiving NSAIAs. Although such reactions are rare, ibuprofen should be discontinued immediately if abnormal liver function test results persist or worsen, if clinical signs and symptoms consistent with liver disease develop, or if systemic manifestations (e.g., eosinophilia, rash) occur. Patients receiving ibuprofen should be informed of the warning signs and symptoms of hepatotoxicity (e.g., nausea, anorexia, fatigue, lethargy, pruritus, jaundice, right upper quadrant tenderness, flu-like syndrome) and advised to discontinue ibuprofen therapy and seek immediate medical care if they experience such symptoms.

Renal Precautions

Renal toxicity has been observed in patients in whom renal prostaglandins have a compensatory role in maintaining renal perfusion. Administration of an NSAIA to such patients may cause a dose-dependent reduction in prostaglandin formation and thereby precipitate overt renal decompensation. Patients at greatest risk of this reaction are those with impaired renal function, heart failure, or hepatic dysfunction; those with extracellular fluid depletion (e.g., patients receiving diuretics); those taking an ACE inhibitor or angiotensin II receptor antagonist concomitantly; and geriatric patients. Patients should be advised to consult their clinician promptly if unexplained weight gain or edema occurs. Fluid depletion should be corrected prior to initiation of ibuprofen therapy, and renal function should be monitored during ibuprofen therapy in patients with renal or hepatic impairment, heart failure, dehydration, or hypovolemia. Recovery of renal function to pretreatment levels usually occurs following discontinuance of NSAIA therapy.

The renal effects of ibuprofen may hasten the progression of renal dysfunction in patients with preexisting renal disease. Patients with preexisting renal disease should be monitored for worsening renal function.

Ibuprofen has not been evaluated in patients with severe renal impairment, and the manufacturers state that use of the drug should be avoided in patients with advanced renal disease unless the benefits of therapy are expected to outweigh the risk of worsening renal function. If ibuprofen is used in patients with advanced renal disease, close monitoring of renal function is recommended.

Ibuprofen lysine is contraindicated in neonates with substantially impaired renal function.

Pharmacogenomic Precautions

In patients with the cytochrome P-450 isoenzyme 2C9 (CYP2C9) poor metabolizer phenotype, metabolism of ibuprofen may be decreased substantially; the half-life of ibuprofen is prolonged and higher plasma concentrations of the drug may increase the likelihood and/or severity of adverse effects. Metabolism of ibuprofen may be moderately reduced in CYP2C9 intermediate metabolizers with a diplotype functional activity score (AS) of 1 and mildly reduced in those with an AS of 1.5. Higher plasma concentrations of the drug in intermediate metabolizers with an AS of 1 may increase the likelihood of adverse effects. The presence of other factors affecting clearance of the drug (e.g., hepatic impairment, advanced age) also may increase the risk of adverse effects in intermediate metabolizers.

Further caution is advised in patients carrying the CYP2C9*2 allele, since this allele is strongly linked to the decreased-function CYP2C8*3 allele, and CYP2C8 also contributes to metabolism of ibuprofen. (See Pharmacogenomic Dosage Considerations under Dosage and Administration and also see Elimination under Pharmacokinetics.) The Clinical Pharmacogenetics Implementation Consortium Guideline (CPIC) for CYP2C9 and Nonsteroidal Anti-Inflammatory Drugs should be consulted for additional information on interpretation of CYP2C9 genotype testing.

Precautions Related to Dermatologic or Hypersensitivity Reactions

Anaphylactoid reactions have been reported in patients receiving NSAIAs. Patients receiving NSAIAs should be informed of the signs and symptoms of an anaphylactoid reaction (e.g., difficulty breathing, swelling of the face or throat) and advised to seek immediate medical attention if an anaphylactoid reaction develops.

Serious skin reactions (e.g., exfoliative dermatitis, Stevens-Johnson syndrome, toxic epidermal necrolysis) can occur in patients receiving NSAIAs. These serious skin reactions may occur without warning; patients should be advised to consult their clinician if skin rash and blisters, fever, or other signs of hypersensitivity reaction (e.g., pruritus) occur. NSAIAs should be discontinued at the first appearance of rash or any other sign of hypersensitivity.

Multi-organ hypersensitivity (also known as drug reaction with eosinophilia and systemic symptoms [DRESS]), a potentially fatal or life-threatening syndrome, has been reported in patients receiving NSAIAs. The clinical presentation is variable, but typically includes eosinophilia, fever, rash, lymphadenopathy, and/or facial swelling, possibly associated with other organ system involvement such as hepatitis, nephritis, hematologic abnormalities, myocarditis, or myositis. Symptoms may resemble those of an acute viral infection. Early manifestations of hypersensitivity, such as fever or lymphadenopathy, may be present in the absence of rash. If such signs or symptoms develop, the NSAIA should be discontinued and the patient evaluated immediately.

Hematologic Precautions

Ibuprofen should be used with caution in patients who may be adversely affected by a prolongation of bleeding time (e.g., patients receiving anticoagulant therapy), since the drug may inhibit platelet function.

NSAIAs, including ibuprofen, may increase the risk of bleeding. Patients with certain coexisting conditions such as coagulation disorders and those receiving concomitant therapy with anticoagulants, antiplatelet agents, or serotonin-reuptake inhibitors may be at increased risk and should be monitored for signs of bleeding. (See Drug Interactions.)

If signs and/or symptoms of anemia occur during therapy with ibuprofen, hemoglobin concentration and hematocrit should be determined.

Premature neonates receiving ibuprofen lysine should be observed closely for bleeding tendencies. Ibuprofen lysine is contraindicated in neonates with active bleeding, such as those with intracranial hemorrhage or GI bleeding, and in neonates with thrombocytopenia or underlying coagulation defect.

Precautions for Self-medication

Adults receiving ibuprofen for *self-medication* should be advised to use the lowest effective dosage and not to exceed the recommended dosage or duration of therapy. Unless otherwise directed by a clinician, adults receiving ibuprofen for *self-medication* should be advised to discontinue the drug and consult a clinician if pain persists for more than 10 days or fever persists for longer than 3 days. Patients should not use ibuprofen for *self-medication* immediately before or after cardiac surgery, or if they have experienced an allergic reaction to any analgesic or antipyretic. Patients receiving ibuprofen for *self-medication* of acute migraine attacks should be advised that headaches may worsen if the drug is used on 10 or more days per month.

Patients receiving ibuprofen for *self-medication* should be advised to consult a clinician before initiating ibuprofen if they have experienced adverse effects associated with any analgesic or antipyretic; if they have hypertension, cardiac disease, asthma, hepatic cirrhosis, or renal disease; if they have had a stroke; if they have a history of bleeding events or GI disorders (e.g., heartburn, peptic ulcer); if they are receiving therapy with a diuretic, an anticoagulant, a corticosteroid,

or any other NSAIA-containing preparation; if they consume 3 or more alcohol-containing drinks per day; or if they are 60 years of age or older. Patients receiving the drug for *self-medication* should consult a clinician or pharmacist before initiating ibuprofen if they are under a clinician's care for any continuing serious medical condition, are taking aspirin for reduction of cardiovascular risk, or are receiving any other drugs.

Patients should be advised to stop taking ibuprofen for *self-medication* and consult their clinician if symptoms of GI bleeding (e.g., faintness, vomiting blood, bloody or black stools, persistent stomach pain) develop; if cardiac symptoms or symptoms of stroke (e.g., chest pain, difficulty breathing, weakness in one part or side of the body, slurred speech, leg swelling) occur; if any new symptoms occur during *self-medication* with the drug; or if redness or swelling is present in the painful area. Patients should be advised that the risk of GI bleeding is increased if they are 60 years of age or older, have a GI disorder (e.g., history of GI bleeding or peptic ulceration), are receiving an anticoagulant or corticosteroid, are receiving another NSAIA (including aspirin) concomitantly, generally consume 3 or more alcohol-containing drinks per day, or exceed the recommended dosage or duration of ibuprofen therapy. In addition, patients should be advised that NSAIAs (except aspirin) increase the risk of myocardial infarction, heart failure, and stroke and that the risk is increased if they exceed the recommended dosage or duration of ibuprofen therapy.

For additional information on use of ibuprofen for *self-medication* in children, see Pediatric Precautions under Cautions.

Other Precautions

Patients receiving long-term NSAIA therapy should have a complete blood cell count and chemistry profile performed periodically.

The possibility that the antipyretic and anti-inflammatory effects of ibuprofen may mask the usual signs and symptoms of infection or other diseases should be considered. Ibuprofen lysine should be used with caution in premature neonates at risk for infection and in those with an existing infection that is adequately controlled. Clinicians should be alert to the masking effect of the drug in these neonates. The drug is contraindicated in neonates with proven or suspected, untreated infection.

Ibuprofen can interfere with the antiplatelet effect of low-dose aspirin. Patients receiving low-dose aspirin for its cardioprotective effects should be informed of this potential interaction and advised about appropriate timing of ibuprofen administration relative to aspirin administration in order to minimize the interaction. (See Nonsteroidal Anti-inflammatory Agents under Drug Interactions.)

Ibuprofen is not a substitute for corticosteroid therapy, and the drug is not effective in the management of adrenal insufficiency. Abrupt withdrawal of corticosteroids may exacerbate corticosteroid-responsive conditions. If corticosteroid therapy is to be discontinued after prolonged therapy, the dosage should be tapered gradually.

Because NSAIAs, including ibuprofen, have caused adverse ocular effects (e.g., blurred or diminished vision, scotoma, changes in color vision), patients who experience such visual disturbances during ibuprofen therapy should discontinue the drug and have an ophthalmologic examination, including testing of central visual fields and color vision.

Ibuprofen should be used with caution in patients with increased total bilirubin because of the potential for ibuprofen to displace bilirubin from albumin binding sites.

Individuals with phenylketonuria (i.e., homozygous genetic deficiency of phenylalanine hydroxylase) and other individuals who must restrict their intake of phenylalanine should be warned that Motrin® chewable tablets contain aspartame (NutraSweet®), which is metabolized in the GI tract to provide 6 mg of phenylalanine for each 100-mg tablet following oral administration and that Advil® Junior Strength chewable tablets contain aspartame, which is metabolized to provide 4.2 mg of phenylalanine for each 100-mg tablet. Diabetic patients should be warned that some commercially available preparations of ibuprofen may contain sucrose.

Contraindications

Ibuprofen is contraindicated in patients with known hypersensitivity (e.g., anaphylaxis, serious dermatologic reactions) to the drug or any ingredient in the formulation. NSAIAs generally are contraindicated in patients in whom asthma, urticaria, or other sensitivity reactions are precipitated by aspirin or other

NSAIAs, since there is potential for cross-sensitivity between NSAIAs and aspirin, and severe, often fatal, anaphylactic reactions may occur in such patients. Although NSAIAs generally are contraindicated in these patients, the drugs have occasionally been used in NSAIA-sensitive patients who have undergone desensitization. Because patients with asthma may have aspirin-sensitivity asthma, patients with asthma but without known aspirin sensitivity who are receiving ibuprofen should be monitored for changes in manifestations of asthma. In patients with asthma, aspirin sensitivity is manifested principally as bronchospasm and usually is associated with nasal polyps; the association of aspirin sensitivity, asthma, and nasal polyps is known as the aspirin triad. Patients who are considering use of ibuprofen for *self-medication* should be advised that ibuprofen is contraindicated in patients who have experienced asthma, urticaria, or other sensitivity reaction to other analgesics or antipyretics. For further discussion of cross-sensitivity of NSAIAs, see Cautions: Sensitivity Reactions, in the Salicylates General Statement 28:08.04.24.

NSAIAs are contraindicated in the setting of CABG surgery.

Ibuprofen lysine is contraindicated in neonates with congenital heart disease when patency of the ductus arteriosus is necessary for adequate pulmonary or systemic blood flow (e.g., neonates with pulmonary atresia, severe tetralogy of Fallot, or severe coarctation of the aorta); in premature neonates with suspected necrotizing enterocolitis; in neonates with proven or suspected, untreated infection; and in neonates with substantially impaired renal function.

● **Pediatric Precautions**

The manufacturers state that the safety and efficacy of oral ibuprofen in children younger than 6 months of age have not been established. Ibuprofen should not be used for *self-medication* in children younger than 6 months of age unless otherwise directed by a clinician. Ibuprofen should not be used for *self-medication* in children immediately before or after cardiac surgery or in children who have experienced an allergic reaction to any analgesic or antipyretic.

Clinicians should be consulted before initiating ibuprofen for *self-medication* in children if the child has experienced adverse effects associated with any analgesic or antipyretic; if the child has hypertension, cardiac disease, asthma, hepatic cirrhosis, or renal disease; if the child has had a stroke; if the child has a history of bleeding events or GI disorders (e.g., heartburn, peptic ulcer) or is receiving therapy with a diuretic, an anticoagulant, a corticosteroid, or any other NSAIA-containing preparation; or if dehydration associated with vomiting, diarrhea, or lack of fluid intake has occurred. A clinician or pharmacist should be consulted before initiating ibuprofen for *self-medication* in children if the child is under a clinician's care for any continuing serious medical condition or is taking any other drugs.

Ibuprofen *self-medication* should be discontinued and a clinician should be contacted if symptoms of GI bleeding (e.g., faintness, vomiting blood, bloody or black stools, persistent stomach pain) develop; if cardiac symptoms or symptoms of stroke (e.g., chest pain, difficulty breathing, weakness in one part or side of the body, slurred speech, leg swelling) occur; if any new symptoms occur during *self-medication* with the drug; if fever worsens during therapy or lasts more than 3 days; if pain worsens during therapy or lasts more than 10 days in adolescents 12 years of age or older or more than 3 days in children younger than 12 years of age; if no relief is observed within the first 24 hours of therapy; or if redness or swelling is present in the painful area. In addition, a clinician should be contacted promptly if the child experiences severe or persistent sore throat or if sore throat is associated with high fever, headache, nausea, or vomiting. Ibuprofen should not be used for *self-medication* of sore throat in children for more than 2 days' duration unless otherwise directed by a clinician, and should not be used for *self-medication* of sore throat in children younger than 3 years of age unless directed by a clinician. The risk of GI bleeding is increased if the child has a GI disorder (e.g., history of GI bleeding or peptic ulceration), is receiving an anticoagulant or corticosteroid, is receiving another NSAIA (including aspirin) concomitantly, or if the recommended dosage or duration of ibuprofen therapy is exceeded. NSAIAs (except aspirin) increase the risk of myocardial infarction, heart failure, and stroke and the risk is increased if the recommended dosage or duration of ibuprofen therapy is exceeded.

Results of a large (about 84,000 children) double-blind, randomized study indicate that risk of hospitalization for GI bleeding, renal failure, anaphylaxis, or Reye's syndrome in febrile children (6 months to 12 years of age) receiving ibuprofen doses of 5 or 10 mg/kg is similar to that in children receiving acetaminophen

doses of 12 mg/kg. These data, however, provide no information on the risks of less severe adverse effects or the risks associated with prolonged use of ibuprofen in children.

Overdosage and toxicity (including death) have been reported in children younger than 2 years of age receiving nonprescription (over-the-counter, OTC) preparations containing antihistamines, cough suppressants, expectorants, and nasal decongestants alone or in combination for relief of symptoms of upper respiratory tract infection. Such preparations also may contain analgesics and antipyretics. There is limited evidence of efficacy for these preparations in this age group, and appropriate dosages (i.e., approved by FDA) have not been established. Therefore, FDA stated that nonprescription cough and cold preparations should not be used in children younger than 2 years of age; the agency continues to assess safety and efficacy of these preparations in older children. Meanwhile, because children 2–3 years of age also are at increased risk of overdosage and toxicity, some manufacturers of oral nonprescription cough and cold preparations have agreed to voluntarily revise the product labeling to state that such preparations should not be used in children younger than 4 years of age. FDA recommends that parents and caregivers adhere to the dosage instructions and warnings on the product labeling that accompanies the preparation if administering to children and consult with their clinician about any concerns. Clinicians should ask caregivers about use of nonprescription cough and cold preparations to avoid overdosage. For additional information on precautions associated with the use of cough and cold preparations in pediatric patients, see Cautions: Pediatric Precautions in Pseudoephedrine 12:12.12.

Pediatric patients receiving ibuprofen dosages exceeding 30 mg/kg daily and those who have had abnormal liver function test results associated with prior NSAIA therapy should be carefully monitored for signs and symptoms of early liver dysfunction.

Safety and efficacy of IV ibuprofen for relief of pain or reduction of fever in pediatric patients 6 months of age and older are supported by evidence of fever reduction from a multicenter, open-label study in hospitalized febrile pediatric patients, safety data from 3 studies in which 143 pediatric patients 6 months of age or older received IV ibuprofen for pain relief or antipyresis, supportive data involving other ibuprofen preparations labeled for use in pediatric patients, and evidence from adequate and well-controlled studies in adults. The most common adverse effects of IV ibuprofen in pediatric patients are infusion site pain, vomiting, nausea, anemia, and headache. Efficacy of IV ibuprofen for relief of pain or reduction of fever has not been established in pediatric patients younger than 6 months of age.

Long-term follow-up (beyond a postconceptional age of 36 weeks) of premature neonates receiving ibuprofen lysine for patent ductus arteriosus (PDA) has not been conducted. The effects of ibuprofen on neurodevelopmental outcome, growth, and other complications of prematurity (e.g., retinopathy of prematurity, chronic lung disease) have not been assessed.

Safety and efficacy of ibuprofen lysine have been established only in premature infants. Ibuprofen lysine is contraindicated in neonates with substantially impaired renal function, thrombocytopenia, coagulation disorders, active bleeding (e.g., intracranial hemorrhage, GI bleeding), known or suspected necrotizing enterocolitis, or proven or suspected infection that is untreated. The drug also is contraindicated in neonates with congenital heart disease when patency of the ductus arteriosus is necessary for adequate pulmonary or systemic blood flow (e.g., neonates with pulmonary atresia, severe tetralogy of Fallot, or severe coarctation of the aorta).

● **Geriatric Precautions**

Geriatric patients are at increased risk for NSAIA-associated serious adverse cardiovascular, GI, and renal effects. Many of the spontaneous reports of fatal adverse GI effects in patients receiving NSAIAs involve geriatric individuals. If the anticipated benefits of ibuprofen therapy outweigh the potential risks, ibuprofen should be initiated at the lower end of the dosing range and patients should be monitored for adverse effects.

Clinical studies of IV ibuprofen did not include sufficient numbers of patients 65 years of age or older to determine whether geriatric patients respond differently than younger adults. Dosage should be selected with caution, starting at the low end of the dosage range, because of the greater frequency of decreased hepatic, renal, and/or cardiac function and concomitant disease and drug therapy observed in the elderly.

● Pregnancy, Fertility, and Lactation

Pregnancy

Use of NSAIAs during pregnancy at about 30 weeks of gestation or later can cause premature closure of the fetal ductus arteriosus, and use at about 20 weeks of gestation or later has been associated with fetal renal dysfunction resulting in oligohydramnios and, in some cases, neonatal renal impairment. Because of these risks, use of NSAIAs should be avoided in pregnant women at about 30 weeks of gestation or later; if NSAIA therapy is necessary between about 20 and 30 weeks of gestation, the lowest effective dosage and shortest possible duration of treatment should be used. Monitoring of amniotic fluid volume via ultrasound examination should be considered if the duration of NSAIA treatment exceeds 48 hours; if oligohydramnios occurs, the drug should be discontinued and follow-up instituted according to clinical practice. Pregnant women should be advised to avoid use of NSAIAs beginning at 20 weeks' gestation unless otherwise advised by a clinician; they should be informed that NSAIAs should be avoided beginning at 30 weeks' gestation because of the risk of premature closure of the fetal ductus arteriosus and that monitoring for oligohydramnios may be necessary if NSAIA therapy is required for longer than 48 hours' duration between about 20 and 30 weeks of gestation.

Known effects of NSAIAs on the human fetus during the third trimester of pregnancy include prenatal constriction of the ductus arteriosus, tricuspid incompetence, and pulmonary hypertension; nonclosure of the ductus arteriosus during the postnatal period (which may be resistant to medical management); and myocardial degenerative changes, platelet dysfunction with resultant bleeding, intracranial bleeding, renal dysfunction or renal failure, renal injury or dysgenesis potentially resulting in prolonged or permanent renal failure, oligohydramnios, GI bleeding or perforation, and increased risk of necrotizing enterocolitis.

Fetal renal dysfunction resulting in oligohydramnios and, in some cases, neonatal renal impairment has been observed, on average, following days to weeks of maternal NSAIA use, although oligohydramnios has been observed infrequently as early as 48 hours after initiation of NSAIA therapy. Oligohydramnios is often, but not always, reversible (generally within 3–6 days) following discontinuance of NSAIA therapy. Complications of prolonged oligohydramnios may include limb contracture and delayed lung maturation. A limited number of case reports have described maternal NSAIA use and neonatal renal dysfunction, in some cases irreversible, without oligohydramnios. Some cases of neonatal renal dysfunction have required treatment with invasive procedures such as exchange transfusion or dialysis. Deaths associated with neonatal renal failure have been reported. Methodologic limitations of these postmarketing studies and case reports include lack of a control group; limited information regarding dosage, duration, and timing of drug exposure; and concomitant use of other drugs. These limitations preclude establishing a reliable estimate of the risk of adverse fetal and neonatal outcomes with maternal NSAIA use. Available data on neonatal outcomes generally involved preterm infants, and the extent to which certain reported risks can be generalized to full-term infants is uncertain.

Animal data indicate that prostaglandins have an important role in endometrial vascular permeability, blastocyst implantation, and decidualization. In animal studies, inhibitors of prostaglandin synthesis, such as ibuprofen, were associated with increased pre- and post-implantation losses. Prostaglandins also have an important role in fetal kidney development. In animal studies, inhibitors of prostaglandin synthesis impaired kidney development at clinically relevant doses.

There are no adequate and well-controlled studies of ibuprofen in pregnant women. In animal reproduction studies, no clear developmental effects were observed in rabbits or rats given ibuprofen throughout the gestational period at dosages up to 0.4 or 0.5 times, respectively, the maximum recommended human dosage (MRHD). An increase in membranous ventricular septal defects was reported in rats given ibuprofen on gestation days 9 and 10 at a dosage of 0.8 times the MRHD.

The effects of ibuprofen on labor and delivery are unknown. In studies in rats, drugs that inhibit prostaglandin synthesis, including NSAIAs, delayed parturition and increased the incidence of stillbirth.

Fertility

Use of NSAIAs, including ibuprofen, may delay or prevent ovarian follicular rupture, which has been associated with reversible infertility in some women. Reversible delays in ovulation have been observed in limited studies in women receiving NSAIAs, and animal studies indicate that inhibitors of prostaglandin synthesis can disrupt prostaglandin-mediated follicular rupture required for ovulation. In animal studies, ibuprofen did not alter male or female fertility or affect litter size in rats; in mice, the drug decreased ovulation in females but did not alter sperm motility or viability in males. Withdrawal of NSAIAs should be considered in women who are experiencing difficulty conceiving or are undergoing evaluation of infertility.

Lactation

Limited data indicate that ibuprofen is distributed into milk, resulting in infant exposures of 0.06–0.6% of the maternal weight-adjusted daily dosage. Adverse effects on breast-fed infants or effects on milk production have not been reported to date. The developmental and health benefits of breast-feeding should be considered along with the mother's clinical need for ibuprofen and any potential adverse effects on the breast-fed infant from the drug or from the underlying maternal condition.

DRUG INTERACTIONS

● Amikacin

Ibuprofen may decrease the clearance of amikacin.

● Anticoagulants and Thrombolytic Agents

The effects of anticoagulants (e.g., warfarin) and NSAIAs on GI bleeding are synergistic. Concomitant use of an NSAIA and anticoagulants is associated with a higher risk of GI bleeding compared with use of either agent alone.

In several short-term, controlled studies, ibuprofen did not have a substantial effect on the prothrombin time of patients receiving oral anticoagulants; however, because ibuprofen may cause GI bleeding, inhibit platelet aggregation, and prolong bleeding time and because bleeding has occurred when ibuprofen and coumarin-derivative anticoagulants were administered concomitantly, the drug should be used with caution and the patient carefully observed for signs of bleeding if the drug is used concomitantly with any anticoagulant (e.g., warfarin) or thrombolytic agent (e.g., streptokinase).

Because reduced CYP2C9 function is associated with an increased risk of major bleeding or supratherapeutic international normalized ratios (INRs) in patients receiving concomitant therapy with warfarin (a CYP2C9 substrate) and NSAIAs, some experts state that concomitant use of warfarin and NSAIAs should be avoided in patients who are CYP2C9 intermediate or poor metabolizers.

● Antihypertensive Agents

Concomitant use of NSAIAs with angiotensin-converting enzyme (ACE) inhibitors, angiotensin II receptor antagonists, or β-adrenergic blocking agents may reduce the blood pressure response to the antihypertensive agent. Therefore, blood pressure should be monitored to ensure that target blood pressure is achieved.

Concomitant use of NSAIAs with ACE inhibitors or angiotensin II receptor antagonists in geriatric patients or patients with volume depletion or renal impairment may result in reversible deterioration of renal function; such patients should be monitored for signs of worsening renal function. Patients receiving concomitant therapy with ibuprofen and ACE inhibitors or angiotensin II receptor antagonists should be adequately hydrated, and renal function should be assessed when concomitant therapy is initiated and periodically thereafter.

● Cyclosporine

Concomitant use of ibuprofen and cyclosporine may increase the nephrotoxic effects of cyclosporine. Patients receiving such concomitant therapy should be monitored for signs of worsening renal function.

● Digoxin

Concomitant use of ibuprofen and digoxin has been reported to result in increased serum concentrations and prolonged half-life of digoxin. Serum digoxin concentrations should be monitored.

● Diuretics

NSAIAs may reduce the natriuretic effect of furosemide or thiazide diuretics, and concomitant use of diuretics and NSAIAs may increase the risk of

NSAIA-associated nephrotoxicity in dehydrated patients. The reduction in natriuretic effect may be related to inhibition of renal prostaglandin synthesis. Patients receiving concomitant NSAIA and diuretic therapy should be monitored for changes in renal function and for adequacy of diuretic and antihypertensive effects.

● *Histamine H$_2$-receptor Antagonists*

In healthy individuals, cimetidine and ranitidine (no longer commercially available in the US) did not substantially alter serum concentrations of ibuprofen. Concomitant administration of ibuprofen (800 mg) and famotidine (40 mg) did not alter the area under the concentration time-curve (AUC) of ibuprofen; peak plasma concentrations of ibuprofen and famotidine and AUC of famotidine were increased by 16, 22, and 16%, respectively.

● *Lithium*

Concomitant use of NSAIAs has been reported to increase mean trough lithium concentrations by 15% and to decrease mean renal lithium clearance by approximately 20%. Ibuprofen has been reported to increase plasma or serum lithium concentrations by 12–67% and to reduce renal lithium clearance. The mechanism involved in the reduction of lithium clearance by NSAIAs (including ibuprofen) is not known, but has been attributed to inhibition of prostaglandin synthesis, which may interfere with the renal elimination of lithium. Some clinicians recommend that patients receiving lithium should not receive ibuprofen. However, if ibuprofen and lithium are used concurrently, the patient should be observed closely for signs of lithium toxicity, and plasma or serum lithium concentrations should be monitored carefully during the initial stages of combined therapy or subsequent dosage adjustment. Dosage of lithium may have to be reduced in some patients; appropriate adjustment of lithium dosage may be required when therapy with ibuprofen is discontinued.

● *Methotrexate*

Concomitant use of NSAIAs and methotrexate may increase the risk for methotrexate toxicity (e.g., neutropenia, thrombocytopenia, renal dysfunction). Patients receiving concomitant ibuprofen and methotrexate therapy should be monitored for methotrexate toxicity. (See Drug Interactions: Nonsteroidal Antiinflammatory Agents, in Methotrexate 10:00.)

● *Nonsteroidal Anti-inflammatory Agents*

In controlled clinical trials, concomitant use of NSAIAs and analgesic dosages of aspirin did not produce any greater therapeutic effect than use of NSAIAs alone. However, concomitant use of aspirin and an NSAIA increases the risk of adverse GI events. Because of the potential for bleeding, concomitant use of ibuprofen with other NSAIAs or with analgesic dosages of aspirin generally is not recommended. Patients should be advised that many nonprescription antipyretic formulations, cough and cold preparations, and sleep aids contain NSAIAs.

In animal studies, blood concentrations of ibuprofen decreased when aspirin and ibuprofen were administered concomitantly. Although limited studies in humans have not shown decreased blood concentrations of ibuprofen when these drugs were administered concurrently, this possibility should be considered.

When ibuprofen is administered with aspirin, protein binding of ibuprofen is reduced, although clearance of the free (unbound) ibuprofen is not altered; the clinical relevance of this interaction has not been established.

Some NSAIAs (e.g., ibuprofen, naproxen) can interfere with the antiplatelet effect of low-dose aspirin. Ibuprofen can antagonize the irreversible inhibition of platelet aggregation induced by aspirin and therefore may limit the cardioprotective effects of aspirin in patients with increased cardiovascular risk. Administration of 400 mg of ibuprofen 3 times daily in patients receiving aspirin 81 mg daily blocked the aspirin-induced inhibition of platelet cyclooxygenase-1 activity as well as the impairment of platelet aggregation achieved with aspirin during prolonged dosing. Administration of aspirin 2 hours before the morning dose of ibuprofen failed to circumvent the interaction with such multiple-dose administration, although such dose timing did effectively obviate the interaction when only single doses of each drug were administered. FDA has recommended that patients taking a single dose of ibuprofen 400 mg for *self-medication* in conjunction with immediate-release, low-dose aspirin therapy be advised to administer the ibuprofen dose at least 8 hours before or at least 30 minutes after administration of aspirin. Data currently are insufficient to support recommendations

regarding the timing of ibuprofen administration relative to that of enteric-coated, low-dose aspirin. The occasional use of ibuprofen is likely to be associated with minimal risk of attenuating the effects of low-dose aspirin. Use of alternative analgesics that do not interfere with the antiplatelet effect of low-dose aspirin (e.g., acetaminophen, opiates) should be considered for patients at high risk of cardiovascular events. Patients receiving ibuprofen should be advised not to take low-dose aspirin without consulting their clinician. Ibuprofen is not a substitute for low-dose aspirin therapy for prophylaxis of cardiovascular events, and patients receiving antiplatelet agents such as aspirin concomitantly with ibuprofen should be monitored closely for bleeding. There is no consistent evidence that use of low-dose aspirin mitigates the increased risk of serious cardiovascular events associated with NSAIAs.

● *Pemetrexed*

Concomitant use of ibuprofen and pemetrexed may increase the risk of pemetrexed-associated myelosuppression, renal toxicity, and GI toxicity. Administration of NSAIAs with short elimination half-lives (e.g., diclofenac, indomethacin) should be avoided beginning 2 days before and continuing through 2 days after pemetrexed administration. In the absence of data regarding potential interactions between pemetrexed and NSAIAs with longer half-lives (e.g., meloxicam, nabumetone), administration of NSAIAs with longer half-lives should be interrupted beginning at least 5 days before and continuing through 2 days after pemetrexed administration. Patients with renal impairment with a creatinine clearance of 45–79 mL/minute should be monitored for myelosuppression, renal toxicity, and GI toxicity if they receive concomitant ibuprofen and pemetrexed therapy.

● *Serotonin-reuptake Inhibitors*

Serotonin release by platelets plays an important role in hemostasis. Results of case-control and epidemiologic cohort studies indicate that concomitant use of NSAIAs and drugs that interfere with serotonin reuptake may potentiate the risk of bleeding beyond that associated with an NSAIA alone. Patients receiving concomitant therapy with ibuprofen and selective serotonin-reuptake inhibitors (SSRIs) or selective serotonin- and norepinephrine-reuptake inhibitors (SNRIs) should be monitored for signs of bleeding.

ACUTE TOXICITY

● *Manifestations*

Limited information is available on the acute toxicity of ibuprofen. Adverse effects associated with overdosage of ibuprofen usually depend on the amount of drug ingested and time elapsed; however, because individual response may vary, each occurrence should be evaluated individually. Occasionally, overdosage of ibuprofen has been associated with severe toxicity, including death.

The most frequent manifestations of ibuprofen overdosage reportedly are abdominal pain, nausea, vomiting, lethargy, and drowsiness. In addition, other adverse effects, including headache, tinnitus, CNS depression, seizures, GI bleeding, hypotension, bradycardia, tachycardia, and atrial fibrillation, may occur. Metabolic acidosis, coma, acute renal failure, hypertension, hyperkalemia, apnea (mainly in young children), respiratory depression, and respiratory failure have been reported rarely. There appears to be little correlation between severity of manifestations associated with ibuprofen overdosage and plasma ibuprofen concentrations.

Drowsiness was the only adverse effect experienced by a child 1 year of age who ingested 1.2 g (120 mg/kg) of the drug even though the blood ibuprofen concentration 90 minutes after ingestion was 700 mcg/mL (nearly 10 times the highest concentration previously recorded in adults following a single oral 800-mg dose of the drug). Signs of acute intoxication or late sequelae also were not present following ingestion of a 120-mg/kg dose of the drug in another child. However, in a 12-kg child who ingested 2.8–4 g of the drug, apnea, cyanosis, and response only to painful stimuli were present about 1.5 hours after ingestion; respiration could be induced by painful stimuli. The blood ibuprofen concentration in this child was about 103 mcg/mL at about 8.5 hours after ingestion and the child appeared to have completely recovered at 12 hours following treatment with oxygen, sodium bicarbonate, and parenteral infusion of dextrose and 0.9% sodium chloride. Dizziness and nystagmus occurred in a 19-year-old who ingested 8 g of the drug over a period of a few hours.

● Treatment

Treatment of acute toxicity associated with ibuprofen overdosage mainly is supportive. When acute overdosage of ibuprofen occurs, the stomach should be emptied by inducing emesis with syrup of ipecac or by lavage, particularly if there is evidence that the drug has been ingested recently (within 30–60 minutes), and standard measures to maintain urine output should be instituted. Administration of activated charcoal may be useful in reducing absorption and reabsorption of ibuprofen. Forced diuresis, alkalinization of urine, hemodialysis, or hemoperfusion may not be useful because of the drug's high protein binding. Management of hypotension, GI bleeding, and acidosis may be necessary.

In children, the estimated amount ingested per unit of body weight may be helpful in predicting the development of toxicity, but each case should be evaluated individually. One manufacturer and some clinicians state that toxicity is unlikely in children who have ingested less than 100 mg/kg of ibuprofen. In children who have ingested 100–200 mg/kg, the stomach should be emptied by inducing emesis and the child observed for at least 4 hours; in children who have ingested 200–400 mg/kg of the drug, the stomach should be emptied and the child observed in a health-care facility for at least 4 hours. Children who have ingested more than 400 mg/kg of ibuprofen require immediate medical referral, careful observation, and appropriate supportive therapy; syrup of ipecac is not recommended in these children because of risk of seizures and potential aspiration of gastric contents. In adults, the amount of ibuprofen ingested does not appear to predict toxicity; therefore, the need for referral and follow-up treatment should be assessed individually. Adults with symptomatic toxicity should be admitted to a health-care facility for observation.

PHARMACOLOGY

Ibuprofen has pharmacologic actions similar to those of other prototypical NSAIAs. Ibuprofen has shown anti-inflammatory, antipyretic, and analgesic activity in both animals and humans. The exact mechanisms of action of the drug have not been clearly established, but many of the actions appear to be associated principally with the inhibition of prostaglandin synthesis. Ibuprofen inhibits synthesis of prostaglandins in body tissues by inhibiting cyclooxygenase; at least 2 isoenzymes, cyclooxygenase-1 (COX-1) and -2 (COX-2) (also referred to as prostaglandin G/H synthase-1 [PGHS-1] and -2 [PGHS-2], respectively), have been identified that catalyze the formation of prostaglandins in the arachidonic acid pathway. Ibuprofen, like other prototypical NSAIAs, inhibits both COX-1 and COX-2. Although the exact mechanisms have not been clearly established, NSAIAs appear to exert anti-inflammatory, analgesic, and antipyretic activity principally through inhibition of the COX-2 isoenzyme; COX-1 inhibition presumably is responsible for the drugs' unwanted effects on GI mucosa and platelet aggregation.

● Anti-inflammatory, Analgesic, and Antipyretic Effects

The anti-inflammatory, analgesic, and antipyretic effects of ibuprofen and other NSAIAs, including selective inhibitors of COX-2 (e.g., celecoxib), appear to result from inhibition of prostaglandin synthesis. While the precise mechanism of the anti-inflammatory and analgesic effects of NSAIAs continues to be investigated, these effects appear to be mediated principally through inhibition of the COX-2 isoenzyme at sites of inflammation with subsequent reduction in the synthesis of certain prostaglandins from their arachidonic acid precursors.

Ibuprofen does not possess glucocorticoid or adrenocorticoid-stimulating properties. Higher doses usually are required for anti-inflammatory effects than for analgesia.

● Genitourinary and Renal Effects

Ibuprofen-induced inhibition of prostaglandin synthesis may result in decreased frequency and intensity of uterine contractility. Prostaglandins E_2 and $F_2\alpha$ increase the amplitude and frequency of uterine contractions in pregnant women; current evidence suggests that primary dysmenorrhea also is mediated by these prostaglandins. Whether the increased production of prostaglandins associated with primary dysmenorrhea is mediated by COX-1 or COX-2 remains to be determined. Therapy with ibuprofen has been effective in relieving menstrual pain probably by inhibiting the formation of these prostaglandins. Administration of ibuprofen during late pregnancy may prolong gestation by inhibiting uterine contractions.

Ibuprofen has been reported to adversely affect renal function. (See Renal Effects under Cautions.) The mechanisms of adverse renal effects of ibuprofen have not been determined, but may involve inhibition of renal synthesis of prostaglandins.

Ibuprofen does not appear to have uricosuric activity.

● GI Effects

Similar to other prototypical NSAIAs, ibuprofen can cause gastric mucosal damage, which may result in ulceration and/or bleeding. (See GI Effects under Cautions.) These gastric effects have been attributed to inhibition of the synthesis of prostaglandins produced by COX-1. Other factors possibly involved in NSAIA-induced gastropathy include local irritation, promotion of acid back-diffusion into gastric mucosa, uncoupling of oxidative phosphorylation, and enterohepatic recirculation of the drugs.

Limited data indicate that ibuprofen, in a dosage of 1.2 or 2.4 g daily, produced less severe gastric mucosal abnormalities (observed with endoscopic examination) than did aspirin in a dosage of 3.6 g daily. In addition, ibuprofen in a dosage of 1.2 g daily produces less severe gastric mucosal damage than indomethacin in a dosage of 100 mg daily.

Epidemiologic and laboratory studies suggest that NSAIAs may reduce the risk of colon cancer. Although the exact mechanism by which NSAIAs may inhibit colon carcinogenesis remains to determined, it has been suggested that inhibition of prostaglandin synthesis may be involved.

● Hematologic Effects

Ibuprofen inhibits platelet aggregation and prolongs bleeding time but does not affect prothrombin time or whole blood clotting time. Similar to aspirin and other prototypical NSAIAs, the effects of ibuprofen on platelets appear to be associated with inhibition of the synthesis of prostaglandins produced by COX-1.

● Cardiovascular Effects

In many premature neonates, administration of ibuprofen results in closure of the persistently patent ductus arteriosus. During fetal life, the ductus arteriosus apparently is maintained in a dilated state by prostaglandins, presumably of the E series, which are produced in the placenta and in the ductus itself. The ductus usually closes within 24 hours after birth, partly as a result of loss of placental prostaglandins and increased pulmonary blood flow. In premature neonates, however, the ductus may not close promptly, perhaps because of increased sensitivity of the immature ductus to prostaglandins; some of these neonates develop cardiopulmonary decompensation because of large left-to-right cardiac shunts. Ibuprofen appears to inhibit the synthesis of the prostaglandins, thereby permitting closure of the ductus. Other factors such as oxygenation and hydration status of the neonate also may contribute to successful ductus closure.

PHARMACOKINETICS

● Absorption

Approximately 80% of an oral dose of ibuprofen is absorbed from the GI tract. Absorption rate is slower and plasma concentrations are reduced when ibuprofen is taken with food; however, the extent of absorption is not affected. When the drug is administered with food, peak plasma ibuprofen concentrations are reduced by 30–50% and time to achieve peak plasma concentrations is delayed by 30–60 minutes. Absorption of ibuprofen does not appear to be affected by concomitant administration of antacids containing aluminum hydroxide or magnesium hydroxide.

In adults, oral bioavailability of ibuprofen (measured by peak plasma concentrations and extent of absorption) is similar following administration of conventional tablets, chewable tablets, or suspension; however, time to reach peak plasma concentrations was reportedly about 120, 62, or 47 minutes following administration of each respective dosage form. Following oral administration of a single 200-mg dose of ibuprofen as chewable tablets, suspension, or conventional tablets in adults, peak plasma concentrations were 15, 19, or 20 mcg/mL, respectively. Following oral administration of ibuprofen in adults, the area under the serum concentration-time curves (AUCs) of total and free drug increase proportionally with single ibuprofen doses of 50–600 and up to 1200 mg, respectively. In febrile children, oral bioavailability (measured by peak plasma concentrations and extent of absorption) of ibuprofen also appears to be similar following administration of the respective dosage form; however, time to reach peak plasma concentrations was reportedly 86 or 58 minutes following administration of chewable tablets or suspension, respectively. Following oral administration of a 200-mg dose in adults or a 10-mg/kg dose in febrile children, peak plasma concentrations and plasma concentration-time curves (AUCs) of ibuprofen appear to be increased in children compared with those achieved in adults; these differences appear to result from age- or fever-related changes in the volume of distribution in children and also to the variability of doses (based on body weight) administered to pediatric patients. Peak plasma or serum ibuprofen concentrations of about 40–55 mcg/mL occur after about 1–1.5 hours in febrile children receiving a single 10-mg/kg dose of ibuprofen suspension or chewable tablets. Following oral administration of ibuprofen suspension in febrile children, AUCs increase with increasing single ibuprofen doses up to 10 mg/kg; it appears that pharmacokinetics of ibuprofen are not affected by age, in children 2 to 11 years of age.

In children, the antipyretic effect of ibuprofen suspension begins within 1 hour after oral administration and peaks within 2-4 hours. The antipyretic effect of single ibuprofen suspension doses of 5 or 10 mg/kg may last up to 6 or 8 hours, respectively. Following oral administration of ibuprofen chewable tablets, onset, peak, and duration of antipyretic effects reportedly are similar to that following oral administration of the suspension. Plasma concentrations required for anti-inflammatory effect are not known. A few days to 2 weeks of therapy are required before therapeutic response occurs.

Following IV administration of 400 or 800 mg of ibuprofen in adults, peak plasma concentrations were 39.2 or 72.6 mcg/mL, respectively. Following IV administration of 10-mg/kg doses of ibuprofen in pediatric patients 6 months to 16 years of age, mean peak plasma concentrations were 59–64 mcg/mL.

● Distribution

Animal studies indicate that ibuprofen distribution varies according to species; human distribution data have not been published. The volume of distribution reportedly is about 0.12 or 0.2 L/kg in adults or febrile children younger than 11 years of age, respectively, suggesting that the volume of distribution may be affected by age or fever; however, the clinical importance of this difference is not known. In pediatric patients 6 months to 16 years of age receiving IV ibuprofen, the apparent volume of distribution during the terminal phase increased with age. In one study in premature neonates receiving IV ibuprofen lysine, the volume of distribution of ibuprofen at birth averaged 0.32 L/kg. Approximately 90–99% of a dose is bound to plasma proteins; protein binding appears to be saturable, and at concentrations exceeding 20 mcg/mL, such binding is nonlinear. Ibuprofen and its metabolites cross the placenta in rats and rabbits. In preliminary studies, ibuprofen was not detected in the milk of nursing women.

● Elimination

Plasma concentrations of ibuprofen appear to decline in a biphasic manner. The terminal elimination half-life of orally administered ibuprofen in children reportedly is similar to that in adults; however, total clearance may be affected by age or fever. It has been suggested that changes in total clearance may result from changes in the volume of distribution in febrile children. The plasma half-life of the drug has been reported to be 2–4 hours. Blood concentrations decline as rapidly after multiple doses as after single doses. In one study in premature neonates receiving IV ibuprofen lysine, clearance of ibuprofen at birth averaged 3 mL/kg per hour. Clearance increased rapidly (by an average of about 0.5 mL/kg per hour each day) as postnatal age increased, and interindividual variability (55%) in clearance was observed. The terminal elimination half-life is at least tenfold longer in premature neonates than in adults. The elimination half-life in pediatric patients receiving IV ibuprofen is shorter than that observed in adults. Following IV administration of 10-mg/kg doses of ibuprofen, the mean half-life was 1.5–1.6 hours in pediatric patients 2–16 years of age and 1.8 hours in those 6 months to less than 2 years of age; the volume of distribution and clearance increased with age.

Ibuprofen is almost completely metabolized, mainly via cytochrome P-450 (CYP)-mediated oxidative metabolism to inactive metabolites. Ibuprofen is metabolized mainly by CYP2C9 and to a lesser extent by CYP2C8. CYP3A4 contributes to ibuprofen clearance at high concentrations; CYP2C19 appears to play a minor role in metabolism of the drug. Approximately 10–15% of an ibuprofen dose is metabolized to ibuprofen acyl glucuronide. Multiple uridine diphosphate-glucuronosyltransferase (UGT) isoenzymes are capable of metabolizing ibuprofen in vitro; however, further study is needed to characterize the relative contributions of individual UGT isoenzymes to ibuprofen metabolism in vivo.

Approximately 37 and 25% of an administered dose of ibuprofen is excreted in urine as the 2 major metabolites, carboxyibuprofen and 2-hydroxyibuprofen (and their corresponding acyl glucuronides), respectively. Small amounts of other hydroxylated metabolites (e.g., 3-hydroxyibuprofen, 1-hydroxyibuprofen) also have been recovered in urine. Little or no unchanged drug is recovered in urine. Excretion of ibuprofen is essentially complete within 24 hours following oral administration. Some biliary excretion of the drug probably occurs in humans. Metabolism and excretion of ibuprofen in premature neonates have not been evaluated.

CHEMISTRY AND STABILITY

● Chemistry

Ibuprofen is a prototypical nonsteroidal anti-inflammatory agent (NSAIA). Ibuprofen is commercially available as the acid and as the potassium salt. Ibuprofen is a racemic mixture of 2 optical isomers. In vivo and in vitro studies indicate that only the *l*-isomer of ibuprofen has clinical activity. However, the *d*-isomer, which is considered clinically inactive, is slowly and incompletely (by about 60%) converted to the *l*-isomer in adults; the degree of such conversion is believed to be similar in children. It also has been suggested that the *d*-isomer serves as a circulating reservoir to maintain concentration of the active drug. Ibuprofen occurs as a white to off-white, crystalline powder having a slight, characteristic odor and is practically insoluble in water and very soluble in alcohol. The apparent pK_a of ibuprofen is about 4.4.

Commercially available ibuprofen lysine injection occurs as a clear sterile solution of the drug in water for injection. Sodium hydroxide or hydrochloric acid may be added during the manufacture of the injection to adjust the pH to 7.

● Stability

Oral preparations containing ibuprofen should be stored in well-closed, light-resistant containers at 20–25°C.

Ibuprofen injection concentrate and the commercially available ibuprofen premixed injection for IV administration should be stored at 20–25°C, but may be exposed to temperatures ranging from 15–30°C. The products contain no preservatives and are intended for single use only; any unused portions should be discarded.

Ibuprofen lysine injection should be stored at 20–25°C; the injection should be stored in the manufacturer's carton until time of use and should be protected from light. The product contains no preservatives and is intended for single use only; any unused portions should be discarded.

PREPARATIONS

Excipients in commercially available drug preparations may have clinically important effects in some individuals; consult specific product labeling for details.

Ibuprofen

Oral

Capsules, liquid-filled	equivalent to 200 mg ibuprofen (as free acid and ibuprofen potassium)*	**Advil® Liqui-Gels®**, GlaxoSmithKline
		Advil® Migraine®, GlaxoSmithKline
		Ibuprofen Liquid-filled Capsules
		Motrin® IB Liquid Gels, McNeil
		Motrin® IB Migraine, McNeil

Suspension	40 mg/mL*	Advil® Infants' Concentrated Drops, GlaxoSmithKline
		Ibuprofen Infants' Concentrated Drops
		Motrin® Infants' Concentrated Drops, McNeil
	100 mg/5 mL*	Advil® Children's Suspension, GlaxoSmithKline
		Ibuprofen Oral Suspension
		Motrin® Children's Suspension, McNeil
Tablets	200 mg*	Ibuprofen Tablets
	400 mg*	Ibuprofen Tablets
	600 mg*	Ibuprofen Tablets
	800 mg*	Ibuprofen Tablets
Tablets, chewable	100 mg*	Advil® Junior Strength Chewable Tablets, GlaxoSmithKline
		Ibuprofen Chewable Tablets
		Motrin® Children's Chewable Tablets, McNeil
Tablets, film-coated	100 mg	Advil® Junior Strength Tablets, GlaxoSmithKline
	200 mg*	Advil® Caplets®, GlaxoSmithKline
		Advil® Gel Caplets, GlaxoSmithKline
		Advil® Tablets, GlaxoSmithKline
		Ibuprofen Film-coated Tablets
		Ibutab®, Cintas
		Motrin® IB Tablets, McNeil
	400 mg*	IBU®, Dr. Reddy's
		Ibuprofen Film-coated Tablets
	600 mg*	IBU®, Dr Reddy's
		Ibuprofen Film-coated Tablets
	800 mg*	IBU®, Dr. Reddy's
		Ibuprofen Film-coated Tablets
Parenteral		
Injection, for IV use	4 mg/mL (800 mg)	Caldolor® in Sterile Water Injection (available in ready-to-use polypropylene bags), Cumberland
Injection concentrate, for IV use	100 mg/mL	Caldolor®, Cumberland

* available from one or more manufacturer, distributor, and/or repackager by generic (nonproprietary) name

Ibuprofen Combinations

Oral		
Capsules, liquid-filled	equivalent to 200 mg ibuprofen (as free acid and ibuprofen potassium) with Diphenhydramine Hydrochloride 25 mg*	Advil® PM Liqui-Gels®, GlaxoSmithKline
		Ibuprofen and Diphenhydramine Hydrochloride Liquid-filled Capsules
Tablets, film-coated	125 mg with Acetaminophen 250 mg	Advil® Dual Action, GlaxoSmithKline
	200 mg with Diphenhydramine Citrate 38 mg*	Advil® PM, GlaxoSmithKline
		Ibuprofen and Diphenhydramine Citrate Film-coated Tablets
		Motrin® PM, McNeil
	200 mg with Hydrocodone Bitrate 2.5 mg*	Hydrocodone Bitartrate and Ibuprofen Film-coated Tablets (C-II),
	200 mg with Hydrocodone Bitartrate 5 mg*	Hydrocodone Bitartrate and Ibuprofen Film-coated Tablets (C-II),
	200 mg with Hydrocodone Bitartrate 7.5 mg*	Hydrocodone Bitartrate and Ibuprofen Film-coated Tablets (C-II),
	200 mg with Hydrocodone Bitartrate 10 mg*	Hydrocodone Bitartrate and Ibuprofen Film-coated Tablets (C-II),
	800 mg with Famotidine 26.6 mg	Duexis®, Horizon

* available from one or more manufacturer, distributor, and/or repackager by generic (nonproprietary) name

Ibuprofen Lysine

Parenteral		
For injection, for IV use only	10 mg/mL (of ibuprofen)*	Ibuprofen Lysine Injection
		NeoProfen®, Recordati Rare Diseases

* available from one or more manufacturer, distributor, and/or repackager by generic (nonproprietary) name

† Use is not currently included in the labeling approved by the US Food and Drug Administration.

Selected Revisions June 10, 2024. © Copyright, July 1, 1975, American Society of Health-System Pharmacists, Inc.w

Ketorolac Tromethamine (Systemic)

28:08.04.04 • REVERSIBLE COX-1/COX-2 INHIBITORS

■ Ketorolac is a prototypical nonsteroidal anti-inflammatory agent (NSAIA) that also exhibits analgesic and antipyretic activity.

USES

● Pain

Ketorolac tromethamine is used parenterally or as a sequential regimen of parenteral followed by oral therapy for the short-term (i.e., up to 5 days) management of moderately severe, acute pain, usually in a postoperative setting, that requires analgesia at the opiate level. Ketorolac tromethamine also is used intranasally for the short-term (i.e., up to 5 days) management of moderate to moderately severe pain that requires analgesia at the opiate level. The manufacturer states that the drug is *not* indicated for use in minor or chronic painful conditions.

The potential benefits and risks of ketorolac therapy as well as alternative therapies should be considered prior to initiating ketorolac therapy. The lowest possible effective dosage and shortest duration of therapy consistent with treatment goals of the patient should be employed.

Ketorolac tromethamine has been used for the symptomatic relief of moderate to severe postoperative pain, including that associated with abdominal, gynecologic, oral, ophthalmologic, orthopedic, urologic, or otolaryngologic surgery. Ketorolac tromethamine should *not* be used in obstetric patients as a preoperative medication or for analgesia during labor since inhibitors of prostaglandin synthesis (e.g., ketorolac tromethamine) may affect uterine contractions and fetal circulation. In addition, ketorolac tromethamine should not be used as a preoperative medication for support of anesthesia, since the drug does not have sedative or anxiolytic effects but may inhibit platelet aggregation and prolong bleeding time. Ketorolac tromethamine also has been used for the relief of acute renal colic, pain associated with trauma, pain associated with vaso-occlusive crisis of sickle-cell disease, and visceral pain associated with cancer. IM ketorolac tromethamine generally produces analgesia comparable to that of moderate IM doses of opiate analgesics. However, unlike opiate agonists, ketorolac tromethamine does not appear to cause respiratory depression and there is no evidence that therapy with ketorolac tromethamine results in physical dependence on the drug.

When used to relieve moderate to severe pain in adults, a single 10-mg IM dose of ketorolac tromethamine has been reported to be more effective than placebo and at least as effective as a single 6-mg IM dose of morphine sulfate, a single 30-mg IM dose of pentazocine, or a single 50- or 100-mg IM dose of meperidine hydrochloride. A single 30-mg IM dose of ketorolac tromethamine has been reported to be more effective than placebo or a single 6-mg IM dose of morphine sulfate and at least as effective as a single 12-mg IM dose of morphine sulfate, a single 30-mg IM dose of pentazocine, or a single 50- to 100-mg IM dose of meperidine hydrochloride. The duration of analgesia produced by single IM doses of ketorolac tromethamine appears to be longer than that of single IM doses of morphine sulfate or meperidine hydrochloride.

In a short-term (up to 5 days) multiple-dose study in adults with moderate to severe postoperative pain, IM ketorolac tromethamine doses of 30 mg were more effective than IM morphine sulfate doses of 6 mg and as effective as IM morphine sulfate doses of 12 mg; the drugs were administered at an average frequency of every 5–6 hours. When used to relieve severe sciatic pain†, IM ketorolac tromethamine dosages of 30 mg 4 times daily have been at least as effective as IM ketoprofen dosages of 100 mg twice daily.

Parenteral ketorolac tromethamine has been used concomitantly with opiate agonist analgesics (e.g., meperidine, morphine) for the management of moderate to severe postoperative pain without apparent adverse drug interactions. Combined use of the drugs can result in reduced opiate analgesic requirements. Ketorolac tromethamine also has been administered concomitantly with non-opiate analgesics (e.g., aspirin, acetaminophen), but the manufacturer states that use of the drug with other NSAIAs is contraindicated because of the potential for additive adverse effects.

In postoperative patients receiving morphine via patient-controlled analgesia, those receiving fixed intermittent doses of IV ketorolac tromethamine (initial dose of 30 mg, followed by 15 mg every 3 hours) required 26% less morphine and achieved superior pain relief compared with those receiving placebo.

Ketorolac tromethamine also is used orally in adults for the symptomatic relief of moderate to severe pain such as postpartum, postoperative (including that associated with oral, orthopedic, or gynecologic surgery), orthopedic (including musculoskeletal strains or sprains), or sciatic pain and for visceral pain associated with cancer. When used to relieve moderate to severe pain in adults, a single 5-mg oral dose of ketorolac tromethamine has been reported to be more effective than placebo and as effective as a single 500-mg or 1-g oral dose of acetaminophen. A single 10-mg oral dose of ketorolac tromethamine has been reported to be more effective than placebo and at least as effective as single oral doses of acetaminophen 500 mg, 600 mg, or 1 g; aspirin 650 mg; pentazocine 100 mg; dihydrocodeine 30 mg; naproxen 550 mg; ibuprofen 400 mg; acetaminophen 600 mg or 1 g with codeine phosphate 60 mg; or propoxyphene napsylate 300 mg with aspirin 700 mg and antipyrine 300 mg. A single 20-mg oral dose of ketorolac tromethamine was more effective than placebo, a single 500- or 600-mg oral dose of acetaminophen, or a single 650-mg oral dose of aspirin and at least as effective as a single 1-g oral dose of acetaminophen, a single 400-mg oral dose of ibuprofen, a single 650-mg oral dose of aspirin with 60 mg of codeine phosphate, or a single 600-mg oral dose of acetaminophen with 60 mg of codeine phosphate.

Oral ketorolac tromethamine dosages of 5 or 10 mg 4 times daily have been as effective as oral diflunisal dosages of 500 mg twice daily. Oral ketorolac tromethamine dosages of 10 mg given up to 4 times daily have been as effective as oral pentazocine dosages of 100 mg given up to 4 times daily, oral dihydrocodeine dosages of 30 mg given up to 4 times daily, or oral acetaminophen dosages of 1 g with oral codeine phosphate dosages of 60 mg given up to 4 times daily. When used to relieve orthopedic (including musculoskeletal strains or sprains) pain, oral ketorolac tromethamine dosages of 10 mg 4 times daily have been at least as effective as oral diclofenac sodium dosages of 50 mg 3 times daily, oral ibuprofen dosages of 400 mg 4 times daily, oral diflunisal dosages of 500 mg twice daily, or oral acetaminophen dosages of 600 mg with oral codeine phosphate dosages of 60 mg 4 times daily.

Long-term† (e.g., up to 1 year) oral ketorolac tromethamine therapy at dosages of 10 mg given up to 4 times daily has been used in adults to relieve chronic pain, including that associated with osteoarthritis, fibromyopathies, fibromyalgias, or tension headaches, and was more effective than chronic aspirin therapy at dosages of 650 mg given up to 4 times daily. However, the manufacturer states that total combined duration of parenteral and oral ketorolac tromethamine therapy in adults should not exceed 5 days, and, therefore, the drug is not indicated for the management of chronic pain.

In adults undergoing elective abdominal or orthopedic surgery, postoperative therapy with ketorolac tromethamine 31.5 mg administered intranasally every 6 or 8 hours reduced postoperative pain intensity over 48 hours compared with placebo; ketorolac-treated patients required 26–36% less morphine administered via patient-controlled analgesia on an as-need basis for pain relief over the 48-hour period than did those receiving placebo.

● Ophthalmic Uses

For ophthalmic uses of ketorolac tromethamine, see 52:08.20.

DOSAGE AND ADMINISTRATION

● Administration

The potential benefits and risks of ketorolac therapy as well as alternative therapies should be considered prior to initiating ketorolac therapy.

Ketorolac tromethamine is administered by IM or IV injection, orally, or intranasally.

Parenteral and Oral Administration

Ketorolac tromethamine is administered by IM or IV injection. The drug also is administered orally. Therapy should be initiated with parenteral (i.e., IV or IM) ketorolac, with the oral formulation used as continuation therapy, as required. The total duration of parenteral and oral ketorolac therapy should *not* exceed 5 days. Patients should be switched to alternate analgesic therapy as soon as clinically possible.

IV administration of ketorolac tromethamine injection must be given over no less than 15 seconds. IM injection of ketorolac should be given slowly, via deep IM injection. While administration with food may delay and reduce peak plasma concentrations following oral administration, the extent of GI absorption of the drug is not affected. Concomitant administration of ketorolac tromethamine and antacids does not appear to affect oral absorption of the NSAIA.

Parenteral solutions of ketorolac tromethamine should be inspected visually for particulate matter and/or discoloration prior to administration whenever solution and container permit.

Intranasal Administration

Ketorolac tromethamine nasal solution is administered using a metered-dose spray pump. Prior to initial use, the spray pump must be primed. The patient instructions provided by the manufacturer should be consulted for use of the nasal spray pump. Because the nasal spray is not an inhalation product, the patient should be instructed not to inhale during administration. Contact of the solution with the eyes should be avoided; if such contact occurs, the affected eye(s) should be rinsed with water or saline, and a clinician should be consulted if ocular irritation persists for more than one hour.

Each bottle should be used for only 24 hours and then discarded; the manufacturer states that the spray pump will not deliver the intended dose after 24 hours.

The total duration of therapy with ketorolac nasal spray alone or sequential therapy that includes the nasal spray and oral or parenteral formulations of ketorolac should not exceed 5 days.

● Dosage

The lowest possible effective dosage and shortest duration of therapy consistent with treatment goals of the patient should be employed.

Current principles of pain management indicate that analgesics, including ketorolac tromethamine, preferably should be administered at regularly scheduled intervals, although the drug also has been administered on an as-needed basis (i.e., withholding subsequent doses until pain returns). The manufacturer states that clinicians should manage breakthrough pain in adults receiving ketorolac tromethamine therapy with supplemental low doses of opiate analgesics (unless contraindicated) as needed rather than considering higher or more frequent dosages of ketorolac tromethamine.

Because there is some evidence of dose-related adverse effects (e.g., GI bleeding), particularly in geriatric patients, the lowest possible effective ketorolac tromethamine dosage should be employed, and total duration of therapy with the drug (including parenteral, oral, and intranasal formulations) should not exceed 5 days. Particular caution and reduced dosage should be employed in geriatric patients, adults weighing less than 50 kg, and those with renal impairment (see Dosage in Renal and Hepatic Impairment under Dosage and Administration). Elimination of the drug generally is slower and sensitivity to adverse renal effects of NSAIAs generally is increased in geriatric patients.

Parenteral and Oral Dosage

For the short-term management of moderately severe, acute pain that requires analgesia at the opiate level in adults, a single IM or IV ketorolac tromethamine dose of 60 or 30 mg, respectively, is recommended by the manufacturer. For geriatric patients (65 years of age or older) and adults weighing less than 50 kg, the manufacturer recommends a single IM or IV dose of 30 or 15 mg, respectively. Such single-dose parenteral ketorolac tromethamine may be followed by oral ketorolac therapy in adults.

The manufacturer recommends that multiple-dose parenteral ketorolac tromethamine therapy be both initiated and continued with IM or IV dosages of 30 mg every 6 hours in adults; the maximum daily dose should not exceed 120 mg. For multiple-dose parenteral therapy in geriatric patients (65 years of age and older) and adults weighing less than 50 kg, the manufacturer recommends 15 mg of ketorolac tromethamine every 6 hours; the maximum daily dose in these patients should not exceed 60 mg.

Adults receiving parenteral ketorolac tromethamine who have experienced pain relief without limiting adverse effects may be switched to oral ketorolac tromethamine therapy, if needed. The manufacturer states that oral ketorolac tromethamine should be used only as continuation therapy following parenteral ketorolac therapy. Adults 17–64 years of age who are being switched from parenteral ketorolac tromethamine to oral therapy with the drug should receive a first oral dose of 20 mg, followed by 10 mg every 4–6 hours as needed. Geriatric patients (65 years of age or older) or adults weighing less than 50 kg who are being switched from parenteral ketorolac tromethamine to oral therapy with the drug should receive 10 mg of ketorolac tromethamine orally every 4–6 hours as needed. The dosing interval should not be shorter than 4–6 hours. The manufacturer states that the daily oral dosage in any patient should not exceed 40 mg in a 24-hour period. Low supplemental doses of an opiate agonist may be administered concomitantly with ketorolac tromethamine if breakthrough pain occurs, unless administration of an opiate agonist is contraindicated.

Intranasal Dosage

Ketorolac tromethamine nasal spray pump delivers 15.75 mg of ketorolac tromethamine per spray and 8 sprays per single-day bottle.

For the short-term management of moderate to moderately severe pain that requires analgesia at the opiate level in adults, the recommended intranasal dosage of ketorolac tromethamine is 31.5 mg (one spray in each nostril) every 6–8 hours; the maximum daily dosage is 126 mg (4 doses). Geriatric patients (65 years of age or older) and adults who weigh less than 50 kg should receive 15.75 mg (one spray in only one nostril) every 6–8 hours; the maximum daily dosage in these patients is 63 mg (4 doses).

● Dosage in Renal and Hepatic Impairment

Renal Impairment

Since ketorolac and its metabolites are excreted mainly by the kidneys, dosage adjustment may be required in geriatric patients and in other patients with reduced renal function.

When ketorolac is used parenterally in adults with renal impairment, the manufacturer recommends a single IM or IV ketorolac tromethamine dose of 30 or 15 mg, respectively. In these patients, multiple-dose parenteral ketorolac tromethamine therapy is administered at a dosage of 15 mg every 6 hours. The daily parenteral dosage in adults with renal impairment should not exceed 60 mg. Subsequent oral ketorolac tromethamine therapy should be administered at a dosage of 10 mg every 4–6 hours as needed. The dosing interval should not be shorter than 4–6 hours. The manufacturer states that the daily oral dosage in any patient should not exceed 40 mg in a 24-hour period. The manufacturer also states that for breakthrough pain, supplemental doses of an opiate agonist may be administered concomitantly with these reduced doses of ketorolac tromethamine, unless opiate agonists are contraindicated.

The recommended intranasal dosage of ketorolac tromethamine in adults with renal impairment is 15.75 mg (one spray in only one nostril) every 6–8 hours; the maximum daily dosage is 63 mg (4 doses). Ketorolac is contraindicated in patients with advanced renal disease.

Hepatic Impairment

Evidence from patients with liver cirrhosis suggests that modification may not be necessary.

CAUTIONS

Ketorolac tromethamine shares the toxic potentials of nonsteroidal anti-inflammatory agents (NSAIAs); when NSAIAs are administered short-term, the incidence of adverse effects is about 10–50% of that associated with chronic administration. Adverse reactions to ketorolac tromethamine usually are mild, dose related, and reportedly occur in about 39% of patients. Ketorolac tromethamine usually is well tolerated. The most common adverse effects associated with short-term IM or oral therapy with the drug are nervous system and GI effects. Results of premarketing studies indicated that short-term IM ketorolac tromethamine therapy was associated with a lower incidence of adverse effects compared with short-term IM morphine therapy. During clinical trials in patients receiving short-term, postoperative, intranasal therapy with ketorolac tromethamine, the most common adverse effects were mild and transient nasal discomfort or irritation, and the most common adverse effects resulting in early discontinuance of therapy were nasal discomfort or nasal pain (rhinalgia).

The manufacturer conducted a postmarketing, nonrandomized, observational study to examine the relative risks and benefits of ketorolac tromethamine and parenteral opiate agonists in a hospital setting. In this study, no attempt was made to assign the drug or dosage employed, and while patients included in the opiate group could not receive NSAIAs concomitantly, there was no limitation on concomitant opiate use by those receiving ketorolac. Interim analysis of data involving 6721 patients in the ketorolac group and 3943 patients in the opiate group revealed an association between mortality rate and age, increasing with age in both groups; the mortality rate was 0.9 and 1.7% for the respective drug groups. In addition, the frequency of GI bleeding, which ranged in severity from occult blood in stools to frank bleeding, also increased with age in both groups but was higher in the ketorolac than opiate group; about half of the reported GI effects involved occult blood in stools only, although death was attributed to GI bleeding in 2 patients (one in each drug group). Final analysis of data accumulated on approximately 10,000 patients revealed that the risk of clinically serious GI bleeding depended on the dose of ketorolac tromethamine; this appeared to be particularly important in geriatric patients who received an average daily dose greater than 60 mg. Serious adverse effects also were associated with long-term ketorolac therapy or therapy in patients with GI bleeding, renal impairment (without appropriate dose modification), or a history of sensitivity reactions to aspirin or other NSAIA-type agents. In addition, through December 4, 1992, the manufacturer had accumulated information on 73 spontaneously reported deaths in patients who received ketorolac.

● **Cardiovascular Effects**

Adverse cardiovascular effects occur in about 4% of patients receiving IM ketorolac tromethamine. Edema occurred in 1–3% of patients receiving the drug IM or orally. Hypertension has been reported in greater than 1% of patients. Vasodilation, pallor, hypotension, flushing, syncope, or palpitation has been reported in 1% or less of patients receiving the drug IM or orally. Bradycardia and hypertension each have been reported in 2% of patients receiving intranasal ketorolac tromethamine.

NSAIAs, including selective cyclooxygenase-2 (COX-2) inhibitors and prototypical NSAIAs, increase the risk of serious adverse cardiovascular thrombotic events, including myocardial infarction and stroke (which can be fatal), in patients with or without cardiovascular disease or risk factors for cardiovascular disease. Use of NSAIAs also is associated with an increased risk of heart failure.

The association between cardiovascular complications and use of NSAIAs is an area of ongoing concern and study. Findings of an FDA review of published observational studies of NSAIAs, a meta-analysis of published and unpublished data from randomized controlled trials of these drugs, and other published information indicate that NSAIAs may increase the risk of serious adverse cardiovascular thrombotic events by 10–50% or more, depending on the drugs and dosages studied. Available data suggest that the increase in risk may occur early (within the first weeks) following initiation of therapy and may increase with higher dosages and longer durations of use. Although the relative increase in cardiovascular risk appears to be similar in patients with or without known underlying cardiovascular disease or risk factors for cardiovascular disease, the absolute incidence of serious NSAIA-associated cardiovascular thrombotic events is higher in those with cardiovascular disease or risk factors for cardiovascular disease because of their elevated baseline risk.

Results from observational studies utilizing Danish national registry data indicated that patients receiving NSAIAs following a myocardial infarction were at increased risk of reinfarction, cardiovascular-related death, and all-cause mortality beginning in the first week of treatment. Patients who received NSAIAs following myocardial infarction had a higher 1-year mortality rate compared with those who did not receive NSAIAs (20 versus 12 deaths per 100 person-years). Although the absolute mortality rate declined somewhat after the first year following the myocardial infarction, the increased relative risk of death in patients who received NSAIAs persisted over at least the next 4 years of follow-up.

In 2 large controlled clinical trials of a selective COX-2 inhibitor for the management of pain in the first 10–14 days following coronary artery bypass graft (CABG) surgery, the incidence of myocardial infarction and stroke was increased. Therefore, NSAIAs are contraindicated in the setting of CABG surgery.

Findings from some systematic reviews of controlled observational studies and meta-analyses of data from randomized studies of NSAIAs suggest that naproxen may be associated with a lower risk of cardiovascular thrombotic events compared with other NSAIAs. However, limitations of these observational studies and the indirect comparisons used to assess cardiovascular risk of the prototypical NSAIAs (e.g., variability in patients' risk factors, comorbid conditions, concomitant drug therapy, drug interactions, dosage, and duration of therapy) affect the validity of the comparisons; in addition, these studies were not designed to demonstrate superior safety of one NSAIA compared with another. Therefore, FDA states that definitive conclusions regarding relative risks of NSAIAs are not possible at this time. (See Cautions: Cardiovascular Effects, in Celecoxib 28:08.04.08.)

Data from observational studies also indicate that use of NSAIAs in patients with heart failure is associated with increased morbidity and mortality. Results from a retrospective study utilizing Danish national registry data indicated that use of selective COX-2 inhibitors or prototypical NSAIAs in patients with chronic heart failure was associated with a dose-dependent increase in the risk of death and an increased risk of hospitalization for myocardial infarction or heart failure. In addition, findings from a meta-analysis of published and unpublished data from randomized controlled trials of NSAIAs indicated that use of selective COX-2 inhibitors or prototypical NSAIAs was associated with an approximate twofold increase in the risk of hospitalization for heart failure. Fluid retention and edema also have been observed in some patients receiving NSAIAs.

There is no consistent evidence that use of low-dose aspirin mitigates the increased risk of serious cardiovascular events associated with NSAIAs.

● **GI Effects**

Adverse GI effects reportedly occur in about 13% of patients receiving IM ketorolac tromethamine. Dyspepsia, nausea, and GI pain are the most common adverse GI effects of ketorolac tromethamine, occurring in about 12–13% of patients receiving the drug. Diarrhea occurs in 3–9% of patients receiving ketorolac tromethamine. Constipation, flatulence, feeling of GI fullness, and vomiting occur in less than 3% of patients receiving ketorolac tromethamine. Melena, peptic ulcer, rectal bleeding, stomatitis, dysgeusia, gastritis, eructation, anorexia, increased appetite, GI bleeding, GI perforation, dry mouth, and excessive thirst occur in 1% or less of patients receiving the drug. GI ulceration has been reported rarely in patients receiving ketorolac tromethamine. Most of these adverse GI effects also have been reported in patients receiving the drug orally but may occur more frequently than in those receiving the drug IM, since the duration of oral therapy often exceeds that of IM therapy. Although a causal relationship to ketorolac tromethamine has not been established, acute pancreatitis has occurred during therapy with the drug.

Usual IM dosages of ketorolac tromethamine reportedly produce fewer adverse GI effects than usual analgesic dosages of aspirin. In healthy individuals, the frequency of GI mucosal lesions observed endoscopically was lower with usual dosages of IM ketorolac tromethamine than with usual analgesic dosages of aspirin; higher than usual dosages of ketorolac tromethamine (i.e., IM dosages of 90 mg 4 times daily) were associated with a frequency of GI mucosal lesions similar to that associated with usual analgesic dosages of aspirin. However, the frequency of adverse GI effects may be increased during long-term administration and, in chronic toxicity studies in animals, GI toxicity (irritation and/or ulceration) was observed with oral but not parenteral ketorolac administration. The incidence of GI ulceration and bleeding in patients receiving long-term oral therapy (10 mg 1–4 times daily for up to 1 year) with the drug occurs at a rate of 1.2–5.4% per year. In one short-term (5 days' duration) study, endoscopically evident ketorolac tromethamine-induced mucosal injury, including GI ulceration, was dose related and independent of the route of administration.

Serious, sometimes fatal, adverse GI effects (e.g., bleeding, ulceration, or perforation of the esophagus, stomach, or small or large intestine) can occur at any time in patients receiving NSAIA therapy, and such effects may *not* be preceded by warning signs or symptoms. Only 1 in 5 patients who develop a serious upper GI adverse event while receiving NSAIA therapy is symptomatic. Therefore, clinicians should remain alert to the possible development of serious GI effects (e.g., bleeding, ulceration) in any patient receiving NSAIA therapy, and such patients should be followed chronically for the development of manifestations of such effects and advised of the importance of this follow-up. In addition, patients should be advised about the signs and symptoms of serious NSAIA-induced GI toxicity and what action to take if they occur. If signs and symptoms of a serious GI event develop, additional evaluation and treatment should be initiated promptly; the NSAIA should be discontinued until appropriate diagnostic studies have ruled out a serious GI event.

Studies to date are inconclusive concerning the relative risk of various prototypical NSAIAs in causing serious GI effects. In patients receiving NSAIAs and observed in clinical studies of several months' to 2 years' duration, symptomatic upper GI ulcers, gross bleeding, or perforation appeared to occur in approximately 1% of patients treated for 3–6 months and in about 2–4% of those treated for 1 year. Longer duration of therapy with an NSAIA increases the likelihood of a serious GI event. However, short-term therapy is not without risk. High dosages of any NSAIA probably are associated with an increased risk of such effects, although controlled studies documenting this probable association are lacking for most NSAIAs. Therefore, whenever use of relatively high dosages (within the recommended dosage range) is considered, sufficient benefit to offset the potential increased risk of GI toxicity should be anticipated.

Studies have shown that patients with a history of peptic ulcer disease and/or GI bleeding who are receiving NSAIAs have a greater than tenfold increased risk for developing GI bleeding than patients without these risk factors. In addition to a history of ulcer disease, pharmacoepidemiologic studies have identified several comorbid conditions and concomitant therapies that may increase the risk for GI bleeding, including concomitant use of oral corticosteroids, aspirin, anticoagulants, or selective serotonin-reuptake inhibitors (SSRIs); longer duration of NSAIA therapy; smoking; alcohol use; older age; and poor general health status. Risk of bleeding also is increased in patients with advanced liver disease and/or coagulopathy. Geriatric or debilitated patients appear to tolerate ulceration and bleeding less well than other individuals, and most spontaneous reports of fatal GI effects have been in such patients.

Results of a postmarketing, nonrandomized, observational study involving approximately 10,000 patients receiving ketorolac tromethamine indicated that the incidence of serious GI bleeding after up to 5 days of therapy with the drug is dose related and that serious GI bleeding occurs most commonly in geriatric patients receiving higher than recommended dosages of the drug. In patients with a history of GI perforation, ulceration, or bleeding, serious GI bleeding occurred in 2.1, 4.6, 7.8, or 15.4% of those younger than 65 years of age receiving total daily IV ketorolac tromethamine dosages of 60 mg or less, 61–90 mg, 91–120 mg, or more than 120 mg, respectively, and in 4.7, 3.7, 2.8, or 25% of those 65 years of age or older receiving these respective dosages. In patients without a history of GI perforation, ulceration, or bleeding, serious GI bleeding occurred in 0.4, 0.4, 0.9, or 4.6% of those younger than 65 years of age receiving total daily IV ketorolac tromethamine dosages of 60 mg or less, 61–90 mg, 91–120 mg, or more than 120 mg, respectively, and in 1.2, 2.8, 2.2, or 7.7% of those 65 years of age or older receiving these respective dosages.

For patients at high risk for complications from NSAIA-induced GI ulceration (e.g., bleeding, perforation), concomitant use of misoprostol can be considered for preventive therapy. (See Misoprostol 56:28.28.) Alternatively, some clinicians suggest that concomitant use of a proton-pump inhibitor (e.g., omeprazole) may be used to decrease the incidence of serious GI toxicity associated with NSAIA therapy.

● Nervous System Effects

Adverse nervous system effects reportedly occur in about 23% of patients receiving IM ketorolac tromethamine. Headache, somnolence or drowsiness, and dizziness have been reported in 17, 3–14, and 3–9%, respectively, of patients receiving ketorolac therapy. Nervousness, abnormal thinking, depression, euphoria, difficulty in concentration, insomnia, CNS stimulation, seizures, tremors, extrapyramidal manifestations, abnormal dreams, hallucinations, vertigo, asthenia, and paresthesia have been reported in 1% or less of patients receiving the drug. Psychosis also has been reported.

Nervousness, hyperkinesia, and asthenia/fatigue have been reported in 1–4% of patients receiving oral ketorolac tromethamine. Euphoria, stupor, and malaise have been reported rarely in patients receiving the drug orally.

● Local and Dermatologic Effects

IM administration of ketorolac tromethamine has produced pain at the injection site in about 2–4% of patients. Ecchymosis, bruising, hematoma or other signs of wound bleeding, and tingling at the injection site have been reported rarely. Adverse local effects may be minimized by applying pressure over the injection site for 15–30 seconds after administration. There has been no evidence (e.g., alterations in serum creatine kinase [CK, creatine phosphokinase, CPK] concentrations) of substantial adverse muscular tissue effects following single or multiple IM injections of ketorolac tromethamine.

Intranasal administration of ketorolac tromethamine has resulted in nasal discomfort or rhinalgia in 13–15% of patients, increased lacrimation or throat irritation in 4–5%, and rhinitis in 2%.

Pruritus occurred in 3–9% of patients receiving ketorolac tromethamine therapy, and sweating has been reported in 1–3% of patients receiving IM ketorolac tromethamine. Rash (may be maculopapular), urticaria, toxic epidermal necrolysis (Lyell's syndrome), and exfoliative dermatitis have been reported in 1% or less of patients receiving the drug IM. These effects also have been reported in patients receiving ketorolac tromethamine orally. Rash also has been reported in 3% of patients receiving intranasal ketorolac tromethamine.

● Sensitivity Reactions

Severe anaphylactoid reactions have been reported in patients receiving ketorolac tromethamine. Anaphylactoid reactions may occur in patients with known hypersensitivity to aspirin or other NSAIA, including ketorolac tromethamine; however, these reactions also have been reported in patients without a history of hypersensitivity or known previous exposure to these drugs. Patients should be questioned carefully before ketorolac tromethamine therapy is initiated about development of allergic reactions (e.g., asthma, nasal polyps, urticaria, hypotension) associated with administration of NSAIAs; if such manifestations occur during therapy, the drug should be discontinued. In premarketing studies in a limited number of patients previously exposed to ketorolac tromethamine but with no history of hypersensitivity to it, there was no evidence that the drug possessed an unusual propensity for causing hypersensitivity reactions. Anaphylaxis, bronchospasm, and laryngeal and/or lingual edema have been reported in 1% or less of patients receiving the drug. Angioedema and anaphylactoid reaction also have been reported.

● Renal, Electrolyte, and Genitourinary Effects

Chronic administration of oral ketorolac tromethamine occasionally has caused impairment of renal function, resulting in hematuria, proteinuria, and transiently increased BUN and serum creatinine concentrations. Increased BUN and serum creatinine concentrations have occurred in about 3 and 2% of patients, respectively, receiving the drug orally for 1 year. Oliguria or decreased urine output has been reported in 2–3% of patients receiving short-term therapy with intranasal ketorolac tromethamine. Oliguria, urinary frequency, urinary retention, hemolytic-uremic syndrome, acute renal failure, flank pain (with or without hematuria and/or azotemia), hyponatremia, and hyperkalemia have occurred in about 1% or less of patients receiving short-term oral or parenteral ketorolac tromethamine therapy. Glomerular nephritis, interstitial nephritis, renal papillary necrosis, and nephrotic syndrome have been reported in patients receiving ketorolac tromethamine; patients at greatest risk of adverse renal effects include those with impaired renal function and geriatric patients. Although a causal relationship to ketorolac tromethamine has not been established, polyuria has occurred during therapy with the drug. As with other NSAIAs, renal papillary necrosis and other evidence of renal toxicity have occurred following prolonged administration of the drug in animals.

● Hepatic Effects

Borderline elevations of one or more liver function test results may occur in up to 15% of patients treated with NSAIAs; meaningful (3 times the upper limit of normal) elevations of serum ALT (SGPT) or AST (SGOT) concentration have occurred in less than 1% of patients receiving oral ketorolac tromethamine in controlled clinical studies. Increased ALT and/or AST concentrations also have been reported in 2% of patients receiving short-term therapy with intranasal ketorolac tromethamine in controlled clinical studies. In addition, liver function abnormalities have been reported in less than 1% of patients receiving short-term, IM therapy with the drug. Such abnormalities may progress, may remain essentially unchanged, or may be transient with continued therapy. Hepatitis, liver failure, and cholestatic jaundice have been reported in 1% or less of patients receiving ketorolac tromethamine.

● *Hematologic Effects*

Purpura has been reported in less than 3% of patients receiving IM ketorolac tromethamine. Ketorolac tromethamine may inhibit platelet adhesion and aggregation and prolong bleeding time (generally by approximately 3 minutes from baseline values). However, the drug has a transient effect on platelet function, and aggregation usually returns to normal within 24–48 hours after discontinuing ketorolac tromethamine. The drug usually does not affect prothrombin time, partial thromboplastin time, or kaolin-cephalin coagulation time. Platelet count may or may not be affected by ketorolac tromethamine; thrombocytopenia (which was not considered clinically important) has been reported rarely in patients receiving the drug IM. Patients who may be affected adversely by a prolongation of bleeding time should be observed carefully during ketorolac tromethamine therapy. (See Hematologic Precautions under Cautions.)

Bleeding at the operative site (rarely requiring blood transfusions) has been reported in 1% or less of patients receiving parenteral ketorolac tromethamine therapy. In controlled clinical trials in patients undergoing major (e.g., orthopedic, abdominal) surgery, serious bleeding or hematoma at the operative site was reported in 1.5% of patients receiving intranasal ketorolac tromethamine. Bleeding has occurred following tonsillectomy in pediatric patients receiving ketorolac tromethamine. In one retrospective analysis of patients undergoing tonsillectomy with or without adenoidectomy, the risk of bleeding was 10.1 or 2.2% in patients receiving ketorolac or an opiate agonist, respectively, for pain management. In pediatric patients 12 years of age or younger, postoperative hemorrhage occurred in 6.5% of those given ketorolac and in 3.3% of those who did not receive the drug. In a prospective study in children 3–9 years of age undergoing tonsillectomy with or without adenoidectomy, the overall incidence of bleeding in children receiving ketorolac (16.3%) was similar to the incidence in children receiving morphine (17%). However, the incidence of bleeding during the first 24 hours after surgery was higher in those receiving ketorolac (14.3%) than in those receiving morphine (4.2%).

Thrombocytopenia, epistaxis, and anemia have been reported in 1% or less of patients receiving the drug. Although a causal relationship to ketorolac tromethamine has not been established, leukopenia and eosinophilia have occurred during therapy with the drug.

● *Ocular and Otic Effects*

Visual disturbances (e.g., blurred vision) have occurred in 1% or less of patients receiving IM ketorolac tromethamine therapy and also have been reported in patients receiving the drug orally. Tinnitus and hearing loss have been reported in 1% or less of patients receiving the drug.

● *Other Adverse Effects*

Dyspnea, infection, pulmonary edema, and myalgia have been reported in 1% or less of patients receiving ketorolac tromethamine IM or orally. Chills occurred in at least one patient receiving the drug IM. Other adverse effects reported rarely in patients receiving oral ketorolac tromethamine include weight gain, generalized pain, and fever. Although a causal relationship to ketorolac tromethamine has not been established, aseptic meningitis, rhinitis, and cough have occurred during therapy with the drug.

● *Precautions and Contraindications*

Ketorolac tromethamine, like other NSAIAs, is not free of potential adverse effects, including some that can cause discomfort; more serious effects (e.g., myocardial infarction, stroke, GI bleeding), which may require hospitalization and may even be fatal, also can occur. The total duration of ketorolac therapy (including parenteral, oral, and intranasal formulations) in adults is *not* to exceed 5 days because of an increased frequency and severity of adverse effects associated with more prolonged therapy; patients should be switched to alternative analgesic agents as soon as clinically possible.

Patients should be advised to read the medication guide for NSAIAs that is provided to the patient each time the drug is dispensed.

Cardiovascular Precautions

NSAIAs increase the risk of serious adverse cardiovascular thrombotic events. (See Cardiovascular Effects under Cautions.) To minimize the potential risk of adverse cardiovascular events, the lowest effective dosage and shortest possible duration of therapy should be employed. Some clinicians suggest that it may be prudent to avoid use of NSAIAs whenever possible in patients with cardiovascular disease. Patients receiving NSAIAs (including those without previous symptoms of cardiovascular disease) should be monitored for the possible development of cardiovascular events throughout therapy. Patients should be informed about the signs and symptoms of serious cardiovascular toxicity (chest pain, dyspnea, weakness, slurring of speech) and instructed to seek immediate medical attention if such toxicity occurs. Ketorolac tromethamine should be avoided in patients with recent myocardial infarction unless the benefits of therapy are expected to outweigh the risk of recurrent cardiovascular thrombotic events; if ketorolac tromethamine is used in such patients, the patient should be monitored for cardiac ischemia.

There is no consistent evidence that concomitant use of low-dose aspirin mitigates the increased risk of serious cardiovascular events associated with NSAIAs. Concomitant use of aspirin and an NSAIA increases the risk for serious GI events. (See Nonsteroidal Anti-inflammatory Agents under Drug Interactions.)

Use of NSAIAs can result in the onset of hypertension or worsening of preexisting hypertension; either of these occurrences may contribute to the increased incidence of cardiovascular events. Patients receiving NSAIAs may have an impaired response to diuretics (i.e., thiazide or loop diuretics), angiotensin-converting enzyme (ACE) inhibitors, angiotensin II receptor antagonists, or β-adrenergic blocking agents. Blood pressure should be monitored closely during initiation of NSAIA therapy and throughout therapy.

Because NSAIAs increase morbidity and mortality in patients with heart failure, the manufacturer states that ketorolac tromethamine should be avoided in patients with severe heart failure unless the benefits of therapy are expected to outweigh the risk of worsening heart failure; if ketorolac tromethamine is used in such patients, the patient should be monitored for worsening heart failure. Some experts state that use of NSAIAs should be avoided whenever possible in patients with reduced left ventricular ejection fraction and current or prior symptoms of heart failure. Patients receiving NSAIAs should be advised to inform their clinician if they experience symptoms of heart failure, including dyspnea, unexplained weight gain, and edema. Use of NSAIAs may diminish the cardiovascular effects of certain drugs used to treat heart failure and edema (e.g., diuretics, ACE inhibitors, angiotensin II receptor antagonists). (See Drug Interactions.)

GI Precautions

Serious GI toxicity (e.g., bleeding, ulceration, perforation), with or without warning symptoms, can occur at any time during ketorolac tromethamine therapy. Studies to date have not identified any subset of patients who are not at risk of NSAIA-associated bleeding or peptic ulceration. Geriatric (i.e., 65 years of age or older) or debilitated patients appear to be more susceptible to such GI bleeding and ulceration and most spontaneous reports of fatal GI events during ketorolac therapy were in these populations.

Use of NSAIAs should be avoided in patients at higher risk (see GI Effects under Cautions) unless the benefits of therapy are expected to outweigh the increased risk of bleeding; for patients who are at high risk, alternate therapy other than an NSAIA should be considered. NSAIAs should be used with great caution in patients with a history of inflammatory bowel disease (ulcerative colitis, Crohn's disease), since these diseases may be exacerbated by NSAIAs. Postmarketing experience with parenterally administered ketorolac suggests that there may be a greater risk of GI ulcerations, bleeding, and perforation in geriatric patients. (See Geriatric Precautions under Cautions.) The incidence and severity of adverse GI effects increase with increasing dose and duration of ketorolac tromethamine therapy. To minimize the potential risk of adverse GI effects, the lowest effective dosage and shortest duration of therapy should be employed, and use of more than one NSAIA at a time should be avoided. (See Nonsteroidal Anti-inflammatory Agents under Drug Interactions.)

In a hospital-based, nonrandomized, observational postmarketing study comparing patients receiving parenteral ketorolac therapy with patients receiving parenteral opiate therapy, higher rates of clinically serious GI bleeding were observed in patients younger than 65 years of age who received an average total daily parenteral ketorolac tromethamine dose of greater than 90 mg. In this same study, patients with a history of peptic ulcer disease also appeared to be at increased risk of developing serious GI complications. The manufacturer states that clinicians should inform their patients of the potential risks of ketorolac tromethamine therapy prior to initiating treatment.

Renal Precautions

Patients receiving ketorolac tromethamine are at risk of developing adverse renal effects, including interstitial nephritis and acute renal failure. Renal toxicity has been observed in patients in whom renal prostaglandins have a compensatory role in maintaining renal perfusion. Administration of an NSAIA to such patients may cause a dose-dependent reduction in prostaglandin formation and thereby precipitate overt renal decompensation. Patients at greatest risk of this reaction include those with impaired renal function, heart failure, or hepatic dysfunction; those with extracellular fluid depletion (e.g., patients receiving diuretics, dehydrated patients); those taking an ACE inhibitor or angiotensin II receptor antagonist concomitantly; and geriatric patients. Recovery of renal function to pretreatment levels usually occurs following discontinuance of NSAIA therapy. The manufacturer recommends that hypovolemia be corrected prior to initiating therapy with ketorolac. Some clinicians recommend that renal function be monitored periodically in patients receiving long-term NSAIA therapy.

The manufacturer states that ketorolac tromethamine should be used with caution in patients with renal impairment or a history of kidney disease, since ketorolac is a potent inhibitor of prostaglandin synthesis and the drug and its metabolites are excreted principally by the kidneys. Such patients should be monitored closely during ketorolac therapy. Because patients with underlying renal insufficiency are at risk of developing acute renal failure, the risks and benefits of ketorolac therapy must be considered before instituting therapy with the drug in these patients. In patients with moderately elevated serum creatinine, the manufacturer recommends that the usual daily dose of parenteral ketorolac tromethamine be halved, and not exceed 60 mg daily in these patients. (See Dosage in Renal and Hepatic Impairment under Dosage and Administration.)

Hepatic Precautions

Elevations in serum ALT concentrations may be the most sensitive indicator of NSAIA-induced liver dysfunction. Patients who experience signs and/or symptoms suggestive of liver dysfunction or an abnormal liver function test result (especially those with a history of hepatic impairment) while receiving ketorolac tromethamine should be evaluated for evidence of the development of a more severe hepatic reaction; the manufacturer states that therapy with the drug should be discontinued in such patients. The manufacturer states that ketorolac tromethamine should be used with caution in patients with a history of hepatic impairment or with a history of liver disease.

Hematologic Precautions

Ketorolac tromethamine should be used very cautiously and with careful monitoring in patients who may be adversely affected by prolongation of bleeding time (e.g., patients receiving anticoagulant therapy, patients with hemophilia, von Willebrand's disease, or platelet deficiency) and *only* when the potential benefits justify the possible risks to the patient, since the drug may inhibit platelet function and hemorrhage is possible. (See Anticoagulants and Thrombolytic Agents under Drug Interactions.) In patients who receive anticoagulants for any reason, there is an increased risk of intramuscular hematoma formation from administration of IM ketorolac tromethamine. In addition, since hematomas and other signs of wound bleeding have been reported in patients receiving ketorolac tromethamine perioperatively, the manufacturer states that postoperative administration of ketorolac tromethamine should be undertaken with caution in any patient in whom hemostasis is critical.

Precautions Related to Sensitivity or Dermatologic Reactions

Anaphylactoid reactions have been reported in patients receiving NSAIAs. Patients receiving ketorolac should be informed of the signs and symptoms of an anaphylactoid reaction (e.g., difficulty breathing, swelling of the face or throat) and advised to seek immediate medical attention if an anaphylactoid reaction develops.

Serious skin reactions (e.g., exfoliative dermatitis, Stevens-Johnson syndrome, toxic epidermal necrolysis) can occur in patients receiving ketorolac. These serious skin reactions may occur without warning; patients should be advised to consult their clinician if skin rash and blisters, fever, or other signs of hypersensitivity reaction (e.g., pruritus) occur. Ketorolac should be discontinued at the first appearance of rash or any other sign of hypersensitivity.

Multi-organ hypersensitivity (also known as drug reaction with eosinophilia and systemic symptoms [DRESS]), a potentially fatal or life-threatening syndrome, has been reported in patients receiving NSAIAs. The clinical presentation is variable, but typically includes eosinophilia, fever, rash, lymphadenopathy, and/or facial swelling, possibly associated with other organ system involvement such as hepatitis, nephritis, hematologic abnormalities, myocarditis, or myositis. Symptoms may resemble those of an acute viral infection. Early manifestations of hypersensitivity, such as fever or lymphadenopathy, may be present in the absence of rash. If such signs or symptoms develop, ketorolac should be discontinued and the patient evaluated immediately.

Other Precautions

In adults who weigh less than 50 kg, the dosage of ketorolac tromethamine should be reduced. (See Dosage under Dosage and Administration.)

The possibility that the antipyretic and anti-inflammatory effects of ketorolac tromethamine may mask the usual signs and symptoms of infection or other diseases should be considered, although some evidence suggests that the likelihood of such an effect may be small.

Ketorolac is not a substitute for corticosteroid therapy, and the drug is not effective in the management of adrenal insufficiency. Abrupt withdrawal of corticosteroids may exacerbate corticosteroid-responsive conditions. If corticosteroid therapy is to be discontinued after prolonged therapy, the dosage should be tapered gradually.

Use of corticosteroids during NSAIA treatment may increase the risk of GI ulceration and the drugs should be used concomitantly with caution.

Ketorolac tromethamine therapy is contraindicated in patients with active peptic ulcer disease, recent GI bleeding or perforation, or a history of peptic ulcer disease or GI bleeding; in patients with advanced renal impairment or patients at risk of renal failure because of volume depletion; in patients with suspected or confirmed cerebrovascular bleeding, hemorrhagic diathesis, or incomplete hemostasis, and in patients at a high risk of bleeding; in the setting of CABG surgery; and in patients receiving concomitant probenecid or pentoxifylline therapy. The manufacturers of oral and parenteral formulations of ketorolac also state that the drug is contraindicated in patients receiving concomitant aspirin or NSAIA therapy, because of the cumulative risk of serious NSAIA-related adverse effects. Use of ketorolac tromethamine as a prophylactic analgesic before any major surgery also is contraindicated. Because of the alcohol content of the parenteral formulations of the drug, epidural or intrathecal administration of ketorolac is contraindicated.

The manufacturers state that ketorolac is contraindicated in patients with known hypersensitivity (e.g., anaphylaxis, serious dermatologic reactions) to the drug or any ingredient in the formulation. In addition, NSAIAs generally are contraindicated in patients in whom asthma, urticaria, or other sensitivity reactions are precipitated by aspirin or other NSAIAs, since there is potential for cross-sensitivity between NSAIAs and aspirin, and severe, often fatal, anaphylactic reactions may occur in such patients. Although NSAIAs generally are contraindicated in these patients, the drugs have occasionally been used in NSAIA-sensitive patients who have undergone desensitization. Because patients with asthma may have aspirin-sensitivity asthma, NSAIAs should be used with caution in patients with asthma. In patients with asthma, aspirin sensitivity is manifested principally as bronchospasm and usually is associated with nasal polyps; the association of aspirin sensitivity, asthma, and nasal polyps is known as the aspirin triad. For a further discussion of cross-sensitivity of NSAIAs, see Cautions: Sensitivity Reactions, in the Salicylates General Statement 28:08.04.24.

● Pediatric Precautions

Safety and efficacy of ketorolac (oral, parenteral, or intranasal) have not been established in pediatric patients younger than 17 years of age. The manufacturer states that ketorolac tromethamine nasal spray should *not* be used in pediatric patients younger than 2 years of age.

Meta-analysis of data from 13 randomized controlled trials that compared postoperative analgesic efficacy of ketorolac (at any dosage and any route of administration) with that of placebo or another active treatment following any type of surgery in pediatric patients up to 18 years of age indicated that available data were inadequate to determine efficacy or assess safety in this population. The studies provided insufficient data regarding postoperative pain intensity or the proportion of patients obtaining at least 50% pain relief and provided only limited data regarding use of rescue medications or opiate analgesics.

Ketorolac tromethamine appears to increase the risk of bleeding following tonsillectomy.

● Geriatric Precautions

Geriatric patients are at increased risk for NSAIA-associated serious adverse cardiovascular, GI, and renal effects. Many of the spontaneous reports of fatal GI effects in patients receiving NSAIAs involve geriatric individuals. Because ketorolac tromethamine may be cleared more slowly in geriatric individuals (i.e., 65 years of age or older) and because this population may be more susceptible to the adverse effects of NSAIA-type drugs, ketorolac therapy must be instituted with extreme caution, with careful clinical monitoring, and at reduced dosages in these patients. The incidence and severity of GI complications increase with increasing dose and duration of ketorolac therapy. If the anticipated benefits of ketorolac therapy outweigh the potential risks, ketorolac should be initiated at the lower end of the dosing range; the total daily parenteral dose of the drug should not exceed 60 mg, and the total daily intranasal dose should not exceed 63 mg. (See Dosage under Dosage and Administration.) The dose and frequency of administration should be adjusted based on response to initial therapy. Ketorolac and its metabolites are substantially excreted by the kidneys, and the risk of adverse effects may be greater in patients with impaired renal function; because geriatric patients are more likely to have decreased renal function, it may be useful to monitor renal function.

● Mutagenicity and Carcinogenicity

No evidence of ketorolac tromethamine-induced mutagenesis was seen in in vitro studies with *Salmonella typhimurium, Saccharomyces cerevisiae*, or *Escherichia coli*. There also was no evidence of mutagenicity when ketorolac tromethamine was tested for chromosome breaks in vivo in the micronucleus assay in mice. Ketorolac was not mutagenic in the Ames microbial mutagen test or in the forward mutation assay; there was no increase in DNA repair when ketorolac tromethamine was tested in an unscheduled DNA synthesis. Ketorolac tromethamine increased chromosomal aberrations in Chinese hamster ovarian cells when they were exposed to the drug at concentrations of 1.59 mg/mL (about 1000 times the average human plasma ketorolac concentrations).

No evidence of carcinogenic potential was seen in an 18-month study in mice receiving oral ketorolac tromethamine dosages up to 2 mg/kg daily (approximately equivalent to the maximum recommended human dosage of IM ketorolac tromethamine). There also was no evidence of carcinogenic potential in a 24-month study in rats receiving oral ketorolac tromethamine dosages up to 5 mg/kg daily (approximately 2.5 times the maximum recommended human dosage of IM ketorolac tromethamine).

● Pregnancy, Fertility, and Lactation

Pregnancy

Use of NSAIAs during pregnancy at about 30 weeks of gestation or later can cause premature closure of the fetal ductus arteriosus, and use at about 20 weeks of gestation or later has been associated with fetal renal dysfunction resulting in oligohydramnios and, in some cases, neonatal renal impairment. Because of these risks, use of NSAIAs should be avoided in pregnant women at about 30 weeks of gestation or later; if NSAIA therapy is necessary between about 20 and 30 weeks of gestation, the lowest effective dosage and shortest possible duration of treatment should be used. Monitoring of amniotic fluid volume via ultrasound examination should be considered if the duration of NSAIA treatment exceeds 48 hours; if oligohydramnios occurs, the drug should be discontinued and follow-up instituted according to clinical practice. Pregnant women should be advised to avoid use of NSAIAs beginning at 20 weeks' gestation unless otherwise advised by a clinician; they should be informed that NSAIAs should be avoided beginning at 30 weeks' gestation because of the risk of premature closure of the fetal ductus arteriosus and that monitoring for oligohydramnios may be necessary if NSAIA therapy is required for longer than 48 hours' duration between about 20 and 30 weeks of gestation.

Known effects of NSAIAs on the human fetus during the third trimester of pregnancy include prenatal constriction of the ductus arteriosus, tricuspid incompetence, and pulmonary hypertension; nonclosure of the ductus arteriosus during the postnatal period (which may be resistant to medical management); and myocardial degenerative changes, platelet dysfunction with resultant bleeding, intracranial bleeding, renal dysfunction or renal failure, renal injury or dysgenesis potentially resulting in prolonged or permanent renal failure, oligohydramnios, GI bleeding or perforation, and increased risk of necrotizing enterocolitis.

Fetal renal dysfunction resulting in oligohydramnios and, in some cases, neonatal renal impairment has been observed, on average, following days to weeks of maternal NSAIA use, although oligohydramnios has been observed infrequently as early as 48 hours after initiation of NSAIA therapy. Oligohydramnios is often, but not always, reversible (generally within 3–6 days) following discontinuance of NSAIA therapy. Complications of prolonged oligohydramnios may include limb contracture and delayed lung maturation. A limited number of case reports have described maternal NSAIA use and neonatal renal dysfunction, in some cases irreversible, without oligohydramnios. Some cases of neonatal renal dysfunction have required treatment with invasive procedures such as exchange transfusion or dialysis. Deaths associated with neonatal renal failure have been reported. Methodologic limitations of these postmarketing studies and case reports include lack of a control group; limited information regarding dosage, duration, and timing of drug exposure; and concomitant use of other drugs. These limitations preclude establishing a reliable estimate of the risk of adverse fetal and neonatal outcomes with maternal NSAIA use. Available data on neonatal outcomes generally involved preterm infants, and the extent to which certain reported risks can be generalized to full-term infants is uncertain.

Animal data indicate that prostaglandins have an important role in endometrial vascular permeability, blastocyst implantation, and decidualization. In animal studies, inhibitors of prostaglandin synthesis, such as ketorolac, were associated with increased pre- and post-implantation losses. Prostaglandins also have an important role in fetal kidney development. In animal studies, inhibitors of prostaglandin synthesis impaired kidney development at clinically relevant doses.

Reproduction studies in rabbits and rats receiving oral ketorolac tromethamine dosages of 3.6 and 10 mg/kg daily, respectively (about 1.8 and 5 times the maximum recommended human parenteral dosage, respectively), during the period of organogenesis have not revealed evidence of harm to the fetus; however, oral dosages exceeding the maximum recommended human parenteral dosage in rats produced delayed parturition and dystocia, probably secondary to inhibition of prostaglandin synthesis.

Use of ketorolac during labor and delivery is contraindicated, since its inhibitory effect on prostaglandin synthesis may adversely affect fetal circulation and inhibit uterine contractions, thus increasing the risk of uterine hemorrhage. In animal studies, NSAIAs, including ketorolac, delayed parturition and increased the incidence of stillbirths.

Fertility

Use of NSAIAs, including ketorolac, may delay or prevent ovarian follicular rupture, which has been associated with reversible infertility in some women. Reversible delays in ovulation have been observed in limited studies in women receiving NSAIAs, and animal studies indicate that inhibitors of prostaglandin synthesis can disrupt prostaglandin-mediated follicular rupture required for ovulation. Therefore, withdrawal of ketorolac tromethamine should be considered in women who are experiencing difficulty conceiving or are undergoing evaluation of infertility.

Reproduction studies in male and female rats using ketorolac tromethamine dosages of 9 or 16 mg/kg daily (about 0.9 or 1.6 times, respectively, the human exposure) have not revealed evidence of impaired fertility.

Lactation

Ketorolac may be distributed into milk in small amounts. (See Distribution under Pharmacokinetics.) The developmental and health benefits of breast-feeding should be considered along with the mother's clinical need for ketorolac and any potential adverse effects on the breast-fed infant from the drug or from the underlying maternal condition.

Caution should be exercised when ketorolac is used in nursing women; although available information has not revealed any specific adverse events in nursing infants, women who are breast-feeding should be advised to contact their infant's clinician if they observe any adverse events.

DRUG INTERACTIONS

• Protein-bound Drugs

Because ketorolac tromethamine is highly protein bound, it could be displaced from binding sites by, or it could displace from binding sites, some other protein-bound drugs. However, the clinical importance of such potential drug interactions has not been established for ketorolac. In vitro studies indicate that salicylates may displace ketorolac from protein-binding sites. (See Nonsteroidal Anti-Inflammatory Agents under Drug Interactions.) In addition, in vitro studies indicate that ketorolac may displace warfarin slightly from protein-binding sites; however, it appears that the NSAIA does not displace digoxin from its protein-binding sites. (See Digoxin under Drug Interactions.) Therapeutic plasma concentrations of digoxin, warfarin, ibuprofen, naproxen, acetaminophen, phenytoin, tolbutamide, or piroxicam do not appear to alter the protein binding of ketorolac.

• Antihypertensive Agents

Concomitant use of NSAIAs with angiotensin-converting enzyme (ACE) inhibitors, angiotensin II receptor antagonists, or β-adrenergic blocking agents may reduce the blood pressure response to the antihypertensive agent. Blood pressure should be monitored to ensure that target blood pressure is achieved.

Concomitant use of ketorolac with ACE inhibitors or angiotensin II receptor antagonists in geriatric patients or patients with volume depletion or renal impairment may result in reversible deterioration of renal function, including possible acute renal failure; such patients should be monitored for signs of worsening renal function. Patients receiving concomitant therapy with ketorolac and ACE inhibitors or angiotensin II receptor antagonists should be adequately hydrated, and renal function should be assessed when concomitant therapy is initiated and periodically thereafter.

• Anticoagulants and Thrombolytic Agents

The effects of warfarin and NSAIAs on GI bleeding are synergistic. Concomitant use of NSAIAs and warfarin is associated with a higher risk of GI bleeding compared with use of either agent alone.

While in vitro studies indicate that protein binding of warfarin may be decreased slightly from 99.5 to 99.3% by ketorolac, a ketorolac dosage of 10 mg daily for 6 days did not substantially alter the pharmacokinetics or pharmacodynamics of a single dose of warfarin in one study in healthy adults. No drug interaction was observed in healthy adults following concomitant administration of heparin (5000 units) and ketorolac tromethamine. However, because ketorolac tromethamine can inhibit platelet function, the drug should be used with extreme caution and prothrombin time should be monitored carefully in patients who may be adversely affected by prolongation of bleeding time (e.g., patients receiving anticoagulant therapy, patients with hemophilia, von Willebrand's disease, or platelet deficiency). Patients receiving therapeutic doses of anticoagulants (e.g., heparin, warfarin) have an increased risk of bleeding complications if ketorolac is administered concomitantly; therefore, the manufacturer recommends that such concomitant therapy be undertaken with extreme caution. The concurrent use of ketorolac tromethamine and prophylactic low-dose heparin (2500–5000 units every 12 hours), warfarin, or dextrans has not been studied extensively, but also associated with an increased risk of bleeding. Until more data are available, the manufacturer recommends that such concomitant therapy be undertaken only very cautiously, and *only* when the potential benefits justify the possible risks to the patient. Patients receiving ketorolac concomitantly with drugs that alter hemostasis should be monitored for signs of bleeding.

• Anticonvulsants

Seizures have been reported rarely in patients receiving concomitant ketorolac and anticonvulsant therapy (e.g., phenytoin, carbamazepine).

• Cyclosporine

Concomitant use of ketorolac and cyclosporine may increase cyclosporine-associated nephrotoxicity. Patients should be monitored for signs of worsening renal function.

• Digoxin

Concomitant use of ketorolac and digoxin has been reported to result in increased serum concentrations and prolonged half-life of digoxin. Serum digoxin concentrations should be monitored.

• Diuretics

Patients receiving diuretics may have an increased risk of developing renal failure secondary to decreased renal blood flow resulting from prostaglandin inhibition by NSAIAs, including ketorolac tromethamine. (See Renal Precautions under Cautions.) In addition, NSAIAs (including ketorolac tromethamine) can reduce the natriuretic effects of furosemide or thiazide diuretics. This effect may be related to inhibition of renal prostaglandin synthesis. Patients receiving concomitant ketorolac and diuretic therapy should be monitored for signs of worsening renal function and for adequacy of diuretic and antihypertensive effects.

• Lithium

NSAIAs appear to decrease renal clearance of lithium, which may lead to an increase in serum or plasma lithium concentrations. Limited reports suggest that concomitant administration of ketorolac tromethamine and lithium results in increased lithium concentrations, with associated symptoms of lithium toxicity (e.g., nausea, vomiting, neurologic effects). NSAIAs reportedly increase mean trough lithium concentrations by 15% and decrease lithium clearance by approximately 20%; these effects have been attributed to inhibition of renal prostaglandin synthesis by NSAIAs. Although such concomitant therapy is not recommended, if patients must receive concomitant ketorolac and lithium therapy, plasma lithium concentrations should be monitored closely, and the patient should be observed for signs and symptoms of lithium toxicity.

• Methotrexate

While the effect of ketorolac tromethamine on clearance of methotrexate has not been evaluated to date, severe, sometimes fatal, toxicity has occurred following administration of an NSAIA concomitantly with methotrexate (principally high-dose therapy) in patients with various malignant neoplasms or rheumatoid arthritis. The toxicity was associated with elevated and prolonged blood concentrations of methotrexate. The exact mechanism of the interaction remains to be established, but it has been suggested that NSAIAs may inhibit renal elimination of methotrexate, possibly by decreasing renal perfusion via inhibition of renal prostaglandin synthesis or by competing for renal elimination. Further studies are needed to evaluate the interaction between NSAIAs and methotrexate. Caution is advised if methotrexate and an NSAIA are administered concomitantly. Patients should be monitored for methotrexate toxicity (e.g., neutropenia, thrombocytopenia, renal dysfunction).

• Nonsteroidal Anti-inflammatory Agents

In vitro studies indicate that therapeutic anti-inflammatory concentrations (e.g., 300 mcg/mL) of salicylates may displace ketorolac from protein binding sites, possibly resulting in elevated plasma concentrations of unbound ketorolac. Protein binding of ketorolac may be decreased from 99.2% to 97.5%, which would represent a potential two-fold increase in plasma concentrations of unbound drug. When NSAIAs were administered with aspirin, protein binding of the NSAIA was reduced but clearance of the free (unbound) NSAIA was not altered. The clinical importance of this interaction is unknown.

In controlled clinical trials, concomitant use of NSAIAs and analgesic dosages of aspirin did not produce any greater therapeutic effect than use of NSAIAs alone. However, concomitant use of aspirin and an NSAIA increases the risk for bleeding and serious GI events. Because of the potential for increased adverse effects, concomitant use of ketorolac and analgesic dosages of aspirin generally is not recommended. Manufacturers of oral and parenteral formulations of ketorolac state that the drug is contraindicated in patients receiving aspirin or other NSAIAs because of the cumulative risk of serious adverse effects.

Patients receiving ketorolac should be advised not to take low-dose aspirin without consulting their clinician. Ketorolac is not a substitute for low-dose aspirin therapy for prophylaxis of cardiovascular events, and patients receiving antiplatelet agents such as aspirin concomitantly with ketorolac should be monitored closely for bleeding. There is no consistent evidence that use of low-dose aspirin mitigates the increased risk of serious cardiovascular events associated with NSAIAs.

● Pemetrexed

Concomitant use of ketorolac and pemetrexed may increase the risk of pemetrexed-associated myelosuppression, renal toxicity, and GI toxicity. Administration of NSAIAs with short elimination half-lives (e. g., diclofenac, indomethacin) should be avoided beginning 2 days before and continuing through 2 days after pemetrexed administration. In the absence of data regarding potential interactions between pemetrexed and NSAIAs with longer half-lives (e.g., meloxicam, nabumetone), administration of NSAIAs with longer half-lives should be interrupted beginning at least 5 days before and continuing through 2 days after pemetrexed administration. Patients with renal impairment with a creatinine clearance of 45–79 mL/minute should be monitored for myelosuppression, renal toxicity, and GI toxicity if they receive concomitant ketorolac and pemetrexed therapy.

● Pentoxifylline

When ketorolac is used concomitantly with pentoxifylline, the risk of bleeding is increased; such concomitant use is contraindicated.

● Probenecid

Concomitant administration of ketorolac tromethamine and probenecid has reportedly decreased clearance and increased plasma concentration, total AUC (by approximately threefold), and half-life (by approximately twofold) of ketorolac. Therefore, the manufacturer states that ketorolac is contraindicated in patients receiving probenecid.

● Psychotherapeutic Agents

Hallucinations have been reported in patients receiving therapy with ketorolac and psychoactive drugs (e.g., fluoxetine, thiothixene, alprazolam). Patients receiving such concomitant therapy should be monitored for hallucinations.

● Serotonin-reuptake Inhibitors

Serotonin release by platelets plays an important role in hemostasis. Results of case-control and epidemiologic cohort studies indicate that concomitant use of NSAIAs and drugs that interfere with serotonin reuptake may potentiate the risk of bleeding beyond that associated with an NSAIA alone. Patients receiving concomitant therapy with ketorolac and selective serotonin-reuptake inhibitors (SSRIs) or selective serotonin- and norepinephrine-reuptake inhibitors (SNRIs) should be monitored for signs of bleeding.

● Skeletal Muscle Relaxants

Results of postmarketing studies indicate that ketorolac tromethamine may potentiate the effects of nondepolarizing skeletal muscle relaxants, resulting in apnea; however, the drug interaction potential of the drugs has not been specifically studied. Patients receiving concomitant therapy with ketorolac and nondepolarizing skeletal muscle relaxants should be monitored for apnea.

● Other Drugs

Ketorolac tromethamine has been administered concomitantly with morphine or meperidine for the management of postoperative pain without apparent adverse interaction. No drug interactions were reported following concomitant administration of ketorolac with some anti-infective agents (e.g., cephalosporins, penicillins, aminoglycosides), antiemetic agents, laxatives, sedatives, anxiolytic agents, corticosteroids, bronchodilators, or hormones.

In individuals with symptomatic allergic rhinitis, the rate and extent of absorption of intranasally administered ketorolac tromethamine (single 31.5-mg dose) were not substantially altered by oxymetazoline hydrochloride nasal spray (single dose administered 30 minutes before ketorolac administration) or by fluticasone propionate nasal spray (200 mcg daily for 7 days).

Evidence from animal or human drug interaction studies suggest that ketorolac is unlikely to interact with the metabolism of itself or other drugs via the hepatic microsomal enzyme system (cytochrome P-450 system).

ACUTE TOXICITY

Limited information is available on the acute toxicity of ketorolac tromethamine. The acute lethal dose of ketorolac tromethamine in humans is not known. The oral LD_{50} of the drug is 200 mg/kg in mice.

Daily parenteral ketorolac tromethamine dosages of 360 mg (3 times the maximum daily recommended dose) for 5 days resulted in abdominal pain and peptic ulcers, which healed after drug discontinuance. Metabolic acidosis following intentional overdosage of ketorolac (amount of drug not specified) also has been reported. Dialysis does not appear to be effective in removing the drug from circulation. In rats, mice, and monkeys, single oral ketorolac tromethamine doses exceeding 100 mg/kg produced diarrhea, pallor, labored breathing, rales, vomiting, and decreased activity.

CHRONIC TOXICITY

Tolerance, psychological dependence, or physical dependence does not appear to occur in patients receiving chronic (for 6 months) oral ketorolac tromethamine. There also was no evidence of manifestations of withdrawal following abrupt discontinuance of IM ketorolac tromethamine. The drug does not appear to affect opiate receptors and does not appear to exhibit opiate agonist or antagonist activity. The most frequent adverse effects observed during chronic toxicity studies in animals were GI irritation and/or ulceration, which at high dosages resulted occasionally in peritonitis, anemia, and death. Renal toxicity also was evident after prolonged therapy at relatively high dosages in animals.

PHARMACOLOGY

Ketorolac tromethamine has pharmacologic actions similar to those of other prototypical NSAIAs. The drug exhibits anti-inflammatory, analgesic, and antipyretic activity. The exact mechanisms have not been clearly established, but many of the actions appear to be associated principally with the inhibition of prostaglandin synthesis. Ketorolac tromethamine inhibits the synthesis of prostaglandins in body tissues by inhibiting cyclooxygenase; at least 2 isoenzymes, cyclooxygenase-1 (COX-1) and -2 (COX-2) (also referred to as prostaglandin G/H synthase-1 [PGHS-1] and -2 [PGHS-2], respectively), have been identified that catalyze the formation of prostaglandins in the arachidonic acid pathway. Ketorolac, like other prototypical NSAIAs, inhibits both COX-1 and COX-2. Although the exact mechanisms have not been clearly established, NSAIAs appear to exert anti-inflammatory, analgesic, and antipyretic activity principally through inhibition of the COX-2 isoenzyme; COX-1 inhibition presumably is responsible for the drugs' unwanted effects on GI mucosa and platelet aggregation.

● Analgesic Effect

The analgesic effect of ketorolac tromethamine appears to result from inhibition of prostaglandin synthesis. While the precise mechanism of the analgesic effect of NSAIAs continues to be investigated, these effects appear to be mediated principally through inhibition of the COX-2 isoenzyme at sites of inflammation with subsequent reduction in the synthesis of certain prostaglandins from their arachidonic acid precursors. Prostaglandins appear to sensitize pain receptors to mechanical stimulation and to other chemical mediators (e.g., bradykinin, histamine). Since many NSAIAs, including ketorolac tromethamine, do not directly alter the pain threshold or prevent pain caused by exogenous or previously synthesized prostaglandins, the drugs may produce analgesia by inhibiting the synthesis of prostaglandins peripherally and possibly centrally. Animal studies suggest that the analgesic activity of ketorolac tromethamine results principally from a peripheral action. In addition, the anti-inflammatory effect of NSAIAs may contribute to their analgesic effect. Ketorolac tromethamine does not appear to affect opiate receptors; however, in one animal study, naloxone decreased the analgesic activity of ketorolac tromethamine. There is no evidence that therapy with ketorolac tromethamine results in physical dependence on the drug.

On a weight basis, the analgesic potency of oral ketorolac tromethamine was about 3–6, 25–50, 180–350, or 180–350 times that of indomethacin, naproxen, aspirin, or phenylbutazone, respectively, as determined by antagonism of phenylbenzoquinone-induced writhing in mice. On a weight basis, as determined by the adjuvant-inflamed paw test in rats, the analgesic potency of oral ketorolac tromethamine was about 500–800 times that of aspirin. The analgesic potency of oral ketorolac tromethamine was similar to that of indomethacin and about 11–25, 30–90, or 100–200 times that of naproxen, phenylbutazone, or aspirin, respectively, as determined by the yeast-inflamed paw test in rats.

● Anti-inflammatory Effect

The anti-inflammatory effect of ketorolac tromethamine and other NSAIAs may result in part from inhibition of prostaglandin synthesis and release during inflammation. While the precise mechanism of the anti-inflammatory effect of NSAIAs continues to be investigated, these effects appear to be mediated principally through inhibition of the COX-2 isoenzyme at sites of inflammation with subsequent reduction in the synthesis of certain prostaglandins from their arachidonic acid precursors. It appears that ketorolac tromethamine does not suppress phagocytic activity of mononuclear macrophages. Ketorolac tromethamine does not possess glucocorticoid or mineralocorticoid activity.

On a weight basis, the anti-inflammatory potency of oral ketorolac tromethamine has been shown to be 2–3 times that of indomethacin or naproxen and about 36 times that of phenylbutazone, as determined by inhibition of carrageenan-induced paw edema in rats. However, when determined by inhibition of cotton pellet-induced granuloma in rats, the anti-inflammatory potency of ketorolac tromethamine was comparable to that of indomethacin. In adjuvant-induced arthritis in rats, the anti-inflammatory activity of oral ketorolac tromethamine was approximately twice that of naproxen. However, there is limited evidence from studies in patients with inflammatory diseases (e.g., rheumatoid arthritis) and in animals that the anti-inflammatory potency of ketorolac is less than the drug's analgesic potency.

● Antipyretic Effect

Ketorolac tromethamine lowers body temperature in animals with antigen-induced fever. Although the mechanism of antipyretic effect of NSAIAs is not known, it has been suggested that suppression of prostaglandin synthesis in the CNS (probably in the hypothalamus) may be involved. In rats, the antipyretic activity of a ketorolac tromethamine dose of 0.1–2.7 mg/kg was similar to that of an aspirin dose of 5–45 mg/kg. However, results of clinical studies on the antipyretic activity of ketorolac tromethamine in humans have been equivocal, and further studies are needed.

● Renal Effects

Ketorolac tromethamine has been reported to adversely affect renal function. (See Renal, Electrolyte and Genitourinary Effects under Cautions.) Although the exact mechanism of adverse renal effects of NSAIAs has not been determined, the effects may be related to inhibition of renal prostaglandin synthesis.

● GI Effects

Ketorolac tromethamine can cause gastric mucosal damage, which may result in ulceration and/or bleeding. (See GI Effects under Cautions.) These gastric effects have been attributed to inhibition of the synthesis of prostaglandins produced by COX-1. Other factors possibly involved in NSAIA-induced gastropathy include local irritation, promotion of acid back-diffusion into gastric mucosa, uncoupling of oxidative phosphorylation, and enterohepatic recirculation of the drugs.

Epidemiologic and laboratory studies suggest that NSAIAs may reduce the risk of colon cancer. Although the exact mechanism by which NSAIAs may inhibit colon carcinogenesis remains to be determined, it has been suggested that inhibition of prostaglandin synthesis may be involved.

● Hematologic Effects

Ketorolac tromethamine can inhibit collagen- and arachidonic acid-induced platelet aggregation and may prolong bleeding time. Information on the effect of the drug on ADP-induced platelet aggregation has been equivocal. It appears that ketorolac tromethamine does not affect thromboxane A_2-induced platelet aggregation, prothrombin time, or partial thromboplastin time; however, serum thromboxane B_2 concentrations are decreased by the drug. In vitro, ketorolac tromethamine is more potent than aspirin in inhibiting collagen-induced platelet aggregation.

Following IM administration of 30 mg of ketorolac tromethamine 4 times daily in healthy adults, bleeding time was prolonged from 4.9 minutes to 7.8 minutes; prolongation of bleeding time was more pronounced in men than in women. In controlled clinical studies, clinically important postoperative bleeding occurred in 0.4 or 0.2% of patients receiving ketorolac tromethamine or opiate analgesics, respectively. In healthy individuals, oral administration of single 2.5- to 200-mg doses of ketorolac tromethamine resulted in 75–100% inhibition of ADP-, collagen-, or arachidonic acid-induced platelet aggregation 3 hours after administration of the drug. Unlike the irreversible action of aspirin on platelets and the resultant prolonged effect on platelet aggregation, ketorolac tromethamine had a transient effect on platelet function, and aggregation returned to normal within 24–48 hours after discontinuance of the drug in individuals receiving oral doses up to 200 mg. Like other prototypical NSAIAs, these effects of ketorolac tromethamine appear to be associated with inhibition of synthesis of prostaglandins produced by COX-1. In healthy adults, ketorolac tromethamine does not produce excessive perioperative bleeding and it appears that prolongation of bleeding time is of little clinical importance in most patients. However, caution is necessary in some patients. (See Hematologic Precautions under Cautions.)

● CNS Effects

In animals, high doses (up to 300 mg/kg) of ketorolac tromethamine did not appear to cause appreciable CNS effects (e.g., CNS depression, EEG disturbances). In mice, ketorolac tromethamine doses of 100 mg/kg did not potentiate barbiturate-induced sleep or protect against drug- or electroshock-induced seizures. Usual doses of ketorolac tromethamine did not appear to cause psychomotor effects in healthy individuals.

● Respiratory Effects

Unlike opiate agonists, ketorolac tromethamine does not appear to cause respiratory depression. In a limited number of patients undergoing surgery, postoperative increases in carbon dioxide tension (PCO_2) were less in patients receiving IM ketorolac tromethamine concomitantly with IM morphine than in patients receiving IM morphine with placebo, although the dose of morphine was higher in patients receiving morphine with placebo. In healthy adults, including some undergoing minor surgery, ketorolac tromethamine did not depress the ventilatory response to carbon dioxide. In patients with chronic obstructive pulmonary disease (COPD), ketorolac tromethamine did not produce substantial decreases in minute ventilation or inspiratory flow.

● Cardiovascular Effects

Usual doses of ketorolac tromethamine do not appear to cause appreciable cardiovascular effects. In healthy individuals, therapeutic doses of the drug did not affect mean arterial blood pressure, heart rate, stroke volume, left ventricular performance, or left ventricular stroke index. It appears that administration of parenteral ketorolac tromethamine does not alter the hemodynamics of anesthetized patients.

● Ocular Effects

Following topical application to the eye, ketorolac tromethamine may reduce some manifestations of ocular inflammation induced by ocular trauma (e.g., ocular surgery) or external agents and also may inhibit corneal neovascularization. The exact mechanism of the ocular effects of the drug has not been clearly established, but these actions appear to be associated principally with the inhibition of ocular prostaglandin synthesis. Topically applied ketorolac tromethamine does not appear to affect intraocular pressure (IOP) nor to worsen bacterial, fungal, or viral ocular infections.

● Other Effects

In a limited number of patients with diabetes mellitus receiving insulin or oral sulfonylurea antidiabetic agents, ketorolac tromethamine did not appear to affect glucose metabolism. Ketorolac tromethamine may exhibit weak anticholinergic and α-adrenergic blocking activity.

PHARMACOKINETICS

The pharmacokinetics of ketorolac after IM, IV, or oral administration are best described by a linear, two-compartment model with first-order absorption and elimination, and pharmacokinetics of the drug after IV administration are best described by a two- or three-compartment model.

● Absorption

Ketorolac tromethamine is rapidly and completely or almost completely absorbed following IM or oral administration, respectively. Bioavailability has been reported to range from 80–100% following oral administration. Bioavailability following intranasal administration is approximately 60% of that achieved with IM injection. At physiologic pH, ketorolac tromethamine is present in dissociated form as ketorolac (anion) and tromethamine (cation). The rate of absorption appears to be slower following IM administration than following oral administration of the drug in fasting, healthy adults; however, the extent of absorption is similar following parenteral or oral routes of administration. Food decreases the rate, but not the extent, of absorption of orally administered ketorolac tromethamine. The rate of absorption from the GI tract also may be decreased in patients with hepatic or renal impairment and in geriatric individuals. The presence of allergic rhinitis does not substantially alter the pharmacokinetics of intranasally administered ketorolac tromethamine.

Following IV administration of 15- or 30-mg doses of ketorolac tromethamine injection in healthy adults, time to peak plasma concentration was about 1 or 3 minutes, respectively. Peak plasma concentration following single-dose IV administration of 15 or 30 mg of ketorolac in healthy adults was approximately 2.5 or 4.7 mcg/mL, respectively. Following IM administration of the drug in adults, plasma concentrations of the drug increase proportionally with increasing doses. Average peak plasma ketorolac concentrations of 0.7–1.4, 2.2–3, 4–4.6 or 6.9 mcg/mL occur within 30–60 minutes following IM administration of a single 10-, 30-, 60-, or 90-mg dose of ketorolac tromethamine, respectively, in healthy adults. Following IM administration of a single 30-, 60-, or 90-mg dose of ketorolac tromethamine in healthy adults, peak plasma *p*-hydroxyketorolac (the principal metabolite of ketorolac) concentrations of about 30, 63, or 102 ng/mL, respectively, occur at about 2 hours. Following oral administration of a single 10- or 30-mg dose of ketorolac tromethamine in healthy adults, average peak plasma ketorolac concentrations of 0.7–1.1 or 2.7 mcg/mL, respectively, occur at about 1 hour (range: 20–60 minutes). Peak plasma *p*-hydroxyketorolac concentrations of about 37 ng/mL occur in about 1 hour following oral administration of a single 30-mg dose of the drug in healthy adults. Following intranasal administration of a 31.5-mg dose, peak ketorolac concentrations of approximately 1.8 mcg/mL occur at about 45 minutes. The area under the plasma concentration-time curves (AUCs) of ketorolac and *p*-hydroxyketorolac increase linearly with single IM ketorolac tromethamine doses of 30–90 mg. AUCs of ketorolac also increase proportionally with oral ketorolac tromethamine doses of 0.8–3.2 mg/kg, and may be increased in adults with renal impairment compared with those in healthy adults.

In healthy adults, steady-state plasma concentrations of ketorolac generally are reached within 24 hours following multiple dosing and average approximately 0.6–0.8 (range: 0.2–1.7) or 1.3–1.5 (range: 0.3–3.5) mcg/mL with IM ketorolac tromethamine dosages of 15 or 30 mg, respectively, 4 times daily. In multiple-dose IV studies, peak plasma steady-state ketorolac concentration following administration of 15- or 30-mg doses 4 times daily in healthy adults was approximately 3.1 or 6.9 mcg/mL, respectively. Mean steady-state plasma concentration following IV ketorolac doses of 15 or 30 mg 4 times daily in healthy adults was approximately 1.1 or 2.2 mcg/mL, respectively. Mean steady-state plasma concentration following oral administration of 10 mg 4 times daily in adults was approximately 0.6 mcg/mL. Steady-state plasma concentrations of ketorolac also generally are reached within 24 hours following multiple dosing with oral ketorolac tromethamine dosages of 12.5 mg 3 times daily; appreciable accumulation of ketorolac does not appear to occur. However, accumulation of ketorolac in special populations (e.g., geriatric, renal failure, or hepatic disease patients) has not been studied.

Following IM administration of ketorolac tromethamine in adults, the onset of analgesic action usually is evident within 10 minutes, and peak analgesia occurs within 75–150 minutes; analgesia may be maintained for up to 6–8 hours. Following oral administration of the drug in adults, onset of analgesic action usually is evident within about 30–60 minutes, peak analgesia occurs within 1.5–4 hours, and analgesia usually is maintained up to 6–8 hours. Although the relationship between plasma ketorolac concentrations and therapeutic effect has not been precisely determined, an estimated therapeutic range of 0.3–5 mcg/mL has been suggested. In adults undergoing dental surgery, pain intensity was reduced by 50% at plasma concentrations of 0.1–0.3 mcg/mL, and adverse effects generally became frequent at concentrations exceeding 5 mcg/mL.

● Distribution

Distribution of ketorolac into human body tissues and fluids has not been fully characterized. Following oral administration in mice, ketorolac is distributed into the kidneys, liver, lungs, heart, muscle, gonads, and spleen, with an average tissue/plasma concentration ratio of about 1.5 for the kidney and less than 1 for the other tissues. However, following oral, IM, or IV administration of ketorolac tromethamine in humans, ketorolac does not appear to be distributed widely. The apparent volume of distribution of ketorolac during the terminal elimination phase in healthy adults is approximately 0.15–0.3 L/kg and the volume of distribution at steady state (V_{ss}) is about 0.11–0.33 L/kg following IV, IM, or oral administration. Following IV administration of a single dose of the drug in children 3–18 years of age, the apparent volume of distribution averaged 0.25–0.26 L/kg. Ketorolac appears to cross the blood-brain barrier poorly; CSF concentrations are reported to be about 0.2% of concurrent plasma concentrations. Following topical application of a ketorolac tromethamine gel to the knee, the drug is distributed into synovial fluid, achieving synovial fluid concentrations approximately 50% of those attained in plasma. Ketorolac is more than 99% bound to plasma proteins; the degree of protein binding appears to be independent of plasma concentration of the drug and constant over the therapeutic range of the drug.

Ketorolac crosses the placenta. In pregnant women receiving single 10-mg IM doses of ketorolac tromethamine during labor, cord blood concentrations averaged about 11.6% (range: 4–25%) of maternal plasma concentrations. Ketorolac is distributed into milk, but in relatively small amounts. Following oral administration of a single 10-mg dose of ketorolac tromethamine in nursing women, peak milk ketorolac concentrations of 7.3 ng/mL occurred within about 2 hours, and the milk-to-plasma ratio was about 0.04. Following oral administration of 10-mg of ketorolac tromethamine 4 times daily for 2 days in nursing women, peak milk ketorolac concentrations 2 hours after dosing on the first or second day were 5.2–7.9 ng/mL and the milk-to-plasma ratio ranged from 0.015–0.037.

Following intranasal administration, most of the ketorolac dose is deposited in the nasal cavity and pharynx; less than 20% of the dose is deposited in the esophagus and stomach, and little or no drug (less than 0.5%) is deposited in the lungs.

● Elimination

Ketorolac tromethamine dissociates into ketorolac (anion) and tromethamine (cation) at physiologic pH. Following single oral, IM, or IV doses of ketorolac tromethamine in healthy adults, plasma concentrations of ketorolac appear to decline in a biphasic manner with a terminal elimination half-life of about 4–6 hours (range: 2.4–9.2 hours). A half-life of approximately 5 hours has been reported following intranasal administration. In a limited number of pediatric patients receiving the drug IV, an elimination half-life of 3.8–6.1 hours has been reported. In geriatric individuals, the elimination half-life was reported to increase to an average of about 5–7 hours (range: 4.3–8.6 hours). The elimination half-life of ketorolac also is prolonged in patients with renal impairment to about 9–10 hours (range: 3.2–19 hours) following oral or IM administration of the drug; in patients undergoing dialysis, elimination half-life of ketorolac tromethamine was about 13.6 hours (range: 8–39.1 hours). There is poor correlation between creatinine clearance and total ketorolac tromethamine clearance in geriatric individuals and in patients with renal impairment. It appears that hepatic impairment (e.g., liver cirrhosis) does not affect substantially the elimination half-life of ketorolac. In patients with liver cirrhosis, elimination half-life of ketorolac was about 5.4 hours (range: 2.2–6.9 hours) and 4.5 hours (range: 1.6–7.6 hours) following IM and oral administration, respectively.

The exact metabolic fate of ketorolac is not clearly established, but the drug undergoes hydroxylation in the liver to form *p*-hydroxyketorolac. This hydroxy metabolite exhibits limited pharmacologic activity, having less than 20 or 1% of the anti-inflammatory or analgesic potency, respectively, of the parent drug. Ketorolac also undergoes conjugation with glucuronic acid. The drug also is metabolized to unidentified polar metabolites, which appear to be pharmacologically inactive probably because of their high polarity and rapid elimination.

Following oral, IM, or IV administration, ketorolac and its metabolites are excreted mainly in urine; only small amounts of the drug and its metabolites are excreted in feces, probably via biliary elimination. Following a single oral or IV dose of ketorolac tromethamine in healthy adults, about 91% of the dose is excreted in urine within 2 days and about 6% in feces within 3 days; most urinary excretion (about 75% of the dose) occurs within about 7 hours. In healthy adults, about 56–60% of a single oral or IV dose is excreted in urine as ketorolac, 20–26% as ketorolac glucuronide, 11–12% as p-hydroxyketorolac, and 6–7% as unidentified polar metabolites.

Following IM, IV, or oral administration of the drug in healthy adults, total plasma clearance of ketorolac averages approximately 0.42–0.55 (range: 0.21–0.83) mL/minute per kg. Following single IV doses of ketorolac tromethamine in children 3–18 years of age, plasma clearance of the drug reportedly averaged 0.7–1.13 mL/minute per kg. Total plasma clearance of ketorolac is decreased in patients with reduced renal function. Following IM or oral administration of ketorolac tromethamine in patients with serum creatinine concentrations of 1.9–5 mg/dL, total apparent plasma ketorolac clearance was reduced to about 0.27 (range: 0.1–0.87) mL/minute per kg. Total plasma clearance reportedly also is decreased in geriatric individuals. In geriatric individuals, total apparent plasma clearance of ketorolac averaged 0.32–0.4 (range: 0.22–0.57) mL/minute per kg. It appears that hepatic impairment does not affect total clearance of ketorolac. In a group of patients with liver cirrhosis, total apparent plasma clearance averaged about 0.5 (range: 0.22–1.1) mL/minute per kg.

The effect of hemodialysis and/or peritoneal dialysis on elimination of ketorolac is not known but probably is minimal secondary to the drug's high protein binding. Limited data indicate that following IM administration of the drug in patients undergoing dialysis total apparent plasma clearance of ketorolac averaged 0.27 (range: 0.05–0.6) mL/minute per kg.

CHEMISTRY AND STABILITY

● Chemistry

Ketorolac, a pyrrolizine carboxylic acid derivative, is a prototypical nonsteroidal anti-inflammatory agent (NSAIA). The drug is structurally and pharmacologically related to tolmetin, zomepirac, and indomethacin, but unlike these pyrrole acetic acid derivatives, ketorolac is a cyclic propionic acid derivative.

Ketorolac is commercially available as the tromethamine salt. The tromethamine moiety enhances the aqueous solubility of ketorolac. Ketorolac tromethamine is commercially available as a racemic mixture. The analgesic and anti-inflammatory activity of the drug results principally from the levorotatory (l) isomer, which has approximately twice the pharmacologic activity of the racemic mixture.

Ketorolac tromethamine occurs as an off-white crystalline powder and has solubilities of 3 mg/mL in alcohol and more than 500 mg/mL in water at 23°C. The pK$_a$ of the drug in water is 3.54.

Ketorolac tromethamine injection is a sterile solution of the drug in alcohol and sterile water for injection. The commercially available injection occurs as a clear, slightly yellow solution; hydrochloric acid and/or sodium hydroxide may be added during manufacture to adjust the pH to 6.9–7.9. About 6.68 or 4.35 mg of sodium chloride is added to each mL of the injection containing 15 or 30 mg of ketorolac tromethamine per mL, respectively, to provide an isotonic solution.

Ketorolac tromethamine nasal spray is commercially available as a preservative-free solution that is administered by spray pump; each 100-μL metered spray delivers 15.75 mg of ketorolac tromethamine, and each bottle contains sufficient solution to deliver 8 sprays.

● Stability

Ketorolac tromethamine injection and oral tablets should be stored at 15–30°C and protected from light. The tablets also should be stored in well-closed containers and protected from excessive humidity. Prolonged exposure of the injection to light may produce discoloration of the solution and also may promote precipitation of the 1-keto derivative (constituting more than 80% of the light-induced degradation products) and, to a lesser extent, the decarboxy and 1-hydroxy derivatives. In commercially available ketorolac tromethamine injections, air has been replaced with nitrogen; the injections have an expiration date of 24 months following the date of manufacture.

Ketorolac tromethamine nasal spray should be stored at 2–8°C prior to opening and protected from light and freezing; during use, bottles of the nasal spray should be stored at 15–20°C out of direct sunlight. The bottle should be discarded within 24 hours after priming the pump.

When stored at 15–30°C, ketorolac tromethamine solutions containing 0.6 mg/mL are chemically and physically compatible for at least 48 hours in the following IV solutions: 0.9% sodium chloride, 5% dextrose, 5% dextrose and 0.9% sodium chloride, Ringer's, lactated Ringer's, or Plasma-Lyte® A.

When admixed in the same syringe to produce the concentrations listed, ketorolac tromethamine (15 mg/mL) is incompatible with solutions of drugs such as opiate agonists (e.g., meperidine hydrochloride [50 mg/mL], morphine sulfate [7.5 mg/mL]), promethazine hydrochloride (25 mg/mL), or hydroxyzine hydrochloride (25 mg/mL) that result in a relatively low pH following admixture since precipitation of the NSAIA can occur. Therefore, ketorolac tromethamine should *not* be administered in the same syringe with any such drug solutions. Specialized references should be consulted for additional compatibility information.

PREPARATIONS

Excipients in commercially available drug preparations may have clinically important effects in some individuals; consult specific product labeling for details.

Ketorolac Tromethamine

Nasal		
Solution	15.75 mg/metered spray	Sprix®, Zyla
Oral		
Tablets, film-coated	10 mg*	Ketorolac Tromethamine Tablets
Parenteral		
Injection, for IM or IV use	15 mg/mL*	Ketorolac Tromethamine Injection
	30 mg/mL*	Ketorolac Tromethamine Injection
Injection, for IM use	30 mg/mL*	Ketorolac Tromethamine Injection

* available from one or more manufacturer, distributor, and/or repackager by generic (nonproprietary) name

† Use is not currently included in the labeling approved by the US Food and Drug Administration.

Meloxicam

28:08.04.04 • REVERSIBLE COX-1/COX-2 INHIBITORS

■ Meloxicam is a nonsteroidal anti-inflammatory agent (NSAIA) exhibiting analgesic, antipyretic, and anti-inflammatory actions that has been referred to as a "preferential" rather than "selective" COX-2 inhibitor.

USES

Meloxicam is used orally for anti-inflammatory and analgesic effects in the symptomatic treatment of osteoarthritis or rheumatoid arthritis in adults and for the management of the signs and symptoms of pauciarticular or polyarticular course juvenile rheumatoid arthritis. Meloxicam also is used parenterally for the relief of moderate to severe pain.

The potential benefits and risks of meloxicam therapy as well as alternative therapies should be considered prior to initiating meloxicam therapy. The lowest possible effective dosage and shortest duration of therapy consistent with treatment goals of the patient should be employed.

● Osteoarthritis

Meloxicam is used orally in the symptomatic treatment of osteoarthritis in adults. Efficacy for the management of the signs and symptoms of osteoarthritis (e.g., pain, stiffness, quality of life) of the knee or hip has been established in controlled studies of 4 weeks' to 6 months' duration in adults. Efficacy of 7.5 or 15 mg once daily (as tablets) was comparable to that of piroxicam 20 mg daily or 100 mg daily of conventional or extended-release diclofenac. Efficacy of meloxicam 5 or 10 mg once daily (as capsules) for the management of pain associated with osteoarthritis of the knee or hip was established in a 12-week placebo-controlled study. Both the 5- and 10-mg daily dosages of meloxicam were superior to placebo for relieving osteoarthritis pain; the proportion of meloxicam-treated patients achieving various percentage reductions in pain intensity from baseline to week 12 was similar for the 5- and 10-mg daily dosages. Meloxicam has not been compared with celecoxib in patients with osteoarthritis. For additional information on the management of osteoarthritis, see Uses: Osteoarthritis, in Celecoxib 28:08.04.08.

● Rheumatoid Arthritis in Adults

Meloxicam is used orally for the management of the signs and symptoms of rheumatoid arthritis in adults. In the management of rheumatoid arthritis in adults, NSAIAs may be useful for initial symptomatic treatment; however, NSAIAs do not alter the course of the disease or prevent joint destruction.

Efficacy of meloxicam for the management of rheumatoid arthritis was established in a placebo-controlled, double-blind study of 12 weeks' duration; the primary measure of clinical response in this study was the American College of Rheumatology criteria for a 20% improvement (ACR 20 response) in measures of disease activity. An ACR 20 response is achieved if the patient experiences a 20% improvement in the number of tender and swollen joints and a 20% or greater improvement in at least 3 of the following criteria: patient pain assessment, patient global assessment, physician global assessment, patient self-assessed disability, or laboratory measures of disease activity (i.e., erythrocyte sedimentation rate [ESR] or C-reactive protein [CRP] level). In this study, meloxicam 7.5 or 15 mg daily was substantially more effective than placebo as evaluated by ACR 20 response; the 22.5-mg daily dosage provided no additional benefit compared with 15 mg daily.

For additional information on the management of rheumatoid arthritis, see Uses: Rheumatoid Arthritis in Adults, in Celecoxib 28:08.04.08.

● Juvenile Arthritis

Meloxicam is used orally for the management of the signs and symptoms of pauciarticular or polyarticular course juvenile rheumatoid arthritis. Efficacy of meloxicam was established in 2 double-blind, active-controlled studies of 12 weeks' duration in pediatric patients 2–16 years of age; response rates were determined according to the American College of Rheumatology pediatric 30% improvement criteria (ACR pediatric 30; a composite of parent and investigator assessments, number of active joints, number of joints with limited range of motion, disability index, and ESR). Results of these studies indicate that meloxicam is as effective as naproxen in the treatment of juvenile rheumatoid arthritis. In one study, response rates (ACR pediatric 30 criteria) of 77, 76, or 74% were achieved at 12 months in children receiving meloxicam 0.125 mg/kg daily, meloxicam 0.25 mg/kg daily, or naproxen 10 mg/kg daily, respectively.

● Pain

Meloxicam is used parenterally for the relief of moderate to severe pain, either alone or in combination with non-NSAIA analgesics. Because of delayed onset of analgesia, use of parenteral meloxicam alone is not recommended when rapid onset of analgesia is required.

Efficacy and safety of IV meloxicam (30 mg once daily for 2 days starting on the day after surgery, with an optional third dose just prior to discharge) were evaluated in 2 randomized, double-blind, placebo-controlled trials (NCT02675907, NCT02678286) in adults with moderate to severe postoperative pain following bunionectomy or abdominoplasty. Mean baseline pain intensity, as measured on an 11-point numeric scale (with higher scores indicating more intense pain), was 6.8–7.3. A difference in the summed pain intensity difference (i.e., the difference between current pain and pain at baseline, multiplied by the interval between ratings and adjusted to account for any rescue analgesics) between the meloxicam and placebo groups was observed in both studies over the first 48 hours of treatment and in one of the studies (abdominoplasty study) over the first 24 hours. A generally consistent separation in pain scores between patients receiving meloxicam and those receiving placebo was observed in both studies from time of onset of pain relief through most of the dosing interval, with narrowing of the difference in pain scores between the meloxicam and placebo groups observed at the end of the first 24-hour dosing interval. In the bunionectomy study, 49–50% of patients receiving either meloxicam or placebo received rescue analgesic within 2 hours of receiving the initial study dose, while in the abdominoplasty study, 78% of patients receiving either meloxicam or placebo received rescue analgesic within 3 hours of receiving the initial study dose. The median time to first use of rescue analgesic (2 hours in patients who underwent bunionectomy, 1 hour in those who underwent abdominoplasty) occurred before the median time to meaningful pain relief in both studies (2 hours in the bunionectomy study, 3 hours in the abdominoplasty study).

● Other Uses

Meloxicam also has been used in the management of ankylosing spondylitis†.

DOSAGE AND ADMINISTRATION

● General

The potential benefits and risks of meloxicam therapy as well as alternative therapies should be considered prior to initiating meloxicam therapy.

● Administration

Meloxicam is administered orally for the management of rheumatoid arthritis, osteoarthritis, and juvenile rheumatoid arthritis and by IV injection for analgesia.

Meloxicam is administered orally once daily without regard to meals.

Meloxicam injection is for IV use only. The drug should be administered by direct ("bolus") IV injection over 15 seconds. To reduce the risk of renal toxicity, patients must be well hydrated prior to administration. The injection should be visually inspected for particulate matter and discoloration prior to administration, and should be discarded if either is present.

● Dosage

The lowest possible effective dosage and shortest duration of therapy consistent with treatment goals of the patient should be employed. Dosage of meloxicam must be carefully adjusted according to individual requirements and response, using the lowest possible effective dosage.

Osteoarthritis, Rheumatoid Arthritis, and Juvenile Arthritis

Meloxicam capsules are not bioequivalent to other oral formulations of the drug and therefore should not be interchanged at similar dosages for other oral meloxicam preparations. (See Description.)

The initial and maintenance dosage of meloxicam for the management of osteoarthritis or rheumatoid arthritis in adults is 7.5 mg once daily (as tablets). Titration to a maximum dosage of 15 mg once daily may provide additional benefit. Higher dosages (e.g., 22.5 mg daily or greater) were associated with increased adverse GI effects, and the manufacturer recommends that the dosage of meloxicam not exceed 15 mg daily.

Alternatively, for the management of osteoarthritis pain in adults, meloxicam may be initiated at a dosage of 5 mg once daily (as capsules). Dosage may be increased to 10 mg once daily in patients who require additional analgesia. The maximum recommended dosage is 10 mg once daily.

For the symptomatic management of juvenile rheumatoid arthritis, the recommended dosage of meloxicam is 0.125 mg/kg (maximum 7.5 mg) once daily; however, an oral suspension of the drug is no longer commercially available in the US, and meloxicam tablets should be used only in pediatric patients who weigh 60 kg or more. In pediatric patients weighing 60 kg or more, the recommended dosage of meloxicam for the treatment of juvenile rheumatoid arthritis is 7.5 mg once daily (as tablets). Higher dosages evaluated in clinical studies were not associated with additional benefit.

Pain

For relief of moderate to severe pain in adults, the recommended IV dosage of meloxicam is 30 mg once daily. Analgesic response should be monitored. Because the median time to meaningful pain relief was 2–3 hours after IV meloxicam administration in clinical trials, patients receiving IV meloxicam may require a non-NSAIA analgesic with a rapid onset of effect (e.g., upon emergence from anesthesia, upon resolution of local or regional anesthetic blocks). In addition, some patients may not experience adequate analgesia for the entire 24-hour dosing interval and may require supplemental use of a short-acting, non-NSAIA, immediate-release analgesic. (See Pain under Uses.)

● Special Populations

Renal Impairment

No dosage adjustment of oral meloxicam is necessary in patients with mild to moderate renal impairment. Use in patients with severe renal impairment is *not* recommended. If meloxicam is used in patients undergoing hemodialysis, the maximum recommended dosage is 5 mg once daily (as capsules) or 7.5 mg once daily (as tablets); additional doses are not required following dialysis. (See Renal Impairment under Cautions.)

Use of IV meloxicam is not recommended in patients with moderate to severe renal impairment and is contraindicated in patients with moderate to severe renal impairment who are at risk for renal failure because of hypovolemia. (See Renal Impairment under Cautions.)

Hepatic Impairment

No dosage adjustment of oral meloxicam is necessary in patients with mild to moderate hepatic impairment. Patients with severe hepatic impairment have not been adequately studied. (See Hepatic Impairment under Cautions.)

IV meloxicam has not been studied in patients with hepatic impairment.

Geriatric Patients

If anticipated benefits of meloxicam outweigh the potential risks, the manufacturers of oral meloxicam state that the drug should be initiated in geriatric patients at the low end of the dosage range. (See Geriatric Use under Cautions.)

CYP2C9 Poor or Intermediate Metabolizers

The manufacturer of IV meloxicam states that dosage reduction should be considered in patients who are known or suspected cytochrome P-450 isoenzyme 2C9 (CYP2C9) poor metabolizers.

Clinical Pharmacogenetics Implementation Consortium (CPIC) guidelines state that use of meloxicam should be avoided in patients who are CYP2C9 poor metabolizers. In patients who are CYP2C9 intermediate metabolizers with a diplotype functional activity score (AS) of 1, meloxicam should be initiated at a dosage that is 50% of the lowest recommended initial dosage and cautiously titrated to a clinically effective dosage, up to a dosage that is 50% of the maximum recommended dosage. Dosage should not be increased until steady-state concentrations are attained (at least 7 days following the initial dose). Patients

who are poor metabolizers should receive an alternative agent that is not metabolized by CYP2C9 or is not substantially affected by CYP2C9 genetic variants in vivo; alternatively, an NSAIA that is metabolized by CYP2C9 but has a shorter half-life could be considered. These alternatives also may be considered for intermediate metabolizers with an AS of 1. Intermediate metabolizers with an AS of 1.5 may receive dosages recommended for normal metabolizers. (See Pharmacogenomic Considerations under Cautions.)

CAUTIONS

● Contraindications

Meloxicam is contraindicated in patients with known hypersensitivity (e.g., anaphylaxis, serious dermatologic reactions) to meloxicam or any ingredient in the formulation; those with a history of asthma, urticaria, or other allergic-type reaction precipitated by aspirin or other nonsteroidal anti-inflammatory agents (NSAIAs); and in the setting of coronary artery bypass graft (CABG) surgery. In addition, parenteral meloxicam is contraindicated in patients with moderate to severe renal impairment who are at risk for renal failure because of hypovolemia.

● Warnings/Precautions

Warnings

Cardiovascular Thrombotic Effects

NSAIAs, including selective cyclooxygenase-2 (COX-2) inhibitors and prototypical NSAIAs, increase the risk of serious adverse cardiovascular thrombotic events, including myocardial infarction and stroke (which can be fatal), in patients with or without cardiovascular disease or risk factors for cardiovascular disease.

Findings of an FDA review of published observational studies of NSAIAs, a meta-analysis of published and unpublished data from randomized controlled trials of these drugs, and other published information indicate that NSAIAs may increase the risk of serious adverse cardiovascular thrombotic events by 10–50% or more, depending on the drugs and dosages studied. Available data suggest that the increase in risk may occur early (within the first weeks) following initiation of therapy and may increase with higher dosages and longer durations of use. Although the relative increase in cardiovascular risk appears to be similar in patients with or without known underlying cardiovascular disease or risk factors for cardiovascular disease, the absolute incidence of serious NSAIA-associated cardiovascular thrombotic events is higher in those with cardiovascular disease or risk factors for cardiovascular disease because of their elevated baseline risk.

Results from observational studies utilizing Danish national registry data indicated that patients receiving NSAIAs following a myocardial infarction were at increased risk of reinfarction, cardiovascular-related death, and all-cause mortality beginning in the first week of treatment. Patients who received NSAIAs following myocardial infarction had a higher 1-year mortality rate compared with those who did not receive NSAIAs (20 versus 12 deaths per 100 person-years). Although the absolute mortality rate declined somewhat after the first year following the myocardial infarction, the increased relative risk of death in patients who received NSAIAs persisted over at least the next 4 years of follow-up. Some clinicians suggest that it may be prudent to avoid use of NSAIAs whenever possible in patients with cardiovascular disease. Meloxicam should be avoided in patients with recent myocardial infarction unless the benefits of therapy are expected to outweigh the risk of recurrent cardiovascular thrombotic events; if meloxicam is used in such patients, the patient should be monitored for cardiac ischemia.

In 2 large controlled clinical trials of a selective COX-2 inhibitor for the management of pain in the first 10–14 days following CABG surgery, the incidence of myocardial infarction and stroke was increased. Therefore, NSAIAs are contraindicated in the setting of CABG surgery.

Findings from some systematic reviews of controlled observational studies and meta-analyses of data from randomized studies of NSAIAs suggest that naproxen may be associated with a lower risk of cardiovascular thrombotic events compared with other NSAIAs. However, limitations of these observational studies and the indirect comparisons used to assess cardiovascular risk of the prototypical NSAIAs (e.g., variability in patients' risk factors, comorbid conditions, concomitant drug therapy, drug interactions, dosage, and duration of therapy) affect the validity of the comparisons; in addition, these studies were not designed to demonstrate superior safety of one NSAIA compared with another.

Therefore, FDA states that definitive conclusions regarding relative risks of NSA-IAs are not possible at this time. (See Cautions: Cardiovascular Effects, in Celecoxib 28:08.04.08.)

To minimize the potential risk of adverse cardiovascular events, NSAIAs should be used at the lowest effective dosage and for the shortest possible duration of therapy. Patients receiving NSAIAs (including those without previous symptoms of cardiovascular disease) should be monitored for the possible development of cardiovascular events throughout therapy.

There is no consistent evidence that concomitant use of low-dose aspirin mitigates the increased risk of serious cardiovascular events associated with NSAIAs.

GI Effects

Serious, sometimes fatal, adverse GI effects (e.g., bleeding, ulceration, perforation of the esophagus, stomach, or small or large intestine) can occur with or without warning symptoms in patients receiving NSAIAs. The risk for GI bleeding is increased more than tenfold in patients with a history of peptic ulcer disease and/or GI bleeding who are receiving NSAIAs compared with patients without these risk factors. Other risk factors for GI bleeding include concomitant use of oral corticosteroids, antiplatelet agents (e.g., aspirin), anticoagulants, or selective serotonin-reuptake inhibitors (SSRIs); longer duration of NSAIA therapy (however, short-term therapy is not without risk); smoking; alcohol use; older age; poor general health status; and advanced liver disease and/or coagulopathy. Most spontaneous reports of fatal adverse GI effects involve geriatric or debilitated patients. The frequency of NSAIA-associated upper GI ulcers, gross bleeding, or perforation is approximately 1% in patients receiving NSAIAs for 3–6 months and 2–4% at one year. In some clinical studies, meloxicam was associated with a lower incidence of adverse GI effects compared with other NSAIAs (e.g., diclofenac, naproxen, piroxicam).

To minimize the risk of adverse GI effects, NSAIAs should be used at the lowest effective dosage for the shortest duration necessary. Use of more than one NSAIA at a time should be avoided. (See Nonsteroidal Anti-inflammatory Agents under Interactions.) Use of NSAIAs should be avoided in patients at higher risk for GI toxicity unless expected benefits outweigh the increased risk of bleeding; alternate therapies other than an NSAIA should be considered in high-risk patients and those with active GI bleeding. Patients receiving NSAIAs should be monitored for GI ulceration and bleeding; even closer monitoring for GI bleeding is recommended in those receiving concomitant low-dose aspirin for cardiac prophylaxis. If a serious adverse GI event is suspected, evaluation of the patient should be initiated promptly and meloxicam should be discontinued until serious adverse GI events have been ruled out.

Other Warnings and Precautions

Hepatic Effects

Borderline elevations of one or more liver function tests may occur in up to 15% of patients treated with NSAIAs, including meloxicam; meaningful (3 times the upper limit of normal) elevations of serum ALT or AST concentration have been reported in approximately 1% of patients receiving other NSAIAs. Severe, sometimes fatal, reactions (e.g., fulminant hepatitis, liver necrosis, hepatic failure) have been reported rarely in patients receiving NSAIAs. If clinical signs and symptoms of liver disease or systemic manifestations (e.g., eosinophilia, rash) occur, meloxicam should be discontinued immediately and the patient should be evaluated.

Hypertension

Use of NSAIAs, including meloxicam, can result in the onset of hypertension or worsening of preexisting hypertension; either of these occurrences may contribute to the increased incidence of cardiovascular events. Patients receiving NSA-IAs may have an impaired response to diuretics (i.e., thiazide or loop diuretics), angiotensin-converting enzyme (ACE) inhibitors, angiotensin II receptor antagonists, or β-adrenergic blocking agents. Blood pressure should be monitored closely during initiation of meloxicam therapy and throughout therapy.

Heart Failure and Edema

Data from observational studies indicate that use of NSAIAs in patients with heart failure is associated with increased morbidity and mortality. Results from a retrospective study utilizing Danish national registry data indicated that use of selective COX-2 inhibitors or prototypical NSAIAs in patients with chronic heart failure was associated with a dose-dependent increase in the risk of death and an increased risk of hospitalization for myocardial infarction or heart failure. In addition, findings from a meta-analysis of published and unpublished data from randomized controlled trials of NSAIAs indicated that use of selective COX-2 inhibitors or prototypical NSAIAs was associated with an approximate twofold increase in the risk of hospitalization for heart failure. Fluid retention and edema also have been observed in some patients receiving NSAIAs. Use of NSAIAs may diminish the cardiovascular effects of certain drugs used to treat these conditions (e.g., diuretics, ACE inhibitors, angiotensin II receptor antagonists). (See Drug Interactions.)

The manufacturer states that meloxicam should be avoided in patients with severe heart failure unless the benefits of therapy are expected to outweigh the risk of worsening heart failure; if meloxicam is used in such patients, the patient should be monitored for worsening heart failure. Some experts state that use of NSAIAs should be avoided whenever possible in patients with reduced left ventricular ejection fraction and current or prior symptoms of heart failure.

Renal Effects

Renal papillary necrosis, renal insufficiency, acute renal failure, and other renal injury may occur with long-term administration of NSAIAs. Overt renal decompensation may occur in patients dependent on renal prostaglandins for maintenance of renal perfusion. Patients at particular risk include those with heart failure, hepatic or renal dysfunction, dehydration, or hypovolemia; those receiving a diuretic, ACE inhibitor, or angiotensin II antagonist; and geriatric patients. Recovery of renal function to pretreatment levels usually occurs following discontinuance of NSAIA therapy.

Fluid depletion should be corrected prior to initiating meloxicam, and renal function should be monitored during therapy in patients with renal or hepatic impairment, heart failure, dehydration, or hypovolemia.

Hyperkalemia

Hyperkalemia has been reported in patients receiving NSAIAs, even in some patients without renal impairment; in such patients, the effect has been attributed to a hyporenin-hypoaldosterone state.

Sensitivity Reactions

Sensitivity reactions, including anaphylactic reactions, are possible in patients with or without prior exposure to meloxicam. Immediate medical intervention and drug discontinuance are required if anaphylaxis occurs. Cross-sensitivity may exist with other NSAIAs. Meloxicam should be avoided in patients with aspirin triad (aspirin sensitivity, asthma, nasal polyps); patients with asthma but without known aspirin sensitivity should be monitored for changes in manifestations of asthma. (See Cautions: Sensitivity Reactions, in the Salicylates General Statement 28:08.04.24.)

Multi-organ hypersensitivity (also known as drug reaction with eosinophilia and systemic symptoms [DRESS]), a potentially fatal or life-threatening syndrome, has been reported in patients receiving NSAIAs. The clinical presentation is variable, but typically includes eosinophilia, fever, rash, lymphadenopathy, and/or facial swelling, possibly associated with other organ system involvement such as hepatitis, nephritis, hematologic abnormalities, myocarditis, or myositis. Symptoms may resemble those of an acute viral infection. Early manifestations of hypersensitivity, such as fever or lymphadenopathy, may be present in the absence of rash. If such signs or symptoms develop, meloxicam should be discontinued and the patient evaluated immediately.

Dermatologic Reactions

Serious, potentially fatal, skin reactions (e.g., exfoliative dermatitis, Stevens-Johnson syndrome, toxic epidermal necrolysis) can occur in patients receiving meloxicam. These serious skin reactions may occur without warning. Meloxicam should be discontinued at the first appearance of rash or any other sign of hypersensitivity.

Hematologic Effects

Anemia has been reported, principally in patients receiving long-term (e.g., 6 months' duration) therapy with meloxicam. Anemia may be due to occult or gross blood loss, fluid retention, or an incompletely described effect on erythropoiesis. If signs and/or symptoms of anemia occur during therapy with meloxicam, hemoglobin concentration or hematocrit should be determined. Notable effects on platelets or bleeding times do not appear to occur.

NSAIAs may increase the risk of bleeding. Patients with certain coexisting conditions (e.g., coagulation disorders) or receiving concomitant therapy with anticoagulants, antiplatelet agents, or serotonin-reuptake inhibitors may be at increased risk; such patients should be monitored for bleeding.

Pharmacogenomic Considerations

In patients with the cytochrome P-450 isoenzyme 2C9 (CYP2C9) poor metabolizer phenotype, metabolism of meloxicam may be decreased substantially; the half-life of meloxicam is prolonged and higher plasma concentrations of the drug may increase the likelihood and/or severity of adverse effects. Metabolism of meloxicam may be moderately reduced in CYP2C9 intermediate metabolizers with a diplotype functional activity score (AS) of 1 and mildly reduced in those with an AS of 1.5. Higher plasma concentrations of the drug in intermediate metabolizers with an AS of 1 may increase the likelihood of adverse effects. The presence of other factors affecting clearance of the drug (e.g., hepatic impairment, advanced age) also may increase the risk of adverse effects in intermediate metabolizers. (See CYP2C9 Poor or Intermediate Metabolizers under Dosage and Administration and also see Description.) The Clinical Pharmacogenetics Implementation Consortium Guideline (CPIC) for CYP2C9 and Nonsteroidal Anti-Inflammatory Drugs should be consulted for additional information on interpretation of CYP2C9 genotype testing.

Other Precautions

NSAIAs may mask certain signs of infection; NSAIAs cannot be used as a substitute for corticosteroid therapy nor used to treat adrenal insufficiency.

Consideration should be given to obtaining a complete blood cell count and chemistry profile periodically during long-term use.

Specific Populations

Pregnancy

Use of NSAIAs during pregnancy at about 30 weeks of gestation or later can cause premature closure of the fetal ductus arteriosus, and use at about 20 weeks of gestation or later has been associated with fetal renal dysfunction resulting in oligohydramnios and, in some cases, neonatal renal impairment. Because of these risks, use of NSAIAs should be avoided in pregnant women at about 30 weeks of gestation or later; if NSAIA therapy is necessary between about 20 and 30 weeks of gestation, the lowest effective dosage and shortest possible duration of treatment should be used. Monitoring of amniotic fluid volume via ultrasound examination should be considered if the duration of NSAIA treatment exceeds 48 hours; if oligohydramnios occurs, the drug should be discontinued and follow-up instituted according to clinical practice. Pregnant women should be advised to avoid use of NSAIAs beginning at 20 weeks' gestation unless otherwise advised by a clinician; they should be informed that NSAIAs should be avoided beginning at 30 weeks' gestation because of the risk of premature closure of the fetal ductus arteriosus and that monitoring for oligohydramnios may be necessary if NSAIA therapy is required for longer than 48 hours' duration between about 20 and 30 weeks of gestation.

Known effects of NSAIAs on the human fetus during the third trimester of pregnancy include prenatal constriction of the ductus arteriosus, tricuspid incompetence, and pulmonary hypertension; nonclosure of the ductus arteriosus during the postnatal period (which may be resistant to medical management); and myocardial degenerative changes, platelet dysfunction with resultant bleeding, intracranial bleeding, renal dysfunction or renal failure, renal injury or dysgenesis potentially resulting in prolonged or permanent renal failure, oligohydramnios, GI bleeding or perforation, and increased risk of necrotizing enterocolitis.

Fetal renal dysfunction resulting in oligohydramnios and, in some cases, neonatal renal impairment has been observed, on average, following days to weeks of maternal NSAIA use, although oligohydramnios has been observed infrequently as early as 48 hours after initiation of NSAIA therapy. Oligohydramnios is often, but not always, reversible (generally within 3–6 days) following discontinuance of NSAIA therapy. Complications of prolonged oligohydramnios may include limb contracture and delayed lung maturation. A limited number of case reports have described maternal NSAIA use and neonatal renal dysfunction, in some cases irreversible, without oligohydramnios. Some cases of neonatal renal dysfunction have required treatment with invasive procedures such as exchange transfusion or dialysis. Deaths associated with neonatal renal failure have been reported. Methodologic limitations of these postmarketing studies and case reports include lack of a control group; limited information regarding dosage, duration, and timing of drug exposure; and concomitant use of other drugs. These limitations preclude establishing a reliable estimate of the risk of adverse fetal and neonatal outcomes with maternal NSAIA use. Available data on neonatal outcomes generally involved preterm infants, and the extent to which certain reported risks can be generalized to full-term infants is uncertain.

Animal data indicate that prostaglandins have an important role in endometrial vascular permeability, blastocyst implantation, and decidualization. In animal studies, inhibitors of prostaglandin synthesis, such as meloxicam, were associated with increased pre- and post-implantation losses. Prostaglandins also have an important role in fetal kidney development. In animal studies, inhibitors of prostaglandin synthesis impaired kidney development at clinically relevant doses.

Embryofetal deaths and an increased incidence of septal heart defects have been observed with meloxicam in animal reproduction studies.

The effects of meloxicam on labor and delivery are unknown. In studies in rats, drugs that inhibit prostaglandin synthesis, including NSAIAs, increased the incidence of dystocia, delayed parturition, and decreased pup survival.

Lactation

Meloxicam is distributed into milk in rats. It is not known whether meloxicam distributes into human milk, affects milk production, or affects nursing infants.

The developmental and health benefits of breast-feeding should be considered along with the mother's clinical need for meloxicam and any potential adverse effects on the breast-fed infant from the drug or from the underlying maternal condition.

Fertility

Use of NSAIAs, including meloxicam, may delay or prevent ovarian follicular rupture, which has been associated with reversible infertility in some women. Reversible delays in ovulation have been observed in limited studies in women receiving NSAIAs, and animal studies indicate that inhibitors of prostaglandin synthesis can disrupt prostaglandin-mediated follicular rupture required for ovulation. Therefore, withdrawal of NSAIAs should be considered in women who are experiencing difficulty conceiving or are undergoing evaluation of infertility.

Meloxicam also may impair fertility in men. Administration of meloxicam to male rats for 35 days at dosages of 0.3 times the maximum recommended human dosage resulted in decreased sperm count and motility and histopathologic evidence of testicular degeneration; it is not known whether these effects on fertility are reversible, and the clinical relevance of the findings is unknown.

Pediatric Use

Safety and efficacy of oral meloxicam have not been established in children younger than 2 years of age. Safety and efficacy of oral meloxicam have been established in pediatric patients 2–17 years of age with juvenile rheumatoid arthritis. The manufacturers state that safety and efficacy of meloxicam capsules and parenteral meloxicam have not been established in pediatric patients.

Geriatric Use

Geriatric patients receiving NSAIAs are at increased risk for serious adverse cardiovascular, GI, and renal effects. Although results from clinical studies of meloxicam revealed no overall differences in efficacy or safety of the drug between geriatric patients and younger individuals, most of the spontaneous reports of fatal adverse GI effects with NSAIAs have been in geriatric or debilitated individuals. If anticipated benefits of meloxicam outweigh the potential risks, the drug should be initiated at the low end of the dosing range and the patient should be monitored for adverse effects.

Hepatic Impairment

Oral meloxicam has not been adequately studied in patients with severe hepatic impairment. Because meloxicam is extensively metabolized in the liver and may cause hepatotoxicity, the drug should be used with caution in patients with hepatic impairment. If anticipated benefits of meloxicam outweigh the potential risks in patients with severe hepatic impairment, the patient should be monitored for signs of worsening liver function. Plasma concentrations of orally administered meloxicam are not substantially altered in patients with mild to moderate hepatic impairment, and the manufacturers of oral meloxicam state that dosage adjustment is not required in these patients.

IV meloxicam has not been studied in patients with hepatic impairment.

Renal Impairment

The renal effects of meloxicam may hasten the progression of renal dysfunction in patients with preexisting renal disease. Because some metabolites of the drug are excreted by the kidneys, patients with preexisting renal disease should be monitored for signs of worsening renal function.

In patients with mild or moderate renal impairment, total plasma concentrations of meloxicam decrease and total clearance increases with the degree of renal impairment, while exposure to the free (unbound) drug is similar across all patient groups. The higher meloxicam clearance in patients with renal impairment may be due to an increased fraction of unbound meloxicam being available for hepatic metabolism and subsequent excretion. Dosage adjustment of oral meloxicam is not necessary in patients with mild to moderate renal impairment.

Oral meloxicam has not been adequately studied in patients with severe renal impairment and use in such patients is not recommended. If meloxicam must be used in patients with advanced renal disease, renal function should be closely monitored.

Meloxicam is not removed by dialysis. Following single-dose administration, peak plasma concentrations of unbound meloxicam were higher in patients with renal failure requiring chronic hemodialysis (free fraction 1%) than in healthy individuals (free fraction 0.3%). (See Renal Impairment under Dosage and Administration.)

Pharmacokinetics of IV meloxicam in geriatric patients with mild renal impairment are similar to those in young healthy individuals. IV meloxicam has not been studied in patients with moderate or severe renal impairment, and use in such patients is not recommended. IV meloxicam is contraindicated in patients with moderate to severe renal impairment who are at risk for renal failure because of hypovolemia.

Common Adverse Effects

Adverse effects occurring in 2% or more of adults receiving oral meloxicam include dyspepsia, headache, nausea, diarrhea, upper respiratory tract infection, abdominal pain or discomfort, dizziness, edema, flatulence, influenza-like illness, musculoskeletal and connective tissue signs and symptoms (back pain, muscle spasms, musculoskeletal pain), and rash. Adverse effects occurring in 2% or more of patients receiving IV meloxicam, with or without rescue opiate analgesics, for postoperative pain and more frequently than with placebo include constipation, increased γ-glutamyltransferase (GGT, γ-glutamyltranspeptidase, GGTP) concentrations, and anemia.

The most common adverse effects reported in pediatric patients receiving oral meloxicam include abdominal pain, vomiting, diarrhea, headache, and pyrexia.

DRUG INTERACTIONS

Drugs Affecting Hepatic Microsomal Enzymes

Meloxicam is extensively metabolized by cytochrome P-450 (CYP) isoenzyme 2C9, with minor contribution by CYP3A4. Concomitant use of CYP2C9 inhibitors (e.g., amiodarone, fluconazole) may result in increased plasma concentrations of meloxicam. Reduction of meloxicam dosage should be considered, and the patient should be monitored for adverse effects.

Antacids

The manufacturer states that meloxicam tablets can be administered without regard to antacid administration since studies indicate that pharmacokinetic interactions are unlikely.

Anticoagulants

Anticoagulants, such as warfarin, and nonsteroidal anti-inflammatory agents (NSAIAs) have synergistic effects on bleeding. Concomitant use of meloxicam and anticoagulants is associated with a higher risk of serious bleeding compared with use of either agent alone. In healthy individuals receiving warfarin (international normalized ratio [INR] 1.2–1.8), meloxicam did not alter warfarin pharmacokinetics or average prothrombin time; however, INR increased from 1.5 to 2.1 in one individual. Caution is advised if meloxicam is used concomitantly with warfarin. Patients receiving such concomitant therapy should be monitored appropriately for signs of bleeding.

Because reduced CYP2C9 function is associated with an increased risk of major bleeding or supratherapeutic INRs in patients receiving concomitant therapy with warfarin (a CYP2C9 substrate) and NSAIAs, some experts state that concomitant use of warfarin and NSAIAs should be avoided in patients who are CYP2C9 intermediate or poor metabolizers.

Antihypertensive Agents

Concomitant use of NSAIAs with angiotensin-converting enzyme (ACE) inhibitors, angiotensin II receptor antagonists, or β-adrenergic blocking agents may reduce the blood pressure response to the antihypertensive agent. Therefore, blood pressure should be monitored to ensure that target blood pressure is achieved.

Concomitant use of meloxicam with ACE inhibitors or angiotensin II receptor antagonists in geriatric patients or patients with volume depletion or renal impairment may result in reversible deterioration of renal function, including possible acute renal failure; such patients should be monitored for signs of worsening renal function. Patients receiving concomitant therapy with meloxicam and ACE inhibitors or angiotensin II receptor antagonists should be adequately hydrated, and renal function should be assessed when concomitant therapy is initiated and periodically thereafter.

Bile Acid Sequestrants

When meloxicam was administered following 4 days of pretreatment with cholestyramine, meloxicam clearance was increased by 50%, half-life was decreased from 19.2 hours to 12.5 hours, and area under the concentration-time curve (AUC) was decreased by 35%. These findings suggest a recirculation pathway for meloxicam in the GI tract. The clinical importance of this interaction has not been established.

Cimetidine

Pharmacokinetic interactions between cimetidine and meloxicam are unlikely.

Cyclosporine

Concomitant use of meloxicam and cyclosporine may increase cyclosporine-associated nephrotoxicity. Patients should be monitored for signs of worsening renal function.

Digoxin

Pharmacokinetic interactions between digoxin and meloxicam are unlikely.

Diuretics

NSAIAs reduce the natriuretic effect of loop diuretics (e.g., furosemide) and thiazide diuretics in some patients. This effect has been attributed to NSAIA inhibition of renal prostaglandin synthesis. Although studies with meloxicam have not demonstrated a reduction in the natriuretic effect of furosemide or an effect of meloxicam on the pharmacokinetics or pharmacodynamics of furosemide, patients receiving concomitant therapy with meloxicam and diuretics should be monitored for signs of worsening renal function and for adequacy of diuretic and antihypertensive effects.

Lithium

NSAIAs can decrease renal clearance of lithium by approximately 20% and increase mean trough lithium concentrations by about 15%. This effect has been attributed to NSAIA inhibition of renal prostaglandin synthesis. In healthy individuals, concomitant administration of meloxicam (15 mg daily) with lithium carbonate (804–1072 mg twice daily) increased lithium exposure by about 21% compared with administration of lithium alone. Patients receiving lithium and meloxicam concomitantly should be monitored closely for signs of lithium toxicity.

● Methotrexate

Concomitant use of NSAIAs and methotrexate may increase the risk for methotrexate toxicity (e.g., neutropenia, thrombocytopenia, renal dysfunction). (See Drug Interactions: Nonsteroidal Anti-inflammatory Agents, in Methotrexate 10:00.) Although no pharmacokinetic interaction was observed in a study of 13 adults with arthritis receiving concomitant methotrexate (weekly) and meloxicam, patients receiving the drugs concomitantly should be monitored for methotrexate toxicity.

● Nonsteroidal Anti-inflammatory Agents

In controlled clinical trials, concomitant use of NSAIAs and analgesic dosages of aspirin did not produce any greater therapeutic effect than use of NSAIAs alone. However, concomitant use of aspirin and an NSAIA increases the risk for serious adverse GI events. Because of the potential for increased adverse effects, concomitant use of meloxicam with other NSAIAs or with low or analgesic dosages of aspirin generally is not recommended.

Patients receiving meloxicam should be advised not to take low-dose aspirin without consulting their clinician. Meloxicam is not a substitute for low-dose aspirin for cardioprophylaxis, and patients receiving antiplatelet agents such as aspirin concomitantly with meloxicam should be monitored closely for bleeding. There is no consistent evidence that use of low-dose aspirin mitigates the increased risk of serious cardiovascular events associated with NSAIAs.

Concomitant administration of aspirin (1 g 3 times daily) and meloxicam in healthy individuals increased the AUC and peak concentration of meloxicam by 10 and 24%, respectively; the clinical importance of this interaction is not known. When NSAIAs were administered with aspirin, protein binding of the NSAIA was reduced but clearance of the free (unbound) NSAIA was not altered.

● Pemetrexed

Concomitant use of meloxicam and pemetrexed may increase the risk of pemetrexed-associated myelosuppression, renal toxicity, and GI toxicity. Administration of NSAIAs with short elimination half-lives (e.g., diclofenac, indomethacin) should be avoided beginning 2 days before and continuing through 2 days after pemetrexed administration. In the absence of data regarding potential interactions between pemetrexed and NSAIAs with longer half-lives (e.g., meloxicam, nabumetone), administration of NSAIAs with longer half-lives should be interrupted beginning at least 5 days before and continuing through 2 days after pemetrexed administration. Patients with renal impairment with a creatinine clearance of 45–79 mL/minute should be monitored for myelosuppression, renal toxicity, and GI toxicity if they receive concomitant meloxicam and pemetrexed therapy. Concomitant use of meloxicam and pemetrexed is not recommended in patients with creatinine clearance less than 45 mL/minute.

● Serotonin-reuptake Inhibitors

Serotonin release by platelets plays an important role in hemostasis. Results of case-control and epidemiologic cohort studies indicate that concomitant use of NSAIAs and drugs that interfere with serotonin reuptake may potentiate the risk of bleeding beyond that associated with an NSAIA alone. Patients receiving concomitant therapy with meloxicam and selective serotonin-reuptake inhibitors (SSRIs) or selective serotonin- and norepinephrine-reuptake inhibitors (SNRIs) should be monitored for signs of bleeding.

DESCRIPTION

Meloxicam, an oxicam derivative that is structurally related to piroxicam, is a nonsteroidal anti-inflammatory agent (NSAIA) exhibiting analgesic, antipyretic, and anti-inflammatory actions. In vitro and in vivo studies indicate that meloxicam inhibits the cyclooxygenase-2 (COX-2) isoform of prostaglandin endoperoxide synthase (prostaglandin G/H synthase [PGHS]) to a greater extent than the COX-1 isoform. However, meloxicam's COX-2 selectivity is dose dependent and is diminished at higher dosages. Therefore meloxicam sometimes has been referred to as a "preferential" rather than "selective" COX-2 inhibitor. For additional information on COX-1 and COX-2, see Pharmacology: Mechanism of Action, in Celecoxib 28:08.04.08.

Meloxicam 10-mg capsules and 15-mg tablets are not bioequivalent. Following administration under fasting conditions, the 33% lower dose of meloxicam in the 10-mg capsules resulted in 33% lower overall systemic exposure to the drug compared with the 15-mg tablets; peak plasma concentrations were comparable with the 10-mg capsules and the 15-mg tablets, and the median time to peak plasma concentration was 2 hours for meloxicam 5- or 10-mg capsules but 4 hours for the 15-mg tablets.

At clinically relevant concentrations, meloxicam is extensively (approximately 99.4%) bound to plasma proteins, mainly to albumin. Protein binding decreases to approximately 99% in patients with renal disease. Following a single oral dose of meloxicam, concentrations of the drug in synovial fluid are 40–50% of plasma concentrations, but the free fraction is 2.5 times higher in synovial fluid than in plasma because of the lower albumin content of synovial fluid.

Meloxicam is extensively metabolized to inactive metabolites in the liver, principally via the cytochrome P-450 (CYP) 2C9 isoenzyme, with minor contribution by CYP3A4. The drug and its metabolites are excreted in urine and feces, and meloxicam undergoes substantial biliary secretion and enterohepatic recirculation. Only trace amounts of an administered dose of meloxicam are excreted unchanged in urine or feces. The elimination half-life of meloxicam reportedly ranges from approximately 15–24 hours. Limited data indicate that meloxicam exposure is increased substantially in individuals with reduced CYP2C9 activity (e.g., CYP2C9*2 and CYP2C9*3 polymorphisms), particularly in poor metabolizers (e.g., individuals with the *3/*3 diplotype), compared with normal metabolizers.

ADVICE TO PATIENTS

Importance of reading the medication guide for NSAIAs that is provided to the patient each time the drug is dispensed.

Risk of serious cardiovascular toxicity (e.g., myocardial infarction, stroke). Importance of seeking immediate medical attention if signs and symptoms of serious cardiovascular toxicity (e.g., chest pain, dyspnea, weakness, slurring of speech) occur.

Risk of GI ulceration or bleeding; importance of reporting any signs or symptoms of GI ulceration or bleeding (e.g., epigastric pain, dyspepsia, melena, hematemesis). Inform patients receiving concomitant low-dose aspirin of the increased risk of GI bleeding.

Risk of hepatotoxicity; advise patients to discontinue taking meloxicam and immediately contact their clinician if signs or symptoms of hepatotoxicity (e.g., nausea, fatigue, lethargy, pruritus, jaundice, right upper quadrant tenderness, flu-like symptoms) occur.

Risk of serious skin reactions, drug reaction with eosinophilia and systemic symptoms (DRESS), and anaphylactic and other sensitivity reactions. Advise patients to discontinue taking meloxicam immediately if they develop any type of rash or fever and to promptly contact their clinician. Importance of seeking immediate medical attention if an anaphylactic reaction occurs.

Risk of heart failure or edema; importance of reporting dyspnea, unexplained weight gain, or edema.

Importance of informing clinicians of existing or contemplated concomitant therapy, including prescription and OTC drugs. Advise patients that concomitant use of other NSAIAs with meloxicam provides little or no increase in efficacy but increases risk of GI toxicity, and is not recommended. Advise patients not to use concomitant low-dose aspirin without consulting their clinician. Alert patients to the presence of NSAIAs in many OTC drugs.

Importance of women informing clinicians if they are or plan to become pregnant or plan to breast-feed. Importance of avoiding use of NSAIAs beginning at 20 weeks' gestation unless otherwise advised by a clinician and of avoiding use beginning at 30 weeks' gestation because of risk of premature closure of the fetal ductus arteriosus; advise pregnant women that monitoring for oligohydramnios may be necessary if NSAIA therapy is required for longer than 48 hours' duration between about 20 and 30 weeks of gestation. Advise women who are trying to conceive that NSAIAs may be associated with a reversible delay in ovulation.

Importance of informing patients of other important precautionary information. (See Cautions.)

PREPARATIONS

Excipients in commercially available drug preparations may have clinically important effects in some individuals; consult specific product labeling for details.

Meloxicam

Oral

Capsules	5 mg*	Meloxicam Capsules
	10 mg*	Meloxicam Capsules

Tablets	7.5 mg*	Meloxicam Tablets
		Mobic®, Boehringer Ingelheim
	15 mg*	Meloxicam Tablets
		Mobic®, Boehringer Ingelheim

Parenteral

Injection, for IV use	30 mg/mL	Anjeso®, Baudax Bio

* available from one or more manufacturer, distributor, and/or repackager by generic (nonproprietary) name

† Use is not currently included in the labeling approved by the US Food and Drug Administration.

Naproxen, Naproxen Sodium

28:08.04.04 • REVERSIBLE COX-1/COX-2 INHIBITORS

■ Naproxen and naproxen sodium are prototypical anti-inflammatory agents (NSAIAs) that also exhibit analgesic and antipyretic activity.

USES

Naproxen and naproxen sodium are used to relieve mild to moderately severe pain. Conventional (immediate-release) and delayed-release (enteric-coated) tablets and suspension formulations of naproxen or naproxen sodium are used for anti-inflammatory and analgesic effects in the symptomatic treatment of rheumatoid arthritis, osteoarthritis, polyarticular juvenile idiopathic arthritis, and ankylosing spondylitis. Conventional (immediate-release) tablets and suspension formulations of naproxen or naproxen sodium also are used for the symptomatic treatment of tendinitis, bursitis, acute gout, pain, and primary dysmenorrhea. Suspension formulations of naproxen are preferred for the management of juvenile arthritis since this formulation provides maximum dosage flexibility. Because of the delayed-release properties of enteric-coated naproxen tablets, this formulation is not recommended for the management of acute pain. Extended-release naproxen sodium tablets are used for the symptomatic treatment of rheumatoid arthritis, osteoarthritis, ankylosing spondylitis, tendinitis, bursitis, acute gout, mild to moderately severe pain, and primary dysmenorrhea. (Naproxen 250 mg is approximately equivalent to naproxen sodium 275 mg.) Naproxen sodium also may be used for *self-medication* for anti-inflammatory and analgesic effects to provide temporary relief of *minor* aches and pains, including those associated with arthritis, and of dysmenorrhea and for its antipyretic effect to reduce fever.

The potential benefits and risks of naproxen therapy as well as alternative therapies should be considered prior to initiating naproxen therapy. The lowest possible effective dosage and shortest duration of therapy consistent with treatment goals of the patient should be employed.

● Inflammatory Diseases

Naproxen and naproxen sodium are used for anti-inflammatory and analgesic effects in the symptomatic treatment of rheumatoid arthritis, osteoarthritis, polyarticular juvenile idiopathic arthritis, and ankylosing spondylitis. Naproxen also is used in fixed combination with esomeprazole magnesium for the symptomatic treatment of rheumatoid arthritis, osteoarthritis, and ankylosing spondylitis in adults and for the symptomatic treatment of juvenile idiopathic arthritis in adolescents 12 years of age and older weighing 38 kg or more who are at risk of developing gastric ulcers associated with NSAIA therapy. For information on the combined use of naproxen and esomeprazole, see Uses: Prevention of Nonsteroidal Anti-inflammatory Agent-induced Ulcers, in Esomeprazole 56:28.36.

Rheumatoid Arthritis, Juvenile Arthritis, and Osteoarthritis

When used in the treatment of rheumatoid arthritis or juvenile idiopathic arthritis, naproxen has relieved pain and stiffness, reduced swelling, and improved mobility and grip strength. In the treatment of osteoarthritis, naproxen has relieved pain and stiffness and improved knee joint function. Naproxen appears to be only palliative in these conditions and has not been shown to permanently arrest or reverse the underlying disease process. Naproxen sodium also may be used for *self-medication* to provide temporary relief of minor aches and pains associated with arthritis.

Most clinical evaluations of naproxen in the management of rheumatoid arthritis or osteoarthritis have shown that the anti-inflammatory and analgesic effects of usual dosages of naproxen are greater than those of placebo and about equal to those of usual dosages of salicylates, indomethacin, fenoprofen, or ibuprofen. The results of a study in patients with osteoarthritis suggested that naproxen (500 mg twice daily) was less effective than tolmetin (800 mg twice daily) in some measures of pain relief, although improvements in functional ability did not differ. In controlled studies in patients with juvenile idiopathic arthritis, the anti-inflammatory and analgesic effects of usual dosages of naproxen were comparable to those of usual dosages of aspirin, indomethacin, or piroxicam. Patient response to oral NSAIAs is variable; patients who do not respond to or cannot tolerate one NSAIA might be successfully treated with a different agent. However, NSAIAs are generally contraindicated in patients in whom sensitivity reactions (e.g., urticaria, bronchospasm, severe rhinitis) are precipitated by aspirin or other NSAIAs. (See Contraindications under Cautions.)

In the management of rheumatoid arthritis in adults, NSAIAs may be useful for initial symptomatic treatment; however, NSAIAs do not alter the course of the disease or prevent joint destruction. Disease-modifying antirheumatic drugs (DMARDs) (e.g., abatacept, hydroxychloroquine, leflunomide, methotrexate, rituximab, sulfasalazine, tocilizumab, tofacitinib, tumor necrosis factor [TNF; TNF-α] blocking agents) have the potential to reduce or prevent joint damage, preserve joint integrity and function, and reduce total health care costs, and all patients with rheumatoid arthritis are candidates for DMARD therapy. DMARDs should be initiated early in the disease course and should not be delayed beyond 3 months in patients with active disease (i.e., ongoing joint pain, substantial morning stiffness, fatigue, active synovitis, persistent elevation of erythrocyte sedimentation rate [ESR] or C-reactive protein [CRP], radiographic evidence of joint damage) despite an adequate regimen of NSAIAs. NSAIA therapy may be continued in conjunction with DMARD therapy or, depending on patient response, may be discontinued. For further information on the treatment of rheumatoid arthritis, see Uses: Rheumatoid Arthritis in Methotrexate 10:00.

Use of naproxen or its salt with aspirin is not recommended by the manufacturers. There is inadequate proof that the combination is more efficacious than either drug alone, and the potential for adverse reactions may be increased. (See Nonsteroidal Anti-inflammatory Agents under Drug Interactions.)

Ankylosing Spondylitis

When used in patients with ankylosing spondylitis, naproxen has relieved night pain, morning stiffness, and pain at rest. In a limited number of controlled studies, the anti-inflammatory and analgesic effects of usual dosages of naproxen in the symptomatic treatment of ankylosing spondylitis were greater than those of placebo and comparable to those of usual dosages of aspirin or phenylbutazone (no longer commercially available in the US).

Other Inflammatory Conditions

Naproxen has been used effectively to relieve pain, fever, redness, swelling, and tenderness in patients with acute gouty arthritis.

When used in the treatment of acute painful shoulder, the anti-inflammatory and analgesic effects of naproxen sodium are greater than those of placebo and about equal to those of indomethacin. When used in the treatment of tendinitis and bursitis, the anti-inflammatory and analgesic effects of usual dosages of naproxen sodium are comparable to those of usual dosages of oxyphenbutazone (no longer commercially available in the US).

● Pain

Naproxen and its salt are used to relieve postoperative pain (including that associated with dental surgery), postpartum pain, primary dysmenorrhea, pain following insertion of an intrauterine contraceptive device, orthopedic pain, headache (including migraine), and visceral pain associated with cancer. Naproxen sodium also may be used in adults and pediatric patients 12 years of age or older for *self-medication* to provide temporary relief of minor aches and pains associated with the common cold, headache, toothache, muscular aches, and backache.

There are few published studies comparing the effectiveness of naproxen and its salt with other analgesics in the relief of nonarthritic pain. In one study, a single 275-mg oral dose of naproxen sodium was as effective as a single 650-mg oral dose of aspirin in the relief of postpartum uterine pain. In another study, when used to relieve postoperative or orthopedic pain, 550 mg of oral naproxen sodium followed by 275 mg every 6 hours was at least as effective as 650 mg of acetaminophen orally every 6 hours or 50 mg of pentazocine orally every 6 hours; in this study, the onset of action appeared to be more rapid for naproxen sodium than for acetaminophen or pentazocine. In another study of patients with postoperative pain, the analgesic effects of 550 mg of oral naproxen sodium and 60 mg of oral codeine sulfate were additive (the combination was more effective than either drug alone).

Some experts state that an NSAIA (e.g., naproxen or its salt) is a reasonable first-line therapy for mild to moderate migraine attacks or for severe attacks that have responded in the past to similar NSAIAs or non-opiate analgesics. When used for prophylaxis† of migraine headache, naproxen and its salt appear to have a modest effect on headache frequency, intensity, and/or duration. For further information on management and classification of migraine headache and on efficacy of concomitant naproxen sodium and sumatriptan therapy, see Uses: Vascular Headaches, in Sumatriptan 28:32.28.

● Dysmenorrhea

When used to relieve dysmenorrhea, including that which develops after insertion of an intrauterine contraceptive device, an oral dosage of 500 mg of naproxen or 550 mg of naproxen sodium followed by 250 mg of naproxen or 275 mg of naproxen sodium every 6 hours, respectively, has been reported to be more effective than placebo or aspirin (650 mg 4 times daily). In a placebo-controlled study of women with primary menorrhagia† or menorrhagia associated with intrauterine contraceptive devices†, administration of naproxen (750 mg daily for the first 2 days of menstrual bleeding followed by 500 mg daily thereafter for up to 7 days) resulted in a reduction of blood loss. In one controlled study in patients with postpartum pain, a single oral dose of 550 mg of naproxen sodium appeared to provide greater pain relief after 4 and 5 hours than 500 mg of naproxen; however, there was no difference in onset of analgesia. Naproxen sodium also may be used for *self-medication* to provide temporary relief of manifestations of dysmenorrhea (e.g., menstrual cramps).

● Fever

Naproxen sodium is used in adults and pediatric patients 12 years of age and older for *self-medication* as an antipyretic. One study indicates that a single oral dose of naproxen (2.5 or 7.5 mg/kg) was at least as effective as a single oral dose of aspirin (15 mg/kg) in the reduction of fever in children. The results of one study suggested that the combination of naproxen sodium and ampicillin was more effective than ampicillin alone in alleviating fever, dyspnea, and coughing associated with acute respiratory infections in children.

● Other Uses

Naproxen has been used in the symptomatic management of osteitis deformans† (Paget's disease of bone) and Bartter's syndrome†.

Results from a large, prospective, population-based cohort study in geriatric individuals indicate a lower prevalence of Alzheimer's disease† among patients who received an NSAIA for 2 years or longer. Similar findings have been reported from some other, but not all, observational studies.

DOSAGE AND ADMINISTRATION

● Administration

The potential benefits and risks of naproxen therapy as well as alternative therapies should be considered prior to initiating naproxen therapy.

Naproxen and naproxen sodium are administered orally. Enteric-coated tablets of naproxen should not be broken, crushed, or chewed, so that the delayed-release properties of this formulation are maintained. Adverse GI effects may be minimized by administering the drugs with meals or milk. When used for *self-medication*, the manufacturer recommends that each dose of naproxen sodium be taken with a full glass of water. Tablets containing naproxen sodium in fixed combination with sumatriptan succinate may be administered without regard to meals; the tablets should not be split, crushed, or chewed. Naproxen oral suspension should be shaken gently prior to use; to ensure accurate measurement of the dose, a calibrated measuring device should always be used to administer the oral suspension. Tablets containing delayed-release naproxen in fixed combination with immediate-release esomeprazole magnesium should be swallowed whole with liquid and administered at least 30 minutes before meals; the tablets should not be split, chewed, crushed, or dissolved.

Because of the delayed-release properties of enteric-coated formulations, enteric-coated preparations of naproxen are not recommended for the management of acute pain. Also, the manufacturer states that because naproxen sodium is absorbed more rapidly than naproxen, the sodium salt conventional tablet formulation is recommended for the management of acute painful conditions when prompt onset of pain relief is desired.

● Dosage

The lowest possible effective dosage and shortest duration of therapy consistent with treatment goals of the patient should be employed. Dosage of naproxen must be carefully adjusted according to individual requirements and response, using the lowest possible effective dosage.

Lower dosages of the drug should be considered in patients with renal or hepatic impairment or in geriatric patients. Use of naproxen or naproxen sodium in patients with moderate to severe renal impairment (creatinine clearance less than 30 mL/minute) is not recommended. Caution is advised when high dosages are required in patients with hepatic impairment. The commercially available preparation containing naproxen in fixed combination with esomeprazole magnesium is not recommended for patients with severe hepatic impairment because the appropriate esomeprazole dosage is not available as a fixed-ratio preparation for twice-daily dosing. In addition, the commercially available preparation containing naproxen sodium in fixed combination with sumatriptan succinate should not be used in patients with hepatic impairment since sumatriptan dosage cannot be appropriately adjusted.

Patients receiving naproxen for *self-medication* should be advised to use the lowest effective dosage and not to exceed the recommended dosage or duration of therapy. (See Precautions for Self-medication under Cautions.)

Each 220, 275, 412.5, 550, or 825 mg of naproxen sodium is approximately equivalent to 200, 250, 375, 500, or 750 mg of naproxen, respectively.

Different dose strengths and formulations are not necessarily bioequivalent, and this should be considered when changing from one strength to another or from one formulation to another.

Inflammatory Diseases
Rheumatoid Arthritis, Osteoarthritis, and Ankylosing Spondylitis

For the symptomatic treatment of osteoarthritis, rheumatoid arthritis, or ankylosing spondylitis, but excluding acute gouty arthritis), the usual adult dosage of naproxen is 250–500 mg (275–550 mg of naproxen sodium) twice daily in the morning and evening. Alternatively, 250 mg of naproxen (275 mg of naproxen sodium) may be given in the morning, and 500 mg (550 mg of the sodium salt) may be given in the evening. It is not necessary to administer either drug more often than twice daily, and morning and evening doses do not have to be equal in size.

The usual adult dosage of extended-release naproxen tablets is 750 mg or 1 g (825 mg or 1.1 g of naproxen sodium) administered once daily. Patients receiving other naproxen dosage forms twice daily may be switched to the extended-release naproxen sodium tablets by replacing their total daily dosage with an equal dosage of the extended-release formulation and then administered once daily.

Subsequent dosage of naproxen or naproxen sodium should be adjusted according to the patient's response and tolerance. In patients who tolerate lower dosages well, the dosage of naproxen may be increased to 1.5 g (1.65 g of naproxen sodium) daily for limited periods of time (up to 6 months) when a greater level of anti-inflammatory and/or analgesic activity is necessary; when a dosage of 1.5 g (1.65 g of the sodium salt) daily is administered, an adequate increase in clinical benefit should be evident to justify potential increased risks associated with this dosage. Symptomatic improvement usually begins within 1 week after beginning therapy; however, 2 weeks of treatment may be required to achieve a therapeutic benefit.

When naproxen is used in fixed combination with esomeprazole magnesium for the symptomatic relief of rheumatoid arthritis, osteoarthritis, or ankylosing spondylitis, the recommended adult dosage of naproxen is 375 or 500 mg twice daily.

For *self-medication* to provide temporary relief of pain associated with arthritis, the recommended adult dosage is 200 mg of naproxen (220 mg of naproxen sodium) every 8–12 hours; therapy may be initiated with a naproxen dosage of 400 mg (440 mg of the sodium salt) within the first hour and 200 mg (220 mg of the sodium salt) 12 hours later. Dosage for *self-medication* should not exceed 400 mg of naproxen (440 mg of naproxen sodium) in any 8- or 12-hour period and 600 mg of naproxen (660 mg of the sodium salt) in any 24-hour period unless otherwise directed by a clinician. Such *self-medication* should not exceed 10 days unless otherwise directed.

Juvenile Arthritis

For the symptomatic treatment of juvenile idiopathic arthritis, the recommended dosage of naproxen is approximately 10 mg/kg daily given in 2 divided doses. Because naproxen and naproxen sodium tablets are not well suited for providing the calculated pediatric dosage of the drug, naproxen oral suspension preferably should be used in this age group. Naproxen tablets should not be used in children weighing less than 50 kg. (See Pediatric Precautions under Cautions.)

When naproxen is used in fixed combination with esomeprazole magnesium for the symptomatic relief of juvenile idiopathic arthritis in adolescents 12 years of age and older weighing 50 kg or more, the recommended dosage of naproxen is 375 or 500 mg twice daily; in those weighing 38 to less than 50 kg, the recommended dosage of naproxen is 375 mg twice daily.

Other Inflammatory Conditions

For the symptomatic treatment of acute gouty arthritis, the usual adult dosage of naproxen is 750 mg (825 mg of naproxen sodium) initially followed by 250 mg (275 mg of naproxen sodium) every 8 hours; therapy is continued until the attack subsides. Alternatively, in the management of acute gout, an initial dosage of 1–1.5 g of naproxen (using extended-release naproxen sodium tablets) may be used (as a single dose) on the first day, followed by 1 g given once daily until the attack subsides. The manufacturer states that delayed-release (enteric-coated) naproxen tablets are not recommended for treatment of acute gout because of the delayed absorption of the drug from this preparation. Relief of pain and tenderness and decreases in heat and swelling have been reported to occur within 24–48 hours.

For the relief of tendinitis or bursitis, the usual initial adult dose of naproxen is 500 mg (550 mg of naproxen sodium), followed by 500 mg (550 mg of the sodium salt) every 12 hours or 250 mg (275 mg of the sodium salt) every 6–8 hours as necessary. Total initial daily dose should not exceed 1.25 g of naproxen (1.375 g of naproxen sodium). Alternatively, the usual adult oral dosage of naproxen from extended-release tablets is 1 g (1.1 g of naproxen sodium) administered once daily. If adequate response does not occur, dosage of the extended-release tablets may be increased to 1.5 g of naproxen daily; however, such dosages should be used for a limited period only. Thereafter, the total daily dose should not exceed 1 g of naproxen (1.1 g of naproxen sodium).

Pain and Dysmenorrhea

For relief of mild to moderate pain or dysmenorrhea, the usual initial adult dose of naproxen is 500 mg (550 mg of naproxen sodium), followed by 500 mg (550 mg of the sodium salt) every 12 hours or 250 mg (275 mg of the sodium salt) every 6–8 hours as necessary. Total initial daily dose should not exceed 1.25 g of naproxen (1.375 g of naproxen sodium). Alternatively, the usual adult oral dosage of naproxen from extended-release tablets is 1 g (1.1 g of naproxen sodium) administered once daily. If adequate response does not occur, dosage of the extended-release tablets may be increased to 1.5 g of naproxen daily; however, such dosages should be used for a limited period only. Thereafter, the total daily dose should not exceed 1 g of naproxen (1.1 g of naproxen sodium).

Alternatively, for self-medication of these conditions in adults and adolescents 12 years of age and older, a naproxen dosage of 200 mg (220 mg of naproxen sodium) every 8–12 hours can be used. Some patients may experience greater relief if therapy is initiated with a dose of 400 mg (440 mg of the sodium salt) within the first hour and then 200 mg (220 mg of the sodium salt) 12 hours later. Regardless of the regimen employed, dosage for self-medication should not exceed 400 mg of naproxen (440 mg of naproxen sodium) in any 8- or 12-hour period and 600 mg of naproxen (660 mg of the sodium salt) in any 24-hour period unless otherwise directed by a clinician. Self-medication of pain should not exceed 10 days unless otherwise directed.

When naproxen sodium is used in fixed combination with sumatriptan succinate for the acute management of migraine attacks in adults, the recommended dosage of naproxen sodium is 500 mg (given in fixed combination with sumatriptan 85 mg) as a single dose. Efficacy of more than 1 dose has not been established. If a second dose is administered, an interval of at least 2 hours should elapse between the first and second doses. No more than 2 doses (total sumatriptan dosage of 170 mg) should be administered in any 24-hour period. The safety of treating an average of more than 5 headaches per 30-day period has not been established.

Fever

For self-medication of fever in adults and adolescents 12 years of age and older, the usual dosage recommended for self-medication of pain can be used. (See Pain and Dysmenorrhea under Dosage and Administration.) Antipyretic therapy with naproxen sodium should not exceed 3 days for self-medication unless otherwise directed by a clinician.

CAUTIONS

● Cardiovascular Effects

Peripheral edema has occurred in patients receiving naproxen; congestive heart failure, palpitations, vasculitis, tachycardia, and dyspnea have occurred less frequently. Increases in blood pressure have been reported in patients receiving naproxen.

Nonsteroidal anti-inflammatory agents (NSAIAs), including selective cyclooxygenase-2 (COX-2) inhibitors and prototypical NSAIAs, increase the risk of serious adverse cardiovascular thrombotic events, including myocardial infarction and stroke (which can be fatal), in patients with or without cardiovascular disease or risk factors for cardiovascular disease. Use of NSAIAs also is associated with an increased risk of heart failure.

The association between cardiovascular complications and use of NSAIAs is an area of ongoing concern and study. Findings of an FDA review of published observational studies of NSAIAs, a meta-analysis of published and unpublished data from randomized controlled trials of these drugs, and other published information indicate that NSAIAs may increase the risk of serious adverse cardiovascular thrombotic events by 10–50% or more, depending on the drugs and dosages studied. Available data suggest that the increase in risk may occur early (within the first weeks) following initiation of therapy and may increase with higher dosages and longer durations of use. Although the relative increase in cardiovascular risk appears to be similar in patients with or without known underlying cardiovascular disease or risk factors for cardiovascular disease, the absolute incidence of serious NSAIA-associated cardiovascular thrombotic events is higher in those with cardiovascular disease or risk factors for cardiovascular disease because of their elevated baseline risk.

Results from observational studies utilizing Danish national registry data indicated that patients receiving NSAIAs following a myocardial infarction were at increased risk of reinfarction, cardiovascular-related death, and all-cause mortality beginning in the first week of treatment. Patients who received NSAIAs following myocardial infarction had a higher 1-year mortality rate compared with those who did not receive NSAIAs (20 versus 12 deaths per 100 person-years). Although the absolute mortality rate declined somewhat after the first year following the myocardial infarction, the increased relative risk of death in patients who received NSAIAs persisted over at least the next 4 years of follow-up.

In 2 large controlled clinical trials of a selective COX-2 inhibitor for the management of pain in the first 10–14 days following coronary artery bypass graft (CABG) surgery, the incidence of myocardial infarction and stroke was increased. Therefore, NSAIAs are contraindicated in the setting of CABG surgery.

Findings from some systematic reviews of controlled observational studies and meta-analyses of data from randomized studies of NSAIAs suggest that naproxen may be associated with a lower risk of cardiovascular thrombotic events compared with other NSAIAs. However, limitations of these observational studies and the indirect comparisons used to assess cardiovascular risk of the prototypical NSAIAs (e.g., variability in patients' risk factors, comorbid conditions, concomitant drug therapy, drug interactions, dosage, and duration of therapy) affect the validity of the comparisons; in addition, these studies were not designed to demonstrate superior safety of one NSAIA compared with another. Therefore, FDA states that definitive conclusions regarding relative risks of NSAIAs are not possible at this time. (See Cautions: Cardiovascular Effects, in Celecoxib 28:08.04.08.)

Data from observational studies also indicate that use of NSAIAs in patients with heart failure is associated with increased morbidity and mortality. Results from a retrospective study utilizing Danish national registry data indicated that use of selective COX-2 inhibitors or prototypical NSAIAs in patients with chronic heart failure was associated with a dose-dependent increase in the risk of death and an increased risk of hospitalization for myocardial infarction or heart failure. In addition, findings from a meta-analysis of published and unpublished data from randomized controlled trials of NSAIAs indicated that use of selective COX-2 inhibitors or prototypical NSAIAs was associated with an approximate twofold increase in the risk of hospitalization for heart failure. Fluid retention and edema also have been observed in some patients receiving NSAIAs.

There is no consistent evidence that use of low-dose aspirin mitigates the increased risk of serious cardiovascular events associated with NSAIAs.

● GI Effects

Adverse reactions to naproxen mainly involve the GI tract. Constipation, heartburn, abdominal pain, and nausea occur in about 3–9% of patients receiving the drug. Less frequently, dyspepsia, diarrhea, stomatitis, vomiting, anorexia, colitis, peptic ulcer, GI bleeding/perforation, hematemesis, and flatulence occur. In patients with rheumatoid arthritis, adverse GI effects appear to be more frequent and more severe at a naproxen dosage of 1.5 g (1.65 g of naproxen sodium) daily than at 750 mg (825 mg of naproxen sodium) daily. The frequency of adverse GI effects in children appears to be similar to that in adults. Adverse GI effects may be minimized by administering naproxen with meals or milk.

Naproxen may reactivate latent peptic ulcer and may cause peptic ulcers in patients with no previous history of ulcers. Hemorrhage and perforation of ulcers may occur, occasionally causing fatalities. Hematemesis, GI bleeding without obvious ulcer formation, and melena also have occurred. Prodromal symptoms do not always precede GI bleeding. Ulcerative stomatitis, esophagitis, and nonpeptic GI ulceration have been reported during postmarketing experience. Although a causal relationship has not been directly determined, one case-control analysis suggests that NSAIAs may contribute to the formation of esophageal stricture in patients with gastroesophageal reflux.

Clinical studies of conventional versus delayed-release (enteric-coated) naproxen tablets demonstrated similar prevalence of minor GI complaints; however, individual patients may prefer one formulation over the other. In a dosage of 500 mg daily, naproxen has been reported to produce fewer adverse GI effects than 3.6–4.8 g of aspirin daily. In one study, a single dose of 550 mg of naproxen sodium produced fewer adverse GI effects than a single dose of 650 mg of aspirin. It is not known whether naproxen causes less peptic ulceration than does aspirin. In one study, the amount of GI bleeding as determined by fecal blood loss and gastroscopic evaluation in healthy adults was reported to be less with 1 g of naproxen or 1.1 g of naproxen sodium daily than with 3.25 g of aspirin daily. In another study in patients with rheumatoid arthritis, fecal blood loss following 750 mg of naproxen daily was less than that following 3.6 g of aspirin daily and no different than that during the control period. The frequency of adverse GI effects in patients receiving 500 mg of naproxen or 550 mg of naproxen sodium daily is reportedly similar to that in patients receiving 1.2 g of ibuprofen daily and less than that in patients receiving 100 mg of indomethacin daily or 2.4 g of fenoprofen daily.

Serious, sometimes fatal, adverse GI effects (e.g., bleeding, ulceration, or perforation of the esophagus, stomach, or small or large intestine) can occur at any time in patients receiving NSAIA therapy, and such effects may *not* be preceded by warning signs or symptoms. Only 1 in 5 patients who develop a serious upper GI adverse event while receiving an NSAIA is symptomatic. Therefore, clinicians should remain alert to the possible development of serious GI effects (e.g., bleeding, ulceration) in any patient receiving NSAIA therapy, and such patients should be followed chronically for the development of manifestations of such effects and advised of the importance of this follow-up. Patients receiving concomitant low-dose aspirin therapy for cardiovascular prophylaxis should be monitored even more closely for evidence of GI bleeding. In addition, patients should be advised about the signs and symptoms of serious NSAIA-induced GI toxicity and what action to take if they occur. If signs and symptoms of a serious GI event develop, additional evaluation and treatment should be initiated promptly; the NSAIA should be discontinued until appropriate diagnostic studies have ruled out a serious GI event.

Results of studies to date are inconclusive concerning the relative risk of various prototypical NSAIAs in causing serious GI effects. In patients receiving NSAIAs and observed in clinical studies of several months' to 2 years' duration, upper GI ulcers, gross bleeding, or perforation appeared to occur in approximately 1% of patients treated for 3–6 months and in about 2–4% of those treated for 1 year. Longer duration of therapy with an NSAIA increases the likelihood of a serious GI event. However, short-term therapy is not without risk. High dosages of any

NSAIA probably are associated with increased risk of such effects, although controlled studies documenting this probable association are lacking for most NSAIAs. Therefore, whenever use of relatively high dosages (within the recommended dosage range) is considered, sufficient benefit to offset the potential increased risk of GI toxicity should be anticipated.

Studies have shown that patients with a history of peptic ulcer disease and/or GI bleeding who are receiving NSAIAs have a greater than tenfold increased risk of developing GI bleeding than patients without these risk factors. In addition to a history of ulcer disease, pharmacoepidemiologic studies have identified several comorbid conditions and concomitant therapies that may increase the risk for GI bleeding, including concomitant use of oral corticosteroids, anticoagulants, aspirin, or selective serotonin-reuptake inhibitors (SSRIs); longer duration of NSAIA therapy; smoking; alcohol use; older age; and poor general health status. Risk of GI bleeding also is increased in patients with advanced liver disease and/or coagulopathy. Patients with rheumatoid arthritis are more likely to experience serious GI complications from NSAIA therapy than are patients with osteoarthritis. In addition, geriatric or debilitated patients appear to tolerate GI ulceration and bleeding less well than other individuals, and most spontaneous reports of fatal GI effects have been in such patients.

For patients at high risk for complications from NSAIA-induced GI ulceration (e.g., bleeding, perforation), concomitant use of misoprostol can be considered for preventive therapy (See Misoprostol 56:28.28.) Alternatively, some clinicians suggest that a proton-pump inhibitor (e.g., esomeprazole, omeprazole) may be used concomitantly to decrease the incidence of serious GI toxicity associated with NSAIA therapy. (See Esomeprazole 56:28.36.) In one study, therapy with high dosages of famotidine (40 mg twice daily) was more effective than placebo in preventing peptic ulcers in NSAIA-treated patients; however, the effect of the drug was modest. In addition, efficacy of usual dosages of H_2-receptor antagonists for the prevention of NSAIA-induced gastric and duodenal ulcers has not been established. Therefore, most clinicians do not recommend use of H_2-receptor antagonists for the prevention of NSAIA-associated ulcers. Another approach in high-risk patients who would benefit from NSAIA therapy is use of an NSAIA that is a selective inhibitor of COX-2 (e.g., celecoxib), since these agents are associated with a lower incidence of serious GI bleeding than are prototypical NSAIAs. However, while celecoxib (200 mg twice daily) was comparably effective to diclofenac sodium (75 mg twice daily) plus omeprazole (20 mg daily) in preventing recurrent ulcer bleeding (recurrent ulcer bleeding probabilities of 4.9 versus 6.4%, respectively, during the 6-month study) in *H. pylori*-negative arthritis (principally osteoarthritis) patients with a recent history of ulcer bleeding, the protective efficacy was unexpectedly low for both regimens and it appeared that neither could completely protect patients at high risk. Additional study is necessary to elucidate optimal therapy for preventing GI complications associated with NSAIA therapy in high-risk patients.

● Nervous System Effects

Adverse nervous system effects of naproxen include headache, drowsiness, and dizziness, which occur in about 3–9% of patients. Vertigo, lightheadedness, inability to concentrate, mental depression, nervousness, irritability, fatigue, malaise, insomnia, sleep disorders, dream abnormalities, and aseptic meningitis may also occur. Although a causal relationship to naproxen has not been definitely established, reversible peripheral neuropathy, cognitive dysfunction, and seizures have occurred rarely in patients receiving the drug. The frequency of adverse nervous system effects in children appears to be similar to that in adults.

● Otic and Ocular Effects

Patients receiving naproxen have experienced tinnitus and, less frequently, other hearing or visual disturbances (e.g., hearing impairment). Corneal opacity, papillitis, papilledema, and retrobulbar optic neuritis have been reported during postmarketing experience.

● Hematologic Effects

Adverse hematologic effects of naproxen include thrombocytopenia, leukopenia, granulocytopenia, and eosinophilia. Although a causal relationship to naproxen has not been established, agranulocytosis, aplastic anemia, and hemolytic anemia have occurred in patients receiving the drug. Naproxen can inhibit platelet aggregation and may prolong bleeding time. The frequency of prolonged bleeding time may be greater in children than in adults. Anemia has occurred in patients receiving NSAIAs and may be due to occult or gross blood loss, fluid retention, or an incompletely described effect on erythropoiesis.

● Renal and Electrolyte Effects

Renal disease, glomerulonephritis, interstitial nephritis, nephrotic syndrome, renal failure, renal papillary necrosis, dysuria, and hyperkalemia have been reported in patients receiving naproxen. Some cases of hyperkalemia in patients receiving NSAIAs have involved individuals without renal impairment; in individuals with normal renal function, hyperkalemia has been attributed to a hyporenin-hypoaldosterone state. Abnormal laboratory findings include hematuria and asymptomatic increases in BUN and serum creatinine. In one patient who developed increased serum creatinine concentration and decreased creatinine clearance during naproxen therapy, these measurements returned to pretreatment values following discontinuance of the drug and remained within normal limits after sulindac therapy was started. Chronic high doses of naproxen have caused nephritis and cortical and papillary necrosis in animals.

● Hepatic Effects

Severe, sometimes fatal, hepatic reactions including fulminant hepatitis, liver necrosis, and hepatic failure have been reported rarely in patients receiving NSAIAs. Jaundice (including cholestatic jaundice which cleared promptly when naproxen was discontinued) and fatal hepatitis have been reported rarely in patients receiving naproxen. Abnormal liver function test results, including mild and generally transient increases in serum alkaline phosphatase, have occurred in some patients.

Borderline (less than 3 times the upper limit of normal) elevations of serum ALT or AST concentration may occur in up to 15% of patients treated with NSAIAs, including naproxen; meaningful (3 or more times the upper limit of normal) elevations of serum ALT or AST concentration have occurred in less than 1% of patients receiving NSAIAs in clinical studies. Naproxen should be discontinued immediately if signs or symptoms consistent with liver disease develop or if systemic manifestations (e.g., eosinophilia, rash) occur, and clinical evaluation of the patient should be performed. (See Hepatic Precautions under Cautions.)

● Dermatologic and Sensitivity Reactions

Pruritus, skin eruptions or rashes, and ecchymoses occur frequently during naproxen administration. Sweating, photosensitive dermatitis, photosensitivity reactions resembling porphyria cutanea tarda and epidermolysis bullosa, and purpura have also occurred occasionally. The frequency of rash may be greater in children than in adults. Toxic epidermal necrolysis, erythema multiforme, Stevens-Johnson syndrome, urticaria, alopecia, erythema nodosum, fixed drug eruption, lichen planus, and pustular reaction have been reported during postmarketing experience. Anaphylactic reactions have been reported in patients with or without known hypersensitivity to the drug, as well as in patients with aspirin-sensitivity asthma.

● Other Adverse Effects

Thirst, myalgia, muscle weakness and cramps, pyrexia, sore throat, eosinophilic pneumonitis or colitis, anaphylactoid reactions, pancreatitis, and menstrual disturbances also have been reported during naproxen therapy. Hypoglycemia, hyperglycemia, angioedema, systemic lupus erythematosus, vasculitis, asthma, pulmonary edema, and female infertility have been reported during postmarketing experience. In a patient receiving naproxen in combination with aspirin, infective symptoms associated with an empyema appeared to be suppressed.

● Precautions and Contraindications

With the exception of precautions related to the sodium content of naproxen sodium, the cautions associated with naproxen sodium use are the same as those for naproxen use. Each 220-, 275-, 412.5-, 550-, or 825-mg naproxen sodium tablet contains about 0.87, 1, 1.5, 2, or 3 mEq of sodium, respectively, and each mL of the commercially available naproxen suspension contains about 0.3 mEq of sodium; this should be considered in patients whose sodium intake must be restricted. Multiple naproxen-containing preparations (e.g., naproxen conventional and delayed-release [enteric-coated] tablets, naproxen suspension, naproxen sodium conventional and extended-release tablets) should not be used concomitantly, as all of these products circulate in the plasma as naproxen anion and may result in naproxen toxicity.

When naproxen or naproxen sodium is used in fixed combination with other drugs (e.g., esomeprazole magnesium, sumatriptan succinate), the usual cautions, precautions, and contraindications associated with the concomitant agent must be considered in addition to those associated with naproxen.

Patients should be advised that naproxen, like other NSAIAs, is not free of potential adverse effects, including some that can cause discomfort, and that more serious effects (e.g., myocardial infarction, stroke, GI bleeding), which may require hospitalization and may even be fatal, can occur.

Patients should be advised to read the medication guide for NSAIAs that is provided to the patient each time the drug is dispensed.

Cardiovascular Precautions

NSAIAs increase the risk of serious adverse cardiovascular thrombotic events. (See Cardiovascular Effects under Cautions.) To minimize the potential risk of adverse cardiovascular events, the lowest effective dosage and shortest possible duration of therapy should be employed. Some clinicians suggest that it may be prudent to avoid use of NSAIAs whenever possible in patients with cardiovascular disease. Patients receiving NSAIAs (including those without previous symptoms of cardiovascular disease) should be monitored for the possible development of cardiovascular events throughout therapy. Patients should be informed about the signs and symptoms of serious cardiovascular toxicity (chest pain, dyspnea, weakness, slurring of speech) and instructed to seek immediate medical attention if such toxicity occurs. Naproxen should be avoided in patients with recent myocardial infarction unless the benefits of therapy are expected to outweigh the risk of recurrent cardiovascular thrombotic events; if naproxen is used in such patients, the patient should be monitored for cardiac ischemia.

There is no consistent evidence that concomitant use of low-dose aspirin mitigates the increased risk of serious cardiovascular events associated with NSAIAs. Concomitant use of aspirin and an NSAIA increases the risk for serious GI events. (See Nonsteroidal Anti-inflammatory Agents under Drug Interactions.)

Use of NSAIAs can result in the onset of hypertension or worsening of preexisting hypertension; either of these occurrences may contribute to the increased incidence of cardiovascular events. Patients receiving NSAIAs may have an impaired response to diuretics (i.e., thiazide or loop diuretics), angiotensin-converting enzyme (ACE) inhibitors, angiotensin II receptor antagonists, or β-adrenergic blocking agents. Blood pressure should be monitored closely during initiation of NSAIA therapy and throughout therapy.

Because NSAIAs increase morbidity and mortality in patients with heart failure, the manufacturer states that naproxen should be avoided in patients with severe heart failure unless the benefits of therapy are expected to outweigh the risk of worsening heart failure; if naproxen is used in such patients, the patient should be monitored for worsening heart failure. Some experts state that use of NSAIAs should be avoided whenever possible in patients with reduced left ventricular ejection fraction and current or prior symptoms of heart failure. Patients receiving NSAIAs should be advised to inform their clinician if they experience symptoms of heart failure, including dyspnea, unexplained weight gain, and edema. Use of NSAIAs may diminish the cardiovascular effects of certain drugs used to treat heart failure and edema (e.g., diuretics, ACE inhibitors, angiotensin II receptor antagonists). (See Antihypertensive Agents and also Diuretics under Drug Interactions.)

GI Precautions

The risk of potentially serious adverse GI effects should be considered in patients receiving naproxen, particularly in patients receiving chronic therapy with the drug. Since peptic ulceration and/or GI bleeding have been reported in patients receiving the drug, patients should be advised to promptly report signs or symptoms of GI ulceration or bleeding to their clinician.

To minimize the potential risk of adverse GI effects, the lowest effective dosage and shortest possible duration of therapy should be employed, and use of more than one NSAIA at a time should be avoided. (See Nonsteroidal Anti-inflammatory Agents under Drug Interactions.) In addition, use of NSAIAs should be avoided in patients at higher risk (see GI Effects under Cautions) unless benefits of therapy are expected to outweigh the increased risk of bleeding; for patients who are at high risk, as well as for those with active GI bleeding, alternative therapy other than an NSAIA should be considered.

Hepatic Precautions

Elevations in serum ALT may be the most sensitive indicator of NSAIA-induced liver dysfunction. Patients who experience signs and/or symptoms suggestive of liver dysfunction or an abnormal liver function test result while receiving naproxen should be evaluated for evidence of the development of a severe hepatic reaction. Severe reactions, including jaundice and/or fatal hepatitis, have occurred during therapy with naproxen. Although such reactions are rare, naproxen should be discontinued immediately if clinical signs and symptoms consistent with liver disease develop or if systemic manifestations (e.g., eosinophilia, rash) occur. Patients receiving naproxen should be informed of the warning signs and symptoms of hepatotoxicity (e.g., nausea, anorexia, fatigue, lethargy, pruritus, jaundice, right upper quadrant tenderness, flu-like syndrome) and advised to discontinue naproxen therapy and seek immediate medical care if they experience such symptoms.

Lower dosages of naproxen should be considered in patients with hepatic impairment. Naproxen has not been evaluated in patients with hepatic impairment, and the manufacturer states that caution is advised when large dosages of the drug are required in patients with hepatic impairment; dosage adjustment may be necessary. Although total plasma concentrations of naproxen are decreased in patients with chronic alcoholic liver disease, concentrations of the unbound drug are increased.

Renal Precautions

Because renal prostaglandins may have a supportive role in maintaining renal perfusion in patients with prerenal conditions, administration of an NSAIA to such patients may cause a dose-dependent reduction in prostaglandin formation and thereby precipitate overt renal decompensation. Patients at greatest risk of this reaction include those with impaired renal function, heart failure, or hepatic dysfunction; those with extracellular fluid depletion (e.g., patients receiving diuretics); those taking an ACE inhibitor or angiotensin II receptor antagonist concomitantly; and geriatric patients. Patients should be advised to consult their clinician promptly if unexplained weight gain or edema occurs. Fluid depletion should be corrected prior to initiation of naproxen therapy, and renal function should be monitored during naproxen therapy in patients with renal or hepatic impairment, heart failure, dehydration, or hypovolemia. Recovery of renal function to pretreatment levels usually occurs following discontinuance of NSAIA therapy. Some clinicians recommend that renal function be monitored periodically in patients receiving long-term NSAIA therapy.

The renal effects of naproxen may hasten the progression of renal dysfunction in patients with preexisting renal disease. Patients with preexisting renal disease should be monitored for worsening renal function.

Lower dosages of naproxen should be considered in patients with renal impairment. Naproxen has not been evaluated in patients with renal impairment; however, naproxen and its metabolites and conjugates are excreted mainly by the kidneys, and the potential exists for naproxen metabolites to accumulate in patients with renal impairment. Elimination of naproxen is decreased in patients with severe renal impairment.

The manufacturers state that use of naproxen in patients with advanced renal disease should be avoided unless the benefits of therapy are expected to outweigh the risk of worsening renal function; use of the drug in those with moderate to severe renal impairment is not recommended. If naproxen is used in patients with advanced renal disease, close monitoring of renal function is recommended.

Precautions Related to Dermatologic or Hypersensitivity Reactions

Anaphylactic reactions have been reported in patients receiving naproxen. Patients receiving naproxen should be informed of the signs and symptoms of an anaphylactic reaction (e.g., difficulty breathing, swelling of the face or throat) and advised to seek immediate medical attention if an anaphylactic reaction develops.

Serious skin reactions (e.g., exfoliative dermatitis, Stevens-Johnson syndrome, toxic epidermal necrolysis) can occur in patients receiving NSAIAs. These serious skin reactions may occur without warning; patients should be advised to consult their clinician if skin rash and blisters, fever, or other signs of hypersensitivity reaction (e.g., pruritus) occur. NSAIAs should be discontinued at the first appearance of rash or any other sign of hypersensitivity.

Multi-organ hypersensitivity (also known as drug reaction with eosinophilia and systemic symptoms [DRESS]), a potentially fatal or life-threatening syndrome, has been reported in patients receiving NSAIAs. The clinical presentation is variable, but typically includes eosinophilia, fever, rash, lymphadenopathy, and/or facial swelling, possibly associated with other organ system involvement such as hepatitis, nephritis, hematologic abnormalities, myocarditis, or myositis. Symptoms may resemble those of an acute viral infection. Early manifestations of hypersensitivity, such as fever or lymphadenopathy, may be present in the absence of rash. If such signs or symptoms develop, naproxen should be discontinued and the patient evaluated immediately.

Hematologic Precautions

NSAIAs, including naproxen, may increase the risk of bleeding. Patients with certain coexisting conditions such as coagulation disorders and those receiving concomitant therapy with anticoagulants, antiplatelet agents, or serotonin-reuptake inhibitors may be at increased risk and should be monitored for signs of bleeding. (See Drug Interactions.)

Since naproxen can inhibit platelet aggregation, patients who may be adversely affected by a prolongation of bleeding time should be carefully observed during naproxen therapy.

If signs and/or symptoms of anemia occur during therapy with naproxen, hemoglobin concentration and hematocrit should be determined. In addition, hemoglobin concentration should be determined periodically during long-term naproxen therapy in individuals with an initial hemoglobin concentration of 10 g/dL or less.

Precautions for Self-medication

Patients receiving naproxen for self-medication should be advised to use the lowest effective dosage and not to exceed the recommended dosage or duration of therapy. Unless otherwise directed by a clinician, patients receiving naproxen for *self-medication* should be advised to discontinue the drug and consult a clinician if pain persists for more than 10 days or fever persists for longer than 3 days. Patients should not use naproxen for *self-medication* immediately before or after cardiac surgery or if they have experienced an allergic reaction to any analgesic or antipyretic.

Patients receiving naproxen for *self-medication* should be advised to consult a clinician before initiating naproxen if they have experienced adverse effects associated with any analgesic or antipyretic; if they have a GI disorder, coagulation disorder, hypertension, cardiac disease, asthma, hepatic cirrhosis, or renal disease; if they have had a stroke; if they have a history of bleeding events or GI disorders (e.g., heartburn, peptic ulcer); if they are receiving therapy with a diuretic, an anticoagulant, a corticosteroid, or any other NSAIA-containing preparation; if they consume 3 or more alcohol-containing drinks per day; or if they are 60 years of age or older. Patients receiving the drug for *self-medication* should consult a clinician or pharmacist before initiating naproxen if they are under a clinician's care for any continuing serious medical condition; are taking aspirin for reduction of cardiovascular risk, or are receiving any other drugs on a regular basis.

Patients should be advised to stop taking naproxen for *self-medication* and consult their clinician if symptoms of GI bleeding (e.g., faintness, vomiting blood, bloody or black stools, persistent stomach pain) develop; if cardiac symptoms or symptoms of stroke (e.g., chest pain, difficulty breathing, weakness in one part or side of the body, slurred speech, leg swelling) occur; if they have difficulty swallowing or feel like a "pill is stuck in their throat"; if any new symptoms occur during *self-medication* with the drug; or if redness or swelling is present in the painful area. Patients should be advised that the risk of GI bleeding is increased if they are 60 years of age or older, have a GI disorder (e.g., history of GI bleeding or peptic ulceration), are receiving an anticoagulant or corticosteroid, are receiving another NSAIA (including aspirin) concomitantly, generally consume 3 or more alcohol-containing drinks per day, or exceed the recommended dosage or duration of naproxen therapy. In addition, patients should be advised that NSAIAs (except aspirin) increase the risk of myocardial infarction, heart failure, and stroke and that the risk is increased if they exceed the recommended dosage or duration of naproxen therapy. Patients receiving low-dose aspirin should be advised that naproxen can interfere with the antiplatelet effect of aspirin.

Other Precautions

Patients receiving long-term NSAIA therapy should have a complete blood cell count and chemistry profile performed periodically.

Naproxen can interfere with the antiplatelet effect of low-dose aspirin. Patients receiving low-dose aspirin for its cardioprotective effects should be informed of this potential interaction. (See Nonsteroidal Anti-inflammatory Agents under Drug Interactions.)

Because NSAIAs have caused adverse ocular effects, patients who experience visual disturbances or changes during naproxen therapy should have an ophthalmologic examination.

The possibility that the antipyretic and anti-inflammatory effects of NSAIAs may mask the usual signs and symptoms of infection or other diseases should be considered.

Contraindications

Naproxen is contraindicated in patients with known hypersensitivity (e.g., anaphylaxis, serious dermatologic reactions) to the drug or any ingredient in the formulation. In addition, NSAIAs, including naproxen, generally are contraindicated in patients in whom asthma, urticaria, or other sensitivity reactions are precipitated by aspirin or other NSAIAs, since there is potential for cross-sensitivity between NSAIAs and aspirin, and severe, rarely fatal, anaphylactic reactions to NSAIAs have been reported in these patients. Although NSAIAs generally are contraindicated in these patients, the drugs have occasionally been used in NSAIA-sensitive patients who have undergone desensitization. Because patients with asthma may have aspirin-sensitivity asthma, patients with asthma but without known aspirin sensitivity who are receiving naproxen should be monitored for changes in manifestations of asthma. In patients with asthma, aspirin sensitivity is manifested principally as bronchospasm and usually is associated with nasal polyps; the association of aspirin sensitivity, asthma, and nasal polyps is known as the aspirin triad. Patients who are considering use of naproxen for *self-medication* should be advised that naproxen is contraindicated in patients who have experienced asthma, urticaria, or other sensitivity reaction to other analgesics or antipyretics. For a further discussion of cross-sensitivity of NSAIAs, see Cautions: Sensitivity Reactions, in the Salicylates General Statement 28:08.04.24.

NSAIAs are contraindicated in the setting of CABG surgery.

● *Pediatric Precautions*

Safety and efficacy of naproxen in children younger than 2 years of age have not been established. Pediatric dosage recommendations for juvenile idiopathic arthritis are based on well-controlled studies. There are no adequate efficacy or dose-response data for other pediatric conditions, but clinical experience in juvenile idiopathic arthritis and other use experience indicate that single doses of 2.5–5 mg/kg with a total daily dose not exceeding 15 mg/kg are safe in children older than 2 years of age. Naproxen sodium should not be used for *self-medication* in children younger than 12 years of age unless otherwise directed by a clinician.

Safety and efficacy of extended-release naproxen sodium tablets in children have not been established.

Overdosage and toxicity (including death) have been reported in children younger than 2 years of age receiving nonprescription (over-the-counter, OTC) preparations containing antihistamines, cough suppressants, expectorants, and nasal decongestants alone or in combination for relief of symptoms of upper respiratory tract infection. Such preparations also may contain analgesics and antipyretics (e.g., naproxen). There is limited evidence of efficacy for these preparations in this age group, and appropriate dosages (i.e., approved by FDA) have not been established. Therefore, FDA stated that nonprescription cough and cold preparations should not be used in children younger than 2 years of age; the agency continues to assess safety and efficacy of these preparations in older children. Meanwhile, because children 2–3 years of age also are at increased risk of overdosage and toxicity, some manufacturers of oral nonprescription cough and cold preparations recently have agreed to voluntarily revise the product labeling to state that such preparations should not be used in children younger than 4 years of age. FDA recommends that parents and caregivers adhere to the dosage instructions and warnings on the product labeling that accompanies the preparation if administering to children and consult with their clinician about any concerns. Clinicians should ask caregivers about use of nonprescription cough and cold preparations to avoid overdosage. For additional information on precautions associated with the use of cough and cold preparations in pediatric patients, see Cautions: Pediatric Precautions in Pseudoephedrine 12:12.12.

● *Geriatric Precautions*

Geriatric patients are at increased risk for NSAIA-associated serious adverse cardiovascular, GI, and renal effects. Geriatric individuals appear to tolerate GI ulceration and bleeding less well than other individuals, and many of the spontaneous reports of fatal adverse GI effects in patients receiving NSAIAs involve geriatric individuals. If the anticipated benefits of naproxen therapy outweigh the potential risks, naproxen should be initiated at the lower end of the dosing range and patients should be monitored for adverse effects.

Lower dosages of naproxen should be considered in geriatric patients. Although the total plasma concentrations of naproxen in geriatric patients are similar to those attained in younger adults, the unbound plasma fraction of the drug is increased in geriatric patients when compared with that in younger adults. The clinical relevance of this finding is unclear, although the increase in unbound naproxen concentrations could be associated with an increase in the frequency of adverse events at any given dosage in some geriatric patients. Naproxen should be used with caution in geriatric patients requiring high dosages; some adjustment of dosage may be needed.

In 2 double-blind clinical trials evaluating hepatic and renal tolerability of naproxen (375 or 750 mg twice daily for up to 6 months), 17% of patients were 65 years of age and older, while less than 2% were 75 years of age and older. Although transient abnormalities in hepatic and renal function test results were observed in some patients, no age-related differences in the frequency of such abnormalities were observed.

Naproxen and its metabolites are eliminated substantially by the kidneys, and individuals with renal impairment may be at increased risk of toxic reactions to the drug. Because geriatric patients frequently have decreased renal function, particular attention should be paid to naproxen dosage, and it may be useful to monitor renal function in these patients.

● *Mutagenicity and Carcinogenicity*

A 2-year study in rats was performed to evaluate the carcinogenic potential of naproxen at 8, 16, or 24 mg/kg daily (50, 100, or 150 mg/m², respectively); the maximum dose used was 0.28 times the human systemic exposure at the recommended dose. There was no evidence of carcinogenicity.

● *Pregnancy, Fertility, and Lactation*

Pregnancy

Use of NSAIAs during pregnancy at about 30 weeks of gestation or later can cause premature closure of the fetal ductus arteriosus, and use at about 20 weeks of gestation or later has been associated with fetal renal dysfunction resulting in oligohydramnios and, in some cases, neonatal renal impairment. Because of these risks, use of NSAIAs should be avoided in pregnant women at about 30 weeks of gestation or later; if NSAIA therapy is necessary between about 20 and 30 weeks of gestation, the lowest effective dosage and shortest possible duration of treatment should be used. Monitoring of amniotic fluid volume via ultrasound examination should be considered if the duration of NSAIA treatment exceeds 48 hours; if oligohydramnios occurs, the drug should be discontinued and follow-up instituted according to clinical practice. Pregnant women should be advised to avoid use of NSAIAs beginning at 20 weeks' gestation unless otherwise advised by a clinician; they should be informed that NSAIAs should be avoided beginning at 30 weeks' gestation because of the risk of premature closure of the fetal ductus arteriosus and that monitoring for oligohydramnios may be necessary if NSAIA therapy is required for longer than 48 hours' duration between about 20 and 30 weeks of gestation.

Known effects of NSAIAs on the human fetus during the third trimester of pregnancy include prenatal constriction of the ductus arteriosus, tricuspid incompetence, and pulmonary hypertension; nonclosure of the ductus arteriosus during the postnatal period (which may be resistant to medical management); and myocardial degenerative changes, platelet dysfunction with resultant bleeding, intracranial bleeding, renal dysfunction or renal failure, renal injury or dysgenesis potentially resulting in prolonged or permanent renal failure, oligohydramnios, GI bleeding or perforation, and increased risk of necrotizing enterocolitis.

Fetal renal dysfunction resulting in oligohydramnios and, in some cases, neonatal renal impairment has been observed, on average, following days to weeks of maternal NSAIA use, although oligohydramnios has been observed infrequently as early as 48 hours after initiation of NSAIA therapy. Oligohydramnios is often, but not always, reversible (generally within 3–6 days) following discontinuance of NSAIA therapy. Complications of prolonged oligohydramnios may include limb contracture and delayed lung maturation. A limited number of case reports have described maternal NSAIA use and neonatal renal dysfunction, in some cases irreversible, without oligohydramnios. Some cases of neonatal renal dysfunction have required treatment with invasive procedures such as exchange transfusion or dialysis. Deaths associated with neonatal renal failure have been reported. Methodologic limitations of these postmarketing studies and case reports include lack of a control group; limited information regarding dosage, duration, and timing of drug exposure; and concomitant use of other drugs. These limitations preclude establishing a reliable estimate of the risk of adverse fetal and neonatal outcomes with maternal NSAIA use. Available data on neonatal outcomes generally involved preterm infants, and the extent to which certain reported risks can be generalized to full-term infants is uncertain.

Animal data indicate that prostaglandins have an important role in endometrial vascular permeability, blastocyst implantation, and decidualization. In animal studies, inhibitors of prostaglandin synthesis, such as naproxen, were associated with increased pre- and post-implantation losses. Prostaglandins also have an important role in fetal kidney development. In animal studies, inhibitors of prostaglandin synthesis impaired kidney development at clinically relevant doses.

Reproduction studies of naproxen in rats at 20 mg/kg daily (125 mg/m^2, 0.23 times the human systemic exposure), rabbits at 20 mg/kg daily (220 mg/m^2, 0.27 times the human systemic exposure), and mice at 170 mg/kg daily (510 mg/m^2, 0.28 times the human systemic exposure) have not revealed evidence of harm to the fetus. Severe hypoxemia due to persistent pulmonary hypertension has occurred in infants whose mothers received naproxen to delay parturition. Neonatal death also has been reported when the drug was used to prevent preterm labor; autopsy of a neonate showed brain hemorrhage, multiple gastric ulcers, extensive GI bleeding, and an adverse cardiovascular effect known to be associated with use of NSAIAs. In addition, severe hyponatremia, water retention, cerebral irritation, and paralytic ileus was reported in a neonate whose mother ingested 5 g of naproxen 8 hours before delivery; it has been suggested that naproxen adversely affected renal function. Renal dysfunction and abnormal prostaglandin E concentrations in premature infants also have been reported.

Effects of naproxen during labor or delivery have not been studied. In animal studies, NSAIAs, including naproxen, inhibited prostaglandin synthesis, delayed parturition, and increased the incidence of stillbirth.

Fertility

Use of NSAIAs may delay or prevent ovarian follicular rupture, which has been associated with reversible infertility in some women. Reversible delays in ovulation have been observed in limited studies in women receiving NSAIAs, and animal studies indicate that inhibitors of prostaglandin synthesis can disrupt prostaglandin-mediated follicular rupture required for ovulation. Therefore, withdrawal of NSAIAs should be considered in women who are experiencing difficulty conceiving or are undergoing evaluation of infertility.

Reproduction studies of naproxen in rats at 20 mg/kg daily (125 mg/m^2, 0.23 times the human systemic exposure), rabbits at 20 mg/kg daily (220 mg/m^2, 0.27 times the human systemic exposure), and mice at 170 mg/kg daily (510 mg/m^2, 0.28 times the human systemic exposure) have not revealed evidence of impaired fertility. Information on the effects of naproxen on fertility in humans is lacking. At least one human case was reported in which ejaculatory dysfunction occurred during naproxen therapy and was reversed upon discontinuing the drug; a definite causal relationship was not established.

Lactation

Naproxen is distributed into milk at concentrations of approximately 1% of peak plasma concentrations of the drug.

The developmental and health benefits of breast-feeding should be considered along with the mother's clinical need for naproxen and any potential adverse effects on the breast-fed infant from the drug or from the underlying maternal condition.

DRUG INTERACTIONS

● Protein-bound Drugs

Because naproxen is highly protein bound, it theoretically could be displaced from binding sites by, or it could displace from binding sites, other protein-bound drugs such as oral anticoagulants, hydantoins, other nonsteroidal anti-inflammatory agents (NSAIAs; including aspirin), sulfonamides, and sulfonylureas. Patients receiving naproxen with any of these drugs should be observed for adverse effects, and dosage should be adjusted as needed.

● Drugs Affecting Gastric pH

Concomitant administration of naproxen and aluminum hydroxide or magnesium oxide antacids may result in delayed absorption of naproxen. However, when delayed-release (enteric-coated) naproxen tablets were administered with antacid (buffering capacity of 54 mEq), peak plasma concentrations of naproxen were unchanged; the mean time to peak concentration was reduced, but not to a substantial extent (from 5.6 hours under fasted conditions to 5 hours with antacid). The manufacturers state that concomitant administration of naproxen and antacids is not recommended.

In a controlled study in healthy adults, concomitant oral administration of naproxen and cimetidine did not appear to alter the pharmacokinetics of either drug and did not affect the inhibition of gastric acid output by cimetidine.

● Anticoagulants and Thrombolytic Agents

The effects of warfarin and NSAIAs on GI bleeding are synergistic. Concomitant use of naproxen and warfarin is associated with a higher risk of GI bleeding compared with use of either agent alone.

Administration of naproxen with warfarin results in a slight increase in free warfarin in serum, but does not affect the hypoprothrombinemic effect of warfarin. Naproxen should be used with caution in patients receiving any anticoagulant or thrombolytic agent (e.g., streptokinase), and patients should be carefully monitored for signs of bleeding.

● Antidiabetic Agents

Results of a study in patients with diabetes mellitus showed no interference by naproxen on the effect of tolbutamide on plasma glucose concentrations.

● Antihypertensive Agents

Concomitant use of NSAIAs with angiotensin-converting enzyme (ACE) inhibitors, angiotensin II receptor antagonists, or β-adrenergic blocking agents may reduce the blood pressure response to the antihypertensive agent. Therefore, blood pressure should be monitored to ensure that target blood pressure is achieved.

Concomitant use of naproxen with ACE inhibitors or angiotensin II receptor antagonists in geriatric patients or patients with volume depletion or renal impairment may result in reversible deterioration of renal function, including possible acute renal failure; such patients should be monitored for signs of worsening renal function. Patients receiving concomitant therapy with naproxen and ACE inhibitors or angiotensin II receptor antagonists should be adequately hydrated, and renal function should be assessed when concomitant therapy is initiated and periodically thereafter.

● Cholestyramine

Concomitant administration of naproxen and cholestyramine may result in delayed absorption of naproxen. Concomitant administration of naproxen and cholestyramine is not recommended.

● Cyclosporine

Concomitant use of naproxen and cyclosporine may increase the nephrotoxic effects of cyclosporine. Patients should be monitored for signs of worsening renal function.

● Digoxin

Concomitant use of naproxen and digoxin has been reported to result in increased serum concentrations and prolonged half-life of digoxin. Serum digoxin concentrations should be monitored.

● *Diuretics*

NSAIAs can reduce the natriuretic effects of furosemide or thiazide diuretics, and concomitant use of diuretics and NSAIAs may increase the risk of NSAIA-associated nephrotoxicity in dehydrated patients. The reduction in natriuretic effect may be related to inhibition of renal prostaglandin synthesis. Patients receiving concomitant NSAIA and diuretic therapy should be monitored for worsening renal function and for adequacy of diuretic and antihypertensive effects.

● *Lithium*

Naproxen may increase serum lithium concentrations and reduce renal lithium clearance. Concomitant use of NSAIAs and lithium has increased trough lithium concentrations by 15% and decreased renal lithium clearance by approximately 20%. If naproxen and lithium are administered concurrently, the patient should be observed closely for signs of lithium toxicity, and serum lithium concentrations should be monitored carefully during the initial stages of combined therapy or subsequent dosage adjustment. In addition, appropriate adjustment of lithium dosage may be required when therapy with naproxen is discontinued.

● *Methotrexate*

Concomitant use of NSAIAs and methotrexate may increase the risk for methotrexate toxicity (e.g., neutropenia, thrombocytopenia, renal dysfunction). Severe, sometimes fatal, toxicity has occurred following administration of an NSAIA concomitantly with methotrexate (principally high-dose therapy) in patients with various malignant neoplasms or rheumatoid arthritis. The toxicity was associated with elevated and prolonged blood concentrations of methotrexate. The exact mechanism of the interaction remains to be established, but it has been suggested that NSAIAs may inhibit renal elimination of methotrexate, possibly by decreasing renal perfusion via inhibition of renal prostaglandin synthesis or by competing for renal elimination. Patients receiving concomitant naproxen and methotrexate therapy should be monitored for methotrexate toxicity. (See Drug Interactions: Nonsteroidal Anti-inflammatory Agents, in Methotrexate 10:00.)

● *Nonsteroidal Anti-inflammatory Agents*

In controlled clinical trials, concomitant use of NSAIAs and analgesic dosages of aspirin did not produce any greater therapeutic effect than use of NSAIAs alone. However, concomitant use of aspirin and an NSAIA increases the risk for bleeding and serious GI events. Because of the potential for increased adverse effects, concomitant use of naproxen with other NSAIAs or with analgesic dosages of aspirin generally is not recommended.

Administration of aspirin with NSAIAs may decrease protein binding of the NSAIA, but clearance of the free (unbound) NSAIA does not appear to be altered. The clinical importance of this pharmacokinetic interaction has not been established.

Some NSAIAs (e.g., ibuprofen, naproxen) can interfere with the antiplatelet effect of low-dose aspirin. Ibuprofen can interfere with the antiplatelet effect of low-dose aspirin (81 mg daily; immediate-release preparation) when the drugs are administered concomitantly. The interaction can be minimized by appropriate timing of ibuprofen administration relative to that of immediate-release, low-dose aspirin. (See Drug Interactions: Nonsteroidal Anti-inflammatory Agents, in Ibuprofen 28:08.04.92.) In one study, concomitant administration of naproxen (500 mg) and low-dose aspirin (100 mg) also interfered with the antiplatelet effect of aspirin. In another study, interference by naproxen sodium (220 mg once or twice daily) with the antiplatelet effect of low-dose, immediate-release aspirin was observed to be most marked during the washout period following discontinuance of naproxen. A similar interaction might be expected with higher (i.e., prescription-strength) dosages of naproxen and enteric-coated, low-dose aspirin, although the timing of peak interference may occur later because of the longer washout period. The observed interaction was greater when naproxen was administered 30 minutes prior to administration of immediate-release, low-dose aspirin and minimal when immediate-release, low-dose aspirin was administered 30 minutes prior to naproxen administration. Because there may be an increased risk of cardiovascular events following discontinuance of naproxen, use of an NSAIA that does not interfere with the antiplatelet effect of aspirin or use of an analgesic other than an NSAIA, when appropriate, should be considered for intermittent analgesic therapy in patients receiving low-dose aspirin.

Naproxen is not a substitute for low-dose aspirin therapy for prophylaxis of cardiovascular events, and patients receiving antiplatelet agents such as aspirin concomitantly with NSAIAs should be monitored closely for bleeding. There is no consistent evidence that use of low-dose aspirin mitigates the increased risk of serious cardiovascular events associated with NSAIAs.

● *Pemetrexed*

Concomitant use of naproxen and pemetrexed may increase the risk of pemetrexed-associated myelosuppression, renal toxicity, and GI toxicity. Administration of NSAIAs with short elimination half-lives (e.g., diclofenac, indomethacin) should be avoided beginning 2 days before and continuing through 2 days after pemetrexed administration. In the absence of data regarding potential interactions between pemetrexed and NSAIAs with longer half-lives (e.g., meloxicam, nabumetone), administration of NSAIAs with longer half-lives should be interrupted beginning at least 5 days before and continuing through 2 days after pemetrexed administration. Patients with renal impairment with a creatinine clearance of 45–79 mL/minute should be monitored for myelosuppression, renal toxicity, and GI toxicity if they receive concomitant naproxen and pemetrexed therapy.

● *Probenecid*

Administration of probenecid with naproxen substantially increases the plasma half-life of naproxen and plasma naproxen concentrations. In one study, the plasma half-life of naproxen increased to an average of 37 hours and plasma naproxen concentrations increased by an average of 50% when the drugs were administered concomitantly. It was suggested that probenecid interfered with the plasma clearance of naproxen by inhibiting the formation of glucuronide conjugates of naproxen, as well as inhibiting its renal clearance. Patients receiving concomitant therapy with probenecid and naproxen should be monitored, and dosage should be adjusted as needed.

● *Serotonin-reuptake Inhibitors*

Serotonin release by platelets plays an important role in hemostasis. Results of case-control and epidemiologic cohort studies indicate that concomitant use of NSAIAs and drugs that interfere with serotonin reuptake may potentiate the risk of bleeding beyond that associated with an NSAIA alone. Patients receiving concomitant therapy with naproxen and selective serotonin-reuptake inhibitors (SSRIs) or selective serotonin- and norepinephrine-reuptake inhibitors (SNRIs) should be monitored for signs of bleeding.

● *Sucralfate*

Concomitant administration of naproxen and sucralfate may result in delayed absorption of naproxen. Concomitant administration of sucralfate with naproxen is not recommended.

● *Other Drugs*

Naproxen should be used cautiously, if at all, with other drugs that might potentiate the adverse GI effects.

LABORATORY TEST INTERFERENCES

Naproxen or its metabolites may cause falsely elevated urinary 17-ketogenic steroid concentrations by interfering with the *m*-dinitrobenzene reagent used in the test. Although 17-hydroxycorticosteroid measurements (Porter-Silber method) are not significantly altered, withdrawal of naproxen for 72 hours before testing has been recommended.

Naproxen may also interfere with some urinary assays of 5-hydroxyindoleacetic acid (5-HIAA).

ACUTE TOXICITY

Limited information is available on the acute toxicity of naproxen or naproxen sodium.

Pathogenesis

The acute dose of naproxen or naproxen sodium associated with life-threatening toxicity in humans is not known. The oral LD_{50} of naproxen is 4110, 1234, more than 1000, and 543 mg/kg in hamsters, mice, dogs, and rats, respectively.

Manifestations

The most frequent manifestations following acute nonsteroidal anti-inflammatory agent (NSAIA) overdosage include lethargy, drowsiness, nausea, vomiting, and epigastric pain. GI bleeding has occurred, and hypertension, acute renal failure, respiratory depression, and coma have occurred rarely. A few patients have experienced seizures, but a causal relationship to the drug is unclear. Because naproxen sodium may be absorbed rapidly, high and early blood concentrations of the drug should be anticipated following naproxen sodium overdosage.

There have been several cases of naproxen overdosage in children which have resulted in acute toxicity. Acute renal failure and hyperkalemia were reported in a 2-year-old child with juvenile arthritis who received a naproxen sodium dosage of 20 mg/kg daily for 1 month. Death occurred in an 8-month-old child following administration of 110–440 mg of naproxen sodium for 5 days for fever and upper respiratory infection. A 2-year-old child recovered after ingesting up to 2 g of naproxen, hydrogen peroxide, and eucalyptus oil and who developed drowsiness, ataxia, and prolonged bleeding time. Another 2-year-old child developed dyspepsia after ingesting 625 mg of naproxen. In addition, seizures were reported in a 5-year-old child who ingested an unknown amount of naproxen sodium.

Most cases of naproxen overdosage have been reported in adults. Adverse GI effects (e.g., heartburn, vomiting) and seizures usually occur in these patients; drowsiness and prolongation of clotting time also may occur. The incidence of adverse effects in adults may differ from those in children since rash and prolonged bleeding time appear to occur more frequently in children while other reactions occur more frequently in adults; the incidence of adverse GI and CNS effects are similar.

One patient who ingested 25 g of naproxen experienced mild nausea and indigestion. Life-threatening adverse effects are uncommon; however, seizures, apnea, metabolic acidosis, and impaired renal function have been reported following overdosage of naproxen. One death due to CNS depression has been attributed to naproxen overdosage.

Treatment

Treatment of acute toxicity associated with naproxen overdosage is mainly supportive. There is no specific antidote. If there is evidence that the drug was ingested recently (within 4 hours) or in large amounts (e.g., 5–10 times the recommended dosage), induction of emesis, administration of activated charcoal, and/or osmotic catharsis should be considered in symptomatic patients. Forced diuresis, alkalinization of urine, hemodialysis, or hemoperfusion may not be useful in enhancing elimination of naproxen because of the high protein binding of the drug.

PHARMACOLOGY

Naproxen has pharmacologic actions similar to those of other prototypical NSAIAs. The drug exhibits anti-inflammatory, analgesic, and antipyretic activity. The exact mechanisms have not been clearly established, but many of the actions appear to be associated principally with the inhibition of prostaglandin synthesis. Naproxen inhibits the synthesis of prostaglandins in body tissues by inhibiting cyclooxygenase; at least 2 isoenzymes, cyclooxygenase-1 (COX-1) and -2 (COX-2) (also referred to as prostaglandin G/H synthase-1 [PGHS-1] and -2 [PGHS-2], respectively), have been identified that catalyze the formation of prostaglandins in the arachidonic acid pathway. Naproxen, like other prototypical NSAIAs, inhibits both COX-1 and COX-2. Although the exact mechanisms have not been clearly established, NSAIAs appear to exert anti-inflammatory, analgesic, and antipyretic activity principally through inhibition of the COX-2 isoenzyme; COX-1 inhibition presumably is responsible for the drugs' unwanted effects on GI mucosa and platelet aggregation.

Anti-inflammatory, Analgesic, and Antipyretic Effects

The anti-inflammatory, analgesic, and antipyretic effects of naproxen and other NSAIAs, including selective inhibitors of COX-2 (e.g., celecoxib, rofecoxib), appear to result from inhibition of prostaglandin synthesis. While the precise mechanism of the anti-inflammatory and analgesic effects of NSAIAs continues to be investigated, these effects appear to be mediated principally through inhibition of the COX-2 isoenzyme at sites of inflammation with subsequent reduction in the synthesis of certain prostaglandins from their arachidonic acid precursors.

Naproxen stabilizes lysosomal membranes and inhibits the response of neutrophils to chemotactic stimuli. The drug does not possess glucocorticoid or adrenocorticoid-stimulating properties.

There is no evidence that long-term therapy with naproxen results in tolerance to or physical dependence on the drug. The drug probably cannot suppress the abstinence syndrome in opiate-dependent patients.

Naproxen lowers body temperature in patients with fever. Although the mechanism of the antipyretic effect of NSAIAs is not known, it has been suggested that suppression of prostaglandin synthesis in the CNS (probably in the hypothalamus) may be involved.

Genitourinary and Renal Effects

Naproxen-induced inhibition of prostaglandin synthesis may result in decreased frequency and intensity of uterine contractility. Prostaglandins E_2 and $F_{2\alpha}$ increase the amplitude and frequency of uterine contractions in pregnant women; current evidence suggests that primary dysmenorrhea is also mediated by these prostaglandins. Whether the increased production of prostaglandins associated with primary dysmenorrhea is mediated by COX-1 or COX-2 remains to be determined. Blood concentrations of a metabolite of prostaglandin $F_{2\alpha}$ have been found to decrease in women with dysmenorrhea who were receiving naproxen. Therapy with naproxen has been effective in relieving menstrual pain and has reduced blood loss in women with menorrhagia, probably by inhibiting the formation of these prostaglandins. Administration of naproxen during late pregnancy may prolong gestation by inhibiting uterine contractions.

Naproxen has been reported to adversely affect renal function. (See Renal and Electrolyte Effects under Cautions.) The mechanisms of adverse renal effects of naproxen have not been determined, but may involve inhibition of renal synthesis of prostaglandins.

Naproxen does not appear to have uricosuric activity.

GI Effects

Naproxen can cause gastric mucosal damage which may result in ulceration and/or bleeding. (See GI Effects under Cautions.) These gastric effects have been attributed to inhibition of the synthesis of prostaglandins produced by COX-1. Other factors possibly involved in NSAIA-induced gastropathy include local irritation, promotion of acid back-diffusion into gastric mucosa, uncoupling of oxidative phosphorylation, and enterohepatic recirculation of the drugs.

Epidemiologic and laboratory studies suggest that NSAIAs may reduce the risk of colon cancer. Although the exact mechanism by which NSAIAs may inhibit colon carcinogenesis remains to be determined, it has been suggested that inhibition of prostaglandin synthesis may be involved.

Hematologic Effects

Although naproxen can inhibit platelet aggregation and may prolong bleeding time, it does not affect prothrombin or whole blood clotting time. (See Hematologic Effects under Cautions.) In one study, the drug inhibited the second phase of platelet aggregation induced by adenosine diphosphate or epinephrine. Like aspirin and other prototypical NSAIAs, the effects of naproxen on platelets appear to be associated with the inhibition of the synthesis of prostaglandins produced by COX-1.

PHARMACOKINETICS

Naproxen pharmacokinetics have not been determined in individuals with renal or hepatic impairment, nor in children younger than 5 years of age.

Pharmacokinetics of the drug in the delayed-release (enteric-coated) formulation have not been determined in individuals younger than 18 years of age.

Absorption

Preparations of naproxen differ in their pattern of absorption, owing to the chemical form of naproxen (i.e., the base or sodium salt) and the formulation used. When administered as the acid or the sodium salt, naproxen is completely absorbed from the GI tract; the sodium salt is absorbed more rapidly than the acid. Oral bioavailability of naproxen is 95%. There appears to be no difference in bioavailability between a single 500-mg conventional tablet and two 250-mg conventional tablets of naproxen. Commercially available formulations of naproxen (i.e., conventional tablets, delayed-release tablets, oral suspension) are bioequivalent in terms of extent of absorption (i.e., area under the curve [AUC]) and peak plasma concentrations; however, the rate of absorption varies depending on the formulation used. When naproxen (either as conventional or delayed-release tablets) or naproxen sodium (either as conventional or extended-release tablets) is taken with food, the rate but not the extent of absorption of the drug is decreased. Studies to date indicate that antacids may have variable, but probably clinically insignificant, effects on absorption of naproxen (either as conventional or delayed-release tablets) or naproxen sodium.

The manufacturers state that peak plasma concentrations of the drug occur in 2–4 hours following oral administration of naproxen as conventional tablets; peak plasma concentration occurs 1–4 hours following administration of the oral suspension. In several studies, following oral administration of a single 500-mg dose of naproxen (as one 500-mg or two 250-mg conventional tablets) to fasting, healthy adults, mean peak plasma concentrations of the drug ranged from 62–96 mcg/mL and occurred at 1.5–2 hours. The manufacturers state that peak plasma concentrations of the drug occur in 1–2 hours following oral administration of naproxen sodium as conventional tablets. Following oral administration of a single 550-mg dose of naproxen sodium as a conventional tablet (equivalent to 500 mg of naproxen) to a group of fasting, healthy adults, mean peak plasma concentrations of the drug were 70 mcg/mL and occurred at about 1 hour. In children 5–16 years of age, plasma naproxen concentrations following a single 5- to 10-mg/kg dose of the suspension are similar to those attained in healthy adults following a 500-mg dose. Steady-state plasma concentrations of naproxen are achieved within 4–5 days.

Commercially available delayed-release (enteric-coated) tablets of naproxen (EC-Naprosyn®) contain the drug within a copolymer coating dispersion. Dissolution of the coating is pH-dependent, with the most rapid dissolution occurring at pH above 6; no dissolution occurs below pH 4. The coating is designed to release the drug in the higher pH environment of the small intestine, avoiding dissolution in the more acidic environment of the stomach. Naproxen is well-absorbed from the enteric-coated formulation. Peak plasma concentration usually is reached about 4–6 (range: 2–12) hours following oral administration of the first dose of the enteric-coated formulation. A crossover study of oral administration of naproxen as conventional or delayed-release tablets in a dosage of 500 mg twice daily in fasted, healthy individuals demonstrated that after one week, only time to peak plasma concentration differed between the two formulations (1.9 versus 4 hours for conventional versus delayed-release tablets, respectively); there were no differences in peak plasma concentration or extent of absorption (i.e., AUC).

Commercially available tablets of naproxen and esomeprazole magnesium (Vimovo®) contain a delayed-release (enteric-coated) naproxen core surrounded by an immediate-release layer of esomeprazole magnesium. The tablet is designed to release esomeprazole in the stomach prior to dissolution of naproxen in the small intestine. At naproxen dosages of 375 or 500 mg twice daily, the fixed-combination tablets are bioequivalent (based on AUC and peak plasma concentration) to enteric-coated preparations of naproxen. Peak steady-state plasma concentrations of naproxen are reached about 3 hours after administration of the fixed-combination tablet. Administration of the fixed-combination tablets with a high-fat meal substantially delays naproxen absorption and modestly decreases peak plasma concentrations of the drug.

Commercially available extended-release tablets of naproxen sodium (Naprelan®) contain an immediate-release component (about 30% of the total dose) and an extended-release component comprised of microparticles that slowly release the drug. The tablet matrix rapidly disintegrates in the stomach, and the microparticles are dispersed throughout the small intestine and into the proximal large intestine allowing absorption of the drug throughout the GI tract. Naproxen is well absorbed from naproxen sodium extended-release tablets, with

a reported bioavailability of about 95%; peak steady-state plasma naproxen concentrations usually are reached in about 3–5 hours following oral administration. The absorption rate from extended-release naproxen sodium tablets is slower than from conventional tablets. Prolonged drug absorption from extended-release tablets allows for once-daily dosing with this formulation.

Following oral administration of fixed-combination tablets containing naproxen sodium 500 mg and sumatriptan 85 mg, peak plasma naproxen concentrations are about 36% lower and the time to peak plasma naproxen concentrations is delayed by about 4 hours compared with oral administration of naproxen sodium as conventional 550-mg tablets; the extent of exposure to naproxen (i.e., AUC) is similar for the 2 formulations. Administration of the fixed-combination tablets with food does not substantially affect the bioavailability of naproxen.

Plasma naproxen concentrations of 30–90 mcg/mL reportedly are required for anti-inflammatory or analgesic effect. In a group of patients with rheumatoid arthritis, the anti-inflammatory effect of naproxen was positively correlated with serum naproxen concentrations, although no such relationship was found for adverse effects. Onset of pain relief can begin within 1 hour in patients receiving naproxen (as conventional tablets) and within 30 minutes in patients receiving naproxen sodium (as conventional tablets), as evidenced by reduction in pain intensity scores, increase in pain relief scores, decrease in the number of patients requiring additional analgesic medication, and delay in time to remedication. In a comparative study in patients with postpartum uterine cramping, there was no difference between the drugs in onset of analgesia; both drugs provided pain relief within 1 hour. Peak analgesia occurs within 1 hour with naproxen sodium and within 2 hours with naproxen. The duration of action of both drugs is generally 7–12 hours. Because of the delayed absorption of enteric-coated naproxen tablets, onset of analgesia may be delayed.

Distribution

The volume of distribution of naproxen is 0.16 L/kg. In one study, the apparent volume of distribution of naproxen averaged about 8.3 L in healthy adults and about 11.9 L in patients with severe renal failure (serum creatinine 5.4–12.5 mg/dL).

After therapeutic doses, naproxen is more than 99% bound to plasma proteins. When naproxen binding sites become saturated (at twice daily doses of 500 mg or more), plasma free drug concentrations increase and may result in increased urinary clearance rates. Therefore, plasma naproxen concentrations tend to plateau when dosage exceeds 500 mg twice daily. In a study in patients with severe renal failure, binding of naproxen to serum proteins was decreased compared to healthy adults; the decreased binding may have accounted for an increase in metabolism and apparent volume of distribution of the drug observed in these patients. In patients with chronic alcoholic liver disease, total plasma concentrations of naproxen are decreased while concentrations of the unbound drug are increased. Total naproxen concentrations are unchanged in geriatric individuals, but concentrations of the unbound drug are increased; the trough concentration of unbound naproxen in geriatric individuals reportedly is 0.12–0.19% of the total naproxen concentration, compared with 0.05–0.075% in younger individuals.

Naproxen crosses the placenta. Naproxen is also distributed into milk in concentrations of about 1% of simultaneous maternal plasma drug concentrations.

Elimination

In healthy adults, the plasma half-life of naproxen reportedly ranges from 12–17 hours. The plasma half-life and elimination of the drug appear to be similar in children and adults. Clearance of naproxen is 0.13 mL/minute per kg.

Naproxen is extensively metabolized in the liver by cytochrome P-450 (CYP) isoenzymes 1A2 and 2C9 to 6-desmethylnaproxen. Approximately 95% of the drug is excreted in urine as unchanged naproxen (less than 1%) and 6-desmethylnaproxen (less than 1%) and their glucuronide or other conjugates (66–92%). Some data suggest that renal excretion of unchanged naproxen may be negligible or absent; previously reported concentrations of unchanged drug may reflect rapid hydrolysis of conjugates during collection, storage, and handling of urine samples. The half-life of naproxen metabolites and conjugates is shorter than 12 hours.

Naproxen metabolites may accumulate in patients with renal impairment. Elimination of naproxen is reduced in patients with severe renal impairment. A small amount (less than 5%) of the drug is excreted in feces.

CHEMISTRY AND STABILITY

● *Chemistry*

Naproxen, a propionic acid derivative, is a prototypical anti-inflammatory agent (NSAIA). The drug is structurally and pharmacologically related to fenoprofen and ibuprofen.

Naproxen is commercially available as the acid and as the sodium salt. Each 275 mg of naproxen sodium is approximately equivalent to 250 mg of naproxen and each 220 mg of naproxen sodium is approximately equivalent to 200 mg of naproxen. The acid occurs as a white to off-white, practically odorless, crystalline powder and is practically insoluble in water at low pH, freely soluble in water at high pH, and freely soluble in alcohol. Naproxen sodium occurs as a white to creamy white, crystalline powder and is freely soluble in water at neutral pH and sparingly soluble in alcohol. The apparent pK_a of naproxen is 4.15. Each 220-, 275-, 412.5-, 550-, or 825-mg tablet of naproxen sodium contains about 0.87, 1, 1.5, 2, or 3 mEq of sodium, respectively, and each 5 mL of the commercially available naproxen suspension contains about 1.5 mEq each of sodium and chloride.

Naproxen is commercially available as conventional tablets, delayed-release (enteric-coated) tablets, and oral suspension. Naproxen sodium is commercially available as conventional tablets, extended-release tablets, and liquid-filled capsules. Extended-release tablets of naproxen sodium (Naprelan®) contain an immediate-release component (about 30% of the total dose) and an extended-release component comprised of microparticles that slowly release the drug. Fixed-combination tablets of naproxen and esomeprazole magnesium contain a delayed-release (enteric-coated) naproxen core surrounded by an immediate-release layer of esomeprazole magnesium.

● *Stability*

Commercially available naproxen conventional and delayed-release (enteric-coated) tablets should be stored in well-closed, light-resistant containers at 15–30°C. Extended-release naproxen sodium tablets should be stored in well-closed containers at 20–25°C but may be exposed to temperatures ranging from 15–30°C. Naproxen oral suspension should be stored in light-resistant containers at 20–25°C but may be exposed to temperatures ranging from 15–30°C; temperatures exceeding 40°C should be avoided. Naproxen sodium conventional tablets should be stored in well-closed containers at 15–30°C. Fixed-combination tablets containing delayed-release naproxen and immediate-release esomeprazole magnesium should be protected from moisture and stored in well-closed containers at 25°C but may be exposed to temperatures ranging from 15–30°C. Fixed-combination tablets containing naproxen sodium and sumatriptan succinate should be stored in the original container with the desiccant packet at 25°C but may be exposed to temperatures ranging from 15–30°C; the tablets should not be repackaged.

Naproxen and naproxen sodium preparations containing the equivalent of 250 mg of naproxen or more per retail package should be stored in child-resistant containers in order to limit the potential toxicity associated with accidental ingestion in children.

PREPARATIONS

Excipients in commercially available drug preparations may have clinically important effects in some individuals; consult specific product labeling for details.

Naproxen

Oral

Suspension	125 mg/5 mL*	**Naprosyn®**, Athena **Naproxen Suspension**
Tablets	250 mg*	**Naproxen Tablets**
	375 mg*	**Naproxen Tablets**
	500 mg*	**Naprosyn®**, Canton **Naproxen Tablets**
Tablets, delayed-release (enteric-coated)	375 mg*	**EC-Naprosyn®**, Canton **Naproxen Delayed-release Tablets**
	500 mg*	**EC-Naprosyn®** (scored), Canton **Naproxen Delayed-release Tablets**

* available from one or more manufacturer, distributor, and/or repackager by generic (nonproprietary) name

Naproxen Combinations

Oral

Tablets, delayed-release core (naproxen only)	375 mg with Esomeprazole Magnesium 20 mg (of esomeprazole)*	**Naproxen and Esomeprazole Magnesium Delayed-release Tablets** **Vimovo®**, Horizon
	500 mg with Esomeprazole Magnesium 20 mg (of esomeprazole)*	**Naproxen and Esomeprazole Magnesium Delayed-release Tablets** **Vimovo®**, Horizon

* available from one or more manufacturer, distributor, and/or repackager by generic (nonproprietary) name

Naproxen Sodium

Oral

Capsules, liquid-filled	220 mg (equivalent to naproxen 200 mg)*	**Aleve®**, Bayer **Naproxen Sodium Capsules**
Tablets	220 mg (equivalent to naproxen 200 mg)*	**Aleve®**, Bayer **Naproxen Sodium Tablets**
Tablets, extended-release	412.5 mg (equivalent to 375 mg naproxen)*	**Naprelan®**, Almatica **Naproxen Sodium Extended-release Tablets**
	550 mg (equivalent to 500 mg naproxen)*	**Naprelan®**, Almatica **Naproxen Sodium Extended-release Tablets**
	825 mg (equivalent to 750 mg naproxen)*	**Naprelan®**, Almatica **Naproxen Sodium Extended-release Tablets**
Tablets, film-coated	275 mg (equivalent to naproxen 250 mg)*	**Naproxen Sodium Film-coated Tablets**
	550 mg (equivalent to naproxen 500 mg)*	**Anaprox® DS** (scored), Canton **Naproxen Sodium Film-coated Tablets**

* available from one or more manufacturer, distributor, and/or repackager by generic (nonproprietary) name

Naproxen Sodium Combinations

Oral

Tablets	220 mg (equivalent to 200 mg naproxen) with Diphenhydramine Hydrochloride 25 mg*	**Aleve® PM**, Bayer **Naproxen Sodium and Diphenhydramine Hydrochloride Tablets**
Tablets, film-coated	500 mg (equivalent to 455 mg naproxen) with Sumatriptan Succinate 85 mg (of sumatriptan)*	**Sumatriptan and Naproxen Sodium Film-coated Tablets** **Treximet®**, Currax

* available from one or more manufacturer, distributor, and/or repackager by generic (nonproprietary) name

† Use is not currently included in the labeling approved by the US Food and Drug Administration.

Selected Revisions June 10, 2024, © Copyright, April 1, 1983, American Society of Health-System Pharmacists, Inc.

Celecoxib

28:08.04.08 • CYCLOOXYGENASE-2 (COX-2) INHIBITORS

■ Celecoxib is a nonsteroidal anti-inflammatory agent (NSAIA) that is a selective inhibitor of cyclooxygenase-2 (COX-2).

REMS

FDA approved a REMS for the fixed combination of celecoxib and tramadol hydrochloride under a shared REMS system (Opioid Analgesic REMS) to ensure that the benefits outweigh the risks. The REMS consists of the following: medication guide and elements to assure safe use. See the FDA REMS page https://www.accessdata.fda.gov/scripts/cder/rems/index.cfm

USES

Celecoxib is used in the management of osteoarthritis, rheumatoid arthritis, juvenile rheumatoid arthritis, pain, ankylosing spondylitis, and dysmenorrhea. There currently is no evidence establishing superiority of selective COX-2 inhibitors relative to prototypical NSAIAs in the management of these conditions, and the principal benefit of selective COX-2 inhibitors is a potential reduction in the incidence of certain adverse effects (e.g., GI toxicity). Both COX-2 inhibitors and prototypical NSAIAs have been associated with an increased risk of cardiovascular events. A decision to use a selective COX-2 inhibitor rather than a prototypical NSAIA usually is based on an individual assessment of the risk of ulcer complications from NSAIA therapy. There is some evidence that therapy with a COX-2 inhibitor may be no more effective in reducing the risk of NSAIA-induced GI complications than a combined regimen of a prototypical NSAIA and a proton-pump inhibitor. (See Uses: Osteoarthritis.) Additional study is planned or under way to establish more definitively the role of COX-2 inhibitors relative to prototypical NSAIAs.

Celecoxib also is used for the acute treatment of attacks of migraine with or without aura.

Celecoxib also has been used to reduce the number of adenomatous colorectal polyps in adults with familial adenomatous polyposis† (FAP).

The potential benefits and risks of celecoxib therapy as well as alternative therapies should be considered prior to initiating therapy with the drug. The lowest possible effective dosage and shortest duration of therapy consistent with treatment goals of the patient should be employed.

● Osteoarthritis

Celecoxib is used for the management of the signs and symptoms of osteoarthritis in adults. Medical management of osteoarthritis of the hip, knee, and/or hand includes both pharmacologic therapy and nonpharmacologic (e.g., educational, behavioral, psychosocial, physical) interventions to reduce pain, maintain and/or improve joint mobility, limit functional impairment, and enhance overall well-being. The American College of Rheumatology (ACR) strongly recommends exercise, weight loss when necessary in patients with osteoarthritis of the knee and/or hip, self-efficacy and self-management programs, tai chi, cane use, hand orthoses, knee bracing, topical NSAIAs for osteoarthritis of the knee, oral NSAIAs, and intra-articular glucocorticoid injections for osteoarthritis of the knee or hip. Other pharmacologic or nonpharmacologic interventions may be recommended conditionally. Interventions and the order of their selection are patient specific. Factors to consider when making decisions regarding therapy for osteoarthritis include patients' values and preferences, the presence of risk factors for serious adverse GI effects, existing comorbidities (e.g., hypertension, heart failure, other cardiovascular disease, chronic kidney disease), injuries, disease severity, surgical history, and access to and availability of the interventions. Pharmacologic therapy should be initiated with treatments resulting in the least systemic exposure or toxicity. For some patients with limited disease, topical NSAIAs may be an appropriate initial choice for pharmacologic therapy; for other patients, particularly those with osteoarthritis of the hip or with polyarticular involvement, oral NSAIAs may be more appropriate.

NSAIAs that are selective inhibitors of COX-2 (e.g., celecoxib) are associated with a lower incidence of adverse GI effects than prototypical NSAIAs. Both COX-2 inhibitors and prototypical NSAIAs have been associated with an increased risk of cardiovascular events. A decision to use a selective COX-2 inhibitor (e.g., celecoxib) rather than a prototypical NSAIA usually is based on an individual assessment of the risk for GI toxicity. If a prototypical NSAIA (e.g., diclofenac, diflunisal, fenoprofen, ibuprofen, indomethacin, ketoprofen, meclofenamate, naproxen, piroxicam, sulindac, tolmetin) is used in osteoarthritis patients at risk for GI complications, concomitant use of misoprostol or a proton-pump inhibitor (e.g., omeprazole) can be considered for preventive therapy. However, in a study comparing the efficacy of celecoxib (200 mg twice daily) versus diclofenac sodium (75 mg twice daily) plus omeprazole (20 mg daily) in preventing recurrent ulcer bleeding in H. pylori-negative arthritis (principally osteoarthritis) patients with a recent history of ulcer bleeding while receiving long-term NSAIA therapy, the protective efficacy was unexpectedly low for both regimens (recurrent ulcer bleeding probabilities of 4.9 versus 6.4%, respectively, during the 6-month study) and it appeared that neither could completely protect patients at high risk.

In several double-blind, placebo-controlled, or comparative studies of up to 12 weeks' duration, celecoxib was at least as effective as naproxen and more effective than placebo in the symptomatic management of osteoarthritis of the knee or hip in patients who experienced exacerbation of symptoms (e.g., pain, joint stiffness) following discontinuance of standard therapy with NSAIAs or other analgesics. While celecoxib and naproxen generally are comparably effective in the management of osteoarthritis, current data suggest that adverse GI effects occur less frequently with celecoxib. (See GI Effects under Cautions.)

In controlled clinical studies in adults with osteoarthritis, therapy with celecoxib (100 mg twice daily or 200 mg once daily) resulted in improvement in the Western Ontario and McMaster Universities (WOMAC) osteoarthritis index; WOMAC is a 24-item questionnaire that measures pain, stiffness, and functioning. Following initiation of celecoxib 100 or 200 mg twice daily in patients with joint pain as a result of symptomatic exacerbation of osteoarthritis, pain relief generally occurs within 24–48 hours and therapy with the drug is associated with greater reductions in joint pain than placebo. In placebo-controlled and comparative studies in patients with symptomatic exacerbation of osteoarthritis of the hip or knee, 31–36% of patients receiving celecoxib 100 mg twice daily for 12 weeks improved as measured by patient and physician assessment of the arthritic condition; improvement occurred in 29–36% of patients receiving celecoxib 200 mg twice daily, 29–37% of patients receiving naproxen 500 mg twice daily, and 17–24% of patients receiving placebo twice daily. Celecoxib dosages of 100 mg twice daily and 200 mg once daily were comparably effective in patients with osteoarthritis as measured by joint pain, disease activity, functionality, and health-related quality of life. Celecoxib dosages of 200 mg twice daily do not appear to provide additional benefit compared with dosages of 100 mg twice daily or 200 mg once daily in these patients.

● Rheumatoid Arthritis in Adults

Celecoxib is used for the management of the signs and symptoms of rheumatoid arthritis in adults. Although current data suggest that the efficacy of celecoxib is similar to that of prototypical NSAIAs but with a lower risk of adverse GI effects, both selective COX-2 inhibitors and prototypical NSAIAs have been associated with an increased risk of cardiovascular events. A decision to use a selective COX-2 inhibitor (e.g., celecoxib) rather than a prototypical NSAIA usually is based on an individual assessment of the risk for GI toxicity. There is some evidence that therapy with a COX-2 inhibitor may be no more effective in reducing the risk of NSAIA-induced GI complications than a combined regimen of a prototypical NSAIA and a proton-pump inhibitor. (See Osteoarthritis under Uses.)

In the management of rheumatoid arthritis in adults, NSAIAs may be useful for initial symptomatic treatment; however, NSAIAs do not alter the course of the disease or prevent joint destruction. Disease-modifying antirheumatic drugs (DMARDs) (e.g., abatacept, hydroxychloroquine, leflunomide, methotrexate, rituximab, sulfasalazine, tocilizumab, tofacitinib, tumor necrosis factor [TNF; TNF-α] blocking agents) have the potential to reduce or prevent joint damage, preserve joint integrity and function, and reduce total health care costs, and all patients with rheumatoid arthritis are candidates for DMARD therapy. DMARDs should be initiated early in the disease course and should not be delayed beyond 3 months in patients with active disease (i.e., ongoing joint pain, substantial morning stiffness, fatigue, active synovitis, persistent elevation of erythrocyte sedimentation rate [ESR] or C-reactive protein [CRP], radiographic evidence of joint damage) despite an adequate regimen of NSAIAs. NSAIA therapy may be continued in conjunction with DMARD therapy or, depending on patient response, may be discontinued.

In double-blind, placebo-controlled studies, therapy with celecoxib was associated with greater reduction in joint tenderness/pain and swelling than placebo. In addition, several double-blind, comparative studies of up to 24 weeks' duration have demonstrated that celecoxib is at least as effective as naproxen or diclofenac in the symptomatic treatment of rheumatoid arthritis but is less likely to cause adverse GI effects. (See GI Effects under Cautions.) Clinical studies of celecoxib generally have included adults receiving standard therapy for rheumatoid arthritis (i.e., NSAIAs with or without DMARDs and/or low-dose oral corticosteroids) who experienced symptomatic exacerbation (symptom "flare") within 2–14 days of discontinuing the NSAIA component of their regimen. Symptom flare was defined as a minimum of 6 *tender* joints *and* an increase of 20% in the number of tender or painful joints or involvement of at least 2 additional joints since discontinuing NSAIA therapy; a minimum of 3 *swollen* joints *and* an increase of 20% in the number of swollen joints or involvement of at least 2 additional joints since discontinuing NSAIA therapy; and either a minimum of 45 minutes of morning stiffness *and* an increase of at least 15 minutes in the duration of morning stiffness *or* an increase in patient-assessed arthritis pain since discontinuing NSAIA therapy.

The American College of Rheumatology criteria for a 20% improvement (ACR 20 response) in measures of disease activity were used as the principal measure of clinical response in studies evaluating the efficacy of celecoxib. An ACR 20 response is achieved if the patient experiences a 20% improvement in the number of tender and swollen joints and a 20% or greater improvement in at least 3 of the following 5 criteria: patient pain assessment; patient global assessment; physician global assessment; patient self-assessed disability; and laboratory measures of disease activity (i.e., ESR or C-reactive protein level). In placebo-controlled and comparative studies in adults with rheumatoid arthritis who had symptom flare, an ACR 20 response was achieved in 30–40% of patients who received celecoxib 100 mg twice daily for 12 weeks, 39–44% of patients who received celecoxib 200 mg twice daily for 12 weeks, 36–42% of patients who received naproxen 500 mg twice daily for 12 weeks, and 23–29% of placebo-treated patients. While celecoxib 100 mg twice daily generally was as effective as celecoxib 200 mg twice daily, some patients experienced additional benefit from the higher dosage. Dosages of 400 mg twice daily provided no additional benefit compared with dosages of 100–200 mg twice daily.

● Juvenile Arthritis

Celecoxib is used for the management of the signs and symptoms of juvenile rheumatoid arthritis in children 2 years of age or older. Efficacy of celecoxib was established in pediatric patients with pauciarticular course, polyarticular course, or systemic onset juvenile rheumatoid arthritis (active systemic disease not present at study entry) in a double-blind, active-controlled study of 12 weeks' duration; pediatric patients 2–17 years of age were randomized to receive celecoxib 3 mg/kg (up to a maximum dose of 150 mg) twice daily, celecoxib 6 mg/kg (up to a maximum dose of 300 mg) twice daily, or naproxen 7.5 mg/kg (up to a maximum dose of 500 mg) twice daily. Response was measured using the juvenile rheumatoid arthritis definition of improvement (i.e., a 30% or greater improvement in at least 3 of 6 and a 30% or greater deterioration in no more than 1 of 6 core set criteria that included physician and patient/parent global assessments, active joint count, limitation of motion, functional assessment, and erythrocyte sedimentation rate: JRA DOI 30). Results of this study indicate that celecoxib is as effective as naproxen in the management of juvenile rheumatoid arthritis. Evaluation at week 12 indicated that clinical response (JRA DOI 30) was achieved in 69, 80, or 67% of pediatric patients receiving celecoxib 3 mg/kg twice daily, celecoxib 6 mg/kg twice daily, or naproxen 7.5 mg/kg twice daily, respectively. The manufacturer states that safety and efficacy of celecoxib therapy beyond 6 months in pediatric patients with juvenile arthritis have not been established.

Clinical trials indicate that either celecoxib or a prototypical NSAIA is effective in the management of juvenile rheumatoid arthritis. Celecoxib may have a lower risk of adverse GI effects compared with prototypical NSAIAs and may be useful in children who have experienced adverse GI effects with prototypical NSAIAs. In addition, celecoxib may be useful in children who have experienced other adverse effects with prototypical NSAIAs (e.g., naproxen-induced pseudoporphyria). It

remains to be determined whether long-term cardiovascular risks in children exposed to celecoxib are similar to those observed in adults receiving celecoxib or other NSAIAs. (See Cardiovascular Effects under Cautions.)

● Ankylosing Spondylitis

Celecoxib is used for the management of the signs and symptoms of ankylosing spondylitis in adults. Clinical trials indicate that either selective COX-2 inhibitors or prototypical NSAIAs are effective for initial symptomatic management of ankylosing spondylitis. Although celecoxib may have a lower risk of adverse GI effects compared with prototypical NSAIAs, both selective COX-2 inhibitors and prototypical NSAIAs have been associated with an increased risk of cardiovascular events. A decision to use a selective COX-2 inhibitor (e.g., celecoxib) rather than a prototypical NSAIA usually is based on an individual assessment of the risk for GI toxicity. There is some evidence that therapy with a COX-2 inhibitor may be no more effective in reducing the risk of NSAIA-induced GI complications than a combined regimen of a prototypical NSAIA and a proton-pump inhibitor. (See Osteoarthritis under Uses.)

In placebo- and active-controlled studies of 6- and 12-weeks' duration in patients with ankylosing spondylitis, celecoxib (100 mg twice daily, 200 mg once daily, or 400 mg once daily) was more effective than placebo, as assessed by global pain intensity and global disease activity (both rated using visual analog scales) and functional impairment (measured using the Bath Ankylosing Spondylitis Functional Index [BASFI]). In the 12-week study, there was no difference in the extent of improvement in those receiving celecoxib 400 mg daily relative to those receiving celecoxib 200 mg daily, but more patients receiving the 400-mg daily dose (53%) than the 200-mg daily dose (44%) were classified as responders (defined as achieving 20% or greater improvement in the Assessment in Ankylosing Spondylitis [ASAS] response criteria). There was no change in responder rates after 6 weeks.

● Colorectal Polyps

Celecoxib has been used to reduce the number of adenomatous colorectal polyps in adults with familial adenomatous polyposis† (FAP) as an adjunct to usual care (e.g., endoscopic surveillance, surgery). Patients with FAP have an inherited mutation in the adenomatous polyposis coli (APC) gene that results in hundreds of adenomatous polyps and an almost 100% risk of colon cancer. Celecoxib previously was FDA-labeled for this use; however, approval was granted under FDA's accelerated approval regulations, and a postapproval study was required to verify clinical benefit. Patient accrual in the study was slow and the manufacturer was unable to provide confirmatory data. Therefore, the labeled indication was withdrawn. Because celecoxib therapy in patients with FAP has involved high-dose, long-term use of the drug, there is concern that potential risks (e.g., GI, cardiovascular) of celecoxib might not be outweighed by the uncertain benefit.

Efficacy of celecoxib in reducing the extent of polyposis has been evaluated in a randomized, placebo-controlled study in adults with FAP. In this study, patients with FAP were randomized to receive a 6-month regimen of celecoxib 400 mg twice daily, celecoxib 100 mg twice daily, or placebo. Patients underwent endoscopy at the beginning and end of the study to determine the number and size of polyps in specified areas (one area of the rectum and up to 4 areas of the colon); response to treatment was expressed as the mean percent change in the number of polyps and in polyp burden (expressed as the sum of polyp diameters). The mean pretreatment number of polyps was 11.5–15.5 and the mean pretreatment polyp burden was 34.8–44.7 mm. At month 6, the mean reduction in the number of polyps was 28% in patients who received celecoxib 400 mg twice daily, 12% in those who received celecoxib 100 mg twice daily, and 5% in those who received placebo; the mean reduction in polyp burden was 30.7, 14.6, and 4.9%, respectively.

Use of celecoxib for the prevention of adenomatous colorectal polyps (colorectal adenomas) in patients without a history of FAP† has been investigated in 2 long-term, National Institute of Health (NIH)-supported, multicenter studies (Adenoma Prevention with Celecoxib [APC]; Prevention of Colorectal Sporadic Adenomatous Polyps [PreSAP]). Patients included in these studies had undergone recent removal of colorectal adenomas and were at high risk of recurrent adenomas. Results of these studies indicate that administration of celecoxib (200 mg twice daily, 400 mg twice daily, or 400 mg once daily) reduces the risk of recurrent colorectal adenomas. The cumulative rate of adenoma detection during up to 3 years of treatment was 33.6–43.2% among patients receiving celecoxib compared with 49.3–60.7% among those receiving placebo. However, some clinicians state that routine use of celecoxib for the prevention of sporadic colorectal adenomas cannot be recommended because of the potential for serious cardiovascular events in celecoxib-treated patients. The studies did not evaluate whether celecoxib alters the risk of a first occurrence of colorectal adenoma or prevents the development of colorectal cancer.

● Pain

Celecoxib is used in the management of acute pain, including postoperative (dental, orthopedic) pain, in adults. In pain studies evaluating the efficacy of celecoxib, the drug was effective in the relief of postoperative dental pain and postoperative orthopedic pain that was described as moderate to severe. Following administration of single doses of celecoxib, the onset of analgesia was 60 minutes. In a single-dose study, celecoxib 100 or 400 mg reportedly was more effective than placebo and as effective as aspirin 650 mg for relief of pain following dental extraction. However, limited data indicate that celecoxib 100 or 200 mg as a single dose may be less effective than single doses of ibuprofen 400 mg or naproxen sodium 550 mg for the acute relief of postoperative dental pain.

Celecoxib in fixed combination with tramadol hydrochloride (celecoxib/tramadol) is used for the management of acute pain in adults that is severe enough to require an opiate analgesic and for which alternative treatments are inadequate; because of the risks of addiction, abuse, and misuse associated with opiates even at recommended dosages, reserve celecoxib/tramadol for use in patients for whom alternative treatment options (e.g., nonopiate analgesics) have not been, or are not expected to be, adequate or tolerated.

● Migraine

Celecoxib is used for the acute treatment of attacks of migraine with or without aura; celecoxib should *not* be used for the prophylaxis of migraine.

In 2 randomized, double-blind, placebo-controlled clinical trials (NCT03009019, NCT03006276), efficacy of celecoxib (120-mg dose given as an oral solution) for the acute treatment of migraine attacks was evaluated in a total of 1253 adults (86% female, 74% White, mean age of 41 years) experiencing a migraine attack causing moderate to severe pain. At 2 hours after treatment, freedom from headache pain was reported by a greater proportion of patients receiving celecoxib compared with those receiving placebo in one study (35 versus 21%) but not in the other study (32 versus 25%). Relief of the patient's most bothersome symptom (i.e., photophobia, nausea, or phonophobia) at 2 hours after treatment was reported by greater proportions of celecoxib recipients in both studies (57–58 versus 44%).

● Dysmenorrhea

Celecoxib is used for the relief of primary dysmenorrhea in adults. In pain studies evaluating the efficacy of celecoxib, the drug was effective in the relief of moderate to severe pain associated with primary dysmenorrhea.

● Other Uses

Celecoxib has no effect on platelet function and is not a substitute for aspirin in the prevention of adverse cardiovascular events (e.g., primary or secondary prevention of myocardial infarction).

Results from a large, prospective, population-based cohort study in geriatric individuals indicate a lower prevalence of Alzheimer's disease† among patients who received an NSAIA for 2 years or longer. Similar findings have been reported from some other, but not all, observational studies.

DOSAGE AND ADMINISTRATION

● Administration

The potential benefits and risks of celecoxib therapy as well as alternative therapies should be considered prior to initiating celecoxib therapy.

Celecoxib is administered orally as a single daily dose or in 2 equally divided doses daily. Once- and twice-daily regimens were equally effective in the management of osteoarthritis. The manufacturer recommends a twice-daily dosing schedule for the management of rheumatoid arthritis and juvenile arthritis. The manufacturer of celecoxib capsules states that dosages up to 200 mg twice

daily may be administered without regard to meals; higher celecoxib dosages (i.e., 400 mg twice daily) should be administered with food to improve absorption. For the acute treatment of migraine attack, celecoxib oral solution may be administered without regard to food. The patient may drink up to 240 mL of water after administering the oral solution.

For patients with difficulty swallowing capsules, the celecoxib capsule may be opened, the contents carefully emptied onto a level teaspoonful of applesauce at room temperature or cooler, and the mixture swallowed immediately with water. This mixture is stable for 6 hours when refrigerated.

Celecoxib oral solution is commercially available in single-dose bottles containing celecoxib 25 mg/mL (120 mg in 4.8 mL). When the intended dose is less than the entire contents of the bottle, use of a calibrated measuring device to accurately measure and deliver the dose is recommended; any remaining solution in the bottle should be discarded. The manufacturer's instructions for use should be consulted for additional information on administration of the drug.

Dispensing and Administration Precautions

Because of similarity in spelling of Celebrex® (celecoxib), Celexa® (citalopram hydrobromide), and Cerebyx® (fosphenytoin sodium), extra care should be exercised in ensuring the accuracy of prescriptions for these drugs.

● Dosage

The lowest possible effective dosage and shortest duration of therapy consistent with treatment goals of the patient should be employed.

When celecoxib is used in the management of arthritis in adults, the dosage of celecoxib should be adjusted according to individual requirements and response, using the lowest possible effective dosage.

Although peak plasma concentrations and area under the plasma concentration-time curve (AUC) were increased 40 and 50%, respectively, in geriatric individuals older than 65 years of age compared with younger adults, dosage adjustment in geriatric adults based solely on age generally is not required. However, for geriatric patients weighing less than 50 kg, celecoxib therapy should be initiated at the lowest recommended dosage.

Osteoarthritis

For the symptomatic treatment of osteoarthritis, the usual adult dosage of celecoxib is 200 mg daily given as a single dose or in 2 equally divided doses. Celecoxib dosages exceeding 200 mg daily (e.g., 200 mg twice daily) do not appear to provide additional therapeutic benefit. Tablets containing celecoxib in fixed combination with amlodipine are available in only one strength of celecoxib (200 mg) and should not be used in patients requiring lower doses of the drug; the manufacturer states that the fixed combination should be administered only once daily in patients requiring celecoxib for symptomatic treatment of osteoarthritis and amlodipine for the management of hypertension.

Rheumatoid Arthritis in Adults

For the symptomatic treatment of rheumatoid arthritis, the usual adult dosage of celecoxib is 100–200 mg twice daily. Although the overall efficacy of celecoxib was similar in patients receiving 100 or 200 mg twice daily, additional benefit was observed in some patients receiving the higher dosage. However, celecoxib dosages of 400 mg twice daily do not appear to provide additional therapeutic benefit compared with dosages of 100–200 mg twice daily.

Juvenile Arthritis

For the symptomatic management of juvenile rheumatoid arthritis in children 2 years of age or older, the recommended dosage of celecoxib for children weighing 10–25 kg is 50 mg twice daily, and the recommended dosage for children weighing more than 25 kg is 100 mg twice daily.

Ankylosing Spondylitis

For the symptomatic treatment of ankylosing spondylitis, the usual initial adult dosage of celecoxib is 200 mg daily given as a single dose or in 2 equally divided doses. If no response is observed after 6 weeks, the dosage may be increased to 400 mg daily. If no response is observed following administration of celecoxib 400 mg daily for 6 weeks, response is unlikely and alternative treatment options should be considered.

Pain and Dysmenorrhea

For the relief of acute pain or dysmenorrhea, the usual initial adult dosage of celecoxib is 400 mg given as a single dose, followed by an additional dose of 200 mg, if necessary, on the first day. For continued relief, 200 mg may be administered twice daily as needed.

Acute Pain

When celecoxib is used in fixed combination with tramadol hydrochloride for the management of acute pain in adults, the recommended dosage is 2 tablets (containing 56 mg of celecoxib and 44 mg of tramadol hydrochloride each) every 12 hours as needed for relief of pain.

Migraine

For the acute treatment of migraine with or without aura, the usual adult dosage of celecoxib is a single 120-mg dose (as oral solution). The maximum recommended dosage is 120 mg per 24-hour period. The efficacy and safety of administering a second dose within a 24-hour period have not been established. Celecoxib should be used on an as-needed basis for the fewest possible number of days per month.

• Dosage in Renal and Hepatic Impairment

Celecoxib has not been studied in patients with severe renal impairment, and is not recommended for use in such patients. However, if celecoxib therapy must be used in patients with severe renal impairment, close monitoring of renal function is recommended. The AUC of celecoxib was 40% lower in adults with chronic renal insufficiency (e.g., glomerular filtration rate [GFR] 35–60 mL/minute) than that reported in adults with normal renal function although no substantial relationship was found between GFR and clearance of the drug. When celecoxib is used for the acute treatment of migraine attacks in patients with mild or moderate renal impairment, no adjustment of the usual recommended dosage is required. The manufacturer makes no specific recommendations for dosage modification in patients with chronic renal insufficiency receiving celecoxib for other indications.

The pharmacokinetics of celecoxib have not been studied in patients with severe hepatic impairment, and the manufacturers state that the drug should not be used in such patients. In addition, the AUC of celecoxib was 40 or 180% higher in adults with mild or moderate hepatic impairment, respectively, compared with that reported in patients with normal hepatic function. In patients with moderate hepatic impairment (Child-Pugh class B), the manufacturer recommends that celecoxib dosage be reduced by approximately 50%. For acute treatment of migraine attacks in patients with moderate hepatic impairment, the recommended and maximum dosage of celecoxib is 60 mg.

• Pharmacogenomic Dosage Considerations

The manufacturer states that, based on experience with other drugs that are substrates of cytochrome P-450 isoenzyme 2C9 (CYP2C9), initial celecoxib dosage should be reduced by 50% in patients who are known or suspected CYP2C9 poor metabolizers with the CYP2C9*3/*3 diplotype. For the acute treatment of migraine attacks in adults who are known or suspected CYP2C9 poor metabolizers, the recommended and maximum dosage of celecoxib is 60 mg. Use of alternatives to celecoxib should be considered in pediatric patients with juvenile rheumatoid arthritis who are known or suspected CYP2C9 poor metabolizers. (See Elimination under Pharmacokinetics.)

Clinical Pharmacogenetics Implementation Consortium (CPIC) guidelines state that, in patients who are CYP2C9 poor metabolizers (i.e., diplotype functional activity score of 0.5 or 0 [e.g., CYP2C9*2/*3, CYP2C9*3/*3]), celecoxib should be initiated at a dosage that is 25–50% of the lowest recommended initial dosage (i.e., 50–75% dosage reduction) and cautiously titrated to a clinically effective dosage, up to a dosage that is 25–50% of the maximum recommended dosage. Dosage should not be increased until steady-state concentrations are attained (at least 8 days following the initial dose in poor metabolizers). Alternatively, a drug that is not metabolized by CYP2C9 or is not substantially affected by CYP2C9 genetic variants in vivo should be considered. In addition, CPIC guidelines state that, in patients who are CYP2C9 intermediate metabolizers with a diplotype functional activity score (AS) of 1, celecoxib may be initiated at the lowest recommended initial dosage and cautiously titrated to a clinically effective dosage, up to the maximum recommended dosage. Intermediate metabolizers with an AS of 1.5 may receive dosages recommended for normal metabolizers. (See Pharmacogenomic Precautions under Cautions.)

Information on the safety of celecoxib has been obtained principally from clinical studies in about 12,000 patients, including those with osteoarthritis, rheumatoid arthritis, or postoperative pain. About 50 or 30% of these patients received the drug for at least 6 months or at least 1 year, respectively; a limited number of patients have received celecoxib for 2 years or longer. Information on the safety of the drug also has been obtained from studies in pediatric patients 2–17 years of age with juvenile rheumatoid arthritis who received the drug for up to 24 weeks and from acute migraine treatment, colorectal adenoma prevention, and Alzheimer's disease prevention studies in adults.

At usual dosages, celecoxib generally is well tolerated. Adverse effects of celecoxib usually are mild and mainly involve the GI tract. During controlled clinical studies in adults receiving celecoxib dosages of 100–800 mg daily, the incidence of celecoxib-associated adverse effects generally was similar to that reported with prototypical nonsteroidal anti-inflammatory agents (NSAIAs) (e.g., diclofenac, ibuprofen, naproxen) or placebo; however, the incidence of endoscopically confirmed GI ulceration and clinically observed upper GI perforations, ulcers, and bleeding was higher in patients receiving a prototypical NSAIA than in those receiving placebo or celecoxib. The adverse effects profile of celecoxib reported in a clinical study in adults with familial adenomatous polyposis (FAP) and in clinical studies in patients with ankylosing spondylitis or acute pain, including postoperative (e.g., dental, orthopedic) pain and primary dysmenorrhea, was similar to that reported in clinical studies in patients with arthritis. About 7.1% of adults receiving celecoxib in clinical studies discontinued therapy because of adverse effects compared with 6.1% of those receiving placebo. The most frequent adverse effects requiring discontinuance of celecoxib include dyspepsia (in about 0.8 or 0.6% of patients receiving celecoxib or placebo, respectively) and abdominal pain (in about 0.7 or 0.6% of patients receiving celecoxib or placebo, respectively).

• Cardiovascular Effects

Peripheral edema has been reported in 2.1% of adults receiving celecoxib in premarketing clinical studies. Angina pectoris, chest pain, coronary artery disorder, hot flushes, myocardial infarction, palpitation, tachycardia, or aggravated hypertension has been reported in 0.1–1.9% of adults receiving the drug. Adverse cardiovascular effects reported in less than 0.1% of adults receiving celecoxib include syncope, congestive heart failure, ventricular fibrillation, pulmonary embolism, cerebrovascular accident, peripheral gangrene, thrombophlebitis, deep-vein thrombosis, and vasculitis. In long-term colorectal polyp prevention studies, deep-vein thrombosis, unstable angina, aortic valve incompetence, coronary artery atherosclerosis, sinus bradycardia, or ventricular hypertrophy occurred in less than 1% of patients receiving celecoxib.

Peripheral edema or hypertension occurred in 4.5 or 2.4%, respectively, of patients receiving celecoxib (400 mg twice daily) in the Celecoxib Long-term Arthritis Safety Study (CLASS). In a substudy of the Prospective Randomized Evaluation of Celecoxib Integrated Safety versus Ibuprofen or Naproxen (PRE-CISION) trial, ambulatory blood pressure monitoring performed 4 months after initiation of therapy indicated a difference between celecoxib and ibuprofen, but not between celecoxib and naproxen, in the effect of the drug on systolic blood pressure. In this study, the mean 24-hour systolic blood pressure decreased by 0.3 mm Hg in patients receiving celecoxib 100 mg twice daily but increased by 3.7 or 1.6 mm Hg in those receiving ibuprofen 600–800 mg 3 times daily or naproxen 375–500 mg twice daily, respectively. Peripheral edema and hypertension also have been described as evidence of adverse renal effects. (See Renal, Electrolyte, and Genitourinary Effects under Cautions.)

Thrombotic Events

NSAIAs, including selective cyclooxygenase-2 (COX-2) inhibitors and prototypical NSAIAs, increase the risk of serious adverse cardiovascular thrombotic events, including myocardial infarction and stroke (which can be fatal), in patients with or without cardiovascular disease or risk factors for cardiovascular disease. Because findings from clinical trials of celecoxib, other selective COX-2 inhibitors, or prototypical NSAIAs of up to 3 years' duration have shown an increased risk of serious cardiovascular thrombotic events, myocardial infarction, and stroke, all NSAIAs are considered to be potentially associated with this risk.

The association between cardiovascular complications and use of NSAIAs is an area of ongoing concern and study. Findings of an FDA review of published observational studies of NSAIAs, a meta-analysis of published and unpublished data from randomized controlled trials of these drugs, and other published information indicate that NSAIAs may increase the risk of serious adverse cardiovascular thrombotic events by 10–50% or more, depending on the drugs and dosages studied. Available data suggest that the increase in risk may occur early (within the first weeks) following initiation of therapy and may increase with higher dosages and longer durations of use. An increase in risk has been observed most consistently at higher NSAIA dosages. Although the relative increase in cardiovascular risk appears to be similar in patients with or without known underlying cardiovascular disease or risk factors for cardiovascular disease, the absolute incidence of serious NSAIA-associated cardiovascular thrombotic events is higher in those with cardiovascular disease or risk factors for cardiovascular disease because of their elevated baseline risk.

Findings from some systematic reviews of controlled observational studies and meta-analyses of data from randomized studies of NSAIAs suggest that naproxen may be associated with a lower risk of cardiovascular thrombotic events compared with other NSAIAs. However, limitations of these observational studies and the indirect comparisons used to assess cardiovascular risk of the prototypical NSAIAs (e.g., variability in patients' risk factors, comorbid conditions, concomitant drug therapy, drug interactions, dosage, and duration of therapy) affect the validity of the comparisons; in addition, these studies were not designed to demonstrate superior safety of one NSAIA compared with another. Therefore, FDA states that definitive conclusions regarding relative risks of NSAIAs are not possible at this time.

Rofecoxib Experience

In September 2004, one selective COX-2 inhibitor, rofecoxib, was voluntarily withdrawn from the world market based on data from a prospective, randomized, placebo-controlled study (Adenomatous Polyp Prevention on Vioxx; APPROVe). This study was designed to evaluate the efficacy of rofecoxib in preventing recurrence of colorectal polyps in patients with a history of colorectal adenomas. The primary efficacy end point was the incidence of colorectal adenoma; safety was monitored on a regular basis by an external board. In this study, there was an increased relative risk of confirmed thrombotic events (e.g., myocardial infarction, unstable angina, sudden death from cardiac causes, ischemic stroke, transient ischemic attack, peripheral arterial thrombosis, peripheral venous thrombosis, pulmonary embolism) in patients receiving rofecoxib compared with those receiving placebo. At study end point, 27 patients had experienced confirmed thrombotic events during 3327 patient-years of placebo use, and 47 had experienced confirmed thrombotic events during 3059 patient-years of rofecoxib use. The relative risk of a confirmed thrombotic event in patients receiving rofecoxib compared with those receiving placebo was 1.89 (95% confidence interval: 1.18–3.04). The difference between the 2 groups was related mainly to an increased number of myocardial infarctions and strokes in patients receiving rofecoxib. The relative risk of an Antiplatelet Trialists' Collaboration end point (death from cardiovascular, hemorrhagic, or unknown causes; nonfatal myocardial infarction; nonfatal ischemic or hemorrhagic stroke) was 2.12 (95% confidence interval: 1.2–3.74). No difference in overall mortality was observed between treatment groups.

Extended posttreatment follow-up data regarding cardiovascular events and mortality were available for approximately 84 and 95%, respectively, of patients in the APPROVe study. The median posttreatment follow-up was 550 or 538 days for rofecoxib-treated patients or placebo recipients, respectively. Over the treatment and extended follow-up periods combined, 59 rofecoxib-treated patients and 34 placebo recipients experienced an Antiplatelet Trialists' Collaboration event (hazard ratio of 1.79; 95% confidence interval: 1.17–2.73). During the first year following discontinuance of the study drug, such events occurred more frequently in patients who had received rofecoxib compared with those who had received placebo (23 versus 12 patients; hazard ratio of 1.95; 95% confidence interval: 0.97–3.93), but no difference was evident after the first posttreatment year.

In a study in adults with rheumatoid arthritis who were randomized to receive rofecoxib (50 mg daily) or naproxen (500 mg twice daily) (Vioxx Gastrointestinal Outcomes Research; VIGOR), the risk of developing a serious cardiovascular thrombotic event was substantially higher in those receiving rofecoxib than in those receiving naproxen; mortality secondary to cardiovascular events was similar in both groups. In addition, information from pooled analyses and database reviews of large populations indicate that use of rofecoxib is associated with an increased risk of major cardiovascular events (e.g., myocardial infarction) relative

to use of celecoxib, prototypical NSAIAs, or no NSAIAs; some evidence indicates that rofecoxib dosages exceeding 25 mg daily are associated with a higher risk of major cardiovascular events than rofecoxib dosages of 25 mg daily or less.

Celecoxib Experience

Data from clinical trials comparing celecoxib with prototypical NSAIAs in patients with osteoarthritis or rheumatoid arthritis and from placebo-controlled trials evaluating use of celecoxib for the prevention of adenomatous polyps or Alzheimer's disease have provided varied estimates of the cardiovascular risk associated with celecoxib. Although data from some large, randomized studies (Prevention of Spontaneous Adenomatous Polyps [PreSAP], Alzheimer's Disease Anti-inflammatory Prevention Trial [ADAPT]) and database reviews of large populations have not shown an increased risk of cardiovascular events in patients receiving celecoxib, an increased incidence of cardiovascular events was observed in patients receiving celecoxib in a colorectal adenoma prevention study (Adenoma Prevention with Celecoxib [APC]).

In a study (CLASS) in adults with osteoarthritis or rheumatoid arthritis who were randomized to receive celecoxib (400 mg twice daily), ibuprofen (800 mg 3 times daily), or diclofenac sodium (75 mg twice daily), no difference in thrombotic events (myocardial infarction, pulmonary embolism, deep-vein thrombosis, unstable angina, transient ischemic attacks, ischemic cardiovascular accidents) was observed between celecoxib and the prototypical NSAIAs used in this study. Although findings from the CLASS study suggested that the risk of cardiovascular events in patients receiving celecoxib was similar to the risk in those receiving prototypical NSAIAs, the study was not designed to establish cardiovascular safety as a primary end point. There are noteworthy differences between the VIGOR and CLASS studies (patient selection relative to cardiac-related factors [e.g., use of low-dose aspirin], indication for use of the selective COX-2 inhibitor, and the active comparator agent), and conclusions regarding differences in risk of cardiovascular events between rofecoxib and celecoxib cannot be made from these studies.

The PRECISION trial also did not show an increased risk for cardiovascular events in patients receiving celecoxib compared with those receiving ibuprofen or naproxen. The PRECISION trial was a randomized, double-blind, controlled, noninferiority trial in 24,081 patients with osteoarthritis or rheumatoid arthritis who had or were at high risk for cardiovascular disease. Randomization was stratified by baseline use of low-dose aspirin. In the intention-to-treat (ITT) population, in which all patients were followed for a maximum of 30 months, the incidence of adverse cardiovascular events (cardiovascular death [including hemorrhagic death], myocardial infarction, stroke) was 2.3, 2.7, or 2.5% in patients receiving celecoxib 100 mg twice daily, ibuprofen 600–800 mg 3 times daily, or naproxen 375–500 mg twice daily, respectively. In the modified ITT (on-treatment) population, in which patients were followed until 30 days following drug discontinuance or for 43 months, whichever occurred first, the incidence of adverse cardiovascular events was 1.7, 1.9, or 1.8% in patients receiving these respective treatments. Because only about 6% of celecoxib-treated patients received a dosage of 200 mg twice daily, the safety of this higher dosage relative to the comparator NSAIAs could not be determined. The mean durations of treatment and follow-up were 20.3 and 34.1 months, respectively.

Additional information on the relationship between use of celecoxib and cardiovascular risk is available from 2 long-term National Institutes of Health (NIH)-supported colorectal adenoma prevention trials and an NIH-supported Alzheimer's disease prevention trial. In one colorectal adenoma prevention trial (APC), an interim analysis of safety data revealed an increased risk of cardiovascular events in patients receiving celecoxib compared with those receiving placebo. The cumulative rates of serious cardiovascular thrombotic events began to differ between those receiving celecoxib and those receiving placebo after about 1 year of treatment. Based on these adverse cardiovascular findings, NIH suspended the study early. Final data for this study became available in 2006, and the findings of the updated safety analysis, which included data for all patients with up to 3 years of follow-up, were similar to those reported in the interim analysis. The final analysis indicated that the risk of serious cardiovascular events (cardiovascular death, myocardial infarction, or stroke) was increased in patients receiving celecoxib 200 mg twice daily (hazard ratio of 2.8; 95% confidence interval: 1.1–7.2) or celecoxib 400 mg twice daily (hazard ratio of 3.4; 95% confidence interval: 1.4–8.5), compared with that in patients receiving placebo; serious cardiovascular events occurred in 2.5 or 3% of patients receiving celecoxib 200 or 400 mg twice daily, respectively, compared with 0.9% of those receiving placebo. The increase in risk with celecoxib compared with placebo was related mainly to an increased incidence of myocardial infarction.

Findings from another colorectal adenoma prevention trial (PreSAP) did not show an increased incidence of adverse cardiovascular events (cardiovascular death, myocardial infarction, stroke) in patients receiving celecoxib 400 mg once daily compared with patients receiving placebo. Serious cardiovascular events (death from cardiovascular causes, myocardial infarction, stroke) occurred in 2.3% of patients receiving celecoxib and in 1.9% of patients receiving placebo (hazard ratio of 1.2; 95% confidence interval: 0.6–2.4). An analysis of pooled data from the APC and PreSAP studies demonstrated an increased risk for death from cardiovascular causes, myocardial infarction, stroke, or heart failure in celecoxib-treated patients.

Analysis of results from ADAPT did not show an increased risk for cardiovascular-related death, myocardial infarction, stroke, or transient ischemic attack, either individually or as composite end points, in patients receiving celecoxib (200 mg twice daily) relative to patients receiving placebo.

Data concerning the risk of cardiovascular events in patients receiving celecoxib continue to be collected and evaluated. Current evidence suggests that cardiovascular risk associated with celecoxib use may be dose related, with dosages exceeding 200 mg daily associated with greater risk. Meta-analyses of data from published and unpublished controlled clinical trials, systematic reviews, and large observational studies have yielded varied estimates of the cardiovascular risks associated with celecoxib use. A systematic review of controlled observational studies that included 11 studies of celecoxib suggested that celecoxib is not associated with an increased risk of cardiovascular events, but because only 3 of these studies provided dose-stratified risk estimates, there were insufficient data to provide stable estimates of the effect of dosage on risk. In an update of this systematic review that included 35 studies of celecoxib, both low (200 mg or less daily) and higher (exceeding 200 mg daily) dosages of celecoxib were associated with an increased risk of cardiovascular events (low dosage: relative risk of 1.26; 95% confidence interval: 1.09–1.47) (higher dosage: 1.69; 1.11–2.57); the increase in the risk estimate at higher dosages compared with lower dosages did not reach conventional levels of significance. In observational studies in patients with prior myocardial infarction, both low and higher dosages of celecoxib were associated with increased cardiovascular risk, but risk appeared to be greater at dosages exceeding 200 mg daily. A pooled analysis of data from 6 randomized placebo-controlled studies evaluating any of 3 higher-dosage regimens of celecoxib suggested that the risk of cardiovascular events was highest for a celecoxib dosage of 400 mg twice daily (hazard ratio of 3.1; 95% confidence interval: 1.5–6.1), intermediate for a dosage of 200 mg twice daily (1.8; 1.1–3.1), and lowest for a dosage of 400 mg once daily (1.1; 0.6–2).

Experience with Other COX-2 Inhibitors

Results of pooled analyses of randomized studies of valdecoxib (no longer commercially available in the US) in patients with rheumatoid arthritis or osteoarthritis and a systematic review of controlled observational studies that included limited data on valdecoxib suggested that such use is not associated with an increased risk of cardiovascular thrombotic events. However, administration of valdecoxib with or without parecoxib (a prodrug of valdecoxib; a parenteral formulation not commercially available in the US) immediately after surgery in patients undergoing coronary artery bypass grafting† (CABG) has been associated with an increase in cardiovascular events compared with CABG patients receiving standard care (e.g., opiate analgesics) for postoperative pain. Therefore, NSAIAs are contraindicated in the setting of CABG surgery.

Findings of pooled analyses and observational studies suggest that use of lumiracoxib or etoricoxib (neither drug commercially available in the US) is associated with an increased risk of major cardiovascular events. Of the 7 NSAIAs studied in one meta-analysis (including celecoxib, diclofenac, etoricoxib, ibuprofen, lumiracoxib, naproxen, and rofecoxib), etoricoxib and diclofenac were associated with the highest risk of cardiovascular death; rofecoxib was associated with the highest risk of myocardial infarction, followed by lumiracoxib; and ibuprofen was associated with the highest risk of stroke, followed by diclofenac, lumiracoxib, and etoricoxib. (See Experience with Prototypical NSAIAs under Cautions.)

Data from long-term studies of lumiracoxib and etoricoxib also are available. In the Therapeutic COX-189 Arthritis Research and Gastrointestinal Event Trial (TARGET), the incidence of myocardial infarction, stroke, or cardiac death in patients receiving lumiracoxib was similar to that in patients receiving a prototypical NSAIA (naproxen or ibuprofen). The study was designed as 2 substudies, and substudy results suggested that lumiracoxib was associated with a slightly, but not significantly, increased risk for cardiovascular events compared with naproxen and a slightly, but not significantly, decreased risk compared with ibuprofen. In the Multinational Etoricoxib and Diclofenac Arthritis Long-term (MEDAL) study, a randomized controlled study designed to evaluate relative cardiovascular thrombotic risk with etoricoxib (60 or 90 mg daily) compared with diclofenac (75 mg twice daily), the risk of a serious cardiovascular event in patients receiving etoricoxib was similar to that in patients receiving diclofenac; the most common cardiovascular event was myocardial infarction.

Experience with Prototypical NSAIAs

Data concerning the risk of cardiovascular events in patients receiving prototypical NSAIAs continue to be collected and evaluated. In some studies (CLASS, MEDAL), the risk of cardiovascular events in patients receiving selective COX-2 inhibitors has been similar to that in patients receiving prototypical NSAIAs (diclofenac, ibuprofen). The risk of cardiovascular events associated with selective COX-2 inhibitors and individual prototypical NSAIAs has been evaluated in several systematic reviews of controlled observational studies and meta-analyses of published and unpublished data from randomized studies.

In one systematic review, 23 observational studies providing data on individual prototypical NSAIAs reported mainly on diclofenac, indomethacin, ibuprofen, naproxen, and piroxicam. A meta-analysis utilizing tabular data from studies found through searches conducted for the period of 1966 to early 2005 provided estimates of cardiovascular risk for 3 of these drugs (diclofenac, ibuprofen, and naproxen, generally at relatively high dosages). In the meta-analysis, the risks associated with these 3 drugs were estimated indirectly relative to placebo (i.e., from studies of prototypical NSAIAs versus selective COX-2 inhibitors and studies of selective COX-2 inhibitors versus placebo) because of insufficient data from randomized placebo-controlled trials of prototypical NSAIAs. Findings from these 2 analyses suggested that use of certain prototypical NSAIAs is associated with an increased risk of cardiovascular events. The findings suggested that use of naproxen does not alter the risk of cardiovascular events (summary relative risk of 0.99; 95% confidence interval: 0.89–1.09; based on data from 16 observational studies) (summary relative risk of 0.92; 95% confidence interval: 0.67–1.26; meta-analysis) but that the risk of cardiovascular events is increased with use of diclofenac (summary relative risk of 1.4; 95% confidence interval: 1.19–1.65; 10 observational studies) (summary relative risk of 1.63; 95% confidence interval: 1.12–2.37; meta-analysis) or indomethacin (summary relative risk of 1.36; 95% confidence interval: 1.15–1.61; 7 observational studies). The findings also suggested that use of ibuprofen may be associated with an increased risk of cardiovascular events, although the reported risk estimates from these 2 analyses did not reach conventional levels of significance (summary relative risk of 1.09; 95% confidence interval: 0.99–1.2; 17 observational studies) (summary relative risk of 1.51; 95% confidence interval: 0.96–2.37; meta-analysis). Few data were available for meloxicam or piroxicam. The available data suggested that use of meloxicam may be associated with an increased risk of cardiovascular events (summary relative risk of 1.24; 95% confidence interval: 1.06–1.45; 4 observational studies); however, the finding of increased risk was based largely on results from one study. The risk ratio reported for piroxicam does not suggest increased risk (summary relative risk of 1.16; 95% confidence interval: 0.86–1.56; 5 observational studies).

The systematic review was subsequently updated to provide updated risk estimates and to evaluate dose-response effects for certain NSAIAs. The updated review included data from 51 controlled observational studies and 43 unique data sets, and provided estimates of cardiovascular risk for 11 NSAIAs. Of the 6 NSAIAs that were evaluated in 10 or more studies (range: 14–41 studies), pooled estimates of overall cardiovascular risk were highest for rofecoxib (pooled relative risk of 1.45; 95% confidence interval: 1.33–1.59) and diclofenac (1.4; 1.27–1.55) and lowest for naproxen (1.09; 1.02–1.16); the pooled risk estimate for indomethacin (1.3; 1.19–1.41) was close to that for diclofenac, and pooled risk estimates for ibuprofen (1.18; 1.11–1.25) and celecoxib (1.17; 1.08–1.27) were somewhat lower. Dose-response data were available from a subset of studies, and analyses utilizing these data indicated that low dosages of rofecoxib (25 mg or less daily), celecoxib (200 mg or less daily), and diclofenac (defined in most studies as 100 mg or less daily) were associated with elevated risk; higher dosages of these drugs were associated with even greater risk, although the increase in risk at higher dosages did not reach conventional levels of significance for celecoxib. With ibuprofen, elevated risk was observed only at high dosages (defined in most studies as more than

1.2 g daily). In this data subset, neither low nor high dosages of naproxen were associated with increased risk. Fewer data were available for etoricoxib, etodolac, meloxicam, piroxicam, and valdecoxib; of these drugs, etoricoxib appeared to be associated with the highest risk of cardiovascular events, followed by etodolac and meloxicam. Pair-wise comparisons suggested that cardiovascular risk was lower with naproxen compared with ibuprofen and was higher with diclofenac compared with celecoxib, ibuprofen, or naproxen; with etoricoxib compared with ibuprofen or naproxen; with indomethacin compared with naproxen; and with meloxicam compared with naproxen. No substantial differences in risk were found for diclofenac compared with rofecoxib, for naproxen compared with celecoxib, or for etodolac compared with diclofenac, ibuprofen, or naproxen.

A meta-analysis from the Coxib and Traditional NSAIDs Trialists' (CNT) Collaboration that utilized data from randomized trials with results available prior to 2011 provided estimates of cardiovascular risk for diclofenac, ibuprofen, and naproxen. Data for individual participants, rather than aggregate tabular data, were utilized when available. The risks associated with diclofenac, ibuprofen, and naproxen relative to placebo were obtained by combining estimates made directly (i.e., from a small number of placebo-controlled trials) or indirectly (i.e., from studies of prototypical NSAIAs versus selective COX-2 inhibitors and studies of selective COX-2 inhibitors versus placebo). The findings suggested that vascular risks of high-dose diclofenac, and possibly those of high-dose ibuprofen, are similar to those of selective COX-2 inhibitors, but high-dose naproxen may be associated with less vascular risk. The prototypical NSAIA regimens all involved high dosages with minimal variations in dosage (diclofenac 150 mg daily, ibuprofen 2.4 g daily, naproxen 1 g daily). The findings suggested that the risk of major vascular events was increased by about one-third by diclofenac (rate ratio of 1.41; 95% confidence interval: 1.12–1.78) or a selective COX-2 inhibitor (1.37; 1.14–1.66), mainly because of an increase in major coronary events (diclofenac: 1.7; 1.19–2.41) (selective COX-2 inhibitors: 1.76; 1.31–2.37). The findings also suggested that ibuprofen increased major coronary events (2.22; 1.1–4.48) but not major vascular events (1.44; 0.89–2.33). Naproxen did not appear to increase major vascular events (0.93; 0.69–1.27) or major coronary events (0.84; 0.52–1.35). In this analysis, the risk of vascular death was increased by diclofenac (1.65; 0.95–2.85) and selective COX-2 inhibitors (1.58; 1–2.49), increased but not to conventional levels of significance by ibuprofen (1.9; 0.56–6.41), but not increased by naproxen (1.08; 0.48–2.47). The estimated excess risks for diclofenac and selective COX-2 inhibitors compared with placebo suggested that diclofenac or a selective COX-2 inhibitor could cause approximately 3 additional major vascular events, including 1 fatal event, per 1000 patients per year.

Another meta-analysis of data from 31 large randomized controlled studies provided estimates of cardiovascular risk for diclofenac, ibuprofen, naproxen, and 4 selective COX-2 inhibitors. The results supported those of other analyses indicating that both prototypical NSAIAs and selective COX-2 inhibitors increase the risk of cardiovascular events. The cardiovascular safety profiles of the individual NSAIAs compared with placebo varied depending on the specific outcome. Of the 7 NSAIAs studied, etoricoxib (rate ratio of 4.07; 95% credibility interval of 1.23–15.7) and diclofenac (3.98; 1.48–12.7) were associated with the highest risk of cardiovascular death; rofecoxib was associated with the highest risk of myocardial infarction (2.12; 1.26–3.56), followed by lumiracoxib (2; 0.71–6.21); and ibuprofen was associated with the highest risk of stroke (3.36; 1–11.6), followed by diclofenac (2.86; 1.09–8.36), lumiracoxib (2.81; 1.05–7.48), and etoricoxib (2.67; 0.82–8.72). Naproxen appeared to have the least harmful cardiovascular effects of the 7 NSAIAs.

Patients with Elevated Cardiovascular Risk

Several observational studies utilizing data from national registries of hospitalization and drug dispensing from pharmacies in Denmark have examined the cardiovascular risk associated with use of NSAIAs in patients with prior myocardial infarction. In these studies, approximately 84,000–99,000 patients who had been hospitalized for a first-time myocardial infarction during the 10 or 13-year study period were identified; approximately 42–44% of these patients subsequently claimed at least one prescription for an NSAIA. Results from these studies indicated that patients who received NSAIAs following a myocardial infarction were at increased risk of reinfarction, cardiovascular-related death, and all-cause mortality beginning in the first week of treatment. Patients who received NSAIAs following myocardial infarction had a higher 1-year mortality rate compared with those who did not receive NSAIAs (20 versus 12 deaths per 100 person-years). Although the absolute mortality rate declined somewhat after the first year

following the myocardial infarction, the increased relative risk of death in patients who received NSAIAs persisted over at least the next 4 years of follow-up. Similar patterns were observed for the composite end point of coronary death or nonfatal recurrent myocardial infarction.

In these Danish registry studies, the most commonly used NSAIAs were ibuprofen and diclofenac, followed by celecoxib, rofecoxib, and naproxen. When analyzed separately, these NSAIAs were associated with increased risk of cardiovascular death and increased risk of coronary death and nonfatal myocardial infarction, but increased risk was evident for ibuprofen and naproxen only at higher dosages (exceeding 1.2 g or 500 mg daily, respectively). Estimated risks were elevated at low dosages of celecoxib (200 mg or less daily), diclofenac (100 mg or less daily), and rofecoxib (25 mg or less daily), but were increased further at higher dosages of these drugs.

In 2 large controlled clinical trials of a selective COX-2 inhibitor for the management of pain in the first 10–14 days following CABG surgery, the incidence of myocardial infarction and stroke was increased. (See Experience with Other COX-2 Inhibitors under Cautions.)

Limited data are available regarding cardiovascular risks associated with use of NSAIAs in patients with stable atherothrombotic disease. A post hoc analysis of data from the International Verapamil Trandolapril Study (INVEST), which compared antihypertensive regimens in patients with stable coronary artery disease and hypertension, indicated an increased risk for the composite end point of death, nonfatal myocardial infarction, or nonfatal stroke in patients who reported long-term NSAIA use compared with patients who did not report long-term use (4.4 versus 3.7 events per 100 patient-years; hazard ratio of 1.47; 95% confidence interval: 1.19–1.82). Results of the PRECISION trial in osteoarthritis or rheumatoid arthritis patients with, or at high risk for, cardiovascular disease indicated that celecoxib was not inferior to ibuprofen or naproxen with respect to risk of cardiovascular events. (See Celecoxib Experience under Cautions.)

Heart Failure

Data from observational studies indicate that use of NSAIAs in patients with heart failure is associated with increased morbidity and mortality. Results from a retrospective study utilizing Danish national registry data indicated that use of selective COX-2 inhibitors or prototypical NSAIAs in patients with chronic heart failure was associated with a dose-dependent increase in the risk of death and an increased risk of hospitalization for myocardial infarction or heart failure. In addition, findings from a meta-analysis of published and unpublished data from randomized controlled trials of NSAIAs indicated that use of selective COX-2 inhibitors or prototypical NSAIAs was associated with an approximate twofold increase in the risk of hospitalization for heart failure. Fluid retention and edema also have been observed in some patients receiving NSAIAs.

In the retrospective study utilizing Danish national registry data, more than 100,000 patients who had survived a first hospitalization for heart failure were identified from the registry; about 34% of these patients claimed at least one prescription for an NSAIA after discharge. Risks associated with the 5 most commonly used NSAIAs were analyzed separately. Low dosages of celecoxib (200 mg or less daily), diclofenac (100 mg or less daily), and rofecoxib (25 mg or less daily) were associated with an increased risk of death; higher dosages of these drugs were associated with even higher levels of risk. With ibuprofen and naproxen, only higher dosages (exceeding 1.2 g or 500 mg daily, respectively) were associated with an increased risk of death. All 5 NSAIAs were associated with an increased risk of hospitalization for myocardial infarction or heart failure.

Cardiovascular Risk Considerations for COX-2 Inhibitors and Prototypical NSAIAs

FDA reviewed the safety of NSAIAs in early 2005 and concluded that the 3 selective COX-2 inhibitors that previously had been marketed in the US or were on the market in the US at that time (celecoxib, rofecoxib, valdecoxib) were associated with an increased risk of serious adverse cardiovascular events compared with placebo. In addition, FDA noted that data from some long-term controlled studies that included both a selective COX-2 inhibitor and a prototypical NSAIA did not clearly demonstrate that use of a selective COX-2 inhibitor was associated with a greater risk of serious adverse cardiovascular events than use of prototypical NSAIAs. Long-term data from placebo-controlled clinical trials were not available to assess the potential for prototypical NSAIAs to increase the risk of serious cardiovascular events. FDA interpreted data on cardiovascular risk available in

2005 as being applicable to all NSAIAs, including selective COX-2 inhibitors and prototypical NSAIAs.

As a result of this analysis, FDA directed manufacturers of all NSAIAs (except aspirin) to add a boxed warning to the labeling of their products to alert clinicians to the increased risk of serious cardiovascular events and GI toxicity. In addition to the boxed warning and other information in the professional labeling, FDA recommended that a patient medication guide explaining the risks and benefits of these drugs be provided to the patient each time the drugs are dispensed.

At that time, short-term use of NSAIAs to relieve acute pain, especially at low dosages, did not appear to be associated with an increased risk of serious cardiovascular events (except immediately following CABG surgery). Therefore, in early 2005, FDA concluded that preparations of NSAIAs that currently were available without a prescription (OTC) had a favorable benefit-to-risk ratio when used according to labeled instructions and determined that these preparations should remain available without a prescription despite the addition of a boxed warning to the professional labeling of prescription-only NSAIA preparations. FDA directed manufacturers of nonprescription NSAIAs to revise the labeling of these preparations to include more specific information on the potential cardiovascular and GI risks and information to assist individuals in the safe use of these agents.

Following completion of additional studies and analyses of pooled study data, FDA again reviewed the cardiovascular risks associated with NSAIAs. Findings of this FDA review of published observational studies of NSAIAs, the CNT meta-analysis of published and unpublished data from randomized controlled trials of these drugs, and other published information indicate that NSAIAs may increase the risk of serious adverse cardiovascular thrombotic events by 10–50% or more, depending on the drugs and dosages studied. Available data now suggest that the increase in risk may occur early (within the first weeks) following initiation of therapy and may increase with higher dosages and longer durations of use. Published observational studies also indicate that use of NSAIAs in patients who have had a myocardial infarction increases the risk of reinfarction and death. Although the relative increase in cardiovascular risk appears to be similar in patients with or without known underlying cardiovascular disease or risk factors for cardiovascular disease, the absolute incidence of serious NSAIA-associated cardiovascular thrombotic events is higher in those with cardiovascular disease or risk factors for cardiovascular disease because of their elevated baseline risk. Therefore, in July 2015, FDA strengthened an existing warning in the labeling of NSAIAs regarding the increased risk of cardiovascular thrombotic events in patients receiving NSAIAs and an existing caution regarding risk in patients with heart failure. FDA directed manufacturers of prescription and nonprescription NSAIA preparations to revise the labeling of these preparations to include updated information regarding cardiovascular risk.

Concomitant Aspirin Therapy

There is no consistent evidence that use of low-dose aspirin mitigates the increased risk of serious cardiovascular events associated with NSAIAs. In several studies (APC, TARGET APPROVe), post hoc analyses or planned subset analyses suggested that the overall risk for cardiovascular events in patients receiving a COX-2 inhibitor versus placebo or a prototypical NSAIA was not influenced by use of low-dose aspirin.

● GI Effects

Dyspepsia, diarrhea, abdominal pain, nausea, or flatulence occurred in 8.8, 5.6, 4.1, 3.5, or 2.2%, respectively, of adults receiving usual dosages of celecoxib in clinical studies. In clinical trials in patients with migraine attacks, dysgeusia occurred in 3% of patients receiving celecoxib oral solution compared with 1% of those receiving placebo. Dry socket (alveolar osteitis) was reported in patients receiving celecoxib for postoperative dental pain in a clinical study. Abdominal pain, nausea, diarrhea, or vomiting has been reported in 3–8% of children receiving celecoxib in an active-controlled clinical study.

GI Risk Considerations for COX-2 Inhibitors and Prototypical NSAIAs

Numerous short-term (12–24 weeks' duration), comparative, randomized, controlled studies using endoscopy have been performed in patients with osteoarthritis or rheumatoid arthritis to evaluate the incidence of celecoxib-associated upper GI ulceration relative to that associated with prototypical NSAIAs. In these studies, the incidence of endoscopically confirmed GI ulceration generally was lower in patients receiving celecoxib than in those receiving a prototypical NSAIA (e.g., diclofenac, ibuprofen, naproxen). Results of two 3-month studies showed that gastroduodenal ulcer occurred in 2.7–5.9% of patients receiving celecoxib (50–400 mg twice daily), 16.2–17.6% of patients receiving naproxen (500 mg twice daily), and 2–2.3% of patients receiving placebo. Celecoxib was associated with a lower incidence of endoscopic ulcers than diclofenac (4% versus 15%) in one 6-month study. No consistent relationship between celecoxib dosage and the incidence of GI ulcers has been established in these studies. The correlation between endoscopic findings and the incidence of clinically important upper GI events remains to be determined.

The incidence of severe adverse upper GI effects in patients receiving celecoxib relative to the incidence in those receiving prototypical NSAIAs has been evaluated in a double-blind, randomized controlled study in patients with osteoarthritis or rheumatoid arthritis (the Celecoxib Long-term Arthritis Safety Study [CLASS]). Patients were randomized to receive celecoxib (400 mg twice daily), ibuprofen (800 mg 3 times daily), or diclofenac (75 twice daily) for up to 65 weeks; patients were allowed to continue aspirin therapy (up to 325 mg daily) for cardiovascular prophylaxis. Published results of the first 6 months of the study indicated that therapy with celecoxib was associated with a lower incidence of symptomatic ulcers and ulcer complications combined than therapy with ibuprofen or diclofenac; the decrease in upper GI toxicity in patients receiving celecoxib generally was observed only in those not receiving concomitant low-dose aspirin. However, results for celecoxib therapy were less favorable at 12 months than at 6 months, since almost all of the ulcer complications reported during the second half of the study occurred in patients receiving celecoxib; however, a greater percentage of patients receiving a prototypical NSAIA (i.e., diclofenac) than patients receiving celecoxib withdrew from the study because of GI intolerance, potentially biasing GI event rates at 12 months. Overall, the incidence of complicated ulcers in patients receiving celecoxib was similar to the incidence in those receiving the comparator agents (i.e., ibuprofen or diclofenac). Patients receiving celecoxib and low-dose aspirin experienced a fourfold higher rate of complicated ulcers compared with those receiving celecoxib alone. The rate of complicated and symptomatic ulcers at 9 months was 0.78 or 2.19% in those receiving celecoxib alone or celecoxib and low-dose aspirin, respectively; the rate of these adverse GI effects was 0.47 or 1.26% in patients younger than 65 years of age or 1.4 or 3.06% in those 65 years of age and older receiving celecoxib alone or celecoxib and low-dose aspirin, respectively. In patients with a history of peptic ulcer disease, the rate of complicated and symptomatic ulcers at 48 weeks was 2.56 or 6.85% in those receiving celecoxib or celecoxib and low-dose aspirin, respectively. Low-dose aspirin did not have a clinically important effect on the rate of upper GI complications in patients receiving prototypical NSAIAs.

Serious, sometimes fatal, adverse GI effects (e.g., bleeding, ulceration, perforation of the stomach, small intestine, or large intestine) can occur at any time in patients receiving NSAIA therapy, and such effects may *not* be preceded by warning signs or symptoms. Only 1 in 5 patients who develop a serious upper GI adverse event while receiving NSAIA therapy is symptomatic. Longer duration of therapy with an NSAIA increases the likelihood of a serious adverse GI event. However, short-term therapy is not without risk. The frequency of NSAIA-associated upper GI ulcers, gross bleeding, or perforation is approximately 1% in patients receiving NSAIA therapy for 3–6 months and approximately 2–4% in those receiving therapy for one year. Therefore, clinicians should remain alert to the possible development of serious adverse GI effects (e.g., bleeding, ulceration) in any patient receiving NSAIA therapy. Patients receiving concomitant low-dose aspirin therapy for cardiac prophylaxis should be monitored even more closely for evidence of GI bleeding. In addition, patients should be advised about the signs and/or symptoms of serious NSAIA-induced GI toxicity and what action to take if such toxicity occurs. In patients with a suspected serious adverse GI event, evaluation should be initiated promptly and celecoxib should be discontinued until a serious adverse GI event is ruled out.

Studies have shown that patients with a history of peptic ulcer disease and/or GI bleeding who are receiving NSAIAs have a greater than tenfold increased risk of developing GI bleeding than patients without these risk factors. In addition to a history of ulcer disease, pharmacoepidemiologic studies have identified several comorbid conditions and concomitant therapies that may increase the risk for GI bleeding, including concomitant use of oral corticosteroids, anticoagulants, aspirin, or selective serotonin-reuptake inhibitors (SSRIs); longer duration of NSAIA therapy; smoking; alcohol use; older age; and poor general health status. Risk of GI bleeding also is increased in patients with advanced liver disease and/or coagulopathy. Patients with rheumatoid arthritis are more likely to experience serious GI complications from NSAIA therapy than are patients with osteoarthritis. In addition, most spontaneous reports of fatal GI effects have been in geriatric or debilitated patients.

For patients at high risk for complications from NSAIA-induced GI ulceration (e.g., bleeding, perforation), concomitant use of misoprostol can be considered for preventive therapy. Alternatively, some clinicians suggest that a proton-pump inhibitor (e.g., omeprazole) may be used concomitantly to decrease the incidence of serious GI toxicity associated with NSAIA therapy. In one study, therapy with high dosages of famotidine (40 mg twice daily) was more effective than placebo in preventing peptic ulcers in NSAIA-treated patients; however, the effect of the drug was modest. In addition, efficacy of usual dosages of H_2-receptor antagonists for the prevention of NSAIA-induced gastric and duodenal ulcers has not been established. Therefore, most clinicians do not recommend use of H_2-receptor antagonists for the prevention of NSAIA-associated ulcers. Another approach in high-risk patients who would benefit from NSAIA therapy is use of an NSAIA that is a selective inhibitor of cyclooxygenase-2 (COX-2) (e.g., celecoxib), since these agents are associated with a lower incidence of serious GI bleeding than are prototypical NSAIAs. However, while celecoxib (200 mg twice daily) was comparably effective to diclofenac sodium (75 mg twice daily) plus omeprazole (20 mg daily) in preventing recurrent ulcer bleeding (recurrent ulcer bleeding probabilities of 4.9 versus 6.4%, respectively, during the 6-month study) in *H. pylori*-negative arthritis (principally osteoarthritis) patients with a recent history of ulcer bleeding, the protective efficacy was unexpectedly low for both regimens and it appeared that neither could completely protect patients at high risk. Additional study is necessary to elucidate optimal therapy for preventing GI complications associated with NSAIA therapy in high-risk patients.

Nervous System Effects

Headache has been reported in about 16% of adults receiving celecoxib in clinical studies, whereas dizziness or insomnia occurred in 2 or 2.3% of these patients, respectively. Headache occurred in 10–13% of children receiving celecoxib in an active-controlled clinical study.

Respiratory Effects

Upper respiratory tract infection, sinusitis, pharyngitis, or rhinitis has occurred in 8.1, 5, 2.3, or 2%, respectively, of adults receiving usual dosages of celecoxib in clinical studies. Cough or nasopharyngitis has been reported in 5–7% of celecoxib-treated children.

Dermatologic and Sensitivity Reactions

Rash occurred in 2.2% of adults receiving celecoxib in clinical studies. Adverse dermatologic effects occurring in 0.1–1.9% of adults receiving celecoxib include alopecia, dermatitis, dry skin, erythematous rash, maculopapular rash, photosensitivity reaction, pruritus, skin disorder, increased sweating, and urticaria.

Anaphylactoid reactions and angioedema have occurred in patients receiving celecoxib. Anaphylactic reactions have been reported in patients with or without known hypersensitivity to the drug, as well as in patients with aspirin-sensitivity asthma.

Hematologic Effects

In contrast to prototypical NSAIAs, including aspirin, usual dosages of celecoxib generally do not appear to inhibit platelet aggregation, serum thromboxane B concentrations, or bleeding time. (See Hematologic Effects under Pharmacology.)

Although comparative studies are limited, therapy with celecoxib is expected to be associated with fewer and less severe episodes of bleeding than therapy with prototypical NSAIAs. However, bleeding events have been reported in postmarketing experience, predominantly in geriatric patients, in association with increased PTs in patients receiving celecoxib concomitantly with warfarin. (See Anticoagulants under Drug Interactions.)

Modest prolongation of the activated partial thromboplastin time (aPTT) with no change in PT has been reported in celecoxib-treated pediatric patients with systemic onset juvenile rheumatoid arthritis.

Renal, Electrolyte, and Genitourinary Effects

Like prototypical NSAIAs, celecoxib has been associated with adverse renal effects. In one study in arthritis (principally osteoarthritis) patients with a recent history of ulcer bleeding while receiving long-term NSAIA therapy, celecoxib therapy (200 mg twice daily) was associated with a 24.3% incidence of adverse renal effects; however, this study defined hypertension as an adverse renal effect, and this was the principal adverse renal effect reported (occurring in 13.9% of treated patients and accounting for 57% of reported renal effects). Peripheral edema also was defined as an adverse renal effect in this study, occurring in 4.9% of treated patients; when its incidence was combined with that of hypertension, these 2 effects accounted for 77% of reported renal effects. The incidence of adverse renal effects was increased in patients with preexisting renal impairment.

In one study in arthritis (principally osteoarthritis) patients receiving celecoxib 200 mg daily, renal failure (a progressive rise in serum creatinine concentration to exceed 2.2 mg/dL) was reported in 5.6% of patients; 25.7% of all celecoxib-treated patients in this study had baseline serum creatinine concentrations exceeding 1.2 mg/dL when therapy with the drug was initiated. Hyperkalemia also has been reported in patients receiving NSAIAs, including in individuals without renal impairment.

Long-term administration of NSAIAs has resulted in renal papillary necrosis and other renal injury.

Musculoskeletal Effects

Back pain has been reported in 2.8% of adults receiving celecoxib. Arthralgia has been reported in 3–7% of children receiving celecoxib in an active-controlled clinical study.

Hepatic Effects

In controlled clinical studies in adults, the incidence of borderline elevations in liver function test results was similar in patients receiving celecoxib or placebo, occurring in 6 or 5% of patients, respectively. Substantial increases in serum concentrations of liver enzymes occurred in approximately 0.2 or 0.3% of patients receiving the drug or placebo, respectively, while borderline elevations of these enzymes occurred in 6 or 5% of patients receiving these respective treatments. Borderline elevations in one or more liver function test results may occur in up to 15% of patients treated with NSAIAs; meaningful (3 times the upper limit of normal) elevations in serum ALT or AST have occurred in approximately 1% of patients receiving NSAIAs in controlled clinical studies. These abnormalities may progress, may remain essentially unchanged, or may be transient with continued therapy. Hepatitis, jaundice, or liver failure has been reported in patients receiving celecoxib during postmarketing surveillance.

Precautions and Contraindications

Patients should be advised that celecoxib, like other NSAIAs, is not free of potential adverse effects, including some that can cause discomfort, and that more serious effects (e.g., myocardial infarction, stroke, GI bleeding), which may require hospitalization and may even be fatal, also can occur.

Patients should be advised to read the medication guide for NSAIAs that is provided to the patient each time the drug is dispensed.

Cardiovascular Precautions

NSAIAs, including selective COX-2 inhibitors and prototypical NSAIAs, increase the risk of serious adverse cardiovascular thrombotic events. (See Cardiovascular Effects under Cautions.) Although findings from some systematic reviews of controlled observational studies and meta-analyses of data from randomized studies of these drugs suggest that naproxen may be associated with a lower risk of cardiovascular thrombotic events compared with other NSAIAs, FDA states that definitive conclusions regarding relative risks of NSAIAs are not possible at this time. Until more data are available, decisions to use an NSAIA, including a selective COX-2 inhibitor (e.g., celecoxib), depend on individual assessment of risk for GI and cardiac toxicity and availability of alternative therapies. Some clinicians have suggested that use of a selective COX-2 inhibitor remains an appropriate choice for patients at low cardiovascular risk who have had serious GI events, especially while receiving a prototypical NSAIA. Some clinicians also suggest that it is prudent to avoid use of NSAIAs whenever possible in patients with cardiovascular disease. Celecoxib should be avoided in patients with recent myocardial infarction unless the benefits of therapy are expected to outweigh the risk of recurrent cardiovascular thrombotic events; if celecoxib is used in such patients, the patient should be monitored for cardiac ischemia. Additional studies, preferably randomized controlled trials, are required to more fully assess cardiovascular risks associated with individual NSAIAs in patients with established cardiovascular disease.

To minimize the potential risk of adverse cardiovascular events in patients receiving NSAIAs, the lowest effective dosage and shortest possible duration of therapy should be employed. Patients receiving NSAIAs (including those without previous symptoms of cardiovascular disease) should be monitored for the possible development of cardiovascular events throughout therapy. Patients should be informed about the signs and symptoms of serious cardiovascular toxicity (chest pain, dyspnea, weakness, slurring of speech) and instructed to seek immediate medical attention if such toxicity occurs.

There is no consistent evidence that concomitant use of low-dose aspirin mitigates the increased risk of serious cardiovascular events associated with NSAIAs. The overall risk for cardiovascular events in patients receiving a COX-2 inhibitor versus placebo or a prototypical NSAIA was not influenced by use of low-dose aspirin. Concomitant use of aspirin and celecoxib increases the risk for serious GI events. (See Nonsteroidal Anti-inflammatory Agents under Drug Interactions.)

Use of NSAIAs, including celecoxib, can result in the onset of hypertension or worsening of preexisting hypertension; either of these occurrences may contribute to the increased incidence of cardiovascular events. Patients receiving NSAIAs may have an impaired response to diuretics (i.e., thiazide or loop diuretics), angiotensin-converting enzyme (ACE) inhibitors, angiotensin II receptor antagonists, or β-adrenergic blocking agents. Blood pressure should be monitored closely during initiation of celecoxib therapy and throughout therapy.

Because NSAIAs increase morbidity and mortality in patients with heart failure, the manufacturer states that celecoxib should be avoided in patients with severe heart failure unless the benefits of therapy are expected to outweigh the risk of worsening heart failure; if celecoxib is used in such patients, the patient should be monitored for worsening heart failure. Some experts state that use of NSAIAs should be avoided whenever possible in patients with reduced left ventricular ejection fraction and current or prior symptoms of heart failure. Patients receiving NSAIAs should be advised to inform their clinician if they experience symptoms of heart failure, including dyspnea, unexplained weight gain, and edema. Use of NSAIAs may diminish the cardiovascular effects of certain drugs used to treat heart failure and edema (e.g., diuretics, ACE inhibitors, angiotensin II receptor antagonists). (See Drug Interactions.)

Use of celecoxib for longer than 6 months in children has not been systematically studied. It remains to be determined whether long-term cardiovascular risks in children exposed to celecoxib are similar to those observed in adults receiving celecoxib or other NSAIAs.

GI Precautions

The risk of potentially serious adverse GI effects should be considered in patients receiving celecoxib, particularly in patients receiving chronic therapy with the drug. (See GI Effects under Cautions.) Because peptic ulceration and/or GI bleeding have been reported in patients receiving the drug, patients should be advised to report promptly signs or symptoms of GI ulceration or bleeding to their clinician.

To minimize the potential risk of adverse GI effects, the lowest effective dosage and shortest possible duration of therapy should be employed, and use of more than one NSAIA at a time should be avoided. (See Nonsteroidal Anti-inflammatory Agents under Drug Interactions.) In addition, use of NSAIAs should be avoided in patients at higher risk (see GI Effects under Cautions) unless the benefits of therapy are expected to outweigh the increased risk of bleeding; for patients who are at high risk, as well as for those with active GI bleeding, alternative therapy other than an NSAIA should be considered.

Use of corticosteroids during NSAIA therapy may increase the risk of GI ulceration, and the drugs should be used concomitantly with caution.

Renal Precautions

Renal toxicity has been observed in patients in whom renal prostaglandins have a compensatory role in maintaining renal perfusion. Administration of an NSAIA to such patients may cause a dose-dependent reduction in prostaglandin formation and thereby precipitate overt renal decompensation. Patients at greatest risk of this reaction are those with impaired renal function, heart failure, or

hepatic dysfunction; those with extracellular fluid depletion (e.g., patients receiving diuretics); those taking an ACE inhibitor or angiotensin II antagonist concomitantly; and geriatric patients. Fluid depletion should be corrected prior to initiation of celecoxib therapy, and renal function should be monitored during celecoxib therapy in patients with renal or hepatic impairment, heart failure, dehydration, or hypovolemia. Patients should be advised to consult their clinician promptly if unexplained weight gain or edema occurs. Recovery of renal function to pretreatment levels usually occurs following discontinuance of NSAIA therapy.

Celecoxib has not been evaluated in patients with severe renal impairment, and the renal effects of the drug may hasten the progression of renal dysfunction in patients with preexisting renal disease. The manufacturers state that use of celecoxib is not recommended in patients with advanced renal disease. If celecoxib therapy must be used in patients with advanced renal disease, close monitoring of renal function is recommended.

Hepatic Precautions

Patients who experience signs and/or symptoms suggestive of liver dysfunction while receiving celecoxib should be evaluated for evidence of the development of a severe hepatic reaction. Severe, sometimes fatal, reactions, including fulminant hepatitis, liver necrosis, and hepatic failure, have been reported rarely in patients receiving NSAIAs. Celecoxib should be discontinued immediately if clinical signs and symptoms consistent with liver disease develop or if systemic manifestations (e.g., eosinophilia, rash) occur. (See Hepatic Effects under Cautions.) Patients receiving celecoxib should be instructed to report to their clinician any early signs or symptoms of possible hepatic dysfunction (e.g., fatigue, lethargy, nausea, pruritus, jaundice, right upper quadrant pain, flu-like symptoms). In addition, patients should be advised to discontinue celecoxib and contact their clinician immediately if any of these manifestations occur.

The manufacturers state that celecoxib has not been evaluated in patients with severe hepatic impairment, and use of the drug in such patients is not recommended.

Pharmacogenomic Precautions

In patients with the cytochrome P-450 isoenzyme 2C9 (CYP2C9) poor metabolizer phenotype, metabolism of celecoxib may be decreased substantially; the half-life of celecoxib is prolonged and higher plasma concentrations of the drug may increase the likelihood and/or severity of adverse effects. Metabolism of celecoxib may be moderately reduced in CYP2C9 intermediate metabolizers with a diplotype functional activity score (AS) of 1 and mildly reduced in those with an AS of 1.5. Higher plasma concentrations of the drug in intermediate metabolizers with an AS of 1 may increase the likelihood of adverse effects. The presence of other factors affecting clearance of the drug (e.g., hepatic impairment, advanced age) also may increase the risk of adverse effects in intermediate metabolizers. (See Pharmacogenomic Dosage Considerations under Dosage and Administration and also see Elimination under Pharmacokinetics.) The Clinical Pharmacogenetics Implementation Consortium Guideline (CPIC) for CYP2C9 and Nonsteroidal Anti-Inflammatory Drugs should be consulted for additional information on interpretation of CYP2C9 genotype testing.

Precautions Related to Dermatologic and Hypersensitivity Reactions

Anaphylactoid reactions have been reported in patients receiving celecoxib. Patients receiving celecoxib should be informed of the signs and symptoms of an anaphylactoid reaction (e.g., difficulty breathing, swelling of the face or throat) and advised to seek immediate medical attention if an anaphylactoid reaction develops.

Serious skin reactions (e.g., exfoliative dermatitis, Stevens-Johnson syndrome, toxic epidermal necrolysis, acute generalized exanthematous pustulosis) can occur in patients receiving celecoxib. These serious skin reactions can occur without warning and in patients without a history of sulfonamide sensitivity reactions; patients should be advised to consult their clinician if skin rash and blisters, fever, or other signs of hypersensitivity reaction (e.g., pruritus) occur. Celecoxib should be discontinued at the first appearance of rash or any other sign of hypersensitivity.

Multi-organ hypersensitivity (also known as drug reaction with eosinophilia and systemic symptoms [DRESS]), a potentially fatal or life-threatening syndrome, has been reported in patients receiving NSAIAs. The clinical presentation is variable, but typically includes eosinophilia, fever, rash, lymphadenopathy, and/or facial swelling, possibly associated with other organ system involvement such as hepatitis, nephritis, hematologic abnormalities, myocarditis, or myositis. Symptoms may resemble those of an acute viral infection. Early manifestations of hypersensitivity, such as fever or lymphadenopathy, may be present in the absence of rash. If such signs or symptoms develop, celecoxib should be discontinued and the patient evaluated immediately.

Hematologic Precautions

Use of NSAIAs, including celecoxib, has been associated with modest prolongation of activated partial thromboplastin time (aPTT) in children with systemic onset juvenile rheumatoid arthritis. Because of the risk of disseminated intravascular coagulation in children with systemic onset juvenile rheumatoid arthritis who are receiving celecoxib, these children should be monitored for clinical signs or symptoms of abnormal clotting or bleeding and with coagulation tests.

NSAIAs, including celecoxib, may increase the risk of bleeding. Patients with certain coexisting conditions such as coagulation disorders and those receiving concomitant therapy with anticoagulants, antiplatelet agents, or serotonin-reuptake inhibitors may be at increased risk and should be monitored for signs of bleeding. (See Drug Interactions.)

If signs and/or symptoms of anemia or blood loss occur during therapy with celecoxib, hemoglobin concentration and hematocrit should be determined.

Other Precautions

The possibility that the anti-inflammatory and, perhaps, antipyretic effects of NSAIAs may mask the usual signs and symptoms of infection should be considered.

Excessive use of drugs indicated for the management of acute migraine attacks (e.g., use of celecoxib, serotonin type 1 [5-HT$_1$] receptor agonists, ergotamine, opiate analgesics, or certain analgesic combinations on a regular basis for 10 or more days per month) may result in migraine-like daily headaches or a marked increase in the frequency of migraine attacks. Detoxification, including withdrawal of the overused drugs and treatment of withdrawal symptoms (which often include transient worsening of headaches), may be necessary. Patients should be encouraged to record the frequency of migraine headaches and medication use and to contact their clinician if the frequency of migraine attacks increases.

Because of similarity in spelling of Celexa® (citalopram hydrobromide), Celebrex® (celecoxib), and Cerebyx® (fosphenytoin sodium), extra care should be exercised in ensuring the accuracy of prescriptions for these drugs.

Patients receiving long-term NSAIA therapy should have a complete blood cell count and chemistry profile performed periodically.

When the fixed combination of celecoxib and amlodipine is used, the cautions, precautions, contraindications, and drug interactions associated with both drugs must be considered. For additional information on precautions and drug interactions related to use of amlodipine, see Amlodipine 24:28.08.

Contraindications

The manufacturer states that celecoxib is contraindicated in patients with known hypersensitivity (e.g., anaphylaxis, serious dermatologic reactions) to the drug or any ingredient in the formulation. In addition, celecoxib should not be given to patients who have experienced allergic-type reactions to sulfonamides. NSAIAs, including celecoxib, generally are contraindicated in patients in whom asthma, urticaria, or other sensitivity reactions are precipitated by aspirin or other NSAIAs, because there is potential for cross-sensitivity between NSAIAs and aspirin, and severe, often fatal, anaphylactic reactions may occur in such patients. Because patients with asthma may have aspirin-sensitivity asthma, patients with asthma but without known aspirin sensitivity who are receiving celecoxib should be monitored for changes in manifestations of asthma. In patients with asthma, aspirin sensitivity is manifested principally as bronchospasm and usually is associated with nasal polyps; the association of aspirin sensitivity, asthma, and nasal polyps is known as the aspirin triad.

Celecoxib is contraindicated in the setting of CABG surgery.

● Pediatric Precautions

Celecoxib is used for the management of the signs and symptoms of juvenile rheumatoid arthritis in children 2 years of age or older; safety and efficacy of celecoxib therapy beyond 6 months in pediatric patients with juvenile arthritis have not

been established. Celecoxib has been evaluated in pediatric patients 2–17 years of age with pauciarticular course, polyarticular course, or systemic onset juvenile rheumatoid arthritis in one clinical study. Celecoxib has not been studied in pediatric patients younger than 2 years of age, those weighing less than 10 kg, or children with active systemic disease. Alternative therapies for juvenile rheumatoid arthritis should be considered in pediatric patients known to be CYP2C9 poor metabolizers.

Safety and efficacy of celecoxib for the acute treatment of attacks of migraine have not been established in pediatric patients. In addition, safety and efficacy of celecoxib in fixed combination with amlodipine have not been established in pediatric patients.

Recommended pediatric dosages of celecoxib should achieve plasma concentrations of the drug that are similar to those achieved in the clinical study that demonstrated efficacy.

In the clinical study in pediatric patients with pauciarticular course, polyarticular course, or systemic onset juvenile rheumatoid arthritis (active systemic disease not present at study entry), children with systemic onset juvenile rheumatoid arthritis appeared to be at risk for the development of abnormal coagulation test results. Use of NSAIAs, including celecoxib, has been associated with modest prolongation of activated partial thromboplastin time (aPTT) in children with systemic onset juvenile rheumatoid arthritis. Because of the risk of disseminated intravascular coagulation in children with systemic onset juvenile rheumatoid arthritis who are receiving celecoxib, these children should be monitored for clinical signs or symptoms of abnormal clotting or bleeding and with coagulation tests.

It remains to be determined whether long-term cardiovascular risks in children exposed to celecoxib are similar to those observed in adults receiving celecoxib or other NSAIAs. (See Cardiovascular Effects under Cautions.)

● Geriatric Precautions

Geriatric patients are at increased risk for NSAIA-associated serious adverse cardiovascular, GI, and renal effects. In clinical trials evaluating celecoxib for acute treatment of migraine attacks, approximately 70 patients were 65 years of age or older, while in clinical trials evaluating celecoxib for other indications, more than 3300 patients were 65–74 years of age and about 1300 were 75 years of age and older. No overall differences in efficacy of celecoxib were observed between geriatric and younger patients. Although results from clinical studies indicated that renal (i.e., glomerular filtration rate, blood urea nitrogen, creatinine) and platelet function (i.e., bleeding time, platelet aggregation) in geriatric individuals receiving celecoxib did not differ from those in younger individuals, more of the spontaneous reports of fatal adverse GI effects and acute renal failure have been in geriatric individuals than in younger individuals. If it is determined that the anticipated benefits of celecoxib therapy outweigh the potential risks, celecoxib should be initiated at the lower end of the dosing range and patients should be monitored for adverse effects; if used for the acute treatment of migraine attacks, celecoxib should be used for the fewest possible number of days per month.

Peak plasma concentration and area under the plasma concentration-time curve (AUC) were increased 40 and 50%, respectively, in geriatric individuals (i.e., older than 65 years of age), but dosage adjustment in this age group based solely on age generally is not required. However, in geriatric patients weighing less than 50 kg, celecoxib therapy should be initiated at the lowest recommended dosage.

● Pregnancy, Fertility, and Lactation

Pregnancy

Use of NSAIAs during pregnancy at about 30 weeks of gestation or later can cause premature closure of the fetal ductus arteriosus, and use at about 20 weeks of gestation or later has been associated with fetal renal dysfunction resulting in oligohydramnios and, in some cases, neonatal renal impairment. Because of these risks, use of NSAIAs should be avoided in pregnant women at about 30 weeks of gestation or later; if NSAIA therapy is necessary between about 20 and 30 weeks of gestation, the lowest effective dosage and shortest possible duration of treatment should be used. Monitoring of amniotic fluid volume via ultrasound examination should be considered if the duration of NSAIA treatment exceeds 48 hours; if oligohydramnios occurs, the drug should be discontinued and follow-up instituted according to clinical practice. Pregnant women should be advised to avoid use of NSAIAs beginning at 20 weeks' gestation unless otherwise advised by a clinician; they should be informed that NSAIAs should be avoided beginning at 30 weeks' gestation because of the risk of premature closure of the fetal ductus arteriosus and that monitoring for oligohydramnios may be necessary if NSAIA therapy is required for longer than 48 hours' duration between about 20 and 30 weeks of gestation.

Known effects of NSAIAs on the human fetus during the third trimester of pregnancy include prenatal constriction of the ductus arteriosus, tricuspid incompetence, and pulmonary hypertension; nonclosure of the ductus arteriosus during the postnatal period (which may be resistant to medical management); and myocardial degenerative changes, platelet dysfunction with resultant bleeding, intracranial bleeding, renal dysfunction or renal failure, renal injury or dysgenesis potentially resulting in prolonged or permanent renal failure, oligohydramnios, GI bleeding or perforation, and increased risk of necrotizing enterocolitis.

Fetal renal dysfunction resulting in oligohydramnios and, in some cases, neonatal renal impairment has been observed, on average, following days to weeks of maternal NSAIA use, although oligohydramnios has been observed infrequently as early as 48 hours after initiation of NSAIA therapy. Oligohydramnios is often, but not always, reversible (generally within 3–6 days) following discontinuance of NSAIA therapy. Complications of prolonged oligohydramnios may include limb contracture and delayed lung maturation. A limited number of case reports have described maternal NSAIA use and neonatal renal dysfunction, in some cases irreversible, without oligohydramnios. Some cases of neonatal renal dysfunction have required treatment with invasive procedures such as exchange transfusion or dialysis. Deaths associated with neonatal renal failure have been reported. Methodologic limitations of these postmarketing studies and case reports include lack of a control group; limited information regarding dosage, duration, and timing of drug exposure; and concomitant use of other drugs. These limitations preclude establishing a reliable estimate of the risk of adverse fetal and neonatal outcomes with maternal NSAIA use. Available data on neonatal outcomes generally involved preterm infants, and the extent to which certain reported risks can be generalized to full-term infants is uncertain.

Animal data indicate that prostaglandins have an important role in endometrial vascular permeability, blastocyst implantation, and decidualization. In animal studies, inhibitors of prostaglandin synthesis, such as celecoxib, were associated with increased pre- and post-implantation losses. Prostaglandins also have an important role in fetal kidney development. In animal studies, inhibitors of prostaglandin synthesis impaired kidney development at clinically relevant doses.

An increased incidence of fetuses with ventricular septal defects, sternebral fusion, rib fusion, and sternebrae abnormality was observed in reproduction studies in rabbits receiving oral celecoxib dosages of 150 mg/kg daily or more throughout organogenesis (exposure approximately twice the usual human dosage of 200 mg twice daily, expressed in terms of AUC [0–24 hours]). A dose-dependent increase in diaphragmatic hernias was observed in rats receiving oral celecoxib dosages of 30 mg/kg or more daily throughout organogenesis (exposure approximately sixfold the usual human dosage of 200 mg twice daily, expressed in terms of AUC [0–24 hours]). Reproduction studies in rats using oral dosages up to 100 mg/kg daily (exposure approximately sevenfold the usual human dosage of 200 mg twice daily, expressed in terms of AUC [0–24 hours]) did not reveal evidence of delayed labor or parturition. In rats receiving oral celecoxib dosages of 50 mg/kg or more daily (exposure approximately sixfold the usual human dosage of 200 mg twice daily, expressed in terms of AUC [0–24 hours]), pre- and post-implantation losses and reduced embryonic/fetal survival were observed.

The effects of celecoxib on labor and delivery are unknown. In studies in rats, drugs that inhibit prostaglandin synthesis, including NSAIAs, increased the incidence of dystocia, delayed parturition, and decreased pup survival.

Fertility

Use of NSAIAs, including celecoxib, may delay or prevent ovarian follicular rupture, which has been associated with reversible infertility in some women. Reversible delays in ovulation have been observed in limited studies in women receiving NSAIAs, and animal studies indicate that inhibitors of prostaglandin synthesis can disrupt prostaglandin-mediated follicular rupture required for ovulation. Therefore, withdrawal of celecoxib should be considered in women who are experiencing difficulty conceiving or are undergoing evaluation of infertility.

Studies in female and male rats using celecoxib dosages up to 600 mg/kg daily (exposure approximately 11-fold the usual human dosage of 200 mg twice daily, expressed in terms of AUC [0–24 hours]) have not revealed evidence of impaired fertility.

Lactation

Celecoxib is distributed into milk in small amounts. Limited data obtained from nursing women receiving celecoxib indicate that the calculated average infant exposure to the drug is 10–40 mcg/kg daily, which is less than 1% of the weight-based therapeutic dosage for a 2-year-old child. Maternal use of celecoxib was not associated with adverse effects in 2 breast-fed infants 17 and 22 months of age. It is not known whether celecoxib affects milk production. The developmental and health benefits of breast-feeding should be considered along with the mother's clinical need for celecoxib and any potential adverse effects on the breast-fed infant from the drug or from the underlying maternal condition.

DRUG INTERACTIONS

● *Drugs Affecting or Metabolized by Hepatic Microsomal Enzymes*

Metabolism of celecoxib is mediated by the cytochrome P-450 (CYP) isoenzyme 2C9, and the possibility exists that drugs that inhibit this enzyme (e.g., fluconazole, fluvastatin, zafirlukast) may affect the pharmacokinetics of celecoxib, thereby increasing celecoxib exposure and toxicity. Drugs that induce CYP2C9 (e.g., rifampin) may reduce efficacy of celecoxib. Adjustment of celecoxib dosage may be required in patients receiving concomitant therapy with CYP2C9 inhibitors or inducers.

In addition, celecoxib inhibits CYP2D6, and the possibility exists that celecoxib may alter the pharmacokinetics of drugs metabolized by this isoenzyme, including various β-adrenergic blocking agents, many tricyclic and other antidepressants, various antipsychotic agents, atomoxetine, and some antiarrhythmics (e.g., encainide, flecainide), potentially increasing exposure to and toxicity of these drugs. Dosage adjustments may be required.

Results of in vitro studies indicate that celecoxib is not a substrate for CYP2D6, and the drug does not inhibit the CYP2C9, CYP2C19, or CYP3A4 isoenzymes.

Fluconazole

Concomitant administration of celecoxib with fluconazole can result in substantially increased plasma concentrations of celecoxib. This pharmacokinetic interaction appears to occur because fluconazole inhibits the CYP2C9 isoenzyme involved in celecoxib metabolism. In one study, concomitant administration of fluconazole (200 mg daily) and celecoxib (a single 200-mg dose) increased plasma concentrations of celecoxib twofold.

Other Drugs Affecting Hepatic Microsomal Enzymes

In clinical studies, concomitant administration of celecoxib with glyburide, ketoconazole, phenytoin, or tolbutamide did not alter the pharmacokinetics and/or pharmacodynamics of these drugs, and no clinically important interactions have been reported.

● *Antacids*

Administration of an antacid containing magnesium or aluminum with celecoxib decreased peak plasma concentrations of celecoxib by 37% and the area under the plasma concentration-time curve (AUC) by 10% in clinical studies. However, the manufacturer makes no specific recommendation for administration of the drug with regard to antacids because these effects are not considered clinically important.

● *Anticoagulants*

Anticoagulants, such as warfarin, and nonsteroidal anti-inflammatory agents (NSAIAs) have synergistic effects on GI bleeding. Concomitant use of celecoxib and anticoagulants is associated with a higher risk of serious bleeding compared with use of either agent alone. In one short-term (7-day) premarketing study in healthy individuals, celecoxib (200 mg twice daily) did not appear to alter the anticoagulant effect of warfarin (2–5 mg daily) as determined by the prothrombin time (PT). However, during postmarketing surveillance, bleeding complications associated with increases in PT were reported in some (mainly geriatric) patients receiving celecoxib concomitantly with warfarin. Therefore, patients receiving such concomitant therapy should be monitored appropriately for changes in anticoagulant activity (e.g., PT), particularly during the first few days after initiating or altering therapy, and for signs of bleeding.

Because reduced CYP2C9 function is associated with an increased risk of major bleeding or supratherapeutic international normalized ratio (INR) in patients receiving concomitant therapy with warfarin (a CYP2C9 substrate) and NSAIAs, some experts state that concomitant use of warfarin and NSAIAs should be avoided in patients who are CYP2C9 intermediate or poor metabolizers.

● Antihypertensive Agents

Concomitant use of NSAIAs with angiotensin-converting enzyme (ACE) inhibitors, angiotensin II receptor antagonists, or β-adrenergic blocking agents may reduce the blood pressure response to the antihypertensive agent. Therefore, blood pressure should be monitored to ensure that target blood pressure is achieved.

Concomitant use of celecoxib with ACE inhibitors or angiotensin II receptor antagonists in geriatric patients or patients with volume depletion or renal impairment may result in reversible deterioration of renal function, including possible acute renal failure; such patients should be monitored for signs of worsening renal function. Patients receiving concomitant therapy with celecoxib and ACE inhibitors or angiotensin II receptor antagonists should be adequately hydrated, and renal function should be assessed when concomitant therapy is initiated and periodically thereafter.

● Corticosteroids

Concomitant use of celecoxib and corticosteroids may increase the risk of GI ulceration or bleeding. Patients should be monitored for signs of bleeding.

● Cyclosporine

Concomitant use of celecoxib and cyclosporine may increase cyclosporine-associated nephrotoxicity. Patients should be monitored for signs of worsening renal function.

● Digoxin

Concomitant use of celecoxib and digoxin has been reported to result in increased serum concentrations and prolonged half-life of digoxin. Serum digoxin concentrations should be monitored.

● Diuretics

NSAIAs may interfere with the natriuretic response to diuretics with activity that depends in part on prostaglandin-mediated alterations in renal blood flow (e.g., furosemide, thiazides). (See Renal, Electrolyte, and Genitourinary Effects under Cautions and also see Renal Effects under Pharmacology.) Patients receiving concomitant celecoxib and diuretic therapy should be monitored for signs of worsening renal function and for adequacy of diuretic and antihypertensive effects.

● Glyburide

In clinical studies, concomitant administration of celecoxib with glyburide did not alter the pharmacokinetics and/or pharmacodynamics of glyburide, and no clinically important interactions have been reported.

● Lithium

Celecoxib and other NSAIAs can decrease renal clearance of lithium, which may lead to increased serum or plasma lithium concentrations. The mechanism involved in the reduction of lithium clearance by NSAIAs is not known, but has been attributed to inhibition of prostaglandin synthesis, which may interfere with the renal elimination of lithium by increasing sodium retention and thus lithium reabsorption; alternatively, inhibition of prostaglandin synthesis may reduce renal blood flow and glomerular filtration rate. In a study in healthy individuals, concomitant administration of celecoxib (200 mg daily) with lithium carbonate (450 mg twice daily) increased the mean steady-state plasma concentrations of lithium by about 17% compared with administration of lithium alone. Patients receiving lithium and celecoxib concomitantly should be monitored for signs of lithium toxicity.

● Methotrexate

Concomitant use of NSAIAs and methotrexate may increase the risk for methotrexate toxicity (e.g., neutropenia, thrombocytopenia, renal dysfunction). Although concomitant administration of celecoxib with methotrexate during clinical studies did not alter the pharmacokinetics of methotrexate, patients receiving concomitant celecoxib and methotrexate therapy should be monitored for methotrexate toxicity.

● Nonsteroidal Anti-inflammatory Agents

In controlled clinical trials, concomitant use of NSAIAs and analgesic dosages of aspirin did not produce any greater therapeutic effect than use of NSAIAs alone. However, concomitant use of aspirin and an NSAIA increases the risk for bleeding and serious GI events. Because of the potential for increased adverse effects, concomitant use of celecoxib with other NSAIAs or with analgesic dosages of aspirin generally is not recommended.

Patients receiving celecoxib should be advised not to take low-dose aspirin without consulting their clinician. Although celecoxib may be used with low doses of aspirin, concomitant use of the 2 NSAIAs may increase the incidence of GI ulceration or other complications compared with that associated with celecoxib alone. (See GI Effects under Cautions.) Celecoxib is not a substitute for low-dose aspirin therapy for prophylaxis of cardiovascular events, and patients receiving antiplatelet agents such as aspirin concomitantly with celecoxib should be monitored closely for bleeding. In studies in healthy individuals and in patients with osteoarthritis and established heart disease, celecoxib (200–400 mg daily) did not interfere with the cardioprotective antiplatelet effect of aspirin (100–325 mg). There is no consistent evidence that use of low-dose aspirin mitigates the increased risk of serious cardiovascular events associated with NSAIAs.

● Pemetrexed

Concomitant use of celecoxib and pemetrexed may increase the risk of pemetrexed-associated myelosuppression, renal toxicity, and GI toxicity. Administration of NSAIAs with short elimination half-lives (e.g., diclofenac, indomethacin) should be avoided beginning 2 days before and continuing through 2 days after pemetrexed administration. In the absence of data regarding potential interactions between pemetrexed and NSAIAs with longer half-lives (e.g., meloxicam, nabumetone), administration of NSAIAs with longer half-lives should be interrupted beginning at least 5 days before and continuing through 2 days after pemetrexed administration. Patients with renal impairment with a creatinine clearance of 45–79 mL/minute should be monitored for myelosuppression, renal toxicity, and GI toxicity if they receive concomitant celecoxib and pemetrexed therapy.

● Serotonin-reuptake Inhibitors

Serotonin release by platelets plays an important role in hemostasis. Results of case-control and epidemiologic cohort studies indicate that concomitant use of NSAIAs and drugs that interfere with serotonin reuptake may potentiate the risk of bleeding beyond that associated with an NSAIA alone. Patients receiving concomitant therapy with celecoxib and selective serotonin-reuptake inhibitors (SSRIs) or selective serotonin- and norepinephrine-reuptake inhibitors (SNRIs) should be monitored for signs of bleeding.

ACUTE TOXICITY

Limited information is available on the acute toxicity of celecoxib in humans. Serious toxicity was not observed in 12 individuals who received celecoxib 2.4 g daily for 10 days.

● Manifestations

Overdosage of NSAIAs can cause lethargy, drowsiness, nausea, vomiting, and epigastric pain; these manifestations generally are reversible with supportive care. GI bleeding also has been reported. Rarely, hypertension, acute renal failure, respiratory depression, and coma may occur.

● Treatment

Treatment of NSAIA overdosage involves symptomatic and supportive care; there is no specific antidote for NSAIA overdosage. During the first 4 hours after overdosage, emesis and/or administration of activated charcoal (60–100 g in adults or 1–2 g/kg in children) and/or an osmotic cathartic may be useful in symptomatic patients or in those who reportedly ingested a large overdosage. It is not known whether celecoxib is removed by hemodialysis, but the drug's extensive protein binding suggests that forced diuresis, alkalinization of urine, hemodialysis, or hemoperfusion is likely to be ineffective in removing substantial amounts of celecoxib from the body.

PHARMACOLOGY

● Mechanism of Action

Celecoxib is a selective inhibitor of the cyclooxygenase-2 (COX-2) isoform of prostaglandin endoperoxide synthase (prostaglandin G/H synthase, PGHS) and exhibits many of the pharmacologic actions of prototypical NSAIAs, including anti-inflammatory, analgesic, and antipyretic activity. NSAIAs appear to inhibit prostaglandin synthesis via inhibition of cyclooxygenase (COX); at least 2 isoenzymes, cyclooxygenase-1 (COX-1) and -2 (COX-2) (also referred to as PGHS-1 and -2, respectively), have been identified that catalyze the formation of prostaglandins in the arachidonic acid pathway. Although the exact mechanisms have not been clearly established, NSAIAs appear to exert anti-inflammatory, analgesic, and antipyretic activity principally through inhibition of the COX-2 isoenzyme; COX-1 inhibition presumably is responsible for the drugs' unwanted effects on GI mucosa. While prototypical NSAIAs are nonselective, inhibiting both COX-1 and COX-2 to varying degrees, celecoxib's highly selective inhibition of COX-2 potentially may be associated with a decreased risk of certain adverse effects (e.g., on GI mucosa); however, additional experience is needed to evaluate fully the adverse effect profile of the drug.

COX-1 is a constitutive enzyme that is expressed in most tissues, blood monocytes, and platelets; COX-1 is involved in thrombogenesis (e.g., promotion of platelet aggregation), maintenance of the gastric mucosal barrier, and renal function (e.g., maintenance of renal perfusion). COX-2 is an inducible enzyme that is found principally at sites of inflammation, although it also is expressed constitutively in the brain, kidney, and reproductive organs. COX-2 is expressed within 2–12 hours in response to cytokines and growth factors. At clinically relevant concentrations, celecoxib inhibits COX-2 in a slow, time-dependent manner involving formation of a tight enzyme-inhibitor complex that is noncovalent but only slowly dissociable. The celecoxib IC_{50}s (concentrations that inhibit enzyme activity by 50%) for COX-1 and COX-2 are 15 and 0.04 μM, respectively; the ED_{50} (dose that results in an effect in 50% of individuals tested) for COX-1 exceeds 200 mg/kg and, for COX-2, 0.2 mg/kg. The ratios of the IC_{50}s and ED_{50}s for COX-1 and COX-2 are 375 and greater than 1000, respectively, indicating that celecoxib is a highly selective COX-2 inhibitor. When celecoxib is administered in the management of osteoarthritis and rheumatoid arthritis, the principal physiologic action of the drug is inhibition of COX-2; celecoxib does not inhibit COX-1 when given in recommended dosages.

● Anti-inflammatory, Analgesic, and Antipyretic Effects

The anti-inflammatory, analgesic, and antipyretic effects of celecoxib and prototypical NSAIAs appear to result from inhibition of prostaglandin synthesis. While the precise mechanism of the anti-inflammatory and analgesic effects of NSAIAs continues to be investigated, these effects appear to be mediated principally through inhibition of the COX-2 isoenzyme at sites of inflammation with subsequent reduction in the synthesis of certain prostaglandins from their arachidonic acid precursors. Evidence supporting the role of COX-2 in inflammation includes up-regulation of COX-2 expression by mediators of inflammation, including cytokines and bacterial endotoxin. In addition, anti-inflammatory glucocorticoids can selectively inhibit cytokine and endotoxin induction of COX-2 while having no effect on expression of COX-1. Selective inhibitors of COX-2 block prostaglandin production and acute tissue inflammation in vivo, and studies in animals suggest that the anti-inflammatory and analgesic properties of selective COX-2 inhibitor NSAIAs are similar to those of prototypical NSAIAs that inhibit both COX-1 and COX-2. Clinical evidence also indicates that COX-2 has an important role in joint inflammation because highly selective COX-2 inhibitor NSAIAs are as effective as prototypical NSAIAs in the management of rheumatoid arthritis and osteoarthritis.

The precise mechanism of action by which celecoxib exerts therapeutic effects in the acute treatment of migraine attacks is not fully understood but may involve inhibition of prostaglandin synthesis, primarily via inhibition of COX-2.

Studies in animals indicate that celecoxib exerts antipyretic activity at concentrations that inhibit COX-2 in vitro.

● Renal Effects

NSAIAs have been associated with reductions in renal blood flow and glomerular filtration rate (GFR) and with sodium retention and hyperkalemia. These effects have been attributed to inhibition of renal prostaglandin synthesis in states of low renal reserve when prostaglandin-related physiologic mechanisms are needed to support renal function. Hyperkalemia also has occurred in some patients without renal impairment, and these effects have been attributed to a hyporenin-hypoaldosterone state.

COX-1 is located in the arteries and arterioles, glomeruli, and collecting ducts of the kidney and is believed to be important in the maintenance of renal blood flow. The location and role of COX-2 in the human kidney remains to be determined, but results of animal studies indicate that COX-2 may be important in the regulation of sodium, volume, and blood pressure homeostasis, and in postnatal renal development. Although the effects of celecoxib on renal function were expected to differ from those of prototypical NSAIAs, results of renal pharmacodynamic and clinical studies indicate that the renal effects of selective inhibitors of COX-2 (e.g., celecoxib) are similar to those of prototypical NSAIAs with respect to renal regulation of sodium excretion, blood pressure, and GFR. In healthy geriatric adults (65–85 years of age), a group likely to have compromised renal function, and in patients with renal impairment (serum creatinine 1.3–3 mg/dL, GFR 40–60 mL/minute per 1.73 m²), celecoxib had minimal effects on renal function.

Current evidence suggests that primary dysmenorrhea is mediated by prostaglandins. Substantially higher concentrations of prostaglandins have been found in the endometrium and menstrual fluid of women with primary dysmenorrhea (painful menses without demonstrable pelvic abnormality) compared with women without primary dysmenorrhea, and the amount of prostaglandin F_2 in menstrual fluid correlates with symptom severity (i.e., cramps, pain). Whether increased production of prostaglandins associated with primary dysmenorrhea is mediated by COX-1 or -2 remains to be determined. Prototypical NSAIAs that inhibit COX-1 and -2 and selective inhibitors of COX-2 (e.g., celecoxib) have been effective in relieving menstrual pain.

Limited evidence indicates that inhibition of COX-2 might interfere with ovulation.

● GI Effects

Therapy with prototypical NSAIAs has been associated with gastric mucosal damage; these effects have been attributed to inhibition of the synthesis of prostaglandins produced by COX-1. Other factors possibly involved in NSAIA-induced gastropathy include local irritation, promotion of acid back-diffusion into gastric mucosa, uncoupling of oxidative phosphorylation, and enterohepatic recirculation of the drugs. Because celecoxib is a selective inhibitor of COX-2, the drug is not expected to produce gastric mucosal damage typical of prototypical NSAIAs. Short-term administration of celecoxib has been associated with a lower incidence of adverse upper GI effects and endoscopically confirmed GI ulcer than prototypical NSAIAs. Whether long-term therapy with celecoxib is associated with a better GI safety profile than therapy with prototypical NSAIAs remains to be established. Limited evidence (e.g., from animal studies) indicates that COX-2 may contribute to healing of GI ulcers and that inhibition of COX-2 might interfere with epithelial cell proliferation, angiogenesis, and maturation of granular tissue at regions of ulcer repair and thus may delay healing of gastric ulcers.

The effect, if any, of selective COX-2 inhibitors in patients with inflammatory bowel disease remains to be established.

Epidemiologic and laboratory studies suggest that NSAIAs may reduce the risk of colon cancer. The exact mechanism by which NSAIAs may inhibit colon carcinogenesis has not been fully determined, and inhibition of COX-1 and/or COX-2 or inhibition of other cellular targets of NSAIAs may be involved. Several lines of evidence suggest that inhibition of COX-2 by NSAIAs may play an important role in this effect, although pathways that do not involve cyclooxygenase also may be involved. Overexpression of COX-2 has been observed in colon tumors in rodents and humans and there is evidence that COX-2 contributes to tumorigenesis. Although the specific cellular pathways responsible for the effects of COX-2 on tumorigenesis remain to be determined, the enzyme apparently mediates mitogenic growth factor signaling and down-regulates apoptosis, thus promoting tumor growth. Biopsy specimens from patients with colorectal cancer (adenocarcinomas) indicate that COX-2 is present in and around colorectal tumors and the degree of expression of COX-2 correlates positively with Duke's stage and tumor size; COX-2 was not present in control tissue from patients without colorectal cancer. The distribution of COX-2 in colorectal tumors suggests that inhibition of COX-2 has the potential to restore apoptosis and prevent proliferation of colon cancer cells. Induction of apoptosis by inhibition of COX-2 may be important in reducing the number of adenomatous colorectal polyps in patients with familial adenomatous polyposis (FAP), a disorder in which apoptosis is believed to be attenuated, and there is some evidence that celecoxib and some other NSAIAs can reduce the size and number of colorectal polyps in patients with FAP. Studies using genetic and carcinogen-induced rodent models of colon cancer indicate that NSAIAs can decrease both the incidence and multiplicity of colon tumors and decrease the overall colon tumor burden and that celecoxib is more effective than prototypical NSAIAs (e.g., aspirin, ibuprofen, piroxicam, sulindac) in these models.

● Hematologic Effects

Unlike prototypical NSAIAs, celecoxib administered in single doses up to 800 mg and in multiple doses of 600 mg twice daily for up to 7 days does not appear to inhibit platelet aggregation or prolong bleeding time. However, bleeding complications have been reported during postmarketing surveillance in some patients with elevated PTs receiving concomitant warfarin therapy. (See Anticoagulants under Drug Interactions.)

It has been postulated that selective COX-2 inhibitors may increase cardiovascular thrombotic risk because they block synthesis of prostacyclin (which is antithrombotic) but leave generation of thromboxane A_2 (which is prothrombotic) unaffected, thereby allowing platelet aggregation and hemostasis to occur unopposed; in contrast, prototypical NSAIAs suppress synthesis of both prostacyclin and thromboxane A_2. However, individual prototypical NSAIAs vary in degree of selectivity for COX-1 relative to COX-2, and both selective COX-2 inhibitors and prototypical NSAIAs have been associated with increased risk of cardiovascular events. Because NSAIAs differ in their selectivity for the COX-2 enzyme and their potency as inhibitors of COX-2, effects of individual NSAIAs on the balance between suppression of prostacyclin and thromboxane A_2 may differ. Rofecoxib is one of the most potent COX-2 inhibitors; rofecoxib also is one of the most selective COX-2 inhibitors in vitro. Celecoxib is less selective than rofecoxib or valdecoxib. The clinical relevance of differences in COX-2 selectivity and potency of individual NSAIAs with regard to cardiovascular thrombotic risk remains to be fully determined.

PHARMACOKINETICS

The pharmacokinetics of celecoxib have been studied principally in healthy adults and in adults with acute pain, rheumatoid arthritis, or osteoarthritis. Certain pharmacokinetic parameters of celecoxib (i.e., peak plasma concentration, area under the plasma concentration-time curve [AUC]) are approximately dose proportional when the drug is administered to fasting adults in dosages up to 200 mg twice daily. However, there is a less-than-proportional increase in peak plasma concentration and AUC when the drug is administered to fasting adults in dosages exceeding 200 mg twice daily; this effect has been attributed to the low aqueous solubility of celecoxib. Limited data indicate that the pharmacokinetics of celecoxib are affected by advanced age, renal and/or hepatic function, and race. (See Absorption under Pharmacokinetics.)

● Absorption

Celecoxib is well absorbed from the GI tract, and peak plasma concentrations of the drug generally are attained within 3 hours after dosing in fasting individuals. Absolute bioavailability of celecoxib has not been determined. Following oral administration of a single 200-mg dose of celecoxib in healthy, fasting adults 19–52 years of age, peak plasma concentrations of the drug averaged 705 ng/mL. Bioavailability (AUC) was increased 10–20% and time to reach peak plasma concentrations of celecoxib was delayed by 1–2 hours when the commercially available 200-mg capsules were administered with a high-fat meal (24 g fat) compared with administration with a medium-fat meal (8 g fat) or under fasting conditions. In addition, AUC and plasma concentration 12 hours after the dose were slightly (about 10%) higher when the drug was given in the evening versus the morning. When a celecoxib capsule is opened and the contents sprinkled over applesauce prior to administration, the pharmacokinetic profile of the drug (i.e., AUC, peak plasma concentration, time to peak plasma concentration, plasma elimination half-life) is similar to that following oral administration of the intact capsule. Following oral administration of celecoxib at recommended dosages (200–400 mg daily), steady-state plasma concentrations are achieved within 5 days. Drug

accumulation has not been observed in individuals receiving celecoxib 400 mg twice daily.

Following oral administration of tablets containing celecoxib in fixed combination with amlodipine, peak concentrations of celecoxib were attained within 2 hours, and the rate and extent of absorption of celecoxib were similar under fed and fasting conditions.

Celecoxib oral solution has a faster rate of absorption and increased bioavailability as compared with celecoxib oral capsules. Following administration of celecoxib 120 mg as an oral solution in healthy, fasting individuals, the median time to peak plasma concentration was 1 hour. When the oral solution was administered with a high-fat meal, the median time to peak plasma concentration was delayed by 2 hours and peak plasma concentration was decreased by approximately 50% compared with administration under fasting conditions, with no change in total exposure (AUC). However, in the principal clinical trials establishing efficacy of celecoxib oral solution for acute treatment of migraine, the drug was administered without regard to food.

Following oral administration of celecoxib capsules at recommended dosages in geriatric individuals older than 65 years of age, peak plasma concentration and AUC were increased 40 and 50%, respectively, compared with younger adults. Peak plasma celecoxib concentration and AUC values were higher in geriatric women than geriatric men, predominantly because of the lower body weight of these women. Analysis of pooled pharmacokinetic data indicates that the AUC of celecoxib, administered as capsules, is about 40% higher in Blacks compared with Whites; the cause and clinical importance of this finding are not known.

Limited information is available on the pharmacokinetics of celecoxib in patients with mild to moderate hepatic and/or renal impairment. AUC of celecoxib at steady state reportedly was increased 40 or 180% in individuals with mild (Child-Pugh class A) or moderate (Child-Pugh class B) hepatic impairment, respectively, receiving celecoxib as capsules compared with that in healthy adults with normal hepatic function. In adults with chronic renal insufficiency (glomerular filtration rates of 35–60 mL/minute), AUC of celecoxib administered as capsules reportedly was 40% lower than that in adults with normal renal function.

● Distribution

Distribution of celecoxib into body tissues and fluids has not been fully characterized. The apparent volume of distribution of celecoxib at steady state is about 400 L (about 7.14 L/kg), suggesting extensive tissue distribution.

At therapeutic plasma concentrations, celecoxib is about 97% bound to plasma proteins, principally albumin and to a lesser extent, α_1-acid glycoprotein. Celecoxib is not preferentially bound to erythrocytes in blood.

It is not known whether celecoxib crosses the placenta in humans. Although it also is not known whether celecoxib is distributed into human milk, the drug is distributed into milk in rats in concentrations similar to those in plasma.

● Elimination

The plasma elimination half-life of celecoxib following oral administration of a single 200-mg dose under fasting conditions is about 11 hours, and the apparent plasma clearance of the drug is about 500 mL/minute; these parameters exhibit wide intraindividual variability, presumably because the low aqueous solubility of celecoxib prolongs absorption. The mean apparent elimination half-life of celecoxib following administration as an oral solution is approximately 6 hours independent of dosing condition and is similar to that observed for celecoxib capsules administered under fed conditions. The half-life of celecoxib is prolonged in patients with renal or hepatic impairment and has been reported to be 13.1 hours in patients with chronic renal insufficiency and 11 or 13.1 hours in patients with mild or moderate hepatic impairment, respectively.

The metabolic fate of celecoxib has not been fully determined, but the drug is metabolized in the liver to inactive metabolites principally by the cytochrome P-450 (CYP) isoenzyme 2C9. Metabolism of celecoxib involves hydroxylation of the 4-methyl group to form a primary alcohol (SC-60613), followed by oxidation of the primary alcohol to the corresponding carboxylic acid (SC-62807), the major metabolite. The carboxylic acid metabolite is conjugated with glucuronic acid to some extent, forming the 1-O-glucuronide. Metabolites of celecoxib do not have pharmacologic activity as cyclooxygenase-1 (COX-1) or COX-2 inhibitors.

In patients with the CYP2C9 poor metabolizer phenotype, the metabolic clearance of celecoxib may be decreased substantially and plasma concentrations may be increased. Metabolism may be moderately or mildly decreased in patients with the CYP2C9 intermediate metabolizer phenotype with a diplotype activity score (AS) of 1 or 1.5, respectively. (See Pharmacogenomic Precautions under Cautions.) Limited data indicate that celecoxib concentrations are increased threefold to sevenfold in individuals with the homozygous CYP2C9*3/*3 diplotype compared with individuals with a diplotype of CYP2C9*1/*1 or CYP2C9*1/*3. Data are lacking in individuals with other CYP2C9 polymorphisms, such as *2, *5, *6, *9, and *11.

Oral clearance of celecoxib appears to increase in a less-than-proportional manner with increasing weight; pediatric patients with juvenile rheumatoid arthritis weighing 10 or 25 kg are predicted to have a 40 or 24% lower clearance, respectively, than a 70-kg adult with rheumatoid arthritis.

Celecoxib is excreted in urine and feces principally as metabolites; less than 3% of the dose is excreted unchanged. Following oral administration of a single 300-mg dose of radiolabeled celecoxib as an oral suspension (not commercially available in the US), approximately 27 and 57% of the dose was excreted in urine and feces, respectively. The principal metabolite in both urine and feces was the carboxylic acid metabolite (73% of the dose); small amounts of the glucuronide metabolite were present in urine.

CHEMISTRY AND STABILITY

● *Chemistry*

Celecoxib, a diaryl substituted pyrazole derivative containing a sulfonamide substituent, is a nonsteroidal anti-inflammatory agent (NSAIA). Celecoxib is a selective inhibitor of cyclooxygenase-2 (COX-2). Because the goal of selective inhibitors of COX-2 is to inhibit COX-2 but not COX-1, the drugs also have been referred to as COX-1-sparing NSAIAs. Celecoxib differs chemically and, to some extent, pharmacologically from prototypical NSAIAs, which inhibit cyclooxygenase-1 (COX-1) and -2 (COX-2).

Celecoxib consists of a central pyrazole ring, 2 substituted aromatic rings, and a benzenesulfonamide attached to one of the rings. Spatial orientation of the 2 aromatic rings relative to the central ring is important for cyclooxygenase inhibitory activity; the 2 aromatic rings must reside at adjacent positions on the central ring for COX-2 activity. Unlike most prototypical NSAIAs, celecoxib does not contain a carboxylate group; it has been postulated that absence of such a group may contribute to the drug's high COX-2 selectivity.

Although the overall structures of COX-1 and COX-2 are similar, a principal difference between the 2 isoforms of cyclooxygenase is the presence of a much larger NSAIA binding site on COX-2 compared with the NSAIA binding site on COX-1. The larger binding site on COX-2 results from the substitution of valine for isoleucine at position 523 in COX-2. It has been postulated that the smaller valine molecule, unlike the larger isoleucine molecule in COX-1, gives access to a side pocket that may be the binding site for many selective COX-2 inhibitors, including celecoxib. It appears that the benzenesulfonamide moiety of celecoxib binds to the side pocket, although diaryl heterocyclic compounds, including celecoxib, may have multiple modes of binding to cyclooxygenases.

Celecoxib occurs as an odorless, white to off-white crystalline powder. The aqueous solubility of celecoxib at a pH less than 9 is about 5 mcg/mL at 5–40°C. Solubility of the drug increases in strongly basic solutions; celecoxib has a solubility of 0.8 mg/mL in water at 40°C and pH 12. The drug has a solubility of 111 mg/mL in alcohol at room temperature.

● *Stability*

Commercially available celecoxib capsules should be stored at 25°C, but may be exposed to temperatures ranging from 15–30°C. When stored as directed, the capsules have an expiration date of 2 years following the date of manufacture. When a celecoxib capsule is opened and the contents mixed with applesauce, the mixture is stable for 6 hours when refrigerated.

The commercially available celecoxib oral solution should be stored at 20–25°C, but may be exposed to temperatures ranging from 15–30°C. The oral solution should not be refrigerated or frozen, and any unused portion remaining in the disposable unit-dose glass bottle should be discarded immediately after use.

Tablets containing celecoxib in fixed combination with amlodipine should be stored at 20–25°C.

PREPARATIONS

Because of similarity in spelling of Celexa® (citalopram hydrobromide), Celebrex® (celecoxib), and Cerebyx® (fosphenytoin sodium), extra care should be exercised in ensuring the accuracy of prescriptions for these drugs.

Excipients in commercially available drug preparations may have clinically important effects in some individuals; consult specific product labeling for details.

Celecoxib

Oral		
Capsules	50 mg*	**CeleBREX®**, Pfizer
		Celecoxib Capsules
	100 mg*	**CeleBREX®**, Pfizer
		Celecoxib Capsules
	200 mg*	**CeleBREX®**, Pfizer
		Celecoxib Capsules
	400 mg*	**CeleBREX®**, Pfizer
		Celecoxib Capsules
Solution	120 mg/4.8 mL	**Elyxyb®**, Dr. Reddy's

* available from one or more manufacturer, distributor, and/or repackager by generic (nonproprietary) name

Celecoxib Combinations

Oral		
Tablets	56 mg with tramadol hydrochloride 44 mg	**Seglentis®** (C-IV), Kowa
	200 mg with Amlodipine Besylate 2.5 mg (of amlodipine)	**Consensi®**, Burke
	200 mg with Amlodipine Besylate 5 mg (of amlodipine)	**Consensi®**, Burke
	200 mg with Amlodipine Besylate 10 mg (of amlodipine)	**Consensi®**, Burke

† Use is not currently included in the labeling approved by the US Food and Drug Administration.

Selected Revisions August 25, 2023, © Copyright, June 01, 1999, American Society of Health-System Pharmacists, Inc.

Salicylates General Statement

28:08.04.24 • SALICYLATES

■ Salicylates (synthetic derivatives of salicylic acid) are nonsteroidal anti-inflammatory agents (NSAIAs); the pharmacologic actions (e.g., analgesia, anti-inflammatory effects) of salicylates appear to result principally from the salicylate moiety.

USES

Salicylates are used principally in the symptomatic treatment of mild to moderate pain, fever, inflammatory diseases, and rheumatic fever. Aspirin, but not other currently available salicylates, is also used in the prevention of arterial thrombosis. (See Uses: Thrombosis, in Aspirin 28:08.04.24.)

Aspirin is the most extensively evaluated and utilized salicylate. Although there are relatively few controlled comparative studies of aspirin and other salicylates (e.g., salicylate salts), the analgesic, antipyretic, and anti-inflammatory effects of other salicylates are generally considered to be comparable to those of aspirin. However, many clinicians prefer aspirin in most patients, at least initially, when a salicylate is indicated. Other salicylates may be particularly useful in patients with GI intolerance to aspirin or in patients in whom interference with normal platelet function by aspirin or other NSAIAs is considered undesirable. Generally, other commercially available salicylates are used only in the symptomatic treatment of rheumatoid arthritis, osteoarthritis, or related inflammatory diseases.

● Pain

Salicylates are generally used to provide temporary analgesia in the treatment of mild to moderate pain, particularly pain associated with inflammation. Salicylates are most effective in relieving low-intensity pain of nonvisceral origin, such as headache, neuralgia, myalgia, and arthralgia; however, the drugs may relieve mild to moderate postoperative pain, postpartum pain, oral surgery and other dental pain, dysmenorrhea, or other visceral pain such as that associated with trauma or cancer. Salicylates have lower maximum analgesic effects than most opiate analgesics and are generally not useful in the treatment of severe acute pain of visceral origin.

In addition to systemic administration, salicylates (e.g., trolamine salicylate) have been applied topically alone or as an adjunct to systemic therapy in the treatment of mild muscle or joint pain, such as that associated with inflammatory disease (e.g., rheumatoid arthritis). A chewing gum formulation or gargle containing aspirin has also been used for topical treatment of sore throat pain. However, the evidence that topical salicylates are effective analgesics is inconclusive.

● Fever

Salicylates are often used to lower body temperature in febrile patients in whom fever may be deleterious or in whom considerable relief is obtained when fever is lowered. However, antipyretic therapy is generally nonspecific, does not influence the course of the underlying disease, and may obscure the course of the patient's illness. For information on salicylates and Reye's syndrome, see Cautions: Pediatric Precautions.

● Inflammatory Diseases

Salicylates are frequently used for anti-inflammatory and analgesic effects in the initial and/or long-term symptomatic treatment of rheumatoid arthritis, juvenile arthritis, and osteoarthritis. Salicylates may also be useful in the symptomatic treatment of other polyarthritic conditions (e.g., psoriatic arthritis, Reiter's syndrome, ankylosing spondylitis), systemic lupus erythematosus, and nonarticular inflammation; however, other NSAIAs may be preferred in the treatment of some of these conditions (e.g., ankylosing spondylitis). Salicylates appear to be only palliative in rheumatic conditions and have not been shown to permanently arrest or reverse the underlying disease process. Salicylates are not effective in the treatment of chronic iridocyclitis in patients with juvenile arthritis.

Rheumatoid Arthritis, Juvenile Arthritis, and Osteoarthritis

When used in the treatment of rheumatoid arthritis or juvenile arthritis, salicylates have relieved pain and stiffness; reduced swelling, fever, tenderness, the duration of morning stiffness, and the number of joints involved; and improved mobility. In patients with rheumatoid arthritis, salicylates have also improved grip strength. When used in the treatment of osteoarthritis, salicylates have relieved pain and stiffness, reduced tenderness, and improved mobility. In the treatment of osteoarthritis, NSAIAs are used principally for their analgesic rather than anti-inflammatory effect, although inflammation may be part of the symptomatology.

Most clinical studies have shown that the anti-inflammatory and analgesic effects of usual dosages of salicylates in the treatment of rheumatoid arthritis, juvenile arthritis, or osteoarthritis are greater than those of placebo and about equal to those of usual dosages of other currently available NSAIAs. Patient response to NSAIAs is variable, however, and patients who do not respond to one agent may be successfully treated with a different agent.

In the management of rheumatoid arthritis in adults, NSAIAs may be useful for initial symptomatic treatment; however, NSAIAs do not alter the course of the disease or prevent joint destruction. Disease modifying antirheumatic drugs (DMARDs) (e.g., azathioprine, cyclosporine, etanercept, oral or injectable gold compounds, hydroxychloroquine, infliximab, leflunomide, methotrexate, minocycline, penicillamine, sulfasalazine) have the potential to reduce or prevent joint damage, preserve joint integrity and function, and reduce total health care costs, and all patients with rheumatoid arthritis are candidates for DMARD therapy. DMARDs should be initiated early in the disease course and should not be delayed beyond 3 months in patients with active disease (i.e., ongoing joint pain, substantial morning stiffness, fatigue, active synovitis, persistent elevation of erythrocyte sedimentation rate [ESR] or C-reactive protein [CRP], radiographic evidence of joint damage. (For further information on the treatment of rheumatoid arthritis, see Uses: Rheumatoid Arthritis, in Methotrexate 10:00.) NSAIA therapy may be continued in conjunction with DMARD therapy or, depending on patient response, may be discontinued.

Psoriatic Arthritis and Reiter's Syndrome

Salicylate therapy may be effective in the treatment of some patients with psoriatic arthritis or Reiter's syndrome but usually only when the disease is mild. Salicylates are also seldom effective in the treatment of ankylosing spondylitis unless the disease is mild.

Systemic Lupus Erythematosus

Some clinicians consider salicylates (particularly aspirin) to be the drugs of choice for the treatment of fever, arthritis, pleurisy, and pericarditis in patients with systemic lupus erythematosus. The anti-inflammatory and analgesic effects of salicylates may also be useful in the symptomatic treatment of nonarticular inflammation such as bursitis and/or tendinitis (e.g., acute painful shoulder) and fibrositis.

● Rheumatic Fever

Salicylates are considered to be the drugs of choice for the symptomatic treatment of patients with rheumatic fever who have only polyarthritis or those (with or without polyarthritis) who develop mild carditis without cardiomegaly or congestive heart failure. Most clinicians consider aspirin to be the salicylate of choice. Although salicylates suppress the acute exudative inflammatory process of rheumatic fever, progression or duration of the disease is usually not altered. Within 1–4 days after an adequate dosage of salicylate has been initiated, there is usually considerable or complete relief of pain, swelling, immobility, local heat, and erythema of the involved joints; fever and heart rate are also decreased.

Although it has not been clearly established by controlled studies, most clinicians prefer corticosteroid therapy to salicylates in the treatment of patients with rheumatic fever who develop carditis with cardiomegaly or congestive heart failure. Corticosteroids control acute manifestations of carditis more rapidly than salicylates and may be life-saving in critically ill patients. However, corticosteroids, like salicylates, cannot prevent valvular damage and are no better than salicylates for long-term treatment. Some clinicians initiate therapy with salicylates in patients with carditis and cardiomegaly; if the disease is not rapidly and adequately controlled, salicylate therapy is discontinued and steroid therapy started immediately. In patients with carditis who are treated with steroids, most clinicians initiate salicylate therapy as steroid therapy is gradually withdrawn, to minimize potential inflammatory rebound. Salicylate therapy is continued for several weeks after steroids are discontinued. Rebound of rheumatic activity after discontinuance of therapy usually subsides within 5–10 days without further treatment.

● Thrombosis

Because of its ability to inhibit platelet aggregation, aspirin is used in the prevention of arterial thrombosis. (See Uses: Thrombosis, in Aspirin 28:08.04.24.) Since other currently available salicylates do not inhibit platelet aggregation, they should not be substituted for aspirin in the prophylaxis of thrombosis.

● Kawasaki Disease

The American Academy of Pediatrics (AAP), the American Heart Association (AHA), and the American College of Chest Physicians (ACCP) recommend aspirin therapy used in conjunction with immune globulin IV (IGIV) for initial treatment of the acute phase of Kawasaki disease†. High-dose aspirin therapy (80–100 mg/kg daily for up to 14 days) combined with a single dose of IGIV (2 g/kg) initiated within 10 days of the onset of fever is more effective than aspirin therapy alone for preventing or reducing the occurrence of coronary artery abnormalities associated with Kawasaki disease; fever and other manifestations of inflammation also may resolve more rapidly with concomitant therapy. Aspirin then is continued alone in lower dosages (i.e., 1–5 mg/kg daily) for antiplatelet effects for 6–8 weeks in those without coronary artery changes or with only transient coronary artery ectasia or dilatation (disappearing within the initial 6–8 weeks of illness). For additional information on initial treatment of Kawasaki disease, see Uses: Kawasaki Disease and see Kawasaki Disease under Dosage and Administration: Dosage for Immune Globulin IV, in Immune Globulin 80:04.

Coronary artery abnormalities develop in 15–25% of children with Kawasaki disease if they are not treated within 10 days of fever onset; 2–4% of patients develop coronary artery abnormalities despite prompt treatment with aspirin and IGIV. Long-term management of those who develop coronary abnormalities depends on the severity of coronary involvement and may include low-dose aspirin (with or without clopidogrel or dipyridamole), anticoagulant therapy with warfarin or low molecular weight heparin, or a combination of antiplatelet and anticoagulant therapy (usually low-dose aspirin and warfarin). If giant coronary aneurysms are present, AHA and ACCP suggest long-term low-dose aspirin therapy in conjunction with warfarin. Specialized references should be consulted for additional information on long-term management of Kawasaki disease in individuals with coronary abnormalities.

● Gout

Because salicylates have a uricosuric effect, they were once used in the treatment of gout. However, other more effective agents are currently available for the treatment of this disease. Indeed, salicylates are generally contraindicated in patients with gout since they may cause uric acid retention (at low to intermediate dosages) and may antagonize the activity of other uricosuric agents. (See Drug Interactions: Uricosuric Agents.)

Other Uses of Aspirin

For information on other uses of aspirin, see Uses in Aspirin 28:08.04.24.

DOSAGE AND ADMINISTRATION

● Administration

Salicylates are usually administered orally, preferably with food or a large quantity (240 mL) of water or milk to minimize gastric irritation. In patients unable to take or retain oral medication, aspirin suppositories may be administered rectally; however, rectal absorption may be slow and incomplete. (See Pharmacokinetics: Absorption.) If gastric irritation and/or symptomatic GI disturbances occur with uncoated oral solid-dosage preparations, these effects may be reduced with enteric-coated tablets, extended-release tablets, or an oral solution of salicylate.

● Dosage

Dosage of salicylates must be carefully adjusted according to individual requirements and response, using the lowest possible effective dosage.

Pain and Fever

For analgesia or antipyresis, salicylates are usually administered in divided doses every 4–6 hours. If a rapid response is required, the more slowly absorbed dosage forms (i.e., enteric-coated tablets, extended-release tablets) should *not* be used.

Salicylates should not be used for *self-medication* of pain for longer than 10 days in adults or 5 days in children, unless directed by a clinician, since pain of such intensity and duration may indicate a pathologic condition requiring medical evaluation and supervised treatment.

Salicylates should not be used in adults or children for *self-medication* of marked fever (greater than 39.5°C), fever persisting longer than 3 days, or recurrent fever, unless directed by a clinician, since such fevers may indicate serious illness requiring prompt medical evaluation and treatment.

To minimize the risk of overdosage, no more than 5 doses of a salicylate preparation should be administered to children for analgesia or antipyresis in any 24-hour period, unless directed by a clinician.

Inflammatory Diseases

For the symptomatic treatment of inflammatory diseases, salicylates are usually administered in 4–6 divided doses daily. If large single doses are tolerated, salicylates can probably be given in 2 or 3 divided doses daily (every 8–12 hours) in many patients during long-term therapy, since the elimination half-life of salicylate is prolonged when high dosages are administered. In some patients, a single daily dose may be effective. At least 5–7 days is generally required to attain steady-state serum salicylate concentrations with high dosages. Therefore, when necessary, dosage is usually increased no more frequently than at weekly intervals.

Dosage should be adjusted according to the patient's response, tolerance, and serum salicylate concentration. Serum salicylate concentrations of 150–300 mcg/mL are usually required for an anti-inflammatory effect. Measurement of serum salicylate concentration should be performed no sooner than 5–7 days after a specific dosage has been initiated (unless toxicity is suspected); blood specimens usually should be obtained approximately 1–3 hours after a dose. In patients with decreased serum albumin concentrations, therapeutic effects may be associated with lower than usual serum salicylate concentrations since the fraction of total drug in serum as free salicylate is increased in these patients; measurement of free salicylate concentration in serum may be useful to guide therapy in such patients.

In the symptomatic treatment of inflammatory diseases, duration of salicylate therapy depends on the specific disease and the patient's response and tolerance; several weeks to months may be required to obtain optimum therapeutic response. In the symptomatic treatment of rheumatoid arthritis, osteoarthritis, or other polyarthritic conditions, therapy is usually continued for as long as a satisfactory response is obtained and no severe or intolerable adverse effect occurs. In the symptomatic treatment of juvenile rheumatoid arthritis, therapy is usually continued for 4–12 months after patients have achieved a complete clinical remission.

Rheumatic Fever

Dosage and duration of salicylate therapy in the symptomatic treatment of rheumatic fever are generally determined by severity and duration of acute manifestations; many clinicians believe that optimum therapeutic effects are associated with serum salicylate concentrations of 250–350 mcg/mL.

In patients with rheumatic fever who have only polyarthritis or those (with or without polyarthritis) who develop mild carditis without cardiomegaly or congestive heart failure, salicylates are usually administered for approximately 4–8 weeks or as long as necessary. Patients who have only polyarthritis are usually asymptomatic after 2–3 weeks of therapy. Some clinicians suggest that salicylate therapy be continued for at least 2 weeks after the patient is asymptomatic and evidence of active inflammation has disappeared.

Patients who have carditis with cardiomegaly or congestive heart failure are usually treated with corticosteroids, and salicylate therapy is initiated as steroid therapy is gradually withdrawn; salicylates are usually administered for approximately 2–4 weeks after steroids are discontinued. High dosages of salicylates should be used with extreme caution in patients with carditis since congestive heart failure or pulmonary edema may be precipitated.

When salicylate therapy is discontinued in patients with rheumatic fever, the drug is withdrawn gradually over 1–2 weeks to minimize the risk of rebound of rheumatic activity. Only extremely severe clinical rebounds of rheumatic activity require reinstitution of therapy, in which case salicylates are administered in the usual dosage for 3–4 additional weeks.

CAUTIONS

● GI Effects

Adverse reactions to salicylates mainly involve the GI tract and include symptomatic GI disturbances, GI bleeding, and/or mucosal lesions (e.g., erosive gastritis, gastric ulcer). These reactions apparently occur more frequently with aspirin than with other currently available salicylates.

Symptomatic GI Disturbances

Symptomatic GI disturbances are manifested most frequently as dyspepsia, heartburn, epigastric distress, or nausea, and less frequently as vomiting, anorexia, or abdominal pain; these disturbances appear to occur more frequently with aspirin than with some other NSAIAs. Symptomatic GI disturbances reportedly occur in about 2–10% of healthy individuals receiving usual analgesic or antipyretic dosages of salicylates, in about 10–30% of patients receiving high dosages (e.g., greater than 3.6 g of aspirin daily), and in about 30–90% of patients with pre-existing peptic ulcer, hemorrhagic gastritis, or duodenitis. Symptomatic GI disturbances frequently occur in the first few days of treatment with high dosages; although these disturbances disappear when therapy is discontinued, they also often subside despite continued treatment and without dosage adjustment. Centrally induced nausea and vomiting occur most often when the plasma salicylate concentration exceeds 270 mcg/mL, but nausea and vomiting may occur at lower concentrations as a result of local gastric irritation.

Symptomatic GI disturbances may be minimized by administering salicylates immediately after meals or with food, antacids, or a large quantity (240 mL) of water or milk. Alternatively, if symptomatic GI disturbances occur with an uncoated tablet, an enteric-coated tablet, extended-release tablet, or an oral solution of salicylate may be better tolerated. If burning in the throat or an unpleasant taste or aftertaste occurs with an uncoated tablet, a film-coated or enteric-coated tablet may be better tolerated. It has not been established that buffered aspirin tablets cause fewer symptomatic GI disturbances than uncoated plain aspirin tablets.

GI Bleeding

Occult GI bleeding, which occurs in most patients receiving salicylates (particularly aspirin), is usually painless and appears to be the result of a local action on GI mucosa. Occult GI blood loss with usual dosages of aspirin appears to be greater than that with usual dosages of most other NSAIAs. There appears to be no correlation between the incidence of salicylate-induced occult GI bleeding and symptomatic GI disturbances. Uncoated plain aspirin tablets in an oral dosage of 1–4.5 g daily produce a blood loss of 2–8 mL daily in about 70% of patients. However, about 10–15% of patients lose 10 mL or more of blood daily, which may result in iron deficiency anemia with long-term therapy; tolerance to salicylate-induced bleeding apparently does not occur. Unlike aspirin, usual oral dosages of salicylate salts or salsalate produce little or no GI blood loss.

The incidence and severity of GI bleeding are generally dose related. GI bleeding is not reduced by administration of salicylates with food. GI bleeding is less in patients with achlorhydria than in healthy individuals with normal gastric acid production, apparently because gastric acid is necessary to produce gastric mucosal injury. There is adequate evidence that sufficient buffering to decrease gastric acidity and increase the pH of gastric contents substantially reduces aspirin-induced GI blood loss; however, concomitant oral administration of high dosages of antacids is necessary to provide sufficient buffering capacity. (See Drug Interactions: Acidifying and Alkalinizing Agents.) It has not been established that the amounts of buffers contained in commercially available buffered aspirin tablets have any effect in reducing GI blood loss. However, GI blood loss is reduced with oral aqueous aspirin solutions. Although single oral doses of highly buffered aqueous aspirin solutions (e.g., Alka-Seltzer®) cause little or no GI blood loss, multiple doses for 2–3 days do cause some GI bleeding; these solutions are not recommended for long-term therapy because of their high buffer and sodium content. Aspirin-induced GI blood loss also may be reduced with enteric-coated tablets, extended-release tablets, or by concomitant oral administration of a histamine H_2-receptor antagonist (e.g., cimetidine hydrochloride).

The risk of GI bleeding is increased in geriatric patients 60 years of age or older and in patients with a history of GI ulcers or bleeding, those receiving an anticoagulant or corticosteroid or taking multiple NSAIAs concomitantly, those consuming 3 or more alcohol-containing beverages daily, and those receiving excessive dosages or prolonged therapy.

In an FDA review of 41 reports of serious bleeding events (site unspecified but severe enough to require hospitalization) associated with use of OTC preparations containing aspirin in fixed combination with antacids (e.g., buffered effervescent tablets administered as oral solutions), 88% of the events occurred in patients with risk factors for bleeding.

Rarely, major upper GI bleeding may occur in patients receiving salicylates (particularly aspirin), regardless of the specific dosage form. A definite relationship between occult GI bleeding and major upper GI bleeding with aspirin therapy has not been established. Patients with active peptic ulcer or those who have recently had major upper GI bleeding do not experience greater occult blood loss after small doses of aspirin than do healthy individuals; however, these patients do have an increased risk of recurrent major bleeding. Most clinicians believe that aspirin and other salicylates can potentiate GI bleeding in patients with GI lesions.

In patients who have undergone tonsillectomy, severe bleeding from tonsillar blood vessels has been reported following topical application of aspirin via gargles or chewing gum tablets.

Mucosal Lesions

Salicylates (especially aspirin) can cause gastric mucosal damage with varying degrees of erythema, petechiae, submucosal bleeding, erosions, and/or ulceration, with or without bleeding, and even in the absence of GI symptoms. Aspirin and other salicylates may also reactivate latent gastric or duodenal ulcers. Although not clearly established, the incidence of gastric mucosal damage may be higher with aspirin than with other NSAIAs. The exact relationships between salicylate-induced gastric mucosal damage and occult GI bleeding or major upper GI bleeding remain to be clearly determined. Microscopic mucosal damage that accompanies endoscopically observed mucosal abnormalities usually resolves within several hours following a single oral dose of aspirin and can be reduced or prevented by concomitant oral administration of sodium bicarbonate (in amounts sufficient to buffer gastric contents) or a histamine $_2$-receptor antagonist (e.g., cimetidine). However, with long-term aspirin therapy, many patients develop persistent gastric erythema and erosions and gastric ulcer (often in the distal antrum). Several studies using endoscopy have indicated that the incidence of aspirin-induced gastric erosions and ulceration is lower with enteric-coated tablets than with buffered or uncoated plain tablets; buffered tablets appear to provide little or no protection against gastric mucosal damage.

Although long-term aspirin therapy has not been clearly associated with the occurrence of duodenal ulceration, duodenal erythema and erosions have been reported to occur frequently in patients receiving aspirin; the incidence of duodenal mucosal damage appears to be lower with enteric-coated tablets than with buffered or uncoated plain tablets.

In patients who develop gastric or duodenal ulcers during treatment with salicylates, salicylate therapy is generally discontinued because of an increased risk of bleeding and/or ulcer perforation; occasionally, another NSAIA is substituted for the salicylate in these patients. However, gastric or duodenal ulcers 1 cm or less in diameter, which are induced by salicylates or other NSAIAs, may heal despite continued treatment with these agents when an oral histamine H_2-receptor antagonist (e.g., cimetidine) and high-dose antacid therapy are administered concomitantly. Although such regimens generally appear to be safe and effective, ulcer perforation has occurred in patients receiving a NSAIA and cimetidine concomitantly; further evaluation of these regimens is necessary.

Uncoated plain aspirin tablets allowed to remain in contact with mucous membranes of the mouth and aspirin chewing gum tablets have produced mucosal erosions and ulcerations of the mouth. Rectally administered aspirin suppositories may rarely cause rectal mucosal irritation, burning pain, rectal bleeding, diarrhea, and tenesmus.

Other Adverse GI Effects

Although a causal relationship has not been established, one case-control analysis suggests that NSAIAs may contribute to the formation of esophageal stricture in patients with gastroesophageal reflux.

Gastric accumulation of enteric-coated aspirin tablets, sometimes resulting in gastric ulceration or salicylate intoxication, has been reported in some patients with gastric outlet obstruction. Removal of accumulated enteric-coated aspirin tablets from the stomach by usual methods (e.g., emesis, gastric lavage) may be unsuccessful in these patients and surgery may be necessary. However, some clinicians have reported successful removal by gastric lavage using an isotonic sodium bicarbonate solution (containing 150 mEq/L) to dissolve the enteric coating and allow dissolution of the aspirin; 300 mL of the solution was instilled into the stomach via a nasogastric tube over 30 minutes and then removed by continuous nasogastric suction for 30 minutes, the regimen being repeated continuously for 24 hours.

● Otic Effects

Tinnitus and hearing loss may occur in patients receiving large dosages of salicylates and/or long-term therapy. These effects are often the initial manifestations of chronic salicylate intoxication in adults. (See Chronic Toxicity: Manifestations.) Tinnitus and hearing loss are rarely noted by young children or patients with preexisting hearing impairment and are therefore usually not useful as indicators of early chronic intoxication in these patients.

Tinnitus and hearing loss are dose related, usually completely reversible (even after administration of large dosages for many years), and are more likely caused by actions on the inner ear than on the CNS. Patients receiving high dosages should be monitored periodically for tinnitus and hearing loss. Tinnitus usually develops only when the serum salicylate concentration exceeds 200 mcg/mL and generally occurs at a concentration of about 300 mcg/mL; however, it may develop only at higher concentrations in some patients. Tinnitus occurs infrequently in patients with preexisting hearing impairment, even at high serum salicylate concentrations (e.g., greater than 400 mcg/mL). Since serum salicylate concentrations of 200–300 mcg/mL are consistent with those considered necessary for anti-inflammatory effects, the occurrence of tinnitus in adults with inflammatory disease can indicate attainment of adequate concentrations, but only in those patients with normal hearing. Because tinnitus can occur over a wide range of concentrations, determinations of serum salicylate concentration are preferred as a guide to adjusting dosage. Tinnitus subsides gradually with reduction of salicylate dosage or usually within 24–48 hours after discontinuance of therapy.

Salicylate-induced hearing impairment involves bilateral loss of pure tone sensitivity for all sound frequencies. Hearing losses generally range from 20–40 decibels, occur initially at a serum salicylate concentration of about 200 mcg/mL, and increase with increasing concentrations. Maximum hearing loss occurs most frequently at a serum salicylate concentration of about 400 mcg/mL. Hearing loss is usually completely reversible, subsiding within 24–72 hours after discontinuance of therapy; rarely, permanent hearing loss has been reported.

● Hepatic Effects

Salicylates occasionally cause acute, reversible hepatotoxicity, particularly in patients with juvenile arthritis, active systemic lupus erythematosus, rheumatic fever, or preexisting hepatic impairment. Therefore, hepatic function should be monitored in these patients. In addition, salicylate therapy has been associated in a few patients with hepatic injury consistent with chronic active hepatitis. Salicylate-induced hepatotoxicity is usually mild, but death or hepatic injury with encephalopathy has occurred in a few patients.

Hepatic injury usually consists of mild, focal, cellular necrosis, eosinophilic degeneration of hepatocytes, and portal inflammation; the exact mechanism is not known. Salicylate-induced hepatotoxicity is manifested principally as elevations in serum aminotransferase concentrations; elevations in serum alkaline phosphatase concentration occur occasionally. Rarely, serum bilirubin concentration may be elevated and/or serum prothrombin concentration may be decreased with a resultant increase in the PT. Although most patients are asymptomatic, some develop nausea, vomiting, anorexia, abdominal distress, loss of taste for cigarettes, liver tenderness, and/or hepatomegaly.

Hepatotoxicity has generally developed after 1–4 weeks of therapy and appears to be related to serum salicylate concentration, occurring principally at concentrations exceeding 200–250 mcg/mL; however, it may occur at lower concentrations. Elevated serum aminotransferase concentrations usually return to pretreatment values within 1–2 weeks after dosage reduction or discontinuance of salicylate therapy; however, they may be transient and return to pretreatment values despite continued therapy and without dosage adjustment.

It is usually not necessary to discontinue salicylate therapy in patients who develop hepatotoxicity, but dosage reduction may be advisable in patients who develop signs of hepatotoxicity and whose serum salicylate concentration exceeds 250 mcg/mL. Some clinicians recommend that the PT be measured periodically in patients with abnormal hepatic function test results and that salicylate therapy be discontinued if prolonged PT occurs.

● Renal Effects

In usual dosages, salicylates rarely cause clinically important adverse renal effects. In overdosage, the drugs may cause a marked reduction in creatinine clearance or acute tubular necrosis with renal failure.

Although the exact mechanism(s) is not known, salicylates cause transient urinary excretion of renal tubular epithelial cells. Albuminuria, proteinuria, and urinary excretion of leukocytes and erythrocytes may also occur. Urinary excretion of renal tubular epithelial cells usually increases markedly in the first several days of continuous therapy and then subsides or continues at a low level with prolonged treatment. Salicylates have also been shown to cause urinary excretion of N-acetyl-β-glucosaminidase 2–4 hours after single doses equivalent in salicylate content to at least 1.95 g of aspirin; the mechanism is not known.

In patients with impaired renal function or systemic lupus erythematosus, aspirin may cause reversible (sometimes marked) decreases in renal blood flow and glomerular filtration rate; as a result, minimal water, sodium, and potassium retention may occur. These effects may also occur in patients with conditions predisposing to sodium and water retention (e.g., congestive heart failure, decompensated hepatic cirrhosis). However, aspirin may have less severe adverse renal effects than other currently available NSAIAs. Renal effects are usually rapidly reversed following discontinuance of aspirin therapy, but they may also subside despite continued treatment. Although these effects on renal function have not been reported to date with salicylates other than aspirin, other salicylates may cause similar effects.

Long-term therapy with aspirin alone or in combination with other analgesic-antipyretic agents (e.g., phenacetin) has been associated with analgesic nephropathy (renal papillary necrosis with subsequent chronic interstitial nephritis); however, evidence to date concerning aspirin alone is conflicting and a causal relationship remains to be clearly established. Several studies indicate that long-term aspirin or salicylate therapy rarely, if ever, causes substantial renal disease; however, some clinicians have reported a high incidence of renal papillary necrosis at autopsy in patients with rheumatoid arthritis who received long-term aspirin therapy. The exact mechanism(s) of renal damage is not known but may include renal medullary ischemia caused by inhibition of renal prostaglandin synthesis and/or a direct cytotoxic effect of the drugs or their metabolites. Further studies are needed to fully evaluate the effects of long-term salicylate therapy on the kidney and renal function.

● Cardiovascular Effects

Salicylates may cause moderate to severe noncardiogenic pulmonary edema, principally with chronic or acute intoxication. Salicylate-induced pulmonary edema may also be precipitated or aggravated by forced alkaline diuresis during the treatment of salicylate overdosage, but fluid volume overload is not necessary for its occurrence. It has been suggested that salicylates cause pulmonary edema by increasing alveolar capillary membrane permeability. Salicylate-induced noncardiogenic pulmonary edema appears to occur most frequently when the serum salicylate concentration exceeds 400 mcg/mL. It is usually manifested as diffuse bilateral infiltrates on chest radiographs, tachypnea or dyspnea, and hypoxemia, and is often associated with proteinuria and adverse neurologic effects such as lethargy or confusion. Patients receiving long-term salicylate therapy or those with a history of smoking appear to have an increased risk of developing pulmonary edema. Treatment of salicylate-induced pulmonary edema is generally supportive and includes measures to increase the excretion of salicylate; an adequate airway should be maintained and assisted pulmonary ventilation may be required. Following treatment, pulmonary edema generally resolves within 1–7 days.

In patients with rheumatic fever who have carditis, congestive heart failure and pulmonary edema may be precipitated with high dosages of salicylates, apparently as a result of increased circulating plasma volume and cardiac workload.

In one placebo-controlled study in a small number of patients with variant angina, aspirin therapy (2 g twice daily) was associated with an increased frequency of angina and an increased risk of exercise-induced angina.

● Hematologic Effects

Although aspirin alters hemostasis through effects on platelet function and high dosages of salicylates can decrease hepatic synthesis of blood coagulation factors (see Pharmacology: Hematologic Effects), salicylates cause few hematologic reactions. Daily aspirin doses of 3–4 g may decrease the hematocrit and plasma iron concentration, and reduce erythrocyte life span. Since the effects of aspirin on platelets are irreversible, ingestion of aspirin or aspirin-containing preparations within 3–5 days of platelet donation generally precludes use of an individual donor as a sole source of platelet preparations for a thrombocytopenic recipient. However, ingestion of aspirin or aspirin-containing preparations does not preclude donation of whole blood. Since other currently available salicylates do not affect platelet aggregation, ingestion of these other salicylates does not preclude donation of platelets or whole blood.

Leukopenia, thrombocytopenia, pancytopenia, eosinopenia, agranulocytosis, aplastic anemia, purpura, eosinophilia associated with aspirin-induced hepatotoxicity, and disseminated intravascular coagulation have been reported rarely in patients receiving salicylates. Leukocytosis has occurred with salicylate overdosage. Increased perioperative and postoperative bleeding, hematomas, and ecchymoses have occurred in patients who ingested aspirin before and for several days after oral surgery. In addition, adverse hematologic effects have been reported in neonates whose mothers ingested aspirin before delivery. (See Cautions: Pregnancy, Fertility, and Lactation.)

Macrocytic anemia associated with folic acid deficiency has been reported in patients abusing analgesic-combination preparations containing aspirin and in patients with rheumatoid arthritis receiving high dosages of aspirin. In one patient, megaloblastic anemia was associated with long-term ingestion of a preparation containing aspirin, salicylamide, and caffeine.

In vitro, salicylates reduce adenosine triphosphate (ATP) concentrations and inhibit hexose-monophosphate shunt activity in erythrocytes of patients with pyruvate kinase deficiency. Although the clinical significance of these effects in vivo is not known, salicylates might cause or aggravate hemolysis in these patients.

Salicylates (especially aspirin) may cause or aggravate hemolysis in patients with glucose-6-phosphate dehydrogenase (G-6-PD) deficiency; however, this has not been clearly established. In a study in patients with G-6-PD deficiency, salicylate did not inhibit hexose-monophosphate shunt activity in erythrocytes from these patients in vitro, and oral doses of aspirin (50 mg/kg daily for 4 days) did not cause hemolysis; however, none of the patients in this study had chronic hemolysis. Some clinicians suggest that aspirin or other salicylates can probably be used safely in most patients with G-6-PD deficiency, but effects of the drugs in patients with rare variants of this enzyme deficiency remain to be fully evaluated.

● Dermatologic Effects

Skin eruptions of a pustular acneiform nature may occur but are usually observed only in patients who have received salicylates continually for longer than 1 week or with overdosage. Erythematous, scarlatiniform, pruritic, eczematoid, or desquamative lesions, which rarely may be bullous or purpuric, have also been reported. Hemorrhage from mucous membranes may occur rarely. Rarely, aspirin has been associated with Stevens-Johnson syndrome and toxic epidermal necrolysis.

● Sensitivity Reactions

Sensitivity reactions to aspirin may occur rarely; sensitivity reactions to other salicylates are extremely rare. Sensitivity reactions manifested principally as bronchospasm appear to be related mainly to inhibition of prostaglandin synthesis. The exact mechanism(s) of sensitivity reactions manifested principally as urticaria and/or angioedema has not been determined; although these reactions may be immune-mediated in some patients, IgE antibodies or specific antibodies have not been detected. If an aspirin (or salicylate) sensitivity reaction occurs, it usually develops within 3 hours of ingestion and is characterized as urticaria, angioedema, bronchospasm, severe rhinitis, or shock. Facial edema also has been reported with aspirin. Lacrimation, complete vasomotor collapse, and loss of consciousness may also occur. Although extremely rare, severe reactions resulting in death have occurred within minutes following ingestion of 325–650 mg of aspirin in individuals with known aspirin sensitivity. If a severe reaction occurs, the drug should be discontinued and the patient given appropriate treatment (e.g., epinephrine, corticosteroids, maintenance of an adequate airway, oxygen) as indicated.

Aspirin sensitivity appears to occur in about 0.3% of the general population, in about 20% of patients with chronic urticaria, in about 4% of patients with asthma, and in about 1.5% of patients with chronic rhinitis. Aspirin sensitivity also appears to occur more frequently in adults 30–60 years of age than in younger adults or children, and more frequently in females.

In patients with asthma, aspirin sensitivity is manifested principally as bronchospasm and is usually associated with the presence of nasal polyps; the association of aspirin sensitivity, asthma, and nasal polyps is known as the aspirin triad. In these patients, nasal symptoms usually precede asthma, and the onset of asthma may precede the development of aspirin sensitivity by many years. Mild to marked bronchospasm of variable duration may occur with oral doses of aspirin as small as 20–30 mg and usually develops within 15–30 minutes after ingestion of the drug.

In one study in patients with asthma, the capacity of aspirin and other NSAIAs to induce bronchospasm was directly correlated with the degree of in vitro inhibition of prostaglandin synthesis caused by the drugs. As an inhibitor of cyclooxygenase, aspirin may alter the synthesis of prostaglandin E (a bronchodilator) and prostaglandin $F_{2\alpha}$ (a bronchoconstrictor), resulting in a predominance of prostaglandin $F_{2\alpha}$ and bronchoconstriction. It has also been suggested that the inhibition of cyclooxygenase favors the formation of leukotrienes that contribute to bronchoconstriction. Patients with aspirin-induced bronchospasm are often cross-sensitive to other inhibitors of prostaglandin synthesis. *Cross-sensitivity in these patients appears to occur most frequently with indomethacin, followed by ibuprofen, mefenamic acid, phenylbutazone, and sodium benzoate; therefore, these drugs and any NSAIA are generally contraindicated in patients with aspirin sensitivity and vice versa.* Patients with aspirin-induced bronchospasm are usually not cross-sensitive to salicylate salts, salicylamide, or acetaminophen. Aspirin desensitization in aspirin-sensitive asthmatic patients has been reported; in some of these patients, cross-desensitization with indomethacin and other NSAIAs was demonstrated. However, continuous aspirin therapy appears to be necessary to maintain desensitization, which disappears gradually over several days when aspirin is withheld. Further evaluation is needed to determine the clinical implications of these findings.

In patients with chronic urticaria or chronic rhinitis, aspirin sensitivity is manifested principally as urticaria and/or angioedema, but bronchospasm and shock may also occur. Patients with aspirin sensitivity who generally have dermatologic reactions to the drug appear to have an increased risk of cross-sensitivity to salicylate salts or acetaminophen.

In general, about 10% of patients with aspirin sensitivity appear to be cross-sensitive to the dye tartrazine (FD&C yellow No. 5) and about 5% appear to be cross-sensitive to acetaminophen; since the incidence of cross-sensitivity to acetaminophen is low, some clinicians state that, if necessary, acetaminophen may be used instead of aspirin for analgesic-antipyretic effects in some patients with aspirin sensitivity.

The manufacturer of salsalate states that patients with aspirin sensitivity are not cross-sensitive to salsalate; although specific data are not available, the manufacturer suggests that patients who have sensitivity reactions to non-salicylate NSAIAs are probably not cross-sensitive to salsalate.

● Precautions and Contraindications

Salicylates (particularly aspirin) should be used with caution in patients with active GI lesions (e.g., erosive gastritis, peptic ulcer) or with a history of recurrent GI lesions, since the drugs may cause or aggravate GI bleeding and/or ulcerations. Patients with ulcers or persistent or recurring stomach disorders (e.g., heartburn, stomach pain, dyspepsia) should contact their clinician prior to initiating therapy with aspirin. If salicylates must be administered, these patients should be closely monitored for signs of GI bleeding or ulcer perforation. For additional information on precautions associated with the use of salicylates in these patients, see Cautions: GI Effects. Use of enteric-coated salicylate preparations in patients with known or suspected gastric outlet obstruction should generally be avoided. When aspirin is used in fixed combination with dipyridamole, the cautions, precautions, and contraindications associated with dipyridamole must be considered in addition to those associated with aspirin.

Patients should be informed that alcohol has a synergistic effect with aspirin in causing GI bleeding. The manufacturers caution that patients who generally consume 3 or more alcohol-containing drinks per day should ask their clinician whether to use salicylates (e.g., aspirin, choline salicylate, magnesium salicylate) or an alternative analgesic for *self-medication* since salicylates may increase the risk of GI bleeding. In addition, the manufacturers caution that patients who generally consume 3 or more alcohol-containing drinks per day should ask their clinician whether to use a salicylate (e.g., aspirin) in fixed combination with acetaminophen or an alternative analgesic for *self-medication* since aspirin in fixed combination with acetaminophen may increase the risk of GI bleeding and hepatotoxicity.

Despite current warnings on OTC product labels, serious bleeding events continue to occur in patients receiving aspirin in fixed combination with antacids (e.g., buffered effervescent tablets administered as oral solutions) for *self-medication*. FDA is evaluating whether additional actions are needed to address this safety concern.

Patients should discontinue aspirin and consult a clinician if they experience erythema or edema in the area being treated for pain or if new symptoms occur.

Because of an increased risk of bleeding, salicylates (particularly aspirin) should be used with extreme caution, if at all, in patients with preexisting hypoprothrombinemia, vitamin K deficiency, thrombocytopenia, thrombotic thrombocytopenic purpura, or severe hepatic impairment, or in patients receiving anticoagulants (see Drug Interactions: Anticoagulants and Thrombolytic Agents). Since salicylates may cause or aggravate hemolysis in patients with pyruvate kinase deficiency or in patients with rare variants of G-6-PD deficiency, the drugs should probably be avoided in these patients. Most clinicians recommend that aspirin therapy be discontinued 5–7 days before surgery to prevent or minimize excessive perioperative bleeding; however, it has not been clearly established that patients receiving aspirin have substantially increased perioperative blood loss. Therapy with salicylates that do not affect platelet aggregation need not be discontinued before surgery.

Because of an increased risk of bleeding, aspirin is contraindicated in patients with bleeding disorders such as hemophilia, von Willebrand's disease, or telangiectasia. If salicylate therapy is considered necessary in patients with bleeding disorders, some clinicians suggest that salicylates which do not inhibit platelet aggregation (e.g., salicylate salts) may be used. Patients with bleeding disorders should contact their clinician prior to initiating therapy with aspirin for *self-medication*.

Because of an increased risk of bleeding, chewing gum tablets or gargles that contain aspirin should be avoided for at least 1 week after tonsillectomy or oral surgery. In addition, tablets containing aspirin should not be chewed before swallowing for at least 1 week after tonsillectomy or oral surgery because of possible injury to oral tissues from prolonged contact with aspirin particles.

Salicylates should be used with caution in patients with impaired renal function and with extreme caution, if at all, in patients with advanced chronic renal insufficiency, since salicylate and its metabolites are excreted almost completely in the urine; in addition, these patients may have an increased risk of developing adverse renal effects.

Hematocrit and renal function should be monitored periodically in patients receiving prolonged salicylate therapy or high dosages since iron deficiency anemia or adverse renal effects may occur. Because of an increased risk of hepatotoxicity, hepatic function should also be monitored in patients with juvenile arthritis, active systemic lupus erythematosus, rheumatic fever, or preexisting hepatic impairment who are receiving high dosages of salicylates.

Because of the high sodium content, highly buffered aspirin solutions (e.g., Alka-Seltzer®) should be used with extreme caution, if at all, in patients with congestive heart failure or other conditions in which a high sodium intake would be harmful; in addition, highly buffered aspirin solutions can result in alkalinization of the urine and enhance urinary excretion of salicylate. Salicylate salts containing magnesium or sodium should be avoided in patients in whom excessive amounts of these electrolytes might be harmful. Patients on a sodium-restricted diet should consult a clinician prior to initiating therapy with aspirin for *self-medication*.

If corticosteroid dosage is decreased during salicylate therapy, it should be done gradually and patients should be observed for adverse effects, including adrenocortical insufficiency or symptomatic exacerbation of the inflammatory condition being treated. In addition, since corticosteroids may increase renal excretion of salicylate or induce its metabolism, reduction of salicylate dosage may be necessary when steroid therapy is discontinued. (See Drug Interactions: Corticosteroids.)

The possibility that the antipyretic and anti-inflammatory effects of NSAIAs may mask the usual signs and symptoms of infection or other diseases should be considered.

Some commercially available formulations of salicylates contain sodium bisulfite, a sulfite that may cause allergic-type reactions, including anaphylaxis and life-threatening or less severe asthmatic episodes, in certain susceptible individuals. The overall prevalence of sulfite sensitivity in the general population is unknown but probably low; such sensitivity appears to occur more frequently in asthmatic than in nonasthmatic individuals. Some commercially available formulations of salicylates contain the dye tartrazine (FD&C yellow No. 5), which may cause allergic reactions including bronchial asthma in certain susceptible individuals. Although the incidence of tartrazine sensitivity is low, it frequently occurs in individuals who are sensitive to aspirin.

A specific salicylate preparation is contraindicated in patients with known hypersensitivity to that preparation or any of the ingredients in the formulation and should be used with extreme caution, if at all, in patients with known hypersensitivity to salicylates. The commercially available preparation containing aspirin in fixed combination with extended-release dipyridamole is contraindicated in patients with hypersensitivity to dipyridamole, aspirin, or any other ingredient in the formulation. Aspirin generally is contraindicated in patients in whom sensitivity reactions (e.g., urticaria, angioedema, bronchospasm, severe rhinitis, shock) are precipitated by any NSAIA and vice-versa, although the drugs have occasionally been used in aspirin- or NSAIA-sensitive patients who have undergone desensitization. Patients with known aspirin sensitivity should be warned to avoid aspirin and aspirin-containing preparations. If an allergic reaction with aspirin occurs, a clinician should be contacted immediately. Patients with asthma should consult their clinician prior to initiating therapy with aspirin. (See Cautions: Sensitivity Reactions.)

● *Pediatric Precautions*

Salicylates should be used with caution in pediatric patients who are dehydrated, since these patients are especially susceptible to salicylate intoxication.

Safety and efficacy of magnesium salicylate in children younger than 12 years of age have not been established. Safety and efficacy of salsalate in children have not been established.

The safety and efficacy of the commercially available preparation containing aspirin in fixed combination with extended-release dipyridamole have not been established in children.

Reye's Syndrome

Use of salicylates (almost exclusively aspirin) in children with varicella infection or influenza-like illnesses reportedly is *associated with* an increased risk of developing Reye's syndrome; however, a *causal relationship* has *not* been established. In several initial epidemiologic studies, children with varicella or influenza-like illnesses who developed Reye's syndrome appeared to receive salicylates more frequently during their antecedent illness than those who did not develop the syndrome; however, the methodology and results of some of these studies have been questioned. Subsequent epidemiologic studies designed and implemented by the US Public Health Service Reye Syndrome Task Force found a *strong association* between development of the syndrome and ingestion of salicylates (almost exclusively aspirin) during the antecedent illness. Most evidence to date, including a decline in the use of aspirin in children accompanied by a continuing decline in reported cases of Reye's syndrome, strongly supports such an association, but some data do not and some controversy still remains. Whether an increased risk of developing the syndrome is associated with aspirin only or with all salicylates has not been adequately evaluated.

The exact pathogenesis of Reye's syndrome and the potential role of aspirin and other salicylates in its pathogenesis remain to be determined. The syndrome has occurred in children who did not receive salicylates and in children who received other medications.

Because of the evidence to date, the US Surgeon General, the American Academy of Pediatrics Committee on Infectious Diseases, the US Food and Drug Administration (FDA), and other authorities currently advise that *salicylates not be used in children and teenagers with varicella or influenza, unless directed by a clinician.* Use of salicylates also generally should be avoided in children and teenagers with suspected varicella or influenza and during presumed outbreaks of influenza, since diagnosis of these diseases may be impossible to establish accurately during the prodromal period; similarly, salicylates should not be used in the management of viral infections in children or adolescents because of the possibility that the infection may be one associated with an increased risk of Reye's syndrome. If antipyretic medication is considered necessary in children or teenagers with known or suspected varicella or influenza or other viral illness, acetaminophen may be used. It is not known whether Reye's syndrome may occur in children who receive salicylates following vaccination with varicella virus vaccine live. (See Drug Interactions: Varicella Virus Vaccine Live.)

● Geriatric Precautions

Geriatric individuals receiving salicylates are more likely than younger individuals to experience adverse effects secondary to age-related decline in renal function and/or increased use of concomitant drug therapy. The risk of GI bleeding is increased in geriatric patients 60 years of age or older. (See Cautions: GI Effects.)

Salicylates are highly protein bound and can be displaced from binding sites by other protein-bound drugs. Because geriatric patients are more likely to be taking multiple drugs than younger patients, geriatric patients are at increased risk of drug interactions mediated by alterations in protein binding (i.e., decrease in protein binding of salicylate and increased concentrations of unbound salicylate). (See Drug Interactions: Protein-bound Drugs.)

● Pregnancy, Fertility, and Lactation

Pregnancy

Although safe use of salicylates during pregnancy has not been established, there is evidence indicating that aspirin is the most frequently used drug during pregnancy either as a single entity or in combination with other drugs. Salicylates have been shown to be teratogenic and embryocidal in animals. In humans, a slight positive association between chronic maternal salicylate ingestion during pregnancy and congenital abnormalities has been reported in some studies, but other studies have found no association. In some studies, chronic maternal salicylate ingestion has also been associated with decreased fetal birth weight; an increased incidence of stillbirth, neonatal mortality, antepartum and postpartum maternal hemorrhage, and complicated deliveries; and prolongation of gestation and spontaneous labor. There have been several reports of adverse hematologic effects (e.g., subconjunctival hemorrhage, hematuria, purpura, petechiae, cephalhematoma) in neonates whose mothers had ingested aspirin before delivery, and at least 2 reports of neonatal salicylate intoxication secondary to salicylate accumulation in utero. In one study, maternal ingestion of aspirin during the week before delivery was associated with an increased incidence of intracranial hemorrhage in premature neonates. In addition, it has been suggested that premature closure of the ductus arteriosus secondary to maternal salicylate ingestion may be one cause of persistent pulmonary hypertension in some infants.

Maternal and fetal hemorrhagic complications observed with maternal ingestion of large doses (e.g., 12–15 g daily) of aspirin generally have not been observed in studies in which low doses (60–150 mg daily) of the drug were used for prevention of complications of pregnancy† (e.g., preeclampsia, recurrent spontaneous abortions, prematurity, intrauterine growth retardation, stillbirth, low birthweight), including those associated with autoimmune disorders such as antiphospholipid syndrome, poor paternal blocking antibody production, or systemic lupus erythematosus. (See Uses: Complications of Pregnancy, in Aspirin 28:08.04.24.) Although current evidence indicates that low dosages of aspirin can be used safely during pregnancy, the possibility of maternal and/or fetal complications (e.g., bleeding) should be considered. At least one case of fatal cerebral hemorrhage has been reported in a woman who was receiving prophylactic therapy with aspirin, heparin, and immune globulin despite no history of recurrent pregnancy loss nor antiphospholipid antibodies; this woman was found to have had a congenital arteriovenous malformation as a predisposing risk for hemorrhage.

Salicylates should be used during pregnancy only when the potential benefits justify the possible risks to the fetus. The drugs (particularly aspirin) generally should be avoided during the last 3 months (although *low* dosages have been useful in the prevention of preeclampsia during this period) of pregnancy (especially during the 1–2 weeks before delivery). Similarly, aspirin in fixed combination with extended-release dipyridamole should be avoided in the third trimester of pregnancy.

If maternal ingestion of aspirin occurs within 1–2 weeks of delivery, the neonate should be closely evaluated for the presence of bleeding.

Fertility

In animals, aspirin has been shown to cause testicular atrophy and inhibit spermatogenesis. Although the effect on fertility is not known, aspirin has been shown to decrease seminal fluid concentrations of prostaglandins E and F in healthy men.

Lactation

Since salicylates are distributed into milk in low concentrations, the drugs should be administered with caution to nursing women. However, maternal consumption of high salicylate dosages potentially may result in adverse effects (e.g., rash, platelet abnormalities, bleeding) in nursing infants. At least one case of salicylate toxicity in an infant has been attributed to breast-feeding; however, some experts consider it unlikely that ingestion of breast milk alone could have resulted in the serum salicylate concentration reported in the infant. In general, nursing should be discontinued during long-term salicylate therapy with high dosages; however, some clinicians state that occasional single doses of salicylates in nursing women appear to be of little risk to nursing infants.

DRUG INTERACTIONS

Numerous drug interactions involving salicylates have been reported but few appear to be clinically important. The salicylate interactions that many clinicians consider to be the most important include those with anticoagulants and thrombolytic agents, uricosuric agents, sulfonylureas, corticosteroids, and methotrexate.

● Protein-bound Drugs

Because salicylate is highly protein bound, it could be displaced from binding sites by, or could displace from binding sites, other protein-bound drugs such as oral anticoagulants, sulfonylureas, hydantoins, penicillins, and sulfonamides; salicylates could also theoretically displace bilirubin in neonates, resulting in hyperbilirubinemia. Patients receiving salicylates with any of these drugs should be observed for adverse effects. The acetylation of albumin by aspirin could alter protein binding of other drugs; acetylated albumin has been shown to have a higher affinity for phenylbutazone.

● Anticoagulants

Salicylates may enhance the hypoprothrombinemic effect of warfarin and other oral anticoagulants and increase the risk of bleeding complications with these agents; several mechanisms may be involved. However, low-dose aspirin (e.g., 75–100 mg daily) may be used in combination with heparin or oral anticoagulants for therapeutic benefit (i.e., additive antithrombotic effects) in selected patients at high risk for thromboembolism (e.g., patients with prosthetic mechanical heart valves).

Although salicylates can cause a dose-dependent hypoprothrombinemia, clinical data are conflicting regarding salicylate enhancement of oral anticoagulant-induced hypoprothrombinemia. In several studies in patients receiving warfarin or other oral anticoagulants, the PT was not affected when aspirin was administered concurrently in dosages up to 3 g daily for 3–14 days. However, in one study in which either a lower or a higher aspirin dosage (1.95 or 3.9 g daily, respectively) was administered concurrently, the PT was substantially increased; patients receiving the higher aspirin dosage also had signs of bleeding. Therefore, it appears that high dosages of salicylates (e.g., greater than 3 g of aspirin daily) may enhance the hypoprothrombinemic effect of oral anticoagulants when administered concurrently. At lower dosages, salicylates may not affect oral anticoagulant-induced hypoprothrombinemia and occasional low doses of salicylates (other than aspirin) can probably be used with caution in patients receiving anticoagulants; however, salicylates should generally be avoided in these patients since they also cause GI bleeding. Patients with preexisting hepatic impairment may have an increased risk of bleeding if salicylates and oral anticoagulants are administered concomitantly. Since aspirin also inhibits platelet aggregation, it should be used with caution in patients receiving anticoagulants. Patients receiving anticoagulants should consult a clinician prior to initiating therapy with aspirin for *self-medication*. If salicylates are indicated for other than their antithrombotic effects in patients receiving anticoagulants, salicylates (e.g., salicylate salts) that do not affect platelet aggregation are preferred to aspirin. In addition, the lowest effective salicylate dosage should be used, the PT should be determined frequently and anticoagulant dosage adjusted accordingly, and patients should be observed closely for adverse effects.

Because aspirin inhibits platelet aggregation and causes GI bleeding, it should be used with caution in patients receiving heparin. Although further documentation is necessary, severe bleeding complications have been reported in some patients with hip fractures who received aspirin in conjunction with heparin as prophylaxis for deep-vein thrombosis.

● Thrombolytic Agents

Aspirin has been administered concomitantly with and/or after therapy with thrombolytic agents (e.g., streptokinase, alteplase) to prevent coronary artery reocclusion and/or reinfarction in patients with acute myocardial infarction. Concomitant administration of low dosages of aspirin with IV streptokinase therapy has been associated with additive reductions in mortality compared with those attributed to streptokinase therapy alone. Although concurrent therapy with aspirin and streptokinase was associated with an increased risk of major bleeding (including a slight increase in the incidence of confirmed intracranial hemorrhage during the first days of therapy) compared with placebo, such therapy appeared to be associated with only a slight increase in minor bleeding complications and no overall increase in serious bleeding episodes compared with streptokinase alone. Concomitant administration of low dosages of oral aspirin and IV heparin with IV alteplase therapy also has been associated with a substantial reduction in acute post-myocardial infarction mortality compared with placebo, but this regimen was accompanied by an apparent increased risk of bleeding complications, notably intracranial hemorrhage. Use after thrombolysis of drugs that affect platelet function should be individualized since these drugs may increase the risk of bleeding complications and have not been shown to be unequivocally effective to date. Further study is needed to elucidate the contribution of anticoagulant and/or platelet-aggregation inhibitor (e.g., aspirin) therapies to mortality reduction and the incidence of hemorrhagic complications observed in patients receiving these agents concomitantly with thrombolytic therapy.

● Uricosuric Agents

The uricosuric effects of salicylates and phenylbutazone, probenecid, or sulfinpyrazone are antagonistic; therefore, salicylates are generally contraindicated during uricosuric therapy. Although the exact mechanism(s) of the interaction has not been established, it appears to involve competition for active renal tubular transport; salicylates may also displace these agents from protein-binding sites. Salicylate-induced uricosuria is inhibited by usual doses of any of these agents. However, probenecid-induced uricosuria appears to be inhibited principally when the serum salicylate concentration exceeds 50 mcg/mL; therefore, occasional doses of salicylates for analgesia or antipyresis in patients receiving probenecid may be insufficient to produce a clinically important interaction. Although high single doses (e.g., greater than 3 g of sodium salicylate) of salicylates inhibit sulfinpyrazone-induced uricosuria, the effect of lower doses has not been determined. Frequent doses of salicylates for analgesia or antipyresis in patients receiving sulfinpyrazone as a uricosuric should probably be avoided. Patients receiving uricosuric agents should consult a clinician prior to initiating therapy with aspirin for *self-medication*. Sulfinpyrazone decreases the renal excretion of salicylate, apparently as a result of preferential tubular secretion of sulfinpyrazone.

● Antidiabetic Agents

The hypoglycemic effect of sulfonylureas (e.g., chlorpropamide, tolbutamide) may be enhanced by salicylates. Although this effect occurs principally with high salicylate dosages, it may occur with serum salicylate concentrations less than 100 mcg/mL. The exact mechanisms of the interaction are not known, but the ability of salicylates to decrease blood glucose concentration in diabetics may be involved. In vitro studies indicate that salicylates displace chlorpropamide and tolbutamide from protein-binding sites. In addition, salicylates may interfere with the renal tubular secretion of chlorpropamide, resulting in increased serum concentrations of the sulfonylurea. Further evaluation of the interaction between salicylates and sulfonylureas is needed. Patients receiving antidiabetic agents should consult a clinician prior to initiation of aspirin for *self-medication*. If salicylates and sulfonylureas are administered concurrently, caution should be exercised. Patients receiving both drugs should be observed closely for signs and symptoms of hypoglycemia and appropriate dosage reduction of either drug should be made accordingly. If reduction in sulfonylurea dosage is necessary when salicylate therapy is initiated, an increase in sulfonylurea dosage may be necessary when salicylate

therapy is discontinued. It is not known whether salicylates have similar effects on insulin.

Although the exact mechanism(s) is not known, aspirin appears to inhibit the flush effect induced by alcohol in some patients receiving chlorpropamide.

● Corticosteroids

Serum salicylate concentrations may decrease when corticosteroids are administered concomitantly. Likewise, when corticosteroids are discontinued in patients receiving salicylates, serum salicylate concentration may increase; salicylate intoxication has been precipitated rarely. Several mechanisms may be involved in this interaction. In one study in healthy individuals and in patients with polyarthritis who received both drugs concomitantly, corticosteroids increased the renal clearance of salicylate, possibly by increasing glomerular filtration rate. Corticosteroids may also induce the metabolism of salicylate. Salicylates and corticosteroids should be used concurrently with caution. Patients with receiving antiarthritic agents should consult a clinician prior to initiating therapy with aspirin for *self-medication*. Patients receiving both drugs should be observed closely for adverse effects of either drug. It may be necessary to increase salicylate dosage when corticosteroids are administered concurrently or decrease salicylate dosage when corticosteroids are discontinued in patients receiving salicylates.

● Methotrexate

Limited clinical data indicate that concurrent administration of salicylates and methotrexate may result in increased serum concentrations of methotrexate and thereby increase the risk of methotrexate toxicity. Salicylates displace methotrexate from plasma protein binding sites and decrease renal excretion of methotrexate by competing with and inhibiting renal tubular secretion of the antineoplastic agent. Several patients receiving both drugs reportedly developed severe pancytopenia; a few of these patients died. Since methotrexate has a low therapeutic index and may produce serious adverse effects, salicylates should be used with extreme caution, if at all, in patients receiving the drug. Geriatric patients and patients with impaired renal function may be at particular risk. If the drugs are administered concurrently, patients should be carefully monitored for signs of adverse effects of methotrexate. Patients receiving methotrexate should be warned to avoid nonprescription preparations containing salicylates.

● Acidifying and Alkalinizing Agents

Since the urinary excretion of salicylate is markedly pH dependent (see Pharmacokinetics: Elimination), concurrent administration of drugs that increase or decrease urine pH may increase or decrease urinary excretion of salicylate, respectively.

In patients receiving high dosages of salicylates, urinary acidifying agents (e.g., ammonium chloride) may increase renal tubular reabsorption of salicylate and possibly increase serum salicylate concentrations. However, if urine is acidic before administration of an acidifying agent, the increase in serum salicylate concentration is likely to be minimal; a substantial increase is likely only in patients who have an initial urine pH greater than 6.5.

Concurrent administration of high dosages of antacids (e.g., 4 g of sodium bicarbonate or at least 60–120 mL of aluminum and magnesium hydroxides suspension daily), or highly buffered aspirin solutions (e.g., Alka-Seltzer®) may increase urine pH and decrease serum salicylate concentrations by decreasing renal tubular reabsorption of salicylate. Although substantial reductions in serum salicylate concentration caused by concomitant antacid therapy have occasionally been reported, a quantitative reduction in serum salicylate concentration cannot be routinely predicted. Patients receiving high dosages of salicylates should be monitored for alterations in serum salicylate concentration if antacid therapy is initiated or discontinued, and salicylate dosage adjusted accordingly when necessary. Except for highly buffered tablets for preparation of an oral solution (Alka-Seltzer®), the amounts of buffer contained in other commercially available solid dosage forms of salicylates are insufficient to alter urine pH.

Carbonic anhydrase inhibitors (e.g., acetazolamide) may also increase urine pH and should generally be avoided in patients receiving high dosages of salicylates. More importantly, however, carbonic anhydrase inhibitors may induce metabolic acidosis and thereby enhance salicylate penetration into the CNS and other tissues, possibly resulting in salicylate intoxication. Likewise, use of a carbonic anhydrase inhibitor to alkalinize the urine in patients with salicylate overdosage may precipitate metabolic acidosis and lead to severe complications. (See

Acute Toxicity: Treatment.) There is evidence from pharmacokinetic studies that salicylates competitively inhibit protein binding of acetazolamide and substantially reduce plasma clearance of the drug, probably by competitively inhibiting renal tubular secretion of the carbonic anhydrase inhibitor. These results and well-documented case reports of toxicity during concomitant administration of acetazolamide and salicylates suggest that the observed toxicity potentially may result from either drug or both, and not necessarily just from the salicylate.

Alcohol

Concomitant ingestion of salicylates (particularly aspirin) and alcohol generally should be avoided since alcohol increases the incidence and severity of salicylate-induced GI bleeding and increases the risk of gastric mucosal erosions and ulceration. In one study, alcohol reportedly enhanced aspirin-induced prolongation of bleeding time in healthy individuals when ingested concomitantly or within at least 36 hours after a single dose of aspirin; the aspirin-induced prolongation of bleeding time was not potentiated when alcohol was ingested 12 hours before the dose of aspirin, and alcohol did not potentiate the effects of aspirin on platelet aggregation. Although further documentation is necessary, some clinicians have suggested that use of aspirin within 8–10 hours of heavy alcohol ingestion should be avoided when possible. The manufacturers caution that patients who generally consume 3 or more alcohol-containing drinks per day should ask their clinician whether to use oral salicylates (e.g., aspirin, choline salicylate, magnesium salicylate) or an alternative analgesic for *self-medication* since salicylates may increase the risk of GI bleeding. In addition, the manufacturers caution that patients who generally consume 3 or more alcohol-containing drinks per day should ask their clinician whether to use a salicylate (e.g., aspirin) in fixed combination with acetaminophen or an alternative analgesic for *self-medication* since salicylates in fixed combination with acetaminophen may increase the risk of GI bleeding and hepatotoxicity.

Nonsteroidal Anti-inflammatory Agents

Salicylates should be used cautiously with non-salicylate NSAIAs. Salicylates appear to have various pharmacokinetic interactions with many other NSAIAs; however, these interactions appear to have little or no clinical importance. Although most of the interactions with other NSAIAs have been studied or detected during concurrent administration of aspirin, the salicylate moiety is probably responsible for the interactions.

Concurrent administration of aspirin may decrease plasma concentrations of diflunisal, fenoprofen, ibuprofen, indomethacin, piroxicam, meclofenamate, and possibly naproxen and the active sulfide metabolite of sulindac; plasma concentrations of free tolmetin may be slightly increased. Aspirin appears to decrease plasma concentrations of indomethacin by decreasing the efficiency of its GI absorption and its renal clearance, and by increasing its biliary clearance. Aspirin apparently decreases GI absorption of meclofenamate sodium. Although the mechanisms of interaction with many of the other NSAIAs remain to be clearly established, salicylates may displace these agents from protein-binding sites, thereby increasing their metabolism and/or excretion. In general, salicylate pharmacokinetics are not affected by other NSAIAs.

Although the pharmacokinetic interactions appear to be of little or no clinical importance, many clinicians recommend that salicylates not be used in conjunction with other NSAIAs, since it has not been established that combination therapy is more efficacious than the individual agents alone and the potential for adverse effects (particularly GI and renal effects) may be increased.

Ibuprofen can antagonize the irreversible inhibition of platelet aggregation induced by aspirin and therefore may limit the cardioprotective effects of aspirin in patients with increased cardiovascular risk. Administration of 400 mg of ibuprofen 3 times daily in patients receiving aspirin 81 mg daily blocked the aspirin-induced inhibition of platelet cyclooxygenase-1 activity as well as the impairment of platelet aggregation achieved with aspirin during prolonged dosing. Administration of aspirin 2 hours before the morning dose of ibuprofen failed to circumvent the interaction with such multiple-dose administration, although such dose timing did effectively obviate the interaction when only single doses of each drug were administered.

The US Food and Drug Administration (FDA) recommends that patients taking a single dose of ibuprofen 400 mg for *self-medication* in conjunction with immediate-release, low-dose aspirin therapy be advised to administer the ibuprofen dose at least 8 hours before or at least 30 minutes after administration of aspirin. Data currently are insufficient to support recommendations regarding the timing of ibuprofen administration relative to that of enteric-coated, low-dose aspirin. The occasional use of ibuprofen is likely to be associated with minimal risk of attenuating the effects of low-dose aspirin. FDA states that other NSAIAs that are used for *self-medication* (e.g., ketoprofen, naproxen) should be viewed as having the potential to interfere with the antiplatelet effect of aspirin unless data are available that indicate otherwise. In one study, concomitant administration of naproxen (500 mg) and low-dose aspirin (100 mg) interfered with the antiplatelet effect of aspirin. Whether ketoprofen interferes with the antiplatelet effect of aspirin has not been investigated. Use of alternative analgesics that do not interfere with the antiplatelet effect of low-dose aspirin (e.g., acetaminophen, opiates) should be considered for patients at high risk of cardiovascular events. Labeling for prescription NSAIAs states that concomitant use of NSAIAs with aspirin is not recommended because of the potential for increased adverse effects. Limited data indicate that administration of diclofenac sodium delayed-release tablets (75 mg twice daily) does not inhibit the antiplatelet effect of aspirin (81 mg daily).

Salicylates

Patients receiving long-term salicylate therapy should be warned to avoid nonprescription preparations containing salicylates to prevent salicylate accumulation and potential toxicity. Results of several studies suggest that repeated doses or maximum recommended dosages of bismuth subsalicylate-containing antidiarrheal preparations (e.g., Pepto-Bismol®) could potentially lead to salicylate intoxication in patients receiving concurrent salicylate therapy.

Anticonvulsants

At high dosages, salicylate appears to displace phenytoin from protein-binding sites; however, it is unlikely that this interaction is clinically important since the increase in serum concentration of free phenytoin is apparently small and transient. However, because the fraction of total drug in serum as free phenytoin is increased, therapeutic effects of phenytoin may be associated with lower than usual total serum phenytoin concentrations in patients receiving both drugs.

Salicylates (particularly aspirin) and valproic acid should be administered concurrently with caution. When aspirin and valproic acid were administered concurrently in one study in children with epilepsy, salicylate apparently displaced valproic acid from serum albumin; the serum concentration and elimination half-life of both free and total valproic acid were increased. Salicylate also appeared to alter the metabolism of valproic acid. Although further evaluation of this interaction is needed, the results of this study suggest that concomitant use of salicylates and valproic acid might result in increased serum concentrations of free valproic acid and thereby increase the risk of adverse effects of the anticonvulsant. In addition to this potential interaction, both salicylates (particularly aspirin) and valproic acid may affect coagulation and their combined use may increase the risk of bleeding complications. If the drugs are administered concurrently, patients should be carefully monitored for adverse effects.

Diuretics

Aspirin has been shown to slightly reduce the natriuretic effect of spironolactone in healthy individuals, possibly by reducing active renal tubular secretion of canrenone, the active metabolite of spironolactone; the antihypertensive effect of spironolactone and its effect on urinary potassium excretion in hypertensive patients are apparently not affected. Until more clinical data are available on this potential interaction, patients receiving both drugs should be monitored for signs and symptoms of decreased clinical response to spironolactone.

Although reports are conflicting, aspirin appears to attenuate the diuretic effect of furosemide, possibly by competing with and inhibiting renal tubular secretion of furosemide. The clinical importance of this potential interaction has not been established; further evaluation is necessary.

Tetracyclines

Because tetracyclines readily chelate divalent and trivalent cations such as aluminum or magnesium, concurrent administration of buffered salicylate preparations containing such cations (e.g., Bufferin®), or concurrent administration of salicylate salts containing magnesium, may decrease absorption of oral tetracyclines. Therefore, such salicylate preparations should be given at least 1 hour before or after the tetracycline.

● Angiotensin-converting Enzyme Inhibitors

Because angiotensin-converting enzyme (ACE) inhibitors may promote kinin-mediated prostaglandin synthesis and/or release, concomitant use of drugs that inhibit prostaglandin synthesis and release, including salicylates, may reduce the blood pressure response to ACE inhibitors (e.g., captopril, enalapril). In addition, salicylates (e.g., aspirin) can attenuate the hemodynamic actions of ACE inhibitors in patients with congestive heart failure. Because ACE inhibitors share and enhance the effects of the compensatory hemodynamic mechanisms of heart failure, with aspirin interacting with the compensatory mechanisms rather than with a given ACE inhibitor per se, these desirable mechanisms are particularly susceptible to the interaction and a subsequent potential loss of clinical benefits. As a result, the more severe the heart failure and the more prominent the compensatory mechanisms, the more appreciable the interaction between aspirin and ACE inhibitors. Even if optimal dosage of an ACE inhibitor is used in the treatment of congestive heart failure, the potential cardiovascular and survival benefit may not be seen if the patient is receiving aspirin concomitantly.

In several multicenter studies, concomitant administration of a single 350-mg dose of aspirin in patients with congestive heart failure inhibited favorable hemodynamic effects associated with ACE inhibitors, attenuating the favorable effects of these drugs on survival and cardiovascular morbidity. However, these findings have not been confirmed by other studies. In one retrospective analysis of pooled data, patients who received an ACE inhibitor concomitantly with aspirin (160–325 mg daily) during the acute phase following myocardial infarction had proportional reductions in 7- and 30-day mortality rates comparable to patients who received an ACE inhibitor alone. Some clinicians have questioned the results of this study because of methodologic concerns (e.g., unsubstantiated assumptions about aspirin therapy [dosage, time of initiation, duration]; disparate distribution of patients).

Although it has been suggested that patients requiring long-term management of heart failure avoid the concomitant use of ACE inhibitors and aspirin (and perhaps substitute another platelet-aggregation inhibitor [e.g., clopidogrel, ticlopidine] for aspirin), many clinicians state that existing data are insufficient to recommend a change in the current prescribing practices of clinicians concerning the use of aspirin in patients receiving therapy with an ACE inhibitor.

● Varicella Virus Vaccine Live

Because of the association between Reye's syndrome, natural varicella infection, and salicylates (see Reye's Syndrome under Cautions: Pediatric Precautions), the manufacturer of varicella virus vaccine live recommends that individuals who receive the vaccine avoid use of salicylates for 6 weeks following vaccination. However, an association between Reye's syndrome, administration of varicella virus vaccine live, and use of salicylates has not been established and the syndrome has not been reported to date in recipients of the vaccine. For children who are receiving long-term salicylate therapy, the American Academy of Pediatrics (AAP) suggests that the theoretical risks associated with the vaccine be weighed against the known risks of the wild-type virus. The ACIP states that, since the risk for serious salicylate-associated complications is likely to be greater in children in whom natural varicella disease develops than in children who receive the vaccine containing attenuated virus, children who have rheumatoid arthritis or other conditions requiring therapeutic salicylate therapy probably should receive varicella virus vaccine live in conjunction with subsequent close monitoring.

● Other Drugs

Salicylates should be used cautiously, if at all, with other drugs that might potentiate the adverse GI effects.

Concurrent administration of salicylates and pyrazinamide may prevent or reduce hyperuricemia which usually occurs with pyrazinamide therapy.

Although there are apparently no published reports to date, the possibility that concurrent administration of salicylates and antiemetics (including antihistamines and phenothiazines) might mask the symptoms of salicylate-induced otic effects should be considered.

LABORATORY TEST INTERFERENCES

At dosages equivalent in salicylate content to 2.4 g or more of aspirin daily, salicylates may cause false-negative results in urinary glucose determinations using glucose oxidase reagent (e.g., Clinistix®, Tes-Tape®) and false-positive results in urinary glucose determinations using the cupric sulfate method (Benedict's solution, Clinitest®). Gentisic acid, a salicylate metabolite, may be responsible for false-negative results with glucose oxidase reagent since it is a potent reducing agent. Although salicylates are generally considered not to substantially affect glucose tolerance tests, some clinicians have reported that 3 g of aspirin daily results in a slightly increased oral glucose tolerance in healthy individuals and in patients with type 2 (non-insulin-dependent) diabetes mellitus.

Salicylates interfere with the Gerhardt test for acetoacetic acid by reacting with ferric chloride to produce a reddish color which, unlike the color produced by acetoacetic acid, persists after boiling.

Salicylates may produce falsely increased or decreased results in urinary vanillylmandelic acid (VMA) determinations, depending on the method used; with the Pisano method, urinary VMA may be falsely decreased. Salicylates should be avoided before and during urine collections for VMA determinations.

Aspirin has been shown to interfere with urinary 5-hydroxyindoleacetic acid (5-HIAA) determinations that use a fluorescent method.

Salicylates may decrease urinary excretion of phenolsulfonphthalein by competing for renal tubular secretion with the diagnostic agent. Therefore, the phenolsulfonphthalein excretion test should not be performed in patients receiving salicylates.

Although the evidence is somewhat conflicting, salicylates probably do not interfere with urinary 17-hydroxycorticosteroid determinations using the Porter-Silber method or with urinary 17-ketosteroid determinations using the Zimmerman color reaction. However, high dosages may cause false decreases in urinary 17-hydroxycorticosteroid determinations which utilize β-glucuronidase to hydrolyze the steroid glucuronides before extraction.

Concurrent administration of aspirin with xylose reportedly reduces urinary excretion of the sugar; the exact mechanism is not known.

At high dosages, salicylates competitively bind to thyroxine-binding globulin and thyroxine-binding prealbumin. As a result, serum protein-bound iodine is decreased; total serum concentrations of thyroxine and triiodothyronine are decreased while the unbound fractions of these hormones are increased. Secretion of thyrotropin, induced by exogenous administration of synthetic thyrotropin-releasing hormone (protirelin), is decreased in patients receiving salicylates, apparently as a result of the increased unbound fraction of thyroid hormones. Resin triiodothyronine uptake may be unchanged or slightly increased in patients receiving salicylates. Although reports are conflicting, 24-hour thyroid uptake of iodine 131 may be reduced following high dosages of salicylates.

Salicylates may falsely increase serum uric acid concentrations determined by colorimetric methods; serum uric acid concentrations determined by the uricase method are not affected.

Salicylates may completely interfere with or falsely decrease plasma theophylline concentrations determined by the Schack and Waxler method.

ACUTE TOXICITY

● Pathogenesis

Acute salicylate overdosage results from ingestion of a single toxic dose. The acute lethal dose of salicylate varies with the specific preparation ingested. Death has occurred in adults who ingested single 10- to 30-g doses of aspirin or sodium salicylate, but one patient survived after ingestion of 130 g of aspirin. In salicylate overdosage resulting from acute ingestion, little or no toxicity generally occurs in individuals ingesting less than 150 mg/kg, mild to moderate toxicity in those ingesting 150–300 mg/kg, severe toxicity in those ingesting 300–500 mg/kg, and potentially lethal toxicity in those ingesting greater than 500 mg/kg.

The pathophysiology of salicylate overdosage is complex because of the variety of toxic effects produced and their resultant manifestations. The principal toxic effects are extensions of pharmacologic actions and include local GI irritation, direct CNS stimulation of respiration, uncoupling of oxidative phosphorylation, altered glucose metabolism through inhibition of Krebs cycle enzymes, stimulation of gluconeogenesis and lipid metabolism, increased tissue glycolysis, inhibition of amino acid metabolism, and interference with hemostatic mechanisms.

● Manifestations

Acute salicylate overdosage produces manifestations similar to those of chronic intoxication, but the effects are often more pronounced and occur in more rapid succession.

Ingestion may cause mild burning pain in the throat and stomach; vomiting, particularly in infants and children, usually begins within 1–8 hours. An asymptomatic interval of several hours may follow these initial manifestations.

In addition to manifestations of chronic intoxication, oliguria or acute renal failure, hyperthermia, restlessness, irritability, garrulity, incoherent speech, apprehension, vertigo, asterixis, tremor, diplopia, confusion, disorientation, delirium, mania, hallucinations, EEG abnormalities, generalized seizures, lethargy, and coma may occur; toxic encephalopathy resembling chorea may also occur. The mental disturbances, sometimes referred to as *salicylate jag*, resemble alcoholic intoxication without euphoria. Pulmonary edema, skin eruptions (see Cautions: Dermatologic Effects), and pancreatitis occur less frequently. Hemorrhagic complications (e.g., petechiae in skin and mucous membranes, GI bleeding, perforated peptic ulcer) or a syndrome resembling inappropriate secretion of antidiuretic hormone (SIADH) occurs rarely. As salicylate intoxication progresses, CNS stimulation is replaced by CNS depression manifested as stupor and coma; respiratory insufficiency and cardiovascular collapse follow, sometimes with asphyxial seizures. Death usually occurs during coma and results from respiratory failure or cardiovascular collapse.

The principal physiologic manifestations of salicylate overdosage are acid-base and electrolyte disturbances, dehydration, hyperpyrexia, and hyperglycemia or hypoglycemia. As with high dosages, single toxic doses of salicylate produce respiratory stimulation by peripheral and central mechanisms, resulting in hyperventilation, hypocapnia, and respiratory alkalosis; compensation for the respiratory alkalosis occurs rapidly. (See Pharmacology: Metabolic Effects.) Hyperventilation usually occurs when the serum salicylate concentration exceeds 350 mcg/mL and begins within 6–12 hours after ingestion of a single toxic dose. Marked hyperpnea usually occurs at a serum concentration of about 500 mcg/mL.

Metabolic acidosis usually follows compensation of respiratory alkalosis; occasionally, respiratory acidosis also occurs, usually only when intoxication progresses and respiration is centrally depressed or when a CNS depressant has been ingested concomitantly. Metabolic acidosis develops principally from accumulation of organic acids (pyruvic, lactic, acetoacetic, and amino acids) secondary to salicylate interference with carbohydrate and amino acid metabolism and increased lipid metabolism; inorganic phosphoric and sulfuric acids also accumulate secondary to salicylate-induced renal impairment. Depletion of buffer capacity as a result of the initial compensatory increase in renal excretion of bicarbonate also contributes to development of metabolic acidosis. Depending on the relative contributions of the metabolic effects, either alkalemia or acidemia and either alkaluria or aciduria may be observed. Early in the course of acute intoxication in most adults and with mild to moderate intoxication in older children, respiratory alkalosis alone or with alkaluria may be present. In adults, alkalemia occurs often and may persist, but a mixed acid-base disturbance (usually metabolic acidosis and respiratory alkalosis) appears to occur most frequently. With acute intoxication in children, metabolic acidosis and respiratory alkalosis are usually present, with acidosis and acidemia predominating. Until adequate salicylate removal from the GI tract has been accomplished, the likelihood of acidosis increases with time elapsed since the ingestion; severe acidosis may not occur for 12–24 hours after acute ingestion.

In general, severity of acidosis increases with decreasing age; metabolic acidosis apparently predominates in young children because they are more susceptible to development of ketosis. The severity of acidosis also generally increases with increasing severity of intoxication and vice versa. Acidosis and acidemia increase the severity of intoxication by enhancing salicylate penetration into the CNS and other tissues (see Pharmacokinetics: Distribution); increased CNS concentrations of salicylate appear to be directly related to CNS dysfunction and death. Therefore, the greater severity of intoxication observed in young children appears to be due in part to the increased frequency and severity of acidosis in these patients. In adults, severe acidosis is associated with impaired consciousness and a poor prognosis.

Toxic effects that result in acid-base disturbances also cause alterations of fluid and electrolyte balance. Increased metabolism and heat production increase cutaneous insensible losses, principally of water, but also of sodium as a result of sweating. During compensation of initial respiratory alkalosis, renal excretion of bicarbonate is accompanied by increased renal excretion of sodium, potassium, and water. As intoxication progresses and metabolic acidosis develops, organic aciduria increases the solute load excreted by the kidney and is also accompanied by increased renal excretion of sodium, potassium, and water. The resultant dehydration and electrolyte imbalance may be enhanced by decreased fluid intake and vomiting, and hyperventilation (increased pulmonary insensible water loss). Electrolyte losses lead to total body depletion of sodium and potassium. However, hypernatremia is usually observed due to dehydration; hyponatremia is uncommon and associated with inappropriate fluid retention (SIADH). Hypokalemia is also usually observed; even if serum potassium concentration is normal, total body potassium depletion is likely. In general, water loss may be as great as 2–3 L/m² with moderate intoxication and 4–6 L/m² with severe intoxication. Oliguria may occur as a result of severe dehydration. Anuria or acute renal failure usually accompanies severe shock, hemorrhage, or cardiovascular collapse.

Hyperthermia, sometimes with rectal temperature as high as 40.5–42.2°C, is secondary to impaired oxidative phosphorylation and the consequent increase in heat production by body tissues. In toxic doses, salicylates appear to decrease efficiency of normal body cooling mechanisms; dehydration enhances this effect. When hyperthermia is present, it contributes to dehydration.

Altered glucose metabolism may result in hyperglycemia or hypoglycemia. Hyperglycemia usually occurs early in the course of intoxication as a result of interference with tissue utilization of glucose. Blood glucose concentration usually does not exceed 200 mg/dL but glucosuria may occur; hyperglycemia may persist for a few hours to a few days. Salicylate-induced hyperglycemia associated with coma, ketoacidosis, dehydration, and hyperventilation closely simulates diabetic ketoacidosis. Eventually, hypoglycemia may occur as a result of glucose depletion. Hypoglycemia may be life-threatening and is most likely to occur in infants or late in the course of intoxication. CNS hypoglycemia may occur despite the absence of systemic hypoglycemia and should be considered in children with seizures, coma, or cardiovascular collapse.

● Treatment

In the treatment of acute salicylate intoxication, intensive symptomatic and supportive therapy should be instituted immediately. Treatment consists principally of removal of salicylate from the GI tract and prevention of further absorption; correction of fluid, electrolyte, and acid-base disturbances; and measures to enhance salicylate elimination.

Assessment of Severity of Intoxication

In acute ingestions, severity of intoxication can be estimated by assessing the amount reported to be ingested, by evaluating the clinical condition of the patient, and by measuring serum salicylate concentration.

Since the apparent volume of distribution of salicylate appears to increase with increasing doses, a specific serum salicylate concentration following acute ingestion of large doses may reflect a higher amount of salicylate in the body than the same serum concentration attained following ingestion of smaller doses; therefore, toxic effects may be more severe than generally anticipated, depending upon the ingested dose.

In overdosage with massive doses, serum salicylate concentration may continue to increase for up to 24 hours. In overdosage with enteric-coated or extended-release salicylate preparations, absorption may be delayed and serum salicylate concentration may continue to increase up to 72 hours after the ingestion. In the event that a serum concentration cannot be obtained or a preliminary estimate is desired, a Phenistix® reagent strip (as used in the diagnosis of phenylketonuria) may be dipped into separated plasma or serum obtained from the intoxicated individual; the reagent strip generally gives a tan color with salicylate concentrations less than 400 mcg/mL, a darker brown color with concentrations of 400–900 mcg/mL, and a purple color with concentrations exceeding 900 mcg/mL.

Measures to Reduce Salicylate Absorption

In acute overdosage, the stomach should be emptied immediately, preferably by ipecac syrup-induced emesis if the patient is alert, or by gastric lavage. These procedures are generally effective up to 3–4 hours after an acute ingestion and may be effective for up to 10 hours following ingestion of massive doses. If the patient is comatose, having seizures, or has lost the gag reflex, gastric lavage may be performed if an endotracheal tube with cuff inflated is in place to prevent aspiration of vomitus. Activated charcoal should be administered since it is extremely effective in reducing salicylate absorption. Activated charcoal is usually administered as an aqueous suspension; adults are usually given 50–100 g and children 30–60 g or 0.5–1 g/kg. *Activated charcoal should not be administered before induction of emesis with ipecac syrup since the emetic is inactivated by activated charcoal.* Administration of a saline cathartic (e.g., magnesium citrate, sodium sulfate) is also usually recommended, with repeated administration until the activated charcoal has been passed rectally. However, the efficacy of saline catharsis in salicylate overdosage remains to be clearly determined. Results of several studies in healthy individuals suggest that saline catharsis in combination with activated charcoal does not further decrease GI absorption of salicylate compared to activated charcoal alone; however, studies in acutely intoxicated patients are needed.

Fluid and Electrolyte Therapy

If hyperthermia and/or dehydration have developed, initial treatment should be directed to their correction and maintenance of normal renal function. Patients with a rectal temperature greater than 40°C should be cooled by cooling devices or by sponging with tepid water. Appropriate fluid and electrolyte therapy should be administered promptly, based on evaluation of the patient's fluid, acid-base, and electrolyte status. Arterial pH and blood gases (Po_2, pCO_2, and total CO_2); serum sodium, potassium, chloride, bicarbonate, and creatinine concentrations; and blood glucose concentration and BUN should be determined immediately. Urinary output should be monitored hourly. The PT should also be monitored. Determinations of acid-base and electrolyte status and renal function should be performed frequently during treatment to guide therapy.

In patients with mild intoxication who have adequate urine output and do not vomit severely, fluids should be administered orally every hour up to a total of 100 mL/kg in the first 24 hours. In more severely intoxicated patients, IV fluid and electrolyte therapy is necessary; fluid requirements usually range from 2–6 L/m² in the first 24 hours. Patients are usually rehydrated initially with an IV solution containing 5–10% dextrose (to prevent hypoglycemia) with 75 mEq of sodium, 50 mEq of chloride, and 25 mEq of bicarbonate per liter; if metabolic acidosis is not present, the bicarbonate is replaced by chloride. This solution is usually administered at a rate of 10–20 mL/kg per hour for 1–2 hours; patients in shock may require more rapid fluid administration. Acidemia should be corrected as rapidly as possible to minimize entry of salicylate into the CNS and other tissues. Just as acidemia enhances intracellular movement of salicylate, correction of acidemia and/or maintenance of an alkaline serum pH facilitate movement of salicylate from intracellular sites to plasma and ultimately to urine. If acidosis is severe (serum pH less than 7.15), patients should receive additional IV sodium bicarbonate, 1–2 mEq/kg every 1–2 hours, as necessary. *Potassium is added to IV fluids to replace losses only after it has been determined that renal function is adequate;* potassium replacement may be necessary to accomplish alkalinization of the urine. Patients should be monitored by ECG and serum potassium determinations during potassium replacement. Subsequent hydration is usually performed with an IV solution containing 5–10% dextrose with 40 mEq of sodium, 35 mEq of potassium, 50 mEq of chloride, and 20 mEq of bicarbonate per liter; if acidosis persists, an additional 15 mEq of sodium bicarbonate is usually added to each liter. This solution is usually administered at a rate of 4–8 mL/kg per hour until the serum salicylate concentration is less than 300 mcg/mL, which may require several hours to several days. Thereafter, IV hydration is continued as necessary, usually with a solution containing 5% dextrose with 25 mEq each of sodium and chloride and 20 mEq each of potassium and bicarbonate per liter; this solution is usually administered at a rate of 2–3 mL/kg per hour.

Other Supportive Therapies

If severe hypotension and/or manifestations of hemorrhagic complications (e.g., petechiae) are initially present, whole blood transfusions (10–15 mL/kg over 1 hour) may be necessary. Plasma transfusions may be beneficial, especially if shock develops. Although routine administration of vitamin K has been suggested in salicylate intoxication, the drug is usually administered only if hemorrhagic complications occur or if the PT is prolonged. Patients with respiratory depression may require assisted pulmonary ventilation and oxygen. CNS depressants (e.g., barbiturates, narcotics) should not be administered to counter salicylate-induced hyperventilation since they may lead to respiratory acidosis and coma. Seizures may usually be controlled by IV administration of a benzodiazepine (e.g., diazepam) or short-acting barbiturate; a short-acting skeletal muscle relaxant (e.g., succinylcholine), assisted pulmonary ventilation, and oxygen may occasionally be necessary.

Measures to Enhance Salicylate Elimination

Although reduction of hyperthermia and appropriate IV fluid and electrolyte therapy constitute adequate treatment for many patients, therapeutic measures (e.g., forced alkaline diuresis, hemodialysis) to enhance salicylate elimination may also be useful and/or necessary, depending on severity of intoxication. Forced alkaline diuresis with IV sodium bicarbonate (and IV furosemide when necessary) may be employed since alkalinization of the urine to pH 7.5 or greater, with maintenance of sufficient urine flow, greatly enhances the rate of urinary salicylate excretion. (See Pharmacokinetics: Elimination.) Sodium bicarbonate should *not* be given orally since it might enhance absorption of salicylate. Forced alkaline diuresis is often employed when the serum salicylate concentration exceeds 500 mcg/mL 6 hours after the ingestion and the patient's condition indicates severe intoxication. However, dehydration must be corrected before the procedure is employed. Forced alkaline diuresis with sodium bicarbonate should be performed with caution, particularly in infants, or in older children and adults with respiratory alkalosis; hypernatremia, pulmonary edema, and severe alkalosis (possibly with tetany and/or hypokalemia) may occur. If forced alkaline diuresis is employed, sufficient urinary output must be maintained, urine and serum pH must be carefully monitored, and dosage of sodium bicarbonate adjusted accordingly; for optimum results, urine pH of 7.5 or greater and serum pH of 7.5 should be maintained. In most children, even high doses of sodium bicarbonate may not produce a sufficiently alkaline urine because the degree of inorganic acid production and resultant aciduria cannot be adequately compensated; in addition, alkalinization of the urine may not be accomplished until potassium depletion is corrected.

Following correction of acidemia with sodium bicarbonate, acetazolamide has been used as an adjunct to alkalinize the urine; *however, its use is dangerous and generally not recommended since it may precipitate metabolic acidosis and lead to severe complications.* (See Drug Interactions: Acidifying and Alkalinizing Agents.) Therefore, if acetazolamide is used at all, it should probably be used only in adults with respiratory alkalosis and only under the supervision of clinicians experienced in the use of the drug in salicylate overdosage. Some clinicians have also suggested that tromethamine may be useful in patients with severe, refractory metabolic acidosis or in patients in whom sodium restriction is necessary; *however, tromethamine should be used with extreme caution, if at all, since the drug produces intracellular as well as extracellular alkalinization and may therefore increase CNS and tissue concentrations of salicylate.*

The most effective measures for removal of salicylate from the body are hemodialysis or hemoperfusion in adults and older children, and peritoneal dialysis or exchange transfusions in young children and infants; however, these measures are rarely necessary. Most clinicians reserve these measures for patients with serum salicylate concentrations of 900–1300 mcg/mL or higher 6 hours after an ingestion, unresponsive acidosis (pH less than 7.1), impaired renal function or renal failure, pulmonary edema, persistent CNS manifestations (e.g., seizures, coma), progressive deterioration despite appropriate therapy, or preexisting disease that prohibits usual therapeutic measures. If any of these conditions occurs, hemodialysis may be useful regardless of serum salicylate concentration. Hemodialysis and hemoperfusion are considered to be equally effective in removing salicylate, but hemodialysis is preferred to hemoperfusion since acid-base and electrolyte disturbances are corrected more rapidly with hemodialysis. In patients with severe intoxication, peritoneal dialysis and exchange transfusions may be instituted while preparations for hemodialysis or hemoperfusion are undertaken. If peritoneal dialysis is employed, 50 g of albumin should be added to each liter of dialysate; binding of salicylate to albumin enhances the efficiency of peritoneal dialysis.

CHRONIC TOXICITY

Since the pathophysiology, manifestations, and treatment of chronic salicylate intoxication are similar to those of acute salicylate intoxication, the Acute Toxicity section should be consulted for additional information.

● Pathogenesis

Chronic salicylate intoxication, also known as *salicylism,* results from high dosages or from prolonged therapy with high dosages. Some clinicians believe that chronic intoxication is generally associated with ingestion of dosages greater than 100 mg/kg daily for 2 days or longer. Severe chronic intoxication has often occurred in infants who were dehydrated as a result of fever and/or illness, and is best prevented by generally avoiding use of salicylates for antipyresis in infants or by limiting dosage in these patients.

● Manifestations

Chronic intoxication is manifested principally as tinnitus, hearing loss, dimness of vision, headache, dizziness, mental confusion, lassitude, drowsiness, sweating, thirst, hyperventilation, increased heart rate, nausea, vomiting, and occasionally diarrhea; however, if intoxication is severe, other manifestations associated with acute intoxication may occur. Chronic salicylate intoxication is sometimes not readily recognized since a preexisting disease or concomitant illness may produce signs and symptoms (e.g., nausea, vomiting, tachypnea, disorientation) that are similar to those of salicylate intoxication.

Tinnitus and hearing loss are the most frequent manifestations of chronic intoxication in adults. (See Cautions: Otic Effects.) In children, the most frequent manifestations are hyperventilation or CNS effects such as giddiness, drowsiness, or behavioral changes; these effects usually occur at serum salicylate concentrations greater than 300 mcg/mL.

The onset of hyperventilation is usually insidious. With chronic intoxication, metabolic acidosis and respiratory alkalosis are usually present, with acidosis and acidemia predominating. Acidosis is usually more severe with chronic intoxication than with ingestion of a single toxic dose. Hypoglycemia, which may be life-threatening, is also likely to occur.

● Treatment

Usually only evaluation of the clinical condition of patients with chronic intoxication is useful in determining the severity of intoxication. Serum salicylate concentrations may be determined but are not as useful in estimating the severity; severe symptomatology has been associated with concentrations as low as 150 mcg/mL.

When chronic intoxication is mild, dosage reduction or discontinuance of salicylates, in conjunction with symptomatic and supportive therapy, usually constitutes adequate treatment. When intoxication is more severe, salicylates are discontinued and intensive symptomatic and supportive therapy, as in the treatment of acute salicylate intoxication, should be instituted immediately. Patients who experience hearing loss of tinnitus during aspirin therapy should discontinue therapy and consult a clinician. Hemodialysis may be particularly useful in chronically intoxicated patients with high serum salicylate concentrations. Regardless of serum salicylate concentration, hemodialysis may also be especially useful in those with unresponsive acidosis (pH less than 7.1), impaired renal function or renal failure, pulmonary edema, persistent CNS manifestations (e.g., seizures, coma), progressive deterioration despite appropriate therapy, or preexisting disease that prohibits usual therapeutic measures.

PHARMACOLOGY

Salicylates mainly exhibit analgesic, anti-inflammatory, and antipyretic activity. These effects appear to result principally from the salicylate moiety. Although aspirin hydrolyzes to salicylate and acetate, it does not require hydrolysis to produce its effects; in addition, aspirin appears to have some pharmacologic effects that are distinct from those of salicylate. The ability of aspirin to acetylate proteins results in some effects, such as inhibition of platelet aggregation, which other currently available salicylates do not exhibit. (See Pharmacology in Aspirin 28:08.04.24.)

The exact mechanisms have not been clearly established, but many actions (e.g., analgesic, anti-inflammatory) of salicylates appear to be associated principally with inhibition of prostaglandin synthesis. Aspirin inhibits the synthesis of prostaglandins in body tissues by irreversibly acetylating and inactivating cyclooxygenase; at least 2 isoenzymes, cyclooxygenase-1 (COX-1) and -2 (COX-2) (also referred to as prostaglandin G/H synthase-1 [PGHS-1] and -2 [PGHS-2], respectively), have been identified that catalyze the formation of prostaglandins in the arachidonic acid pathway. Salicylate only minimally inhibits cyclooxygenase in vitro but is as active as aspirin in vivo in decreasing prostaglandin synthesis. Salicylate may be a reversible inhibitor of cyclooxygenase, but this has not been clearly established. Inhibition of prostaglandin synthesis by aspirin and salicylate may also involve other mechanisms.

Although aspirin and other salicylates inhibit cyclooxygenase and thereby decrease production of prostaglandins, they apparently do not inhibit

lipoxygenase, an enzyme involved in the formation of 12-hydroperoxyarachidonic acid (12-HPETE) and leukotrienes from arachidonic acid. Since cyclooxygenase and lipoxygenase appear to compete for the metabolism of arachidonic acid, the inhibition of cyclooxygenase by aspirin and other salicylates may actually result in increased formation of 12-HPETE and leukotrienes. In platelets, 12-HPETE increases lipoxygenase activity (thereby increasing its own formation) and inhibits cyclooxygenase. Therefore, in the presence of salicylate, increased formation of 12-HPETE via lipoxygenase may contribute to the inhibition of cyclooxygenase. In addition, high concentrations of aspirin or salicylate have been reported to reversibly inhibit the conversion of 12-HPETE to 12-hydroxyarachidonic acid (12-HETE) via peroxidase. By inhibiting this conversion, salicylates may also increase concentrations of 12-HPETE and thereby indirectly inhibit cyclooxygenase. However, further evaluation of these effects is needed.

● Analgesic Effect

The analgesic effect of salicylates may result from inhibition of prostaglandin synthesis. Prostaglandins appear to sensitize pain receptors to mechanical stimulation or to other chemical mediators (e.g., bradykinin, histamine). Since salicylates do not directly alter the pain threshold or prevent pain caused by exogenous or previously synthesized endogenous prostaglandins, the drugs may produce analgesia by inhibiting the formation of prostaglandins involved in pain. The analgesic effect of salicylates appears to result from mainly a peripheral action, but the drugs may also have similar activity and/or other mechanisms of action in the CNS, possibly in the hypothalamus. In addition, the anti-inflammatory effect of the drugs may contribute to their analgesic effect. There is no evidence that long-term therapy with salicylates results in tolerance to or physical dependence on the drugs.

● Anti-inflammatory Effect

Due in part to the complexity of the inflammatory response, the exact mechanisms of the anti-inflammatory effect of salicylates have not been fully elucidated. Since prostaglandins appear to mediate many inflammatory effects and have been shown to directly produce many of the signs and symptoms of inflammation, the anti-inflammatory effect of salicylates may be due in part to inhibition of prostaglandin synthesis and release during inflammation. The anti-inflammatory effect of salicylates and other NSAIAs generally appears to be positively correlated with their ability to inhibit prostaglandin synthesis; however, the relative contributions of this and other mechanisms of action remain to be determined.

Although aspirin and other salicylates inhibit cyclooxygenase and thereby decrease production of prostaglandins, they apparently do not inhibit the formation of leukotrienes. The exact roles of leukotrienes in inflammation have not been fully elucidated, but they may contribute to the inflammatory response. Inhibition of cyclooxygenase by aspirin and other salicylates, while reducing prostaglandin synthesis and release, may actually result in the increased formation of leukotrienes. However, the clinical importance of such an effect remains to be determined.

Although high concentrations of aspirin or salicylate have been reported to reversibly inhibit the conversion of 12-HPETE to 12-HETE, a compound that appears to be a chemotactic stimulus for polymorphonuclear leukocytes, it is not clear whether salicylates enhance or inhibit migration of leukocytes into inflamed tissue. Salicylates have been shown to stabilize lysosomal membranes in vitro; therefore, they may prevent the release of lysosomal substances which contribute to inflammation. The anti-inflammatory action of the drugs may also involve effects on other cellular and immunologic processes in mesenchymal and connective tissues. Salicylates may inhibit lymphocyte activation, and by inhibiting cyclooxygenase, salicylates and other NSAIAs may interfere with prostaglandin-mediated formation of autoantibodies that are involved in the inflammatory process. High serum concentrations of salicylates may also suppress antigen-antibody reactions, but the contribution of this effect to the anti-inflammatory action of salicylates has not been established. Although the mechanism is not known, salicylates have been shown to enhance monocyte-mediated cytotoxicity and thereby increase antigen removal. Salicylates may also alter the composition, synthesis, and metabolism of connective tissue mucopolysaccharides related to the ground substance that helps prevent spread of inflammation.

● Antipyretic Effect

Salicylates lower body temperature in patients with fever; the drugs rarely decrease body temperature in afebrile patients. Salicylates decrease body temperature principally by inhibiting the synthesis and release of prostaglandins that mediate the effect of endogenous pyrogen in the hypothalamus; however, other mechanisms may be involved. Although heat production is not directly inhibited by salicylates, centrally mediated dilation of peripheral blood vessels and sweating enhance dissipation of heat. Paradoxically, toxic doses of salicylates may increase body temperature by increasing oxygen consumption and metabolic rate, apparently as a result of salicylate-induced uncoupling of oxidative phosphorylation.

● **Hematologic Effects**

Aspirin, but not other currently available salicylates, inhibits platelet aggregation and prolongs bleeding time. (See Pharmacology: Hematologic Effects, in Aspirin 28:08.04.24.)

Salicylates alter the hepatic synthesis of blood coagulation factors VII, IX, and X, apparently by interfering with the action of vitamin K; this effect appears to be dose-dependent and occurs principally when serum salicylate concentration exceeds 300 mcg/mL. At usual dosages (e.g., 1.3–6 g of aspirin daily), the prothrombin time (PT) may rarely be increased by 2–3 seconds; larger increases in the PT may occur at higher dosages or in patients with fever or increased metabolic rate. The increased PT is due mainly to a deficiency in factor VII and can be reversed by administration of phytonadione (vitamin K_1) or discontinuance of salicylate therapy; in some patients, the PT may return to normal even if salicylate therapy is continued.

Although salicylates usually do not alter the leukocyte or erythrocyte count, the drugs may decrease leukocytosis and erythrocyte sedimentation rate in patients with rheumatic fever; the mechanisms of these effects are not known. Although reports are conflicting, salicylates also apparently increase fibrinolysis, possibly by enhancing the fibrinolytic action of leukocytes.

● **Genitourinary and Renal Effects**

Salicylates produce various effects on the uterus, apparently by inhibiting prostaglandin synthesis. Prostaglandins E_2 and F_{2a} increase the amplitude and frequency of uterine contractions in pregnant women; current evidence suggests that primary dysmenorrhea is also mediated by these prostaglandins. In some patients with primary dysmenorrhea, salicylate therapy has produced analgesic effects and has been associated with decreased synthesis of prostaglandin F_{2a}. Administration of salicylates during late pregnancy may prolong gestation and labor by inhibiting the formation of prostaglandins involved in these processes.

Salicylates have dose-related effects on urinary excretion of uric acid. In large dosages (e.g., 1.3 g of aspirin 4 times daily), salicylates enhance urinary excretion of uric acid and decrease serum uric acid concentration by inhibiting reabsorption of uric acid in the proximal renal tubule. Intermediate dosages (e.g., 650 mg to 1 g of aspirin 3 times daily) inhibit secretion of uric acid in the distal renal tubule but only slightly inhibit its reabsorption; therefore, urinary uric acid excretion is usually not altered. Low dosages (e.g., 325 mg of aspirin 3 times daily or less) inhibit renal tubular secretion of uric acid and therefore may decrease urinary uric acid excretion and increase serum uric acid concentration. In general, serum uric acid concentrations are increased when plasma salicylate concentrations are less than 100 mcg/mL and decreased when plasma salicylate concentrations are greater than 100 mcg/mL. Salicylates antagonize the activity of other uricosuric agents. (See Drug Interactions: Uricosuric Agents.)

Although salicylates generally do not alter renal function in healthy individuals, aspirin has been reported to cause reversible (sometimes marked) decreases in renal blood flow and glomerular filtration rate (which may be accompanied by minimal water, sodium, and potassium retention) in sodium-restricted, otherwise healthy individuals and in patients with impaired renal function, systemic lupus erythematosus, or other conditions predisposing to sodium and water retention. (See Cautions: Renal Effects.) These effects appear to be associated with inhibition of renal synthesis of prostaglandins such as prostaglandin E_2 and prostacyclin (epoprostenol, PGI_2); these prostaglandins increase renal blood flow and help to maintain renal function. Aspirin-induced renal impairment has been directly correlated with decreased urinary excretion of immunoreactive prostaglandin E. In addition, aspirin has been associated with analgesic nephropathy. (See Cautions: Renal Effects.)

● **GI Effects**

Salicylates (especially aspirin) can cause gastric mucosal damage which may result in ulceration and/or bleeding. (See Cautions: GI Effects.) The damage is generally believed to be the result of a local action; however, IV administration of salicylates has also been reported to cause gastric mucosal lesions and bleeding.

The mechanism of salicylate-induced gastric mucosal damage is complex. Gastric mucosal effects have been attributed to inhibition of the synthesis of prostaglandins produced by COX-1. Salicylates appear to selectively increase permeability of the gastric mucosa to cations, and thus, enhance back diffusion of hydrogen ions; the increased entry of acid into the mucosa causes cellular damage. The resultant cellular damage leads to additional alterations in gastric mucosal permeability. Salicylates may also alter mucosal permeability by disrupting metabolism in gastric mucosal cells.

Salicylates cause nausea and vomiting as a result of local gastric irritation and/or by CNS stimulation.

● **Cardiovascular Effects**

Salicylates generally have no direct cardiovascular effects; however, large single doses (e.g., 2.4 g of aspirin) may result in dilation of peripheral blood vessels by a direct effect on smooth muscle. In patients receiving large dosages of salicylates, such as those with rheumatic fever, circulating plasma volume may increase by about 20% (with resultant hemodilution) and cardiac workload and output may also increase. The increase in plasma volume may be due to sodium and water retention secondary to salicylate-induced renal impairment. In overdosage, salicylates may directly suppress cardiac conduction and may cause circulatory depression and possibly collapse, both directly and through central vasomotor paralysis.

● **Metabolic Effects**

In high dosages (e.g., greater than 6 g of aspirin daily) or in the initial phase of overdosage, salicylates produce respiratory stimulation by peripheral and central mechanisms, with resultant changes in acid-base balance and electrolytes. Peripherally, salicylates uncouple oxidative phosphorylation, principally in skeletal muscle; the resultant increased production of carbon dioxide stimulates alveolar ventilation so that carbon dioxide tension is not changed. This increase in alveolar ventilation is characterized as an increase in depth of respiration and a slight increase in rate of respiration. As salicylates enter the CNS, the drugs directly stimulate the respiratory center in the medulla, resulting in marked hyperventilation that is characterized as an increase in depth of respiration and a pronounced increase in rate of respiration. Plasma carbon dioxide tension decreases, and intracellular and extracellular respiratory alkalosis develops. Compensation for respiratory alkalosis occurs rapidly and includes increased renal excretion of bicarbonate, sodium, potassium, and water; as a result, plasma bicarbonate concentration is decreased and blood pH returns toward normal. If substantial potassium depletion occurs, the kidneys retain potassium and excrete hydrogen ions instead, regardless of blood pH; therefore, a paradoxical aciduria can occur in the presence of salicylate-induced systemic alkalosis. These changes in acid-base balance and electrolytes are most often observed in adults receiving high dosages; more severe alterations in acid-base balance (e.g., metabolic acidosis) and electrolytes generally occur only in overdosage.

Salicylates produce a variety of other metabolic effects. The effects on carbohydrate metabolism are complex and involve numerous mechanisms, often with opposing results on blood glucose concentration. High dosages may cause hyperglycemia and glycosuria by interfering with tissue utilization of glucose; however, blood glucose concentration may be decreased in diabetics. It has been suggested that this effect in diabetics may result from increased uptake of glucose by muscle, increased rate of tissue glycolysis, and decreased synthesis of glucose from noncarbohydrate precursors, all of which may be due in part to uncoupling of oxidative phosphorylation. It has also been suggested that salicylates stimulate insulin secretion. In high dosages, or with long-term therapy or overdosage, salicylates eventually decrease aerobic metabolism of glucose and cause depletion of liver and muscle glycogen; hypoglycemia may occur. Depletion of liver glycogen may be caused by an increased rate of glycogenolysis and a decreased rate of glycogen synthesis; these effects may also be related to the uncoupling action of salicylates. In vitro studies have shown that salicylates also inhibit aldose reductase, the enzyme that catalyzes the formation of sorbitol. In overdosage, salicylates decrease synthesis and increase catabolism of proteins which results in a negative nitrogen balance characterized as aminoaciduria. Salicylates may also decrease fatty acid synthesis, increase metabolism of fatty acids and oxidation of ketone bodies, and decrease plasma concentrations of phospholipids and free fatty acids.

With a dosage equivalent in salicylate content to at least 5 g of aspirin daily, plasma concentrations of cholesterol may be decreased.

Salicylates inhibit uptake of ascorbic acid by leukocytes and platelets. As a result, leukocyte and plasma concentrations of ascorbic acid are decreased to concentrations slightly higher than those associated with tissue depletion of the vitamin; however, there is no evidence to date that salicylate therapy precipitates ascorbic acid deficiency. Although concomitant administration of ascorbic acid supplements increases plasma ascorbic acid concentrations, leukocyte ascorbic acid concentrations are not increased and tissue stores of the vitamin may not be increased. Therefore, routine administration of ascorbic acid supplements to patients receiving salicylates is not warranted; however, patients receiving high dosages of salicylates who exhibit any signs or symptoms of ascorbic acid deficiency should be evaluated for such a deficiency.

Aspirin has been shown to inhibit osteolytic activity of human breast carcinoma in vitro, apparently by inhibiting the synthesis of prostaglandins that may mediate this activity. Supporting evidence for this effect and its mechanism has been obtained in patients with certain types of solid tumors (e.g., lung carcinoma) who developed hypercalcemia; in some of these patients, aspirin therapy has resulted in normalization of serum calcium concentrations and has been associated with a reduction in the urinary excretion of a metabolite of prostaglandin E.

Toxic doses of salicylates may stimulate corticosteroid secretion by the adrenal cortex through an effect on the hypothalamus and may transiently increase plasma concentrations of free corticosteroids by displacement from plasma proteins; however, the anti-inflammatory action of salicylates is not dependent on these effects.

PHARMACOKINETICS

● Absorption

In general, salicylates are rapidly and well absorbed from the GI tract following oral administration. Although some absorption occurs from the stomach, salicylates are absorbed primarily from the upper small intestine via passive diffusion of un-ionized molecules (e.g., salicylic acid).

The rate of absorption of an orally administered salicylate depends on many factors, including dosage form and its formulation characteristics, gastric and intestinal pH, gastric emptying time, and the presence of food in the GI tract. The rate of absorption is generally most rapid with effervescent and noneffervescent aqueous solutions, followed by uncoated tablets (plain or with buffers) or film-coated tablets, and capsules; however, clinically significant therapeutic differences between these dosage forms or specific preparations have not been established. The rate of absorption is slowest for enteric-coated tablets, followed by extended-release tablets.

Dissolution is usually the rate-limiting process in the absorption of tablets containing salicylate; however, the in vitro dissolution rate of a specific preparation does not necessarily reflect the in vivo absorption rate. Dissolution depends on several factors such as pH in the GI tract and formulation characteristics of the preparation. An increase in gastric pH (e.g., as a result of concomitant administration of an antacid) enhances dissolution by increasing solubility of salicylate, but it may also decrease gastric absorption by increasing the degree of ionization of salicylate and decreasing gastric emptying time. The buffers contained in buffered aspirin tablets may increase pH in the microenvironment of aspirin particles and thereby increase solubility of the drug in surrounding GI fluids; as a result, the dissolution rate of the tablets may be increased. (See Pharmacokinetics: Absorption, in Aspirin 28:08.04.24.) Although the increased pH in the small intestine also increases dissolution and degree of ionization of salicylate, the high degree of ionization does not appear to limit the absorption of salicylate from the small intestine, probably because of the large surface area of the small intestine.

Other formulation characteristics of tablets (e.g., particle size, compression pressure) may have varied effects on the rate of absorption. In general, the smaller the particle size, the faster the absorption rate since the resultant increase in surface area of dissolving drug enhances the rate of dissolution. Since enteric-coated tablets are formulated to resist dissolution in the stomach and thereby lessen gastric irritation, the rate of absorption from this dosage form is usually decreased

compared to uncoated tablets. Absorption of aspirin from extended-release tablets is delayed and prolonged. Since salicylates are absorbed primarily from the upper small intestine, the rate of absorption is generally slower when gastric emptying time is increased, and faster when gastric emptying time is decreased (e.g., by metoclopramide or when gastric pH is increased by concomitant administration of an antacid). Gastric emptying time may be partially dependent on salicylate dosage; in overdosage, there is some evidence that salicylates may remain in the stomach for as long as 10 hours if not removed. Food delays absorption and decreases the rate, but not the extent, of absorption of orally administered salicylates.

In general, solid oral dosage forms of aspirin are 80–100% absorbed. Although well-designed bioavailability studies are generally lacking, solid oral dosage forms of most other salicylates also appear to be 80–100% absorbed. Oral aqueous solutions of aspirin or other salicylates appear to be completely absorbed. There is some evidence that absorption of salicylate following oral administration may be substantially impaired or is highly variable during the febrile phase of Kawasaki disease. Following rectal administration, salicylates are slowly and variably absorbed; the extent of absorption increases with increasing rectal retention time. Methyl salicylate, salicylic acid, and trolamine salicylate are rapidly and well absorbed percutaneously following topical application.

Salicylates are detected in serum within 5–30 minutes after oral administration of rapidly absorbed dosage forms (e.g., aqueous solutions, uncoated or film-coated tablets), and peak serum salicylate concentrations are usually attained within 0.25–2 hours, depending on dosage form and specific formulation. Although some rapidly absorbed dosage forms (e.g., aqueous solutions) may produce slightly higher peak serum salicylate concentrations than others (e.g., uncoated tablets), clinically significant therapeutic differences between such dosage forms or between specific preparations have not been established. However, if a rapid response is required (e.g., analgesic effect), the more slowly absorbed dosage forms (i.e., enteric-coated tablets, extended-release tablets) should not be used.

In general, analgesic and antipyretic effects of single oral doses of rapidly absorbed salicylates begin within 30 minutes, peak at 1–3 hours, and persist for 3–6 hours. Following rectal administration of aspirin as a suppository, the antipyretic effect generally begins within 1–2 hours, peaks at 4–5 hours, and may persist 7 or more hours. In patients with inflammatory diseases, the onset of anti-inflammatory effect generally occurs within 1–4 days of continuous oral salicylate therapy. The time required to achieve optimum anti-inflammatory effect depends principally on the attainment and maintenance of adequate serum salicylate concentrations; several weeks or longer may be required in some patients.

Onset, intensity, and duration of analgesic, antipyretic, and anti-inflammatory effects of single doses of salicylates do not directly coincide with the time course of serum salicylate concentrations; however, these effects appear to be related to total (protein-bound and free) serum salicylate concentration. The usual total serum salicylate concentration associated with analgesia and antipyresis is 30–100 mcg/mL. The usual total serum salicylate concentration required for anti-inflammatory effect is 150–300 mcg/mL; however, in the treatment of rheumatic fever, many clinicians believe a total serum salicylate concentration of 250–350 mcg/mL is associated with optimum therapeutic effects. Although many adverse effects are not well correlated with serum salicylate concentrations, most patients experience toxicity when the total serum salicylate concentration exceeds 300–350 mcg/mL. Because of large interindividual and intraindividual variations in the saliva to serum salicylate concentration ratio, salivary salicylate concentrations are generally not useful.

There is limited evidence from animal studies that the pharmacologic effects of salicylates are produced by free salicylate; however, serum concentrations of free salicylate are technically difficult to obtain and have not been clearly correlated with therapeutic effects. Measurements of serum free salicylate concentration may be useful in some patients with documented or suspected alterations in salicylate protein-binding (e.g., patients with extremely low serum albumin concentrations).

● Distribution

Salicylates are rapidly distributed throughout extracellular fluid and into most body tissues and fluids, with high concentrations in the liver and kidneys. During absorption from the stomach, salicylate concentrations in gastric mucosal cells may be 15–20 times higher than concentrations within the gastric lumen. Salicylate can be detected in synovial, peritoneal, and cerebrospinal fluids.

The apparent volume of distribution of salicylate is generally 0.15–0.2 L/kg at usual therapeutic concentrations but may be higher in neonates. The volume of distribution appears to increase with increasing doses and/or serum concentration of salicylate. This increase with increasing doses and/or serum concentration may be due in part to decreased binding of salicylate to serum proteins. The volume of distribution is decreased in patients with decreased serum albumin concentrations and is also affected by plasma and tissue pH.

Distribution of salicylate occurs principally by pH-dependent processes; studies in animals have shown that the tissue-to-plasma distribution ratio of salicylate is increased when plasma pH is greater than that of tissue and decreased when plasma pH is less than that of tissue. Since a large fraction of salicylate in blood is ionized at normal pH, it usually crosses the blood-brain barrier slowly. However, when blood pH is decreased from 7.4 to 7.2, the amount of un-ionized salicylate in blood increases about twofold. Since acidosis often occurs in salicylate overdosage, pH-dependent distribution of salicylate into the CNS and other tissues must be considered. Salicylate is actively transported out of CSF across the choroid plexus by a low-capacity, saturable process.

Salicylate is rapidly distributed into synovial fluid. The principal mechanism of distribution from blood into synovial fluid appears to be passive diffusion. Following single oral doses, salicylate concentrations attained in synovial fluid are about 50–75% of peak serum concentrations. At steady-state, free salicylate concentrations in synovial fluid and serum are approximately equal; however, the total salicylate concentration in synovial fluid is slightly less than in serum because of decreased protein binding of salicylate in synovial fluid.

Salicylate is variably bound to serum proteins, mainly albumin. The fraction bound to serum proteins depends on both the serum salicylate and serum albumin concentrations; even with comparable serum albumin concentrations at a specific serum salicylate concentration, there are interindividual differences in the amount of drug bound. In healthy individuals, salicylate is approximately 90–95% bound to serum proteins at serum salicylate concentrations up to 100 mcg/mL; approximately 70–85% bound to serum proteins at serum salicylate concentrations of 100–400 mcg/mL; and possibly as little as 25–60% bound to serum proteins at higher serum salicylate concentrations. As a result of decreased serum albumin concentrations, serum protein binding of salicylate is decreased and the free fraction is increased in pregnant women, neonates, anephric patients, patients with impaired renal function, and patients with inflammatory diseases. In pregnant women, anephric patients, and patients with impaired renal function, salicylate may be displaced from serum proteins by accumulating endogenous compounds. Protein binding of salicylate is lower in synovial fluid than in serum, possibly as a result of decreased concentrations of albumin in synovial fluid and/or decreased affinity of salicylate for binding sites on synovial fluid proteins.

Salicylate readily crosses the placenta and fetal serum salicylate concentrations may exceed maternal serum concentrations. During chronic oral administration, salicylate may be distributed throughout fetal tissues in concentrations higher than those in the mother.

Salicylate is distributed into milk; however, the extent of distribution into milk is not clearly established. In one study, peak concentrations of salicylate in milk were only 2–5% of peak maternal plasma concentrations. In another study, peak salicylate concentrations in milk were 170–480 mcg/mL at 5–8 hours following maternal ingestion of a single 650-mg dose of aspirin; concurrent maternal plasma concentrations were not reported.

● *Elimination*

Salicylate is metabolized principally in the liver by the microsomal enzyme system. Salicylate is predominantly conjugated with glycine to form salicyluric acid (salicylurate). Salicylate is also conjugated with glucuronic acid to form salicyl phenolic glucuronide and salicyl acyl glucuronide. In addition, small amounts of salicylate are hydroxylated to form 2,5-dihydroxybenzoic acid (gentisic acid), 2,3-dihydroxybenzoic acid, and 2,3,5-trihydroxybenzoic acid. Gentisuric acid, formed either by conjugation of gentisic acid with glycine or by hydroxylation of salicyluric acid, has also been identified as a minor metabolite. Of the salicylate metabolites, only gentisic acid appears to be active; although gentisic acid is a potent inhibitor of prostaglandin synthesis, its contribution to the clinical effects of salicylate is generally considered insignificant because only small amounts are formed. Salicyluric acid and salicyl phenolic glucuronide are formed

by capacity-limited (saturable) processes which can be characterized by Michaelis-Menten kinetics. Other salicylate metabolites appear to be formed by first-order processes.

As a result of the capacity-limited processes, steady-state serum salicylate concentrations increase more than proportionally with increasing doses. The time required to attain steady-state concentrations also increases with increasing doses since the apparent serum half-life of salicylate increases with increasing serum salicylate concentration. With low doses (e.g., 325 mg of aspirin), elimination of salicylate is a first-order process and serum salicylate half-life is approximately 2–3 hours; however, with higher doses, elimination of salicylate is capacity limited and the apparent serum salicylate half-life may increase to 15–30 hours. Because of decreased serum protein binding, the effect of increasing doses is more pronounced on the free serum salicylate concentration than on the total serum salicylate concentration. However, in healthy adults, it has been shown that total serum salicylate clearance remains relatively constant at serum salicylate concentrations of 100–300 mcg/mL. The following pharmacokinetic parameters for adults, expressed in concentrations of salicylate and amounts of salicylate metabolized, have been reported for the Michaelis-Menten variables that characterize the capacity-limited metabolism of salicylate: the Michaelis-Menten constant (K_m) for salicyluric acid formation is approximately 5 mg/L; the maximum rate (V_{max}) of salicyluric acid formation is approximately 800–900 mcg/kg per hour (but may increase with long-term therapy, possibly as a result of enzyme induction); the Michaelis-Menten constant (K_m) for salicyl phenolic glucuronide formation is approximately 9 mg/L; and the maximum rate (V_{max}) of salicyl phenolic glucuronide formation is approximately 400 mcg/kg per hour. Specialized references should be consulted for more specific information on salicylate pharmacokinetics.

Genetically determined differences in salicylate metabolism have been reported. There is some evidence that salicylate may induce its own metabolism, as suggested by increased formation of salicyluric acid and decreased serum salicylate concentrations during long-term therapy. Although not clearly established, it has been reported that salicylate is eliminated more slowly by women. The elimination rate of salicylate is reduced in neonates compared to adults, apparently because neonatal metabolic and excretory pathways are incompletely developed; however, prolonged fetal exposure to salicylate resulting from chronic maternal ingestion of salicylate during pregnancy may increase the rate of development of fetal mechanisms of salicylate elimination.

Salicylate and its metabolites are rapidly and almost completely excreted in urine. Trace amounts of salicylate are also excreted in sweat, saliva, and feces. In patients with normal renal function, 80–100% of a single dose is excreted in the urine within 24–72 hours. The relative amounts of salicylate and its metabolites excreted in the urine are extremely variable, being dependent on the dose administered and urine pH. Following a single oral dose of salicylate of less than 10 mg/kg in patients with normal renal function, about 10% of the dose is excreted in urine as unchanged salicylate, 75% as salicyluric acid, 10% as salicyl phenolic glucuronide, 5% as salicyl acyl glucuronide, and less than 1% as gentisic acid and gentisuric acid. With higher single doses or long-term therapy, the proportions excreted in urine as unchanged salicylate, salicyl acyl glucuronide, and gentisic acid generally increase as a result of capacity-limited formation of salicyluric acid and salicyl phenolic glucuronide.

Unchanged salicylate and its metabolites are excreted in the urine via glomerular filtration and renal tubular secretion; since unchanged salicylate also undergoes renal tubular reabsorption, its urinary excretion is markedly pH dependent. As urine pH increases from 5 to 8, the urinary excretion rate of salicylate is greatly increased and the fraction of a single dose excreted in the urine as unchanged salicylate may increase from 5–10% to 85%. Therefore, concomitant administration of drugs that alter urine pH may have substantial effects on serum salicylate concentrations. (See Drug Interactions: Acidifying and Alkalinizing Agents.)

In patients with normal renal function, salicylate metabolites are excreted in the urine as rapidly as they are formed. Although anephric patients appear to eliminate small doses of salicylate (e.g., 650 mg of sodium salicylate) as rapidly as healthy individuals, the pharmacokinetics of salicylate in patients with severe renal impairment have not been clearly established and salicylates are usually avoided in these patients.

Salicylate and its metabolites are readily removed by hemodialysis and, to a lesser extent, by peritoneal dialysis.

CHEMISTRY AND STABILITY

● *Chemistry*

Salicylates are nonsteroidal anti-inflammatory agents (NSAIAs) that are synthetic derivatives of salicylic acid. The drugs hydrolyze or dissociate to salicylate (ionized salicylic acid) in vivo. Salicylic acid is not used systemically because of its severe irritating effect on GI mucosa and other tissues; therefore, better tolerated chemical derivatives have been prepared for systemic use.

The pharmacologic actions of salicylates appear to result principally from the salicylate moiety. The carboxyl group and an adjacent hydroxyl group on salicylic acid are necessary for activity; either or both groups may have substituents. The currently available salicylates are either esters of organic acids derived by substitution at the hydroxyl group of salicylic acid, or esters or salts of salicylic acid derived by substitution at the carboxyl group. Aspirin, the prototype of the salicylates, is the salicylate ester of acetic acid; the drug hydrolyzes to salicylate and acetate. Salsalate is the salicylate ester of salicylic acid; the drug hydrolyzes to 2 molecules of salicylate. Many commercially available salicylate preparations contain salts of salicylic acid (e.g., choline salicylate, magnesium salicylate, sodium salicylate, trolamine salicylate) which dissociate to form salicylate. Although related to the salicylates structurally and pharmacologically, diflunisal, salicylamide, and probably sodium thiosalicylate are not hydrolyzed to salicylate; therefore, these drugs are not considered true salicylates and are not included in this discussion.

Salicylic acid occurs as white crystals, usually in fine needles, or as a fluffy, white, crystalline powder. The drug has a sweetish taste and an acrid aftertaste and is slightly soluble in water and freely soluble in alcohol. The synthetic form is white and odorless; when prepared from natural methyl salicylate, the drug may have a slightly yellow or pink tint and a faint, mint-like odor. Salicylic acid has pK_as of 2.97 and 13.4. Most salicylates occur as white, crystalline powders and are practically insoluble to very soluble in water and soluble to freely soluble in alcohol.

● *Stability*

Aqueous solutions of salicylates slowly darken in color due to oxidation; however, the color change appears to have no effect on efficacy or toxicity. Darkening of solutions of salicylates is delayed by the presence of 0.1% of sodium bisulfite, sodium sulfite, sodium thiosulfate, or sodium hypophosphite, or 0.5% sodium citrate. Addition of mineral acids to aqueous solutions of salicylates results in precipitation of salicylic acid.

For specific dosages and additional information on chemistry and stability, pharmacology, pharmacokinetics, uses, and cautions, see the individual monographs on Aspirin, Salicylate Salts, and Salsalate in 28:08.04.24.

† Use is not currently included in the labeling approved by the US Food and Drug Administration.

Aspirin

28:08.04.24 • SALICYLATES

■ Aspirin (the prototype of the salicylates) is a nonsteroidal anti-inflammatory agent (NSAIA) and also exhibits antithrombotic, analgesic, and antipyretic activity.

USES

Aspirin is used extensively in the treatment of mild to moderate pain, fever, and inflammatory diseases. Aspirin is also used in the prevention of arterial and venous thrombosis. Aspirin, however, should be used with extreme caution, if at all, in patients in whom urticaria, angioedema, bronchospasm, severe rhinitis, or shock is precipitated by other salicylates or other NSAIAs. (See Cautions: Sensitivity Reactions in the Salicylates General Statement 28:08.04.24.)

● **Pain**

Aspirin is used to relieve headache, neuralgia, myalgia, arthralgia, and other low-intensity pain of nonvisceral origin, particularly pain associated with inflammation. Aspirin may also relieve mild to moderate postoperative pain, postpartum pain, oral surgery or other dental pain, dysmenorrhea, or other visceral pain such as that associated with trauma or cancer. Many studies have shown that the analgesic effects of aspirin are greater than those of placebo in the treatment of these types of pain. The drug, however, does not usually relieve severe acute pain of visceral origin. In addition, use of chewing gum tablets or gargles containing aspirin has not been shown to be effective in relieving sore throat pain.

The analgesic effect of aspirin appears to increase with increasing single oral doses up to at least 1.2 g; however, single oral doses of aspirin exceeding 650 mg apparently do not result in a greater incidence or degree of pain relief in most patients. Multiple oral doses of aspirin exceeding 650 mg each have not been shown to be more effective in relieving pain than multiple oral doses of 650 mg.

When used to relieve postoperative pain, 600-mg oral doses of aspirin appear to be as effective as 60-mg oral doses of codeine or 50-mg oral doses of pentazocine. When used to relieve oral surgery pain, 650-mg oral doses of aspirin appear to be more effective than 30-mg oral doses of codeine, as effective as 650-mg oral doses of acetaminophen, and less effective than 250-mg, 500-mg, or 1-g oral doses of diflunisal.

In the treatment of postpartum uterine pain, the analgesic effect of 650-mg oral doses of aspirin is about equal to that of 300- or 600-mg oral doses of naproxen or 275-mg oral doses of naproxen sodium and greater than that of 60-mg oral doses of codeine or codeine sulfate. When used to relieve episiotomy pain, several studies have shown that 600-mg to 1.2-g oral doses of aspirin are more effective than placebo; in one study, the analgesic effect of 900-mg oral doses of aspirin was about equal to that of 300- or 900-mg oral doses of ibuprofen. In another study, the analgesic effect of 600-mg oral doses of aspirin was less than that of 500-mg oral doses of diflunisal.

In the treatment of nonspecific pain associated with cancer, 650-mg oral doses of aspirin appear to be at least as effective as 650-mg oral doses of acetaminophen, 65-mg oral doses of codeine, 250-mg oral doses of mefenamic acid, or 50-mg oral doses of pentazocine, and more effective than 75-mg oral doses of ethoheptazine citrate or 65-mg oral doses of propoxyphene hydrochloride (no longer commercially available in the US). When used to relieve nonspecific pain associated with cancer, 650-mg oral doses of aspirin in combination with oral doses of codeine (65 mg), oxycodone (976 mcg), or pentazocine hydrochloride (25 mg) appear to be more effective than 650-mg oral doses of aspirin alone or in combination with oral doses of caffeine (65 mg), ethoheptazine citrate (75 mg), pentobarbital sodium (25 mg), promazine hydrochloride (25 mg), or propoxyphene napsylate (100 mg) (no longer commercially available in the US).

Results of studies comparing aspirin (500–650 mg 4 times daily) with placebo to relieve primary dysmenorrhea have been inconsistent. Although the effects of higher dosages of aspirin remain to be evaluated, most clinicians consider aspirin to be one of the *least* effective NSAIAs currently available for the treatment of primary dysmenorrhea.

In several double-blind placebo-controlled studies with small numbers of patients with migraine, prophylactic therapy with aspirin (650 mg twice daily) alone or aspirin (300 mg twice daily) with dipyridamole (25 mg 3 times daily) has reportedly been effective in reducing the frequency of headache; however, further evaluation is needed. In addition, aspirin in fixed combination with acetaminophen and caffeine (aspirin 500 mg, acetaminophen 500 mg, and caffeine 130 mg per dose) is used for the temporary relief of mild to moderate pain associated with migraine headache. Some experts state that an NSAIA (e.g., aspirin alone or in fixed combination with acetaminophen and caffeine) is a reasonable first-line therapy for mild to moderate migraine attacks or for severe attacks that have responded in the past to similar NSAIAs or non-opiate analgesics. The efficacy of oral aspirin in fixed combination with acetaminophen and caffeine for the management of mild to moderate pain associated with migraine headache was established by 3 double-blind, randomized, parallel-group, placebo-controlled studies (one of them a population-based study) in adults who had migraine with aura or migraine without aura as defined by criteria established by the International Headache Society (IHS). The efficacy of therapy for management of pain associated with migraine headache in these studies was evaluated in terms of a reduction in headache severity as rated by the patient (i.e., a reduction in pain from at least moderate to mild or to absent 2 hours after dosing using a 4-point scale). Pooled analysis of data from the 3 studies indicated that about 59% of patients receiving 500 mg of aspirin in fixed combination with acetaminophen 500 mg and caffeine 130 mg attained relief of pain associated with migraine headache (i.e., mild or no headache) within 2 hours compared with about 33% of placebo recipients; at 6 hours, about 79 and 52%, respectively, of drug- and placebo-treated patients had mild or no headache pain. In addition, about 21% of patients receiving the combination were pain-free 2 hours after dosing versus about 7% of those receiving placebo, while at 6 hours, 51% of drug-treated patients were pain-free versus 24% of those receiving placebo. It appears that this combination also may relieve manifestations of migraine other than headache, including nausea, vomiting, photophobia, and phonophobia. Patients in whom pain associated with migraine headache is not relieved by aspirin in fixed combination with acetaminophen and caffeine should consult their clinician about possible alternatives (e.g., use of prescription drugs including ergot alkaloids or vascular serotonin type 1-like receptor agonists) based on evaluation of their medical condition. In several double-blind controlled studies in patients with acute migraine headache, aspirin 900 or 1000 mg given as a single dose with or without metoclopramide 10 mg (as an antiemetic) was more effective than placebo and had efficacy generally similar to that of sumatriptan 50 or 100 mg for relief of pain and associated symptoms of migraine (nausea, vomiting, photophobia, phonophobia). For further information on management and classification of migraine headache, see General Principles in Migraine Therapy under Uses: Vascular Headaches, in Sumatriptan 28:32.28.

Aspirin has been used in the treatment of pain in various combinations with acetaminophen, caffeine, opiates, salicylamide, and/or other agents. However, combinations of aspirin with agents such as acetaminophen, caffeine, or salicylamide have not been clearly shown to have greater analgesic effect than an optimal dose of aspirin alone. In addition, there is little evidence that such combinations cause fewer adverse effects than higher doses of the individual agents alone. In one study, the simultaneous administration of 325- or 650-mg oral doses of acetaminophen with 650-mg oral doses of aspirin resulted in increased blood concentrations of unhydrolyzed aspirin compared with 650-mg oral doses of aspirin alone; however, the clinical importance of such an effect remains to be established. Aspirin (650-mg oral doses) in combination with oral doses of an opiate (e.g., codeine, oxycodone) produces greater analgesic effect than that produced by either aspirin or higher doses of the opiate alone. There is also some evidence that aspirin/opiate combinations may cause fewer adverse effects than equianalgesic doses of the individual drugs alone.

● **Fever**

Aspirin is used frequently to lower body temperature in febrile patients in whom fever may be deleterious or in whom considerable relief is obtained when fever is lowered. However, antipyretic therapy is generally nonspecific, does not influence the course of the underlying disease, and may obscure the course of the patient's illness. For information on salicylates and Reye's syndrome, see Cautions: Pediatric Precautions, in the Salicylates General Statement 28:08.04.24.

Aspirin and acetaminophen are equally effective as antipyretics. In one study in febrile children, the combination of oral doses of aspirin and acetaminophen was at least as effective in reducing fever as either drug alone, and the duration of fever reduction was longer with the combination than with the individual drugs. However, because of the study design, it could not be concluded that the combination had additive effects. Many clinicians use regimens of alternating doses of aspirin and acetaminophen; however, combined overdosage with both drugs has occurred with such a regimen and the efficacy and safety of these regimens remain to be established.

Several clinical studies have shown that the antipyretic effect of usual dosages of aspirin is about equal to that of usual dosages of mefenamic acid and naproxen, and less than that of usual dosages of indomethacin. However, efficacy of these other NSAIAs as antipyretics remains to be clearly established and they should not be used for routine treatment of fever because of their potential adverse effects.

● Inflammatory Diseases

Aspirin is used for anti-inflammatory and analgesic effects in the initial and/or long-term symptomatic treatment of rheumatoid arthritis, juvenile arthritis, and osteoarthritis. Aspirin may also be useful in the treatment of other polyarthritic conditions (e.g., psoriatic arthritis, Reiter's syndrome, ankylosing spondylitis), systemic lupus erythematous, and nonarticular inflammation; however, other NSAIAs may be preferred in the treatment of some of these conditions (e.g., ankylosing spondylitis).

Rheumatoid Arthritis, Juvenile Arthritis, and Osteoarthritis

Most clinical studies have shown that the anti-inflammatory and analgesic effects of usual dosages of aspirin in the treatment of rheumatoid arthritis or osteoarthritis are greater than those of placebo and about equal to those of usual dosages of fenoprofen calcium, ibuprofen, indomethacin, meclofenamate sodium, naproxen, piroxicam, sulindac, and tolmetin sodium. In the treatment of juvenile arthritis, the anti-inflammatory and analgesic effects of usual dosages of aspirin are about equal to those of usual dosages of fenoprofen, naproxen, or tolmetin sodium. Patient response to NSAIAs is variable, however, and patients who do not respond to one agent may be successfully treated with a different agent.

Aspirin has been used in conjunction with other NSAIAs in the treatment of some patients with rheumatoid arthritis, but such combination therapy is generally not recommended because there is inadequate proof that such combination therapy is more efficacious than the individual agents alone and the potential for adverse reactions may be increased. In addition, there is evidence that aspirin alters plasma concentrations of some other NSAIAs.

Psoriatic Arthritis and Reiter's Syndrome

Aspirin may be effective in the treatment of some patients with psoriatic arthritis or Reiter's syndrome but usually only when the disease is mild. Aspirin is seldom effective in the treatment of ankylosing spondylitis unless the disease is mild. In one study in patients with ankylosing spondylitis, the anti-inflammatory and analgesic effects of aspirin were less than those of indomethacin or phenylbutazone.

Systemic Lupus Erythematous

Some clinicians consider aspirin to be a drug of first choice for the treatment of fever, arthritis, pleurisy, and pericarditis in patients with systemic lupus erythematous (SLE). In one study in patients with SLE, the anti-inflammatory and analgesic effects of aspirin were greater than those of ibuprofen. The anti-inflammatory and analgesic effects of aspirin may also be useful in the symptomatic treatment of nonarticular inflammation such as bursitis and/or tendinitis (e.g., acute painful shoulder) and fibrositis.

● Rheumatic Fever

Most clinicians consider aspirin to be the salicylate of choice when salicylate therapy is indicated in the treatment of rheumatic fever†. For information on salicylate therapy in the treatment of rheumatic fever, see Uses: Rheumatic Fever, in the Salicylates General Statement 28:08.04.24.

● Thrombosis

Generally accepted indications for prophylactic aspirin therapy include its use for reducing the risk of recurrent vascular events (e.g., recurrent stroke, death) in men and women who have had single or multiple transient ischemic attacks (TIAs)† or ischemic stroke†, for reducing the risk of vascular mortality in patients with suspected acute myocardial infarction† (MI), for reducing the risk of recurrent nonfatal MI and/or death in patients with previous MI or unstable angina†, for

reducing the risk of MI and sudden death in patients with chronic stable angina pectoris†, and for reducing cardiovascular risks in patients undergoing percutaneous coronary intervention [PCI] or certain revascularization procedures (e.g., coronary artery bypass grafting [CABG]). Aspirin also has been used to prevent thrombosis in patients undergoing percutaneous transluminal angioplasty (PTA) of the lower extremities†, and for postoperative thromboprophylaxis in children undergoing surgery for placement of modified Blalock-Taussig shunts†, surgery for univentricular heart lesions (i.e., Fontan procedure†), surgery for placement of ventricular assist devices†, or surgery for hypoplastic left heart (i.e., Norwood procedure)†. Aspirin also has been used to prevent thromboembolism in patients with atrial fibrillation† or atrial flutter†, valvular heart disease† (e.g., mitral valve prolapse), chronic limb ischemia (e.g., intermittent claudication)†, or prosthetic heart valves†.

Transient Ischemic Attacks and Acute Ischemic Stroke

Aspirin is used for *secondary prevention* of vascular events (e.g., recurrent stroke, death) in patients who have had an acute ischemic stroke or TIAs. The American College of Chest Physicians (ACCP), the American Stroke Association (ASA), the American Heart Association (AHA), and other clinicians recommend antiplatelet therapy over oral anticoagulation (e.g., warfarin) for *secondary prevention* of ischemic atherothrombotic (noncardioembolic) stroke or TIAs in patients with prior TIAs or ischemic stroke who do not have atrial fibrillation.

AHA and ASA recommend aspirin for *primary prevention* or *secondary prevention* of ischemic stroke in high-risk women (i.e., women with established coronary heart disease, cerebrovascular disease, peripheral arterial disease, abdominal aortic aneurysm, end-stage or chronic kidney disease, diabetes mellitus, or a 10-year Framingham risk exceeding 20%). AHA and ASA also suggest that low-dose aspirin therapy can be useful in women 65 years of age or older in whom the benefits for ischemic stroke and MI prevention are likely to outweigh the risk of GI bleeding and hemorrhagic stroke and may be reasonable to consider in women younger than 65 years of age in whom the benefits for ischemic stroke prevention are likely to outweigh the adverse effects of aspirin. Results of several trials suggest that use of aspirin therapy for *primary prevention* of stroke in men without a history of TIAs or stroke may be associated with a slightly increased risk of stroke, particularly hemorrhagic stroke, and aspirin is not recommended for *primary prevention* of ischemic stroke in men.

Restoring perfusion (e.g., with thrombolytic therapy) is the principal goal of acute stroke therapy, with the second goal being prevention of early recurrence of cerebrovascular events with anticoagulants and antiplatelet agents. Unless contraindicated or unless too much time (i.e., more than 3–4.5 hours†) has elapsed since the event, thrombolytic therapy generally is preferred for the acute treatment of ischemic stroke. (See Uses: Acute Ischemic Stroke, in Alteplase 20:12.20.) In patients with acute ischemic stroke or TIA in whom thrombolytic therapy is contraindicated or not appropriate, early aspirin therapy (160–325 mg initially, followed by 75–100 mg daily to reduce bleeding risk) is recommended. Aspirin should be initiated within 48 hours of stroke onset. The rationale for antithrombotic therapy such as aspirin in patients with acute ischemic stroke is to reduce the risk of stroke progression or recurrent cerebral thromboembolism and prevent thromboembolic complications. Current evidence indicates that aspirin therapy initiated within 48 hours of stroke onset is relatively safe and can produce a small but definite net benefit by reducing both stroke recurrence risk and mortality.

For *secondary prevention* of ischemic stroke in patients with cerebrovascular disease, including patients with a history of TIAs or previous ischemic stroke, aspirin is the most widely studied and used antiplatelet agent. Secondary prevention with aspirin has been shown to reduce the combined endpoint of stroke, MI, and/or vascular death by 13–25%. Data from numerous clinical studies have shown that aspirin reduces the risk of these cardiovascular events in a wide variety of patients at high risk for these atherosclerotic outcomes.

Because there is evidence from clinical studies to support the efficacy of low dosages of aspirin (e.g., 50–325 mg daily) in patients with a history of TIAs or cerebral ischemia and considerable evidence supporting the antithrombotic efficacy of such dosages in patients with MI, these dosages have supplanted the moderate- to high-dose regimens employed in the past. Further supporting this change in dosage recommendations is evidence that efficacy is not compromised with low-dosage regimens, but patient tolerance is improved. Although early evidence supporting the beneficial effects of aspirin in patients with TIAs came from studies that included mainly men, more recent studies have shown numerically similar results for men and women, and favorable trends generally have been seen in both genders. Current data suggest that an aspirin dosage of 75–81 mg daily may be sufficient for long-term cardiovascular prevention and is associated with less GI bleeding risk.

Aspirin in fixed combination with extended-release dipyridamole is used to reduce the risk of recurrent stroke in patients who have had TIAs or completed ischemic stroke caused by noncardioembolic thrombosis (e.g., atherothrombotic, lacunar, cryptogenic). In a randomized, comparative, placebo-controlled study, patients who had experienced either an ischemic stroke or TIAs were assigned to receive treatment with aspirin (25 mg twice daily), extended-release dipyridamole (200 mg twice daily), aspirin plus extended-release dipyridamole (25 and 200 mg twice daily, respectively), or placebo. All active treatments reduced the risk of the primary end points of stroke (nonfatal or fatal) or stroke and/or death compared with placebo. Aspirin plus dipyridamole reduced the risk of stroke by about 23% compared with aspirin alone and by about 25% compared with dipyridamole alone at 2 years of follow-up; the effects of combined therapy on risk reductions with aspirin and dipyridamole were additive but not synergistic. Aspirin, dipyridamole, and the combination also reduced the incidence of TIAs and other vascular events in a manner consistent with these treatments' effects on the risk of stroke. None of the treatments had a statistically significant effect on the end point of death (i.e., no effect on survival). Headache and GI events were the most common adverse effects in this study, occurring more frequently in the dipyridamole-treated groups, while bleeding from the GI tract or from any site was more common in the aspirin-treated groups.

In another randomized, placebo-controlled, open-label study (European/Australasian Stroke Prevention in Reversible ischemia Trial [ESPRIT]) in patients who had experienced a TIA or minor stroke within the previous 6 months, treatment with aspirin (median dosage 75 mg daily, range 30–325 mg daily) in combination with dipyridamole (200 mg twice daily) resulted in a reduction in the overall risk of the composite primary outcome (death from all vascular causes, nonfatal stroke, nonfatal MI, major bleeding complication) compared with that in patients receiving aspirin alone. Approximately 34% of patients discontinued treatment with the aspirin-dipyridamole combination during the study because of adverse effects, principally headache. Results from other trials evaluating combination therapy with aspirin (900 mg to 1.3 g daily) and dipyridamole (150–300 mg daily) also have been reported to reduce the risk of cerebral infarction in patients with TIAs or mild stroke. A meta-analysis of data from the ESPRIT and several prior studies comparing aspirin with or without dipyridamole in patients with cerebral ischemia of presumed arterial origin demonstrated an overall reduction of 18% in the incidence of primary outcome events with combined aspirin and dipyridamole treatment compared with aspirin alone.

ACCP, ASA, AHA, and other clinicians recommend long-term antiplatelet therapy for *secondary prevention* of ischemic atherothrombotic (noncardioembolic) stroke or TIAs in patients with prior TIAs or stroke. In such patients, ACCP states that aspirin, clopidogrel, the combination of aspirin and dipyridamole, or cilostazol are all acceptable options for long-term antithrombotic therapy. Based on a somewhat greater risk reduction for stroke, ACCP suggests that clopidogrel or the combination of aspirin and dipyridamole may be preferred over the other options for secondary prevention of noncardioembolic stroke. When selecting an appropriate antiplatelet regimen for the secondary prevention of noncardioembolic stroke, factors such as the patient's individual risk for recurrent stroke, tolerance, and cost of the different agents should be considered. Oral anticoagulation (e.g., warfarin) rather than antiplatelet therapy is recommended for the secondary prevention of cardioembolic stroke in patients with a history of ischemic stroke or TIA and concurrent atrial fibrillation; however, in patients who cannot take or choose not to take warfarin (e.g., those with difficulty maintaining stable international normalized ratios [INRs], compliance issues, dietary restrictions, cost limitations), dual antiplatelet therapy with aspirin and clopidogrel is recommended.

In children with acute arterial ischemic stroke†, aspirin is recommended as one of the options for initial antithrombotic therapy until cerebral arterial dissection and embolic causes have been excluded. Once dissection and cardioembolic causes have been excluded, secondary prevention with aspirin therapy (in prophylactic dosages for at least 2 years) is suggested. Children who experience recurrent arterial ischemic stroke or TIAs despite aspirin therapy may be switched to clopidogrel or anticoagulant therapy with a low molecular weight heparin or warfarin.

Coronary Artery Disease and Myocardial Infarction

ST-Segment-Elevation Myocardial Infarction

The current standard of care in patients with ST-segment-elevation MI (STEMI) is timely reperfusion (with primary PCI or thrombolytic therapy). Adjunctive therapy with anticoagulant (e.g., heparin) and antiplatelet (e.g., aspirin and clopidogrel) agents should be used during and after successful coronary artery reperfusion for the prevention of early reocclusion and death, unless contraindicated. Aspirin reduces the risk of stroke, recurrent infarction, and death in adults with STEMI and should be administered in all such patients regardless of the reperfusion strategy. Aspirin in a dose of 162–325 mg, initiated as soon as possible after the clinical impression of an evolving acute STEMI is formed and continued indefinitely at a dosage of 81–325 mg daily, also is strongly recommended for the acute management of all patients (unless contraindicated) with suspected STEMI, regardless of whether thrombolytic therapy is to be given. Some experts prefer the use of a maintenance dosage of 81 mg daily because of a decreased risk of bleeding and lack of definitive evidence demonstrating that higher dosages confer greater benefit in this setting. A P2Y12 platelet adenosine diphosphate (ADP)-receptor antagonist (e.g., clopidogrel, prasugrel, ticagrelor) should be administered in conjunction with aspirin in patients with STEMI.

In a large, multicenter study (Second International Study of Infarct Survival; ISIS-2) of patients with an evolving STEMI allocated to treatment early (within 24 hours of symptom onset), therapy with aspirin 162.5 mg daily for 1 month was shown conclusively to be associated with a vascular mortality reduction at 5 weeks of 23% compared with placebo. In this study, a statistically significant difference in both vascular and all-cause mortality, which persisted for at least a median of 15 months after treatment, was observed. Patients receiving aspirin had fewer nonfatal reinfarctions and nonfatal strokes compared with those given placebo and, when given concomitantly with IV streptokinase therapy, aspirin appeared to prevent the increase in reinfarction observed with streptokinase treatment alone. Compared with placebo, aspirin treatment resulted in a small increase in the incidence of minor bleeding complications but no increase in major bleeding (e.g., intracranial hemorrhage). When aspirin is combined with thrombolytic therapy (streptokinase), the reduction in mortality associated with acute STEMI is even greater, being reported as a 42% reduction. Pooled analysis of clinical studies indicates that aspirin reduces coronary reocclusion and recurrent ischemic events after thrombolytic therapy with streptokinase or alteplase. At doses of at least 160 mg, aspirin produces a rapid clinical antithrombotic effect via immediate and near-total inhibition of thromboxane A_2. As a result, aspirin is an important therapy in the early management of suspected acute STEMI.

In patients with STEMI who have indications for anticoagulation (e.g., atrial fibrillation, left ventricular dysfunction, cerebral emboli, extensive wall-motion abnormality, mechanical heart valves), many experts recommend the addition of warfarin (INR 2–3) to antiplatelet therapy; in some cases, triple antithrombotic therapy (warfarin, low-dose aspirin, and clopidogrel) is suggested, such as in patients with an anterior STEMI and left ventricular thrombosis undergoing PCI with coronary artery stent implantation. However, triple-drug antithrombotic regimens are associated with an increased risk of bleeding. (See Uses: ST-Segment Elevation Myocardial Infarction, in Warfarin 20:12.04.08.)

Secondary Prevention of Cardiovascular Events

Unless contraindicated, therapy with low-dose aspirin currently is recommended by AHA and the American College of Cardiology Foundation (ACCF) for all patients with coronary artery disease in order to reduce the risk of vascular events (*secondary prevention*). ACCP recommends long-term, single-drug antiplatelet therapy with aspirin or clopidogrel in patients with established coronary artery disease (i.e., 1 year after ACS with prior revascularization, coronary stenosis greater than 50% by coronary angiogram, and/or evidence of cardiac ischemia on diagnostic testing). The efficacy of aspirin for secondary prevention of cardiovascular events does not appear to be influenced by gender or age. The American Diabetes Association (ADA) currently recommends low-dose aspirin (e.g., 75–162 mg daily) for secondary prevention of cardiovascular events (e.g., MI) in patients with diabetes mellitus and a history of atherosclerotic cardiovascular disease (ASCVD).

Primary Prevention of Ischemic Cardiac Events

The beneficial effects of aspirin for secondary prevention of cardiovascular disease are well established; however, use of aspirin for *primary prevention* of cardiovascular disease remains controversial. Low-dose aspirin (e.g., 75–162 mg daily) has been used to reduce the risk of a first cardiac event (*primary prevention*†) in patients with at least a moderate risk factor for a coronary event. However, recent evidence suggests that aspirin therapy should not be used routinely for *primary prevention* of cardiovascular disease because of a lack of net benefit.

Most clinical studies that demonstrated the beneficial effect of aspirin for primary prevention of cardiovascular disease (e.g., the US Physicians' Health Study [men 40–84 years of age without a history of ischemic heart disease], the British Doctors' Study [men younger than 60 up to 79 years of age without ischemic heart disease], the Medical Research Council's Thrombosis Prevention Trial [men 45–69 years of age with an increased risk of ischemic heart disease], the Hypertension Optimal Treatment [HOT] trial [men and women 50–80 years with hypertension], the Primary Prevention Project [PPP] [patients at least 50 years of age who had at least one major cardiovascular risk factor]) were conducted prior to modern preventative and therapeutic practices (i.e., emphasis on stricter blood pressure control, smoking cessation, and cholesterol reduction). While low-dose aspirin may still confer benefits in selected patients, there is less certainty regarding the drug's widespread use for primary prevention. In 3 recently conducted randomized, placebo-controlled primary prevention studies evaluating the use of low-dose aspirin regimens (100 mg once daily in all 3 studies) in various patient populations, there was no substantial net clinical benefit with low-dose aspirin therapy largely because of an increased risk of bleeding with aspirin use. In the ARRIVE (Aspirin to Reduce Risk of Initial Vascular Events) study, which included patients 55 years of age or older without diabetes mellitus and with a low to moderate cardiovascular risk, low-dose aspirin did not substantially reduce the combined outcome of first MI, stroke, cardiovascular death, unstable angina, or transient ischemic attack but was associated with an increased risk of GI bleeding. In the ASCEND (A Study of Cardiovascular Events In Diabetes) study, which included patients 40 years of age or older with type 1 or type 2 diabetes mellitus who did not have known cardiovascular disease, the use of low-dose aspirin for 7.4 years was associated with a 12% reduction in the rate of serious vascular events at the cost of a 29% increase in major bleeding. In this study, there was no substantial difference in all-cause mortality among patients who received aspirin therapy and those who did not. In the ASPREE (ASPirin in Reducing Events in the Elderly) study, which included healthy patients 65 years of age and older without cardiovascular disease, low-dose aspirin use resulted in a substantially higher risk of major hemorrhage (composite of hemorrhagic stroke, symptomatic intracranial bleeding, or clinically important extracranial bleeding) and did not substantially reduce the risk of cardiovascular disease.

Based on available evidence including the results of these recent clinical studies, experts from the American College of Cardiology and American Heart Association (ACC/AHA) recommend that low-dose aspirin (e.g., 75–100 mg daily) for *primary prevention* be reserved for adults 40–70 years of age who have a higher risk of cardiovascular disease without an increased risk of bleeding (e.g., patients with a history of previous GI bleed, peptic ulcer disease, thrombocytopenia, coagulopathy, chronic kidney disease, concomitant use of drugs that increase bleeding risk [e.g., nonsteroidal anti-inflammatory drugs, corticosteroids, direct oral anticoagulants, warfarin]). When determining a patient's risk for ASCVD, these experts state that the totality of patient risk factors should be considered (e.g., strong family history of premature MI; inability to achieve lipid, blood pressure, or blood glucose targets; substantial elevation in coronary artery calcium score) in conjunction with patient and clinician preferences. High-risk patients also include adults 40–70 years of age without diabetes mellitus who have a 10-year ASCVD risk of at least 20% and those with diabetes mellitus who have a 10-year ASCVD risk of at least 10%. Low-dose aspirin for *primary prevention* is not recommended for adults with a low ASCVD risk, and the routine use of aspirin for *primary prevention* is not recommended in patients younger than 40 years of age or older than 70 years of age. In addition, such experts state that it is unclear whether low-dose aspirin should be *continued* in patients already taking aspirin who turn 70 years of age. Additional studies are needed to clarify aspirin's role in the primary prevention of cardiovascular disease.

Based on a systematic review of evidence, the US Preventive Services Task Force (USPSTF) has concluded that the beneficial effects of aspirin for primary prevention of cardiovascular disease are modest and occur at daily dosages of 100 mg or less; subpopulation analyses suggest a greater relative benefit for MI prevention in older age groups.

The ADA states that the use of aspirin for *primary prevention* of cardiovascular disease should be carefully considered and generally may not be recommended. ADA states that *primary prevention* with low-dose aspirin may be considered in patients with type 1 or type 2 diabetes mellitus who are at high risk for cardiovascular events (i.e., familial history of premature ASCVD, smoking, hypertension, chronic kidney disease/albuminuria, elevated blood cholesterol or triglyceride concentrations) and have a low bleeding risk. ADA also states that aspirin use is not recommended for patients at low risk of ASCVD (e.g., men and women younger than 50 years of age with diabetes mellitus and no other major risk factors) as the risk of bleeding is likely to outweigh the small benefit. For patients older than 70 years of age (with or without diabetes mellitus), the risks associated with the use of low-dose aspirin appear to outweigh any potential benefits

Non-ST-Segment-Elevation Acute Coronary Syndromes

Aspirin is used to reduce the risk of death and/or nonfatal MI in patients with non-ST-segment-elevation acute coronary syndromes (NSTE ACS). Patients with NSTE ACS have either unstable angina or non-ST-segment-elevation MI (NSTEMI); because these conditions are part of a continuum of acute myocardial ischemia and have indistinguishable clinical features upon presentation, the same initial treatment strategies are recommended. The American Heart Association/American College of Cardiology (AHA/ACC) guideline for the management of patients with NSTE ACS recommends an early invasive strategy (angiographic evaluation with the intent to perform revascularization procedures such as PCI with coronary artery stent implantation or CABG) or an ischemia-guided strategy (initial medical management followed by cardiac catheterization and revascularization if indicated) in patients with definite or likely NSTE ACS; standard medical therapies for all patients should include a β-adrenergic blocking agent (β-blocker), antiplatelet agents, anticoagulant agents, nitrates, and analgesic agents regardless of the initial management approach. Aspirin is the mainstay of antiplatelet therapy in patients with NSTE ACS and should be administered in all such patients unless contraindicated; a loading dose of aspirin should be administered as soon as possible after diagnosis, followed by a maintenance dosage that should be continued indefinitely unless such therapy is not tolerated or contraindicated. A P2Y12-receptor antagonist (e.g., clopidogrel, ticagrelor) should be administered in conjunction with aspirin for up to 12 months unless contraindicated.

Aspirin therapy has been shown to substantially reduce the rates of total mortality or cardiac death and nonfatal MI in patients with NSTE ACS. Several randomized, placebo-controlled studies indicate that prophylactic aspirin therapy is associated with a reduction of at least 50% in the risk of death and/or nonfatal MI in men and women with NSTE ACS. In another randomized, controlled study in men with NSTE ACS who received 75 mg of aspirin daily, the risk of MI and death was reduced by 57–69% at least 5 days after initiation of therapy.

Chronic Stable Angina

In patients with chronic stable angina, low-dose aspirin is used to reduce the risk of MI and sudden death. Experts recommend that aspirin therapy (75–162 mg daily) be continued indefinitely in patients with stable ischemic heart disease who do not have contraindications. There is some evidence suggesting that an aspirin dosage not exceeding 75–81 mg daily may be sufficient for long-term cardiovascular prevention and is associated with less GI bleeding risk. Clopidogrel may be used as an alternative to aspirin in patients with symptomatic chronic stable angina who cannot tolerate aspirin.

Evidence from a large, randomized, placebo-controlled study in patients with stable chronic angina pectoris showed that aspirin (75 mg daily) combined with sotalol therapy is associated with 34% reduction in the primary endpoint of fatal or nonfatal MI and sudden death and a 22–32% reduction in secondary endpoints (vascular events, vascular death, all-cause mortality, stroke). There also was a reduction in nonfatal MI, the principal component of benefit of the primary end point. Although not significantly different from placebo, aspirin therapy also was associated with a favorable trend in decreasing vascular deaths and all-cause mortality when considered separately. Because all patients in this study received sotalol concomitantly, this study did not establish whether aspirin alone is effective in patients with chronic stable angina. However, the ability of aspirin to decrease the rate of thrombotic vascular events in various conditions has not depended on concomitant β-blocker therapy to date, and therefore it is likely that aspirin therapy would be beneficial in patients with chronic stable angina pectoris regardless of concomitant β-blocker therapy.

Percutaneous Coronary Intervention and Revascularization Procedures

Aspirin is used to reduce early ischemic complications in patients with ACS undergoing PCI (e.g., coronary angioplasty, coronary stent implantation). ACCF, AHA, and the Society for Cardiovascular Angiography and Interventions (SCAI) recommend pretreatment with aspirin (81–325 mg in those already receiving long-term aspirin therapy, otherwise 325 mg as non-enteric-coated aspirin) at least 2, and preferably 24, hours before the procedure. In addition to aspirin, a loading dose of a P2Y12-receptor antagonist (clopidogrel, prasugrel, or ticagrelor) is recommended in patients undergoing PCI with stent placement. Aspirin should be continued indefinitely after PCI, while a P2Y12-receptor antagonist generally should be continued for at least 12 months following stent placement.

In patients with anterior MI and left ventricular thrombus (or at high risk for left ventricular thrombus) who undergo stent placement, ACCP suggests the use of warfarin and clopidogrel in addition to aspirin therapy; the recommended duration of such triple antithrombotic therapy is dependent on whether the patient has a bare-metal or drug-eluting stent. However, such triple antithrombotic regimens are associated with an increased risk of bleeding.

An increased incidence of late stent thrombosis has been reported in patients with drug-eluting stents, often coincident with discontinuance of clopidogrel after initially recommended durations of dual-drug antiplatelet therapy. Stent thrombosis can be a catastrophic event leading to MI and/or death, and a broad range of experts currently recommend that dual-drug therapy with aspirin and a P2Y12-receptor antagonist (e.g., clopidogrel, prasugrel, ticagrelor) be continued for at least 12 months in patients with any type of coronary artery stent (drug-eluting or bare-metal) who are not at high risk of bleeding. Some evidence suggests that an even longer duration of dual antiplatelet therapy (more than 12 months) may be beneficial in some patients with drug-eluting stents, but such prolonged therapy may be associated with a higher risk of bleeding and other adverse effects. (See Uses: Prevention of Stent Thrombosis, in Clopidogrel 20:12.18.)

Aspirin is used to prevent reocclusion of the aortocoronary bypass graft in patients undergoing coronary revascularization procedures (e.g., CABG), and there is some evidence indicating that early (within 48 hours) administration of aspirin (75–325 mg daily) after CABG also is associated with a substantially reduced risk of both fatal and nonfatal (e.g., ischemic complications) outcomes in patients undergoing saphenous vein CABG. In a multicenter, prospective, longitudinal study, data on nonfatal and fatal outcomes (e.g., MI, heart failure, stroke, renal dysfunction or failure, GI ischemia or infarction) were recorded for patients with CHD who were refractory to medical therapy and who underwent CABG. Use of aspirin (total dose of 80–650 mg) within the first 48 hours following CABG was associated with a reduction in overall mortality during hospitalization of about 68% and reductions of 48, 50, 74, and 62% in the incidences of MI, stroke, renal failure, and bowel infarction, respectively. Duration of hospitalization also was shorter in patients receiving aspirin compared to those who did not (9.5 versus 11.5 days, respectively). Aspirin use was not associated with an increased risk of bleeding, gastritis, infection, or impaired wound healing. Subset analysis of data suggested that discontinuance of aspirin use prior to CABG and institution of hemostatic therapies (e.g., platelet transfusions, antifibrinolytic agents) during the perioperative period (i.e., during reperfusion following CABG) was associated with an increased risk of mortality and ischemic complications.

Some clinicians suggest that early administration of aspirin now be considered standard therapy in all patients undergoing CABG, including internal mammary artery bypass grafting, unless specifically contraindicated. AHA and ACCF recommend that aspirin therapy be initiated within 6 hours after CABG and continued for up to 1 year to reduce saphenous vein graft closure; aspirin dosages of 100–325 mg daily appear to be effective for this use. For long-term therapy after 1 year, ACCP recommends the use of low-dose aspirin in all patients with established coronary artery disease, including those with prior CABG. There are some data suggesting that an aspirin dosage not exceeding 75–81 mg daily may be sufficient for long-term cardiovascular prevention and is associated with less GI bleeding risk.

Aspirin has been used in combination with dipyridamole to prevent thrombosis in vein grafts in patients who undergo aortocoronary-artery bypass. However, dipyridamole does not appear to enhance the efficacy of aspirin, regardless of aspirin dosage, in patients receiving saphenous vein or internal mammary artery grafts.

Embolism Associated with Atrial Fibrillation

Antiplatelet agents (e.g., aspirin) have been used as an alternative or adjunct to warfarin therapy to reduce the incidence of thromboembolic episodes in selected patients with chronic atrial fibrillation†. ACC, AHA, ACCP, ASA, and other experts currently recommend that antithrombotic therapy be administered to all patients with nonvalvular atrial fibrillation (i.e., atrial fibrillation in the absence of rheumatic mitral stenosis, a prosthetic heart valve, or mitral valve repair) who are considered to be at increased risk of stroke, unless such therapy is contraindicated.

Recommendations regarding choice of antithrombotic therapy in patients with atrial fibrillation are based on the patient's risk for stroke and bleeding. In general, oral anticoagulant therapy (traditionally warfarin) is recommended in patients with atrial fibrillation who have a high risk for stroke and acceptably low risk of bleeding, while aspirin or no antithrombotic therapy may be considered in patients at low risk of stroke. Although many risk stratification methods have been used, patients considered to be at increased risk of stroke generally include those with prior ischemic stroke or TIA, advanced age (e.g., 75 years or older), history of hypertension, diabetes mellitus, or congestive heart failure. In addition, population-based studies suggest that female sex is an important risk factor for stroke in patients with atrial fibrillation, particularly in patients 75 years of age or older, and AHA and ASA recommend the use of risk stratification tools that account for age- and sex-specific differences in stroke risk. One such tool is the CHA_2DS_2-VASc score, an extension of the $CHADS_2$ system (which considers the risk factors congestive heart failure, hypertension, age 75 years or older, diabetes mellitus, and prior stroke/TIA) that adds extra points for female sex (1 point); previous MI, peripheral arterial disease, or aortic plaque (1 point); and age 65–74 years (1 point) or 75 years or older (2 points). Pooled analyses of data from a number of comparative studies evaluating therapy with a coumarin derivative (e.g., warfarin) or aspirin suggest that warfarin therapy is more effective than aspirin in reducing thromboembolic complications (e.g., TIAs, ischemic stroke) in patients with atrial fibrillation. However, the anticipated greater benefit of warfarin compared with aspirin must be weighed against the greater risk of bleeding with warfarin. Because the net clinical benefit with warfarin relative to aspirin appears to be greatest in patients with a high (and possibly also intermediate) risk of stroke, ACCP and other experts recommend the use of warfarin (target INR 2–3) over aspirin in such patients. Some experts also suggest that a non-vitamin K antagonist oral anticoagulant (e.g., apixaban, dabigatran, rivaroxaban) may provide certain advantages over warfarin (e.g., rapid onset of action, predictable anticoagulant effect, no requirement for coagulation monitoring, less potential for drug-drug and drug-food interactions) and may be considered as alternative therapy to warfarin in selected patients. (See Uses: Embolism Associated with Atrial Fibrillation, in Apixaban 20:12.04.14.) For patients at low risk of stroke, the expected benefits of warfarin may not outweigh the risks of bleeding, and thus, aspirin is preferred.

Results of a study comparing dual antiplatelet therapy (clopidogrel and aspirin) with aspirin in patients with atrial fibrillation who had an increased risk of stroke but were unable to take warfarin showed that the combination of clopidogrel and aspirin was more effective than aspirin in reducing the risk of stroke; however, such dual antiplatelet therapy was associated with an increased risk of bleeding. Based on these findings, ACCP and other experts recommend the use of clopidogrel and aspirin rather than aspirin alone as an alternative to warfarin in patients with atrial fibrillation at increased risk of stroke who cannot take or choose not to take warfarin (e.g., those with difficulty maintaining stable INRs).

The risk of thromboembolism in patients with atrial flutter is not as well established as it is in those with atrial fibrillation. In addition, many patients with atrial flutter have alternating periods of atrial fibrillation. Experts state that antithrombotic therapy in patients with atrial flutter generally should be managed in the same manner as in patients with atrial fibrillation.

Peripheral Arterial Disease

Aspirin also has been used for primary and secondary prophylaxis of cardiovascular events in patients with peripheral arterial disease, including those with intermittent claudication or carotid artery stenosis and those undergoing revascularization procedures (peripheral artery percutaneous transluminal angioplasty or peripheral arterial bypass graft surgery, carotid endarterectomy). ACCP recommendations for the use of aspirin in patients with peripheral arterial disease are largely similar to those in patients with coronary arterial disease. In general, aspirin is suggested in patients with asymptomatic disease (primary prevention) because of some evidence demonstrating a slight reduction in total mortality when the drug is taken over a period of 10 years. For patients with symptomatic peripheral arterial disease or those undergoing revascularization procedures, single-drug antiplatelet therapy with aspirin or clopidogrel is recommended; dual antiplatelet therapy with aspirin and clopidogrel generally is not suggested except in patients receiving below-the-knee prosthetic bypass grafts. AHA and ASA state that unless contraindicated, aspirin is recommended in patients who are to undergo carotid endarterectomy because aspirin was used in every trial that demonstrated the efficacy of this procedure. Aspirin or the combination of aspirin and dipyridamole also are recommended as 2 of several options for long-term antiplatelet therapy in patients with symptomatic carotid stenosis†, including those who have undergone recent carotid endarterectomy.

Although aspirin has generally been ineffective in preventing thrombosis after arterial catheterization, a single 600-mg oral dose the evening before surgery has been reported to reduce the incidence of thrombosis following radial-artery catheterization for surgery.

Valvular Heart Disease

In selected patients with mitral valve prolapse and atrial fibrillation (i.e., those younger than 65 years of age who have no history of mitral valve regurgitation, hypertension, or heart failure), aspirin therapy (e.g., 75–325 mg daily) is recommended by ACC and AHA. Aspirin also is recommended for symptomatic patients with mitral valve prolapse who experience a TIA.

Prosthetic Heart Valves

Aspirin is used for the prevention of thromboembolism in selected patients with prosthetic heart valves†. Warfarin generally is recommended in patients with *mechanical* heart valves because of the high risk of thromboembolism associated with these valves. In patients with a *bioprosthetic* heart valve in the aortic position who are in sinus rhythm and who have no other indications for warfarin, ACCP and ACC/AHA suggest the use of low-dose aspirin (50–100 mg daily) for initial (i.e., first 3 months after valve insertion) and long-term antithrombotic therapy. Warfarin therapy is suggested by ACCP in patients with bioprosthetic heart valves in the mitral position, at least for the first 3 months after valve insertion; after the first 3 months, aspirin may be substituted for warfarin therapy, provided the patient is in normal sinus rhythm.

Because warfarin therapy alone does not completely prevent thrombosis in patients with prosthetic mechanical heart valves†, aspirin has been used in conjunction with warfarin to reduce the incidence of thrombosis in these patients. The combination of aspirin and warfarin appears to be more effective than warfarin alone in patients with prosthetic mechanical valves, but the risk of bleeding complications may be increased. Pooled analysis of several randomized, controlled studies comparing combined therapy with an antiplatelet agent (aspirin or dipyridamole) and an oral anticoagulant (e.g., warfarin) versus oral anticoagulant monotherapy in patients who had received mechanical prosthetic heart valves showed that combined therapy substantially reduced systemic thromboembolism (principally manifested as stroke) and overall mortality compared with oral anticoagulant therapy alone; however, the risk of bleeding complications (e.g., hemorrhage, major GI hemorrhage) also was increased with combined therapy. In this analysis, it was estimated that for every 1.6 patients who had stroke prevented by combined therapy, there was an excess of one major GI bleeding episode, suggesting that the benefits derived from enhanced antithrombotic activity outweigh the risks resulting from enhanced bleeding potential. Subgroup analyses also showed that such benefits occur when only studies in which combined aspirin and oral anticoagulant therapy were considered, but that the increased risk of bleeding occurred mainly in patients receiving an oral anticoagulant combined with aspirin rather than with dipyridamole. Of 4 studies involving aspirin, 3 employed moderate (500 mg daily) or high (1 g daily) aspirin dosages, with the remaining one employing a low dosage of 100 mg daily.

Based on current evidence, ACCP and other experts recommend the addition of an antiplatelet agent such as low-dose aspirin to warfarin therapy in all patients with mechanical heart valves who are at low risk of bleeding. Combination therapy with aspirin and warfarin also is recommended by ACC/AHA in patients with bioprosthetic heart valves who have additional risk factors for thrombosis (e.g., atrial fibrillation, previous thromboembolism, left ventricular dysfunction, hypercoagulable condition).

In pregnant women with prosthetic heart valves, a low molecular weight heparin or unfractionated heparin is substituted for warfarin because of concerns about warfarin embryopathy. Based on extrapolation of data from nonpregnant patients with prosthetic heart valves, aspirin (75–100 mg daily) may be added to therapy with a low molecular weight heparin or unfractionated heparin in pregnant women with prosthetic heart valves who are at high risk for thrombosis.

In patients with a prosthetic heart valve receiving long-term oral antithrombotic therapy (warfarin and/or aspirin) who require surgical procedures, the risk of perioperative bleeding should be weighed against the increased risk of thromboembolism that may occur as a result of temporary discontinuance of oral antithrombotic therapy. Oral antithrombotic therapy generally should not be discontinued for procedures in which bleeding is unlikely or inconsequential, such as minor dental, dermatologic, or ophthalmologic procedures.

Thrombosis Associated with Heart Surgery in Children

ACCP recommends aspirin (1–5 mg/kg daily) or unfractionated heparin followed by warfarin for the prevention of thromboembolic complications in children undergoing Fontan surgery† (the definitive palliative surgical treatment for most congenital univentricular heart lesions). However, despite even aggressive antithrombotic therapy in children who have undergone the Fontan procedure, thromboembolic events associated with the procedure result in a high mortality rate and respond to therapy in less than 50% of patients. There currently is no consensus on the optimal type or duration of antithrombotic therapy following Fontan surgery, and a wide variety of prophylactic regimens currently are in use.

Venous Thromboembolism

Thromboprophylaxis in Orthopedic Surgery

Aspirin has been used for the prevention of venous thromboembolism in patients undergoing major orthopedic surgery (total-hip replacement†, total-knee replacement†, or hip-fracture surgery†). Although aspirin generally is not considered the drug of choice for this use, there is some evidence suggesting that aspirin may provide some benefit over placebo or no antithrombotic prophylaxis in patients undergoing major orthopedic surgery. (See Hip-Replacement, Knee-Replacement, or Hip-Fracture Surgery under Venous Thromboembolism: Prophylaxis, in Uses in Enoxaparin 20:12.04.16.) Results of a large, randomized placebo-controlled study (The Randomized Placebo-controlled Pulmonary Embolism Prevention [PEP] Trial) in patients undergoing hip-fracture surgery or elective arthroplasty showed that aspirin was associated with a modest reduction in the risk of symptomatic deep-vein thrombosis at the expense of a possible increased risk of major bleeding and nonfatal MI. Based on these findings, ACCP considers the use of aspirin to be an acceptable option for pharmacologic thromboprophylaxis in patients undergoing major orthopedic surgery. When selecting an appropriate thromboprophylaxis regimen, ACCP states that factors such as relative efficacy and bleeding risk as well as logistics and compliance issues should be considered. For additional information on the prevention of venous thromboembolism in patients undergoing major orthopedic surgery, consult the most recent ACCP Evidence-based Clinical Practice Guidelines on Antithrombotic Therapy and Prevention of Thrombosis available at http://www.chestnet.org.

Thromboprophylaxis in General Surgery

Aspirin also has been used for thromboprophylaxis in patients undergoing general (e.g., abdominal) surgery who are at high risk of venous thromboembolism. If pharmacologic prophylaxis is indicated in such patients undergoing general surgery, ACCP states that a low molecular weight heparin or low-dose unfractionated heparin is preferred, but when these agents are contraindicated or not available, aspirin or fondaparinux may be considered.

For additional information on the prevention of venous thromboembolism in patients undergoing surgery, consult the most recent ACCP Evidence-based Clinical Practice Guidelines on Antithrombotic Therapy and Prevention of Thrombosis available at http://www.chestnet.org.

Pericarditis

In addition to its use for reducing the risk of death and/or nonfatal recurrent MI (secondary prevention) (see Coronary Artery Disease and Myocardial Infarction under Uses: Thrombosis), aspirin also is used for the treatment of pain associated with acute pericarditis that develops after an acute MI.

ACCF and AHA recommend that pericarditis be considered in the differential diagnosis of recurrent chest pain after STEMI. Pericarditis probably is not responsible for clinically important chest pain during the initial 24 hours after infarction and may not become evident for up to several weeks after an acute MI. Recurrent pain occurring during the initial 12 hours after onset of infarction usually is considered related to the original infarction itself. Pericarditis in acute MI occurs with extension of myocardial necrosis throughout the epicardial wall. The Multicenter Investigation of the Limitation of Infarct Size (MILIS) study found that pericarditis (defined as presence of pericardial friction rub) occurred in about 20% of patients following acute MI. In patients not treated with thrombolytic therapy, pericarditis occurs in about 25% of patients as evidenced by either typical symptoms or pericardial friction rub, but the incidence averages only 14% when the presence of a friction rub is required for diagnosis. Patients with pericarditis have larger infarcts, lower ejection fractions, and a higher incidence of congestive heart failure. Although anterior chest discomfort mimicking ischemia can occur with pericarditis, pericardial pain usually exhibits distinguishing characteristics, including pleural or positional discomfort; radiation to the left shoulder, scapula, or trapezius muscle; and a pericardial rub, ECG J-point elevation with concave upward ST-segment elevation, and PR depression. It is important to distinguish between pain caused by pericarditis and that caused by ischemia since management will differ. On occasion, pericarditis may be a clinical clue to the presence of subacute myocardial rupture. Although pericarditis is not an absolute contraindication to anticoagulation, ACCF and AHA state that anticoagulation therapy should be used with caution due to the potential for hemorrhagic conversion.

In one study, the effects of 2.6 g of oral aspirin daily were comparable to those of 100–200 mg of oral indomethacin daily, with either drug relieving symptoms within 48 hours. Although other NSAIAs (e.g., indomethacin, ibuprofen) or corticosteroids also can provide symptomatic relief, these drugs may be associated with adverse cardiac effects (e.g., increased coronary vascular resistance, thinning of the developing scar, myocardial rupture). The possibility that cardiac rupture, which occurs in about 1–4% of patients hospitalized for acute MI, may account for recurrent pain should be considered since use of NSAIAs may be a risk factor in its development. ACCF and AHA state the administration of acetaminophen, colchicine, or opiate analgesics may be reasonable if pain relief with aspirin therapy is ineffective.

Kawasaki Disease

The American Academy of Pediatrics (AAP), AHA, and ACCP recommend aspirin therapy used in conjunction with immune globulin IV (IGIV) for initial treatment of the acute phase of Kawasaki disease†; aspirin also is used alone or in conjunction with other antiplatelet agents or anticoagulants for follow-up treatment.

High-dose aspirin therapy (80–100 mg/kg daily for up to 14 days) combined with a single dose of IGIV (2 g/kg) initiated within 10 days of the onset of fever is more effective than aspirin therapy alone for preventing or reducing the occurrence of coronary artery aneurysms associated with Kawasaki disease; fever and other manifestations of inflammation also may resolve more rapidly with concomitant therapy. Aspirin then is continued alone in lower dosages (i.e., 1–5 mg/kg daily) for antiplatelet effects for 6–8 weeks in those without coronary artery changes or with only transient coronary artery ectasia or dilatation (disappearing within the initial 6–8 weeks of illness). For additional information on initial treatment of Kawasaki disease, see Uses: Kawasaki Disease and also see Kawasaki Disease under Dosage and Administration: Dosage for Immune Globulin IV, in Immune Globulin 80:04.

Coronary artery abnormalities develop in 15–25% of children with Kawasaki disease if they are not treated within 10 days of onset of fever; 2–4% of patients develop coronary artery abnormalities despite prompt treatment with aspirin and IGIV. Long-term management of those who develop coronary abnormalities depends on the severity of coronary involvement and may include low-dose aspirin (with or without clopidogrel or dipyridamole), anticoagulant therapy with warfarin or low molecular weight heparin, or a combination of antiplatelet and anticoagulant therapy (usually low-dose aspirin and warfarin). If giant coronary aneurysms are present, AHA and ACCP suggest long-term low-dose aspirin therapy in conjunction with warfarin for primary thromboprophylaxis. Specialized references should be consulted for additional information on long-term management of Kawasaki disease in individuals with coronary abnormalities.

Complications of Pregnancy

Aspirin should be used during pregnancy only when clearly needed, weighing carefully the potential benefits versus the possible risks to the mother and fetus. (See Cautions: Pregnancy, Fertility, and Lactation, in the Salicylates General Statement 28:08.04.24.)

Aspirin has been used alone or in combination with other drugs (e.g., unfractionated heparin, low molecular weight heparins, corticosteroids, immune globulin) for the prevention of complications of pregnancy† (e.g., preeclampsia, pregnancy loss in women with a history of antiphospholipid syndrome and recurrent fetal loss). Maternal and fetal hemorrhagic complications observed with maternal ingestion of large dosages (e.g., 12–15 g daily) of aspirin generally have not been observed in studies in which dosages of 50–150 mg daily of the drug were used during the second and third trimesters for prevention of complications of pregnancy (e.g., preeclampsia, recurrent spontaneous abortions, prematurity, intrauterine growth retardation, stillbirth, low birthweight), including those associated with autoimmune disorders such as antiphospholipid syndrome, poor paternal blocking antibody production, or systemic lupus erythematosus.

Results of several controlled studies suggest that low dosages of aspirin administered from preconception through delivery alone or in combination with heparin or corticosteroids in high-risk women may prevent the development of preeclampsia and fetal growth retardation and reduce perinatal death, possibly by suppressing thromboxane A_2-mediated vasospasm, ischemia, and thrombosis. The presence of maternal antiphospholipid antibodies is associated with an increased risk of thrombosis and pregnancy loss. Data from several small comparative studies indicate that combined prophylaxis with heparin and low dosages of aspirin may be more effective than aspirin alone or aspirin combined with a corticosteroid in preventing recurrent pregnancy loss (fetal death, miscarriage), preeclampsia, or premature delivery in women with antiphospholipid syndrome (Hughes syndrome). In at least one study in women with antiphospholipid antibodies and at least 2 prior pregnancy losses, combined aspirin (100 mg daily) and corticosteroid (prednisone 0.5–0.8 mg/kg daily) therapy was not effective in promoting live birth and was associated with an increased risk of prematurity. The beneficial effect of prophylactic therapy with aspirin and heparin may result from aspirin-induced suppression of thromboxane$_2$-mediated vasospasm, ischemia, and thrombosis in the placental vasculature and by heparin-induced anticoagulation combined with binding to phospholipid antibodies that protects the trophoblast from antibody attack and thus promotes successful implantation in early pregnancy.

Women with antiphospholipid syndrome and a history of multiple pregnancy losses are candidates for prophylactic therapy†, and most experts currently recommend combined prophylactic therapy with low dosages of aspirin and unfractionated heparin or low molecular weight heparin, followed by postpartum warfarin therapy. ACCP states that women with antiphospholipid antibody (APLA) syndrome and a history of multiple pregnancy losses (at least 3) should receive antepartum prophylaxis with low-dose aspirin in combination with subcutaneous unfractionated heparin or a low molecular weight heparin. (See Uses: Thromboembolism Occurring During Pregnancy, in Enoxaparin 20:12.04.16.)

Because of experience in women with antiphospholipid syndrome, aspirin and heparin (often combined with immune globulin) also have been used to prevent venous thromboembolism and early pregnancy loss in women who have undergone in vitro fertilization†. However, current evidence suggests that the overall absolute risk of symptomatic thrombosis appears to be low in women undergoing in vitro fertilization. Therefore, ACCP recommends against routine thromboprophylaxis in most women undergoing assisted reproduction.

Aspirin in low dosages throughout pregnancy also has been used to prevent preeclampsia† in pregnant women at high risk, including those with pregestational diabetes mellitus, obesity, age exceeding 40 years, chronic hypertension, nulliparity, multifetal gestations, preexisting vascular disease, collagen vascular disease, renal disease, and/or antiphospholipid syndrome (see preceding discussion), and those with a history of preeclampsia during prior pregnancy. The rationale for aspirin prophylaxis is that hypertension and coagulation abnormalities in preeclampsia are caused in part by an imbalance between vasodilating and vasoconstricting prostaglandins (prostacyclin and thromboxane A_2, respectively); by preferentially inhibiting thromboxane A_2 production at low doses, aspirin was postulated to provide some protection against the abnormalities associated with preeclampsia. Some clinicians have suggested that prophylaxis with low dosages of aspirin be considered in selected high-risk women (e.g., those with chronic hypertension, a history of early or recurrent preeclampsia, diabetes mellitus, underlying renal disease, high body mass index, those 35 years of age or older) who do not have thrombophilia.

Systematic reviews involving large numbers of patients have suggested beneficial effects of low-dose aspirin on preeclampsia and its complications. In a systematic review based on pooled data in more than 12,000 women with historical risk factors for preeclampsia, aspirin prophylaxis (generally 50–150 mg daily) was associated with a reduction of about 15% in the risk of preeclampsia and also some benefit on perinatal death, spontaneous preterm birth, and birth weight. Another systematic review in more than 30,000 women receiving prophylaxis with antiplatelet drugs (usually aspirin in a dosage of up to 75 mg daily) demonstrated similar findings. Neither of these reviews found evidence of a harmful effect of aspirin prophylaxis in these women. ACCP, AHA, and ASA recommend the use of low-dose aspirin during pregnancy (starting from the second trimester) in women who are at high risk for preeclampsia, including those with chronic primary or secondary hypertension or previous pregnancy-related hypertension.

Prevention of Cancer

While data principally from observational studies suggest that aspirin or other NSAIAs may reduce the risk of various cancers† (e.g., colorectal, breast, gastric), results of several randomized, placebo-controlled studies generally have not confirmed these observations. A large, long-term randomized study (Women's Health Study) in women with no history of cancer or cardiovascular disease indicated *no* reduction in the risk of developing cancer overall or at specific sites, including breast, colorectal, or lung cancer, with use of low dosages of aspirin (100 mg every other day). In this study, approximately 40,000 predominantly middle-aged (mean age 54.6 years at study entry) women received aspirin or placebo in a 2 x 2 factorial design (patients also were randomized to receive vitamin E or placebo as part of the study; no effect of the vitamin E treatment arm was noted on the aspirin results); patients received aspirin for an average of 10 years. Aspirin use also was not associated with a reduction in overall cancer mortality, including deaths due to breast or colorectal cancer. However, a statistically significant reduction in lung cancer *mortality* and a trend toward a reduction in the risk of lung cancer were noted in patients taking aspirin. Given the variability of aspirin's effects on lung cancer reported in other trials, it has been suggested that the positive findings in this study may be due to chance; however, data from this study cannot rule out a protective effect of aspirin on lung cancer.

Observational studies and a few randomized, placebo-controlled trials in patients with a history of colorectal adenomas have shown a reduction in the risk of recurrent colorectal adenomas† with regular (e.g., daily) use of aspirin or other NSAIAs. However, evidence that aspirin and other NSAIAs prevent colorectal *cancer* itself currently is based principally on observational studies, and available data suggest that beneficial effects on cancer may only be evident following at least a decade of regular aspirin therapy. Almost all evidence indicates that the beneficial effects of NSAIAs in reducing colorectal cancer risk dissipate following discontinuance of NSAIA therapy. Current data suggest that the potential clinical benefits of aspirin for primary or secondary prevention of colorectal cancer may be small considering the efficacy of screening and removal of colorectal adenomas in preventing cancer and the risks of bleeding complications associated with long-term aspirin therapy in patients at average risk for colorectal cancer. Therefore, most clinicians state that such preventive therapy with aspirin currently is not recommended and, because randomized trials indicate that aspirin does not completely eliminate adenomas, it should not be considered a replacement for colorectal cancer screening and surveillance. Further studies are necessary to determine whether aspirin therapy can lessen the required intensity or frequency of such surveillance measures. Certain other NSAIAs, particularly selective inhibitors of cyclooxygenase-2 (COX-2) (e.g., celecoxib), currently are used as adjunctive therapy to reduce the number of colorectal polyps in patients with familial adenomatous polyposis; such patients are at particularly high risk for developing colorectal cancer. (See Uses: Colorectal Polyps, in Celecoxib 28:08.04.08.)

Epidemiologic studies have consistently demonstrated a 40–50% reduction in the risk of colorectal neoplasia with aspirin use that is not explained by differences in study design, study populations, patterns of aspirin use, or outcomes. The mechanism by which aspirin and other NSAIAs prevent the development of colorectal adenomas or neoplasms has not been fully elucidated, but some evidence suggests that NSAIAs may restore apoptosis in adenomatous colorectal polyps and/or inhibit angiogenesis, both through COX-2 inhibition and COX-independent mechanisms. (See Pharmacology: GI Effects, in Celecoxib

28:08.04.08.) Since most colorectal cancers arise from benign adenomas but have a long latency period (e.g., 5–10 years), prevention of adenomas has been used as a surrogate end point in clinical prevention trials of colorectal cancer. Several randomized, placebo-controlled trials involving patients with prior colorectal neoplasia have demonstrated reductions in the incidence of recurrent colorectal adenomas with regular use of aspirin.

DOSAGE AND ADMINISTRATION

● Administration

Aspirin is usually administered orally, preferably with food or a large quantity (240 mL) of water (unless the patient is fluid restricted) or milk to minimize gastric irritation. In patients unable to take or retain oral medication, aspirin suppositories may be administered rectally; however, rectal absorption may be slow and incomplete. (See Pharmacokinetics: Absorption.) *Aspirin tablets should not be administered rectally, since they are likely to cause irritation and erosion of the rectal mucosa.* Aspirin preparations should not be used if a strong vinegar-like odor is present. (See Chemistry and Stability: Stability.)

If an unpleasant taste or aftertaste, burning in the throat, or difficulty in swallowing occurs with uncoated aspirin-containing tablets, these effects may be reduced with film-coated tablets. Although specific data are not available, these effects are also likely to be reduced with enteric-coated tablets. If gastric irritation and/or symptomatic GI disturbances occur with uncoated aspirin-containing tablets, these effects may be reduced with enteric-coated tablets or extended-release tablets. If a liquid dosage form of aspirin is desired for short-term treatment of pain, an oral solution may be prepared from commercially available effervescent tablets (e.g., Alka-Seltzer®) by dissolving tablets in 120 mL of water; ingest the entire solution to ensure adequate dosing.

In addition to potentially reducing adverse GI effects, some clinicians suggest that enteric-coated tablets may be swallowed more easily by children receiving chronic therapy with the drug and may therefore result in increased compliance.

Aspirin or buffered aspirin preparations should not be chewed before swallowing for at least 7 days following tonsillectomy or oral surgery because of possible injury to oral tissues from prolonged contact with aspirin particles. In addition, aspirin or buffered aspirin tablets should not be placed directly on a tooth or gum surface because of possible injury to tissues.

Capsules containing the fixed combination of aspirin and extended-release dipyridamole should be swallowed whole and should not be chewed.

Chewable aspirin tablets may be chewed, crushed, and/or dissolved in a liquid, or swallowed whole, followed by approximately 120 mL of water, milk, or fruit juice immediately after administration of the drug.

For information on the concomitant administration of aspirin with nonsteroidal anti-inflammatory agents (NSAIAs), see Drug Interactions: Nonsteroidal Anti-inflammatory Agents, in the Salicylates General Statement 28:08.04.24.

● Dosage

Dosage of aspirin must be carefully adjusted according to individual requirements and response, using the lowest possible effective dosage. When used at high (e.g., anti-inflammatory) dosages, the development of tinnitus can be used as a sign of elevated serum salicylate concentrations, except in patients with high-frequency hearing impairment.

When preparations containing aspirin in fixed combination with other drugs are used, the cautions, precautions, and contraindications applicable to each ingredient must be considered.

Pain and Fever

Aspirin should not be used for *self-medication* of pain for longer than 10 days in adults or 5 days in children, unless directed by a physician, since pain of such intensity and duration may indicate a pathologic condition requiring medical evaluation and supervised treatment. Aspirin, including chewing gum pieces, should not be used for *self-medication* of sore throat pain for longer than 2 days in adults or children, unless directed by a physician, since prolonged use could cause mucosal erosions in the mouth. Patients should be warned that the risk of GI bleeding is increased in geriatric patients 60 years of age or older, in patients with a history of GI ulcers or bleeding, when recommended dosages and durations of *self-medication* are exceeded, when anticoagulants or corticosteroids are used concomitantly, in patients receiving more than one NSAIA, and in those consuming 3 or more alcohol-containing beverages daily. (See Cautions: GI Effects, in the Salicylates General Statement 28:08.04.24)

Aspirin should not be used in adults or children for *self-medication* of marked fever (exceeding 39.5°C), fever persisting longer than 3 days, or recurrent fever, unless directed by a physician, since such fevers may indicate serious illness requiring prompt medical evaluation.

Aspirin should not be used in adults or children for *self-medication* of sore throat for longer than 2 days, and should be discontinued and a clinician consulted if sore throat persists or is accompanied by fever, headache, rash, nausea, or vomiting.

To minimize the risk of overdosage, no more than 5 doses of aspirin should be administered to children for analgesia or antipyresis in any 24-hour period, unless directed by a physician.

For analgesia or antipyresis in adults or children older than 12 years of age, the usual oral or rectal dosage of aspirin is 324–650 mg every 4 hours as necessary, but should not exceed 3.9 g daily; higher single doses (e.g., 975 mg or 1 g) may be useful for analgesia in some patients. If a rapid response is required, the more slowly absorbed dosage forms (i.e., enteric-coated, extended-release tablets) should not be used. In children 2–11 years of age, the usual oral or rectal dosage for analgesia or antipyresis is 1.5 g/m² daily, administered in 4–6 divided doses; total daily rectal dosage should not exceed 2.5 g/m². Alternatively, children may receive the following *approximate* oral or rectal doses every 4 hours as necessary: children 11–12 years of age, 320–480 mg; children 9–11 years of age, 320–400 mg; children 6–7 years of age, 320–325 mg; children 4–6 years of age, 240 mg; and children 2–4 years of age, 160 mg. Dosage in children younger than 2 years of age must be individualized.

The usual dosage of aspirin (as chewing gum pieces) for analgesia and antipyresis in adults and children older than 12 years of age is 454 mg, repeated every 4 hours as necessary (maximum 3.632 g daily). The chewing gum pieces should be thoroughly chewed for about 15 minutes to ensure adequate dosing and then the gum should be expelled from the mouth and discarded. Children 6–12 years of age may be given 227–454 mg, repeated as necessary up to 4 times daily. Children 3–6 years of age may be given 227 mg, repeated as necessary up to 3 times daily. Aspirin chewing gum pieces should not be used in children younger than 3 years of age unless directed by a physician; dosage must be individualized.

The usual oral dosage of aspirin as a highly buffered effervescent solution (Alka-Seltzer® Original, Lemon-Lime) for analgesia in adults and children 12 years of age or older is 650 mg every 4 hours as necessary; total dosage in any 24-hour period should not exceed 2.6 g. Alternatively, in adults and children 12 years of age or older, the usual dosage of Alka-Seltzer Extra Strength is 1 g every 6 hours; total dosage in any 24-hour period should not exceed 3.5 g Because of the high sodium content of this preparation (approximately 24 mEq of sodium per 325 mg of aspirin), it should be used with extreme caution, if at all, in patients in whom excessive amounts of sodium may be harmful. The usual oral dosage of aspirin (Alka-Seltzer® lemon-Lime or Original) for patients 60 years of age or older is 650 mg every 4 hours as necessary, not to exceed 1.3 g in any 24-hour period. The usual dosage of aspirin (Alka-Seltzer® Extra Strength) for patients 60 years of age or older is 1 g every 6 hours; total dosage in any 24-hour period should not exceed 2 g. The manufacturer states that the preparation should not be used in children younger than 12 years of age unless directed by a physician. In addition, higher than usually recommended dosages of this preparation should not be used unless directed by a physician.

The usual oral dosage of aspirin (as 650-mg extended-release tablets) for analgesia in adults is 650 mg to 1.3 g every 8 hours as necessary, not to exceed 3.9 g daily. For patients who have difficulty swallowing the 650-mg tablets whole, the tablets may be gently broken or crumbled before administration (or in the mouth), but they must *not* be ground up if they are to retain the property of extended release. An 800-mg extended-release aspirin tablet is also commercially available but is indicated for use only in the symptomatic treatment of inflammatory disease; the 800-mg tablet *cannot* be broken or crumbled and must be swallowed whole. Most clinicians believe that extended-release aspirin tablets offer no therapeutic advantage over other types of aspirin tablets; this is particularly true at high dosages since the elimination half-life of salicylate is dose dependent and prolonged at high dosages. However, symptomatic GI disturbances and/or occult GI bleeding may be reduced with extended-release tablets.

For *self-medication* for the temporary relief of mild to moderate pain associated with migraine headache in adults, the recommended oral aspirin dosage is 500 mg (combined with 500 mg of acetaminophen and 130 mg of caffeine) as a single dose of an immediate-release (conventional) preparation taken with a full glass of water; no more than 500 mg of aspirin (in combination with 500 mg of acetaminophen and 130 mg of caffeine) should be taken in a 24-hour period unless directed by a clinician. Individuals younger than 18 years of age should consult their clinician before using this combination preparation. Patients receiving the combination for *self-medication* should be advised to discontinue the drug and consult a clinician if an allergic reaction occurs, if migraine headache pain worsens or persists after the first dose, or if new or unexpected symptoms, including tinnitus (ringing in the ears) or hearing loss, occur.

For temporary relief of acute migraine headache pain and associated symptoms (nausea, vomiting, photophobia, phonophobia) in adults, aspirin 900 or 1000 mg has been given as a single dose with or without metoclopramide 10 mg (as an antiemetic).

Inflammatory Diseases

For the symptomatic treatment of rheumatoid arthritis, osteoarthritis, or other polyarthritic or inflammatory conditions (e.g., spondyloarthropathies, arthritis and pleurisy of systemic lupus erythematosus [SLE]), the usual initial adult dosage of aspirin is 2.4–3.6 g daily, administered in divided doses. When necessary, dosage is generally increased by 325 mg to 1.2 g daily at intervals of 1 week or more. The usual adult maintenance dosage is 3.6–5.4 g daily; however, higher dosages may be necessary. Dosage should be adjusted according to the patient's response, tolerance, and serum salicylate concentration. (See Dosage: Inflammatory Diseases under Dosage and Administration, in the Salicylates General Statement 28:08.04.24.)

For the symptomatic treatment of juvenile arthritis, the usual initial dosage is 60–130 mg/kg daily in children weighing 25 kg or less, or 2.4–3.6 g daily in children weighing more than 25 kg, administered in divided doses. Alternatively, some clinicians recommend an initial dosage of 1.5 g/m² daily, administered in divided doses. When necessary, dosage is generally increased by 10 mg/kg daily no more frequently than at weekly intervals. The usual maintenance dosage is 80–100 mg/kg daily; up to 130 mg/kg daily may be required in some children. Although some clinicians have reported a high incidence of chronic intoxication in children receiving 90–100 mg/kg daily, this has not been found by many others. However, it appears that dosages of at least 100 mg/kg daily should not be used in children weighing more than 25 kg. Based on body surface area, dosage should generally not exceed 3 g/m² daily. Dosage should be adjusted according to the patient's response, tolerance, and serum salicylate concentration. (See Dosage: Inflammatory Diseases under Dosage and Administration, in the Salicylates General Statement 28:08.04.24.)

Because of the prolonged elimination half-life of salicylate at high dosages, at least 5–7 days are generally required to achieve steady-state serum salicylate concentrations in the treatment of inflammatory diseases. Therefore, some clinicians have suggested that loading-dose regimens of aspirin may be useful to more rapidly attain serum concentrations associated with an anti-inflammatory effect. In one small study, healthy individuals were given oral dosages of 650 mg of aspirin every 4 hours for 4 days (conventional-dose regimen) or two 1.3-g doses 4 hours apart followed 2 hours later by initiation of a maintenance dosage of 650-mg oral doses every 4 hours through 4 days (loading-dose regimen). In this study, the time required to reach a serum salicylate concentration of 150 mcg/mL was approximately 15 hours with the loading-dose regimen and approximately 48 hours with the conventional-dose regimen; serum salicylate concentrations were higher during the first 36 hours with the loading-dose regimen. However, the actual clinical importance of any difference between these regimens in patients with inflammatory diseases is not known; further evaluation of loading-dose regimens in such patients is needed.

Rheumatic Fever

For the symptomatic treatment of rheumatic fever†, dosage and duration of aspirin therapy are generally determined by the severity and duration of acute manifestations. For maximal suppression of acute inflammation, the usual initial dosage of aspirin is 4.9–7.8 g daily in adults and 90–130 mg/kg daily in children, administered in divided doses every 4–6 hours. Patients with only polyarthritis and fever usually respond to lower dosages. Subsequent dosage should be adjusted according to the patient's response, tolerance, and serum salicylate concentration.

The initial dosage is generally administered for up to 1–2 weeks, then decreased to approximately 60–70 mg/kg daily for 1–6 weeks or as long as necessary, and then gradually withdrawn over 1–2 weeks. Various aspirin regimens have been suggested depending on the severity of acute manifestations, and the clinician should consult published protocols for more information on specific dosages and schedules of administration.

In patients with carditis and cardiomegaly or congestive heart failure who are treated with corticosteroids, aspirin therapy is usually initiated as steroid therapy is gradually withdrawn. In these patients, some clinicians recommend an aspirin dosage of 60 mg/kg daily, administered in divided doses. High dosages should be used with caution in patients with carditis since congestive heart failure or pulmonary edema may be precipitated. Aspirin is usually administered for approximately 2–4 weeks after steroids are discontinued. Only extremely severe clinical rebounds of rheumatic activity require reinstitution of therapy, in which case aspirin is administered in the usual dosage for 3–4 additional weeks.

Thrombosis

Transient Ischemic Attacks and Acute Ischemic Stroke

For secondary prevention of vascular events (e.g., death, recurrent stroke) in patients with transient ischemic attacks (TIAs) or stroke, the usual oral dosage of aspirin in adults is 50–325 mg daily, continued long term. In patients with non-cardioembolic ischemic stroke or TIA, the American College of Chest Physicians (ACCP) recommends an aspirin dosage of 75–100 mg daily, continued long term. While dosages up to 1.3 g daily, administered in 2 or 4 divided doses, have been recommended, there is little evidence supporting superiority of such dosages relative to currently recommended low dosages, and the risk of adverse effects (e.g., GI intolerance, bleeding) is increased with increasing dosage. Current data suggest that an aspirin dosage not exceeding 75–81 mg daily may be sufficient for long-term cardiovascular prevention and is associated with less GI bleeding risk.

For the acute treatment of ischemic stroke in patients who are not receiving a thrombolytic agent, the usual oral dosage of aspirin when given as monotherapy in adults is 150–325 mg initiated within 24–48 hours of stroke onset. In children with acute arterial ischemic stroke†, aspirin 1–5 mg/kg daily is recommended as an option for initial anticoagulation until dissection and embolic causes have been excluded. When cerebral arterial dissection and cardioembolic causes have been excluded, the usual suggested dosage of aspirin for secondary prevention in such children is 1–5 mg/kg daily for a minimum of 2 years. If aspirin is used in children with acute arterial ischemic stroke secondary to non-Moyamoya vasculopathy, ACCP recommends at least 3 months of therapy; ongoing antithrombotic therapy should be determined by repeat cerebrovascular imaging.

When aspirin is given in combination with dipyridamole to reduce the risk of stroke in patients who have had noncardioembolic stroke or TIAs, the usual dosage of aspirin in fixed combination with extended-release dipyridamole (200 mg) is 25 mg (1 capsule) twice daily in the morning and evening.

The American Heart Association (AHA) and American Stroke Association (ASA) state that unless contraindicated, an aspirin dosage of 75–325 mg daily is recommended for *secondary prevention* of ischemic stroke in high-risk women and is reasonable in selected women (e.g., those with diabetes mellitus) for *primary prevention* of ischemic stroke†. (See Transient Ischemic Attacks and Acute Ischemic Stroke under Uses: Thrombosis for definition of high risk.) If the benefit of aspirin for the prevention of ischemic stroke or myocardial infarction (MI) in women is considered to outweigh the risks of therapy, a dosage of 81 mg daily or 100 mg every *other* day has been suggested by AHA and ASA.

Coronary Artery Disease

For the secondary prevention of cardiovascular events in patients with coronary artery disease, a low dosage of aspirin (e.g., 75–162 mg daily) generally is recommended. ACCP recommends long-term, single-drug antiplatelet therapy with aspirin 75–100 mg daily in patients with established coronary artery disease (i.e., 1 year after ACS with prior revascularization, coronary stenosis greater than 50% by coronary angiogram, and/or evidence of cardiac ischemia on diagnostic testing).

ST-Segment-Elevation Myocardial Infarction

As an adjunct in the acute management of suspected acute ST-segment-elevation MI (STEMI), the usual initial adult oral dose of aspirin for prevention of early recurrence or extension of infarction and mortality reduction is 162–325 mg. Such acute aspirin therapy should be initiated as soon as possible after the clinical impression of an evolving acute STEMI is formed, preferably by chewing and/or swallowing a conventional tablet.

Aspirin therapy for the management of STEMI should be continued indefinitely at a dosage of 81–325 mg daily. Some experts prefer the use of a maintenance dosage of 81 mg daily because of a decreased risk of bleeding and lack of definitive evidence demonstrating that higher dosages confer greater benefit. Although higher dosages of aspirin have been used in patients surviving an MI (900 mg to 1.5 g daily in divided doses), lower-dosage regimens appear to be equally effective and may minimize adverse GI effects. Some data suggest that 75–81 mg of aspirin daily is sufficient for long-term cardiovascular disease prevention and is associated with less GI bleeding risk.

In patients with STEMI who have indications for anticoagulation (e.g., atrial fibrillation, left ventricular dysfunction, cerebral emboli, extensive wall-motion abnormality, mechanical heart valves), warfarin (INR 2–3) should be administered in addition to aspirin therapy; in some cases (e.g., patients with an anterior STEMI and left ventricular thrombosis undergoing percutaneous coronary intervention [PCI] with stenting), both warfarin (INR 2–3) and clopidogrel 75 mg daily may be added to aspirin therapy (triple antithrombotic therapy).

For primary prevention† to reduce the risk of atherosclerotic cardiovascular disease (ASCVD), including first STEMI in patients 40–70 years of age at increased risk for ASCVD but without an increased bleeding risk, the usual oral dosage of aspirin is 75–162 mg daily. The efficacy of dosages lower than 75 mg daily has not been established. An oral aspirin dosage of 325 mg every other day has been used but is no longer preferred.

Non-ST-Segment-Elevation Acute Coronary Syndromes

In patients with non-ST-segment-elevation acute coronary syndromes (NSTE ACS), the American College of Cardiology (ACC) and AHA recommend an initial aspirin dose of 162–325 mg as soon as possible after presentation, unless such therapy is contraindicated, followed by a maintenance dosage of 81–325 mg daily. Aspirin should be used in conjunction with a P2Y12-receptor antagonist (e.g., clopidogrel, ticagrelor) for up to 12 months. When used in conjunction with ticagrelor, aspirin should be administered in a maintenance dosage of 75–100 mg daily since aspirin dosages exceeding 100 mg daily have been associated with reduced efficacy of ticagrelor.

Percutaneous Coronary Intervention and Revascularization Procedures

To reduce the incidence of early ischemic complications in patients undergoing PCI (e.g., coronary angioplasty, coronary stent placement), ACCF, AHA, and the Society for Cardiovascular Angiography and Interventions (SCAI) recommend pretreatment with 81–325 mg of aspirin, initiated at least 2, and preferably 24, hours before the procedure. In patients not already receiving long-term aspirin therapy, an aspirin dose of 325 mg (as the non-enteric-coated formulation) initiated at least 2, and preferably 24, hours prior to PCI is recommended.

In addition to aspirin, a loading dose of a P2Y12-receptor antagonist (clopidogrel, prasugrel, or ticagrelor) should be administered in patients with ACS undergoing PCI with stent placement (bare-metal or drug-eluting). Aspirin should be continued indefinitely after PCI, while a P2Y12-receptor antagonist generally should be continued for at least 12 months following placement of an intracoronary stent.

In patients with anterior MI and left ventricular thrombus (or at high risk for left ventricular thrombus) undergoing stent placement, ACCP suggests the use of warfarin (INR 2–3) and clopidogrel 75 mg daily in addition to aspirin therapy; the recommended duration of such triple antithrombotic therapy is dependent on whether the patient has a bare-metal or drug-eluting stent.

When aspirin is used to prevent reocclusion in adults undergoing coronary artery bypass grafting (CABG), ACCF/AHA recommends a dosage of 100–325 mg daily; aspirin should be initiated within 6 hours after surgery and continued for up to 1 year. For long-term therapy after 1 year, ACCP recommends aspirin 75–100 mg daily. There are some data suggesting that an aspirin dosage not exceeding 75–81 mg daily may be sufficient for long-term cardiovascular prevention and is associated with less GI bleeding risk.

Managing Antiplatelet Therapy in Patients Undergoing Invasive Procedures

Temporary interruption of long-term aspirin therapy generally is not necessary for patients undergoing surgery or other invasive procedures. In patients receiving dual antiplatelet therapy (e.g., with aspirin and clopidogrel) who require surgery within 6 weeks of bare-metal stent implantation or within 6 months of drug-eluting stent implantation, ACCP suggests continuation of dual antiplatelet therapy during the periprocedural period. In patients receiving dual antiplatelet therapy (e.g., with aspirin and clopidogrel) who require CABG, interruption of clopidogrel therapy is recommended 5 days prior to surgery; however, aspirin may be continued around the time of surgery in such patients. For additional information on the perioperative management of antithrombotic therapy, consult the most recent ACCP Evidence-based Clinical Practice Guidelines on Antithrombotic Therapy and Prevention of Thrombosis available at http://www.chestnet.org.

Embolism Associated with Atrial Fibrillation

When aspirin is used for the prevention of thromboembolism in patients with atrial fibrillation†, a dosage of 75–325 mg daily has been suggested.

Experts recommend that atrial flutter† generally be managed in the same manner as atrial fibrillation.

Valvular Heart Disease

Aspirin therapy at a dosage of 75–325 mg daily is recommended by ACC and AHA for selected patients with mitral valve prolapse† (i.e., symptomatic patients who experience a TIA or patients younger than 65 years of age with concurrent atrial fibrillation and no history of mitral valve regurgitation, hypertension, or heart failure).

Peripheral Arterial Disease

To reduce vascular morbidity and mortality in patients with asymptomatic peripheral arterial disease (*primary prevention*), ACCP suggests that aspirin be given a dosage of 75–100 mg daily.

For *secondary prevention* of cardiovascular events in patients with symptomatic peripheral arterial disease, ACCP recommends aspirin 75–100 mg daily. In patients with refractory intermittent claudication, ACCP suggests the use of cilostazol in addition to aspirin therapy.

Peripheral Artery Bypass Graft Surgery

To reduce graft occlusion in patients undergoing peripheral artery bypass graft surgery, aspirin 75–100 mg daily is recommended by ACCP; aspirin should be initiated preoperatively and continued long term. ACCP suggests the addition of clopidogrel 75 mg daily to aspirin therapy in patients undergoing below-the-knee prosthetic graft bypass surgery.

Prosthetic Heart Valves

In patients with a bioprosthetic heart valve† in the aortic position who are in sinus rhythm and who have no other indications for warfarin therapy, ACCP suggests aspirin 50–100 mg daily for initial (i.e., first 3 months after valve insertion) and long-term antithrombotic therapy. Aspirin 50–100 mg daily also may be used for long-term antithrombotic therapy after an initial 3 months of treatment with warfarin in patients with bioprosthetic heart valves in the mitral position. In all patients with a mechanical heart valve who are at low risk of bleeding, ACCP suggests the addition of low-dose aspirin (50–100 mg daily) to warfarin anticoagulation. Combination therapy with aspirin and warfarin also is recommended by ACC/AHA for patients with bioprosthetic heart valves with additional risk factors for thromboembolism.

In pregnant women with prosthetic heart valves who are at high risk for thromboembolism, aspirin (75–100 mg daily) may be added to therapy with a low molecular weight heparin or unfractionated heparin.

Thrombosis Associated with Heart Surgery in Children

Following the Fontan procedure† in children, aspirin in a dosage of 1–5 mg/kg daily is recommended by ACCP; the optimal duration of therapy in such patients is unknown.

Kawasaki Disease

For initial treatment of the acute phase of Kawasaki disease†, the American Academy of Pediatrics (AAP), AHA, and ACCP recommend that aspirin therapy be initiated as soon as possible (optimally within 7–10 days of illness) and given in a dosage of 80–100 mg/kg daily in 4 equally divided doses for up to 14 days; a single dose (2 g/kg) of immune globulin IV (IGIV) also should be administered as soon as possible (optimally within 7–10 days of illness). Although absorption of aspirin may be impaired or is highly variable during the initial phase of the illness, AAP states that it is not necessary to monitor aspirin concentrations in most patients.

After the patient has been afebrile for 48 hours or longer (usually about day 14 of illness), the aspirin dosage should be decreased to 1–5 mg/kg once daily to provide antiplatelet effects for prevention of coronary aneurysm, thrombosis, and subsequent infarction. In patients without coronary artery changes or with only transient coronary artery ectasia or dilatation (disappearing within the initial 6–8 weeks of illness), low-dose aspirin therapy usually is discontinued at 6–8 weeks. In those with coronary abnormalities, long-term low-dose aspirin therapy (with or without anticoagulants) may be indicated. (See Uses: Kawasaki Disease.)

Complications of Pregnancy

In women with antiphospholipid antibody (APLA) syndrome† and a history of multiple pregnancy losses (at least 3), ACCP recommends antepartum administration of aspirin (75–100 mg daily) plus prophylactic- or intermediate-dose subcutaneous unfractionated heparin or prophylactic-dose low molecular weight heparin.

In women at high risk for preeclampsia, including those with chronic primary or secondary hypertension or previous pregnancy-related hypertension, ACCP, AHA, and the American Stroke Association (ASA) recommend low-dose aspirin during pregnancy, starting from the second trimester.

PHARMACOLOGY

Aspirin exhibits analgesic, anti-inflammatory, and antipyretic activity. Although aspirin hydrolyzes to salicylate and acetate, the drug does not require hydrolysis to produce its effects and appears to have some pharmacologic effects that are distinct from those of salicylate. The ability of aspirin to acetylate proteins (e.g., platelet proteins, hormones, DNA, hemoglobin) results in some effects, such as inhibition of platelet aggregation, that other currently available salicylates do not exhibit.

Aspirin acetylates prostaglandin endoperoxide synthase (prostaglandin G/H-synthase) and irreversibly inhibits its cyclooxygenase (COX) activity. The enzyme catalyzes the conversion of arachidonic acid to PGH_2, the first committed step in prostanoid biosynthesis. Two isoforms of prostaglandin endoperoxide synthase exist, PGHS-1 and PGHS-2 (also referred to as COX-1 and COX-2, respectively). PGHS-1 (COX-1) is expressed constitutively in most cell types, including platelets. PGHS-2 (COX-2) is undetectable in most mammalian cells, but its expression can be induced rapidly in response to mitogenic and inflammatory stimuli. Aspirin is a relatively selective inhibitor of platelet PGHS-1 (cyclooxygenase-1, COX-1). The existence of 2 isoenzymes with different aspirin sensitivities, coupled with extremely different recovery rates of their cyclooxygenase (COX) activity following inactivation by aspirin, at least partially explains the different dosage requirements and durations of aspirin effects on platelet function versus the drug's analgesic and anti-inflammatory effects. Human platelets and vascular endothelial cells process PGH_2 to produce thromboxane A_2 and prostacyclin (epoprostenol, PGI_2), respectively. Thromboxane A_2 induces platelet aggregation and vasoconstriction, while prostacyclin inhibits platelet aggregation and induces vasodilation. Aspirin is antithrombotic in a wide range of doses inhibiting thromboxane A_2 and prostacyclin. (See Pharmacology: Antithrombotic Effects.)

● Analgesic, Anti-inflammatory, and Antipyretic Effects

While unhydrolyzed aspirin has been shown to be more potent than sodium salicylate in relieving pain in animals, it remains to be clearly established that aspirin has greater analgesic effect than salicylate in humans. A direct correlation between onset, intensity, or duration of analgesia and the time course of serum aspirin (or salicylate) concentrations or peak serum aspirin (or salicylate) concentrations also remains to be established. There are relatively few controlled comparative studies of aspirin and other salicylates (e.g., salicylate salts), but the analgesic, anti-inflammatory, and antipyretic effects of aspirin and other salicylates are generally considered to be comparable. However, in terms of antipyretic activity, aspirin is approximately 1.6 times as potent as sodium salicylate on an equimolar basis.

For further information on analgesic, anti-inflammatory, antipyretic, and other effects of aspirin, see Pharmacology in the Salicylates General Statement 28:08.04.24.

● *Hematologic Effects*

At usual dosages (e.g., 1.3–6 g daily), aspirin may rarely prolong the prothrombin time (usually only by 2–3 seconds) by inhibiting hepatic synthesis of blood coagulation factors VII, IX, and X.

Aspirin (but not other salicylates) inhibits platelet aggregation induced by epinephrine or low concentrations of collagen but not that induced by thrombin or high concentrations of collagen. Aspirin inhibits the second phase of platelet aggregation by preventing release of adenosine diphosphate (ADP) from platelets. The drug also prevents release of platelet factor 4 from platelets. Mean bleeding time may be prolonged by several minutes (approximately doubled) in healthy individuals and longer in children or in patients with bleeding disorders (e.g., hemophilia). In healthy individuals receiving a single 325-mg oral dose of aspirin, bleeding time may increase to a maximum within 12 hours and generally return to normal within 24 hours; any increase is usually of little clinical significance. Some clinicians have reported that mean bleeding time is progressively prolonged with increasing single doses of up to 1 g, but may be only slightly prolonged or unaffected by higher single doses; however, this has not been consistently found. The effect on bleeding time depends on the measurement method (e.g., Duke, Ivy, Mielke) used and technical variables (e.g., venostasis), and this may partially account for conflicting reports.

Like the analgesic and anti-inflammatory effects, the effects of aspirin on platelets appear to be mainly associated with inhibition of prostaglandin synthesis. Aspirin irreversibly acetylates and inactivates cyclooxygenase in circulating platelets and possibly in megakaryocytes. A single 325-mg oral dose of the drug results in about 90% inhibition of the enzyme in circulating platelets. This inactivation prevents platelet synthesis of prostaglandin endoperoxides and thromboxane A_2, compounds which induce platelet aggregation and constrict arterial smooth muscle. Since cyclooxygenase in platelets is not resynthesized, this effect of aspirin on platelet function persists for the life span of platelets (4–7 days). When approximately 20% of circulating platelets have not been exposed to aspirin (about 36 hours after the last dose), the hemostatic function of the platelet pool generally returns to normal; however, altered hemostasis has been reported to persist longer in some patients receiving long-term therapy.

● *Antithrombotic Effects*

Because of its ability to inhibit platelet aggregation via platelet cyclooxygenase inhibition, aspirin has been extensively investigated for potential therapeutic effects in the prevention of thrombosis (particularly arterial thrombosis). (See Uses: Thrombosis.) Aspirin has also been found to inactivate cyclooxygenase in venous endothelium and thereby inhibit venous synthesis of prostacyclin (epoprostenol, PGI_2). Since prostacyclin inhibits platelet aggregation and causes vasodilation, it appears to oppose the effects of thromboxane A_2 (and prostaglandin endoperoxides) on hemostasis. Therefore, it has been suggested that the relative extent to which the formation of these compounds is inhibited by aspirin might result in an increased or decreased likelihood of thrombosis. It has not been established whether interruption of prostacyclin formation is a sufficient stimulus to initiate the thrombotic process, but studies in mice deficient in the gene that encodes the prostacyclin receptor support the importance of this prostanoid in the prevention of arterial thrombosis. Although prostacyclin is synthesized by arterial endothelium and in vitro studies suggest that arterial cyclooxygenase is less sensitive to inhibition by aspirin than venous cyclooxygenase, the actual effects of aspirin on arterial synthesis of prostacyclin in healthy or diseased human arteries remain to be established.

In some clinical studies that evaluated the effect of aspirin in preventing thrombosis, the dosages of aspirin (900 mg to 1.5 g daily in divided doses) probably inhibited the synthesis of prostacyclin as well as that of thromboxane A_2.

Although concomitant inhibition of prostacyclin synthesis by aspirin may potentially decrease the antithrombotic efficacy of the drug, it is unlikely that this effect increases the risk of thrombosis since an increased risk has not been observed in these studies or in patients with rheumatoid arthritis receiving higher dosages of the drug. Cyclooxygenase in both platelets and venous endothelium has been found to be inhibited by single oral aspirin doses of 80–300 mg. However, at these doses, the duration of inhibition of thromboxane A_2 synthesis in platelets (about 48–96 hours) is longer than inhibition of prostacyclin synthesis in venous endothelium (about 24–48 hours), apparently because cyclooxygenase is resynthesized in venous endothelium but not in platelets. Since cyclooxygenase in platelets appears to be more sensitive to inactivation than cyclooxygenase in venous endothelium, it has been suggested that low dosages of aspirin might prevent thrombosis by selectively inhibiting prostaglandin endoperoxide and thromboxane A_2 synthesis. In addition, limited data indicate that modifying the absorption rate of aspirin to limit its systemic availability may result in such selective effects. Uncoated or film-coated, plain aspirin or buffered aspirin tablets or capsules have been used in most studies in which aspirin has been shown to prevent thrombosis, and limited data indicate that differences in the systemic availability of unhydrolyzed aspirin may be associated with different effects of the drug on thromboxane A_2 and prostacyclin synthesis, which might theoretically affect antithrombotic efficacy. In a comparative study in healthy men, administration of aspirin 75 mg daily as a controlled-release matrix formulation designed to release 10 mg of drug per hour produced essentially complete suppression of thromboxane A_2 formation (as determined by thromboxane B_2 concentrations) while having only modest effects on basal or bradykinin-stimulated prostacyclin synthesis. Suppression of thromboxane A_2 production and prolongation of template bleeding time in individuals receiving the controlled-release preparation daily for 28 days were comparable to those produced by immediate-release aspirin given as 162.5 mg daily or 325 mg every other day. Doses as low as 50–80 mg of enteric-coated aspirin have been shown to produce near-maximal inhibition of thromboxane A_2 synthesis, and some studies demonstrate that enteric-coated and controlled-release aspirin produce similar, although somewhat delayed, inhibition of cyclooxygenase activity and platelet aggregation compared with the same doses of plain or buffered aspirin. However, an optimum aspirin dose and administration schedule required to achieve these selective effects have not been clearly determined, and the actual clinical importance of such a selective inhibitory effect remains to be clearly established. In addition, salicylate appears to competitively inhibit the effect of aspirin on platelets; the relevance of this effect to the prevention of thrombosis is not known.

PHARMACOKINETICS

Since both unhydrolyzed aspirin and its metabolite, salicylate, are pharmacologically active, the pharmacokinetics of both compounds must be considered. For additional information on the distribution and elimination of *salicylate*, see Pharmacokinetics in the Salicylates General Statement 28:08.04.24.

● *Absorption*

Approximately 80–100% of an oral dose of aspirin is absorbed from the GI tract. However, the actual bioavailability of the drug as unhydrolyzed aspirin is lower since aspirin is partially hydrolyzed to salicylate in the GI mucosa during absorption and on first pass through the liver. There are relatively few studies of the bioavailability of unhydrolyzed aspirin. In one study in which aspirin was administered IV and as an oral aqueous solution, it was shown that the solution was completely absorbed but only about 70% reached the systemic circulation as unhydrolyzed aspirin. In another study in which aspirin was administered IV and orally as capsules, only about 50% of the oral dose reached the systemic circulation as unhydrolyzed aspirin. There is some evidence that the bioavailability of unhydrolyzed aspirin from slowly absorbed dosage forms (e.g., enteric-coated tablets) may be substantially decreased. Food does not appear to decrease the bioavailability of unhydrolyzed aspirin or salicylate; however, absorption is delayed and peak serum aspirin or salicylate concentration may be decreased. There is some evidence that absorption of salicylate following oral administration may be substantially impaired or is highly variable during the febrile phase of Kawasaki disease.

Most studies reported to date determined the bioavailability of aspirin preparations in terms of salicylate. Effervescent or noneffervescent oral aqueous solutions of aspirin appear to be completely absorbed. Oral buffered aspirin tablets, uncoated plain aspirin tablets, and methylcellulose film-coated (non-enteric) plain aspirin tablets are approximately 80–100% absorbed. Erratic and incomplete absorption of some enteric-coated aspirin tablets (particularly those with shellac coatings) has been reported, but recent studies indicate that the extent of absorption of currently available enteric-coated aspirin tablets is similar to that of buffered, uncoated plain, and film-coated plain aspirin tablets. Although well-designed studies are lacking, the extent of absorption of extended-release aspirin tablets appears to be similar to that of uncoated plain aspirin tablets. There are apparently no published studies on the bioavailability of aspirin capsules. Following rectal administration as a suppository, aspirin is slowly and variably absorbed; the extent of absorption increases with increasing rectal retention time. In general, 20–60% of the dose is absorbed if the suppository is retained for 2–4 hours and 70–100% is absorbed if the suppository is retained for at least 10 hours.

The rate of absorption of aspirin depends on the same factors that determine the rate of absorption of other salicylates and the relative rates of absorption from various oral aspirin dosage forms are generally the same as for oral dosage forms of other salicylates (e.g., aqueous solutions are the most rapidly absorbed). As with other salicylates, dissolution is usually the rate-limiting process in the absorption of tablets containing aspirin; however, the in vitro dissolution rate of a specific preparation does not necessarily reflect the in vivo absorption rate. According to the manufacturer, the in vitro dissolution of film-coated aspirin tablets does not differ from that of uncoated plain tablets; however, the film-coated tablet does not undergo dissolution in the mouth during administration.

● Buffered Aspirin

There has been controversy over the relative rates of absorption of buffered aspirin tablets and uncoated plain aspirin tablets and their relative potential for producing gastric irritation and analgesia.

The buffers contained in buffered aspirin tablets may increase the pH in the microenvironment of aspirin particles and thereby increase solubility of the drug in surrounding GI fluids; as a result, the dissolution rate of the tablets may be increased. However, it cannot be stated that *all* buffered aspirin tablets are dissolved and absorbed more rapidly than *all* uncoated plain aspirin tablets. The types and amounts of buffers affect dissolution rate, and claims for a specific preparation should be substantiated by appropriate data. Conflicting reports of the relative rates of absorption of buffered or uncoated plain aspirin tablets are most likely due to differences in the specific preparations studied. Some studies have shown that, like aqueous aspirin solutions, some buffered aspirin tablet preparations may be absorbed slightly more rapidly than some uncoated plain aspirin tablet preparations and may produce slightly higher peak serum salicylate concentrations; however, clinically important differences in the onset or intensity of analgesia produced by these dosage forms or specific preparations have not been established. Crossover studies directly comparing peak serum concentrations of unhydrolyzed aspirin attained with these dosage forms are lacking.

It has been suggested that buffered aspirin tablets cause less gastric irritation than uncoated plain aspirin tablets since the potentially more rapid dissolution of the former may reduce contact time between aspirin particles and gastric mucosa. However, several recent, well-designed studies indicate that buffered aspirin tablets do not cause less gastric irritation than uncoated plain aspirin tablets.

● Rapidly Absorbed Dosage Forms

Following oral administration of single doses of rapidly absorbed aspirin dosage forms, salicylate is detected in serum within 5–30 minutes, and peak serum salicylate concentrations are attained within 0.25–2 hours, depending on dosage form and specific formulation. Clinically important differences in the onset or intensity of analgesia produced by rapidly absorbed dosage forms or specific preparations have not been established.

Following oral administration of a single 650-mg dose of aspirin as an effervescent or noneffervescent aqueous solution in healthy adults, average peak plasma aspirin concentrations of about 13 mcg/mL are attained within 15–40 minutes and average peak plasma salicylate concentrations of about 40–55 mcg/mL are attained within 30–60 minutes. After a single 650-mg oral dose of aspirin (as two 325-mg uncoated plain tablets) in fasting healthy adults, average peak plasma aspirin concentrations of about 7–9 mcg/mL occur within 25–40 minutes and average peak plasma salicylate concentrations of about 35–50 mcg/mL

occur within 1.5–2 hours. Following oral administration of a single 650-mg dose of buffered aspirin (as 2 tablets, each containing 325 mg of aspirin), average peak plasma salicylate concentrations of about 40–60 mcg/mL are attained within 45–60 minutes.

In one study in healthy fasting adults given a single 975-mg oral dose of aspirin (as three 325-mg uncoated plain tablets), peak serum salicylate concentrations averaged 60–75 mcg/mL and occurred within 2 hours. In another study in fasting rheumatoid arthritis patients given a single 1.95-g oral dose of aspirin (as six 325-mg uncoated plain tablets), peak plasma aspirin concentrations of about 12–16 mcg/mL occurred within 1 hour and peak plasma salicylate concentrations of about 110–160 mcg/mL occurred within 4 hours. When these patients were given the same dose of buffered aspirin (as 6 tablets, each containing 325 mg of aspirin), peak plasma aspirin concentrations of about 14–18 mcg/mL occurred within 1–2 hours and peak plasma salicylate concentrations of about 140–160 mcg/mL occurred within 1–2 hours.

● Enteric-Coated Aspirin

There are few published studies reporting plasma aspirin or salicylate concentrations after single oral doses of enteric-coated aspirin tablets. In one crossover study, following single 975-mg oral doses (three 325-mg tablets) of 2 commercially available enteric-coated aspirin preparations in healthy adults, average peak serum salicylate concentrations of 48 mcg/mL occurred at 8 hours with one preparation, and average peak serum salicylate concentrations of 25 mcg/mL occurred at 14 hours with the other preparation. In one study in fasting rheumatoid arthritis patients given a single 1.92-g oral dose (as six 320-mg enteric-coated tablets), peak plasma aspirin concentrations of about 4–7 mcg/mL occurred within about 4 hours and average peak plasma salicylate concentrations of about 70 mcg/mL occurred within about 8 hours.

● Extended-Release Aspirin

There are few published studies reporting plasma aspirin or salicylate concentrations after single oral doses of extended-release aspirin tablets. Combining data from several small studies, some clinicians report that following a single 1.3-g oral dose of aspirin as two 650-mg extended-release tablets, an average peak serum aspirin concentration of about 3 mcg/mL was attained within 1 hour and peak serum salicylate concentrations of about 70–80 mcg/mL were attained within 4 hours; the serum aspirin concentration declined to less than 1 mcg/mL by 3 hours and the serum salicylate concentration was about 60 mcg/mL at 8 hours, 45 mcg/mL at 12 hours, and 25 mcg/mL at 16 hours. Following a single 1.6-g oral dose (as two 800-mg tablets) of one commercially available extended-release aspirin preparation in healthy adults in one crossover study, an average peak plasma aspirin concentration of about 1 mcg/mL was attained within 2 hours and average peak plasma salicylate concentrations of about 22 mcg/mL were attained within 8–12 hours; the plasma salicylate concentration declined to about 15 mcg/mL by 24 hours.

● Suppositories

In one study in children given a rectal dose of 150–300 mg of aspirin as a suppository, peak serum salicylate concentrations of 20–140 mcg/mL generally occurred within 3–4 hours.

● Distribution

Aspirin is rapidly and widely distributed, apparently into most body tissues and fluids. The volume of distribution of aspirin is approximately the same as that of salicylate and is generally 0.15–0.2 L/kg.

In one study in patients with rheumatic disease who received a single 650-mg oral dose of buffered aspirin, aspirin was detected in synovial fluid within 10–30 minutes and salicylate was detected in synovial fluid within 15–35 minutes. In this study, peak aspirin concentrations in synovial fluid occurred after an average of 1.3 hours and were about 75% of peak blood concentrations; peak salicylate concentrations in synovial fluid occurred after an average of 2.2 hours and were about 60% of peak blood concentrations.

Aspirin is poorly bound to plasma proteins; the unhydrolyzed drug is 33% bound at a serum salicylate concentration of 120 mcg/mL. However, aspirin acetylates serum albumin at the E-amino group of lysine; the acetylation may alter binding of other drugs (e.g., phenylbutazone) to the protein. Acetylation of serum albumin by aspirin is inhibited by salicylate.

● Elimination

The elimination half-life of aspirin in plasma is approximately 15–20 minutes. Unlike salicylate, unhydrolyzed aspirin does not undergo capacity-limited metabolism and does not accumulate in plasma following multiple doses.

Following oral administration, aspirin is partially hydrolyzed to salicylate during absorption by esterases in the GI mucosa. Following absorption, unhydrolyzed aspirin is rapidly and almost completely hydrolyzed by esterases principally in the liver but also in plasma, erythrocytes, and synovial fluid; hydrolysis occurs more slowly in synovial fluid apparently because the amounts of esterases in synovial fluid are lower. It has been reported that aspirin may be hydrolyzed more slowly in women because women apparently have lower amounts of plasma aspirin esterases.

Only about 1% of an oral dose of aspirin is excreted unhydrolyzed in urine. The remainder is excreted in urine as salicylate and its metabolites.

CHEMISTRY AND STABILITY

● Chemistry

Aspirin, the prototype of the salicylates, is a nonsteroidal anti-inflammatory agent (NSAIA). Aspirin is the salicylate ester of acetic acid. In vivo, the drug rapidly hydrolyzes to salicylate and acetate. Aspirin occurs as white crystals, which are usually tabular or needle-like, or as a white, crystalline powder. Aspirin is available in fixed combination with dipyridamole as a hard gelatin capsule containing dipyridamole as extended-release pellets and aspirin as an immediate-release tablet. The drug may have a faint odor, is slightly soluble in water and freely soluble in alcohol, and has a pK_a of 3.5. Each gram of aspirin contains approximately 760 mg of salicylate.

● Stability

Aspirin is stable in dry air. However, in moist air or in aqueous or hydroalcoholic solutions, the drug gradually hydrolyzes to salicylate and acetate and emits a strong vinegar-like odor; the rate of hydrolysis is increased by heat and is pH dependent.

In aqueous solutions, aspirin is most stable at a pH of 2–3, less stable at a pH of 4–8, and least stable at a pH less than 2 or exceeding 8. In a saturated aqueous solution at a pH of 5–7, aspirin is almost completely hydrolyzed within 1 week at 25°C. If a liquid dosage form of aspirin is desired for short-term treatment of pain, an oral solution may be prepared from commercially available buffered effervescent tablets (Alka-Seltzer®). Following dissolution of 1 Alka-Seltzer® tablet in approximately 90 mL of water, the solution has a pH of 6–7. In the resultant solution, aspirin is about 99% ionized and is at least 90% unhydrolyzed for approximately 10 hours at room temperature and about 90 hours at 5°C.

Chewable aspirin tablets containing 81 mg of the drug should be stored in child-resistant containers holding not more than 36 tablets each in order to limit the potential toxicity associated with accidental ingestion in children. Aspirin extra-strength (Anacin®) tablets should be stored at 20–25°C and protected from moisture. Aspirin (Bayer products, excluding Alka-Seltzer® products) tablets or caplets should be stored at room temperature; high humidity and excessive heat (40°C) should be avoided. Aspirin effervescent antacid and pain relief tablets (Alka-Seltzer® products) should be protected from excessive heat. Aspirin gum should be stored at 15–25°C and protected from excessive moisture. Aspirin suppositories should be stored at 2–15°C. The fixed-combination preparation of extended-release dipyridamole with aspirin should be stored at 25°C and protected from excessive moisture, but may be exposed to temperatures ranging from 15–30 degrees.

PREPARATIONS

Excipients in commercially available drug preparations may have clinically important effects in some individuals; consult specific product labeling for details.

Aspirin

Oral		
Pieces, chewing gum	227 mg	**Aspergum®**, Heritage, Schering Plough
Tablets	81 mg*	**Aspirin Tablets**
	325 mg*	**Aspirin Tablets**
		Norwich® Aspirin, Chattem
	500 mg*	**Aspirin Tablets**
		Norwich® Aspirin Maximum Strength, Chattem
	650 mg*	**Aspirin Tablets**
Tablets, chewable	81 mg*	**Aspirin Chewable Tablets**
		Bayer® Children's Chewable Aspirin, Bayer
		St. Joseph® Aspirin Adult Low Strength Chewable®, McNeil
Tablets, delayed-release (enteric-coated)	81 mg*	**Aspirin Delayed-release (Enteric-coated) Tablets**
		Bayer® Aspirin Regimen Adult Low Strength, Bayer
		Ecotrin® Adult Low Strength, GlaxoSmithKline
		Halfprin®, Kramer
		St. Joseph® Adult Low Strength Enteric Coated Tablets, McNeil
	162 mg	**Halfprin®**, Kramer
	325 mg*	**Aspirin Delayed-release (Enteric-coated) Tablets**
		Bayer® Aspirin Regimen Regular Strength Caplets®, Bayer
		Ecotrin® Regular Strength, GlaxoSmithKline
		Genacote®, Teva
	500 mg*	**Aspirin Delayed-release (Enteric-coated) Tablets**
		Ecotrin® Maximum Strength, GlaxoSmithKline
	650 mg*	**Aspirin Delayed-release (Enteric-coated) Tablets**
	975 mg	**Easprin®**, Harvest
Tablets, extended-release	800 mg	**ZORprin®**, Par
Tablets, film-coated	325 mg*	**Aspirin Film-coated Tablets**
		Bayer® Aspirin Caplets®, Bayer
		Genuine Bayer® Aspirin Tablets, Bayer
	500 mg	**Bayer® Aspirin Extra Strength Caplets®**, Bayer
		Bayer® Aspirin Extra Strength Gelcaplets®, Bayer
		Bayer® Aspirin Extra Strength Tablets, Bayer
Rectal		
Suppositories	60 mg*	**Aspirin Suppositories**,
	120 mg*	**Aspirin Suppositories**
	200 mg*	**Aspirin Suppositories**
	300 mg*	**Aspirin Suppositories**
	600 mg*	**Aspirin Suppositories**

* available from one or more manufacturer, distributor, and/or repackager by generic (nonproprietary) name

Aspirin with Buffers

Oral

Tablets	325 mg with buffers*	**Aspirin with Buffers Tablets**
Tablets, enteric-coated	81 mg with buffers*	**Aspirin with Buffers Enteric-coated Tablets**
	325 mg with buffers	**Ascriptin® Enteric Regular Strength**, Novartis
Tablets, film-coated		81 mg with buffers
		Bayer® Women's Aspirin Plus Calcium Caplets®, Bayer
	325 mg with buffers	**Ascriptin® Regular Strength**, Novartis
		Ascriptin® Arthritis Pain Caplets®, Novartis
		Bufferin® Tablets, Novartis Consumer Health
	500 mg with buffers	**Ascriptin® Maximum Strength Caplets®**, Novartis
		Bayer® Aspirin Plus Buffered Extra Strength Caplets®, Bayer
		Bufferin® Arthritis Strength Caplets®, Bristol-Myers
		Bufferin® Extra Strength, Novartis Consumer Health
Tablets, for solution	325 mg	**Alka-Seltzer® Effervescent Pain Reliever and Antacid**, Bayer
		Alka-Seltzer® Lemon-Lime Effervescent Pain Reliever and Antacid, Bayer
	500 mg	**Alka-Seltzer® Extra Strength Effervescent Pain Reliever and Antacid**, Bayer

*available from one or more manufacturer, distributor, and/or repackager by generic (nonproprietary) name

Acetaminophen and Aspirin

Oral

For solution	325 mg/packet Acetaminophen and Aspirin 500 mg/packet	**Goody's® Back & Body Pain Powder**, Prestige
Tablets, film-coated	250 mg Acetaminophen, Aspirin 250 mg, and buffer	**Excedrin® Back and Body Caplets**, Novartis

Acetaminophen, Aspirin, and Caffeine

Oral

Capsules, gel-coated	250 mg Acetaminophen, Aspirin 250 mg, and Caffeine 65 mg*	**Acetaminophen, Aspirin, and Caffeine Gelcaps**
		Excedrin® Menstrual Complete Gelcaps, Novartis
For solution	260 mg/packet Acetaminophen, Aspirin 520 mg/packet, and Caffeine 32.5 mg/packet	**Goody's® Extra Strength Headache Powder**, Prestige
	325 mg/packet Acetaminophen, Aspirin 500 mg/packet, and Caffeine 65 mg/packet	**Goody's® Cool Orange Extra Strength Powder**, Prestige
Tablets, film-coated	194 mg Acetaminophen, Aspirin 227 mg, Caffeine 33 mg, and buffers	**Vanquish® Caplets**, Moberg
	250 mg Acetaminophen, Aspirin 250 mg, and Caffeine 65 mg	**Excedrin® Extra Strength Caplets**, Novartis
		Excedrin® Migraine Caplets, Novartis
		Goody's® Extra Strength Caplets, Prestige
		Pamprin® Max, Chattem

*available from one or more manufacturer, distributor, and/or repackager by generic (nonproprietary) name

Oxycodone and Aspirin

Oral

Tablets	4.8355 mg Oxycodone Hydrochloride and Aspirin 325 mg*	**Endodan®** (C-II), Qualitest
		Oxycodone Hydrochloride and Aspirin Tablets (C-II)
		Percodan® (C-II; scored), Endo

*available from one or more manufacturer, distributor, and/or repackager by generic (nonproprietary) name

Other Aspirin Combinations

Oral

Capsules	325 mg with Butalbital 50 mg and Caffeine 40 mg*	**Butalbital, Aspirin, and Caffeine Capsules** (C-III)
		Fiorinal® (C-III), Actavis
	325 mg with Butalbital 50 mg, Caffeine 40 mg, and Codeine Phosphate 30 mg*	**Butalbital, Aspirin, Caffeine, and Codeine Phosphate Capsules** (C-III)
		Fiorinal® with Codeine (C-III), Actavis
	356.4 mg with Caffeine 30 mg and Dihydrocodeine Bitartrate 16 mg	**Synalgos®-DC** (C-III), Leitner
Capsules, extended-release core (dipyridamole only)	25 mg with Dipyridamole 200 mg	**Aggrenox®**, Boehringer Ingelheim
For solution	845 mg/packet with Caffeine 65 mg/packet	**BC® Powder**, Prestige
		Stanback® Powder, Prestige
	1000 mg/packet with Caffeine 65 mg/packet	**BC® Powder Arthritis Strength**, Prestige
Tablets	325 mg with Butalbital 50 mg and Caffeine 40 mg*	**Butalbital, Aspirin, and Caffeine Tablets** (C-III)
		Fortabs® (C-III), United Research
	325 mg with Carisoprodol 200 mg*	**Carisoprodol and Aspirin Tablets** (C-IV)
		Soma® Compound (C-IV), Meda
	325 mg with Carisoprodol 200 mg and Codeine Phosphate 16 mg*	**Carisoprodol, Aspirin, and Codeine Phosphate Tablets** (C-III)
		Soma® Compound with Codeine (C-III), Meda
	325 mg with Meprobamate 200 mg	**Equagesic®** (C-IV; scored), Leitner
		Micrainin® (C-IV), Wallace
	385 mg with Caffeine 30 mg and Orphenadrine Citrate 25 mg*	**Norgesic®**, 3M
		Orphenadrine Citrate, Aspirin, and Caffeine Tablets,
	400 mg with Caffeine 32 mg	**P-A-C® Analgesic**, Lee
	770 mg with Caffeine 60 mg and Orphenadrine Citrate 50 mg*	**Norgesic® Forte** (scored), 3M
		Orphenadrine Citrate, Aspirin, and Caffeine Tablets
Tablets, film-coated	400 mg with Caffeine 32 mg	**Anacin® Caplets®**, Wyeth
		Anacin® Tablets, Wyeth
	421 mg with Caffeine 32 mg and buffers	**Cope®**, Lee
	500 mg with Caffeine 32 mg	**Anacin® Maximum Strength**, Wyeth
	500 mg with Caffeine 32.5 mg	**Extra Strength Bayer® Back and Body Pain**, Bayer
Tablets, for solution	500 mg with Caffeine 65 mg	**Alka Seltzer® Morning Relief**, Bayer

*available from one or more manufacturer, distributor, and/or repackager by generic (nonproprietary) name

† Use is not currently included in the labeling approved by the US Food and Drug Administration.

Selected Revisions September 10, 2024, © Copyright, January 1, 1983, American Society of Health-System Pharmacists, Inc.

Opioid Agonists General Statement

28:08.08 · OPIOID AGONISTS

■ Opiate agonists encompass a group of naturally occurring, semisynthetic, and synthetic drugs that stimulate opiate receptors and effectively relieve pain without producing loss of consciousness.

USES

● Pain

Opiate agonists are generally used to provide temporary analgesia in the symptomatic treatment of moderate to severe pain such as that associated with acute and some chronic medical disorders including renal or biliary colic, myocardial infarction (MI), acute trauma, postoperative pain, and terminal cancer. Opiate analgesics increasingly have been used for the management of chronic noncancer pain despite uncertainty over the long-term benefits of such therapy. The drugs may also be used to provide analgesia during diagnostic and orthopedic procedures and during labor. In patients with acute pulmonary edema, opiate agonists are used for their cardiovascular effects and to relieve anxiety associated with this condition. The drugs are also used to provide preoperative sedation and as a supplement to anesthesia. Although most of the opiate agonists produce similar analgesia in equianalgesic doses, such factors as oral effectiveness, duration of action, other CNS effects such as euphoria or sedation, degree of action on smooth muscle, and individual variation in patient response should be considered in the selection of a specific opiate agonist.

Some opiates have been used in the treatment of pain in various combinations with nonsteroidal anti-inflammatory agents (NSAIAs), acetaminophen, and/or caffeine. Opiates (e.g., codeine, oxycodone, hydrocodone) given orally in combination with acetaminophen or NSAIAs may produce a greater analgesic effect than that produced by either drug used individually. There also is some evidence that acetaminophen or NSAIAs in combination with oral doses of an opiate may cause fewer adverse effects than equianalgesic doses of the individual drugs alone.

Various extended-release and long-acting opiate analgesics are used for the management of pain that is severe enough to require long-term, daily, around-the-clock use of an opiate analgesic. Because of the risks of addiction, abuse, and misuse associated with opiates, even at recommended doses, and because of the greater risks of overdose and death with extended-release and long-acting opiate formulations, these extended-release and long-acting opiate analgesics should be reserved for use in patients for whom alternative treatment options (e.g., nonopiate analgesics or immediate-release opiates) are inadequate or not tolerated. These preparations are not indicated for use on an as-needed ("prn") basis. Some extended-release or long-acting preparations or dosage strengths should be used only in opiate-tolerant patients (see the individual monographs in 28:08.08). Patients are considered opiate tolerant if they have been receiving opiate therapy consisting of at least 60 mg of morphine sulfate daily, 25 mcg of transdermal fentanyl per hour, 30 mg of oral oxycodone daily, 8 mg of oral hydromorphone hydrochloride daily, 25 mg of oxymorphone hydrochloride daily, or an equianalgesic dosage of another opiate daily for at least 1 week.

Because of the risks associated with opiate overdosage, clinicians should routinely discuss the availability of the opiate antagonist naloxone with all patients receiving new or reauthorized prescriptions for opiate analgesics. Clinicians should consider prescribing naloxone for patients receiving opiate analgesics who are at increased risk of opiate overdosage or who have household members, including children, or other close contacts who are at risk for accidental ingestion or overdosage. (See Cautions: Precautions and Contraindications.)

Chronic Pain

Chronic Noncancer Pain

In patients with chronic pain (generally defined as pain lasting longer than 3 months or past the time of normal tissue healing) that is not associated with active cancer treatment, palliative care, or end-of-life care (also referred to as chronic noncancer pain), opiate analgesics generally should be used only if other appropriate pain management strategies (nonpharmacologic and nonopiate pharmacologic therapies) have been ineffective and the expected benefits of opiate analgesics for both pain relief and functional improvement are anticipated to outweigh the risks. If opiate analgesics are used, they should be part of an integrated approach that also includes appropriate nonpharmacologic modalities (e.g., cognitive-behavioral therapy, relaxation techniques, biofeedback, functional restoration, exercise therapy, certain interventional procedures) and other appropriate pharmacologic therapies (e.g., nonopiate analgesics, analgesic adjuncts such as selected anticonvulsants and antidepressants for certain neuropathic pain conditions).

Use of opiate analgesics for the management of chronic noncancer pain has increased despite uncertainty over the long-term benefits of such therapy. Clinical trials of opiate analgesics in the symptomatic treatment of chronic pain generally have been of short duration, and available evidence is insufficient to determine whether long-term opiate therapy results in sustained pain relief or improvements in function and quality of life. In addition, evidence that opiate analgesics are superior to other pharmacologic or nonpharmacologic treatments for chronic pain generally is lacking. However, use of opiate analgesics is associated with serious risks (e.g., opiate use disorder, overdose). Prior to initiation of opiate therapy for chronic noncancer pain, patients should undergo thorough evaluation, including assessment of risk factors for misuse, abuse, and addiction. Clinicians should establish treatment goals with all patients, including realistic goals for pain and function, and should consider how therapy will be discontinued if benefits do not outweigh risks. Initial opiate therapy for chronic noncancer pain should be regarded as a therapeutic trial that will be continued only if there are clinically meaningful improvements in pain and function that outweigh the risks of therapy. Prior to and periodically during therapy, clinicians should discuss with patients known risks and realistic benefits of such therapy and patient and clinician responsibilities for managing therapy.

Although specific recommendations for the management of opiate therapy for chronic noncancer pain vary across clinical practice guidelines, common elements include risk mitigation strategies, upper dosage thresholds, careful dosage titration, and consideration of risks associated with particular opiates and formulations, coexisting diseases, and concomitant drug therapy.

Some experts recommend that opiate therapy for chronic noncancer pain be initiated with conventional (immediate-release) opiate analgesics prescribed at the lowest effective dosage. Opiate selection, initial dosage, and dosage titration should be individualized according to the patient's health status, prior opiate use, attainment of therapeutic goals, and predicted or observed harms. Experts generally agree that methadone should be prescribed for the management of chronic pain only by clinicians who are knowledgeable about its risks (e.g., QT-interval prolongation) and pharmacokinetic properties, and should not be the first choice for an extended-release or long-acting opiate analgesic. Similarly, fentanyl transdermal system should be prescribed only by clinicians who are familiar with the absorption characteristics and dosing of this formulation.

Benefits and harms of opiate analgesic therapy should be evaluated within 1–4 weeks following initiation of therapy or an increase in dosage and reevaluated on an ongoing basis (e.g., at least every 3 months) throughout therapy. Monitoring should include documentation of pain intensity and level of functioning, assessment of progress toward therapeutic goals, presence of adverse effects, and adherence to prescribed therapies. Common opiate-related adverse effects (e.g., constipation, nausea and vomiting, cognitive and psychomotor impairment) should be anticipated and appropriately managed. If benefits do not outweigh harms, other therapies should be optimized and opiate therapy should be tapered to a lower dosage or tapered and discontinued.

When repeated increases in dosage are required, potential causes should be evaluated and the relative benefits and risks reassessed. Although evidence is limited, some experts state that a trial of opiate rotation may be considered in patients experiencing intolerable adverse effects or inadequate benefit despite increases in dosage. Although the dosage level that constitutes high-dose therapy varies across clinical practice guidelines, there is agreement that use of higher dosages requires particular caution, including more frequent and intensive monitoring or referral to a specialist. (See Dosage and Administration: Dosage.) Greater benefits of high-dose opiate therapy for chronic pain have not been established in controlled clinical studies, and higher dosages have been associated with increased risks of motor vehicle accidents, overdosage, and opiate use disorder.

Various strategies for managing risks associated with opiate therapy for chronic noncancer pain have been recommended, including written treatment agreements or plans (e.g., "contracts"), urine drug testing, review of state prescription drug monitoring program (PDMP) data, and risk assessment and monitoring tools. Although precise recommendations may vary, recent clinical practice guidelines generally recommend such monitoring in all patients receiving opiate therapy for chronic noncancer pain, although the frequency and intensity of monitoring may vary depending on risk assessments. Urine drug testing may be used at baseline and periodically during therapy to assess adherence to the treatment plan and to screen for use of other prescription or illicit drugs. Baseline and periodic review of the patient's history of controlled substance prescriptions using state PDMP data also may assist in reducing prescription drug abuse and in identifying opiate dosages or drug combinations (e.g., benzodiazepines) that increase the risk for overdosage. (See Drug Interactions: Benzodiazepines and Other CNS Depressants.) Opiate therapy should be tapered and discontinued in patients who engage in serious or repeated aberrant drug-related behaviors or drug abuse or diversion. Clinicians should offer or arrange treatment for patients with opiate use disorder.

Chronic Cancer Pain

In the management of severe, chronic pain associated with a terminal illness such as cancer, the principal goal of analgesic therapy is to make the patient relatively pain-free while maintaining as good a quality of life as possible. Analgesic therapy must be individualized and titrated according to patient response and tolerance. When nonopiate or combinations of nonopiate and opiate analgesics are ineffective, oral administration of an opiate agonist on a regular schedule generally will provide adequate relief of severe, chronic pain and the fear of its recurrence. Extended-release and long-acting preparations are used orally for the management of such pain when it is severe enough to require long-term, daily, around-the-clock use of an opiate analgesic and when alternative treatment options (e.g., nonopiate analgesics or immediate-release opiates) are inadequate or not tolerated. Although consideration of the dependence potential of opiate agonists has often limited their effective use by many clinicians in terminally ill patients with severe, chronic pain, such consideration is irrelevant in the context of terminal illness. When oral opiate agonists no longer provide adequate relief or in patients unable to swallow or tolerate oral drugs, alternative methods of administration such as subcutaneous, rectal, continuous IV infusion, patient-controlled IV infusion, epidural, intrathecal, or transdermal systems should be considered.

Acute Pain

In the symptomatic treatment of acute pain, opiate analgesics generally should be reserved for pain resulting from severe injuries or medical conditions, surgical procedures, or when nonopiate alternatives for relieving pain and restoring function are expected to be ineffective or are contraindicated. Concomitant use of other appropriate therapies should be optimized. Because long-term opiate use often begins with the treatment of acute pain, conventional (immediate-release) opiates should be used in the smallest effective dosage and for the shortest possible duration when opiate analgesia is required for symptomatic treatment of acute pain. When sufficient for pain management, lower-potency opiate analgesics given in conjunction with acetaminophen or an NSAIA on an as-needed ("prn") basis have been recommended. The prescribed quantity of opiate analgesics should be limited to the amount needed for the expected duration of pain severe enough to require opiate analgesia, generally 3 days or less, and rarely more than 7 days, for acute pain not related to trauma or surgery. Clinicians should not prescribe larger quantities of opiate analgesics for use in the event that pain continues longer than expected; instead, patients should be reevaluated if severe acute pain does not remit.

When opiate analgesics are used to alleviate moderate to severe postoperative pain, opiate therapy should be provided as part of a multimodal regimen that also includes acetaminophen and/or NSAIAs and other pharmacologic

(e.g., certain anticonvulsants, regional local anesthetic techniques) and non-pharmacologic therapy as appropriate. In the management of postoperative pain, scheduled administration of nonopiate analgesics is recommended to reduce use of opiate analgesics and provide more-consistent analgesia. Oral administration of conventional opiate analgesics generally is preferred over IV administration in patients who can tolerate oral therapy. Scheduled (around-the-clock) dosing of opiate analgesics frequently is required during the immediate postoperative period or following major surgery. When repeated parenteral administration is required, IV patient-controlled analgesia (PCA) generally is recommended. Routine use of continuous (basal) IV infusions of opiates in opiate-naive patients receiving PCA is not recommended. IM administration of opiate analgesics is discouraged because IM injections can cause pain and are associated with unreliable absorption, resulting in inconsistent postoperative analgesia.

Pain that will likely be of short duration, such as that associated with diagnostic procedures or orthopedic manipulation, should be controlled with a short-acting opiate agonist such as fentanyl. Severe but intermittent pain such as may occur in patients with renal colic should also be treated with an opiate agonist providing short-duration analgesia. In bronchoscopy, a drug with good antitussive activity such as morphine may be preferred. Opiate agonists have been used in the treatment of pain of biliary or pancreatic origin. Although it may seem illogical to treat pain of biliary origin with drugs that increase biliary pressure and spasm, these biliary effects do not always occur with therapeutic doses and sedation produced by opiate agonists may contribute to relief of pain.

When administered during labor, opiate agonists should effectively relieve pain without interfering with the progress of labor or normal respiration in the neonate. The closer to delivery the drug is given, the greater the possibility of respiratory depression in the neonate.

Acute Coronary Syndromes

Opiate agonists, principally morphine, are used to relieve pain and anxiety associated with acute coronary syndromes (ACS). Although morphine usually is considered the drug of choice in relieving pain associated with MI, other strong opiate agonists such as meperidine, hydromorphone, and levorphanol tartrate also have been used.

Because of its ability to alleviate the work of breathing, reduce anxiety, and favorably affect ventricular loading conditions, morphine is considered the analgesic agent of choice in patients with ST-segment-elevation MI (STEMI). In addition to its potent analgesic and anxiolytic effects, morphine also exhibits favorable hemodynamic effects by causing venodilation and modest reductions in heart rate and systolic blood pressure. These properties also may be beneficial in patients with non-ST-segment-elevation ACS (NSTE ACS; unstable angina or non-ST-segment-elevation MI [NSTEMI]); although randomized controlled studies specifically evaluating the use of morphine in patients with NSTE ACS have not been conducted, experts state that it may be reasonable to administer IV morphine in such patients who have continued pain despite treatment with maximally tolerated anti-ischemic drugs (e.g., nitrates). However, use of morphine should not preclude the use of other anti-ischemic drugs with proven benefit. Patients with acute MI typically exhibit overactivity of the sympathetic nervous system, which adversely increases myocardial oxygen demand via acceleration of heart rate, elevation in arterial blood pressure, augmentation of cardiac contractility, and heightened tendency to develop ventricular tachyarrhythmias. This increased sympathetic activity results from combined ischemic-type chest discomfort and anxiety, and the principal objective of therapy is to administer sufficient doses of an analgesic such as morphine to relieve what many patients describe as a feeling of impending doom. The dose of morphine sulfate needed to achieve adequate pain control is dependent upon several factors such as patient age (e.g., lower doses are recommended in geriatric patients), body size, blood pressure, and heart rate. In patients with STEMI, an initial morphine sulfate dose of 4–8 mg IV is recommended, with additional doses of 2–8 mg administered every 5–15 minutes as needed. In patients with NSTE ACS, experts state that a morphine sulfate dose of 1–5 mg IV may be administered during IV nitroglycerin therapy and repeated every 5–30 minutes to relieve symptoms and maintain patient comfort.

Pain in Critically Ill Patients

Opiate agonists may be used in combination with sedative agents to maintain an optimal level of comfort and safety in patients in a critical care setting. Some clinicians state that pain assessment and subsequent documentation using standard assessment tools (e.g., numeric rating scale) should be performed regularly to monitor the patient's response to analgesic therapy. If patients are unable to communicate, their pain should be assessed by subjective observations of pain-related behaviors (e.g., movement, facial expression, posturing) and physiologic indicators (e.g., heart rate, blood pressure, respiratory rate). To ensure consistent analgesic therapy, a therapeutic plan and goal of analgesia should be established for each patient and communicated to all caregivers. Analgesics, including opiate agonists, should be administered on a continuous or scheduled intermittent basis, with supplemental doses given as required. If IV administration is required, some clinicians state that fentanyl, hydromorphone, or morphine are the recommended agents. In addition, fentanyl is recommended for use in acutely distressed patients because of its rapid onset of analgesia, and morphine or hydromorphone is preferred for intermittent therapy because of their longer duration of action. Fentanyl or hydromorphone also is recommended for use in critically ill patients who have hemodynamic instability or renal insufficiency. The potential for withdrawal symptoms should be considered in patients receiving high dosages of opiate agonists or longer than 7 days of continuous opiate agonist therapy and the dosage should be tapered systematically to prevent manifestations of opiate withdrawal.

Vascular Headaches

Opiate agonists are not recommended for routine use in the management of acute migraine attacks because evidence of superiority over other standard therapies (e.g., serotonin type 1 [5-HT$_1$] receptor agonists [triptans], NSAIAs) generally is lacking and because of the risk of medication overuse headache with frequent use, risk of dependence and abuse, and potential for opiate withdrawal syndrome following drug discontinuance. Some clinicians state that infrequent use of a short-acting opiate or fixed-combination preparation (e.g., acetaminophen and tramadol, codeine-containing fixed combinations) may be considered for abortive therapy of moderate to severe acute migraine attacks when standard therapies are ineffective or not tolerated or as rescue therapy when the patient's usual therapy fails. For further information on management and classification of migraine headache, see Vascular Headaches: General Principles in Migraine Therapy, under Uses in Sumatriptan 28:32.28.

• Delirium

The American Psychiatric Association (APA) states that opiate agonists, including morphine, may be used in the palliative management of delirium which may have been aggravated by pain. However, some opiate agonists (e.g., fentanyl, meperidine) can exacerbate delirium, because their metabolites may exhibit anticholinergic activity. For information on the management of delirium, see Uses: Delirium, in Haloperidol 28:16.08.08.

• Acute Pulmonary Edema

Morphine and other strong opiate agonists including meperidine, oxymorphone, and hydromorphone have been used to relieve anxiety in patients with dyspnea associated with acute pulmonary edema and acute left ventricular failure. These drugs should *not* be used in the treatment of pulmonary edema resulting from a chemical respiratory irritant. Opiate agonists cause pooling of blood in the extremities by decreasing peripheral resistance. This effect results in decreases in venous return, cardiac work, and pulmonary venous pressure, and blood is shifted from the central to peripheral circulation.

• Preoperative Sedation

Routine use of opiate agonists for preoperative sedation in patients without pain is not recommended. Preoperative use of opiate agonists may cause serious complications, usually involving the respiratory or circulatory systems, during surgery and increases the incidence of adverse effects after surgery. The usefulness of mixtures of opiate agonists and antagonists in preanesthetic medication, during surgery, or postoperatively to prevent respiratory depression has not been confirmed by well-controlled clinical studies.

• Cough

Some opiate agonists, notably codeine and its derivative hydrocodone, are used as cough suppressants. For a discussion of opiate agonists as antitussive agents, see Codeine 48:08 and Hydrocodone 48:08. Diphenoxylate and opium preparations are used mainly as antidiarrheal agents (see 56:08).

• Detoxification and Maintenance of Opiate Dependence

Methadone is used in detoxification treatment as an oral substitute for heroin or other morphine-like drugs to suppress the opiate-agonist abstinence syndrome in patients who are dependent on these drugs. If more prolonged suppressive therapy is necessary, methadone or buprenorphine hydrochloride can be used as oral substitutes for maintenance treatment of opiate dependence (opiate use disorder [OUD]). Levomethadyl acetate also has been used for the management of opiate dependence but is no longer commercially available in the US because of potentially severe adverse cardiac effects. (See Chronic Toxicity, see Cautions: Precautions and Contraindications, and also see Methadone Hydrochloride 28:08.08 and Buprenorphine Hydrochloride 28:02.12.)

• Neonatal Opiate Withdrawal

Opiate agonists, including morphine and methadone, have been used to manage manifestations of opiate abstinence syndrome (i.e., postnatal withdrawal) in neonates† exposed to opiates in utero. Opiates are recommended as first-line pharmacologic therapy when environmental and supportive measures (e.g., minimization of external stimuli, maximization of mother-infant contact [e.g., parental "rooming in"], breast-feeding when not contraindicated, swaddling and gentle handling) are inadequate. Other adjunctive therapy (e.g., clonidine, phenobarbital) may be added if the response to opiates is inadequate, or phenobarbital may be added if the neonate was exposed to additional substances in utero. Approximately 60–80% of neonates with opiate abstinence syndrome may require pharmacologic treatment for withdrawal symptoms. While morphine has been used more extensively than other opiates in the management of neonatal opiate abstinence syndrome, some studies suggest that use of methadone or buprenorphine (an opiate partial agonist) may be associated with shorter treatment durations and hospital stays compared with morphine use. However, additional study is needed to establish optimal dosage schedules and preferred opiate drugs and to evaluate longer-term (e.g., neurodevelopmental) outcomes.

Use of standardized protocols for identification, evaluation, and treatment of neonatal opiate abstinence syndrome is recommended since use of such protocols has been shown to improve overall response, including shorter hospital stays and durations of pharmacologic treatment. Some evidence suggests that use of a standardized protocol may be more important than use of a specific opiate agonist (e.g., methadone versus morphine) in improving outcomes. Protocols generally utilize assessment tools that were developed to quantify severity of withdrawal in term neonates to facilitate decisions regarding initiation, titration, and tapering of therapy. (See Oral Dosage for Neonatal Opiate Withdrawal under Dosage and Administration: Dosage, in Morphine Sulfate 28:08.08 and also see Neonatal Opiate Withdrawal under Dosage and Administration: Dosage, in Methadone Hydrochloride 28:08.08.)

DOSAGE AND ADMINISTRATION

• Administration

Opiate agonists may be administered orally, rectally, IM, subcutaneously, or IV. The parenteral route is usually used for relief of severe pain, and for relief of surgical or postoperative pain and pain during labor. IV administration is used to relieve acute, unbearable pain, and as a supplement to anesthesia. The drugs should also be administered IV in patients with shock or hypothermia in whom absorption is likely to be delayed following subcutaneous or IM injection. If opiate agonists are administered IV, usual dosage should generally be reduced and the solution should be injected slowly. An opiate antagonist and facilities for administration of oxygen and control of respiration should be immediately available during and immediately following IV administration of opiate agonists. A preservative-free preparation of morphine sulfate may also be administered epidurally or intrathecally. Morphine sulfate extended-release liposomal injection is administered epidurally. Fentanyl also may be administered percutaneously (by topical application of a transdermal system or iontophoretic transdermal system) or transmucosally (intrabuccally, sublingually, intranasally).

When therapy with an extended-release or long-acting opiate formulation is initiated, all other around-the-clock opiate analgesics should be discontinued.

Oral extended-release tablets or capsules should be swallowed whole, one at a time, with enough water to ensure complete swallowing of the tablet or capsule immediately after it is placed in the mouth; crushing, chewing, or dissolving the capsules or tablets will result in uncontrolled delivery of the opiate agonist and can result in overdosage and death.

● Dosage

Current principles of pain management indicate that opiate analgesics should be used in conjunction with appropriate nonopiate pharmacologic therapy and/or nonpharmacologic modalities in the symptomatic treatment of both acute and chronic pain. Because of the potential harms associated with opiate therapy, care is required to prevent inappropriate transition from short-term therapy for acute pain to chronic opiate therapy when other treatment modalities may be more appropriate. The lowest effective dosage and shortest duration of therapy consistent with treatment goals of the patient should be employed. Dosage of opiate agonists must be carefully adjusted according to the severity of pain and the response of the patient. Standard pain assessment tools adjusted to the patient's age and cognitive development may be employed to help the patient communicate pain intensity and to guide treatment. During long-term therapy of chronic noncancer pain, both pain intensity and functional status should be assessed regularly using validated tools, and progress toward therapeutic goals, adherence to the treatment plan, and presence of adverse effects should be monitored; when opiate therapy fails to provide clinically meaningful improvements in pain and functional status or when the risks of such therapy outweigh the benefits, other treatment approaches should be optimized and opiate analgesic therapy should be tapered and discontinued. Reduced dosage is indicated in poor-risk patients, in patients with substantial hepatic impairment, in patients with renal impairment, and in very young or very old patients. If concomitant therapy with other CNS depressants is required, the lowest effective dosages and shortest possible duration of concomitant therapy should be used. (See Drug Interactions: Benzodiazepines and Other CNS Depressants.) Following parenteral administration, adverse effects such as nausea, vomiting, dizziness, and hypotension may be alleviated by maintaining the patient in a supine position and elevating his legs. In surgical patients, dosage of opiate agonists should be based on response of the patient, premedication or concomitant medication, the anesthetics which are being used, and the nature and duration of the operation.

The following doses administered orally or IM provide analgesia comparable to that produced by 30 mg of oral morphine sulfate or 10 mg of IM morphine sulfate:

TABLE 1. Comparative Opiate Agonist Dosage with Oral or Parenteral Administration

Opiate Agonist	Equianalgesic Dose (in mg)[a]	
	Oral	IM[b]
Morphine	30	10
Hydrocodone	30	–
Hydromorphone	7.5	1.5
Oxycodone	20	–
Methadone	20 (acute)	10 (acute)
Levorphanol	4 (acute)	2 (acute)
	1 (chronic)	1 (chronic)
Fentanyl	–	0.1
Oxymorphone	10	1
Meperidine	300	75

[a] For specific dosages for these opiate agonists, see the individual monographs in 28:08.08.

[b] These are standard IM doses for acute pain in adults and also can be used to convert doses for IV infusions and repeated small IV doses ("boluses"). For single IV doses ("boluses"), use half the IM dose.

These equivalencies were based principally on single-dose studies comparing oral and IM doses of these drugs in cancer patients and patients with postoperative pain. When such comparisons are used to convert patients already receiving opiate therapy to therapy using a different opiate agonist or a different administration route, the equianalgesic dosage estimate should be adjusted based on consideration of the clinical situation (e.g., response to the previous regimen, adverse effects) and characteristics of the specific drugs involved (e.g., elimination half-life). In patients receiving chronic opiate therapy, the calculated equianalgesic dosage of the new opiate agonist generally should be reduced by about 25–50% in order to avoid inadvertent overdosage. Equivalencies based on single-dose studies may overestimate dosage requirements for methadone during chronic therapy; such comparisons should not be used to convert patients already receiving chronic opiate therapy to therapy with methadone. For further information about transferring patients from another opiate agonist to therapy with methadone, see Dosage and Administration in Methadone Hydrochloride 28:08.08.

Orally administered oxycodone in a dose of 4.88 mg produces analgesia comparable to 30 mg of oral codeine. Orally administered oxycodone also has been described as being 7–9.5 times as potent as oral codeine. Oxycodone hydrochloride extended-release tablets are reported to be 1.5–2 times as potent as morphine sulfate extended-release tablets (MS Contin®).

When repeated increases in dosage are required, potential causes should be evaluated and the relative benefits and risks reassessed. Use of higher dosages requires particular caution, including more frequent and intensive monitoring or consultation with or referral to a pain management specialist. (See Chronic Noncancer Pain under Pain: Chronic Pain, in Uses.) The US Centers for Disease Control and Prevention (CDC) guideline for primary care clinicians who prescribe opiates for chronic noncancer pain states that clinicians should carefully reassess individual benefits and risks before prescribing dosages equivalent to 50 mg or more of morphine sulfate daily and should avoid dosages equivalent to 90 mg or more of morphine sulfate daily or carefully justify their decision to titrate dosage to such levels. Other experts have stated that a pain management specialist should be consulted before exceeding an opiate dosage equivalent to 80–120 mg of morphine sulfate daily. In contrast, guidelines developed several years earlier tended to suggest higher dosage thresholds (e.g., equivalent to 200 mg or more of morphine sulfate daily) for more frequent and intensive monitoring or consultation or referral. Clinicians should be aware that some states have established dosage thresholds for opiate prescribing (e.g., maximum daily dosages that can be prescribed, dosage thresholds at which consultation with a specialist is mandated or recommended) or have mandated certain risk-management strategies (e.g., review of state prescription drug monitoring program [PDMP] data prior to prescribing).

Extended-release and Long-acting Formulations for the Management of Chronic Pain

Appropriate dosage selection and titration are essential to reduce the risk of respiratory depression associated with use of extended-release or long-acting formulations of opiate analgesics. The initial dosage must be individualized, taking into account the patient's prior analgesic use and risk factors for addiction, abuse, and misuse. Patients should be monitored closely for respiratory depression, especially during the first 24–72 hours of therapy and following any increase in dosage. Use of higher than recommended initial dosages in patients who are not opiate tolerant may result in fatal respiratory depression. Some extended-release or long-acting preparations or dosage strengths should be used only in opiate-tolerant patients. In patients who are being transferred from other oral opiates to therapy with an extended-release or long-acting opiate analgesic, all other around-the-clock opiate analgesics should be discontinued when therapy with the extended-release or long-acting formulation is initiated. Dosage must be carefully individualized since overestimation of the initial dosage in opiate-tolerant patients can result in fatal overdosage with the first dose. Because there is substantial interpatient variability in the relative potency of opiate analgesics and formulations, it is preferable to underestimate the patient's 24-hour opiate requirements and provide "rescue" therapy with an immediate-release opiate analgesic than to overestimate the requirements and manage an adverse reaction. For recommended initial dosages and titration schedules, see the individual monographs in 28:08.08.

Extended-release and long-acting formulations should be prescribed only by clinicians who are knowledgeable in the use of potent opiates for the management of chronic pain. Following transfer from other opiate analgesics to an extended-release or long-acting opiate analgesic, patients should be monitored for manifestations of opiate withdrawal and for oversedation or toxicity. Particularly close monitoring is required when patients are switched from methadone, since conversion ratios between methadone and other opiate analgesics vary widely depending on extent of prior methadone exposure and because methadone has a long half-life and tends to accumulate in plasma. Dosage of the extended-release or long-acting opiate agonist should be titrated to a level that provides adequate analgesia with minimal adverse effects. Patients should be reevaluated continually for adequacy of pain control and for adverse effects, as well as for the development of addiction, abuse, or misuse. Patients who experience breakthrough pain may require an increase in dosage of the extended-release or long-acting opiate agonist or "rescue" therapy with an appropriate dose of an immediate-release analgesic. If the pain intensity increases after dosage stabilization, an attempt should be made to identify the source of increased pain before increasing the dosage. Frequent communication is important among the prescriber, other members of the healthcare team, the patient, and the patient's caregiver or family during periods of changing analgesic requirements, including the initial dosage titration period. During long-term therapy, the continued need for opiate analgesics should be continually reevaluated.

CAUTIONS

Respiratory depression and, to a lesser degree, circulatory depression (including orthostatic hypotension) are the chief hazards of opiate agonist therapy. Respiratory arrest, shock, and cardiac arrest have occurred. Rapid IV administration of opiate agonists increases the incidence of these serious adverse effects.

● Respiratory Depression

Respiratory depression is produced even with therapeutic analgesic doses of opiate agonists, but it is usually not clinically important in patients with normal respiratory capacity. It is probable that equianalgesic doses of individual opiate agonists produce similar degrees of respiratory depression; they may differ in the duration of the depressant effects they produce. Since opiate agonists may depress deep breathing and the reflex to sigh, these drugs may induce atelectasis, especially in patients with pulmonary disorders. If opiate agonists are necessary for the relief of severe pain in these patients, breathing exercises or use of forced deep inspiration with bag and mask should be encouraged. Neonates should be observed closely for signs of respiratory depression if the mother has received opiate agonists during labor.

Modified-release (e.g., extended-release) opiate agonists are associated with a greater risk of overdose and death because of the larger amount of drug contained in each dosage unit. Serious, life-threatening, or fatal respiratory depression has been reported even when these formulations were used as recommended. Although respiratory depression can occur at any time during therapy, the risk is greatest during initiation of therapy or following an increase in dosage.

● Nervous System Effects

Adverse CNS effects of opiate agonists include dizziness, visual disturbances, mental clouding or depression, sedation, coma, euphoria, dysphoria, weakness, faintness, agitation, restlessness, nervousness, seizures, and, rarely, delirium and insomnia. Opiate agonists may interfere with evaluation of CNS function, especially relative to consciousness levels, pupillary changes, and respiratory depression, thereby masking the patient's clinical course. Ambulatory patients and those patients not experiencing severe pain seem to have a higher incidence of adverse effects such as dizziness, nausea, vomiting, and hypotension than those who are in a supine position or who have severe pain. Patients with reduced blood volume, as may occur with hemorrhage or hemorrhagic shock, may be more sensitive than other patients to the hypotensive effect of opiate agonists. Although controlled studies are lacking, patients with hyperthyroidism appear to be more tolerant to the depressant effects of opiate agonists than patients with normal thyroid function.

● GI Effects

Adverse GI effects of opiate agonists include nausea, vomiting, and constipation. The use of morphine and its congeners in patients with chronic ulcerative colitis may stimulate motility in the colon; in patients with acute ulcerative colitis, toxic

dilation may occur. Opiate agonist-induced increase in intraluminal pressure may endanger surgical anastomosis. Opiate agonists may obscure the diagnosis or clinical course in patients with acute abdominal conditions.

Opiate agonist-induced increase in biliary tract pressure may result in biliary spasm or colic, especially in the sphincter of Oddi. This spasm is usually accompanied by increased plasma concentrations of amylase and lipase. Because of this effect, plasma amylase and lipase determinations should not be performed within 24 hours after an opiate agonist has been given.

● Cardiovascular Effects

Several cases of QT-interval prolongation and severe cardiac arrhythmias, including torsades de pointes, have been reported during postmarketing surveillance of levomethadyl acetate hydrochloride (no longer commercially available in the US) and also have been reported in patients receiving methadone hydrochloride, especially in individuals receiving higher dosages. QT-interval prolongation also has been observed in healthy individuals receiving oliceridine or extended-release hydrocodone bitartrate. (For further information, see the individual monographs for Methadone Hydrochloride, Hydrocodone Bitartrate, and Oliceridine Fumarate in 28:08.08.) In addition, cardiac arrest, ST segment elevation, ventricular tachycardia, myocardial infarction, angina pectoris, and syncope have been reported during postmarketing surveillance of levomethadyl acetate hydrochloride. In a study evaluating safety, tolerability, and electrocardiographic (ECG) effects of propoxyphene (no longer commercially available in the US) in healthy individuals, QT-interval prolongation, widening of the QRS complex, and prolongation of the PR interval were observed at therapeutic dosages of the drug.

● Genitourinary and Endocrine Effects

Opiate agonists may cause urinary retention and oliguria. Patients with prostatic hypertrophy or urethral stricture may be more prone to these effects. Opiate agonists may increase the risk of water intoxication in postoperative patients because of stimulation of the release of vasopressin.

Opiate agonists inhibit release of corticotropin as reflected by a decrease in plasma and urinary concentrations of 17-hydroxysteroids and 17-ketosteroids; rarely, secondary adrenocortical hypofunction or adrenal hypertrophy associated with hyperplasia of the reticular zone may follow chronic opiate agonist therapy. Onset of adrenal insufficiency in patients receiving opiate agonists or opiate partial agonists generally has occurred after at least 1 month of opiate agonist or partial agonist use, although the time to onset has ranged from within 1 day to more than 1 year. Manifestations of adrenal insufficiency are nonspecific and may include nausea, vomiting, anorexia, fatigue, weakness, dizziness, and hypotension. In many of the reported cases, patients required hospitalization. If adrenal insufficiency is suspected, appropriate laboratory testing should be performed promptly and physiologic (replacement) dosages of corticosteroids provided; therapy with the opiate agonist or partial agonist should be tapered and discontinued to allow recovery of adrenal function. If the opiate agonist or partial agonist can be discontinued, follow-up assessment of adrenal function should be performed to determine if corticosteroid replacement therapy can be discontinued. In some patients, switching to a different opiate improved symptoms.

Hypogonadism and androgen deficiency have been reported in patients receiving long-term opiate agonist or opiate partial agonist therapy, although a causal relationship has not been established. Suppression of gonadotropic function produced by opiate agonists may cause impotence and a decline in libido, possibly accompanied by decreased plasma and urinary concentrations of 17-ketosteroids. Patients receiving long-term opiate agonist or partial agonist therapy who present with manifestations of hypogonadism (e.g., decreased libido, impotence, erectile dysfunction, amenorrhea, infertility) should undergo laboratory evaluation.

● Cholinergic Effects

Bradycardia and other cholinergic effects which may occur following administration of opiate agonists may be controlled with atropine. In contrast to cholinergic effects produced by other opiates, meperidine or its congeners may produce anticholinergic effects such as dry mouth, palpitation, and tachycardia; uncoordinated jerky movements, muscle tremors and twitches, delirium with disorientation, hallucinations, and, occasionally, tonic-clonic (grand mal) seizures may also occur.

● Other Adverse Effects

Opiate agonists can release histamine (see Pharmacology: Effects on Histamine) and may produce sweating, flushing, or warmness of the face, neck, and upper thorax; pruritus; and urticaria. True anaphylactic reactions are extremely rare. Wheals, phlebitis, and pain may occur at the site of injection and local tissue irritation and induration are common following repeated subcutaneous administration of some opiate agonists. Reversible thrombocytopenia has been reported in an opiate-dependent patient with underlying chronic hepatitis who was receiving methadone.

● Precautions and Contraindications

Concomitant use of opiate agonists and benzodiazepines or other CNS depressants (e.g., anxiolytics, sedatives, hypnotics, tranquilizers, muscle relaxants, general anesthetics, antipsychotics, other opiate agonists, alcohol) may result in profound sedation, respiratory depression, coma, and death. Concomitant use of opiate analgesics and benzodiazepines or other CNS depressants should be reserved for patients in whom alternative treatment options are inadequate; the lowest effective dosages and shortest possible duration of concomitant therapy should be used, and the patient should be monitored closely for respiratory depression and sedation. Opiate antitussives should be avoided in patients receiving CNS depressants. Patients receiving opiate agonists and/or their caregivers should be apprised of the risks associated with concomitant therapeutic or illicit use of benzodiazepines, alcohol, or other CNS depressants. Concomitant use with alcohol should be avoided. (See Drug Interactions: Benzodiazepines and Other CNS Depressants.)

Because the morbidity and mortality associated with untreated opiate addiction (opiate use disorder [OUD]) can outweigh the serious risks associated with concomitant use of opiates and benzodiazepines or other CNS depressants, FDA states that therapy with opiate agonists or partial agonists (e.g., methadone, buprenorphine) for opiate addiction (i.e., medication-assisted treatment [MAT]) should not be withheld from patients receiving benzodiazepines or other CNS depressants. These drugs should be tapered and discontinued, if possible, in patients receiving MAT. However, excluding or discharging patients from MAT because of benzodiazepine or CNS depressant use is not likely to prevent such concomitant use and may lead to use outside the treatment setting, which could result in more severe outcomes. Careful management can reduce the risks associated with such concomitant use. (See Cautions in Methadone Hydrochloride 28:08.08.)

Because exposure to opiate agonists may be increased in patients with renal or hepatic impairment, use of conservative initial dosages followed by slow dosage titration generally is recommended; patients should be monitored closely for respiratory and CNS depression, particularly during dosage titration.

Opiate agonists also should be used with caution in cachectic, debilitated, or geriatric patients, since pharmacokinetics of the drugs may be altered and these patients may be at increased risk for respiratory depression. These patients should be monitored closely, particularly during initiation of therapy and dosage titration and when other drugs with respiratory depressant effects are used concomitantly.

Opiate agonists are contraindicated in patients with substantial respiratory depression or with acute or severe bronchial asthma or hypercarbia in unmonitored settings or in the absence of resuscitative equipment. Opiate agonists should be used with extreme caution in patients with preexisting respiratory depression and in those with conditions accompanied by hypoxia, hypercapnia, or decreased respiratory reserve, such as asthma, chronic obstructive pulmonary disease, cor pulmonale, severe obesity, sleep apnea, myxedema, kyphoscoliosis, CNS depression, or coma. In such patients, even therapeutic doses of opiate agonists may decrease respiratory drive while simultaneously increasing airway resistance to the point of apnea. Alternative analgesics without opiate agonist activity should be considered, and opiate agonists should be used only with close monitoring and at the lowest effective dosage in such patients. The risk of respiratory depression also is increased in geriatric, cachectic, or debilitated patients; following large initial doses of opiate agonists in patients who are not opiate tolerant; and in patients receiving other agents with respiratory depressant effects.

Clinicians should routinely discuss the availability of the opiate antagonist naloxone with all patients receiving new or reauthorized opiate prescriptions for pain management or new or reauthorized prescriptions for medications for treatment of OUD. Clinicians should consider prescribing naloxone for patients receiving opiate analgesics who are at increased risk of opiate overdosage (e.g., those receiving concomitant therapy with benzodiazepines or other CNS depressants, those with a history of opiate or substance use disorder, those with medical conditions that could increase sensitivity to opiate effects, those who have experienced a prior opiate overdose) and should strongly consider prescribing naloxone for all patients receiving medications for treatment of OUD. Clinicians also should consider prescribing naloxone when patients receiving opiates for pain management or for treatment of OUD have household members, including children, or other close contacts who are at risk for accidental ingestion or overdosage. Even if patients are not receiving an opiate for pain management or medication for treatment of OUD, a naloxone prescription should be considered if the patient is at increased risk of opiate overdosage (e.g., those with a current or past diagnosis of OUD, those who have experienced a prior opiate overdose). (See Naloxone Hydrochloride 28:10.)

Opiate agonists may cause severe hypotension in patients whose ability to maintain blood pressure has been compromised by blood volume depletion or concomitant use of certain drugs (e.g., general anesthetics, phenothiazines). Because opiate agonists may cause vasodilation that can further reduce cardiac output and blood pressure in patients with circulatory shock, the drugs should be used with caution in these patients; use of extended-release opiate agonists generally should be avoided in such patients. Opiate agonists may cause orthostatic hypotension and syncope in ambulatory patients.

The respiratory depressant effects of opiate agonists promote carbon dioxide retention, which results in elevation of intracranial pressure. The ability of opiate agonists to increase intracranial pressure may be markedly exaggerated in patients with head injury, other intracranial lesions, or preexisting elevated intracranial pressure. Opiate agonists also produce effects (e.g., pupillary changes, altered consciousness) that may obscure the clinical course and neurologic signs of further increases in intracranial pressure in patients with head injuries. Patients who may be particularly susceptible to the effects of carbon dioxide retention (e.g., those with elevated intracranial pressure, brain tumors, or impaired consciousness or coma) should be monitored closely. Use of long-acting or extended-release opiate agonists generally should be avoided in patients with impaired consciousness or coma.

Serotonin syndrome has been reported during concomitant use of opiate agonists and serotonergic drugs at recommended dosages. Manifestations of serotonin syndrome may include mental status changes (e.g., agitation, hallucinations, coma), autonomic instability (e.g., tachycardia, labile blood pressure, hyperthermia), neuromuscular aberrations (e.g., hyperreflexia, incoordination, rigidity), and/or GI symptoms (e.g., nausea, vomiting, diarrhea). Symptom onset generally occurs within several hours to a few days of concomitant use, but may occur later, particularly after dosage increases. (See Drug Interactions: Drugs Associated with Serotonin Syndrome.)

Opiate agonists are contraindicated in patients with known or suspected paralytic ileus and GI obstruction. Opiate agonists should be used with caution in patients at risk for ileus. Because opiate agonists diminish propulsive peristaltic waves in the GI tract and decrease bowel motility, postoperative patients receiving opiate analgesia should be monitored for decreased bowel motility. Chronic use of opiate agonists may result in obstructive bowel disease, especially in patients with underlying intestinal motility disorders. Opiate agonists may cause or aggravate constipation. Opiate agonists may obscure the diagnosis or clinical course of patients with acute abdominal conditions. Because opiate agonists may cause spasm of the sphincter of Oddi and diminish biliary and pancreatic secretions, patients with biliary tract disease, including those with acute pancreatitis, should be monitored for worsening symptoms.

Because of their cholinergic effects, opiate agonists should be used with caution in patients with cardiac arrhythmias.

Opiate agonists may aggravate preexisting seizures in patients with seizure disorders and may induce or aggravate seizures in some clinical settings. During long-term opiate agonist therapy, patients with seizure disorders should be monitored for worsening of seizure control.

Opiate agonists also should be used with caution in patients with hypothyroidism, adrenocortical insufficiency (e.g., Addison's disease), prostatic hyperplasia or urethral stricture, toxic psychosis, acute alcoholism, or delirium tremens.

Individuals who perform hazardous tasks requiring mental alertness or physical coordination should be warned about possible adverse CNS effects of opiate agonists.

Patients who are unable to tolerate one agent may be able to tolerate a different agent. Opiate agonists are contraindicated in patients with known hypersensitivity to the particular drug.

Pediatric Precautions

Serious adverse events, including deaths, have been reported in pediatric patients receiving codeine or tramadol for management of pain; in some of these cases, ultrarapid or extensive metabolism of cytochrome P-450 (CYP) isoenzyme 2D6 substrates was confirmed or suspected. (See Pharmacogenomics under Pharmacokinetics: Elimination.) Because of the potential for serious or fatal adverse effects in pediatric patients, use of codeine or tramadol for the management of pain is *contraindicated* in children younger than 12 years of age; tramadol and codeine also are *contraindicated* in pediatric patients younger than 18 years of age for the management of postoperative pain following tonsillectomy and/or adenoidectomy. FDA also states that use of codeine or tramadol for pain management is *not* recommended in children 12–18 years of age who are obese or have conditions such as obstructive sleep apnea or compromised respiratory function, since they may be susceptible to the respiratory depressant effects of the drug. (See Codeine 28:08.08 and Tramadol Hydrochloride 28:08.08.)

Serious adverse events, including deaths, also have been reported in pediatric patients receiving opiate agonists for the management of cough and cold. For information on precautions and contraindications associated with use of codeine or hydrocodone as antitussives in pediatric patients, see Cautions: Pediatric Precautions, in Codeine 48:08 and in Hydrocodone Bitartrate 48:08.

Geriatric Precautions

Geriatric patients are more likely than younger individuals to experience adverse effects, especially respiratory depressant effects, of opiate agonists and may be more sensitive to the analgesic effects of these drugs. Geriatric adults also are more likely to have prostatic hyperplasia or obstruction and renal impairment and thus may be at increased risk of opiate agonist-induced urinary retention. Clearance of opiate agonists may be decreased in geriatric patients, resulting in longer durations of action. Care should be exercised, and appropriate dosage adjustments (e.g., lower initial doses, longer dosing intervals) should be considered.

Some clinicians recommend that methadone and other opiate agonists with long elimination half-lives be used with caution in geriatric patients because of the greater frequency of decreased renal and hepatic function observed in these individuals. Meperidine should be used with caution in geriatric patients, and dosage adjustment should be considered because of the potential for adverse CNS effects (e.g., anxiety, excitation, tremors, myoclonus, seizures) secondary to accumulation of the toxic metabolite normeperidine, especially in those with decreased renal and hepatic function. Because of this risk, many experts recommend that alternative opiates be used in patients with renal impairment and in other individuals requiring large or repeated doses of opiate agonists.

Pregnancy, Fertility, and Lactation

Pregnancy

Analysis of data from the National Birth Defects Prevention Study, a large population-based, case-control study, suggests that therapeutic maternal use of opiate agonists during the period of organogenesis is associated with a low absolute risk of birth defects, including heart defects, spina bifida, and gastroschisis. Although there are no adequate and controlled studies to date in humans, some opiate agonists (e.g., morphine) have been shown to be teratogenic in animals. Therefore, opiate agonists should be used during pregnancy only when the potential benefits justify the possible risks to the fetus.

Prolonged maternal use of opiate agonists during pregnancy can result in neonatal opiate withdrawal syndrome with manifestations of irritability, hyperactivity and abnormal sleep pattern, high-pitched cry, tremor, vomiting, diarrhea, and failure to gain weight. In contrast to adults, the withdrawal syndrome in neonates may be life-threatening if not recognized and treated, and requires management according to protocols developed by neonatology experts. Women who require prolonged opiate agonist therapy during pregnancy should be advised of the risk of neonatal opiate withdrawal syndrome, and availability of appropriate treatment should be ensured. The onset, duration, and severity of the syndrome vary depending on the specific opiate agonist used, duration of use, timing and amount of last maternal use, and rate of drug elimination by the neonate. Use of

standardized protocols for identification and management of opiate withdrawal syndrome has been shown to improve overall response, including reductions in hospital stay and duration of pharmacologic treatment. When environmental and supportive measures are inadequate, opiates are recommended as first-line pharmacologic therapy. (See Uses: Neonatal Opiate Withdrawal.)

Use of opiate agonists during late pregnancy can result in neonatal respiratory depression.

Use of long-acting or extended-release opiate agonist analgesics is not recommended immediately before or during labor, when shorter-acting analgesics or other analgesic techniques may be more appropriate. Opiate agonists may prolong labor through actions that temporarily reduce the strength, duration, and frequency of uterine contractions. However, this effect is inconsistent and may be offset by an increased rate of cervical dilatation, which tends to shorten labor.

Lactation

Higher than expected concentrations of morphine (the active metabolite of codeine) may be distributed into breast milk of women taking codeine who are ultrarapid metabolizers of CYP2D6 substrates. (See Pharmacogenomics under Pharmacokinetics: Elimination.) Because of the potential for serious adverse effects in nursing infants, especially if the infant's mother is an ultrarapid metabolizer of CYP2D6 substrates, use of codeine is not recommended in nursing women. (See Codeine 48:08 and also see Codeine 28:08.08.) Because tramadol is distributed into milk and has similar risks as codeine in ultrarapid metabolizers of CYP2D6 substrates, use of tramadol also is not recommended in nursing women. (See Cautions in Tramadol Hydrochloride 28:08.08.)

DRUG INTERACTIONS

Benzodiazepines and Other CNS Depressants

Concomitant use of opiate agonists and benzodiazepines or other CNS depressants including other opiate agonists, anxiolytics, general anesthetics, tranquilizers, sedatives, hypnotics, muscle relaxants, antipsychotics, and alcohol can increase the risk of respiratory depression, hypotension, profound sedation, coma, and death. Opiate analgesics frequently are implicated as contributing to fatal overdoses involving other CNS depressants, and epidemiologic studies have shown that a substantial proportion of fatal opiate overdoses involve the concurrent use of benzodiazepines, alcohol, or other CNS depressants.

Whenever possible, concomitant use of opiate agonists and benzodiazepines should be avoided. Alcohol also should be avoided in patients receiving opiate agonists. Concomitant use of opiate analgesics and benzodiazepines or other CNS depressants should be reserved for patients in whom alternative treatment options are inadequate, and opiate antitussive agents should be avoided in patients receiving CNS depressant therapy. If a decision is made to prescribe opiate analgesics and CNS depressants concomitantly, the lowest effective dosages and shortest possible duration of concomitant therapy should be used, and the patient should be monitored closely for sedation, hypotension, and respiratory depressant effects. If a benzodiazepine or other CNS depressant is required for any indication other than epilepsy in a patient receiving opiate therapy for analgesia, the drug should be initiated at a lower dosage than indicated in the absence of opiate therapy and titrated based on clinical response. In patients receiving a CNS depressant, opiate analgesics, if required, should be initiated at a reduced dosage and titrated based on clinical response.

Because the morbidity and mortality associated with untreated opiate addiction can outweigh the serious risks associated with concomitant use of opiates and benzodiazepines or other CNS depressants, FDA states that therapy with opiates (e.g., methadone) for opiate addiction (i.e., medication-assisted treatment [MAT]) should not be withheld from patients receiving benzodiazepines or other CNS depressants. Clinicians should develop treatment plans that minimize the risks associated with such concomitant use. If possible, benzodiazepines or other CNS depressants should be tapered and discontinued. (See Cautions in Methadone Hydrochloride 28:08.08.)

Clinicians should consider prescribing the opiate antagonist naloxone for patients receiving opiates who are at increased risk of opiate overdosage, including those receiving benzodiazepines or other CNS depressants concomitantly. (See Cautions: Precautions and Contraindications.)

When considering use of extended-release or long-acting opiate agonist therapy in a patient already receiving another CNS depressant, the duration of use and response to the CNS depressant, including the degree of tolerance to CNS depressant effects, as well as the patient's use of alcohol or any illicit CNS depressants, should be evaluated. Concomitant use of alcohol with some oral extended-release opiate agonist formulations can result in increased plasma concentrations of the opiate agonist and potentially fatal overdosage.

● **Antidepressants**

Opiate agonists may potentiate the effects of tricyclic antidepressants and monoamine oxidase (MAO) inhibitors, including procarbazine hydrochloride; therefore, opiate agonists should be used with great caution and in reduced dosage when used in conjunction with such drugs. Virtually all the reported incidents of opiate agonist interaction with MAO inhibitors have occurred in patients receiving meperidine. (See Meperidine Hydrochloride 28:08.08.) Because MAO inhibitors may potentiate the effects of opiate agonists and because these effects may be severe and unpredictable, use of opiate agonists during or within 14 days following treatment with an MAO inhibitor is not recommended. Meperidine is contraindicated in patients receiving MAO inhibitors. Some manufacturers state that if an opiate agonist is required in patients receiving MAO inhibitors, a sensitivity test should be performed with small increments of morphine or the opiate agonist administered over a period of several hours while the patient is kept under close medical observation.

● **Drugs Associated with Serotonin Syndrome**

Serotonin syndrome may occur in patients receiving opiate agonists in conjunction with other serotonergic drugs, including serotonin (5-hydroxytryptamine; 5-HT) type 1 receptor agonists ("triptans"), selective serotonin-reuptake inhibitors (SSRIs), selective serotonin- and norepinephrine-reuptake inhibitors (SNRIs), tricyclic antidepressants, antiemetics that are 5-HT$_3$ receptor antagonists, buspirone, cyclobenzaprine, dextromethorphan, lithium, St. John's wort (*Hypericum perforatum*), tryptophan, other serotonin modulators (e.g., mirtazapine, nefazodone, trazodone, vilazodone), and MAO inhibitors (both those used to treat psychiatric disorders and others, such as linezolid, methylene blue, and selegiline). Serotonin syndrome may occur within the recommended dosage ranges for these drugs. Manifestations of serotonin syndrome may include mental status changes (e.g., agitation, hallucinations, coma), autonomic instability (e.g., tachycardia, labile blood pressure, hyperthermia), neuromuscular aberrations (e.g., hyperreflexia, incoordination, rigidity), and/or GI symptoms (e.g., nausea, vomiting, diarrhea). Symptom onset generally occurs within several hours to a few days of concomitant use, but may occur later, particularly after dosage increases.

If concurrent therapy with opiate agonists and serotonergic drugs is warranted, patients should be monitored for serotonin syndrome, particularly during initiation of therapy and dosage increases. If serotonin syndrome is suspected, treatment with opiate agonists and any concurrently administered serotonergic agents should be discontinued.

For further information on serotonin syndrome, including manifestations and treatment, see Drug Interactions: Serotonergic Drugs, in Fluoxetine Hydrochloride 28:16.04.20.

● **Opiate Antagonists and Opiate Partial Agonists**

Withdrawal symptoms may occur in patients receiving opiate agonists concomitantly with opiate antagonists (e.g., naloxone, naltrexone) or opiate partial agonists (e.g., buprenorphine, butorphanol, nalbuphine, pentazocine). Partial agonists should not be administered in patients receiving opiate agonists as they may reduce the analgesic effect and/or precipitate withdrawal symptoms.

● **Drugs Affecting Hepatic Microsomal Enzymes**

Metabolism of some opiates (e.g., codeine, fentanyl, hydrocodone, methadone, oliceridine, oxycodone, tramadol) is mediated by the cytochrome P-450 (CYP) microsomal enzyme system. Metabolism of methadone is mediated mainly by CYP isoenzymes 2B6, 2C19, and 3A4, and, to a lesser extent, by CYP isoenzymes 2C9 and 2D6. Fentanyl, hydrocodone, and oxycodone are metabolized mainly by CYP3A4, although CYP2D6 also is involved in the metabolism of hydrocodone and oxycodone. Codeine and tramadol are metabolized by CYP2D6 and CYP3A4. Oliceridine also is metabolized mainly by CYP2D6 and CYP3A4, with minor contributions from CYP2C9 and CYP2C19. Concomitant use of these opiates with drugs that induce or inhibit these isoenzymes may alter metabolism and clearance of the opiate. For further information, see Drug Interactions in the individual monographs in 28:08.08.

● **Drugs Affecting the P-glycoprotein Transport System**

Some opiate agonists (e.g., hydromorphone, morphine, tapentadol) are eliminated mainly as glucuronide conjugates. Concomitant use of morphine with P-glycoprotein inhibitors has been shown to increase systemic exposure to morphine.

● **Drugs that Prolong QT Interval**

Because of the potential for prolongation of the QT interval or serious cardiac arrhythmias, methadone should be used with extreme caution in patients receiving drugs that are known to prolong the QT interval or drugs that may result in electrolyte disturbances (e.g., hypokalemia, hypomagnesemia) that may prolong the QT interval. For further information on cardiovascular effects of methadone and associated drug interactions, see Methadone Hydrochloride 28:08.08.

● **Anticholinergic Agents**

Concomitant use of opiate agonists and drugs with anticholinergic activity may increase the risk of urinary retention or severe constipation, which can lead to paralytic ileus. Patients receiving such concomitant therapy should be monitored for signs or symptoms of urinary retention and reduced GI motility.

● **Neuromuscular Blocking Agents**

Opiate agonists may enhance the neuromuscular-blocking action of skeletal muscle relaxants.

● **Amphetamines**

Dextroamphetamine may enhance opiate agonist analgesia.

● **Diuretics**

Opiate agonists may decrease the effects of diuretics by inducing the release of vasopressin (antidiuretic hormone).

ACUTE TOXICITY

● **Manifestations**

Opiate agonist overdosage usually produces CNS depression ranging from stupor to a profound coma; respiratory depression which may progress to Cheyne-Stokes respiration and/or cyanosis; cold, clammy skin and/or hypothermia; flaccid skeletal muscles; bradycardia; and hypotension. In patients with severe overdosage, particularly following rapid IV administration of an opiate agonist, apnea, circulatory collapse, cardiac arrest, respiratory arrest, and death may occur. Complications such as pneumonia, shock, and/or pulmonary edema may also prove fatal. Although miosis is characteristic of overdosage with morphine derivatives and methadone, mydriasis may occur in terminal narcosis or severe hypoxia. Overdosage of meperidine or its congeners may produce mydriasis rather than miosis. Toxic effects of meperidine and its derivatives may be excitatory, especially in patients who have developed tolerance to the depressant effects of the drug. These patients may exhibit dry mouth, increased muscular activity, muscle tremors and twitches, tachycardia, delirium with disorientation, hallucinations, and, occasionally, tonic-clonic seizures.

Overdosage may be caused inadvertently by delayed absorption when repeated doses of opiate agonists are administered IM or subcutaneously to a patient with hypothermia, shock, hypotension, or any other condition that might impair circulation. When circulation is restored in these patients, large amounts of the opiate agonist are absorbed into the blood stream. Therefore, such patients should receive IV rather than subcutaneous or IM injections with the consideration that IV administration may increase the already severe cardiorespiratory impairment.

Modified-release (e.g., extended-release) opiate agonists are associated with a greater risk of overdosage and death because of the larger amount of drug contained in each dosage unit. Abuse or misuse of extended-release dosage forms by crushing or chewing the extended-release capsules or tablets, snorting the contents, or injecting the dissolved contents or by intentionally compromising the transdermal system (e.g., by swallowing, snorting, or injecting drug extracted from the system) will result in uncontrolled delivery of the opiate agonist and can result in overdosage and death. Inadvertent exposure to or ingestion of these formulations, especially by a child, also can result in respiratory depression and fatal overdosage.

Neonates whose mothers have received opiate agonists during labor should be closely observed for signs of respiratory depression and treatment for opiate agonist overdosage should be instituted if necessary.

● Treatment

In the treatment of opiate agonist overdosage, especially in the presence of apnea, primary attention should be given to reestablishment of adequate respiratory exchange by maintaining an adequate, patent airway, using assisted or controlled respiration and oxygen as necessary. Opiate agonist-induced respiratory depression may be treated with naloxone hydrochloride (an opiate antagonist) (see 28:10); however, the duration of respiratory depression following overdosage of an opiate agonist may be longer than the duration of action of the opiate antagonist and other more immediate supportive and symptomatic treatment should also be initiated. In addition, it should be considered that use of an opiate antagonist in patients physically dependent on opiate agonists may precipitate an acute withdrawal syndrome that cannot be readily suppressed while the action of the antagonist persists. The safety and efficacy of naltrexone hydrochloride in the management of acute opiate toxicity have not been established. If respiratory depression is associated with muscular rigidity, administration of a neuromuscular blocking agent may be necessary to facilitate assisted or controlled respiration. Muscular rigidity may also respond to opiate antagonist therapy. Gastric lavage may be effective even many hours after drug ingestion since pylorospasm produced by the opiate agonist may cause much of the drug to be retained in the stomach for an extended period of time.

● Chronic Toxicity

Opiate agonists have the potential to produce physical dependence and are subject to control under the Federal Controlled Substances Act of 1970. (See Preparations in the individual monographs.) Because of the drugs' opiate agonist activity at μ-receptors, tapentadol and tramadol also can produce dependence. The abuse potential of tapentadol is similar to that of hydromorphone, and tapentadol is subject to control under the Federal Controlled Substances Act of 1970. Although tramadol was *not* originally subject to control as a scheduled drug, current data suggest that the abuse potential of tramadol is less than that of morphine or oxycodone but similar to that of propoxyphene, and tramadol became subject to control under the Act effective August 18, 2014.

Tolerance, psychological dependence, and physical dependence may occur in patients receiving opiate agonists. Addiction can occur at recommended dosages or may be associated with misuse or abuse. Each patient's risk for addiction, abuse, or misuse should be assessed prior to prescribing opiate analgesics and all patients receiving the drugs should be monitored regularly for the development of these behaviors or conditions. Risks are increased in patients with a personal or family history of substance abuse (including drug or alcohol addiction or abuse) or mental illness (e.g., major depression). The potential for these risks should not prevent appropriate use of opiate agonists for the management of pain; however, use of the drugs in patients at increased risk necessitates intensive counseling about the risks and proper use, along with intensive monitoring for signs of addiction, abuse, and misuse.

Surveillance data suggest a parallel relationship between the number of opiate analgesic prescriptions dispensed in the US and the diversion and abuse of these drugs and associated adverse outcomes. Prescriptions for opiate analgesics in the US increased substantially (nearly tripling) from 1991 to 2011, and then plateaued or decreased slightly from 2011 through 2013; rates of diversion and abuse of prescription opiate analgesics followed similar patterns. Deaths associated with the use of prescription opiate analgesics increased sharply from 1999 to 2006, plateaued for several years, decreased slightly through 2013, but then increased again in 2014. From 2001 to 2014, deaths associated with the use of prescription opiate analgesics increased 3.4-fold. Fatal overdoses of heroin (diacetylmorphine, which is not available on the legitimate commercial market) have increased since 2007,

with substantial increases observed each year from 2011 through 2014. Fatal heroin overdoses in 2013 were nearly quadruple the rate in the early 2000s, with most of the increase occurring after 2010. From 2001 to 2014, the number of heroin-related deaths increased sixfold. Although data suggest that only a very small proportion of individuals who abuse prescription opiate analgesics transition to heroin use, prescription opiate abuse has emerged as a growing risk factor for heroin use. In a survey of individuals entering treatment programs for heroin addiction, 80% of those who began abusing opiates in the 1960s reported that heroin was their first opiate of abuse, whereas 75% of those who began abusing opiates in the 2000s reported that their first opiate of abuse was a prescription drug. Factors that have been cited as potentially contributing to the upsurge in heroin use include the lower cost and greater accessibility of high-purity heroin, the introduction of abuse-deterrent prescription formulations, and flattening of opiate prescribing rates.

Tolerance to the analgesic, respiratory depressant, sedative, and euphoric effects of opiate agonists usually develops during prolonged therapy; however, overdosage even in patients who have developed tolerance will cause respiratory depression and death. Tolerance to all effects of opiate agonists does not develop uniformly. Meperidine-dependent patients, for example, receiving 3–4 g of the drug daily, do not develop substantial tolerance to the excitant and anticholinergic actions of meperidine and may develop stimulatory symptoms of acute meperidine toxicity.

Development of tolerance seems to depend on the degree of opiate agonist-induced CNS depression and the extent to which this depression is continued by frequent or prolonged opiate agonist administration and may occur as a result of prolonged medical use or intentional abuse. Development of tolerance in patients receiving meperidine has been reported to be more gradual than in those receiving morphine; tolerance to methadone may develop more slowly than to meperidine. Patients who have developed tolerance to one opiate agonist usually exhibit cross-tolerance to other opiate agonists. Cross-tolerance among opiate agonists may be incomplete (see Cautions in Methadone Hydrochloride 28:08.08).

Continued administration of opiate agonists may lead to physical dependence which is closely related to tolerance. Individuals who are physically dependent on opiate agonists may remain relatively asymptomatic as long as they are able to maintain their daily opiate agonist requirement. Individuals who are morphine dependent will usually continue to exhibit miosis while those who are dependent on methadone may develop some tolerance to miosis. Physical dependence results in withdrawal symptoms in patients who abruptly discontinue the drug or receive an opiate antagonist. The abstinence syndrome varies in severity according to the specific drug and the amount of drug the patient has been taking. If the abstinence syndrome is precipitated by the parenteral administration of naloxone, symptoms will be apparent within a few minutes and maximal within 30 minutes after administration; effects will usually be more severe than those following withdrawal of the opiate agonist. (Induction of methadone abstinence in this manner is especially severe.) Because of naltrexone's long duration of antagonist effect, withdrawal precipitated by the drug may be prolonged. Until the antagonist has been eliminated, large doses of opiate agonists will only partially suppress these symptoms.

In patients who have taken up to 80 mg of morphine sulfate daily for up to one month, withdrawal symptoms are usually slight and require little or no treatment. A severe abstinence syndrome occurs if the patient has received 240 mg or more of morphine sulfate for 30 days or longer. Severe opiate agonist abstinence syndrome is characterized by restlessness, lacrimation, rhinorrhea, yawning, perspiration, gooseflesh, restless sleep or "yen," and mydriasis during the first 24 hours. As the syndrome progresses, these symptoms become more severe and may be accompanied by twitching and spasms of muscles; kicking movements; severe aches in back, abdomen, and legs; abdominal and muscle cramps; hot and cold flashes; insomnia; nausea, vomiting, and diarrhea; coryza and severe sneezing; and increases in body temperature, blood pressure, respiratory rate, and heart rate. These symptoms reach peak intensity 36–72 hours following withdrawal of morphine sulfate. In addition, marked increase in urinary 17-ketosteroid concentrations and leukocytosis with leukocyte counts above 14,000/mm³ occur frequently. Because of the excessive loss of fluids through sweating, vomiting and diarrhea, there is usually marked weight loss, dehydration, ketosis, and disturbances in acid-base balance. Cardiovascular collapse may occur especially in aged or debilitated patients. Administration of an opiate agonist will readily suppress most withdrawal symptoms except those resulting from fluid deficiency. If no treatment is given, most observable symptoms disappear in 5–14 days; however, there appears to be a phase of secondary or chronic abstinence which may last for 2–6 months after withdrawal of the drug. This phase is associated with gradually decreasing insomnia, irritability, and muscular aches. In addition, the patient may have miosis and a slight lowering of blood pressure, pulse rate, and body temperature; respiratory centers exhibit a decreased response to the stimulatory effects of carbon dioxide.

In patients who are physically dependent on meperidine, abstinence symptoms usually occur 3–4 hours after the last dose of the drug, reaching maximal intensity within 8–12 hours. Although symptoms associated with meperidine withdrawal are generally milder than those of morphine withdrawal, during the period of maximal intensity, muscle twitching, restlessness and nervousness may be worse than with morphine. Symptoms of meperidine withdrawal decline until few are apparent after 4–5 days.

Because of the cumulative effects of methadone, abstinence symptoms following its withdrawal are less intense and more prolonged than those following withdrawal of other opiate agonists and may not be manifested until 3 or 4 days after the last dose. Peak intensity of symptoms occurs on the sixth day and may include weakness, anxiety, anorexia, insomnia, abdominal discomfort, headache, sweating, and hot and cold flashes. Few symptoms are apparent after 10–14 days, although patients may exhibit lethargy and anorexia for longer periods. Other opiate agonists produce abstinence syndromes similar to those described previously. In general, the shorter the onset and duration of action of the drug, the greater the intensity and rapidity of onset of withdrawal symptoms. Those drugs which are eliminated slowly produce a mild, prolonged abstinence syndrome.

In the treatment of physical dependence, the patient may be detoxified by gradual reduction of daily opiate agonist dosage. If abstinence symptoms become severe, the patient may receive methadone (see Methadone Hydrochloride 28:08.08). Temporary administration of tranquilizers and sedatives may aid in reducing patient anxiety and opiate agonist craving. Symptoms involving GI disturbance or dehydration should be treated accordingly. Supportive social, vocational, psychiatric, and educational services should be available to the patient. For some patients, maintenance treatment with relatively stable doses of methadone or buprenorphine for relatively long periods may be necessary in the management of opiate dependence. (See Methadone Hydrochloride 28:08.08 and Buprenorphine Hydrochloride 28:08.12.) Therapy with naltrexone, an opiate antagonist, may be a useful adjunct in the maintenance of opiate cessation in some individuals formerly physically dependent on opiates who have successfully undergone detoxification. (See Naltrexone Hydrochloride 28:10.)

Alternatively, rapid detoxification has been used in the management of opiate withdrawal in opiate-dependent individuals, both in inpatient and outpatient settings. Rapid opiate detoxification involves the administration of opiate antagonists such as naloxone and naltrexone to shorten the time period of detoxification. The reported advantage of this technique is to minimize the risk of relapse and to initiate maintenance therapy with naltrexone and psychosocial interventions more quickly. Ultrarapid detoxification is similar, but involves the administration of opiate antagonists while the patient is sedated or under general anesthesia. However, the risk of adverse respiratory and cardiovascular effects associated with this procedure must be considered as well as the costs of general anesthesia and hospitalization. Safety and efficacy of these therapies have not been established and further study is needed.

Neonates born to mothers physically dependent on opiate agonists may also be opiate dependent and usually exhibit withdrawal symptoms from 1–4 days after birth. These symptoms include generalized tremors and hypertonicity with any form of tactile stimuli, hyperalertness, sleeplessness, excessive crying, vomiting, diarrhea, yawning, and, occasionally, fever. (See Pregnancy under Cautions: Pregnancy and Lactation and also see Uses: Neonatal Opiate Withdrawal.)

PHARMACOLOGY

● Nervous System Effects

Opiate agonists exert their principal pharmacologic effect on the CNS and on the intestines. The drugs interact as agonists at specific receptor binding sites in the CNS and other tissues. Opiate receptors are present in highest concentration in the limbic system, thalamus, striatum, hypothalamus, midbrain, and spinal cord. Several subtypes of opiate receptors have been described including the μ-receptor, which is localized in pain modulating regions of the CNS; the κ-receptor, which is localized in the deep layers of the cerebral cortex; the δ-receptor, which is localized in the limbic regions of the CNS; and the σ-receptor, which is thought to mediate the dysphoric and psychotomimetic effects of some opiate partial agonists (e.g., pentazocine). Morphine, the prototype opiate agonist, has agonist activity at the μ- and κ-receptors but has little, if any, activity at the σ-receptor; the drug is a more potent agonist at the μ- than κ-receptor. Morphine may also have some agonist activity at the δ-receptor. Agonist activity at the μ- or κ-receptor can result in analgesia, miosis, and/or decreased body temperature. Agonist activity at the μ-receptor can also result in suppression of opiate withdrawal, whereas antagonist activity can result in precipitation of withdrawal. Respiratory depression may be mediated by μ-receptors, possibly μ_2-receptors (which may be distinct from μ_1-receptors involved in analgesia); κ- and δ-receptors may also be involved in respiratory depression. Cough-suppressant opiate receptors have also been suggested.

Opiate agonists act at several sites within the CNS involving several systems of neurotransmitters to produce analgesia, but the precise mechanism of action has not been fully elucidated. Opiate agonists do not alter the threshold or responsiveness of afferent nerve endings to noxious stimuli nor the conduction of impulses along peripheral nerves; instead, the drugs alter the perception of pain at the spinal cord and higher levels in the CNS (substantia gelatinosa, spinal trigeminal nucleus, periaqueductal gray, periventricular gray, medullary raphe nuclei, hypothalamus) and the patient's emotional response to pain.

In addition to analgesia, the effects of opiate agonists on the CNS cause suppression of the cough reflex, respiratory depression, drowsiness, sedation, change in mood, euphoria, dysphoria, mental clouding, nausea, vomiting, and EEG changes. Dosages higher than usual analgesic dosages result in anesthesia; however, prevention of awareness during and recall after opiate-agonist anesthesia may require supplementation with other agents (e.g., benzodiazepines), since awareness and recall of the surgical procedure have been reported by some patients even at high doses of an opiate agonist alone. Large doses of opiate agonists may induce excitation or seizures. Morphine and its congeners and methadone depress the cough reflex by a direct effect on the cough centers in the medulla; antitussive effects may occur with doses lower than those required for analgesia. Meperidine and its congeners generally have appreciable antitussive activity only in analgesic doses. Opiate agonists produce respiratory depression by a direct effect on the respiratory centers in the brain stem resulting in decreased sensitivity and responsiveness to increases in serum carbon dioxide tension (Pco_2). These drugs depress the pontine and medullary centers which regulate respiratory rhythm and may also alter voluntary control of respiration. Depressed respiration produces an increase in arterial Pco_2 resulting in cerebral vasodilation and a consequential rise in cerebral blood flow and CSF pressure. Increased CSF pressure is more likely to occur following IV administration of opiate agonists than following other routes of administration. Nausea is probably caused by stimulation of the chemoreceptor trigger zone (CTZ) in the medulla oblongata or by the occurrence of orthostatic hypotension. Vomiting may result from stimulation of the CTZ. In addition, the opiate agonists depress the vomiting center; therefore, subsequent doses of the drugs are unlikely to produce vomiting. Increase in vestibular sensitivity may also contribute to the high incidence of nausea and vomiting in ambulatory patients.

● Ocular Effects

Morphine and its congeners and, to a lesser extent, methadone cause miosis which is antagonized by atropine. Some reports state that meperidine and its congeners also produce miosis, whereas others indicate that these drugs tend to produce mydriasis or no pupillary change. Therapeutic doses of morphine and its congeners increase accommodation and sensitivity to light reflex and decrease intraocular tension in both normal and glaucomatous eyes. Opiate agonists decrease the response of the hypothalamus to afferent stimulation; slight hypothermia may also occur.

● GI Effects

Gastric, biliary, and pancreatic secretions are decreased by opiate agonists and the drugs delay digestion. Although the precise action of clinical doses of opiate agonists on GI smooth muscle tone is controversial, the ultimate result is constipation. Morphine congeners, meperidine and its congeners, and methadone are less constipating than morphine. Opiate agonists increase smooth muscle tone in the antral portion of the stomach, the small intestine (particularly the duodenum), the large intestine, and the sphincters. It has been generally believed that tone increases to the point of spasm. Although intensity and frequency of propulsive contractions are decreased, amplitude of nonpropulsive rhythmic contractions may be enhanced. Vigorous spasms that occur in the smooth muscle of intestinal walls and sphincters may be partially blocked by atropine. Although meperidine and its congeners have some anticholinergic properties, these drugs produce smooth muscle spasms to a similar or lesser degree than does morphine.

Tone is increased in the biliary tract, and spasms (particularly of the sphincter of Oddi) and an increase in biliary tract pressure may result. Morphine produces a greater increase in biliary pressure than does meperidine; meperidine produces a greater effect than does codeine. These biliary effects do not always occur with therapeutic doses; some patients may have no change in bile duct diameter or pressure. Biliary spasms may result in plasma amylase and lipase concentrations as much as 2–15 times the normal values.

● Genitourinary Effects

Opiate agonists increase smooth muscle tone in the urinary tract and induce spasms. Although the response of the ureters is quite variable, the drugs may increase tone and amplitude of contractions, especially of the lower third of the ureter. In the urinary bladder, tone of the detrusor muscle is increased, possibly resulting in urinary urgency. Opiate agonists also increase tone of the vesical sphincter which may make urination difficult. These effects, in conjunction with the central effect of the drugs on release of vasopressin, may produce oliguria; however, results of one study suggest that decreased urine output may occur without any apparent release of vasopressin and may be attributed to decreased rate of glomerular filtration and solute excretion. Some clinicians have attributed decreased urine output to decreased renal plasma flow or increased reabsorption. Large doses of opiate agonists may cause bronchoconstriction, but this effect is rarely seen with therapeutic doses.

Morphine and its congeners in therapeutic doses may prolong labor. There are conflicting reports on the effect of meperidine on the progress of labor. Generally, the effect of opiate agonists on the pregnant uterus appears to depend on the time of administration; administration of the drugs during the latent phase of the first stage of labor or before cervical dilation of 4–5 cm has occurred will probably hamper the progress of labor. In the uterus made hyperactive by oxytocics, morphine tends to restore uterine tone and contractions to a normal level. Although meperidine may have little effect on the normal contracting uterus late in pregnancy, if oxytocics have been administered, meperidine tends to increase uterine tone and contractions.

● Cardiovascular Effects

Most opiate agonists have little cardiovascular effect when given in therapeutic doses to supine patients. When the supine patient who has received an opiate agonist assumes a head-up position, however, orthostatic hypotension and fainting may occur as a result of peripheral vasodilation, particularly in volume-depleted patients. Dilation of peripheral blood vessels may be caused by opiate agonist-induced release of histamine or by depression of the vasomotor center in the medulla. Large doses of opiate agonists may produce hypotension, even in the supine patient. In addition, large doses and/or rapid administration of opiate agonists may produce bradycardia as a result of stimulation of medullary vagal nuclei. Meperidine may produce either bradycardia or tachycardia.

● Effects on Histamine

Although meperidine and its congeners may have some antihistaminic activity, these drugs also cause histamine release although it may be less than that produced by morphine. Sufentanil and fentanyl are less potent stimulators of histamine release than are meperidine or morphine. Manifestations of histamine release and/or peripheral dilation also include flushing, pruritus, red eyes, and sweating.

● Endocrine Effects

Opiate agonists exert endocrinologic effects, some of which may be related to CNS effects. The drugs generally stimulate release of vasopressin. Although opiate agonists have been reported to stimulate the release of corticotropin in animals, the drugs generally inhibit the stress-induced (e.g., associated with surgery) release of corticotropin and the release of gonadotropins (i.e., luteinizing

hormone, follicle-stimulating hormone) from the pituitary resulting in decreased plasma and urinary 17-hydroxycorticosteroid and 17-ketosteroid concentrations; however, the functions of the adrenal gland and sex organs are not necessarily suppressed and usually exhibit a normal response to administration of exogenous corticotropin and chorionic gonadotropin. The drugs inhibit the release of thyrotropin from the adenohypophysis leading to a decrease in release of thyroid hormone. Opiate agonists may produce hyperglycemia by an action on paraventricular receptor sites near the foramen of Monro or by stimulating release of epinephrine. Basal metabolic rate may be decreased by 10–20% in patients receiving opiate agonists.

● Other Effects

Opiate agonists may also decrease olfactory and auditory acuity.

PHARMACOKINETICS

● Absorption and Distribution

Some opiate agonists are well absorbed following oral or rectal administration, but others must be administered parenterally. Individual opiate agonists differ in onset and duration of action. Following subcutaneous administration, rates of absorption and onset of action differ because of differences in solubility and/or rate of dissolution. Opiate agonists are rapidly removed from the blood stream and distributed in decreasing order of concentration into skeletal muscle, kidneys, liver, intestinal tract, lungs, spleen, and brain. The drugs readily penetrate the placental barrier.

● Elimination

Opiate agonists are metabolized mainly in the liver, the microsomes in the endoplasmic reticulum being the major site of metabolism. The drugs are also metabolized in the CNS, kidneys, lungs, and placenta. Opiate agonists undergo conjugation with glucuronic acid, hydrolysis, oxidation, and/or N- or O-dealkylation. The drugs are excreted principally in urine in the unchanged form and as metabolites; small amounts are excreted in the feces.

Some opiate agonists (e.g., codeine, fentanyl, hydrocodone, methadone, oxycodone, tramadol) undergo metabolism via the cytochrome P-450 (CYP) microsomal enzyme system. Methadone is metabolized mainly by CYP isoenzymes 2B6, 2C19, and 3A4, and, to a lesser extent, by CYP isoenzymes 2C9 and 2D6. Fentanyl, hydrocodone, and oxycodone are metabolized mainly by CYP3A4, although CYP2D6 also is involved in the metabolism of hydrocodone and oxycodone. Codeine and tramadol are metabolized by CYP2D6 and CYP3A4. Oliceridine also is metabolized mainly by CYP2D6 and CYP3A4, with minor contributions from CYP2C9 and CYP2C19. Other opiate agonists (e.g., hydromorphone, morphine, tapentadol) are eliminated mainly via hepatic metabolism to glucuronide conjugates that are excreted in urine.

● Pharmacogenomics

Genetic polymorphism of CYP2D6 may cause variations in individual drug response and should be considered as a factor when differences in efficacy or toxicity of drugs metabolized by this pathway are observed. Serious adverse reactions have been reported in individuals who are ultrarapid metabolizers of codeine because they convert codeine to morphine (its active metabolite) at a higher rate. (See Codeine 48:08 and also see Codeine 28:08.08.)

CHEMISTRY

Opiate agonists encompass a group of naturally occurring, semisynthetic, and synthetic drugs that stimulate opiate receptors and effectively relieve pain without producing loss of consciousness.

The term "opiate" has been used in the medical literature to describe drugs that are opium derivatives, and "opioid" has been used to describe opium derivatives as well as drugs that are not opium derivatives but are, at least to some extent, opium- or morphine-like in their effects and to describe endogenous peptides (e.g., enkephalins) that have morphine-like activity. Using these definitions, drugs with pharmacologic effects that result in part from agonist activity at opiate receptors but that are not opium derivatives nor semisynthetic derivatives of morphine or thebaine (e.g., tapentadol, tramadol) would not be considered an "opiate" but would be considered an "opioid." However, the terms "opiate" and "opioid" also have been used interchangeably to describe the receptors and associated agonist and antagonist activity of drugs (e.g., morphine) and other mediators at these receptors. In the AHFS Pharmacologic-Therapeutic Classification©, the term "opiate agonist" is applied to any drug, regardless of chemical origin, whose pharmacologic and/or toxicologic effects result to an important degree from agonist activity at opiate receptors. The emphasis in the AHFS Classification is on the actual effects of the drugs rather than on chemical derivation. While the term "opioid agonist" also has been applied to drugs that stimulate opiate receptors, the AHFS Pharmacologic-Therapeutic Classification© employs "opiate" rather than "opioid" as the modifier for agonist (and antagonist) activity since *true* opiate receptors, not opiate-*like* (i.e., opi-*oid*) receptors, are affected. Therefore, although drugs like tapentadol and tramadol do not fit the classic definition of an opiate (i.e., if they are not opium derivatives nor semisynthetic derivatives), these drugs *are* classified as opiate agonists in *AHFS Drug Information* because they possess agonist activity at opiate receptors.

Chemically, opiate agonists generally may be classified as phenanthrene derivatives, phenylpiperidine derivatives, or diphenylheptane derivatives. Oliceridine is structurally unrelated to morphine or other μ-opiate receptor agonists.

● Phenanthrene Derivatives

codeine	levorphanol tartrate
concentrated opium alkaloids hydrochlorides	morphine sulfate
hydrocodone bitartrate	oxycodone
hydromorphone hydrochloride	oxymorphone hydrochloride

Morphine is the prototype of the phenanthrene-derivative opiate agonists. Etherification of the 3-hydroxyl group (e.g., codeine) decreases analgesic activity. Oxidation of the 6-hydroxyl group (e.g., hydromorphone, oxymorphone) increases analgesic activity. Although levorphanol is a morphinan derivative, it is structurally similar to the phenanthrene-derivative opiate agonists. Most phenanthrene derivatives are analgesics; however, naloxone hydrochloride and naltrexone

hydrochloride are essentially pure opiate antagonists (see 28:10), which have little or no analgesic activity. Hydrocodone bitartrate is also used as an antitussive (see 48:08).

● Phenylpiperidine Derivatives

anileridine hydrochloride	meperidine hydrochloride
fentanyl citrate	sufentanil citrate

Meperidine is the prototype of the phenylpiperidine-derivative opiate agonists. Replacement of the *N*-methyl group of meperidine with a large rigid aralkyl group (e.g., anileridine) increases analgesic activity. Replacement of the *N*-methyl group of meperidine with a diphenylcyanopropyl group produces diphenoxylate, a compound which is devoid of analgesic activity but has good antidiarrheal activity (see 56:08).

● Diphenylheptane Derivatives

methadone hydrochloride	levomethadyl acetate hydrochloride

Methadone hydrochloride is the prototype of the diphenylheptane-derivative opiate agonists. Levomethadyl acetate hydrochloride (no longer commercially available in the US because of potentially severe adverse cardiac effects) is a synthetic congener of methadone with a delayed onset of action and prolonged duration of effect. Propoxyphene (no longer commercially available in the US), which is closely related structurally to methadone, has mild analgesic activity.

Most opiate agonists are basic in reaction and readily react with acids to form water-soluble salts. Such salts have a wide range of water solubility.

For specific dosages and additional information on chemistry and stability, pharmacology, pharmacokinetics, uses, cautions, and drug interactions of the opiate agonists, see the individual monographs in 28:08.08.

† Use is not currently included in the labeling approved by the US Food and Drug Administration.

Selected Revisions April 19, 2023, © Copyright, September 01, 1972, American Society of Health-System Pharmacists, Inc.

Codeine Phosphate, Codeine Sulfate

28:08.08 • OPIOID AGONISTS

■ Codeine is a phenanthrene-derivative opiate agonist.

REMS

FDA approved a REMS for codeine to ensure that the benefits outweigh the risk. The REMS may apply to one or more preparations of codeine and consists of the following: medication guide and elements to assure safe use. See the FDA REMS page (http://www.accessdata.fda.gov/scripts/cder/rems/index.cfm).

USES

Codeine is a mild analgesic used in the relief of mild to moderately severe pain that is not relieved by a nonopiate analgesic. Because of differing mechanisms of action, codeine and aspirin or acetaminophen in combination probably produce additive analgesic effects. Combinations containing codeine, aspirin, and caffeine are effective but produce no more analgesia than a combination of aspirin and codeine. For further information on the role of opiate analgesics in the management of acute or chronic pain, see Uses: Pain, in the Opiate Agonists General Statement 28:08.08.

For use of codeine as an antitussive agent, see 48:08.

DOSAGE AND ADMINISTRATION

● Administration

Codeine sulfate and codeine phosphate are administered orally.

● Dosage

Codeine salts should be given at the lowest effective dosage and for the shortest duration of therapy consistent with the treatment goals of the patient. Reduced dosage is indicated in poor-risk patients and in very old patients. If concomitant therapy with other CNS depressants is required, the lowest effective dosages and shortest possible duration of concomitant therapy should be used.

When opiate analgesics are administered in fixed combination with nonopiate analgesics, the opiate dosage may be limited by the nonopiate component. Because commercially available preparations contain codeine and nonopiate analgesics in various fixed ratios and because these nonopiate analgesics also are available in many other prescription and OTC preparations, care should be taken to ensure that therapy is not duplicated and that dosage of the nonopiate drug does not exceed maximum recommended dosages.

The initial dosage must be individualized, taking into account the patient's prior opiate use; concurrent drug therapy; degree of opiate tolerance; medical condition; type and severity of pain; and risk factors for addiction, abuse, and misuse.

For the relief of mild to moderate pain in adults, the usual oral dosage of codeine phosphate or codeine sulfate is 30 mg every 4 hours as necessary; the usual dose range is 15–60 mg. Adult dosage should not exceed 360 mg daily.

Children may receive 3 mg/kg or 100 mg/m² daily in 6 divided doses. Alternatively, children may be given 0.5 mg/kg or 15 mg/m² every 4–6 hours. (See Cautions: Pediatric Precautions.)

For acute pain not related to trauma or surgery, the prescribed quantity should be limited to the amount needed for the expected duration of pain severe enough to require opiate analgesia (generally 3 days or less and rarely more than 7 days). When opiate analgesics are used for the management of chronic noncancer pain, the US Centers for Disease Control and Prevention (CDC) recommends that primary care clinicians carefully reassess individual benefits and risks before prescribing dosages equivalent to 50 mg or more of morphine sulfate daily (approximately 330 mg or more of codeine phosphate or codeine sulfate daily) and avoid dosages equivalent to 90 mg or more of morphine sulfate daily or carefully justify their decision to titrate the dosage to such levels. Other experts recommend consulting a pain management specialist before exceeding a dosage equivalent to 80–120 mg of morphine sulfate daily. For further information on the management of opiate analgesic therapy, see Dosage and Administration: Dosage, in the Opiate Agonists General Statement 28:08.08.

CAUTIONS

● Precautions and Contraindications

Codeine shares the toxic potentials of the opiate agonists, and the usual precautions of opiate agonist therapy should be observed. (See Cautions in the Opiate Agonists General Statement 28:08.08.)

Codeine is contraindicated in children younger than 12 years of age for the management of pain and in pediatric patients younger than 18 years of age for the management of postoperative pain following tonsillectomy and/or adenoidectomy. In addition, FDA states that use of codeine for the management of pain is *not* recommended in pediatric patients 12–18 years of age who are obese or have conditions such as obstructive sleep apnea or compromised respiratory function. (See Cautions: Pediatric Precautions.)

Individuals who are ultrarapid metabolizers of cytochrome P-450 (CYP) 2D6 substrates are likely to have higher than expected serum concentrations of morphine, the active metabolite of codeine; therefore, FDA states that codeine should *not* be used in such patients. (See Pharmacokinetics: Pharmacogenomics.)

FDA also states that use of codeine is *not* recommended in nursing women, especially those who have evidence of ultrarapid metabolism of CYP2D6 substrates. Serious adverse events (e.g., excessive sedation, difficulty nursing, respiratory depression), including death, have been reported in nursing infants exposed to codeine. One case of opiate toxicity resulting in neonatal death has been reported in the nursing infant of a woman receiving codeine; genetic testing of the woman indicated that she was an ultrarapid metabolizer of codeine. (See Pharmacokinetics: Pharmacogenomics.) Higher than expected concentrations of morphine were found in breast milk and in the blood of the infant. Somnolence also has been reported more frequently in nursing infants whose mothers received codeine in combination with acetaminophen compared with those whose mothers received acetaminophen alone; evidence of ultrarapid metabolism of CYP2D6 substrates was identified in some of these women. Concentrations of morphine in breast milk are low and dose dependent in women who are normal metabolizers of codeine. Although not routinely used in clinical practice, FDA-approved tests (e.g., AmpliChip° CYP450 Test) are available to identify an individual's CYP2D6 genotype. However, testing alone may not adequately predict the risk of adverse reactions. Infants exposed to codeine through breast milk should be monitored closely for clinical manifestations of opiate toxicity (e.g., sedation, difficulty breast-feeding or breathing, hypotonia). If such manifestations occur, caregivers should seek immediate medical treatment for the infant.

When preparations containing codeine in fixed combination with other drugs are administered, the cautions, precautions, and contraindications applicable to each ingredient must be considered.

● Pediatric Precautions

Pediatric patients receiving codeine for the management of pain, especially those who are obese, have obstructive sleep apnea or severe lung disease, or have evidence of ultrarapid metabolism of CYP2D6 substrates, are at increased risk of respiratory depression. Serious adverse events, including deaths, have been reported during postmarketing experience in pediatric patients receiving codeine. Between January 1969 and May 2015, the FDA Adverse Event Reporting System (AERS) received 64 reports of respiratory depression, including 24 reports of death, worldwide that were associated with codeine use in pediatric patients younger than 18 years of age; in all 10 of the reports that provided information about CYP2D6 metabolizer status, the patients were ultrarapid or extensive metabolizers of CYP2D6 substrates. (See Pharmacokinetics: Pharmacogenomics.) Most of the cases of respiratory depression, including most of the deaths, occurred in children younger than 12 years of age. Respiratory depression may occur despite serum concentrations of codeine or morphine being within the therapeutic range; one patient who had concentrations within the therapeutic range died following use of codeine for management of pain after tonsillectomy and adenoidectomy.

To minimize the risk of serious adverse events in pediatric patients, FDA states that codeine-containing preparations must *not* be used for the management of pain in children younger than 12 years of age or for the management of postoperative pain following tonsillectomy and/or adenoidectomy in pediatric patients younger than 18 years of age, and that use of codeine for the management of pain is *not* recommended in pediatric patients 12–18 years of age who are obese or have conditions such as obstructive sleep apnea or compromised respiratory function (because of potentially greater susceptibility to the respiratory depressant effects of the drug). If codeine is used for the management of pain in pediatric patients 12–18 years of age, caregivers should closely monitor the child for clinical manifestations of opiate toxicity (e.g., shallow, difficult, or noisy breathing; confusion; unusual sleepiness) and seek immediate medical treatment for the child if such manifestations occur.

Serious adverse events, including deaths, also have been reported in children receiving codeine for relief of symptoms of upper respiratory tract infection. For additional information on precautions and contraindications associated with the use of codeine as an antitussive in pediatric patients, see Cautions: Pediatric Precautions, in Codeine 48:08.

PHARMACOLOGY

Equianalgesic parenteral doses of codeine phosphate and morphine sulfate have produced similar degrees of respiratory depression. Codeine has good antitussive activity, although on a weight basis antitussive activity of codeine is less than that of morphine.

PHARMACOKINETICS

Codeine and its salts are well absorbed following oral administration. Following oral administration, onset of action occurs in 15–30 minutes and analgesia is maintained for 4–6 hours. Codeine is distributed into milk. Codeine is metabolized mainly in the liver where it undergoes O-demethylation (by cytochrome P-450 [CYP] isoenzyme 2D6), N-demethylation (by CYP3A4), and partial conjugation with glucuronic acid; the drug is excreted mainly in urine as norcodeine and free and conjugated morphine. Negligible amounts of codeine and its metabolites are found in feces.

Codeine is metabolized by the CYP microsomal enzyme system, principally by CYP3A4, and to a lesser extent by CYP2D6 (debrisoquine hydroxylase). Although the CYP2D6 isoenzyme accounts for only 10% of the metabolism of codeine, it plays an essential role in converting the drug to its active O-demethylated metabolite, morphine.

Pharmacogenomics: Metabolism of certain drugs, including codeine, is influenced by CYP2D6 polymorphism. Individuals who lack functional alleles of the CYP2D6 gene are described as poor metabolizers, those with 1 or 2 functional alleles are described as extensive metabolizers, and those who carry a duplicate or amplified gene are described as ultrarapid metabolizers. Genetically determined differences in drug metabolism can affect an individual's response to a drug or risk of having an adverse event. Individuals who are poor metabolizers experience no analgesic effects of codeine; individuals who are ultrarapid metabolizers are likely to have higher than expected serum concentrations of morphine.

Variations in CYP2D6 polymorphism occur at different frequencies among subpopulations of different ethnic or racial origin. Approximately 1–7% of Caucasians and 10–30% of Ethiopians and Saudi Arabians carry the genotype associated with ultrarapid metabolism of CYP2D6 substrates.

CHEMISTRY AND STABILITY

● Chemistry

Codeine is a phenanthrene-derivative opiate agonist. Codeine occurs as colorless or white crystals or as a white, crystalline powder; the drug is slightly soluble in water and freely soluble in alcohol. Codeine phosphate occurs as fine, white, needle-shaped crystals or as a white, crystalline powder and is freely soluble in water and slightly soluble in alcohol. Codeine sulfate occurs as white crystals, usually needle-like, or as a white, crystalline powder and is soluble in water and very slightly soluble in alcohol.

● Stability

Codeine sulfate tablets should be stored in well-closed, light-resistant containers at a temperature less than 40°C, preferably between 15–30°C.

For further information on chemistry, pharmacology, uses, cautions, chronic toxicity, acute toxicity, drug interactions, and dosage and administration of codeine, see the Opiate Agonists General Statement 28:08.08.

PREPARATIONS

Codeine preparations are subject to control under the Federal Controlled Substances Act of 1970.

Excipients in commercially available drug preparations may have clinically important effects in some individuals; consult specific product labeling for details.

Codeine Phosphate

Crystal

Powder

Acetaminophen and Codeine Phosphate

Oral		
Solution	120 mg/5 mL Acetaminophen and Codeine Phosphate 12 mg/5 mL*	Acetaminophen and Codeine Phosphate Oral Solution (C-V)
Tablets	300 mg Acetaminophen and Codeine Phosphate 15 mg*	Acetaminophen and Codeine Phosphate Tablets (C-III)
	300 mg Acetaminophen and Codeine Phosphate 30 mg*	Acetaminophen and Codeine Phosphate Tablets (C-III)
		Tylenol® with Codeine No. 3 (C-III), Janssen
	300 mg Acetaminophen and Codeine Phosphate 60 mg*	Acetaminophen and Codeine Phosphate Tablets (C-III)
		Tylenol® with Codeine No. 4 (C-III), Janssen

* available from one or more manufacturer, distributor, and/or repackager by generic (nonproprietary) name

Other Codeine Phosphate Combinations

Oral		
Capsules	30 mg with Acetaminophen 300 mg, Butalbital 50 mg, and Caffeine 40 mg*	Butalbital, Acetaminophen, Caffeine, and Codeine Phosphate Capsules (C-III)
		Fioricet® with Codeine (C-III), Actavis
	30 mg with Acetaminophen 325 mg, Butalbital 50 mg, and Caffeine 40 mg*	Butalbital, Acetaminophen, Caffeine, and Codeine Phosphate Capsules (C-III)
	30 mg with Aspirin 325 mg, Butalbital 50 mg, and Caffeine 40 mg*	Ascomp® with Codeine (C-III), Nexgen
		Butalbital, Aspirin, Caffeine, and Codeine Phosphate Capsules (C-III)
		Fiorinal® with Codeine (C-III), Allergan

| Tablets | 16 mg with Aspirin 325 mg and Carisoprodol 200 mg* | **Carisoprodol, Aspirin, and Codeine Phosphate Tablets (C-III)** |
| | | **Soma® Compound with Codeine (C-III), Meda** |

* available from one or more manufacturer, distributor, and/or repackager by generic (nonproprietary) name

Codeine Sulfate

Oral

Tablets	15 mg*	**Codeine Sulfate Tablets (C-II)**
	30 mg*	**Codeine Sulfate Tablets (C-II)**
	60 mg*	**Codeine Sulfate Tablets (C-II)**

* available from one or more manufacturer, distributor, and/or repackager by generic (nonproprietary) name

Selected Revisions April 19, 2023, © Copyright, September 01, 1972, American Society of Health-System Pharmacists, Inc.

fentaNYL, fentaNYL Citrate

28:08.08 • OPIOID AGONISTS

REMS

FDA approved a REMS for fentanyl transdermal systems under a shared REMS system (Opioid Analgesic REMS) to ensure that the benefits outweigh the risks. The REMS may apply to one or more preparations of fentanyl and consists of the following: medication guide and elements to assure safe use. See the FDA REMS page (https://www.accessdata.fda.gov/scripts/cder/rems/index.cfm).

FDA approved a REMS for transmucosal immediate-release fentanyl (TIRF) products under a shared REMS system (TIRF REMS) to ensure that the benefits outweigh the risks. The REMS may apply to one or more preparations of fentanyl and consists of the following: medication guide, elements to assure safe use, and implementation system. See the FDA REMS page (https://www.accessdata.fda.gov/scripts/cder/rems/index.cfm

■ Fentanyl is a synthetic phenylpiperidine-derivative opiate agonist.

USES

● *Pain*

Fentanyl is a strong analgesic used for the management of severe pain. The drug is commercially available in various dosage forms and formulations including immediate-release transmucosal preparations (buccal tablet, transmucosal lozenge), long-acting/extended-release transdermal systems, and a parenteral formulation; FDA-labeled indications and patient populations vary based on the specific preparation.

Pain needs to be appropriately and effectively treated, regardless of whether opioids are part of the treatment regimen. Treatment should be individualized, patient-centered, and include multimodal approaches. Opioids can be essential in the management of pain but are associated with considerable potential harm, including opioid use disorder and overdose. Therefore, safer and more effective treatments should be considered prior to initiating opioid therapy. There are multiple nonpharmacologic treatments (e.g., exercise, physical therapy, psychological therapies) and nonopioid drugs (e.g., serotonin and norepinephrine reuptake inhibitors [SNRIs], gabapentinoids, nonsteroidal anti-inflammatory agents [NSAIAs]) that have been shown to be at least as effective as opioids for many types of common pain conditions. These nonopioid treatments are generally preferred to opioids in most situations. If opioids are used, clinicians should carefully evaluate the risk of opioid-related harms and work with the patient to incorporate appropriate risk-mitigation strategies into the treatment plan, including offering naloxone.

The Centers for Disease Control and Prevention (CDC) clinical guideline for prescribing opioids for pain provides recommendations for the management of acute (duration <1 month), subacute (duration 1–3 months), and chronic (duration >3 months) pain in adults in the outpatient setting. The CDC guideline addresses the following areas: 1) determining whether or not to initiate opioids for pain, 2) selecting opioids and determining opioid dosages, 3) deciding duration of initial opioid prescription and conducting follow-up, and 4) assessing risk and addressing potential harms of opioid use.

Other clinical practice guidelines provide recommendations for the management of specific types of pain including postoperative pain, cancer-related pain, sickle-cell pain, and pain associated with palliative care; although specific recommendations for the management of opioid therapy vary across the guidelines, common elements include risk mitigation strategies, careful dosage titration, and consideration of risks and benefits.

Acute Pain

Fentanyl citrate preservative-free injection is indicated for IV or IM use to provide short durations of analgesia prior to, during, or following surgical procedures. The drug should be administered only by clinicians specifically trained in the use of IV anesthetics and management of the respiratory effects of potent opioids, and in appropriate settings where an opiate antagonist, resuscitative equipment, and oxygen are readily available.

Because of the risk of life-threatening respiratory depression, fentanyl transdermal systems and transmucosal immediate-release preparations (buccal tablets, transmucosal lozenges) are contraindicated in the management of acute or postoperative pain.

CDC guidelines state that nonopioid therapies are at least as effective as opioids for many common types of acute pain (e.g., low back pain, neck pain, pain related to other musculoskeletal injuries). Use of nonpharmacologic therapies (e.g., ice, heat, elevation, rest, immobilization, exercise) and nonopioid pharmacologic therapies (e.g., topical or oral NSAIAs, acetaminophen) should be maximized as appropriate for the specific condition and patient.

Chronic Pain

Fentanyl transdermal system is used for the management of severe and persistent pain in opioid-tolerant patients (adults and pediatric patients 2 through 18 years of age) who require extended treatment with a daily opioid analgesic and for which alternative treatment options are inadequate. Patients are considered opioid-tolerant if they have been receiving at least 60 mg oral morphine per day, 25 mcg transdermal fentanyl per hour, 30 mg oral oxycodone per day, 8 mg oral hydromorphone per day, 25 mg oral oxymorphone per day, 60 mg oral hydrocodone per day, or an equianalgesic dose of another opioid for at least 1 week. Fentanyl transdermal system is a long-acting (extended-release) formulation of fentanyl with complex absorption and pharmacodynamic properties, which can increase the risk of fatal overdose if not used appropriately. Because of the greater risks of overdose and death with extended-release opiate formulations, therapy with fentanyl transdermal system should be reserved for use in patients for whom alternative treatment options (e.g., nonopiate analgesics, immediate-release opiates) are inadequate or not tolerated. Fentanyl transdermal system is contraindicated in patients who are not opiate tolerant, in those who require opiate analgesia for a short period of time, and for the management of acute, mild, intermittent, or postoperative pain. Fentanyl transdermal systems should be prescribed only by qualified clinicians who are experienced in the use of extended-release/long-acting opioids and management of associated risks.

CDC guidelines state that in patients with chronic or subacute pain not associated with active cancer treatment, palliative care, or end-of-life care (also referred to as chronic noncancer pain), nonopioid therapies are preferred. There is insufficient evidence to determine the long-term benefits of opioid therapy for chronic pain, and there is an increased risk for serious harms related to long-term opioid therapy that appears to be dose dependent. Use of opioid analgesics for the management of chronic noncancer pain increased four-fold in the US from 1999 to 2010, along with a parallel increase in overdose deaths, despite uncertainty over the long-term benefits of such therapy. In addition, evidence that opioid analgesics are superior to other pharmacologic or nonpharmacologic treatments for chronic pain generally is lacking. Opioid analgesics should be considered only if other pain management strategies (nonpharmacologic [e.g., exercise, physical therapy] and nonopioid drugs [e.g., NSAIAs, select antidepressants or anticonvulsants, gabapentinoids, lidocaine and capsaicin patches for neuropathic pain]) have been maximized as appropriate for the specific condition and patient, and the expected benefits of opioid analgesics are anticipated to outweigh the risks. If opioid analgesics are used, they should be part of an integrated approach that also includes appropriate nonpharmacologic modalities (e.g., cognitive behavioral therapy, relaxation techniques, biofeedback, functional restoration, exercise therapy, certain interventional procedures) and other appropriate pharmacologic therapies. The lowest-effective dosage of an immediate-release preparation should be used. Clinicians should work with patients to establish treatment goals and also consider how opioid therapy wll be discontinued if the benefits do not outweigh the risks.

The benefits and risks of opioid analgesic therapy should be evaluated within 1–4 weeks following initiation of therapy or an increase in dosage, and reevaluated on an ongoing basis throughout therapy. Monitoring should include documentation of pain intensity and level of functioning, assessment of progress toward therapeutic goals, presence of adverse effects, and adherence to prescribed therapies. Common opioid-related adverse effects (e.g., constipation, nausea and vomiting, cognitive and psychomotor impairment) should be anticipated and appropriately managed.

Patients should be closely monitored for adverse effects and other risks of therapy, including opioid use disorder. Various strategies for managing risks associated with opioid therapy for chronic noncancer pain have been recommended, including written treatment agreements or plans (e.g., "contracts"), urine drug testing, review of state prescription drug monitoring program (PDMP) data, and risk assessment and monitoring tools. Clinicians should offer or arrange treatment for patients with opioid use disorder.

Cancer Pain

The American Society of Clinical Oncology (ASCO) states that opioids should be offered to patients with moderate-to-severe pain associated with cancer or active cancer treatment, unless contraindicated. Prior to initiating opioid therapy, it is useful to assess the mechanism for the pain syndrome (imaging may be required), the response to nonopioid analgesics (e.g., acetaminophen or NSAIAs), and the presence of risk factors such as a history of misuse of alcohol, recreational substances, or prescription drugs. Opioids should be initiated as an immediate-release formulation and as needed to establish an effective dosage. The lowest possible dosage should be used to achieve acceptable analgesia and patient goals, and patients should be assessed early with frequent dosage titration. In patients receiving opioids around the clock, an immediate-release opioid at a dose of 5–20% of the regular morphine equivalent daily dose should be prescribed for breakthrough pain. Evidence remains insufficient to recommend a specific, short-acting opioid for breatkthrough pain.

Fentanyl transdermal system is indicated for the management of severe and persistent pain in opioid tolerant patients (adults and pediatric patients 2 through 18 years of age) who require extended treatment with a daily opioid analgesic, and has been used for pain control in patients with cancer. (See Chronic Pain under Uses.) In clinical studies in patients with cancer, fentanyl transdermal system was administered at dosages of 25–600 mcg/hour for variable periods of time (i.e., periods exceeding 30 days, 4 months, or 1 year in 56, 28, or 10% of patients, respectively, and extending up to 866 days in individual patients). At 1 month following initiation of transdermal fentanyl therapy, pain intensity generally was less than that reported with the oral morphine regimen used prior to the study.

Fentanyl citrate immediate-release transmucosal formulations (buccal tablets, transmucosal lozenges) are indicated for the management of breakthrough pain in cancer patients who are already being treated with, and are tolerant of, opiates used around the clock for persistent cancer pain. The fentanyl preparation labeled as Fentora® is indicated for use in adults 18 years of age or older, and the fentanyl preparation labeled as Actiq® is labeled for use in patients 16 years of age or older. Patients are considered opiate tolerant if they have been receiving around-the-clock opiate therapy consisting of at least 60 mg of oral morphine sulfate daily, 25 mcg of transdermal fentanyl per hour, 30 mg of oral oxycodone daily, 8 mg of oral hydromorphone hydrochloride daily, 25 mg of oral oxymorphone hydrochloride daily, or an equianalgesic dosage of another opiate daily for at least 1 week. Patients must continue around-the-clock opiate analgesic therapy while receiving these transmucosal immediate-release preparations for the relief of breakthrough pain. Because of the risk of fatal or life-threatening respiratory depression, fentanyl citrate buccal tablets and transmucosal lozenges are contraindicated in the management of acute or postoperative pain and in patients who are not opiate tolerant. In addition, these formulations should be administered only under the supervision of qualified clinicians who are trained in the use of IV anesthetics and management of respiratory effects of potent opioids. *Substantial pharmacokinetic differences exist among these transmucosal immediate-release formulations of fentanyl, and between these formulations and other preparations of the drug; these differences could result in clinically important differences in the rate and extent of absorption. Therefore, these fentanyl products should not be used interchangeably (e.g., on a mcg-per-mcg basis) or substituted with any other fentanyl products.* Fatal overdosage may occur if these formulations are substituted on a mcg-per-mcg basis for any other fentanyl preparation.

In clinical studies in opiate-tolerant adults with breakthrough cancer pain, transmucosal immediate-release fentanyl formulations have been shown to provide substantially more pain relief than placebo. In studies with fentanyl citrate buccal tablets and transmucosal lozenges, approximately 65–70% of patients successfully achieved an adequate dose during the titration period. Fentanyl doses evaluated in these studies ranged from 100–800 mcg as the buccal tablets and 200–1600 mcg as the transmucosal lozenges.

Pain in Critically Ill Patients

Fentanyl also has been used for the management of pain in critically ill patients in the intensive care unit (ICU). Opioid agonists may be used in combination with sedative agents to maintain an optimal level of comfort and safety in patients in a critical care setting. To ensure consistent analgesic therapy, a therapeutic plan and goal of analgesia should be established for each patient. There are important safety concerns with opioids, such as sedation, delirium, respiratory depression, ileus, and immunosuppression, that should be considered in ICU patients. A multimodal analgesic approach generally is used to reduce opioid requirements and optimize patient outcomes and has included the use of nonopioid analgesics such as acetaminophen, ketamine, lidocaine, neuropathic agents, and NSAIAs.

• Anesthesia

Fentanyl citrate preservative-free injection is indicated for IV or IM use as an adjunct in the maintenance of general or regional anesthesia. When attenuation of the response to surgical stress is especially important, fentanyl citrate may be administered with oxygen and a skeletal muscle relaxant to provide anesthesia without the use of additional anesthetic agents. Fentanyl citrate injection should be administered only by clinicians specifically trained in the use of IV anesthetics and management of the respiratory effects of potent opioids, and in appropriate settings where resuscitative equipment and oxygen are readily available.

DOSAGE AND ADMINISTRATION

• General

Pretreatment Screening

- Prior to initiation, carefully evaluate risks and benefits of opioid therapy, and assess for opioid-related harms (e.g., addiction, abuse, misuse). Incorporate risk mitigation strategies into the treatment plan, including offering naloxone. Consider a discontinuation plan in case treatment needs to be withdrawn if benefits do not outweigh risks.

- Review the patient's history of controlled substance prescriptions using state prescription drug monitoring program (PDMP) data to determine whether the patient is receiving opioid dosages or combinations that put the patient at high risk for overdose.

- Screen patients for sleep-related breathing disorders including central sleep apnea and sleep-related hypoxemia.

Patient Monitoring

- When opioids are used for subacute or chronic pain, evaluate the benefits and risks within 1–4 weeks following initiation of therapy or an increase in dosage, and re-evaluate on an ongoing basis.

- Monitor patients closely for signs of sedation and respiratory depression, particularly when initiating therapy and following dosage increases.

- Monitor and manage common adverse effects of opioid therapy (e.g., constipation, nausea and vomiting, cognitive and psychomotor impairment).

Dispensing and Administration Precautions

- Based on the Institute for Safe Medication Practices (ISMP) fentanyl is a high-alert medication that has a heightened risk of causing significant patient harm when used in error.

Handling and Disposal

- Advise patients to store opioids in a secure and preferably locked location and discuss options for safe disposal of unused opioids. Accidental ingestion or exposure has resulted in fatal overdose.

Administration Precautions for Transmucosal Immediate-release Fentanyl (TIRF) Preparations

- Do not convert patients on a mcg-per-mcg basis from any other fentanyl products and do not substitute with any other fentanyl products.

Administration Precautions for Fentanyl Transdermal System

- Should be prescribed only by healthcare providers knowledgeable about the use of extended-release/long-acting opioids and how to manage associated risks.

- Exposure of the fentanyl transdermal system application site and surrounding area to direct external heat sources has resulted in fatal overdose of fentanyl. Warn patients to avoid exposing the application site and surrounding area to direct external heat sources.

REMS

TIRF REMS

- Because of the risk of accidental exposure, misuse, abuse, addiction, and overdosage, transmucosal immediate-release fentanyl (TIRF) preparations (transmucosal lozenges, buccal tablets) are available only through a restricted distribution program under the TIRF REMS Access program.

- Outpatients who receive transmucosal immediate-release fentanyl preparations, clinicians who prescribe these preparations, and pharmacies, wholesalers, and distributors that dispense or distribute these preparations must enroll in the program. Prescribers must document opioid tolerance and outpatient pharmacies must verify such documentation with each prescription; inpatient pharmacies must develop policies and procedures to verify opioid tolerance in patients who require these preparations while hospitalized.

- Additional information available at https://www.tirfremsaccess.com or 866-822-1483.

Opioid Analgesic REMS

- FDA approved a REMS for fentanyl transdermal system under a shared REMS system (Opioid Analgesic REMS).

- The goals are to reduce the occurrence of addiction, unintentional overdosage, and death resulting from inappropriate prescribing, misuse, and abuse of opioid analgesics.

- The REMS program consists of educational programs for healthcare professionals, a patient counseling guide, and a product-specific medication guide for patients.

- Additional information available at https://opioidanalgesicrems.com or 1-800-503-0784.

● Administration

Fentanyl citrate injection is administered parenterally (IV or IM).

Fentanyl citrate buccal tablets and transmucosal lozenges are administered intrabuccally. Once an effective dose is determined, the buccal tablets may be administered sublingually as an alternate route of administration.

Fentanyl transdermal systems are applied topically to the skin.

Parenteral Administration

Fentanyl citrate injection is administered parenterally (IV or IM). The drug also has been administered by continuous IV infusion† or via patient controlled analgesia (PCA)†.

Preservative-free injections of fentanyl citrate also have been administered epidurally†; specialized techniques are required for administration of the drug by this route, and such administration should be performed only by qualified individuals familiar with the techniques of administration, dosages, and special patient management problems associated with epidural fentanyl citrate administration.

An opiate antagonist and facilities for administration of oxygen and respiratory support should be available during and immediately following IV administration of fentanyl.

Standardize 4 Safety

Standardized concentrations for fentanyl have been established through Standardize 4 Safety (S4S), a national patient safety initiative to reduce medication errors, especially during transitions of care. Multidisciplinary expert panels were convened to determine recommended standard concentrations. Because recommendations from the S4S panels may differ from the manufacturer's prescribing

information, caution is advised when using concentrations that differ from labeling, particularly when using rate information from the label. For additional information on S4S (including updates that may be available), see https://www.ashp.org/pharmacy-practice/standardize-4-safety-initiative

TABLE 1. Standardize 4 Safety Continuous IV Infusion Standard Concentrations for Fentanyl

Patient Population	Concentration Standards	Dosing Units
Adults[a]	10 mcg/mL	mcg/hour
	50 mcg/mL	
Pediatric patients (<50 kg)	10 mcg/mL[b]	mcg/kg/hour
	50 mcg/mL	

[a] These concentrations are for continuous infusions not delivered by a PCA device
[b] Babies under 500 g may require a lower concentration

TABLE 2. Standardize 4 Safety PCA Standard Concentrations for Fentanyl

Patient Population	Concentration Standards	Dosing Units
Adults	10 mcg/mL	mcg/kg/hour
	50 mcg/mL	
Pediatric patients (<50 kg)	10 mcg/mL	mcg/kg/hour
	50 mcg/mL	

TABLE 3. Standardize 4 Safety Epidural Standard Concentrations for Fentanyl as a Single Drug

Patient Population	Concentration standard
Adults	2 mcg/mL
	5 mcg/mL
	10 mcg/mL
Pediatric patients (<50 kg)	0.3 mcg/mL
	2 mcg/mL
	5 mcg/mL

TABLE 4. Standardize 4 Safety ADULT Epidural Combination Drug Standard Concentrations for Fentanyl

Drug Combinations	Anesthetic Concentration	Narcotic Concentration	Alpha Agonist Concentration
Bupivacaine with fentanyl	1. Bupivacaine 0.0625%	1. Fentanyl 2 mcg/mL	
	2. Bupivacaine 0.0625%	2. Fentanyl 5 mcg/mL	
	3. Bupivacaine 0.125%	3. Fentanyl 2 mcg/mL	
	4. Bupivacaine 0.125%	4. Fentanyl 5 mcg/mL	
Bupivacaine with fentanyl and clonidine	1. Bupivacaine 0.0625%	1. Fentanyl 2 mcg/mL	1. Clonidine 1 mcg/mL
	2. Bupivacaine 0.0625%	2. Fentanyl 5 mcg/mL	2. Clonidine 1 mcg/mL
	3. Bupivacaine 0.125%	3. Fentanyl 2 mcg/mL	3. Clonidine 1 mcg/mL
	4. Bupivacaine 0.125%	4. Fentanyl 5 mcg/mL	4. Clonidine 1 mcg/mL

TABLE 4. Continued

Drug Combinations	Anesthetic Concentration	Narcotic Concentration	Alpha Agonist Concentration
Ropivacaine with fentanyl	1. Ropivacaine 0.1%	1. Fentanyl 2 mcg/mL	
	2. Ropivacaine 0.1%	2. Fentanyl 5 mcg/mL	
	3. Ropivacaine 0.2%	3. Fentanyl 2 mcg/mL	
	4. Ropivacaine 0.2%	4. Fentanyl 5 mcg/mL	
Ropivacaine with fentanyl and clonidine	1. Ropivacaine 0.1%	1. Fentanyl 2 mcg/mL	1. Clonidine 0.3 mcg/mL
	2. Ropivacaine 0.1%	2. Fentanyl 2 mcg/mL	2. Clonidine 0.5 mcg/mL
	3. Ropivacaine 0.2%	3. Fentanyl 2 mcg/mL	3. Clonidine 0.3 mcg/mL
	4. Ropivacaine 0.2%	4. Fentanyl 2 mcg/mL	4. Clonidine 0.5 mcg/mL

TABLE 5. Standardize 4 Safety PEDIATRIC (<50 kg) Epidural Combination Drug Standard Concentrations for Fentanyl

Drug Combinations	Anesthetic Concentration	Narcotic Concentration	Alpha Agonist Concentration
Bupivacaine with fentanyl	1. Bupivacaine 0.0625%	1. Fentanyl 2 mcg/mL	
	2. Bupivacaine 0.0625%	2. Fentanyl 5 mcg/mL	
	3. Bupivacaine 0.125%	3. Fentanyl 2 mcg/mL	
	4. Bupivacaine 0.125%	4. Fentanyl 5 mcg/mL	
Bupivacaine with fentanyl and clonidine	1. Bupivacaine 0.0625%	1. Fentanyl 2 mcg/mL	1. Clonidine 0.3 mcg/mL
	2. Bupivacaine 0.0625%	2. Fentanyl 2 mcg/mL	2. Clonidine 0.5 mcg/mL
	3. Bupivacaine 0.125%	3. Fentanyl 2 mcg/mL	3. Clonidine 0.3 mcg/mL
	4. Bupivacaine 0.125%	4. Fentanyl 2 mcg/mL	4. Clonidine 0.5 mcg/mL
Ropivacaine with fentanyl	1. Ropivacaine 0.1%	1. Fentanyl 2 mcg/mL	
	2. Ropivacaine 0.1%	2. Fentanyl 5 mcg/mL	
	3. Ropivacaine 0.2%	3. Fentanyl 2 mcg/mL	
	4. Ropivacaine 0.2%	4. Fentanyl 5 mcg/mL	
Ropivacaine with fentanyl and clonidine	1. Ropivacaine 0.1%	1. Fentanyl 2 mcg/mL	1. Clonidine 0.3 mcg/mL
	2. Ropivacaine 0.1%	2. Fentanyl 2 mcg/mL	2. Clonidine 0.5 mcg/mL
	3. Ropivacaine 0.2%	3. Fentanyl 2 mcg/mL	3. Clonidine 0.3 mcg/mL
	4. Ropivacaine 0.2%	4. Fentanyl 2 mcg/mL	4. Clonidine 0.5 mcg/mL

Intrabuccal Administration

Transmucosal Lozenges

When fentanyl citrate transmucosal lozenges are used, the package should be cut open with scissors just prior to administration. The lozenge should be placed in the patient's mouth (between the cheek and the lower gum) using the handle and the patient should be instructed to suck, and *not* bite or chew, the lozenge; efficacy may be reduced if the lozenge is chewed and swallowed rather than being administered as directed. The lozenge occasionally may be moved from one side to the other using the handle. Transmucosal lozenges of fentanyl citrate usually should be consumed over a period of 15 minutes; longer or shorter consumption times may result in reduced efficacy compared with that reported in clinical trials.

If signs of excessive opiate effects develop before the transmucosal lozenge is consumed completely, the remaining portion should be removed from the patient's mouth immediately, and future doses should be decreased.

After consumption of a lozenge unit is complete and the lozenge matrix is totally dissolved, the handle should be disposed of in a trash container that is out of the reach of children; any drug matrix remaining on the handle can be removed by placing the handle under hot running tap water until the drug matrix is completely dissolved. While all units should be disposed of immediately after use, unused portions of the preparation represent a special risk, since they are no longer protected by the child-resistant blister package, and they still may contain sufficient amounts of the drug to be fatal to a child. If unused portions of the drug cannot be disposed of immediately, they should be stored in a temporary storage bottle (supplied by the manufacturer). Consult manufacturer's prescribing information for additional details on proper storage and disposal.

Buccal Tablets

When fentanyl citrate buccal tablets are used, separate a single blister unit by bending and tearing along the blister card perforations immediately prior to administration. Peel back the blister backing to expose the tablet. The buccal tablet should not be pushed through the blister, since this may damage the buccal tablet. The buccal tablet should be placed in the patient's buccal cavity (above a rear molar, between the upper cheek and gum); alternatively, once an effective dose has been established, the tablet may be administered sublingually. The patient should be instructed *not* to split, crush, suck, chew, or swallow the tablet; efficacy may be reduced if the buccal tablet is not administered as directed. The buccal tablet should be left between the patient's upper cheek and gum or under the tongue until it has disintegrated (generally 14–25 minutes); the disintegration time does not appear to affect early systemic exposure to the drug. If the buccal tablet has not completely disintegrated after 30 minutes, the remnants may be swallowed with a glass of water. Patients should be instructed to alternate sides of the mouth with each intrabuccal dose.

If signs of excessive opiate effects develop before the buccal tablet has disintegrated completely, the remaining portion should be removed from the patient's mouth immediately, and future doses should be decreased.

Consult manufacturer's prescribing information for additional details on proper storage and disposal.

Sublingual Administration

The manufacturer states that fentanyl citrate buccal tablets also may be administered sublingually once an effective dose of the drug has been established.

Transdermal Administration

Patients receiving fentanyl transdermal systems should be carefully instructed in the proper use and disposal of the transdermal system.

To expose the adhesive surface of the system, the protective-liner covering should be peeled and discarded just prior to application. The transdermal system is applied to a dry, intact, nonirritated, nonirradiated flat surface on the chest, back, flank, or upper arm by firmly pressing the system with the palm of the hand for 30 seconds with the adhesive side touching the skin and ensuring that contact is complete, particularly around the edges. When the transdermal system is applied to young children or to individuals with cognitive impairment, the system should be placed on the upper back to reduce the risk that the system could be removed and placed in the mouth. The transdermal system should *not* be used if the seal of the package is broken or if the system is cut, damaged, or altered in any way.

Hair at the application site should be clipped, not shaved, prior to application of the transdermal system. If the site must be cleansed prior to application, only clear water should be used. Soaps, oils, lotions, alcohol, or any other agents that could irritate the skin or alter its characteristics should *not* be used.

Patients or caregivers who apply the transdermal system should wash their hands with soap and water immediately after application. Contact with unwashed or unclothed application sites can result in secondary exposure to the drug and should be avoided. If a transdermal system accidentally adheres to the skin of another person, the system should be removed immediately, the area should be washed with water, and medical attention for the exposed person should be sought immediately.

Patients may bathe, shower, or swim while wearing a transdermal system. However, they should be advised to avoid sunbathing, taking hot baths, engaging in strenuous exercise that increases core body temperature, or exposing the application site and surrounding area to direct external heat sources (e.g., heating pads, electric blankets, heat or tanning lamps, saunas, hot tubs, heated water beds) while wearing the transdermal system, since temperature-dependent increases in percutaneous absorption of fentanyl from the system are possible under such conditions and may result in fatal overdosage.

Each fentanyl transdermal system may be worn continuously for 72 hours; subsequent systems should be applied to a different site after removal of the previous system. If a system should inadvertently come off during the period of use, a new system may be applied to a different skin site and left in place for 72 hours. Patients who experience difficulty with system adhesion should be advised that they may tape the edges of the system in place with first-aid tape. If adhesion problems persist, patients may apply a transparent adhesive film dressing (e.g., Bioclusive®, Askina®) over the system.

● Dosage

Dosage of fentanyl and fentanyl citrate is expressed in terms of fentanyl. The drug should be given at the lowest effective dosage and for the shortest duration of therapy consistent with the treatment goals of the patient. Reduced dosage is indicated initially in poor-risk patients and geriatric patients. Dosage of fentanyl should be titrated carefully in geriatric patients. If concomitant therapy with other CNS depressants is required, the lowest effective dosages and shortest possible duration of concomitant therapy should be used.

Parenteral Dosage

For use as a preoperative medication in adults, 50–100 mcg of fentanyl may be administered IM 30–60 minutes prior to surgery.

As an adjunct to general anesthesia, fentanyl may be given in low-dose, moderate-dose, or high-dose regimens. In the low-dose regimen, which is used for minor but painful surgical procedures, an IV dose of 2 mcg/kg is administered; additional doses are usually not necessary. In the moderate-dose regimen, which is used in more major surgical procedures, an initial IV dose of 2–20 mcg/kg is administered; additional doses of 25–100 mcg may be given IV or IM as necessary. In the high-dose regimen, which may be used during open heart surgery or certain complicated neurosurgical or orthopedic procedures where surgery is more prolonged, an initial IV dose of 20–50 mcg/kg may be given; additional doses ranging from 25 mcg to one-half the initial dose may be administered as necessary.

To provide general anesthesia without additional anesthetic agents when attenuation of the response to surgical stress is especially important, fentanyl doses of 50–100 mcg/kg may be administered IV in conjunction with oxygen and a skeletal muscle relaxant; in some cases, doses up to 150 mcg/kg may be required.

As an adjunct to regional anesthesia, 50–100 mcg of fentanyl may be administered by IM injection or by slow IV injection over 1–2 minutes when additional analgesia is required.

For the control of postoperative pain, restlessness, tachypnea, and emergence delirium, 50–100 mcg of the drug may be administered IM every 1–2 hours as needed.

During the induction and maintenance phases of general anesthesia in children 2–12 years of age, the manufacturer recommends an IV fentanyl dose of 2–3 mcg/kg. Other experts suggest a 2–3 mcg/kg IV bolus, followed by a 1-3 mcg/kg/hour continuous IV infusion.

For analgesia in children <50 kg, experts recommend a pediatric dosage of 0.5–1 mcg/kg IV or IM, repeated every 1–2 hours as needed, or continuous IV infusion of 0.5–1.5 mcg/kg per hour. For children >50 kg, a dose of 0.5–1 mcg/kg IV or IM, repeated every 1–2 hours as needed, or continuous IV infusion of 0.5–1.5 mcg/kg per hour is recommended.

Intrabuccal Dosage
Transmucosal Lozenges

Dosage of transmucosal fentanyl citrate lozenges (Actiq®, generic oral transmucosal fentanyl citrate lozenge) should be individualized based on clinical response to provide adequate analgesia and to minimize adverse effects.

When transmucosal lozenges of fentanyl citrate are used for the management of breakthrough cancer pain in adults who are already receiving and are tolerant of opiates used for chronic cancer pain, the initial recommended dose is 200 mcg (of fentanyl) in all patients. Because of differences in pharmacokinetic properties, patients should not be switched on a mcg-per-mcg basis from any other fentanyl preparation, including fentanyl citrate transmucosal tablets (Fentora®), to the transmucosal lozenges, since the transmucosal lozenges are not equivalent to other fentanyl preparations and are not a generic version of the buccal tablets. The manufacturer recommends that a total of 6 lozenges be prescribed initially and that all 6 lozenges be used before the dose of fentanyl is increased. Until the appropriate dose of fentanyl citrate is attained, it may be necessary to use more than one lozenge per episode of breakthrough cancer pain; the additional lozenge may be administered 15 minutes after the previous lozenge has been consumed (i.e., 30 minutes after the first lozenge initially was placed in the mouth). The manufacturer states that, during the dosage titration phase, a maximum of 2 lozenges per breakthrough pain episode may be given, if necessary. If several consecutive breakthrough cancer pain episodes occur that require the use of more than one lozenge per episode, the dose should be increased to the next higher available strength, again prescribing only 6 lozenges.

During the titration phase, each new dose should be evaluated over several breakthrough cancer pain episodes to determine efficacy and tolerability of the drug. Patients should be instructed to record their use of transmucosal lozenges over several episodes of breakthrough pain and to discuss their experience with their clinician to decide whether dosage adjustment is warranted. To reduce the risk of overdosage, patients should have only one strength of the transmucosal lozenges available for use at any one time.

Once the patient has been titrated to an adequate fentanyl dose (average breakthrough pain episode is treated with a single lozenge), the patient should use only one lozenge of the appropriate strength per episode of breakthrough pain. On occasion during maintenance therapy, when a breakthrough pain episode is not relieved within 15 minutes after the previous lozenge was consumed (i.e., 30 minutes after the first lozenge initially was placed in the mouth), the patient may take only one additional dose of the same strength during that episode of breakthrough pain.

Patients should be instructed that, after treating one episode of breakthrough pain with fentanyl citrate transmucosal lozenges, they must wait at least 4 hours before taking an additional dose of the transmucosal lozenges to treat a subsequent episode of breakthrough pain.

During maintenance therapy, dosage adjustment may be necessary to ensure that an appropriate dosage is maintained; however, dosage generally should be increased only if several consecutive episodes require administration of more than one lozenge of the current dose for pain relief. If the patient experiences more than 4 breakthrough pain episodes daily, the dosage of the maintenance opioid used around the clock for persistent cancer pain should be reevaluated.

When opioid therapy is no longer required, consider discontinuing the transmucosal lozenges along with a gradual downward tapering (titration) of other opioids to minimize possible withdrawal effects. In patients who continue to take their chronic opioid therapy for persistent pain but no longer require treatment for breakthrough pain, therapy with the transmucosal lozenges can usually be discontinued immediately.

In clinical trials, geriatric patients (older than 65 years of age) were titrated to an adequate dose of fentanyl citrate transmucosal lozenges that generally was about 200 mcg (of fentanyl) lower than the dose required in younger patients.

Buccal Tablets

For the management of breakthrough pain in adults who are already receiving and are tolerant of opiates used for the management of chronic cancer pain, the recommended initial dose of fentanyl citrate buccal tablets (Fentora®) is 100 mcg in all patients except those being switched from fentanyl citrate transmucosal lozenges (Actiq®). In patients being switched from the transmucosal lozenges to the buccal tablets, the initial dose of the buccal tablets should be based on the current transmucosal lozenge dose. Because of differences in pharmacokinetic properties, patients should not be switched on a mcg-per-mcg basis from any other fentanyl preparation to the buccal tablets, since the buccal tablets are not equivalent to other fentanyl preparations. For opiate-tolerant adults who are being transferred from fentanyl citrate transmucosal lozenges to fentanyl citrate buccal tablets for the management of breakthrough cancer pain, the increased bioavailability of the buccal tablets must be considered. Fatal overdosage may occur if the preparations are substituted on a mcg-per-mcg basis or substituted with any other fentanyl preparation.

The manufacturer's dosage conversion recommendations for patients being transferred from the transmucosal lozenges to the buccal tablets are shown in Table 6. The manufacturer states that these doses should be considered starting doses for the buccal tablets and are not intended to represent equianalgesic doses. If the patient previously received 600 mcg or more of fentanyl daily as the transmucosal lozenges, therapy with the buccal tablets should be initiated using the 200-mcg strength of buccal tablets, and dosage should be titrated in multiples of this tablet strength. Patients being transferred from the transmucosal lozenges to the buccal tablets should be instructed to discontinue use of the transmucosal lozenges and to dispose of any remaining lozenges.

TABLE 6. Initial Dosage Recommendations for Adults Being Transferred from Fentanyl Citrate Transmucosal Lozenges to Fentanyl Citrate Buccal Tablets for Management of Breakthrough Cancer Pain

Current Fentanyl Dose Administered as Transmucosal Lozenge	Initial Fentanyl Dose Administered as Buccal Tablet
200 mcg	100 mcg (as one 100-mcg tablet)
400 mcg	100 mcg (as one 100-mcg tablet)
600 mcg	200 mcg (as one 200-mcg tablet)
800 mcg	200 mcg (as one 200-mcg tablet)
1200 mcg	400 mcg (as two 200-mcg tablets)
1600 mcg	400 mcg (as two 200-mcg tablets)

If breakthrough pain is not relieved within 30 minutes following the initial dose of fentanyl citrate buccal tablets, the patient may take *only one* additional dose of the same strength during that episode of breakthrough pain. Patients should be instructed that, after treating one episode of breakthrough pain with fentanyl citrate buccal tablets, they must wait at least 4 hours before treating a subsequent episode of breakthrough pain with the buccal tablets.

Dosage should be titrated with close monitoring to a level that provides adequate analgesia with acceptable adverse effects. Patients should be instructed to record their use of buccal tablets over several episodes of breakthrough pain and to discuss their experience with their clinician to decide whether dosage adjustment is warranted. Patients receiving an initial dose of 100 mcg who require titration to a higher dosage level may be instructed to increase the dose to 200 mcg (two 100-mcg tablets, with one tablet placed on each side of the mouth in the buccal cavity) with the next episode of breakthrough pain. Patients who require a further increase in dosage may be instructed to place two 100-mcg tablets on each side of the mouth in the buccal cavity (total of four 100-mcg tablets). If doses exceeding 400 mcg (i.e., doses of 600 or 800 mcg) are required, dosage should be titrated using multiples of 200-mcg tablets. During dosage titration, one dose may include administration of 1–4 tablets of the same strength. No more than 4 tablets should be administered simultaneously. The manufacturer states that the only time that patients should take more than one tablet as a single dose (e.g., two 100-mcg tablets for a single 200-mcg dose) is during dosage titration.

During the dosage titration period, if breakthrough pain is not relieved within 30 minutes following the initial dose of fentanyl citrate buccal tablets, the patient may take *only one* additional dose of the same strength during that episode of breakthrough pain. The manufacturer states that no more than 2 doses of the buccal tablet formulation may be given during a single episode of breakthrough pain, even if the patient continues to experience pain after the second dose is administered. To reduce the risk of overdosage during titration, patients should be strongly advised to use or discard all the buccal tablets of one strength prior to obtaining tablets of a different strength. During the dosage titration phase, each new dose should be evaluated over several breakthrough cancer pain episodes to determine efficacy and tolerability of the drug.

Once the patient has been titrated to an adequate fentanyl dose, breakthrough pain episodes generally should be treated effectively with a single buccal tablet. The manufacturer states that sublingual administration of the buccal tablets is an alternative to intrabuccal administration once an effective dose has been established. On occasion during maintenance therapy, when a breakthrough pain episode is not relieved within 30 minutes after the first intrabuccal dose, the patient may take *only one* additional dose of the same strength during that episode of breakthrough pain. Some patients may require adjustment of the intrabuccal fentanyl dosage to maintain effective analgesia for breakthrough pain episodes; however, dosage generally should be increased only if several consecutive episodes require administration of more than one intrabuccal dose for pain relief. Patients should be instructed that, after treating one episode of breakthrough pain with fentanyl citrate buccal tablets, they must wait at least 4 hours before taking an additional dose of the buccal tablets to treat a subsequent episode of breakthrough cancer pain. If after increasing the dosage, unacceptable opioid-related adverse reactions are observed (including an increase in pain after dosage increase), consider reducing the dosage. Adjust the dosage to obtain an appropriate balance between management of pain and opioid-related adverse reactions. If the patient experiences more than 4 breakthrough pain episodes daily, the dosage of opiates used around the clock for chronic cancer pain should be reevaluated.

For patients no longer requiring opioid therapy, consider discontinuing fentanyl citrate buccal tablets along with a gradual downward tapering (titration) of other opioids to minimize possible withdrawal effects. In patients who continue to take their chronic opioid therapy for persistent pain but no longer require treatment for breakthrough pain, fentanyl citrate buccal tablets therapy can usually be discontinued immediately.

In a limited number of patients, the presence of grade 1 mucositis did not appear to substantially alter fentanyl absorption or adverse effects following intrabuccal administration of the tablets.

In clinical trials, the dosage of fentanyl citrate buccal tablets (following titration to an adequate dose) tended to be slightly lower in geriatric (older than 65 years of age) patients than in younger patients.

Transdermal Dosage

Transdermal System

Appropriate dosage selection and titration of fentanyl transdermal systems are essential to reduce the risk of respiratory depression. The initial dosage must be individualized, taking into account the patient's prior analgesic use and risk factors for addiction, abuse, and misuse.

The manufacturers provide specific dosage recommendations for switching opiate-tolerant children and adults from therapy with certain oral or parenteral opiates to therapy with fentanyl transdermal system (see Table 7 and Table 8).

TABLE 7. Dosage of Fentanyl Transdermal System Based on Current Oral Opiate Dosage

Daily Dosage of Oral Opiate (in mg/day)	Transdermal Fentanyl (in mcg/hr)
Morphine sulfate	
60–134	25
135–224	50
225–314	75
315–404	100
Oxycodone hydrochloride	
30–67	25
67.5–112	50
112.5–157	75
157.5–202	100

TABLE 7. Continued

Daily Dosage of Oral Opiate (in mg/day)	Transdermal Fentanyl (in mcg/hr)
Codeine phosphate	
150–447	25
Hydromorphone hydrochloride	
8–17	25
17.1–28	50
28.1–39	75
39.1–51	100
Methadone hydrochloride	
20–44	25
45–74	50
75–104	75
105–134	100

TABLE 8. Dosage of Fentanyl Transdermal System Based on Current Parenteral Opiate Dosage

Daily Dosage of Parenteral Opiate (in mg/day)	Transdermal Fentanyl (in mcg/hr)
Morphine sulfate IV/IM	
10–22	25
23–37	50
38–52	75
53–67	100
Hydromorphone hydrochloride IV	
1.5–3.4	25
3.5–5.6	50
5.7–7.9	75
8–10	100
Meperidine hydrochloride IM	
75–165	25
166–278	50
279–390	75
391–503	100

Alternatively, to switch patients who currently are receiving other opiate therapy or dosages that are not listed in Table 7 or 8 to therapy with fentanyl transdermal system, the manufacturers state that the opiate analgesic requirements during the previous 24 hours should be calculated, an equianalgesic 24-hour dosage of oral morphine sulfate should be calculated using a reliable source, and the initial dosage of fentanyl transdermal system should be determined using Table 9. For transdermal dosages exceeding labeled delivery rates of 100 mcg/hour, multiple systems can be applied at different sites simultaneously.

TABLE 9. Dosage of Fentanyl Transdermal System Based on Daily Oral Morphine Equivalence

Oral 24-hr Morphine Sulfate (in mg/day)	Transdermal Fentanyl (in mcg/hr)
60–134	25
135–224	50
225–314	75
315–404	100
405–494	125
495–584	150
585–674	175
675–764	200
765–854	225
855–944	250
945–1034	275
1035–1124	300

The manufacturers consider the recommended initial dosages of transdermal fentanyl in Tables 7, 8, and 9 to be conservative estimates. *The dosage conversion guidelines in these tables should not be used to switch patients from therapy with fentanyl transdermal system to therapy with oral or parenteral opiates, since dosage of oral or parenteral opiates may be overestimated.* In clinical trials, the dosage conversion guidelines in these tables were used as a basis for switching patients to therapy with fentanyl transdermal system.

Dosage of transdermal fentanyl should be titrated to a level that provides adequate analgesia and minimizes adverse effects. Patients should be reevaluated continually for adequacy of pain control and for adverse effects, as well as for the development of addiction, abuse, or misuse. Frequent communication is important among the prescriber, other members of the healthcare team, the patient, and the patient's caregiver or family during periods of changing analgesic requirements, including the initial dosage titration period. During long-term therapy, the continued need for opiate analgesics should be continually reevaluated.

Most patients maintain adequate pain control with fentanyl transdermal systems applied at 72-hour intervals, although some patients may require application of the systems at 48-hour intervals. However, dosing intervals of less than 72 hours have not been evaluated in children and adolescents and therefore cannot be recommended for use in this population. Before shortening the dosing interval in patients not responding adequately to a given dosage, an increase in dosage should be evaluated so that patients can be maintained on a 72-hour regimen if possible. Supplemental doses of a short-acting opiate analgesic should be used as needed during the initial application period and subsequently thereafter as necessary to relieve breakthrough pain.

The initial transdermal dosage may be increased after 3 days based on the daily dose of supplemental opiate analgesics during the second or third day after initial application. Because subsequent equilibrium with an increased dose may require up to 6 days to achieve, the manufacturers recommend that further upward titration in dosage based on supplemental opiate analgesic requirements be made no more frequently than every 6 days (i.e., after two 72-hour application periods with a given dosage). The manufacturers recommend that conversion of supplemental opiate requirements to transdermal fentanyl dosage be based on a ratio of 45 mg of oral morphine sulfate (during a 24-hour period) to each 12-mcg/hour of transdermal fentanyl. If unacceptable adverse effects are observed, subsequent dosage should be decreased. Adjust the dose to obtain an appropriate balance between management of pain and opioid-related adverse reactions.

Do not abruptly discontinue fentanyl transdermal system in patients who may be physically dependent on opioids as rapid discontinuation has resulted in serious withdrawal symptoms, uncontrolled pain, and suicide. Rapid discontinuation has also been associated with attempts to find other sources of opioid analgesics, which may be confused with drug seeking for abuse.

When a decision has been made to decrease the dose or discontinue therapy in an opioid-dependent patient using fentanyl transdermal system, consider the total daily dose of opioid (including fentanyl transdermal system) the patient has been using, the duration of treatment, the type of pain being treated, and the physical and psychological attributes of the patient. When opioid analgesics are being discontinued due to a suspected substance use disorder, evaluate and treat the patient, or refer for evaluation and treatment of the substance use disorder. Treatment should include evidence-based approaches, such as medication assisted treatment of opioid use disorder; complex patients with comorbid pain and substance use disorders may benefit from referral to a specialist.

There are no standard opioid tapering schedules that are suitable for all patients. Good clinical practice dictates a patient-specific plan to taper the dose of the opioid gradually. For patients on fentanyl transdermal system who are physically opioid-dependent, initiate the taper by a small enough increment (e.g., no greater than 25% of the total daily dose) to avoid withdrawal symptoms, and proceed with dose-lowering at an interval of every 2 to 4 weeks. Patients who have been taking opioids for briefer periods of time may tolerate a more rapid taper.

It may be necessary to provide the patient with a lower dosage strength to accomplish a successful taper. Reassess the patient frequently to manage pain and withdrawal symptoms (restlessness, lacrimation, rhinorrhea, yawning, perspiration, chills, myalgia, and mydriasis), should they emerge. Other signs and symptoms also may develop, including irritability, anxiety, backache, joint pain, weakness, abdominal cramps, insomnia, nausea, anorexia, vomiting, diarrhea, or increased blood pressure, respiratory rate, or heart rate. If withdrawal symptoms arise, it may be necessary to pause the taper for a period of time or raise the dose of the opioid analgesic to the previous dose, and then proceed with a slower taper. In addition, evaluate patients for any changes in mood, emergence of suicidal thoughts, or use of other substances.

When managing patients taking opioid analgesics, particularly those who have been treated for an extended period of time and/or with high doses for chronic pain, ensure that a multimodal approach to pain management, including mental health support (if needed), is in place prior to initiating an opioid analgesic taper.

● **Special Populations**

Hepatic Impairment

In patients with mild to moderate hepatic impairment, the initial dosage of fentanyl transdermal system should be reduced by 50%, and such patients should be monitored closely for sedation and respiratory depression, including after each increase in dosage. Because of the long half-life of fentanyl when administered as fentanyl transdermal system, the manufacturers state that this formulation should be avoided in patients with severe hepatic impairment.

The manufacturers of transmucosal immediate-release fentanyl preparations (fentanyl citrate transmucosal lozenges, buccal tablets) state that insufficient information is available to make recommendations regarding use of these preparations in patients with hepatic impairment. Caution is advised if these preparations are used in patients with hepatic impairment.

Renal Impairment

In patients with mild to moderate renal impairment, the initial dosage of fentanyl transdermal system should be reduced by 50%, and such patients should be monitored closely for sedation and respiratory depression, including after each dosage increase. Because of the long half-life of fentanyl when administered as the transdermal system, the manufacturers state that this formulation should be avoided in patients with severe renal impairment.

The manufacturers of transmucosal immediate-release fentanyl preparations (transmucosal lozenges, buccal tablets) state that insufficient information is available to make recommendations regarding use of these preparations in patients with renal impairment. Caution is advised if these preparations are used in patients with renal impairment.

Geriatric Patients

Geriatric patients may have increased sensitivity to fentanyl. In general, use caution when selecting a dosage for an elderly patient, usually starting at the low end of the dosing range, reflecting the greater frequency of decreased hepatic, renal, or cardiac function and of concomitant disease or other drug therapy.

CAUTIONS

● *Contraindications*

● *Opioid non-tolerant patients*: Life-threatening respiratory depression and death could occur at any dose.

● Significant respiratory depression.

● Patients with substantial respiratory depression, especially in settings where adequate monitoring and equipment for resuscitation are not available; in patients with acute or severe bronchial asthma; and in those with known or suspected paralytic ileus.

● Known hypersensitivity to fentanyl or any ingredient or component of the respective formulation.

● *Fentanyl Transdermal Systems*:: Managment of mild pain, acute or intermittent pain, or in patients that require analgesia for a short period of time.

● *Fentanyl Transdermal Systems, Transmucosal Lozenges, and Buccal Tablets*: Acute or postoperative pain including headache/migraine and dental pain, or acute pain in the emergency department.

● *Warnings/Precautions*

Warnings

Addiction, Abuse, and Misuse

As an opioid, fentanyl exposes users to the risks of addiction, abuse, and misuse. A boxed warning about this risk is including in the prescribing information for fentanyl. Although the risk of addiction in any individual is unknown, it can occur in patients with appropriate prescribing. Addiction can occur at recommended dosages and if the drug is misused or abused.

Assess each patient's risk for opioid addiction, abuse, or misuse prior to prescribing, and reassess all patients receiving the drug for the development of these behaviors and conditions. Risks are increased in patients with a personal or family history of substance abuse (including drug or alcohol abuse or addiction) or mental illness (e.g., major depression). The potential for these risks should not, however, prevent the proper management of pain in any given patient. Patients at increased risk may be prescribed opioids but use in such patients necessitates intensive counseling about the risks and proper use along with frequent reevaluation for signs of addiction, abuse, and misuse.

Opioids are sought for nonmedical use and are subject to diversion from legitimate prescribed use. Consider these risks when prescribing or dispensing. Strategies to reduce these risks include prescribing the drug in the smallest appropriate quantity and advising the patient on careful storage of the drug during treatment and proper disposal of unused drug. Contact local state professional licensing board or state-controlled substances authority for information on how to prevent and detect abuse or diversion of this product.

Respiratory Depression

Serious, life-threatening, or fatal respiratory depression has been reported with the use of opioids, even when used as recommended. A boxed warning about this risk is included in the prescribing information for fentanyl. Respiratory depression, if not immediately recognized and treated, may lead to respiratory arrest and death.

While serious, life-threatening, or fatal respiratory depression can occur at any time during fentanyl use, the risk is greatest during the initiation of therapy or following a dosage increase. To reduce the risk of respiratory depression, proper dosing and titration of fentanyl is essential.

Patients with significant chronic obstructive pulmonary disease or cor pulmonale, and those with a substantially decreased respiratory reserve, hypoxia, hypercapnia, or preexisting respiratory depression are at increased risk of decreased respiratory drive including apnea, even at recommended dosages of parenteral fentanyl.

Transmuccosal immediate-release fentanyl and fentanyl transdermal systems could be fatal to individuals for whom it is not prescribed and for those who are not opioid-tolerant.

Educate patients and caregivers on how to recognize respiratory depression and emphasize the importance of calling 911 or getting emergency medical help right away in the event of a known or suspected fentanyl overdose.

Opioids can cause sleep-related breathing disorders including central sleep apnea (CSA) and sleep-related hypoxemia. Opioid use increases the risk of CSA in a dose-dependent fashion. In patients who present with CSA, consider decreasing fentanyl dosage using best practices for tapering the drug.

Discuss the availability of naloxone for the emergency treatment of opioid overdose with the patient and caregiver and assess the potential need for access to naloxone, both when initiating and renewing treatment.

Increased Risk of Overdose in Children Due to Accidental Ingestion or Exposure

Death has been reported in children who have accidentally ingested transmucosal immediate-release fentanyl products. Death and other serious problems also have been reported when children and adults were accidentally exposed to fentanyl transdermal system. A boxed warning about this risk is included in the prescribing information for fentanyl transmucosal products.

Patients and their caregivers must be informed that transmucosal immediate-release fentanyl products contains a medicine in an amount which can be fatal to a child. Patients and their caregivers must be instructed to keep both used and unused dosage units out of the reach of children. While all units should be disposed of immediately after use, partially consumed units represent a special risk to children. If a unit is not completely consumed it must be properly disposed as soon as possible.

Placing a fentanyl transdermal system in the mouth, chewing it, swallowing it, or using it in ways other than indicated may cause choking or overdose that could result in death. A boxed warning about this risk has been included in the prescribing information for fentanyl transdermal system. Improper disposal of fentanyl transdermal system in the trash has resulted in accidental exposures and deaths as a considerable amount of active fentanyl remains in fentanyl transdermal system even after use as directed. Advise patients about strict adherence to the recommended handling and disposal instructions in order to prevent accidental exposure to fentanyl transdermal system.

Risks from Concomitant Use with Benzodiazepines or Other CNS Depressants

Profound sedation, respiratory depression, coma, and death may result from the concomitant use of fentanyl with benzodiazepines and/or other CNS depressants, including alcohol (e.g., non-benzodiazepine sedatives/hypnotics, anxiolytics, tranquilizers, muscle relaxants, general anesthetics, antipsychotics, other opioids). A boxed warning about this risk has been included in the prescribing information for fentnayl. Because of these risks, reserve concomitant prescribing of these drugs for use in patients for whom alternative treatment options are inadequate.

Clinical studies have demonstrated that concomitant use of opioid analgesics and benzodiazepines increased the risk of drug-related mortality compared to use of opioid analgesics alone. Because of similar pharmacological properties, it is reasonable to expect similar risk with the concomitant use of other CNS depressant drugs with opioid analgesics.

If concomitant use of a benzodiazepine or other CNS depressant with fentanyl is necessary, prescribe the lowest effective dosages and minimum durations of concomitant use. In patients already receiving fentanyl, prescribe a lower initial dose of the benzodiazepine or other CNS depressant than indicated in the absence of an opioid, and titrate based on clinical response. If an opioid analgesic is initiated in a patient already taking a benzodiazepine or other CNS depressant, prescribe a lower initial dose of the opioid analgesic such as fentanyl, and titrate based on clinical response. Inform patients and caregivers of this potential interaction and educate them on the signs and symptoms of respiratory depression (including sedation). If concomitant use is warranted, consider prescribing naloxone for the emergency treatment of opioid overdose.

Advise both patients and caregivers about the risks of respiratory depression and sedation when fentanyl transdermal system is used with benzodiazepines or other CNS depressants (including alcohol and illicit drugs). Also advise patients not to drive or operate heavy machinery until the effects of concomitant use of the benzodiazepine or other CNS depressant have been determined.

Risks of Concomitant Use or Discontinuation of Cytochrome P450 3A4 Inhibitors and Inducers

Concomitant use of fentanyl with a CYP3A4 inhibitor, such as macrolide antibiotics (e.g., erythromycin), azole antifungals (e.g., ketoconazole), and protease inhibitors (e.g., ritonavir), may increase plasma concentrations of fentanyl and prolong opioid adverse reactions, which may cause potentially fatal respiratory depression, particularly when the inhibitor is added after a stable dose is achieved. Similarly, discontinuation of a CYP3A4 inducer, such as rifampin, carbamazepine, and phenytoin, in fentanyl-treated patients may increase fentanyl plasma concentrations and prolong opioid adverse reactions. A boxed warning about these risks has been included in the prescribing information for fentanyl. When using fentanyl with CYP3A4 inhibitors or discontinuing CYP3A4 inducers, evaluate patients at frequent intervals and consider dosage reduction of fentanyl until stable drug effects are achieved. Concomitant use of fentanyl with CYP3A4 inducers or discontinuation of a CYP3A4 inhibitor could decrease fentanyl plasma concentrations, decrease opioid efficacy or, possibly, lead to a withdrawal syndrome in a patient who had developed physical dependence to fentanyl. When using fentanyl with CYP3A4 inducers or discontinuing CYP3A4 inhibitors, evaluate patients at frequent intervals and consider increasing the opioid dosage if needed to maintain adequate analgesia or if symptoms of opioid withdrawal occur.

Risk of Medication Errors

Do not convert patients to transmucosal immediate-release fentanyl (TIRF) preparations from any other fentanyl product based on dosage amounts as these products are not equivalent on a mcg-per-mcg basis. A boxed warning about this risk is included in the prescribing information for fentanyl transmucosal products.

TIRF preparations are not generic versions of other TIRF formulations. When dispensing, do not substitute these prescriptions for any other TIRF formulation under any circumstances as substantial differences exist in the pharmacokinetic profile compared to other fentanyl products, including other TIRF formulations. Differences in the rate and extent of absorption of fentanyl may result in a fatal overdose.

There are no safe conversion directions available for patients on any other fentanyl products (e.g., oral, transdermal, or parenteral formulations of fentanyl) except the conversion of Actiq® to Fentora®. Therefore, for opioid-tolerant patients, the initial starting dose should be prescribed and dosage should be titrated to provide adequate analgesia while minimizing side effects.

Neonatal Opioid Withdrawal Syndrome

Use of fentanyl transdermal system and transmucosal immediate release products for an extended period of time during pregnancy can result in withdrawal in the neonate. A boxed warning about this risk has been included in the prescribing information for fentanyl. Neonatal opioid withdrawal syndrome, unlike opioid withdrawal syndrome in adults, may be life-threatening if not recognized and treated, and requires management according to protocols developed by neonatology experts.

Observe newborns for signs of neonatal opioid withdrawal syndrome and manage accordingly. Advise pregnant women using opioids for an extended period of time of the risk of neonatal opioid withdrawal syndrome and ensure that appropriate treatment will be available.

Risk of Increased Fentanyl Absorption with Application of External Heat

Exposure to heat may increase fentanyl absorption from transdermal systems and there have been reports of overdose and death from exposure to heat. A boxed warning about this risk has been included in the prescribing information for fentanyl transdermal system. A clinical pharmacology study conducted in healthy adult subjects has shown that the application of heat over the fentanyl transdermal system increased fentanyl exposure.

Warn patients to avoid exposing the fentanyl transdermal system application site and surrounding area to direct external heat sources.

Other Warnings and Precautions

Risks of Muscle Rigidity and Skeletal Muscle Movement

Fentanyl citrate injection may cause muscle rigidity, particularly involving the muscles of respiration. The incidence and severity of muscle rigidity are dose-related and also related to the speed of injection. Skeletal muscle rigidity has been reported to occur or recur infrequently in the extended postoperative period, usually following high dose administration. In addition, skeletal muscle movements of various groups in the extremities, neck, and external eye have been reported during induction of anesthesia with fentanyl citrate injection; these reported movements have, on rare occasions, been strong enough to pose patient management problems. These effects can be reduced by: 1) administration of up to 1/4 of the full paralyzing dose of a nondepolarizing neuromuscular blocking agent just prior to administration of fentanyl citrate injection; 2) administration of a full paralyzing dose of a neuromuscular blocking agent following loss of eyelash reflex when fentanyl citrate injection is used in anesthetic doses titrated by slow IV infusion; or, 3) simultaneous administration of fentanyl citrate injection and a full paralyzing dose of a neuromuscular blocking agent when fentanyl citrate injection is used in rapidly administered anesthetic dosages.

Severe Cardiovascular Depression

Fentanyl citrate injection may cause severe bradycardia, severe hypotension, including orthostatic hypotension, and syncope. There is increased risk in patients whose ability to maintain blood pressure has already been compromised by a reduced blood volume or concurrent administration of certain CNS depressants (e.g., phenothiazines or general anesthetics). In patients with circulatory shock, fentanyl citrate injection may cause vasodilation that can further reduce cardiac output and blood pressure. Monitor these patients for signs of hypotension after initiating or titrating the dosage.

Opioid-Induced Hyperalgesia and Allodynia

Opioid-induced hyperalgesia (OIH) occurs when an opioid analgesic paradoxically causes an increase in pain, or an increase in sensitivity to pain. This condition differs from tolerance, which is the need for increasing doses of opioids to maintain a defined effect. Symptoms of OIH include (but may not be limited to) increased levels of pain upon opioid dosage increase, decreased levels of pain upon opioid dosage decrease, or pain from ordinarily non-painful stimuli (allodynia) if there is no evidence of underlying disease progression, opioid tolerance, opioid withdrawal, or addictive behavior. Cases of OIH have been reported, both with short- and longer-term use of opioid analgesics.

If a patient is suspected to be experiencing OIH, carefully consider appropriately decreasing the dose of the current opioid analgesic or opioid rotation (safely switching the patient to a different opioid moiety).

Serotonin Syndrome with Concomitant Use of Serotonergic Drugs

Cases of serotonin syndrome, a potentially life-threatening condition, have been reported during concomitant use of fentanyl with serotonergic drugs. Serotonergic drugs include selective serotonin reuptake inhibitors (SSRIs), serotonin and norepinephrine reuptake inhibitors (SNRIs), tricyclic antidepressants (TCAs), triptans, 5-HT$_3$ receptor antagonists, drugs that affect the serotonergic neurotransmitter system (e.g., mirtazapine, trazodone, tramadol), certain muscle relaxants (i.e., cyclobenzaprine, metaxalone), and drugs that impair metabolism of serotonin (including MAO inhibitors, both those intended to treat psychiatric disorders and also others, such as linezolid and IV methylene blue). This may occur within the recommended dosage range. Serotonin syndrome symptoms may include mental status changes (e.g., agitation, hallucinations, coma), autonomic instability (e.g., tachycardia, labile blood pressure, hyperthermia), neuromuscular aberrations (e.g., hyperreflexia, incoordination, rigidity), and/or GI symptoms (e.g., nausea, vomiting, diarrhea) and can be fatal. The onset of symptoms generally occurs within several hours to a few days of concomitant use but may occur later. Discontinue fentanyl citrate injection if serotonin syndrome is suspected.

Life-Threatening Respiratory Depression in Patients with Chronic Pulmonary Disease or in Elderly, Cachectic, or Debilitated Patients

The use of fentanyl transdermal systems and transmucosal immediate release products in patients with acute or severe bronchial asthma in an unmonitored setting or in the absence of resuscitative equipment is contraindicated. Patients with chronic pulmonary disease such as those with significant chronic obstructive pulmonary disease or cor pulmonale, and those with a substantially decreased respiratory reserve, hypoxia, hypercapnia, or pre-existing respiratory depression are at increased risk of decreased respiratory drive including apnea, even at recommended dosages. Additionally, life-threatening respiratory depression is more likely to occur in elderly, cachectic, or debilitated patients because they may have

altered pharmacokinetics or altered clearance compared to younger, healthier patients.

Regularly evaluate patients, particularly when initiating and titrating fentanyl and when given concomitantly with other drugs that depress respiration. Alternatively, consider the use of non-opioid analgesics in these patients.

Adrenal Insufficiency

Cases of adrenal insufficiency have been reported with opioid use, more often following greater than one month of use. Presentation of adrenal insufficiency may include nonspecific symptoms and signs including nausea, vomiting, anorexia, fatigue, weakness, dizziness, and low blood pressure. If adrenal insufficiency is suspected, confirm the diagnosis with diagnostic testing as soon as possible. If adrenal insufficiency is diagnosed, treat with physiologic replacement doses of corticosteroids. Taper the opioid to allow adrenal function to recover and continue corticosteroid treatment until adrenal function recovers. Other opioids may be tried as some cases reported use of a different opioid without recurrence of adrenal insufficiency; however, available information does not identify any particular opioids as being more likely to be associated with adrenal insufficiency.

Severe Hypotension

Fentanyl transdermal systems and transmucosal immediate release products may cause severe hypotension including orthostatic hypotension and syncope in ambulatory patients. There is increased risk in patients whose ability to maintain blood pressure has already been compromised by a reduced blood volume or concurrent administration of certain CNS depressants (e.g. phenothiazines or general anesthetics). Regularly evaluate these patients for signs of hypotension after initiating or titrating the dosage. May cause vasodilation in patients with circulatory shock that can further reduce cardiac output and blood pressure; avoid use in patients with circulatory shock.

Risks of Use in Patients with Increased Intracranial Pressure, Brain Tumors, or Head Injury

In patients who may be susceptible to the intracranial effects of carbon dioxide retention (e.g., those with evidence of increased intracranial pressure or brain tumors), fentanyl may reduce respiratory drive, and the resultant carbon dioxide retention can further increase intracranial pressure. Monitor such patients for signs of sedation and respiratory depression, particularly when initiating therapy.

Opioids may also obscure the clinical course in a patient with a head injury. Avoid use in patients with impaired consciousness or coma.

Risks of Use in Patients with GI Conditions

Fentanyl is contraindicated in patients with known or suspected GI obstruction, including paralytic ileus. Fentanyl may cause spasm of the sphincter of Oddi. Opioids may cause increases in serum amylase. Regularly evaluate patients with biliary tract disease, including acute pancreatitis, for worsening symptoms.

Seizures

Fentanyl may increase the frequency of seizures in patients with seizure disorders, and may increase the risk of seizures occurring in other clinical settings associated with seizures. Regularly evaluate patients with a history of seizure disorders for worsened seizure control during therapy.

CNS Effects

May impair the mental or physical abilities needed to perform potentially hazardous activities such as driving a car or operating machinery. Warn patients not to drive or operate dangerous machinery unless they are tolerant to the effects and know how they will react to the medication.

Application Site Reactions

Application site reactions occurred in 10% of patients in clinical trials and ranged from paresthesia to ulceration and bleeding in patients using fentanyl transdermal systems.

Risks due to Interaction with Neuroleptic Agents

Elevated blood pressure, with and without pre-existing hypertension, has been reported following administration of fentanyl citrate injection combined with a neuroleptic. This might be due to unexplained alterations in sympathetic activity following large doses; however, it is also frequently attributed to anesthetic and surgical stimulation during light anesthesia.

ECG monitoring is indicated when a neuroleptic agent is used in conjunction with fentanyl citrate injection as an anesthetic premedication, for the induction of anesthesia, or as an adjunct in the maintenance of general or regional anesthesia. When used with a neuroleptic and an EEG is used for postoperative monitoring, the EEG pattern may return to normal slowly.

Risk of Increased Fentanyl Absorption with Elevated Body Temperature

Pharmacokinetic modeling suggests that serum fentanyl concentrations could theoretically increase by approximately one-third for patients with a body temperature of 40°C (104°F) due to temperature-dependent increases in fentanyl released from the system and increased skin permeability. Monitor patients wearing fentanyl transdermal systems who develop fever closely for sedation and respiratory depression and reduce the fentanyl transdermal system dose, if necessary.

Withdrawal

Do not abruptly discontinue fentanyl transdermal system in a patient physically dependent on opioids. When discontinuing fentanyl transdermal system in a physically dependent patient, gradually taper the dosage. Rapid tapering of fentanyl transdermal system in a patient physically dependent on opioids may lead to a withdrawal syndrome and return of pain.

Additionally, avoid the use of mixed agonist/antagonist (e.g., pentazocine, nalbuphine, and butorphanol) or partial agonist (e.g., buprenorphine) analgesics in patients receiving a full opioid agonist analgesic, including fentanyl transdermal system. In these patients, mixed agonist/antagonist and partial agonist analgesics may reduce the analgesic effect and/or may precipitate withdrawal symptoms.

Specific Populations

Pregnancy

Available data in pregnant women are insufficient to inform a drug-associated risk for major birth defects and miscarriage.

In animal reproduction studies, fentanyl administration to pregnant rats during organogenesis was embryocidal at doses within the range of the human recommended dosing and when administered during gestation through lactation resulted in reduced pup survival and developmental delays at doses within the range of the human recommended dosing. No evidence of malformations noted in animal studies completed to date.

Opioids cross the placenta and may produce respiratory depression and psychophysiologic effects in neonates. There are insufficient data to support the use of fentanyl in labor or delivery and therefore such use is not recommended.

Transient neonatal muscular rigidity reported in infants whose mothers received IV fentanyl during labor.

Prolonged maternal use of opioids during pregnancy can result in neonatal opioid withdrawal syndrome; withdrawal syndrome in neonates may be life-threatening and requires management according to protocols developed by neonatology experts. Syndrome presents with irritability, hyperactivity and abnormal sleep pattern, high-pitched cry, tremor, vomiting, diarrhea, and failure to gain weight.

Lactation

Fentanyl is distributed into human milk.

Manufacturers of fentanyl transdermal system and transmucosal immediate-release fentanyl preparations (used only in opioid-tolerant patients) state these preparations should not be used in nursing women because of the potential for serious adverse effects in nursing infants.

There is a potential risk of sedation and respiratory depression in nursing infants; monitor breastfeeding infants for excess sedation and respiratory depression. Withdrawal symptoms can occur in breastfed infants when maternal administration of an opioid analgesic is stopped, or when breastfeeding is stopped.

Females and Males of Reproductive Potential

Use of opioids for an extended period of time may cause reduced fertility in females and males of reproductive potential. It is not known whether these effects on fertility are reversible.

Pediatric Use

Safety and efficacy of parenteral fentanyl citrate and fentanyl transdermal systems have not been established in pediatric patients <2 years of age.

Safety and efficacy of transmucosal lozenges have not been established in pediatric patients <16 years of age. Safety and efficacy of buccal tablets have not been established in pediatric patients <18 years of age.

To reduce the potential for accidental ingestion, carefully select application sites in young children receiving transdermal fentanyl therapy and monitor the system for proper adhesion over the period of application. Transdermal systems and transmucosal immediate-release preparations (transmucosal lozenges, buccal tablets) contain fentanyl in amounts that can be fatal to a child. Fatal respiratory depression can occur if a transdermal system is accidentally or deliberately applied or ingested by a child or adolescent; choking can occur if the system is ingested. There is a high risk of respiratory depression if a child accidentally ingests a transmucosal immediate-release preparation.

Geriatric Use

Pharmacokinetics of fentanyl may be altered in geriatric patients, increasing risk of life-threatening respiratory depression. Monitor closely for sedation and respiratory depression, particularly during initiation or titration of therapy and when other respiratory depressants are used concomitantly.

Use caution when titrating dosage. Renal clearance of fentanyl may be reduced. Geriatric patients may be more sensitive to effects of fentanyl.

Clinical studies of fentanyl transdermal system did not include sufficient numbers of patients 65 years of age and older to determine whether they respond differently from younger subjects. However, a study reported that the pharmacokinetics of fentanyl transdermal system in geriatric patients are not substantially different than that in younger adults, although peak serum concentrations tended to be lower and mean half-life was prolonged in geriatric patients. Dosages of transmucosal lozenges (following titration) are generally about 200 mcg lower in geriatric patients than in younger adults. Dosages of buccal tablets (following titration) are slightly lower in geriatric patients than in younger adults. Increased frequency of certain adverse effects (e.g., vomiting, constipation, abdominal pain) reported in geriatric patients compared with younger adults receiving buccal tablets.

Hepatic Impairment

Exercise caution and reduce initial parenteral dosage and monitor closely for signs of respiratory depression, sedation, and hypotension. Reduce initial dosage of fentanyl transdermal system by one-half in patients with mild to moderate hepatic impairment; monitor closely for sedation and respiratory depression, including after each increase in dosage. Because of the long half-life of transdermal systems, avoid use in patients with severe hepatic impairment. Insufficient information is available to support recommendations regarding use of transmucosal immediate-release preparations; if used, caution advised.

Renal Impairment

Exercise caution and reduce initial parenteral dosage and monitor closely for signs of respiratory depression, sedation, and hypotension. Reduce initial dosage of fentanyl transdermal system by one-half in patients with mild to moderate renal impairment; monitor closely for sedation and respiratory depression, including after each increase in dosage. Because of the long half-life of this formulation, avoid use in patients with severe renal impairment. Insufficient information is available to support recommendations regarding use of transmucosal immediate-release preparations; if used, caution advised.

Patients with Cardiac Diseases

IV administered fentanyl may produce bradycardia. Use fentanyl transdermal systems and transmucosal immediate release products with caution in patients with bradyarrhythmias.

● Common Adverse Effects

The most common adverse effects reported with parenteral administration of fentanyl include respiratory depression, apnea, rigidity, and bradycardia.

The most common adverse effects reported with use of fentanyl transdermal system (≥5% incidence) include nausea, vomiting, somnolence, dizziness, insomnia, constipation, hyperhidrosis, fatigue, feeling cold, anorexia, headache, and diarrhea.

The most common adverse effects reported with use of fenanyl buccal tablets (≥10% incidence) include nausea, dizziness, vomiting, fatigue, anemia, constipation, peripheral edema, asthenia, dehydration, and headache.

The most common adverse effects reported with use of fentanyl transmucosal lozenges (≥5% incidence) include nausea, dizziness, somnolence, vomiting, asthenia, headache, dyspnea, constipation, anxiety, confusion, depression, rash, and insomnia.

DRUG INTERACTIONS

● Drugs Affecting or Metabolized by Hepatic Microsomal Enzymes

Because fentanyl undergoes metabolism via cytochrome P-450 (CYP) isoenzyme 3A4 in the liver and the intestinal mucosa, concomitant use of inhibitors of CYP3A4 (e.g., macrolide antibiotics [e.g., erythromycin, clarithromycin], azole-antifungal agents [e.g., ketoconazole, itraconazole, fluconazole], protease inhibitors [e.g., nelfinavir, ritonavir, fosamprenavir], amiodarone, amprenavir, diltiazem, nefazodone, verapamil, grapefruit juice) may increase plasma concentrations of fentanyl, possibly resulting in increased or prolonged opiate effects, including potentially fatal respiratory depression.

Conversely, concomitant use of drugs that induce CYP3A4 (e.g., rifampin, carbamazepine, phenytoin) may reduce plasma concentrations of fentanyl, possibly resulting in decreased analgesic efficacy and/or development of opiate withdrawal. If concomitant use of fentanyl with CYP3A4 inducers is necessary, patients should be monitored for opiate withdrawal and dosage adjustments should be considered until stable drug effects are achieved. Discontinuance of a concomitantly used CYP3A4 inducer may result in increased plasma concentrations of fentanyl, possibly resulting in increased or prolonged therapeutic or adverse effects, including sedation or potentially fatal respiratory depression. Patients receiving fentanyl who discontinue therapy with, or decrease the dosage of, a CYP3A4 inducer should be monitored for increased opiate effects and the fentanyl dosage should be adjusted as necessary.

● Benzodiazepines and Other CNS Depressants

Concomitant use of opiate agonists and benzodiazepines or other CNS depressants, including other opiate agonists, anxiolytics, sedatives, hypnotics, muscle relaxants, general anesthetics, antipsychotics, and alcohol, may result in hypotension, profound sedation, respiratory depression, coma, and death.

Concomitant use of parenteral fentanyl and benzodiazepines or other CNS depressants also may result in decreased pulmonary arterial pressure; even relatively small dosages of diazepam may cause cardiovascular depression when used with high or anesthetic dosages of fentanyl. Clinicians should consider the potential for such concomitant therapy to decrease pulmonary arterial pressure when performing diagnostic or surgical procedures where interpretation of pulmonary arterial pressure measurements might determine patient management. If hypotension occurs, the possibility of hypovolemia should be considered and managed with appropriate fluid therapy. When operative conditions permit, repositioning of the patient to improve venous return to the heart should be considered. Because of the potential for orthostatic hypotension, care should be exercised when moving and repositioning the patient. If volume expansion and other countermeasures do not correct hypotension, administration of a pressor agent (other than epinephrine, which may cause a reduction in blood pressure in patients receiving a neuroleptic with alpha-adrenergic blocking activity) should be considered. If used parenterally for postoperative analgesia in conjunction with a benzodiazepine or other CNS depressant, fentanyl should be initiated at a reduced dosage and titrated based on clinical response, and the patient should be monitored closely for respiratory depression, sedation, and hypotension. Fluids or other measures to counteract hypotension should be available.

● Drugs Associated with Serotonin Syndrome

Serotonin syndrome has occurred in patients receiving opiate agonists, including fentanyl, in conjunction with other serotonergic drugs, including serotonin (5-hydroxytryptamine; 5-HT) type 1 receptor agonists ("triptans"), selective serotonin-reuptake inhibitors (SSRIs), selective serotonin- and norepinephrine-reuptake inhibitors (SNRIs), tricyclic antidepressants, antiemetics that are 5-HT₃ receptor antagonists, other serotonin modulators (e.g., mirtazapine, nefazodone, trazodone, tramadol), and monoamine oxidase (MAO) inhibitors (both those used to treat psychiatric disorders and others, such as linezolid and methylene blue). Serotonin syndrome may occur within the recommended dosage ranges for these drugs. Manifestations of serotonin syndrome may include mental status changes (e.g., agitation, hallucinations, coma), autonomic instability (e.g., tachycardia, labile blood pressure, hyperthermia), neuromuscular aberrations (e.g., hyperreflexia, incoordination, rigidity), and/or GI symptoms (e.g., nausea, vomiting, diarrhea). Symptom onset generally occurs within several hours to a few days of concomitant use, but may occur later, particularly after dosage increases.

If concurrent therapy with opiate agonists and serotonergic drugs is warranted, patients should be monitored for serotonin syndrome, particularly during initiation of therapy and dosage increases. If serotonin syndrome is suspected, treatment with fentanyl, other opiate therapy, and/or any concurrently administered serotonergic agents should be discontinued.

● Anticholinergic Agents

Concomitant use of anticholinergic drugs may increase the risk of urinary retention and/or severe constipation, which may lead to paralytic ileus Patients should be monitored for signs of urinary retention or decreased GI motility when fentanyl preparations are used concomitantly with anticholinergic drugs.

● Diuretics

Concomitant use of opioids with diuretics may decrease diuretic efficacy by inducing the release of antidiuretic hormone. Evaluate patients for signs of diminished diuresis and/or effects on blood pressure and increase the dosage of the diuretic as needed.

● Mixed Agonist/Antagonist and Partial Agonist Opioids

The use of mixed agonist/antagonist and partial agonist opioid analgesics (e.g., butorphanol, nalbuphine, pentazocine, buprenorphine) may reduce the analgesic effect of fentanyl and/or precipitate withdrawal symptoms. Concomitant use should be avoided.

● Monoamine Oxidase Inhibitors (MAOIs)

Monoamine oxidase inhibitors (e.g., phenelzine, tranylcypromine) may interact with opioids and manifest as serotonin syndrome or opioid toxicity (e.g., respiratory depression, coma). The use of fentanyl preparations is not recommended for patients taking MAOIs or within 14 days of stopping such treatment.

● Muscle Relaxants

Concomitant use may enhance the neuromuscular blocking action of skeletal muscle relaxants and produce an increased degree of respiratory depression. Use with parenteral fentanyl may decrease pulmonary arterial pressure and cause hypotension.

Because respiratory depression may be greater than otherwise expected, decrease the dosage of fentanyl and/or the muscle relaxant as necessary. Due to the risk of respiratory depression with concomitant use of skeletal muscle relaxants and opioids, consider prescribing naloxone for the emergency treatment of opioid overdose.

DESCRIPTION

Fentanyl is a potent analgesic that shares the actions of the opiate agonists. Fentanyl interacts predominately with the opioid mu receptor; mu receptor binding sites are distributed in the human brain, spinal cord, and other tissues. The agonist activity of fentanyl at the mu receptor can also result in suppression of opioid withdrawal (and antagonist activity can result in precipitation of withdrawal).

Fentanyl mediates respiratory depression by direct action on brain stem respiratory centers. Fentanyl also causes a reduction in motility associated with an increase in smooth muscle tone in the antrum of the stomach and in the duodenum. Other opioid-related effects may include a reduction in biliary and pancreatic secretions, spasm of the sphincter of Oddi, and transient elevations in serum amylase. Cardiovascular effects of fentanyl include peripheral vasodilation, which may result in orthostatic hypotension or syncope. Manifestations of histamine release and/or peripheral vasodilation may include pruritus, flushing, red eyes, sweating, and/or orthostatic hypotension. Opioid agonists have been shown to have a variety of effects on the secretion of hormones including adrenocorticotropic hormone (ACTH), cortisol, luteinizing hormone (LH), prolactin, growth hormone (GH), insulin, glucagon, and thyroid stimulating hormone (TSH). Use of opioids for an extended period of time may influence the hypothalamic-pituitary-gonadal axis, leading to androgen deficiency that may manifest as low libido, impotence, erectile dysfunction, amenorrhea, or infertility.

Fentanyl is well absorbed percutaneously following topical application of fentanyl transdermal system to a flat surface on the upper torso. The amount of fentanyl released from the system is proportional to the surface area of the system; however, the actual amount of drug delivered to the skin exhibits interindividual variation. Peak concentration is attained within 20–72 hours after initial application. Serum concentrations increase with the first 2 transdermal system applications; steady state is reached by the end of the second 72-hour application and is maintained during continued use at the same dosage. Application of heat over the transdermal system increases mean exposure and peak plasma concentrations by 120 and 61%, respectively. Following use of fentanyl transdermal system in non-opioid-tolerant children, plasma fentanyl concentrations in children 1.5–5 years of age were about twice the concentrations achieved in adults; however, pharmacokinetic parameters in older children were similar to those in adults.

Fentanyl is well absorbed transmucosally following intrabuccal administration as fentanyl citrate transmucosal lozenge or buccal tablet. Substantial pharmacokinetic differences exist among the transmucosal immediate-release preparations; these preparations must not be substituted on a mcg-for-mcg basis. Bioavailability of the transmucosal lozenge averages about 50%; generally, approximately 25% of the drug is absorbed rapidly from the buccal mucosa and the remaining portion is swallowed with saliva and then absorbed slowly from the GI tract. Bioavailability of the buccal tablet averages about 65%. Generally, approximately 50% of the drug is absorbed rapidly from the buccal mucosa and the remaining portion is swallowed with saliva and then absorbed slowly from the GI tract. The time required for the buccal tablet to fully disintegrate does not appear to affect early systemic drug exposure. When fentanyl is administered as a buccal tablet rather than a transmucosal lozenge, a larger fraction of the administered dose is absorbed transmucosally (48% versus 22%), peak plasma concentration is achieved earlier (47 versus 91 minutes), and systemic exposure is approximately 30–50% greater.

The onset of action following IV administration of fentanyl is rapid; peak analgesia occurs within several minutes and the duration of analgesia is 30–60 minutes after a single dose of up to 100 mcg. Following IM administration of fentanyl citrate, the onset of action occurs within about 7–15 minutes and the duration of action is 1–2 hours. Respiratory depressant effects may persist longer than analgesia. Residual effects of one dose of fentanyl citrate may potentiate the effects of subsequent doses. It has been suggested that redistribution is the main cause of the brief analgesic effect of fentanyl.

Fentanyl is highly lipophilic. Fentanyl crosses the placenta and is distributed into breast milk. Approximately 80–85% of the drug is protein-bound, principally to α1-acid glycoprotein. Fentanyl is metabolized extensively in the liver and the intestinal mucosa via cytochrome P-450 (CYP) 3A4 to norfentanyl and other inactive metabolites. Transdermally administered fentanyl does not appear to be metabolized in the skin. Fentanyl is principally eliminated in urine, as inactive metabolites and to a lesser extent (<10%) as unchanged drug. The terminal half-life of the transmucosal lozenges is about 7 hours. The terminal elimination half-life of parenteral fentanyl is 219 minutes.

ADVICE TO PATIENTS

- Inform patients that the use of fentanyl, even when taken as recommended, can result in addiction, abuse, and misuse, which can lead to overdose and death. Instruct patients not to share the drug with others and to take steps to protect it from theft or misuse.

- Inform patients that the risk of life-threatening respiratory depression is most likely to occur following initiation of therapy or an increase in dosage; may also occur at recommended dosages. Educate patients and caregivers on how to recognize respiratory depression and emphasize the importance of calling 911 or getting emergency medical help right away in the event of a known or suspected overdose.

- Inform patients and caregivers not to increase opioid dosage without first consulting a clinician. Advise patients to inform their healthcare provider if they experience symptoms of hyperalgesia, including worsening pain, increased sensitivity to pain, or new pain.

- Inform patients that opioids could cause a rare but potentially life-threatening condition called serotonin syndrome resulting from concomitant administration of serotonergic drugs. Warn patients of the symptoms of serotonin syndrome and to seek medical attention right away if symptoms develop after discharge from the hospital. Instruct patients to inform their healthcare provider if they are taking, or plan to take serotonergic medications.

- Advise patients of the potential for severe constipation, including management instructions and when to seek medical attention.

- Strongly warn patients and/or caregivers to keep new, used, and partially used preparations in a secure location out of the reach of children and to strictly adhere to instructions for storage, handling, and disposal of unused and partially or fully used fentanyl preparations. Inform patients that leaving preparations unsecured can pose a deadly risk to others in the home. Advise patients and caregivers that when medicines are no longer needed, they should be disposed of promptly. Inform patients that they can visit https://www.fda.gov/drugdisposal for a complete list of medicines recommended for disposal by flushing, as well as additional information on disposal of unused medicines.

- Discuss with the patient and caregiver the availability of naloxone for the emergency treatment of opioid overdose, both when initiating and renewing treatment. Inform patients and caregivers about the various ways to obtain naloxone as permitted by individual state naloxone dispensing and prescribing requirements or guidelines (e.g., by prescription, directly from a pharmacist, or as part of a community-based program). Educate patients and caregivers on how to recognize the signs and symptoms of an overdose. Explain to patients and caregivers that naloxone's effects are temporary, and that they must call 911 or get emergency medical help right away in all cases of known or suspected opioid overdose, even if naloxone is administered.

- Inform patients that potentially fatal additive effects may occur if used with benzodiazepines or other CNS depressants, including alcohol, and not to use these concomitantly unless supervised by a healthcare provider.

- Inform patients to avoid taking fentanyl while using any drugs that inhibit monoamine oxidase (MAO). Patients should not start MAOIs while taking fentanyl preparations.

- Inform patients that fentanyl may impair the ability to perform potentially hazardous activities such as driving a car or operating heavy machinery. Advise patients not to perform such tasks until they know how they will react to the medication.

- Inform patients that opioids could cause adrenal insufficiency, a potentially life-threatening condition. Adrenal insufficiency may present with nonspecific symptoms and signs such as nausea, vomiting, anorexia, fatigue, weakness, dizziness, and low blood pressure. Advise patients to seek medical attention if they experience these symptoms.

- Inform patients that fentanyl may cause orthostatic hypotension and syncope. Instruct patients how to recognize symptoms of low blood pressure and how to reduce the risk of serious consequences should hypotension occur (e.g., sit or lie down, carefully rise from a sitting or lying position).

- Inform patients that anaphylaxis has been reported with ingredients contained in fentanyl preparations. Advise patients how to recognize such a reaction and when to seek medical attention.

- Advise women to inform their clinicians if they are or plan to become pregnant. Inform women that long-term use during pregnancy may result in neonatal opioid withdrawal syndrome, which can be life-threatening if not recognized and treated.

- Advise women to inform their clinicians if they are or plan to breast-feed. Advise nursing mothers to carefully observe infants for increased sleepiness (more than usual), breathing difficulties, or limpness. Instruct nursing mothers to seek immediate medical care if they notice these symptoms.

- Inform patients that use of opioids for an extended period of time may cause reduced fertility. It is not known whether these effects on fertility are reversible.

- Advise patients to inform their clinician of existing or contemplated concomitant therapy, including prescription and OTC drugs and dietary and herbal supplements, as well as any concomitant illnesses.

- Inform patients of other important precautionary information.

Transmucosal Immediate-release Fentanyl Preparations

- Inform patients of the importance of understanding the requirements of the TIRF REMS Access program and of signing the patient-prescriber agreement mandated by the program.

- Inform patients on the importance of using transmucosal immediate-release preparations (transmucosal lozenges, buccal tablets) exactly as prescribed and only if opioid tolerant. Inform patients of the importance of not using these preparations for acute, postoperative, or short-term pain. Advise patients that if around-the-clock therapy with opioid analgesics is discontinued, they must stop taking transmucosal immediate-release fentanyl preparations for management of breakthrough pain.

- Advise patients with diabetes mellitus that fentanyl citrate transmucosal lozenges contain approximately 2 g of sugar per lozenge. Frequent consumption may also increase the risk of dental decay. The occurrence of dry mouth associated with the use of opioid medications (such as fentanyl) may add to this risk. Advise patients to consult their dentist to ensure appropriate oral hygiene. Inform patients that buccal tablets are not to be swallowed whole; this will reduce the effectiveness of the medication. Tablets are to be placed between the cheek and gum above a molar tooth or under the tongue and allowed to dissolve. If remnants of the tablet still remain after 30 minutes, patients may swallow it with a glass of water.

- Advise patients to talk to their healthcare provider if breakthrough pain is not alleviated or worsens after taking their medicine as directed.

Fentanyl Transdermal Systems

- Inform patients that accidental exposure, especially in children, may result in respiratory depression or death. Fentanyl transdermal system can be accidentally transferred to children. Instruct patients to take special precautions to avoid accidental contact when holding or caring for children. Instruct patients that, if the patch dislodges and accidentally sticks to the skin of another person, to immediately take the patch off, wash the exposed area with water, and seek medical attention for the accidentally exposed individual as accidental exposure may lead to death or other serious medical problems.

- Advise patients never to change the dose of fentanyl transdermal system or the number of patches applied to the skin unless instructed to do so by the prescribing healthcare professional.

- Advise patients to avoid strenuous exertion that can increase core body temperature and to avoid exposing the application site or surrounding area to direct external heat sources (e.g., heating pads, electric blankets, heat or tanning lamps, saunas, hot tubs, hot baths, heated water beds, sunbathing) while wearing the transdermal system since temperature-dependent increases in percutaneous absorption of fentanyl from the system are possible under such conditions. Stress importance of contacting clinician if a high fever occurs during transdermal fentanyl therapy.

- Instruct patients not to discontinue fentanyl transdermal system without first discussing a tapering plan with the prescriber, in order to avoid developing withdrawal symptoms.

PREPARATIONS

Fentanyl and fentanyl citrate preparations are subject to control under the Federal Controlled Substances Act of 1970 as schedule II (C-II) drugs.

Distribution of transmucosal immediate-release fentanyl preparations is restricted.

Excipients in commercially available drug preparations may have clinically important effects in some individuals; consult specific product labeling for details.

fentaNYL

Topical

Transdermal System	12 mcg/hour (total fentanyl content and transdermal system size may vary by manufacturer)*	fentaNYL Transdermal System (C-II)
	25 mcg/hour (total fentanyl content and transdermal system size may vary by manufacturer)*	fentaNYL Transdermal System (C-II)
	37.5 mcg/hour (total fentanyl content and transdermal system size may vary by manufacturer)*	fentaNYL Transdermal System (C-II)
	50 mcg/hour (total fentanyl content and transdermal system size may vary by manufacturer)*	fentaNYL Transdermal System (C-II)
	62.5 mcg/hour (total fentanyl content and transdermal system size may vary by manufacturer)*	fentaNYL Transdermal System (C-II)
	75 mcg/hour (total fentanyl content and transdermal system size may vary by manufacturer)*	fentaNYL Transdermal System (C-II)
	87.5 mcg/hour (total fentanyl content and transdermal system size may vary by manufacturer)*	fentaNYL Transdermal System (C-II)
	100 mcg/hour (total fentanyl content and transdermal system size may vary by manufacturer)*	fentaNYL Transdermal System (C-II)

* available from one or more manufacturer, distributor, and/or repackager by generic (nonproprietary) name

fentaNYL Citrate

Buccal-transmucosal

Transmucosal Lozenge (solid drug matrix on a handle)	200 mcg (of fentanyl)*	Actiq® (C-II), Cephalon Oral Transmucosal fentaNYL Citrate (C-II)
	400 mcg (of fentanyl)*	Actiq® (C-II), Cephalon Oral Transmucosal fentaNYL Citrate (C-II)
	600 mcg (of fentanyl)*	Actiq® (C-II), Cephalon Oral Transmucosal fentaNYL Citrate (C-II)
	800 mcg (of fentanyl)*	Actiq® (C-II), Cephalon Oral Transmucosal fentaNYL Citrate (C-II)
	1200 mcg (of fentanyl)*	Actiq® (C-II), Cephalon Oral Transmucosal fentaNYL Citrate (C-II)
	1600 mcg (of fentanyl)*	Actiq® (C-II), Cephalon Oral Transmucosal fentaNYL Citrate (C-II)

Tablet	100 mcg (of fentanyl)	Fentora® (C-II), Cephalon
	200 mcg (of fentanyl)	Fentora® (C-II), Cephalon
	400 mcg (of fentanyl)	Fentora® (C-II), Cephalon
	600 mcg (of fentanyl)	Fentora® (C-II), Cephalon
	800 mcg (of fentanyl)	Fentora® (C-II), Cephalon Teva
Parenteral		
Injection	50 mcg (of fentanyl) per mL*	**fentaNYL Citrate Injection** (C-II)

* available from one or more manufacturer, distributor, and/or repackager by generic (nonproprietary) name

† Use is not currently included in the labeling approved by the US Food and Drug Administration.

Selected Revisions September 10, 2024, © Copyright, March 1, 1979, American Society of Health-System Pharmacists, Inc.

HYDROcodone Bitartrate

28:08.08 · OPIOID AGONISTS

■ Hydrocodone bitartrate is a phenanthrene-derivative opiate agonist that is used as an analgesic and antitussive agent.

REMS

FDA approved a REMS for hydrocodone to ensure that the benefits outweigh the risks. The REMS may apply to one or more preparations of hydrocodone and consists of the following: medication guide and elements to assure safe use. See the FDA REMS page (https://www.accessdata.fda.gov/scripts/cder/rems/index.cfm).

USES

Extended-release hydrocodone bitartrate is used for the relief of pain that is severe enough to require long-term, daily, around-the-clock use of an opiate analgesic. Because of the risks of addiction, abuse, and misuse associated with opiates, even at recommended dosages, and because of the greater risks of overdose and death associated with extended-release opiate formulations, extended-release hydrocodone bitartrate should be reserved for use in patients for whom alternative treatment options (e.g., nonopiate analgesics or immediate-release opiates) are inadequate or not tolerated. Extended-release hydrocodone bitartrate is *not* indicated for use on an as-needed ("prn") basis.

Efficacy of hydrocodone bitartrate extended-release capsules (Zohydro® ER) was established in patients with moderate to severe chronic low back pain requiring chronic opiate therapy; the currently prescribed opiate was switched to the extended-release hydrocodone bitartrate capsules and the dosage was titrated to a stable level (up to 100 mg twice daily) during an initial open-label phase of the study; over a subsequent 12-week, randomized, placebo-controlled withdrawal phase, hydrocodone was associated with reductions in pain intensity compared with placebo.

Efficacy of extended-release tablets of hydrocodone bitartrate (Hysingla® ER) also was established in patients with moderate to severe chronic low back pain. The currently prescribed opiate and/or nonopiate analgesic(s) were switched to extended-release hydrocodone bitartrate tablets and the dosage was titrated to a stable level (20–120 mg once daily) during an initial open-label phase of the study; over a subsequent 12-week, randomized, placebo-controlled withdrawal phase, hydrocodone provided greater analgesia compared with placebo.

Hydrocodone bitartrate in fixed combination with acetaminophen is used for the relief of moderate to moderately severe pain.

Hydrocodone bitartrate in fixed combination with ibuprofen is used short term (generally for less than 10 days) for the relief of acute pain. Efficacy was established in single-dose studies in patients with postoperative (abdominal, gynecologic, orthopedic) pain. Hydrocodone bitartrate in fixed combination with ibuprofen is not indicated for the management of pain associated with such chronic conditions as osteoarthritis or rheumatoid arthritis.

For further information on the role of opiate analgesics in the management of acute or chronic pain, see Uses: Pain, in the Opiate Agonists General Statement 28:08.08.

For use of hydrocodone as an antitussive agent, see 48:08.

DOSAGE AND ADMINISTRATION

● Administration

Hydrocodone bitartrate is administered orally. Patients receiving hydrocodone should avoid alcohol; concomitant use may result in profound sedation, respiratory depression, coma, or death.

Hydrocodone bitartrate extended-release capsules are administered twice daily (every 12 hours). The extended-release capsules must be taken whole; crushing, breaking, cutting, chewing, or dissolving the capsules will result in uncontrolled delivery of hydrocodone and can result in overdosage and death. Patients should be advised that they must *not* consume alcoholic beverages or take prescription or nonprescription preparations containing alcohol during therapy, since concomitant ingestion of alcohol with hydrocodone bitartrate extended-release capsules may result in increased plasma concentrations of the drug and a potentially fatal overdose. (See Drug Interactions: Alcohol.)

Hydrocodone bitartrate extended-release tablets are administered once daily (every 24 hours) without regard to meals. Multiple tablets of lower-dose strengths that provide the desired total daily dosage can be taken as a once-daily dose. If a dose is missed, the next dose should be taken at the scheduled time on the following day. The extended-release tablets must be taken whole, one tablet at a time, with enough water to ensure complete swallowing of the tablet immediately after it is placed in the mouth. The tablets should not be wet (e.g., soaked, licked) before they are placed in the mouth for swallowing, since wetting the tablets results in formation of a gelatinous mass that may be difficult to swallow. (See Cautions.) Crushing, chewing, or dissolving the tablets will result in uncontrolled delivery of hydrocodone and can result in overdosage and death.

● Dosage

Hydrocodone bitartrate should be given at the lowest effective dosage and for the shortest duration of therapy consistent with the treatment goals of the patient. Reduced dosage is indicated in poor-risk and geriatric patients. If concomitant therapy with other CNS depressants is required, the lowest effective dosages and shortest possible duration of concomitant therapy should be used.

For acute pain not related to trauma or surgery, the prescribed quantity should be limited to the amount needed for the expected duration of pain severe enough to require opiate analgesia (generally 3 days or less and rarely more than 7 days). When opiate analgesics are used for the management of chronic noncancer pain, the US Centers for Disease Control and Prevention (CDC) recommends that primary care clinicians carefully reassess individual benefits and risks before prescribing dosages equivalent to 50 mg or more of morphine sulfate daily (approximately 50 mg or more of hydrocodone bitartrate daily) and avoid dosages equivalent to 90 mg or more of morphine sulfate daily (approximately 90 mg or more of hydrocodone bitartrate daily) or carefully justify their decision to titrate the dosage to such levels. Other experts recommend consulting a pain management specialist before exceeding a dosage equivalent to 80–120 mg of morphine sulfate daily. For further information on the management of opiate analgesic therapy, see Dosage and Administration: Dosage, in the Opiate Agonists General Statement 28:08.08.

Extended-release Capsules

To reduce the risk of respiratory depression in patients receiving hydrocodone bitartrate extended-release capsules, appropriate dosage selection and titration are essential. The initial dosage must be individualized, taking into account the patient's prior analgesic use and risk factors for addiction, abuse, and misuse. Patients should be monitored closely for respiratory depression, especially during the first 24–72 hours of therapy and following any increase in dosage.

For the management of severe pain requiring long-term, around-the-clock analgesia in adults who are not opiate tolerant or not currently receiving opiate analgesics, therapy with extended-release hydrocodone bitartrate capsules (Zohydro® ER) should be initiated at a dosage of 10 mg every 12 hours. Use of higher initial dosages in patients who are not opiate tolerant may result in fatal respiratory depression. A single dose exceeding 40 mg, the 50-mg extended-release hydrocodone bitartrate capsules, or a total daily dosage exceeding 80 mg should be used only in patients in whom tolerance to an opiate of comparable potency has been established. Patients are considered opiate tolerant if they have been receiving at least 60 mg of oral morphine sulfate daily, 25 mcg of transdermal fentanyl per hour, 30 mg of oral oxycodone hydrochloride daily, 8 mg of oral hydromorphone hydrochloride daily, 25 mg of oral oxymorphone hydrochloride daily, or an equianalgesic dose of another opiate daily for at least 1 week.

In adults who are being transferred from other oral opiates to therapy with extended-release hydrocodone bitartrate capsules, all other around-the-clock opiate analgesics should be discontinued when therapy with the extended-release capsules is initiated. Dosage must be carefully individualized since overestimation of the initial dosage in opiate-tolerant patients can result in fatal overdosage. The manufacturer states that the conversion factors in Table 1 may be used as a guide for selecting an initial dosage of extended-release hydrocodone bitartrate capsules for patients being transferred from therapy with one of the oral opiates listed in the table. The manufacturer cautions that the doses in Table 1 are not equianalgesic doses and the table cannot be used to transfer patients from extended-release hydrocodone bitartrate capsules to another opiate, as this will result in overestimation of the dosage of the new opiate and possible fatal overdosage. For patients receiving a single opiate analgesic, the current total daily dosage of the opiate should be multiplied by the appropriate conversion factor in Table 1 to calculate the approximate daily dosage of extended-release hydrocodone bitartrate capsules; the calculated daily dosage should then be divided in half for administration every 12 hours. For patients receiving more than one opiate analgesic, the approximate daily dosage of extended-release hydrocodone bitartrate should be calculated for each opiate and then those totals should be summed to obtain the approximate total daily dosage of extended-release hydrocodone bitartrate capsules; the calculated total daily dosage should then be divided in half for administration every 12 hours. For patients receiving analgesics containing opiates and nonopiates in a fixed ratio, only the opiate component should be considered in the conversion. Calculated doses that do not correspond to an available capsule strength should always be rounded down to the nearest whole capsule.

TABLE 1. Conversion Factors for Transfer from Other Oral Opiates to Extended-release Hydrocodone Bitartrate Capsules (Zohydro® ER)

Prior Oral Opiate	Oral Dose (mg)	Approximate Oral Conversion Factor
Hydrocodone	10	1
Oxycodone	10	1
Methadone	10	1
Oxymorphone	5	2
Hydromorphone	3.75	2.67
Morphine	15	0.67
Codeine	100	0.1

Following transfer from other opiate analgesics to extended-release hydrocodone bitartrate, patients should be monitored for manifestations of opiate withdrawal and for oversedation or toxicity. Particularly close monitoring is required when patients are switched from methadone, since conversion ratios between methadone and other opiates vary widely depending on extent of prior methadone exposure and because methadone has a long half-life and tends to accumulate in plasma.

In adults who are being transferred from transdermal fentanyl to extended-release hydrocodone bitartrate capsules, therapy with the extended-release capsules can be initiated 18 hours following removal of the transdermal fentanyl system at a conservative hydrocodone bitartrate dosage of approximately 10 mg every 12 hours for each 25 mcg/hour of transdermal fentanyl. Patients should be monitored closely, as there is limited experience with this conversion.

Dosage of extended-release hydrocodone bitartrate capsules should be adjusted gradually, every 3–7 days in increments of 10 mg every 12 hours, to provide adequate analgesia and to minimize adverse effects. If discontinuance of therapy is required, gradual tapering of the dosage every 2–4 days is recommended to avoid manifestations associated with abrupt withdrawal. Patients should be monitored closely for manifestations of withdrawal, which may indicate the need for slower tapering. In a phase 3 clinical trial, dosage of extended-release hydrocodone bitartrate capsules in patients reassigned to receive placebo was tapered according to the schedule in Table 2; dosages exceeding 100 mg twice daily were not evaluated in the clinical trial.

TABLE 2. Dosage Taper Used in Clinical Trial of Extended-release Hydrocodone Bitartrate Capsules (Zohydro® ER)

Stable Dosage at Time of Taper Initiation	Taper Schedule
20–30 mg every 12 hours	10 mg every 12 hours for 2 days, then discontinue on day 3
40–70 mg every 12 hours	40 mg every 12 hours for 2 days, 20 mg every 12 hours for 2 days, 10 mg every 12 hours for 2 days, then discontinue on day 7
80–100 mg every 12 hours	80 mg every 12 hours for 2 days, 60 mg every 12 hours for 2 days, 40 mg every 12 hours for 2 days, 20 mg every 12 hours for 2 days, 10 mg every 12 hours for 2 days, then discontinue on day 11

Extended-release Tablets

To reduce the risk of respiratory depression in patients receiving hydrocodone bitartrate extended-release tablets, appropriate dosage selection and titration are essential. The initial dosage must be individualized, taking into account the patient's prior analgesic use and risk factors for addiction, abuse, and misuse. Patients should be monitored closely for respiratory depression, especially during the first 24–72 hours of therapy and following any increase in dosage.

For the management of severe pain requiring long-term, around-the-clock analgesia in adults who are not opiate tolerant or not currently receiving opiate analgesics, therapy with extended-release hydrocodone bitartrate tablets (Hysingla® ER) should be initiated at a dosage of 20 mg every 24 hours. Use of higher initial dosages in patients who are not opiate tolerant may result in fatal respiratory depression. Dosages of 80 mg or more daily should be used only in opiate-tolerant patients. Patients are considered opiate tolerant if they have been receiving at least 60 mg of oral morphine sulfate daily, 25 mcg of transdermal fentanyl per hour, 30 mg of oral oxycodone hydrochloride daily, 8 mg of oral hydromorphone hydrochloride daily, 25 mg of oral oxymorphone hydrochloride daily, or an equianalgesic dose of another opiate daily for at least 1 week.

Patients being transferred from other oral hydrocodone-containing formulations to the extended-release tablets should receive the same total daily dosage of hydrocodone bitartrate administered once daily.

In adults who are being transferred from other oral opiates to therapy with extended-release hydrocodone bitartrate tablets, all other around-the-clock opiate analgesics should be discontinued when therapy with the extended-release tablets is initiated. Dosage must be carefully individualized since overestimation of the initial dosage in opiate-tolerant patients can result in fatal overdosage. The conversion factors in Table 3 may be used as a guide for selecting an initial dosage of extended-release hydrocodone bitartrate tablets for patients being transferred from therapy with one of the oral opiates listed in the table. The manufacturer cautions that the doses in Table 3 are not equianalgesic doses and the table cannot be used to transfer patients from extended-release hydrocodone bitartrate tablets to another opiate, as this will result in overestimation of the dosage of the new opiate and possible fatal overdosage. For patients receiving a single opiate analgesic, the current total daily dosage of the opiate should be multiplied by the appropriate conversion factor in Table 3 to calculate the approximate daily dosage of oral hydrocodone bitartrate; for patients receiving more than one opiate analgesic, the approximate daily dosage of oral hydrocodone bitartrate should be calculated for each opiate and then those totals should be summed to obtain the approximate daily dosage of oral hydrocodone bitartrate. *Initial oral hydrocodone bitartrate dosages calculated using the conversion factors in Table 3 should be reduced by 25% to account for interpatient variability in the relative potency of different opiates.* For patients receiving analgesics containing opiates and nonopiates in a fixed ratio, only the opiate component should be considered in the conversion. Calculated doses that do not correspond to an available tablet strength should always be rounded down to the nearest whole tablet. If the calculated dose is less than 20 mg, therapy should be initiated at a dosage of 20 mg once daily.

TABLE 3. Conversion Factors for Transfer from Other Oral Opiates to Extended-release Hydrocodone Bitartrate Tablets (Hysingla® ER)

Prior Oral Opiate	Oral Dose (mg)	Approximate Oral Conversion Factor
Codeine	133	0.15
Hydromorphone	5	4
Methadone	13.3	1.5
Morphine	40	0.5
Oxycodone	20	1
Oxymorphone	10	2
Tramadol	200	0.1

Following transfer from other opiate analgesics to extended-release hydrocodone bitartrate, patients should be monitored for manifestations of opiate withdrawal and for oversedation or toxicity. Particularly close monitoring is required when patients are switched from methadone, since conversion ratios between methadone and other opiates vary widely depending on extent of prior methadone exposure and because methadone has a long half-life and tends to accumulate in plasma.

In adults who are being transferred from transdermal fentanyl to extended-release hydrocodone bitartrate tablets, therapy with the extended-release tablets can be initiated 18 hours following removal of the transdermal fentanyl system at a conservative hydrocodone bitartrate dosage of approximately 20 mg every 24 hours for each 25 mcg/hour of transdermal fentanyl. Patients should be monitored closely, as there is limited experience with this conversion.

Adults receiving transdermal buprenorphine at a dosage of 20 mg or less per hour should be switched to extended-release hydrocodone bitartrate tablets at a dosage of 20 mg every 24 hours. Patients should be monitored closely, as there is limited experience with this conversion.

Dosage of extended-release hydrocodone bitartrate tablets should be adjusted gradually, every 3–5 days in increments of 10–20 mg every 24 hours, to provide adequate analgesia and to minimize adverse effects. If discontinuance of therapy is required, gradual tapering of the dosage every 2–4 days is recommended to avoid manifestations associated with abrupt withdrawal. As the dosage is tapered, each new dose should be at least 50% of the prior dose; once the dosage has been reduced to 20 mg daily for 2–4 days, therapy can be discontinued.

Immediate-release Fixed-combination Preparations

The usual adult dosage of hydrocodone bitartrate when used in fixed combination with acetaminophen for relief of moderate to moderately severe pain is 5–10 mg every 4–6 hours as necessary. When used in fixed combination with ibuprofen for relief of acute pain, the usual adult dosage of hydrocodone bitartrate is 2.5–10 mg every 4–6 hours as needed, generally given for no longer than 10 days; the manufacturers state that the total daily dosage should not exceed 5 tablets (each providing from 2.5–10 mg of hydrocodone bitartrate and 200 mg of ibuprofen). Dosage should be adjusted according to the severity of the pain and the response and tolerance of the patient. When opiate analgesics are administered in fixed combination with nonopiate analgesics, the opiate dosage may be limited by the nonopiate component. Because commercially available preparations contain hydrocodone bitartrate and nonopiate analgesics in various fixed ratios and because these nonopiate analgesics also are available in many other prescription and OTC preparations, care should be taken to ensure that therapy is not duplicated and that dosage of the nonopiate drug does not exceed maximum recommended dosages.

● Dosage in Renal and Hepatic Impairment

No adjustment of initial hydrocodone bitartrate dosage is required in patients with mild or moderate hepatic impairment. Because of the potential for increased drug exposure, the manufacturer states that therapy with hydrocodone bitartrate extended-release capsules should be initiated at a dosage of 10 mg every 12 hours in patients with severe hepatic impairment. The manufacturer of hydrocodone bitartrate extended-release tablets states that dosage of this formulation should be reduced by 50% in patients with severe hepatic impairment. Patients with severe hepatic impairment should be monitored closely for adverse effects (e.g., respiratory depression, sedation).

Because of the potential for increased drug exposure, the manufacturer states that therapy with hydrocodone bitartrate extended-release capsules should be initiated at a low dose in patients with renal impairment. The manufacturer of hydrocodone bitartrate extended-release tablets states that dosage of this formulation should be reduced by 50% in patients with moderate or severe renal impairment (including end-stage renal disease); the manufacturer states that the extended-release tablets may be used without dosage adjustment in patients with mild renal impairment. Patients with renal impairment should be monitored closely for adverse effects (e.g., respiratory depression, sedation).

CAUTIONS

Hydrocodone bitartrate shares the toxic potentials of the opiate agonists, and the usual precautions of opiate agonist therapy should be observed. (See Cautions in the Opiate Agonists General Statement 28:08.08.) For further information on cautions, precautions, and contraindications associated with the use of hydrocodone, see also Cautions in Hydrocodone Bitartrate 48:08. When hydrocodone is used as a fixed-combination preparation that includes acetaminophen or ibuprofen, the cautions, precautions, and contraindications associated with these drugs must be considered in addition to those associated with hydrocodone.

Because some patients have reported difficulty in swallowing hydrocodone bitartrate extended-release tablets, the tablets should be administered one at a time with enough water to ensure that each tablet is completely swallowed immediately after it is placed in the mouth; the extended-release tablets should not be wet (e.g., soaked, licked) before they are placed in the mouth for swallowing. Choking, dysphagia, and esophageal obstruction (in at least one case requiring medical intervention to remove the tablet) have been reported. Patients with underlying GI disorders (e.g., esophageal or colon cancer) associated with a narrow GI lumen are at greater risk of developing these complications. Use of an alternative analgesic should be considered for patients who have difficulty swallowing and in those at risk for underlying GI disorders associated with a narrow GI lumen. Because the extended-release tablets gradually form a gelatinous mass when exposed to fluids, pediatric patients may be at increased risk of esophageal obstruction, dysphagia, and choking because of their smaller GI lumen if they ingest the tablets.

Prolongation of the corrected QT (QT_c) interval was observed in healthy individuals receiving hydrocodone bitartrate 160 mg daily (as extended-release tablets). This observation should be considered when making decisions regarding patient monitoring (e.g., periodic monitoring of ECGs and electrolyte concentrations) when hydrocodone bitartrate extended-release tablets are used in patients with congestive heart failure, bradyarrhythmias, or electrolyte abnormalities or in those who are receiving drugs that are known to prolong the QT_c interval. The manufacturer states that use of the extended-release tablets should be avoided in patients with congenital long QT syndrome. If prolongation of the QT_c interval occurs, reduction of hydrocodone bitartrate dosage by 33–50% or use of an alternative analgesic should be considered.

● Misuse and Abuse

Because of the challenges associated with providing access to an adequate array of options for management of chronic pain while simultaneously preventing prescription opiate abuse and misuse, the decision by the US Food and Drug Administration (FDA) to approve hydrocodone bitartrate extended-release capsules (Zohydro® ER) was controversial, as the formulation lacks tamper-resistant features that might deter abuse and, like other extended-release opiates, some strengths contain substantial amounts of the drug (up to 50 mg). Hydrocodone bitartrate extended-release tablets (Hysingla® ER; containing up to 120 mg of the drug) are formulated with physical and chemical properties that are intended to make this dosage form more difficult to manipulate for IV or intranasal abuse and misuse, and some extended-release characteristics are retained if the tablets are physically compromised. In vitro studies indicate that exposing the tablets to water results in formation of a viscous hydrogel that resists passage through a needle; the tablets also are resistant to crushing, breaking, and dissolution by various tools and solvents. Results of clinical abuse potential studies suggest a reduced potential for intranasal abuse (compared with powdered hydrocodone bitartrate) or oral abuse by chewing the tablets (compared with hydrocodone bitartrate solution). However, the potential for IV, intranasal, and oral abuse still exists.

Modified-release (e.g., extended-release) opiates are associated with a greater risk of overdose and death because of the larger amount of drug contained in each dosage unit. Abuse or misuse of hydrocodone bitartrate extended-release dosage forms by cutting, breaking, crushing, chewing, or dissolving the capsules or tablets, snorting the contents, or injecting the dissolved contents will result in uncontrolled delivery of the drug and can result in overdosage and death. Inadvertent ingestion of even one dose of extended-release hydrocodone bitartrate capsules or tablets, especially by a child, also can result in a fatal overdose. Intake of alcohol with the extended-release capsules may result in increased peak plasma concentrations of hydrocodone and ingestion of a potentially toxic dose of the drug. (See Drug Interactions: Alcohol.) Extended-release preparations of hydrocodone bitartrate should be prescribed only by clinicians who are knowledgeable in the use of potent opiates for the management of chronic pain.

Hydrocodone in fixed combination with other analgesics (e.g., acetaminophen, nonsteroidal anti-inflammatory agents) is used widely in the management of pain. Hydrocodone also is used in antitussive preparations for the management of cough. Depending on the formulation, many of these fixed-combination analgesic and antitussive preparations previously were subject to control under the Federal Controlled Substances Act of 1970 as schedule III (C-III) drugs. However, because of increasing concerns about misuse, abuse, and diversion of these preparations, the US Department of Health and Human Services (HHS) recommended on December 16, 2013, that these preparations be rescheduled to schedule II (C-II) in response to an evidence-based analysis by FDA. This recommendation subsequently was accepted by the US Drug Enforcement Administration (DEA) and became effective October 6, 2014. Preparations containing hydrocodone in fixed combination with other analgesics have a clinically important and legitimate role in the management of moderate to moderately severe pain. Hydrocodone-containing combination preparations also have a clinically important and legitimate role in the symptomatic treatment of cough and upper respiratory symptoms associated with allergy and cold when they combine hydrocodone with other antitussives or antihistamines.

The conclusions of FDA and DEA considered a number of factors such as abuse potential, pharmacologic effects, history and current patterns of abuse, public health risk, dependence liability, and scope, duration, and significance of abuse. In recent years, hydrocodone-containing preparations have become the most frequently prescribed products in the US. In 2011, 131 million prescriptions totaling up to 8 billion or more tablets for fixed-combination hydrocodone analgesic preparations were prescribed and dispensed in the US to over 47 million patients, representing about 4 times the number of prescriptions written for fixed-combination oxycodone preparations and about 10 times the number of prescriptions for codeine-containing preparations. In 2011, approximately 5 million prescriptions were dispensed for hydrocodone-containing combination antitussives.

Data from 2012 showed that 37 million Americans had used analgesics nonmedically (misuse and abuse) in their lifetime, and that roughly 70% of these individuals reported lifetime nonmedical use of fixed-combination hydrocodone preparations. Further, hydrocodone is associated with substantial numbers of reports of overdose, suicide, abuse, and dependence. While the addition of nonopiate analgesic ingredients decreases the abuse potential and the rates of abuse for hydrocodone-containing combination analgesic preparations are lower than those for oxycodone-containing preparations, hydrocodone-containing combinations have a high potential for abuse that is considered similar to that of schedule II oxycodone-containing combination preparations. There also is evidence to suggest that individuals are taking sufficient amounts of hydrocodone to create a hazard to their health or the safety of others or the community, that there is considerable diversion from legitimate channels, and that individuals are taking the drug on their own initiative rather than on the basis of medical advice. Similar to the pattern for abuse are the risks of psychological and physical dependence, which can be severe. Considering this and other evidence, a decision to reschedule these hydrocodone-containing combination preparations

to C-II was made. However, because of concerns about the impact of this scheduling change on public health, particularly access to effective pain management, FDA recommended that the impact of this action be assessed through close continued monitoring.

● Pregnancy, Fertility, and Lactation

Analysis of data from the National Birth Defects Prevention Study, a large population-based, case-control study, suggests that therapeutic use of opiates in pregnant women during the period of organogenesis is associated with a low absolute risk of birth defects, including heart defects, spina bifida, and gastroschisis. Oral hydrocodone bitartrate was not teratogenic in rats or rabbits at dosages or 25 or 50 mg/kg daily (equivalent to 2 or 10 times, respectively, a human dosage of 100 mg daily on a mg/m² basis). In studies in rats, oral administration of hydrocodone bitartrate 10 mg/kg daily (approximately equivalent to a human dosage of 100 mg daily) during gestation and lactation was associated with reduced fetal viability (increase in stillborn pups and decrease in pup survival). At a dosage of 25 mg/kg daily, reduced nursing behavior and decreased pup body weight were observed; minimal maternal toxicity was observed at this dosage. In studies in rabbits, an increase in umbilical hernias, irregularly shaped bones, and delayed fetal skeletal maturation were observed at a maternally toxic dosage of 75 mg/kg daily (equivalent to 15 times a human dosage of 100 mg daily). An oral hydrocodone bitartrate dosage of 25 mg/kg daily (equivalent to approximately 5 times a human dosage of 100 mg daily) was associated with reduced fetal weights.

No effects on fertility were observed in male rats receiving hydrocodone bitartrate at dosages equivalent to 10 times a human dosage of 100 mg daily, although decreased weight of male reproductive organs was observed at dosages equivalent to 2.4 times a human dosage of 100 mg daily. Reductions in female fertility indices observed at a dosage equivalent to twice the human dosage of 100 mg daily are not thought to be clinically relevant to humans.

Hydrocodone is distributed into breast milk. The manufacturers state that a decision should be made whether to discontinue nursing or the drug, taking into account the importance of the drug to the woman. Infants exposed to hydrocodone through breast milk should be observed for excessive sedation, respiratory depression, GI effects, and altered feeding patterns. Symptoms of withdrawal can occur in opiate-dependent infants when maternal administration of opiates is discontinued or breast-feeding is stopped.

DRUG INTERACTIONS

● Drugs Affecting Hepatic Microsomal Enzymes

Because hydrocodone is metabolized by the cytochrome P-450 (CYP) microsomal enzyme system, principally by isoenzyme 3A4, concomitant use of hydrocodone with drugs that inhibit CYP3A4 activity may result in reduced clearance and increased plasma concentrations of the drug, possibly resulting in increased or prolonged opiate effects, including an increased risk of fatal respiratory depression. Concomitant administration of hydrocodone bitartrate (single 20-mg dose as extended-release tablets) and the potent CYP3A4 inhibitor ketoconazole (200 mg twice daily for 6 days) increased mean area under the concentration-time curve (AUC) and peak plasma concentration of hydrocodone by 135 and 78%, respectively. Conversely, concomitant use of hydrocodone with CYP3A4 inducers may result in increased clearance and decreased plasma concentrations of hydrocodone, with possible lack of efficacy or development of opiate withdrawal. If concomitant therapy with a CYP3A4 inducer is discontinued, an increase in plasma hydrocodone concentrations may occur, potentially increasing or prolonging therapeutic and adverse effects of the drug and increasing the risk of fatal overdosage. Therefore, caution should be exercised and patients who require concomitant therapy with a CYP3A4 inhibitor or inducer, or who have recently discontinued such therapy, should be monitored closely at frequent intervals, and dosage adjustments should be considered until stable drug effects are achieved.

Hydrocodone is metabolized to a lesser extent by CYP2D6; however, concomitant administration of hydrocodone bitartrate (single 20-mg dose as extended-release tablets) and the CYP2D6 inhibitor paroxetine (20 mg once daily for 12 days) did not alter systemic exposure to hydrocodone.

• Alcohol

Alcohol and hydrocodone may cause additive CNS depression and may result in hypotension, profound sedation, coma, respiratory depression, and death. Patients receiving hydrocodone should be instructed to avoid alcohol, including alcoholic beverages and prescription or nonprescription preparations containing alcohol.

In addition to such additive depressant effects, concomitant use of alcohol with extended-release hydrocodone bitartrate capsules can result in increased plasma concentrations of the opiate and potentially fatal overdosage. Administration of extended-release hydrocodone bitartrate capsules (Zohydro® ER) 50 mg with 40% alcohol in the fasted state increased the rate of hydrocodone absorption, increased peak plasma concentrations of the drug by an average of 2.4-fold (up to 3.9-fold in one individual), and increased the extent of absorption by an average of 1.2-fold (up to 1.7-fold in one individual).

• Laxatives

Concomitant use of hydrocodone bitartrate extended-release tablets with strong laxatives that rapidly increase GI motility (e.g., lactulose) may result in decreased absorption and decreased plasma concentrations of the opiate. Patients receiving such concomitant therapy should be monitored closely for adverse events and changing analgesic requirements.

For further information about drug interactions involving opiate agonists (including hydrocodone bitartrate), see Drug Interactions in the Opiate Agonists General Statement 28:08.08.

PHARMACOKINETICS

Overall systemic exposure or bioavailability of hydrocodone bitartrate following administration as extended-release capsules (Zohydro® ER) or tablets (Hysingla® ER) is similar to that observed following administration of immediate-release fixed-combination preparations containing the drug in the same or similar dosage; however, peak plasma concentrations of the drug are lower with the extended-release formulations. Peak plasma concentrations of hydrocodone are attained approximately 1.3–1.7 hours after administration as an immediate-release preparation, 5 hours after administration as extended-release capsules, and 6–30 hours (median: 14–16 hours) after administration as extended-release tablets.

After administration of the extended-release capsules for 7 days, area under the plasma concentration-time curve (AUC) and peak concentrations of hydrocodone are approximately twofold higher than values attained on the first day of administration. At doses of up to 50 mg, the pharmacokinetics of extended-release hydrocodone bitartrate are independent of dose. Administration of the extended-release capsules with food does not substantially affect the extent of absorption, although peak plasma hydrocodone concentrations were increased by 27% following administration of a 20-mg dose of the extended-release capsules with a high-fat meal.

After single-dose administration of hydrocodone bitartrate extended-release tablets, peak concentrations and AUC of the drug increased linearly and in a slightly more than dose-proportional manner over the dose range of 20–120 mg. With once-daily dosing, peak plasma concentrations and AUC were 1.1- and 1.3-fold higher at steady state. Higher doses (80 or 120 mg versus 30 mg) produced larger fluctuations in peak-to-trough plasma concentrations of the drug. Although administration of the 120-mg extended-release tablets with a high-fat meal increased peak plasma concentrations by 54% compared with administration in the fasted state, AUC was increased by only 20% and the manufacturer states that the extended-release tablets may be administered without regard to meals.

Hydrocodone is about 36% bound to plasma proteins.

Hydrocodone is metabolized by N-demethylation, O-demethylation, and 6-keto reduction to the corresponding 6-α- and 6-β-hydroxy metabolites. Hydrocodone is metabolized principally by cytochrome P-450 (CYP) isoenzyme 3A4 to form norhydrocodone (N-demethylation) and to a lesser extent by CYP2D6 to form hydromorphone (O-demethylation). Hydrocodone also may be metabolized to a small extent by CYP2B6 and CYP2C19. Hydromorphone accounts for less than 3% of the circulating parent drug, but may contribute to

the total analgesic effect of hydrocodone. Hydrocodone and its metabolites are eliminated mainly in urine; only about 6.5% of an administered dose is excreted as unchanged drug. About 99% of an administered dose is eliminated within 72 hours. The mean plasma half-life of the drug is 3.8–4.5 hours after oral administration as an immediate-release preparation and approximately 7–9 hours after oral administration as extended-release capsules or tablets.

Following oral administration of a single 20-mg dose of hydrocodone bitartrate as extended-release capsules, peak plasma concentrations of the drug were 15, 48, or 41% higher and AUC was 15, 57, or 44% higher in patients with mild, moderate, or severe renal impairment, respectively, compared with individuals with normal renal function. Following oral administration of a single 20-mg dose of hydrocodone bitartrate as extended-release capsules, peak plasma concentrations of the drug were 8–10% higher and AUC was 10 or 26% higher in patients with mild or moderate hepatic impairment, respectively, compared with individuals with normal hepatic function; pharmacokinetics of the drug were not evaluated in patients with severe hepatic impairment. Population analyses indicated that the pharmacokinetics of the drug were not substantially affected by gender or age of 65 years or older.

Following oral administration of a single 20-mg dose of hydrocodone bitartrate as extended-release tablets, peak plasma concentrations and AUC of the drug reportedly were 6 and 14% lower, respectively, in patients with mild hepatic impairment; 5 and 13% higher, respectively, in patients with moderate hepatic impairment; and 5 and 4% higher, respectively, in patients with severe hepatic impairment compared with individuals with normal hepatic function. Hepatic impairment did not substantially alter plasma protein binding of the drug. Following oral administration of a single 60-mg dose of the drug as extended-release tablets, peak plasma concentrations reportedly were 14, 23, or 11% higher and AUC was 13, 61, or 57% higher in patients with mild, moderate, or severe renal impairment, respectively, compared with individuals with normal renal function; among patients with end-stage renal disease requiring dialysis, peak plasma concentrations of the drug reportedly were decreased by 13% and AUC was increased by 4% compared with values in individuals with normal renal function.

Age (65 years or older) and gender do not appear to substantially alter exposure to hydrocodone.

CHEMISTRY AND STABILITY

• Chemistry

Hydrocodone bitartrate is a phenanthrene-derivative opiate agonist that is used as an analgesic and antitussive agent. Hydrocodone is a hydrogenated-ketone derivative of codeine. Hydrocodone bitartrate occurs as fine, white crystals or as a crystalline powder and is soluble in water and slightly soluble in alcohol.

• Stability

Hydrocodone bitartrate is affected by light. Hydrocodone bitartrate preparations should be stored in tight, light-resistant containers at 15–30°C.

For further information on the chemistry, pharmacology, pharmacokinetics, uses, cautions, chronic toxicity, acute toxicity, drug interactions, and dosage and administration of hydrocodone bitartrate, see the Opiate Agonists General Statement 28:08.08 and Hydrocodone Bitartrate 48:08.

PREPARATIONS

Single-entity hydrocodone bitartrate preparations are subject to control under the Federal Controlled Substances Act of 1970 as schedule II (C-II) drugs; when available as a fixed-combination preparation in a concentration of 15 mg or less per dosage unit or 5 mL combined with a therapeutic amount of one or more non-opiate drugs or with a fourfold or greater quantity of isoquinolone opium alkaloid, hydrocodone previously was subject to control as a schedule III (C-III) drug. However, because of increasing concerns about misuse, abuse, and diversion, hydrocodone-containing preparations that previously were subject to control as schedule III drugs have been rescheduled and, effective October 6, 2014, are subject to control as schedule II (C-II) drugs. (See Cautions: Misuse and Abuse.)

Preparations containing hydrocodone in combination with more than 325 mg of acetaminophen per dosage unit have been discontinued to minimize the risk of inadvertent acetaminophen overdosage; some of these preparations may have been reformulated to limit the amount of acetaminophen to 325 mg or less per dosage unit.

Excipients in commercially available drug preparations may have clinically important effects in some individuals; consult specific product labeling for details.

HYDROcodone Bitartrate

Oral

Capsules, extended-release	10 mg	**Zohydro® ER** (C-II), Zogenix
	15 mg	**Zohydro® ER** (C-II), Zogenix
	20 mg	**Zohydro® ER** (C-II), Zogenix
	30 mg	**Zohydro® ER** (C-II), Zogenix
	40 mg	**Zohydro® ER** (C-II), Zogenix
	50 mg	**Zohydro® ER** (C-II), Zogenix
Tablets, extended-release, film-coated	20 mg	**Hysingla® ER** (C-II), Purdue Pharma
	30 mg	**Hysingla® ER** (C-II), Purdue Pharma
	40 mg	**Hysingla® ER** (C-II), Purdue Pharma
	60 mg	**Hysingla® ER** (C-II), Purdue Pharma
	80 mg	**Hysingla® ER** (C-II), Purdue Pharma
	100 mg	**Hysingla® ER** (C-II), Purdue Pharma
	120 mg	**Hysingla® ER** (C-II), Purdue Pharma

HYDROcodone Bitartrate Combinations

Oral

Solution	2.5 mg/5 mL with Acetaminophen 108 mg/5 mL*	**HYDROcodone Bitartrate and Acetaminophen Oral Solution** (C-II)
	3.3 mg/5 mL with Acetaminophen 100 mg/5 mL*	**HYDROcodone Bitartrate and Acetaminophen Oral Solution** (C-II) **Lortab® Elixir** (C-II), ECR
	3.3 mg/5 mL with Acetaminophen 108 mg/5 mL*	**HYDROcodone Bitartrate and Acetaminophen Oral Solution** (C-II)

Tablets	2.5 mg with Acetaminophen 325 mg*	**HYDROcodone Bitartrate and Acetaminophen Tablets** (C-II)
	5 mg with Acetaminophen 300 mg*	**HYDROcodone Bitartrate and Acetaminophen Tablets** (C-II) **Vicodin®** (C-II; scored), AbbVie
	5 mg with Acetaminophen 325 mg*	**HYDROcodone Bitartrate and Acetaminophen Tablets** (C-II) **Lortab®** (C-II; scored), UCB **Norco®** (C-II; scored), Actavis
	7.5 mg with Acetaminophen 300 mg*	**HYDROcodone Bitartrate and Acetaminophen Tablets** (C-II) **Vicodin ES®** (C-II); scored, AbbVie
	7.5 mg with Acetaminophen 325 mg*	**HYDROcodone Bitartrate and Acetaminophen Tablets** (C-II) **Lortab®** (C-II; scored), UCB **Norco®** (C-II; scored), Actavis
	10 mg with Acetaminophen 300 mg*	**HYDROcodone Bitartrate and Acetaminophen Tablets** (C-II) **Vicodin HP®** (C-II; scored), AbbVie
	10 mg with Acetaminophen 325 mg*	**HYDROcodone Bitartrate and Acetaminophen Tablets** (C-II) **Lortab®** (C-II; scored), UCB **Norco®** (C-II; scored), Actavis
Tablets, film-coated	2.5 mg with Ibuprofen 200 mg*	**HYDROcodone Bitartrate and Ibuprofen Film-coated Tablets** (C-II) **Reprexain®** (C-II), Gemini
	5 mg with Ibuprofen 200 mg*	**HYDROcodone Bitartrate and Ibuprofen Film-coated Tablets** (C-II) **Reprexain®** (C-II), Gemini
	7.5 mg with Ibuprofen 200 mg*	**HYDROcodone Bitartrate and Ibuprofen Film-coated Tablets** (C-II) **Vicoprofen®** (C-II), AbbVie
	10 mg with Ibuprofen 200 mg*	**HYDROcodone Bitartrate and Ibuprofen Film-coated Tablets** (C-II) **Reprexain®** (C-II), Gemini

* available from one or more manufacturer, distributor, and/or repackager by generic (nonproprietary) name

HYDROmorphone Hydrochloride

28:08.08 · OPIOID AGONISTS

■ Hydromorphone is a semisynthetic phenanthrene-derivative opiate agonist.

REMS

FDA approved a REMS for hydromorphone to ensure that the benefits outweigh the risks. The REMS may apply to one or more preparations of hydromorphone and consists of the following: medication guide and elements to assure safe use. See the FDA REMS page (https://www.accessdata.fda.gov/scripts/cder/rems/index.cfm).

USES

Hydromorphone hydrochloride injection and conventional oral preparations of the drug (immediate-release tablets, oral solution) are used for the relief of pain that is severe enough to require an opiate analgesic. The injection containing 10 mg of the drug per mL is a highly concentrated parenteral formulation of the drug that should be used *only* in *opiate-tolerant* patients who require higher dosages of opiate analgesics; during treatment with this formulation, patients must remain on around-the-clock opiate therapy. Patients are considered opiate tolerant if they have been receiving at least 60 mg of oral morphine sulfate daily, 25 mcg of transdermal fentanyl per hour, 30 mg of oral oxycodone hydrochloride daily, 60 mg of oral hydrocodone bitartrate daily, 8 mg of oral hydromorphone hydrochloride daily, 25 mg of oral oxymorphone hydrochloride daily, or an equianalgesic dosage of another opiate daily for at least 1 week. Because of the risks of addiction, abuse, and misuse associated with opiates even at recommended dosages, parenteral and conventional oral formulations of hydromorphone should be reserved for use in patients for whom alternative treatment options (e.g., nonopiate analgesics, opiate-containing fixed combinations) have not been, or are not expected to be, adequate or tolerated.

Extended-release tablets of hydromorphone hydrochloride are used orally in opiate-tolerant patients for the management of pain that is severe enough to require long-term, daily, around-the-clock use of an opiate analgesic; because of the risks of addiction, abuse, and misuse associated with opiates even at recommended dosages, and because of the greater risks of overdosage and death associated with extended-release opiate formulations, extended-release hydromorphone should be reserved for use in patients for whom alternative treatment options (e.g., nonopiate analgesics, immediate-release opiates) are inadequate or not tolerated. Extended-release hydromorphone is *not* intended for use on an as-needed ("prn") basis.

For further information on the role of opiate analgesics in the management of acute or chronic pain, see Uses: Pain, in the Opiate Agonists General Statement 28:08.08.

DOSAGE AND ADMINISTRATION

● *Administration*

Hydromorphone hydrochloride may be administered by subcutaneous, IM, or slow IV injection; the drug also may be administered orally as conventional (immediate-release) or extended-release tablets or as an oral solution. If rapid onset and shorter duration of analgesia are required, the drug may be given IV at a very slow rate (over at least 2–3 minutes depending on the dose) with special attention to the possibility of respiratory depression and hypotension. Hydromorphone hydrochloride has been administered as a continuous subcutaneous or IV infusion in selected opiate-tolerant patients with chronic pain conditions;

extreme caution is advised when administering continuous infusions of opiates to patients with no prior exposure to opiate analgesics. The drug also has been administered IV via a controlled-delivery device for patient-controlled analgesia (PCA). Hydromorphone hydrochloride also has been administered epidurally†.

Parenteral Administration

Parenteral preparations of hydromorphone hydrochloride are commercially available in various concentrations (0.2, 1, 2, 4, and 10 mg/mL). Preparations containing lower concentrations of the drug (0.2, 1, 2, or 4 mg/mL) should be used to initiate parenteral hydromorphone therapy in opiate-naive patients. **The highly concentrated (10-mg/mL) injection is intended for use only in patients who are tolerant to and already receiving high dosages of opiate agonists.** (See Uses and also Cautions.) **Confusion between the different concentrations or between mg and mL can result in accidental overdosage and/or death. To avoid such dosing errors, care should be taken to ensure that correct dosages are prescribed and dispensed.** The highly concentrated injection should be used only when the volume required for the intended dose can be accurately measured; this injection should not be used when low doses are required. The highly concentrated injection should be reserved for use in patients who require the reduced total volume and higher concentration of this formulation.

When the single-dose 10-mg/mL vial containing 500 mg of hydromorphone hydrochloride is used for preparation of IV infusion solutions, the appropriate amount should be withdrawn for preparation of a single large-volume parenteral solution and any unused portion of the vial should be discarded. Hydromorphone hydrochloride has been diluted (e.g., to a concentration of 1 mg/mL) in 5% dextrose or 0.9% sodium chloride injection for continuous IV infusion in critically ill adults. Hydromorphone hydrochloride injection has been self-administered intermittently as needed ("prn") via a controlled-delivery device for PCA with usual lockout intervals (minimum time between self-administered doses programmed into device) of 5–10 minutes.

IM administration of opiate analgesics is discouraged; IM injections can cause pain and are associated with unreliable absorption, resulting in inconsistent analgesia.

Standardize 4 Safety

Standardized concentrations for hydromorphone have been established through Standardize 4 Safety (S4S), a national patient safety initiative to reduce medication errors, especially during transitions of care. Multidisciplinary expert panels were convened to determine recommended standard concentrations. Because recommendations from the S4S panels may differ from the manufacturer's prescribing information, caution is advised when using concentrations that differ from labeling, particularly when using rate information from the label. For additional information on S4S (including updates that may be available), see http://www.ashp.org/pharmacy-practice/standardize-4-safety-initiative.

TABLE 1. Standardize 4 Safety Standards for Hydromorphone Continuous IV Infusions

Patient Population	Concentration Standard[a]	Dosing Units
Adults	0.2 mg/mL	mg/hour
	1 mg/mL	
	5 mg/mL (based on high dose requirements)	
Pediatric patients (<50 kg)	0.2 mg/mL	mg/kg/hr
	1 mg/mL	
	5 mg/mL	

[a] Concentration standard for adults is for continuous infusions *not* delivered by a PCA device. Concentration standard for pediatric patients also is for continuous infusions and *not* for delivery via PCA device.

TABLE 2. Standardize 4 Safety PCA Standard Concentrations for Hydromorphone

Patient Population	Concentration Standard	Dosing Units
Adults	0.2 mg/mL	mg
	1 mg/mL (caution is advised if both hydromorphone and morphine are used to avoid confusion in selection as both have the same concentration)	
	10 mg/mL (sub-Q only)	
Pediatric patients (<50 kg)	0.05 mg/mL	mg/kg/hr
	0.2 mg/mL	
	1 mg/mL (caution is advised if both hydromorphone and morphine are used to avoid confusion in selection as both have the same concentration)	

TABLE 3. Standardize 4 Safety Epidural Single Drug Standard Concentrations for Hydromorphone

Patient Population	Concentration Standard
Adults	10 mcg/mL
Pediatric patients (<50 kg)	5 mcg/mL
	10 mcg/mL

TABLE 4. Standardize 4 Safety ADULT Epidural Combination Drug Standard Concentrations for Hydromorphone

Drug Combinations	Anesthetic Concentration	Narcotic Concentration
Bupivacaine with hydromorphone	1. Bupivacaine 0.0625%	1. Hydromorphone 10 mcg/mL
	2. Bupivacaine 0.125%	2. Hydromorphone 10 mcg/mL
Ropivacaine with hydromorphone	1. Ropivacaine 0.2%	1. Hydromorphone 10 mcg/mL

TABLE 5. Standardize 4 Safety PEDIATRIC Epidural Combination Drug Standard Concentrations for Hydromorphone

Drug Combinations	Anesthetic Concentration	Narcotic Concentration
Bupivacaine with hydromorphone	1. Bupivacaine 0.0625%	1. Hydromorphone 5 mcg/mL
	2. Bupivacaine 0.0625%	2. Hydromorphone 10 mcg/mL
	3. Bupivacaine 0.125%	3. Hydromorphone 5 mcg/mL
	4. Bupivacaine 0.125%	4. Hydromorphone 10 mcg/mL
Ropivacaine with hydromorphone	1. Ropivacaine 0.1%	1. Hydromorphone 5 mcg/mL
	2. Ropivacaine 0.1%	2. Hydromorphone 10 mcg/mL
	3. Ropivacaine 0.2%	3. Hydromorphone 5 mcg/mL
	4. Ropivacaine 0.2%	4. Hydromorphone 10 mcg/mL

Oral Administration

Commercially available conventional (immediate-release) tablets and oral solutions of hydromorphone hydrochloride are bioequivalent. Although food may decrease the rate and extent of absorption of hydromorphone hydrochloride conventional tablets (see Pharmacokinetics), the manufacturer states that these effects may not be clinically important. Patients receiving hydromorphone should avoid alcohol; concomitant use may result in profound sedation, respiratory depression, coma, and death.

Extended-release tablets of hydromorphone hydrochloride should be prescribed only by clinicians who are knowledgeable in the use of potent opiates for the management of chronic pain. When therapy with extended-release hydromorphone hydrochloride is initiated, all other extended-release opiates should be discontinued. Extended-release tablets of hydromorphone hydrochloride should be administered once every 24 hours. The tablets should be swallowed intact and should *not* be broken, crushed, dissolved, or chewed; ingestion of broken, crushed, chewed, or dissolved tablets may result in rapid release of the drug from the preparation and absorption of a potentially fatal dose of hydromorphone hydrochloride. Extended-release tablets of hydromorphone hydrochloride may be administered without regard to food. Intake of alcohol with the extended-release tablets may result in increased peak plasma concentrations of hydromorphone and ingestion of a potentially toxic dose of the drug.

Caution should be exercised when prescribing or dispensing oral hydromorphone hydrochloride to avoid inadvertent interchange of the 8-mg extended-release tablets and the 8-mg conventional tablets and to avoid confusion between mg and mL of the oral solution. Prescriptions for the oral solution should specify the intended total dose of the drug (in mg) along with the corresponding total volume (in mL). To ensure accurate measurement of the dose, a calibrated measuring device should always be used to administer the oral solution; household teaspoons and tablespoons should not be used.

● Dosage

Hydromorphone hydrochloride should be given at the lowest effective dosage and for the shortest duration of therapy consistent with the treatment goals of the patient. Reduced dosage is indicated in geriatric or debilitated patients and in patients with hepatic or renal impairment. If concomitant therapy with other CNS depressants is required, the lowest effective dosages and shortest possible duration of concomitant therapy should be used.

For acute pain not related to trauma or surgery, the prescribed quantity should be limited to the amount needed for the expected duration of pain severe enough to require opiate analgesia (generally 3 days or less and rarely more than 7 days). When opiate analgesics are used for the management of chronic non-cancer pain, the US Centers for Disease Control and Prevention (CDC) recommends that primary care clinicians carefully reassess individual benefits and risks before prescribing dosages equivalent to 50 mg or more of morphine sulfate daily (approximately 12.5 mg or more of hydromorphone hydrochloride daily) and avoid dosages equivalent to 90 mg or more of morphine sulfate daily (approximately 22.5 mg or more of hydromorphone hydrochloride daily) or carefully justify their decision to titrate the dosage to such levels. Other experts recommend consulting a pain management specialist before exceeding a dosage equivalent to 80–120 mg of morphine sulfate daily. For further information on the management of opiate analgesic therapy, see Dosage and Administration: Dosage, in the Opiate Agonists General Statement 28:08.08.

Dosage of hydromorphone hydrochloride should be individualized to provide adequate analgesia and to minimize adverse effects. When selecting an initial dosage, consideration should be given to the severity of the patient's pain, patient response, prior analgesic treatment experience, and risk factors for addiction, abuse, and misuse. There is substantial interpatient variability in the relative potency of opiate analgesics and analgesic formulations; therefore, in patients who are being transferred to hydromorphone from other opiate therapy, it is preferable to underestimate the patient's 24-hour opiate requirements than to overestimate the requirements and manage an adverse reaction.

Appropriate dosage selection and titration are essential to reduce the risk of respiratory depression. Patients should be monitored closely for respiratory depression, especially during the first 24–72 hours of therapy and following any increase in dosage.

Patients receiving opiate analgesia should be reevaluated continually for adequacy of pain control and for adverse effects, as well for the development of addiction, abuse, or misuse. During long-term therapy, the continued need for opiate analgesics should be periodically reevaluated. Frequent communication among the prescriber, other members of the healthcare team, the patient, and the patient's caregiver or family is important during periods of changing analgesic requirements, including the initial dosage titration period. If the level of pain increases after dosage stabilization, an attempt should be made to identify the source of increased pain before increasing the hydromorphone hydrochloride dosage.

Parenteral Dosage

The manufacturer states that the usual initial parenteral dosage of hydromorphone hydrochloride in opiate-naive adults is 1–2 mg every 2–3 hours as needed by subcutaneous or IM injection, or 0.2–1 mg every 2–3 hours by slow (i.e., over at least 2–3 minutes depending on the dose) IV injection. Lower initial subcutaneous or IM dosages may be appropriate in some opiate-naive patients. The initial IV dose should be reduced in geriatric or debilitated patients, and may be reduced to 0.2 mg. The dose and/or frequency of administration should be adjusted gradually based on patient response. In critically ill adults in an intensive care unit (ICU) setting, an IV loading dose of 0.2–0.6 mg followed by a maintenance continuous IV infusion of 0.5–3 mg/hour has been used. Hydromorphone hydrochloride also has been administered in intermittent IV doses of 10–30 mcg/kg every 1–2 hours or as a continuous IV infusion of 7–15 mcg/kg per hour in critically ill adults.

To switch patients who currently are receiving other opiate therapy to therapy with parenteral hydromorphone hydrochloride, the total daily dosage of the current opiate should be converted to an equivalent daily dosage of hydromorphone hydrochloride. The manufacturer states that the estimated parenteral dosage of hydromorphone hydrochloride should then be reduced by one-half because of the possibility of incomplete cross-tolerance and administered in divided doses. Dosage of parenteral hydromorphone hydrochloride should then be adjusted based on patient response.

The manufacturer states that when parenteral hydromorphone hydrochloride therapy is discontinued in a patient who may be physically dependent on opiates, the dosage should be reduced by 25–50% every 2–4 days. If manifestations of withdrawal occur, the dosage should be increased to the prior level and tapered more slowly (i.e., by increasing the interval between dosage reductions and/or reducing the amount of each incremental change in dose).

Although safety and efficacy of parenteral hydromorphone hydrochloride have not been established in pediatric patients†, some clinicians recommend an initial parenteral dosage of 0.015 mg/kg every 3–6 hours as needed in children who weigh less than 50 kg and an initial parenteral dosage of 0.2–0.6 mg IV every 2–4 hours or 0.8–1 mg by IM or subcutaneous injection every 4–6 hours as needed in children and adolescents who weigh 50 kg or more.

Oral Dosage
Conventional Preparations

The usual initial oral dosage of hydromorphone hydrochloride in non-opiate-tolerant adults is 2–4 mg as conventional (immediate-release) tablets every 4–6 hours or 2.5–10 mg as oral solution every 3–6 hours as needed. For adults with severe pain, initial oral doses of 4–8 mg have been used. The dose and/or frequency of administration should be adjusted gradually based on patient response. For management of chronic pain, conventional oral preparations of the drug should be administered at regularly scheduled intervals ("around the clock"); supplemental doses equivalent to 5–15% of the total daily dosage may be administered every 2 hours as needed for breakthrough pain.

To switch patients who currently are receiving other opiate therapy to therapy with conventional oral preparations of hydromorphone hydrochloride, the manufacturer states that it is generally safest to initiate hydromorphone hydrochloride therapy at one-half the usual initial dose administered every 3–6 hours as oral solution or every 4–6 hours as conventional tablets. The dose and/or frequency of administration of oral hydromorphone hydrochloride should then be adjusted based on patient response.

Although safety and efficacy of conventional oral preparations of hydromorphone hydrochloride have not been established in pediatric patients†, some clinicians recommend an initial oral hydromorphone hydrochloride dosage of 0.03–0.08 mg/kg every 3–4 hours as needed in children who weigh less than 50 kg and a usual initial oral dosage of 1–2 mg every 3–4 hours as needed in children

and adolescents who weigh 50 kg or more. For children with severe pain, initial oral doses of 0.06 mg/kg have been used.

Extended-release Tablets

When hydromorphone hydrochloride extended-release tablets are used in opiate-tolerant patients, dosage must be carefully individualized since overestimation of the initial dosage can result in fatal overdosage. Patients are considered opiate tolerant if they have been receiving at least 60 mg of oral morphine sulfate daily, 25 mcg of transdermal fentanyl per hour, 30 mg of oral oxycodone hydrochloride daily, 60 mg of oral hydrocodone bitartrate daily, 8 mg of oral hydromorphone hydrochloride daily, 25 mg of oral oxymorphone hydrochloride daily, or an equianalgesic dosage of another opiate daily for at least 1 week. All other around-the-clock opiate analgesics should be discontinued when therapy with hydromorphone hydrochloride extended-release tablets is initiated.

Adults being transferred from conventional (immediate-release) oral hydromorphone hydrochloride preparations to the extended-release tablets should receive the same total daily dosage administered once every 24 hours.

When transferring adults from other oral opiates to extended-release hydromorphone hydrochloride, the approximate oral conversion factors in Table 6 may be used to calculate the estimated daily hydromorphone hydrochloride requirement. The recommended initial dosage is 50% of the calculated estimated daily requirement administered once daily (e.g., for a patient receiving a total daily oral oxycodone hydrochloride dosage of 60 mg, the estimated daily oral hydromorphone hydrochloride requirement would be 24 mg, and the approximate initial dosage of hydromorphone hydrochloride extended-release tablets would be 12 mg once daily). For patients receiving more than one opiate, the approximate oral hydromorphone hydrochloride dosage should be calculated for each opiate separately and then the totals should be summed; for patients receiving fixed-combination analgesics, only the opiate component should be considered. The calculated dosage should always be rounded down, when necessary, to an appropriate available tablet strength.

Table 6 is not a table of equianalgesic doses. The conversion factors in the table should be used only to switch patients from one of the listed oral opiate analgesics to hydromorphone hydrochloride extended-release tablets, and cannot be used to switch patients from hydromorphone hydrochloride extended-release tablets to another opiate, as this will result in overestimation of the dosage of the new opiate and possible fatal overdosage.

Particularly close monitoring is required when patients are switched from methadone therapy, since equianalgesic conversion ratios between methadone and other opiates vary widely depending on extent of prior methadone exposure (see Dosage and Administration: Dosage, in Methadone Hydrochloride 28:08.08).

TABLE 6. Approximate Oral Conversion Factors for Determining Hydromorphone Hydrochloride Requirements When Converting from Oral Opiate Agonists to Extended-release Hydromorphone Hydrochloride

Opiate Agonist	Approximate Oral Conversion Factor
Hydromorphone hydrochloride	1
Codeine phosphate	0.06
Hydrocodone bitartrate	0.4
Methadone hydrochloride	0.6
Morphine sulfate	0.2
Oxycodone hydrochloride	0.4
Oxymorphone hydrochloride	0.6

For conversion from transdermal fentanyl, the estimated equianalgesic dosage of extended-release hydromorphone hydrochloride is 12 mg every 24 hours for each 25-mcg/hour increment in fentanyl transdermal dosage. In general, dosage of extended-release hydromorphone hydrochloride should be initiated at 50% of the calculated total daily dosage. The calculated dosage should always be rounded down, when necessary, to an appropriate available tablet strength. Therapy with the extended-release tablets can be initiated 18 hours following removal of the fentanyl transdermal system.

Patients who experience breakthrough pain may require dosage adjustment or supplemental analgesia (i.e., "rescue" therapy with an immediate-release analgesic). Dosage of hydromorphone hydrochloride extended-release tablets can be titrated in increments of 4–8 mg every 3–4 days based on patient response. Dosage of extended-release hydromorphone hydrochloride in clinical trials ranged from 12–64 mg daily.

Discontinuance of Therapy

When oral hydromorphone hydrochloride therapy is discontinued in a patient who may be physically dependent on opiates, dosage generally should be reduced by no more than 10–25% daily every 2–4 weeks. Patients who have been taking opiates for briefer periods of time may tolerate a more rapid taper. If manifestations of withdrawal occur, it may be necessary to pause the taper or to increase the dosage to the prior level before tapering the dosage more slowly. When opiate dosage is tapered, patients should be monitored for adequacy of pain control, changes in mood, and emergence of suicidal thoughts, as well as for manifestation of opiate withdrawal. A multimodal approach to pain management should be in place prior to initiation of an opiate taper, particularly for patients receiving high dosages and/or long-term opiate therapy for chronic pain.

● Dosage in Renal and Hepatic Impairment

Because of the potential for increased drug exposure, dosage of hydromorphone hydrochloride should be reduced in patients with renal or hepatic impairment based on the degree of impairment. Patients with hepatic or renal impairment should be closely monitored during initiation of therapy and dosage titrations.

Hepatic Impairment

In patients with hepatic impairment, the initial oral dosage of hydromorphone hydrochloride administered as conventional preparations (immediate-release tablets, oral solution) should be reduced to one-fourth to one-half the usual recommended dosage depending on the degree of impairment; the initial dosage should be reduced in patients with moderate hepatic impairment (Child-Pugh class B), and even more conservative initial dosages should be used in patients with severe hepatic impairment (Child-Pugh class C).

Initial dosage of hydromorphone hydrochloride extended-release tablets in patients with moderate hepatic impairment should be reduced to one-fourth the usual recommended dosage; use of alternative analgesic preparations is recommended in those with severe hepatic impairment.

When hydromorphone hydrochloride injection is used in patients with moderate hepatic impairment, the manufacturer recommends that the initial dosage be reduced to one-fourth to one-half the usual recommended dosage; the likelihood that systemic exposure to hydromorphone will be further increased in patients with severe hepatic impairment should be taken into account when selecting an initial dosage.

Renal Impairment

In patients with renal impairment, the initial oral dosage of hydromorphone hydrochloride administered as conventional preparations (immediate-release tablets, oral solution) should be reduced to one-fourth to one-half the usual recommended dosage depending on the degree of impairment; the initial dosage should be reduced in patients with moderate renal impairment (creatinine clearance of 40–60 mL/minute) and even further reduced in those with severe renal impairment (creatinine clearance less than 30 mL/minute).

Initial dosage of hydromorphone hydrochloride extended-release tablets in patients with moderate renal impairment should be reduced to one-half the usual recommended dosage; because the extended-release preparation of the drug is intended only for once-daily administration, the manufacturer recommends that an alternative analgesic regimen with a more flexible dosing interval should be considered in patients with severe renal impairment.

When hydromorphone hydrochloride injection is used in patients with renal impairment, the manufacturer states that the initial dosage be reduced to one-fourth to one-half the usual recommended dosage depending on the degree of renal impairment.

CAUTIONS

Hydromorphone shares the toxic potentials of the opiate agonists, and the usual precautions of opiate agonist therapy should be observed. (See Cautions in the Opiate Agonists General Statement 28:08.08.) Mild to severe seizures and myoclonus have been reported in critically ill patients receiving high doses of parenterally administered hydromorphone.

Nausea, vomiting, constipation, and euphoria may be less marked with hydromorphone than with morphine.

Some commercially available preparations of hydromorphone hydrochloride contain sulfites that may cause allergic-type reactions, including anaphylaxis and life-threatening or less severe asthmatic episodes, in certain susceptible individuals. The overall prevalence of sulfite sensitivity in the general population is unknown but probably low; such sensitivity appears to occur more frequently in asthmatic than in nonasthmatic individuals.

Some packaging components of some hydromorphone hydrochloride products may contain natural latex proteins in the form of dry natural rubber and/or natural rubber latex (see the manufacturers' labeling). Some individuals may be hypersensitive to natural latex proteins found in a wide range of medical devices, including such packaging components, and the level of sensitivity may vary depending on the form of natural rubber present; rarely hypersensitivity reactions to natural latex proteins have been fatal. Therefore, while the specific risk cannot necessarily be predicted, health-care professionals should take appropriate precautions when administration of such hydromorphone preparations is considered for individuals with a history of natural latex sensitivity.

Because hydromorphone hydrochloride extended-release tablets are nondeformable and do not appreciably change shape in the GI tract, they are contraindicated in patients with GI obstruction or with severe narrowing of the GI tract due to any pathologic or iatrogenic condition (e.g., esophageal motility disorders, small bowel inflammatory disease, short-gut syndrome due to adhesions or decreased transit time, history of peritonitis, cystic fibrosis, chronic intestinal pseudo-obstruction, Meckel's diverticulum). Obstructive symptoms have been reported in patients with strictures or at risk for strictures (e.g., because of prior GI surgery) who ingested nondeformable extended-release drug formulations.

Hydromorphone hydrochloride extended-release tablets may be visible on abdominal radiographs under certain circumstances, especially when digital enhancing techniques are utilized.

Hydromorphone hydrochloride extended-release tablets should only be used in patients who are tolerant to opiate agonists; use of this formulation in patients who are not opiate tolerant may result in fatal respiratory depression.

Patients receiving hydromorphone should avoid alcohol; intake of alcohol with the extended-release tablets may result in increased peak plasma concentrations of hydromorphone and ingestion of a potentially toxic dose of the drug.

In clinical studies, hydromorphone hydrochloride injection containing 10 mg of the drug per mL was not associated with local tissue irritation or induration at the site of subcutaneous injection but pain and/or burning occurred rarely; mild erythema occurred rarely at the site of IM injection. Because local irritation and induration have been reported with other opiate agonists, the possibility that they could occur with hydromorphone hydrochloride injection should be considered. The highly concentrated (10 mg/mL) injection should be used *only* in patients who are tolerant to opiate agonists (see Uses); use of this injection in patients who are *not* tolerant to opiate agonists may result in overdosage and/or death. Extreme caution should be taken to avoid confusing the highly concentrated injection with the less concentrated injections of the drug.

● Pediatric Precautions

Safety and efficacy of hydromorphone hydrochloride in children have not been established; however, conventional preparations of hydromorphone have been used in children.

● Geriatric Precautions

Because of the greater frequency of decreased hepatic, renal, and/or cardiac function and of concomitant disease and drug therapy in geriatric patients, the manufacturers suggest that patients in this age group receive initial dosages of the drug in the lower end of the usual range. It may be useful to monitor renal function since hydromorphone is substantially excreted by the kidneys and the risk of adverse reactions may be increased in patients with impaired renal function.

● Pregnancy, Fertility, and Lactation

Pregnancy

Safe use of hydromorphone in pregnancy has not been established. Results of animal studies suggest the potential for fetal risk. In animal studies, neural tube defects were observed in hamsters, soft tissue and skeletal abnormalities were observed in mice, and reduced postnatal survival of pups, developmental delays, and altered behavioral responses were observed in rats following subcutaneous injection, continuous subcutaneous infusion, or oral administration of hydromorphone hydrochloride in these respective species at dosages of 4.8, 2.3, or 2.1 times, respectively, a human dosage of 32 mg daily. No malformations were observed in rats or rabbits at dosages of 2.1 or 17 times, respectively, this human dosage.

The manufacturers state that hydromorphone hydrochloride should not be used during and immediately prior to labor and delivery.

Lactation

Low concentrations of hydromorphone have been detected in human milk. The developmental and health benefits of breast-feeding should be considered along with the mother's clinical need for hydromorphone and any potential adverse effects on the breast-fed infant from the drug or from the underlying maternal condition. The manufacturer states that women receiving hydromorphone hydrochloride extended-release tablets should not breast-feed infants.

DRUG INTERACTIONS

In vitro data suggest that hydromorphone has minimal potential to inhibit the activity of hepatic cytochrome P-450 (CYP) enzymes, including CYP isoenzymes 1A2, 2C9, 2C19, 2D6, 3A4, and 4A11, at clinically relevant concentrations.

For further information about drug interactions involving opiate agonists (including hydromorphone), see Drug Interactions in the Opiate Agonists General Statement 28:08.08.

PHARMACOKINETICS

● Absorption

Hydromorphone hydrochloride is well absorbed following oral, rectal, or parenteral administration. Hydromorphone has a more rapid onset and may have a shorter duration of action than does morphine. The onset of action of hydromorphone with conventional (immediate-release) preparations is usually 15–30 minutes and analgesia is maintained for 4–5 hours, depending on the route of administration.

Hydromorphone undergoes extensive first-pass metabolism following oral administration. Bioavailability following oral administration of a single 8-mg conventional tablet of the drug is approximately 24%, and peak plasma concentrations generally are attained within 0.5–1 hour following administration. Systemic exposure to hydromorphone is dose proportional over a hydromorphone hydrochloride dose range of 2–8 mg. Commercially available conventional tablets and oral solutions of hydromorphone hydrochloride are bioequivalent.

Following oral administration of hydromorphone hydrochloride as conventional tablets given 4 times daily or as extended-release tablets given once daily at the same total daily dosage, steady-state plasma concentrations of the drug are maintained within the same concentration range; however, the extended-release preparation produces less fluctuation between peak and trough concentrations. Following administration of the extended-release tablets, peak plasma concentrations of hydromorphone occur about 12–16 hours after a dose. Steady state is reached after 3–4 days of once-daily dosing of the extended-release tablets.

Administration of hydromorphone hydrochloride extended-release tablets with food does not alter the pharmacokinetics of the drug. Oral administration of a single 8-mg dose of hydromorphone hydrochloride (as conventional tablets) with food decreased peak plasma concentrations and increased systemic exposure of the drug by 25 and 35%, respectively, and delayed peak plasma concentrations by 0.8 hour.

● Distribution

At therapeutic plasma concentrations, hydromorphone is approximately 8–19% bound to plasma proteins.

● Elimination

Hydromorphone is metabolized primarily in the liver where it undergoes conjugation with glucuronic acid (more than 95% of an administered dose) and is excreted principally in the urine as the glucuronide conjugate. Minor amounts of 6-hydroxy reduction metabolites also are formed. The terminal elimination half-life of hydromorphone is about 2.3 hours following IV administration and 2.6–2.8 hours following oral administration as conventional preparations. The mean half-life of the extended-release formulation is approximately 11 hours (range: 8–15 hours).

Following oral administration of a single 4-mg dose of conventional hydromorphone hydrochloride tablets, systemic exposure to the drug was increased twofold in individuals with moderate renal impairment (creatinine clearance of 40–60 mL/minute), threefold to fourfold in individuals with severe renal impairment (creatinine clearance less than 30 mL/minute), and fourfold in individuals with moderate hepatic impairment (Child-Pugh class B). In addition, the elimination half-life of hydromorphone was prolonged (40 hours) in patients with severe renal impairment.

Pharmacokinetics of hydromorphone are not substantially altered by age or sex. In patients receiving hydromorphone hydrochloride extended-release tablets, systemic exposure to the drug was increased by approximately 11% in patients 65–75 years of age compared with those 65 years of age or younger. Females receiving conventional preparations of the drug reportedly have 25% higher peak concentrations compared with males, but AUC is comparable. Following administration as extended-release tablets, peak concentrations and AUC reportedly are increased by about 10% in females compared with males.

CHEMISTRY AND STABILITY

● Chemistry

Hydromorphone is a semisynthetic phenanthrene-derivative opiate agonist. The drug differs structurally from morphine in the substitution of an oxygen for the 6-hydroxyl group and hydrogenation of the 7-8 double bond of the morphine molecule. Hydromorphone is commercially available as the hydrochloride salt. Hydromorphone hydrochloride occurs as a fine, white or practically white, crystalline powder and is freely soluble in water and sparingly soluble in alcohol. Hydromorphone hydrochloride injection has a pH of 3.5–5.5.

● Stability

Hydromorphone hydrochloride is affected by light; although hydromorphone hydrochloride injection may develop a slight yellowish discoloration, this change apparently does not indicate loss of potency. Hydromorphone hydrochloride injection should be protected from light and stored at a controlled room temperature of 20–25°C, but may be exposed to temperatures ranging from 15–30°C. Hydromorphone hydrochloride immediate-release tablets and oral solution should be protected from light and stored at 20–25°C. The extended-release tablets should also be stored at 20–25°C.

Hydromorphone hydrochloride injection reportedly is physically and chemically stable for at least 24 hours in most common IV infusion solutions when protected from light at 25°C. Specialized references should be consulted for specific solution and drug compatibility information.

PREPARATIONS

Hydromorphone hydrochloride preparations are subject to control under the Federal Controlled Substances Act of 1970 as schedule II (C-II) drugs.

Excipients in commercially available drug preparations may have clinically important effects in some individuals; consult specific product labeling for details.

HYDROmorphone Hydrochloride

Oral

Solution	5 mg/5 mL*	**Dilaudid®** (C-II), Rhodes
		HYDROmorphone Hydrochloride Solution (C-II)
Tablets	2 mg*	**Dilaudid®** (C-II), Rhodes
		HYDROmorphone Hydrochloride Tablets (C-II)
	4 mg*	**Dilaudid®** (C-II), Rhodes
		HYDROmorphone Hydrochloride Tablets (C-II)
	8 mg*	**Dilaudid®** (C-II; scored), Rhodes
		HYDROmorphone Hydrochloride Tablets (C-II)
Tablets, extended-release	8 mg*	**HYDROmorphone Hydrochloride Extended-release Tablets** (C-II)
	12 mg*	**HYDROmorphone Hydrochloride Extended-release Tablets** (C-II)
	16 mg*	**HYDROmorphone Hydrochloride Extended-release Tablets** (C-II)
	32 mg*	**HYDROmorphone Hydrochloride Extended-release Tablets** (C-II)

Parenteral

Injection	0.2 mg/mL	**Dilaudid®** (C-II), Fresenius Kabi
	1 mg/mL*	**Dilaudid®** (C-II), Fresenius Kabi
		HYDROmorphone Hydrochloride Injection (C-II)
	2 mg/mL*	**Dilaudid®** (C-II), Fresenius Kabi
		HYDROmorphone Hydrochloride Injection (C-II)
	4 mg/mL*	**HYDROmorphone Hydrochloride Injection** (C-II)
	10 mg/mL (10, 50, or 500 mg)*	**HYDROmorphone Hydrochloride High-Potency Formulation Injection** (C-II)

* available from one or more manufacturer, distributor, and/or repackager by generic (nonproprietary) name

† Use is not currently included in the labeling approved by the US Food and Drug Administration.

Selected Revisions June 10, 2024, © Copyright, September 1, 1972, American Society of Health-System Pharmacists, Inc.

Methadone Hydrochloride

28:08.08 · OPIOID AGONISTS

■ Methadone hydrochloride is a synthetic diphenylheptane-derivative opiate agonist.

REMS

FDA approved a REMS for methadone hydrochloride to ensure that the benefits outweigh the risk. The REMS may apply to one or more preparations of methadone hydrochloride and consists of the following: medication guide and elements to assure safe use. See the FDA REMS page (https://www.accessdata.fda.gov/scripts/cder/rems/index.cfm).

USES

Methadone is used in the relief of pain. Methadone also may be used in detoxification and maintenance treatment. Although the drug has antitussive activity, methadone is no longer approved by the US Food and Drug Administration for this indication.

● Pain

Methadone is a strong analgesic used parenterally for the treatment of moderate to severe pain that has not responded to non-opiate analgesics. Methadone is used orally for relief of moderate to severe pain when a continuous, around-the-clock analgesic is needed for an extended period of time. Methadone is used for relief of chronic pain in both opiate-naive patients and in individuals being switched to methadone therapy from other opiate agonists because of inadequate pain relief or adverse effects from the previous drug (opiate rotation). Most clinical studies evaluating methadone in the management of pain have involved individuals with chronic malignant pain. The manufacturers state that oral preparations of the drug are not indicated for relief of acute (including postoperative) pain, for relief of pain that is mild or is not expected to persist for an extended period of time, or for use on an as-needed ("prn") basis.

Clinical studies suggest that methadone may have efficacy similar to that of morphine and other opiates in patients with chronic malignant pain. However, experts generally agree that methadone should be prescribed for chronic pain management only by clinicians knowledgeable about its risks (e.g., QT-interval prolongation) and pharmacokinetics, and should not be the first choice for an extended-release or long-acting opiate analgesic. Benefits associated with the use of methadone for management of chronic pain include the commercial availability of multiple dosage forms of the drug, good oral bioavailability, rapid onset of action, reduced dosing frequency (because of the drug's long half-life), low cost, and lack of active metabolites. Incomplete cross-tolerance between methadone and other opiate agonists has been reported; some patients who were previously refractory to high doses of other opiate agonists have experienced pain relief with methadone therapy. This incomplete cross-tolerance may allow for successful pain relief in patients who previously were refractory to or who experienced adverse effects from increasing dosages of other opiate agonists. Disadvantages associated with the use of methadone include its increased potential for accumulation with repeated doses (which may result in toxicity), considerable interindividual variability in pharmacokinetic parameters, the potential for drug interactions, challenges associated with methadone dosage titration and with the transfer of patients from therapy with other opiate agonists to therapy with methadone, and the commercial availability and relative ease of use of extended-release preparations of other opiate agonists. (See Cautions.)

For further information on the role of opiate analgesics in the management of chronic pain, see Uses: Pain, in the Opiate Agonists General Statement 28:08.08.

● Detoxification and Maintenance of Opiate Dependence

Methadone is used in detoxification treatment and maintenance treatment as an oral substitute for heroin or other morphine-like drugs to suppress the opiate-agonist abstinence syndrome in patients who are dependent on these drugs. The success of such treatment programs is dependent on the selection of properly motivated patients and on the availability of social, psychologic, vocational, and educational as well as medical supportive services. In **detoxification treatment**, methadone is administered in decreasing doses over a period not exceeding either 30 days (*short-term detoxification*) or 180 days (*long-term detoxification*) in order to withdraw use of opiate agonist(s); previously (prior to enactment of Public Law 98-509 in 1984), detoxification treatment with methadone could not exceed 21 days. Patients of any age may undergo detoxification treatment. Methadone is approved by the US Food and Drug Administration (FDA) for **detoxification treatment of opiate dependence** and for **maintenance treatment of opiate dependence** (opiate use disorder [OUD]). Buprenorphine hydrochloride is approved by the FDA for the management of opiate dependence. Levomethadyl acetate (LAAM, ORLAAM®) also has been approved by the FDA for the management of opiate dependence but is no longer commercially available in the US because of potentially severe adverse cardiac effects.

Maintenance treatment consists of administration of stable doses of methadone or buprenorphine for relatively long periods (i.e., exceeding 21 days). **Maintenance treatment** with methadone is provided as *comprehensive maintenance*, which is provided in conjunction with a comprehensive range of appropriate medical and rehabilitative services, or *interim maintenance*, which is provided in conjunction with appropriate medical services while the patient is awaiting transfer to comprehensive maintenance. **Maintenance treatment** with buprenorphine is provided as office-based outpatient therapy. Office-based treatment with buprenorphine is an innovative model intended to increase access to opiate dependence treatment and may be appropriate for individuals who may not otherwise seek methadone maintenance treatment (comprehensive maintenance), do not meet enrollment criteria, do not have access to such programs, or have chosen to opt out of such programs for another reason. In the office-based treatment model, specially trained physicians prescribe buprenorphine as a take-home medication. As with detoxification treatment, the eventual goal of maintenance therapy is withdrawal of the drug.

According to federal regulations, only patients who have demonstrated current physiologic dependence on opiate drugs and at least a 1-year history of this dependence can be admitted to *comprehensive* maintenance programs. If clinically appropriate, the 1-year history of dependence can be waived for individuals released within the previous 6 months from a penal institution, pregnant women, or previously treated individuals (up to 2 years after discharge from treatment).

Detoxification or maintenance treatment with methadone is permitted to be undertaken only by opiate-dependency treatment programs certified by the Substance Abuse and Mental Health Services Administration (SAMHSA) and approved by the designated state authority; however, this does not preclude detoxification or maintenance treatment of an addict who is hospitalized or is admitted to a long-term care facility for medical conditions other than addiction and who requires detoxification or maintenance treatment during his hospitalization or stay in the long-term care facility, nor does it exclude administration of opiates for up to 72 hours (emergency treatment to relieve acute withdrawal symptoms) while care in an opiate-dependency treatment program is being sought. For information on the use of methadone for detoxification and maintenance treatment in children younger than 18 years of age and during pregnancy, see Cautions: Pediatric Precautions and also Pregnancy and Lactation.

Because of the risk of acquiring human immunodeficiency virus (HIV) infection from illicit IV drug use, the conditions for use of methadone in maintenance treatment were revised (effective January 6, 1993) to facilitate more rapid entry into treatment programs of increased numbers of opiate-dependent patients more rapidly. The revisions permit programs to provide minimum service (*interim*) maintenance treatment (which is aimed at helping to alleviate the human suffering of opiate-dependent individuals, including the risk of HIV infection, and to reduce the abuse of IV drugs) in addition to *comprehensive* maintenance treatment (which already existed). There is some evidence that the revised conditions for treatment of opiate dependence can reduce substantially the illicit use of IV drugs (and hence needles) by dependent individuals and that such reductions in IV use of these drugs will decrease the spread of HIV within this population. In addition, the revised conditions for use of methadone in detoxification and in maintenance treatment require provision of counseling for preventing HIV transmission and exposure and provision of information on the availability of, and ensuring access to, HIV testing; mandatory HIV testing is *not* a requirement of opiate-dependency treatment programs, but such testing must be made available, either on site or at another facility, to any patient requesting it.

The minimum service program serves as interim treatment until a patient can be admitted into a comprehensive program; however, such treatment cannot exceed 120 days in any 12-month period. In general, the requirements for comprehensive maintenance treatment or detoxification treatment apply to interim maintenance treatment, although the provision of a comprehensive range of services is *not* required during interim maintenance treatment. Comprehensive medical, vocational rehabilitative, employment, educational, and counseling services (e.g., formation and periodic evaluation of treatment plans, primary counselor assignments) are *not* required during interim maintenance. However, some services are required (e.g., medical treatment referrals, prenatal care referrals, HIV counseling), and sufficient counseling staff should be available to provide such services and to respond to emergencies. In addition to initial drug screening, interim programs must provide a minimum of 2 additional drug screenings to assist in assessing patient needs and priorities for transfer into comprehensive programs. Patients admitted to an interim maintenance program are required to be administered each daily methadone dose while being closely observed; take-home medication is *not* permitted. Both admission to interim treatment programs and transfer to comprehensive treatment programs are to be provided preferentially to pregnant women. Interim maintenance treatment programs can be implemented by existing maintenance programs, provided the program has filed for and received federal authorization (formerly from FDA but as of May 18, 2001, from SAMHSA) and authorization from the appropriate local (e.g., state) authority.

Federal regulations (effective May 18, 2001) concerning use of opiates in detoxification and maintenance programs transferred oversight for such programs from FDA to SAMHSA and altered the nature of the regulatory system from one that relied on inspection for compliance with process-oriented regulations to a system based on program accreditation and subsequent certification by SAMHSA. Standards for treatment programs also were modified to permit greater flexibility and professional judgment in treatment. The requirement that programs use only liquid oral formulations was modified to allow for use of either liquid or solid oral dosage forms. The requirement that treatment programs administer methadone hydrochloride dosages exceeding 100 mg daily under direct supervision at least 6 days per week regardless of length of time in the program (unless prior approval for take-home dosages exceeding 100 mg had been obtained from FDA and the state authority) was eliminated, and a more flexible schedule for unsupervised administration was allowed (see Maintenance under Dosage: Detoxification and Maintenance of Opiate Dependence, in Dosage and Administration).

Other federal initiatives were undertaken in 2000 to expand access to treatment and to involve office-based physicians in the care of opiate-dependent individuals. These initiatives were taken in response to limitations in the heavily regulated comprehensive maintenance programs and the increasing heroin use and high rates of HIV and hepatitis C virus transmission among illicit users of IV drugs. The Drug Addiction Treatment Act (DATA) of 2000 allows qualifying physicians to prescribe and dispense opiates in schedules III, IV, and V of the Federal Controlled Substances Act that have been approved by the FDA for detoxification or maintenance treatment of opiate dependence. With the approval of buprenorphine and buprenorphine in fixed combination with naloxone for the management of opiate dependence, treatment of opiate

dependence can be undertaken in a system that resembles care provided for other chronic medical conditions.

● *Neonatal Opiate Withdrawal*

Methadone has been used to manage manifestations of opiate abstinence syndrome (i.e., postnatal withdrawal) in neonates† exposed to opiates in utero. Opiates are recommended as first-line pharmacologic therapy when environmental and supportive measures (e.g., minimization of external stimuli, maximization of mother-infant contact [e.g., parental "rooming in"], breast-feeding when not contraindicated, swaddling and gentle handling) are inadequate. Other adjunctive therapy (e.g., clonidine, phenobarbital) may be added if the response to opiates is inadequate, or phenobarbital be added if the neonate was exposed to additional substances in utero. Approximately 60–80% of neonates with opiate abstinence syndrome may require pharmacologic treatment for withdrawal symptoms. While morphine has been used more extensively than other opiates in the management of neonatal opiate abstinence syndrome, some studies suggest that use of methadone or buprenorphine (an opiate partial agonist) may be associated with shorter treatment durations and hospital stays compared with morphine use. However, additional study is needed to establish optimal dosage schedules and preferred opiate drugs and to evaluate longer-term (e.g., neurodevelopmental) outcomes. Conflicting findings to date may be related in part to differences in study design, nonpharmacologic care, concomitant in utero drug exposures, the stringency of institutional protocols for care, and optimization of dosage schedules.

Use of standardized protocols for identification, evaluation, and treatment of neonatal opiate withdrawal syndrome is recommended since use of such protocols has been shown to improve overall response, including shorter hospital stays and durations of pharmacologic treatment. Some evidence suggests that use of a standardized protocol may be more important than use of a specific opiate agonist (e.g., methadone versus morphine) in improving outcomes. Protocols generally utilize assessment tools that were developed to quantify severity of withdrawal in term neonates (e.g., Finnegan or modified Finnegan scoring tools) to facilitate decisions regarding initiation, titration, and tapering of therapy.

DOSAGE AND ADMINISTRATION

● *Administration*

Methadone hydrochloride may be administered orally as tablets, solution, concentrated solution, or dispersible tablets or by subcutaneous, IM, or IV injection.

Methadone hydrochloride dispersible tablets are intended for dispersion in a liquid prior to oral administration. Dispersible tablets of the drug contain insoluble excipients and therefore must *not* be used to prepare solutions for injection. Each 40-mg dispersible tablet can be divided in half or in quarters; the desired dose should be dispersed in approximately 120 mL of water, orange juice, Tang®, citrus-flavored Kool-Aid®, or other acidic fruit beverage immediately prior to administration. Complete tablet dispersion occurs within 1 minute; dispersion time is slightly increased when a cold and/or acidic vehicle is used. If any residue remains in the cup after initial administration, a small amount of liquid should be added and the resulting mixture administered. Because the dispersible tablets can be administered only in increments of 10 mg, this dosage form may not be appropriate in many patients for initial dosing during detoxification and maintenance treatment or for gradual dosage reduction following short-term detoxification or a period of maintenance treatment.

When the 10-mg/mL oral concentrate solution is used for the treatment of pain, the dose must be diluted with water or other suitable liquid (e.g., Kool-Aid®, Tang®, apple juice, Crystal Light® [with aspartame]) to at least 30 mL prior to administration.

Absorption of methadone following subcutaneous or IM injection may be unpredictable and has not been fully characterized; local tissue reactions may occur.

Methadone hydrochloride also has been administered rectally† and by epidural injection†.

Restricted Distribution

Manufacturers of methadone hydrochloride 40-mg dispersible tablets and the Drug Enforcement Administration (DEA) have agreed to restrict distribution of this preparation to authorized opiate-dependency treatment programs and to hospitals. This restriction is in response to reports of serious adverse effects such as cardiotoxicity and death in patients receiving methadone (see Cautions). Methadone hydrochloride 40-mg dispersible tablets are used in detoxification and maintenance treatment of opiate addiction; this preparation is *not* labeled by the US Food and Drug Administration (FDA) for the treatment of pain.

● *Dosage*

Dosage of methadone hydrochloride must be carefully individualized because repeated doses may result in substantial accumulation of the drug, prolonging its duration of action and possibly resulting in adverse effects, and because there is considerable interindividual variability in absorption, metabolism, and relative analgesic potency of the drug. Patients should be carefully monitored during initiation of therapy, dosage titration, and conversion from one opiate agonist to another. Steady-state plasma concentrations and full analgesic effects of methadone generally are not achieved until completion of 3–5 days of therapy.

Pain

When selecting an initial dosage of methadone hydrochloride for management of pain, consideration should be given to the type, severity, and expected duration of the patient's pain; the age, general condition, and medical status of the patient; concurrent drug therapy (see Drug Interactions); and the acceptable balance between pain relief and adverse effects. In addition, in patients who are being transferred to methadone from other opiate therapy, consideration should be given to the daily dosage, potency, and specific characteristics (e.g., elimination half-life) of the previously administered opiate; adverse effects of and response to the previous regimen; degree of opiate tolerance; and the relative potency estimate used to calculate an equianalgesic dosage of methadone hydrochloride. Appropriate dosage selection and titration are essential to prevent overdosage.

A high degree of opiate tolerance does not preclude the possibility of unintended methadone overdosage. Failure to individualize dosage has resulted in serious adverse effects, including death, in opiate-tolerant patients during conversion to methadone therapy. (See Cautions.) Overestimation of the methadone dosage when transferring patients from other opiate therapy to methadone therapy can result in fatal overdosage with the first dose.

Published equianalgesic dosage conversion ratios between methadone hydrochloride and other opiate agonists are imprecise. Dose equivalencies that are obtained from commonly used tables generally are based on single-dose studies in patients who are not opiate tolerant. When transferring patients to methadone from other opiate agonist therapy, use of single-dose equivalency tables may *overestimate* dosage requirements for methadone hydrochloride during chronic therapy, since methadone may accumulate with repeated doses secondary to the long elimination half-life of the drug (see Pharmacokinetics: Elimination). Therefore, estimates of methadone hydrochloride dosage that are based on single-dose studies should *not* be used for conversion in patients receiving chronic opiate therapy. In addition, equianalgesic dosage conversion ratios between morphine sulfate and methadone hydrochloride have been reported to vary substantially depending on the dosage of the previously administered morphine regimen; the morphine sulfate-to-methadone hydrochloride equianalgesic dosage conversion ratio has been reported to be lower in patients receiving prior opiate therapy at a lower morphine sulfate dosage and higher in those receiving prior therapy at a higher morphine sulfate dosage.

Regardless of the strategy employed to determine initial methadone dosage, methadone hydrochloride therapy is most safely initiated using small initial doses and gradual dosage adjustments. Some clinicians recommend a transition period of at least 3 days for patients being transferred from therapy with another opiate agonist to therapy with methadone; during the transition period, the dosage of the previous opiate agonist is gradually tapered while the dosage of methadone hydrochloride is slowly increased. Other clinicians state that patients receiving *low* dosages of another opiate agonist may be transferred to methadone therapy in 1 day.

As an analgesic, methadone hydrochloride should be given at the lowest effective dosage and for the shortest duration of therapy consistent with the treatment goals of the patient. Reduced dosage is indicated in poor-risk patients such as very young, very old, or debilitated patients. If concomitant therapy with other CNS depressants is required, the lowest effective dosages and shortest possible duration of concomitant therapy should be used. (See Drug Interactions: Benzodiazepines and Other CNS Depressants.)

When opiate analgesics are used for the management of chronic noncancer pain, the US Centers for Disease Control and Prevention (CDC) recommends that primary care clinicians carefully reassess individual benefits and risks before prescribing dosages equivalent to 50 mg or more of morphine sulfate daily and avoid dosages equivalent to 90 mg or more of morphine sulfate daily or carefully justify their decision to titrate the dosage to such levels. Other experts recommend consulting a pain management specialist before exceeding a dosage equivalent to 80–120 mg of morphine sulfate daily. For further information on the management of opiate analgesic therapy, see Dosage and Administration: Dosage, in the Opiate Agonists General Statement 28:08.08.

Parenteral Dosage

For the relief of moderate to severe pain, the manufacturer recommends a usual initial methadone hydrochloride dosage in opiate-naive adults of 2.5–10 mg administered IV every 8–12 hours. Dosage may be increased as necessary to provide adequate analgesia, but should be increased slowly to avoid accumulation of the drug and potential toxicity. More frequent administration may be required during initiation of therapy in order to maintain adequate analgesia, but caution is necessary to avoid overdosage.

In patients being switched from oral to parenteral methadone hydrochloride, parenteral methadone hydrochloride should be initiated at a parenteral-to-oral dosage ratio of 1:2 (e.g., 5 mg of parenteral methadone hydrochloride in patients previously receiving 10 mg of oral methadone hydrochloride).

When patients are transferred from chronic therapy with another oral or parenteral opiate to therapy with parenteral methadone hydrochloride, dosage must be selected carefully, since cross-tolerance between methadone and other opiate agonists is incomplete, dosage conversion ratios are imprecise, and substantial interindividual variability exists. The dosage conversion methods recommended by the manufacturer for converting to IV methadone hydrochloride (See Tables 1 and 2) are based on comparisons with morphine. The manufacturer states that these estimates provide a safe starting point for opiate conversion; however, the IV methadone hydrochloride dosage obtained from these comparisons must be individualized (e.g., based on prior opiate use, medical condition, concurrent drug therapy, anticipated use of analgesics for breakthrough pain). The total daily dosage should be administered in divided doses (e.g., at 8-hour intervals) based on individual patient requirements. For patients being transferred from therapy with opiate agonists other than morphine, a comparative opiate agonist dosage table (such as the table in the Opiate Agonists General Statement 28:08.08) may be consulted to determine the equivalent morphine dosage.

TABLE 1. Conversion of Oral Morphine Sulfate to IV Methadone Hydrochloride (for Chronic Administration)

Baseline Total Daily *Oral* Morphine Sulfate Dosage	Estimated Daily *IV* Methadone Hydrochloride Dosage (as % of Total Daily Morphine Sulfate Dosage)
<100 mg	10–15%
100–300 mg	5–10%
300–600 mg	4–6%
600–1000 mg	3–5%
>1000 mg	<3%

TABLE 2. Conversion of Parenteral Morphine Sulfate to IV Methadone Hydrochloride (for Chronic Administration)[a]

Baseline Total Daily *Parenteral* Morphine Sulfate Dosage	Estimated Daily *IV* Methadone Hydrochloride Dosage (as % of Total Daily Morphine Dosage)
10–30 mg	40–66%
30–50 mg	27–66%
50–100 mg	22–50%
100–200 mg	15–34%
200–500 mg	10–20%

[a] Derived from Table 1 assuming a 3:1 oral-to-parenteral morphine ratio.

Oral Dosage

When oral methadone hydrochloride is used for the relief of moderate to severe pain in opiate-naive adults who require a continuous, around-the-clock analgesic for an extended period of time, therapy should be initiated with small doses of no more than 2.5–10 mg given every 8–12 hours. Dosage must be carefully individualized according to patient response. Dosage may be titrated to provide adequate analgesia, but should be increased slowly to avoid accumulation of the drug and potential toxicity. The dosage interval during methadone therapy may range from 4–12 hours, since the duration of analgesia is relatively short during the first days of therapy but increases substantially with continued administration. Clinicians and patients must be prepared to markedly reduce the methadone hydrochloride dose and/or increase the dosing interval after the first few doses based on assessments of pain relief, sedation, and other adverse effects. Some clinicians experienced with the use of methadone may elect to initiate opiate therapy by administering methadone hydrochloride on an as-needed basis for the first 3–7 days and then establishing an around-the-clock dosage schedule based on the duration of action reported by the patient. Opiate therapy also may be initiated with a short-acting opiate agonist and then switched to methadone once adequate analgesia is established.

In patients being switched from parenteral to oral methadone hydrochloride, oral methadone hydrochloride should be initiated at an oral-to-parenteral dosage ratio of 2:1 (e.g., 10 mg of oral methadone hydrochloride in patients previously receiving 5 mg of parenteral methadone hydrochloride).

When patients are transferred to oral methadone from chronic therapy with other oral or parenteral opiates, dosage must be selected carefully because cross-tolerance between methadone hydrochloride and other opiate agonists is incomplete, dosage conversion ratios are imprecise, and considerable interindividual variability exists. The dosage conversion method shown in Table 3 is based on comparison with morphine sulfate. The oral methadone hydrochloride dosage obtained from this comparison must be individualized (e.g., based on prior opiate use, medical condition, concurrent drug therapy, anticipated use of analgesics for breakthrough pain). The total daily dosage should be administered in divided doses (e.g., at 8-hour intervals) based on individual patient requirements. For patients being transferred from therapy with opiate agonists other than morphine, a comparative opiate agonist dosage table (such as the table in the Opiate Agonists General Statement 28:08.08) may be consulted to determine the equivalent morphine dosage.

Dosage adjustments may be made at intervals of 1–2 days with close monitoring to achieve adequate analgesia with minimal adverse effects. Patients who experience breakthrough pain may require dosage adjustment or rescue therapy with a small dose of an immediate-release analgesic. If excessive opiate-related adverse effects are observed, the next dose of methadone hydrochloride may be reduced; if adverse effects are intolerable, either the dose or dosing interval of the drug may be adjusted. If discontinuance of opiates is required, gradual tapering of the dosage every 2–4 days is recommended to avoid manifestations of abrupt withdrawal.

TABLE 3. Conversion of Oral Morphine Sulfate to Oral Methadone Hydrochloride (for Chronic Administration)

Baseline Total Daily *Oral* Morphine Sulfate Dosage	Estimated Daily *Oral* Methadone Hydrochloride Dosage (as % of Total Daily Morphine Sulfate Dosage)
<100 mg	20–30%
100–300 mg	10–20%
300–600 mg	8–12%
600–1000 mg	5–10%
>1000 mg	<5%

Detoxification and Maintenance of Opiate Dependence

In detoxification and maintenance treatment, methadone hydrochloride may be administered or dispensed only as an oral preparation (e.g., tablet, dispersible tablet, liquid) that is formulated and packaged in such a way as to reduce potential for parenteral abuse and accidental ingestion. Hospitalized patients being treated for a medical or surgical condition may receive methadone parenterally if necessary. The dosage of methadone used for detoxification or maintenance treatment should be adjusted to control abstinence symptoms without causing respiratory depression or marked sedation. Any substantial deviations from the FDA-approved labeling for methadone hydrochloride (e.g., concerning dose, frequency of administration, or conditions of use) must be documented in the patient's medical record.

If at any time during detoxification or maintenance the patient cannot tolerate oral medication because of nausea or vomiting associated with acute complicating illness, he should be hospitalized and methadone hydrochloride may be continued by the parenteral route. The patient should receive 2 injections daily by the subcutaneous or IM route; each dose should be about one-fourth of the total oral daily dosage.

Detoxification

Detoxification treatment is initiated when there are substantial opiate-agonist abstinence symptoms. The initial dose of methadone hydrochloride should be based on the opiate tolerance of the patient. A single oral dose of 20–30 mg of methadone hydrochloride will often suppress withdrawal symptoms. The initial dose should not exceed 30 mg. Initial doses should be lower for patients whose tolerance is expected to be low at treatment initiation. Loss of tolerance should be considered if more than 5 days have elapsed since the patient took opiates. Initial doses should not be based on those used during prior treatment episodes or on the patient's expenditures for illicit drugs. If there is any doubt, it is usually safer to start with a smaller dose and keep the patient under observation. Additional doses of methadone hydrochloride may be necessary if withdrawal symptoms are not suppressed or if they reappear. The manufacturer states that if same-day dosage adjustments are to be made, the patient should be reevaluated 2–4 hours after the previous dose, since peak plasma concentrations of methadone will have been attained. If an additional dose is required to suppress withdrawal symptoms, an additional 5–10 mg of methadone hydrochloride may be administered. The total dose on the first day should not exceed 40 mg unless it is documented that this total dose does not suppress withdrawal symptoms.

Dosage adjustments should be made over the first week of methadone therapy based on assessments of withdrawal-symptom suppression at times of expected peak activity (i.e., 2–4 hours after a methadone hydrochloride dose). Dosage adjustments should be cautious, in order to avoid overdosage. With continued dosing, symptoms will be suppressed for longer periods of time as the drug accumulates in body tissues. In most patients, a daily dosage of 40 mg of methadone hydrochloride in single or divided doses will usually constitute an adequate stabilizing dosage level, but higher dosage may be required. When the patient has been stabilized (i.e., substantial symptoms of withdrawal are absent) for 2 or 3 days, dosage of methadone hydrochloride can be gradually decreased daily or at 2-day intervals. Dosage must be individualized and adjusted to keep withdrawal symptoms at a tolerable level. In hospitalized patients, dosage can usually be reduced by 20% daily, but a more gradual reduction may be required in ambulatory patients.

For short-term detoxification, methadone must be administered daily while the patient is under close observation in reducing dosages over a period not exceeding 30 days. For long-term detoxification, methadone must be administered in a regimen designed to reach a drug-free state within 180 days or less. Take-home medication may be allowed during long-term detoxification if certain conditions are met (see Maintenance under Dosage: Detoxification and Maintenance of Opiate Dependence, in Dosage and Administration). Individuals with 2 or more unsuccessful detoxification episodes within a 12-month period should be evaluated for alternative forms of treatment. An opiate-dependency treatment program may not admit an individual for more than 2 detoxification treatments within one year.

Maintenance

Interim (minimum service) maintenance treatment is that which is provided in conjunction with appropriate medical services while a patient is awaiting transfer to comprehensive maintenance treatment. A maintenance program that is unable to place a patient requesting treatment into a comprehensive maintenance treatment program within 14 days of application for admission and within a reasonable geographic area may place the patient in an interim maintenance treatment program until placement in a comprehensive program is possible. A patient may *not* continue in an interim treatment program for longer than 120 days in any 12-month period, and must be transferred to a comprehensive program after 120 days in an interim program if still in need of treatment. A patient admitted to an interim maintenance program is required to be administered each daily methadone dose while being closely observed, and take-home medication is *not* allowed. Although most requirements for comprehensive maintenance treatment apply to interim maintenance treatment, some do *not* apply. (See Uses: Detoxification and Maintenance of Opiate Dependence.)

When methadone hydrochloride is used to initiate maintenance treatment, the initial dose should be based on the opiate tolerance of the patient. A single oral dose of 20–30 mg of methadone hydrochloride will often suppress withdrawal symptoms. The initial dose should not exceed 30 mg. Initial doses should be lower for patients whose tolerance is expected to be low at treatment initiation. Loss of tolerance should be considered if more than 5 days have elapsed since the patient took opiates. Initial doses should not be based on those used during prior treatment episodes or on the patient's expenditures for illicit drugs. If there is any doubt, it is usually safer to start with a smaller dose and keep the patient under observation. Additional doses of methadone hydrochloride may be necessary if withdrawal symptoms are not suppressed or if they reappear. The manufacturer states that if same-day dosage adjustments are to be made, the patient should be reevaluated 2–4 hours after the previous dose, since peak plasma concentrations of methadone will have been attained. If an additional dose is required to suppress withdrawal symptoms, an additional 5–10 mg of methadone hydrochloride may be administered. The total dose on the first day should not exceed 40 mg unless it is documented that this total dose does not suppress withdrawal symptoms.

Subsequent dosage should be adjusted according to the requirements and response of the patient. Dosage adjustments should be made over the first week of methadone treatment based on assessments of withdrawal-symptom suppression at times of expected peak activity (i.e., 2–4 hours after a methadone hydrochloride dose). Dosage adjustments should be cautious, in order to avoid overdosage. With continued dosing, symptoms will be suppressed for longer periods of time as the drug accumulates in body tissues. Dosage should be titrated to a level at which opiate symptoms are prevented for 24 hours, drug craving is reduced, the euphoric effects of self-administered opiates are blocked or attenuated, and tolerance to the sedative effect of methadone is evident. It has been suggested that trough plasma methadone concentrations exceeding 100–200 ng/mL may be necessary to optimize the success of methadone maintenance, particularly during the first 6 months of treatment. Stabilization of maintenance dosage usually occurs at 80–120 mg daily, although higher dosage is sometimes required. A single dose of methadone daily usually adequately maintains the patient and there generally is no apparent advantage to divided doses. However, rapid metabolizers of methadone may not maintain adequate plasma methadone concentrations with usual

dosing regimens. Highly motivated patients may be maintained on dosage as low as 20–30 mg daily.

Because levomethadyl acetate hydrochloride is no longer commercially available in the US, patients receiving maintenance treatment with the drug should be transferred to alternative treatments. Patients maintained on levomethadyl acetate hydrochloride can be transferred to methadone. Methadone hydrochloride can be initiated at a daily dose that is 80% of the levomethadyl acetate hydrochloride dose; the initial methadone dose must be given no sooner than 48 hours after the last levomethadyl acetate hydrochloride dose. Subsequent doses of methadone hydrochloride may be increased or decreased in increments of 5–10 mg daily to control manifestations of withdrawal or excess sedation according to clinical observation.

Experience with the transfer of patients from methadone maintenance to buprenorphine is limited.

Any individual in a comprehensive maintenance treatment program, including long-term detoxification treatment, may receive one daily dose of methadone to take at home for a day that the clinic is closed. Decisions to allow additional unsupervised administration by these individuals should be based on the following factors: absence of recent abuse of drugs (including alcohol), regularity of clinic attendance, absence of serious behavioral problems at the clinic, absence of known recent criminal activity, stability of the individual's home environment and social relationships, length of time in the program, assurance that the drug can be safely stored in the individual's home, and assessment of whether the rehabilitative benefit derived from decreased clinic attendance outweighs potential risks of diversion. Individuals meeting these criteria may be permitted to receive additional supplies of the drug to take at home each week, in the following amounts: 1-day supply during the first 90 days of treatment, 2-day supply during the second 90 days, and 3-day supply during the third 90 days (each in addition to the one dose allowed for clinic closure). All other doses must be administered while the individual is closely observed. During the remainder of the first year of treatment, individuals may receive a maximum 6-day supply of methadone and must visit the clinic once weekly. After 1 year of continuous treatment, individuals may receive a maximum 2-week supply of methadone and must make twice monthly visits. After 2 years of continuous treatment, the individual may receive a maximum 1-month supply of the drug and must make monthly visits.

Maintenance dosage requirements should be reviewed regularly and reduced as indicated. In patients desiring medically supervised withdrawal from methadone maintenance treatment, there is considerable variability in the appropriate rate of methadone dosage reduction; dosage generally should be reduced at intervals of 10–14 days by an amount that is less than 10% of the established tolerance or maintenance dosage. All patients in a maintenance program should be given careful consideration for discontinuance of methadone therapy, especially after reaching a dosage of 10–20 mg daily.

Neonatal Opiate Withdrawal

For the management of neonatal opiate abstinence syndrome†, use of standardized protocols that base initiation, adjustment, and tapering of methadone hydrochloride dosage on standardized patient assessments performed at regular intervals is recommended. The most commonly used tool for assessing severity of withdrawal in term neonates is the Finnegan scoring system (original or modified versions) performed every 3–4 hours. Treatment with methadone hydrochloride oral solution generally is initiated at a dose of 0.05–0.1 mg/kg based on Finnegan score (e.g., score is 8 or greater on 2 or 3 occasions, a single score or 2 consecutive scores are 12 or greater). However, protocols vary in initial dosing frequency, incremental changes and thresholds for dosage adjustment, and tapering strategies. In general, dosage may be escalated if Finnegan score remains elevated (e.g., 2 consecutive scores are 8 or greater, one score is 12 or greater), and dosage is tapered once patients are stable (e.g., no score exceeds 8 or average score is less than 8 for 24 hours).

Some protocols are based on pharmacokinetic modeling of methadone in neonates and utilize a stepwise approach to dosage escalation and tapering. Under such protocols, methadone hydrochloride may be administered at an initial dose of 0.1 mg/kg; dosing intervals are shorter during the initial steps of the protocol, but then are lengthened to and maintained at 12 hours while the dose is tapered, if tolerated, by a modest amount every 24 hours until the dosage of the drug has been reduced to 0.01 mg/kg once daily. The drug may then be discontinued. Such protocols increase early exposure to the drug, and limited experience suggests that such an approach may allow for shorter treatment durations and hospital stays. Other clinicians have recommended administration of methadone hydrochloride at an initial dosage of 0.05–0.1 mg/kg every 12 hours; dosage increases, when indicated, in increments of 0.02–0.05 mg/kg per dose or 10%; a maximum dosage of 1 mg/kg daily; and/or tapering schedules of 10–20% per week. Following discontinuance of methadone, neonates should be monitored for 48–72 hours. Specialized protocols should be consulted for further information on methadone hydrochloride dosage and monitoring of Finnegan scores in neonates with opiate abstinence syndrome. Further study is needed to define optimal dosing strategies.

CAUTIONS

Methadone shares the toxic potentials of the opiate agonists, and the usual precautions of opiate agonist therapy should be observed. (See Cautions in the Opiate Agonists General Statement 28:08.08.)

Death and life-threatening adverse effects, including respiratory depression and cardiac arrhythmias, have occurred during initiation of methadone for the treatment of pain and in patients being transferred to methadone from other opiate therapy, possibly as a result of inadvertent overdosage, drug interactions, and adverse cardiac effects of the drug.

While serious, life-threatening, or fatal respiratory depression can occur at any time during therapy, the risk is greatest during initiation of therapy and following dosage increases. In some cases, respiratory depression has occurred when methadone was used as recommended and was not misused or abused. Deaths have been reported in patients being transferred to methadone from chronic therapy with high dosages of other opiate analgesics; deaths also have been reported during initiation of methadone maintenance treatment for opiate dependence (opiate use disorder [OUD]) in individuals who previously used high dosages of other opiates. An understanding of methadone's pharmacokinetic and pharmacodynamic properties is crucial for safe use of the drug. Methadone's elimination half-life (8–59 hours) is substantially longer than the duration of its analgesic action (4–8 hours); in addition, peak respiratory depressant effects of the drug typically occur later and persist longer than its peak analgesic effect, particularly during the early dosing period. The full analgesic effect usually is not attained for 3–5 days. These properties can contribute to inadvertent overdosage, particularly during treatment initiation and dosage adjustment. Methadone should be prescribed only by clinicians who are experienced in the use of potent opiates for the treatment of chronic pain. Methadone dosage should be selected carefully and titrated slowly, even in opiate-tolerant patients, and patients should be monitored carefully during treatment initiation, transfer to methadone from other opiate therapy, and dosage titration.

Prolongation of the QT interval and serious cardiac arrhythmias, including torsades de pointes, have been reported in patients receiving methadone. Most of the reported cases have occurred in patients receiving methadone at relatively high dosages (more than 200 mg daily) for the treatment of chronic pain, but cases also have been reported in patients receiving methadone maintenance therapy at lower dosages. In most cases involving patients receiving usual methadone maintenance dosages, concomitant drug therapy and/or conditions such as hypokalemia were identified as contributing factors. Methadone should be used for pain management only when the potential benefit from the drug outweighs the possible risk of QT-interval prolongation that has been reported with higher methadone dosages. Patients should be monitored closely for changes in cardiac rhythm during initiation of therapy and following increases in dosage. In addition, methadone should be used with caution and careful monitoring in patients who may be at risk for development of prolonged QT syndrome (e.g., those with cardiac hypertrophy, hypokalemia, or hypomagnesemia; those receiving methadone at relatively high dosages or receiving concomitant therapy with a drug that may cause electrolyte disturbances or prolong the QT interval [see Drug Interactions: Drugs that Prolong QT Interval]). If prolongation of the QT interval occurs in a patient receiving methadone, the patient's drug regimen should be evaluated to identify drugs that may prolong the QT interval, cause electrolyte abnormalities, or inhibit metabolism of methadone. Use of methadone in patients with known prolongation of the QT interval has not been systematically evaluated.

Profound sedation, respiratory depression, coma, and death may occur when opiate agonists are used concomitantly with benzodiazepines or other CNS depressants. Concomitant use of opiate analgesics and other CNS depressants should be reserved for patients in whom alternative treatment options are inadequate; the lowest effective dosages and shortest possible duration of concomitant therapy should be used, and the patient should be monitored closely for respiratory depression and sedation. Patients receiving methadone and/or their caregivers should be apprised of the risks associated with concomitant therapeutic or illicit use of benzodiazepines, alcohol, or other CNS depressants. Concomitant use with alcohol should be avoided. (See Drug Interactions: Alcohol and also see Drug Interactions: Benzodiazepines and Other CNS Depressants.)

Because the morbidity and mortality associated with untreated opiate addiction can outweigh the serious risks associated with concomitant use of opiates and benzodiazepines or other CNS depressants, FDA states that methadone treatment for opiate addiction (i.e., medication-assisted treatment [MAT]) should not be withheld from patients receiving benzodiazepines or other CNS depressants. These drugs should be tapered and discontinued, if possible, in patients receiving MAT. However, excluding or discharging patients from MAT because of benzodiazepine or CNS depressant use is not likely to prevent such concomitant use and may lead to use outside the treatment setting, which could result in more severe outcomes. Careful management can reduce the risks associated with concomitant use of benzodiazepines or other CNS depressants in patients receiving methadone treatment for opiate addiction. FDA states that benzodiazepines are not the treatment of choice for anxiety or insomnia in patients receiving methadone treatment for opiate addiction; other pharmacologic or nonpharmacologic therapies should be considered. FDA also states that current evidence does not support dose limitations or other arbitrary limits on methadone as a strategy for addressing concomitant benzodiazepine or other CNS depressant use in patients receiving MAT. However, in patients who are sedated at the time of a scheduled methadone dose, the cause of sedation should be evaluated and omission or reduction of the methadone dose may be appropriate.

Precautions recommended by FDA for minimizing risks associated with concomitant use of benzodiazepines or other CNS depressants in patients receiving MAT include the following:

- Patient education upon initiation of MAT regarding the risks associated with concomitant use of benzodiazepines or other CNS depressants;

- Development of strategies upon initiation of MAT for managing any prescribed or illicit use of benzodiazepines or other CNS depressants;

- Verification of the diagnosis in any patient receiving prescribed benzodiazepines or other CNS depressants for anxiety or insomnia, and consideration of other treatment options for these conditions;

- Recognition that MAT may be required indefinitely and should be continued for as long as the patient derives benefit and MAT contributes to the intended treatment goals;

- Coordination of care to minimize risks and ensure that other prescribers are aware that the patient is receiving methadone treatment; and

- Toxicology screening to monitor for prescribed or illicit drug use.

Because of the risks associated with opiate overdosage, clinicians should routinely discuss the availability of the opiate antagonist naloxone with all patients receiving new or reauthorized opiate prescriptions for pain management or new or reauthorized prescriptions for medications for treatment of OUD. Clinicians should consider prescribing naloxone for patients receiving opiate analgesics who are at increased risk of opiate overdosage (e.g., those receiving concomitant therapy with benzodiazepines or other CNS depressants, those with a history of opiate or substance use disorder, those with medical conditions that could increase sensitivity to opiate effects, those who have experienced a prior opiate overdose) and should strongly consider prescribing naloxone for all patients receiving medications for treatment of OUD. Clinicians also should consider prescribing naloxone when patients receiving opiates for pain management or for treatment of OUD have household members, including children, or other close contacts who are at risk for accidental ingestion or overdosage. Even if patients are not receiving an opiate for pain management or medication for treatment of OUD, a naloxone prescription should be considered if the patient is at increased risk of opiate overdosage (e.g., those with a current or past diagnosis of OUD, those who have experienced a prior opiate overdose). (See Naloxone Hydrochloride 28:10.)

Patients should be instructed to take methadone exactly as prescribed and advised not to initiate or discontinue use of other drugs or dietary supplements without consulting their clinician; patients also should be informed of the signs and symptoms of overdosage and symptoms suggestive of a cardiac arrhythmia, and advised to seek immediate medical attention if such manifestations occur.

Serotonin syndrome has been reported during concomitant use of opiate agonists, including methadone, and serotonergic drugs at recommended dosages. Manifestations of serotonin syndrome may include mental status changes (e.g., agitation, hallucinations, coma), autonomic instability (e.g., tachycardia, labile blood pressure, hyperthermia), neuromuscular aberrations (e.g., hyperreflexia, incoordination, rigidity), and/or GI symptoms (e.g., nausea, vomiting, diarrhea). Symptom onset generally occurs within several hours to a few days of concomitant use, but may occur later, particularly after dosage increases. (See Drug Interactions: Drugs Associated with Serotonin Syndrome.)

Patients who are tolerant to other opiate agonists may have incomplete tolerance to methadone; therefore, methadone should be used with caution and at appropriately adjusted dosages in patients being transferred to methadone from other opiate therapy. Overdosage of methadone (sometimes fatal) has been reported in patients being transferred from chronic, high-dose therapy with other opiate analgesics to therapy with methadone. Pharmacokinetic parameters must be carefully considered during initiation and titration of methadone therapy in patients who previously received chronic opiate agonist therapy. (See Dosage and Administration: Dosage.)

Inadvertent ingestion of methadone, particularly by children, may result in fatal overdosage.

Deaths associated with illicit use of methadone frequently have involved concomitant abuse of benzodiazepines.

Methadone overdosage has been reported to induce pulmonary edema. During methadone maintenance treatment, most adverse effects disappear over a period of several weeks; however, constipation and excessive sweating often persist.

In patients receiving methadone maintenance treatment for opiate dependence, abrupt discontinuance of the drug can result in withdrawal symptoms and may increase the risk of relapse to illicit drug use. Anxiety in a patient receiving methadone maintenance treatment should not be confused with withdrawal syndrome and should not be treated with an increase in methadone dosage.

Patients receiving methadone maintenance treatment for opiate dependence who experience physical trauma or other acute (e.g., postoperative) pain should not be expected to derive adequate analgesia from their stable methadone regimen. Such patients should receive analgesics, including opiates, that would be appropriate for other patients experiencing similar nociceptive stimulation. Opiate doses may be somewhat higher or dosing intervals somewhat shorter than those used in non-opiate-tolerant patients.

Use of methadone has not been extensively evaluated in patients with renal or hepatic impairment. Because methadone is metabolized in the liver, patients with hepatic impairment may be at risk for accumulation of the drug with repeated administration.

● Pediatric Precautions

The manufacturers state that safety, efficacy, and pharmacokinetics of methadone in pediatric patients younger than 18 years of age have not been established.

Short- or long-term *detoxification* treatment using methadone is not subject to any age limitation. However, the effects of prolonged methadone use on the physiologic and psychologic development of children are not known; therefore, *maintenance* treatment with the drug should not be initiated indiscriminately in children younger than 18 years of age. Children younger than 18 years of age are eligible to receive maintenance treatment with methadone provided they have undergone at least 2 documented attempts at detoxification or drug-free treatment within a 12-month period and the program physician has documented that the child continues to be, or is again, physiologically dependent on opiates. In addition, signed informed consent must be obtained from a parent, legal guardian, or responsible adult designated by the appropriate local (e.g., state) authority (e.g., via emancipated minor laws).

● Pregnancy, Fertility, and Lactation

Pregnancy

Methadone should be used during pregnancy only when the potential benefits justify the possible risks. Because of the drug's long duration of effect, use of methadone for obstetric analgesia is not recommended since there may be an increased risk of neonatal respiratory depression.

Untreated opiate addiction during pregnancy is associated with adverse obstetrical outcomes, including preeclampsia, fetal growth restriction, preterm birth, spontaneous abortion, and fetal death. In addition, untreated opiate addiction often results in continued or relapsing illicit opiate use and engagement in high-risk behaviors. The recommended treatment of opiate dependence in pregnant women is maintenance treatment with methadone or buprenorphine; this approach is superior to medically supervised withdrawal (i.e., detoxification) because withdrawal is associated with high relapse rates and poorer outcomes.

Short- or long-term *detoxification* treatment using methadone is *not* recommended during pregnancy. However, pregnant women, regardless of age, are eligible for admission into a comprehensive *maintenance* treatment program using methadone if they have a history of documented opiate dependence and are considered at risk of possibly returning to such dependence (and all its attendant risks) during pregnancy. For such women, evidence of *current* physiologic dependence is not necessary, provided the program physician certifies the pregnancy and considers such therapy medically justified using reasonable clinical judgment. All pregnant women admitted into a maintenance program with methadone must be given the opportunity for prenatal care either by the program or by referral to an appropriate health-care provider. Such women should be advised of the possible risks to them and their fetus from continued use of illicit drugs and from the use and withdrawal of methadone as part of maintenance or detoxification treatment.

Pharmacokinetic data from a limited number of pregnant women suggest that methadone clearance may be increased, trough plasma concentrations of the drug may be lower, and half-life of the drug may be decreased during the second and third trimesters of pregnancy compared with pharmacokinetic values determined for the same women postpartum or for nonpregnant opiate-dependent women. If methadone is used during pregnancy, dosage adjustment (i.e., increased dose or decreased dosing interval) may be necessary.

Studies of methadone use during pregnancy generally have compared benefits of methadone maintenance treatment with the risks of untreated dependence on illicit drugs; the relevance of these findings to use of methadone as an analgesic during pregnancy is unclear. Pregnant women in methadone maintenance programs receive better prenatal care, with fewer obstetric and fetal complications and reduced neonatal morbidity and mortality, compared with women using illicit drugs. Available data suggest that maternal use of methadone during pregnancy as part of a supervised therapeutic regimen is unlikely to pose a substantial teratogenic risk; however, data are insufficient to fully exclude such risk. Most information regarding pregnancy outcomes involves methadone exposure after the first trimester, and information on methadone dosage and duration of use during pregnancy is limited. Interpretation of available information on pregnancy outcomes also is complicated by maternal factors such as illicit drug use, nutritional status, presence of infections, and psychosocial circumstances.

In a double-blind, randomized, controlled trial (Maternal Opioid Treatment: Human Experimental Research [MOTHER]), outcomes, principally opiate withdrawal effects, were assessed in neonates born to women who received methadone or buprenorphine treatment for opiate dependence during pregnancy. Enrollment in the study occurred at an average gestational age of 18.7 weeks. Prior to the end of pregnancy, 18% of methadone-treated women and 33% of buprenorphine-treated women discontinued treatment; outcomes were evaluated for the neonates whose mothers remained in treatment until delivery. No difference was observed between methadone- and buprenorphine-exposed neonates in the proportion of neonates requiring treatment for opiate withdrawal syndrome or the peak severity of the syndrome. Buprenorphine-exposed neonates required a lower total mean morphine sulfate dosage for treatment of withdrawal (1.1 versus 10.4 mg), had shorter hospital stays (10 versus 17.5 days), and shorter duration of treatment for withdrawal (4.1 versus 9.9 days) compared with methadone-exposed neonates. The groups did not differ in other outcome measures (head circumference, weight and length at birth, preterm birth, gestational age at delivery, and 1- and 5-minute Apgar scores) or in the rates of serious maternal or neonatal adverse events. The imbalance in treatment discontinuance rates between methadone- and buprenorphine-treated women complicate interpretation of the study findings.

A retrospective review of pregnancy outcomes for women who underwent inpatient methadone detoxification did not reveal any increase in the risk of spontaneous abortion during the second trimester or premature delivery during the third trimester, although other studies have suggested an increased risk of premature delivery in opiate-dependent women who received methadone during pregnancy. Several studies have suggested that use of methadone in opiate-dependent women during pregnancy results in decreased fetal growth (with reduced birth weight, length, and/or head circumference), but this growth deficit does not appear to persist into later childhood. However, mild but persistent deficits in psychometric and behavioral test performance have been observed in children who were exposed to methadone in utero. In addition, several studies have suggested that the risk of visual developmental anomalies may be increased in children born to opiate-dependent women who received methadone during pregnancy. There are conflicting reports on whether maternal use of methadone during pregnancy is associated with a higher incidence of sudden infant death syndrome. During late pregnancy, results of fetal nonstress tests reportedly are more likely to be abnormal when the tests are performed 1–2 hours after a maintenance dose of methadone than when they are performed in control subjects.

Methadone has been detected in cord blood and amniotic fluid at concentrations proportional to maternal plasma concentrations.

Prolonged maternal use of opiate agonists during pregnancy can result in neonatal opiate withdrawal syndrome with manifestations of irritability, hyperactivity and abnormal sleep pattern, high-pitched cry, tremor, vomiting, diarrhea, and failure to gain weight. In contrast to adults, the withdrawal syndrome in neonates may be life-threatening if not recognized and treated, and requires management according to protocols developed by neonatology experts. Women who require prolonged opiate agonist therapy during pregnancy should be advised of the risk of neonatal opiate withdrawal syndrome, and availability of appropriate treatment should be ensured. The onset, duration, and severity of the syndrome vary depending on the specific opiate agonist used, duration of use, timing and amount of last maternal use, and rate of drug elimination by the neonate. Use of standardized protocols for identification and management of opiate withdrawal syndrome has been shown to improve overall response, including reductions in hospital stay and duration of pharmacologic treatment. When environmental and supportive measures are inadequate, opiates (e.g., methadone) are recommended as first-line pharmacologic therapy. (See Uses: Neonatal Opiate Withdrawal.)

Although no teratogenic effects were observed in rats or rabbits given methadone, administration of large doses of the drug in guinea pigs, hamsters, and mice resulted in teratogenic effects including exencephaly and cranioschisis. When male rodents were given methadone prior to mating, their offspring exhibited decreased weight gain after weaning, increased neonatal mortality, reduced thymus weight (male progeny), increased adrenal weight (female progeny), and physiologic and behavioral changes; increased embryolethality and preimplantation deaths also have been reported. Perinatal exposure to methadone in rats has been associated with alterations in learning ability, motor activity, thermal regulation, nociceptive responses, and sensitivity to other drugs. Animal data also indicate neurochemical changes in the brains of methadone-treated offspring, including changes to the cholinergic, dopaminergic, noradrenergic, and serotonergic systems.

Lactation

Methadone is distributed into human milk. Peak concentrations in milk reportedly occur approximately 4–5 hours after an oral dose of the drug. In 2 studies in 22 nursing women who were receiving methadone maintenance treatment, methadone was present in low concentrations in milk, but no adverse effects on breast-fed infants were observed. At maternal oral dosages of 10–80 mg daily, reported concentrations of methadone in milk were 50–570 ng/mL; in most of the milk samples, methadone concentrations were lower than maternal steady-state serum concentrations of the drug. At maternal oral dosages of 20–80 mg daily, the mean infant dosage of the drug, calculated based on an assumed average milk consumption of 150 mL/kg daily, was approximately 17.4 mcg/kg daily, which was approximately 2–3.5% of the oral maternal dosage. Methadone has been detected in very low plasma concentrations in some infants whose mothers were receiving methadone. Cases of sedation and respiratory depression in infants exposed to methadone through breast milk have been reported rarely.

Experts recommend that women who are stable on methadone treatment for opiate dependence, are not using other illicit drugs, and have no contraindications to nursing be encouraged to breast-feed their infants; to lower the risk of return to substance use, women receiving methadone should be encouraged to continue treatment during the postpartum period. Breast-feeding has been associated with decreased severity of neonatal opiate withdrawal syndrome, decreased need for pharmacotherapy, and shorter hospital stays for the neonate. The manufacturers state that the benefits of breast-feeding should be considered along with the mother's clinical need for the drug and any potential adverse effects on the breast-fed infant from either the drug or the underlying maternal condition. Women who are receiving methadone and are breast-feeding or wish to breast-feed should be advised that the drug distributes into human milk, should be instructed to recognize respiratory depression and sedation in infants and to know when to seek medical care, and should be informed that nursing should be discontinued gradually (not abruptly) in order to prevent withdrawal (neonatal abstinence syndrome) in the infant.

DRUG INTERACTIONS

● *Drugs Affecting Hepatic Microsomal Enzymes*

Methadone is metabolized principally by the cytochrome P-450 (CYP) microsomal enzyme system, mainly by isoenzymes 3A4, 2B6, and 2C19 and to a lesser extent by isoenzymes 2C9 and 2D6. Concomitant use of methadone with drugs that induce CYP isoenzymes may result in increased metabolism and decreased plasma concentrations of methadone. Conversely, administration of methadone with drugs that inhibit CYP3A4 and/or CYP2C9 may result in decreased metabolism and increased plasma concentrations of methadone. Therefore, methadone should be used with caution in patients receiving drugs that inhibit or induce these CYP isoenzymes, and patients receiving such drugs concomitantly should be monitored carefully.

Alcohol

Chronic consumption of alcohol has been reported to increase metabolism of methadone and reduce serum concentrations of the drug; however, acute consumption of alcohol has been reported to increase the area under the plasma concentration-time curve (AUC) of methadone, resulting in an increased potential for adverse effects. Concomitant use of opiate agonists and CNS depressants, including alcohol, may result in profound sedation, respiratory depression, coma, and death. (See Drug Interactions: Benzodiazepines and Other CNS Depressants.)

Anticonvulsants

Administration of phenytoin, phenobarbital, or carbamazepine in patients receiving methadone may result in increased metabolism of methadone secondary to induction of CYP3A4. Concomitant use of phenytoin (250 mg twice daily for 24 hours followed by 300 mg daily for 3–4 days) in patients receiving methadone maintenance therapy reduced plasma concentrations of methadone by 50% and resulted in withdrawal symptoms. Withdrawal symptoms also may occur in patients receiving methadone concomitantly with phenobarbital or carbamazepine.

Antidepressants

Concomitant use of certain selective serotonin-reuptake inhibitors (SSRIs) (e.g., sertraline, fluoxetine, fluvoxamine) may increase serum methadone concentrations and increase opiate effects secondary to inhibition of methadone metabolism.

Concomitant use of desipramine with methadone may result in increased serum desipramine concentrations. Opiate agonists (including methadone) may potentiate the effects of tricyclic antidepressants (see Drug Interactions: Antidepressants, in the Opiate Agonists General Statement 28:08.08).

Concomitant use of methadone and antidepressants also may result in serotonin syndrome. (See Drug Interactions: Drugs Associated with Serotonin Syndrome.)

Antifungals

Administration of azole antifungal agents that are known to inhibit the CYP3A4 isoenzyme (e.g., fluconazole, ketoconazole, itraconazole, voriconazole) in patients receiving methadone may result in decreased clearance of methadone. Administration of fluconazole (200 mg daily) has been shown to increase the AUC and peak plasma concentrations of methadone by 35 and 27%, respectively. Administration of voriconazole increased steady-state peak plasma concentrations and AUC of the pharmacologically active *R*-isomer of methadone by 31 and 47%, respectively, in individuals receiving methadone maintenance treatment (30–100 mg daily). Because of the potential for increased or prolonged opiate agonist effects, patients receiving these agents concomitantly should be carefully monitored and methadone dosage should be adjusted as necessary.

Antimycobacterials

Administration of rifampin in patients receiving methadone therapy has reduced serum methadone concentrations and resulted in withdrawal symptoms.

Antiretrovirals

Approximately 25–30% of patients receiving methadone maintenance therapy are HIV-positive, and numerous drug interactions have been reported in HIV-positive patients receiving antiretroviral agents concomitantly with methadone. Clinicians should monitor patients carefully for potential adverse effects when antiretroviral agents are used concomitantly with methadone.

Abacavir

Concomitant use of methadone and abacavir increased methadone clearance by 22%. Some experts state that dosage adjustment is not necessary in patients receiving the drugs concomitantly. The manufacturer states that patients receiving concomitant therapy with abacavir and methadone should be monitored closely for opiate withdrawal, and methadone dosage should be increased as clinically indicated.

Atazanavir

Concomitant use of methadone and atazanavir does not substantially alter plasma concentrations of either drug. No dosage adjustment is necessary.

Concomitant use of methadone and *ritonavir-boosted* atazanavir decreased plasma concentrations of *R*-methadone by about 16–18%. Opiate withdrawal is unlikely but may occur. Patients should be monitored for opiate withdrawal, and methadone dosage should be increased as clinically indicated.

Darunavir

Concomitant use of methadone and *ritonavir-boosted* darunavir decreased the AUC of methadone by 16%. Opiate withdrawal is unlikely but may occur. Patients should be carefully monitored for opiate withdrawal, and methadone dosage should be increased as clinically indicated.

Delavirdine

Concomitant use of delavirdine and methadone may increase plasma concentrations of methadone. Patients receiving concomitant delavirdine and methadone therapy should be closely monitored for methadone toxicity; methadone dosage may need to be reduced.

Didanosine

Concomitant use of methadone and buffered didanosine preparations appears to decrease bioavailability of didanosine. In a limited number of individuals, concomitant use of methadone and buffered didanosine resulted in a 66% decrease in the peak serum concentration and 63% decrease in the AUC of didanosine; trough concentrations of methadone did not appear to be affected. Concomitant use of methadone and didanosine delayed-release capsules does not affect the pharmacokinetics of didanosine; dosage adjustments are not necessary with this preparation.

Efavirenz

Administration of methadone hydrochloride (35–100 mg daily) and efavirenz (600 mg daily for 14–21 days) in HIV-infected individuals with a history of drug dependence decreased the peak plasma concentration and AUC of methadone by 45 and 52%, respectively, and resulted in manifestations of opiate withdrawal. The maintenance dosage of methadone hydrochloride was increased by an average of 22% to alleviate withdrawal symptoms.

Individuals receiving concurrent methadone and efavirenz therapy should be informed of this potential interaction and closely monitored for signs of opiate withdrawal; an increase in the maintenance dosage of methadone frequently is necessary in such individuals.

Elvitegravir, Cobicistat, Tenofovir, and Emtricitabine

Concomitant use of methadone and the fixed combination of elvitegravir, cobicistat, tenofovir, and emtricitabine does not substantially affect plasma concentrations of any of the concomitantly administered drugs. No dosage adjustment is necessary.

Etravirine

Concomitant use of etravirine and methadone does not appear to affect plasma concentrations of either drug. Dosage adjustment is not needed.

Fosamprenavir

Concomitant use of methadone and amprenavir (no longer commercially available in the US) decreased trough plasma concentrations of *R*-methadone by 21% but did not substantially alter the AUC of methadone. Because fosamprenavir is metabolized to amprenavir, interactions reported with amprenavir are expected to occur in patients receiving fosamprenavir. Patients receiving methadone concomitantly with fosamprenavir should be carefully monitored and methadone dosage should be adjusted as necessary.

Concomitant use of methadone and *ritonavir-boosted* fosamprenavir decreased the AUC of *R*-methadone by 18%. Opiate withdrawal is unlikely but may occur. Patients should be monitored for opiate withdrawal, and methadone dosage should be increased as clinically indicated.

Indinavir

Concomitant use of methadone and indinavir does not appear to substantially affect exposure to either drug.

Lopinavir

Concomitant use of methadone and the fixed combination of lopinavir and ritonavir (lopinavir/ritonavir) decreased the AUC of methadone by 26–53%; opiate withdrawal symptoms may occur. Patients should be monitored closely for opiate withdrawal, and methadone dosage should be increased as clinically indicated.

Maraviroc

No data are available regarding concomitant use of maraviroc and methadone. Some experts state that maraviroc is considered safe for use in patients receiving methadone.

Nelfinavir

Concomitant use of methadone and nelfinavir may result in decreased plasma concentrations of methadone; opiate withdrawal occurs rarely. Individuals receiving concomitant methadone and nelfinavir therapy should be closely monitored for signs of opiate withdrawal; an increase in the maintenance dosage of methadone may be necessary.

Nevirapine

There have been reports of opiate withdrawal and subtherapeutic or decreased serum methadone concentrations following initiation of nevirapine therapy in individuals who were receiving long-term methadone treatment for opiate addiction. nevirapine has been reported to decrease the AUC of methadone by 37–51%.

Individuals receiving concomitant methadone and nevirapine therapy should be informed of this potential interaction, and should be closely monitored for signs of opiate withdrawal when nevirapine therapy is initiated; an increase in the maintenance dosage of methadone frequently is necessary. If methadone dosage is increased during nevirapine therapy, patients should be monitored for methadone overdosage when the antiretroviral agent is discontinued.

Raltegravir

Concomitant use of methadone and raltegravir does not substantially affect plasma concentrations of either drug. Dosage adjustment is not necessary in patients receiving the drugs concomitantly.

Rilpivirine

Rilpivirine has been reported to decrease the AUC of methadone by 16%. No dosage adjustment is necessary, but patients should be monitored for withdrawal symptoms.

Ritonavir

Administration of a single 5-mg dose of methadone hydrochloride and ritonavir (500 mg every 12 hours for 15 days) decreased the AUC of methadone by 36%. There has been at least one report of opiate withdrawal and subtherapeutic or decreased serum methadone concentrations following initiation of ritonavir therapy in an HIV-infected patient who was receiving long-term methadone treatment for opiate addiction.

Methadone should be administered with caution in patients receiving ritonavir, especially when used in combination with other drugs that may decrease plasma concentrations of methadone. Individuals receiving concomitant methadone and ritonavir therapy should be informed of this potential interaction, and should be closely monitored for manifestations of opiate withdrawal when ritonavir therapy is initiated; an increase in the maintenance dosage of methadone may be necessary. If methadone dosage is increased during ritonavir therapy, patients should be monitored for methadone overdosage when the antiretroviral agent is discontinued.

Saquinavir

Concomitant use of methadone and *ritonavir-boosted* saquinavir decreased the AUC of *R*-methadone by 19%. Opiate withdrawal is unlikely but may occur. Patients should be monitored closely for opiate withdrawal, and methadone dosage should be increased as clinically indicated.

Stavudine

Concomitant use of stavudine and methadone appears to decrease bioavailability of stavudine. In a limited number of individuals, concomitant use of stavudine and methadone resulted in a 44% decrease in peak concentrations and a 25% decrease in the AUC of stavudine; trough concentrations of methadone did not appear to be affected. Dosage adjustment is not necessary in patients receiving the drugs concomitantly.

Tenofovir

Concomitant use of tenofovir and methadone does not appear to affect plasma concentrations of either drug.

Tipranavir

Concomitant use of methadone and *ritonavir-boosted* tipranavir decreased peak plasma concentrations and AUC of *R*-methadone by 46 and 48%, respectively. Patients should be monitored closely for opiate withdrawal, and methadone dosage should be increased as clinically indicated.

Zidovudine

In one study in IV drug abusers with HIV infection who were receiving long-term methadone hydrochloride treatment for opiate addiction (30–90 mg daily), initiation of zidovudine therapy (200 mg orally every 4 hours) did not appear to have any clinically important effects on the pharmacokinetics of methadone and did not result in any evidence of opiate withdrawal. However, the AUC of zidovudine was increased about 43% in patients receiving concomitant methadone compared with those receiving zidovudine alone. In another study in HIV-infected individuals who had been receiving methadone treatment for approximately 2 months, concomitant use of oral or IV zidovudine increased the zidovudine AUC by 29 or 41%, respectively, and reduced the clearance of zidovudine by about 26%. While the mechanism of this interaction requires further study, limited data indicate that methadone inhibits zidovudine glucuronidation and also reduces renal clearance of zidovudine.

Based on the results of these studies, it appears that the maintenance dosage of methadone probably does not need to be adjusted when zidovudine therapy is initiated in patients receiving long-term methadone treatment; however, the clinical importance of the increased zidovudine AUC during concomitant therapy is unclear. Patients receiving concomitant zidovudine and methadone therapy should be monitored for dose-related zidovudine toxicity.

Macrolide Antibiotics

Administration of macrolide anti-infectives that are known to inhibit CYP3A4 (e.g., clarithromycin, erythromycin, telithromycin) may result in decreased clearance of methadone. Patients receiving methadone concomitantly with macrolide anti-infectives should be carefully monitored and methadone dosage should be adjusted as necessary.

Smoking

Some evidence indicates that cigarette smoking increases CYP1A2 activity and may reduce plasma methadone concentrations.

St. John's Wort

Manifestations of opiate withdrawal may occur in patients receiving methadone and St. John's wort (*Hypericum perforatum*) concomitantly, since St. John's wort may increase metabolism of methadone via induction of CYP3A4. Patients receiving methadone concomitantly with St. John's wort should be carefully monitored, and methadone dosage should be adjusted as necessary.

Concomitant use of methadone and St. John's wort also may result in serotonin syndrome. (See Drug Interactions: Drugs Associated with Serotonin Syndrome.)

• Benzodiazepines and Other CNS Depressants

Concomitant use of opiate agonists, including methadone, and benzodiazepines or other CNS depressants (e.g., anxiolytics, sedatives, hypnotics, tranquilizers, muscle relaxants, general anesthetics, antipsychotics, other opiate agonists, alcohol) may result in profound sedation, respiratory depression, coma, and death. (See Drug Interactions: Benzodiazepines and Other CNS Depressants, in the Opiate Agonists General Statement 28:08.08.) Concomitant use of opiate analgesics and other CNS depressants should be reserved for patients in whom alternative treatment options are inadequate; the lowest effective dosages and shortest possible duration of concomitant therapy should be used, and the patient should be monitored closely for respiratory depression and sedation. Concomitant use with alcohol should be avoided.

If a benzodiazepine or other CNS depressant is required for any indication other than epilepsy in a patient receiving methadone for analgesia, the drug should be initiated at a lower dosage than indicated in the absence of opiate therapy and titrated based on clinical response. In patients receiving a benzodiazepine or other CNS depressant, methadone, if required for analgesia, should be initiated at a reduced dosage and titrated based on clinical response.

Because the morbidity and mortality associated with untreated opiate addiction can outweigh the serious risks associated with concomitant use of opiates and benzodiazepines or other CNS depressants, FDA states that methadone treatment for opiate addiction (i.e., medication-assisted treatment [MAT]) should not be withheld from patients receiving benzodiazepines or other CNS depressants. Clinicians should develop treatment plans that minimize the risks associated with concomitant use. If possible, benzodiazepines or other CNS depressants should be tapered and discontinued. (See Cautions.)

Clinicians should consider prescribing the opiate antagonist naloxone for patients receiving opiates who are at increased risk of opiate overdosage, including those receiving benzodiazepines or other CNS depressants concomitantly. (See Cautions.)

• Drugs Associated with Serotonin Syndrome

Serotonin syndrome has occurred in patients receiving opiate agonists, including methadone, in conjunction with other serotonergic drugs, including serotonin (5-hydroxytryptamine; 5-HT) type 1 receptor agonists ("triptans"), selective serotonin-reuptake inhibitors (SSRIs), selective serotonin- and norepinephrine-reuptake inhibitors (SNRIs), tricyclic antidepressants, antiemetics that are 5-HT$_3$ receptor antagonists, buspirone, cyclobenzaprine, dextromethorphan, lithium, St. John's wort, tryptophan, other serotonin modulators (e.g., mirtazapine, nefazodone, trazodone, vilazodone), and monoamine oxidase (MAO) inhibitors (both those used to treat psychiatric disorders and others, such as linezolid, methylene blue, and selegiline). Serotonin syndrome may occur within the recommended dosage ranges for these drugs. Manifestations of serotonin syndrome may include mental status changes (e.g., agitation, hallucinations, coma), autonomic instability (e.g., tachycardia, labile blood pressure, hyperthermia), neuromuscular aberrations (e.g., hyperreflexia, incoordination, rigidity), and/or GI symptoms (e.g., nausea, vomiting, diarrhea). Symptom onset generally occurs within several hours to a few days of concomitant use, but may occur later, particularly after dosage increases.

If concurrent therapy with opiate agonists and serotonergic drugs is warranted, patients should be monitored for serotonin syndrome, particularly during initiation of therapy and dosage increases. If serotonin syndrome is suspected, treatment with methadone, other opiate therapy, and/or any concurrently administered serotonergic agents should be discontinued.

For further information on serotonin syndrome, including manifestations and treatment, see Drug Interactions: Serotonergic Drugs, in Fluoxetine Hydrochloride 28:16.04.20.

● Drugs that Prolong QT Interval

Drugs known to prolong the QT interval (e.g., class I or III antiarrhythmic agents, calcium-channel blocking agents, some antipsychotic agents, tricyclic antidepressants) should be used with extreme caution in patients receiving methadone because of the risk of severe and potentially life-threatening cardiac arrhythmias. Methadone also should be used with caution in patients receiving drugs (e.g., diuretics, laxatives, corticosteroid hormones with mineralocorticoid activity) that may result in electrolyte disorders (e.g., hypomagnesemia, hypokalemia) that may prolong the QT interval.

● Risperidone

There have been reports of opiate withdrawal following the initiation of risperidone therapy in patients receiving methadone.

For further information about drug interactions involving opiate agonists (including methadone hydrochloride), see Drug Interactions in the Opiate Agonists General Statement 28:08.08.

LABORATORY TEST INTERFERENCES

Chlorpromazine, clomipramine, diphenhydramine, doxylamine, quetiapine, thioridazine, and verapamil may produce false-positive results for urine screening tests for methadone.

PHARMACOLOGY

In equianalgesic doses, methadone hydrochloride may produce a similar or slightly greater degree of respiratory depression than does morphine sulfate. A single dose of methadone may produce less sedation and euphoria than does morphine; however, because of the cumulative effect of methadone, marked sedation occurs after repeated administration. Methadone causes less constipation than does morphine. Methadone has antitussive activity. Methadone inhibits cardiac potassium channels and prolongs the QT interval.

PHARMACOKINETICS

● Absorption

Methadone is well absorbed from the GI tract. Following oral administration, bioavailability is approximately 80%; however, there is considerable interindividual variability in oral bioavailability (range: 36–100%). Following IM or subcutaneous administration of a single dose of methadone, onset and duration of analgesic effect are similar to those of morphine; duration is approximately 4–8 hours. Oral administration delays the onset as compared to parenteral administration. Peak plasma concentrations of the drug occur 1–7.5 hours following oral administration. Steady-state plasma concentrations and full analgesic effects usually are not attained until completion of 3–5 days of therapy.

With repeated methadone dosing, storage in and slow release of the drug from the liver and other tissues may prolong the duration of action of methadone despite the presence of low plasma concentrations. Peak respiratory depressant effects of methadone typically occur later and persist longer than the drug's peak analgesic effects, particularly during the early dosing period. The drug has an extended duration of action in patients who are physically dependent on oral methadone. Duration of action increases with repeated administration and is approximately 22–48 hours following oral administration in patients on methadone maintenance. Depressant effects after overdosage may also continue for 36–48 hours.

● Distribution

Methadone is highly lipophilic and is widely distributed in body tissues. Because of its lipophilicity, methadone may persist in the liver and other tissues. Slow release of methadone from these sites may prolong the duration of action of the drug despite the presence of low plasma concentrations.

Methadone is highly bound (85–90%) to plasma proteins, mainly α_1-acid glycoprotein.

Methadone crosses the placenta and is distributed into milk.

● Elimination

In clinical studies, the terminal elimination half-life of methadone ranged from 8–59 hours. In clinical use, the elimination half-life of methadone has varied considerably, ranging from 9–87 hours in postoperative patients, from 8.5–75 hours in opiate-dependent patients, and up to 120 hours in outpatients receiving therapy for chronic malignant pain. In one study in 5 patients receiving 100 or 120 mg of oral methadone hydrochloride daily for maintenance treatment of opiate addiction, the drug had an apparent plasma half-life of 13–47 hours, with an average of 25 hours.

Methadone is extensively metabolized, principally by cytochrome P-450 (CYP) isoenzymes 3A4, 2B6, and 2C19 and to a lesser extent by CYP isoenzymes 2C9 and 2D6. The drug undergoes N-demethylation to an inactive metabolite, 2-ethylidene-1,5-dimethyl-3,3-diphenylpyrrolidine (EDDP), and other metabolites with little or no pharmacologic activity. Although methadone appears to be a substrate of the P-glycoprotein transport system, its pharmacokinetics do not appear to be substantially altered by P-glycoprotein polymorphism or inhibition.

Methadone and its metabolites are excreted to varying degrees in urine and feces. Methadone is excreted by glomerular filtration and undergoes renal reabsorption. Reabsorption of methadone decreases as urinary pH decreases. Urinary excretion of methadone and its metabolic end products is dose dependent and comprises the major route of excretion only in dosages exceeding 55 mg daily. Methadone metabolites are also excreted in the feces via the bile.

CHEMISTRY AND STABILITY

● Chemistry

Methadone hydrochloride is a synthetic diphenylheptane-derivative opiate agonist. The drug occurs as colorless crystals or a white, crystalline powder and is soluble in water and freely soluble in alcohol. Dispersible tablets of methadone hydrochloride are specially formulated with insoluble excipients to deter use of the drug by injection. Methadone hydrochloride injection has a pH of 3–6.5. Methadone hydrochloride oral concentrate has a pH of 1–6.

● Stability

Methadone hydrochloride preparations should be stored in tight, light-resistant containers. Methadone hydrochloride oral concentrate and oral solution should be stored at 15–30°C; the tablets and injection should be stored at a controlled room temperature of 25°C, but may be exposed to temperatures ranging from 15–30°C.

Methadone hydrochloride injection has been reported to be physically or chemically incompatible with solutions containing aminophylline, ammonium chloride, amobarbital sodium, chlorothiazide sodium, phenytoin sodium, heparin sodium, methicillin sodium (no longer commercially available in the US), nitrofurantoin sodium, pentobarbital sodium, phenobarbital sodium, sodium bicarbonate, and thiopental sodium (no longer commercially available in the US). Specialized references should be consulted for more specific compatibility information.

For further information on chemistry, pharmacology, pharmacokinetics, uses, cautions, chronic toxicity, acute toxicity, drug interactions, and dosage and administration of methadone hydrochloride, see the Opiate Agonists General Statement 28:08.08.

PREPARATIONS

Methadone hydrochloride is subject to control under the Federal Controlled Substances Act of 1970 as a schedule II (C-II) drug and, in addition, is subject to US Food and Drug Administration regulations (21 CFR 291.505) for drugs that require special studies, records, and reports when used for detoxification and maintenance of opiate dependence.

Distribution of methadone hydrochloride 40-mg dispersible tablets is restricted. (See Restricted Distribution under Dosage and Administration: Administration.)

Excipients in commercially available drug preparations may have clinically important effects in some individuals; consult specific product labeling for details.

Methadone Hydrochloride

Oral

Solution	5 mg/5 mL*	Methadone Hydrochloride Oral Solution (C-II)
	10 mg/5 mL*	Methadone Hydrochloride Oral Solution (C-II)

Solution, concentrate	10 mg/mL*	Methadone Hydrochloride Intensol® (C-II), Roxane
		Methadone Hydrochloride Oral Concentrate (C-II)
		Methadose® Oral Concentrate (C-II), Mallinckrodt
Tablets	5 mg*	Dolophine® Hydrochloride (C-II; scored), Roxane
		Methadone Hydrochloride Tablets (C-II)
		Methadose® (C-II; scored), Mallinckrodt
	10 mg*	Dolophine® Hydrochloride (C-II; scored), Roxane
		Methadone Hydrochloride Tablets (C-II)
		Methadose® (C-II; scored), Mallinckrodt
Tablets, dispersible	40 mg*	Methadone Hydrochloride Diskets® (C-II; scored), Roxane
		Methadose® (C-II; scored), Mallinckrodt

Parenteral

Injection	10 mg/mL*	Methadone Hydrochloride Injection (C-II)

* available from one or more manufacturer, distributor, and/or repackager by generic (nonproprietary) name

† Use is not currently included in the labeling approved by the US Food and Drug Administration.

Selected Revisions April 19, 2023, © Copyright, April 01, 1973, American Society of Health-System Pharmacists, Inc.

Morphine Sulfate

28:08.08 · OPIOID AGONISTS

REMS

FDA approved a REMS for morphine under a shared REMS system (Opioid Analgesic REMS) to ensure that the benefits outweigh the risks. The REMS may apply to one or more preparations of morphine and consists of the following: medication guide and elements to assure safe use. See the FDA REMS page (https://www.accessdata.fda.gov/scripts/cder/rems/index.cfm).

- Morphine sulfate is a phenanthrene-derivative opioid agonist; morphine is the principal alkaloid of opium and considered to be the prototype of the opioid agonists.

USES

● *Pain*

Morphine sulfate is used in the management of acute or chronic pain severe enough to require an opioid analgesic and for which alternative treatments are inadequate. Because of the risks of addiction, abuse, and misuse with opioids, which can occur at any dosage or duration, reserve use in patients for whom alternative treatment options (e.g., non-opioid analgesics or opioid combination products) have not been tolerated (or not expected to be tolerated) or have not provided (or not expected to provide) adequate analgesia. Morphine sulfate should not be used for an extended period of time unless the pain remains severe enough to require an opioid analgesic and for which alternative treatment options continue to be inadequate.

Morphine sulfate is commercially available in various preparations and formulations. Currently available preparations include immediate-release tablets, oral solution, extended-release tablets, extended-release capsules, rectal suppositories, and injection solutions for IV, IM, epidural, or intrathecal use.

Preservative-free injection solutions of morphine sulfate are indicated for IV, epidural, or intrathecal use. Epidural or intrathecal administration can provide pain relief without attendant loss of motor, sensory, or sympathetic function. The preservative-free concentrated morphine sulfate injection (Infumorph®) is indicated for use only in continuous microinfusion devices as an epidural or intrathecal infusion; this formulation has been designated an orphan drug by the FDA for intraspinal administration using microinfusion devices in the treatment of intractable chronic pain.

Extended-release oral morphine sulfate preparations may be used in patients with severe and persistent pain requiring extended treatment with a daily opioid analgesic and for which alternative treatment options are inadequate. Extended-release preparations should not be used on an as-needed ("prn") basis.

Pain needs to be appropriately and effectively treated, regardless of whether opioids are part of the treatment regimen. Treatment should be individualized, patient-centered, and include multimodal approaches. Opioids can be essential in the management of pain but are associated with considerable potential harm, including opioid use disorder and overdose. Therefore, safer and more effective treatments should be considered prior to initiating opioid therapy. There are multiple nonpharmacologic treatments (e.g., exercise, physical therapy, psychological therapies) and nonopioid drugs (e.g., serotonin and norepinephrine reuptake inhibitors [SNRIs], gabapentinoids, nonsteroidal anti-inflammatory agents [NSAIAs]) that have been shown to be at least as effective as opioids for many types of common pain conditions. These nonopioid treatments are generally preferred to opioids in most situations. If opioids are used, clinicians should carefully evaluate the risk of opioid-related harms and work with the patient to incorporate appropriate risk-mitigation strategies into the treatment plan, including offering naloxone.

The Centers for Disease Control and Prevention (CDC) clinical guideline for prescribing opioids for pain provides recommendations for the management of acute (duration <1 month), subacute (duration 1–3 months), and chronic pain

(duration >3 months) in adults in the outpatient setting. The CDC guideline addresses the following areas: 1) determining whether or not to initiate opioids for pain, 2) selecting opioids and determining opioid dosages, 3) deciding duration of initial opioid prescription and conducting follow-up, and 4) assessing risk and addressing potential harms of opioid use.

Other clinical practice guidelines provide recommendations for the management of specific types of pain including postoperative pain, cancer-related pain, sickle-cell pain, and pain associated with palliative care; although specific recommendations for the management of opioid therapy vary across the guidelines, common elements include risk mitigation strategies, careful dosage titration, and consideration of risks and benefits.

Chronic or Subacute Pain

In patients with chronic or subacute pain not associated with active cancer treatment, palliative care, or end-of-life care (also referred to as chronic noncancer pain), nonopioid therapies are preferred. There is insufficient evidence to determine the long-term benefits of opioid therapy for chronic pain, and there is an increased risk for serious harms related to long-term opioid therapy that appears to be dose dependent. Use of opioid analgesics for the management of chronic noncancer pain increased four-fold in the US from 1999 to 2010, along with a parallel increase in overdose deaths, despite uncertainty over the long-term benefits of such therapy. In addition, evidence that opioid analgesics are superior to other pharmacologic or nonpharmacologic treatments for chronic pain generally is lacking. Opioid analgesics should be considered only if other pain management strategies (nonpharmacologic [e.g., exercise, physical therapy] and nonopioid drugs [e.g., NSAIAs, select antidepressants or anticonvulsants, gabapentinoids, lidocaine and capsaicin patches for neuropathic pain) have been maximized as appropriate for the specific condition and patient, and the expected benefits of opioid analgesics are anticipated to outweigh the risks. If opioid analgesics are used, they should be part of an integrated approach that also includes appropriate nonpharmacologic modalities (e.g., cognitive behavioral therapy, relaxation techniques, biofeedback, functional restoration, exercise therapy, certain interventional procedures) and other appropriate pharmacologic therapies. The lowest-effective dosage of an immediate-release preparation should be used. Clinicians should work with patients to establish treatment goals and also consider how opioid therapy wll be discontinued if the benefits do not outweigh the risks.

The benefits and risks of opioid analgesic therapy should be evaluated within 1–4 weeks following initiation of therapy or an increase in dosage, and reevaluated on an ongoing basis throughout therapy. Monitoring should include documentation of pain intensity and level of functioning, assessment of progress toward therapeutic goals, presence of adverse effects, and adherence to prescribed therapies. Common opioid-related adverse effects (e.g., constipation, nausea and vomiting, cognitive and psychomotor impairment) should be anticipated and appropriately managed.

If opioids are continued for chronic or subacute pain, clinicians should use caution when prescribing opioids at any dosage and should generally avoid dosage increases when possible. Many patients do not experience benefit in pain or function from increasing opioid dosages to ≥50 morphine mg equivalent/day but are exposed to progressive increases in risk as dosage increases.

Patients should be closely monitored for adverse effects and other risks of therapy, including opioid use disorder. Various strategies for managing risks associated with opioid therapy for chronic noncancer pain have been recommended, including written treatment agreements or plans (e.g., "contracts"), urine drug testing, review of state prescription drug monitoring program (PDMP) data, and risk assessment and monitoring tools. Clinicians should offer or arrange treatment for patients with opioid use disorder.

Acute Pain

Nonopioid therapies are at least as effective as opioids for many common types of acute pain (e.g., low back pain, neck pain, pain related to other musculoskeletal injuries). Use of nonpharmacologic therapies (e.g., ice, heat, elevation, rest, immobilization, exercise) and nonopioid pharmacologic therapies (e.g., topical or oral NSAIAs, acetaminophen) should be maximized as appropriate for the specific condition and patient. In the symptomatic treatment of acute pain, opioid analgesics have an important role in the management of pain resulting from traumatic injuries, invasive surgeries, or other severe acute pain when nonopioid alternatives are expected to be ineffective or are contraindicated. However, opioid therapy should be considered for acute pain only if the benefits are anticipated to outweigh the risks. If opioid therapy is warranted, immediate-release preparations are recommended at the lowest effective dosage. The prescribed quantity should be limited to the amount needed for the expected duration of pain severe enough to require opioid analgesia. For the treatment of acute pain, opioids should be prescribed only as needed rather than on a scheduled basis. Because short-term opioid use can lead to unintended long-term use, clinicians should work with patients to develop a plan for discontinuation as soon as feasible.

When opioid analgesics are used for the management of postoperative pain, opioid therapy should be provided as part of a multimodal regimen that also includes acetaminophen and/or NSAIAs and other pharmacologic and nonpharmacologic therapy as appropriate. Because of the availability of effective nonopioid analgesics and nonpharmacologic therapies for postoperative pain, it is suggested that clinicians routinely incorporate these therapies into pain management regimens. Systemic opioids may not be required in all patients. If opioid therapy is required, oral administration of a short-acting opioid generally is preferred over IV administration in patients who can tolerate oral therapy. Scheduled (around-the-clock) dosing of opioid analgesics frequently is required during the immediate postoperative period or following major surgery. When parenteral administration is required, some experts recommend that IV patient-controlled analgesia (PCA) be used for postoperative systemic analgesia. Routine use of basal IV infusions of opioids in opioid-naïve patients receiving PCA is not recommended. IM administration of analgesics for the management of postoperative pain is discouraged because IM injections can cause pain and are associated with unreliable absorption, which may result in inconsistent analgesia.

Cancer Pain

The American Society of Clinical Oncology (ASCO) states that opioids should be offered to patients with moderate-to-severe pain associated with cancer or active cancer treatment, unless contraindicated. In a recent review of 17 studies of patients receiving oral morphine for cancer pain, 96% of morphine-treated patients (362 of 377) achieved an outcome of no worse than mild pain. Prior to initiating opioid therapy, it is useful to assess the mechanism for the pain syndrome (imaging may be required), the response to nonopioid analgesics (e.g., acetaminophen or NSAIAs), and the presence of risk factors such as a history of misuse of alcohol, recreational substances, or prescription drugs. Opioids should be initiated as an immediate-release formulation and as needed to establish an effective dosage. The lowest possible dosage should be used to achieve acceptable analgesia and patient goals, and patients should be assessed early with frequent dosage titration. In patients receiving opioids around the clock, an immediate-release opioid at a dose of 5–20% of the regular morphine equivalent daily dose should be prescribed for breakthrough pain. When opioids are no longer indicated, they should be weaned or tapered.

Sickle Cell Pain

Pain associated with sickle cell disease can manifest as both acute intermittent pain, chronic daily pain, and acute-on-chronic pain. Management of acute and chronic pain must be individualized and include multimodal treatment approaches. Opioids may potentially be used as part of the treatment regimen to manage acute pain in adults and children with sickle cell disease; selection of an appropriate dosage should consider baseline opioid therapy and prior effective therapy, and the lowest effective dosage should be prescribed. For adults and children with emerging and/or recently developed chronic pain related to sickle cell disease, experts suggest against the initiation of chronic opioid therapy unless pain is refractory to multiple other treatments. Clinicians should be aware that patients may inadvertently be treated with opioids chronically if episodic pain is frequent. Efforts should be made to reduce or eliminate scheduled opioid doses between acute episodic pain events to reduce the likelihood of unintentional chronic opioid therapy.

Palliative Care

Palliative care is defined as care that provides relief from pain and other symptoms, supports quality of life, and is focused on patients with serious advanced illness and their families. Palliative care may begin early in the course of treatment for a serious illness and may be delivered in a number of ways across the continuum of health care settings, including in the home, nursing homes, long-term acute care facilities, acute care hospitals, and outpatient clinics.

Palliative care guidelines address the use of opioids for pain management in this setting. The ongoing care of patients being treated with opioids for physical symptoms, such as pain and dyspnea, includes documentation of treatment goals,

ongoing risk assessments for opioid misuse, and frequency of re-assessments. The interdisciplinary care team should regularly conduct pain assessments and evaluate the effectiveness of treatments after initiation and upon any changes to the therapeutic regimen. The guidelines also recommend that palliative care clinicians receive training on safe and appropriate use of opioids and how to assess risk for opioid use disorder, monitor for signs of opioid abuse and diversion, and manage pain in patients at risk for substance abuse.

● Acute Coronary Syndrome

Morphine is used to relieve pain and anxiety associated with acute coronary syndrome (ACS). Because of its ability to alleviate the work of breathing, reduce anxiety, and favorably affect ventricular loading conditions, morphine is considered the analgesic agent of choice in patients with ST-segment-elevation myocardial infarction (STEMI). In addition to its potent analgesic and anxiolytic effects, morphine also exhibits favorable hemodynamic effects by causing venodilation and modest reductions in heart rate and systolic blood pressure.

These properties also may be beneficial in patients with non-ST-segment-elevation ACS (NSTE ACS; unstable angina or non-ST-segment-elevation myocardial infarction [NSTEMI]); although randomized controlled studies specifically evaluating the use of morphine in patients with NSTE ACS have not been conducted, experts state that it may be reasonable to administer IV morphine in such patients who have continued pain despite treatment with maximally tolerated anti-ischemic drugs (e.g., nitrates). However, use of morphine should not preclude the use of other anti-ischemic drugs with proven benefit.

● Neonatal Opioid Withdrawal

Morphine has been used to manage manifestations of opioid abstinence syndrome (i.e., postnatal withdrawal) in neonates† exposed to opioids in utero. Opioids are recommended as first-line pharmacologic therapy when environmental and supportive measures (e.g., minimization of external stimuli, maximization of mother-infant contact [e.g., parental "rooming in"], breast-feeding when not contraindicated, swaddling and gentle handling) are inadequate. Other adjunctive therapy (e.g., clonidine, phenobarbital) may be added if the response to opioids is inadequate; currently, clonidine is recommended over phenobarbital until further study of long-term effects of phenobarbital are known. Approximately 60–80% of neonates with opioid abstinence syndrome may require pharmacologic treatment for withdrawal symptoms. While morphine has been used more extensively than other opioids in the management of neonatal opioid abstinence syndrome, some studies suggest that use of methadone or buprenorphine (an opioid partial agonist) may be associated with shorter treatment durations and hospital stays compared with morphine use, but caution is advised if the preparation has a high alcohol content. Additional study is needed to establish optimal dosage schedules and preferred opioid drugs and to evaluate longer-term (e.g., neurodevelopmental) outcomes. Conflicting findings to date may be related in part to differences in study design, nonpharmacologic care, concomitant in utero drug exposures, the stringency of institutional protocols for care, and optimization of dosage schedules.

Use of standardized protocols for identification, evaluation, and treatment of neonatal opioid withdrawal syndrome is recommended since use of such protocols has been shown to improve overall response, including shorter hospital stays and durations of pharmacologic treatment. Some evidence suggests that use of a standardized protocol may be more important than use of a specific opioid agonist (e.g., morphine versus methadone) in improving outcomes. Protocols generally utilize assessment tools that were developed to quantify severity of withdrawal in term neonates (e.g., Finnegan or modified Finnegan scoring tools) to facilitate decisions regarding initiation, titration, and tapering of therapy.

DOSAGE AND ADMINISTRATION

● General

Pretreatment Screening

● Prior to initiation, carefully evaluate risks and benefits of opioid therapy, and assess for opioid-related harms (e.g., addiction, abuse, misuse). Incorporate risk mitigation strategies into the treatment plan, including offering naloxone. Consider a discontinuation plan in case treatment needs to be withdrawn if benefits do not outweigh risks.

- Review the patient's history of controlled substance prescriptions using state prescription drug monitoring program (PDMP) data to determine whether the patient is receiving opioid dosages or combinations that put the patient at high risk for overdose.

- Screen patients for sleep-related breathing disorders including central sleep apnea and sleep-related hypoxemia.

Patient Monitoring

- When opioids are used for subacute or chronic pain, evaluate the benefits and risks within 1–4 weeks following initiation of therapy or an increase in dosage, and re-evaluate on an ongoing basis.

- Monitor patients closely for signs of sedation and respiratory depression, particularly when initiating therapy and following dosage increases.

- Monitor and manage common adverse effects of opioid therapy (e.g., constipation, nausea and vomiting, cognitive and psychomotor impairment).

Dispensing and Administration Precautions

- Based on the Institute for Safe Medication Practices (ISMP), morphine is a high-alert medication that has a heightened risk of causing significant patient harm when used in error.

Handling and Disposal

- Advise patients to store opioids in a secure and preferably locked location and discuss options for safe disposal of unused opioids.

Administration Precautions for Oral Solution

- Ensure accuracy when prescribing, dispensing, and administering morphine sulfate oral solution to avoid dosing errors due to confusion between mg and mL, and with other morphine sulfate oral solutions of different concentrations, which could result in accidental overdose and death. Ensure the proper dose is communicated and dispensed. When writing prescriptions, include both the total dose in mg and the total dose in volume.

- Instruct patients and caregivers on how to accurately measure and administer the correct dose of morphine sulfate oral solution.

- Strongly advise patients and caregivers to always use a graduated oral syringe when administering morphine sulfate oral solution to ensure the dose is measured and administered accurately.

Administration Precautions for Parenteral Preparations

- Dosing errors can result in accidental overdose and death. Avoid dosing errors that may result from confusion between mg and mL and with morphine injections of different concentrations when prescribing, dispensing, and administering morphine sulfate injection. Ensure that the dose is communicated and dispensed accurately.

- Use parenteral preparations only for the intended, labeled route of administration (e.g., IV injection, continuous infusion, epidural, intrathecal) and with the appropriate infusion device (e.g., microinfusion, patient-controlled analgesia [PCA]).

- Epidural or intrathecal morphine should be administered by or under the direction of a physician experienced in the techniques of epidural or intrathecal administration.

- Because of the risk of severe adverse reactions when preservative-free morphine sulfate injection is administered by the epidural or intrathecal route, patients must be observed in a fully equipped and staffed environment for at least 24 hours after the initial dose.

REMS

- FDA approved a REMS for morphine under a shared REMS system (Opioid Analgesic REMS).

- The goals are to reduce the occurrence of addiction, unintentional overdosage, and death resulting from inappropriate prescribing, misuse, and abuse of opioid analgesics.

- The REMS program consists of educational programs for health professionals, a patient counseling guide, and a product-specific medication guide for patients.

● Administration

Morphine sulfate is administered by the oral, rectal, IV, IM, intrathecal, or epidural routes.

Parenteral Administration

Morphine sulfate is administered by IM or slow IV injection, or by IV infusion. The preservative-free injections may also be administered epidurally or intrathecally via intermittent injection or continuous infusion. Morphine sulfate also has been administered subcutaneously†.

Morphine sulfate 2, 4, 5, 8, and 10 mg/mL injections are available in single-dose prefilled syringes for direct IV or IM injection. IV injections should be administered slowly; rapid IV administration may result in chest wall rigidity.

Morphine sulfate 50 mg/mL injection is for continuous IV infusion only and should not be injected directly. The commercially available injection should be diluted in 5% dextrose or 0.9% sodium chloride injection to a concentration of 0.1–5 mg/mL. The rate of continuous IV infusion of the drug must be individualized according to response and patient tolerance.

Morphine sulfate 0.5 and 1 mg/mL preservative-free injections may be administered IV, epidurally, or intrathecally. The Duramorph® preparation is not for use in continuous microinfusion devices.

Morphine sulfate 10 and 25 mg/mL preservative-free injections are intended for use only with a continuous microinfusion device for intrathecal or epidural infusion.

Highly concentrated preservative-free morphine sulfate injections intended for continuous epidural or intrathecal infusion via a controlled-microinfusion device (e.g., Infumorph® 10 or 25 mg/mL) are not recommended for IV, IM, or subcutaneous administration of individual doses of the drug because of the large amount of morphine sulfate contained in each ampul (200 mg/20 mL, 500 mg/20 mL) and the attendant risk of substantial overdosage.

Morphine sulfate 1 mg/mL preservative-free injection is intended for use only with a compatible infusion device for PCA.

When morphine sulfate is administered IM, IV, epidurally, or intrathecally, an opioid antagonist and facilities for administration of oxygen and control of respiration should be available. Because single-dose neuraxial administration may result in acute or delayed respiratory depression, such administration should occur in a setting where adequate monitoring is possible and patients should be observed for at least 24 hours after the initial dose. When morphine is administered via continuous, controlled microinfusion, such precautions should be continued for at least 24 hours after administration of each test dose and for several days after surgical implantation of the catheter as appropriate for additional monitoring and dosage adjustment. An opioid antagonist and resuscitative equipment also should be immediately available whenever the reservoir of the microinfusion device is refilled with morphine sulfate or is otherwise being manipulated. Facilities, drugs, and equipment necessary for the management of inadvertent intravascular injection during attempted epidural or intrathecal injection should also be readily available.

Parenteral solutions of morphine sulfate injection should be inspected visually prior to administration whenever container and solution permit. Unopened solutions should be discarded if they contain a precipitate that does not disappear with shaking. In addition, solutions that are not colorless or pale yellow (outside any amber container) should be discarded.

Morphine sulfate injections are subject to substantial risk of overdosage if used inappropriately and to diversion and abuse; therefore, special control measures should be implemented within the institution, including restricted access, rigid accounting, and rigorous control of waste disposal.

Store morphine sulfate injection solutions at 20-25°C; protect from light and do not freeze.

Store preservative-free morphine sulfate injection solutions at 20-25°C, with excursions permitted from 15-30°C; do not freeze.

Epidural and Intrathecal Administration

Specialized techniques are required for epidural or intrathecal administration of morphine sulfate; the drug should be administered via these routes only by qualified individuals familiar with the techniques of administration and patient management problems associated with these routes of administration. Epidural or intrathecal administration should be limited to the lumbar region since administration in the thoracic region has been associated with a substantially increased frequency of early and late respiratory depression, even at low doses. Because epidural administration of the drug has been associated with a lower potential for immediate and delayed adverse effects than intrathecal administration, the epidural rather than intrathecal route should be used whenever possible. For additional information on epidural administration, consult the prescribing information for individual morphine sulfate preparations.

Highly concentrated, preservative-free morphine sulfate injections intended for continuous epidural or intrathecal infusion via a controlled-microinfusion device (e.g., Infumorph® 10 or 25 mg/mL) should not be used for individual-dose epidural or intrathecal injection since less-concentrated, preservative-free injections can be employed more reliably for the small doses required.

Standardize 4 Safety

Standardized concentrations for morphine have been established through Standardize 4 Safety (S4S), a national patient safety initiative to reduce medication errors, especially during transitions of care. Multidisciplinary expert panels were convened to determine recommended standard concentrations. Because recommendations from the S4S panels may differ from the manufacturer's prescribing information, caution is advised when using concentrations that differ from labeling, particularly when using rate information from the label. For additional information on S4S (including updates that may be available), see http://www.ashp.org/pharmacy-practice/standardize-4-safety-initiative.

TABLE 1. Standardize 4 Safety Continuous IV Infusion Standards for Morphine

Patient Population	Concentration Standard	Dosing Units
Adults[a]	1 mg/mL	mg/hr
	5 mg/mL (based on high dose requirements)	
Pediatric patients (<50 kg)	0.2 mg/mL	mg/kg/hr
	0.5 mg/mL	
	1 mg/mL	

[a] The S4S panel recommends trying to standardize dosing units but understand some protocols may use "flat" dosing while others may require weight-based dosing.

TABLE 2. Standardize 4 Safety PCA Standard Concentrations for Morphine

Patient Population	Concentration Standard	Dosing Units
Adults	**1 mg/mL** (caution is advised if both hydromorphone and morphine are used to avoid confusion in selection as both have the same concentration)	mg
	5 mg/mL	
	10 mg/mL	
Pediatric patients (<50 kg)	0.25 mg/mL	mg/kg/hr
	1 mg/mL (caution is advised if both hydromorphone and morphine are used to avoid confusion in selection as both have the same concentration)	
	5 mg/mL	

TABLE 3. Standardize 4 Safety Epidural Single Drug Standard Concentrations for Morphine

Patient Population	Concentration Standard
Adults	0.5 mg/mL
	1 mg/mL
Pediatric patients (<50 kg)	0.5 mg/mL
	1 mg/mL

TABLE 4. Standardize 4 Safety ADULT Epidural Combination Drug Standard Concentrations for Morphine

Drug Combinations	Anesthetic Concentration	Narcotic Concentration
Bupivacaine with morphine	1. Bupivacaine 0.0625%	1. Morphine 0.5 mg/mL
	2. Bupivacaine 0.125%	2. Morphine 1 mg/mL
Ropivacaine with morphine	1. Ropivacaine 0.1%	1. Morphine 0.5 mg/mL
	2. Ropivacaine 0.2%	2. Morphine 1 mg/mL

TABLE 5. Standardize 4 Safety PEDIATRIC Epidural Combination Drug Standard Concentrations for Morphine

Drug Combinations	Anesthetic Concentration	Narcotic Concentration
Bupivacaine with morphine	1. Bupivacaine 0.0625%	1. Morphine 0.5 mg/mL
	2. Bupivacaine 0.125%	2. Morphine 0.5 mg/mL
Ropivacaine with hydromorphone	1. Ropivacaine 0.1%	1. Morphine 0.5 mg/mL

Oral Administration

Morphine sulfate is administered orally as a solution, immediate-release tablets, or extended-release preparations.

Store immediate-release tablets and oral solution at 20-25°C. Store extended-release tablets and extended-release capsules at 25°C with excursions permitted between 15-30°C.

Extended-release Preparations

Extended-release morphine sulfate tablets should be swallowed intact and should not be broken, crushed, or chewed; intake of a broken, crushed, or chewed tablet may result in too rapid a release of the drug from the preparation and absorption of a potentially toxic dose of morphine.

Morphine sulfate extended-release capsules may be swallowed whole or the entire contents of the capsules may be sprinkled on a small amount of applesauce, at room temperature or cooler, immediately prior to administration. The patient should swallow the entire mixture. The pellets should not be crushed, chewed, or dissolved; intake of crushed, chewed, or dissolved beads or pellets may result in too rapid a release of the drug from the preparation and absorption of a potentially fatal dose of morphine sulfate. Following administration, the patient should drink a glass of water to rinse the mouth and ensure that the pellets are swallowed. The mixture of applesauce and pellets should not be stored for future use. The contents of the extended-release capsules should not be administered through a nasogastric or gastric tube.

Oral Solution

Morphine sulfate oral solution is commercially available in various concentrations (2 mg/mL, 4 mg/mL, and 20 mg/mL). Serious adverse events and deaths have occurred as a result of inadvertent overdosage of concentrated morphine oral solutions. In most of these cases, the oral solutions prescribed in mg were mistakenly interchanged for mL of the concentrated preparation, resulting in 20-fold overdoses.

The 20 mg/mL concentration is indicated for use only in patients who are opioid tolerant (i.e., individuals who have been receiving ≥60 mg of oral morphine sulfate daily, ≥30 mg of oral oxycodone daily, ≥8 mg of hydromorphone hydrochloride daily, or an equianalgesic dosage of another opioid daily for ≥1 week) and have been titrated to a stable analgesic dosage using a preparation containing a lower concentration of morphine sulfate. A graduated oral syringe is supplied by the manufacturer with the 20 mg/mL oral solution; always use this oral syringe to ensure that the dose is measured and administered accurately.

To avoid medication errors, prescriptions for morphine sulfate oral solution should clearly specify the concentration of oral solution to be dispensed and, in the directions for use, indicate the intended dose of morphine in mg along with the corresponding volume in mL (in parentheses). It is important that the prescription be filled with the proper concentration of morphine sulfate oral solution to prevent potential medication errors.

Provide careful instructions to patients receiving morphine oral solutions.

Rectal Administration

Morphine sulfate is also administered rectally as suppositories. Administer carefully according to manufacturer's instructions.

Store rectal suppositories at 20-25°C.

Extemporaneously Compounded Oral Solution

An extemporaneously compounded oral solution of morphine containing 0.4 mg/mL has been prepared.

Standardize 4 Safety

Standardized concentrations for an extemporaneously prepared oral liquid formulation of morphine have been established through Standardize 4 Safety (S4S), a national patient safety initiative to reduce medication errors, especially during transitions of care. Multidisciplinary expert panels were convened to determine recommended standard concentrations. Because recommendations from the S4S panels may differ from the manufacturer's prescribing information, caution is advised when using concentrations that differ from labeling, particularly when using rate information from the label. For additional information on S4S (including updates that may be available), see https://www.ashp.org/pharmacy-practice/standardize-4-safety-initiative.

TABLE 6. Standardize 4 Safety Compounded Oral Liquid Standards for Morphine

Concentration Standards
400 mcg/mL

● Dosage

Morphine Sulfate Conversions
Common Conversions

Common opioid medications and their doses in morphine mg equivalents (MME) are provided in Table 7. These conversions are intended as a guide to help inform clinician-patient decision-making; dosage should be individualized based on the patient and clinical setting.

TABLE 7. Morphine Mg Equivalent Doses for Commonly Prescribed Opioids for Pain Management

Opioid Agonist	Conversion Factor[a]
Codeine	0.15
Fentanyl transdermal (in mcg/hr)	2.4
Hydrocodone	1
Hydromorphone	5
Methadone	4.7
Morphine	1
Oxycodone	1.5
Oxymorphone	3
Tapentadol[b]	0.4
Tramadol[c]	0.2

[a] Multiply the dose for each opioid by the conversion factor to determine the dose in MMEs. For example, tablets containing hydrocodone 5 mg and acetaminophen 325 mg taken 4 times a day would contain a total of 20 mg of hydrocodone daily, equivalent to 20 MME daily; extended-release tablets containing oxycodone 10 mg and taken twice a day would contain a total of 20 mg of oxycodone daily, equivalent to 30 MME daily. The following cautions should be noted: 1) All doses are in mg/day except for fentanyl, which is mcg/hr. 2) Equianalgesic dose conversions are only estimates and cannot account for individual variability in genetics and pharmacokinetics. 3) Do not use the calculated dose in MMEs to determine the doses to use when converting one opioid to another; when converting opioids, the new opioid is typically dosed at a substantially lower dose than the calculated MME dose to avoid overdose because of incomplete cross-tolerance and individual variability in opioid pharmacokinetics. 4) Use caution with methadone dose conversions because methadone has a long and variable half-life, and peak respiratory depressant effect occurs later and lasts longer than peak analgesic effect. 5) Use caution with transdermal fentanyl because it is dosed in mcg/hr instead of mg/day, and its absorption is affected by heat and other factors. 6) Buprenorphine products approved for the treatment of pain are not included in the table because of their partial μ-receptor agonist activity and resultant ceiling effects compared with full μ-receptor agonists. 7) These conversion factors should not be applied to dosage decisions related to the management of opioid use disorder.

[b] Tapentadol is a μ-receptor agonist and norepinephrine reuptake inhibitor. MMEs are based on degree of μ-receptor agonist activity; however, it is unknown whether tapentadol is associated with overdose in the same dose-dependent manner as observed with medications that are solely μ-receptor agonists.

[c] Tramadol is a μ-receptor agonist and norepinephrine and serotonin reuptake inhibitor. MMEs are based on degree of μ-receptor agonist activity; however, it is unknown whether tramadol is associated with overdose in the same dose-dependent manner as observed with medications that are solely μ-receptor agonists.

Conversion from Other Opioids to Morphine Sulfate Immediate-release Products

There is inter-patient variability in the potency of opioid drugs and opioid formulations. Therefore, a conservative approach is advised when determining the total daily dosage of morphine sulfate immediate-release tablets and oral solution. It is safer to underestimate a patient's 24-hour tablet or oral solution dosage than to overestimate the 24-hour dosage and manage an adverse reaction due to overdose.

Conversion from Morphine Sulfate Immediate-release Preparations to Extended-Release Morphine

For a given dose, the same total amount of morphine sulfate is available from morphine sulfate immediate-release tablets and extended-release morphine formulations. The extended duration of release of morphine sulfate from extended-release formulations results in reduced maximum and increased minimum plasma morphine concentrations than with shorter acting morphine sulfate products. Conversion from morphine sulfate tablets to the same total daily dose of an extended-release formulation could lead to excessive sedation at peak serum levels.

Conversion from Other Oral Morphine Preparations to Morphine Sulfate Extended-release Tablets

Patients receiving other oral morphine preparations may be converted to morphine sulfate extended-release tablets by administering one-half of the patient's 24-hour requirement as morphine sulfate extended-release tablets on an every 12-hour schedule or by administering one-third of the patient's daily requirement as morphine sulfate extended-release tablets on an every-8-hour schedule.

Conversion from Other Oral Morphine Preparations to Morphine Sulfate Extended-Release Capsules

Patients receiving other oral morphine formulations may be converted to morphine sulfate extended-release capsules by administering the patient's total daily oral morphine dose as morphine sulfate extended-release capsules once-daily. Monitor patients closely when initiating morphine sulfate extended-release capsule therapy and adjust the dosage as needed. Morphine sulfate extended-release capsules should not be given more frequently than every 24 hours.

Conversion from Parenteral Morphine to Oral Morphine Sulfate Preparations

For conversion from parenteral morphine to oral morphine sulfate preparations, anywhere from 3 to 6 mg of oral morphine sulfate may be required to provide pain relief equivalent to 1 mg of parenteral morphine.

Discontinuation of Morphine

Do not abruptly discontinue morphine in patients who may be physically dependent on opioids. Rapid discontinuation of opioid analgesics in patients who are physically dependent on opioids has resulted in serious withdrawal symptoms, uncontrolled pain, and suicide. Rapid discontinuation has also been associated with attempts to find other sources of opioid analgesics, which may be confused with drug-seeking for abuse. Patients may also attempt to treat their pain or withdrawal symptoms with illicit opioids, such as heroin, and other substances.

Common withdrawal symptoms include restlessness, lacrimation, rhinorrhea, yawning, perspiration, chills, myalgia, and mydriasis. Other signs and symptoms may develop, including irritability, anxiety, backache, joint pain, weakness, abdominal cramps, insomnia, nausea, anorexia, vomiting, diarrhea, or increased blood pressure, respiratory rate, or heart rate. If withdrawal symptoms arise, it may be necessary to pause the taper for a period of time or raise the dose of the opioid analgesic to the previous dose, and then proceed with a slower taper. In addition, evaluate patients for any changes in mood, emergence of suicidal thoughts, or use of other substances.

When managing patients taking opioid analgesics, particularly those who have been treated for an extended period, and/or with high doses for chronic pain, ensure that a multimodal approach to pain management, including mental health support (if needed), is in place prior to initiating an opioid analgesic taper. A multimodal approach to pain management may optimize the treatment of chronic pain, as well as assist with the successful tapering of the opioid analgesic.

Oral Morphine Sulfate Preparations

When a decision has been made to decrease the dose or discontinue therapy in an opioid-dependent patient taking oral morphine sulfate preparations, there are a variety of factors that should be considered, including the total daily dose of opioids the patient has been taking, the duration of treatment, the type of pain being treated, and the physical and psychological attributes of the patient. It is important to ensure ongoing care of the patient and to agree on an appropriate tapering schedule and follow-up plan so that patient and clinician goals and expectations are clear and realistic. When opioid analgesics are being discontinued due to a suspected substance use disorder, evaluate and treat the patient, or refer for evaluation and treatment of the substance use disorder. Treatment should include evidence-based approaches, such as medication-assisted treatment. Complex patients with co-morbid pain and substance use disorders may benefit from referral to a specialist.

There is no standard opioid tapering schedule that is suitable for all patients. Experts recommend a patient-specific plan to taper the dose of the opioid gradually. For patients taking morphine sulfate who are physically opioid-dependent, initiate the taper by a small enough increment (e.g., no greater than 10% to 25% of the total daily dose) to avoid withdrawal symptoms, and proceed with

dose-lowering at an interval of every 2 to 4 weeks. Patients who have been taking opioids for briefer periods of time may tolerate a more rapid taper.

It may be necessary to provide the patient with a lower dosage preparation strength to accomplish a successful taper. Reassess the patient frequently to manage pain and withdrawal symptoms, should they emerge.

Rectal Morphine

When a patient who has been taking morphine sulfate suppositories regularly and may be physically dependent no longer requires therapy with the suppositories, taper the dose gradually, by 25% to 50% every 2 to 4 days, while monitoring carefully for signs and symptoms of withdrawal. If the patient develops signs or symptoms of withdrawal, increase the dose to the previous level and taper more slowly, either by increasing the interval between decreases, decreasing the amount of change in dose, or both.

Parenteral Morphine

For patients receiving parenteral morphine sulfate regularly and may be physically dependent or no longer requires therapy, taper the dose gradually, by 25% to 50% every 2 to 4 days, while monitoring carefully for signs and symptoms of withdrawal. If the patient develops these signs or symptoms, raise the dose to the previous level and taper more slowly, either by increasing the interval between decreases, decreasing the amount of change in dose, or both.

Dosage for Pain

Morphine sulfate should be given at the lowest effective dosage and for the shortest duration of therapy consistent with the treatment goals of the patient.

Titrate the dose based on the individual patient's response to their initial dose of morphine sulfate to a dose that provides adequate analgesia and minimizes adverse reactions. Continually re-evaluate patients to assess the maintenance of pain control, signs and symptoms of opioid withdrawal, and other adverse reactions as well as to reassess for the development of addiction, abuse, or misuse.

If the level of pain increases after dosage stabilization, attempt to identify the source of increased pain before increasing the dosage. If after increasing the dosage, unacceptable opioid-related adverse reactions are observed (including an increase in pain after dosage increase), consider reducing the dosage. Adjust the dosage to obtain an appropriate balance between management of pain and opioid-related adverse reactions.

Oral Dosage

Immediate-release tablets in adults: The recommended initial adult dosage of morphine sulfate immediate-release tablets is 15–30 mg orally every 4 hours as needed for pain; the lowest effective dosage should be used.

Immediate-release tablets in pediatric patients: The recommended initial dosage of morphine sulfate immediate-release tablets in pediatric patients weighing at least 50 kg is 15 mg every 4 hours as needed for pain; the lowest effective dosage should be used. Morphine sulfate immediate-release tablets are not recommended for pediatric patients weighing less than 50 kg.

Oral solution in adults: The recommended initial adult dosage of morphine sulfate oral solution is 10–20 mg every 4 hours as needed for pain; the lowest effective dosage should be used. Titrate the dose based upon the individual patient's response to their initial dose of morphine sulfate oral solution.

Oral solution in pediatric patients: The recommended initial dosage in pediatric patients 2 years of age and older is 0.15-0.3 mg/kg every 4 hours as needed for pain; the lowest effective dosage should be used.

Extended-release capsules: The recommended initial dose of morphine sulfate extended-release capsules in adult opioid-naïve patients or in those who are not opioid tolerant is 30 mg orally every 24 hours. Adjust the dosage in increments no greater than 30 mg every 3 to 4 days. Patients who experience breakthrough pain may require a dosage increase or may need rescue medication with an appropriate dose of an immediate-release analgesic. If the level of pain increases after dosage stabilization, attempt to identify the source of increased pain before increasing the dosage of morphine sulfate. Because steady-state plasma concentrations are approximated within 2 to 3 days, dosage may be adjusted every 3 to 4 days. The daily dosage of morphine sulfate extended-release capsules must be limited to a maximum of 1600 mg/day; higher amounts contain a quantity of fumaric acid that has not been demonstrated to be safe, and which may result in serious renal toxicity.

Extended-release tablets: The recommended initial dose of morphine sulfate extended-release tablets in adult opioid-naïve patients is 15 mg every 8 or 12 hours. The recommended initial dose of morphine sulfate extended-release tablets in adult opioid non-tolerant patients is 15 mg every 12 hours. Patients who experience breakthrough pain may require a dosage increase of morphine sulfate extended-release tablets, or may need rescue medication with an appropriate dose of an immediate-release analgesic. If the level of pain increases after dosage stabilization, attempt to identify the source of increased pain before increasing the morphine dosage. Because steady-state plasma concentrations are approximated in 1 day, morphine sulfate extended-release tablets dosage adjustments may be adjusted every 1 to 2 days.

Rectal Dosage

The recommended initial adult dosage of morphine sulfate rectal suppositories is 10–20 mg every 4 hours as needed for pain and at the lowest dose necessary to achieve analgesia.

IV Injection Dosage

The usual starting dosage of morphine sulfate injection in adults is 0.1–0.2 mg/kg every 4 hours as needed by slow IV injection.

An initial adult IV dosage range of 2 –10 mg based on a patient's weight of 70 kg has been recommended by some manufacturers.

Continous IV Infusion

The recommended initial dosage of morphine sulfate injection administered by continuous IV infusion in adults is 0.02 to 0.1 mg/kg per hour as needed. The dosage should be titrated according to the patient's response. For opioid-naïve patients, a maximum dosing rate of 10 mg/hour should not be exceeded. For opioid-tolerant patients, including patients who, because of their condition, have a high analgesic requirement (e.g., terminal cancer pain), dosing rates as high as 30 mg/hour or higher may be required to manage pain.

The recommended initial dosage of morphine sulfate injection administered by continuous IV infusion in pediatric patients ≥1 year of age weighing at least 50 kg is 1,500 mcg/hour (1.5 mg/hour). The recommended initial dosage in pediatric patients ≥1 year of age weighing less than 50 kg is 20 to 30 mcg/kg per hour (0.02 to 0.03 mg/kg per hour). The recommended initial dosage in pediatric patients less than 1 year of age, including neonates, is 0.005 to 0.01 mg/kg per hour. The dosage should be titrated according to the patient's response. For opioid-tolerant patients, including patients with a high analgesic requirement (e.g., terminal cancer pain, sickle-cell disease crisis), higher initial doses may be required. The recommended maintenance dosage in pediatric patients ≥1 year of age weighing less than 60 kg is 10 to 60 mcg/kg per hour (0.01 to 0.06 mg/kg per hour). For pediatric patients ≥1 year of age weighing at least 60 kg, the recommended maintenance dosage is 0.8 to 3 mg/hour.

PCA

When morphine sulfate is administered by multiple, slow IV injections for patient-controlled analgesia (PCA), dosage is adjusted according to the severity of the pain and response of the patient; the operator's manual for the patient-controlled infusion device should be consulted for directions on administering the drug at the desired rate of infusion. For adults, the usual dose of PCA with morphine sulfate is a 1 mg bolus, with a range of 0.2 to 3 mg for each incremental dose. The recommended time between doses is 6 minutes (lockout period). Patients with a high degree of opioid tolerance may require a larger bolus size to be comfortable without excessively frequent triggering of the device. In such patients, a bolus dose of 2-3 mg is usually adequate, although up to a 5 mg bolus has been used in opioid-tolerant patients in some studies. For opioid-naïve patients, the combination of dosing rate and lockout should not permit a maximal dosing rate greater than 10 mg/hour (1 mg possible every 6 minutes), while for opioid-tolerant patients maximal dosing rates up to 30 mg/hour are common (3 mg every 6 minutes) and greater rates may be needed in selected patients.

IM Dosage

The initial IM dose of morphine sulfate is 10 mg every 4 hours as needed to manage pain (based on a 70 kg adult).

Epidural Dosage

When the 0.5 mg/mL or 1 mg/mL morphine sulfate injection is administered epidurally, the recommended initial injection of 5 mg in the lumbar region may provide satisfactory pain relief for up to 24 hours. If adequate pain relief is not achieved within 1 hour, carefully administer incremental doses of 1 to 2 mg at intervals sufficient to assess effectiveness. Do not administer more than 10 mg per 24 hours.

When the 10 mg/mL or 25 mg/mL morphine sulfate injection is administered as a continuous epidural infusion, the recommended initial dosage in adults who are not tolerant to opioids is 3.5–7.5 mg/day. Based on limited experience, the usual initial epidural dosage for continuous infusion in adults with some degree of opioid tolerance is 4.5–10 mg/day. Epidural dosage requirements may increase substantially during chronic therapy, frequently to 20–30 mg daily; the upper daily limit must be individualized for each patient.

Intrathecal Dosage

When the 0.5 mg/mL or 1 mg/mL morphine sulfate injection is administered intrathecally, the recommended initial injection of 0.2–1 mg may provide satisfactory pain relief for up to 24 hours. For the morphine sulfate injection (Duramorph®) preparation, this is only 0.4 to 2 mL of the 5 mg/10 mL ampul or 0.2 to 1 mL of the 10 mg/10 mL ampul. Do not inject more than 2 mL of the 5 mg/10 mL ampul or 1 mL of the 10 mg/10 mL ampul intrathecally. Repeated intrathecal injections are not recommended. If pain recurs, consider alternative routes of administration. A constant IV infusion of naloxone 0.6 mg/hr for 24 hours after intrathecal injection may be used to reduce the incidence of potential side effects.

When the 10 mg/mL or 25 mg/mL morphine sulfate injection is administered as a continuous intrathecal infusion, the recommended initial lumbar intrathecal dose range in adult patients with no tolerance to opioids is 0.2 to 1 mg/day. The published range of doses for individuals who have some degree of opioid tolerance varies from 1 to 10 mg/day. The upper daily dosage limit for each patient must be individualized.

Dosage for Acute Coronary Syndrome (ACS)

To relieve pain in adults with ST-segment-elevation myocardial infarction (STEMI), an initial morphine sulfate dose of 2–4 mg IV is recommended; additional doses of 2–8 mg may be administered every 5–15 minutes as needed. In patients with non-ST-segment-elevation acute coronary syndromes (NSTE ACS) who continue to experience pain despite maximally tolerated anti-ischemic therapy, experts state that a morphine sulfate dose of 1–5 mg IV may be administered during IV nitroglycerin therapy; additional doses may be given every 5–30 minutes to relieve symptoms and maintain patient comfort.

Dosage for Neonatal Opioid Withdrawal

For the management of neonatal opiate abstinence syndrome†, use of protocols that base initiation, adjustment, and tapering of morphine sulfate dosage on standardized patient assessments performed at regular intervals is recommended. The most commonly used tool for assessing severity of withdrawal in term neonates is the Finnegan scoring system (original or modified versions) performed every 3–4 hours. Treatment protocols vary in recommended dosages, thresholds for initiation of therapy, incremental changes and thresholds for dosage adjustment, and tapering strategies.

Under various protocols, treatment with morphine sulfate oral solution is initiated at a dosage of 0.04–0.05 mg/kg every 3–4 hours based on Finnegan score (e.g., score exceeds 8 on at least 2 or 3 occasions, the sum of 3 consecutive scores is 24 or greater, a single score or 2 consecutive scores are 12 or greater); under other protocols, initial dosage may vary depending on the severity of withdrawal manifestations, with higher initial dosages recommended for neonates with higher Finnegan scores. Some clinicians state that initial dosage usually ranges from 0.03–0.1 mg/kg every 3–4 hours. If Finnegan score remains elevated (e.g., a single score or 2 consecutive scores are 12 or greater, 2 consecutive scores are 8 or greater, the sum of 3 scores is 24 or greater), dosage may be increased, generally by 0.02–0.05 mg/kg per dose or by 10–20% depending on the protocol and/or Finnegan score, to achieve stabilization. Some clinicians have recommended a usual maximum dosage of 1.2–1.3 mg/kg daily or 0.2 mg/kg per dose. Once patients are stable (generally, no score exceeds 8) for at least 48 hours, morphine sulfate dosage typically is tapered in decrements of approximately 0.02 mg/kg per dose or approximately 10% of the highest (stabilization) dose at intervals of approximately 24–48 hours. Protocols vary in terms of the dosage at which morphine sulfate can be discontinued. However, neonates should be monitored for at least 48 hours after the drug has been discontinued. Specialized protocols should be consulted for further information on morphine sulfate dosage and monitoring of Finnegan scores in neonates with opiate abstinence syndrome. Further study is needed to define optimal dosing strategies.

● Special Populations

Hepatic Impairment

Morphine pharmacokinetics have been reported to be significantly altered in patients with cirrhosis. Start these patients with a lower than usual dosage of morphine sulfate and titrate slowly while regularly evaluating for signs of respiratory depression, sedation, and hypotension.

Renal Impairment

Morphine pharmacokinetics are altered in patients with renal failure. Start these patients with a lower than usual dosage of morphine sulfate and titrate slowly while regularly evaluating for signs of respiratory depression, sedation, and hypotension.

Geriatric Patients

Elderly patients (65 years of age or older) may have increased sensitivity to morphine. In general, use caution when selecting a dose for an elderly patient, usually starting at the low end of the dosing range, reflecting the greater frequency of decreased hepatic, renal, or cardiac function and of concomitant disease or other drug therapy. Titrate the dosage of morphine sulfate slowly in geriatric patients and frequently reevaluate the patient for signs of central nervous system and respiratory depression.

The pharmacodynamic effects of neuraxial morphine in the elderly are more variable than in the younger population. Patients will vary widely in the effective initial dose, rate of development of tolerance and the frequency and magnitude of associated adverse effects as the dosage is increased. Initial doses should be based on careful clinical observation following "test doses", after making allowances for the effects of the patient's age and infirmity on his/her ability to clear the drug, particularly in patients receiving epidural morphine.

Pharmacogenomic Considerations

There are no therapeutic recommendations for dosing opioids, such as morphine, based on either *OPRM1* (the gene coding for the mu opioid receptor mu1) or COMT (the enzyme responsible for the methylconjugation of catecholamines) genotype. Genetic variability studies have not shown UDP-glucuronosyltransferase (UGT) metabolism to alter production of main metabolites or patient response to morphine.

CAUTIONS

● Contraindications

- Significant respiratory depression.
- Acute or severe bronchial asthma in an unmonitored setting or in the absence of resuscitative equipment.
- Concurrent use of monoamine oxidase inhibitors (MAOIs) or use of MAOIs within the last 14 days.
- Known or suspected GI obstruction, including paralytic ileus.
- Hypersensitivity to morphine (e.g., anaphylaxis).
- Neuraxial administration of morphine sulfate injection (Duramorph®) in patients with infection at the injection microinfusion site, concomitant anticoagulant therapy, uncontrolled bleeding diathesis, or the presence of any other concomitant therapy or medical condition which would render epidural or intrathecal administration especially hazardous.

● Warnings/Precautions

Warnings

Addiction, Abuse, and Misuse

As an opioid agonist, morphine sulfate exposes users to the risks of addiction, abuse, and misuse. A boxed warning regarding this risk has been included in the prescribing information for morphine. Although the risk of addiction in any individual is unknown, it can occur in patients appropriately prescribed morphine

sulfate. Addiction can occur at recommended dosages and if the drug is misused or abused. Because extended-release products deliver the drug over a prolonged period of time, there is a greater risk for overdose and death due to the larger amount of morphine present.

Assess each patient's risk for opioid addiction, abuse, or misuse prior to prescribing morphine sulfate and reassess all patients receiving the drug for the development of these behaviors or conditions. Risks are increased in patients with a personal or family history of substance abuse (including drug or alcohol abuse or addiction) or mental illness (e.g., major depression). The potential for these risks should not, however, prevent the proper management of pain in any given patient. Patients at increased risk may be prescribed opioid agonists such as morphine sulfate but use in such patients necessitates intensive counseling about the risks and proper use of the drug along with frequent reevaluation for signs of addiction, abuse, and misuse. Consider prescribing naloxone for the emergency treatment of opioid agonist overdose.

Abuse or misuse of extended-release products (e.g., MS-Contin®) by crushing, chewing, snorting, or injecting the dissolved product will result in the uncontrolled delivery of morphine and can result in overdose and death.

Opioid agonists are sought for nonmedical use and are subject to diversion from legitimate prescribed use; consider these risks when prescribing or dispensing morphine sulfate. Strategies to reduce these risks include prescribing the drug in the smallest appropriate quantity and advising the patient on careful storage of the drug during treatment and proper disposal of unused drug. Contact a state professional licensing board or state-controlled substances authority for information on how to prevent and detect abuse or diversion.

Life-threatening Respiratory Depression

Serious, life-threatening, or fatal respiratory depression has been reported with the use of opioid agonists, even when used as recommended. A boxed warning regarding this risk has been included in the prescribing information for morphine. Respiratory depression, if not immediately recognized and treated, may lead to respiratory arrest and death. Management of respiratory depression may include close observation, supportive measures, and use of opioid antagonists, depending on the patient's clinical status. Carbon dioxide (CO_2) retention from opioid-induced respiratory depression can exacerbate the sedating effects of opioids.

While serious, life-threatening, or fatal respiratory depression can occur at any time during the use of morphine, the risk is greatest during the initiation of therapy or following a dosage increase. Certain morphine sulfate preparations also have an increased risk of serious, life-threatening, or fatal respiratory depression.

Morphine sulfate oral solution 20 mg/mL is for use only in opioid-tolerant adult patients. Administration of this formulation may cause fatal respiratory depression when administered to patients who are not tolerant to the respiratory depressant effects of opioid agonists.

Rapid IV administration of morphine sulfate injection can cause a delay (30 minutes) in the maximum CNS effect and result in overdosing. The respiratory depression may be severe and could require intervention.

Neuraxial administration of morphine as a single dose may result in acute or delayed respiratory depression for periods at least as long as 24 hours. Intrathecal use has been associated with a higher incidence of respiratory depression than epidural use. Thoracic administration has been shown to dramatically increase the incidence of early and late respiratory depression even at doses of 1 to 2 mg. Because of the risk of severe adverse effects when the epidural or intrathecal route of administration is employed, patients must be observed in a fully equipped and staffed environment for at least 24 hours after the initial dose. The facility must be able to resuscitate patients with severe opioid overdosage, and the personnel must be familiar with the use and limitations of specific opioid antagonists (naloxone, naltrexone) in such cases.

Improper or erroneous substitution of concentrated morphine sulfate injection (Infumorph® 200 or 500 [10 or 25 mg/mL, respectively]) for conventional morphine injection (e.g., Duramorph® 0.5 or 1 mg/mL) is likely to result in serious overdosage, leading to seizures, respiratory depression, and death.

Monitor patients closely for respiratory depression, especially within the first 24–72 hours of initiating therapy and following dosage increases. To reduce the risk of respiratory depression, proper dosing and titration of morphine are essential.

Overestimating the dosage when converting patients from another opioid agonist product can result in a fatal overdose with the first dose.

Accidental ingestion of even one dose of morphine sulfate, especially by children, can result in respiratory depression and death due to an overdose of morphine. Educate patients and caregivers on how to recognize respiratory depression and emphasize the importance of calling 911 or seeking emergency medical assistance immediately in the event of a known or suspected overdose.

Opioid agonists can cause sleep-related breathing disorders including central sleep apnea and sleep-related hypoxemia. Opioid use increases the risk of central sleep apnea in a dose-dependent fashion. In patients who present with central sleep apnea, consider decreasing the opioid agonist dosage using best practices for opioid taper.

Patient Access to Naloxone for Emergency Treatment of Opioid Overdose

Discuss the availability of naloxone for the emergency treatment of opioid agonist overdose with the patient and caregiver and assess the potential need for access to naloxone, both when initiating and renewing treatment with morphine sulfate preparations. Inform patients and caregivers about the various ways to obtain naloxone as permitted by individual state naloxone dispensing and prescribing requirements or guidelines (e.g., by prescription, directly from a pharmacist, or as part of a community-based program). Educate patients and caregivers on how to recognize respiratory depression and emphasize the importance of calling 911 or seeking emergency medical help, even if naloxone is administered.

Consider prescribing naloxone, based on the patient's risk factors for overdose, such as concomitant use of CNS depressants, history of opioid use disorder, or prior opioid agonist overdose. The presence of risk factors for overdose should not prevent the proper management of pain in any given patient. Also consider prescribing naloxone if the patient has household members (including children) or other close contacts at risk for accidental ingestion or overdose. If naloxone is prescribed, educate patients and caregivers on use of the drug.

Risks from Concomitant Use with Benzodiazepines or Other CNS Depressants

Profound sedation, respiratory depression, coma, and death may result from concomitant use of morphine with benzodiazepines and/or other CNS depressants, including alcohol (e.g., non-benzodiazepine sedatives/hypnotics, anxiolytics, tranquilizers, muscle relaxants, general anesthetics, antipsychotics, other opioids). A boxed warning regarding this risk has been included in the prescribing information for morphine. Because of these risks, reserve concomitant prescribing of these drugs for patients in whom alternative treatment options are inadequate.

Use of neuroleptics in conjunction with neuraxial administration of morphine may increase the risk of respiratory depression.

Observational studies have demonstrated that concomitant use of opioid analgesics and benzodiazepines increases the risk of drug-related mortality compared to use of opioid analgesics alone. Because of similar pharmacological properties, it is reasonable to expect similar risk with concomitant use of other CNS depressant drugs with opioid analgesics.

If the decision is made to prescribe a benzodiazepine or other CNS depressant concomitantly with an opioid analgesic, prescribe the lowest effective dosages and minimum durations of concomitant use. In patients already receiving an opioid analgesic, prescribe a lower initial dose of the benzodiazepine or other CNS depressant than indicated in the absence of an opioid, and titrate based on clinical response. If an opioid analgesic is initiated in a patient already taking a benzodiazepine or other CNS depressant, prescribe a lower initial dosage of the opioid analgesic, and titrate based on clinical response. In clinical settings, monitor patients closely for signs and symptoms of respiratory depression and sedation. For ambulatory use, inform patients and caregivers of this potential interaction and educate them on the signs and symptoms of respiratory depression (including sedation). If concomitant use is warranted, consider prescribing naloxone for the emergency treatment of opioid overdose.

Advise both patients and caregivers about the risks of respiratory depression and sedation when morphine is used with benzodiazepines or other CNS depressants (including alcohol and illicit drugs). Advise patients not to drive or operate heavy machinery until the effects of concomitant use of the benzodiazepine or other CNS depressant have been determined. Screen patients for risk of substance use disorders, including opioid abuse and misuse, and warn them of the risk for overdose and death associated with the use of additional CNS depressants including alcohol and illicit drugs.

Patients must not consume alcoholic beverages or prescription or non-prescription products containing alcohol while receiving treatment with morphine sulfate extended-release capsules. The concomitant use of alcohol with morphine sulfate extended-release capsules may result in increased plasma levels and a potentially fatal overdose of morphine.

Neonatal Opioid Withdrawal Syndrome

Use of morphine for an extended period during pregnancy can result in withdrawal in the neonate. A boxed warning regarding this risk has been included in the prescribing information for morphine. Neonatal opioid withdrawal syndrome, unlike opioid withdrawal syndrome in adults, may be life-threatening if not recognized and treated, and requires management according to protocols developed by neonatology experts. Observe newborns for signs of neonatal opioid withdrawal syndrome and manage accordingly. Advise pregnant women using opioids for an extended period of the risk of neonatal opioid withdrawal syndrome and ensure that appropriate treatment will be available.

Risk of Accidental Overdose and Death due to Medication Errors

Dosing errors can result in accidental overdose and death. A boxed warning regarding this risk has been included in the prescribing information for morphine. Avoid dosing errors that may result from confusion between mg and mL and confusion with morphine sulfate oral solutions of different concentrations, when prescribing, dispensing, and administering morphine sulfate oral solution. Ensure that the dose is communicated clearly and dispensed accurately.

Instruct patients and caregivers on how to measure and take or administer the correct dose of morphine sulfate oral solution and to use extreme caution when measuring the dose. Instruct patients and caregivers to always use a graduated oral syringe when administering the oral solution to ensure the dose is measured and administered accurately. Instruct patients to never use a household teaspoon or tablespoon to measure a dose because these are not adequate measuring devices.

Parenteral administration of narcotics in patients receiving epidural or intrathecal morphine may result in overdosage.

Other Warnings and Precautions
Opioid-Induced Hyperalgesia and Allodynia

Opioid-induced hyperalgesia (OIH) occurs when an opioid analgesic paradoxically causes an increase in pain, or an increase in sensitivity to pain; however, this condition differs from tolerance, which is the need for increasing doses of opioids to maintain a defined effect. Symptoms of OIH may include increased levels of pain upon opioid dosage increase, decreased levels of pain upon opioid dosage decrease, or pain from ordinarily non-painful stimuli (allodynia). Evidence of underlying disease progression, opioid tolerance, opioid withdrawal, or addictive behavior should be ruled out to suggest a diagnosis of OIH based on these symptoms.

Cases of OIH have been reported, both with short-term and longer-term use of opioid analgesics. Though the mechanism of OIH is not fully understood, multiple biochemical pathways have been implicated. There is evidence suggesting a strong biologic plausibility between opioid analgesics and OIH and allodynia. If OIH is suspected, carefully consider appropriately decreasing the dose of the current opioid analgesic or safely switch the patient to a different opioid drug.

Life-Threatening Respiratory Depression in Patients with Chronic Pulmonary Disease or in Elderly, Cachectic, or Debilitated Patients

The use of morphine sulfate in patients with acute or severe bronchial asthma in an unmonitored setting or in the absence of resuscitative equipment is contraindicated.

Patients with significant chronic obstructive pulmonary disease or cor pulmonale, and those with a substantially decreased respiratory reserve, hypoxia, hypercapnia, or pre-existing respiratory depression receiving morphine sulfate are at increased risk of decreased respiratory drive including apnea, even at recommended dosages. Life-threatening respiratory depression is also more likely to occur in elderly, cachectic, or debilitated patients because they may have altered pharmacokinetics or altered clearance compared to younger, healthier patients.

Regularly evaluate or monitor patients, particularly when initiating and titrating morphine sulfate and when morphine sulfate is given concomitantly with other drugs that depress respiration. Alternatively, consider the use of non-opioid analgesics in these patients.

Interaction with Monoamine Oxidase Inhibitors

Monoamine oxidase inhibitors (MAOIs) may potentiate the effects of morphine, including respiratory depression, coma, and confusion. Morphine sulfate should not be used in patients taking MAOIs or within 14 days of stopping such treatment. (See Drug Interactions.)

Adrenal Insufficiency

Cases of adrenal insufficiency have been reported with opioid use, generally after more than 1 month of use. Presentation of adrenal insufficiency may include non-specific symptoms and signs including nausea, vomiting, anorexia, fatigue, weakness, dizziness, and low blood pressure.

If adrenal insufficiency is suspected, confirm the diagnosis as soon as possible. If adrenal insufficiency is diagnosed, treat with physiologic replacement doses of corticosteroids. Wean the patient from the opioid to allow adrenal function to recover and continue corticosteroid treatment until recovery. Use of opioids other than morphine may be tried as some cases reported use of a different opioid without recurrence of adrenal insufficiency. Current evidence does not identify any particular opioid as being more likely to be associated with adrenal insufficiency.

Severe Hypotension

Morphine may cause severe hypotension, including orthostatic hypotension and syncope in ambulatory patients. There is increased risk in patients whose ability to maintain blood pressure has already been compromised by reduced blood volume or concurrent administration of certain CNS depressant drugs (e.g., phenothiazines, general anesthetics). Regularly evaluate patients for signs of hypotension after initiating or titrating the dosage of morphine sulfate. In patients with circulatory shock, morphine may cause vasodilation that can further reduce cardiac output and blood pressure; avoid use in such patients.

In ambulatory patients with reduced circulating blood volume, impaired myocardial function, or on sympatholytic drugs receiving single-dose neuraxial morphine, monitor for orthostatic hypotension.

Risks of Use in Patients with Increased Intracranial Pressure, Brain Tumors, Head Injury, or Impaired Consciousness

In patients who may be susceptible to the intracranial effects of CO_2 retention (e.g., those with evidence of increased intracranial pressure or brain tumors), morphine may reduce respiratory drive, and the resultant CO_2 retention can further increase intracranial pressure. Monitor patients for signs of sedation and respiratory depression, particularly when initiating therapy. Opioids may also obscure the clinical course in patients with head injuries. Avoid the use of morphine in patients with impaired consciousness or coma.

Risks in Patients with GI Conditions

Morphine is contraindicated in patients with GI obstruction, including paralytic ileus, as the drug may cause spasm of the sphincter of Oddi. Opioids may cause increases in serum amylase. Monitor patients with biliary tract disease, including acute pancreatitis for worsening symptoms.

Risk of Seizures

Morphine may increase the frequency of seizures in patients with seizure disorders and may increase the risk of seizures occurring in other clinical settings associated with seizures. Regularly evaluate patients with a history of seizure disorders for worsened seizure control during morphine therapy.

Excitation of the CNS, resulting in convulsions, may accompany high doses of morphine given by IV administration.

Withdrawal

Do not abruptly discontinue morphine in a patient physically dependent on opioids, but rather gradually taper the dosage. Rapid tapering in a physically dependent patient may lead to withdrawal symptoms and return of pain.

Avoid the use of mixed agonist/antagonist (e.g., pentazocine, nalbuphine, and butorphanol) or partial agonist (e.g., buprenorphine) analgesics in patients receiving a full opioid agonist analgesic, such as morphine. In these patients, mixed agonist/antagonist and partial agonist analgesics may reduce the analgesic effect and/or may precipitate withdrawal symptoms.

Risks of Driving and Operating Machinery

Morphine may impair the mental or physical abilities needed to perform potentially hazardous activities such as driving a car or operating machinery. Warn patients not to drive or operate dangerous machinery unless they are tolerant to the effects of morphine and know how they will react to the medication.

Risk of Tolerance and Myoclonic Activity

Patients sometimes manifest unusual acceleration of neuraxial morphine requirements, which may cause concern regarding systemic absorption and the hazards of large doses; these patients may benefit from hospitalization and detoxification. Myoclonic-like spasm of the lower extremities in patients receiving more than 20 mg/day of intrathecal morphine have been reported. After detoxification, it might be possible to resume treatment at lower doses, and some patients have been successfully switched from continuous epidural morphine to continuous intrathecal morphine. Repeat detoxification may be indicated at a later date. The upper daily dosage limit for each patient during continuous treatment must be individualized.

Cardiovascular Instability

While low doses of IV administered morphine have little effect on cardiovascular stability, high doses are excitatory, resulting from sympathetic hyperactivity and increase in circulatory catecholamines. Ensure that naloxone and resuscitative equipment are immediately available for use in case of life-threatening or intolerable side effects and whenever IV morphine is being initiated.

Risks with Neuraxial Administration

In the case of epidural or intrathecal administration, morphine sulfate injection should be administered by or under the direction of a physician experienced in the techniques and familiar with the patient management problems associated with epidural or intrathecal drug administration. The physician should be familiar with patient conditions such as infection at the injection site, bleeding diathesis, and anticoagulant therapy, which require special evaluation of benefit versus risk.

Because epidural administration has been associated with less potential for immediate or late adverse effects than intrathecal administration, the epidural route should be used whenever possible. Administration of morphine sulfate injection by the epidural or intrathecal routes should be limited to the lumbar area. Thoracic epidural administration has been shown to dramatically increase the incidence of early and late respiratory depression even with doses of 1 to 2 mg.

Chest Wall Rigidity

Rapid IV administration of morphine sulfate may result in chest wall rigidity.

Risks in Patients with Urinary System Disorders

Urinary retention, which may persist 10 to 20 hours following a single epidural or intrathecal administration, is frequently associated with neuraxial opioid administration and must be anticipated, more frequently in male than female patients. Urinary retention may also occur during the first several days of hospitalization for the initiation of continuous intrathecal or epidural morphine therapy. Early recognition of difficulty in urination and prompt intervention in cases of urinary retention is indicated. Patients who develop urinary retention have responded to cholinomimetic treatment and/or judicious use of catheters.

CNS Toxicity

Dysphoric reactions may occur after any size dose and toxic psychoses have been reported with use of morphine.

Exposure, Hypothermia, Immersion and Shock

Caution must be used when injecting any opioid intramuscularly into chilled areas or in patients with hypotension or shock, since impaired perfusion may prevent complete absorption; if repeated injections are administered, an excessive amount may be suddenly absorbed if normal circulation is re-established.

Risk of Inflammatory Masses

Inflammatory masses such as granulomas, some of which have resulted in serious neurologic impairment including paralysis, have been reported to occur in patients receiving continuous infusion of opioid analgesics including morphine sulfate injection (Infumorph®) via indwelling intrathecal catheters. Patients receiving continuous infusion of morphine sulfate injection (Infumorph®) via an indwelling intrathecal catheter should be carefully monitored for new neurologic signs or symptoms. Further assessment or intervention should be based on the clinical condition of the individual patient.

Patient-controlled Analgesia (PCA)

Although self-administration of opioids by PCA may allow each patient to individually titrate to an acceptable level of analgesia, PCA administration has resulted in adverse outcomes and episodes of respiratory depression. Healthcare providers and family members monitoring patients receiving PCA analgesia should be instructed in the need for appropriate monitoring for excessive sedation, respiratory depression, or other adverse effects of opioid medications.

Specific Populations

Pregnancy

There are no available data with morphine use in pregnant women to inform a drug-associated risk for major birth defects and miscarriage. Clinical studies of morphine use during pregnancy have not reported a clear association between morphine and major birth defects. Based on findings from animal studies, advise pregnant women of the potential risk to a fetus.

Opioids cross the placenta and may produce respiratory depression and psycho-physiologic effects in neonates. An opioid antagonist, such as naloxone, must be available for reversal of opioid-induced respiratory depression in the neonate. Morphine is not recommended for use in women during and immediately prior to labor, when use of shorter-acting analgesics or other analgesic techniques are more appropriate. Opioid analgesics, including morphine, can prolong labor through actions that temporarily reduce the strength, duration, and frequency of uterine contractions. However, this effect is not consistent and may be offset by an increased rate of cervical dilatation, which may shorten labor. Monitor neonates exposed to opioid analgesics during labor for signs of excessive sedation and respiratory depression.

Use of opioid analgesics for an extended period during pregnancy for medical or nonmedical purposes can result in physical dependence in the neonate and neonatal opioid withdrawal syndrome shortly after birth. Neonatal opioid withdrawal syndrome presents as irritability, hyperactivity and abnormal sleep pattern, high pitched cry, tremor, vomiting, diarrhea, and failure to gain weight. Observe newborns for signs of neonatal opioid withdrawal syndrome and manage accordingly.

Lactation

Morphine should be used with caution in nursing women, since the drug has been reported to distribute into human milk.

The developmental and health benefits of breastfeeding should be considered along with the mother's clinical need for morphine and any potential adverse effects on the breastfed infant from the drug or from the underlying maternal condition. Because of the potential for serious adverse reactions, including excessive sedation and respiratory depression in a breastfed infant, advise patients that breastfeeding is not recommended during treatment with morphine sulfate extended-release capsules or tablets.

Monitor infants exposed to morphine through breast milk for excess sedation and respiratory depression. Withdrawal symptoms can occur in breastfed infants when maternal administration of morphine is stopped, or when breastfeeding is stopped.

Females and Males of Reproductive Potential

Use of opioids for an extended period of time may cause reduced fertility in females and males of reproductive potential. It is not known whether these effects on fertility are reversible. In animal studies, morphine sulfate administration adversely effected fertility and reproductive endpoints in male rats and prolonged estrus cycle in female rats.

Pediatric Use

Safety and effectiveness of morphine in pediatric patients vary based on the route of administration and characteristics of the preparation.

The safety and effectiveness of immediate-release morphine sulfate tablets administered orally have been established for the management of pediatric patients weighing at least 50 kg with acute pain severe enough to require an opioid analgesic when alternative treatments are inadequate. Use of the immediate-release tablets in this age group is supported by clinical evidence in adults and supportive data from an open-label, safety and pharmacokinetic study in pediatric patients 2 through 17 years of age with postoperative acute pain. The safety and effectiveness of immediate-release morphine sulfate tablets have not been established in pediatric patients weighing less than 50 kg because the recommended dosage cannot be achieved with available tablet strengths. Consider use of another morphine sulfate product in patients who cannot swallow oral tablets or who weigh less than 50 kg.

The safety and effectiveness of morphine sulfate oral solution (2 mg/mL and 4 mg/mL) have been established for the management of pediatric patients 2 to 17 years of age with acute pain severe enough to require an opioid analgesic when alternative treatments are inadequate. The safety and effectiveness of the oral solution have not been established in pediatric patients younger than 2 years of age. The safety and effectiveness of morphine sulfate oral solution 20 mg/mL have not been established in pediatric patients. The safety and effectiveness of morphine sulfate oral solution have not been established for the management of pediatric patients 2 years of age and older with chronic pain severe enough to require an opioid analgesic when alternative treatments are inadequate.

The safety and effectiveness of continuous IV infusion of morphine have been established for the management of pain in pediatric patients of all age groups. Such use is supported by evidence from randomized controlled studies in pediatric patients. Monitor cardiorespiratory function in children younger than 3 months of age. Adjust the infusion rate based on clinical signs of inadequate pain relief and/or increased somnolence. For premature infants and former premature infants with chronic lung disease and up to 5 to 6 months of age, careful monitoring for depressed hypoxic drive is required following continuous IV infusion of the opioid.

Safety and efficacy of morphine sulfate suppositories in pediatric patients have not been established.

Safety and efficacy of epidural or intrathecal injection of morphine in pediatric patients have not been established and such injections are not recommended. Safety and efficacy of patient-controlled analgesia (PCA) have not been established in pediatric patients.

Safety and efficacy of morphine sulfate extended-release capsules in children younger than 18 years of age have not been established. In addition, the manufacturers state that commercially available strengths of morphine sulfate extended-release capsules are not appropriate for children and that the contents of the capsules should not be sprinkled onto applesauce for administration to children.

Safety and efficacy of morphine sulfate extended-release tablets in children have not been established.

Geriatric Use

Patients 65 years of age or older may have increased sensitivity to morphine. In general, use caution when selecting dosage for an elderly patient, usually starting at the low end of the dosing range, reflecting the greater frequency of decreased hepatic, renal, or cardiac function and of concomitant disease or other drug therapy.

Respiratory depression is the main risk for geriatric patients treated with opioids and has occurred after administration of large initial doses in patients who were not opioid-tolerant or when opioids were co-administered with other drugs that depress respiration. Titrate the dosage of morphine sulfate slowly in geriatric patients and frequently reevaluate the patient for signs of CNS and respiratory depression.

Morphine is known to be substantially excreted by the kidney, and the risk of adverse reactions to this drug may be greater in patients with impaired renal function. Because elderly patients are more likely to have decreased renal function, care should be taken in dose selection; regular evaluation of renal function should occur.

Hepatic Impairment

Morphine pharmacokinetics have been reported to be significantly altered in patients with cirrhosis. Initiate treatment in these patients with a lower than usual dosage and titrate slowly while regularly evaluating for signs of respiratory depression, sedation, and hypotension.

Renal Impairment

Morphine pharmacokinetics are altered in patients with renal failure. Initiate treatment in these patients with a lower than usual dosage and titrate slowly while regularly evaluating for signs of respiratory depression, sedation, and hypotension.

● Common Adverse Effects

Common adverse effects reported in adults receiving morphine include constipation, nausea, somnolence, lightheadedness, dizziness, sedation, vomiting, headache, and sweating. Serious adverse effects include apnea, circulatory depression, respiratory depression or arrest, shock, and cardiac arrest.

Common adverse effects reported in pediatric patients (>5%) receiving morphine include nausea, vomiting, constipation, decreased oxygen saturation, and flatulence.

DRUG INTERACTIONS

Morphine is not significantly metabolized by cytochrome P-450 (CYP) isoenzyme 3A4; the drug does not induce or inhibit CYP enzymes. Morphine is a substrate of the efflux transporter P-glycoprotein (P-gp). Morphine is mainly metabolized by UDP-glucuronosyltransferases (UGTs) with a specific affinity for the UGT2B7 isoenzyme.

● Drugs Affecting or Affected by Transport Systems

Concomitant use of morphine and P-gp inhibitors (e.g., quinidine, verapamil) can increase exposure to morphine by two-fold and can increase the risk of hypotension, respiratory depression, profound sedation, coma, and death. Evaluate patients for signs of respiratory depression that may be greater than otherwise expected and decrease the dosage of morphine sulfate tablets and/or the P-gp inhibitor as necessary.

Studies have shown that drugs that inhibit the UGT2B7 pathway may alter the amount of metabolites available from morphine metabolism. Drugs that are the most potent inhibitors of this pathway include tamoxifen, diclofenac, naloxone, carbamazepine, tricyclic and heterocyclic antidepressants, and benzodiazepines.

● Alcohol

Concomitant use of alcohol with morphine sulfate extended-release capsules can result in increased morphine plasma levels and potentially fatal overdose. Instruct patients not to consume alcoholic beverages or use prescription or non-prescription products containing alcohol while receiving the extended-release capsules.

● Anticholinergic Drugs

Concomitant use of morphine and anticholinergic drugs may increase the risk of urinary retention and/or severe constipation, which may lead to paralytic ileus. Evaluate patients for signs of urinary retention or reduced gastric motility when these drugs are used concomitantly.

● Benzodiazepines and Other CNS Depressants

Due to additive pharmacologic effect, concomitant use of morphine with benzodiazepines or other CNS depressants (other sedatives/hypnotics, anxiolytics, tranquilizers and muscle relaxants, general anesthetics, antipsychotics, other opioids, and alcohol) can increase the risk of hypotension, respiratory depression, profound sedation, coma, and death.

Reserve concomitant use for patients for whom alternative treatment options are inadequate. Limit dosages and durations to the minimum required. Inform patients and caregivers of this potential interaction and educate them on the signs and symptoms of respiratory depression (including sedation).

If concomitant use is warranted, consider prescribing naloxone for the emergency treatment of opioid overdose.

● Cimetidine

Concomitant use of morphine and cimetidine has been reported to precipitate apnea, confusion, and increase the risk of hypotension, respiratory depression, profound sedation, coma, and death. Monitor patients for increased respiratory and CNS depression when morphine is used concomitantly with cimetidine and decrease dosage of the drugs as necessary.

● Diuretics

Opioids can reduce the efficacy of diuretics by inducing the release of antidiuretic hormone. Evaluate patients for signs of diminished diuresis and/or effects on blood pressure and increase the dosage of the diuretic as needed.

● Mixed Agonist/Antagonist and Partial Agonist Opioid Analgesics

Mixed agonist/antagonist and partial agonist opioid analgesics (butorphanol, nalbuphine, pentazocine, buprenorphine) may reduce the analgesic effect of morphine and/or precipitate withdrawal symptoms. Avoid concomitant use.

● Monamine Oxidase (MAO) Inhibitors

Interactions between opioids and MAO inhibitors (e.g., phenelzine, tranylcypromine, linezolid, IV methylene blue) may manifest as serotonin syndrome or opioid toxicity (e.g., respiratory depression, coma). Do not use morphine in patients taking MAOIs or within 14 days of stopping such treatment.

● Muscle Relaxants

Morphine may enhance the neuromuscular blocking action of skeletal muscle relaxants (e.g., cyclobenzaprine, metaxalone) and produce an increased degree of respiratory depression. Because respiratory depression may be greater than otherwise expected, decrease the dosage of morphine and/or the muscle relaxant as necessary. Due to the risk of respiratory depression with concomitant use of skeletal muscle relaxants and opioids, consider prescribing naloxone for the emergency treatment of opioid overdose.

● P2Y12 Inhibitors

Co-administration of oral P2Y12 inhibitors (e.g., clopidogrel, prasugrel, ticagrelor) and IV morphine sulfate can decrease the absorption and peak concentration of the P2Y12 inhibitor and delay the onset of the antiplatelet effect. Consider the use of a parenteral antiplatelet agent in the setting of acute coronary syndrome (ACS) requiring co-administration of IV morphine sulfate.

● Serotonergic Drugs

Concomitant use of opioids with other drugs that affect the serotonergic neurotransmitter system (e.g., selective serotonin reuptake inhibitors [SSRIs], serotonin and norepinephrine reuptake inhibitors [SNRIs], tricyclic antidepressants [TCAs], triptans, 5-HT3 receptor antagonists, drugs that affect the serotonin neurotransmitter system [e.g., mirtazapine, trazodone, tramadol]) has resulted in serotonin syndrome. If concomitant use is warranted, frequently evaluate the patient, particularly during treatment initiation and dose adjustment. Discontinue morphine therapy if serotonin syndrome is suspected.

DESCRIPTION

Morphine is a phenanthrene-derivative opioid agonist. The drug is the principal alkaloid of opium and considered to be the prototype of the opioid agonists. Morphine is a full opioid agonist and is relatively selective for the mu-opioid receptor, although it can bind to other opioid receptors at higher doses.

The principal therapeutic action of morphine is analgesia. Like all full opioid agonists, there is no ceiling effect for analgesia with morphine. Clinically, dosage is titrated to provide adequate analgesia and may be limited by adverse reactions, including respiratory and CNS depression. The precise mechanism of the analgesic action is unknown. However, specific CNS opioid receptors for endogenous compounds with opioid-like activity have been identified throughout the brain and spinal cord and are thought to play a role in the analgesic effects of the drug.

Morphine sulfate is about two-thirds absorbed from the GI tract. The oral bioavailability of morphine is 20–40% but exhibits large inter-individual variability due to extensive pre-systemic metabolism. The extent of absorption from immediate-release and extended-release oral preparations is essentially the same, but time to peak plasma concentrations is longer and peak plasma concentrations are lower with extended-release preparations.Food may decrease the rate of GI absorption of morphine sulfate administered orally as either immediate-release or extended-release preparations, but extent of absorption is unchanged. Peak plasma concentrations of morphine are achieved 5–30 minutes after IM injection, 30 minutes after conventional tablet administration, 60 minutes after rectal administration, about 90 minutes after administration of extended-release preparations, and within 5–10 minutes after epidural or intrathecal administration. Although the primary site of action is the CNS, only about 40–50% of the dose crosses the blood-brain barrier due to poor lipid solubility, protein binding, rapid conjugation with glucuronic acid, and ionization of the drug at a physiologic pH. Morphine is metabolized by demethylation and glucuronidation; glucuronidation is the predominant mode of metabolism, producing morphine-6 glucuronide (M6G), morphine-3 glucuronide (M3G), and a demethylated normorphine metabolite. M6G has been shown to have analgesic activity but crosses the blood-brain barrier poorly, while M3G has no significant analgesic activity. Protein binding is low and reported to be 20–36%. Morphine is generally excreted in the urine as M3G and M6G, with smaller amounts excreted unchanged. Elimination half-life in patients with normal renal function is 1.5 to 2 hours.

ADVICE TO PATIENTS

- Inform patients that the use of morphine, even when taken as recommended, can result in addiction, abuse, and misuse, which can lead to overdose and death. Instruct patients not to share morphine preparations with others and to take steps to protect the drug from theft or misuse.

- Inform patients of the risk of life-threatening respiratory depression, including information that the risk is greatest when starting morphine or when the dosage is increased, and that it can occur even at recommended dosages. Educate patients and caregivers on how to recognize respiratory depression and emphasize the importance of calling 911 or seeking emergency medical assistance immediately in the event of a known or suspected overdose.

- Advise patients and caregivers not to increase opioid dosage without first consulting a clinician. Advise patients to seek medical attention if they experience symptoms of hyperalgesia, including worsening pain, increased sensitivity to pain, or new pain.

- Inform patients that opioids could cause a rare but potentially life-threatening condition called serotonin syndrome resulting from concomitant administration of serotonergic drugs. Warn patients of the symptoms of serotonin syndrome and to seek medical attention right away if symptoms develop. Instruct patients to inform their physicians if they are taking, or plan to take, serotonergic medications.

- Inform patients not to take morphine sulfate preparations while using any drugs that inhibit monoamine oxidase. Patients also should not start taking monoamine oxidase inhibitors (MAOIs) while taking morphine sulfate preparations.

- Inform patients that morphine may impair the ability to perform potentially hazardous activities such as driving a car or operating heavy machinery. Advise patients not to perform such tasks until they know how they will react to the medication.

- Advise patients of the potential for severe constipation, including management instructions and when to seek medical attention.

- Inform patients that opioids could cause adrenal insufficiency, a potentially life-threatening condition. Adrenal insufficiency may present with non-specific symptoms and signs such as nausea, vomiting, anorexia, fatigue, weakness, dizziness, and low blood pressure. Advise patients to seek medical attention if they experience a constellation of these symptom.

- Inform patients that morphine sulfate preparations may cause orthostatic hypotension and syncope. Instruct patients on how to recognize symptoms of low blood pressure and reduce the risk of serious consequences should hypotension occur (e.g., sit or lie down, carefully rise from a sitting or lying position).

- Inform patients that anaphylaxis has been reported with ingredients contained in morphine sulfate. Advise patients how to recognize such a reaction and when to seek medical attention.

- Advise patients to inform their clinician of existing or contemplated concomitant therapy, including prescription and OTC drugs and dietary or herbal supplements, as well as any concomitant illnesses.

- Advise women to inform their clinician if they are or plan to become pregnant. Inform patients of reproductive potential that use of morphine for an extended period of time during pregnancy can result in neonatal opioid withdrawal syndrome, which may be life-threatening if not recognized and treated.

- Inform patients that use of opioids for an extended period of time may cause reduced fertility. It is not known whether these effects on fertility are reversible.

- Advise woment to inform their clinicians if they are breastfeeding. Advise nursing mothers to carefully observe infants for increased sleepiness (more than usual), breathing difficulties, or limpness. Instruct nursing mothers to seek immediate medical care if they notice these signs. Breastfeeding is not recommended during treatment with morphine sulfate extended-release tablets (e.g., MS Contin®) or capsules.

- Inform patients of other important precautionary information.

Patient Advice Related to Outpatient Use of Morphine

- Advise patients to store morphine prescriptions securely, out of sight and reach of children, and in a location not accessible by others, including visitors to the home because of the risks associated with accidental ingestion, misuse, and abuse. Inform patients that leaving morphine unsecured can pose a deadly risk to others in the home.

- Advise patients and caregivers that when medicines are no longer needed, they should be disposed of promptly. Expired, unwanted, or unused morphine preparations should be disposed of by flushing the unused medication down the toilet if a drug take-back option is not readily available. Inform patients that they can visit https://www.fda.gov/drugdisposal for a complete list of medicines recommended for disposal by flushing, as well as additional information on disposal of unused medicines.

- Inform patients that accidental ingestion, especially by children, may result in respiratory depression or death.

- Inform patients and caregivers that potentially fatal additive effects may occur if morphine preparations are used with benzodiazepines or other CNS depressants, including alcohol, and not to use these concomitantly unless supervised by a healthcare provider.

- Discuss with the patient and caregiver the availability of naloxone for the emergency treatment of opioid overdose, both when initiating and renewing treatment with a morphine preparation. Inform patients and caregivers about the various ways to obtain naloxone as permitted by individual state naloxone dispensing and prescribing requirements or guidelines (e.g., by prescription, directly from a pharmacist, or as part of a community-based program). Educate patients and caregivers on how to recognize the signs and symptoms of an overdose and how to use naloxone in the event of a suspected overdose. Explain to patients and caregivers that naloxone's effects are temporary, and that they must call 911 or get emergency medical help right away in all cases of known or suspected opioid overdose, even if naloxone is administered.

- Instruct patients how to properly take morphine. Advise patients not to adjust the dose without consulting a physician or other healthcare professional.

- Instruct patients not to discontinue morphine without first discussing a tapering plan with the prescriber.

Patient Advice Related to Oral Solution

- Strongly advise patients and caregivers to always use a graduated oral syringe when administering morphine sulfate oral solution to correctly measure the prescribed amount of medication.

- Instruct patients and caregivers to never use household teaspoons or tablespoons to measure morphine sulfate oral solution.

- Morphine sulfate oral solution 20 mg/mL: Inform patients that the 20 mg/mL formulation is only for adult patients who are already receiving opioid therapy and have demonstrated opioid tolerance. Use of this formulation may cause fatal respiratory depression when administered to patients who have not had previous exposure to opioids. Instruct patients and caregivers how to measure and take or administer the correct dose of morphine oral solution 20 mg/mL using the enclosed graduated oral syringe.

- Morphine sulfate oral solution 2 mg/mL and 4 mg/mL: Strongly advise patients and caregivers to always use a graduated oral syringe with metric units of measurement (i.e., mL) to correctly measure the prescribed amount of medication. Inform patients that oral syringes may be obtained from their pharmacy.

Patient Advice Related to Extended-release Preparations

- Instruct patients to swallow morphine sulfate extended-release tablets or capsules whole.

- Advise patients to not crush or chew the extended-release tablets or capsules and not dissolve the extended-release tablets or pellets in the extended-release capsules.

- Instruct patient to use morphine sulfate extended-release tablets or capsules exactly as prescribed to reduce the risk of life-threatening adverse reactions (e.g., respiratory depression).

PREPARATIONS

Subject to control under the Federal Controlled Substances Act of 1970 as a schedule II (C-II) drug.

Excipients in commercially available drug preparations may have clinically important effects in some individuals; consult specific product labeling for details.

Morphine Sulfate

Oral

Capsules, extended-release (containing pellets)	30 mg*	Morphine Sulfate Extended-release Capsules (C-II)
	45 mg*	Morphine Sulfate Extended-release Capsules (C-II)
	60 mg*	Morphine Sulfate Extended-release Capsules (C-II)
	75 mg*	Morphine Sulfate Extended-release Capsules (C-II)
	90 mg*	Morphine Sulfate Extended-release Capsules (C-II)
	120 mg*	Morphine Sulfate Extended-release Capsules (C-II)
Solution	10 mg/5 mL*	Morphine Sulfate Oral Solution (C-II)
	20 mg/5 mL*	Morphine Sulfate Oral Solution (C-II)
	100 mg/5 mL*	Morphine Sulfate Oral Solution (C-II; with graduated oral syringe)
Tablets	15 mg*	Morphine Sulfate Tablets (C-II; scored)
	30 mg*	Morphine Sulfate Tablets (C-II; scored)

Tablets, extended-release, film-coated	15 mg*	Morphine Sulfate Tablets ER (C-II) MS Contin® (C-II), Rhodes
	30 mg*	Morphine Sulfate Tablets ER (C-II) MS Contin® (C-II), Rhodes
	60 mg*	Morphine Sulfate Tablets ER (C-II) MS Contin® (C-II), Rhodes
	100 mg*	Morphine Sulfate Tablets ER (C-II), MS Contin® (C-II), Rhodes
	200 mg*	Morphine Sulfate Tablets ER (C-II), MS Contin® (C-II), Rhodes

Parenteral

Injection, for IV or IM use	2 mg/mL*	Morphine Sulfate Injection (C-II),
	4 mg/mL*	Morphine Sulfate Injection (C-II),
	5 mg/mL*	Morphine Sulfate Injection (C-II),
	8 mg/mL*	Morphine Sulfate Injection (C-II),
	10 mg/mL*	Morphine Sulfate Injection (C-II),
Injection, for epidural, intrathecal, or IV use	0.5 mg/mL*	Duramorph® (C-II), Hikma Preservative-free Morphine Sulfate Injection (C-II),
	1 mg/mL*	Duramorph® (C-II), Hikma Preservative-free Morphine Sulfate Injection (C-II),
Injection, for epidural or intrathecal use via continuous microinfusion device only	10 mg/mL	Infumorph® (C-II), Hikma
	25 mg/mL*	Infumorph® (C-II), Hikma Morphine Sulfate Injection(C-II)
Injection, for IV infusion via compatible patient-controlled infusion device only	1 mg/mL*	Morphine Sulfate Preservative-free Injection (C-II),
Injection, for IV infusion	50 mg/mL*	Morphine Sulfate Injection (C-II),

Rectal

Suppositories	5 mg*	Morphine Sulfate Suppositories (C-II),
	10 mg*	Morphine Sulfate Suppositories (C-II),
	20 mg*	Morphine Sulfate Suppositories (C-II),
	30 mg*	Morphine Sulfate Suppositories (C-II),

* available from one or more manufacturer, distributor, and/or repackager by generic (nonproprietary) name

† Use is not currently included in the labeling approved by the US Food and Drug Administration.

Selected Revisions August 10, 2024, © Copyright, September 1, 1972, American Society of Health-System Pharmacists, Inc.

Oxycodone, Oxycodone Hydrochloride, oxyCODONE Myristate

28:08.08 • OPIOID AGONISTS

■ Oxycodone is a synthetic phenanthrene-derivative opiate agonist.

REMS

FDA approved a REMS for oxycodone to ensure that the benefits outweigh the risk. The REMS may apply to one or more preparations of oxycodone and consists of the following: medication guide and elements to assure safe use. See the FDA REMS page (https://www.accessdata.fda.gov/scripts/cder/rems/index.cfm).

USES

● Pain

Conventional preparations of oxycodone hydrochloride are used orally for the management of moderate to severe acute or chronic pain when use of an opiate analgesic is appropriate.

Oxycodone hydrochloride extended-release tablets and oxycodone myristate extended-release capsules are used orally for the relief of pain that is severe enough to require long-term, daily, around-the-clock use of an opiate analgesic. Because of the risks of addiction, abuse, and misuse associated with opiates even at recommended dosages, and because of the greater risks of overdose and death associated with extended-release opiate formulations, these extended-release preparations of oxycodone hydrochloride or oxycodone myristate should be reserved for use in patients for whom alternative treatment options (e.g., nonopiate analgesics, immediate-release opiates) are inadequate or not tolerated. Oxycodone hydrochloride extended-release tablets may be used for the relief of such pain in pediatric patients 11 years of age or older who are opiate tolerant and already receiving and tolerating opiate agonist therapy at a dosage equivalent to 20 mg or more of oxycodone hydrochloride daily. The manufacturer states that safety and efficacy of oxycodone myristate extended-release capsules have not been established in patients younger than 18 years of age. Oxycodone hydrochloride extended-release tablets and oxycodone myristate extended-release capsules are *not* intended for use on an as-needed ("prn") basis.

Extended-release tablets containing oxycodone hydrochloride in fixed combination with acetaminophen are used for the relief of acute pain that is severe enough to require opiate therapy and for which alternative treatments (e.g., nonopiate analgesics) are inadequate or not tolerated.

For further information on the role of opiate analgesics in the management of acute or chronic pain, see Uses: Pain, in the Opiate Agonists General Statement 28:08.08.

● Misuse and Abuse

Oxycodone has emerged as one of the most problematic abused opiate agonists in the US; therefore, patients should be advised about the risk of theft, and clinicians should be informed about abuse and diversion issues. (See Cautions.)

DOSAGE AND ADMINISTRATION

● Administration

Oxycodone is administered orally as the hydrochloride salt, often in combination with nonopiate analgesics (e.g., acetaminophen), or as the myristate salt.

Conventional Oxycodone Hydrochloride Formulations

Some manufacturers state that their formulations of oxycodone hydrochloride conventional tablets should not be crushed and dissolved. These formulations should not be administered via gastric, nasogastric, or other feeding tube since they can obstruct the tube. Instead, these tablets should be administered intact with sufficient water to ensure that each tablet is completely swallowed immediately after it is placed in the mouth. The respective manufacturer's labeling should be consulted for specific recommendations.

Oxycodone hydrochloride is commercially available as a 5-mg/5-mL oral solution and as a 100-mg/5-mL oral concentrate solution; confusion between the different concentrations or between mg and mL can result in accidental overdosage and/or death. The oral concentrate solution should be used only in opiate-tolerant patients. Caution is required when prescribing, dispensing, and administering oral solutions of the drug to avoid dosing errors. Care should be taken to ensure that the appropriate dose is communicated and dispensed. Prescriptions should specify the intended total dose of the drug (in mg) along with the corresponding total volume (in mL). The calibrated measuring device provided with the particular formulation should always be used to ensure that the dose is measured and administered accurately.

Oxycodone Hydrochloride and Acetaminophen Fixed-combination Extended-release Tablets

Extended-release tablets containing oxycodone hydrochloride in fixed combination with acetaminophen should be swallowed whole and should *not* be broken, chewed, crushed, cut, or dissolved, since such physical alteration of the tablets could result in rapid release of the drug and absorption of a potentially toxic dose. The fixed-combination extended-release tablets should be administered one at a time with enough water to ensure that each tablet is completely swallowed immediately after it is placed in the mouth; extended-release tablets should not be wet (e.g., soaked, licked) before they are placed in the mouth for swallowing. The tablets may be administered without regard to food. This formulation should not be used for administration through a nasogastric, gastric, or other feeding tube.

Oxycodone Hydrochloride Extended-release Tablets

Oxycodone hydrochloride extended-release tablets should be swallowed whole and should *not* be broken, chewed, crushed, cut, split, or dissolved, since such physical alteration of the tablets could result in rapid release of the drug and absorption of a potentially toxic dose. Extended-release tablets should be administered one at a time with enough water to ensure that each tablet is completely swallowed immediately after it is placed in the mouth; extended-release tablets should not be wet (e.g., soaked, licked) before they are placed in the mouth for swallowing. Oxycodone hydrochloride extended-release tablets should not be administered rectally because of increased bioavailability and peak plasma concentrations compared with oral administration. (See Pharmacokinetics.) Food does not substantially affect the extent of oral absorption of oxycodone hydrochloride extended-release tablets.

Oxycodone Myristate Extended-release Capsules

Oxycodone myristate extended-release capsules *must* be administered orally with food. Each dose should be administered with approximately the same amount of food (whether given as an intact capsule or as capsule contents sprinkled on food or directly in the mouth) in order to ensure that consistent plasma concentrations of the drug are achieved. (See Pharmacokinetics.) For patients who have difficulty swallowing, the capsules may be opened and the contents sprinkled onto a small amount of soft food (e.g., applesauce, pudding, yogurt, ice cream, jam) or into a cup and then administered directly into the mouth. The capsule contents should be swallowed immediately, and the mouth should be rinsed to ensure that the entire dose has been swallowed.

Alternatively, the capsule contents may be administered through a nasogastric or gastrostomy tube. The tube should first be flushed with water and then the capsule should be opened and the contents carefully poured directly into the tube; the capsule contents should not be premixed with the liquid that will be used to flush the tube. Following administration, the tube should be flushed with 15 mL of liquid (water, milk, or liquid nutritional supplement) and then flushed 2 more times, each time with 10 mL of liquid, to ensure that the entire dose is delivered.

● *Dosage*

Dosage of oxycodone hydrochloride is expressed in terms of the salt; dosage of oxycodone myristate is expressed in terms of oxycodone base.

Oxycodone should be given at the lowest effective dosage and for the shortest duration of therapy consistent with the treatment goals of the patient. Reduced dosage is indicated in debilitated patients and in very young or very old patients. If concomitant therapy with other CNS depressants is required, the lowest effective dosages and shortest possible duration of concomitant therapy should be used. Some manufacturers recommend that initial dosages of 33–50% of the usual dosage be employed when therapy with oxycodone hydrochloride extended-release tablets is initiated in patients receiving other CNS depressants. When therapy with extended-release tablets containing oxycodone hydrochloride in fixed combination with acetaminophen is initiated in patients receiving other CNS depressants, the manufacturer states that the initial oxycodone hydrochloride dosage should be reduced by 50% (i.e., to 7.5 mg twice daily).

For acute pain not related to trauma or surgery, the prescribed quantity should be limited to the amount needed for the expected duration of pain severe enough to require opiate analgesia (generally 3 days or less and rarely more than 7 days). When opiate analgesics are used for the management of chronic noncancer pain, the US Centers for Disease Control and Prevention (CDC) recommends that primary care clinicians carefully reassess individual benefits and risks before prescribing dosages equivalent to 50 mg or more of morphine sulfate daily (approximately 33 mg or more of oxycodone hydrochloride daily) and avoid dosages equivalent to 90 mg or more of morphine sulfate daily (approximately 60 mg or more of oxycodone hydrochloride daily) or carefully justify their decision to titrate the dosage to such levels. Other experts recommend consulting a pain management specialist before exceeding a dosage equivalent to 80–120 mg of morphine sulfate daily.

Patients receiving long-term, daily, around-the-clock opiate analgesia should be reevaluated continually for adequacy of pain control and for adverse effects, as well as for manifestations of opiate withdrawal and for the development of addiction, abuse, or misuse. To reduce the risk of respiratory depression, appropriate dosage selection and titration are essential. The initial dosage of oxycodone must be individualized, taking into account the patient's severity of pain, response, prior analgesic use, and risk factors for addiction, abuse, and misuse. Because there is substantial interpatient variability in the relative potency of opiate analgesics and analgesic formulations, it is preferable to underestimate the patient's 24-hour opiate requirements and provide "rescue" therapy with an immediate-release opiate analgesic than to overestimate the requirements and manage an adverse reaction. Patients should be monitored closely for respiratory depression, especially during the first 24–72 hours of therapy and following any increase in dosage.

In patients requiring long-term around-the-clock opiate analgesia, dosage of oxycodone should be titrated to a level that provides adequate analgesia and minimizes adverse effects. Frequent communication among the prescriber, other members of the healthcare team, the patient, and the patient's caregiver or family is important during periods of changing analgesic requirements, including the initial dosage titration period. Patients who experience breakthrough pain may require dosage adjustment or supplemental analgesia (i.e., "rescue" therapy with an immediate-release analgesic). If the level of pain increases after dosage stabilization, an attempt should be made to identify the source of increased pain before increasing the oxycodone dosage. During long-term therapy, the continued need for opiate analgesics should be continually reevaluated. If discontinuance of opiate therapy is required, the dosage should be tapered gradually to avoid manifestations of abrupt withdrawal.

For further information on the management of opiate analgesic therapy, see Dosage and Administration: Dosage, in the Opiate Agonists General Statement 28:08.08.

Conventional (Immediate-release) Preparations

For the management of moderate to severe pain in patients who have not been receiving opiate analgesic therapy, the usual initial adult dosage of conventional oxycodone hydrochloride preparations is 5–15 mg every 4–6 hours as needed. Although safety and efficacy of conventional oxycodone hydrochloride preparations have not been established in children, the drug has been recommended for use in pediatric patients. For the management of moderate to severe pain in

children, some experts have suggested a dosage of 0.05–0.15 mg/kg (up to 5 mg) every 4–6 hours as needed.

Dosage should be adjusted based on the response and tolerance of the patient. Patients with chronic pain may require around-the-clock rather than as-needed dosing. Because opiate analgesics given on a fixed dosage schedule have a narrow therapeutic index in certain patient populations, especially when used concomitantly with other drugs, fixed dosage schedules should be reserved for patients for whom the benefits of opiate analgesia outweigh the risks of respiratory depression, altered mental state, and orthostatic hypotension. In patients switching from other opiates or opiate formulations to therapy with conventional oxycodone hydrochloride preparations, the potency of the prior opiate relative to that of oxycodone should be considered, keeping in mind that published dosage conversion ratios are only approximations. Conservative initial dosages, patient monitoring, and dosage adjustment based on response are essential when the opiate or opiate formulation is switched.

When opiate analgesics are administered in fixed combination with nonopiate analgesics, the opiate dosage may be limited by the nonopiate component. Because commercially available preparations contain oxycodone and nonopiate analgesics in various fixed ratios and because these nonopiate analgesics also are available in many other prescription and OTC preparations, care should be taken to ensure that therapy is not duplicated and that dosage of the nonopiate drug does not exceed maximum recommended dosages.

When therapy with conventional preparations of oxycodone hydrochloride is discontinued following long-term opiate therapy, dosage generally can be reduced by 25–50% per day. If symptoms of withdrawal occur, the dosage should be increased to the prior level and tapered more slowly.

Oxycodone Hydrochloride and Acetaminophen Fixed-combination Extended-release Tablets

When extended-release tablets containing oxycodone hydrochloride in fixed combination with acetaminophen are used for the management of acute pain in adults, the recommended oxycodone hydrochloride dosage is 15 mg (given in fixed combination with 650 mg of acetaminophen) every 12 hours. The second dose may be administered as soon as 8 hours after the initial dose if required for adequate analgesia, but all subsequent doses should be administered at 12-hour intervals. When therapy with this formulation is discontinued in a patient who may be opiate dependent, the dosage should be tapered gradually (i.e., reduced by 50% every 2–4 days) to avoid manifestations of abrupt withdrawal.

When opiate analgesics are administered in fixed combination with acetaminophen, the opiate dosage may be limited by the acetaminophen component. Because acetaminophen also is available in many other prescription and OTC preparations, care should be taken to ensure that therapy is not duplicated and that dosage of acetaminophen does not exceed maximum recommended dosages.

Oxycodone Hydrochloride Extended-release Tablets
Adult Dosage

For the management of pain severe enough to require daily, around-the-clock, long-term opiate analgesia in adults who are *not* opiate tolerant, therapy with oxycodone hydrochloride extended-release tablets should be initiated at a dosage of 10 mg every 12 hours. The manufacturers state that use of higher initial dosages in patients who are not opiate tolerant may result in fatal respiratory depression. A single dose exceeding 40 mg, total daily dosages exceeding 80 mg, and 60- and 80-mg extended-release tablets should be used only in adults in whom tolerance to an opiate of comparable potency has been established. Adults are considered opiate tolerant if they have been receiving opiate therapy consisting of at least 60 mg of morphine sulfate daily, 25 mcg of transdermal fentanyl per hour, 30 mg of oral oxycodone hydrochloride daily, 8 mg of oral hydromorphone hydrochloride daily, 25 mg of oxymorphone hydrochloride daily, or an equianalgesic dosage of another opiate daily for at least 1 week.

In patients who are being switched from other opiates to oxycodone hydrochloride extended-release tablets, all other around-the-clock opiate analgesics should be discontinued when therapy with the extended-release tablets is initiated. For patients receiving conventional oxycodone preparations, the total daily dosage of the drug should be calculated and given as oxycodone hydrochloride extended-release tablets in 2 divided doses at 12-hour intervals.

For patients receiving conventional formulations of other opiates, the recommended initial dosage of oxycodone hydrochloride extended-release tablets is 10 mg every 12 hours, since dosage conversion factors have not been established in clinical trials. Particularly close monitoring is required when patients are switched from methadone, since conversion ratios between methadone and other opiates vary widely depending on extent of prior methadone exposure and because methadone has a long half-life and tends to accumulate in plasma.

Patients receiving fentanyl transdermal systems may receive oxycodone hydrochloride extended-release tablets beginning 18 hours after removal of the transdermal system. The manufacturers state that an initial oxycodone hydrochloride dosage of approximately 10 mg every 12 hours as extended-release tablets can be substituted for each 25-mcg/hour increment in fentanyl transdermal system dosage; however, patients should be monitored closely, since clinical experience with this dosage conversion ratio is limited.

Dosage adjustments in adults generally may be made in increments of 25–50% of the total daily dosage at intervals of 1–2 days, to a level that provides adequate analgesia and minimizes adverse effects. Safety and efficacy of dosing intervals shorter than 12 hours have not been established.

The manufacturer states that usual doses and dosing intervals for oxycodone hydrochloride extended-release tablets may be appropriate for geriatric patients, since no unexpected adverse effects were observed in geriatric patients receiving this preparation in clinical trials with appropriate initiation of therapy and dosage titration. However, the manufacturer recommends that initial dosages of 33–50% of the usual dosage be employed when therapy with oxycodone hydrochloride extended-release tablets is initiated in non-opiate-tolerant, debilitated geriatric patients. Dosage in geriatric patients should be titrated cautiously.

Pediatric Dosage

Extended-release oxycodone hydrochloride tablets should be used only in opiate-tolerant pediatric patients 11 years of age and older; such patients must be receiving and tolerating opiate analgesics for at least 5 consecutive days, and at a dosage of at least 20 mg of oxycodone hydrochloride (or equivalent) daily for at least 2 days immediately prior to initiation of therapy with oxycodone hydrochloride extended-release tablets. All other around-the-clock opiate analgesics should be discontinued when therapy with the extended-release tablets is initiated.

In pediatric patients who are being switched from other opiate therapy to oxycodone hydrochloride extended-release tablets, the manufacturer states that the conversion factors in Table 1 may be used as a guide for selecting an initial dosage of the extended-release tablets. The manufacturer cautions that the doses in Table 1 are not equianalgesic doses and the table cannot be used to switch patients from oxycodone hydrochloride extended-release tablets to another opiate, as this will result in overestimation of the dosage of the new opiate and possible fatal overdosage. For patients receiving a single opiate analgesic, the current total daily dosage of the opiate should be multiplied by the appropriate conversion factor in Table 1 to calculate the approximate daily dosage of oxycodone hydrochloride extended-release tablets; the calculated daily dosage should then be divided in half for administration every 12 hours. For patients receiving more than one opiate analgesic, the approximate daily dosage of extended-release oxycodone hydrochloride should be calculated for each opiate and then those totals should be summed to obtain the approximate total daily dosage of oxycodone hydrochloride extended-release tablets; the calculated total daily dosage should then be divided in half for administration every 12 hours. For patients receiving analgesics containing opiates and nonopiates in a fixed ratio, only the opiate component should be considered in the conversion. Calculated doses that do not correspond to an available tablet strength should always be rounded down to the nearest whole tablet when initiating therapy; if the calculated total daily dosage is less than 20 mg, patients should *not* be switched to the extended-release formulation.

Dosage adjustments in pediatric patients may be made in increments of 25% of the total daily dosage at intervals of 1–2 days, to a level that provides adequate analgesia and minimizes adverse effects. Safety and efficacy of dosing intervals shorter than 12 hours have not been established.

In patients receiving asymmetric dosing, the higher dose should be taken in the morning and the lower dose in the evening.

TABLE 1. Conversion Factors When Switching Pediatric Patients 11 Years of Age or Older to Oxycodone Hydrochloride Extended-release Tablets

Prior Opiate	Conversion Factor	
	Oral	Parenteral[a]
Oxycodone	1	
Hydrocodone	0.9	–
Hydromorphone	4	20
Morphine	0.5	3
Tramadol	0.17	0.2

[a] For patients receiving high-dose parenteral opiates, a more conservative conversion is warranted (e.g., for high-dose parenteral morphine, use 1.5 instead of 3 as a multiplication factor).

Pediatric patients receiving fentanyl transdermal systems may receive oxycodone hydrochloride extended-release tablets beginning 18 hours after removal of the transdermal system. The manufacturers state that an initial oxycodone hydrochloride dosage of approximately 10 mg every 12 hours as extended-release tablets can be substituted for each 25-mcg/hour increment in fentanyl transdermal system dosage; however, patients should be monitored closely, since clinical experience with this dosage conversion ratio is limited.

Oxycodone Myristate Extended-release Capsules

Adult Dosage

For the management of pain that is severe enough to require long-term, daily, around-the-clock analgesia in adults who are not currently receiving opiate analgesics or are not opiate tolerant, therapy with oxycodone myristate extended-release capsules should be initiated at a dosage of 9 mg of oxycodone (equivalent to 10 mg of oxycodone hydrochloride) every 12 hours. Use of higher initial dosages in patients who are not opiate tolerant may result in fatal respiratory depression. A single dose exceeding 36 mg of oxycodone (equivalent to 40 mg of oxycodone hydrochloride) or total daily dosages exceeding 72 mg of oxycodone (equivalent to 80 mg of oxycodone hydrochloride) should be used only in patients in whom tolerance to an opiate of comparable potency has been established. Patients are considered opiate tolerant if they have been receiving at least 60 mg of oral morphine sulfate daily, 25 mcg of transdermal fentanyl per hour, 30 mg of oral oxycodone hydrochloride daily, 8 mg of oral hydromorphone hydrochloride daily, 25 mg of oral oxymorphone hydrochloride daily, 60 mg of oral hydrocodone bitartrate daily, or an equianalgesic dose of another opiate daily for at least 1 week.

In adults who are being transferred from other oral opiates to therapy with oxycodone myristate extended-release capsules, all other around-the-clock opiate analgesics should be discontinued when therapy with the extended-release capsules is initiated. Dosage must be carefully individualized since overestimation of the initial dosage in opiate-tolerant patients can result in fatal overdosage. For adults receiving other oral oxycodone preparations, the total daily dosage of the drug should be calculated and given as oxycodone myristate extended-release capsules in 2 divided doses at 12-hour intervals; because oxycodone myristate extended-release capsules are not bioequivalent to other extended-release preparations of the drug, dosage adjustment may be necessary. For patients receiving other opiate analgesics, the recommended initial dosage of oxycodone myristate extended-release capsules is 9 mg of oxycodone every 12 hours, since dosage conversion factors have not been established in clinical trials. Particularly close monitoring is required when patients are switched from methadone, since conversion ratios between methadone and other opiates vary widely depending on extent of prior methadone exposure and because methadone has a long half-life and tends to accumulate in plasma.

Adults receiving therapy with fentanyl transdermal system may receive oxycodone myristate extended-release capsules beginning 18 hours after removal of the transdermal system. The manufacturer states that a conservative initial oxycodone dosage of approximately 9 mg every 12 hours as extended-release capsules can be substituted for each 25-mcg/hour increment in transdermal fentanyl system dosage; however, patients should be monitored closely, since clinical experience with this dosage conversion ratio is limited.

Dosage adjustments generally may be made in increments of 25–50% of the total daily dosage at intervals of 1–2 days, to a level that provides adequate analgesia and minimizes adverse effects. Safety and efficacy of dosing intervals shorter than 12 hours have not been established. The maximum recommended dosage of oxycodone myristate extended-release capsules is 288 mg of oxycodone daily (eight 36-mg capsules), since safety of excipients in the formulation at dosages exceeding 288 mg daily has not been established.

The manufacturer states that usual doses and dosing intervals for oxycodone myristate extended-release capsules may be appropriate for geriatric patients, since no unexpected adverse effects were observed in geriatric patients receiving this preparation in a clinical trial with appropriate initiation of therapy and dosage titration. Nevertheless, dosage should be selected with caution because of the greater frequency of decreased hepatic, renal, and/or cardiac function and of concomitant disease and drug therapy observed in geriatric patients and titrated slowly because of the risk of respiratory depression.

● Dosage in Renal and Hepatic Impairment

In patients with impaired hepatic function, initial oxycodone dosages should be conservative and adjusted according to the clinical situation. The manufacturers recommend that therapy with oxycodone hydrochloride extended-release tablets or oxycodone myristate extended-release capsules be initiated at 33–50% of the usual dosage and titrated carefully. When extended-release tablets containing oxycodone hydrochloride in fixed combination with acetaminophen are used for the management of acute pain in patients with hepatic impairment, the manufacturer recommends an initial oxycodone hydrochloride dose of 7.5 mg (given in fixed combination with 325 mg of acetaminophen); dosage should be adjusted as needed with close monitoring for respiratory depression.

In patients with impaired renal function (creatinine clearance less than 60 mL/minute), initial oxycodone dosages should be conservative and adjusted according to the clinical situation. When extended-release tablets containing oxycodone hydrochloride in fixed combination with acetaminophen are used for the management of acute pain in patients with renal impairment, the manufacturer recommends an initial oxycodone hydrochloride dose of 7.5 mg (given in fixed combination with 325 mg of acetaminophen); dosage should be adjusted as needed with close monitoring for respiratory depression.

If the required dose of oxycodone myristate extended-release capsules is less than 9 mg of oxycodone, an alternative analgesic should be selected.

CAUTIONS

Although adverse effects are milder than those of morphine, addiction liability of oxycodone is about the same as that of morphine; oxycodone shares the toxic potentials of the opiate agonists, and the usual precautions of opiate agonist therapy should be observed. (See Cautions in the Opiate Agonists General Statement 28:08.08.) When preparations containing oxycodone in combination with other drugs are administered, the cautions applicable to each ingredient must be considered.

Because oxycodone hydrochloride is commercially available as an oral solution (5 mg/5 mL) and as an oral concentrate solution (100 mg/5 mL), confusion between the different concentrations or between mg and mL can result in accidental overdosage and/or death. Caution is required to avoid confusing the formulations. (See Conventional Oxycodone Hydrochloride Formulations under Dosage and Administration: Administration.) The oral concentrate solution should be used only in opiate-tolerant patients.

Extended-release opiates are associated with a greater risk of overdose and death because of the larger amount of drug contained in each dosage unit. Oxycodone has been intentionally abused by crushing extended-release preparations and "snorting" the powder or dissolving the contents in water and injecting the solution IV.

Abuse by chewing extended-release preparations also has been reported.

Breaking, chewing, crushing, or dissolving of extended-release tablets containing oxycodone hydrochloride results in immediate release of the opiate and the risk of a potentially fatal overdose.

Snorting or injecting the dissolved contents of oxycodone myristate extended-release capsules also can result in a potentially fatal overdose. The risk of toxicity is increased when oxycodone is used concomitantly with alcohol or other CNS depressants, including other opiates.

Oxycodone hydrochloride extended-release tablets (OxyContin®) and oxycodone myristate extended-release capsules (Xtampza® ER) are formulated with physical and chemical properties that are intended to make these dosage forms more difficult to manipulate for IV or intranasal abuse and misuse. However, abuse by these routes, as well as by the oral route, is still possible.

Because some patients have reported difficulty in swallowing oxycodone hydrochloride extended-release tablets, the tablets should be administered one at a time with enough water to ensure that each tablet is completely swallowed immediately after it is placed in the mouth; the extended-release tablets should not be wet (e.g., soaked, licked) before they are placed in the mouth for swallowing. Choking, gagging, regurgitation, tablets stuck in the throat, and, rarely, intestinal obstruction and exacerbation of diverticulitis (sometimes requiring medical intervention to remove the tablet) have been reported. Patients with underlying GI disorders (e.g., esophageal or colon cancer) associated with a narrow GI lumen are at greater risk of developing these complications. Use of an alternative analgesic should be considered for patients who have difficulty swallowing and in those at risk for underlying GI disorders associated with a narrow GI lumen. Because extended-release tablets containing oxycodone hydrochloride in fixed combination with acetaminophen swell and become sticky when wet, the same precautions apply to this formulation.

Some commercially available formulations of oxycodone hydrochloride contain sodium metabisulfite, a sulfite that may cause allergic-type reactions, including anaphylaxis and life-threatening or less severe asthmatic episodes, in certain susceptible individuals. The overall prevalence of sulfite sensitivity in the general population is unknown but probably low; such sensitivity appears to occur more frequently in asthmatic than in nonasthmatic individuals.

The presence of oxycodone is not reliably detected by all urine drug tests for opiates, especially those designed for in-office use, and laboratories may report urine drug concentrations below a specified value as negative results. If urine testing for oxycodone is used in patient management, the limitations of such testing should be considered and appropriate assay sensitivity and specificity should be ensured.

Oxycodone is distributed into milk. Because of the possibility of sedation or respiratory depression in breast-fed infants, use of oxycodone in nursing women should be avoided. Infants exposed to oxycodone through breast milk should be observed for GI effects, excessive sedation, respiratory depression, and changes in feeding patterns. Symptoms of withdrawal can occur in opiate-dependent breast-fed infants when maternal administration of opiates is discontinued or breast-feeding is stopped.

DRUG INTERACTIONS

● Drugs Affecting Hepatic Microsomal Enzymes

Because oxycodone is metabolized by the cytochrome P-450 (CYP) microsomal enzyme system, principally by isoenzyme 3A4, concomitant use of oxycodone with drugs that inhibit CYP3A4 activity (e.g., macrolide antibiotics [e.g., erythromycin], azole antifungals [e.g., ketoconazole, voriconazole], protease inhibitors [e.g., ritonavir]) may result in reduced clearance and increased plasma concentrations of oxycodone, possibly resulting in increased or prolonged opiate effects, including an increased risk of fatal respiratory depression. These effects could be more pronounced with concomitant use of oxycodone and inhibitors of both CYP2D6 and CYP3A4 (see Pharmacokinetics), particularly when an inhibitor is added after a stable oxycodone dosage has been achieved. Concomitant administration of oxycodone hydrochloride (single 10-mg dose as extended-release tablets) and the potent CYP3A4 inhibitor ketoconazole (200 mg twice daily) increased area under the plasma concentration-time curve (AUC) and peak plasma concentration of oxycodone by 170 and 100%, respectively, while concomitant administration of voriconazole with oxycodone increased the AUC and peak plasma concentration of oxycodone by 3.6- and 1.7-fold, respectively.

However, inhibition of the CYP2D6 pathway alone has not been shown to result in clinically important interactions. If concomitant therapy with a CYP3A4 inhibitor is discontinued, a decrease in plasma oxycodone concentrations may occur, potentially decreasing analgesic efficacy or resulting in withdrawal effects.

Concomitant use of oxycodone with CYP3A4 inducers (e.g., carbamazepine, phenytoin, rifampin) may result in increased clearance and decreased plasma concentrations of oxycodone, with possible lack of efficacy or development of opiate withdrawal. Concomitant administration of oxycodone and the CYP3A4 inducer rifampin decreased AUC and peak plasma concentration of oxycodone by 86 and 63%, respectively. If concomitant therapy with a CYP3A4 inducer is discontinued, an increase in plasma oxycodone concentrations may occur, potentially increasing or prolonging therapeutic and adverse effects of the drug and increasing the risk of serious respiratory depression.

Therefore, caution should be exercised and patients who require concomitant therapy with a CYP3A4 inhibitor or inducer, or who have recently discontinued such therapy, should be monitored closely at frequent intervals, and dosage adjustments should be considered until stable drug effects are achieved.

For further information about drug interactions involving opiate agonists (including oxycodone), see Drug Interactions in the Opiate Agonists General Statement 28:08.08.

PHARMACOKINETICS

Following oral administration of conventional preparations of oxycodone, the analgesic effect occurs within 10–15 minutes, reaches its maximum in 30–60 minutes, and persists for 3–6 hours. Following oral administration of oxycodone as an extended-release tablet, the onset of analgesia occurred within 1 hour in most patients. Oxycodone is extensively metabolized to noroxycodone, oxymorphone, and noroxymorphone and their glucuronide conjugates, with the formation of noroxycodone and oxymorphone mediated by cytochrome P-450 (CYP) isoenzymes 3A and 2D6, respectively; oxycodone and its metabolites are excreted principally in urine. Because oxymorphone is present in plasma in only low concentrations following oxycodone administration, it is not thought to contribute substantially to analgesic effects of the drug.

The oral bioavailability of oxycodone is 60–87%. The relative oral bioavailability of extended-release tablets of oxycodone hydrochloride compared with conventional oral preparations is 100%. The extended-release tablets are formulated to provide controlled delivery of oxycodone over 12 hours. Release of the drug from the extended-release tablets is pH independent. Following rectal administration of oxycodone hydrochloride extended-release tablets in healthy adults, the area under the plasma concentration-time curve (AUC) and peak plasma concentration were increased by 39 and 9%, respectively, compared with oral administration. With multiple oral dosing, steady-state plasma concentrations usually are achieved within 24–36 hours in healthy individuals receiving extended-release tablets of oxycodone hydrochloride. Administration of the extended-release tablets with food does not substantially affect the extent of absorption. The apparent elimination half-life following oral administration of the extended-release tablets or conventional preparations is 4.5 or 3.2 hours, respectively.

Oxycodone myristate extended-release capsules also are formulated to provide delivery of oxycodone over 12 hours but are not bioequivalent to oxycodone hydrochloride extended-release tablets. Under fasting conditions, both peak serum concentrations and AUC are lower for the extended-release capsules; under fed conditions, peak serum concentrations are lower, but AUC is similar to values for the extended-release tablets. Mean peak serum concentrations of oxycodone are lower (73 and 43% lower for administration under fasting and fed conditions, respectively) and the median time to peak serum concentration is approximately 3 hours longer when the drug is administered as extended-release capsules compared with administration as an oral solution in the fasting state. The relative oral bioavailability of oxycodone myristate extended-release capsules compared with an oral solution of the drug is lower in the fasting state (75%) but comparable in the fed state (114%). The time to peak plasma concentrations is approximately 4.5 hours following administration of the extended-release capsules under fed conditions. With repeated administration in healthy individuals, steady-state concentrations are achieved within 24–36 hours. The apparent elimination half-life following oral administration of the extended-release capsules under fed conditions is 5.6 hours, compared with 3.2 hours following administration of conventional preparations of the drug.

Bioavailability of oxycodone myristate extended-release capsules is increased by administration with food and is dependent on the content of the meal. When the extended-release capsules are administered following a high-fat, high-calorie meal rather than in the fasted state, peak concentrations and AUC are increased by 100–150 and 50–60%, respectively; when the extended-release capsules are administered following a medium-fat, medium-calorie meal, peak concentrations and AUC are increased by 84 and 28%, respectively. When the extended-release capsules are administered following a low-fat, low-calorie meal, peak concentrations are 19% higher and AUC is comparable to values following administration under fasting conditions. The pharmacokinetic profile for the capsule contents sprinkled on food is equivalent to that for the intact capsule administered with food.

Extended-release tablets containing oxycodone hydrochloride in fixed combination with acetaminophen are available as a bilayer formulation in which a portion of the labeled oxycodone hydrochloride and acetaminophen doses is contained in an immediate-release layer and the remaining portion is contained in a layer that slowly releases the drugs. Following single or multiple doses of this formulation, the bioavailability (dose-normalized AUC and peak plasma concentration) of oxycodone is comparable to that of conventional preparations of the drug. Oxycodone is detectable in plasma within 30 minutes following administration of the fixed-combination extended-release tablets; peak concentrations are achieved in 3–4 hours. Following administration every 12 hours, steady-state concentrations are attained within 24 hours. Administration of this fixed-combination extended-release formulation with a low-fat or high-fat meal delayed peak concentrations by 1 or 2 hours, respectively; increased mean AUC by 15–16%; and increased peak concentrations by 12–25%. The apparent elimination half-life of oxycodone following oral administration of the fixed-combination extended-release tablets is 4.5 hours, compared with 3.9 hours following administration of conventional preparations of the drug.

Following oral administration of oxycodone hydrochloride extended-release tablets in patients with renal impairment (creatinine clearance less than 60 mL/minute), peak plasma concentrations of the drug and its noroxycodone metabolite were 50 and 20% higher, respectively, and AUCs of oxycodone, noroxycodone, and oxymorphone were 60, 50, and 40% higher, respectively, than values in individuals with normal renal function. The elimination half-life of oxycodone was increased by 1 hour in patients with renal impairment compared with individuals with normal renal function.

Administration of oxycodone hydrochloride extended-release tablets to patients with mild to moderate hepatic impairment resulted in increases in peak plasma concentrations and AUCs of oxycodone (50 and 95%, respectively) and noroxycodone (20 and 65%, respectively) but decreases in peak plasma concentrations and AUC of oxymorphone (30 and 40%, respectively). The elimination half-life of oxycodone was increased by 2.3 hours in patients with mild to moderate hepatic impairment compared with individuals with normal hepatic function.

CHEMISTRY AND STABILITY

● Chemistry

Oxycodone is a synthetic phenanthrene-derivative opiate agonist. The drug differs structurally from hydrocodone only in the attachment of a hydroxyl group to carbon 14 on the phenanthrene nucleus. Oxycodone occurs as long rods or as tautomeric, strongly refringent scales and is insoluble in water and soluble in alcohol. Oxycodone is commercially available as the hydrochloride or myristate salt; the hydrochloride salt is freely soluble in water and slightly soluble in alcohol. Oxycodone hydrochloride oral solution has a pH of 1.4–4.

Oxycodone myristate extended-release capsules contain extended-release microspheres in which oxycodone is present as a solid solution of a fatty acid salt (oxycodone myristate) in a hydrophobic matrix that also contains waxes. Homogeneous dispersion of the drug in the form of a solid solution in fatty acid and waxes imparts extended-release properties.

Extended-release tablets containing oxycodone hydrochloride in fixed combination with acetaminophen are available as a bilayer formulation in which a portion of the labeled oxycodone hydrochloride and acetaminophen doses is contained in an immediate-release layer and the remaining portion is contained in a layer that slowly releases the drugs. The tablets are designed to swell in gastric fluid and gradually release the extended-release components.

● *Stability*

Oxycodone preparations should be stored in tight containers and generally should be protected from light and stored at 15–30°C.

For further information on chemistry, pharmacology, pharmacokinetics, uses, cautions, chronic toxicity, acute toxicity, drug interactions, and dosage and administration of oxycodone, see the Opiate Agonists General Statement 28:08.08.

PREPARATIONS

Oxycodone preparations are subject to control under the Federal Controlled Substances Act of 1970 as schedule II (C-II) drugs.

Preparations containing oxycodone in combination with more than 325 mg of acetaminophen per dosage unit have been discontinued to minimize the risk of inadvertent acetaminophen overdosage.

Excipients in commercially available drug preparations may have clinically important effects in some individuals; consult specific product labeling for details.

oxyCODONE Hydrochloride

Oral

Capsules	5 mg*	oxyCODONE Hydrochloride Capsules (C-II)
Solution	5 mg/5 mL*	oxyCODONE Hydrochloride Oral Solution (C-II)
	100 mg/5 mL*	oxyCODONE Hydrochloride Oral Concentrate Solution (C-II)
Tablets	5 mg*	Oxaydo® (C-II), Egalet
		Oxecta® (C-II), Pfizer
		oxyCODONE Hydrochloride Tablets (C-II)
		Roxicodone® (C-II; scored), Mallinckrodt
	7.5 mg	Oxaydo® (C-II), Egalet
		Oxecta® (C-II), Pfizer
	10 mg*	oxyCODONE Hydrochloride Tablets (C-II)
	15 mg*	oxyCODONE Hydrochloride Tablets (C-II)
		Roxicodone® (C-II; scored), Mallinckrodt
	20 mg*	oxyCODONE Hydrochloride Tablets (C-II)
	30 mg*	oxyCODONE Hydrochloride Tablets (C-II)
		Roxicodone® (C-II), Mallinckrodt
Tablets, extended-release	10 mg	OxyCONTIN® (C-II), Purdue
	15 mg	OxyCONTIN® (C-II), Purdue
	20 mg	OxyCONTIN® (C-II), Purdue
	30 mg	OxyCONTIN® (C-II), Purdue
	40 mg	OxyCONTIN® (C-II), Purdue
	60 mg	OxyCONTIN® (C-II), Purdue
	80 mg	OxyCONTIN® (C-II), Purdue

* available from one or more manufacturer, distributor, and/or repackager by generic (nonproprietary) name

oxyCODONE and Acetaminophen

Oral

Solution	5 mg/5 mL Oxycodone Hydrochloride and Acetaminophen 325 mg/5 mL	Roxicet® (C-II), Roxane
Tablets	2.5 mg Oxycodone Hydrochloride and Acetaminophen 300 mg*	oxyCODONE Hydrochloride and Acetaminophen Tablets (C-II)
	2.5 mg Oxycodone Hydrochloride and Acetaminophen 325 mg*	oxyCODONE Hydrochloride and Acetaminophen Tablets (C-II)
		Percocet® (C-II), Endo
	5 mg Oxycodone Hydrochloride and Acetaminophen 300 mg*	oxyCODONE Hydrochloride and Acetaminophen Tablets
		Primlev® (C-II), Akrimax
	5 mg Oxycodone Hydrochloride and Acetaminophen 325 mg*	Endocet® (C-II; scored), Qualitest
		oxyCODONE Hydrochloride and Acetaminophen Tablets (C-II)
		Percocet® (C-II; scored), Endo
	7.5 mg Oxycodone Hydrochloride and Acetaminophen 300 mg*	oxyCODONE Hydrochloride and Acetaminophen Tablets (C-II)
		Primlev® (C-II), Akrimax
	7.5 mg Oxycodone Hydrochloride and Acetaminophen 325 mg*	Endocet® (C-II), Qualitest
		oxyCODONE Hydrochloride and Acetaminophen Tablets (C-II)
		Percocet® (C-II), Endo
	10 mg Oxycodone Hydrochloride and Acetaminophen 300 mg*	oxyCODONE Hydrochloride and Acetaminophen Tablets (C-II)
		Primlev® (C-II), Akrimax
	10 mg Oxycodone Hydrochloride and Acetaminophen 325 mg*	Endocet® (C-II), Qualitest
		oxyCODONE Hydrochloride and Acetaminophen Tablets (C-II)
		Percocet® (C-II), Endo
Tablets, extended-release, film-coated	7.5 mg Oxycodone Hydrochloride and Acetaminophen 325 mg	Xartemis® XR (C-II), Mallinckrodt

* available from one or more manufacturer, distributor, and/or repackager by generic (nonproprietary) name

oxyCODONE and Aspirin

Oral

Tablets	4.835 mg Oxycodone Hydrochloride and Aspirin 325 mg*	Endodan® (C-II; scored), Endo
		oxyCODONE Hydrochloride and Aspirin Tablets (C-II)

* available from one or more manufacturer, distributor, and/or repackager by generic (nonproprietary) name

Other oxyCODONE Hydrochloride Combinations

Oral

Tablets, film-coated	5 mg with Ibuprofen 400 mg*	oxyCODONE Hydrochloride and Ibuprofen Film-coated Tablets (C-II)

* available from one or more manufacturer, distributor, and/or repackager by generic (nonproprietary) name

oxyCODONE Myristate

Oral

Capsules, extended-release	9 mg (of oxycodone [equivalent to 10 mg oxycodone hydrochloride])	**Xtampza® ER** (C-II), Collegium
	13.5 mg (of oxycodone [equivalent to 15 mg oxycodone hydrochloride])	**Xtampza® ER** (C-II), Collegium
	18 mg (of oxycodone [equivalent to 20 mg oxycodone hydrochloride])	**Xtampza® ER** (C-II), Collegium
	27 mg (of oxycodone [equivalent to 30 mg oxycodone hydrochloride])	**Xtampza® ER** (C-II), Collegium
	36 mg (of oxycodone [equivalent to 40 mg oxycodone hydrochloride])	**Xtampza® ER** (C-II), Collegium

Selected Revisions April 19, 2023, © Copyright, January 01, 1973, American Society of Health-System Pharmacists, Inc.

traMADol Hydrochloride

28:08.08 • OPIOID AGONISTS

■ Tramadol hydrochloride is a synthetic opiate agonist and inhibitor of norepinephrine and serotonin uptake.

REMS

FDA approved a REMS for tramadol under a shared REMS system (Opioid Analgesic REMS) to ensure that the benefits outweigh the risks. The REMS may apply to one or more preparations of tramadol and consists of the following: medication guide and elements to assure safe use. See the FDA REMS page (https://www.accessdata.fda.gov/scripts/cder/rems/index.cfm).

USES

● Pain

Tramadol hydrochloride conventional tablets are used orally for the relief of pain that is severe enough to require an opiate analgesic; because of the risks of addiction, abuse, and misuse associated with opiates even at recommended dosages, conventional preparations of tramadol should be reserved for use in patients for whom alternative treatment options (e.g., nonopiate analgesics) have not been, or are not expected to be, adequate or tolerated. Comparative and noncomparative clinical studies have shown that tramadol is an effective analgesic agent in the treatment of moderately severe acute or chronic pain, including postoperative, gynecologic, and obstetric pain, as well as pain of various other origins, including cancer.

Tramadol hydrochloride extended-release capsules and tablets are used for the relief of pain that is severe enough to require long-term, daily, around-the-clock use of an opiate analgesic. Because of the risks of addiction, abuse, and misuse associated with opiates even at recommended dosages, and because of the greater risks of overdose and death associated with extended-release opiate formulations, these extended-release preparations of tramadol should be reserved for use in patients for whom alternative treatment options (e.g., nonopiate analgesics, immediate-release opiates) are inadequate or not tolerated. These extended-release preparations of tramadol are *not* intended for use on an as-needed ("prn") basis.

Tramadol hydrochloride in fixed combination with acetaminophen (tramadol/acetaminophen) is used for the short-term (5 days or less) management of acute pain that is severe enough to require an opiate analgesic; because of the risks of addiction, abuse, and misuse associated with opiates even at recommended dosages, reserve tramadol/acetaminophen for use in patients for whom alternative treatment options (e.g., nonopiate analgesics) have not been, or are not expected to be, adequate or tolerated.

Tramadol hydrochloride in fixed combination with celecoxib (celecoxib/tramadol) is used for the management of acute pain in adults that is severe enough to require an opiate analgesic and for which alternative treatments are inadequate; because of the risks of addiction, abuse, and misuse associated with opiates even at recommended dosages, reserve celecoxib/tramadol for use in patients for whom alternative treatment options (e.g., nonopiate analgesics) have not been, or are not expected to be, adequate or tolerated.

Single oral doses of tramadol hydrochloride ranging from 50–200 mg (as conventional tablets) have provided relief of postoperative pain in patients who have undergone various types of surgery, including orthopedic, gynecologic, and cesarean section, and in oral surgical procedures (e.g., extraction of impacted molars). In controlled clinical studies of postoperative pain, tramadol hydrochloride administered as a single oral dose of 150 mg was comparable to, or more effective than, the combination of acetaminophen 650 mg and propoxyphene napsylate 100 mg. In patients undergoing oral surgery, a single oral tramadol hydrochloride dose of 50 or 75 mg provided analgesia in some patients, and a single oral dose of 100 mg provided analgesia that was superior to that provided by 60 mg of codeine sulfate but inferior to the combination of codeine phosphate 60 mg and aspirin

650 mg. In a study of patients undergoing dental extraction, a single oral dose of tramadol hydrochloride 75 or 150 mg was more effective than codeine phosphate 60 mg, and tramadol hydrochloride 150 mg was more effective (while tramadol hydrochloride 75 mg was less effective) than acetaminophen 650 mg and propoxyphene napsylate 100 mg.

In several long-term controlled clinical studies of patients with chronic pain (e.g., low back pain, cancer pain, neuropathic pain, pain associated with orthopedic and joint disorders), tramadol hydrochloride dosages averaging 250 mg daily administered in divided doses as conventional tablets were as effective as acetaminophen 300 mg or aspirin 325 mg administered with codeine phosphate 30 mg 5 times daily or acetaminophen 500 mg administered with oxycodone hydrochloride 5 mg 2 or 3 times daily. Tramadol also may be useful in the management of cancer pain when nonopiate-agonist analgesics are no longer effective (i.e., step 2 of the WHO guidelines for cancer pain treatment). In a study of cancer patients with severe chronic pain, tramadol hydrochloride conventional tablets provided effective analgesia but were less effective than an extended-release morphine dosage form; however, patients receiving tramadol experienced only mild adverse effects, none of which resulted in patient withdrawal from the study, while about 23% of patients receiving extended-release morphine withdrew from the study because of severe adverse effects.

Tolerance to tramadol-induced adverse effects may be increased by initiating therapy with a dosage titration regimen. In clinical studies, the rate of discontinuation of tramadol therapy (as conventional tablets) secondary to adverse effects was decreased by utilizing a 10- or 16-day dosage titration regimen for initiating therapy. Fewer patients discontinued therapy because of dizziness or vertigo when the dosage was titrated over 10 days rather than 4 days; similarly, if the dosage was titrated over 16 days rather than 10 days, fewer patients discontinued therapy because of nausea or vomiting, or any cause. When tramadol hydrochloride conventional tablets are used, the manufacturers currently recommend a dosage titration regimen in patients not requiring rapid onset of analgesic effect. (See Dosage and Administration.)

The onset and peak of analgesia occur within 1 and 2–4 hours, respectively, after oral administration of tramadol hydrochloride conventional tablets; peak plasma concentrations of racemic tramadol and its O-desmethyl metabolite (M1) are achieved about 2 and 3 hours, respectively, after oral administration, corresponding to the time of peak analgesic effect. The duration of analgesia produced by a single oral dose of tramadol hydrochloride conventional tablets has been reported to be about 3–6 hours. Following oral administration of the drug as extended-release tablets, peak plasma concentrations of tramadol and its M1 metabolite are achieved about 12 and 15 hours, respectively, after a dose. Following oral administration of the drug as extended-release capsules, peak plasma concentrations of tramadol and its M1 metabolite are achieved about 6 and 11 hours, respectively, after a dose.

Efficacy and safety of tramadol hydrochloride extended-release tablets have been evaluated in clinical studies in adults with chronic, moderate to moderately severe pain associated with osteoarthritis and/or low back pain. Adequate evidence of efficacy was demonstrated in 2 of 4 clinical studies. In a placebo-controlled clinical study of 12 weeks' duration in patients with moderate to moderately severe pain associated with osteoarthritis of the knee or hip, therapy with tramadol hydrochloride extended-release tablets (100 and 200 mg daily) was more effective than placebo as evaluated by changes from baseline in the Western Ontario and McMasters Universities (WOMAC) pain subscale. In a placebo-controlled, flexible-dose study of 12 weeks' duration in patients with osteoarthritis of the knee, therapy with tramadol hydrochloride extended-release tablets (average dose: 270 mg daily) was more effective than placebo as measured by change from baseline on the Arthritis Pain Intensity Visual Analog Scale. Efficacy of tramadol hydrochloride extended-release capsules (which are bioequivalent to the extended-release tablets under fasting conditions) has been evaluated in 4 randomized, placebo-controlled clinical studies of 12 weeks' duration. These studies failed to demonstrate efficacy but differed in design from the clinical studies evaluating the extended-release tablets. In 2 clinical studies, tramadol hydrochloride extended-release capsules were evaluated at dosages of 100, 200, and 300 mg daily in patients with moderate to moderately severe osteoarthritis pain of the hip and knee; the other 2 studies were similar in design, but evaluated only a fixed dosage of 300 mg daily (even in patients who responded to a lower dosage).

A variety of drugs have been used for management of pain in patients with osteoarthritis, including oral agents (e.g., acetaminophen, nonsteroidal anti-inflammatory agents [NSAIAs], tramadol), intra-articular agents (e.g., gluco-corticoids, sodium hyaluronate), and topical agents (e.g., capsaicin, methylsalicy-late). Factors to consider when making treatment decisions for the management of pain in patients with osteoarthritis include the presence of risk factors for seri-ous adverse GI effects or renal toxicity (which may affect decisions regarding use of NSAIAs), existing comorbidities and concomitant therapy, and the adverse effects profiles and costs of specific therapies.

Because there is evidence that acetaminophen can be effective and because of its relative safety and low cost, the American College of Rheumatology (ACR) rec-ommends use of the drug as the initial analgesic for many osteoarthritis patients. Acetaminophen appears to be as effective as NSAIAs for relief of mild to moder-ate joint pain in many patients with osteoarthritis; however, the drug is not effec-tive in all patients and may not provide adequate relief in those with moderate to severe pain or when joint inflammation is present. An NSAIA can be considered an alternative initial drug of choice for patients with osteoarthritis, especially for those who have moderate to severe pain and signs of joint inflammation, and also can be considered in patients who fail to obtain adequate symptomatic relief with acetaminophen. Tramadol can be considered in patients in whom NSAIAs are contraindicated (e.g., those with renal impairment) or in whom acetaminophen or NSAIAs have not produced an adequate response.

In controlled single-dose studies in patients with acute pain following oral surgery, analgesia provided by tramadol hydrochloride (75 mg) in fixed combina-tion with acetaminophen (650 mg) was comparable to that provided by ibuprofen 400 mg, and superior to that provided by monotherapy with tramadol hydrochlo-ride 75 mg or acetaminophen 650 mg or by placebo. Onset of pain relief occurred in about 17 minutes in patients receiving the fixed combination of tramadol and acetaminophen and about 15 minutes in those receiving acetaminophen alone. Onset of pain relief occurred in about 30 minutes in patients receiving either tra-madol alone or ibuprofen. Duration of pain relief was about 5 hours in patients receiving either tramadol in fixed combination with acetaminophen or ibuprofen, but was about 2 hours with administration of tramadol alone and 3 hours with acetaminophen alone.

For further information on the role of opiate analgesics in the management of acute or chronic pain, see Uses: Pain, in the Opiate Agonists General State-ment 28:08.08.

DOSAGE AND ADMINISTRATION

● Administration

Tramadol hydrochloride alone or in fixed combination with acetaminophen or celecoxib is administered orally.

Since food does not affect substantially the rate or extent of absorption of tra-madol hydrochloride administered alone as conventional tablets, the manufactur-ers state that conventional tablets of the drug can be taken without regard to food. Food may decrease the rate and extent of absorption of tramadol when the drug is administered as extended-release tablets (delaying peak plasma concentrations by about 3 hours and decreasing the extent of absorption by about 16%); the manu-facturer states that although tramadol hydrochloride extended-release tablets may be administered once daily without regard to food, the extended-release tablets should be administered in a consistent manner relative to food intake. The man-ufacturer also recommends that tramadol hydrochloride extended-release cap-sules be administered in a consistent manner relative to food intake, although the rate and extent of absorption are similar following oral administration with or without food. Food delays absorption of tramadol hydrochloride and acetamino-phen administered in fixed combination, increasing times to peak plasma concen-trations by about 35 and 60 minutes, respectively. However, food does not affect peak plasma concentrations achieved or the extent of absorption of the drugs, and the clinical importance of the delays in absorption is unknown. The manufac-turers make no specific recommendation regarding administration of the fixed-combination preparation with food.

Tramadol hydrochloride extended-release tablets or capsules should be swal-lowed whole and should not be broken, crushed, chewed, split, or dissolved, since such physical alteration of the tablets or capsules could result in rapid release of the drug and absorption of a potentially fatal overdose. The extended-release preparations should not be used concomitantly with other tramadol-containing preparations.

For patients receiving tramadol hydrochloride conventional tablets alone for the relief of moderate to moderately severe pain and not requiring rapid onset of analgesic effect, the manufacturers recommend a dosage titration regimen to decrease the likelihood of discontinuance secondary to adverse effects (e.g., nau-sea, vomiting, dizziness, vertigo) associated with administration at higher initial dosages.

● Dosage

Opiate agonists should be given at the lowest effective dosage and for the shortest duration of therapy consistent with the treatment goals of the patient. The initial dosage of tramadol must be individualized, taking into account the patient's sever-ity of pain, response, prior analgesic use, and risk factors for addiction, abuse, and misuse. Dosage should be titrated to a level that provides adequate analgesia and minimizes adverse effects. If concomitant therapy with other CNS depressants is required, the lowest effective dosages and shortest possible duration of con-comitant therapy should be used. (See Concomitant Use with Benzodiazepines or Other CNS Depressants under Cautions: Precautions and Contraindications.)

Because of the greater frequency of decreased hepatic, renal, and/or cardiac function and of concomitant disease and/or drug therapy in geriatric patients, care should be taken in dosage selection for such patients. The manufacturers rec-ommend that geriatric patients receive initial dosages of tramadol hydrochloride alone in the lower end of the usual range and that the dosage not exceed 300 mg daily in those older than 75 years of age. Dosage of tramadol hydrochloride should be titrated slowly in geriatric patients, with close monitoring for CNS and respi-ratory depression.

Appropriate dosage selection and titration are essential to reduce the risk of respiratory depression. Patients should be monitored closely for respiratory depression, especially during the first 24–72 hours of therapy and following any increase in dosage.

Patients receiving opiate analgesics should be reevaluated continually for ade-quacy of pain control and for adverse effects, as well as for manifestations of opi-ate withdrawal and for the development of addiction, abuse, or misuse. During long-term therapy, the continued need for opiate analgesics should be continually reevaluated. Frequent communication among the prescriber, other members of the healthcare team, the patient, and the patient's caregiver or family is important during periods of changing analgesic requirements, including the initial dosage titration period. Patients with chronic pain who experience episodes of break-through pain may require dosage adjustment or supplemental analgesia (i.e., "res-cue" therapy with an immediate-release analgesic). If the level of pain increases after dosage stabilization, an attempt should be made to identify the source of increased pain before increasing the dosage.

For acute pain not related to trauma or surgery, the prescribed quantity should be limited to the amount needed for the expected duration of pain severe enough to require opiate analgesia (generally 3 days or less and rarely more than 7 days).

When opiate analgesics are used for the management of chronic noncancer pain, the US Centers for Disease Control and Prevention (CDC) recommends that primary care clinicians carefully reassess individual benefits and risks before prescribing dosages equivalent to 50 mg or more of morphine sulfate daily and avoid dosages equivalent to 90 mg or more of morphine sulfate daily or carefully justify their decision to titrate the dosage to such levels. Other experts recommend consulting a pain management specialist before exceeding a dosage equivalent to 80–120 mg of morphine sulfate daily.

If discontinuance of opiate therapy is required in a patient who may be physi-cally dependent on opiates, the dosage should be tapered gradually to avoid man-ifestations of abrupt withdrawal. When tramadol therapy is discontinued in such patients, dosage generally can be reduced by 25–50% every 2–4 days. If manifes-tations of withdrawal occur, the dosage should be increased to the prior level and tapered more slowly (i.e., by increasing the interval between dosage reductions and/or reducing the amount of each incremental change in dose).

For further information on the management of opiate analgesic therapy, see Dosage and Administration: Dosage, in the Opiate Agonists General Statement 28:08.08.

Conventional (Immediate-release) Tablets

Adults with moderate to moderately severe chronic pain not requiring rapid onset of analgesic effect may initially receive tramadol hydrochloride conventional tablets using a dosage titration regimen; the manufacturers recommend an initial dosage of 25 mg daily in the morning, increased by increments of 25 mg every 3 days as separate doses up to a dosage of 25 mg 4 times daily. Thereafter, daily dosage of conventional tablets may be increased as tolerated by 50 mg every 3 days, up to 50 mg 4 times daily. Following titration, 50–100 mg of conventional tablets may be administered every 4–6 hours as needed. Dosages exceeding 400 mg daily are not recommended by the manufacturers.

Adults requiring rapid onset of analgesia, and in whom the benefit of rapid onset of analgesia outweighs the risk of drug discontinuance secondary to adverse effects associated with higher initial dosage, may receive tramadol hydrochloride conventional tablets in a dosage of 50–100 mg every 4–6 hours. Dosages exceeding 400 mg daily are not recommended by the manufacturers.

Tramadol Hydrochloride in Fixed Combination with Acetaminophen

When tramadol hydrochloride is used in fixed combination with acetaminophen for the short-term (5 days or less) management of acute pain in adults, the usual dosage is 75 mg of tramadol hydrochloride every 4–6 hours as needed, up to a maximum of 300 mg daily.

Tramadol Hydrochloride in Fixed Combination with Celecoxib

When tramadol hydrochloride is used in fixed combination with celecoxib for the management of acute pain in adults, the recommended dosage is 2 tablets (containing 56 mg of celecoxib and 44 mg of tramadol hydrochloride each) every 12 hours as needed for relief of pain.

Extended-release Tablets and Capsules

When tramadol hydrochloride extended-release tablets or capsules are used in the management of chronic pain in adults who are not currently receiving tramadol, the recommended initial dosage is 100 mg once daily. The daily dosage may be increased in 100-mg increments every 5 days as needed and tolerated. Dosages exceeding 300 mg daily are not recommended by the manufacturers.

Because ratios for conversion from other opiate analgesics to extended-release preparations of tramadol hydrochloride have not been established in clinical trials, the manufacturers state that patients being switched from therapy with other opiate agonists should receive an initial tramadol hydrochloride dosage of 100 mg daily as extended-release tablets or capsules. For patients receiving conventional tramadol hydrochloride preparations, the total daily dosage of the drug should be calculated and rounded down to the next lower 100-mg increment for administration as the extended-release tablets or capsules; the dosage may then be adjusted according to patient requirements. Patients being switched from immediate-release to extended-release preparations of tramadol should be monitored closely for sedation and respiratory depression since data establishing the relative bioavailability of these formulations are lacking. Because of limitations in dose selection, some patients may not be successfully switched from immediate-release to extended-release preparations of the drug. All other around-the-clock opiate analgesics should be discontinued when therapy with the extended-release preparation is initiated.

● Dosage in Renal and Hepatic Impairment

Dosage of tramadol hydrochloride (as conventional tablets) should be reduced in certain patients with renal or hepatic impairment by decreasing the frequency of administration. Adults with creatinine clearances less than 30 mL/minute may receive oral tramadol hydrochloride conventional tablets in a dosage of 50–100 mg every 12 hours, not to exceed 200 mg daily. Since less than 7% of a dose of tramadol hydrochloride is removed by hemodialysis, patients undergoing dialysis may receive their usual dosage on the day of dialysis. Adults with hepatic cirrhosis may receive the conventional tablets in a dosage of 50 mg every 12 hours.

Tramadol hydrochloride extended-release oral formulations should not be used in patients with severe renal impairment (creatinine clearances less than 30 mL/minute) or severe hepatic impairment (Child-Pugh class C). The available tablet or capsule strengths and once-daily dosing of these formulations do not provide sufficient dosing flexibility for safe use in these patients.

Adults with creatinine clearances of less than 30 mL/minute may receive tramadol hydrochloride in fixed combination with acetaminophen at a dosing interval of every 12 hours; in such patients, the dosage of tramadol hydrochloride

administered as the fixed combination should not exceed 75 mg every 12 hours. Tramadol hydrochloride in fixed combination with acetaminophen should *not* be used in patients with impaired hepatic function.

CAUTIONS

At recommended dosages, tramadol generally is well tolerated. Adverse effects usually have been mild and similar in incidence to active controls (i.e., acetaminophen 300 mg with codeine phosphate 30 mg and aspirin 325 mg with codeine phosphate 30 mg). The frequency of some adverse effects may be related to dose and route of administration. The most common adverse effects observed with tramadol in controlled clinical trials and open-label extension periods enrolling patients with chronic nonmalignant pain were nervous system effects (e.g., dizziness) and GI disturbances.

● Nervous System Effects

The most frequent adverse nervous system effect of tramadol is dizziness or vertigo, which occurred in 26, 31, and 33% of patients receiving tramadol hydrochloride conventional tablets for up to 7, 30, and 90 days, respectively, in clinical studies. In patients receiving tramadol hydrochloride as extended-release tablets in clinical studies, dizziness was reported in about 16, 20, 23, or 28% of patients receiving the drug in a dosage of 100, 200, 300, or 400 mg once daily, respectively. In patients receiving tramadol hydrochloride as extended-release capsules in clinical studies, dizziness was reported in about 10, 12, or 14% of patients receiving the drug in a dosage of 100, 200, or 300 mg once daily, respectively. The incidence of dizziness may be dose related.

Headache occurred in 18, 26, and 32% of patients, and somnolence occurred in 16, 23, and 25% of patients receiving the conventional tablets for up to 7, 30, and 90 days, respectively. Headache was reported in up to 16 or 23% of patients receiving tramadol hydrochloride as extended-release tablets or extended-release capsules, respectively, at recommended dosages (100–300 mg daily) in clinical studies. Somnolence or insomnia occurred in up to 11 or 9%, respectively, of patients receiving recommended dosages of tramadol hydrochloride extended-release tablets and in up to 16 or 5%, respectively, of patients receiving recommended dosages of tramadol hydrochloride extended-release capsules in clinical studies. Weakness has been reported in up to 4% of patients receiving the extended-release tablets in recommended dosages.

CNS stimulation (a composite of nervousness, anxiety, agitation, tremor, spasticity, euphoria, emotional lability, and hallucinations) occurred in 7, 11, and 14% of patients receiving tramadol hydrochloride conventional tablets for up to 7, 30, and 90 days, respectively. Asthenia occurred in 6, 11, and 12% of patients, and sweating occurred in 6, 7, and 9% of patients receiving the conventional tablets for up to 7, 30, and 90 days, respectively. Sweating may be more common following rapid IV injection. Asthenia or increased sweating was reported in up to 7 or 4%, respectively, of patients receiving recommended dosages of tramadol hydrochloride extended-release tablets in clinical studies. Asthenia or increased sweating was reported in up to 9% or 7%, respectively, of patients receiving recommended dosages of the extended-release capsules in clinical studies.

● GI Effects

Constipation is the most common adverse GI effect of tramadol, occurring in 24, 38, and 46% of patients receiving tramadol hydrochloride conventional tablets for up to 7, 30, and 90 days, respectively, in clinical studies. Nausea occurred in 24, 34, and 40% of patients, and vomiting occurred in 9, 13, and 17% of patients receiving conventional tablets of the drug for up to 7, 30, and 90 days, respectively. Nausea, constipation, vomiting, or anorexia has been reported in up to 26, 22, 9, or 5%, respectively, of patients receiving recommended dosages of tramadol hydrochloride extended-release tablets (100–300 mg daily) in clinical studies. Nausea, constipation, vomiting, or anorexia has been reported in up to 25, 21, 10, or 6%, respectively, of patients receiving recommended dosages of the extended-release capsules (100–300 mg daily) in clinical studies. Nausea and vomiting may occur more frequently with higher doses and following rapid IV injection.

Other adverse GI effects reported in patients receiving conventional tablets of the drug include dyspepsia, which occurred in 5, 9, and 13% of patients, dry mouth, which occurred in 5, 9, and 10%, and diarrhea, which occurred in 5, 6, and

10% of patients receiving tramadol for up to 7, 30, and 90 days, respectively. Dry mouth or diarrhea was reported in up to 10 or 9%, respectively, of patients receiving recommended dosages of tramadol hydrochloride extended-release tablets in clinical studies. Dry mouth also was reported in up to 13% of patients receiving recommended dosages of the extended-release capsules in clinical studies.

● Sensitivity Reactions

Pruritus occurred in 8, 10, and 11% of patients receiving tramadol hydrochloride conventional tablets for up to 7, 30, and 90 days, respectively; in up to 9% of patients receiving the extended-release tablets in recommended dosages (100–300 mg daily); and in up to 7% of patients receiving the extended-release capsules in recommended dosages (100–300 mg daily). Rash or dermatitis was reported in 1% to less than 5% of patients receiving the drug in clinical trials. Serious and rarely fatal anaphylactoid reactions, often occurring after the initial dose, have been reported in patients receiving tramadol. (See Cautions: Precautions and Contraindications.) Urticaria, bronchospasm, and angioedema have occurred.

● Cardiovascular Effects

Vasodilation has been reported in 1% to less than 5% of patients receiving tramadol hydrochloride conventional tablets in clinical trials. Postural hypotension or flushing occurred in up to 4 or 10%, respectively, of patients receiving tramadol hydrochloride extended-release tablets in recommended dosages (100–300 mg daily) in clinical studies.

● Genitourinary and Endocrine Effects

Hypoglycemia has been reported very rarely in patients receiving tramadol, mainly in patients with predisposing risk factors (e.g., diabetes mellitus, renal insufficiency) or in geriatric patients. Increased blood glucose concentrations have occurred in patients receiving tramadol hydrochloride extended-release tablets.

Adrenal insufficiency has been reported in patients receiving opiate agonists or opiate partial agonists. Manifestations of adrenal insufficiency are nonspecific and may include nausea, vomiting, anorexia, fatigue, weakness, dizziness, and hypotension. The onset generally has occurred after at least 1 month of opiate agonist or partial agonist use, although the time to onset has ranged from within 1 day to more than 1 year. In many of the reported cases, patients required hospitalization. If adrenal insufficiency is suspected, appropriate laboratory testing should be performed promptly and physiologic (replacement) dosages of corticosteroids provided; therapy with the opiate agonist or partial agonist should be tapered and discontinued to allow recovery of adrenal function. If the opiate agonist or partial agonist can be discontinued, follow-up assessment of adrenal function should be performed to determine if corticosteroid replacement therapy can be discontinued. In some patients, switching to a different opiate improved symptoms.

Hypogonadism and androgen deficiency have been reported in patients receiving long-term opiate agonist or opiate partial agonist therapy, although a causal relationship has not been established. Patients receiving long-term opiate agonist or partial agonist therapy who present with manifestations of hypogonadism (e.g., decreased libido, impotence, erectile dysfunction, amenorrhea, infertility) should undergo laboratory evaluation.

● Acute Toxicity

Manifestations

Tramadol taken in excessive doses, either alone or in combination with other CNS depressants, is a cause of drug-related deaths. Fatalities associated with both intentional and unintentional overdose have been reported. Estimates of ingested dose in non-US fatalities ranged from 3–5 g. A 3-g intentional overdose by a patient enrolled in a clinical trial produced emesis and no sequelae. The lowest tramadol hydrochloride dose reportedly associated with fatality was possibly between 0.5–1 g in a 40-kg woman, but details of the case are not completely known. Tramadol is intended for oral use only. Crushing, cutting, breaking, or chewing tramadol hydrochloride extended-release tablets or capsules, "snorting" the powder, or injecting dissolved contents of the tablets or capsules results in uncontrolled delivery of tramadol and poses a risk of a potentially fatal overdose. The risk of a fatal overdose is increased when tramadol is misused concurrently with other CNS depressants (e.g., alcohol, other opiates). Manifestations of overdosage are similar to those of other opiate agonists, with the most serious potential consequences being respiratory depression, lethargy, skeletal muscle flaccidity, coma,

seizure, bradycardia, hypotension, pulmonary edema, partial or complete airway obstruction, cardiac arrest, cardiac collapse, and death. Death may occur within 1 hour of overdosage. Other manifestations may include miosis, vomiting, cold and clammy skin, and atypical snoring. Marked mydriasis (rather than miosis) may be observed in patients with hypoxia.

Treatment

When treating tramadol overdosage, primary attention should be given to maintaining adequate ventilation along with general supportive treatment (including administration of oxygen and vasopressors as clinically indicated). Tramadol hydrochloride extended-release tablets or capsules will continue to release the drug for 24–48 hours or longer following ingestion, necessitating prolonged monitoring. An opiate antagonist should be administered if clinically important respiratory or circulatory depression is present, but should not be administered in the absence of such manifestations. Although an opiate antagonist (e.g., naloxone, nalmefene) will reverse some, but not all, manifestations of tramadol overdosage, the risk of seizures also is increased with naloxone administration. In animals, seizures following the administration of toxic tramadol doses could be suppressed with barbiturates or benzodiazepines but were increased with naloxone. Naloxone administration did not change the lethality of an overdose in mice. Hemodialysis is unlikely to be helpful in a tramadol overdosage because it removes less than 7% of the administered dose in a 4-hour dialysis period.

● Precautions and Contraindications

General Opiate Agonist Precautions

Administration of tramadol may cause effects similar to those produced by other opiate agonist drugs, and the usual precautions of opiate agonist therapy should be observed. (See Description and the manufacturers' labeling.)

Extended-release preparations of tramadol should be prescribed only by clinicians who are knowledgeable in the use of potent opiates for the management of chronic pain.

Addiction, Abuse, and Misuse

Tramadol exposes patients and other users to the risks of opiate addiction (opiate use disorder [OUD]), abuse, and misuse, which can lead to overdosage and death. The abuse potential of tramadol is less than that of morphine or oxycodone but similar to that of propoxyphene (see Description). Addiction can occur with appropriately prescribed or illicitly obtained opiates, and at recommended dosages or with misuse or abuse. Concurrent abuse of alcohol or other CNS depressants increases the risk of toxicity. Each patient's risk for addiction, abuse, and misuse should be assessed prior to initiating tramadol therapy, and all patients receiving the drug should be monitored for development of these behaviors or conditions. Personal or family history of substance abuse (drug or alcohol addiction or abuse) or mental illness (e.g., major depression) increases risk. The potential for addiction, abuse, and misuse should not prevent opiate prescribing for appropriate pain management, but does necessitate intensive counseling about risks and proper use and intensive monitoring for signs of addiction, abuse, and misuse. Tramadol should be prescribed in the smallest appropriate quantity and the patient should be instructed on secure storage and proper disposal to prevent theft.

Extended-release opiates are associated with a greater risk of overdosage and death because of the larger amount of drug contained in each dosage unit. Abuse or misuse of tramadol extended-release tablets or capsules by splitting, crushing, breaking, cutting, or chewing the tablets or capsules, snorting the contents, or injecting the dissolved contents will result in uncontrolled delivery of tramadol and can result in a fatal overdosage. IV injection of excipients in these formulations can result in local tissue necrosis, infection, pulmonary granulomas, embolism, and death and increase the risk of endocarditis and valvular heart injury.

Respiratory Depression

Serious, life-threatening, or fatal respiratory depression can occur in patients receiving opiates, even when used as recommended. Although respiratory depression can occur at any time during therapy, the risk is greatest during initiation of therapy and following an increase in dosage; therefore, patients receiving tramadol should be monitored closely for respiratory depression, especially during the first 24–72 hours of therapy and following any increase in dosage. Appropriate dosage selection and titration are essential to reduce the risk of respiratory depression. Large initial doses in nontolerant patients, overestimation of the initial tramadol dosage when transferring patients from another opiate analgesic, or accidental ingestion of even one dose of tramadol, especially by a child, can result in respiratory depression and death. For clinically important respiratory depression resulting from tramadol overdosage, an opiate antagonist should be administered. (See Treatment under Cautions: Acute Toxicity.)

Geriatric, cachectic, or debilitated patients are at increased risk of life-threatening respiratory depression. In patients with chronic obstructive pulmonary disease or cor pulmonale, substantially decreased respiratory reserve, hypoxia, hypercapnia, or preexisting respiratory depression, even recommended doses of tramadol may decrease respiratory drive to the point of apnea. Such patients should be monitored closely, particularly following initiation of therapy, during dosage titration, and during concomitant therapy with other respiratory depressants. Alternatively, use of nonopiate analgesics should be considered in such patients. Use of tramadol in patients with substantial respiratory depression or in those with severe bronchial asthma in unmonitored settings or in the absence of resuscitative equipment is contraindicated.

Because of the risks associated with opiate overdosage, clinicians should routinely discuss the availability of the opiate antagonist naloxone with all patients receiving new or reauthorized prescriptions for opiate analgesics, including tramadol. Clinicians should consider prescribing naloxone for patients receiving opiate analgesics who are at increased risk of opiate overdosage (e.g., those receiving concomitant therapy with benzodiazepines or other CNS depressants, those with a history of opiate or substance use disorder, those with medical conditions that could increase sensitivity to opiate effects, those who have experienced a prior opiate overdose) or who have household members, including children, or other close contacts who are at risk for accidental ingestion or overdosage. Even if patients are not receiving an opiate analgesic, a naloxone prescription should be considered if the patient is at increased risk of opiate overdosage (e.g., those with a current or past diagnosis of OUD, those who have experienced a prior opiate overdose). (See Naloxone Hydrochloride 28:10.)

Drugs Affecting Hepatic Microsomal Enzymes

Because orally administered tramadol undergoes extensive hepatic metabolism, including metabolism by cytochrome P-450 (CYP) isoenzymes 2D6 and 3A4, concomitant use of drugs that inhibit or induce CYP3A4 or inhibit CYP2D6 requires careful consideration of the effects on tramadol and its active O-desmethyl metabolite (M1) (see Description).

Because formation of M1 is dependent on CYP2D6 activity, concomitant use of tramadol and CYP2D6 inhibitors (e.g., amiodarone, bupropion, fluoxetine, paroxetine, quinidine) may result in increased plasma concentrations of tramadol and decreased concentrations of M1, particularly when the CYP2D6 inhibitor is initiated after a stable dosage of tramadol has been achieved. The increase in tramadol concentrations can result in increased or prolonged therapeutic effects and an increased risk of serious adverse effects, including seizures and serotonin syndrome, while the decrease in M1 concentrations may result in reduced therapeutic effects and, in patients physically dependent on opiates, manifestations of opiate withdrawal. Discontinuance of the CYP2D6 inhibitor may result in a decrease in plasma concentrations of tramadol and an increase in M1 concentrations, which could increase or prolong therapeutic effects or manifestations of opiate toxicity and potentially cause fatal respiratory depression. If concomitant therapy with tramadol and a CYP2D6 inhibitor is required, patients should be monitored closely for serious tramadol-related adverse effects (including seizures and serotonin syndrome) and manifestations of opiate toxicity or opiate withdrawal. If concomitant therapy with a CYP2D6 inhibitor is discontinued, the patient should be monitored closely for adverse effects, including respiratory depression and sedation, and consideration should be given to reducing the tramadol dosage until stable drug effects are achieved.

Concomitant use of tramadol and CYP3A4 inhibitors, such as macrolide antibiotics (e.g., erythromycin), azole antifungals (e.g., ketoconazole), or HIV protease inhibitors (e.g., ritonavir), can increase plasma concentrations of tramadol, which may result in larger amounts of parent drug being metabolized by CYP2D6 and higher concentrations of M1. If concomitant therapy with tramadol and a CYP3A4 inhibitor is required, patients should be monitored closely for serious adverse effects (including seizures and serotonin syndrome) and for manifestations of opiate toxicity (including sedation and potentially fatal respiratory depression), particularly when the CYP3A4 inhibitor is initiated after a stable

dosage of tramadol has been achieved, and consideration should be given to reducing the tramadol dosage until stable drug effects are achieved. If concomitant therapy with a CYP3A4 inhibitor is discontinued, the patient should be monitored for manifestations of opiate withdrawal, and consideration should be given to increasing the tramadol dosage until stable drug effects are achieved.

Concomitant use of tramadol and CYP3A4 inducers (e.g., carbamazepine, phenytoin, rifampin) can decrease plasma concentrations of tramadol, resulting in decreased efficacy and, in patients who are physically dependent on opiates, manifestations of opiate withdrawal. Discontinuance of the CYP3A4 inducer may result in increased plasma concentrations of tramadol, which could increase or prolong both the therapeutic and adverse effects of tramadol and may cause seizures, serotonin syndrome, and potentially fatal respiratory depression. If concomitant therapy with tramadol and a CYP3A4 inducer is required, patients should be monitored for manifestations of opiate withdrawal, and consideration should be given to increasing the tramadol dosage until stable drug effects are achieved. If concomitant therapy with a CYP3A4 inducer is discontinued, patients should be monitored for seizures, serotonin syndrome, sedation, and respiratory depression, and consideration should be given to decreasing the tramadol dosage until stable drug effects are achieved.

Concomitant use of tramadol with carbamazepine is not recommended because carbamazepine increases tramadol metabolism and substantially reduces tramadol's analgesic effect, and because tramadol is associated with increased risk of seizures.

Concomitant Use with Benzodiazepines or Other CNS Depressants

Tramadol may potentiate the respiratory and CNS depressant effects of other CNS depressants. Concomitant use of tramadol with benzodiazepines or other CNS depressants (e.g., anxiolytics, sedatives, hypnotics, tranquilizers, muscle relaxants, general anesthetics, antipsychotics, other opiate agonists, alcohol) may result in profound sedation, respiratory depression, hypotension, coma, and death. (See Cautions: Acute Toxicity.) Concomitant use of such drugs should be reserved for patients in whom alternative treatment options are inadequate; the lowest effective dosages and shortest possible duration of concomitant therapy should be used, and the patient should be monitored closely for respiratory depression and sedation. Concomitant use with alcohol should be avoided. Clinicians should consider prescribing the opiate antagonist naloxone for patients receiving opiates who are at increased risk of opiate overdosage, including those receiving benzodiazepines or other CNS depressants concomitantly. (See Drug Interactions: Benzodiazepines and Other CNS Depressants, in the Opiate Agonists General Statement 28:08.08.)

If a benzodiazepine or other CNS depressant is required for any indication other than epilepsy in a patient receiving tramadol, the drug should be initiated at a lower dosage than indicated in the absence of opiate therapy and titrated based on clinical response. In patients receiving a CNS depressant, tramadol, if required, should be initiated at a reduced dosage and titrated based on clinical response.

Serotonin Syndrome

Potentially life-threatening serotonin syndrome may occur with tramadol, particularly with concurrent use of other serotonergic drugs, drugs that impair the metabolism of serotonin (e.g., monoamine oxidase [MAO] inhibitors), or drugs that impair the metabolism of tramadol (e.g., inhibitors of CYP2D6 and CYP3A4). Manifestations of serotonin syndrome may include mental status changes (e.g., agitation, hallucinations, coma), autonomic instability (e.g., tachycardia, labile blood pressure, hyperthermia), neuromuscular aberrations (e.g., hyperreflexia, incoordination, rigidity), and/or GI symptoms (e.g., nausea, vomiting, diarrhea). Symptom onset generally occurs within several hours to a few days of concomitant use, but may occur later, particularly after dosage increases. (See Drugs Associated with Serotonin Syndrome under Cautions: Precautions and Contraindications.)

Seizures

Seizures have occurred during tramadol therapy with recommended dosages. Spontaneous postmarketing reports indicate that seizure risk is increased with tramadol doses above the recommended range. Seizures can occur following the first dose. The manufacturers warn that tramadol increases the seizure risk in patients taking selective serotonin-reuptake inhibitors (SSRIs), selective serotonin- and norepinephrine-reuptake inhibitors (SNRIs), anorectic agents, tricyclic antidepressants or other tricyclic compounds (e.g., cyclobenzaprine, promethazine), or other opiate agonists. The manufacturers also warn that the drug may enhance the risk of seizure in those receiving MAO inhibitors, antipsychotic agents, or other drugs that decrease the seizure threshold. Patients with epilepsy, those with a history of seizures, or patients with a recognized risk for seizure (e.g., head trauma, metabolic disorders, alcohol and drug withdrawal, CNS infections) may be at increased risk of seizure. Naloxone administration in patients with tramadol overdose also may increase the risk of seizure.

Suicide

Tramadol should not be prescribed for individuals who are suicidal or prone to addiction. Tramadol should be used with caution in patients with a history of misuse, patients receiving concomitant therapy with CNS-active drugs including tranquilizers or antidepressants, individuals with excessive alcohol consumption, and patients with emotional disturbances or depression. The use of alternative analgesics without opiate agonist activity should be considered in suicidal or depressed patients. (See Cautions: Acute Toxicity.)

Monoamine Oxidase Inhibitors

Concomitant use of opiates with MAO inhibitors (e.g., linezolid, phenelzine, tranylcypromine) may increase the risk of serotonin syndrome, seizures, and opiate toxicity (e.g., respiratory depression, coma). Use of tramadol is contraindicated in patients who are currently receiving or have recently (within 14 days) received an MAO inhibitor.

Pharmacogenomics

Tramadol is metabolized by the CYP microsomal enzyme system, principally by CYP2D6 to its active M1 metabolite. Metabolism of certain drugs, including tramadol, is influenced by CYP2D6 polymorphism. Individuals who lack functional alleles of the CYP2D6 gene are described as poor metabolizers, those with one or two functional alleles are described as extensive metabolizers, and those who carry a duplicate or amplified gene are described as ultrarapid metabolizers. Population pharmacokinetic analysis of phase 1 studies of tramadol hydrochloride conventional tablets in healthy individuals indicated that concentrations of tramadol were approximately 20% higher and those of M1 were 40% lower in poor metabolizers compared with extensive metabolizers.

Genetically determined differences in drug metabolism can affect an individual's response to a drug or risk of having an adverse event. Individuals who are poor metabolizers may experience reduced analgesic effects of tramadol; individuals who are ultrarapid metabolizers are likely to have higher than expected serum concentrations of M1. To minimize the risk of adverse events in individuals who are ultrarapid metabolizers of CYP2D6, FDA states that tramadol should *not* be used in such patients. Variations in CYP2D6 polymorphism occur at different frequencies among subpopulations of different ethnic or racial origin. Approximately 1–7% of Caucasians and 10–30% of Ethiopians and Saudi Arabians carry the genotype associated with ultra-rapid metabolism of CYP2D6 substrates.

Drugs Associated with Serotonin Syndrome

Serotonin syndrome may occur when tramadol is used concurrently with other serotonergic drugs, including serotonin (5-hydroxytryptamine; 5-HT) type 1 (5-HT$_1$) receptor agonists ("triptans"), SSRIs, SNRIs, tricyclic antidepressants, antiemetics that are 5-HT$_3$ receptor antagonists, buspirone, cyclobenzaprine, dextromethorphan, lithium, St. John's wort (*Hypericum perforatum*), tryptophan, other serotonin modulators (e.g., mirtazapine, nefazodone, trazodone, vilazodone), and MAO inhibitors (both those used to treat psychiatric disorders and others, such as linezolid, methylene blue, and selegiline). Serotonin syndrome may occur within the recommended dosage ranges for these drugs. Serotonin syndrome has been reported during postmarketing experience in patients receiving tramadol concomitantly with MAO inhibitors, SSRIs, SNRIs, or α$_2$-adrenergic blocking agents. Tramadol decreases the synaptic reuptake of the monoamine neurotransmitters norepinephrine and serotonin, and animal studies have shown increased deaths with combined administration of tramadol and MAO inhibitors. Manifestations of serotonin syndrome may include mental status changes (e.g., agitation, hallucinations, coma), autonomic instability (e.g., tachycardia, labile blood pressure, hyperthermia), neuromuscular aberrations (e.g., hyperreflexia,

incoordination, rigidity), and/or GI symptoms (e.g., nausea, vomiting, diarrhea). Symptom onset generally occurs within several hours to a few days of concomitant use, but may occur later, particularly after dosage increases.

If concomitant use of other serotonergic drugs is warranted, great caution is advised and patients should be monitored for serotonin syndrome, particularly during initiation of therapy and dosage increases. If serotonin syndrome is suspected, treatment with tramadol, other opiate therapy, and/or any concurrently administered serotonergic agents should be discontinued.

For further information on serotonin syndrome, including manifestations and treatment, see Drug Interactions: Serotonergic Drugs, in Fluoxetine Hydrochloride 28:16.04.20.

Hypotension

Tramadol may cause severe hypotension, including orthostatic hypotension and syncope, in ambulatory patients. Because the risk of severe hypotension is increased in patients whose ability to maintain blood pressure has been compromised by blood volume depletion or concomitant use of certain CNS depressants (e.g., phenothiazines, general anesthetics), such patients should be monitored for hypotension following initiation of tramadol therapy or an increase in tramadol dosage. Use of tramadol should be avoided in patients with circulatory shock since the drug may cause vasodilation that can further reduce cardiac output and blood pressure.

Increased Intracranial Pressure or Head Injury

The respiratory depressant effects of opiate agonists promote carbon dioxide retention, which can result in elevation of intracranial pressure. Patients who may be particularly susceptible to these effects (e.g., those with evidence of elevated intracranial pressure or brain tumors) should be monitored closely for sedation and respiratory depression, particularly during initiation of therapy. Opiates also may obscure the clinical course in patients with head injuries. Use of tramadol should be avoided in patients with impaired consciousness or coma.

GI Conditions

Opiates may increase serum amylase concentrations and cause spasm of the sphincter of Oddi. Patients with biliary tract disease, including those with acute pancreatitis, should be monitored for worsening symptoms. Tramadol is contraindicated in patients with known or suspected GI obstruction, including paralytic ileus.

Sensitivity Reactions

Serious and rarely fatal anaphylactoid reactions have been reported in patients receiving tramadol. These reactions often occur following the first dose. Other reported hypersensitivity reactions include pruritus, urticaria, angioedema, bronchospasm, toxic epidermal necrolysis, and Stevens-Johnson syndrome. The manufacturers warn that patients with a history of anaphylactoid reactions to codeine or other opiate agonists may be at increased risk and therefore should not receive tramadol. If anaphylaxis or other hypersensitivity reaction occurs, tramadol should be discontinued immediately and permanently.

Dependence and Tolerance

Both tolerance and physical dependence can develop during long-term opiate therapy. Tolerance may not develop uniformly to all opiate effects.

In patients who are physically dependent on opiates, abrupt discontinuance of tramadol or a substantial reduction in dosage may result in manifestations of withdrawal (e.g., restlessness, lacrimation, rhinorrhea, yawning, sweating, chills, myalgia, mydriasis, irritability, anxiety, backache, joint pain, weakness, abdominal cramps, insomnia, nausea, anorexia, vomiting, diarrhea, increases in blood pressure, respiratory rate, or heart rate). When tramadol therapy is discontinued in a patient who may be physically dependent on opiates, the dosage should be tapered gradually. Infants born to women who are physically dependent on opiates also will be physically dependent. (See Cautions: Pregnancy, Fertility, and Lactation.)

Concomitant use of opiate partial agonists (e.g., buprenorphine, butorphanol, nalbuphine, pentazocine) should be avoided since they may reduce the analgesic effect of tramadol and/or precipitate withdrawal symptoms.

CNS Depression

Tramadol may impair mental alertness and/or physical coordination required to perform potentially hazardous activities such as driving or operating machinery; patients should be warned about possible adverse CNS effects of the drug.

Warfarin

Prolongation of the international normalized ratio (INR) and prothrombin time and extensive ecchymoses have been reported in patients receiving tramadol and warfarin concomitantly. Therefore, tramadol should be used with caution in patients receiving warfarin; the INR should be closely monitored in those receiving the combination, and the warfarin dosage should be adjusted as needed.

Digoxin

Digoxin toxicity has been reported rarely during postmarketing experience in patients receiving digoxin and tramadol concomitantly. Patients receiving such concomitant therapy should be monitored for digoxin toxicity, and digoxin dosage should be adjusted as needed.

Renal and Hepatic Impairment

Impaired renal function results in a decreased rate and extent of excretion of tramadol and its active *O*-desmethyl metabolite (M1). Therefore, in patients with creatinine clearance less than 30 mL/minute, the manufacturers recommend dosage reduction when tramadol is used alone as conventional tablets or in fixed combination with acetaminophen. Tramadol hydrochloride extended-release tablets and capsules should *not* be used in patients with severe renal impairment (i.e., creatinine clearance less than 30 mL/minute); the available tablet and capsule strengths and once-daily dosing do not provide sufficient dosing flexibility for safe use in these patients. (See Dosage and Administration: Dosage in Renal and Hepatic Impairment.)

Tramadol and M1 metabolism are reduced in patients with advanced hepatic cirrhosis. When tramadol hydrochloride conventional tablets are used in adults with cirrhosis, dosage adjustment is recommended. Tramadol hydrochloride extended-release tablets and capsules should *not* be used in patients with severe hepatic impairment (Child-Pugh class C); the available tablet and capsule strengths and once-daily dosing do not provide sufficient dosing flexibility for safe use in these patients. The manufacturers state that pharmacokinetics and safety of tramadol in fixed combination with acetaminophen have not been studied in patients with impaired hepatic function. Therefore, because both tramadol and acetaminophen are extensively metabolized by the liver, the fixed-combination preparation should *not* be used in patients with hepatic impairment. (See Dosage and Administration: Dosage in Renal and Hepatic Impairment.)

With the prolonged half-life of tramadol in patients with renal or hepatic impairment, achievement of steady-state plasma concentrations is delayed, and it may take several days for elevated plasma concentrations to occur.

Advice to Patients

Patients should be advised to read the manufacturer's patient information (e.g., medication guide) for tramadol before initiating therapy with the drug and each time the prescription is refilled. Patients should be informed that use of tramadol, even when taken as recommended, can result in addiction, abuse, and misuse, which can lead to overdosage and death. Patients also should be informed that accidental ingestion of tramadol, especially by a child, may result in respiratory depression or death. Patients should be instructed not to share the drug with others, to take steps to protect the drug from theft or misuse, to securely store the drug, to keep the drug out of reach of children, and to properly dispose of any unused drug.

Patients should be advised of the risk of life-threatening respiratory depression and instructed to seek immediate medical attention if manifestations of respiratory depression occur. Patients receiving tramadol and/or their caregivers should be advised that concomitant therapeutic or illicit use of benzodiazepines or other CNS depressants, including alcohol, can result in potentially fatal additive effects (e.g., profound sedation, respiratory depression, coma); patients should be advised to avoid concomitant use of alcohol and to avoid concomitant use of other CNS depressants unless such use is supervised by a clinician. Patients should be advised of the benefits of naloxone administration following an overdose and of their options for obtaining the drug.

Patients should be informed of the risk of opiate toxicity in children, especially those who are obese, have respiratory diseases, or have evidence of ultrarapid metabolism of tramadol and advised that tramadol should *not* be given to children younger than 12 years of age for pain relief or to children younger than 18 years of age for pain relief following tonsillectomy or adenoidectomy. (See Cautions: Pediatric Precautions.)

Patients should be advised that tramadol may cause seizures and/or serotonin syndrome, particularly when used concurrently with serotonergic drugs or drugs that substantially decrease the metabolism of tramadol. (See Drugs Associated with Serotonin Syndrome and also Drugs Affecting Hepatic Microsomal Enzymes under Cautions: Precautions and Contraindications.) Patients should be advised that tramadol may impair mental or physical abilities required for the performance of potentially hazardous tasks such as driving a car or operating machinery. Patients should be advised of the importance of informing clinicians of existing or contemplated concomitant therapy, including prescription and OTC drugs, as well as any concomitant illnesses; patients should be advised that tramadol should not be used concomitantly with MAO inhibitors. Patients also should be advised that severe hypersensitivity reactions have occurred and that the drug may cause orthostatic hypotension and syncope. Because opiates can cause severe constipation, patients should be advised on appropriate management of constipation. Because of the potential risk of adrenal insufficiency, patients should be advised to immediately contact a clinician if manifestations of adrenal insufficiency (e.g., nausea, vomiting, loss of appetite, fatigue, weakness, dizziness, hypotension) develop. Although a causal relationship between hypogonadism or androgen deficiency and long-term opiate agonist use has not been established, patients should be advised of this potential risk and instructed to inform their clinician if decreased libido, impotence, erectile dysfunction, amenorrhea, or infertility occurs.

Women of childbearing potential should be instructed to inform their clinician if they are or plan to become pregnant and should be advised that use of tramadol is not recommended in nursing women. Women of childbearing potential should be advised that tramadol may cause fetal harm and that prolonged use of opiates during pregnancy may result in neonatal opiate withdrawal syndrome, which can be life-threatening if not recognized and treated. (See Cautions: Pregnancy, Fertility, and Lactation.)

Clinicians should be certain that patients understand the single-dose and 24-hour dose limit, and the recommended interval between doses of tramadol administered alone or in fixed combination with acetaminophen, since exceeding these recommendations can result in respiratory depression, seizures, acetaminophen-associated hepatic toxicity, and death. Patients receiving therapy with tramadol hydrochloride extended-release tablets or capsules should be advised that the tablets or capsules should be swallowed whole and should not be crushed, chewed, broken, split, or dissolved. Because of the risk of withdrawal syndrome, patients should be advised not to abruptly discontinue therapy with the drug without consulting their clinician.

Contraindications

Tramadol is contraindicated in patients with substantial respiratory depression; acute or severe bronchial asthma in unmonitored settings or in the absence of resuscitative equipment; known or suspected GI obstruction, including paralytic ileus; or known hypersensitivity (e.g., anaphylaxis) to the drug, other opiates, or any ingredient in the formulation. Tramadol also is contraindicated during or within 14 days following treatment with an MAO inhibitor.

Tramadol is contraindicated in children younger than 12 years of age for the management of pain and in those younger than 18 years of age for the management of postoperative pain following tonsillectomy and/or adenoidectomy. (See Cautions: Pediatric Precautions.)

● *Pediatric Precautions*

Children receiving tramadol for the management of pain, especially those who are obese, have obstructive sleep apnea or severe lung disease, or have evidence of ultrarapid metabolism of CYP2D6 substrates, are at increased risk of respiratory depression. Between January 1969 and May 2016, the FDA Adverse Event Reporting System (AERS) received 9 reports of respiratory depression, including 3 deaths, worldwide that were associated with tramadol use in children younger than 18 years of age. Respiratory depression generally occurred within the first 24 hours of dosing and required medical intervention (e.g., naloxone). All 3 of the fatal cases occurred outside of the US in children younger than 6 years of age receiving tramadol hydrochloride oral solution for postoperative analgesia or management of fever. One 5-year-old child with obstructive sleep apnea experienced severely slowed and difficult breathing requiring emergency intervention and hospitalization after receiving a single 20-mg dose of tramadol hydrochloride oral solution (approximately 1 mg/kg) for pain relief following tonsillectomy and adenoidectomy. The child was resuscitated and later found to be a CYP2D6 ultra-rapid metabolizer and to have a high concentration of the active O-desmethyl metabolite (M1). In the other 8 reported cases, the CYP2D6 metabolizer status was unknown.

To minimize the risk of serious adverse events in children, FDA states that tramadol-containing preparations must *not* be used for the management of pain in children younger than 12 years of age or for the management of postoperative pain following tonsillectomy and/or adenoidectomy in children younger than 18 years of age. FDA also states that use of tramadol for the management of pain is *not* recommended in children 12–18 years of age who are obese or have conditions such as obstructive sleep apnea or compromised respiratory function (because of potentially greater susceptibility to the respiratory depressant effects of the drug). If tramadol is used for the management of pain in children 12–18 years of age, caregivers should closely monitor the child for clinical manifestations of opiate toxicity (e.g., slow, shallow, difficult, or noisy breathing; confusion; unusual sleepiness) and seek immediate medical treatment for the child if such manifestations occur.

The manufacturers state that safety and efficacy of tramadol hydrochloride conventional tablets have not been established in children younger than 16 years of age. Safety and efficacy of tramadol hydrochloride extended-release tablets and capsules and of tablets containing tramadol hydrochloride in fixed combination with acetaminophen have not been established in children younger than 18 years of age. The manufacturers state that use of tramadol in pediatric patients is not recommended.

Geriatric Precautions

In general, tramadol dosage should be titrated carefully in geriatric patients, usually initiating therapy at the low end of the dosage range, considering the greater frequency of decreased hepatic, renal, and/or cardiac function and of concomitant disease and drug therapy observed in the elderly. (See Dosage and Administration: Dosage.) Because respiratory depression is the chief risk for geriatric patients receiving opiates, dosage should be titrated slowly and geriatric patients should be monitored closely for CNS and respiratory depression. Tramadol is substantially excreted by the kidneys, and the risk of adverse effects may be increased in patients with impaired renal function. Because geriatric patients may have decreased renal function, dosage should be selected carefully; it may be useful to monitor renal function in such patients.

In controlled clinical trials of tramadol hydrochloride conventional tablets, 455 patients who received the drug were 65 years of age or older, while 145 patients were 75 years of age or older. In patients older than 75 years of age receiving conventional tablets of the drug, maximum serum tramadol concentrations are elevated (208 ng/mL) and the elimination half-life is prolonged (7 hours) compared with patients 65–75 years of age (162 ng/mL and 6 hours, respectively). In clinical studies including geriatric patients receiving tramadol hydrochloride conventional tablets, treatment-limiting adverse GI effects occurred in 30% of patients older than 75 years of age compared with 17% of those younger than 65 years of age, and constipation resulted in discontinuance of treatment in 10% of those older than 75 years of age.

In clinical trials of tramadol hydrochloride extended-release tablets, 901 patients who received the drug were 65 years of age or older, while 156 patients were 75 years of age or older. In these studies, the incidence of adverse effects was higher in patients older than 65 years of age compared with younger adults; adverse effects reported more frequently in older adults include constipation, fatigue, weakness, postural hypotension, and dyspepsia. Tramadol hydrochloride extended-release tablets should be used with caution in patients older than 65 years of age and with even greater caution in those older than 75 years of age.

In clinical trials of tramadol hydrochloride extended-release capsules, 812 patients who received the drug were 65 years of age or older, while 240 patients were 75 years of age or older. In these studies, the incidence of adverse effects was higher in patients older than 65 years of age compared with younger adults; adverse effects reported more frequently in older adults include nausea, constipation, somnolence, dizziness, dry mouth, vomiting, asthenia, pruritus, anorexia, sweating, fatigue, weakness, postural hypotension, and dyspepsia. Tramadol hydrochloride extended-release capsules should be used with great caution in geriatric patients older than 75 years of age.

Limited data from a study of patients with chronic pain receiving tramadol in fixed combination with acetaminophen indicated that there were no substantial changes in pharmacokinetics of tramadol or acetaminophen in patients 65 years of age and older with normal renal and hepatic function compared with younger adults.

Pregnancy, Fertility, and Lactation
Pregnancy

Prolonged maternal use of opiate agonists during pregnancy can result in neonatal opiate withdrawal syndrome with manifestations of irritability, hyperactivity and abnormal sleep pattern, high-pitched cry, tremor, vomiting, diarrhea, and failure to gain weight. In contrast to adults, the withdrawal syndrome in neonates may be life-threatening if not recognized and treated, and requires management according to protocols developed by neonatology experts. Women who require prolonged opiate agonist therapy during pregnancy should be advised of the risk of neonatal opiate withdrawal syndrome, and availability of appropriate treatment should be ensured. The onset, duration, and severity of the syndrome vary depending on the specific opiate agonist used, duration of use, timing and amount of last maternal use, and rate of drug elimination by the neonate. Neonatal seizures, neonatal withdrawal syndrome, fetal death, and stillbirth have been reported with tramadol during postmarketing experience. The effect of tramadol, if any, on the later growth, development, and functional maturation of the child is unknown.

Use of opiates in pregnant women during labor can result in neonatal respiratory depression. Use of tramadol is not recommended immediately before or during labor, when other analgesic techniques may be more appropriate. Opiate agonists may prolong labor through actions that temporarily reduce the strength, duration, and frequency of uterine contractions. However, this effect is inconsistent and may be offset by an increased rate of cervical dilatation, which tends to shorten labor. Neonates exposed to opiates during labor should be monitored for excessive sedation and respiratory depression. An opiate antagonist must be available for reversal of opiate-induced respiratory depression.

Tramadol has been shown to cross the placenta. The mean ratio of serum tramadol in the umbilical veins compared with maternal veins was 0.83 for women given tramadol during labor.

Analysis of data from the National Birth Defects Prevention Study, a large population-based, case-control study, suggests that therapeutic maternal use of opiate agonists during the period of organogenesis is associated with a low absolute risk of birth defects, including heart defects, spina bifida, and gastroschisis. The manufacturers state that available data regarding use of tramadol in pregnant women are insufficient to establish the risk of major birth defects and spontaneous abortion with the drug.

Based on animal data, women of childbearing potential should be advised of the potential for tramadol to cause fetal harm.

Although there are no adequate and controlled studies to date in humans, tramadol has been shown to be embryotoxic and fetotoxic in mice, rats, and rabbits at maternally toxic doses 1.4, 0.6, and 3.6 times, respectively, the maximum daily human dosage (120 mg/kg in mice, 25 mg/kg in rats, and 75 mg/kg in rabbits). Embryo and fetal toxicity consisted mainly of decreased fetal weights, decreased skeletal ossification, and increased supernumerary ribs at maternally toxic dose levels. Transient delays in developmental or behavioral parameters also were seen in pups from rat dams allowed to deliver. Embryo and fetal lethality was reported in only one rabbit study, in which rabbits received tramadol hydrochloride 300 mg/kg, a dose that would cause extreme maternal toxicity in rabbits.

Embryotoxicity and fetotoxicity have been demonstrated in rats when tramadol and acetaminophen were administered in fixed combination at maternally toxic doses of 50 and 434 mg/kg, respectively, or 1.6 times the maximum daily human dosages of these drugs. Embryonic and fetal toxicity consisted of decreased fetal weights and increased supernumerary ribs.

Tramadol was not teratogenic in mice, rats, and rabbits at maternally toxic doses 1.4, 0.6, and 3.6 times, respectively, the maximum human daily dosage (120 mg/kg in mice, 25 mg/kg in rats, and 75 mg/kg in rabbits). No drug-related teratogenic effects were observed in progeny of mice, rats, or rabbits receiving tramadol (up to 140, 80, or 300 mg/kg or 1.7, 1.9, or 14.6 times, respectively, the maximum daily human dosage) by various routes.

Tramadol and acetaminophen in fixed combination was not teratogenic in rats at a maternally toxic dose of 50 and 434 mg/kg, respectively, or 1.6 times the maximum daily human dosages of these drugs.

In perinatal and postnatal studies in rats, progeny of dams receiving oral (gavage) tramadol hydrochloride doses of 50 mg/kg or higher had decreased weights, and pup survival was decreased early in lactation at tramadol hydrochloride doses of 80 mg/kg (1.2–1.6 or 1.9–2.6 times, respectively, the maximum human dose). No toxicity was observed for progeny of dams receiving doses of 8, 10, 20, 25, or 40 mg/kg. Maternal toxicity was observed at all dose levels, but effects on progeny were evident only at higher dose levels where maternal toxicity was more severe.

Fertility

Long-term use of opiates may reduce fertility in females and males of reproductive potential. It is not known whether these effects are reversible. (See Cautions: Genitourinary and Endocrine Effects.)

No effects on fertility were observed in male rats receiving oral tramadol hydrochloride doses up to 50 mg/kg or in female rats receiving oral tramadol hydrochloride doses up to 75 mg/kg or 1.2 or 1.8 times, respectively, the maximum daily human dosage based on body surface area.

Lactation

Tramadol is distributed into milk. Following a single IV tramadol dose of 100 mg, the cumulative distribution into milk within 16 hours after dosing was 100 mcg of tramadol (0.1% of the maternal dose) and 27 mcg of M1.

Because the safety of tramadol in infants and neonates has not been established, the drug is not recommended for obstetrical preoperative medication or for use in nursing women, including use for post-delivery analgesia. FDA review of available medical literature did not reveal evidence of an increased frequency of adverse effects in nursing infants of women receiving tramadol; however, because the drug is distributed into milk and has similar risks as codeine in ultrarapid metabolizers of CYP2D6 substrates, FDA recommends that tramadol *not* be used in nursing women. (See Pharmacogenomics under Cautions: Precautions and Contraindications. Also see Cautions: Precautions and Contraindications, in Codeine Phosphate and Codeine Sulfate 28:08.08.) Infants exposed to tramadol through breast milk should be monitored closely for clinical manifestations of opiate toxicity (e.g., sedation, difficulty breast-feeding or breathing, hypotonia). If clinical manifestations of opiate toxicity occur, caregivers should seek immediate medical treatment for the infant.

Symptoms of withdrawal can occur in opiate-dependent infants when maternal administration of opiates is discontinued or breast-feeding is stopped.

DESCRIPTION

Tramadol hydrochloride is a synthetic, centrally active analgesic. The drug (and its active *O*-desmethyl metabolite [M1]) acts as an opiate agonist, apparently by selective activity at the μ-receptor. In addition to opiate agonist activity, tramadol inhibits reuptake of certain monoamines (norepinephrine, serotonin), which appears to contribute to the drug's analgesic effect. Although the relative contribution of tramadol versus its M1 metabolite to analgesia in humans is unknown, the metabolite is 6 times more potent than the parent drug in producing analgesia in animal models and 200 times more potent in μ-receptor binding. The antinociceptic effect of tramadol is antagonized only partially by naloxone in some tests in animals and healthy individuals.

Although the pharmacologic effects of tramadol result in part from agonist activity at opiate receptors, the drug is not an opium derivative nor a semisynthetic derivative of morphine or thebaine. However, because tramadol is an agonist of *true* opiate receptors, not opiate-*like* (i.e., opi-*oid*) receptors, the drug is classified as an opiate agonist in the AHFS Pharmacologic-Therapeutic Classification®. (See Chemistry in the Opiate Agonists General Statement 28:08.08.)

Because of the drug's opiate agonist activity at μ-receptors, tramadol also can produce dependence. Although tramadol and tramadol in fixed combination with acetaminophen were *not* originally subject to control under the Federal Controlled Substances Act of 1970 as scheduled drugs, these preparations became subject to such control as schedule IV (C-IV) drugs effective August 18, 2014. Current data suggest that the abuse potential of tramadol is less than that of morphine or oxycodone but similar to that of propoxyphene. Tolerance and manifestations of withdrawal also can occur, although such effects are relatively mild compared with those of other opiate agonists.

Tramadol shares many of the other pharmacologic and toxicologic effects of opiate agonists, including dizziness, somnolence, nausea, constipation, dry mouth, sweating, and pruritus. The respiratory depressant effects of the drug are less than those of morphine, and usually are not clinically important at usual oral doses. At relatively high doses (e.g., those administered parenterally), tramadol can produce respiratory depression, and even usual oral doses should be employed cautiously in patients at risk for respiratory depression. At usual oral doses, the drug exhibits minimal cardiovascular effects, although hypotension, syncope, and tachycardia can occur occasionally.

PREPARATIONS

Effective August 18, 2014, tramadol hydrochloride preparations are subject to control under the Federal Controlled Substances Act of 1970 as schedule IV (C-IV) drugs. (See Description.)

Excipients in commercially available drug preparations may have clinically important effects in some individuals; consult specific product labeling for details.

traMADol Hydrochloride

Oral

Capsules, extended-release	100 mg (with extended-release 75 mg and immediate-release 25 mg)	Conzip® (C-IV), Vertical
	200 mg (with extended-release 150 mg and immediate-release 50 mg)	Conzip® (C-IV), Vertical
	300 mg (with extended-release 250 mg and immediate-release 50 mg)	Conzip®, (C-IV), Vertical
Tablets, extended-release	100 mg*	traMADol Hydrochloride Extended-Release Tablets (C-IV)
	200 mg*	traMADol Hydrochloride Extended-Release Tablets (C-IV)
	300 mg*	traMADol Hydrochloride Extended-Release Tablets (C-IV)
Tablets, film-coated	50 mg*	traMADol Hydrochloride Tablets (C-IV)

* available from one or more manufacturer, distributor, and/or repackager by generic (nonproprietary) name

traMADol Hydrochloride Combinations

Oral

Tablets, film-coated	44 mg with celecoxib 56 mg	Seglentis® (C-IV), Kowa
	37.5 with Acetaminophen 325 mg*	traMADol Hydrochloride and Acetaminophen Tablets (C-IV)

* available from one or more manufacturer, distributor, and/or repackager by generic (nonproprietary) name

† Use is not currently included in the labeling approved by the US Food and Drug Administration.

Selected Revisions September 10, 2024, © Copyright, September 1, 1995, American Society of Health-System Pharmacists, Inc.

Buprenorphine, Buprenorphine Hydrochloride

28:08.12 • OPIOID PARTIAL AGONISTS

■ Buprenorphine is a synthetic opiate partial agonist analgesic.

REMS

FDA approved a REMS for buprenorphine to ensure that the benefits outweigh the risk. (See Risk Evaluation and Mitigation Strategies under Dosage and Administration: Administration.) The REMS may apply to one or more preparations of buprenorphine. See the FDA REMS page (https://www.accessdata.fda.gov/scripts/cder/rems/index.cfm).

USES

Buprenorphine hydrochloride is used parenterally for the relief of pain that is severe enough to require opiate analgesia and for which alternative treatment options are inadequate. Buprenorphine hydrochloride also is used buccally and buprenorphine is used transdermally for the management of pain that is severe enough to require daily, around-the-clock, long-term opiate analgesia and for which alternative treatment options are inadequate.

In the management of opiate dependence (opiate use disorder [OUD]), buprenorphine is used parenterally as an extended-release subcutaneous injection, buprenorphine hydrochloride is used sublingually or as a subdermal implant, and buprenorphine hydrochloride in fixed combination with naloxone hydrochloride is used sublingually or buccally.

● Pain

Parenteral Therapy

Buprenorphine hydrochloride is used parenterally as an analgesic for the relief of pain that is severe enough to require an opiate analgesic and for which alternate treatments are inadequate; because of the risks of addiction, abuse, and misuse associated with opiates even at recommended dosages, parenteral buprenorphine should be reserved for use in patients for whom alternative treatment options (e.g., nonopiate analgesics, opiate-containing fixed combinations) have not been, or are not expected to be, adequate or tolerated. The analgesic activity of 0.3 mg of parenteral buprenorphine is about equal to that of 10 mg of parenteral morphine sulfate or 75–100 mg of parenteral meperidine. In equianalgesic doses, parenteral buprenorphine generally appears to be as effective as or possibly slightly more effective than parenteral morphine, meperidine, or pentazocine in relieving moderate to severe pain. The duration of analgesia produced by a single dose of parenteral buprenorphine is generally longer than that produced by a single parenteral dose of meperidine or pentazocine and is comparable to and, in some patients, may be longer than that produced by a single parenteral dose of morphine.

Buprenorphine is used parenterally in the management of postoperative pain in patients who have undergone various types of surgery, including neurologic, cardiovascular (e.g., coronary artery bypass, valve replacement), cesarean section, gynecologic, abdominal (e.g., cholecystectomy, bowel resection), urologic, general (e.g., head and neck, breast), and orthopedic (e.g., total hip replacement, spinal fusion). Because of its limited cardiovascular effects, buprenorphine may be safer than morphine when used as an analgesic in patients with compromised cardiac function undergoing cardiovascular surgery. The drug has also been administered by epidural injection† in the management of postoperative pain in total dosages substantially less than the equivalent morphine dosages necessary to produce a comparable analgesic effect. Buprenorphine has also been used to provide preoperative sedation and analgesia† and as an adjunct to surgical anesthesia†; however, the drug should be used with caution in patients undergoing surgery of the biliary tract.

Buprenorphine has been used parenterally as an analgesic for the relief of moderate to severe pain associated with cancer and trigeminal neuralgia. The drug has also been used as an analgesic in critically ill patients for the relief of moderate to severe pain resulting from accidental trauma and as an analgesic for the relief of moderate to severe pain resulting from ureteral calculi. Buprenorphine has also been used as an analgesic for the relief of moderate to severe pain associated with myocardial infarction.

Transdermal Therapy

Buprenorphine is used transdermally for the management of pain that is severe enough to require daily, around-the-clock, long-term opiate analgesia and for which alternative treatment options are inadequate. Because of the risks of addiction, abuse, and misuse associated with opiates, even at recommended dosages, and because of the greater risks of overdosage and death associated with extended-release opiate formulations, transdermal buprenorphine should be reserved for use in patients for whom alternative treatment options (e.g., nonopiate analgesics, immediate-release opiates) are inadequate or not tolerated. Transdermal buprenorphine is *not* intended for use on an as-needed ("prn") basis.

The safety and efficacy of transdermal buprenorphine have been evaluated in 4 double-blind, controlled trials of 12 weeks' duration. Two studies, one in patients with chronic low back pain and one in patients with osteoarthritis, failed to show efficacy for either transdermal buprenorphine or the active comparators. Efficacy and safety of transdermal buprenorphine were established in 2 studies in patients with moderate to severe chronic low back pain, including one study in adults not previously receiving opiates and one study in adults receiving chronic opiate therapy at a dosage equivalent to 30–80 mg daily of oral morphine sulfate. Chronic opiate regimens were tapered prior to initiating buprenorphine. Both studies utilized an initial open-label dose titration period of up to 3–4 weeks; buprenorphine was initiated at a dosage of 5 mcg/hour (or 10 mcg/hour in those previously receiving opiate treatment) and increased at intervals of at least 72 hours to a maximum dosage of 20 mcg/hour. Patients who achieved adequate analgesia with tolerable adverse effects (approximately 53–57% of patients) during this phase were randomized to 12 weeks of double-blind treatment. In patients who had not previously received opiates for analgesia, transdermal buprenorphine was more effective than placebo in reducing 24-hour average pain scores (measured on an 11-point numeric rating scale). Patients who previously had received opiates for analgesia also achieved greater reductions in 24-hour average pain scores with 20 mcg/hour of transdermal buprenorphine when compared with 5 mcg/hour of transdermal buprenorphine (low-dose control).

Oral Transmucosal Therapy

Buprenorphine is used buccally for the management of pain that is severe enough to require daily, around-the-clock, long-term opiate analgesia and for which alternative treatment options are inadequate. Because of the risks of addiction, abuse, and misuse associated with opiates, even at recommended dosages, and because of the greater risks of overdosage and death associated with long-acting opiate formulations, intrabuccal buprenorphine should be reserved for use in patients for whom alternative treatment options (e.g., nonopiate analgesics, immediate-release opiates) are inadequate or not tolerated. Intrabuccal buprenorphine is *not* intended for use on an as-needed ("prn") basis.

The safety and efficacy of intrabuccal buprenorphine have been evaluated in 3 double-blind, controlled trials of 12 weeks' duration in patients with moderate to severe, chronic low back pain. One study failed to show efficacy. Efficacy and safety of intrabuccal buprenorphine were established in 2 studies, including one study in adults not previously receiving opiates and one study in adults receiving long-term opiate therapy at a dosage equivalent to 30–160 mg daily of oral morphine sulfate. Opiate regimens were tapered to a dosage equivalent to 30 mg daily of oral morphine sulfate prior to initiating buprenorphine. Both studies utilized an initial open-label dose-titration period with buprenorphine of up to 8 weeks' duration. Patients who achieved adequate analgesia with tolerable adverse effects (61–63% of patients) during this phase were randomized to 12 weeks of double-blind treatment with buprenorphine or placebo. In patients who had not previously received opiates for analgesia, intrabuccal buprenorphine was more effective than placebo in reducing mean pain scores (as measured on an 11-point numeric rating scale), and a greater proportion of buprenorphine-treated patients compared with placebo recipients achieved at least a 30% reduction in pain score (62 versus 47%) or at least a 50% reduction in pain score (41 versus 33%) from baseline (prior to the open-label titration period) to end of study. In patients who previously had received opiates for analgesia, intrabuccal buprenorphine also was more effective than placebo in reducing mean pain scores, and a greater proportion of buprenorphine-treated patients compared with placebo recipients achieved at least a 30% reduction in pain score (64 versus 31%) or at least a 50% reduction in pain score (39 versus 17%) from baseline (prior to the open-label titration period) to end of study.

Oral transmucosal formulations of buprenorphine or buprenorphine in fixed combination with naloxone that are intended for use in the treatment of opiate dependence should *not* be used for analgesia. Fatal overdosage has been reported following administration of 2 mg of sublingual buprenorphine for analgesia in opiate-naive individuals.

For further information on the role of opiate analgesics in the management of acute or chronic pain, see Uses: Pain, in the Opiate Agonists General Statement 28:08.08.

● *Opiate Dependence*

Buprenorphine is used parenterally as an extended-release subcutaneous injection, buprenorphine hydrochloride is used sublingually or as a subdermal implant, and buprenorphine hydrochloride in fixed combination with naloxone hydrochloride is used sublingually or buccally for the treatment of opiate dependence (opiate use disorder [OUD]); buprenorphine has been designated an orphan drug by FDA for this indication. Safety and efficacy of transdermal buprenorphine for the management of opiate dependence have not been established. In the treatment of opiate dependence, buprenorphine should be used as part of a comprehensive treatment program that includes counseling and psychosocial support.

Buprenorphine and buprenorphine in fixed combination with naloxone (buprenorphine/naloxone) are available in the US for office-based outpatient medication-assisted treatment (MAT) of opiate dependence. The Drug Addiction Treatment Act of 2000 (DATA 2000) allows qualifying physicians to prescribe and dispense opiates in schedules III, IV, and V of the Federal Controlled Substances Act that have been approved by FDA for the management of opiate dependence. Prior to passage of this law, opiate dependence treatment could be provided only at specially registered clinics. The Comprehensive Addiction and Recovery Act of 2016 (CARA 2016) expands the categories of practitioners recognized under DATA 2000 to include qualifying nurse practitioners and physician assistants. Office-based treatment with buprenorphine is intended to increase access to opiate dependence treatment. Expansion of the categories of qualifying practitioners is intended to further bridge the gap between MAT providers and individuals seeking such treatment, a particular problem in rural areas. In the office-based treatment model, specially trained clinicians may prescribe buprenorphine as a take-home medication.

The choice between buprenorphine and methadone for maintenance treatment of opiate dependence should take into consideration the patient's preferences; the patient's medical, psychiatric, substance use, and treatment histories; and treatment availability and setting. Buprenorphine is preferred for many patients because it can be prescribed in an office-based setting and is considered to have a better safety profile than methadone. Methadone may be preferred for patients who would benefit from daily supervised dosing in an opiate treatment program and for those who do not have access to, or have not benefited from, buprenorphine therapy. Office-based treatment may not be suitable for patients with other concurrent substance use disorders or for those routinely using other CNS depressants.

Oral Transmucosal Therapy for Induction and Maintenance Treatment

Buprenorphine and buprenorphine/naloxone are used sublingually or buccally for the treatment of opiate dependence. Although buprenorphine traditionally has been considered the preferred drug for the initial (i.e., induction) phase of treatment, additional experience indicates that either buprenorphine or buprenorphine/naloxone may be used for induction therapy in patients dependent on heroin or other short-acting opiates. Use of buprenorphine/naloxone for the induction phase of treatment in patients dependent on long-acting opiates has not been evaluated to date in adequate and well-controlled studies, and the manufacturers and some experts still recommend use of buprenorphine alone for induction in these patients. Following induction, buprenorphine/naloxone is the preferred drug for

maintenance treatment when use includes unsupervised administration since the presence of naloxone (an opiate antagonist) in the formulation should discourage parenteral misuse of the oral transmucosal preparation. Administration of buprenorphine without naloxone in an unsupervised setting should be limited to pregnant women and patients who cannot tolerate naloxone.

Sublingual buprenorphine and buprenorphine/naloxone have been evaluated in several placebo- and active-controlled studies in patients physically dependent on opiates. In these studies, buprenorphine therapy has been used in conjunction with psychosocial counseling as part of a comprehensive addiction treatment program. When administered sublingually, buprenorphine and buprenorphine/naloxone have similar clinical effects. Results of a dose-ranging study indicate that sublingual administration of buprenorphine dosages of 6–24 mg daily are effective in the treatment of opiate dependence. Buprenorphine and buprenorphine/naloxone were more effective than placebo in reducing illicit opiate use, as determined by urine tests for other opiates, in one placebo-controlled study that included patients randomized to receive buprenorphine 8 mg or placebo on day 1, buprenorphine 16 mg or placebo on day 2, and then buprenorphine 16 mg daily, buprenorphine 16 mg in fixed combination with naloxone 4 mg daily, or placebo daily for 4 weeks. In another study that included a 16- to 17-week maintenance phase and a 7- to 8-week detoxification phase, buprenorphine generally was more effective than low dosages of methadone hydrochloride (20 mg daily) and as effective as high dosages of methadone hydrochloride (60 mg daily) in reducing illicit opiate use and retaining patients in the program. In another comparative study, buprenorphine, levomethadyl acetate (no longer commercially available in the US because of potentially severe adverse cardiac effects), and high-dose methadone hydrochloride (60–100 mg daily) were more effective than low-dose methadone hydrochloride (20 mg daily) in reducing illicit opiate use.

Induction therapy with sublingual buprenorphine/naloxone has been evaluated in 2 blinded, randomized noninferiority studies in a total of 1068 opiate-dependent adults. In both studies, treatment retention rates at day 3 were compared following induction therapy with buprenorphine/naloxone sublingual tablets (Zubsolv®; total induction dosage of buprenorphine 5.7 mg and naloxone 1.4 mg on day 1 followed by either buprenorphine 5.7 mg and naloxone 1.4 mg or buprenorphine 11.4 mg and naloxone 2.8 mg on day 2) or generic buprenorphine sublingual tablets (total induction dosage of 8 mg on day 1 followed by 8 or 16 mg on day 2). On day 1, patients received an initial supervised dose of the assigned drug (buprenorphine 1.4 mg and naloxone 0.36 mg or buprenorphine 2 mg); at the investigator's discretion, the remainder of the day 1 dosage was administered in 1 dose or, if the first dose precipitated withdrawal manifestations, in 3 divided doses at intervals of 1–2 hours. Because of its higher bioavailability, a Zubsolv® sublingual tablet containing buprenorphine 5.7 mg and naloxone 1.4 mg provides equivalent buprenorphine exposure and 12% lower naloxone exposure as a Suboxone® sublingual tablet containing buprenorphine 8 mg and naloxone 2 mg. In the first study, the treatment retention rate at day 3 was 93% for patients receiving buprenorphine/naloxone compared with 92% for those receiving buprenorphine alone; in the second study, treatment retention rates at day 3 were 85 and 95%, respectively. The lower retention rate observed with the fixed-combination preparation compared with buprenorphine alone in the second study may have been related to infrequent use of divided dosing in this study (5%) compared with the first study (22%).

Maintenance Treatment with Buprenorphine Extended-release Subcutaneous Injection

Buprenorphine extended-release subcutaneous injection is used for the treatment of moderate to severe opiate dependence in patients who have initiated treatment with an oral transmucosal buprenorphine-containing preparation followed by dosage adjustment for a minimum of 7 days.

Buprenorphine extended-release subcutaneous injection has been evaluated in an opiate challenge study and in a randomized, double-blind, placebo-controlled clinical trial.

In the opiate challenge study, efficacy of buprenorphine extended-release subcutaneous injection in blocking subjective opiate effects following hydromorphone challenge was assessed in 39 individuals with moderate to severe opiate use disorder who were not seeking treatment. Following stabilization on sublingual buprenorphine/naloxone over one week, study participants received two 300-mg subcutaneous doses of extended-release buprenorphine given 4 weeks apart. "Drug liking" scores (measured on a 100-mm visual analog scale) following challenge with placebo and hydromorphone hydrochloride (IM doses of 6 and 18 mg) were recorded weekly for 12 weeks after the first buprenorphine injection. At weeks 1–4, neither hydromorphone dose was substantially more likeable than placebo. Full blockade of the subjective effects of hydromorphone was observed at both dosage levels during each of the 12 weeks of the study, although substantial variability in isolated measurements from individual study participants was observed.

In the randomized double-blind study, 504 patients seeking treatment for moderate to severe opiate use disorder were randomized to receive buprenorphine extended-release subcutaneous injection (300 mg monthly for 6 months or 300 mg monthly for 2 months followed by 100 mg monthly for 4 months) or placebo following stabilization on buprenorphine/naloxone sublingually dissolving strips. Supplemental sublingual doses of buprenorphine/naloxone were not permitted during the study. All patients received psychosocial counseling at least weekly. Efficacy was evaluated over weeks 5–24 by means of urine drug testing and self-reports of illicit opiate use. Treatment success, defined as opiate-free status for 80% or more of the weeks during the evaluation period, was attained by 28–29% of buprenorphine-treated patients compared with 2% of placebo recipients.

Maintenance Treatment with Buprenorphine Subdermal Implants

Buprenorphine hydrochloride subdermal implants are used for maintenance treatment of opiate dependence in patients who have achieved and maintained prolonged clinical stability on a low to moderate dosage of an oral transmucosal buprenorphine-containing preparation (i.e., a transmucosal dosage that provides blood buprenorphine concentrations comparable to or lower than those provided by the subdermal implants). Examples of appropriate dosages of oral transmucosal buprenorphine-containing preparations include the following: Subutex® sublingual tablets (or generic equivalent; branded formulation no longer commercially available in the US) at a dosage not exceeding buprenorphine 8 mg daily, Suboxone® sublingual tablets (or generic equivalent; branded formulation no longer commercially available in the US) at a dosage not exceeding buprenorphine 8 mg and naloxone 2 mg daily, Bunavail® buccally dissolving strips at a dosage not exceeding buprenorphine 4.2 mg and naloxone 0.7 mg daily, and Zubsolv® sublingual tablets at a dosage not exceeding buprenorphine 5.7 mg and naloxone 1.4 mg daily. Buprenorphine subdermal implants are not appropriate for individuals just initiating treatment for opiate dependence or for those who have not achieved and sustained prolonged clinical stability on a low to moderate oral transmucosal dosage of the drug.

Efficacy of buprenorphine subdermal implants for the maintenance treatment of opiate dependence was established in a randomized, double-blind study in 177 patients who were clinically stable while receiving a sublingual buprenorphine dosage of 8 mg daily or less (as Suboxone® sublingual tablets or equivalent). Patients were randomized to receive 4 buprenorphine hydrochloride 80-mg subdermal implants (with daily placebo sublingual tablets) or daily treatment with buprenorphine/naloxone sublingual tablets administered at the prerandomization dosage (with 4 placebo subdermal implants). Supplemental doses of sublingual buprenorphine/naloxone tablets were permitted as clinically indicated. In the sublingual treatment group, supplemental dosing was considered consistent with usual treatment, whereas in the implant treatment group, supplemental dosing was interpreted as indicating that the implant dosage was inadequate. Efficacy assessments were based on urine drug testing and self-reports of illicit opiate use. During 6 months of treatment, 63% of patients with subdermal buprenorphine implants (without supplemental sublingual therapy) had no evidence of illicit opiate use, compared with 64% of patients receiving usual sublingual buprenorphine therapy. In addition, 11 patients with buprenorphine implants required supplemental sublingual dosing but had no evidence of illicit opiate use; one of these patients required supplemental dosing only at the end of the implantation period, potentially indicating the need for early implant replacement.

Two additional studies in patients who had not previously received buprenorphine therapy suggested that buprenorphine subdermal implants should not be used for patients who are new to buprenorphine treatment or who have not achieved and sustained prolonged clinical stability while receiving a low to moderate dosage of an oral transmucosal buprenorphine-containing preparation; the implant dosage appears to be too low to be effective in these populations.

● Other Uses

Buprenorphine has been used in a limited number of patients as an antagonist to reverse fentanyl-induced anesthesia† and provide subsequent analgesia; however, buprenorphine-induced reversal of fentanyl anesthesia may occur slowly, and usefulness of the drug in situations when rapid recovery from fentanyl anesthesia is desirable may therefore be limited.

Buprenorphine has caused substantial clinical improvement in a limited number of patients with refractory endogenous depression† when administered as a sublingual tablet for several days.

DOSAGE AND ADMINISTRATION

● Administration

Risk Evaluation and Mitigation Strategies

FDA required and approved a REMS for oral transmucosal formulations of buprenorphine alone or in fixed combination with naloxone (buprenorphine/naloxone) that are used for treatment of opiate dependence (opiate use disorder), for opiate analgesics used in the outpatient setting (including buprenorphine transdermal systems and buprenorphine buccally dissolving strips), for buprenorphine subdermal implants, and for buprenorphine extended-release subcutaneous injection. (See REMS.)

The REMS program for buprenorphine-containing oral transmucosal preparations (i.e., sublingual tablets and sublingually or buccally dissolving strips) used for the treatment of opiate dependence include a medication guide requirement and outline steps to ensure documentation of safe use conditions and proper monitoring for each patient receiving the drug. The REMS requirement does not apply when buprenorphine-containing oral transmucosal preparations are dispensed to patients admitted to an opiate treatment program. The goals are to reduce the risk of accidental overdosage, misuse, and abuse and to inform prescribers, pharmacists, and patients of the serious risks associated with these preparations. Additional information about the REMS programs for buprenorphine-containing oral transmucosal preparations can be obtained at http://www.btodrems.com.

The Sublocade® REMS program is intended to reduce the risk of serious harm or death that could result from IV self-administration by ensuring that buprenorphine extended-release subcutaneous injection is dispensed by certified health care settings and pharmacies directly to health care providers for administration by a health care professional. The REMS includes a redistricted distribution program. Additional information about the program can be obtained at http://www.sublocaderems.com.

The goals of the Probuphine® REMS are to reduce the risks of complications of buprenorphine subdermal implant migration, protrusion, or expulsion; nerve damage associated with implant insertion and removal; and accidental overdosage, misuse, and abuse if an implant is expelled or protrudes from the skin. The program includes requirements for certification of pharmacies that dispense the implant, clinicians who prescribe the implant, and clinicians who insert the implants; monitoring and documentation of implant removal; restriction of distribution to settings with a certified prescriber; and a medication guide for patients. Additional information about the program can be obtained at http://probuphinerems.com.

FDA also has approved a REMS program for opiate analgesics used in the outpatient setting and not covered by other REMS programs, including buprenorphine transdermal system (Butrans®) and buprenorphine buccally dissolving strips (Belbuca®). The goals of this program are to reduce the occurrence of addiction, unintentional overdosage, and death resulting from inappropriate prescribing, misuse, and abuse of opiate analgesics. The program consists of educational programs for health professionals, a patient counseling guide, and a product-specific medication guide for patients. Additional information about the program can be obtained at http://opioidanalgesicrems.com.

In addition to the restricted distribution systems established for certain buprenorphine-containing preparations (extended-release subcutaneous injection, subdermal implants) under REMS programs, buprenorphine and buprenorphine/naloxone may be prescribed for the treatment of opiate dependence only by clinicians who meet certain requirements, have notified the Secretary of the US Department of Health and Human Services (HHS) of their intent to prescribe these preparations for this indication, and have been assigned a unique identification number that must be included on each prescription for the drug.

Parenteral Administration

Conventional Injection for Pain Management

For the relief of pain severe enough to require opiate analgesia and for which alternative treatments are inadequate, buprenorphine hydrochloride is administered by IM or slow (over a period of at least 2 minutes) IV injection. The drug has also been administered by continuous IV infusion†, by IM or IV injection using a patient-controlled infusion device†, and by epidural injection†.

For continuous IV infusion†, buprenorphine hydrochloride injection has been diluted to a concentration of 15 mcg/mL in 0.9% sodium chloride and administered via a controlled-infusion device. For continuous IV infusion†, the drug should be administered only by qualified individuals familiar with the technique and patient management problems (i.e., respiratory depression) associated with buprenorphine administration. For epidural injection†, buprenorphine hydrochloride injection has been diluted to a concentration of 6–30 mcg/mL in 0.9% sodium chloride.

Buprenorphine hydrochloride injection and diluted solutions of the drug should be inspected visually for particulate matter and discoloration prior to administration whenever solution and container permit.

If accidental dermal exposure occurs, any contaminated clothing should be removed and the affected area rinsed with water.

Extended-release Subcutaneous Injection for Opiate Dependence

For the management of opiate dependence in patients who have initiated buprenorphine therapy with an oral transmucosal buprenorphine-containing preparation followed by dosage adjustment for at least 7 days, buprenorphine extended-release injection is administered by subcutaneous injection into the abdomen at monthly intervals (minimum of 26 days between injections); this formulation is for subcutaneous injection *only* and should *not* be administered IV or IM. A clinician must prepare and administer the injection.

Buprenorphine extended-release injection should be removed from the refrigerator and allowed to reach room temperature (over at least 15 minutes) prior to administration. Each injection should be administered using the manufacturer-provided syringe and safety needle. The foil pouch containing the syringe should not be opened until the patient has arrived for the injection, and the safety needle should not be attached until just prior to administration. The injection should be inspected visually for discoloration and particulate matter prior to administration; the injection should appear clear, viscous, and colorless to yellow to amber. The injection should be discarded if stored at room temperature for longer than 7 days. Injections should be made into the abdomen between the transpyloric and transtubercular planes at a site with adequate subcutaneous tissue that is free of skin conditions (e.g., nodules, lesions, excessive pigmentation). Injections should not be made into areas that are irritated, reddened, bruised, infected, or scarred. It is recommended that injections be made with the patient in the supine position. Injection sites should be rotated.

Following administration, the injection forms a solid depot from which buprenorphine is gradually released. Patients should be advised that a lump may be present at the injection site for several weeks and that it will decrease in size over time. Patient should be instructed that they should not rub or massage the injection site or allow belts or waistbands to rub the site. Injection sites should be monitored for signs of infection and for evidence of tampering or attempted depot removal. A depot can be excised surgically, if necessary, under local anesthesia within 14 days of injection.

Subdermal Implants for Opiate Dependence

For maintenance treatment of opiate dependence in patients who have achieved and maintained prolonged clinical stability on a low to moderate dosage of an oral transmucosal buprenorphine-containing preparation, buprenorphine hydrochloride implants are inserted subdermally in the inner aspect of the upper arm. Clinicians must successfully complete required training and become certified prior to prescribing buprenorphine implant therapy; those performing implant insertion or removal procedures must successfully complete training on these procedures and be certified to perform implant insertion. Patients must be monitored to ensure that buprenorphine implants are removed by a clinician with appropriate certification, and clinicians must maintain documentation of implant insertion and removal in each patient's medical record. A surgical specialist consulted to assist with a difficult implant removal does not require certification.

Each buprenorphine dose consists of 4 implants that are intended to be left in place for 6 months and then removed by the end of the sixth month. If continued implant therapy is desired at the time the initial implants are removed, new implants may be inserted subdermally in the contralateral arm. After one insertion in each arm, most patients should be transitioned back to oral transmucosal buprenorphine therapy, since experience is lacking with insertion of implants into other sites in the arm or with insertion of new implants at prior administration sites. The manufacturer's prescribing information should be consulted for proper methods of implant insertion and removal and associated precautions. The presence of each implant should always be verified by palpation or, if necessary, by ultrasound or magnetic resonance imaging (MRI) immediately after insertion and prior to attempted removal.

Proper implant placement is essential to avoid serious complications and to facilitate removal. The implant site should be examined one week following insertion for signs of infection, adequacy of wound healing, and evidence of implant extrusion. If an implant is expelled spontaneously, the expelled portion should be measured to ensure that it is intact; any partial implant remaining in the patient's arm should be removed, and the incision site should be examined for infection and to determine whether the remaining implants should be removed. A replacement for the expelled implant may be inserted in the same arm medially or laterally to the existing implants or, alternatively, in the contralateral arm.

Sublingual Administration

Sublingual Preparations for Opiate Dependence

For management of opiate dependence, buprenorphine hydrochloride is administered sublingually as a single agent (as sublingual tablets) or in fixed combination with naloxone hydrochloride (as sublingual tablets and sublingually dissolving strips). Buprenorphine/naloxone sublingually dissolving strips (Suboxone®) may be administered either sublingually or buccally during maintenance treatment of opiate dependence; however, sublingual administration of this formulation is recommended during induction therapy to minimize exposure to naloxone and reduce the risk of withdrawal.

Buprenorphine or buprenorphine/naloxone sublingual tablets are placed under the tongue and allowed to dissolve. Drinking warm fluids prior to administration may aid dissolution. For doses requiring multiple tablets, patients are advised to place all the tablets under the tongue at once. Alternatively, patients may place 2 tablets under the tongue at a time if they are unable to place more than 2 tablets comfortably under the tongue. Patients should continue to hold the tablets under the tongue until the tablets dissolve. If sequential administration is preferred, patients should adhere to the same manner of dosing with continued use to ensure consistent bioavailability. The median dissolution time for buprenorphine/naloxone (Zubsolv®) sublingual tablets is 5 minutes.

Buprenorphine/naloxone sublingually dissolving strips are placed under the tongue, on either side near the base of the tongue. The strip(s) should be kept under the tongue until completely dissolved; drinking water prior to administration may aid dissolution. Up to 2 strips may be administered at one time and should be placed under opposite sides of the tongue in a way that minimizes overlapping. When more than 2 strips are required to complete the dose, additional strips may be administered after the first 2 strips have dissolved. Strips should not be moved after placement.

To ensure consistency in bioavailability, patients should follow a consistent manner of administration. Proper administration technique should be demonstrated to the patient. The sublingual tablet or strip must be administered whole and should not be cut. Patients should not eat or drink until the tablet or strip is completely dissolved. Talking while the tablet or strip is dissolving, chewing the tablet or strip, or swallowing the tablet or strip may affect absorption and, therefore, efficacy of the drug and should be avoided. Patients should be advised to keep unused sublingual tablets or strips containing buprenorphine out of sight and reach of children. After completion of sublingual buprenorphine therapy, patients should be advised to discard any remaining tablets or strips by removing the tablets or strips from their packaging and then flushing them down the toilet.

Buccal Administration

Buccal Preparations for Pain Management

For the relief of pain severe enough to require daily, around-the-clock, long-term opiate analgesia and for which alternative treatment options are inadequate, buprenorphine hydrochloride is administered buccally every 12 hours as buccally dissolving strips (Belbuca®). The manufacturer states that this formulation is for buccal use only.

Immediately prior to administering buprenorphine buccally dissolving strips (Belbuca®), the patient must wet the inside of the cheek with the tongue or rinse the mouth with water to wet the area for placement. The strip is then applied immediately after removal from the individually sealed package with the yellow side of the strip placed against the inside of the cheek, where it will adhere to the moist mucosa. The entire strip should be held in place with clean, dry fingers for 5 seconds and then left in place until fully dissolved (usually within 30 minutes). The strip should not be applied to areas of the mouth with open sores or lesions. The strip should not be manipulated with the tongue or fingers; eating and drinking should be avoided until the strip has dissolved. Chewing or swallowing the strip may result in lower peak plasma concentrations and reduced bioavailability of the drug. The strip should not be used if the package seal is broken or the strip is cut, damaged, or altered in any way. Proper administration technique should be demonstrated to the patient.

Patients should be advised to keep the strips out of sight and reach of children. Any strips that are no longer needed should be removed from their packaging and flushed down the toilet.

Buccal Preparations for Opiate Dependence

For the management of opiate dependence, buprenorphine/naloxone is administered buccally as buccally dissolving strips (Bunavail®). Sublingually dissolving strips containing buprenorphine/naloxone (Suboxone®) may be administered either sublingually or buccally during maintenance treatment of opiate dependence; however, sublingual administration of this formulation is recommended during induction therapy to minimize exposure to naloxone and reduce the risk of withdrawal. To ensure consistency in bioavailability, patients should follow a consistent manner of administration.

Immediately prior to administering buprenorphine/naloxone buccally dissolving strips (Bunavail®), the patient should wet the inside of the cheek with the tongue or rinse the mouth with water to moisten the area for placement. The strip is then applied immediately after removal from the individually sealed package. The strip should be held by clean, dry fingers with the text on the strip facing up and then placed against the inside of the cheek with the text side against the cheek; the strip should be pressed in place for 5 seconds. If a second strip is required to complete the dose, it should be placed on the inside of the other cheek immediately after the first strip is administered. When multiple strips are required, no more than 2 strips should be applied to the inside of one cheek at a time. The strip should not be manipulated with the tongue or fingers; eating and drinking should be avoided until the strip has dissolved. The strip must be administered whole and should not be cut or torn. Chewing or swallowing the strip may alter absorption and should be avoided.

For buccal administration of buprenorphine/naloxone sublingually dissolving strips (Suboxone®), one strip is placed on the inside of the right or left cheek. If a second strip is required to complete the dose, it is placed on the inside of the opposite cheek. If a third strip is required, it is placed on the inside of the right or left cheek after the first 2 strips have dissolved. Strips should not be moved after placement and must be left in place on the inside of the cheek until completely dissolved. Eating and drinking should be avoided until the strip has completely dissolved. The strip must be administered whole and should not be cut. Talking while the strip is dissolving, chewing the strip, or swallowing the strip may affect absorption and, therefore, efficacy of the drug and should be avoided.

Patients should be advised to keep the strips out of sight and reach of children. Any strips that are no longer needed should be removed from their packaging and flushed down the toilet.

Transdermal Administration

Transdermal System for Pain Management

For the relief of pain severe enough to require daily, around-the-clock, long-term opiate analgesia and for which alternative treatment options are inadequate, buprenorphine is administered transdermally. Each buprenorphine transdermal system is intended to be worn continuously for 7 days; subsequent systems should be applied to a different site after removal of the previous system. The manufacturer recommends an interval of at least 21 days between applications to a particular site, since more frequent application at the same site may result in variable absorption. Rotation among 8 recommended application sites (4 on each side of the body) is advised.

Patients receiving buprenorphine transdermal systems should be carefully instructed in the proper use and disposal of the transdermal system. The transdermal system should not be used if the seal of the package is broken or if the system is cut, damaged, or altered in any way. The transdermal system should be removed from the sealed pouch and the protective-liner covering should be peeled and discarded just prior to application of the system. The transdermal system should be applied to a dry, intact, nonirritated, hairless or nearly hairless surface on the upper chest, upper back, side of chest, or upper outer arm on either side of the body by firmly pressing the system by hand for 15 seconds with the adhesive side touching the skin and ensuring that contact is complete, particularly around the edges. If 2 systems are applied for a single dose, the systems should be applied adjacently at the same site and should always be applied and removed at the same time. If needed, hair at the application site should be clipped, not shaved, prior to application of the transdermal system. If the site must be cleansed prior to application, only water should be used. Soaps, oils, lotions, alcohol, or abrasive devices could alter the absorption of buprenorphine and should not be used.

If a system should inadvertently come off during the period of use, a new system may be applied to a different skin site and left in place for 7 days. Patients who experience difficulty with system adhesion should be advised that they may tape the edges of the system in place with first-aid tape. If adhesion problems persist, patients may apply a transparent, waterproof or semipermeable adhesive film dressing that is suitable for 7 days of wear (e.g., Bioclusive®, Tegaderm®) over the system.

Although incidental exposure to water (e.g., while showering or bathing) is acceptable, the transdermal system should not be exposed to external heat sources, hot water, or prolonged direct sunlight. Patients should be advised to avoid sunbathing, taking hot baths, or exposing the application site and surrounding area to direct external heat sources (e.g., heating pads, electric blankets, heat or tanning lamps, saunas, hot tubs, heated water beds) while wearing the transdermal system, since temperature-dependent increases in percutaneous absorption of buprenorphine from the system are possible under such conditions and may result in fatal overdosage.

Patients should be advised to keep both used and unused buprenorphine transdermal systems out of the reach of children. The manufacturer states that immediately following removal, used systems should be properly discarded. In addition, following completion of a course of transdermal buprenorphine therapy, any unused systems should be removed from the package and properly discarded. Systems to be discarded should be folded carefully so that the adhesive side adheres to itself and then should be flushed down the toilet; transdermal systems may be disposed in the trash only after the system has been sealed in the manufacturer-supplied disposal unit. If the drug-containing adhesive matrix accidentally contacts the skin, the affected area should be washed with water; soap, alcohol, or other solvents should not be used to cleanse the area since they actually may enhance percutaneous absorption of buprenorphine. Patients or caregivers should always wash their hands after applying or handling a buprenorphine transdermal system.

● Dosage

Dosage of buprenorphine and buprenorphine hydrochloride usually is expressed in terms of buprenorphine. Dosage of buprenorphine hydrochloride subdermal implants may be expressed as either the salt or the base.

Pain

Opiate analgesics should be given at the lowest effective dosage and for the shortest duration of therapy consistent with the treatment goals of the patient. Initial dosage of buprenorphine should be individualized according to severity of pain, response, prior analgesic use, and risk factors for addiction, abuse, and misuse. Appropriate dosage selection and titration are essential to reduce the risk of respiratory depression. Overestimation of the dosage of buprenorphine when transferring patients from other opiate therapy to buprenorphine therapy can result in fatal overdosage with the first dose. Patients should be monitored closely for respiratory depression, especially during the first 24–72 hours of therapy and following any increase in dosage, and dosage should be adjusted accordingly. If concomitant therapy with other CNS depressants is required, the lowest effective dosages and shortest possible duration of concomitant therapy should be used.

For acute pain not related to trauma or surgery, the prescribed quantity should be limited to the amount needed for the expected duration of pain severe enough to require opiate analgesia (generally 3 days or less and rarely more than 7 days).

When opiate analgesics are used for the management of chronic noncancer pain, the US Centers for Disease Control and Prevention (CDC) recommends that primary care clinicians carefully reassess individual benefits and risks before prescribing dosages equivalent to 50 mg or more of morphine sulfate daily and avoid dosages equivalent to 90 mg or more of morphine sulfate daily or carefully justify their decision to titrate the dosage to such levels. Other experts recommend consulting a pain management specialist before exceeding a dosage equivalent to 80–120 mg of morphine sulfate daily. Some states have set prescribing limits (e.g., maximum daily dosages that can be prescribed, dosage thresholds at which consultation with a specialist is mandated or recommended).

Parenteral Dosage

For the relief of pain that is severe enough to require opiate analgesia and for which alternative treatments are inadequate, the usual IM or IV dosage of buprenorphine in patients 13 years of age and older is 0.3 mg given at intervals of up to every 6 hours as necessary. The initial dose (up to 0.3 mg) may be repeated once in 30–60 minutes, if needed. The dose should be limited to the minimum amount required in high-risk patients (e.g., geriatric or debilitated patients, those with respiratory disease) and in patients receiving other CNS depressants, including patients in the immediate postoperative period. Particular caution is necessary if the drug is administered IV, especially with initial doses. In some patients, it may be necessary to increase the dose up to 0.6 mg, but the manufacturer recommends that such relatively high doses *only* be administered IM and *only* to adults who are not considered high-risk patients. In some patients, a dosing interval greater than 6 hours may be adequate. Alternatively, a regimen including an initial dose of 0.3 mg of buprenorphine followed by another 0.3-mg dose repeated in 3 hours has been shown to be as effective as a single 0.6-mg dose in relieving postoperative pain. There are insufficient clinical data to recommend single doses greater than 0.6 mg for long-term use.

Although children 2–12 years of age have received parenteral buprenorphine dosages of 2–6 mcg/kg every 4–6 hours, longer dosing intervals (e.g., every 6–8 hours) may be sufficient for some children, and a fixed around-the-clock dosing interval should not be used until an adequate dosing interval has been established by clinical observation of the patient. In addition, the manufacturer states that there are insufficient data in children 2–12 years of age to recommend buprenorphine doses exceeding 6 mcg/kg or administration of a repeat dose within 30–60 minutes of the initial dose.

When buprenorphine has been administered by continuous IV infusion† in the management of postoperative pain, dosages of 25–250 mcg/hour have been used in adults.

Buprenorphine has been administered epidurally† in the management of postoperative pain in single doses of 60 mcg, up to a mean total dose of 180 mcg administered over a 48-hour period. Buprenorphine has also been administered epidurally† in a dose of 0.3 mg as a supplement to surgical anesthesia with a local anesthetic. In the management of severe, chronic pain (e.g., in terminally ill patients), buprenorphine doses of 0.15–0.3 mg have been administered epidurally as frequently as every 6 hours up to a mean total daily dose of 0.86 mg (range: 0.15–7.2 mg).

The manufacturer states that data are insufficient to recommend a parenteral buprenorphine dosage for infants younger than 2 years of age. In children 9 months to 9 years of age† undergoing circumcision, some clinicians have used an initial IM buprenorphine dose of 3 mcg/kg as an adjunct to surgical anesthesia followed by additional 3-mcg/kg doses as necessary to provide analgesia postoperatively.

Transdermal Dosage

Buprenorphine transdermal system should be prescribed only by clinicians who are knowledgeable in the use of potent opiates for the management of chronic pain. Dosages of 7.5, 10, 15, and 20 mcg/hour should be reserved for patients who are opiate experienced (i.e., have been receiving oral morphine sulfate dosages of

up to 80 mg or more daily [or equivalent] for one week or longer) and have developed tolerance to an opiate of comparable potency.

In opiate-naive adults with pain that is severe enough to require daily, around-the-clock, long-term opiate analgesia and for which alternative treatments are inadequate, treatment with transdermal buprenorphine should be initiated at a dosage of 5 mcg/hour.

When patients currently receiving opiate agonist therapy are switched to transdermal buprenorphine, there is a potential for buprenorphine to precipitate withdrawal. In these patients, the current opiate regimen should be tapered over a period of up to 7 days to a total 24-hour dosage equivalent to 30 mg or less of oral morphine sulfate. For patients whose prior total daily dosage of opiates was less than 30 mg of oral morphine sulfate (or equivalent), transdermal buprenorphine may be initiated at a dosage of 5 mcg/hour. For patients whose prior total daily dosage was 30–80 mg of oral morphine sulfate (or equivalent), transdermal buprenorphine may be initiated at a dosage of 10 mcg/hour. Patients may receive supplemental short-acting analgesics as needed until adequate analgesia is attained. For patients whose prior total daily dosage exceeded 80 mg of oral morphine sulfate (or equivalent), buprenorphine 20 mcg/hour may not provide adequate analgesia and an alternative analgesic should be considered. When therapy with a buprenorphine transdermal system is initiated, all other around-the-clock opiate analgesics should be discontinued. Buprenorphine may be initiated at the next dosing interval following discontinuance of the current opiate regimen. Particularly close monitoring is required when patients are switched from methadone, since conversion ratios between methadone and other opiates vary widely depending on extent of prior methadone exposure and because methadone has a long half-life and tends to accumulate in plasma.

Buprenorphine dosage may be titrated upward at minimum intervals of 72 hours to a level that provides adequate analgesia and minimizes adverse effects. The maximum recommended transdermal dosage of buprenorphine is 20 mcg/hour, since higher dosages have been shown to prolong the QT interval. Dosage may be adjusted in increments of 5, 7.5, or 10 mcg/hour by simultaneously applying no more than two 5-, 7.5-, or 10-mcg/hour systems; the total combined dosage of the 2 transdermal systems should not exceed 20 mcg/hour.

Patients should be reevaluated continually for adequacy of pain control and for adverse effects, as well as for the development of addiction, abuse, or misuse. Patients who experience episodes of breakthrough pain may require dosage adjustment or supplemental analgesia (i.e., "rescue" therapy with an immediate-release analgesic). If the level of pain increases after dosage stabilization, an attempt should be made to identify the source of increased pain before increasing the dosage. Frequent communication is important among the prescriber, other members of the healthcare team, the patient, and the patient's caregiver or family during periods of changing analgesic requirements, including the initial dosage titration period. During long-term therapy, the continued need for opiate analgesics should be periodically reevaluated. If unacceptable adverse effects are observed, dosage reduction should be considered.

When the patient no longer requires buprenorphine therapy, the dosage should be tapered gradually every 7 days to prevent symptoms of opiate withdrawal. The use of an appropriate short-acting opiate may be considered during the tapering process. Therapy with buprenorphine transdermal system should not be discontinued abruptly.

Buccal Dosage

Buprenorphine hydrochloride buccally dissolving strips (Belbuca®) should be prescribed only by clinicians who are knowledgeable in the use of potent opiates for the management of chronic pain.

For the management of pain that is severe enough to require daily, around-the-clock, long-term opiate analgesia and for which alternative treatments are inadequate, treatment with buprenorphine bucally dissolving strips should be initiated at a dosage of 75 mcg once daily or, if tolerated, 75 mcg every 12 hours in adults who are opiate-naive or are not tolerant to opiates. After at least 4 days at this initial dosage, dosage may be increased to 150 mcg every 12 hours. Use of higher initial dosages in patients who are not opiate tolerant may cause fatal respiratory depression.

When patients currently receiving opiate agonist therapy are switched to intrabuccal buprenorphine, there is a potential for buprenorphine to precipitate withdrawal. In these patients, the current opiate regimen should be tapered to a total 24-hour dosage equivalent to 30 mg or less of oral morphine sulfate. For patients whose prior total daily dosage of opiates was less than 30 mg of oral morphine sulfate (or equivalent), intrabuccal buprenorphine may be initiated at a dosage of 75 mcg once daily or 75 mcg every 12 hours. For patients whose prior total daily dosage was 30–89 mg of oral morphine sulfate (or equivalent), intrabuccal buprenorphine may be initiated at a dosage of 150 mcg every 12 hours. For those whose prior total daily dosage was 90–160 mg of oral morphine sulfate (or equivalent), intrabuccal buprenorphine may be initiated at a dosage of 300 mcg every 12 hours. Patients may receive supplemental short-acting analgesics as needed until adequate analgesia is attained. For patients whose prior total daily dosage exceeded 160 mg of oral morphine sulfate (or equivalent), buprenorphine buccally dissolving strips may not provide adequate analgesia and an alternative analgesic should be considered. When therapy with buprenorphine buccally dissolving strips is initiated, all other around-the-clock opiate analgesics should be discontinued. Particularly close monitoring is required when patients are switched from methadone, since conversion ratios between methadone and other opiates vary widely depending on extent of prior methadone exposure and because methadone has a long half-life and tends to accumulate in plasma.

Buprenorphine dosage may be titrated upward in increments of no more than 150 mcg every 12 hours at minimum intervals of 4 days to a level that provides adequate analgesia and minimizes adverse effects. Doses of 600, 750, and 900 mcg should be used only following titration from lower intrabuccal dosages. Dosages of up to 450 mcg every 12 hours were studied in opiate-naive patients in clinical trials. The maximum recommended intrabuccal dosage is 900 mcg every 12 hours because of the risk of QT-interval prolongation; if this dosage fails to provide adequate analgesia, an alternative analgesic should be considered.

Patients should be reevaluated continually for adequacy of pain control and for adverse effects, as well as for the development of addiction, abuse, or misuse. Patients who experience episodes of breakthrough pain may require dosage adjustment or supplemental analgesia (i.e.," rescue" therapy with an immediate-release analgesic). If the level of pain increases after dosage stabilization, an attempt should be made to identify the source of increased pain before increasing the dosage. Frequent communication is important among the prescriber, other members of the healthcare team, the patient, and the patient's caregiver or family during periods of changing analgesic requirements, including the initial dosage titration period. During long-term therapy, the continued need for opiate analgesics should be periodically reevaluated. If unacceptable adverse effects are observed, dosage should be adjusted to obtain an appropriate balance between pain control and adverse effects.

In patients with known or suspected mucositis, the usual initial dosage and each incremental dosage during titration should be reduced by one-half because of the potential for higher peak concentrations and systemic exposure to the drug.

When the patient no longer requires buprenorphine therapy, the dosage should be tapered gradually to prevent symptoms of opiate withdrawal. Intrabuccal therapy with buprenorphine should not be discontinued abruptly. If manifestations of withdrawal occur, the dosage should be increased to the prior level and tapered more slowly by increasing the interval between dosage reductions and/or reducing the amount of each incremental change in dose.

For further information on the management of opiate analgesic therapy, see Dosage and Administration: Dosage, in the Opiate Agonists General Statement 28:08.08.

Opiate Dependence

Buprenorphine and buprenorphine/naloxone are prescribed and distributed in the management of opiate dependence (opiate use disorder [OUD]) under a restricted distribution program.

Oral transmucosal preparations containing buprenorphine or buprenorphine/naloxone may be used during induction and/or maintenance phases of treatment, while buprenorphine extended-release subcutaneous injection and buprenorphine subdermal implants are used only during maintenance. Because all oral transmucosal formulations are *not* bioequivalent, dosage recommendations vary according to differences in bioavailability. Recommended dosage ranges (based on the buprenorphine component) are the same for generic buprenorphine sublingual tablets (i.e., generic equivalents of Subutex® sublingual tablets [branded formulation no longer commercially available in the US]), generic

buprenorphine/naloxone sublingual tablets (i.e., generic equivalents of Suboxone® sublingual tablets [branded formulation no longer commercially available in the US]), and buprenorphine/naloxone sublingually dissolving strips (Suboxone®), although some strengths and dose combinations of these preparations are not bioequivalent. Dosage ranges for certain other oral transmucosal buprenorphine/naloxone preparations (i.e., Bunavail® buccally dissolving strips, Zubsolv® sublingual tablets) are lower, reflecting the greater bioavailability of these preparations. Although generic buprenorphine/naloxone sublingual tablets are labeled in the US only for maintenance treatment, this formulation also has been used (similarly to other oral transmucosal buprenorphine/naloxone preparations) in the induction† phase of treatment.

Presence of naloxone, an opiate antagonist, in the fixed-combination preparation is intended to deter parenteral abuse of buprenorphine by individuals dependent on other opiates since a sufficient amount of the opiate antagonist is present in the formulation to precipitate opiate withdrawal if administered parenterally (but not sublingually). When administered sublingually, systemic naloxone concentrations are insufficient to elicit clinically important effects; in addition, sublingual administration of buprenorphine and buprenorphine/naloxone has been shown to elicit similar clinical, physiologic, and subjective effects.

Although buprenorphine traditionally has been considered the preferred drug for the initial (i.e., induction) phase of treatment, additional experience indicates that either buprenorphine or buprenorphine/naloxone may be used for induction in patients dependent on heroin or other short-acting opiates. Use of buprenorphine/naloxone for the induction phase of treatment in patients dependent on long-acting opiates has not been evaluated to date in adequate and well-controlled studies; the manufacturers and some experts still recommend use of buprenorphine alone for induction in these patients. Following induction, buprenorphine/naloxone is the preferred drug for maintenance treatment when use includes unsupervised administration. Administration of buprenorphine without naloxone in an unsupervised setting should be limited to pregnant women and patients who cannot tolerate naloxone.

Prior to induction, the type of opiate dependence (i.e., long- or short-acting opiate), time since last opiate use, and degree of opiate dependence should be considered. Abuse of long-acting formulations by manipulation of the dosage form (e.g., crushing and snorting or injecting extended-release oral dosage forms) may cause these formulations to act as short-acting drugs. To avoid precipitating withdrawal, the first dose of buprenorphine or buprenorphine/naloxone should be given when objective and clear signs of opiate withdrawal are evident.

In individuals dependent on heroin or other short-acting opiates, the manufacturers state that the first dose of buprenorphine or buprenorphine/naloxone should be administered at least 4 or 6 hours, respectively, after the last use of the opiate. Some experts recommend waiting at least 6–12 hours after last use of short-acting opiates and recommend use of an opiate withdrawal scale (e.g., Clinical Opioid Withdrawal Scale [COWS] score of approximately 11–12 or higher) to establish that withdrawal is sufficient to allow for safe and comfortable induction. Administration of a low initial dose of buprenorphine or buprenorphine/naloxone also reduces the risk of precipitated withdrawal. Because gradual titration of buprenorphine dosage over several days has been associated with a high dropout rate during the induction phase in clinical studies, an adequate treatment dosage, titrated to clinical effectiveness, should be achieved as rapidly as possible once it has been established that the initial dose of the drug was well tolerated.

Patients dependent on methadone or other long-acting opiates may be more susceptible than those who are dependent on short-acting opiates to precipitated and prolonged withdrawal during induction. Therefore, the first dose of buprenorphine should be given when objective and clear signs of opiate withdrawal are evident, generally not less than 24 hours after the last use of the opiate. Controlled experience with the transfer of patients from methadone maintenance to buprenorphine is limited. Withdrawal symptoms appear to be more likely in those receiving higher dosages of methadone hydrochloride (greater than 30 mg daily) and when the first dose of buprenorphine is given shortly after the last methadone dose. Thus, dosage of methadone hydrochloride should be tapered to approximately 30–40 mg daily or less and maintained at this level for at least a week prior to induction. Experts state that the first dose of buprenorphine may be administered at least 24–72 hours or longer after last use of long-acting opiates such as methadone and recommend use of an opiate withdrawal scale (e.g., COWS score of approximately 11–12 or higher) to establish that withdrawal is sufficient to allow for safe and comfortable induction.

Induction in the prescribing clinician's office is recommended to reduce the risk of precipitated withdrawal; unsupervised administration may then be initiated as the patient's clinical stability allows. Although large, randomized, controlled studies are lacking, experts state that at-home induction (with early in-office follow-up) by patients dependent on short-acting opiates may be considered depending on the patient's circumstances if the patient and/or clinician is experienced with the use of buprenorphine and the patient can rate withdrawal symptoms, fully understand induction dosing instructions, and can and will contact the clinician as needed.

Patients receiving maintenance treatment should be seen at reasonable intervals (e.g., at least weekly during the first months of therapy) based on the individual's circumstances; once patients are receiving a stable buprenorphine dosage and are progressing toward treatment goals, less frequent (e.g., monthly) visits may be reasonable. Prescription quantities for unsupervised administration should take into account the patient's clinical stability, home situation, and ability to manage take-home medication. Authorization of multiple refills is not advised early in treatment or without appropriate follow-up visits. Review of state prescription drug monitoring program (PDMP) data for other prescribed drugs of concern, urine drug testing, and recall visits for "pill" counts also are recommended. If treatment goals are not being achieved, the appropriateness of the current therapy should be reevaluated. Unstable patients (e.g., those who are abusing or are dependent on various drugs or are unresponsive to psychosocial interventions) may require referral for more intensive treatment.

For the maintenance treatment of opiate dependence, oral transmucosal preparations of buprenorphine/naloxone are labeled only for once-daily administration; however, other dosage regimens (i.e., administration every other day† or 3 times weekly† at a dose higher than the individually titrated daily dose) have been used once satisfactory stabilization has been achieved.

Dosage of Lower-bioavailability Oral Transmucosal Formulations for Induction and Maintenance

When generic buprenorphine sublingual tablets (i.e., generic equivalents of Subutex® sublingual tablets), generic buprenorphine/naloxone sublingual tablets (i.e., generic equivalents of Suboxone® sublingual tablets), or buprenorphine/naloxone sublingually dissolving strips (Suboxone®) are used for induction therapy, the recommended induction dosage of buprenorphine on day 1 is up to 8 mg (alone or in fixed combination with up to 2 mg of naloxone). Induction should be initiated on day 1 with a buprenorphine dose of 2 or 4 mg (alone or in fixed combination with naloxone 0.5 or 1 mg, respectively), with additional doses of 2 or 4 mg administered at approximately 2-hour intervals if there are continued withdrawal symptoms and sedation is not observed. Use of an opiate withdrawal scale (e.g., COWS) during induction can be helpful in assessing the effects of administered doses. On day 2, a single dose of up to 16 mg of buprenorphine (alone or in fixed combination with up to 4 mg of naloxone) is given. Other induction dosages that also employ a low initial dose with rapid titration to an effective maintenance dosage have been used.

For oral transmucosal maintenance treatment, buprenorphine/naloxone is preferred over buprenorphine alone. (See initial paragraphs of Opiate Dependence under Dosage and Administration: Dosage.) From day 3 onward, buprenorphine/naloxone dosage should be adjusted in increments or decrements of 2 or 4 mg of buprenorphine in fixed combination with 0.5 or 1 mg, respectively, of naloxone daily to a dosage that suppresses opiate withdrawal symptoms and ensures that the patient continues buprenorphine treatment. The maintenance buprenorphine/naloxone dosage generally ranges from 4–24 mg of buprenorphine in fixed combination with 1–6 mg of naloxone daily. The recommended buprenorphine/naloxone target dosage during maintenance treatment is 16 mg of buprenorphine and 4 mg of naloxone as a single daily dose. Dosages exceeding 24 mg of buprenorphine in fixed combination with 6 mg of naloxone daily have not been shown to provide any additional clinical advantage.

Zubsolv® Dosage for Induction and Maintenance

When Zubsolv® sublingual tablets are used for induction and maintenance treatment, the recommended induction dosage on day 1 is up to 5.7 mg of buprenorphine in fixed combination with up to 1.4 mg of naloxone. Induction should be initiated with a buprenorphine/naloxone dose of 1.4 mg of buprenorphine in fixed combination with 0.36 mg of naloxone, with the remainder of the day 1 dosage (up to 4.2 mg of buprenorphine and up to 1.08 mg of naloxone) administered in divided doses as 1 or 2 tablets containing buprenorphine 1.4 mg and naloxone

0.36 mg at intervals of 1.5–2 hours. Some patients (e.g., those who recently received buprenorphine) may tolerate up to 3 tablets containing buprenorphine 1.4 mg and naloxone 0.36 mg as a single second dose. On day 2, a single dose of up to 11.4 mg of buprenorphine and 2.9 mg of naloxone is recommended.

From day 3 onward, buprenorphine/naloxone dosage should be adjusted in increments or decrements of no more than 2.9 mg of buprenorphine and 0.71 mg of naloxone to a level that suppresses opiate withdrawal symptoms and ensures that the patient continues buprenorphine treatment. After induction and stabilization, the maintenance buprenorphine/naloxone dosage generally ranges from 2.9–17.2 mg of buprenorphine in fixed combination with 0.71–4.2 mg of naloxone daily. The recommended buprenorphine/naloxone target dosage during maintenance treatment is 11.4 mg of buprenorphine and 2.9 mg of naloxone as a single daily dose. Dosages exceeding 17.2 mg of buprenorphine in fixed combination with 4.2 mg of naloxone daily have not been shown to provide any additional clinical advantage.

Bunavail® Dosage for Induction and Maintenance

When Bunavail® buccally dissolving strips are used for induction and maintenance treatment, the recommended induction dosage on day 1 is up to 4.2 mg of buprenorphine in fixed combination with up to 0.7 mg of naloxone. Induction should be initiated with a buprenorphine/naloxone dose of 2.1 mg of buprenorphine in fixed combination with 0.3 mg of naloxone; a second dose of the same strength is administered approximately 2 hours later based on control of acute withdrawal symptoms. On Day 2, a single dose of up to 8.4 mg of buprenorphine in fixed combination with 1.4 mg of naloxone is recommended.

From day 3 onward, buprenorphine/naloxone dosage should be adjusted in increments or decrements of 2.1 mg of buprenorphine and 0.3 mg of naloxone to a level that suppresses opiate withdrawal symptoms and ensures that the patient continues buprenorphine treatment. After induction and stabilization, the maintenance buprenorphine/naloxone dosage generally ranges from 2.1–12.6 mg of buprenorphine in fixed combination with 0.3–2.1 mg of naloxone daily. The recommended buprenorphine/naloxone target dosage during maintenance treatment is 8.4 mg of buprenorphine and 1.4 mg of naloxone as a single daily dose. Dosages exceeding 12.6 mg of buprenorphine in fixed combination with 2.1 mg of naloxone daily have not been shown to provide any additional clinical advantage.

Dosage Adjustments When Switching Between Oral Transmucosal Strengths and Preparations

Not all formulations, strengths, or dose combinations of oral transmucosal buprenorphine/naloxone preparations are bioequivalent.

Patients who currently are receiving generic buprenorphine or buprenorphine/naloxone sublingual tablets (i.e., generic equivalents of Subutex® or Suboxone® sublingual tablets) and are switching to buprenorphine/naloxone sublingually dissolving strips (Suboxone®), or vice versa, should continue to receive the same drug dosage. However, not all strengths and dose combinations of the strips and sublingual tablets are bioequivalent. Because of potentially greater bioavailability with the strips relative to the tablets, patients should be monitored for underdosage (e.g., manifestations of withdrawal) or overdosage when switching between sublingual dosage forms and the dosage should be adjusted when indicated.

The 4 strengths of Suboxone® sublingually dissolving strips differ in size and buprenorphine and naloxone concentrations (on a % [w/w] basis). Switching between various combinations of lower- and higher-strength strips to obtain the same total dose may result in changes in systemic exposure to buprenorphine and naloxone and require that the patient be monitored for underdosage or overdosage. Therefore, substitution of one or more strip strengths for another without the prescriber's approval is not recommended. Because systemic exposure to naloxone is somewhat higher after buccal compared with sublingual administration of the strips, sublingual administration is recommended during induction to minimize the risk of precipitated withdrawal. However, exposure to buprenorphine is similar following either buccal or sublingual administration, and once induction is complete, patients can switch between buccal and sublingual administration without substantial risk of underdosage or overdosage.

Bunavail® and Zubsolv® have different bioavailabilities than Suboxone® (or generic equivalent) sublingual tablets. Patients switching between these preparations should receive a different dosage strength (see Table 1 and Table 2) and should be monitored for underdosage or overdosage. Dosage adjustments may be necessary. Systemic buprenorphine exposure following administration of one Suboxone® sublingual tablet containing buprenorphine 8 mg and naloxone 2 mg is equivalent to that achieved following administration of one Bunavail® buccally dissolving strip containing buprenorphine 4.2 mg and naloxone 0.7 mg or one Zubsolv® sublingual tablet containing buprenorphine 5.7 mg and naloxone 1.4 mg.

TABLE 1. Corresponding Doses and Strengths of Suboxone® Sublingual Tablets and Bunavail® Buccally Dissolving Strips

Suboxone® Sublingual Dose or Tablet Strength	Corresponding Bunavail® Strip Strength
Buprenorphine 4 mg and naloxone 1 mg	Buprenorphine 2.1 mg and naloxone 0.3 mg
Buprenorphine 8 mg and naloxone 2 mg	Buprenorphine 4.2 mg and naloxone 0.7 mg
Buprenorphine 12 mg and naloxone 3 mg	Buprenorphine 6.3 mg and naloxone 1 mg

TABLE 2. Corresponding Dosage Strengths of Suboxone® Sublingual Tablets (or Generic Equivalent) and Zubsolv® Sublingual Tablets

Suboxone® (or Generic Equivalent) Sublingual Dose (Tablet Strength)	Corresponding Zubsolv® Sublingual Tablet Strength
Buprenorphine 2 mg and naloxone 0.5 mg (as one 2-mg/0.5-mg tablet)	One 1.4-mg/0.36-mg tablet
Buprenorphine 4 mg and naloxone 1 mg (as two 2-mg/0.5-mg tablets)	One 2.9-mg/0.71-mg tablet
Buprenorphine 8 mg and naloxone 2 mg (as one 8-mg/2-mg tablet)	One 5.7-mg/1.4-mg tablet
Buprenorphine 12 mg and naloxone 3 mg (as one 8-mg/2-mg tablet and two 2-mg/0.5-mg tablets)	One 8.6-mg/2.1-mg tablet
Buprenorphine 16 mg and naloxone 4 mg (as two 8-mg/2-mg tablets)	One 11.4-mg/2.9-mg tablet

Extended-release Subcutaneous Injection Dosage for Maintenance Treatment

Maintenance treatment with buprenorphine extended-release subcutaneous injection may be initiated in patients who have initiated buprenorphine induction therapy with an oral transmucosal buprenorphine-containing preparation followed by dosage adjustment over a least 7 days to an oral transmucosal buprenorphine dosage of 8–24 mg daily (as Subutex® or Suboxone® [or equivalent generic buprenorphine or buprenorphine/naloxone preparation]) or a dosage of another oral transmucosal preparation that provides equivalent buprenorphine exposure. One Bunavail® buccally dissolving strip containing buprenorphine 4.2 mg and naloxone 0.7 mg or one Zubsolv® sublingual tablet containing buprenorphine 5.7 mg and naloxone 1.4 mg provides equivalent buprenorphine exposure as one Suboxone® sublingual tablet containing buprenorphine 8 mg and naloxone 2 mg or one Subutex® sublingual tablet containing buprenorphine 8 mg.

The recommended dosage of buprenorphine extended-release subcutaneous injection following induction and dosage adjustment with oral transmucosal buprenorphine is 300 mg monthly for the first 2 months followed by a maintenance dosage of 100 mg monthly. The maintenance dosage may be increased to 300 mg monthly in patients who tolerate the 100-mg monthly dosage but do not achieve a satisfactory clinical response, as evidenced by self-reports or urine drug test results indicating illicit opiate use. If a dose is missed, the dose should be administered as soon as possible, with the following dose given no less than

26 days later. Occasional delays in dosing of up to 2 weeks are not expected to substantially alter the treatment effect. If a subcutaneous depot of the drug must be surgically excised, the patient should be monitored for manifestations of withdrawal and appropriate treatment (e.g., an oral transmucosal preparation of the drug) should be instituted as clinically indicated.

Implant Dosage for Maintenance Treatment

Maintenance treatment with buprenorphine subdermal implants may be initiated in patients who have achieved and maintained prolonged clinical stability on oral transmucosal buprenorphine therapy; are currently receiving an oral transmucosal buprenorphine maintenance dosage of 8 mg daily or less (as Subutex® or Suboxone® [or equivalent generic buprenorphine or buprenorphine/naloxone preparation] or a dosage of another oral transmucosal preparation that provides comparable blood buprenorphine concentrations [e.g., Bunavail® buccally dissolving strips at a dosage of buprenorphine 4.2 mg and naloxone 0.7 mg daily or less, Zubsolv® sublingual tablets at a dosage of buprenorphine 5.7 mg and naloxone 1.4 mg daily or less]); and have received a stable oral transmucosal buprenorphine maintenance dosage of 8 mg daily or less for at least 3 months without the need for supplemental doses of the drug or dosage adjustments. The dosage of oral transmucosal buprenorphine should not be tapered to this dosage level solely for the purpose of transitioning to implant therapy. The 8-mg oral transmucosal dosage provides blood buprenorphine concentrations that are similar to or less than those provided by the recommended implant dosage.

Each buprenorphine dose consists of 4 implants (each containing 80 mg of buprenorphine hydrochloride [equivalent to 74.2 mg of the base]) inserted subdermally in the inner aspect of the upper arm; the implants are intended to be left in place for 6 months and then removed by the end of the sixth month. If continued implant therapy is desired at the time the initial implants are removed, new implants may be inserted subdermally in the contralateral arm. If new implants are not inserted on the same day that the current ones are removed, patients should receive their previous dosage of oral transmucosal buprenorphine (i.e., the dosage they received prior to initiation of implant therapy) prior to additional implant therapy. After one insertion in each arm, most patients should be transitioned back to oral transmucosal buprenorphine therapy, since experience is lacking with insertion of implants at other sites in the arm or with insertion of new implants at prior administration sites (where potential effects of scarring and fibrosis on efficacy and safety are unknown).

Although some patients may require occasional supplemental dosing with buprenorphine, the manufacturer states that patients should not be provided with prescriptions for oral transmucosal buprenorphine-containing preparations for use on as-needed basis. Instead, patients who feel the need for supplemental dosing should be evaluated promptly by a clinician. An ongoing need for supplemental dosing indicates that the amount of buprenorphine delivered by the implants is not adequate for stable maintenance treatment; use of an alternative buprenorphine preparation for maintenance treatment should be considered. If an implant is expelled spontaneously, the patient should be carefully monitored until the implant is replaced for withdrawal manifestations or other indications that supplemental oral transmucosal dosing may be required.

Discontinuance

The decision to discontinue therapy with buprenorphine or buprenorphine/naloxone after a period of maintenance or brief stabilization should be made as part of a comprehensive treatment plan. Oral transmucosal dosage should be tapered to reduce the occurrence of withdrawal manifestations. Dosage generally is tapered over several months with close monitoring and a plan for sustaining recovery.

If therapy with buprenorphine extended-release subcutaneous injection is discontinued, the patient should be monitored for several months for manifestations of withdrawal, since the onset of any withdrawal manifestations may be delayed; if treatment of withdrawal manifestations is required, use of oral transmucosal buprenorphine should be considered. In clinical trials, withdrawal manifestations were not observed during the first month following discontinuance of treatment with buprenorphine extended-release subcutaneous injection. Plasma concentrations of buprenorphine may be detectable for 12 months or longer if therapy with this formulation is discontinued after steady state has been achieved (4–6 months of treatment); the correlation between plasma and detectable urine concentrations of buprenorphine is not known.

If therapy with buprenorphine implants is discontinued, the patient should be monitored for manifestations of withdrawal and use of a tapering dosage of oral transmucosal buprenorphine should be considered.

Other Uses

To reverse fentanyl-induced anesthesia† and provide subsequent analgesia in adults, IV or IM buprenorphine doses of 0.3–0.8 mg have been administered 1–4 hours following induction of anesthesia and about 30 minutes prior to the end of surgery.

● *Restricted Distribution Program for Buprenorphine Treatment of Opiate Dependence*

The Drug Addiction Treatment Act of 2000 (DATA 2000) allows qualifying physicians to prescribe and dispense narcotics in schedules III, IV, and V of the Federal Controlled Substances Act that have been approved by FDA for detoxification or maintenance treatment of opiate dependence. The Comprehensive Addiction and Recovery Act of 2016 (CARA 2016) expands the categories of practitioners through October 1, 2021, to include qualifying nurse practitioners and physician assistants. Prior to passage of DATA 2000, opiate dependence treatment could be provided only at specially registered clinics. Under DATA 2000 and CARA 2016, prescription use of buprenorphine and buprenorphine/naloxone in the treatment of opiate dependence is limited to practitioners who meet certain requirements, have notified the Secretary of the US Department of Health and Human Services (HHS) of their intent to prescribe these preparations for this indication, and have been assigned a unique identification number that must be included on each prescription for the drug.

Prescribers

DATA 2000 limited office-based use of buprenorphine and buprenorphine/naloxone for the management of opiate dependence to physicians who meet special training criteria and can provide appropriate services. CARA 2016 expanded the categories of practitioners to include qualifying nurse practitioners and physician assistants. To qualify, physicians must meet one or more of the following training requirements: hold a subspecialty board certification in addiction psychiatry from the American Board of Medical Specialties; hold subspecialty board certification in addiction medicine from the American Osteopathic Association; hold an addiction certification from the American Society of Addiction Medicine; have completed not less than 8 hours of authorized training on the management or treatment of opiate-dependent patients; have participated as an investigator in one or more clinical trials leading to the approval of a schedule III, IV, or V opiate for maintenance or detoxification treatment; and/or have other training or experience that is deemed by HHS or the state medical licensing board to demonstrate the physician's ability to treat and manage opiate-dependent patients. To quality, nurse practitioners and physician assistants must meet all of the following requirements: be authorized under state law to prescribe schedule III, IV, or V drugs for pain management; work in collaboration with or be supervised by a qualifying physician if so required by state law; and have completed not less than 24 hours of authorized initial training. In addition, practitioners must have the capacity to provide or to refer patients for needed ancillary services (i.e., psychosocial therapy) and must agree to prescribe schedule III, IV, or V drugs for management of opiate dependence for a limited number of patients. Before prescribing buprenorphine or buprenorphine/naloxone, practitioners who meet these criteria must notify the HHS Substance Abuse and Mental Health Services Administration (SAMHSA) of their intention to prescribe these agents.

Initially, each qualifying practitioner, whether practicing individually or in a group practice, can treat no more than 30 patients at one time. Practitioners who have been certified to treat opiate dependence with buprenorphine for at least 1 year can apply to treat up to 100 patients at one time. Those who have been eligible to treat up to 100 patients at a time for at least one year without interruption can apply to increase the limit to 275 patients if they have additional credentialing or practice in a qualified setting. In addition, practitioners who currently are eligible to treat up to 100 patients but who otherwise are not eligible to increase their patient limit to 275 may request a temporary increase in certain emergency situations.

The US Drug Enforcement Administration (DEA) will issue qualifying practitioners a unique identification number; this number indicates that the practitioner is qualified under DATA 2000 or CARA 2016 to prescribe buprenorphine for the management of opiate dependence and is intended to preserve the confidentiality of the patient. The SAMHSA Center for Substance Abuse Treatment will inform the practitioner of the new DEA identification number in writing via email. The DEA requires inclusion of the new identification number along with the practitioner's usual DEA number on all prescriptions issued for the treatment of opiate dependence. Although it is anticipated that most prescribers will obtain DEA identification numbers before prescribing buprenorphine or buprenorphine/naloxone for such use, DATA 2000 allows practitioners with qualifying credentials and/or training to write prescriptions for these agents before the DEA identification number is issued if the practitioner has notified SAMHSA of their intention to begin treating a patient immediately and has verified that SAMHSA received the notification form. Immediate treatment is limited to one patient per notification form, and no more than one form may be submitted on a given day.

Practitioners should be aware that there are special federal regulations concerning confidentiality of substance abuse treatment records and the privacy of health records. Any patient-identifying information pertaining to treatment of substance abuse must be handled with a greater degree of confidentiality than patients' general medical information. Before a prescriber can disclose any information to a third party about a patient's treatment for substance abuse, that prescriber must obtain the patient's signed consent. Each disclosure made with the patient's consent must be accompanied by a statement indicating that unauthorized disclosure is prohibited.

Dispensing Pharmacies

Each time a pharmacist fills a prescription for buprenorphine or buprenorphine/naloxone, the pharmacist is expected to verify that the prescription is from a prescriber who is in compliance with the provisions of DATA 2000. Practitioners who are qualified to prescribe buprenorphine and buprenorphine/naloxone and are in compliance with DATA 2000 are issued a *unique* DEA identification number; the new identification number along with the practitioner's usual DEA number is required on all prescriptions issued for the treatment of opiate dependence. If a prescription is phoned to the pharmacy, pharmacists must ensure that both numbers are on the prescription record. Pharmacists may utilize SAMHSA's online look-up tool (at https://www.samhsa.gov/bupe/lookup-form) or contact 866-287-2728 to verify whether a prescriber is in compliance with the provisions of DATA 2000.

If a pharmacist receives a prescription for buprenorphine or buprenorphine/naloxone that does not include the *unique* DEA identification number, the pharmacist should contact the prescriber for clarification and to confirm that the prescriber has notified SAMHSA of their intention to prescribe the drug. Pharmacists also may contact SAMHSA (at infobuprenorphine@samhsa.hhs.gov or 866-287-2728). It is anticipated that most prescribers will obtain DEA identification numbers before prescribing buprenorphine or buprenorphine/naloxone. However, DATA 2000 allows practitioners with qualifying credentials and/or training to write prescriptions for these agents before the DEA identification number is issued if the practitioner has notified SAMHSA of their intention to begin treating a patient immediately.

Pharmacists should be aware that there are special federal regulations concerning confidentiality of substance abuse treatment records and the privacy of health records. Any patient-identifying information pertaining to treatment of substance abuse must be handled with a greater degree of confidentiality than patients' general medical information. Before a prescriber can disclose any information to a third party about a patient's treatment for substance abuse, the prescriber must obtain the patient's signed consent. When a prescriber directly transmits a prescription for a buprenorphine-containing preparation for treatment of substance abuse to a pharmacy, the patient's signed consent must be obtained before any patient-identifying information is further disclosed by the pharmacy.

With the availability of buprenorphine for outpatient management of opiate dependence, many pharmacists have the opportunity to provide services that focus on ensuring appropriate drug administration, monitoring for adverse effects, alleviating withdrawal symptoms, treating intercurrent illnesses, minimizing diversion, and aiding in the prevention of relapse.

A potential problem with take-home outpatient opiate agonist treatment is diversion. While the addition of naloxone is intended to decrease the potential for parenteral abuse of the combination preparations, the possibility of diversion exists because the drug may be used by opiate-dependent individuals in an attempt to attenuate withdrawal symptoms when illicit substances (e.g., heroin) are not available. In addition, individuals who are not opiate dependent may acquire buprenorphine for the purpose of getting high. To address diversion, patients may be asked on a random, unannounced basis to return to the clinic or pharmacy for verification of tablet counts. Since diversion is a concern, pharmacists should be alert for signs of this activity, including presentation of simultaneous prescriptions for the same patient from multiple prescribers, requests for additional doses or refills prior to the appropriate date, calls from opiate-dependent individuals who are not patients, and accidental loss or destruction of the drug. It is important to report any suspicion of diversion to the appropriate authorities.

● Dosage in Hepatic Impairment

Transdermal buprenorphine has not been studied in patients with severe hepatic impairment; use of an alternative analgesic regimen that allows for greater dosage flexibility should be considered in these patients.

When buprenorphine buccally dissolving strips (Belbuca®) are used for analgesia in patients with severe hepatic impairment (i.e., Child-Pugh class C), the usual initial dosage should be reduced and each incremental change in dosage during titration should be reduced by one-half (i.e., from 150 mcg to 75 mcg). No dosage adjustment is required in patients with moderate hepatic impairment, but patients with either moderate or severe hepatic impairment should be monitored for overdosage and toxicity.

When buprenorphine or buprenorphine/naloxone is used sublingually or buccally for the management of opiate dependence in patients with mild hepatic impairment, plasma concentrations and half-lives of the drugs are not substantially altered. However, in individuals with moderate or severe hepatic impairment, plasma concentrations of both buprenorphine and naloxone are increased and half-lives of the drugs are prolonged. Naloxone is affected to a greater degree than buprenorphine, and the magnitude of the difference in effect is greater in individuals with severe hepatic impairment than in those with moderate hepatic impairment. (See Pharmacokinetics: Elimination.) This may result in an increased risk of precipitated withdrawal during induction and interference with buprenorphine's efficacy throughout treatment. Buprenorphine/naloxone should be avoided in patients with severe hepatic impairment and may not be appropriate for those with moderate hepatic impairment. In patients with moderate hepatic impairment, buprenorphine/naloxone is not recommended for induction therapy but may be used with caution and careful monitoring for maintenance treatment following induction therapy with buprenorphine alone. The manufacturer states that the initial dose and titration increments of buprenorphine administered as the single-entity sublingual tablets should be reduced by one-half in patients with severe hepatic impairment and recommends that patients with either moderate or severe hepatic impairment be monitored for buprenorphine overdosage or toxicity.

Use of buprenorphine extended-release subcutaneous injection or buprenorphine subdermal implants is not recommended in patients with preexisting moderate to severe hepatic impairment since the extended-release injection does not allow for rapid adjustment of plasma buprenorphine concentrations and the implant dosage cannot be titrated.

CAUTIONS

Adverse effects of buprenorphine are qualitatively similar to those of morphine, meperidine, and the opiate partial agonists (e.g., pentazocine, nalbuphine); however, the frequency of specific adverse effects produced by buprenorphine may differ from that of the various opiate agonists and partial agonists. Certain adverse effects of buprenorphine, including nausea, vomiting, CNS effects, and respiratory depression, appear to be dose and plasma concentration related. In opiate-tolerant patients, this relationship may be altered by the development of tolerance to opiate-related adverse effects; however, tolerance to opiate effects does not develop uniformly.

When administered sublingually, the adverse effect profile of buprenorphine is similar to that of buprenorphine in fixed combination with naloxone (buprenorphine/naloxone). Sublingually dissolving strips and sublingual tablets containing buprenorphine/naloxone generally have similar adverse effect profiles. Following buccal administration of buprenorphine/naloxone sublingually dissolving strips, the adverse effect profile is similar to that observed following sublingual administration.

● Nervous System Effects

Buprenorphine may cause CNS depression, including somnolence, dizziness, alterations in judgment, and alterations in levels of consciousness, including coma.

Sedation (e.g., drowsiness) is the most common adverse effect of parenteral buprenorphine, occurring in approximately two-thirds of patients; however, patients reportedly are easily aroused to an alert state. Dizziness and vertigo have been reported in about 5–10% of patients receiving parenteral buprenorphine. Headache has been reported in about 1–5% of these patients. Confusion, euphoria, weakness, fatigue, nervousness, mental depression, slurred speech, paresthesia, dreaming, psychosis, malaise, hallucinations, depersonalization, and coma have been reported in less than 1% of patients receiving parenteral buprenorphine for pain relief. Lightheadedness, insomnia, and disorientation have also occurred. Seizures, muscle twitching, lack of muscle coordination, ataxia, dysphoria, and agitation have been reported rarely. Psychotomimetic effects occur less frequently in patients receiving buprenorphine than in patients receiving pentazocine but more frequently than in patients receiving morphine.

Buprenorphine has the potential to lower the seizure threshold and may aggravate seizure disorders and induce seizures in some clinical settings.

Frequent adverse CNS effects reported in clinical trials in patients receiving transdermal buprenorphine include headache and dizziness (each occurring in about 5–15% of patients) and somnolence (occurring in up to 15% of patients). Fatigue, asthenia, insomnia, hypoesthesia, paresthesia, tremor, migraine, anxiety, and depression have been reported in about 1–5% of patients receiving transdermal buprenorphine. Other adverse nervous system effects reported in less than 1% of patients receiving transdermal buprenorphine include affect lability, agitation, apathy, confusional state, abnormal coordination, depersonalization, depressed mood, disorientation, attention disturbance, dysarthria, euphoric mood, gait disturbance, hallucination, loss of consciousness, depressed level of consciousness, malaise, memory impairment, mental impairment, mental status changes, nervousness, nightmare, psychotic disorder, restlessness, sedation, and vertigo.

In clinical trials in patients receiving buprenorphine buccally dissolving strips for pain relief, fatigue, headache, dizziness, and somnolence were reported in at least 5% of patients receiving the buccally administered drug; anxiety, insomnia, and depression were reported in 1 to less than 5% of patients; and asthenia, hypoesthesia, lethargy, migraine, and tremor were reported in less than 1% of patients.

Adverse nervous system effects reported in clinical trials in patients receiving sublingual buprenorphine or buprenorphine/naloxone for the treatment of opiate dependence include headache, insomnia, anxiety, depression, irritability, restlessness, asthenia, dizziness, nervousness, and somnolence. Intoxication and disturbance in attention also have been reported. In clinical trials in patients receiving buprenorphine/naloxone buccally dissolving strips, headache and lethargy were reported in at least 5% of patients, and insomnia, somnolence, and fatigue were reported in more than 1 to less than 5% of patients.

In phase 3 clinical trials, headache, fatigue, somnolence, sedation, and dizziness were reported in less than 10% of patients receiving buprenorphine extended-release subcutaneous injection.

In phase 3 clinical trials, headache and depression were reported in 6–13% and dizziness, somnolence, fatigue, asthenia, migraine, sedation, and paresthesia were reported in less than 5% of patients with buprenorphine subdermal implants.

● GI Effects

Nausea occurs in about 5–10% of patients receiving parenteral buprenorphine for pain relief and is accompanied by vomiting in about 1–5% of patients. Vomiting alone occurs in about 1–5% of these patients. Dry mouth, constipation, dyspepsia, abdominal cramps, and flatulence have occurred in less than 1% of patients receiving parenteral buprenorphine. Anorexia and diarrhea have been reported rarely.

In clinical trials in patients receiving transdermal buprenorphine, the most frequent adverse GI effects were nausea (10–25% of patients), constipation (5–15%), vomiting (5–10%), and dry mouth (6%). Diarrhea, dyspepsia, stomach discomfort, anorexia, and upper abdominal pain have been reported in about 1–5% of patients receiving transdermal buprenorphine. Other adverse GI effects reported in less than 1% of patients receiving transdermal buprenorphine include abdominal distension, abdominal pain, diverticulitis, dysgeusia, dysphagia, flatulence, and ileus.

In clinical trials in patients receiving buprenorphine buccally dissolving strips for pain relief, nausea, constipation, vomiting, diarrhea, and dry mouth were reported in at least 5% of patients receiving the buccally administered drug; abdominal pain, decreased appetite, and gastroenteritis were reported in 1 to less than 5% of patients; and abdominal discomfort, dyspepsia, toothache, and tooth abscess were reported in less than 1% of patients.

Nausea, abdominal pain, constipation, vomiting, diarrhea, dyspepsia, and stomach discomfort have occurred in patients receiving sublingual buprenorphine or buprenorphine/naloxone for the treatment of opiate dependence in clinical trials. Oral hypoesthesia, glossodynia, glossitis, stomatitis, blistering and ulceration of the mouth or tongue, and oral mucosal erythema also have occurred with sublingual use of the drug. Constipation and oral mucosal erythema have been reported in less than 5% of patients receiving buprenorphine/naloxone buccally dissolving strips.

In phase 3 clinical trials, constipation, nausea, and vomiting were reported in about 5–9% of patients receiving buprenorphine extended-release subcutaneous injection.

Nausea, vomiting, constipation, upper abdominal pain, flatulence, and toothache were reported in phase 3 clinical trials in 1–6% of patients with buprenorphine subdermal implants.

● Hepatic Effects

Cytolytic hepatitis and hepatitis with jaundice have occurred in individuals receiving buprenorphine for the treatment of opiate dependence in clinical trials and during postmarketing experience. Adverse hepatic effects that have occurred in these individuals include transient asymptomatic elevations in serum hepatic aminotransferase concentrations, hepatic failure, hepatic necrosis, hepatorenal syndrome, and hepatic encephalopathy. In some individuals, preexisting hepatic enzyme abnormalities, hepatitis B virus (HBV) or hepatitis C virus (HCV) infection, concomitant use of potentially hepatotoxic drugs, or ongoing illicit use of injectable drugs may have contributed to or caused these adverse hepatic events. Data were insufficient in some cases to determine the etiology of the adverse event. The possibility exists that buprenorphine had a causative or contributory role in some of these adverse hepatic events.

Increased ALT concentrations have been reported in clinical trials in less than 1% of patients receiving transdermal buprenorphine.

In clinical trials in patients receiving buprenorphine buccally dissolving strips for pain relief, increased AST concentration and liver function test abnormality were reported in less than 1% of patients receiving the buccally administered drug.

In phase 3 clinical trials, increased concentrations of ALT, AST, and γ-glutamyltransferase (GGT, γ-glutamyltranspeptidase, GGTP) were reported in about 1–5% of patients receiving buprenorphine extended-release subcutaneous injection.

● Cardiovascular Effects

Buprenorphine has the potential to prolong the QT interval. In a randomized, double-blind, placebo-controlled, single-dose study in 132 healthy adults, the effect of transdermal buprenorphine on the QT interval corrected for heart rate (QT_c) was evaluated under steady-state conditions (i.e., on day 3 of treatment with buprenorphine 10 mcg/hour and day 4 of treatment with buprenorphine 40 mcg/hour). Although the 10-mcg/hour dosage had no clinically meaningful effect on the QT_c interval, the 40-mcg/hour dosage prolonged the QT_c interval by a maximum of 9.2 msec. Therefore, the maximum recommended dosage of transdermal buprenorphine is 20 mcg/hour. In controlled and open-label clinical trials, prolongation of the QT_c interval (corrected for heart rate using Fridericia's formula) to 450–480 msec occurred in 2% of patients with chronic pain receiving buprenorphine buccally dissolving strips at dosages up to 900 mcg every 12 hours, which is the maximum recommended dosage of buccally dissolving strips.

Hypotension has reportedly occurred in about 1–5% of patients receiving parenteral buprenorphine for pain relief. Other adverse cardiovascular effects, including hypertension, tachycardia, bradycardia, and ECG abnormalities manifested as Wenckebach period, have occurred in less than 1% of patients receiving parenteral buprenorphine for pain relief. Shock has occurred rarely.

Peripheral edema and hypertension have been reported in clinical trials in about 1–5% of patients receiving transdermal buprenorphine. Other adverse cardiovascular effects reported in less than 1% of patients receiving transdermal

buprenorphine include hypotension, orthostatic hypotension, angina pectoris, bradycardia, palpitation, syncope, tachycardia, and vasodilation. Hypotension may be severe, especially in patients with blood volume depletion and those receiving concomitant therapy with dugs that may compromise vasomotor tone (e.g., phenothiazines).

In clinical trials in patients receiving buprenorphine buccally dissolving strips for pain relief, hypertension and peripheral edema were reported in 1 to less than 5% of patients receiving the buccally administered drug, and increased blood pressure and QT-interval prolongation were reported less than 1% of patients.

Vasodilation has occurred in patients receiving sublingual buprenorphine or buprenorphine/naloxone for the treatment of opiate dependence in clinical trials. Peripheral edema and palpitations also have been reported.

● Respiratory Effects

Respiratory depression (decreased rate and depth of respiration) may occur occasionally in patients receiving parenteral buprenorphine. Respiratory depression requiring active treatment has occurred in less than 1% of patients receiving parenteral buprenorphine for pain relief. Hypoventilation has been reported in about 1–5% of these patients. Dyspnea, cyanosis, and apnea have been reported in less than 1% of these patients. Hypoxemia has occurred rarely.

Dyspnea, cough, pharyngolaryngeal pain, upper respiratory infection, nasopharyngitis, influenza, sinusitis, and bronchitis have been reported in clinical trials in about 1–5% of patients receiving transdermal buprenorphine. Other adverse respiratory effects reported in less than 1% of patients receiving transdermal buprenorphine include aggravated asthma, rhinitis, hyperventilation, hypoventilation, abnormal respiration, respiratory depression, respiratory distress, respiratory failure, and wheezing.

In clinical trials in patients receiving buprenorphine buccally dissolving strips for pain relief, upper respiratory infection was reported in at least 5% of patients receiving the buccally administered drug; nasopharyngitis, sinusitis, bronchitis, oropharyngeal pain, and sinus congestion were reported in at least 1% of patients; and acute sinusitis, cough, dyspnea, nasal congestion, and rhinorrhea were reported in less than 1% of patients.

Rhinitis, rhinorrhea, increased cough, and pharyngitis have occurred in patients receiving sublingual buprenorphine or buprenorphine/naloxone for the treatment of opiate dependence in clinical trials. In clinical trials in patients receiving buprenorphine/naloxone buccally dissolving strips, rhinorrhea was reported in more than 1 to less than 5% of patients.

Oropharyngeal pain, cough, and dyspnea were reported in phase 3 clinical trials in 1–5% of patients with buprenorphine subdermal implants.

Naloxone and doxapram have been used to reverse buprenorphine-induced respiratory depression, but these agents may be only partially effective and, rarely, completely ineffective. Consequently, the principal management of respiratory depression induced by the drug should be assisted or controlled respiration and administration of oxygen as necessary.

● Sensitivity Reactions

Acute and chronic hypersensitivity reactions have been reported in patients receiving buprenorphine. Rash, urticaria, and pruritus are the most common manifestations of these hypersensitivity reactions. Bronchospasm, angioedema, and anaphylactic shock also have occurred in patients receiving the drug.

Angioedema, hypersensitivity reaction, facial edema, and urticaria have been reported in clinical trials in less than 1% of patients receiving transdermal buprenorphine.

● Ocular Effects

Miosis occurs in about 1–5% of patients receiving parenteral buprenorphine. Blurred vision, diplopia, amblyopia, mydriasis, other visual abnormalities, and conjunctivitis have been reported in less than 1% of patients receiving parenteral buprenorphine for pain relief.

Dry eye, miosis, blurred vision, and visual disturbance have been reported in clinical trials in less than 1% of patients receiving transdermal buprenorphine.

Runny eyes, increased lacrimation, and blurred vision have been reported in patients receiving sublingual buprenorphine or buprenorphine/naloxone for the treatment of opiate dependence.

● **Dermatologic Effects**

Adverse dermatologic effects, including pruritus, reactions at the injection site, and rash, have occurred in less than 1% of patients receiving parenteral buprenorphine for pain relief. Urticaria has been reported rarely. Stevens-Johnson syndrome occurred in at least one patient receiving concomitant radiation and drug therapy that included parenteral buprenorphine; however, a causal relationship to buprenorphine was not established.

Application site reactions, including pruritus, erythema, rash, and irritation, have been reported in about 5–15% of patients receiving transdermal buprenorphine in clinical trials. Severe application site reactions with marked inflammation, characterized by burning, discharge, or vesicles occurring days to months after initiation of therapy, also have occurred rarely. Application site dermatitis, contact dermatitis, and dry skin have been reported in less than 1% of patients receiving transdermal buprenorphine.

In clinical trials in patients receiving buprenorphine buccally dissolving strips for pain relief, pruritus and rash were reported in 1 to less than 5% of patients receiving the buccally administered drug, and cellulitis was reported in less than 1% of patients.

In phase 3 clinical trials in patients receiving buprenorphine extended-release subcutaneous injection, the most frequent injection site reactions were pain, pruritus, and erythema (each occurring in about 5–7% of patients); induration at the injection site was reported in 1.4% of patients; and bruising, swelling, discomfort, cellulitis, and infection at the injection site were reported in less than 1% of patients.

Pain, pruritus, erythema, hematoma, hemorrhage, and edema at the implant site were reported in phase 3 clinical trials in 5–13% of patients with buprenorphine subdermal implants. Rash and skin lesion were reported in 1–2% of patients with buprenorphine implants.

● **Genitourinary and Endocrine Effects**

Urinary retention and decreased libido have been reported in less than 1% of patients receiving parenteral buprenorphine for pain relief. Flushing, hot flush, decreased libido, sexual dysfunction, urinary hesitancy, and urinary incontinence have been reported in less than 1% of patients receiving transdermal buprenorphine.

In clinical trials in patients receiving buprenorphine buccally dissolving strips for pain relief, urinary tract infection and hot flush were reported in 1 to less than 5% of patients receiving the buccally administered drug, and decreased blood testosterone concentration was reported in less than 1% of patients.

Adrenal insufficiency has been reported in patients receiving opiate agonists or opiate partial agonists. Manifestations of adrenal insufficiency are nonspecific and may include nausea, vomiting, anorexia, fatigue, weakness, dizziness, and hypotension. The onset generally has occurred after at least 1 month of opiate agonist or partial agonist use, although the time to onset has ranged from within 1 day to more than 1 year. In many of the reported cases, patients required hospitalization. If adrenal insufficiency is suspected, appropriate laboratory testing should be performed promptly and physiologic (replacement) dosages of corticosteroids provided; therapy with the opiate agonist or partial agonist should be tapered and discontinued to allow recovery of adrenal function. If the opiate agonist or partial agonist can be discontinued, follow-up assessment of adrenal function should be performed to determine if corticosteroid replacement therapy can be discontinued. In some patients, switching to a different opiate improved symptoms.

Hypogonadism and androgen deficiency have been reported in patients receiving long-term opiate agonist or opiate partial agonist therapy, although a causal relationship has not been established. Patients receiving long-term opiate agonist or partial agonist therapy who present with manifestations of hypogonadism (e.g., decreased libido, impotence, erectile dysfunction, amenorrhea, infertility) should undergo laboratory evaluation.

● **Other Adverse Effects**

Diaphoresis occurs in about 1–5% of patients receiving parenteral buprenorphine for pain relief. Other adverse effects reported in less than 1% of these patients include flushing and a sensation of warmth, tremor, chills and a sensation of cold, hiccups, tinnitus, and pallor. Increased pressure in the common bile duct has occurred in some patients receiving parenteral buprenorphine for pain relief. Decreases in erythrocyte count, hemoglobin, hematocrit, sedimentation rate, and total serum protein concentration have been reported during prolonged

administration of buprenorphine (1–2 months), but these effects were reversible upon discontinuance of the drug. Serum alkaline phosphatase concentrations also decreased during prolonged buprenorphine therapy and were not reversible upon discontinuance; however, values remained within the normal range.

Hyperhidrosis, falls, pain (including pain in extremity, back, neck, or chest), pyrexia, urinary tract infection, joint swelling, arthralgia, muscle spasm, musculoskeletal pain, and myalgia have been reported in clinical trials in about 1–5% of patients receiving transdermal buprenorphine. Accidental injury, chills, dehydration, hiccups, muscle weakness, tinnitus, and weight loss have been reported in less than 1% of patients receiving transdermal buprenorphine.

In clinical trials in patients receiving buprenorphine buccally dissolving strips for pain relief, anemia, contusion, falls, hyperhidrosis, muscle spasm, back pain, and pyrexia were reported in 1 to less than 5% of patients receiving the buccally administered drug, and chills, excoriation, laceration, musculoskeletal pain, and neck pain were reported in less than 1% of patients.

Pain (including back pain), sweating, cold sweat, chills, fever, infection, abscess, flu syndrome, arthralgia, piloerection, and accidental injury have been reported in patients receiving sublingual buprenorphine or buprenorphine/naloxone for the treatment of opiate dependence in clinical trials. In clinical trials in patients receiving buprenorphine/naloxone buccally dissolving strips, chills and hyperhidrosis were reported in more than 1 to less than 5% of patients.

In clinical trials, increased creatine kinase (CK, creatine phosphokinase, CPK) concentration was reported in up to about 5% of patients receiving buprenorphine extended-release subcutaneous injection.

In phase 3 clinical trials, pain (including pain in back, chest, or extremity), pyrexia, chills, feeling cold, local swelling, laceration, excoriation, and scratch were reported in 1–6% of patients with buprenorphine subdermal implants.

● **Opiate Withdrawal**

Because of buprenorphine's antagonist activity, the drug may precipitate mild to moderate signs and symptoms of withdrawal in some patients physically dependent on opiates. Signs and symptoms of mild withdrawal may also appear following discontinuance of prolonged therapy with buprenorphine alone.

● **Precautions and Contraindications**

When the fixed-combination preparation containing buprenorphine and naloxone is used, the usual cautions, precautions, and contraindications associated with naloxone should be considered in addition to those associated with buprenorphine.

Addiction, Abuse, and Misuse

Buprenorphine exposes patients and other users to the risks of opiate addiction, abuse, and misuse, which can lead to overdosage and death. Addiction can occur with appropriately prescribed or illicitly obtained opiate analgesics, and at recommended dosages or with misuse or abuse. Concurrent abuse of alcohol or other CNS depressants increases the risk of toxicity. Each patient's risk for addiction, abuse, and misuse should be assessed prior to initiating buprenorphine for analgesia, and all patients receiving the drug should be monitored for development of these behaviors or conditions. Personal or family history of substance abuse (drug or alcohol addiction or abuse) or mental illness (e.g., major depression) increases risk. The potential for addiction, abuse, and misuse should not prevent opiate prescribing for appropriate pain management, but does necessitate intensive counseling about risks and proper use and intensive monitoring for signs of addiction, abuse, and misuse. Buprenorphine should be prescribed for analgesia in the smallest appropriate quantity, and the patient should be instructed on secure storage and proper disposal to prevent theft.

When used for treatment of opiate dependence (opiate use disorder [OUD]), buprenorphine should be prescribed and dispensed with appropriate precautions to minimize risk of misuse, abuse, or diversion, and to ensure appropriate protection from theft, including in the patient's home. Patients should be monitored for progression of opiate use disorder and addictive behaviors. Clinical monitoring appropriate to the patient's level of stability is essential. Multiple refills should not be authorized early in treatment or without appropriate patient follow-up visits.

Extended-release opiates (e.g., buprenorphine transdermal system) are associated with a greater risk of overdosage and death because of the larger amount of drug contained in each dosage unit. Abuse or misuse of the transdermal system by placing it in the mouth, chewing it, swallowing it, or using it in other unintended ways may cause choking, overdosage, and death.

Abuse or misuse of buprenorphine buccally dissolving strips by swallowing the strips may cause choking, overdosage, and death.

Buprenorphine subdermal implants that protrude from the skin or have been expelled are subject to misuse and abuse.

Respiratory and CNS Depression

Serious, life-threatening, or fatal respiratory depression may occur in patients receiving opiates, including buprenorphine, even when used as recommended. Although respiratory depression can occur at any time during therapy, the risk is greatest during initiation of therapy and following an increase in dosage; therefore, patients receiving buprenorphine should be monitored closely for respiratory depression, especially during the first 24–72 hours of therapy and following any increase in dosage. Appropriate dosage selection and titration are essential to reduce the risk of respiratory depression. Large initial doses in nontolerant patients, overestimation of the initial buprenorphine dosage when transferring patients from another opiate analgesic, or accidental exposure to buprenorphine, especially by a child, can result in respiratory depression and death.

The risk of respiratory depression is increased when opiates, including buprenorphine, are used concomitantly with other agents that cause respiratory depression. Many postmarketing reports of coma and death have involved misuse of buprenorphine by self-injection or were associated with the concomitant use of buprenorphine and benzodiazepines or other CNS depressants, including alcohol.

Carbon dioxide retention from opiate-induced respiratory depression can exacerbate the drug's sedative effects and, in certain patients, can lead to elevated intracranial pressure.

Geriatric, cachectic, or debilitated patients are at increased risk of life-threatening respiratory depression. In patients with chronic obstructive pulmonary disease or cor pulmonale, substantially decreased respiratory reserve, hypoxia, hypercapnia, or preexisting respiratory depression, even recommended doses of buprenorphine may decrease respiratory drive to the point of apnea. Such patients should be monitored closely, particularly following initiation of therapy, during dosage titration, and during concomitant therapy with other respiratory depressants. Alternatively, use of nonopiate analgesics should be considered in such patients. Use of buprenorphine formulations labeled for analgesic use is contraindicated in patients with substantial respiratory depression and in those with severe bronchial asthma in unmonitored settings or in the absence of resuscitative equipment.

If therapy with buprenorphine extended-release subcutaneous injection is discontinued because of compromised respiratory function, the patient should be monitored for continued buprenorphine effects for several months.

Because of the risks associated with opiate overdosage, clinicians should routinely discuss the availability of the opiate antagonist naloxone with all patients receiving new or reauthorized opiate prescriptions for pain management or new or reauthorized prescriptions for medications for treatment of OUD. Clinicians should consider prescribing naloxone for patients receiving opiate analgesics who are at increased risk of opiate overdosage (e.g., those receiving concomitant therapy with benzodiazepines or other CNS depressants, those with a history of opiate or substance use disorder, those with medical conditions that could increase sensitivity to opiate effects, those who have experienced a prior opiate overdose) and should strongly consider prescribing naloxone for all patients receiving medications for treatment of OUD. Clinicians also should consider prescribing naloxone when patients receiving opiates for pain management or for treatment of OUD have household members, including children, or other close contacts who are at risk for accidental ingestion or overdosage. Even if patients are not receiving an opiate for pain management or medication for treatment of OUD, a naloxone prescription should be considered if the patient is at increased risk of opiate overdosage (e.g., those with a current or past diagnosis of OUD, those who have experienced a prior opiate overdose).

Since naloxone and doxapram may be only partially effective in reversing buprenorphine-induced respiratory depression, the use of assisted or controlled respiration may be necessary and should be considered the principal method of management.

Concomitant Use of Benzodiazepines or Other CNS Depressants

Concomitant use of opiate agonists or opiate partial agonists and benzodiazepines or other CNS depressants (e.g., anxiolytics, sedatives, hypnotics, tranquilizers,

muscle relaxants, general anesthetics, antipsychotics, other opiates, alcohol) may result in profound sedation, respiratory depression, coma, and death. Concomitant use of opiate analgesics and benzodiazepines or other CNS depressants should be reserved for patients in whom alternative treatment options are inadequate; the lowest effective dosages and shortest possible duration of concomitant therapy should be used, and the patient should be monitored closely for respiratory depression and sedation. Patients receiving buprenorphine and/or their caregivers should be apprised of the risks associated with concomitant therapeutic or illicit use of benzodiazepines, alcohol, or other CNS depressants. Concomitant use with alcohol should be avoided.

Because the morbidity and mortality associated with untreated opiate addiction can outweigh the serious risks associated with concomitant use of opiate agonists or partial agonists and benzodiazepines or other CNS depressants, buprenorphine treatment for opiate addiction (i.e., medication-assisted treatment [MAT]) should not be categorically withheld from patients receiving benzodiazepines or other CNS depressants. These drugs should be tapered and discontinued, if possible, in patients receiving MAT. However, excluding or discharging patients from MAT because of benzodiazepine or CNS depressant use is not likely to prevent such concomitant use and may lead to use outside the treatment setting, which could result in more severe outcomes. Careful management can reduce the risks associated with concomitant use of benzodiazepines or other CNS depressants in patients receiving buprenorphine treatment for opiate addiction. Benzodiazepines are not the treatment of choice for anxiety or insomnia in patients receiving buprenorphine treatment for opiate addiction; other pharmacologic or nonpharmacologic therapies should be considered. Current evidence does not support dose limitations or other arbitrary limits on buprenorphine as a strategy for addressing concomitant benzodiazepine or other CNS depressant use in patients receiving MAT. However, in patients who are sedated at the time of a scheduled buprenorphine dose, the cause of sedation should be evaluated and omission or reduction of the buprenorphine dose may be appropriate.

Precautions for minimizing risks associated with concomitant use of benzodiazepines or other CNS depressants in patients receiving MAT include the following:

- Patient education upon initiation of MAT regarding the risks associated with concomitant use of benzodiazepines or other CNS depressants;

- Development of strategies upon initiation of MAT for managing any prescribed or illicit use of benzodiazepines or other CNS depressants;

- Verification of the diagnosis in any patient receiving prescribed benzodiazepines or other CNS depressants for anxiety or insomnia, and consideration of other treatment options for these conditions;

- Possible adjustment of induction procedures and more intensive monitoring;

- Recognition that MAT may be required indefinitely and should be continued for as long as the patient derives benefit and MAT contributes to the intended treatment goals;

- Coordination of care to minimize risks and ensure that other prescribers are aware that the patient is receiving buprenorphine treatment; and

- Measures to confirm that prescribed drugs are being used as intended and are not being diverted or supplemented with illicit drugs;

- Toxicology screening to monitor for prescribed or illicit drug use.

Selection of an Appropriate Formulation

Oral transmucosal preparations of buprenorphine that are intended for use in the treatment of opiate dependence should *not* be used for analgesia. Fatal overdosage has been reported following administration of 2 mg of sublingual buprenorphine for analgesia in opiate-naive individuals. Buprenorphine extended-release subcutaneous injection also should not be used in opiate-naive individuals. Safety and efficacy of transdermal buprenorphine for the management of opiate dependence have not been established.

Accidental Exposure

Accidental exposure to buprenorphine can cause severe, possibly fatal, respiratory depression in children. Buprenorphine-containing preparations are involved in a disproportionate share of unsupervised prescription drug and opiate ingestions by children younger than 6 years of age. From 2004–2011, buprenorphine was involved in an estimated 24% of emergency department visits involving accidental opiate ingestion by children 1–5 years of age. Other surveillance data for 2010–2011 indicate that buprenorphine was involved in approximately 30% of emergency department visits and 60% of emergent hospitalizations involving opiate ingestion by children younger than 6 years of age. The surveillance data for 2010–2011 also indicate that approximately 96% of the reported emergency department visits involving buprenorphine ingestion in this age group involved buprenorphine/naloxone. Buprenorphine-containing preparations should be stored out of the sight and reach of children. Used transdermal systems and any drug that is no longer needed should be disposed of appropriately. Any subdermal implant that has been expelled from the skin should be kept away from others, especially from children.

QT-Interval Prolongation

Prolongation of the QT interval corrected for heart rate (QT_c) has occurred in some patients receiving buprenorphine in clinical trials. In controlled and open-label clinical trials, prolongation of the QT_c interval (corrected for rate using Fridericia's formula) to 450–480 msec occurred in 2% of patients with chronic pain receiving buprenorphine buccally dissolving strips at dosages up to 900 mcg every 12 hours. In healthy adults, transdermal buprenorphine given in a dosage of 40 mcg/hour prolonged the QT interval. These findings should be taken into account when considering buprenorphine therapy in patients with hypokalemia, hypomagnesemia, or clinically unstable cardiac disease (e.g., unstable atrial fibrillation, symptomatic bradycardia, unstable congestive heart failure, active myocardial ischemia). Periodic ECG monitoring is recommended in such patients. Use of buprenorphine should be avoided in patients with a personal or family (i.e., immediate family member) history of long QT syndrome and in patients who are receiving class IA (e.g., quinidine, procainamide, disopyramide) or class III (e.g., sotalol, amiodarone, dofetilide) antiarrhythmic agents or other drugs known to prolong the QT interval. The maximum dosage of transdermal buprenorphine should not exceed 20 mcg/hour, and the maximum dosage of buprenorphine administered as buccally dissolving strips (Belbuca®) should not exceed 900 mcg every 12 hours.

Opiate Withdrawal

Misuse of oral transmucosal preparations of buprenorphine/naloxone via parenteral injection by individuals who are physically dependent on opiates is likely to produce marked and intense opiate withdrawal symptoms.

Because of buprenorphine's opiate antagonist activity, it may precipitate withdrawal in patients physically dependent on opiates if administered before the agonistic effects of the full opiate agonist have subsided. To avoid precipitating withdrawal symptoms in patients currently receiving opiate analgesia, the dosage of the current opiate analgesic should be tapered to a dosage equivalent to no more than 30 mg daily of oral morphine sulfate prior to switching to buprenorphine. In patients initiating buprenorphine therapy for opiate dependence, induction therapy should be initiated when objective and clear signs of opiate withdrawal are evident. Prior to receiving therapy with buprenorphine implants or buprenorphine extended-release subcutaneous injection, patients should be stabilized on oral transmucosal therapy with the drug.

Because abrupt discontinuance of buprenorphine or rapid reduction in dosage may result in withdrawal symptoms in patients who are physically dependent on the drug, dosage should be tapered gradually when therapy with the drug is discontinued.

Prolonged maternal use of opiates during pregnancy can result in neonatal opiate withdrawal syndrome.

Hepatic Impairment

Since buprenorphine is metabolized in the liver, the activity of the drug may be increased and/or prolonged in patients with hepatic impairment. Buprenorphine injection should be used with caution in patients with severe hepatic impairment. When buprenorphine buccally dissolving strips are used for analgesia, dosage adjustment is recommended in patients with severe hepatic impairment, and patients with either moderate or severe hepatic impairment should be monitored for toxicity or overdosage. Because buprenorphine transdermal system is intended for 7-day application, use of an alternative analgesic regimen that allows for greater dosage flexibility should be considered in patients with severe hepatic impairment.

When oral transmucosal preparations of buprenorphine or buprenorphine/naloxone are used for the management of opiate dependence in patients with moderate or severe hepatic impairment, plasma concentrations of buprenorphine and naloxone are increased and half-lives of the drugs are prolonged. Naloxone is affected to a greater degree than buprenorphine, and the magnitude of the difference in effect is greater in individuals with severe hepatic impairment than in those with moderate hepatic impairment. This may result in an increased risk of precipitated withdrawal during the induction phase of treatment and interference with buprenorphine's efficacy throughout treatment. Buprenorphine/naloxone should be avoided in patients with severe hepatic impairment and may not be appropriate for those with moderate hepatic impairment. In patients with moderate hepatic impairment, buprenorphine/naloxone is not recommended for induction therapy but may be used with caution and careful monitoring for maintenance treatment following induction therapy with buprenorphine alone. Dosage adjustment of sublingual buprenorphine is recommended in patients with severe hepatic impairment, and patients with either moderate or severe hepatic impairment who are receiving the single-entity sublingual tablets should be monitored for toxicity or overdosage.

Use of buprenorphine extended-release subcutaneous injection or buprenorphine subdermal implants is not recommended in patients with moderate to severe hepatic impairment since the extended-release injection does not allow for rapid adjustment of plasma buprenorphine concentrations and the implant dosage cannot be titrated.

If moderate or severe hepatic impairment develops during therapy with buprenorphine extended-release subcutaneous injection or buprenorphine subdermal implants, the patient should be monitored for manifestations of toxicity or overdosage. If such manifestations occur in patients with buprenorphine implants, removal of the implants may be required. Patients who have received the extended-release subcutaneous injection should be monitored for several months; if manifestations of overdosage or toxicity occur within 2 weeks following an injection, the depot containing buprenorphine may be surgically excised, if necessary.

Hepatotoxicity

Serious adverse hepatic events have occurred in patients receiving buprenorphine for the treatment of opiate dependence. While some individuals had risk factors for such adverse events (i.e., preexisting hepatic enzyme abnormalities, HBV or HCV infection, concomitant use of potentially hepatotoxic drugs, ongoing illicit use of injectable drugs), the possibility exists that buprenorphine had a causative or contributory role in some of these adverse hepatic events. In patients with opiate dependence, evaluation of liver function prior to initiation of buprenorphine therapy and periodically during treatment is recommended. The manufacturer of buprenorphine extended-release subcutaneous injection recommends monthly monitoring of liver function during treatment with this formulation, particularly in patients receiving the 300-mg dosage. Liver function also should be evaluated prior to initiation of buprenorphine therapy for analgesia and periodically during such treatment in patients at increased risk of hepatotoxicity (e.g., patients with a history of excessive alcohol intake, IV drug abuse, or liver disease). Careful biologic and etiologic evaluation is recommended in the event of an adverse hepatic event. In some patients, withdrawal of buprenorphine has resulted in amelioration of acute hepatitis; in other patients, no dosage reduction was necessary. If a decision is made to discontinue buprenorphine therapy, the drug should be discontinued carefully to prevent withdrawal symptoms and, in patients being treated for opiate dependence, the return to illicit drug use; strict monitoring of the patient should be initiated.

Hypotension

Buprenorphine may cause severe hypotension, including orthostatic hypotension and syncope, in ambulatory patients. Because the risk of severe hypotension is increased in patients whose ability to maintain blood pressure has been compromised by blood volume depletion or concomitant use of certain CNS depressants (e.g., phenothiazines, general anesthetics), such patients should be monitored for hypotension following initiation of buprenorphine therapy or an increase in buprenorphine dosage. Use of buprenorphine should be avoided in patients with circulatory shock since the drug may cause vasodilation that can further reduce cardiac output and blood pressure.

Increased Intracranial Pressure or Head Injury

The respiratory depressant effects of opiates promote carbon dioxide retention, which can result in elevation of intracranial pressure. Patients who may be particularly susceptible to these effects (e.g., those with evidence of elevated intracranial pressure or brain tumors) should be monitored closely for sedation and respiratory depression, particularly during initiation of therapy. Opiates also may obscure the clinical course in patients with head injuries. Use of buprenorphine should be avoided in patients with impaired consciousness or coma.

Seizures

Buprenorphine may increase the frequency of seizures in patients with seizure disorders and may increase the risk of seizures in some clinical settings associated with seizures. Patients with seizure disorders should be monitored for worsening of seizure control during buprenorphine therapy.

GI Conditions

Opiates may increase serum amylase concentrations and cause spasm of the sphincter of Oddi. Patients with biliary tract disease, including those with acute pancreatitis, should be monitored for worsening symptoms. Buprenorphine formulations labeled for analgesic use are contraindicated in patients with known or suspected GI obstruction, including paralytic ileus.

Like other opiates, buprenorphine may obscure the diagnosis and/or clinical course of acute abdominal conditions.

Anesthesia and Analgesia in Patients Receiving Extended-release Injection or Implant Therapy for Opiate Dependence

When patients with buprenorphine subdermal implants or those who have received buprenorphine extended-release subcutaneous injection within the prior 6 months require anesthesia or analgesia for acute pain, nonopiate analgesics should be used whenever possible. Those patients requiring opiate analgesia may receive a high-affinity, full opiate agonist under clinician supervision, with particular attention given to respiratory function. Because higher doses may be required for analgesia, the potential for toxicity is increased. If opiates are a required component of anesthesia, patients should be continuously monitored in an anesthesia care setting by persons not involved in the conduct of the surgical or diagnostic procedure. Opiate therapy must be provided by individuals trained in the use of anesthetic drugs and the management of respiratory effects of potent opiates, specifically the establishment and maintenance of a patent airway and assisted ventilation.

Implant Complications

Improper insertion of buprenorphine subdermal implants may result in rare but serious complications including nerve damage and implant migration resulting in embolism and death. Local migration, protrusion, and expulsion of implants also may occur. Protrusion or expulsion may be caused by incomplete insertion or infection at the insertion site and may result in accidental exposure to the drug. Buprenorphine implants should be inserted in accordance with the manufacturer's instructions. It is essential for each implant to be inserted subdermally so that it is palpable following insertion and for proper placement to be confirmed by palpation immediately after insertion.

Neural or vascular injury may occur if buprenorphine implants are inserted into muscle or fascia. If an implant is inserted too deeply, cannot be palpated, or has migrated, removal may be complicated. Additional surgical procedures may be required to remove an implant that was inserted too deeply and cannot be readily localized. Injury to deeper neural or vascular structures may occur when deeply inserted implants are removed.

Excessive palpation shortly after insertion or improper removal may increase the risk of infection at the implant site.

Because of the risks associated with implant insertion and removal, buprenorphine implants are available only through a restricted distribution program (Probuphine® REMS).

Extended-release Subcutaneous Injection

Because buprenorphine extended-release subcutaneous injection forms a solid mass upon contact with body fluids, IV administration could result in death or serious complications (e.g., venous occlusion, local tissue damage, thromboembolic events including life-threatening pulmonary embolism). The extended-release subcutaneous injection should *not* be administered IV or by IM injection. Because of the risks associated with IV self-administration, the extended-release subcutaneous injection is available only through a restricted distribution program (Sublocade® REMS).

Transdermal Therapy

Patients receiving transdermal buprenorphine therapy who develop severe reactions with marked inflammation (e.g., burning, discharge, vesicles) at the application site should be advised to consult their clinician promptly about the need to remove the transdermal system.

Because the absorption of topically applied buprenorphine from the transdermal system depends in part on the temperature of the skin and increases with increased temperature, patients who develop a fever while using the transdermal system and individuals whose core body temperature increases as a result of strenuous exercise should be observed closely for manifestations of opiate toxicity, and dosage of the drug should be adjusted if respiratory or CNS depression occurs. In addition, patients wearing a transdermal system of the drug should be advised to avoid exposing the application site or surrounding area to direct external heat sources.

Dental Complications Associated with Transmucosal Buprenorphine Preparations

Adverse dental events, sometimes severe, have been reported following the use of transmucosal buprenorphine-containing preparations (i.e., tablets and films dissolved under the tongue or placed against the inside of the cheek available as single-ingredient products or in combination with naloxone). FDA has issued a drug safety communication about this risk.

Since initial approval of buprenorphine, 305 cases of dental problems associated with the use of transmucosal buprenorphine have been reported to FDA or published in the medical literature; 131 cases were classified as serious. Reported events included cavities/tooth decay, including rampant caries; dental abscesses/infection; tooth erosion; fillings falling out; and, in some cases, total tooth loss. These dental complications have been reported in patients with or without prior history of dental issues. The average age of patients was 42 years, and the median time to diagnosis was 24.25 months. Most cases were reported in patients using buprenorphine for OUD; however, 28 cases occurred in patients receiving the drugs for pain treatment. Tooth extraction or removal was required in 71 cases; other dental interventions included root canals, dental surgery, crowns, and implants.

Screen patients for oral disease and assess oral health history prior to prescribing transmucosal buprenorphine. Counsel patients about the potential for dental problems and the importance of taking extra steps after the drug has completely dissolved to reduce this risk, including gently rinsing teeth and gums with water and then swallowing. Advise patients to wait at least 1 hour before brushing their teeth. Refer patients to a dentist as soon as possible after starting transmucosal buprenorphine for a baseline dental evaluation and caries risk assessment and preventive plan; encourage regular dental checkups. Advise patients to not stop taking buprenorphine without first discussing with their health care professional as it could lead to serious consequences, including relapse to opioid misuse or abuse that could result in overdose and death. The benefits of buprenorphine clearly outweigh its risks.

Buccal Buprenorphine in Cancer Patients with Mucositis

Cancer patients with oral mucositis may absorb buprenorphine from buccally dissolving strips (Belbuca®) more rapidly than intended and are likely to achieve higher plasma concentrations of the drug. Dosage reduction and careful monitoring for toxicity or overdosage is recommended in patients with known or suspected mucositis receiving this formulation of the drug.

Patient Advice

Patients should be advised to read the manufacturer's patient information (e.g., medication guide and any instructions for use of the prescribed formulation) for buprenorphine before initiating therapy with the drug and each time the prescription is refilled. Patients should be informed that use of buprenorphine, even when taken as recommended, can result in addiction, abuse, and misuse, which can lead to overdosage and death. Patients also should be informed that accidental exposure to buprenorphine, especially by a child, may result in respiratory depression or death. Patients should be instructed not to share the drug with others, to take steps to protect the drug from theft or misuse, to securely store the drug, to keep the drug out of reach of children, and to properly dispose of any unused drug.

Patients should be advised of the risk of life-threatening respiratory depression and instructed to seek immediate medical attention if manifestations of respiratory depression occur. They also should be advised of the benefits of naloxone administration following an overdose and of their options for obtaining the drug. Patients receiving buprenorphine and/or their caregivers should be advised that concomitant therapeutic or illicit use of benzodiazepines or other CNS depressants, including alcohol, can result in potentially fatal additive effects (e.g., profound sedation, respiratory depression, coma); patients should be advised to avoid concomitant use of alcohol and to avoid concomitant use of other CNS depressants unless such use is supervised by a clinician. Patients should be advised that self-administration of benzodiazepines while taking buprenorphine is extremely dangerous.

Patients should be advised of the importance of informing clinicians of existing or contemplated concomitant therapy, including prescription and OTC drugs, and herbal supplements, as well as any concomitant illnesses. Patients should be advised that buprenorphine should not be used concomitantly with or within 14 days following a monoamine oxidase (MAO) inhibitor and that concomitant use of buprenorphine and serotonergic drugs may cause serotonin syndrome.

Patients should be advised that buprenorphine may impair mental or physical abilities required to perform potentially hazardous tasks such as driving a car or operating machinery and that they should avoid such activities until they know how the drug affects them. Patients also should be advised that severe hypersensitivity reactions (e.g., anaphylaxis) have occurred and that the drug may cause orthostatic hypotension and syncope. Because opiates can cause severe constipation, patients should be advised on appropriate management of constipation. Because of the potential risk of adrenal insufficiency, patients should be advised to immediately contact a clinician if manifestations of adrenal insufficiency (e.g., nausea, vomiting, anorexia, fatigue, weakness, dizziness, hypotension) develop. Although a causal relationship between hypogonadism or androgen deficiency and long-term opiate use has not been established, patients should be advised of this potential risk and instructed to inform their clinician if decreased libido, impotence, erectile dysfunction, amenorrhea, or infertility occurs.

Women of childbearing potential should be instructed to inform their clinician if they are or plan to become pregnant or plan to breast-feed. Risks and benefits of buprenorphine therapy should be discussed with pregnant and nursing women in the context of the intended use (pain management, treatment of opiate dependence). Women of childbearing potential should be advised that prolonged use of opiates during pregnancy may result in neonatal opiate withdrawal syndrome, which can be life-threatening if not recognized and treated. Nursing women should be advised to monitor their breast-fed infants for drowsiness or difficulty breathing.

Patients should be instructed on proper administration of the prescribed dosage form and instructed not to alter the dosage without consulting their clinician. Patients receiving oral transmucosal therapy with buprenorphine or buprenorphine/naloxone for treatment of opiate dependence should be instructed that if a dose of the drug is missed, the missed dose should be taken as soon as it is remembered; however, if it is almost time for the next dose, the missed dose should be skipped and the regular schedule resumed with the next dose.

Patients should be informed that buprenorphine can cause physical dependence and that gradual tapering of the dosage may be required to prevent withdrawal symptoms when the drug is discontinued. Patients receiving buprenorphine or buprenorphine/naloxone for maintenance treatment of opiate dependence should be advised of the potential for relapse to illicit drug use upon discontinuance of maintenance treatment.

Patients receiving buprenorphine as an analgesic should be instructed to inform their clinician of any breakthrough pain or adverse effects that occur, so that therapy may be adjusted based on individual patient requirements.

Patients receiving buprenorphine or buprenorphine/naloxone for treatment of opiate dependence should be advised to instruct their family members that, in the event of an emergency, they should inform the treating clinician or emergency department staff that the patient is physically dependent on opiates and is receiving treatment with an oral transmucosal or long-acting formulation of the drug.

Patients receiving therapy with buprenorphine extended-release subcutaneous injection should be informed that the drug may be detectable for a prolonged time after administration and that drug effects and other associated precautions and considerations (e.g., risk of drug interactions, risks associated with treatment of emergent acute pain) may persist for several months after the last injection. Patients should be informed that a lump may develop at the injection site and that it will gradually diminish in size. Patients should be instructed not to tamper with

or attempt to remove the solid depot containing buprenorphine and should be advised that the extended-release subcutaneous injection is available only under a restricted distribution program because of the risk of serious harm or death if the formulation is self-administered IV.

Patients receiving buprenorphine subdermal implants should be instructed on appropriate care of the incision and should be advised of potential complications resulting from insertion or removal procedures, including neural or vascular injury, infection, and implant migration with the potential for embolism or nerve damage. Patients should be informed that complications may be more likely during removal if the implants were inserted too deeply or were manipulated by the patient or if the patient has gained substantial weight following insertion. Patients also should be informed that implant removal carries risks inherent to other minor surgical procedures, improper removal may result in infection, and premature removal may induce withdrawal symptoms. Patients should be informed that there is a risk to others of accidental overdosage, misuse, and abuse if an implant protrudes from the skin or is expelled; patients should be instructed on safety precautions that they must follow prior to seeing their clinician for such events. Patients should be advised that buprenorphine implants are available only under a restricted distribution program and must be inserted and removed in the facility of a certified prescriber.

Patients receiving buprenorphine transdermal systems should be advised to avoid exposing the application site or surrounding area to direct external heat sources, hot water, or prolonged direct sunlight since such exposure can increase absorption of the drug.

Contraindications

Buprenorphine is contraindicated in patients with known hypersensitivity to the drug or any components of the formulation. In addition, buprenorphine/naloxone is contraindicated in patients with known hypersensitivity to naloxone. Buprenorphine formulations labeled for analgesic use are contraindicated in patients with known or suspected GI obstruction (including paralytic ileus), substantial respiratory depression, or acute or severe bronchial asthma in an unmonitored setting or in the absence of resuscitative equipment.

● Pediatric Precautions

Safety and efficacy of buprenorphine conventional injection in children 2–12 years of age is supported by evidence from adequate and well-controlled trials in adults, with additional data from studies including 960 children and adolescents 9 months to 18 years of age; data are available from a pharmacokinetic study, several controlled clinical trials, and several large postmarketing studies and case series. The manufacturer states that there is reasonable evidence of safety in children 2–12 years of age and efficacy similar to that observed in adults. Safety and efficacy of buprenorphine injection for pain relief in children younger than 2 years of age have not been established.

Safety and efficacy of buprenorphine buccally dissolving strips for pain relief in pediatric patients have not been established. Safety and efficacy of transdermal buprenorphine for pain relief in patients younger than 18 years of age have not been established.

Safety and efficacy of buprenorphine sublingual tablets, buprenorphine/naloxone sublingual tablets, or buprenorphine/naloxone buccally or sublingually dissolving strips for the management of opiate dependence in pediatric patients have not been established. Naloxone-containing preparations are not appropriate for management of neonatal opiate withdrawal syndrome.

Safety and efficacy of buprenorphine extended-release subcutaneous injection for the treatment of opiate dependence in pediatric patients have not been established. Safety and efficacy of buprenorphine subdermal implants for treatment of opiate dependence have not been established in pediatric patients younger than 16 years of age.

● Geriatric Precautions

When the total number of patients studied in clinical trials of transdermal buprenorphine or buprenorphine buccally dissolving strips for pain relief is considered, approximately 25 or 16%, respectively, were 65 years of age or older, while about 8 or 2%, respectively, were 75 years of age and older. The pharmacokinetic profiles of these analgesic formulations in geriatric adults appear to be similar to those in younger adults. The safety profile of transdermal buprenorphine in healthy geriatric individuals appears to be similar to that in younger adults; however, constipation and urinary retention may occur more frequently in geriatric individuals. In clinical trials of buprenorphine buccally dissolving strips in patients with chronic pain, some adverse effects also occurred more frequently in geriatric patients. Other reported clinical experience with buprenorphine has not identified differences in responses between geriatric and younger adults. While specific dosage adjustments of transdermal buprenorphine or buprenorphine buccally dissolving strips are not necessary based on age, buprenorphine should be used with caution in geriatric patients. Because geriatric patients may have increased sensitivity to the drug, the manufacturer of buprenorphine injection states that dosage in geriatric patients should be selected with caution, usually starting at the low end of the dosing range, reflecting the greater frequency of decreased hepatic, renal, and/or cardiac function and of concomitant disease or other drug therapy. Because respiratory depression is the chief risk for geriatric patients receiving opiate analgesics, buprenorphine dosage should be titrated slowly and the patient should be monitored closely for CNS and respiratory depression.

Clinical studies of buprenorphine subdermal implants for the treatment of opiate dependence did not include patients older than 65 years of age and clinical studies of buprenorphine sublingual tablets, buprenorphine/naloxone sublingual tablets, buprenorphine/naloxone buccally or sublingually dissolving strips, and buprenorphine extended-release subcutaneous injection did not include sufficient numbers of patients 65 years of age or older to determine whether geriatric patients respond differently than younger adults. However, other reported clinical experience with buprenorphine has not revealed age-related differences in response. Because of age-related decreases in hepatic, renal, and/or cardiac function and the potential for concomitant disease and drug therapy, the decision to use buprenorphine or buprenorphine/naloxone for the treatment of opiate dependence in patients 65 years of age or older should be made cautiously, and these patients should be monitored for toxicity or overdosage.

● *Pregnancy, Fertility, and Lactation*

Pregnancy

Animal Reproduction Studies

Reproduction studies in rats and rabbits using IM or subcutaneous buprenorphine dosages up to 5 mg/kg daily (3 and 6 times, respectively, the human exposure on a mg/m² basis of a sublingual dosage of 16 mg daily), transdermal dosages of 20 mcg/hour in rats and 80 mcg/hour in rabbits (110 times the human exposure at a transdermal dosage of 20 mcg/hour), oral dosages of 160 mg/kg daily in rats or 25 mg/kg daily in rabbits (approximately 95 or 30 times, respectively, a human sublingual dosage of 16 mg daily), and IV dosages up to 0.8 mg/kg daily in rats and rabbits (0.5 and 1 times, respectively, the human exposure on a mg/m² basis of a sublingual dosage of 16 mg daily) have not revealed evidence of teratogenicity, although an increase in skeletal abnormalities (e.g., extra rib formation) occurred in rats receiving a subcutaneous dosage of 1 mg/kg daily (0.6 times the human exposure on a mg/m² basis of a sublingual dosage of 16 mg daily).

Studies in rats and rabbits using buprenorphine (in a 1:1 ratio with naloxone) at oral dosages up to 250 mg/kg daily in rats and 40 mg/kg daily in rabbits (approximately 150 and 50 times, respectively, the human exposure on a mg/m² basis of a sublingual dosage of 16 mg daily) have not revealed evidence of teratogenicity. Studies in rats and rabbits using buprenorphine (in a 3:2 ratio with naloxone) at IM dosages of up to 30 mg/kg daily (20 and 35 times, respectively, the human exposure on a mg/m² basis of a sublingual dosage of 16 mg daily) have not revealed definitive drug-related teratogenic effects; acephalus was observed in one rabbit fetus from the low-dose group, omphalocele was observed in 2 rabbit fetuses from the same litter in the medium-dose group, and no teratogenic effects were observed in fetuses from the high-dose group.

Buprenorphine has been shown to increase pregnancy loss in rats and rabbits. Dose-related postimplantation loss occurred in rats at oral dosages of 10 mg/kg daily (approximately 6 times the human exposure on a mg/m² basis of a sublingual dosage of 16 mg daily); postimplantation loss also occurred in rats at IM dosages of 30 mg/kg daily. In rabbits, increased preimplantation loss occurred at oral dosages of 1 mg/kg daily and increased postimplantation loss occurred at IV dosages of 0.2 mg/kg daily (both approximately 0.3 times the human exposure on a mg/m² basis of a sublingual dosage of 16 mg daily). Increased postimplantation loss also was observed in rabbits at oral dosages of 40 mg/kg daily and IM dosages of 30 mg/kg daily.

Transdermal or subcutaneous buprenorphine caused maternal toxicity in rats and increased the number of stillborns, reduced litter size, and reduced offspring

growth at maternal rat exposure levels that were approximately 10 times those observed with a human transdermal dosage of 20 mcg/hour. Dystocia occurred in pregnant rats receiving IM dosages of 5 mg/kg daily (approximately 3 times the human sublingual dosage of 16 mg daily on a mg/m² basis). An increase in rat neonatal mortality was observed with oral, IM, or subcutaneous dosages of 0.8, 0.5, or 0.1 mg/kg daily (approximately 0.5, 0.3, or 0.06 times, respectively, the human sublingual dosage of 16 mg daily on a mg/m² basis). An apparent lack of milk production during reproduction studies in rats likely contributed to decreased pup survival. Oral dosages of 80 mg/kg daily (approximately 50 times the human sublingual dosage of 16 mg daily on a mg/m² basis) were associated with delayed occurrence of the righting reflex and startle response in rat pups.

In studies in rats using a solvent (*N*-methyl-2-pyrrolidone; NMP) contained in the Atrigel® vehicle of buprenorphine extended-release subcutaneous injection (Sublocade®), preimplantation loss, delayed ossification, reduced fetal weight, and developmental delays and impaired cognitive function in pups born to NMP-exposed animals occurred at inhaled NMP dosages approximately equivalent to the amount of NMP provided by the recommended human dose of the Sublocade® formulation; fetal malformations and resorption occurred at oral NMP dosages approximately 3 times that provided by the human dose of this buprenorphine formulation. Decreased pup survival occurred at oral maternal NMP dosages of 1.8 times that provided by the maximum recommended human dose of the Sublocade® formulation. In rabbits, postimplantation loss and increased cardiovascular and skull malformations occurred at oral NMP dosages of 3.2 times the amount of NMP provided by the maximum recommended human dose of this formulation.

In studies in rats using the Sublocade® formulation at subcutaneous buprenorphine dosages of approximately 38 times the maximum recommended human dosage, embryolethality (which appeared to be attributable principally to the vehicle), reduced fetal body weight, and increased visceral and skeletal (principally skull) malformations occurred. These effects also were observed with the Atrigel® vehicle alone, but the skeletal and visceral malformations appeared to be at least partially attributable to buprenorphine. In studies in rabbits using the Sublocade® formulation, increased skeletal malformations (which appeared to be related to buprenorphine) occurred at a subcutaneous buprenorphine dosage of 7 times the maximum recommended human dosage. Increased malformations (external malformations, visceral malformations, skeletal malformations and variations), embryolethality, and decreased fetal body weight occurred at a subcutaneous buprenorphine dosage of approximately 15 times the maximum recommended human dosage and appeared to be attributable to the vehicle.

Clinical Experience

Limited data from clinical trials, observational studies, case series, and case reports on use of buprenorphine during pregnancy do not indicate an increased risk of major malformations specifically due to the drug. However, interpretation is complicated by maternal factors such as illicit drug use, late presentation for prenatal care, poor nutritional status, presence of infections, poor compliance, and psychosocial circumstances and by the lack of comparative data for untreated opiate-dependent pregnant women. Comparisons generally have been made to women receiving a different opiate for medication-assisted treatment of opiate dependence or to women in the general population, who may differ from buprenorphine-treated women in their risk factors for poor pregnancy outcomes.

In a double-blind, randomized, controlled trial (Maternal Opioid Treatment: Human Experimental Research [MOTHER]), outcomes, principally opiate withdrawal effects, were assessed in neonates born to women who received buprenorphine or methadone treatment for opiate dependence during pregnancy. Enrollment in the study occurred at an average gestational age of 18.7 weeks. Prior to the end of pregnancy, 33% of buprenorphine-treated women and 18% of methadone-treated women discontinued treatment; outcomes were evaluated for the neonates whose mothers remained in treatment until delivery. No difference was observed between buprenorphine- and methadone-exposed neonates in the proportion of neonates requiring treatment for opiate withdrawal syndrome or the peak severity of the syndrome. Buprenorphine-exposed neonates required a lower total mean morphine sulfate dosage for treatment of withdrawal (1.1 versus 10.4 mg), had shorter hospital stays (10 versus 17.5 days), and shorter duration of treatment for withdrawal (4.1 versus 9.9 days) compared with methadone-exposed neonates. The groups did not differ in other outcome measures (head circumference, weight and length at birth, preterm birth, gestational age at delivery, and 1- and 5-minute Apgar scores) or in the rates of serious maternal or neonatal adverse events. The imbalance in treatment discontinuance rates between buprenorphine- and methadone-treated women complicate interpretation of the study findings.

Untreated opiate addiction during pregnancy is associated with adverse obstetrical outcomes, including preeclampsia, fetal growth restriction, preterm birth, spontaneous abortion, and fetal death. In addition, untreated opiate addiction often results in continued or relapsing illicit opiate use and engagement in high-risk behaviors. The recommended treatment of opiate dependence in pregnant women is maintenance treatment with buprenorphine or methadone; this approach is superior to medically supervised withdrawal because withdrawal is associated with high relapse rates and poorer outcomes.

Use of a single-entity buprenorphine preparation is recommended during pregnancy to protect the fetus from any potential exposure to naloxone, especially if the fixed-combination preparation is injected, and also to avoid precipitated withdrawal in the event of IV injection. However, expert opinion regarding use of buprenorphine versus buprenorphine/naloxone during pregnancy appears to be evolving. Recent studies suggest that neonatal outcomes are similar with buprenorphine/naloxone or buprenorphine; if additional safety data confirm these findings, buprenorphine/naloxone use during pregnancy may increase, since the single-entity preparation has a higher risk for misuse and diversion. The manufacturers of buprenorphine/naloxone preparations currently state that the extremely limited data on sublingual naloxone exposure in pregnancy are not sufficient to evaluate a drug-associated risk.

The manufacturer states that buprenorphine extended-release subcutaneous injection should be used during pregnancy only if the potential benefits justify the potential risks to the fetus. Based on animal data, pregnant women should be advised of the potential risk of this formulation to the fetus. There are no adequate and well-controlled studies to date with use of buprenorphine subdermal implants in pregnant women.

Dosage adjustments of buprenorphine may be required during pregnancy, even if the patient was receiving a stable dosage prior to pregnancy. Pregnant women receiving buprenorphine should be monitored closely for withdrawal manifestations and the dosage adjusted as necessary.

Opiate-dependent women receiving buprenorphine maintenance therapy may require additional analgesia during labor. When opiate analgesics are required during the intrapartum period, higher than usual dosages generally are needed to achieve adequate analgesia because of tolerance to the maintenance treatment dosage.

Opiate analgesics, including buprenorphine, cross the placenta and may produce respiratory depression in neonates. The manufacturer states that safety of buprenorphine injection when administered during labor and delivery has not been established. Opiate analgesics, including buprenorphine, may prolong labor through actions that temporarily reduce the strength, duration, and frequency of uterine contractions. However, this effect is inconsistent and may be offset by an increased rate of cervical dilatation, which tends to shorten labor. Transdermal buprenorphine and buprenorphine buccally dissolving strips should not be used for pain relief in women immediately prior to or during labor, when use of shorter-acting analgesics or other analgesic techniques is more appropriate. Neonates exposed to opiates during labor should be monitored for respiratory depression. An opiate antagonist must be available for reversal of opiate-induced respiratory depression.

Prolonged maternal use of opiates, including buprenorphine, during pregnancy can result in physical dependence in the neonate and neonatal opiate withdrawal syndrome. Manifestations may include irritability, hyperactivity and abnormal sleep pattern, high-pitched cry, tremor, vomiting, diarrhea, and failure to gain weight. In contrast to adults, the withdrawal syndrome in neonates may be life-threatening if not recognized and treated, and requires management according to protocols developed by neonatology experts. Women who require prolonged opiate agonist therapy during pregnancy should be advised of the risk of neonatal opiate withdrawal syndrome, and availability of appropriate treatment should be ensured. The onset, duration, and severity of the syndrome vary depending on the specific opiate agonist used, duration of use, timing and amount of last maternal use, and rate of drug elimination by the neonate. In neonates who have been exposed to buprenorphine, the onset of neonatal withdrawal symptoms generally occurs in the first 1–2 days after birth. Neonates born to women taking opiates chronically should be closely observed for signs of withdrawal.

Fertility

Long-term use of opiates may reduce fertility in females and males of reproductive potential. It is not known whether these effects on fertility are reversible. Long-term use of opiates may influence the hypothalamic-pituitary-gonadal axis, resulting in androgen deficiency that may be manifested as low libido, impotence, erectile dysfunction, amenorrhea, or infertility. The causal role of opiates in hypogonadism is unknown because studies to date have not adequately controlled for other potential influences on gonadal hormone levels (e.g., medical or physical factors, lifestyle, psychological stressors).

Reproduction studies in rats using IM and subcutaneous buprenorphine have not revealed evidence of impaired fertility. Reduced conception rates were observed in female rats receiving dietary buprenorphine dosages of approximately 47 mg/kg daily (approximately 28 times the human exposure on a mg/m² basis of a sublingual dosage of 16 mg daily). No evidence of impaired fertility or reproductive performance was observed in rats receiving transdermal buprenorphine in dosages resulting in AUCs up to 65 (in females) or 100 (in males) times the exposure level in humans receiving a transdermal dosage of 20 mcg/hour.

However, adverse effects on sperm (low motility, low sperm count, and higher percentage of abnormal sperm) were observed in rats at a buprenorphine dose of 600 mg/kg (as buprenorphine extended-release subcutaneous injection [Sublocade®]) and with the corresponding dose of the Atrigel® vehicle contained in the drug injection. No effects on female mating, fertility, or fecundity indices were observed at subcutaneous extended-release buprenorphine dosages up to 900 mg/kg (approximately 38 times the maximum recommended human dose based on AUC comparison). Adverse effects on testes and male fertility also have been observed in rats receiving a solvent (N-methyl-2-pyrrolidone; NMP) contained in the Atrigel® vehicle for 10 weeks at a daily oral dosage greater than 11.6 times the amount of solvent delivered by the maximum recommended human dosage.

Lactation

Buprenorphine is distributed into milk in humans. In 2 studies that included 13 nursing women receiving maintenance treatment with sublingual buprenorphine (2.4–24 mg daily) for opiate dependence, buprenorphine and its metabolite norbuprenorphine were present in low concentrations in milk and in the breast-fed infant's urine; the infants were exposed to less than 1% of the maternal daily buprenorphine dosage. In the first study in 6 women receiving buprenorphine (median dosage of 0.29 mg/kg daily) at 5–8 days postpartum, breast milk provided a median infant dosage of 0.42 mcg/kg daily of buprenorphine and 0.33 mcg/kg daily of norbuprenorphine (0.2 and 0.12%, respectively, of the maternal weight-adjusted dosage). In the other study in 7 women receiving buprenorphine (median dosage of 7 mg daily) at an average of 1.12 months postpartum, mean milk concentrations of buprenorphine and norbuprenorphine were 3.65 and 1.94 mcg/L, respectively; based on the results of this study, an exclusively breast-fed infant consuming 150 mL/kg daily of milk would receive a mean estimated dosage of 0.55 mcg/kg daily of buprenorphine and 0.29 mcg/kg daily of norbuprenorphine (0.38 and 0.18%, respectively, of the maternal weight-adjusted dosage). Adverse reactions in nursing infants were not observed.

Experts recommend that women who are stable on buprenorphine or buprenorphine/naloxone treatment for opiate dependence, are not using other illicit drugs, and have no contraindications to nursing be encouraged to breast-feed their infants; to lower the risk of return to substance use, women receiving buprenorphine should be encouraged to continue treatment during the postpartum period. Breast-feeding has been associated with decreased severity of neonatal opiate withdrawal syndrome, decreased need for pharmacotherapy, and shorter hospital stays for the neonate. The manufacturers of buprenorphine-containing preparations used for treatment of opiate dependence state that developmental and health benefits of breast-feeding should be considered along with the mother's clinical need for buprenorphine or buprenorphine/naloxone and any potential adverse effects on the breast-fed child from the drug or from the underlying maternal condition. Because of the potential for serious adverse reactions, including excess sedation and respiratory depression in nursing infants, the manufacturers of buprenorphine preparations labeled for use as analgesics state that women should be advised not to nurse an infant while receiving the drug. Infants who are exposed to buprenorphine through breast milk should be monitored for excess sedation and respiratory depression.

Symptoms of withdrawal can occur in opiate-dependent infants when maternal administration of opiates is discontinued or breast-feeding is stopped.

DRUG INTERACTIONS

Drug interactions that reportedly occur with other opiate agonists may also potentially occur during administration of buprenorphine.

● Benzodiazepines and Other CNS Depressants

Concomitant use of opiate agonists or opiate partial agonists, including buprenorphine, and benzodiazepines or other CNS depressants (e.g., anxiolytics, sedatives or hypnotics, tranquilizers, muscle relaxants, general anesthetics, antipsychotics, other opiates, alcohol) may result in profound sedation, respiratory depression, hypotension, coma, and death. Opiate analgesics frequently are implicated as contributing to fatal overdoses involving other CNS depressants, and epidemiologic studies have shown that a substantial proportion of fatal opiate overdoses involve the concurrent use of benzodiazepines, alcohol, or other CNS depressants. Whenever possible, concomitant use of opiates and benzodiazepines should be avoided. Alcohol also should be avoided in patients receiving opiates. Concomitant use of opiate analgesics and benzodiazepines or other CNS depressants should be reserved for patients in whom alternative treatment options are inadequate; the lowest effective dosages and shortest possible duration of concomitant therapy should be used, and the patient should be monitored closely for respiratory depression and sedation.

If a benzodiazepine or other CNS depressant is required for any indication other than epilepsy in a patient receiving buprenorphine for analgesia, the drug should be initiated at a lower dosage than indicated in the absence of opiate therapy and titrated based on clinical response. In patients receiving a CNS depressant, buprenorphine, if required for analgesia, should be initiated at a reduced dosage and titrated based on clinical response.

Because the morbidity and mortality associated with untreated opiate addiction can outweigh the serious risks associated with concomitant use of opiate agonists or partial agonists and benzodiazepines or other CNS depressants, buprenorphine treatment for opiate addiction (i.e., medication-assisted treatment [MAT]) should not be categorically withheld from patients receiving benzodiazepines or other CNS depressants. Clinicians should develop treatment plans that minimize the risks associated with concomitant use. If possible, benzodiazepines or other CNS depressants should be tapered and discontinued. (See Concomitant Use of Benzodiazepines or Other CNS Depressants under Cautions: Precautions and Contraindications.)

Clinicians should consider prescribing the opiate antagonist naloxone for patients receiving opiates who are at increased risk of opiate overdosage, including those receiving benzodiazepines or other CNS depressants concomitantly. (See Respiratory and CNS Depression under Cautions: Precautions and Contraindications.)

There have been reports of death or coma when buprenorphine was misused, often via self-injection of crushed tablets, or used concomitantly with benzodiazepines or other CNS depressants, including alcohol. In addition, results of preclinical studies indicate that the combination of benzodiazepines and buprenorphine may alter the usual ceiling on buprenorphine-induced respiratory depression, making the respiratory-depressant effects of buprenorphine, an opiate partial agonist, appear similar to those of opiate agonists. Patients receiving treatment with buprenorphine should be warned of the potential danger of self-administration of benzodiazepines or other CNS depressants, including IV self-administration.

Respiratory and cardiovascular collapse has occurred in several patients receiving usual doses of IV buprenorphine and oral diazepam concomitantly; the patients recovered following treatment that included assisted respiration and IV doxapram. Bradycardia, respiratory depression, and prolonged drowsiness occurred following IV administration of buprenorphine during surgery in a patient who had received oral lorazepam preoperatively. The patient recovered following treatment that included IV atropine and assisted respiration; however, drowsiness persisted for more than 12 hours, and lack of awareness and recall of the surgical procedure (amnesia) reportedly lasted for 48 hours.

Concomitant administration of buprenorphine and fentanyl produced satisfactory analgesia of prolonged duration, minimal respiratory depression, and allowed the patient to be aroused quickly and easily following surgery.

Concomitant administration of buprenorphine and droperidol produced satisfactory analgesia during and after surgery and also in a terminally ill patient with severe, chronic pain that was previously unresponsive to buprenorphine therapy

alone. In a group of patients who received a single, high dose of buprenorphine before undergoing cholecystectomy with balanced anesthesia and experienced pain in the immediate postoperative phase, addition of naloxone reportedly resulted in adequate analgesia, possibly by counteracting dominant antagonistic effects of buprenorphine.

● Drugs Affecting Hepatic Microsomal Enzymes

Buprenorphine metabolism is mediated principally by cytochrome P-450 (CYP) isoenzyme 3A4. Buprenorphine and its major metabolite (norbuprenorphine) also undergo conjugation with glucuronic acid.

CYP3A4 Inhibitors

Concomitant use of buprenorphine with drugs that inhibit CYP3A4 (e.g., macrolide antibiotics [e.g., erythromycin], azole antifungals [e.g., ketoconazole], protease inhibitors [e.g., ritonavir]) may increase plasma concentrations of buprenorphine, possibly resulting in increased or prolonged opiate effects, particularly when an inhibitor is added after a stable buprenorphine dosage has been achieved. If concomitant use of buprenorphine with drugs that inhibit CYP3A4 is necessary, patients should be monitored at frequent intervals for respiratory depression and sedation, and dosage adjustments should be considered until stable drug effects are achieved. Discontinuance of a concomitantly used CYP3A4 inhibitor may result in decreased plasma concentrations of buprenorphine, possibly resulting in decreased opiate effects and/or development of opiate withdrawal. Patients receiving buprenorphine who discontinue therapy with a CYP3A4 inhibitor should be monitored for opiate withdrawal, and dosage adjustments should be considered until stable drug effects are achieved.

Patients who initiate therapy with buprenorphine subdermal implants or buprenorphine extended-release subcutaneous injection after being stabilized on oral transmucosal buprenorphine administered concurrently with a CYP3A4 inhibitor should be monitored to ensure that the plasma buprenorphine concentrations provided by the implants or subcutaneous injection are adequate. Patients already receiving therapy with buprenorphine implants or buprenorphine extended-release subcutaneous injection who initiate therapy with a CYP3A4 inhibitor should be monitored for manifestations of excessive buprenorphine dosage; if there is evidence of buprenorphine toxicity or overdosage and dosage reduction or discontinuance of the concomitant CYP3A4 inhibitor is not feasible, removal of the buprenorphine implants or subcutaneous drug depot and initiation of a buprenorphine formulation that permits dosage adjustments may be necessary. Conversely, if a CYP3A4 inhibitor is discontinued following stable concomitant therapy with either the implants or extended-release subcutaneous injection, the patient should be monitored for manifestations of withdrawal; if the dosage of buprenorphine from the implants or subcutaneous depot is inadequate in the absence of the CYP3A4 inhibitor, the patient should be switched to a buprenorphine formulation that permits dosage adjustments.

The potential for interactions may depend in part on the route of buprenorphine administration. The manufacturer of transdermal buprenorphine states that the pharmacokinetics of buprenorphine administered by the transdermal route are not expected to be affected by concomitant use of CYP3A4 inhibitors.

CYP3A4 Inducers

Although specific drug interaction studies have not been performed, concomitant use of drugs that induce CYP3A4 (e.g., carbamazepine, phenytoin, rifampin) may reduce plasma concentrations of buprenorphine, possibly resulting in decreased analgesic efficacy and/or development of opiate withdrawal. If concomitant use of buprenorphine with CYP3A4 inducers is necessary, patients should be monitored for opiate withdrawal, and dosage adjustments should be considered until stable drug effects are achieved. Discontinuance of a concomitantly used CYP3A4 inducer may result in increased plasma concentrations of buprenorphine, possibly resulting in increased or prolonged therapeutic or adverse effects, including serious respiratory depression. Patients receiving buprenorphine who discontinue therapy with a CYP3A4 inducer should be monitored for respiratory depression, and the buprenorphine dosage should be adjusted as necessary.

Patients who initiate therapy with buprenorphine subdermal implants or buprenorphine extended-release subcutaneous injection after being stabilized on oral transmucosal buprenorphine administered concurrently with a CYP3A4 inducer should be monitored to ensure that the plasma buprenorphine concentrations provided by the implants or subcutaneous injection are adequate but not excessive. Patients already receiving therapy with buprenorphine implants or buprenorphine extended-release subcutaneous injection who initiate therapy with a CYP3A4 inducer should be monitored for manifestations of withdrawal; if the dosage of buprenorphine from the implants or subcutaneous injection is inadequate and dosage reduction or discontinuance of the concomitant CYP3A4 inducer is not feasible, the patient should be switched to a buprenorphine formulation that permits dosage adjustments. Conversely, if a CYP3A4 inducer is discontinued following stable concomitant therapy with either the implants or extended-release subcutaneous injection, the patient should be monitored for manifestations of excessive buprenorphine dosage; if the dosage of buprenorphine from the implants or subcutaneous injection is excessive in the absence of the CYP3A4 inducer, removal of the buprenorphine implants or subcutaneous drug depot and initiation of a buprenorphine formulation that permits dosage adjustments may be necessary.

The potential for interactions may depend in part on the route of buprenorphine administration.

Antifungals

Administration of ketoconazole 400 mg daily in patients receiving stable sublingual doses of buprenorphine in fixed combination with naloxone (buprenorphine/naloxone) increased peak plasma concentrations of buprenorphine by 100% and mean area under the plasma concentration-time curve (AUC) by 75–100% from baseline. However, concomitant use of ketoconazole 200 mg twice daily for 11 days and transdermal buprenorphine 10 mcg/hour for 7 days did not affect the pharmacokinetics of buprenorphine.

Antiretrovirals

Some human immunodeficiency virus (HIV) protease inhibitors (PIs) with CYP3A4 inhibitory activity (i.e., lopinavir in fixed combination with ritonavir [lopinavir/ritonavir], nelfinavir, ritonavir) have been shown to have minimal pharmacokinetic and no clinically important pharmacodynamic interactions with buprenorphine. However, concomitant use of buprenorphine and other PIs with CYP3A4 inhibitory activity (i.e., *unboosted* atazanavir, *ritonavir-boosted* atazanavir) has resulted in increased plasma concentrations of buprenorphine and norbuprenorphine and excessive opiate effects. While concomitant use of *ritonavir-boosted* atazanavir and buprenorphine is not expected to affect the pharmacokinetics of atazanavir, concomitant use of *unboosted* atazanavir and buprenorphine may result in decreased plasma atazanavir concentrations. The manufacturers of buprenorphine state that patients receiving buprenorphine concomitantly with atazanavir (with or without ritonavir) should be monitored; buprenorphine dosage reduction may be warranted. The manufacturer of atazanavir states that concomitant use of *unboosted* atazanavir and buprenorphine is not recommended. If therapy with *ritonavir-boosted* or *unboosted* atazanavir must be initiated in a patient already receiving therapy with buprenorphine subdermal implants or extended-release subcutaneous injection, the patient should be monitored for manifestations of excessive buprenorphine dosage; removal of the buprenorphine implants or subcutaneous drug depot and initiation of an alternative buprenorphine formulation that permits dosage adjustments may be necessary.

Nonnucleoside reverse transcriptase inhibitors (NNRTIs) are metabolized principally by CYP3A4, and certain NNRTIs may either inhibit (e.g., delavirdine) or induce (e.g., efavirenz, etravirine, nevirapine) CYP3A enzymes. Pharmacokinetic interactions have been observed with concomitant use of buprenorphine and certain NNRTIs (i.e., efavirenz, delavirdine). However, these interactions did not result in substantial pharmacodynamic effects. Patients receiving chronic buprenorphine therapy who begin therapy with an NNRTI should have their buprenorphine dosage monitored.

Nucleoside reverse transcriptase inhibitors (NRTIs) do not appear to induce or inhibit CYP enzymes, and interactions with buprenorphine are not expected.

● Drugs Metabolized by Hepatic Microsomal Enzymes

In vitro studies indicate that buprenorphine inhibits activity of CYP2D6 and CYP3A4 and its major metabolite, norbuprenorphine, is a moderate inhibitor of CYP2D6. However, the relatively low plasma concentrations of buprenorphine and norbuprenorphine resulting from therapeutic doses of the drug are not expected to result in clinically important interactions.

● Drugs that Prolong the QT Interval

Because of the risk of QT-interval prolongation, buprenorphine should be avoided in patients receiving class IA (e.g., quinidine, procainamide, disopyramide) or class III (e.g., sotalol, amiodarone, dofetilide) antiarrhythmic agents or other drugs known to prolong the QT interval. (See Cautions: Cardiovascular Effects.)

● Drugs Associated with Serotonin Syndrome

Serotonin syndrome may occur in patients receiving opiate partial agonists concomitantly with other serotonergic drugs, including serotonin (5-hydroxytryptamine; 5-HT) type 1 receptor agonists ("triptans"), selective serotonin-reuptake inhibitors (SSRIs), selective serotonin- and norepinephrine-reuptake inhibitors (SNRIs), tricyclic antidepressants, antiemetics that are 5-HT₃ receptor antagonists, buspirone, cyclobenzaprine, dextromethorphan, lithium, St. John's wort (*Hypericum perforatum*), tryptophan, other serotonin modulators (e.g., mirtazapine, nefazodone, trazodone, vilazodone), and monoamine oxidase (MAO) inhibitors (both those used to treat psychiatric disorders and others, such as linezolid, methylene blue, and selegiline). Serotonin syndrome may occur within the recommended dosage ranges for these drugs. Manifestations of serotonin syndrome may include mental status changes (e.g., agitation, hallucinations, coma), autonomic instability (e.g., tachycardia, labile blood pressure, hyperthermia), neuromuscular aberrations (e.g., hyperreflexia, incoordination, rigidity), and/or GI symptoms (e.g., nausea, vomiting, diarrhea). Symptom onset generally occurs within several hours to a few days of concomitant use, but may occur later, particularly after dosage increases.

If concomitant use of other serotonergic drugs is warranted, patients should be monitored for serotonin syndrome, particularly during initiation of therapy and dosage increases. If serotonin syndrome is suspected, treatment with buprenorphine, other opiate agonist or partial agonist therapy, and/or any concurrently administered serotonergic agents should be discontinued.

● Drugs Affecting Hepatic Blood Flow

When buprenorphine is administered concomitantly with a drug(s) that may reduce hepatic blood flow (e.g., halothane) and thereby reduce hepatic elimination of the partial opiate agonist, the activity of buprenorphine may be increased and/or prolonged. If such concomitant therapy is administered, buprenorphine should be used with caution and dosage of at least one of the drugs should be reduced.

● Anticholinergic Agents

Concomitant use of buprenorphine and drugs with anticholinergic activity may increase the risk of urinary retention and/or severe constipation, which can lead to paralytic ileus. Patients receiving such concomitant therapy should be monitored for signs or symptoms of urinary retention and reduced GI motility.

● Diuretics

Opiates may decrease the effects of diuretics by inducing the release of vasopressin (antidiuretic hormone). Patients receiving such concomitant therapy should be monitored for decreased diuretic or hypotensive effects; dosage of the diuretic may be increased if clinically indicated.

● Local Anesthetics

Buprenorphine may potentiate the effects of local anesthetics (e.g., bupivacaine hydrochloride, mepivacaine hydrochloride), and concomitant administration of the drugs may result in a more rapid onset and prolonged duration of analgesia.

● Monoamine Oxidase Inhibitors

Because concomitant use of opiates with MAO inhibitors (e.g., linezolid, phenelzine, tranylcypromine) may result in serotonin syndrome or manifestations of opiate toxicity (e.g., respiratory depression, coma), use of buprenorphine is not recommended in patients who are receiving or have recently (i.e., within 2 weeks) received an MAO inhibitor.

● Neuromuscular Blocking Agents

Buprenorphine may enhance the neuromuscular blocking action and increase the respiratory depressant effect of neuromuscular blocking agents. Patients receiving such concomitant therapy should be monitored for a greater than expected degree of respiratory depression; dosage of one or both drugs should be decreased as needed.

● Opiate Agonists and Partial Agonists

Opiate partial agonists (e.g., butorphanol, nalbuphine, pentazocine) may reduce the analgesic effect of buprenorphine and/or precipitate withdrawal symptoms; such concomitant use should be avoided.

Buprenorphine, which has high affinity but weaker agonistic effects at μ-opiate receptors, can displace full agonists from these receptors, with a resultant reduction in opiate agonist effects; therefore, initiation of buprenorphine therapy in individuals dependent on full opiate agonists before the agonistic effects of the opiate have subsided may precipitate withdrawal. Dosage of the full opiate agonist should be tapered before buprenorphine is initiated for analgesia. Induction therapy with buprenorphine-containing preparations for opiate dependence should be initiated only when clear and objective signs of withdrawal are evident.

ACUTE TOXICITY

● Manifestations

Acute overdosage of buprenorphine may produce respiratory depression, CNS depression with somnolence progressing to stupor or coma, cardiovascular manifestations including bradycardia and hypotension, skeletal muscle flaccidity, cold and clammy skin, pinpoint pupils, partial or complete airway obstruction, pulmonary edema, atypical snoring, and death. Marked mydriasis (rather than miosis) may be observed in patients with hypoxia.

● Treatment

In acute buprenorphine overdosage, the patient's respiratory and cardiac status should be monitored carefully. Primary attention should be given to reestablishment of adequate respiratory exchange by maintaining an adequate, patent airway and using assisted or controlled respiration. Other supportive measures, such as oxygen and IV fluids and vasopressors, should also be used as necessary. While doxapram and naloxone may be of value in the management of buprenorphine overdosage, they also may be ineffective in, and therefore should *not* be relied on for, reversing buprenorphine-induced respiratory depression; instead, the use of assisted or controlled respiration and administration of oxygen may be necessary and should be considered the principal method of management of buprenorphine overdosage. When naloxone is used to reverse respiratory depression in patients receiving buprenorphine, larger than usual doses and repeated administration may be necessary.

An opiate antagonist (e.g., naloxone, nalmefene) should not be administered in the absence of clinically important respiratory or circulatory depression secondary to buprenorphine overdosage. In patients physically dependent on opiates, administration of the usual dose of an opiate antagonist will precipitate acute withdrawal. If a decision is made to treat serious respiratory depression in a physically dependent patient with an opiate antagonist, administration should be initiated with care and by titration using smaller than usual doses.

In cases of acute overdosage involving transdermal buprenorphine, the transdermal system should be removed immediately and the pharmacokinetic profile of transdermal administration should be considered. While patients may appear to improve with appropriate supportive measures, there is the possibility of extended buprenorphine effects as the drug continues to be absorbed from the skin. After removal of the buprenorphine transdermal system, plasma drug concentrations decrease by 50% in approximately 12 hours (range 10–24 hours) and the apparent terminal half-life is approximately 26 hours. The duration of action of transdermal buprenorphine may exceed the duration of action of the opiate antagonist used to treat the overdose. Patients may require monitoring and treatment for at least 24 hours after the buprenorphine transdermal system is removed.

In cases of overdosage potentially involving multiple agents, the potential contribution of buprenorphine versus other CNS depressants should be considered in deciding whether buprenorphine subdermal implants should be removed. In an emergency situation, the implants may be removed by a surgeon who is not REMS certified. In patients who have received buprenorphine extended-release subcutaneous injection, clinical data are limited regarding possible surgical removal of the subcutaneous drug depot.

CHRONIC TOXICITY

Patients may develop psychological dependence to the opiate agonist activity of buprenorphine; however, animal studies suggest that the reinforcing efficacy of buprenorphine may be less than that of the opiate agonists, morphine and codeine, and less than that of the other opiate partial agonists, butorphanol, nalbuphine, and pentazocine. Limited physical dependence also may occur, although

infrequently, and the potential for development of tolerance to the drug's opiate agonist activity is limited. Studies in animals have suggested that cross-tolerance between buprenorphine and other opiate agonists (i.e., morphine) may develop. Studies in animals and humans have also suggested that buprenorphine may have a lesser physical dependence liability than morphine or pentazocine; however, buprenorphine has been misused by drug abusers and patients physically dependent on opiates in an attempt to substitute the drug for opiate agonists.

Administration of naloxone in a group of patients who received prolonged therapy with buprenorphine (1–2 months) and who were formerly physically dependent on opiates did not produce withdrawal. In a group of patients physically dependent on opiates who had substituted buprenorphine for the opiate agonist, discontinuance of buprenorphine slowly over several days resulted in a complete absence of signs and symptoms of withdrawal during the 30-day observation period. An initial 0.4-mg IV dose of naloxone produced no evidence of withdrawal in an individual with a history of parenteral misuse of opiate agonists who had substituted IV buprenorphine for the opiate agonist for a 6-month period and in whom a urinalysis confirmed the absence of opiate agonists in the urine; however, additional 2-mg doses of naloxone injected IV every 5 minutes up to a total dose of 10 mg precipitated signs and symptoms of opiate withdrawal which were relieved by administration of IV morphine.

Signs and symptoms of acute withdrawal following discontinuance of buprenorphine are similar to, but less intense than, those produced by morphine or methadone and may include abdominal pain, nausea, vomiting, restlessness, insomnia, diarrhea, chills, hot flushes (flashes), general aches and pains, hypertension, anorexia, malaise, tachycardia, lacrimation, rhinorrhea, diaphoresis, and piloerection. Similar signs and symptoms of withdrawal reportedly occurred following administration of naloxone in an individual with a history of buprenorphine abuse. Following abrupt discontinuance of buprenorphine after prolonged use (1–2 months), signs and symptoms of acute withdrawal were delayed and gradually appeared over 3–10 days, reached a peak after about 14 days, and continued for an additional 7–14 days.

PHARMACOLOGY

● Opiate Agonist and Antagonist Properties

Buprenorphine is an opiate partial agonist and shares many of the actions of opiate agonists. The drug exhibits analgesic and opiate antagonist activities. Buprenorphine is thought to act as a partial agonist at μ-opiate receptors in the CNS and peripheral tissues. The drug also is an antagonist at κ-opiate receptors and an agonist at δ-opiate receptors.

Buprenorphine appears to have a high affinity for both μ- and κ-receptors, and low to moderate intrinsic activity at μ- and κ-receptors; in contrast, the drug appears to have low to high affinity for and low intrinsic activity at δ-receptors. Buprenorphine binds slowly with and dissociates slowly from the μ-receptor. It is thought that the high affinity of buprenorphine for the μ-receptor and its slow binding to and dissociation from the receptor may account for the prolonged duration of analgesia and possibly in part for the limited physical dependence potential observed with the drug.

The opiate agonist and antagonist activities of buprenorphine appear to be dose related. At doses of up to 1 mg subcutaneously, buprenorphine has a potent analgesic effect; at doses greater than 1 mg subcutaneously, the opiate agonist activity of the drug decreases and the opiate antagonist activity predominates. Following IM administration, the opiate antagonist activity of buprenorphine occurs principally at doses greater than 0.8 mg. The drug may antagonize its own opiate agonist activity when administered at doses within the opiate antagonist range.

Animal studies have shown that antagonism of the opiate agonist activity of buprenorphine by other opiate antagonists may not occur once buprenorphine binds to opiate receptors in the CNS. In animals not physically dependent on opiates, administration of an opiate antagonist (e.g., naloxone) prior to or concomitantly with administration of buprenorphine results in a reduction or complete block of buprenorphine-induced opiate agonist activity. When buprenorphine is administered prior to an opiate antagonist, the agonist activity of buprenorphine is dominant. Similarly, administration of naloxone in a group of patients receiving prolonged therapy with buprenorphine (1–2 months) did not precipitate withdrawal.

On a weight basis, the opiate antagonist activity of buprenorphine is reportedly equal to or up to 3 times greater than that of naloxone when both drugs are compared as antagonists of morphine. Buprenorphine may precipitate mild to moderate withdrawal in some patients physically dependent on opiates. In patients who have received single subcutaneous morphine doses of up to 120 mg during chronic buprenorphine therapy, buprenorphine produces a block of the pharmacologic effects of morphine. Buprenorphine reportedly does not antagonize respiratory depression produced by non-opiate analgesics and other drugs.

Repeated exposure to short-acting opiates appears to result in neurobiologic changes in cellular and molecular systems; these changes include perturbations in opiate-receptor kinetics, transmembrane signaling, postreceptor signal transduction, and intracellular messengers. The physiologic dependence and addictive behavior that are characteristic of opiate dependence result from these neurobiologic changes and are the basis for use of opiate agonists for the treatment of opiate dependence. Opiate agonists stabilize brain neurochemistry by replacing short-acting euphorigenic opiates (e.g., heroin) with long-acting noneuphorigenic opiates (e.g., buprenorphine, levomethadyl acetate hydrochloride [no longer commercially available in the US], methadone). The mechanism(s) of action of these long-acting noneuphorigenic opiates include cross-tolerance at the opiate receptor, thus preventing opiate withdrawal, and competition for opiate-receptor binding sites, thus blocking the effects of exogenously administered opiates.

Like opiate agonists such as methadone or hydromorphone, sublingual administration of buprenorphine produces typical opiate agonist effects, which are limited by a ceiling effect. In individuals who were not opiate dependent, administration of a single sublingual dose of buprenorphine produced opiate agonist effects; these effects were maximal at doses of 8–16 mg. The effect of buprenorphine 16 mg was similar to that of an equivalent dose of buprenorphine given in fixed combination with naloxone.

Administration of single doses of buprenorphine produce physiologic and subjective effects that are similar to those produced by equivalent doses of buprenorphine administered in fixed combination with naloxone. When administered sublingually, the naloxone in fixed combination with buprenorphine does not have any clinically important pharmacologic effects. Buprenorphine in fixed combination with naloxone is recognized as an opiate agonist in opiate-dependent individuals when the preparation is given sublingually. However, parenteral administration of buprenorphine in conjunction with naloxone results in opiate antagonist actions similar to those of naloxone. IV administration of buprenorphine in conjunction with naloxone precipitates opiate withdrawal symptoms in opiate-dependent individuals.

● CNS Effects

Like other opiate agonists, buprenorphine produces dose-related analgesia. The exact mechanism has not been fully elucidated, but analgesia appears to result from a high affinity of buprenorphine for μ- and possibly κ-opiate receptors in the CNS. The drug may also alter the pain threshold (threshold of afferent nerve endings to noxious stimuli). On a weight basis, the analgesic potency of parenteral buprenorphine appears to be about 25–50, 200, and 600 times that of parenteral morphine, pentazocine, and meperidine, respectively. Buprenorphine may produce sex-related differences in analgesia, with females requiring substantially less drug than males to produce adequate analgesia. Following IV doses of 4 mcg/kg and higher, the drug may produce amnesia.

In patients physically dependent on opiates, buprenorphine produces many of the subjective and objective effects of opiates; however, the drug may not be a satisfactory substitute for opiate agonists for pain relief in all patients physically dependent on opiates. The potential for development of tolerance to the drug's opiate agonist activity is limited.

Buprenorphine may produce psychological dependence. Buprenorphine may also produce limited physical dependence, although infrequently. Signs and symptoms of mild withdrawal may appear following discontinuance of prolonged therapy with the drug alone. (See Chronic Toxicity.) Because buprenorphine binds slowly with and dissociates slowly from the μ-receptor, elimination of the drug from the CNS is prolonged following abrupt discontinuance; consequently, signs and symptoms of acute withdrawal are less intense than those produced by morphine and delayed in appearance. Buprenorphine is a partial opiate agonist with behavioral and psychic effects similar to morphine, and, unlike pentazocine, it rarely causes psychotomimetic effects.

Like other opiate agonists, buprenorphine may produce increases in intracranial pressure.

In rats, buprenorphine produces dose-related changes in the EEG pattern, and changes appear to be maximal at doses of 1 mg/kg. Increasing doses up to 1 mg/kg

produce intense stupor and continuous high-voltage bursting activity, while doses of 0.3 and 10 mg/kg produce less intense stupor and intermittent bursting activity. In rabbits, buprenorphine produces EEG patterns characterized by increases in delta and theta wave activity. When administered in daily subcutaneous doses of 2 mg in individuals formerly receiving methadone, buprenorphine therapy was associated with EEG patterns characterized by an increase in alpha wave activity; however, the increase in activity may have resulted from a return of normal EEG patterns following discontinuance of methadone. Upon discontinuance of buprenorphine, the EEG pattern was characterized by a decrease in alpha wave activity; an increase in alpha wave activity was subsequently observed about 20 days following discontinuance of buprenorphine.

● Cardiovascular Effects

Buprenorphine generally produces few cardiovascular effects. In healthy individuals, cardiovascular effects induced by parenteral buprenorphine are similar to those following equivalent parenteral doses of morphine, including decreases in heart rate and systolic and diastolic blood pressures. Cardiovascular effects of buprenorphine appear to be of minor clinical importance in most patients, including patients with compromised cardiac function who have undergone surgery or patients who are recovering from myocardial infarction. In a limited number of patients, buprenorphine has been reported to inhibit cardiovascular effects that occur during surgery (e.g., increases in heart rate and systolic blood pressure).

Buprenorphine may decrease heart rate and systolic and/or diastolic blood pressure. The drug has also been shown to increase heart rate and blood pressure (principally systolic pressure) in some patients. Stroke volume and cardiac output may be slightly increased or decreased. Buprenorphine produces peripheral vasodilation, which may result in orthostatic hypotension or syncope. Cardiovascular effects of buprenorphine, including changes in heart rate, stroke volume, and systolic blood pressure, may be dose related; in several studies, buprenorphine-induced cardiovascular effects were not apparent at IV doses of 1.5 mcg/kg but appeared at IV doses of 2 mcg/kg and higher.

Prolongation of the QT interval was observed in healthy individuals receiving transdermal buprenorphine at dosages of 40 mcg/hour; dosages of 10 mcg/hour did not result in clinically relevant changes in the QT interval. Prolongation of the QT interval also was observed in patients receiving buprenorphine buccally dissolving strips at dosages of up to 900 mcg every 12 hours.

● Respiratory Effects

Usual parenteral doses of buprenorphine potentially may depress respiration to the same degree as 10 mg of parenteral morphine sulfate. The onset of buprenorphine-induced respiratory depression is slower than that of morphine-induced respiratory depression and the duration appears to be more prolonged. Respiratory depression may be severe in individuals with compromised respiratory function or those receiving other respiratory depressant drugs concomitantly.

Buprenorphine-induced respiratory depression is dose related in single parenteral doses of up to 1.2 mg. Unlike morphine, there appears to be a ceiling to buprenorphine-induced respiratory depression in most patients, so that higher doses of the drug do not necessarily produce a proportionate increase in respiratory depression. Changes in frequency, depth, and pattern of respiration and changes in arterial blood gas values do not appear to be clinically important in most patients. However, in animal studies, concomitant use of buprenorphine with benzodiazepines appeared to alter the usual ceiling on buprenorphine-induced respiratory depression, resulting in respiratory depressant effects similar to those of full opiate agonists.

Buprenorphine-induced respiratory depression is characterized by decreases in arterial P_{O_2} and rate of respiration and increases in arterial P_{CO_2}.

IV naloxone hydrochloride has been used to reverse signs of buprenorphine-induced respiratory depression; however, in usual doses, naloxone is substantially less effective in reversing buprenorphine-induced respiratory depression than in reversing morphine-induced respiratory depression and is occasionally only partially effective and, rarely, completely ineffective in reversing buprenorphine-induced respiratory depression. When naloxone is used to reverse signs of respiratory depression in patients receiving buprenorphine, larger than usual doses may be necessary. Doxapram has also been used with some success in reversing buprenorphine-induced respiratory depression.

The effect of buprenorphine on the cough reflex in humans has not been studied; however, in guinea pigs, the drug suppresses experimentally induced cough.

● Endocrine Effects

Like other opiate agonists, buprenorphine has been shown to decrease plasma concentrations of luteinizing hormone (LH) and increase plasma concentrations of prolactin. Buprenorphine has been reported to prevent the stress-induced increase in plasma cortisol concentration that occurs during surgery; however, the drug has also been reported to lack an inhibitory effect on surgery-induced increases in plasma cortisol in other patients and to increase plasma cortisol in healthy individuals. In some patients, the drug did not inhibit increases in plasma glucose concentration, but in other patients it reportedly prevented increases in plasma glucose concentration. Buprenorphine has been shown to reverse surgery-induced increases in plasma growth hormone (GH) and insulin concentrations, but the drug has produced increases in plasma GH concentration in healthy individuals.

● GI Effects

Buprenorphine produces minimal GI effects, including nausea, vomiting, and constipation. Like other opiate agonists, buprenorphine may produce an increase in pressure within the common bile duct, which may be followed by a rapid decrease in pressure. In healthy individuals, the drug did not alter baseline pressure of the sphincter of Oddi, and flow of biliary and pancreatic fluids was unaffected.

● Other Effects

Buprenorphine causes dose-related miosis, with peak miotic effects occurring at 6 hours and miosis continuing for about 72 hours after parenteral administration.

Buprenorphine produces urinary retention in some patients.

PHARMACOKINETICS

● Absorption

Some pharmacokinetic data indicate that a relationship between plasma buprenorphine concentrations and a given analgesic effect does not exist.

Buprenorphine Hydrochloride Conventional Injection

Buprenorphine hydrochloride is rapidly and approximately 40–90% absorbed systemically following IM administration.

Following IV administration of a single 0.3-mg dose of buprenorphine, mean peak plasma drug concentrations of 18 ng/mL occurred within 2 minutes; plasma concentrations declined to 9 and 0.4 ng/mL after 5 minutes and 3 hours, respectively. Following IM administration of a second 0.3-mg dose 3 hours after the initial IV dose, mean peak plasma buprenorphine concentrations of 3.6 ng/mL occurred within 2–5 minutes and declined to 0.4 ng/mL after 3 hours. Approximately 10 minutes after administration, plasma concentrations of buprenorphine are similar following IV or IM injection. Plasma concentrations of buprenorphine may be increased slightly by concomitant administration of a general anesthetic (e.g., halothane) as a result of anesthesia-induced decrease in hepatic blood flow and hepatic clearance of the drug.

Following IM or IV administration of a single dose of buprenorphine, onset of analgesia is similar to that following IM or IV administration of morphine, respectively; the time of peak analgesia is similar to that of parenteral morphine, meperidine, or pentazocine. The onset of analgesia and time to peak analgesia are shorter following IV administration of buprenorphine than IM administration. The duration of analgesia produced by parenteral buprenorphine is longer than that produced by parenteral meperidine or pentazocine and is comparable to and, in some patients, may be longer than that produced by parenteral morphine. The duration of analgesia may vary according to the route of administration, with a more prolonged duration following IV or epidural administration than IM administration. The duration of analgesia may be prolonged with higher doses of buprenorphine; however, duration of analgesia did not differ substantially in a group of patients receiving 0.15- to 0.4-mg doses of the drug. The duration of analgesia induced by buprenorphine may also be affected by patient age, with the duration slightly prolonged in older patients. Following parenteral administration of single doses of 0.15–0.6 mg or 2–12 mcg/kg of buprenorphine in postoperative patients, the onset of analgesia usually occurs within 10–30 minutes, and peak analgesia usually occurs within 60 minutes; however, peak analgesia may occur within as little as 15 minutes in some patients. The mean duration of analgesia generally is

6 hours following single IM or IV doses of 0.2–0.3 mg or 2–4 mcg/kg; however, in some studies, the mean duration of analgesia reportedly ranged from 4–10 hours following single IM doses of 0.2–0.6 mg and 2–24 hours following single IV doses of 0.3 mg or 2–15 mcg/kg.

Buprenorphine Transdermal System

When administered transdermally, buprenorphine has an absolute bioavailability of approximately 15%. Following application of a single transdermal system delivering buprenorphine 5, 10, or 20 mcg/hour, peak plasma concentrations of buprenorphine average 0.176, 0.191, or 0.471 ng/mL, respectively. Quantifiable buprenorphine concentrations are detectable approximately 17 hours after placement of the 10-mcg/hour transdermal system, with steady-state concentrations attained by the third day of treatment. Blood concentrations of buprenorphine increased by 26–55% when heat was applied directly to a transdermal system designed to deliver the drug at a dosage of 10 mcg/hour; concentrations returned to normal within 5 hours after the heat source was removed.

Oral Transmucosal Formulations Used for Analgesia

Following administration of a single dose of buprenorphine (75–1200 mcg) as a buccally dissolving strip (Belbuca®), absolute bioavailability is 46–65% and peak plasma concentrations and AUC increase in a linear manner. Following single doses of 75, 300, or 1200 mcg, peak plasma concentrations of buprenorphine average 0.17, 0.47, or 1.43 ng/mL, respectively, and are achieved at a median of 2.5–3 hours. Following repeated administration at a dosage of 60–240 mcg every 12 hours, steady-state plasma concentrations are attained prior to the sixth dose, and steady-state peak plasma concentrations and AUC are proportional to dose.

Ingestion of cold, hot, or room-temperature water during buccal administration of the strips decreased systemic exposure to buprenorphine by 23–27%; concurrent ingestion of a low-pH liquid such as decaffeinated cola decreased systemic exposure to the drug by approximately 37%.

In cancer patients with grade 3 mucositis, absorption of buprenorphine from the buccally dissolving strips was more rapid and peak plasma concentrations and AUC were approximately 79 and 56% higher, respectively, compared with healthy controls.

Oral Transmucosal Formulations Used for Treatment of Opiate Dependence

Not all formulations, strengths, or dose combinations of oral transmucosal preparations containing buprenorphine in fixed combination with naloxone (buprenorphine/naloxone) are bioequivalent.

Following sublingual administration of generic buprenorphine or buprenorphine/naloxone sublingual tablets (i.e., generic equivalents of Subutex® or Suboxone® sublingual tablets [branded formulations no longer commercially available in the US]), there is substantial interindividual variability in absorption of the drugs, but intraindividual variability is low. Peak plasma concentrations and AUC of buprenorphine increase with increasing dose (over the range of 4–16 mg), but the increase is not directly proportional to dose. Following sublingual administration of buprenorphine sublingual tablets at a dose of 2, 8, or 16 mg, peak plasma buprenorphine concentrations average 1.25, 2.88, or 4.7 ng/mL, respectively. Following sublingual administration of a single tablet containing buprenorphine 2 mg and naloxone 0.5 mg or containing buprenorphine 8 mg and naloxone 2 mg, peak plasma buprenorphine concentrations average 0.78 or 2.58 ng/mL, respectively. In most individuals, quantifiable amounts of naloxone are not detected in plasma beyond 2 hours after sublingual administration of buprenorphine/naloxone at naloxone doses of 1–4 mg; mean peak plasma concentrations of naloxone at these doses range from 0.11–0.28 ng/mL.

Not all strengths and combinations of buprenorphine/naloxone (Suboxone®) sublingually dissolving strips are bioequivalent to Suboxone® sublingual tablets administered at the same total dose. A dose consisting of one or two strips, each containing buprenorphine 2 mg and naloxone 0.5 mg, administered sublingually or buccally showed comparable relative bioavailability to sublingual tablets providing the same total dose. However, at a strength of buprenorphine 8 mg in fixed combination with naloxone 2 mg or a strength of buprenorphine 12 mg in fixed combination with naloxone 3 mg, a single strip administered sublingually or buccally showed higher relative bioavailability for both buprenorphine and naloxone compared with sublingual tablets providing the same total dose. A combination of one strip containing buprenorphine 8 mg and naloxone 2 mg and two strips containing buprenorphine 2 mg and naloxone 0.5 mg (total dose of buprenorphine 12 mg and naloxone 3 mg) administered sublingually showed comparable relative bioavailability as sublingual tablets providing the same total dose; however, when the strips were administered buccally, relative bioavailability was higher than that of the sublingual tablets. Pharmacokinetic parameters and systemic exposures are generally comparable following either buccal or sublingual administration of buprenorphine/naloxone strips, although systemic exposure to naloxone may be somewhat higher after buccal administration.

Buprenorphine/naloxone (Zubsolv®) sublingual tablets are not bioequivalent to Suboxone® sublingual tablets. One Zubsolv® sublingual tablet containing buprenorphine 5.7 mg and naloxone 1.4 mg provides 12% lower naloxone exposure and equivalent buprenorphine exposure as one Suboxone® sublingual tablet containing buprenorphine 8 mg and naloxone 2 mg. Although there is substantial interindividual variability in absorption of buprenorphine and naloxone from Zubsolv® sublingual tablets, intraindividual variability is low. Peak plasma concentrations and AUC of buprenorphine increase with increasing dose (over the range of 1.4–11.4 mg), but the increase is not directly proportional to dose.

Buprenorphine/naloxone (Bunavail®) buccally dissolving strips are not bioequivalent to Suboxone® sublingual tablets. One buccally dissolving strip containing buprenorphine 4.2 mg and naloxone 0.7 mg provides 33% lower naloxone exposure and equivalent buprenorphine exposure as one sublingual tablet containing buprenorphine 8 mg and naloxone 2 mg. Although there is substantial interindividual variability in buccal absorption of buprenorphine and naloxone from Bunavail® strips, intraindividual variability is low. Peak plasma concentrations and AUC of buprenorphine increase with increasing dose (over the range of 0.875–6.3 mg), but the increase is not directly proportional to dose. Administration of liquids with the strips reduces systemic exposure to both buprenorphine and naloxone by as much as 59 and 76%, respectively, depending on the pH of the liquid.

Concomitant administration of naloxone and buprenorphine does not affect the pharmacokinetics of buprenorphine.

Buprenorphine Extended-release Subcutaneous Injection

Following subcutaneous administration of buprenorphine extended-release injection, a solid depot forms and the drug is released via diffusion from and biodegradation of the depot. Following administration of single doses of 50–200 mg and repeated doses of 50–300 mg at 28-day intervals, initial peak plasma concentrations of the drug were attained at a median of 24 hours after injection; concentrations then decreased slowly to a plateau, and steady-state concentrations were achieved at 4–6 months. Mean steady-state plasma concentrations attained following 6 doses of the extended-release subcutaneous injection (a series of two 300-mg doses followed by four 100-mg doses or a series of six 300-mg doses) administered at 28-day intervals were 3.21 or 6.54 ng/mL, respectively, compared with 2.91 ng/mL following stabilization on a buprenorphine dosage of 24 mg daily as sublingual tablets. At steady state, mean trough plasma concentrations achieved with both subcutaneous dosages and the mean peak concentration achieved with the higher-dosage subcutaneous regimen exceeded those attained with the sublingual dosage; the peak concentration attained with the lower-dosage subcutaneous regimen was approximately 59% of that attained with the sublingual dosage. Pharmacokinetic simulations suggest that therapeutic concentrations of the drug persist for 2–5 months, depending on the dosage (100 or 300 mg monthly), following the last injection of the drug.

Buprenorphine Hydrochloride Subdermal Implants

Following insertion of buprenorphine hydrochloride subdermal implants, initial peak plasma concentrations of the drug were attained at a median of 12 hours after insertion; concentrations then decreased slowly, and steady-state concentrations were achieved by approximately week 4. Mean steady-state plasma concentrations of approximately 0.5–1 ng/mL were maintained for approximately 20 weeks (weeks 4–24) and were comparable to the steady-state trough buprenorphine concentrations attained with a sublingual buprenorphine dosage of 8 mg daily. In one study in patients who received sublingual buprenorphine (16 mg daily for at least 5 days) followed by insertion of 4 implants (total buprenorphine hydrochloride dose of 320 mg), overall peak plasma concentrations of buprenorphine were markedly lower after implant insertion compared with the sublingual dosing lead-in period. On day 28 of implant therapy, the steady-state AUC was 31% of the steady-state AUC achieved with the sublingual dosage, and the mean

steady-state drug concentration was approximately 0.82 ng/mL (8% of the peak concentration and 52% of the trough concentration achieved at steady state with the sublingual dosage).

● Distribution

Distribution of buprenorphine into human body tissues and fluids has not been well characterized. Following oral or IM administration in rats, buprenorphine distributes into the liver, brain, placenta, and GI tract; highest concentrations were attained in the liver within 10 or 40 minutes following oral or IM administration, respectively. The hepatic extraction ratio of buprenorphine (E_H) is approximately 1. The drug and its metabolites are distributed into bile. Following IV administration in humans, the drug rapidly distributes into CSF (within several minutes). CSF buprenorphine concentrations appear to be approximately 15–25% of concurrent plasma concentrations.

The volume of distribution of buprenorphine following IV administration in adults is approximately 430 L.

Buprenorphine is approximately 96% bound to plasma proteins, mainly to α- and β-globulins.

Buprenorphine crosses the placenta and distributes into milk.

● Elimination

Plasma concentrations of buprenorphine generally appear to decline in a triphasic manner. Following IV administration of a single dose in postoperative patients with normal renal and hepatic function, the plasma half-life of buprenorphine reportedly averages 2 minutes in the initial (distribution) phase, 11 minutes in the second (redistribution) phase, and 2.2 hours (range: 1.2–7.2 hours) in the terminal (elimination) phase. Some pharmacokinetic data indicate that plasma concentrations of buprenorphine may decline in a biphasic manner in some patients.

Buprenorphine reportedly has a mean elimination half-life of 31–35 hours following sublingual administration as buprenorphine sublingual tablets, 24–42 hours following sublingual administration as buprenorphine/naloxone sublingual tablets or sublingual or buccal administration as buprenorphine/naloxone sublingually dissolving strips, 16–28 hours following buccal administration as buprenorphine/naloxone buccally dissolving strips, and 28 hours following buccal administration as buprenorphine buccally dissolving strips. Following transdermal administration, the terminal elimination half-life of buprenorphine is approximately 26 hours. Following administration as an extended-release subcutaneous injection, buprenorphine has an apparent elimination half-life of 43–60 days as a result of slow release from the subcutaneous depot.

Buprenorphine is almost completely metabolized in the liver, principally by N-dealkylation, to form norbuprenorphine (N-dealkylbuprenorphine). The N-dealkylation pathway is mediated by the cytochrome P-450 (CYP) 3A4 isoenzyme. Buprenorphine and norbuprenorphine also undergo conjugation with glucuronic acid. Buprenorphine is conjugated by uridine diphosphate-glucuronosyltransferase (UGT) isoenzymes, mainly UGT 1A1 and 2B7, to form buprenorphine 3-O-glucuronide; norbuprenorphine also is conjugated, mainly by UGT 1A3. Following oral administration, buprenorphine appears to undergo extensive first-pass metabolism in the GI mucosa and liver. Following transdermal administration, buprenorphine undergoes negligible metabolism in the skin.

Norbuprenorphine binds to opiate receptors in vitro, but it is not known whether norbuprenorphine contributes to the overall effects of buprenorphine. The AUC ratio of norbuprenorphine to buprenorphine is reportedly 0.2–0.4 at steady state following administration of buprenorphine extended-release subcutaneous injection and approximately 0.36–0.45 following sublingual administration of buprenorphine sublingual tablets. A norbuprenorphine half-life of 12–21 hours has been reported following sublingual administration of buprenorphine sublingual tablets.

Buprenorphine and its metabolites are excreted principally in feces (about 69%) via biliary elimination and also in urine (about 30%), almost entirely as unchanged drug, norbuprenorphine, and 2 unidentified metabolites. Most of the buprenorphine and norbuprenorphine excreted in urine is conjugated (buprenorphine: 1% unconjugated and 9.4% conjugated; norbuprenorphine: 2.7% unconjugated and 11% conjugated), whereas most of the buprenorphine and norbuprenorphine excreted in feces is unconjugated (buprenorphine: 33% unconjugated and 5% conjugated; norbuprenorphine: 21% unconjugated and 2% conjugated). Buprenorphine and its metabolites are believed to undergo enterohepatic circulation. Following IM administration of a 2-mcg/kg dose of buprenorphine, approximately 70% of the dose is excreted in feces and 27% in urine within 7 days. Following IV administration of a 0.6-mg dose, about 30% of the dose is excreted in urine within 7 days; approximately 9 and 8% of the dose are excreted in urine as buprenorphine (almost completely as conjugated drug) and norbuprenorphine (mainly as conjugated norbuprenorphine), respectively, within 4 days.

Reductions in hepatic blood flow induced by some general anesthetics (e.g., halothane) and other drugs may result in a decreased rate of hepatic elimination of buprenorphine. Plasma clearance of the drug is substantially reduced to 0.9 L/minute following IV administration of a single 0.3-mg dose in patients undergoing nitrous oxide and halothane anesthesia.

Limited data indicate that there is considerable interindividual variability in buprenorphine pharmacokinetics in children; however, clearance of the drug appears to be increased in children (e.g., those 5–7 years of age) compared with that in adults. Optimal dosing interval of buprenorphine may have to be decreased in pediatric patients.

No substantial relationship between estimated creatinine clearance and steady-state buprenorphine concentrations has been observed. Following IV administration, no differences in pharmacokinetics of buprenorphine have been observed between patients with renal impairment or renal failure requiring dialysis and those with normal renal function. In dialysis-dependent patients receiving transdermal buprenorphine, predialysis and postdialysis concentrations of the drug were not substantially different.

Following sublingual administration of a single buprenorphine/naloxone sublingual tablet (buprenorphine 2 mg and naloxone 0.5 mg) in patients with hepatic impairment, no clinically important changes in peak plasma concentrations, systemic exposures, and half-lives of buprenorphine or naloxone were observed in those with mild hepatic impairment. However, pharmacokinetics of the drugs were altered in patients with moderate or severe hepatic impairment; naloxone was affected to a greater degree than buprenorphine, and the magnitude of the difference in effect was greater in individuals with severe hepatic impairment than in those with moderate hepatic impairment. In those with moderate hepatic impairment, peak plasma concentrations of buprenorphine and naloxone were increased by 8 and 170%, respectively; AUC was increased by 64 and 218%, respectively; and half-life was increased by 35 and 165%, respectively, compared with individuals with normal hepatic function. In those with severe hepatic impairment, peak plasma concentrations of buprenorphine and naloxone were increased by 72 and 1030%, respectively; AUC was increased by 181 and 1302%, respectively; and half-life was increased by 57 and 122%, respectively.

The effects of hepatic impairment on the pharmacokinetics of buprenorphine administered as a 0.3-mg IV infusion have been evaluated in a limited number of patients with mild or moderate hepatic impairment (Child-Pugh class A or B). Exposure to buprenorphine and norbuprenorphine was not increased in such patients when compared with patients with normal hepatic function. Buprenorphine transdermal system and buprenorphine buccally dissolving strips have not been evaluated in patients with severe hepatic impairment (Child-Pugh class C). Data are lacking on the effects of hepatic impairment on the pharmacokinetics of buprenorphine administered as subdermal implants or as an extended-release subcutaneous injection.

In patients with hepatitis C virus (HCV) infection without evidence of hepatic impairment, no clinically important changes in peak plasma concentrations, systemic exposure, and half-lives of buprenorphine or naloxone were observed.

CHEMISTRY AND STABILITY

● Chemistry

Buprenorphine is a synthetic partial opiate agonist analgesic that is structurally related to morphine and pharmacologically similar to other currently available opiate partial agonists.

Buprenorphine hydrochloride occurs as a white, crystalline powder and has solubilities of 17 mg/mL in water (pH 4.4) at 25°C and 42 mg/mL in alcohol at room temperature. The drug has pK$_a$s of 8.24–8.42 (amine) and 9.92–10 (phenol). Commercially available buprenorphine hydrochloride injection is a sterile

solution of the drug in 5% dextrose injection. The injection occurs as a clear solution and has an osmolality of 297 mOsm/kg.

Potency of buprenorphine hydrochloride is expressed in terms of buprenorphine, calculated on the anhydrous basis.

The Sublocade® extended-release subcutaneous injection contains buprenorphine (18% by weight) dissolved in a biodegradable vehicle (Atrigel®) containing poly(D,L-lactide coglycolide) polymer and N-methyl-2-pyrrolidone (NMP) solvent in a 50:50 ratio. Following subcutaneous injection, precipitation of the polymer results in formation of a solid depot; buprenorphine is released from the depot at a controlled rate over one month via diffusion from and biodegradation of the depot.

Each Probuphine® implant is a soft, flexible rod (26 mm in length and 2.5 mm in diameter) that contains 80 mg of buprenorphine hydrochloride (equivalent to 74.2 mg of the base) and ethylene vinyl acetate. It is designed to be implanted subdermally and to provide sustained delivery of the drug for up to 6 months.

The Butrans® transdermal system consists of an outer web backing layer, an adhesive rim that does not contain buprenorphine, a separating layer over the buprenorphine-containing adhesive matrix, and a buprenorphine-containing adhesive matrix. The adhesive layer is covered by a protective strip that is removed prior to application. The amount of buprenorphine released from each system per hour is proportional to the surface area; release of the drug is designed to occur at an average rate of 5 mcg/hour per 6.25 cm². The total buprenorphine content in each 5-, 7.5-, 10-, 15-, and 20-mcg/hour system is 5, 7.5, 10, 15, and 20 mg, respectively.

● Stability

Buprenorphine hydrochloride injection should be protected from prolonged exposure to light and stored at a temperature of 20–25°C, but may be exposed to temperatures ranging from 15–30°C.

Oral transmucosal preparations of buprenorphine hydrochloride (sublingual tablets, buccally dissolving strips) or buprenorphine hydrochloride in fixed combination with naloxone hydrochloride (sublingual tablets, sublingually dissolving strips, buccally dissolving strips) should be stored at room temperature (generally 20–25°C, but may be exposed to temperatures ranging from 15–30°C). Sublingually or buccally dissolving strips should be used immediately after removal from the individually sealed package; strips that have been altered (e.g., torn, cut, damaged) should not be used. Bunavail® buccally dissolving strips should be protected from freezing and moisture.

Buprenorphine extended-release subcutaneous injection should be stored at 2–8°C. After removal from the refrigerator, the injection may be stored in its original package at 15–30°C for up to 7 days prior to administration; if not used within 7 days, the injection should be discarded.

Kits containing buprenorphine hydrochloride implants should be stored at 20–25°C, but may be exposed to temperatures ranging from 15–30°C.

Buprenorphine transdermal systems should be stored at 25°C, but may be exposed to temperatures ranging from 15–30°C. The system should be applied to the skin immediately after removal from the individually sealed package, and should be discarded if the seal was previously broken. Transdermal systems that have been cut, damaged, or altered in any way should be discarded since use of such systems may expose the patient or caregiver to the contents of the system and result in a potentially lethal overdose of the drug.

Buprenorphine preparations should be stored in a secure place to prevent access by children.

PREPARATIONS

Buprenorphine and buprenorphine hydrochloride are subject to control under the Federal Controlled Substances Act of 1970 as schedule III (C-III) drugs.

Under the Drug Addiction Treatment Act of 2000 (DATA 2000) and Comprehensive Addiction and Recovery Act of 2016 (CARA 2016), use of buprenorphine hydrochloride and buprenorphine hydrochloride in fixed combination with naloxone hydrochloride for the treatment of opiate dependence is restricted to physicians, nurse practitioners, and physician assistants who meet certain qualifying requirements; have notified the US Department of Health and

Human Services (HHS) Substance Abuse and Mental Health Services Administration (SAMHSA) of their intention to prescribe these preparations for this indication; and have been assigned a unique identification number that must be included on each prescription for the drug. (See Dosage and Administration: Restricted Distribution Program for Buprenorphine Treatment of Opiate Dependence.)

Distribution of buprenorphine hydrochloride subdermal implants and buprenorphine extended-release subcutaneous injection is further restricted under risk evaluation and mitigation strategies. (See Risk Evaluation and Mitigation Strategies under Dosage and Administration: Administration.)

Excipients in commercially available drug preparations may have clinically important effects in some individuals; consult specific product labeling for details.

Buprenorphine

Parenteral

Injection, extended-release, for subcutaneous use	100 mg/0.5 mL	**Sublocade®** (C-III; available as single-use prefilled syringe), Indivior
	300 mg/1.5 mL	**Sublocade®** (C-III; available as single-use prefilled syringe), Indivior

Topical

Transdermal System	5 mcg/hour (5 mg/6.25 cm²)	**Butrans®** (C-III), Purdue Pharma
	7.5 mcg/hour (7.5 mg/9.375 cm²)	**Butrans®** (C-III), Purdue Pharma
	10 mcg/hour (10 mg/12.5 cm²)	**Butrans®** (C-III), Purdue Pharma
	15 mcg/hour (15 mg/18.75 cm²)	**Butrans®** (C-III), Purdue Pharma
	20 mcg/hour (20 mg/25 cm²)	**Butrans®** (C-III), Purdue Pharma

Buprenorphine Hydrochloride

Buccal

Strips, buccally dissolving	75 mcg (of buprenorphine)	**Belbuca®** (C-III), BioDelivery Sciences
	150 mcg (of buprenorphine)	**Belbuca®** (C-III), BioDelivery Sciences
	300 mcg (of buprenorphine)	**Belbuca®** (C-III), BioDelivery Sciences
	450 mcg (of buprenorphine)	**Belbuca®** (C-III), BioDelivery Sciences
	600 mcg (of buprenorphine)	**Belbuca®** (C-III), BioDelivery Sciences
	750 mcg (of buprenorphine)	**Belbuca®** (C-III), BioDelivery Sciences
	900 mcg (of buprenorphine)	**Belbuca®** (C-III), BioDelivery Sciences

Parenteral

Implant, for subdermal use	80 mg (equivalent to buprenorphine 74.2 mg) per implant	**Probuphine®** (C-III; available as a kit containing 4 implants and 1 disposable applicator), Braeburn
Injection	0.3 mg (of buprenorphine) per mL*	**Buprenex®** (C-III), Reckitt Benckiser
		Buprenorphine Hydrochloride Injection (C-III)

Sublingual

Tablets	2 mg (of buprenorphine)*	**Buprenorphine Hydrochloride Sublingual Tablets** (C-III)
	8 mg (of buprenorphine)*	**Buprenorphine Hydrochloride Sublingual Tablets** (C-III)

Buprenorphine Hydrochloride Combinations

Buccal

Strips, buccally dissolving	2.1 mg (of buprenorphine) with Naloxone Hydrochloride 0.3 mg (of naloxone)	**Bunavail®** (C-III), BioDelivery Sciences
	4.2 mg (of buprenorphine) with Naloxone Hydrochloride 0.7 mg (of naloxone)	**Bunavail®** (C-III), BioDelivery Sciences
	6.3 mg (of buprenorphine) with Naloxone Hydrochloride 1 mg (of naloxone)	**Bunavail®** (C-III), BioDelivery Sciences

Sublingual

Strips, sublingually dissolving	2 mg (of buprenorphine) with Naloxone Hydrochloride 0.5 mg (of naloxone)	**Suboxone®** (C-III), Indivior
	4 mg (of buprenorphine) with Naloxone Hydrochloride 1 mg (of naloxone)	**Suboxone®** (C-III), Indivior
	8 mg (of buprenorphine) with Naloxone Hydrochloride 2 mg (of naloxone)	**Suboxone®** (C-III), Indivior
	12 mg (of buprenorphine) with Naloxone Hydrochloride 3 mg (of naloxone)	**Suboxone®** (C-III), Indivior
Tablets	0.7 mg (of buprenorphine) with Naloxone Hydrochloride 0.18 mg (of naloxone)	**Zubsolv®** (C-III), Orexo
	1.4 mg (of buprenorphine) with Naloxone Hydrochloride 0.36 mg (of naloxone)	**Zubsolv®** (C-III), Orexo
	2 mg (of buprenorphine) with Naloxone Hydrochloride 0.5 mg (of naloxone)*	**Buprenorphine Hydrochloride and Naloxone Hydrochloride Sublingual Tablets** (C-III)
	2.9 mg (of buprenorphine) with Naloxone Hydrochloride 0.71 mg (of naloxone)	**Zubsolv®** (C-III), Orexo
	5.7 mg (of buprenorphine) with Naloxone Hydrochloride 1.4 mg (of naloxone)	**Zubsolv®** (C-III), Orexo
	8 mg (of buprenorphine) with Naloxone Hydrochloride 2 mg (of naloxone)*	**Buprenorphine Hydrochloride and Naloxone Hydrochloride Sublingual Tablets** (C-III)
	8.6 mg (of buprenorphine) with Naloxone Hydrochloride 2.1 mg (of naloxone)	**Zubsolv®** (C-III), Orexo
	11.4 mg (of buprenorphine) with Naloxone Hydrochloride 2.9 mg (of naloxone)	**Zubsolv®** (C-III), Orexo

* available from one or more manufacturer, distributor, and/or repackager by generic (nonproprietary) name

† Use is not currently included in the labeling approved by the US Food and Drug Administration.

Selected Revisions April 19, 2023, © Copyright, June 01, 1987, American Society of Health-System Pharmacists, Inc.

Acetaminophen

28:08.16 • NON-OPIOID ANALGESICS

■ Acetaminophen is a synthetic nonopiate derivative of *p*-aminophenol that produces analgesia and antipyresis.

USES

Acetaminophen is used extensively in the treatment of mild to moderate pain and fever.

● Pain

Acetaminophen is used to provide temporary analgesia in the treatment of mild to moderate pain. Acetaminophen also is used in fixed combination with other agents (e.g., chlorpheniramine, dextromethorphan, diphenhydramine, doxylamine, guaifenesin, phenylephrine, pseudoephedrine) for short-term relief of minor aches and pain, headache, and/or other symptoms (e.g., rhinorrhea, sneezing, lacrimation, itching eyes, oronasopharyngeal itching, nasal congestion, cough) associated with seasonal allergic rhinitis (e.g., hay fever), other upper respiratory allergies, or the common cold.

Acetaminophen is most effective in relieving low intensity pain of nonvisceral origin. Acetaminophen does *not* have antirheumatic effects. Unlike salicylates and prototypical nonsteroidal anti-inflammatory agents (NSAIAs), acetaminophen does not usually depress prothrombin levels. In addition, acetaminophen produces a lower incidence of gastric irritation, erosion, or bleeding than do salicylates or prototypical NSAIAs. Acetaminophen is a desirable alternative in patients who require a mild analgesic or antipyretic but in whom salicylates or prototypical NSAIAs are contraindicated or not tolerated. Because of its efficacy, relative safety at recommended dosages, and low cost, many experts recommend use of the drug as the initial analgesic for many patients. However, the risk of inadvertent overdosage and resultant acute liver failure must be considered, and patients should be counseled about the importance of not exceeding recommended dosages or combining acetaminophen-containing preparations.

Acetaminophen has been used in the treatment of pain in various combinations with aspirin, caffeine, opiates, and/or other agents. Acetaminophen (650-mg oral doses) in combination with oral doses of an opiate (e.g., codeine, oxycodone) produces greater analgesic effect than that produced by either acetaminophen or higher doses of the opiate alone. In patients with moderate to severe postoperative pain, single or repeated IV doses of acetaminophen (650 mg every 4 hours or 1 g every 6 hours) reduced pain intensity and rescue opiate requirements compared with placebo, but clinical benefits of the lower opiate dosages (e.g., reduction in opiate-related adverse effects) have not been established. Although some evidence suggests that the combination of acetaminophen, aspirin, and caffeine is more effective than acetaminophen alone for the treatment of tension-type headache, combinations of acetaminophen with aspirin or caffeine generally have not been shown to have greater analgesic effect than an optimal dose of acetaminophen alone. In addition, there is little evidence that such combinations cause fewer adverse effects than higher doses of the individual agents alone. In one study, the simultaneous administration of 325- or 650-mg oral doses of acetaminophen with 650-mg oral doses of aspirin resulted in increased blood concentrations of unhydrolyzed aspirin compared with 650-mg oral doses of aspirin alone; however, the clinical importance of such an effect remains to be established.

Pain Associated with Migraine Headache

Acetaminophen in fixed combination with aspirin and caffeine (containing 250 mg of acetaminophen, 250 mg of aspirin, and 65 mg of caffeine) is used for the temporary relief of mild to moderate pain associated with migraine headache. Some experts state that this combination also may be used for the treatment of severe migraine headache if previous attacks have responded to similar nonopiate analgesics or nonsteroidal anti-inflammatory agents (NSAIAs). The efficacy of oral acetaminophen in fixed combination with aspirin and caffeine for the management of mild to moderate pain associated with migraine headache was established by 3 double-blind, randomized, parallel group, placebo-controlled (one of them a population-based study) studies in adult patients who had migraine with

aura or migraine without aura as defined by criteria established by International Headache Society (IHS). The efficacy of therapy for management of pain associated with migraine headache in these studies was evaluated in terms of a reduction in headache severity as rated by the patient (i.e., a reduction in pain from at least moderate to mild or to absent 2 hours after dosing using a 4-point scale). Pooled analysis of data from the 3 studies indicate that about 59% of patients receiving 500 mg of acetaminophen in fixed combination with aspirin and caffeine attained relief of pain associated with migraine headache within 2 hours compared with about 33% of placebo recipients; at 6 hours, about 79 and 52%, respectively, of drug- and placebo-treated patients had mild or no headache pain. In addition, 2 hours after dosing about 21% of patients receiving the combination were pain free versus about 7% receiving placebo, and at 6 hours 51% of drug-treated patients were pain free versus 24% receiving placebo. It appears that the drug also relieves manifestations of migraine other than headache, including nausea, vomiting, photophobia, and phonophobia. Patients in whom pain associated with migraine headache is not relieved by acetaminophen in fixed combination with aspirin and caffeine should consult their clinician about possible alternatives (e.g., use of prescription drugs including ergot alkaloids or vascular serotonin type 1-like receptor agonists) based on evaluation of their medical condition. Efficacy of oral acetaminophen alone for the treatment of acute migraine headache has not been established. For further information on management and classification of migraine headache, see Vascular Headaches: General Principles in Migraine Therapy, under Uses in Sumatriptan 28:32.28.

Pain Associated with Osteoarthritis

Acetaminophen is used in the symptomatic treatment of pain associated with osteoarthritis and is considered an initial drug of choice for pain management in osteoarthritis patients. Medical management of osteoarthritis of the hip and knee includes both pharmacologic therapy to reduce pain and nonpharmacologic therapy to maintain and/or improve joint mobility and limit functional impairment (e.g., patient education, weight loss when necessary, aerobic and muscle-strengthening exercise programs, physical therapy and range-of-motion exercises, assistive devices for ambulation and activities of daily living, patellar taping, appropriate footwear or bracing). Pain management is considered an adjunct to nonpharmacologic measures and is most effective when combined with nonpharmacologic strategies.

A variety of drugs have been used for management of pain in patients with osteoarthritis, including oral agents (e.g., acetaminophen, NSAIAs, tramadol), intraarticular agents (e.g., glucocorticoids, sodium hyaluronate), and topical agents (e.g., capsaicin, methylsalicylate). Factors to consider when making treatment decisions for the management of pain in patients with osteoarthritis include the presence of risk factors for serious adverse GI effects or renal toxicity (which may affect decisions regarding use of NSAIAs), existing comorbidities and concomitant therapy, and the adverse effects profiles and costs of specific therapies. Because there is evidence that acetaminophen can be effective, because of its relative safety when used at recommended dosages, and because of its low cost, the American College of Rheumatology (ACR) and other clinicians recommended use of the drug as the initial analgesic for many osteoarthritis patients.

Acetaminophen appears to be as effective as NSAIAs for relief of mild to moderate joint pain in many patients with osteoarthritis; however, the drug is not effective in all patients and may not provide adequate relief in those with moderate to severe pain or when joint inflammation is present. A NSAIA can be considered an alternative initial drug of choice for patients with osteoarthritis, especially for those who have moderate to severe pain and signs of joint inflammation, and also can be considered in patients who fail to obtain adequate symptomatic relief with acetaminophen. Because NSAIAs that selectively inhibit COX-2 (e.g., celecoxib) are associated with a lower incidence of serious adverse GI effects than prototypical NSAIAs and, unlike prototypical NSAIAs, do not affect platelet aggregation and bleeding time, one of these selective inhibitors of COX-2 may be preferred when a NSAIA is being considered for management of pain in osteoarthritis patients at risk for GI complications. (See Uses: Osteoarthritis, in Celecoxib 28:08.04.08.) In patients with osteoarthritis of the knee who have moderate to severe pain and signs of joint inflammation, some clinicians suggest that joint aspiration accompanied by intraarticular glucocorticoid injections or use of an oral NSAIA can be considered for initial therapy.

In patients with osteoarthritis of the knee who fail to respond to adequate regimens of acetaminophen or other appropriate oral analgesics given in conjunction with nonpharmacologic therapy, intraarticular sodium hyaluronate therapy may be indicated; this alternative may be especially advantageous when oral NSAIAs are contraindicated or ineffective. Intraarticular glucocorticoid injections can be used as an adjunct to oral therapy with acetaminophen or other appropriate oral analgesic or as monotherapy in selected patients with osteoarthritis of the knee; these injections also are used occasionally in patients with osteoarthritis of the hip. Intraarticular glucocorticoid injections are of value and may be particularly beneficial in patients with osteoarthritis of the knee who have signs of local inflammation with joint effusion. Use of topical analgesics can be considered as either adjunctive treatment or monotherapy in patients with osteoarthritis of the knee who have mild to moderate pain and have failed to obtain adequate symptomatic relief with acetaminophen and cannot or prefer not to receive other systemic analgesics; topical agents have not been evaluated for pain management in patients with osteoarthritis of the hip and are of questionable value in these patients because of the depth of the hip joint.

● Fever

Acetaminophen is used frequently to lower body temperature in febrile patients in whom fever may be deleterious or in whom considerable relief is obtained when fever is lowered. However, antipyretic therapy is generally nonspecific, does not influence the course of the underlying disease, and may obscure the patient's illness. Parents and caregivers of pediatric patients should be reassured that while some parental anxiety over fever is understandable, the principal reason for treating fever is for patient comfort and that complete normalization of body temperature is not necessary and may not be possible. To minimize the risk of acetaminophen overdosage, alternative antipyretics should be considered for children at increased risk of developing toxicity and in those with refractory fever.

Acetaminophen is used in fixed combination with other agents (e.g., chlorpheniramine, dextromethorphan, diphenhydramine, doxylamine, guaifenesin, phenylephrine, pseudoephedrine) for short-term relief of fever and/or other symptoms (e.g., rhinorrhea, sneezing, lacrimation, itching eyes, oronasopharyngeal itching, nasal congestion, cough) associated with seasonal allergic rhinitis (e.g., hay fever), other upper respiratory allergies, or the common cold.

If an antipyretic is considered necessary in children or teenagers with known or suspected varicella, influenza-like illness, or other viral illness, use of acetaminophen (not aspirin) is recommended because use of salicylates in these pediatric patients may be associated with an increased risk of developing Reye's syndrome. (See Cautions: Pediatric Precautions, in the Salicylates General Statement 28:08.04.24.) In the treatment of influenza in young children, control of fever with acetaminophen or other appropriate antipyretic may be important because the fever and other symptoms of influenza could exacerbate underlying chronic conditions.

Acetaminophen and aspirin are equally effective as antipyretics. In one study in febrile children, the combination of oral doses of acetaminophen and aspirin was at least as effective in reducing fever as either drug alone, and the duration of fever reduction was longer with the combination than with the individual drugs. However, because of the study design, it could not be concluded that the combination had additive effects. Many clinicians use regimens of alternating doses of acetaminophen and aspirin; however, combined overdosage with both drugs has occurred with such a regimen and the efficacy and safety of these regimens remain to be established.

To minimize the risk of acetaminophen overdosage, some clinicians have used pediatric regimens of alternating doses of acetaminophen and ibuprofen; however, the efficacy and safety of these regimens remain to be established. In addition, although some such clinicians have alternated acetaminophen and ibuprofen at 2-hour intervals (i.e., with each drug administered every 4 hours) in pediatric patients, there is no pharmacokinetic rationale to support such a regimen; longer alternating dosing intervals would seem more appropriate if an alternating regimen is considered, but additional study and experience are necessary.

Febrile Seizures

Because febrile seizures occur only in conjunction with a fever, it has been postulated that aggressive intermittent antipyretic therapy might prevent such seizures. However, there currently is no evidence to substantiate that aggressive antipyretic therapy can prevent recurrent febrile seizures. In one study in a limited number of children, 25% of patients in whom antipyretic therapy was initiated when any rectal temperature exceeded 37.2°C (99°F) experienced seizure recurrence compared with 5% of those who received continuous phenobarbital prophylaxis. In

another study comparing low-dose diazepam, acetaminophen, and placebo, there was no evidence that acetaminophen prevented recurrent febrile seizures; acetaminophen was administered in a dosage of 10 mg/kg 4 times daily. In children hospitalized after a simple febrile seizure, administration of aggressive antipyretic therapy with acetaminophen 15–20 mg/kg every 4 hours was no more effective than sporadic acetaminophen use in preventing a second febrile seizure during that admission; the 2 treatment groups also had a similar frequency, duration, and magnitude of temperature elevations.

DOSAGE AND ADMINISTRATION

● Administration

Acetaminophen is administered orally, rectally as suppositories, and by IV infusion over 15 minutes.

Acetaminophen preparations for *self-medication* should not be used unless seals on the tamper-resistant packaging are intact.

Oral Administration

Acetaminophen usually is administered orally. Extended-release acetaminophen tablets should not be crushed, chewed, or dissolved in liquid. Orally disintegrating tablets containing acetaminophen (e.g., Tylenol® Meltaways) should be allowed to dissolve in the mouth or should be chewed before swallowing.

Rectal Administration

In patients who cannot tolerate oral medication, acetaminophen may be administered rectally as suppositories; however, the rectal dose required to produce the same plasma concentrations may be higher than the oral dose and rectal absorption can be erratic. Dividing suppositories in an attempt to administer lower dosages may not provide a predictable dose.

Some experts state that rectal preparations of acetaminophen should not be used for *self-medication* in children unless such use is specifically discussed with a clinician and parents or caregivers are instructed to adhere to dosage and administration recommendations; poor or variable absorption of acetaminophen following rectal administration may be associated with inadequate therapy or may result in toxicity following frequent or excessive doses.

IV Administration

Acetaminophen is administered by IV infusion over 15 minutes. The commercially available acetaminophen injection may be administered without further dilution. Each vial containing 1 g/100 mL is intended for single use only; any unused portions must be discarded.

Acetaminophen doses of 1 g should be administered by inserting a vented IV set through the septum of the 100-mL vial. Doses of less than 1 g must be withdrawn from the vial and placed in a separate container for IV infusion in order to avoid inadvertent administration of the total volume of the commercially available vial. The appropriate dose of acetaminophen should be withdrawn aseptically from an intact sealed vial and transferred to an empty sterile container (e.g., glass bottle, plastic container, syringe); small-volume (up to 60 mL) pediatric doses should be drawn into a syringe and administered using a syringe pump. Once the vacuum seal of the vial has been penetrated or the vial contents have been transferred to another container, the dose of acetaminophen should be administered within 6 hours. The end of the infusion should be monitored in order to prevent the possibility of air embolism, especially when the acetaminophen solution is the primary infusion.

Acetaminophen should not be admixed with any other drugs. Acetaminophen solution should be inspected visually for particulate matter and discoloration prior to preparation and administration; if either is present, the solution should be discarded.

● Dosage

Acetaminophen is relatively safe when used at recommended dosages. However, acetaminophen overdosage has been the leading cause of acute liver failure in the US, United Kingdom, and most of Europe, with about 50% of US cases in recent years resulting from inadvertent overdosage (e.g., in patients not recognizing the presence of the drug in multiple over-the-counter [OTC] and/or prescription products that they may be taking). Therefore, patients should be warned about the importance of determining whether acetaminophen is present in their medications (e.g., by examining labels carefully, by consulting their clinician and pharmacist) and of not exceeding recommended dosages or combining acetaminophen-containing preparations.

Acetaminophen should not be used for *self-medication* of pain for longer than 10 days (in adults or children 12 years of age and older) or 5 days (in children 2–11 years of age), unless directed by a clinician because pain of such intensity and duration may indicate a pathologic condition requiring medical evaluation and supervised treatment.

Acetaminophen should not be used in adults or children for *self-medication* of marked fever (greater than 39.5°C), fever persisting longer than 3 days, or recurrent fever, unless directed by a clinician because such fevers may indicate serious illness requiring prompt medical evaluation.

Acetaminophen should not be used in adults or children for *self-medication* of sore throat pain (pharyngitis, laryngitis, tonsillitis) for longer than 2 days.

To minimize the risk of overdosage, recommended age-appropriate daily dosages of acetaminophen should not be exceeded. Because severe liver toxicity and death have occurred in children who received multiple excessive doses of acetaminophen as part of therapeutic administration, parents or caregivers should be instructed to use weight-based dosing for acetaminophen, to use only the calibrated measuring device provided with the particular acetaminophen formulation for measuring dosage, to ensure that the correct number of tablets required for the intended dose is removed from the package, and not to exceed the recommended daily dosage because serious adverse effects could result. In addition, patients should be warned that the risk of overdosage and severe liver damage is increased if more than one preparation containing acetaminophen are used concomitantly.

Pharmacists have an important role in preventing acetaminophen-induced hepatotoxicity by advising consumers about the risk of failing to recognize that a wide variety of OTC and prescription preparations contain acetaminophen. Failure to recognize acetaminophen as an ingredient may be particularly likely with prescription drugs because the label of the dispensed drug may not clearly state its presence. Educating consumers about the risk of exceeding recommended acetaminophen dosages also is important. The US Food and Drug Administration (FDA) recommends that pharmacists receiving prescriptions for fixed-combination preparations containing more than 325 mg of acetaminophen per dosage unit contact the prescriber to discuss use of a preparation containing no more than 325 mg of the drug per dosage unit. (See Preparations.)

Clinicians should exercise caution when prescribing, preparing, and administering IV acetaminophen to avoid dosing errors that could result in accidental overdosage and death. In particular, clinicians should ensure that the dose (in mg) and the volume (in mL) are not confused, the dose for patients weighing less than 50 kg is based on body weight, the infusion pump is programmed correctly, and the total daily dosage of acetaminophen from all sources does not exceed the maximum recommended daily dosage.

Adult Dosage
Pain and Fever

For analgesia or antipyresis in adults or children 12 years of age or older, the usual oral dosage of acetaminophen as an immediate-release (conventional) preparation is 650 mg every 4–6 hours or 1 g every 6 hours as necessary. An oral acetaminophen dosage of 1.3 g as extended-release tablets every 8 hours can be used for the management of pain in adults. The currently recommended maximum dosage of acetaminophen is 4 g daily. Some experts recommend a maximum dosage of 3 g daily when the drug is used for long-term therapy (e.g., 2 or more weeks). The FDA is reviewing available data to determine whether it is possible to identify subgroups of patients with increased susceptibility to acetaminophen-associated hepatotoxicity and to determine whether data support establishing a lower (i.e., less than 4 g daily) maximum daily dosage for certain patients. (See Cautions: Precautions and Contraindications.) To minimize the risk of inadvertent overdosage, some manufacturers (e.g., McNeil, Tylenol®) have voluntarily revised their labeling to recommend less frequent dosing and lower total daily dosages of acetaminophen. These manufacturers now recommend that dosages in adults and children 12 years of age and older not exceed 1 g every 6 hours up to a maximum of 3 g daily.

For analgesia or antipyresis in adults or children 12 years of age or older, the usual rectal dosage of acetaminophen is 325–650 mg every 4 hours as necessary; dosage should not exceed 4 g daily.

Acetaminophen may be given IV as a single dose or as repeated doses for analgesia or antipyresis. No dosage adjustment is required when an adult or adolescent who weighs 50 kg or more is switched between oral and IV acetaminophen. The recommended IV dosage of acetaminophen for analgesia or antipyresis in adults and adolescents 13 years of age or older who weigh 50 kg or more is 1 g every 6 hours or 650 mg every 4 hours; the maximum recommended single dose is 1 g, the minimum dosing interval is 4 hours, and the maximum daily dosage is 4 g per 24-hour period, including all routes of administration and all acetaminophen-containing preparations, including fixed combinations. In adults and adolescents 13 years of age or older who weigh less than 50 kg, the recommended dosage is 15 mg/kg every 6 hours or 12.5 mg/kg every 4 hours; the maximum single dose is 15 mg/kg, the minimum dosing interval is 4 hours, and the maximum daily dosage is 75 mg/kg per 24-hour period, including all routes of administration and all acetaminophen-containing preparations, including fixed combinations.

Patients receiving acetaminophen in fixed combination with an opiate analgesic may develop tolerance to the opiate and increase the dosage of the combination not realizing the risk of inadvertent acetaminophen overdosage. Therefore, to minimize the risk of inadvertent acetaminophen overdosage, FDA has requested manufacturers to reformulate prescription combination preparations to limit the amount of acetaminophen to 325 mg or less per dosage unit. (See Preparations.) FDA also recommends that health care providers stop prescribing and dispensing prescription combination preparations containing more than 325 mg of acetaminophen per dosage unit. FDA states that doses consisting of either 1 or 2 dosage units (i.e., 325 or 650 mg of acetaminophen per dose) may be prescribed as clinically appropriate for the patient; to ensure appropriate dosages of each component of the fixed combination, the strength of each component (generally acetaminophen and an opiate analgesic) must be considered. FDA states that there are no data indicating that use of prescription combination preparations containing more than 325 mg of acetaminophen per dosage unit provides additional benefit that would outweigh the increased risk of liver injury resulting from inadvertent overdosage.

Pain Associated with Migraine Headache

For *self-medication* for the temporary relief of mild to moderate pain associated with migraine headache in adults, the recommended oral dosage is 500 mg of acetaminophen (combined with 500 mg of aspirin and 130 mg of caffeine) as a single dose of an immediate-release (conventional) preparation taken with a full glass of water; no more than 500 mg of acetaminophen (in combination with 500 mg of aspirin and 130 mg of caffeine) should be taken in any 24-hour period, unless directed by a clinician. Individuals younger than 18 years of age should consult their clinician before using this combination preparation.

Pain Associated with Osteoarthritis

For the treatment of pain associated with osteoarthritis, many clinicians recommend acetaminophen dosages in adults up to 1 g administered 4 times daily as an immediate-release (conventional) preparation. Alternatively, 1.3 g as extended-release tablets every 8 hours can be used. Some experts recommend a maximum dosage of 3 g daily when the drug is used for long-term therapy (e.g., 2 or more weeks). FDA is reviewing available data to determine whether it is possible to identify subgroups of patients with increased susceptibility to acetaminophen-associated hepatotoxicity and to determine whether data support establishing a lower (i.e., less than 4 g daily) maximum daily dosage for certain patients. (See Cautions: Precautions and Contraindications.) To minimize the risk of inadvertent overdosage, some manufacturers (e.g., McNeil, Tylenol®) have voluntarily revised their labeling to recommend less frequent dosing and lower total daily dosages of acetaminophen. These manufacturers now recommend that dosages in adults not exceed 1 g every 6 hours up to a maximum of 3 g daily.

Pediatric Dosage
Pain and Fever

For analgesia and antipyresis in children 12 years of age or older, the usual oral dosage of acetaminophen as an immediate-release (conventional) preparation is 650 mg every 4–6 hours or 1 g every 6 hours as necessary. The currently recommended maximum dosage of acetaminophen in children 12 years of age and older is 4 g daily; however, some manufacturers recommend that dosage of acetaminophen not exceed 3 g daily in such patients. For analgesia and antipyresis, children may receive the following oral doses of acetaminophen every 4–6 hours as necessary (up to 5 times in 24 hours) as an immediate-release (conventional) preparation: children 11 years of age (33–43 kg), 480 mg; children 9–10 years of age (27–32 kg), 400 mg; children 6–8 years of age (22–27 kg), 320 mg; children 4–5 years of age (16–21 kg), 240 mg; children 2–3 years of age (11–16 kg), 160 mg; children 12–23 months of age (8–11 kg), 120 mg; children 4–11 months of age (5–8 kg), 80 mg; and children up to 3 months of age (2.7–5 kg), 40 mg. (See Cautions: Pediatric Precautions.)

For analgesia and antipyresis in children 12 years of age or older, the usual rectal dosage of acetaminophen is 325–650 mg every 4 hours as necessary; dosage should not exceed 4 g daily. For analgesia and antipyresis, children may receive the following rectal doses of acetaminophen every 4 hours as necessary (up to 5 times in 24 hours): children 11–12 years of age, 320–480 mg; children 9–11 years of age, 320–400 mg; children 6–9 years of age, 320 mg; children 4–6 years of age, 240 mg; children 2–4 years of age, 160 mg. Rectal dosages in children younger than 2 years of age must be individualized, and the possibility of erratic systemic absorption should be considered.

Acetaminophen may be given IV as a single dose or as repeated doses for analgesia or antipyresis. The recommended IV dosage of acetaminophen for analgesia or antipyresis in children 2–12 years of age is 15 mg/kg every 6 hours or 12.5 mg/kg every 4 hours; the maximum single dose is 15 mg/kg, the minimum dosing interval is 4 hours, and the maximum daily dosage is 75 mg/kg per 24-hour period, including all routes of administration and all acetaminophen-containing preparations, including fixed combinations.

● Dosage in Renal and Hepatic Impairment

In patients with hepatic impairment or active liver disease, reduction of the total daily dosage of acetaminophen may be warranted. In patients with severe renal impairment (creatinine clearance of 30 mL/minute or less), longer dosing intervals and a reduced total daily dosage of acetaminophen may be warranted. (See Cautions: Precautions and Contraindications.)

CAUTIONS

Acetaminophen is relatively nontoxic in therapeutic doses when taken as directed. However, acetaminophen overdosage has been the leading cause of acute liver failure (with encephalopathy and coagulopathy) in the US, United Kingdom, and most of Europe, with about 50% of US cases in recent years resulting from inadvertent overdosage (e.g., in patients not recognizing the presence of the drug in multiple over-the-counter (OTC) and/or prescription products that they may be taking). Therefore, patients should be warned about the importance of determining whether acetaminophen is present in their medications (e.g., by examining labels carefully, by consulting their clinician and pharmacist) and of not exceeding recommended dosages or combining acetaminophen-containing preparations.

Many OTC drug products and prescription preparations contain acetaminophen. In fact, acetaminophen, alone or in combination, is one of the most commonly used drugs in the US. Simultaneous use of more than one preparation containing acetaminophen can result in adverse consequences (e.g., acetaminophen overdose). Patients should be advised not to take multiple acetaminophen-containing preparations concomitantly.

When acetaminophen is used in fixed combination with other agents (e.g., antihistamines, aspirin, caffeine, dextromethorphan, guaifenesin, nasal decongestants, opiate agonists), the usual cautions, precautions, and contraindications associated with these agents must be considered in addition to those associated with acetaminophen.

The most common adverse effects reported in clinical trials in patients receiving IV acetaminophen were nausea, vomiting, headache, and insomnia in adults and nausea, vomiting, constipation, pruritus, agitation, and atelectasis in pediatric patients.

● Dermatologic and Sensitivity Reactions

Serious, potentially fatal dermatologic reactions, including Stevens-Johnson syndrome, toxic epidermal necrolysis, and acute generalized exanthematous pustulosis, have been reported rarely in patients receiving acetaminophen. In several published cases, serious dermatologic reactions recurred following rechallenge with the drug; in other published cases, acetaminophen was the only drug administered prior to the reaction, or hypersensitivity to acetaminophen was demonstrated by skin testing or by other means. In addition to these published cases, the US Food and Drug Administration (FDA) identified 107 cases of Stevens-Johnson syndrome, toxic epidermal necrolysis, or acute generalized exanthematous pustulosis that had been reported to the FDA Adverse Event Reporting System (AERS) from 1969–2012 and were considered possibly or probably related to acetaminophen; 67 of the patients described in these reports were hospitalized and 12 patients died. Serious dermatologic reactions may occur at any time during acetaminophen therapy. Results of case-control studies suggest that the risk of Stevens-Johnson syndrome or toxic epidermal necrolysis associated with acetaminophen use generally is independent of the effects of other drugs. Although other analgesic and antipyretic agents (e.g., nonsteroidal anti-inflammatory agents [NSAIAs]) may cause similar reactions, cross-sensitivity with acetaminophen does not appear to occur. Acetaminophen should be discontinued immediately at the first appearance of rash or any other manifestation of hypersensitivity (e.g., urticaria, rash, pruritus, respiratory distress, swelling of the face, mouth, or throat). Patients should be advised to discontinue acetaminophen and seek immediate medical attention if rash or other manifestations of dermatologic or hypersensitivity reactions occur during therapy with the drug. Individuals with a history of such reactions should be advised *not* to take any acetaminophen-containing preparations.

Other dermatologic reactions including pruritic maculopapular rash, urticaria, rash, and periorbital edema also have been reported, and other sensitivity reactions including laryngeal edema, angioedema, and anaphylactoid reactions may occur rarely.

● Hematologic Effects

Thrombocytopenia, leukopenia, and pancytopenia have been associated with the use of *p*-aminophenol derivatives, especially with prolonged administration of large doses. Neutropenia, anemia, and thrombocytopenic purpura have been reported with acetaminophen use. Rarely, agranulocytosis has been reported in patients receiving acetaminophen.

● Hepatic Effects

Hepatotoxicity can result from ingestion of a single toxic dose or multiple excessive doses of acetaminophen, and overdosage of acetaminophen is the leading cause of acute liver failure (ALF) in adults in the US; in most cases, overdosage was inadvertent rather than intentional. (See Acute Toxicity and also see Chronic Toxicity.) While most patients who develop acetaminophen-induced acute liver failure survive without liver transplantation (60%), 9% require transplantation and 30% die.

Substantial elevations in ALT occurred in healthy individuals receiving oral acetaminophen in a dosage of 4 g daily in one randomized study. Study participants (58–59% Hispanic American, 28–31% Caucasian, 12–13% African American) were randomized to receive 4 g of acetaminophen daily (alone or in combination with an opiate) or placebo for 14 days; the study was conducted at an inpatient clinical pharmacology unit. Maximum ALT values exceeding 3 times the upper limit of normal (ULN) occurred in 38 or 31–44% of individuals receiving acetaminophen or acetaminophen in combination with an opiate, respectively; substantial elevations in ALT (i.e., values exceeding 3 times the ULN) were not observed in individuals given placebo. In clinical trials evaluating IV acetaminophen, increased AST concentrations have been reported in adults and increased hepatic enzyme concentrations have been reported in pediatric patients receiving the drug.

● Other Adverse Effects

Nausea, vomiting, headache, and insomnia were reported in clinical trials in 34, 15, 10, and 7%, respectively, of adults receiving IV acetaminophen compared with 31, 11, 9, and 5%, respectively, of placebo recipients. Other adverse effects reported in clinical trials in adults receiving IV acetaminophen include abnormal breath sounds, anxiety, dyspnea, fatigue, hypertension, hypokalemia, hypotension, infusion site pain, muscle spasms, peripheral edema, and trismus.

Adverse effects reported in clinical trials in pediatric patients receiving IV acetaminophen include cardiovascular effects (hypertension, hypotension, tachycardia), GI effects (abdominal pain, diarrhea), nervous system effects (headache, insomnia), respiratory effects (hypoxia, pleural effusion, pulmonary edema, stridor, wheezing), hypoalbuminemia, hypokalemia, hypomagnesemia, hypophosphatemia, hypervolemia, injection site pain, muscle spasm, oliguria, pain in extremity, peripheral edema, and pyrexia.

● Precautions and Contraindications

Some commercially available formulations of acetaminophen contain sulfites that may cause allergic-type reactions, including anaphylaxis and life-threatening or less severe asthmatic episodes, in certain susceptible individuals. The overall prevalence of sulfite sensitivity in the general population is unknown but probably low; such sensitivity appears to occur more frequently in asthmatic than in nonasthmatic individuals. Acetaminophen should be discontinued if hypersensitivity reactions occur.

Although psychologic dependence on acetaminophen may occur, tolerance and physical dependence do not appear to develop even with prolonged use.

The antipyretic effects of acetaminophen may mask the presence of fever.

Because concomitant administration of acetaminophen (especially when administered in high dosages or for prolonged periods) with oral anticoagulants may potentiate the effects of the oral anticoagulant, additional monitoring of prothrombin time (PT)/international normalized ratio (INR) values has been suggested for patients receiving oral anticoagulants following initiation of, or during sustained therapy with, large doses of acetaminophen. The manufacturer of acetaminophen injection states that more frequent monitoring of the INR also may be appropriate when patients receiving oral anticoagulants require short-term IV acetaminophen therapy, since the effects of such concomitant use have not been established. (See Drug Interactions: Oral Anticoagulants.)

Acetaminophen should be used with caution in patients with hepatic impairment or active liver disease and is contraindicated in those with severe hepatic impairment or severe active liver disease. Acetaminophen also should be used with caution in patients with alcoholism, chronic malnutrition, severe hypovolemia (e.g., resulting from dehydration or blood loss), or severe renal impairment (creatinine clearance of 30 mL/minute or less). Dosage reduction may be warranted in patients with hepatic impairment, active liver disease, or severe renal impairment. (See Dosage and Administration: Dosage in Renal and Hepatic Impairment.)

Because chronic, excessive consumption of alcohol may increase the risk of acetaminophen-induced hepatotoxicity, chronic alcoholics should be cautioned to avoid regular or excessive use of acetaminophen, or alternatively, to avoid chronic ingestion of alcohol. The manufacturers currently caution that patients who generally consume 3 or more alcohol-containing drinks per day should ask their clinician whether to use acetaminophen or an alternative analgesic for self-medication. However, FDA has proposed eliminating this statement from the labeling of OTC acetaminophen-containing preparations and adding a new warning that would highlight the potential for severe liver damage to occur in individuals who consume 3 or more alcohol-containing drinks per day while taking acetaminophen, in those who use more than one acetaminophen-containing product concomitantly, and in those who exceed the recommended daily dosage of the drug. FDA also has proposed revising the labeling of OTC acetaminophen-containing preparations to include a statement that patients should consult a clinician prior to use if they have liver disease. FDA is reviewing available data to determine whether it is possible to identify subgroups of patients with increased susceptibility to acetaminophen-associated hepatotoxicity and to determine whether data support establishing a lower (i.e., less than 4 g daily) maximum daily dosage for certain patients (e.g., those who chronically ingest alcohol).

Acetaminophen is contraindicated in patients with known hypersensitivity to the drug or any ingredient in the formulation.

● Pediatric Precautions

Because severe liver toxicity and death have occurred in children who received multiple excessive doses of acetaminophen as part of therapeutic administration (i.e., with therapeutic intent), parents or caregivers should be instructed to use weight-based dosing for acetaminophen, to use only the calibrated measuring device provided with the particular acetaminophen formulation for measuring dosage, to ensure that the correct number of tablets required for the intended dose is removed from the package, and not to exceed the recommended daily dosage because serious adverse effects could result. Parents also should be cautioned not to use other acetaminophen-containing products (e.g., some cold and cough

products) concomitantly with acetaminophen in children because of the potential for overdoses.

Because acetaminophen therapy usually is begun without the direct advice of a clinician and carries the risk of potential overdosage, instruction regarding appropriate pain and fever therapy preferably should be incorporated into well-child visits. Optimally, clinicians should provide parents and/or caregivers with written, specific advice as part of well-child visits, which should be reviewed during subsequent visits. Parents and caregivers should be advised about the appropriate dose, frequency, duration of therapy, and specific strength and formulation for an individual pediatric patient. They also should be advised of the danger of substituting alternative dosage forms, particularly adult for pediatric formulations. Parents and caregivers should be warned not to exceed recommended acetaminophen dosages and cautioned that children should not be allowed to administer the drug themselves. They also should be warned to read the labeled contents of over-the-counter (OTC) preparations, particularly those recommended for cold, cough, fever, headache, and general ache and pain because simultaneous use of more than one preparation containing acetaminophen could be dangerous. In addition, they should be warned not to substitute extended-release formulations for immediate-release (conventional) ones without making appropriate changes in the dosing interval. A clinician should be contacted for advice if fever and/or other signs and symptoms amenable to acetaminophen persist.

Inadvertent acetaminophen overdosage, possibly resulting in hepatic failure and death, has been reported following confusion over different concentrations of the drug (e.g., 80 mg/0.8 mL, 80 mg/mL, 160 mg/5 mL) contained in various pediatric preparations. To minimize dosing confusion, a recommendation was made in June 2009 during a joint meeting between several FDA advisory committees to have only one concentration of liquid acetaminophen be available for self-medication (OTC use) in all pediatric patients. As a result, some manufacturers have decided to voluntarily change the concentration of the infants' formulation to be the same as that of the children's formulation (i.e., from 80 mg/0.8 mL or 80 mg/mL to 160 mg/5 mL). On December 22, 2011, FDA announced that a new liquid preparation marketed for infants, containing the lower concentration of acetaminophen (160 mg/5 mL), was available. This change in concentration affects the amount of liquid acetaminophen given to an infant, and should be especially noted if parents or caregivers have been accustomed to using the 80-mg/0.8-mL or 80-mg/mL concentration of liquid acetaminophen. The new preparation may be packaged with an oral syringe instead of a dropper. Because reformulation of the infants' preparation was voluntary, older, more-concentrated liquid acetaminophen preparations marketed for infants may remain available. To avoid confusion and the potential for dosing errors, clinicians should advise caregivers on product differences; clinicians also should specify both the concentration and dose of liquid acetaminophen when providing directions for use in children. Consumers, parents, and caregivers should be advised to carefully read the product labeling to identify the concentration of acetaminophen (in mg/mL), dosage, and directions for use. Parents and caregivers also should be advised to use only the measuring device provided with the particular preparation and not to mix and match measuring devices; if use of the measuring device seems confusing, or if there is any uncertainty in the proper use of the device, a clinician should be contacted. It should be noted that older, more-concentrated preparations of liquid acetaminophen (80 mg/0.8 mL or 80 mg/mL), if not expired, are safe and effective if used according to the directions specified on the product labeling that accompanies the preparation.

Overdosage and toxicity (including death) have been reported in children younger than 2 years of age receiving OTC preparations containing antihistamines, cough suppressants, expectorants, and nasal decongestants alone or in combination for relief of symptoms of upper respiratory tract infection. Such preparations also may contain analgesics and antipyretics (e.g., acetaminophen). There is limited evidence of efficacy for these preparations in this age group, and appropriate dosages (i.e., approved by FDA) have not been established. FDA recommends that parents and caregivers adhere to the dosage instructions and warnings on the product labeling that accompanies the preparation if administering to children and consult with their clinician about any concerns. Clinicians should ask caregivers about use of nonprescription cough and cold preparations to avoid overdosage. For additional information on precautions associated with the use of cough and cold preparations in pediatric patients, see Cautions: Pediatric Precautions in Pseudoephedrine 12:12.12.

Use of IV acetaminophen for analgesia or antipyresis in pediatric patients 2 years of age and older is supported by evidence from adequate and well-controlled studies of IV acetaminophen in adults and additional safety and pharmacokinetic data from 355 pediatric patients ranging in age from premature neonates (postmenstrual age of at least 32 weeks) to adolescents. Efficacy of IV acetaminophen for analgesia and antipyresis has not been established in pediatric patients younger than 2 years of age.

● Geriatric Precautions

When the total number of patients studied in clinical trials of IV acetaminophen is considered, 15% were 65 years of age or older, while 5% were 75 years of age and older. Although no overall differences in efficacy or safety were observed between geriatric and younger patients, and other clinical experience revealed no evidence of age-related differences, the possibility that some older patients may exhibit increased sensitivity to IV acetaminophen cannot be ruled out.

● Mutagenicity and Carcinogenicity

Acetaminophen was not mutagenic in the bacterial reverse mutation assay (Ames test), but positive results were observed in vitro in the mouse lymphoma assay and the chromosomal aberration assay using human lymphocytes. The drug has been reported to be clastogenic in rats at a dosage equivalent to 3.6 times the maximum recommended human daily dosage (4 g daily, based on body surface area comparison) but was not clastogenic at a dosage equivalent to 1.8 times the maximum recommended human daily dosage; these results suggest a threshold effect.

In 2-year studies in rats and mice fed a diet containing acetaminophen (up to 6000 ppm), there was no evidence of carcinogenicity in male rats or in mice given acetaminophen at dosages equivalent to 0.7 or 1.2–1.4 times, respectively, the maximum recommended human daily dosage (based on body surface area comparison). In female rats, there was equivocal evidence of carcinogenic activity based on an increased incidence of mononuclear cell leukemia at dosages equivalent to 0.8 times the maximum recommended human daily dosage.

● Pregnancy, Fertility, and Lactation

Pregnancy

Epidemiologic data regarding oral acetaminophen use in pregnant women have shown no increased risk of major congenital malformations in infants exposed in utero to the drug. In a large population-based prospective cohort study involving more than 26,000 women with live-born singleton infants who were exposed to oral acetaminophen during the first trimester of pregnancy, no increase in the risk of congenital malformations was observed in exposed children compared with a control group of unexposed children; the rate of congenital malformations (4.3%) was similar to the rate in the general population. A population-based, case-control study from the National Birth Defects Prevention Study also found no increase in the risk of major birth defects in a group of 11,610 children who had been exposed to acetaminophen during the first trimester of pregnancy compared with a control group of 4500 children.

Animal reproduction studies in pregnant rats given oral acetaminophen during organogenesis at dosages up to 0.85 times the maximum recommended human daily dosage (4 g daily, based on body surface area comparison) showed evidence of fetotoxicity (reduced fetal weight and length) and a dose-related increase in bone variations (reduced ossification and rudimentary rib changes); the offspring showed no evidence of external, visceral, or skeletal malformations. When pregnant rats received oral acetaminophen throughout gestation at a dosage of 1.2 times the maximum recommended human daily dosage, areas of necrosis occurred in both the liver and kidney of pregnant rats and fetuses; these effects did not occur in animals given acetaminophen at dosages of 0.3 times the maximum recommended human dosage.

In a continuous breeding study in which pregnant mice were given acetaminophen at dosages approximately equivalent to 0.43, 0.87, or 1.7 times the maximum recommended human daily dosage (based on body surface area comparison), a dose-related reduction in body weight of the fourth and fifth litter offspring of the treated mating pair occurred during lactation and following weaning at all dosages studied. Animals receiving the highest dosage had a reduced number of litters per mating pair, male offspring with an increased percentage of abnormal sperm, and reduced birth weights in the next-generation pups.

Acetaminophen is commonly used during all stages of pregnancy for its analgesic and antipyretic effects. Although acetaminophen has been thought not to be associated with risk in offspring, some recent reports have questioned this

assessment, especially with frequent maternal use or in cases involving genetic variability. FDA reviewed data on a possible association between acetaminophen use during pregnancy and risk of attention deficit hyperactivity disorder (ADHD) in children and announced in January 2015 that the data were inconclusive. Some experts state that as with all drug use during pregnancy, *routine* use of acetaminophen should be avoided.

The manufacturer states that there are no studies of IV acetaminophen in pregnant women and animal reproduction studies have not been conducted with this preparation. Therefore, the manufacturer states that IV acetaminophen should be used during pregnancy only when clearly needed.

Because there are no adequate and well-controlled studies of IV acetaminophen during labor and delivery, the manufacturer states that IV acetaminophen should be used in this setting only after careful assessment of potential benefits and risks.

Fertility

In a continuous breeding study in mice, no effects on fertility were observed in mice given acetaminophen at dosages up to 1.7 times the maximum recommended human daily dosage (based on body surface area comparison). In mice receiving acetaminophen at a dosage of 1.7 times the maximum recommended human daily dosage, no effect on sperm motility or sperm density in the epididymis was observed, but the percentage of abnormal sperm was increased and the number of mating pairs producing a fifth litter was reduced, suggesting the potential for cumulative toxicity with chronic administration of acetaminophen near the upper limit of daily dosing.

Other studies in rodents indicate that oral administration of acetaminophen at doses equivalent to at least 1.2 times the maximum recommended human daily dosage (based on body surface area comparison) results in decreased testicular weights, reduced spermatogenesis, and reduced fertility in males and reduced implantation sites in females. These effects appeared to increase with duration of treatment. The clinical relevance of these findings is not known.

Lactation

Acetaminophen is distributed into human milk in small quantities after oral administration. Data from more than 15 nursing women suggest that approximately 1–2% of the maternal daily dosage would be ingested by a nursing infant. A case of maculopapular rash in a breast-fed infant has been reported; the rash resolved when the mother discontinued acetaminophen use and recurred when she resumed acetaminophen therapy. The American Academy of Pediatrics and other experts state that acetaminophen is an acceptable choice for use in nursing women. The manufacturer states that IV acetaminophen should be used with caution in nursing women.

DRUG INTERACTIONS

● Drugs Affecting Hepatic Microsomal Enzymes

Drugs that induce or regulate hepatic cytochrome P-450 isoenzyme 2E1 (CYP2E1) may alter the metabolism of acetaminophen and increase its hepatotoxic potential. (See Pharmacokinetics: Elimination.) The clinical importance of such effects has not been established to date.

● Alcohol

The effects of alcohol on acetaminophen pharmacokinetics are complex; although excessive alcohol use can induce hepatic cytochromes, alcohol also competitively inhibits the metabolism of acetaminophen. Because there is some evidence that chronic, excessive consumption of alcohol may increase the risk of acetaminophen-induced hepatotoxicity, chronic alcoholics should be cautioned to avoid regular or excessive use of acetaminophen, or alternatively, to avoid chronic ingestion of alcohol. The manufacturers currently caution that patients who generally consume 3 or more alcohol-containing drinks per day should ask their clinician whether to use acetaminophen or an alternative analgesic for *self-medication* because acetaminophen may increase the risk of hepatotoxicity. However, the US Food and Drug Administration (FDA) has proposed eliminating this statement from the labeling of OTC acetaminophen-containing preparations and adding a new warning that would highlight the potential for severe liver damage to occur under certain circumstances, including in individuals who consume 3 or more alcohol-containing drinks per day while taking acetaminophen. (See Cautions: Precautions and Contraindications.)

● Anticonvulsants

Anticonvulsants (including phenytoin, barbiturates, carbamazepine) that induce hepatic microsomal enzymes may increase acetaminophen-induced liver toxicity because of increased conversion of the drug to hepatotoxic metabolites. The risk of acetaminophen-induced hepatic toxicity is substantially increased in patients ingesting larger than recommended dosages of acetaminophen while receiving anticonvulsants. Usually, no dosage reduction is required in patients receiving concomitant administration of therapeutic dosages of acetaminophen and anticonvulsants; however, patients should limit self-medication with acetaminophen while receiving anticonvulsants.

● Aspirin

Limited data indicate that administration of acetaminophen (1 g daily) does not inhibit the antiplatelet effect of aspirin (81 mg daily).

● Isoniazid

Concomitant administration of isoniazid with acetaminophen may result in an increased risk of hepatotoxicity, but the exact mechanism of this interaction has not been established. The risk of hepatic toxicity is substantially increased in patients ingesting larger than recommended dosages of acetaminophen while receiving isoniazid. Therefore, patients should limit self-medication with acetaminophen while receiving isoniazid.

● Oral Anticoagulants

Chronic ingestion of large doses of acetaminophen has been reported to potentiate the effects of coumarin- and indandione-derivative anticoagulants, although conflicting data exist and the clinical importance of any such interaction has been questioned. The results of an observational study in patients stabilized on warfarin therapy indicate an association between ingestion of even low to moderate dosages of acetaminophen (7 or more 325-mg tablets weekly) and excessively high international normalized ratio (INR) values, and some clinicians suggest that additional monitoring of INR values may be prudent in patients receiving warfarin therapy following initiation of, and during sustained therapy with, large doses of acetaminophen.

In a case-control study, patients receiving warfarin who had an INR exceeding 6 (target INR: 2–3) were more likely to have taken acetaminophen during the week preceding the INR than patients who had actual INRs of 1.7–3.3 (i.e., controls) on warfarin therapy; this association was dose-dependent in that case patients reported ingesting greater amounts of acetaminophen in the week preceding the INR (approximately 21 acetaminophen 325-mg tablets) than did controls (approximately 9 acetaminophen 325-mg tablets). For most of these patients, the elevated INR represented a recent deterioration in control of anticoagulation. Patients who reported taking about 1.3 g of acetaminophen daily for longer than 1 week had a tenfold increase in the risk of having an INR exceeding 6 compared with those not reporting acetaminophen use. Such risk decreased with lower acetaminophen dosages (4.6 up to 9.1 g weekly) and reached baseline values at acetaminophen dosages of about 2 g weekly or less. Although the precise mechanism of the described interaction is not known, it has been suggested that acetaminophen (particularly when administered in large doses) can inhibit metabolism of warfarin probably via inhibition of the cytochrome P-450 microsomal enzyme system, resulting in increased blood concentrations of warfarin. There is controversy concerning the design of this study (e.g., presence of possibly confounding risk factors, lack of causality assessment), and some clinicians doubt the clinical importance of these findings.

Pending completion of randomized, controlled studies to assess causality and more fully determine the clinical importance of this interaction, acetaminophen generally remains preferable to nonsteroidal anti-inflammatory agents (NSAIAs) as a mild analgesic or antipyretic in patients receiving warfarin because of the potential for serious adverse effects (e.g., bleeding) associated with concomitant warfarin and NSAIA therapy. Some clinicians suggest that when long-term therapy with acetaminophen (e.g., 3–4 g daily, as may be required for pain in patients with osteoarthritis) is initiated in patients receiving warfarin, the INR or prothrombin time (PT) should be determined about 7–14 days after beginning acetaminophen therapy. As with other drugs that may interact with warfarin, when concomitant acetaminophen therapy is initiated or discontinued or acetaminophen dosage is modified, the INR or PT should be monitored more frequently and warfarin dosage adjusted if necessary until these values have stabilized.

The manufacturer of acetaminophen injection states that more frequent monitoring of the INR may also be appropriate when patients receiving oral anticoagulants require short-term IV acetaminophen therapy, since the effects of such concomitant use have not been established.

● Phenothiazines

The possibility of severe hypothermia should be considered in patients receiving concomitant phenothiazine and antipyretic (e.g., acetaminophen) therapy.

LABORATORY TEST INTERFERENCES

Acetaminophen may produce false-positive test results for urinary 5-hydroxyindoleacetic acid.

ACUTE TOXICITY

● Pathogenesis

The toxicity of acetaminophen is closely linked to the drug's metabolism. With therapeutic dosing, acetaminophen is metabolized principally by sulfate and glucuronide conjugation. Small amounts (5–10%) usually are oxidized by cytochrome P-450 (CYP)-dependent pathways (mainly CYP2E1) to a toxic metabolite, N-acetyl-p-benzoquinoneimine (NAPQI). NAPQI is detoxified by glutathione and eliminated in urine and/or bile, and any remaining toxic metabolite may bind to hepatocytes and cause cellular necrosis. Because of the relatively small amount of NAPQI usually formed and the adequate supply of glutathione that usually is present in the body, acetaminophen generally has an excellent safety profile. However, with acetaminophen overdosage and occasionally with usual dosages in susceptible individuals (e.g., those with nutritional [malnutrition] or drug interactions, those consuming alcohol chronically, those with predisposing medical conditions, those with a genetic metabolic predisposition), hepatotoxic concentrations of NAPQI may accumulate.

● Manifestations

Acetaminophen toxicity may result from a single toxic dose, from repeated ingestion of large doses of acetaminophen (e.g., 7.5–10 g daily for 1–2 days), or from chronic ingestion of the drug. (See Chronic Toxicity.) Dose-dependent, hepatic necrosis is the most serious acute toxic effect associated with overdosage and is potentially fatal.

Acetaminophen toxicity usually involves 4 phases: 1) anorexia, nausea, vomiting, malaise, and diaphoresis (which inappropriately may prompt administration of additional acetaminophen); 2) resolution of phase-1 manifestations and replacement with right upper quadrant pain or tenderness, liver enlargement, elevated bilirubin and hepatic enzyme concentrations, prolongation of prothrombin time, and occasionally oliguria; 3) anorexia, nausea, vomiting, and malaise recur (usually 3–5 days after initial symptom onset) and signs of hepatic failure (e.g., jaundice, hypoglycemia, coagulopathy, encephalopathy) and possibly renal failure and cardiomyopathy develop; and 4) recovery or progression to fatal complete liver failure.

Nausea, vomiting, and abdominal pain usually occur within 2–3 hours after ingestion of toxic doses of the drug. Unlike salicylates, acetaminophen does not usually cause acid/base changes in toxic doses. In severe poisoning, CNS stimulation, excitement, and delirium may occur initially. This may be followed by CNS depression; stupor; hypothermia; marked prostration; rapid, shallow breathing; rapid, weak, irregular pulse; low blood pressure; and circulatory failure. Vascular collapse results from the relative hypoxia and from a central depressant action that occurs only with massive doses. Shock may develop if vasodilation is marked. Fatal asphyxial seizures may occur. Coma usually precedes death, which may occur suddenly or may be delayed for several days.

Fulminant, fatal hepatic failure may occur in chronic alcoholics following overdosage of acetaminophen. p-Aminophenol derivatives may elevate serum bilirubin concentrations, and jaundice may develop within 2–6 days after ingestion of one of the drugs. In adults, hepatic toxicity rarely has occurred with acute overdoses of less than 10 g, although hepatotoxicity has been reported in fasting patients ingesting 4–10 g of acetaminophen. (See Pharmacokinetics: Elimination.) Fatalities are rare with less than 15 g. However, the risk of severe and possibly fatal hepatic injury following acetaminophen overdosage cannot be accurately assessed based on the amount of acetaminophen ingested. Although some discordance in evidence exists, the overwhelming weight of existing evidence currently supports a relationship between chronic, excessive consumption of alcohol and an increased risk of acetaminophen-induced hepatotoxicity. When an individual has ingested a toxic dose of acetaminophen, the individual should be hospitalized for several days of observation, even if there are no apparent ill effects, because maximum liver damage usually does not become apparent until 2–4 days after ingestion of the drug. Transient azotemia and renal tubular necrosis have been reported in patients with acetaminophen poisoning; renal failure is often associated with fatality. There have been reports of acute myocardial necrosis and pericarditis in individuals with acetaminophen poisoning. Maximum cardiotoxic effects of these drugs appear to be delayed in a manner similar to hepatotoxic effects. Hypoglycemia, which can progress to coma, and metabolic acidosis have been reported in patients ingesting toxic doses of acetaminophen and cerebral edema occurred in one patient.

Young children appear to be less likely to develop hepatotoxic effects than adults, apparently because of age-related differences in acetaminophen metabolism. However, cases of severe hepatotoxicity and death have been reported in children who apparently received acetaminophen dosages exceeding those recommended (10–15 mg/kg per dose with a maximum of 5 doses per day) for children. Factors contributing to overdosage and toxicity of acetaminophen in children appear to include improper interpretation by the parent or caregiver of dosing information or failure to read such information, use of adult-strength acetaminophen preparations because of unavailability of pediatric formulations, use of excessive dosing because of the perception that desired therapeutic effects had not been achieved, and lack of knowledge about the potential toxicity of acetaminophen in excessive dosage. Current data suggest that the outcome after multiple excessive doses of acetaminophen in children under conditions of therapeutic intent may differ from the outcome observed after acute intoxications where as few as 1% of children have developed serious liver toxicity, which was successfully managed. Diagnosis and treatment may be made more difficult in cases of multiple overdoses because the parent or caregiver may not recognize acetaminophen overdose as a factor in the child's symptoms or may not accurately recall the dosage administered. The mechanism of acetaminophen toxicity in pediatric patients after multiple supratherapeutic doses remains to be elucidated. It has been suggested that certain individuals may be more susceptible to cellular injury induced by acetaminophen, and the combination of supratherapeutic doses, disease (e.g., diabetes mellitus, viral infection, febrile illness accompanied by acute malnourishment), nutritional factors (e.g., obesity, chronic undernutrition, prolonged fasting), metabolic factors (e.g., polymorphism in expression of the cytochrome P-450 enzyme system, alternate metabolic pathways under conditions of drug accumulation after multiple doses, enzyme induction), and stage of development may result in enhanced acetaminophen toxicity in these individuals. Whether hepatic injury resulting from other underlying conditions (e.g., viral infections, metabolic diseases) is exacerbated by acetaminophen has not been established.

Low prothrombin levels have been reported in patients with acetaminophen poisoning and in one patient fatal GI hemorrhage was attributed to hypoprothrombinemia. Thrombocytopenia also has been reported. Toxic doses of p-aminophenol derivatives may produce skin reactions of an erythematous or urticarial nature which may be accompanied by fever and oral mucosal lesions.

● Treatment

In all cases of suspected acetaminophen overdosage, a regional poison control center at 800-222-1212 may be contacted immediately for assistance in diagnosis and for directions in the use of acetylcysteine as an antidote.

Management of acetaminophen acute overdosage includes determination of the magnitude of the ingestion, classification of risk, and measures to reduce morbidity and mortality. Early recognition and treatment of overdosage are essential to prevent morbidity and mortality.

If acetaminophen has been recently ingested, activated charcoal may reduce acetaminophen absorption and should be administered as soon as possible (preferably within 1 hour of ingestion). Other methods of gastric decontamination

(i.e., syrup of ipecac) are less effective and generally are not recommended. Management of acetaminophen overdose also includes general physiologic supportive measures such as control of respiration and fluid and electrolyte therapy.

Because reported or estimated quantity of acetaminophen ingestion often is inaccurate and is not a reliable guide to the therapeutic management of the overdose, the preferred method to assess the risk of toxicity after acetaminophen ingestion usually is measurement of plasma or serum acetaminophen concentrations. Plasma or serum acetaminophen concentrations should be determined as soon as possible, but no sooner than 4 hours after ingestion (to ensure that peak concentrations have occurred). If an extended-release preparation of acetaminophen was ingested, it may be appropriate to obtain an additional sample of plasma or serum 4–6 hours after the initial sample for determination of drug concentrations. Plasma or serum acetaminophen concentrations are used in conjunction with a nomogram that follows to estimate the potential for hepatotoxicity and the necessity of acetylcysteine therapy (https://www.merckmanuals.com/professional/multimedia/image/rumack-matthew-nomogram-for-single-acute-acetaminophen-ingestions). If the initial acetaminophen concentration falls on or above the top line in the nomogram, hepatotoxicity is probable (in the absence of acetylcysteine therapy), and if the initial concentration falls on the bottom line or between the top and bottom lines, hepatotoxicity is possible (in the absence of acetylcysteine therapy). (To allow error on the side of safety, the bottom line is plotted 25% below the line indicating probable toxicity). If the initial plasma or serum acetaminophen concentration is below the bottom line on the nomogram, there is minimal risk of hepatotoxicity.

A full course of acetylcysteine therapy is indicated if initial plasma or serum acetaminophen concentrations fall on or above the bottom line on the nomogram. Results are optimal if acetylcysteine therapy is initiated within 8–16 hours of ingestion, but acetylcysteine is effective when given more than 24 hours after ingestion. If plasma or serum acetaminophen concentrations cannot be obtained, it should be assumed that the overdosage is potentially toxic, and acetylcysteine therapy should be initiated. Acetylcysteine may be withheld until acetaminophen assay results are available provided initiation of acetylcysteine is not delayed beyond 8 hours after acetaminophen ingestion. If more than 8 hours has elapsed since acetaminophen ingestion, acetylcysteine therapy should be started immediately.

When indicated (e.g., in patients in whom the initial acetaminophen concentration is toxic on the nomogram or in those in whom a toxic dose is suspected and the time of ingestion is unknown, 8 hours have elapsed since ingestion, acetaminophen concentrations cannot be obtained, or acetaminophen concentration values will not be available within 8 hours of ingestion), acetylcysteine therapy is initiated as soon as possible with an oral or IV loading dose in adults and pediatric patients. In the event that a loading dose of acetylcysteine is administered before plasma or serum acetaminophen concentration values are available, the initial plasma or serum concentration (obtained at least 4 hours after ingestion) is used in conjunction with the nomogram to determine the necessity of completing a full course of acetylcysteine therapy. In such situations, administration of a full course of acetylcysteine therapy is indicated if initial plasma or serum acetaminophen concentrations fall on or above the bottom line on the nomogram; acetylcysteine therapy is discontinued if initial acetaminophen concentrations fall below the bottom line on the nomogram.

When acetylcysteine is administered orally, a loading dose of 140 mg/kg is administered; the loading dose is followed by oral maintenance doses of 70 mg/kg every 4 hours for 17 doses (full course of therapy). Alternatively, when acetylcysteine is administered IV, a loading dose of 150 mg/kg is infused over 60 minutes; the loading dose is followed by an IV maintenance dose of 50 mg/kg infused over 4 hours and then 100 mg/kg infused over 16 hours (for a full course consisting of 300 mg/kg administered IV over 21 hours).

If a patient receiving oral acetylcysteine vomits a loading or maintenance dose within 1 hour of administration, the dose should be repeated. If the patient is persistently unable to retain orally administered acetylcysteine, the drug may be administered via a duodenal tube. Antiemetic therapy also may be used for persistent vomiting. The usual dosage of oral acetylcysteine is appropriate in patients given activated charcoal; higher dosages are not necessary in these patients.

Because acetylcysteine therapy may be useful even when instituted more than 24 hours after an overdose, a full course of acetylcysteine therapy is recommended for patients presenting 24 or more hours postingestion with measurable plasma or serum acetaminophen concentrations or biochemical evidence of hepatic injury. In a few patients with fulminant hepatic failure, IV administration of acetylcysteine has been associated with increased oxygen delivery and consumption resulting in beneficial effects on survival in such patients.

Because there is some evidence that excessive consumption of alcohol may increase the risk of acetaminophen-induced hepatotoxicity, some clinicians recommend that plasma or serum acetaminophen concentrations on the nomogram indicating the necessity for acetylcysteine therapy be lowered (by 25–70%) in chronic alcoholic patients. Some clinicians recommend that following overdosage of acetaminophen, plasma or serum acetaminophen concentrations on the nomogram indicating the necessity for acetylcysteine therapy also be lowered in patients receiving drugs that may interfere with the hepatic metabolism of acetaminophen (e.g., isoniazid; anticonvulsants including phenytoin, phenobarbital, primidone, valproic acid, carbamazepine) because the risk of acetaminophen-induced hepatotoxicity also may be increased in these patients. It has been suggested that when acetaminophen toxicity results from repeated ingestion of large doses of acetaminophen (e.g., 7.5–10 g daily for 1 or 2 days), acetylcysteine therapy should be considered irrespective of plasma or serum acetaminophen concentrations. Some experts state that early therapy with acetylcysteine should be considered when acetaminophen toxicity is a likely contributor to hepatic dysfunction. In addition, some clinicians state that if an extended-release preparation of acetaminophen has been ingested, the usefulness of the current nomogram (which is based on ingestion of immediate-release preparations) may be limited. Although area under the plasma concentration-time curve (AUC) may be increased following ingestion of an extended-release preparation, delayed absorption and decreased peak plasma acetaminophen concentrations may occur, which may lead to an underestimation of the need for antidotal therapy. Some clinicians suggest that higher than usual doses of acetylcysteine may be necessary in patients ingesting an overdosage of acetaminophen extended-release preparations. However, the manufacturer states that the standard nomogram may be used for acetaminophen extended-release tablets, but that an additional determination of plasma or serum acetaminophen concentrations from a sample obtained 4–6 hours after the initial sample also should be evaluated using the nomogram. In cases where it is unclear whether high doses of the drug were ingested as extended-release tablets or as conventional preparations of acetaminophen, the manufacturer suggests that overdosage of the drug be managed as if extended-release preparations were ingested.

In addition to plasma or serum acetaminophen concentrations, baseline prothrombin time, BUN, blood glucose concentration, and serum AST (SGOT), ALT (SGPT), bilirubin, creatinine, and electrolyte concentrations should be determined. Prothrombin time, blood glucose concentration, and serum AST, ALT, bilirubin, and electrolyte concentrations should be determined at 24-hour intervals for at least 96 hours after the time of ingestion; if toxicity is evident, these parameters should continue to be monitored at least daily as necessary. Fluid and electrolyte balance should be maintained; use of diuretics and forced diuresis should be avoided. Hypoglycemia should be treated as necessary. If the prothrombin time is greater than 1.5 times the control value, phytonadione should be administered; if the prothrombin time is greater than 3 times the control value, fresh frozen plasma should be given. If hepatic or renal impairment develops, appropriate laboratory parameters should be monitored until values return toward normal. A serum bilirubin concentration greater than 4 mg/dL and a prothrombin time greater than 2.2 times the control value may indicate impending hepatic encephalopathy. Hemodialysis or charcoal hemoperfusion generally are not useful in enhancing the elimination of acetaminophen from the body. Peritoneal dialysis is ineffective.

CHRONIC TOXICITY

While some evidence from animal studies suggests that tolerance to acetaminophen may occur when the dose is increased gradually, continued increases presumably will eventually exceed a threshold resulting in toxicity that is similar in acuity and severity to single time-point overdoses. Unintentional overdosage and resultant acute liver failure often may go unrecognized for several days. Despite long-term acetaminophen ingestion histories associated with unintentional acetaminophen overdosages, such overdosage still is associated with acute hepatic injury that is indistinguishable from intentional (suicidal) ingestions. This experience suggests that there may not be a true chronic form of toxicity but instead a safety threshold that may be breached with devastating consequences.

Three hundred and seven cases of liver injury associated with acetaminophen use were reported to the US Food and Drug Administration (FDA) from January 1998 to July 2001. Sixty percent of these adverse events were categorized as severe life-threatening injury with liver failure (category 4); 40% of patients died. Review of these case reports indicates that use of higher than recommended daily dosages of acetaminophen results in adverse hepatotoxic effects more often than use of recommended dosages.

Twenty-five of these case reports involved pediatric patients 12 years of age or younger and 84% (21) of these cases involved medication errors. Administration of higher than recommended dosages of acetaminophen has occurred as a result of parents or caregivers misunderstanding the directions provided on the product label or given by a clinician. An added source of confusion is the different concentrations of acetaminophen available in pediatric preparations (e.g., acetaminophen drops 100 mg/mL, acetaminophen suspension 160 mg/5 mL). Based on information from 10 of these reports, the dosage range of acetaminophen in these children was 106–375 mg/kg daily. The maximum recommended pediatric dosage is 75 mg/kg daily. Limited information indicates that the daily dosage of acetaminophen was higher in children who experienced serious hepatic injury (category 4) compared with those who experienced less severe hepatic effects.

The mean and median daily dosage of acetaminophen was 6.5 and 5 g daily, respectively, in the 282 adults who experienced liver toxicity. Although the maximum recommended adult dosage of 4 g daily is tolerated in most patients without clinically important liver injury, there are varying views on the specific threshold dosage for toxicity. Reversible aminotransferase (transaminase) elevations were reported in one study to occur in 40% of patients receiving 4 g daily over several days, and rare cases of acute liver failure have been associated with dosages lower than 2.5 g daily. In addition, liver toxicity has occurred at a lower acetaminophen dosage in adults who reported alcohol use compared with adults who did not report alcohol use. Concomitant use of other drugs also may contribute to hepatotoxicity in some patients. In one study, prescription labeling for 64 of 74 drugs taken concomitantly with acetaminophen in patients experiencing liver toxicity contained information on hepatotoxic events; 10 drugs had warnings or precautions concerning hepatic failure. Adding to concerns about currently recommended maximum daily dosages of acetaminophen is evidence that patients routinely and knowingly take more than recommended maximum dosages of OTC analgesics. FDA's Acetaminophen Hepatotoxicity Working Group recently recommended that the maximum daily acetaminophen dosage be reduced to 3.25 g daily (5 single 650-mg doses daily), and some manufacturers (e.g., McNeil, Tylenol®) have voluntarily revised their labeling to recommend less frequent dosing and lower total daily dosages of acetaminophen in adults to not exceed 1 g every 6 hours up to a maximum of 3 g daily.

In contrast to acute acetaminophen overdosage, guidelines for the treatment of ingestions involving multiple higher-than-recommended doses of acetaminophen currently are not available. In addition, it can be difficult to recognize the onset of liver injury, with symptom onset taking several days in some patients, even in severe cases. Symptoms also may not be specific, mimicking flu symptoms, which can result in patients continuing to take acetaminophen after symptoms emerge. Some poison centers use plasma aspartate aminotransferase (AST) and/or alanine aminotransferase (ALT) concentrations and plasma or serum acetaminophen concentrations to estimate the potential for hepatotoxicity and necessity of acetylcysteine therapy. In cases of repeated supratherapeutic ingestion of acetaminophen, a regional poison center (800-222-1222) or an assistance line for acetaminophen overdosage (800-525-6115) can be contacted.

Chronic ingestion of large doses of analgesics (e.g., 1 kg or more of phenacetin [no longer commercially available in the US] and/or salicylate over any period of time) has been associated with analgesic nephropathy which is characterized by papillary necrosis and subsequent chronic interstitial nephritis, with or without pyelonephritis. Analgesic nephropathy frequently has been associated with ingestion of large amounts of combinations of aspirin, phenacetin, and caffeine (combinations containing phenacetin no longer are commercially available in the US). Because phenacetin previously was a component of many analgesic drug mixtures, this drug has been implicated as the causative agent of renal damage. Many clinicians, however, believe that nephropathy may be caused by a combination of several analgesics rather than a single drug. Cancer of the renal pelvis has been reported in patients with analgesic nephropathy and in patients following chronic ingestion of phenacetin-containing analgesic mixtures. Splenomegaly has also been associated with abuse of phenacetin-containing mixtures.

PHARMACOLOGY

Acetaminophen produces analgesia and antipyresis by a mechanism similar to that of salicylates. Unlike salicylates, however, acetaminophen does not have uricosuric activity. There is some evidence that acetaminophen has weak anti-inflammatory activity in some nonrheumatoid conditions (e.g., in patients who have had oral surgery). In equal doses, the degree of analgesia and antipyresis produced by acetaminophen is similar to that produced by aspirin.

Acetaminophen lowers body temperature in patients with fever but rarely lowers normal body temperature. The drug acts on the hypothalamus to produce antipyresis; heat dissipation is increased as a result of vasodilation and increased peripheral blood flow.

The effects of acetaminophen on cyclooxygenase activity have not been fully determined. Acetaminophen is a weak, reversible, isoform-nonspecific cyclooxygenase inhibitor at dosages of 1 g daily. The inhibitory effect of acetaminophen on cyclooxygenase-1 is limited, and the drug does not inhibit platelet function.

Therapeutic doses of acetaminophen appear to have little effect on cardiovascular and respiratory systems; however, toxic doses may cause circulatory failure and rapid, shallow breathing.

PHARMACOKINETICS

● Absorption

Acetaminophen is rapidly and almost completely absorbed from the GI tract following oral administration. In healthy men, steady-state oral bioavailability of 1.3-g doses of extended-release tablets of acetaminophen administered every 8 hours for a total of 7 doses was equal to 1-g doses of conventional tablets of acetaminophen given every 6 hours for a total of 7 doses. Food may delay slightly absorption of extended-release tablets of acetaminophen. Following oral administration of immediate- or extended-release acetaminophen preparations, peak plasma concentrations are attained within 10–60 or 60–120 minutes, respectively. Following oral administration of a single 500-mg conventional tablet or a single 650-mg extended-release tablet, average plasma acetaminophen concentrations of 2.1 or 1.8 μg/mL, respectively, occur at 6 or 8 hours, respectively. In addition, dissolution of the extended-release tablets may depend slightly on the gastric or intestinal pH. Dissolution appears to be slightly faster in the alkaline pH of the intestines compared with the acidic pH of the stomach; however, this is of no clinical importance. Following administration of conventional preparations of acetaminophen, only small amounts of the drug are detectable in plasma after 8 hours. The extended-release tablets of acetaminophen release the drug for up to 8 hours, but in vitro data indicate that at least 95% of the dose is released within 5 hours.

Following rectal administration of acetaminophen, there is considerable variation in peak plasma concentrations attained, and time to reach peak plasma concentrations is substantially longer than after oral administration.

Following IV administration of single 500-mg, 650-mg, and 1-g doses of acetaminophen in adults, the pharmacokinetics of the drug are proportional to the dose administered. The peak plasma concentration of acetaminophen occurs at the end of the 15-minute IV infusion and is up to 70% higher than peak concentrations observed following oral administration of the same dose; however, systemic exposure to the drug is similar following IV or oral administration. Following IV administration of a single dose of 15 mg/kg in pediatric patients or 1 g in adults, systemic exposure to acetaminophen in children and adolescents is similar to that in adults, but exposure is higher in neonates and infants. Dosing simulations using pharmacokinetic data from infants and neonates suggest that dose reductions of 33% in infants 1 month to less than 2 years of age and 50% in neonates up to 28 days of age, with a minimum dosing interval of 6 hours, would result in systemic exposures similar to those observed in children 2 years of age and older.

● Distribution

Acetaminophen is rapidly and uniformly distributed into most body tissues except fat. Acetaminophen crosses the placenta and is distributed into human milk in small quantities following oral administration. About 10–25% of acetaminophen in blood is bound to plasma proteins.

● Elimination

Acetaminophen has been reported to have a plasma half-life of 1.25–3 hours. Following IV administration of a single dose of 15 mg/kg in pediatric patients or 1 g in adults, plasma half-lives of 2.4 hours in adults, 2.9–3 hours in children and adolescents, 4.2 hours in infants, and 7 hours in neonates have been reported. Plasma half-life of acetaminophen may be prolonged following toxic doses or in patients with liver damage, although limited data indicate that following overdosage of acetaminophen the terminal plasma half-life of the drug reported with extended-release tablets is comparable to that reported with standard-release preparations.

About 80–85% of the acetaminophen in the body undergoes conjugation principally with glucuronic acid and to a lesser extent with sulfuric acid. Acetaminophen also is metabolized by microsomal enzyme systems in the liver.

In vitro and animal data indicate that small quantities of acetaminophen are metabolized by cytochrome P-450 (CYP) microsomal enzymes, mainly CYP2E1, to a reactive intermediate metabolite (N-acetyl-p-benzoquinoneimine, N-acetylimidoquinone, NAPQI) which is further metabolized via conjugation with glutathione and ultimately excreted in urine as a mercapturic acid. It has been suggested that this intermediate metabolite is responsible for acetaminophen-induced liver necrosis and that high doses of acetaminophen may deplete glutathione so that inactivation of this toxic metabolite is decreased. At high doses, the capacity of metabolic pathways for conjugation with glucuronic acid and sulfuric acid may be exceeded, resulting in increased metabolism of acetaminophen by alternative pathways. In addition, it also has been suggested that in fasting individuals conjugation of high doses of acetaminophen with glucuronic acid may be reduced, secondary to decreased hepatic carbohydrate reserves and microsomal oxidation may be increased, resulting in increased risk of hepatotoxicity. Drugs that potentially modify these metabolic processes are used (e.g., acetylcysteine) or are being studied (e.g., cysteine, mercaptamine) as antidotes for acetaminophen-induced hepatotoxicity.

Acetaminophen is excreted in urine principally as acetaminophen glucuronide with small amounts of acetaminophen sulfate and mercaptate and unchanged drug. Approximately 85% of a dose of acetaminophen is excreted in urine as free and conjugated acetaminophen within 24 hours after ingestion. Administration of acetaminophen to patients with moderate to severe renal impairment may result in accumulation of acetaminophen conjugates.

CHEMISTRY AND STABILITY

● Chemistry

Acetaminophen is a synthetic nonopiate derivative of p-aminophenol that produces analgesia and antipyresis. Acetaminophen is a major metabolite of phenacetin. Phenacetin, another derivative of p-aminophenol, has been associated with analgesic nephropathy (renal papillary necrosis with subsequent chronic interstitial nephritis) and no longer is commercially available in the US. Acetaminophen occurs as a white, crystalline powder with a slightly bitter taste. Acetaminophen is soluble in boiling water and freely soluble in alcohol.

Acetaminophen oral solution has a pH of 3.8–6.1, and the oral suspension has a pH of 4–6.9. Although an official USP acetaminophen elixir that contained 6.5–10.5% alcohol was previously available under this title, USP combined the official descriptions for the elixir and solution to just acetaminophen oral solution in 1990 to simplify compendial standards for these liquid oral dosage forms. Therefore, both preparations, regardless of whether they contain alcohol, currently are titled oral solutions; those that contain alcohol are differentiated from those that do not only by specifying the alcohol content on the labeling.

Acetaminophen 650-mg extended-release tablets (e.g., Tylenol® Arthritis Pain Extended Release, Tylenol® 8 Hour Extended-Release) are bilayer (immediate-release and extended-release layers) tablets.

Acetaminophen injection is a sterile, clear, colorless, nonpyrogenic, isotonic aqueous solution containing 10 mg of acetaminophen per mL. Hydrochloric acid and/or sodium hydroxide may be added to adjust pH to approximately 5.5. The commercially available injection also contains mannitol, cysteine hydrochloride monohydrate, and dibasic sodium phosphate and has an osmolality of approximately 290 mOsm/kg.

● *Stability*

Oral acetaminophen preparations should be stored at a controlled room temperature of 20–25°C; freezing of the oral solution or suspension should be avoided. Acetaminophen suppositories should be stored at room temperature or in a refrigerator.

Acetaminophen injection should be stored at a temperature of 20–25°C and should not be refrigerated or frozen. The injection should be used within 6 hours after the vacuum seal of the vial has been penetrated or the vial contents have been transferred to another container. Acetaminophen injection is incompatible with acyclovir sodium, diazepam, and chlorpromazine hydrochloride.

PREPARATIONS

To minimize the risk of inadvertent acetaminophen overdosage in pediatric patients, FDA has recommended that only one concentration of liquid acetaminophen be available for *self-medication* (over-the-counter [OTC] use) in all pediatric patients. As a result, some manufacturers have decided to voluntarily change the concentration of the infants' formulation to be the same as that of the children's formulation. (See Cautions: Pediatric Precautions.) However, because this change is voluntary, older, more-concentrated liquid acetaminophen preparations marketed for infants may remain available.

To minimize the risk of inadvertent acetaminophen overdosage, FDA has requested manufacturers to reformulate prescription combination preparations containing the drug to limit the acetaminophen amount to 325 mg or less per dosage unit. FDA no longer considers prescription combination preparations containing more than 325 mg of acetaminophen per dosage unit to be safe. As of March 26, 2014, all manufacturers of such preparations had discontinued marketing of the preparations, although some had not withdrawn the drug applications. FDA intends to withdraw approval of those applications if they are not voluntarily withdrawn. Therefore, availability of combination preparations with higher concentrations of acetaminophen per dose will diminish over time. Some prescription combination preparations that previously contained more than 325 mg of acetaminophen per dosage unit may have been reformulated to contain a smaller amount of acetaminophen. Pharmacists are encouraged to return any prescription combination preparations containing more than 325 mg of acetaminophen per dosage unit to the wholesaler or manufacturer. FDA has stated that the agency intends to address nonprescription acetaminophen-containing preparations in a separate regulatory action.

Excipients in commercially available drug preparations may have clinically important effects in some individuals; consult specific product labeling for details.

Acetaminophen

Oral		
Capsules, gel-coated	500 mg*	**Acetaminophen Extra Strength Gel-coated Capsules**
Solution	167 mg/5 mL*	**Tylenol® Extra-Strength Adult**, McNeil
Suspension	160 mg/5 mL*	**Tylenol® Oral Suspension Children's**, McNeil
		Tylenol® Oral Suspension Infant's, McNeil
Tablets	325 mg*	**Tylenol® Regular Strength (scored)**, McNeil
Tablets, extended-release, film-coated	650 mg*	**Tylenol® Arthritis Pain Extended-Release Caplets**, McNeil
		Tylenol® 8 HR Extended-Release Caplets®, McNeil
Tablets, film-coated	500 mg*	**Tylenol® Extra Strength Caplets**, McNeil
Tablets, orally disintegrating	80 mg*	**Tylenol® Meltaways Children's**, McNeil
	160 mg*	**Tylenol® Meltaways Junior Strength**, McNeil

Parenteral		
Injection, for IV infusion	10 mg/mL (1 g)	**Ofirmev®**, Mallinckrodt
Rectal		
Suppositories	80 mg	**FeverAll® Infants'**, Taro
	120 mg*	**Acephen®**, G&W
		FeverAll® Children's, Taro
	325 mg	**Acephen®**, G&W
		FeverAll® Junior Strength, Taro
	650 mg*	**Acephen®**, G&W

* available from one or more manufacturer, distributor, and/or repackager by generic (nonproprietary) name

Acetaminophen and Aspirin

Oral		
For solution	325 mg/packet Acetaminophen and Aspirin 500 mg/packet	**Goody's® Back & Body Pain Powder**, Prestige
Tablets, film-coated	250 mg Acetaminophen, Aspirin 250 mg, and buffer	**Excedrin® Back and Body Caplets**, Novartis

Acetaminophen, Aspirin, and Caffeine

Oral		
Capsules, gel-coated	250 mg Acetaminophen, Aspirin 250 mg, and Caffeine 65 mg*	**Excedrin® Menstrual Complete Gelcaps**, Novartis
For solution	260 mg/packet Acetaminophen, Aspirin 520 mg/packet, and Caffeine 32.5 mg/packet	**Goody's® Extra Strength Headache Powder**, Prestige
	325 mg/packet Acetaminophen, Aspirin 500 mg/packet, and Caffeine 65 mg/packet	**Goody's® Cool Orange Extra Strength Powder**, Prestige
Tablets, film-coated	194 mg Acetaminophen, Aspirin 227 mg, Caffeine 33 mg, and buffers	**Vanquish® Caplets**, Moberg
	250 mg Acetaminophen, Aspirin 250 mg, and Caffeine 65 mg	**Excedrin® Extra Strength Caplets**, Novartis
		Excedrin® Migraine Caplets, Novartis
		Goody's® Extra Strength Caplets, Prestige
		Pamprin® Max, Chattem

* available from one or more manufacturer, distributor, and/or repackager by generic (nonproprietary) name

Acetaminophen and Codeine Phosphate

Oral		
Solution	120 mg/5 mL Acetaminophen and Codeine Phosphate 12 mg/5 mL*	**Acetaminophen and Codeine Phosphate Oral Solution**(C-V),
Suspension	120 mg/5 mL Acetaminophen and Codeine Phosphate 12 mg/5 mL	**Capital® and Codeine** (C-V), Valeant
Tablets	300 mg Acetaminophen and Codeine Phosphate 15 mg*	**Acetaminophen and Codeine Phosphate Tablets**(C-III),
	300 mg Acetaminophen and Codeine Phosphate 30 mg*	**Tylenol® with Codeine No. 3** (C-III), Janssen
	300 mg Acetaminophen and Codeine Phosphate 60 mg*	**Tylenol® with Codeine No. 4** (C-III), Janssen

* available from one or more manufacturer, distributor, and/or repackager by generic (nonproprietary) name

Acetaminophen and Diphenhydramine Citrate

Oral

For solution	500 mg/packet Acetaminophen and Diphenhydramine Citrate 38 mg/packet	**Goody's® PM Powder**, Prestige
Tablets, film-coated	500 mg Acetaminophen and Diphenhydramine Citrate 38 mg*	**Excedrin PM® Caplets**, Novartis
		Excedrin PM® Geltabs, Novartis
		Midol® PM Caplets, Bayer

* available from one or more manufacturer, distributor, and/or repackager by generic (nonproprietary) name

Oxycodone and Acetaminophen

Oral

Solution	5 mg/5 mL Oxycodone Hydrochloride and Acetaminophen 325 mg/5 mL	**Roxicet®** (C-II), Roxane
Tablets	2.5 mg Oxycodone Hydrochloride and Acetaminophen 300 mg*	**Oxycodone Hydrochloride and Acetaminophen Tablets** (C-II),
	2.5 mg Oxycodone Hydrochloride and Acetaminophen 325 mg*	**Percocet®** (C-II), Endo
	5 mg Oxycodone Hydrochloride and Acetaminophen 300 mg*	**Primlev®** (C-II), Akrimax
	5 mg Oxycodone Hydrochloride and Acetaminophen 325 mg*	**Endocet®** (C-II; scored), Qualitest
		Percocet® (C-II; scored), Endo
	7.5 mg Oxycodone Hydrochloride and Acetaminophen 300 mg*	**Primlev®** (C-II), Akrimax
	7.5 mg Oxycodone Hydrochloride and Acetaminophen 325 mg*	**Endocet®** (C-II), Qualitest
		Percocet® (C-II), Endo
	10 mg Oxycodone Hydrochloride and Acetaminophen 300 mg*	**Primlev®** (C-II), Akrimax
	10 mg Oxycodone Hydrochloride and Acetaminophen 325 mg*	**Endocet®** (C-II), Qualitest
		Percocet® (C-II), Endo

* available from one or more manufacturer, distributor, and/or repackager by generic (nonproprietary) name

Other Acetaminophen Combinations

Oral

Capsules	300 mg with Butalbital 50 mg and Caffeine 40 mg*	**Fioricet®**, Actavis
	300 mg with Butalbital 50 mg, Caffeine 40 mg, and Codeine Phosphate 30 mg*	**Fioricet® with Codeine** (C-III), Actavis
	320.5 mg with Caffeine 30 mg and Dihydrocodeine Bitartrate 16 mg	**Trezix®** (C-III), WraSer
	325 mg with Butalbital 50 mg and Caffeine 40 mg*	**Capacet®** Magna
	325 mg with Butalbital 50 mg, Caffeine 40 mg, and Codeine Phosphate 30 mg*	**Butalbital, Acetaminophen, Caffeine, and Codeine Phosphate Capsules** (C-III),
Capsules, gel-coated	500 mg with Caffeine 60 mg and Pyrilamine Maleate 15 mg	**Midol® Complete Gelcaps**, Bayer
	500 mg with Caffeine 65 mg*	**Acetaminophen with Caffeine Gelcaps**

Solution	83 mg/5 mL with Caffeine 5.4 mg/5 mL	**Goody's® Headache Relief Shot**, Prestige
	100 mg/5 mL with Hydrocodone Bitartrate 3.3 mg/5 mL*	**Lortab® Elixir** (C-II), ECR
	108 mg/5 mL with Butalbital 16.7 mg/5 mL and Caffeine 13.3 mg/5 mL*	**Alagesic LQ®**, Poly Pharmaceuticals
	108 mg/5 mL with Hydrocodone Bitartrate 2.5 mg/5 mL*	**Hydrocodone Bitartrate and Acetaminophen Oral Solution** (C-II),
	108 mg/5 mL with Hydrocodone Bitartrate 3.3 mg/5 mL*	**Hydrocodone Bitartrate and Acetaminophen Oral Solution** (C-II),
Tablets	300 mg with Butalbital 50 mg	**Bupap®**, ECR
	300 mg with Hydrocodone Bitartrate 5 mg*	**Vicodin®** (C-II; scored), AbbVie
	300 mg with Hydrocodone Bitartrate 7.5 mg*	**Vicodin ES®** (C-II; scored), AbbVie
	300 mg with Hydrocodone Bitartrate 10 mg*	**Vicodin HP®** (C-II; scored), AbbVie
	325 mg with Butalbital 50 mg	**Butapap®**, Mikart
		Phrenilin® (scored), Valeant
	325 mg with Butalbital 50 mg and Caffeine 40 mg*	**Butalbital, Acetaminophen, and Caffeine Tablets**
	325 mg with Hydrocodone Bitartrate 2.5 mg*	**Hydrocodone and Acetaminophen Tablets** (C-II),
	325 mg with Hydrocodone Bitartrate 5 mg*	**Lortab®** (C-II; scored), UCB
		Norco® (C-II; scored), Actavis
	325 mg with Hydrocodone Bitartrate 7.5 mg*	**Lortab®** (C-II; scored), UCB
		Norco® (C-II; scored), Actavis
	325 mg with Hydrocodone Bitartrate 10 mg*	**Lortab®** (C-II; scored), UCB
		Norco® (C-II; scored), Actavis
Tablets, film-coated	325 mg with Diphenhydramine Hydrochloride 12.5 mg*	**Percogesic® Original Strength**, Prestige
	325 mg with Tramadol Hydrochloride 37.5 mg*	**Ultracet®** (C-IV), Janssen
	500 mg with Caffeine 60 mg and Pyrilamine Maleate 15 mg*	**Midol® Complete Caplets**, Bayer
	500 mg with Caffeine 65 mg*	**Excedrin® Tension Headache Caplets**, Novartis
	500 mg with Diphenhydramine Hydrochloride 12.5 mg	**Percogesic® Extra Strength Caplets®**, Prestige
	500 mg with Diphenhydramine Hydrochloride 25 mg*	**Tylenol® PM Extra Strength Caplets**, McNeil
		Tylenol® PM Extra Strength Geltabs®, McNeil
	500 mg with Pamabrom 25 mg	**Midol® Teen Caplets®**, Bayer
	500 mg with Pamabrom 25 mg and Pyrilamine Maleate 15 mg	**Pamprin® Multi-Symptom Caplets**, Chattem
		Premsyn PMS® Caplets, Chattem

* available from one or more manufacturer, distributor, and/or repackager by generic (nonproprietary) name

† Use is not currently included in the labeling approved by the US Food and Drug Administration.

Selected Revisions June 10, 2024, © Copyright, April 1, 1973, American Society of Health-System Pharmacists, Inc.

Naloxone Hydrochloride

28:10 • OPIOID ANTAGONISTS

On March 29, 2023, FDA approved naloxone hydrochloride nasal spray 4 mg (Narcan®) for nonprescription (OTC) use. The timeline for availability and price of this OTC product will be determined by the manufacturer. Manufacturers of generic naloxone nasal spray products will be required to submit a supplement to their applications to effectively switch their products to OTC status. This approval may also affect the status of other brand-name naloxone nasal spray products of 4 mg or less, but determinations will be made on a case-by-case basis.

On July 28, 2023, FDA announced the approval of a second OTC naloxone hydrochloride nasal spray product (RiVive®) for the emergency treatment of known or suspected opioid overdose. The timeline for availability and price of this OTC product will be determined by the manufacturer. Also in July 2023, FDA approved the first generic OTC naloxone nasal spray.

■ Naloxone hydrochloride is an opioid antagonist.

USES

● *Opioid-induced Depression and Acute Opioid Overdosage*

Naloxone is used for the complete or partial reversal of opioid-induced depression, including respiratory depression, caused by natural and synthetic opioids (e.g., codeine, diphenoxylate, fentanyl citrate, heroin, hydromorphone, levorphanol, meperidine, methadone, morphine, oxymorphone, concentrated opium alkaloids, propoxyphene) and certain opioid partial agonists (e.g., butorphanol, nalbuphine, pentazocine). Reversal of respiratory depression resulting from overdosage of opioid partial agonists (e.g., buprenorphine, pentazocine) may be incomplete and require higher or more frequent doses of naloxone.

The availability of naloxone as prefilled syringes and as nasal spray formulations facilitates administration by family members or other caregivers; such treatment is *not* a substitute for emergency medical care. Administration of naloxone should be accompanied by other resuscitative measures such as administration of oxygen, mechanical ventilation, or artificial respiration. When administering naloxone outside of a supervised medical setting, always seek emergency medical assistance after the first dose is administered.

Naloxone is used in both adults and pediatric adults (including neonates) to reverse the effects of opioids. Naloxone has been given to the mother shortly before delivery†, but it is preferable to administer the drug directly to the neonate if needed after delivery.

Naloxone hydrochloride injection containing 5 mg per 0.5 mL (Zimhi®) is a higher concentration of the drug for IM or subcutaneous use in adults and pediatric patients for emergency treatment of known or suspected opioid overdose. The preparation is commercially available as single-dose prefilled syringes that are administered using a delivery device. Naloxone hydrochloride 5 mg/0.5 mL was developed in response to increasing reports indicating that multiple 2-mg doses of naloxone have been required in resuscitations. Efficacy of this preparation for community use is supported by pharmacokinetic bridging studies.

Clinical Perspective

Deaths associated with the use of prescription opioid analgesics increased in the US from 1999 through 2019, with nearly 69,000 deaths involving any opioid occurring in 2020; approximately 16,000 of these deaths involved prescription opioids. Deaths due to opioid overdose can be prevented with the use of naloxone, and distribution of naloxone through community-based programs that provide overdose education has been associated with decreased opioid-related mortality rates. When administered at usual doses for opioid overdose, serious adverse effects of naloxone are rare.

The 2022 Centers for Disease Control and Prevention (CDC) clinical practice guideline on prescribing opioids for pain recommends that clinicians discuss the risk of opioid-related harms with their patients, including risk mitigation strategies such as naloxone for overdose reversal. Many experts including CDC recommend the administration of naloxone in the event of a known or suspected opioid overdose. Clinicians should offer naloxone and provide overdose prevention education to patients receiving opioid analgesics who are at increased risk of opioid overdosage (e.g., those receiving concomitant therapy with benzodiazepines or other CNS depressants, those with a history of opioid or substance use disorder, those with medical conditions that could increase sensitivity to opioid effects, those who have experienced a prior opioid overdose, those taking higher dosages of opioids [e.g., ≥50 morphine mg equivalents/day, and those at risk of returning to a high dose to which they have lost tolerance [e.g., patients undergoing tapering or recently released from prison]). Naloxone also should be offered when patients receiving opioids have household members who are at risk for accidental ingestion or overdosage.

Although naloxone historically has been administered mainly by trained medical personnel in hospitals or ambulances, naloxone increasingly is being administered by nonmedical personnel in community (nonmedical) settings for emergency treatment of known or suspected opioid overdosage, as manifested by respiratory and/or CNS depression. Experts recommend that additional first responders (e.g., other emergency medical service personnel, police officers, fire fighters) be trained and authorized to administer naloxone following known or suspected opioid overdosage and support greater access to naloxone by workers in settings where opioid overdoses may be witnessed (e.g., nursing homes, home visiting nurses, school nurses and college campuses, outreach programs, substance abuse treatment programs, halfway houses, homeless shelters, correctional facilities). Commercially available naloxone prefilled syringes and nasal spray formulations facilitate administration of the drug by family members or other caregivers in such settings and are available for community use; however, such treatment is *not* a substitute for emergency medical care.

● *Diagnosis of Suspected or Known Acute Opioid Overdosage*

Naloxone is used for the diagnosis of suspected or known acute opioid overdosage.

● *Septic Shock*

Naloxone hydrochloride injection is FDA-labeled for adjunctive use in the management of septic shock. Naloxone has been shown to produce a rise in blood pressure that may last up to several hours in some cases of septic shock; however, use of the drug in this setting has not resulted in improved survival and has been associated with adverse effects (e.g., agitation, nausea, vomiting, pulmonary edema, hypotension, cardiac arrhythmias, seizures). Because of limited experience with this use, optimal dosage and treatment regimens have not been established.

Naloxone therapy is not included in the current Surviving Sepsis Campaign International Guidelines for Management of Sepsis and Septic Shock; fluid resuscitation and vasopressors (e.g., norepinephrine, vasopressin) are used first-line in hemodynamic management. If a decision is made to use naloxone for management of septic shock, the manufacturers state that the drug should be used with caution, particularly in patients who may have underlying pain or have previously received opioid therapy and may have developed opioid tolerance.

● *Naloxone Challenge Test*

To avoid precipitating opioid withdrawal following administration of naltrexone, naloxone has been used as a screening test (naloxone challenge test†) to document the absence of physiological dependence and reduce the risk of precipitated withdrawal. The naloxone challenge test is not recommended in pregnant patients.

● *Other Uses*

A combination of pentazocine hydrochloride and naloxone hydrochloride in a ratio of 100:1 is commercially available for oral use as an analgesic. (See Pentazocine 28:08.12.) Combinations of buprenorphine hydrochloride and naloxone hydrochloride in a ratio of 4:1 for sublingual administration or approximately 6:1 for intrabuccal administration are commercially available for use in the management of opioid dependence. (See Buprenorphine 28:08.12.)

Naloxone has been used in the prevention of opioid-induced pruritus† in children and adolescents.

DOSAGE AND ADMINISTRATION

● General

Patient Monitoring

- Carefully monitor patients who have responded to naloxone; the duration of action of most opioids may exceed that of naloxone and may result in recurrent respiratory and CNS depression. Administer repeated doses of naloxone when necessary.

- Monitor pediatric patients who have responded to naloxone for at least 24 hours.

- Monitor for development of opioid withdrawal symptoms (e.g., abdominal cramps, body aches, diarrhea, fever, increased blood pressure, nausea or vomiting, nervousness, runny nose, piloerection, restlessness or irritability, shivering or trembling, sneezing, sweating, tachycardia, weakness, yawning).

Other General Considerations

- Resuscitative measures such as maintenance of a patent airway, artificial ventilation, cardiac massage, and vasopressor agents should be available and employed when necessary in the treatment of opioid overdose.

- State naloxone laws vary, and may permit prescribing and dispensation to patients with risk factors for overdose or to lay persons (including nonmedical first responders, potential bystanders, and family and friends of opioid users). Consult state law for further information.

- Carefully instruct patients and their family members or close contacts regarding clinical manifestations requiring naloxone administration, proper administration technique, and the importance of seeking emergency care immediately following administration of the initial dose. Advise caregivers, household members, and other close contacts of where naloxone is stored, and to ensure the location is easily accessible during an emergency (e.g., naloxone should not be stored in a locked container with the opioid).

- Advise patients taking doses of opioid analgesics when away from home to carry naloxone with them and to advise individuals who are with them of the availability of the drug and its proper use.

● Administration

Naloxone may be administered by IV, subcutaneous, or IM injection; by IV infusion; or intranasally. The drug also has been administered via endotracheal tube† and by intraosseous† (IO) injection.

Parenteral Administration

Naloxone may be administered via IV, IM, or subcutaneous routes, depending on the product formulation. The American Academy of Pediatrics (AAP) does not endorse subcutaneous or IM administration for emergency medical management of opioid intoxication in children or neonates since hypotension, hypoperfusion, and/or peripheral vasoconstriction may result in erratic or delayed absorption of the drug.

Continuous IV infusions of naloxone may be most appropriate in patients who require higher doses, continue to experience recurrent respiratory or CNS depression after effective therapy with repeated doses, and/or in whom the effects of long-acting opioids are being antagonized. For continuous IV infusion, the manufacturers state that 2 mg of naloxone hydrochloride may be diluted in 500 mL of 0.9% sodium chloride or 5% dextrose injection to produce a solution containing 0.004 mg/mL (4 mcg/mL). Titrate the rate of IV infusion in accordance with the patient's response. Other concentrations have been recommended (see Standardize 4 Safety under Dosage and Administration). Following dilution in 5% dextrose or 0.9% sodium chloride injection to a concentration of 0.004 mg/mL (4 mcg/mL), naloxone solutions are stable for 24 hours; after 24 hours, discard any unused solution.

Naloxone hydrochloride 5 mg/0.5 mL injection (Zimhi®) is administered by IM or subcutaneous injection into the anterolateral aspect of the thigh, through clothing if necessary, using the prefilled syringes and accompanying delivery device. When administered to pediatric patients younger than 1 year of age, pinch the thigh muscle while administering the prefilled syringe. This preparation is intended to be administered by individuals ≥12 years of age since younger individuals with limited hand strength may find the device difficult to use.

Prior to administration, carefully inspect parenteral solutions of naloxone for the presence of particulate matter or discoloration.

Store vials, ampuls, and prefilled syringes containing naloxone hydrochloride injection at 20–25°C and protect from light.

Intranasal Administration

Naloxone may be administered intranasally for the emergency treatment of known or suspected opioid overdose. To administer the intranasal formulation, place the patient in a supine position and then remove the nasal spray unit from the carton and blister package. Tilt the patient's head back, with one hand supporting the neck. Do not prime or test the device prior to administration. Gently insert the tip of the nasal spray unit into one nostril until the fingers on either side of the nozzle are against the patient's nose, and press the device plunger firmly to administer the dose. Remove the nozzle from the nostril following administration of the drug, place the patient in the recovery position, and closely monitor. If additional doses are required, administer each dose into alternate nostrils using a new nasal spray unit. Call for emergency medical assistance immediately after administration of the first dose of naloxone nasal spray. Consult the prescribing information for formulation-specific administration instructions.

Store naloxone nasal spray (Narcan®) below 25°C (excursions permitted up to 40°C). Store naloxone nasal spray (Kloxxado®) at 20–25°C (excursions permitted at 5–40°C). Do not freeze or expose intranasal naloxone to temperatures above 40°C. Protect from light. If the nasal spray freezes (e.g., if stored below -15°C), the device will not spray. If this occurs, do not wait for the nasal spray to thaw; seek emergency medical help immediately. Naloxone nasal spray may still be used if it has been thawed after previously being frozen.

Endotracheal and Intraosseous Administration

When IV access cannot be established in emergency situations, naloxone can also be administered effectively via an endotracheal tube† in adults or pediatric patients or by IO† injection for opioid overdosage in pediatric patients.

Standardize 4 Safety

Standardize 4 safety (S4S) is a national patient safety initiative to standardize drug concentrations to reduce medication errors, especially during transitions of care. Multidisciplinary expert panels were convened to determine recommended standard concentrations. Because recommendations from the S4S panels may differ from the manufacturer's prescribing information, caution is advised when using concentrations that differ from labeling, particularly when using rate information from the label. For additional information on S4S (including updates that may be available), see https://www.ashp.org/pharmacy-practice/standardize-4-safety-initiative.

TABLE 1. Standardize 4 Safety Continuous IV Infusion Standard Concentrations for Naloxone Hydrochloride

Patient Population	Concentration standard[a]	Dosing units
Pediatric patients (<50 kg)	16 mcg/mL	mcg/kg/hr
	40 mcg/mL	
	400 mcg/mL	
Adults	16 mcg/mL	mg/hr[b]
	40 mcg/mL	mcg/kg/hr - pruritus†

[a] The panel recognizes that 40 and 400 mcg/mL concentrations listed in the pediatric standards are 10× different; however, these are the only two concentrations studied for stability.

[b] Dosing units differ from concentration units

● Dosage

Naloxone is commercially available as naloxone hydrochloride; dosage is expressed in terms of the salt.

Postoperative Opioid Depression in Pediatric Patients
Parenteral

When naloxone hydrochloride is used to partially reverse opioid depression following the use of opioids during surgery in pediatric patients, the usual initial dosage recommended by the manufacturers is 0.005–0.01 mg IV, given at 2- to 3-minute intervals until the desired response (i.e., adequate ventilation and alertness without substantial pain or discomfort) is obtained. Additional doses may be necessary at 1- to 2-hour intervals depending on the response of the patient and the dosage and duration of action of the opioid administered.

Opioid-induced Depression in Neonates
Parenteral

When used to reverse opioid-induced depression in neonates, the usual initial dosage of naloxone hydrochloride is 0.01 mg/kg, administered IV, IM, or subcutaneously at 2- to 3-minute intervals to the desired degree of reversal.

Known or Suspected Opioid Overdosage in Children
Parenteral

Children may receive an initial IV naloxone hydrochloride dose of 0.01 mg/kg; if this dose does not produce the desired degree of response, a subsequent dose of 0.1 mg/kg may be administered.

Since the duration of action of the opioid is often longer than that of naloxone, the depressant effects of the opioid may return as the effects of naloxone diminish, and additional doses of naloxone may be required.

The dosage delivered by the initial dose of naloxone hydrochloride prefilled syringes for IM or subcutaneous use (Zimhi®) is 5 mg; if the desired response is not obtained after 2 or 3 minutes of administration, an additional dose may be administered every 2 to 3 minutes until emergency medical assistance arrives. Observe the patient closely and seek emergency care immediately following administration of the initial dose. If necessary, perform supportive and/or resuscitative measures until emergency care arrives.

Intranasal

The recommended initial dose of naloxone hydrochloride nasal spray in pediatric patients is one spray (2, 4, or 8 mg) administered intranasally into one nostril. If the patient fails to respond or responds but subsequently relapses back into respiratory depression before emergency assistance arrives, administer additional doses every 2–3 minutes using a new nasal spray unit into the alternating nostril until emergency personnel arrive.

The requirement for repeat doses depends upon the amount, type, and route of administration of the opioid being antagonized.

Reversal of respiratory depression by partial agonists or mixed agonist/antagonists, such as buprenorphine and pentazocine, may be incomplete and require higher doses of naloxone hydrochloride or repeated administration using a new nasal spray.

Endotracheal, Intraosseous

Some experts suggest an endotracheal† or IO† dose of 0.1 mg/kg in pediatric patients younger than 5 years of age or weighing 20 kg or less or a dose of 2 mg in pediatric patients 5 years of age or older or weighing more than 20 kg; however, the optimum dose of naloxone administered via an endotracheal tube† remains to be established and higher (e.g., double or triple) doses may be necessary.

Postoperative Opioid Depression in Adults
Parenteral

When naloxone hydrochloride is used to partially reverse opioid depression following the use of opioids during surgery in adults, the usual initial dosage recommended by the manufacturers is 0.1–0.2 mg IV, given at 2- to 3-minute intervals until the desired response (i.e., adequate ventilation and alertness without substantial pain or discomfort) is obtained. Additional doses may be necessary at

1- to 2-hour intervals depending on the response of the patient and the dosage and duration of action of the opioid administered.

The manufacturers state that supplemental IM doses of naloxone produce a more prolonged effect than repeated IV doses of the drug. For continuous IV infusion, titrate the rate of IV infusion in accordance with the patient's response.

Known or Suspected Opioid Overdosage in Adults
Parenteral

For the treatment of known or suspected opioid overdosage, the usual initial adult dosage of naloxone hydrochloride is 0.4–2 mg IV, administered at 2- to 3-minute intervals if necessary; if no response is observed after a total of 10 mg of the drug has been administered, the depressive condition may be caused by a drug or disease process not responsive to naloxone. Naloxone hydrochloride 2 mg may also be administered IM or subcutaneously using naloxone prefilled syringes.

Since the duration of action of the opioid is often longer than that of naloxone, the depressant effects of the opioid may return as the effects of naloxone diminish, and additional doses of naloxone may be required.

The dosage delivered by the initial dose of naloxone hydrochloride prefilled syringes for IM or subcutaneous administration (Zimhi®) is 5 mg; if the desired response is not obtained after 2 or 3 minutes of administration, an additional dose may be administered every 2 to 3 minutes until emergency medical assistance arrives.

Intranasal

The recommended initial dose of naloxone hydrochloride nasal spray in adults is one spray (2, 4, or 8 mg) administered intranasally into one nostril. If the patient fails to respond or responds but subsequently relapses into respiratory depression before emergency personnel arrive, administer additional 2-, 4-, or 8-mg doses using a new nasal spray unit every 2–3 minutes into alternating nostrils until emergency personnel arrive. Prescribe the 2-mg strength for opioid-dependent patients expected to be at risk for severe opioid withdrawal only when the risk for accidental or intentional opioid exposure by household contacts is low.

Endotracheal

The optimal dosage of most drugs, including naloxone, via endotracheal administration is not established; however, the typical dose given by the endotracheal route is 2–2.5 times the recommended IV dose.

Diagnosis of Suspected or Known Acute Opioid Overdosage

The manufacturers make no specific recommendations at this time for dosage in diagnosis of suspected or known acute opioid overdosage. However, if no response is observed after administration of 10 mg of naloxone, the diagnosis of opioid-induced toxicity should be questioned.

Septic Shock

Because of the limited number of patients who have been treated, optimal dosage and treatment regimens have not been established.

Naloxone Challenge Test

Administration of naloxone hydrochloride 0.4–0.8 mg before initiating treatment with naltrexone may assist in documenting the absence of physiological dependence and minimizing the risk for withdrawal.

Opioid-induced Pruritus

When naloxone hydrochloride was used in the prevention of opioid-induced pruritus† in children and adolescents, dosages ranged from 0.25–1.0 mcg/kg per hour via continuous IV infusion.

● Special Populations

Hepatic Impairment

The manufacturers make no specific dosage recommendations for patients with hepatic impairment.

Renal Impairment

The manufacturers recommend using caution when administering naloxone injection to patients with renal impairment.

Geriatric Patients

The manufacturers recommend using caution when selecting a dose of naloxone for geriatric patients.

CAUTIONS

• Contraindications

• Patients with known hypersensitivity to the drug or any ingredient in the formulation.

• Warnings/Precautions

Other Resuscitative Measures

When naloxone is used in the management of acute opioid overdosage, other resuscitative measures (e.g., maintenance of an adequate airway, artificial respiration, cardiac massage, vasopressor agents) should be readily available and used when necessary.

Excessive Doses in Postoperative Patients

Following the use of opioids during surgery, excessive doses of naloxone hydrochloride may result in significant reversal of analgesia and cause agitation.

Use in Patients with Cardiovascular Disorders

Hypotension, hypertension, ventricular tachycardia and fibrillation, pulmonary edema, and cardiac arrest have been reported in postoperative patients receiving naloxone, sometimes resulting in death, coma, or encephalopathy. These events have been observed mainly in patients with preexisting cardiovascular disorders or who were receiving other drugs with similar adverse cardiovascular effects.

Use naloxone with caution in patients with preexisting cardiovascular disease or in those receiving potentially cardiotoxic drugs; monitor such patients for hypotension, ventricular tachycardia or fibrillation, and pulmonary edema.

Limited Efficacy with Partial Agonists or Mixed Agonist/Antagonists

Reversal of respiratory depression resulting from overdosage of opioid partial agonists (e.g., buprenorphine, pentazocine) may be incomplete and require higher or repeated doses of naloxone.

Precipitation of Severe Opioid Withdrawal

Administer naloxone with caution to patients known or suspected to be physically dependent on opioids (including neonates born to women who are opioid dependent), particularly in patients with cardiovascular disease, because the drug may precipitate severe withdrawal symptoms.

Abrupt postoperative reversal of opioid effects may induce nausea, vomiting, sweating, tremor, tachycardia, increased blood pressure, hypotension, hypertension, seizures, ventricular tachycardia and fibrillation, pulmonary edema, and cardiac arrest, which may result in death. These events have been observed mainly in patients with preexisting cardiovascular disorders or who were receiving other drugs with similar adverse cardiovascular effects. (See Use in Patients with Cardiovascular Disorders under Cautions.)

Risk of Recurrent Respiratory and CNS Depression

The duration of action of most opioids may exceed that of naloxone resulting in a return of respiratory and/or CNS depression after an initial improvement. Carefully monitor patients and administer repeated doses of naloxone when necessary. Some experts state that while a brief observation period may be adequate following overdosage of certain opioids with a shorter duration of action (morphine, heroin), patients who have presented with life-threatening overdosage of a long-acting or extended-release opioid may require longer periods of observation. The manufacturers state that pediatric patients who have responded to naloxone must be carefully monitored for at least 24 hours.

Risk of Accidental Needlestick Injury

After using naloxone prefilled syringes for IM or subcutaneous injection (Zimhi®), the needle is exposed until the safety guard is deployed. A needlestick injury could occur during use in emergency situations. If an accidental needlestick occurs, seek medical attention. Seek immediate evaluation by a medical professional for potential exposure to blood borne pathogens (e.g., HIV, hepatitis B virus, hepatitis C virus). Stress to patients the importance of familiarizing themselves with the device and its operation prior to experiencing an emergency situation.

Specific Populations

Pregnancy

There are limited data to date on use of naloxone in pregnant women. Naloxone should be used during pregnancy only when clearly needed. Reproduction studies in mice and rats using naloxone hydrochloride dosages of 4 and 8 times, respectively, a human dosage of 10 mg daily in a 50-kg individual demonstrated no embryotoxic or teratogenic effects. Furthermore, no adverse effects were reported in the offspring of rats receiving naloxone hydrochloride subcutaneously at dosages of 2 or 10 mg/kg (up to 12 times a human dosage of 8 mg daily) from gestation day 15 to postnatal day 21. No embryotoxic or teratogenic effects were observed in mice and rats during the period of organogenesis with the 8 mg/0.1 mL nasal spray at doses 3 and 6 times a human dose of 16 mg.

The risk-benefit ratio must be considered before naloxone is administered to a pregnant woman who is known or suspected to be dependent on opioids, since maternal dependence may often be accompanied by fetal dependence. Naloxone crosses the placenta and may precipitate withdrawal symptoms in both the fetus and the pregnant woman. Use of naloxone in opioid-dependent pregnant women should be accompanied by monitoring for fetal distress.

It is not known if naloxone affects the duration of labor and/or delivery. However, published reports indicate that administration of naloxone during labor did not adversely affect maternal or neonatal status. Carefully monitor patients with mild to moderate hypertension who receive naloxone during labor, as severe hypertension may occur.

Lactation

It is not known whether naloxone is distributed into milk or has any effect on the breast-fed infant or on milk production; use naloxone with caution in nursing women. The drug does not affect prolactin or oxytocin concentrations in nursing women, and oral bioavailability of naloxone is minimal.

Females and Males of Reproductive Potential

Animal studies revealed no evidence of impaired fertility. Reproduction studies in mice and rats using naloxone hydrochloride dosages of 4 and 8 times, respectively, a human dosage of 10 mg daily in a 50-kg individual (based on body surface area) revealed no evidence of impaired fertility. In addition, studies in rats using intranasal naloxone hydrochloride dosages of 2 or 10 mg/kg (up to 12 times a human dosage of 8 mg daily) administered for 60 days prior to mating in males or administered for 14 days prior to mating and then throughout gestation in females revealed no evidence of impaired fertility. Studies using the 8 mg/0.1 mL nasal spray in mice and rats at doses 3 and 6 times, respectively, a human dose of 16 mg/day demonstrated no adverse effects on fertility.

Pediatric Use

Naloxone hydrochloride injection may be used to reverse the effects of opioids in pediatric patients, including neonates. In addition, safety and efficacy of naloxone hydrochloride prefilled syringes for IM or subcutaneous use (Zimhi®) or nasal spray (e.g., Narcan®, Kloxxado®) have been established in pediatric patients of all ages for the emergency treatment of known or suspected opioid overdosage manifested by respiratory and/or CNS depression. Use of naloxone for reversal of opioid effects in pediatric patients is supported by adult bioequivalence studies and evidence from the safe and effective use of other naloxone hydrochloride products.

As in adults, naloxone may precipitate opiate withdrawal in pediatric patients who are physically dependent on opiates; however, unlike opiate withdrawal in adults, neonatal opiate withdrawal may be life-threatening and should be treated according to protocols developed by neonatology experts. To avoid abrupt precipitation of neonatal opiate withdrawal syndrome, use of a naloxone preparation that can be dosed based on weight and titrated to effect may be preferred over a preparation that delivers a fixed dose of the drug (e.g., auto-injector, nasal spray) in neonates with known or suspected exposure to maternally administered opiates.

Absorption of naloxone following intranasal administration or IM or subcutaneous injection in pediatric patients may be erratic or delayed. Pediatric patients who have responded to naloxone must be carefully monitored for at least 24 hours, since relapse may occur as the opioid antagonist is metabolized.

Safety and efficacy of naloxone hydrochloride injection in the management of hypotension associated with septic shock have not been established in pediatric patients. In a study of 2 neonates with septic shock, treatment with naloxone produced a positive pressor response; however, one patient subsequently died after intractable seizures.

Geriatric Use

Clinical studies of naloxone did not include sufficient numbers of patients 65 years of age and older to determine whether geriatric patients respond differently than younger patients. While other clinical experience has not revealed age-related differences in response, drug dosage generally should be titrated carefully in geriatric patients, usually initiating therapy at the low end of the dosage range. The greater frequency of decreased hepatic, renal, and/or cardiac function and of concomitant disease and drug therapy observed in the elderly also should be considered.

Hepatic Impairment

Safety and efficacy of naloxone in patients with hepatic impairment have not been established in well-controlled clinical trials. Use naloxone with caution in these patients.

Renal Impairment

Safety and efficacy of naloxone in patients with renal impairment have not been established in well-controlled clinical trials. Use naloxone with caution in these patients.

• Common Adverse Effects

Intranasal naloxone: Adverse effects reported in clinical trials of intranasally administered naloxone include abdominal pain, asthenia, dizziness, headache, increased blood pressure, constipation, toothache, muscle spasms, musculoskeletal pain, nasal congestion, nasal discomfort, nasal dryness, nasal edema, nasal inflammation, presyncope, rhinalgia, and xeroderma.

Parenteral naloxone: Adverse effects, including serious and fatal cases, reported in clinical trials of parenterally administered naloxone for postoperative patients include cardiac arrest, dyspnea, hypotension, hypertension, pulmonary edema, and ventricular tachycardia and fibrillation. Excessive doses of naloxone in postoperative patients may result in agitation caused by significant reversal of analgesia. Adverse effects reported in clinical trials of parenterally administered naloxone after abrupt reversal of dependence are related to acute withdrawal syndrome, which may include the following signs and symptoms: abdominal cramps, body aches, diarrhea, fever, increased blood pressure, nausea or vomiting, nervousness, runny nose, piloerection, restlessness or irritability, shivering or trembling, sneezing, sweating, tachycardia, weakness, yawning. Abrupt reversal of opioid depression may result in cardiac arrest, increased blood pressure, nausea, pulmonary edema, seizures, sweating, tachycardia, tremulousness, ventricular tachycardia and fibrillation, and vomiting. In the neonate, opioid withdrawal may also include convulsions, excessive crying, and hyperactive reflexes. Adverse effects reported in clinical trials of naloxone hydrochloride injection for IM or subcutaneous use (Zimhi®) included dizziness, elevated bilirubin, lightheadedness, and nausea.

DRUG INTERACTIONS

Naloxone is metabolized in the liver primarily by glucuronide conjugation.

• Buprenorphine

Buprenorphine has a long duration of action; therefore, large doses of naloxone are required to antagonize buprenorphine.

• Methohexital

Methohexital appears to block the acute onset of withdrawal symptoms induced by naloxone in patients with opioid addiction.

DESCRIPTION

Naloxone hydrochloride is an opioid antagonist. The precise mechanism of action of the drug's opioid antagonist effects is not fully understood. Naloxone is thought to act as a competitive antagonist at μ, κ, and σ opiate receptors in the CNS; it is thought that the drug has the highest affinity for the μ receptor.

Naloxone can reverse the psychotomimetic and dysphoric effects of agonist-antagonists such as pentazocine. Because the duration of action of naloxone is generally shorter than that of the opioid, the effects of the opioid may return as the effects of naloxone dissipate.

Naloxone does not produce tolerance or physical or psychological dependence. In patients who are dependent on opioids, parenteral administration of naloxone will precipitate opioid withdrawal symptoms, which may appear within minutes of naloxone administration and subside in about 2 hours. The severity and duration of the withdrawal symptoms are related to the dose of naloxone and the degree and type of opioid dependence.

The onset of action of naloxone is within 2 minutes following parenteral administration, and is shorter for IV compared to IM or subcutaneous routes of administration. The duration of action depends on the dose and route of administration and is more prolonged following IM administration than after IV administration.

Following intranasal administration of naloxone hydrochloride (2, 4, or 8 mg) nasal spray in healthy adults, the median time to peak plasma concentration was similar to that observed following IM injection of a 0.4-mg dose of the drug and the dose-normalized bioavailability relative to that of the IM injection ranged from 43–54%. Peak plasma concentrations and AUC of naloxone were substantially higher following intranasal administration of a 2-mg dose as a single spray in one nostril (approximately 3.3- and 2.6-fold higher, respectively), a 4-mg dose as a single spray in one nostril (approximately 5.5- and 4.4-fold higher, respectively), a 4-mg dose as one 2-mg spray in each nostril (approximately 7.2- and 5.4-fold higher, respectively), or an 8-mg dose as one 4-mg spray in each nostril (approximately 11- and 8.7-fold higher, respectively) than following IM injection of a 0.4-mg dose.

Following intranasal administration of naloxone hydrochloride (Kloxxado®) 8 mg (single spray) in healthy adults, the median time to peak plasma concentration was similar to that observed following IM injection of a 0.4-mg dose of the drug and the dose-normalized bioavailability relative to that of the IM injection ranged from 42–47%. Peak plasma concentrations and AUC of naloxone were substantially higher following intranasal administration of an 8-mg dose (approximately 12- to 13-fold and 17- to 19-fold higher, respectively) than following IM injection of a 0.4-mg dose.

Following parenteral administration, naloxone is rapidly distributed into body tissues and fluids. Naloxone is weakly bound to plasma proteins (mainly albumin). In humans, the drug readily crosses the placenta. It is not known whether naloxone is distributed into breast milk. The half-life of naloxone has been reported to be 30–81 minutes in adults and about 3 hours in neonates. The mean plasma half-life of naloxone was 1.5 hours following IM or subcutaneous injection of naloxone 5 mg using a prefilled syringe (Zimhi®). Following intranasal administration, naloxone exhibits a slightly longer half-life compared with the IM route (1.8–2.7 versus 1.2–1.4 hours). Naloxone is rapidly metabolized in the liver, principally by conjugation with glucuronic acid. The major metabolite is naloxone-3-glucuronide. Limited studies with radiolabeled naloxone indicate that 25–40% of an oral or IV dose of the drug is excreted as metabolites in urine in 6 hours, about 50% in 24 hours, and 60–70% in 72 hours.

ADVICE TO PATIENTS

- Advise patients, family members, and caregivers to read the FDA-approved patient labeling and to become familiar with all information related to appropriate administration of the provided naloxone formulation.

- Instruct patients and family members or close contacts regarding clinical manifestations requiring naloxone administration, proper administration technique, and the importance of seeking emergency care immediately following administration of the initial dose.

- Advise caregivers, household members, and other close contacts of where naloxone is stored, and to ensure the location is easily accessible during an emergency (e.g., naloxone should not be stored in a locked container with the opioid).

- Instruct patients and their family members or caregivers on recognition of signs and symptoms of opioid overdose (e.g., extreme somnolence, respiratory depression, miosis, bradycardia, hypotension).

- Advise patients of the risk of recurrent respiratory and CNS depression, and to seek immediate emergency medical assistance after the first dose of naloxone and to continually monitor the patient.

- Advise patients of the potential limited efficacy of naloxone administration when used to reverse respiratory depression caused by partial agonists or mixed agonists/antagonists such as buprenorphine and pentazocine, and that higher doses or additional administration of naloxone may be required.

- Instruct patients that administration of naloxone in patients who are opioid-dependent may precipitate severe opioid withdrawal accompanied by symptoms such as body aches, diarrhea, tachycardia, fever, runny nose, sneezing, piloerection, sweating, yawning, nausea or vomiting, nervousness, restlessness or irritability, shivering or trembling, abdominal cramps, weakness, and hypertension. Instruct patients that opioid withdrawal may be life-threatening in neonates if not recognized and properly treated; instruct patients on these signs and symptoms (e.g., convulsions, excessive crying, hyperactive reflexes).

- Advise patients to inform their clinician of existing or contemplated concomitant therapy, including prescription and OTC drugs and dietary or herbal supplements, as well as any concomitant illnesses.

- Advise women to inform clinicians if they are or plan to become pregnant or plan to breast-feed.

- Inform patients of other important precautionary information.

PREPARATIONS

To facilitate timely administration of naloxone following opioid overdosages occurring in community (nonmedical) settings, many states have taken steps to make naloxone available to first responders, community-based organizations, and laypersons (e.g., through legislation permitting prescribing to third parties, prescribing by standing order, or pharmacist prescribing or dispensing in accordance with protocols or standing orders) and to limit adverse legal consequences to prescribers and to laypersons who administer the drug.

Excipients in commercially available drug preparations may have clinically important effects in some individuals; consult specific product labeling for details.

Naloxone Hydrochloride

Intranasal		
Solution	2 mg/0.1 mL	Narcan®, Emergent Devices
	4 mg/0.1 mL*	Naloxone Hydrochloride Nasal Spray
		Narcan®, Emergent Devices
	8 mg/0.1 mL	Kloxxado®, Hikma

Parenteral		
Injection	0.4 mg/mL*	Naloxone Hydrochloride Injection (available in single-dose vials or ampuls and multiple-dose vials)
	1 mg/mL*	Naloxone Hydrochloride Injection (available in prefilled syringes)
	10 mg/mL	Zimhi®, Adamis Pharmaceuticals

* available from one or more manufacturer, distributor, and/or repackager by generic (nonproprietary) name

Pentazocine and Naloxone Hydrochlorides

Oral		
Tablets	Pentazocine Hydrochloride 50 mg (of pentazocine) and Naloxone Hydrochloride 0.5 mg (of naloxone)*	Pentazocine and Naloxone Hydrochlorides Tablets (C-IV)

* available from one or more manufacturer, distributor, and/or repackager by generic (nonproprietary) name

Naloxone Hydrochloride Dihydrate Combinations

Sublingual		
Strips, sublingually dissolving	0.5 mg (of naloxone) with Buprenorphine Hydrochloride 2 mg (of buprenorphine)*	Naloxone Sublingual Strips Suboxone® (C-III), Indivior
	1 mg (of naloxone) with Buprenorphine Hydrochloride 4 mg (of buprenorphine)*	Naloxone Sublingual Strips Suboxone® (C-III), Indivior
	2 mg (of naloxone) with Buprenorphine Hydrochloride 8 mg (of buprenorphine)*	Naloxone Sublingual Strips Suboxone® (C-III), Indivior
	3 mg (of naloxone) with Buprenorphine Hydrochloride 12 mg (of buprenorphine)*	Naloxone Sublingual Strips Suboxone® (C-III), Indivior
Tablets	0.18 mg (of naloxone) with Buprenorphine Hydrochloride 0.7 mg (of buprenorphine)	Zubsolv® (C-III), Orexo
	0.36 mg (of naloxone) with Buprenorphine Hydrochloride 1.4 mg (of buprenorphine)	Zubsolv® (C-III), Orexo
	0.5 mg (of naloxone) with Buprenorphine Hydrochloride 2 mg (of buprenorphine)*	Buprenorphine Hydrochloride and Naloxone Hydrochloride Sublingual Tablets (C-III)
	0.71 mg (of naloxone) with Buprenorphine Hydrochloride 2.9 mg (of buprenorphine)	Zubsolv® (C-III), Orexo
	1.4 mg (of naloxone) with Buprenorphine Hydrochloride 5.7 mg (of buprenorphine)	Zubsolv® (C-III), Orexo
	2 mg (of naloxone) with Buprenorphine Hydrochloride 8 mg (of buprenorphine)*	Buprenorphine Hydrochloride and Naloxone Hydrochloride Sublingual Tablets (C-III)
	2.1 mg (of naloxone) with Buprenorphine Hydrochloride 8.6 mg (of buprenorphine)	Zubsolv® (C-III), Orexo
	2.9 mg (of naloxone) with Buprenorphine Hydrochloride 11.4 mg (of buprenorphine)	Zubsolv® (C-III), Orexo

* available from one or more manufacturer, distributor, and/or repackager by generic (nonproprietary) name

† Use is not currently included in the labeling approved by the US Food and Drug Administration.

Selected Revisions June 10, 2024, © Copyright, November 1, 1976, American Society of Health-System Pharmacists, Inc.

Naltrexone
Naltrexone Hydrochloride

28:10 • OPIOID ANTAGONISTS

■ Naltrexone is essentially a pure opiate antagonist.

USES

● Opiate Dependence

Naltrexone hydrochloride is designated an orphan drug by the US Food and Drug Administration (FDA) and is used orally for its opiate antagonist effects as an adjunct to a medically supervised behavior modification program in the maintenance of opiate cessation (opiate-free state) in individuals formerly physically dependent on opiates and who have successfully undergone detoxification. Behavior modification is an integral component in maintaining opiate cessation when naltrexone is used, and such modification involves supervised programs of counseling, psychologic support and therapy, and education, and changes in life-style (social rehabilitation). The theoretical rationale for using naltrexone as an adjunct in opiate cessation therapy is that the drug may diminish or eliminate opiate-seeking behavior by blocking the euphoric reinforcement produced by self-administration of opiates and by preventing the conditioned abstinence syndrome (i.e., heightened sensitivity to stimuli, abnormal autonomic responses, dysphoria, and intense opiate craving) that occurs following opiate withdrawal. There are no data that unequivocally demonstrate a beneficial effect of naltrexone on the tendency to relapse (recidivism) to drug abuse in detoxified, former opiate-dependent individuals; however, by blocking opiate-induced euphoria and potentially preventing the redevelopment of opiate dependence (opiate use disorder [OUD]), naltrexone therapy in conjunction with a medically supervised behavior modification program may contribute to the prevention of relapse in the post-addiction period.

In individuals formerly dependent on opiates, naltrexone reportedly decreases opiate craving within 3–5 weeks of initiation of therapy; however, decreased opiate craving has occurred during the first week of naltrexone therapy in some individuals, with further decreases occurring in subsequent weeks. The efficacy of opiate cessation therapy that includes naltrexone on long-term cessation rates appears to be low, and poor compliance appears to be the major limiting factor in opiate cessation therapy that includes naltrexone. Because noncompliance with naltrexone therapy, unlike methadone or levomethadyl acetate (LAAM; no longer commercially available in the US because of potentially severe adverse cardiac effects) maintenance therapy, is not associated with unpleasant symptoms of withdrawal, compliance with opiate cessation therapy that includes naltrexone depends more on the voluntary efforts of the individual, and successful cessation appears to be more likely in highly motivated individuals. Repeated attempts at opiate cessation therapy may increase efficacy in terms of the amount of time the individual remains opiate-free; complete cessation may not be an obtainable goal in some individuals, and cycles of relapse to opiate use and cessation may be likely. Because of the potential risk of relapse to opiate use and subsequent opiate overdosage, clinicians should routinely discuss the availability of the opiate antagonist naloxone with all patients receiving new or reauthorized prescriptions for medications for treatment of OUD and should strongly consider prescribing naloxone for use in the event of an overdose in all such patients. (See Naloxone Hydrochloride 28:10.)

Behavioral therapy, as a component of opiate cessation therapy, allows the patient to undergo a social and psychologic rehabilitation that will aid in maintaining opiate cessation. Naltrexone therapy in combination with behavioral therapy has been shown to be more effective than naltrexone or behavioral therapy alone in prolonging opiate cessation in patients formerly physically dependent on opiates. Individuals who are highly motivated, employed, and in a stable married or other relationship appear to be most successful with naltrexone therapy and able to maintain opiate cessation. Strong external support from family and/or employer also contributes to the success of opiate cessation therapy that includes naltrexone. Because naltrexone is used as an adjunct to the individual's own cessation efforts, individuals should be highly motivated to develop a life-style free of opiate dependence. Individuals who are psychologically healthier generally are

more successful in opiate cessation than those with more baseline psychologic disturbances, including mood disorders. Potential candidates for opiate cessation therapy that involves naltrexone include former opiate-dependent individuals who are employed and socially functioning, were recently detoxified from methadone maintenance, are leaving prison or residential treatment settings, are sporadically abusing opiates but are not yet dependent, are physically dependent on opiates secondary to medical use of the drugs, and/or are ineligible for methadone maintenance; naltrexone therapy may also be useful when the waiting period for admission into a methadone maintenance program is long. Naltrexone may be particularly useful as maintenance therapy in the prevention of relapse in former opiate-dependent individuals during times of stress when relapse to drug abuse may be most likely. Adolescents who have only recently become physically dependent on opiates may benefit particularly well from opiate cessation therapy that includes naltrexone. Opiate cessation therapy that includes naltrexone may also be especially beneficial in health-care professionals physically dependent on opiates. However, individuals may differ in their specific needs for behavioral therapy (e.g., psychotherapy, counseling) or additional pharmacologic support (e.g., sedatives and hypnotics, GI drugs). Individuals from lower socioeconomic groups who have recently been detoxified from methadone maintenance appear to benefit less from naltrexone therapy than health-care professionals and white-collar workers; however, behavioral therapy in the form of strong family external support improves the beneficial results of naltrexone therapy observed in individuals from lower socioeconomic groups.

Most clinical experience with naltrexone therapy in detoxified, former opiate-dependent individuals has been reported to date in uncontrolled studies. In controlled studies, patients receiving naltrexone therapy generally appeared to decrease their consumption of opiates, participated in opiate cessation programs longer, and had greater decreases in craving for opiates than did patients receiving placebo.

Opiate antagonists (e.g., naltrexone, naloxone) have been used for rapid or ultrarapid detoxification in the management of opiate withdrawal† in opiate-dependent individuals, both in inpatient and outpatient settings. Rapid opiate detoxification involves the administration of opiate antagonists such as naltrexone and/or naloxone to shorten the time period of detoxification. When used for this purpose, naltrexone sometimes has been given in combination with clonidine, guanabenz, or lofexidine (not currently available in the US). The reported advantage of rapid detoxification is to minimize the risk of relapse and to initiate maintenance therapy with naltrexone and psychosocial interventions more quickly. Ultrarapid detoxification is similar, but involves the administration of opiate antagonists (i.e., naltrexone, naloxone) while the patient is sedated or under general anesthesia. However, the risk of adverse respiratory and cardiovascular effects associated with this procedure must be considered as well as the costs of general anesthesia and hospitalization. Safety and efficacy of these therapies have not been established and further study is needed.

Parenteral naltrexone is not approved for use for its opiate antagonist effects or for the treatment of OUD.

● Alcohol Dependence

Naltrexone is used orally or IM in the management of alcohol dependence in conjunction with a comprehensive management program that includes psychosocial support. Naltrexone is used IM in patients with alcohol dependence who are able to abstain from alcohol in an outpatient setting prior to initiation of naltrexone therapy and are abstinent at the time such therapy is initiated.Individuals who are willing to use pharmacologic therapy as part of their treatment for alcohol dependence are candidates for naltrexone therapy. A comprehensive management program is an integral component in maintaining alcohol cessation when naltrexone is used, since the drug has not been shown to provide any therapeutic benefit except as part of an appropriate plan of addiction management. These programs involve evaluation, counseling, psychologic support and therapy, and education. Although psychosocial programs alone (i.e., without drug therapy) may be associated with moderate improvement in complete cessation rates and substantial initial rates of alcohol cessation, long-term cessation rates are low, with 50% of patients undergoing intensive inpatient and/or outpatient behavior modification usually relapsing within the first 3 months. When pharmacologic therapy (e.g., naltrexone) is used in conjunction with a comprehensive management program, benefits of such programs may be prolonged.

In general, the goals of pharmacologic therapy in alcohol dependence are to consistently reduce craving for alcohol and to reduce the motivation to drink by blunting pleasant feelings associated with alcohol consumption. In addition, pharmacologic therapy for alcohol dependence should not interact with alcohol or have addictive potential. Factors associated with positive outcomes in clinical trials in alcohol-dependent patients receiving naltrexone for alcohol dependence include type, intensity, and duration of pharmacologic therapy; use of community-based support groups; appropriate management of conditions accompanying alcoholism; and good medication compliance.

When used in conjunction with a comprehensive management program, naltrexone reportedly decreases alcohol craving, reduces alcohol consumption, decreases the number of drinking days, maintains abstinence from alcohol ingestion, and prevents, decreases, or ameliorates the severity of relapse. However, naltrexone therapy is not uniformly effective, and the expected effect is a modest improvement in the outcome of conventional therapy. The theoretical rationale for using naltrexone as an adjunct in alcohol dependence therapy is that the drug may diminish alcohol consumption by blocking the rewarding, pleasurable effects associated with alcohol ingestion. (See Pharmacology: Opiate Antagonist Effects).

In one controlled study in alcohol-dependent patients, reported abstinence rates for naltrexone hydrochloride (50 mg orally once daily for 12 weeks) compared with placebo were 51 vs 23%, while relapse (defined as consumption of 4 or 5 drinks per occasion for women or men, respectively) within 12 weeks of the study period occurred in 31 vs 60% of patients receiving the drug or placebo, respectively. In this study, psychologic behavior modification consisted either of learning coping skills to prevent relapse or of abstinence supportive therapy without coping skills training. Further analysis of these data indicates that rates of abstinence for naltrexone vs placebo were 61 vs 19% in patients receiving supportive therapy in addition to naltrexone or placebo, respectively, while in patients undergoing coping skills training, abstinence rates were 28 vs 21% in those receiving additional naltrexone or placebo therapy, respectively.

In another controlled study in alcohol-dependent patients that evaluated oral naltrexone, rates of abstinence for naltrexone vs placebo were 54 vs 43%, respectively. Although relapse (defined as drinking during 5 or more days within 1 week, having 5 or more drinks per drinking occasion, or having an alcohol blood concentration exceeding 100 mg/dL) in this study was reported in 23 or 54% of patients receiving naltrexone hydrochloride (50 mg orally once daily for 12 weeks) or placebo, respectively, reanalysis by the manufacturer found relapse rates of 21 or 41% in patients receiving the drug or placebo, respectively. In patients who reportedly had consumed at least one drink while undergoing the study, relapse occurred in 50 or 95% of patients receiving naltrexone or placebo, respectively. Results of this study also indicate that patients receiving naltrexone experienced less pleasure after alcohol ingestion and had fewer drinking days and less alcohol craving than those receiving placebo. In an uncontrolled, large multicenter study in patients with alcohol dependence, including those with psychiatric conditions, those physically dependent on other substances, and those with human immunodeficiency virus (HIV) infection, abstinence and relapse rates were similar to those in the controlled studies.

In a study in 627 US veterans (almost all men) with chronic, severe alcoholism (history of heavy drinking at least twice in a week during the previous 30 days and a DSM-IV diagnosis of alcohol dependence but who were sober for at least 5 days prior to study entry), oral naltrexone hydrochloride therapy (50 mg daily) was not effective as an adjunct to standard psychosocial therapy in the management of alcohol dependence as evidenced by no apparent benefit after 13 weeks on days to relapse (mean: 72.3 vs 62.4 days for naltrexone and placebo, respectively) nor at 52 weeks on the percentage of days on which drinking occurred or the number of drinks per drinking day. As a result, it was concluded that the use of adjunctive naltrexone therapy could not be supported in men with chronic, severe alcoholism. Whether these findings can be extrapolated to patients with less severe or less chronic alcoholism or to women or non-veterans remains to be established. Patients in this study relative to other studies typically were older, had been drinking for longer periods, and were less likely to be married or living with a partner; although employment data were not reported, about one-third were receiving disability pensions, which may have negatively affected their motivation to stop drinking. Pending further accumulation of data, some experts recommend that naltrexone continue to be prescribed for patients considered likely to benefit from such therapy such as those who have been drinking heavily for no longer than 20 years and who have stable social support and living situations.

Efficacy of oral naltrexone therapy for alcohol dependence has been established in short-term (up to 12 weeks) clinical studies involving a limited number of patients with alcohol dependence, and the long-term safety and efficacy of the drug for the management of this condition have not been established.

Efficacy of an injectable extended-release formulation of naltrexone has been evaluated in a 6-month study in individuals with alcohol dependence. Adults were randomized to receive naltrexone 380 mg, naltrexone 190 mg, or placebo administered IM monthly in conjunction with 12 sessions of psychosocial intervention. Treatment with 380 mg of naltrexone was associated with a greater reduction in days of heavy drinking (defined as 5 or more alcohol-containing drinks per day for men and 4 or more alcohol-containing drinks per day for women) than treatment with placebo. Individuals receiving 380 mg of naltrexone reported a 25% greater reduction in the rate of heavy drinking relative to placebo-treated individuals. Treatment with 190 mg of naltrexone generally was not associated with a substantial reduction in the rate of heavy drinking. Subgroup analyses suggested that treatment effects were greater in men than in women and also were greater in individuals with lead-in abstinence (about 8% of the study population) than in those who drank during the lead-in phase. Naltrexone-associated reductions in heavy drinking were observed in men and individuals with lead-in abstinence, but the same effects were not observed in women or individuals who drank during the lead-in period.

Studies sponsored by the National Institute of Alcohol Abuse and Alcoholism (NIAAA) are ongoing in an attempt to identify which alcohol-dependent patients are most likely to benefit from naltrexone therapy, to determine optimum duration and dosage of naltrexone, and to identify potential combination therapies that are most effective for use with naltrexone in these patients. *Routine* use of naltrexone in the management of alcohol dependence currently is not recommended.

● Obesity

For use of naltrexone hydrochloride in fixed combination with bupropion hydrochloride for weight management, see Naltrexone Hydrochloride and Bupropion Hydrochloride 28:20.08.92.

● Other Uses

Naltrexone has been used in dosages up to 800 mg daily for the treatment of schizophrenic disorder,† since elevated endorphin concentrations have been observed in patients with this disorder and naltrexone may inhibit the effects of endogenous endorphins. Although a few patients with schizophrenic disorder have shown some clinical improvement during naltrexone therapy, patients generally showed no improvement and psychoses worsened in some patients. Naltrexone has also been used in a patient with a psychoneurologic syndrome of unknown etiology† that included some signs and symptoms similar to those associated with mast cell disease, carcinoid disease, and dermatitis herpetiformis; the drug reversed and/or suppressed flush and organic psychosis and associated mood alterations, anxiety, and severe skin, bone, and abdominal pain in this patient.

There is preliminary evidence that opiate antagonists (i.e., naloxone, naltrexone) may cause some clinical improvement in patients with dementia of the Alzheimer's type (Alzheimer's disease), but additional study of the efficacy of these drugs in this disease is necessary. In one study in a limited number of patients, there was little evidence of cognitive or behavioral improvement following oral naltrexone dosages up to 100 mg daily.

DOSAGE AND ADMINISTRATION

● Reconstitution and Administration

Naltrexone hydrochloride is administered orally. Adverse GI effects may be minimized by taking the drug with food or antacids or after meals.

Naltrexone extended-release injection is administered by deep IM injection into the upper outer quadrant of the gluteal muscle every 4 weeks or once a month. Subsequent injections should be made in alternate buttocks. To avoid inadvertent injection of the suspension into a blood vessel, the plunger of the syringe should be drawn back prior to IM administration to ensure that blood is not aspirated. The IM preparation should *not* be administered by IV or subcutaneous injection; the IM preparation should *not* be inadvertently administered into fatty tissue. Inadvertent subcutaneous injection may increase the likelihood of severe injection site reactions. Therefore, the patient's body habitus should be evaluated prior to each injection to ensure that the length of the needle supplied by the manufacturer (1.5 inches) is adequate for gluteal IM injection in that patient. Because the IM preparation must be administered using the manufacturer-provided needle, alternative treatment should be considered for any patient whose body habitus (i.e., thickness of gluteal adipose tissue) precludes IM injection with the provided needle. Patients should be instructed to monitor the injection site and to notify the clinician if injection site reactions (i.e., pain, swelling, tenderness, induration, bruising, pruritus, redness) worsen or if they do not improve within 2 weeks following injection. Patients should be advised to notify the clinician promptly if intense or prolonged pain, swelling, skin color changes, or signs of necrosis (e.g., hard nodule, blistering, open wound, dark scab) are present at the injection site. Patients with signs of abscess, cellulitis, necrosis, or extensive swelling at the injection site should be promptly evaluated to determine if referral to a surgeon is warranted.

Naltrexone for extended-release injectable suspension should be reconstituted prior to administration using the components of the dose pack supplied by the manufacturer. The dose pack should be allowed to reach room temperature prior to reconstitution of the injection. The preparation should be reconstituted using only the diluent supplied by the manufacturer and administered with the needle supplied by the manufacturer. The vial labeled as containing 380 mg of naltrexone extended-release microspheres should be reconstituted with 3.4 mL of diluent and shaken vigorously for 1 minute. The resulting suspension should be administered immediately. The manufacturer's prescribing information should be consulted for further details on the reconstitution and administration of this preparation.

Patients should be advised not to attempt self-administration of opiates during therapy with the drug. (See Cautions: Precautions and Contraindications.)

The US Food and Drug Administration (FDA) required and approved a Risk Evaluation and Mitigation Strategy (REMS) for parenteral naltrexone. The REMS requires that a medication guide be given to the patient each time parenteral naltrexone is dispensed. The goal of the REMS is to inform patients about serious risks associated with parenteral naltrexone (see Cautions: Precautions and Contraindications). Patients should be advised to read the medication guide prior to initiating parenteral naltrexone therapy and before each injection of the drug. Clinicians should advise patients about the risks and benefits of parenteral naltrexone therapy prior to initiating such therapy and ensure that patients understand the risks.

● *Dosage*

Prior to initiation of naltrexone therapy in patients physically dependent on opiates, detoxification should be completed. Because of the risk of precipitating opiate withdrawal (see Cautions: Opiate Withdrawal), the manufacturers recommend that a period of at least 7–10 days elapse between discontinuance of opiates and initiation of naltrexone therapy. This period varies depending on the dose and duration of the opiate used, and some clinicians recommend at least 7 days in patients using relatively short-acting opiates (e.g., heroin, hydromorphone, meperidine, morphine) and at least 10–14 days in those using longer-acting opiates (e.g., methadone). Because of the risk of relapse to drug abuse during this period, shorter periods of opiate abstinence (e.g., 2–5 days) prior to initiation of naltrexone therapy have been used in some patients. Alternatively, clonidine has been used concomitantly with naltrexone during initiation of therapy to minimize symptoms of opiate withdrawal. Some clinicians have cautiously precipitated withdrawal using repeated naloxone injections and then rapidly initiated naltrexone therapy with incremental doses of the drug; this procedure can reduce the transition period from opiate dependence to naltrexone maintenance and generally is well accepted by patients. Detoxification from opiates may be accomplished in an outpatient or supervised (e.g., hospital) setting. Detoxification in a supervised setting permits closer monitoring of patients during withdrawal, control over access to illicit drugs, and the opportunity to initiate naltrexone therapy during the period when the tendency to relapse to drug abuse may be greatest. Regardless of the setting for detoxification, it generally is preferable to detoxify the patient from all drugs on which they are dependent before initiating naltrexone therapy. In addition to patient verification of abstinence from opiates, urinalysis should be performed after the minimum 7- to 10-day waiting period, but prior to administration of naltrexone, to confirm the absence of opiates. If urinary determination is negative, a naloxone challenge test should be performed prior to administering naltrexone if the clinician believes there is a risk of precipitating a withdrawal reaction following administration of naltrexone.

Naloxone Challenge Test

To avoid precipitating opiate withdrawal following administration of naltrexone, the naloxone challenge test should be performed prior to induction of naltrexone therapy in patients formerly physically dependent on opiates who have completed detoxification and in those suspected of having been dependent on opiates. *The naloxone challenge test should not be performed in patients who are exhibiting signs and/or symptoms of opiate withdrawal, those whose urine shows evidence of opiates, or those in whom there is a high degree of suspicion that opiates are still being used, since naloxone may precipitate potentially severe opiate withdrawal. If signs and/or symptoms of opiate withdrawal are evident following administration of the naloxone challenge test, naltrexone therapy should not be attempted;* the naloxone challenge test may be repeated in 24 hours in these patients.

The manufacturer of naltrexone recommends that the naloxone challenge test be performed by administering naloxone by IV or subcutaneous injection. For IV or subcutaneous administration of the test, a sterile syringe containing 0.8 mg of naloxone hydrochloride should be used. For IV administration, the manufacturer of naltrexone recommends that an initial 0. 2-mg dose of the drug be injected IV and, while the needle remains in the vein, the patient should be observed for 30 seconds for evidence of opiate withdrawal. Alternatively, some clinicians recommend that an initial 0. 2-mg dose of naloxone hydrochloride be injected IV and the patient observed for 15 minutes for evidence of withdrawal. Signs and symptoms of withdrawal include, but are not limited to, nasal stuffiness, rhinorrhea, lacrimation, yawning, sweating, tremor, abdominal cramps, vomiting, piloerection, myalgia, and skin crawling. (See Chronic Toxicity in the Opiate Agonists General Statement 28:08.08.) If no evidence of withdrawal is observed, the remaining 0. 6-mg dose of naloxone hydrochloride should be injected IV and the patient observed for an additional 20 minutes for evidence of withdrawal. Some clinicians recommend that a total IV dose of 2 mg be used in the test since withdrawal has been precipitated by the first oral dose of naltrexone despite a negative naloxone challenge test using lower doses and a false-negative test rarely occurs with the 2-mg naloxone hydrochloride dose. For subcutaneous administration, the entire 0. 8-mg dose should be injected subcutaneously and the patient observed for 20 minutes for evidence of opiate withdrawal. For further information on the chemistry and stability, pharmacology, pharmacokinetics, uses, cautions, and dosage and administration of naloxone, see Naloxone Hydrochloride 28:10.

During the appropriate period (i.e., 20 or 45 minutes) in the naloxone challenge test, the patient should be closely monitored for the appearance of signs and symptoms of opiate withdrawal and vital signs should be monitored. Although the naloxone challenge test may precipitate opiate withdrawal in a patient physically dependent on opiates, signs and symptoms will be milder and of shorter duration than those precipitated by naltrexone. If signs and/or symptoms of opiate withdrawal are evident following administration of the naloxone challenge test, a potential risk for precipitating more severe and prolonged withdrawal with naltrexone exists and naltrexone therapy should *not* be initiated; if evidence of withdrawal is absent, naltrexone therapy may be initiated. (See Induction of Therapy for Opiate Cessation in Dosage and Administration: Dosage.) Some clinicians caution that even minor and/or transient GI symptoms following naloxone challenge be considered evidence of withdrawal since patients with such symptoms will often develop severe and disturbing GI symptoms if naltrexone therapy is then initiated. If evidence of opiate withdrawal is present, naltrexone therapy should be delayed and the naloxone challenge test repeated in 24 hours with the 0. 8-mg dose and every 24 hours until results are negative.

Opiate Dependence

Induction of Therapy for Opiate Cessation

Following completion of opiate detoxification and verification that the patient is free of opiates, oral naltrexone therapy is initiated with an induction regimen. Naltrexone therapy should be initiated carefully by slowly titrating the dose; an initial 25-mg dose of naltrexone hydrochloride is recommended by the manufacturer. Following administration of the initial dose, the patient should be observed for 1 hour for the development of opiate withdrawal. If no evidence of withdrawal is present, the usual oral dosage of 50 mg once daily can be started the next day. Alternatively, some clinicians have induced therapy by administering an initial 10- or 12. 5-mg dose of naltrexone hydrochloride, followed by incremental increases of 10 or 12.5 mg daily until the usual dosage of 50 mg daily has been achieved. Therapy has also been induced by administering an initial 5-mg dose, followed by incremental increases of 10 mg hourly until the usual total daily dose of 50 mg has been achieved.

Maintenance Therapy for Opiate Cessation

Following induction of therapy, an oral maintenance dosage of 50 mg of naltrexone hydrochloride daily produces adequate antagonist activity to block the pharmacologic effects of parenterally administered opiates (e.g., a 25-mg IV dose of heroin). Flexible naltrexone dosing schedules in which the dose and/or frequency of administration of the drug are altered in an attempt to improve compliance have been suggested. The manufacturer states that naltrexone hydrochloride may be administered in dosages of 50 mg daily Monday through Friday and 100 mg on Saturday, 100 mg every other day, or 150 mg every third day. Alternatively, the drug has been administered in a regimen of 100 mg on Monday and Wednesday and 150 mg on Friday or in a regimen of 150 mg on Monday and 200 mg on Thursday. Although the opiate antagonist activity may be somewhat reduced by the administration of larger doses of naltrexone hydrochloride at longer intervals, improved patient compliance may result from administration of the drug every 48–72 hours rather than daily. Most clinicians suggest that observed ingestion of the drug in a clinic setting or by a responsible family member generally be used to ensure compliance, in which case, regimens requiring less frequent visits may be more acceptable to the patient. Some patients, particularly those who are employed, may remain in opiate cessation programs longer if they are permitted take-home doses once they are doing well in the program. Some clinicians suggest that random testing of urine for naltrexone and 6-β-naltrexol or for the presence of opiates may be used to monitor patient compliance.

The optimum duration of naltrexone maintenance therapy has not been established, but should be based on individual requirements and response. In general, patients formerly physically dependent on opiates need a minimum of 6 months to make the behavioral changes necessary to maintain opiate cessation, and naltrexone therapy may be beneficial during this period. For patients unable to successfully deal with the temptation of opiate use, maintenance naltrexone therapy may be necessary throughout the course of a comprehensive opiate cessation program. For other patients, short-term maintenance therapy with naltrexone during the early transition from opiate use to abstinence may be all that is necessary. For other patients who are able to remain abstinent for prolonged periods after an initial period of treatment but who may revert to opiate use during a crisis or get occasional irresistible cravings for opiates, additional naltrexone therapy may only be necessary during these periods. In patients who discontinue naltrexone therapy prematurely and then desire to resume therapy following a relapse to opiate abuse, urinalysis for the presence of opiates and, if necessary, a naloxone challenge test should be performed prior to resuming naltrexone therapy; if there is evidence of opiate dependence, detoxification should be conducted prior to reinitiation of naltrexone therapy.

Management of Opiate Withdrawal

In studies of naltrexone for the management of opiate withdrawal†, various dosage regimens of the drug have been used for rapid or ultrarapid detoxification of opiate dependence. In one study evaluating naltrexone in combination with clonidine, an initial 0. 005-mg/kg dose of clonidine hydrochloride was administered on the first day of detoxification to attenuate opiate withdrawal; clonidine dosage was then titrated according to the severity of withdrawal and the adverse effects induced by clonidine. The highest mean dose of clonidine hydrochloride was 2.3 mg daily, administered on the third day of detoxification. Naltrexone therapy was initiated on the second day of detoxification and administered every 4 hours on the second and third days; the initial dose of naltrexone hydrochloride was 1 mg and was increased by 1- and 2-mg increments during the daytime on the second and third days of detoxification, respectively. Clonidine was also administered every 4 hours on the second and third days to attenuate the withdrawal induced by naltrexone; however, after the third day, clonidine was administered only as needed to reduce signs and symptoms of withdrawal. Naltrexone hydrochloride was administered at a dosage of 10 mg 3 times daily on the fourth day, and as single 50-mg daily doses thereafter.

Alcohol Dependence

Following verification that the patient is free of opiates (see Dosage: Naloxone Challenge Test, in Dosage and Administration), oral naltrexone hydrochloride therapy may be initiated for alcohol dependence. A dosage of 50 mg once daily has been recommended for patients with alcohol dependence. Since about 5–15% of patients reportedly have experienced adverse effects (mainly GI effects) with this dosage, some clinicians have recommended an initial dose of 25 mg, dividing the daily dosage, or adjusting the time of dosing in an effort to minimize such effects; however, naltrexone-associated adverse effects did not appear to be alleviated by such alterations in the recommended dosage. Safety and efficacy of naltrexone hydrochloride for alcohol dependence have been established only in short-term (up to 12 weeks) clinical studies using an oral naltrexone hydrochloride dosage of 50 mg daily, and the optimum duration of naltrexone therapy for this condition currently is not known.

When naltrexone extended-release injection is used for the treatment of alcohol dependence in patients who are free of opiates (See Dosage: Naloxone Challenge Test, in Dosage and Administration), the recommended dosage is 380 mg of naltrexone IM every 4 weeks or once a month. The IM preparation should *not* be administered by IV or subcutaneous injection; the IM preparation should not be inadvertently administered into fatty tissue (see Dosage and Administration: Reconstitution and Administration).

If the patient misses a dose, the next dose should be administered as soon as possible. Dosage adjustment is not needed in patients with mild to moderate (Child-Pugh class A or B) hepatic impairment or mild renal impairment (creatinine clearance of 50–80 mL/minute). Patients initiating therapy with naltrexone for alcohol dependence may initiate therapy with the parenteral preparation; it is not necessary to initiate therapy with oral naltrexone and then switch to the parenteral preparation. Information regarding reinitiation of naltrexone therapy in patients who discontinued such therapy is lacking; data needed to support recommendations for switching patients from oral to parenteral naltrexone therapy have not been systematically collected.

CAUTIONS

At usual oral dosages, adverse effects of naltrexone are generally mild to moderate in severity and usually subside within a few days. Because of the potential for naltrexone to precipitate or exacerbate withdrawal in patients formerly physically dependent on opiates and who are not completely free of the drugs, adverse effects associated with naltrexone in some patients may have been secondary to opiate withdrawal. Many adverse effects reported during administration of naltrexone have occurred prior to as well as during administration of the drug and may be the result of alcohol and drug abuse and poor nutrition; in some patients, adverse effects improved or resolved during administration of the drug. Therefore, a causal relationship for many adverse reactions to naltrexone has not been clearly established.

When administered to opiate-free individuals in usual oral dosages (i.e., 50 mg daily), naltrexone generally has not caused serious adverse effects or abnormal laboratory test results (e.g., liver function). In several controlled studies, the incidence of naltrexone-associated adverse effects was similar to that reported with placebo. In addition, in uncontrolled studies, the incidence of naltrexone-induced adverse effects (e.g., lymphocytosis, increases in serum aminotransferase [transaminase] concentrations, GI effects) was similar to that expected in individuals not receiving the drug.

In controlled studies in alcohol-dependent patients receiving oral therapy with naltrexone hydrochloride 50 mg daily for 12 weeks, the drug was well tolerated. In these studies, nausea required discontinuance of therapy in about 5% of patients; however, no serious adverse effects were reported.

Adverse effects reported in patients with alcohol dependence receiving naltrexone extended-release IM injection generally have been described as mild to moderate. The most common adverse effects associated with IM therapy with the drug are injection site reactions, nausea, and headache. (See Cautions: Precautions and Contraindications.)

● GI Effects

The most frequent adverse effects reported in individuals receiving oral naltrexone are GI effects. Abdominal pain and cramps, nausea, and vomiting reportedly occur in more than 10% of patients receiving naltrexone for opiate dependence and may occasionally be severe enough to require discontinuance of the drug. Adverse GI effects reported in 1–10% of patients receiving the drug for opiate dependence include constipation and anorexia. Other adverse GI effects reported in less than 1% of patients receiving the drug for opiate dependence include diarrhea, flatulence, upset stomach, hemorrhoids, epigastric pain or heartburn, and ulcer. Nausea and vomiting were reported in 10 and 3%, respectively, of patients receiving naltrexone for the management of alcohol dependence, and were among the most common adverse effects reported in these patients.

Nausea (most commonly following the initial dose), vomiting, or diarrhea occurred in 33, 14, or 13%, respectively, of individuals receiving naltrexone extended-release IM injection in a dosage of 380 mg every 4 weeks in clinical studies. Abdominal pain, dry mouth, or anorexia (appetite disorder) was reported in 11, 5, or 14%, respectively, of these individuals. Nausea has required discontinuance of the drug in about 2% of patients.

● Hepatic Effects

Naltrexone reportedly can cause dose-related hepatocellular injury, manifested as increases in serum hepatic enzyme concentrations. Liver function abnormalities have been observed mainly in patients receiving high dosages (e.g., 300 mg daily) of the drug investigationally for the treatment of obesity or dementia of the Alzheimer's type (Alzheimer's disease), but increases in serum aminotransferase concentrations have also occurred following administration of dosages 2 times that recommended for blockade of pharmacologic effects of opiates. Following naltrexone hydrochloride dosages of 300 mg daily for 3–8 weeks in obese patients in one placebo-controlled study, serum ALT (SGPT) concentrations increased to up to 3–19 times the baseline values in about 20% of patients receiving the drug, but not in those receiving placebo, and decreased to or near baseline values within several weeks following discontinuance of the drug. In another placebo-controlled study in obese patients, increases in serum ALT, AST (SGOT), and/or LDH concentrations occurred in about 15% of patients receiving 50 or 100 mg of naltrexone hydrochloride daily for 8 weeks and in about 25% of those receiving placebo; in the naltrexone-treated group, hepatic enzymes decreased to at or less than baseline values over several weeks to months following discontinuance of the drug. Clinical symptoms of hepatotoxicity generally were not present in patients with liver function abnormalities. Mild liver function abnormalities are common in very obese patients, probably secondary to fatty infiltration of the liver, and were present in about 50% of obese patients at baseline in one naltrexone study. Increases in serum aminotransferase concentrations have also occurred in several patients with a history of alcohol dependence or of hepatitis.

The manufacturer states that naltrexone-induced hepatocellular injury appears to be a direct toxic rather than an idiosyncratic effect of the drug. However, some clinicians suggest that liver function abnormalities associated with naltrexone use may be caused by noroxymorphone, a minor metabolite of naltrexone that has opiate agonist activity, since opiate agonists have been shown to cause increases in serum hepatic enzyme concentrations and hepatocellular injury in animals and humans. In addition, opiate antagonists, including naltrexone, have been shown to block the increases in serum hepatic enzymes and hepatocellular injury caused by opiates. Therefore, additional study to more fully elucidate the hepatotoxic potential of naltrexone and its metabolites and any possible dose relationship is necessary.

Hepatotoxicity reportedly has not occurred at dosages recommended for blockade of pharmacologic effects of opiates, and serum concentrations of liver enzymes observed following recommended dosages of the drug have been reported to be similar to those observed in the same patients prior to administration of naltrexone. In one short-term study, the incidence of serum AST elevations in individuals receiving parenteral naltrexone was similar to the incidence in those receiving oral naltrexone (1.5% each) and higher than the incidence in those receiving placebo (0.9%). Deterioration in pretreatment liver function abnormalities in former opiate-dependent patients has not been reported to date following initiation of naltrexone therapy. However, the manufacturers state that the margin between therapeutic and hepatotoxic dosages may be less than fivefold, and the hepatotoxic potential of naltrexone must be considered prior to initiation of and during therapy with the drug. (See Cautions: Precautions and Contraindications.)

● Nervous System Effects

Adverse nervous system effects reported in more than 10% of patients receiving oral naltrexone for opiate dependence include headache, lassitude, low energy, difficulty sleeping, anxiety, and nervousness. Increased energy, mental depression, irritability, and dizziness have been reported in 1–10% of patients receiving oral naltrexone for opiate dependence. Other adverse nervous system effects reported in less than 1% of patients receiving the drug for opiate dependence include paranoia, akathisia, fatigue, restlessness, confusion, dysphoria, disorientation, hallucinations, lightheadedness, nightmares and bad dreams, talkativeness, yawning, drowsiness or somnolence, and malaise. In some patients receiving the drug for opiate dependence, severe lethargy and somnolence have developed after only one or two doses of naltrexone and persisted for 12–36 hours; several such patients were receiving a phenothiazine antipsychotic agent (thioridazine) concomitantly.

Depression, suicide, attempted suicide, and suicidal ideation (possibly associated with substance abuse) have been reported in patients receiving oral naltrexone for opiate or alcohol dependence, but the risk of suicide is known to be increased in substance abusers with or without depression, and a causal relationship to the drug has not been established. Clinicians should consider that naltrexone has not been associated with a decrease in the risk of suicide. Depression has been reported in up to 15% of patients receiving oral naltrexone for alcohol

dependence. Suicidal ideation or attempted suicide has been reported in up to 1% of these individuals. Headache occurred in 7% and dizziness, nervousness, fatigue, insomnia, anxiety, and somnolence have been reported in 2–4% of patients receiving oral naltrexone for the treatment of alcohol dependence.

Headache, dizziness, and somnolence have occurred in 25, 13, and 4%, respectively, of individuals receiving naltrexone extended-release IM injection in a dosage of 380 mg every 4 weeks in clinical studies. Insomnia or sleep disorder, anxiety, and depression have been reported in 14, 12, and 8–10%, respectively, of these individuals. Headache has required discontinuance of the drug in about 1% of patients. Suicidality (i.e., suicidal ideation, suicide attempt, completed suicide) was reported more frequently in individuals receiving parenteral naltrexone than in those receiving placebo (1 versus 0%). Two completed suicides, both in naltrexone-treated individuals, occurred in controlled clinical studies.

● Musculoskeletal Effects

Joint and muscle pain reportedly occur in more than 10% of patients receiving oral or parenteral naltrexone. Other adverse musculoskeletal effects reported in less than 1% of patients receiving oral naltrexone include tremors, twitching, and painful shoulders, legs, or knees. Back pain or stiffness and muscle cramps have occurred in 6–8% of patients receiving parenteral naltrexone in the recommended dosage.

● Dermatologic Effects

Rash has been reported in 1–10% of patients receiving oral naltrexone. Oily skin, pruritus, acne, athlete's foot, cold sores, and alopecia have been reported in less than 1% of these patients.

● Local Reactions

Injection site reactions, including tenderness, induration, pain, pruritus, ecchymosis, nodules, and swelling, have been reported in 65% of patients receiving parenteral naltrexone in the recommended dosage and have required discontinuance of the drug in about 3% of patients. Cellulitis, hematoma, abscess, sterile abscess, and necrosis also have been reported during postmarketing surveillance of parenteral naltrexone. Some injection site reactions may be very severe, result in substantial scarring, or require surgical intervention, including debridement of necrotic tissue. Injection site reactions have occurred predominantly in females. Inadvertent subcutaneous injection may increase the likelihood of a severe injection reaction. (See Cautions: Precautions and Contraindications and see Dosage and Administration: Reconstitution and Administration.)

● Respiratory and Cardiovascular Effects

Respiratory symptoms, including nasal congestion, rhinorrhea, sneezing, sore throat, excessive mucus or phlegm production, sinus trouble, labored breathing, hoarseness, cough, epistaxis, and dyspnea, have been reported in less than 1% of patients receiving oral naltrexone. Adverse cardiovascular effects reported in less than 1% of these patients include phlebitis, edema, increased systolic and/or diastolic blood pressures, nonspecific ECG changes, palpitation, and tachycardia. Systolic pressures have returned to pretreatment levels after the first week of therapy in some patients.

Upper respiratory tract infection and pharyngitis have occurred in 11–13% of patients receiving the recommended dosage of parenteral naltrexone. Eosinophilic pneumonia has been reported in at least one individual receiving parenteral naltrexone. Clinicians should consider eosinophilic pneumonia in the differential diagnosis of patients with pneumonia that has not responded to anti-infective therapy.

● Opiate Withdrawal

Naltrexone may precipitate mild to severe signs and symptoms of withdrawal in some patients physically dependent on opiates. The manufacturers recommend that a period of at least 7–10 days elapse between discontinuance of opiates and initiation of naltrexone therapy, and patients should be adequately evaluated to confirm that they are free of opiates prior to initiating therapy with the drug. (See Cautions: Precautions and Contraindications.)

Accidental ingestion of naltrexone has precipitated severe withdrawal in some patients physically dependent on opiates; signs and symptoms of withdrawal usually appeared within 5 minutes of ingestion of naltrexone and continued for up to 48 hours. Signs and symptoms of opiate withdrawal vary in severity depending on the specific opiate used, its dose and duration of use, and individual physiologic and psychologic characteristics of the patient. Signs and symptoms of opiate withdrawal reported in patients receiving naltrexone have included drug craving, confusion, drowsiness, visual hallucinations, abdominal pain, and vomiting and diarrhea which resulted in substantial fluid loss requiring IV fluid replacement therapy in some patients. Other signs and symptoms of withdrawal included fever, chills, tachypnea, perspiration, salivation, lacrimation, rhinorrhea, and mydriasis. Opiate-like withdrawal symptoms, including lacrimation, nasal symptoms, mild nausea, abdominal cramps, restlessness, bone or joint pain, and myalgia have been reported in a few healthy individuals and alcohol-dependent patients receiving naltrexone. It is not known if these symptoms were associated with occult opiate use or with naltrexone therapy. For additional information on opiate withdrawal, including its management, see Chronic Toxicity in the Opiate Agonists General Statement 28:08.08.

● *Other Adverse Effects*

Chills have been reported in less than 10% of patients receiving oral naltrexone. Increased thirst reportedly occurs in more than 1% of these patients.

Other adverse effects of oral naltrexone reportedly occur in less than 1% of patients. Adverse genitourinary effects include urinary frequency and dysuria. Adverse ocular effects include blurred vision, sensitivity to light, burning, swelling, and aching and strained eyes. Adverse otic effects include congestion, tinnitus, and aching ears. Other adverse effects include lymphocytosis, decreased hematocrit, increased appetite, weight loss or gain, fever, diaphoresis, dry mouth, throbbing head, inguinal pain, swollen glands, cold feet, and hot flushes (flashes).

Idiopathic thrombocytopenic purpura reportedly occurred in one patient receiving oral naltrexone; however, the patient improved without additional complications following discontinuance of the drug and initiation of corticosteroid therapy. Although the patient may have developed hypersensitivity to naltrexone during previous therapy, standard antigen-antibody studies failed to clearly establish a causal relationship to the drug.

A hypersensitivity reaction, characterized by an allergic rash, occurred in one patient receiving oral naltrexone but disappeared 5 days after discontinuance of the drug; palmar erythema, pruritus, and exfoliative dermatitis reappeared upon rechallenge with low doses of the drug.

Altered plasma proteins and increases in IgM, IgA, and IgG levels have been reported in patients receiving oral naltrexone but may have been the result of alcohol abuse or a history of hepatitis.

Asthenia has occurred in 23% of patients receiving the recommended dosage of parenteral naltrexone.

Although the manufacturers state that a dose-related causal relationship between naltrexone and abnormal liver function test results has been established (see Cautions: Hepatic Effects), other abnormal laboratory test results observed during oral naltrexone therapy have not been directly attributed to the drug. Increases in eosinophil counts (which returned to normal over several months with continued use of the drug), decreases in platelet count not associated with bleeding, and serum creatine kinase (CK, creatine phosphokinase, CPK) abnormalities have occurred in individuals receiving parenteral naltrexone. Changes in baseline concentrations of some hypothalamic, pituitary, adrenal, or gonadal hormones have occurred in patients receiving opiate antagonists; however, the clinical importance of such changes has not been established.

● *Precautions and Contraindications*

Naltrexone reportedly can cause dose-related hepatotoxicity. (See Cautions: Hepatic Effects.) Baseline determinations of liver function should be performed in all patients prior to initiation of naltrexone. The manufacturers state that the potential benefits of naltrexone therapy should be weighed carefully against the possible hepatotoxic risks of the drug in patients with active liver disease (e.g., liver function test values exceeding 3 times the upper limit of normal). However, some clinicians have questioned the need for considering withholding naltrexone therapy in most opiate or alcohol-dependent individuals with marginal evidence of hepatic injury or disease, since baseline serum concentrations of liver enzymes are frequently elevated in opiate- or alcohol-dependent individuals and evidence of hepatotoxic risk of naltrexone therapy at usual dosages has not been demonstrated in these individuals. Naltrexone is contraindicated in patients with acute hepatitis or liver failure. Naltrexone should be discontinued if manifestations of acute hepatitis (e.g., abdominal pain lasting more than a few days, light-colored [e.g., white] stools, dark urine, yellowing of the eyes) develop. Patients receiving naltrexone therapy should be instructed

to contact a clinician if such manifestations occur and to discontinue therapy with the drug (if receiving oral therapy). Although naltrexone-associated hepatic failure has not been reported, clinicians are advised to consider the risk of naltrexone-associated hepatic failure and to use the drug with caution similar to that employed with other drugs that may cause hepatic injury. In addition, some clinicians state that the possibility that naltrexone might have synergistic toxic effects in patients with alcohol-induced hepatic disease has not been ruled out. The manufacturer of oral naltrexone recommends that liver function be monitored at regular intervals in all patients during naltrexone therapy to detect hepatic injury or disease that may develop secondary to the drug. The manufacturer states that the risk of naltrexone-induced toxicity may be increased when flexible naltrexone hydrochloride dosing schedules that involve administration of single doses greater than 50 mg (e.g., 100 mg every other day, 150 mg every third day) are used, and clinicians should balance the benefits of improved patient compliance against possible risks.

Naltrexone may precipitate mild to severe withdrawal in patients physically dependent on opiates. (See Cautions: Opiate Withdrawal.) If signs and/or symptoms of withdrawal are precipitated by naltrexone in a patient physically dependent on opiates, the patient should be closely monitored and therapy adjusted according to individual requirements and response. To minimize the risk of developing acute withdrawal, opiate-dependent individuals who are candidates for naltrexone therapy should be instructed to remain free of opiates for a minimum of 7–10 days prior to initiating therapy with the drug. A urinalysis to confirm the absence of opiates should be performed after the minimum 7- to 10-day waiting period but prior to administration of naltrexone; however, the absence of opiates in urine is frequently insufficient evidence that a patient is free of opiates, and, if opiates are absent, a naloxone challenge test should also be performed prior to administering naltrexone if the clinician believes there is a risk of precipitating a withdrawal reaction following administration of naltrexone. (See Naloxone Challenge Test in Dosage and Administration: Dosage.)

Although naltrexone is a potent opiate antagonist with a dose-dependent duration of activity that ranges from 24–72 hours following oral administration, the opiate antagonist activity produced by oral or parenteral naltrexone can be overcome by administration of opiates; overcoming the blockade of pharmacologic effects produced by naltrexone may be useful in certain patients in whom opiate analgesia is necessary. Generally, if analgesia is necessary in patients receiving naltrexone, a nonopiate analgesic, regional analgesia, conscious sedation with a benzodiazepine, or general anesthesia should be used whenever possible. In an emergency situation when adequate analgesia can only be achieved by administration of an opiate agonist in naltrexone-treated patients, cautious administration of an opiate may afford adequate analgesia, but higher than usual dosages may be required. If an opiate agonist is used in these patients, the possibility that the respiratory depression produced by the opiate may be deeper and more prolonged should be considered. If an opiate is required as a component of anesthesia or analgesia, the patient should be continuously monitored in an anesthesia care setting by individuals who are trained in the use of anesthetic agents and in the management of respiratory depressant effects of potent opiates and who are not involved in the conduct of the surgical or diagnostic procedure. In addition, patients receiving naltrexone and analgesic therapy with opiate agonists may also experience apparent non-opiate receptor-induced effects such as facial swelling, pruritus, generalized erythema, or bronchoconstriction that are probably caused by opiate-induced histamine release and/or other mechanisms. Since methods for reversing opiate overdosage in patients receiving naltrexone have not been established, use of a short-acting opiate with minimal respiratory depression is preferable and dosage of the opiate agonist should be carefully adjusted according to individual requirements and response. However, regardless of the opiate agonist used, the patient should be closely monitored in a setting equipped and staffed by health-care personnel appropriately trained in cardiopulmonary resuscitation. Prior to elective surgery in which analgesia can only be achieved by administration of an opiate, oral naltrexone should be discontinued at least 48 hours prior to the surgical procedure. Use of other opiate-agonist-containing preparations such as those used for the management of cough or diarrhea should generally be avoided, since adequate therapeutic benefit may be difficult to achieve with an opiate.

Self-administration of large doses of opiates may produce serum opiate concentrations sufficient to overcome the antagonist effects of naltrexone and may produce signs and symptoms of acute opiate overdosage, including respiratory arrest, circulatory collapse, and possibly death. For a complete discussion of opiate overdosage, see Acute Toxicity in the Opiate Agonists General Statement 28:08.08.

Self-administration of smaller doses of opiate agonists than previously used may produce signs and symptoms of opiate overdosage and toxicity.

Patients undergoing naltrexone therapy should be carefully instructed that naltrexone has been prescribed as part of a comprehensive program for the treatment of their drug dependence and to carry some form of medical identification that can alert medical personnel that they are taking a long-acting opiate antagonist. Patients should be instructed to take oral naltrexone as directed; patients receiving parenteral naltrexone should be advised of the frequency of administration. Patients should be warned of the serious consequences of self-administration of opiates in an attempt to overcome the antagonist activity of naltrexone. They should be advised that self-administration of small doses of opiates (e.g., heroin) during naltrexone therapy will not result in any pharmacologic effect and that large doses may result in serious pharmacologic effects, including coma and death. Patients also should be advised that if they previously self-administered opiates, they may be more sensitive to lower doses of opiates after naltrexone therapy is discontinued. Because of the potential for relapse to opiate use and subsequent opiate overdosage to occur, patients should be advised of the benefits of naloxone administration following an opiate overdose and of their options for obtaining the drug.

Because naltrexone and its metabolites are eliminated principally in urine, naltrexone should be used with caution in patients with moderate to severe renal impairment.

Injection site reactions have been reported in patients receiving parenteral naltrexone. Patients should be instructed to monitor the injection site and to notify the clinician if injection site reactions (i.e., pain, swelling, tenderness, induration, bruising, pruritus, redness) worsen or if they do not improve within 2 weeks following injection. Patients should be advised to notify the clinician promptly if intense or prolonged pain, swelling, skin color changes, or signs of necrosis (e.g., hard nodule, blistering, open wound, dark scab) are present at the injection site. Patients with signs of abscess, cellulitis, necrosis, or extensive swelling at the injection site should be promptly evaluated to determine if referral to a surgeon is warranted.

As with any preparation administered IM, parenteral naltrexone should be used with caution in patients with thrombocytopenia or other coagulation disorder (e.g., hemophilia).

Because eosinophilic pneumonia has been reported rarely in patients receiving parenteral naltrexone, patients receiving this preparation should be advised to seek medical attention if symptoms of pneumonia develop.

Depression and suicidality have occurred in naltrexone-treated individuals. Patients receiving naltrexone should be closely monitored for symptoms of depression and suicidal thinking and should be advised to contact their clinician immediately if they experience new or worsening symptoms of depression or suicidal thoughts.

Because naltrexone may cause dizziness, patients should be advised to avoid driving or operating heavy machinery until they know how the drug affects them.

The US Food and Drug Administration (FDA) required and approved a Risk Evaluation and Mitigation Strategy (REMS) for parenteral naltrexone. The REMS requires that a medication guide be given to the patient each time parenteral naltrexone is dispensed. The goal of the REMS is to inform patients about serious risks associated with parenteral naltrexone. Patients should be advised to read the medication guide prior to initiating parenteral naltrexone therapy and before each injection of the drug. Clinicians should advise patients about the risks and benefits of parenteral naltrexone therapy prior to initiating such therapy and ensure that patients understand the risks.

Naltrexone is contraindicated in patients receiving opiate agonists (except for emergency situations), nondetoxified patients physically dependent on opiates (including those receiving methadone), patients experiencing acute opiate withdrawal, patients who experience opiate withdrawal following administration of the naloxone challenge test, and patients in whom urinalysis for the presence of opiates is positive. Naltrexone is also contraindicated in patients with acute hepatitis or hepatic failure and in patients with known hypersensitivity to the drug or any ingredient in the formulation. It is not known whether cross-sensitivity exists between naltrexone and naloxone or phenanthrene-derivative opiate agonists (e.g., codeine, morphine, oxymorphone).

● **Pediatric Precautions**

Safety of naltrexone in children younger than 18 years of age has not been established.

● **Geriatric Precautions**

Clinical studies of parenteral naltrexone did not include sufficient numbers of patients 65 years of age or older to determine whether geriatric patients respond differently than younger adults.

● **Mutagenicity and Carcinogenicity**

Mutagenic changes and chromosomal damage have occurred in vitro in human lymphocytes and Chinese hamster ovarian cells, in the Drosophila recessive lethal assay, and in nonspecific DNA repair tests with *Escherichia coli* and WI-38 cells. However, the importance of these findings has not been determined and naltrexone did not show evidence of mutagenic potential in many other tests using bacterial, mammalian, or tissue culture systems.

In a 2-year study of the carcinogenic potential of naltrexone, there was an increase in the frequency of mesotheliomas in male rats and tumors of vascular origin in both male and female rats. No evidence of carcinogenicity was observed in several other 2-year studies in mice or rats receiving naltrexone dosages of 30 or 100 mg/kg daily (47 or 150 times greater than the usual dosage in humans), respectively.

The possible mutagenic and carcinogenic effects of 6-β-naltrexol (an active metabolite) are unknown.

● **Pregnancy, Fertility, and Lactation**

Pregnancy

In reproduction studies in rats and rabbits, oral naltrexone was shown to increase the incidence of early fetal loss. There are no adequate and controlled studies to date using naltrexone in pregnant women, and the drug should be used during pregnancy only when the potential benefits justify the possible risks to the fetus. It is not known whether naltrexone affects the duration of labor and delivery.

Fertility

Naltrexone dosages of 100 mg/kg daily in rats (about 16 times the usual human oral dosage based on body surface area) produced an increase in pseudopregnancy and a decrease in the pregnancy rate in mated rats, but the relevance of these findings to human fertility is not known. Use of the drug has been associated with delayed ejaculation and decreased or increased sexual potency in less than 10% of patients. Increased (see Pharmacology: Other Effects) or decreased libido has been reported in less than 1% of patients.

Lactation

Naltrexone and its major metabolite, 6-β-naltrexol, are distributed into human milk. Because of the potential for serious adverse effects in nursing infants, a decision should be make whether to discontinue nursing or the drug, taking into account the importance of the drug to the woman.

DRUG INTERACTIONS

The manufacturer states that concomitant administration of naltrexone with drugs other than opiate agonists has not been studied; therefore, naltrexone should be used with caution in patients receiving other drugs.

● **Opiate Agonists**

Patients receiving naltrexone may not benefit therapeutically from opiate-containing preparations, including those used for the management of cough and cold, diarrhea, and pain. Use of these preparations should generally be avoided during naltrexone therapy. (See Cautions: Precautions and Contraindications.) Because naltrexone can precipitate potentially severe opiate withdrawal, naltrexone should not be used in patients receiving opiates or in nondetoxified patients physically dependent on opiates (including those receiving methadone maintenance treatment).

● **Effects on Hepatic Clearance of Drugs**

Since naltrexone is metabolized principally in the liver, other drugs that alter hepatic metabolism may increase or decrease serum naltrexone concentrations. In animals and in vitro, naltrexone and 6-β-naltrexol (an active metabolite) have been shown to inhibit hepatic metabolism of aminopyrine and aniline via hepatic microsomal mixed-function oxidase enzymes; the importance of this effect on metabolism of other drugs in humans requires further study. Naltrexone reportedly does not induce its own metabolism.

● Other Drugs

Naltrexone has been administered concurrently with non-opiate drugs (e.g., disulfiram, antidepressants, lithium) frequently used in the treatment of drug dependence without evidence of unusual adverse effects; however, these drug interactions have not been examined closely under a controlled clinical environment.

Because the safety and efficacy of concomitant use of naltrexone and disulfiram currently are not known but potentially hepatotoxic drugs usually are not administered concomitantly, the manufacturer recommends that the drugs be used together only if the potential benefits justify the possible risks to the patient. Augmentation of naltrexone-induced lethargy and somnolence have been reported following initial doses of naltrexone in several patients stabilized on phenothiazine therapy (thioridazine). (See Cautions: Nervous System Effects.)

In a study in healthy individuals, concomitant use of acamprosate (1 g every 12 hours) and naltrexone hydrochloride (50 mg orally once daily) resulted in an increase in the rate and extent of absorption of acamprosate but did not alter the pharmacokinetics of naltrexone or 6-β-naltrexol. Area under the plasma concentration-time curve (AUC) and peak plasma concentration of acamprosate were increased by 25 and 33%, respectively, and time to peak plasma concentration was reduced by 33% when acamprosate and naltrexone were given concomitantly. Cognitive testing indicated that, although each drug alone was associated with some adverse effects on cognitive performance, combined use of the drugs did not appear to enhance these effects.

Following abrupt discontinuance of methadone, concomitant administration of naltrexone and clonidine hydrochloride has attenuated withdrawal symptoms generally precipitated or exacerbated by naltrexone. Clonidine alone reduces the severity of opiate withdrawal symptoms by stimulation of presynaptic α_2-adrenergic receptors resulting in attenuation of rebound increases in noradrenergic activity in the CNS, which may be responsible for the behavioral symptoms of opiate withdrawal. Concomitant administration of clonidine and naltrexone may reduce the duration of opiate withdrawal by decreasing opiate-induced postsynaptic supersensitivity.

LABORATORY TEST INTERFERENCES

Naltrexone reportedly does not interfere with the determination of urinary morphine, methadone, or quinine using thin-layer (TLC), gas-liquid (GLC), or high-pressure liquid (HPLC) chromatography. Naltrexone may interfere with some immunoassay or enzymatic methods used for the detection of urinary opiates.

ACUTE TOXICITY

The manufacturers state that there has been limited experience to date with overdosage of naltrexone in humans.

● Pathogenesis

The oral LD$_{50}$ of naltrexone has been reported to be 1.1–1.55, 1.45, 1.49, and 3 g/kg in mice, rats, guinea pigs, and monkeys, respectively; death usually occurred within 4 hours after administration. The IV LD$_{50}$ has been reported to be 180 mg/kg in mice, and the subcutaneous LD$_{50}$ has been reported to be 550–590, 1930, and 200 mg/kg in mice, rats, and dogs, respectively. Acute toxicity from naltrexone in mice, rats, and dogs resulted in death secondary to tonic-clonic seizures and/or respiratory failure. Weight loss occurred in monkeys following subcutaneous administration of 100-mg/kg doses, and prostration, seizures, and death occurred following subcutaneous administration of 300-mg/kg doses. Hypoactivity, salivation, and emesis occurred in monkeys following oral administration of 1-g/kg doses, and seizures and death occurred following oral administration of 3-g/kg doses.

Patients receiving 800 mg of naltrexone hydrochloride daily for up to 1 week in one study showed no evidence of toxicity. However, lower dosages reportedly have been hepatotoxic in some patients. (See Cautions: Hepatic Effects.) No serious adverse effects were observed following administration of single naltrexone doses of up to 784 mg (as the extended-release IM injection) in several healthy individuals.

● Treatment

There has been limited experience to date in the treatment of naltrexone overdosage, but supportive and symptomatic treatment should be initiated as necessary. When the drug has been ingested orally, usual measures to decrease GI absorption of the drug (e.g., induction of emesis, gastric lavage) should also be employed. Clinicians should consider contacting a poison control center for the most current information on treatment of naltrexone overdosage.

PHARMACOLOGY

● Opiate Antagonist Effects

Naltrexone hydrochloride is essentially a pure opiate antagonist. In contrast to levallorphan or nalorphine but like naloxone, naltrexone generally has little or no agonist activity. The opiate antagonist activity of naltrexone on a weight basis is reportedly 2–9 times that of naloxone, 17 times that of nalorphine, and about one-tenth that of cyclazocine (not currently available in the US). The major metabolite of naltrexone, 6-β-naltrexol, is also an opiate antagonist and may contribute to the antagonist activity of the drug. (See Pharmacokinetics: Elimination.) When administered in usual doses to patients who have not recently received opiates, naltrexone exhibits little or no pharmacologic effect. At oral doses of 30–50 mg daily, naltrexone generally produces minimal analgesia, only slight drowsiness, and no respiratory depression. Psychotomimetic effects or circulatory changes are generally absent following administration of naltrexone. However, pharmacologic effects, including psychotomimetic effects, increased systolic and/or diastolic blood pressure, respiratory depression, and decreased oral temperature, which are suggestive of opiate agonist activity, have reportedly occurred in a few individuals. The drug has also occasionally produced a small degree of miosis in some individuals, suggesting some opiate agonist activity, but the exact mechanism of this effect is not known. It has been suggested that a metabolite of naltrexone (e.g., noroxymorphone) may be responsible for any opiate agonist activity observed with the drug. (See Pharmacokinetics: Elimination.)

In patients who have received single or repeated large doses of morphine or other opiate agonists, naltrexone attenuates or produces a complete but reversible block of the pharmacologic effects (e.g., physical dependence, analgesia, euphoria, tolerance) of the opiate. The drug antagonizes most of the subjective and objective effects of opiates, including respiratory depression, miosis, euphoria, and drug craving. Like naloxone, naltrexone probably also antagonizes the psychotomimetic effects of opiate partial agonists (e.g., pentazocine). Because the duration of action of naltrexone may be shorter than that of the opiate, the effects of the opiate may return as the effects of naltrexone dissipate. The degree of opiate antagonism produced by naltrexone depends on the dose and the time elapsed since the last dose of naltrexone and the dose of the opiate. Doses of up to 3 g daily of oral naloxone are necessary to produce the degree of antagonist activity produced by 30- to 50-mg daily doses of oral naltrexone.

Naltrexone does not produce physical or psychologic dependence, and tolerance to the drug's opiate antagonist activity reportedly does not develop. Naltrexone may precipitate mild to potentially severe withdrawal in individuals physically dependent on opiates or pentazocine.

The precise mechanism of the opiate antagonist effects of naltrexone is not known. However, naltrexone reportedly shares the actions of naloxone and is thought to act as a competitive antagonist at μ, κ, and δ receptors in the CNS; the drug appears to have the highest affinity for the μ receptor. The drug may displace opiates from opiate-occupied receptor sites by competitive binding at the receptors, and displacement of naltrexone from these receptors by opiates is also reportedly possible. In one study in dogs, naltrexone failed to antagonize the agonist effect of N-allylnormetazocine at the Σ receptor. Naltrexone may antagonize the pharmacologic effects of endorphins, but the effect of the drug on endorphins has not been fully elucidated. Sensitivity to the analgesic effects of morphine and the number of opiate receptors in the CNS has reportedly increased in rats following chronic subcutaneous administration of naltrexone for 8 days; sensitivity and number of receptors returned to pretreatment levels within 6 days after withdrawal of naltrexone.

The mechanism of action of naltrexone in alcohol dependence is not known. Evidence from studies in animals suggests that alcohol ingestion stimulates release of endogenous opiate agonists, which may increase some of the rewarding effects associated with alcohol ingestion through agonist activity at opiate (e.g., μ) receptors. In animals and humans, opiate antagonists (e.g., naltrexone) that competitively bind to opiate receptors may reduce alcohol consumption by blocking the effects of endogenous opiates and thus making alcohol ingestion less pleasurable. In addition, naltrexone appears to decrease substantially the subjective alcohol "high" and increase the negative or dysphoric effects associated with alcohol consumption. The drug also may decrease alcohol-associated stimulant effects and increase alcohol-associated sedative effects without altering psychomotor performance in individuals receiving an intoxicating dose of alcohol. Naltrexone does not cause disulfiram-like reactions following ingestion of alcohol.

● *Endocrine Effects*

Like naloxone, naltrexone has been shown to increase plasma concentrations of luteinizing hormone (LH), corticotropin (ACTH), and cortisol. Since corticotropin has been shown to have partial antagonist activity at opiate receptors, it has been suggested that increases in plasma concentrations of corticotropin and cortisol following administration of naltrexone may result from displacement of corticotropin and endorphins from opiate receptors by naltrexone, although other mechanisms may be responsible (e.g., naltrexone-induced release of adrenocorticotropic releasing factor). Naltrexone has been shown to have little, if any, effect on plasma concentrations of follicle-stimulating hormone (FSH) and to produce minimal increases in serum testosterone concentrations. It is believed that naltrexone may influence plasma concentrations of LH by enhancing the secretion of gonadotropin releasing hormone. When administered prior to heroin (diacetylmorphine), naltrexone prevents the decrease in plasma concentrations of LH and testosterone usually produced by heroin. However, in one study, chronic administration of naltrexone in obese individuals was shown to have little, if any, effect on plasma concentrations of LH, FSH, testosterone, estradiol, cortisol, prolactin, glucose, or insulin. Like naloxone, naltrexone generally has been shown to have little, if any, effect on plasma growth hormone (GH) or serum prolactin concentrations.

Naloxone does not affect serum concentrations of basal or stimulated glucagon. The drug does not affect serum concentrations of basal or stimulated thyrotropin (TSH) or TSH concentrations in hypothyroid patients; in animals, naltrexone has reversed the decrease in plasma TSH concentrations usually observed following exposure to acute or chronic stress. Naloxone and naltrexone indirectly block the effect of thyrotropin releasing hormone (TRH) on GI transit and fluid accumulation in rabbits and rats, presumably by blocking TRH-induced release of serotonin.

Naltrexone has increased sensory-stimulated release of acetylcholine (ACh) from the cerebral cortex in rats, but spontaneous release of ACh was unaffected by the drug. The effect of naltrexone on antidiuretic hormone (ADH, vasopressin) in humans has not been studied; in animals, naltrexone did not affect changes in plasma ADH concentrations induced by most stimuli (i.e., nicotine, osmotic stimuli, hypovolemia, hemorrhage, tail pinch, overhydration). Basal plasma concentrations of ADH have not been affected by high doses (10 mg) of naloxone. The effect of naltrexone on GI secretions has not been studied; however, naloxone has reduced basal and meal-stimulated gastric acid secretion but not postprandial gastric acid secretion or basal, meal-stimulated, or postprandial gastrin and pancreatic polypeptide secretion.

● *Other Effects*

The effect of naltrexone on catecholamines in humans has not been studied; however, in rats, naltrexone produced a decrease in the midbrain and hippocampal concentrations of norepinephrine. Increased plasma concentrations of epinephrine and norepinephrine have been reported following high (10 mg) but not low (0.4 mg) doses of naloxone.

Naltrexone has produced recurrent, spontaneous sexual arousal (i.e., penile erections) associated with dysphoric sexual ideation in several individuals. However, one study failed to confirm this finding.

In a limited number of schizophrenic patients, naltrexone hydrochloride reportedly enhanced electrical evoked potentials to somatosensory stimuli and visual evoked potentials; following administration of naltrexone (average daily dose of 500 mg at time of testing) for 8 days in schizophrenic patients, electrical evoked potentials were characterized by larger amplitude at higher stimulus intensities. These effects on evoked potentials may result from the drug's inhibition of the effects of endogenous endorphins and reversal of endorphin suppression of noradrenergic activity in the CNS.

Naltrexone, in single doses of 50 or 100 mg in healthy individuals, produced EEG patterns characterized by alpha waves of decreased frequency; in addition,

1 hour after administration of 100 mg of the drug, the EEG pattern in the fast frequency band was characterized by less power than after placebo.

Inhibition of weight gain or decreased food consumption has occurred in rats following administration of naltrexone hydrochloride in single doses ranging from 0.3–10 mg/kg or daily doses of 100 mg/kg for 1–8 weeks. Anorexia and/or weight loss have occurred in several patients following oral administration of usual dosages of naltrexone for the treatment of opiate addiction. Although the exact mechanism of the anorexic effect has not been fully determined, the drug may inhibit the effects of endogenous endorphins, and decreased concentrations of endorphins in the CNS have been associated with fasting and starvation. It has also been suggested that the anorexic effect of the drug may be characteristic of withdrawal from chronic use of opiates rather than secondary to a direct effect of naltrexone. Naltrexone, administered to mice in doses of 10 mg/kg, blocked the lack of weight gain and growth inhibition produced by 5- to 20-mg/kg doses of pentazocine administered daily for 3 weeks; in these same animals, naltrexone alone did not produce growth inhibition. In the same study, protein synthesis in brain, liver, and muscle was substantially depressed by pentazocine but was unaffected by naltrexone.

Like naloxone, naltrexone increases mean arterial pressure, cardiac output, stroke volume, and left ventricular contractility in dogs with hypovolemic shock following administration of naltrexone hydrochloride doses ranging from 2.5–10 mg/kg as a rapid IV injection or 2 mg/kg rapidly IV followed by an IV infusion of 2 mg/kg per hour for 4 hours. Pretreatment with naltrexone has blocked the potentiating effect of morphine in mice with anaphylactic shock. The effects of naltrexone in shock in humans requires further study.

Bradycardia has occurred following IV naltrexone hydrochloride doses of 5–80 mcg/kg in unanesthetized dogs; respiratory rate, blood pressure, arterial blood gases, and EEG remained unchanged throughout the dose range. Within 20 minutes of 1-mg/kg IV doses in cats, total brain oxygen consumption decreased by about 48% and blood flow to the entire brain and the pons decreased by about 40%; however, the effect of naltrexone on total oxygen consumption and blood flow in humans has not been determined.

PHARMACOKINETICS

● *Absorption*

Naltrexone hydrochloride is rapidly and almost completely (about 96%) absorbed from the GI tract following oral administration, but the drug undergoes extensive first-pass metabolism in the liver. (See Pharmacokinetics: Elimination.) Only 5–40% of an orally administered dose reaches systemic circulation unchanged. Considerable interindividual variation in absorption of the drug during the first 24 hours after a single dose has been reported. The bioavailability of naltrexone hydrochloride tablets is reportedly similar to that of an oral solution of the drug (not commercially available in the US).

Peak plasma concentrations of naltrexone and 6-β-naltrexol (the major metabolite of naltrexone) usually occur within 1 hour following oral administration of the tablets and 0.6 hours following oral administration of the solution. Because orally administered naltrexone undergoes substantial first-pass metabolism, plasma concentrations of 6-β-naltrexol following oral administration are substantially higher than corresponding concentrations of naltrexone. Following oral administration, the area under the serum concentration-time curve (AUC) for 6-β-naltrexol is 10–30 times greater than the AUC for naltrexone. Following single- or multiple-dose (i.e., once daily) oral administration of naltrexone hydrochloride 50 mg in healthy individuals, peak plasma concentrations of naltrexone and 6-β-naltrexol averaged 10.6–13.7 and 109–139 ng/mL, respectively.

Plasma concentrations of naltrexone and 6-β-naltrexol increase with increasing doses of the drug. The AUC and peak plasma concentrations of naltrexone and 6-β-naltrexol increase proportionally with single naltrexone hydrochloride doses of 50–200 mg. Following oral administration of single doses of a 50-mg tablet, two 50-mg tablets, or 100 mg of a solution in a study in healthy individuals, mean peak plasma naltrexone concentrations were 8.6, 19.6, or 20.7 ng/mL, and mean peak plasma concentrations of 6-β-naltrexol were 99.3, 206.8, or 206.2 ng/mL, respectively.

Little, if any, accumulation of naltrexone and/or 6-β-naltrexol appears to occur following chronic administration of the drug. Following chronic administration of naltrexone, plasma concentrations of 6-β-naltrexol are at least 40%

higher than those following administration of a single dose of the drug; however, plasma concentrations of naltrexone and 6-β-naltrexol 24 hours after each dose of chronically administered drug are similar to concentrations 24 hours after a single dose of the drug in most patients.

The onset of opiate antagonism following oral administration of naltrexone has been reported to be 15–30 minutes in a limited number of patients who had been receiving morphine chronically. Administration of a single 15-mg oral dose of naltrexone hydrochloride immediately following a single 30-mg subcutaneous dose of morphine has been reported to produce opiate antagonism that is prominent within 6 hours, maximal within 12 hours, and persists for at least 24 hours. The extent and duration of antagonist activity of naltrexone appear to be directly related to plasma and tissue concentrations of the drug. Plasma naltrexone concentrations of 2 ng/mL have been reported to be associated with an 87% blockade of the pharmacologic effects of a 25-mg IV dose of heroin. In one study in former opiate-dependent individuals receiving 100 mg of naltrexone hydrochloride daily and subsequently challenged with a 25-mg IV dose of heroin, the extent of blockade of the effects of heroin was 96, 87, and 47% at 24, 48, and 72 hours after naltrexone, respectively; corresponding plasma naltrexone concentrations were 2.4, 2, and 1.7 ng/mL, respectively.

The duration of the opiate antagonist activity of naltrexone appears to be dose dependent and is longer than that of equipotent doses of naloxone. A single 50-mg oral dose of naltrexone hydrochloride effectively antagonizes the pharmacologic effects of 25 mg of IV heroin or subcutaneous morphine for up to 24 hours. Increasing the dose of naltrexone hydrochloride to 100 or 150 mg reportedly antagonizes the effects of 25 mg of IV heroin for up to 48 or 72 hours, respectively.

Bioavailability of orally administered naltrexone is altered in individuals with hepatic impairment. Following oral administration of naltrexone in patients with compensated (Child-Pugh class A or B) or decompensated liver cirrhosis (Child-Pugh class C), naltrexone AUC values are fivefold or tenfold higher, respectively, than values in individuals with normal hepatic function. Although peak plasma concentrations of 6-β-naltrexol were delayed in patients with hepatic impairment, systemic exposure to the metabolite in these patients was not altered substantially compared with that in healthy individuals.

Following IM administration of naltrexone extended-release injection, the drug is released slowly and gradually from the microspheres by diffusion and erosion as the polylactide co-glycolide polymer degrades. Following IM administration of naltrexone 380 mg, peak plasma naltrexone concentrations of 12.9 ng/mL occur in 2–3 days (there is a transient initial peak 2 hours after injection); plasma concentrations start to decline after 14 days but remain detectable for 1 month or longer. Following IM administration of naltrexone 380 mg, peak plasma concentrations of 6-β-naltrexol (the major metabolite of naltrexone) generally occur in 3 days. Exposure to 6-β-naltrexol is about twofold higher than the corresponding naltrexone exposure. Following administration of a single IM dose of naltrexone 380 mg, total naltrexone exposure is threefold to fourfold higher and 6-β-naltrexol exposure is 3.4-fold lower than exposure following oral administration of naltrexone 50 mg daily for 28 days. Steady-state plasma concentrations of naltrexone and 6-β-naltrexol are attained by the end of the dosing interval after the first injection. Minimal accumulation of naltrexone and/or 6-β-naltrexol appears to occur following repeated IM administration.

Following IM administration of naltrexone extended-release injection, plasma concentrations of naltrexone and 6-β-naltrexol achieved in individuals with mild to moderate hepatic impairment (Child-Pugh class A and B) are similar to those in healthy individuals with normal hepatic function.

● Distribution

Naltrexone hydrochloride is widely distributed throughout the body, but considerable interindividual variation in distribution parameters during the first 24 hours following a single oral dose has been reported. Following subcutaneous administration of radiolabeled drug in rats, the drug distributes into CSF within 30 minutes. In animals, CSF naltrexone concentrations are reported to be approximately 30% of concurrent peak plasma concentrations. The drug and its metabolites have been shown to distribute into saliva and erythrocytes following oral administration in humans. Following IV injection of a single 1-mg dose of the drug in healthy adults with normal renal and hepatic function, the volume of distribution of naltrexone was estimated to be 1350 L. The volume of distribution of the drug in former opiate-dependent individuals with normal renal and hepatic

function reportedly averages 16.1 L/kg following oral administration of a single 100-mg dose and 14.2 L/kg following oral administration of 100 mg daily for at least 18 days.

Naltrexone is approximately 21–28% protein bound.

It is not known if naltrexone and/or its metabolites cross the placenta. Naltrexone and its major metabolite, 6-β-naltrexol, are distributed into human milk.

● Elimination

Plasma concentrations of naltrexone and 6-β-naltrexol, the major metabolite, appear to decline in a biphasic manner during the first 24 hours following a single oral dose or during chronic administration of the drug. Following oral administration of single or multiple doses of naltrexone hydrochloride, the plasma half-lives of naltrexone and 6-β-naltrexol in the initial phase ($t_{\frac{1}{2}\alpha}$) average 1.1–3.9 and 2.3–3.1 hours, respectively, and the plasma half-lives in the terminal phase ($t_{\frac{1}{2}\beta}$) average 9.7–10.3 and 11.4–16.8 hours, respectively. Plasma concentrations of naltrexone and 6-β-naltrexol have also been reported to decline in a triphasic manner following oral administration, with a terminal elimination half-life after the first 24 hours of 96 hours for naltrexone and 18 hours for 6-β-naltrexol, possibly resulting from initial distribution into body tissues and subsequent redistribution into systemic circulation.

Naltrexone is metabolized in the liver principally by reduction of the 6-keto group of naltrexone to 6-β-naltrexol (6-β-hydroxynaltrexone). Naltrexone also undergoes metabolism by catechol-O-methyl transferase (COMT) to form 2-hydroxy-3-methoxy-6-β-naltrexol (HMN) and 2-hydroxy-3-methoxynaltrexone. Several minor metabolites have also been identified, including noroxymorphone and 3-methoxy-6-β-naltrexol. Because oral but not IM administration of naltrexone results in substantial first-pass hepatic metabolism of the drug, 6-β-naltrexol concentrations following IM administration are substantially lower than concentrations of the metabolite obtained following oral administration. Naltrexone does not appear to inhibit or induce its own metabolism following chronic administration. Cytochrome P-450 (CYP) isoenzymes are not involved in the metabolism of naltrexone. Naltrexone and its metabolites undergo conjugation with glucuronic acid. The major fraction of total drug and metabolites in both plasma and urine consists of conjugated metabolites. The drug and its metabolites may undergo enterohepatic circulation.

Metabolites of naltrexone may contribute to the opiate antagonist activity of the drug. Like naltrexone, 6-β-naltrexol is an essentially pure opiate antagonist, with a potency of 6–8% that of naltrexone in precipitating withdrawal symptoms in dogs physically dependent on morphine and 1.25–2% that of naltrexone in mice. Because of its weak affinity for opiate receptors, HMN may not contribute appreciably to the opiate antagonist activity of naltrexone; however, the in vivo opiate antagonist activity of HMN or 2-hydroxy-3-methoxynaltrexone has not been studied. Noroxymorphone, a minor metabolite of naltrexone, is a potent opiate agonist and may be responsible for the agonist activity (e.g., miosis) that occurs infrequently in individuals receiving naltrexone.

Naltrexone and its metabolites (unconjugated and conjugated) are excreted principally in urine via glomerular filtration; 6-β-naltrexol, conjugated 6-β-naltrexol, and conjugated naltrexone are also excreted via tubular secretion. Naltrexone may also undergo partial reabsorption by the renal tubules. Following single- or multiple-dose oral administration of naltrexone hydrochloride, respectively, approximately 38–60 or 70% of a dose has been recovered in urine, principally as 6-β-naltrexol (conjugated and unconjugated). Most urinary excretion of naltrexone occurs within the first 4 hours after oral administration. Less than 2% of an orally administered dose is excreted unchanged in urine within 24 hours. Approximately 5–10, 19–35, 7–16, 3.5–4.6, and 0.45% of an oral dose are excreted in urine as conjugated naltrexone, 6-β-naltrexol, conjugated 6-β-naltrexol, HMN, and 2-hydroxy-3-methoxynaltrexone, respectively, within 24 hours. Less than 5% of a dose is excreted in feces, principally as 6-β-naltrexol, within 24 hours following single- or multiple-dose oral administration of the drug. Following oral administration of 50 mg of radiolabeled naltrexone in one patient, approximately 93% of the radiolabeled dose was excreted within 133 hours; about 79 and 14% were excreted in urine and feces, respectively.

Following oral administration of a single 100-mg dose in individuals formerly dependent on opiates and in healthy individuals, renal clearance of naltrexone and 6-β-naltrexol is reported to be 67–137 and 283–318 mL/minute, respectively. Renal clearance of naltrexone and 6-β-naltrexol is reported to be 30 and 369 mL/minute, respectively, following administration of 100 mg daily for at least 18 days.

Total body clearance of naltrexone following oral administration is reported to be 1.5 L/minute, while systemic clearance following IV administration reportedly is about 3.5 L/minute. Since systemic clearance exceeds hepatic blood flow, it appears that the drug also is metabolized at extrahepatic sites.

Following IM administration of naltrexone extended-release injection, the half-life of naltrexone and 6-β-naltrexol is 5–10 days.

Pharmacokinetics of parenterally administered naltrexone do not appear to be substantially altered in patients with mild renal impairment (creatinine clearance of 50–80 mL/minute).

Limited data suggest that orally administered naltrexone is not removed by hemodialysis.

CHEMISTRY AND STABILITY

● Chemistry

Naltrexone is a synthetic opiate antagonist that is derived from thebaine. Naltrexone differs structurally from oxymorphone only in that the methyl group on the nitrogen atom of oxymorphone is replaced by a cyclopropylmethyl group. This structural modification results in naltrexone having essentially pure opiate antagonist activity, rather than the pure opiate agonist activity of oxymorphone. Naltrexone differs structurally from naloxone, another opiate antagonist, in that the allyl group on the nitrogen atom of naloxone is replaced by a cyclopropylmethyl group. This structural modification results in increased oral activity and duration of action of naltrexone compared with naloxone.

Naltrexone hydrochloride occurs as white crystals having a bitter taste and has a solubility of 100 mg/mL in water at 25°C. The drug has a pK$_a$ of 8.13 at 37°C.

Commercially available naltrexone for extended-release injectable suspension (Vivitrol®) contains naltrexone incorporated into microspheres composed of polylactide co-glycolide, a biodegradable polymer matrix. Following reconstitution with the diluent provided by the manufacturer, naltrexone suspension is milky white, does not contain clumps, and moves freely down the wall of the vial. The diluent provided by the manufacturer provides an appropriate vehicle for reconstitution and delivery of the drug and contains carboxymethylcellulose sodium, polysorbate 20, and sodium chloride in sterile water for injection.

● Stability

Naltrexone hydrochloride tablets should be stored in well-closed containers at 15–30°C.

The entire dose pack containing naltrexone for extended-release injectable suspension should be refrigerated at 2–8°C; the dose pack can be stored at room temperature (i.e., room temperatures not exceeding 25°C) for up to 7 days. Storage at temperatures above 25°C or freezing should be avoided.

PREPARATIONS

Excipients in commercially available drug preparations may have clinically important effects in some individuals; consult specific product labeling for details.

Naltrexone

Parenteral		
For injectable suspension, extended-release, for IM use	380 mg	Vivitrol® (available as a dose pack containing naltrexone microspheres, diluent, needles), Alkermes

Naltrexone Hydrochloride

Oral		
Tablets	50 mg*	Naltrexone Hydrochloride
Tablets, film-coated	50 mg*	Naltrexone Hydrochloride ReVia® (scored), Duramed

* available from one or more manufacturer, distributor, and/or repackager by generic (nonproprietary) name

† Use is not currently included in the labeling approved by the US Food and Drug Administration.

Selected Revisions July 19, 2021, © Copyright, November 1, 1985, American Society of Health-System Pharmacists, Inc.

clonazePAM

28:12.08 • BENZODIAZEPINES

■ Clonazepam is a benzodiazepine derivative that is used both as an anticonvulsant and for the treatment of panic disorder with or without agoraphobia.

USES

● Seizure Disorders

Clonazepam is used in the prophylactic management of Lennox-Gastaut syndrome (petit mal variant epilepsy) and akinetic and myoclonic seizures. The drug also may be used in the management of absence (petit mal) seizures in patients who have not responded to succinimides. In some patients, use of clonazepam may permit reduction in dosage or discontinuance of other anticonvulsants; however, paradoxical increases in seizure activity also have occurred. (See Cautions: Precautions and Contraindications.) A decreased response to the drug may occur after several months or years of clonazepam therapy; however, seizures may be less severe than those before clonazepam therapy. In some patients, dosage adjustment may restore efficacy.

Most studies to date on the use of clonazepam have been uncontrolled and have involved patients with seizures refractory to other anticonvulsants. In addition, clonazepam has been used mainly as an adjunct to other drugs. For these reasons, determination of the precise role of clonazepam in the management of seizure disorders must await the results of well-controlled comparative studies.

Clonazepam has been used with some success in other refractory seizures†, including partial seizures with complex symptomatology (psychomotor seizures) and other partial (focal) seizures and some cases of infantile spasms. Clonazepam also has been useful in some patients with tonic-clonic (grand mal) seizures†; however, when used in patients with multiple types of seizure disorders, the drug may increase the frequency of or precipitate tonic-clonic seizures in some patients. If this occurs, addition of another anticonvulsant and/or increase in dosage may be required.

IV clonazepam has been used with good results in the management of status epilepticus†; however, a parenteral dosage form of the drug is not currently commercially available in the US.

● Panic Attacks and Disorder

Clonazepam is used in the treatment of panic disorder with or without agoraphobia. Panic disorder is characterized by the occurrence of unexpected panic attacks and associated concern about having additional attacks, worry about the implications or consequences of the attacks, and/or a clinically important change in behavior related to the attacks.

According to DSM-IV, panic disorder is characterized by recurrent unexpected panic attacks, which consist of a discrete period of intense fear or discomfort in which 4 (or more) of the following symptoms develop abruptly and reach a peak within 10 minutes: palpitations, pounding heart, or accelerated heart rate; sweating; trembling or shaking; sensations of shortness of breath or smothering; feeling of choking; chest pain or discomfort; nausea or abdominal distress; feeling dizzy, unsteady, lightheaded, or faint; derealization (feelings of unreality) or depersonalization (being detached from oneself); fear of losing control; fear of dying; paresthesias (numbness or tingling sensations); and chills or hot flushes.

The efficacy of clonazepam for the management of panic disorder has been established by 2 multicenter, double-blind, placebo-controlled studies of 6–9 weeks' duration in adult outpatients who had a primary diagnosis of panic disorder (DSM-IIIR) with or without agoraphobia. In these studies, clonazepam was found to be superior to placebo on the following measures of efficacy: change from baseline in panic attack frequency, the Clinician's Global Impression Severity of Illness Score, and the Clinician's Global Impression Improvement Score.

The first study was a fixed-dose study of 9 weeks' duration involving clonazepam dosages of 0.5, 1, 2, 3, or 4 mg daily. This study was conducted in 4 phases: a 1-week placebo run-in phase, a 3-week phase of upward titration of the dosage, a 6-week fixed-dosage maintenance phase, and a 7-week discontinuance

phase. A substantial difference from placebo was observed consistently only in the group receiving 1 mg of clonazepam daily; the difference between the reduction from baseline in the number of full panic attacks was approximately 1 per week in patients receiving clonazepam 1 mg daily compared with placebo. At the study end point (the end of the fixed-dosage maintenance phase), 74% of patients receiving clonazepam 1 mg daily were free of panic attacks compared to 56% of patients receiving placebo. Daily dosages exceeding 1 mg were less effective and more commonly associated with adverse effects (e.g., somnolence and ataxia) in this study.

The second study was of 6 weeks' duration and used a flexible dosing schedule involving clonazepam dosages ranging from 0.5–4 mg daily. The study was conducted in 3 phases: a 1-week placebo run-in phase, a 6-week optimal dose-finding phase, and a 6-week discontinuance phase. The mean clonazepam dosage during the optimal dosing period was 2.3 mg daily. The difference between the reduction from baseline in the number of full panic attacks was approximately 1 per week in patients receiving clonazepam compared with placebo. At the study end point, 62% of patients receiving clonazepam were free of panic attacks compared with 37% of patients receiving placebo.

Subgroup analysis from these 2 controlled studies for possible race- or gender-related effects on treatment outcome did not suggest any difference in efficacy based on either the race or gender of the patient.

The manufacturer states that the efficacy of clonazepam for long-term use (i.e., longer than 9 weeks) has not been systematically evaluated in controlled studies. However, limited information from follow-up studies of patients with panic disorder who responded favorably to benzodiazepine therapy indicates that the benefits observed during short-term therapy are usually maintained for longer periods (e.g., up to several years) without increases in dosage. In an open study in which patients with panic disorder were treated with clonazepam over a 2-year period, clonazepam produced and maintained a therapeutic benefit without evidence of tolerance development (as manifested by dosage escalation or worsening of clinical status). The manufacturer states that there is insufficient experience concerning how long patients with panic disorder who are treated with clonazepam should remain on the drug. However, some clinicians state that panic disorder is a chronic condition; therefore, it may be reasonable to continue therapy in responding patients. If clonazepam is used for extended periods, the need for continued therapy with the drug should be reassessed periodically. (See Dosage and Administration: Dosage.)

Panic disorder can be treated with cognitive behavioral psychotherapy and/or pharmacologic therapy. Currently, there are several classes of drugs that appear to be effective in the pharmacologic management of panic disorder, including tricyclic antidepressants (e.g., imipramine, clomipramine), monoamine oxidase inhibitors (e.g., phenelzine), selective serotonin-reuptake inhibitors (e.g., citalopram, escitalopram, fluoxetine, fluvoxamine, paroxetine, sertraline), selective serotonin-and norepinephrine-reuptake inhibitors (e.g., venlafaxine), and benzodiazepines (e.g., alprazolam, clonazepam). When choosing among the available drugs in the treatment of panic disorder, clinicians should consider their acceptance and tolerability by patients; their ability to reduce or eliminate panic attacks, reduce clinically important anxiety and disability secondary to phobic avoidance, and ameliorate other common comorbid conditions (such as depression); their cost; and their ability to prevent relapse during long-term therapy.

Because of their better tolerability when compared with other agents (such as the tricyclic antidepressants, monoamine oxidase inhibitors, and benzodiazepines) and the lack of physical dependence problems commonly associated with benzodiazepines, some clinicians currently prefer selective serotonin-reuptake inhibitors as first-line therapy in the management of panic disorder. However, benzodiazepines such as clonazepam have a more rapid onset of action often with immediate reduction of panic symptoms, whereas antidepressants may require several weeks or more for therapeutic effect. Therefore, benzodiazepines can be used for early symptom control (usually in combination with another form of treatment such as cognitive behavioral therapy or antidepressant therapy) and are useful in relieving anticipatory anxiety. Benzodiazepines also can be used to treat surges of anxiety or panic, although some experts state that this as-needed use of benzodiazepines should not replace the use of adequate daily dosages when clinically necessary. In addition, some clinicians consider the anxiolytic effect of benzodiazepines advantageous in reducing anxiety between panic attacks. The most serious risk factor associated with benzodiazepines in panic disorder is physical dependence; withdrawal symptoms or a recurrence of panic symptoms may occur during drug tapering or following abrupt discontinuation of therapy. Therefore, gradual discontinuance of clonazepam therapy is advised. (See Chronic Toxicity and see also Dosage and Administration.) In addition, as with other benzodiazepines, clonazepam can produce sedation and psychomotor impairment and potentially may interact with alcohol if it is not restricted. (See Cautions: Precautions and Contraindications.)

● Schizophrenia

Clonazepam also has been used in patients who experience akathisia† while receiving antipsychotic drugs (e.g., for management of schizophrenia) and for the treatment of acute catatonic reactions†, whether associated with schizophrenia or other conditions. (See Uses: Schizophrenia, in the Benzodiazepines General Statement 28:24.08.)

● Other Uses

The efficacy of clonazepam as a hypnotic† has not been fully evaluated.

DOSAGE AND ADMINISTRATION

● Administration

Clonazepam is administered orally.

Clonazepam conventional tablets should be administered with water and swallowed whole. The orally disintegrating tablets should be administered immediately after opening the pouch and peeling back the blister; do *not* push the tablet through the foil. The orally disintegrating tablet should be removed with a dry hand and placed on the tongue, where it disintegrates rapidly in saliva, and then subsequently can be swallowed with or without water.

In the treatment of seizure disorders, the manufacturer states that daily dosage usually is given in 3 equally divided doses. The largest dose should be given at bedtime if doses are not equally divided.

In the treatment of panic disorder, the daily dosage of clonazepam may be given in 2 equally divided doses. Alternatively, the drug may be given as one dose at bedtime to reduce the inconvenience of somnolence.

Clonazepam also has been administered IV†, but a parenteral dosage form is not currently commercially available in the US.

Patients who are currently receiving or beginning therapy with clonazepam and/or any other anticonvulsant for any indication should be closely monitored for the emergence or worsening of depression, suicidal thoughts or behavior (suicidality), and/or any unusual changes in mood or behavior. (See Cautions: CNS Effects and Cautions: Precautions and Contraindications, in the Anticonvulsants General Statement 28:12.)

● Dosage

Dosage of clonazepam must be carefully and slowly adjusted according to individual requirements and response. Clonazepam should be withdrawn slowly, and abrupt discontinuance of the drug should be avoided, especially during long-term, high-dose therapy to avoid precipitating seizures, status epilepticus, or withdrawal symptoms. If clonazepam is to be discontinued in patients who have received prolonged therapy with the drug, it is recommended that dosage be tapered gradually. Addiction-prone patients (e.g., alcoholic patients, individuals known to have been dependent on other drugs) should be carefully monitored while receiving clonazepam or other psychotropic therapy because of the predisposition of these patients to habituation and addiction. During clonazepam withdrawal, simultaneous substitution of another anticonvulsant may be indicated.

Seizure Disorders

Various clonazepam dosage regimens have been used in published studies. The manufacturer states that the usual initial dosage for infants and children up to 10 years of age or weighing up to 30 kg is 0.01–0.03 mg/kg daily. Initial pediatric dosage should not exceed 0.05 mg/kg daily given in 2 or 3 divided doses. Dosage may be increased by no more than 0.5 mg every third day until seizure control is achieved with minimal adverse effects. Pediatric maintenance dosage should not exceed 0.2 mg/kg daily.

Initial adult dosage of clonazepam should not exceed 1.5 mg daily given in 3 equally divided doses. Dosage may be increased in increments of 0.5–1 mg every

third day until seizure control is achieved with minimal adverse effects. Adult maintenance dosage should not exceed 20 mg daily.

Panic Disorder

For the management of panic disorder in adults, the recommended initial dosage of clonazepam is 0.25 mg twice daily. An increase to the target dose for most patients of 1 mg daily may be made after 3 days. The manufacturer states that the recommended dosage of 1 mg daily is based on the results of a fixed-dose study in which the optimal therapeutic effect was seen at this dosage. In this study, higher dosages of 2, 3, and 4 mg daily were found to be less effective than the 1 mg daily dosage and more commonly associated with adverse effects (e.g., somnolence and ataxia). Some clinicians recommend a dosage of 1–2 mg daily in patients with panic disorder and the manufacturer states that certain individual patients may benefit from dosages up to a maximum of 4 mg daily. In such cases, the dosage of clonazepam may be increased in increments of 0.125–0.25 mg twice daily every 3 days until panic disorder is controlled or until adverse effects make further increases in dosage undesirable.

The manufacturer states that the efficacy of clonazepam for long-term use (i.e., longer than 9 weeks) has not been systematically evaluated in controlled studies. However, limited information from follow-up studies of patients with panic disorder who responded favorably to benzodiazepine therapy indicate that the benefits observed during short-term therapy usually are maintained for longer periods without increases in dosage. In an open study in which patients with panic disorder were treated with clonazepam over a 2-year period, clonazepam produced and maintained a therapeutic benefit without evidence of tolerance development (as manifested by dosage escalation or worsening of clinical status). The manufacturer states that there is insufficient experience concerning how long patients with panic disorder who are treated with clonazepam should remain on the drug. However, some clinicians state that panic disorder is a chronic condition; therefore, it may be reasonable to continue therapy in responding patients. If clonazepam is used for extended periods, the need for continued therapy with the drug should be reassessed periodically.

When clonazepam therapy is to be discontinued in patients with panic disorder, the manufacturer states that therapy should be gradually discontinued by decreasing the dosage by 0.125 mg twice daily every 3 days until the drug is completely withdrawn.

● Dosage in Renal and Hepatic Impairment

The effect of renal impairment on clonazepam elimination is not known.

The possibility that clonazepam dosage adjustment may be necessary in patients with hepatic impairment should be considered.

CAUTIONS

A boxed warning has been included in the prescribing information for all benzodiazepines describing the risks of abuse, misuse, addiction, physical dependence, and withdrawal reactions associated with all drugs in this class. Abuse and misuse can result in overdose or death, especially when benzodiazepines are combined with other medicines, such as opioid pain relievers, alcohol, or illicit drugs. Frequent follow-up with patients receiving benzodiazepines is important. Reassess patients regularly to manage their medical conditions and any withdrawal symptoms. Clinicians should assess a patient's risk of abuse, misuse, and addiction. Standardized screening tools are available (https://nida.nih.gov/nidamed-medical-health-professionals/screening-tools-resources/chart-screening-tools). To reduce the risk of acute withdrawal reactions, use a gradual dose taper when reducing the dosage or discontinuing benzodiazepines. Take precautions when benzodiazepines are used in combination with opioid medications.

● Nervous System Effects

The most frequent adverse effects of clonazepam are sedation or drowsiness, ataxia or hypotonia, and behavioral disturbances (principally in children) including aggressiveness, irritability, agitation, and hyperkinesis. In one study, some patients experienced euphoria that was followed by dysphoria. Tolerance to clonazepam varies considerably among patients and is not necessarily dose related. Behavioral disturbances are most likely to occur in patients with preexisting brain damage and/or mental retardation or a history of behavioral or psychiatric disturbances; however, the precise role of clonazepam in inducing behavioral changes in these patients is difficult to assess. It has been suggested that methylphenidate or amphetamines may be useful to control behavioral disturbances if they occur. Drowsiness, ataxia, and behavioral disturbances are most severe during initial therapy and frequently decrease or disappear during continued therapy. It has been suggested that these adverse effects may be minimized by starting with low dosages and gradually increasing dosage over a 2-week period and by administering the drug in divided doses daily. In some patients, however, these adverse effects have necessitated discontinuance of clonazepam.

Adverse neurologic effects of clonazepam include abnormal eye movements, aphonia, choreiform movements, coma, diplopia, dysarthria, dysdiadochokinesis, glassy-eyed appearance, headache, hemiparesis, nystagmus, respiratory depression, slurred speech, tremor, dizziness, and vertigo. Clonazepam also may cause confusion, mental depression, forgetfulness, hallucinations, hysteria, increased libido, insomnia, psychosis, or suicidal tendencies. (See Cautions: Precautions and Contraindications.) Muscle weakness and pains also may occur.

● Respiratory Effects

Increased salivation, hypersecretion in upper respiratory passages, chest congestion, rhinorrhea, and shortness of breath may occur in patients receiving clonazepam. In one study, increased salivation, mucous obstruction of the nasopharynx and bronchi, and difficulty in swallowing occurred in infants receiving the drug. The investigator reported that these effects occurred most frequently when clonazepam was used in conjunction with phenobarbital.

● Dermatologic Effects

Dermatologic reactions, including hair loss, hirsutism, skin rash, and ankle and facial edema, have been reported in patients receiving clonazepam. Rarely, abnormal skin pigmentation has been reported in patients receiving clonazepam and phenytoin.

● GI Effects

Adverse GI effects of clonazepam include constipation, diarrhea, encopresis, gastritis, increased or decreased appetite, weight gain or loss, dyspepsia, nausea, coated tongue, dry mouth, abnormal thirst, and sore gums.

● Genitourinary Effects

Adverse genitourinary effects of clonazepam include dysuria, enuresis, nocturia, and urinary retention.

● Hematologic Effects

Adverse hematologic effects of clonazepam include anemia, leukopenia, thrombocytopenia, and eosinophilia.

● Hepatic Effects

Hepatomegaly and transient elevations of serum aminotransferase and alkaline phosphatase concentrations may occur in patients receiving clonazepam.

● Other Adverse Effects

Other reported adverse effects include palpitations, dehydration, general deterioration, fever, and lymphadenopathy. Abnormal retinal vascularization without visual impairment was reported in one patient who received clonazepam and other anticonvulsants.

● Precautions and Contraindications

Clonazepam shares the toxic potential of other benzodiazepines, and the usual cautions, precautions, and contraindications of benzodiazepine therapy should be followed. (See Cautions in the Benzodiazepines General Statement 28:24.08.)

Concomitant use of benzodiazepines, including clonazepam, and opiate agonists or opiate partial agonists may result in profound sedation, respiratory depression, coma, and death. Patients receiving clonazepam and/or their caregivers should be apprised of the risks associated with concomitant therapeutic or illicit use of benzodiazepines and opiates. (See Opiate Agonists and Opiate Partial Agonists under Drug Interactions: CNS Depressants.)

Benzodiazepines have the potential to impair judgment, thinking, or motor skills. Therefore, patients receiving clonazepam should be cautioned that the drug may impair their ability to perform activities requiring mental alertness or physical coordination (e.g., operating machinery, driving a motor vehicle) and to avoid such activities until they experience how the drug affects them.

Patients receiving clonazepam should be advised to avoid alcohol while receiving the drug. In addition, they should be advised to notify their clinician if they are taking or plan to take nonprescription (over-the-counter) or prescription medications or alcohol-containing beverages or preparations.

Clinicians should inform patients, their families, and caregivers about the potential for an increased risk of suicidal thinking and behavior (suicidality) associated with anticonvulsant therapy. For a complete discussion, see Cautions: CNS Effects and Cautions: Precautions and Contraindications, in the Anticonvulsants General Statement 28:12.

When used in patients in whom several different types of seizure disorders coexist, clonazepam may increase the incidence or precipitate the onset of generalized tonic-clonic (grand mal) seizures. This may require the addition of appropriate anticonvulsants or an increase in their dosages. The concomitant use of valproic acid and clonazepam may produce absence status.

Because clonazepam may increase salivation, it should be used with caution in patients in whom increased secretions might be harmful. The manufacturer states that the drug also should be used with caution in patients with chronic respiratory disease or impaired renal function. Periodic blood counts and liver function tests should be performed in patients receiving long-term clonazepam therapy.

The manufacturer states that clonazepam is contraindicated in patients with clinical or biochemical evidence of significant hepatic impairment or a history of sensitivity to benzodiazepines. The manufacturer states that the drug is contraindicated in patients with acute angle-closure glaucoma, but it may be used with caution in patients with open-angle glaucoma who are receiving appropriate therapy.

● Pediatric Precautions

The effect of long-term administration of clonazepam on physical and mental development in children has not been established. Therefore, the drug should not be administered to pediatric patients with seizure disorders unless the potential benefits outweigh the possible risks.

The manufacturer states that the safety and efficacy of clonazepam in pediatric patients with panic disorder younger than 18 years of age have not been established. Clonazepam has been effective in a limited number of adolescents with panic disorder; however, controlled studies are needed to confirm these preliminary findings.

● Pregnancy, Fertility, and Lactation

Pregnancy

Safe use of clonazepam during pregnancy has not been established. Adverse fetal effects have been observed in reproduction studies in rats and rabbits. Although several reports suggest an association between use of anticonvulsants in pregnant, epileptic women and an increased incidence of birth defects in children born to these women, a causal relationship to many of these drugs has not been established. The manufacturer states that the majority of women receiving anticonvulsant therapy deliver normal infants. Clonazepam should be used in pregnant women or women who might become pregnant only if the drug is considered essential in the management of their seizures. Anticonvulsants should *not* be discontinued in pregnant women in whom the drugs are administered to prevent major seizures because of the strong possibility of precipitating status epilepticus with attendant hypoxia and threat to life. In individual cases, when the severity and frequency of the seizure disorder are such that discontinuance of therapy does not pose a serious threat to the patient, discontinuance of the drugs may be considered prior to and during pregnancy; however, it cannot be said with any certainty that even minor seizures do not pose some hazard to the fetus. The clinician should carefully weigh these considerations in treating or counseling epileptic women of childbearing potential.

Lactation

Safe use of clonazepam during lactation has not been established. The manufacturer states that it is inadvisable for women receiving clonazepam to nurse infants.

DRUG INTERACTIONS

• CNS Depressants

Additive CNS depression may occur when clonazepam is administered concomitantly with other CNS depressants, including alcohol, opiate agonists, barbiturates, anxiolytics, sedatives and hypnotics, some antipsychotic agents, monoamine oxidase (MAO) inhibitors, tricyclic antidepressants, and other anticonvulsants. If clonazepam is used concomitantly with other CNS depressants, caution should be used to avoid excessive CNS depression. Patients also should be advised to avoid alcohol while receiving clonazepam therapy.

Opiate Agonists and Opiate Partial Agonists

Concomitant use of benzodiazepines, including clonazepam, and opiate agonists or opiate partial agonists may result in profound sedation, respiratory depression, coma, and death. Whenever possible, such concomitant use should be avoided. Opiate antitussive agents should be avoided in patients receiving benzodiazepines, and concomitant use of opiate analgesics and benzodiazepines should be reserved for patients in whom alternative treatment options are inadequate. The lowest effective dosages and shortest possible duration of concomitant therapy should be used, and the patient should be monitored closely for respiratory depression and sedation.

If clonazepam is required for any indication other than epilepsy in a patient receiving opiate therapy, the drug should be initiated at a lower dosage than indicated in the absence of opiate therapy and titrated based on clinical response. If an opiate analgesic is required in a patient receiving clonazepam, the opiate analgesic should be initiated at a reduced dosage and titrated based on clinical response. For further information on potential interactions between benzodiazepines and opiates, see Opiate Agonists and Opiate Partial Agonists under Drug Interactions: CNS Agents, in the Benzodiazepines General Statement 28:24.08.

• Phenytoin

In one study, increased serum phenytoin concentrations were reported to occur when clonazepam and phenytoin were administered concomitantly. In another study, plasma clonazepam concentrations decreased when the two drugs were administered. Although the clinical importance of these reports has not been established, it may be desirable to monitor serum concentrations of both drugs during initial concomitant therapy, making dosage adjustments as necessary.

ACUTE TOXICITY

• Manifestations

Overdosage of clonazepam may produce somnolence, confusion, ataxia, diminished reflexes, or coma.

• Treatment

Treatment of clonazepam intoxication consists of general supportive therapy. Flumazenil, a benzodiazepine antagonist, can be used in the management of benzodiazepine overdosage, but the drug is an adjunct to, not a substitute for, appropriate supportive and symptomatic therapy. (See Flumazenil 28:92.) The possibility that the antagonist could precipitate withdrawal in benzodiazepine-dependent individuals should be weighed carefully against the possible benefits. Clinicians should be aware of the risk of seizure in association with flumazenil administration, particularly in patients receiving long-term benzodiazepine therapy or following tricyclic antidepressant overdosage. The risks of flumazenil therapy should be weighed carefully when multiple-drug overdosage is possible. Flumazenil is *not* indicated in patients with epilepsy who have been treated with benzodiazepines. Antagonism of the benzodiazepine's effects in such patients may provoke seizures.

If ingestion of the benzodiazepine is recent and the patient is fully conscious, emesis should be induced. If the patient is comatose, gastric lavage may be performed if an endotracheal tube with cuff inflated is in place to prevent aspiration of gastric contents. Activated charcoal and a saline cathartic may be administered after gastric lavage and/or emesis to remove any remaining drug. The patient's

heart rate, blood pressure, and respiration should be monitored and the patient closely observed. IV fluids should be administered and an adequate airway maintained. Hypotension may be controlled, if necessary, by IV administration of norepinephrine or metaraminol. Although some manufacturers of benzodiazepines recommend use of caffeine and sodium benzoate to combat CNS depression, most authorities believe caffeine and other analeptic agents should *not* be used, because these drugs have questionable benefit and transient action. Instead, administration of flumazenil, if indicated, generally would be preferred. As in overdosage with other benzodiazepines, dialysis is of no known value in clonazepam overdosage.

• Chronic Toxicity

The possibility of physical or psychological dependence should be considered, particularly when clonazepam is administered to alcoholic patients or to those known to have been dependent on other drugs. Abrupt withdrawal of clonazepam following prolonged administration has resulted in severe withdrawal symptoms including seizures, psychosis, hallucinations, behavioral disturbances, tremors, abdominal and muscle cramps, vomiting, sweating, irritability, restlessness, sleeplessness, and hand tremors. In one study, patients who experienced some of these withdrawal symptoms had plasma 7-aminoclonazepam concentrations 3–4 times greater than those who did not have withdrawal symptoms. In addition, milder withdrawal symptoms such as dysphoria and insomnia have been reported following abrupt discontinuance of benzodiazepines in patients receiving therapeutic dosages for several months. Because clonazepam has a long half-life, withdrawal symptoms may not occur until several days after the drug has been discontinued.

PHARMACOLOGY

The pharmacologic actions of clonazepam are qualitatively similar to those of other benzodiazepine derivatives.

In animal studies, clonazepam has been shown to protect against seizures induced by pentylenetetrazol and, to a lesser extent, electrical stimulation. Clonazepam also appears to antagonize seizures produced by photic stimulation in animals. In humans, clonazepam can suppress the spike and wave discharge in absence seizures (petit mal) and can decrease the frequency, amplitude, duration, and spread of discharge in minor motor seizures. Clonazepam also has been shown to produce a taming effect, muscle weakness, and hypnosis in animals.

The exact mechanism(s) by which clonazepam exerts its anticonvulsant, sedative, and antipanic effects is unknown. However, it is believed to be related at least in part to the drug's ability to enhance the activity of γ-aminobutyric acid (GABA), the principal inhibitory neurotransmitter in the central nervous system.

PHARMACOKINETICS

• Absorption

Clonazepam is rapidly and well absorbed from the GI tract. The absolute bioavailability is approximately 90%. In one study, peak blood concentrations of 6.5–13.5 ng/mL were usually reached within 1–2 hours following a single 2-mg oral dose of micronized clonazepam in healthy adults. In some individuals, however, peak blood concentrations were reached at 4–8 hours. Although the plasma concentration of clonazepam required for anticonvulsant effects has not been definitely established, some studies indicate it may be 20–80 ng/mL. Plasma concentrations in this range have been reported to be maintained in adults receiving 6 mg of clonazepam daily in 3 divided doses and in children 6–13 years of age receiving 1.5–4 mg of the drug daily in 3 divided doses. The onset of anticonvulsant action usually occurs within 20–60 minutes, and the duration of action usually is 6–8 hours in infants and young children and up to 12 hours in adults.

• Distribution

There is little information on the distribution of clonazepam. Clonazepam is approximately 85% bound to plasma proteins. Like other benzodiazepines, the drug apparently crosses the blood-brain barrier and the placenta.

● Elimination

The elimination half-life of clonazepam has been reported to be 18.7–39 hours.

Clonazepam is extensively metabolized in the liver to several metabolites including 7-aminoclonazepam, 7-acetaminoclonazepam, and 3-hydroxy derivatives of these metabolites and clonazepam. Clonazepam metabolites are excreted in urine by first-order kinetics, principally as their glucuronide and/or sulfate conjugates. Only very small amounts of the drug (less than 2%) are excreted unchanged.

CHEMISTRY AND STABILITY

● Chemistry

Clonazepam is a benzodiazepine derivative that is used both as an anticonvulsant and for the treatment of panic disorder with or without agoraphobia. The drug is structurally and pharmacologically related to diazepam and other benzodiazepines. Clonazepam occurs as an off-white to light yellow, crystalline powder with a faint odor and is insoluble in water and slightly soluble in alcohol. Clonazepam has pK$_a$s of 1.5 and 10.5.

● Stability

Clonazepam tablets and orally disintegrating tablets should be stored in air-tight, light-resistant containers at 25°C, but may be exposed to temperatures ranging from 15–30°C. The commercially available conventional tablets have an expiration date of 5 years following the date of manufacture.

For further information on uses, cautions, and dosage and administration of clonazepam, see the Anticonvulsants General Statement 28:12 and the Benzodiazepines General Statement 28:24.08.

PREPARATIONS

Clonazepam is subject to control under the Federal Controlled Substances Act of 1970 as a schedule IV (C-IV) drug.

Excipients in commercially available drug preparations may have clinically important effects in some individuals; consult specific product labeling for details.

clonazePAM

Oral		
Tablets	0.5 mg*	clonazePAM Tablets (C-IV)
		KlonoPIN® (C-IV; scored), Genentech
	1 mg*	clonazePAM Tablets (C-IV)
		KlonoPIN® (C-IV), Genentech
	2 mg*	clonazePAM Tablets (C-IV)
		KlonoPIN® (C-IV), Genentech
Tablets, orally disintegrating	0.125 mg*	clonazePAM Orally Disintegrating Tablets (C-IV)
	0.25 mg*	clonazePAM Orally Disintegrating Tablets (C-IV)
	0.5 mg*	clonazePAM Orally Disintegrating Tablets (C-IV)
	1 mg*	clonazePAM Orally Disintegrating Tablets (C-IV)
	2 mg*	clonazePAM Orally Disintegrating Tablets (C-IV)

† Use is not currently included in the labeling approved by the US Food and Drug Administration.

* available from one or more manufacturer, distributor, and/or repackager by generic (nonproprietary) name

Gabapentin, Gabapentin Enacarbil

28:12.28 • GABA-MEDIATED ANTICONVULSANTS

■ Gabapentin is an anticonvulsant structurally related to the inhibitory CNS neurotransmitter γ -aminobutyric acid (GABA); the drug also possesses analgesic activity. Gabapentin enacarbil is a prodrug of gabapentin.

USES

Conventional (immediate-release) preparations of gabapentin are used in the management of seizure disorders. Conventional preparations also may be used in the treatment of postherpetic neuralgia (PHN). Gabapentin also is commercially available as a gastroretentive tablet formulation (Gralise®) for once-daily administration in the treatment of PHN. Because of differences in pharmacokinetic properties, gabapentin gastroretentive tablets are *not* interchangeable with other gabapentin preparations.

Gabapentin enacarbil, a prodrug of gabapentin, is commercially available as an extended-release tablet formulation (Horizant®) for once-daily administration in the treatment of PHN or primary restless legs syndrome. Because of differences in pharmacokinetic properties, gabapentin enacarbil extended-release tablets are *not* interchangeable with other gabapentin preparations.

● Seizure Disorders

Gabapentin (as conventional preparations) is used as adjunctive therapy (i.e., in combination with other anticonvulsants) in the management of partial seizures with or without secondary generalization. Clinical studies establishing efficacy of gabapentin for this indication were conducted with conventional (immediate-release) preparations of the drug; efficacy of gabapentin gastroretentive tablets (Gralise®) and gabapentin enacarbil (Horizant®) have not been established in patients with seizure disorders. The anticonvulsant potential of conventional gabapentin has been established in studies in which the drug was compared to placebo in adults and children 3 years of age or older with refractory partial seizures; comparative efficacy of therapeutically effective dosages of gabapentin versus other anticonvulsants remains to be established.

In several placebo-controlled studies, gabapentin (administered as conventional preparations) was effective in reducing seizure frequency, including that of secondarily generalized tonic-clonic seizures, in 17–26% of patients with partial seizures refractory to therapy with other anticonvulsant drugs (e.g., phenytoin, carbamazepine, phenobarbital, valproic acid). Patients in these studies had a history of at least 4 partial seizures (with or without secondary tonic-clonic generalization) per month despite optimum therapy with one or more anticonvulsants and were eligible for study entry if they continued to have at least 2–4 seizures per month during a 12-week baseline period while receiving their established anticonvulsant regimen. Efficacy of gabapentin in these studies was evaluated principally in terms of the percentage of patients with a reduction in seizure frequency of 50% or greater compared with baseline values (i.e., responder rate) and the change in seizure frequency associated with the addition of gabapentin or placebo to existing anticonvulsant treatment (i.e., response ratio, calculated as treatment seizure frequency minus baseline seizure frequency divided by the sum of the treatment and baseline seizure frequencies). Combined analysis of these response parameters in patients receiving various dosages of gabapentin (600, 900, 1200, or 1800 mg in 3 divided doses daily as conventional preparations) or placebo indicated a dose-related reduction in the frequency of partial seizures with gabapentin, although a dose-response relationship was not consistently found in the individual studies. The efficacy of adjunctive therapy with gabapentin for the management of partial seizures does not appear to be affected by patient gender or age, although the influence of these characteristics on efficacy has not been studied systematically.

Efficacy of gabapentin (as conventional preparations) in children 3–12 years of age with partial seizures was established in a multicenter randomized controlled trial. Response ratios were substantially better in patients receiving gabapentin 25–35 mg/kg daily (as conventional preparations) compared with those

receiving placebo; for the same population, the responder rate for the drug (21%) was not substantially different from placebo (18%). Another study in children 1 month to 3 years of age reported no substantial difference in either the response ratio or responder rate for those receiving gabapentin compared with those receiving placebo.

● Neuropathic Pain

Postherpetic Neuralgia

Gabapentin and gabapentin enacarbil are used in the management of postherpetic neuralgia (PHN) in adults.

Efficacy of conventional (immediate-release) preparations of gabapentin for the management of PHN was established in 2 placebo-controlled studies of 7–8 weeks' duration in patients who were continuing to experience pain for longer than 3 months after healing of their herpes zoster rash. In these studies, gabapentin was titrated over several weeks up to a target dosage of 1.8, 2.4, or 3.6 g daily (administered in 3 divided doses as conventional preparations). Gabapentin substantially reduced weekly mean pain scores from baseline compared with placebo (assessed by an 11-point numeric rating scale); improvement was noted at 1 week and maintained throughout the duration of these studies. In addition, a greater proportion of patients receiving gabapentin compared with placebo achieved at least a 50% reduction in pain from baseline, and this was observed at all dosages evaluated.

Efficacy of gabapentin gastroretentive tablets (Gralise®) for the management of PHN was established in an 11-week double-blind, placebo-controlled study in patients who were experiencing persistent pain for at least 6 months after healing of their herpes zoster rash. Gabapentin (at a dosage of 1.8 g once daily as gastroretentive tablets) was substantially more effective than placebo in improving average pain scores from baseline; the extent of improvement was similar to that achieved with the conventional (immediate-release) formulation of the drug. In this study, the proportion of patients who experienced at least a 50% reduction in pain with gabapentin (29.5%) was not substantially different from placebo (22.6%).

Efficacy of gabapentin enacarbil for the management of PHN was established in a 12-week randomized, double-blind, placebo-controlled multicenter study that evaluated 3 different dosages of the drug (600 mg, 1.2 g, or 1.8 g twice daily as extended-release tablets) in patients who were experiencing persistent pain for at least 3 months after healing of their herpes zoster rash. Compared with placebo, treatment with gabapentin enacarbil substantially reduced mean pain scores and increased the proportion of patients with at least a 50% reduction in pain intensity from baseline; improvements were noted as early as 1 week following initiation of therapy and were maintained throughout the duration of the study. Although benefits of gabapentin enacarbil were observed at all dosages evaluated, the 1.2-g daily dosage (administered as 600 mg twice daily) appeared to provide the greatest benefit-to-risk ratio.

Results of a systematic review of 8 randomized controlled studies in patients with PHN indicated that treatment with gabapentin (administered orally as gabapentin or gabapentin enacarbil preparations at dosages of at least 1.2 g daily) provided substantial benefit (i.e., reduction in pain intensity by at least 50% or a score of "very much improved" on the Patient Global Impression of Change [PGIC] scale) in 32% of patients who received the drug compared with 17% of those who received placebo; a moderate benefit (i.e., reduction in pain intensity by at least 30% or a PGIC score of "much or very much improved") was observed in 46% of patients who received the drug compared with 25% of those who received placebo. However, the strength of evidence was considered moderate because of uncertainties and differences between dosage regimens, formulations, and statistical methods used in the studies.

Although gabapentin is considered by many experts to be one of several first-line therapies for PHN, the evidence suggests that only a small proportion of patients will derive a clinically meaningful benefit from the drug. Other drugs that have been recommended for the management of PHN include pregabalin, tricyclic antidepressants, and topical lidocaine. When selecting an appropriate regimen, clinicians should consider the relative efficacy and safety of the specific drugs as well as individual patient-related factors (e.g., age, preference, tolerability, contraindications, comorbid conditions, concomitant medications).

Diabetic Peripheral Neuropathy

Gabapentin also has been used for the treatment of pain associated with diabetic peripheral neuropathy (DPN)†. The drug has been shown in a number of clinical studies to be more effective than placebo in relieving pain in patients with DPN; however, mixed results have been reported and when a benefit was observed, the effect size tended to be small. In a systematic review of 6–7 randomized controlled studies in patients with DPN, gabapentin (administered orally as gabapentin or gabapentin enacarbil formulations at dosages of at least 1.2 g daily) provided substantial benefit (i.e., reduction in pain intensity by at least 50% or a score of "very much improved" on the PGIC scale) in 38% of patients who received the drug compared with 23% of those who received placebo; a moderate benefit (i.e., reduction in pain intensity by at least 30% or a PGIC score of "much or very much improved") was achieved in 52% of patients who received the drug compared with 37% of those who received placebo. However, the strength of evidence was considered moderate because of uncertainties and differences between dosage regimens, formulations, and statistical methods used in the studies.

Although gabapentin is considered by many experts to be one of several first-line therapies for DPN, the evidence suggests that only a small proportion of patients will derive a clinically meaningful benefit from the drug. Other drugs that have been recommended for the management of DPN include pregabalin, tricyclic antidepressants, and serotonin- and norepinephrine-reuptake inhibitors (e.g., duloxetine, venlafaxine). Although comparative data are limited, studies generally have not found any substantial differences among the available treatments. When selecting an appropriate regimen, clinicians should consider the relative efficacy, safety, pharmacokinetics, drug interaction potential, and cost of the specific drugs in addition to individual patient-related factors (e.g., contraindications, comorbid conditions, concomitant medications).

Other Types of Neuropathic Pain

Gabapentin also has been used for the management of other types of neuropathic pain†, including central neuropathic pain associated with spinal cord injury†, complex regional pain syndrome† (CRPS), cancer-related neuropathic pain†, pain associated with multiple sclerosis†, phantom limb pain†, radicular pain†, and HIV-related peripheral neuropathy†. Results of controlled studies have been negative or equivocal in many cases, and the evidence remains extremely limited for the use of gabapentin in neuropathic pain conditions other than PHN and DPN†. Although the majority of studies evaluating gabapentinoids (i.e., gabapentin and pregabalin) for chronic neuropathic pain were conducted in patients with PHN or DPN, the evidence is often extrapolated to other neuropathic pain conditions and many experts recommend these drugs as first-line agents for all types of neuropathic pain (except for trigeminal neuralgia). However, additional study and experience are needed to further elucidate the role of gabapentin in the management of these other neuropathic pain conditions.

● Restless Legs Syndrome

Gabapentin enacarbil is used for the symptomatic treatment of moderate-to-severe primary restless legs syndrome in adults. The drug is not recommended in patients who are required to sleep during the daytime and remain awake at night.

Restless legs syndrome (also known as Ekbom syndrome) is a sensorimotor disorder characterized by a distressing urge to move the legs accompanied by sensations deep in the limbs that have been variously described as tingling, pulling, itching, aching, or jittering. These symptoms are present at rest, especially in the evening and at night, and are relieved by movement. Dopamine receptor agonists (e.g., pramipexole, ropinirole) traditionally have been considered the drugs of choice for patients with restless legs syndrome, particularly those with symptoms that occur nightly. Current evidence from randomized placebo-controlled studies also supports the use of gabapentin enacarbil for this condition. Although direct comparison studies have not been conducted to date, efficacy of gabapentin enacarbil appears to be comparable to that of the dopamine receptor agonists.

Efficacy of gabapentin enacarbil for the management of restless legs syndrome was established in 2 randomized, placebo-controlled studies of 12 weeks' duration in adults with moderate-to-severe restless legs syndrome (defined as a score of at least 15 on the International Restless Legs Syndrome [IRLS] scale, and a history of symptoms for at least 15 days in the month prior to screening). The primary measure of efficacy in these studies was a composite of the change from baseline in IRLS total score and the proportion of patients considered to be responders (i.e., those with a "much improved" or "very much improved" rating on the Clinical Global Impression-Global Improvement [CGI-I] scale) at

12 weeks. Gabapentin enacarbil (600 mg or 1.2 g once daily as extended-release tablets) substantially improved both measures of efficacy compared with placebo; improvements were noted as early as 1 week and were maintained throughout the duration of the studies. At 12 weeks, the mean change in IRLS score was a reduction of 13–13.8 with gabapentin enacarbil (versus a reduction of 8.8–9.8 with placebo), and 73–77% of patients receiving gabapentin enacarbil compared with 39–45% of those receiving placebo were described as responders. The 1.2-g daily dosage of gabapentin enacarbil appeared to provide no additional benefit over the 600-mg daily dosage, and was associated with an increased incidence of adverse effects.

Gabapentin also has been used in the treatment of restless legs syndrome†; however, the drug (unlike gabapentin enacarbil) currently is not labeled by the FDA for this use. Although evidence supporting the use of gabapentin for restless legs syndrome alone generally is insufficient, some experts state that the analgesic effects of the drug may provide some benefit in patients with both restless legs syndrome and pain.

● Vasomotor Symptoms

Gabapentin has been used for the management of vasomotor symptoms† in women with breast cancer and in postmenopausal women. Therapy with the drug has improved both the frequency and severity of vasomotor symptoms (e.g., hot flushes or flashes) in these women.

Most women receiving systemic antineoplastic therapy for breast cancer experience vasomotor symptoms, particularly those receiving tamoxifen therapy. In a randomized, double-blind, placebo-controlled study in 420 women with breast cancer (68–75% were receiving tamoxifen) who were experiencing 2 or more episodes of hot flushes daily, the percentage reductions in hot flush severity score at 4 and 8 weeks of treatment were 21 and 15%, respectively, for placebo; 33 and 31%, respectively, for gabapentin 300 mg daily (100 mg 3 times daily); and 49 and 46%, respectively, for gabapentin 900 mg daily (300 mg 3 times daily). Comparisons among treatment groups showed that only the 900-mg daily dosage was associated with a statistically significant reduction in hot flush frequency and severity. Whether higher dosages will provide further reductions in vasomotor symptoms remains to be determined. The role of gabapentin in managing vasomotor symptoms in women with breast cancer relative to other nonhormonal therapies (e.g., selective serotonin-reuptake inhibitors [SSRIs], selective serotonin- and norepinephrine-reuptake inhibitors [SNRIs]) remains to be determined. Well-designed, comparative studies are needed to establish optimum nonhormonal therapy, both in terms of efficacy and patient tolerance of adverse effects, in these women.

Because of the risks associated with hormone replacement therapy (HRT) for vasomotor symptoms in perimenopausal and postmenopausal women, alternative nonhormonal therapies are being investigated. In a randomized, double-blind, placebo-controlled study in 59 postmenopausal women who were experiencing 7 or more hot flushes daily, intent-to-treat analysis revealed that 12 weeks of gabapentin 900 mg daily (300 mg 3 times daily) was associated with a 45% reduction in hot flush frequency and a 54% reduction in composite hot flush score (frequency and severity). In a continuation open-label phase in which patients were permitted upward titration of dosage as needed to a maximum of 2.7 g daily (25% received 900 mg or less daily, 61% received 900 mg–1.8 g daily, 14% received 1.8–2.7 g daily), the associated reductions in hot flush frequency and composite score were 54 and 67%, respectively. The role of gabapentin therapy relative to other nonhormonal therapies (e.g., SSRIs, SNRIs) for postmenopausal vasomotor symptoms, both in terms of efficacy and safety, as well as the optimum dosage remain to be established.

Current evidence indicates that gabapentin is effective and well tolerated in the short-term treatment of vasomotor symptoms associated with breast cancer treatment and with menopause. The principal adverse effects associated with gabapentin therapy in women with vasomotor symptoms have been somnolence, fatigue, dizziness, and rash (with or without peripheral edema). Additional study and experience are needed to further elucidate the role of gabapentin relative to other nonhormonal therapies, and to establish longer-term (i.e., beyond 17 weeks) efficacy and safety.

The possible role of gabapentin in the management of vasomotor symptoms† associated with antiandrogenic therapy in men with prostate cancer remains to be established. Current evidence of efficacy is limited; well-designed, controlled studies are under way in this population.

DOSAGE AND ADMINISTRATION

● Administration

Gabapentin and gabapentin enacarbil are administered orally.

If discontinuance of gabapentin or gabapentin enacarbil therapy is required, gradual tapering of the dosage generally is recommended to avoid manifestations of abrupt withdrawal. (See Dosage and Administration: Dosage, and also see Cautions: Precautions and Contraindications.)

Patients who are currently receiving or beginning therapy with gabapentin, gabapentin enacarbil, and/or any other anticonvulsant for any indication should be closely monitored for the emergence or worsening of depression, suicidal thoughts or behavior (suicidality), and/or any unusual changes in mood or behavior. (See Suicidality under Cautions: Nervous System Effects and see Cautions: Precautions and Contraindications.)

Gabapentin

Gabapentin is commercially available as conventional (immediate-release) capsules, tablets, or oral solution (e.g., Neurontin®). The drug also is available as a gastroretentive tablet (Gralise®) for once-daily administration in the treatment of postherpetic neuralgia (PHN). Although the gastroretentive tablet is not considered by FDA to be an extended-release formulation, it is sometimes referred to in this manner because of similar pharmacokinetic properties to an extended-release dosage form (see Description). Because of differences in pharmacokinetics that affect frequency of administration, gabapentin gastroretentive tablets are *not* interchangeable with other gabapentin preparations.

Conventional (immediate-release) preparations of gabapentin should be administered orally in divided doses (3 times daily) without regard to meals; food does not substantially affect the bioavailability of gabapentin when administered as an immediate-release formulation. Gabapentin capsules should be swallowed whole with water. If film-coated scored tablets containing 600 or 800 mg of gabapentin are divided to allow administration of a 300- or 400-mg dose, the remaining half tablet should be used for the next dose; half tablets that are not used within 28 days should be discarded.

Gabapentin gastroretentive tablets should be administered orally once daily with the evening meal; food increases the rate and extent of absorption of gabapentin when administered as the gastroretentive formulation. The gastroretentive tablets should be swallowed intact and not chewed, crushed, or split.

If use of an antacid containing aluminum hydroxide and magnesium hydroxide is necessary in a patient receiving gabapentin, it is recommended that gabapentin be administered at least 2 hours after the antacid.

Gabapentin Enacarbil

Gabapentin enacarbil is commercially available as extended-release tablets (Horizant®) for administration once or twice daily depending on the indication. When used for the treatment of restless legs syndrome, the drug should be administered once daily at about 5 p.m.; if a dose is missed, the next dose should be taken the following day as scheduled. When used for the management of PHN, gabapentin enacarbil extended-release tablets should be administered twice daily; if a dose is missed, the dose should be skipped and the next dose taken at the regularly scheduled time. Gabapentin enacarbil extended-release tablets should be swallowed intact and not crushed, chewed, or cut.

Because of differences in pharmacokinetics that affect frequency of administration, gabapentin enacarbil extended-release tablets are *not* interchangeable with other gabapentin preparations.

● Dosage

Seizure Disorders

For adjunctive therapy in the management of partial seizures with or without secondary generalization in adults and children 12 years of age or older, the manufacturer recommends an initial gabapentin dosage of 300 mg 3 times daily and a maintenance dosage of 300–600 mg 3 times daily (as conventional preparations). Dosages up to 2.4 g daily have been well tolerated in long-term clinical studies, and a small number of patients have tolerated dosages of 3.6 g daily for short periods. When administered 3 times daily, the interval between doses should not exceed 12 hours.

In pediatric patients 3–11 years of age, the recommended initial dosage of gabapentin (as conventional preparations) for the management of partial seizures is 10–15 mg/kg daily in 3 divided doses. Dosage should be titrated upward over a period of approximately 3 days until an effective maintenance dosage is achieved. The recommended maintenance dosage of conventional gabapentin in pediatric patients 5–11 years of age is 25–35 mg/kg daily administered in 3 divided doses; for children 3–4 years of age, the recommended maintenance dosage is 40 mg/kg daily administered in 3 divided doses. Dosages up to 50 mg/kg daily have been well tolerated by pediatric patients 3–12 years of age in a long-term clinical study. When administered 3 times daily, the interval between doses should not exceed 12 hours.

Gabapentin may be used concomitantly with other anticonvulsant agents without concern for alterations in plasma drug concentrations; therapeutic plasma concentration monitoring is not necessary during such concomitant therapy.

If gabapentin dosage reduction or discontinuance or substitution of an alternative anticonvulsant is necessary, such changes in therapy should be made gradually over a period of at least 1 week.

Postherpetic Neuralgia

For the management of PHN in adults, the initial dosage of gabapentin as conventional (immediate-release) preparations is 300 mg once daily on the first day, 300 mg twice daily on the second day, and 300 mg 3 times daily on the third day. Subsequently, the dosage may be increased as needed for pain relief up to a total dosage of 1.8 g daily administered in 3 divided doses. In clinical studies evaluating gabapentin for the treatment of PHN, dosages of the drug ranging from 1.8–3.6 g daily were effective, but there was no evidence that dosages exceeding 1.8 g daily provided any additional benefit. If gabapentin dosage reduction or discontinuance or substitution of an alternative drug is necessary, such changes in therapy should be made gradually over a period of at least 1 week.

The recommended dosage of gabapentin as the gastroretentive preparation in adults with PHN is 1.8 g once daily; dosage should be titrated gradually over 2 weeks up to the recommended maintenance dosage as follows: 300 mg once daily on the first day, 600 mg once daily on the second day, 900 mg once daily on days 3–6, 1.2 g once daily on days 7–10, 1.5 g once daily on days 11–14, and 1.8 g once daily on day 15. If gabapentin dosage reduction or discontinuance or substitution of an alternative drug is necessary, such changes in therapy should be made gradually over a period of at least 1 week.

If gabapentin enacarbil extended-release tablets are used for the management of PHN in adults, the recommended dosage is 600 mg twice daily; dosage should be initiated at 600 mg once daily in the morning for 3 days, then increased to 600 mg twice daily. In the principal efficacy study of gabapentin enacarbil in patients with PHN, dosages exceeding 1.2 g daily provided no additional benefit and were associated with an increased incidence of adverse effects. When discontinuing gabapentin enacarbil therapy, patients receiving a dosage of 600 mg twice daily should reduce their dosage to 600 mg once daily for 1 week prior to withdrawing therapy. (See Cautions: Precautions and Contraindications.)

Restless Legs Syndrome

For the treatment of restless legs syndrome, the recommended adult dosage of gabapentin enacarbil extended-release tablets is 600 mg once daily, administered at approximately 5 p.m. In clinical studies, a higher dosage of 1.2 g daily provided no additional benefit and was associated with an increased incidence of adverse effects.

When discontinuing gabapentin enacarbil therapy in patients with restless legs syndrome, gradual tapering of the dosage is not necessary in patients receiving a daily dosage of 600 mg or less; however, in patients receiving higher than recommended dosages, dosage should be reduced to 600 mg once daily for 1 week prior to withdrawing therapy. (See Cautions: Precautions and Contraindications.)

Diabetic Neuropathy

For the symptomatic treatment of diabetic neuropathy† in adults, initial gabapentin dosages of 300 mg to 1.2 g daily (usually administered in divided doses; as conventional [immediate-release] preparations) have been used; gradual dosage titration is recommended based on patient response and tolerability. Target daily dosages from 1.2 g up to a maximum of 3.6 g (administered in divided doses; given as conventional preparations) often are required for adequate pain relief in such patients.

In a systematic review of gabapentin in chronic neuropathic pain, including diabetic neuropathy, in adults, some benefit was observed with gabapentin dosages of at least 1.2 g daily (administered orally as gabapentin or gabapentin enacarbil formulations).

Vasomotor Symptoms

Although the optimum dosage remains to be established, a gabapentin dosage of 300 mg 3 times daily (as conventional [immediate-release] preparations) has been effective in reducing both the severity and frequency of vasomotor symptoms† in women with breast cancer and in postmenopausal women. Some clinicians recommend that therapy be initiated with a dosage of 300 mg once daily at bedtime. If needed, the dosage can be increased to 300 mg twice daily, and then to 300 mg 3 times daily, at 3- to 4-day intervals. A dosage of 100 mg 3 times daily appears to be no more effective than placebo, whereas dosages exceeding 900 mg daily (e.g., up to 2.7 g daily administered as 900 mg 3 times daily) may provide additional benefit in some women.

● *Dosage in Renal Impairment*

Gabapentin

In adults and children 12 years of age or older with impaired renal function or undergoing hemodialysis, dosage of gabapentin (as conventional preparations) should be reduced from the effective dosages for each indication based on the patient's creatinine clearance (see Table 1). In patients with a creatinine clearance of less than 15 mL/minute, dosage should be reduced in proportion to creatinine clearance (e.g., a patient with a creatinine clearance of 7.5 mL/minute should receive one-half the dosage that a patient with a creatinine clearance of 15 mL/minute should receive). Patients undergoing hemodialysis should receive a supplemental dose of gabapentin 125–350 mg immediately following each 4-hour hemodialysis session in addition to their renally adjusted daily dosage of the drug. The use of gabapentin conventional preparations in children younger than 12 years of age with impaired renal function has not been evaluated.

TABLE 1. Dosage Adjustments for Renal Impairment in Adults and Children 12 Years of Age or Older Receiving Conventional (Immediate-release) Gabapentin

Creatinine Clearance (mL/minute)	Adjusted Dosage Regimen
>30 to 59	200–700 mg twice daily (i.e., up to a total dosage of 1.4 g daily)
>15 to 29	200–700 mg once daily
15	100–300 mg once daily

If gabapentin gastroretentive tablets are used in adults with a creatinine clearance of 30–60 mL/minute, dosage of the drug should be reduced to a target daily dosage between 600 mg and 1.8 g once daily; dosage must be initiated at 300 mg once daily in these patients and may be titrated according to the same schedule recommended for those with normal renal function based on individual patient response and tolerability. Gabapentin gastroretentive tablets should not be used in patients with a creatinine clearance of less than 30 mL/minute or in those undergoing hemodialysis.

Gabapentin Enacarbil

In patients with renal impairment, dosage of gabapentin enacarbil should be modified based on the degree of impairment as assessed by creatinine clearance (see Tables 2 or 3 depending on indication).

TABLE 2. Dosage Adjustments for Renal Impairment in Adults Receiving Gabapentin Enacarbil for Postherpetic Neuralgia

Creatinine Clearance (mL/minute)	Titration Schedule	Maintenance Dosage	Tapering Schedule
30–59	300 mg once daily in the morning for 3 days	300 mg twice daily; increase to 600 mg twice daily as necessary based on patient response and tolerability	Reduce maintenance dosage to once daily in the morning for 1 week
15–29	300 mg once daily in the morning on days 1 and 3	300 mg once daily in the morning; increase to 300 mg twice daily if necessary based on patient response and tolerability	In patients currently receiving a maintenance dosage of 300 mg twice daily, reduce to 300 mg once daily in the morning for 1 week; in patients currently receiving a maintenance dosage of 300 mg once daily, no taper needed
<15 not on hemodialysis	None	300 mg every other day in the morning; increase to 300 mg once daily if necessary based on patient response and tolerability	None
<15 on hemodialysis	None	300 mg following each hemodialysis session; increase to 600 mg following each hemodialysis session if necessary based on patient response and tolerability	None

TABLE 3. Dosage Adjustments for Renal Impairment in Adults Receiving Gabapentin Enacarbil for Restless Legs Syndrome

Creatinine Clearance (mL/minute)	Target Dosage
30–59	Initiate at 300 mg once daily, then increase to 600 mg once daily as needed
15–29	300 mg once daily
<15 not on hemodialysis	300 mg every other day
<15 on hemodialysis	Use not recommended

CAUTIONS

Gabapentin generally is well tolerated, and adverse effects of the drug usually are mild to moderate in severity and may be self-limiting. CNS effects are the most frequently reported adverse affects of gabapentin and those most frequently requiring discontinuance of the drug.

The most common adverse effects reported in clinical studies of conventional (immediate-release) gabapentin as adjunctive therapy for seizures in adults and children older than 12 years of age were somnolence, dizziness, ataxia, fatigue, and nystagmus. Discontinuance of gabapentin because of adverse effects was required in 7% of these patients, most frequently due to somnolence (1.2%), ataxia (0.8%), fatigue (0.6%), nausea and/or vomiting (0.6%), and dizziness (0.6%). The most common adverse effects reported in clinical studies of conventional (immediate-release) gabapentin as adjunctive therapy of seizures in children 3–12 years of age were viral infection, fever, nausea and/or vomiting, somnolence, and hostility. Discontinuance of gabapentin because of adverse effects was required in approximately 7% of these patients, most frequently due to emotional lability (1.6%), hostility (1.3%), and hyperkinesia (1.1%). Because clinical trials of gabapentin in the treatment of partial seizures involved specific patient populations and use of the drug as adjunctive therapy, it is difficult to determine whether a causal relationship exists for many reported adverse effects, to compare adverse effect frequencies with other clinical reports, and/or to extrapolate the adverse effect experience from controlled clinical trials to usual clinical practice.

In placebo-controlled studies of gabapentin for the management of postherpetic neuralgia (PHN), adverse effects most frequently reported in adults receiving conventional (immediate-release) preparations of the drug were dizziness, somnolence, and peripheral edema. Discontinuance of gabapentin because of adverse effects was required in 16% of these patients, most frequently due to dizziness, somnolence, and nausea. In placebo-controlled studies using the gastroretentive formulation of gabapentin, dizziness was reported as the most frequent adverse effect (10.9%); in these trials, 9.7% of patients required premature discontinuance of therapy because of adverse effects, the most common of which was dizziness.

Similar to gabapentin, the most frequently reported adverse effects of gabapentin enacarbil are CNS effects. In the principal efficacy study of gabapentin enacarbil for the management of PHN, the most common adverse effects were dizziness, somnolence, and headache. Adverse effects resulted in discontinuance of gabapentin enacarbil therapy in 6% of these patients. The most common adverse effects observed in patients receiving gabapentin enacarbil for the treatment of restless legs syndrome in placebo-controlled trials were somnolence/sedation, and dizziness; in these trials, 7% of patients required premature discontinuance of therapy because of adverse effects.

● Nervous System Effects

In controlled clinical trials of conventional (immediate-release) gabapentin as adjunctive therapy of seizures in adults and children older than 12 years of age, somnolence was the most frequent adverse CNS effect, occurring in about 19% of those receiving the drug; the incidence and severity of somnolence appear to be dose related. Dose-related dizziness or ataxia was reported in about 17 or 13%, respectively, of patients receiving gabapentin in these trials. Fatigue was reported in 11%, nystagmus in 8%, tremor in 7%, dysarthria in 2%, amnesia in 2%, depression in 2%, abnormal thinking in 2%, and abnormal coordination in 1% of patients receiving the drug.

In controlled clinical trials of conventional gabapentin as adjunctive therapy of seizures in children 3–12 years of age, somnolence, hostility (including aggressive behavior), and emotional lability were reported in 8, 8, and 4%, respectively, of patients receiving the drug. Fatigue, hyperkinesia, and dizziness each were reported in 3% of these patients. Headache and convulsions were reported in more than 2%, and thought disorders (e.g., concentration difficulty, change in school performance) were reported in 1.7% of these children.

In controlled clinical trials of conventional gabapentin for the management of PHN in adults, dizziness was reported in 28%, somnolence in 21%, asthenia in 6%, ataxia in 3%, and abnormal thinking in 3% of patients receiving the drug. Abnormal gait and incoordination occurred in 2% of these patients. Pain, tremor, and neuralgia were reported in greater than 1% of patients receiving gabapentin for PHN in clinical studies but occurred with equal or greater frequency in patients receiving placebo. Dizziness, somnolence, headache, and lethargy were reported in about 11, 5, 4, and 1%, respectively, of adults receiving gabapentin gastroretentive tablets for PHN in controlled clinical studies; vertigo occurred in about 1% of patients receiving the drug.

In the placebo-controlled study of gabapentin enacarbil for the management of PHN, dizziness was reported in 17–30%, somnolence was reported in 10–14%, and headache was reported in 7–10% of patients receiving the drug. Fatigue or asthenia occurred in 4–10% and insomnia occurred in 3–7% of these patients. Somnolence/sedation (20–27%) and dizziness (13–22%) were the most common adverse effects reported in patients receiving gabapentin enacarbil for the treatment of restless legs syndrome in placebo-controlled studies. Headache occurred in 12–15%, fatigue in 6–7%, and irritability in 4% of patients receiving the drug;

1–3% of these patients reported feeling intoxicated. Depression and decreased libido were reported in up to 3% and up to 2% of these patients, respectively.

The effect of gabapentin enacarbil on driving performance was evaluated in several driving simulation studies. In one study in healthy individuals, gabapentin enacarbil (600 mg once daily for 5 days) did not appear to affect driving performance (as assessed by lane position variability) when tested at various time points after dosing. However, results of another driving simulation study in patients with moderate-to-severe primary restless legs syndrome showed evidence of substantial driving impairment with gabapentin enacarbil (1.2 or 1.8 g daily); patients receiving the drug had greater lane position variability and a higher incidence of simulated crashes compared with those receiving placebo or an active comparator (diphenhydramine). There is some evidence, however, that patients with restless legs syndrome may have impaired driving ability in the absence of medication.

Suicidality

An increased risk of suicidality (suicidal behavior or ideation) was observed in an analysis of studies using various anticonvulsants, including gabapentin, compared with placebo. The analysis of suicidality reports from 199 placebo-controlled studies involving 11 anticonvulsants (carbamazepine, felbamate, gabapentin, lamotrigine, levetiracetam, oxcarbazepine, pregabalin, tiagabine, topiramate, valproate, and zonisamide) in patients with epilepsy, psychiatric disorders (e.g., bipolar disorder, depression, anxiety), and other conditions (e.g., migraine, neuropathic pain) found that patients receiving anticonvulsants had approximately twice the risk of suicidal behavior or ideation (0.43%) compared with patients receiving placebo (0.24%). The increased suicidality risk was observed as early as 1 week after beginning therapy. Because most of these studies did not extend beyond 24 weeks, the suicidality risk beyond 24 weeks is not known. The results were generally consistent among the 11 drugs studied. Although patients who were treated for epilepsy, psychiatric disorders, and other conditions were all found to be at increased risk for suicidality when compared with placebo, the relative risk for suicidality was higher in patients with epilepsy compared with those receiving anticonvulsants for other conditions. (See Cautions: Precautions and Contraindications.)

● GI Effects

Dyspepsia, dry mouth or throat, constipation, and dental abnormalities each occurred in 2% of adults and children older than 12 years of age receiving conventional (immediate-release) gabapentin as adjunctive therapy for seizures in controlled clinical trials.

Nausea and/or vomiting was reported in 8% of children 3–12 years of age receiving conventional (immediate-release) gabapentin as adjunctive therapy for seizures in controlled clinical trials. Diarrhea and anorexia were reported in more than 2% of children 3–12 years of age receiving the drug in these trials.

Diarrhea was reported in 6%, dry mouth in 5%, constipation in 4%, nausea in 4%, and vomiting in 3% of adults receiving conventional (immediate-release) gabapentin for the management of PHN in controlled clinical trials. Dyspepsia was reported in greater than 1% of patients receiving conventional gabapentin for the management of PHN in clinical studies, but occurred with equal or greater frequency in patients receiving placebo. In controlled clinical trials evaluating gabapentin gastroretentive tablets for the management of PHN, diarrhea was reported in 3.3%, dry mouth in 2.8%, constipation in 1.4%, and dyspepsia in 1.4% of adults receiving the drug.

In the principal efficacy study of gabapentin enacarbil in the management of PHN, nausea occurred in 4–9% of adults receiving the drug. Nausea, dry mouth, and flatulence were reported in 6–7%, 3–4%, and 2–3%, respectively, of patients receiving gabapentin enacarbil in placebo-controlled studies of the drug for restless legs syndrome.

● Cardiovascular Effects

Peripheral edema was reported in 2% and vasodilation in 1% of adults and children older than 12 years of age receiving conventional (immediate-release) gabapentin as adjunctive therapy for seizures in controlled clinical trials.

Peripheral edema was reported in 8% of adults receiving conventional (immediate-release) gabapentin and in 3.9% of adults receiving gabapentin gastroretentive tablets for the management of PHN in controlled clinical trials.

In controlled clinical studies, peripheral edema was reported in 6–7% of adults receiving gabapentin enacarbil for the management of PHN and in up to 3% of adults receiving the drug for restless legs syndrome.

● Respiratory Effects

Pharyngitis occurred in 3% and coughing in 2% of adults and children older than 12 years of age receiving conventional (immediate-release) gabapentin as adjunctive therapy for seizures in controlled clinical trials.

Bronchitis and respiratory infection each were reported in 3% of children 3–12 years of age receiving conventional (immediate-release) gabapentin as adjunctive therapy for seizures in controlled clinical trials. Pharyngitis, upper respiratory infection, rhinitis, and coughing were reported in more than 2% of these children receiving the drug in these studies.

Pharyngitis was reported in 1% of adults receiving conventional (immediate-release) gabapentin for the management of PHN in controlled clinical trials; dyspnea was reported in greater than 1% of patients receiving the drug, but occurred with equal or greater frequency in patients receiving placebo. Nasopharyngitis was reported in 2.5% of adults receiving gabapentin gastroretentive tablets for PHN in controlled clinical trials.

Respiratory Depression

Serious, life-threatening, or fatal respiratory depression has been reported in patients receiving gabapentinoids (i.e., gabapentin and pregabalin). In the majority of cases, the drugs were used in combination with an opiate analgesic (or other CNS depressant), in patients with preexisting respiratory risk factors (e.g., COPD), or in geriatric patients. During a 5-year period between 2012 and 2017, 49 cases of respiratory depression associated with gabapentinoid use (15 cases with gabapentin and 34 cases with pregabalin) were reported to the FDA, including 12 fatalities. Most of the cases (92%) reported either concomitant use of another CNS depressant or a respiratory risk factor, including age-related decreases in lung function. In all of the fatal cases, patients had at least one risk factor for developing respiratory depression or were receiving a CNS depressant concomitantly. In addition, there is evidence from small randomized studies in healthy individuals and observational studies in postoperative patients suggesting that use of gabapentinoids alone or in conjunction with opiate analgesics may increase the risk of respiratory depression. In one study, gabapentin increased the apnea-hypopnea index in men 60 years of age or older who did not have preexisting sleep apnea. Although findings from these studies as well as animal data suggest that gabapentinoids may have an independent respiratory depressant effect, there is less evidence supporting the risk of serious respiratory complications when these drugs are used alone in otherwise healthy individuals. (See Cautions: Precautions and Contraindications.)

● Ocular and Otic Effects

Diplopia was reported in 6% and amblyopia in 4% of adults and children older than 12 years of age receiving conventional (immediate-release) gabapentin as adjunctive therapy for seizures in controlled clinical trials.

Otitis media was reported in more than 2% of children 3–12 years of age receiving conventional gabapentin as adjunctive therapy for seizures in clinical studies.

Amblyopia occurred in 3%, and conjunctivitis, diplopia, and otitis media each occurred in 1% of adults receiving conventional (immediate-release) gabapentin for the management of PHN in controlled clinical trials. In the placebo-controlled study of gabapentin enacarbil for the management of PHN, blurred vision occurred in 2–5% of adults receiving the drug.

● Musculoskeletal Effects

Back pain was reported in 2% of adults and children older than 12 years of age receiving conventional (immediate-release) gabapentin as adjunctive therapy for seizures in controlled clinical trials.

Elevated creatine kinase, rhabdomyolysis, and movement disorders have been reported during postmarketing experience with conventional gabapentin; however, the manufacturers state that data are insufficient to provide an estimate of the incidence of such effects or to establish a causal relationship to the drug.

Back pain was reported in greater than 1% of adults receiving conventional (immediate-release) gabapentin in clinical studies for the management of PHN but occurred with equal or greater frequency in patients receiving placebo. Back pain and extremity pain were reported in 1.7 and 1.9%, respectively, of adults receiving gabapentin gastroretentive tablets for PHN in controlled clinical trials.

● Genitourinary Effects

Impotence was reported in 2% of patients receiving conventional (immediate-release) gabapentin as adjunctive therapy for seizures in controlled clinical trials.

● Dermatologic and Sensitivity Reactions

Anaphylaxis and angioedema, sometimes requiring emergency treatment, have been reported in patients receiving conventional (immediate-release) gabapentin. Reported signs and symptoms include difficulty breathing; swelling of the lips, throat, and tongue; and hypotension.

Abrasion occurred in 1% of adults and children older than 12 years of age receiving conventional gabapentin as adjunctive therapy for seizures in controlled clinical trials.

Erythema multiforme and Stevens-Johnson syndrome have been reported during postmarketing experience with conventional gabapentin; however, the manufacturers state that data are insufficient to provide an estimate of the incidence of such effects or to establish a causal relationship to gabapentin.

Drug reaction with eosinophilia and systemic symptoms (DRESS), also known as multiorgan hypersensitivity, has been reported in patients receiving anticonvulsants, including gabapentin. The clinical presentation is variable, but typically includes fever, rash, eosinophilia, and/or lymphadenopathy in association with other organ system involvement (e.g., hepatitis, nephritis, hematologic abnormalities, myositis, myocarditis). In some cases, these reactions have been life-threatening or fatal. Early manifestations of hypersensitivity (e.g., fever, lymphadenopathy) may be present even if a rash is not evident.

● Hepatic Effects

Elevated liver function test results and jaundice have been reported during postmarketing experience with conventional (immediate-release) gabapentin; however, the manufacturers state that data are insufficient to provide an estimate of the incidence of such effects or to establish a causal relationship to gabapentin.

● Electrolyte and Metabolic Effects

Weight gain has been reported in 3% of patients receiving conventional (immediate-release) gabapentin as adjunctive therapy for seizures in clinical trials.

Weight gain and hyperglycemia were reported in 2 and 1%, respectively, of adults receiving conventional gabapentin for the management of PHN in controlled clinical trials. In studies evaluating gabapentin gastroretentive tablets for the management of PHN, weight gain was reported in about 2% of adults receiving the drug.

Fluctuation in blood glucose concentrations and hyponatremia have been reported during postmarketing experience with conventional gabapentin; however, the manufacturers state that data are insufficient to provide an estimate of the incidence of such effects or to establish a causal relationship to the drug.

Weight increase was reported in 3% of children 3–12 years of age receiving conventional gabapentin in controlled clinical trials.

In placebo-controlled studies of gabapentin enacarbil for the treatment of restless legs syndrome, weight gain occurred in 2–3% and increased appetite occurred in 2% of patients receiving the drug; weight gain was reported in 3–5% of patients receiving gabapentin enacarbil for the management of PHN in the principal efficacy study.

● Other Adverse Effects

Breast enlargement has been reported during postmarketing experience with conventional (immediate-release) gabapentin; however, the manufacturers state that data are insufficient to provide an estimate of the incidence of such an effect or to establish a causal relationship to the drug.

Viral infection and fever were reported in 11 and 10%, respectively, of children 3–12 years of age receiving conventional gabapentin as adjunctive therapy for seizures in controlled clinical trials.

Infection and accidental injury were reported in 5 and 3%, respectively, of adults receiving conventional gabapentin for the management of PHN in controlled clinical trials. Flu syndrome was reported in greater than 1% of patients receiving conventional gabapentin for the management of PHN, but occurred with equal or greater frequency in patients receiving placebo. In controlled clinical trials evaluating gabapentin gastroretentive tablets for the management of PHN, urinary tract infection was reported in 1.7% of adults receiving the drug.

In placebo-controlled studies of gabapentin enacarbil for the treatment of restless legs syndrome, up to 3% of patients reported feeling abnormal.

● Precautions and Contraindications

An increased risk of suicidality (suicidal behavior or ideation) has been observed with various anticonvulsants, including gabapentin. (See Suicidality under Cautions: Nervous System Effects.) Because gabapentin enacarbil is a prodrug of gabapentin, a similar risk with gabapentin enacarbil cannot be ruled out. Patients who are currently receiving or beginning therapy with any anticonvulsant for any indication should be closely monitored for the emergence or worsening of depression, suicidal thoughts or behavior (suicidality), and/or any unusual changes in mood or behavior. Clinicians should inform patients, their families, and caregivers of the potential for an increased risk of suicidality with anticonvulsant therapy and advise them to pay close attention to any day-to-day changes in mood, behavior, and actions; since changes can happen very quickly, it is important to be alert to any sudden differences. In addition, patients, family members, and caregivers should be aware of common warning signs that may signal suicide risk (e.g., talking or thinking about wanting to hurt oneself or end one's life, withdrawing from friends and family, becoming depressed or experiencing worsening of existing depression, becoming preoccupied with death and dying, giving away prized possessions). If these or any new and worrisome behaviors occur, the responsible clinician should be contacted immediately. Clinicians who prescribe gabapentin or any other anticonvulsant should balance the risk for suicidality with the risk of untreated illness. Epilepsy and many other illnesses for which anticonvulsants are prescribed are themselves associated with an increased risk of morbidity and mortality and an increased risk of suicidal thoughts and behavior. If suicidal thoughts and behavior emerge during anticonvulsant therapy, the clinician must consider whether the emergence of these symptoms in any given patient may be related to the illness being treated.

Because serious and potentially fatal respiratory depression can occur when gabapentinoids (i.e., gabapentin and pregabalin) are used in combination with opiate analgesics or other CNS depressants (e.g., benzodiazepines), in the setting of underlying respiratory impairment, or in geriatric patients, patients should be monitored for respiratory depression and sedation in these situations. (See Cautions: Respiratory Effects.) Consideration should be given to initiating gabapentin therapy at the lowest dosage and titrating the dosage carefully; appropriate dosage adjustments should be made in patients with renal impairment and those undergoing hemodialysis. (See Dosage in Renal Impairment under Dosage and Administration: Dosage.) Patients and caregivers should be advised to seek immediate medical attention if signs or symptoms of respiratory depression occur (e.g., slow, shallow, or difficult breathing; confusion or disorientation; unusual dizziness or lightheadedness; extreme sleepiness or lethargy; bluish-colored or tinted skin, especially on the lips, fingers, and toes; unresponsiveness). Management of respiratory depression may include close observation, supportive measures, and reduction or withdrawal of CNS depressants, including gabapentin. If the decision is made to discontinue gabapentin, dosage should be reduced gradually.

Because of the possibility of increased seizure frequency and other withdrawal symptoms (e.g., anxiety, insomnia, nausea), gabapentin and gabapentin enacarbil should not be discontinued suddenly; any changes in therapy (e.g., discontinuance, dosage reduction, substitution with an alternative drug) should be done gradually. (See Dosage and Administration: Dosage.) In controlled studies of gabapentin as conventional (immediate-release) formulations, the incidence of status epilepticus was 0.6% in adults and children older than 12 years of age receiving gabapentin and 0.5% in those receiving placebo. In all (uncontrolled and controlled) clinical studies of gabapentin as adjunctive therapy in adults and children older than 12 years of age, the incidence of status epilepticus was 1.5%. Because adequate historical data are unavailable for comparison, it has not been established whether the incidence of status epilepticus in patients with epilepsy treated with gabapentin is higher or lower than would be expected in a similar population of patients not treated with the drug.

During the premarketing development of conventional (immediate-release) gabapentin, 8 sudden and unexplained deaths were reported among a cohort of 2203 patients with epilepsy (2103 patient-years of exposure). Although the rate of these deaths exceeds that expected to occur in a healthy (nonepileptic) population matched for age and gender, this rate was similar to that occurring in a similar population of epileptic patients not receiving gabapentin. This evidence suggests, but does not prove that the incidence of sudden, unexplained death observed with adjunctive gabapentin therapy may be reflective of the population itself rather than the effects of gabapentin.

Gabapentin can produce drowsiness and dizziness, and patients should be cautioned that the drug may impair their ability to perform hazardous activities requiring mental alertness or physical coordination (e.g., operating machinery, driving a motor vehicle) or cause accidental injury (e.g., falls). Gabapentin enacarbil has been shown to cause substantial impairment in driving performance, which may be related to somnolence or other CNS effects of the drug; the duration of such impairment following administration of the drug is not known. Patients should not drive a car (or operate other complex machinery) until they have gained sufficient experience with these drugs; clinicians should consider that a patient's ability to assess their performance on these tasks or their degree of somnolence may not be reliable.

Patients should be evaluated immediately if manifestations of multiorgan hypersensitivity (or DRESS) occur during gabapentin or gabapentin enacarbil therapy; the drug should be discontinued if an alternative etiology cannot be identified.

Anaphylaxis and angioedema may occur after the first dose of gabapentin or at any time during therapy. Patients should be instructed to discontinue gabapentin and seek immediate medical attention if they develop any manifestations of anaphylaxis or angioedema.

Concomitant use of alcohol or other drugs that can cause sedation or dizziness can potentiate the CNS effects of gabapentin and generally should be avoided. In addition, alcohol can increase the rate of drug release from gabapentin enacarbil extended-release tablets and should be avoided in patients receiving this formulation. Concomitant use of opiate analgesics in patients receiving gabapentin may result in increased plasma concentrations of gabapentin and increase the risk of adverse CNS effects and respiratory depression; dosage adjustments may be required with such concomitant use.

Gabapentin is contraindicated in patients with known hypersensitivity to the drug or any ingredient in the formulation. The manufacturer of gabapentin enacarbil states that there are no known contraindications to the use of this preparation.

● Pediatric Precautions

Safety and efficacy of conventional (immediate-release) gabapentin as adjunctive therapy in the management of partial seizures in children younger than 3 years of age have not been established. Safety and efficacy of conventional gabapentin in the management of PHN have not been established in pediatric patients. Safety and efficacy of gabapentin gastroretentive tablets and gabapentin enacarbil have not been established in pediatric patients.

● Geriatric Precautions

Safety and efficacy of conventional (immediate-release) gabapentin in the management of partial seizures in geriatric patients have not been evaluated systematically, and clinical trials did not include sufficient numbers of patients 65 years of age and older to determine whether they respond differently than do younger patients. However, in clinical studies of the drug in patients ranging from 20–80 years of age, gabapentin plasma clearance, renal clearance, and renal clearance adjusted for body surface area declined with age. Although safety and efficacy of conventional gabapentin in geriatric patients with PHN have not been established specifically, 30% of the patients receiving the drug in clinical studies were 65–74 years of age and 50% were 75 years of age and older. In these studies, gabapentin appeared to be more effective for the management of PHN in patients older than 75 years of age than in younger patients. The manufacturers state that the apparent greater efficacy in geriatric patients may be related to decreased renal function in this age group. Although adverse effects reported in older patients receiving conventional gabapentin generally were similar to those reported in younger adults, the incidence of peripheral edema and ataxia appeared to increase with age. Among patients receiving the gastroretentive formulation of gabapentin in clinical studies, 63% were 65 years of age or older. Adverse effects reported in these studies generally were similar across all age groups except for the incidence of peripheral edema, which tended to increase with age.

Clinical trials of gabapentin enacarbil for the treatment of restless legs syndrome did not include sufficient numbers of patients 65 years of age or older to determine whether they respond differently than younger patients. In the principal efficacy study of gabapentin enacarbil for the treatment of PHN, 37% of the patients were 65–74 years of age and 13% were 75 years of age and older. No overall differences in safety and efficacy were observed between these geriatric patients and younger patients.

FDA warns that geriatric patients receiving gabapentinoids are at increased risk of potentially serious, life-threatening, or fatal respiratory depression; gabapentin therapy should be initiated at the lowest dosage and titrated carefully with close monitoring in such patients. The manufacturers state that if gabapentin or gabapentin enacarbil is used in geriatric patients, dosage reduction may be required because of age-related compromised renal function; caution should be exercised since renal, hepatic, and cardiovascular dysfunction and concomitant disease or other drug therapy are more common in this age group than in younger patients. (See Dosage and Administration: Dosage in Renal Impairment.)

● Mutagenicity and Carcinogenicity

Gabapentin has not been shown to be mutagenic or genotoxic in various in vitro and in vivo tests.

An increased incidence of pancreatic acinar cell tumors was observed with gabapentin and gabapentin enacarbil in rat carcinogenicity studies; the clinical importance of these findings to humans is not known. In clinical studies of gabapentin in patients older than 12 years of age with seizure disorders, new tumors or worsening of preexisting tumors was reported in 21 patients (based on 2085 patient-years of exposure); however, a causal relationship to the drug has not been established.

● Pregnancy, Fertility, and Lactation

Pregnancy

Although there are no adequate and controlled studies to date in pregnant women, gabapentin and gabapentin enacarbil have been shown to cause developmental toxicity when administered to pregnant animals during the period of organogenesis at doses similar to or lower than those used clinically. Such effects include skeletal abnormalities, hydroureter and hydronephrosis, and increased embryofetal mortality. In addition, abnormal or decreased synaptic formation was observed in neonatal mice exposed to intraperitoneal injections of gabapentin during the first postnatal week (corresponding to the last trimester of pregnancy in humans); the clinical importance of these findings is not known.

Gabapentin and gabapentin enacarbil should be used during pregnancy only when the potential benefits justify the possible risks to the fetus. Women who become pregnant while receiving gabapentin should be encouraged to enroll in the North American Antiepileptic Drug (NAAED) Pregnancy Registry by calling 888-233-2334; registry information also is available on the website at https://www.aedpregnancyregistry.org.

Fertility

Animal reproduction studies revealed no adverse effects on fertility or reproduction with gabapentin exposure levels 8 times those achieved in humans at the maximum recommended dosages.

Lactation

Gabapentin is distributed into milk following oral administration. Because of the potential for serious adverse reactions to gabapentin in nursing infants, the drug should be administered to nursing women only if the potential benefits justify the risk to the infant. The manufacturer of gabapentin enacarbil states that a decision should be made whether to discontinue nursing or the drug, taking into account the importance of the drug to the woman.

DESCRIPTION

Gabapentin is an anticonvulsant agent structurally related to the inhibitory CNS neurotransmitter γ-aminobutyric acid (GABA). Gabapentin enacarbil is a prodrug of gabapentin that is rapidly converted to gabapentin following oral administration; the therapeutic effects of gabapentin enacarbil are attributed to gabapentin. Although gabapentin was developed as a structural analog of GABA that would penetrate the blood-brain barrier (unlike GABA) and mimic the action of GABA at inhibitory neuronal synapses, the drug has no direct GABA-mimetic action and its precise mechanism of action has not been elucidated.

Results of some studies in animals indicate that gabapentin protects against seizure and/or tonic extensions induced by the GABA antagonists picrotoxin and bicuculline or by GABA synthesis inhibitors (e.g., 3-mercaptopropionic acid, isonicotinic acid, semicarbazide). However, gabapentin does not appear to bind to GABA receptors nor affect GABA reuptake or metabolism and does not act as a precursor of GABA or of other substances active at GABA receptors. Gabapentin also has no affinity for binding sites on common neuroreceptors (e.g., benzodiazepine; glutamate; quisqualate; kainate; strychnine-insensitive or -sensitive glycine; α_1-, α_2-, or β-adrenergic; adenosine A_1 or A_2; cholinergic [muscarinic or nicotinic]; dopamine D_1 or D_2; histamine H_1; type 1 or 2 serotonergic [5-HT_1 or 5-HT_2]; opiate μ, δ, or κ) or ion channels (e.g., voltage-sensitive calcium channel sites labeled with nitrendipine or diltiazem, voltage-sensitive sodium channel sites labeled with batrachotoxin A 20α-benzoate). Conflicting results have been reported in studies of gabapentin affinity for and activity at N-methyl-D-aspartic acid (NMDA) receptors.

In animal test systems, gabapentin exhibits anticonvulsant activity similar to that of other commonly used anticonvulsant drugs. The drug protects against seizures induced in animals by electrical stimulation or pentylenetetrazole, suggesting that it may be effective in the management of tonic-clonic (grand mal) and partial seizures or absence (petit mal) seizures, respectively. However, available data in animals and humans are conflicting regarding the effect of gabapentin on EEG spike and wave activity associated with absence (petit mal) seizures. Gabapentin also prevents seizures in some animals with congenital epilepsy and protects against audiogenic tonic extensions and clonic seizures in mice.

Although the exact mechanism by which gabapentin exerts its analgesic effects is not known, the drug has been shown to prevent allodynia (pain-related behavior in response to normally innocuous stimuli) and hyperalgesia (exaggerated response to painful stimuli) in several models of neuropathic pain. Gabapentin also has been shown to decrease pain-related responses after peripheral inflammation in animals; however, the drug has not altered immediate pain-related behaviors. The clinical relevance of these findings is not known. In vitro studies demonstrate that gabapentin binds to the $\alpha_2\delta$ subunit of voltage-activated calcium channels; however, the clinical importance of this effect is not known.

The pharmacokinetic properties of gabapentin vary based on the specific formulation of the drug. (See Dosage and Administration: Administration.) Following oral administration, gabapentin is absorbed principally in the proximal small intestine via a saturable L-amino acid transport system; as a result, the bioavailability of the drug decreases with increasing doses. Gabapentin gastroretentive tablets are specifically formulated to swell upon contact with gastric fluid to a size that promotes gastric retention for approximately 8–10 hours when taken with a meal; this allows for gradual and slow release of the drug to the proximal small intestine, its principal site of absorption. Following administration of gabapentin gastroretentive tablets in healthy individuals, time to peak plasma concentrations of the drug was increased (about 4–6 hours longer), peak plasma concentrations were increased, and systemic exposure was decreased relative to conventional (immediate-release) gabapentin. Gabapentin enacarbil, a prodrug of gabapentin, is rapidly and efficiently converted to gabapentin by first-pass hydrolysis following oral administration. Unlike gabapentin, gabapentin enacarbil is absorbed via high-capacity transporters throughout the GI tract and is not affected by saturable absorption; this improves bioavailability of the drug and allows for dose-proportional exposure. Food has only a minimal effect on the pharmacokinetics of conventional (immediate-release) formulations of gabapentin, but increases the bioavailability of gabapentin gastroretentive tablets. Administration of gabapentin enacarbil extended-release tablets with food also increases systemic exposure of the drug compared with exposure under fasted conditions. Gabapentin does not bind to plasma proteins, is not appreciably metabolized, does not induce hepatic enzyme activity, and does not appear to alter the pharmacokinetics of commonly used anticonvulsant drugs (e.g., carbamazepine, phenytoin, valproate, phenobarbital, diazepam) or oral contraceptives. In addition, the pharmacokinetics of gabapentin are not altered substantially by concomitant administration of other anticonvulsant drugs.

PREPARATIONS

Excipients in commercially available drug preparations may have clinically important effects in some individuals; consult specific product labeling for details.

Gabapentin

Oral

Capsules	100 mg*	Gabapentin Capsules Neurontin®, Pfizer
	300 mg*	Gabapentin Capsules Neurontin®, Pfizer
	400 mg*	Gabapentin Capsules Neurontin®, Pfizer
Solution	250 mg/5 mL*	Neurontin®, Pfizer
Tablets	100 mg*	Gabapentin Tablets
	300 mg*	Gabapentin Tablets Gralise®, Depomed
	400 mg*	Gabapentin Tablets
	600 mg*	Gabapentin Tablets Gralise®, Depomed
	800 mg*	Gabapentin Tablets
Tablets, film-coated	600 mg*	Gabapentin Tablets Neurontin®, Pfizer
	800 mg*	Gabapentin Tablets Neurontin®, Pfizer

* available from one or more manufacturer, distributor, and/or repackager by generic (nonproprietary) name

Gabapentin Enacarbil

Oral

Tablets, extended-release	300 mg	Horizant®, Arbor
	600 mg	Horizant®, Arbor

† Use is not currently included in the labeling approved by the US Food and Drug Administration.

Selected Revisions June 10, 2024, © Copyright, June 1, 1993, American Society of Health-System Pharmacists, Inc.

Pregabalin

28:12.28 • GABA-MEDIATED ANTICONVULSANTS

■ Pregabalin is an anticonvulsant structurally related to the inhibitory CNS neurotransmitter γ-aminobutyric acid (GABA); the drug also possesses analgesic activity.

USES

● Seizure Disorders

Pregabalin is used as adjunctive therapy (i.e., in combination with other anticonvulsant agents) for the management of partial seizures in adults and pediatric patients 1 month of age or older. Clinical studies establishing efficacy of pregabalin for this indication were conducted with conventional (immediate-release) preparations of the drug; efficacy of the extended-release preparation has not been established in patients with partial seizures.

Efficacy of pregabalin conventional preparations for adjunctive therapy of partial seizures in adults was established in three 12-week, multicenter, randomized, double-blind, placebo-controlled studies in patients with refractory partial onset seizures with or without secondary generalization who were receiving a regimen of 1–3 anticonvulsants, but were continuing to have seizures (based on a prespecified number of partial seizures experienced during a baseline period). In these studies, patients receiving pregabalin 150, 300, or 600 mg daily (administered in 2 or 3 divided doses as conventional preparations) experienced a median decrease in seizure frequency of 17–35, 37, or 36–51%, respectively, while those receiving placebo experienced no appreciable change in seizure frequency. In one study, 31, 40, or 51% of patients receiving pregabalin 150, 300, or 600 mg daily, respectively, and 14% of those receiving placebo experienced at least a 50% reduction in seizure frequency; in another study, 43 or 49% of those receiving pregabalin 600 mg daily in 2 or 3 divided doses, respectively, and 9% of those receiving placebo experienced at least a 50% reduction in seizure frequency.

Efficacy of pregabalin conventional preparations for adjunctive therapy of partial seizures in pediatric patients was established in 2 multicenter, randomized, double-blind, placebo-controlled studies (one 12-week study in patients 4–16 years of age and one 14-day study in patients 1 month to less than 4 years of age). Both studies included patients with partial onset seizures with or without secondary generalization who were receiving 1–3 concurrent anticonvulsant agents at baseline, but were continuing to have seizures (based on a prespecified number of partial-onset seizures experienced during a baseline period). In the 12-week study, patients were randomized to receive pregabalin 2.5 mg/kg daily (maximum of 150 mg daily), pregabalin 10 mg/kg daily (maximum of 600 mg daily), or placebo in 2 divided doses. Because of higher clearance in patients weighing less than 30 kg, the daily dosage of pregabalin for these patients was increased to 3.5 or 14 mg/kg daily. In this study, patients receiving pregabalin 10 mg/kg daily experienced a 21% greater reduction in partial seizure frequency relative to placebo. Although patients receiving the 2.5-mg/kg daily dosage had a reduction in partial seizure frequency of about 10.5% compared with placebo, the difference was not statistically significant. Approximately 41 or 29% of patients receiving pregabalin 10 or 2.5 mg/kg daily, respectively, and 23% of those receiving placebo in this study experienced at least a 50% reduction in seizure frequency. In the 14-day study, patients were randomized to receive pregabalin (7 or 14 mg/kg daily in 3 divided doses) or placebo. Pregabalin 14 mg/kg daily reduced partial seizure frequency by 43.9% compared with placebo. Approximately 54% of patients receiving pregabalin 14 mg/kg daily experienced at least a 50% reduction in seizure frequency compared with 42% of those receiving placebo. The 7-mg/kg daily dosage of pregabalin was not more effective than placebo in this study.

● Neuropathic Pain

Postherpetic Neuralgia

Pregabalin is used for the management of postherpetic neuralgia (PHN) in adults.

Efficacy of pregabalin conventional preparations for the management of PHN has been established in 3 multicenter, double-blind, placebo-controlled studies in adults with neuralgia persisting for at least 3 months following healing of herpes zoster rash. In these studies, mean pain scores (assessed on an 11-point numerical rating scale) at the end of 8 or 13 weeks of treatment were improved in patients receiving pregabalin compared with those receiving placebo; in addition, a greater proportion of patients receiving pregabalin, compared with those receiving placebo, achieved at least a 50% reduction in pain score from baseline. In these studies, pregabalin was administered at dosages of 150 or 300 mg daily in patients with renal impairment (i.e., creatinine clearance of 30–60 mL/minute) and at dosages of 150, 300, or 600 mg daily in patients with normal renal function (i.e., creatinine clearance greater than 60 mL/minute).

Efficacy of extended-release pregabalin for the management of PHN is based on studies conducted with conventional preparations of the drug in addition to a randomized withdrawal study in adults with persistent pain for more than 3 months after healing of their herpes zoster rash. In the randomized withdrawal study, pregabalin daily doses of 82.5, 165, 247.5, 330, 495, and 660 mg as extended-release tablets were compared with placebo. Patients who experienced at least a 50% reduction in mean pain scores during a 6-week single-blind treatment phase were randomized to receive pregabalin or placebo. Mean pain scores were substantially improved in patients receiving pregabalin compared with those receiving placebo; in addition, a greater proportion of patients receiving pregabalin, compared with those receiving placebo, achieved at least a 50% reduction in pain scores from baseline.

Pregabalin is considered by many experts to be one of several first-line therapies for PHN; although the drug has been shown to be more effective than placebo in reducing pain associated with PHN, the evidence suggests that only a small proportion of patients will derive a clinically meaningful benefit from the drug. Other drugs that have been recommended for the management of PHN include gabapentin, tricyclic antidepressants, and topical lidocaine. When selecting an appropriate regimen, clinicians should consider the relative efficacy and safety of the specific drugs as well as individual patient-related factors (e.g., age, preference, tolerability, contraindications, comorbid conditions, concomitant medications).

Diabetic Neuropathy

Pregabalin is used for the management of pain associated with diabetic peripheral neuropathy (DPN) in adults.

Efficacy of pregabalin conventional preparations for the management of DPN has been established in 3 multicenter, double-blind, placebo-controlled studies in adults with type 1 or 2 diabetes mellitus and painful distal symmetrical sensorimotor polyneuropathy of 1–5 years' duration. In 2 studies that excluded patients with renal impairment (i.e., creatinine clearance of 60 mL/minute or less), treatment with pregabalin 300 mg daily (given in 3 divided doses) for 5 or 8 weeks improved the mean pain score (assessed on an 11-point numeric rating scale) compared with placebo; in addition, a greater proportion of patients receiving pregabalin 300 mg daily, compared with those receiving placebo, achieved at least a 50% reduction in pain score from baseline. One of these studies also evaluated pregabalin at dosages of 75 and 600 mg daily. The 600-mg daily dosage did not provide additional benefit, but was associated with an increased risk of dose-dependent adverse effects when compared with the 300-mg daily dosage. The 75-mg daily dosage was not effective.

Efficacy of extended-release pregabalin for the management of DPN is based on studies conducted with conventional preparations of the drug in addition to a randomized withdrawal study in adults with PHN. (See Postherpetic Neuralgia under Uses: Neuropathic Pain.)

Pregabalin also has been evaluated in other randomized controlled studies for the management of DPN. The overall evidence indicates that the drug is more effective than placebo in relieving pain associated with DPN, but the effect size is small and not all studies found a benefit with the drug. A dose-related effect has been observed in which higher dosages of pregabalin are associated with greater efficacy and a more rapid onset of pain relief, but the increase in efficacy is accompanied by an increased risk of adverse effects.

Although pregabalin is considered by many experts to be one of several first-line therapies for DPN, the evidence suggests that only a small proportion of patients will derive a clinically meaningful benefit from the drug. Other drugs that have been recommended for the management of DPN include gabapentin, tricyclic antidepressants, and serotonin- and norepinephrine-reuptake inhibitors (e.g., duloxetine, venlafaxine). When selecting an appropriate regimen, clinicians should consider the relative efficacy, safety, pharmacokinetics, drug interaction potential, and cost of the specific drugs in addition to individual patient-related factors (e.g., contraindications, comorbid conditions, concomitant medications).

Neuropathic Pain Associated with Spinal Cord Injury

Pregabalin is used for the management of neuropathic pain associated with spinal cord injury in adults. Clinical studies establishing efficacy of pregabalin for this indication were conducted with conventional (immediate-release) preparations of the drug.

Efficacy of pregabalin for neuropathic pain associated with spinal cord injury was established in 2 multicenter, double-blind, placebo-controlled studies in adults with such pain that persisted continuously for at least 3 months or relapsed/remitted for at least 6 months. Patients were randomized to receive flexible-dose pregabalin in the range of 150–600 mg daily or placebo for 12 or 16 weeks. Patients were allowed to continue their existing pain management therapy (e.g., opiates, nonopiate analgesics, anticonvulsants, muscle relaxants, antidepressants) if the dosages were stable for at least 30 days prior to screening; acetaminophen and nonsteroidal anti-inflammatory drugs could be used as needed during the studies.

In both studies, treatment with pregabalin 150–600 mg daily substantially improved weekly mean pain scores. In addition, the percentages of patients achieving at least a 30 or 50% reduction in pain scores from baseline were substantially greater in the pregabalin compared with placebo groups. Some patients experienced a decrease in pain as early as 1 week, which was sustained throughout the studies.

Other Types of Neuropathic Pain

Pregabalin also has been evaluated for the management of other types of neuropathic pain, including central post-stroke pain†, HIV-related peripheral neuropathy†, and cancer-related neuropathy. Although the majority of studies evaluating gabapentinoids (i.e., gabapentin and pregabalin) for chronic neuropathic pain were conducted in patients with PHN or DPN, the evidence is often extrapolated to other neuropathic pain conditions and many experts recommend these drugs as first-line agents for all types of neuropathic pain (except for trigeminal neuralgia). However, controlled studies generally have shown only limited benefit or no benefit of pregabalin for these other neuropathic conditions.

● Fibromyalgia

Pregabalin is used for the management of fibromyalgia in adults. Clinical studies establishing efficacy of pregabalin for this indication were conducted with conventional (immediate-release) preparations of the drug; efficacy of the extended-release preparation has not been established in patients with fibromyalgia.

Efficacy of pregabalin conventional preparations for the management of fibromyalgia has been established in a 14-week multicenter, randomized, double-blind, placebo-controlled study and a 6-month, randomized, withdrawal study in adults with a diagnosis of fibromyalgia based on the American College of Rheumatology (ACR) classification criteria (i.e., history of widespread pain for 3 months and pain present at 11 or more of the 18 specific tender point sites). In the 14-week study, treatment with pregabalin 300, 450, or 600 mg daily (administered in 2 divided doses) improved the mean end-of-treatment pain score compared with placebo; in addition, a greater proportion of patients receiving pregabalin at all 3 dosages, compared with those receiving placebo, achieved at least a 30 and 50% reduction in pain score from baseline. However, the 600-mg daily dosage did not appear to provide additional improvement in pain scores when compared with the 450-mg daily dosage, but dose-dependent adverse effects were observed.

In the 6-month withdrawal study, patients who responded to treatment with pregabalin 300, 450, or 600 mg daily (i.e., at least 50% reduction in pain score and a self-rating of overall improvement on the Patient Global Impression of Change [PGIC] scale of "much improved" or "very much improved") during a 6-week, open-label, dose optimization period were randomized to a 26-week, double-blind treatment period to remain on their optimal pregabalin dosage or receive placebo. In the double-blind treatment period, patients receiving pregabalin had a longer time to loss of therapeutic response than did those receiving placebo.

Results of a systematic review of 5 randomized controlled studies indicated that treatment with pregabalin (at dosages of 300–600 mg daily over 12–26 weeks) provided substantial benefit (i.e., reduction in pain intensity by at least 50%) in about 22–24% of patients who received the drug compared with 14% of those who received placebo; a moderate benefit (i.e., reduction in pain intensity by at least 30%) was reported in 39–43% of patients who received the drug compared

with 28% of those who received placebo. The majority of patients in these studies experienced adverse effects from pregabalin. Overall findings from these studies suggest that pregabalin may be effective in reducing pain in a small proportion of patients with fibromyalgia.

DOSAGE AND ADMINISTRATION

● Administration

Pregabalin is administered orally as conventional (immediate-release) capsules or oral solution. The drug also is available as extended-release tablets for the treatment of postherpetic neuralgia (PHN) or diabetic peripheral neuropathy (DPN) in adults; efficacy of this preparation has not been established for other indications. Pregabalin capsules and oral solution are administered orally without regard to food; the extended-release tablets should be administered once daily after the evening meal. The extended-release tablets should be swallowed whole and not split, crushed, or chewed.

When switching from conventional preparations of pregabalin to the extended-release tablets, patients should take their usual morning dose of conventional capsules or oral solution, and initiate therapy with the extended-release tablets after the evening meal. The appropriate dose conversion should be performed according to the table below (see Table 1).

TABLE 1. Dose Conversion from Conventional to Extended-release Pregabalin

Conventional Pregabalin Total Daily Dose	Extended-release Pregabalin Dose
75 mg daily (given 2 or 3 times daily)	82.5 mg once daily
150 mg daily (given 2 or 3 times daily)	165 mg once daily
225 mg daily (given 2 or 3 times daily)	247.5 mg once daily
300 mg daily (given 2 or 3 times daily)	330 mg once daily
450 mg daily (given 2 or 3 times daily)	495 mg once daily
600 mg daily (given 2 or 3 times daily)	660 mg once daily

When discontinuing therapy, pregabalin should be withdrawn gradually by tapering the dosage over at least 1 week. (See Discontinuance of Therapy under Cautions: Warnings/Precautions.)

Patients currently receiving or beginning therapy with pregabalin and/or any other anticonvulsant for any indication should be closely monitored for the emergence or worsening of depression, suicidal thoughts or behavior (suicidality), and/or any unusual changes in mood or behavior. (See Suicidality Risk under Cautions: Warnings/Precautions.)

● Dosage
Seizure Disorders

For adjunctive therapy of partial seizures in adults, pregabalin therapy generally is initiated at a dosage of 150 mg daily, administered in 2 or 3 divided doses as conventional preparations; based on individual patient response and tolerability, dosage may be increased at approximately weekly intervals up to a maximum daily dosage of 600 mg. Dosage adjustments are required in patients with renal impairment. (See Dosage and Administration: Special Populations.)

Dosage of pregabalin for adjunctive therapy of partial seizures in pediatric patients is based on body weight. In pediatric patients 1 month of age or older who weigh less than 30 kg, the recommended initial dosage of pregabalin as conventional preparations is 3.5 mg/kg daily (administered in 3 divided doses for patients 1 month to less than 4 years of age, or in 2 or 3 divided doses for patients 4 years of age or older); dosage may be increased at approximately weekly intervals based on individual patient response and tolerability up to a maximum of 14 mg/kg daily. In pediatric patients 1 month of age or older who weigh 30 kg or more, the recommended initial dosage of pregabalin is 2.5 mg/kg daily (administered in 2 or 3 divided doses as conventional preparations); dosage may be increased at approximately weekly intervals based on individual patient response and tolerability up to a maximum of 10 mg/kg daily (not to exceed 600 mg daily). In clinical studies, the 2.5-mg/kg daily dosage of pregabalin was not substantially more effective than placebo in reducing seizure frequency; however, additional support for this dosage can be derived from adult studies and pharmacokinetic data.

Both the efficacy and adverse effects of pregabalin are dose related, but the effect of the dosage escalation rate on tolerability of the drug has not been specifically studied.

The manufacturer states that dosage recommendations for the use of pregabalin in conjunction with gabapentin are not available because such regimens have not been evaluated in controlled clinical studies.

Neuropathic Pain

Postherpetic Neuralgia

For the management of PHN in adults, the recommended dosage range of pregabalin (as conventional preparations) is 150–300 mg daily, administered in 2 or 3 divided doses. Therapy is generally initiated at a dosage of 150 mg daily (75 mg twice daily or 50 mg 3 times daily); dosage may be increased to 300 mg daily (administered in 2 or 3 divided doses) within 1 week based on efficacy and tolerability. In patients who are tolerating the drug but not experiencing adequate pain relief following 2–4 weeks of treatment with pregabalin 300 mg daily as conventional tablets, dosage may be increased up to a maximum of 600 mg daily (administered in 2 or 3 divided doses). Because of dose-dependent adverse reactions, dosages exceeding 300 mg daily should be reserved for patients who have continuing pain and are tolerating the drug.

If the extended-release tablets are used, the recommended initial adult dosage is 165 mg once daily after the evening meal; dosage may be increased to 330 mg once daily within 1 week based on individual patient response and tolerability. In patients who are tolerating the drug but not experiencing adequate pain relief following 2–4 weeks of treatment with pregabalin 330 mg daily as extended-release tablets, dosage may be increased up to a maximum of 660 mg once daily. Because of dose-dependent adverse reactions, dosages exceeding 330 mg daily should be reserved for patients who have continuing pain and are tolerating the 330-mg daily dosage.

Dosage adjustments are required in patients with renal impairment. (See Dosage and Administration: Special Populations.)

When switching from conventional to extended-release preparations of pregabalin, the manufacturer's dose conversion guidelines in Table 1 should be followed. (See Dosage and Administration: Administration.)

Diabetic Neuropathy

For the management of pain associated with DPN in adults, the initial dosage of pregabalin (as conventional preparations) is 150 mg daily administered in 3 divided doses; dosage may be increased within 1 week based on efficacy and tolerability to the maximum recommended daily dosage of 300 mg. If the extended-release tablets are used, the recommended initial adult dosage is 165 mg once daily after the evening meal; dosage may be increased to the maximum recommended dosage of 330 mg once daily within 1 week based on individual patient response and tolerability. Although higher dosages of pregabalin (e.g., 600 mg daily) were evaluated in clinical studies, there is no evidence that these dosages provide additional benefit and may increase the risk of adverse effects.

Dosage adjustments are required in patients with renal impairment. (See Dosage and Administration: Special Populations.)

When switching from conventional to extended-release preparations of pregabalin, the manufacturer's dose conversion guidelines in Table 1 should be followed. (See Dosage and Administration: Administration.)

Neuropathic Pain Associated with Spinal Cord Injury

For the management of neuropathic pain associated with spinal cord injury in adults, the recommended dosage range of pregabalin is 150–600 mg daily (administered in 2 divided doses as conventional preparations). An initial dosage of 150 mg daily (75 mg twice daily) is recommended; dosage may be increased to 300 mg daily (150 mg twice daily) within 1 week based on efficacy and tolerability. In patients who are tolerating the drug but not experiencing adequate pain relief after 2–3 weeks of treatment with a dosage of 300 mg daily, dosage may be further increased to 600 mg daily (300 mg twice daily).

Dosage adjustments are required in patients with renal impairment. (See Dosage and Administration: Special Populations.)

Fibromyalgia

For the management of fibromyalgia in adults, the recommended dosage of pregabalin is 300–450 mg daily (as conventional preparations). An initial dosage of 150 mg daily (administered as 75 mg twice daily) is recommended; dosage may be increased to 300 mg daily (150 mg twice daily) within 1 week based on efficacy and tolerability. Patients who do not experience adequate benefit with pregabalin 300 mg daily may have their dosage further increased to the maximum recommended dosage of 450 mg daily (225 mg twice daily). Clinical studies in patients with fibromyalgia indicate that higher pregabalin dosages (e.g., 600 mg daily) provide no additional benefit but may increase the risk of adverse effects; therefore, dosages exceeding 450 mg daily are not recommended.

Dosage adjustments are required in patients with renal impairment. (See Dosage and Administration: Special Populations.)

● Special Populations

In patients with renal impairment (creatinine clearance of less than 60 mL/minute), dosage of pregabalin should be modified based on creatinine clearance (see Tables 2 or 3 based on the preparation of drug used). Patients with a creatinine clearance of less than 30 mL/minute or who are undergoing hemodialysis should not receive the extended-release formulation of pregabalin; in these patients, conventional preparations of the drug should be used.

TABLE 2. Dosage Adjustment of Pregabalin Conventional Preparations in Patients with Renal Impairment

Usual Dosage Regimen (for Patients with Creatinine Clearances of ≥60 mL/minute)	Creatinine Clearance (mL/minute)	Adjusted Dosage Regimen
150 mg daily given in 2 or 3 divided doses	30–60	75 mg daily given in 2 or 3 divided doses
	15–30	25–50 mg daily given as a single dose or in 2 divided doses
	<15	25 mg once daily
300 mg daily given in 2 or 3 divided doses	30–60	150 mg daily given in 2 or 3 divided doses
	15–30	75 mg daily given as a single dose or in 2 divided doses
	<15	25–50 mg once daily
450 mg daily given in 2 or 3 divided doses	30–60	225 mg daily given in 2 or 3 divided doses
	15–30	100–150 mg daily given as a single dose or in 2 divided doses
	<15	50–75 mg once daily
600 mg daily given in 2 or 3 divided doses	30–60	300 mg daily given in 2 or 3 divided doses
	15–30	150 mg daily given as a single dose or in 2 divided doses
	<15	75 mg once daily

Because pregabalin is removed by hemodialysis, in addition to the adjusted daily dosage, patients undergoing hemodialysis should receive a supplemental dose of the drug (as a conventional [immediate-release] preparation) immediately following each 4-hour dialysis session. Individuals receiving the 25-mg once daily dosage regimen should receive a supplemental dose of 25 or 50 mg, those receiving the 25- to 50-mg once daily dosage regimen should receive a supplemental dose of 50 or 75 mg, those receiving the 50- to 75-mg once daily dosage regimen should receive a supplemental dose of 75 or 100 mg, and those receiving the 75-mg once daily dosage regimen should receive a supplemental dose of 100 or 150 mg. The extended-release preparation of pregabalin is not recommended in patients undergoing hemodialysis.

TABLE 3. Dosage Adjustment of Pregabalin Extended-release Tablets in Patients with Renal Impairment

Usual Dosage Regimen (for Patients with Creatinine Clearances ≥60 mL/minute)	Creatinine Clearance (mL/minute)	Adjusted Dosage Regimen
165 mg daily	30–60	82.5 mg daily
	<30 or receiving hemodialysis	Use conventional pregabalin preparations
330 mg daily	30–60	165 mg daily
	<30 or receiving hemodialysis	Use conventional pregabalin preparations
495 mg daily	30–60	247.5 mg daily
	<30 or receiving hemodialysis	Use conventional pregabalin preparations
660 mg daily	30–60	330 mg daily
	<30 or receiving hemodialysis	Use conventional pregabalin preparations

CAUTIONS

● Contraindications

Known hypersensitivity to pregabalin or any ingredient in the formulation.

● Warnings/Precautions

Sensitivity Reactions

Angioedema

Angioedema, including life-threatening cases with respiratory compromise requiring emergency treatment, has been reported during postmarketing surveillance in patients receiving initial and chronic pregabalin therapy. Specific symptoms included swelling of the face, mouth (e.g., tongue, lips, gums), and neck (e.g., throat, larynx). Pregabalin should be immediately discontinued in patients with these symptoms. Caution is advised if the drug is used in patients who have had a previous episode of angioedema. Patients receiving concomitant drugs associated with angioedema (e.g., angiotensin-converting enzyme [ACE] inhibitors) may be at increased risk of developing angioedema.

Hypersensitivity Reactions

Hypersensitivity reactions (i.e., skin redness, blisters, hives, rash, dyspnea, wheezing) have been reported during postmarketing surveillance in patients shortly after initiation of pregabalin therapy. Pregabalin should be immediately discontinued in patients with symptoms of hypersensitivity.

Suicidality Risk

An increased risk of suicidality (suicidal behavior or ideation) has been observed in an analysis of studies using various anticonvulsants, including pregabalin, compared with placebo. The analysis of suicidality reports from placebo-controlled studies involving 11 anticonvulsants (i.e., carbamazepine, felbamate, gabapentin, lamotrigine, levetiracetam, oxcarbazepine, pregabalin, tiagabine, topiramate, valproate, zonisamide) in patients with epilepsy, psychiatric disorders (e.g., bipolar disorder, depression, anxiety), and other conditions (e.g., migraine, neuropathic pain) found that patients receiving anticonvulsants had approximately twice the risk of suicidal behavior or ideation (0.43%) compared with patients receiving placebo (0.24%). This increased suicidality risk was consistent among anticonvulsants with varying mechanisms of action and across a range of indications, and was observed as early as 1 week after beginning therapy. Because most of these studies did not extend beyond 24 weeks, the suicidality risk beyond 24 weeks is not known. Although patients treated with an anticonvulsant for epilepsy, psychiatric disorders, and other conditions were all found to have an increased suicidality risk compared with those receiving placebo, the relative suicidality risk was higher for patients with epilepsy compared to those receiving anticonvulsants for other conditions.

Clinicians should inform patients, their families, and caregivers of the potential for an increased risk of suicidality with anticonvulsant therapy. All patients currently receiving or beginning therapy with any anticonvulsant should be closely monitored for notable changes that may indicate the emergence or worsening of suicidal thoughts or behavior or depression.

Clinicians who prescribe pregabalin or any other anticonvulsant should balance the risk of suicidality with the risk of untreated illness. Epilepsy and many other illnesses for which anticonvulsants are prescribed are themselves associated with morbidity and mortality and an increased risk of suicidal thoughts and behavior. If suicidal thoughts or behavior emerge during anticonvulsant therapy, the clinician should consider whether these symptoms may be related to the illness being treated. (See Advice to Patients.)

Respiratory Depression

Serious, life-threatening, or fatal respiratory depression has been reported in patients receiving gabapentinoids (i.e., gabapentin and pregabalin). In the majority of cases, the drugs were used in combination with an opiate analgesic (or other CNS depressant), in patients with preexisting respiratory risk factors (e.g., COPD), or in geriatric patients. During a 5-year period between 2012 and 2017, 49 cases of respiratory depression associated with gabapentinoid use (15 cases with gabapentin and 34 cases with pregabalin) were reported to the FDA, including 12 fatalities. Most of the cases (92%) reported either concomitant use of another CNS depressant or a respiratory risk factor, including age-related decreases in lung function. In all of the fatal cases, patients had at least one risk factor for developing respiratory depression or were receiving a CNS depressant concomitantly. In addition, there is evidence from small randomized studies in healthy individuals and observational studies in postoperative patients suggesting that use of gabapentinoids alone or in conjunction with opiate analgesics may increase the risk of respiratory depression. Although findings from these studies as well as animal data suggest that gabapentinoids may have an independent respiratory depressant effect, there is less evidence supporting the risk of serious respiratory complications when these drugs are used alone in otherwise healthy individuals.

Because of the risk of respiratory depression when gabapentinoids are used in combination with opiate analgesics or other CNS depressants (e.g., benzodiazepines) or in the setting of underlying respiratory impairment, patients should be monitored for respiratory depression and sedation in these situations. Consideration should be given to initiating pregabalin therapy at the lowest dosage and titrating the dosage carefully; appropriate dosage adjustments should be made in patients with renal impairment and those undergoing hemodialysis. (See Dosage and Administration: Special Populations.) Patients should be advised to seek immediate medical attention if signs or symptoms of respiratory depression occur. (See Advice to Patients.) Management of respiratory depression may include supportive measures and reduction or withdrawal of CNS depressants, including pregabalin. If the decision is made to discontinue pregabalin, dosage should be reduced gradually. (See Discontinuance of Therapy under Cautions: Warnings/Precautions.)

Dizziness and Somnolence

Pregabalin may cause dizziness and somnolence. (See Advice to Patients.) In controlled studies, approximately 24–30% of adults who received pregabalin experienced dizziness and approximately 16–23% of the patients experienced somnolence. Dizziness and somnolence were the most frequent adverse effects requiring discontinuance of the drug in these studies. In controlled studies in pediatric patients with partial seizures, somnolence was reported in 15–21% of the patients who received pregabalin. These adverse effects occurred more frequently at higher doses and, in some cases, persisted throughout therapy.

Discontinuance of Therapy

As with all anticonvulsant agents, there is a potential for increased seizure frequency when pregabalin therapy is withdrawn abruptly. When discontinuing pregabalin therapy, dosage should be reduced gradually over at least 1 week. Abrupt or rapid discontinuance of pregabalin has been associated with symptoms suggestive of physical dependence (e.g., insomnia, nausea, headache, anxiety, hyperhidrosis, diarrhea).

Peripheral Edema

Pregabalin may cause peripheral edema. In short-term clinical trials of patients without clinically important cardiac or peripheral vascular disease, there was no apparent association between peripheral edema and cardiovascular complications (e.g., hypertension, congestive heart failure). Peripheral edema was not associated with deterioration of renal or hepatic function. In controlled clinical studies, peripheral edema was reported in about 5–6% of adults receiving pregabalin.

Concomitant use of pregabalin with a thiazolidinedione antidiabetic agent has been associated with a greater risk of developing weight gain and peripheral edema than use of either drug alone. (See Drug Interactions: Antidiabetic Agents.)

Because there are limited data regarding use of pregabalin in patients with New York Heart Association (NYHA) class III or IV heart failure, the drug should be used with caution in these patients.

Weight Gain

Pregabalin may cause weight gain. Pregabalin-associated weight gain appeared to be related to dosage and duration of exposure; however, weight gain did not appear to be associated with baseline body mass index (BMI), gender, or age and was not limited to patients with edema.

Although weight gain was not associated with clinically important changes in blood pressure in short-term controlled studies, the long-term cardiovascular effects of such weight gain have not been elucidated. In addition, while the effects of pregabalin-associated weight gain on glycemic control have not been systematically assessed in controlled and longer-term open label clinical trials in diabetic patients, pregabalin therapy did not appear to be associated with loss of glycemic control.

Carcinogenicity

Possible carcinogenicity of pregabalin (e.g., hemangiosarcoma) has been demonstrated in animals.

In clinical studies across various patient populations, comprising 6396 patient-years of exposure in those 12 years of age or older, new or worsening-preexisting tumors were reported in 57 patients; however, a causal relationship to the drug has not been established.

Ocular Effects

In controlled studies in adults, blurred vision was reported in about 5–7% of patients receiving pregabalin and resolved in the majority of cases with continued dosing. In addition, decreased visual acuity was reported in 7% of patients receiving pregabalin, while visual field and funduscopic changes were detected in 13 and 2%, respectively, of patients receiving the drug. However, these ocular effects occurred at a similar incidence to placebo and the clinical importance of these findings has not been elucidated.

Patients receiving pregabalin should inform their clinician if any changes in vision occur. If visual disturbance persists, further ophthalmologic assessment should be considered, while more frequent assessment should be considered in patients who already are monitored for ocular conditions.

Creatine Kinase Elevations

In clinical trials in adults, increases in serum creatinine kinase (CK, creatine phosphokinase, CPK) concentrations at least 3 times the upper limit of normal have been reported in 1.5 or 0.7% of patients receiving pregabalin or placebo, respectively.

Rhabdomyolysis has been reported rarely in premarketing clinical trials. However, a definite causal relationship between these musculoskeletal effects and the drug has not been fully elucidated because the cases had documented factors that may have caused or contributed to these events.

Pregabalin treatment should be discontinued if myopathy is diagnosed or suspected or if markedly elevated CK (CPK) concentrations occur.

Thrombocytopenia

In controlled clinical trials in adults, potentially clinically important decreases in platelet count (thrombocytopenia; defined as 20% below baseline value and less than 150,000/mm^3) have been reported in 3 or 2% of patients receiving pregabalin or placebo, respectively. Pregabalin-treated patients experienced a mean maximal decrease in platelet count of 20,000/mm^3 compared with 11,000/mm^3 in placebo recipients. Severe thrombocytopenia with a platelet count less than 20,000/mm^3 has been reported in at least one patient who received pregabalin. In randomized controlled trials, pregabalin was not associated with an increase in bleeding-related adverse effects.

PR Interval Prolongation

Prolongation of the PR interval (mean increase: 3–6 msec) has been reported in adults receiving pregabalin dosages of at least 300 mg daily. Subgroup analyses in a limited number of patients suggest that those with preexisting PR prolongation at baseline or those receiving drugs that prolong the PR interval do not appear to have an increased risk for developing prolongation of the PR interval.

Abuse Potential and Dependence

In controlled clinical studies using conventional pregabalin, 4 or 1% of patients receiving the drug or placebo, respectively, reported euphoria as an adverse event; in some patient populations studied, the rate of euphoria was higher and ranged from 1–12%. In clinical studies, abrupt or rapid discontinuance of pregabalin has resulted in withdrawal symptoms (e.g., insomnia, nausea, headache, diarrhea). (See Discontinuance of Therapy under Cautions: Warnings/Precautions.)

Pregabalin is not known to be active at receptor sites associated with drugs of abuse. However, the drug is subject to control as a schedule V (C-V) drug.

As with any CNS active drug, clinicians should carefully evaluate patients for a history of drug abuse and observe them for signs of pregabalin misuse or abuse (e.g., development of tolerance, dose escalation, drug-seeking behavior).

Specific Populations

Pregnancy

Women who are pregnant while receiving pregabalin should be encouraged to enroll in the North American Antiepileptic Drug (NAAED) Pregnancy Registry at 888-233-2334 (for patients); registry information also is available on the website https://www.aedpregnancyregistry.org/.

There are no adequate and well-controlled studies of pregabalin in pregnant women; however, based on animal studies, pregabalin may cause fetal harm. In animal reproductive studies, pregabalin produced developmental toxicity (e.g., fetal structural abnormalities, skeletal malformations, retarded ossification, decreased fetal body weight) when administered orally to pregnant animals during the period of organogenesis at exposure levels 16 times higher than those associated with the maximum recommended human dosage of 600 mg daily. When pregabalin was administered to female rats throughout the period of gestation and lactation, growth retardation, impairment to the nervous and reproductive systems, and decreased survival were observed in the offspring.

Lactation

Pregabalin is distributed into human milk at steady-state concentrations approximately 76% of those in maternal plasma. Following administration of maternal dosages of 300 mg daily, the estimated average infant dose of pregabalin from breast milk is 0.31 mg/kg daily (approximately 7% of the maternal dose). Because of the potential for tumorigenicity (see Carcinogenicity under Cautions: Warnings/Precautions), breastfeeding is not recommended during pregabalin therapy.

Pediatric Use

Safety and efficacy of pregabalin conventional preparations for adjunctive treatment of partial seizures have not been established in children younger than 1 month of age. Use of conventional pregabalin in older children is supported by evidence from 2 randomized placebo-controlled studies. (See Uses: Seizure Disorders.) Although the youngest patient evaluated in these studies was 3 months of age, use of pregabalin in infants 1–3 months of age can be supported by additional pharmacokinetic data.

Clearance of pregabalin (normalized for body weight) is approximately 40% higher in patients weighing less than 30 kg. For children weighing less than 30 kg, a dosage increase is required to achieve comparable exposure to those weighing 30 kg or more.

Safety and efficacy of pregabalin for the treatment of fibromyalgia, diabetic peripheral neuropathy (DPN), postherpetic neuralgia (PHN), or neuropathic pain associated with spinal cord injury have not been established in pediatric patients.

Safety and efficacy of pregabalin extended-release tablets have not been established in pediatric patients.

Geriatric Use

The manufacturer states that no substantial differences in safety and efficacy have been observed in geriatric patients relative to younger adults; however, increased sensitivity to pregabalin in certain individuals cannot be ruled out. In controlled clinical studies of patients with fibromyalgia, neurological adverse reactions including dizziness, blurred vision, balance disorder, tremor, confusional state, abnormal coordination, and lethargy occurred more frequently in patients 65 years of age and older than in younger adults. In addition, FDA warns that geriatric patients receiving gabapentinoids are at increased risk of potentially serious, life-threatening, or fatal respiratory depression; pregabalin therapy should be initiated at the lowest dosage and titrated carefully with close monitoring in such patients.

It should be considered that pregabalin is substantially excreted by the kidneys, and the risk of adverse reactions to the drug may be increased in patients with impaired renal function. The dosage should be adjusted for geriatric patients with renal impairment. Monitoring renal function in geriatric patients may be helpful. (See Dosage and Administration: Special Populations.)

Renal Impairment

Pregabalin is eliminated renally. Dosage of pregabalin should be modified in adults according to the degree of renal impairment. (See Dosage and Administration: Special Populations.) The drug has not been evaluated in pediatric patients with renal impairment.

Pregabalin is removed from plasma by hemodialysis. Plasma pregabalin concentrations are reduced by approximately 50% following a 4-hour hemodialysis treatment. (See Dosage and Administration: Special Populations.)

● Common Adverse Effects

The most common adverse effects in adults receiving conventional pregabalin preparations across indications in clinical trials (occurring in 5% or more of patients and more frequently than placebo) include dizziness, somnolence, dry mouth, edema, blurred vision, weight gain, and abnormal thinking (primarily difficulty with concentration/attention). The most common adverse effects in pediatric patients receiving conventional pregabalin for the treatment of partial seizures (occurring in 5% or more of patients and more frequently than placebo) include somnolence, weight gain, and increased appetite.

The most common adverse effects in adults receiving extended-release pregabalin in clinical studies include dizziness, somnolence, headache, fatigue, peripheral edema, nausea, blurred vision, dry mouth, and weight gain.

Other adverse effects commonly reported in adults receiving conventional pregabalin in combination with other anticonvulsant agents in the management of partial seizures include ataxia, tremor, amnesia, speech disorder, increased appetite, peripheral edema, diplopia, and accidental injury.

Other adverse effects commonly reported in adults receiving conventional pregabalin for the management of PHN include headache, ataxia, constipation, peripheral edema, infection, and pain.

Other adverse effects commonly reported in adults receiving conventional pregabalin for the management of DPN include asthenia and peripheral edema.

Other adverse effects commonly reported in adults receiving conventional pregabalin for the management of fibromyalgia include headache, euphoric mood, attention disturbance, balance disorder, constipation, fatigue, peripheral edema, increased appetite, and sinusitis.

Other adverse effects commonly reported in adults receiving conventional pregabalin for the management of neuropathic pain associated with spinal cord injury include fatigue, peripheral edema, constipation, nasopharyngitis, and muscle weakness.

DRUG INTERACTIONS

Specific drug interaction studies conducted with pregabalin extended-release tablets are limited; the information presented below is derived principally from studies with conventional preparations of pregabalin. Similar pharmacokinetic interactions are expected with the various preparations of pregabalin.

● Drugs Affecting Hepatic Microsomal Enzymes

Based on results of in vitro studies, pregabalin does not appear to inhibit cytochrome P-450 (CYP) isoenzymes 1A2, 2A6, 2C9, 2C19, 2D6, 2E1, and 3A4 or induce CYP1A2 or CYP3A4.

The manufacturer states that increased metabolism of concomitantly administered CYP1A2 substrates (e.g., caffeine, theophylline) or CYP3A4 substrates (e.g., midazolam, testosterone) is not anticipated.

Since pregabalin undergoes negligible metabolism in humans, pharmacokinetics of the drug are unlikely to be affected by other agents through metabolic interactions.

● Drugs that Cause Constipation

Concomitant use of pregabalin and drugs that can cause constipation (e.g., opiate analgesics) has been associated with adverse events related to reduced lower GI tract function (e.g., intestinal obstruction, paralytic ileus, constipation).

● Protein-bound Drugs

Because pregabalin does not bind to plasma proteins, pharmacokinetic interactions with drugs that are highly protein bound are unlikely.

● Alcohol

Although a pharmacokinetic interaction has not been observed with pregabalin and alcohol, additive effects on cognitive and gross motor functioning have occurred; however, concomitant use of pregabalin and alcohol did not result in any clinically important effects on respiration. Use of alcohol should be avoided in patients receiving pregabalin.

● Angiotensin-converting Enzyme Inhibitors

Potential pharmacologic interaction with angiotensin-converting enzyme (ACE) inhibitors (e.g., increased risk of developing angioedema).

● Anticonvulsants

Pharmacokinetic interactions have not been observed when pregabalin was used concomitantly with phenytoin, carbamazepine, valproate, lamotrigine, phenobarbital, or topiramate.

Concomitant administration of gabapentin with pregabalin did not alter pharmacokinetics of gabapentin, although the rate, but not extent, of absorption of pregabalin was decreased slightly.

Tiagabine does not appear to affect the pharmacokinetics of pregabalin.

● Antidiabetic Agents

Glyburide, insulin, and metformin do not appear to affect the pharmacokinetics of pregabalin.

Concomitant use of pregabalin and thiazolidinediones may increase the risk of weight gain and peripheral edema, possibly exacerbating or causing heart failure. Caution is advised when these drugs are used concomitantly.

● CNS Depressants

Additive CNS and respiratory depressant effects can occur with concurrent use of pregabalin and CNS depressants, including opiates and benzodiazepines. If pregabalin is used concomitantly with other CNS depressants, pregabalin should be initiated with the lowest dosage and titrated carefully. (See Respiratory Depression under Cautions: Warnings/Precautions.)

● Erythromycin

Concomitant administration of a single dose of pregabalin (as the extended-release tablet) and erythromycin resulted in a 17% decrease in systemic exposure of pregabalin.

● *Furosemide*

Furosemide does not appear to affect the pharmacokinetics of pregabalin.

● *Lorazepam*

Although a pharmacokinetic interaction has not been observed, additive effects on cognitive and gross motor functioning have occurred when pregabalin was administered concomitantly with lorazepam; concomitant use of these drugs did not result in any clinically important effects on respiration. (See Drug Interactions: CNS Depressants.)

● *Opiates*

Additive CNS and respiratory depressant effects can occur with concurrent use of pregabalin and opiates. If pregabalin is used concomitantly with opiates, pregabalin should be initiated with the lowest dosage and titrated carefully. (See Respiratory Depression under Cautions: Warnings/Precautions.)

In addition, events related to reduced lower GI function (e.g., intestinal obstruction, paralytic ileus, constipation) have been reported during postmarketing experience in patients taking pregabalin concomitantly with drugs that have the potential to produce constipation, such as opiates.

Oxycodone

Although a pharmacokinetic interaction has not been observed, additive effects on cognitive and gross motor functioning have occurred when pregabalin was administered concomitantly with oxycodone; concomitant use of these drugs did not result in any clinically important effects on respiration.

● *Oral Contraceptives*

Concomitant administration of pregabalin and an oral contraceptive containing norethindrone and ethinyl estradiol in healthy individuals did not affect the pharmacokinetics of either component of the oral contraceptive.

DESCRIPTION

Pregabalin is an anticonvulsant that is structurally related to the inhibitory CNS neurotransmitter γ-aminobutyric acid (GABA). Pregabalin also has demonstrated analgesic activity. Although pregabalin was developed as a structural analog of GABA, the drug does not bind directly to $GABA_A$, $GABA_B$, or benzodiazepine receptors; does not augment $GABA_A$ responses in cultured neurons; and does not alter brain concentrations of GABA in rats or affect GABA uptake or degradation. However, in cultured neurons, prolonged application of pregabalin increases the density of GABA transporter protein and increases the rate of functional GABA transport.

Pregabalin binds with high affinity to the α_2-δ site (an auxiliary subunit of voltage-gated calcium channels) in CNS tissues. Although the exact mechanism of action of pregabalin has not been elucidated, binding to the α_2-δ subunit may be involved in pregabalin's analgesic and anticonvulsant effects. In vitro, pregabalin reduces the calcium-dependent release of several neurotransmitters, including glutamate, norepinephrine, calcitonin gene-related peptide, and substance P, possibly by modulation of calcium channel function.

Pregabalin is well absorbed following oral administration and exhibits linear pharmacokinetics; peak plasma concentrations are attained within 1.5 or 12 hours with conventional or extended-release preparations, respectively. Steady-state concentrations are achieved within 24–48 hours following repeated administration of conventional pregabalin and within 48–72 hours following repeated administration of the extended-release tablets. In pediatric patients receiving conventional pregabalin, peak plasma concentrations of the drug are achieved within 0.5–2 hours in the fasted state. The oral bioavailability of pregabalin (administered as the conventional preparation) is at least 90% and is independent of dose. Bioavailability of the extended-release tablets administered once daily following an evening meal is equivalent to that of comparable doses of the conventional preparation administered without food twice daily. Administration of conventional preparations of pregabalin with food has been shown to delay the time to peak concentration and decrease peak plasma concentrations of the drug by approximately 25–30%, but does not affect the extent of absorption. Administration of the extended-release tablets in the fasted state reduces systemic exposure of pregabalin by approximately 30% compared with administration following an evening meal. Pregabalin is not appreciably metabolized. Following administration of a single radiolabeled dose of pregabalin, approximately 90% of the administered dose was recovered in urine as unchanged drug. Clearance of pregabalin is nearly proportional to creatinine clearance in both adults and pediatric patients. In pediatric patients, the weight-normalized clearance of pregabalin is approximately 40% higher in those weighing less than 30 kg. (See Pediatric Use under Warnings/Precautions: Specific Populations, in Cautions.) The mean elimination half-life of pregabalin is 6.3 hours in adults with normal renal function, 3–4 hours in children up to 6 years of age, and 4–6 hours in children 7 years of age or older.

ADVICE TO PATIENTS

Importance of advising patients or caregivers to read the manufacturer's patient information (medication guide) before the start of therapy and each time the prescription is refilled.

Importance of patients, family members, and caregivers being aware that anticonvulsants, including pregabalin, may increase the risk of having suicidal thoughts or actions in a very small number of people (about 1 in 500). Advise patients, family members, and caregivers to pay close attention to any day-to-day changes in mood, behavior, and actions; these changes can happen very quickly. They also should be aware of common warning signs that may signal suicide risk (e.g., talking or thinking about wanting to hurt oneself or end one's life, withdrawing from friends and family, becoming depressed or experiencing worsening of existing depression, becoming preoccupied with death and dying, giving away prized possessions). Advise patients, family members, and caregivers to contact the responsible clinician immediately if these or any other new and worrisome behaviors occur.

Risk of angioedema (e.g., swelling of the face, mouth [e.g., tongue, lips, gums], and neck [e.g., throat, larynx] with or without life-threatening respiratory compromise) and other hypersensitivity reactions (e.g., wheezing, dyspnea, rash, hives, blisters); importance of discontinuing the drug and seeking immediate medical attention if such reactions occur. Concomitant administration with an angiotensin-converting enzyme (ACE) inhibitor may increase such risk.

Importance of taking pregabalin only as prescribed. Importance of advising patients or caregivers to consult their clinician before changing the dosage of or abruptly discontinuing the drug. Patients or caregivers should be informed that abrupt or rapid discontinuance of pregabalin can result in increased risk of seizures in patients with epilepsy or withdrawal symptoms such as insomnia, nausea, headache, anxiety, hyperhidrosis, or diarrhea.

Risk of respiratory depression; concomitant use of CNS depressants (e.g., opiates) increases the risk. Risk also is increased in patients with underlying respiratory impairment and in geriatric patients. Importance of patients seeking immediate medical attention if signs or symptoms of respiratory depression occur (e.g., slow, shallow, or difficult breathing; confusion or disorientation; unusual dizziness or lightheadedness; extreme sleepiness or lethargy; bluish-colored or tinted skin, especially on the lips, fingers, and toes; unresponsiveness).

Risk of dizziness, somnolence, blurred vision, and other neuropsychiatric effects. Avoid driving or operating machinery while taking pregabalin until experience is gained with the drug's effects.

Inform patients that concomitant use of CNS depressants and pregabalin (e.g., opiates or benzodiazepines) may result in additive CNS effects such as respiratory depression, somnolence, and dizziness.

Avoid alcohol-containing beverages or products; pregabalin may potentiate impairment of motor skills and sedation associated with ingestion of alcohol.

Advise patients that if a dose of pregabalin (as conventional preparations) is missed, the missed dose should be taken as soon as possible; if it is almost time for the next dose, the missed dose should be skipped and the next dose should be taken at the regularly scheduled time. Patients should not take 2 doses at the same time.

Advise patients that if a dose of pregabalin (as extended-release tablets) is missed after an evening meal, the dose should be taken prior to bedtime following a snack. If they miss the dose prior to bedtime, then they should take their usual dose the next morning following breakfast. If they miss taking the dose following the morning meal, they should take their usual dose at the regularly scheduled time after the evening meal.

Risk of edema and weight gain; concomitant administration with a thiazolidinedione antidiabetic agent may increase such risk. In patients with preexisting cardiac conditions, risk of heart failure may be increased.

Risk of visual disturbances. Importance of informing clinician if changes in vision occur.

Importance of patients promptly informing clinicians of any unexplained muscle pain, tenderness, or weakness, particularly if accompanied by malaise or fever.

Advise diabetic patients to watch for skin damage while receiving pregabalin therapy, since increased risk of skin ulcerations associated with pregabalin therapy has been observed in animal studies.

Importance of women informing clinicians if they are or plan to become pregnant or plan to breast-feed. Importance of clinicians informing women about the existence of and encouraging enrollment in the North American Antiepileptic Drug Pregnancy Registry (see Pregnancy under Warnings/Precautions: Specific Populations, in Cautions). Women should be advised that breastfeeding is not recommended during treatment with pregabalin.

Advise patients of male-mediated teratogenicity. Importance of men informing clinicians if they plan to father a child.

Importance of informing clinicians of existing or contemplated concomitant therapy, including prescription and OTC drugs, as well as any concomitant illnesses. Potential for additive CNS effects if used concomitantly with other CNS depressants (e.g., opiates, benzodiazepines).

Importance of informing patients of other important precautionary information. (See Cautions.)

PREPARATIONS

Pregabalin is subject to control under the Federal Controlled Substances Act of 1970 as a schedule V (C-V) drug. (See Abuse Potential and Dependence under Cautions: Warnings/Precautions.)

Excipients in commercially available drug preparations may have clinically important effects in some individuals; consult specific product labeling for details.

Pregabalin

Oral		
Capsules	25 mg	Lyrica® (C-V), Pfizer
	50 mg	Lyrica® (C-V), Pfizer
	75 mg*	Lyrica® (C-V), Pfizer
		Pregabalin Capsules
	100 mg*	Lyrica® (C-V), Pfizer
		Pregabalin Capsules
	150 mg*	Lyrica® (C-V), Pfizer
		Pregabalin Capsules
	200 mg*	Lyrica® (C-V), Pfizer
		Pregabalin Capsules
	225 mg*	Lyrica® (C-V), Pfizer
		Pregabalin Capsules
	300 mg*	Lyrica® (C-V), Pfizer
		Pregabalin Capsules
Solution	20 mg/mL*	Lyrica® (C-V), Pfizer
		Pregabalin Oral Solution
Tablets, extended-release	82.5 mg	Lyrica® CR (C-V), Pfizer
	165 mg	Lyrica® CR (C-V), Pfizer
	330 mg	Lyrica® CR (C-V), Pfizer

* available from one or more manufacturer, distributor, and/or repackager by generic (nonproprietary) name

† Use is not currently included in the labeling approved by the US Food and Drug Administration.

Selected Revisions October 10, 2024, © Copyright, March 1, 2006, American Society of Health-System Pharmacists, Inc.

lamoTRIgine

28:12.92 · ANTICONVULSANTS, MISCELLANEOUS

■ Lamotrigine is a phenyltriazine anticonvulsant.

USES

● Seizure Disorders

Lamotrigine immediate-release formulations (conventional tablets, tablets for oral suspension [previously referred to as chewable dispersible tablets], and orally disintegrating tablets) are used as monotherapy or adjunctive therapy for management of seizure disorders or maintenance treatment of bipolar disorder. Extended-release lamotrigine tablets are used in the management of seizure disorders.

Partial-onset Seizures

Immediate-release Lamotrigine

Lamotrigine (administered as conventional tablets, tablets for oral suspension, or orally disintegrating tablets) is used as adjunctive therapy in the management of partial-onset seizures in adults and children 2 years of age or older. Immediate-release lamotrigine also may be used as monotherapy for partial-onset seizures in adults (16 years of age and older) who are converting from single-agent anticonvulsant therapy with phenytoin, carbamazepine, phenobarbital, primidone, or valproate. Safety and efficacy of lamotrigine have not been established for conversion to monotherapy from single-agent therapy with other anticonvulsants, for simultaneous conversion to monotherapy from 2 or more concomitant anticonvulsants, or as initial monotherapy.

In 3 multicenter, double-blind, placebo-controlled studies, adjunctive therapy with lamotrigine (administered as conventional [immediate-release] formulations) was effective in reducing seizure frequency in adults with partial-onset seizures refractory to therapy with one or more anticonvulsant drugs (e.g., phenytoin, carbamazepine, phenobarbital, valproate); the median reduction in seizure frequency was 20–36% depending on the dosage of lamotrigine administered. In a multicenter, double-blind, placebo-controlled study in children 2–16 years of age with partial-onset seizures, the median reduction in seizure frequency was 36 or 7% in patients receiving immediate-release lamotrigine or placebo, respectively, in addition to their current therapy with up to 2 anticonvulsant drugs.

The effectiveness of lamotrigine monotherapy (given as immediate-release formulations) in adults with partial-onset seizures who are converting from monotherapy with a hepatic enzyme-inducing anticonvulsant drug (e.g., phenytoin, carbamazepine, phenobarbital, primidone) was established in a controlled clinical study of patients who experienced at least 4 simple or complex partial seizures, with or without secondary generalization, during each of 2 consecutive 4-week baseline periods; during the baseline periods, patients were receiving either phenytoin or carbamazepine monotherapy. Patients were randomized to lamotrigine (target dosage of 500 mg daily) or valproate (1000 mg daily), which was added to their baseline regimen over a 4-week period. Patients were then converted to either lamotrigine or valproate monotherapy. Study end points were either successful completion of the 12-week monotherapy period or meeting a study "escape" criterion, relative to baseline. Escape criteria were defined as doubling of the mean monthly seizure count; doubling of the highest consecutive 2-day seizure frequency; emergence of a new seizure type (defined as a seizure that did not occur during the 8-week baseline period) that was more severe than the other seizure types occurring during the study period; or clinically important prolongation of generalized tonic-clonic seizures. The proportion of lamotrigine- or valproate-treated patients meeting escape criteria was 42 or 69%, respectively; no differences in efficacy were detected based on age, race, or sex. Patients in the valproate arm were treated intentionally with a relatively low dosage of the drug because the study was designed to establish the effectiveness of lamotrigine monotherapy; therefore, the study results cannot be interpreted to imply the superiority of lamotrigine therapy to an adequate dosage of valproate.

Extended-release Lamotrigine

Lamotrigine (extended-release tablets) is used as adjunctive therapy in the management of partial-onset seizures, with or without secondary generalization, in adults and children 13 years of age or older. In a multicenter, double-blind, placebo-controlled study in such patients with partial seizures receiving 1 or 2 anticonvulsants, adjunctive treatment with extended-release lamotrigine (target dosage of 200–500 mg daily) substantially reduced the median weekly seizure frequency compared with placebo (by 47 versus 25%, respectively).

Extended-release lamotrigine also may be used as monotherapy for the treatment of partial-onset seizures in patients 13 years of age or older who are converting from single-agent anticonvulsant therapy. The manufacturer states that safety and efficacy of the drug have not been established as initial monotherapy or for simultaneous conversion to monotherapy from 2 or more concomitant anticonvulsants. The effectiveness of extended-release lamotrigine for this use was established in a historically controlled study in 223 adults with partial-onset seizures who were receiving valproate or a nonenzyme-inducing anticonvulsant agent. The historical control group was derived from the control groups of 8 similarly-designed studies which utilized a subtherapeutic dosage of a comparator anticonvulsant drug. Extended-release lamotrigine was added to the patient's current regimen over a 6–7 week period followed by gradual withdrawal of the previous anticonvulsant and continuance of lamotrigine monotherapy (250 or 300 mg once daily) for 12 weeks. Lamotrigine demonstrated statistical superiority to the historical control group based on the proportion of patients meeting an escape criteria that was similar to the criteria used in the 8 controlled studies from which the historical group was derived. Efficacy of extended-release lamotrigine as monotherapy is further supported with studies using immediate-release formulations.

Primary Generalized Tonic-Clonic Seizures

Immediate-release Lamotrigine

Lamotrigine (administered as conventional tablets, tablets for oral suspension, or orally disintegrating tablets) is used as adjunctive therapy in the management of primary generalized tonic-clonic seizures in adults and children 2 years of age and older. Efficacy of the drug for this indication was established in a placebo-controlled trial in adults and pediatric patients at least 2 years of age who had experienced at least 3 primary generalized tonic-clonic seizures during an 8-week baseline phase. Patients were randomized to receive either placebo or immediate-release lamotrigine in a fixed-dose regimen (target dosage of 200–400 mg daily in adults and 3–12 mg/kg daily in children) for 19–24 weeks, which was added to their current anticonvulsant regimen of up to 2 anticonvulsant drugs. Patients receiving lamotrigine experienced a substantially greater median reduction in seizure frequency from baseline than did patients receiving placebo (66 and 34%, respectively).

Extended-release Lamotrigine

Extended-release lamotrigine is used as adjunctive therapy in the management of primary generalized tonic-clonic seizures in adults and adolescents 13 years of age and older. Efficacy of extended-release lamotrigine as adjunctive therapy was established in a multicenter, double-blind, placebo-controlled trial in adults and pediatric patients at least 13 years of age who had experienced at least 3 primary generalized tonic-clonic seizures during an 8-week baseline phase. Patients were randomized to receive either placebo or extended-release lamotrigine in a fixed-dose regimen (target dosage of 200–500 mg daily based on concomitant anticonvulsant therapy) for 19 weeks, which was added to their current anticonvulsant regimen of up to 2 anticonvulsant drugs. Patients receiving extended-release lamotrigine experienced a substantially greater median reduction in seizure frequency compared with baseline than did patients receiving placebo (75 and 32%, respectively).

Seizures Associated with Lennox-Gastaut Syndrome

Immediate-release Lamotrigine

Lamotrigine (administered as immediate-release formulations) is used as adjunctive therapy in the management of generalized seizures associated with Lennox-Gastaut syndrome in adults and pediatric patients 2 years of age or older. Efficacy of the drug for this indication was established in a placebo-controlled trial in adults and pediatric patients 3–25 years of age. Patients were randomized to receive either placebo or immediate-release lamotrigine in a fixed-dose regimen (target dosage of 5 mg/kg daily [maximum of 200 mg daily] in patients taking valproate and 15 mg/kg daily [maximum of 400 mg daily] in patients not taking valproate) for 16 weeks in addition to their current anticonvulsant regimen of up to 3 anticonvulsant drugs. Adjunctive therapy with immediate-release lamotrigine resulted in a 32, 34, and 36% decrease in major motor seizures, drop attacks, and tonic-clonic seizures, respectively.

● *Bipolar Disorder*

Immediate-release Lamotrigine

Lamotrigine (administered as immediate-release formulations) is used for maintenance therapy of bipolar I disorder to delay the occurrence of mood episodes (e.g., depression, mania, hypomania, mixed episodes) in adults following standard treatment of an acute depressive or manic episode. Lamotrigine should not be used to treat acute manic or mixed episodes; the manufacturer states that the effectiveness of lamotrigine in the acute treatment of mood episodes has not been established.

Efficacy of lamotrigine in patients with bipolar disorder has been established in 2 multicenter, double-blind, placebo-controlled trials in adults who met DSM-IV criteria for bipolar I disorder. Patients were titrated to a target lamotrigine dosage of 200 mg daily (alone or as adjunctive therapy), and other psychotropic therapies were withdrawn over 8–16 weeks during an open-label period. Patients were subsequently randomized in a double-blind manner to receive monotherapy with lamotrigine or placebo for up to 18 months. Lamotrigine was superior to placebo in delaying the time to occurrence of a mood episode (depression, mania, hypomania, or a mixed episode) in these studies; combined analysis of the trials suggests that the effects may be more robust for depression (versus mania). Although a lamotrigine dosage of 400 mg daily as monotherapy also was evaluated, no additional benefit was observed with this higher dosage.

The American Psychiatric Association (APA) considers lamotrigine an alternative to lithium and valproate for maintenance treatment of bipolar disorder. Although the manufacturer states that efficacy of lamotrigine in the acute treatment of mood episodes has yet to be fully established, APA guidelines state that lamotrigine may be added when optimal dosages of first-line medications do not adequately treat an acute depressive episode of bipolar disorder. Lamotrigine also has been used in the management of patients with rapid cycling bipolar disorder.

DOSAGE AND ADMINISTRATION

● *Administration*

Lamotrigine is administered orally as immediate-release formulations (conventional tablets, tablets for oral suspension, orally disintegrating tablets) or as extended-release tablets. Immediate-release formulations of the drug (Lamictal®, generics) are administered once or twice daily; the extended-release tablets (Lamictal® XR) are administered once daily. Lamotrigine may be administered without regard to meals.

Lamotrigine conventional tablets should be swallowed whole.

Lamotrigine tablets for oral suspension may be swallowed whole, chewed (and consumed with a small amount of water or diluted fruit juice to aid swallowing), or dispersed in water or diluted fruit juice. To disperse the tablets, they should be added to a small volume (i.e., 5 mL or enough to cover the tablet) of liquid and allowed to disperse completely (over approximately 1 minute); the solution should then be swirled and consumed immediately. Administration of partial quantities of the dispersed tablets should *not* be attempted; calculated doses that do not correspond to available strengths of whole tablets should be rounded down to the nearest whole tablet.

Lamotrigine orally disintegrating tablets should be placed on the tongue and moved around in the mouth; the tablets should disintegrate rapidly in saliva, and then subsequently swallowed with or without water.

Lamotrigine extended-release tablets should be swallowed whole and *not* chewed, crushed, or divided.

Patients who are currently receiving or beginning therapy with lamotrigine and/or any other anticonvulsant for any indication should be closely monitored for the emergence or worsening of depression, suicidal thoughts or behavior (suicidality), and/or any unusual changes in mood or behavior. (See Suicidality Risk under Cautions.)

Conversion from Immediate-release Lamotrigine to Extended-release Lamotrigine

Adults and adolescents 13 years of age or older may be converted directly from immediate-release formulations to extended-release lamotrigine tablets (Lamictal® XR). The initial dosage of extended-release lamotrigine should be the same as the total daily dosage of immediate-release lamotrigine. However, some patients receiving concomitant therapy with enzyme-inducing drugs may have lower plasma concentrations of lamotrigine after conversion and should be monitored. Following conversion to extended-release lamotrigine, all patients (particularly those receiving drugs that induce lamotrigine glucuronidation) should be closely monitored for seizure control. Depending on the therapeutic response following conversion, the total daily dosage of extended-release lamotrigine may require adjustment within the recommended dosing guidelines.

Dispensing and Administration Precautions

Dispensing errors have occurred because of product name confusion between Lamictal® and other commonly used drugs. Medication errors also may occur between the different formulations of lamotrigine (Lamictal®, Lamictal® XR, generic lamotrigine tablets). Therefore, extra care should be exercised in ensuring the accuracy of both oral and written prescriptions for lamotrigine and these other drugs. (See Possible Prescribing and Dispensing Errors under Cautions.)

● *Dosage*

General Dosing Considerations

Dosage of lamotrigine depends on whether valproate, glucuronidation-inducing anticonvulsant drugs (e.g., carbamazepine, phenobarbital, phenytoin, primidone), other drugs that induce lamotrigine glucuronidation (e.g., rifampin, estrogen-containing oral contraceptives, fixed combination of lopinavir and ritonavir [lopinavir/ritonavir], *ritonavir-boosted* atazanavir [atazanavir/ritonavir]), or a combination of these drugs is administered concomitantly. The addition of glucuronidation-inducing drugs may be expected to increase the clearance (i.e., reduce plasma concentrations) of lamotrigine; conversely, discontinuance of these drugs may decrease clearance and increase plasma concentrations of lamotrigine. Addition of valproate (a glucuronidation-inhibiting drug) to lamotrigine therapy may decrease clearance and increase plasma concentrations of lamotrigine. Therefore, clinicians should be aware that addition of glucuronidation-inducing drugs or valproate to, or their discontinuance from, an anticonvulsant regimen including lamotrigine may require modification of the dosage of lamotrigine and/or the other drug.

Exceeding the recommended initial dosage and subsequent dosage escalations of lamotrigine may increase the risk of developing a rash and is *not* recommended. (See Dermatologic and Sensitivity Reactions under Cautions.) In patients who discontinue lamotrigine because of a rash, the manufacturer recommends that the drug not be restarted unless the benefits of therapy outweigh risks (e.g., severe life-threatening rash). Assessment of initial dosing recommendations is required if lamotrigine is restarted in a patient who discontinues therapy because of a rash. If the interval of time since the last dose is greater than 5 half-lives of the drug, the manufacturer recommends that the initial dosage and subsequent dosage escalation guidelines be followed.

Concomitant Use with Oral Contraceptives

Estrogen-containing oral contraceptives may increase the clearance of lamotrigine. The manufacturers state that no dosage adjustment to the recommended dosage escalation guidelines for lamotrigine should be necessary based solely on concomitant use of estrogen-containing oral contraceptives. Dosage escalation should follow the recommended guidelines for initiating adjunctive lamotrigine therapy based on the concomitant anticonvulsant(s) or other concomitant medications.

In women currently receiving estrogen-containing oral contraceptives and not receiving carbamazepine, phenobarbital, phenytoin, primidone, or other drugs that induce lamotrigine glucuronidation (e.g., rifampin, lopinavir/ritonavir, atazanavir/ritonavir), it usually is necessary to increase the maintenance dosage of lamotrigine as much as twofold over the recommended target maintenance dosage in order to maintain a consistent plasma lamotrigine concentration.

In women starting estrogen-containing oral contraceptives who are receiving a stable dosage of lamotrigine, but not receiving carbamazepine, phenobarbital, phenytoin, primidone, or other drugs that induce lamotrigine glucuronidation (e.g., rifampin, lopinavir/ritonavir, atazanavir/ritonavir), it usually is necessary to increase the maintenance dosage of lamotrigine as much as twofold in order to maintain a consistent plasma lamotrigine concentration. The dosage increases should begin at the same time that the oral contraceptive is added and continue, based on clinical response, no more rapidly than by 50–100 mg daily every week. Dosage increases should not be made more frequently than recommended unless plasma lamotrigine concentrations or clinical response supports larger increases. Gradual transient increases in plasma lamotrigine concentrations may occur during the week of inactive hormonal preparation (i.e., the "pill-free" week); these increases will be greater if dosage increases are made during the days before or during the week of the inactive hormonal preparation. Such increased lamotrigine levels could potentially result in additional adverse effects (e.g., dizziness, ataxia, diplopia). If such adverse effects consistently occur during the "pill-free" week, dosage adjustments to the overall maintenance dosage may be necessary; however, dosage adjustments limited to the "pill-free" week are not recommended.

In women starting estrogen-containing oral contraceptives and receiving lamotrigine in addition to carbamazepine, phenobarbital, phenytoin, primidone, or other drugs that induce lamotrigine glucuronidation (e.g., rifampin, lopinavir/ritonavir, atazanavir/ritonavir), no adjustment to the lamotrigine dosage should be necessary.

When discontinuing estrogen-containing oral contraceptives in women not concurrently receiving carbamazepine, phenobarbital, phenytoin, primidone, or other drugs that induce lamotrigine glucuronidation (e.g., rifampin, lopinavir/ritonavir, atazanavir/ritonavir), the maintenance dosage of lamotrigine will in most cases need to be decreased by as much as 50% in order to maintain a consistent plasma lamotrigine concentration. The decrease in lamotrigine dosage should not exceed 25% of the total daily dosage per week over a 2-week period unless clinical response or plasma lamotrigine concentrations indicate otherwise. In women receiving lamotrigine in addition to carbamazepine, phenobarbital, phenytoin, primidone, or other drugs that induce lamotrigine glucuronidation (e.g., rifampin, lopinavir/ritonavir, atazanavir/ritonavir), adjustment of the maintenance dosage of lamotrigine should not be necessary upon discontinuance of the estrogen-containing oral contraceptive.

The effects of other hormonal contraceptive preparations or hormone replacement therapy on the pharmacokinetics of lamotrigine have not been systematically evaluated. Ethinyl estradiol, but not progestins, reportedly increased lamotrigine clearance up to twofold, and progestin-only formulations did not affect lamotrigine plasma concentrations. Therefore, adjustment of lamotrigine dosage in patients receiving progestins alone is unlikely to be necessary.

Concomitant Use with Atazanavir/Ritonavir

Atazanavir/ritonavir can induce lamotrigine glucuronidation and decrease plasma concentrations of lamotrigine. The manufacturers state that no adjustment to the recommended dosage escalation guidelines for lamotrigine should be necessary based solely on concomitant use of atazanavir/ritonavir. Dosage escalation should follow the recommended guidelines for initiating adjunctive lamotrigine therapy based on the concomitant anticonvulsant(s) or other concomitant medications. In patients already receiving maintenance dosage of lamotrigine who are not taking drugs that induce glucuronidation, dosage of lamotrigine may need to be increased or decreased if atazanavir/ritonavir is added or discontinued, respectively.

Concomitant Use with Rifampin or Lopinavir/Ritonavir

Patients being treated with rifampin or lopinavir/ritonavir should receive lamotrigine dosages recommended for individuals receiving anticonvulsants that induce glucuronidation (i.e., carbamazepine, phenobarbital, phenytoin, or primidone).

Discontinuing Therapy

Discontinuance of lamotrigine therapy should be done gradually over at least 2 weeks, in a step-wise fashion (e.g., achieving a 50% reduction in the daily dosage of lamotrigine each week). However, concerns for patient safety with continued use of lamotrigine may require more rapid withdrawal of the drug.

Seizure Disorders

Adjunctive Therapy Using Immediate-release Formulations

Recommended initial dosages and dosage escalations for lamotrigine administered as immediate-release formulations (conventional tablets, tablets for oral suspension, orally disintegrating tablets) are based on the patient's concomitant anticonvulsant regimens and other concomitant therapies. Dosage recommendations for adjunctive therapy of partial-onset seizures, primary generalized tonic-clonic seizures, or Lennox-Gastaut syndrome in patients taking valproate (Table 1), in patients not taking carbamazepine, phenytoin, phenobarbital, primidone, or valproate (Table 2), or in patients taking carbamazepine, phenytoin, phenobarbital, or primidone but not valproate (Table 3) are presented in the tables below.

TABLE 1. Recommended Dosages of Immediate-release Lamotrigine When Added to Anticonvulsant Regimens Containing Valproate

Week of Therapy	Children 2–12 Years of Age [a]	Adults and Children >12 Years of Age
Weeks 1 and 2	0.15 mg/kg daily in 1 dose or 2 divided doses	25 mg every other day
Weeks 3 and 4	0.3 mg/kg daily in 1 dose or 2 divided doses	25 mg daily
Week 5 onward	Increase dosage in increments of 0.3 mg/kg daily every 1–2 weeks until an effective maintenance dosage is reached	Increase dosage in increments of 25–50 mg daily every 1–2 weeks until an effective maintenance dosage is reached
Usual maintenance dosage [b]	1–5 mg/kg daily (maximum 200 mg daily in 1 dose or 2 divided doses)	100–400 mg daily in 1 dose or 2 divided doses if added to an anticonvulsant regimen containing valproate and other drugs that induce glucuronidation
	1–3 mg/kg daily if added to anticonvulsant regimen containing valproate alone	100–200 mg daily if added to an anticonvulsant regimen containing valproate alone

[a] Round dosage down to the nearest whole tablet.

[b] In patients weighing <30 kg, may need to increase maintenance dosage by as much as 50% based on clinical response, regardless of age or concomitant anticonvulsant(s).

TABLE 2. Recommended Dosages of Immediate-release Lamotrigine When Added to Anticonvulsant Regimens NOT Containing Carbamazepine, Phenobarbital, Phenytoin, Primidone, or Valproate

Week of Therapy	Children 2–12 Years of Age [a]	Adults and Children >12 Years of Age
Weeks 1 and 2	0.3 mg/kg daily in 1 dose or 2 divided doses	25 mg daily
Weeks 3 and 4	0.6 mg/kg daily in 2 divided doses	50 mg daily
Week 5 onward	Increase dosage in increments of 0.6 mg/kg daily every 1–2 weeks until an effective maintenance dosage is reached	Increase dosage in increments of 50 mg daily every 1–2 weeks until an effective maintenance dosage is reached
Usual maintenance dosage [b]	4.5–7.5 mg/kg daily (maximum 300 mg daily in 2 divided doses)	225–375 mg daily in 2 divided doses

[a] Round dosage down to the nearest whole tablet.

[b] In patients weighing <30 kg, may need to increase maintenance dosage by as much as 50% based on clinical response, regardless of age or concomitant anticonvulsant(s).

TABLE 3. Recommended Dosages of Immediate-release Lamotrigine When Added to Anticonvulsant Regimens Containing Carbamazepine, Phenobarbital, Phenytoin, or Primidone (*Without* Valproate)

Week of Therapy	Children 2–12 Years of Age [a]	Adults and Children >12 Years of Age
Weeks 1 and 2	0.6 mg/kg daily in 2 divided doses	50 mg daily
Weeks 3 and 4	1.2 mg/kg daily in 2 divided doses	100 mg daily in 2 divided doses
Week 5 onward	Increase dosage in increments of 1.2 mg/kg daily every 1–2 weeks until an effective maintenance dosage is reached	Increase dosage in increments of 100 mg daily every 1–2 weeks until an effective maintenance dosage is reached
Usual maintenance dosage [b]	5–15 mg/kg daily (maximum 400 mg daily in 2 divided doses)	300–500 mg daily in 2 divided doses

[a] Round dosage down to the nearest whole tablet.

[b] In patients weighing <30 kg, may need to increase maintenance dosage by as much as 50% based on clinical response, regardless of age or concomitant anticonvulsant(s).

Although maintenance dosages of immediate-release lamotrigine as high as 700 mg daily have been used in anticonvulsant drug regimens that included carbamazepine, phenytoin, phenobarbital, or primidone (without valproate), or as high as 200 mg daily in drug regimens that included valproate alone, the benefit of using dosages above those recommended by the manufacturer has not been established in controlled trials.

Adjunctive Therapy Using Extended-release Lamotrigine

The recommended dosage of extended-release lamotrigine for adjunctive therapy in the management of partial-onset seizures or primary generalized tonic-clonic seizures in adults and adolescents 13 years of age or older is based on the patient's concomitant drugs and is presented in Table 4.

TABLE 4. Recommended Dosage of Extended-release Lamotrigine (Adults and Adolescents 13 Years of Age and Older)

Week of Therapy	Regimens Containing Valproate	Regimens NOT containing Carbamazepine, Phenobarbital, Phenytoin, Primidone, or Valproate	Regimens Containing Carbamazepine, Phenobarbital, Phenytoin, or Primidone (Without Valproate)
Weeks 1 and 2	25 mg every other day	25 mg daily	50 mg daily
Weeks 3 and 4	25 mg daily	50 mg daily	100 mg daily
Week 5	50 mg daily	100 mg daily	200 mg daily
Week 6	100 mg daily	150 mg daily	300 mg daily
Week 7	150 mg daily	200 mg daily	400 mg daily
Usual maintenance dosage (Week 8 onward)	200–250 mg daily [a]	300–400 mg daily [a]	400–600 mg daily [a]

[a] Dosage increases from week 8 or later should not exceed 100 mg daily at weekly intervals.

Monotherapy for Partial-onset Seizures

For lamotrigine monotherapy in adults (16 years of age or older) with partial-onset seizures converting from monotherapy with carbamazepine, phenytoin, phenobarbital, or primidone, the recommended maintenance dosage of lamotrigine given as immediate-release formulations (conventional tablets, tablets for oral suspension, orally disintegrating tablets) is 500 mg daily given in 2 divided doses. The transition regimen for converting patients from these drugs to lamotrigine monotherapy is a 2-step process; the goal is to ensure adequate seizure control while minimizing the possibility of developing a serious rash associated with the rapid titration of lamotrigine. In the first step of the process, immediate-release lamotrigine therapy is added to the current drug regimen (which should be maintained at a fixed dosage) at a dosage of 50 mg once daily for 2 weeks, followed by 100 mg daily in 2 divided doses for 2 weeks; the daily dosage is then increased by 100 mg every 1–2 weeks until the maintenance dosage of 500 mg daily (in 2 divided doses) is reached. Once the maintenance lamotrigine dosage is reached, the concomitant drug can then be withdrawn gradually over a period of 4 weeks; based on experience from the controlled clinical trial, the concomitant drug was withdrawn by 20% decrements each week over a 4-week period.

For lamotrigine monotherapy in adults (16 years of age or older) with partial-onset seizures converting from monotherapy with valproate, the recommended maintenance dosage of lamotrigine given as immediate-release formulations (conventional tablets, tablets for oral suspension, orally disintegrating tablets) is 500 mg daily given in 2 divided doses. The transition regimen for converting patients from valproate to lamotrigine monotherapy is summarized in Table 5.

TABLE 5. Conversion from Adjunctive Therapy with Valproate to Immediate-release Lamotrigine Monotherapy (Adults 16 Years of Age and Older)

Step	Lamotrigine	Valproate
1	Achieve a dosage of 200 mg daily according to guidelines in Table 1 (if not already receiving 200 mg daily)	Maintain established stable dosage
2	Maintain at 200 mg daily	Decrease to 500 mg daily in decrements no greater than 500 mg daily every week and then maintain dosage of 500 mg daily for 1 week
3	Increase to 300 mg daily and maintain for 1 week	Simultaneously decrease to 250 mg daily and maintain for 1 week
4	Increase in increments of 100 mg daily every week to achieve maintenance dosage of 500 mg daily	Discontinue

In patients converting from adjunctive therapy with carbamazepine, phenobarbital, phenytoin, or primidone to monotherapy with extended-release lamotrigine, dosage of lamotrigine should be titrated until a maintenance dosage of 500 mg daily is reached (see dosage guidelines in Table 4); the concomitant anticonvulsant should then be withdrawn by 20% decrements each week over a 4-week period. Two weeks after withdrawal of the concomitant anticonvulsant drug is completed, lamotrigine dosage may be decreased by no more than 100 mg daily each week until a monotherapy maintenance dosage of 250–300 mg daily is reached.

In patients converting from adjunctive therapy with valproate to monotherapy with extended-release lamotrigine, the conversion regimen in Table 6 should be followed.

TABLE 6. Conversion from Valproate to Extended-release Lamotrigine Monotherapy (Adults and Adolescents 13 Years of Age and Older)

Step	Lamotrigine (Extended-release)	Valproate
1	Achieve a dosage of 150 mg daily according to guidelines in Table 4	Maintain established stable dosage
2	Maintain at 150 mg daily	Decrease to 500 mg daily in decrements no greater than 500 mg daily every week and then maintain dosage of 500 mg daily for 1 week
3	Increase to 200 mg daily	Simultaneously decrease to 250 mg daily and maintain for 1 week
4	Increase to 250 or 300 mg daily	Discontinue

In patients converting from adjunctive therapy with an anticonvulsant other than carbamazepine, phenytoin, phenobarbital, primidone, or valproate to monotherapy with extended-release lamotrigine, dosage of lamotrigine should be titrated until a maintenance dosage of 250-300 mg daily is reached (see dosage guidelines in Table 4); the concomitant anticonvulsant should then be withdrawn by 20% decrements each week over a 4-week period.

Bipolar Disorder

The recommended dosage of immediate-release lamotrigine for maintenance treatment of bipolar disorder in adults is based on the patient's concomitant drugs and is summarized in Table 7.

The optimum duration of lamotrigine therapy for the management of bipolar disorder has not been established, and the usefulness of the drug during prolonged therapy (i.e., longer than 18 months) should be reevaluated periodically.

TABLE 7. Immediate-release Lamotrigine Dosage Titration Regimen for Adults with Bipolar Disorder

Week of Therapy	For Patients NOT Receiving Carbamazepine, Phenobarbital, Phenytoin, Primidone, Rifampin, or Valproate	For Patients Receiving Valproate	For Patients Receiving Carbamazepine, Phenobarbital, Phenytoin, Primidone, or Rifampin (Without Valproate)
Weeks 1 and 2	25 mg daily	25 mg every other day	50 mg daily
Weeks 3 and 4	50 mg daily	25 mg daily	100 mg daily in divided doses
Week 5	100 mg daily	50 mg daily	200 mg daily in divided doses
Week 6	200 mg daily	100 mg daily	300 mg daily in divided doses
Week 7 (target dosages)	200 mg daily	100 mg daily	Up to 400 mg daily in divided doses

Addition of concomitant drugs (e.g., carbamazepine, phenobarbital, phenytoin, primidone, valproate) may require modification of the dosage of lamotrigine and/or the concomitant drug. In pivotal clinical studies, dosages of lamotrigine were halved immediately following the addition of valproate to treat an acute mood episode and maintained at that dosage as long as valproate was administered concomitantly with lamotrigine. Following addition of carbamazepine or other glucuronidation-inducing drugs to treat an acute mood episode, dosages of lamotrigine were gradually doubled (e.g., over a period of at least 3 weeks) and maintained at that dosage as long as these drugs were administered concomitantly with lamotrigine. Following the addition of other psychotropic agents with no known clinical pharmacokinetic interactions with lamotrigine, patients were maintained at current maintenance dosages of lamotrigine.

Discontinuance of glucuronidation-inducing (e.g., carbamazepine) or glucuronidation-inhibiting (e.g., valproate) drugs from a regimen including lamotrigine may require modification of the dosage of lamotrigine. For patients discontinuing carbamazepine, phenytoin, phenobarbital, primidone, or other drugs such as rifampin, lopinavir/ritonavir, and atazanavir/ritonavir that induce lamotrigine glucuronidation, lamotrigine dosage should remain constant for the first week and then should be decreased in 100-mg daily increments at weekly intervals until an effective maintenance dosage of 200 mg daily is reached. For patients discontinuing valproate following resolution of the acute mood episode and achievement of a maintenance lamotrigine dosage, lamotrigine dosage should be increased in 50-mg daily increments at weekly intervals until an effective maintenance dosage of 200 mg daily is reached.

● **Dosage in Renal and Hepatic Impairment**

The manufacturers state that lamotrigine should be used with caution in patients with severe renal impairment because there is insufficient information from controlled clinical studies to establish the safety and efficacy of the drug in such patients. The initial dosage of lamotrigine in patients with renal impairment should be based on the patient's existing anticonvulsant drug regimen. The manufacturers state that a reduced maintenance dosage of lamotrigine may be effective in patients with substantial renal impairment.

The manufacturers state that experience with lamotrigine therapy in patients with hepatic impairment is limited. Based on a clinical pharmacology study of the drug in a small number of patients with moderate to severe hepatic dysfunction, the manufacturers make the general recommendation that initial, escalation, and maintenance dosages of lamotrigine therapy should be decreased by approximately 25% in patients with moderate (e.g., Child-Pugh class B) or severe (e.g., Child-Pugh class C) hepatic impairment without ascites and by 50% in patients with severe hepatic impairment with ascites. Escalation and maintenance dosages should be adjusted according to clinical response. Dosage adjustment is not necessary in patients with mild (e.g., Child-Pugh class A) hepatic impairment.

CAUTIONS

Lamotrigine generally is well tolerated. However, there have been rare reports of serious dermatologic reactions (including some fatalities) in adults and children receiving lamotrigine. Nervous system and dermatologic effects are among the most frequently reported adverse effects of lamotrigine and among those most frequently requiring discontinuance of the drug.

The most frequently occurring adverse effects associated with lamotrigine as adjunctive anticonvulsant therapy in adults in controlled clinical trials include dizziness, ataxia, somnolence, headache, diplopia, blurred vision, nausea, vomiting, and rash. Discontinuance of lamotrigine because of adverse effects was required in about 11% of adult patients receiving immediate-release lamotrigine as adjunctive therapy in uncontrolled and controlled clinical trials; adverse effects most frequently associated with discontinuance of therapy were rash, dizziness, and headache. In children receiving immediate-release lamotrigine as adjunctive anticonvulsant therapy in controlled clinical trials, the most commonly reported adverse effects were infection, vomiting, rash, fever, somnolence, accidental injury, dizziness, diarrhea, abdominal pain, nausea, ataxia, tremor, asthenia, bronchitis, flu syndrome, and diplopia. Approximately 11.5% of these children discontinued the drug because of an adverse effect, most frequently due to rash, aggravated reaction, or ataxia.

The most common adverse effects associated with extended-release lamotrigine as adjunctive anticonvulsant therapy in adults and adolescents 13 years of age or older in 2 controlled clinical trials include dizziness, tremor/intention tremor, vomiting, and diplopia. Discontinuance of lamotrigine because of adverse effects was required in 5% of these patients, most frequently due to dizziness, rash, headache, nausea, or nystagmus.

The most common adverse effects associated with immediate-release lamotrigine as monotherapy in adults in the controlled clinical trial were vomiting, coordination abnormality, dyspepsia, nausea, dizziness, rhinitis, anxiety, insomnia, infection, pain, weight decrease, chest pain, and dysmenorrhea; during the conversion period (i.e., when lamotrigine was initially added on to an existing monotherapy regimen consisting of a hepatic enzyme-inducing anticonvulsant drug), the most commonly reported adverse effects were dizziness, headache, nausea, asthenia, coordination abnormality, vomiting, rash, somnolence, diplopia, ataxia, accidental injury, tremor, blurred vision, insomnia, nystagmus, diarrhea, lymphadenopathy, pruritus, and sinusitis. The adverse effects most commonly associated with discontinuance of the drug in this trial were rash (4.5% of patients), headache (3.1% of patients), and asthenia (2.4% of patients).

The most common adverse effects associated with immediate-release lamotrigine in adults with bipolar disorder include nausea, insomnia, somnolence, back pain, fatigue, rash, rhinitis, abdominal pain, and xerostomia.

The adverse effect profiles and rates of drug discontinuance in males and females in clinical trials of immediate-release lamotrigine were similar and were independent of age. In general, females receiving adjunctive therapy with immediate-release lamotrigine or placebo in controlled trials were more likely to report adverse effects than were males; however, dizziness was the only adverse effect reported with at least 10% greater frequency (i.e., 16.5% greater frequency) in females than in males (without a corresponding difference by gender with placebo) in controlled trials.

● Nervous System Effects

Nervous system effects were among the most frequent adverse effects reported in patients receiving lamotrigine as adjunctive anticonvulsant therapy in controlled clinical trials. Dizziness, headache, and ataxia were the most frequent adverse nervous system effects, occurring in 38, 29, and 22% of adults, respectively, in controlled trials of immediate-release lamotrigine adjunctive therapy. The frequency of dizziness and ataxia and the rate of discontinuance of lamotrigine because of these adverse effects were dose related in clinical trials; in a dose-response study, dizziness occurred in 54, 31, or 27% of patients receiving lamotrigine 500 mg/day, lamotrigine 300 mg/day, or placebo, respectively, while ataxia occurred in 28, 10, or 10% of those receiving these respective regimens. Limited data also suggest an increased incidence of adverse nervous system effects in patients receiving carbamazepine concomitantly with lamotrigine. (See Drug Interactions under Cautions.)

Somnolence or insomnia occurred in 14 or 6%, respectively, of adults receiving immediate-release lamotrigine as adjunctive therapy in controlled clinical trials. Incoordination or tremor was reported in 6 or 4%, respectively, of lamotrigine-treated adults; limited evidence suggests that incoordination and tremor may be dose related, and tremor may occur more frequently with concomitant administration of valproate and lamotrigine. Depression occurred in 4%, anxiety in 4%, irritability in 3%, speech disorder in 3%, and concentration disturbance in 2% of adults receiving lamotrigine as adjunctive therapy in controlled clinical trials. Seizure or seizure exacerbation has been reported in 3 or 2% of adults, respectively, receiving lamotrigine as adjunctive therapy in controlled trials; an increase in seizure frequency also has been reported with lamotrigine therapy. Treatment-emergent seizures diagnosed unequivocally as status epilepticus were reported in 7 of 2343 adults receiving adjunctive therapy with immediate-release lamotrigine in clinical trials; however, the manufacturers state that valid estimates of the incidence of treatment-emergent status epilepticus are difficult to obtain because of variations in the definitions used by different investigators to identify such cases.

Coordination abnormality, dizziness, anxiety, and insomnia occurred in 7, 7, 5, and 5%, respectively, of adults receiving immediate-release lamotrigine as monotherapy in a controlled trial; amnesia, ataxia, asthenia, depression, hypesthesia, libido increase, decreased or increased reflexes, nystagmus, and irritability each occurred in 2% of such patients. Paresthesia or asthenia occurred in more than 1% of adults receiving lamotrigine as adjunctive therapy in controlled clinical trials but with equal or greater frequency in those receiving placebo.

Somnolence occurred in 17%, dizziness in 14%, ataxia in 11%, tremor in 10%, and asthenia in 8% of children receiving immediate-release lamotrigine as adjunctive therapy in controlled clinical trials. Emotional lability, gait abnormality, thinking abnormality, seizures, nervousness, and vertigo each occurred in 2-4% of children receiving lamotrigine as adjunctive therapy in controlled clinical trials.

Insomnia and somnolence occurred in 10 and 9%, respectively, of adults receiving immediate-release lamotrigine for bipolar disorder in controlled clinical trials. Dizziness and headache each occurred in more than 5% of adults receiving

immediate-release lamotrigine as monotherapy in clinical trials. Amnesia, depression, agitation, abnormal dreams, emotional lability, dyspraxia, abnormal thinking, or hypoesthesia each occurred in at least 1% but less than 5% of such patients.

Aseptic Meningitis

Lamotrigine therapy increases the risk of developing aseptic meningitis. FDA states that a total of 40 cases of aseptic meningitis have been identified in pediatric and adult lamotrigine-treated patients from December 1994 through November 2009. Symptoms in these cases included headache, fever, nausea, vomiting, nuchal rigidity, skin rash, photophobia, myalgia, chills, altered consciousness, and/or somnolence and occurred 1-42 days (mean of 16 days) after beginning therapy with the drug. There was one death reported; however, the death was not thought to be caused by aseptic meningitis. Hospitalization was required in 35 of the patients. In most of the cases, symptoms resolved following discontinuance of lamotrigine. In 15 cases, however, symptoms rapidly returned (within 0.5-24 hours; mean: 5 hours) following reinitiation of lamotrigine. In these rechallenge cases, symptoms were frequently more severe following reexposure to the drug. CSF findings that were available in 25 cases were characterized by mild to moderate pleocytosis, normal glucose concentrations, and mild to moderate increases in protein. CSF white blood cell differentials showed a predominance of neutrophils in the majority of cases; however, a predominance of lymphocytes was reported in approximately one-third of the cases. Some of the lamotrigine-treated patients who developed aseptic meningitis had underlying diagnoses of systemic lupus erythematosus or other autoimmune diseases. In addition, some of the patients had new onset of signs and symptoms of other organ involvement (predominantly hepatic and renal involvement), which may suggest that in these cases, the aseptic meningitis was part of a hypersensitivity reaction.

Patients receiving lamotrigine should be instructed to immediately contact their clinician if they experience headache, fever, chills, nausea, vomiting, stiff neck, rash, abnormal sensitivity to light, myalgia, drowsiness, and/or confusion. If meningitis is suspected, patients should be evaluated and treated, as indicated, for other possible causes of meningitis. Discontinuance of lamotrigine should be considered if no other clear cause of meningitis is identified.

● Immune System Effects

Hemophagocytic Lymphohistiocytosis

Hemophagocytic lymphohistiocytosis (HLH), a rare but potentially life-threatening condition involving pathologic activation of the immune system, has been reported in adults and children receiving lamotrigine. If not recognized and treated promptly, HLH is associated with high mortality. HLH can occur within days to weeks after starting lamotrigine therapy and is characterized by clinical signs and symptoms of uncontrolled systemic inflammation; manifestations include, but are not limited to, persistent fever (usually greater than 101°F), rash, hepatosplenomegaly, lymphadenopathy, neurologic effects (e.g., seizures, visual disturbances, difficulty ambulating), cytopenias, hepatic dysfunction, high serum ferritin concentrations, and coagulation abnormalities. Diagnosis may be difficult because early signs and symptoms (particularly fever and rash) are nonspecific and may be confused with other immune-related adverse reactions such as drug reaction with eosinophilia and systemic symptoms (DRESS). (See Multiorgan Hypersensitivity under Cautions.) Since 1994, at least 8 cases of confirmed or suspected HLH have been reported among patients receiving lamotrigine worldwide; serious outcomes included hospitalization in all cases and death in one patient. In the reported cases, a temporal relationship was observed between administration of lamotrigine and development of HLH, with symptoms presenting 8-24 days following initiation of the drug.

Patients receiving lamotrigine should be advised to seek immediate medical attention if they develop any manifestations suggestive of HLH (e.g., fever, usually exceeding 101°F; rash; enlarged liver and lymph nodes; unusual bleeding; yellowing of the skin or eyes; neurologic effects including seizures, difficulty walking, and visual disturbances). An evaluation for possible HLH should be performed based on published international diagnostic criteria. Unless an alternative etiology for the observed signs or symptoms can be established, lamotrigine should be discontinued.

● GI Effects

GI effects were among the most frequent adverse effects reported in adults receiving immediate-release lamotrigine as adjunctive therapy in controlled clinical trials. Nausea was the most frequent adverse GI effect, occurring in 19% of adults in controlled clinical trials; vomiting was reported in 9% of patients in these trials. The frequency of nausea and vomiting appears to be dose related; in a dose-response study, nausea occurred in 25, 18, or 11% of patients receiving lamotrigine 500 mg daily, lamotrigine 300 mg daily, or placebo, respectively, while vomiting occurred in 18, 11, or 4% of those receiving these respective regimens. Diarrhea occurred in 6%, dyspepsia in 5%, abdominal pain in 5%, constipation in 4%, tooth disorder in 3%, and anorexia in 2% of adults receiving lamotrigine as adjunctive therapy in controlled clinical trials. Flatulence was reported in more than 1% of adults receiving lamotrigine as adjunctive therapy in controlled clinical trials but occurred with equal or greater frequency in patients receiving placebo. Vomiting, dyspepsia, and nausea occurred in 9, 7, and 7%, respectively, of adults receiving lamotrigine as monotherapy in a controlled trial; anorexia, dry mouth, rectal hemorrhage, and peptic ulcer each occurred in 2% of such patients.

Vomiting occurred in 20%, diarrhea in 11%, abdominal pain in 10%, and nausea in 10% of children receiving immediate-release lamotrigine as adjunctive therapy in controlled clinical trials. Constipation, dyspepsia, and tooth disorder each occurred in 2–4% of children receiving lamotrigine as adjunctive therapy in controlled clinical trials.

● Dermatologic and Sensitivity Reactions

Serious and sometimes fatal dermatologic reactions (e.g., Stevens-Johnson syndrome, toxic epidermal necrolysis, angioedema, rash associated with multiorgan hypersensitivity) have been reported in adults and children receiving lamotrigine therapy. A black box warning about the risk of serious skin rashes is included in the prescribing information for all formulations of the drug.

The incidence of severe rash associated with lamotrigine appears to be higher in pediatric patients than in adults; severe rash, including Stevens-Johnson syndrome, has been reported in approximately 0.3–0.8% of children 2–17 years of age and in 0.08–0.3% of adults receiving immediate-release lamotrigine in clinical trials. The risk of serious rashes associated with extended-release lamotrigine therapy is not expected to differ from that with the immediate-release formulations of the drug; however, the relatively limited treatment experience makes it difficult to characterize the incidence and risk of such rashes with the extended-release formulation.

There is evidence that most cases of rash associated with lamotrigine therapy are associated with transiently high plasma concentrations of the drug occurring during the initial weeks of therapy or with high plasma concentrations occurring during concomitant valproate therapy. Cases of life-threatening rashes associated with lamotrigine almost always have occurred within 2–8 weeks of treatment initiation; however, severe rashes rarely have presented following prolonged treatment (e.g., 6 months). Lamotrigine-associated rashes do not appear to have distinguishing features. Because it is not possible to distinguish benign rashes from those that may become severe and/or life-threatening, lamotrigine generally should be discontinued at the first sign of rash (unless the rash is known not to be drug related). However, a rash may become life-threatening or permanently disabling or disfiguring despite discontinuance of the drug. The potential for development of a rash at the beginning of lamotrigine therapy may be decreased by employing low initial dosages and by gradual escalation of dosage to avoid initially high plasma concentrations of the drug.

A history of hypersensitivity or rash to other anticonvulsant drugs may increase the risk of developing a rash with lamotrigine. In addition, the risk of serious and potentially life-threatening rash with lamotrigine appears to be increased in patients receiving concomitant valproate (including valproic acid and divalproex sodium). Valproate can decrease clearance and increase plasma concentrations of lamotrigine more than twofold. Exceeding the recommended initial dosage of lamotrigine or the subsequent recommended schedule for escalation of lamotrigine dosage, particularly in patients receiving valproate, may increase the incidence of serious rash. In clinical trials, 1% of adults and 1.2% of children receiving a drug regimen including immediate-release lamotrigine concomitantly with valproate experienced a serious rash, while 0.16% of adults and 0.6% of children who did not receive concomitant valproate experienced a serious rash. (See Serious Skin Rash under Cautions.)

Lamotrigine also can cause benign rashes and other adverse dermatologic effects.

Multiorgan Hypersensitivity

Multiorgan hypersensitivity (also known as drug reaction with eosinophilia and systemic symptoms [DRESS]), a potentially fatal or life-threatening reaction, has been reported with lamotrigine. The clinical presentation is variable, but typically includes eosinophilia, fever, rash, and/or lymphadenopathy associated with other organ system involvement such as hepatitis, nephritis, hematologic abnormalities, myocarditis, or myositis. However, signs and symptoms associated with other organ systems may occur. Fatalities associated with acute multiorgan failure and various degrees of hepatic failure have been reported in some adults and pediatric patients who received lamotrigine in epilepsy clinical trials. Isolated liver failure without a rash or involvement of other organs also has been reported.

Prior to initiating lamotrigine therapy, patients should be instructed that a rash or other signs of hypersensitivity may indicate a serious event and advised to immediately contact their clinician if any such signs occur. If signs or symptoms of DRESS occur during lamotrigine therapy, patients should be evaluated immediately; if an alternative cause cannot be identified, the drug should be discontinued. Early manifestations of hypersensitivity (e.g., fever, lymphadenopathy) may be present even if a rash is not evident.

● Cardiovascular Effects

Hemorrhage was reported in 2% of pediatric patients receiving immediate-release lamotrigine as adjunctive therapy in controlled clinical trials. Chest pain occurred in more than 1% of adults receiving lamotrigine as adjunctive therapy in controlled clinical trials but occurred with equal or greater frequency in patients receiving placebo. Chest pain also occurred in 5% of adults receiving lamotrigine as monotherapy in a controlled clinical trial.

Cardiac Arrhythmias

FDA has received reports of abnormal ECG findings and other serious manifestations (e.g., chest pain, loss of consciousness, cardiac arrest) in patients receiving lamotrigine, and is currently evaluating whether other drugs in the same class have similar cardiac effects. In vitro studies indicate that lamotrigine exhibits Class IB antiarrhythmic activity at therapeutically relevant concentrations, which can be life-threatening in patients with clinically important structural or functional heart disorders (i.e., those with heart failure, valvular heart disease, congenital heart disease, conduction system disease, ventricular arrhythmias, cardiac channelopathies [e.g., Brugada syndrome], clinically important ischemic heart disease, or multiple risk factors for coronary artery disease). In patients with clinically important structural or functional heart disease, the expected or observed benefits of lamotrigine must be carefully weighed against the risk of serious arrhythmias and/or death. The risk of arrhythmias may be increased with concomitant use of other sodium channel blockers (e.g., carbamazepine, cenobamate, eslicarbazepine, fosphenytoin, lacosamide, oxcarbazepine, phenytoin, rufinamide, topiramate, zonisamide).

● Respiratory Effects

Rhinitis occurred in 14%, pharyngitis in 10%, increased cough in 8%, and flu-like syndrome in 7% of adults receiving immediate-release lamotrigine as adjunctive therapy in controlled clinical trials. Respiratory disorder was reported in more than 1% of adults receiving lamotrigine as adjunctive therapy in controlled clinical trials but occurred with equal or greater frequency in patients receiving placebo. Rhinitis occurred in 7% of adults receiving lamotrigine as monotherapy in a controlled trial; epistaxis, bronchitis, and dyspnea each occurred in 2% of such patients. Pharyngitis, bronchitis, and increased cough occurred in 14, 7, and 7%, respectively, of children receiving immediate-release lamotrigine as adjunctive therapy in controlled clinical trials. Sinusitis and bronchospasm each were reported in 2% of children in these trials.

● Ocular and Otic Effects

Ocular effects were among the most frequent adverse effects reported in patients receiving lamotrigine as adjunctive therapy in controlled clinical trials. Diplopia was the most frequent adverse ocular effect reported in adults receiving immediate-release lamotrigine as adjunctive therapy in controlled trials, occurring in 28% of such patients, and blurred vision occurred in 16% of patients. The frequency of diplopia and blurred vision appears to be dose related; in a dose-response study, diplopia occurred in 49, 24, or 8% of patients receiving lamotrigine 500 mg daily, lamotrigine 300 mg daily, or placebo, respectively, while blurred vision occurred in 25, 11, or 10% of patients receiving these respective regimens. Limited data also indicate an increased incidence of some adverse effects, including diplopia and blurred vision, in patients receiving carbamazepine concomitantly with lamotrigine.

Vision abnormality occurred in 3% of adults receiving immediate-release lamotrigine as adjunctive therapy in controlled clinical trials and in 2% of adults receiving immediate-release lamotrigine as monotherapy in a controlled trial. Diplopia, blurred vision, or vision abnormality occurred in 5, 4, or 2%, respectively, of children receiving lamotrigine as adjunctive therapy in controlled clinical trials.

Ear disorder was reported in 2% of children receiving immediate-release lamotrigine as adjunctive therapy in controlled clinical trials.

● Musculoskeletal Effects

Neck pain and arthralgia each occurred in 2% of adults receiving immediate-release lamotrigine as adjunctive therapy in controlled clinical trials. Back pain or myalgia occurred in more than 1% of patients receiving lamotrigine as adjunctive therapy in controlled trials but with equal or greater frequency in patients receiving placebo.

● Genitourinary Effects

Dysmenorrhea occurred in 7%, vaginitis in 4%, and amenorrhea in 2% of women receiving immediate-release lamotrigine as adjunctive therapy in controlled clinical trials. Dysmenorrhea occurred in 5% of women receiving lamotrigine as monotherapy in a controlled trial. Menstrual disorder or urinary tract infection occurred in more than 1% of adults receiving adjunctive lamotrigine therapy in controlled trials but with equal or greater frequency in patients receiving placebo. Urinary tract infection occurred in 3% of children receiving lamotrigine as adjunctive therapy in controlled clinical trials; penis disorder was reported in 2% of male pediatric patients receiving lamotrigine in these trials.

● Endocrine and Metabolic Effects

Weight decrease occurred in 5% of adults receiving lamotrigine as monotherapy in a controlled trial. Edema occurred in 2% of children receiving lamotrigine as adjunctive therapy in controlled clinical trials.

● Hepatic Effects

Fatalities associated with multiorgan failure and various degrees of hepatic failure have been reported rarely with lamotrigine. Multiorgan hypersensitivity (also known as DRESS), which may have a hepatic component, also has been reported with lamotrigine. (See Multiorgan Hypersensitivity under Cautions.) Isolated liver failure without rash or other organ involvement also has been reported.

● Hematologic Effects

Blood dyscrasias that may or may not be associated with multiorgan hypersensitivity (also known as DRESS), including neutropenia, leukopenia, anemia, thrombocytopenia, pancytopenia, and rarely, aplastic anemia and pure red cell aplasia (PRCA), have been reported with lamotrigine. Lymphadenopathy occurred in 2% of children receiving immediate-release lamotrigine as adjunctive therapy in controlled clinical trials.

● Precautions and Contraindications
Withdrawal Seizures

Because of the possibility of increased seizure frequency, anticonvulsant drugs, including lamotrigine, should not be discontinued suddenly, particularly in patients with preexisting seizure disorders. Unless safety concerns dictate a more rapid withdrawal of the drug, discontinuance of lamotrigine should be done gradually over a period of at least 2 weeks. (See Dosage under Dosage and Administration.) Seizure exacerbation and/or status epilepticus have been reported in patients receiving lamotrigine as adjunctive therapy in the management of seizure disorders, although the incidence of these adverse effects has been difficult to determine conclusively. (See Nervous System Effects under Cautions.) The use and dosage of all anticonvulsant drugs in a regimen including lamotrigine should

be reevaluated if there is a change in seizure control or appearance or worsening of adverse effects, and patients should be instructed to report immediately any worsening of seizure control.

Suicidality Risk

An increased risk of suicidality (suicidal behavior or ideation) was observed in an analysis of 199 randomized, placebo-controlled studies evaluating 11 anticonvulsants (carbamazepine, felbamate, gabapentin, lamotrigine, levetiracetam, oxcarbazepine, pregabalin, tiagabine, topiramate, valproate, and zonisamide) in patients with epilepsy, psychiatric disorders (e.g., bipolar disorder, depression, anxiety), and other conditions (e.g., migraine, neuropathic pain). The analysis revealed that patients receiving these anticonvulsants had approximately twice the risk of suicidal behavior or ideation (0.43%) compared with patients receiving placebo (0.24%); this increased suicidality risk was observed as early as one week after beginning therapy and continued through 24 weeks. The results were generally consistent among the 11 drugs studied. Patients who were treated for epilepsy, psychiatric disorders, and other conditions were all found to be at increased risk for suicidality when compared with placebo; there did not appear to be a specific demographic subgroup of patients to which the increased risk could be attributed. However, the relative risk for suicidality was found to be higher in patients with epilepsy compared with patients who were given one of the drugs for psychiatric or other conditions.

All patients who are currently receiving or beginning therapy with any anticonvulsant for any indication should be closely monitored for the emergence or worsening of depression, suicidal thoughts or behavior (suicidality), and/or unusual changes in mood or behavior. Clinicians should inform patients, their families, and caregivers of the potential for an increased risk of suicidality so that they are aware and able to notify their clinician of any unusual behavioral changes. Patients, family members, and caregivers also should be advised not to make any changes to the anticonvulsant regimen without first consulting with the responsible clinician. They should pay close attention to any day-to-day changes in mood, behavior, and actions; since changes can happen very quickly, it is important to be alert to any sudden differences. In addition, patients, family members, and caregivers should be aware of common warning signs that may signal suicide risk (e.g., talking or thinking about wanting to hurt oneself or end one's life, withdrawing from friends and family, becoming depressed or experiencing worsening of existing depression, becoming preoccupied with death and dying, giving away prized possessions). If these or any new and worrisome behaviors occur, the responsible clinician should be contacted immediately. Clinicians who prescribe lamotrigine or any other anticonvulsant should balance the risk for suicidality with the risk of untreated illness. Epilepsy and many other illnesses for which anticonvulsants are prescribed are themselves associated with an increased risk of morbidity and mortality and an increased risk of suicidal thoughts and behavior. If suicidal thoughts and behavior emerge during anticonvulsant therapy, the clinician must consider whether the emergence of these symptoms in any given patient may be related to the illness being treated.

Sudden Death in Epilepsy

During the premarketing development of lamotrigine, 20 sudden and unexplained deaths were reported among a cohort of 4700 patients with epilepsy receiving adjunctive therapy with immediate-release lamotrigine (5747 patient-years of exposure). Although the rate of these deaths exceeds that expected to occur in a healthy (nonepileptic) population matched for age and gender, this rate was similar to that occurring in a similar population of epileptic patients receiving a chemically unrelated anticonvulsant agent. This evidence suggests, but does not prove, that the incidence of sudden, unexplained death observed with lamotrigine adjunctive therapy may be reflective of the population itself rather than the effects of lamotrigine.

Serious Skin Rash

Cases of serious and sometimes life-threatening rashes, including Stevens-Johnson syndrome and toxic epidermal necrolysis, have occurred in patients receiving lamotrigine. (See Dermatologic and Sensitivity Reactions under Cautions.) Some evidence suggests that use of lamotrigine concomitantly with valproate increases the risk of serious rash. The incidence of rash also appears to increase with the magnitude of the initial dosage of lamotrigine and the subsequent rate of dosage escalation; exceeding the recommended dosage of lamotrigine at initiation of therapy appears to increase the risk of rash requiring withdrawal of therapy.

A benign initial appearance of a rash in a patient receiving lamotrigine therapy cannot predict an entirely benign outcome. Patients receiving lamotrigine, especially in conjunction with valproate, should be cautioned that rash, in some cases potentially life-threatening, may occur, and that any occurrence of rash should immediately be reported by the patient to their clinician.

Drug Interactions

Anticonvulsants

Concomitant use of valproate or glucuronidation-inducing anticonvulsant drugs (e.g., carbamazepine, phenobarbital, phenytoin, primidone) can increase or decrease the metabolism and elimination of lamotrigine, respectively, requiring dosage adjustments to maintain efficacy and/or avoid toxicity. (See Dosage under Dosage and Administration.)

Addition of valproate to lamotrigine therapy reduces lamotrigine clearance and increases steady-state plasma lamotrigine concentrations by slightly more than 50% whether or not hepatic enzyme-inducing anticonvulsant drugs are given concomitantly. Conversely, steady-state plasma concentrations of lamotrigine are decreased by about 40% when carbamazepine, phenobarbital, or primidone is added to lamotrigine therapy and by about 45–54% when phenytoin is added to lamotrigine therapy; the magnitude of the effect with phenytoin is dependent on the total daily dosage of phenytoin (from 100–400 mg daily). Discontinuance of an enzyme-inducing anticonvulsant drug can be expected to increase, and discontinuance of valproate can be expected to decrease, the elimination half-life and plasma concentrations of lamotrigine. Although the manufacturers state that a therapeutic plasma concentration range has not been established for lamotrigine and that dosage should be based on therapeutic response, the change in plasma lamotrigine concentrations resulting from addition or discontinuance of glucuronidation-inducing anticonvulsant drugs or valproate should be considered when these drugs are added to or withdrawn from an existing anticonvulsant drug regimen that includes lamotrigine.

Addition of lamotrigine to existing therapy with phenytoin or carbamazepine generally does not appreciably alter the steady-state plasma concentrations of these concomitantly administered drugs. Addition of lamotrigine to carbamazepine therapy reportedly has resulted in increased plasma concentrations of a pharmacologically active metabolite of carbamazepine (carbamazepine-10,11-epoxide) and an increased incidence of some adverse effects (e.g., dizziness, headache, diplopia, blurred vision, ataxia, nausea, nystagmus). However, elevations in carbamazepine-10,11-epoxide plasma concentrations and/or increased toxicity have not been consistently observed with concomitant administration of lamotrigine and carbamazepine, and the mechanism of the interaction between these drugs remains unclear.

Addition of lamotrigine to valproate therapy in healthy individuals resulted in a 25% reduction in trough steady-state plasma concentrations of valproate over a 3-week period, followed by stabilization of these concentrations.

The effects of adding lamotrigine to an existing regimen including valproate, phenytoin, and/or carbamazepine may be expected to be similar to those associated with addition of each drug independently (i.e., valproate concentrations decrease, phenytoin and carbamazepine concentrations do not change).

Oral Contraceptives

Some estrogen-containing oral contraceptives have been shown to decrease plasma concentrations of lamotrigine. Therefore, dosage adjustment of lamotrigine will be necessary in most patients who begin or stop estrogen-containing oral contraceptives while receiving lamotrigine therapy. (See Concomitant use with Oral Contraceptives under Dosage and Administration.) During the week of inactive hormonal preparation (i.e., "pill-free" week) of oral contraceptive therapy, plasma lamotrigine concentrations are expected to increase by as much as twofold by the end of the week. Adverse effects associated with elevated plasma lamotrigine concentrations (such as dizziness, ataxia, and diplopia) may occur.

Folate Inhibitors

Lamotrigine is a weak inhibitor of dihydrofolate reductase. Although clinically important alterations in blood folate concentrations or hematologic parameters have not been documented in clinical studies of lamotrigine therapy of at least 5 years duration, the manufacturers state that clinicians should be aware of this effect when prescribing other drugs that inhibit folate metabolism.

Somnolence and Dizziness

Lamotrigine can produce drowsiness and dizziness, and patients should be cautioned that the drug may impair their ability to perform hazardous activities requiring mental alertness or physical coordination (e.g., operating machinery, driving a motor vehicle).

Renal Impairment

Limited information indicates that the elimination half-life of immediate-release lamotrigine is prolonged in patients with severe chronic renal failure (mean creatinine clearance of 13 mL/minute) not receiving other anticonvulsant drugs. In a study of a limited number of patients and healthy individuals receiving a single 100-mg dose of immediate-release lamotrigine, the mean plasma half-life of the drug was 42.9 hours in patients with chronic renal failure, 57.4 hours between treatments in dialysis patients, and 26.2 hours in healthy individuals. The mean plasma half-life of lamotrigine was decreased to 13 hours during hemodialysis; an average of 20% (range: 5.6–35.1%) of the total body load of lamotrigine was eliminated during a 4-hour hemodialysis treatment. (See Dosage in Renal and Hepatic Impairment under Dosage and Administration.)

Hepatic Impairment

The manufacturers state that experience with use of lamotrigine in patients with impaired liver function is limited. Following a single 100-mg dose of immediate-release lamotrigine, the mean half-life of the drug in patients with hepatic impairment that was mild (Child-Pugh class A), moderate (Child-Pugh class B), severe (Child-Pugh class C) without ascites, or severe with ascites was 46, 72, 67, or 100 hours, respectively, compared with 33 hours in healthy individuals. The manufacturers recommend reduction of initial, escalation, and maintenance dosages of lamotrigine in patients with moderate or severe hepatic impairment. (See Dosage in Renal and Hepatic Impairment under Dosage and Administration.)

Concomitant Diseases

Because lamotrigine is transformed in the liver principally to glucuronide metabolites that are eliminated renally, the drug should be used with caution in patients with diseases or conditions (e.g., renal, hepatic, or cardiac impairment) that could affect metabolism and/or elimination of the drug. In dogs, lamotrigine is extensively metabolized to its 2-N-methyl metabolite, which has caused dose-dependent prolongations of the PR interval, widening of the QRS complex, and at high dosages, complete AV block. There have been no consistent effects of lamotrigine metabolites on cardiac conduction in humans. Trace amounts of the 2-N-methyl metabolite of lamotrigine have been found in urine, but not in plasma, with chronic dosing of lamotrigine in humans. However, the manufacturers state that it is possible that increased plasma concentrations of the 2-N-methyl metabolite could occur in patients with hepatic disease who have decreased ability to glucuronidate lamotrigine.

Binding to Melanin-Rich Tissues

Lamotrigine binds to melanin-containing ocular tissue in pigmented rats and cynomolgus monkeys, but evidence of this manifestation has not been reported in humans. Although ophthalmologic testing was conducted in one controlled clinical trial of lamotrigine therapy, the manufacturers state that it was inadequate to detect subtle effects or injury resulting from long-term administration of lamotrigine and that the ability of available tests to detect potentially adverse effects associated with the binding of lamotrigine to melanin is unknown. The manufacturers further state that while no specific recommendations for periodic ophthalmologic monitoring of patients receiving long-term lamotrigine therapy can be provided, prolonged administration of the drug could potentially result in its accumulation and possible toxic effects in melanin-rich tissues, including those of the eye, and that clinicians should be aware of possible adverse ophthalmologic effects occurring as a result of binding of the drug to melanin.

Possible Prescribing and Dispensing Errors

Medication errors involving lamotrigine have occurred because of similarity in spelling between Lamictal® (the trade name for lamotrigine) and the names of other commonly used medications. These medication errors may be associated with serious adverse events either due to lack of appropriate therapy for seizures (e.g., in patients not receiving the prescribed anticonvulsant, lamotrigine, which may lead to status epilepticus) or, alternatively, to the risk of developing adverse effects (e.g., serious rash) associated with the use of lamotrigine in patients for whom the drug was not prescribed and consequently was not properly titrated. Therefore, extra care should be exercised in ensuring the accuracy of both oral and written prescriptions for Lamictal® and these other drugs. When appropriate, clinicians might consider including the intended use of the particular drug on the prescription in addition to alerting patients to carefully check the drug they receive and promptly bring any question or concern to the attention of the dispensing pharmacist. The manufacturer of Lamictal® also recommends that pharmacists assess various measures of avoiding dispensing errors and implement them as appropriate (e.g., by computerized filling and handling of prescriptions, patient counseling). Medication errors also may occur between the different formulations of lamotrigine. Depictions of Lamictal® conventional tablets, tablets for oral suspension, and orally disintegrating tablets, Lamictal® XR extended-release tablets, and generic lamotrigine tablets may be found in the medication guide; patients are strongly advised to verify the correct drug as well as the correct formulation every time they fill their prescription.

Contraindications

Lamotrigine is contraindicated in patients with known hypersensitivity to the drug or any ingredient in the formulation.

● Pediatric Precautions

Safety and efficacy of immediate-release formulations of lamotrigine for adjunctive therapy of seizures have not been established in pediatric patients younger than 2 years of age. Safety and efficacy of immediate-release lamotrigine have not been established for monotherapy in pediatric patients younger than 16 years of age.

Safety and efficacy of extended-release lamotrigine tablets have not been established in pediatric patients younger than 13 years of age.

Safety and efficacy of immediate-release lamotrigine for the management of bipolar disorder in patients younger than 18 years of age have not been established.

The incidence of severe rashes appears to be higher in pediatric patients compared with adults. (See Dermatologic and Sensitivity Reactions under Cautions.)

Analyses of population pharmacokinetic data for children 2–18 years of age demonstrated that lamotrigine clearance is influenced mainly by total body weight and concomitant anticonvulsant therapy. Oral clearance of lamotrigine is higher in children than adults when calculated on the basis of body weight; patients weighing less than 30 kg have a higher clearance on a weight-adjusted basis than patients weighing more than 30 kg and may require increases in maintenance dosage.

● Geriatric Precautions

The manufacturers state that clinical trials of lamotrigine in epilepsy and in bipolar disorder did not include sufficient numbers of patients older than 65 years of age to determine whether they respond differently than younger patients or exhibit a different safety profile than that of younger patients. Because of the greater frequency of decreased hepatic, renal, and/or cardiac function and of concomitant diseases and drug therapy in geriatric patients, the manufacturers recommend cautious dosage selection in patients in this age group, usually beginning at the lower end of the usual range.

● Pregnancy, Fertility, and Lactation

Pregnancy

There are no adequate and well-controlled studies of lamotrigine in pregnant women. Women who are pregnant while receiving lamotrigine should be encouraged to enroll in the North American Antiepileptic Drug (NAAED) Pregnancy Registry at 888-233-2334 or http://www.aedpregnancyregistry.org/.

Data from several prospective pregnancy exposure registries and epidemiological studies of pregnant women have not detected an increased frequency of major congenital malformations or a consistent pattern of malformations among women exposed to lamotrigine compared with the general population. The majority of lamotrigine pregnancy exposure data are from women with epilepsy.

In animal reproduction studies, lamotrigine produced developmental toxicity (e.g., increased mortality, decreased body weight, increased structural variation, neurobehavioral abnormalities) when administered to pregnant animals at doses lower than those used clinically.

Lamotrigine decreased fetal folate concentrations in rats, an effect known to be associated with adverse pregnancy outcomes in animals and humans.

Although preliminary information from the NAAED Pregnancy Registry suggested a possible association between exposure to lamotrigine monotherapy during the first trimester of pregnancy and an increased incidence of cleft lip or cleft palate in infants, this finding has not be observed in other international registries.

The effect of lamotrigine on labor and delivery in humans is unknown.

Physiologic changes during pregnancy may affect plasma lamotrigine concentrations and/or therapeutic effect. Decreased lamotrigine concentrations during pregnancy and restoration of prepartum concentrations after delivery have been reported. Dosage adjustment of lamotrigine may be necessary to maintain clinical response.

Lactation

Lamotrigine is distributed into human milk. There is some evidence that lamotrigine plasma concentrations in breast-fed infants may be as high as 50% of maternal serum levels. Exposure to lamotrigine in these infants may be further increased due to the immaturity of the infant glucuronidation process required for drug clearance. Apnea, drowsiness, and poor sucking have been reported in nursing infants whose mothers were receiving lamotrigine, although it is not known whether these effects were caused by lamotrigine. It is not known whether lamotrigine can affect milk production.

The known benefits of breast-feeding should be considered along with the mother's clinical need for lamotrigine and any potential adverse effects on the breast-fed infant from the drug or underlying condition.

DESCRIPTION

Lamotrigine is a phenyltriazine anticonvulsant agent. The drug differs structurally from other currently available anticonvulsant agents. Although the precise mechanism of anticonvulsant action of lamotrigine is unknown, studies in animals indicate that the drug may stabilize neuronal membranes by blocking voltage-sensitive sodium channels, which inhibits the release of excitatory amino acid neurotransmitters (e.g., glutamate, aspartate) that play a role in the generation and spread of epileptic seizures. In animal test systems, lamotrigine exhibits anticonvulsant activity similar to that of phenytoin, phenobarbital, and carbamazepine. The drug protects against seizures induced by electrical stimulation or pentylenetetrazole, suggesting that it may be effective in the management of tonic-clonic (grand mal) and partial seizures or absence (petit mal) seizures, respectively. Lamotrigine also is active in electrically evoked after-discharge tests, indicating activity against simple and complex partial seizures, and in rat cortical kindling tests, which may indicate activity against complex partial seizures. The mechanism(s) of action of lamotrigine in bipolar disorder has not been established.

In vitro studies indicate that lamotrigine has weak inhibitory effects on type 3 serotonergic (5-HT$_3$) receptors, and does not exhibit high affinity for type 2 serotonergic (5-HT$_2$), adenosine A$_1$ or A$_2$, α$_1$- or α$_2$-adrenergic, β-adrenergic, dopamine D$_1$ or D$_2$, γ-aminobutyric acid (GABA) A or B, histamine H$_1$, opiate κ, or cholinergic muscarinic receptors. The drug has weak agonist effects at opiate σ receptors. Lamotrigine apparently has no effect on dihydropyridine-sensitive calcium channels or N-methyl-d-aspartate (NMDA) receptors and does not inhibit the uptake of norepinephrine, dopamine, serotonin, or aspartic acid.

PREPARATIONS

Excipients in commercially available drug preparations may have clinically important effects in some individuals; consult specific product labeling for details.

lamoTRIgine

Oral

Tablets	25 mg*	LaMICtal® (scored), GlaxoSmithKline LamoTRIgine Tablets
	100 mg*	LaMICtal® (scored), GlaxoSmithKline LamoTRIgine Tablets
	150 mg*	LaMICtal® (scored), GlaxoSmithKline LamoTRIgine Tablets
	200 mg*	LaMICtal® (scored), GlaxoSmithKline LamoTRIgine Tablets
Tablets, extended-release, film-coated	25 mg	LaMICtal® XR, GlaxoSmithKline
	50 mg	LaMICtal® XR, GlaxoSmithKline
	100 mg	LaMICtal® XR, GlaxoSmithKline
	200 mg	LaMICtal® XR, GlaxoSmithKline
	250 mg	LaMICtal® XR, GlaxoSmithKline
	300 mg	LaMICtal® XR, GlaxoSmithKline
Tablets, for oral suspension	2 mg	LaMICtal®, GlaxoSmithKline
	5 mg*	LaMICtal®, GlaxoSmithKline LamoTRIgine Tablets for Oral Suspension
	25 mg*	LaMICtal®, GlaxoSmithKline Lamotrigine Tablets for Oral Suspension
Tablets, orally disintegrating	25 mg*	LaMICtal® ODT, GlaxoSmithKline lamoTRIgine Orally Disintegrating Tablets
	50 mg*	LaMICtal® ODT, GlaxoSmithKline lamoTRIgine Orally Disintegrating Tablets
	100 mg*	LaMICtal® ODT, GlaxoSmithKline lamoTRIgine Orally Disintegrating Tablets
	200 mg*	LaMICtal® ODT, GlaxoSmithKline lamoTRIgine Orally Disintegrating Tablets

* available from one or more manufacturer, distributor, and/or repackager by generic (nonproprietary) name

levETIRAcetam

28:12.92 • ANTICONVULSANTS, MISCELLANEOUS

> On November 28, 2023, FDA issued a drug safety communication about the risk of DRESS (Drug Reaction with Eosinophilia and Systemic Symptoms) with levetiracetam. DRESS is a rare, but serious hypersensitivity reaction that may start as a rash but can quickly progress to organ injury resulting in hospitalization and/or death. Early symptoms of DRESS such as fever or swollen lymph nodes can be present even when a rash cannot be seen. FDA's analysis of case reports and the published literature identified a total of 32 serious cases of DRESS reported worldwide through March 2023 in patients receiving levetiracetam; reported signs and symptoms included skin rash, fever, eosinophilia, lymph node swelling, atypical lymphocytes, and injury to organs including the liver, lungs, kidneys, and gallbladder. Most patients in these cases required hospitalization and medical treatment; 2 patients treated with levetiracetam died. Patients should seek immediate attention if unexplained rash, fever, or swollen lymph nodes develop while receiving the drug. For the full FDA safety communication see https://www.fda.gov/media/174157/download?attachment

■ Levetiracetam, a pyrrolidine derivative, is an anticonvulsant.

USES

● Seizure Disorders

Levetiracetam is used orally in combination with other anticonvulsants in the management of partial onset, myoclonic, and primary generalized tonic-clonic seizures. The drug also is commercially available as an IV formulation for the management of such seizure disorders when oral therapy is temporarily not feasible. Efficacy of IV levetiracetam is supported by studies using oral formulations of the drug since the oral and parenteral formulations are bioequivalent.

Partial Seizures

Levetiracetam conventional (immediate-release) tablets, oral solution, and injection are used in combination with other anticonvulsants in the management of partial onset seizures in adults and pediatric patients 1 month of age and older with epilepsy.

Efficacy of levetiracetam for this use was established in 3 double-blind, placebo-controlled trials in patients who had refractory partial onset seizures with or without secondary generalization while receiving a stable regimen of 1 or 2 anticonvulsants and had experienced at least 2 partial seizures during each 4-week interval of the baseline period (8–12 weeks). Patients received levetiracetam (1, 2, or 3 g daily as a conventional oral preparation) or placebo for 12 weeks after a 4- to 6-week titration period. The weekly frequency of partial seizures was reduced in patients receiving levetiracetam relative to placebo. More patients receiving levetiracetam experienced a reduction in seizure frequency of 50% or greater from baseline (i.e., responder rate) compared with placebo-treated patients. Clinical benefit was evident within 2 weeks in one study.

Data from open-label extension periods of phase 1, 2, and 3 studies with oral levetiracetam (as conventional preparations) in 1422 adult patients with epilepsy indicate that 39% of patients experienced a 50% or greater decrease in seizure frequency, while 13 and 8% of patients were seizure-free for at least 6 and 12 months, respectively, during therapy with the drug. Continuation rates for levetiracetam therapy in these patients were estimated to be 60, 37, and 32% after 1, 3, and 5 years, respectively.

Efficacy of levetiracetam as adjunctive therapy in pediatric patients with partial onset seizures was established in 2 randomized, double-blind, placebo-controlled studies. The first study was conducted in children 4–16 years of age who had refractory partial onset seizures with or without secondary generalization while receiving a stable regimen of 1 or 2 anticonvulsants and had experienced at least 4 partial seizures during the 4 weeks prior to screening as well as at least 4 partial seizures during each of the two 4-week baseline periods. Patients received levetiracetam (20–60 mg/kg daily as a conventional oral preparation) or placebo for 10 weeks after a 4-week titration period. Pediatric patients receiving levetiracetam experienced a reduction of 26.8% in mean weekly partial seizure frequency relative to placebo. The second study was conducted in infants and children 1 month to less than 4 years of age with refractory partial onset seizures (with or without secondary generalization). Seizures were assessed in this study using video electroencephalography (EEG). Patients who had experienced at least 2 partial seizures during a 48-hour baseline period while receiving a stable regimen of 1 or 2 anticonvulsants were randomized to receive levetiracetam oral solution (20–50 mg/kg daily based on age) or placebo; after an initial 1-day dose titration period, treatment was continued for an additional 4 days. The responder rate (i.e., proportion of patients experiencing a reduction in seizure frequency of 50% or greater from baseline) was substantially higher in pediatric patients receiving levetiracetam (43.1%) compared with those receiving placebo (19.6%), and these results were consistent across age groups in this study.

Levetiracetam also is commercially available as extended-release tablets for once-daily administration in the management of partial onset seizures in adults and pediatric patients 12 years of age and older. Efficacy of levetiracetam (as extended-release tablets) was established in a double-blind, placebo-controlled study in patients 12–70 years of age who had refractory partial onset seizures with or without secondary generalization. Patients who had experienced at least 8 partial seizures during an 8-week baseline period and at least 2 seizures during each 4-week interval of the baseline period while receiving a stable regimen of 1–3 anticonvulsants were randomized to receive levetiracetam 1 g daily (as extended-release tablets) or placebo for 12 weeks. The median percent reduction in weekly seizure frequency from baseline was 46.1% in patients receiving levetiracetam compared with 33.4% in those receiving placebo.

Myoclonic Seizures

Levetiracetam conventional (immediate-release) tablets, oral solution, and injection are used in combination with other anticonvulsants in the management of myoclonic seizures in adults and adolescents 12 years of age and older with juvenile myoclonic epilepsy.

Efficacy of levetiracetam for this use was established in a randomized, double-blind, placebo-controlled study in patients who had myoclonic seizures while receiving a stable regimen of 1 anticonvulsant and had experienced at least one myoclonic seizure daily for at least 8 days during the 8-week baseline period. Patients received levetiracetam 3 g daily (as a conventional oral preparation) or placebo for 12 weeks after a 4-week titration period. More patients receiving levetiracetam (60.4%) experienced a reduction in seizure frequency of 50% or greater from baseline (i.e., responder rate) compared with placebo-treated patients (23.7%).

Primary Generalized Tonic-Clonic Seizures

Levetiracetam conventional (immediate-release) tablets, oral solution, and injection are used in combination with other anticonvulsants in the management of primary generalized tonic-clonic seizures in adults and children 6 years of age and older with idiopathic generalized epilepsy.

Efficacy of levetiracetam for this use was established in a randomized, double-blind, placebo-controlled study in patients who had primary generalized tonic-clonic seizures while receiving a stable regimen of 1 or 2 anticonvulsants and had experienced at least 3 primary generalized tonic-clonic seizures during the 8-week combined baseline period (4-week pre-prospective baseline period and 4-week prospective baseline period). Patients received levetiracetam 3 g daily (adult dosage) or 60 mg/kg daily (pediatric dosage) as a conventional oral preparation or placebo for 20 weeks after a 4-week titration period. The median percent reduction in weekly seizure frequency from baseline was 77.6% in patients receiving levetiracetam compared with 44.6% in those receiving placebo. In addition, more patients receiving levetiracetam (72.2%) experienced a reduction in seizure frequency of 50% or greater from baseline (i.e., responder rate) compared with placebo-treated patients (45.2%).

DOSAGE AND ADMINISTRATION

● Administration

Levetiracetam is administered orally (as immediate-release tablets, extended-release tablets, or oral solution). The drug also may be administered by IV infusion in patients in whom oral therapy is temporarily not feasible.

Commercially available levetiracetam conventional (immediate-release) tablets, extended-release tablets, oral solution, and IV formulations have been shown to be bioequivalent.

Patients currently receiving or beginning therapy with levetiracetam and/or any other anticonvulsant for any indication should be closely monitored for the emergence or worsening of depression, suicidal thoughts or behavior (suicidality), and/or any unusual changes in mood or behavior.

Oral Administration

Levetiracetam immediate-release tablets and oral solution are administered orally twice daily without regard to meals. The immediate-release tablets should be swallowed whole and not chewed or crushed. A calibrated dosing device (e.g., medicine dropper, medicine cup) should be used to measure and administer doses of the oral solution; a household teaspoon or tablespoon is not an adequate measuring device.

Levetiracetam extended-release tablets are administered once daily; the tablets must be swallowed intact and not chewed, broken, or crushed.

IV Administration

For IV administration, levetiracetam is commercially available as an injection concentrate that must be diluted prior to use and as a premixed solution in sodium chloride injection that is administered without further dilution; the premixed injection is indicated for use only in adults 16 years of age or older.

When using the injection concentrate, the appropriate dose should be diluted in 100 mL of a compatible IV solution (e.g., 0.9% sodium chloride injection, lactated Ringer's, 5% dextrose injection) and administered by IV infusion over 15 minutes. A smaller volume of diluent may be used (e.g., in pediatric patients or patients who may be susceptible to fluid volume overload), but the final concentration of the diluted solution should not exceed 15 mg/mL. Following dilution, the infusion solution may be stored in polyvinyl chloride (PVC) bags for up to 4 hours at controlled room temperature (15–30°C). Unused contents of the levetiracetam injection vial should be discarded after use.

When using the premixed solution, a single 100-mL bag containing 500 mg, 1 g, or 1.5 g of levetiracetam in sodium chloride 0.82, 0.75, or 0.54%, respectively, should be administered by IV infusion over 15 minutes without further dilution. Doses that are not commercially available as a premixed solution (e.g., 250 or 750 mg) should be prepared by transferring the appropriate volume of solution from an intact commercial infusion bag into a separate sterile, empty infusion bag; any unused contents of the original infusion bag should be discarded and should not be reused or stored. Levetiracetam in sodium chloride injection should not be used in series connections.

Levetiracetam injection and diluted solutions of the drug should be inspected visually for particulate matter and discoloration prior to administration whenever solution and container permit. Levetiracetam injection solutions may be mixed with diazepam, lorazepam, or valproate sodium.

Dispensing and Administration Precautions

Because of similarity in spelling between Keppra® (a trade name for levetiracetam) and Kaletra® (the trade name for the fixed combination of lopinavir and ritonavir, both antiretroviral agents), the potential exists for dispensing errors involving these drugs. Therefore, extra care should be exercised in ensuring the accuracy of both oral and written prescriptions for Keppra® and Kaletra®. The manufacturer of Keppra® recommends that clinicians consider including the intended use of the particular drug on the prescription, in addition to alerting patients to carefully check the drug they receive and promptly bring any question or concern to the attention of the dispensing pharmacist. Some experts also recommend that pharmacists assess various measures of avoiding dispensing errors and implement them as appropriate (e.g., by verifying all orders for these drugs by spelling both the trade and generic names to prescribers, using computerized name alerts, attaching reminders to drug containers and pharmacy shelves, separating the drugs on pharmacy shelves, employing independent checks in the dispensing process, counseling patients).

● Dosage

Levetiracetam therapy should not be discontinued abruptly. The manufacturer recommends that oral levetiracetam be withdrawn gradually (e.g., by reducing the dosage by 1 g daily at 2-week intervals).

When switching from oral to IV levetiracetam therapy, the initial total daily dosage of IV levetiracetam should be equivalent to the daily dose and frequency of oral levetiracetam. At the completion of the IV treatment period, the patient may be switched back to oral levetiracetam at the equivalent daily dose and frequency that was administered IV.

Partial Seizures

Adult Dosage

In adults 16 years of age and older, the recommended initial oral dosage of levetiracetam for adjunctive therapy of partial seizures is 1 g daily (administered as 500 mg twice daily as conventional tablets or oral solution, or 1 g once daily as extended-release tablets). Dosage may be increased in increments of 1 g daily at 2-week intervals up to the maximum recommended dosage of 3 g daily. However, some clinicians reportedly have initiated therapy with oral dosages of 2–4 g daily. Dosages exceeding 3 g daily have been used in open-label studies for periods of 6 months or longer; however, the manufacturers state that there is no evidence that these higher dosages provide additional therapeutic benefit.

When oral therapy is temporarily not feasible, levetiracetam may be administered by IV infusion at the same dosages recommended for conventional oral preparations.

Pediatric Dosage

When conventional oral preparations of levetiracetam are used in pediatric patients, the manufacturer recommends that children weighing 20 kg or less receive the oral solution; children weighing more than 20 kg may receive either the immediate-release tablets or oral solution. Extended-release levetiracetam tablets are indicated for use only in pediatric patients 12 years of age and older.

In pediatric patients 1 to younger than 6 months of age, the recommended initial oral dosage of levetiracetam for adjunctive therapy of partial seizures is 14 mg/kg daily, administered as 7 mg/kg twice daily (as immediate-release preparations). Dosage should be increased in increments of 14 mg/kg daily at 2-week intervals up to the recommended dosage of 42 mg/kg daily, given as 21 mg/kg twice daily. In the clinical trial, the mean daily dosage was 35 mg/kg in this age group; efficacy of lower dosages has not been established.

In pediatric patients 6 months to younger than 4 years of age, the recommended initial oral dosage of levetiracetam is 20 mg/kg daily, administered as 10 mg/kg twice daily (as immediate-release preparations). Dosage should be increased in increments of 20 mg/kg daily at 2-week intervals up to the recommended dosage of 50 mg/kg daily, given as 25 mg/kg twice daily. Dosage may be reduced if the patient is unable to tolerate a dosage of 50 mg/kg daily. In the clinical trial, the mean daily dosage was 47 mg/kg in this age group.

In pediatric patients 4 years to younger than 16 years of age, the recommended initial oral dosage of levetiracetam is 20 mg/kg daily, administered as 10 mg/kg twice daily (as immediate-release preparations). Dosage should be increased in increments of 20 mg/kg daily at 2-week intervals up to the recommended dosage of 60 mg/kg daily, given as 30 mg/kg twice daily. Dosage may be reduced if the patient is unable to tolerate a dosage of 60 mg/kg daily. In the clinical trial, the mean daily dosage was 44 mg/kg and the maximum daily dosage was 3 g daily. If levetiracetam immediate-release tablets are used in pediatric patients weighing 20–40 kg, the recommended initial dosage is 500 mg daily, given as 250 mg twice daily; dosage may be increased in increments of 500 mg daily every 2 weeks up to a maximum of 1.5 g daily, given as 750 mg twice daily. If levetiracetam immediate-release tablets are used in pediatric patients weighing more than 40 kg, the recommended initial dosage is 1 g daily, given as 500 mg twice daily; dosage may be increased in increments of 1 g daily every 2 weeks up to a maximum of 3 g daily, given as 1.5 g twice daily.

In pediatric patients 12 years of age and older, the recommended initial dosage of levetiracetam (as extended-release tablets) is 1 g once daily. Dosage may be increased in increments of 1 g daily at 2-week intervals up to the maximum recommended dosage of 3 g daily.

When oral therapy is temporarily not feasible, levetiracetam may be administered by IV infusion at the same dosages recommended for conventional oral preparations.

Myoclonic Seizures

The recommended initial dosage of oral levetiracetam as adjunctive therapy for myoclonic seizures in patients 12 years of age and older is 1 g daily, given as 500 mg twice daily (as immediate-release preparations). Dosage should be increased in increments of 1 g daily at 2-week intervals up to the recommended dosage of 3 g daily, given as 1.5 g twice daily. Efficacy of dosages lower than 3 g daily has not been established.

When oral therapy is temporarily not feasible, levetiracetam may be administered by IV infusion at the same dosages recommended above.

Primary Generalized Tonic-Clonic Seizures

Adult Dosage

The recommended initial dosage of oral levetiracetam as adjunctive therapy for primary generalized tonic-clonic seizures in adults 16 years of age and older is 1 g daily, given as 500 mg twice daily (as immediate-release preparations). Dosage should be increased in increments of 1 g daily at 2-week intervals up to the recommended dosage of 3 g daily, given as 1.5 g twice daily. Efficacy of dosages lower than 3 g daily has not been established.

When oral therapy is temporarily not feasible, levetiracetam may be administered by IV infusion at the same dosages recommended above.

Pediatric Dosage

The recommended initial dosage of oral levetiracetam as adjunctive therapy for primary generalized tonic-clonic seizures in pediatric patients 6 to younger than 16 years of age is 20 mg/kg daily, given as 10 mg/kg twice daily (as immediate-release preparations). Children weighing 20 kg or less should receive the oral solution; children weighing more than 20 kg may receive either the tablets (administered whole) or the oral solution. Dosage should be increased in increments of 20 mg/kg daily at 2-week intervals up to the recommended dosage of 60 mg/kg daily, given as 30 mg/kg twice daily. Efficacy of dosages lower than 60 mg/kg daily has not been established.

When oral therapy is temporarily not feasible, levetiracetam may be administered by IV infusion at the same dosages recommended above.

● Special Populations

In adults with impaired renal function, dosage of levetiracetam must be modified according to the degree of impairment. Dosage should be based on the patient's creatinine clearance adjusted for body surface area. (See Tables 1 and 2.)

TABLE 1. Immediate-release Levetiracetam Dosage Adjustment in Adults with Impaired Renal Function

Renal Function	Creatinine Clearance (mL/minute per 1.73 m²)	Dosage (mg)	Interval (hours)
Normal	>80	500–1500	12
Mild	50–80	500–1000	12
Moderate	30–50	250–750	12
Severe	<30	250–500	12
Patients with end-stage renal disease undergoing dialysis	–	500–1000	24ᵃ

ᵃ Following dialysis, a 250–500 mg supplemental dose is recommended.

TABLE 2. Extended-release Levetiracetam Dosage Adjustment in Adults with Impaired Renal Function

Renal Function	Creatinine Clearance (mL/minute per 1.73 m²)	Dosage (mg)	Interval (hours)
Normal	>80	1000–3000	24
Mild	50–80	1000–2000	24
Moderate	30–50	500–1500	24
Severe	<30	500–1000	24

Dosage should be selected carefully and renal function monitoring should be considered in geriatric patients 65 years of age and older because of the greater frequency of decreased renal function observed in this age group. Total body clearance was reduced by 38% and half-life was increased by 2.5 hours in geriatric patients with creatinine clearances of 30–74 mL/minute.

No dosage adjustment is necessary in patients with hepatic impairment. Levetiracetam pharmacokinetics were unchanged in patients with mild (Child-Pugh class A) to moderate (Child-Pugh class B) hepatic impairment. Total body clearance was reduced by 50% in patients with severe hepatic impairment (Child-Pugh class C), principally because of decreased renal clearance.

CAUTIONS

● Contraindications

Levetiracetam is contraindicated in patients with known hypersensitivity to the drug.

● Warnings/Precautions

Warnings

Nervous System Effects

Adverse neuropsychiatric effects reported during levetiracetam therapy are classified into 3 categories: somnolence and fatigue, coordination difficulties, and behavioral/psychiatric abnormalities. Patients should be monitored for these adverse effects during therapy. In addition, patients should be advised not to drive or operate machinery until the effects of levetiracetam are known.

In controlled studies in adults, approximately 15% of patients with partial onset seizures who received levetiracetam (as an oral conventional preparation) experienced somnolence compared with 8% of placebo-treated patients, and about 3% of levetiracetam-treated patients discontinued treatment because of somnolence. Pediatric patients and adults with other seizure types who receive levetiracetam appear to experience similar rates of somnolence and fatigue. In controlled studies in adults, asthenia was reported in about 15% of patients who received levetiracetam (as conventional preparations) compared with 9% of placebo-treated patients, and 0.8% of levetiracetam-treated patients discontinued treatment because of asthenia. Coordination difficulties (e.g., ataxia, abnormal gait, incoordination) were experienced by 3.4% of patients receiving levetiracetam (as conventional preparations) compared with 1.6% of placebo-treated patients. Somnolence, asthenia, and coordination difficulties occurred most frequently within the first 4 weeks of treatment. In studies with extended-release levetiracetam, somnolence was reported in 8% of patients receiving the drug compared with 3% of patients receiving placebo; however, the number of patients exposed to the extended-release preparation is considerably less than that of the immediate-release preparation.

In clinical studies, psychotic symptoms were reported in 1% of adults, 2% of children 4–16 years of age, and 17% of children younger than 4 years of age receiving conventional levetiracetam preparations compared with 0.2, 2, and 5% of the corresponding age groups receiving placebo, respectively. At least 2 adults who received levetiracetam in these studies were hospitalized as a result of psychosis. Nonpsychotic behavioral symptoms (e.g., aggression, agitation, anger, anxiety, apathy, depersonalization, depression, emotional lability, hostility, hyperkinesias, irritability, nervousness, neurosis, personality disorder) were reported in 13% of adults and 38% of children 4–16 years of age receiving conventional levetiracetam preparations in clinical studies compared with 6 and 19% of placebo-treated patients, respectively. Exploratory analysis of a placebo-controlled study that evaluated neurocognitive and behavioral effects of conventional levetiracetam in children 4–16 years of age indicated possible worsening of aggression in pediatric patients receiving the drug. Increased irritability was reported in clinical studies of younger children (1 month to younger than 4 years of age). In studies with extended-release levetiracetam, behavioral abnormalities (irritability and aggression) were reported in 7% of patients receiving the drug compared with none of the patients receiving placebo; however, the number of patients exposed to the extended-release preparation is considerably less than that of the immediate-release preparation.

Suicidality Risk

The FDA has alerted healthcare professionals about an increased risk of suicidality (suicidal behavior or ideation) observed in an analysis of studies using various anticonvulsants, including levetiracetam, compared with placebo. The analysis of suicidality reports from placebo-controlled studies involving 11 anticonvulsants (i.e., carbamazepine, felbamate, gabapentin, lamotrigine, levetiracetam, oxcarbazepine, pregabalin, tiagabine, topiramate, valproate, zonisamide) in patients with epilepsy, psychiatric disorders (e.g., bipolar disorder, depression, anxiety), and other conditions (e.g., migraine, neuropathic pain) found that patients receiving anticonvulsants had approximately twice the risk of suicidal behavior or ideation (0.43%) compared with patients receiving placebo (0.24%). This increased suicidality risk was observed as early as one week after beginning therapy and continued through 24 weeks. Although patients treated with an anticonvulsant for epilepsy, psychiatric disorders, and other conditions were all found to have an increased suicidality risk compared with those receiving placebo, the relative suicidality risk was higher for patients with epilepsy compared with those receiving anticonvulsants for other conditions.

Based on the current analysis of the available data, FDA recommends that clinicians inform patients, their families, and caregivers about the potential for an increase in the risk of suicidality with anticonvulsant therapy and that all patients currently receiving or beginning therapy with any anticonvulsant for any indication be closely monitored for the emergence or worsening of depression, suicidal thoughts or behavior (suicidality), and/or unusual changes in mood or behavior. Symptoms such as anxiety, agitation, hostility, hypomania, and mania may be precursors to emerging suicidality.

Clinicians who prescribe levetiracetam or any other anticonvulsant should balance the risk of suicidality with the risk of untreated illness. Epilepsy and many other illnesses for which anticonvulsants are prescribed are themselves associated with an increased risk of morbidity and mortality and an increased risk of suicidal thoughts and behavior. If suicidal thoughts and behavior emerge during anticonvulsant therapy, the clinician should consider whether these symptoms may be related to the illness being treated.

Dermatologic Reactions

Serious dermatologic reactions, including Stevens-Johnson syndrome and toxic epidermal necrolysis, have been reported in both adults and pediatric patients receiving levetiracetam. The median time of onset is reported to be between 14 and 17 days, although cases have occurred at least 4 months after initiation of therapy.

Levetiracetam should be discontinued at the first sign of a rash, unless the rash is clearly not drug-related. If manifestations suggestive of Stevens-Johnson syndrome or toxic epidermal necrolysis occur, levetiracetam therapy should be permanently discontinued and alternative therapy considered.

Discontinuance of Therapy

Because of the possibility of increased seizure frequency, anticonvulsant drugs, including levetiracetam, should not be discontinued suddenly. The manufacturer recommends that oral levetiracetam be withdrawn gradually by reducing the dosage by 1 g daily at 2-week intervals.

Hematologic Effects

Hematologic abnormalities (e.g., decreased red blood cell, white blood cell, and neutrophil counts) were reported in patients receiving levetiracetam in clinical studies. Agranulocytosis, leukopenia, neutropenia, pancytopenia, and thrombocytopenia also have occurred during postmarketing experience.

A complete blood count (CBC) is recommended in patients who experience any signs or symptoms of hematologic abnormalities (e.g., severe weakness, pyrexia, recurrent infections, coagulation disorders) during levetiracetam therapy.

Increased Blood Pressure

In a study of pediatric patients 1 month to younger than 4 years of age, increased diastolic blood pressure was observed in levetiracetam-treated patients (17%) compared with those receiving placebo (2%). However, there was no overall difference in mean diastolic blood pressure between the treatment groups. These findings were not observed in older children or adults receiving the drug.

Pediatric patients younger than 4 years of age should be monitored for increased diastolic blood pressure during levetiracetam therapy.

Seizure Control During Pregnancy

Physiologic changes that occur during pregnancy may gradually decrease plasma levels of levetiracetam in pregnant women. This effect is most notable during the third trimester.

Patients should be closely monitored during pregnancy and throughout the postpartum period, especially if levetiracetam dosage is adjusted during pregnancy.

Sensitivity Reactions
Anaphylaxis and Angioedema

Anaphylaxis and angioedema, in some cases life-threatening and/or requiring emergency treatment, have been reported during postmarketing experience in patients receiving levetiracetam.(See Cautions: Contraindications.) Manifestations have included hypotension, hives, rash, respiratory distress, facial swelling, and swelling of the tongue, throat, and feet. Such reactions can occur at any time during therapy.

If any signs or symptoms of anaphylaxis or angioedema occur, patients should discontinue levetiracetam immediately and seek medical attention. Levetiracetam therapy should be permanently discontinued if an alternative etiology cannot be identified.

General Precautions
Dispensing and Administration Precautions

Because of similarity in spelling between Keppra® (a trade name for levetiracetam) and Kaletra® (the trade name for the fixed combination of lopinavir and ritonavir, both antiretroviral agents), the potential exists for dispensing errors involving these drugs. These medication errors may be associated with serious adverse events (e.g., status epilepticus) due to lack of appropriate therapy for seizures or with the risk of developing adverse effects associated with the use of levetiracetam or lopinavir and ritonavir in patients for whom the drug was not prescribed. Therefore, extra care should be exercised in ensuring the accuracy of both oral and written prescriptions for these drugs. The manufacturer of Keppra® recommends that clinicians consider including the intended use of the particular drug on the prescription in addition to alerting patients to carefully check the drug they receive and promptly bring any question or concern to the attention of the dispensing pharmacist. Some experts also recommend that pharmacists assess various measures of avoiding dispensing errors and implement them as appropriate (e.g., by verifying all orders for these drugs by spelling both the trade and generic names to prescribers, using computerized name alerts, attaching reminders to drug containers and pharmacy shelves, separating the drugs on pharmacy shelves, employing independent checks in the dispensing process, counseling patients).

Dispensing errors involving Keppra® and Kaletra® should be reported to the manufacturers, the USP Medication Errors Reporting Program by phone (800-233-7767), or directly to the FDA MedWatch program by phone (800-FDA-1088), fax (800-FDA-0178), internet (http://www.fda.gov/Safety/MedWatch/default.htm), or mail.

Specific Populations
Pregnancy

Seizure control during pregnancy should be carefully monitored.

North American Antiepileptic Drug (NAAED) Pregnancy Registry at 888-233-2334 (for patients); NAAED registry information also available at http://www.aedpregnancyregistry.org.

The effect of levetiracetam on labor and delivery is unknown.

Lactation

Levetiracetam is distributed into milk. Because of the potential for serious adverse reactions to levetiracetam in nursing infants, a decision should be made whether to discontinue nursing or the drug, taking into account the importance of the drug to the woman.

Pediatric Use

Safety and efficacy of levetiracetam immediate-release tablets, oral solution, and injection for the management of partial onset seizures have not been established in pediatric patients younger than 1 month of age. Behavioral abnormalities (e.g., paranoia, confusional state, increased aggression) have been observed in pediatric patients 4–16 years of age with partial onset seizures receiving the drug.

Safety and efficacy of levetiracetam immediate-release tablets, oral solution, and injection for the management of myoclonic seizures have not been established in pediatric patients younger than 12 years of age.

Safety and efficacy of levetiracetam immediate-release tablets, oral solution, and injection for the management of primary generalized tonic-clonic seizures have not been established in pediatric patients younger than 6 years of age.

Safety and efficacy of extended-release levetiracetam tablets have not been established in pediatric patients younger than 12 years of age. Use of the extended-release tablets in children 12 years of age and older is supported by a placebo-controlled study using the immediate-release preparation in patients 4–16 years of age.

Safety and efficacy of levetiracetam in sodium chloride injection have not been established in pediatric patients younger than 16 years of age.

Geriatric Use

Controlled clinical studies evaluating levetiracetam have not included sufficient numbers of patients 65 years of age and older to determine whether geriatric patients respond differently than younger adults. No substantial differences in safety have been observed in geriatric patients relative to younger adults.

Renal Impairment

Dosage adjustment is recommended for patients with decreased creatinine clearance.

Hepatic Impairment

Safety and efficacy of levetiracetam have been demonstrated in a limited number of epileptic patients with chronic liver disease. No dosage adjustment is necessary in patients with hepatic impairment.

● Common Adverse Effects

Adverse effects occurring in 1% or more of adults receiving oral levetiracetam (as conventional preparations) for adjunctive management of partial seizures include somnolence, asthenia, headache, infection, dizziness, pain, pharyngitis, depression, nervousness, rhinitis, anorexia, ataxia, vertigo, amnesia, anxiety, emotional lability, hostility, paresthesia, increased cough, sinusitis, and diplopia.

Adverse effects occurring in 2% or more of pediatric patients older than 4 years of age receiving oral levetiracetam (as conventional preparations) for adjunctive management of partial seizures include headache, vomiting, nasopharyngitis, somnolence, fatigue, aggression, upper abdominal pain, cough, nasal congestion, decreased appetite, dizziness, pharyngolaryngeal pain, abnormal behavior, dizziness, irritability, diarrhea, lethargy, insomnia, head injury, anorexia, agitation, constipation, influenza, contusion, fall, depression, altered mood, ear pain, conjunctivitis, gastroenteritis, rhinitis, joint sprain, arthralgia, neck pain, sedation, labile affect, anxiety, confusional state, and mood swing. The most common adverse effects in patients younger than 4 years of age were somnolence and irritability.

The adverse effect profile of levetiracetam (as conventional preparations) in patients with myoclonic seizures or primary generalized tonic-clonic seizures is generally similar to that of patients with partial seizures.

Adverse effects occurring in 5% or more of patients receiving extended-release levetiracetam tablets for adjunctive management of partial seizures include influenza, somnolence, irritability, nasopharyngitis, dizziness, and nausea.

Adverse effects associated with IV levetiracetam generally appear to be consistent with those associated with oral administration of the drug.

DRUG INTERACTIONS

● Drugs Affecting or Metabolized by Hepatic Microsomal Enzymes

Because levetiracetam is neither a substrate nor inhibitor of cytochrome P-450 (CYP), pharmacokinetic interactions are unlikely with drugs affecting or metabolized by CYP isoenzymes.

● Anticonvulsants

Clinically important pharmacokinetic interactions are unlikely when levetiracetam is administered concomitantly with other anticonvulsants (e.g., carbamazepine, gabapentin, lamotrigine, phenobarbital, phenytoin, primidone, valproic acid).

In pediatric patients, an approximate 22% increase in levetiracetam clearance was observed when the drug was administered concurrently with hepatic enzyme-inducing anticonvulsants (e.g., carbamazepine); however, dosage adjustment is not recommended by the manufacturer. Levetiracetam did not alter plasma concentrations of carbamazepine, lamotrigine, topiramate, or valproic acid in pediatric patients with epilepsy.

● Digoxin

Levetiracetam does not appear to affect the pharmacokinetics or pharmacodynamics (e.g., cardiac rhythm effects) of digoxin; digoxin also does not affect the pharmacokinetics of levetiracetam.

● Oral Contraceptives

Pharmacokinetic interactions are unlikely when levetiracetam is coadministered with oral contraceptives.

● Probenecid

When levetiracetam was administered concomitantly with probenecid, no effect on levetiracetam pharmacokinetics was observed, but steady-state plasma concentrations of the principal inactive metabolite were approximately doubled due to a 60% reduction in renal clearance. The manufacturer states, however, that this effect is not clinically important.

● Protein-bound Drugs

Pharmacokinetic interactions are unlikely with protein-bound drugs.

● Warfarin

Levetiracetam does not appear to affect the pharmacokinetics or pharmacodynamics (e.g., prothrombin time) of warfarin; warfarin also does not affect the pharmacokinetics of levetiracetam.

DESCRIPTION

Levetiracetam, a pyrrolidine derivative, is an anticonvulsant agent that is structurally unrelated to other currently available anticonvulsants. The mechanism of anticonvulsant action of levetiracetam is unknown. In animal models, levetiracetam conferred no protection against single seizures induced by electrical current or different chemoconvulsants and offered only limited protection in submaximal stimulation and threshold tests. Protection was observed against secondarily generalized activity from focal seizures induced by 2 chemoconvulsants known to induce seizures that mimic some features of human complex partial seizures with secondary generalization. Levetiracetam also showed inhibitory properties in the kindling model in rats, another model of human complex partial seizures.

Levetiracetam does not exhibit binding affinity for benzodiazepine, γ-aminobutyric acid (GABA), glycine, or N-methyl-D-aspartate (NMDA) receptors, reuptake sites, or second messenger systems. Levetiracetam does not appear to directly facilitate GABA-mediated neurotransmission or have an effect on neuronal voltage-gated sodium or T-type calcium currents. However, the drug has been shown to oppose the activity of negative modulators of GABA- and glycine-gated currents in neuronal cell culture.

Levetiracetam is not extensively metabolized in humans, with 66% of an administered dose excreted unchanged in urine. About 24% of an administered dose is metabolized to an inactive metabolite by enzymatic hydrolysis of the acetamide group, which does not depend on hepatic cytochrome P-450 (CYP) isoenzymes. Levetiracetam is not a high-affinity substrate for or inhibitor of CYP isoenzymes.

ADVICE TO PATIENTS

Importance of providing copy of written patient information (medication guide) each time levetiracetam is dispensed.

Risk of adverse neuropsychiatric effects (e.g., somnolence, fatigue, dizziness, coordination difficulties, behavioral changes), especially during the initial weeks of therapy. Avoid driving, operating machinery, or performing hazardous tasks while taking levetiracetam until the drug's effects on the individual are known.

Importance of patients, family members, and caregivers being aware that anticonvulsants, including levetiracetam, may increase the risk of having suicidal thoughts or actions in a very small number of people (about 1 in 500). Advise patients, family members, and caregivers to pay close attention to any day-to-day changes in mood, behavior, and actions; these changes can happen very quickly. They should also be aware of common warning signs that may signal suicide risk (e.g., talking or thinking about wanting to hurt oneself or end one's life, withdrawing from friends and family, becoming depressed or experiencing worsening of existing depression, becoming preoccupied with death and dying, giving away prized possessions). Advise patients, family members, and caregivers to contact the responsible clinician immediately if these or any new and worrisome behaviors occur.

Risk of serious dermatologic reactions. Importance of patients immediately notifying their clinician if a rash develops.

Risk of anaphylaxis and angioedema. Importance of patients discontinuing therapy and seeking medical care if any signs and symptoms of these reactions occur.

Importance of adhering to prescribed directions for use. Importance of not discontinuing levetiracetam abruptly. Levetiracetam is used in combination with other anticonvulsants, not as monotherapy.

Importance of informing patients who are taking levetiracetam oral solution not to use a household teaspoon or tablespoon to measure the dose; a calibrated measuring device (such as a medicine dropper, spoon, cup, or syringe) should be obtained and used when administering the oral solution.

Importance of women informing clinicians if they are or plan to become pregnant or plan to breast-feed. Importance of clinicians informing women about the existence of and encouraging enrollment in pregnancy registries.

Importance of informing clinicians of existing or contemplated concomitant therapy, including prescription and OTC drugs, dietary supplements, and/or herbal products, as well as any concomitant illness (e.g., renal disease).

Importance of informing patients of other important precautionary information.

PREPARATIONS

Excipients in commercially available drug preparations may have clinically important effects in some individuals; consult specific product labeling for details.

levETIRAcetam

Oral			
Solution	100 mg/mL*	Keppra® Oral Solution, UCB
		Levetiracetam Oral Solution
Tablets, film-coated	250 mg*	Keppra® (scored), UCB
		Levetiracetam Tablets
	500 mg*	Keppra® (scored), UCB
		Levetiracetam Tablets
	750 mg*	Keppra® (scored), UCB
		Levetiracetam Tablets
	1 g*	Keppra® (scored), UCB
		Levetiracetam Tablets
Tablets, extended-release, film-coated	500 mg*	Keppra XR®, UCB
		Levetiracetam Extended-release Tablets
	750 mg*	Keppra XR®, UCB
		Levetiracetam Extended-release Tablets
Parenteral			
Concentrate, for injection, for IV infusion	100 mg/mL*	Keppra®, UCB
		Levetiracetam Injection

* available from one or more manufacturer, distributor, and/or repackager by generic (nonproprietary) name

levETIRAcetam in Sodium Chloride

Parenteral		
Injection, for IV infusion	5 mg/mL (500 mg in 0.82% sodium chloride injection)*	Levetiracetam in Sodium Chloride Injection
	10 mg/mL (1 g in 0.75% sodium chloride injection)*	Levetiracetam in Sodium Chloride Injection
	15 mg/mL (1.5 g in 0.54% sodium chloride injection)*	Levetiracetam in Sodium Chloride Injection

* available from one or more manufacturer, distributor, and/or repackager by generic (nonproprietary) name

† Use is not currently included in the labeling approved by the US Food and Drug Administration.

Selected Revisions December 17, 2023, © Copyright, June 1, 2000, American Society of Health-System Pharmacists, Inc.

Topiramate

28:12.92 • ANTICONVULSANTS, MISCELLANEOUS

■ Topiramate, a sulfamate-substituted derivative of D-fructose, is an anti-convulsant and antimigraine agent.

USES

● Seizure Disorders

Topiramate is used as *initial* monotherapy or as adjunctive therapy (i.e., in combination with other anticonvulsants) in the management of seizure disorders. Efficacy of the drug in the management of seizure disorders has been evaluated principally using topiramate immediate-release tablets. Efficacy of the extended-release capsules is based on experience with immediate-release topiramate and studies demonstrating pharmacokinetic equivalence between the formulations. Efficacy of topiramate oral solution is based on experience with topiramate tablets and sprinkle capsules and studies demonstrating comparable bioavailability between these dosage forms.

Initial Monotherapy

Partial Seizures or Primary Generalized Tonic-Clonic Seizures

Topiramate is used as *initial* monotherapy in the management of partial-onset seizures or primary generalized tonic-clonic seizures in adults and pediatric patients 2 years of age or older (6 years of age or older for Trokendi XR® only).

Safety and efficacy of topiramate as initial monotherapy of seizures in adults and pediatric patients 10 years of age or older have been established in a randomized, double-blind study in 487 patients (age range: 6–83 years) with epilepsy who had 1 or 2 well-documented seizures within 3 months prior to enrollment and were not receiving anticonvulsant therapy at the time of randomization. Of those enrolled, 49% had no prior treatment with anticonvulsant drugs. During an initial open-label phase, all patients received an initial topiramate dosage of 25 mg daily for 7 days (as an immediate-release preparation). This was followed by a double-blind phase, in which patients were randomized to receive topiramate (titrated to a target maintenance dosage of 50 or 400 mg daily or the maximum tolerated dosage) for a median of 9 months. Patients randomized to the target dosage of 400 mg daily received a mean of 275 mg daily; 58% of patients achieved the maximum dosage of 400 mg daily for at least 2 weeks. In this study, the 400-mg daily dosage was superior to the 50-mg daily dosage in delaying time to first seizure. Substantial differences in efficacy between the 2 treatment groups were observed at day 14, when patients randomized to receive target dosages of 400 or 50 mg daily were actually receiving 100 or 25 mg daily, respectively. At 6 months following initiation of treatment, 83% of patients randomized to the 400-mg daily dosage target were seizure free, compared with 71% of those randomized to the 50-mg daily dosage target. At 12 months, 76 or 59% of patients randomized to the 400- or 50-mg daily dosage targets, respectively, were seizure free. Treatment effects were consistent across various patient subgroups defined by age, gender, geographic region, baseline body weight, baseline seizure type, time since diagnosis, and baseline anticonvulsant use.

Topiramate's efficacy as initial monotherapy in pediatric patients 2–9 years of age with partial seizures or primary generalized tonic-clonic seizures was concluded based on a pharmacometric bridging approach using data from controlled epilepsy studies conducted with an immediate-release formulation of the drug. This approach consisted of first demonstrating that the exposure-response relationships in pediatric patients (as young as 2 years of age) and adults were similar when immediate-release topiramate was given as adjunctive therapy; similarity of the exposure-response was then demonstrated in pediatric patients (6 to younger than 16 years of age) and adults when topiramate was used as initial monotherapy. Specific dosage recommendations in children 2–9 years of age were derived from simulations using plasma exposure ranges observed in pediatric and adult patients receiving topiramate as initial monotherapy.

Adjunctive Therapy

Partial Seizures

Topiramate is used as adjunctive therapy (i.e., in combination with other anticonvulsants) in the management of partial-onset seizures in adults and pediatric patients 2 years of age or older (6 years of age or older for Trokendi XR® only).

Efficacy of topiramate as adjunctive therapy in adults with partial seizures with or without secondarily generalized tonic-clonic seizures has been established in 6 controlled clinical studies. In these studies, patients initially were stabilized with optimum dosages of 1 or 2 anticonvulsant drugs (e.g., carbamazepine, clonazepam, phenobarbital, phenytoin, primidone, valproic acid) during a 4- to 12-week baseline period; those experiencing a prespecified minimum number of partial seizures during this baseline period were randomized to receive topiramate (as an immediate-release preparation) or placebo during a dosage titration period of 3–6 weeks followed by a 4-, 8-, or 12-week stabilization period during which the maximally achieved dosage of topiramate or placebo was maintained. Efficacy of topiramate in these studies principally was evaluated in terms of the change in seizure frequency (i.e., median percent decrease or increase in average monthly seizure rate) and the responder rate (i.e., percentage of patients with at least a 50% reduction in seizure frequency).

Patients receiving topiramate 200 mg daily or placebo in 2 of the studies experienced a decrease in seizure frequency of 27–44 or 12–20%, respectively, and the responder rate was 24–45 or 18–24%, respectively. In 2 of the studies, patients receiving topiramate 400 mg daily or placebo experienced a decrease in seizure frequency of 41–48 or 1–13%, respectively, and the responder rate was 35–47 or 8–18%, respectively. Patients receiving 600 mg of topiramate daily in 3 of the studies experienced a decrease in seizure frequency of 41–46%, and patients receiving placebo experienced a decrease in seizure frequency of 1–13% in 2 of the studies, and an *increase* in seizure frequency of 12% in the third study. In the 3 studies in which patients received topiramate 600 mg daily or placebo, 40–47 or 9–18%, respectively, were considered responders. Patients receiving topiramate 800 mg daily in 2 studies experienced a decrease in seizure frequency of 24–41%, and patients receiving placebo experienced a decrease in monthly seizure rate of 1–2% in one study and an 18–21% *increase* in seizure frequency in the other study. In the studies of patients receiving topiramate 800 mg daily or placebo, 40–43 or 0–9%, respectively, were considered responders. Patients receiving 1 g of topiramate or placebo daily in one study experienced a decrease in seizure frequency of 36–38 or 1–2%, respectively, and 36–38 or 8–9% of patients, respectively, were reported to be responders. Overall, topiramate dosages exceeding 600 mg daily did not result in substantially improved efficacy, although individual patients may have benefited from such relatively high dosages.

Efficacy of topiramate as adjunctive therapy in pediatric patients (2–16 years of age) with partial seizures with or without secondarily generalized seizures has been established in a multicenter, randomized controlled trial. In this study, patients initially were stabilized with optimum dosages of 1 or 2 anticonvulsant drugs; patients who experienced 6 or more partial seizures with or without secondary generalization during an 8-week baseline period were randomized to receive topiramate (as an immediate-release preparation) or placebo. Target dosages were assigned based on the patient's body weight to approximate a dosage of 6 mg/kg daily (corresponding to daily dosages of 125, 175, 225, or 400 mg daily); after titration to the target dosage, patients were treated for an additional 8 weeks. Patients receiving topiramate 6 mg/kg daily or placebo experienced a decrease in seizure frequency of 33 or 11%, respectively, and the responder rate was 39 or 20%, respectively.

Efficacy of topiramate extended-release capsules (Qudexy® XR) was evaluated in a double-blind, placebo-controlled study (PREVAIL) in adults with partial-onset seizures with or without secondary generalization who were experiencing at least 8 partial seizures during an 8-week baseline period while receiving stable dosages of 1–3 anticonvulsant agents. Topiramate was administered at an initial dosage of 50 mg once daily (as extended-release capsules) and increased at weekly intervals during a 3-week titration period up to a dosage of 200 mg daily; the maintenance dosage was continued for an additional 8 weeks. Patients receiving topiramate experienced a substantial reduction in seizure frequency from baseline compared with those receiving placebo (mean percent reduction of 40 versus 22%). This reduction in seizure frequency was sustained over 1 year in an open-label extension study of PREVAIL (PREVAIL OLE).

Primary Generalized Tonic-Clonic Seizures

Topiramate is used as adjunctive therapy (i.e., in combination with other anticonvulsants) in the management of primary generalized tonic-clonic seizures in adults and pediatric patients 2 years of age or older (6 years of age or older for Trokendi XR®).

Efficacy of topiramate for this seizure type has been established in a multicenter, double-blind, randomized controlled trial. In this study, patients (age range: 3–59 years) initially were stabilized on optimum dosages of 1 or 2 anticonvulsant drugs during an 8-week baseline period; patients who experienced 3 or more primary generalized tonic-clonic seizures were randomized to receive topiramate (as an immediate-release preparation) or placebo. Target dosages were assigned based on the patient's body weight to approximate a dosage of 6 mg/kg daily (corresponding to daily dosages of 175, 225, or 400 mg daily); after titration to the target dosage, patients were treated for an additional 12 weeks. Efficacy of topiramate was evaluated in terms of the change in seizure frequency (i.e., median percent reduction in primary generalized tonic-clonic seizures) and by the responder rate (i.e., percentage of patients with at least a 50% reduction in seizure frequency). Patients receiving topiramate 6 mg/kg daily or placebo experienced a decrease in seizure frequency of 57 or 9%, respectively, and the responder rate was 56 or 20%, respectively. Preliminary data from the open-label extension period of a double-blind, placebo-controlled study in a limited number of patients with resistant primary generalized seizures indicate that 92% of patients experienced a 50% or greater decrease in seizures, while 58% of patients were seizure-free during this extension period.

Seizures Associated with Lennox-Gastaut Syndrome

Topiramate is used as adjunctive therapy (i.e., in combination with other anticonvulsants) in the management of seizures associated with Lennox-Gastaut syndrome in adults and pediatric patients 2 years of age or older (6 years of age or older for Trokendi XR® only).

Efficacy of topiramate for this seizure type has been established in a multicenter, double-blind, randomized controlled trial. In this study, patients (age range: 2–42 years) who were experiencing 60 or more seizures per month prior to study entry were stabilized on optimum dosages of 1 or 2 anticonvulsant drugs during a 4-week baseline period. Patients were then randomized to receive adjunctive therapy with topiramate (administered as an immediate-release preparation and titrated to a target dosage of 6 mg/kg daily) or placebo; after titration to the target dosage, patients were treated for an additional 8 weeks. Efficacy of topiramate was evaluated in terms of the change in seizure frequency (i.e., median percent reduction in drop attacks), the responder rate (i.e., percentage of patients with at least a 50% reduction in seizure frequency), and the overall improvement in seizure severity as rated by the caregiver. Patients receiving topiramate 6 mg/kg daily experienced a median reduction in seizure frequency of 15%, while those receiving placebo experienced an *increase* of 5%. Overall improvement in seizure severity was reported in more patients receiving topiramate (52%) than in those receiving placebo (28%). Responder rates were not significantly different between patients receiving topiramate (28%) and those receiving placebo (14%). An open-label, long-term extension study of this trial found sustained efficacy of topiramate for 3 or more years.

Seizures Associated with Dravet Syndrome

Topiramate has been used as adjunctive therapy in the treatment of seizures associated with Dravet syndrome†. Although evidence from controlled studies is limited, experts generally recommend initial treatment with either clobazam† or valproic acid†, followed by a combination of both drugs; however, adequate seizure control is rarely achieved with these drugs alone, and most patients will require additional anticonvulsant agents. Topiramate has been recommended as a second-line anticonvulsant option in patients with Dravet syndrome. Results of several small, open-label prospective and retrospective studies indicate that about 35–78% of patients respond with a greater than 50% reduction in seizures and about 8–17% of patients achieve seizure freedom.

Clinical Perspective

Current drugs or drug classes used in the management of focal (partial onset) and/or generalized seizures include benzodiazepines, lamotrigine, levetiracetam, perampanel, phenobarbital, topiramate, sodium valproate, zonisamide, brivaracetam, carbamazepine, eslicarbazepine, gabapentin, lacosamide, oxcarbazepine, phenytoin, pregabalin, tiagabine, and vigabatrin. Selection of appropriate treatment should be individualized and consider factors such as the specific seizure type, epilepsy syndrome, drug efficacy and adverse effects, and comorbid conditions.

In a joint 2018 guideline from the American Academy of Neurology (AAN) and the American Epilepsy Society, topiramate is classified as possibly effective for the management of adults with new-onset epilepsy with focal epilepsy or unclassified generalized tonic-clonic seizures; however, the guideline states that efficacy should be further evaluated in randomized controlled studies with doses commonly used in clinical practice. For pediatric patients with new-onset epilepsy with focal epilepsy or unclassified generalized tonic-clonic seizures, the guideline states that no recommendations can be made regarding the use of topiramate monotherapy due to inappropriate dosing of the drug in clinical trials.

Guidelines on management of treatment-resistant epilepsy from the AAN and the American Epilepsy Society include recommendations for use of topiramate as monotherapy for focal epilepsy in adults and as adjunctive treatment for focal epilepsy in adults and pediatric patients in addition to use for treatment of idiopathic generalized epilepsy and Lennox-Gastaut syndrome. No recommendation is made for use of monotherapy to manage treatment-resistant focal epilepsy in pediatric patients due to a lack of data.

● Migraine Prophylaxis

Topiramate is used for the prevention of migraine headaches in adults and adolescents 12 years of age or older.

Efficacy of topiramate for migraine prophylaxis in adults has been established in 2 randomized, double-blind, placebo-controlled trials in over 900 patients with at least a 6-month history of migraine headaches, with or without associated aura, who were experiencing 3–12 migraines over a 4-week baseline period; patients with cluster headaches or basilar, ophthalmoplegic, hemiplegic, or transformed migraine headaches were excluded from the studies. In both studies, patients were randomized to receive topiramate (as an immediate-release preparation and titrated to a target dosage of 50, 100, or 200 mg daily or the maximum tolerated dosage) or placebo for 26 weeks. Efficacy of topiramate was evaluated in terms of the reduction in migraine headache frequency, as measured by the change in 4-week migraine headache rate from baseline to the double-blind treatment period in each topiramate treatment group compared with placebo. The mean migraine headache frequency at baseline in all treatment groups in both studies was approximately 5.5 migraines per 28 days. In the first study, the reduction in mean 4-week migraine headache frequency from baseline was 1.3, 2.1, or 2.2 for topiramate dosages of 50, 100, or 200 mg daily, respectively, and 0.8 for placebo. In the second study, the reduction in mean 4-week migraine headache frequency from baseline was 1.4, 2.1, or 2.4 for topiramate dosages of 50, 100, or 200 mg daily, respectively, and 1.1 for placebo. In both studies, there were no apparent differences in treatment effect with respect to age or gender. Because most patients were white, there are insufficient data to determine whether there are any treatment differences based on race. A long-term, open-label extension study that included patients from both randomized controlled trials of topiramate for migraine prophylaxis found the reduction in migraine frequency to be sustained for up to 14 months.

Efficacy of topiramate for the prevention of migraine headaches in adolescents has been established in a randomized, double-blind, parallel-group study in patients 12–17 years of age with episodic migraine headaches with or without aura. Patients who experienced 3–12 migraines with no more than 14 headache days (including nonmigraine headaches) over a 4-week baseline period were randomized to receive topiramate (administered as an immediate-release preparation and titrated to a dosage of 50 or 100 mg daily) or placebo for 16 weeks. Patients receiving topiramate 100 mg daily experienced a substantially greater reduction in monthly migraine attacks from baseline compared with placebo (median reduction of 72 versus 44%); however, there was no difference in the monthly attack rate between topiramate 50 mg daily and placebo.

Clinical Perspective

Preventive treatment of migraine should be considered in patients with frequent attacks or attacks that interfere with daily life; patients with adverse effects or contraindications to acute treatments; and those who fail or overuse acute treatments. Patient preference should also factor into the decision-making process. Prior to establishing a preventive treatment plan, appropriate use of acute treatments should be evaluated and lifestyle modifications initiated. Several guidelines on the management of migraines have been published by experts including the American Academy of Neurology (AAN) and the American Headache Society (AHS). Drugs with established efficacy for migraine prevention based on reliable evidence supporting efficacy and safety include several oral agents (e.g., divalproex sodium, sodium valproate, topiramate, metoprolol, propranolol, timolol, frovatriptan) and parenteral agents (e.g., eptinezumab, erenumab, fremanezumab, galcanezumab, onabotulinumtoxinA). The existing evidence is not sufficient to support superiority of one agent over another; therefore, selection of an appropriate agent should be individualized and take into consideration drug efficacy, tolerability, cost, patient comorbidities, and other patient-specific factors. Combining preventive drugs from different classes may be useful when there is a suboptimal response or dose-limiting adverse effects of a particular agent.

Guidelines on pediatric migraine prevention from the AAN and AHS suggest that preventive treatments may be considered in pediatric patients with frequent headaches, disability related to migraine, or medication overuse; however, the existing evidence is limited and many trials failed to show a benefit with preventive treatments over placebo. Although topiramate has been shown to decrease the frequency of migraine, it is not clear whether the effects achieved are clinically meaningful in children and adolescents.

● Alcohol Dependence

Topiramate has been used successfully in adults for the management of alcohol dependence†. Efficacy of the drug in this condition has been evaluated in 2 randomized, double-blind, placebo-controlled studies in adults who met Diagnostic and Statistical Manual of Mental Disorders (DSM-IV) criteria for alcohol dependence; the initial trial was of 12 weeks' duration and was conducted at a single site, while the subsequent trial was of 14 weeks' duration and was conducted at multiple sites. Patients in both studies received escalating dosages of topiramate (initially, 25 mg daily and gradually increased up to 300 mg daily) or placebo in conjunction with a weekly medication compliance intervention. Topiramate was found to be more effective than placebo in improving self-reported drinking outcomes (e.g., number of drinks per day, number of drinks per drinking day, percentage of heavy drinking days, percentage of days abstinent) as well as the objective laboratory measure of alcohol consumption (reduced plasma γ-glutamyltransferase) in both of these studies. In addition, topiramate was shown to reduce self-reported alcohol craving to a greater extent than placebo in the 12-week study. Additional analyses of these 2 studies found topiramate to be more effective than placebo at improving physical and psychosocial well-being and some aspects of quality of life in these alcoholic individuals. In an open-label, longer-term study comparing topiramate with naltrexone in alcohol-dependent patients, topiramate was found to be at least as effective at reducing drinking behaviors as naltrexone during 6 months of therapy and appeared superior to naltrexone at reducing alcohol-related cravings.

Topiramate is one of several drugs currently recommended by the National Institute of Alcohol Abuse and Alcoholism (NIAAA) for treating alcohol dependence; however, unlike the other recommended drugs (naltrexone, acamprosate, disulfiram), topiramate has not been approved by the FDA for this indication. Topiramate also differs from the other recommended drug therapies because it has been administered to patients who were still drinking alcohol, and a period of abstinence from alcohol does not appear to be necessary before starting therapy with the drug. Additional studies, including longer-term trials, are needed to more clearly determine topiramate's efficacy, safety, and potential role in treating alcohol dependence, including its use in different populations and alcoholic subtypes, its potential use in combination with other drugs, and the optimal dosage and duration of therapy.

Topiramate has been effective in the management of alcohol withdrawal† in a limited number of patients in uncontrolled studies; however, larger, well-controlled studies are needed to confirm these initial findings.

● Antipsychotic-induced Weight Gain

Topiramate has been effective for moderate weight loss and prevention of weight gain from second-generation antipsychotics in patients with schizophrenia†. Guidelines from the American Psychiatric Association (APA) state that pharmacologic weight management with topiramate can be considered in such patients based on a modest benefit seen in several small studies evaluating the efficacy of topiramate for this indication; however, this benefit should be weighed against the potential risk of adverse effects.

● Binge Eating Disorder

Topiramate has been evaluated in randomized controlled trials and found to be effective for the treatment of binge eating disorder†, by reducing the number of binge episodes and binge days per week; however, its use may be precluded by the potential for adverse effects. Guidelines from the APA support the use of topiramate for this indication.

● Essential Tremor

Topiramate has been found to be effective for the treatment of essential tremor (ET)†, by improving functional disability, based on low-quality evidence from randomized controlled trials. Patients receiving topiramate for this indication were also significantly more likely to withdraw from treatment due to adverse effects including paresthesia, weight loss, decreased appetite, and cognitive dysfunction.

Guidelines from the AAN recommend primidone and propranolol as first-line treatments for limb tremor in ET based on established evidence of efficacy; topiramate is listed among agents that are probably effective for this condition based on a lower level of evidence. Recommendations from the International Parkinson and Movement Disorder Society also conclude that topiramate (when dosed higher than 200 mg per day), primidone, and propranolol are all efficacious and clinically useful for treatment of limb tremor.

DOSAGE AND ADMINISTRATION

● General

Pretreatment Screening

- Measure serum bicarbonate prior to initiating treatment with topiramate.

Patient Monitoring

- Closely monitor patients who are currently receiving or beginning therapy with topiramate and/or any other anticonvulsant for any indication for the emergence or worsening of depression, suicidal thoughts or behavior (suicidality), and/or any unusual changes in mood or behavior.

- Monitor height and weight in pediatric patients receiving long-term treatment with topiramate.

- Measure serum bicarbonate periodically during treatment with topiramate.

- Closely monitor patients, particularly pediatric patients, for evidence of decreased sweating and increased body temperature, especially in hot weather.

- Monitor for seizures/increased seizure frequency when rapid withdrawal of topiramate is medically required.

- Monitor for signs of hyperammonemic encephalopathy in patients who develop unexplained lethargy, vomiting, or changes in mental status.

Dispensing and Administration Precautions

- Because of similarity in spelling between Topamax® (the trade name for topiramate) and Toprol-XL® (a trade name for metoprolol succinate, a β-adrenergic blocking agent), the potential exists for dispensing or prescribing errors involving these drugs. These medication errors have been associated with serious adverse events sometimes requiring hospitalization as a result of either lack of the intended medication (e.g., seizure or hypertension recurrence) or exposure to the wrong drug (e.g., bradycardia in a patient erroneously receiving metoprolol). Therefore, extra care should be exercised to ensure the accuracy of both oral and written prescriptions for these drugs. Patients should be advised to carefully check their medications and to bring any questions or concerns to the attention of the dispensing pharmacist.

- Dispensing errors involving Topamax® (topiramate) and Toprol-XL® (metoprolol succinate) should be reported to the manufacturers, the USP/

ISMP (Institute for Safe Medication Practices) Medication Errors Reporting Program by phone (800-233-7767), or directly to the FDA MedWatch program by phone (800-FDA-1088), fax (800-FDA-0178), or internet (https://www.fda.gov/Safety/MedWatch/default.htm).

● Administration

Topiramate is administered orally; the drug is commercially available in various dosage forms for oral administration, including immediate-release tablets, sprinkle capsules, extended-release capsules, and an oral solution.

Store topiramate tablets at 15–30°C and topiramate sprinkle capsules at or below 25°C. Store Qudexy® XR extended-release capsules at 20–25°C (excursions permitted between 15–30°C). Store Trokendi XR® extended-release capsules at 25°C (excursions permitted between 15–30°C). Store Eprontia® oral solution at 20–25°C (excursions permitted between 15–30°C). Protect topiramate tablets, sprinkle capsules, and extended-release capsules from moisture during storage; additionally, protect Trokendi XR® from light during storage.

Oral Administration

Topiramate is administered orally as immediate-release tablets, sprinkle capsules, extended-release capsules, or an oral solution. The immediate-release tablets, sprinkle capsules, and oral solution are administered in 2 divided doses; the extended-release capsules are administered once daily.

The manufacturer states that the sprinkle capsule formulation of topiramate is bioequivalent to the immediate-release tablet and may be substituted as a therapeutic equivalent. At steady state, the extended-release capsules administered once daily are bioequivalent to the immediate-release tablets administered twice daily. Because the bioavailability of topiramate is not affected by food, the drug may be administered without regard to meals.

Because of the bitter taste, immediate-release tablets of topiramate should be swallowed intact and *not* broken or chewed. For patients experiencing difficulty in swallowing the tablets, contents of the capsule/sprinkle formulation may be sprinkled on a small amount of food as described below.

The sprinkle capsule formulation of topiramate may be taken whole, or may be administered by opening the capsule and sprinkling the entire contents on a small amount (e.g., a teaspoonful) of soft food (e.g., applesauce, custard, ice cream, oatmeal, pudding, yogurt). The patient should swallow the entire spoonful of the sprinkle/food mixture immediately; chewing should be avoided. It may be helpful to have the patient drink fluids immediately after administration in order to make sure that all of the mixture is swallowed. The sprinkle/food mixture must not be stored for use at a later time.

Qudexy® XR extended-release capsules may be swallowed whole or may be administered by opening the capsule and sprinkling the contents on a small amount of soft food; the sprinkle/food mixture should be swallowed immediately and not chewed, crushed, or stored for later use.

Trokendi XR® extended-release capsules must be swallowed whole and may not be sprinkled on food, crushed, or chewed; because of these limitations, Trokendi XR® is not recommended for use in children younger than 6 years of age. The manufacturer of Trokendi XR® states that patients should completely avoid consumption of alcohol at least 6 hours prior to and 6 hours after administration of the drug.

A calibrated measuring device is recommended for use with Eprontia® to ensure accurate measurement of the dose. A household tablespoon or teaspoon should not be used to measure the dose. Discard any unused portion of Eprontia® oral solution within 30 days after opening.

Extemporaneously Compounded Oral Liquid

An extemporaneously compounded oral liquid formulation of topiramate has been prepared.

Standardize 4 Safety

Standardized concentrations for an extemporaneously prepared oral liquid preparation of topiramate has been established through Standardize 4 Safety (S4S), a national patient safety initiative to reduce medication errors, especially during transitions of care. Multidisciplinary expert panels were convened to determine recommended standard concentrations. Because recommendations from the S4S panels may differ from the manufacturer's prescribing information, caution is advised when using concentrations that differ from labeling, particularly when using rate information from the label. For additional information on S4S (including updates that may be available), see https://www.ashp.org/pharmacy-practice/standardize-4-safety-initiative.

Standardize 4 Safety Compounded Oral Liquid Standards for Topiramate[a]

Concentration Standard
20 mg/mL

[a] The topiramate concentration is copyright protected by USP and can be used for internal purposes only.

● Dosage

Dosage of topiramate must be adjusted carefully and individualized according to patient response and tolerance and the condition being treated. The manufacturer states that titration of topiramate dosages too rapidly (e.g., over 3–6 weeks) to achieve target dosages and/or excessive target dosages may have contributed to an unnecessarily high incidence of adverse effects in clinical studies.

In patients with or without a history of seizures or epilepsy, anticonvulsant drugs, including topiramate, should be withdrawn gradually to minimize the risk of seizures or increased seizure frequency. In clinical studies for seizure disorders, daily dosages of topiramate were decreased in weekly intervals by 50–100 mg in adults and over a 2–8 week period in pediatric patients; transition to a new anticonvulsant regimen was permitted when clinically indicated. In clinical studies for migraine prophylaxis, daily dosages were decreased in weekly intervals by 25–50 mg. However, in situations where more rapid withdrawal of topiramate is clinically necessary, the manufacturers recommend appropriate monitoring.

Seizure Disorders

The manufacturers state that it is not necessary to monitor plasma topiramate concentrations to achieve optimal clinical effect with the drug.

Addition or withdrawal of phenytoin and/or carbamazepine during adjunctive therapy may require adjustment of topiramate dosage. Addition of topiramate to an anticonvulsant regimen containing phenytoin may require adjustment of the dosage of phenytoin.

Initial Monotherapy

The recommended dosage of topiramate as initial monotherapy for management of partial-onset seizures or primary generalized tonic-clonic seizures in adults and pediatric patients 10 years of age or older is 400 mg daily (administered in 2 divided doses as immediate-release tablets, sprinkle capsules, or oral solution, or once daily as extended-release capsules). The dosage of topiramate should be titrated using the schedule in Table 1 or 2 depending on the dosage form used.

TABLE 1. Topiramate (Immediate-release Tablets, Sprinkle Capsules, and Oral Solution) Dosage Titration Schedule for Monotherapy of Partial Seizures or Primary Generalized Tonic-Clonic Seizures in Adults and Pediatric Patients 10 Years of Age or Older

Week	Morning Dose	Evening Dose
1	25 mg	25 mg
2	50 mg	50 mg
3	75 mg	75 mg
4	100 mg	100 mg
5	150 mg	150 mg
6	200 mg	200 mg

TABLE 2. Topiramate (Extended-release Capsules) Dosage Titration Schedule for Monotherapy of Partial Seizures or Primary Generalized Tonic-Clonic Seizures in Adults and Pediatric Patients 10 Years of Age or Older

Week	Dosage
1	50 mg once daily
2	100 mg once daily
3	150 mg once daily
4	200 mg once daily
5	300 mg once daily
6	400 mg once daily

In a controlled study evaluating safety and efficacy of topiramate (titrated up to 50 or 400 mg daily as an immediate-release preparation) as initial monotherapy, approximately 58% of patients randomized to receive the 400-mg daily dosage achieved this maximum dosage. Because a therapeutic effect emerges during titration, the investigators of this study recommend that topiramate dosages should be titrated in a stepwise fashion with intermediate stopping points (e.g., 100 mg daily) to evaluate patient response and achieve the optimal maintenance dosage, and to avoid possibly exceeding an appropriate dosage for an individual patient.

Dosage of topiramate as initial monotherapy for the management of partial-onset seizures or primary generalized tonic-clonic seizures in pediatric patients 2–9 years of age (or 6–9 years of age if using Trokendi XR®) is based on body weight. During the titration period, the recommended initial dosage of topiramate is 25 mg daily (administered in the evening) for the first week. Based on tolerability, dosage can be increased to 50 mg daily (administered in 2 divided doses as immediate-release tablets, sprinkle capsules, or oral solution, or once daily as extended-release capsules) during the second week. The total daily dosage can then be increased by 25–50 mg daily each subsequent week as tolerated. Titration to the minimum recommended dosage (see Table 3) should be attempted over 5–7 weeks of the total titration period. Based upon tolerability and seizure control, additional titration to a higher dosage (up to the maximum recommended maintenance dosage) can be attempted in weekly increments of 25–50 mg daily. The total daily dosage of topiramate should not exceed the maximum recommended maintenance dosage for each range of body weight (see Table 3).

TABLE 3. Target Maintenance Topiramate Dosage for Monotherapy of Partial Seizures or Primary Generalized Tonic-Clonic Seizures in Pediatric Patients 2–9 Years of Age

Weight (kg)	Minimum Total Daily Dosage (mg/day)*	Maximum Total Daily Dosage (mg/day)*
Up to 11	150	250
12–22	200	300
23–31	200	350
32–38	250	350
>38	250	400

*Administered in 2 equally divided doses if using the immediate-release tablets, sprinkle capsule, or oral solution formulation of the drug.

Adjunctive Therapy

In adults, the recommended dosage of topiramate as adjunctive therapy for management of partial-onset seizures or Lennox-Gastaut Syndrome is 200–400 mg daily (administered in 2 divided doses as immediate-release tablets, sprinkle capsules, or oral solution, or once daily as extended-release capsules). The recommended adult dosage for adjunctive management of primary generalized tonic-clonic seizures is 400 mg daily (administered in 2 divided doses as immediate-release tablets, sprinkle capsules, or oral solution, or once daily as extended-release capsules). Topiramate therapy should be initiated at 25–50 mg daily, titrating the daily dosage upward in increments of 25–50 mg at weekly intervals to an optimal level, but generally not exceeding 400 mg daily. Limited data indicate that upward titration in increments of 25 mg per week may delay the time to reach an effective dosage; however, such a titration schedule appears to be associated with a lower incidence of neurocognitive and/or psychiatric adverse effects and a lower discontinuance rate. Maintenance dosages less than 400 mg daily may be optimally effective in some patients and therefore dosage should be individualized; however, results from clinical studies in adults with partial-onset seizures indicate that a daily dosage of 200 mg may produce inconsistent effects and appears to be less effective than a daily dosage of 400 mg. Dosages exceeding 400 mg daily have not been shown to improve responses in adults with partial-onset seizures.

In pediatric patients 2–16 years of age (or 6–16 years of age if using Trokendi XR®), the recommended dosage of topiramate as adjunctive therapy for the management of partial-onset seizures, primary generalized tonic-clonic seizures, or seizures associated with Lennox-Gastaut syndrome is approximately 5–9 mg/kg daily (administered in 2 divided doses as immediate-release tablets, sprinkle capsules, or oral solution, or once daily as extended-release capsules). An initial dose of 25 mg (or less, based on a range of 1–3 mg/kg daily) should be given nightly for the first week. The dosage should then be increased at 1- or 2-week intervals in increments of 1–3 mg/kg daily (administered in 2 divided doses as immediate-release tablets, sprinkle capsules, or oral solution, or once daily as extended-release capsules) to achieve optimal clinical response. Dosage titration should be guided by clinical outcome; some manufacturers recommend that the total daily dose should not exceed 400 mg. Alternatively, some clinicians recommend that the initial topiramate dosage should range from 0.5–1 mg/kg daily and that the drug should be titrated slowly (e.g., followed by incremental increases of 1–3 mg/kg every other week or incremental increases of 0.5–1 mg/kg per week) to obtain optimal efficacy with minimal adverse effects.

Dravet Syndrome

For the adjunctive treatment of seizures associated with Dravet syndrome† in children, dosages of topiramate are similar to those of other epilepsy types; typical starting dosage ranges from 0.5 to 2 mg/kg daily (in divided doses) and is increased to a target dosage of 5–12 mg/kg daily.

Migraine Prophylaxis

The recommended dosage of topiramate for prophylaxis of migraine headache in adults and adolescents 12 years of age or older is 100 mg daily (administered in 2 divided doses as immediate-release tablets, sprinkle capsules, or oral solution, or once daily as extended-release capsules). The dosage of topiramate should be titrated using the schedule in Table 4 or 5 depending on the dosage form used.

TABLE 4. Topiramate (Immediate-release Tablets, Sprinkle Capsules, or Oral Solution) Dosage Titration Schedule for Migraine Prophylaxis in Adults and Adolescents

Week	Morning Dose	Evening Dose
1	None	25 mg
2	25 mg	25 mg
3	25 mg	50 mg
4	50 mg	50 mg

TABLE 5. Topiramate (Extended-release Capsules) Dosage Titration Schedule for Migraine Prophylaxis in Adults and Adolescents

Week	Dosage
1	25 mg once daily
2	50 mg once daily
3	75 mg once daily
4	100 mg once daily

Titration of topiramate dosage should be guided by clinical outcome. If required, longer intervals between dosage adjustments can be used.

Alcohol Dependence

The optimal dosage regimen of topiramate for the management of alcohol dependence† remains to be established; however, initial dosages of 25 mg given once daily in the afternoon or evening (e.g., at bedtime) followed by gradual dosage titration (e.g., increasing dosage in increments of 25–50 mg daily each week, given in 2 divided doses) to target maintenance dosages of 200–300 mg daily were found to be effective in short-term, controlled clinical trials in adults and have been recommended by some authorities.

Results from clinical studies in alcohol dependence suggest that a more gradual titration (e.g., over 8 weeks) to achieve target dosages of 200–300 mg daily may be better tolerated than more rapid titration (e.g., over 6 weeks). A period of abstinence from alcohol prior to initiating topiramate therapy for alcohol dependence does not appear to be necessary.

● Special Populations

Hepatic Impairment

Although topiramate clearance may decrease in patients with hepatic impairment, the manufacturers make no specific recommendations for dosage adjustment in such patients.

Renal Impairment

Dosage of topiramate should be adjusted according to the degree of renal impairment. In patients with creatinine clearance less than 70 mL/minute per 1.73 m², the daily dosage of topiramate should be decreased by 50%. Dosage adjustment also may be required in patients undergoing hemodialysis since clearance of topiramate is 4–6 times faster in such patients. To avoid rapid decreases in plasma topiramate concentrations in patients undergoing hemodialysis, a supplemental dose of the drug may be required; selection of the supplemental dose should take into account the duration of dialysis, clearance rate of the dialysis system being used, and the patient's effective renal clearance of topiramate.

Geriatric Patients

The manufacturers make no specific dosage recommendations for geriatric patients.

CAUTIONS

● Contraindications

- There are no known contraindications to the use of immediate-release topiramate and Qudexy® XR extended-release topiramate capsules. Trokendi XR® extended-release topiramate capsules are contraindicated in patients with recent alcohol use (i.e., within 6 hours prior to or 6 hours after topiramate use).

● Warnings/Precautions

Acute Myopia and Secondary Closure Glaucoma Syndrome

A syndrome consisting of acute myopia associated with secondary angle-closure glaucoma has been reported in some adults and pediatric patients receiving topiramate. This syndrome may be associated with supraciliary effusion, resulting in anterior displacement of the lens and iris and, subsequently, secondary angle-closure glaucoma. Symptoms include acute onset of decreased visual acuity and/or ocular pain and typically occur within one month of initiating topiramate therapy. Ophthalmologic findings include myopia, mydriasis, anterior chamber shallowing, ocular hyperemia, choroidal detachments, retinal pigment epithelial detachments, macular striae, and increased intraocular pressure. Untreated elevations in intraocular pressure can lead to serious sequelae including permanent vision loss.

If any adverse ocular effects or visual problems occur during topiramate therapy, discontinue the drug as rapidly as possible; additional supportive measures may also be indicated.

Visual Field Defects

Visual field defects not associated with elevated intraocular pressure also have been reported in patients receiving topiramate in clinical trials and during postmarketing experience. If visual problems occur during treatment with topiramate, consider discontinuing the drug. Manifestations generally resolve after drug is discontinued.

Oligohidrosis and Hyperthermia

Oligohidrosis, which rarely may require hospitalization, has been reported in patients receiving topiramate; most cases have occurred in pediatric patients. Manifestations include decreased sweating and an elevation in body temperature above normal (hyperthermia). Some cases occurred following exposure to elevated environmental temperatures. Closely monitor patients, particularly pediatric patients, receiving topiramate for evidence of decreased sweating and increased body temperature, especially in hot weather. Caution is advised if topiramate is used concomitantly with other drugs that predispose patients to heat-related disorders (e.g., carbonic anhydrase inhibitors, drugs with anticholinergic activity).

Metabolic Acidosis

Hyperchloremic, non-anion gap, metabolic acidosis (i.e., decreased serum bicarbonate concentrations to below the normal reference range in the absence of chronic respiratory alkalosis) has been reported in adults and pediatric patients receiving immediate-release topiramate. Such electrolyte imbalance can occur at any time during therapy. Metabolic acidosis is caused by renal bicarbonate loss due to the inhibitory effect of topiramate on carbonic anhydrase. Decreases in serum bicarbonate concentrations usually are mild to moderate (average decrease of 4 mEq/L at daily topiramate dosages of 400 mg in adults and approximately 6 mg/kg daily in pediatric patients); marked decreases in serum bicarbonate concentrations (to below 10 mEq/L) may rarely occur. Manifestations of acute or chronic metabolic acidosis may include hyperventilation, nonspecific symptoms such as fatigue and anorexia, or more severe sequelae including cardiac arrhythmias or stupor.

Because chronic, untreated metabolic acidosis may have potentially serious sequelae (e.g., increased risk of nephrolithiasis or nephrocalcinosis, development of osteomalacia and/or osteoporosis with an increased risk for fractures, reduced growth rates in pediatric patients), the manufacturers state that serum bicarbonate concentrations should be measured at baseline and periodically during topiramate therapy. If metabolic acidosis develops and persists, consider reducing the dosage or discontinuing topiramate therapy (by gradually tapering the dosage). If a decision is made to continue topiramate therapy in the presence of persistent acidosis, consider alkali treatment.

Interaction with Alcohol

Use of Trokendi XR® is contraindicated in patients with recent alcohol use (i.e., within 6 hours prior to or 6 hours after topiramate use). In vitro data indicate that in the presence of alcohol, plasma concentrations of Trokendi XR® extended-release topiramate capsules may be markedly increased soon after dosing and become subtherapeutic later in the day.

Suicidal Behavior and Ideation

An increased risk of suicidality (suicidal behavior or ideation) was observed in an analysis of studies using various anticonvulsants compared with placebo. The analysis of suicidality reports from 199 placebo-controlled studies involving

11 anticonvulsants (carbamazepine, felbamate, gabapentin, lamotrigine, levetiracetam, oxcarbazepine, pregabalin, tiagabine, topiramate, valproate, and zonisamide) in patients with epilepsy, psychiatric disorders (e.g., bipolar disorder, depression, anxiety), and other conditions (e.g., migraine, neuropathic pain) found that patients receiving anticonvulsants had approximately twice the risk of suicidal behavior or ideation (0.43%) compared with patients receiving placebo (0.24%); this increased suicidality risk was observed as early as 1 week after beginning therapy and continued through 24 weeks. Although patients treated with an anticonvulsant for epilepsy, psychiatric disorders, and other conditions were all found to be at increased risk for suicidality compared with those receiving placebo, the relative risk for suicidality was found to be higher in patients with epilepsy compared with those receiving anticonvulsants for other conditions.

Clinicians who prescribe topiramate or any other anticonvulsant should balance the risk for suicidality with the risk of untreated illness. Epilepsy and many other illnesses for which anticonvulsants are prescribed are themselves associated with an increased risk of morbidity and mortality and an increased risk of suicidal thoughts and behavior. If suicidal thoughts and behavior emerge during anticonvulsant therapy, the clinician should consider whether these symptoms may be related to the illness being treated.

Cognitive/Neuropsychiatric Adverse Events

Immediate-release formulations of topiramate have been associated with cognitive and neuropsychiatric adverse effects; thus, these adverse effects are also expected to be associated with extended-release preparations of topiramate. Adverse CNS effects are frequently reported with topiramate and generally can be classified into 3 categories: cognitive-related dysfunction (e.g., confusion, psychomotor slowing, difficulty with concentration or attention, difficulty with memory, speech or language problems, particularly word-finding difficulties); psychiatric or behavioral disturbances (e.g., depression, mood problems); and somnolence or fatigue.

The risk of adverse cognitive effects is increased with rapid titration and higher initial dosages of topiramate.

Somnolence and fatigue were the most commonly reported adverse effects in patients receiving topiramate for adjunctive therapy of seizure disorders. In patients receiving topiramate as initial monotherapy for seizure disorders, the incidence of somnolence appeared to be dose related. In patients receiving topiramate as adjunctive therapy for seizure disorders, the incidence of fatigue appeared to be dose related. In patients receiving topiramate for migraine prophylaxis, both somnolence and fatigue appeared to be dose related and occurred more frequently during the titration phase.

Psychiatric or behavioral disturbances reported with topiramate in the adjunctive epilepsy and migraine populations were dose related. Suicide attempts also have been reported in patients receiving the drug.

Other common adverse psychiatric effects reported with topiramate include nervousness, anxiety, aggression, insomnia, decreased libido, personality disorder, and anorexia; other frequently reported CNS effects include dizziness, ataxia, paresthesia, hypoesthesia, nystagmus, tremor, and abnormal gait or coordination.

Fetal/Neonatal Morbidity and Mortality

Topiramate can cause fetal harm when administered to pregnant patients. Exposure to the drug in utero has been associated with an increased risk of oral clefts (cleft lip and/or palate) and for neonates being small for gestational age (SGA). Structural malformations, including craniofacial defects, and reduced fetal weights have occurred in the offspring of pregnant animals exposed to topiramate at clinically relevant dosages.

Carefully consider the benefits and risks of topiramate therapy when use of the drug in females of reproductive potential is contemplated, particularly for conditions not usually associated with permanent injury or death. Inform all females of reproductive potential of the potential risks to the fetus from exposure to topiramate.

Withdrawal of Antiepileptic Drugs

In patients with or without a history of seizures or epilepsy, anticonvulsant drugs, including topiramate, should be gradually withdrawn to minimize the potential for seizures or increased seizure frequency. The manufacturers recommend appropriate monitoring in situations where more rapid withdrawal of topiramate is required.

Decrease in Bone Mineral Density

The results from a one-year, active-controlled trial in pediatric patients treated with topiramate monotherapy found statistically significant decreases in bone mineral density in both the lumbar spine and total body less head among patients treated with topiramate. Of 63 pediatric patients in the trial, 21% of patients treated with topiramate experienced decreases in Z score of at least −0.5 from baseline compared with 0% of patients in the control group. These bone mineral density changes occurred most commonly among patients aged 6–9 years, although they occurred across all age groups in the trial. The potential impact of topiramate on fracture risk cannot be determined due to the small sample size and short duration of the trial. Decreases in bone mineral density in the lumbar spine were correlated with decreases in serum bicarbonate; these decreases are reflective of metabolic acidosis, which is known to occur during treatment with topiramate and is associated with increased resorption of bone. Patients treated with topiramate also had small reductions in markers of bone metabolism (e.g., alkaline phosphatase, calcium, phosphorus, and 1,25-dihydroxyvitamin D), larger reductions in markers of bone metabolism (e.g., parathyroid hormone and 25-hydroxyvitamin D), and increased urinary calcium excretion.

Negative Effects on Growth (Height and Weight)

A one-year, active-controlled study of 63 pediatric patients treated with topiramate found statistically significant reductions in mean annual change from baseline in body weight compared to control; similar reductions in height velocity and change in height from baseline were also observed. These negative effects on height and weight were observed across all included age groups. Carefully monitor height and weight in pediatric patients receiving long-term therapy with topiramate.

Serious Skin Reactions

Serious skin reactions, including Stevens-Johnson syndrome and toxic epidermal necrolysis, have been reported in patients treated with topiramate. Discontinue topiramate at the first sign of a rash, unless it is clearly unrelated to the drug. If signs or symptoms of Stevens-Johnson syndrome or toxic epidermal necrolysis occur, do not resume therapy with topiramate and consider alternative treatment.

Hyperammonemia and Encephalopathy (without and with Concomitant Valproic Acid)

Dose-related hyperammonemia with or without encephalopathy has been reported in patients receiving topiramate in clinical studies and during postmarketing experience. In adolescents 12–17 years of age who received topiramate monotherapy in migraine prophylaxis studies, hyperammonemia was reported in 26, 14, or 9% of those receiving topiramate 100 mg daily, topiramate 50 mg daily, or placebo, respectively. In some cases, ammonia concentrations were markedly increased in patients receiving the highest dosage of 100 mg daily. Concomitant administration of topiramate and valproic acid also has been associated with hyperammonemia with or without encephalopathy in patients who have previously tolerated either drug alone. Although topiramate is not labeled for use in pediatric patients 1–24 months of age, dose-related hyperammonemia was observed in such patients who were receiving topiramate and valproic acid concomitantly in partial-onset seizure studies. Although some patients may be asymptomatic, manifestations of hyperammonemic encephalopathy include acute alterations in the level of consciousness and/or cognitive function with lethargy or vomiting; in most cases, manifestations abated after discontinuance of therapy. Patients with inborn errors of metabolism or reduced hepatic mitochondrial activity may be at an increased risk for hyperammonemia with or without encephalopathy. Although not studied, it is possible that an interaction between topiramate and valproic acid may exacerbate existing defects or unmask deficiencies in susceptible individuals. If unexplained lethargy, vomiting, or changes in mental status occur, hyperammonemic encephalopathy should be considered, and an ammonia concentration should be measured.

Kidney Stones

Formation of kidney stones has been reported in approximately 1.5% of adults receiving topiramate in clinical trials. As in the general population, the incidence of kidney stone formation among topiramate-treated patients appears to be higher in men than in women; kidney stones also have been reported in pediatric patients receiving topiramate. Because topiramate is a carbonic anhydrase inhibitor, the drug may promote stone formation by reducing urinary citrate excretion and increasing urinary pH. The manufacturers state that use of topiramate in patients on a ketogenic diet or concomitant use of the drug with other drugs that produce metabolic acidosis may increase the risk of kidney stone formation and, therefore, should be avoided. Increased fluid intake may increase urinary output and reduce the concentration of substances involved in stone formation. Instruct patients receiving topiramate, particularly those with predisposing factors, to maintain adequate hydration to prevent kidney stone formation. In a one-year, active controlled trial of pediatric patients, an increase in urinary calcium and a marked decrease in urinary citrate were observed among patients treated with topiramate; this increased ratio increases the risk for kidney stones and nephrocalcinosis.

Hypothermia with Concomitant Valproic Acid

Hypothermia (defined as an unintentional drop in body core temperature to less than 35°C), both in conjunction with and in the absence of hyperammonemia, has been reported in patients receiving concurrent topiramate and valproic acid therapy. Hypothermia may be manifested by a variety of clinical abnormalities including lethargy, confusion, coma, and substantial alterations in other major organ systems such as the cardiovascular and respiratory systems. Hypothermia may occur after initiating topiramate therapy or following a dosage increase. Consider discontinuance of topiramate or valproic acid therapy in patients who develop hypothermia. Since hypothermia also may be a manifestation of hyperammonemia, clinical management and assessment of hypothermia should include determination of plasma ammonia concentrations.

Specific Populations
Pregnancy

Topiramate can cause fetal harm when administered to pregnant patients. Exposure to the drug in utero has been associated with an increased risk of oral clefts (cleft lip and/or palate) and for neonates being SGA (i.e., birth weight less than 10th percentile). Data from pregnancy registries, including the North American Antiepileptic Drug (NAAED) pregnancy registry, indicate that infants exposed to topiramate in utero have a higher prevalence of oral cleft birth defects than those with no such exposure. The prevalence of oral clefts among infants in the NAAED registry who were exposed to topiramate in utero was 1.1% compared with a prevalence of 0.36% in infants exposed to a reference anticonvulsant and a prevalence of 0.12% in infants born to women without epilepsy and without exposure to anticonvulsant agents. For comparison, the estimated background rate of oral clefts in the US as estimated by the US Centers for Disease Control and Prevention (CDC) is 0.17%. Based on NAAED data, the relative risk of developing an oral cleft defect in topiramate-exposed pregnancies was 9.6 compared with the risk in a background population of untreated women. The United Kingdom Epilepsy and Pregnancy Registry reported a similarly increased prevalence of oral clefts of 3.2% among infants exposed in utero to topiramate monotherapy; the reported rate was 16 times higher than the background rate in the United Kingdom, which is approximately 0.2%.

Data from the NAAED registry indicate that 19.7% of infants who were exposed to topiramate in utero were SGA compared with 7.9% of infants exposed to a reference anticonvulsant and 5.4% of infants born to women without epilepsy and without exposure to anticonvulsant agents. In another population-based birth registry, 25% of topiramate-exposed infants were SGA compared with 9% of infants who were not exposed to anticonvulsants. The prevalence of this adverse effect is higher in infants born to women who received higher dosages of topiramate during pregnancy or who continued to receive topiramate through the third trimester. SGA has been observed at all dosages of topiramate and appears to be dose dependent; however, the long-term consequences of these findings are not known.

Topiramate has demonstrated selective developmental toxicity, including teratogenicity and embryotoxicity, in multiple species of animals (rats, rabbits, mice). Structural malformations, including craniofacial defects, and reduced fetal weights have occurred in the offspring of pregnant animals exposed to topiramate at clinically relevant dosages in the absence of maternal toxicity. However, there also was some evidence of maternal toxicity (e.g., decreased maternal body weight gain, increased mortality).

Topiramate therapy can cause metabolic acidosis. The effect of topiramate-induced metabolic acidosis has not been specifically studied during pregnancy;

however, metabolic acidosis from other causes during pregnancy can result in decreased fetal growth, decreased fetal oxygenation, and fetal death, and also may affect the ability of the fetus to tolerate labor. Therefore, pregnant women receiving topiramate should be monitored and treated for metabolic acidosis in the same manner as nonpregnant patients. In addition, neonates born to women treated with topiramate should be monitored for metabolic acidosis because of possible drug transfer to the fetus and possible occurrence of transient metabolic acidosis following birth.

The benefits and risks of topiramate therapy should be carefully considered when use of the drug in females of reproductive potential is contemplated, particularly for conditions not usually associated with permanent injury or death. All females of reproductive potential should be informed of the potential risks to the fetus from exposure to topiramate. Alternative options should be considered in patients who are planning a pregnancy. If a decision is made to use topiramate in a female of reproductive potential who is not planning a pregnancy, clinicians should recommend use of effective contraception. The potential for decreased efficacy of estrogen-containing oral contraceptives should be considered.

Women who become pregnant while receiving topiramate should be encouraged to enroll in the NAAED pregnancy registry; patients can enroll by calling 888-233-2334. Information on the registry also can be found on the website https://www.aedpregnancyregistry.org.

Lactation

Limited data indicate that topiramate distributes into human milk at concentrations similar to those in maternal plasma. The effects of topiramate on milk production are not known. Diarrhea and somnolence have been reported in breast-fed infants whose mothers were receiving topiramate treatment. The known benefits of breast-feeding should be considered along with the clinical importance of the drug to the mother and any potential adverse effects on the breast-fed infant from topiramate or the underlying maternal condition.

Females and Males of Reproductive Potential

All females of reproductive potential should be informed of the potential risks to the fetus from exposure to topiramate. Alternative options should be considered in patients who are planning a pregnancy. If a decision is made to use topiramate in a female of reproductive potential who is not planning a pregnancy, clinicians should recommend use of effective contraception. The potential for decreased efficacy of estrogen-containing oral contraceptives should be considered.

Pediatric Use

Safety and efficacy of topiramate for the management of seizure disorders have not been established in children younger than 2 years of age. In a randomized, double-blind, placebo-controlled study in infants 1–24 months of age, topiramate in fixed dosages of 5, 15, and 25 mg/kg daily was not shown to be more effective than placebo in controlling seizures after 20 days of treatment. Results of this study in addition to a long-term open-label study in infants and toddlers suggest that very young children may experience adverse effects not previously observed in older pediatric patients and adults or that occur with greater frequency or severity than in these older age groups. Such adverse effects included growth/length retardation, changes in certain laboratory parameters (e.g., increased serum creatinine concentrations, increased BUN, increased protein concentrations, decreased potassium concentrations, increased eosinophil count, increased alkaline phosphatase concentrations), and impairment of adaptive behavior. Although other preparations of topiramate may be used in children as young as 2 years of age for the management of seizure disorders, use of Trokendi XR® extended-release capsules is recommended only in children 6 years of age or older because this capsule formulation must be swallowed whole and cannot be sprinkled on food, crushed, or chewed.

Safety and efficacy of topiramate for migraine prophylaxis have not been established in pediatric patients younger than 12 years of age. In a controlled study in pediatric patients 6–16 years of age, topiramate 2–3 mg/kg daily was not more effective than placebo for preventing migraine headaches.

As in adults, cognitive/neuropsychiatric effects are commonly reported in pediatric patients receiving topiramate, although the incidence appears to be lower than that observed in adults. Such effects include psychomotor slowing, difficulty with concentration or attention, speech disorders, and language problems. The most common adverse CNS effects reported in pediatric patients receiving topiramate as initial monotherapy for seizure disorders include dizziness, headache, anorexia, and somnolence. The most common adverse CNS effects reported in pediatric patients receiving the drug as adjunctive therapy for seizure disorders include somnolence and fatigue. In migraine prophylaxis studies in pediatric patients 12–17 years of age, difficulty with concentration/attention was the most commonly reported adverse CNS effect. Adverse cognitive effects observed in pediatric migraine studies were dose dependent and occurred with greater frequency in younger (6–11 years of age) compared with older (12–17 years of age) children. Topiramate may cause psychomotor slowing and decreased verbal fluency based on results of a standard neuropsychological test that was administered to adolescents 12–17 years of age.

Hyperchloremic, non-anion gap, metabolic acidosis (i.e., decreased serum bicarbonate concentrations to below the normal reference range in the absence of chronic respiratory alkalosis) has been reported in pediatric patients receiving topiramate. In pediatric studies evaluating topiramate as adjunctive therapy for refractory partial-onset seizures or Lennox-Gastaut syndrome, the incidence of decreased serum bicarbonate concentrations was as high as 67 or 10% for patients receiving topiramate (approximately 6 mg/kg daily) or placebo, respectively. *Markedly* abnormally low serum bicarbonate concentrations (defined as concentrations of less than 17 mEq/L and a decrease from pretreatment values exceeding 5 mEq/L) were observed in up to 11% of patients receiving topiramate in these studies compared with no more than 2% of those receiving placebo. Similar reductions in serum bicarbonate were reported in an open-label, active-controlled study of pediatric patients treated with topiramate monotherapy for partial-onset seizures. Markedly low serum bicarbonate concentrations and persistent metabolic acidosis were reported in 35 and 76% of patients treated with topiramate, respectively. Chronic, untreated metabolic acidosis may have potentially serious sequelae, including development of osteomalacia (rickets), reduction of growth rates, and a decrease in maximal height achieved in pediatric patients. Although the effects of topiramate on growth and bone-related sequelae have not been systematically evaluated in long-term, placebo-controlled trials, results of an open-label study demonstrated that pediatric patients 1–24 months old who received topiramate for up to 1 year had reduced length, weight, and head circumference compared with age- and sex-matched normative data; reductions in length and weight were correlated with the degree of acidosis. Because of the potential risk of metabolic acidosis, the manufacturers state that serum bicarbonate concentrations should be measured at baseline and periodically during topiramate therapy.

Reductions in bone mineral density and growth have been reported in a 1-year active-controlled study of pediatric patients receiving monotherapy with topiramate for treatment of partial-onset seizures. In an open-label, active-controlled study of pediatric patients aged 4–15 years with partial-onset seizures, statistically significant reductions in weight and bone mineral density in the lumbar spine and total body less head were reported among patients treated with topiramate monotherapy compared to those treated with levetiracetam monotherapy.

Oligohidrosis (decreased sweating) and hyperthermia have been reported in clinical trials and during postmarketing surveillance of topiramate. Because oligohidrosis and hyperthermia typically occurred in children and may have potentially serious sequelae, the manufacturers state that patients, particularly pediatric patients, receiving topiramate should be monitored closely for evidence of decreased sweating and increased body temperature, especially in hot weather.

Clearance of topiramate is higher in pediatric patients than in adults, and also higher in younger versus older pediatric patients, presumably because of age-related changes in the rate of drug metabolism. Pediatric patients (2 to younger than 16 years of age) receiving adjunctive therapy with topiramate exhibited higher oral topiramate clearance than those receiving topiramate monotherapy; the observed difference was presumably due to concomitant use of enzyme-inducing anticonvulsant agents.

Geriatric Use

While clinical studies evaluating topiramate did not include sufficient numbers of adults 65 years of age or older to determine whether geriatric patients respond differently than younger adults, approximately 3% of patients receiving the drug in clinical trials were older than 60 years of age. Although no age-related differences in efficacy or safety were evident in these patients, pharmacokinetic data from one controlled clinical study revealed a decreased clearance of topiramate in geriatric

patients with reduced renal function (i.e., creatinine clearance reduced by 20% compared with that in younger adults). Following administration of a single 100-mg dose of topiramate in these patients, plasma clearance and renal clearance of topiramate were reduced by 21 and 19%, respectively; half-life was prolonged by 13%; and peak plasma concentrations and area under the plasma concentration-time curve (AUC) were increased by 23 or 25%, respectively, compared with younger adults. Therefore, the manufacturers state that it may be useful to monitor renal function in geriatric patients; dosage adjustment may be necessary in geriatric patients with impaired renal function (i.e., creatinine clearance less than 70 mL/minute per 1.73 m^2).

Hepatic Impairment

Pharmacokinetic studies have shown that plasma clearance of topiramate decreases by an average of 26% in patients with moderate to severe hepatic impairment; however, the manufacturer does not make specific recommendations for dosage adjustment in patients with hepatic impairment.

Renal Impairment

Pharmacokinetic studies have shown a decrease in clearance of topiramate by 42 and 54% in patients with moderate (creatinine clearance of 30 to less than 70 mL/minute per 1.73 m^2), and severe (creatinine clearance less than 30 mL/minute per 1.73 m^2) renal impairment, respectively, compared to patients with normal renal function. Administration of hemodialysis with a high-efficiency, counter-flow, single pass-dialysate procedure cleared topiramate at a rate of 120 mL/minute with blood flow through the dialyzer at 400 mL/minute; this rate of clearance will remove a substantial amount of topiramate over a typical hemodialysis session. In patients with creatinine clearance less than 70 mL/minute per 1.73 m^2, the daily dosage of topiramate should be decreased by 50%. Dosage adjustment also may be required in patients undergoing hemodialysis since clearance of topiramate is 4–6 times faster in such patients.

● Common Adverse Effects

The most common adverse effects reported in adults and pediatric patients receiving topiramate for epilepsy (≥10% incidence and occurring more frequently with the drug than placebo) include paresthesia, anorexia, weight loss, speech disorders or other related speech problems, fatigue, dizziness, somnolence, nervousness, psychomotor slowing, abnormal vision, and fever.

The most common adverse effects reported in adults and pediatric patients receiving topiramate for migraine prophylaxis (5% or greater incidence and occurring more frequently with the drug than with placebo) include paresthesia, anorexia, weight loss, difficulty with memory, taste perversion, diarrhea, hypoesthesia, nausea, abdominal pain, and upper respiratory tract infection.

In controlled clinical trials evaluating topiramate for alcohol dependence†, paresthesia, taste perversion, fatigue, anorexia, insomnia, concentration and attention difficulties, memory impairment, nervousness, somnolence, diarrhea, dizziness, and pruritus were reported more frequently in patients receiving topiramate than in patients receiving placebo.

DRUG INTERACTIONS

● Drugs Metabolized by Hepatic Microsomal Enzymes

In vitro studies indicate that topiramate is a mild inhibitor of cytochrome P-450 (CYP) isoenzyme 2C19 and a mild inducer of CYP3A4. Pharmacokinetic interactions with drugs metabolized by these isoenzymes, including some anticonvulsants, CNS depressants, and oral contraceptives, are therefore possible. Topiramate does not inhibit CYP1A2, 2A6, 2B6, 2C9, 2D6, 2E1, or 3A4/5.

● Amitriptyline

In healthy individuals, concomitant administration of topiramate (200 mg daily) and amitriptyline (25 mg daily) increased both peak plasma concentrations and area under the plasma concentration-time curve (AUC) of amitriptyline by 12%. Because some patients may experience a large increase in amitriptyline concentrations in the presence of topiramate, any adjustments in amitriptyline dosage should be made according to the patient's clinical response and not on the basis of plasma concentrations.

● Anticonvulsants

Clinically important decreases in plasma concentrations of topiramate have been observed in patients receiving concomitant therapy with phenytoin or carbamazepine. Plasma concentrations of topiramate were reduced by 48% when administered concomitantly with phenytoin. Plasma concentrations of phenytoin increased by 25% in some patients (generally in those receiving a twice-daily dosage regimen of phenytoin) and did not change substantially in others who received these drugs in combination. Concomitant administration of carbamazepine and topiramate decreased plasma concentrations of topiramate by 40%, but did not substantially alter plasma concentrations of carbamazepine or its active metabolite, carbamazepine epoxide. Neither phenytoin nor carbamazepine alters the protein binding of topiramate.

Concomitant administration of valproic acid and topiramate decreased topiramate plasma concentrations by 14% and valproic acid plasma concentrations by 11%. In addition, concomitant use of topiramate and valproic acid has been associated with hyperammonemia with or without encephalopathy in patients who have previously tolerated either drug alone.. Although not studied, the interaction between valproic acid and topiramate may exacerbate existing defects or unmask deficiencies in susceptible patients. Concomitant use of topiramate with valproic acid also has been associated with hypothermia (with and without hyperammonemia). Discontinuance of topiramate or valproic acid therapy should be considered in patients who develop hypothermia. Valproic acid (at concentrations 5–10 times higher than therapeutic concentrations) decreases protein binding of topiramate from 23 to 13%; topiramate does not affect protein binding of valproic acid.

Concomitant administration of topiramate and phenobarbital or primidone altered plasma concentrations of the concomitantly administered anticonvulsant by less than 10%; the effects of phenobarbital or primidone on the pharmacokinetics of topiramate were not evaluated.

Plasma concentrations of lamotrigine were altered by less than 10% when topiramate was dosed at up to 400 mg per day; plasma topiramate concentrations were decreased by 13% when the drugs were administered concomitantly.

● Antidiabetic Agents

Concomitant administration of topiramate and glyburide in patients with type 2 diabetes mellitus decreased steady-state peak plasma concentrations and AUC of glyburide by 22 and 25%, respectively. Systemic exposure of the active metabolites, 4-*trans*-hydroxyglyburide and 3-*cis*-hydroxyglyburide, also were reduced by 13 and 15%, respectively. Steady-state pharmacokinetics of topiramate were not affected by concomitant glyburide administration.

Concurrent administration of topiramate and pioglitazone in healthy individuals resulted in a nonsignificant decrease in steady-state pioglitazone AUC with no change in peak plasma concentrations. Decreases in systemic exposure to the active hydroxy- and keto-metabolites of pioglitazone were observed; however, the clinical importance of these findings is not known. When topiramate therapy is initiated in patients receiving pioglitazone or vice versa, careful attention should be given to the routine monitoring of patients for adequate glycemic control.

In healthy individuals, mean peak plasma concentrations and AUC of metformin were increased by 18 and 25%, respectively, following concomitant administration of topiramate; however, time to reach peak plasma concentrations of metformin was not affected. Oral clearance of topiramate appears to be reduced when administered in conjunction with metformin. The clinical importance of these pharmacokinetic interactions is not known. However, topiramate can cause metabolic acidosis, a condition for which the use of metformin is contraindicated.

● Drugs Predisposing to Heat-related Disorders

Increased risk of hyperthermia is possible with concomitant use of topiramate and drugs that predispose patients to heat-related disorders (e.g., carbonic anhydrase inhibitors, drugs with anticholinergic activity); caution is advised when topiramate is used in combination with such drugs.

● Carbonic Anhydrase Inhibitors

Concomitant use of topiramate with other carbonic anhydrase inhibitors (e.g., acetazolamide, dichlorphenamide, zonisamide) may increase the risk or severity of metabolic acidosis and may also increase the risk of kidney stone formation.

If topiramate is used concomitantly with another carbonic anhydrase inhibitor, the patient should be monitored for the onset or worsening of metabolic acidosis.

● CNS Depressants

Concomitant administration of topiramate and CNS depressants (including alcohol) has not been evaluated in clinical studies. Because of the potential for topiramate to cause CNS depression as well as other cognitive and/or neuropsychiatric adverse effects, the drug should be used with extreme caution if administered concurrently with alcohol or other CNS depressants.

In vitro data indicate that in the presence of alcohol, plasma concentrations of Trokendi XR® extended-release topiramate capsules may be markedly increased soon after dosing and become subtherapeutic later in the day. Use of Trokendi XR® is contraindicated in patients with recent alcohol use (i.e., within 6 hours prior to or 6 hours after topiramate use).

● Digoxin

Serum digoxin AUC was decreased by 12% with concomitant use of topiramate in a single-dose study; however, the clinical importance of this interaction is unknown.

● Dihydroergotamine

Concomitant administration of topiramate and a single dose of dihydroegotamine (1 mg subcutaneously) in healthy individuals did not affect the pharmacokinetics of either drug.

● Diltiazem

Concomitant administration of topiramate and diltiazem decreased peak plasma concentrations and AUC of diltiazem by 10 and 25%, respectively. Systemic exposure to deacetyldiltiazem also was decreased, but there was no effect on *N*-monodesmethyldiltiazem. Diltiazem increased peak plasma concentrations and AUC of topiramate by 16 and 19%, respectively.

● Haloperidol

Pharmacokinetics of haloperidol were not affected by topiramate in healthy individuals.

● Hydrochlorothiazide

In healthy individuals, peak plasma concentrations and AUC of topiramate increased by 27 and 29%, respectively, following concomitant administration of hydrochlorothiazide. Steady-state pharmacokinetics of hydrochlorothiazide were not substantially altered by topiramate. Although the clinical importance of this interaction is not known, a reduction in topiramate dosage may be necessary when hydrochlorothiazide is initiated.

In addition, both topiramate and hydrochlorothiazide have been shown to decrease serum potassium concentrations, and the decrease is greater when the drugs are given in combination.

● Lithium

Although the pharmacokinetics of lithium were not affected during concurrent administration of topiramate at a dosage of 200 mg daily, peak concentrations and AUC of lithium increased by 27 and 26%, respectively during concurrent administration of topiramate dosages up to 600 mg daily. Serum lithium concentrations should therefore be monitored in patients receiving concurrent lithium and high-dose topiramate therapy.

● Oral Contraceptives

In healthy individuals, mean exposure to either component of an oral contraceptive containing 35 mcg of ethinyl estradiol and 1 mg of norethindrone was not substantially altered by concomitant administration of topiramate (given in the absence of other drugs). However, substantially decreased exposure to ethinyl estradiol was observed in patients receiving an oral contraceptive containing ethinyl estradiol and norethindrone in conjunction with topiramate and valproic acid therapy; exposure to norethindrone was not substantially affected.

The possibility of contraceptive failure and increased breakthrough bleeding should be considered in patients receiving combination oral contraceptives with topiramate. Such patients should be advised to report any changes in bleeding patterns to a clinician; contraceptive efficacy can be decreased even in the absence of breakthrough bleeding.

• Propranolol

Concomitant administration of topiramate and propranolol in healthy individuals did not affect the pharmacokinetics of either drug.

• Risperidone

Risperidone systemic exposure was decreased by 16 and 33% during concomitant topiramate therapy at dosages of 250 and 400 mg daily, respectively; no alterations of 9-hydroxyrisperidone (active metabolite) concentrations were observed. Concurrent administration of topiramate and risperidone increased peak plasma concentrations and AUC of topiramate by 14 and 12%, respectively. There were no clinically important changes in the systemic exposure of risperidone plus 9-hydroxyrisperidone or of topiramate; therefore, this interaction is unlikely to be clinically important.

• Sumatriptan

In healthy individuals, topiramate did not affect the pharmacokinetics of single-dose sumatriptan.

• Venlafaxine

Concomitant administration of topiramate and venlafaxine in healthy individuals did not affect the pharmacokinetics of venlafaxine, O-desmethylvenlafaxine (active metabolite), or topiramate.

• Warfarin

Concomitant use of topiramate and warfarin has resulted in decreased international normalized ratio (INR) or prothrombin time (PT).

DESCRIPTION

Topiramate, a sulfamate-substituted derivative of the monosaccharide D-fructose, is an anticonvulsant agent that is also used for prophylaxis of migraine headache and management of alcohol dependence. The drug differs structurally from other currently available anticonvulsant agents. The spectrum of topiramate's anticonvulsant activity resembles that of carbamazepine and phenytoin, although differences in certain animal models have been observed and additive effects appear to occur when the drug is combined with these anticonvulsants.

Although the precise mechanism of action of topiramate is unknown, data from electrophysiologic and biochemical studies have revealed 4 properties that may contribute to the drug's efficacy for seizure disorders and migraine prophylaxis. At pharmacologically relevant concentrations, topiramate blocks voltage-dependent sodium channels; augments the activity of γ-aminobutyric acid (GABA) at some subtypes of the GABA-A receptor; antagonizes the AMPA/kainate subtype of the glutamate receptor; and inhibits carbonic anhydrase (particularly the CA-II and CA-IV isoenzymes).

Topiramate exhibits effects on cultured neurons similar to those observed with phenytoin and carbamazepine, and such effects are suggestive of an inactive state-dependent block of voltage-dependent sodium channels. Topiramate reduces the duration of epileptiform bursts of neuronal firing and decreases the number of action potentials in studies of cultured rat hippocampal neurons with spontaneous epileptiform burst activity. Topiramate also decreases the frequency of action potentials elicited by depolarizing electric current in cultured rat hippocampal neurons. During a partial seizure, neurons characteristically undergo high-frequency depolarization and firing of action potentials which is uncommon during normal physiologic neuronal activity. Some anticonvulsant drugs (e.g., phenytoin, carbamazepine) preferentially bind to voltage-dependent sodium channels during their inactivated state, slow the rate of recovery of sodium channels from their period of inactivation, and limit the ability of the neuron to depolarize and fire at high frequencies.

Topiramate enhances the activity of the inhibitory neurotransmitter GABA at a nonbenzodiazepine site on GABA$_A$ receptors. Activation of the postsynaptic GABA$_A$ receptor by GABA causes inhibition by increasing the inward flow of chloride ions, resulting in hyperpolarization of the postsynaptic cell; in chloride ion-depleted murine cerebellar granule cells, therapeutic concentrations of topiramate (in combination with GABA) enhance GABA-evoked inward flux of chloride ions in a concentration-dependent manner. Benzodiazepines act at GABA$_A$ receptors to enhance GABA-evoked inward flow of chloride ions, but the benzodiazepine antagonist flumazenil does not appear to inhibit topiramate enhancement of GABA-evoked currents in GABA$_A$ cortical neuronal receptors. Topiramate also does not appear to increase duration of chloride ion channel opening. Therefore, topiramate may potentiate GABA$_A$-evoked chloride ion flux by a mechanism other than GABA$_A$-receptor modulation.

Topiramate antagonizes a non-N-methyl-d-aspartate (NMDA) glutamate receptor and the kainate/α-amino-3-hydroxy-5-methylisoxazole-4-propionic acid (AMPA) receptor subtype. Although topiramate had no apparent effect on glutamate receptors of the NMDA subtype in cultured rat hippocampal neurons, topiramate antagonized the ability of kainate to activate the kainate/AMPA glutamate receptor subtype, and these effects were shown to be concentration dependent. Glutamate, the principal excitatory neurotransmitter amino acid in the brain, interacts with specific neuronal membrane receptors, including ion channel coupled (ionotropic) (e.g., NMDA, kainate/AMPA, kainate) receptor subtypes and with G-protein coupled (metabotropic) receptors that modulate intracellular second-messengers. The pathogenesis of seizures is thought to be mediated at least in part through excessive stimulation of glutamate receptors. In spontaneously epileptic rats, topiramate has reduced extracellular hippocampal concentrations of both glutamate and aspartate, and a correlation existed between reduction in glutamate concentrations and suppression of tonic seizures.

In animals, topiramate exhibits anticonvulsant activity in the maximal electroshock seizure (MES) test, suggesting that, like phenytoin, it may be effective in the management of partial and tonic-clonic (grand mal) seizures in humans. Topiramate also exhibited dose-dependent inhibition of absence-like seizures, which was antagonized by pretreatment with haloperidol. In animals, topiramate was ineffective or weakly effective in blocking clonic seizures induced by pentylenetetrazole, indicating that the drug may not enhance GABA inhibitory activity substantially.

Although the precise mechanism(s) of action of topiramate in the management of alcohol dependence is unclear, topiramate enhances GABA-mediated inhibitory neurotransmission and inhibits glutamatergic stimulatory neurotransmission; such changes appear to decrease dopaminergic activity in the mesocorticolimbic areas of the brain, which have been associated with alcohol dependence.

Topiramate is rapidly absorbed; peak plasma concentrations occur about 2 hours following an oral dose of 400 mg (as an immediate-release formulation) or approximately 20–24 hours following a single oral dose of 200 mg (as an extended-release formulation). The sprinkle capsule formulation of the drug is bioequivalent to the immediate-release tablet and, therefore, may be substituted as a therapeutic equivalent. The relative bioavailability of topiramate from the tablet formulation is about 80% compared with a solution. At steady state, the extended-release capsules administered once daily are bioequivalent to the immediate-release tablets administered twice daily. Topiramate exhibits linear, dose-proportional increases in plasma concentration over the dosage ranges evaluated (50 mg to 1.4 g daily depending on the formulation). Food may affect time to peak concentrations of the drug (depending on the formulation), but does not appear to affect systemic exposure. Approximately 15–41% of topiramate is bound to plasma proteins, with the fraction of protein binding decreasing as blood concentration increases.

The mean elimination half-life of topiramate is 21 hours following single or multiple doses of the drug as immediate-release formulations; the mean elimination half-life of Trokendi XR® extended-release capsules is approximately 31 hours following multiple doses, and the mean effective half-life of Qudexy® XR extended-release capsules is 56 hours. Approximately 70% of an administered dose is eliminated principally in urine as unchanged drug. Topiramate is not extensively metabolized; six minor metabolites have been identified, none of which constitutes more than 5% of an administered dose.

In patients with moderate (creatinine clearance 30–69 mL/minute per 1.73 m²) or severe (creatinine clearance less than 30 mL/minute per 1.73 m²) renal impairment, clearance of topiramate was reduced by 42 or 54%, respectively. However, since topiramate also undergoes substantial tubular reabsorption, the manufacturers state that creatinine clearance may not always predict clearance of topiramate. Geriatric patients with age-related renal impairment also may exhibit reduced clearance of the drug. In patients undergoing hemodialysis, clearance of topiramate is 4–6 times more rapid than in healthy individuals.

Although the mechanism is not well understood, patients with hepatic impairment may have decreased clearance of topiramate.

Changes in topiramate clearance also have been observed in pediatric patients.

ADVICE TO PATIENTS

- Advise the patient to read the FDA-approved patient labeling (Medication Guide).
- Counsel patients to swallow Qudexy® XR capsules whole or carefully open and sprinkle the entire contents on a spoonful of soft food. The drug/food mixture should be swallowed immediately and not chewed. Do not store drug/food mixture for future use. Counsel patients to swallow Trokendi XR® capsules whole and intact. Trokendi XR® should not be sprinkled on food, chewed or crushed.
- Counsel patients that Eprontia® may be taken with or without food. Advise patients that the dosage of Eprontia® should be measured using a calibrated measuring device and not a household teaspoon and an oral dosing syringe may be obtained from their pharmacist. Instruct patients to discard any unused Eprontia® after 30 days of first opening the bottle.
- Advise patients to completely avoid consumption of alcohol at least 6 hours prior to and 6 hours after taking Trokendi XR®.
- Instruct patients taking topiramate to seek immediate medical attention if they experience blurred vision, visual disturbances, or periorbital pain.
- Closely monitor patients treated with topiramate, especially pediatric patients, for evidence of decreased sweating and increased body temperature, especially in hot weather. Counsel patients to contact their healthcare professionals immediately if they develop a high or persistent fever, or decreased sweating.
- Warn patients about the potential significant risk for metabolic acidosis that may be asymptomatic and may be associated with adverse effects on kidneys (e.g., kidney stones, nephrocalcinosis), bones (e.g., osteoporosis, osteomalacia, and/or rickets in children), and growth (e.g., growth delay/retardation) in pediatric patients, and on the fetus.
- Counsel patients, their caregivers, and families that antiepileptic drugs, including topiramate, may increase the risk of suicidal thoughts and behavior, and advise of the need to be alert for the emergence or worsening of the signs and symptoms of depression, any unusual changes in mood or behavior or the emergence of suicidal thoughts, or behavior or thoughts about self-harm. Instruct patients to immediately report behaviors of concern to their healthcare providers.
- Warn patients about the potential for somnolence, dizziness, confusion, difficulty concentrating, or visual effects, and advise patients not to drive or operate machinery until they have gained sufficient experience on topiramate to gauge whether it adversely affects their mental performance, motor performance, and/or vision.
- Even when taking topiramate or other anticonvulsants, some patients with epilepsy will continue to have unpredictable seizures. Therefore, advise all patients taking topiramate for epilepsy to exercise appropriate caution when engaging in any activities where loss of consciousness could result in serious danger to themselves or those around them (including swimming, driving a car, climbing in high places, etc.). Some patients with refractory epilepsy will need to avoid such activities altogether. Discuss the appropriate level of caution with patients, before patients with epilepsy engage in such activities.
- Inform pregnant patients and females of reproductive potential that use of topiramate during pregnancy can cause fetal harm, including an increased risk for cleft lip and/or cleft palate (oral clefts), which occur early in pregnancy before many people know they are pregnant. Also inform patients that infants exposed to topiramate monotherapy in utero may be small for gestational age. There may also be risks to the fetus from chronic metabolic acidosis with use of topiramate during pregnancy. When appropriate, counsel pregnant patients and females of reproductive potential about alternative therapeutic options.
- Advise females of reproductive potential who are not planning a pregnancy to use effective contraception while using topiramate, keeping in mind that there is a potential for decreased contraceptive efficacy when using estrogen-containing birth control with topiramate.
- Encourage pregnant patients using topiramate to enroll in the North American Antiepileptic Drug (NAAED) Pregnancy Registry. The registry is collecting information about the safety of antiepileptic drugs during pregnancy.
- Inform the patient or caregiver that long-term treatment with topiramate can decrease bone formation and increase bone resorption in children.
- Discuss with the patient or caregiver that long-term topiramate treatment may attenuate growth as reflected by slower height increase and weight gain in pediatric patients.
- Inform patients about the signs of serious skin reactions. Instruct patients to immediately inform their healthcare provider at the first appearance of skin rash.
- Warn patients about the possible development of hyperammonemia with or without encephalopathy. Although hyperammonemia may be asymptomatic, clinical symptoms of hyperammonemic encephalopathy often include acute alterations in level of consciousness and/or cognitive function with lethargy and/or vomiting. This hyperammonemia and encephalopathy can develop with topiramate treatment alone or with topiramate treatment with concomitant valproic acid. Instruct patients to contact their physician if they develop unexplained lethargy, vomiting, or changes in mental status.
- Instruct patients, particularly those with predisposing factors, to maintain an adequate fluid intake in order to minimize the risk of kidney stone formation.
- Counsel patients taking extended-release forms of topiramate that these formulations can cause a reduction in body temperature, which can lead to alterations in mental status. If they note such changes, they should call their health care professional and measure their body temperature. Patients taking concomitant valproic acid should be specifically counseled on this potential adverse reaction.
- Instruct patients that if they miss a single dose of immediate-release topiramate, it should be taken as soon as possible. However, if a patient is within 6 hours of taking the next scheduled dose, tell the patient to wait until then to take the usual dose of topiramate and to skip the missed dose. Tell patients that they should not take a double dose in the event of a missed dose. Advise patients to contact their healthcare provider if they have missed more than one dose.
- Advise female patients to inform their clinician if they are or plan to become pregnant or plan to breast-feed.
- Advise patients to inform their clinician of existing or contemplated concomitant therapy, including prescription and OTC drugs and dietary and herbal supplements, as well as any concomitant illnesses.
- Advise patients of other important precautionary information. (See Cautions.)

PREPARATIONS

Excipients in commercially available drug preparations may have clinically important effects in some individuals; consult specific product labeling for details.

Topiramate

Oral

Capsules (containing coated particles)	15 mg*	**Topamax® Sprinkle Capsules**, Janssen **Topiramate Sprinkle Capsules**
	25 mg*	**Topamax® Sprinkle Capsules**, Janssen **Topiramate Sprinkle Capsules**
Capsules, extended-release	25 mg*	**Qudexy® XR**, Upsher-Smith **Topiramate Extended-release Capsules**
		Trokendi XR®, Supernus

	50 mg*	**Qudexy® XR**, Upsher-Smith
		Topiramate Extended-release Capsules
		Trokendi XR®, Supernus
	100 mg*	**Qudexy® XR**, Upsher-Smith
		Topiramate Extended-release Capsules
		Trokendi XR®, Supernus
	150 mg*	**Qudexy® XR**, Upsher-Smith
		Topiramate Extended-release Capsules
	200 mg*	**Qudexy® XR**, Upsher-Smith
		Topiramate Extended-release Capsules
		Trokendi XR®, Supernus
Solution	25 mg/mL	**Eprontia®**, Azurity
Tablets, film-coated	25 mg*	**Topamax®**, Janssen
		Topiramate Tablets
	50 mg*	**Topamax®**, Janssen
		Topiramate Tablets
	100 mg*	**Topamax®**, Janssen
		Topiramate Tablets
	200 mg*	**Topamax®**, Janssen
		Topiramate Tablets

* available from one or more manufacturer, distributor, and/or repackager by generic (nonproprietary) name

† Use is not currently included in the labeling approved by the US Food and Drug Administration.

Selected Revisions June 10, 2024, © Copyright, June 1, 1997, American Society of Health-System Pharmacists, Inc.

Monoamine Oxidase Inhibitors General Statement

28:16.04.12 • MONOAMINE OXIDASE INHIBITORS

■ Nonselective monoamine oxidase inhibitors block oxidative deamination of naturally occurring monoamines and are used as antidepressants.

USES

● Major Depressive Disorder

Monoamine oxidase (MAO) inhibitors with antidepressant action (phenelzine, tranylcypromine) are used in the treatment of major depressive disorder. A major depressive episode implies a prominent and relatively persistent depressed or dysphoric mood that usually interferes with daily functioning (nearly every day for at least 2 weeks). According to DSM-IV criteria, a major depressive episode includes at least 5 of the following 9 symptoms (with at least one of the symptoms being depressed mood or loss of interest or pleasure): depressed mood most of the day as indicated by subjective report (e.g., feels sad or empty) or observation made by others; markedly diminished interest or pleasure in all, or almost all, activities most of the day; significant weight loss (when not dieting) or weight gain (e.g., a change of more than 5% of body weight in a month) or decrease or increase in appetite; insomnia or hypersomnia; psychomotor agitation or retardation (observable by others, not merely subjective feelings of restlessness or being slowed down); fatigue or loss of energy; feelings of worthlessness or excessive or inappropriate guilt (not merely self-reproach or guilt about being sick); diminished ability to think or concentrate or indecisiveness (either by subjective account or as observed by others); and recurrent thoughts of death, recurrent suicidal ideation without a specific plan, or a suicide attempt or specific plan for committing suicide.

Treatment of major depressive disorder generally consists of an acute phase (to induce remission), a continuation phase (to preserve remission), and a maintenance phase (to prevent recurrence). Various interventions (e.g., psychotherapy, antidepressant drug therapy, electroconvulsive therapy [ECT]) are used alone or in combination to treat major depressive episodes. Treatment should be individualized and the most appropriate strategy for a particular patient is determined by clinical factors such as severity of depression (e.g., mild, moderate, severe), presence or absence of certain psychiatric features (e.g., suicide risk, catatonia, psychotic or atypical features, alcohol or substance abuse or dependence, panic or other anxiety disorder, cognitive dysfunction, dysthymia, personality disorder, seasonal affective disorder), and concurrent illness (e.g., asthma, cardiac disease, dementia, seizure disorder, glaucoma, hypertension). Demographic and psychosocial factors as well as patient preference also are used to determine the most effective treatment strategy.

While use of psychotherapy alone may be considered as an initial treatment strategy for patients with mild to moderate major depressive disorder (based on patient preference and presence of clinical features such as psychosocial stressors), combined use of antidepressant drug therapy and psychotherapy may be useful for initial treatment of patients with moderate to severe major depressive disorder with psychosocial issues, interpersonal problems, or a comorbid axis II disorder. In addition, combined use of antidepressant drug therapy and psychotherapy may be beneficial in patients who have a history of poor compliance or only partial response to adequate trials of either antidepressant drug therapy or psychotherapy alone.

Antidepressant drug therapy can be used alone for initial treatment of patients with mild major depressive disorder (if preferred by the patient) and usually is indicated alone or in combination with psychotherapy for initial treatment of patients with moderate to severe major depressive disorder (unless ECT is planned). ECT is not generally used for initial treatment of uncomplicated major depression, but is recommended as first-line treatment for severe major depressive disorder when it is coupled with psychotic features, catatonic stupor, severe suicidality, food refusal leading to nutritional compromise, or other situations when a rapid antidepressant response is required. ECT also is recommended for patients who have previously shown a positive response or a preference for this treatment modality

and can be considered for patients with moderate or severe depression who have not responded to or cannot receive antidepressant drug therapy. In certain situations involving severely depressed patients unresponsive to adequate trials of individual antidepressant agents, adjunctive therapy with another agent (e.g., buspirone, lithium) or concomitant use of a second antidepressant agent (e.g., bupropion) has been used; however, such combination therapy is associated with an increased risk of adverse reactions, may require dosage adjustments, and (if not contraindicated) should be undertaken only after careful consideration of the relative risks and benefits. (See Drug Interactions: Drugs Associated with Serotonin Syndrome and see Drug Interactions: Tricyclic Antidepressants.)

A variety of antidepressant drugs are available for the treatment of major depressive disorder, including selective serotonin-reuptake inhibitors (SSRIs) (e.g., citalopram, escitalopram, fluoxetine, paroxetine, sertraline), tricyclic antidepressants (e.g., amitriptyline, amoxapine, desipramine, doxepin, imipramine, nortriptyline, protriptyline, trimipramine), MAO inhibitors (e.g., phenelzine, tranylcypromine), and other antidepressants (e.g., bupropion, duloxetine, maprotiline, nefazodone, trazodone, venlafaxine). Most clinical studies have shown that the antidepressant effect of usual dosages of various antidepressant agents in patients with major depression are similar. Therefore, the choice of antidepressant agent for a given patient depends principally on other factors such as potential adverse effects, safety or tolerability of these adverse effects in the individual patient, psychiatric and medical history, patient or family history of response to specific therapies, patient preference, quantity and quality of available clinical data, cost, and relative acute overdose safety. No single antidepressant can be recommended as optimal for all patients because of substantial heterogeneity in individual responses and in the nature, likelihood, and severity of adverse effects. In addition, patients vary in the degree to which certain adverse effects and other inconveniences of drug therapy (e.g., cost, dietary restrictions) affect their preferences.

Because of the potential for serious adverse effects, MAO inhibitors generally are not used as initial therapy in the management of depression, but are reserved for patients who do not respond adequately to other antidepressant agents (e.g., SSRIs, tricyclic antidepressants) or in whom other therapies are contraindicated. It has been suggested that patients most likely to respond to MAO inhibitors are those who have depression with atypical features, including those who exhibit reactivity of mood and weight gain or increased appetite, sleep, and libido; those with a history of agoraphobia with secondary depression or agoraphobia with panic attacks; those with primary depression in whom pain or other somatic discomfort is the major complaint; and those with psychogenic pain or hypochondriasis and secondary depression. Phenelzine has been found to be effective in depressed patients clinically characterized as atypical, nonendogenous, or neurotic (these patients often have mixed anxiety and depression and phobic or hypochondriacal features), but there is less conclusive evidence that phenelzine is useful in severely depressed patients with endogenous features. Tranylcypromine is indicated for the treatment of major depressive episodes without melancholia, and effectiveness of the drug in patients who have major depressive episodes with melancholia (endogenous features) has not been established. MAO inhibitors appear to be particularly effective in reducing psychomotor retardation and morbid preoccupation. Somatic signs and symptoms associated with depression, including sleep and eating disturbances, also are reduced during MAO inhibitor therapy.

For further information on treatment of major depressive disorder and considerations in choosing the most appropriate antidepressant agent for a particular patient, including considerations related to patient tolerance, patient age, and cardiovascular, sedative, and suicidal risks, see Considerations in Choosing Antidepressants under Uses: Major Depressive Disorder, in the Tricyclic Antidepressants General Statement 28:16.04.28.

● Parkinsonian Syndrome

Certain MAO inhibitors that have increased selectivity for MAO-B (i.e., rasagiline, safinamide, selegiline) are used for the symptomatic treatment of parkinsonian syndrome (e.g., parkinsonism, Parkinson disease [paralysis agitans]); these drugs generally are *not* used for the management of major depressive disorder. For additional information on the use of MAO-B inhibitors in the management of parkinsonian syndrome, see the individual monographs for Rasagiline Mesylate, Safinamide Mesylate, and Selegiline Hydrochloride in 28:36.32.

● Eating Disorders

MAO inhibitors (e.g., phenelzine) have been used with some success in the management of bulimia nervosa†. However, MAO inhibitors potentially are dangerous in patients with chaotic binge eating and purging behaviors and the American Psychiatric Association (APA) states that MAO inhibitors should be used with caution in the management of bulimia nervosa. For information on the diagnosis and treatment of bulimia nervosa and other eating disorders, see Uses: Eating Disorders, in Fluoxetine Hydrochloride 28:16.04.20.

DOSAGE AND ADMINISTRATION

● Administration

Monoamine oxidase (MAO) inhibitors are administered orally.

● Dosage

There is a wide range of individual requirements for MAO inhibitor dosage, and dosage must be carefully adjusted according to individual requirements and response, using the lowest possible effective dosage. The initial dosage may be increased gradually according to the patient's tolerance and therapeutic response; however, because therapeutic response to the drugs may be delayed for several days to up to 4 weeks or more, sufficient time should be allowed between increases in dosage. Some manufacturers recommend that at least 1–2 weeks elapse between dosage adjustments. Dosage should be increased more gradually in debilitated, emaciated, or geriatric patients.

Patients receiving MAO inhibitors should be monitored for possible worsening of depression, suicidality, or unusual changes in behavior, especially at the beginning of therapy or during periods of dosage adjustment. (See Worsening of Depression and Suicidality Risk under Cautions: Precautions and Contraindications.)

CAUTIONS

The potential adverse effects of monoamine oxidase (MAO) inhibitors are more varied and potentially more serious than those reported for most other classes of antidepressant agents. Because monoamine oxidase is widely distributed throughout the body, MAO inhibitor therapy can be expected to cause diverse pharmacologic effects. Many adverse effects of MAO inhibitors are mild to moderate in severity and often subside as therapy is continued. However, serious reactions requiring discontinuance of therapy can occur and usually involve the cardiovascular, CNS, and hepatic systems. Some of the most serious adverse effects reported with MAO inhibitors (e.g., hypertensive crisis, serotonin syndrome) have occurred when MAO inhibitors were administered concomitantly with certain foods or prescription or nonprescription (OTC) drugs.

The adverse effect profiles of phenelzine and tranylcypromine are similar; reports of differences among the individual MAO inhibitors have been poorly substantiated.

● Cardiovascular Effects

Orthostatic Hypotension

Orthostatic hypotension is a common adverse effect of MAO inhibitors. Although it has been reported most frequently in patients with preexisting hypertension, it also has occurred in normotensive and hypotensive patients. Hypertensive patients may occasionally experience a transient moderate rise in blood pressure while receiving MAO inhibitors, but these patients more commonly exhibit symptoms of orthostatic hypotension. Unlike hypotension reported with tricyclic antidepressants, hypotension related to MAO inhibitors affects both supine and postural blood pressure changes.

Orthostatic hypotension reported with MAO inhibitors is dose related, and may result in syncope at high doses. In patients who show some hypotensive response during initiation of MAO inhibitor therapy, dosage should be increased gradually. Postural hypotension may be relieved by having the patient lie down until blood pressure returns to normal. If orthostatic hypotension persists or is severe, dosage should be reduced or therapy with the drugs discontinued.

Hypertensive Crisis

One of the most serious adverse effects associated with MAO inhibitor therapy is hypertensive crisis, which has been fatal in some patients. Several cases of spontaneous hypertension or significant increases in supine blood pressure without similar changes in standing blood pressure have been reported in patients receiving phenelzine or tranylcypromine, and it has been suggested that a family history of hypertension may be a risk factor for MAO inhibitor-induced hypertensive events. However, most reported cases of hypertensive crisis in patients receiving MAO inhibitor therapy usually have occurred when the drugs were used concomitantly with certain food or prescription or nonprescription drugs. (See Drug Interactions: Food and Drugs Associated with Hypertensive Crisis.)

Hypertensive crisis is characterized by severe headache (occipital headache which may radiate frontally); palpitation; neck stiffness or soreness; nausea or vomiting; sweating (sometimes with fever and sometimes with cold, clammy skin); and mydriasis and/or visual disturbances such as photophobia. Tachycardia or bradycardia may be present, and associated constricting chest pain and dilated pupils may occur. Intracranial hemorrhage, which may be fatal, has also been reported to occur in some patients with hypertensive crisis.

If a hypertensive crisis or prodromal signs of a hypertensive crisis occur, MAO inhibitor therapy should be discontinued and appropriate therapy to lower blood pressure should be instituted immediately. Phentolamine has been considered the hypotensive drug of choice for the management of MAO inhibitor-induced hypertensive crisis. Phentolamine should be given by IV injection; the drug should be administered slowly to avoid producing an excessive hypotensive effect. The usual adult dose of phentolamine for the treatment of hypertensive crisis is 5 mg. In general, headache tends to subside as blood pressure is lowered. Fever should be managed by external cooling. Other symptomatic and supportive measures may be necessary in some patients; however, administration of parenteral reserpine should be avoided. (See Sympathomimetic Agents and Catecholamine-releasing Agents under Drug Interactions: Food and Drugs Associated with Hypertensive Crisis.)

● Nervous System Effects

The most common adverse CNS effects of MAO inhibitors include dizziness, headache (without increases in blood pressure), drowsiness, sleep disturbances (e.g., insomnia, hypersomnia), fatigue, weakness, tremors, twitching, myoclonic movements, and hyperreflexia. In addition, confusion, disorientation, memory loss, palilalia, euphoria, nystagmus, akinesia, and paresthesias have been reported.

Hyperexcitability, increased anxiety, agitation, restlessness, manic symptoms, and precipitation of schizophrenia, have occurred in some patients receiving high dosages of MAO inhibitors. If these symptoms occur, dosage should be reduced or a phenothiazine agent should be administered concomitantly.

Worsening of depression and/or emergence of suicidal ideation and behavior (suicidality) or unusual changes in behavior may occur with antidepressants. (See Worsening of Depression and Suicidality Risk under Cautions: Precautions and Contraindications.)

Rarely, ataxia, shock-like coma, toxic delirium, manic reactions, seizures, and acute anxiety reaction have occurred in patients receiving MAO inhibitors.

Serotonin syndrome has occurred rarely in patients receiving MAO inhibitors when other drugs that increase serotonin availability were used concomitantly. Although serotonin syndrome occurs only rarely, it has the potential to cause fatalities. (See Drug Interactions: Drugs Associated with Serotonin Syndrome.)

● GI Effects

Adverse GI effects reported with MAO inhibitors include constipation, dry mouth, and GI disturbances. Anorexia, nausea, vomiting, arthralgia, increased appetite, and weight gain also have been reported.

● Hepatic Effects

Although the potential for hepatotoxicity with commercially available MAO inhibitors is lower than with prototypical MAO inhibitors (iproniazid), such toxicities, when they do occur, can be serious because the hydrazine derivatives cause cellular damage to the hepatic parenchyma. A carefully controlled study has shown that patients with impaired liver function may be especially sensitive to tranylcypromine. The manufacturers of commercially available MAO inhibitors report that the most common adverse hepatic effect is elevated plasma transaminase concentrations (without accompanying signs or symptoms of hepatotoxicity). Reversible jaundice and fatal progressive necrotizing hepatocellular damage have been reported rarely.

● Genitourinary Effects

Impotence, ejaculatory disturbances, and anorgasmia have been reported in patients receiving phenelzine or tranylcypromine. Urinary frequency, urinary retention, and urinary incontinence also have been reported in patients receiving MAO inhibitors.

● Dermatologic Effects

Although a causal relationship to MAO inhibitors has not been established, localized scleroderma, flare-up of cystic acne, rash, pruritus, urticaria, purpura, increased sweating, and photosensitivity have been reported in patients receiving MAO inhibitors.

● Metabolic Effects

A hypermetabolic syndrome, which may include, but is not limited to, hyperpyrexia, tachycardia, tachypnea, muscular rigidity, elevated creatine kinase (CK, creatine phosphokinase, CPK) concentrations, metabolic acidosis, hypoxia, and coma and may resemble an overdose, has been described in patients receiving MAO inhibitors.

● Ocular Effects

Rarely, therapy with MAO inhibitors has been associated with adverse ocular effects (e.g., amblyopia, visual disturbances, blurred vision). Aggravation of glaucoma has also occurred. Retinal degradation, retinal scarring, cataracts, and loss of photoreceptor cells have been observed in animal toxicity studies with safinamide.

● Hematologic Effects

A normocytic, normochromic anemia has reportedly developed in some patients receiving MAO inhibitors. Leukopenia, agranulocytosis, and thrombocytopenia also have been reported.

● Other Effects

Other adverse effects of MAO inhibitors include arthralgia, lupus-like syndrome, edema of the glottis, fissuring in the corner of the mouth, and impaired water excretion resembling syndrome of inappropriate secretion of antidiuretic hormone (SIADH).

● Precautions and Contraindications

MAO inhibitors can cause potentially serious adverse effects, and should only be used in carefully selected patients who can be closely supervised and only by clinicians who are completely familiar with the proper use, potential adverse effects, and associated precautions and contraindications of the drugs. MAO inhibitors generally are not used as initial therapy in the management of depression, but are reserved for patients who do not respond adequately to other antidepressant agents (e.g., selective serotonin-reuptake inhibitors [SSRIs], tricyclic antidepressants) or in whom other therapies are contraindicated.

Hypertensive Crisis

Potentially fatal hypertensive crisis has been reported in patients receiving MAO inhibitors, and blood pressure should be monitored closely in all patients to detect any evidence of a pressor response; however, full reliance should not be placed on blood pressure determinations alone. The patient's clinical status should be observed frequently, particularly for signs and symptoms of hypertension. In addition, all patients receiving MAO inhibitors should be warned to contact their clinician promptly if headache or other unusual symptoms occur (e.g., palpitation and/or tachycardia, a sense of constriction of the throat or chest, sweating, dizziness, neck stiffness, nausea or vomiting). If palpitation or frequent or severe headaches occur during MAO inhibitor therapy, the drug should be discontinued immediately, since these may be prodromal symptoms of a hypertensive reaction. (See Cautions: Cardiovascular Effects.)

Because hypertensive crisis may occur if MAO inhibitors are used concomitantly with certain foods that contain large amounts of tyramine or tryptophan, patients receiving MAO inhibitors should be warned against eating food that has a high tyramine or tryptophan content and also should be advised not to consume alcohol (since tyramine is present in certain alcoholic beverages) or excessive amounts of caffeine in any form. (See Drug Interactions: Food and Drugs Associated with Hypertensive Crisis.)

Because of the potential for hypertensive crisis, concomitant use of MAO inhibitors and some sympathomimetic agents (e.g., amphetamines, dopamine, epinephrine, norepinephrine, methylphenidate) or related substances (e.g., methyldopa, levodopa, L-tryptophan, L-tyrosine, phenylalanine) is contraindicated. In addition, patients receiving MAO inhibitors should be cautioned not to take prescription or nonprescription (OTC) cold, hay fever, or weight-reducing preparations unless under the direction of a clinician, since many of these preparations contain pressor agents. (See Drug Interactions: Food and Drugs Associated with Hypertensive Crisis.) To help avoid possible drug interactions, patients receiving MAO inhibitors should be instructed to inform their other clinicians and their dentist that they are receiving an MAO inhibitor.

MAO inhibitors are contraindicated in patients with pheochromocytoma. The drugs also are contraindicated in patients with confirmed or suspected cerebrovascular or cardiovascular disease, including hypertension and congestive heart failure. Since headache may be the first symptom of a hypertensive reaction during MAO inhibitor therapy, the drugs should not be used in patients with a history of severe or frequent headaches.

Worsening of Depression and Suicidality Risk

Worsening of depression and/or the emergence of suicidal ideation and behavior (suicidality) or unusual changes in behavior may occur in both adult and pediatric (see Cautions: Pediatric Precautions) patients with major depressive disorder or other psychiatric disorders, whether or not they are taking antidepressants. This risk may persist until clinically important remission occurs. Suicide is a known risk of depression and certain other psychiatric disorders, and these disorders themselves are the strongest predictors of suicide. However, there has been a long-standing concern that antidepressants may have a role in inducing worsening of depression and the emergence of suicidality in certain patients during the early phases of treatment. Pooled analyses of short-term, placebo-controlled studies of antidepressants (i.e., selective serotonin-reuptake inhibitors and other antidepressants) have shown an increased risk of suicidality in children, adolescents, and young adults (18–24 years of age) with major depressive disorder and other psychiatric disorders. An increased suicidality risk was not demonstrated with antidepressants compared with placebo in adults older than 24 years of age, and a reduced risk was observed in adults 65 years of age or older. It is currently unknown whether the suicidality risk extends to longer-term use (i.e., beyond several months); however, there is substantial evidence from placebo-controlled maintenance trials in adults with major depressive disorder that antidepressants can delay the recurrence of depression.

The US Food and Drug Administration (FDA) recommends that all patients being treated with antidepressants for any indication be appropriately monitored and closely observed for clinical worsening, suicidality, and unusual changes in behavior, particularly during initiation of therapy (i.e., the first few months) and during periods of dosage adjustments. Families and caregivers of patients being treated with antidepressants for major depressive disorder or other indications, both psychiatric and nonpsychiatric, also should be advised to monitor patients on a daily basis for the emergence of agitation, irritability, or unusual changes in behavior, as well as the emergence of suicidality, and to report such symptoms immediately to a health-care provider.

Although a causal relationship between the emergence of symptoms such as anxiety, agitation, panic attacks, insomnia, irritability, hostility, aggressiveness, impulsivity, akathisia, hypomania, and/or mania and either the worsening of depression and/or the emergence of suicidal impulses has not been established, there is concern that such symptoms may represent precursors to emerging suicidality. Consequently, consideration should be given to changing the therapeutic regimen or discontinuing therapy in patients whose depression is persistently worse or in patients experiencing emergent suicidality or symptoms that might be precursors to worsening depression or suicidality, particularly if such manifestations are severe, abrupt in onset, or were not part of the patient's presenting symptoms. FDA also recommends that the drugs be prescribed in the smallest quantity consistent with good patient management, in order to reduce the risk of overdosage.

Bipolar Disorder

It is generally believed (though not established in controlled trials) that treating a major depressive episode with an antidepressant alone may increase the likelihood of precipitating a mixed or manic episode in patients at risk for bipolar disorder. Therefore, patients should be adequately screened for bipolar disorder prior to initiating treatment with an antidepressant; such screening should include a detailed psychiatric history (e.g., family history of suicide, bipolar disorder, and depression). MAO inhibitors are *not* approved for use in treating bipolar depression in adults.

When MAO inhibitors are used in patients with bipolar disorder, there may be a mood swing to mania. If such a mood swing occurs, MAO inhibitor therapy should be temporarily withheld and subsequently resumed at a reduced dosage.

Other Precautions and Contraindications

Since MAO inhibitors may suppress anginal pain that would otherwise serve as a warning sign of myocardial ischemia, patients with angina pectoris or coronary artery disease should be warned against overexertion.

MAO inhibitors should be used with caution in patients with impaired renal function, since the drugs may accumulate in plasma in these patients.

Since MAO inhibitors have a variable effect on the seizure threshold, the drugs should be used with caution in patients with a history of seizures.

Nonselective MAO inhibitors should be used with caution in patients with parkinsonian syndrome, since the drugs may increase the frequency and severity of signs and symptoms associated with this disorder. Selective MAO-B inhibitors (e.g., rasagiline, safinamide, selegiline), on the other hand, have been used principally for the management of parkinsonian syndrome.

Since hepatic damage (e.g., progressive necrotizing hepatocellular damage) has occurred in some patients receiving MAO inhibitors (e.g., isocarboxazid [no longer commercially available in the US], phenelzine), periodic evaluation of liver function (i.e., bilirubin, serum alkaline phosphatase, serum aminotransferases [transaminases]) is recommended in patients receiving high dosages and in those receiving prolonged therapy with the drugs. MAO inhibitors are contraindicated in patients with a history of liver disease or abnormal liver function tests.

There is conflicting evidence regarding whether MAO inhibitors affect glucose metabolism or potentiate antidiabetic agents. Use of MAO inhibitors in patients receiving insulin or oral antidiabetic agents has been associated with hypoglycemic episodes. MAO inhibitors should be used with caution in diabetic patients who are receiving insulin or oral antidiabetic agents.

MAO inhibitors should be used with caution in patients with hyperthyroidism, since these patients have an increased sensitivity to pressor amines.

Since inhibition of monoamine oxidase may persist for several days following discontinuance of therapy, it is suggested that MAO inhibitors be discontinued for at least 10 days prior to elective surgery to allow time for recovery of enzymatic activity before general anesthetics are used. (See Drug Interactions: Anesthetics.)

MAO inhibitors are contraindicated in patients currently receiving, or having recently received, SSRIs or tricyclic antidepressants. (See Drug Interactions: Drugs Associated with Serotonin Syndrome and see Drug Interactions: Tricyclic Antidepressants.)

MAO inhibitors are contraindicated in patients who are hypersensitive to the drugs or any ingredients in the formulations.

● Pediatric Precautions

Safety and efficacy of phenelzine in children younger than 16 years of age have not been established. Safety and efficacy of tranylcypromine in pediatric patients have not been established.

FDA warns that antidepressants increase the risk of suicidal thinking and behavior (suicidality) in children and adolescents with major depressive disorder and other psychiatric disorders. The risk of suicidality for these drugs was identified in a pooled analysis of data from a total of 24 short-term (4–16 weeks), placebo-controlled studies of 9 antidepressants (i.e., bupropion, citalopram, fluoxetine, fluvoxamine, mirtazapine, nefazodone, paroxetine, sertraline, venlafaxine) in over 4400 children and adolescents with major depressive disorder, obsessive-compulsive disorder (OCD), or other psychiatric disorders. The analysis revealed a greater risk of adverse events representing suicidal behavior or thinking (suicidality) during the first few months of treatment in pediatric patients receiving antidepressants than in those receiving placebo. The average risk of such events was 4% among children and adolescents receiving these drugs, twice the risk (2%) that was observed among those receiving placebo. However, a more recent meta-analysis of 27 placebo-controlled trials of 9 antidepressants (SSRIs and others) in patients younger than 19 years of age with major depressive disorder, OCD, or non-OCD anxiety disorders suggests that the benefits of antidepressant therapy in treating these conditions may outweigh the risks of suicidal behavior or suicidal ideation. No suicides occurred in these pediatric trials.

The risk of suicidality in FDA's pooled analysis differed across the various psychiatric indications, with the highest incidence observed in the major depressive disorder studies. In addition, although there was considerable variation in risk among the antidepressants, a tendency toward an increase in suicidality risk in younger patients was found for almost all drugs studied. It is currently unknown whether the suicidality risk in pediatric patients extends to longer-term use (i.e., beyond several months).

As a result of this analysis and public discussion of the issue, FDA has directed manufacturers of all antidepressants to add a boxed warning to the labeling of their products to alert clinicians of this suicidality risk in children and adolescents and to recommend appropriate monitoring and close observation of patients receiving these agents. (See Worsening of Depression and Suicidality Risk under Cautions: Precautions and Contraindications.) The drugs that are the focus of the revised labeling are all drugs included in the general class of antidepressants, including those that have not been studied in controlled clinical trials in pediatric patients, since the available data are not adequate to exclude any single antidepressant from an increased risk. In addition to the boxed warning and other information in professional labeling on antidepressants, FDA currently recommends that a patient medication guide explaining the risks associated with the drugs be provided to the patient each time the drugs are dispensed.

Anyone considering the use of antidepressants in a child or adolescent for any clinical use must balance the potential risk of therapy with the clinical need.

● Geriatric Precautions

Clinical experience to date with MAO inhibitors in geriatric patients has not identified any differences in responses between geriatric and younger adults. However, geriatric patients appear to be more susceptible to adverse effects of MAO inhibitors (e.g., episodes of hypertension, malignant hyperthermia) than younger patients, and these adverse effects are associated with increased morbidity in geriatric patients since they have less compensatory reserve to cope with any serious adverse reactions. Therefore, MAO inhibitor therapy should be initiated cautiously in geriatric patients using a low initial dosage and patients observed closely since renal, hepatic, and cardiovascular dysfunction and concomitant disease or other drug therapy are more common in this age group than in younger patients.

In pooled data analyses, a *reduced* risk of suicidality was observed in adults 65 years of age or older with antidepressant therapy compared with placebo. (See Precautions and Contraindications: Worsening of Depression and Suicidality Risk, in Cautions.)

● Pregnancy, Fertility, and Lactation

Pregnancy

Safety of MAO inhibitors during pregnancy has not been established. Administration of phenelzine to pregnant mice resulted in a decrease in the number of viable offspring, and the growth of young dogs and rats has been retarded by phenelzine dosages exceeding the maximum human dosage. Tranylcypromine has been shown to cross the placenta in rats. It is not known whether MAO inhibitors can cause fetal harm when administered to pregnant women, and the drugs should be used during pregnancy only when the potential benefits justify the possible risks to the fetus.

Fertility

The effect of MAO inhibitors on fertility in humans is not known. Sexual disturbances including impotence and delayed ejaculation have occurred in some individuals during MAO inhibitor therapy.

Lactation

It is not known if MAO inhibitors are distributed into human milk; however, tranylcypromine is distributed into the milk of lactating dogs. MAO inhibitors should be used with caution in nursing women.

DRUG INTERACTIONS

● Food and Drugs Associated with Hypertensive Crisis

Concomitant use of MAO inhibitors and certain food or prescription or nonprescription (over-the-counter, OTC) drugs can result in interactions that have the potential to cause hypertensive crisis due to the release and potentiation of catecholamines similar to that experienced in pheochromocytoma. The severity and consequences of such interactions vary among individuals. If only minor increases in blood pressure occur, patients may be unaware of the interactions. However, if substantial and rapid increases in blood pressure (an increase of 30 mm Hg or more in systolic blood pressure within 20 minutes) occur, patients may experience symptoms associated with subarachnoid hemorrhage or cardiac failure (sudden severe occipital headache, palpitations) if the cerebral vasculature or cardiac musculature are already weakened. (See Hypertensive Crisis under Cautions: Cardiovascular Effects.)

Food

Hypertensive crises have occurred following ingestion of foods containing large amounts of tyramine or tryptophan in some patients receiving MAO inhibitors. In general, patients should avoid protein foods that have undergone protein breakdown by aging, fermentation, pickling, smoking, or bacterial contamination; protein extracts and liquid or powdered dietary supplements also should be avoided. Patients should be specifically instructed not to eat foods such as cheese, particularly strong or aged varieties (e.g., cheddar, Camembert, Stilton) and processed cheese; sour cream; wine, especially chianti, champagne, and alcohol-free or reduced-alcohol wine products; beer, including alcohol-free and reduced-alcohol beers; pickled herring; anchovies; caviar; shrimp paste; liver, especially chicken liver; dry sausage (e.g., Genoa salami, hard salami, pepperoni, Lebanon bologna); figs, particularly if overripe, or canned figs; raisins; bananas or avocados, particularly if overripe; chocolate; soy sauce; bean curd; yeast extracts (including brewer's yeast in large quantities); yogurt; papaya products, including certain meat tenderizers; and pods of broad beans (e.g., fava beans). Excessive amounts of caffeine may also reportedly precipitate hypertensive crisis. Specialized references on food constituents or a dietician should be consulted for more specific information on the tyramine content of foods and beverages.

Sympathomimetic Agents and Catecholamine-releasing Agents

Because some patients appear to be particularly sensitive to the hypertensive effects of sympathomimetic agents during MAO inhibitor therapy, centrally acting sympathomimetic agents (e.g., amphetamines) or peripherally acting sympathomimetic agents, including prescription or nonprescription cold, hay fever, or weight-reducing preparations that contain pressor agents (e.g., ephedrine) generally should not be administered concomitantly with an MAO inhibitor. The manufacturer of rasagiline states that concomitant use of the drug with sympathomimetic agents should be employed with caution. The manufacturer of safinamide states that concomitant use of the drug with methylphenidate or amphetamines is contraindicated and that patients receiving safinamide in conjunction with other prescription or nonprescription sympathomimetics should be monitored for hypertension.

Parenteral or oral administration of reserpine or guanethidine in patients receiving MAO inhibitors may cause a severe pressor response as a result of a sudden release of accumulated catecholamines. Therefore, the manufacturers of MAO inhibitors do not recommend concomitant use of guanethidine in patients receiving an MAO inhibitor and also recommend that reserpine be administered cautiously in patients receiving MAO inhibitors.

Levodopa and other Catecholamines

Hypertension, headache, hyperexcitability, and related symptoms reportedly have occurred in patients receiving MAO inhibitors concurrently with methyldopa, dopamine, or levodopa. It has been suggested that use of a decarboxylase inhibitor (e.g., carbidopa) with levodopa may prevent hypertensive reactions during concomitant therapy with an MAO inhibitor.

● *Drugs Associated with Serotonin Syndrome*

Serotonin syndrome may occur in patients receiving MAO inhibitors in combination with other serotonergic drugs. Although the syndrome appears to be relatively uncommon and usually mild in severity, serious complications, including seizures, disseminated intravascular coagulation, respiratory failure, severe hyperthermia, and death occasionally have been reported. The precise mechanism of the syndrome is not fully understood; however, it appears to result from excessive serotonergic activity in the CNS, probably mediated by activation of serotonin 5-HT_{1A} receptors. The possible involvement of dopamine and 5-HT_2 receptors also has been suggested, although their roles remain unclear.

The syndrome most commonly occurs when 2 or more serotonergic agents with different mechanisms of action are administered either concurrently or in close succession. Serotonergic agents include those that increase serotonin synthesis (e.g., the serotonin precursor tryptophan), stimulate synaptic serotonin release (e.g., some amphetamines, dexfenfluramine [no longer commercially available in the US], fenfluramine [no longer commercially available in the US]), inhibit the reuptake of serotonin after release (e.g., selective serotonin-reuptake inhibitors [SSRIs], tricyclic antidepressants, trazodone, dextromethorphan, meperidine, tramadol), decrease the metabolism of serotonin (e.g., MAO inhibitors), have direct serotonin postsynaptic receptor activity (e.g., buspirone), or nonspecifically induce increases in serotonergic neuronal activity (e.g., lithium salts).

The combination of MAO inhibitors and SSRI antidepressants (e.g., fluoxetine) appears to be responsible for most of the recent case reports of serotonin syndrome. The syndrome also has been reported when MAO inhibitors have been combined with tricyclic antidepressants, tryptophan, meperidine, or dextromethorphan. In rare cases, serotonin syndrome reportedly has occurred with the recommended dosage of a single serotonergic agent (e.g., clomipramine) or during accidental overdosage (e.g., sertraline intoxication in a child). Some other drugs that have been implicated in certain circumstances include buspirone, bromocriptine, dextropropoxyphene, methylenedioxymethamphetamine (MDMA; "ecstasy"), and selegiline (a selective MAO-B inhibitor). Other drugs that have been associated with the syndrome but for which less convincing data are available include carbamazepine, fentanyl, and pentazocine.

Clinicians should be aware of the potential for serious, possibly fatal reactions associated with serotonin syndrome in patients receiving 2 or more drugs that increase the availability of serotonin in the CNS, even if no such interactions with the specific drugs have been reported to date in the medical literature. Pending further data, all drugs with serotonergic activity should be used cautiously in combination and such combinations avoided whenever clinically possible. Some clinicians state that patients who have experienced serotonin syndrome may be at higher risk for recurrence of the syndrome upon reinitiation of serotonergic drugs. Pending further experience in such cases, some clinicians recommend that therapy with serotonergic agents be limited following recovery. In cases in which the potential benefit of the drug is thought to outweigh the risk of serotonin syndrome, lower potency agents and reduced dosages should be used, combination serotonergic therapy should be avoided, and patients should be monitored carefully for symptoms of serotonin syndrome. For further information on serotonin syndrome, including manifestations and treatment, see Serotonin Syndrome under Drug Interactions: Drugs Associated with Serotonin Syndrome, in Fluoxetine Hydrochloride 28:16.04.20.

Selective Serotonin-reuptake Inhibitors

Concurrent use of SSRIs and MAO inhibitors potentially is hazardous and may result in serotonin syndrome. Probably because of its extensive clinical use and the prolonged elimination half-life of both fluoxetine and norfluoxetine, fluoxetine has been the SSRI most commonly implicated in serotonin syndrome when combined with MAO inhibitor therapy. In at least 2 cases, serotonin syndrome has developed when MAO inhibitor therapy has been initiated after the discontinuance of fluoxetine therapy. Shivering, diplopia, nausea, confusion, and anxiety reportedly occurred in one patient 6 days after discontinuance of fluoxetine therapy and 4 days after initiation of tranylcypromine therapy; signs and symptoms resolved without apparent sequelae within 24 hours following discontinuance of the MAO inhibitor in this patient. In another case, the initiation of tranylcypromine therapy more than 5 weeks after discontinuance of fluoxetine reportedly resulted in serotonin syndrome. The manufacturer of fluoxetine, the manufacturers of MAO inhibitors, and some clinicians state that concurrent use of fluoxetine with MAO inhibitors is contraindicated or generally should be avoided. Because both fluoxetine and its principal metabolite have relatively long half-lives, the manufacturer of fluoxetine, the manufacturers of MAO inhibitors, and some clinicians recommend that at least 5 weeks elapse between discontinuance of fluoxetine therapy and initiation of MAO inhibitor therapy, since administration of an MAO inhibitor prior to elapse of this time may increase the risk of serious adverse effects. Although the manufacturers of some MAO inhibitors (i.e., phenelzine) recommend that at least 10 days elapse following discontinuance of MAO inhibitor therapy prior to initiation of fluoxetine therapy, based on clinical experience with concurrent administration of tricyclic antidepressants and MAO inhibitors, the manufacturers of fluoxetine and the manufacturers of some MAO inhibitors (e.g., selegiline, tranylcypromine) recommend that at least 2 weeks elapse following discontinuance of an MAO inhibitor prior to initiation of fluoxetine therapy.

Other SSRI antidepressants, including sertraline and citalopram, also have been associated with serotonin syndrome when given in combination with MAO inhibitors. Because of the potential risk of serotonin syndrome when SSRIs are combined with MAO inhibitor therapy, the manufacturers of fluvoxamine, paroxetine, and sertraline currently recommend that a drug-free interval of at least 2 weeks elapse when switching from an MAO inhibitor to these agents or when switching from these agents to an MAO inhibitor. The manufacturer of the selective MAO-B inhibitor safinamide states that if safinamide is used concomitantly with an SSRI, the lowest effective dosage of the SSRI should be used.

Moclobemide, a selective and reversible MAO-A inhibitor (not commercially available in the US), also has been associated with serotonin syndrome and such reactions have been fatal in several cases in which the drug was given in combination with citalopram or with clomipramine. Pending further experience with such combinations, some clinicians recommend that concurrent therapy with moclobemide and SSRIs be used only with extreme caution and that the SSRI should have been discontinued for some time (depending on the elimination half-lives of the drug and its active metabolites) before initiating moclobemide therapy.

Tryptophan

Although tryptophan sometimes has been used to enhance the antidepressant activity of MAO inhibitors, serotonin syndrome, which was fatal in at least one case, has been reported in a limited number of patients receiving these drugs in combination either with or without concurrent lithium therapy. While the mechanism for this interaction has not been fully elucidated, it has been suggested that these adverse effects resemble serotonin syndrome and therefore may result from a marked increase in serotonin availability in the CNS when these agents are administered concurrently. Behavioral and neurologic syndromes, including disorientation, confusion, amnesia, delirium, agitation, hypomanic signs, ataxia, myoclonus, hyperreflexia, shivering, ocular oscillations, and Babinski signs, also have been reported in patients receiving MAO inhibitors and tryptophan concomitantly. Pending further evaluation of this potential interaction, clinicians should be aware that toxic reactions may occur when MAO inhibitors and tryptophan are administered concomitantly.

Buspirone

Elevations in blood pressure have been observed in several patients receiving an MAO inhibitor and buspirone concomitantly; no adverse sequelae were associated with these elevations. Buspirone may have been partially responsible for a case of serotonin syndrome that resulted in the death of a patient receiving buspirone, an MAO inhibitor (tranylcypromine), and fluoxetine concomitantly. Pending accumulation of additional data, it is recommended that MAO inhibitors not be used concomitantly with buspirone. Some manufacturers recommend that at least 10 days elapse between discontinuance of MAO inhibitor therapy and administration of buspirone.

● Tricyclic Antidepressants

Concomitant use of MAO inhibitors with tricyclic antidepressants is contraindicated or generally should be avoided, and it generally is recommended that at least 2 weeks should elapse between discontinuance of tricyclic antidepressant therapy or MAO inhibitor therapy and initiation of therapy with the other class of drugs. Serious, sometimes fatal, reactions including hyperpyrexia, confusion, diaphoresis, myoclonus, rigidity, seizures, cardiovascular disturbances, and coma have occurred in patients who received an MAO inhibitor and a tricyclic antidepressant concomitantly. Patients receiving therapeutic dosages of an oral MAO inhibitor and an oral tricyclic antidepressant concomitantly generally have experienced nonfatal hyperpyrexia, hypertension, tachycardia, confusion, and seizures; most reported cases of hyperpyretic crises, severe seizures, or death occurred following overdosage or parenteral administration of one or both drugs. Although the mechanism has not been clearly established, these reactions resemble serotonin syndrome and may be caused by excessive serotonergic activity in CNS. (See Drug Interactions: Drugs Associated with Serotonin Syndrome.)

● CNS Depressants

Several manufacturers caution that MAO inhibitors may be additive with, or may potentiate the action of, CNS depressants such as opiates or other analgesics, barbiturates or other sedatives, anesthetics, or alcohol. CNS depressants should be administered cautiously to patients receiving MAO inhibitors in order to avoid excessive sedation and acute hypotension; a reduction in dosage of the CNS depressant agent(s) may be necessary. One manufacturer recommends that, if emergency surgery is necessary in a patient receiving an MAO inhibitor, the dose of opiate, sedative, analgesic, and other premedication be reduced to one-fourth to one-fifth the usual dose.

Meperidine

Meperidine should *not* be used in patients receiving MAO inhibitors since severe, generally immediate reactions, including excitation, sweating, rigidity, and hypertension, suggestive of serotonin syndrome, have occurred. Circulatory collapse and death have also occurred following administration of a single dose of meperidine in some patients receiving an MAO inhibitor.

Dextromethorphan

Concomitant use of MAO inhibitors and dextromethorphan (ingested as a lozenge) has been reported to cause brief episodes of psychosis or bizarre behavior.

Cases of apparent serotonin syndrome, including at least 2 fatalities, have been reported in patients receiving concurrent MAO inhibitor and dextromethorphan therapy. Dextromethorphan preparations should *not* be used in patients receiving an MAO inhibitor.

● Bupropion

Studies in animals using phenelzine have shown that the acute toxicity of bupropion is enhanced by the MAO inhibitor. Concomitant use of an MAO inhibitor and bupropion is contraindicated, and it is suggested that at least 14 days elapse between discontinuance of MAO inhibitor therapy and initiation of bupropion therapy.

● Anesthetics

The hypotensive and CNS depressant effects of general anesthetics may be exaggerated in patients receiving MAO inhibitors. Since inhibition of monoamine oxidase may persist for several days following discontinuance of therapy, some manufacturers suggest that MAO inhibitors be discontinued for at least 7–14 days prior to elective surgery to allow time for recovery of enzymatic activity before general anesthetics are used. If emergency surgery is necessary in a patient receiving an MAO inhibitor, the dose of the general anesthetic should be carefully adjusted.

Patients receiving MAO inhibitors should not be given cocaine or local anesthetics that contain sympathomimetic vasoconstrictors, since hypertension may result.

Because MAO inhibitors may potentiate the hypotensive effect of local anesthetics used in spinal anesthesia, these agents should be used with caution in patients receiving MAO inhibitors.

● Disulfiram

MAO inhibitors should probably be used with caution in patients receiving disulfiram. In one study in animals receiving large intraperitoneal doses of disulfiram and the *d*- or *l*-isomer of tranylcypromine, severe toxicity, including seizures and death, occurred. However, in other studies in animals receiving large oral doses of disulfiram and racemic tranylcypromine, no adverse interaction was reported.

● Diuretics and Hypotensive Agents

In general, MAO inhibitor antidepressants should not be administered concomitantly with diuretics or hypotensive agents since a marked hypotensive effect may occur.

● Drugs with Anticholinergic Activity

Some manufacturers state that anticholinergic antiparkinsonian drugs should be used with caution in patients receiving MAO inhibitors, since severe reactions have reportedly occurred when these drugs were used concurrently; however, additional information is needed to determine the clinical importance of this potential interaction. It also should be considered that MAO inhibitors may prolong and intensify some anticholinergic effects (e.g., dryness) of antihistamines.

ACUTE TOXICITY

● Manifestations

In general, overdosage of monoamine oxidase (MAO) inhibitors may be expected to produce effects that are extensions of common adverse reactions. Patients with early or mild intoxication may experience drowsiness, dizziness (sometimes severe), ataxia, headache (sometimes severe), insomnia, restlessness, anxiety, and irritability. Other reported effects associated with severe overdosage include mental confusion, incoherence, tachycardia, rapid and irregular pulse, hypotension, coma, seizures, respiratory depression, hyporeflexia or hyperreflexia, fever, diaphoresis (sometimes perfuse and associated with cool, clammy skin), precordial pain, and shock. A few patients have developed hypertension, which rarely may be associated with twitching or myoclonic fibrillation of skeletal muscles and with hyperpyrexia, sometimes progressing to generalized rigidity and coma. In addition, trismus and opisthotonus have been reported to occur in some patients. Hyperactivity with marked agitation may occur. Signs and symptoms following acute overdosage may be delayed for 12–24 hours. Although signs and symptoms usually resolve within 3–4 days, they may persist for up to 2 weeks in some patients. Careful observation of patients for at least 1 week after overdosage is generally recommended.

● Treatment

Treatment of MAO inhibitor overdosage generally involves symptomatic and supportive care; there is no specific antidote for intoxication. In acute overdosage, the stomach should be emptied immediately by inducing emesis or by gastric lavage with instillation of charcoal slurry. If the patient is comatose, having seizures, or lacks the gag reflex, gastric lavage may be performed if an endotracheal tube with cuff inflated is in place to prevent aspiration of gastric contents. Hemodialysis, peritoneal dialysis, and charcoal hemoperfusion may be of value in cases of massive overdosage, but data are insufficient to recommend the routine use of these procedures in MAO inhibitor overdosage.

Because of the potential for interactions with other drugs, extreme caution should be used in the management of patients following MAO inhibitor overdosage. Conservative measures to maintain normal body temperature (e.g., external cooling), respiration, and blood pressure and to correct fluid and electrolyte abnormalities have generally been successful. Appropriate therapy (e.g., volume expansion) should be instituted if hypotension occurs; however, administration of pressor amines (e.g., norepinephrine) may be of limited value and should be used with caution, since the hypertensive effects of these agents may be potentiated by MAO inhibitors (see Sympathomimetic Agents and Catecholamine-releasing Agents under Drug Interactions: Food and Drugs Associated with Hypertensive Crisis). Appropriate therapy should be instituted if severe hypertension (i.e., hypertensive crisis) occurs. For the management of hypertensive crisis, see Hypertensive Crisis under Cautions: Cardiovascular Effects. Signs and symptoms of CNS stimulation, including seizures, should be treated with diazepam. Appropriate therapy should be instituted if excessive sedation occurs. Phenothiazines and CNS stimulants should be avoided (see Sympathomimetic Agents and Catecholamine-releasing Agents under Drug Interactions: Food and Drugs Associated with Hypertensive Crisis). Evaluation of liver function is recommended at the time of overdosage and for 4–6 weeks following recovery.

CHRONIC TOXICITY

Although MAO inhibitors are not usually associated with dependence and addiction, drug dependence has occurred in some patients receiving tranylcypromine doses substantially in excess of the usual therapeutic range. Some of these patients had a history of previous substance abuse. Following discontinuance of the drug, symptoms of withdrawal, including restlessness, anxiety, depression, confusion, hallucinations, headache, weakness, and diarrhea have occurred. A withdrawal syndrome also has been reported to occur infrequently after abrupt discontinuance of phenelzine. In reported cases, signs and symptoms of withdrawal ranging from vivid nightmares with agitation to frank psychosis and seizures have been evident within 24–72 hours after phenelzine was discontinued; the syndrome generally responds to reinitiation of MAO inhibitor therapy followed by cautious downward titration and discontinuance.

PHARMACOLOGY

The discovery of monoamine oxidase (MAO) inhibitors resulted from a search for derivatives of isoniazid (isonicotinic acid hydrazide) with antitubercular activity. During clinical trials with these hydrazine derivatives, a rather consistent beneficial effect of mood elevation was noted in depressed patients with tuberculosis receiving the drugs. Iproniazid, the first derivative synthesized, was found to be too toxic (principally hepatotoxicity) at the dosage level required for antitubercular activity. Although its antidepressant effect was still pronounced at lower dosage, toxicity was also eventually observed at the lower dosage level and use of iproniazid was finally discontinued. However, the antidepressant activity of iproniazid prompted a search for other MAO inhibitors and resulted in the synthesis of several agents, both hydrazine and nonhydrazine compounds, that were relatively less toxic than iproniazid.

Monoamine oxidase, an enzyme found mainly in nerve tissue and in the liver and lungs, catalyzes the oxidative deamination of various amines, including epinephrine, norepinephrine, dopamine, and serotonin (5-HT). There appear to be at least 2 isoforms of monoamine oxidase, monoamine oxidase-A (MAO-A) and monoamine oxidase-B (MAO-B), with differences in substrate preference, inhibitor specificity, tissue distribution, immunologic properties, and amino acid sequence. MAO-A substrates include serotonin; MAO-B substrates include phenylethylamine. Tyramine, epinephrine, norepinephrine, and dopamine are substrates for both MAO-A and MAO-B. Inhibition of monoamine oxidase results in increased concentrations of these amines. Currently available MAO inhibitor antidepressants (phenelzine, tranylcypromine) are considered nonselective inhibitors of MAO. Phenelzine binds irreversibly to monoamine oxidase; tranylcypromine binds reversibly to the enzyme. Selective inhibitors of monoamine oxidase-A (e.g., clorgiline) are being investigated. Rasagiline, safinamide, and selegiline are considered selective MAO-B inhibitors and are used for the symptomatic treatment of parkinsonian

syndrome. (See Rasagiline Mesylate 28:36.32, see Safinamide Mesylate 28:36.32, and see Selegiline Hydrochloride 28:36.32.)

Although the precise mechanism of antidepressant action of MAO inhibitors is unclear, it has been suggested that the increase in free serotonin and norepinephrine and/or alterations in other amine concentrations within the CNS are mainly responsible for the antidepressant effect of the drugs. Although this concept offers a useful working hypothesis, it should be remembered that definite proof of the mode of action of MAO inhibitors is lacking. Attempts have been made to correlate inhibition of platelet monoamine oxidase (a possible index of a drug's effect on brain monoamine oxidase) with therapeutic effect; preliminary evidence suggests that a dose-related effect of phenelzine on platelet monoamine oxidase correlates with a beneficial effect on mood in depressed patients.

MAO inhibitors may cause hypotension or hypertension, probably by the same mechanism of action. The reduction in blood pressure induced by MAO inhibitors is mainly an orthostatic (postural) effect; reduction in supine blood pressure is minimal in most patients. Although the precise mechanism of hypotensive action of MAO inhibitors is not fully understood, it has been postulated that this paradoxical effect may result from gradual accumulation of false neurotransmitters (phenylethylamines) in peripheral adrenergic neurons. Phenylethylamines (e.g., tyramine) are usually oxidatively deaminated in the GI tract and liver; however, inhibition of monoamine oxidase in the GI tract and liver may result in substantial systemic absorption of these indirect-acting amines. Gradual accumulation of octopamine in the adrenergic neurons may result from MAO inhibition in the neurons with subsequent alternate hydroxylation of tyramine to octopamine. It has been suggested that octopamine gradually displaces norepinephrine from storage granules. Stimulation of norepinephrine release may result in release of some norepinephrine and some octopamine, the latter amine having minimal activity at α- or β-adrenergic receptors. Thus, gradual MAO inhibitor-induced displacement of norepinephrine from adrenergic neurons may result in a functional block of sympathetic neurotransmission. Similarly, MAO inhibitors may cause severe hypertension when foods containing large amounts of tyramine are ingested. (See Drug Interactions: Food and Drugs Associated with Hypertensive Crisis.) Following systemic absorption of large amounts of tyramine, there may be a rapid, massive displacement and release of norepinephrine from adrenergic neurons resulting in severe hypertension. It has been suggested that selective inhibitors of monoamine oxidase-B (e.g., rasagiline, selegiline) may be less likely than nonselective MAO inhibitors to cause hypertension; however, hypertensive reactions have been reported rarely with selegiline at recommended doses as a result of dietary influences.

MAO inhibitors interfere with the hepatic metabolism of many drugs and may potentiate the actions of such agents as general anesthetics, barbiturates, morphine, alcohol, corticosteroids, and atropine. (See Drug Interactions.)

The pharmacologic effects of MAO inhibitors are cumulative; a latent period of a few days to several months may occur before the onset of antidepressant or hypotensive activity, and effects may persist for up to 3 weeks following discontinuance of therapy.

CHEMISTRY

Monoamine oxidase (MAO) inhibitors are a chemically heterogeneous group of drugs that can block oxidative deamination of naturally occurring monoamines. Various MAO inhibitors have been found to have antidepressant action (e.g., isocarboxazid, iproniazid, phenelzine, tranylcypromine); however, the only MAO inhibitors currently commercially available in the US for use as antidepressant agents are phenelzine and tranylcypromine.

Based on their structure, MAO inhibitors can be classified as hydrazines (e.g., phenelzine) and nonhydrazines (e.g., tranylcypromine). Although no longer used clinically, the prototype hydrazine MAO inhibitor is iproniazid. (See Pharmacology.) MAO inhibitors also can be classified according to their ability to selectively or nonselectively inhibit monoamine oxidase. (See Pharmacology.)

For further information on chemistry and stability, pharmacology, pharmacokinetics, uses, cautions, and dosage and administration of MAO inhibitors, see the individual monographs on Phenelzine Sulfate and Tranylcypromine Sulfate in 28:16.04.12 and see Rasagiline Mesylate, Safinamide Mesylate, and Selegiline Hydrochloride in 28:36.32.

---

† Use is not currently included in the labeling approved by the US Food and Drug Administration.

Desvenlafaxine, Desvenlafaxine Succinate

28:16.04.16 • SELECTIVE SEROTONIN- AND NOREPINEPHRINE-REUPTAKE INHIBITORS

■ Desvenlafaxine and its succinate salt (desvenlafaxine succinate) are selective serotonin- and norepinephrine-reuptake inhibitors (SNRIs); desvenlafaxine is the principal active metabolite of venlafaxine.

USES

● Major Depressive Disorder

Desvenlafaxine is used in the treatment of major depressive disorder in adults.

Clinical Experience

The antidepressant efficacy of desvenlafaxine has been established in 4 randomized, double-blind, placebo-controlled, fixed-dose studies of 8 weeks' duration in adult outpatients who met DSM-IV criteria for major depressive disorder. In all of these studies, patients receiving desvenlafaxine (50–400 mg daily as extended-release tablets) demonstrated greater improvement in the 17-item Hamilton Rating Scale for Depression (HAMD-17) total score than did patients receiving placebo. Patients receiving desvenlafaxine also demonstrated greater overall improvement as measured by the Clinical Global Impressions Scale-Improvement (CGI-I) compared with placebo recipients in 3 out of 4 of these studies. In the 2 studies that directly compared 50 mg and 100 mg of desvenlafaxine given once daily, there was no evidence of a greater therapeutic effect at the higher 100-mg dosage. In addition, adverse effects and drug discontinuances were reported more frequently at higher dosages of the drug in these studies. No age- or gender-related differences in efficacy were noted in these studies; data were insufficient to determine whether there were race-related differences in efficacy.

Longer-term studies with desvenlafaxine have also been conducted. In one trial, adults with major depressive disorder who responded to 8 weeks of open-label desvenlafaxine (50 mg per day) and subsequently remained stable on treatment for 12 weeks were randomized in a double-blind manner to continue desvenlafaxine or switch to placebo for up to 26 weeks. Patients were monitored for relapse of depression (defined as HAMD-17 score ≥16 at any visit, discontinuation of treatment due to lack of efficacy, hospitalization for depression, suicide attempt, or suicide). Compared to placebo, patients who continued on desvenlafaxine had a longer time to relapse. At 26 weeks, 14.3 or 30.2% of patients had a relapse of depression with desvenlafaxine or placebo, respectively.

In another longer-term trial, adults with major depressive disorder responding to 12 weeks of treatment with desvenlafaxine were randomized in a double-blind manner to continue the same dose of desvenlafaxine (200 or 400 mg per day) or switch to placebo for up to 26 weeks. Relapse was defined as a HAMD-17 score ≥16 at any visit, CGI-I score ≥6 at any visit, or discontinuation of study drug due to unsatisfactory response. At 26 weeks, the rate of relapse was 29 or 49% with desvenlafaxine or placebo, respectively.

A postmarketing randomized double-blind trial evaluated the efficacy of desvenlafaxine 25 or 50 mg versus placebo in 699 adult patients with major depressive disorder. Based on the primary efficacy measure (change from baseline in HAMD-17 total score), desvenlafaxine 50 mg was superior to placebo, but desvenlafaxine 25 mg was not. Change in HAMD-17 score from baseline was -10.02, -8.98, or -8.52 for desvenlafaxine 50 mg, desvenlafaxine 25 mg, or placebo, respectively.

Clinical Perspective

Treatment options for major depressive disorder include pharmacologic and non-pharmacologic (e.g., psychotherapy) approaches. Several classes of antidepressant drugs are available for the treatment of major depressive disorder. In general, these drugs have shown similar effectiveness; therefore, treatment is guided by specific patient and drug-related factors.

A legacy practice guideline from the American Psychiatric Association (APA) published in 2010 states that the effectiveness of antidepressants in the treatment of major depressive disorder is generally comparable between and within classes of medications, including selective serotonin reuptake inhibitors (SSRIs), selective serotonin- and norepinephrine-reuptake inhibitors (SNRIs), tricyclic antidepressants (TCAs), monoamine oxidase inhibitors (MAOIs), and other antidepressants (e.g., bupropion, mirtazapine, trazodone). Therefore, the initial selection of an antidepressant can be based mainly on the following factors: patient preference; response to prior therapies; safety, tolerability, and anticipated adverse effects; concurrent psychiatric and medical conditions; specific properties of the medication (e.g., half-life, cytochrome P-450 [CYP] interactions, other drug interactions); and cost.

The Department of Veterans Affairs and Department of Defense developed more current guidelines for the management of major depressive disorder. These guidelines state that treatment of uncomplicated major depressive disorder can be initiated with either psychotherapy (e.g., cognitive behavioral therapy) or pharmacotherapy, depending on patient preference; for patients with severe, persistent, or recurrent major depressive disorder, a combination of pharmacotherapy and psychotherapy is suggested. When pharmacotherapy is used as initial therapy, either bupropion, mirtazapine, a selective serotonin reuptake inhibitor (SSRI), a SNRI, trazodone, vilazodone, or vortioxetine is suggested. No evidence is available to suggest superiority of one agent over another. The guidelines recommend against using esketamine, ketamine, MAOIs, nefazodone, or TCAs as initial therapy. For patients not responding to initial therapy, recommendations include switching to another antidepressant (including MAOIs or TCAs), switching to or augmenting with psychotherapy, or augmenting with a second-generation antipsychotic.

● Vasomotor Symptoms

Like some other SNRIs and SSRIs, desvenlafaxine succinate has been studied for the management of vasomotor symptoms† in postmenopausal women.

Guidelines from the North American Menopause Society recommend several treatments for vasomotor symptoms associated with menopause, including cognitive-behavioral therapy, SNRIs (including desvenlafaxine), SSRIs, fezolinetant, and gabapentin.

DOSAGE AND ADMINISTRATION

● General

Pretreatment Screening

- Perform a detailed psychiatric history (including family history of suicide, bipolar disorder, and depression) to assess risk of bipolar disorder prior to starting desvenlafaxine.

- Control preexisting hypertension before initiating desvenlafaxine therapy; use caution in patients with preexisting hypertension, cardiovascular, or cerebrovascular conditions that may be compromised by blood pressure increases.

- Inquire about sexual function prior to initiation of desvenlafaxine.

Patient Monitoring

- Monitor for worsening depression, suicidality, or unusual changes in behavior, especially at the beginning of therapy or during periods of dosage adjustment.

- Monitor blood pressure regularly.

- Monitor for development of serotonin syndrome.

- In patients receiving concomitant warfarin, monitor coagulation indices and look for signs of bleeding during initiation, titration, or discontinuance of desvenlafaxine.

- When discontinuing desvenlafaxine, monitor for discontinuance symptoms (e.g., nausea, sweating, dysphoric mood, irritability, agitation, dizziness, sensory disturbances, tremor, anxiety, confusion, headache, lethargy, emotional lability, insomnia, hypomania, tinnitus, seizures).

- Inquire about changes in sexual function during treatment.

Dispensing and Administration Precautions

- To avoid medication errors, the Institute for Safe Medication Practices (ISMP) recommends that prescribers communicate both the brand and generic names for desvenlafaxine succinate (Pristiq®) on the prescription order form.

Other General Considerations

- Acute episodes of major depressive disorder typically require pharmacologic treatment for several months or longer; reassess patients periodically to determine need for continued treatment.

- When discontinuing therapy, reduce dosage gradually and monitor for possible withdrawal symptoms; avoid abrupt discontinuance whenever possible. Some patients require discontinuation over a period of several months. If intolerable symptoms occur following dosage reduction or upon discontinuance of therapy, consider resuming therapy at the previously prescribed dosage and decreasing the dosage at a more gradual rate.

- If switching to desvenlafaxine from a monoamine oxidase inhibitor (MAOI) intended to treat psychiatric disorders, allow 14 days to elapse between discontinuation of the MAOI and initiation of desvenlafaxine. Conversely, if switching from desvenlafaxine to an MAOI, allow 7 days to elapse between discontinuation of desvenlafaxine and initiation of the MAOI.

- When switching from another antidepressant to desvenlafaxine, it may be necessary to taper the dosage of the previous antidepressant to minimize discontinuance symptoms.

- Do not initiate desvenlafaxine in patients receiving linezolid or IV methylene blue; if urgent treatment with linezolid or IV methylene blue is required in a patient receiving desvenlafaxine, stop desvenlafaxine and monitor for symptoms of serotonin syndrome for 7 days or until 24 hours after the last dose of linezolid or IV methylene blue (whichever comes first). Resume desvenlafaxine 24 hours after the last dose of linezolid or IV methylene blue.

● Administration

Desvenlafaxine and desvenlafaxine succinate are administered orally and are available as extended-release tablets.

Administer desvenlafaxine and desvenlafaxine succinate with or without food at approximately the same time each day. Extended-release tablets should be swallowed whole with fluid and should not be divided, crushed, chewed, or dissolved.

Store at 20-25°C (excursions permitted between 15–30°C).

● Dosage

Dosage of desvenlafaxine succinate is expressed in terms of desvenlafaxine.

Major Depressive Disorder

For the management of major depressive disorder in adults, the recommended dosage of desvenlafaxine is 50 mg once daily. Although efficacy has been established at dosages of 50–400 mg once daily in clinical studies, no additional benefit was observed with dosages greater than 50 mg once daily, and adverse effects and discontinuances were more frequent at higher dosages. The 25-mg per day dose is intended for gradual reduction in dose when discontinuing treatment.

Vasomotor Symptoms

For the management of vasomotor symptoms in postmenopausal women†, guidelines suggest an initial desvenlafaxine dosage of 25–50 mg daily; the dosage may be titrated up by that amount each day. The effective dosage range is usually 100–150 mg daily.

● Special Populations

Hepatic Impairment

The manufacturers make no specific dosage recommendations in mild hepatic impairment. In patients with moderate to severe hepatic impairment (Child-Pugh score 7–15), the recommended desvenlafaxine dosage is 50 mg given once daily. Dosages exceeding 100 mg daily are not recommended.

Renal Impairment

The manufacturers make no specific dosage recommendations in mild renal impairment (creatinine clearance >50 mL/minute based on Cockcroft-Gault). In patients with moderate renal impairment (creatinine clearance of 30–50 mL/minute), the maximum recommended desvenlafaxine dosage is 50 mg given once daily. The maximum recommended dosage in patients with severe renal impairment (creatinine clearance 15–29 mL/minute) or end-stage renal disease (creatinine clearance <15 mL/minute) is 25 mg once daily or 50 mg given every other day. Supplemental doses should not be administered to patients after dialysis.

Geriatric Patients

Although there are no specific dosage recommendations for desvenlafaxine in geriatric patients, the possibility of reduced renal clearance of the drug should be considered when determining dosage.

CAUTIONS

● Contraindications

- Known hypersensitivity to desvenlafaxine, venlafaxine hydrochloride, or any ingredient in the formulation.

- Concurrent or recent (i.e., within 14 days) therapy with a monoamine oxidase inhibitor (MAOI) intended to treat psychiatric disorders. Use of an MAOI intended to treat psychiatric disorders within 7 days of desvenlafaxine discontinuance.

- Initiation of desvenlafaxine therapy in patients receiving MAOIs such as linezolid or IV methylene blue.

● Warnings/Precautions

Warnings

Suicidal Thoughts and Behaviors

A boxed warning regarding an increased risk of suicidal thoughts and behaviors in children, adolescents, and young adults is included in the prescribing information for desvenlafaxine. Worsening of depression and/or the emergence of suicidal ideation and behavior (suicidality) or unusual changes in behavior may occur in both adult and pediatric patients with major depressive disorder, whether or not they are taking antidepressants. This risk may persist until clinically important remission occurs. Suicide is a known risk of depression and certain other psychiatric disorders, and these disorders themselves are the strongest predictors of suicide. However, there has been a long-standing concern that antidepressants may have a role in inducing worsening of depression and the emergence of suicidality in certain patients during the early phases of treatment. Pooled analyses of short-term, placebo-controlled studies of antidepressants (i.e., selective serotonin reuptake inhibitors [SSRIs] and other antidepressants) have shown an increased risk of suicidality in children, adolescents, and young adults (18–24 years of age) with major depressive disorder and other psychiatric disorders. An increased suicidality risk was not demonstrated with antidepressants compared with placebo in adults older than 24 years of age, and a reduced risk was observed in adults ≥65 years of age. All patients being treated with antidepressants for any indication should be appropriately monitored and closely observed for clinical worsening, suicidality, and unusual changes in behavior, particularly during initiation of therapy (i.e., the first few months) and during periods of dosage adjustments. Families and caregivers of patients being treated with antidepressants for major depressive disorder or other indications, both psychiatric and nonpsychiatric, also should be advised to monitor patients on a daily basis for the emergence of agitation, irritability, or unusual changes in behavior as well as the emergence of suicidality, and to report such symptoms immediately to a health-care provider. Although a causal relationship between the emergence of symptoms such as anxiety, agitation, panic attacks, insomnia, irritability, hostility, aggressiveness, impulsivity, akathisia, hypomania, and/or mania and either the worsening of depression and/or the emergence of suicidal impulses has not been established, there is concern that such symptoms may represent precursors to emerging suicidality. Consequently, consideration should be given to changing the therapeutic regimen or discontinuing therapy in patients whose depression is persistently worse or in patients experiencing emergent suicidality or symptoms that might be precursors to worsening depression or suicidality, particularly if such manifestations are severe, abrupt in onset, or were not part of the patient's presenting symptoms. It is also recommended that the drugs be prescribed in the smallest quantity consistent with good patient management, in order to reduce the risk of overdosage. Because bipolar disorder may initially present as a major depressive episode, screen patients with depressive symptoms to determine the risk of bipolar disorder prior to initiating desvenlafaxine. Screening should include a detailed psychiatric history (including family history of suicide, bipolar disorder, and depression). Although not established in controlled clinical studies, it is thought that treatment of bipolar disorder with an antidepressant alone may precipitate the development of a mixed/manic episode in patients at risk for bipolar disorder. Desvenlafaxine is not indicated for use in the treatment of bipolar disorder.

Other Warnings and Precautions

Serotonin Syndrome

Potentially life-threatening serotonin syndrome has been reported with SSRIs and serotonin- and norepinephrine-reuptake inhibitors (SNRIs) alone, including desvenlafaxine, but particularly with concurrent use of other serotonergic drugs (including serotonin [5-hydroxytryptamine; 5-HT] type 1 receptor agonists ["triptans"], tricyclic antidepressants, fentanyl, lithium, tramadol, meperidine, methadone, tryptophan, buspirone, amphetamines, St. John's Wort [*Hypericum perforatum*]) and drugs that impair the metabolism of serotonin (e.g., MAOIs). Signs and symptoms of serotonin syndrome may include mental status changes (e.g., agitation, hallucinations, delirium, coma), autonomic instability (e.g., tachycardia, labile blood pressure, dizziness, diaphoresis, flushing, hyperthermia), neuromuscular symptoms (e.g., tremor, rigidity, myoclonus, hyperreflexia, incoordination), seizures, and/or GI symptoms (e.g., nausea, vomiting, diarrhea). Patients receiving desvenlafaxine should be monitored for the development of serotonin syndrome. If use of desvenlafaxine with other serotonergic drugs is warranted, inform patients of the risk for serotonin syndrome, and monitor for symptoms.

Concurrent or recent (i.e., within 14 days) therapy with MAOIs used for treatment of psychiatric disorders is contraindicated. Desvenlafaxine should not be initiated in patients receiving MAOIs such linezolid or IV methylene blue. If an MAOI such as linezolid or IV methylene blue is necessary in a patient receiving desvenlafaxine, discontinue desvenlafaxine before initiating the MAOI and monitor for serotonin syndrome for 7 days or until 24 hours after the last dose of the MAOI (whichever comes first).

If serotonin syndrome occurs, immediately discontinue treatment with desvenlafaxine and any concurrently administered serotonergic agents, and initiate supportive symptomatic treatment.

Elevated Blood Pressure

Because of observed increases in blood pressure in clinical studies of desvenlafaxine, regular monitoring of blood pressure is recommended in patients receiving the drug.

Sustained blood pressure increases could have adverse consequences in patients receiving the drug. Therefore, the manufacturers recommend that preexisting hypertension be controlled before initiating desvenlafaxine therapy. Desvenlafaxine should be used cautiously in patients with preexisting hypertension, cardiovascular, or cerebrovascular conditions that may be compromised by increases in blood pressure. Dosage reduction or drug discontinuance should be considered in patients who experience a sustained increase in blood pressure during therapy.

Increased Risk of Bleeding

SSRIs and SNRIs, including desvenlafaxine, may increase the risk of bleeding events. Concurrent administration of aspirin, nonsteroidal anti-inflammatory agents, warfarin, and other anticoagulants may add to this risk. Case reports and epidemiologic studies have demonstrated an association between the use of drugs that interfere with serotonin reuptake and the occurrence of GI bleeding. Observational data indicate that exposure to SNRIs, has been associated with a less than 2-fold increase in the risk of postpartum hemorrhage, particularly during the month before delivery.

The manufacturers recommend that patients be advised of the risk of bleeding associated with the concomitant use of desvenlafaxine and antiplatelet agents or anticoagulants. For patients receiving warfarin therapy, careful coagulation

monitoring is recommended during initiation, titration, and discontinuation of desvenlafaxine.

Angle Closure Glaucoma

Many antidepressant drugs, including desvenlafaxine, may cause pupillary dilation, which can trigger an angle closure attack in patients with anatomically narrow angles who do not have a patent iridectomy. Avoid use of desvenlafaxine and other antidepressants in patients with untreated anatomically narrow angles.

Activation of Mania/Hypomania

Mania was reported in approximately 0.02% of desvenlafaxine-treated patients during clinical studies for major depressive disorder. Activation of mania/hypomania has also been reported in some patients treated with other antidepressants. Use with caution in patients with a personal or family history of mania or hypomania.

Discontinuation Syndrome

Abrupt discontinuance of serotonergic antidepressants has been associated with the appearance of adverse effects, including nausea, sweating, dysphoric mood, irritability, agitation, dizziness, sensory disturbances (e.g., paresthesia), tremor, anxiety, confusion, headache, lethargy, emotional lability, insomnia, hypomania, tinnitus, and seizures.

There have also been postmarketing reports of serious discontinuation symptoms with desvenlafaxine, some protracted and severe. Completed suicide, suicidal thoughts, and severe aggression have been reported during desvenlafaxine dosage reduction and discontinuation. Visual changes (i.e., blurred vision, trouble focusing) and increased blood pressure have also been reported after stopping or reducing the dosage of desvenlafaxine. Therefore, patients should be monitored for possible withdrawal symptoms when discontinuing desvenlafaxine therapy. A gradual reduction in dosage rather than abrupt cessation is recommended whenever possible. If intolerable symptoms occur following dosage reduction or discontinuance, consider reinstituting previously prescribed dosage, then resume more gradual dosage reductions. Some patients may require discontinuation of desvenlafaxine over a period of several months.

Seizures

Seizures have been reported in premarketing clinical studies of desvenlafaxine. Desvenlafaxine has not been systematically evaluated in patients with seizure disorders; such patients were excluded from premarketing clinical studies. The manufacturers state that the drug should be used with caution in patients with a seizure disorder.

Hyponatremia

Treatment with SSRIs and SNRIs, including desvenlafaxine, may result in hyponatremia. In many cases, hyponatremia appears to be due to the syndrome of inappropriate antidiuretic hormone secretion (SIADH). Cases with serum sodium concentrations lower than 110 mmol/L have been reported. Geriatric individuals and patients receiving diuretics or who are otherwise volume depleted may be at greater risk of developing hyponatremia. Signs and symptoms of hyponatremia include headache, difficulty concentrating, memory impairment, confusion, weakness, and unsteadiness, which may lead to falls; more severe and/or acute cases have been associated with hallucinations, syncope, seizures, coma, respiratory arrest, and death. Initiate appropriate medical intervention and consider drug discontinuance in patients with symptomatic hyponatremia.

Interstitial Lung Disease and Eosinophilic Pneumonia

Interstitial lung disease and eosinophilic pneumonia associated with venlafaxine (the parent drug of desvenlafaxine) have been reported rarely. The possibility of such adverse effects should be considered in patients treated with desvenlafaxine who present with progressive dyspnea, cough, or chest discomfort. Such patients should be evaluated promptly and discontinuation of desvenlafaxine should be considered.

Sexual Dysfunction

Sexual dysfunction can occur with the use of SNRIs, including desvenlafaxine; this can include ejaculatory delay or failure, decreased libido, or erectile dysfunction in males, and decreased libido or delayed/absent orgasm in females.

Providers should inquire about sexual function prior to initiation and during treatment with desvenlafaxine, since sexual function may not be spontaneously reported. Obtaining a detailed history, including time of symptom onset, is important when evaluating changes in sexual function, since sexual symptoms can have other causes (including the underlying psychiatric disorder). Potential management strategies should be discussed to support patients in making informed treatment decisions.

Specific Populations

Pregnancy

The National Pregnancy Registry for Antidepressants monitors pregnancy outcomes in women exposed to desvenlafaxine during pregnancy. Clinicians are encouraged to register patients by calling the National Pregnancy Registry for Antidepressants at 1-844-405-6185.

No published studies are available on desvenlafaxine use in pregnancy; however, available epidemiologic data with venlafaxine (parent compound) in pregnant women have not found a clear association between venlafaxine and adverse developmental outcomes.

There are risks associated with both untreated depression and exposure to SNRIs or SSRIs during pregnancy. A longitudinal study of women with a history of major depression who discontinued antidepressants during pregnancy found that these women were more likely to experience a relapse of major depression compared to women who continued treatment.

The risk of preeclampsia may be increased with desvenlafaxine exposure in mid to late pregnancy. Observational data indicate that exposure to SNRIs, particularly during the month before delivery, has been associated with a less than 2-fold increase in the risk of postpartum hemorrhage.

Some neonates exposed to SNRIs or SSRIs late in the third trimester of pregnancy have developed complications that have sometimes been severe and required prolonged hospitalization, respiratory support, and tube feeding. Such complications may arise immediately upon delivery. Clinical findings reported to date in neonates have included respiratory distress, cyanosis, apnea, seizures, temperature instability, feeding difficulty, vomiting, hypoglycemia, hypotonia, hypertonia, hyperreflexia, tremor, jitteriness, irritability, and constant crying. These clinical features appear to be consistent with either a direct toxic effect of the SNRI or SSRI or, possibly, a drug withdrawal syndrome. It should be noted that, in some cases, the clinical picture was consistent with serotonin syndrome. Neonates exposed to desvenlafaxine during the third trimester of pregnancy should be monitored for discontinuation syndrome.

Lactation

Desvenlafaxine is excreted into human milk at low levels, and adverse reactions have not been detected in breast-fed infants exposed to desvenlafaxine through breast milk. It is not known if desvenlafaxine affects milk production. Consider the developmental and health benefits of breastfeeding, the mother's clinical need for the drug, and the potential for adverse effects on the breast-fed infant from exposure to desvenlafaxine or the underlying maternal condition.

Pediatric Use

Safety and effectiveness of desvenlafaxine for major depressive disorder in pediatric patients younger than 18 years of age have not been established. Desvenlafaxine failed to demonstrate efficacy for major depressive disorder in patients 7–17 years of age in 2 randomized studies conducted over an 8-week period.

A greater risk of suicidal thinking or behavior (suicidality) is associated with antidepressant treatment in children and adolescents with major depressive disorder. Decreases in body weight were also observed in short-term pediatric clinical trials of desvenlafaxine, with a ≥3.5% weight loss from baseline occurring in 22% and 14% of patients receiving low dose and high dose desvenlafaxine, respectively, compared to 7% of patients receiving placebo. Six-month extension studies of desvenlafaxine in pediatric patients 7–17 years of age with major depressive disorder demonstrated mean changes in weight similar to the expected changes in pediatric patients based on age and sex.

Desvenlafaxine exposure was approximately 30% higher in pediatric patients 7–11 years of age compared to adult patients receiving the same dose. Desvenlafaxine exposure was similar in adolescents 12–17 years of age and adult patients.

Geriatric Use

In clinical studies of desvenlafaxine, 6% of patients were ≥65 years of age. Although no overall differences in safety or efficacy were observed between geriatric and younger patients in these studies, a higher incidence of systolic orthostatic hypotension was reported in patients ≥65 years of age compared with younger patients who received desvenlafaxine. Consider possible reduced renal clearance of the drug in geriatric patients when determining dosage.

SSRIs and SNRIs, including desvenlafaxine, have been associated with clinically important hyponatremia in geriatric patients, who may be at greater risk for this adverse effect.

Hepatic Impairment

In patients with moderate to severe (Child-Pugh score 7–15) hepatic impairment, AUC of desvenlafaxine was increased by approximately 31–35%. The recommended desvenlafaxine dosage in patients with moderate to severe hepatic impairment is 50 mg daily; dosages exceeding 100 mg daily are not recommended in such patients.

Renal Impairment

In patients with moderate or severe renal impairment (creatinine clearance 15–50 mL/minute based on Cockcroft-Gault) or end-stage renal disease (creatinine clearance <15 mL/minute based on Cockcroft Gault), clearance of desvenlafaxine was decreased, resulting in potentially clinically significant increases in drug exposure. Dosage adjustment is necessary in such patients. In pharmacokinetic studies, AUC was increased approximately 42% in mild renal impairment (creatinine clearance 50–80 mL/minute based on Cockcroft-Gault), 56% in moderate renal impairment (creatinine clearance 30–49 mL/minute), 108% in severe renal impairment (creatinine clearance 15–29 mL/minute), and approximately 116% in patients with end-stage renal disease (creatinine clearance <15 mL/minute), compared to the reference population.

● Common Adverse Effects

Adverse effects reported in at least 5% of patients with major depressive disorder receiving desvenlafaxine (50 or 100 mg daily) and at an incidence of at least twice that reported with placebo in short-term clinical studies include nausea, dizziness, insomnia, hyperhidrosis, constipation, somnolence, decreased appetite, anxiety, and sexual function disorders in males.

DRUG INTERACTIONS

Desvenlafaxine is principally metabolized by uridine diphosphoglucuronosyltransferase (UGT) isoenzymes and, to a lesser extent, by cytochrome P-450 (CYP) 3A4 isoenzyme. The drug does not inhibit CYP1A2, 2A6, 2C8, 2C9, 2C19, or 2D6 isoenzymes. Desvenlafaxine is not an inhibitor or inducer of CYP3A4.

Desvenlafaxine is not a substrate or an inhibitor of the P-glycoprotein transporter in vitro.

● Drugs Metabolized by Hepatic Microsomal Enzymes

Concomitant use of desvenlafaxine with drugs primarily metabolized by CYP2D6 (e.g., desipramine, atomoxetine, dextromethorphan, metoprolol, nebivolol, perphenazine, tolterodine) may result in higher peak plasma concentrations and total exposure of the substrate drug, which may lead to an increased risk of toxicity. Concurrent administration of desvenlafaxine 100 mg and desipramine, a CYP2D6 substrate, increased peak plasma concentrations and AUC of desipramine by approximately 25 and 17%, respectively; coadministration of desvenlafaxine 400 mg and desipramine increased peak plasma concentrations and AUC of desipramine by approximately 52 and 90%, respectively. The manufacturers state that when desvenlafaxine dosages of 100 mg daily or lower are used concomitantly with a CYP2D6 substrate, no dosage adjustment of the CYP2D6 substrate is needed. However, when desvenlafaxine dosages of 400 mg daily are used concurrently with a CYP2D6 substrate, dosage of the CYP2D6 substrate should be reduced by up to 50%.

Desvenlafaxine does not inhibit or induce the CYP3A4 isoenzyme in vitro. Concurrent administration of desvenlafaxine 400 mg and midazolam, a CYP3A4 substrate, decreased AUC and peak plasma concentrations of midazolam by approximately 31 and 16%, respectively. The manufacturers state that no dosage adjustment is necessary when drugs mainly metabolized by CYP3A4 (e.g., midazolam) are used concomitantly with desvenlafaxine.

No dosage adjustment of drugs metabolized by both CYP2D6 and CYP3A4 (e.g., tamoxifen, aripiprazole) is needed when used concomitantly with desvenlafaxine. Concurrent administration of desvenlafaxine 100 mg and tamoxifen did not substantially impact peak plasma concentrations or AUC of tamoxifen or its active metabolites (4-hydroxytamoxifen and endoxifen). Concurrent administration of desvenlafaxine 100 mg and aripiprazole did not substantially impact peak plasma concentrations or AUC of aripiprazole or its active metabolite (dehydroaripiprazole).

● Drugs Affecting Hepatic Microsomal Enzymes

CYP3A4 is a minor pathway for the metabolism of desvenlafaxine. Concomitant administration of ketoconazole, a CYP3A4 inhibitor, resulted in a 43% increase in AUC and an 8% increase in peak plasma concentrations of desvenlafaxine.

Clinically important pharmacokinetic interactions are unlikely with inhibitors of CYP isoenzymes 1A1, 1A2, 2A6, 2D6, 2C8, 2C9, 2C19, and 2E1.

● Drugs Affecting Hemostasis

Potential pharmacologic interaction (increased risk of bleeding) if used concurrently with antiplatelet or anticoagulant drugs (e.g., aspirin, nonsteroidal anti-inflammatory agents, warfarin). This increased risk of bleeding is potentially caused by the effect of desvenlafaxine on the release of serotonin by platelets.

The manufacturers recommend carefully monitoring in patients receiving an antiplatelet or anticoagulant drug during initiation and discontinuance of desvenlafaxine therapy.

● Alcohol

In a clinical study, desvenlafaxine did not increase the impairment of mental and motor skills caused by alcohol. However, the manufacturers recommend avoiding concomitant alcohol consumption during desvenlafaxine therapy.

● Monoamine Oxidase Inhibitors

Concomitant use of SSRIs and SNRIs, including desvenlafaxine, with MAOIs increases the risk of serotonin syndrome. Concomitant use of desvenlafaxine with MAOIs (e.g. selegiline, tranylcypromine, isocarboxazid, phenelzine, linezolid, methylene blue) is contraindicated.

At least 14 days should elapse between discontinuance of an MAOI intended to treat psychiatric disorders and initiation of desvenlafaxine, and at least 7 days should elapse between discontinuance of desvenlafaxine and initiation of an MAOI intended to treat psychiatric disorders.

Do not initiate desvenlafaxine in patients receiving linezolid or IV methylene blue; if urgent treatment with linezolid or IV methylene blue is required in a patient receiving desvenlafaxine, stop desvenlafaxine and monitor for symptoms of serotonin syndrome for 7 days or until 24 hours after the last dose of linezolid or IV methylene blue (whichever comes first). Resume desvenlafaxine 24 hours after the last dose of linezolid or IV methylene blue.

● Serotonergic Drugs

Concomitant use of desvenlafaxine and other drugs affecting serotonergic neurotransmission (e.g., SNRIs, SSRIs, triptans, tricyclic antidepressants, opioids, lithium, buspirone, amphetamines, tryptophan, St. John's wort [Hypericum perforatum]) increases the risk of serotonin syndrome. Monitor for serotonin syndrome if serotonergic agents are used concomitantly with desvenlafaxine. If serotonin syndrome occurs, consider discontinuation of desvenlafaxine and any concurrently administered serotonergic agents.

● Laboratory Tests

Due to a lack of specificity in screening tests, false-positive urine immunoassay screening tests for phencyclidine (PCP) and amphetamine have been reported in patients receiving desvenlafaxine. False-positive tests can be expected for several days following discontinuance of desvenlafaxine. Gas chromatography/mass spectrometry can be used for confirmatory testing to distinguish desvenlafaxine from PCP and amphetamine.

DESCRIPTION

Desvenlafaxine, a selective serotonin- and norepinephrine-reuptake inhibitor (SNRI), is an antidepressant. The drug is the principal active metabolite of venlafaxine.

The exact mechanism of antidepressant action of desvenlafaxine has not been fully elucidated but appears to be associated with the drug's potentiation of serotonergic and noradrenergic activity in the CNS. Desvenlafaxine is a potent inhibitor of neuronal serotonin and norepinephrine reuptake; however, inhibition of dopamine reuptake at concentrations that inhibit serotonin and norepinephrine reuptake appears unlikely in most patients. The drug does not inhibit monoamine oxidase (MAO) and has not demonstrated significant affinity for muscarinic cholinergic, H₁-histaminergic, α₁-adrenergic, dopaminergic, γ-aminobutyric acid (GABA), glutamate, and opiate receptors in vitro.

The pharmacokinetics of desvenlafaxine are linear and dose proportional over a single-dose range of 50–600 mg (1–12 times the recommended dosage) per day. Following repeated once-daily dosing, steady state serum concentrations of desvenlafaxine are attained in approximately 4–5 days. Following oral administration of desvenlafaxine, the absolute oral bioavailability is about 80%. Peak plasma concentrations are increased approximately 16% when administered with a high-fat meal (800–1000 calories) compared to the fasted state, with no effect on the AUC. Desvenlafaxine is 30% protein-bound, which is independent of plasma concentrations. It is principally metabolized via conjugation by UGT isoenzymes and, to a lesser extent, through oxidation (by the cytochrome P-450 [CYP] 3A4 isoenzyme). Approximately 45% of a single oral dose of desvenlafaxine is eliminated unchanged in the urine at 72 hours; approximately 19% of the dose is excreted as the glucuronide metabolite, and less than 5% is excreted as the oxidative metabolite (N,O-didesmethylvenlafaxine).

In female patients, peak plasma concentrations were approximately 26% higher compared to the reference population, with no substantial change in AUC. In geriatric patients 65–75 years of age, there was no substantial change in peak plasma concentrations, but AUC was increased approximately 32% compared to the reference population. In geriatric patients >75 years of age, peak plasma concentrations increased approximately 32%, and AUC increased 56% compared to the reference population. There were no clinically significant differences in desvenlafaxine exposure based on ethnicity (White, Black, Hispanic).

ADVICE TO PATIENTS

● Risk of suicidality; advise patients, family, and caregivers to look for and immediately report emergence of suicidality, especially during the first few months of therapy and during periods of dosage adjustment.

● Advise patients about the importance of reading the patient information before taking desvenlafaxine and each time the prescription is refilled.

● Inform patients of potential risk of serotonin syndrome, particularly with concurrent use of 5-HT1 receptor agonists (also called triptans), tricyclic antidepressants, opioids, lithium, tryptophan, buspirone, amphetamines, St. John's Wort (Hypericum perforatum), and other serotonergic agents. Patients should immediately contact their clinician if signs and symptoms of serotonin syndrome develop.

● Advise patients not to concurrently take other products containing desvenlafaxine or venlafaxine.

● Instruct patients not to take desvenlafaxine with a MAOI or within 14 days of stopping the drug, and to allow at least 7 days after stopping desvenlafaxine before starting therapy with an MAOI.

● Risk of discontinuance symptoms when switching from other antidepressants, including venlafaxine, to desvenlafaxine. Advise patients that tapering of the previous antidepressant may be necessary to minimize the risk of such symptoms.

● Advise patients that they should have regular monitoring of blood pressure while taking desvenlafaxine.

● Advise patients, their families, and caregivers to observe desvenlafaxine-treated patients for signs of activation of mania/hypomania.

- Advise patients to notify their clinician if they develop any allergic signs or symptoms during therapy (e.g., rash, hives, swelling, difficulty breathing).

- Risk of cognitive and motor impairment; advise patients to exercise caution while operating hazardous machinery, including automobile driving, until they are reasonably certain that desvenlafaxine therapy does not adversely affect their ability to engage in such activities.

- Risk of sexual dysfunction in male and female patients; advise patients to discuss any changes in sexual function and potential management strategies with their clinician.

- Advise patients to avoid alcohol during desvenlafaxine therapy.

- Advise patients to inform their clinician of existing or contemplated concomitant therapy, including prescription and OTC drugs and dietary and herbal supplements, as well as any concomitant illnesses.

- Advise patients about the risk of bleeding associated with concomitant use of desvenlafaxine and aspirin, nonsteroidal anti-inflammatory agents, other antiplatelet drugs, warfarin, or other anticoagulants.

- Advise women to inform their clinician if they are or plan to become pregnant or plan to breast-feed. Advise patients that there is a pregnancy exposure registry that monitors pregnancy outcomes in patients exposed to desvenlafaxine during pregnancy.

- Advise patients not to stop taking desvenlafaxine without first talking with their clinician. Advise patients that discontinuance effects may occur when stopping the drug.

- Inform patients that they may notice an inert matrix tablet passing in the stool or via colostomy, and that the active medication has already been absorbed by the time the patient sees the inert matrix tablet.

- Inform patients of other important precautionary information.

PREPARATIONS

Excipients in commercially available drug preparations may have clinically important effects in some individuals; consult specific product labeling for details.

Desvenlafaxine Succinate

Oral

Tablet, extended-release, film-coated	25 mg (of desvenlafaxine)*	Desvenlafaxine Succinate Extended-release Tablets
		Pristiq®, Pfizer
	50 mg (of desvenlafaxine)*	Desvenlafaxine Succinate Extended-release Tablets
		Pristiq®, Pfizer
	100 mg (of desvenlafaxine)*	Desvenlafaxine Succinate Extended-release Tablets
		Pristiq®, Pfizer

* available from one or more manufacturer, distributor, and/or repackager by generic (nonproprietary) name

Desvenlafaxine

Oral

| Tablets, extended-release, film-coated | 50 mg* | Desvenlafaxine Extended-release Tablets |
| | 100 mg* | Desvenlafaxine Extended-release Tablets |

* available from one or more manufacturer, distributor, and/or repackager by generic (nonproprietary) name

† Use is not currently included in the labeling approved by the US Food and Drug Administration.

Selected Revisions September 10, 2024, © Copyright, August 1, 2008, American Society of Health-System Pharmacists, Inc.

DULoxetine Hydrochloride

28:16.04.16 • SELECTIVE SEROTONIN- AND NOREPINEPHRINE-
REUPTAKE INHIBITORS

■ Duloxetine hydrochloride, a selective serotonin- and norepinephrine-
reuptake inhibitor (SNRI), is an antidepressant and anxiolytic agent.

USES

● Major Depressive Disorder

Duloxetine hydrochloride is used for the acute and maintenance treatment of
major depressive disorder in adults.

Clinical Experience

Efficacy of duloxetine for the acute treatment of major depression has been established in 4 double-blind, placebo-controlled studies of 8–9 weeks' duration in outpatient settings in adults. In these studies, patients receiving duloxetine (40–120
mg daily) had greater improvements in the 17-item Hamilton depression rating
scale (HAMD-17) total score than did patients receiving placebo. No age-, race-,
or gender-related differences in efficacy were noted in these studies.

Efficacy of duloxetine for the maintenance treatment of major depressive
disorder has been established in a randomized, placebo-controlled, relapse prevention study in which 533 adult outpatients who met DSM-IV criteria for
major depressive disorder initially received duloxetine 60 mg once daily in a
12-week, open-label, acute phase. Patients who responded to treatment during
the acute phase were then randomized to continue receiving duloxetine at the
same dosage or to receive placebo for 26 weeks in the continuation phase. The
duloxetine-treated patients experienced a longer time to relapse of depression
compared with the placebo recipients. In addition, more placebo recipients
relapsed compared with patients receiving duloxetine (approximately 29% and
17%, respectively).

Clinical Perspective

Treatment options for major depressive disorder include pharmacologic and nonpharmacologic (e.g., psychotherapy) approaches. Several classes of antidepressant
drugs are available for the treatment of major depressive disorder. In general, these
drugs have shown similar effectiveness; therefore, treatment is guided by specific
patient and drug-related factors.

A legacy practice guideline from the American Psychiatric Association (APA)
published in 2010 states that the effectiveness of antidepressants in the treatment
of major depressive disorder is generally comparable between and within classes
of medications, including selective serotonin reuptake inhibitors (SSRIs), selective
serotonin- and norepinephrine-reuptake inhibitors (SNRIs), tricyclic antidepressants (TCAs), monoamine oxidase inhibitors (MAOIs), and other antidepressants
(e.g., bupropion, mirtazapine, trazodone). Therefore, the initial selection of an
antidepressant can be based mainly on the following factors: patient preference;
nature of prior response to medication; safety, tolerability, and anticipated adverse
effects; concurrent psychiatric and medical conditions; specific properties of the
medication (e.g., half-life, cytochrome P-450 [CYP] interactions, other drug interactions); and cost.

The Department of Veterans Affairs and Department of Defense developed
more current guidelines for management of major depressive disorder. These
guidelines state that treatment of uncomplicated major depressive disorder can be
initiated with either psychotherapy (e.g., cognitive behavioral therapy) or pharmacotherapy, depending on patient preference; for patients with severe, persistent,
or recurrent major depressive disorder, a combination of pharmacotherapy and
psychotherapy is suggested. When pharmacotherapy is used as initial therapy,
either bupropion, mirtazapine, a SSRI, SNRI, trazodone, vilazodone, or vortioxetine is suggested. No evidence is available to suggest superiority of one agent over
another. The guidelines recommend against using esketamine, ketamine, MAOIs,
nefazodone, or TCAs as initial therapy. For patients not responding to initial therapy, recommendations include switching to another antidepressant (including

MAOIs or TCAs), switching to or augmenting with psychotherapy, or augmenting with a second-generation antipsychotic.

● Generalized Anxiety Disorder

Duloxetine hydrochloride is used for the acute management of generalized anxiety disorder in adults and pediatric patients ≥7 years of age.

The manufacturer states that the anxiolytic efficacy of duloxetine for long-
term use (i.e., exceeding 10 weeks) has not been established by controlled studies
to date. If duloxetine is used for extended periods, the need for continued therapy
should be reassessed periodically.

Clinical Experience

Efficacy of duloxetine for the treatment of generalized anxiety disorder in adults
has been established in 3 placebo-controlled trials of 9–10 weeks' duration in outpatient settings in adults who met DSM-IV criteria for generalized anxiety disorder. In these studies, patients receiving duloxetine (60–120 mg daily) had greater
improvements in the Hamilton anxiety scale (HAM-A) total score and the Sheehan Disability Scale (SDS) global functional impairment score than did patients
receiving placebo. No age- or gender-related differences in efficacy were noted in
these studies.

Another trial, which included a 26-week, open-label, flexible-dose (up to
120 mg daily) acute treatment phase followed by a 26-week, double-blind, placebo-
controlled, continuation phase, evaluated the efficacy of duloxetine for prevention of relapse in patients with generalized anxiety disorder. Patients responding
to acute treatment (≥50% reduction in HAM-A score and Clinical Global Impressions of Improvement (CGI-I) rating of much or very much improved) with
duloxetine were randomly re-assigned to treatment with either duloxetine at
the same dosage or placebo. Of 887 patients in the acute phase, 429 entered the
double-blind phase. Relapse was defined as an increase of ≥2 points in the Clinical
Global Impressions of Improvement-Severity (CGI-S) score to ≥4 and a Mini-In-
ternational Neuropsychiatric Interview diagnosis of generalized anxiety disorder
or discontinuation of treatment due to lack of efficacy. The relapse rate was 13.7
or 41.8% for duloxetine- or placebo-treated patients, respectively. Time to relapse
was also longer with duloxetine as compared to placebo.

Efficacy of duloxetine for the treatment of generalized anxiety disorder was also
evaluated in geriatric patients (≥65 years of age) in a randomized, double-blind,
placebo-controlled, phase 4 trial. A total of 288 patients were treated with either
duloxetine (30 mg with increases up to 120 mg per day) or placebo for 10 weeks, followed by a 2-week taper-off period. Response to treatment was assessed by a ≥50%
reduction from baseline in HAM-A total score; remission was a HAM-A total score
of ≤7. Improvement in HAM-A scores from baseline was substantially greater with
duloxetine compared to placebo (-15.9 or -11.7 for duloxetine or placebo, respectively). Response and remission rates for duloxetine were 71.3 and 44.8%, respectively, compared to 45.5 and 29.5%, respectively, for placebo.

Efficacy of duloxetine for the treatment of generalized anxiety disorder in
pediatric patients was evaluated in a flexible dose, randomized, double-blind,
placebo controlled study. A total of 272 patients 7–17 years of age with generalized anxiety disorder were randomized to treatment with duloxetine (30 mg with
increases up to 120 mg once daily) or placebo for 10 weeks. After the acute treatment phase, all patients were treated with duloxetine (30–120 mg once daily) in
an 18-week extension phase. At 10 weeks, duloxetine treatment resulted in greater
improvement in the Pediatric Anxiety Rating Scale (PARS) for anxiety severity
compared to placebo. At 28 weeks, duloxetine also resulted in improvements in
CGI-S scores, anxiety symptom severity, and Children's Global Assessment Scale
(CGAS) scores.

Clinical Perspective

First-line treatments for generalized anxiety disorder in adults include cognitive
behavioral therapy, pharmacotherapy (SSRIs or SNRIs), or a combination of both.
Pregabalin and buspirone are considered second-line or add-on therapies. SSRIs
approved for use in generalized anxiety disorder include paroxetine, sertraline,
and escitalopram; approved SNRIs include venlafaxine and duloxetine.

Among children and adolescents, anxiety disorders have a lifetime prevalence
of 20–30% in the US. Similar to treatment for adults, guidelines from the American Academy of Child and Adolescent Psychiatry (AACAP) recommend cognitive behavioral therapy or an SSRI for patients 6–18 years of age with generalized

anxiety. The guidelines suggest that combination treatment (cognitive behavioral therapy plus an SSRI) could be offered preferentially to either therapy alone. SNRIs can also be considered.

● Neuropathic Pain

Duloxetine hydrochloride is used for the management of neuropathic pain associated with diabetic peripheral neuropathy in adults.

Clinical Experience

Efficacy of duloxetine for the management of diabetic peripheral neuropathy has been established in 2 randomized, controlled, 12-week studies in adults with type 1 or 2 diabetes mellitus and a diagnosis of painful distal symmetrical sensorimotor polyneuropathy for at least 6 months. Patients were excluded from the studies if they met DSM-IV-TR criteria for major depressive disorder and dysthymia. Patients were randomized to receive duloxetine 60 mg once daily, 60 mg twice daily, or placebo in study 1 and to duloxetine 20 or 60 mg once daily, 60 mg twice daily, or placebo in study 2. In both studies, the primary outcome was the reduction in weekly mean pain scores. A total of 791 patients were enrolled. Duloxetine 60 mg once or twice daily resulted in greater improvement in mean pain scores and a greater percentage of patients achieving a ≥50% reduction in pain scores from baseline over placebo (26–27% for placebo versus 41–53% for duloxetine). Some patients in the study experienced a decrease in pain as early as week 1, which persisted throughout the study.

Clinical Perspective

The American Diabetes Association (ADA) standards of care on diabetic neuropathy stress the importance of optimal glucose, serum lipid, and blood pressure control along with lifestyle changes to help prevent or delay the development of diabetic neuropathies. However, no treatment is currently available to reverse the underlying nerve damage resulting from the neuropathy. Symptoms of diabetic neuropathy can vary, depending on the sensory fibers affected, but most commonly include pain (burning or stabbing), numbness, and tingling. For pain, the ADA pharmacologic recommendations include gabapentinoids, SNRIs, sodium channel blockers, and tricyclic antidepressants. The guidelines do not state a preference for one agent over another. The use of opioid agents for chronic neuropathic pain is not recommended.

● Fibromyalgia

Duloxetine hydrochloride is used for the management of fibromyalgia in adults and pediatric patients ≥13 years of age.

Clinical Experience

Efficacy of duloxetine for the management of fibromyalgia in adults has been established in 2 randomized, double-blind, placebo-controlled, fixed-dose studies; the studies included patients with a diagnosis of fibromyalgia based on the American College of Rheumatology (ACR) criteria (i.e., history of widespread pain for 3 months and pain present in 11 or more of the 18 specific tender point sites). The first study (FM-1) was 3 months in duration and enrolled female patients only, while the second study (FM-2) was 6 months in duration and enrolled both male and female patients. Approximately 25% of the patients had concurrent major depressive disorder. Both of these studies compared duloxetine 60 mg once daily or 120 mg daily (given in divided doses in FM-1 and as a single daily dose in FM-2) with placebo. In addition, FM-2 compared duloxetine 20 mg daily with placebo during the initial 3 months of the 6-month study; after 3 months, the duloxetine dosage was titrated up to 60 mg once daily for the remainder of the study. In these studies, duloxetine therapy in dosages of 60 or 120 mg daily significantly improved the endpoint mean pain scores from baseline and increased the number of patients who had at least a 50% reduction in pain score compared with baseline. Although pain reduction was observed in patients both with and without major depressive disorder, the degree of pain reduction may be greater in patients with major depressive disorder. Some patients experienced a reduction in pain as early as week 1, which persisted throughout the study. Improvement also was noted on measures of function as well as on the Patient Global Impression of Improvement (PGI) scale. Neither study demonstrated an additional therapeutic benefit with a dosage of 120 mg daily compared with 60 mg daily, and the higher dosage was associated with more frequent adverse effects and early discontinuance of therapy.

The efficacy of duloxetine in the treatment of fibromyalgia in pediatric patients 13–17 years of age was evaluated in a 13-week, placebo-controlled trial in 184 patients. Patients with a diagnosis of juvenile-onset fibromyalgia and a baseline score of ≥4 on the Brief Pain Inventory (BPI)-Modified Short Form were randomized to treatment with duloxetine (initial dosage of 30 mg once daily for 1 week then 60 mg daily) or placebo. Patients with rheumatologic disorders (e.g., arthritis or an autoimmune disorder) were excluded. The primary outcome was mean change from baseline in pain severity based on BPI ratings. Baseline BPI pain severity was 5.7. At 13 weeks, greater improvement was seen in BPI pain severity from baseline with duloxetine compared to placebo; however, the difference was not statistically different (-1.62 versus -0.97).

Clinical Perspective

The Centers for Disease Control and Prevention (CDC) guidelines on the use of opioids address treatment approaches to chronic pain, including pain resulting from fibromyalgia. Nonpharmacologic therapies (e.g., exercise, cognitive behavioral therapy, massage) are initially recommended to manage chronic pain. Nonopioid analgesics can be used if nonpharmacologic approaches are not sufficient for pain relief; opioids should not be considered first-line treatments for chronic pain conditions in most situations. In patients with fibromyalgia, the CDC guidelines state that tricyclic and SNRI antidepressants (including duloxetine), NSAIAs, and the gabapentinoids are used to improve pain, function, and quality of life. Selection of an appropriate regimen should be individualized.

● Chronic Musculoskeletal Pain

Duloxetine hydrochloride is used for the treatment of chronic musculoskeletal pain in adults.

Clinical Experience

Efficacy of duloxetine for the management of chronic musculoskeletal pain has been established in several randomized, double-blind, placebo-controlled studies in adults with chronic low back pain or chronic pain from osteoarthritis.

Three double-blind, placebo-controlled studies enrolled adult patients with chronic low back pain who were randomized to treatment with duloxetine 20, 60, or 120 mg daily or placebo. Two studies (CLBP-1 and CLPB-2) treated patients for 13 weeks; the third study (CLBP-3) was 12 weeks in duration.

Study CLBP-1 enrolled 236 adult patients with chronic low back pain who were randomized to treatment with either duloxetine 60 mg or placebo for 13 weeks. In patients not responding to duloxetine 60 mg (<30% reduction in pain at 7 weeks), dosage was increased to 120 mg daily in a double-blind fashion. The primary outcome was reduction in pain intensity (PI) as measured by the BPI 24-hour average pain ratings. Baseline mean pain rating was 6 on a scale of 0–10. Patients treated with duloxetine experienced greater pain reduction than placebo; at 13 weeks, the mean change from baseline in pain rating was -2.32 or -1.50 for duloxetine or placebo, respectively.

Study CLBP-2 randomized 404 adult patients with chronic low back pain to treatment with either a fixed-dose of duloxetine (20, 60, or 120 mg daily) or placebo for 13 weeks. The primary outcome was reduction in PI, defined as the weekly mean of the 24-h average pain ratings. At baseline, weekly mean PI pain ratings ranged from 6.1–6.4 on a scale of 0–10. At 13 weeks, no difference in pain reduction was seen between duloxetine and placebo.

Study CLBP-3 enrolled 401 adult patients with chronic low back pain who were randomized to receive either duloxetine 60 mg or placebo daily for 12 weeks. The primary outcome was reduction in pain intensity as measured by the BPI 24-hour average pain ratings at week 12. Baseline pain intensity was 6 on a scale of 0–10 for both groups. At 12 weeks, 48.7 or 34.7% of patients treated with duloxetine or placebo had a 50% reduction in BPI average pain score from baseline. Duloxetine was also associated with a greater reduction in average pain ratings compared to placebo (-2.25 versus -1.65).

Two double-blind, 13-week clinical trials (OA-1 and OA-2) evaluated the efficacy of duloxetine in adults for treatment of chronic pain due to osteoarthritis of the knee. Patients were randomly assigned to treatment with either duloxetine (60 or 120 mg once daily) or placebo. In Study OA-1, duloxetine was initiated at 30 mg daily for 1 week, then increased to 60 mg daily; for patients with <30% pain reduction at week 7, dosage of duloxetine was increased to 120 mg daily for the remainder of the study. In Study OA-2, duloxetine was started at 30 mg daily for 1 week, then increased to 60 mg daily for 7 weeks; patients were then re-randomized to either duloxetine 60 or 120 mg daily. Study OA-1 enrolled 256 patients, and Study OA-2 enrolled 231 patients. The primary outcome assessed was reduction from baseline in weekly 24-hour average pain severity. At baseline, patients in both studies had a mean pain rating of 6 on a scale of 0–10.

In Study OA-1, duloxetine resulted in a greater reduction in pain rating compared with placebo (-2.32 versus -1.73, respectively). A 50% reduction in pain was reported by 37.9 or 22.2% of patients treated with duloxetine (60 or 120 mg) or placebo, respectively. In study OA-2, duloxetine did not provide greater pain relief than placebo.

Clinical Perspective

The Centers for Disease Control and Prevention (CDC) guidelines on the use of opioids address treatment approaches to chronic pain, including pain resulting from osteoarthritis or low back pain. Nonpharmacologic therapies (e.g., exercise, weight loss) are initially recommended to manage chronic pain. Nonopioid analgesics can be used if nonpharmacologic approaches are not sufficient for pain relief; opioids should not be considered as first-line treatment for chronic pain conditions in most situations. In patients with osteoarthritis or chronic low back pain who have an insufficient response to nonpharmacologic interventions, CDC guidelines state that topical NSAIAs, systemic NSAIAs, or duloxetine may be considered. Selection of an appropriate regimen should be individualized.

● Stress Urinary Incontinence

Duloxetine has been used for the management of moderate to severe stress urinary incontinence (SUI)† in women. In a number of placebo-controlled clinical trials involving women with predominantly SUI receiving duloxetine or placebo for up to 12 weeks, duloxetine was significantly better than placebo in reducing the frequency of incontinence episodes (which were reduced by approximately 50% in patients receiving duloxetine) and improving patients' quality of life (as assessed by Incontinence Quality of Life questionnaire scores). Therapy with the drug generally was well tolerated in these studies, with nausea being the most commonly reported adverse effect.

Data from one subsequent analysis suggest that the beneficial effects of duloxetine in women with SUI are maintained for up to 30 months. In addition, some data suggest that combining duloxetine and pelvic floor muscle training exercises may be more effective than either treatment alone. The potential role of duloxetine therapy relative to other forms of treatment (including pelvic floor muscle training, management of fluid intake and voiding, weight loss, devices, and surgery) remains to be established and requires additional study.

● Chemotherapy-induced Peripheral Neuropathy

Duloxetine has been used for the management of chemotherapy-induced peripheral neuropathy†. Guidelines from the American Society of Clinical Oncology (ASCO) recommend that clinicians assess and discuss with patients the appropriateness of dosage reduction, dosage delay, or use of an alternate chemotherapy in patients who develop intolerable neuropathy during administration of neurotoxic chemotherapy. Duloxetine may be offered to patients with painful chemotherapy-induced peripheral neuropathy who have completed neurotoxic chemotherapy. This recommendation is based on the results of clinical trials evaluating duloxetine versus venlafaxine, pregabalin, or vitamin B12.

DOSAGE AND ADMINISTRATION

● General

Pretreatment Screening

- Screen patients with depressive symptoms for a personal or family history of suicide, bipolar disorder, and depression.

- Assess blood pressure prior to initiating therapy.

Patient Monitoring

- Monitor blood pressure periodically during duloxetine therapy.

- Monitor patients for possible worsening of depression, suicidality, or unusual changes in behavior, especially at the beginning of therapy or during periods of dosage adjustment.

- Monitor patients for serotonin syndrome.

- Regular monitoring of weight and growth is also recommended in pediatric patients receiving duloxetine.

Other General Considerations

- If patient is being transitioned to duloxetine therapy from a monoamine oxidase (MAO) inhibitor intended to treat psychiatric disorders, allow 14 days to elapse between discontinuation of the MAO inhibitor and initiation of duloxetine. Conversely, if switching from duloxetine to an MAO inhibitor, allow 5 days to elapse between discontinuation of duloxetine and initiation of the MAO inhibitor.

- Do not initiate duloxetine in patients receiving linezolid or IV methylene blue; if urgent treatment with linezolid or IV methylene blue is required, stop duloxetine and monitor for symptoms of serotonin syndrome for 5 days or until 24 hours after the last dose of linezolid or IV methylene blue (whichever comes first). Resume duloxetine 24 hours after the last dose of linezolid or IV methylene blue.

- When duloxetine therapy is discontinued, dosage should be tapered gradually and the patient carefully monitored to reduce the risk of withdrawal symptoms.

● Administration

Duloxetine hydrochloride is administered orally without regard to meals. The delayed-release capsules should be swallowed whole and *not* chewed or crushed; the contents should not be sprinkled on food or mixed with liquids.

If a dose is missed, take the missed dose as soon as it is remembered. If it is almost time for the next scheduled dose, skip the missed dose and resume regular dosing. Do not take 2 doses of duloxetine at the same time.

Store duloxetine capsules at 25°C; excursions are permitted to 15—30°C.

● Dosage

Dosage of duloxetine hydrochloride is expressed in terms of duloxetine.

Because withdrawal effects may occur, abrupt discontinuance of duloxetine should be avoided. When duloxetine therapy is discontinued, dosage should be tapered gradually and the patient carefully monitored to reduce the risk of withdrawal symptoms. If intolerable symptoms occur following dosage reduction or upon discontinuance of treatment, duloxetine therapy may be reinstituted at the previously prescribed dosage until such symptoms abate. Clinicians may resume dosage reductions at that time but at a more gradual rate.

Pediatric Dosage

Generalized Anxiety Disorder

For the management of generalized anxiety disorder in pediatric patients ≥7 years of age, the recommended initial dosage of duloxetine is 30 mg once daily. After 2 weeks, the dosage may be increased to 60 mg once daily. The manufacturer states the recommended dosage range is 30-60 mg once daily; however, some patients may benefit from dosages higher than 60 mg once daily. If the decision is made to increase the dosage beyond 60 mg once daily, increase dosage in increments of 30 mg once daily (up to a maximum dosage of 120 mg daily).

Fibromyalgia

For the management of fibromyalgia in pediatric patients ≥13 years of age, the recommended initial dosage of duloxetine is 30 mg once daily. Based on response and tolerability, the manufacturer states that dosage may be increased up to 60 mg once daily.

Adult Dosage

Major Depressive Disorder

For the management of major depressive disorder, the recommended initial dosage of duloxetine in adults is 40 mg daily (given as 20 mg twice daily) to 60 mg daily (given either as 60 mg once daily or 30 mg twice daily). In some patients, it may be desirable to initiate therapy with a dosage of 30 mg once daily for 1 week to allow patients to adjust to duloxetine before increasing to 60 mg once daily.

The manufacturer recommends a maintenance duloxetine dosage of 60 mg once daily in adults. Although duloxetine dosages of 120 mg daily have been effective, there is no evidence that dosages exceeding 60 mg daily provide additional therapeutic benefit. The usefulness of duloxetine therapy and the appropriate dosage should be reevaluated periodically in patients receiving long-term therapy.

Generalized Anxiety Disorder

For the management of generalized anxiety disorder in adults <65 years of age, the recommended initial dosage of duloxetine is 60 mg once daily. In some patients, it may be desirable to initiate therapy with a dosage of 30 mg once daily for 1 week to allow patients to adjust to duloxetine before increasing to 60 mg once daily. Dosage may be increased in increments of 30 mg once daily (up to a maximum dosage of 120 mg once daily). However, no additional benefit has been demonstrated from duloxetine dosages exceeding 60 mg once daily. The usefulness of duloxetine therapy and the appropriate dosage should be reevaluated periodically in patients receiving prolonged therapy.

For the management of generalized anxiety disorder in adults ≥65 years of age, the recommended initial dosage of duloxetine is 30 mg once daily. Dosage may be increased after 2 weeks to a target dosage of 60 mg once daily. If the decision is made to increase above 60 mg once daily, increase dosage in increments of 30 mg once daily (up to a maximum dosage of 120 mg once daily).

Neuropathic Pain

For the management of neuropathic pain associated with diabetic peripheral neuropathy, the recommended adult dosage of duloxetine is 60 mg once daily. Duloxetine dosages exceeding 60 mg daily do not appear to provide substantially greater therapeutic benefit and are less well tolerated. For patients in whom tolerability is a concern, a lower initial dosage may be considered. Because renal disease is often present in patients with diabetes, consider initiating duloxetine at a reduced starting dosage and then gradually increasing the dosage.

Fibromyalgia

For the management of fibromyalgia, the recommended adult dosage of duloxetine is 60 mg once daily. The manufacturer states that treatment should be initiated at 30 mg once daily for 1 week to allow patients to adjust to the drug before increasing the dosage to 60 mg once daily. Some patients may respond to the initial dosage of 30 mg once daily. Duloxetine dosages exceeding 60 mg daily do not appear to provide greater therapeutic benefit, even in patients not responding to a dosage of 60 mg daily, and are associated with a higher incidence of adverse effects.

Chronic Musculoskeletal Pain

For the management of chronic musculoskeletal pain, the recommended adult dosage of duloxetine is 60 mg once daily. The manufacturer states that treatment should be initiated at 30 mg once daily for 1 week to allow patients to adjust to the drug before increasing to 60 mg once daily. Duloxetine dosages exceeding 60 mg daily do not appear to provide greater therapeutic benefit, even in patients not responding to a dosage of 60 mg daily, and are associated with a higher incidence of adverse effects.

Stress Urinary Incontinence

Although the optimum dosage and duration of duloxetine therapy for the treatment of stress urinary incontinence† in women remain to be established, the most commonly used dosage in controlled trials has been 80 mg daily, usually given as 40 mg twice daily (dosage range: 20–120 mg daily). Some patients may benefit (i.e., reduced risk of nausea and dizziness) from initiating therapy with a duloxetine dosage of 20 mg twice daily for 2 weeks before increasing to the usual dosage of 40 mg twice daily. If adverse effects are bothersome during the first few weeks of therapy at the usual dosage, the dosage may be reduced to 20 mg twice daily. The safety of higher dosages (i.e., 120 mg daily), which have been used in a limited number of women with more severe cases of stress urinary incontinence, requires additional study.

● Special Populations

Hepatic Impairment

The manufacturer makes no specific dosage recommendations for patients with hepatic impairment. Use of duloxetine should be avoided in patients with chronic liver disease or cirrhosis.

Renal Impairment

The manufacturer makes no specific dosage recommendations for patients with mild or moderate renal impairment. Use of duloxetine should be avoided in patients with severe renal impairment (creatinine clearance <30 mL/minute).

Geriatric Patients

The manufacturer recommends initiating duloxetine therapy at a dosage of 30 mg once daily for 2 weeks before considering a dosage increase when treating generalized anxiety disorder in geriatric patients ≥65 years of age.

Consider dosage reduction or discontinuation if symptomatic orthostatic hypotension, falls, or syncope occur. Geriatric patients typically have a greater fall risk due to the use of multiple medications and increased presence of comorbid conditions and gait disturbances.

CAUTIONS

● Contraindications

- Concurrent or recent (i.e., within 14 days) therapy with a monoamine oxidase (MAO) inhibitor intended to treat psychiatric disorders. Use of an MAO inhibitor intended to treat psychiatric disorders within 5 days of duloxetine discontinuance.

- Initiation of duloxetine in a patient receiving MAO inhibitors such as linezolid or IV methylene blue.

● Warnings/Precautions

Warnings

Suicidal Thoughts and Behaviors

A boxed warning is included in the prescribing information for duloxetine about the increased risk of suicidal thoughts and behaviors in children, adolescents, and young adults taking antidepressants. Worsening of depression and/or the emergence of suicidal ideation and behavior (suicidality) or unusual changes in behavior may occur in both adult and pediatric patients with major depressive disorder or other psychiatric disorders, whether or not they are taking antidepressants. This risk may persist until clinically important remission occurs. Suicide is a known risk of depression and certain other psychiatric disorders, and these disorders themselves are the strongest predictors of suicide. However, there has been a long-standing concern that antidepressants may have a role in inducing worsening of depression and the emergence of suicidality in certain patients during the early phases of treatment. Pooled analyses of short-term, placebo-controlled studies of antidepressants (i.e., selective serotonin-reuptake inhibitors [SSRIs] and other antidepressants) have shown an increased risk of suicidality in children, adolescents, and young adults (18–24 years of age) with major depressive disorder and other psychiatric disorders. An increased suicidality risk was not demonstrated with antidepressants compared with placebo in adults older than 24 years of age and a reduced risk was observed in adults 65 years of age or older.

All patients being treated with antidepressants for any indication should be appropriately monitored and closely observed for clinical worsening, suicidality, and unusual changes in behavior, particularly during initiation of therapy (i.e., the first few months) and during periods of dosage adjustments. Families and caregivers of patients being treated with antidepressants for major depressive disorder or other indications, both psychiatric and nonpsychiatric, also should be advised to monitor patients on a daily basis for the emergence of agitation, irritability, or unusual changes in behavior as well as the emergence of suicidality, and to report such symptoms immediately to a health-care provider.

Although a causal relationship between the emergence of symptoms such as anxiety, agitation, panic attacks, insomnia, irritability, hostility, aggressiveness, impulsivity, akathisia, hypomania, and/or mania and either the worsening of depression and/or the emergence of suicidal impulses has not been established, there is concern that such symptoms may represent precursors to emerging suicidality. Consequently, consideration should be given to changing the therapeutic regimen or discontinuing therapy in patients whose depression is persistently worse or in patients experiencing emergent suicidality or symptoms that might be precursors to worsening depression or suicidality, particularly if such manifestations are severe, abrupt in onset, or were not part of the patient's presenting symptoms. It is also recommended that the drugs be prescribed in the smallest quantity consistent with good patient management, in order to reduce the risk of overdosage.

Because bipolar disorder may initially present as a major depressive episode, screen patients with depressive symptoms to determine the risk of bipolar disorder prior to initiating duloxetine. Screening should include taking a detailed psychiatric history (including family history of suicide, bipolar disorder, and depression). Although not established in controlled clinical studies, treatment of bipolar disorder with an antidepressant alone may precipitate the development of a mixed/manic episode in patients at risk for bipolar disorder. Duloxetine is not indicated for use in the treatment of bipolar disorder.

Other Warnings and Precautions

Hepatotoxicity

Hepatic failure, sometimes fatal, has been reported in duloxetine-treated patients. The cases presented as hepatitis accompanied by abdominal pain, hepatomegaly, and markedly elevated serum transaminase concentrations (more than 20 times the upper limit of normal [ULN]) with or without jaundice, reflecting a mixed or hepatocellular pattern of hepatic injury. Duloxetine should be discontinued in any patient who develops jaundice or other evidence of clinically important hepatic dysfunction; therapy should not be resumed unless another cause for the hepatic dysfunction can be established.

Cases of cholestatic jaundice with minimal elevation of serum transaminase concentrations also have been reported. Postmarketing reports indicate that elevated serum transaminase, bilirubin, and alkaline phosphatase concentrations have occurred in duloxetine-treated patients with chronic hepatic disease or cirrhosis.

Duloxetine has been shown to increase the risk of serum transaminase elevations in clinical trials; such elevations resulted in discontinuance of the drug in 0.3% of patients. The median time to detection of the transaminase elevation was about 2 months. In placebo-controlled trials, elevations in serum ALT concentrations to more than 3 times the ULN occurred in 1.25% of duloxetine-treated patients compared with 0.45% of those receiving placebo. There was evidence of a dose-response relationship for ALT and AST elevations.

Because of the possibility that duloxetine and alcohol may interact to cause hepatic injury or that duloxetine may aggravate preexisting hepatic disease, duloxetine should not be prescribed to patients with substantial alcohol consumption or evidence of chronic hepatic disease.

Orthostatic Hypotension, Falls, and Syncope

Orthostatic hypotension and syncope have been reported with therapeutic dosages of duloxetine; although these effects tend to occur within the first week of therapy, they may occur at any time, particularly following increases in dosage. Falls resulting in serious injury also have been reported in patients receiving duloxetine. The degree of orthostatic decrease in blood pressure appears related to the risk of falling, as well as other factors that may increase the underlying fall risk. A higher rate of falls was reported in clinical trials with duloxetine compared to placebo. The risk of decreased blood pressure may be greater in patients receiving concomitant treatment with other drugs that produce orthostatic hypotension (such as antihypertensive agents); in patients receiving potent inhibitors of the cytochrome P-450 (CYP) 1A2 isoenzyme; or in those receiving duloxetine dosages exceeding 60 mg daily. Dosage reduction or discontinuance of duloxetine should be considered in patients experiencing symptomatic orthostatic hypotension and/or syncope during therapy.

Fall risk appears to be proportional to a patient's underlying fall risk, and appears to increase with increasing age. Geriatric patients typically have a greater underlying fall risk due to the increased prevalence of multiple medications and the increased presence of comorbid conditions and gait disturbances.

Serotonin Syndrome

Potentially life-threatening serotonin syndrome has been reported with selective serotonin- and norepinephrine-reuptake inhibitors (SNRIs alone), including duloxetine, but particularly with concurrent administration of other serotonergic drugs (e.g., serotonin [5-hydroxytryptamine; 5-HT] type 1 receptor agonists ["triptans"]), tricyclic antidepressants, fentanyl, lithium, tramadol, meperidine, methadone, tryptophan, buspirone, amphetamines, and St. John's Wort [*Hypericum perforatum*]) and drugs that impair serotonin metabolism (e.g., MAO inhibitors). Signs and symptoms of serotonin syndrome may include mental status changes (e.g., agitation, hallucinations, delirium, coma), autonomic instability (e.g., tachycardia, labile blood pressure, dizziness, diaphoresis, flushing, hyperthermia), neuromuscular symptoms (e.g., tremor, rigidity, myoclonus, hyperreflexia, incoordination), seizures, and/or GI symptoms (e.g., nausea, vomiting, diarrhea).

Concurrent therapy with MAO inhibitors used for treatment of depression is contraindicated. Duloxetine should not be initiated in patients receiving MAO inhibitors such as linezolid or IV methylene blue. If an MAO inhibitor such as linezolid or IV methylene blue is necessary in a patient receiving duloxetine, discontinue duloxetine before initiating the MAO inhibitor.

Monitor all patients receiving duloxetine for serotonin syndrome. If serotonin syndrome occurs, immediately discontinue treatment with duloxetine and any concurrently administered serotonergic agents and initiate supportive symptomatic treatment.

Bleeding

Drugs that inhibit serotonin reuptake, including duloxetine, may increase the risk of bleeding events. Concurrent administration of aspirin, nonsteroidal anti-inflammatory agents (NSAIAs), warfarin, and other anticoagulants may add to this risk. Case reports and epidemiologic studies have demonstrated an association between the use of drugs that interfere with serotonin reuptake and the occurrence of GI bleeding. A postmarketing study found an increased incidence of postpartum hemorrhage in mothers receiving duloxetine. Bleeding events related to SSRI and SNRI use have ranged from ecchymoses, hematomas, epistaxis, and petechiae to life-threatening hemorrhages. Advise patients of the risk of bleeding associated with concomitant use of duloxetine and aspirin or other NSAIAs, warfarin, or other drugs that affect coagulation.

Severe Skin Reactions

Severe skin reactions such as erythema multiforme and Stevens-Johnson Syndrome (SJS) can occur with duloxetine. The rate of reported cases of SJS associated with duloxetine is greater than the incidence reported in the general population (1 to 2 cases per million person-years). Discontinue duloxetine at the first appearance of blisters, peeling rash, mucosal erosions, or other signs of hypersensitivity if not attributed to another condition.

Discontinuation Syndrome

Because withdrawal effects (e.g., dysphoric mood, irritability, agitation, nausea/vomiting, dizziness, sensory disturbances, anxiety, confusion, headache, lethargy, emotional lability, insomnia, nightmares, hypomania, tinnitus, seizures) may occur, abrupt discontinuance of duloxetine should be avoided. Gradually reduce dosage when discontinuing therapy.

If intolerable symptoms occur following dosage reduction or discontinuance, reinstitute previously prescribed dosage until symptoms abate, then resume more gradual dosage reductions.

Activation of Mania/Hypomania

Activation of mania and hypomania has occurred in patients with major depressive disorder receiving duloxetine. Use the drug with caution in patients with a history of mania.

Angle-closure Glaucoma

Antidepressant drugs such as duloxetine may cause pupillary dilation, which can trigger an angle closure attack in patients without a patent iridectomy with anatomically narrow angles.

Seizures

Use of duloxetine has not been systematically evaluated in patients with seizures, but seizures have been reported in patients receiving the drug; therefore, duloxetine should be used with caution in patients with a history of seizures.

Elevated Blood Pressure

Duloxetine may increase blood pressure. Monitor blood pressure prior to and periodically during duloxetine therapy.

Clinically Important Drug Interactions

Because cytochrome P-450 (CYP)1A2 and CYP2D6 are responsible for duloxetine metabolism, the potential exists for clinically important drug interactions when duloxetine is used concomitantly with CYP1A2 inhibitors, CYP2D6 inhibitors, and CYP2D6 substrates.

Concurrent therapy with MAO inhibitors used for the treatment of depression is contraindicated.

Because of the possibility that duloxetine and alcohol may interact to cause hepatic injury, duloxetine should not be prescribed to patients with a history of substantial alcohol use.

Caution is advised when duloxetine is given with or substituted for other centrally acting drugs, including those with a similar mechanism of action.

Hyponatremia

Treatment with SSRIs and SNRIs, including duloxetine, may result in hyponatremia. In many cases, hyponatremia appears to be due to the syndrome of inappropriate antidiuretic hormone (SIADH). Cases with serum sodium concentrations lower than 110 mmol/L have been reported and hyponatremia appeared reversible when duloxetine was discontinued. Geriatric individuals and patients receiving diuretics or who are otherwise volume depleted may be at greater risk of developing hyponatremia. Signs and symptoms of hyponatremia include headache, difficulty concentrating, memory impairment, confusion, weakness, and unsteadiness, which may lead to falls; more severe and/or acute cases have been associated with hallucinations, syncope, seizures, coma, respiratory arrest, and death. Initiate appropriate medical intervention and consider drug discontinuance in patients with symptomatic hyponatremia.

Use in Patients with Concomitant Illnesses

Experience with duloxetine in patients with concomitant diseases is limited.

Because alterations in gastric motility may affect the stability of the enteric coating of the pellets contained in duloxetine capsules, the drug should be used with caution in patients with conditions that may slow gastric emptying (e.g., in some patients with diabetes mellitus).

Duloxetine has not been systematically evaluated in patients with a recent history of myocardial infarction or unstable coronary artery disease; such patients were generally excluded from clinical studies.

Duloxetine worsens glycemic control in some patients with diabetes. In the 12-week acute treatment phase of 3 clinical studies in patients with diabetic peripheral neuropathy, small increases in fasting blood glucose were observed in duloxetine-treated patients compared with those receiving placebo. In the extension phase of these studies, which lasted up to 52 weeks, fasting blood glucose increased by 12 mg/dL in duloxetine-treated patients and decreased by 11.5 mg/dL in the routine care group; increases in glycosylated hemoglobin (hemoglobin A_{1c}) were observed in both groups of patients although the average increase was 0.3% greater in the duloxetine-treated patients compared with those receiving routine care.

Urinary Hesitation and Retention

Duloxetine belongs to a class of drugs known to affect urethral resistance. If symptoms of urinary hesitation develop during therapy, consider possibility that they may be drug-related.

Cases of urinary retention have been reported during postmarketing experience; in some of these cases, hospitalization and/or catheterization has been necessary.

Sexual Dysfunction

Sexual dysfunction, resulting in ejaculatory delay or failure, decreased libido, or erectile dysfunction in males, and decreased libido or absent orgasm in females, can occur with the use of SNRIs, including duloxetine.

Providers should inquire about sexual function prior to initiation and during treatment with duloxetine, since sexual function may not be spontaneously reported. Obtaining a detailed history, including time to symptom onset, is important when evaluating changes in sexual function, since sexual symptoms can have other causes, including the underlying psychiatric disorder. Potential management strategies should be discussed to support patients in making informed treatment decisions.

Specific Populations

Pregnancy

A National Pregnancy Registry for Antidepressants is available that monitors pregnancy outcomes in women exposed to antidepressants, including duloxetine, during pregnancy. Clinicians are encouraged to register patients by calling the National Pregnancy Registry for Antidepressants at 1-866-961-2388.

Available evidence has not identified a clear drug-associated risk of major birth defects or adverse developmental outcomes with duloxetine. There are risks associated with untreated depression and fibromyalgia and also the exposure to SNRIs or SSRIs during pregnancy. A prospective, longitudinal study of 201 euthymic women receiving antidepressants with a history of major depressive disorder showed that the discontinuation of antidepressants during pregnancy or the postpartum period was associated with a greater likelihood of a relapse of major depression. The risks of untreated depression when discontinuing or adjusting treatment during pregnancy or during the postpartum period should be considered. Fibromyalgia during pregnancy is also associated with an increased risk of adverse maternal and infant outcomes (preterm premature rupture of membranes, preterm birth, small for gestational age, intrauterine growth restriction, placental disruption, venous thrombosis), although it is not known if these outcomes are directly associated with fibromyalgia or other comorbid factors.

Data from a post-marketing cohort study suggests that duloxetine use in the month before delivery is associated with an increased risk of postpartum hemorrhage.

Some neonates exposed to SNRIs or SSRIs late in the third trimester of pregnancy have developed complications that have sometimes been severe and required prolonged hospitalization, respiratory support, and tube feeding. Such complications can arise immediately upon delivery. Clinical findings reported to date in these neonates have included respiratory distress, cyanosis, apnea, seizures, temperature instability, feeding difficulty, vomiting, hypoglycemia, hypotonia, hypertonia, hyperreflexia, tremor, jitteriness, irritability, and constant crying. These clinical features appear to be consistent with either a direct toxic effect of the SNRI or SSRI or, possibly, a drug withdrawal syndrome. It should be noted that, in some cases, the clinical picture was consistent with serotonin syndrome.

Lactation

Duloxetine is distributed into human milk. Because exposure to duloxetine through breast milk has resulted in cases of sedation, poor feeding, and poor weight gain in breast-fed infants, breast-fed infants exposed to duloxetine should be monitored for these symptoms.

Following the administration of duloxetine 40 mg once daily in 6 lactating women for 3.5 days, the resulting amount of duloxetine in the breast milk was approximately 7 mcg/day, which is an estimated daily infant dose of approximately 2 mcg/kg/day, less than 1% of the maternal dose. Peak concentrations of duloxetine in the breast milk occurred a median of 3 hours after the dose was administered. The presence of duloxetine metabolites in the breast milk has not been evaluated.

It is not known if duloxetine affects milk production. Consider the developmental and health benefits of breast-feeding, the mother's clinical need for the drug, and the potential for adverse effects on the nursing infant from exposure to duloxetine or to the untreated underlying maternal condition.

Pediatric Use

Safety and efficacy of duloxetine have been established in children 7-17 years of age for the treatment of generalized anxiety disorder, and in adolescents 13-17 years of age for the treatment of juvenile fibromyalgia syndrome. Safety and efficacy of duloxetine have not been established in pediatric patients with major depressive disorder, diabetic peripheral neuropathic pain, or chronic musculoskeletal pain.

Use of duloxetine for the treatment of generalized anxiety disorder in children 7-17 years of age is supported by one 10-week, placebo-controlled clinical trial. Safety and efficacy of duloxetine for the treatment of generalized anxiety disorder in children <7 years of age have not been established.

Use of duloxetine for the treatment of fibromyalgia in adolescents 13-17 years of age is supported by one 13-week, placebo-controlled clinical trial. Safety and efficacy of duloxetine for the treatment of fibromyalgia in pediatric patients <13 years of age have not been established.

Safety and efficacy of duloxetine for major depressive disorder have not been established in pediatric patients. In two 10-week, placebo-controlled trials, duloxetine failed to establish superiority for major depressive disorder compared to placebo.

A greater risk of suicidal thinking or behavior (suicidality) occurred during the first few months of antidepressant treatment compared with placebo in children and adolescents with major depressive disorder, obsessive-compulsive disorder (OCD), or other psychiatric disorders based on pooled analyses of 24 short-term, placebo-controlled trials of 9 antidepressant drugs (SSRIs and other antidepressants). No suicides occurred in these pediatric trials.

Monitor all pediatric patients receiving antidepressant therapy for clinical worsening and the development of suicidal thinking or behavior, especially during the first few months of treatment and during dosage changes. Decreased appetite and loss of weight have been observed with use of SSRIs and SNRIs. Regular monitoring of weight and growth is also recommended in pediatric patients receiving duloxetine.

Geriatric Use

Approximately 6, 21, 41, 33, and 8% of patients studied in clinical trials of duloxetine for major depressive disorder, chronic low back pain, osteoarthritis, diabetic peripheral neuropathy, and fibromyalgia, respectively, were 65 years of age or older. Although no overall differences in efficacy or safety were observed between geriatric and younger adult patients in the major depressive disorder, generalized anxiety disorder, diabetic peripheral neuropathic pain, fibromyalgia, osteoarthritis, and chronic low back pain clinical trials, and other clinical experience has not revealed any evidence of age-related differences, the possibility that some older patients may exhibit increased sensitivity to the drug cannot be ruled out.

Clinically important hyponatremia has been reported in geriatric patients, who may be at greater risk for this adverse effect.

In placebo-controlled trials, patients receiving duloxetine reported a higher rate of falls. Fall risk appears to be proportional to the patient's underlying fall risk, and appears to increase with increasing age. The impact of age itself on fall risk is unknown, as geriatric patients typically have greater underlying fall risk due to the increased prevalence of multiple medications and the increased presence of comorbid conditions and gait disturbances. Falls with serious consequences (fractures, hospitalization) have been reported with duloxetine.

Hepatic Impairment

Because duloxetine can aggravate underlying liver dysfunction and interact with alcohol to cause liver injury, duloxetine should not be prescribed to patients with substantial alcohol use or evidence of chronic liver disease.

In 6 cirrhotic patients with moderate liver impairment (Child-Pugh Class B), administration of a single 20-mg duloxetine dose resulted in a mean plasma clearance approximately 15% that of age- and gender-matched controls, and mean exposure (based on AUC) was increased 5-fold. Although peak plasma concentrations were not changed, the elimination half-life of duloxetine was increased 3-fold.

Renal Impairment

In patients with end-stage renal disease (requiring dialysis), AUC and peak plasma concentrations of duloxetine and its metabolites are increased. Use of duloxetine is not recommended in patients with severe renal impairment (creatinine clearance less than 30 mL/minute).

Population pharmacokinetic analyses suggest that mild to moderate (estimated creatinine clearance 30-80 mL/minute) renal impairment has no clinically important effect on duloxetine apparent clearance.

● Common Adverse Effects

Adverse effects reported in 5% or more of adults receiving duloxetine include nausea, dry mouth, somnolence, constipation, decreased appetite, and increased sweating.

Adverse effects reported in 5% or more of pediatric patients receiving duloxetine include decreased weight, decreased appetite, nausea, vomiting, fatigue, and diarrhea.

DRUG INTERACTIONS

Duloxetine is metabolized by cytochrome P-450 (CYP) isoenzymes, principally CYP2D6 and CYP1A2. Duloxetine is a moderate inhibitor of CYP2D6 and also inhibits CYP1A2. In vitro studies indicate that duloxetine does not inhibit CYP2C9, CYP3A, or CYP2C19. In vitro studies indicate that duloxetine does not induce CYP1A2 or CYP3A.

● Drugs Metabolized by Hepatic Microsomal Enzymes

Substrates of CYP2D6 (e.g., tricyclic antidepressants [TCAs; amitriptyline, desipramine, imipramine, nortriptyline], phenothiazines, class IC antiarrhythmics [flecainide, propafenone]): increased AUC of the substrate is possible. Use with caution. Consider monitoring plasma TCA concentrations and reducing the TCA dosage if used concomitantly with duloxetine.

● Drugs Affecting Hepatic Microsomal Enzymes

Potent inhibitors of CYP1A2 (e.g., fluvoxamine, some quinolone anti-infective agents [e.g., ciprofloxacin, enoxacin]): increased plasma duloxetine concentrations are possible. Avoid concomitant use.

Potent inhibitors of CYP2D6 (e.g., fluoxetine, paroxetine, quinidine) isoenzymes: increased plasma duloxetine concentrations are possible.

Concomitant administration of duloxetine and fluvoxamine, a dual CYP1A2 and CYP2D6 inhibitor, in poor CYP2D6 metabolizers resulted in a sixfold increase in duloxetine AUC and peak plasma concentrations.

● Drugs Affecting Hemostasis

Altered anticoagulant effects, including increased bleeding, have been reported when selective serotonin-reuptake inhibitors (SSRIs) or selective serotonin- and norepinephrine-reuptake inhibitors (SNRIs), including duloxetine, were concurrently administered with warfarin. Because of the potential effect of duloxetine on platelets, the manufacturer recommends careful monitoring of patients receiving warfarin during initiation and discontinuance of duloxetine therapy.

Concomitant administration of duloxetine (60 or 120 mg once daily) and warfarin (2-9 mg once daily) in healthy subjects for up to 2 weeks did not result in significant changes in the international normalized ratio (INR) from baseline; the pharmacokinetics of either protein-bound and free drug concentrations of R- and S-warfarin were not affected by concomitant use of duloxetine.

An increased risk of bleeding is possible when duloxetine is used concomitantly with aspirin or other nonsteroidal anti-inflammatory agents; use with caution.

● Drugs that Affect Gastric Acidity

The bioavailability of duloxetine may be altered if administered with drugs that increase gastric pH. However, no clinically important effect was demonstrated when duloxetine was administered with aluminum- and magnesium-containing antacids or famotidine.

Whether the concomitant administration of proton-pump inhibitors affects duloxetine absorption is currently unknown.

● Alcohol

An increased risk of hepatotoxicity is possible when duloxetine is used with alcohol; avoid concomitant use in patients with substantial alcohol use.

Duloxetine has not been shown to potentiate the impairment of mental and motor skills caused by alcohol.

● Antihypertensive Agents

An increased risk of hypotension and syncope is possible when duloxetine is used with antihypertensive agents.

● Benzodiazepines

Lorazepam does not appear to affect the pharmacokinetics of duloxetine.

Temazepam does not appear to affect the pharmacokinetics of duloxetine.

● CNS-active Drugs

A potential pharmacologic interaction is possible when duloxetine is given with or substituted for other centrally acting drugs, including those with a similar mechanism of action; use with caution.

● Monoamine Oxidase (MAO) Inhibitors

Potentially fatal serotonin syndrome may occur if duloxetine is used concomitantly with MAO inhibitors; concomitant use is contraindicated. The manufacturer recommends that at least 2 weeks should elapse between discontinuance of an MAO inhibitor and initiation of duloxetine and that at least 5 days elapse between discontinuance of duloxetine therapy and initiation of MAO inhibitor therapy.

Duloxetine should not be initiated in patients receiving MAO inhibitors such as linezolid or IV methylene blue. For those patients who require more urgent psychiatric treatment, consider other interventions such as hospitalization.

In patients already receiving duloxetine, some situations may require urgent treatment with linezolid or IV methylene blue. Duloxetine should be immediately discontinued in patients who are deemed to have no acceptable alternatives to linezolid or IV methylene blue and in whom the benefits of linezolid or IV methylene blue therapy are judged to outweigh the potential risks of serotonin syndrome. In these patients, monitor for symptoms of serotonin syndrome for 5 days or until 24 hours after the last dose of linezolid or IV methylene blue, whichever occurs earlier. Resumption of duloxetine may occur 24 hours after the last dose of linezolid or IV methylene blue.

The risk of serotonin syndrome with administration of methylene blue via non-IV routes (e.g., oral tablets, local injection) or at IV doses <1 mg/kg in patients receiving duloxetine is unclear; however, the provider should be aware of the potential for emergent symptoms of serotonin syndrome when such agents are used concomitantly.

● *Serotonergic Drugs*

Potentially life-threatening serotonin syndrome may occur if duloxetine is used concomitantly with drugs affecting serotonergic neurotransmission, including other SNRIs, SSRIs, triptans, TCAs, opioids, lithium, buspirone, amphetamines, tryptophan, and St. John's wort (*Hypericum perforatum*); use with caution.

Monitor all patients receiving duloxetine for serotonin syndrome, particularly during treatment initiation and with increases in dosage. If serotonin syndrome occurs, consider discontinuation of duloxetine and any concurrently administered serotonergic agents.

● *Smoking*

Smoking reduces duloxetine bioavailability by about one-third. The manufacturer states that routine dosage adjustment is not necessary.

● *Theophylline*

Small increases (averaging from 7–20%) in theophylline AUCs have been reported during concurrent administration of theophylline and duloxetine.

● *Thioridazine*

Increased plasma thioridazine concentrations have been observed in patients receiving duloxetine, resulting in increased risk of serious ventricular arrhythmias and sudden death; concomitant use is not recommended.

DESCRIPTION

Duloxetine hydrochloride, a selective serotonin- and norepinephrine-reuptake inhibitor (SNRI), is an antidepressant and anxiolytic agent. The drug also has demonstrated analgesic activity in animal models of chronic and persistent pain and in clinical trials evaluating the drug's activity in conditions associated with chronic pain (e.g., neuropathic pain, fibromyalgia).

The exact mechanisms of the antidepressant, anxiolytic, and central pain inhibitory actions of duloxetine have not been fully elucidated, but appear to be associated with the drug's potentiation of serotonergic and noradrenergic activity in the CNS. Duloxetine is a potent inhibitor of neuronal serotonin and norepinephrine reuptake and a less potent inhibitor of dopamine reuptake. Duloxetine does not inhibit monoamine oxidase (MAO) and has not demonstrated significant affinity for dopaminergic, adrenergic, cholinergic, γ-aminobutyric acid (GABA), glutamate, histaminergic, and opiate receptors in vitro.

Duloxetine is well absorbed following oral administration, with peak plasma concentrations usually attained in 6 hours. With evening administration, there is a 3 hour delay in absorption and a 33% increase in clearance of the drug compared to morning administration. Food increases the time to peak plasma concentrations from 6 to 10 hours, and marginally decreases the extent (about 10%) of absorption. Duloxetine pharmacokinetics are dose-proportional over the

therapeutic dosing range (30-120 mg daily). Steady state plasma concentrations are attained after 3 days of once daily dosing. Mean duloxetine concentrations at steady state are about 30% lower in pediatric patients 7-17 years of age relative to adult patients, and are considered comparable between these age groups. Duloxetine is extensively metabolized in the liver, principally via oxidation by the cytochrome P-450 (CYP) 2D6 and 1A2 isoenzymes. Major circulating metabolites do not significantly contribute to the pharmacologic activity of duloxetine. Duloxetine is a moderate inhibitor of CYP2D6 and a somewhat weak inhibitor of CYP1A2. The drug is not an inhibitor of CYP2C9, CYP2C19, or CYP3A, nor is it an inducer of CYP1A2 or CYP3A. Duloxetine is highly bound (>90%) to human plasma proteins, which is not affected by renal or hepatic impairment. The interaction potential of duloxetine with other highly protein bound drugs has not been fully elucidated. Duloxetine is excreted principally in the urine as metabolites (about 70%) and unchanged drug (<1%), and in feces (20%). The elimination half-life of duloxetine is approximately 12 hours (range: 8-17 hours). The bioavailability of duloxetine is decreased by approximately 33% in smokers. Pharmacokinetics of duloxetine are not affected by sex; half-life is similar in men and women. The impact of race on duloxetine pharmacokinetics has not been evaluated.

ADVICE TO PATIENTS

- Risk of suicidality; stress importance of patients, family, and caregivers being alert to and immediately reporting emergence of suicidality, worsening depression, or unusual changes in behavior, especially during the first few months of therapy or during periods of dosage adjustment. Advise patients to read the FDA-approved patient information (medication guide).

- Advise patients to promptly report any manifestations of liver dysfunction (e.g., pruritus, dark urine, jaundice, right upper quadrant tenderness) to their clinician. Instruct patients that they should talk to their healthcare provider about alcohol consumption.

- Inform patients of risk of severe liver injury associated with concomitant use of duloxetine and heavy alcohol intake.

- Risk of psychomotor impairment; stress importance of exercising caution while operating hazardous machinery, including automobile driving, until patient gains experience with the drug's effects.

- Advise patients of risk of orthostatic hypotension and syncope, particularly during initial therapy and subsequent dosage escalation and during concomitant therapy with drugs that may potentiate these effects.

- Inform patients of the risk of serotonin syndrome with concurrent use of duloxetine and other serotonergic agents including SNRIs, SSRIs, triptans, TCAs, opioids, lithium, buspirone, amphetamines, tryptophan, and St. John's wort (*Hypericum perforatum*). Stress importance of seeking immediate medical attention if symptoms of serotonin syndrome develop.

- Inform patients of the risk of serious skin reactions that can be severe and life-threatening. Stress importance of seeking immediate medical attention if skin blisters, peeling rash, mouth sores, hives, or other allergic reactions occur.

- Inform patients that discontinuation of duloxetine can be associated with symptoms of dizziness, headache, nausea, diarrhea, paresthesia, irritability, vomiting, insomnia, anxiety, hyperhidrosis, and fatigue. Advise patients of the importance of not discontinuing treatment or altering the dosage regimen until speaking with their healthcare provider.

- Advise patients of the importance of taking medication exactly as prescribed by the clinician. Stress importance of swallowing the capsule whole, without chewing, crushing, sprinkling on food, or mixing with liquids.

- Advise patients of the importance of adequately screening for risk of bipolar disorder (e.g., family history of suicide, bipolar disorder, and depression) prior to initiating duloxetine. Inform patients that they should report any symptoms of a manic reaction (e.g., great increases in energy, significant issues sleeping, racing thoughts, reckless behavior, excessive talking or talking faster than usual, unusual grand ideas, excessive happiness or irritability).

- Inform patients of the risk of mild pupillary dilation, which can cause angle-closure glaucoma in susceptible individuals.

- Advise patients to inform their clinicians of a history of seizure disorder.

- Inform patients that duloxetine may increase blood pressure.

- Inform patients that hyponatremia has been reported with duloxetine.

- Instruct patients to report any changes in urine flow.

- Inform patients that duloxetine can cause sexual dysfunction, and to discuss any changes and potential management strategies with their healthcare provider.

- Advise women to inform their clinicians if they are or plan to become pregnant or plan to breast-feed. Inform patients that duloxetine use can increase the risk of neonatal complications that necessitate prolonged hospitalization, respiratory support, and tube feeding. Inform pregnant women of the risk of major depression relapse with discontinuation of duloxetine. Inform patients of the pregnancy exposure registry that monitors outcomes in women exposed to duloxetine. Advise breastfeeding women to monitor infants for sedation, poor feeding, and poor weight gain and to seek medical attention if these symptoms occur.

- Advise patients to inform their clinicians of existing or contemplated concomitant therapy, including prescription and OTC drugs, as well as any concomitant illnesses (e.g., bipolar disorder, liver disease) or family history of suicidality or bipolar disorder. Advise patients of the risk of bleeding associated with concomitant use of duloxetine with aspirin or other nonsteroidal anti-inflammatory agents, warfarin, or other drugs that affect coagulation.

- Inform patients of other important precautionary information.

PREPARATIONS

Excipients in commercially available drug preparations may have clinically important effects in some individuals; consult specific product labeling for details.

DULoxetine Hydrochloride

Oral

Capsules, delayed-release (containing enteric-coated pellets)	20 mg (of duloxetine)*	**Cymbalta®**, Lilly
		Duloxetine Delayed-release Capsules
	30 mg (of duloxetine)*	**Cymbalta®**, Lilly
		Duloxetine Delayed-release Capsules
	60 mg (of duloxetine)*	**Cymbalta®**, Lilly
		Duloxetine Delayed-release Capsules

* available from one or more manufacturer, distributor, and/or repackager by generic (nonproprietary) name

† Use is not currently included in the labeling approved by the US Food and Drug Administration.

Citalopram Hydrobromide

28:16.04.20 • SELECTIVE SEROTONIN-REUPTAKE INHIBITORS

■ Citalopram hydrobromide, a selective serotonin-reuptake inhibitor (SSRI), is an antidepressant.

USES

Citalopram hydrobromide is used in the treatment of major depressive disorder. In addition, citalopram has been used for the treatment of obsessive-compulsive disorder†, panic disorder†, social phobia† (social anxiety disorder), alcohol dependence†, premenstrual dysphoric disorder†, premature ejaculation†, eating disorders†, diabetic neuropathy†, and posttraumatic stress disorder†.

● Major Depressive Disorder

Citalopram hydrobromide is used in the treatment of major depressive disorder. A major depressive episode implies a prominent and relatively persistent depressed or dysphoric mood that usually interferes with daily functioning (nearly every day for at least 2 weeks). According to DSM-IV criteria, a major depressive episode includes at least 5 of the following 9 symptoms (with at least one of the symptoms being either depressed mood or loss of interest or pleasure): depressed mood most of the day as indicated by subjective report (e.g., feels sad or empty) or observation made by others; markedly diminished interest or pleasure in all, or almost all, activities most of the day; significant weight loss (when not dieting) or weight gain (e.g., a change of more than 5% of body weight in a month), or decrease or increase in appetite; insomnia or hypersomnia; psychomotor agitation or retardation (observable by others, not merely subjective feelings of restlessness or being slowed down); fatigue or loss of energy; feelings of worthlessness or excessive or inappropriate guilt (not merely self-reproach or guilt about being sick); diminished ability to think or concentrate or indecisiveness (either by subjective account or as observed by others); and recurrent thoughts of death, recurrent suicidal ideation without a specific plan, or a suicide attempt or specific plan for committing suicide.

Treatment of major depressive disorder generally consists of an acute phase (to induce remission), a continuation phase (to preserve remission), and a maintenance phase (to prevent recurrence). Various interventions (e.g., psychotherapy, antidepressant drug therapy, electroconvulsive therapy [ECT]) are used alone or in combination to treat major depressive episodes. Treatment should be individualized, and the most appropriate strategy for a particular patient is determined by clinical factors such as severity of depression (e.g., mild, moderate, severe), presence or absence of certain psychiatric features (e.g., suicide risk, catatonia, psychotic or atypical features, alcohol or substance abuse or dependence, panic or other anxiety disorder, cognitive dysfunction, dysthymia, personality disorder, seasonal affective disorder), and concurrent illness (e.g., asthma, cardiac disease, dementia, seizure disorder, glaucoma, hypertension). Demographic and psychosocial factors as well as patient preference also are used to determine the most effective treatment strategy.

While use of psychotherapy alone may be considered as an initial treatment strategy for patients with mild to moderate major depressive disorder (based on patient preference and presence of clinical features such as psychosocial stressors), combined use of antidepressant drug therapy and psychotherapy may be useful for initial treatment of patients with moderate to severe major depressive disorder with psychosocial issues, interpersonal problems, or a comorbid axis II disorder. In addition, combined use of antidepressant drug therapy and psychotherapy may be beneficial in patients who have a history of poor compliance or only partial response to adequate trials of either antidepressant drug therapy or psychotherapy alone.

Antidepressant drug therapy can be used alone for initial treatment of patients with mild major depressive disorder (if preferred by the patient) and usually is indicated alone or in combination with psychotherapy for initial treatment of patients with moderate to severe major depressive disorder (unless ECT is planned). ECT is not generally used for initial treatment of uncomplicated major depression, but is recommended as first-line treatment for severe major depressive disorder when it is coupled with psychotic features, catatonic stupor, severe suicidality, food refusal leading to nutritional compromise, or other situations when a rapid antidepressant response is required. ECT also is recommended for patients who have

previously shown a positive response to or a preference for this treatment modality and can be considered for patients with moderate or severe depression who have not responded to or cannot receive antidepressant drug therapy. In certain situations involving depressed patients unresponsive to adequate trials of several individual antidepressant agents, adjunctive therapy with another agent (e.g., buspirone, lithium) or concomitant use of a second antidepressant agent (e.g., bupropion) has been used; however, such combination therapy is associated with an increased risk of adverse reactions, may require dosage adjustments, and (if not contraindicated) should be undertaken only after careful consideration of the relative risks and benefits. (See Drug Interactions: Serotonergic Drugs, Tricyclic and Other Antidepressants under Drug Interactions: Drugs Undergoing Hepatic Metabolism or Affecting Hepatic Microsomal Enzymes, and Drug Interactions: Lithium.)

The efficacy of citalopram for the management of major depression has been established in short-term (4–6 weeks' duration), placebo-controlled studies in outpatients 18–66 years of age who met DSM-III or -III-R criteria for major depressive disorder. In a 6-week study in which patients received fixed citalopram dosages of 10, 20, 40, or 60 mg daily, the drug was effective at dosages of 40 and 60 mg daily as measured by the Hamilton Depression Rating Scale (HAM-D) Total Score, the HAM-D Depressed Mood Item (Item 1), the Montgomery Asberg Depression Rating Scale, and the Clinical Global Impression (CGI) Severity Scale. This study showed no clear antidepressant effect of the 10 or 20 mg daily dosages, and the 60 mg daily dosage was not more effective than the 40 mg daily dosage.

In a 4-week, placebo-controlled study in depressed adult patients, of whom 85% met criteria for melancholia, those who were treated with citalopram (at an initial dosage of 20 mg daily, titrated to the maximum tolerated dosage or to a maximum daily dosage of 80 mg) showed greater improvement than patients receiving placebo on the HAM-D Total Score, HAM-D Item 1, and the CGI Severity score. In 3 additional placebo-controlled depression trials, the difference in response to treatment between patients receiving citalopram and patients receiving placebo was not statistically significant, possibly due at least in part to a high spontaneous response rate, a high placebo response rate, small sample size, or, in the case of one study, too low a dosage.

In 2 placebo-controlled studies, depressed adult patients who had responded to an initial 6- to 8-week course of citalopram (fixed dosage of 20 or 40 mg daily in one study and flexible dosages ranging from 20–60 mg daily in the second study) were randomized to continue receiving citalopram or placebo for up to 6 months. In both of these studies, patients receiving citalopram experienced substantially lower relapse rates over the subsequent 6 months compared with those receiving placebo. In the fixed-dose study, the decreased rate of depression relapse was similar in patients receiving 20 or 40 mg daily of citalopram. An analysis of these data for possible age-, gender-, and race-related effects on treatment outcome did not suggest any difference in antidepressant efficacy based on the age, gender, and race of the patient. In a placebo-controlled trial, citalopram also was shown to help prevent recurrences of depression in patients with recurrent major depression receiving the drug for up to 6–18 months.

While the optimum duration of citalopram therapy has not been established, many experts state that acute depressive episodes require several months or longer of sustained antidepressant therapy. In addition, some clinicians recommend that long-term antidepressant therapy be considered in certain patients at risk for recurrence of depressive episodes (such as those with highly recurrent unipolar depression). In placebo-controlled studies, citalopram has been shown to be effective for the long-term (e.g., up to 18 months) management of depression. In addition, the drug has been used in some patients for longer periods (e.g., up to 28 months) without apparent loss of clinical effect or increased toxicity. However, when citalopram is used for extended periods, the need for continued therapy should be reassessed periodically. (See Dosage and Administration: Dosage.)

The manufacturer states that efficacy of citalopram as an antidepressant in hospital settings has not been studied adequately to date; however, the drug has been shown to be effective in hospitalized patients with depression, including severe depression, in several studies.

As with other antidepressants, the possibility that citalopram may precipitate hypomanic or manic attacks in patients with bipolar or other major affective disorder should be considered. Citalopram is *not* approved for use in treating bipolar depression.

Considerations in Choosing an Antidepressant

A variety of antidepressant drugs are available for the treatment of major depressive disorder, including selective serotonin-reuptake inhibitors (SSRIs; e.g., citalopram, fluoxetine, paroxetine, sertraline), selective serotonin- and norepinephrine-re-uptake inhibitors (SNRIs; e.g., desvenlafaxine, duloxetine, venlafaxine), tricyclic antidepressants (e.g., amitriptyline, amoxapine, desipramine, doxepin, imipramine, nortriptyline, protriptyline, trimipramine), monoamine oxidase (MAO) inhibi-tors (e.g., phenelzine, tranylcypromine), and other antidepressants (e.g., bupropion, maprotiline, nefazodone, trazodone, vilazodone). Most clinical studies have shown that the antidepressant effect of usual dosages of citalopram in patients with depres-sion is greater than that of placebo and comparable to that of usual dosages of tri-cyclic antidepressants (e.g., amitriptyline, imipramine, clomipramine), other SSRIs (e.g., fluoxetine, fluvoxamine, paroxetine, sertraline), and other antidepressants (e.g., mirtazapine, venlafaxine). Escitalopram, the active S-enantiomer of citalo-pram, also is commercially available for the treatment of depression. Although there is some evidence that escitalopram may offer some clinical advantages compared with citalopram or other SSRIs (e.g., increased efficacy, more rapid onset of thera-peutic effect, fewer adverse effects), additional studies are needed to confirm these initial findings. The onset of antidepressant action of citalopram appears to be com-parable to that of tricyclic antidepressants and other SSRIs, although there is some evidence that the onset of action may occur slightly earlier with citalopram than with some other antidepressants, including sertraline. However, additional study is needed to confirm these findings.

In general, response rates in patients with major depression are similar for cur-rently available antidepressants, and the choice of antidepressant agent for a given patient depends principally on other factors such as potential adverse effects, safety or tolerability of these adverse effects in the individual patient, psychiat-ric and medical history, patient or family history of response to specific therapies, patient preference, quantity and quality of available clinical data, cost, and relative acute overdose safety. No single antidepressant can be recommended as optimal for all patients because of substantial heterogeneity in individual responses and in the nature, likelihood, and severity of adverse effects. In addition, patients vary in the degree to which certain adverse effects and other inconveniences of drug ther-apy (e.g., cost, dietary restrictions) affect their preferences.

In the large-scale Sequenced Treatment Alternatives to Relieve Depression (STAR*D) effectiveness trial, patients with major depressive disorder who did not respond to or could not tolerate citalopram therapy were randomized to switch to extended-release ("sustained-release") bupropion, sertraline, or extended-release venlafaxine as a second step of treatment (level 2). Remission rates as assessed by the 17-item Hamilton Rating Scale for Depression (HRSD-17) and the Quick Inventory of Depressive Symptomatology—Self Report (QIDS-SR-16) were approximately 21 and 26% for extended-release bupropion, 18 and 27% for sertraline, and 25 and 25% for extended-release venlafaxine therapy, respectively; response rates as assessed by the QIDS-SR-16 were 26, 27, and 28% for extended-release bupropion, sertraline, and extended-release venlafaxine therapy, respectively. These results suggest that after unsuccessful initial treatment of depressed patients with an SSRI, approxi-mately 25% of patients will achieve remission after therapy is switched to another antidepressant, and either another SSRI (e.g., sertraline) or an agent from another class (e.g., bupropion, venlafaxine) may be reasonable alternative antidepressants in patients not responding to initial SSRI therapy.

Patient Tolerance Considerations

Because of differences in the adverse effect profile between selective serotonin-re-uptake inhibitors and tricyclic antidepressants, particularly less frequent anti-cholinergic effects, cardiovascular effects, and/or weight gain with selective serotonin-reuptake inhibitors, these drugs may be preferred in patients in whom such effects are not tolerated or are of potential concern. The decreased incidence of anticholinergic effects associated with citalopram and other selective serotonin-re-uptake inhibitors compared with tricyclic antidepressants is a potential advantage, since such effects may result in discontinuance of the drug early during therapy in unusually sensitive patients. In addition, some anticholinergic effects may become troublesome during long-term tricyclic antidepressant therapy (e.g., persistent dry mouth may result in tooth decay). Although selective serotonin-reuptake inhibi-tors share the same overall tolerability profile, certain patients may tolerate one drug in this class better than another. Antidepressants other than selective serotonin-re-uptake inhibitors may be preferred in patients in whom certain adverse GI effects (e.g., nausea, anorexia), nervous system effects (e.g., anxiety, nervousness, insom-nia), and/or weight loss are not tolerated or are of concern, since such effects appear to occur more frequently with citalopram and other drugs in this class.

Pediatric Considerations

The clinical presentation of depression in children and adolescents† can differ from that in adults and generally varies with the age and developmental stages of the child. Younger children may exhibit behavioral problems such as social with-drawal, aggressive behavior, apathy, sleep disruption, and weight loss; adolescents may present with somatic complaints, self-esteem problems, rebelliousness, poor performance in school, or a pattern of engaging in risky or aggressive behavior.

Only limited data are available to date from controlled clinical studies evaluat-ing various antidepressant agents in children and adolescents, and many of these studies have methodologic limitations (e.g., nonrandomized or uncontrolled, small sample size, short duration, nonspecific inclusion criteria). However, there is some evidence that the response to antidepressants in pediatric patients may differ from that seen in adults, and caution should be used in extrapolating data from adult studies when making treatment decisions for pediatric patients.

Results of several studies evaluating tricyclic antidepressants (e.g., amitrip-tyline, desipramine, imipramine, nortriptyline) in preadolescent and adolescent patients with major depression indicate a lack of overall efficacy in this age group. Based on the lack of efficacy data regarding use of tricyclic antidepressants and MAO inhibitors in pediatric patients and because of the potential for life-threat-ening adverse effects associated with the use of these drugs, many experts con-sider selective serotonin-reuptake inhibitors, including citalopram, the drugs of choice when antidepressant therapy is indicated for the treatment of major depressive disorder in children and adolescents. However, the US Food and Drug Administration (FDA) states that, while efficacy of fluoxetine has been established in pediatric patients, efficacy of other newer antidepressants (i.e., citalopram, des-venlafaxine, duloxetine, escitalopram, fluvoxamine, mirtazapine, nefazodone, paroxetine, sertraline, venlafaxine) was not conclusively established in clinical tri-als in pediatric patients with major depressive disorder. In addition, FDA now warns that antidepressants increase the risk of suicidal thinking and behavior (sui-cidality) in children and adolescents with major depressive disorder and other psychiatric disorders. (See Cautions: Pediatric Precautions.) FDA currently states that anyone considering using an antidepressant in a child or adolescent for any clinical use must balance the potential risk of therapy with the clinical need. (See Cautions: Precautions and Contraindications.)

Geriatric Considerations

The response to antidepressants in depressed geriatric patients without dementia is similar to that reported in younger adults, but depression in geriatric patients often is not recognized and is not treated. In geriatric patients with major depres-sive disorder, SSRIs appear to be as effective as tricyclic antidepressants but may cause fewer overall adverse effects than these other agents. Geriatric patients appear to be especially sensitive to anticholinergic (e.g., dry mouth, constipation, vision disturbance), cardiovascular, orthostatic hypotensive, and sedative effects of tricyclic antidepressants. The low incidence of anticholinergic effects associ-ated with citalopram and other SSRIs compared with tricyclic antidepressants is a potential advantage in geriatric patients, since such effects (e.g., constipation, dry mouth, confusion, memory impairment) may be particularly troublesome in these patients. However, SSRI therapy may be associated with other troublesome adverse effects (e.g., nausea and vomiting, agitation and akathisia, parkinsonian adverse effects, sexual dysfunction, weight loss, and hyponatremia). Some clini-cians state that SSRIs including citalopram may be preferred for treating depres-sion in geriatric patients in whom the orthostatic hypotension associated with many antidepressants (e.g., tricyclics) potentially may result in injuries (such as severe falls). However, despite the fewer cardiovascular and anticholinergic effects associated with SSRIs, these drugs did not show any advantage over tricyclic anti-depressants with regard to hip fracture in a case-control study. In addition, there was little difference in the rates of falls between nursing home residents receiv-ing SSRIs and those receiving tricyclic antidepressants in a retrospective study. Therefore, all geriatric patients receiving either type of antidepressant should be considered at increased risk of falls and appropriate measures should be taken. In addition, clinicians prescribing SSRIs in geriatric patients should be aware of the many possible drug interactions associated with these drugs, including those involving metabolism of the drugs through the cytochrome P-450 system. (See Drug Interactions.)

Patients with dementia of the Alzheimer's type (Alzheimer's disease, presenile or senile dementia) often present with depressive symptoms, such as depressed mood, appetite loss, insomnia, fatigue, irritability, and agitation. Most experts rec-ommend that patients with dementia of the Alzheimer's type who present with clinically significant and persistent depressive symptoms be considered as candi-dates for pharmacotherapy even if they fail to meet the criteria for a major depres-sive syndrome. The goals of such therapy are to improve mood, functional status (e.g., cognition), and quality of life. Treatment of depression also may reduce other neuropsychiatric symptoms associated with depression in patients with dementia, including aggression, anxiety, apathy, and psychosis. Although patients may present with depressed mood alone, the possibility of more extensive depressive symptomatology should be considered. Therefore, patients should be evaluated and monitored carefully for indices of major depression, suicidal ideation, and neurovegetative signs since safety measures (e.g., hospitalization for suicidal ideations) and more vigorous and aggressive therapy (e.g., relatively high dosages, multiple drug trials) may be needed in some patients.

Although placebo-controlled trials of antidepressants in depressed patients with concurrent dementia have shown mixed results, the available evidence and experience with the use of antidepressants in patients with dementia of the Alzheimer's type and associated depressive manifestations indicate that depressive symptoms (including depressed mood alone and with neurovegetative changes) in such patients are responsive to antidepressant therapy. In some patients, cognitive deficits may partially or fully resolve during antidepressant therapy, but the extent of response will be limited to the degree of cognitive impairment that is directly related to depression. SSRIs such as citalopram, escitalopram, fluoxetine, paroxetine, or sertraline generally are considered first-line agents in the treatment of depressed patients with dementia since they usually are better tolerated than some other antidepressants (e.g., tricyclic antidepressants, monoamine oxidase inhibitors). Some possible alternative agents to SSRIs include bupropion, mirtazapine, and venlafaxine. Some geriatric patients with dementia and depression may be unable to tolerate the antidepressant dosages needed to achieve full remission. When a rapid antidepressant response is not critical, some experts therefore recommend a very gradual dosage titration to increase the likelihood that a therapeutic dosage of the SSRI or other antidepressant will be reached and tolerated. In a controlled study comparing citalopram and placebo in elderly patients with dementia, citalopram was found to improve depression as well as cognitive and emotional functioning more than placebo. In an open study in a limited number of patients with dementia and behavioral disturbances, citalopram was found to improve the behavioral complications associated with dementia†.

Cardiovascular Considerations

Clinical studies of citalopram for the management of depression generally did not include individuals with cardiovascular disease (e.g., those with a recent history of myocardial infarction or unstable cardiovascular disease).

Citalopram causes dose-dependent QT_c-interval prolongation, and torsades de pointes, ventricular tachycardia, and sudden death have been reported in postmarketing experience in patients receiving the drug. Patients with congenital long QT syndrome, uncompensated heart failure, bradyarrhythmias, recent acute myocardial infarction, or hypokalemia or hypomagnesemia or who are receiving other drugs that prolong the QT interval are at higher risk of developing torsades de pointes. (See Cautions: Cardiovascular Effects, Cautions: Precautions and Contraindications, and Drug Interactions: Drugs that Prolong the QT Interval.)

Sedative Considerations

Because citalopram and other selective serotonin-reuptake inhibitors generally are less sedating than some other antidepressants (e.g., tricyclics), some clinicians state that these drugs may be preferable in patients who do not require the sedative effects associated with many antidepressant agents or in patients who are prone to accidents; however, an antidepressant with more prominent sedative effects (e.g., trazodone) may be preferable in certain patients (e.g., those with insomnia).

Suicidal Risk Considerations

Suicide is a known risk of depression and certain other psychiatric disorders, and these disorders themselves are the strongest predictors of suicide. However, there has been a long-standing concern that antidepressants may have a role in inducing worsening of depression and the emergence of suicidal thinking and behavior (suicidality) in certain patients during the early phases of treatment. FDA states that antidepressants increased the risk of suicidality in short-term studies in children, adolescents, and young adults (18–24 years of age) with major depressive disorder and other psychiatric disorders. (See Cautions: Pediatric Precautions.) An increased suicidality risk was not demonstrated with antidepressants compared with placebo in adults older than 24 years of age and a reduced risk was observed in adults 65 years of age or older. It currently is unknown whether the suicidality risk extends to longer-term antidepressant use (i.e., beyond several months); however, there is substantial evidence from placebo-controlled maintenance trials in adults with major depressive disorder that antidepressants can delay the recurrence of depression. Because the risk of suicidality in depressed patients may persist until substantial remission of depression occurs, appropriate monitoring and close observation of patients of all ages who are receiving antidepressant therapy are recommended. (See Cautions: Precautions and Contraindications.)

Other Considerations

Citalopram has been effective in patients with moderate to severe depression, endogenous depression, post-stroke depression and pathologic crying, and depression associated with chronic hepatitis C virus infection.

In an open study in a limited number of patients with bipolar depression† (mainly bipolar I disorder), citalopram was effective and well tolerated when added to monotherapy or combined therapy with lithium, divalproex sodium, and/or carbamazepine. Controlled studies are needed to confirm these preliminary findings. The manufacturer states that citalopram is *not* approved for use in treating bipolar depression, and that the possibility that the drug may precipitate hypomanic or manic attacks in patients with bipolar or other major affective disorder should be considered. For detailed information on bipolar disorder, including its management, see Uses: Bipolar Disorder, in Lithium Salts 28:28.

In patients with refractory depression, citalopram was more effective when given in combination with buspirone in one placebo-controlled study. However, combined citalopram and buspirone therapy was not found to be more effective than citalopram monotherapy in another placebo-controlled study. In the Sequenced Treatment Alternatives to Relieve Depression (STAR*D) level 2 trial, patients with major depressive disorder who did not respond to or could not tolerate citalopram therapy were randomized to receive either extended-release ("sustained-release") bupropion or buspirone therapy in addition to citalopram. Although both extended-release bupropion and buspirone were found to produce similar remission rates, extended-release bupropion produced a greater reduction in the number and severity of symptoms and a lower rate of drug discontinuance than buspirone in this large-scale effectiveness trial. These results suggest that augmentation of SSRI therapy with extended-release bupropion may be useful in some patients with refractory depression. The addition of lithium to citalopram in depressed patients not responding to citalopram alone also has been found to be effective and well tolerated in a double-blind, placebo-controlled trial. (See Drug Interactions: Lithium.)

In a limited number of depressed patients not responding to citalopram alone, the addition of carbamazepine was effective and well tolerated in an open study. However, the possibility of serotonin syndrome and drug interactions should be considered pending further clinical experience with this combination. (See Drug Interactions: Serotonergic Drugs and Carbamazepine under Drug Interactions: Drugs Undergoing Hepatic Metabolism or Affecting Hepatic Microsomal Enzymes.)

Citalopram was found to improve personality disturbances† (decrease in anxiety and aggression-related symptoms and increase in social desirability and socialization) in depressed patients in one study.

● Obsessive-Compulsive Disorder

Citalopram has been used in the treatment of obsessive-compulsive disorder†. In a large, double-blind, placebo-controlled trial evaluating citalopram (20, 40, or 60 mg daily for 12 weeks) in adults with obsessive-compulsive disorder, the drug was more effective than placebo as measured by Yale-Brown Obsessive-Compulsive Scale score changes at all 3 dosages. The highest response rate (65%) was observed in those who received 60 mg daily; this compared with 52 or 57% in those receiving 40 or 20 mg daily, respectively. An analysis of predictors of response to citalopram therapy from this trial suggested that patients with a longer duration of obsessive-compulsive disorder, more severe symptoms, or a history of previous selective serotonin-reuptake inhibitor therapy were less likely to respond to therapy with citalopram. In an open trial, 76% of patients with obsessive-compulsive disorder receiving citalopram therapy (usually 40 or 60 mg daily) for 24 weeks demonstrated improved symptoms associated with this condition. In another open study, citalopram (40 mg daily) was effective in a limited number of patients with refractory obsessive-compulsive disorder who had failed to respond to therapy with other selective serotonin-reuptake inhibitors. Clinical experience to date indicates that citalopram is well tolerated in patients with obsessive-compulsive disorder. Additional study is needed to determine the long-term efficacy of citalopram in the treatment of this condition.

For additional information on the use of selective serotonin-reuptake inhibitors in the treatment of obsessive-compulsive disorder, see Uses: Obsessive-Compulsive Disorder, in Sertraline Hydrochloride 28:16.04.20.

● Panic Disorder

Citalopram has been used in the treatment of panic disorder with or without agoraphobia†. In a randomized, single-blind study comparing citalopram and paroxetine in adults with panic disorder, both drugs were found to be effective and well tolerated, with 86% of the citalopram-treated patients and 84% of the paroxetine-treated patients responding well to 2 months of therapy. In a limited number of adults with panic disorder, citalopram therapy (20–60 mg daily) produced a full remission in 66% of the patients and improved symptomatology.

In a large, double-blind, placebo-controlled trial evaluating the efficacy and tolerability of long-term therapy (up to 1 year) with citalopram at 3 dosages (10–15 mg daily, 20–30 mg daily, 40–60 mg daily) or clomipramine in adult outpatients with panic disorder with or without agoraphobia, both drugs were more effective than placebo. Citalopram was more effective than placebo at all dosages studied, with a dosage of 20–30 mg daily being the most effective maintenance dosage in most patients.

For additional information on the use of selective serotonin-reuptake inhibitors in the treatment of panic disorder, see Uses: Panic Disorder, in Sertraline Hydrochloride 28:16.04.20.

● Social Phobia

Like some other selective serotonin-reuptake inhibitors, citalopram has been used in the treatment of social phobia† (social anxiety disorder). However, additional evidence from well-designed studies is needed to more fully elucidate the role of the drug in this disorder.

In an open study in a limited number of patients with social phobia, 86% of patients responded to citalopram 40 mg daily after 12 weeks as rated by the Clinical Global Impressions (CGI) score and the Liebowitz Social Anxiety Scale (LSAS).

In an open, flexible-dose study in patients with social anxiety disorder with comorbid major depression, response rates after 12 weeks of citalopram therapy (mean dosage: 38 mg daily) were approximately 67 and 76% for social anxiety disorder and depression, respectively. However, the depression symptoms responded more rapidly and completely than the social anxiety symptoms after 12 weeks of citalopram therapy, suggesting that a longer duration of therapy may be necessary to fully assess the clinical efficacy of the drug in such patients.

In a randomized, open trial comparing citalopram and moclobemide (not commercially available in the US) in patients with social phobia, similar improvements in the CGI-improvement score and LSAS were noted with these drugs. Clinical experience to date suggests that citalopram generally is well tolerated in patients with social phobia. However, well controlled studies are needed to confirm the efficacy and safety and to determine the optimal dosage of citalopram in patients with this condition.

● Alcohol Dependence

Like some other selective serotonin-reuptake inhibitors (fluoxetine, zimelidine [not commercially available in the US]), citalopram has been used in the management of alcohol dependence†. In clinical studies, citalopram has been shown to reduce alcohol consumption in alcohol-dependent, nondepressed drinkers receiving short-term therapy with 40 mg of the drug daily. In clinical studies conducted to date with selective serotonin-reuptake inhibitors in alcoholic patients, considerable interindividual variability in response has been observed, with reduction in alcohol consumption ranging from 10 to more than 70%. Several factors, including gender, alcoholic subtype, presence or absence of depression, and extent of drinking, appear to affect the clinical efficacy of selective serotonin-reuptake inhibitors in the management of alcohol dependence. Additional study is required to fully determine the safety and efficacy of citalopram in the management of alcohol dependence. (See Pharmacology: Effects on Alcohol Intake and also see Drug Interactions: Alcohol.)

● Premenstrual Dysphoric Disorder

Like some other selective serotonin-reuptake inhibitors (e.g., fluoxetine, paroxetine, sertraline), citalopram has been used in a limited number of women with premenstrual dysphoric disorder† (previously late luteal phase dysphoric disorder). Clinical experience to date suggests that the onset of action of serotonin-reuptake inhibitors in women with premenstrual dysphoric disorder is more rapid than when used for other psychiatric conditions; therefore, administration only during the luteal phase of the menstrual cycle may potentially be effective in this condition.

In a placebo-controlled trial, intermittent administration of citalopram (10–30 mg daily during the luteal phase) for 3 menstrual cycles appeared to be more effective than continuous (10–30 mg daily throughout the menstrual cycle) or semi-intermittent administration (5 mg daily during the follicular phase and 10–30 mg daily during the luteal phase) of the drug and substantially more effective than placebo. Citalopram was well tolerated in all 3 regimens, and adverse effects generally were mild and transient. Additional controlled studies are needed to determine whether the efficacy of the drug is sustained during longer-term, maintenance therapy in women with this condition.

● Premature Ejaculation

Like some other selective serotonin-reuptake inhibitors, citalopram has been used for the treatment of premature ejaculation†. However, studies with citalopram to date have only involved a limited number of patients and there is some evidence that the drug may be less effective than certain other selective serotonin-reuptake inhibitors (e.g., paroxetine). In a double-blind study in men with premature ejaculation, citalopram 20 mg daily delayed ejaculation to a slight degree (1. 8-fold increase in intravaginal ejaculation latency time) compared with a marked increase (8. 9-fold increase) with paroxetine 20 mg daily following 6 weeks of therapy. These preliminary findings suggest that paroxetine may be more effective than citalopram in the treatment of premature ejaculation.

● Eating Disorders

Citalopram has been used in a limited number of patients for the treatment of bulimia nervosa† or anorexia nervosa†. Although citalopram reportedly has been effective in some patients with these eating disorders, underweight patients with anorexia nervosa who received citalopram in conjunction with psychotherapy did worse (i.e., experienced greater weight loss) than those receiving psychotherapy alone in one open-label study. Because of limited evidence and experience to date, the role if any of citalopram in the management of eating disorders remains to be elucidated. For information on the use of selective serotonin-reuptake inhibitors in the treatment of eating disorders, see Uses: Eating Disorders, in Fluoxetine Hydrochloride 28:16.04.20.

● Diabetic Neuropathy

Tricyclic antidepressants generally have been considered a mainstay of therapy for the treatment of diabetic neuropathy. However, because of potentially improved patient tolerability, therapy with selective serotonin-reuptake inhibitors or selective serotonin- and norepinephrine-reuptake inhibitors (e.g., duloxetine, venlafaxine) has been attempted as an alternative. In a double-blind, placebo-controlled trial, citalopram (40 mg daily) substantially reduced the symptoms associated with diabetic neuropathy† (pain, paresthesia, and dysesthesia) in a limited number of patients and generally was well tolerated. When compared with earlier results obtained with imipramine in the management of this condition, selective serotonin-reuptake inhibitors such as citalopram, fluoxetine, paroxetine, and sertraline appear to be less effective but better tolerated overall. Additional study and experience are needed to elucidate the relative roles of selective serotonin-reuptake inhibitors versus tricyclic antidepressants, selective serotonin- and norepinephrine-reuptake inhibitors, anticonvulsants (e.g., pregabalin, gabapentin), and other forms of treatment in the management of this condition.

● Posttraumatic Stress Disorder

Citalopram has been used in a limited number of adults with civilian- or combat-related posttraumatic stress disorder† (PTSD). In an open study, patients treated with citalopram for 8 weeks showed marked improvement in PTSD manifestations (reexperiencing, hyperarousal, and avoidance) as well as in depression and anxiety. Well-designed, controlled studies are needed to confirm these preliminary findings.

For additional information on the use of selective serotonin-reuptake inhibitors in the treatment of PTSD, see Uses: Posttraumatic Stress Disorder, in Prazosin Hydrochloride 24:20, Paroxetine 28:16.04.20, and Sertraline Hydrochloride 28:16.04.20.

DOSAGE AND ADMINISTRATION

● Administration

Citalopram hydrobromide is administered orally. Citalopram also has been administered by IV infusion†, but a parenteral dosage form is not commercially available in the US.

Citalopram usually is administered once daily in the morning or evening. Since food does not substantially affect the absorption of citalopram, the drug may be administered without regard to meals.

Hypokalemia and hypomagnesemia, if present, should be corrected prior to initiation of citalopram therapy and electrolytes should be monitored periodically during therapy as needed. (See Cautions: Cardiovascular Effects and also see Cautions: Precautions and Contraindications.)

Dispensing and Administration Precautions

Because of similarity in spelling of Celexa® (citalopram hydrobromide), Celebrex® (celecoxib), and Cerebyx® (fosphenytoin sodium), extra care should be exercised in ensuring the accuracy of prescriptions for these drugs.

● Dosage

Dosage of citalopram hydrobromide is expressed in terms of citalopram.

Patients receiving citalopram should be monitored for possible worsening of depression, suicidality, or unusual changes in behavior, especially at the beginning of therapy or during periods of dosage adjustment. (See Cautions: Precautions and Contraindications.)

The manufacturers state that at least 2 weeks must elapse between discontinuance of a monoamine oxidase (MAO) inhibitor intended to treat psychiatric disorders and initiation of citalopram therapy and that at least 2 weeks must elapse between discontinuance of citalopram and initiation of MAO inhibitor therapy intended to treat psychiatric disorders. For additional information on potentially serious drug interactions that may occur between citalopram and MAO inhibitors or other serotonergic agents, see Cautions: Precautions and Contraindications and also see Drug Interactions: Serotonergic Drugs.

Because withdrawal effects may occur with discontinuance of citalopram, other selective serotonin-reuptake inhibitors (SSRIs), and selective serotonin- and norepinephrine-reuptake inhibitors (SNRIs), abrupt discontinuance of these drugs should be avoided whenever possible. When citalopram therapy is discontinued, the dosage should be reduced gradually (e.g., over a period of several weeks) and the patient monitored for possible withdrawal symptoms. If intolerable symptoms occur following a dosage reduction or upon discontinuance of therapy, the drug may be reinstituted at the previously prescribed dosage. Subsequently, the clinician may continue decreasing the dosage, but at a more gradual rate. (See Cautions: Nervous System Effects and see Chronic Toxicity.)

Major Depressive Disorder

For the management of major depressive disorder in adults, the recommended initial dosage of citalopram is 20 mg once daily, with an increase to a maximum dosage of 40 mg once daily at an interval of not less than 1 week. Previously, the prescribing information for citalopram stated that certain patients may require a dosage of 60 mg daily. However, *citalopram dosages above 40 mg once daily no longer are recommended because of the risk of QT-interval prolongation* (see Cautions: Cardiovascular Effects and see also Cautions: Precautions and Contraindications) and because they provide no additional therapeutic benefit. A dose-response study did not show the 60-mg daily dosage to be more effective than the 40-mg daily dosage overall. Although antidepressant effects may be evident within 1 week in some patients, the full antidepressant effect of citalopram may not be observed for several weeks.

While the optimum duration of citalopram therapy has not been established, many experts state that acute depressive episodes require several months or longer of sustained antidepressant therapy. In addition, some clinicians recommend that long-term antidepressant therapy be considered in certain patients at risk for recurrence of depressive episodes (such as those with highly recurrent unipolar depression). Whether the dosage of citalopram required to induce remission is identical to the dosage needed to maintain and/or sustain euthymia is unknown. In placebo-controlled studies, the antidepressant efficacy of citalopram was maintained for up to 8 months in patients receiving 20–60 mg daily. In addition, the drug has been used in some patients for longer periods (e.g., up to 28 months) without apparent loss of clinical effect or increased toxicity.

If troublesome adverse effects occur during maintenance therapy, the manufacturer states that a decrease in dosage to 20 mg daily can be considered. If citalopram is used for extended periods, the need for continued therapy should be reassessed periodically.

Obsessive-Compulsive Disorder

For the management of obsessive-compulsive disorder† in adults, citalopram usually has been given orally in an initial dosage of 20 mg daily and the dosage was then gradually increased according to clinical response. The usual maintenance dosage in adults has been 40 or 60 mg daily; however, citalopram dosages exceeding 40 mg daily no longer are recommended due to the risk of QT prolongation.

Panic Disorder

For the management of panic disorder† in adults, the usual initial dosage of citalopram is 10 mg daily. After an interval of at least 1 week, the dosage may be gradually increased in increments of 10–20 mg up to a dosage of 20–40 mg daily, depending on individual patient response and tolerability. The usual maintenance dosage in adults has been 20–30 mg daily. Citalopram dosages exceeding 40 mg daily no longer are recommended due to the risk of QT prolongation.

● Dosage in Geriatric Patients
Major Depressive Disorder

For the management of depression in geriatric patients over 60 years of age, the maximum recommended citalopram dosage is 20 mg once daily due to the risk of QT-interval prolongation. (See Cautions: Cardiovascular Effects.)

For the management of depressive symptoms associated with dementia of the Alzheimer's type in geriatric patients, some experts recommend a lower initial citalopram dosage of 5–10 mg once daily. The dosage may then be gradually increased at intervals of at least several weeks up to the maximum recommended dosage of 20 mg once daily.

● Dosage in Hepatic and Renal Impairment

In depressed patients with hepatic impairment, the maximum recommended citalopram dosage is 20 mg once daily due to the risk of QT-interval prolongation. (See Cautions: Cardiovascular Effects and also see Pharmacokinetics: Elimination.)

Dosage adjustment is not necessary in depressed patients with mild to moderate renal impairment. Severe renal failure did not substantially affect the pharmacokinetics of citalopram in one study, suggesting that dosage adjustment also may be unnecessary in patients with severe renal impairment. However, the manufacturer recommends that the drug be used with caution in patients with severe renal impairment. (See Pharmacokinetics: Elimination.)

● Dosage in Poor CYP2C19 Metabolizers or Patients Receiving CYP2C19 Inhibitors

For the management of major depressive disorder in patients who are poor metabolizers of the cytochrome P-450 (CYP) isoenzyme 2C19 and in patients receiving cimetidine or another CYP2C19 inhibitor, the maximum recommended dosage of citalopram is 20 mg once daily due to the risk of QT-interval prolongation. (See CYP2C19 Inhibitors under Drug Interactions: Drugs Undergoing Hepatic Metabolism or Affecting Hepatic Microsomal Enzymes and see also Pharmacokinetics: Elimination.)

● Treatment of Pregnant Women during the Third Trimester

Some neonates exposed to citalopram and other SSRIs or SNRIs late in the third trimester of pregnancy have developed severe complications. When treating pregnant women with citalopram during the third trimester, the clinician should carefully consider the potential risks and benefits of therapy. (See Pregnancy under Cautions: Pregnancy, Fertility, and Lactation.)

CAUTIONS

The adverse effect profile of citalopram is similar to that of other selective serotonin-reuptake inhibitors (SSRIs) (e.g., escitalopram, fluoxetine, fluvoxamine, paroxetine, sertraline). Because citalopram is a highly selective serotonin-reuptake inhibitor with little or no effect on other neurotransmitters, the incidence of some adverse effects commonly associated with tricyclic antidepressants, such as anticholinergic effects (e.g., dry mouth, constipation), certain cardiovascular effects (e.g., orthostatic hypotension), drowsiness, and weight gain, is lower in patients receiving citalopram. However, certain adverse GI (e.g., nausea, anorexia), nervous system (e.g., somnolence, anxiety, nervousness, insomnia), and sexual function effects appear to occur more frequently with citalopram and other SSRIs than with tricyclic antidepressants.

In controlled studies, the most common adverse effects occurring more frequently in patients receiving citalopram than in those receiving placebo included nervous system effects such as somnolence, insomnia, anxiety, agitation, fatigue, tremor, and yawning; GI effects such as nausea, dry mouth, diarrhea, dyspepsia, anorexia, vomiting, and abdominal pain; sweating; ejaculation dysfunction (principally ejaculation delay) and impotence in male patients, decreased libido, and dysmenorrhea; fever, arthralgia, and myalgia; and upper respiratory tract infection, rhinitis, and sinusitis.

The results of a fixed-dose clinical study in depressed patients suggest that somnolence, insomnia, increased sweating, fatigue, impotence, and yawning are dose-related adverse effects of citalopram.

In short-term, placebo-controlled trials (6 weeks or less), discontinuance of citalopram therapy was required in approximately 16% of depressed patients, principally because of adverse psychiatric (e.g., insomnia, somnolence, agitation), other nervous system (e.g., dizziness, asthenia), or GI (e.g., nausea, vomiting, dry mouth) effects.

• Nervous System Effects

Somnolence and insomnia, which appear to be dose related, are the most common adverse nervous system effects of citalopram, occurring in approximately 18 and 15% of depressed patients, respectively, receiving the drug and in approximately 10 and 14% of those receiving placebo, respectively, in short-term controlled clinical trials. Insomnia or somnolence required discontinuance of therapy in about 3 or 2% of patients, respectively. However, because insomnia is a symptom also associated with depression, relief of insomnia and improvement in sleep patterns may occur when clinical improvement in depression becomes apparent during antidepressant therapy. Sleep disorders have been reported in at least 2% of citalopram-treated patients in clinical trials, although a causal relationship to the drug has not been established.

Fatigue, which appeared to be dose related, occurred in approximately 5% of patients receiving citalopram in short-term clinical studies. Asthenia has been reported in at least 2% of citalopram-treated patients in clinical trials and required discontinuance of therapy in about 1% of patients.

Tremor occurred in about 8%, anxiety in about 4%, and agitation in about 3% of patients receiving citalopram in short-term clinical studies; agitation resulted in discontinuance of therapy in about 1% of patients receiving the drug. Nervousness, headache, yawning, and dizziness have been reported in at least 2% of citalopram-treated patients in clinical trials. Yawning appeared to be dose related. Dizziness required discontinuance of therapy in 2% of patients.

Impaired concentration, amnesia, apathy, depression and aggravated depression, confusion, paresthesia, and migraine each have been reported in at least 1% of patients receiving citalopram; however, these adverse effects have not been definitely attributed to the drug.

Adverse nervous system effects reported in at least 0.1% of patients receiving citalopram include aggressive reaction, paroniria (disagreeable or terrifying dreams), depersonalization, hallucinations, euphoria, psychotic depression, delusion, paranoid reaction, emotional lability, panic reaction, psychosis, vertigo, neuralgia, abnormal gait, hyperkinesia, hypertonia, hypoesthesia, and ataxia; a causal relationship to the drug has not been clearly established.

Seizures occurred in 0.3% of patients receiving citalopram and in 0.5% of patients receiving placebo in clinical studies. A causal relationship to citalopram remains to be established in these cases. (See Cautions: Precautions and Contraindications.) Nonconvulsive status epilepticus also has been reported in a geriatric patient receiving citalopram for poststroke depression. In addition, involuntary muscle contractions have been reported in less than 1% of patients receiving the drug.

Activation of mania and hypomania have occurred in 0.2% of depressed patients receiving citalopram in placebo-controlled trials; some of these trials included patients with bipolar disorder. In an analysis of postmarketing clinical trials, manic episodes were reported in 0.62% of unipolar depressed patients. (See Cautions: Precautions and Contraindications.) Such reactions have been reported in patients receiving other antidepressant agents and may be caused by antidepressant-induced functional increases in catecholamine activity within the CNS, resulting in a "switch" from depressive to manic behavior. There is some evidence that patients with bipolar disorder may be more likely to experience antidepressant-induced hypomanic or manic reactions than patients without evidence of this disorder. In addition, limited evidence suggests that such reactions may occur

more frequently in bipolar depressed patients receiving tricyclics and tetracyclics (e.g., maprotiline, mianserin [not commercially available in the US]) than in those receiving selective serotonin-reuptake inhibitors (e.g., citalopram, escitalopram, fluoxetine, fluvoxamine, paroxetine, sertraline). However, further studies are needed to confirm these findings.

Extrapyramidal reactions associated with citalopram, which are uncommon, appear to be a class effect of selective serotonin-reuptake inhibitors and dose related. Reactions occurring early during therapy with the drug may be secondary to preexisting parkinsonian syndrome and/or concomitant therapy. Although a causal relationship to citalopram has not been established, extrapyramidal symptoms reported in at least 0.1% of patients receiving the drug include tremor, hypokinesia, and dystonia. Choreoathetosis also has been reported rarely. Pending further clinical experience, some clinicians recommend that extrapyramidal reactions developing in patients receiving selective serotonin-reuptake inhibitors be managed by reducing the dosage or discontinuing the drug; if necessary, the symptoms appear to respond to the same treatment as antipsychotic-induced extrapyramidal reactions.

Adverse nervous system effects reported in less than 0.1% of patients receiving citalopram include abnormal coordination, hyperesthesia, melancholia, catatonic reaction, and stupor. Although a causal relationship to the drug has not been established, serotonin syndrome also has been reported in patients receiving citalopram, other selective serotonin-reuptake inhibitors (SSRIs), and selective serotonin- and norepinephrine-reuptake inhibitors (SNRIs). (See Cautions: Precautions and Contraindications, Drug Interactions: Serotonergic Drugs, and see also Acute Toxicity.)

Withdrawal Reactions

Withdrawal symptoms, including dysphoric mood, irritability, agitation, dizziness, sensory disturbances (e.g., paresthesias such as electric shock sensations), anxiety, confusion, headache, lethargy, emotional lability, insomnia, hypomania, tinnitus, and seizures, have been reported upon discontinuance of citalopram, other SSRIs, and SNRIs, particularly when discontinuance of these drugs is abrupt. While these reactions are generally self-limiting, there have been reports of serious discontinuance symptoms. Therefore, patients should be monitored for such symptoms when discontinuing citalopram therapy. A gradual reduction in the dosage rather than abrupt cessation is recommended whenever possible. (See Dosage and Administration: Dosage.)

Withdrawal reactions have been reported rarely in citalopram-treated patients following discontinuance of the drug. Data from a controlled study evaluating citalopram in preventing depression relapse suggest that the symptoms associated with abrupt discontinuance of therapy generally are mild and transient. Overall clinical experience to date suggests that the risk of withdrawal effects may be somewhat lower with citalopram, fluoxetine, and sertraline compared with paroxetine. These differences may be due at least in part to the prolonged elimination half-lives of the parent drugs and/or their active metabolites. In addition, drug dependence has been reported in at least 0.1% of patients receiving citalopram, although a causal relationship to the drug remains to be established. (See Chronic Toxicity.)

Suicidality

Suicide and suicide attempts have been reported in less than 1% of depressed adults receiving citalopram. The US Food and Drug Administration (FDA) has determined that antidepressants increase the risk of suicidal thinking and behavior (suicidality) in children, adolescents, and young adults (18–24 years of age) with major depressive disorder and other psychiatric disorders. Patients, therefore, should be appropriately monitored and closely observed for clinical worsening, suicidality, and unusual changes in behavior, particularly during initiation of citalopram therapy (i.e., the first few months) and during periods of dosage adjustments. (See Cautions: Precautions and Contraindications, see Cautions: Pediatric Precautions, and see also Acute Toxicity.)

• GI Effects

Like other selective serotonin-reuptake inhibitors (e.g., escitalopram, fluoxetine, fluvoxamine, paroxetine, sertraline), citalopram therapy is associated with a relatively high incidence of GI disturbances, principally nausea, dry mouth, diarrhea, dyspepsia, anorexia, vomiting, and abdominal pain. The most frequent adverse GI effect associated with citalopram therapy is nausea, which occurred in about 21% of patients receiving the drug in controlled clinical trials. Nausea generally is mild to moderate in severity. In clinical trials, nausea required discontinuance of citalopram in about 4% of patients and was the most frequent adverse effect requiring discontinuance of the drug. While the mechanism(s) of citalopram-induced GI effects has not been fully elucidated, such effects appear to arise at least in part because of increased serotonergic activity in the GI tract (which may result in stimulation of small intestine motility and inhibition of gastric and large intestine motility) and possibly because of the drug's effect on central serotonergic type 3 (5-HT$_3$) receptors.

Dry mouth occurred in about 20%, diarrhea in about 8%, and dyspepsia in about 5% of patients receiving citalopram in short-term controlled clinical trials. Other adverse GI effects associated with citalopram therapy include vomiting and anorexia, which both occurred in 4% of patients, and abdominal pain, which occurred in about 3% of patients receiving the drug in short-term controlled clinical trials. Vomiting and dry mouth each resulted in discontinuance of citalopram in about 1% of patients. Constipation was reported in at least 2% of citalopram-treated patients in clinical trials.

As with some other selective serotonin-reuptake inhibitors, bruxism (involuntary clenching or grinding of the teeth) has been reported in at least 0.1% of patients receiving citalopram. The cases of bruxism reported to date with citalopram and other serotonin-reuptake inhibitors suggest that bruxism may be dose dependent and that buspirone therapy may be helpful in relieving this symptom.

Although a causal relationship to citalopram has not been established, increased salivation and flatulence have been reported in at least 1% of patients receiving the drug. Gastritis, gastroenteritis, stomatitis, eructation, hemorrhoids, dysphagia, gingivitis, and esophagitis have been reported in at least 0.1% of patients receiving citalopram. However, a causal relationship to the drug has not been established for these effects.

Epidemiologic case-control and cohort design studies have suggested that selective serotonin-reuptake inhibitors may increase the risk of upper GI bleeding. Although the precise mechanism for this increased risk remains to be clearly established, serotonin release by platelets is known to play an important role in hemostasis, and selective serotonin-reuptake inhibitors decrease serotonin uptake from the blood by platelets thereby decreasing the amount of serotonin in platelets. In addition, concurrent use of aspirin or other nonsteroidal anti-inflammatory agents was found to substantially increase the risk of GI bleeding in patients receiving selective serotonin-reuptake inhibitors in 2 of these studies. Although these studies focused on upper GI bleeding, there is some evidence suggesting that bleeding at other sites may be similarly potentiated. Further clinical studies are needed to determine the clinical importance of these findings. (See Cautions: Hematologic Effects and see also Drug Interactions: Drugs Affecting Hemostasis.)

Colitis, gastric ulcer, duodenal ulcer, cholecystitis, cholelithiasis, gastroesophageal reflux, glossitis, diverticulitis, and rectal hemorrhage have been reported in less than 0.1% of patients receiving citalopram. However, these adverse effects have not been definitely attributed to the drug.

● Dermatologic and Sensitivity Reactions

Increased sweating, which appears to be dose related, occurred in approximately 11% of patients receiving citalopram in short-term clinical studies. Rash and pruritus have been reported in at least 1% of patients receiving citalopram; however, these adverse effects have not been definitely attributed to the drug.

Photosensitivity reaction, urticaria, acne, skin discoloration, eczema, alopecia, dermatitis, dry skin, and psoriasis have been reported in less than 1% of patients receiving citalopram; however, these adverse effects have not been definitely attributed to the drug.

Hypertrichosis, decreased sweating, melanosis, keratitis, cellulitis, pruritus ani, hay fever, and facial edema have occurred in less than 0.1% of citalopram-treated patients, although a causal relationship to the drug has not been established. Allergic reactions, anaphylaxis, and angioedema also have been reported in patients receiving citalopram, although a causal relationship to the drug has not been established.

Severe adverse dermatologic effects such as erythema multiforme and epidermal necrolysis have occurred rarely in patients receiving citalopram. In addition, a case of extensive papular and purpuric erythema with keratinocytes, necrosis, and dermal leukocytoclastic vasculitis has been reported in a patient receiving citalopram; improvement occurred slowly following discontinuance of the drug.

● Metabolic and Endocrine Effects

Weight loss and weight gain each occurred in at least 1% of patients receiving citalopram in controlled clinical trials; obesity has occurred rarely. Increased appetite also has been reported in at least 1% of patients receiving the drug, although

a causal relationship has not been established. While clinically important weight loss may occur in some patients receiving citalopram, only minimal weight loss (averaging 0.5 kg) generally occurred in patients receiving the drug in controlled clinical trials. In addition, while decreased appetite was reported in about 4% of patients receiving citalopram in short-term clinical trials, the drug, unlike fluoxetine, does not appear to exhibit clinically important anorectic effects nor to produce clinically important long-term weight changes. In addition, short-term citalopram therapy did not produce substantial weight loss in severely obese individuals in one study.

Taste perversion has occurred in more than 1% of patients, and thirst and abnormal glucose tolerance have been reported in less than 1% of citalopram-treated patients, although a causal relationship to the drug has not been established. Taste loss has been reported rarely. Adverse metabolic and endocrine effects reported in less than 0.1% of patients receiving the drug include hypoglycemia, hypothyroidism, and goiter.

● Ocular and Otic Effects

Vision abnormalities occurred in about 2% and abnormality of accommodation in at least 1% of patients receiving citalopram in short-term controlled clinical trials. Ocular dryness, conjunctivitis, and ocular pain have been reported in less than 1% of citalopram-treated patients, although a causal relationship to the drug has not been established. Mydriasis, photophobia, diplopia, ptosis, abnormal lacrimation, and cataract have been reported in less than 0.1% of patients receiving the drug; these adverse effects have not been definitely attributed to the drug. Angle-closure glaucoma (narrow-angle glaucoma) also has been reported in citalopram-treated patients. (See Cautions: Precautions and Contraindications.)

Tinnitus occurred in less than 1% of patients receiving citalopram; this adverse effect has not been definitely attributed to the drug.

● Cardiovascular Effects

Citalopram does not exhibit clinically important anticholinergic activity, and current evidence suggests that the drug generally is less cardiotoxic than many older antidepressants (e.g., tricyclic antidepressants, monoamine oxidase inhibitors) at the usual recommended dosages.

No clinically important changes in vital signs (systolic and diastolic blood pressure and heart rate) were observed in patients receiving citalopram in controlled trials.

Citalopram causes dose-dependent prolongation of the corrected QT (QT$_c$) interval, an ECG abnormality that has been associated with torsades de pointes, ventricular tachycardia, and sudden death, all of which have been reported in postmarketing experience in patients receiving the drug. In a study of the effects of citalopram on the QT interval, use of the drug was associated with a dose-dependent increase in the corrected QT$_c$ interval. In this placebo-controlled study, a change from baseline in QT$_c$F (Fridericia's formula) greater than 60 msec occurred in 1.9% of patients receiving citalopram compared with 1.2% of patients receiving placebo. None of the patients receiving placebo had a post-dose QT$_c$F greater than 500 msec compared with 0.5% of patients receiving citalopram. The incidence of tachycardic and bradycardic outliers was 0.5 and 0.9% in the citalopram group, respectively, and 0.4% in the placebo group. Individually corrected QT$_c$ (QT$_c$Ni) interval was evaluated in a randomized, double-blind, placebo- and active-controlled, crossover study in healthy individuals. In this study, the maximum mean differences from placebo were 8.5 and 18.5 msec for daily dosages of 20 and 60 mg of citalopram, respectively. Based on these results, the predicted QT$_c$Ni for citalopram 40 mg daily is 12.6 msec. ECG changes, including QT-interval prolongation, also have been reported in individuals receiving overdosages of the drug (more than 400–600 mg). (See Dosage and Administration: Dosage, Cautions: Precautions and Contraindications, and see also Acute Toxicity.)

Palpitation was reported in at least 2% of citalopram-treated patients in clinical trials, although a causal relationship to the drug remains to be established. A comparison of supine and standing vital signs in depressed patients receiving citalopram indicated that the drug generally does not produce orthostatic changes such as hypotension. Although postural hypotension and hypotension occurred in at least 1% of patients receiving citalopram in short-term controlled clinical trials, a causal relationship to the drug has not been established.

Tachycardia, hypertension, bradycardia, peripheral edema, syncope, angina pectoris, extrasystoles, cardiac failure, flushing and hot flushes, myocardial infarction, cerebrovascular accident, myocardial ischemia, transient ischemic attack, phlebitis, atrial fibrillation, ventricular arrhythmia, cardiac arrest, and bundle branch block have been reported in premarketing studies of citalopram or during postmarketing surveillance; these adverse effects have not been definitely attributed to the drug.

● **Musculoskeletal Effects**

Arthralgia and myalgia each occurred in about 2% of patients receiving citalopram in short-term controlled clinical trials. In addition, back pain was reported in at least 2% of citalopram-treated patients in clinical trials, although a causal relationship to the drug remains to be established.

Arthritis, muscle weakness, leg cramps, and skeletal pain have been reported in at least 0.1% of citalopram-treated patients; these adverse effects have not been definitely attributed to the drug. Bursitis and osteoporosis have been reported in less than 0.1% of patients receiving citalopram, although a causal relationship has not been established.

● **Hematologic Effects**

Purpura, anemia, leukocytosis, and leukopenia have been reported in at least 0.1% of patients receiving citalopram, although a causal relationship to the drug has not been established.

Adverse hematologic effects reported in less than 0.1% of patients receiving citalopram include pulmonary embolism, granulocytopenia, lymphocytosis, lymphopenia, hypochromic anemia, coagulation disorders, and gingival bleeding; however, a causal relationship to the drug has not been established. In addition, thrombocytopenia has been reported.

Bleeding complications (e.g., ecchymosis, purpura, menorrhagia, rectal bleeding) have been reported infrequently in patients receiving citalopram and other selective serotonin-reuptake inhibitors. Although the precise mechanism for these reactions has not been established, it has been suggested that impaired platelet aggregation and prolonged bleeding time may be due at least in part to inhibition of serotonin reuptake into platelets and/or that increased capillary fragility and vascular tone may contribute to these cases. (See Cautions: GI Effects and see also Drug Interactions: Drugs Affecting Hemostasis.)

● **Respiratory Effects**

Respiratory disorders have been reported in patients receiving citalopram in short-term controlled clinical trials. Upper respiratory tract infections and rhinitis both have been reported in about 5% of citalopram-treated patients and sinusitis has occurred in about 3% of patients receiving the drug. Yawning and pharyngitis each occurred in about 2% of patients receiving citalopram. In addition, coughing has been reported in at least 1% of citalopram-treated patients.

Adverse respiratory effects reported in at least 0.1% of patients receiving citalopram in controlled trials include bronchitis, dyspnea, epistaxis, and pneumonia; however, a causal relationship to the drug remains to be established. Other adverse effects reported in less than 0.1% of citalopram-treated patients include asthma, laryngitis, bronchospasm, pneumonitis, and increased sputum; these adverse effects have not been definitely attributed to the drug.

● **Renal, Electrolyte, and Genitourinary Effects**
Sexual Dysfunction

Like other selective serotonin-reuptake inhibitors, adverse effects on sexual function have been reported in both men and women receiving citalopram. Although changes in sexual desire, sexual performance, and sexual satisfaction often occur as manifestations of a psychiatric disorder, they also may occur as the result of pharmacologic therapy. It is difficult to determine the true incidence and severity of adverse effects on sexual function during citalopram therapy, in part because patients and clinicians may be reluctant to discuss these effects. Therefore, incidence data reported in product labeling and earlier studies are most likely underestimates of the true incidence of adverse sexual effects. Recent reports indicate that up to 50% of patients receiving selective serotonin-reuptake inhibitors describe some form of sexual dysfunction during treatment and the actual incidence may be even higher.

Ejaculatory disturbances (principally ejaculatory delay) are the most common adverse urogenital effects associated with citalopram in males, occurring in about 6% of male patients receiving the drug compared with 1% of depressed patients receiving placebo in controlled clinical studies. However, the adverse effect of ejaculatory delay associated with serotonin-reuptake inhibitors has been used for therapeutic benefit in the treatment of premature ejaculation. (See Uses: Premature Ejaculation.) Results of some (but not all) studies in men and women suggest

that paroxetine may be associated with a higher incidence of sexual dysfunction than some other currently available selective serotonin-reuptake inhibitors, including citalopram and sertraline. Since it is difficult to know the precise risk of sexual dysfunction associated with citalopram and other serotonin-reuptake inhibitors, clinicians should routinely inquire about such possible adverse effects in patients receiving these drugs.

Decreased libido was reported in about 4% of depressed male patients receiving citalopram in short-term placebo-controlled studies compared with less than 1% of patients receiving placebo. In these studies, impotence, which appears to be dose related, was reported in about 3% of male patients receiving citalopram compared with less than 1% of males receiving placebo. In female patients receiving citalopram in controlled clinical studies for the treatment of depression, decreased libido and anorgasmia were reported in about 1% of those receiving citalopram. Increased libido has been reported in up to 1% of patients receiving citalopram. Priapism also has been reported during postmarketing surveillance in male patients, and clitoral priapism has been reported in at least 3 female patients receiving the drug.

The long-term effects of selective serotonin-reuptake inhibitors on sexual function have not been fully determined to date. In a double-blind study evaluating 6 months of citalopram or sertraline therapy in depressed patients, sexual desire and overall sexual functioning (as measured on the UKU Side Effect Scale) substantially improved in women and sexual desire improved in men. In men, no change in orgasmic dysfunction, erectile dysfunction, or overall sexual functioning was reported after 6 months of therapy with citalopram or sertraline, although there was a trend toward worsening of ejaculatory dysfunction. However, in the subgroups of women and men reporting no sexual problems at baseline, approximately 12% of women reported decreased sexual desire and 14% reported orgasmic dysfunction after 6 months of citalopram therapy; the corresponding figures in the same subgroup of men were approximately 17 and 19%, respectively, and as many as 25% experienced ejaculatory dysfunction after 6 months. No substantial differences between citalopram and sertraline were reported in this study.

Management of sexual dysfunction caused by selective serotonin-reuptake inhibitor therapy includes waiting for tolerance to develop; using a lower dosage of the drug; using drug holidays; delaying administration of the drug until after coitus; or changing to another antidepressant. Although further study is needed, there is some evidence that adverse sexual effects of the selective serotonin-reuptake inhibitors may be reversed by concomitant use of certain drugs, including buspirone, 5-hydroxytryptamine-2 (5-HT$_2$) receptor antagonists (e.g., nefazodone), 5-HT$_3$ receptor inhibitors (e.g., granisetron), or α_2-adrenergic receptor antagonists (e.g., yohimbine), selective phosphodiesterase (PDE) inhibitors (e.g., sildenafil), or dopamine receptor agonists (e.g., amantadine, dextroamphetamine, pemoline [no longer commercially available in the US], methylphenidate). In most patients, sexual dysfunction is fully reversed 1–3 days after discontinuance of the antidepressant.

Other Renal, Electrolyte, and Genitourinary Effects

Treatment with SSRIs, including citalopram, or selective serotonin- and norepinephrine-reuptake inhibitors (SNRIs) may result in hyponatremia. In many cases, this hyponatremia appeared to be due to the syndrome of inappropriate antidiuretic hormone secretion (SIADH) and was reversible when citalopram was discontinued. Cases with serum sodium concentrations lower than 110 mmol/L have been reported. Prolonged coma caused by hyponatremia has been reported in a patient with multiple sclerosis receiving citalopram therapy. Severe postoperative hyponatremia has been reported in an elderly female patient receiving the drug. Hyponatremia and SIADH usually develop an average of 2 weeks after initiating therapy (range: 3–120 days). Geriatric individuals and patients receiving diuretics or who are otherwise volume depleted may be at greater risk of developing hyponatremia during therapy with SSRIs or SNRIs. Discontinuance of citalopram should be considered in patients with symptomatic hyponatremia and appropriate medical intervention should be instituted. Because geriatric patients may be at increased risk for hyponatremia associated with these drugs, clinicians prescribing citalopram in such patients should be aware of the possibility that such reactions may occur. In addition, periodic monitoring of serum sodium concentrations (particularly during the first several months) in geriatric patients receiving selective serotonin-reuptake inhibitors has been recommended by some clinicians.

Hypokalemia and dehydration have occurred in less than 0.1% of patients receiving citalopram; these adverse effects have not been definitely attributed to the drug.

Urinary disorders (e.g., micturition disorders) have been reported in at least 2% of patients receiving citalopram in short-term controlled trials. In addition, polyuria has been reported in at least 1% of patients receiving the drug. Although a definite causal relationship to citalopram has not been established, urinary frequency, urinary incontinence, urinary retention, and dysuria have been reported in at least 0.1% of patients receiving the drug. Other adverse urologic effects reported in less than 0.1% of citalopram-treated patients include hematuria, oliguria, pyelonephritis, renal calculus, and renal pain; these adverse effects have not been definitely attributed to the drug.

Dysmenorrhea has been reported in at least 3% of female patients receiving citalopram in short-term controlled trials. In addition, amenorrhea has been reported in at least 1% of patients receiving the drug. Galactorrhea, breast pain, breast enlargement, and vaginal hemorrhage have been reported in less than 1% of patients receiving citalopram, and spontaneous abortion has been reported rarely; however, these adverse effects have not been definitely attributed to the drug. Breast enlargement also has been reported in some women receiving chronic therapy with other selective serotonin-reuptake inhibitors. In one study, approximately 40% of patients receiving selective serotonin-reuptake inhibitors (e.g., fluoxetine, paroxetine, sertraline) or venlafaxine reported some degree of breast enlargement; most patients with breast enlargement also experienced weight gain. In addition, serum prolactin concentrations were increased in the women receiving other selective serotonin-reuptake inhibitors in this study. Gynecomastia has been reported rarely.

● **Hepatic Effects**

Abnormal liver function test results, including elevations in serum hepatic enzyme concentrations, and increased serum alkaline phosphatase concentrations have been reported in at least 0.1% of patients receiving citalopram. Hepatitis, jaundice, and hyperbilirubinemia have been reported in less than 0.1% of patients receiving citalopram; however, these adverse effects have not been definitely attributed to the drug. Hepatic necrosis has also been reported during postmarketing surveillance in citalopram-treated patients.

● **Other Adverse Effects**

Fever occurred in about 2% of patients receiving citalopram in short-term controlled clinical trials. Rigors, alcohol intolerance, lymphadenopathy, and influenza-like symptoms have been reported in less than 1% of patients receiving citalopram; however, these adverse effects have not been definitely attributed to the drug. Pancreatitis also has occurred in association with citalopram, although a causal relationship to the drug has not been clearly established.

● **Precautions and Contraindications**

Worsening of depression and/or the emergence of suicidal ideation and behavior (suicidality) or unusual changes in behavior may occur in both adult and pediatric (see Cautions: Pediatric Precautions) patients with major depressive disorder or other psychiatric disorders, whether or not they are taking antidepressants. This risk may persist until clinically important remission occurs. Suicide is a known risk of depression and certain other psychiatric disorders, and these disorders themselves are the strongest predictors of suicide. However, there has been a long-standing concern that antidepressants may have a role in inducing worsening of depression and the emergence of suicidality in certain patients during the early phases of treatment. Pooled analyses of short-term, placebo-controlled studies of antidepressants (i.e., selective serotonin-reuptake inhibitors and other antidepressants) have shown an increased risk of suicidality in children, adolescents, and young adults (18–24 years of age) with major depressive disorder and other psychiatric disorders. An increased suicidality risk was not demonstrated with antidepressants compared with placebo in adults older than 24 years of age and a reduced risk was observed in adults 65 years of age or older. It currently is unknown whether the suicidality risk extends to longer-term use (i.e., beyond several months); however, there is substantial evidence from placebo-controlled maintenance trials in adults with major depressive disorder that antidepressants can delay the recurrence of depression.

The US Food and Drug Administration (FDA) recommends that all patients being treated with antidepressants for any indication be appropriately monitored and closely observed for clinical worsening, suicidality, and unusual changes in behavior, particularly during initiation of therapy (i.e., the first few months) and during periods of dosage adjustments. Families and caregivers of patients being treated with antidepressants for major depressive disorder or other indications, both psychiatric and nonpsychiatric, also should be advised to monitor patients on a daily basis for the emergence of agitation, irritability, or unusual changes in behavior as well as the emergence of suicidality, and to report such symptoms immediately to a health-care provider. (See Suicidality under Cautions: Nervous System Effects, in Paroxetine 28:16.04.20.)

Although a causal relationship between the emergence of symptoms such as anxiety, agitation, panic attacks, insomnia, irritability, hostility, aggressiveness, impulsivity, akathisia, hypomania, and/or mania and either the worsening of depression and/or the emergence of suicidal impulses has not been established, there is concern that such symptoms may represent precursors to emerging suicidality. Consequently, consideration should be given to changing the therapeutic regimen or discontinuing therapy in patients whose depression is persistently worse or in patients experiencing emergent suicidality or symptoms that might be precursors to worsening depression or suicidality, particularly if such manifestations are severe, abrupt in onset, or were not part of the patient's presenting symptoms. If a decision is made to discontinue therapy, citalopram dosage should be tapered as rapidly as is feasible but with recognition of the risks of abrupt discontinuance. (See Dosage and Administration: Dosage.) FDA also recommends that the drugs be prescribed in the smallest quantity consistent with good patient management, in order to reduce the risk of overdosage.

Citalopram causes dose-dependent QT_c-interval prolongation, an ECG abnormality that has been associated with torsades de pointes, ventricular tachycardia, and sudden death, all of which have been reported in postmarketing experience in patients receiving the drug. On August 24, 2011, the US Food and Drug Administration (FDA) notified healthcare professionals that *citalopram should no longer be used at dosages exceeding 40 mg daily due to the risk of QT-interval prolongation and torsades de pointes*; previously, the prescribing information for the drug stated that certain patients may require a dosage of 60 mg daily. On March 28, 2012, the FDA provided the following revised recommendations for citalopram use related to the potential risk of abnormal heart rhythms associated with higher dosages of the drug. The FDA advised that citalopram therapy is not recommended in patients with congenital long QT syndrome, bradycardia, hypokalemia or hypomagnesemia, recent acute myocardial infarction, or uncompensated heart failure. The FDA also stated that citalopram should not be used in patients receiving other drugs known to prolong the QT_c interval. Such drugs include class IA (e.g., quinidine, procainamide) or class III (e.g., amiodarone, sotalol) antiarrhythmic agents, certain antipsychotic agents (e.g., chlorpromazine, thioridazine), some anti-infective agents (e.g., gatifloxacin, moxifloxacin), and other drugs (e.g., pentamidine, levomethadyl acetate, methadone). In addition, the *maximum* dosage of citalopram should be limited to 20 mg once daily in patients who are poor metabolizers of the cytochrome P-450 (CYP) isoenzyme 2C19; patients receiving cimetidine or another CYP2C19 inhibitor; patients with hepatic impairment; and in patients older than 60 years of age; higher citalopram exposures in such patients increase the risk of QT-interval prolongation and torsades de pointes. Furthermore, electrolyte and/or ECG monitoring is recommended in certain situations. Patients being considered for citalopram therapy who are at risk for clinically important electrolyte disturbances should have baseline measurements of serum potassium and magnesium concentrations with subsequent periodic monitoring. Because hypokalemia and/or hypomagnesemia may increase the risk of QT_c-interval prolongation and arrhythmias, hypokalemia and hypomagnesemia should be corrected prior to citalopram administration and serum concentrations of these electrolytes should be periodically monitored. In addition, ECG monitoring is recommended in patients for whom citalopram use is not recommended but nevertheless considered essential, including those with the above-mentioned cardiovascular conditions (e.g., congenital long QT syndrome, bradycardia, recent acute myocardial infarction, uncompensated heart failure) and those concurrently receiving other drugs that may prolong the QT_c interval. Citalopram should be discontinued in any patient who has persistent QT_c measurements exceeding 500 msec. Patients receiving citalopram should be informed of the possible symptoms of QT-interval prolongation and torsades de pointes (e.g., chest pain, irregular heartbeat, shortness of breath, dizziness or fainting) and advised to seek immediate medical attention should such symptoms occur. If a citalopram-treated patient experiences such symptoms, further evaluation should be initiated, including cardiac monitoring.

It is generally believed (though not established in controlled trials) that treating a major depressive episode with an antidepressant alone may increase the likelihood of precipitating a mixed or manic episode in patients at risk for bipolar disorder. Therefore, patients should be adequately screened for bipolar disorder prior to initiating treatment with an antidepressant; such screening should include a detailed psychiatric history (e.g., family history of suicide, bipolar disorder, and depression).

Potentially life-threatening serotonin syndrome has been reported with SSRIs, including citalopram, and selective serotonin- and norepinephrine-reuptake inhibitors (SNRIs) when used alone, but particularly with concurrent use of other serotonergic drugs (including serotonin [5-hydroxytryptamine; 5-HT] type 1 receptor agonists ["triptans"], tricyclic antidepressants, buspirone, fentanyl, lithium, tramadol, tryptophan, and St. John's wort [*Hypericum perforatum*]) and with drugs that impair the metabolism of serotonin (particularly monoamine oxidase [MAO] inhibitors, both those used to treat psychiatric disorders and others, such as linezolid and methylene blue). Manifestations of serotonin syndrome may include mental status changes (e.g., agitation, hallucinations, delirium, coma), autonomic instability (e.g., tachycardia, labile blood pressure, dizziness, diaphoresis, flushing, hyperthermia), neuromuscular symptoms (e.g., tremor, rigidity, myoclonus, hyperreflexia, incoordination), seizures, and/or GI symptoms (e.g., nausea, vomiting, diarrhea). Patients receiving citalopram should be monitored for the development of serotonin syndrome.

Concomitant use of citalopram and MAO inhibitors intended to treat psychiatric disorders is contraindicated. Citalopram also should not be initiated in patients who are being treated with other MAO inhibitors such as linezolid or IV methylene blue. In patients who require more urgent treatment of a psychiatric condition, other interventions, including hospitalization, should be considered. Citalopram may be started 24 hours after the last dose of linezolid or IV methylene blue.

If concurrent therapy with citalopram and other serotonergic drugs is clinically warranted, the patient should be made aware of the potential increased risk for serotonin syndrome, particularly during initiation of therapy or when dosage is increased. If manifestations of serotonin syndrome occur, treatment with citalopram and any concurrently administered serotonergic agents should be discontinued immediately and supportive and symptomatic treatment should be initiated. (See Drug Interactions: Serotonergic Drugs.) For further information on serotonin syndrome, including manifestations and treatment, see Drug Interactions: Serotonergic Drugs, in Fluoxetine Hydrochloride 28:16.04.20.

The pupillary dilation (mydriasis) that occurs following the use of many antidepressant agents, including citalopram, may trigger an acute attack of angle-closure glaucoma (narrow-angle glaucoma) in patients with anatomically narrow angles who do not have a patent iridectomy. Possible symptoms of angle-closure glaucoma include eye pain, vision changes, and swelling or redness in or around the eye. Preexisting glaucoma is almost always open-angle glaucoma since angle-closure glaucoma can be treated definitively with iridectomy when diagnosed; open-angle glaucoma is not a risk factor for angle-closure glaucoma. Patients should be advised that citalopram can cause mild pupillary dilation, which can lead to an episode of angle-closure glaucoma in susceptible individuals. In addition, patients may wish to be examined to determine whether they are susceptible to angle-closure glaucoma and have a prophylactic procedure (e.g., iridectomy) if they are susceptible.

Citalopram should be used with caution and a lower maximum dosage (20 mg once daily) is recommended in patients with hepatic impairment, since decreased clearance and increased plasma concentrations of the drug may occur in such patients. (See Dosage and Administration: Dosage in Hepatic and Renal Impairment and see also Pharmacokinetics: Elimination.)

Because citalopram is extensively metabolized, excretion of unchanged drug in urine is a minor route of elimination. Severe renal failure did not markedly affect the pharmacokinetics of citalopram in one study, suggesting that dosage adjustment may not be necessary in patients with severe renal impairment. However, until long-term citalopram therapy has been more fully evaluated in such patients, citalopram should be used with caution in patients with severe renal impairment. (See Dosage and Administration: Dosage in Hepatic and Renal Impairment and see also Pharmacokinetics: Elimination.)

Because of the potential for adverse drug interactions, patients receiving citalopram should be advised to notify their clinician if they are taking or plan to take nonprescription (over-the-counter) or prescription medications. Although citalopram has not been shown to potentiate the impairment of mental and motor skills caused by alcohol, patients should be advised to avoid alcohol while receiving the drug.

Citalopram generally is less sedating than many other currently available antidepressants and does not appear to produce substantial impairment of cognitive or psychomotor function nor to potentiate psychomotor impairment induced by other CNS depressants (e.g., alcohol). However, patients should be cautioned that citalopram may impair their ability to perform activities requiring mental alertness or physical coordination (e.g., operating machinery, driving a motor vehicle) and to avoid such activities until they gain experience with the drug's effects.

Patients receiving citalopram should be advised that while they may notice improvement within 1–4 weeks after starting therapy, they should continue therapy with the drug as directed by their clinician.

Although anticonvulsant effects have been observed in animal studies with citalopram, the drug has not been systematically evaluated in patients with a seizure disorder. In addition, patients with seizure disorders were excluded from premarketing clinical trials with the drug. In clinical studies of citalopram,

seizures occurred in 0.3% of patients receiving citalopram and in 0.5% of patients receiving placebo; a causal relationship to the drug remains to be established. However, as with other antidepressants, citalopram should be initiated and used with caution in patients with a history of seizures.

Activation of mania and hypomania have occurred in patients receiving therapeutic dosages of citalopram. The drug should be used with caution in patients with a history of mania. (See Cautions: Nervous System Effects.)

Treatment with SSRIs, including citalopram, or SNRIs may result in hyponatremia. In many cases, this hyponatremia appears to be due to the syndrome of inappropriate antidiuretic hormone secretion (SIADH) and was reversible when the SSRI or SNRI was discontinued. Geriatric individuals and patients receiving diuretics or who are otherwise volume depleted may be at greater risk of developing hyponatremia during therapy with SSRIs or SNRIs. Signs and symptoms of hyponatremia include headache, difficulty concentrating, memory impairment, confusion, weakness, and unsteadiness, which may lead to falls; more severe and/or acute cases have been associated with hallucinations, syncope, seizures, coma, respiratory arrest, and death. Discontinuance of citalopram should be considered in patients with symptomatic hyponatremia and appropriate medical intervention should be instituted. (See Cautions: Renal, Electrolyte, and Genitourinary Effects and see also see Cautions: Geriatric Precautions.)

Because of similarity in spelling of Celexa® (citalopram hydrobromide), Celebrex® (celecoxib), and Cerebyx® (fosphenytoin sodium), extra care should be exercised in ensuring the accuracy of prescriptions for these drugs.

Use of citalopram is contraindicated in patients who are currently receiving or have recently (i.e., within 2 weeks) received therapy with an MAO inhibitor intended to treat psychiatric disorders because of an increased risk of serotonin syndrome. Conversely, use of an MAO inhibitor intended to treat psychiatric disorders is contraindicated within 2 weeks of citalopram discontinuance. (See Drug Interactions: Serotonergic Drugs.)

Initiation of citalopram therapy in patients receiving MAO inhibitors such as linezolid or IV methylene blue also is contraindicated because of an increased risk of serotonin syndrome. (See Drug Interactions: Serotonergic Drugs.)

Concurrent use of citalopram in patients receiving pimozide is contraindicated. (See Drug Interactions: Pimozide.)

Citalopram is contraindicated in patients who are hypersensitive to the drug, escitalopram, or any ingredient in the formulation.

● *Pediatric Precautions*

Safety and efficacy of citalopram in pediatric patients have not been established. Two placebo-controlled trials involving 407 children and adolescents with major depressive disorder have been conducted with citalopram; the results of these trials were not sufficient to support a claim of efficacy for use of the drug in pediatric patients with this condition. (See Pediatric Considerations under Uses: Major Depressive Disorder.)

Decreased appetite and weight loss have been observed in patients receiving SSRIs. Therefore, regular monitoring of weight and growth should be performed in children and adolescents receiving citalopram therapy.

FDA warns that antidepressants increase the risk of suicidal thinking and behavior (suicidality) in children and adolescents with major depressive disorder and other psychiatric disorders. The risk of suicidality for these drugs was identified in a pooled analysis of data from a total of 24 short-term (4–16 weeks), placebo-controlled studies of 9 antidepressants (i.e., citalopram, bupropion, fluoxetine, fluvoxamine, mirtazapine, nefazodone, paroxetine, sertraline, venlafaxine) in over 4400 children and adolescents with major depressive disorder, obsessive-compulsive disorder (OCD), or other psychiatric disorders. The analysis revealed a greater risk of adverse events representing suicidal behavior or thinking (suicidality) during the first few months of treatment in pediatric patients receiving antidepressants than in those receiving placebo. However, a more recent meta-analysis of 27 placebo-controlled trials of 9 antidepressants (SSRIs and others) in patients younger than 19 years of age with major depressive disorder, OCD, or non-OCD anxiety disorders suggests that the benefits of antidepressant therapy in treating these conditions may outweigh the risks of suicidal behavior or suicidal ideation. No suicides occurred in these pediatric trials.

The risk of suicidality in the FDA's pooled analysis differed across the different psychiatric indications, with the highest incidence observed in the major depressive disorder studies. In addition, although there was considerable variation in risk among the antidepressants, a tendency toward an increase in suicidality risk in younger patients was found for almost all drugs studied. It currently is unknown whether the suicidality risk in pediatric patients extends to longer-term use (i.e., beyond several months). (See Suicidality under Cautions: Nervous System Effects, in Paroxetine 28:16.04.20.)

As a result of this analysis and public discussion of the issue, FDA has directed manufacturers of all antidepressants to add a boxed warning to the labeling of their products to alert clinicians of this suicidality risk in children and adolescents and to recommend appropriate monitoring and close observation of patients receiving these agents. (See Cautions: Precautions and Contraindications.) The drugs that are the focus of the revised labeling are all drugs included in the general class of antidepressants, including those that have not been studied in controlled clinical trials in pediatric patients, since the available data are not adequate to exclude any single antidepressant from an increased risk. In addition to the boxed warning and other information in professional labeling on antidepressants, FDA currently recommends that a patient medication guide explaining the risks associated with the drugs be provided to the patient each time the drugs are dispensed. Caregivers of pediatric patients whose depression is persistently worse or who are experiencing emergent suicidality or symptoms that might be precursors to worsening depression or suicidality during antidepressant therapy should consult their clinician regarding the best course of action (e.g., whether the therapeutic regimen should be changed or the drug discontinued). *Patients should not discontinue use of selective serotonin-reuptake inhibitors without first consulting their clinician; it is very important that the drugs not be abruptly discontinued, as withdrawal effects may occur.* (See Dosage and Administration: Dosage.)

Anyone considering the use of citalopram in a child or adolescent for any clinical use must balance the potential risk of therapy with the clinical need.

● Geriatric Precautions

While safety and efficacy of citalopram in geriatric patients have not been established specifically, approximately 31% of patients receiving the drug for depression in clinical trials were 60 years of age or older, approximately 23% were 65 years of age or older, and approximately 10% were 75 years of age or older.

Although no overall differences in the efficacy or adverse effect profile of citalopram were observed between geriatric and younger patients and other clinical experience revealed no evidence of age-related differences in response, pharmacokinetic studies in healthy geriatric individuals and depressed patients 60 years of age or older have revealed higher areas under the plasma concentration-time curve (AUC) values and longer elimination half-lives compared with those in younger individuals. (See Pharmacokinetics: Absorption and Elimination.) Therefore, the manufacturer and some clinicians recommend a maximum citalopram dosage of 20 mg once daily for geriatric patients older than 60 years of age with major depressive disorder. (See Dosage and Administration: Dosage in Geriatric Patients.)

In pooled data analyses, a *reduced* risk of suicidality was observed in adults 65 years of age or older with antidepressant therapy compared with placebo. (See Cautions: Precautions and Contraindications.)

Limited evidence suggests that geriatric patients also may be more likely than younger patients to develop citalopram-induced hyponatremia and transient syndrome of inappropriate secretion of antidiuretic hormone (SIADH). Therefore, clinicians prescribing citalopram in geriatric patients should be aware of the possibility that such reactions may occur. In addition, periodic monitoring (especially during the first several months) of serum sodium concentrations in geriatric patients receiving selective serotonin-reuptake inhibitors has been recommended by some clinicians.

In a double-blind, multicenter trial, citalopram (20 or 40 mg daily) was found to be as effective as and better tolerated than amitriptyline in depressed geriatric patients. In a small study comparing citalopram and nortriptyline in depressed geriatric patients, citalopram was found to be somewhat less effective but better tolerated than nortriptyline.

In a controlled study comparing citalopram and placebo in elderly patients with dementia†, citalopram (20–30 mg daily) was found to improve depression as well as cognitive and emotional functioning more than placebo. In an open study in a limited number of patients with dementia and behavioral disturbances†, citalopram was found to improve the behavioral complications associated with dementia†.

As with other psychotropic drugs, geriatric patients receiving antidepressants appear to have an increased risk of hip fracture. Despite the decreased incidence of cardiovascular and anticholinergic effects associated with selective serotonin-reuptake inhibitors, these drugs did not show any advantage over tricyclic antidepressants with regard to hip fracture in a case-control study. In addition, there was little difference in the rates of falls between nursing home residents receiving selective serotonin-reuptake inhibitors and those receiving tricyclic antidepressants in a retrospective study. Therefore, all geriatric individuals receiving either type of antidepressant should be considered at increased risk of falls, and appropriate measures should be taken.

● Mutagenicity and Carcinogenicity

Citalopram was mutagenic in the in vitro bacterial reverse mutation assay (Ames test) in 2 out of 5 bacterial strains (Salmonella TA98 and TA1537) in the absence of metabolic activation. In the in vitro Chinese hamster lung cell assay for chromosomal aberrations, citalopram was clastogenic in the presence and absence of metabolic activation. The drug was not mutagenic in the in vitro mammalian forward gene mutation assay (HPRT) in mouse lymphoma cells or in a coupled in vitro/in vivo unscheduled DNA synthesis (UDS) assay in rat liver. Citalopram was not found to be clastogenic in the in vitro chromosomal aberration assay in human lymphocytes or in 2 in vivo mouse micronucleus assays.

Studies to determine the carcinogenic potential of citalopram were performed in mice receiving oral dosages of up to 240 mg/kg daily for 18 months and in rats receiving 8 or 24 mg/kg daily for 24 months. These dosages were approximately 20 times the maximum recommended human daily dosage of 60 mg on a surface area (mg/m^2) basis in mice and approximately 1.3 and 4 times the maximum recommended human daily dosage on a mg/m^2 basis in rats, respectively. No evidence of carcinogenicity was found in the mice. In rats receiving 8 or 24 mg/kg daily of citalopram, an increased incidence of small intestine carcinoma was reported. The manufacturer states that a no-effect dosage for this finding was not established; the relevance of this finding to humans is not known.

● Pregnancy, Fertility, and Lactation

Pregnancy

Some neonates exposed to citalopram and other selective serotonin-reuptake inhibitors (SSRIs) or selective serotonin- and norepinephrine-reuptake inhibitors (SNRIs) late in the third trimester of pregnancy have developed complications that have sometimes been severe and required prolonged hospitalization, respiratory support, enteral nutrition, and other forms of supportive care in special-care nurseries. Such complications can arise immediately upon delivery and usually last several days or up to 2–4 weeks. Clinical findings reported to date in the neonates have included respiratory distress, cyanosis, apnea, seizures, temperature instability or fever, feeding difficulty, dehydration, excessive weight loss, vomiting, hypoglycemia, hypotonia, hypertonia, hyperreflexia, tremor, jitteriness, irritability, lethargy, reduced or lack of reaction to pain stimuli, and constant crying. These clinical features appear to be consistent with either a direct toxic effect of the SSRI or SNRI or, possibly, a drug withdrawal syndrome. It should be noted that, in some cases, the clinical picture was consistent with serotonin syndrome (see Drug Interactions: Serotonergic Drugs).

Infants exposed to SSRIs in late pregnancy may have an increased risk of persistent pulmonary hypertension of the newborn (PPHN). PPHN is a rare heart and lung condition occurring in an estimated 1–2 infants per 1000 live births in the general population; it occurs when a neonate does not adapt to breathing outside the womb. Some experts have suggested that respiratory distress in neonates exposed to SSRIs may occur along a spectrum of seriousness in association with maternal use of SSRIs, with PPHN among the most serious consequences. Neonates with PPHN may require intensive care support, including mechanical ventilation; in severe cases, multiple organ damage, including brain damage, and even death may occur. Although several epidemiologic studies have suggested an increased risk of PPHN with SSRI use during pregnancy, other studies did not demonstrate a statistically significant association. Thus, the FDA states that it is currently unclear whether use of SSRIs, including citalopram, during pregnancy can cause PPHN and recommends that clinicians not alter their current clinical practice of treating depression during pregnancy.

Clinicians should consider that in a prospective longitudinal study of 201 women with a history of recurrent major depression who were euthymic in the context of antidepressant therapy at the beginning of pregnancy, women who discontinued their antidepressant medication (SSRIs, tricyclic antidepressants, or others) during pregnancy were found to be substantially more likely to have a relapse of depression than were women who continued to receive their antidepressant therapy while pregnant. When treating a pregnant woman with citalopram, the clinician should carefully consider the potential risks of taking an SSRI along with the established benefits of treating depression with an antidepressant; this decision can only be made on a case-by-case basis. (See Dosage and Administration: Treatment of Pregnant Women during the Third Trimester.)

For additional information on the management of depression in women prior to conception and during pregnancy, including treatment algorithms, the FDA advises clinicians to consult the joint American Psychiatric Association and American College of Obstetricians and Gynecologists guidelines (at https://www.ncbi.nlm.nih.gov/pmc/articles/PMC3103063/pdf/nihms293836.pdf).

Most epidemiologic studies of pregnancy outcome following first-trimester exposure to SSRIs, including citalopram, conducted to date have not revealed evidence of an increased risk of major congenital malformations. Analysis of data collected in 531 Swedish women who received SSRIs during early pregnancy (citalopram accounted for 375 of these exposures) found that no increase in congenital abnormalities was observed during the neonatal period compared with the general population. In a prospective, controlled, multicenter study, maternal use of several SSRIs (fluvoxamine, paroxetine, sertraline) did not appear to increase the risk of congenital malformation, miscarriage, stillbirth, or premature delivery when used during pregnancy at recommended dosages. Birth weight and gestational age in neonates exposed to the drugs were similar to those in the control group. In another small study based on medical records review, the incidence of congenital anomalies reported in infants born to women who were treated with several other SSRIs (fluoxetine, paroxetine, sertraline) during pregnancy was comparable to that observed in the general population.

Citalopram and its metabolites have been shown to cross the placenta in humans. In 11 women who received 20–40 mg of citalopram daily during pregnancy, trough plasma citalopram, demethylcitalopram, and didemethylcitalopram concentrations in the infants at the time of delivery were found to be 64, 66, and 68%, respectively, of maternal concentrations. No significant difference in pregnancy outcome was observed between the group of women who received citalopram during pregnancy and a similar control group of pregnant women who did not receive the drug. In addition, the body weight and neurologic status of the infants in both groups were all assessed as normal after 12 months. However, the results of epidemiologic studies indicate that exposure to paroxetine during the first trimester of pregnancy may increase the risk for congenital malformations, particularly cardiovascular malformations. (See Pregnancy, under Cautions: Pregnancy, Fertility, and Lactation, in Paroxetine 28:16.04.20.) Additional epidemiologic studies are needed to more thoroughly evaluate the relative safety of citalopram and other SSRIs during pregnancy, including their potential teratogenic risks and possible effects on neurobehavioral development.

There are no adequate and well-controlled studies to date using citalopram in pregnant women and the drug should be used during pregnancy only when the potential benefits justify the potential risks to the fetus. Women should be advised to notify their clinician if they become pregnant or plan to become pregnant during therapy with the drug. FDA states that women who are pregnant or thinking about becoming pregnant should not discontinue any antidepressant, including citalopram, without first consulting their clinician. The decision whether or not to continue antidepressant therapy should be made only after careful consideration of the potential benefits and risks of antidepressant therapy for each individual pregnant patient. If a decision is made to discontinue treatment with citalopram or other SSRIs before or during pregnancy, discontinuance of therapy should be done in consultation with the clinician in accordance with the prescribing information for the antidepressant, and the patient should be closely monitored for possible relapse of depression.

The effect of citalopram on labor and delivery is not known.

In animal reproduction studies, citalopram has been shown to have adverse effects on embryo/fetal and postnatal development, including teratogenic effects, when administered at dosages that exceeded the recommended human dosage. Teratogenic effects were observed in rats receiving dosages of citalopram that were toxic to the dams but were not observed in rabbits. In 2 rat embryo/fetal development studies, oral administration of citalopram dosages of 32, 56, or 112 mg/kg daily to pregnant animals during the period of organogenesis resulted in decreased embryo/fetal growth and survival and an increased incidence of fetal abnormalities, including cardiovascular and skeletal defects, at the highest dosage (equivalent to approximately 18 times the maximum recommended human daily dosage on a mg/m^2 basis). This dosage also was associated with maternal toxicity. The developmental no-effect dosage was 56 mg/kg daily, which is approximately 9 times the maximum recommended human daily dosage on a mg/m^2 basis. No adverse effects on embryo/fetal development were observed in rabbits receiving citalopram dosages of up to 16 mg/kg daily (equivalent to approximately 5 times the maximum recommended human dosage on a mg/m^2 basis).

In female rats receiving citalopram dosages of 4.8, 12.8, or 32 mg/kg daily from late gestation through weaning, increased offspring mortality during the first 4 days following birth and persistent offspring growth retardation were observed at the highest dosage, which is equivalent to approximately 5 times the maximum recommended human dosage on a mg/m^2 basis. The no-effect dosage of 12.8 mg/kg daily is approximately 2 times the maximum recommended human dosage on a mg/m^2 basis. Similar effects on offspring mortality and growth were seen when dams were treated with the drug throughout gestation and early lactation at daily dosages of 24 mg/kg or more (approximately 4 or more times the maximum recommended human dosage on a mg/m^2 basis). A no-effect dosage was not determined in this study.

Fertility

In reproduction studies in male and female rats receiving oral citalopram dosages of 16/24 (males/females), 32, 48, and 72 mg/kg daily, decreased mating was observed at all dosages. Fertility was decreased at daily dosages of 32 mg/kg or more (approximately 5 times the maximum recommended human dosage on a mg/m^2 basis). Gestation duration was increased in rats receiving 48 mg/kg daily of the drug, which is equivalent to approximately 8 times the maximum recommended human dosage.

Lactation

Like other SSRIs, citalopram and its principal metabolite, demethylcitalopram, are distributed into milk. (See Pharmacokinetics: Distribution.) Limited data indicate that milk-to-plasma ratios of citalopram and demethylcitalopram range from 1.7–3. Available data indicate that citalopram and fluoxetine are the serotonin-reuptake inhibitors with the highest relative exposure for breast-fed infants. Excessive somnolence, decreased feeding, and weight loss were reported in 2 nursing infants whose mothers received citalopram. In one of these cases, the infant reportedly recovered completely upon discontinuance of citalopram by its mother, and in the second case, no follow-up information is available. Disturbed sleep has been reported in another breast-feeding infant whose mother was receiving citalopram 40 mg daily. The infant's sleep normalized once the citalopram dosage was reduced and 2 breast-feedings were replaced with artificial nutrition.

Women should be advised to notify their clinician if they plan to breast-feed. Because of the potential for adverse reactions to citalopram in nursing infants, a decision should be made whether to discontinue nursing or the drug, taking into account the importance of the drug to the woman. If a decision is made to continue citalopram therapy in a nursing woman, some clinicians recommend that the lowest effective dosage of citalopram be used and that breast-feeding during the period of drug absorption be avoided.

DRUG INTERACTIONS

• Drugs that Prolong the QT Interval

Citalopram use is not recommended in patients concurrently receiving other drugs known to prolong the QT$_c$ interval, including class IA (e.g., quinidine, procainamide) or class III (e.g., amiodarone, sotalol) antiarrhythmic agents, certain antipsychotic agents (e.g., chlorpromazine, thioridazine), some anti-infective agents (e.g., gatifloxacin, moxifloxacin), and other drugs (e.g., pentamidine, levomethadyl acetate, methadone). However, if citalopram therapy is considered essential in such patients, ECG monitoring is recommended. (See Cautions: Cardiovascular Effects and see Drug Interactions: Pimozide.)

• Serotonergic Drugs

Use of selective serotonin-reuptake inhibitors (SSRIs) such as citalopram concurrently or in close succession with other drugs that affect serotonergic neurotransmission may result in potentially life-threatening serotonin syndrome. Manifestations of serotonin syndrome may include mental status changes (e.g., agitation, hallucinations, delirium, coma), autonomic instability (e.g., tachycardia, labile blood pressure, dizziness, diaphoresis, flushing, hyperthermia), neuromuscular symptoms (e.g., tremor, rigidity, myoclonus, hyperreflexia, incoordination), seizures, and/or GI symptoms (e.g., nausea, vomiting, diarrhea). The precise mechanism of serotonin syndrome is not fully understood; however, it appears to result from excessive serotonergic activity in the CNS, probably mediated by activation of serotonin 5-HT$_{1A}$ receptors. The possible involvement of dopamine and 5-HT$_2$ receptors also has been suggested, although their roles remain unclear.

Serotonin syndrome most commonly occurs when 2 or more drugs that affect serotonergic neurotransmission are administered either concurrently or in close succession. Serotonergic agents include those that increase serotonin synthesis (e.g., the serotonin precursor tryptophan), stimulate synaptic serotonin release (e.g., some amphetamines, dexfenfluramine [no longer commercially available in the US], fenfluramine [no longer commercially available in the US]), inhibit the reuptake of serotonin after release (e.g., SSRIs, selective serotonin- and norepinephrine-reuptake inhibitors [SNRIs], tricyclic antidepressants, trazodone, dextromethorphan, meperidine, tramadol), decrease the metabolism of serotonin (e.g., monoamine oxidase [MAO] inhibitors), have direct serotonin postsynaptic receptor activity (e.g., buspirone), or nonspecifically induce increases in serotonergic neuronal activity (e.g., lithium salts). Selective agonists of serotonin (5-hydroxytryptamine; 5-HT) type 1 ($5-HT_1$) receptors ("triptans") and dihydroergotamine, agents with serotonergic activity used in the management of migraine headache, and St. John's wort (*Hypericum perforatum*) also have been implicated in cases of serotonin syndrome.

The combination of SSRIs and MAO inhibitors may result in serotonin syndrome. Such reactions also have been reported in patients receiving SSRIs concomitantly with tryptophan, lithium, dextromethorphan, sumatriptan, or dihydroergotamine. In rare cases, serotonin syndrome reportedly has occurred in patients receiving the recommended dosage of a single serotonergic agent (e.g., clomipramine) or during accidental overdosage (e.g., sertraline intoxication in a child). Some other drugs that have been implicated in precipitating symptoms suggestive of serotonin syndrome include buspirone, bromocriptine, dextropropoxyphene, linezolid, methylene blue, methylenedioxymethamphetamine (MDMA; "ecstasy"), selegiline (a selective MAO-B inhibitor), and sibutramine (an SNRI used for the management of obesity [no longer commercially available in the US]). Other drugs that have been associated with the syndrome but for which less convincing data are available include carbamazepine, fentanyl, and pentazocine.

Clinicians should be aware of the potential for serious, possibly fatal reactions associated with serotonin syndrome in patients receiving 2 or more drugs that affect serotonergic neurotransmission, even if no such interactions with the specific drugs have been reported to date in the medical literature. Such patients should be monitored for the emergence of serotonin syndrome. Serotonin syndrome may be more likely to occur when initiating therapy, increasing the dosage, or following the addition of another serotonergic drug. Some clinicians state that patients who have experienced serotonin syndrome may be at higher risk for recurrence of the syndrome upon reinitiation of serotonergic drugs. Pending further experience in such cases, some clinicians recommend that therapy with serotonergic agents be limited following recovery. If concomitant use of citalopram and other serotonergic drugs is clinically warranted, patients should be advised of the increased risk for serotonin syndrome, particularly during treatment initiation and dosage increases. If manifestations of serotonin syndrome occur, treatment with citalopram and any concurrently administered serotonergic agents should be discontinued immediately and supportive and symptomatic treatment should be initiated.

For further information on serotonin syndrome, including manifestations and treatment, see Drug Interactions: Serotonergic Drugs, in Fluoxetine Hydrochloride 28:16.04.20.

Monoamine Oxidase Inhibitors

Concomitant use of citalopram and MAO inhibitors, both those used to treat psychiatric disorders and others such as linezolid and methylene blue, is associated with a risk of potentially life-threatening serotonin syndrome. Such reactions also have been reported in patients who recently have discontinued an SSRI and have initiated therapy with an MAO inhibitor.

Because of the potential risk of serotonin syndrome, concomitant use of citalopram and MAO inhibitors intended to treat psychiatric disorders is contraindicated. At least 2 weeks should elapse between discontinuance of MAO inhibitors intended to treat psychiatric disorders and initiation of citalopram therapy and vice versa.

Linezolid

Linezolid, an anti-infective agent that is a nonselective and reversible MAO inhibitor, has been associated with drug interactions resulting in serotonin syndrome, including some associated with SSRIs. Because of this potential risk, linezolid generally should *not* be used in patients receiving citalopram. However, certain life-threatening or urgent situations may necessitate immediate linezolid treatment in a patient receiving a serotonergic drug, including citalopram. In such emergency situations, the availability of acceptable alternative anti-infectives should be considered and the benefits of linezolid should be weighed against the risk of serotonin syndrome. If linezolid is indicated in such emergency situations, citalopram must be immediately discontinued and the patient monitored for symptoms of serotonin syndrome for 2 weeks or until 24 hours after the last

linezolid dose, whichever comes first. Treatment with citalopram may be resumed 24 hours after the last linezolid dose.

If nonemergency use of linezolid is being planned for a patient receiving citalopram, citalopram should be withheld for at least 2 weeks prior to initiating linezolid.

Initiation of citalopram in a patient receiving linezolid is contraindicated; when necessary, citalopram may be started 24 hours after the last linezolid dose. (See Drug Interactions: Serotonergic Drugs, in Linezolid 8:12.28.24.)

Methylene Blue

Methylene blue, a potent and reversible inhibitor of MAO-A, has been associated with drug interactions resulting in serotonin syndrome, including some associated with SSRIs. All of the reports of serotonin syndrome with methylene blue that provided information on the route of administration involved IV administration of doses of 1–8 mg/kg (e.g., when used as a diagnostic [visualizing] dye† during parathyroid surgery); none of the reports to date involved administration of methylene blue by other routes (such as oral tablets or by local tissue injection) or at lower doses. Because of this potential risk, methylene blue generally should *not* be used in patients receiving citalopram. However, certain life-threatening or urgent situations may necessitate immediate IV methylene blue administration in a patient receiving a serotonergic drug, including citalopram. In such emergency situations, the availability of acceptable alternatives to methylene blue should be considered and the benefits of IV methylene blue should be weighed against the risk of serotonin syndrome. If methylene blue is indicated in such emergency situations, citalopram must be immediately discontinued and the patient monitored for symptoms of serotonin syndrome for 2 weeks or until 24 hours after the last methylene blue dose, whichever comes first. Treatment with citalopram may be resumed 24 hours after the last methylene blue dose.

If nonemergency use of methylene blue is being planned for a patient receiving citalopram, citalopram should be withheld for at least 2 weeks prior to initiating methylene blue treatment.

Initiation of citalopram in a patient receiving IV methylene blue is contraindicated; when necessary, citalopram may be started 24 hours after the last IV methylene blue dose.

Moclobemide

Moclobemide (not commercially available in the US), a selective and reversible MAO-A inhibitor, has been associated with serotonin syndrome, and such reactions have been fatal in several cases in which the drug was given in combination with citalopram or with clomipramine. Pending further experience with such combinations, some clinicians recommend that concurrent therapy with moclobemide and a selective serotonin-reuptake inhibitor be used only with extreme caution and serotonin-reuptake inhibitors should have been discontinued for some time (depending on the elimination half-lives of the drug and its active metabolites) before initiating moclobemide therapy.

Selegiline

Selegiline, a selective MAO-B inhibitor used in the management of parkinsonian syndrome, has been reported to cause serotonin syndrome when given concurrently with selective serotonin-reuptake inhibitors (e.g., fluoxetine, paroxetine, sertraline). Although selegiline is a selective MAO-B inhibitor at therapeutic dosages, the drug appears to lose its selectivity for the MAO-B enzyme at higher dosages (e.g., those exceeding 10 mg/kg), thereby increasing the risk of serotonin syndrome in patients receiving higher dosages of the drug either alone or in combination with other serotonergic agents.

In a double-blind, placebo-controlled study in healthy individuals receiving citalopram and selegiline concurrently, no clinically important differences in vital signs or in the frequency of adverse events between the study groups were reported. In addition, no evidence of a clinically relevant pharmacokinetic interaction between the 2 drugs was found. Pending further accumulation of data, the manufacturer of selegiline recommends avoiding concurrent selegiline and selective serotonin-reuptake inhibitor therapy. In addition, the manufacturer of selegiline recommends that at least 2 weeks elapse between discontinuance of selegiline and initiation of selective serotonin-reuptake inhibitor therapy.

Isoniazid

Isoniazid, an antituberculosis agent, appears to have some MAO-inhibiting activity. In addition, iproniazid (not commercially available in the US), another antituberculosis agent structurally related to isoniazid that also possesses MAO-inhibiting activity, reportedly has resulted in serotonin syndrome in at least 2 patients when given in combination with meperidine. Pending further experience, clinicians should be aware of the potential for serotonin syndrome when isoniazid is given in conjunction with selective serotonin-reuptake inhibitor therapy (such as citalopram) or other serotonergic agents.

Tryptophan

An interaction between paroxetine (another SSRI) and tryptophan (a serotonin precursor) has been reported during concurrent use. Adverse reactions reported to date during combined therapy with these drugs resemble serotonin syndrome and have consisted principally of headache, nausea, sweating, and dizziness. If concomitant use of citalopram and tryptophan is clinically warranted, patients should be advised of the increased risk for serotonin syndrome, particularly during treatment initiation and dosage increases. If serotonin syndrome manifestations occur, treatment with citalopram, tryptophan, and any other concurrently administered serotonergic agents should be discontinued immediately and supportive and symptomatic treatment should be initiated. (See Cautions: Precautions and Contraindications.)

5-HT$_1$ Receptor Agonists ("Triptans")

Weakness, hyperreflexia, and incoordination have been reported rarely during postmarketing surveillance in patients receiving sumatriptan concomitantly with an SSRI (e.g., citalopram, escitalopram, fluoxetine, fluvoxamine, paroxetine, sertraline); these reactions resembled serotonin syndrome. Oral or subcutaneous sumatriptan and SSRIs were used concomitantly in some clinical studies without unusual adverse effects. However, an increase in the frequency of migraine attacks and a decrease in the effectiveness of sumatriptan in relieving migraine headache have been reported in a patient receiving subcutaneous injections of sumatriptan intermittently while undergoing fluoxetine therapy.

Clinicians prescribing triptans, SSRIs, and SNRIs should consider that triptans often are used intermittently and that either the triptan, SSRI, or SNRI may be prescribed by a different clinician. Clinicians also should weigh the potential risk of serotonin syndrome with the expected benefit of using a triptan concurrently with SSRI or SNRI therapy. If concomitant treatment with a triptan and citalopram is clinically warranted, patients should be advised of the increased risk of serotonin syndrome, particularly during treatment initiation and dosage increases. If serotonin syndrome manifestations occur, treatment with citalopram, the triptan, and any other concurrently administered serotonergic agents should be discontinued immediately and supportive and symptomatic treatment should be initiated. (See Cautions: Precautions and Contraindications.)

Other Selective Serotonin-reuptake Inhibitors and Selective Serotonin- and Norepinephrine-reuptake Inhibitors

Concomitant use of citalopram and other SSRIs or SNRIs potentially may result in serotonin syndrome. If concomitant use of citalopram and other SSRIs or SNRIs is clinically warranted, patients should be advised of the increased risk for serotonin syndrome, particularly during treatment initiation and dosage increases. If serotonin syndrome manifestations occur, treatment with citalopram, the other SSRI or SNRI, and any other concurrently administered serotonergic agents should be discontinued immediately and supportive and symptomatic treatment should be initiated. (See Cautions: Precautions and Contraindications.)

Clinical experience regarding the optimal timing of switching from other SSRIs to citalopram therapy is limited. Therefore, care and prudent medical judgment should be exercised when switching from other SSRIs to citalopram, particularly from long-acting agents (e.g., fluoxetine). Because some adverse reactions resembling serotonin syndrome have developed when fluoxetine therapy has been abruptly discontinued and therapy with another SSRI (sertraline) was initiated immediately afterward, a washout period may be advisable when transferring a patient from fluoxetine to another SSRI. However, the appropriate duration of the washout period when switching from other SSRIs to citalopram has not been clearly established. Pending further experience in patients being transferred from therapy with another SSRI to citalopram and as the clinical situation permits, it generally is recommended that the previous antidepressant be discontinued according to the recommended guidelines for the specific SSRI prior to initiation of citalopram therapy.

Drugs Undergoing Hepatic Metabolism or Affecting Hepatic Microsomal Enzymes

In vitro enzyme inhibition data did not reveal an inhibitory effect of citalopram on cytochrome P-450 (CYP) isoenzyme 3A4, 2C9, or 2E1 but did suggest that it is a weak inhibitor of 1A2, 2D6, and 2C19. Citalopram would be expected to have little inhibitory effect on in vivo metabolism mediated by these isoenzymes. However, in vivo data to address this question are very limited.

In vitro studies have indicated that CYP3A4 and CYP2C19 are the principal isoenzymes involved in the metabolism of citalopram. Therefore, it is expected that potent inhibitors of CYP3A4 (e.g., ketoconazole, itraconazole, macrolide antibiotics) and potent inhibitors of CYP2C19 (e.g., omeprazole) might decrease the clearance of citalopram. However, concurrent administration of citalopram and ketoconazole, a potent inhibitor of CYP3A4, did not substantially affect the pharmacokinetics of citalopram. (See Ketoconazole under Drug Interactions: Drugs Undergoing Hepatic Metabolism or Affecting Hepatic Microsomal Enzymes.)

Steady-state plasma citalopram concentrations were not substantially different in healthy individuals with poor or extensive CYP2D6 metabolizer phenotypes following multiple-dose administration of citalopram, suggesting that coadministration of citalopram with a drug that inhibits CYP2D6 is unlikely to have clinically important effects on citalopram metabolism.

Carbamazepine

Concurrent administration of citalopram (40 mg daily for 14 days) and carbamazepine (titrated up to 400 mg daily for a total of 35 days) in healthy individuals did not significantly affect the pharmacokinetics of carbamazepine, a CYP3A4 substrate. Trough plasma citalopram concentrations were unaffected in this study, which suggests that the initiation of citalopram therapy in patients stabilized on carbamazepine should not produce clinically important changes in plasma carbamazepine concentrations. However, in an open study in depressed patients, the addition of carbamazepine to citalopram therapy resulted in a decrease in the plasma concentrations of escitalopram, the active enantiomer with the 1-(S) absolute configuration. In addition, 2 cases of increased plasma citalopram concentrations and altered antidepressant response have been reported when carbamazepine was discontinued. Because of the enzyme-inducing properties of carbamazepine, the possibility that carbamazepine might increase the clearance of citalopram should be considered if the 2 drugs are administered concomitantly or if carbamazepine therapy is initiated or discontinued in a patient receiving citalopram.

CYP2C19 Inhibitors

Cimetidine is known to inhibit many CYP oxidative enzymes, including CYP2C19, and can affect the pharmacokinetics of citalopram. In a study in which oral citalopram (40 mg daily) was given for 3 weeks, the area under the plasma concentration-time curve (AUC) and peak plasma concentrations of citalopram were increased by approximately 43 and 39%, respectively, during concomitant use of oral cimetidine (400 mg daily) for the final 8 days. The possible effects of citalopram on the pharmacokinetics of cimetidine have not been studied.

Because of the potential risk of QT-interval prolongation and torsades de pointes, the maximum recommended dosage of citalopram is 20 mg once daily in patients concomitantly receiving citalopram and cimetidine or other CYP2C19 inhibitors.

Ketoconazole

In a randomized, double-blind study, concurrent administration of single doses of citalopram (40 mg) and ketoconazole (200 mg), a potent inhibitor of CYP3A4, in healthy individuals decreased the peak plasma ketoconazole concentrations and AUC by 21 and 10%, respectively. The pharmacokinetics of citalopram and demethylcitalopram were not substantially affected during concomitant administration of these two drugs in this study. Therefore, citalopram dosage adjustment is unlikely to be necessary in patients receiving ketoconazole concurrently.

Triazolam

Concurrent administration of citalopram (titrated to 40 mg daily for 28 days) and a single dose of triazolam (0.25 mg), a CYP3A4 substrate, in healthy individuals did not substantially affect the pharmacokinetics of either drug. However, triazolam appeared to be absorbed slightly more quickly during citalopram coadministration.

Tricyclic and Other Antidepressants

The extent to which selective serotonin-reuptake inhibitor interactions with tricyclic antidepressants may pose clinical problems depends on the degree of inhibition and the pharmacokinetics of the serotonin-reuptake inhibitor involved. In vitro studies suggest that citalopram is a relatively weak inhibitor of CYP2D6 and CYP2C19. In one study in healthy adults receiving citalopram (40 mg once daily for 10 days), concurrent administration of a single 100-mg dose of imipramine hydrochloride, a CYP2D6 and CYP2C19 substrate, did not substantially affect the plasma concentrations of either citalopram or imipramine. However, the plasma concentration of the principal imipramine metabolite, desipramine, increased by approximately 50%; the clinical importance of this change is not known. The manufacturer of citalopram recommends that caution be exercised during concurrent use of tricyclic antidepressants with citalopram.

In addition, concomitant use of citalopram and tricyclic antidepressants potentially may result in serotonin syndrome. If concomitant use of citalopram and a tricyclic antidepressant is clinically warranted, patients should be advised of the increased risk for serotonin syndrome, particularly during treatment initiation and dosage increases. If serotonin syndrome manifestations occur, treatment with citalopram, the tricyclic antidepressant, and any concurrently administered serotonergic agents should be discontinued immediately and supportive and symptomatic treatment should be initiated. (See Cautions: Precautions and Contraindications and also see Drug Interactions: Serotonergic Drugs.)

Clinical experience regarding the optimal timing of switching from other antidepressants to citalopram therapy is limited. Therefore, care and prudent medical judgment should be exercised when switching from other antidepressants to citalopram. Pending further experience in patients being transferred from therapy with another antidepressant to citalopram and as the clinical situation permits, it generally is recommended that the previous antidepressant be discontinued according to the recommended guidelines for the specific antidepressant prior to initiation of citalopram therapy.

● Alcohol

Citalopram has not been shown to potentiate the impairment of mental and motor skills caused by alcohol. However, the drug's ability to reduce alcohol consumption in animals and humans suggests that there may be a serotonergically mediated, pharmacodynamic interaction between citalopram and alcohol within the CNS. (See Pharmacology: Effects on Alcohol Intake, and also see Uses: Alcohol Dependence.) The manufacturer recommends that patients be advised to avoid alcohol while receiving citalopram.

● Lithium

The manufacturer states that coadministration of lithium and citalopram did not substantially affect the pharmacokinetics of either drug in healthy individuals. In a placebo-controlled trial in depressed patients refractory to citalopram therapy alone, there also was no evidence of a pharmacokinetic interaction when lithium therapy (800 mg daily) was added; the combination was found to be well tolerated. However, pending further accumulation of data, the manufacturer of citalopram recommends that plasma lithium concentrations be monitored in patients receiving citalopram concurrently and that the lithium dosage be adjusted accordingly. Lithium also may enhance the serotonergic effects of citalopram, potentially resulting in serotonin syndrome. Caution should be exercised in patients receiving these two drugs concomitantly. (See Drug Interactions: Serotonergic Drugs.)

● Drugs Affecting Hemostasis

Warfarin

The administration of a single, 25-mg dose of warfarin, a CYP3A4 substrate, in healthy individuals receiving citalopram 40 mg daily for 15 days did not affect the pharmacokinetics of warfarin. However, the prothrombin time increased by an average of 5% compared with baseline. The clinical importance, if any, of these findings is not known.

Other Drugs that Interfere with Hemostasis

Epidemiologic case-control and cohort design studies that have demonstrated an association between selective serotonin-reuptake inhibitor therapy and an increased risk of upper GI bleeding also have shown that concurrent use of aspirin or other nonsteroidal anti-inflammatory agents substantially increases the risk of GI bleeding. Although these studies focused on upper GI bleeding, there is some evidence suggesting that bleeding at other sites may be similarly potentiated. The precise mechanism for this increased risk remains to be clearly established;

however, serotonin release by platelets is known to play an important role in hemostasis, and selective serotonin-reuptake inhibitors decrease serotonin uptake from the blood by platelets, thereby decreasing the amount of serotonin in platelets. Patients receiving citalopram should be cautioned about the concomitant use of drugs that interfere with hemostasis, including aspirin and other nonsteroidal anti-inflammatory agents.

● Pimozide

In a controlled study, concurrent administration of a single 2-mg dose of pimozide in individuals receiving citalopram (40 mg once daily for 11 days) was associated with mean increases in the QT, interval of approximately 10 msec compared with pimozide given alone. Citalopram did not substantially affect the mean AUC or peak plasma concentrations of pimozide. The mechanism for this potential pharmacodynamic interaction is not known. In addition, concomitant use of citalopram and pimozide rarely may result in potentially serious, sometimes fatal serotonin syndrome.

The manufacturers of citalopram hydrobromide state that concurrent administration of citalopram and pimozide is contraindicated.

● Other CNS-active Agents

The manufacturers state that, given the primary CNS effects of citalopram, caution should be used when it is given concurrently with other centrally acting drugs.

● Digoxin

In healthy adults who received citalopram (40 mg daily for 3 weeks), the concurrent administration of a single, 1-mg dose of digoxin did not significantly affect the pharmacokinetics of citalopram or digoxin. Concurrent administration of the 2 drugs was well tolerated, with no serious adverse events and no clinically important ECG changes reported. These data suggest that concomitantly administered citalopram is unlikely to substantially affect serum digoxin concentrations in patients who are receiving chronic digoxin therapy.

● Diuretics

Concomitant use of citalopram and diuretics may increase the risk of hyponatremia. (See Other Renal, Electrolyte, and Genitourinary Effects under Cautions: Renal, Electrolyte, and Genitourinary Effects.)

● Electroconvulsive Therapy

The manufacturer states that there are no clinical studies on the concurrent use of citalopram and electroconvulsive therapy (ECT). In a limited number of depressed women given either citalopram 20 mg or placebo before their third and fourth ECT sessions, no adverse effects were reported after citalopram administration and the length of the electrically induced seizures and neurohormonal responses did not substantially differ between the 2 groups. However, additional studies are needed to confirm the safety and efficacy of ECT in patients receiving citalopram.

● Metoprolol

Administration of citalopram 40 mg daily for 22 days resulted in a twofold increase in the plasma concentrations of metoprolol in one study. Increased plasma concentrations of metoprolol have been associated with decreased cardioselectivity. Concurrent administration of citalopram and metoprolol had no clinically important effects on blood pressure or heart rate.

● Theophylline

In an open, multiple-dose study, concurrent administration of citalopram (40 mg daily) for 21 days and theophylline (single, 300-mg dose), a CYP1A2 substrate, in healthy individuals did not substantially affect the pharmacokinetics of theophylline. Therefore, some clinicians state that dosage adjustment of theophylline may not be necessary in patients receiving citalopram concurrently. The effect of theophylline on the pharmacokinetics of citalopram was not evaluated.

● Cyclosporine

Limited evidence suggests that citalopram does not substantially affect the pharmacokinetics of cyclosporine; further study is needed to confirm these preliminary findings.

ACUTE TOXICITY

Limited information is available on the acute toxicity of citalopram.

The acute lethal dose of citalopram in humans is not known. The manufacturer states that no fatalities were reported among patients taking overdosages of up to 2 g during clinical trials. However, postmarketing reports of citalopram overdosage have included ingestions of up to 6 g; as with other selective serotonin-reuptake inhibitors, fatalities have been reported rarely following citalopram overdosage.

● **Manifestations**

In general, overdosage of citalopram may be expected to produce effects that are extensions of the drug's pharmacologic and adverse effects. Case reports in humans indicate that the possible effects of citalopram overdosage (either alone or in combination with other drugs and/or alcohol) include dizziness, sweating, nausea, vomiting, tremor, somnolence, and sinus tachycardia. In rare cases, observed symptoms have included amnesia, confusion, coma, seizures, hyperventilation, cyanosis, and rhabdomyolysis.

ECG changes, including QT_c prolongation, sinus bradycardia, nodal rhythm, ventricular arrhythmias, left bundle branch block, and torsades de pointes, have been reported rarely in citalopram overdosage. In a young, healthy female who ingested 400 mg of citalopram, QT_c prolongation was reported. In most cases of pure citalopram overdosage at doses exceeding 600 mg, ECG changes, including QT prolongation and sinus bradycardia, gradually resolved 12–24 hours following the intoxication. However, severe sinus bradycardia developed within about 4 hours following ingestion of 800 mg of citalopram alone in one female patient and lasted up to 6 days during intensive care unit (ICU) treatment; hypotension and syncope also occurred but no QT-interval prolongation was observed. A temporary pacemaker was necessary for treatment of this patient. In another case, a woman developed life-threatening cardiac toxicity, including torsades de pointes with cardiac arrest, approximately 32 hours following ingestion of 1 g of citalopram; her corrected QT interval remained abnormal for 24 hours after presentation.

Manifestations resembling serotonin syndrome also have been reported following citalopram overdosage either alone or in combination with other serotonergic drugs (e.g., moclobemide [not commercially available in the US]). (See Cautions: Precautions and Contraindications and also see Drug Interactions: Serotonergic Drugs.)

In one fatal case involving a 47-year-old man who ingested an unknown amount of citalopram in combination with other drugs, postmortem citalopram concentrations were 0.88 mg/L in femoral blood, 1.16 mg/L in heart blood, and 0.9 mg/L in urine. In another fatal case involving a 53-year-old woman who ingested an unknown amount of citalopram and trimipramine, postmortem analysis revealed a citalopram concentration of 4.81 mg/L and a trimipramine concentration of 2.33 mg/L in femoral blood. The citalopram to demethylcitalopram ratios were 1.96 and 2.02 in femoral blood and hepatic tissue, respectively.

● **Treatment**

Because fatalities and severe toxicity have been reported following overdosage of citalopram and other selective serotonin-reuptake inhibitors, particularly in large overdosage and when taken with other drugs or alcohol, some clinicians recommend that any overdosage involving these drugs be managed aggressively. Because suicidal ingestion often involves more than one drug, clinicians treating citalopram overdosage should be alert to possible manifestations caused by drugs other than citalopram.

Clinicians also should consider the possibility of serotonin syndrome in patients presenting with similar clinical features and a recent history of citalopram ingestion and/or ingestion of other serotonergic agents. (See Cautions: Precautions and Contraindications and also see Drug Interactions: Serotonergic Drugs.)

Management of citalopram overdosage generally requires symptomatic and supportive care. A patent airway should be established and maintained, and adequate oxygenation and ventilation should be ensured. An ECG should be obtained and monitoring of cardiac function instituted. Frequent vital sign monitoring and close observation of the patient is necessary. Clinicians should consider that development of cardiac toxicity following citalopram overdosage may be delayed. There is no specific antidote for citalopram intoxication.

Following recent (i.e., within 4 hours) ingestion of a potentially toxic amount of citalopram and in the absence of signs and symptoms of cardiac toxicity, the stomach should be emptied immediately by inducing emesis or by gastric lavage. However, some clinicians recommend avoidance of emesis in patients who have ingested overdoses of selective serotonin-reuptake inhibitors because of the potential for unexpected changes in mental status. If the patient is comatose, having seizures, or lacks the gag reflex, gastric lavage may be performed if an endotracheal tube with cuff inflated is in place to prevent aspiration of gastric contents. However, some clinicians note that gastric lavage generally is not necessary because of the low

incidence of fatalities associated with selective serotonin-reuptake inhibitor overdoses. In one study, activated charcoal alone or gastric lavage followed by activated charcoal demonstrated similar efficacy in preventing the absorption of citalopram. In another study, single-dose activated charcoal administration given an average of 2.1 hours after citalopram ingestion was found to be effective in reducing the risk of QT-interval prolongation associated with overdosage of the drug. Since administration of activated charcoal (which may be used in conjunction with sorbitol) may be as or more effective than induction of emesis or gastric lavage, its use has been recommended either in the initial management of selective serotonin-reuptake inhibitor overdosage or following induction of emesis or gastric lavage in patients who have ingested a potentially toxic quantity of these drugs.

Because of the large volume of distribution of citalopram, hemodialysis, peritoneal dialysis, forced diuresis, hemoperfusion, and/or exchange transfusion are unlikely to be effective in removing substantial amounts of citalopram from the body.

Clinicians should consult a poison control center for additional information on the management of citalopram overdosage.

CHRONIC TOXICITY

The results of animal studies suggest that the abuse potential for citalopram is low. Citalopram has not been studied systematically in humans to determine whether therapy with the drug is associated with abuse, tolerance, or physical dependence.

The premarketing clinical experience with citalopram did not reveal any drug-seeking behavior. However, these observations were not systematic, and it is not possible to accurately predict from the limited data currently available the extent to which a CNS-active drug like citalopram will be misused, diverted, and/or abused.

Experience with citalopram, other selective serotonin-reuptake inhibitors (SSRIs), and selective serotonin- and norepinephrine-reuptake inhibitors (SNRIs) suggests that a withdrawal syndrome may occur within several days following discontinuance of these drugs, particularly when abrupt. The most commonly observed manifestations are those that resemble influenza, such as fatigue, lethargy, GI complaints (e.g., nausea), dizziness or lightheadedness, impaired sleep, tremor, anxiety, insomnia, chills, sweating, and incoordination. Other reported manifestations include dysphoric mood, irritability, emotional lability, hypomania, memory impairment, sensory disturbances (such as paresthesias, including electric shock-like sensations), confusion, headache, palpitations, agitation, and aggression. Although the mechanism(s) for such withdrawal reactions is not fully understood, it has been suggested that they may be caused by a sudden decrease in serotonin availability at the synapse or cholinergic rebound; other neurotransmitters (e.g., dopamine, norepinephrine, GABA) also may be involved. These manifestations may in some cases be mistaken for physical illness or relapse into depression. While these reactions generally appear to be self-limiting and improve over one to several weeks, there have been reports of serious discontinuance symptoms. Manifestations of withdrawal also may be improved by restarting therapy with citalopram or another antidepressant with a similar pharmacologic profile.

Withdrawal reactions have been reported rarely in citalopram-treated patients. Data from a controlled study evaluating citalopram in preventing depression relapse indicate that the symptoms associated with abrupt discontinuance of therapy generally are mild and transient. Overall clinical experience to date suggests that the risk of withdrawal effects may be somewhat lower with citalopram, fluoxetine, and sertraline compared with paroxetine. These differences may be due at least in part to the prolonged elimination half-lives of the parent drugs and/or their active metabolites. The manufacturer and some clinicians recommend that citalopram, like other SSRIs, be discontinued gradually (e.g., over a period of several weeks) rather than abruptly whenever possible to prevent the possible development of withdrawal reactions.

As with other CNS-active drugs, clinicians should carefully evaluate patients for a history of substance abuse prior to initiating citalopram therapy. If citalopram therapy is initiated in patients with a history of substance abuse, such patients should be monitored closely for signs of misuse or abuse of the drug (e.g., development of tolerance, use of increasing doses, drug-seeking behavior).

PHARMACOLOGY

The pharmacology of citalopram is complex and in many ways resembles that of other antidepressant agents, particularly those agents (e.g., escitalopram, fluoxetine, fluvoxamine, paroxetine, sertraline, clomipramine, trazodone) that predominantly potentiate the pharmacologic effects of serotonin (5-hydroxytryptamine

[5-HT]). Like other selective serotonin-reuptake inhibitors (SSRIs), citalopram is a potent and highly selective inhibitor of serotonin reuptake and has little or no effect on other neurotransmitters.

● *Nervous System Effects*

The precise mechanism of antidepressant action of citalopram is unclear, but the drug has been shown to selectively inhibit the reuptake of serotonin at the presynaptic neuronal membrane. Citalopram-induced inhibition of serotonin reuptake causes increased synaptic concentrations of serotonin in the CNS, resulting in numerous functional changes associated with enhanced serotonergic neurotransmission. Like other selective serotonin-reuptake inhibitors (e.g., fluoxetine, fluvoxamine, paroxetine, sertraline), citalopram appears to have only very weak effects on the reuptake of norepinephrine or dopamine and does not exhibit clinically important anticholinergic, antihistaminic, or adrenergic (α_1, α_2, β) blocking activity at usual therapeutic dosages.

Although the mechanism of antidepressant action of antidepressant agents may involve inhibition of the reuptake of various neurotransmitters (e.g., serotonin, norepinephrine) at the presynaptic neuronal membrane, it has been suggested that postsynaptic receptor modification is mainly responsible for the antidepressant action observed during long-term administration of antidepressant agents. During long-term therapy with most antidepressants (e.g., tricyclic antidepressants, monoamine oxidase [MAO] inhibitors), these adaptive changes mainly consist of subsensitivity of the noradrenergic adenylate cyclase system in association with a decrease in the number of β-adrenergic receptors; such effects on noradrenergic receptor function are commonly referred to as "down regulation." However, selective serotonin-reuptake inhibitors have not consistently demonstrated the ability to downregulate β-adrenergic receptors despite being effective antidepressant agents clinically. Thus, downregulation of β-adrenergic receptors does not appear to be an absolute prerequisite for antidepressant action. Long-term administration of desipramine but not citalopram substantially decreased β-adrenergically mediated cyclic adenosine monophosphate accumulation. In addition, some antidepressants (e.g., amitriptyline) reportedly decreased the number of serotonergic binding sites following chronic administration.

The exact mechanism of action of citalopram in panic disorder has not been fully elucidated but appears to involve at least in part changes in serotonergic neurotransmission.

The precise mechanism of action that is responsible for the efficacy of citalopram in the treatment of obsessive-compulsive disorder is unclear. However, because of the potency of clomipramine and other selective serotonin-reuptake inhibitors (e.g., fluoxetine, fluvoxamine, paroxetine, sertraline) in inhibiting serotonin reuptake and their efficacy in the treatment of obsessive-compulsive disorder, a serotonin hypothesis has been developed to explain the pathogenesis of the condition. The hypothesis postulates that a dysregulation of serotonin is responsible for obsessive-compulsive disorder and that citalopram and these other agents are effective because they correct this imbalance. Although considerable evidence supports the serotonergic hypothesis of obsessive-compulsive disorder, additional studies are necessary to confirm this hypothesis. Regardless of the precise pathogenesis of obsessive-compulsive disorder, the clinical efficacy of long-term therapy with selective serotonin-reuptake inhibitors such as citalopram appears to be due at least in part to alterations in serotonergic neurotransmission.

Serotonergic mechanisms also appear to be involved at least in part in a number of other pharmacologic effects associated with selective serotonin-reuptake inhibitors, including citalopram, such as decreased alcohol intake and regulation of food intake.

Serotonergic Effects

Citalopram is a highly selective inhibitor of serotonin reuptake at the presynaptic neuronal membrane. Citalopram-induced inhibition of serotonin reuptake causes increased synaptic concentrations of the neurotransmitter, resulting in numerous functional changes associated with enhanced serotonergic neurotransmission.

Based on in vitro studies, the relative potency of citalopram as an inhibitor of serotonin reuptake compared with norepinephrine and dopamine reuptake inhibition is 3400 and 22,000, respectively, making the drug the most selective serotonin-reuptake inhibitor currently available. These findings have been confirmed by the results of in vivo and ex vivo studies demonstrating that citalopram inhibits the uptake of serotonin without appreciably inhibiting the uptake of norepinephrine or dopamine. In an initial study in rats, tolerance to the serotonin-reuptake

inhibiting effect was not induced following long-term (14 days) citalopram administration.

Citalopram occurs as a racemic mixture and data from in vitro and in vivo studies indicate that the serotonin-reuptake blocking activity of citalopram is principally due to escitalopram, the (+)-enantiomer with the 1-(S) absolute configuration. Escitalopram is at least 100-fold more potent as an inhibitor of the reuptake of serotonin at the presynaptic membranes and the 5-HT neuronal firing rate than the R-enantiomer and is twice as potent as the racemic mixture. However, further studies are needed to determine whether these differences result in any clinical superiority of escitalopram. For additional information on escitalopram, see Escitalopram Oxalate 28:16.04.20.

Unlike some other serotonin-reuptake inhibitors, the demethylated metabolites of citalopram, demethylcitalopram and didemethylcitalopram, are substantially less active than the parent compound as inhibitors of serotonin reuptake and have negligible affinity for various neurotransmitter receptor-binding sites. In vitro studies have shown that citalopram is at least 8 times more potent than its metabolites in inhibiting serotonin reuptake; therefore, the drug's metabolites are unlikely to contribute to the clinical activity of the drug.

At therapeutic dosages in humans, citalopram has been shown to inhibit the reuptake of serotonin into platelets.

Like other selective serotonin-reuptake inhibitors, in vitro data have demonstrated that citalopram has no or very low affinity for serotonergic receptor subtypes (5-HT$_{1A}$ and 5-HT$_{2A}$ receptors).

Effects on Other Neurotransmitters

The results of in vitro and in vivo studies indicate that citalopram has little effect on the neuronal reuptake of norepinephrine and dopamine. In addition, in vivo and in vitro data suggest that citalopram does not substantially inhibit MAO. However, citalopram has demonstrated some inhibitory activity towards MAO-A and MAO-B, with clear selectivity for MAO-B, in one in vivo study.

Unlike tricyclic and some other antidepressants, citalopram does not exhibit clinically important anticholinergic, α- or β-adrenergic blocking, or antihistaminic activity at usual therapeutic dosages. As a result, the incidence of adverse effects commonly associated with blockade of muscarinic cholinergic receptors (e.g., dry mouth, blurred vision, urinary retention, constipation, confusion), α-adrenergic receptors (e.g., orthostatic hypotension), and histamine H$_1$- and H$_2$-receptors (e.g., sedation) is lower in citalopram-treated patients. In vitro studies have demonstrated that citalopram possesses no or very low affinity for α_1- or α_2-adrenergic, β-adrenergic, histaminergic (H$_1$), GABA, muscarinic, benzodiazepine, dopamine D$_1$ and D$_2$, or opiate receptors.

Effects on Sleep

Like tricyclic and most other antidepressants, citalopram suppresses rapid eye movement (REM) sleep. In animals, citalopram has been shown to suppress REM sleep and increase deep slow wave sleep. In one study in humans, single doses of the drug suppressed REM sleep in a dose-dependent manner while chronic therapy produced more sustained REM sleep inhibition. Single doses of citalopram resulted in only minor changes in non-REM sleep as well as in non-REM EEG power spectral density in this study. However, chronic administration of the drug resulted in a major shift from slow-wave sleep stage 2 to slow-wave sleep stage 1. In another study, citalopram prolonged REM latency and increased non-REM stage 2 sleep.

Although not clearly established, there is some evidence that the REM-suppressing effects of antidepressant agents may contribute to the antidepressant activity of these drugs. Although the precise mechanism has not been fully elucidated, available data suggest that citalopram's effects on REM sleep may be serotonergically mediated.

Effects on EEG

Limited data currently are available regarding the effects of citalopram on the EEG. In animals, EEG studies have revealed an activating effect associated with behavioral arousal. In healthy individuals receiving single 20- and 40-mg doses, citalopram decreased slow-wave EEG activity in one study. However, the overall EEG changes were considered minimal in this study, particularly following repeated doses of the drug. EEG changes in healthy individuals receiving single, 10- to 50-mg oral doses of citalopram were dose-related and similar to those produced by desipramine, protriptyline, and fluvoxamine in another study.

Effects on Psychomotor Function

Citalopram generally does not appear to cause clinically important sedation and generally does not adversely affect psychomotor performance. In studies in healthy individuals, citalopram did not produce impairment of psychomotor function or intellectual function when given in doses of 40 mg daily. In one controlled study, improved psychomotor responses to sensory stimuli and sustained attention, with substantial decreases in movement times of the choice reaction time test and an increase in critical flicker fusion threshold, were reported in healthy individuals receiving single doses of the drug.

● *Cardiovascular Effects*

No clinically important changes in vital signs (systolic and diastolic blood pressure and heart rate) were observed in patients receiving citalopram in controlled trials. In addition, a comparison of supine and standing vital signs in depressed patients receiving citalopram indicated that the drug generally does not produce orthostatic changes. Adverse cardiovascular effects, including QT-interval prolongation and torsades de pointes, have occasionally been reported in healthy individuals and in depressed patients receiving citalopram. (See Cautions: Cardiovascular Effects and see also Cautions: Precautions and Contraindications.)

In a thorough QT study, citalopram was associated with a dose-dependent increase in the corrected QT (QT$_c$) interval. In a placebo-controlled study, a change from baseline in QT$_c$F (Fridericia's formula) greater than 60 msec occurred in 1.9% of patients receiving citalopram compared with 1.2% of patients receiving placebo. None of the patients receiving placebo had a post-dose QT$_c$F greater than 500 msec compared with 0.5% of patients receiving citalopram. The incidence of tachycardic and bradycardic outliers was 0.5 and 0.9% in the citalopram group, respectively, and 0.4% in the placebo group. ECG changes also have been reported in individuals receiving overdosages of the drug. (See Acute Toxicity.)

Citalopram did not induce any substantial change in cardiovascular autonomic function tests (such as heart rate variability) in a limited number of healthy individuals receiving the drug.

● *Effects on Appetite and Body Weight*

Citalopram appears to possess some anorexigenic activity, although to a lesser degree than certain other serotonergic agents (e.g., fenfluramine [no longer commercially available in the US], fluoxetine, sertraline, zimelidine [not commercially available in the US]). Although the precise mechanism has not been clearly established, results from animal studies indicate that the appetite-inhibiting action of these drugs may result at least in part from serotonin-reuptake blockade and enhancement of serotonin release thereby increasing serotonin availability at the neuronal synapse.

Only minimal weight loss (averaging 0.5 kg) generally occurred in patients receiving citalopram in controlled clinical trials. In addition, while decreased appetite was reported in about 4% of patients receiving citalopram in short-term clinical trials, the drug, unlike fluoxetine, does not appear to exhibit clinically important anorectic effects nor to produce clinically important long-term weight changes. Short-term citalopram therapy did not produce substantial weight loss in severely obese individuals in one study. Paradoxical weight gain and obesity also have been reported in some patients receiving the drug.

● *Effects on Alcohol Intake*

Like some other serotonergic agents, citalopram produces a substantial decrease in voluntary alcohol intake in animals; however, development of tolerance to this effect has been reported. Like some other serotonin-reuptake inhibitors (fluoxetine, zimelidine), citalopram also has been shown to reduce alcohol consumption in alcohol-dependent, nondepressed drinkers receiving short-term therapy with 40 mg of the drug daily. Because serotonin appears to be involved in the regulation of alcohol intake, it has been suggested that selective serotonin-reuptake inhibitors may attenuate alcohol consumption via enhanced serotonergic neurotransmission. (See Uses: Alcohol Dependence and see Drug Interactions: Alcohol.)

● *Neuroendocrine Effects*

Limited data currently are available regarding the effects of citalopram on the neuroendocrine system. In a controlled study in healthy individuals, plasma prolactin concentrations reportedly were increased by 40% following 10 days of treatment with citalopram 20 mg daily. In addition, in healthy individuals receiving low-dose IV citalopram (parenteral dosage form not commercially available in the US), plasma prolactin and cortisol concentrations increased in a dose-dependent manner.

● *Other Effects*

Like some other antidepressants that are amphiphilic cationic compounds, citalopram has been found to cause a generalized lipidosis in animal studies. Lipidosis-like changes in lymph nodes, adrenal cortex and medulla, kidney, lung, and sympathetic ganglia have been noted in animals receiving 140 mg/kg daily of the drug for 7 weeks; however, the clinical importance of these findings remains to be established.

Limited data in animals suggest that citalopram may possess anticonvulsant activity during chronic administration.

PHARMACOKINETICS

In all human studies described in the Pharmacokinetics section, citalopram was administered as the hydrobromide salt; dosages and concentrations are expressed in terms of citalopram.

A concentration of 1 nmol/L of citalopram is approximately equivalent to 0.32 ng/mL.

● *Absorption*

Like other selective serotonin-reuptake inhibitors, citalopram is a highly lipophilic compound that appears to be rapidly and well absorbed from the GI tract following oral administration. Following a single 40-mg oral dose of citalopram as a tablet, the manufacturer states that peak plasma concentrations averaging approximately 44 ng/mL occur at about 4 hours.

The absolute bioavailability of citalopram is approximately 80% relative to an IV dose. The oral tablets and solution of citalopram reportedly are bioequivalent. Food does not substantially affect the absorption of citalopram.

The single- and multiple-dose pharmacokinetics of citalopram are linear and dose-proportional in a dosage range of 10–60 mg daily. With once-daily dosing, steady-state plasma concentrations are achieved within approximately 1 week. In one study, the steady-state plasma concentrations ranged from about 30–230 ng/mL in depressed patients receiving dosages of 30–60 mg daily and agreed well with predicted values. The mean plasma concentration was approximately 80 ng/mL at the usual dosage of 40 mg daily. At steady state, the extent of accumulation of citalopram in plasma, based on the half-life, is expected to be about 2.5 times higher than the plasma concentrations observed after a single dose of the drug.

In depressed patients receiving 20–60 mg daily of citalopram, steady-state plasma concentrations of racemic citalopram and demethylcitalopram, a principal metabolite, ranged from 9–200 ng/mL and 10–105 ng/mL, respectively. When using a stereoselective analysis method, plasma concentrations ranged from 9–106 ng/mL for escitalopram (S-citalopram), 20–186 ng/mL for R-citalopram, 4–38 ng/mL for S-demethylcitalopram, and 3–75 ng/mL for R-demethylcitalopram in depressed patients receiving citalopram therapy (20–80 mg daily). The mean ratio between R-citalopram and escitalopram was 0.56 (range: 0.32–0.97).

The effect of age on the pharmacokinetics of citalopram has not been fully elucidated. Studies in healthy individuals and depressed patients 60 years of age or older have found higher areas under the plasma concentration-time curves (AUC) and longer elimination half-lives compared with those in younger individuals. (See Pharmacokinetics: Elimination.) In healthy individuals 60 years of age or older, the AUC of citalopram was increased by an average of approximately 30% in a single-dose study and by an average of approximately 23% in a multiple-dose study. Steady-state plasma citalopram concentrations were up to 4 times higher in geriatric patients receiving 20 mg of the drug once daily in one multiple-dose study than expected based on data in younger patients and healthy individuals. (See Dosage and Administration: Dosage in Geriatric Patients and see Cautions: Geriatric Precautions.)

The effect of gender on the pharmacokinetics of citalopram has not been fully elucidated to date. The manufacturer states that in 3 pharmacokinetic studies, the AUC of citalopram in women was 1.5–2 times higher than that found in men; however, this difference was not observed in 5 other pharmacokinetic studies performed with the drug. In clinical studies, no differences in steady-state plasma citalopram concentrations were observed between men and women. In addition, there were no gender differences in the pharmacokinetics of the principal metabolites of citalopram, demethylcitalopram and didemethylcitalopram. Therefore, the manufacturer states that no adjustment of citalopram dosage on the basis of gender is necessary.

The onset of antidepressant activity following oral administration of citalopram hydrobromide usually occurs within 1–4 weeks.

As with other selective serotonin-reuptake inhibitors, the relationship between plasma citalopram concentrations and the therapeutic and/or toxic effects of the drug has not been clearly established. Since citalopram is administered as a racemic mixture with the pharmacologic effect of the drug associated mainly with escitalopram, the S-enantiomer, it may be important to take the stereoselective metabolism of the drug into account when evaluating the relationship between the clinical effect of the drug and plasma concentrations of citalopram.

• Distribution

Distribution of citalopram and its metabolites into human body tissues and fluids has not been fully characterized. However, limited pharmacokinetic data suggest that the drug, which is highly lipophilic, is widely distributed in body tissues.

The volume of distribution of citalopram is approximately 12 L/kg. The drug crosses the blood-brain barrier in humans and animals.

The binding of citalopram, demethylcitalopram, and didemethylcitalopram to human plasma proteins in vitro is about 80%.

Citalopram and demethylcitalopram are distributed into milk and also cross the placenta. In a study involving 7 lactating women who received median oral citalopram doses of 0.36 mg/kg daily for the treatment of depression, mean milk-to-plasma AUC values of 1.8 were calculated for both citalopram and demethylcitalopram. Depending on the method of calculation, mean infant exposure was estimated to be 3.2 or 3.7% for citalopram and 1.2 or 1.4% for demethylcitalopram in this study. In 9 lactating women receiving 20–40 mg daily of citalopram in another study, maternal milk-to-plasma ratios of the drug ranged from approximately 2–3; however, plasma citalopram concentrations in the neonates were found to be very low or below the limit of detection. In a lactating woman receiving 40 mg daily of citalopram, concentrations of the drug in milk and serum were about 205 ng/mL and 99 ng/mL, respectively, and the drug concentration in the infant's serum was about 13 ng/mL. In another lactating woman receiving 20 mg daily of citalopram, peak milk concentrations of the drug occurred 3–9 hours following maternal drug intake; the milk-to-serum concentration ratio was approximately 3 for both citalopram and demethylcitalopram. Accordingly, the infant received approximately 5% of the mother's dose when adjusted for weight. (See Cautions: Pregnancy, Fertility, and Lactation.)

• Elimination

The elimination half-life of citalopram averages approximately 35 hours in adults with normal renal and hepatic function.

The exact metabolic fate of citalopram has not been fully elucidated; however, metabolism of citalopram is mainly hepatic and involves N-demethylation. Citalopram is metabolized to demethylcitalopram, didemethylcitalopram, citalopram-N-oxide, and a deaminated propionic acid derivative. In vitro studies have indicated that cytochrome P-450 (CYP) 3A4 and 2C19 isoenzymes are the principal enzymes involved in the N-demethylation of citalopram to demethylcitalopram and that demethylcitalopram is further N-demethylated to didemethylcitalopram by CYP2D6. Because citalopram is metabolized by multiple enzyme systems, inhibition of a single enzyme is unlikely to appreciably decrease the clearance of citalopram. Unlike some other selective serotonin-reuptake inhibitors, the demethylated metabolites of citalopram, demethylcitalopram and didemethylcitalopram, are substantially less active than the parent compound as inhibitors of serotonin reuptake. Thus, citalopram's metabolites are unlikely to contribute to the antidepressant and other clinical actions of the drug.

In humans, unchanged citalopram is the predominant compound in plasma. At steady state, the concentrations of demethylcitalopram and didemethylcitalopram in plasma are approximately one-half and one-tenth, respectively, that of the parent drug. Following IV (parenteral dosage form not commercially available in the US) administration of citalopram, the fraction of drug recovered in urine as citalopram and demethylcitalopram was about 10 and 5%, respectively.

Following oral administration of a single, radiolabeled dose of citalopram in healthy individuals, approximately 75% of the dose was excreted in urine and approximately 10% was eliminated in feces within 17 days. An analysis of the urinary composition showed that besides the known metabolites of citalopram, 3 glucuronides were present. The relative amounts of citalopram, demethylcitalopram, didemethylcitalopram, and the N-oxide metabolite present in urine collected for 7 days were 26, 19, 9, and 7%, respectively, with glucuronidated metabolites accounting for the remainder.

Following IV administration, the mean systemic clearance of citalopram is approximately 330 mL/minute, with approximately 20% of that due to renal clearance.

The effect of age on the elimination of citalopram has not been fully elucidated. Studies in healthy geriatric individuals and depressed geriatric patients have found higher AUC values and longer elimination half-lives compared with younger individuals. (See Pharmacokinetics: Absorption.) In healthy individuals 60 years of age or older, the elimination half-life of citalopram was increased by 50% in a single-dose study and by 30% in a multiple-dose study. It has been suggested that these differences in pharmacokinetic parameters may reflect declining liver and kidney function. In addition, the stereoselective metabolism of the enantiomers for citalopram and demethylcitalopram in older individuals appears to differ from that reported in younger patients, suggesting possible age-associated changes in CYP2C19 activities. (See Dosage and Administration: Dosage in Geriatric Patients and see Cautions: Geriatric Precautions.)

Because citalopram is extensively metabolized in the liver, hepatic impairment can affect the elimination of the drug. Following oral administration, the clearance of citalopram in patients with impaired hepatic function was reduced by 37% and the elimination half-life was increased twofold compared with that in healthy individuals. Therefore, the manufacturer recommends that in depressed patients with hepatic impairment, the maximum recommended dosage of citalopram is 20 mg once daily due to the risk of QT-interval prolongation. (See Dosage and Administration: Dosage in Hepatic and Renal Impairment and see Cautions: Precautions and Contraindications.)

In poor metabolizers of CYP2C19, steady-state peak concentrations and AUC values of citalopram increased by 68 and 107%, respectively. Therefore, the manufacturer recommends that in poor metabolizers of CYP2C19, the maximum recommended dosage of citalopram is 20 mg once daily due to the risk of QT-interval prolongation. (See Dosage and Administration: Dosage in Poor CYP2C19 Metabolizers or Patients Receiving CYP2C19 Inhibitors and see Cautions: Precautions and Contraindications.) Steady-state plasma citalopram concentrations were not substantially different in healthy individuals with poor or extensive CYP2D6 metabolizer phenotypes following multiple-dose administration of the drug.

The effect of renal impairment on the pharmacokinetics of citalopram has not been fully evaluated to date. In patients with moderate renal impairment, the renal clearance of citalopram and its 2 principal metabolites was reduced and the elimination half-life of citalopram was slightly prolonged to an average of about 50 hours. In a study comparing the pharmacokinetics of citalopram in a limited number of patients with severe renal failure undergoing hemodialysis and in healthy individuals, no substantial differences were found between the 2 groups in any of the pharmacokinetic parameters, with the exception of the renal clearance of citalopram, which was significantly lower in the renal failure group than in the control group (1.7 mL/minute versus 66 mL/minute). Therefore, moderate to severe renal failure does not appear to markedly affect the pharmacokinetics of citalopram suggesting that dosage adjustment in such patients may not be necessary. Additional studies evaluating long-term citalopram therapy in patients with severe renal impairment are necessary to confirm these findings. (See Dosage and Administration: Dosage in Hepatic and Renal Impairment.)

Limited data indicate that citalopram and demethylcitalopram are not appreciably removed by hemodialysis. In a limited number of patients, hemodialysis cleared only about 1% of an oral dose of citalopram as the parent drug and 1% as demethylcitalopram. Because of the large volume of distribution of citalopram, hemodialysis, peritoneal dialysis, forced diuresis, hemoperfusion, and/or exchange transfusion also are unlikely to be effective in removing substantial amounts of citalopram from the body.

CHEMISTRY AND STABILITY

• Chemistry

Citalopram hydrobromide, a selective serotonin-reuptake inhibitor (SSRI), is a bicyclic phthalane-derivative antidepressant. The drug differs structurally from most other selective serotonin-reuptake inhibitors (e.g., fluoxetine, fluvoxamine, paroxetine, sertraline) and also differs structurally and pharmacologically from tricyclic and tetracyclic antidepressants. The commercially available drug is a 50:50 racemic mixture of the R- and S-enantiomers. The inhibition of serotonin reuptake by citalopram is principally due to the S-enantiomer, escitalopram (see Escitalopram Oxalate 28:16.04.20).

Citalopram hydrobromide occurs as a fine white to off-white powder that is sparingly soluble in water and soluble in ethanol. The drug has a pK$_a$ of 9.5.

Citalopram hydrobromide is commercially available for oral administration as tablets and as an oral solution. Commercially available citalopram hydrobromide oral solution is a clear, colorless solution with a peppermint flavor and contains 10 mg of citalopram per 5 mL. Citalopram hydrobromide oral solution contains methylparabens and propylparabens as preservatives. Citalopram also is commercially available in some countries as an IV injection†; however, this dosage form currently is not available in the US.

● *Stability*

Citalopram hydrobromide tablets should be stored at a temperature of 25°C but may be exposed to temperatures ranging from 15–30°C. When stored as directed, the tablets have an expiration date of 2 years following the date of manufacture.

Citalopram hydrobromide oral solution should be stored at 20–25°C but may be exposed to temperatures ranging from 15–30°C.

PREPARATIONS

Because of similarity in spelling of Celexa® (citalopram hydrobromide), Celebrex® (celecoxib), and Cerebyx® (fosphenytoin sodium), extra care should be exercised in ensuring the accuracy of prescriptions for these drugs.

Excipients in commercially available drug preparations may have clinically important effects in some individuals; consult specific product labeling for details.

Citalopram Hydrobromide

Oral		
Tablets, film-coated	10 mg (of citalopram)*	**CeleXA®**, Forest
		Citalopram Hydrobromide Tablets
	20 mg (of citalopram)*	**CeleXA®** (scored), Forest
		Citalopram Hydrobromide Tablets
	40 mg (of citalopram)*	**CeleXA®** (scored), Forest
		Citalopram Hydrobromide Tablets
Solution	10 mg (of citalopram) per 5 mL*	**Citalopram Hydrobromide Oral Solution**

* available from one or more manufacturer, distributor, and/or repackager by generic (nonproprietary) name

† Use is not currently included in the labeling approved by the US Food and Drug Administration.

Escitalopram Oxalate

28:16.04.20 • SELECTIVE SEROTONIN-REUPTAKE INHIBITORS

■ Escitalopram, the *S*-enantiomer of citalopram, is a selective serotonin-reuptake inhibitor (SSRI) and an antidepressant.

USES

• Major Depressive Disorder

Escitalopram oxalate is used for the acute and maintenance treatment of major depressive disorder in adults and adolescents 12–17 years of age.

Efficacy of escitalopram for the acute management of major depression in adults was established in 3 placebo-controlled studies of 8 weeks' duration in adult outpatients who met DSM-IV criteria for major depressive disorder. In these studies, 10- and 20-mg daily dosages of escitalopram were more effective than placebo in improving scores on the Montgomery Asberg Depression Rating Scale (MADRS), the Hamilton Rating Scale for Depression (HAM-D), and the Clinical Global Impression Improvement and Severity of Illness Scale. Escitalopram also was more effective than placebo in improving other aspects of depressive disorder, including anxiety, social functioning, and overall quality of life. Substantial improvement in MADRS and HAM-D scores was noted in patients receiving either dosage of escitalopram compared with those receiving placebo after 1–2 weeks of therapy. In addition, escitalopram dosages of 10–20 mg daily appeared to be at least as effective as racemic citalopram dosages of 20–40 mg daily. No age-, race-, or gender-related differences in efficacy were noted in these studies.

Efficacy of escitalopram for the acute management of major depressive disorder in adolescents 12–17 years of age was established in an 8-week, flexible-dose, placebo-controlled study in outpatients who met DSM-IV criteria for major depressive disorder. Escitalopram-treated patients in this study demonstrated substantially greater improvement on the Children's Depression Rating Scale–Revised (CDRS-R) compared with those receiving placebo. Efficacy of escitalopram in the acute treatment of major depressive disorder in adolescents was also established on the basis of extrapolation from an 8-week, flexible-dose, placebo-controlled study with racemic citalopram 20–40 mg daily. In this outpatient study conducted in children and adolescents 7–17 years of age who met DSM-IV criteria for major depressive disorder, citalopram-treated patients demonstrated substantially greater improvement on the CDRS-R compared with those receiving placebo; the positive results in this trial came largely from the adolescent subgroup. Two additional flexible-dose, placebo-controlled depression studies (one for escitalopram in patients 7–17 years of age and one for citalopram in adolescents) did not demonstrate efficacy.

In a longer-term study, 274 adults with major depressive disorder who had responded to escitalopram 10 or 20 mg daily during an initial 8-week, open-label, flexible dosage treatment phase were randomized to continue escitalopram at the same dosage or receive placebo for up to 36 weeks of observation for relapse in the double-blind phase. Relapse during the double-blind phase was defined as an increase in the MADRS total score to 22 or greater or discontinuance due to insufficient clinical response. Escitalopram-treated patients experienced a substantially longer time to relapse of depression compared with those receiving placebo. In addition, more placebo recipients relapsed compared with patients receiving escitalopram (cumulative relapse rates were approximately 40 and 26%, respectively).

Although efficacy of escitalopram as maintenance therapy in adolescent patients has not been systematically evaluated, such efficacy can be extrapolated from adult data along with comparisons of escitalopram pharmacokinetic parameters in adults and adolescent patients.

The manufacturers state that if escitalopram is used for extended periods, the need for continued therapy should be reassessed periodically.

There is some evidence that escitalopram may offer some clinical advantages compared with citalopram or other selective serotonin-reuptake inhibitors (e.g., increased efficacy, more rapid onset of therapeutic effect, fewer adverse effects); however, additional studies are needed to confirm these initial findings.

For further information on use of SSRIs in the treatment of major depressive disorder and considerations in choosing the most appropriate antidepressant agent for a particular patient, see Uses: Major Depressive Disorder, in Citalopram Hydrobromide 28:16.04.20.

• Generalized Anxiety Disorder

Escitalopram is used in the management of generalized anxiety disorder in adults. Efficacy for the management of generalized anxiety disorder was established in 3 multicenter, flexible-dose, placebo-controlled studies of 8-weeks' duration in adult outpatients who met DSM-IV criteria for generalized anxiety disorder. In these studies, patients receiving 10–20 mg daily of escitalopram had substantially greater mean improvements in scores on the Hamilton Anxiety Scale (HAM-A) than those receiving placebo.

For further information on the treatment of generalized anxiety disorder, see Uses: Anxiety Disorders, in Paroxetine 28:16.04.20.

DOSAGE AND ADMINISTRATION

• Administration

Escitalopram oxalate is administered orally once daily, in the morning or evening, without regard to meals. Commercially available escitalopram oxalate tablets and oral solution are bioequivalent.

Patients receiving escitalopram should be monitored for possible worsening of depression, suicidality, or unusual changes in behavior, especially at the beginning of therapy or during periods of dosage adjustment. (See Worsening of Depression and Suicidality Risk under Warnings/Precautions: Warnings, in Cautions.)

The manufacturers recommend that at least 2 weeks elapse between discontinuance of a monoamine oxidase (MAO) inhibitor and initiation of escitalopram and vice versa. (See Serotonin Syndrome or Neuroleptic Malignant Syndrome-like Reactions under Warnings/Precautions: Other Warnings and Precautions, in Cautions and also see Drug Interactions: Monoamine Oxidase Inhibitors.)

• Dosage

Dosage of escitalopram oxalate is expressed in terms of escitalopram.

Major Depressive Disorder

For the acute management of major depressive disorder in adults, the recommended initial dosage of escitalopram is 10 mg once daily. Although efficacy has been established at dosages of 10 or 20 mg once daily, no additional benefit was observed with the 20-mg dosage in a fixed-dose study. If a dosage exceeding 10 mg daily is considered necessary, dosage may be increased to 20 mg daily after a minimum of 1 week.

For the acute management of major depressive disorder in adolescents 12–17 years of age, the recommended initial dosage of escitalopram is 10 mg once daily. Efficacy has been established at dosages of 10–20 mg daily in a flexible-dose study. If dosage is increased to 20 mg daily, this should occur after a minimum of 3 weeks.

While the optimum duration of escitalopram oxalate therapy has not been established, many experts state that acute depressive episodes require several months or longer of sustained antidepressant therapy. In addition, some clinicians recommend that long-term antidepressant therapy be considered in certain patients at risk for recurrence of depressive episodes (such as those with highly recurrent unipolar depression). Whether the dosage of escitalopram oxalate required to induce remission is identical to the dosage needed to maintain and/or sustain euthymia is unknown. Systematic evaluation of escitalopram oxalate has shown that its antidepressant efficacy is maintained for periods of up to 36 weeks in adults receiving 10–20 mg daily. Nevertheless, the manufacturers recommend that the usefulness of escitalopram be reevaluated periodically in patients receiving long-term therapy.

Generalized Anxiety Disorder

For the management of generalized anxiety disorder in adults, the recommended initial dosage of escitalopram is 10 mg once daily. If no clinical improvement is apparent, dosage may be increased to 20 mg daily after a minimum of 1 week.

Although the manufacturers state that the efficacy of escitalopram for long-term therapy (i.e., longer than 8 weeks) has not been demonstrated in controlled studies to date, generalized anxiety disorder is a chronic condition. If escitalopram is used for extended periods, the need for continued therapy with the drug should be reassessed periodically.

Discontinuance of Therapy

Because withdrawal effects may occur with discontinuance of escitalopram and other SSRIs and selective serotonin- and norepinephrine-reuptake inhibitors (SNRIs), abrupt discontinuance should be avoided whenever possible. When escitalopram therapy is discontinued, the dosage should be reduced gradually and the patient monitored for possible withdrawal symptoms. If intolerable symptoms occur following dosage reduction or upon discontinuance of therapy, the drug may be reinstituted at the previously prescribed dosage. Subsequently, the clinician may continue decreasing the dosage, but at a more gradual rate. (See Withdrawal of Therapy under Warnings/Precautions: Other Warnings and Precautions, in Cautions.)

● **Special Populations**

The recommended dosage of escitalopram in most geriatric patients and those with hepatic impairment is 10 mg once daily.

Dosage adjustment in patients with mild to moderate renal impairment is not necessary, but the drug should be used with caution in those with severe renal impairment.

CAUTIONS

● **Contraindications**

Concurrent or recent (i.e., within 2 weeks) therapy with a monoamine oxidase (MAO) inhibitor. At least 14 days should elapse between discontinuance of escitalopram and initiation of MAO inhibitor therapy and vice versa. (See Serotonin Syndrome or Neuroleptic Malignant Syndrome-like Reactions under Warnings/Precautions: Other Warnings and Precautions, in Cautions and also see Drug Interactions: Monoamine Oxidase Inhibitors.)

Concomitant use with pimozide. (See Drug Interactions: Antipsychotic Agents and Other Dopamine Antagonists.)

Known hypersensitivity to escitalopram, citalopram, or any ingredient in the formulation.

● **Warnings/Precautions**

Warnings

Worsening of Depression and Suicidality Risk

Worsening of depression and/or the emergence of suicidal ideation and behavior (suicidality) or unusual changes in behavior may occur in both adult and pediatric (see Pediatric Use under Warnings/Precautions: Specific Populations, in Cautions) patients with major depressive disorder or other psychiatric disorders, whether or not they are taking antidepressants. This risk may persist until clinically important remission occurs. Suicide is a known risk of depression and certain other psychiatric disorders, and these disorders themselves are the strongest predictors of suicide. However, there has been a long-standing concern that antidepressants may have a role in inducing worsening of depression and the emergence of suicidality in certain patients during the early phases of treatment. Pooled analyses of short-term, placebo-controlled studies of antidepressants (i.e., selective serotonin-reuptake inhibitors [SSRIs] and other antidepressants) have shown an increased risk of suicidality in children, adolescents, and young adults (18–24 years of age) with major depressive disorder and other psychiatric disorders. An increased suicidality risk was not demonstrated with antidepressants compared with placebo in adults older than 24 years of age and a reduced risk was observed in adults 65 years of age or older.

The US Food and Drug Administration (FDA) recommends that all patients being treated with antidepressants for any indication be appropriately monitored and closely observed for clinical worsening, suicidality, and unusual changes in behavior, particularly during initiation of therapy (i.e., the first few months) and during periods of dosage adjustments. Families and caregivers of patients being treated with antidepressants for major depressive disorder or other indications, both psychiatric and nonpsychiatric, also should be advised to monitor patients on a daily basis for the emergence of agitation, irritability, or unusual changes in behavior as well as the emergence of suicidality, and to report such symptoms immediately to a health-care provider.

Although a causal relationship between the emergence of symptoms such as anxiety, agitation, panic attacks, insomnia, irritability, hostility, aggressiveness, impulsivity, akathisia, hypomania, and/or mania and either the worsening of depression and/or the emergence of suicidal impulses has not been established, there is concern that such symptoms may represent precursors to emerging suicidality. Consequently, consideration should be given to changing the therapeutic regimen or discontinuing therapy in patients whose depression is persistently worse or in patients experiencing emergent

suicidality or symptoms that might be precursors to worsening depression or suicidality, particularly if such manifestations are severe, abrupt in onset, or were not part of the patient's presenting symptoms. If a decision is made to discontinue therapy, taper escitalopram dosage as rapidly as is feasible but consider the risks of abrupt discontinuance. (See Discontinuance of Therapy, under Dosage and Administration: Dosage.) FDA also recommends that the drugs be prescribed in the smallest quantity consistent with good patient management, in order to reduce the risk of overdosage.

Other Warnings and Precautions

Serotonin Syndrome or Neuroleptic Malignant Syndrome-like Reactions

Potentially life-threatening serotonin syndrome or neuroleptic malignant syndrome (NMS)-like reactions have been reported with SSRIs, including escitalopram, and selective serotonin- and norepinephrine-reuptake inhibitors (SNRIs) alone, but particularly with concurrent use of other serotonergic drugs (including serotonin [5-hydroxytryptamine; 5-HT] type 1 receptor agonists ["triptans"]), drugs that impair the metabolism of serotonin (e.g., MAO inhibitors), or antipsychotics or other dopamine antagonists. Manifestations of serotonin syndrome may include mental status changes (e.g., agitation, hallucinations, coma), autonomic instability (e.g., tachycardia, labile blood pressure, hyperthermia), neuromuscular aberrations (e.g., hyperreflexia, incoordination), and/or GI symptoms (e.g., nausea, vomiting, diarrhea). In its most severe form, serotonin syndrome may resemble NMS, which is characterized by hyperthermia, muscle rigidity, autonomic instability with possible rapid fluctuation in vital signs, and mental status changes. Patients receiving escitalopram should be monitored for the development of serotonin syndrome or NMS-like signs and symptoms. (See Contraindications and also see Drug Interactions.)

Concurrent or recent (i.e., within 2 weeks) therapy with MAO inhibitors intended to treat depression is contraindicated. (See Contraindications and also see Drug Interactions: Monoamine Oxidase Inhibitors.)

If concurrent therapy with escitalopram and a 5-HT₁ receptor agonist (triptan) is clinically warranted, the patient should be observed carefully, particularly during initiation of therapy, when dosage is increased, or when another serotonergic agent is initiated.

Concomitant use of escitalopram and serotonin precursors (e.g., tryptophan) is not recommended.

If signs and symptoms of serotonin syndrome or NMS occur, treatment with escitalopram and any concurrently administered serotonergic or antidopaminergic agents, including antipsychotic agents, should be immediately discontinued and supportive and symptomatic treatment initiated.

Withdrawal of Therapy

Withdrawal symptoms, including dysphoric mood, irritability, agitation, dizziness, sensory disturbances (e.g., paresthesias such as electric shock sensations), anxiety, confusion, headache, lethargy, emotional lability, insomnia, hypomania, tinnitus, and seizures, have been reported upon discontinuance of escitalopram and other SSRIs and SNRIs, particularly when discontinuance of these drugs is abrupt. While these reactions are generally self-limiting, there have been reports of serious discontinuance symptoms. Therefore, patients should be monitored for such symptoms when discontinuing escitalopram therapy. A gradual reduction in dosage rather than abrupt cessation is recommended whenever possible. (See Discontinuance of Therapy under Dosage and Administration: Dosage.)

If intolerable symptoms occur following dosage reduction or discontinuance of escitalopram, the previously prescribed dosage should be reinstituted until symptoms abate; dosage reductions may then be resumed at a more gradual rate.

Seizures

Although anticonvulsant effects of racemic citalopram have been observed in animal studies, escitalopram has not been systematically evaluated in patients with seizure disorders. Seizures have been reported in patients receiving escitalopram in clinical trials; therefore, as with other antidepressants, escitalopram therapy should be initiated with caution in patients with a history of seizure disorder.

Activation of Mania/Hypomania

Activation of mania and hypomania has occurred in patients receiving escitalopram or citalopram. Escitalopram should be used with caution in patients with a history of mania.

Hyponatremia/Syndrome of Inappropriate Antidiuretic Hormone Secretion

Treatment with SNRIs and SSRIs, including escitalopram, may result in hyponatremia. In many cases, hyponatremia appears to be due to the syndrome of inappropriate antidiuretic hormone secretion (SIADH). Cases with serum sodium concentrations lower than 110 mEq/L have been reported. Geriatric individuals and patients receiving diuretics or who are otherwise volume depleted may be at greater risk of developing hyponatremia. Signs and symptoms of hyponatremia include headache, difficulty concentrating, memory impairment, confusion, weakness, and unsteadiness, which may lead to falls; more severe and/or acute cases have been associated with hallucinations, syncope, seizures, coma, respiratory arrest, and death. Discontinuance of escitalopram should be considered and appropriate medical intervention should be initiated in patients with symptomatic hyponatremia.

Abnormal Bleeding

SNRIs and SSRIs, including escitalopram, may increase the risk of bleeding events. Concurrent use of aspirin, nonsteroidal anti-inflammatory agents (NSAIAs), warfarin, and other anticoagulants may add to this risk. Case reports and epidemiologic studies have demonstrated an association between the use of drugs that interfere with serotonin reuptake and the occurrence of GI bleeding. Bleeding events related to SNRI and SSRI use have ranged from ecchymoses, hematomas, epistaxis, and petechiae to life-threatening hemorrhages. The manufacturers recommend that patients be advised of the risk of bleeding associated with the concomitant use of escitalopram and aspirin or other NSAIAs, warfarin, or other drugs that affect coagulation. (See Drug Interactions: Drugs Affecting Hemostasis.)

Interference with Cognitive and Motor Performance

In a study in healthy volunteers, escitalopram 10 mg daily did not impair intellectual function or psychomotor performance. However, because any psychoactive drug may impair judgment, thinking, or motor skills, caution patients about operating hazardous machinery, including driving a motor vehicle, until they are reasonably certain that the drug does not affect their ability to engage in such activities.

Concomitant Illnesses

Experience with escitalopram in patients with certain concomitant diseases is limited. (See Renal Impairment and see Hepatic Impairment under Warnings/Precautions: Specific Populations, in Cautions.)

Escitalopram has not been systematically evaluated in patients with a recent history of myocardial infarction or unstable cardiovascular disease; such patients were generally excluded from clinical studies. The drug should be used with caution in patients with diseases or conditions that produce altered metabolism or hemodynamic responses.

Concomitant use of SSRIs and MAO inhibitors has been associated with serious, sometimes fatal, reactions, including hyperthermia, rigidity, myoclonus, autonomic instability, and mental status changes; these reactions have resembled serotonin syndrome or NMS. (See Contraindications and Serotonin Syndrome or Neuroleptic Malignant Syndrome-like Reactions under Warnings/Precautions: Other Warnings and Precautions, in Cautions and see also Drug Interactions: Monoamine Oxidase Inhibitors.)

Specific Populations
Pregnancy

Category C. (See Users Guide.)

Some neonates exposed to serotonergic antidepressants (e.g., SSRIs, SNRIs) late in the third trimester of pregnancy have developed complications that have sometimes been severe and required prolonged hospitalization, respiratory support, enteral nutrition, and other forms of supportive care in special-care nurseries. Such complications may arise immediately upon delivery and usually last several days or up to 2–4 weeks. Clinical findings reported in the neonates have included respiratory distress, cyanosis, apnea, seizures, temperature instability or fever, feeding difficulty, dehydration, excessive weight loss, vomiting, hypoglycemia, hypotonia, hypertonia, hyperreflexia, tremor, jitteriness, irritability, and constant crying. These features appear to be consistent with either a direct toxic effect of serotonergic antidepressants or, possibly, a drug withdrawal syndrome. In some cases, the clinical picture was consistent with serotonin syndrome.

Infants exposed to SSRIs in late pregnancy may have an increased risk of persistent pulmonary hypertension of the newborn (PPHN), a rare heart and lung condition associated with substantial neonatal morbidity and mortality. Although several epidemiologic studies have suggested an increased risk of PPHN with SSRI use during pregnancy, other studies did not demonstrate a statistically significant association. The US Food and Drug Administration (FDA) states that it is currently unclear whether the use of SSRIs, including escitalopram, during pregnancy can cause PPHN and recommends that clinicians not alter their current clinical practice of treating depression during pregnancy.

For additional information on the management of depression in women prior to conception and during pregnancy, including treatment algorithms, clinicians may consult the joint American Psychiatric Association and American College of Obstetricians and Gynecologists guidelines (at https://www.ncbi.nlm.nih.gov/pmc/articles/PMC3103063/pdf/nihms293836.pdf).

Lactation

Escitalopram is distributed into human milk. Because of the potential for serious adverse effects (e.g., excessive somnolence, decreased feeding, weight loss) in nursing infants, caution should be exercised and nursing infants should be observed for adverse reactions when escitalopram is administered to a nursing woman.

Pediatric Use

Safety and efficacy of escitalopram have not been established in pediatric patients younger than 12 years of age with major depressive disorder. Safety and effectiveness have been established in adolescents 12–17 years of age for the acute treatment of major depressive disorder. Although efficacy of escitalopram as maintenance therapy in adolescent patients with major depressive disorder has not been systematically evaluated, such efficacy can be extrapolated from adult data along with comparisons of pharmacokinetic parameters in adults and adolescent patients. (See Uses: Major Depressive Disorder.)

Safety and efficacy of escitalopram have not been established in pediatric patients younger than 18 years of age with generalized anxiety disorder.

Decreased appetite and weight loss have been observed in association with the use of SSRIs. Therefore, regular monitoring of weight and growth should be performed in children and adolescents treated with an SSRI such as escitalopram.

FDA warns that a greater risk of suicidal thinking or behavior (suicidality) occurred during first few months of antidepressant treatment compared with placebo in children and adolescents with major depressive disorder, obsessive-compulsive disorder (OCD), or other psychiatric disorders based on pooled analyses of 24 short-term, placebo-controlled trials of 9 antidepressant drugs (SSRIs and other antidepressants). However, a more recent meta-analysis of 27 placebo-controlled trials of 9 antidepressants (SSRIs and others) in patients younger than 19 years of age with major depressive disorder, OCD, or non-OCD anxiety disorders suggests that the benefits of antidepressant therapy in treating these conditions may outweigh the risks of suicidal behavior or suicidal ideation. No suicides occurred in these pediatric trials. These findings should be carefully considered when assessing potential benefits and risks of escitalopram in a child or adolescent for any clinical use. (See Worsening of Depression and Suicidality Risk under Warnings/Precautions: Warnings, in Cautions.)

Geriatric Use

Approximately 6% of patients studied in clinical trials of escitalopram for major depressive disorder and generalized anxiety disorder were 60 years of age or older; geriatric patients in these trials received daily dosages of 10–20 mg daily. Experience in geriatric patients in these trials was insufficient to determine whether they respond differently from younger adults; however, increased sensitivity cannot be ruled out.

In 2 pharmacokinetic studies, the mean area under the plasma concentration-time curve (AUC) and elimination half-life of escitalopram were increased by approximately 50% in geriatric individuals compared with younger individuals and peak escitalopram concentrations were unchanged. Therefore, the manufacturers state that the recommended dosage of escitalopram in geriatric patients is 10 mg once daily.

SNRIs and SSRIs, including escitalopram, have been associated with clinically important hyponatremia in geriatric patients, who may be at greater risk for this adverse effect. (See Hyponatremia/Syndrome of Inappropriate Antidiuretic Hormone Secretion under Warnings/Precautions: Other Warnings and Precautions, in Cautions.)

In pooled data analyses, a *reduced* risk of suicidality was observed in adults 65 years of age or older with antidepressant therapy compared with placebo. (See Worsening of Depression and Suicidality Risk under Warnings/Precautions: Warnings, in Cautions.)

Renal Impairment

Escitalopram should be used with caution in patients with severe renal impairment (i.e., creatinine clearance less than 20 mL/minute). (See Dosage and Administration: Special Populations.)

Hepatic Impairment

In clinical studies, clearance of racemic citalopram was decreased by 37% and elimination half-life was doubled relative to that in patients with normal hepatic function. Dosage reduction is recommended for patients with hepatic impairment. (See Dosage and Administration: Special Populations.)

● Common Adverse Effects

Adverse effects reported in approximately 5% or more of patients with generalized anxiety or major depressive disorder receiving escitalopram and with an incidence of at least twice that of placebo include insomnia, nausea, increased sweating, sexual dysfunction (ejaculation disorder [primarily ejaculatory delay], decreased libido, anorgasmia), fatigue, and somnolence.

DRUG INTERACTIONS

● Drugs Affecting or Metabolized by Hepatic Microsomal Enzymes

Inhibitors or inducers of cytochrome P-450 (CYP) 3A4 (e.g., carbamazepine, ketoconazole, ritonavir, triazolam) and 2C19 isoenzymes: clinically important pharmacokinetic interaction unlikely since escitalopram is metabolized by multiple enzyme systems. However, possibility that carbamazepine may increase clearance of escitalopram should be considered.

Substrates of CYP2D6 isoenzyme (e.g., desipramine, metoprolol): potential pharmacokinetic (increased peak plasma concentrations and AUC of the substrate) interactions. Use with caution. Increased plasma concentrations of metoprolol have been associated with decreased cardioselectivity.

● Drugs Affecting Hemostasis

Pharmacokinetics of warfarin were not affected by racemic citalopram; however, prothrombin time increased by 5%. The effects of escitalopram have not been evaluated, and the clinical importance of this interaction is unknown.

Altered anticoagulant effects, including increased bleeding, have been reported when SSRIs or selective serotonin- and norepinephrine-reuptake inhibitors (SNRIs) were concurrently administered with warfarin or other anticoagulants. The manufacturers of escitalopram recommend carefully monitoring patients receiving warfarin during initiation and discontinuance of escitalopram therapy.

Potential pharmacologic (increased risk of bleeding) interaction with aspirin or other nonsteroidal anti-inflammatory agents (NSAIAs); escitalopram and drugs that affect hemostasis should be used concomitantly with caution.

● Antipsychotic Agents and Other Dopamine Antagonists

Potential pharmacologic interaction (potentially serious, sometimes fatal serotonin syndrome or NMS-like reactions) if used concurrently with antipsychotic agents or other dopamine antagonists. If signs and symptoms of serotonin syndrome or NMS occur, immediately discontinue treatment with escitalopram and any concurrently administered antidopaminergic or serotonergic agents and initiate supportive and symptomatic treatment. (See Serotonin Syndrome or Neuroleptic Malignant Syndrome-like Reactions under Warnings/Precautions: Other Warnings and Precautions, in Cautions.)

Pimozide

In a controlled study, concurrent administration of a single, 2-mg dose of pimozide in individuals receiving citalopram (40 mg once daily for 11 days) was associated with mean increases in the corrected QT (QT$_c$) interval of approximately 10 msec compared with pimozide given alone. Citalopram did not substantially affect the mean area under the plasma concentration-time curve (AUC) or peak plasma concentrations of pimozide. The mechanism for this potential pharmacodynamic interaction is not known. In addition, concomitant use of citalopram and pimozide rarely may result in potentially serious, sometimes fatal serotonin syndrome or NMS-like reactions. The manufacturers of escitalopram state that concurrent use of escitalopram and pimozide is contraindicated.

● 5-HT$_1$ Receptor Agonists ("Triptans")

Potential pharmacologic interaction (potentially serious, sometimes fatal serotonin syndrome or NMS-like reactions) if used concurrently with 5-HT$_1$ receptor agonists (e.g., almotriptan, eletriptan, frovatriptan, naratriptan, rizatriptan, sumatriptan, zolmitriptan). If concomitant use is clinically warranted, the patient should be observed carefully, particularly during treatment initiation, when dosage is increased, or when another serotonergic agent is initiated. (See Serotonin Syndrome or Neuroleptic Malignant Syndrome-like Reactions under Warnings/Precautions: Other Warnings and Precautions, in Cautions.)

● Monoamine Oxidase Inhibitors

Potential pharmacologic interaction (potentially serious, sometimes fatal serotonin syndrome or NMS-like reactions). Concomitant use of monoamine oxidase (MAO) inhibitors with escitalopram is contraindicated. In addition, at least 2 weeks should elapse between discontinuance of an MAO inhibitor and initiation of escitalopram and vice versa. (See Serotonin Syndrome or Neuroleptic Malignant Syndrome-like Reactions under Warnings/Precautions: Other Warnings and Precautions, in Cautions.)

Isoniazid

Potential pharmacologic interaction (potentially serious serotonin syndrome) when isoniazid, an antituberculosis agent that appears to have some MAO-inhibiting activity, is used concomitantly with escitalopram.

● Linezolid

Linezolid, an anti-infective agent that is also a reversible MAO inhibitor, has been associated with drug interactions resulting in serotonin syndrome, including some associated with SSRIs. Because of this potential risk, linezolid generally should not be used in patients receiving escitalopram. However, the FDA states that certain life-threatening or urgent situations may necessitate immediate linezolid treatment in a patient receiving a serotonergic drug. In such emergency situations, the availability of alternative anti-infectives should be considered and the benefits of linezolid should be weighed against the risk of serotonin syndrome. If linezolid is indicated in such emergency situations, escitalopram must be immediately discontinued and the patient monitored for symptoms of CNS toxicity for 2 weeks or until 24 hours after the last linezolid dose, whichever comes first. Treatment with escitalopram may be resumed 24 hours after the last linezolid dose. If nonemergency use of linezolid is being planned for a patient receiving escitalopram, escitalopram should be withheld for at least 2 weeks prior to initiating linezolid. Treatment with escitalopram should not be initiated in a patient receiving linezolid; when necessary, escitalopram may be started 24 hours after the last linezolid dose. (See Drug Interactions: Serotonergic Drugs, in Linezolid 8:12.28.24.)

● Selective Serotonin-reuptake Inhibitors and Selective Serotonin- and Norepinephrine-reuptake Inhibitors

Potential pharmacologic interaction (potentially serious, sometimes fatal serotonin syndrome or NMS-like reactions); concurrent administration not recommended. (See Serotonin Syndrome or Neuroleptic Malignant Syndrome-like Reactions under Warnings/Precautions: Other Warnings and Precautions, in Cautions.)

● Other Serotonergic Drugs

Potential pharmacologic interaction (potentially serious, sometimes fatal serotonin syndrome or NMS-like reactions) with drugs affecting serotonergic neurotransmission, including tramadol and St. John's wort (Hypericum perforatum); use concomitantly with caution. If signs and symptoms of serotonin syndrome or NMS occur, immediately discontinue treatment with escitalopram and any concurrently administered serotonergic or antidopaminergic agents and initiate supportive and symptomatic treatment. Concurrent administration of escitalopram and serotonin precursors (such as tryptophan) is not recommended. (See Serotonin Syndrome or Neuroleptic Malignant Syndrome-like Reactions under Warnings/Precautions: Other Warnings and Precautions, in Cautions.)

● Alcohol

Concomitant use not recommended.

● Cimetidine

Potential pharmacokinetic interaction (increased AUC and peak plasma concentrations of citalopram have been observed); effects on escitalopram have not been evaluated. Clinical importance of this interaction is unknown.

● *Citalopram*

Potential pharmacologic interaction (potentially serious, sometimes fatal serotonin syndrome or NMS-like reactions).

Because escitalopram is the more active isomer of racemic citalopram, the 2 agents should not be used concomitantly.

● *CNS-active Drugs*

Potential pharmacologic interaction when given with other centrally acting drugs; use concomitantly with caution.

● *Digoxin*

Pharmacokinetic interaction unlikely based on studies with racemic citalopram.

● *Lithium*

Concurrent administration of racemic citalopram and lithium did not substantially affect the pharmacokinetics of either drug. However, pending further accumulation of data, the manufacturers of escitalopram recommend that plasma lithium concentrations be monitored in patients concurrently receiving escitalopram and that lithium dosage be adjusted accordingly.

Potential pharmacologic interaction (enhanced serotonergic effects of escitalopram and potentially serious, sometimes fatal serotonin syndrome or NMS-like reactions); use concomitantly with caution.

● *Ritonavir*

Combined administration of a single 600-mg dose of ritonavir, a CYP3A4 substrate and potent inhibitor of CYP3A4, and escitalopram 20 mg did not substantially affect the pharmacokinetics of either drug.

● *Sibutramine*

Potential pharmacologic interaction (potentially serious, sometimes fatal serotonin syndrome or NMS-like reactions). Use concomitantly with caution.

● *Theophylline*

Pharmacokinetics of theophylline were not affected by racemic citalopram. The effect of theophylline on the pharmacokinetics of racemic citalopram, however, has not been evaluated.

● *Electroconvulsive Therapy*

The combined use of electroconvulsive therapy and escitalopram has not been evaluated.

DESCRIPTION

Escitalopram, a selective serotonin-reuptake inhibitor (SSRI), is a bicyclic phthalane-derivative antidepressant. Escitalopram is the *S*-enantiomer of citalopram, an SSRI that occurs as a 50:50 racemic mixture of the *R*- and *S*-enantiomers. Escitalopram and citalopram differ structurally from other SSRIs (e.g., fluoxetine, fluvoxamine, paroxetine, sertraline) and other currently available antidepressants (e.g., monoamine oxidase inhibitors, tricyclic and tetracyclic antidepressants). Escitalopram is at least 100-fold more potent as an inhibitor of the reuptake of serotonin (5-hydroxytryptamine [5-HT]) at the presynaptic membranes and the 5-HT neuronal firing rate than the *R*-enantiomer and is twice as potent as the racemic mixture. However, further studies are needed to determine whether these differences result in any clinical superiority of escitalopram compared with citalopram.

Like other SSRIs, escitalopram's antidepressant effect is believed to involve potentiation of serotonin activity in the CNS. Escitalopram appears to have little or no effect on reuptake of other neurotransmitters such as norepinephrine and dopamine. In vitro studies also have demonstrated that escitalopram possesses little or no affinity for α- or β-adrenergic, dopamine D_{1-5}, histamine H_{1-3}, GABA-benzodiazepine, muscarinic M_{1-5}, or $5\text{-}HT_{1-7}$ receptors or various ion channels (e.g., calcium, chloride, potassium, sodium channels).

Escitalopram is extensively metabolized, principally by the hepatic cytochrome P-450 (CYP) 2C19 and 3A4 isoenzymes. The principal metabolites are less potent inhibitors of serotonin reuptake, suggesting that the metabolites do not substantially contribute to the antidepressant activity of escitalopram.

ADVICE TO PATIENTS

Importance of providing a copy of written patient information (medication guide) each time escitalopram is dispensed. Importance of advising patients to read the patient information before taking escitalopram and each time the prescription is refilled.

Risk of suicidality; importance of patients, family, and caregivers being alert to and immediately reporting emergence of suicidality, worsening depression, or unusual changes in behavior, especially during the first few months of therapy or during periods of dosage adjustment. (See Worsening of Depression and Suicidality Risk under Warnings/Precautions: Warnings, in Cautions.)

Importance of informing patients of potential risk of serotonin syndrome and neuroleptic malignant syndrome (NMS)-like reactions, particularly with concurrent use of escitalopram and $5\text{-}HT_1$ receptor agonists (also called triptans), tramadol, tryptophan, other serotonergic agents, or antipsychotic agents. Importance of immediately contacting clinician if signs and symptoms of these syndromes develop (e.g., restlessness, hallucinations, loss of coordination, fast heart beat, increased body temperature, muscle stiffness, labile blood pressure, diarrhea, coma, nausea, vomiting, confusion).

Risk of psychomotor impairment; importance of exercising caution while operating hazardous machinery, including driving a motor vehicle, until the drug's effects on the individual are known.

Importance of patients being aware that withdrawal effects may occur when stopping escitalopram, especially with abrupt discontinuance of the drug.

Risks associated with concomitant use of escitalopram with alcohol or racemic citalopram.

Importance of informing clinicians of existing or contemplated concomitant therapy, including prescription and OTC drugs or herbal supplements, as well as any concomitant illnesses (e.g., bipolar disorder) or personal or family history of suicidality or bipolar disorder. Importance of advising patients about the risk of bleeding associated with concomitant use of escitalopram with aspirin or other nonsteroidal anti-inflammatory agents, warfarin, or other drugs that affect coagulation.

Importance of women informing clinicians if they are or plan to become pregnant or plan to breast-feed.

Importance of advising patients that, although they may notice improvement with escitalopram therapy within 1–4 weeks, they should continue therapy as directed.

Importance of informing patients of other important precautionary information. (See Cautions.)

PREPARATIONS

Excipients in commercially available drug preparations may have clinically important effects in some individuals; consult specific product labeling for details.

Escitalopram Oxalate

Oral		
Solution	5 mg (of escitalopram) per 5 mL	Lexapro®, Forest
Tablets, film-coated	5 mg (of escitalopram)*	**Escitalopram Oxalate Tablets**
		Lexapro®, Forest
	10 mg (of escitalopram)*	**Escitalopram Oxalate Tablets**
		Lexapro® (scored), Forest
	20 mg (of escitalopram)*	**Escitalopram Oxalate Tablets**
		Lexapro® (scored), Forest

* available from one or more manufacturer, distributor, and/or repackager by generic (nonproprietary) name

Selected Revisions December 6, 2012, © Copyright, December 1, 2002, American Society of Health-System Pharmacists, Inc.

FLUoxetine Hydrochloride

28:16.04.20 • SELECTIVE SEROTONIN-REUPTAKE INHIBITORS

■ Fluoxetine, a selective serotonin-reuptake inhibitor (SSRI), is an antidepressant.

USES

Fluoxetine is used in the treatment of major depressive disorder, obsessive-compulsive disorder, premenstrual dysphoric disorder, bulimia nervosa, and panic disorder with or without agoraphobia. In addition, fluoxetine has been used for the treatment of depression associated with bipolar disorder†; obesity†; anorexia nervosa†; myoclonus†; cataplexy†; alcohol dependence†; and premature ejaculation†.

● *Major Depressive Disorder*

Fluoxetine is used in the acute and maintenance treatment of major depressive disorder in adults and pediatric patients 8 years of age and older. If fluoxetine is used for extended periods, the need for continued therapy should be reassessed periodically.

A major depressive episode implies a prominent and relatively persistent depressed or dysphoric mood that usually interferes with daily functioning (nearly every day for at least 2 weeks). According to DSM-IV criteria, a major depressive episode includes at least 5 of the following 9 symptoms (with at least one of the symptoms being either depressed mood or loss of interest or pleasure): depressed mood most of the day as indicated by subjective report (e.g., feels sad or empty) or observation made by others; markedly diminished interest or pleasure in all, or almost all, activities most of the day; significant weight loss (when not dieting) or weight gain (e.g., a change of more than 5% of body weight in a month), or decrease or increase in appetite; insomnia or hypersomnia; psychomotor agitation or retardation (observable by others, not merely subjective feelings of restlessness or being slowed down); fatigue or loss of energy; feelings of worthlessness or excessive or inappropriate guilt (not merely self-reproach or guilt about being sick); diminished ability to think or concentrate or indecisiveness (either by subjective account or as observed by others); and recurrent thoughts of death, recurrent suicidal ideation without a specific plan, or a suicide attempt or specific plan for committing suicide.

Treatment of major depressive disorder generally consists of an acute phase (to induce remission), a continuation phase (to preserve remission), and a maintenance phase (to prevent recurrence). Various interventions (e.g., psychotherapy, antidepressant drug therapy, electroconvulsive therapy [ECT]) are used alone or in combination to treat major depressive episodes. Treatment should be individualized and the most appropriate strategy for a particular patient is determined by clinical factors such as severity of depression (e.g., mild, moderate, severe), presence or absence of certain psychiatric features (e.g., suicide risk, catatonia, psychotic or atypical features, alcohol or substance abuse or dependence, panic or other anxiety disorder, cognitive dysfunction, dysthymia, personality disorder, seasonal affective disorder), and concurrent illness (e.g., asthma, cardiac disease, dementia, seizure disorder, glaucoma, hypertension). Demographic and psychosocial factors as well as patient preference also are used to determine the most effective treatment strategy.

While use of psychotherapy alone may be considered as an initial treatment strategy for patients with mild to moderate major depressive disorder (based on patient preference and presence of clinical features such as psychosocial stressors), combined use of antidepressant drug therapy and psychotherapy may be useful for initial treatment of patients with moderate to severe major depressive disorder with psychosocial issues, interpersonal problems, or a comorbid axis II disorder. In addition, combined use of antidepressant drug therapy and psychotherapy may be beneficial in patients who have a history of poor compliance or only partial response to adequate trials of either antidepressant drug therapy or psychotherapy alone.

Antidepressant drug therapy can be used alone for initial treatment of patients with mild major depressive disorder (if preferred by the patient) and usually is indicated alone or in combination with psychotherapy for initial treatment

of patients with moderate to severe major depressive disorder (unless ECT is planned). ECT is not generally used for initial treatment of uncomplicated major depression, but is recommended as first-line treatment for severe major depressive disorder when it is coupled with psychotic features, catatonic stupor, severe suicidality, food refusal leading to nutritional compromise, or other situations when a rapid antidepressant response is required. ECT also is recommended for patients who have previously shown a positive response or a preference for this treatment modality and can be considered for patients with moderate or severe depression who have not responded to or cannot receive antidepressant drug therapy. In certain situations involving depressed patients unresponsive to adequate trials of several individual antidepressant agents, adjunctive therapy with another agent (e.g., buspirone, lithium) or concomitant use of a second antidepressant agent (e.g., bupropion) has been used; however, such combination therapy is associated with an increased risk of adverse reactions, may require dosage adjustments, and (if not contraindicated) should be undertaken only after careful consideration of the relative risks and benefits. (See Drug Interactions: Serotonergic Drugs, see Drug Interactions: Tricyclic and Other Antidepressants, and see Drug Interactions: Lithium.)

Efficacy of fluoxetine for the management of major depression has been established principally in outpatient settings. Most patients evaluated in clinical studies with fluoxetine had major depressive episodes of at least moderate severity, had no evidence of bipolar disorder, and had experienced either single or recurrent episodes of depressive illness. Limited evidence suggests that mildly depressed patients may respond less well to fluoxetine than moderately depressed patients. There also is some evidence that patients with atypical depression (which usually is characterized by atypical signs and symptoms such as hypersomnia and hyperphagia), a history of poor response to prior antidepressant therapy, chronic depressive symptomatology with or without episodic worsening of depressive symptoms, a longer duration of depression in the current episode, and/or a younger age of onset of depression may be more likely to respond to fluoxetine than to tricyclic antidepressant therapy.

As with other antidepressants, the possibility that fluoxetine may precipitate hypomanic or manic attacks in patients with bipolar or other major affective disorder should be considered. Fluoxetine monotherapy is *not* approved for use in treating depressive episodes associated with bipolar disorder. However, fluoxetine is used in combination with olanzapine for the treatment of acute depressive episodes in patients with bipolar disorder. (See Uses: Bipolar Disorder.)

Considerations in Choosing Antidepressants

A variety of antidepressant drugs are available for the treatment of major depressive disorder, including selective serotonin-reuptake inhibitors (SSRIs; e.g., citalopram, escitalopram, fluoxetine, paroxetine, sertraline), selective serotonin- and norepinephrine-reuptake inhibitors (SNRIs; e.g., desvenlafaxine, duloxetine, venlafaxine), tricyclic antidepressants (e.g., amitriptyline, amoxapine, desipramine, doxepin, imipramine, nortriptyline, protriptyline, trimipramine), monoamine oxidase (MAO) inhibitors (e.g., phenelzine, tranylcypromine), and other antidepressants (e.g., bupropion, maprotiline, nefazodone, trazodone, vilazodone). Most clinical studies have shown that the antidepressant effect of usual dosages of fluoxetine in patients with moderate to severe depression is greater than that of placebo and comparable to that of usual dosages of tricyclic antidepressants, maprotiline, other selective serotonin-reuptake inhibitors (e.g., paroxetine, sertraline), and other antidepressants (e.g., trazodone). Fluoxetine appears to be as effective as tricyclic antidepressants in reducing most of the signs and symptoms associated with major depressive disorder, including depression, anxiety, cognitive disturbances, and somatic symptoms. However, in some studies, the drug did not appear to be as effective as tricyclic antidepressants or trazodone in reducing sleep disturbances associated with depression. In geriatric patients with major depressive disorder, fluoxetine appears to be as effective as and to cause fewer overall adverse effects than doxepin. The onset of action of fluoxetine appears to be comparable to that of tricyclic antidepressants, although the onset of action has been variably reported to be somewhat faster or slower than that of tricyclic antidepressants in some studies.

Because response rates in patients with major depression are similar for most currently available antidepressants, the choice of antidepressant agent for a given patient depends principally on other factors such as potential adverse effects, safety or tolerability of these adverse effects in the individual patient, psychiatric and medical history, patient or family history of response to specific therapies, patient preference, quantity and quality of available clinical data, cost, and relative acute overdose safety. No single antidepressant can be recommended as optimal for all patients because of substantial heterogeneity in individual responses and in the nature, likelihood, and severity of adverse effects. In addition, patients vary in the degree to which certain adverse effects and other inconveniences of drug therapy (e.g., cost, dietary restrictions) affect their preferences.

In the large-scale Sequenced Treatment Alternatives to Relieve Depression (STAR*D) effectiveness trial, patients with major depressive disorder who did not respond to or could not tolerate therapy with one SSRI (citalopram) were randomized to switch to extended-release ("sustained-release") bupropion, sertraline, or extended-release venlafaxine as a second step of treatment (level 2). Remission rates as assessed by the 17-item Hamilton Rating Scale for Depression (HRSD-17) and the Quick Inventory of Depressive Symptomatology—Self Report (QIDS-SR-16) were approximately 21 and 26% for extended-release bupropion, 18 and 27% for sertraline, and 25 and 25% for extended-release venlafaxine therapy, respectively; response rates as assessed by the QIDS-SR-16 were 26, 27, and 28% for extended-release bupropion, sertraline, and extended-release venlafaxine therapy, respectively. These results suggest that after unsuccessful initial treatment of depressed patients with an SSRI, approximately 25% of patients will achieve remission after therapy is switched to another antidepressant, and either another SSRI (e.g., sertraline) or an agent from another class (e.g., bupropion, venlafaxine) may be reasonable alternative antidepressants in patients not responding to initial SSRI therapy.

Patient Tolerance Considerations

Because of differences in the adverse effect profile between selective serotonin-reuptake inhibitors and tricyclic antidepressants, particularly less frequent anticholinergic effects, cardiovascular effects, and weight gain with selective serotonin-reuptake inhibitors, these drugs may be preferred in patients in whom such effects are not tolerated or are of potential concern. The decreased incidence of anticholinergic effects associated with fluoxetine and other selective serotonin-reuptake inhibitors compared with tricyclic antidepressants is a potential advantage, since such effects may result in discontinuance of the drug early during therapy in unusually sensitive patients. In addition, some anticholinergic effects may become troublesome during long-term tricyclic antidepressant therapy (e.g., persistent dry mouth may result in tooth decay). Although selective serotonin-reuptake inhibitors share the same overall tolerability profile, certain patients may tolerate one drug in this class better than another. In an open study, most patients who had discontinued fluoxetine therapy because of adverse effects subsequently tolerated sertraline therapy. Antidepressants other than selective serotonin-reuptake inhibitors may be preferred in patients in whom certain adverse GI effects (e.g., nausea, anorexia) or nervous system effects (e.g., anxiety, nervousness, insomnia, weight loss) are not tolerated or are of concern, since such effects appear to occur more frequently with fluoxetine and other drugs in this class.

Pediatric Considerations

The clinical presentation of depression in children and adolescents can differ from that in adults and generally varies with the age and developmental stages of the child. Younger children may exhibit behavioral problems such as social withdrawal, aggressive behavior, apathy, sleep disruption, and weight loss; adolescents may present with somatic complaints, self esteem problems, rebelliousness, poor performance in school, or a pattern of engaging in risky or aggressive behavior.

Data from controlled clinical studies evaluating various antidepressant agents in children and adolescents are less extensive than with adults, and many of these studies have methodologic limitations (e.g., nonrandomized or uncontrolled, small sample size, short duration, nonspecific inclusion criteria). However, there is some evidence that the response to antidepressants in pediatric patients may differ from that seen in adults, and caution should be used in extrapolating data from adult studies when making treatment decisions for pediatric patients. Results of several studies evaluating tricyclic antidepressants (e.g., amitriptyline, desipramine, imipramine, nortriptyline) in preadolescent and adolescent patients with major depression indicate a lack of overall efficacy in this age group.

Based on the lack of efficacy data regarding use of tricyclic antidepressants and MAO inhibitors in pediatric patients and because of the potential for life-threatening adverse effects associated with the use of these drugs, many experts consider selective serotonin-reuptake inhibitors, including fluoxetine, the drugs of choice when antidepressant therapy is indicated for the treatment of major

depressive disorder in children and adolescents. However, the US Food and Drug Administration (FDA) states that, while efficacy of fluoxetine has been established in pediatric patients, efficacy of other newer antidepressants (i.e., citalopram, desvenlafaxine, duloxetine, escitalopram, fluvoxamine, mirtazapine, nefazodone, paroxetine, sertraline, venlafaxine) was not conclusively established in clinical trials in pediatric patients with major depressive disorder. In addition, FDA now warns that antidepressants increase the risk of suicidal thinking and behavior (suicidality) in children and adolescents with major depressive disorder and other psychiatric disorders. (See Cautions: Pediatric Precautions.) FDA currently states that anyone considering using an antidepressant in a child or adolescent for any clinical use must balance the potential risk of therapy with the clinical need. (See Cautions: Precautions and Contraindications.)

Geriatric Considerations

The response to antidepressants in depressed geriatric patients without dementia is similar to that reported in younger adults, but depression in geriatric patients often is not recognized and is not treated. In geriatric patients with major depressive disorder, SSRIs appear to be as effective as tricyclic antidepressants (e.g., amitriptyline) but may cause fewer overall adverse effects than these other agents. Geriatric patients appear to be especially sensitive to anticholinergic (e.g., dry mouth, constipation, vision disturbance), cardiovascular, orthostatic hypotensive, and sedative effects of tricyclic antidepressants. The low incidence of anticholinergic effects associated with fluoxetine and other SSRIs compared with tricyclic antidepressants is a potential advantage in geriatric patients, since such effects (e.g., constipation, dry mouth, confusion, memory impairment) may be particularly troublesome in these patients. However, SSRI therapy may be associated with other troublesome adverse effects (e.g., nausea and vomiting, agitation and akathisia, parkinsonian adverse effects, sexual dysfunction, weight loss, hyponatremia). Some clinicians state that SSRIs including fluoxetine may be preferred for treating depression in geriatric patients in whom the orthostatic hypotension associated with many antidepressants (e.g., tricyclics) potentially may result in injuries (such as severe falls). However, despite the fewer cardiovascular and anticholinergic effects associated with SSRIs, these drugs did not show any advantage over tricyclic antidepressants with regard to hip fracture in a case-control study. In addition, there was little difference in the rates of falls between nursing home residents receiving SSRIs and those receiving tricyclic antidepressants in a retrospective study. Therefore, all geriatric individuals receiving either type of antidepressant should be considered at increased risk of falls and appropriate measures should be taken. In addition, clinicians prescribing SSRIs in geriatric patients should be aware of the many possible drug interactions associated with these drugs, including those involving metabolism of the drugs through the cytochrome P-450 system. (See Drug Interactions.)

Patients with dementia of the Alzheimer's type (Alzheimer's disease, presenile or senile dementia) often present with depressive symptoms, such as depressed mood, appetite loss, insomnia, fatigue, irritability, and agitation. Most experts recommend that patients with dementia of the Alzheimer's type who present with clinically important and persistent depressive symptoms be considered as candidates for pharmacotherapy even if they fail to meet the criteria for a major depressive syndrome. The goals of such therapy are to improve mood, functional status (e.g., cognition), and quality of life. Treatment of depression also may reduce other neuropsychiatric symptoms associated with depression in patients with dementia, including aggression, anxiety, apathy, and psychosis. Although patients may present with depressed mood alone, the possibility of more extensive depressive symptomatology should be considered. Therefore, patients should be evaluated and monitored carefully for indices of major depression, suicidal ideation, and neurovegetative signs since safety measures (e.g., hospitalization for suicidality) and more vigorous and aggressive therapy (e.g., relatively high dosages, multiple drug trials) may be needed in some patients.

Although placebo-controlled trials of antidepressants in depressed patients with concurrent dementia have shown mixed results, the available evidence and experience with the use of antidepressants in patients with dementia of the Alzheimer's type and associated depressive manifestations indicate that depressive symptoms (including depressed mood alone and with neurovegetative changes) in such patients are responsive to antidepressant therapy. In some patients, cognitive deficits may partially or fully resolve during antidepressant therapy, but the extent of response will be limited to the degree of cognitive impairment that is directly related to depression. SSRIs such as fluoxetine, citalopram, escitalopram, paroxetine, or sertraline are generally considered as first-line agents in the treatment of depressed patients with dementia since they are usually better tolerated than some other antidepressants (e.g., tricyclic antidepressants, monoamine oxidase inhibitors). Some possible alternative agents to SSRIs include bupropion, mirtazapine, and venlafaxine. Some geriatric patients with dementia and depression may be unable to tolerate the antidepressant dosages needed to achieve full remission. When a rapid antidepressant response is not critical, some experts therefore recommend a very gradual dosage increase to increase the likelihood that a therapeutic dosage of the SSRI or other antidepressant will be reached and tolerated. In a randomized, double-blind study comparing fluoxetine and amitriptyline in a limited number of patients with major depression complicating Alzheimer's disease, fluoxetine and amitriptyline were found to be equally effective; however, fluoxetine was better tolerated.

Cardiovascular Considerations

The relatively low incidence of adverse cardiovascular effects, including orthostatic hypotension and conduction disturbances, associated with fluoxetine and most other selective serotonin-reuptake inhibitors may be advantageous in patients in whom cardiovascular effects associated with tricyclic antidepressants may be hazardous. However, most clinical studies of fluoxetine for the management of depression did not include individuals with cardiovascular disease (e.g., those with a recent history of myocardial infarction or unstable heart disease), and further experience in such patients is necessary to confirm the reported relative lack of cardiotoxicity with the drug. (See Cautions: Precautions and Contraindications.)

Sedative Considerations

Because fluoxetine and other SSRIs generally are less sedating than some other antidepressants (e.g., tricyclics), some clinicians state that these drugs may be preferable in patients who do not require the sedative effects associated with many antidepressant agents; however, an antidepressant with more prominent sedative effects (e.g., trazodone) may be preferable in some patients (e.g., those with insomnia).

Suicidal Risk Considerations

Suicide is a known risk of depression and certain other psychiatric disorders, and these disorders themselves are the strongest predictors of suicide. However, there has been a long-standing concern that antidepressants may have a role in inducing worsening of depression and the emergence of suicidal thinking and behavior (suicidality) in certain patients during the early phases of treatment. FDA states that antidepressants increased the risk of suicidality in short-term studies in children, adolescents, and young adults (18–24 years of age) with major depressive disorder and other psychiatric disorders. (See Cautions: Pediatric Precautions.) An increased suicidality risk was not demonstrated with antidepressants compared with placebo in adults older than 24 years of age and a reduced risk was observed in adults 65 years of age or older. It currently is unknown whether the suicidality risk extends to longer-term antidepressant use (i.e., beyond several months); however, there is substantial evidence from placebo-controlled maintenance trials in adults with major depressive disorder that antidepressants can delay the recurrence of depression. Because the risk of suicidality in depressed patients may persist until substantial remission of depression occurs, appropriate monitoring and close observation of patients of all ages who are receiving antidepressant therapy are recommended. (See Cautions: Precautions and Contraindications.)

Dosing Interval Considerations

Fluoxetine can be administered once weekly as delayed-release capsules for continuing management of major depressive disorder. Whether the weekly regimen is equivalent to daily therapy with conventional preparations for preventing relapse has not been established. In a double-blind study in adults who responded to daily fluoxetine therapy for major depressive disorder, the relapse rate for continuing therapy with fluoxetine 20-mg conventional capsules administered daily, fluoxetine 90-mg delayed-release capsules administered once weekly, or placebo was 26, 37, or 50%, respectively.

Other Considerations

Fluoxetine has been effective for the treatment of depression in adults with human immunodeficiency virus (HIV) infection. In one randomized, placebo-controlled study, analysis of patients who completed the study showed a statistically significant benefit in patients receiving fluoxetine compared with those receiving placebo.

However, results of intent-to-treat analysis did not show a statistically significant benefit in those receiving the antidepressant, possibly because of a high attrition rate and substantial placebo response. There was no evidence that the degree of immunosuppression affected the response to antidepressant therapy.

Fluoxetine has been effective when used in combination with lithium in a limited number of patients with refractory depression who had not responded to prior therapy (including tricyclic antidepressants and MAO inhibitors administered alone or in combination with lithium), suggesting that lithium may potentiate the antidepressant activity of fluoxetine. (See Drug Interactions: Lithium.) In the Sequenced Treatment Alternatives to Relieve Depression (STAR*D) level 2 trial, patients with major depressive disorder who did not respond to or could not tolerate therapy with citalopram (another SSRI) were randomized to receive either extended-release ("sustained-release") bupropion or buspirone therapy in addition to citalopram. Although both extended-release bupropion and buspirone were found to produce similar remission rates, extended-release bupropion produced a greater reduction in the number and severity of symptoms and a lower rate of drug discontinuance than buspirone in this large-scale, effectiveness trial. These results suggest that augmentation of SSRI therapy with extended-release bupropion may be useful in some patients with refractory depression.

Fluoxetine has been used safely for the management of depression in at least one patient with established susceptibility to malignant hyperthermia, suggesting that the drug may be useful in depressed patients susceptible to malignant hyperthermia and in whom tricyclics and MAO inhibitors are potentially hazardous; however, additional experience is necessary to confirm this preliminary finding.

Because fluoxetine possesses anorectic and weight-reducing properties, some clinicians state that the drug may be preferred in obese patients and/or patients in whom the increase in appetite, carbohydrate craving, and weight gain associated with tricyclic antidepressant therapy may be undesirable (e.g., potentially hazardous to the patient's health; result in possible discontinuance of or noncompliance with therapy). However, the possibility that some patients with concurrent eating disorders or those who may desire to lose weight may misuse fluoxetine for its anorectic and weight-reducing effects should be considered. (See Uses: Eating Disorders and also see Chronic Toxicity.)

● Obsessive-Compulsive Disorder

Fluoxetine is used in the acute and maintenance treatment of obsessive-compulsive disorder in adults and pediatric patients 7 years of age and older when the obsessions or compulsions cause marked distress, are time consuming, or interfere substantially with social or occupational functioning. Obsessions are recurrent and persistent ideas, thoughts, impulses, or images that, at some time during the disturbance, are experienced as intrusive and inappropriate (i.e., "ego dystonic") and that cause marked anxiety or distress but that are not simply excessive worries about real-life problems. Compulsions are repetitive, intentional behaviors (e.g., hand washing, ordering, checking) or mental acts (e.g., praying, counting, repeating words silently) performed in response to an obsession or according to rules that must be applied rigidly (e.g., in a stereotyped fashion). Although the behaviors or acts are aimed at preventing or reducing distress or preventing some dreaded event or situation, they either are not connected in a realistic manner with what they are designed to neutralize or prevent or are clearly excessive. At some time during the course of the disturbance, the patient, if an adult, recognizes that the obsessions or compulsions are excessive or unreasonable; children may not make such a recognition.

The efficacy of fluoxetine for the management of obsessive-compulsive disorder has been established in several multicenter, placebo-controlled studies, including 2 studies of 13 weeks' duration in adults and one study of 13 weeks' duration in children and adolescents 7–17 years of age. Patients in these studies had moderate to severe obsessive-compulsive disorder with average baseline total scores on the Yale-Brown Obsessive-Compulsive Scale (YBOCS) of 22–26 in adults and 25–26 in children and adolescents (measured on the Children's Yale-Brown Obsessive-Compulsive Scale [CY-BOCS]).

In 2 fixed-dose studies of 13 weeks' duration, adults receiving fluoxetine dosages of 20, 40 and 60 mg daily experienced substantially greater reductions in the YBOCS total score than those receiving placebo. Mean reductions in total scores on the YBOCS in fluoxetine-treated patients were approximately 4–6 units in one study and 4–9 units in the other study compared with a 1-unit reduction in patients receiving placebo. In these 2 studies, a positive clinical response (much or very much improved on the Clinical Global Impressions improvement scale) occurred in 36–47 or 11% of patients receiving fluoxetine or placebo, respectively.

While there was no indication of a dose-response relationship for effectiveness in one study, a dose-response relationship was observed in the other study, with numerically better responses in patients receiving 40 or 60 mg of fluoxetine daily compared with those receiving 20 mg of the drug daily. No age- or gender-related differences in outcome were noted in either of these studies.

In another randomized, placebo-controlled study of 13 weeks' duration, children and adolescents 7–17 years of age with obsessive-compulsive disorder who received mean fluoxetine dosages of approximately 25 mg daily (range: 10–60 mg daily) demonstrated substantially greater reductions in the CY-BOCS total score than those receiving placebo. In this study, a positive clinical response (much or very much improved on the Clinical Global Impressions improvement scale) occurred in approximately 55–58 or 9–19% of patients receiving fluoxetine or placebo, respectively. In addition, 49% of patients who received fluoxetine were classified as responders (i.e., patients with a 40% or greater reduction in their CY-BOCS total score from baseline) compared with 25% of those who received placebo. Subgroup analyses on outcome did not suggest any differential responsiveness on the basis of age or gender.

Results from comparative studies to date suggest fluoxetine and other selective serotonin-reuptake inhibitors (SSRIs; e.g., fluvoxamine, paroxetine, sertraline) are as effective or somewhat less effective than clomipramine in the management of obsessive-compulsive disorder. In a pooled analysis of separate short-term (10–13 weeks) studies comparing clomipramine, fluoxetine, fluvoxamine, or sertraline with placebo, clomipramine was calculated as being more effective (as determined by measures on the YBOC scale) than SSRIs, although all drugs were superior to placebo.

Many clinicians consider an SSRI (e.g., fluoxetine, fluvoxamine, paroxetine, sertraline) or clomipramine to be the drugs of choice for the pharmacologic treatment of obsessive-compulsive disorder. The decision whether to initiate therapy with an SSRI or clomipramine often is made based on the adverse effect profile of these drugs. For example, some clinicians prefer clomipramine in patients who may not tolerate the adverse effect profile of SSRIs (e.g., nausea, headache, overstimulation, sleep disturbances) while SSRIs may be useful alternatives in patients unable to tolerate the adverse effects associated with clomipramine therapy (e.g., anticholinergic effects, cardiovascular effects, sedation). Consideration of individual patient characteristics (age, concurrent medical conditions), pharmacokinetics of the drug, potential drug interactions, and cost of therapy may also influence decisions regarding use of SSRIs or clomipramine as first-line therapy in patients with obsessive-compulsive disorder. Although not clearly established, it has been suggested that the mechanism of action of fluoxetine and other drugs (e.g., clomipramine) used in the management of obsessive-compulsive disorder may be related to their serotonergic activity.

Other Disorders with an Obsessive-Compulsive Component

Experience in a limited number of patients suggests that fluoxetine also reduces obsessive-compulsive symptoms associated with Tourette's disorder† (Gilles de la Tourette's syndrome); however, the drug did not appear to be effective in suppressing motor and vocal tics associated with the condition.

Trichotillomania† (an urge to pull out one's hair) has some features in common with those of obsessive-compulsive disorder and some studies have suggested that antiobsessional agents such as SSRIs and clomipramine may be useful in treating this condition. Successful treatment with fluoxetine has been reported in some patients with trichotillomania, including in 2 short-term, open studies in which dosages of up to 80 mg daily were given. However, fluoxetine's efficacy in the management of this disorder was not demonstrated in 2 double-blind, placebo-controlled, crossover studies. In addition, behavioral therapy was found to be more effective than fluoxetine in treating trichotillomania in a short-term, controlled study. Further studies are needed to more clearly determine the role of fluoxetine and other serotonin-reuptake blockers in the management of this condition.

● *Premenstrual Dysphoric Disorder*

Fluoxetine is used in the treatment of premenstrual dysphoric disorder (previously late luteal phase dysphoric disorder). DSM-IV criteria for premenstrual dysphoric disorder (PMDD) require that in most menstrual cycles of the previous year at least 5 of the following 11 symptoms must have been present for most of the time during the last week of the luteal phase (with at least one of the symptoms being the first 4 listed): marked depressed mood, feelings of hopelessness, or self-deprecating thoughts; marked anxiety, tension, feelings of being "keyed up" or on "edge"; marked affective lability (e.g., feeling suddenly sad or tearful or increased sensitivity to rejection); persistent and marked anger or irritability or increased interpersonal conflicts; decreased interest in usual activities (e.g., work, school, friends, hobbies); a subjective sense of difficulty in concentrating;

lethargy, easy fatigability, or marked lack of energy; marked change in appetite, overeating, or specific food cravings; hypersomnia or insomnia; a subjective sense of being overwhelmed or out of control; and other physical symptoms, such as breast tenderness or swelling, headaches, joint or muscle pain, or a sensation of "bloating" or weight gain. Such symptoms should begin to remit within a few days of the onset of menses (follicular phase) and are always absent in the week following menses. The presence of this cyclical pattern of symptoms must be confirmed by at least 2 consecutive months of prospective daily symptom ratings. PMDD should be distinguished from the more common premenstrual syndrome (PMS) by prospective daily ratings and the strict criteria listed above.

There is some evidence that serotonergic agents (e.g., fluoxetine, paroxetine) have greater efficacy compared with non-serotonergic agents (e.g., bupropion, maprotiline) in relieving the physical and/or emotional symptoms of PMDD. In published studies, the response rates to fluoxetine therapy in women with PMDD appear to be similar to those described in patients with depression, panic disorder, and obsessive-compulsive disorder. However, unlike the onset of action of fluoxetine in other psychiatric conditions (6–8 weeks), some clinicians have observed a rapid onset of response to fluoxetine (approximately 2–4 weeks) in women with PMDD, suggesting that the mechanism of action of these agents in PMDD is not mediated by the drug's antidepressant or anti-obsessive effects. In addition, use of fluoxetine in the treatment of PMDD does not appear to produce the sustained remission typically seen in the treatment of major depressive disorder. PMDD symptoms recur soon after discontinuance of fluoxetine therapy (e.g., within 2 menstrual cycles), even in women who have received the drug for more than 1 year. It has been suggested that a past history of major depression may be associated with a partial or absent response to lower dosages of fluoxetine therapy. Because patients on oral contraceptives were excluded from most clinical studies to date, efficacy of fluoxetine used in conjunction with oral contraceptives for the treatment of PMDD has not been determined.

The efficacy of fluoxetine for the management of PMDD has been established in 3 randomized, placebo-controlled (1 intermittent- and 2 continuous-dosing) studies of 3 or 6 months' duration in adult women who met DSM-III-R or DSM-IV criteria for PMDD. One study involved over 300 women (20–40 years of age) who were randomized to receive either fluoxetine (at fixed dosages of 20 or 60 mg daily) or placebo continuously throughout the full menstrual cycle, beginning on the first day of their cycle. In this study, fixed doses of fluoxetine were shown to be substantially more effective than placebo in decreasing the mean total of 3 visual analog scale scores (tension, irritability, dysphoria); total scores decreased by 36–39% on 20 or 60 mg of fluoxetine and 7% on placebo. However, marked (greater than 50% reduction from baseline) improvement in total luteal phase visual analog scale scores occurred only in 18% of patients receiving 60 mg of fluoxetine and in 6 or 4% of those receiving 20 mg of fluoxetine or placebo, respectively. Fluoxetine therapy appeared to be well tolerated in patients receiving dosages of 20 mg daily, but approximately 33% of women receiving 60 mg daily discontinued the drug because of adverse reactions and 86% of those receiving this dosage who remained in the study reported one or more adverse effects attributable to the drug.

In a second double-blind, placebo-controlled, crossover study, women with PMDD who received flexible doses of fluoxetine (20–60 mg daily; mean dosage of 27 mg daily) throughout the menstrual cycle for a total of 3 cycles had an average visual analog scale total score (follicular to luteal phase increase) that was 3.8 times lower than that of patients receiving placebo. However, results of another double-blind, parallel study indicated that the response rate in women receiving fluoxetine 20 mg daily or bupropion 300 mg daily continuously for 2 cycles was not substantially superior to placebo on the Clinical Global Impressions scale.

The efficacy of intermittent dosing (defined as initiation of daily dosage 14 days prior to the anticipated onset of menstruation and continuing through the first full day of menses) was established in a double-blind, parallel group study of 3 months' duration. In this study, women receiving intermittent dosing of 20 mg daily dosages of fluoxetine had substantially greater improvements on the Daily Record of Severity of Problems, a patient-rated instrument that mirrors the diagnostic criteria for PMDD as identified in the DSM-IV, than those receiving placebo. Further studies are needed to evaluate the comparative efficacy of continuous and intermittent dosing regimens.

● *Eating Disorders*

Fluoxetine is used in the acute and maintenance treatment of bulimia nervosa in adults; the drug also has been used in a limited number of patients with other eating disorders (e.g., anorexia nervosa).

Although DSM-IV criteria provide guidelines for establishing a diagnosis of a specific eating disorder, the symptoms frequently occur along a continuum between those of anorexia nervosa and bulimia nervosa. The primary features in both anorexia nervosa and bulimia nervosa are weight preoccupation and excessive self-evaluation (i.e., disturbed perception) of body weight and shape, and many patients exhibit a mixture of both anorexic and bulimic behaviors.

The American Psychiatric Association (APA) states that psychiatric management forms the foundation of treatment for patients with eating disorders and should be instituted for all patients in combination with other specific treatment modalities (e.g., nutritional rehabilitation and pharmacotherapy). Because patients with eating disorders often exhibit comorbid conditions and/or associated psychiatric features that may compromise clinical outcome, treatment programs should identify and address all comorbid conditions before initiating therapy. Clinicians should recognize that patients with concurrent diabetes mellitus often underdose their insulin in order to lose weight, and that pregnant patients with disturbed eating behaviors (e.g., inadequate nutritional intake, binge eating, purging, abuse of teratogenic medications) may be at high risk for fetal or maternal complications. Results from several studies indicate that patients with associated psychiatric features such as substance abuse/dependence or personality disorder may require longer-term therapy than those without these comorbid conditions. Although the presence of depression at initial presentation has no predictive value for treatment outcome, many clinicians suggest that severe depression can impair the patient's involvement in and/or response to psychotherapy, and such patients should receive initial pharmacologic therapy to improve mood symptoms.

Bulimia Nervosa

Fluoxetine is used in the acute and maintenance treatment of binge-eating and self-induced vomiting behaviors in patients with moderate to severe bulimia nervosa (e.g., at least 3 bulimic episodes per week for 6 months).

According to DSM-IV, bulimia nervosa is characterized by recurrent episodes of binge eating and recurrent inappropriate compensatory behaviors to prevent weight gain (e.g., self-induced vomiting; misuse of laxatives, diuretics, enemas, or other medications; fasting; excessive exercise) and binge eating and compensatory behaviors both occur at least twice a week for 3 months.

Treatment strategies for bulimia nervosa include psychosocial interventions, nutritional counseling and rehabilitation, and pharmacotherapy. The primary goals in treating bulimia nervosa are to reduce binge eating and purging. Although antidepressants initially were used only in bulimic patients who were clinically depressed, evidence from recent studies indicates that nondepressed patients also respond to these agents, and that the presence of depression is not predictive of therapeutic response. Therefore, antidepressants are included as one component of initial treatment regimens for patients with bulimia nervosa. Because selective serotonin-reuptake inhibitors have a more favorable adverse effects profile, these drugs usually are preferred and may be especially useful for patients with symptoms of depression, anxiety, obsessions, or certain impulse disorder symptoms or for those who previously failed to achieve optimal response to psychosocial therapy. Other antidepressants also may be used to reduce the symptoms of binge eating and purging and help prevent relapse. However, the APA cautions against the use of tricyclic antidepressants in patients who are suicidal and cautions against use of MAO inhibitors in those with chaotic binge eating and purging.

The APA states that in patients who fail to respond to initial antidepressant therapy, it may be necessary to assess whether the patient has taken the drug shortly before vomiting or to determine whether effective drug concentrations have been achieved. Although only limited data are available regarding use of antidepressants for maintenance therapy, there appears to be a high rate of relapse during the treatment phase and an even higher rate following discontinuance of therapy. However, limited data indicate that the rate of relapse appears to correlate with the time at which drug therapy is initiated. In one small, open-label study, patients who received drug treatment within 13 weeks of diagnosis were more likely to exhibit sustained recovery during the first year than those who did not receive pharmacotherapy. Furthermore, continuing cognitive behavior therapy following discontinuance of drug therapy appears to prevent relapse in patients with bulimia nervosa. Additional study is needed to determine the effects of sequential use of psychotherapy and pharmacotherapy in the treatment of bulimia nervosa.

The efficacy of fluoxetine for the management of bulimia nervosa has been established in several multicenter, placebo-controlled studies, including 2 studies of 8 weeks' duration (using fluoxetine dosages of 20 or 60 mg daily) and one study of 16 weeks' duration (using fluoxetine dosages of 60 mg once daily) in patients with moderate to severe bulimia nervosa with median binge eating and self-induced vomiting of 7–10 and 5–9 times a week, respectively. In these studies, fluoxetine given in dosages of 60 mg daily (but not in dosages of 20 mg daily) was substantially more effective than placebo in reducing the number of binge-eating and self-induced vomiting episodes weekly. The superiority of fluoxetine compared with placebo was evident as early as within 1 week of therapy and persisted throughout each study period. The drug-related reduction in bulimic episodes appeared to be independent of baseline depression as assessed by the Hamilton Depression Rating Scale. The beneficial effect of fluoxetine therapy (compared with placebo), as measured by median reductions in the frequency of bulimic behaviors at the end of therapy compared with baseline, ranged from 1–2 and 2–4 episodes per week for binge eating and self-induced vomiting, respectively. The magnitude of clinical effect was related to baseline frequency of bulimic behaviors since greater reductions in such behaviors were observed in patients with higher baseline frequencies. Although binge eating and purging resolved completely in some patients who received fluoxetine therapy, the majority of fluoxetine-treated patients only experienced a partial reduction in the frequency of bulimic behaviors.

In an uncontrolled study in patients with bulimia nervosa, fluoxetine substantially reduced the frequency of binge eating and self-induced vomiting but did not affect bodily dissatisfaction in patients receiving 60–80 mg of the drug for 4 weeks; in several patients, therapeutic effects of the drug appeared to be maintained during chronic therapy. In another uncontrolled study, fluoxetine reduced the frequency of binge eating and self-induced vomiting in several patients with bulimia nervosa who were unresponsive to previous therapy with imipramine. The drug also reportedly improved bulimic symptoms, expanded food preferences, and resulted in weight gain in one underweight patient with anorexia nervosa and bulimia who was unresponsive to or unable to tolerate previous therapy for her eating disorder (including tricyclic antidepressants, monoamine oxidase inhibitors, bupropion, nomifensine, or lithium). In addition, fluoxetine used in combination with lithium was effective in improving bulimic symptoms in a patient with major depression and bulimia who was unresponsive to prior therapy.

The efficacy of fluoxetine for long-term use in the treatment of bulimia nervosa has been established in a placebo-controlled study of up to 52 weeks' duration in patients who responded to an initial single-blind, 8-week acute treatment phase with fluoxetine 60 mg daily for bulimia nervosa. In this study, fluoxetine decreased the likelihood of relapse and improved the clinical outcome. However, symptoms of bulimia gradually worsened over time in patients in both the fluoxetine and placebo groups in this study, suggesting that fluoxetine alone may not be an adequate maintenance treatment after acute response in some patients with bulimia nervosa. Additional management strategies, such as psychotherapy, may be required to augment or to sustain initial improvement in this condition.

Pending further accumulation of data, most clinicians recommend that antidepressant therapy, including fluoxetine, be continued for at least 6–12 months in patients with bulimia nervosa before attempting to discontinue therapy. If fluoxetine is used for extended periods, the need for continued therapy with the drug should be reassessed periodically.

Anorexia Nervosa

Fluoxetine has been used in a limited number of patients with anorexia nervosa†. According to DSM-IV, anorexia nervosa is characterized by refusal to maintain body weight at or above a minimally normal weight for age and height (e.g., weight loss leading to maintenance of body weight less than 85% of that expected or failure to make expected weight gain during periods of growth, leading to body weight less than 85% of that expected); intense fear of gaining weight or becoming fat (even though underweight); disturbance in the perception of body weight and shape, undue influence of body weight or shape on self-evaluation, or denial of the seriousness of the current low body weight; and amenorrhea in postmenarchal females (i.e., absence of at least 3 consecutive menstrual cycles). Patients with anorexia nervosa often exhibit depressive (e.g., depressed mood, social withdrawal, irritability, insomnia, and diminished interest in sex) and obsessive-compulsive symptoms that may be associated with or exacerbated by undernutrition.

The APA recommends that a program of nutritional rehabilitation, including vitamin (e.g., potassium and phosphorus) supplementation, be established for all patients who are significantly underweight. The APA states that pharmacologic measures (e.g., antidepressants) may be considered in patients with anorexia nervosa to maintain weight and normal eating behaviors; to treat psychiatric symptoms associated with the disorder (e.g., depression, anxiety, or obsessive-compulsive symptoms); and to prevent relapse. However, such therapy should not be used as the sole or primary treatment for anorexia nervosa. Because associated psychiatric symptoms of anorexia nervosa (e.g., depression) often improve with weight gain, the APA states that the decision to initiate antidepressant therapy should be deferred until weight gain has been restored, and that the choice of an antidepressant agent depends on the remaining symptoms. According to the APA, selective serotonin-reuptake inhibitors commonly are considered in patients with anorexia nervosa whose depressive, obsessive, or compulsive symptoms persist in spite of or in the absence of weight gain.

Although there are few well-controlled, clinical studies of antidepressants for the treatment of anorexia nervosa, data from one study indicate that weight-restored patients with anorexia nervosa who received fluoxetine (40 mg daily) after hospital discharge had less weight loss, depression, and fewer rehospitalizations for anorexia nervosa during the subsequent year than those who received placebo. However, it should be noted that fluoxetine has been misused for its anorectic and weight-reducing effects in a patient with a history of chronic depression, anorexia nervosa, and laxative abuse who was receiving the drug for the treatment of depression; therefore, the misuse potential of fluoxetine in depressed patients with concurrent eating disorders or in other patients who may desire to lose weight should be considered. (See Chronic Toxicity.)

● Panic Disorder

Fluoxetine is used in the acute treatment of panic disorder with or without agoraphobia in adults. Panic disorder is characterized by the occurrence of unexpected panic attacks and associated concern about having additional attacks, worry about the implications or consequences of the attacks, and/or a clinically important change in behavior related to the attacks.

According to DSM-IV, panic disorder is characterized by recurrent unexpected panic attacks, which consist of a discrete period of intense fear or discomfort in which 4 (or more) of the following symptoms develop abruptly and reach a peak within 10 minutes: palpitations, pounding heart, or accelerated heart rate; sweating; trembling or shaking; sensations of shortness of breath or smothering; feeling of choking; chest pain or discomfort; nausea or abdominal distress; feeling dizzy, unsteady, lightheaded, or faint; derealization (feelings of unreality) or depersonalization (being detached from oneself); fear of losing control; fear of dying; paresthesias (numbness or tingling sensations); and chills or hot flushes.

The efficacy of fluoxetine for the management of panic disorder with or without agoraphobia has been established by 2 randomized, double-blind, placebo-controlled studies in adult outpatients who met DSM-IV criteria for panic disorder with or without agoraphobia. These studies were of 12 weeks' duration and used a flexible dosing schedule. Fluoxetine therapy in both studies was initiated in a dosage of 10 mg daily for the first week and then the dosage was escalated to 20–60 mg daily depending on clinical response and tolerability. In these studies, 42–62% of patients receiving fluoxetine were free from panic attacks at week 12 compared with 28–44% of those receiving placebo. The mean fluoxetine dosage in one of these studies was approximately 30 mg daily.

The optimum duration of fluoxetine therapy required to prevent recurrence of panic disorder has not been established to date. The manufacturer states that the efficacy of fluoxetine for long-term use (i.e., longer than 12 weeks) has not been demonstrated in controlled studies. However, in a 10-week, placebo-controlled, fixed-dose study, patients responding to fluoxetine 10 or 20 mg daily were randomized to receive continued therapy with their previous fluoxetine dosage or placebo during a 6-month continuation phase. The patients who received an additional 6 months of fluoxetine therapy in this study demonstrated continued clinical improvement.. The manufacturer and some clinicians state that panic disorder is a chronic condition and requires several months or longer of sustained therapy. Therefore, it is reasonable to continue therapy in responding patients. The manufacturer recommends, however, that patients be reassessed periodically to determine the need for continued therapy.

Panic disorder can be treated with cognitive and behavioral psychotherapy and/or pharmacologic therapy. There are several classes of drugs that appear to be effective in the pharmacologic management of panic disorder, including tricyclic antidepressants (e.g., imipramine, clomipramine), monoamine oxidase (MAO) inhibitors (e.g., phenelzine), selective serotonin-reuptake inhibitors (SSRIs), and benzodiazepines (e.g., alprazolam, clonazepam). When choosing among the available drugs, clinicians should consider their acceptance and tolerability by patients; their ability to reduce or eliminate panic attacks, reduce clinically important anxiety and disability secondary to phobic avoidance, and ameliorate other common comorbid conditions (such as depression); and their ability to prevent relapse during long-term

therapy. Because of their better tolerability when compared with other agents (such as the tricyclic antidepressants and benzodiazepines), the lack of physical dependence problems commonly associated with benzodiazepines, and efficacy in panic disorder with comorbid conditions (e.g., depression, other anxiety disorders such as obsessive-compulsive disorder, alcoholism), many clinicians prefer SSRIs as first-line therapy in the management of panic disorder. If SSRI therapy is ineffective or is not tolerated, use of a tricyclic antidepressant or a benzodiazepine is recommended.

● Bipolar Disorder

Fluoxetine monotherapy has been used for the short-term treatment of acute depressive episodes† in a limited number of patients with bipolar depression† (bipolar disorder, depressed). In one poorly controlled study, fluoxetine was more effective than imipramine, and each drug was more effective than placebo in the management of depression in patients with bipolar disorder; fluoxetine appeared to be particularly effective in reducing anxiety and somatic symptoms in these patients. However, because the drug has been reported to cause manic reactions in some patients, the possibility that hypomanic or manic attacks may be precipitated in patients with bipolar disorder must be considered. In addition, some experts have reported an association between use of antidepressants and the development of rapid cycling and mixed affective states in patients with bipolar disorder, suggesting that such use may worsen the overall course of bipolar disorder in these patients. Consequently, the American Psychiatric Association (APA) does not recommend use of antidepressant monotherapy in patients with bipolar disorder. Initiation or optimization of dosages of maintenance agents (i.e., lithium, lamotrigine) are considered first-line therapies for the management of acute episodes of depression in patients with bipolar disorder. While the addition of either lamotrigine, bupropion, or paroxetine currently is recommended as the next step for patients who fail to respond to optimum dosages of maintenance agents, the APA states that other SSRIs (e.g., fluoxetine) can be used as an alternative to these agents. For further information on the management of bipolar disorder, see Uses: Bipolar Disorder, in Lithium Salts 28:28.

Fluoxetine also is used in combination with olanzapine for the treatment of acute depressive episodes in patients with bipolar I disorder. In 2 randomized, double-blind studies of 8 weeks' duration comparing a fixed combination of fluoxetine and olanzapine with olanzapine monotherapy and placebo, the fixed combination (flexible daily dosages of 6 mg olanzapine and 25 or 50 mg of fluoxetine or of 12 mg of olanzapine and 50 mg of fluoxetine) was more effective than olanzapine monotherapy (5–20 mg daily) or placebo in improvement in depressive symptoms as assessed by the Montgomery-Asberg Depression Rating Scale (MADRS). Although the manufacturer states that efficacy beyond 8 weeks' duration remains to be established, patients have received the fixed combination for up to 24 weeks in clinical trials. Clinicians who elect to extend therapy beyond 8 weeks should reevaluate the risks and benefits of continued therapy periodically.

● Obesity

Fluoxetine has been used in a limited number of patients for the short-term management of exogenous obesity†. In a controlled study, obese (i.e., more than 20% overweight), nondepressed individuals receiving fluoxetine (average dosage: 64.9 mg daily), benzphetamine hydrochloride (average dosage: 97 mg daily), or placebo concurrently with reduced food intake and increased exercise for 8 weeks lost an average of about 4.8, 4, and 1.7 kg, respectively. Fluoxetine-treated patients who usually experienced carbohydrate cravings reportedly lost more weight during this study than those who did not experience such cravings. (See Pharmacology: Effects on Appetite and Body Weight.)

In a study evaluating the safety of fluoxetine therapy in the management of exogenous obesity, the drug was generally well tolerated. The adverse effect profile of the drug in nondepressed obese patients appeared to differ somewhat from that in depressed patients receiving similar dosages of the drug; obese patients reportedly had a higher incidence of fatigue and a lower incidence of nausea, anxiety, and tremor. Unlike amphetamines, the potential for addiction to or abuse of fluoxetine appears to be minimal (see Chronic Toxicity), and tolerance to the drug's anorectic and weight-reducing effects has not been reported to date following short-term administration. However, long-term studies are necessary to fully determine whether tolerance develops during chronic fluoxetine therapy and to fully establish the relative efficacy and safety of fluoxetine in the management of exogenous obesity.

● Cataplexy

Fluoxetine has been used for the symptomatic management of cataplexy† in a limited number of patients with cataplexy and associated narcolepsy. In one study, the drug appeared to be as effective as clomipramine in reducing the number of cataplexy attacks in patients concurrently receiving CNS stimulants (e.g., dextro-amphetamine) for the symptomatic management of associated narcolepsy.

● Alcohol Dependence

Like some other selective serotonin-reuptake inhibitors (SSRIs; e.g., citalopram, zimeldine [not commercially available in the US]), fluoxetine has been used in the management of alcohol dependence†. However, studies of SSRIs have generally shown modest effects on alcohol consumption. In a limited number of early-stage problem drinkers (who drank an average of about 8 drinks daily prior to therapy), alcohol consumption was reduced by an average of 17% in patients receiving 60 mg of fluoxetine daily; however, response showed considerable interindividual variability, and alcohol consumption was not altered substantially in problem drinkers receiving 40 mg of the drug daily. It has been suggested that the clinical effects of SSRIs in the management of alcohol dependence may only be transient. In patients with mild to moderate alcohol dependence, alcohol consumption is substantially decreased for only the first 1–4 weeks of fluoxetine therapy or first 12 weeks of citalopram therapy. Additional study is required to fully determine the safety and efficacy of fluoxetine in the management of alcohol dependence. (See Pharmacology: Effects on Alcohol Intake and also see Drug Interactions: Alcohol.)

● Myoclonus

Fluoxetine has been used for the management of intention myoclonus†, including postanoxic action myoclonus† and progressive action myoclonus†, in a limited number of patients. Although fluoxetine alone was not effective in improving myoclonus, speech abnormalities, gait abnormalities, or overall performance on neurological examination in such patients, the drug did appear to potentiate the therapeutic effects of combined oxitriptan (l-5-hydroxytryptophan, l-5HTP) and carbidopa therapy in some patients. In addition, fluoxetine reportedly reduced the dosage requirement of oxitriptan and the incidence of adverse GI effects (e.g., diarrhea, abdominal cramps) associated with such therapy. Fluoxetine used in combination with oxitriptan also has exhibited antimyoclonic activity in animals. (See Pharmacology: Other Effects.) However, because toxic effects have been reported in some patients concurrently receiving fluoxetine and tryptophan, a serotonergic agent that is structurally similar to oxitriptan (see Tryptophan and Other Serotonin Precursors under Drug Interactions: Serotonergic Drugs), further study and experience are needed to fully determine the safety and efficacy of combined therapy with fluoxetine and oxitriptan-carbidopa in the management of intention myoclonus.

● Premature Ejaculation

Like some other SSRIs, fluoxetine has been used with some success in the treatment of premature ejaculation†. In a placebo-controlled study, fluoxetine produced substantial improvements compared with placebo in time to ejaculation and was well tolerated in most patients. However, in a comparative study, patients receiving either clomipramine or sertraline reported a greater increase in mean intravaginal ejaculation latency time and a greater patient sexual satisfaction rating than those receiving either fluoxetine or placebo. Although the mechanism of action of SSRIs in delaying ejaculation is unclear, it has been suggested that these drugs may be particularly useful in patients who fail or refuse behavioral or psychotherapeutic treatment or when partners are unwilling to cooperate with such therapy.

DOSAGE AND ADMINISTRATION

● Administration

Fluoxetine hydrochloride is administered orally without regard to meals.

Fluoxetine hydrochloride conventional capsules, tablets, and solution are administered once or twice daily; the delayed-release capsules are administered once weekly. For the initial management of depression, obsessive-compulsive disorder, premenstrual dysphoric disorder, or bulimia nervosa, the drug generally is administered once daily in the morning. If the dosage exceeds 20 mg daily, the manufacturer and some clinicians state that fluoxetine should be administered in 2 divided doses daily (preferably in the morning and at noon). However, limited evidence suggests that no clinically important differences in either the efficacy or incidence of adverse effects exist with once-daily (in the morning) versus twice-daily (in the morning and at noon) administration of the drug. If sedation occurs during fluoxetine therapy, administering the second dose at bedtime rather than at noon may be useful. Because fluoxetine and its principal active metabolite have relatively long half-lives, the drug has been administered less frequently than once daily (e.g., every 2–7 days), particularly during maintenance therapy. Fluoxetine delayed-release capsules are administered once weekly as maintenance therapy in the management of major depressive disorder in patients who have responded to daily administration of the drug. Some clinicians have suggested that conventional fluoxetine preparations administered less frequently than once daily (i.e., three 20-mg capsules once weekly) may also be effective as maintenance therapy in the management of major depressive disorder, but such dosing regimens should be considered investigational at this time and require additional study to confirm their safety and efficacy.

Because of the prolonged elimination of fluoxetine and its active metabolite from the body, missing a dose of the drug once steady-state concentrations have been achieved is unlikely to result in substantial alterations in plasma fluoxetine or norfluoxetine concentrations.

● Dosage

Dosage of fluoxetine hydrochloride is expressed in terms of fluoxetine.

In titrating dosage of or discontinuing fluoxetine therapy, the prolonged elimination half-life of fluoxetine and norfluoxetine should be considered. Several weeks will be required before the full effect of such alterations is realized.

The manufacturers and some clinicians recommend that an interval of at least 5 weeks elapse between discontinuance of fluoxetine therapy and initiation of monoamine oxidase (MAO) inhibitor therapy, and that at least 2 weeks elapse following discontinuance of an MAO inhibitor prior to initiation of fluoxetine therapy. For additional information on potentially serious drug interactions that may occur between fluoxetine and MAO inhibitors or other serotonergic agents, see Cautions: Precautions and Contraindications and also see Drug Interactions: Serotonergic Drugs.

Because withdrawal effects may occur with discontinuance of fluoxetine, other selective serotonin-reuptake inhibitors (SSRIs), and selective serotonin- and norepinephrine-reuptake inhibitors (SNRIs), abrupt discontinuance of these drugs should be avoided whenever possible. When fluoxetine therapy is discontinued, the dosage should be reduced gradually (e.g., over a period of several weeks) and the patient monitored for possible withdrawal symptoms. If intolerable symptoms occur following a dosage reduction or upon discontinuance of therapy, the drug may be reinstituted at the previously prescribed dosage. Subsequently, the clinician may continue decreasing the dosage, but at a more gradual rate. Plasma concentrations of fluoxetine and norfluoxetine (the principal metabolite) decline gradually after cessation of therapy, which may minimize the risk of withdrawal symptoms. (See Withdrawal Reactions under Cautions: Nervous System Effects and also see Chronic Toxicity.)

Patients receiving fluoxetine should be monitored for possible worsening of depression, suicidality, or unusual changes in behavior, especially at the beginning of therapy or during periods of dosage adjustment. (See Cautions: Precautions and Contraindications.)

Major Depressive Disorder

Adult Dosage

For the management of major depression, the recommended initial dosage of fluoxetine in adults is 20 mg daily administered in the morning. However, some clinicians suggest that fluoxetine therapy be initiated with lower dosages (e.g., 5 mg daily or 20 mg every 2 or 3 days). Although symptomatic relief may be apparent within the first 1–3 weeks of fluoxetine therapy, optimum antidepressant effect usually requires at least 4 weeks or more of therapy with the drug. If insufficient clinical improvement is apparent after several weeks of fluoxetine therapy at 20 mg daily, an increase in dosage may be considered. Efficacy of fluoxetine for major depression was demonstrated in clinical trials employing 10–80 mg daily. Studies comparing fluoxetine 20, 40, and 60 mg daily to placebo indicate that a dosage of 20 mg daily is sufficient to obtain a satisfactory response in most adults with major depression. Fluoxetine dosages up to 80 mg daily have been administered in some patients, and dosages as low as 5 mg daily may be effective in some patients with depression. In addition, in a study in moderately depressed patients, increasing the dosage of fluoxetine from 20 mg to 40 or 60 mg daily did not result in substantial improvement in depression but was associated with an increase in certain adverse effects (e.g., nausea, anxiety, diarrhea, dry mouth, weight loss). The manufacturer states that the maximum dosage of fluoxetine in adults with major depression should not exceed 80 mg daily; however, somewhat higher dosages (e.g., 100–120 mg daily) occasionally have been used in patients who did not respond adequately to lower dosages.

When fluoxetine hydrochloride delayed-release capsules are used for the continuing management of major depressive disorder, the recommended dosage of fluoxetine is 90 mg once weekly beginning 7 days after the last dose of fluoxetine 20 mg daily. If a satisfactory response is not maintained with once weekly administration, consideration may be given to reestablishing a daily dosage schedule.

As with the use of fluoxetine for other indications, lower dosages or less frequent dosing regimens should be considered for geriatric patients, patients with concurrent disease, and patients receiving multiple concomitant drug therapies.

Pediatric Dosage

For the management of major depressive disorder in children and adolescents 8–18 years of age, the recommended initial dosage of fluoxetine is 10 or 20 mg daily. If therapy is initiated at 10 mg daily, it should be increased after 1 week to 20 mg daily. Because higher plasma fluoxetine concentrations occur in lower weight children, the manufacturer states that both the initial and target dosage in lower weight children may be 10 mg daily. An increase in dosage to 20 mg daily may be considered after several weeks in lower weight children if insufficient clinical improvement is observed. Because a rare but serious drug interaction may occur in depressed children and adolescents with comorbid attention-deficit hyperactivity disorder (ADHD) who receive stimulants and selective serotonin-reuptake inhibitors concomitantly, some experts recommend a maximum fluoxetine dosage of 20 mg daily in such patients. (See Tramadol and Other Serotonergic Drugs under Drug Interactions: Serotonergic Drugs.)

Duration of Therapy

The optimum duration of fluoxetine therapy required to prevent recurrence of depressive symptoms has not been established to date. However, many experts state that acute depressive episodes require several months or longer of sustained antidepressant therapy. Systematic evaluation of fluoxetine has shown that its antidepressant efficacy is maintained for periods of up to approximately 9 months following 3 months of open-label acute treatment (12 months total) in adults receiving 20 mg daily as conventional fluoxetine capsules or for periods of up to approximately 6 months with once-weekly dosing of the 90 mg delayed-release fluoxetine capsules following 3 months of open-label treatment with 20 mg once daily as conventional fluoxetine capsules. However, the therapeutic equivalence of once-weekly administration of the 90-mg delayed-release capsules with that of once-daily administration of the 20-mg conventional preparations for delaying time to relapse has not been established. In addition, it has not been determined to date whether the dosage of the antidepressant necessary to treat acute symptoms of depression is the same as the dosage necessary to prevent recurrence of such symptoms. If therapy with the drug is prolonged, the need for continued therapy should be reassessed periodically.

Switching To or From Other Antidepressants

Because concurrent use of fluoxetine and a tricyclic antidepressant may result in greater than two- to 10-fold elevations in plasma tricyclic antidepressant concentrations, dosage of the tricyclic antidepressant may need to be reduced and plasma tricyclic concentrations may need to be monitored temporarily when fluoxetine is administered concurrently or has been recently discontinued. (See Drug Interactions: Tricyclic and Other Antidepressants.)

Because of the potential risk of serotonin syndrome, the manufacturer recommends that an interval of at least 2 weeks elapse when switching a patient from a monoamine oxidase (MAO) inhibitor to fluoxetine. Because both fluoxetine and its principal metabolite have relatively long half-lives, the manufacturers and some clinicians recommend that at least 5 weeks elapse between discontinuance of fluoxetine therapy and initiation of MAO inhibitor therapy. (See Drug Interactions: Serotonergic Drugs.)

Obsessive-Compulsive Disorder
Adult Dosage

For the management of obsessive-compulsive disorder, the recommended initial dosage of fluoxetine in adults is 20 mg daily administered in the morning. Because a possible dose-response relationship for effectiveness was suggested in one clinical study, an increase in dosage may be considered following several weeks of therapy if insufficient clinical improvement is observed. The manufacturer recommends fluoxetine dosages of 20–60 mg daily for the treatment of obsessive-compulsive disorder; dosages up to 80 mg daily have been well tolerated in clinical studies evaluating the drug in adults with obsessive-compulsive disorder. The manufacturer states that fluoxetine dosage should not exceed 80 mg

daily. Like fluoxetine's antidepressant effect, the full therapeutic effect of the drug in patients with obsessive-compulsive disorder may be delayed until 5 weeks of fluoxetine therapy or longer.

Pediatric Dosage

For the management of obsessive-compulsive disorder, the recommended initial dosage of fluoxetine in children and adolescents 7–17 years of age is 10 mg once daily. In adolescents and higher weight children, the dosage should be increased to 20 mg daily after 2 weeks; additional dosage increases may be considered after several more weeks if insufficient clinical improvement is observed. In lower weight children, dosage increases may be considered after several weeks if insufficient clinical improvement is observed. The manufacturer recommends fluoxetine dosages of 20–60 mg daily for adolescents and higher weight children and fluoxetine dosages of 20–30 mg daily for lower weight children for the treatment of obsessive-compulsive disorder. In lower weight children, the manufacturer states that clinical experience with fluoxetine dosages exceeding 20 mg daily is minimal and that there is no experience with dosages exceeding 60 mg daily in such patients.

Duration of Therapy

Although the efficacy of fluoxetine for long-term use (i.e., longer than 13 weeks) has not been demonstrated in controlled studies, patients have been continued on the drug under double-blind conditions for up to an additional 6 months without loss of benefit. The manufacturer and many experts state that obsessive-compulsive disorder is chronic and requires several months or longer of sustained therapy. Therefore, it is reasonable to continue therapy in responding patients. If fluoxetine is used for extended periods, dosage should be adjusted so that the patient is maintained on the lowest effective dosage, and the need for continued therapy with the drug should be reassessed periodically.

Premenstrual Dysphoric Disorder

For the management of premenstrual dysphoric disorder (previously late luteal phase dysphoric disorder), the recommended dosage of fluoxetine is 20 mg once daily given continuously throughout the menstrual cycle or intermittently (i.e., only during the luteal phase, starting 14 days prior to the anticipated onset of menstruation and continuing through the first full day of menses). The intermittent dosing regimen is then repeated with each new menstrual cycle. Decisions regarding which dosing regimen to use should be individualized. In a clinical study evaluating continuous dosing of fluoxetine dosages of 20 or 60 mg once daily for the treatment of premenstrual dysphoric disorder (PMDD), both dosages were effective but there was no evidence that the higher dosage provided any additional benefit. The manufacturer states that dosages exceeding 60 mg daily have not been systematically studied in patients with PMDD and that 80 mg daily is the maximum dosage of fluoxetine for the management of PMDD.

Clinical studies using fluoxetine dosages of 20 mg daily given intermittently or continuously have shown that the efficacy of the drug in the treatment of PMDD is maintained for up to 3 or 6 months, respectively. Patients should be periodically reassessed to determine the need for continued treatment. Discontinuance of the drug (even after more than 1 year of therapy) has resulted in relapse of PMDD within approximately 2 menstrual cycles.

Eating Disorders
Bulimia Nervosa

For the management of bulimia nervosa in adults, the recommended dosage of fluoxetine is 60 mg daily, administered as a single dose in the morning. The manufacturer states that in some patients, oral dosage of the drug may be carefully titrated up to the recommended initial dosage over a period of several days. However, since 60-mg doses of fluoxetine were found to be well tolerated, the APA states that many clinicians initiate treatment for bulimia nervosa at the higher dosage, titrating downward as necessary to minimize adverse effects. Fluoxetine dosages exceeding 60 mg daily have not been evaluated in patients with bulimia.

Systematic evaluation of fluoxetine has demonstrated that its efficacy in the treatment of bulimia nervosa is maintained for periods of up to 12 months following 2 months of acute treatment in patients receiving 60 mg daily as conventional fluoxetine capsules. Pending further accumulation of data, most clinicians recommend that antidepressant therapy, including fluoxetine, be continued for at least 6–12 months in patients with bulimia nervosa before attempting to discontinue therapy. If fluoxetine is used for extended periods, the manufacturer states that the need for continued therapy should be reassessed periodically.

Anorexia Nervosa

Although safety and efficacy of fluoxetine for the management of anorexia nervosa† and optimal dosage of the drug for this disorder have not been established, fluoxetine has been given in a dosage of 40 mg daily in weight-restored patients with anorexia nervosa.

Panic Disorder

For the management of panic disorder, the recommended initial dosage of fluoxetine in adults is 10 mg daily. After 1 week, the dosage should be increased to 20 mg once daily. If no clinical improvement is apparent after several weeks of fluoxetine therapy at 20 mg daily, an increase in dosage may be considered. Efficacy of the drug was demonstrated in clinical trials employing 10–60 mg daily. However, the most frequently administered dosage in flexible-dose clinical studies was 20 mg daily. As with the use of fluoxetine for other indications, lower dosages or less frequent dosing regimens should be considered for geriatric patients and patients with concurrent disease or those receiving multiple concomitant drug therapies. The manufacturer states that fluoxetine dosages exceeding 60 mg daily have not been systematically evaluated in patients with panic disorder.

The optimum duration of fluoxetine therapy required to prevent recurrence of panic disorder has not been established to date. The manufacturer states that the efficacy of fluoxetine beyond 12 weeks of therapy has not been demonstrated in controlled studies. However, the manufacturer and some clinicians state that panic disorder is chronic and requires several months or longer of sustained therapy. Therefore, it is reasonable to continue therapy in responding patients. The manufacturer recommends, however, that patients be reassessed periodically to determine the need for continued therapy.

Bipolar Disorder

Monotherapy

For the short-term treatment of acute depressive episodes in patients with bipolar disorder†, fluoxetine has been given in a dosage of 20–60 mg daily. Because of the risk of developing manic episodes associated with antidepressant therapy in patients with bipolar disorder, many clinicians recommend using the lowest effective dosage of fluoxetine for the shortest time necessary using the antidepressant in conjunction with a mood-stabilizing agent (e.g., lithium).

Combination Therapy

When used in fixed combination with olanzapine for acute depressive episodes associated with bipolar I disorder, fluoxetine is administered once daily in the evening, usually initiating therapy with a dosage of 6 mg of olanzapine and 25 mg of fluoxetine. A dosage of 3 mg of olanzapine and 25 mg of fluoxetine or 6 mg of olanzapine and 25 mg of fluoxetine should be used as initial therapy in patients with a predisposition to hypotensive reactions, patients with hepatic impairment, those with a combination of factors that may slow metabolism of the drugs(s) (e.g., female gender, geriatric age, nonsmoking status), or those patients who may be pharmacodynamically sensitive to olanzapine; when indicated, dosage should be escalated with caution. In other patients, dosage can be increased according to patient response and tolerance as indicated. In clinical trials, antidepressive efficacy was demonstrated at olanzapine dosages ranging from 6–12 mg daily and fluoxetine dosages ranging from 25–50 mg daily. Dosages exceeding 18 mg of olanzapine and 75 mg of fluoxetine have not been evaluated in clinical studies.

Alternatively, when using fluoxetine and olanzapine in combination as the single-ingredient components for acute depressive episodes associated with bipolar I disorder, the drugs should be given once daily in the evening, generally initiating therapy with 5 mg of olanzapine and 20 mg of fluoxetine. When indicated, dosage adjustments may be made within the dosage ranges of 20–50 mg for fluoxetine and 5–12.5 mg for olanzapine. An initial dosage of 2.5–5 mg of olanzapine with fluoxetine 20 mg should be used in patients with a predisposition to hypotensive reactions, patients with hepatic impairment, those with a combination of factors that may slow metabolism of the drugs(s) (e.g., female gender, geriatric age, nonsmoking status), or those patients who may be pharmacodynamically sensitive to olanzapine; when indicated, dosage increases should be escalated with caution.

Cataplexy

For the management of cataplexy†, fluoxetine has been given in a dosage of 20 mg once or twice daily in conjunction with CNS stimulant therapy (e.g., methylphenidate, dextroamphetamine).

Alcohol Dependence

For the management of alcohol dependence†, fluoxetine has been given in a dosage of 60 mg daily. Studies have shown that reductions in alcohol intake occur only with dosages of selective serotonin-reuptake inhibitors that are higher than the average therapeutic dosages used in depression. Alcohol intake in patients receiving lower dosages of fluoxetine (40 mg daily) was comparable to that of patients receiving placebo.

● Dosage in Renal and Hepatic Impairment

In depressed patients on hemodialysis, chronic fluoxetine administration produced steady-state plasma fluoxetine and norfluoxetine concentrations that were comparable with those observed in patients with normal renal function. The manufacturer therefore states that a reduction in dosage and/or frequency of administration of fluoxetine is not routinely required in patients with renal impairment. Supplemental doses of fluoxetine during hemodialysis also do not appear to be necessary since the drug and its active metabolite norfluoxetine are not removed substantially by hemodialysis. (See Pharmacokinetics: Elimination.)

Since fluoxetine is extensively metabolized in the liver, elimination may be prolonged in patients with hepatic impairment. Therefore, the manufacturer and some clinicians recommend a reduction in dosage and/or frequency of administration of fluoxetine in patients with hepatic impairment. Some clinicians recommend a 50% reduction in initial fluoxetine dosage for patients with well-compensated cirrhosis; however, patients with more substantial hepatic impairment, particularly those with severe disease, will require careful individualization of dosage. Subsequent dosage adjustment based on the tolerance and therapeutic response of the patient has been recommended in patients with hepatic impairment.

● Treatment of Pregnant Women during the Third Trimester

Because some neonates exposed to fluoxetine and other SSRIs or selective serotonin- and norepinephrine-reuptake inhibitors (SNRIs) late in the third trimester of pregnancy have developed severe complications, consideration may be given to cautiously tapering fluoxetine therapy in the third trimester prior to delivery if the drug is administered during pregnancy. (See Pregnancy under Cautions: Pregnancy, Fertility, and Lactation.)

CAUTIONS

The adverse effect profile of fluoxetine is similar to that of other selective serotonin-reuptake inhibitors (SSRIs; e.g., citalopram, escitalopram, fluvoxamine, paroxetine, sertraline). Because fluoxetine is a highly selective serotonin-reuptake inhibitor with little or no effect on other neurotransmitters, the incidence of some adverse effects commonly associated with tricyclic antidepressants, such as anticholinergic effects (dry mouth, dizziness, constipation), adverse cardiovascular effects, drowsiness, and weight gain, is lower in patients receiving fluoxetine. However, certain adverse GI (e.g., nausea) and nervous system (e.g., anxiety, nervousness, insomnia) effects appear to occur more frequently during fluoxetine therapy than during therapy with tricyclic antidepressants.

In controlled studies, the most common adverse reactions occurring more frequently in adults receiving fluoxetine than in those receiving placebo included nervous system effects such as anxiety, nervousness, insomnia, somnolence, asthenia, tremor, and abnormal dreams; GI effects such as anorexia, nausea, diarrhea, and dyspepsia; abnormal ejaculation, decreased libido, and impotence; dry mouth; flu syndrome; pharyngitis; rash; sinusitis; sweating; vasodilation; and yawn. Discontinuance of fluoxetine therapy was required principally because of adverse psychiatric (e.g., nervousness, anxiety, insomnia) and dermatologic (e.g., rash) effects. Because of the relatively long elimination half-lives of fluoxetine and its principal metabolite norfluoxetine, the possibility that some adverse effects may resolve slowly following discontinuance of the drug should be considered.

In controlled clinical trials, adverse effects reported in adults with weekly administration of fluoxetine delayed-release capsules were similar to those reported with daily administration of conventional capsules. Diarrhea and cognitive problems occurred more frequently with the delayed-release formulation compared with the conventional capsules.

Common adverse effects associated with fluoxetine therapy for major depressive disorder or obsessive-compulsive disorder in children and adolescents 7 years of age and older are generally similar to those observed in adults and include nausea, tiredness, nervousness, dizziness, and difficulty concentrating. However, manic reactions, including mania and hypomania, were the most common adverse events associated with discontinuance of the drug in 3 pivotal, pediatric, placebo-controlled studies. These reactions occurred in 2.6% of pediatric patients receiving fluoxetine compared with 0% of those receiving placebo and resulted in the discontinuance of fluoxetine in 1.8% of the patients during the acute phases of the studies combined. Consequently, regular monitoring for the occurrence of mania and hypomania in pediatric patients is recommended by the manufacturer.

The usual cautions and precautions of olanzapine should be observed when fluoxetine is used in fixed combination with the antipsychotic.

● Nervous System Effects

Headache has occurred in approximately 21% of patients receiving fluoxetine. Nervousness and anxiety have occurred in about 13 and 12% of patients, respectively, and insomnia has occurred in about 19% of patients receiving the drug; such effects appear to be dose-related and have required discontinuance of therapy in approximately 1–2% of fluoxetine-treated patients. The manufacturer and some clinicians state that a sedative (e.g., a short-acting benzodiazepine) may be administered to patients who experience insomnia or nervousness early in therapy; however, the possibility that fluoxetine may interact with some benzodiazepines (e.g., diazepam) should be considered. (See Drug Interactions: Benzodiazepines.)

Drowsiness or somnolence and asthenia reportedly occur in about 12 and 11%, respectively, of patients receiving fluoxetine therapy. Tremor and dizziness have both occurred in about 9% of patients; the incidence of dizziness may be dose-related. Abnormal thinking and abnormal dreams have been reported in about 2 and 1–5% of patients receiving fluoxetine therapy, respectively, and emotional lability has been reported in at least 1% of patients treated with the drug.

Hypomania, mania, and manic reaction have been reported in 1% or less of patients receiving fluoxetine, including those with depression or obsessive-compulsive disorder. In addition, mania reportedly occurred following administration of a higher than recommended dosage (140 mg daily) in a patient with major depression refractory to conventional antidepressant therapy; this patient subsequently responded to a fluoxetine dosage of 60 mg daily without apparent adverse effects. Such reactions have occurred in patients receiving other antidepressant agents and may be caused by antidepressant-induced functional increases in catecholamine activity within the CNS, resulting in a "switch" from depressive to manic behavior. There is some evidence that patients with bipolar disorder may be more likely to experience antidepressant-induced hypomanic or manic reactions than patients without evidence of this disorder. In addition, limited evidence suggests that such reactions may occur more frequently in bipolar depressed patients receiving tricyclics and tetracyclics (e.g., maprotiline, mianserin [not commercially available in the US]) than in those receiving SSRIs (e.g., citalopram, escitalopram, fluoxetine, fluvoxamine, paroxetine, sertraline). However, further studies are needed to confirm these findings.

Extrapyramidal reactions, including acute dystonic reactions, torticollis, dyskinesia (including buccolingual and buccoglossal syndrome), hypertonia, and akathisia, have occurred in 1% or less of patients receiving fluoxetine. An extrapyramidal reaction consisting of torticollis, jaw rigidity, cogwheel rigidity, and loss of fluid motion in gait reportedly occurred in one patient several days after initiation of fluoxetine therapy, but responded rapidly to an anticholinergic antiparkinsonian agent (i.e., trihexyphenidyl) and did not recur despite continued fluoxetine therapy. Serum prolactin concentrations were increased and CSF 3-methoxy-4-hydroxyphenylacetic acid (homovanillic acid, HVA) concentrations were decreased in this patient, suggesting that a decrease in dopaminergic activity (possibly as a result of enhanced serotonergic neurotransmission) may have contributed to the reaction.

Although a causal relationship to the drug has not been established, serotonin syndrome and neuroleptic malignant syndrome (NMS)-like reactions also have been reported rarely in patients receiving fluoxetine, other SSRIs, and selective serotonin- and norepinephrine-reuptake inhibitors (SNRIs). (See Cautions: Precautions and Contraindications and also see Drug Interactions: Serotonergic Drugs.)

The incidence of seizures during fluoxetine therapy appears to be similar to that observed during therapy with most other currently available antidepressants. Seizures or events that were described as possible seizures have been reported in approximately 0.2% of patients receiving fluoxetine therapy to date. (See Cautions: Precautions and Contraindications.) In addition, seizures have occurred following acute overdosage of the drug (see Acute Toxicity) and in at least one patient undergoing electroconvulsive therapy (ECT) concomitantly.

Adverse nervous system effects occurring in less than 1% of fluoxetine-treated patients include ataxia, balance disorder, and bruxism; however, a causal relationship to the drug has not been established. Depersonalization, euphoria, myoclonus, and paranoid reaction also have been reported in less than 1% of patients receiving the drug and delusions have been reported rarely, although these adverse effects have not been definitely attributed to fluoxetine. Rarely reported adverse nervous system effects for which a causal relationship has not been established include violent behavior, precipitation or worsening of depression, hypertonia, myoclonus, dyskinesia, and exacerbation of multiple sclerosis. Interference with facial nerve conduction, manifesting as ocular tics and impaired hearing, and memory impairment also have been reported. In some patients developing movement disorders with fluoxetine, there were underlying risk factors such as predisposing drug therapy and/or the disorder was an exacerbation of a preexisting disorder.

Withdrawal Reactions

Withdrawal symptoms, including dysphoric mood, irritability, agitation, dizziness, sensory disturbances (e.g., paresthesias such as electric shock sensations), anxiety, confusion, headache, lethargy, emotional lability, insomnia, and hypomania, have been reported upon discontinuance of fluoxetine, other SSRIs, and SNRIs, particularly when discontinuance of these drugs is abrupt. While these reactions are generally self-limiting, there have been reports of serious discontinuance symptoms. Therefore, patients should be monitored for such symptoms when discontinuing fluoxetine therapy. A gradual reduction in the dosage rather than abrupt cessation is recommended whenever possible. Plasma concentrations of fluoxetine and norfluoxetine (the principal metabolite) decline gradually after cessation of therapy, which may minimize the risk of withdrawal symptoms. (See Dosage and Administration: Dosage and also see Chronic Toxicity.)

Suicidality

Suicide attempts have been reported in less than 1% of fluoxetine-treated patients in clinical trials. The US Food and Drug Administration (FDA) has determined that antidepressants increase the risk of suicidal thinking and behavior (suicidality) in children, adolescents, and young adults (18–24 years of age) with major depressive disorder and other psychiatric disorders. Suicidal ideation, which can manifest as persistent, obsessive, and violent suicidal thoughts, has emerged occasionally in adults receiving fluoxetine. In a report of several fluoxetine-associated cases, severe suicidal ideation developed within 2–7 weeks after initiation of fluoxetine therapy and resolved within several days to months after discontinuance of the drug; however, the patients were unresponsive to fluoxetine and had received monoamine oxidase inhibitor therapy previously, and most had a history of suicidal ideation, were receiving relatively high dosages (60–80 mg daily) of fluoxetine, and were receiving other psychotropic therapy concomitantly. Suicidal ideation also has been reported in patients who reportedly had no history of such ideation, but the drug also has been used without recurrence of suicidal ideation in a few patients in whom such ideation emerged during tricyclic antidepressant therapy. Because of the possibility of suicidality, patients should be appropriately monitored and closely observed for clinical worsening, suicidality, and unusual changes in behavior, particularly during initiation of fluoxetine therapy (i.e., the first few months) and during periods of dosage adjustments. (See Cautions: Precautions and Contraindications and see Cautions: Pediatric Precautions and see Acute Toxicity.)

● GI Effects

The most frequent adverse effect associated with fluoxetine therapy is nausea, which occurs in about 22% of patients. Nausea generally is mild, occurs early in therapy, and usually subsides after a few weeks of continued therapy with the drug. Limited evidence suggests that the incidence of nausea may be dose-related, but additional experience with the drug is necessary to confirm this finding. Although the incidence of vomiting appears to be similar in patients receiving fluoxetine or tricyclic antidepressants (e.g., imipramine), the incidence of nausea appears to be higher with fluoxetine. While the mechanism(s) of fluoxetine-induced GI effects has not been fully elucidated, serotonin has been shown to have complex effects on the GI tract (e.g., stimulation of small intestine motility, inhibition of gastric and large intestine motility).

Diarrhea occurs in about 11%, anorexia in about 10%, and dyspepsia in about 8% of patients receiving fluoxetine; limited evidence suggests that the incidence of anorexia may be dose-related. Other adverse GI effects associated with fluoxetine therapy include vomiting and flatulence, which both reportedly occur in about 3% of patients receiving the drug. Change in taste perception has been reported in at least 1% of fluoxetine-treated patients.

Other adverse GI effects, including dysphagia, gastritis, gastroenteritis, melena, and stomach ulcer, have been reported in less than 1% of fluoxetine-treated patients; however, a causal relationship to the drug has not been established. Bloody diarrhea, duodenal or esophageal ulcer, GI hemorrhage, hematemesis, hepatitis, peptic ulcer, and stomach ulcer hemorrhage have occurred rarely, but have not been definitely attributed to fluoxetine.

Epidemiologic case-control and cohort design studies have suggested that selective serotonin-reuptake inhibitors may increase the risk of upper GI bleeding. Although the precise mechanism for this increased risk remains to be clearly established, serotonin release by platelets is known to play an important role in hemostasis, and selective serotonin-reuptake inhibitors decrease serotonin uptake from the blood by platelets thereby decreasing the amount of serotonin in platelets. In addition, concurrent use of aspirin or other nonsteroidal anti-inflammatory agents was found to substantially increase the risk of GI bleeding in patients receiving selective serotonin-reuptake inhibitors in 2 of these studies. Although these studies focused on upper GI bleeding, there is some evidence suggesting that bleeding at other sites may be similarly potentiated. Further clinical studies are needed to determine the clinical importance of these findings. (See Cautions: Hematologic Effects and also see Drug Interactions: Drugs Affecting Hemostasis.)

● Dermatologic and Sensitivity Reactions

Rash (including purpuric rash and erythema multiforme) and/or urticaria occurs in about 7% and pruritus occurs in about 3% of patients receiving fluoxetine. Adverse dermatologic effects, principally rash and pruritus, generally occur during the first few weeks of therapy and have required discontinuance of the drug in approximately 1% of patients.

Fluoxetine-induced rash and/or urticaria have been associated with systemic signs or symptoms such as fever, leukocytosis, arthralgia, edema, carpal tunnel syndrome, respiratory distress, lymphadenopathy, proteinuria, and mild elevation in serum aminotransferase (transaminase) concentrations in some patients. Serious systemic illnesses have developed rarely in patients with fluoxetine-induced dermatologic reactions to date. Although the diagnosis was equivocal in at least 2 of these patients, one patient was diagnosed as having a leukocytoclastic vasculitis and the other patient exhibited a severe desquamating syndrome that was variably diagnosed as either vasculitis or erythema multiforme. In addition, serum sickness reactions have developed in several other patients who experienced adverse dermatologic effects in association with fluoxetine therapy. Additional cases of systemic reactions possibly related to vasculitis have been reported in patients with rash. Although systemic reactions appear to occur rarely in patients receiving fluoxetine, such reactions may be serious and potentially may involve the lung, kidney, or liver; death reportedly has occurred in association with such reactions.

Anaphylactoid reactions (including bronchospasm, angioedema, and/or urticaria) have been reported in fluoxetine-treated patients; adverse pulmonary effects (including inflammatory processes of varying histopathology and/or fibrosis), which have occurred with dyspnea as the only preceding symptom, have been reported rarely. It has not been established whether the systemic reactions and associated skin rash in fluoxetine-treated patients share a common underlying cause or are due to different etiologies or pathogenic processes; in addition, a specific, underlying immunologic basis for these effects has not been identified. However, such systemic reactions are of potential concern since zimeldine (another selective serotonin-reuptake inhibitor that previously was commercially available outside the US) reportedly was associated with the development of Guillain-Barré syndrome following flu-like, hypersensitivity reactions to the drug; because of such reactions, zimeldine no longer is commercially available. Most patients with fluoxetine-induced rash and/or urticaria improve soon after discontinuance of therapy and/or administration of an antihistamine or corticosteroid, and most patients with such reactions to date have recovered completely without serious adverse sequelae. In addition, several patients who developed hypersensitivity reactions while receiving zimeldine subsequently received fluoxetine with no recurrence of a similar reaction. However, because of associated severe adverse systemic effects with fluoxetine and pharmacologically similar antidepressants (e.g., zimeldine), it is recommended that fluoxetine be discontinued if rash and/or other possible manifestations of hypersensitivity (e.g., fever, flu-like symptoms), for which alternative etiologies cannot be identified, occur during therapy with the drug.

Sweating occurs in about 7% of patients receiving fluoxetine. Adverse dermatologic and hypersensitivity reactions occurring in less than 1% of patients receiving fluoxetine include dry skin, alopecia, and photosensitivity reaction; however, these effects have not been definitely attributed to the drug. Although a causal relationship has not been established, erythema nodosum, epidermal necrolysis, exfoliative dermatitis, and Stevens-Johnson syndrome have also been reported.

● Metabolic Effects

Weight loss occurs in approximately 2% of patients receiving fluoxetine therapy. Normal-weight and overweight (i.e., body mass index exceeding 25 kg/m^2) depressed patients lost an average of 0.9–1.8 kg and 1.8 kg, respectively, following 6 weeks of therapy with the drug. Weight loss associated with fluoxetine therapy appears to be reversible, with a gradual increase in body weight occurring following discontinuance of the drug. Such weight loss appears to result from decreased food consumption rather than adverse GI effects associated with the drug; there is some evidence that fluoxetine-induced weight loss may be dose-related. (See Pharmacology: Effects on Appetite and Body Weight.) In addition, weight loss appears to occur independent of the antidepressant effect of the drug. Although weight loss is commonly associated with fluoxetine therapy, less than 1% of patients discontinue the drug because of this effect. In some cases, however, substantial weight loss may be an undesirable effect of therapy with the drug, particularly in underweight depressed or bulimic patients.

Fluoxetine potentially may alter blood glucose concentrations. Hypoglycemia has occurred during fluoxetine therapy. In addition, hyperglycemia has developed following discontinuance of the drug. Therefore, the possibility that insulin and/or oral antidiabetic agent dosage adjustments may be necessary when fluoxetine therapy is initiated or discontinued in patients with diabetes mellitus should be considered.

● Ocular Effects

Vision abnormalities, including blurred vision, occur in approximately 2% of patients receiving fluoxetine. In addition, cataract and optic neuritis have been reported in patients treated with fluoxetine, although a causal relationship to the drug remains to be established.

Mydriasis has been reported in less than 1% of patients receiving fluoxetine. (See Cautions: Precautions and Contraindications.)

● Cardiovascular Effects

Current evidence suggests that fluoxetine is less cardiotoxic than most antidepressant agents (e.g., tricyclic antidepressants, monoamine oxidase inhibitors). Unlike tricyclic antidepressants, which may cause characteristic ECG changes such as prolongation of PR, QRS, and QT intervals and ST-segment and T-wave abnormalities, clinically important ECG changes (such as conduction abnormalities) have not been commonly reported during controlled studies in fluoxetine-treated patients without preexisting cardiac disease. In addition, while tricyclic antidepressants commonly cause an increase in heart rate, heart rate reportedly is reduced by an average of approximately 3 beats/minute in patients receiving fluoxetine. (See Pharmacology: Cardiovascular Effects.)

Vasodilation has been reported in approximately 2% and palpitations have been reported in at least 1% of patients receiving fluoxetine. Unlike tricyclic antidepressants, fluoxetine has been associated with hypotension relatively infrequently. Cardiac arrhythmia also has occurred infrequently in fluoxetine-treated patients. Atrial fibrillation, ventricular tachycardia (including torsades de pointes-type arrhythmias), QT-interval prolongation, cardiac arrest, pulmonary hypertension, and cerebrovascular accident have occurred rarely, but these adverse effects have not been definitely attributed to the drug.

● Hematologic Effects

Ecchymosis has been reported in less than 1% of patients receiving fluoxetine. Lymphadenopathy and anemia also have been reported in patients receiving fluoxetine. Blood dyscrasia, leukopenia, pancytopenia, aplastic anemia, immune-related hemolytic anemia, petechiae, and purpura have occurred rarely, although a causal relationship to the drug has not been established. Thrombocytopenia and thrombocytopenic purpura also have been reported.

SNRIs and SSRIs, including fluoxetine, may increase the risk of bleeding events. Concomitant use of aspirin, nonsteroidal anti-inflammatory agents, warfarin, and other anticoagulants may add to this risk. Bleeding complications (e.g., ecchymosis, purpura, menorrhagia, rectal bleeding) have been reported infrequently in patients receiving SSRIs. Although the precise mechanism for these reactions has not been established, it has been suggested that impaired platelet aggregation and prolonged bleeding time may be due at least in part to inhibition of serotonin reuptake into platelets and/or that increased capillary fragility and vascular tone may contribute to these cases. (See Cautions: GI Effects and also see Drug Interactions: Drugs Affecting Hemostasis.)

● Respiratory Effects

Flu-like syndrome (see Cautions: Dermatologic and Sensitivity Reactions), pharyngitis, and sinusitis have occurred in approximately 1–11% of patients receiving fluoxetine in controlled clinical trials. Adverse respiratory effects reportedly occurring in at least 1% of patients but not directly attributable to the drug include rhinitis and yawning. Laryngeal edema has occurred rarely in patients receiving fluoxetine. Pulmonary fibrosis, pulmonary embolism, and eosinophilic pneumonia also have been reported in fluoxetine-treated patients; however, these adverse effects have not been definitely attributed to the drug.

● Renal, Electrolyte, and Genitourinary Effects
Sexual Dysfunction

Like other SSRIs, adverse effects on sexual function have been reported in both men and women receiving fluoxetine. Although changes in sexual desire, sexual performance, and sexual satisfaction often occur as manifestations of a psychiatric disorder, they also may occur as the result of pharmacologic therapy. It is difficult to determine the true incidence and severity of adverse effects on sexual function during fluoxetine therapy, in part because patients and clinicians may be reluctant to discuss these effects. Therefore, incidence data reported in product labeling and earlier studies are most likely underestimates of the true incidence of adverse sexual effects. Recent reports indicate that up to 50% of patients receiving SSRIs describe some form of sexual dysfunction during treatment and the actual incidence may be even higher.

Ejaculatory disturbances (principally ejaculatory delay) are the most common adverse urogenital effects associated with fluoxetine in men, occurring in up to 7% of men receiving the drug compared with less than 1% of those receiving placebo in controlled clinical studies for the treatment of obsessive-compulsive disorder or bulimia. In some cases, the adverse effect of ejaculatory delay has been used for therapeutic benefit in the treatment of premature ejaculation. (See Uses: Premature Ejaculation.) Other genital disorders reported in patients receiving the drug include impotence, increased libido, penile (of the glans) anesthesia, and anorgasmy (in both males and females). Decreased libido also reportedly occurs in up to 11% of patients. In addition, clitoral engorgement, sexual arousal, and orgasm reportedly occurred in at least one female patient receiving fluoxetine.

Management of sexual dysfunction caused by selective SSRI therapy includes waiting for tolerance to develop; using a lower dosage of the drug; using drug holidays; delaying administration of the drug until after coitus; or changing to another antidepressant. Although further study is needed, there is some evidence that adverse sexual effects of the SSRIs may be reversed by concomitant use of certain drugs, including buspirone, 5-hydroxytryptamine-2 (5-HT$_2$) receptor antagonists (e.g., nefazodone), 5-HT$_3$ receptor inhibitors (e.g., granisetron), or α$_2$-adrenergic receptor antagonists (e.g., yohimbine), selective phosphodiesterase (PDE) inhibitors (e.g., sildenafil), or dopamine receptor agonists (e.g., amantadine, dextroamphetamine, pemoline [no longer commercially available in the US], methylphenidate). In most patients, sexual dysfunction is fully reversed 1–3 days after discontinuance of the antidepressant. Ejaculatory dysfunction associated with fluoxetine therapy also has responded to concomitant cyproheptadine therapy in a few patients.

Other Renal, Electrolyte, and Genitourinary Effects

Treatment with SSRIs, including fluoxetine, and SNRIs may result in hyponatremia. In many cases, this hyponatremia appears to be due to the syndrome of inappropriate antidiuretic hormone secretion (SIADH) and was reversible when fluoxetine was discontinued. Cases with serum sodium concentrations lower than 110 mEq/L have been reported. Geriatric individuals and patients receiving diuretics or who are otherwise volume depleted may be at greater risk of developing hyponatremia during therapy with SSRIs or SNRIs. Signs and symptoms of hyponatremia include headache, difficulty concentrating, memory impairment, confusion, weakness, and unsteadiness, which may lead to falls; more severe and/or acute cases have been associated with hallucinations, syncope, seizures, coma, respiratory arrest, and death. Discontinuance of fluoxetine should be considered

in patients with symptomatic hyponatremia and appropriate medical intervention should be instituted. Because geriatric patients may be at increased risk for hyponatremia associated with these drugs, clinicians prescribing fluoxetine in such patients should be aware of the possibility that such reactions may occur. In addition, periodic monitoring of serum sodium concentrations (particularly during the first several months) in geriatric patients receiving SSRIs has been recommended by some clinicians.

Micturition disorder has occurred in at least 1% of patients receiving fluoxetine. Gynecological bleeding and dysuria have been reported in less than 1% of fluoxetine-treated patients, although these adverse effects have not been definitely attributed to the drug. Menorrhagia, gynecomastia, uterine hemorrhage, vaginal hemorrhage, and vaginal bleeding also have occurred, although a causal relationship to the drug has not been established.

● Anticholinergic Effects

Although bothersome anticholinergic effects occur commonly in patients receiving tricyclic antidepressant agents, such effects occur less frequently with fluoxetine. Dry mouth, dizziness, and constipation have been reported in about 9, 9, and 5% of patients receiving the drug, respectively. Blurred vision also has been reported.

● Other Adverse Effects

Chills have occurred in more than 1% of patients receiving fluoxetine. (See Cautions: Dermatologic and Sensitivity Reactions.)

Abnormal liver function test results, lymphadenopathy, and epistaxis have been reported in less than 1% of fluoxetine-treated patients, although such effects have not been definitely attributed to the drug. Adverse effects occurring rarely in patients receiving fluoxetine include hepatitis, jaundice (including cholestatic jaundice), acute abdominal syndrome, serum sickness, and lupus erythematosus syndrome. Pancreatitis and hyperprolactinemia also have occurred in patients receiving the drug. Although a causal relationship to fluoxetine has not been established for these effects, serotonin has been implicated as a possible physiologic factor in the release of prolactin. (See Pharmacology: Neuroendocrine Effects.)

● Precautions and Contraindications

Worsening of depression and/or the emergence of suicidal ideation and behavior (suicidality) or unusual changes in behavior may occur in both adult and pediatric (see Cautions: Pediatric Precautions) patients with major depressive disorder or other psychiatric disorders, whether or not they are taking antidepressants. This risk may persist until clinically important remission occurs. Suicide is a known risk of depression and certain other psychiatric disorders, and these disorders themselves are the strongest predictors of suicide. However, there has been a long-standing concern that antidepressants may have a role in inducing worsening of depression and the emergence of suicidality in certain patients during the early phases of treatment. Pooled analyses of short-term, placebo-controlled studies of antidepressants (i.e., selective serotonin-reuptake inhibitors [SSRIs] and other antidepressants) have shown an increased risk of suicidality in children, adolescents, and young adults (18–24 years of age) with major depressive disorder and other psychiatric disorders. An increased suicidality risk was not demonstrated with antidepressants compared with placebo in adults older than 24 years of age, and a reduced risk was observed in adults 65 years of age or older. It currently is unknown whether the suicidality risk extends to longer-term use (i.e., beyond several months); however, there is substantial evidence from placebo-controlled maintenance trials in adults with major depressive disorder that antidepressants can delay the recurrence of depression.

The US Food and Drug Administration (FDA) recommends that all patients being treated with antidepressants for any indication be appropriately monitored and closely observed for clinical worsening, suicidality, and unusual changes in behavior, particularly during initiation of therapy (i.e., the first few months) and during periods of dosage adjustments. Families and caregivers of patients being treated with antidepressants for major depressive disorder or other indications, both psychiatric and nonpsychiatric, also should be advised to monitor patients on a daily basis for the emergence of agitation, irritability, or unusual changes in behavior, as well as the emergence of suicidality, and to report such symptoms immediately to a health care provider.

Although a causal relationship between the emergence of symptoms such as anxiety, agitation, panic attacks, insomnia, irritability, hostility, aggressiveness, impulsivity, akathisia, hypomania, and/or mania and either the worsening of depression and/or the emergence of suicidal impulses has not been established, there is concern that such symptoms may represent precursors to emerging suicidality. Consequently, consideration should be given to changing the therapeutic regimen or discontinuing therapy in patients whose depression is persistently worse or in patients experiencing emergent suicidality or symptoms that might be precursors to worsening depression or suicidality, particularly if such manifestations are severe, abrupt in onset, or were not part of the patient's presenting symptoms. FDA also recommends that the drugs be prescribed in the smallest quantity consistent with good patient management, in order to reduce the risk of overdosage.

It is generally believed (though not established in controlled trials) that treating a major depressive episode with an antidepressant alone may increase the likelihood of precipitating a mixed or manic episode in patients at risk for bipolar disorder. Therefore, patients should be adequately screened for bipolar disorder prior to initiating treatment with an antidepressant; such screening should include a detailed psychiatric history (e.g., family history of suicide, bipolar disorder, and depression).

Potentially life-threatening serotonin syndrome or neuroleptic malignant syndrome (NMS)-like reactions have been reported with SSRIs, including fluoxetine, and selective serotonin- and norepinephrine-reuptake inhibitors (SNRIs) alone, but particularly with concurrent administration of other serotonergic drugs (including serotonin [5-hydroxytryptamine; 5-HT] type 1 receptor agonists [triptans]), drugs that impair the metabolism of serotonin (e.g., monoamine oxidase [MAO] inhibitors), or antipsychotic agents or other dopamine antagonists. Symptoms of serotonin syndrome may include mental status changes (e.g., agitation, hallucinations, coma), autonomic instability (e.g., tachycardia, labile blood pressure, hyperthermia), neuromuscular aberrations (e.g., hyperreflexia, incoordination), and/or GI symptoms (e.g., nausea, vomiting, diarrhea). In its most severe form, serotonin syndrome may resemble NMS, which is characterized by hyperthermia, muscle rigidity, autonomic instability with possible rapid fluctuation in vital signs, and mental status changes. Patients receiving fluoxetine should be monitored for the development of serotonin syndrome or NMS-like signs and symptoms.

Fluoxetine is contraindicated in patients who currently are receiving or recently (i.e., within 2 weeks) have received therapy with MAO inhibitors used for treatment of depression. If concurrent therapy with fluoxetine and a 5-HT$_1$ receptor agonist (triptan) is clinically warranted, the patient should be observed carefully, particularly during initiation of therapy, when dosage is increased, or when another serotonergic agent is initiated. Concomitant use of fluoxetine and serotonin precursors (e.g., tryptophan) is not recommended. If signs and symptoms of serotonin syndrome or NMS develop during therapy, treatment with fluoxetine and any concurrently administered serotonergic or antidopaminergic agents, including antipsychotic agents, should be discontinued immediately and supportive and symptomatic treatment should be initiated. (See Drug Interactions: Serotonergic Drugs.)

Because clinical experience with fluoxetine in patients with concurrent systemic disease, including cardiovascular disease, hepatic impairment, and renal impairment, is limited, caution should be exercised when fluoxetine is administered to patients with any systemic disease or condition that may alter metabolism of the drug or adversely affect hemodynamic function. (See Dosage and Administration: Dosage.) Fluoxetine should be used with caution in patients with hepatic impairment, since prolonged elimination of the drug and its principal metabolite has been reported to occur in patients with liver cirrhosis. Because the safety of long-term fluoxetine therapy in patients with severe renal impairment has not been adequately evaluated to date, fluoxetine also should be used with caution in patients with severe renal impairment. (See Dosage and Administration: Dosage in Renal and Hepatic Impairment.) Although current evidence suggests that fluoxetine is less cardiotoxic than most older antidepressant agents (see Cautions: Cardiovascular Effects), the safety of fluoxetine in patients with a recent history of myocardial infarction or unstable cardiovascular disease has not been adequately evaluated to date.

Patients receiving fluoxetine should be advised to notify their clinician if they are taking or plan to take nonprescription (over-the-counter), including herbal supplements, or prescription medications or alcohol-containing beverages or products. (See Drug Interactions.)

Patients receiving fluoxetine should be cautioned about the concurrent use of nonsteroidal anti-inflammatory agents (including aspirin), warfarin, or other drugs that affect coagulation since combined use of SSRIs and these drugs has been associated with an increased risk of bleeding. Patients should be advised to contact their physician if they experience any increased or unusual bruising or bleeding while taking fluoxetine. (See Cautions: GI Effects and also see Drug Interactions: Drugs Affecting Hemostasis.)

Fluoxetine generally is less sedating than many other currently available antidepressants and does not appear to produce substantial impairment of cognitive or psychomotor function. However, patients should be cautioned that fluoxetine may impair their ability to perform activities requiring mental alertness or physical coordination (e.g., operating machinery, driving a motor vehicle) and to avoid such activities until they experience how the drug affects them.

Patients receiving fluoxetine should be advised to notify their clinician if they develop a rash or other possible signs of an allergic reaction during therapy with the drug. Pending further accumulation of data, monitoring for such effects is particularly important since these effects have been associated with the development of potentially serious systemic reactions in patients receiving fluoxetine or pharmacologically similar antidepressants (e.g., zimeldine). (See Cautions: Dermatologic and Sensitivity Reactions.)

Seizures have been reported in patients receiving therapeutic dosages and following acute overdosage of fluoxetine. Because of limited experience with fluoxetine in patients with a history of seizures, therapy with the drug should be initiated with caution in such patients.

Because fluoxetine may alter blood glucose concentrations in patients with diabetes mellitus (see Cautions: Metabolic Effects), the possibility that insulin and/or oral antidiabetic agent dosage adjustments may be necessary when fluoxetine therapy is initiated or discontinued should be considered.

Because fluoxetine therapy has been commonly associated with anorexia and weight loss, the drug should be used with caution in patients who may be adversely affected by these effects (e.g., underweight or bulimic patients).

Because mydriasis has been reported in association with fluoxetine therapy (see Cautions: Ocular Effects), the drug should be used with caution in patients elevated intraocular pressure or those at risk of acute narrow-angle glaucoma.

Treatment with SSRIs, including fluoxetine, or SNRIs may result in hyponatremia. In many cases, this hyponatremia appears to be due to the syndrome of inappropriate antidiuretic hormone secretion (SIADH) and was reversible when the SSRI or SNRI was discontinued. Cases with serum sodium concentrations lower than 110 mEq/L have been reported. Geriatric individuals and patients receiving diuretics or who are otherwise volume depleted may be at greater risk of developing hyponatremia during therapy with SSRIs or SNRIs. Signs and symptoms of hyponatremia include headache, difficulty concentrating, memory impairment, confusion, weakness, and unsteadiness, which may lead to falls; more severe and/or acute cases have been associated with hallucinations, syncope, seizures, coma, respiratory arrest, and death. Discontinuance of fluoxetine should be considered in patients with symptomatic hyponatremia and appropriate medical intervention should be instituted. (See Cautions: Renal, Electrolyte, and Genitourinary Effects and also see Cautions: Geriatric Precautions.)

Fluoxetine therapy is contraindicated in patients concurrently receiving thioridazine therapy. The manufacturer recommends that an interval of at least 5 weeks elapse between discontinuance of fluoxetine therapy and initiation of thioridazine. In addition, concurrent use of fluoxetine in patients receiving pimozide is contraindicated. (See Thioridazine and also see Pimozide under Drug Interactions: Antipsychotic Agents.)

● **Pediatric Precautions**

Safety and efficacy of fluoxetine in pediatric patients have not been established in children younger than 8 years of age for the management of major depressive disorder (see Pediatric Considerations under Uses: Major Depressive Disorder) or in children younger than 7 years of age for the management of obsessive-compulsive disorder.

FDA warns that antidepressants increase the risk of suicidal thinking and behavior (suicidality) in children and adolescents with major depressive disorder and other psychiatric disorders. The risk of suicidality for these drugs was identified in a pooled analysis of data from a total of 24 short-term (4–16 weeks), placebo-controlled studies of 9 antidepressants (i.e., fluoxetine, bupropion, citalopram, fluvoxamine, mirtazapine, nefazodone, paroxetine, sertraline, venlafaxine) in over 4400 children and adolescents with major depressive disorder, obsessive-compulsive disorder (OCD), or other psychiatric disorders. The analysis revealed a greater risk of adverse events representing suicidal behavior or thinking (suicidality) during the first few months of treatment in pediatric patients receiving antidepressants than in those receiving placebo. However, a more recent meta-analysis of 27 placebo-controlled trials of 9 antidepressants (SSRIs and others) in patients younger than 19 years of age with major depressive disorder, OCD, or non-OCD anxiety disorders suggests that the benefits of antidepressant therapy in treating these conditions may outweigh the risks of suicidal behavior or suicidal ideation. No suicides occurred in these pediatric trials.

The risk of suicidality in FDA's pooled analysis differed across the different psychiatric indications, with the highest incidence observed in the major depressive disorder studies. In addition, although there was considerable variation in risk among the antidepressants, a tendency toward an increase in suicidality risk in younger patients was found for almost all drugs studied. It is currently unknown whether the suicidality risk in pediatric patients extends to longer-term use (i.e., beyond several months).

As a result of this analysis and public discussion of the issue, FDA has directed manufacturers of all antidepressants to add a boxed warning to the labeling of their products to alert clinicians of this suicidality risk in children and adolescents and to recommend appropriate monitoring and close observation of patients receiving these agents. (See Cautions: Precautions and Contraindications.) The drugs that are the focus of the revised labeling are all drugs included in the general class of antidepressants, including those that have not been studied in controlled clinical trials in pediatric patients, since the available data are not adequate to exclude any single antidepressant from an increased risk. In addition to the boxed warning and other information in professional labeling on antidepressants, FDA currently recommends that a patient medication guide explaining the risks associated with the drugs be provided to the patient each time the drugs are dispensed. Caregivers of pediatric patients whose depression is persistently worse or who are experiencing emergent suicidality or symptoms that might be precursors to worsening depression or suicidality during antidepressant therapy should consult their clinician regarding the best course of action (e.g., whether the therapeutic regimen should be changed or the drug discontinued). *Patients should not discontinue use of selective serotonin-reuptake inhibitors without first consulting their clinician; it is very important that the drugs not be abruptly discontinued, as withdrawal effects may occur.* (See Dosage and Administration: Dosage.)

Anyone considering the use of fluoxetine in a child or adolescent for any clinical use must balance the potential risks of therapy with the clinical need.

Important toxicity, including myotoxicity, long-term neurobehavioral and reproductive toxicity, and impaired bone development, has been observed following exposure of juvenile animals to fluoxetine; some of these effects occurred at clinically relevant exposures to the drug. In a study in which fluoxetine (3, 10, or 30 mg/kg) was orally administered to young rats from weaning (postnatal day 21) through adulthood (day 90), male and female sexual development was delayed at all dosages, and growth (body weight gain, femur length) was decreased during the dosing period in animals receiving the highest dosage. At the end of the treatment period, serum levels of creatine kinase (a marker of muscle damage) were increased in animals receiving the intermediate and highest dosage, and abnormal muscle and reproductive organ histopathology (skeletal muscle degeneration and necrosis, testicular degeneration and necrosis, epididymal vacuolation and hypospermia) was observed at the highest dosage. When animals were evaluated after a recovery period (up to 11 weeks after drug cessation), neurobehavioral abnormalities (decreased reactivity at all dosages and learning deficit at the highest dosage) and reproductive functional impairment (decreased mating at all dosages and impaired fertility at the highest dosage) were noted; testicular and epididymal microscopic lesions and decreased sperm concentrations were observed in the high-dosage group indicating that the reproductive organ effects seen at the end of treatment were irreversible. Reversibility of fluoxetine-induced muscle damage was not assessed in this study. Adverse effects similar to those observed in rats treated with fluoxetine during the juvenile period have not been reported after administration of fluoxetine to adult animals. Plasma exposures (AUC) to fluoxetine in juvenile rats receiving the low, intermediate, and high dosages in this study were approximately 0.1–0.2, 1–2, and 5–10 times, respectively, the average exposure in pediatric patients receiving the maximum recommended dosage of 20 mg daily. Exposures to norfluoxetine, the principal active metabolite of fluoxetine, in rats were approximately 0.3–0.8, 1–8, and 3–20 times the pediatric exposure at the maximum recommended dosage, respectively.

A specific effect of fluoxetine on bone development has been reported in mice treated with fluoxetine during the juvenile period. In mice treated with fluoxetine (5 or 20 mg/kg given intraperitoneally) for 4 weeks beginning at 4 weeks of age, bone formation was reduced resulting in decreased bone mineral content and density. These dosages did not affect overall growth (e.g., body weight gain or femoral length). The dosages given to juvenile mice in this study were approximately 0.5 and 2 times the maximum recommended dose for pediatric patients on a mg/m^2 basis.

In a study conducted in mice, fluoxetine administration (10 mg/kg intraperitoneally) during early postnatal development (postnatal days 4 to 21) produced abnormal emotional behaviors (decreased exploratory behavior in elevated plus-maze, increased shock avoidance latency) in adulthood (12 weeks of age). The dosage used in this study was approximately equal to the pediatric maximum recommended dosage on a mg/m^2 basis. Because of the early dosing period in this study, the clinical importance of these findings for the labeled pediatric use in humans is unknown.

As with other SSRIs, decreased weight gain has been observed in association with the use of fluoxetine in children and adolescents. In one clinical trial in pediatric patients 8–17 years of age, height gain averaged about 1.1 cm less and weight gain averaged about 1 kg less after 19 weeks of fluoxetine therapy relative to placebo-treated patients. In addition, fluoxetine therapy was associated with a decrease in plasma alkaline phosphatase concentrations. Because the safety of fluoxetine in pediatric patients has not been systematically assessed for chronic therapy longer than several months in duration and studies that directly evaluate the long-term effects of fluoxetine on the growth, development, and maturation of children and adolescents are lacking, height and weight should be monitored periodically in pediatric patients receiving fluoxetine. The clinical importance of these findings on long-term growth currently is not known, but the manufacturer will conduct a phase IV study to evaluate any potential impact of fluoxetine therapy on long-term pediatric growth. For further information on adverse effects associated with the use of fluoxetine in pediatric patients, see the opening discussion in Cautions.

● *Geriatric Precautions*

The efficacy of fluoxetine has been established in clinical studies in geriatric patients. Although no overall differences in efficacy or safety were observed between geriatric and younger patients, the possibility that some older patients particularly those with systemic disease or those who are receiving other drugs concomitantly (see Pharmacokinetics: Elimination and also see Uses: Major Depressive Disorder) may exhibit increased sensitivity to the drug cannot be ruled out.

In pooled data analyses, a *reduced* risk of suicidality was observed in adults 65 years of age or older with antidepressant therapy compared with placebo. (See Cautions: Precautions and Contraindications.)

Limited evidence suggests that geriatric patients may be more likely than younger patients to develop fluoxetine-induced hyponatremia and transient syndrome of inappropriate secretion of antidiuretic hormone (SIADH). Therefore, clinicians prescribing fluoxetine in geriatric patients should be aware of the possibility that such reactions may occur. In addition, periodic monitoring (especially during the first several months) of serum sodium concentrations in geriatric patients receiving the drug has been recommended by some clinicians.

As with other psychotropic drugs, geriatric patients receiving antidepressants appear to have an increased risk of hip fracture. Despite the fewer cardiovascular and anticholinergic effects associated with SSRIs, these drugs did not show any advantage over tricyclic antidepressants with regard to hip fracture in a case-control study. In addition, there was little difference in the rates of falls between nursing home residents receiving SSRIs and those receiving tricyclic antidepressants in a retrospective study. Therefore, all geriatric individuals receiving either type of antidepressant should be considered at increased risk of falls, and appropriate measures should be taken.

● *Mutagenicity and Carcinogenicity*

Fluoxetine and norfluoxetine did not exhibit mutagenic activity in vitro in mammalian cell (e.g., mouse lymphoma, rat hepatocyte DNA repair) or microbial (the *Salmonella* microbial mutagen [Ames]) test systems, or with the in vivo sister chromatid-exchange assay in Chinese hamster bone marrow cells. No evidence of carcinogenesis was seen in rats or mice receiving oral fluoxetine dosages of about 7.5 or 9 times the maximum recommended human dosage of the drug, respectively, for 24 months.

● *Pregnancy, Fertility, and Lactation*

Pregnancy

Some neonates exposed to fluoxetine and other selective serotonin-reuptake inhibitors (SSRIs) or selective serotonin- and norepinephrine-reuptake inhibitors (SNRIs) late in the third trimester of pregnancy have developed complications that have sometimes been severe and required prolonged hospitalization, respiratory support, enteral nutrition, and other forms of supportive care in special care nurseries. Such complications can arise immediately upon delivery and usually last several days or up to 2–4 weeks. Clinical findings reported to date in the neonates have included respiratory distress, cyanosis, apnea, seizures, temperature instability or fever, feeding difficulty, dehydration, excessive weight loss, vomiting, hypoglycemia, hypotonia, hypertonia, hyperreflexia, tremor, jitteriness, irritability, lethargy, reduced or lack of reaction to pain stimuli, and constant crying. These clinical features appear to be consistent with either a direct toxic effect of the SSRI or SNRI or, possibly, a drug withdrawal syndrome. It should be noted that, in some cases, the clinical picture was consistent with serotonin syndrome (see Drug Interactions: Serotonergic Drugs).

Infants exposed to SSRIs in late pregnancy may have an increased risk of persistent pulmonary hypertension of the newborn (PPHN). PPHN is a rare heart and lung condition occurring in an estimated 1–2 infants per 1000 births in the general population; it occurs when a neonate does not adapt to breathing outside the womb. Some experts have suggested that respiratory distress in neonates exposed to SSRIs may occur along a spectrum of seriousness in association with maternal use of SSRIs, with PPHN among the most serious consequences. Neonates with PPHN may require intensive care support, including mechanical ventilation; in severe cases, multiple organ damage, including brain damage, and even death may occur. Although several epidemiologic studies have suggested an increased risk of PPHN with SSRI use during pregnancy, other studies did not demonstrate a statistically significant association. Thus, the FDA states that it is currently unclear whether the use of SSRIs, including fluoxetine, during pregnancy can cause PPHN and recommends that clinicians not alter their current clinical practice of treating depression during pregnancy.

When treating a pregnant woman with fluoxetine, the clinician should carefully consider the potential risks and benefits of such therapy. Clinicians should consider that in a prospective longitudinal study of 201 women with a history of recurrent major depression who were euthymic in the context of antidepressant therapy at the beginning of pregnancy, women who discontinued their antidepressant medication (SSRIs, tricyclic antidepressants, or others) during pregnancy were found to be substantially more likely to have a relapse of depression than were women who continued to receive their antidepressant therapy while pregnant. Consideration may be given to cautiously tapering fluoxetine therapy in the third trimester prior to delivery if the drug is administered during pregnancy. (See Dosage and Administration: Treatment of Pregnant Women during the Third Trimester.)

Fluoxetine and its principal metabolite norfluoxetine have been shown to cross the placenta in animals. There are no adequate and controlled studies to date using fluoxetine in pregnant women, and the drug should be used during pregnancy only if the potential benefit justifies the potential risk to the fetus. Women should be advised to notify their clinician if they are or plan to become pregnant. FDA states that women who are pregnant or thinking about becoming pregnant should not discontinue any antidepressant, including fluoxetine, without first consulting their clinician. The decision whether or not to continue antidepressant therapy should be made only after careful consideration of the potential benefits and risks of antidepressant therapy for each individual pregnant patient. If a decision is made to discontinue treatment with fluoxetine or other SSRIs before or during pregnancy, discontinuance of therapy should be done in consultation with the clinician in accordance with the prescribing information for the antidepressant, and the patient should be closely monitored for possible relapse of depression. In addition, the prolonged elimination of the drug and its active metabolite from the body after discontinuance of therapy should be considered when a woman of childbearing potential receiving fluoxetine plans to become pregnant.

For additional information on the management of depression in women prior to conception and during pregnancy, including treatment algorithms, the FDA advises clinicians to consult the joint American Psychiatric Association and American College of Obstetricians and Gynecologists guidelines (at https://www.ncbi.nlm.nih.gov/pmc/articles/PMC3103063/pdf/nihms293836.pdf).

Results of a number of epidemiologic studies assessing the risk of fluoxetine exposure during the first trimester of pregnancy have demonstrated inconsistent results. Although more than 10 cohort studies and case-control studies failed to demonstrate an increased risk of congenital malformations with fluoxetine overall, one prospective cohort study conducted by the European Network of Teratology Information Services reported an increased risk of cardiovascular malformations in infants born to women exposed to fluoxetine during the first trimester of pregnancy compared with those born to women who were not exposed to the drug. There was no specific pattern of cardiovascular malformations

observed in this trial. Overall, a causal relationship between fluoxetine exposure during early pregnancy and congenital malformations has not been established. However, the results of epidemiologic studies indicate that exposure to paroxetine during the first trimester of pregnancy may increase the risk for congenital malformations, particularly cardiovascular malformations. (See Pregnancy, under Cautions: Pregnancy, Fertility, and Lactation, in Paroxetine 28:16.04.20.) Additional epidemiologic studies are needed to more thoroughly evaluate the relative safety of fluoxetine and other SSRIs during pregnancy, including their potential teratogenic risks and possible effects on neurobehavioral development.

The effect of fluoxetine on labor and delivery is not known.

Fertility

Reproduction studies in rats using fluoxetine dosages 5–9 times the maximum recommended human daily dosage have not revealed evidence of impaired fertility. However, a slight decrease in neonatal survival that probably was related to reduced maternal food consumption and suppressed weight gain was reported in the offspring. Like some other SSRIs, pretreatment with fluoxetine inhibits methoxydimethyltryptamine-induced ejaculation in rats; this effect is blocked by metergoline, a serotonin antagonist. Alterations in sexual function also have been reported in patients receiving the drug. (See Sexual Dysfunction under Cautions: Renal, Electrolyte, and Genitourinary Effects and also see Cautions: Pediatric Precautions.)

Lactation

Fluoxetine and its metabolites distribute into human milk. Limited data indicate that fluoxetine and norfluoxetine concentrations are 20–30% of concurrent maternal plasma drug concentrations. Crying, sleep disturbance, vomiting, and watery stools developed in an infant who nursed from a woman receiving fluoxetine; plasma fluoxetine and norfluoxetine concentrations in the infant on the second day of feeding were 340 and 208 ng/mL, respectively. Therefore, fluoxetine should not be used in nursing women, and women should be advised to notify their physician if they plan to breast-feed. In addition, the slow elimination of fluoxetine and norfluoxetine from the body after discontinuance of the drug should be considered.

DRUG INTERACTIONS

As with other drugs, the possibility that fluoxetine may interact with any concomitantly administered drug by a variety of mechanisms, including pharmacodynamic and pharmacokinetic interactions, should be considered. The potential for interactions exists not only with concomitantly administered drugs but also with drugs administered for several weeks after discontinuance of fluoxetine therapy due to the prolonged elimination of fluoxetine and its principal metabolite, norfluoxetine. (See Pharmacokinetics: Elimination.)

● *Serotonergic Drugs*

Use of selective serotonin-reuptake inhibitors (SSRIs) such as fluoxetine concurrently or in close succession with other drugs that affect serotonergic neurotransmission may result in serotonin syndrome or neuroleptic malignant syndrome (NMS)-like reactions. Symptoms of serotonin syndrome may include mental status changes (e.g., agitation, hallucinations, coma), autonomic instability (e.g., tachycardia, labile blood pressure, hyperthermia), neuromuscular aberrations (e.g., hyperreflexia, incoordination), and/or GI symptoms (e.g., nausea, vomiting, diarrhea). Although the syndrome appears to be relatively uncommon and usually mild in severity, serious and potentially life-threatening complications, including seizures, disseminated intravascular coagulation, respiratory failure, and severe hyperthermia, as well as death occasionally have been reported. In its most severe form, serotonin syndrome may resemble NMS, which is characterized by hyperthermia, muscle rigidity, autonomic instability with possible rapid fluctuation in vital signs, and mental status changes. The precise mechanism of these reactions is not fully understood; however, they appear to result from excessive serotonergic activity in the CNS, probably mediated by activation of serotonin 5-HT$_{1A}$ receptors. The possible involvement of dopamine and 5-HT$_2$ receptors also has been suggested, although their roles remain unclear.

Serotonin syndrome most commonly occurs when 2 or more drugs that affect serotonergic neurotransmission are administered either concurrently or in close succession. Serotonergic agents include those that increase serotonin synthesis (e.g., the serotonin precursor tryptophan), stimulate synaptic serotonin release (e.g., some amphetamines, dexfenfluramine [no longer commercially available in the US], fenfluramine [no longer commercially available in the US]), inhibit the reuptake of serotonin after release (e.g., SSRIs, selective serotonin- and nor-epinephrine-reuptake inhibitors [SNRIs], tricyclic antidepressants, trazodone, dextromethorphan, meperidine, tramadol), decrease the metabolism of sero-tonin (e.g., monoamine oxidase [MAO] inhibitors), have direct serotonin post-synaptic receptor activity (e.g., buspirone), or nonspecifically induce increases in serotonergic neuronal activity (e.g., lithium salts). Selective agonists of sero-tonin (5-hydroxytryptamine; 5-HT) type 1 receptors ("triptans") and dihydroer-gotamine, agents with serotonergic activity used in the management of migraine headache, and St. John's wort (*Hypericum perforatum*) also have been implicated in serotonin syndrome.

The combination of SSRIs and MAO inhibitors may result in serotonin syn-drome or NMS-like reactions. Such reactions have also been reported when SSRIs have been used concurrently with tryptophan, lithium, dextromethorphan, sumatriptan, dihydroergotamine, or antipsychotics or other dopamine antagonists. In rare cases, the serotonin syndrome reportedly has occurred in patients receiv-ing the recommended dosage of a single serotonergic agent (e.g., clomipramine) or during accidental overdosage (e.g., sertraline intoxication in a child). Some other drugs that have been implicated in precipitating symptoms suggestive of serotonin syndrome or NMS-like reactions include buspirone, bromocriptine, dextroprop-oxyphene, linezolid, methylene blue, methylenedioxymethamphetamine (MDMA; "ecstasy"), selegiline (a selective MAO-B inhibitor), and sibutramine (an SNRI used for the management of obesity [no longer commercially available in the US]). Other drugs that have been associated with the syndrome but for which less convincing data are available include carbamazepine, fentanyl, and pentazocine.

Clinicians should be aware of the potential for serious, possibly fatal reactions associated with serotonin syndrome or NMS-like reactions in patients receiving 2 or more drugs that affect serotonergic neurotransmission, even if no such interac-tions with the specific drugs have been reported to date in the medical literature. Pending further accumulation of data, serotonergic drugs should be used cau-tiously in combination and such combinations avoided whenever clinically possi-ble. Serotonin syndrome may be more likely to occur when initiating therapy with a serotonergic agent, increasing the dosage, or following the addition of another serotonergic drug. Some clinicians state that patients who have experienced sero-tonin syndrome may be at higher risk for recurrence of the syndrome upon reini-tiation of serotonergic drugs. Pending further experience in such cases, some clinicians recommend that therapy with serotonergic agents be limited follow-ing recovery. In cases in which the potential benefit of the drug is thought to out-weigh the risk of serotonin syndrome, lower potency agents and reduced dosages should be used, combination serotonergic therapy should be avoided, and patients should be monitored carefully for manifestations of serotonin syndrome. If signs and symptoms of serotonin syndrome or NMS develop during therapy, treatment with fluoxetine and any concurrently administered serotonergic or antidopami-nergic agents, including antipsychotic agents, should be discontinued immedi-ately and supportive and symptomatic treatment should be initiated.

Serotonin Syndrome
Manifestations

Serotonin syndrome is characterized by mental status and behavioral changes, altered muscle tone or neuromuscular activity, autonomic instability with rapid fluctuations of vital signs, hyperthermia, and diarrhea. Some clinicians have stated that the diagnosis of serotonin syndrome can be made based on the pres-ence of at least 3 of the following manifestations: mental status changes (e.g., confusion, hypomania), agitation, myoclonus, hyperreflexia, fever, shivering, tremor, diaphoresis, ataxia, and diarrhea in the setting of a recent addition or an increase in dosage of a serotonergic agent; the absence of other obvious causes of mental status changes and fever (e.g., infection, metabolic disorders, sub-stance abuse or withdrawal); and no recent initiation or increase in dosage of an antipsychotic agent prior to the onset of the signs and symptoms (in order to rule out NMS). In some cases, features of the serotonin syndrome have resem-bled those associated with NMS, which may occur in patients receiving phe-nothiazines or other antipsychotic agents. (See Extrapyramidal Reactions in Cautions: Nervous System Effects, in the Phenothiazines General Statement 28:16.08.24.)

Other signs and symptoms associated with serotonin syndrome have included restlessness, irritability, insomnia, aggressive behavior, headache, drowsiness, diz-ziness, disorientation, loss of coordination, anxiety, euphoria, hallucinations, dilated pupils, nystagmus, paresthesias, rigidity, clonus, seizures, and coma.

Nausea, vomiting, abdominal cramping, flushing, hypertension, hypotension, tachycardia, tachypnea, and hyperventilation also have occurred.

The onset of the serotonin syndrome can range from minutes after initiating therapy with a second serotonergic agent to several weeks after receiving a sta-ble dosage. Preliminary evidence to date suggests that neither the occurrence nor the severity of serotonin syndrome is related to the dose or duration of serotoner-gic drug therapy.

The incidence of serotonin syndrome is unknown, but it is likely that the syn-drome is underreported because it is not recognized or appears in various degrees of severity (mild, moderate, or severe). In addition, serotonin syndrome may be confused with or resemble NMS in some cases.

Treatment

Mild cases of serotonin syndrome generally respond within 12–24 hours to the immediate discontinuance of serotonergic agents and general supportive therapy. Symptoms rarely last more than 72–96 hours in the absence of complications. Supportive therapy in such cases may include hospitalization, adequate hydration, control of myoclonus and hyperreflexia with benzodiazepines such as clonazepam (and possibly propranolol), and control of fever with acetaminophen and external cooling, if necessary. Other possible causes of altered mental status and fever also should be considered and treated accordingly.

Patients with severe hyperthermia (i.e., a temperature of more than 40.5°C) are considered to have more severe cases of serotonin syndrome which are asso-ciated with more serious complications and mortality. Muscular rigidity often accompanies hyperthermia and may respond to benzodiazepine therapy. Such patients should be managed with aggressive cooling measures, including exter-nal cooling, the institution of muscular paralysis (to decrease body temperature, help prevent rhabdomyolysis and disseminated intravascular coagulation from muscular rigidity refractory to benzodiazepines, and facilitate intubation), and maintenance of a patent airway with endotracheal intubation. Seizures may be treated with benzodiazepines and, if necessary, other anticonvulsants (e.g., bar-biturates). Patients who develop hypertension, cardiac arrhythmias, and other serious complications such as disseminated intravascular coagulation or rhabdo-myolysis associated with serotonin syndrome should receive appropriate therapy for these conditions.

Although there is no specific therapy for serotonin syndrome, nonspecific serotonin (5-HT$_1$ and 5-HT$_2$) receptor antagonists such as cyproheptadine and methysergide and drugs with 5-HT$_{1A}$ receptor affinity such as propranolol have been used with some success in a limited number of patients whose symptoms persisted or were unusually severe. Dantrolene, bromocriptine, and chlorprom-azine (for sedation, to help reduce fever, and because of its 5-HT-receptor block-ing activity) also have been used in a limited number of patients with serotonin syndrome but with inconsistent results; the possibility that chlorpromazine may lower the seizure threshold in this setting should be considered.

Monoamine Oxidase Inhibitors

Potentially serious, sometimes fatal serotonin syndrome or NMS-like reactions have been reported in patients receiving serotonin-reuptake inhibitors in combi-nation with an MAO inhibitor. Such reactions also have been reported in patients who recently have discontinued a selective serotonin-reuptake inhibitor and have been started on an MAO inhibitor.

Probably because of its extensive clinical use and the prolonged elimination half-life of both fluoxetine and norfluoxetine, fluoxetine has been the selective serotonin-reuptake inhibitor most commonly implicated in serotonin syndrome. In at least 2 cases, serotonin syndrome developed when MAO inhibitor therapy was initiated after the discontinuance of fluoxetine therapy. Shivering, diplopia, nausea, confusion, and anxiety reportedly occurred in one patient 6 days after dis-continuance of fluoxetine therapy and 4 days after initiation of tranylcypromine therapy; signs and symptoms resolved without apparent sequelae within 24 hours following discontinuance of the MAO inhibitor in this patient. In another case, the initiation of tranylcypromine therapy more than 5 weeks after discontinuance of fluoxetine reportedly resulted in serotonin syndrome.

Concurrent administration of fluoxetine and MAO inhibitors is contraindi-cated. Because both fluoxetine and its principal metabolite have relatively long half-lives, at least 5 weeks should elapse between discontinuance of fluoxetine therapy and initiation of MAO inhibitor therapy, since administration of an MAO inhibitor prior to elapse of this time may increase the risk of serious adverse effects. Based on clinical experience with concurrent administration of tricyclic antidepressants and MAO inhibitors, at least 2 weeks should elapse following discontinuance of an MAO inhibitor prior to initiation of fluoxetine therapy.

Linezolid

Linezolid, an anti-infective agent that is a nonselective and reversible MAO inhibitor, has been associated with drug interactions resulting in serotonin syndrome, including some associated with SSRIs, and potentially may also cause NMS-like reactions. Because of the risk of serotonin syndrome, linezolid generally should *not* be used in patients receiving fluoxetine. The US Food and Drug Administration (FDA) states that certain life-threatening or urgent situations may necessitate immediate linezolid treatment in a patient receiving a serotonergic drug, including SSRIs. In such emergency situations, the availability of alternative anti-infectives should be considered and the benefits of linezolid should be weighed against the risk of serotonin syndrome. If linezolid is indicated in such emergency situations, fluoxetine must be immediately discontinued and the patient monitored for symptoms of CNS toxicity (e.g., mental changes, muscle twitching, excessive sweating, shivering/shaking, diarrhea, loss of coordination, fever) for 5 weeks or until 24 hours after the last linezolid dose, whichever comes first. Treatment with fluoxetine may be resumed 24 hours after the last linezolid dose. If nonemergency use of linezolid is being planned for a patient receiving fluoxetine, fluoxetine should be withheld for at least 5 weeks prior to initiating linezolid. Treatment with fluoxetine should not be initiated in a patient receiving linezolid; when necessary, fluoxetine may be started 24 hours after the last linezolid dose. (See Drug Interactions: Serotonergic Drugs, in Linezolid 8:12.28.24.)

Methylene Blue

There have been case reports of serotonin syndrome in patients who received methylene blue, which is a potent and selective inhibitor of MAO-A, while receiving serotonergic drugs, including SSRIs (e.g., citalopram, escitalopram, fluoxetine, fluvoxamine, paroxetine, sertraline). Therefore, methylene blue generally should *not* be used in patients receiving fluoxetine. However, the FDA states that certain emergency situations (e.g., methemoglobinemia, ifosfamide-induced encephalopathy†) may necessitate immediate use of methylene blue in a patient receiving fluoxetine.

Moclobemide

Moclobemide, a selective and reversible MAO-A inhibitor (not commercially available in the US), also has been associated with serotonin syndrome and such reactions have been fatal in several cases in which the drug was given in combination with the selective serotonin-reuptake inhibitor citalopram or with clomipramine. Pending further experience with such combinations, some clinicians recommend that concurrent therapy with moclobemide and selective serotonin-reuptake inhibitors be used only with extreme caution and serotonin-reuptake inhibitors should have been discontinued for some time (depending on the elimination half-lives of the drug and its active metabolites) before initiating moclobemide therapy.

Selegiline

Selegiline, a selective MAO-B inhibitor used in the management of parkinsonian syndrome, also has been reported to cause serotonin syndrome when given concurrently with selective serotonin-reuptake inhibitors (fluoxetine, paroxetine, sertraline). Although selegiline is a selective MAO-B inhibitor at therapeutic dosages, the drug appears to lose its selectivity for the MAO-B enzyme at higher dosages (e.g., those exceeding 10 mg/kg), thereby increasing the risk of serotonin syndrome in patients receiving higher dosages of the drug either alone or in combination with other serotonergic agents. The manufacturer of selegiline recommends avoiding concurrent selegiline and selective serotonin-reuptake inhibitor therapy. In addition, the manufacturer of selegiline recommends that a drug-free interval of at least 2 weeks elapse between discontinuance of selegiline and initiation of selective serotonin-reuptake inhibitor therapy. Because of the long half-lives of fluoxetine and its principal metabolite, at least 5 weeks should elapse or even longer (particularly if fluoxetine has been prescribed chronically and/or at higher dosages) between discontinuance of fluoxetine and initiation of selegiline therapy.

Isoniazid

Isoniazid, an antituberculosis agent, appears to have some MAO-inhibiting activity. In addition, iproniazid (not commercially available in the US), another antituberculosis agent structurally related to isoniazid that also possesses MAO-inhibiting activity, reportedly has resulted in serotonin syndrome in at least 2 patients when given in combination with meperidine. Pending further experience, clinicians should be aware of the potential for serotonin syndrome when isoniazid is given in combination with selective serotonin-reuptake inhibitor therapy or other serotonergic agents.

Tryptophan and Other Serotonin Precursors

Adverse nervous system effects (e.g., agitation, restlessness, aggressive behavior, insomnia, poor concentration, headache, paresthesia, incoordination, worsening of symptoms of obsessive-compulsive disorder), adverse GI effects (e.g., nausea, abdominal cramps, diarrhea), palpitation, and/or chills reportedly have occurred in a limited number of patients receiving fluoxetine concurrently with tryptophan, a serotonin precursor. Such symptoms generally resolved within several weeks following discontinuation of tryptophan despite continued fluoxetine therapy. Although the mechanism for this interaction has not been fully elucidated, it has been suggested that these adverse effects resemble the serotonin syndrome observed in animals and therefore may result from a marked increase in serotonin availability when tryptophan and potent serotonin-reuptake inhibitors such as fluoxetine are administered concurrently. Because of the potential risk of serotonin syndrome or NMS-like reactions, concurrent use of tryptophan or other serotonin precursors should be avoided in patients receiving fluoxetine.

Sibutramine

Because of the possibility of developing potentially serious, sometimes fatal serotonin syndrome or NMS-like reactions, sibutramine (no longer commercially available in the US) should be used with caution in patients receiving fluoxetine.

5-HT$_1$ Receptor Agonists ("Triptans")

Weakness, hyperreflexia, and incoordination have been reported rarely during postmarketing surveillance in patients receiving sumatriptan concomitantly with an SSRI (e.g., fluoxetine, citalopram, escitalopram, fluvoxamine, paroxetine, sertraline). Oral or subcutaneous sumatriptan and SSRIs were used concomitantly in some clinical studies without unusual adverse effects. However, an increase in the frequency of migraine attacks and a decrease in the effectiveness of sumatriptan in relieving migraine headache have been reported in a patient receiving subcutaneous injections of sumatriptan intermittently while undergoing fluoxetine therapy.

Clinicians prescribing 5-HT$_1$ receptor agonists, SSRIs, and SNRIs should consider that triptans often are used intermittently and that either the 5-HT$_1$ receptor agonist, SSRI, or SNRI may be prescribed by a different clinician. Clinicians also should weigh the potential risk of serotonin syndrome or NMS-like reactions with the expected benefit of using a triptan concurrently with SSRI or SNRI therapy. If concomitant treatment with fluoxetine and a triptan is clinically warranted, the patient should be observed carefully, particularly during treatment initiation, dosage increases, and following the addition of other serotonergic agents. Patients receiving concomitant triptan and fluoxetine therapy should be informed of the possibility of serotonin syndrome or NMS-like reactions and advised to immediately seek medical attention if they experience symptoms of these syndromes.

Other Selective Serotonin-reuptake Inhibitors and Selective Serotonin- and Norepinephrine-reuptake Inhibitors

Concomitant administration of fluoxetine with other SSRIs or SNRIs potentially may result in serotonin syndrome or NMS-like reactions and is therefore not recommended.

Antipsychotic Agents and Other Dopamine Antagonists

Concomitant use of antipsychotic agents and other dopamine antagonists with fluoxetine potentially may result in serotonin syndrome or NMS-like reactions. If signs and symptoms of serotonin syndrome or NMS occur, treatment with fluoxetine and any concurrently administered antidopaminergic or serotonergic agents should be immediately discontinued and supportive and symptomatic treatment initiated. (See Drug Interactions: Antipsychotic Agents.)

Tramadol and Other Serotonergic Drugs

Because of the potential risk of serotonin syndrome or NMS-like reactions, caution is advised whenever SSRIs, including fluoxetine, and SNRIs are concurrently administered with other drugs that may affect serotonergic neurotransmitter systems, including tramadol and St. John's wort (*Hypericum perforatum*).

Pentazocine, an opiate partial agonist analgesic, has been reported to cause transient symptoms of diaphoresis, ataxia, flushing, and tremor suggestive of the serotonin syndrome when used concurrently with fluoxetine.

Serotonin syndrome rarely may occur following concomitant use of fluoxetine and stimulants because stimulants can release serotonin, and amphetamine is metabolized by the cytochrome P-450 (CYP) 2D6 isoenzyme, which is inhibited by some SSRIs (e.g., fluoxetine, paroxetine).

● *Drugs Undergoing Metabolism by Hepatic Microsomal Enzymes*

Drugs Metabolized by Cytochrome P-450 (CYP) 2D6

Fluoxetine, like many other antidepressants (e.g., other selective serotonin-reuptake inhibitors, many tricyclic antidepressants), is metabolized by the drug-metabolizing cytochrome P-450 (CYP) 2D6 isoenzyme (debrisoquine hydroxylase). In addition, like many other drugs metabolized by CYP2D6, fluoxetine inhibits the activity of CYP2D6 and potentially may increase plasma concentrations of concomitantly administered drugs that also are metabolized by this enzyme. Fluoxetine may make normal CYP2D6 metabolizers resemble "poor metabolizers". Although similar interactions are possible with other selective serotonin-reuptake inhibitors, there is considerable variability among the drugs in the extent to which they inhibit CYP2D6; fluoxetine and paroxetine appear to be more potent in this regard than sertraline.

Concomitant use of fluoxetine with other drugs metabolized by CYP2D6 has not been systematically studied. The extent to which this potential interaction may become clinically important depends on the extent of inhibition of CYP2D6 by the antidepressant and the therapeutic index of the concomitantly administered drug. The drugs for which this potential interaction is of greatest concern are those that are metabolized principally by CYP2D6 and have a narrow therapeutic index, such as tricyclic antidepressants, class IC antiarrhythmics (e.g., propafenone, flecainide, encainide), vinblastine, and some phenothiazines (e.g., thioridazine).

Caution should be exercised whenever concurrent therapy with fluoxetine and other drugs metabolized by CYP2D6 is considered. If fluoxetine therapy is initiated in a patient already receiving a drug metabolized by CYP2D6, the need for decreased dosage of that drug should be considered. In addition, a low initial dosage should be used whenever a drug that is predominantly metabolized by CYP2D6 and has a relatively narrow therapeutic margin (e.g., tricyclic antidepressants, class IC antiarrhythmics) is initiated in a patient who is receiving or has received fluoxetine during the previous 5 weeks. Because of the risk of serious ventricular arrhythmias and sudden death potentially associated with increased plasma concentrations of thioridazine, thioridazine is contraindicated in any patient who is receiving or has received fluoxetine during the previous 5 weeks. (See Thioridazine under Drug Interactions: Antipsychotic Agents.)

Drugs Metabolized by Cytochrome P-450 (CYP) 3A4

Although fluoxetine can inhibit the cytochrome P-450 (CYP) 3A4 isoenzyme, results of in vitro and in vivo studies indicate that the drug is a much less potent inhibitor of this enzyme than many other drugs. In one in vivo drug interaction study, concomitant administration of single doses of the CYP3A4 substrate terfenadine (no longer commercially available in the US) and fluoxetine did not increase plasma concentrations of terfenadine. In addition, in vitro studies have shown that ketoconazole, a potent inhibitor of CYP3A4 activity, is at least 100 times more potent than fluoxetine or norfluoxetine as an inhibitor of several substrates of this enzyme (e.g., astemizole [no longer commercially available in the US], cisapride, midazolam). Some clinicians state that concomitant use of fluoxetine with astemizole or terfenadine is not recommended since substantially increased plasma concentrations of unchanged astemizole or terfenadine could occur, resulting in an increased risk of serious adverse cardiac effects. However, the manufacturer of fluoxetine states that the extent of fluoxetine's inhibition of CYP3A4 activity is unlikely to be of clinical importance.

● *Tricyclic and Other Antidepressants*

Concurrent administration of fluoxetine and a tricyclic antidepressant (e.g., nortriptyline, desipramine, imipramine) reportedly has resulted in adverse effects associated with tricyclic toxicity (including sedation, decreased energy, lightheadedness, psychomotor retardation, dry mouth, constipation, memory impairment).

In patients receiving imipramine or desipramine, initiation of fluoxetine therapy reportedly resulted in plasma concentrations of these tricyclic antidepressants that were at least 2–10 times higher; this effect persisted for 3 weeks or longer after fluoxetine was discontinued. Elevated plasma trazodone concentrations and adverse effects possibly associated with trazodone toxicity (e.g., sedation, unstable gait) also have been reported during concomitant fluoxetine and trazodone therapy. Although the mechanism for this possible interaction has not been established, it has been suggested that fluoxetine may inhibit the hepatic metabolism of tricyclic antidepressants. (See Drugs Metabolized by Cytochrome P-450 [CYP] 2D6 under Drug Interactions: Drugs Undergoing Metabolism by Hepatic Microsomal Enzymes.) Further study of this potential interaction is needed, but current evidence suggests that patients receiving fluoxetine and a tricyclic antidepressant or trazodone concomitantly should be closely observed for adverse effects; monitoring of plasma tricyclic or trazodone concentrations also should be considered and their dosage reduced as necessary. Because fluoxetine may increase plasma concentrations and prolong the elimination half-life of tricyclic antidepressants, the need for more prolonged monitoring following combined tricyclic and fluoxetine overdose should be considered. In addition, because of the prolonged elimination of fluoxetine and norfluoxetine, the possibility that the drug may interact with tricyclic antidepressants after recent discontinuance of fluoxetine also should be considered.

● *Antipsychotic Agents*

Concomitant use of antipsychotic agents with fluoxetine potentially may result in serotonin syndrome or NMS-like reactions. If signs and symptoms of serotonin syndrome or NMS occur, treatment with fluoxetine and any concurrently administered antipsychotic agent should be immediately discontinued and supportive and symptomatic treatment initiated. (See Drug Interactions: Serotonergic Drugs.)

Some clinical data suggest a possible pharmacodynamic and/or pharmacokinetic interaction between SSRIs, including fluoxetine, and some antipsychotic agents.

Clozapine

Concomitant use of fluoxetine and clozapine can increase plasma concentrations of clozapine and enhance clozapine's pharmacologic effects secondary to suspected inhibition of clozapine metabolism by fluoxetine. Increased plasma clozapine concentrations also have been reported in patients receiving other SSRIs (e.g., fluvoxamine, paroxetine). There has been at least one fatality related to clozapine toxicity following ingestion of clozapine, fluoxetine, and alcohol. The manufacturer of clozapine states that caution should be used and patients closely monitored if clozapine is used in patients receiving SSRIs, and a reduction in clozapine dosage should be considered.

Haloperidol

Elevated plasma concentrations of haloperidol have been observed in patients receiving concomitant fluoxetine therapy. Severe extrapyramidal symptoms (e.g., tongue stiffness, parkinsonian symptoms, akathisia), which required hospitalization and were refractory to conventional therapy (including anticholinergic antiparkinsonian agents, diphenhydramine, and diazepam), reportedly occurred in a patient receiving fluoxetine and haloperidol concurrently; this patient previously had experienced only mild adverse extrapyramidal effects with haloperidol therapy alone. The extrapyramidal symptoms gradually abated following discontinuance of both drugs, and the patient subsequently tolerated haloperidol therapy with evidence of only a slight parkinsonian gait. The clinical importance of this possible interaction has not been established, and additional study is required to determine the safety of combined fluoxetine and antipsychotic therapy.

Olanzapine

Concomitant administration of fluoxetine (60 mg as a single dose or 60 mg daily for 8 days) with a single 5-mg dose of oral olanzapine caused a small increase in peak plasma olanzapine concentrations (averaging 16%) and a small decrease (averaging 16%) in olanzapine clearance; the elimination half-life was not substantially affected. Fluoxetine is an inhibitor of CYP2D6, and thereby may affect a minor metabolic pathway for olanzapine. Although the changes in pharmacokinetics are statistically significant when olanzapine and fluoxetine are given concurrently, the changes are unlikely to be clinically important in comparison to the overall variability observed between individuals; therefore, routine dosage adjustment is not recommended.

When fluoxetine is used in fixed combination with olanzapine, the drug interactions associated with olanzapine also should be considered. (See Drug Interactions in Olanzapine 28:16.08.04.)

Pimozide

Clinical studies evaluating pimozide in combination with other antidepressants have demonstrated an increase in adverse drug interactions or QT$_c$ prolongation during combined therapy. In addition, rare case reports have suggested possible additive cardiovascular effects of fluoxetine and pimozide, resulting in bradycardia. Marked changes in mental status (e.g., stupor, inability to think clearly) and hypersalivation also were reported in one woman who received both drugs concurrently. Although a specific study evaluating concurrent fluoxetine and pimozide therapy has not been performed to date, concurrent use of these drugs is contraindicated because of the potential for adverse drug interactions or QT$_c$ prolongation.

Risperidone

Extrapyramidal symptoms followed by persistent tardive dyskinesia (dyskinetic tongue movements) have occurred in one 18-year-old who received risperidone concomitantly with fluoxetine; however, a causal relationship has not been established. The AUC of risperidone increased during concomitant fluoxetine therapy in one study in psychotic patients, and the AUC of active drug (risperidone plus 9-hydroxyrisperidone) increased in poor and extensive metabolizers (determined by CYP2D6 genotyping); there was no evidence of increased severity or incidence of extrapyramidal symptoms in this 30-day study.

Thioridazine

Although specific drug interaction studies evaluating concomitant use of fluoxetine and thioridazine are not available, concomitant use of other SSRIs (e.g., fluvoxamine) has resulted in increased plasma concentrations of the antipsychotic agent. Because of the risk of serious ventricular arrhythmia and sudden death associated with elevated plasma concentrations of thioridazine, thioridazine is contraindicated in any patient who is receiving or has received fluoxetine during the previous 5 weeks. (See Drugs Metabolized by Cytochrome P-450 [CYP] 2D6 under Drug Interactions: Drugs Undergoing Metabolism by Hepatic Microsomal Enzymes.)

● Benzodiazepines

Fluoxetine appears to inhibit the metabolism of diazepam, as evidenced by increases in the elimination half-life and plasma concentration of diazepam and decreases in diazepam clearance and the rate of formation of desmethyldiazepam (an active metabolite of diazepam) during concomitant use of the drugs. Although clinically important increase in psychomotor impairment has not been noted when fluoxetine and diazepam were administered concomitantly as compared with administration of diazepam alone, concomitant administration of alprazolam and fluoxetine has resulted in increased plasma concentrations of alprazolam and further psychomotor performance impairments. Pending further accumulation of data, the possibility that a clinically important interaction could occur in geriatric or other susceptible patients should be considered.

● Buspirone

Buspirone has serotonergic activity and may have been partially responsible for a case of serotonin syndrome that resulted in the death of a patient receiving fluoxetine, buspirone, and an MAO inhibitor (tranylcypromine) concomitantly. (See Drug Interactions: Serotonergic Drugs.)

In a patient with depression, generalized anxiety disorder, and panic attacks who was receiving concomitant buspirone and trazodone therapy, an increase in anxiety symptoms to a level comparable to that observed prior to buspirone therapy occurred when fluoxetine was added to the regimen. Although the mechanism of this possible interaction has not been established, it was suggested that fluoxetine may have either directly antagonized the therapeutic activity of buspirone or may have precipitated the anxiety symptoms through a separate mechanism. However, combined use of the drugs also has been reported to potentiate therapeutic efficacy in patients with obsessive-compulsive disorder.

● Lithium

Fluoxetine and lithium have been used concurrently in a limited number of patients without apparent adverse effects. However, both increased and decreased serum lithium concentrations and adverse neuromuscular effects possibly associated with lithium toxicity and/or serotonin syndrome (e.g., ataxia, dizziness, dysarthria, stiffness of the extremities) have been reported during combined therapy with the drugs. Lithium appears to have some serotonergic activity, and serotonin syndrome has been reported following the initiation of lithium therapy in at least one patient receiving fluoxetine. (See Drug Interactions: Serotonergic Drugs.) The

clinical importance of this potential interaction remains to be determined and further substantiation is required; however, caution should be exercised when fluoxetine and lithium are administered concurrently. It is recommended that serum lithium concentrations be monitored closely during concomitant fluoxetine therapy.

● Anticonvulsants

Carbamazepine

Fluoxetine can increase plasma carbamazepine and carbamazepine 10,11-epoxide (CBZ-E, an active metabolite) concentrations, and carbamazepine toxicity (e.g., ocular changes, vertigo, tremor) has been reported in some patients maintained on carbamazepine following initiation of fluoxetine. It has been suggested that fluoxetine-induced inhibition of hepatic metabolism (e.g., inhibition of epoxide hydrolase) of carbamazepine and/or CBZ-E may be principally responsible for such increases; alteration in protein binding does not appear to be principally responsible for this interaction. The patient and plasma concentrations of carbamazepine and its metabolite should be monitored closely whenever fluoxetine therapy is initiated or discontinued; carbamazepine dosage should be adjusted accordingly.

Phenytoin

Initiation of fluoxetine in patients stabilized on phenytoin has resulted in increased plasma phenytoin concentrations and clinical manifestations of phenytoin toxicity.

● β-Adrenergic Blocking Agents

Concomitant use of fluoxetine and a β-adrenergic blocking agent has resulted in increased plasma concentrations that have enhanced the β-adrenergic blocking effects of the drug, possibly resulting in cardiac toxicity. Metoprolol is metabolized by the CYP2D6 isoenzyme and fluoxetine is known to potently inhibit this enzyme. Although specific data are lacking, β-adrenergic blocking agents that are renally eliminated (e.g., atenolol) may be a safer choice. Patients who were previously stabilized on propranolol or metoprolol should be monitored for toxicity (e.g., bradycardia, conduction defects, hypotension, heart failure, central nervous system disturbances) following initiation of fluoxetine therapy.

● Protein-bound Drugs

Because fluoxetine is highly protein bound, the drug theoretically could be displaced from binding sites by, or it could displace from binding sites, other protein-bound drugs such as oral anticoagulants and digitoxin (no longer commercially available in the US). Pending further accumulation of data, patients receiving fluoxetine with any highly protein-bound drug should be observed for potential adverse effects associated with such therapy. (See Drug Interactions: Drugs Affecting Hemostasis.)

● Drugs Affecting Hemostasis

Warfarin

Concomitant use of fluoxetine and warfarin has resulted in altered anticoagulant effects, including increased bleeding. Therefore, patients receiving warfarin should be carefully monitored whenever fluoxetine is initiated or discontinued.

Other Drugs that Interfere with Hemostasis

Epidemiologic case-control and cohort design studies that have demonstrated an association between selective serotonin-reuptake inhibitor therapy and an increased risk of upper GI bleeding also have shown that concurrent use of aspirin or other nonsteroidal anti-inflammatory agents substantially increases the risk of GI bleeding. Although these studies focused on upper GI bleeding, there is some evidence suggesting that bleeding at other sites may be similarly potentiated. The precise mechanism for this increased risk remains to be clearly established; however, serotonin release by platelets is known to play an important role in hemostasis, and selective serotonin-reuptake inhibitors decrease serotonin uptake from the blood by platelets, thereby decreasing the amount of serotonin in platelets. Patients receiving fluoxetine should be cautioned about the concomitant use of drugs that interfere with hemostasis, including aspirin and other nonsteroidal anti-inflammatory agents.

● Alcohol

Concurrent administration of single or multiple doses of fluoxetine and alcohol does not appear to alter blood or Breathalyzer® alcohol, plasma fluoxetine, or plasma norfluoxetine concentrations in healthy individuals, suggesting that there is no pharmacokinetic interaction between fluoxetine and alcohol. In addition, fluoxetine does not appear to potentiate the psychomotor and cognitive impairment or cardiovascular effects induced by alcohol. However, the drug's ability to reduce alcohol consumption in animals and humans suggests that there may be a serotonergically mediated, pharmacodynamic interaction between fluoxetine and alcohol within the CNS. (See Pharmacology: Effects on Alcohol Intake, and also see Uses: Alcohol Dependence.)

● *Electroconvulsive Therapy*

The effects of fluoxetine in conjunction with electroconvulsive therapy (ECT) for the management of depression have not been evaluated to date in clinical studies. Prolonged seizures reportedly have occurred rarely during concurrent use of fluoxetine and ETC.

● *Antidiabetic Agents*

Fluoxetine potentially may alter blood glucose concentrations in patients with diabetes mellitus. (See Cautions: Metabolic Effects.) Therefore, dosage adjustments of insulin and/or oral antidiabetic agents may be necessary when fluoxetine therapy is initiated or discontinued in such patients.

ACUTE TOXICITY

Limited information is available on the acute toxicity of fluoxetine.

● *Pathogenesis*

The acute lethal dose of fluoxetine in humans is not known. The median oral LD_{50} of fluoxetine has been reported to be approximately 452 and 248 mg/kg in rats and mice, respectively. In animals, oral administration of single large doses of the drug has resulted in hyperirritability and seizures. Tonic-clonic seizures occurred in 5 of 6 dogs given a toxic dose of fluoxetine orally; the seizures ceased immediately after IV administration of diazepam. In these dogs, the lowest plasma fluoxetine concentration at which seizures occurred reportedly was only twice the maximum plasma concentration reported in humans receiving 80 mg of the antidepressant daily during long-term therapy. Single large oral doses of fluoxetine reportedly do not cause QT- or PR-interval prolongation or widening of the QRS complex in dogs, although tachycardia and an increase in blood pressure have occurred.

The risk of fluoxetine overdosage may be increased in patients with a genetic deficiency in the cytochrome P-450 (CYP) isoenzyme 2D6.

● *Manifestations*

In general, overdosage of fluoxetine may be expected to produce effects that are extensions of the drug's pharmacologic and adverse effects. Animal studies and case reports in humans indicate that possible effects of overdosage include agitation, restlessness, hypomania, vertigo, insomnia, tremor, and other signs of CNS excitation; nausea and vomiting; and tachycardia and/or increased blood pressure. Seizures have been reported in at least one patient after overdosage of fluoxetine. Acute overdosage of fluoxetine alone reportedly has resulted in nystagmus, drowsiness, coma, urticaria, spontaneous emesis, and ST-segment depression. Nausea and vomiting appear to occur commonly following acute ingestion of relatively large single doses of the drug.

Several fatalities following fluoxetine overdosage have been reported to date. One of the deaths occurred in a patient who reportedly ingested 1.8 g of fluoxetine and an unknown quantity of maprotiline; plasma fluoxetine and maprotiline concentrations in this patient were approximately 4570 and 4180 ng/mL, respectively. Another patient died after concomitantly ingesting fluoxetine, codeine, and temazepam; plasma fluoxetine, norfluoxetine, codeine, and temazepam concentrations in this patient reportedly were 1930, 1110, 1800, and 3800 ng/mL, respectively. A fatal overdose also has been reported in a patient ingesting fluoxetine and alcohol concomitantly. There also are a few reported cases of overdose in which fatality was attributed to fluoxetine alone. In one such case, death was associated with extracted blood fluoxetine and norfluoxetine concentrations of 6000 and 5000 ng/mL, respectively, and biliary concentrations of 13,000 ng/mL each for the drug and metabolite. A patient enrolled in a clinical study of fluoxetine reportedly died following intentional ingestion of an unknown quantity of amitriptyline, clobazam, and pentazocine; however, it is not known whether this patient also ingested fluoxetine with the other drugs.

A patient with a history of seizures who reportedly ingested 3 g of fluoxetine and an unknown quantity of aspirin experienced 2 tonic-clonic seizures, tachycardia, dizziness, blurred vision, unsustained clonus, and ECG changes. The seizures

occurred about 9 hours post-ingestion, lasted approximately 2–3 minutes, and remitted spontaneously without anticonvulsant therapy. Although the actual amount of fluoxetine absorbed by this patient may have been less than expected because of vomiting and gastric lavage, the plasma fluoxetine concentration reportedly was 2461 ng/mL when seizures occurred; the patient recovered with no apparent sequelae. Another patient reported that he experienced sleepiness and nausea that lasted for several days following the intentional ingestion of 840 mg of fluoxetine with alcohol; this patient did not seek medical treatment. Drowsiness, lethargy, and nausea occurred in a patient who reportedly ingested 1.4 g of fluoxetine and 15 mg of clonazepam. No ECG abnormalities were reported in 2 patients who intentionally ingested 200 mg and 1 g of fluoxetine.

A child with a genetic deficiency in the CYP2D6 isoenzyme died following prolonged therapy with fluoxetine, methylphenidate, and clonidine. Autopsy findings revealed blood, brain, and other tissue concentrations of fluoxetine and norfluoxetine that were several-fold higher than expected. Poor metabolism of fluoxetine via CYP2D6 was the likely cause of fluoxetine intoxication in this child.

● *Treatment*

Because fatalities and severe toxicity have been reported following overdosage of selective serotonin-reuptake inhibitors, particularly in large overdosage and when taken with other drugs or alcohol, some clinicians recommend that any overdosage involving these drugs be managed aggressively. Because suicidal ingestion often involves more than one drug, clinicians treating fluoxetine overdosage should be alert to possible toxic manifestations caused by drugs other than fluoxetine.

Clinicians also should consider the possibility of serotonin syndrome or NMS-like reactions in patients presenting with similar clinical features and a recent history of fluoxetine ingestion and/or ingestion of other serotonergic and/or antipsychotic agents or other dopamine antagonists. (See Cautions: Precautions and Contraindications and also see Drug Interactions: Serotonergic Drugs.)

Management of fluoxetine overdosage generally involves symptomatic and supportive care. A patent airway should be established and maintained, and adequate oxygenation and ventilation should be assured. ECG and vital sign monitoring is recommended following acute overdosage with the drug, although the value of ECG monitoring in predicting the severity of fluoxetine-induced cardiotoxicity is not known. (See Acute Toxicity: Manifestations, in the Tricyclic Antidepressants General Statement.) There is no specific antidote for fluoxetine intoxication.

Following recent (i.e., within 4 hours) ingestion of a potentially toxic amount of fluoxetine and in the absence of signs and symptoms of cardiac toxicity, the stomach should be emptied immediately by inducing emesis or by gastric lavage. If the patient is comatose, having seizures, or lacks the gag reflex, gastric lavage may be performed if an endotracheal tube with cuff inflated is in place to prevent aspiration of gastric contents. Since administration of activated charcoal (which may be used in conjunction with sorbitol or a saline cathartic) may be as effective or more effective than induction of emesis or gastric lavage, its use has been recommended either in the initial management of fluoxetine overdosage or following induction of emesis or gastric lavage in patients who have ingested a potentially toxic quantity of the drug.

Based on data from animal studies, IV diazepam should be considered for the management of fluoxetine-induced seizures that do not remit spontaneously. If seizures are not controlled or recur following administration of diazepam, administration of phenytoin or phenobarbital has been recommended by some clinicians.

Fluoxetine and norfluoxetine are not substantially removed by hemodialysis. Because of the large volume of distribution and extensive protein binding of the drug and its principal metabolite, peritoneal dialysis, forced diuresis, hemoperfusion, and/or exchange transfusion probably are also ineffective in removing substantial amounts of fluoxetine and norfluoxetine from the body. Clinicians should consider consulting a poison control center for additional information on the management of fluoxetine overdosage.

CHRONIC TOXICITY

Fluoxetine has not been studied systematically in animals or humans to determine whether therapy with the drug is associated with tolerance or psychologic and/or physical dependence. One patient receiving the drug for the management of obesity reportedly experienced nervousness 2 days following discontinuance of fluoxetine therapy. However, it is unclear whether this adverse effect represented a withdrawal reaction since both the parent drug and its principal metabolite have relatively long half-lives, and withdrawal reactions following discontinuance of fluoxetine therapy may therefore be more delayed. Although clinical experience to date has not revealed substantial evidence of drug-seeking behavior or a withdrawal syndrome associated with discontinuance of fluoxetine therapy, it is difficult to predict from the limited data currently available the extent to which a CNS-active drug like fluoxetine may be misused, diverted, and/or abused.

Despite the lack of substantial evidence for abuse potential or dependence liability, clinicians should carefully evaluate patients for a history of substance abuse prior to initiating fluoxetine therapy. If fluoxetine therapy is initiated in patients with a history of substance abuse, such patients should be monitored closely for signs of misuse or abuse of the drug (e.g., development of tolerance, use of increasing doses, drug-seeking behavior).

The potential for misuse of fluoxetine by depressed patients with concurrent eating disorders and/or those who may seek the drug for its appetite-suppressant effects also should be considered. One patient with an undisclosed history of anorexia nervosa and laxative abuse who was given fluoxetine for depression ingested larger-than-prescribed doses (e.g., 90–120 mg/day) and lost 9.1 kg within 2 months; this patient falsely claimed mood improvement in order to continue receiving the drug for its anorectic and weight-reducing effects.

Fluoxetine has produced phospholipidosis following long-term administration in animals; however, no evidence of phospholipidosis has been reported in humans receiving the drug to date. Additional study is needed to determine the clinical importance of these findings in patients receiving long-term fluoxetine therapy. (See Pharmacology: Effects on Phospholipids.)

PHARMACOLOGY

The pharmacology of fluoxetine is complex and in many ways resembles that of other antidepressant agents, particularly those agents (e.g., citalopram, clomipramine, escitalopram, fluvoxamine, paroxetine, sertraline, trazodone) that predominantly potentiate the pharmacologic effects of serotonin (5-HT). Like other selective serotonin-reuptake inhibitors (SSRIs), fluoxetine is a potent and highly selective reuptake inhibitor of serotonin and has little or no effect on other neurotransmitters.

● Nervous System Effects

The precise mechanism of antidepressant action of fluoxetine is unclear, but the drug has been shown to selectively inhibit the reuptake of serotonin at the presynaptic neuronal membrane. Fluoxetine-induced inhibition of serotonin reuptake causes increased synaptic concentrations of serotonin in the CNS, resulting in numerous functional changes associated with enhanced serotonergic neurotransmission. Like other selective serotonin-reuptake inhibitors (fluvoxamine, paroxetine, sertraline), fluoxetine appears to have minimal or no effect on the reuptake of norepinephrine or dopamine and does not exhibit clinically important anticholinergic, antihistaminic, or α_1-adrenergic blocking activity at usual therapeutic dosages.

Although the mechanism of antidepressant action of antidepressant agents may involve inhibition of the reuptake of various neurotransmitters (i.e., norepinephrine, serotonin) at the presynaptic neuronal membrane, it has been suggested that postsynaptic receptor modification is mainly responsible for the antidepressant action observed during long-term administration of antidepressant agents. During long-term therapy with most antidepressants (e.g., tricyclic antidepressants, monoamine oxidase [MAO] inhibitors), these adaptive changes generally consist of subsensitivity of the noradrenergic adenylate cyclase system in association with a decrease in the number of β-adrenergic receptors; such effects on noradrenergic receptor function commonly are referred to as "down-regulation." In addition, some antidepressants reportedly decrease the number of 5-HT binding sites following chronic administration. Fluoxetine may exert its antidepressant activity by somewhat different mechanisms than those usually associated with tricyclic and some other antidepressants. Although some evidence indicates that long-term administration of fluoxetine does not substantially decrease the number of β-adrenergic binding sites or reduce the sensitivity of β-adrenergic receptors, a decrease in the number of β-adrenergic binding sites in the brain has been reported in at least one study in animals. Data regarding the effects of fluoxetine on the number of serotonin (5-HT$_1$ and/or 5-HT$_2$) binding sites have been conflicting, with either no change or a reduction in the number of binding sites being reported during chronic administration of the drug. Increased postsynaptic receptor binding of GABA B also has been reported following prolonged

administration of many antidepressants, including fluoxetine. The clinical importance of these findings for fluoxetine has not been fully elucidated to date, and further study is needed to determine the role, if any, of binding site alteration in the antidepressant action of fluoxetine and other antidepressants.

The precise mechanism of action responsible for the efficacy of fluoxetine in the treatment of obsessive-compulsive disorder is unclear. However, based on the efficacy of other selective serotonin-reuptake inhibitors (e.g., fluvoxamine, paroxetine, sertraline) and clomipramine in the treatment of obsessive-compulsive disorder and the potency of these drugs in inhibiting serotonin reuptake, a serotonergic hypothesis has been developed to explain the pathogenesis of the condition. The hypothesis postulates that a dysregulation of serotonin is responsible for obsessive-compulsive disorder and that fluoxetine and these other agents are effective because they correct this imbalance. Although the available evidence supports the serotonergic hypothesis of obsessive-compulsive disorder, additional studies are necessary to confirm this hypothesis.

Serotonergic Effects

Fluoxetine is a highly selective inhibitor of serotonin reuptake at the presynaptic neuronal membrane. In addition, the potency and selectivity of serotonin-reuptake inhibition exhibited by fluoxetine's principal metabolite, norfluoxetine, appear to be similar to those of the parent drug. Fluoxetine- and norfluoxetine-induced inhibition of serotonin reuptake causes increased synaptic concentrations of serotonin, resulting in numerous functional changes associated with enhanced serotonergic neurotransmission.

Data from in vitro studies suggest that fluoxetine is approximately equivalent to or less potent than clomipramine as a serotonin-reuptake inhibitor; however, in vivo studies indicate that the serotonin-reuptake inhibiting effect of fluoxetine may be more potent than that of clomipramine on a weight as well as an equimolar basis. This apparent discrepancy may be explained at least in part by the relatively long elimination half-lives of fluoxetine and norfluoxetine. In addition, metabolism via N-demethylation decreases the potency and specificity of serotonin-reuptake inhibition of clomipramine but not fluoxetine. Data from both in vivo and in vitro studies indicate that fluoxetine also is a more potent serotonin-reuptake inhibitor than other currently available antidepressant agents, including imipramine and trazodone. Fluoxetine appears to have practically no affinity for serotonin (e.g., 5-HT$_1$ and 5-HT$_2$) receptors in vitro, although limited in vivo data suggest that the drug may bind to low-affinity sites on 5-HT receptors.

Fluoxetine appears to decrease the turnover of serotonin in the CNS, probably as a result of a decrease in the rate of serotonin synthesis. The drug reportedly decreases brain concentrations of 5-hydroxyindoleacetic acid (5-HIAA), the principal metabolite of serotonin; reduces the uptake of radiolabeled tryptophan by synaptosomes; and reduces the rate of conversion of tryptophan to serotonin. Fluoxetine also inhibits spontaneous firing of serotonergic neurons in the dorsal raphe nucleus.

Like other serotonin-reuptake inhibitors, administration of fluoxetine alone does not produce the serotonin behavioral syndrome (a characteristic behavioral pattern caused by central stimulation of serotonin activity) in animals. However, the drug potentiates the serotonin behavioral syndrome induced by oxitriptan (l-5-hydroxytryptophan, l-5HTP), MAO inhibitors, and MAO inhibitors combined with tryptophan.

Effects on Other Neurotransmitters

Like other selective serotonin-reuptake inhibitors, fluoxetine appears to have little or no effect on the reuptake of other neurotransmitters such as norepinephrine or dopamine. In addition, the drug appears to have a substantially higher selectivity ratio of serotonin-to-norepinephrine reuptake inhibiting activity than tricyclic antidepressant agents, including clomipramine.

Unlike tricyclic and some other antidepressants, fluoxetine does not exhibit clinically important anticholinergic, α_1-adrenergic blocking, or antihistaminic activity at usual therapeutic dosages. As a result, the incidence of adverse effects commonly associated with blockade of muscarinic cholinergic receptors (e.g., dry mouth, blurred vision, urinary retention, constipation, confusion), α_1-adrenergic receptors (e.g., orthostatic hypotension), and histamine H$_1$- and H$_2$-receptors (e.g., sedation) is lower in fluoxetine-treated patients. In vitro studies have demonstrated that the drug possesses only weak affinity for α_1- and α_2-adrenergic, β-adrenergic, H$_1$ and H$_2$, muscarinic, opiate, GABA-benzodiazepine, and dopamine receptors.

Effects on Sleep

Like tricyclic and most other antidepressants, fluoxetine suppresses rapid eye movement (REM) sleep. Although not clearly established, there is some evidence that the REM-suppressing effects of antidepressant agents may contribute to the antidepressant activity of these drugs. In animal studies, fluoxetine produces a dose-related suppression of REM sleep; the drug generally appears to reduce the amount of REM sleep by increasing REM latency (the time to onset of REM sleep) and by decreasing the number rather than the duration of REM episodes. Limited data in animals suggest that REM rebound does not occur following discontinuance of fluoxetine. The precise mechanism has not been fully elucidated, but results of animal studies indicate that fluoxetine's effects on REM sleep are serotonergically mediated. Like other specific serotonin-reuptake inhibitors (e.g., zimeldine [previously zimelidine]), the effects of fluoxetine on non-REM sleep reported to date have been variable and do not appear to be as clearly defined as those of tricyclic antidepressants, which usually increase slow-wave sleep.

Effects on EEG

Limited data currently are available regarding the effects of fluoxetine on the EEG. Substantial EEG changes did not occur following oral administration of single 30-mg doses of the drug in healthy individuals. An increase in alpha activity and a decrease in fast beta activity and slow activity were noted following single oral 60-mg doses in this study; such changes are characteristic of desipramine-type antidepressants and appear to indicate increased vigilance. Single 75-mg doses of fluoxetine produced an increase in slow and fast activity and a decrease in alpha activity; such EEG changes are similar to those observed with amitriptyline and imipramine and suggest possible sedative activity.

Effects on Psychomotor Function

Fluoxetine does not appear to cause clinically important sedation and does not interfere with psychomotor performance. Controlled studies in healthy young adults 21–45 of years and in adults with major depression did not demonstrate any adverse effects on psychomotor performance in those receiving the drug. No adverse effects on psychomotor performance or cognitive function were observed in men with depression older than 60 years of age who received 20-mg doses of fluoxetine in a controlled study. Results of this study showed that overall cognition, as assessed by the critical flicker fusion thresholds test, generally was better in patients receiving fluoxetine than in those receiving amitriptyline (a tricyclic antidepressant); however, less sedating tricyclic antidepressants (e.g., desipramine) were not included in the study and it is possible that fluoxetine may not have such an advantage over these other agents. In a controlled study evaluating the effects of fluoxetine (20 mg daily for 22 days) on psychomotor performance and car driving in healthy adults, the drug did not affect the highway driving or the car following tests but slightly impaired performance in correctly detecting changes in visual signals was evident in the sustained attention test.

Analgesic Effects

Like other serotonin-reuptake inhibitors (e.g., zimeldine), fluoxetine exhibits analgesic activity in some analgesic test systems when administered alone in animals, but the lack of such effects observed in other test systems suggests that demonstration of analgesic activity may be test-dependent. Fluoxetine has potentiated opiate agonist-induced analgesia in most but not all studies, possibly as a result of the drug's ability to enhance serotonergic neurotransmission. The clinical importance of these effects in the management of acute and chronic pain remains to be determined.

Effects on Respiration

Usual therapeutic dosages of fluoxetine do not appear to affect respiration substantially in humans; however, the effect of higher dosages of the drug on respiratory function remains to be established. In animals, administration of single 20-mg/kg doses of fluoxetine reportedly increased blood Po_2 concentrations but did not alter blood Pco_2 concentrations. The drug also has been shown to attenuate morphine-induced respiratory depression, although the precise mechanism for this effect has not been established.

Effects on Thermoregulation

Data are conflicting regarding the effect of fluoxetine on thermoregulation. In animals, fluoxetine has produced dose-dependent hypothermia in some studies, suggesting that serotonin may play a role in thermoregulation, but the drug has produced only slight or minimal hypothermia in other studies.

The drug has been used safely in at least one patient with established susceptibility to malignant hyperthermia; however, additional experience with the drug is needed to confirm the safety of fluoxetine in patients known to be susceptible to this condition.

• Cardiovascular Effects

The cardiovascular effects of fluoxetine have been studied in animals and to a limited extent in humans. Unlike some other antidepressant agents (e.g., tricyclic antidepressants, MAO inhibitors), fluoxetine has been associated with only minimal cardiovascular effects. The absence of substantial anticholinergic activity, α_1-adrenergic blocking activity, catecholamine-potentiating effects, and quinidine-like cardiotoxic effects appears to be the principal reason for the general lack of cardiovascular effects associated with fluoxetine.

Fluoxetine does not exhibit clinically important α_1-adrenergic blocking activity and does not inhibit catecholamine reuptake. Unlike tricyclic antidepressants, fluoxetine does not block the neuronal reuptake of norepinephrine and therefore does not potentiate the pressor response associated with administration of norepinephrine. In addition, the drug does not inhibit the reuptake of and has no effect on the pressor response to tyramine.

Fluoxetine does not appear to have substantial arrhythmogenic activity; however, safety of the drug in patients with a recent history of myocardial infarction or unstable cardiovascular disease has not been adequately evaluated to date. Fluoxetine generally does not appear to affect cardiac conduction, and clinically important ECG changes have not been reported in patients without preexisting heart disease receiving therapeutic dosages of the drug. Unlike tricyclic antidepressants, which commonly cause an increase in heart rate, fluoxetine reportedly reduces heart rate by an average of about 3 beats/minute in patients receiving usual therapeutic dosages of the antidepressant. (See Cautions: Cardiovascular Effects.) Unlike tricyclics, the drug does not appear to exhibit direct quinidine-like cardiotoxic activity, although the cardiovascular effects associated with fluoxetine overdosage have not been fully established to date. (See Acute Toxicity.)

• Effects on Appetite and Body Weight

Like some other serotonergic agents (e.g., fenfluramine [no longer commercially available in the US], zimeldine), fluoxetine possesses anorectic activity. Although the precise mechanism has not been clearly established, results of animal studies indicate that the drug's appetite-inhibiting action may result from serotonin-reuptake blockade and the resultant increase in serotonin availability at the neuronal synapse. Following administration of single and multiple doses of fluoxetine in both meal-fed and free-feeding animals, a reduction in food intake usually occurs, particularly at relatively high doses of the drug (i.e., 10 mg/kg). The anorectic effect of fluoxetine appears to be potentiated by oxitriptan. Tolerance to the anorectic effect of fluoxetine has not developed following short-term administration in humans and animals; however, long-term studies in humans are necessary to fully determine whether tolerance develops during chronic therapy with the drug.

In animal studies, fluoxetine has been shown to suppress palatability-induced food consumption (as determined by the volume of sweetened versus plain water ingested). Like fenfluramine, fluoxetine also appears to selectively suppress carbohydrate and overall food intake while maintaining protein intake. Such carbohydrate intake-suppressing and protein-sparing effects may be of potential clinical importance in the management of obesity; however, additional study is necessary. (See Uses: Obesity.) Fluoxetine therapy also has resulted in decreases in body weight in normal-weight and obese animals as well as in depressed, nondepressed, and obese individuals receiving the drug. (See Uses: Obesity and also see Cautions: Metabolic Effects.)

• Effects on Alcohol Intake

Like some other serotonergic agents, fluoxetine produces a dose-dependent decrease in voluntary alcohol intake in normal and alcohol-preferring animals. Like some other serotonin-reuptake inhibitors (e.g., citalopram, zimeldine), fluoxetine has been shown to reduce alcohol consumption in a limited number of heavy drinkers receiving 60 mg of the drug daily. Because serotonin appears to be involved in the regulation of alcohol intake, it has been suggested that fluoxetine may attenuate alcohol consumption via enhanced serotonergic neurotransmission. In addition, there is some evidence that such effects may be at least partially mediated by the renin-angiotensin-aldosterone system. (See Uses: Alcohol Dependence and see Drug Interactions: Alcohol.)

● Neuroendocrine Effects

Fluoxetine affects the endocrine system. Like other selective inhibitors of serotonin reuptake, the drug has produced a dose-related increase in serum corticosterone concentrations in animals. Fluoxetine also reportedly potentiates oxitriptan-induced elevation in serum corticosterone concentrations. Such effects appear to be serotonergically mediated. Following parenteral administration of fluoxetine in animals, the elevation in serum corticosterone concentration generally lasts only a few hours, although fluoxetine-induced inhibition of serotonin reuptake is known to persist for longer than 24 hours. Therefore, it has been suggested that other compensatory mechanisms, possibly including decreased firing of serotonergic neurons, may contribute to the restoration of normal hypothalamic-pituitary-adrenal (HPA) axis function despite prolonged blockade of serotonin reuptake by the drug. Fluoxetine also has increased corticotropin (ACTH) and vasopressin (antidiuretic hormone, ADH) concentrations in peripheral plasma and has increased corticotropin and corticotropin-releasing factor (CRF, corticoliberin) concentrations in hypophysial portal blood. These effects may represent the initial step in fluoxetine-induced elevation of plasma corticosterone concentrations.

The effects of fluoxetine on serum prolactin concentrations have not been clearly established. In some animal studies, fluoxetine potentiated tryptophan-induced increases in serum prolactin concentrations, although administration of the drug alone in animals and humans usually does not substantially alter prolactin concentrations. However, administration of fluoxetine alone reportedly increased serum prolactin concentrations in young but not old male rats in one study. Fluoxetine-induced effects on prolactin secretion appear to be serotonergically mediated.

● Effects on Phospholipids

Like many other cationic, amphiphilic drugs (e.g., amiodarone, fenfluramine, imipramine, ranitidine), fluoxetine reportedly increases tissue phospholipid concentrations following chronic administration in animal studies; however, such effects have not been demonstrated in humans receiving fluoxetine to date. Histologic examination following long-term (i.e., 1–12 months) fluoxetine administration in animals has revealed the presence of characteristic concentric, lamellar inclusion bodies associated with phospholipidosis in alveolar macrophages of the lung, Kupffer cells of the liver, and adrenal cortical cells; an increase in phospholipid content of the lung also has been reported. Fluoxetine-induced phospholipid accumulation in these animals was reversible within 1–2 months following discontinuance of the drug.

Studies in humans receiving fluoxetine have not revealed biochemical or clinical evidence of drug-induced phospholipidosis to date. There was no evidence of increased phospholipid content or changes in lamellar inclusion bodies in peripheral blood lymphocytes of either healthy individuals receiving 1 month of fluoxetine therapy or depressed patients receiving long-term (0.9–2.6 years) therapy with the drug. In addition, ophthalmologic examination and chest radiographs in patients receiving fluoxetine during clinical studies have not revealed evidence of phospholipidosis induced by the drug. Although data from clinical studies suggest that fluoxetine-induced phospholipidosis is unlikely to occur in humans receiving long-term therapy with the drug, further study is needed to fully determine whether the phospholipidosis observed in animal studies is clinically important in humans receiving therapeutic dosages of the drug.

● Other Effects

Fluoxetine has demonstrated some antimyoclonic activity in animals and humans when used in combination with oxitriptan. Although the mechanism of fluoxetine's antimyoclonic activity has not been fully elucidated, some forms of myoclonus appear to be related to impaired serotonergic neurotransmission. Therefore, it has been suggested that fluoxetine-induced enhancement of serotonergic neurotransmission via serotonin-reuptake blockade potentially may contribute to oxitriptan-induced increases in CNS serotonin concentrations in the management of this condition. (See Uses: Myoclonus.)

Fluoxetine also has reduced cataplexy in both humans and animals. (See Uses: Cataplexy.)

Fluoxetine reportedly has produced a dose-related elevation in plasma β-endorphin and β-lipotropin concentrations in healthy individuals receiving single oral doses of the drug.

PHARMACOKINETICS

In all human studies described in the Pharmacokinetics section, fluoxetine was administered as the hydrochloride salt.

● Absorption

Fluoxetine hydrochloride appears to be well absorbed from the GI tract following oral administration. The oral bioavailability of fluoxetine in humans has not been fully elucidated to date, but at least 60–80% of an oral dose appears to be absorbed. However, the relative proportion of an oral dose reaching systemic circulation unchanged currently is not known. The conventional and delayed-release capsules, tablets, and solution of fluoxetine hydrochloride reportedly are bioequivalent. However, onset of absorption of fluoxetine hydrochloride delayed-release capsules (Prozac® Weekly®) is delayed 1–2 hours relative to the onset of absorption when the drug is administered as a conventional preparation. Limited data from animals suggest that the drug may undergo first-pass metabolism and extraction in the liver and/or lung following oral administration. In these animals (beagles), approximately 72% of an oral dose reached systemic circulation unchanged. Food appears to cause a slight decrease in the rate, but not the extent, of absorption of fluoxetine in humans.

Peak plasma fluoxetine concentrations usually occur within 4–8 hours (range: 1.5–12 hours) after oral administration of conventional preparations. Following oral administration of a single 40-mg dose of the drug in healthy fasting adults, peak plasma concentrations of approximately 15–55 ng/mL are attained. Peak plasma fluoxetine concentrations following administration of single oral doses of 20–80 mg are approximately proportional and are linearly related to dose, although there appears to be considerable interindividual variation in plasma concentrations attained with a given dose. The manufacturer states that the peak plasma concentrations achieved following weekly administration of fluoxetine 90-mg delayed-release capsules are in the range of the average concentrations achieved following daily administration of 20-mg conventional preparations; however, average trough concentrations are reported to be lower following weekly administration of the delayed-release preparation. Peak-to-trough fluctuations in plasma concentrations of fluoxetine and norfluoxetine (the principal metabolite) reportedly are greater following weekly administration of the delayed-release capsules (164 and 43%, respectively) compared with daily administration of conventional preparations (24 and 17%, respectively).

Preliminary data suggest that fluoxetine may exhibit nonlinear accumulation following multiple dosing. (See Pharmacokinetics: Elimination.) The relatively slow elimination of fluoxetine and its active metabolite, norfluoxetine, leads to clinically important accumulation of these active species in chronic use and delayed attainment of steady state, even when a fixed dose is used. In healthy adults receiving 40 mg of fluoxetine daily for 30 days, plasma concentrations of 91–302 and 72–258 ng/mL of fluoxetine and norfluoxetine, respectively, were attained. These plasma concentrations of fluoxetine were higher than those predicted by single-dose studies because fluoxetine's metabolism is not proportional to dose. In addition, prolonged administration of the drug and/or patient's disease states did not appear to affect steady-state concentrations. In one study, steady-state plasma fluoxetine and norfluoxetine concentrations did not differ substantially among healthy individuals receiving 4 weeks of fluoxetine therapy, depressed patients receiving 5 weeks of fluoxetine therapy, or depressed patients receiving more than a year of fluoxetine therapy.

Average steady-state fluoxetine and norfluoxetine concentrations, however, were affected by patient age. In pediatric patients with major depressive disorder or obsessive-compulsive disorder (OCD) who received fluoxetine 20 mg daily for up to 62 days, average steady-state concentrations of fluoxetine and norfluoxetine in children 6–12 years of age were 2- and 1.5-fold higher, respectively, than in adolescents 13–17 years of age who received the same fluoxetine regimen. These results are consistent with those observed in another study in 94 pediatric patients 8–17 years of age diagnosed with major depressive disorder, and can be almost entirely explained by differences in children's weight. Higher average steady-state fluoxetine and norfluoxetine concentrations also were observed in children relative to adults; however, these concentrations were within the range of concentrations observed in the adult population. As in adults, fluoxetine and norfluoxetine accumulated extensively following multiple oral dosing. Following daily oral administration of the drug, steady-state plasma fluoxetine and norfluoxetine concentrations generally are achieved within about 2–4 weeks.

The manufacturer states that average steady-state plasma fluoxetine concentrations are approximately 50% lower with weekly administration of the 90-mg delayed-release capsules compared with daily administration of a 20-mg conventional preparation. In patients being switched from daily therapy with fluoxetine 20-mg conventional preparations to weekly therapy with fluoxetine 90-mg delayed-release capsules, peak plasma fluoxetine concentrations reportedly were

1.7 times higher with the weekly regimen than with the established daily regimen when there was no transition period (i.e., therapy with delayed-release fluoxetine was initiated the day after the last daily dose of fluoxetine 20 mg). When weekly therapy was initiated one week after the last daily dose of fluoxetine 20 mg, peak plasma fluoxetine concentrations for the 2 regimens were similar. (See Dosage and Administration: Dosage.)

The onset of antidepressant activity following oral administration of fluoxetine hydrochloride usually occurs within the first 1–3 weeks of therapy, but optimum therapeutic effect usually requires 4 weeks or more of therapy with the drug. Maximal EEG changes and behavioral changes on psychometric tests reportedly occur about 8–10 hours after single oral doses of the drug; the delay in maximal CNS effects compared with achievement of peak plasma fluoxetine concentrations may relate to formation of an active metabolite or to delayed distribution of the parent drug and its principal metabolite into the CNS.

The relationship between plasma fluoxetine and norfluoxetine concentrations and the therapeutic and/or toxic effects of the drug has not been clearly established. In a group of patients receiving fluoxetine for the management of major depressive disorder, there was no correlation between plasma fluoxetine, norfluoxetine, or total fluoxetine plus norfluoxetine concentrations and either the antidepressant response or the weight-reducing effect of the drug.

● **Distribution**

Distribution of fluoxetine and its metabolites into human body tissues and fluids has not been fully characterized. Limited pharmacokinetic data obtained during long-term administration of fluoxetine to animals suggest that the drug and some of its metabolites, including norfluoxetine, are widely distributed in body tissues, with highest concentrations occurring in the lungs and liver. The drug crosses the blood-brain barrier in humans and animals. In animals, fluoxetine:norfluoxetine ratios reportedly were similar in the cerebral cortex, corpus striatum, hippocampus, hypothalamus, brain stem, and cerebellum 1 hour after administration of a single dose of the drug.

The apparent volumes of distribution of fluoxetine and norfluoxetine in healthy adults each reportedly average 20–45 L/kg. Limited data suggest that the volume of distribution of fluoxetine is not altered substantially following multiple dosing. The apparent volume of distribution of norfluoxetine reportedly is higher in patients with cirrhosis than in healthy individuals, although this difference may reflect decreases in the rates of formation and elimination of the metabolite rather than changes in volume of distribution. The volumes of distribution of fluoxetine and norfluoxetine do not appear to be altered substantially in patients with renal impairment.

At in vitro plasma concentrations of 200–1000 ng/mL, fluoxetine is approximately 94.5% bound to plasma proteins, including albumin and α_1-acid glycoprotein (α_1-AGP); the extent of protein binding appears to be independent of plasma concentration. The extent of fluoxetine protein binding does not appear to be altered substantially in patients with hepatic cirrhosis or renal impairment, including those undergoing hemodialysis.

It is not known whether fluoxetine or its metabolites cross the placenta in humans, but fluoxetine and norfluoxetine reportedly cross the placenta in rats following oral administration. Fluoxetine and norfluoxetine are distributed into milk. Limited data indicate that concentrations of the drug and this metabolite in milk are about 20–30% of concurrent plasma concentrations.

● **Elimination**

Fluoxetine and norfluoxetine, the principal metabolite, are eliminated slowly. Following a single oral dose of fluoxetine in healthy adults, the elimination half-life of fluoxetine reportedly averages approximately 2–3 days (range: 1–9 days) and that of norfluoxetine averages about 7–9 days (range: 3–15 days). The plasma half-life of fluoxetine exhibits considerable interindividual variation, which may be related to genetic differences in the rate of N-demethylation of the drug in the liver. The absence of either a bimodal or trimodal distribution of clearance values suggests that the rate of such metabolism may be under polygenic control. The half-life of fluoxetine reportedly is prolonged (to approximately 4–5 days) after administration of multiple versus single doses, suggesting a nonlinear pattern of drug accumulation during long-term administration. Norfluoxetine appears to exhibit dose-proportional pharmacokinetics following multiple dosing, although limited data indicate that the rate of formation of the metabolite is decreased slightly once steady-state plasma concentrations have been achieved.

Following oral administration of single doses of fluoxetine in healthy individuals, total apparent plasma clearances of fluoxetine and norfluoxetine average

approximately 346 mL/minute (range: 94–703 mL/minute) and 145 mL/minute (range: 61–284 mL/minute), respectively. Limited data suggest that plasma clearance of fluoxetine decreases by approximately 75% following multiple oral doses of the drug once steady-state plasma fluoxetine concentrations have been achieved. Plasma clearances of fluoxetine and norfluoxetine also reportedly are decreased in patients with chronic liver disease (e.g., cirrhosis). Evidence from single-dose studies indicates that clearances of the drug and its principal metabolite are not altered substantially in patients with renal impairment.

The exact metabolic fate of fluoxetine has not been fully elucidated. The drug appears to be metabolized extensively, probably in the liver, to norfluoxetine and several other metabolites. Norfluoxetine (desmethylfluoxetine), the principal metabolite, is formed by N-demethylation of fluoxetine, which may be under polygenic control. The potency and selectivity of norfluoxetine's serotonin-reuptake inhibiting activity appear to be similar to those of the parent drug. Both fluoxetine and norfluoxetine undergo conjugation with glucuronic acid in the liver, and limited evidence from animals suggests that both the parent drug and its principal metabolite also undergo O-dealkylation to form p-trifluoromethylphenol, which subsequently appears to be metabolized to hippuric acid.

Following oral administration, fluoxetine and its metabolites are excreted principally in urine. In healthy individuals, approximately 60% of an orally administered, radiolabeled dose of fluoxetine is excreted in urine within 35 days, with approximately 72.8% of excreted drug as unidentified metabolites, 10% as norfluoxetine, 9.5% as norfluoxetine glucuronide, 5.2% as fluoxetine glucuronide, and 2.5% as unchanged drug. Approximately 12% of the dose was eliminated in feces within 28 days following oral administration, but the relative proportion of unabsorbed versus absorbed drug that is excreted in feces (e.g., via biliary elimination) is not known.

The effect of age on the elimination of fluoxetine has not been fully elucidated. Single-dose studies suggest that the pharmacokinetics of fluoxetine in healthy geriatric individuals do not differ substantially from those in younger adults. However, because the drug has a relatively long half-life and nonlinear disposition following multiple-dose administration, single-dose studies are not sufficient to exclude the possibility of altered pharmacokinetics in geriatric individuals, particularly those with systemic disease and/or in those receiving multiple medications concomitantly. The elimination half-lives of fluoxetine and norfluoxetine may be prolonged in patients with hepatic impairment. Following a single oral dose of the drug in patients with hepatic cirrhosis, the elimination half-lives of fluoxetine and norfluoxetine reportedly average approximately 7 and 12 days, respectively.

The elimination half-lives of fluoxetine and norfluoxetine do not appear to be altered substantially in patients with renal impairment following oral administration of single doses of fluoxetine. In addition, chronic fluoxetine administration in depressed patients on hemodialysis produced steady-state plasma fluoxetine and norfluoxetine concentrations that were comparable with those observed in patients with normal renal function.

Fluoxetine and norfluoxetine are not removed substantially by hemodialysis. Because of the large volume of distribution and extensive protein binding of the drug and its principal metabolite, peritoneal dialysis, forced diuresis, hemoperfusion, and/or exchange transfusion also are likely to be ineffective in removing substantial amounts of fluoxetine and norfluoxetine from the body.

CHEMISTRY AND STABILITY

● **Chemistry**

Fluoxetine, a selective serotonin-reuptake inhibitor (SSRI) antidepressant, is a phenylpropylamine-derivative. The drug differs structurally from other selective serotonin-reuptake inhibitor antidepressants (e.g., citalopram, paroxetine, sertraline) and also differs structurally and pharmacologically from other currently available antidepressant agents (e.g., tricyclic antidepressants, monoamine oxidase inhibitors).

Fluoxetine contains a p-trifluoromethyl substituent that appears to contribute to the drug's high selectivity and potency for inhibiting serotonin reuptake, possibly as a result of its electron-withdrawing effect and lipophilicity. The commercially available drug is a racemic mixture of 2 optical isomers. Limited in vivo and in vitro data suggest that the pharmacologic activities of the optical isomers do not differ substantially, although the dextrorotatory isomer appears to have slightly greater serotonin-reuptake inhibiting activity and a longer duration of action than the levorotatory isomer.

Fluoxetine is commercially available as the hydrochloride salt, which occurs as a white to off-white crystalline solid and has a solubility of 14 mg/mL in water.

● *Stability*

Fluoxetine hydrochloride conventional and delayed-release capsules should be stored at 15–30°C and protected from light. Fluoxetine hydrochloride tablets and oral solution should be stored at 20–25°C and protected from light.

PREPARATIONS

Excipients in commercially available drug preparations may have clinically important effects in some individuals; consult specific product labeling for details.

FLUoxetine Hydrochloride

Oral		
Capsules	10 mg (of fluoxetine)*	**FLUoxetine Hydrochloride Capsules**
		PROzac® Pulvules®, Dista
		Sarafem® Pulvules®, Lilly
	20 mg (of fluoxetine)*	**FLUoxetine Hydrochloride Capsules**
		PROzac® Pulvules®, Dista
		Sarafem® Pulvules®, Lilly
	40 mg (of fluoxetine)*	**FLUoxetine Hydrochloride Capsules**
		PROzac® Pulvules®, Dista
Capsules, delayed-release (containing enteric-coated pellets)	90 mg (of fluoxetine)	**PROzac® Weekly**, Dista
Solution	20 mg (of fluoxetine) per 5 mL*	**FLUoxetine Hydrochloride Oral Solution**

Tablets	10 mg (of fluoxetine)*	**FLUoxetine Hydrochloride Tablets**
		Sarafem®, Warner Chilcott
	15 mg (of fluoxetine)*	**Sarafem®**, Warner Chilcott
	20 mg (of fluoxetine)*	**FLUoxetine Hydrochloride Tablets**
		Sarafem®, Warner Chilcott
	60 mg (of fluoxetine)*	**FLUoxetine Hydrochloride Tablets**

* available from one or more manufacturer, distributor, and/or repackager by generic (nonproprietary) name

FLUoxetine Hydrochloride Combinations

Oral		
Capsules	25 mg (of fluoxetine) with Olanzapine 3 mg*	**Symbyax®**, Lilly
	25 mg (of fluoxetine) with Olanzapine 6 mg*	**Symbyax®**, Lilly
	25 mg (of fluoxetine) with Olanzapine 12 mg*	**Symbyax®**, Lilly
	50 mg (of fluoxetine) with Olanzapine 6 mg*	**Symbyax®**, Lilly
	50 mg (of fluoxetine) with Olanzapine 12 mg*	**Symbyax®**, Lilly

* available from one or more manufacturer, distributor, and/or repackager by generic (nonproprietary) name

† Use is not currently included in the labeling approved by the US Food and Drug Administration.

Selected Revisions October 3, 2014, © Copyright, July 1, 1989, American Society of Health-System Pharmacists, Inc.

Sertraline Hydrochloride

28:16.04.20 • SELECTIVE SEROTONIN-REUPTAKE INHIBITORS

■ Sertraline, a selective serotonin-reuptake inhibitor (SSRI), is an antidepressant agent.

USES

● Major Depressive Disorder

Sertraline is used in the treatment of major depressive disorder. A major depressive episode implies a prominent and relatively persistent depressed or dysphoric mood that usually interferes with daily functioning (nearly every day for at least 2 weeks). According to DSM-IV criteria, a major depressive episode includes at least 5 of the following 9 symptoms (with at least one of the symptoms being either depressed mood or loss of interest or pleasure): depressed mood most of the day as indicated by subjective report (e.g., feels sad or empty) or observation made by others; markedly diminished interest or pleasure in all, or almost all, activities most of the day; significant weight loss (when not dieting) or weight gain (e.g., a change of more than 5% of body weight in a month), or decrease or increase in appetite; insomnia or hypersomnia; psychomotor agitation or retardation (observable by others, not merely subjective feelings of restlessness or being slowed down); fatigue or loss of energy; feelings of worthlessness or excessive or inappropriate guilt (not merely self-reproach or guilt about being sick); diminished ability to think or concentrate or indecisiveness (either by subjective account or as observed by others); and recurrent thoughts of death, recurrent suicidal ideation without a specific plan, or a suicide attempt or specific plan for committing suicide.

Treatment of major depressive disorder generally consists of an acute phase (to induce remission), a continuation phase (to preserve remission), and a maintenance phase (to prevent recurrence). Various interventions (e.g., psychotherapy, antidepressant drug therapy, electroconvulsive therapy [ECT]) are used alone or in combination to treat major depressive episodes. Treatment should be individualized and the most appropriate strategy for a particular patient is determined by clinical factors such as severity of depression (e.g., mild, moderate, severe), presence or absence of certain psychiatric features (e.g., suicide risk, catatonia, psychotic or atypical features, alcohol or substance abuse or dependence, panic or other anxiety disorder, cognitive dysfunction, dysthymia, personality disorder, seasonal affective disorder), and concurrent illness (e.g., asthma, cardiac disease, dementia, seizure disorder, glaucoma, hypertension). Demographic and psychosocial factors as well as patient preference also are used to determine the most effective treatment strategy.

While use of psychotherapy alone may be considered as an initial treatment strategy for patients with mild to moderate major depressive disorder (based on patient preference and presence of clinical features such as psychosocial stressors), combined use of antidepressant drug therapy and psychotherapy may be useful for initial treatment of patients with moderate to severe major depressive disorder with psychosocial issues, interpersonal problems, or a comorbid axis II disorder. In addition, combined use of antidepressant drug therapy and psychotherapy may be beneficial in patients who have a history of poor compliance or only partial response to adequate trials of either antidepressant drug therapy or psychotherapy alone.

Antidepressant drug therapy can be used alone for initial treatment of patients with mild major depressive disorder (if preferred by the patient) and usually is indicated alone or in combination with psychotherapy for initial treatment of patients with moderate to severe major depressive disorder (unless ECT is planned). ECT is not generally used for initial treatment of uncomplicated major depression, but is recommended as first-line treatment for severe major depressive disorder when it is coupled with psychotic features, catatonic stupor, severe suicidality, food refusal leading to nutritional compromise, or other situations when a rapid antidepressant response is required. ECT also is recommended for patients who have previously shown a positive response or a preference for this treatment modality and can be considered for patients with moderate or severe depression who have not responded to or cannot receive antidepressant drug therapy. In certain situations involving depressed patients unresponsive to adequate trials of several individual antidepressant agents, adjunctive therapy with another agent (e.g., buspirone, lithium) or concomitant use of a second antidepressant agent (e.g., bupropion) has been used; however,

such combination therapy is associated with an increased risk of adverse reactions, may require dosage adjustments, and (if not contraindicated) should be undertaken only after careful consideration of the relative risks and benefits. (See Drug Interactions: Serotonergic Drugs, Drug Interactions: Tricyclic and Other Antidepressants, and Drug Interactions: Lithium.)

The efficacy of sertraline for the acute treatment of major depression has been established by 2 placebo-controlled studies in adult outpatients who met DSM-III criteria for major depression. In the first study of 8 weeks' duration, sertraline was administered with flexible dosing in a range of 50–200 mg daily; the mean daily dosage for patients completing the study was 145 mg daily. In the second study of 6 weeks' duration, sertraline was administered in fixed doses of 50, 100, and 200 mg daily. Overall, these 2 studies demonstrated that sertraline was superior to placebo in improving scores on the Hamilton Depression Rating Scale and the Clinical Global Impression Severity and Improvement Scales. However, the second study was not readily interpretable regarding whether there was a dose-response relationship for the drug's efficacy.

In a third study, depressed outpatients who had responded by the end of an initial 8-week open treatment phase to sertraline 50–200 mg daily were randomized to continue sertraline in the same dosage range or placebo for 44 weeks in a double-blind manner. The mean daily dosage of sertraline in those who completed this long-term study was 70 mg daily, and the relapse rate in the sertraline-treated patients was substantially lower than in those who received placebo.

An analysis of these 3 controlled studies for possible gender-related effects on treatment outcome did not suggest any difference in efficacy based on the gender of the patient.

While the optimum duration of sertraline therapy has not been established, many experts state that acute depressive episodes require several months or longer of sustained antidepressant therapy. In addition, some clinicians recommend that long-term antidepressant therapy be considered in certain patients at risk for recurrence of depressive episodes (such as those with highly recurrent unipolar depression). The efficacy of sertraline in maintaining an antidepressant response for up to 1 year without increased toxicity has been demonstrated in a controlled setting. The manufacturers state that the usefulness of the drug in patients receiving prolonged therapy should be reevaluated periodically. (See Dosage and Administration: Dosage.)

The manufacturers state that the drug's antidepressant efficacy in hospital settings has not been adequately studied to date.

As with certain other antidepressants, the possibility that sertraline may precipitate hypomanic or manic attacks in patients with bipolar or other major affective disorder should be considered. Sertraline is *not* approved for use in treating bipolar depression in adults.

Considerations in Choosing an Antidepressant

A variety of antidepressant drugs is available for the treatment of major depressive disorder, including selective serotonin-reuptake inhibitors (SSRIs; e.g., citalopram, escitalopram, fluoxetine, paroxetine, sertraline), selective serotonin- and norepinephrine-reuptake inhibitors (SNRIs; e.g., desvenlafaxine, duloxetine, venlafaxine), tricyclic antidepressants (e.g., amitriptyline, amoxapine, desipramine, doxepin, imipramine, nortriptyline, protriptyline, trimipramine), monoamine oxidase (MAO) inhibitors (e.g., phenelzine, tranylcypromine), and other antidepressants (e.g., bupropion, maprotiline, nefazodone, trazodone, vilazodone). Most clinical studies have shown that the antidepressant effect of usual dosages of sertraline in patients with depression is greater than that of placebo and comparable to that of usual dosages of tricyclic antidepressants (e.g., amitriptyline), other SSRIs (e.g., fluoxetine), and other antidepressants (e.g., nefazodone). In geriatric patients with major depression, sertraline appears to be as effective as amitriptyline. The onset of action of sertraline appears to be comparable to that of tricyclic antidepressants.

In general, response rates in patients with major depression are similar for currently available antidepressants, and the choice of antidepressant agent for a given patient depends principally on other factors such as potential adverse effects, safety or tolerability of these adverse effects in the individual patient, psychiatric and medical history, patient or family history of response to specific therapies, patient preference, quantity and quality of available clinical data, cost, and relative acute overdose safety. No single antidepressant can be recommended as optimal for all patients because of substantial heterogeneity in individual responses and in the nature, likelihood, and severity of adverse effects. In addition, patients vary in the degree to which certain adverse effects and other inconveniences of drug therapy (e.g., cost, dietary restrictions) affect their preferences.

In the large-scale Sequenced Treatment Alternatives to Relieve Depression (STAR*D) effectiveness trial, patients with major depressive disorder who did not respond to or could not tolerate therapy with one SSRI (citalopram) were randomized to switch to extended-release ("sustained-release") bupropion, sertraline, or extended-release venlafaxine as a second step of treatment (level 2). Remission rates as assessed by the 17-item Hamilton Rating Scale for Depression (HRSD-17) and the Quick Inventory of Depressive Symptomatology—Self Report (QIDS-SR-16) were approximately 21 and 26% for extended-release bupropion, 18 and 27% for sertraline, and 25 and 25% for extended-release venlafaxine therapy, respectively; response rates as assessed by the QIDS-SR-16 were 26, 27, and 28% for extended-release bupropion, sertraline, and extended-release venlafaxine therapy, respectively. These results suggest that after unsuccessful initial treatment of depressed patients with an SSRI, approximately 25% of patients will achieve remission after therapy is switched to another antidepressant and that either another SSRI (e.g., sertraline) or an agent from another class (e.g., bupropion, venlafaxine) may be reasonable alternative antidepressants in patients not responding to initial SSRI therapy.

Patient Tolerance Considerations

Because of differences in the adverse effect profile between SSRIs and tricyclic antidepressants, particularly less frequent anticholinergic effects, cardiovascular effects, and weight gain with SSRIs, these drugs may be preferred in patients in whom such effects are not tolerated or are of potential concern. The decreased incidence of anticholinergic effects associated with sertraline and other SSRIs compared with tricyclic antidepressants is a potential advantage, since such effects may result in discontinuance of the drug early during therapy in unusually sensitive patients. In addition, some anticholinergic effects may become troublesome during long-term tricyclic antidepressant therapy (e.g., persistent dry mouth may result in tooth decay). Although SSRIs share the same overall tolerability profile, certain patients may tolerate one drug in this class better than another. In an open study, most patients who had discontinued fluoxetine therapy because of adverse effects subsequently tolerated sertraline therapy. Antidepressants other than SSRIs may be preferred in patients in whom certain adverse GI effects (e.g., nausea, anorexia), nervous system effects (e.g., anxiety, nervousness, insomnia), and/or weight loss are not tolerated or are of concern, since such effects appear to occur more frequently with this class of drugs.

Pediatric Considerations

The clinical presentation of depression in children and adolescents can differ from that in adults and generally varies with the age and developmental stages of the child. Younger children may exhibit behavioral problems such as social withdrawal, aggressive behavior, apathy, sleep disruption, and weight loss; adolescents may present with somatic complaints, self esteem problems, rebelliousness, poor performance in school, or a pattern of engaging in risky or aggressive behavior.

Only limited data are available to date from controlled clinical studies evaluating various antidepressant agents in children and adolescents, and many of these studies have methodologic limitations (e.g., nonrandomized or uncontrolled, small sample size, short duration, nonspecific inclusion criteria). However, there is some evidence that the response to antidepressants in pediatric patients may differ from that seen in adults, and caution should be used in extrapolating data from adult studies when making treatment decisions for pediatric patients. Results of several studies evaluating tricyclic antidepressants (e.g., amitriptyline, desipramine, imipramine, nortriptyline) in preadolescent and adolescent patients with major depression indicate a lack of overall efficacy in this age group. Based on the lack of efficacy data regarding use of tricyclic antidepressants and MAO inhibitors in pediatric patients and because of the potential for life-threatening adverse effects associated with the use of these drugs, many experts consider selective serotonin-reuptake inhibitors, including sertraline, the drugs of choice when antidepressant therapy is indicated for the treatment of major depressive disorder in children and adolescents. However, the US Food and Drug Administration (FDA) states that, while efficacy of fluoxetine has been established in pediatric patients, efficacy of other newer antidepressants (i.e., sertraline, citalopram, desvenlafaxine, duloxetine, escitalopram, fluvoxamine, mirtazapine, nefazodone, paroxetine, venlafaxine) was not conclusively established in clinical trials in pediatric patients with major depressive disorder. In addition, FDA now warns that antidepressants increase the risk of suicidal thinking and behavior (suicidality) in children and adolescents with major depressive disorder and other psychiatric disorders. (See Cautions: Pediatric Precautions.) FDA currently states that anyone considering using an antidepressant in a child or adolescent for any clinical use must balance the potential risk of therapy with the clinical need. (See Cautions: Precautions and Contraindications.)

Geriatric Considerations

The response to antidepressants in depressed geriatric patients without dementia is similar to that reported in younger adults, but depression in geriatric patients often is not recognized and is not treated. In geriatric patients with major depressive disorder, selective serotonin-reuptake inhibitors (SSRIs) appear to be as effective as tricyclic antidepressants (e.g., amitriptyline) but generally are associated with fewer overall adverse effects than these other agents. Geriatric patients appear to be especially sensitive to anticholinergic (e.g., dry mouth, constipation, vision disturbance), cardiovascular, orthostatic hypotensive, and sedative effects of tricyclic antidepressants. The low incidence of anticholinergic effects associated with sertraline and other SSRIs compared with tricyclic antidepressants also is a potential advantage in geriatric patients, since such effects (e.g., constipation, dry mouth, confusion, memory impairment) may be particularly troublesome in these patients. However, SSRI therapy may be associated with other troublesome adverse effects (e.g., nausea and vomiting, agitation and akathisia, parkinsonian adverse effects, sexual dysfunction, weight loss, hyponatremia). Some clinicians state that SSRIs such as sertraline may be preferred for treating depression in geriatric patients in whom the orthostatic hypotension associated with many antidepressants (e.g., tricyclics) potentially may result in injuries (such as severe falls). However, despite the fewer cardiovascular and anticholinergic effects associated with SSRIs, these drugs did not show any advantage over tricyclic antidepressants with regard to hip fracture in a case-control study. In addition, there was little difference in the rates of falls between nursing home residents receiving SSRIs and those receiving tricyclic antidepressants in a retrospective study. Therefore, all geriatric individuals receiving either type of antidepressant should be considered at increased risk of falls and appropriate measures should be taken. In addition, clinicians prescribing SSRIs in geriatric patients should be aware of the many possible drug interactions associated with these drugs, including those involving metabolism of the drugs through the cytochrome P-450 system. (See Drug Interactions.)

Patients with dementia of the Alzheimer's type (Alzheimer's disease, presenile or senile dementia) often present with depressive symptoms, such as depressed mood, appetite loss, insomnia, fatigue, irritability, and agitation. Most experts recommend that patients with dementia of the Alzheimer's type who present with clinically important and persistent depressive symptoms be considered as candidates for pharmacotherapy even if they fail to meet the criteria for a major depressive syndrome. The goals of such therapy are to improve mood, functional status (e.g., cognition), and quality of life. Treatment of depression also may reduce other neuropsychiatric symptoms associated with depression in patients with dementia, including aggression, anxiety, apathy, and psychosis. Although patients may present with depressed mood alone, the possibility of more extensive depressive symptomatology should be considered. Therefore, patients should be evaluated and monitored carefully for indices of major depression, suicidal ideation, and neurovegetative signs since safety measures (e.g., hospitalization for suicidality) and more vigorous and aggressive therapy (e.g., relatively high dosages, multiple drug trials) may be needed in some patients.

Although placebo-controlled trials of antidepressants in depressed patients with concurrent dementia have shown mixed results, the available evidence and experience with the use of antidepressants in patients with dementia of the Alzheimer's type and associated depressive manifestations indicate that depressive symptoms (including depressed mood alone and with neurovegetative changes) in such patients are responsive to antidepressant therapy. In some patients, cognitive deficits may partially or fully resolve during antidepressant therapy, but the extent of response will be limited to the degree of cognitive impairment that is directly related to depression. SSRIs such as sertraline, citalopram, escitalopram, fluoxetine, or paroxetine are generally considered as first-line agents in the treatment of depressed patients with dementia since they are better tolerated than some other antidepressants (e.g., tricyclic antidepressants, monoamine oxidase inhibitors). Some possible alternative agents to SSRIs include bupropion, mirtazapine, and venlafaxine. Some geriatric patients with dementia and depression may be unable to tolerate the antidepressant dosages needed to achieve full remission. When a rapid antidepressant response is not critical, some experts therefore recommend a very gradual dosage increase to increase the likelihood that a therapeutic dosage of the SSRI or other antidepressant will be reached and tolerated. In a randomized, placebo-controlled study in a limited number of patients with major depression and Alzheimer's disease, sertraline was found to be superior to placebo; depression reduction in this study was accompanied by lessened behavior disturbance and improved activities of daily living but not improved cognition.

Cardiovascular Considerations

The relatively low incidence of adverse cardiovascular effects, including orthostatic hypotension and conduction disturbances, associated with sertraline and most other SSRIs may be advantageous in patients in whom the cardiovascular effects associated with tricyclic antidepressants may be hazardous. Patients with a recent history of myocardial infarction or unstable cardiovascular disease were excluded from premarketing clinical studies with sertraline. However, the cardiovascular safety of sertraline (50–200 mg daily for 24 weeks; mean dosage of 89 mg daily) was evaluated in a postmarketing, double-blind, placebo-controlled study in adult outpatients with major depressive disorder and a recent history of myocardial infarction or unstable angina pectoris requiring hospitalization but who were otherwise free of life-threatening medical conditions. When therapy was initiated during the acute phase of recovery (within 30 days after a myocardial infarction or hospitalization for unstable angina), sertraline therapy did not differ from placebo on the following cardiovascular end points at week 16: left ventricular ejection fraction and total cardiovascular events (angina, chest pain, edema, palpitations, syncope, postural dizziness, chronic heart failure, myocardial infarction, tachycardia, bradycardia, blood pressure changes). Although not statistically significant, approximately 20% fewer major cardiovascular events involving death or requiring hospitalization (e.g., for myocardial infarction, chronic heart failure, stroke, angina) occurred in the sertraline-treated patients compared with those receiving placebo. (See Cautions: Cardiovascular Effects and also see Cautions: Precautions and Contraindications.)

Sedative Considerations

Because sertraline and other SSRIs are generally less sedating than some other antidepressants (e.g., tricyclics), some clinicians state that these drugs may be preferable in patients who do not require the sedative effects associated with many antidepressant agents; however, an antidepressant with more prominent sedative effects (e.g., trazodone) may be preferable in certain patients (e.g., those with insomnia).

Suicidal Risk Considerations

Suicide is a known risk of depression and certain other psychiatric disorders, and these disorders themselves are the strongest predictors of suicide. However, there has been a long-standing concern that antidepressants may have a role in inducing worsening of depression and the emergence of suicidal thinking and behavior (suicidality) in certain patients during the early phases of treatment. FDA states that antidepressants increased the risk of suicidality in short-term studies in children, adolescents, and young adults (18–24 years of age) with major depressive disorder and other psychiatric disorders. (See Cautions: Pediatric Precautions.) An increased suicidality risk was not demonstrated with antidepressants compared with placebo in adults older than 24 years of age and a reduced risk was observed in adults 65 years of age or older. It currently is unknown whether the suicidality risk extends to longer-term antidepressant use (i.e., beyond several months); however, there is substantial evidence from placebo-controlled maintenance trials in adults with major depressive disorder that antidepressants can delay the recurrence of depression. Because the risk of suicidality in depressed patients may persist until substantial remission of depression occurs, appropriate monitoring and close observation of all patients who are receiving antidepressant therapy is recommended. (See Cautions: Precautions and Contraindications.)

Other Considerations

Sertraline has been effective in patients with moderate to severe depression.

In the Sequenced Treatment Alternatives to Relieve Depression (STAR*D) level 2 trial, patients with major depressive disorder who did not respond to or could not tolerate therapy with citalopram (another SSRI) were randomized to receive either extended-release ("sustained-release") bupropion or buspirone therapy in addition to citalopram. Although both extended-release bupropion and buspirone were found to produce similar remission rates, extended-release bupropion produced a greater reduction in the number and severity of symptoms and a lower rate of drug discontinuance than buspirone in this large-scale, effectiveness trial. These results suggest that augmentation of SSRI therapy with extended-release bupropion may be useful in some patients with refractory depression.

Sertraline has been effective in patients with depression and concurrent human immunodeficiency virus (HIV) infection and depression with anxiety.

In a double-blind, placebo-controlled study, both sertraline and imipramine were found to be more effective than placebo in reducing the depressive symptoms and improving psychosocial functioning in patients with dysthymia† without concurrent major depression; moreover, fewer patients treated with sertraline than those treated with imipramine or placebo discontinued therapy because of adverse effects. The results of several other studies, both controlled and uncontrolled, also suggest that sertraline may be effective in patients with dysthymia. Because dysthymia is a chronic condition and requires prolonged antidepressant therapy, the good tolerability demonstrated in clinical studies to date may be advantageous. Sertraline also has been used in the treatment of anger attacks associated with atypical depression and dysthymia† in a limited number of patients.

● Obsessive-Compulsive Disorder

Sertraline is used in the treatment of obsessive-compulsive disorder when the obsessions or compulsions cause marked distress, are time consuming (take longer than 1 hour daily), or interfere substantially with the patient's normal routine, occupational or academic functioning, or usual social activities or relationships. Obsessions are recurrent and persistent ideas, thoughts, impulses, or images that, at some time during the disturbance, are experienced as intrusive and inappropriate (i.e., "ego dystonic") and that cause marked anxiety or distress but that are not simply excessive worries about real-life problems. Compulsions are repetitive, intentional behaviors (e.g., hand washing, ordering, checking) or mental acts (e.g., praying, counting, repeating words silently) performed in response to an obsession or according to rules that must be applied rigidly (e.g., in a stereotyped fashion). Although the behaviors or acts are aimed at preventing or reducing distress or preventing some dreaded event or situation, they either are not connected in a realistic manner with what they are designed to neutralize or prevent or are clearly excessive. At some time during the course of the disturbance, the patient, if an adult, recognizes that the obsessions or compulsions are excessive or unreasonable; children may not make such a recognition.

The efficacy of sertraline for the management of obsessive-compulsive disorder has been established in several multicenter, placebo-controlled studies, including one study of 8 weeks' duration and 2 studies of 12 weeks' duration in adults and one study of 12 weeks' duration in children and adolescents 6–17 years of age. Patients in these studies had moderate to severe obsessive-compulsive disorder with mean baseline total scores on the Yale-Brown Obsessive-Compulsive Scale (YBOCS) of 23–25 in adults and 22 in children and adolescents (measured in the Children's Yale-Brown Obsessive-Compulsive Scale [CY-BOCS]). In the 8-week study with flexible dosing, adult patients received sertraline in dosages ranging from 50–200 mg daily; the mean dosage for those completing the study was 186 mg daily. Total scores on the YBOCS decreased by an average of approximately 4 points in sertraline-treated patients and 2 points in patients receiving placebo; this difference was statistically significant.

In a fixed-dose study of 12 weeks' duration involving sertraline dosages of 50, 100, and 200 mg daily, adult patients receiving 50 and 200 mg of the drug daily experienced substantially greater reductions in the YBOCS total score than those receiving placebo (approximately 6 to approximately 3 points, respectively). In a 12-week study with flexible dosing in the range of 50–200 mg daily, the mean sertraline dosage in adult patients completing the study was 185 mg daily. YBOCS total scores in the sertraline-treated patients were reduced by a mean of approximately 7 points, which was better than the mean reduction of approximately 4 points reported in the placebo-treated patients.

In a 12-week study with flexible dosing, sertraline therapy was initiated at dosages of 25 or 50 mg daily in children 6–12 years of age or adolescents 13–17 years of age, respectively. Subsequent dosage was titrated according to individual tolerance over the first 4 weeks to a maximum dosage of 200 mg daily; the mean dosage for those completing the study was 178 mg daily. The drug produced substantially greater reductions in scores in the Children's Yale-Brown Obsessive-Compulsive Scale (CY-BOCS), the National Institute of Mental Health Global Obsessive-Compulsive Scale (NIMH-OC), and the Clinical Global Impressions (CGI) Improvement Scale; total scores on the CY-BOCS decreased by an average of approximately 7 units in sertraline-treated patients and 3 units in patients receiving placebo. An analysis of these controlled studies for possible age- and gender-related effects on treatment outcome did not suggest any difference in efficacy based on either the age or gender of the patient.

In addition, in an uncontrolled 6-week study with flexible dosing (50–200 mg daily) in children or adolescents 6–17 years of age with obsessive-compulsive disorder or major depression†, those with a diagnosis of obsessive-compulsive disorder had mean baseline total scores on the CY-BOCS, NIMH-OC, and CGI of about 24.9, 10.2, and 5.2, respectively. Sertraline produced substantial reductions in all 3 of the scales; total scores on CY-BOCS, NIMH-OC, and CGI decreased to 12.9, 6.7, and 3.4, respectively. In another uncontrolled, 6-week study employing a sertraline dosage that was escalated from 25 to 200 mg daily over 3 weeks, the drug combined with behavioral therapy was effective in a limited number of adolescents 13–17 years of age with obsessive-compulsive disorder refractory to other therapies; total scores on the CY-BOCS at the end of the study decreased by 11 points (from 25.4 to 14.4).

Results from comparative studies to date suggest sertraline and other selective serotonin-reuptake inhibitors (SSRIs; e.g., fluoxetine, fluvoxamine, paroxetine) are as effective or somewhat less effective than clomipramine and more effective than tricyclic antidepressants (e.g., amitriptyline, desipramine, imipramine, nortriptyline) in the management of obsessive-compulsive disorder. In a pooled analysis of separate short-term (10–13 weeks) studies comparing clomipramine, fluoxetine, fluvoxamine, or sertraline with placebo, clomipramine was calculated as being more effective (as determined by measures on the YBOC scale) than SSRIs, although all drugs were superior to placebo. Like clomipramine, SSRIs reduce but do not completely eliminate obsessions and compulsions.

Many clinicians consider an SSRI (e.g., sertraline, fluoxetine, fluvoxamine, paroxetine) or clomipramine to be the drugs of choice for the pharmacologic treatment of obsessive-compulsive disorder. The decision whether to initiate therapy with an SSRI or clomipramine often is made based on the adverse effect profile of these drugs. For example, some clinicians prefer clomipramine in patients who may not tolerate the adverse effect profile of SSRIs (nausea, headache, overstimulation, sleep disturbances) while SSRIs may be useful alternatives in patients unable to tolerate the adverse effects (anticholinergic effects, cardiovascular effects, sedation) associated with clomipramine therapy. Consideration of individual patient characteristics (age, concurrent medical conditions), pharmacokinetics of the drug, potential drug interactions, and cost of therapy may also influence clinicians when selecting between SSRIs and clomipramine as first-line therapy in patients with obsessive-compulsive disorder. Although not clearly established, it has been suggested that the mechanism of action of sertraline and other potent serotonin-reuptake inhibitors (e.g., clomipramine, fluoxetine, fluvoxamine, paroxetine) used in the management of obsessive-compulsive disorder may be related to their serotonergic activity.

● Panic Disorder

Sertraline is used in the treatment of panic disorder with or without agoraphobia. Panic disorder is characterized by the occurrence of unexpected panic attacks and associated concern about having additional attacks, worry about the implications or consequences of the attacks, and/or a clinically important change in behavior related to the attacks.

According to DSM-IV, panic disorder is characterized by recurrent unexpected panic attacks, which consist of a discrete period of intense fear or discomfort in which 4 (or more) of the following symptoms develop abruptly and reach a peak within 10 minutes: palpitations, pounding heart, or accelerated heart rate; sweating; trembling or shaking; sensations of shortness of breath or smothering; feeling of choking; chest pain or discomfort; nausea or abdominal distress; feeling dizzy, unsteady, lightheaded, or faint; derealization (feelings of unreality) or depersonalization (being detached from oneself); fear of losing control; fear of dying; paresthesias (numbness or tingling sensations); and chills or hot flushes.

The efficacy of sertraline for the management of panic disorder has been established by 3 double-blind, placebo-controlled studies in adult outpatients who met DSM-III-R criteria for panic disorder with or without agoraphobia. The first 2 studies were of 10 weeks' duration and used a flexible dosing schedule. Sertraline therapy was initiated in a dosage of 25 mg daily for the first week and then dosage was escalated to 50–200 mg daily depending on clinical response and tolerability. The mean sertraline dosages for completers were 131 and 144 mg daily for the first 2 studies. Overall, these 2 studies demonstrated that sertraline was superior to placebo in decreasing the frequency of panic attacks and in improving scores on the Clinical Global Impression Severity of Illness and Global Improvement Scales. The difference between sertraline and placebo in reduction in the number of full panic attacks per week compared with baseline was approximately 2 in both studies.

The third study was a fixed-dose study of 12 weeks' duration. Sertraline was given in dosages of 50, 100, and 200 mg daily. The patients receiving sertraline demonstrated a substantially greater reduction in panic attack frequency than patients receiving placebo. However, the results of this study were not readily interpretable regarding a dose-response relationship for efficacy in this condition.

An analysis of these 3 controlled studies for possible age-, race-, or gender-related effects on treatment outcome did not suggest any difference in efficacy based on these patient characteristics.

Panic disorder can be treated with cognitive and behavioral psychotherapy and/or pharmacologic therapy. There are several classes of drugs that appear to be effective in the pharmacologic management of panic disorder, including tricyclic antidepressants, MAO inhibitors (e.g., phenelzine), selective serotonin-reuptake inhibitors (SSRIs; e.g., citalopram, fluoxetine, paroxetine, sertraline), and benzodiazepines (e.g., alprazolam, clonazepam). When choosing among the available drugs, clinicians should consider their acceptance and tolerability by patients; their ability to reduce or eliminate panic attacks, reduce clinically important anxiety and disability secondary to phobic avoidance, and ameliorate other common comorbid conditions (such as depression); and their ability to prevent relapse during long-term therapy. Because of their better tolerability when compared with other agents (such as the tricyclic antidepressants and benzodiazepines), the lack of physical dependence problems commonly associated with benzodiazepines, and efficacy in panic disorder with comorbid conditions (e.g., depression, other anxiety disorders such as obsessive-compulsive disorder, alcoholism), many clinicians prefer SSRIs as first-line therapy in the management of panic disorder. If SSRI therapy is ineffective or not tolerated, use of a tricyclic antidepressant or a benzodiazepine is recommended.

Sertraline has improved chronic idiopathic urticaria† associated with panic disorder in at least one patient, but further study is needed to determine whether serotonin is involved in the pathogenesis of urticaria and whether SSRIs are effective in this condition.

● Posttraumatic Stress Disorder

Sertraline is used in the treatment of posttraumatic stress disorder (PTSD). PTSD is an anxiety disorder that involves the development of certain characteristic symptoms following personal exposure to an extreme traumatic stressor. According to DSM-IV, PTSD requires exposure to a traumatic event(s) that involved actual or threatened death or serious injury, or threat to the physical integrity of self or others, and the response to the event must involve intense fear, helplessness, or horror (in children the response may be expressed by disorganized or agitated behavior). PTSD is characterized by persistent symptoms of *reexperiencing* the trauma (e.g., intrusive distressing recollections of the event; recurrent distressing dreams of the event; acting or feeling as if the event were recurring including illusions, hallucinations, or flashbacks; intense distress at exposure to internal or external cues that symbolize or resemble an aspect of the event; physiologic reactivity on exposure to internal or external cues that symbolize or resemble an aspect of the event), persistent *avoidance* of stimuli associated with the trauma and numbing of general responsiveness (e.g., efforts to avoid thoughts, feelings, or conversations related to the event; efforts to avoid activities, places, or people that arouse recollections of the event; inability to recall an important aspect of the event; markedly diminished interest or participation in significant activities; feeling of detachment or estrangement from others; restricted emotions and/or range of affect not present before the event; sense of a foreshortened future), and persistent symptoms of *increased arousal* (e.g., difficulty sleeping; irritability/outbursts of anger; difficulty concentrating; hypervigilance; exaggerated startle response). According to DSM-IV, a PTSD diagnosis requires the presence of 1 or more symptoms of *reexperiencing*, 3 or more symptoms of *avoidance*, and 2 or more symptoms of *increased arousal*, all of which must be present for at least one month and cause clinically important distress or impairment in social, occupational, or other important areas of functioning. PTSD, like other anxiety disorders, rarely occurs alone, and patients with PTSD often present with comorbid disorders (e.g., major depressive disorder, substance abuse disorders, panic disorder, generalized anxiety disorders, obsessive-compulsive disorder, social phobia); it is unknown whether these comorbid disorders precede or follow the onset of PTSD.

Psychotherapy alone or in combination with pharmacotherapy generally is considered the treatment of choice for PTSD. Pharmacologic therapy may be indicated in addition to psychotherapy for initial treatment of PTSD in patients who have comorbid disorders (e.g., major depressive disorder, bipolar disorder, other anxiety disorders) and also may be indicated in those who do not respond to initial treatment with psychotherapy alone. If pharmacotherapy is indicated in patients with PTSD, selective serotonin-reuptake inhibitors (SSRIs; e.g., sertraline, fluoxetine, paroxetine) usually are considered the drugs of choice (except in patients with bipolar disorder who require treatment with mood stabilizing agents).

The efficacy of sertraline for the management of PTSD has been established in 2 placebo-controlled studies of 12 weeks' duration in adult outpatients (76% women) who met DSM-III-R criteria for chronic PTSD (duration of symptoms 3 months or longer). The mean duration of PTSD for these patients was approximately 12 years and 44% of patients had secondary depressive disorders. Sertraline therapy was initiated at a dosage of 25 mg daily for the first week and then dosage was escalated (using a flexible dosage schedule) to 50–200 mg daily based on clinical response and tolerability. The mean sertraline dosage for patients who completed studies 1 and 2 was 146 mg and 151 mg daily, respectively. Overall, these 2 studies showed that sertraline was superior to placebo in improving scores on the Clinician-Administered PTSD Scale Part 2 total severity scale (a measure of the intensity and frequency of all 3 PTSD diagnostic symptom clusters [reexperiencing/intrusion, avoidance/numbing, and hyperarousal]), Impact of Event Scale (a patient rated measurement of the intrusion and avoidance symptoms), and the Clinical Global Impressions Severity of Illness and Global Improvement Scales.

However, in 2 additional placebo-controlled studies of similar design and duration, the difference in response to treatment on key assessment scales between patients receiving sertraline and those receiving placebo was not statistically significant. In one study of mostly female patients who met the DSM-III-R criteria for PTSD related to sexual/physical trauma, those receiving placebo experienced substantially greater improvement on the Impact of Event Scale than those receiving sertraline therapy. Although this study enrolled a higher proportion of patients with comorbid anxiety disorders and a higher proportion of patients receiving placebo with a successful response to previous psychotropic therapies than the studies demonstrating efficacy of the drug, it is unknown whether these factors alone account for the high placebo response in the study.

Efficacy of sertraline for the management of PTSD related to war or combat was evaluated in a study involving primarily white men in a VA medical center outpatient setting (mean duration of PTSD approximately 18 years). At the end of this study, patients receiving sertraline did not differ from those receiving placebo on any of the key efficacy assessment scales (e.g., Clinician-Administered PTSD scale, Davidson Self-Rating Trauma scale, Impact of Event Scale). In addition, the mean change from baseline for both treatment groups in this study was of a lesser magnitude than those of patients receiving placebo in the other reported studies. The lack of response to sertraline treatment in these combat veterans is consistent with controlled studies evaluating other selective serotonin-reuptake inhibitors (e.g., fluoxetine, brofaromine [not commercially available in the US]) in Vietnam veterans with PTSD. Some experts suggest that patients with combat- or war-related PTSD may be less responsive to treatment than patients with PTSD related to other traumatic events (e.g., sexual assault, accidents, natural disasters) because of some factor inherent in combat- or war-related trauma. However, other experts suggest that the poor treatment response in studies evaluating use in veterans may be the result of sampling error since veterans receiving treatment at VA hospitals may constitute a self-selected group of patients with chronic PTSD who have multiple impairments (comorbid disorders, substance abuse) that make them less responsive to treatment.

Since PTSD is a more common disorder in women than men, the majority (76%) of patients in reported studies were women. A retrospective analysis of pooled data has shown a substantial difference between sertraline and placebo on key efficacy assessment scales (e.g., Clinician-Administered PTSD scale, Impact of Event Scale, Clinical Global Impressions Severity of Illness Scale) in women (regardless of a baseline diagnosis of comorbid depression), but essentially no effect in the limited number of men studied. The clinical importance of this apparent gender effect is unknown; however, only limited data are available to date regarding use of SSRIs in men who have PTSD related to noncombat-related trauma (e.g., sexual assault, accidents, natural disasters). There are insufficient data to date to determine whether race or age has any effect on the efficacy of sertraline in the management of PTSD.

For additional information on the use of SSRIs in the treatment of PTSD, see Uses: Posttraumatic Stress Disorder, in Prazosin Hydrochloride 24:20 and Paroxetine 28:16.04.20.

Premenstrual Dysphoric Disorder

Sertraline is used in the treatment of premenstrual dysphoric disorder (previously late luteal phase dysphoric disorder). DSM-IV criteria for premenstrual dysphoric disorder (PMDD) require that in most menstrual cycles of the previous year at least 5 of the following 11 symptoms must have been present for most of the time during the last week of the luteal phase (with at least one of the symptoms being one of the first 4 listed): marked depressed mood, feelings of hopelessness, or self-deprecating thoughts; marked anxiety, tension, feelings of being "keyed up" or on "edge"; marked affective lability (e.g., feeling suddenly sad or tearful or increased sensitivity to rejection); persistent and marked anger or irritability or increased interpersonal conflicts; decreased interest in usual activities

(e.g., work, school, friends, hobbies); a subjective sense of difficulty in concentrating; lethargy, easy fatigability, or marked lack of energy; marked change in appetite, overeating, or specific food cravings; hypersomnia or insomnia; a subjective sense of being overwhelmed or out of control; and other physical symptoms, such as breast tenderness or swelling, headaches, joint or muscle pain, or a sensation of "bloating" or weight gain. Such symptoms should begin to remit within a few days of the onset of menses (follicular phase) and are always absent in the week following menses. The presence of this cyclical pattern of symptoms must be confirmed by at least 2 consecutive months of prospective daily symptom ratings. PMDD should be distinguished from the more common premenstrual syndrome (PMS) by prospective daily ratings and the strict criteria listed above.

The efficacy of sertraline for the management of PMDD has been established in 2 randomized, placebo-controlled studies over 3 menstrual cycles in adult women who met DSM-III-R or DSM-IV criteria for PMDD. In these studies, flexible dosages (range: 50–150 mg daily) of sertraline administered continuously throughout the menstrual cycle or during the luteal phase only (i.e., for 2 weeks prior to the onset of menses) were shown to be substantially more effective than placebo in improving scores from baseline on the Daily Record of Severity of Problems (DRSP), the Clinical Global Impression of Severity of Illness (CGI-S) and Improvement (CGI-I), and/or the Hamilton Depression Rating Scales (HAMD-17). The mean dosage of sertraline in patients completing these trials was 102 or 74 mg daily for those receiving continuous or luteal-phase dosing of the drug, respectively.

When given in a flexible dosage of 50–150 mg daily in a separate double-blind, placebo-controlled study, sertraline was substantially better than placebo in improving symptoms (depressive symptoms, physical symptoms, anger/irritability) and functional impairment associated with this disorder. The beneficial effect of the drug was apparent by the first treatment cycle. In an open study comparing sertraline and desipramine in the treatment of premenstrual dysphoric disorder, sertraline and possibly desipramine were found to be effective; however, sertraline was better tolerated than desipramine. Additional controlled studies are needed to determine whether the efficacy of the drug is sustained during longer-term, maintenance therapy in women with this condition. In addition, efficacy of sertraline used in conjunction with oral contraceptives for the treatment of PMDD has not been determined since patients receiving oral contraceptives were excluded from most clinical studies to date.

Social Phobia

Sertraline is used in the treatment of social phobia (social anxiety disorder). According to DSM-IV, social phobia is characterized by a marked and persistent fear of one or more social or performance situations in which the person is exposed to unfamiliar people or to possible scrutiny by others. Exposure to the feared situation almost invariably provokes anxiety, which may approach the intensity of a panic attack. The feared situations are avoided or endured with intense anxiety or distress. The avoidance, fear, or anxious anticipation of encountering the social or performance situation interferes significantly with the person's daily routine, occupational or academic functioning, or social activities or relationships, or there is marked distress about having the phobias. Lesser degrees of performance anxiety or shyness generally do not require psychotherapy or pharmacologic treatment.

The efficacy of sertraline in the treatment of social phobia has been established in 2 multicenter, placebo-controlled studies in adult outpatients who met DSM-IV criteria for social phobia. In one study of 12 weeks' duration, 47% of patients receiving flexible dosages of sertraline (50–200 mg daily; mean dosage of 144 mg daily) were characterized as responders (defined as a score of 1 or 2 on the Clinical Global Impressions [CGI] Global Improvement Scale) compared with 26% of those receiving placebo (intent-to-treat analysis). Sertraline also was found to be superior to placebo on the Liebowitz Social Anxiety Scale (LSAS), a 24-item clinician administered measure of fear, anxiety, and avoidance of social and performance situation, and on most secondary efficacy measures, including the Duke Brief Social Phobia Scale (BSPS) total score, fear and avoidance subscales of BSPS, and fear/anxiety and avoidance subscales of LSAS. These results were similar to those seen in a flexible-dose study of 20 weeks' duration, in which a score of 1 ("very much improved") or 2 ("much improved") on the CGI Global Improvement Scale was attained by the end of the treatment period by 53 or 29% of patients receiving sertraline (50–200 mg daily; mean dosage of 147 mg daily) or placebo, respectively (intent-to-treat analysis). Sixty-five patients in this study subsequently were enrolled in a separate controlled study, including 50 patients who had responded to sertraline in the initial study and then were randomized to receive either continued treatment with sertraline or placebo in the subsequent study and 15 patients who had responded to placebo in the initial study and continued to receive placebo in the subsequent study. Based on an intent-to-treat analysis, 4% of patients who continued treatment with sertraline, 36% of patients randomized to receive placebo, and 27% of those who continued treatment with placebo relapsed (defined as an increase of 2 or more points from baseline in the CGI Severity of Illness score or discontinuance of the study drug because of lack of efficacy) at the end of the 24-week treatment period. Similar to results of pivotal, short-term clinical studies, sertraline also was shown to be substantially more effective than placebo on the CGI Severity of Illness Scale, Marks Fear Questionnaire (MFQ) Social Phobia subscale, and BSPS total score.

Subgroup analysis of short-term, controlled studies in adult outpatients with social anxiety disorder did not reveal any evidence of gender-related differences in treatment outcome. There was insufficient information to determine the effect of race or age on treatment outcome. Safety and efficacy of sertraline for the treatment of social phobia in children or adolescents have not been established to date.

● Premature Ejaculation

Like some other serotonin-reuptake inhibitors, sertraline has been used with some success in the treatment of premature ejaculation†. In a placebo-controlled study, sertraline produced substantial improvements compared with placebo in time to ejaculation, number of successful attempts at intercourse, and incidence of ejaculation during foreplay, as well as overall clinical judgment of improvement. In addition, the drug was well tolerated in most patients. A trial with drug therapy may be particularly useful in patients who fail or refuse behavioral or psychotherapeutic treatment or when partners are unwilling to cooperate with such therapy.

● Other Uses

Sertraline has been used in a limited number of patients with various types of headache† with variable results; however, its use in this condition may be limited by frequent adverse effects.

DOSAGE AND ADMINISTRATION

● Administration

Sertraline is administered orally. The drug usually is administered once daily in the morning or evening. The extent of GI absorption of sertraline reportedly may be increased slightly, the peak concentration increased by about 25%, and the time to peak concentration after a dose decreased from about 8 to 5.5 hours when the drug is administered with food, but such changes do not appear to be clinically important.

When sertraline hydrochloride concentrate for oral solution (Zoloft®) is used, doses of the drug should be measured carefully using the calibrated dropper provided by the manufacturer. The appropriate dose of the oral solution should be diluted in 120 mL of water, ginger ale, lemon/lime soda, lemonade, or orange juice before administration. The diluted solution containing sertraline hydrochloride should be mixed and administered immediately and should not be allowed to stand before administration. A slight haze may occasionally appear in the diluted oral solution, but the manufacturer states that this is normal.

● Dosage

Dosage of sertraline hydrochloride is expressed in terms of sertraline.

Patients receiving sertraline should be monitored for possible worsening of depression, suicidality, or unusual changes in behavior, especially at the beginning of therapy or during periods of dosage adjustment. (See Cautions: Precautions and Contraindications.)

Because withdrawal effects may occur with discontinuance of sertraline, other selective serotonin-reuptake inhibitors (SSRIs), and selective serotonin- and norepinephrine-reuptake inhibitors (SNRIs), abrupt discontinuance of these drugs should be avoided whenever possible. In addition, patients may experience a worsening of psychiatric status when the drug is discontinued abruptly. When sertraline therapy is discontinued, the dosage should be reduced gradually (e.g., over a period of several weeks) and the patient monitored for possible withdrawal symptoms. If intolerable symptoms occur following a dosage reduction or upon discontinuance of therapy, the drug may be reinstituted at the previously prescribed dosage. Subsequently, the clinician may continue decreasing the dosage, but at a more gradual rate. (See Cautions: Nervous System Effects and see Chronic Toxicity.)

The manufacturers recommend that an interval of at least 2 weeks elapse when switching a patient from a monoamine oxidase (MAO) inhibitor to sertraline or when switching from sertraline to an MAO inhibitor. For additional information on potentially serious drug interactions that may occur between sertraline and

MAO inhibitors or other serotonergic agents, see Cautions: Precautions and Contraindications and also see Drug Interactions: Serotonergic Drugs.

Clinical experience regarding the optimal timing of switching from other drugs used in the treatment of major depressive disorder, obsessive-compulsive disorder, panic disorder, posttraumatic stress disorder, premenstrual dysphoric disorder, and social anxiety disorder to sertraline therapy is limited. Therefore, the manufacturers recommend that care and prudent medical judgment be exercised when switching from other drugs to sertraline, particularly from long-acting agents (such as fluoxetine). Because some adverse reactions resembling serotonin syndrome have developed when fluoxetine therapy was discontinued abruptly and sertraline therapy was initiated immediately afterward, a washout period appears to be advisable when transferring a patient from fluoxetine to sertraline therapy. However, the appropriate duration of the washout period when switching from one selective serotonin-reuptake inhibitor to another has not been clearly established. Pending further experience in patients being transferred from therapy with another antidepressant to sertraline, it generally is recommended that the previous antidepressant be discontinued according to the recommended guidelines for the specific antidepressant prior to initiation of sertraline therapy. (See Drug Interactions: Serotonergic Drugs and see Drug Interactions: Tricyclic and Other Antidepressants.)

Major Depressive Disorder

For the management of major depressive disorder in adults, the recommended initial dosage of sertraline is 50–100 mg once daily. If no clinical improvement is apparent, dosage may be increased at intervals of not less than 1 week up to a maximum of 200 mg daily. Clinical experience with the drug to date suggests that many patients will respond to 50–100 mg of the drug once daily. While a relationship between dose and antidepressant effect has not been established, efficacy of the drug was demonstrated in clinical trials employing 50–200 mg daily.

While the optimum duration of sertraline therapy has not been established, many experts state that acute depressive episodes require several months or longer of sustained antidepressant therapy. In addition, some clinicians recommend that long-term antidepressant therapy be considered in certain patients at risk for recurrence of depressive episodes (such as those with highly recurrent unipolar depression). Whether the dose of sertraline required to induce remission is identical to the dose needed to maintain and/or sustain euthymia is unknown. Systematic evaluation of sertraline has shown that its antidepressant efficacy is maintained for periods of up to 1 year in patients receiving 50–200 mg daily (mean dose of 70 mg daily). The usefulness of the drug in patients receiving prolonged therapy should be reevaluated periodically.

Obsessive-Compulsive Disorder

For the management of obsessive-compulsive disorder in adults and adolescents 13–17 years of age, the recommended initial dosage of sertraline is 50 mg once daily. In children 6–12 years of age, the recommended initial dosage of sertraline is 25 mg once daily. If no clinical improvement is apparent, dosage may be increased at intervals of not less than 1 week up to a maximum of 200 mg daily. However, it should be considered that children usually have a lower body weight than adults and particular care should be taken to avoid excessive dosage in children. While a relationship between dose and efficacy in obsessive-compulsive disorder has not been established, efficacy of the drug was demonstrated in clinical trials employing 50–200 mg daily in adults and 25–200 mg daily in children and adolescents.

While the optimum duration of sertraline therapy required to prevent recurrence of obsessive-compulsive symptoms has not been established to date, the manufacturer and many experts state that this disorder is chronic and requires several months or longer of sustained therapy. Whether the dose of sertraline required to induce remission is identical to the dose needed to maintain and/or sustain remission in patients with this disorder is unknown. Systematic evaluation of sertraline has shown that its efficacy in the management of obsessive-compulsive disorder is maintained for periods of up to 28 weeks in patients receiving 50–200 mg daily. The usefulness of the drug in patients receiving prolonged therapy should be reevaluated periodically.

Panic Disorder

For the management of panic disorder in adults, the recommended initial dosage of sertraline is 25 mg once daily. After 1 week, the dosage should be increased to 50 mg once daily. If no clinical improvement is apparent, dosage may then be increased at intervals of not less than 1 week up to a maximum of 200 mg daily.

While the optimum duration of sertraline therapy required to prevent recurrence of panic disorder has not been established to date, the manufacturer and many experts state that this disorder is chronic and requires several months or longer of sustained therapy. Whether the dose of sertraline required to induce remission is identical to the dose needed to maintain and/or sustain remission in patients with this disorder is unknown. Systematic evaluation of sertraline has shown that its efficacy in the management of panic disorder is maintained for periods of up to 28 weeks in patients receiving 50–200 mg daily. The usefulness of the drug in patients receiving prolonged therapy should be reevaluated periodically.

Posttraumatic Stress Disorder

For the management of posttraumatic stress disorder (PTSD) in adults, the recommended initial dosage of sertraline is 25 mg once daily. After 1 week, dosage should be increased to 50 mg once daily. If no clinical improvement is apparent, dosage may then be increased at intervals of not less than 1 week up to a maximum of 200 mg daily.

While the optimum duration of sertraline therapy required to prevent recurrence of PTSD has not been established to date, this disorder is chronic and it is reasonable to continue therapy in responding patients. Whether the dose of sertraline required to induce remission is identical to the dose needed to maintain and/or sustain remission in patients with this disorder is unknown. Systematic evaluation of sertraline has shown that its efficacy in the management of posttraumatic stress disorder is maintained for periods of up to 28 weeks in patients receiving 50–200 mg daily. The usefulness of the drug in patients receiving prolonged therapy should be reevaluated periodically.

Premenstrual Dysphoric Disorder

For the treatment of premenstrual dysphoric disorder (previously late luteal phase dysphoric disorder), the recommended initial dosage of sertraline is 50 mg daily given continuously throughout the menstrual cycle or given during the luteal phase only (i.e., starting 2 weeks prior to the anticipated onset of menstruation and continuing through the first full day of menses). If no clinical improvement is apparent, dosage may be increased in 50-mg increments at the onset of each new menstrual cycle up to a maximum of 150 mg daily when administered continuously or 100 mg daily when administered during the luteal phase only. If a dosage of 100 mg daily has been established with luteal phase dosing, dosages should be increased gradually over the first 3 days of each luteal phase dosing period. While a relationship between dose and effect in premenstrual dysphoric disorder (PMDD) has not been established, efficacy of the drug was demonstrated in clinical trials employing 50–150 mg daily.

The optimum duration of sertraline therapy required to treat PMDD has not been established to date. The manufacturer states that the efficacy of sertraline therapy beyond 3 menstrual cycles has not been demonstrated in controlled studies. However, because women commonly report that symptoms of PMDD worsen with age until relieved by the onset of menopause, the manufacturer recommends that long-term sertraline therapy be considered in responding women. Dosage adjustments, which may include transfers between dosing regimens (e.g., continuous versus luteal phase dosing), may be needed to maintain the patient on the lowest effective dosage, and patients should be periodically reassessed to determine the need for continued treatment.

Social Phobia

For the management of social phobia in adults, the recommended initial dosage of sertraline is 25 mg once daily. After 1 week, the dosage should be increased to 50 mg once daily. If no clinical improvement is apparent, dosage may then be increased at intervals of not less than 1 week up to a maximum of 200 mg daily.

While the optimum duration of sertraline therapy required to prevent recurrence of social phobia symptoms has not been established to date, the manufacturer states that this disorder is chronic and requires several months or longer of sustained therapy. Whether the dose of sertraline required to induce remission is identical to the dose needed to maintain and/or sustain remission in patients with this disorder is unknown. Systematic evaluation of sertraline has shown that its efficacy in the management of social phobia is maintained for periods of up to 24 weeks following 20 weeks of therapy at dosages of 50–200 mg daily. Dosages should be adjusted so that the patient is maintained on the lowest effective dosage, and patients should be reassessed periodically to determine the need for continued therapy.

Premature Ejaculation

For the management of premature ejaculation†, sertraline has been given in a dosage of 25–50 mg daily. Alternatively, patients have taken sertraline on an "as needed" basis using doses of 25–50 mg daily.

● Dosage in Geriatric Patients

Major Depressive Disorder

For the management of depressive symptoms associated with dementia of the Alzheimer's type in geriatric patients, some experts recommend an initial sertraline dosage of 12.5–25 mg once daily. The dosage may then be gradually increased at intervals of 1–2 weeks up to a maximum dosage of 150–200 mg once daily.

● Dosage in Renal and Hepatic Impairment

The manufacturers state that, based on the pharmacokinetics of sertraline, there is no need for dosage adjustment in patients with renal impairment. Because sertraline does not appear to be removed substantially by dialysis, supplemental doses of the drug probably are unnecessary after dialysis.

Because sertraline is metabolized extensively by the liver, hepatic impairment can affect the elimination of the drug. (See Pharmacokinetics: Elimination.) Therefore, the manufacturers recommend that sertraline be administered with caution and in a reduced dosage or less frequently in patients with hepatic impairment.

● Treatment of Pregnant Women during the Third Trimester

Because some neonates exposed to sertraline and other SSRIs or SNRIs late in the third trimester of pregnancy have developed severe complications, consideration may be given to cautiously tapering sertraline therapy in the third trimester prior to delivery if the drug is administered during pregnancy. (See Pregnancy, under Cautions: Pregnancy, Fertility, and Lactation.)

CAUTIONS

The adverse effect profile of sertraline is similar to that of other selective serotonin-reuptake inhibitors (SSRIs) (e.g., citalopram, escitalopram, fluoxetine, fluvoxamine, paroxetine). Because sertraline is a highly selective serotonin-reuptake inhibitor with little or no effect on other neurotransmitters, the incidence of some adverse effects commonly associated with tricyclic antidepressants, such as anticholinergic effects (dry mouth, constipation), certain cardiovascular effects (e.g., orthostatic hypotension), drowsiness, and weight gain, is lower in patients receiving sertraline. However, certain adverse GI (e.g., nausea, diarrhea, anorexia) and nervous system (e.g., tremor, insomnia) effects appear to occur more frequently with sertraline and other SSRIs than with tricyclic antidepressants.

Overall, the adverse effect profile of sertraline in adults with depression, obsessive-compulsive disorder, or panic disorder appears to be similar. In controlled studies, the most common adverse effects occurring more frequently in adults receiving sertraline than in those receiving placebo included GI effects such as nausea, diarrhea or loose stools, dyspepsia, and dry mouth; nervous system effects such as somnolence, dizziness, insomnia, and tremor; sexual dysfunction in males (principally ejaculatory delay); and sweating. Discontinuance of sertraline therapy was required in about 15% of adults in clinical trials, principally because of adverse psychiatric (e.g., somnolence, insomnia, agitation, tremor), other nervous system (e.g., dizziness, headache), GI (e.g., nausea, diarrhea or loose stools, anorexia), or male sexual dysfunction (e.g., ejaculatory delay) effects or because of fatigue.

● Nervous System Effects

Headache is the most common adverse nervous system effect of sertraline, occurring in approximately 26% of patients receiving the drug in controlled clinical trials; headache occurred in 23% of those receiving placebo in these trials. Somnolence or drowsiness occurred in about 14% of patients receiving sertraline in controlled clinical trials. Headache or somnolence each required discontinuance of therapy in about 2% of patients. Fatigue has been reported in approximately 12% of patients receiving the drug in clinical trials and required discontinuance of therapy in about 1% of patients; this effect was reported in 8% of those receiving placebo in these trials.

Dizziness occurred in about 13% of patients receiving sertraline in controlled clinical trials and required discontinuance of therapy in less than 1% of patients. Insomnia occurred in about 22% of patients receiving the drug in controlled clinical trials. However, because insomnia is a symptom also associated with depression, relief of insomnia and improvement in sleep patterns may occur when clinical improvement in depression becomes apparent during antidepressant therapy. In clinical trials, about 2% of patients discontinued sertraline because of insomnia.

Tremor occurred in about 9%, nervousness in about 6%, anxiety (which occasionally may be severe [e.g., panic]) in about 4%, paresthesia in about 3%, and agitation in about 6% of patients receiving sertraline in controlled clinical trials. Tremor, agitation, and nervousness resulted in discontinuance of sertraline in about 1% of patients while anxiety resulted in discontinuance in less than 1% of patients in clinical trials. Agitation and anxiety may subside with continued therapy. Hypoesthesia, hypertonia, or malaise occurred in at least 1% of patients receiving sertraline in clinical trials. Impaired concentration, dystonia, or twitching occurred in approximately 0.1–1% of patients receiving sertraline, although these adverse effects have not been definitely attributed to the drug.

The incidence of seizures during sertraline therapy appears to be similar to or less than that observed during therapy with most other currently available antidepressants. Seizures occurred in less than 0.1% of patients receiving sertraline in clinical trials. (See Cautions: Precautions and Contraindications.)

Hypomania and mania have been reported in approximately 0.4% of patients receiving sertraline in controlled clinical trials, which is similar to the incidence reported in patients receiving active control agents (i.e., other antidepressants). In at least 2 patients, hypomanic symptoms occurred after they were receiving sertraline 200 mg daily for approximately 9 weeks. In both patients, the adverse reaction was obviated by a reduction in sertraline dosage. (See Cautions: Precautions and Contraindications.) Such reactions have occurred in patients receiving other antidepressant agents and may be caused by antidepressant-induced functional increases in catecholamine activity within the CNS, resulting in a "switch" from depressive to manic behavior. There is some evidence that patients with bipolar disorder may be more likely to experience antidepressant-induced hypomanic or manic reactions than patients without evidence of this disorder. In addition, limited evidence suggests that such reactions may occur more frequently in bipolar depressed patients receiving tricyclics and tetracyclics (e.g., maprotiline, mianserin [not commercially available in the US]) than in those receiving SSRIs (e.g., citalopram, escitalopram, fluoxetine, paroxetine, sertraline). However, further studies are needed to confirm these findings.

Asthenia has been reported in at least 1% of patients receiving sertraline; however, a causal relationship to the drug has not been established. Confusion, migraine, abnormal coordination, abnormal gait, hyperesthesia, ataxia, depersonalization, hallucinations, hyperkinesia, hypokinesia, nystagmus, vertigo, abnormal dreams, aggressive reaction, amnesia, apathy, paroniria, delusion, depression or aggravated depression, emotional lability, euphoria, abnormal thinking, or paranoid reaction have been reported in 0.1–1% of patients receiving the drug, although these adverse effects have not been definitely attributed to sertraline.

Adverse nervous system effects reported in less than 0.1% of patients receiving sertraline include dysphoria, choreoathetosis, dyskinesia, coma, dysphonia, hyperreflexia, hypotonia, ptosis, somnambulism, and illusion; these effects have not been definitely attributed to the drug. Although a causal relationship has not been established, psychosis, extrapyramidal symptoms, and oculogyric crisis have been reported during postmarketing surveillance. Forgetfulness, panic attacks, and unspecified pain also have been reported rarely, although a causal relationship to sertraline has not been established. Sertraline also has been reported to precipitate or exacerbate "flashbacks" in patients who previously had used lysergic acid diethylamide (LSD).

Serotonin syndrome and neuroleptic malignant syndrome (NMS)-like reactions have been reported in patients receiving sertraline, other SSRIs, and selective serotonin- and norepinephrine-reuptake inhibitors (SNRIs). (See Cautions: Precautions and Contraindications, Drug Interactions: Serotonergic Drugs, and Acute Toxicity.)

Extrapyramidal reactions, including akathisia, stuttering (which may be a speech manifestation of akathisia), bilateral jaw stiffness, and torticollis, have been reported rarely with sertraline use, and such reactions appear to be a class effect of SSRIs and dose related. Reactions occurring *early* during therapy with these drugs may be secondary to preexisting parkinsonian syndrome and/or concomitant therapy.

Withdrawal Reactions

Withdrawal symptoms, including dysphoric mood, irritability, agitation, dizziness, sensory disturbances (e.g., paresthesias such as electric shock sensations), anxiety, confusion, headache, lethargy, emotional lability, insomnia, and hypomania, have been reported upon discontinuance of sertraline, other SSRIs, and SNRIs, particularly when discontinuance of these drugs is abrupt. While these reactions are generally self-limiting, there have been reports of serious discontinuance symptoms. Therefore, patients should be monitored for such symptoms when discontinuing sertraline therapy. A gradual reduction in the dosage rather than abrupt cessation is recommended whenever possible. (See Dosage and Administration: Dosage.)

A withdrawal syndrome has been reported in less than 0.1% of sertraline-treated patients. Fatigue, severe abdominal cramping, memory impairment, and influenza-like symptoms were reported 2 days following abrupt discontinuance of sertraline in one patient; when sertraline was restarted, the symptoms remitted. Electric shock-like sensations occurred in another patient 1 day after the last administered dose of sertraline; these sensations became less intense and eventually disappeared 13 weeks after sertraline therapy was discontinued. (See Chronic Toxicity.)

Suicidality

Suicidal ideation has been reported in less than 0.1% of adults receiving sertraline. The US Food and Drug Administration (FDA) has determined that antidepressants increase the risk of suicidal thinking and behavior (suicidality) in children, adolescents, and young adults (18–24 years of age) with major depressive disorder and other psychiatric disorders. (See Suicidality, under Cautions: Nervous System Effects, in Paroxetine 28:16.04.20.) Patients, therefore, should be appropriately monitored and closely observed for clinical worsening, suicidality, and unusual changes in behavior, particularly during initiation of sertraline therapy (i.e., the first few months) and during periods of dosage adjustments. (See Cautions: Precautions and Contraindications and see Cautions: Pediatric Precautions.)

● GI Effects

Like other selective serotonin-reuptake inhibitors (e.g., citalopram, escitalopram, fluoxetine, fluvoxamine, paroxetine), sertraline therapy is associated with a relatively high incidence of GI disturbances, principally nausea, dry mouth, and diarrhea/loose stools. The most frequent adverse effect associated with sertraline therapy is nausea, which occurred in about 28% of patients receiving the drug in controlled clinical trials. In clinical trials, nausea required discontinuance of sertraline in about 4% of patients. In general, the incidence of nausea associated with selective serotonin-reuptake inhibitors appears to be higher when therapy is initiated with high doses but decreases as therapy with these drugs is continued. While the mechanism(s) of sertraline-induced GI effects has not been fully elucidated, they appear to arise at least in part because of increased serotonergic activity in the GI tract (which may result in stimulation of small intestine motility and inhibition of gastric and large intestine motility) and possibly because of the drug's effect on central serotonergic type 3 (5-HT$_3$) receptors.

Diarrhea or loose stools occurred in about 20%, dry mouth in about 15%, constipation in about 7%, dyspepsia in about 8%, or anorexia in about 6% of patients receiving sertraline in controlled clinical trials. Other adverse GI effects associated with sertraline therapy include vomiting which occurred in about 4% and flatulence which occurred in about 3% of patients receiving the drug in controlled clinical trials. Abdominal pain was reported in approximately 2% and taste perversion in about 1% of patients receiving sertraline. In clinical trials, diarrhea or loose stools required discontinuance of sertraline in about 3% of patients and dry mouth required discontinuance of therapy in about 1% of patients.

Epidemiologic case-control and cohort design studies have suggested that selective serotonin-reuptake inhibitors may increase the risk of upper GI bleeding. Although the precise mechanism for this increased risk remains to be clearly established, serotonin release by platelets is known to play an important role in hemostasis, and selective serotonin-reuptake inhibitors decrease serotonin uptake from the blood by platelets thereby decreasing the amount of serotonin in platelets. In addition, concurrent use of aspirin or other nonsteroidal anti-inflammatory drugs was found to substantially increase the risk of GI bleeding in patients receiving selective serotonin-reuptake inhibitors in 2 of these studies. Although these studies focused on upper GI bleeding, there is some evidence suggesting that bleeding at other sites may be similarly potentiated. Further clinical studies are needed to determine the clinical importance of these findings. (See Cautions: Hematologic Effects and also see Drug Interactions: Drugs Affecting Hemostasis.)

Although a causal relationship to sertraline has not been established, dysphagia, esophagitis, aggravation of dental caries, gastroenteritis, eructation, and increased salivation have been reported in 0.1–1% of patients receiving the drug. Aphthous stomatitis, ulcerative stomatitis, stomatitis, tongue ulceration or edema, glossitis, diverticulitis, gastritis, hemorrhagic peptic ulcer, rectal hemorrhage, colitis, proctitis, fecal incontinence, melena, or tenesmus has been reported in less than 0.1% of patients receiving sertraline; however, these adverse effects have not been definitely attributed to the drug. Pancreatitis also has been reported rarely in association with sertraline; however, a causal relationship to the drug has not been clearly established.

Although a causal relationship has not been established, nocturnal bruxism (clenching and/or grinding of the teeth during sleep) has developed within 2–4 weeks following initiation of sertraline or fluoxetine therapy in several patients. The bruxism remitted upon reduction in dosage of the serotonin-reuptake inhibitor and/or the addition of buspirone therapy.

Speech blockage also has been reported in at least one sertraline-treated patient.

Dermatologic and Sensitivity Reactions

Sweating occurred in about 7% of patients receiving sertraline in controlled clinical trials.

Rash, which may be erythematous, follicular, maculopapular, or pustular, has been reported in about 3% of patients receiving sertraline in controlled clinical trials. Adverse dermatologic effects reported in 0.1–1% of patients receiving sertraline in controlled clinical trials include acne, alopecia, dry skin, urticaria, pruritus, and photosensitivity reaction (which may be severe); however, these adverse effects have not been definitely attributed to sertraline. Bullous eruption, eczema, contact dermatitis, skin discoloration, and hypertrichosis have been reported in less than 0.1% of patients receiving the drug, although a causal relationship to sertraline has not been established. Allergy, allergic reaction, and angioedema also have been reported rarely.

Other dermatologic and sensitivity events, which can be severe and potentially may be fatal, reported during the postmarketing surveillance of sertraline have included anaphylactoid reaction, angioedema, Stevens-Johnson syndrome, erythema multiforme, and vasculitis.

Metabolic Effects

Thirst has been reported in 0.1–1% of patients receiving sertraline in controlled clinical trials.

Weight loss occurred in 0.1–1% of patients receiving sertraline. In controlled clinical trials, patients lost an average of about 0.45–0.9 kg while receiving sertraline. Rarely, weight loss has required discontinuance of therapy. Like fluoxetine, sertraline exhibits anorexigenic activity and can cause anorexia, which may be more pronounced in overweight patients and those with carbohydrate craving. Anorexia occurred in about 3% of patients receiving sertraline in controlled clinical trials and required discontinuance in at least 1% of patients. Increased appetite and weight gain have been reported in at least 1% of patients receiving sertraline in controlled clinical trials, although a causal relationship to the drug has not been established. (See Cautions: Pediatric Precautions.)

Sertraline use has been associated with small mean decreases (approximately 7%) in serum uric acid concentration as a result of a weak uricosuric effect; the clinical importance is not known and there have been no cases of acute renal failure associated with the drug. Small mean increases in serum total cholesterol (about 3%) and triglyceride (about 5%) concentrations also have been reported in patients receiving sertraline. Hypercholesterolemia has been reported in less than 0.1% of patients. Other adverse effects reported in less than 0.1% of patients receiving the drug include dehydration and hypoglycemia. These adverse effects have not been definitely attributed to sertraline.

Ocular and Otic Effects

Abnormal vision (including blurred vision) occurred in about 4% of patients receiving sertraline in controlled clinical trials. Adverse ocular effects reported in 0.1–1% of patients receiving sertraline include abnormality of accommodation, conjunctivitis, and ocular pain. Although a causal relationship to sertraline has not been established, anisocoria, abnormal lacrimation, xerophthalmia, diplopia, scotoma, visual field defect, exophthalmos, hemorrhage of the anterior chamber of the eye, or photophobia has been reported in less than 0.1% of patients receiving the drug. Other adverse ocular effects reported during postmarketing surveillance of sertraline have included blindness, optic neuritis, and cataract; however, a causal relationship to the drug has not been established.

SSRIs, including sertraline, may have an effect on pupil size resulting in mydriasis. This mydriatic effect potentially can narrow the eye angle resulting in increased intraocular pressure and angle-closure glaucoma, particularly in predisposed patients. Mydriasis has been reported in 0.1–1% of patients receiving sertraline and glaucoma has been reported in less than 0.1% of patients receiving the drug. (See Cautions: Precautions and Contraindications.)

Tinnitus occurred in at least 1% of patients receiving sertraline in controlled clinical trials. Earache has been reported in 0.1–1% of patients, and hyperacusis and labyrinthine disorder have been reported in less than 0.1% of patients.

Cardiovascular Effects

Sertraline does not exhibit clinically important anticholinergic activity, and current evidence suggests that sertraline is less cardiotoxic than many antidepressant agents (e.g., tricyclic antidepressants, monoamine oxidase inhibitors). (See Cardiovascular Considerations in Uses: Major Depressive Disorder and also see Pharmacology: Cardiovascular Effects.) However, bradycardia, AV block, atrial arrhythmias, QT-interval prolongation, and ventricular tachycardia (including torsades de pointes-type arrhythmias) have been reported during postmarketing surveillance evaluations of the drug.

Hot flushes occurred in about 2% of patients receiving sertraline in controlled clinical trials. Palpitation and chest pain have been reported in at least 1% of patients receiving sertraline in controlled clinical trials. In one patient with underlying coronary artery disease, chest pain developed suddenly and was relieved with sublingual nitroglycerin but was not associated with ECG changes; the mechanism of this effect, particularly regarding any potential cardiovascular effect, is unclear and alternative mechanisms (e.g., GI) for the chest pain have been proposed.

Unlike tricyclic antidepressants, sertraline has been associated with hypotension (e.g., orthostatic) infrequently; in controlled clinical trials, postural effects (e.g., dizziness, hypotension [which can also be nonpostural]) occurred in 0.1–1% of patients receiving sertraline. Syncope also occurred in at least 0.1% of patients.

Hypertension, peripheral ischemia, and tachycardia have been reported in 0.1–1% of patients receiving the drug, although a definite causal relationship to sertraline has not been established. Precordial or substernal chest pain, aggravated hypertension, myocardial infarction, pallor, vasodilation, and cerebrovascular disorder have been reported in less than 0.1% of patients receiving sertraline; these adverse effects have not been definitely attributed to the drug. Cerebrovascular spasm (including reversible cerebral vasoconstriction syndrome and Call-Fleming Syndrome) also has been reported during postmarketing experience with sertraline.

Generalized, dependent, periorbital, or peripheral edema has been reported in at least 0.1% of patients receiving sertraline, and facial edema has been reported rarely. However, a causal relationship to the drug has not been established.

Musculoskeletal Effects

Myalgia or back pain occurred in at least 1% of patients receiving sertraline in controlled clinical trials. Arthralgia, arthrosis, leg or other muscle cramps, or muscle weakness has been reported in 0.1–1% of patients receiving sertraline; these adverse effects have not been definitely attributed to the drug.

Hematologic Effects

Purpura, aplastic anemia, pancytopenia, leukopenia, thrombocytopenia, and abnormal bleeding have been reported occasionally in patients receiving sertraline; however, these adverse effects have not been definitely attributed to the drug.

Altered platelet function and/or abnormal platelet laboratory results have been reported rarely, but a causal relationship to sertraline remains to be established. In addition, in at least one patient with idiopathic thrombocytopenic purpura, sertraline therapy was associated with an increase in platelet counts. Anemia has been reported in less than 0.1% of patients receiving sertraline, although a causal relationship to the drug has not been established. Neutropenia also has been reported rarely with sertraline use and has been a reason for drug discontinuance. Agranulocytosis and septic shock developed in a geriatric woman who had been receiving sertraline for about 1 month in addition to atenolol, bendroflumethiazide, and thioridazine; the patient responded to anti-infective and granulocyte colony-stimulating factor therapy and made a full recovery within 10 days.

Bleeding complications (e.g., ecchymosis, purpura, menorrhagia, rectal bleeding) have been reported infrequently in patients receiving selective serotonin-reuptake inhibitors. Although the precise mechanism for these reactions has not been established, it has been suggested that impaired platelet aggregation and prolonged bleeding time may be due at least in part to inhibition of serotonin reuptake into platelets and/or that increased capillary fragility and vascular tone may contribute to these cases. (See Cautions: GI Effects and also see Drug Interactions: Drugs Affecting Hemostasis.)

● Respiratory Effects

Rhinitis or yawning has been reported in at least 1% of patients receiving sertraline in controlled clinical trials. Adverse respiratory effects reported in 0.1–1% of patients receiving the drug include bronchospasm, dyspnea, epistaxis, upper respiratory tract infection, sinusitis, and coughing; however, a definite causal relationship to sertraline has not been established. Adverse respiratory effects reported in less than 0.1% of patients receiving sertraline include bradypnea, hypoventilation, hyperventilation, apnea, stridor, hiccups, hemoptysis, bronchitis, laryngismus, and laryngitis. Pulmonary hypertension also has been reported during postmarketing surveillance evaluations of the drug. However, these adverse effects have not been definitely attributed to the drug.

● Renal, Electrolyte, and Genitourinary Effects

Sexual Dysfunction

Like other selective serotonin-reuptake inhibitors, adverse effects on sexual function have been reported in both men and women receiving sertraline. Although changes in sexual desire, sexual performance, and sexual satisfaction often occur as manifestations of a psychiatric disorder, they also may occur as the result of pharmacologic therapy. It is difficult to determine the true incidence and severity of adverse effects on sexual function during sertraline therapy, in part because patients and clinicians may be reluctant to discuss these effects. Therefore, incidence data reported in product labeling and earlier studies are most likely underestimates of the true incidence of adverse sexual effects. Recent reports indicate that up to 50% of patients receiving selective serotonin-reuptake inhibitors describe some form of sexual dysfunction during treatment and the actual incidence may be even higher.

Sexual dysfunction (principally ejaculatory delay) is the most common adverse urogenital effect of sertraline in males, occurring in about 14% of male patients receiving the drug in controlled clinical trials. In some cases, this effect has been used for therapeutic benefit in the treatment of premature ejaculation. (See Uses: Premature Ejaculation.) Impotence has occurred in at least 1% of male patients receiving sertraline in controlled trials, and priapism has been reported rarely. Female sexual dysfunction (e.g., anorgasmia) has been reported in at least 1% of female patients receiving the drug in controlled clinical trials. Decreased libido has been reported in males and females, occurring in 6% of patients in controlled clinical studies. Sexual dysfunction (principally ejaculatory delay) required discontinuance of therapy in at least 1% of patients in controlled clinical trials. Increased libido has been reported in less than 1% of patients receiving the drug.

Results of some (but not all) studies in men and women suggest that paroxetine may be associated with a higher incidence of sexual dysfunction than some other currently available selective serotonin-reuptake inhibitors, including sertraline and citalopram. Since it is difficult to know the precise risk of sexual dysfunction associated with serotonin-reuptake inhibitors, clinicians should routinely inquire about such possible adverse effects in patients receiving these drugs.

The long-term effects of selective serotonin-reuptake inhibitors on sexual function have not been fully determined to date. In a double-blind study evaluating 6 months of sertraline or citalopram therapy in depressed patients, sexual desire and overall sexual functioning (as measured on the UKU Side Effect Scale) substantially improved in women and sexual desire improved in men. In men, no change in orgasmic dysfunction, erectile dysfunction, or overall sexual functioning was reported after 6 months of therapy with sertraline or citalopram, although there was a trend toward worsening of ejaculatory dysfunction. However, in the subgroups of women and men reporting no sexual problems at baseline, approximately 12% of women reported decreased sexual desire and 14% reported orgasmic dysfunction after 6 months of citalopram therapy; the corresponding figures in the same subgroup of men were approximately 17 and 19%, respectively, and as many as 25% experienced ejaculatory dysfunction after 6 months. No substantial differences between sertraline and citalopram were reported in this study.

Management of sexual dysfunction caused by selective serotonin-reuptake inhibitor therapy includes waiting for tolerance to develop; using a lower dosage of the drug; using drug holidays; delaying administration of the drug until after coitus; or changing to another antidepressant. Although further study is needed, there is some evidence that adverse sexual effects of the selective serotonin-reuptake inhibitors may be reversed by concomitant use of certain drugs, including buspirone, 5-hydroxytryptamine-2 (5-HT$_2$) receptor antagonists (e.g., nefazodone), 5-HT$_3$ receptor inhibitors (e.g., granisetron), or α_2-adrenergic receptor antagonists (e.g., yohimbine), selective phosphodiesterase (PDE) inhibitors (e.g., sildenafil), or dopamine receptor agonists (e.g., amantadine, dextroamphetamine, pemoline [no longer commercially available in the US], methylphenidate). In most patients, sexual dysfunction is fully reversed 1–3 days after discontinuance of the antidepressant.

Other Renal, Electrolyte, and Genitourinary Effects

Although a definite causal relationship to sertraline has not been established, menstrual disorders, dysmenorrhea, intermenstrual bleeding, amenorrhea, vaginal hemorrhage, and leukorrhea have been reported in 0.1–1% of patients receiving sertraline. In addition, menorrhagia, breast enlargement, female breast pain or tenderness, acute mastitis in females, gynecomastia, and atrophic vaginitis have been reported in less than 0.1% of patients receiving sertraline; however, a causal relationship to the drug has not been clearly established.

Treatment with SSRIs, including sertraline, and selective serotonin- and norepinephrine-reuptake inhibitors (SNRIs) may result in hyponatremia. In many cases, this hyponatremia appears to be due to the syndrome of inappropriate antidiuretic hormone secretion (SIADH) and was reversible when the SSRI or SNRI was discontinued. Cases with serum sodium concentrations lower than 110 mEq/L have been reported. Hyponatremia and SIADH in patients receiving SSRIs usually develop an average of 2 weeks after initiating therapy (range: 3–120 days). Geriatric individuals and patients receiving diuretics or who are otherwise volume depleted may be at greater risk of developing hyponatremia during therapy with SSRIs or SNRIs. Discontinuance of sertraline should be considered in patients with symptomatic hyponatremia and appropriate medical intervention should be instituted. Because geriatric patients may be at increased risk for hyponatremia associated with these drugs, clinicians prescribing sertraline in such patients should be aware of the possibility that such reactions may occur. In addition, periodic monitoring of serum sodium concentrations (particularly during the first several months) in geriatric patients receiving SSRIs has been recommended by some clinicians.

A variety of urinary disorders, including urinary frequency, polyuria, urinary hesitancy and/or retention, dysuria, nocturia, and urinary incontinence, has been reported in 0.1–1% of patients receiving sertraline; however, these effects have not been definitely attributed to the drug. In addition, cystitis, oliguria, pyelonephritis, hematuria, renal pain, strangury, and balanoposthitis have been reported in less than 0.1% of patients receiving sertraline, although a causal relationship to the drug has not been clearly established.

● Hepatic Effects

Impaired hepatic function has been reported in less than 1% of patients receiving sertraline in controlled clinical trials; in most cases, such reactions appeared to be reversible upon discontinuance of sertraline therapy. Asymptomatic elevations in serum AST (SGOT) and ALT (SGPT) concentrations have been reported in approximately 0.8% of patients receiving the drug and occasionally have been a reason for drug discontinuance. Elevations in aminotransferase concentrations usually occurred within the first 1–9 weeks of sertraline therapy and were rapidly reversible following discontinuance of the drug. In addition, in at least 2 patients, elevated liver enzymes returned to normal levels with continued therapy.

Increased serum alkaline phosphatase and bilirubin concentrations occurred rarely in patients receiving sertraline in clinical trials and required discontinuance of therapy in some cases. Other clinical features associated with adverse hepatic reactions that have been reported in at least one patient include hepatitis, hepatomegaly, jaundice, abdominal pain, vomiting, hepatic failure, and death. However, these effects have not been definitely attributed to the drug.

● Endocrine Effects

Low levels of total thyroxine developed in a depressed adolescent who had been receiving sertraline therapy; however, it appears that sertraline only displaced the bound fraction of total thyroxine but was not associated with true hypothyroidism. In a limited number of hypothyroid patients receiving thyroxine therapy, elevated serum thyrotropin and reduced serum thyroxine concentrations have been observed following the initiation of sertraline therapy.

Hypothyroidism also has been reported. (See Cautions: Precautions and Contraindications.)

Diabetes mellitus, hyperglycemia, hyperprolactinemia, and galactorrhea have been reported rarely in sertraline-treated patients; however, a causal relationship to the drug has not been established.

● Other Adverse Effects

Cold clammy skin, flushing, fever, or rigors has been reported in 0.1–1% of patients receiving the drug, although a causal relationship to sertraline has not been established. In addition, lupus-like syndrome and serum sickness have been reported during postmarketing surveillance evaluations of the drug; however, a causal relationship has not been definitively established.

● Precautions and Contraindications

Worsening of depression and/or the emergence of suicidal ideation and behavior (suicidality) or unusual changes in behavior may occur in both adult and pediatric (see Cautions: Pediatric Precautions) patients with major depressive disorder or other psychiatric disorders, whether or not they are taking antidepressants. This risk may persist until clinically important remission occurs. Suicide is a known risk of depression and certain other psychiatric disorders, and these disorders themselves are the strongest predictors of suicide. However, there has been a long-standing concern that antidepressants may have a role in inducing worsening of depression and the emergence of suicidality in certain patients during the early phases of treatment. Pooled analyses of short-term, placebo-controlled studies of antidepressants (i.e., selective serotonin-reuptake inhibitors [SSRIs] and other antidepressants) have shown an increased risk of suicidality in children, adolescents, and young adults (18–24 years of age) with major depressive disorder and other psychiatric disorders. An increased suicidality risk was not demonstrated with antidepressants compared to placebo in adults older than 24 years of age and a reduced risk was observed in adults 65 years of age or older. It currently is unknown whether the suicidality risk extends to longer-term use (i.e., beyond several months); however, there is substantial evidence from placebo-controlled maintenance trials in adults with major depressive disorder that antidepressants can delay the recurrence of depression.

The US Food and Drug Administration (FDA) recommends that all patients being treated with antidepressants for any indication be appropriately monitored and closely observed for clinical worsening, suicidality, and unusual changes in behavior, particularly during initiation of therapy (i.e., the first few months) and during periods of dosage adjustments. Families and caregivers of patients being treated with antidepressants for major depressive disorder or other indications, both psychiatric and nonpsychiatric, also should be advised to monitor patients on a daily basis for the emergence of agitation, irritability, or unusual changes in behavior as well as the emergence of suicidality, and to report such symptoms immediately to a health-care provider. (See Suicidality under Cautions: Nervous System Effects, in Paroxetine 28:16.04.20.)

Although a causal relationship between the emergence of symptoms such as anxiety, agitation, panic attacks, insomnia, irritability, hostility, aggressiveness, impulsivity, akathisia, hypomania, and/or mania and either the worsening of depression and/or the emergence of suicidal impulses has not been established, there is concern that such symptoms may represent precursors to emerging suicidality. Consequently, consideration should be given to changing the therapeutic regimen or discontinuing therapy in patients whose depression is persistently worse or in patients experiencing emergent suicidality or symptoms that might be precursors to worsening depression or suicidality, particularly if such manifestations are severe, abrupt in onset, or were not part of the patient's presenting symptoms. If a decision is made to discontinue therapy, sertraline dosage should be tapered as rapidly as is feasible but with recognition of the risks of abrupt discontinuance. (See Dosage and Administration: Dosage.) FDA also recommends that the drugs be prescribed in the smallest quantity consistent with good patient management, in order to reduce the risk of overdosage.

It is generally believed (though not established in controlled trials) that treating a major depressive episode with an antidepressant alone may increase the likelihood of precipitating a mixed or manic episode in patients at risk for bipolar disorder. Therefore, patients should be adequately screened for bipolar disorder prior to initiating treatment with an antidepressant; such screening should include a detailed psychiatric history (e.g., family history of suicide, bipolar disorder, and depression).

Potentially life-threatening serotonin syndrome or neuroleptic malignant syndrome (NMS)-like reactions have been reported with SSRIs, including sertraline, and selective serotonin- and norepinephrine-reuptake inhibitors (SNRIs) alone, but particularly with concurrent administration of other serotonergic drugs (including serotonin [5-hydroxytryptamine; 5-HT] type 1 receptor agonists ["triptans"]), drugs that impair the metabolism of serotonin (e.g., monoamine oxidase [MAO] inhibitors), or antipsychotic agents or other dopamine antagonists. Symptoms of serotonin syndrome may include mental status changes (e.g., agitation, hallucinations, coma), autonomic instability (e.g., tachycardia, labile blood pressure, hyperthermia), neuromuscular aberrations (e.g., hyperreflexia, incoordination), and/or GI symptoms (e.g., nausea, vomiting, diarrhea). In its most severe form, serotonin syndrome may resemble NMS, which is characterized by hyperthermia, muscle rigidity, autonomic instability with possible rapid fluctuation in vital signs, and mental status changes. Patients receiving sertraline should be monitored for the development of serotonin syndrome or NMS-like signs and symptoms.

Concurrent or recent (i.e., within 2 weeks) therapy with MAO inhibitors used for treatment of depression is contraindicated in patients receiving sertraline and vice versa. If concurrent therapy with sertraline and a 5-HT$_1$ receptor agonist (triptan) is clinically warranted, the patient should be observed carefully, particularly during initiation of therapy, when dosage is increased, or when another serotonergic agent is initiated. Concomitant use of sertraline and serotonin precursors (e.g., tryptophan) is not recommended. If signs and symptoms of serotonin syndrome or NMS develop during sertraline therapy, treatment with sertraline and any concurrently administered serotonergic or antidopaminergic agents, including antipsychotic agents, should be discontinued immediately and supportive and symptomatic treatment should be initiated. (See Drug Interactions: Serotonergic Drugs.)

The dropper dispenser provided with Zoloft® oral solution contains natural latex proteins in the form of dry natural rubber which may cause sensitivity reactions in susceptible individuals.

Because clinical experience with sertraline in patients with certain concurrent systemic disease, including cardiovascular disease and renal impairment, is limited, caution should be exercised when sertraline is administered to patients with any systemic disease or condition that may alter metabolism of the drug or adversely affect hemodynamic function. (See Dosage and Administration: Dosage.)

Sertraline should be used with caution in patients with hepatic impairment, since prolonged elimination of the drug has been reported to occur in patients with liver cirrhosis. (See Pharmacokinetics: Elimination and see Dosage and Administration: Dosage in Renal and Hepatic Impairment.)

The manufacturers recommend that patients receiving sertraline be advised to notify their clinician if they are taking or plan to take nonprescription (over-the-counter) or prescription medications or alcohol-containing beverages or preparations. Although no interactions with nonprescription medications have been reported to date, the potential for such adverse drug interactions exists. Therefore, the use of any nonprescription medication should be initiated cautiously according to the directions of use provided on the nonprescription medication. Although sertraline has not been shown to potentiate the impairment of mental and motor skills caused by alcohol, the manufacturers recommend that patients be advised to avoid alcohol while receiving the drug.

Sertraline generally is less sedating than most other currently available antidepressants and does not appear to produce substantial impairment of cognitive or psychomotor function. However, patients should be cautioned that sertraline may impair their ability to perform activities requiring mental alertness or physical coordination (e.g., operating machinery, driving a motor vehicle) and to avoid such activities until they experience how the drug affects them. Because the risk of using sertraline concomitantly with other CNS active drugs has not been evaluated systematically to date, the manufacturers recommend that such therapy be employed cautiously.

Seizures have been reported in patients receiving therapeutic dosages of sertraline. Because of limited experience with sertraline in patients with a history of seizures, the drug should be used with caution in such patients.

Activation of mania and hypomania has occurred in patients receiving therapeutic dosages of sertraline. The drug should be used with caution in patients with a history of mania or hypomania.

Treatment with SSRIs, including sertraline, and selective serotonin- and norepinephrine-reuptake inhibitors (SNRIs) may result in hyponatremia. In many cases, this hyponatremia appears to be due to the syndrome of inappropriate antidiuretic hormone secretion (SIADH) and was reversible when sertraline was discontinued. Cases with serum sodium concentrations lower than 110 mEq/L have been reported. Geriatric individuals and patients receiving diuretics or who are otherwise volume depleted may be at greater risk of developing hyponatremia during therapy with SSRIs or SNRIs. Signs and symptoms of hyponatremia include headache, difficulty concentrating, memory impairment, confusion, weakness, and unsteadiness, which may lead to falls; more severe and/or acute cases have been associated with hallucinations, syncope, seizures, coma, respiratory arrest, and death. Discontinuance of sertraline should be considered in patients with symptomatic hyponatremia and appropriate medical intervention should be instituted. (See Cautions: Renal, Electrolyte, and Genitourinary Effects and also see Cautions: Geriatric Precautions.)

Altered platelet function has been reported rarely in patients receiving sertraline. In addition, use of the drug has been associated with several reports of abnormal bleeding or purpura. While a causal relationship to sertraline remains to be established, pending such establishment, the drug should be used with caution in patients with an underlying coagulation defect since the possible effects on hemostasis may be exaggerated in such patients. (See Cautions: Hematologic Effects.)

SSRIs, including sertraline, may have an effect on pupil size resulting in mydriasis. This mydriatic effect potentially can narrow the eye angle resulting in increased intraocular pressure and angle-closure glaucoma, particularly in predisposed patients. Sertraline should therefore by used with caution in patients with angle-closure glaucoma or a history of glaucoma.

Sertraline has a weak uricosuric effect. (See Cautions: Metabolic Effects.) Pending further elucidation of the clinical importance, if any, of this effect, the drug should be used with caution in patients who may be adversely affected (e.g., those at risk for acute renal failure).

Because sertraline therapy has been associated with anorexia and weight loss (see Cautions: Metabolic Effects), the drug should be used with caution in patients who may be adversely affected by these effects (e.g., underweight patients).

Like many other antidepressant drugs, sertraline has been associated with hypothyroidism, elevated serum thyrotropin, and/or reduced serum thyroxine concentrations in a limited number of patients. Because of reports with other antidepressant agents and the complex interrelationship between the hypothalamic-pituitary-thyroid axis and affective (mood) disorders, at least one manufacturer recommends that thyroid function be reassessed periodically in patients with thyroid disease who are receiving sertraline.

Commercially available sertraline hydrochloride oral solution (Zoloft®) contains alcohol. Therefore, concomitant use of sertraline hydrochloride oral solution and disulfiram is contraindicated.

Sertraline is contraindicated in patients concurrently receiving pimozide. (See Drug Interactions: Pimozide.)

Sertraline also is contraindicated in patients who are hypersensitive to the drug or any ingredient in the formulation.

● Pediatric Precautions

Safety and efficacy of sertraline in children with obsessive-compulsive disorder (OCD) younger than 6 years of age have not been established. Safety and efficacy of sertraline in pediatric patients with other disorders (e.g., major depressive disorder, panic disorder, posttraumatic stress disorder, premenstrual dysphoric disorder, social phobia) have not been established. The overall adverse effect profile of sertraline in over 600 pediatric patients who received sertraline in controlled and uncontrolled clinical trials was generally similar to that seen in the adult clinical studies. As with other SSRIs, decreased appetite and weight loss have been observed in association with sertraline therapy.

Efficacy of sertraline in pediatric patients with major depressive disorder was evaluated in 2 randomized, 10-week, double-blind, placebo-controlled, flexible-dose (50–200 mg daily) trials in 373 children and adolescents with major depressive disorder, but data from these studies were not sufficient to establish efficacy in pediatric patients. In a safety analysis of the pooled data from these 2 studies, a difference in weight change between the sertraline and placebo groups was noted of approximately 1 kg for both pediatric patients (6–11 years of age) and adolescents (12–17 years of age) representing a slight weight loss for those receiving sertraline and a slight weight gain for those receiving placebo. In addition, a larger difference was noted in children than in adolescents between the

sertraline and placebo groups in the proportion of outliers for clinically important weight loss; about 7% of the children and about 2% of the adolescents receiving sertraline in these studies experienced a weight loss of more than 7% of their body weight compared with none of those receiving placebo.

A subset of patients who completed these controlled trials was continued into a 24-week, flexible-dose, open-label, extension study. A mean weight loss of approximately 0.5 kg was observed during the initial 8 weeks of treatment for those pediatric patients first exposed to sertraline during the extension study, which was similar to the weight loss observed among sertraline-treated patients during the first 8 weeks of the randomized controlled trials. The patients continuing in the extension study began gaining weight relative to their baseline weight by week 12 of sertraline therapy, and patients who completed the entire 34 weeks of therapy with the drug had a weight gain that was similar to that expected using data from age-adjusted peers. The manufacturers state that periodic monitoring of weight and growth is recommended in pediatric patients receiving long-term therapy with sertraline or other selective serotonin-reuptake inhibitors (SSRIs).

FDA warns that antidepressants increase the risk of suicidal thinking and behavior (suicidality) in children and adolescents with major depressive disorder and other psychiatric disorders. The risk of suicidality for these drugs was identified in a pooled analysis of data from a total of 24 short-term (4–16 weeks), placebo-controlled studies of 9 antidepressants (i.e., sertraline, bupropion, citalopram, fluoxetine, fluvoxamine, mirtazapine, nefazodone, paroxetine, venlafaxine) in over 4400 children and adolescents with major depressive disorder, OCD, or other psychiatric disorders. The analysis revealed a greater risk of adverse events representing suicidal behavior or thinking (suicidality) during the first few months of treatment in pediatric patients receiving antidepressants than in those receiving placebo. However, a more recent meta-analysis of 27 placebo-controlled trials of 9 antidepressants (SSRIs and others) in patients younger than 19 years of age with major depressive disorder, OCD, or non-OCD anxiety disorders suggests that the benefits of antidepressant therapy in treating these conditions may outweigh the risks of suicidal behavior or suicidal ideation. No suicides occurred in these pediatric trials.

The risk of suicidality in FDA's pooled analysis differed across the different psychiatric indications, with the highest incidence observed in the major depressive disorder studies. In addition, although there was considerable variation in risk among the antidepressants, a tendency toward an increase in suicidality risk in younger patients was found for almost all drugs studied. It is currently unknown whether the suicidality risk in pediatric patients extends to longer-term use (i.e., beyond several months). (See Suicidality, under Cautions: Nervous System Effects, in Paroxetine 28:16.04.20.)

As a result of this analysis and public discussion of the issue, FDA has directed manufacturers of all antidepressants to add a boxed warning to the labeling of their products to alert clinicians of this suicidality risk in children and adolescents and to recommend appropriate monitoring and close observation of patients receiving these agents. (See Cautions: Precautions and Contraindications.) The drugs that are the focus of the revised labeling are all drugs included in the general class of antidepressants, including those that have not been studied in controlled clinical trials in pediatric patients, since the available data are not adequate to exclude any single antidepressant from an increased risk. In addition to the boxed warning and other information in professional labeling on antidepressants, FDA currently recommends that a patient medication guide explaining the risks associated with the drugs be provided to the patient each time the drugs are dispensed. Caregivers of pediatric patients whose depression is persistently worse or who are experiencing emergent suicidality or symptoms that might be precursors to worsening depression or suicidality during antidepressant therapy should consult their clinician regarding the best course of action (e.g., whether the therapeutic regimen should be changed or the drugs discontinued). *Patients should not discontinue use of selective serotonin-reuptake inhibitors without first consulting their clinician; it is very important that the drugs not be abruptly discontinued (see Dosage and Administration: Dosage), as withdrawal effects may occur.*

Anyone considering the use of sertraline in a child or adolescent for any clinical use must balance the potential risk of therapy with the clinical need.

● Geriatric Precautions

In clinical studies in geriatric patients, 660 patients receiving sertraline for the treatment of depression were 65 years of age or older, and 180 were 75 years of age or older. No overall differences in efficacy or adverse effects were observed for geriatric patients in these studies relative to younger patients, and other clinical experience has revealed no evidence of age-related differences in safety. In addition, no adverse effects on psychomotor performance were observed in geriatric individuals who received the drug in one controlled study. However, the possibility that older patients may exhibit increased sensitivity to the drug cannot be excluded. (See Dosage in Geriatric Patients under Dosage and Administration.)

Limited evidence suggests that geriatric patients may be more likely than younger patients to develop sertraline-induced hyponatremia and transient syndrome of inappropriate secretion of antidiuretic hormone (SIADH). Therefore, clinicians prescribing sertraline in geriatric patients should be aware of the possibility that such reactions may occur. Periodic monitoring (especially during the first several months) of serum sodium concentrations in geriatric patients receiving the drug has been recommended by some clinicians. (See Cautions: Precautions and Contraindications.)

As with other psychotropic drugs, geriatric patients receiving antidepressants appear to have an increased risk of hip fracture. Despite the fewer cardiovascular and anticholinergic effects associated with selective serotonin-reuptake inhibitors (SSRIs), these drugs did not show any advantage over tricyclic antidepressants with regard to hip fracture in a case-control study. In addition, there was little difference in the rates of falls between nursing home residents receiving SSRIs and those receiving tricyclic antidepressants in a retrospective study. Therefore, all geriatric individuals receiving either type of antidepressant should be considered to be at increased risk of falls and appropriate measures should be taken.

In pooled data analyses, a *reduced* risk of suicidality was observed in adults 65 years of age or older with antidepressant therapy compared with placebo. (See Cautions: Precautions and Contraindications.)

Plasma clearance of sertraline may be decreased in geriatric patients; plasma clearance of the less active metabolite, *N*-desmethylsertraline, also may be decreased in older males.

● *Mutagenicity and Carcinogenicity*

Sertraline was not mutagenic, with or without metabolic activation, in several in vitro tests including the bacterial mutation assay and the mouse lymphoma mutation assay. Sertraline also was not mutagenic in tests for cytogenetic aberrations in vivo in mouse bone marrow and in vitro in human lymphocytes.

Lifetime studies to determine the carcinogenic potential of sertraline were performed in CD-1 mice and Long-Evans rats receiving dosages up to 40 mg/kg daily. This dosage corresponded to 1 and 2 times the maximum recommended human dose on a mg/m² basis in mice and rats, respectively. There was a dose-related increase in the incidence of hepatic adenomas in male mice receiving sertraline dosages of 10–40 mg/kg (0.25–1 times the maximum recommended human dose on a mg/m² basis). No increase was seen in female mice or in rats of either gender receiving the same dosages, nor was there an increase in hepatocellular carcinomas. Hepatic adenomas have a variable rate of spontaneous occurrence in this strain of mice, and the relevance of this finding to humans is not known. There was an increase in follicular adenomas of the thyroid, not accompanied by thyroid hyperplasia, in female rats receiving a sertraline dosage of 40 mg/kg (2 times the maximum recommended human dose on a mg/m² basis). There also was an increase in uterine adenocarcinomas in rats receiving sertraline dosages of 10–40 mg/kg (0.5–2 times the maximum recommended human dose on a mg/m² basis); however, this effect could not be directly attributed to the drug.

● *Pregnancy, Fertility, and Lactation*
Pregnancy

Some neonates exposed to sertraline and other SSRIs or SNRIs late in the third trimester of pregnancy have developed complications that have sometimes been severe and required prolonged hospitalization, respiratory support, enteral nutrition, and other forms of supportive care in special-care nurseries. Such complications can arise immediately upon delivery and usually last several days or up to 2–4 weeks. Clinical findings reported in the neonates have included respiratory distress, cyanosis, apnea, seizures, temperature instability or fever, feeding difficulty, dehydration, excessive weight loss, vomiting, hypoglycemia, hypotonia, hypertonia, hyperreflexia, tremor, jitteriness, irritability, lethargy, reduced or lack of reaction to pain stimuli, and constant crying. These clinical features appear to be consistent with either a direct toxic effect of the SSRI or SNRI or, possibly, a drug withdrawal syndrome. It should be noted that in some cases the clinical picture was consistent with serotonin syndrome (see Drug Interactions: Serotonergic Drugs).

Infants exposed to SSRIs in late pregnancy may have an increased risk of persistent pulmonary hypertension of the newborn (PPHN). PPHN is a rare heart and lung condition occurring in an estimated 1–2 infants per 1000 live births in the general population; it occurs when a neonate does not adapt to breathing outside the womb. Some experts have suggested that respiratory distress in neonates exposed to SSRIs may occur along a spectrum of seriousness in association with maternal use of SSRIs, with PPHN among the most serious consequences. Neonates with PPHN may require intensive care support, including mechanical ventilation; in severe cases, multiple organ damage, including brain damage, and even death may occur. Although several epidemiologic studies have suggested an increased risk of PPHN with SSRI use during pregnancy, other studies did not demonstrate a statistically significant association. Thus, the FDA states that it is currently unclear whether use of SSRIs, including sertraline, during pregnancy can cause PPHN and recommends that clinicians not alter their current clinical practice of treating depression during pregnancy.

When treating a pregnant woman with sertraline during the third trimester of pregnancy, the clinician should carefully consider the potential risks and benefits of such therapy. Clinicians should consider that in a prospective longitudinal study of 201 women with a history of recurrent major depression who were euthymic in the context of antidepressant therapy at the beginning of pregnancy, women who discontinued their antidepressant medication (SSRIs, tricyclic antidepressants, or others) during pregnancy were found to be substantially more likely to have a relapse of depression than were women who continued to receive their antidepressant therapy while pregnant. Consideration may be given to cautiously tapering sertraline therapy in the third trimester prior to delivery if the drug is administered during pregnancy. (See Treatment of Pregnant Women during the Third Trimester under Dosage and Administration: Dosage.)

For additional information on the management of depression in women prior to conception and during pregnancy, including treatment algorithms, the FDA advises clinicians to consult the joint American Psychiatric Association and American College of Obstetricians and Gynecologists guidelines (at https://www.ncbi.nlm.nih.gov/pmc/articles/PMC3103063/pdf/nihms293836.pdf).

Most epidemiologic studies of pregnancy outcome following first-trimester exposure to SSRIs, including sertraline, conducted to date have not revealed evidence of an increased risk of major congenital malformations. In a prospective, controlled, multicenter study, maternal use of several SSRIs (sertraline, fluvoxamine, paroxetine) in a limited number of pregnant women did not appear to increase the risk of congenital malformation, miscarriage, stillbirth, or premature delivery when used during pregnancy at recommended dosages. Birth weight and gestational age in neonates exposed to the drugs were similar to those in the control group. In another small study based on medical records review, the incidence of congenital anomalies reported in infants born to women who were treated with sertraline and other SSRIs during pregnancy was comparable to that observed in the general population. However, the results of epidemiologic studies indicate that exposure to paroxetine during the first trimester of pregnancy may increase the risk for congenital malformations, particularly cardiovascular malformations. (See Cautions: Pregnancy, Fertility, and Lactation, in Paroxetine 28:16.04.20.) Additional epidemiologic studies are needed to more thoroughly evaluate the relative safety of sertraline and other SSRIs during pregnancy, including their potential teratogenic risks and possible effects on neurobehavioral development.

The manufacturers state that there are no adequate and controlled studies to date using sertraline in pregnant women, and the drug should be used during pregnancy only when the potential benefits justify the potential risks to the fetus. Women should be advised to notify their clinician if they become pregnant or plan to become pregnant during therapy with the drug. FDA states that women who are pregnant or thinking about becoming pregnant should not discontinue any antidepressant, including sertraline, without first consulting their clinician. The decision whether or not to continue antidepressant therapy should be made only after careful consideration of the potential benefits and risks of antidepressant therapy for each individual pregnant patient. If a decision is made to discontinue treatment with sertraline or other SSRIs before or during pregnancy, discontinuance of therapy should be done in consultation with the clinician in accordance with the prescribing information for the antidepressant and the patient should be closely monitored for possible relapse of depression.

Reproduction studies in rats using sertraline dosages up to 80 mg/kg daily and in rabbits using dosages up to 40 mg/kg daily have not revealed evidence of teratogenicity; these dosages correspond to approximately 4 times the maximum recommended human dosage on a mg/m² basis. No evidence of teratogenicity was observed at any dosage studied. When pregnant rats and rabbits were given sertraline during the period of organogenesis, delayed ossification was observed in fetuses at doses of 10 mg/kg (0.5 times the maximum recommended human dose on a mg/m² basis) in rats and 40 mg/kg (4 times the maximum recommended human dose on a mg/m² basis) in rabbits. When female rats received sertraline during the last third of gestation and throughout lactation, there was an increase in the number of stillborn pups and in the number of pups dying during the first 4 days after birth. The body weights of the pups also were decreased during the first 4 days after birth. These effects occurred at a dose of 20 mg/kg (approximately the same as the maximum recommended human dose on a mg/m² basis). At 10 mg/kg (0.5 times the maximum recommended human dose on a mg/m² basis), no effect on rat pup mortality was observed. The decrease in pup survival was shown to result from in utero exposure to the drug. The clinical importance of these effects is not known.

The effect of sertraline on labor and delivery is not known.

Fertility

A decrease in fertility was observed in 1 of 2 reproduction studies in rats using sertraline dosages of 80 mg/kg (4 times the maximum recommended human dose on a mg/m² basis).

Lactation

Sertraline and its principal metabolite, *N*-desmethylsertraline, are distributed into milk. Sertraline should be used with caution in nursing women, and women should be advised to notify their physician if they plan to breast-feed.

DRUG INTERACTIONS

● *Serotonergic Drugs*

Use of selective serotonin-reuptake-inhibitors (SSRIs) such as sertraline concurrently or in close succession with other drugs that affect serotonergic neurotransmission may result in serotonin syndrome or neuroleptic malignant syndrome (NMS)-like reactions. Symptoms of serotonin syndrome may include mental status changes (e.g., agitation, hallucinations, coma), autonomic instability (e.g., tachycardia, labile blood pressure, hyperthermia), neuromuscular aberrations (e.g., hyperreflexia, incoordination), and/or GI symptoms (e.g., nausea, vomiting, diarrhea). Although the syndrome appears to be relatively uncommon and usually mild in severity, serious and potentially life-threatening complications, including seizures, disseminated intravascular coagulation, respiratory failure, and severe hyperthermia as well as death occasionally have been reported. In its most severe form, serotonin syndrome may resemble NMS, which is characterized by hyperthermia, muscle rigidity, autonomic instability with possible rapid fluctuation in vital signs, and mental status changes. The precise mechanism of these reactions is not fully understood; however, they appear to result from excessive serotonergic activity in the CNS, probably mediated by activation of serotonin 5-HT$_{1A}$ receptors. The possible involvement of dopamine and 5-HT$_2$ receptors also has been suggested, although their roles remain unclear.

Serotonin syndrome most commonly occurs when 2 or more drugs that affect serotonergic neurotransmission are administered either concurrently or in close succession. Serotonergic agents include those that increase serotonin synthesis (e.g., the serotonin precursor tryptophan), stimulate synaptic serotonin release (e.g., some amphetamines, dexfenfluramine [no longer commercially available in the US], fenfluramine [no longer commercially available in the US]), inhibit the reuptake of serotonin after release (e.g., SSRIs, selective serotonin- and norepinephrine-reuptake inhibitors [SNRIs], tricyclic antidepressants, trazodone, dextromethorphan, meperidine, tramadol), decrease the metabolism of serotonin (e.g., MAO inhibitors), have direct serotonin postsynaptic receptor activity (e.g., buspirone), or nonspecifically induce increases in serotonergic neuronal activity (e.g., lithium salts). Selective agonists of serotonin (5-hydroxytryptamine; 5-HT) type 1 receptors ("triptans") and dihydroergotamine, agents with serotonergic activity used in the management of migraine headache, and St. John's wort (*Hypericum perforatum*) also have been implicated in serotonin syndrome.

The combination of SSRIs and MAO inhibitors may result in serotonin syndrome or NMS-like reactions. Such reactions have also been reported in patients receiving SSRIs concomitantly with tryptophan, lithium, dextromethorphan, sumatriptan, dihydroergotamine, or antipsychotics or other dopamine antagonists. In rare cases, serotonin syndrome reportedly has occurred in patients receiving the recommended dosage of a single serotonergic agent (e.g., clomipramine) or during accidental overdosage (e.g., sertraline intoxication in a child). Some other drugs that have been implicated in precipitating symptoms suggestive of serotonin syndrome or NMS-like reactions include buspirone, bromocriptine, dextropropoxyphene, linezolid, methylene blue, methylenedioxymethamphetamine (MDMA; "ecstasy"), selegiline (a selective MAO-B inhibitor),

and sibutramine (an SNRI used for the management of obesity [no longer commercially available in the US]). Other drugs that have been associated with the syndrome but for which less convincing data are available include carbamazepine, fentanyl, and pentazocine.

Clinicians should be aware of the potential for serious, possibly fatal reactions associated with serotonin syndrome or NMS-like reactions in patients receiving 2 or more drugs that affect serotonergic neurotransmission, even if no such interactions with the specific drugs have been reported to date in the medical literature. Pending further accumulation of data, serotonergic drugs should be used cautiously in combination and such combinations avoided whenever clinically possible. Serotonin syndrome may be more likely to occur when initiating therapy, increasing the dosage, or following the addition of another serotonergic drug. Some clinicians state that patients who have experienced serotonin syndrome may be at higher risk for recurrence of the syndrome upon reinitiation of serotonergic drugs. Pending further experience in such cases, some clinicians recommend that therapy with serotonergic agents be limited following recovery. In cases in which the potential benefit of the drug is thought to outweigh the risk of serotonin syndrome, lower potency agents and reduced dosages should be used, combination serotonergic therapy should be avoided, and patients should be monitored carefully for manifestations of serotonin syndrome. If signs and symptoms of serotonin syndrome or NMS develop during therapy, treatment with sertraline and any concurrently administered serotonergic or antidopaminergic agents, including antipsychotic agents, should be discontinued immediately and supportive and symptomatic treatment should be initiated.

For further information on serotonin syndrome, including manifestations and treatment, see Drug Interactions: Serotonergic Drugs, in Fluoxetine Hydrochloride 28:16.04.20.

Monoamine Oxidase Inhibitors

Potentially serious, sometimes fatal serotonin syndrome or NMS-like reactions have been reported in patients receiving SSRIs, including sertraline, in combination with an MAO inhibitor. Severe serotonin syndrome reaction developed several hours after initiating sertraline in a woman already receiving phenelzine, lithium, thioridazine, and doxepin. Such reactions also have been reported in patients who recently have discontinued an SSRI and have been started on an MAO inhibitor.

Because of the potential risk of serotonin syndrome or NMS-like reactions, concomitant use of sertraline and MAO inhibitors is contraindicated. At least 2 weeks should elapse between discontinuance of MAO inhibitor therapy and initiation of sertraline therapy and vice versa.

Linezolid

Linezolid, an anti-infective agent that is a nonselective and reversible MAO inhibitor, has been associated with drug interactions resulting in serotonin syndrome, including some associated with SSRIs, and potentially may also cause NMS-like reactions. Because of the risk of serotonin syndrome, linezolid generally should *not* be used in patients receiving sertraline. The US Food and Drug Administration (FDA) states that certain life-threatening or urgent situations may necessitate immediate linezolid treatment in a patient receiving a serotonergic drug, including SSRIs. In such emergency situations, the availability of alternative anti-infectives should be considered and the benefits of linezolid should be weighed against the risk of serotonin syndrome. If linezolid is indicated in such emergency situations, sertraline must be immediately discontinued and the patient monitored for symptoms of CNS toxicity (e.g., mental changes, muscle twitching, excessive sweating, shivering/shaking, diarrhea, loss of coordination, fever) for 2 weeks or until 24 hours after the last linezolid dose, whichever comes first. Treatment with sertraline may be resumed 24 hours after the last linezolid dose.

If nonemergency use of linezolid is being planned for a patient receiving sertraline, sertraline should be withheld for at least 2 weeks prior to initiating linezolid.

Treatment with sertraline should not be initiated in a patient receiving linezolid; when necessary, sertraline may be started 24 hours after the last linezolid dose. (See Drug Interactions: Serotonergic Drugs, in Linezolid 8:12.28.24.)

Methylene Blue

There have been case reports of serotonin syndrome in patients who received methylene blue, which is a potent and selective inhibitor of MAO-A, while receiving serotonergic drugs, including SSRIs (e.g., citalopram, escitalopram, fluoxetine, fluvoxamine, paroxetine, sertraline). Therefore, methylene blue generally should *not* be used in patients receiving sertraline. The FDA states that certain emergency situations (e.g., methemoglobinemia, ifosfamide-induced encephalopathy†) may necessitate immediate use of methylene blue in a patient receiving sertraline. In such emergency situations, the availability of alternative interventions should be considered and the benefits of methylene blue should be weighed against the risk of serotonin syndrome. If methylene blue is indicated in such emergency situations, sertraline must be immediately discontinued and the patient monitored for symptoms of CNS toxicity (e.g., mental changes, muscle twitching, excessive sweating, shivering/shaking, diarrhea, loss of coordination, fever) for 2 weeks or until 24 hours after the last methylene blue dose, whichever come first. Treatment with sertraline may be resumed 24 hours after the last methylene blue dose.

If nonemergency use of methylene blue is being planned for a patient receiving sertraline, sertraline should be withheld for at least 2 weeks prior to initiating methylene blue.

Treatment with sertraline should not be initiated in a patient receiving methylene blue; when necessary, sertraline may be started 24 hours after the last methylene blue dose.

Moclobemide

Moclobemide (not commercially available in the US), a selective and reversible MAO-A inhibitor, has been associated with serotonin syndrome, and such reactions have been fatal in several cases in which the drug was given in combination with the SSRI citalopram or with clomipramine. Pending further experience with such combinations, some clinicians recommend that concurrent therapy with moclobemide and SSRIs be used only with extreme caution and that SSRIs should have been discontinued for some time (depending on the elimination half-lives of the drug and its active metabolites) before initiating moclobemide therapy.

Selegiline

Selegiline, a selective MAO-B inhibitor used in the management of parkinsonian syndrome, has been reported to cause serotonin syndrome when given concurrently with SSRIs (e.g., fluoxetine, paroxetine, sertraline). Although selegiline is a selective MAO-B inhibitor at therapeutic dosages, the drug appears to lose its selectivity for the MAO-B enzyme at higher dosages (e.g., those exceeding 10 mg/kg), thereby increasing the risk of serotonin syndrome in patients receiving higher dosages of the drug either alone or in combination with other serotonergic agents. The manufacturer of selegiline recommends avoiding concurrent selegiline and SSRI therapy. In addition, the manufacturer of selegiline recommends that at least 2 weeks elapse between discontinuance of selegiline and initiation of SSRI therapy.

Isoniazid

Isoniazid, an antituberculosis agent, appears to have some MAO-inhibiting activity. In addition, iproniazid (not commercially available in the US), another antituberculosis agent structurally related to isoniazid that also possesses MAO-inhibiting activity, reportedly has resulted in serotonin syndrome in at least 2 patients when given in combination with meperidine. Pending further experience, clinicians should be aware of the potential for serotonin syndrome when isoniazid is given in combination with SSRI therapy (such as sertraline) or other serotonergic agents.

Tryptophan and Other Serotonin Precursors

Because of the potential risk of serotonin syndrome or NMS-like reactions, concurrent use of tryptophan or other serotonin precursors should be avoided in patients receiving sertraline.

5-HT$_1$ Receptor Agonists ("Triptans")

Weakness, hyperreflexia, and incoordination have been reported rarely during postmarketing surveillance in patients receiving sumatriptan concomitantly with an SSRI (e.g., citalopram, escitalopram, fluoxetine, fluvoxamine, paroxetine, sertraline); these reactions resembled serotonin syndrome. Oral or subcutaneous sumatriptan and SSRIs were used concomitantly in some clinical studies without unusual adverse effects. However, an increase in the frequency of migraine attacks and a decrease in the effectiveness of sumatriptan in relieving migraine headache have been reported in a patient receiving subcutaneous injections of sumatriptan intermittently while undergoing fluoxetine therapy.

Clinicians prescribing 5-HT$_1$ receptor agonists, SSRIs, and SNRIs should consider that 5-HT$_1$ receptor agonists often are used intermittently and that either the 5-HT$_1$ receptor agonist, SSRI, or SNRI may be prescribed by a different clinician. Clinicians also should weigh the potential risk of serotonin syndrome or NMS-like reactions with the expected benefit of using a 5-HT$_1$ receptor agonist concurrently with SSRI or SNRI therapy. If concomitant treatment with sumatriptan or another 5-HT$_1$ receptor agonist and sertraline is clinically warranted, the patient should be observed carefully, particularly during treatment initiation, dosage increases, and following the addition of other serotonergic agents. Patients receiving concomitant 5-HT$_1$ receptor agonist and SSRI or SNRI therapy should be informed of the possibility of serotonin syndrome or NMS-like reactions and advised to immediately seek medical attention if they experience signs or symptoms of these syndromes.

Sibutramine

Because of the possibility of developing potentially serious, sometimes fatal serotonin syndrome or NMS-like reactions, sibutramine (no longer commercially available in the US) should be used with caution in patients receiving sertraline.

Other Selective Serotonin-reuptake Inhibitors and Selective Serotonin- and Norepinephrine-reuptake Inhibitors

Concomitant administration of sertraline with other SSRIs or SNRIs potentially may result in serotonin syndrome or NMS-like reactions and is therefore not recommended. (See Dosage and Administration: Dosage.)

Antipsychotic Agents and Other Dopamine Antagonists

Concomitant use of antipsychotic agents and other dopamine antagonists with sertraline rarely may result in potentially serious, sometimes fatal serotonin syndrome or NMS-like reactions. If signs and symptoms of serotonin syndrome or NMS occur, treatment with sertraline and any concurrently administered antidopaminergic or serotonergic agents should be immediately discontinued and supportive and symptomatic treatment initiated. (See Drug Interactions: Clozapine and also see Drug Interactions: Pimozide.)

Tramadol and Other Serotonergic Drugs

Because of the potential risk of serotonin syndrome or NMS-like reactions, caution is advised whenever SSRIs, including sertraline, and SNRIs are concurrently administered with other drugs that may affect serotonergic neurotransmitter systems, including tramadol and St. John's wort (*Hypericum perforatum*).

● Drugs Undergoing Hepatic Metabolism or Affecting Hepatic Microsomal Enzymes

Animal studies have demonstrated that sertraline induces hepatic microsomal enzymes. In humans, microsomal enzyme induction by sertraline was minimal as determined by a small (5%) but statistically significant decrease in antipyrine half-life following sertraline administration (200 mg daily) for 21 days. The manufacturers state that this small change in antipyrine half-life reflects a clinically unimportant change in hepatic metabolism. Nonetheless, caution should be exercised when sertraline is given to patients receiving drugs that are hepatically metabolized and that have a low therapeutic ratio, such as warfarin. (See Drug Interactions: Protein-bound Drugs and also see Anticoagulants under Drug Interactions: Drugs Affecting Hemostasis.)

Drugs Metabolized by Cytochrome P-450 (CYP) 2D6

Sertraline, like many other antidepressants (e.g., other SSRIs, many tricyclic antidepressants) is metabolized by the drug-metabolizing cytochrome P-450 (CYP) 2D6 isoenzyme (debrisoquine hydroxylase). In addition, like many other drugs metabolized by CYP2D6, sertraline inhibits the activity of CYP2D6 and potentially may increase plasma concentrations of concomitantly administered drugs that also are metabolized by this isoenzyme. Although similar interactions are possible with other SSRIs, there is considerable variability among the drugs in the extent to which they inhibit CYP2D6. At lower doses, sertraline has demonstrated a less prominent inhibitory effect on CYP2D6 than some other SSRIs. Nevertheless, even sertraline has the potential for clinically important CYP2D6 inhibition.

Concomitant use of sertraline with other drugs metabolized by CYP2D6 has not been systematically studied. The extent to which this potential interaction may become clinically important depends on the extent of inhibition of CYP2D6 by the antidepressant and the therapeutic index of the concomitantly administered drug. The drugs for which this potential interaction is of greatest concern are those that are metabolized principally by CYP2D6 and have a narrow therapeutic index, such as tricyclic antidepressants, class IC antiarrhythmics (e.g., propafenone, flecainide, encainide), and some phenothiazines (e.g., thioridazine).

Caution should be used whenever concurrent therapy with sertraline and other drugs metabolized by CYP2D6 is considered. Because concomitant use of sertraline and thioridazine may result in increased plasma concentrations of the phenothiazine and increase the risk of serious, potentially fatal, adverse cardiac effects (e.g., cardiac arrhythmias), the manufacturer of thioridazine states that the drug should not be used concomitantly with any drug that inhibits the CYP2D6 isoenzyme. The manufacturers of sertraline state that concurrent use of a drug metabolized by CYP2D6 may necessitate the administration of dosages of the other drug that are lower than those usually prescribed. Furthermore, whenever sertraline therapy is discontinued (and plasma concentrations of sertraline are decreased) during concurrent therapy with another drug metabolized by CYP2D6, an increased dosage of the concurrently administered drug may be necessary.

Drugs Metabolized by Cytochrome P-450 (CYP) 3A4

Although sertraline can inhibit the cytochrome P-450 (CYP) 3A4 isoenzyme, results of in vitro and in vivo studies indicate that the drug is a much less potent inhibitor of this enzyme than many other drugs. In an in vivo drug interaction study, concomitant use of sertraline and the CYP3A4 substrate, carbamazepine, under steady-state conditions had no effect on plasma concentrations of carbamazepine. The manufacturers of sertraline state that these data suggest that the extent of sertraline's inhibition of CYP3A4 activity is unlikely to be of clinical importance. However, a marked increase in plasma concentrations (ranging from 80–250%) and bone marrow suppression developed within 1–2 months of initiating sertraline in a patient previously stabilized on carbamazepine and flecainide therapy. Although the precise mechanism for this possible interaction and the role of the cytochrome P-450 enzyme system are unclear, some clinicians recommend that carbamazepine concentrations be monitored during concomitant sertraline therapy.

Results of an in vivo drug interaction study with cisapride indicate that concomitant use of sertraline (200 mg daily) induces the metabolism of cisapride; peak plasma concentrations and area under the plasma concentration-time curve (AUC) of cisapride were decreased by about 35% in the study. However, the manufacturers of sertraline state that the extent of sertraline's inhibition of CYP3A4 activity is unlikely to be of clinical importance.

Results of another drug interaction study in which sertraline was used concomitantly with terfenadine (no longer commercially available in the US), a drug metabolized principally by the cytochrome P-450 microsomal enzyme system (mainly by the CYP3A4 isoenzyme), indicate that concurrent use of sertraline did not increase plasma concentrations of terfenadine and, therefore, the manufacturers state that these data suggest that the extent of sertraline's inhibition of CYP3A4 activity is unlikely to be of clinical importance. However, the manufacturer of astemizole (no longer commercially available in the US) and some clinicians state that until the clinical importance of these findings is established, concomitant use of sertraline with astemizole or terfenadine is not recommended since substantially increased plasma concentrations of unchanged astemizole or terfenadine could occur resulting in an increased risk of serious adverse cardiac effects.

Tricyclic and Other Antidepressants

The extent to which SSRI interactions with tricyclic antidepressants may pose clinical problems depends on the degree of inhibition and the pharmacokinetics of the serotonin-reuptake inhibitor involved. In healthy individuals, sertraline has been shown to substantially reduce the clearance of two tricyclic antidepressants, desipramine and imipramine. This interaction appears to result from sertraline-induced inhibition of CYP2D6. Thus, the manufacturers and some clinicians recommend that caution be exercised during concurrent use of tricyclics with sertraline since sertraline may inhibit the metabolism of the tricyclic antidepressant. In addition, plasma tricyclic concentrations may need to be monitored and the dosage of the tricyclic reduced during concomitant administration. (See Dosage and Administration: Dosage and also see Drugs Metabolized by Cytochrome P-450 [CYP] 2D6 under Drug Interactions: Drugs Undergoing Hepatic Metabolism or Affecting Hepatic Microsomal Enzymes.)

Clinical experience regarding the optimal timing of switching from other antidepressants to sertraline therapy is limited. Therefore, the manufacturers recommend that care and prudent medical judgment be exercised when switching from

other antidepressants to sertraline, particularly from long-acting agents (e.g., fluoxetine). Pending further experience in patients being transferred from therapy with another antidepressant to sertraline and as the clinical situation permits, it generally is recommended that the previous antidepressant be discontinued according to the recommended guidelines for the specific antidepressant prior to initiation of sertraline therapy. (See Drug Interactions: Serotonergic Drugs.)

Protein-bound Drugs

Because sertraline is highly protein bound, the drug theoretically could be displaced from binding sites by, or it could displace from binding sites, other protein-bound drugs such as oral anticoagulants or digitoxin. In vitro studies to date have shown that sertraline has no effect on the protein binding of 2 other highly protein-bound drugs, propranolol or warfarin; these findings also have been confirmed in clinical studies. However, pending further accumulation of data, patients receiving sertraline concomitantly with any highly protein-bound drug should be observed for potential adverse effects associated with combined therapy. (See Anticoagulants under Drug Interactions: Drugs Affecting Hemostasis.)

Drugs Affecting Hemostasis
Anticoagulants

In a study comparing prothrombin time AUC (0–120 hour) following a dose of warfarin (0.75 mg/kg) or placebo prior to and after 21 days of either sertraline (50–200 mg daily) or placebo, prothrombin time increased by an average of 8% compared with baseline in the sertraline group and decreased by an average of 1% in those receiving placebo. In addition, the normalization of prothrombin time was slightly delayed in those receiving sertraline when compared with those receiving placebo. Because the clinical importance of these findings is not known, prothrombin time should be monitored carefully whenever sertraline therapy is initiated or discontinued in patients receiving anticoagulants. (See Drug Interactions: Protein-bound Drugs.)

Other Drugs That Interfere with Hemostasis

Epidemiologic case-control and cohort design studies that have demonstrated an association between selective serotonin-reuptake inhibitor therapy and an increased risk of upper GI bleeding also have shown that concurrent use of aspirin or other nonsteroidal anti-inflammatory agents substantially increases the risk of GI bleeding. Although these studies focused on upper GI bleeding, there is some evidence suggesting that bleeding at other sites may be similarly potentiated. The precise mechanism for this increased risk remains to be clearly established; however, serotonin release by platelets is known to play an important role in hemostasis, and selective serotonin-reuptake inhibitors decrease serotonin uptake from the blood by platelets, thereby decreasing the amount of serotonin in platelets. Patients receiving sertraline should be cautioned about the concomitant use of drugs that interfere with hemostasis, including aspirin and other nonsteroidal anti-inflammatory agents.

Alcohol

Sertraline administration did not potentiate the cognitive and psychomotor effects induced by alcohol in healthy individuals. In addition, no apparent additive CNS depressant effects were observed in geriatric patients receiving sertraline together with moderate amounts of alcohol. Nonetheless, the manufacturers state that concurrent use of sertraline and alcohol is not recommended.

Electroconvulsive Therapy

The effects of sertraline in conjunction with electroconvulsive therapy (ECT) have not been evaluated to date in clinical studies.

Cimetidine

In a study evaluating the effect of the addition of a single dose of sertraline (100 mg) on the second of 8 days of cimetidine administration (800 mg daily), the mean AUC, peak concentration, and elimination half-life of sertraline increased substantially (by 50, 24, and 26%, respectively) compared with the placebo group. The clinical importance of these changes is unknown.

Benzodiazepines

In a study comparing the disposition of diazepam administered IV before and after 21 days of sertraline therapy (dosage titrated from 50–200 mg daily) or placebo, there was a 32% decrease in diazepam clearance in the sertraline recipients and a 19% decrease in those receiving placebo when compared with baseline. There was a 23% increase in the time to maximal plasma concentration for desmethyldiazepam in the sertraline group compared with a 20% decrease in the placebo group. The clinical importance of these findings is unknown; however, they suggest that sertraline and *N*-desmethylsertraline are not likely to substantially inhibit the CYP2C19 and CYP3A3/4 hepatic isoenzymes involved in the metabolism of diazepam.

● Clozapine

Concomitant use of SSRIs such as sertraline in patients receiving clozapine can increase plasma concentrations of the antipsychotic agent. In a study in schizophrenic patients receiving clozapine under steady-state conditions, initiation of paroxetine therapy resulted in only minor changes in plasma concentrations of clozapine and its metabolites; however, initiation of fluvoxamine therapy resulted in increases that were threefold compared with baseline. In other published reports, concomitant use of clozapine and SSRIs (fluvoxamine, paroxetine, sertraline) resulted in modest increases (less than twofold) in clozapine and metabolite concentrations. The manufacturer of clozapine states that caution should be exercised and patients closely monitored if clozapine is used in patients receiving SSRIs, and a reduction in clozapine dosage should be considered. (See Antipsychotic Agents and Other Dopamine Antagonists under Drug Interactions: Serotonergic Drugs.)

● Lithium

In a placebo-controlled trial, the administration of 2 doses of sertraline did not substantially alter steady-state plasma lithium concentrations or the renal clearance of lithium. Pending further accumulation of data, however, the manufacturers recommend that plasma lithium concentrations be monitored following initiation of sertraline in patients receiving lithium and that lithium dosage be adjusted accordingly. In addition, because of the potential risk of serotonin syndrome or NMS-like reactions, caution is advised during concurrent sertraline and lithium use. (See Drug Interactions: Serotonergic Drugs.)

● Hypoglycemic Drugs

In a placebo-controlled study in healthy male volunteers, sertraline administration for 22 days (including 200 mg daily for the final 13 days) caused a small but statistically significant decrease (16%) in the clearance of a 1-g IV dose of tolbutamide compared with baseline values and an increase in the terminal elimination half-life (from 6.9 to 8.6 hours). The decrease in clearance was not accompanied by any substantial changes in the plasma protein binding or the apparent volume of distribution of tolbutamide, which suggests that the change in tolbutamide clearance may be caused by a slight inhibition of the cytochrome P-450 isoenzyme CYP2C9/10 when sertraline is given in the maximum recommended dosage. The clinical importance of these findings remains to be determined.

● Digoxin

In a placebo-controlled trial in healthy volunteers, sertraline administration for 17 days (including 200 mg daily for the final 10 days) did not alter serum digoxin concentrations or renal clearance of digoxin. The results of this study suggest that dosage adjustment of digoxin may not be necessary in patients receiving concomitant sertraline.

● Atenolol

In a double-blind, placebo-controlled, randomized, crossover study, a single, 100-mg dose of sertraline had no effect on the β-adrenergic blocking activity of atenolol when administered to a limited number of healthy males.

● Amiodarone

A decrease in the plasma concentrations of amiodarone and its active metabolite, desmethylamiodarone, to 82 and 85% of the baseline values, respectively, occurred in one patient following the discontinuance of sertraline and carbamazepine therapy, suggesting that sertraline may have been inhibiting the metabolism of amiodarone by CYP3A4.

● Phenytoin

In a randomized, double-blind, placebo-controlled trial, chronic administration of high dosages of sertraline (200 mg daily) did not substantially affect the pharmacokinetics or pharmacodynamics of phenytoin when the 2 drugs were given concurrently in healthy volunteers. However, substantial reductions in plasma sertraline concentrations have been observed in sertraline-treated patients concurrently

receiving phenytoin; it was suggested that induction of the cytochrome P-450 isoenzymes may be responsible. In addition, concurrent administration of sertraline and phenytoin reportedly resulted in elevated phenytoin concentrations in 2 geriatric patients. Pending further accumulation of data, the manufacturers and some clinicians recommend that plasma phenytoin concentrations be monitored following initiation of sertraline therapy and that phenytoin dosage should be adjusted as necessary, particularly in patients with multiple underlying medical conditions and/or those receiving multiple concomitant drugs.

● Pimozide

Concomitant use of sertraline and pimozide has resulted in substantial increases in peak plasma concentrations and area under the plasma concentration-time curve (AUC) of pimozide. In one controlled study, administration of a single 2-mg dose of pimozide in individuals receiving sertraline 200 mg daily resulted in a mean increase in pimozide AUC and peak plasma concentrations of about 40%, but was not associated with changes in ECG parameters. The effects on QT interval and pharmacokinetic parameters of pimozide administered in higher doses (i.e., doses exceeding 2 mg) in combination with sertraline are as yet unknown. Concomitant use of sertraline and pimozide is contraindicated because of the low therapeutic index of pimozide and because the reported interaction between the 2 drugs occurred at a low dose of pimozide. The mechanism of this interaction is as yet unknown. (See Antipsychotic Agents and Other Dopamine Antagonists under Drug Interactions: Serotonergic Drugs.)

● Valproic Acid

The effect of sertraline on plasma valproic acid concentrations remains to be evaluated in clinical studies. In the absence of such data, the manufacturers recommend monitoring plasma valproic acid concentrations following initiation of sertraline therapy and adjusting the dosage of valproic acid as necessary.

ACUTE TOXICITY

● Pathogenesis

The acute lethal dose of sertraline in humans is not known. One patient who ingested 13.5 g of sertraline alone subsequently recovered. However, death occurred in another patient who ingested 2.5 g of the drug alone.

In general, overdosage of sertraline may be expected to produce effects that are extensions of the drug's pharmacologic and adverse effects. The most common signs and symptoms associated with nonfatal sertraline overdosage include somnolence, nausea, vomiting, tachycardia, dizziness, agitation, and tremor. Other adverse events observed in patients who received overdosages of sertraline (alone or in combination with other drugs) include bradycardia, bundle branch block, coma, seizures, delirium, hallucinations, hypertension, hypotension, manic reaction, pancreatitis, QT-interval prolongation, serotonin syndrome, stupor, and syncope. Prolonged tachycardia, hypertension, hallucinations, hyperthermia, tremors of the extremities, and skin flushing have occurred in a child after accidental sertraline ingestion; the reaction resembled serotonin syndrome. Flushing, anger, emotional lability, and distractability developed 1 hour after an adult female ingested 2 g of sertraline; recovery was uneventful apart from watery bowel movements.

● Treatment

Because fatalities and severe toxicity have been reported when sertraline was ingested alone or in combination with other drugs and/or alcohol, the manufacturers and some clinicians recommend that any overdosage involving sertraline be managed aggressively. Clinicians also should consider the possibility of serotonin syndrome or NMS-like reactions in patients presenting with similar clinical features and a recent history of sertraline and/or ingestion of other serotonergic agents and/or antipsychotic agents or other dopamine antagonists. (See Cautions: Precautions and Contraindications and also see Drug Interactions: Serotonergic Drugs.)

Management of sertraline overdosage generally involves symptomatic and supportive care. A patent airway should be established and maintained, and adequate oxygenation and ventilation should be ensured. ECG and vital sign monitoring is recommended following acute overdosage with the drug, although the value of ECG monitoring in predicting the severity of sertraline-induced cardiotoxicity is not known. (See Acute Toxicity: Manifestations, in the Tricyclic Antidepressants General Statement 28:16.04.28.) There is no specific antidote for sertraline intoxication. Because suicidal ingestion often involves more than one drug, clinicians treating sertraline overdosage should be alert to possible manifestations caused by drugs other than sertraline.

If the patient is comatose, having seizures, or lacks the gag reflex, gastric lavage may be performed if an endotracheal tube with cuff inflated is in place to prevent aspiration of gastric contents. Since administration of activated charcoal (which may be used in conjunction with sorbitol) may be as effective as or more effective than induction of emesis or gastric lavage, its use has been recommended either in the initial management of sertraline overdosage or following induction of emesis or gastric lavage in patients who have ingested a potentially toxic quantity of the drug.

Limited data indicate that sertraline is not appreciably removed by hemodialysis. Because of the large volume of distribution of sertraline and its principal metabolite, peritoneal dialysis, forced diuresis, hemoperfusion, and/or exchange transfusion also are likely to be ineffective in removing substantial amounts of sertraline and N-desmethylsertraline from the body.

Clinicians should consult a poison control center for additional information on the management of sertraline overdosage.

CHRONIC TOXICITY

Sertraline has not been studied systematically in animals or humans to determine whether therapy with the drug is associated with abuse, tolerance, or physical dependence.

The premarketing clinical experience with sertraline did not reveal any tendency for a withdrawal syndrome or any drug-seeking behavior. However, fatigue, severe abdominal cramping, memory impairment, and influenza-like symptoms were reported 2 days following abrupt discontinuance of sertraline in one patient; when sertraline was restarted, the symptoms remitted. Electric shock-like sensations occurred in another patient 1 day after the last administered dose of sertraline; these sensations became less intense and eventually disappeared 13 weeks after sertraline therapy was discontinued. When evaluating these cases and those reported with other serotonin-reuptake inhibitors, it appears that a withdrawal syndrome may occur within several days following abrupt discontinuance of these drugs. The most commonly observed symptoms are those that resemble influenza, such as fatigue, stomach complaints (e.g., nausea), dizziness or lightheadedness, tremor, anxiety, chills, sweating, and incoordination. Other reported symptoms include memory impairment, insomnia, paresthesia, shock-like sensations, headache, palpitations, agitation, or aggression. Such reactions appear to be self-limiting and improve over 1 to several weeks. Pending further experience, sertraline therapy should be discontinued gradually to prevent the possible development of withdrawal reactions.

As with other CNS-active drugs, clinicians should carefully evaluate patients for a history of substance abuse prior to initiating sertraline therapy. If sertraline therapy is initiated in patients with a history of substance abuse, such patients should be monitored closely for signs of misuse or abuse of the drug (e.g., development of tolerance, use of increasing doses, drug-seeking behavior).

The potential for misuse of sertraline in patients with concurrent eating disorders and/or those who may seek the drug for its appetite-suppressant effects also may be considered.

PHARMACOLOGY

The pharmacology of sertraline is complex and in many ways resembles that of other antidepressant agents, particularly those agents (e.g., fluoxetine, fluvoxamine, paroxetine, clomipramine, trazodone) that predominantly potentiate the pharmacologic effects of serotonin (5-HT). Like other selective serotonin-reuptake inhibitors (SSRIs), sertraline is a potent and highly selective reuptake inhibitor of serotonin and has little or no effect on other neurotransmitters.

● Nervous System Effects

The precise mechanism of antidepressant action of sertraline is unclear, but the drug has been shown to selectively inhibit the reuptake of serotonin at the presynaptic neuronal membrane. Sertraline-induced inhibition of serotonin reuptake causes increased synaptic concentrations of serotonin in the CNS, resulting in numerous functional changes associated with enhanced serotonergic neurotransmission. Like other SSRIs (e.g., fluoxetine, fluvoxamine, paroxetine), sertraline appears to have only very weak effects on the reuptake of norepinephrine or dopamine and does not exhibit clinically important anticholinergic, antihistaminic, or adrenergic (α_1, α_2, β) blocking activity at usual therapeutic dosages.

Although the mechanism of antidepressant action of antidepressant agents may involve inhibition of the reuptake of various neurotransmitters (i.e.,

serotonin, norepinephrine) at the presynaptic neuronal membrane, it has been suggested that postsynaptic receptor modification is mainly responsible for the antidepressant action observed during long-term administration of antidepressant agents. During long-term therapy with most antidepressants (e.g., tricyclic antidepressants, monoamine oxidase [MAO] inhibitors), these adaptive changes mainly consist of subsensitivity of the noradrenergic adenylate cyclase system in association with a decrease in the number of β-adrenergic receptors; such effects on noradrenergic receptor function are commonly referred to as "down regulation." In animal studies, long-term administration of sertraline has been shown to downregulate noradrenergic receptors in the CNS as has been observed with many other clinically effective antidepressants. In addition, some antidepressants (e.g., amitriptyline) reportedly decrease the number of serotonergic (5-HT) binding sites following chronic administration. Although changes in the density of type 2 serotonergic (5-HT$_2$) binding sites were not observed during chronic administration of sertraline in animals in one study, the drug caused desensitization of the 5-HT$_2$ receptor transmembrane signaling system; the clinical importance of these findings requires further study.

The precise mechanism of action that is responsible for the efficacy of sertraline in the treatment of obsessive-compulsive disorder is unclear. However, because of the potency of clomipramine and other selective serotonin-reuptake inhibitors (e.g., fluoxetine, fluvoxamine, paroxetine) in inhibiting serotonin reuptake and their efficacy in the treatment of obsessive-compulsive disorder, a serotonin hypothesis has been developed to explain the pathogenesis of the condition. The hypothesis postulates that a dysregulation of serotonin is responsible for obsessive-compulsive disorder and that sertraline and these other agents are effective because they correct this imbalance. Although the available evidence supports the serotonergic hypothesis of obsessive-compulsive disorder, additional studies are necessary to confirm this hypothesis.

Serotonergic mechanisms also appear to be involved at least in part in a number of other pharmacologic effects associated with selective serotonin-reuptake inhibitors, including sertraline, such as decreased food intake and altered food selection as well as decreased alcohol intake.

Serotonergic Effects

Sertraline is a highly selective inhibitor of serotonin reuptake at the presynaptic neuronal membrane. Sertraline-induced inhibition of serotonin reuptake causes increased synaptic concentrations of the neurotransmitter, resulting in numerous functional changes associated with enhanced serotonergic neurotransmission.

Data from in vitro studies suggest that sertraline is more potent than fluvoxamine, fluoxetine, or clomipramine as a serotonin-reuptake inhibitor. Like some other serotonin-reuptake inhibitors, sertraline undergoes metabolism via N-demethylation to form N-desmethylsertraline, the principal metabolite. Data from in vivo and in vitro studies have shown that N-desmethylsertraline is approximately 5–10 times less potent as an inhibitor of serotonin reuptake than sertraline; however, the metabolite retains selectivity for serotonin reuptake compared with either norepinephrine or dopamine reuptake.

At therapeutic dosages (50–200 mg daily) in healthy individuals, sertraline has been shown to inhibit the reuptake of serotonin into platelets in a dose-dependent manner. Like other serotonin-reuptake inhibitors, sertraline inhibits the spontaneous firing of serotonergic neurons in the dorsal raphe nucleus. In vitro data have demonstrated that sertraline has substantial affinity for serotonergic (5-HT$_{1A}$, 5-HT$_{1B}$, 5-HT$_2$) receptors.

Effects on Other Neurotransmitters

Like other serotonin-reuptake inhibitors, sertraline has been shown to have little or no activity in inhibiting the reuptake of norepinephrine. In addition, the drug has demonstrated a substantially higher selectivity ratio of serotonin-to-norepinephrine reuptake inhibiting activity than fluoxetine or tricyclic antidepressant agents, including clomipramine.

Although sertraline has only weak activity in inhibiting the reuptake of dopamine, the relative selectivity of sertraline for inhibiting serotonin reuptake relative to dopamine reuptake appears to be somewhat less than that of fluoxetine, fluvoxamine, zimelidine, or clomipramine. In addition, sertraline does not inhibit monoamine oxidase.

Unlike tricyclic and some other antidepressants, sertraline does not exhibit clinically important anticholinergic, α- or β-adrenergic blocking, or antihistaminic activity at usual therapeutic dosages. As a result, the incidence of adverse effects commonly associated with blockade of muscarinic cholinergic receptors (e.g., dry mouth, blurred vision, urinary retention, constipation, confusion), α-adrenergic receptors (e.g., orthostatic hypotension), and histamine H$_1$- and H$_2$-receptors (e.g., sedation) is lower in sertraline-treated patients. In vitro studies have demonstrated that sertraline does not possess clinically important affinity for α₁- or α₂-adrenergic, β-adrenergic, histaminergic, muscarinic, GABA, benzodiazepine, or dopamine receptors.

Effects on Sleep

Like tricyclic and most other antidepressants, sertraline suppresses rapid eye movement (REM) sleep. Although not clearly established, there is some evidence that the REM-suppressing effects of antidepressant agents may contribute to the antidepressant activity of these drugs. In animal studies, sertraline suppressed REM sleep; the drug appears to reduce the amount of REM sleep by decreasing the number as well as the duration of REM episodes. Although the precise mechanism has not been fully elucidated, results of animal studies indicate that sertraline's effects on REM sleep are serotonergically mediated.

Effects on EEG

Limited data currently are available regarding the effects of sertraline on the EEG. EEG changes in healthy individuals receiving single, 100-mg doses of sertraline resembled the EEG profiles of patients receiving desipramine-type antidepressants (increased alpha and decreased but accelerated delta activity) and suggest improved vigilance and psychometric performance. In individuals receiving higher single doses (200 and 400 mg) of the drug, sertraline produced EEG changes similar to imipramine-type antidepressants (reduced alpha and low beta activity and increased theta and fast beta activity), which reflect vigilance changes of the dissociative type and therefore possible sedative activity.

Effects on Psychomotor Function

Sertraline does not appear to cause clinically important sedation and does not interfere with psychomotor performance. The drug did not appear to have any adverse effects on psychomotor performance when given to healthy women in single doses up to 100 mg. In healthy individuals over 50 years of age, single, 100-mg doses of sertraline increased the critical flicker fusion frequency slightly and the subjective perception of sedation; however, the drug had no depressant effect on objective tests of psychomotor performance. In addition, no adverse effects on psychomotor performance were observed in geriatric individuals who received the drug in a controlled study.

● Cardiovascular Effects

Sertraline appears to have little effect on the ECG. Data from controlled studies indicate sertraline does not produce clinically important changes in heart rate, cardiac conduction, or other ECG parameters in depressed patients.

● Effects on Appetite and Body Weight

Like some other serotonergic agents (e.g., fenfluramine [no longer commercially available in the US], fluoxetine, zimelidine), sertraline possesses anorexigenic activity. Limited data from animal studies suggest that fenfluramine has been the most effective inhibitor of food intake followed by fluoxetine and then sertraline. Although the precise mechanism has not been clearly established, results from animal studies indicate that sertraline's appetite-inhibiting action may result at least in part from serotonin-reuptake blockade and the resultant increase in serotonin availability at the neuronal synapse. Because sertraline's anorexigenic activity was not antagonized by prior administration of serotonergic antagonists, other mechanisms also may be involved but require further study. Following administration of single doses of sertraline in meal-fed animals, food intake was reduced in a dose-dependent manner. At a dose of 3 mg/kg, the reduction in food intake was substantially reduced and higher doses of 10 or 30 mg/kg reduced food intake by 45 or 74%, respectively.

Sertraline therapy has resulted in dose-dependent decreases in body weight in animals receiving the drug for 3 days; the weight loss was not accompanied by any overt signs of behavioral abnormality. Sertraline therapy also has resulted in decreases in body weight in individuals receiving the drug. However, weight loss is usually minimal and averaged about 0.45–0.9 kg in individuals treated with the drug in controlled clinical trials. (See Cautions: Metabolic Effects and see also Cautions: Pediatric Precautions.) Rarely, weight loss has required discontinuance of therapy.

● Effects on Alcohol Intake

Like some other serotonergic agents, sertraline produces a substantial decrease in voluntary alcohol intake in animals. Because serotonin appears to be involved in the regulation of alcohol intake, it has been suggested that selective serotonin-reuptake inhibitors may attenuate alcohol consumption via enhanced serotonergic neurotransmission. (See Cautions.)

● Neuroendocrine Effects

Limited data currently are available regarding the effects of sertraline on the endocrine system. In one animal study, sertraline did not demonstrate substantial neuroendocrine effects at a dose that substantially reduced gross activity.

Although a causal relationship has not been established, hypothyroidism, decreased serum thyroxine concentrations, and/or increased serum thyrotropin (thyroid-stimulating hormone, TSH) concentrations have been reported in a limited number of sertraline patients, some of whom were receiving thyroxine concurrently. (See Cautions: Other Adverse Effects and also see Precautions and Contraindications.)

● Other Effects

Sertraline appears to have a weak uricosuric effect; mean decreases in serum uric acid of approximately 7% have been reported in patients receiving the drug. The clinical importance of these findings is unknown, and there have been no reports of acute renal failure associated with the drug. (See Cautions: Precautions and Contraindications.)

PHARMACOKINETICS

In all human studies described in the Pharmacokinetics section, sertraline was administered as the hydrochloride salt; dosages and concentrations are expressed in terms of sertraline.

● Absorption

Sertraline appears to be slowly but well absorbed from the GI tract following oral administration. The oral bioavailability of sertraline in humans has not been fully elucidated to date because a preparation for IV administration is not available. However, the relative proportion of an oral dose that reaches systemic circulation unchanged appears to be relatively small because sertraline undergoes extensive first-pass metabolism. In animals, the oral bioavailability of sertraline ranges from 22–36%. The manufacturers state that the bioavailability of a single dose of sertraline hydrochloride tablets is approximately equal to that of an equivalent dose of sertraline hydrochloride oral solution. In a study in healthy adults who received a single 100-mg dose of sertraline as a tablet or oral solution, the solution to tablet ratios of the mean geometric AUC and peak plasma concentration were 114.8 and 120.6%, respectively.

The effect of food on the absorption of sertraline hydrochloride given as tablets or the oral solution has been studied in single-dose studies. Administration of a sertraline hydrochloride tablet with food slightly increased the area under the concentration-time curve (AUC) of sertraline, increased peak plasma concentrations by approximately 25%, and decreased the time to achieve peak plasma concentrations from about 8 to 5.5 hours. Administration of sertraline hydrochloride oral solution with food increased the time to achieve peak plasma concentrations from 5.9 to 7.0 hours.

Peak plasma sertraline concentrations usually occur within 4.5–8.4 hours following oral administration of 50–200 mg once daily for 14 days. Peak plasma sertraline concentrations following administration of single oral doses of 50–200 mg are proportional and linearly related to dose. Peak plasma concentrations and bioavailability are increased in geriatric individuals.

Following multiple dosing, steady-state plasma sertraline concentrations should be achieved after approximately 1 week of once-daily dosing. When compared with a single dose, there is an approximate twofold accumulation of sertraline after multiple daily dosing in dosages ranging from 50–200 mg daily. N-Desmethylsertraline, sertraline's principal metabolite, exhibits time-related, dose-dependent increases in AUC (0–24 hour), peak plasma concentrations, and trough plasma concentrations with about a 5- to 9-fold increase in these parameters between day 1 and 14.

As with other serotonin-reuptake inhibitors, the relationship between plasma sertraline and N-desmethylsertraline concentrations and the therapeutic and/or toxic effects of the drug has not been clearly established.

● Distribution

Distribution of sertraline and its metabolites into human body tissues and fluids has not been fully characterized. However, limited pharmacokinetic data suggest that the drug and some of its metabolites are widely distributed in body tissues. Although the apparent volume of distribution of sertraline has not been determined in humans, values exceeding 20 L/kg have been reported in rats and dogs. The drug crosses the blood-brain barrier in humans and animals.

At in vitro plasma concentrations ranging from 20–500 ng/mL, sertraline is approximately 98% bound to plasma proteins, principally to albumin and α_1-acid glycoprotein. Protein binding is independent of plasma concentrations from 20–2000 mcg/mL. However, sertraline and N-desmethylsertraline did not alter the plasma protein binding of 2 other highly protein bound drugs, warfarin or propranolol, at concentrations of 300 and 200 ng/mL, respectively.

Sertraline and N-desmethylsertraline are distributed into milk. In a study involving 12 lactating women who received oral dosages of sertraline ranging from 25–200 mg daily, both sertraline and N-desmethylsertraline were present in all breast milk samples, with the highest concentrations observed in hind milk 7–10 hours after the maternal dose. Detectable concentrations of sertraline were found in 3 and N-desmethylsertraline in 6, respectively, out of 11 nursing infants.

● Elimination

The elimination half-life of sertraline averages approximately 25–26 hours and that of desmethylsertraline averages about 62–104 hours. In geriatric adults elimination half-life may be increased (e.g., to about 36 hours); however, such prolongation does not appear clinically important and does not warrant dosing alterations.

The exact metabolic fate of sertraline has not been fully elucidated. Sertraline appears to be extensively metabolized, probably in the liver, to N-desmethylsertraline and several other metabolites. Like some other serotonin-reuptake inhibitors, sertraline undergoes metabolism via N-demethylation to form N-desmethylsertraline, the principal metabolite. Unlike some other serotonin-reuptake inhibitors, the drug metabolizing isoenzyme CYP2D6 (a cytochrome P-450 isoenzyme implicated in the sparteine/debrisoquine polymorphism) does not appear to have a major role in the conversion of sertraline to N-desmethylsertraline. Nonetheless, sertraline has the potential for clinically important inhibition of this enzyme. (See Drug Interactions: Drugs Undergoing Hepatic Metabolism or Affecting Hepatic Microsomal Enzymes.) In vitro, the conversion of sertraline to N-desmethylsertraline correlates more with CYP3A3/4 activity than with CYP2D6 activity. Data from in vivo and in vitro studies have shown that N-desmethylsertraline is approximately 5–10 times less potent as an inhibitor of serotonin reuptake than sertraline; however, the metabolite retains selectivity for serotonin reuptake compared with either norepinephrine or dopamine reuptake. Both sertraline and desmethylsertraline undergo oxidative deamination and subsequent reduction, hydroxylation, and glucuronide conjugation. Desmethylsertraline has an elimination half-life approximately 2.5 times that of sertraline.

Following oral administration, sertraline and its metabolites are excreted in both urine and feces. Following oral administration of a single, radiolabeled dose in 2 healthy males, unchanged sertraline accounted for less than 5% of plasma radioactivity. Approximately 40–45% of the radiolabeled dose was excreted in urine within 9 days. Unchanged sertraline was not detectable in urine. During the same period, approximately 40–45% of the radiolabeled drug was eliminated in feces, including 12–14% of unchanged sertraline.

The effect of age on the elimination of sertraline has not been fully elucidated. Plasma clearance of sertraline was approximately 40% lower in a group of 16 geriatric patients (8 males and 8 females) who received 100 mg of the drug for 14 days than that reported in a similar study involving younger individuals (from 25–32 years of age). Based on these results, the manufacturers state that steady-state should be achieved in about 2–3 weeks in older individuals. In addition, decreased clearance of N-desmethylsertraline was noted in older males but not in older females. (See Dosage and Administration: Dosage in Geriatric Patients.)

Because sertraline is extensively metabolized by the liver, hepatic impairment can affect the elimination of the drug. In one study in patients with chronic mild hepatic impairment (Child-Pugh scores of 5–8) who received 50 mg of sertraline daily for 21 days, sertraline clearance was reduced resulting in a 2–3 times greater exposure to the drug and its metabolite (desmethylsertraline) than that reported for age-matched individuals without hepatic impairment. In a single-dose study in patients with mild, stable cirrhosis, the elimination half-life of sertraline was prolonged to a mean of 52 hours compared with 22 hours in individuals without hepatic disease. In addition, peak plasma concentrations and AUC values for sertraline were 1.7- and 4.4-fold higher, respectively, in patients with hepatic impairment when compared with healthy individuals without liver disease, reflecting decreased clearance of the drug. The pharmacokinetics of sertraline have not been studied to date in patients with moderate and severe hepatic impairment; therefore, the manufacturers recommend that sertraline be administered with caution and in reduced dosage or less frequently in patients with hepatic impairment. (See Cautions: Precautions and Contraindications and see Dosage and Administration: Dosage in Renal and Hepatic Impairment.)

Because sertraline is extensively metabolized in the liver and renal clearance of the drug is negligible, the manufacturers state that clinically important decreases in sertraline clearance are not anticipated if the drug is used in patients with renal impairment. Results of a multiple-dose study indicate that the pharmacokinetics of sertraline are not affected by renal impairment. In this study, individuals with mild to moderate renal impairment (creatinine clearance: 30–60 mL/minute), moderate to severe renal impairment (creatinine clearance: 10–29 mL/minute), or severe renal impairment (undergoing hemodialysis) received 200 mg of sertraline daily for 21 days; the pharmacokinetics and protein binding of the drug in these patients were similar to those reported for age-matched individuals without renal impairment. (See Cautions: Precautions and Contraindications and see Dosage and Administration: Dosage in Renal and Hepatic Impairment.)

Limited data indicate that sertraline is not appreciably removed by hemodialysis. Because of the large volume of distribution of sertraline and its principal metabolite, peritoneal dialysis, forced diuresis, hemoperfusion, and/or exchange transfusion also are likely to be ineffective in removing substantial amounts of sertraline and N-desmethylsertraline from the body.

CHEMISTRY AND STABILITY

● Chemistry

Sertraline, a selective serotonin-reuptake inhibitor antidepressant agent, is a naphthalenamine (naphthylamine)-derivative. Sertraline differs structurally from other selective serotonin-reuptake inhibitor antidepressants (e.g., citalopram, fluoxetine, paroxetine) and also differs structurally and pharmacologically from other currently available antidepressants (e.g., tricyclic antidepressants, monoamine oxidase inhibitors). Like most other serotonin-reuptake inhibitors, sertraline contains an asymmetric carbon; therefore, there are 2 existing optical isomers of the drug. However, only one of the optical isomers is present in the commercially available form of the drug.

Sertraline is commercially available as the hydrochloride salt, which occurs as a white, crystalline powder that is slightly soluble in water and isopropyl alcohol and sparingly soluble in ethanol. Commercially available sertraline hydrochloride oral solution is a clear, colorless solution with a menthol scent containing 20 mg of sertraline per mL and 12% alcohol.

● Stability

Commercially available sertraline hydrochloride tablets and oral solution should be stored at 25°C, but may be exposed to temperatures ranging from 15–30°C. Sertraline hydrochloride oral solution should be diluted only in the liquids specified by the manufacturer, and should be used immediately after dilution.

PREPARATIONS

Excipients in commercially available drug preparations may have clinically important effects in some individuals; consult specific product labeling for details.

Sertraline Hydrochloride

Oral

For solution, concentrate	20 mg (of sertraline) per mL*	Sertraline Hydrochloride Oral Solution
		Zoloft® (with calibrated dropper dispenser containing latex rubber), Pfizer
Tablets, film-coated	25 mg (of sertraline)*	Sertraline Hydrochloride Tablets
		Zoloft® (scored), Pfizer
	50 mg (of sertraline)*	Sertraline Hydrochloride Tablets
		Zoloft® (scored), Pfizer
	100 mg (of sertraline)*	Sertraline Hydrochloride Tablets
		Zoloft® (scored), Pfizer
	150 mg (of sertraline)*	Sertraline Hydrochloride Tablets, Ranbaxy
	200 mg (of sertraline)*	Sertraline Hydrochloride Tablets, Ranbaxy

* available from one or more manufacturer, distributor, and/or repackager by generic (nonproprietary) name

† Use is not currently included in the labeling approved by the US Food and Drug Administration.

Amitriptyline Hydrochloride

28:16.04.28 • TRICYCLICS AND OTHER NOREPINEPHRINE-REUPTAKE INHIBITORS

■ Amitriptyline hydrochloride is a dibenzocycloheptene-derivative tricyclic antidepressant.

DOSAGE AND ADMINISTRATION

● Administration

Amitriptyline hydrochloride is given orally. Although amitriptyline has been administered in up to 4 divided doses throughout the day, it is long-acting and the entire oral daily dose may be administered at one time. Administration of the entire daily dose at bedtime may reduce daytime sedation.

In patients who were unwilling or unable to take amitriptyline orally, the drug also has been given IM. However, a parenteral dosage form is no longer commercially available in the US. Oral therapy should replace IM administration as soon as possible.

● Dosage

There is a wide range of oral amitriptyline hydrochloride dosage requirements, and dosage must be carefully individualized.

Patients should be monitored for possible worsening of depression, suicidality, or unusual changes in behavior, especially at the beginning of therapy or during periods of dosage adjustment. (See Cautions: Precautions and Contraindications, in the Tricyclic Antidepressants General Statement 28:16.04.28.)

Initial dosages should be low and generally range from 75–100 mg daily, depending on the severity of the condition being treated. Dosage may be gradually adjusted (preferably the late-afternoon and/or bedtime doses) to the level that produces maximal therapeutic effect with minimal toxicity and may range from 150–300 mg daily. Alternatively, the manufacturers recommend an initial amitriptyline hydrochloride dosage of 50–100 mg daily at bedtime. Dosage then can be increased by 25 or 50 mg as necessary to a suggested maximum of 150 mg daily. Hospitalized patients under close supervision may generally be given higher dosages than outpatients. Hospitalized patients generally may receive an initial amitriptyline dosage of 100 mg daily; dosage may be increased gradually to 200 mg daily as needed. Some patients may require dosages as high as 300 mg daily. Geriatric and adolescent patients should usually be given lower than average dosages. Manufacturers state that these patients may obtain satisfactory improvement with 10 mg of amitriptyline hydrochloride 3 times daily plus 20 mg at bedtime. Maximum antidepressant effects may not occur for 30 days after therapy is begun.

After symptoms are controlled, dosage should be gradually reduced to the lowest level that will maintain relief of symptoms. If maintenance therapy is necessary, the manufacturers recommend 50–100 mg of amitriptyline hydrochloride daily; however, 25–40 mg daily may be sufficient for some patients. During maintenance therapy, the total daily dosage may be administered as a single daily dose, preferably at bedtime. The manufacturers recommend that maintenance therapy be continued for at least 3 months to prevent relapse. To avoid the possibility of precipitating withdrawal symptoms, amitriptyline should not be terminated abruptly in patients who have received a high dosage for prolonged periods.

When amitriptyline is used in conjunction with a phenothiazine, commercially available fixed-ratio combination preparations should not be used initially. Dosage should first be adjusted by administering each drug separately. If it is determined that the optimum maintenance dosage corresponds to the ratio in a commercial combination, such a preparation may be used. However, whenever dosage adjustment is necessary, the drugs should be administered separately.

CAUTIONS

Amitriptyline shares the pharmacologic actions, uses, and toxic potentials of the tricyclic antidepressants, and the usual precautions of tricyclic antidepressant

administration should be observed. Patients should be fully advised about the risks, especially suicidal thinking and behavior (suicidality), associated with tricyclic antidepressant therapy. For a complete discussion, see Cautions: Precautions and Contraindications and Cautions: Pediatric Precautions, in the Tricyclic Antidepressants General Statement 28:16.04.28.

● Pediatric Precautions

Safety and efficacy of amitriptyline in children younger than 12 years of age have not been established. Therefore, the manufacturers state that the drug should not be used in this age group.

The US Food and Drug Administration (FDA) has determined that antidepressants increase the risk of suicidal thinking and behavior (suicidality) in children and adolescents with major depressive disorder and other psychiatric disorders, However, the FDA also states that depression and certain other psychiatric disorders are themselves associated with an increased risk of suicide. Anyone considering the use of amitriptyline in a child or adolescent for any clinical use must therefore balance the potential risk of therapy with the clinical need. (See Cautions: Precautions and Contraindications and Cautions: Pediatric Precautions, in the Tricyclic Antidepressants General Statement 28:16.04.28.)

PHARMACOKINETICS

● Absorption

Amitriptyline hydrochloride is rapidly absorbed from the GI tract and from parenteral sites. Peak plasma concentrations occur within 2–12 hours after oral or IM (a parenteral dosage form no longer is commercially available in the US) administration.

● Distribution

Amitriptyline and its active metabolite, nortriptyline, are distributed into milk. Amitriptyline and nortriptyline concentrations in milk appear to be similar to or slightly greater than those present in maternal serum. It is estimated that a nursing infant would ingest less than 1% of the daily maternal dose of amitriptyline, and the drug was not detected in the serum of several nursing infants whose mothers were receiving 75–100 mg daily.

● Elimination

The plasma half-life of amitriptyline ranges from 10–50 hours. Amitriptyline is metabolized via the same pathways as are other tricyclic antidepressants; nortriptyline, its N-monodemethylated metabolite, is pharmacologically active. Approximately 25–50% of a dose of amitriptyline is excreted in urine as inactive metabolites within 24 hours; small amounts are excreted in feces via biliary elimination.

CHEMISTRY AND STABILITY

● Chemistry

Amitriptyline hydrochloride is a dibenzocycloheptene-derivative tricyclic antidepressant. Amitriptyline hydrochloride occurs as a white or practically white, odorless or practically odorless, crystalline powder or small crystals with a bitter, burning taste and is freely soluble in water and in alcohol. The drug has a pK_a of 9.4.

● Stability

Amitriptyline hydrochloride tablets should be stored in well-closed containers at a temperature preferably between 15–30°C; exposure to temperatures exceeding 30°C should be avoided. Perphenazine and amitriptyline hydrochloride tablets should be stored at 2–25°C; in addition, unit-dose packages of these tablets should be protected from excessive moisture. Following the date of manufacture, amitriptyline hydrochloride preparations have expiration dates of 3–5 years depending on the manufacturer and dosage form.

For further information on chemistry, pharmacology, pharmacokinetics, uses, cautions, acute toxicity, drug interactions, and dosage and administration of amitriptyline, see the Tricyclic Antidepressants General Statement 28:16.04.28.

PREPARATIONS

Excipients in commercially available drug preparations may have clinically important effects in some individuals; consult specific product labeling for details.

Amitriptyline Hydrochloride

Oral

Tablets, film-coated	10 mg*	**Amitriptyline Hydrochloride Film-coated Tablets**
	25 mg*	**Amitriptyline Hydrochloride Film-coated Tablets**
	50 mg*	**Amitriptyline Hydrochloride Film-coated Tablets**
	75 mg*	**Amitriptyline Hydrochloride Film-coated Tablets**
	100 mg*	**Amitriptyline Hydrochloride Film-coated Tablets**
	150 mg*	**Amitriptyline Hydrochloride Film-coated Tablets**

* available from one or more manufacturer, distributor, and/or repackager by generic (nonproprietary) name

Chlordiazepoxide and Amitriptyline Hydrochloride

Oral

Tablets, film-coated	5 mg Chlordiazepoxide and Amitriptyline Hydrochloride 12.5 mg (of amitriptyline)*	**Chlordiazepoxide and Amitriptyline Hydrochloride Tablets** (C-IV) **Limbitrol®** (C-IV), Valeant
	10 mg Chlordiazepoxide and Amitriptyline Hydrochloride 25 mg (of amitriptyline)*	**Chlordiazepoxide and Amitriptyline Hydrochloride Tablets** (C-IV) **Limbitrol® DS** (C-IV), Valeant

* available from one or more manufacturer, distributor, and/or repackager by generic (nonproprietary) name

Perphenazine and Amitriptyline Hydrochloride

Oral

Tablets, film-coated	2 mg Perphenazine and Amitriptyline Hydrochloride 10 mg*	**Perphenazine and Amitriptyline Hydrochloride Tablets**
	2 mg Perphenazine and Amitriptyline Hydrochloride 25 mg*	**Perphenazine and Amitriptyline Hydrochloride Tablets**
	4 mg Perphenazine and Amitriptyline Hydrochloride 10 mg*	**Perphenazine and Amitriptyline Hydrochloride Tablets**
	4 mg Perphenazine and Amitriptyline Hydrochloride 25 mg*	**Perphenazine and Amitriptyline Hydrochloride Tablets**
	4 mg Perphenazine and Amitriptyline Hydrochloride 50 mg*	**Perphenazine and Amitriptyline Hydrochloride Tablets**

* available from one or more manufacturer, distributor, and/or repackager by generic (nonproprietary) name

Bupropion Hydrobromide

28:16.04.92 • ANTIDEPRESSANTS, MISCELLANEOUS

■ Bupropion is an aminoketone-derivative antidepressant and smoking deterrent.

USES

● Major Depressive Disorder

Bupropion is used in the treatment of major depressive disorder as defined by the Diagnostic and Statistical Manual (DSM). Efficacy of conventional bupropion hydrochloride tablets for long-term use (i.e., >6 weeks) as an antidepressant has not been established by controlled studies; if conventional or extended-release tablets of the drug are used for extended periods, the need for continued therapy should be reassessed periodically. Systematic evaluation of bupropion hydrochloride extended-release tablets has shown that antidepressant efficacy is maintained for periods of up to 44 weeks in patients receiving a dosage of 150 mg twice daily.

For information on the use of bupropion in fixed combination with dextromethorphan for the treatment of major depressive disorder in adults, see Dextromethorphan Hydrobromide and Bupropion Hydrochloride 28:16.04.92.

Clinical Experience

Efficacy of bupropion for the management of major depression has been established in a controlled outpatient study of approximately 6 weeks' duration and in 2 controlled inpatient studies of approximately 4 weeks' duration. Bupropion hydrochloride was administered as conventional tablets in these studies, and the dosage received by 78% of the patients in one of the studies of 4 weeks' duration was ≤450 mg daily, although the dosage was titratable to 600 mg daily. Efficacy of bupropion in these studies was demonstrated by improvement in total score on the Hamilton rating scale for depression (HAM-D), in item 1 of the HAM-D that measures depressed mood, and in the Clinical Global Impressions of Severity of Illness (CGI-S) scale. Patients received 300 or 450 mg daily of bupropion hydrochloride in the second study of 4 weeks' duration, which demonstrated efficacy only of the higher dosage, as indicated by improvement in total score on the HAM-D and in the CGI-S scale. However, in the study of 6 weeks' duration that evaluated the efficacy of 300 mg daily of bupropion hydrochloride, the drug was superior to placebo in improvement of total score on the HAM-D, which was the primary measure of efficacy. In addition, depressed mood, as measured by item 1 on the HAM-D, was improved in patients treated with bupropion. The drug also was superior to placebo in improvement of scores on the Montgomery-Asberg Depression Rating Scale, the CGI-S scale, and the Clinical Global Impressions of Improvement (CGI-I) scale. Although clinical studies specifically establishing the efficacy of extended-release tablets of bupropion in the management of major depression have not been performed to date, the extended-release, film-coated tablet (e.g., Wellbutrin® SR) has been shown to be bioequivalent at steady state to conventional tablets of bupropion, and antidepressant efficacy was maintained for up to 44 weeks in a placebo-controlled study. In addition, the extended-release tablet (Wellbutrin® XL) has been shown to be bioequivalent to the conventional and the extended-release, film-coated tablets. Bupropion hydrochloride extended-release, 450-mg tablets (Forfivo XL®) and bupropion hydrochloride extended-release tablets (Aplenzin®) have been shown to be bioequivalent to bupropion hydrochloride extended-release tablets (e.g., Wellbutrin® XL). Bupropion hydrobromide doses of 174, 348, or 522 mg are equivalent to bupropion hydrochloride doses of 150, 300, or 450 mg, respectively.

Clinical studies have shown that the antidepressant effect of usual dosages of bupropion in patients with moderate to severe depression is greater than that of placebo and comparable to that of usual dosages of tricyclic antidepressants, fluoxetine, or trazodone. Bupropion generally was not distinguishable from these antidepressant agents in measures of efficacy that included the HAM-D scale, the CGI-S scale, the CGI-I scale, and the Hamilton rating scale for anxiety (HAM-A). However, other antidepressants were associated with greater improvement on the HAM-D rating scale during some weeks of the evaluations principally because of greater improvement in the sleep factor of this scale observed with tricyclic antidepressants or trazodone in comparison to bupropion.

Because of differences in the adverse effect profile between bupropion and tricyclic antidepressants, particularly less frequent anticholinergic effects, cardiovascular effects, antihistaminic effects, and weight gain with bupropion therapy, bupropion may be preferred for patients in whom such effects are not tolerated or are of potential concern. In a study that compared bupropion with doxepin, discontinuance of therapy because of adverse effects resulted mainly from anticholinergic effects, particularly drowsiness, in patients treated with doxepin but from a variety of adverse effects in patients treated with bupropion. After 13 weeks of therapy, patients who received doxepin had gained 2.73 kg while those who received bupropion had lost 1.36 kg. Orthostatic hypotension that required discontinuance of the antidepressant agent occurred with some frequency with imipramine but not with bupropion. In addition, in a large 102-center prospective study, 54% of patients who responded poorly to previous antidepressant therapy responded to bupropion therapy, and 63% of patients who poorly tolerated previous antidepressant therapy tolerated bupropion; 81% of patients who completed an initial 8-week treatment phase in this study elected to receive maintenance therapy with bupropion. Although the possibility of bupropion-induced seizures should be considered in weighing the benefits versus risks compared with alternative therapies, the risk of seizures appears to be within clinically acceptable parameters in patients without preexisting risk.

Bupropion also may be preferable because of its minimal adverse effects and possibly beneficial effects on sexual functioning. Most men with depression who experienced sexual dysfunction (e.g., decreased libido, partial erectile failure) during therapy with another antidepressant (e.g., tricyclic antidepressant, maprotiline, trazodone, tranylcypromine) did not have such impairment with bupropion. In a study comparing the adverse sexual effects of bupropion with those of certain selective serotonin-reuptake inhibitors (SSRIs; i.e., fluoxetine, paroxetine, and sertraline), statistically significant increases in libido, sexual arousal, intensity of orgasm, and/or duration of orgasm were reported in most bupropion-treated patients compared with those reported before the onset of illness, while SSRI therapy significantly reduced these aspects of sexual functioning in most of the patients studied. In another study, dysfunctional orgasm resolved when antidepressant therapy was changed from fluoxetine to bupropion in most men and women who developed orgasm failure and/or delay with fluoxetine. Libido and satisfaction with overall sexual functioning also were improved with bupropion. Limited experience suggests that bupropion also may be useful in the management of sexual dysfunction associated with fluoxetine. Sexual dysfunction (e.g., decreased libido, erectile and orgasmic impairment) associated with fluoxetine was reported to respond to concomitant administration of 75 mg daily of bupropion hydrochloride.

Bupropion administered alone or concurrently with other antidepressant agents may be useful in patients with refractory depression. In the large-scale Sequenced Treatment Alternatives to Relieve Depression (STAR*D) effectiveness trial, patients with major depressive disorder who did not respond to or could not tolerate citalopram (an SSRI) were randomized to switch to extended-release ("sustained-release") bupropion, sertraline (another SSRI), or extended-release venlafaxine (a selective serotonin- and norepinephrine-reuptake inhibitor) as a second step of treatment (level 2). Remission rates as assessed by the 17-item Hamilton Rating Scale for Depression (HRSD-17) and the Quick Inventory of Depressive Symptomatology—Self Report (QIDS-SR-16) were approximately 21 and 26% for extended-release bupropion, 18 and 27% for sertraline, and 25 and 25% for extended-release venlafaxine therapy, respectively; response rates as assessed by the QIDS-SR-16 were 26%, 27%, and 28% for extended-release bupropion, sertraline, and extended-release venlafaxine therapy, respectively. These results suggest that after unsuccessful initial treatment of depressed patients with an SSRI, approximately 25% of patients will achieve remission after therapy is switched to another antidepressant, and either another SSRI (e.g., sertraline) or an agent from another class (e.g., bupropion, venlafaxine) may be reasonable alternative antidepressants in patients not responding to initial SSRI therapy.

In a second STAR*D level 2 trial, patients with major depressive disorder who did not respond to or could not tolerate SSRI therapy (citalopram) were randomized to receive either extended-release ("sustained-release") bupropion or buspirone therapy in addition to citalopram. Although both extended-release bupropion and buspirone were found to produce similar remission rates, extended-release bupropion produced a greater reduction in the number and severity of symptoms and a lower rate of drug discontinuance than buspirone in this large-scale, effectiveness trial. These results suggest that augmentation of SSRI therapy with extended-release bupropion may be useful in some patients with refractory depression.

Clinical Perspective

The American Psychiatric Association (APA) has published clinical guidelines for the treatment of major depressive disorder in adults. According to these guidelines, the goals of treatment are to induce remission of the major depressive episode and achieve a full return to the patient's baseline level of functioning. Data on comparative efficacy of various antidepressants show generally comparable effectiveness between and within classes of antidepressant agents. The choice of agent should be directed by symptoms, past treatment response, patient preference, cost and availability, comorbid conditions/contraindications, concomitant drug therapy/interactions, and potential adverse effects. For most patients, bupropion is recommended as an option for first-line pharmacologic therapy for major depressive disorder.

Patients in whom bupropion may be a particularly good option include those also seeking assistance with smoking cessation; patients concerned about weight gain or who have experienced weight gain with other antidepressants; patients experiencing adverse sexual effects with other antidepressants; patients who are sensitive to anticholinergic effects (e.g., patients with dementia); patients experiencing fatigue or sleepiness; and, possibly, patients with Parkinson's disease. Bupropion may be less well tolerated than other antidepressants in patients with severe anxiety, and the drug should be used cautiously in patients with a history of psychotic disorders. In addition, bupropion is contraindicated in patients with a history of anorexia nervosa, bulimia, or seizure disorders and in patients undergoing abrupt discontinuation of alcohol, benzodiazepines, barbiturates, or antiepileptic drugs.

● *Seasonal Affective Disorder*

Bupropion hydrochloride extended-release tablets (Wellbutrin® XL) and bupropion hydrobromide extended-release tablets (Aplenzin®) are used for the prevention of seasonal major depressive episodes in patients with a diagnosis of seasonal affective disorder (SAD). SAD is characterized by recurrent major depressive episodes, most commonly occurring during the autumn and/or winter months. Although patients with SAD may have depressive episodes during other times of the year, the number of seasonal episodes should substantially outnumber the number of nonseasonal episodes during the individual's lifetime for a diagnosis of SAD to be considered.

Efficacy of bupropion for the prevention of seasonal major depressive episodes associated with SAD has been established in 3 double-blind, placebo-controlled trials in adult outpatients with a history of major depressive disorder with an autumn-winter seasonal pattern (as defined by DSM-IV criteria). Bupropion therapy was initiated prior to symptom onset during the autumn (September to November), continued through the winter months, and discontinued following a 2-week tapering period beginning the first week of spring (the fourth week of March), which resulted in a treatment duration of approximately 4–6 months for the majority of patients. Patients were randomized to receive either placebo or 150 mg of bupropion hydrochloride as extended-release tablets once daily for 1 week, then the dosage was titrated upward to 300 mg once daily. Patients judged by the investigator to be unlikely or unable to tolerate the 300-mg daily dosage were allowed to continue to receive 150 mg daily or to have their dosage reduced to 150 mg once daily; mean dosages in the 3 studies ranged from 257–280 mg once daily. In these 3 trials, a substantially higher percentage of patients receiving bupropion extended-release tablets were depression-free at the end of treatment compared with those receiving placebo (81.4 vs 69.7%, 87.2 vs 78.7%, and 84 vs 69%, respectively, for studies 1, 2, and 3, respectively); the depression-free rate for the 3 studies combined was 84.3% for extended-release bupropion tablets and 72% for placebo.

● *Smoking Cessation*

Bupropion hydrochloride extended-release (SR) 150-mg tablets are used as an adjunct in the cessation of smoking. Such therapy may be combined with nicotine replacement therapy if necessary. However, the manufacturer states that before patients receive this combination of therapies, the labeling for both bupropion and nicotine should be consulted and recommends that patients who receive bupropion and nicotine concurrently be monitored for the development of hypertension related to such therapy.

Clinical Experience

The efficacy of bupropion extended-release tablets as adjunctive therapy for smoking cessation has been established in controlled studies of smokers of ≥15 cigarettes daily, who did not have an underlying depressive disorder. Patients were treated with bupropion in conjunction with individual counseling. Cessation of smoking was defined as total abstinence, as determined with patients' daily diaries and verified by measurement of expiratory carbon monoxide, during the fourth through seventh week of treatment. Treatment over 7 weeks with bupropion hydrochloride or placebo resulted in 1-year cessation of smoking in a greater proportion of patients treated with the drug at a dosage of 150 or 300 mg daily but not in those receiving 100 mg daily. Cessation of smoking was achieved at the end of 7 weeks of treatment in 36–44, 27–39, or 17–19% of patients who received 300 mg daily of bupropion hydrochloride, 150 mg daily of the drug, or placebo, respectively. Maintenance of abstinence was observed with bupropion hydrochloride at a dosage of 300 mg daily. At follow-up during the twelfth week, abstinence continued in 25–30 or 14% of patients who had received bupropion hydrochloride at 300 mg daily or placebo, respectively, and at follow-up during the twenty-sixth week, abstinence continued in 19–27 or 11–16% of patients who had received bupropion hydrochloride at 300 mg daily or placebo, respectively.

Treatment over 9 weeks with bupropion hydrochloride at a dosage of 300 mg daily, transdermal nicotine at a dosage of 21 mg/24 hours, the combination of 300 mg daily of bupropion hydrochloride and transdermal nicotine at 21 mg/24 hours, or placebo resulted in cessation of smoking in a greater proportion of patients treated with bupropion, transdermal nicotine, or the combination of bupropion and transdermal nicotine than in those receiving placebo. Cessation of smoking was achieved during weeks 4–7 in 49, 36, 58, or 23% of patients who received bupropion, transdermal nicotine, the combination of bupropion and transdermal nicotine, or placebo, respectively. At follow-up during the tenth week, abstinence was observed in 46, 32, 51, or 20% of patients who had received bupropion, transdermal nicotine, the combination of bupropion and transdermal nicotine, or placebo, respectively. Additionally, when these patients were assessed at 26 weeks, cessation of smoking continued to be observed in 30, 33, and 13% of patients who received bupropion, the combination of bupropion and transdermal nicotine, or placebo, respectively. A final assessment was performed at 52 weeks and abstinence continued to be observed in 23, 28, and 8% of patients who received bupropion, the combination of bupropion and nicotine, or placebo, respectively. The manufacturer states that because the comparisons between bupropion extended-release tablets, transdermal nicotine, or the combination of these products have not been replicated, these data should not be interpreted as demonstrating superiority of any individual treatment protocol.

Another clinical study also reviewed long-term maintenance treatment with bupropion. Patients received bupropion hydrochloride extended-release tablets at a dosage of 300 mg daily for 7 weeks; therapy was continued in the patients who achieved cessation of smoking at 7 weeks with either bupropion hydrochloride extended-release tablets or placebo. At 6-month follow-up, abstinence continued in 55% of patients receiving bupropion compared with 44% of patients who received placebo therapy.

The safety and efficacy of bupropion extended-release tablets as adjunctive therapy for smoking cessation in patients with chronic obstructive pulmonary disease (COPD) was established in a clinical trial in adults with mild to moderate COPD ($FEV_1 \geq 35\%$, $FEV_1/FVC \leq 70\%$) and a diagnosis of chronic bronchitis, emphysema, and/or small airways disease. Treatment over a 12 week period with bupropion or placebo resulted in cessation of smoking during the final four weeks of the study in 22 or 12% of patients, respectively.

Since efficacy in clinical studies is influenced by the population selected, a lower rate of cessation of smoking is possible with use of bupropion in an unselected population. The reported cessation rates in patients receiving bupropion were similar in patients who had and had not previously received nicotine replacement therapy for the cessation of smoking. Withdrawal symptoms, especially irritability, frustration, anger, anxiety, difficulty concentrating, restlessness, and depressed mood or negative affect, were reduced with bupropion compared with placebo. Craving for cigarettes or urge to smoke appeared to be reduced with bupropion compared with placebo.

Clinical Perspective

The US Public Health Service (USPHS) guideline for the treatment of tobacco use and dependence recommends bupropion (as extended-release tablets) as one of several first-line drugs that may reliably increase long-term smoking abstinence rates. Nicotine (tobacco) dependence is a chronic relapsing disorder that requires ongoing assessment and often repeated intervention. Because effective nicotine dependence therapies are available, every patient should be offered effective treatment, and those who are unwilling to attempt cessation should be provided at least brief interventions designed to increase their motivation to stop tobacco use. Delineated in the current USPHS guideline for the treatment of tobacco use and dependence are 5 brief strategies of intervention that can be provided by any clinician; these strategies consist of asking patients if they use tobacco, advising those who use tobacco to quit, assessing their willingness to quit, assisting those who attempt to quit, and arranging follow-up to prevent relapse. Also included in the USPHS guideline are recommendations for the use of pharmacotherapy in general, first-line drugs (i.e., extended-release bupropion, buccal [gum or lozenge] nicotine polacrilex, transdermal nicotine, nicotine nasal spray, nicotine oral inhaler, varenicline) that should be considered initially as part of treatment for tobacco dependence, unless contraindicated, and second-line drugs (i.e., clonidine, nortriptyline). Clinicians should encourage all patients attempting to quit smoking to use effective pharmacotherapy, except when contraindicated or in specific populations for which there is insufficient evidence of efficacy (e.g., pregnant women, smokeless tobacco users, light smokers [e.g., <10 cigarettes daily], adolescents).

Bupropion hydrochloride (extended-release) may be particularly useful in patients greatly concerned about gaining weight after cessation of smoking since therapy with the drug has been shown to result in a delay in such weight gain. Nicotine dependence therapy with an antidepressant such as bupropion also may be particularly useful when a depressive disorder is included in the current or past history of patients attempting to quit smoking. Although it is not necessary to assess for possible comorbid psychiatric disorders prior to initiating therapy for nicotine dependence, awareness of such comorbidity is important in the assessment and treatment of nicotine-dependent patients since psychiatric disorders are common in this population and smoking cessation or nicotine withdrawal may exacerbate the comorbid condition; bupropion and varenicline therapy also have been associated with worsening of preexisting psychiatric disorders in some cases, and patients with psychiatric comorbidities have an increased risk for relapse to smoking after a cessation attempt.

It should be considered that serious neuropsychiatric adverse effects (including but not limited to depression, suicidal ideation, suicide attempt, and completed suicide) have been reported during postmarketing experience in patients being treated with bupropion or varenicline (another smoking cessation drug). The possible risk of serious adverse effects during bupropion therapy should always be weighed against the significant health benefits of its use for smoking cessation, including a reduction in the risk of developing pulmonary disease, cardiovascular disease, and cancer.

Patients should begin receiving bupropion while they are still smoking since steady-state plasma concentrations of the drug are not achieved until after about 1 week. A date on which patients quit smoking (cessation date) should be scheduled within the first 2 weeks of therapy with bupropion and generally should be set for the second week (e.g., day 8). Counseling and support are important interventions for patients to receive throughout therapy with bupropion and for a period after its discontinuance. Achievement of cessation of smoking and maintenance of abstinence are more likely with frequent follow-ups and the provision of support by the clinician and other health-care professionals. The importance of participation in behavioral therapies, counseling, and/or support services to which bupropion is adjunctive therapy should be discussed with the patient. The overall program of interventions to enable cessation of smoking should be reviewed by clinicians. The choice of adjunctive therapy (e.g., nicotine replacement, bupropion) should consider factors such as ease of administration, compliance, and potential adverse effects and risks.

● Depression Associated with Bipolar Disorder

Bupropion has been used for the treatment of bipolar depression† (bipolar disorder, depressive episode). Lithium preferably or lamotrigine alternatively are considered first-line agents by the American Psychiatric Association (APA) for the treatment of acute depressive episode of bipolar disorder, and lamotrigine (if not used initially), bupropion, or paroxetine are considered second-line agents when first-line agents are ineffective or not tolerated. If bupropion was effective for the management of an acute depressive episode, including during the continuation phase, then maintenance therapy with the drug should be considered to prevent recurrences of major depressive episodes. In a comparative study, bupropion hydrochloride (mean dosage of 358 mg daily) was as effective as desipramine (mean dosage of 140 mg daily) in the management of depression in patients with bipolar disorder. Hypomania or mania occurred less frequently with bupropion

than with desipramine in patients treated for up to 1 year with either drug and concomitant lithium, carbamazepine, or valproate sodium.

Because bupropion may be less likely than some other antidepressants to cause a switch to mania or rapid cycling in patients with bipolar disorder, many experts consider bupropion a preferred antidepressant for use in combination with a mood-stabilizing agent in patients with severe (nonpsychotic) depression that is unresponsive to therapy with mood-stabilizing agents alone. However, the possibility that manic attacks may be precipitated in patients with bipolar disorder who receive bupropion still must be considered. To reduce the risk of developing mania, antidepressants should not be used alone in patients with depression associated with bipolar disorder and the lowest effective dosage of the antidepressant should be used for the shortest time necessary.

● Attention Deficit Hyperactivity Disorder (ADHD)

Bupropion has been used in a limited number of children with attention deficit hyperactivity disorder† (ADHD). Although stimulants (e.g., methylphenidate, dextroamphetamine) usually are considered the drugs of first choice when pharmacotherapy is indicated as an adjunct to psychological, educational, social, and other remedial measures in the treatment of ADHD in children, some clinicians recommend use of bupropion or tricyclic antidepressants as second-line therapy when there has been no response to at least 2 stimulants or when the patient is intolerant of stimulants. In controlled studies, bupropion was more effective than placebo and comparably effective to methylphenidate. In addition, in a comparative study, bupropion hydrochloride (mean dosage of 3.3 mg/kg daily; range: 1.4–5.7 mg/kg daily) was comparably effective to methylphenidate hydrochloride (mean dosage of 31 mg daily; range: 20–60 mg daily) in overall improvement of symptoms, as evaluated with the Iowa-Conners Abbreviated Parent and Teacher Questionnaire, although a trend favoring methylphenidate was noted in almost all rating scales.

Bupropion also has been used in a limited number of adults with ADHD. In an uncontrolled study in adults, bupropion hydrochloride (mean dosage of 359 mg daily; range: 150–450 mg daily) administered for 6–8 weeks reduced the severity of signs and symptoms of ADHD, as evaluated with the Targeted Attention Deficit Disorder Symptoms Scale. Additional study and experience are needed to establish the role of antidepressants versus CNS stimulants in the treatment of this disorder.

● Panic Disorder

Bupropion does not appear to be effective in the treatment of panic disorder and concomitant phobic disorder†. However, the drug generally improves symptoms of panic and depression in patients with major depression who have superimposed panic symptoms.

DOSAGE AND ADMINISTRATION

● General

Pretreatment Screening

● Assess blood pressure before initiating bupropion.

● Screen for history of bipolar disorder and risk factors for bipolar disorder (e.g., family history of suicide, bipolar disorder, depression) prior to initiating therapy.

Patient Monitoring

● Appropriately monitor and closely observe all patients receiving bupropion for any indication of clinical worsening, suicidality, or unusual changes in behavior, particularly during initial therapy or following any change (increase or decrease) in dosage.

● Monitor all patients receiving bupropion for smoking cessation for serious neuropsychiatric symptoms or worsening of preexisting psychiatric illness.

● Monitor blood pressure periodically.

● Consider monitoring renal function in geriatric patients.

● Closely monitor patients with renal impairment (glomerular filtration rate <90 mL/minute) for adverse reactions that could indicate high exposures of bupropion or its metabolites.

● Administration

Bupropion is administered orally with or without food. Do not chew, divide, or crush conventional tablets or extended-release tablets; tablets should be swallowed whole.

As conventional tablets, bupropion hydrochloride initially is administered orally twice daily in the morning and evening, then increased to 3 times daily, with ≥6 hours separating doses. Dosages ≥300 mg should be administered as divided doses of ≤150 mg.

As extended-release, film-coated tablets (e.g., Wellbutrin® SR), bupropion hydrochloride initially is administered orally once daily in the morning, then increased to twice daily, in the morning and evening. Dosages >150 mg should be administered as divided doses twice daily, with ≥8 hours separating the doses.

Avoiding bedtime administration of the evening dose of bupropion hydrochloride conventional tablets or extended-release, film-coated tablets may lessen the occurrence of insomnia.

As extended-release tablets (Aplenzin®, Wellbutrin® XL), bupropion is administered orally once daily in the morning. The shell of the extended-release tablet (Aplenzin®, Wellbutrin® XL) does not dissolve and may be passed in the stool.

As extended-release, 450-mg tablets (Forfivo XL®), bupropion hydrochloride is administered once daily. If insomnia occurs, avoid administration close to bedtime.

● Dosage

Dosage of bupropion hydrobromide and bupropion hydrochloride is expressed in terms of the salt. Bupropion hydrobromide doses of 174, 348, or 522 mg are equivalent to bupropion hydrochloride doses of 150, 300, or 450 mg, respectively.

Major Depression

Increase bupropion dosage *gradually* and avoid exceeding recommended maximum individual doses or daily dosages to minimize the risk of seizures.

For the management of depressive disorder in adults, the recommended initial dosage of bupropion hydrochloride as conventional tablets is 100 mg twice daily. Alternatively, dosage also has been initiated at 75 mg 3 times daily. To minimize the risk of seizures, bupropion hydrochloride dosage as conventional tablets should not be increased by >100 mg daily every 3 days. After 3 days of dosing, dosage may be increased to 100 mg 3 times daily as conventional tablets. Bupropion hydrochloride dosages >300 mg daily can be achieved using the 75- or 100-mg tablets to avoid any individual doses of >150 mg and should not be considered until several weeks of therapy at 300 mg daily have been completed. Beyond this time, if no clinical improvement is apparent, dosage of the conventional preparation may be increased to a maximum of 450 mg daily as divided doses ≤150 mg each.

If extended-release, film-coated tablets of bupropion hydrochloride (e.g., Wellbutrin® SR) are used for the management of depression in adults, the recommended initial dosage is 150 mg once daily given as a single dose. If the initial dosage is tolerated adequately, it may be increased to the target dosage of 150 mg twice daily (with ≥8 hours between doses) as early as the fourth day of therapy. Caution is recommended when increasing dosages to minimize the risk of bupropion-induced seizures. For patients not exhibiting clinical improvement after several weeks of treatment with 300 mg daily, dosage of the extended-release, film-coated tablets may be increased to a maximum of 400 mg daily, given as divided doses of 200 mg twice daily (with ≥8 hours between doses). To avoid high peak concentrations of bupropion and/or its metabolites, do not exceed 200 mg in any single dose.

Alternatively, for management of depression in adults, extended-release tablets of bupropion hydrochloride (Wellbutrin® XL) may be used. The recommended initial adult dosage of Wellbutrin® XL extended-release tablets is 150 mg given as a single dose once daily in the morning. If the initial dosage is tolerated adequately, the dosage may be increased after 4 days of therapy to the target dosage of 300 mg once daily given as a single dose.

If therapy is to be switched from conventional bupropion hydrochloride (e.g., Wellbutrin®) or from the extended-release, film-coated tablets (e.g., Wellbutrin® SR) to the once-daily Wellbutrin® XL extended-release tablets, the same total daily dosage should be given when possible, but as a single daily dose.

Bupropion hydrochloride extended-release 450-mg tablets (Forfivo XL®) may be used for the management of depression in adults but are not appropriate as initial treatment. In patients receiving 300 mg daily of another bupropion hydrochloride formulation for ≥2 weeks who require a dosage of 450 mg daily, or in patients currently receiving 450 mg daily of another bupropion hydrochloride formulation, Forfivo XL® may be administered as 450 mg once daily. When discontinuing therapy with Forfivo XL®, use another bupropion formulation to taper the dose prior to discontinuance of bupropion.

Bupropion hydrobromide extended-release tablets (Aplenzin®) also may be used for the management of depression in adults. The recommended initial adult dosage of Aplenzin® extended-release tablets is 174 mg once daily in the morning. After 4 days of dosing, the dosage may increased to the target dosage of 348 mg once daily in the morning. When discontinuing therapy in patients receiving bupropion hydrobromide 348 mg once daily, taper dosage to 174 mg once daily prior to discontinuance.

Although the optimum duration of bupropion therapy has not been established, acute depressive episodes are thought to require several months or longer of sustained antidepressant therapy. In addition, some clinicians recommend that long-term antidepressant therapy be considered in certain patients at risk for recurrence of depressive episodes (such as those with highly recurrent unipolar depression). Whether the dosage of bupropion required to induce remission is identical to the dosage needed to maintain and/or sustain euthymia is unknown. Systematic evaluation of bupropion hydrochloride extended-release, film-coated tablets (Wellbutrin® SR) has shown that antidepressant efficacy is maintained for periods of up to 44 weeks in patients receiving 150 mg twice daily. Efficacy of bupropion hydrochloride conventional tablets beyond 6 weeks has not been established systematically in controlled studies. The usefulness and dosage of the drug in patients receiving prolonged therapy with conventional or extended-release tablets should be reevaluated periodically.

Seasonal Affective Disorder

For the prevention of seasonal major depressive episodes associated with seasonal affective disorder in adults, therapy with extended-release tablets of bupropion hydrochloride (Wellbutrin® XL) or bupropion hydrobromide (Aplenzin®) generally should be initiated in the autumn prior to the onset of depressive symptoms; treatment should continue through the winter season and should be tapered and discontinued in the early spring. The timing of initiation and duration of treatment should be individualized based on the patient's historical pattern of seasonal major depressive episodes.

The recommended initial adult dosage of bupropion hydrochloride, as extended-release tablets (Wellbutrin® XL), is 150 mg once daily in the morning. If the 150-mg once-daily dosage is adequately tolerated, the dosage may be increased to the target dosage of 300 mg once daily after 7 days of dosing. For patients receiving 300 mg of bupropion hydrochloride as extended-release tablets once daily during the autumn-winter season, the dosage should be tapered to 150 mg once daily prior to discontinuance. Dosages >300 mg daily as extended-release bupropion hydrochloride tablets have not been studied for prevention of episodes of seasonal major depression.

The recommended initial adult dosage of bupropion hydrobromide, as extended-release tablets (Aplenzin®), is 174 mg once daily. After 7 days of dosing, the dosage may be increased to the target dosage of 348 mg once daily in the morning. For patients receiving 348 mg of bupropion hydrobromide as extended-release tablets once daily during the autumn-winter season, the dosage should be tapered to 174 mg once daily prior to discontinuance.

Smoking Cessation

For use in adults as an adjunct in smoking cessation, the initial dosage of bupropion hydrochloride, as extended-release (SR) tablets is 150 mg daily for the first 3 days of therapy. The dosage subsequently is increased in most patients to the usual recommended dosage of 150 mg twice daily (with ≥8 hours between doses), which also is the maximum recommended dosage. Dosages >300 mg daily should not be used for smoking cessation because of the risk of seizures. Because steady-state plasma concentrations of the drug are not achieved for about 1 week, bupropion therapy for smoking cessation should be initiated 1–2 weeks prior to discontinuance of cigarette smoking. Patients should continue to receive bupropion hydrochloride for 7–12 weeks; the need for more prolonged therapy should be individualized depending on benefits and risks to the patient.

For some patients, it may be appropriate to continue pharmacotherapy with bupropion for smoking cessation for periods longer than usually recommended since nicotine dependence is a chronic condition. Use of bupropion hydrochloride as an adjunct in smoking cessation has been studied systematically as maintenance therapy at 150 mg twice daily for up to 6 months. The decision to continue therapy beyond 12 weeks for smoking cessation must be individualized. Although weaning should be encouraged for all smoking cessation pharmacotherapies, continued use of such therapy is clearly preferable to a return to smoking with respect to health consequences.

Patients have received the combination of bupropion hydrochloride, as extended-release tablets, and transdermal nicotine. Patients treated with this combination have been started on bupropion hydrochloride at a dosage of 150 mg daily, while they were still smoking. After 3 days, the dosage of bupropion hydrochloride was increased to 150 mg twice daily. Patients received concomitant transdermal nicotine therapy at a dosage of 21 mg/24 hours after about 1 week of therapy with bupropion, when the date scheduled for patients to stop smoking was reached. The dosage of transdermal nicotine was tapered to 14 and 7 mg/24 hours during the eighth and ninth weeks of therapy, respectively.

Complete smoking abstinence is the goal of therapy with bupropion hydrochloride. Cessation of smoking is unlikely in patients who do not show substantial progress toward abstinence after receiving bupropion hydrochloride for 7 weeks, so such therapy probably should be discontinued at that time in these patients. Unsuccessful patients may benefit from interventions to enhance the possibility for success on the next attempt. Such patients should be evaluated to determine why failure occurred, and another attempt to quit smoking should be encouraged by a more favorable context that includes elimination or reduction of the factors responsible for failure.

Depression Associated With Bipolar Disorder†

While comparative efficacy of various dosages in the usual range have not been established in the management of depression associated with bipolar disorder†, some experts recommend that dosages of antidepressants, including bupropion, be titrated to levels comparable to those used in the treatment of unipolar depression. In clinical studies in patients with depression associated with bipolar disorder, bupropion hydrochloride has been given in a dosage of 75–400 mg daily in conjunction with a mood-stabilizing agent (e.g., carbamazepine, lithium, valproate). Antidepressants should be used in these patients for the shortest time necessary.

ADHD†

For the treatment of attention deficit hyperactivity disorder† (ADHD) in adults, bupropion hydrochloride therapy has been initiated with a dosage of 150 mg daily as conventional tablets. Dosage was then titrated to a maximum daily dosage of 450 mg as conventional tablets. Bupropion hydrochloride as extended-release tablets also has been used at dosages of 150–450 mg daily.

Although safety and efficacy of bupropion hydrochloride in pediatric patients <18 years of age have not been established, if bupropion is used for the treatment of ADHD in children†, some experts recommend that those weighing ≥20 kg or more receive an initial dosage of 1 mg/kg daily in 2–3 divided doses. This initial dosage should be given for the first 3 days of therapy, then dosage should be titrated up to 3 mg/kg daily in 2–3 divided doses by day 7 and up to 6 mg/kg daily in 2–3 divided doses or 300 mg (whichever is smaller) by the third week of therapy. Alternatively, some experts suggest that pediatric patients with ADHD receive bupropion hydrochloride beginning with an initial dosage of 37.5 mg or 50 mg twice daily with dosage titration over 2 weeks up to a maximum dosage of 250 mg daily (300–400 mg daily in adolescents). Up to 4 weeks of bupropion therapy may be necessary to attain maximum effects of the drug. Pediatric dosage for ADHD generally has ranged from 50–100 mg 3 times daily. If extended-release tablets are used for ADHD, the pediatric dosage generally has ranged from 100–150 mg twice daily.

● Special Populations

Hepatic Impairment

Because substantial increases in peak plasma bupropion concentrations and accumulation of the drug may occur in patients with moderate or severe hepatic impairment (Child-Pugh score: 7–15), bupropion should be used with caution in these patients. Dosage of the drug in these patients should not exceed 75 mg

once daily as conventional bupropion hydrochloride tablets, 100 mg once daily or 150 mg every other day as extended-release, film-coated bupropion hydrochloride tablets (e.g., Wellbutrin® SR), 150 mg every other day as Wellbutrin® XL extended-release bupropion hydrochloride tablets or extended-release (SR) bupropion hydrochloride tablets, or 174 mg every other day as extended-release bupropion hydrobromide tablets (Aplenzin®). The drug should also be used with caution in patients with mild hepatic impairment (Child-Pugh score: 5–6) and a reduction in dose and/or frequency of administration of bupropion should be considered in these patients.

Bupropion hydrochloride extended-release 450-mg tablets (Forfivo XL®) are not recommended for use in patients with hepatic impairment.

Renal Impairment

Bupropion should be used with caution in patients with renal impairment (creatinine clearance <90 mL/minute), and a reduction in dosage and/or frequency of administration should be considered. Although bupropion is extensively metabolized in the liver to active metabolites, its active metabolites are renally excreted and may accumulate to a greater extent in patients with renal impairment than in those with normal renal function. Therefore, patients with renal impairment should be closely monitored for possible adverse effects (e.g., seizures) that could indicate higher than recommended drug or metabolite concentration and necessitate a reduction in dose and/or frequency of administration of bupropion. Based on limited pharmacokinetic data obtained in a single-dose study, some clinicians suggest that patients undergoing hemodialysis should receive 150 mg of bupropion hydrochloride as extended-release tablets every 3 days instead of daily for smoking cessation; a multiple-dose study is needed to confirm these findings.

Bupropion hydrochloride extended-release 450-mg tablets (Forfivo XL®) are not recommended for use in patients with renal impairment.

CAUTIONS

● Contraindications

- Seizure disorders.

- Current or past diagnosis of anorexia nervosa or bulimia.

- Patients receiving any other bupropion formulation because risk of seizures is dose-dependent.

- Patients undergoing abrupt discontinuance of alcohol, benzodiazepines, barbiturates, or antiepileptic drugs.

- Patients currently receiving, or having recently received (i.e., within 14 days), MAO inhibitor therapy.

- Patients currently receiving a reversible MAO inhibitor (e.g., linezolid, IV methylene blue).

- Hypersensitivity to the drug or any ingredient in the formulation.

● Warnings/Precautions

Warnings

Suicidal Thoughts and Behaviors in Children, Adolescents, and Young Adults

Worsening of depression and/or the emergence of suicidal ideation and behavior (suicidality) or unusual changes in behavior may occur in both adult and pediatric patients with major depressive disorder or other psychiatric disorders, whether or not they are taking antidepressants. This risk may persist until clinically important remission occurs. Suicide is a known risk of depression and certain other psychiatric disorders, and these disorders themselves are the strongest predictors of suicide. However, there has been a long-standing concern that antidepressants may have a role in inducing worsening of depression and the emergence of suicidality in certain patients during the early phases of treatment. A boxed warning about the risk of suicidal thoughts and behaviors is included in the prescribing information for bupropion.

Pooled analyses of short-term, placebo-controlled studies of antidepressants (i.e., selective serotonin-reuptake inhibitors [SSRIs] and other antidepressants) have shown an increased risk of suicidality in children, adolescents, and young adults (18–24 years of age) with major depressive disorder and other psychiatric disorders. An increased suicidality risk was not demonstrated with antidepressants compared with placebo in adults >24 years of age, and a reduced risk was observed in adults ≥65 years of age. It is currently unknown whether the suicidality risk extends to longer-term use (i.e., beyond several months); however, there is substantial evidence from placebo-controlled maintenance trials in adults with major depressive disorder that antidepressants can delay the recurrence of depression.

The risk of suicidality for these drugs was identified in a pooled analysis of data from a total of 24 short-term (4–16 weeks), placebo-controlled studies of 9 antidepressants (i.e., bupropion, citalopram, fluoxetine, fluvoxamine, mirtazapine, nefazodone, paroxetine, sertraline, venlafaxine) in >4400 children and adolescents with major depressive disorder, obsessive-compulsive disorder (OCD), or other psychiatric disorders. The analysis revealed a greater risk of adverse events representing suicidal behavior or thinking (suicidality) during the first few months of treatment in pediatric patients receiving antidepressants than in those receiving placebo. However, a later meta-analysis of 27 placebo-controlled trials of 9 antidepressants (SSRIs and others) in patients <19 years of age with major depressive disorder, OCD, or non-OCD anxiety disorders suggests that the benefits of antidepressant therapy in treating these conditions may outweigh the risks of suicidal behavior or suicidal ideation. No suicides occurred in these pediatric trials. There were suicides reported in the adult trials; however, the number was not sufficient to reach any conclusion about drug effect on suicide.

The risk of suicidality in FDA's pooled analysis differed across the different psychiatric indications, with the highest incidence observed in the major depressive disorder studies. In addition, although there was considerable variation in risk among the antidepressants, a tendency toward an increase in suicidality risk in younger patients was found for almost all drugs studied.

FDA recommends that all patients being treated with antidepressants for any indication be appropriately monitored and closely observed for clinical worsening, suicidality, and unusual changes in behavior, particularly during initiation of therapy (i.e., the first few months) and during periods of dosage adjustments. Families and caregivers of patients being treated with antidepressants for major depressive disorder or other indications, both psychiatric and nonpsychiatric, also should be advised to monitor patients on a daily basis for the emergence of agitation, irritability, or unusual changes in behavior, as well as the emergence of suicidality, and to report such symptoms immediately to a health-care provider.

Although a causal relationship between the emergence of symptoms such as anxiety, agitation, panic attacks, insomnia, irritability, hostility, aggressiveness, impulsivity, akathisia, hypomania, and/or mania and either the worsening of depression and/or the emergence of suicidal impulses has not been established, there is concern that such symptoms may represent precursors to emerging suicidality. Consequently, consideration should be given to changing the therapeutic regimen or discontinuing therapy in patients whose depression is persistently worse or in patients experiencing emergent suicidality or symptoms that might be precursors to worsening depression or suicidality, particularly if such manifestations are severe, abrupt in onset, or were not part of the patient's presenting symptoms. FDA also recommends that the drugs be prescribed in the smallest quantity consistent with good patient management, in order to reduce the risk of overdosage.

Sensitivity Reactions

Hypersensitivity Reactions

Anaphylactoid/anaphylactic reactions (e.g., pruritus, urticaria, angioedema, dyspnea) have been reported that may require medical treatment; however, causality has not been established. Postmarketing reports include erythema multiforme, Stevens-Johnson syndrome, and anaphylactic shock.

Arthralgia, myalgia, and fever with rash and other symptoms suggestive of delayed hypersensitivity reported.

Advise patients to discontinue bupropion and contact their clinician if symptoms of a possible hypersensitivity reaction occur.

Other Warnings and Precautions

Neuropsychiatric Symptoms and Suicidality in Smoking Cessation Treatment

Serious neuropsychiatric symptoms, including mood changes (e.g., depression, mania), psychosis, hallucinations, paranoia, delusions, homicidal ideation,

hostility, agitation, aggression, anxiety, and panic as well as suicidal ideation, suicide attempt, and completed suicide, have been reported in patients receiving bupropion or varenicline for smoking cessation; such events have occurred in patients with or without psychiatric history. Some patients with preexisting psychiatric conditions have experienced worsening of their psychiatric illnesses while receiving bupropion for smoking cessation. Some patients who stopped smoking may have been experiencing symptoms of nicotine withdrawal, including depressed mood. Depression, including suicidal ideation in rare cases, has been reported in smokers undergoing a smoking cessation attempt without medication. However, some of these adverse events have been observed in patients receiving bupropion who continued to smoke.

Additional analyses and studies, including a large randomized controlled study in >8000 patients, indicate that risk is lower than previously thought and comparable to nicotine replacement therapy or placebo. However, there is evidence indicating patients with a preexisting psychiatric illness (e.g., depression, anxiety disorder, schizophrenia) may be more likely to experience such events.

Although risk remains, particularly in individuals with current or past psychiatric illnesses, patients generally do not experience serious consequences (e.g., hospitalization); therefore, benefits of smoking cessation (e.g., reduced risk of developing pulmonary disease, cardiovascular disease, and cancer) continue to outweigh risks of these cessation drugs.

Monitor patients for neuropsychiatric symptoms or for worsening of preexisting psychiatric conditions. Advise patients to discontinue bupropion and contact their clinician immediately if they develop agitation, hostility, depressed mood, or changes in behavior or thinking that are not typical for the patient or suicidal ideation/suicidal behavior. The clinician should evaluate the severity of the adverse events and the extent to which the patient is responding to treatment and should consider options, including continued treatment under closer monitoring or discontinuance of treatment. In many postmarketing cases, resolution of symptoms after discontinuance of bupropion was reported; however, symptoms persisted in some cases. Provide ongoing monitoring and supportive care until symptoms resolve.

Seizures

Bupropion is associated with a dose-related increase in the risk of seizures. To reduce the risk of seizures, dosage of bupropion should be increased gradually, and the recommended daily and single dosage recommendations should not be exceeded. The daily dosage of bupropion hydrochloride as conventional tablets should not exceed 450 mg (as 150 mg 3 times daily). The dosage of bupropion hydrochloride extended-release, film-coated tablets (e.g., Wellbutrin® SR) should not exceed 400 mg daily (as 200 mg twice daily). The dosage of bupropion hydrochloride extended-release (SR) tablets for smoking cessation should not exceed 300 mg daily (as 150 mg twice daily). The dosage of bupropion hydrochloride extended-release tablets (e.g., Wellbutrin® XL) should not exceed 300 mg once daily. The dosage of bupropion hydrochloride extended-release 450-mg tablets (Forfivo XL®) should not exceed 450 mg once daily. The dosage of bupropion hydrobromide extended-release tablets (Aplenzin®) should not exceed 522 mg once daily.

Seizures have been reported in approximately 0.4% of patients receiving dosages not exceeding 450 mg daily of bupropion hydrochloride as conventional tablets. The estimated seizure incidence increases almost 10-fold between daily bupropion hydrochloride doses of 450 and 650 mg. Seizures reportedly occurred in about 0.1% of patients treated with the extended-release, film-coated tablets of bupropion hydrochloride (as Wellbutrin® SR) at dosages of 100–300 mg daily, and the incidence increased to approximately 0.4% in patients receiving the maximum recommended dosage of 400 mg daily.

Bupropion is contraindicated in patients with a seizure disorder, anorexia nervosa or bulimia, or undergoing abrupt discontinuation of alcohol, benzodiazepines, barbiturates, or antiepileptic drugs. Risk factors for seizure also include patient-related factors (e.g., history of severe head trauma, arteriovenous malformation, CNS tumor, CNS infection, severe stroke), clinical situations (excessive use of alcohol, benzodiazepines, sedative hypnotic agents, or opiates; use of anorectics; use of illicit drugs [e.g., cocaine]; abuse or misuse of prescription drugs [e.g., CNS stimulants]; metabolic disorders [e.g., hypoglycemia, hyponatremia, severe hepatic impairment, hypoxia]; diabetes treated with oral hypoglycemics or insulin), and concomitant drugs that lower seizure threshold (e.g., other bupropion-containing drugs, antipsychotics, tricyclic antidepressants, theophylline, systemic corticosteroids).

If patients experience a seizure during therapy, permanently discontinue bupropion.

Hypertension

Hypertension (sometimes severe) has occurred with bupropion therapy either alone or in combination with transdermal nicotine in patients with and without preexisting hypertension. The risk of hypertension is increased if bupropion is used concomitantly with MAO inhibitors (contraindicated) or other dopaminergic or noradrenergic drugs. The risk of hypertension also appears to be increased in patients receiving concomitant treatment with transdermal nicotine therapy.

The safety of bupropion therapy in patients with recent history of MI or unstable heart disease has not been established.

Assess blood pressure before initiating bupropion and monitor blood pressure periodically during therapy, especially in patients receiving concomitant nicotine replacement therapy.

Activation of Mania or Hypomania

Precipitation of manic, mixed, or hypomanic manic episodes may occur in patients receiving bupropion; the risk appears to be increased in patients with bipolar disorder or in patients with risk factors for bipolar disoder.

Bupropion is *not* FDA-labeled for use in treating bipolar depression. Screen patients for a history of bipolar disorder or risk factors for bipolar disorder (e.g., family history of suicide, bipolar disorder, depression) prior to initiating therapy.

Psychosis and Other Neuropsychiatric Effects in Patients Treated for Depression

Neuropsychiatric manifestations, including confusion, delusions, hallucinations, psychosis, disturbances in concentration, and paranoia, have been reported in patients receiving bupropion in depression trials. Some of these patients had a diagnosis of bipolar disorder. In some cases, symptoms diminished with dosage reduction or withdrawal of therapy. Similar types of neuropsychiatric manifestations have been reported during postmarketing experience in patients receiving the drug for smoking cessation.

Advise patients to contact a clinician if adverse neuropsychiatric effects occur. Discontinue bupropion extended-release tablets (e.g., Wellbutrin® XL, Forfivo XL®, Aplenzin®) if such reactions occur.

Angle-closure Glaucoma

The pupillary dilation (mydriasis) that occurs following the use of many antidepressant agents, including bupropion, may trigger an acute attack of angle-closure glaucoma (narrow-angle glaucoma) in patients with anatomically narrow angles who do not have a patent iridectomy.

Laboratory Test Interferences

False-positive results for urine immunoassay screening tests for amphetamines have been reported in patients receiving bupropion and following discontinuance of the drug. Confirmatory tests (e.g., gas chromatography/mass spectrometry) can distinguish bupropion from amphetamines.

Specific Populations

Pregnancy

Data from epidemiologic studies, including the international bupropion pregnancy registry (675 first-trimester exposures) and a retrospective cohort study using the United Healthcare database (1213 first-trimester exposures), have not shown an overall increased risk for congenital malformations associated with bupropion. The pregnancy registry was not designed or powered to evaluate specific defects; however, a possible increase in cardiac malformations was identified. There also are risks to the mother associated with untreated depression in pregnancy.

When bupropion was administered to pregnant rats during organogenesis at doses up to approximately 11 times the maximum recommended human dose (MRHD) of 400 mg daily, no evidence of fetal malformations was observed. When administered to pregnant rabbits during organogenesis at doses greater than or approximately equal to the MRHD, non-dose-related increases in the incidence of fetal malformations, and skeletal variations, were observed; decreased fetal weights were observed at doses ≥2 times the MRHD.

The National Pregnancy Registry for Antidepressants, an independent pregnancy exposure registry that monitors pregnancy outcomes in women exposed to antidepressants during pregnancy, is available at 844-405-6185 or https://womensmentalhealth.org/research/pregnancyregistry/antidepressants.

Consider the risks to the mother of untreated depression and potential effects on the fetus when discontinuing or changing treatment with antidepressant medications during pregnancy and postpartum.

Pregnant smokers should be encouraged to attempt smoking cessation using educational and behavioral interventions before drug approaches are used. Bupropion extended-release (SR) tablets should be used during pregnancy only if the potential benefit justifies the potential risk to the fetus.

Lactation

Bupropion and its metabolites are distributed into human milk. The effects of bupropion or its metabolites on milk production are not known.

Limited data from postmarketing reports of bupropion use in nursing women have not identified a clear association of adverse reactions in the breast-fed infant. Postmarketing reports have described seizures in breast-fed infants; however, the relationship of bupropion exposure and these seizures is unclear.

Consider the developmental and health benefits of breast-feeding along with the mother's clinical need for bupropion and any potential adverse effects on the breast-fed child from the drug or the underlying maternal condition.

Pediatric Use

Safety and efficacy of bupropion have not been established in children <18 years of age.

FDA warns that a greater risk of suicidal thinking or behavior (suicidality) occurred during first few months of antidepressant treatment compared with placebo in children and adolescents with major depressive disorder, obsessive-compulsive disorder (OCD), or other psychiatric disorders based on pooled analyses of 24 short-term, placebo-controlled trials of 9 antidepressant drugs (SSRIs and others). However, a later meta-analysis of 27 placebo-controlled trials of 9 antidepressants (SSRIs and others) in patients <19 years of age with major depressive disorder, OCD, or non-OCD anxiety disorders suggests that the benefits of antidepressant therapy in treating these conditions may outweigh the risks of suicidal behavior or suicidal ideation. No suicides occurred in these pediatric trials.

Carefully consider these findings when assessing potential benefits and risks of bupropion in a child or adolescent for any clinical use.

Bupropion has been used in a limited number of children 7–16 years of age for attention deficit disorder† without unusual adverse effect.

Geriatric Use

Of the approximately 6000 patients studied in clinical trials of extended-release bupropion hydrochloride for smoking cessation or depression, 275 were ≥65 years of age, while 47 were ≥75 years of age. In addition, several hundred patients ≥65 years of age participated in clinical studies using conventional bupropion hydrochloride tablets for depression. Although no overall differences in efficacy or safety were observed between geriatric and younger patients, and other clinical experience revealed no evidence of age-related differences, the possibility that some older patients may exhibit increased sensitivity to the drug cannot be ruled out. In general, smoking cessation interventions that have been shown to be effective in the general population also have been shown to be effective in adults ≥50 years of age.

The risk of adverse reactions may be increased in patients with impaired renal function. The possibility of decreased renal function in geriatric patients should be considered in dose selection; consider monitoring renal function in geriatric patients.

In pooled data analyses, a *reduced* risk of suicidality was observed in adults ≥65 years of age with antidepressant therapy compared with placebo.

Hepatic Impairment

Dosage reduction is required in patients with severe hepatic impairment (Child-Pugh score: 7–15). In patients with mild hepatic impairment (Child-Pugh score: 5–6), consider reducing the frequency of administration and/or dosage.

Use of bupropion hydrochloride extended-release, 450-mg tablets (Forfivo XL®) is not recommended in patients with hepatic impairment.

Renal Impairment

Use bupropion with caution in patients with renal impairment; the drug and its active metabolites may accumulate. Monitor closely for adverse effects that could indicate high bupropion or metabolite exposures; consider a reduction in dosage and/or frequency of administration in patients with renal impairment (glomerular filtration rate <90 mL/minute).

Use of bupropion hydrochloride extended-release, 450-mg tablets (Forfivo XL®) is not recommended in patients with renal impairment.

● Common Adverse Effects

Adverse effects reported in ≥5% of patients receiving conventional bupropion hydrochloride tablets include agitation, dry mouth, constipation, headache/migraine, nausea/vomiting, dizziness, excessive sweating, tremor, insomnia, blurred vision, tachycardia, confusion, rash, hostility, cardiac arrhythmias, and auditory disturbance.

Adverse effects reported in ≥5% of patients receiving bupropion hydrochloride extended-release, film-coated tablets (e.g., Wellbutrin® SR) include headache, dry mouth, nausea, insomnia, dizziness, pharyngitis, constipation, agitation, anxiety, abdominal pain, tinnitus, tremor, palpitation, myalgia, sweating, rash, and anorexia.

Adverse effects reported in ≥5% of patients receiving bupropion hydrochloride extended-release (SR) tablets for smoking cessation include insomnia, rhinitis, dry mouth, dizziness, nervous disturbance, anxiety, nausea, constipation, and arthralgia.

Adverse effects reported in ≥5% of patients receiving bupropion hydrochloride extended-release tablets (e.g., Wellbutrin® XL, Forfivo XL®) include dry mouth, nausea, insomnia, dizziness, pharyngitis, abdominal pain, agitation, anxiety, tremor, palpitation, sweating, tinnitus, myalgia, anorexia, urinary frequency, and rash.

Adverse effects reported in ≥5% of patients receiving bupropion hydrobromide extended-release tablets (e.g., Aplenzin®) include dry mouth, nausea, insomnia, dizziness, pharyngitis, abdominal pain, agitation, anxiety, tremor, palpitation, sweating, tinnitus, myalgia, anorexia, urinary frequency, and rash.

DRUG INTERACTIONS

Bupropion is metabolized to hydroxybupropion, principally by cytochrome P-450 (CYP) isoenzyme 2B6; CYP isoenzymes are not involved in the formation of other bupropion metabolites.

Bupropion and its metabolites (erythrohydrobupropion, threohydrobupropion, hydroxybupropion) inhibit CYP2D6.

● Drugs Affecting Hepatic Microsomal Enzymes

Concomitant use of bupropion with CYP2B6 inducers or inhibitors may result in altered serum concentrations of bupropion.

● Drugs Metabolized by Hepatic Microsomal Enzymes

Concomitant use of bupropion with substrates of CYP2D6 may result in increased plasma concentrations of the CYP2D6 substrate. Caution should be exercised if bupropion and drugs that are metabolized by the CYP2D6 isoenzyme, including certain antidepressants (e.g., nortriptyline, imipramine, desipramine, paroxetine, fluoxetine, sertraline, venlafaxine), antipsychotic agents (e.g., haloperidol, risperidone, thioridazine), β-adrenergic blocking agents (e.g., metoprolol), and class IC antiarrhythmic agents (e.g., propafenone, flecainide), are used concomitantly. When drugs that are metabolized by CYP2D6 are added to existing bupropion therapy or if bupropion is added to the treatment regimen of a patient already receiving one of these drugs, a reduction in dosages of the drugs that are metabolized by CYP2D6 should be considered, particularly for those with a narrow therapeutic index.

In a clinical trial of 15 male subjects who were extensive CYP2D6 metabolizers, bupropion 300 mg daily (150 mg twice a day) followed by a single 50-mg dose of desipramine increased the peak concentration, AUC, and elijimination half-life of desipramine by an average of approximately 2-, 5-, and 2-fold, respectively; the

effect was present for at least 7 days after the last dose of bupropion. Concomitant use of bupropion with other drugs metabolized by CYP2D6 has not been formally studied.

For prodrugs dependent on CYP2D6 for activation (e.g., tamoxifen), concomitant therapy with bupropion may reduce the clinical efficacy of the prodrug. An increase in dosage of the prodrug may be necessary in patients receiving bupropion.

● Drugs Affecting the Seizure Threshold

Extreme caution should be observed with concurrent administration of bupropion and drugs (e.g., other antidepressants, other bupropion-containing drugs, antipsychotic agents, theophylline, systemic corticosteroids) or treatment regimens (e.g., abrupt discontinuance of benzodiazepines) that lower the seizure threshold. Therapy should be initiated with low doses and dosage should be increased gradually.

● Smoking Cessation

Smoking, via enzyme induction, can increase the metabolism of some drugs. Therefore, cessation of smoking (with or without adjunctive use of bupropion) may result in decreased enzyme induction and altered metabolism of some drugs (e.g., theophylline, warfarin, insulin); consider dosage adjustment.

● Alcohol

Adverse neuropsychiatric events or reduced alcohol tolerance have been reported rarely in patients who ingested alcohol during bupropion therapy. Patients receiving the drug should be advised to minimize or avoid alcohol consumption.

● Antiretroviral Agents

Concomitant treatment with antiretroviral agents that induce CYP2B6 (e.g., efavirenz, lopinavir, ritonavir) can decrease bupropion and hydroxybupropion exposure. Administration of ritonavir 100 mg twice daily in healthy subjects reduced the AUC and peak concentration of bupropion by 22% and 21%, respectively. Exposures of hydroxybupropion, threohydrobupropion, and erythrohydrobupropion were decreased by 23, 38, and 48%, respectively. Administration of ritonavir 600 mg twice daily in healthy subjects decreased AUC and peak concentration of bupropion by 66% and 62%, respectively. Exposures of hydroxybupropion, threohydrobupropion, and erythrohydrobupropion were decreased by 78, 50, and 68%, respectively. Administration of lopinavir 400 mg/ritonavir 100 mg twice daily in healthy subjects decreased bupropion AUC and peak concentration by 57%; the AUC and peak concentration of hydroxybupropion were decreased by 50% and 31%, respectively. Administration of efavirenz 600 mg once daily for 2 weeks in healthy volunteers reduced the AUC and peak concentration of bupropion by approximately 55% and 34%, respectively; the AUC of hydroxybupropion was unchanged, and peak concentration of hydroxybupropion was increased by 50%. An increase in bupropion dosage may be necessary in patients receiving concomitant treatment with antiretroviral agents that induce CYP2B6; however, the maximum recommended dosage of bupropion should not be exceeded.

In vitro studies suggest that nelfinavir may inhibit hydroxylation of bupropion.

● Benzodiazepines

Concurrent administration of single doses of bupropion and diazepam to healthy individuals did not result in potentiation of the mental impairment induced by diazepam. The impairment of performance on the auditory vigilance test observed with diazepam alone was absent with the combination of diazepam and bupropion. Individuals did not feel more drowsy with the combination of diazepam and bupropion than with placebo or bupropion alone but subjective assessment indicated an increase in drowsiness with diazepam alone.

Use with extreme caution; initiate therapy with lower dosages of bupropion and increase gradually.

● Carbamazepine

Concomitant treatment with carbamazepine may increase metabolism of bupropion. An increase in bupropion dosage may be necessary; however, the maximum recommended dosage of bupropion should not be exceeded.

● Cimetidine

Concomitant administration of bupropion and cimetidine resulted in 16% increases in the 24-hour area under the combined plasma concentration-time curve (AUC) and 32% increases in combined peak plasma concentration of the erythro- and threo-amino metabolites of bupropion. However, the pharmacokinetics of bupropion and hydroxybupropion were not affected.

● Digoxin

Concomitant treatment with bupropion may decrease plasma concentrations of digoxin. Decreased digoxin exposure has been reported following administration of a single oral dose of 0.5-mg digoxin 24 hours after a single oral dose of extended-release 150-mg bupropion hydrochloride in healthy subjects.

Monitor plasma concentrations of digoxin in patients receiving concomitant treatment with bupropion.

● Dopaminergic Drugs

Adverse CNS effects (e.g., restlessness, agitation, tremor, ataxia, gait disturbance, vertigo, dizziness), presumably related to cumulative dopamine agonist effects, have been reported in patients receiving bupropion concomitantly with amantadine or levodopa. Caution should be exercised if bupropion therapy is used concomitantly with levodopa or amantadine.

● Monoamine Oxidase Inhibitors

Concomitant use of bupropion and monoamine oxidase (MAO) inhibitors is associated with an increased risk of hypertensive reactions. In animals, phenelzine enhanced the acute toxicity of bupropion.

Concomitant administration of bupropion with an MAO inhibitor is contraindicated; ≥14 days should elapse between discontinuation of an MAO inhibitor and initiation of treatment with bupropion. Conversely, ≥14 days should elapse between discontinuance of bupropion and initiation of an MAO inhibitor.

● Nicotine

The manufacturer states that patients can receive bupropion concomitantly with transdermal nicotine therapy if indicated for smoking cessation. In a clinical study, concurrent use of bupropion extended-release tablets and nicotine transdermal systems resulted in similar plasma concentrations of bupropion and its active metabolites compared with patients receiving only bupropion extended-release tablets. However, the manufacturer reported a possible increased risk of hypertension during combined use, and the possibility of treatment-emergent hypertension should be considered when bupropion is used concomitantly with nicotine replacement therapy.

● Phenobarbital

Concomitant use of bupropion with phenobarbital may increase metabolism of bupropion. An increase in bupropion dosage may be necessary; however, the maximum recommended dosage of bupropion should not be exceeded.

● Phenytoin

Concomitant use of bupropion with phenytoin may increase metabolism of bupropion. An increase in bupropion dosage may be necessary; however, the maximum recommended dosage of bupropion should not be exceeded.

● Platelet-aggregation Inhibitors

Concomitant use of platelet-aggregation inhibitors that inhibit CYP2B6 (e.g., clopidogrel, ticlopidine) may increase bupropion exposure but decrease hydroxybupropion exposure. Administration of clopidogrel 75 mg once daily or ticlopidine 250 mg twice daily in healthy subjects increased bupropion peak concentration and AUC by 40% and 60%, respectively, for clopidogrel, and by 38% and 85%, respectively, for ticlopidine. The peak concentration and AUC of hydroxybupropion were decreased by 50% and 52%, respectively, by clopidogrel, and 78% and 84%, respectively, by ticlopidine. This effect is thought to be due to inhibition of CYP2B6, which catalyzes hydroxylation of bupropion. Administration of prasugrel, a weak CYP2B6 inhibitor, in healthy subjects increased bupropion peak concentration and AUC by 14% and 18%, respectively, and decreased peak concentration and AUC of hydroxybupropion by 32% and 24%, respectively.

Based on clinical response, dosage adjustment of bupropion may be necessary when used concomitantly with these drugs.

● Reversible MAO Inhibitors

Administration of bupropion with a reversible MAO inhibitor (e.g., linezolid, IV methylene blue) may increase the risk of hypertensive reactions; therefore, initiation of bupropion is not recommended in patients receiving treatment with a reversible MAO inhibitor. In a patient who requires more urgent treatment of a psychiatric condition, non-pharmacologic interventions, including hospitalization, should be considered.

Urgent treatment with linezolid or IV methylene blue may in some cases be necessary in a patient already receiving therapy with bupropion. If acceptable alternatives to linezolid or IV methylene blue treatment are not available and the potential benefits of linezolid or IV methylene blue treatment are thought to outweigh the risks of hypertensive reactions in a particular patient, bupropion should be discontinued promptly, and linezolid or IV methylene blue can then be administered. The patient should be monitored for 2 weeks or until 24 hours after the last dose of linezolid or IV methylene blue, whichever comes first. Therapy with bupropion may be resumed 24 hours after the last dose of linezolid or IV methylene blue.

● Serotonin Reuptake Inhibitors and Serotonin/Norepinephrine Reuptake Inhibitors

In vitro studies suggest that paroxetine, sertraline, norfluoxetine, and fluvoxamine may inhibit hydroxylation of bupropion.

● Tamoxifen

Concomitant use of bupropion with tamoxifen may reduce the efficacy of tamoxifen due to decreased metabolism of tamoxifen to its active form. Increased dosage of tamoxifen may be necessary when used concomitantly with bupropion.

● Warfarin

Concomitant use of bupropion with warfarin has resulted in altered prothrombin time/international normalized ratio (INR) that has been rarely associated with hemorrhagic or thrombotic complications.

DESCRIPTION

Bupropion hydrochloride is an aminoketone-derivative antidepressant agent that is chemically unrelated to tricyclic, tetracyclic, or other currently available antidepressants (e.g., selective serotonin-reuptake inhibitors) and also is chemically unrelated to nicotine or other agents currently used in the treatment of nicotine dependence.

The precise mechanism of antidepressant action of bupropion is unclear, although noradrenergic and/or dopaminergic pathways appear to be principally involved. Bupropion is a relatively weak inhibitor of the neuronal reuptake of norepinephrine and dopamine; bupropion does not inhibit monoamine oxidase or reuptake of serotonin.

The precise mechanism of action responsible for the efficacy of bupropion as an adjunct in the cessation of smoking is unclear, although noradrenergic and/or dopaminergic effects presumably are involved. It has been suggested that CNS effects of dopamine might be involved in the reinforcement properties of addictive drugs and that nicotine withdrawal manifestations may involve the absence of CNS effects of norepinephrine that are mediated by nicotine. Efficacy of bupropion in smoking cessation does not appear to depend on the presence of underlying depression.

Bupropion produces less frequent anticholinergic effects, cardiovascular effects, antihistaminic effects, and weight gain compared with tricyclic antidepressants at usual dosages.

Bupropion hydrochloride extended-release, 450-mg tablets (Forfivo XL®) and bupropion hydrobromide extended-release tablets (Aplenzin®) are bioequivalent to bupropion hydrochloride extended-release tablets (e.g., Wellbutrin® XL). Bupropion hydrobromide doses of 174, 348, or 522 mg are equivalent to bupropion hydrochloride doses of 150, 300, or 450 mg, respectively.

Bupropion hydrochloride appears to be well absorbed from the GI tract following oral administration. The absolute oral bioavailability of bupropion in humans has not been elucidated because a preparation for IV administration is not available. However, the relative proportion of an oral dose reaching systemic circulation unchanged appears likely to be small. In animals, the oral bioavailability of bupropion varies from 5–20%. Food does not appear to affect substantially the peak plasma concentration or area under the plasma concentration-time curve of bupropion achieved with extended-release tablets of the drug.

Peak plasma bupropion concentrations usually occur within 2, 3, or 5 hours after oral administration of conventional or extended-release bupropion hydrochloride tablets of Wellbutrin® SR or Wellbutrin® XL, respectively. Peak plasma concentrations occur within approximately 5 or 12 hours under fasted or fed conditions, respectively, after oral administration of extended-release, 450-mg bupropion hydrochloride tablets (Forfivo XL®). Peak plasma concentrations occur within approximately 5 hours after oral administration of extended-release bupropion hydrobromide tablets (Aplenzin®). Steady-state plasma concentrations of bupropion are achieved within 8 days. Bupropion and its metabolites are distributed into milk. Bupropion is 84% bound to human albumin at in vitro plasma concentrations ≤200 mcg/mL. The half-life of bupropion in the terminal phase averages about 14 hours following single doses; with multiple dosing, the elimination half-life reportedly averages 21 hours. Bupropion is extensively metabolized in the liver to 3 active metabolites: hydroxybupropion (principally by CYP2B6), threohydrobupropion, and erythrohydrobupropion. CYP isoenzymes are not involved in the formation of the threohydrobupropion and erythrohydrobupropion metabolites. Approximately 87 and 10% of an orally administered, radiolabeled dose of bupropion are excreted in urine and feces, respectively. Unchanged drug comprises 0.5% of the dose excreted. Hepatic impairment can decrease elimination of the drug. Renal impairment may decrease elimination of the major metabolites.

ADVICE TO PATIENTS

- Advise patients to swallow tablets whole and do not crush, chew, or divide the tablets.

- Advise patients to take conventional bupropion hydrochloride tablets in 3-4 divided doses daily, with ≥6 hours between subsequent doses.

- Instruct patients to take bupropion hydrochloride film-coated extended-release tablets in 2 divided doses, preferably with ≥8 hours between successive doses, when doses are >150 mg daily to minimize the risk of seizures.

- Instruct patients to take bupropion hydrochloride extended-release tablets (e.g., Wellbutrin® XL) once daily in the morning.

- Instruct patients that if they miss a dose, they should not take an extra tablet to make up for the missed dose and should take the next tablet at the regular time because of the dose-related risk of seizure.

- Risk of suicidality with antidepressants; instruct patients, families, and caregivers to be alert to the emergence of anxiety, agitation, panic attacks, insomnia, irritability, hostility, aggressiveness, impulsivity, akathisia (psychomotor restlessness), hypomania, mania, other unusual changes in behavior, suicidality, or worsening depression, especially during the first few months of therapy or during periods of dosage adjustment. Advise families and caregivers of patients to observe for the emergence of such symptoms on a day-to-day basis, since changes may be abrupt; such symptoms should be reported to the patient's clinician, especially if they are severe, abrupt in onset, or were not part of the patient's presenting symptoms. Such symptoms may be associated with an increased risk for suicidal thinking and behavior and indicate a need for very close monitoring and possibly changes in medication.

- Risk of serious neuropsychiatric symptoms, including changes in mood (e.g., depression, mania), psychosis, hallucinations, paranoia, delusions, homicidal ideation, aggression, hostility, agitation, anxiety, and panic as well as suicidal ideation, suicide attempt, and completed suicide, when used for smoking cessation. Instruct patients to discontinue bupropion and contact a clinician if they experience such symptoms.

- Risk of hypersensitivity reactions. Advise patients to stop taking bupropion and notify their clinician if they develp signs of a severe allergic reaction.

- Risk of seizures. Advise patients to permanently stop taking the drug and immediately notify their clinician if they have a seizure. Advise patients that excessive use or abrupt discontinuation of alcohol, benzodiazepines, antiepileptic drugs, or sedative hypnotic drugs can increase the risk of seizure. Advise patients to minimize or avoid use of alcohol.

- Risk of angle-closure glaucoma in susceptible individuals secondary to mild pupillary dilation associated with bupropion. Patients may wish to be examined to determine whether they are suscetible to angle closure, and have a prophylactic procedure (e.g., iridectomy) if they are susceptible.

- Importance of avoiding concomitant therapy with preparations containing bupropion for use as an adjunct in smoking cessation and preparations used for treatment of major depressive disorder or seasonal affective disorder.

- May impair patient's ability to perform tasks requiring judgment or motor and cognitive skills. Advise patients to avoid operating machinery or driving a motor vehicle until the effects on the individual are known. May decrease alcohol tolerance.

- Importance of minimizing or avoiding consumption of alcohol; excessive use of alcohol or abrupt cessation of use may alter the seizure threshold.

- Importance of informing patients that the shell of certain extended-release tablets (e.g., Aplenzin®, Wellbutrin® XL) does not dissolve and may be passed in the stool.

- Advise patients that bupropion hydrochloride extended-release tablets (e.g., Wellbutrin® SR) may have an odor.

- Advise patients to inform their clinician of existing or contemplated concomitant therapy, including prescription and OTC drugs and dietary or herbal supplements, as well as any concomitant illnesses.

- Importance of women notifying clinicians if they are or plan to become pregnant or plan to breast-feed. Advise patients of any pregnancy exposure registry that monitors pregnancy outcomes in women exposed to bupropion during pregnancy. Advise patients that bupropion is distributed into milk in small amounts.

- Inform patients of other important precautionary information.

PREPARATIONS

Excipients in commercially available drug preparations may have clinically important effects in some individuals; consult specific product labeling for details.

buPROPion Hydrobromide

Oral

Tablets, extended-release	174 mg	Aplenzin®, Bausch Health US
	348 mg	Aplenzin®, Bausch Health US
	522 mg	Aplenzin®, Bausch Health US

buPROPion Hydrochloride

Oral

Tablets, extended-release	150 mg*	buPROPion Hydrochloride Extended-release Tablets (SR)
		Wellbutrin® XL, Bausch Health US
	300 mg*	Wellbutrin® XL, Bausch Health US
	450 mg	Forfivo XL®, Almatica Pharma
Tablets, extended-release, film-coated	100 mg*	buPROPion Hydrochloride Extended-release Tablets
		Wellbutrin® SR, GlaxoSmithKline
	150 mg*	buPROPion Hydrochloride Extended-release Tablets
		Wellbutrin® SR, GlaxoSmithKline
	200 mg*	buPROPion Hydrochloride Extended-release Tablets
		Wellbutrin® SR, GlaxoSmithKline

| Tablets, film-coated | 75 mg* | buPROPion Hydrochloride Tablets |
| | 100 mg* | buPROPion Hydrochloride Tablets |

* available from one or more manufacturer, distributor, and/or repackager by generic (nonproprietary) name

† Use is not currently included in the labeling approved by the US Food and Drug Administration.

Selected Revisions September 10, 2024, © Copyright, January 1, 1996, American Society of Health-System Pharmacists, Inc.

ARIPiprazole

28:16.08.04 • ATYPICAL ANTIPSYCHOTICS

■ Aripiprazole is considered an atypical or second-generation antipsychotic agent.

USES

Aripiprazole is used orally for the symptomatic management of psychotic disorders (e.g., schizophrenia). Aripiprazole also is used orally for the treatment of bipolar I disorder, as an adjunct to antidepressants for the acute treatment of major depressive disorder, for the acute treatment of irritability associated with autistic disorder, and for the treatment of Tourette's syndrome (Gilles de la Tourette's syndrome). Short-acting (immediate-release) aripiprazole injection (Abilify*; no longer commercially available in the US) has been used IM for the management of acute agitation in patients with bipolar disorder or schizophrenia. Extended-release aripiprazole injection (Abilify Maintena®) is used IM for the treatment of schizophrenia and maintenance treatment of bipolar I disorder. Extended-release aripiprazole lauroxil injection (Aristada®; available as prefilled syringes in 441-mg, 662-mg, 882-mg, and 1064-mg strengths) is used IM for the treatment of schizophrenia; the 675-mg strength of extended-release aripiprazole lauroxil injection (Aristada Initio®) is used IM in combination with oral aripiprazole for the initiation of extended-release aripiprazole lauroxil therapy for the treatment of schizophrenia.

Aripiprazole tablets with sensor (Abilify MyCite®) is part of a digital ingestion tracking system intended to provide objective data on drug ingestion. (See Tablets with Sensor under Administration: Oral Administration, in Dosage and Administration and also see Description: Aripiprazole Tablets with Sensor.) The ability of the system to improve patient compliance or help guide aripiprazole dosage adjustments has not been established. The manufacturer states that the use of Abilify MyCite® to track drug ingestion in "real time" or during an emergency is not recommended because detection of tablet ingestion may be delayed or may not occur. Abilify MyCite® is used orally for the treatment of schizophrenia, for the treatment of bipolar I disorder, and as an adjunct to antidepressants for the treatment of major depressive disorder.

● *Psychotic Disorders*

Aripiprazole is used orally and parenterally for the symptomatic management of psychotic disorders (e.g., schizophrenia). Drug therapy is integral to the management of acute psychotic episodes in patients with schizophrenia and generally is required for long-term stabilization to sustain symptom remission or control and to minimize the risk of relapse. Antipsychotic agents are the principal class of drugs used for the management of all phases of schizophrenia. Patient response and tolerance to antipsychotic agents are variable, and patients who do not respond to or tolerate one drug may be successfully treated with an agent from a different class or with a different adverse effect profile.

Schizophrenia

Aripiprazole is used orally for the acute and maintenance treatment of schizophrenia. In addition, extended-release formulations of aripiprazole (Abilify Maintena®) and aripiprazole lauroxil (Aristada®, Aristada Initio®) are used IM for the treatment of schizophrenia. Schizophrenia is a major psychotic disorder that frequently has devastating effects on various aspects of the patient's life and carries a high risk of suicide and other life-threatening behaviors. Manifestations of schizophrenia involve multiple psychologic processes, including perception (e.g., hallucinations), ideation, reality testing (e.g., delusions), emotion (e.g., flatness, inappropriate affect), thought processes (e.g., loose associations), behavior (e.g., catatonia, disorganization), attention, concentration, motivation (e.g., avolition, impaired intention and planning), and judgment. The principal manifestations of this disorder usually are described in terms of positive and negative (deficit) symptoms and, more recently, disorganized symptoms. Positive symptoms include hallucinations, delusions, bizarre behavior, hostility, uncooperativeness, and paranoid ideation, while negative symptoms include restricted range and intensity of emotional expression (affective flattening), reduced thought and speech productivity (alogia), anhedonia, apathy, and decreased initiation of goal-directed behavior (avolition). Disorganized symptoms include disorganized speech (thought disorder) and behavior and poor attention.

Short-term efficacy of oral aripiprazole monotherapy in the acute treatment of schizophrenia in adults was evaluated in 5 placebo-controlled studies of 4 and 6 weeks' duration principally in acutely relapsed, hospitalized patients who predominantly met DSM-III/IV criteria for schizophrenia. Four of the 5 studies were able to distinguish aripiprazole from placebo, but the smallest study did not. In the 4 positive studies, assessment of improvement in manifestations of schizophrenia was based on results of psychiatric rating scales, including the Positive and Negative Syndrome Scale (PANSS), the PANSS positive subscale, the PANSS negative subscale, and the Clinical Global Impressions (CGI) scale. Aripiprazole generally was found to be superior to placebo in improving both positive and negative manifestations in acute exacerbations of schizophrenia in these 4 studies. Efficacy of 10-, 15-, 20-, and 30-mg daily dosages of aripiprazole was established in 2 studies for each dosage; however, there was no evidence that higher dosages offered any therapeutic advantage over lower dosages in these studies. Active controls (haloperidol or risperidone) were used in addition to placebo controls in 3 of these studies, but study design did not allow for comparison between aripiprazole and the active controls. An examination of population subgroups did not reveal any clear evidence of differential responsiveness to the drug based on age, gender, or race.

In a longer-term study, adult inpatients or outpatients who met DSM-IV criteria for schizophrenia and who were, by history, symptomatically stable on other antipsychotic agents for at least 3 months were discontinued from those other agents and randomized to receive either oral aripiprazole 15 mg daily or placebo for up to 26 weeks of observation for relapse in the double-blind phase. Relapse was based on results of the CGI-Improvement and PANSS psychiatric rating scales. Patients receiving aripiprazole experienced a significantly longer time to relapse over the subsequent 26 weeks compared with those receiving placebo. In addition, pooled data from 2 double-blind, multicenter studies in acutely ill patients with schizophrenia in whom therapy with aripiprazole or haloperidol was continued for 52 weeks demonstrated a substantially higher rate of symptomatic remission across 52 weeks in the aripiprazole-treated patients compared with the haloperidol-treated patients; improved tolerability with aripiprazole may have contributed to the higher overall remission rates observed in this pooled analysis.

Short-term efficacy of oral aripiprazole in the acute treatment of schizophrenia in adolescents 13–17 years of age was evaluated in a double-blind, placebo-controlled trial of 6 weeks' duration in 302 outpatients who met DSM-IV criteria for schizophrenia and had a PANSS total score of 70 or more at baseline. Patients were randomized to receive a fixed dosage of aripiprazole 10 mg daily or 30 mg daily or to receive placebo. Both dosages of aripiprazole were found to be superior to placebo in reducing the PANSS total score, which was the primary efficacy measure; the 10-mg daily dosage also demonstrated superiority over placebo on the PANSS negative subscale score at the study end point. However, the 30-mg daily dosage failed to demonstrate superiority over the 10-mg daily dosage. The drug was generally well tolerated.

Short-term efficacy of the extended-release IM formulation of aripiprazole (Abilify Maintena®) in the treatment of schizophrenia in adults was established in a multicenter, double-blind, placebo-controlled study of 12 weeks' duration in acutely relapsed inpatients who met DSM-IV-TR criteria for schizophrenia and who were experiencing an acute psychotic episode. Patients in this study were randomized to receive IM injections of extended-release aripiprazole (400 mg) or placebo every 4 weeks. Patients receiving extended-release IM aripiprazole were also given oral aripiprazole (10–20 mg daily) for 14 days beginning on the day of the first injection to provide therapeutic plasma concentrations, which may take longer to achieve in some patients; patients who received placebo injections were given placebo tablets for the first 14 days. The IM dosage of extended-release aripiprazole could be adjusted down to 300 mg and increased back to 400 mg on a one-time basis. The primary efficacy measure in this study was the change in PANSS total score from baseline to end point (week 10). Patients treated with extended-release IM aripiprazole injection demonstrated substantially greater improvement in mean PANSS total scores compared with those receiving placebo.

In a longer-term maintenance study, adults who met DSM-IV-TR criteria for schizophrenia and who were receiving at least one antipsychotic agent were treated with open-label oral aripiprazole for 4–6 weeks followed by extended-release aripiprazole (Abilify Maintena®) 400 mg IM once every 4 weeks with oral aripiprazole continued for the first 2 weeks after the initial injection. The IM extended-release aripiprazole dosage could be adjusted down to 300 mg based on tolerability and increased back to 400 mg on a one-time basis. Patients who remained stable on the extended-release IM injection for at least 12 weeks were then randomized either to continue receiving extended-release IM aripiprazole at the same dosage or to receive placebo injection IM every 4 weeks for up to 52 weeks and observed for relapse in the double-blind withdrawal phase. The primary efficacy measure was the time from randomization to relapse, and patients who received extended-release IM aripiprazole had a substantially longer time to relapse than those who received placebo.

Efficacy of extended-release aripiprazole lauroxil IM injection (Aristada®) in the treatment of schizophrenia was established, in part, based on extrapolation of efficacy data from clinical trials with oral aripiprazole. In addition, efficacy was established in a multicenter, double-blind, placebo-controlled, fixed-dose study of 12 weeks' duration in adults who met DSM-IV-TR criteria for schizophrenia and were experiencing an acute exacerbation or relapse. Patients were randomized to receive extended-release aripiprazole lauroxil 441 mg, aripiprazole lauroxil 882 mg, or placebo by IM injection every 4 weeks. After establishing tolerability to oral aripiprazole, patients concomitantly received oral aripiprazole 15 mg daily (if randomized to aripiprazole) or placebo for the first 3 weeks. The primary efficacy measure in this study was the change in PANSS total score from baseline to end point (week 12). At the study end point, both dosages of extended-release aripiprazole lauroxil injection resulted in substantially greater improvement in the PANSS total score compared with placebo. Substantial improvements in the PANSS total score were evident as early as day 8 with extended-release aripiprazole lauroxil therapy and continued through the end of the treatment period. The secondary efficacy end point was the Clinical Global Impression-Improvement (CGI-I) score on day 85. Both groups of patients receiving extended-release aripiprazole lauroxil therapy demonstrated substantially better CGI-I scores compared with the placebo group. An examination of population subgroups did not reveal any clear evidence of differential responsiveness to the drug based on age, gender, race, or body weight.

Aripiprazole tablets with sensor (Abilify MyCite®) is part of a digital ingestion tracking system intended to provide objective data on drug ingestion. (See Tablets with Sensor under Administration: Oral Administration, in Dosage and Administration and also see Description: Aripiprazole Tablets with Sensor.) The usability (i.e., ease of use, helpfulness) of this digital ingestion tracking system was evaluated in a multicenter, open-label study in 67 adults with a primary diagnosis of schizophrenia. Patients who had been stabilized on oral aripiprazole therapy were switched to the same dosage of aripiprazole tablets with sensor (Abilify MyCite®) for 8 weeks. Patients received training at baseline and weekly as needed for the first 3 weeks then were instructed to change the wearable sensor and pair it with their mobile device independently or with the assistance of a caregiver weekly for the next 5 weeks. The majority of patients in this study were male (74.6%) and black or African-American (76.1%), and 70.1% had mild disease (i.e., Clinical Global Impression-Severity [CGI-S] score of 3) and a higher range of function (indicated by relatively high mean scores on the Instrumental Activities of Daily Living and Personal and Social Performance scales). Forty-nine patients (73.1%) completed the 8-week study; by the end of the study period or at the time of withdrawal from the study, 55.2% of patients were able to apply and pair a wearable sensor with their mobile device independently and 82.1% completed the tasks independently or with minimal assistance (as rated by a clinician using a standardized scale). Of the 60 patients who rated the ease of use and helpfulness of the digital ingestion tracking system at the end of study or at the time of withdrawal from the study, 78% reported that they were somewhat satisfied to extremely satisfied with the digital ingestion tracking system, 70% rated the system as at least somewhat helpful in management of their condition, 77% rated the system as at least somewhat helpful in improving discussions with their healthcare provider, and 65% rated the system as somewhat easy to extremely easy to use.

Although the efficacy of oral aripiprazole as maintenance therapy in pediatric patients with schizophrenia has not been systematically evaluated, the manufacturer states that such efficacy can be extrapolated from adult data in addition to comparisons of aripiprazole pharmacokinetic parameters in adult and pediatric patients.

If aripiprazole is used for extended periods as maintenance therapy for schizophrenia, the need for continued therapy should be reassessed periodically. (See Dosage and Administration: Dosage and see also Pediatric Use under Warnings/Precautions: Specific Populations, in Cautions.)

The American Psychiatric Association (APA) considers most atypical antipsychotic agents first-line drugs for the management of the acute phase of schizophrenia (including first psychotic episodes), principally because of the decreased risk of adverse extrapyramidal effects and tardive dyskinesia, with the understanding that the relative advantages, disadvantages, and cost-effectiveness of conventional and atypical antipsychotic agents remain controversial. The APA states that, with the possible exception of clozapine for the management of treatment-resistant symptoms, there currently is no definitive evidence that one atypical antipsychotic agent will have superior efficacy compared with another agent in the class, although meaningful differences in response may be observed in individual patients. Conventional antipsychotic agents may be considered first-line therapy in patients who have been treated successfully in the past with or who prefer conventional agents. The choice of an antipsychotic agent should be individualized, considering past response to therapy, adverse effect profile (including the patient's experience of subjective effects such as dysphoria), and the patient's preference for a specific drug, including route of administration.

For additional information on the symptomatic management of schizophrenia, including treatment recommendations, see Schizophrenia and Other Psychotic Disorders under Uses: Psychotic Disorders, in the Phenothiazines General Statement 28:16.08.24.

● Bipolar Disorder

Aripiprazole is used orally as monotherapy or as an adjunct to either lithium or valproate for the acute treatment of manic or mixed episodes associated with bipolar I disorder with or without psychotic features. The drug also is used orally as monotherapy or as adjunctive therapy with lithium or valproate for the maintenance treatment of bipolar I disorder. Extended-release aripiprazole injection (Abilify Maintena®) is used IM as monotherapy for the maintenance treatment of bipolar I disorder. According to DSM-IV criteria, manic episodes are distinct periods lasting 1 week or longer (or less than 1 week if hospitalization is required) of abnormally and persistently elevated, expansive, or irritable mood accompanied by at least 3 (or 4 if the mood is only irritability) of the following 7 symptoms: grandiosity, reduced need for sleep, pressure of speech, flight of ideas, distractability, increased goal-directed activity (either socially, at work or school, or sexually) or psychomotor agitation, and engaging in high-risk behavior (e.g., unrestrained buying sprees, sexual indiscretions, foolish business investments).

Efficacy of oral aripiprazole monotherapy in the treatment of acute manic and mixed episodes has been demonstrated in 4 short-term (i.e., 3 weeks' duration), placebo-controlled trials in hospitalized adults who met DSM-IV criteria for bipolar I disorder with manic or mixed episodes. These studies included patients with or without psychotic features and 2 of the studies also included patients with or without a rapid cycling course. The principal rating instrument used for assessing manic symptoms in these trials was the Young Mania Rating Scale (Y-MRS), an 11-item clinician-rated scale traditionally used to assess the degree of manic symptomatology in a range from 0 (no manic features) to 60 (maximum score). The main secondary rating instrument used in these trials was the Clinical Global Impression-Bipolar (CGI-BP) scale. In these trials, aripiprazole 15–30 mg once daily (with an initial dosage of 15 mg daily in 2 studies and an initial dosage of 30 mg daily in the other 2 studies) was found to be superior to placebo in the reduction of the Y-MRS total score and the CGI-BP Severity of Illness score (mania). In the 2 studies with an initial aripiprazole dosage of 15 mg daily, 48 and 44% of patients were receiving 15 mg daily at the study end point; in the 2 studies with an initial dosage of 30 mg daily, 86 and 85% of patients were receiving 30 mg daily at end point.

Aripiprazole is used orally as monotherapy for the acute treatment of manic and mixed episodes associated with bipolar I disorder with or without psychotic features in pediatric patients 10–17 years of age. Efficacy of aripiprazole in the acute treatment of manic and mixed episodes has been demonstrated in a double-blind, placebo-controlled study of 4 weeks' duration in pediatric outpatients who met DSM-IV criteria for bipolar I disorder manic or mixed episodes (with or without psychotic features) and who had Y-MRS scores of 20 or greater at baseline. Patients in this study received aripiprazole 10 mg daily, aripiprazole 30 mg daily, or placebo. Aripiprazole was initiated at a dosage of 2 mg daily, then titrated to 5 mg daily after 2 days, and to the target dosage of 10 mg daily in 5 days or 30 mg daily in 13 days. Both dosages of aripiprazole were found to be superior to placebo in the reduction of the Y-MRS total score from baseline to week 4.

Efficacy of oral aripiprazole as an adjunct to lithium or valproate in the treatment of acute manic and mixed episodes has been demonstrated in a placebo-controlled study of 6 weeks' duration in adult outpatients who met DSM-IV criteria for bipolar I disorder manic or mixed type (with or without psychotic features). Patients initially received open-label lithium (dosage producing a serum lithium concentration of 0.6–1 mEq/L) or valproate (dosage producing a serum valproic acid concentration of 50–125 mcg/mL) monotherapy for 2 weeks during the lead-in phase. At the end of 2 weeks, patients demonstrating an inadequate response to lithium or valproate were randomized to receive either aripiprazole (15 mg daily or increased to 30 mg daily as early as day 7) or placebo as adjunctive therapy with open-label lithium or valproate during the 6-week, placebo-controlled phase. Patients who received adjunctive aripiprazole with lithium or valproate demonstrated greater reductions in the Y-MRS total score and the CGI-BP Severity of Illness score (mania) compared with patients who received adjunctive placebo with lithium or valproate.

The use of oral aripiprazole as an adjunct to lithium or valproate in the acute treatment of manic or mixed episodes associated with bipolar I disorder has not been evaluated in the pediatric population. However, the manufacturer states that such efficacy can be extrapolated from adult data in addition to comparisons of aripiprazole pharmacokinetic parameters in adult and pediatric patients.

For the initial management of less severe manic or mixed episodes in patients with bipolar disorder, current APA recommendations state that monotherapy with lithium, valproate (e.g., valproate sodium, valproic acid, divalproex), or an antipsychotic such as olanzapine may be adequate. For more severe manic or mixed episodes, combination therapy with an antipsychotic and lithium or valproate is recommended as first-line therapy. For further information on the management of bipolar disorder, see Uses: Bipolar Disorder, in Lithium Salts 28:28.

Efficacy of oral aripiprazole as monotherapy for the maintenance treatment of bipolar I disorder was evaluated in a 26-week, double-blind, placebo-controlled trial in patients with a recent manic or mixed episode who had been stabilized on open-label aripiprazole monotherapy (15–30 mg daily); patients who maintained clinical response with the drug for at least 6 weeks were randomized to either continue aripiprazole at the same dosage or be switched to placebo and monitored for manic or depressive relapse. In this study, time to relapse to any mood episode, particularly manic episode, was substantially longer and there were fewer manic relapses among patients receiving aripiprazole than in those receiving placebo. There were no differences between aripiprazole and placebo in time to relapse to depressive or mixed episodes or in the number of depressive episodes. A 74-week extension of the study also found that time to relapse to any mood episode, particularly manic episode, was substantially longer with aripiprazole than placebo at 100 weeks of treatment; however, the design and interpretation of these study findings suggesting aripiprazole's efficacy in the maintenance therapy of bipolar disorder have been criticized (i.e., insufficient duration to demonstrate prophylactic efficacy, use of an "enriched" patient sample consisting of aripiprazole responders, abrupt discontinuance of aripiprazole in patients randomized to placebo, and low study completion rate). Time to relapse to depressive episode was not substantially different between treatment groups during the 74-week extension phase.

Oral aripiprazole as adjunctive maintenance therapy in adults with bipolar I disorder was evaluated in a double-blind, placebo-controlled trial in patients with a recent manic or mixed episode. Patients in this study had received lithium or valproate therapy for at least 2 weeks, and those with an inadequate response to the mood stabilizer also received adjunctive aripiprazole therapy (10–30 mg daily) and were maintained on the combined regimen for at least 12 weeks. Patients who maintained clinical response with aripiprazole and a mood stabilizer during this period were randomized to either continue aripiprazole or be switched to placebo (combined with lithium or valproate therapy) and monitored for manic, mixed, or depressive relapse for a maximum of 52 weeks. Patients receiving adjunctive aripiprazole therapy with lithium or valproate experienced a significant delay in time to relapse to any mood episode compared with those receiving placebo plus lithium or valproate, particularly for relapse to manic episode; no difference between the treatment groups was observed for time to relapse to depressive episode.

Efficacy of extended-release IM aripiprazole injection (Abilify Maintena®) as monotherapy for the maintenance treatment of bipolar I disorder has been established in a randomized, double-blind, placebo-controlled withdrawal study of 52 weeks' duration in adults with bipolar I disorder. This study included patients currently experiencing a manic episode and who had experienced at least 1 prior manic or mixed episode with manic symptoms necessitating treatment (e.g., hospitalization, mood stabilizer, antipsychotic agent) who were converted to oral aripiprazole monotherapy over 4–6 weeks. Patients successfully converted to oral aripiprazole monotherapy or patients already receiving oral aripiprazole monotherapy continued

receiving the drug orally for a stabilization phase of 2–8 weeks at a target dosage of 15–30 mg daily, and those who remained stable were subsequently converted to extended-release aripiprazole 400 mg IM once every 4 weeks for 12–28 weeks. Oral aripiprazole was continued for the first 2 weeks after the initial injection during the stabilization phase. Patients who remained stable on the extended-release IM injection for at least 8 consecutive weeks were then randomized either to continue receiving extended-release IM aripiprazole at the same dosage or placebo for up to 52 weeks during the double-blind withdrawal phase. The monthly IM aripiprazole dosage could be adjusted down to 300 mg based on tolerability and increased back to 400 mg on a one-time basis. The primary efficacy measure was the time from randomization to recurrence of any mood episode, which was defined as hospitalization for any mood episode; Y-MRS total score 15 or higher; Montgomery-Asberg Depression Rating Scale (MADRS) total score 15 or higher; CGI-BP scale overall score over 4; worsening of bipolar I disorder; withdrawal from the study because of lack of efficacy, adverse event, or worsening disease; clinical worsening with the need for addition of a mood stabilizer, antidepressant, or antipsychotic agent, and/or increase in benzodiazepine dosage above the highest permitted dosage (i.e., exceeding 2 mg of lorazepam or equivalent per day); or active suicidality. Patients who received extended-release IM aripiprazole had a substantially longer time to recurrence of any mood episode than those who received placebo. Time to recurrence of manic or mixed episodes was substantially longer in patients receiving extended-release IM aripiprazole compared with those receiving placebo; no difference between the treatment groups was observed for time to relapse to depressive episodes.

● Major Depressive Disorder

Aripiprazole is used orally as an adjunct to antidepressants for the treatment of major depressive disorder. The adjunctive efficacy of aripiprazole has been demonstrated in 2 short-term, double-blind, placebo-controlled trials of 6 weeks' duration in adults who met DSM-IV criteria for major depressive disorder and who had an inadequate response to previous antidepressant therapy (1–3 courses) in the current episode and who had also demonstrated an inadequate response during a prospective treatment period to 8 weeks of antidepressant therapy with extended-release paroxetine, extended-release venlafaxine, fluoxetine, escitalopram, or sertraline. The primary instrument used for assessing depressive symptoms was the MADRS, a 10-item clinician-rated scale used to assess the degree of depressive symptomatology. The principal secondary instrument was the Sheehan Disability Scale (SDS), a 3-item self-rated instrument used to assess the impact of depression on three domains of functioning (work/school, social life, and family life), with each item scored from 0 (not at all) to 10 (extreme). In both of these trials, aripiprazole was found to be superior to placebo in reducing mean MADRS total scores; aripiprazole was also superior to placebo in reducing the mean SDS score in one study. Patients in both trials initially received an aripiprazole dosage of 5 mg daily; subsequent dosage adjustments, based on efficacy and tolerability, could be made in 5-mg increments 1 week apart. Allowable aripiprazole dosages were 2, 5, 10, and 15 mg daily; patients who were not receiving the potent cytochrome P-450 (CYP) isoenzyme 2D6 inhibitors fluoxetine and paroxetine could also receive 20 mg daily.

An analysis of population subgroups did not reveal evidence of differential response based on age, choice of prospective antidepressant, or race. With regard to gender, a smaller mean reduction in the MADRS total score was observed in males than in females.

● Irritability Associated with Autistic Disorder

Aripiprazole is used orally for the acute treatment of irritability associated with autistic disorder. Efficacy of aripiprazole was established in 2 double-blind, placebo-controlled trials of 8 weeks' duration in pediatric patients 6–17 years of age who met DSM-IV criteria for autistic disorder and demonstrated behaviors such as aggression towards others, self-injurious behavior, quickly changing moods, or a combination of these behaviors. Over 75% of the enrolled patients were under 13 years of age. The primary instruments used for assessing clinical efficacy were the Aberrant Behavior Checklist (ABC) and the Clinical Global Impression-Improvement (CGI-I) scale. The primary outcome measure in both trials was the change from baseline to end point in the irritability subscale of the ABC (ABC-I). In one of the trials, 98 children and adolescents with autistic disorder received flexible daily dosages of aripiprazole ranging from 2–15 mg daily, starting at 2 mg daily with increases allowed up to 15 mg daily based on clinical response, and placebo. In this trial, aripiprazole improved scores on both the ABC-I subscale and on the CGI-I scale compared with placebo. The mean daily dosage of aripiprazole at the end of the 8-week treatment period was approximately 9 mg daily.

In the other trial, 218 children and adolescents with autistic disorder received one of 3 fixed dosages of aripiprazole (5, 10, or 15 mg daily) or placebo. Aripiprazole therapy was started at 2 mg daily and was increased to 5 mg daily after 1 week. After the second week, the dosage was increased to 10 mg daily for patients in the 10- and 15-mg daily dosage arms; after the third week, the dosage was increased to 15 mg daily in the 15-mg daily treatment arm. Patients receiving all 3 aripiprazole dosages in this study demonstrated improved ABC-I subscale and CGI-I scores compared with placebo.

● Tourette's Syndrome

Aripiprazole is used orally for the treatment of Tourette's syndrome (Gilles de la Tourette's syndrome). Efficacy of aripiprazole was established in 2 controlled trials (one 8-week and one 10-week) in pediatric patients who met DSM-IV criteria for Tourette's disorder and who had a total tic score (TTS) of at least 20–22 on the Yale Global Tic Severity Scale (YGTSS). The YGTSS is a fully validated scale that measures current tic severity. The primary outcome measure in both trials was the change from baseline to end point in the TTS on the YGTSS (YGTSS TTS). Over 65% of the enrolled patients were under 13 years of age.

In the 8-week, placebo-controlled, fixed-dose trial, 133 patients 7–17 years of age were randomized to receive high-dose aripiprazole (target daily dosage of 10 mg for patients weighing less than 50 kg and 20 mg for those weighing 50 kg or more), low-dose aripiprazole (target daily dosage of 5 mg for those weighing less than 50 kg and 10 mg for those weighing 50 kg or more), or placebo. Aripiprazole was initiated at 2 mg daily and increased to 5 mg after 2 days with subsequent increases of 5 mg on day 7 and weekly thereafter when the target dosage was 10 mg daily or higher. Patients receiving aripiprazole in both the high-dose and low-dose groups demonstrated substantially improved scores on the YGTSS TTS compared with patients receiving placebo.

In the 10-week, placebo-controlled, flexible-dose study, which was conducted in Korea, 61 patients 6–18 years of age with Tourette's syndrome were randomized to receive flexible daily dosages of aripiprazole, starting at 2 mg daily with increases allowed up to 20 mg daily based on clinical response, or placebo. The aripiprazole-treated patients in this study demonstrated substantially improved scores on the YGTSS TTS compared with patients receiving placebo. The mean daily dosage of aripiprazole at the end of the 10-week treatment period was approximately 6.5 mg daily.

For further information on Tourette's syndrome, including clinical manifestations, diagnosis, and management of the disorder, see Uses: Tourette's Syndrome, in Pimozide 28:16.08.92.

● Agitation Associated with Schizophrenia or Bipolar Mania

Aripiprazole has been used IM for the acute management of agitation associated with schizophrenia or bipolar disorder, manic or mixed, in patients for whom treatment with aripiprazole is appropriate and who require an IM antipsychotic agent for rapid control of behaviors that interfere with diagnosis and care (e.g., threatening behaviors, escalating or urgently distressing behavior, self-exhausting behavior). However, immediate-release aripiprazole IM injection (Abilify®) has been discontinued by the manufacturer and is no longer commercially available in the US.

DOSAGE AND ADMINISTRATION

● Administration

Aripiprazole is administered orally or by IM injection. Aripiprazole lauroxil is administered *only* by IM injection.

Patients receiving aripiprazole should be monitored for possible worsening of depression, suicidality, or unusual changes in behavior, especially at the beginning of therapy or during periods of dosage adjustment. (See Worsening of Depression and Suicidality Risk under Warnings/Precautions: Warnings, in Cautions.)

Oral Administration

Aripiprazole conventional tablets, tablets with sensor (Abilify MyCite®), orally disintegrating tablets, and oral solution are administered orally once daily without regard to meals.

Orally Disintegrating Tablets

Patients receiving aripiprazole orally disintegrating tablets should be instructed not to remove a tablet from the blister package until just prior to dosing. The tablet should not be pushed through the foil, since this may damage the tablet. With dry hands, the blister package should be peeled open to expose a tablet. The tablet should then be removed and placed on the tongue, where it rapidly disintegrates in saliva. The manufacturer recommends that the orally disintegrating tablets be taken without liquid; however, they may be taken with liquid, if necessary. Aripiprazole orally disintegrating tablets should *not* be split.

Tablets with Sensor

Aripiprazole is available as part of a digital ingestion tracking system comprised of the following components: aripiprazole tablets embedded with an ingestible event marker sensor (IEM; Abilify MyCite®); a wearable sensor (MyCite® patch), which detects the signal from the IEM sensor after ingestion and transmits data to a compatible mobile device (i.e., a smart phone); a software application (app) for compatible mobile devices (e.g., smart phones; MyCite® App), which displays information for the patient; and a web-based portal for healthcare professionals and caregivers.

Prior to initial patient use of the Abilify MyCite® system, use of the combination product and its components (patch, app, portal) should be facilitated. Clinicians should ensure that patients are capable and willing to use a mobile device (e.g., smart phone) and the software application (app). Before using any component of the system, clinicians should instruct patients to download the mobile software application and follow all the instructions for use and to ensure that the software is compatible with their specific mobile device.

Aripiprazole tablets with sensor are administered orally once daily without regard to meals; tablets with sensor should be swallowed whole and *not* divided, crushed, or chewed.

Prior to use of the software application, the patient's mobile device should be powered on and Bluetooth® enabled. The accompanying wearable sensor should be applied when prompted by the mobile software application; the application will instruct patients to apply and remove the sensor correctly. Patients should confirm that their mobile device is paired with the wearable sensor prior to use; the mobile software application will display a status icon on the mobile device to indicate that the wearable sensor is properly adhered and functioning. For further information, clinicians and patients may refer to the information provided in the product packaging as well as the instructions for use within the mobile software application.

Most ingestions of aripiprazole tablets with sensor will be detected within 30 minutes following ingestion; however, it may take up to 2 hours for the smart phone application and web portal to detect the ingestion of the tablet with sensor. In some cases, ingestion of the tablet with sensor may not be detected. If the tablet with sensor is not detected following ingestion, the dose should *not* be repeated.

The wearable sensor should be applied topically to the left side of the body just above the lower edge of the rib cage. Application to areas where the skin is scraped, cracked, inflamed, or irritated or areas overlapping the area of the most recently removed wearable sensor should be avoided. The wearable sensor should be changed weekly or sooner as needed; the mobile software application will remind patients when to change the sensor. Patients should be instructed keep the sensor in place while showering, swimming, or exercising. However, the sensor should be removed before undergoing magnetic resonance imaging (MRI) and replaced with a new sensor as soon as possible following the procedure. If skin irritation occurs, the wearable sensor should be removed. (See Skin Irritation associated with Abilify MyCite® Wearable Sensor under Warnings/Precautions: Other Warnings and Precautions, in Cautions.)

IM Administration

Clinicians should be aware that there are several different IM formulations of aripiprazole with different indications, dosages, and dosing frequencies. A short-acting, immediate-release IM formulation of aripiprazole (Abilify®) has been used for agitation associated with schizophrenia and bipolar mania, but is no longer commercially available in the US. The extended-release IM formulation of aripiprazole (Abilify Maintena®) is available in 300- and 400-mg vials and prefilled syringes and is used for the treatment of schizophrenia and maintenance monotherapy of bipolar I disorder. The extended-release IM formulation of aripiprazole lauroxil (Aristada®) is available in 441-, 662-, 882-, and 1064-mg prefilled syringes and is used for the treatment of schizophrenia.

Extended-release aripiprazole lauroxil injection also is available in 675-mg prefilled syringes (Aristada Initio®), which are used IM as a single dose to initiate treatment of schizophrenia or to re-initiate therapy following a missed dose; this formulation is not intended for repeated dosing.

Aristada Initio® is not interchangeable with Aristada® because of their different pharmacokinetic profiles.

Extended-release aripiprazole injection and extended-release aripiprazole lauroxil injection are administered *only* by IM injection by a healthcare professional. Extended-release aripiprazole injection (Abilify Maintena®) is administered monthly. The 441- and 662-mg doses of extended-release aripiprazole lauroxil injection (Aristada®) are administered monthly, the 882-mg dose may be administered every month or every 6 weeks, and the 1064-mg dose is administered every 2 months. Extended-release aripiprazole lauroxil injection available in 675-mg prefilled syringes (Aristada Initio®) is used as a single dose only and is not intended for repeated dosing.

The manufacturers state that tolerability with oral aripiprazole therapy should be established prior to initiating IM therapy with extended-release formulations of the drug.

Extended-release Aripiprazole Injection

Extended-release aripiprazole injection (Abilify Maintena®) is administered by deep IM injection monthly into the deltoid or gluteal muscle. The manufacturer states that at least 26 days should elapse between doses. Each injection should be administered only by IM injection by a healthcare professional.

Aripiprazole extended-release IM injection must be reconstituted with sterile water for injection prior to administration. The drug is commercially available in 2 types of kits that contain aripiprazole lyophilized powder in either single-use vials or prefilled dual-chamber syringes with all the components required for reconstitution and administration (e.g., sterile water for injection diluent, needles, syringes). Because the entire contents of the prefilled syringe should be administered following reconstitution, only vials of the drug should be used for dosages smaller than 300 mg (e.g., for the 160- and 200-mg dosage adjustments recommended in patients concurrently receiving certain cytochrome P-450 [CYP] isoenzyme inhibitors or inducers; see Dosage and Administration: Special Populations). Kits containing prefilled dual-chamber syringes should be stored below 30°C and not frozen; the syringe should be protected from light by storing in the original package until the time of use. Kits containing single-use vials should be stored at 25°C, but may be exposed to temperatures ranging from 15–30°C. The manufacturer's instructions for use should be consulted for specific information on the preparation, reconstitution, and administration of aripiprazole extended-release injection using these single-use kits.

Following reconstitution, the prefilled syringe or vial should be shaken vigorously for 20 or 30 seconds, respectively, to ensure a uniform suspension. The reconstituted suspension should be inspected visually for particulate matter and discoloration prior to administration; the suspension should appear to be a uniform, homogeneous suspension that is opaque and milky-white in color. If using vials, the appropriate dose of aripiprazole should be drawn from the vial into the syringe supplied by the manufacturer and injected immediately. If a vial of reconstituted suspension is not administered immediately, the vial should be shaken vigorously for at least 60 seconds to resuspend the drug; reconstituted suspension should not be stored in a syringe. If using prefilled syringes, the entire contents of the prefilled syringe should be injected immediately following reconstitution; the manufacturer states that the contents of the prefilled syringe should be administered within 30 minutes of reconstitution.

Extended-release aripiprazole should be administered slowly by deep IM injection into the deltoid or gluteal muscle using the appropriate length needle (based on body type and injection site) supplied by the manufacturer. Injection sites should be rotated between the 2 deltoid or gluteal muscles. Following IM administration, the injection site should *not* be massaged.

Extended-release Aripiprazole Lauroxil Injection

Both formulations of extended-release aripiprazole lauroxil injectable suspension (Aristada® and Aristada Initio®) are administered by IM injection into the deltoid (441- and 675-mg doses only) or gluteal muscle (441-, 662-, 675-, 882-, or 1064-mg doses). The 441-, 662-, and 882-mg doses are administered

monthly; the 882-mg dose also may be administered every 6 weeks; and the 1064-mg dose is administered every 2 months. The manufacturer states that if a dose of Aristada® is given earlier than the scheduled time, at least 14 days should elapse between doses. Each injection should be administered only by IM injection by a healthcare professional.

Extended-release aripiprazole lauroxil injection in 675-mg prefilled syringes (Aristada Initio®) is used *only* as a single dose to initiate treatment of schizophrenia or to re-initiate therapy following a missed dose; this formulation is *not* intended for repeated dosing. *Aristada Initio® is not interchangeable with Aristada® because of their different pharmacokinetic profiles.*

Aripiprazole lauroxil injectable suspension (Aristada® and Aristada Initio®) is commercially available in a kit containing the drug in a prefilled syringe and safety needles for IM injection. The kit should be stored at room temperature. Prior to use, the prefilled syringe should be tapped at least 10 times to dislodge any material that may have settled. The syringe should then be shaken vigorously for at least 30 seconds to ensure a uniform suspension. If the drug is not administered within 15 minutes, the syringe should be shaken again for 30 seconds.

The entire contents of the syringe should be administered rapidly and continuously by IM injection into either the deltoid (for 441- and 675-mg doses only) or gluteal muscle (for 441-, 662-, 675-, 882-, and 1064-mg doses) using the appropriate length needle supplied by the manufacturer. The manufacturer states that the longer needles provided should be used in patients with a larger amount of subcutaneous tissue over the injection site muscle. Concurrent administration of the 2 different aripiprazole lauroxil injection formulations (Aristada Initio® and Aristada®) in the same muscle should be avoided.

For patients receiving aripiprazole lauroxil injection 441 mg monthly, supplementation with oral aripiprazole is *not* required if the time elapsed since the last injection does not exceed 6 weeks; however, if the time elapsed since the last injection exceeds 6 weeks, but not 7 weeks, oral aripiprazole should be given for 7 days, and if the time elapsed since the last injection exceeds 7 weeks, oral aripiprazole should be given for 21 days. In patients receiving aripiprazole lauroxil injection 662 mg monthly, 882 mg monthly, or 882 mg every 6 weeks, supplementation with oral aripiprazole is *not* required if the time elapsed since the last injection does not exceed 8 weeks; however, if the time elapsed since the last injection exceeds 8 weeks, but not 12 weeks, oral aripiprazole should be given for 7 days, and if the time elapsed since the last injection exceeds 12 weeks, oral aripiprazole should be given for 21 days. In patients receiving aripiprazole lauroxil injection 1064 mg every 2 months, supplementation with oral aripiprazole is *not* required if the time elapsed since the last injection does not exceed 10 weeks; however, if the time elapsed since the last injection exceeds 10 weeks, but not 12 weeks, oral aripiprazole should be given for 7 days, and if the time elapsed since the last injection exceeds 12 weeks, oral aripiprazole should be given for 21 days. The dosage of oral aripiprazole supplementation should be the same as when the patient started receiving aripiprazole lauroxil injection. (See IM Dosage of Aripiprazole Lauroxil under Dosage: Schizophrenia, in Dosage and Administration.)

● Dosage

Aripiprazole oral solution may be given at the same dose on a mg-per-mg basis as the tablet strengths of the drug up to a dose of 25 mg. However, if the oral solution is used in patients who were receiving aripiprazole 30 mg as tablets, a dose of 25 mg of the oral solution should be used.

Conventional tablets and orally disintegrating tablets of aripiprazole are bioequivalent; therefore, dosing for the orally disintegrating tablets is the same as for the conventional tablets.

Dosage of aripiprazole lauroxil is expressed in terms of aripiprazole lauroxil.

Extended-release aripiprazole lauroxil (Aristada®) doses of 441, 662, 882, and 1064 mg correspond to aripiprazole doses of 300, 450, 600, and 724 mg, respectively.

Schizophrenia
Oral Dosage

For the management of schizophrenia in adults, the recommended initial and target dosage of aripiprazole is 10 or 15 mg orally once daily. Although dosages ranging from 10–30 mg daily administered as conventional tablets were effective in clinical trials, the manufacturer states that dosages exceeding 10–15 mg daily did not result in greater efficacy. The maximum recommended dosage is 30 mg daily. Because steady-state plasma concentrations of aripiprazole and dehydro-aripiprazole, its active metabolite, may not be attained for 2 weeks, dosage adjustments generally should be made at intervals of not less than 2 weeks.

For the management of schizophrenia in adolescents 13–17 years of age, the recommended target dosage of aripiprazole is 10 mg orally once daily. Therapy was initiated in a dosage of 2 mg once daily in these patients, with subsequent titration to 5 mg once daily after 2 days and to the target dosage of 10 mg once daily after 2 additional days. The manufacturer recommends that any subsequent dosage increases be made in 5-mg, once-daily increments. Although aripiprazole dosages of 10 and 30 mg once daily administered as conventional tablets have been studied in adolescents, the 30-mg daily dosage was not found to be more effective than the 10-mg daily dosage.

The optimum duration of oral aripiprazole therapy in patients with schizophrenia currently is not known, but maintenance therapy with aripiprazole 15 mg once daily as conventional tablets has been shown to be effective in preventing relapse for up to 26 weeks in adults. In addition, a combined analysis of data from 2 double-blind, multicenter studies indicates that maintenance therapy with the drug may be effective for up to 52 weeks in adults.

Although the efficacy of oral aripiprazole as maintenance therapy in pediatric patients with schizophrenia has not been systematically evaluated, the manufacturer states that such efficacy can be extrapolated from adult data in addition to comparisons of aripiprazole pharmacokinetic parameters in adult and pediatric patients.

The American Psychiatric Association (APA) states that prudent long-term treatment options in patients with schizophrenia with remitted first episodes or multiple episodes include either indefinite maintenance therapy or gradual discontinuance of the antipsychotic agent with close follow-up and a plan to reinstitute treatment upon symptom recurrence. Discontinuance of antipsychotic therapy should be considered only after a period of at least 1 year of symptom remission or optimal response while receiving the antipsychotic agent. In patients who have had multiple previous psychotic episodes or 2 psychotic episodes within 5 years, indefinite maintenance antipsychotic treatment is recommended.

The manufacturer states that the need for continued therapy with the drug should be reassessed periodically.

There are no systematically collected data to specifically address switching patients with schizophrenia from other antipsychotic agents to aripiprazole or concerning concomitant administration with other antipsychotic agents. Immediate discontinuance of the previous antipsychotic agent may be acceptable in some patients with schizophrenia, and more gradual discontinuance may be most appropriate for other patients. In all patients, the period of overlapping antipsychotic administration should be minimized.

IM Dosage of Aripiprazole (Abilify Maintena®)

In patients who have never received aripiprazole, the manufacturer recommends that tolerability with oral aripiprazole be established prior to initiating IM therapy with extended-release aripiprazole injection (Abilify Maintena®). Because of the half-life of oral aripiprazole, it may take up to 2 weeks to fully assess tolerability.

For the treatment of schizophrenia in adults, the recommended dosage of extended-release aripiprazole injection (Abilify Maintena®) is 400 mg administered by IM injection every month (no sooner than 26 days following the previous injection). In patients experiencing adverse effects, a reduction in dosage to 300 mg every month may be considered.

To maintain therapeutic antipsychotic concentrations during initiation of therapy with extended-release aripiprazole injection, oral aripiprazole at a dosage of 10–20 mg daily or another oral antipsychotic agent (for patients already stable on another oral antipsychotic agent and known to tolerate aripiprazole) should be given after the first IM injection of extended-release aripiprazole and continued for 14 days.

If a dose of extended-release aripiprazole injection is missed, the next dose should be administered as soon as possible. Supplementation with oral aripiprazole may be required depending on the time elapsed. If the second or third doses are missed, supplementation with oral aripiprazole is *not* required if the time elapsed since the last injection does not exceed 5 weeks; however, if the time elapsed since the last injection exceeds 5 weeks, supplementation with oral aripiprazole should be given for 14 days with the next administered injection. If the fourth or subsequent doses are missed, supplementation with oral aripiprazole is *not* required if the time elapsed since the last injection does not exceed 6 weeks; however, if the time elapsed since the last injection exceeds 6 weeks, supplementation with oral aripiprazole should be given for 14 days with the next administered injection.

IM Dosage of Aripiprazole Lauroxil (Aristada®)

In patients who have never received aripiprazole, the manufacturer recommends that tolerability with oral aripiprazole therapy be established prior to initiating IM therapy with extended-release aripiprazole lauroxil (Aristada®). Because of the half-life of oral aripiprazole, it may take up to 2 weeks to fully assess tolerability.

For the treatment of schizophrenia in adults, extended-release aripiprazole lauroxil injection (Aristada®) may be initiated at a dosage of 441, 662, or 882 mg every month; 882 mg every 6 weeks; or 1064 mg every 2 months by IM injection. Oral aripiprazole should be administered with the first IM injection of aripiprazole lauroxil and continued for 21 days.

For *patients established on oral aripiprazole 10 mg daily*, the recommended IM dosage of extended-release aripiprazole lauroxil is 441 mg every month.

For *patients established on oral aripiprazole 15 mg daily*, the recommended IM dosage of extended-release aripiprazole lauroxil is 662 mg every month, 882 mg every 6 weeks, or 1064 mg every 2 months.

For *patients established on oral aripiprazole 20 mg or higher daily*, the recommended IM dosage of extended-release aripiprazole lauroxil is 882 mg every month.

Subsequent dosage adjustments may be made if needed. If dosage adjustments are required, the manufacturer states that the pharmacokinetics and prolonged-release characteristics of extended-release aripiprazole lauroxil injection should be considered when making dosage and dosing interval adjustments.

If a dose of aripiprazole lauroxil injection is missed, the next dose should be administered as soon as possible. Supplementation with oral aripiprazole and/or a 675-mg IM dose of extended-release aripiprazole lauroxil (Aristada Initio®) may be required depending on the dosage and the time elapsed (see Tables 1 and 2).

TABLE 1. Recommended Oral Aripiprazole Supplementation Following Missed Doses of Extended-release Aripiprazole Lauroxil Injection (Aristada®).[a]

Dosage of Patient's Last Injection	No Oral Supplementation Required	Supplement with Oral Aripiprazole for 7 Days	Supplement with Oral Aripiprazole for 21 Days
441 mg monthly	≤6 weeks since last injection	>6 and ≤7 weeks since last injection	>7 weeks since last injection
662 mg monthly	≤8 weeks since last injection	>8 and ≤12 weeks since last injection	>12 weeks since last injection
882 mg monthly	≤8 weeks since last injection	>8 and ≤12 weeks since last injection	>12 weeks since last injection
882 mg every 6 weeks	≤8 weeks since last injection	>8 and ≤12 weeks since last injection	>12 weeks since last injection
1064 mg every 2 months	≤10 weeks since last injection	>10 and ≤12 weeks since last injection	>12 weeks since last injection

[a] Dosage of oral aripiprazole supplementation should be same as when patient began extended-release aripiprazole lauroxil therapy.

TABLE 2. Recommended IM Aripiprazole Lauroxil Supplementation with Aristada Initio® Following Missed Doses of Extended-release Aripiprazole Lauroxil Injection (Aristada®).

Dose of Patient's Last Injection	No IM Supplementation Required	Supplement with a Single 675-mg IM Dose of Aripiprazole Lauroxil	Reinitiate with a Single 675-mg IM Dose of Aripiprazole Lauroxil and a Single 30-mg Dose of Oral Aripiprazole
441 mg	≤6 weeks since last injection	>6 and ≤7 weeks since last injection	>7 weeks since last injection
662 mg	≤8 weeks since last injection	>8 and ≤12 weeks since last injection	>12 weeks since last injection
882 mg	≤8 weeks since last injection	>8 and ≤12 weeks since last injection	>12 weeks since last injection
1064 mg	≤10 weeks since last injection	>10 and ≤12 weeks since last injection	>12 weeks since last injection

IM Dosage of Aripiprazole Lauroxil (Aristada Initio®)

In patients who have never received aripiprazole, the manufacturer recommends that tolerability with oral aripiprazole therapy be established prior to initiating IM therapy with extended-release aripiprazole lauroxil (Aristada Initio®). Because of the half-life of oral aripiprazole, it may take up to 2 weeks to fully assess tolerability.

The 675-mg strength of extended-release aripiprazole lauroxil injection (Aristada Initio®) is *only* used as a single dose to initiate aripiprazole lauroxil therapy or as a single dose to reinitiate therapy following a missed dose of extended-release aripiprazole lauroxil injection (Aristada®). The 675-mg strength of extended-release aripiprazole lauroxil injection (Aristada Initio®) is *not* used for repeated dosing of the drug.

For the initiation of aripiprazole lauroxil therapy for the treatment of schizophrenia in adults and after establishing tolerability with oral aripiprazole, the first IM injection of aripiprazole lauroxil (Aristada®; 441 mg, 662 mg, 882 mg, or 1064 mg) may be administered in conjunction with *both* one 675-mg IM injection of aripiprazole lauroxil (Aristada Initio®) into the deltoid or gluteal muscle (this dosage is equivalent to 459 mg of aripiprazole) and one 30-mg dose of oral aripiprazole.

The first dosage of aripiprazole lauroxil (Aristada®) may be administered on the same day as Aristada Initio® or up to 10 days thereafter. Clinicians should avoid injecting both IM formulations of aripiprazole lauroxil concurrently into the same deltoid or gluteal muscle.

For re-initiation of aripiprazole lauroxil (Aristada®) therapy following a missed dose, the next injection of aripiprazole lauroxil (Aristada®) should be administered as soon as possible. Depending on the time elapsed since the last Aristada® injection, the next Aristada® injection may be supplemented as recommended in Table 2.

Bipolar Disorder

Oral Dosage

For the acute management of manic and mixed episodes associated with bipolar I disorder in adults, the recommended initial aripiprazole dosage is 15 mg given orally once daily as monotherapy or 10–15 mg given orally once daily as adjunctive therapy with lithium or valproate. The recommended target dosage of aripiprazole is 15 mg daily whether the drug is given as monotherapy or as adjunctive therapy with lithium or valproate. Based on clinical response, the dosage can be increased to the maximum recommended dosage of 30 mg daily. Safety of aripiprazole dosages exceeding 30 mg daily has not been established in clinical trials.

For the acute management of manic and mixed episodes associated with bipolar I disorder in pediatric patients 10–17 years of age, the recommended initial aripiprazole dosage when given as monotherapy is 2 mg orally once daily, with subsequent titration to 5 mg once daily after 2 days and to the target dosage of 10 mg once daily after 2 additional days. The recommended dosage when aripiprazole is given as adjunctive therapy with lithium or valproate is the same as that for monotherapy. Subsequent increases in the daily dosage of aripiprazole, if necessary, should be made in 5-mg increments. In pediatric clinical studies, oral aripiprazole dosages of 10 and 30 mg daily were effective.

IM Dosage of Aripiprazole

In patients who have never received aripiprazole, the manufacturer recommends that tolerability with oral aripiprazole be established prior to initiating IM therapy with extended-release aripiprazole injection (Abilify Maintena®). Because of the half-life of oral aripiprazole, it may take up to 2 weeks to fully assess tolerability.

For the maintenance treatment of bipolar I disorder in adults, the recommended dosage of extended-release aripiprazole injection (Abilify Maintena®) is 400 mg administered by IM injection every month (no sooner than 26 days following the previous injection). In patients experiencing adverse effects, a reduction in dosage to 300 mg every month may be considered.

To maintain therapeutic antipsychotic concentrations during initiation of therapy with extended-release aripiprazole injection, oral aripiprazole at a dosage of 10–20 mg daily or another oral antipsychotic agent (for patients already stable on another oral antipsychotic agent and known to tolerate aripiprazole) should be given after the first IM injection of extended-release aripiprazole and continued for 14 days.

If a dose of extended-release aripiprazole injection is missed, the next dose should be administered as soon as possible. Supplementation with oral aripiprazole may be required depending on the time elapsed. If the second or third doses are missed, supplementation with oral aripiprazole is *not* required if the time elapsed since the last injection does not exceed 5 weeks; however, if the time elapsed since the last injection exceeds 5 weeks, supplementation with oral

aripiprazole should be given for 14 days with the next administered injection. If the fourth or subsequent doses are missed, supplementation with oral aripiprazole is *not* required if the time elapsed since the last injection does not exceed 6 weeks; however, if the time elapsed since the last injection exceeds 6 weeks, supplementation with oral aripiprazole should be given for 14 days with the next administered injection.

Major Depressive Disorder

For adjunctive management of major depressive disorder in adults already receiving an antidepressant, the manufacturer recommends an initial aripiprazole dosage of 2–5 mg orally once daily for acute treatment. Subsequent dosage adjustments of up to 5 mg daily should occur gradually at intervals of at least 1 week; the recommended dosage range is 2–15 mg once daily. The maximum recommended dosage is 15 mg daily. Efficacy of the drug was established within a dosage range of 2–15 mg daily in clinical studies; mean maintenance dosage in these studies was approximately 11 mg daily.

The manufacturer states that if aripiprazole is used for maintenance therapy, the need for continued therapy with the drug should be reassessed periodically.

Irritability Associated with Autistic Disorder

For the treatment of irritability associated with autistic disorder in pediatric patients 6–17 years of age, efficacy of oral aripiprazole was established within a dosage range of 5–15 mg daily in clinical studies. Dosing should be initiated at 2 mg daily, then increased to 5 mg daily, with subsequent increases to 10 mg daily or 15 mg daily, if necessary. Dosage increases should be gradual, at intervals of at least 1 week.

The manufacturer states that the need for continued therapy with the drug should be reassessed periodically.

Tourette's Syndrome

For the treatment of Tourette's syndrome in pediatric patients 6–18 years of age, the recommended dosage range of oral aripiprazole is 5–20 mg once daily.

In pediatric patients weighing less than 50 kg, therapy should be initiated at 2 mg once daily, then increased to the recommended target dosage of 5 mg once daily after 2 days. In patients who do not achieve optimal control of tics, the dosage may be increased to 10 mg once daily. Dosage adjustments should be made gradually at intervals of at least 1 week.

In pediatric patients weighing 50 kg or more, therapy should be initiated at 2 mg once daily for 2 days and then increased to 5 mg once daily for 5 days, with a recommended target dosage of 10 mg once daily on day 8. In patients who do not achieve optimal control of tics, the dosage may be increased up to 20 mg once daily. Dosage adjustments should be made gradually in increments of 5 mg daily at intervals of at least 1 week.

The manufacturer states that the need for continued maintenance therapy with aripiprazole should be reassessed periodically.

● Special Populations

No dosage adjustment is necessary in patients with renal or hepatic impairment or in geriatric patients. In addition, no dosage adjustment is recommended based on gender, race, or smoking status.

Pharmacogenomics and Poor CYP2D6 Metabolizer Phenotype

Patients who are known poor metabolizers of cytochrome P-450 isoenzyme 2D6 (CYP2D6) should receive one-half (50%) of the usual oral aripiprazole dosage. Such patients who are also taking a potent CYP3A4 inhibitor should receive 25% of the usual oral aripiprazole dosage. (See Drug Interactions: Drugs Affecting Hepatic Microsomal Enzymes.) Dosage adjustment is *not* necessary when oral aripiprazole is used as adjunctive treatment of major depressive disorder.

The manufacturer of aripiprazole extended-release injection (Abilify Maintena®) recommends a dosage of 300 mg every month in patients who are poor CYP2D6 metabolizers. In such patients who are also receiving a potent CYP3A4 inhibitor for longer than 14 days, a dosage of 200 mg every month is recommended.

Dosage of extended-release aripiprazole lauroxil injection (Aristada®) in patients who are poor CYP2D6 metabolizers should be based on the patient's established oral aripiprazole dosage. In such patients receiving a concomitant potent CYP3A4 inhibitor for longer than 2 weeks, dosage should be reduced to 441 mg every month; in patients already receiving 441 mg every month, no dosage adjustment is necessary, if tolerated. If the potent CYP3A4 inhibitor is used for less than 2 weeks, this dosage adjustment is not necessary. No further dosage adjustment is necessary in patients who are poor CYP2D6 metabolizers receiving a concomitant potent CYP2D6 inhibitor.

Extended-release aripiprazole lauroxil injection (Aristada Initio®) is only available in a single strength (675 mg) in a single-dose prefilled syringe; therefore, dosage adjustments in patients who are poor CYP2D6 metabolizers are not possible. Use of this extended-release formulation should therefore be avoided in patients who are poor CYP2D6 metabolizers.

Drugs Affecting Hepatic Microsomal Enzymes

In patients receiving concomitant therapy with potent CYP3A4 inhibitors (e.g., clarithromycin, itraconazole, ketoconazole) *or* potent CYP2D6 inhibitors (e.g., quinidine, fluoxetine, paroxetine), dosage of oral aripiprazole should be reduced to 50% of the usual dosage, except when oral aripiprazole is used in the adjunctive treatment of major depressive disorder. Dosage adjustment is *not* necessary when oral aripiprazole is used as adjunctive treatment of major depressive disorder.

In patients receiving concomitant therapy with potent CYP3A4 *or* CYP2D6 inhibitors for longer than 14 days, dosage of extended-release aripiprazole injection (Abilify Maintena®) should be reduced from 400 mg to 300 mg every month, or from 300 mg to 200 mg every month. In such patients, dosage of extended-release aripiprazole lauroxil injection (Aristada®) should be reduced to the next available lower strength; in patients tolerating the 441-mg dosage, dosage reduction is not necessary. A dosage of 882 mg every 6 weeks or 1064 mg every 2 months should be reduced to 441 mg every 4 weeks. If the potent CYP3A4 or 2D6 inhibitor is used for less than 14 days, dosage adjustment of extended-release aripiprazole or aripiprazole lauroxil injection is *not* necessary.

In patients receiving concomitant therapy with potent CYP3A4 inhibitors *and* potent CYP2D6 inhibitors, oral aripiprazole dosage should be reduced to 25% of the usual dosage, except when aripiprazole is used in the adjunctive treatment of major depressive disorder. Dosage adjustment is *not* necessary when oral aripiprazole is used as adjunctive treatment of major depressive disorder.

In patients receiving concomitant therapy with potent CYP3A4 inhibitors *and* potent CYP2D6 inhibitors for longer than 14 days, dosage of extended-release aripiprazole injection (Abilify Maintena®) should be reduced from 400 mg to 200 mg every month, or from 300 mg to 160 mg every month. In such patients tolerating the 441-mg dosage of extended-release aripiprazole lauroxil injection (Aristada®), dosage adjustment is not necessary; however, the manufacturer states that concomitant therapy with potent CYP2D6 inhibitors *and* potent CYP3A4 inhibitors for longer than 2 weeks should be avoided in patients receiving 662-, 882-, or 1064-mg dosages of extended-release aripiprazole lauroxil injection. If such therapy is used for less than 14 days, dosage adjustment of extended-release aripiprazole or aripiprazole lauroxil injection is *not* necessary.

Dosage of oral aripiprazole should be reduced to 25% of the usual dosage in patients receiving aripiprazole concurrently with a combination of potent, moderate, or weak inhibitors of CYP3A4 and CYP2D6 (e.g., a potent CYP3A4 inhibitor and a moderate CYP2D6 inhibitor or a moderate CYP3A4 inhibitor and a moderate CYP2D6 inhibitor). The oral aripiprazole dosage may then be adjusted based on clinical response. (See Drug Interactions: Drugs Affecting Hepatic Microsomal Enzymes.)

Aripiprazole dosages should be increased back to the original dosage when the CYP2D6 and/or CYP3A4 inhibitor is discontinued.

In patients receiving potent CYP3A4 inducers (e.g., carbamazepine, rifampin), dosage of oral aripiprazole should be doubled over 1–2 weeks of concomitant therapy. When the CYP3A4 inducer is discontinued, the dosage should be reduced back to the original dosage over 1–2 weeks. (See Drug Interactions: Drugs Affecting Hepatic Microsomal Enzymes.)

The manufacturer recommends avoiding use of potent CYP3A4 inducers for longer than 14 days in patients receiving extended-release aripiprazole injection (Abilify Maintena®).

In patients receiving extended-release aripiprazole lauroxil injection (Aristada®), if a potent CYP3A4 inducer is used for longer than 2 weeks, dosage of aripiprazole lauroxil should be increased from 441 mg to 662 mg every month; dosage adjustment is *not* necessary in patients receiving 662-, 882-, or 1064-mg dosages. If a potent CYP3A4 inducer is used for less than 2 weeks, dosage adjustment is *not* necessary.

Extended-release aripiprazole lauroxil injection (Aristada Initio®) is only available in a single strength (675 mg); therefore, dosage adjustments in patients

receiving potent CYP3A4 inhibitors, potent CYP2D6 inhibitors, or potent CYP3A4 inducers are not possible. Use of this extended-release formulation of the drug should be avoided in such patients. (See Drug Interactions: Drugs Affecting Hepatic Microsomal Enzymes.)

CAUTIONS

● *Contraindications*

Known hypersensitivity to aripiprazole; hypersensitivity reactions have ranged from pruritus/urticaria to anaphylaxis. (See Sensitivity Reactions under Cautions: Warnings/Precautions.)

● *Warnings/Precautions*

Warnings

Increased Mortality in Geriatric Patients with Dementia-related Psychosis

Geriatric patients with dementia-related psychosis treated with antipsychotic drugs are at an increased risk of death. Analyses of 17 placebo-controlled trials (modal duration of 10 weeks) revealed a 1.6- to 1.7-fold increase in mortality among geriatric patients receiving atypical antipsychotic drugs (i.e., aripiprazole, olanzapine, quetiapine, risperidone) compared with that observed in patients receiving placebo. Over the course of a typical 10-week controlled trial, the rate of death in drug-treated patients was about 4.5% compared with a rate of about 2.6% in the placebo group. Although the causes of death were varied, most of the deaths appeared to be either cardiovascular (e.g., heart failure, sudden death) or infectious (e.g., pneumonia) in nature. Observational studies suggest that, similar to atypical antipsychotics, treatment with conventional (first-generation) antipsychotics may increase mortality; the extent to which the findings of increased mortality in observational studies may be attributed to the antipsychotic drug as opposed to some characteristic(s) of the patients remains unclear.

The manufacturers state that aripiprazole is *not* approved for the treatment of patients with dementia-related psychosis. If the clinician elects to treat such patients with aripiprazole, patients should be assessed for the emergence of difficulty swallowing or excessive somnolence, which could predispose to accidental injury or aspiration. (See Adverse Cerebrovascular Events, including Stroke, in Geriatric Patients with Dementia-related Psychosis and see Dysphagia under Warnings/Precautions: Other Warnings and Precautions, in Cautions, and also see Geriatric Use under Warnings/Precautions: Specific Populations, in Cautions.)

Worsening of Depression and Suicidality Risk

Worsening of depression and/or the emergence of suicidal ideation and behavior (suicidality) or unusual changes in behavior may occur in both adult and pediatric (see Pediatric Use under Warnings/Precautions: Specific Populations, in Cautions) patients with major depressive disorder or other psychiatric disorders, whether or not they are taking antidepressants. This risk may persist until clinically important remission occurs. Suicide is a known risk of depression and certain other psychiatric disorders, and these disorders themselves are the strongest predictors of suicide. However, there has been a long-standing concern that antidepressants may have a role in inducing worsening of depression and the emergence of suicidality in certain patients during the early phases of treatment. Pooled analyses of short-term, placebo-controlled studies of antidepressants (i.e., selective serotonin-reuptake inhibitors [SSRIs] and other antidepressants) have shown an increased risk of suicidality in children, adolescents, and young adults (18–24 years of age) with major depressive disorder and other psychiatric disorders. An increased suicidality risk was not demonstrated with antidepressants compared with placebo in adults older than 24 years of age and a reduced risk was observed in adults 65 years of age or older.

The US Food and Drug Administration (FDA) recommends that all patients being treated with antidepressants for any indication be appropriately monitored and closely observed for clinical worsening, suicidality, and unusual changes in behavior, particularly during initiation of therapy (i.e., the first few months) and during periods of dosage adjustments. Families and caregivers of patients being treated with antidepressants for major depressive disorder or other indications, both psychiatric and nonpsychiatric, also should be advised to monitor patients on a daily basis for the emergence of agitation, irritability, or unusual changes in behavior as well as the emergence of suicidality, and to report such symptoms immediately to a health-care provider.

Although a causal relationship between the emergence of symptoms such as anxiety, agitation, panic attacks, insomnia, irritability, hostility, aggressiveness, impulsivity, akathisia, hypomania, and/or mania and either the worsening of depression and/or the emergence of suicidal impulses has not been established, there is concern that such symptoms may represent precursors to emerging suicidality. Consequently, consideration should be given to changing the therapeutic regimen or discontinuing therapy in patients whose depression is persistently worse or in patients experiencing emergent suicidality or symptoms that might be precursors to worsening depression or suicidality, particularly if such manifestations are severe, abrupt in onset, or were not part of the patient's presenting symptoms. FDA also recommends that the drugs be prescribed in the smallest quantity consistent with good patient management, in order to reduce the risk of overdosage.

It is generally believed (though not established in controlled trials) that treating a major depressive episode with an antidepressant alone may increase the likelihood of precipitating a mixed or manic episode in patients at risk for bipolar disorder. Therefore, patients with depressive symptoms should be adequately screened for bipolar disorder prior to initiating treatment with an antidepressant; such screening should include a detailed psychiatric history (e.g., family history of suicide, bipolar disorder, and depression).

Aripiprazole is not approved for use in treating depression in the pediatric population. (See Pediatric Use under Warnings/Precautions: Specific Populations, in Cautions.)

Sensitivity Reactions

Allergic and sensitivity reactions (e.g., anaphylactic reaction, angioedema, laryngospasm, pruritus/urticaria, photosensitivity, rash, oropharyngeal spasm) have been reported in patients receiving aripiprazole. (See Cautions: Contraindications.)

Other Warnings and Precautions

Adverse Cerebrovascular Events, including Stroke, in Geriatric Patients with Dementia-related Psychosis

An increased incidence of adverse cerebrovascular events (cerebrovascular accidents and transient ischemic attacks), including fatalities, has been observed in geriatric patients with dementia-related psychosis treated with oral aripiprazole in several placebo-controlled studies (2 flexible-dose studies and one fixed-dose study). A statistically significant dose-response relationship for adverse cerebrovascular events was observed in patients receiving oral aripiprazole in the fixed-dose study. The manufacturers state that aripiprazole is *not* approved for the treatment of patients with dementia-related psychosis. (See Increased Mortality in Geriatric Patients with Dementia-related Psychosis under Warnings/Precautions: Warnings, and also see Geriatric Use under Warnings/Precautions: Specific Populations, in Cautions.)

Potential for Dosing and Medication Errors

Medication errors, including substitution and dispensing errors, may occur between the 2 different extended-release IM formulations of aripiprazole lauroxil (e.g., Aristada Initio® and Aristada®).

Aristada Initio® is for single-dose administration only. Aristada Initio® should not be substituted for Aristada® because of their different pharmacokinetic profiles.

Neuroleptic Malignant Syndrome

Neuroleptic malignant syndrome (NMS), a potentially fatal syndrome requiring immediate discontinuance of the drug and intensive symptomatic treatment, has been reported in patients receiving antipsychotic agents, including rare cases associated with aripiprazole therapy. (See Advice to Patients.) For additional information on NMS, see Neuroleptic Malignant Syndrome under Cautions: Nervous System Effects, in the Phenothiazines General Statement 28:16.08.24.

Tardive Dyskinesia

Because use of antipsychotic agents, including aripiprazole, may be associated with tardive dyskinesia (a syndrome of potentially irreversible, involuntary, dyskinetic movements), aripiprazole should be prescribed in a manner that is most likely to minimize the occurrence of this syndrome. Chronic antipsychotic treatment generally should be reserved for patients who suffer from a chronic illness that is known to respond to antipsychotic agents, and for whom alternative, equally effective, but potentially less harmful treatments are not available or appropriate. In patients who do require chronic treatment, the lowest dosage and the shortest

duration of treatment producing a satisfactory clinical response should be sought, and the need for continued treatment should be reassessed periodically.

The American Psychiatric Association (APA) currently recommends that patients receiving atypical antipsychotic agents be assessed clinically for abnormal involuntary movements every 12 months and that patients considered to be at increased risk for tardive dyskinesia be assessed every 6 months. If signs and symptoms of tardive dyskinesia appear in an aripiprazole-treated patient, aripiprazole discontinuance should be considered; however, some patients may require continued treatment with the drug despite the presence of the syndrome. For additional information on tardive dyskinesia, see Tardive Dyskinesia under Cautions: Nervous System Effects, in the Phenothiazines General Statement 28:16.08.24.

Metabolic Changes

Atypical antipsychotic agents have been associated with metabolic changes, including hyperglycemia and diabetes mellitus, dyslipidemia, and body weight gain. While all of these drugs produce some metabolic changes, each drug has its own specific risk profile. (See Hyperglycemia and Diabetes Mellitus, see Dyslipidemia, and also see Weight Gain under Warnings/Precautions: Other Warnings and Precautions, in Cautions.)

Hyperglycemia and Diabetes Mellitus

Hyperglycemia, sometimes severe and associated with ketoacidosis, hyperosmolar coma, or death, has been reported in patients receiving atypical antipsychotic agents. Hyperglycemia has been reported in patients treated with aripiprazole. In short- and longer-term clinical trials in adult and pediatric patients, clinically important differences between oral aripiprazole and placebo in mean change from baseline to end point in fasting glucose concentrations were not observed. While confounding factors such as an increased background risk of diabetes mellitus in patients with schizophrenia and the increasing incidence of diabetes mellitus in the general population make it difficult to establish with certainty the relationship between use of agents in this drug class and glucose abnormalities, epidemiologic studies suggest an increased risk of treatment-emergent hyperglycemia-related adverse events in patients treated with atypical antipsychotic agents.

Patients with preexisting diabetes mellitus in whom therapy with an atypical antipsychotic is initiated should be periodically monitored for worsening of glucose control; those with risk factors for diabetes (e.g., obesity, family history of diabetes) should undergo fasting blood glucose testing upon therapy initiation and periodically throughout treatment. Any patient who develops manifestations of hyperglycemia (including polydipsia, polyuria, polyphagia, and weakness) during treatment with an atypical antipsychotic should undergo fasting blood glucose testing. (See Advice to Patients.) In some cases, patients who developed hyperglycemia while receiving an atypical antipsychotic have required continuance of antidiabetic treatment despite discontinuance of the atypical antipsychotic; in other cases, hyperglycemia resolved with discontinuance of the antipsychotic.

For further information on managing the risk of hyperglycemia and diabetes mellitus associated with atypical antipsychotic agents, see Hyperglycemia and Diabetes Mellitus under Cautions: Precautions and Contraindications, in Clozapine 28:16.08.04.

Dyslipidemia

Undesirable changes in lipid parameters have been observed in patients treated with some atypical antipsychotic agents; however, aripiprazole generally does not appear to adversely affect the lipid profile in patients receiving the drug. Pooled data from short- and longer-term clinical studies in adult and pediatric patients indicate no clinically important differences from baseline to end point in the proportion of patients with changes in fasting/nonfasting total cholesterol, fasting triglycerides, fasting low-density lipoprotein (LDL)-cholesterol, and fasting/nonfasting high-density lipoprotein (HDL)-cholesterol between aripiprazole-treated patients and those receiving placebo.

Weight Gain

Weight gain has been observed with atypical antipsychotic therapy. Clinical monitoring of weight is recommended in patients receiving aripiprazole.

In an analysis of 13 placebo-controlled monotherapy studies in adults primarily with schizophrenia or bipolar disorder, mean weight gain in aripiprazole-treated patients was 0.3 kg compared with a loss of 0.1 kg in those receiving placebo (with a median exposure of 21–25 days); at 24 weeks, patients receiving aripiprazole or placebo lost an average of 1.5 or 0.2 kg, respectively. In 2 placebo-controlled trials in pediatric patients with schizophrenia or bipolar disorder, mean weight gain was 1.6 kg in patients receiving oral aripiprazole and 0.3 kg in those receiving placebo (with a median exposure of 42–43 days); at 24 weeks, mean weight gain was 5.8 and 1.4 kg in aripiprazole- and placebo-treated patients, respectively.

For additional information on metabolic effects associated with atypical antipsychotic agents, see Hyperglycemia and Diabetes Mellitus under Warnings/Precautions: Other Warnings and Precautions, in Cautions.

Pathological Gambling and Other Compulsive Behaviors

Serious impulse-control and compulsive behaviors, particularly pathological gambling, have been reported rarely in adult and pediatric patients treated with aripiprazole. In May 2016, FDA reported that a total of 184 cases of impulse-control problems associated with aripiprazole use have been identified since November 2002; most of these cases (89%) involved pathological gambling. Other impulse-control and compulsive behaviors reported less frequently than gambling include compulsive or binge eating, compulsive spending or shopping, and compulsive sexual behaviors. The majority of patients in these cases had no history of compulsive behaviors and experienced the uncontrollable urges only after beginning treatment with aripiprazole. Impulse-control symptoms may also be associated with the underlying disorder. The results of a large pharmacoepidemiologic study suggest that patients with bipolar disorder who are receiving aripiprazole have a higher risk of gambling compared with patients with bipolar disorder who are not receiving aripiprazole. In some, but not all, cases, these uncontrollable urges reportedly stopped within days to weeks when the aripiprazole dosage was reduced or the drug was discontinued; recurrence of compulsive behaviors following rechallenge with the drug has been reported.

Aripiprazole-associated compulsive behaviors may result in harm to the patient or others if not recognized. Because patients may not recognize such behaviors as abnormal, clinicians should specifically ask patients or caregivers whether any new or intense gambling urges, compulsive sexual urges, compulsive shopping, binge or compulsive eating, or other urges have developed during treatment with the drug. If a patient develops new or increased impulsive or compulsive behaviors while receiving aripiprazole, consideration should be given to reducing the dosage or discontinuing the drug. (See Advice to Patients.)

Orthostatic Hypotension

Orthostatic hypotension and associated adverse effects (e.g., postural dizziness, syncope, tachycardia) have been reported in patients receiving oral or IM aripiprazole and IM aripiprazole lauroxil, perhaps because of the drug's α_1-adrenergic blocking activity. The risk of orthostatic hypotension generally appears to be greatest during initiation of therapy and dosage titration. The drug should be used with caution in patients with known cardiovascular disease (e.g., heart failure, history of myocardial infarction or ischemia, conduction abnormalities), cerebrovascular disease, and/or conditions that would predispose patients to hypotension (e.g., dehydration, hypovolemia, concomitant antihypertensive therapy), as well as in patients who are antipsychotic naive. In such patients, the manufacturer of extended-release IM aripiprazole lauroxil states that use of a lower initial dosage of the drug and monitoring of vital signs should be considered.

Falls

Aripiprazole therapy may cause somnolence, postural hypotension, and motor and sensory instability, which may lead to falls; as a consequence, fractures or other injuries may occur. For patients with diseases or conditions or receiving other drugs that could exacerbate these effects, fall risk assessments should be completed when initiating antipsychotic treatment and periodically during long-term therapy.

Leukopenia, Neutropenia, and Agranulocytosis

In clinical trial and/or postmarketing experience, leukopenia and neutropenia have been temporally related to antipsychotic agents, including aripiprazole. Agranulocytosis also has been reported.

Possible risk factors for leukopenia and neutropenia include preexisting low leukocyte count and a history of drug-induced leukopenia and neutropenia. Patients with a preexisting low leukocyte count or a history of drug-induced leukopenia or neutropenia should have their complete blood count monitored frequently during the first few months of therapy. Aripiprazole should be discontinued at the first sign of a decline in leukocyte count in the absence of other causative factors.

Patients with clinically significant neutropenia should be carefully monitored for fever or other signs or symptoms of infection and promptly treated if such signs and symptoms occur. In patients with severe neutropenia (absolute neutrophil count [ANC] less than 1000/mm³), aripiprazole should be discontinued and the leukocyte count monitored until recovery occurs. Lithium has reportedly been used successfully in the treatment of several cases of leukopenia associated with aripiprazole, clozapine, and some other drugs; however, further clinical experience is needed to confirm these anecdotal findings.

Seizures

As with other antipsychotic agents, aripiprazole may cause seizures. Seizures have occurred in 0.1% of adult and pediatric patients (6–18 years of age) treated with oral aripiprazole. Aripiprazole should be used with caution in patients with a history of seizures or other conditions that may lower the seizure threshold; conditions that lower the seizure threshold may be more prevalent in geriatric patients 65 years of age or older.

Cognitive and Motor Impairment

Like other antipsychotic agents, aripiprazole potentially may impair judgment, thinking, or motor skills. In short-term clinical trials, somnolence (including sedation) was reported in 11% of adults treated with oral aripiprazole compared with 6% of those receiving placebo. In pediatric patients 6–17 years of age, somnolence (including sedation) was reported in 24% of aripiprazole-treated patients compared with 6% of those receiving placebo. (See Advice to Patients.)

Body Temperature Regulation

Disruption of the body's ability to reduce core body temperature has been attributed to antipsychotic agents. The manufacturers recommend appropriate caution when aripiprazole is used in patients who will be experiencing conditions that may contribute to an elevation in core body temperature (e.g., strenuous exercise, extreme heat, concomitant use of agents with anticholinergic activity, dehydration).

Suicide

Attendant risk with psychotic illnesses, bipolar disorder, and major depressive disorder; high-risk patients should be closely supervised. Aripiprazole should be prescribed in the smallest quantity consistent with good patient management to reduce the risk of overdosage. (See Worsening of Depression and Suicidality Risk under Warnings/Precautions: Warnings, in Cautions.)

Dysphagia

Esophageal dysmotility and aspiration have been associated with the use of antipsychotic agents, including aripiprazole. Aspiration pneumonia is a common cause of morbidity and mortality in geriatric patients, particularly in those with advanced Alzheimer's dementia. Aripiprazole should be used with caution in patients at risk for aspiration pneumonia. (See Increased Mortality in Geriatric Patients with Dementia-related Psychosis under Warnings/Precautions: Warnings, in Cautions.)

Phenylketonuria

Individuals with phenylketonuria (i.e., homozygous genetic deficiency of phenylalanine hydroxylase) and other individuals who must restrict their intake of phenylalanine should be warned that each aripiprazole 10- or 15-mg orally disintegrating tablet contains aspartame, which is metabolized in the GI tract to provide about 1.12 or 1.68 mg of phenylalanine, respectively, following oral administration. Aripiprazole conventional tablets and oral solution do not contain aspartame.

Skin Irritation associated with Abilify MyCite® Wearable Sensor

Symptoms of skin irritation (e.g., rash, pruritus, skin discoloration) may occur at the application site of the wearable sensor (MyCite® patch). In clinical studies, 12.4% of the patients receiving aripiprazole tablets with sensor experienced rashes at the site of wearable sensor placement. If skin irritation occurs, the manufacturer states that the wearable sensor should be removed.

Specific Populations

Pregnancy

Neonates exposed to antipsychotic agents during the third trimester of pregnancy are at risk for extrapyramidal and/or withdrawal symptoms following delivery. Symptoms reported to date have included agitation, hypertonia, hypotonia, tardive dyskinetic-like symptoms, tremor, somnolence, respiratory distress, and feeding disorder. Neonates exhibiting such symptoms should be monitored. The complications have varied in severity; some neonates recovered within hours to days without specific treatment, while others have required intensive care unit support and prolonged hospitalization. For further information on extrapyramidal and withdrawal symptoms in neonates, see Cautions: Pregnancy, Fertility, and Lactation, in the Phenothiazines General Statement 28:16.08.24.

National Pregnancy Registry for Atypical Antipsychotics: 866-961-2388 and http://womensmentalhealth.org/clinical-and-research-programs/pregnancyregistry/atypicalantipsychotic/.

Lactation

Aripiprazole is distributed into milk in humans. However, data are insufficient to determine the amount present in human milk, the effects of the drug on breast-fed infants, or the effects on milk production. Because of the potential for serious adverse reactions to aripiprazole in nursing infants, the manufacturer of aripiprazole tablets states that a decision should be made whether to discontinue nursing or the drug, taking into consideration the importance of the drug to the woman. The manufacturers of extended-release IM formulations of aripiprazole and aripiprazole lauroxil state that the benefit of aripiprazole therapy to the woman as well as the benefits of breast-feeding to the infant should be weighed against the potential risk to the infant resulting from exposure to the drug or from the underlying maternal condition.

Pediatric Use

Safety and efficacy of aripiprazole tablets with sensor have not been established in pediatric patients.

Safety and efficacy of oral aripiprazole have not been established in pediatric patients with major depressive disorder.

Safety and efficacy of extended-release IM formulations of aripiprazole and aripiprazole lauroxil have not been evaluated in pediatric patients younger than 18 years of age.

Safety and efficacy of oral aripiprazole for the acute management of schizophrenia in pediatric patients 13–17 years of age have been established in a placebo-controlled study of 6 weeks' duration. Although the efficacy of oral aripiprazole for maintenance treatment of schizophrenia in pediatric patients has not been systematically evaluated, the manufacturer states that such efficacy can be extrapolated from adult data in addition to comparisons of aripiprazole pharmacokinetic parameters in adult and pediatric patients. (See Schizophrenia under Uses: Psychotic Disorders.)

Safety and efficacy of oral aripiprazole monotherapy for the acute management of bipolar mania in pediatric patients 10–17 years of age have been established in a placebo-controlled study of 4 weeks' duration.

The efficacy of oral aripiprazole as an adjunct to lithium or valproate for the acute treatment of manic or mixed episodes associated with bipolar disorder in pediatric patients has not been systematically evaluated. However, efficacy can be extrapolated from adult data in addition to pharmacokinetic comparisons of aripiprazole between adult and pediatric populations.

Safety and efficacy of oral aripiprazole for the treatment of irritability associated with autistic disorder have been established in 2 placebo-controlled clinical trials of 8 weeks' duration in pediatric patients 6–17 years of age. Efficacy of the drug as maintenance therapy for irritability associated with autistic disorder was not established in a longer-term, placebo-controlled relapse prevention trial in pediatric patients 6–17 years of age.

Safety and efficacy of oral aripiprazole for the treatment of Tourette's syndrome have been established in one 8-week, placebo-controlled trial in pediatric patients 7–17 years of age and one 10-week, placebo-controlled trial in pediatric patients 6–18 years of age. Efficacy of the drug as maintenance therapy in pediatric patients with Tourette's syndrome has not been systematically evaluated. (See Uses: Tourette's Syndrome.)

The pharmacokinetics of aripiprazole and dehydro-aripiprazole in pediatric patients 10–17 years of age are similar to those in adults after correcting for differences in body weight.

Mean weight gain of 1.6 kg was reported in pediatric patients with schizophrenia or bipolar disorder receiving oral aripiprazole compared with a gain of 0.3 kg in those receiving placebo in 2 short-term studies. After 24 weeks of therapy, the mean change from baseline in body weight in the aripiprazole-treated patients was 5.8 kg compared with 1.4 kg in placebo recipients. Similar gains in weight were observed in short-term studies in pediatric patients with irritability associated with autistic disorder and Tourette's syndrome.

FDA warns that a greater risk of suicidal thinking or behavior (suicidality) occurred during the first few months of antidepressant treatment compared with placebo in children and adolescents with major depressive disorder, obsessive-compulsive disorder (OCD), or other psychiatric disorders based on pooled analyses of 24 short-term, placebo-controlled trials of 9 antidepressant drugs (SSRIs and other antidepressants). However, a more recent meta-analysis of 27 placebo-controlled trials of 9 antidepressants (SSRIs and others) in patients younger than 19 years of age with major depressive disorder, OCD, or non-OCD anxiety disorders suggests that the benefits of antidepressant therapy in treating these conditions may outweigh the risks of suicidal behavior or suicidal ideation. No suicides occurred in these pediatric trials. These findings should be carefully considered when assessing potential benefits and risks of aripiprazole in a child or adolescent for any clinical use. (See Worsening of Depression and Suicidality Risk under Warnings/Precautions: Warnings, in Cautions.)

Geriatric Use

In clinical studies, approximately 8% of over 13,000 patients treated with oral aripiprazole were 65 years of age or older and approximately 6% were 75 years of age or older. Experience from placebo-controlled trials with oral aripiprazole in patients with schizophrenia, bipolar mania, or major depressive disorder who are 65 years of age and older is insufficient to determine whether they respond differently than younger adults.

The manufacturer of oral and extended-release IM formulations of aripiprazole states that dosage adjustment is not necessary in geriatric patients on the basis of age alone. The manufacturer of extended-release IM aripiprazole lauroxil states that the safety and efficacy of the drug have not been evaluated in patients older than 65 years of age and makes no specific dosage recommendations for geriatric patients.

Geriatric patients with dementia-related psychosis treated with antipsychotic agents are at an increased risk of death. In addition, an increased incidence of adverse cerebrovascular events (cerebrovascular accidents and transient ischemic attacks), including fatalities, has been observed in geriatric patients with dementia-related psychosis treated with aripiprazole in placebo-controlled studies. Aripiprazole is *not* approved for the treatment of dementia-related psychosis. (See Increased Mortality in Geriatric Patients with Dementia-related Psychosis under Warnings/Precautions: Warnings, in Cautions and see also Adverse Cerebrovascular Events, including Stroke, in Geriatric Patients with Dementia-related Psychosis and see Dysphagia under Warnings/Precautions: Other Warnings and Precautions, in Cautions.) For additional information on the use of antipsychotic agents in the management of dementia-related psychosis, see Geriatric Considerations under Uses: Psychotic Disorders, in the Phenothiazines General Statement 28:16.08.24.

In pooled data analyses, a *reduced* risk of suicidality was observed in adults 65 years of age or older with antidepressant therapy compared with placebo. (See Worsening of Depression and Suicidality Risk under Warnings/Precautions: Warnings, in Cautions.)

Pharmacogenomics and Poor CYP2D6 Metabolizers

Because higher concentrations of aripiprazole have been observed in poor metabolizers of cytochrome P-450 (CYP) isoenzyme 2D6 than in normal CYP2D6 metabolizers, dosage adjustment of the drug is recommended in patients known to be poor metabolizers of CYP2D6. Approximately 8% of Caucasians and 3–8% of Blacks/African Americans cannot metabolize CYP2D6 substrates and are classified as poor CYP2D6 metabolizers. (See Pharmacogenomics and Poor CYP2D6 Metabolizer Phenotype under Dosage and Administration: Special Populations.)

● Common Adverse Effects

Adverse effects occurring in 10% or more of adults receiving oral aripiprazole in clinical trials include nausea, vomiting, constipation, headache, dizziness, akathisia, anxiety, insomnia, and restlessness.

Adverse effects occurring in 10% or more of pediatric patients receiving oral aripiprazole in clinical trials include somnolence, headache, vomiting, extrapyramidal disorder, fatigue, increased appetite, insomnia, nausea, nasopharyngitis, and increased weight.

In clinical trials with aripiprazole tablets with sensor and other components of the digital ingestion tracking system (Abilify MyCite®), skin rash localized at the application site of the wearable sensor (patch) was reported in 12.4% of patients. Other symptoms of skin irritation (e.g., pruritus, skin discoloration) have also been reported.

Adverse effects occurring in 5% or more of adults receiving extended-release IM aripiprazole injection (Abilify Maintena®) for schizophrenia in clinical trials and at an incidence at least twice that for placebo include increased weight, akathisia, injection site pain, and sedation.

In patients receiving extended-release IM aripiprazole lauroxil injection (Aristada®) in clinical trials, akathisia was the only adverse effect that occurred in 5% of more of patients and at an incidence at least twice that for placebo. Other extrapyramidal adverse effects (e.g., parkinsonism, dystonia) and injection site reactions (e.g., pain) were reported in 5–7% and 4–5% of patients in the clinical trials, respectively.

DRUG INTERACTIONS

● Drugs Affecting Hepatic Microsomal Enzymes

Cytochrome P-450 (CYP) isoenzyme 3A4 (CYP3A4) inducers (e.g., carbamazepine, rifampin), CYP3A4 inhibitors (e.g., clarithromycin, itraconazole, ketoconazole), or CYP2D6 inhibitors (e.g., fluoxetine, paroxetine, quinidine): Potential pharmacokinetic interaction (altered aripiprazole metabolism); dosage adjustment generally is recommended. (See Drugs Affecting Hepatic Microsomal Enzymes under Dosage and Administration: Special Populations.)

Inhibitors or inducers of CYP isoenzymes 1A1, 1A2, 2A6, 2B6, 2C8, 2C9, 2C19, or 2E1: Pharmacokinetic interaction is unlikely.

Ketoconazole and Other CYP3A4 Inhibitors

Concurrent oral administration of aripiprazole and ketoconazole, a potent CYP3A4 inhibitor, substantially increased peak serum concentrations and area under the plasma concentration-time curve (AUC) values of aripiprazole and its active metabolite, dehydro-aripiprazole. Concomitant use of aripiprazole with other potent CYP3A4 inhibitors (e.g., clarithromycin, itraconazole) would also be expected to result in substantially increased systemic exposure to aripiprazole.

Except when used in the adjunctive treatment of major depressive disorder, dosage of oral aripiprazole should be reduced by 50% when used concurrently with potent CYP3A4 inhibitors. IM dosages of extended-release aripiprazole (Abilify Maintena®) and aripiprazole lauroxil (Aristada®) should be reduced when used concurrently with potent CYP3A4 inhibitors for longer than 14 days. When the potent CYP3A4 inhibitor is withdrawn from combined therapy, the aripiprazole dosage should be increased. Use of the 675-mg strength of extended-release aripiprazole lauroxil injection (Aristada Initio®) should be avoided in patients receiving potent CYP3A4 inhibitors. (See Dosage and Administration: Special Populations.)

Quinidine and Other CYP2D6 Inhibitors

Concurrent oral administration of aripiprazole and quinidine, a potent CYP2D6 inhibitor, substantially increased the AUC of aripiprazole but decreased the AUC of its active metabolite, dehydro-aripiprazole. Concomitant use of aripiprazole with other potent CYP2D6 inhibitors (e.g., fluoxetine, paroxetine) would also be expected to result in substantially increased systemic exposure to aripiprazole.

Except when used in the adjunctive treatment of major depressive disorder, dosage of oral aripiprazole should be reduced by 50% when used concurrently with potent CYP2D6 inhibitors. IM dosages of extended-release aripiprazole (Abilify Maintena®) and aripiprazole lauroxil (Aristada®) should be reduced when used concurrently with potent CYP2D6 inhibitors for longer than 14 days. When the potent CYP2D6 inhibitor is withdrawn from combined therapy, the aripiprazole dosage should be increased. Use of the 675-mg strength of extended-release aripiprazole lauroxil injection (Aristada Initio®) should be avoided in patients receiving potent CYP2D6 inhibitors. (See Dosage and Administration: Special Populations.)

Carbamazepine and Other CYP3A4 Inducers

Concurrent administration of aripiprazole and carbamazepine, a potent CYP3A4 inducer, substantially decreased peak plasma concentrations and AUC of aripiprazole and its active metabolite, dehydro-aripiprazole. Concomitant use of aripiprazole with other potent CYP3A4 inducers (e.g., rifampin) may result in substantially decreased systemic exposure to aripiprazole.

Oral aripiprazole dosage should be doubled over 1–2 weeks of concurrent use with potent CYP3A4 inducers. Concurrent use of CYP3A4 inducers and extended-release aripiprazole injection (Abilify Maintena®) should be avoided since aripiprazole concentrations may fall below therapeutic concentrations. The 441-mg dose of extended-release aripiprazole lauroxil (Aristada®) should be increased

to 662 mg when used concurrently with potent CYP3A4 inducers for longer than 2 weeks; dosage adjustment is not required in patients receiving 662-, 882-, or 1064-mg doses of the drug. When the potent CYP3A4 inducer is withdrawn from combined therapy, the aripiprazole dosage should be reduced to the original dosage over 1–2 weeks. Use of the 675-mg strength of extended-release aripiprazole lauroxil injection (Aristada Initio®) should be avoided in patients receiving potent CYP3A4 inducers. (See Dosage and Administration: Special Populations.)

● Drugs Metabolized by Hepatic Microsomal Enzymes

Substrates of CYP isoenzymes 2C9, 2C19, 2D6, and 3A4: Clinically important pharmacokinetic interaction is unlikely; dosage adjustment is not necessary.

● Anticholinergic Agents

Potential pharmacologic interaction (possible disruption of body temperature regulation); aripiprazole should be used with caution in patients concurrently receiving drugs with anticholinergic activity. (See Body Temperature Regulation under Warnings/Precautions: Other Warnings and Precautions, in Cautions.)

● Hypotensive Agents

Potential pharmacologic interaction (additive hypotensive effects due to α-adrenergic antagonism); aripiprazole should be used with caution in patients receiving hypotensive agents. During concomitant use, blood pressure should be monitored and antihypertensive dosage(s) adjusted accordingly.

● Lorazepam and Other Benzodiazepines

Clinically important pharmacokinetic changes have not been reported during concurrent administration of lorazepam and aripiprazole. The manufacturers state that routine dosage adjustment of aripiprazole or lorazepam is not necessary when the drugs are concurrently administered. However, increased sedative and orthostatic hypotensive effects have been reported in patients receiving these drugs in combination. If aripiprazole therapy in conjunction with a benzodiazepine is considered necessary, the patient should be carefully monitored for excessive sedation and orthostatic hypotension and dosage of the drug(s) adjusted, if necessary. (See Orthostatic Hypotension and see also Cognitive and Motor Impairment under Warnings/Precautions: Other Warnings and Precautions, in Cautions.)

● Alcohol

Concomitant administration of ethanol and oral aripiprazole in healthy individuals did not have clinically important effects on gross motor skills or stimulus response compared with administration of ethanol with placebo. The manufacturer of the extended-release IM formulation of aripiprazole (Abilify Maintena®) states that alcohol should be avoided during therapy. The manufacturers of other commercially available formulations of aripiprazole and aripiprazole lauroxil do not provide specific recommendations concerning alcohol use in the prescribing information for the drugs.

● Dextromethorphan

Clinically important pharmacokinetic interaction is unlikely. Dosage adjustment of dextromethorphan (a CYP2D6 and CYP3A4 substrate) is not necessary when administered concomitantly with aripiprazole.

● Escitalopram

Concurrent administration of aripiprazole 10 mg orally daily for 14 days in healthy individuals did not substantially alter the steady-state pharmacokinetics of 10 mg daily of escitalopram, a CYP2C19 and CYP3A4 substrate. Dosage adjustment of escitalopram is not necessary when administered concurrently with aripiprazole.

● Famotidine

Concomitant use of aripiprazole and famotidine may result in decreased peak plasma concentrations and systemic exposure of aripiprazole and its active metabolite, dehydro-aripiprazole; however, a clinically important pharmacokinetic interaction between the drugs appears unlikely. No dosage adjustment of aripiprazole is necessary when administered concurrently with famotidine.

● Fluoxetine, Paroxetine, and Sertraline

A population pharmacokinetic analysis in patients with major depressive disorder did not demonstrate substantial changes in the pharmacokinetics of fluoxetine, paroxetine, or sertraline (dosed to steady state) following the addition of aripiprazole therapy. Therefore, dosage adjustment of fluoxetine, paroxetine, and sertraline is not necessary in patients concomitantly receiving aripiprazole therapy.

However, fluoxetine and paroxetine are potent inhibitors of CYP2D6 and the manufacturer recommends that oral aripiprazole dosage be reduced to one-half the usual dosage in patients receiving concomitant therapy with potent inhibitors of CYP2D6, including fluoxetine and paroxetine. When fluoxetine or paroxetine is withdrawn from combined therapy with aripiprazole, the aripiprazole dosage should be increased back to the original dosage. When adjunctive aripiprazole is concurrently administered to patients with major depressive disorder receiving fluoxetine or paroxetine, aripiprazole should be given without dosage adjustment. (See Dosage and Administration: Special Populations.)

● **Lamotrigine**

Combined aripiprazole and lamotrigine therapy appears to be well tolerated in patients with bipolar disorder. Pharmacokinetic interaction is unlikely; no dosage adjustment of lamotrigine is necessary when aripiprazole is administered concurrently.

● **Lithium**

Clinically important pharmacokinetic interaction is unlikely; no dosage adjustment of aripiprazole or lithium is necessary during concurrent administration.

● **Omeprazole**

Clinically important pharmacokinetic interaction is unlikely; dosage adjustment of omeprazole is not necessary when administered concurrently with aripiprazole.

● **Valproate**

Clinically important pharmacokinetic interaction is unlikely; no dosage adjustment of aripiprazole or valproate is necessary during concurrent administration.

● **Venlafaxine**

Concurrent administration of oral aripiprazole (10–20 mg daily for 14 days) in healthy individuals did not substantially alter the steady-state pharmacokinetics of venlafaxine and O-desmethylvenlafaxine following 75 mg daily of extended-release venlafaxine, a CYP2D6 substrate. Dosage adjustment of venlafaxine is not necessary during concurrent use of aripiprazole.

● **Warfarin**

Concurrent administration of aripiprazole did not substantially affect warfarin pharmacokinetics, suggesting a lack of a clinically important effect of aripiprazole on CYP2C9 and CYP2C19 metabolism. Warfarin dosage adjustment is not necessary when administered concurrently with aripiprazole.

DESCRIPTION

Aripiprazole is a quinolinone derivative antipsychotic agent that differs chemically from other currently available antipsychotic agents (e.g., butyrophenones, phenothiazines) and has been referred to as an atypical or second-generation antipsychotic agent. The exact mechanism of action of aripiprazole in schizophrenia, bipolar disorder, major depressive disorder, irritability associated with autistic disorder, Tourette's syndrome, and agitation associated with schizophrenia or bipolar mania has not been fully elucidated but, like that of other drugs with efficacy in these conditions (e.g., olanzapine, risperidone, ziprasidone), may involve the drug's activity at dopamine D_2 and serotonin type 1 (5-HT$_{1A}$) and type 2 (5-HT$_{2A}$) receptors. However, aripiprazole appears to differ from other atypical antipsychotic agents because the drug demonstrates partial agonist activity at D_2 and 5-HT$_{1A}$ receptors and antagonist activity at 5-HT$_{2A}$ receptors. Antagonism at other receptors (e.g., α_1-adrenergic receptors, histamine H_1 receptors) may contribute to other therapeutic and adverse effects (e.g., orthostatic hypotension, somnolence) observed with aripiprazole.

Aripiprazole is well absorbed following oral administration; peak plasma concentrations following oral administration of conventional tablets occur within 3–5 hours. Administration with a high-fat meal does not affect peak plasma concentration or systemic exposure of aripiprazole or dehydro-aripiprazole. Absolute oral bioavailability of conventional tablets is 87%. Following administration of the oral solution, plasma aripiprazole concentrations are higher than those after administration of equivalent dosages of the conventional tablets. Steady-state plasma concentrations of both aripiprazole and dehydro-aripiprazole are achieved within 14 days with oral administration. Aripiprazole is extensively metabolized in the liver principally via dehydrogenation, hydroxylation, and N-dealkylation by the cytochrome P-450 (CYP) 2D6 and 3A4 isoenzymes. The major active metabolite of aripiprazole, dehydro-aripiprazole, exhibits affinity for D_2 receptors similar to that of the parent compound and represents approximately 40% of aripiprazole area under the concentration-time curve (AUC) in plasma. Poor CYP2D6 metabolizers have substantially increased aripiprazole and dehydro-aripiprazole exposures compared with extensive metabolizers (see Dosage and Administration: Special Populations). Approximately 18% of an orally administered dose of aripiprazole is excreted unchanged in feces and less than 1% is excreted unchanged in urine.

Following IM administration of immediate-release aripiprazole injection (no longer commercially available in the US), peak plasma concentrations were achieved within 1–3 hours and were an average of 19% higher than those achieved following oral administration of conventional tablets. Systemic exposure is similar following IM and oral administration of aripiprazole; however, in the first 2 hours after administration, AUC was 90% higher following IM administration of the injection compared with oral administration of the conventional tablets.

Following IM administration of extended-release aripiprazole (Abilify Maintena®), the low solubility of aripiprazole particles results in prolonged aripiprazole absorption. Following multiple IM doses, peak plasma aripiprazole concentrations occur after a median of 4 or 5–7 days when administered into the deltoid or gluteal muscle, respectively. Single IM injections into the deltoid result in 31% higher peak plasma concentrations compared with the gluteal site; however, aripiprazole systemic exposures and peak plasma concentrations at steady state were similar for both injection sites. Dose-proportional increases in aripiprazole and dehydro-aripiprazole systemic exposures were observed following extended-release aripiprazole IM doses of 300 or 400 mg given every 4 weeks. Steady-state plasma concentrations of aripiprazole are achieved by the fourth dose of extended-release aripiprazole for both sites of administration. Following gluteal administration of multiple 300- or 400-mg doses of extended-release aripiprazole every 4 weeks, the mean terminal half-life of aripiprazole is 29.9 or 46.5 days, respectively.

Aripiprazole lauroxil is a prodrug of aripiprazole. Following IM injection, aripiprazole lauroxil is probably converted by enzyme-mediated hydrolysis to N-hydroxymethyl aripiprazole, which is then hydrolyzed to aripiprazole. Following IM administration of extended-release aripiprazole lauroxil (Aristada®), aripiprazole begins to appear in the systemic circulation in 5–6 days and is continually released for an additional 36 days. Plasma concentrations of aripiprazole increase with consecutive doses and reach steady-state concentrations following the fourth monthly injection. When administered with oral aripiprazole for 21 days following the first injection, therapeutic plasma concentrations of aripiprazole are achieved within 4 days. IM injection of extended-release aripiprazole lauroxil (441 mg) into the deltoid and gluteal areas results in similar systemic exposure; therefore, these injection sites are considered interchangeable. In addition, IM administration of aripiprazole lauroxil 882 mg every 6 weeks or 1064 mg every 2 months results in plasma aripiprazole concentrations that are within the established therapeutic range for dosages of 441 and 882 mg once monthly. The mean terminal half-life of aripiprazole ranges from about 54–57 days following monthly, every 6 week, or every 2 month injections of extended-release aripiprazole lauroxil.

● **Aripiprazole Tablets with Sensor**

Aripiprazole is available as part of a digital ingestion tracking system comprised of the following components: aripiprazole tablets embedded with an ingestible event marker sensor (IEM; Abilify MyCite®); a wearable sensor (MyCite® patch), which detects the signal from the IEM sensor after ingestion and transmits data to a compatible mobile device (i.e., a smart phone); a software application (app) for compatible mobile devices (e.g., smart phones; MyCite® App), which displays information for the patient; and a web-based portal for healthcare professionals and caregivers.

Following oral administration of aripiprazole tablets with sensor, magnesium and cuprous chloride within the sensor react with gastric fluid to activate and power the sensor. Once activated, the ingestible sensor communicates with the wearable sensor within a 9-foot proximity using Bluetooth® technology. The wearable sensor records the date and time of ingestions and transmits the data to the mobile software application. The mobile software application records and displays ingestion data for patients to review; subjective data such as activity level, mood, and quality of rest also may be reported to the software application.

Healthcare professionals, caregivers, and/or family members may access ingestion data shared by the patient through a web-based portal or dashboard. The manufacturer states that this access is granted by the patient and may be withdrawn by the patient at any time.

Most ingestions of aripiprazole tablets with sensor are detected within 30 minutes of oral administration; however, it may take up to 2 hours for the mobile device and web portal to detect ingestion of the sensor and, in some cases, the ingestion may not be detected at all. In a study to assess accuracy and latency of post-ingestion detection of the ingestible sensor in 29 healthy individuals, a wearable sensor was placed and paired with a mobile device provided and monitored by investigators. Placebo tablets with embedded ingestible sensors were then administered under observation every 2 hours for 4 doses without regard to food. The overall ingestion detection rate was 96.6%; approximately 90% of ingestions were detected by the mobile software application within 30 minutes of ingestion. Mean time from ingestion to detection by the wearable sensor was 1.1–1.3 minutes and from detection by the wearable sensor to detection on the cloud-based server was 6.2–10.3 minutes.

ADVICE TO PATIENTS

Importance of providing copy of written patient information (medication guide) each time aripiprazole is dispensed. Importance of advising patients to read the patient information before taking aripiprazole and each time the prescription is refilled.

Importance of advising patients and caregivers that geriatric patients with dementia-related psychosis treated with antipsychotic agents are at an increased risk of death. Patients and caregivers also should be informed that aripiprazole is *not* approved for treating geriatric patients with dementia-related psychosis.

Risk of suicidality; importance of patients, family, and caregivers being alert to and immediately reporting emergence of suicidality, worsening depression, manic or hypomanic symptoms, irritability, agitation, or unusual changes in behavior, especially during the first few months of therapy or during periods of dosage adjustment. (See Worsening of Depression and Suicidality Risk under Warnings/Precautions: Warnings, in Cautions.)

Because somnolence and impairment of judgment, thinking, or motor skills may be associated with aripiprazole, avoid driving, operating machinery, or performing hazardous tasks while taking aripiprazole until the drug's effects on the individual are known.

Importance of avoiding alcohol during extended-release IM aripiprazole (Abilify Maintena®) therapy.

Importance of informing patients and caregivers about the risk of neuroleptic malignant syndrome (NMS); importance of immediately contacting clinician or seeking emergency medical attention if signs and symptoms of this rare but potentially life-threatening syndrome develop (e.g., high fever, muscle stiffness, sweating, fast or irregular heart beat, change in blood pressure, confusion, kidney damage).

Importance of clinicians informing patients in whom chronic aripiprazole use is contemplated of risk of tardive dyskinesia. Importance of informing patients to report any muscle movements that cannot be stopped to a healthcare professional.

Risk of leukopenia, neutropenia, and agranulocytosis. Importance of advising patients with a preexisting low leukocyte count or a history of drug-induced leukopenia/neutropenia that they should have their complete blood cell (CBC) count monitored during aripiprazole therapy.

Importance of informing patients about the risk of metabolic changes (e.g., hyperglycemia and diabetes mellitus, dyslipidemia, weight gain), how to recognize symptoms of hyperglycemia and diabetes mellitus, and the need for specific monitoring, including blood glucose, lipids, and weight, for such changes during therapy.

Risk of pathological gambling and other compulsive behaviors. Importance of advising patients and caregivers of the possibility that they may experience compulsive urges to shop, intense urges to gamble, compulsive sexual urges, binge eating, and/or other compulsive urges and the inability to control these urges during aripiprazole therapy. In some cases, but not all, the urges reportedly stopped when the dosage was reduced or the drug was discontinued. Importance of advising patients or their caregivers to contact a clinician promptly if they experience any such urges that seem out of the ordinary;

importance of also advising patients not to abruptly stop taking aripiprazole without first consulting their clinician.

Importance of informing patients about the risk of orthostatic hypotension and syncope, especially when initiating or reinitiating treatment or increasing the dosage.

Importance of informing clinicians of existing or contemplated concomitant therapy, including prescription and OTC drugs and dietary or herbal supplements, as well as any concomitant illnesses (e.g., cardiovascular or cerebrovascular disease, diabetes mellitus, seizures).

Importance of women informing clinicians if they are or plan to become pregnant or plan to breast-feed. Importance of clinicians informing patients about the benefits and risks of taking antipsychotics during pregnancy, including that third trimester use of aripiprazole may cause extrapyramidal and/or withdrawal symptoms in a neonate, and about the pregnancy exposure registry (see Pregnancy under Warnings/Precautions: Specific Populations, in Cautions). Importance of advising patients not to stop taking aripiprazole if they become pregnant without consulting their clinician; abruptly discontinuing antipsychotic agents may cause complications. Importance of advising patients that aripiprazole can pass into breast milk and to consult with their clinician about the best way to feed their infant during aripiprazole therapy.

Importance of avoiding overheating or dehydration.

For patients taking aripiprazole orally disintegrating tablets, importance of not removing a tablet from the blister package until just before administering a dose; importance of peeling blister open with dry hands and placing tablet on tongue to dissolve and be swallowed with saliva.

Importance of informing patients with phenylketonuria that aripiprazole orally disintegrating 10- and 15-mg tablets (Abilify Discmelt®) contain 1.12 and 1.68 mg of phenylalanine, respectively.

Importance of informing patients of other important precautionary information. (See Cautions.)

Aripiprazole Tablets with Sensor

Importance of instructing patients to download the MyCite® App prior to initial use of aripiprazole tablets with sensor and ensure that the software is compatible with their mobile device (i.e., smart phone). Patients should refer to the information provided by the manufacturer and within the MyCite® App for instructions regarding applying and changing the wearable sensor (i.e., MyCite® patch) and pairing the wearable sensor to their mobile device. Importance of advising patients that initial use of the MyCite® system should be facilitated by a healthcare professional.

Importance of advising patients that most ingestions of the tablets with sensor will be detected within 30 minutes; however, it may sometimes take over 2 hours for the mobile device and web portal to detect the ingestion of the tablet with sensor, and, in some cases, ingestion may not be detected at all. Importance of advising patients not to repeat a dose if the tablet with sensor is not detected after ingestion.

Importance of advising patients that if their mobile device is lost, impaired, or otherwise rendered unusable, patients should change the wearable sensor immediately and connect to a new mobile device using their current account information. Inform patients that some data collected by the system may be lost; however, data that have been previously synchronized to the patient's account will be available.

Importance of informing patients that in order for the wearable sensor to communicate with the mobile device, the device must be powered on and Bluetooth®-enabled. Importance of advising patients that the wearable sensor will communicate with a paired device when it is within a 9-foot proximity. Advise patients to keep the wearable sensor in place while showering, swimming, or exercising since it is intended to tolerate exposure to water and perspiration. However, the wearable sensor should be removed before magnetic resonance imaging (MRI) and replaced with a new wearable sensor as soon as possible following the MRI. Importance of advising patients to remove the wearable sensor if skin irritation occurs. (See Tablets with Sensor under Administration: Oral Administration, in Dosage and Administration.)

Importance of instructing patients to swallow aripiprazole tablets with sensor whole. Do not divide, crush, or chew the tablets.

PREPARATIONS

Excipients in commercially available drug preparations may have clinically important effects in some individuals; consult specific product labeling for details.

ARIPiprazole

Oral

Solution	5 mg/5 mL	Aripiprazole Oral Solution
Tablets	2 mg*	Abilify®, Otsuka
	5 mg*	Abilify®, Otsuka
	10 mg*	Abilify®, Otsuka
	15 mg*	Abilify®, Otsuka
	20 mg*	Abilify®, Otsuka
	30 mg*	Abilify®, Otsuka
Tablets, orally disintegrating	10 mg*	Abilify Discmelt®, Otsuka
	15 mg*	Abilify Discmelt®, Otsuka
Tablets with sensor	2 mg	Abilify MyCite® (available as kit containing 30 tablets embedded with sensor and 7 wearable sensor patches), Otsuka
	5 mg	Abilify MyCite® (available as kit containing 30 tablets embedded with sensor and 7 wearable sensor patches), Otsuka
	10 mg	Abilify MyCite® (available as kit containing 30 tablets embedded with sensor and 7 wearable sensor patches), Otsuka
	15 mg	Abilify MyCite® (available as kit containing 30 tablets embedded with sensor and 7 wearable sensor patches), Otsuka
	20 mg	Abilify MyCite® (available as kit containing 30 tablets embedded with sensor and 7 wearable sensor patches), Otsuka
	30 mg	Abilify MyCite® (available as kit containing 30 tablets embedded with sensor and 7 wearable sensor patches), Otsuka

Parenteral

For injectable suspension, extended-release, for IM use	300 mg	Abilify Maintena® (available as kit containing either a single-dose vial, sterile water for injection, needles, and syringe or a prefilled dual-chamber syringe, sterile water for injection, and needles), Otsuka (also promoted by Lundbeck)
	400 mg	Abilify Maintena® (available as kit containing either a single-dose vial, sterile water for injection, needles, and syringe or a prefilled dual-chamber syringe, sterile water for injection, and needles), Otsuka (also promoted by Lundbeck)

* available from one or more manufacturer, distributor, and/or repackager by generic (nonproprietary) name

ARIPiprazole Lauroxil

Parenteral

Injectable suspension, extended-release, for IM use	441 mg/1.6 mL	Aristada® (available as kit containing prefilled syringe and needles), Alkermes
	662 mg/2.4 mL	Aristada® (available as kit containing prefilled syringe and needles), Alkermes
	675 mg/2.4 mL	Aristada Initio® (available as kit containing prefilled syringe and needles), Alkermes
	882 mg/3.2 mL	Aristada® (available as kit containing prefilled syringe and needles), Alkermes
	1064 mg/3.9 mL	Aristada® (available as kit containing prefilled syringe and needles), Alkermes

Brexpiprazole

28:16.08.04 · ATYPICAL ANTIPSYCHOTICS

■ Brexpiprazole is considered an atypical or second-generation antipsychotic agent.

USES

● Adjunctive Therapy of Major Depressive Disorder

Brexpiprazole is used orally as an adjunct to antidepressants for the treatment of major depressive disorder.

The adjunctive antidepressant efficacy of brexpiprazole was established in 2 short-term, double-blind, placebo-controlled, fixed-dose studies of 6 weeks' duration (studies 1 and 2) in adults who met DSM-IV-TR criteria for major depressive disorder with or without symptoms of anxiety and who had an inadequate response to previous antidepressant therapy (1–3 courses) in the current episode and had also demonstrated an inadequate response during an 8-week prospective treatment period of antidepressant therapy with delayed-release duloxetine, escitalopram, fluoxetine, extended-release paroxetine, sertraline, or extended-release venlafaxine. The primary efficacy end point in these studies was change from baseline to week 6 on the Montgomery-Asberg Depression Rating Scale (MADRS) total score. In study 1, patients were randomized to receive either brexpiprazole 2 mg once daily or placebo in addition to their antidepressant therapy; in study 2, patients were randomized to receive brexpiprazole 1 or 3 mg once daily or placebo as adjunctive therapy. Brexpiprazole therapy was initiated at a dosage of 0.5 mg once daily in all patients, then the dosage was increased to 1 mg once daily at week 2 in all treatments groups; the dosage was then either maintained at 1 mg once daily or increased to 2 or 3 mg once daily, based on treatment assignment, from week 3 onward. In studies 1 and 2, brexpiprazole at a dosage of 2 or 3 mg daily was superior to placebo in reducing mean MADRS total scores at week 6 and was generally well tolerated. An analysis of population subgroups did not reveal evidence of differential response to adjunctive brexpiprazole therapy based on age, gender, race, or choice of prospective antidepressant.

The manufacturer states that the need for continued therapy and appropriate dosage of brexpiprazole should be reassessed periodically in patients with major depressive disorder. (See Dosage under Dosage and Administration.)

● Schizophrenia

Brexpiprazole is used for the treatment of schizophrenia. Schizophrenia is a chronic major psychotic disorder that frequently has devastating effects on various aspects of the patient's life and is associated with an increased risk of suicide and increased overall mortality. The principal manifestations of schizophrenia usually are described in terms of positive, negative, and cognitive symptoms. Positive (i.e., psychotic) symptoms include hallucinations and delusions, while negative symptoms include decreases in emotional expression, initiation of goal-directed behavior (avolition), speech productivity (alogia), ability to experience pleasure from external stimuli (anhedonia), and apparent interest in social interactions (asociality). Cognitive symptoms include impairments in attention, concentration, and memory. Diagnostic criteria for schizophrenia also may include disorganized speech (e.g., frequent derailment or incoherence) or grossly disorganized or catatonic behavior.

Short-term efficacy of oral brexpiprazole monotherapy in the acute treatment of schizophrenia has been established in 2 randomized, multicenter, double-blind, placebo-controlled, fixed-dose studies of 6 weeks' duration (studies 3 and 4) in adults who met DSM-IV-TR criteria for schizophrenia and were experiencing an acute exacerbation of psychotic symptoms. Both studies evaluated fixed brexpiprazole dosages of 2 or 4 mg once daily. Brexpiprazole therapy was initiated at a dosage of 1 mg once daily, given on days 1 through 4, then the dosage was increased to 2 mg once daily on days 5 to 7; the dosage was then either maintained at 2 mg once daily or increased to 4 mg once daily, based on treatment assignment, for 5 weeks. The primary efficacy end point in these studies was the change from baseline to week 6 on the Positive and Negative Syndrome Scale (PANSS) total score. In both studies, brexpiprazole 4 mg once daily was found to be more effective than placebo in improving the PANSS total score at week 6; the 2-mg daily dosage of brexpiprazole was more effective than placebo only in study 3. An

examination of population subgroups did not reveal any clear evidence of differential responsiveness to the drug based on age, gender, or race.

Efficacy and safety of brexpiprazole in the maintenance treatment of schizophrenia have been established in a randomized, multicenter withdrawal study (study 5). Adults with schizophrenia were stabilized for at least 12 weeks on 1–4 mg daily of brexpiprazole and were then randomized in the double-blind treatment phase to either continue brexpiprazole at their achieved stable dosage or to switch to placebo for up to 52 weeks. The primary efficacy end point in this study was time from randomization to impending relapse during the double-blind phase. A prespecified interim analysis demonstrated a substantially longer time to relapse in patients randomized to brexpiprazole therapy compared with the placebo recipients. The study was therefore terminated early because maintenance of efficacy had been demonstrated. Long-term brexpiprazole therapy also was found to be well tolerated in this study.

Antipsychotic therapy is integral to the management of patients with schizophrenia, both for management of acute psychotic symptoms and for maintenance treatment to prevent symptom recurrence. The American Psychiatric Association (APA) and other experts consider antipsychotic agents (i.e., first- and second-generation antipsychotic agents) to be first-line drugs for the management of schizophrenia (including first psychotic episodes). The APA states that, with the possible exception of clozapine for the management of treatment-resistant symptoms, there currently is no definitive evidence that one antipsychotic agent will have superior efficacy compared with another agent, although meaningful differences in response may be observed in individual patients. Therefore, initial choice of an antipsychotic agent should be individualized, and generally be made in the context of shared decision-making, taking into consideration multiple patient- and drug-related factors, including adverse effect profiles, concurrent medical conditions or risk factors, potential for drug interactions, and potential pharmacogenomic considerations, as well as the patient's preferences, prior responses to treatment, available formulations, and cost. Patient response and tolerance to antipsychotic agents are variable, and patients who do not respond to or tolerate one drug may be successfully treated with another drug with different receptor binding or adverse effect profile.

The APA recommends that patients with schizophrenia whose symptoms have improved with an antipsychotic agent continue to receive such therapy. The APA also suggests that patients whose symptoms have improved with an antipsychotic agent continue to be treated with the same antipsychotic agent; however, some circumstances (e.g., patient preferences, drug availability, adverse effects) may necessitate a change in antipsychotic agent. Drug therapy should be used as part of a comprehensive, patient-centered treatment plan that includes evidence-based nonpharmacologic and pharmacologic treatments for schizophrenia. Clinicians may consult APA's Practice Guideline for the Treatment of Patients with Schizophrenia (available at https://psychiatryonline.org/doi/book/10.1176/appi.books.9780890424841) for additional information on the treatment of schizophrenia.

For additional information on the symptomatic management of schizophrenia, including treatment recommendations, see Schizophrenia and Other Psychotic Disorders under Uses: Psychotic Disorders, in the Phenothiazines General Statement 28:16.08.24.

DOSAGE AND ADMINISTRATION

● Administration

Brexpiprazole is commercially available as tablets, which are administered orally once daily without regard to meals. (See Description.)

Patients receiving brexpiprazole should be monitored for possible worsening of depression and emergence of suicidal thoughts or behaviors, especially at the beginning of therapy or during periods of dosage adjustments. (See Suicidal Thoughts and Behaviors in Children, Adolescents, and Young Adults under Cautions.)

● Dosage

Adjunctive Therapy of Major Depressive Disorder

For adjunctive treatment of major depressive disorder in adults already receiving an antidepressant, the recommended initial dosage of brexpiprazole is 0.5 or 1 mg orally once daily. The dosage should be titrated to 1 mg once daily and then up to the target dosage of 2 mg once daily; dosage adjustments should be made at weekly intervals based on individual patient response and tolerability. The maximum recommended dosage of brexpiprazole for the adjunctive treatment of major depressive disorder is 3 mg daily.

The manufacturer states that the need for continued therapy with brexpiprazole and the appropriate dosage of the drug should be reassessed periodically.

Schizophrenia

For the management of schizophrenia in adults, the recommended initial dosage of brexpiprazole is 1 mg orally once daily on days 1–4, followed by an increase in dosage to 2 mg once daily on days 5–7. Based on individual patient response and tolerability, the dosage may be increased to 4 mg once daily on day 8. The recommended target dosage of brexpiprazole for the treatment of schizophrenia is 2–4 mg once daily. The maximum recommended dosage of the drug for the treatment of schizophrenia is 4 mg daily.

In patients with schizophrenia whose symptoms have improved with an antipsychotic agent, continued treatment (i.e., maintenance therapy) with an antipsychotic agent is recommended to reduce the risk of relapse. The APA suggests that such patients continue to be treated with the same antipsychotic agent that was effective during acute treatment. Some experts have recommended maintenance antipsychotic therapy for at least 1–2 years after the first psychotic episode and for 2–5 years or longer following recurrent episodes. Indefinite maintenance antipsychotic treatment may be necessary in many cases; however, the benefits and risks of continued antipsychotic therapy should be assessed periodically in the context of shared decision-making, taking into consideration each patient's risk of relapse, drug-associated adverse effects, course of disease, and the specific goals and needs of each patient.

• Special Populations

In patients with moderate, severe, or end-stage renal impairment (creatinine clearance less than 60 mL/minute), the maximum recommended dosage of brexpiprazole is 2 mg once daily for adjunctive treatment of major depressive disorder and 3 mg once daily for the treatment of schizophrenia. (See Renal Impairment under Cautions.)

The manufacturer does not provide any specific dosage recommendations for brexpiprazole in patients with mild hepatic impairment. In patients with moderate to severe hepatic impairment (Child-Pugh score of 7 or higher), the maximum recommended dosage of brexpiprazole is 2 mg once daily for adjunctive treatment of major depressive disorder and 3 mg once daily for the treatment of schizophrenia. (See Hepatic Impairment under Cautions.)

In geriatric patients, the manufacturer states that dosage selection of brexpiprazole should be cautious, usually starting at the lower end of the recommended dosage range, reflecting the greater frequency of decreased hepatic, renal, and cardiac function and concomitant illness and other drug therapy in this population. (See Geriatric Use under Cautions.)

Dosage adjustment is not required based on gender, race, or smoking status.

Hepatic Microsomal Enzyme Considerations

Dosage adjustments of brexpiprazole are recommended in patients who are known poor metabolizers of the cytochrome P-450 (CYP) isoenzyme 2D6 and in patients concomitantly receiving CYP3A4 and/or CYP2D6 inhibitors or potent CYP3A4 inducers. (See Drugs Affecting Hepatic Microsomal Enzymes under Drug Interactions.)

Patients who are known CYP2D6 poor metabolizers should receive 50% of the usual brexpiprazole dosage, since CYP2D6 poor metabolizers have higher concentrations of brexpiprazole than extensive metabolizers (see Description). Such patients who are also taking moderate or potent CYP3A4 inhibitors should receive 25% of the usual brexpiprazole dosage.

For the treatment of schizophrenia, brexpiprazole dosage should be reduced to 50% of the usual dosage when used concurrently with potent CYP2D6 inhibitors (e.g., fluoxetine, paroxetine, quinidine). When the potent CYP2D6 inhibitor is withdrawn from combined therapy, the original brexpiprazole dosage may be resumed. For adjunctive therapy of major depressive disorder, brexpiprazole dosage adjustment is *not* necessary when used concomitantly with potent CYP2D6 inhibitors because CYP-related considerations have already been taken into account for the general dosage recommendations. (See Adjunctive Therapy of Major Depressive Disorder under Dosage and Administration and also see Drugs Affecting Hepatic Microsomal Enzymes under Drug Interactions.)

Brexpiprazole dosage should be reduced to 50% of the usual dosage when used concurrently with potent CYP3A4 inhibitors (e.g., clarithromycin, itraconazole, ketoconazole). When the potent CYP3A4 inhibitor is withdrawn from combined therapy, the original brexpiprazole dosage may be resumed.

When used concurrently with a combination of moderate or potent CYP2D6 inhibitors and moderate or potent CYP3A4 inhibitors, brexpiprazole dosage should be reduced to 25% of the usual dosage. When the moderate or potent CYP2D6 inhibitor(s) and moderate or potent CYP3A4 inhibitor(s) are withdrawn from combined therapy, the original brexpiprazole dosage may be resumed.

If brexpiprazole is used concurrently with potent CYP3A4 inducers (e.g., rifampin, St. John's wort [*Hypericum perforatum*]), the usual brexpiprazole dosage should be doubled over 1–2 weeks, with further dosage adjustments based on clinical response. When the potent CYP3A4 inducer is withdrawn from combined therapy, the original brexpiprazole dosage may be resumed over 1–2 weeks.

CAUTIONS

• Contraindications

Known hypersensitivity to brexpiprazole or any components in the formulation. Rash, facial swelling, urticaria, and anaphylaxis have been reported in patients receiving brexpiprazole.

• Warnings/Precautions

Warnings

Increased Mortality in Geriatric Patients with Dementia-related Psychosis

Geriatric patients with dementia-related psychosis treated with antipsychotic drugs are at an increased risk of death. Analyses of 17 placebo-controlled trials (modal duration of 10 weeks) revealed a 1.6- to 1.7-fold increase in mortality among geriatric patients who were mainly receiving atypical antipsychotic drugs (i.e., aripiprazole, olanzapine, quetiapine, risperidone) compared with that observed in patients receiving placebo. Over the course of a typical 10-week controlled trial, the rate of death in drug-treated patients was about 4.5% compared with a rate of about 2.6% in the placebo group. Although the causes of death were varied, most of the deaths appeared to be either cardiovascular (e.g., heart failure, sudden death) or infectious (e.g., pneumonia) in nature. The manufacturer states that brexpiprazole is *not* approved for the treatment of patients with dementia-related psychosis. (See Adverse Cerebrovascular Events, including Stroke, in Geriatric Patients with Dementia-related Psychosis, and also see Geriatric Use under Cautions.)

Suicidal Thoughts and Behaviors in Children, Adolescents, and Young Adults

Antidepressants may increase the risk of suicidal thoughts and behaviors in children, adolescents, and young adults. Pooled analyses of short-term, placebo-controlled studies of antidepressants (i.e., selective serotonin-reuptake inhibitors [SSRIs] and other antidepressants) have shown an increased risk of suicidal thoughts and behaviors in children, adolescents, and young adults (24 years of age or younger) receiving antidepressants for major depressive disorder and other indications. Although the risk varied considerably between drugs, an increased risk was identified for most antidepressants studied. Differences in absolute risk of suicidal thoughts and behaviors were seen across the different indications, with the highest incidence in patients with major depressive disorder. An increased risk of suicidal thoughts and behaviors was not demonstrated with antidepressants compared with placebo in adults older than 24 years of age, and a reduced risk was observed in adults 65 years of age or older. Because the studies analyzed were short-term, it is not known whether the increased risk of suicidal thoughts or behaviors in such patients continues with longer-term antidepressant treatment (i.e., beyond 4 months). However, substantial evidence from placebo-controlled maintenance studies in adults with major depressive disorder indicates that antidepressants delay the recurrence of depression. Safety and efficacy of brexpiprazole have not been established in pediatric patients.

All patients being treated with antidepressants for any indication should be closely monitored for worsening of depression and emergence of suicidal thoughts and behaviors, particularly during initiation of therapy (i.e., the first few months) and during periods of dosage adjustments. Family members and caregivers of patients being treated with antidepressants also should be advised to monitor patients for changes in behavior and to alert a health-care provider if such changes occur. Consideration should be given to changing the therapeutic regimen or discontinuing therapy in patients whose depression is persistently worse or who are experiencing emergent suicidal thoughts or behaviors.

Other Warnings and Precautions

Adverse Cerebrovascular Events, including Stroke, in Geriatric Patients with Dementia-related Psychosis

In placebo-controlled studies in geriatric patients with dementia, patients randomized to risperidone, aripiprazole, and olanzapine had a higher incidence of adverse cerebrovascular events (cerebrovascular accidents and transient ischemic attacks), including fatalities. The manufacturer states that brexpiprazole is *not* approved for the treatment of patients with dementia-related psychosis. (See Increased Mortality in Geriatric Patients with Dementia-related Psychosis and also see Geriatric Use under Cautions.)

Neuroleptic Malignant Syndrome

Neuroleptic malignant syndrome (NMS), a potentially fatal syndrome characterized by hyperpyrexia, muscle rigidity, altered mental status, and autonomic instability, has been reported with antipsychotic agents, including brexpiprazole. If NMS is suspected, antipsychotic therapy should be immediately discontinued and intensive symptomatic treatment and monitoring should be provided. (See Advice to Patients.) For additional information on NMS, see Neuroleptic Malignant Syndrome under Cautions: Nervous System Effects, in the Phenothiazines General Statement 28:16.08.24.

Tardive Dyskinesia

Because use of antipsychotic agents, including brexpiprazole, may be associated with tardive dyskinesia (a syndrome consisting of potentially irreversible, involuntary, dyskinetic movements), brexpiprazole should be prescribed in a manner that is most likely to reduce the risk of this syndrome. Chronic antipsychotic treatment generally should be reserved for patients who suffer from a chronic illness that is known to respond to antipsychotic agents, and for whom alternative, effective, but potentially less harmful treatments are not available or appropriate. In patients who do require chronic treatment, the lowest dosage and the shortest duration of treatment needed to achieve a satisfactory clinical response should be used, and the need for continued treatment should be reassessed periodically.

The American Psychiatric Association (APA) currently recommends that patients with schizophrenia who are receiving antipsychotic agents be assessed clinically for abnormal involuntary movements at baseline and at each follow-up visit and that assessment with a structured instrument (e.g., the Abnormal Involuntary Movement Scale [AIMS], Dyskinesia Identification System: Condensed User Scale [DISCUS]) occur at least every 6 months in patients considered at high risk for tardive dyskinesia (including patients older than 55 years of age; women; individuals with a mood disorder, substance use disorder, intellectual disability, or CNS injury; individuals with high cumulative exposure to antipsychotic medications, particularly high-potency dopamine D_2 receptor antagonists; and patients who experience acute dystonic reactions, clinically significant parkinsonism, or akathisia) or at least every 12 months in other patients as well as if a new onset or exacerbation of preexisting movements is observed at any follow-up visit. In some jurisdictions, the frequency of monitoring for involuntary movements in individuals receiving antipsychotic agents may also be subject to local regulations.

If signs and symptoms of tardive dyskinesia appear in a brexpiprazole-treated patient, brexpiprazole discontinuance should be considered; however, some patients may require continued treatment with the drug despite the presence of the syndrome.

APA recommends that patients who have moderate to severe or disabling tardive dyskinesia associated with antipsychotic therapy be treated with a vesicular monoamine transporter 2 (VMAT2) inhibitor (e.g., deutetrabenazine, valbenazine, tetrabenazine); such treatment may also be considered for patients with mild tardive dyskinesia based on factors such as patient preference, associated impairment, and effect on psychosocial functioning. (See Deutetrabenazine 28:56, Tetrabenazine 28:56, and Valbenazine 28:56.)

For additional information on tardive dyskinesia, see Tardive Dyskinesia under Cautions: Nervous System Effects, in the Phenothiazines General Statement 28:16.08.24.

Metabolic Changes

Atypical antipsychotic agents, including brexpiprazole, have caused metabolic changes, including hyperglycemia and diabetes mellitus, dyslipidemia, and body weight gain. While all of these drugs produce some metabolic changes, each drug has its own specific risk profile. (See Hyperglycemia and Diabetes Mellitus, see Dyslipidemia, and also see Weight Gain under Cautions.)

Hyperglycemia and Diabetes Mellitus

Hyperglycemia, sometimes severe and associated with ketoacidosis, hyperosmolar coma, or death, has been reported in patients receiving atypical antipsychotic agents. Hyperglycemia has been reported in patients treated with brexpiprazole. While confounding factors such as an increased background risk of diabetes mellitus in patients with schizophrenia and the increasing incidence of diabetes mellitus in the general population make it difficult to establish with certainty the relationship between use of agents in this drug class and glucose abnormalities, epidemiologic studies suggest an increased risk of treatment-emergent hyperglycemia-related adverse events in patients treated with atypical antipsychotic agents. In short-term clinical studies, clinically important differences between brexpiprazole and placebo in the proportion of patients experiencing an increase in fasting glucose concentrations were not observed. In longer-term studies, 9–10% of brexpiprazole-treated patients with normal or borderline fasting glucose concentrations experienced shifts to high fasting glucose concentrations.

Patients with preexisting diabetes mellitus in whom therapy with an atypical antipsychotic is initiated should be periodically monitored for worsening of glucose control; those with risk factors for diabetes (e.g., obesity, family history of diabetes) should undergo fasting blood glucose testing upon therapy initiation and periodically throughout treatment. Any patient who develops manifestations of hyperglycemia (including polydipsia, polyuria, polyphagia, and weakness) during treatment with an atypical antipsychotic should undergo fasting blood glucose testing. (See Advice to Patients.) In some cases, patients who developed hyperglycemia while receiving an atypical antipsychotic have required continuance of antidiabetic treatment despite discontinuance of the atypical antipsychotic; in other cases, hyperglycemia resolved with discontinuance of the antipsychotic.

For further information on managing the risk of hyperglycemia and diabetes mellitus associated with atypical antipsychotic agents, see Hyperglycemia and Diabetes Mellitus under Cautions, in Clozapine 28:16.08.04.

Dyslipidemia

Atypical antipsychotics cause adverse alterations in lipid parameters. In short-term clinical studies, a higher incidence of hypertriglyceridemia was reported with brexpiprazole than with placebo while changes in fasting total cholesterol, low-density lipoprotein (LDL)-cholesterol, and high-density lipoprotein (HDL)-cholesterol were similar between brexpiprazole-treated patients and those receiving placebo. In uncontrolled, longer-term depression studies, 14% of brexpiprazole-treated patients experienced a shift from normal baseline HDL-cholesterol concentrations to low HDL-cholesterol concentrations and 17% of brexpiprazole-treated patients with normal baseline triglyceride concentrations experienced shifts to high and 0.2% experienced shifts to very high triglyceride concentrations. In uncontrolled, longer-term schizophrenia studies, 13% of brexpiprazole-treated patients with normal baseline triglyceride concentrations experienced shifts to high and 0.4% experienced shifts to very high triglyceride concentrations.

Weight Gain

Weight gain has been observed with atypical antipsychotic therapy. Monitoring of weight at baseline and frequently thereafter is recommended in patients receiving brexpiprazole.

Brexpiprazole generally appears to be associated with moderate weight gain. Mean weight gain during short-term studies in patients receiving brexpiprazole for depression or schizophrenia was 1–1.6 kg compared with 0.2–0.3 kg in those receiving placebo. In longer-term, open-label studies, 20–30% of brexpiprazole-treated patients gained 7% or more of their baseline body weight while 4–10% of patients receiving the drug lost 7% or more.

For additional information on metabolic effects associated with atypical antipsychotic agents, see Hyperglycemia and Diabetes Mellitus under Cautions.

Pathological Gambling and Other Compulsive Behaviors

Postmarketing case reports have suggested that patients receiving brexpiprazole may experience intense urges, particularly for gambling, and the inability to control these urges. Other compulsive urges reported include sexual urges, shopping, eating or binge eating, and other impulsive or compulsive behaviors. In some, but not all, cases, these uncontrollable urges reportedly stopped when the brexpiprazole dosage was reduced or the drug was discontinued.

Brexpiprazole-associated compulsive behaviors may result in harm to the patient or others if not recognized. Because patients may not recognize such behaviors as abnormal, clinicians should specifically ask patients or caregivers whether any new or intense gambling urges, compulsive sexual urges, compulsive shopping, binge or compulsive eating, or other urges have developed during treatment with the drug. If a patient develops such urges or other compulsive behaviors while receiving brexpiprazole, consideration should be given to reducing the dosage or discontinuing the drug. (See Advice to Patients.)

Leukopenia, Neutropenia, and Agranulocytosis

Leukopenia and neutropenia have been reported during therapy with antipsychotic agents. Agranulocytosis (including fatal cases) has been reported with other antipsychotic agents.

Possible risk factors for leukopenia and neutropenia include preexisting low leukocyte count or absolute neutrophil count (ANC) or a history of drug-induced leukopenia or neutropenia. Patients with a preexisting low leukocyte count or ANC or a history of drug-induced leukopenia or neutropenia should have their complete blood count monitored frequently during the first few months of therapy. Brexpiprazole should be discontinued at the first sign of a clinically important decline in leukocyte count in the absence of other causative factors.

Patients with neutropenia should be carefully monitored for fever or other signs or symptoms of infection and promptly treated if such signs and symptoms occur. In patients with severe neutropenia (ANC less than 1000/mm³), brexpiprazole should be discontinued and the leukocyte count monitored until recovery occurs. Lithium reportedly has been used successfully in the treatment of several cases of leukopenia associated with aripiprazole, clozapine, and some other drugs; however, further clinical experience is needed to confirm these anecdotal findings.

Orthostatic Hypotension and Syncope

Atypical antipsychotic agents cause orthostatic hypotension and syncope, perhaps because of their α_1-adrenergic blocking activity. The risk of these adverse effects generally is greatest during initial dosage titration and when the dosage is increased.

In short-term depression studies, dizziness and orthostatic hypotension were reported as adverse events in 2 and 0.1%, respectively, of patients receiving brexpiprazole with an antidepressant compared with 2% and none, respectively, of patients receiving placebo with an antidepressant. In short-term schizophrenia studies, dizziness, orthostatic hypotension, and syncope were reported in 2 and 2%, 0.4 and 0.2%, and 0.1% and none of the patients receiving brexpiprazole or placebo, respectively.

The manufacturer recommends monitoring orthostatic vital signs in patients who are susceptible to hypotension (e.g., geriatric patients, patients with dehydration or hypovolemia, patients receiving concomitant antihypertensive therapy), patients with known cardiovascular disease (e.g., history of myocardial infarction, ischemic heart disease, heart failure, or conduction abnormalities), and patients with cerebrovascular disease. The manufacturer states that brexpiprazole has not been evaluated in patients with a recent history of myocardial infarction or unstable cardiovascular disease. Such patients were excluded from premarketing clinical trials.

Falls

Brexpiprazole therapy may cause somnolence, postural hypotension, and motor and sensory instability, which may lead to falls; as a consequence, fractures or other injuries may occur. For patients with diseases or conditions or receiving other drugs that could exacerbate these effects, fall risk assessments should be completed when initiating antipsychotic treatment and periodically during long-term therapy.

Seizures

As with other antipsychotic agents, brexpiprazole may cause seizures. The risk of seizures is greatest in patients with a history of seizures or with conditions that lower the seizure threshold; such conditions may be more prevalent in older patients.

Body Temperature Dysregulation

Atypical antipsychotics may disrupt the body's ability to reduce core body temperature. The manufacturer recommends using brexpiprazole with caution in patients who may experience conditions that contribute to an elevation in core body temperature (e.g., strenuous exercise, extreme heat, dehydration, concomitant use of agents with anticholinergic activity). (See Advice to Patients.)

Dysphagia

Esophageal dysmotility and aspiration have been associated with the use of antipsychotic agents. Brexpiprazole should be used with caution in patients at risk for aspiration pneumonia.

Cognitive and Motor Impairment

Like other antipsychotic agents, brexpiprazole potentially may impair judgment, thinking, or motor skills. In short-term major depressive disorder studies, somnolence (including sedation and hypersomnia) was reported in 4% of patients receiving brexpiprazole with an antidepressant compared with 1% of patients receiving placebo with an antidepressant. In short-term, placebo-controlled schizophrenia studies, somnolence (including sedation and hypersomnia) was reported in 5% of patients receiving brexpiprazole compared with 3% of placebo recipients. (See Advice to Patients.)

Specific Populations

Pregnancy

There are no adequate and well-controlled studies to date of brexpiprazole use in pregnant women. In animals, brexpiprazole was not teratogenic but increased perinatal death in pups at dosages much higher than the maximum recommended human dosage.

Neonates exposed to antipsychotic agents during the third trimester of pregnancy are at risk for extrapyramidal and/or withdrawal symptoms following delivery. Symptoms reported to date have included agitation, hypertonia, hypotonia, tremor, somnolence, respiratory distress, and feeding disorder. Neonates exhibiting such symptoms should be monitored. The complications have varied in severity; some neonates recovered within hours to days without specific treatment while others have required intensive care unit support and prolonged hospitalization. For further information on extrapyramidal and withdrawal symptoms in neonates, see Cautions: Pregnancy, Fertility, and Lactation, in the Phenothiazines General Statement 28:16.08.24.

National Pregnancy Registry for Atypical Antipsychotics: 866-961-2388 and https://womensmentalhealth.org/research/pregnancyregistry/.

Lactation

It is not known whether brexpiprazole is distributed into milk in humans. The drug is distributed into milk in rats. The effects of brexpiprazole on nursing infants and on milk production also are unknown. The benefits of brexpiprazole therapy to the woman as well as the benefits of breast-feeding to the infant should be weighed against the potential risk to the infant resulting from exposure to the drug or from the underlying maternal condition.

Pediatric Use

Safety and efficacy of brexpiprazole in pediatric patients have not been established.

Antidepressants may increase the risk of suicidal thoughts and behaviors in children, adolescents, and young adults. (See Suicidal Thoughts and Behaviors in Children, Adolescents, and Young Adults under Cautions.)

Geriatric Use

Clinical trials of the efficacy of brexpiprazole did not include any patients 65 years of age and older to determine whether they respond differently than younger adults. In a safety, tolerability, and pharmacokinetics study in geriatric patients (70–85 years of age) with major depressive disorder, the pharmacokinetics of brexpiprazole were similar to those observed in younger adults.

The manufacturer of brexpiprazole states that dosage selection for geriatric patients should be cautious, usually starting at the lower end of the dosage range, reflecting the greater incidence of decreased hepatic, renal, and cardiac function and concomitant illness and other drug therapy in this population.

Geriatric patients with dementia-related psychosis treated with antipsychotic agents are at an increased risk of death. In addition, an increased incidence of adverse cerebrovascular events (cerebrovascular accidents and transient isch-emic attacks), including fatalities, has been observed in geriatric patients with dementia-related psychosis treated with certain atypical antipsychotic agents (aripiprazole, olanzapine, risperidone) in placebo-controlled studies. Brexpipra-zole is *not* approved for the treatment of patients with dementia-related psycho-sis (see Increased Mortality in Geriatric Patients with Dementia-related Psychosis under Cautions). For additional information on the use of antipsychotic agents in the management of dementia-related psychosis, see Geriatric Considerations under Uses: Psychotic Disorders, in the Phenothiazines General Statement 28:16.08.24.

Hepatic Impairment

Brexpiprazole is extensively metabolized in the liver. In individuals with mild, moderate, or severe hepatic impairment, brexpiprazole exposures were 26, 73, or 4% higher, respectively, than those in patients with normal hepatic function. Because greater exposure to the drug may increase the risk of adverse effects, a reduction in the maximum recommended dosage of brexpiprazole is recom-mended for patients with moderate or severe hepatic impairment (Child-Pugh score of 7 or higher). (See Special Populations under Dosage and Administration.)

Renal Impairment

Following a single 3-mg dose, brexpiprazole exposure was 72% higher in patients with severe renal impairment than in patients with normal renal function. In a population pharmacokinetic analysis, brexpiprazole exposures were similar between patients with mild renal impairment and those with normal renal func-tion but exposure to the drug was 71% higher in patients with moderate renal impairment. Because greater exposure to the drug may increase the risk of adverse effects, a reduction in the maximum recommended dosage of brexpiprazole is recommended in patients with moderate or severe renal impairment (creatinine clearance less than 60 mL/minute) or end-stage renal disease. (See Special Popu-lations under Dosage and Administration.)

Hemodialysis is not expected to affect plasma concentrations of brexpiprazole because the drug is highly bound to plasma proteins.

CYP2D6 Poor Metabolizers

Because higher concentrations of brexpiprazole have been observed in poor metabolizers of cytochrome P-450 (CYP) isoenzyme 2D6 than in extensive metabolizers, dosage adjustment of the drug is recommended in patients known to be CYP2D6 poor metabolizers. Approximately 8% of Caucasians and 3–8% of Blacks/African Americans cannot metabolize CYP2D6 substrates and are classi-fied as CYP2D6 poor metabolizers. (See Hepatic Microsomal Enzyme Consider-ations under Dosage and Administration.)

● Common Adverse Effects

Adverse effects occurring in 2% or more of patients receiving brexpiprazole as adjunctive therapy for major depressive disorder and at a higher frequency than reported with placebo include akathisia, headache, weight gain, extrapyramidal symptoms (excluding akathisia), somnolence, nasopharyngitis, tremor, anxiety, increased appetite, dizziness, fatigue, restlessness, constipation, and decreased blood cortisol concentration. Akathisia and restlessness were found to be dose related in placebo-controlled studies.

Adverse effects occurring in 2% or more of patients receiving brexpiprazole for treatment of schizophrenia and at a higher frequency than reported with pla-cebo include akathisia, extrapyramidal symptoms (excluding akathisia), weight gain, diarrhea, dyspepsia, tremor, increased serum creatine kinase (CK, creatine phosphokinase, CPK) concentrations, and sedation.

DRUG INTERACTIONS

Brexpiprazole is metabolized principally by cytochrome P-450 (CYP) isoenzymes 3A4 and 2D6.

In vitro studies indicate that brexpiprazole and its principal major metabo-lite, DM-3411, are not potent inhibitors and/or inducers of CYP isoenzymes 1A2, 2A6, 2B6, 2C8, 2C9, 2C19, 2D6, 2E1, or 3A4/5.

In vitro studies indicate that brexpiprazole and its principal metabolite, DM-3411, are not clinically relevant substrates or inhibitors of the efflux trans-porters P-glycoprotein (P-gp) and breast cancer resistance protein (BCRP),

organic anion transport proteins (OATP) 1B1 and 1B3, organic anion transporter 3 (OAT3), organic cation transporter 2 (OCT2), and multidrug and toxic com-pound extrusion (MATE) 1 and MATE2K.

● Drugs Affecting Hepatic Microsomal Enzymes

Clinically important pharmacokinetic interactions with brexpiprazole are possi-ble with drugs that inhibit or induce CYP3A4 or CYP2D6.

Inhibitors of CYP3A4

Concomitant use of brexpiprazole with potent inhibitors of CYP3A4 (e.g., clar-ithromycin, itraconazole, ketoconazole) may result in substantially increased systemic exposure (area under the concentration-time curve [AUC]) of brexpi-razole. When the potent CYP3A4 inhibitor ketoconazole was administered con-comitantly with brexpiprazole (single 2-mg dose), peak plasma concentrations and AUC of brexpiprazole were increased by approximately 1.2-fold and twofold, respectively.

Brexpiprazole dosage should be reduced by 50% of the usual dosage when used concurrently with potent CYP3A4 inhibitors. When the potent CYP3A4 inhibitor is withdrawn from combined therapy, the original brexpiprazole dos-age may be resumed. Brexpiprazole dosage should be reduced to 25% of the usual dosage when used concurrently with moderate or potent CYP3A4 inhibitors in patients who are CYP2D6 poor metabolizers. In patients taking moderate or potent CYP3A4 inhibitors (e.g., clarithromycin, fluconazole, itraconazole) *and* moderate or potent CYP2D6 inhibitors (e.g., duloxetine, paroxetine, quinidine), brexpiprazole dosage also should be reduced to 25% of the usual dosage. Brexpi-razole dosage should be increased back to the original dosage when the CYP2D6 and CYP3A4 inhibitors are discontinued. (See Hepatic Microsomal Enzyme Con-siderations under Dosage and Administration.)

Ketoconazole

Concomitant administration of ketoconazole, a potent CYP3A4 inhibitor, and brexpiprazole (single 2-mg dose) increased peak plasma concentrations and AUC of brexpiprazole by approximately 1.2-fold and twofold, respectively, com-pared with administration of brexpiprazole alone. Brexpiprazole dosage should be reduced by 50% when used concurrently with ketoconazole.

Inhibitors of CYP2D6

Concomitant use of brexpiprazole with potent CYP2D6 inhibitors (e.g., fluoxe-tine, paroxetine, quinidine) may result in substantially increased systemic expo-sure to brexpiprazole. Brexpiprazole dosage should be reduced by 50% when used concurrently with potent CYP2D6 inhibitors. This dosage reduction is not neces-sary in patient receiving brexpiprazole for adjunctive treatment of major depres-sive disorder because CYP considerations have been taken into account for the general dosage recommendations. In patients taking moderate or potent CYP3A4 inhibitors (e.g., clarithromycin, fluconazole, itraconazole) *and* moderate or potent CYP2D6 inhibitors (e.g., duloxetine, paroxetine, quinidine), brexpiprazole dos-age should be reduced to 25% of the usual dosage. Brexpiprazole dosage should be increased back to the original dosage when the CYP2D6 and CYP3A4 inhibitors are discontinued. (See Hepatic Microsomal Enzyme Considerations under Dos-age and Administration.)

Quinidine

Concomitant administration of quinidine, a potent CYP2D6 inhibitor, and brex-piprazole (single 2-mg dose) increased peak plasma concentration and AUC of brexpiprazole by approximately 1.1- and 1.9-fold, respectively, compared with administration of brexpiprazole alone. Except when used in the adjunctive treat-ment of major depressive disorder, brexpiprazole dosage should be reduced by 50% when used concurrently with quinidine.

Inducers of CYP3A4

Concomitant use of brexpiprazole with potent CYP3A4 inducers (e.g., rifampin, St. John's wort [*Hypericum perforatum*]) may result in substantially decreased sys-temic exposure of brexpiprazole. The usual brexpiprazole dosage should there-fore be doubled over 1–2 weeks during concurrent therapy with potent CYP3A4 inducers; further dosage adjustment should be based on clinical response. If the potent CYP3A4 inducer is discontinued, the brexpiprazole dosage should be reduced back to the original dosage over 1–2 weeks. (See Hepatic Microsomal Enzyme Considerations under Dosage and Administration.)

Rifampin

Concomitant administration of rifampin, a potent CYP3A4 inducer, and brexpiprazole (single 4-mg dose) decreased peak serum concentration and AUC of brexpiprazole by 40 and 73%, respectively. Brexpiprazole dosage should be doubled when used concomitantly with potent CYP3A4 inducers. (See Hepatic Microsomal Enzyme Considerations under Dosage and Administration.)

● *Drugs Metabolized by Hepatic Microsomal Enzymes*

The manufacturer states that no dosage adjustments are necessary if brexpiprazole is used concomitantly with substrates of CYP isoenzymes 3A4, 2B6, or 2D6.

Bupropion

Concomitant administration of brexpiprazole (2 mg daily for 11 days) with the CYP2B6 substrate bupropion did not substantially affect the pharmacokinetics of bupropion.

Dextromethorphan

Concomitant administration of brexpiprazole (2 mg daily for 11 days) with the CYP2D6 substrate dextromethorphan did not substantially affect the metabolism of dextromethorphan.

Lovastatin

Concomitant administration of brexpiprazole (2 mg daily for 11 days) with the CYP3A4 substrate lovastatin did not substantially affect the pharmacokinetics of lovastatin.

● *Drugs Affecting Gastric pH*

Concomitant administration of brexpiprazole (single 4-mg dose) with omeprazole did not have a clinically important effect on the pharmacokinetics of brexpiprazole.

Drugs that increase gastric pH (e.g., antacids, histamine H_2-receptor antagonists, proton-pump inhibitors) are not expected to substantially affect the absorption of brexpiprazole following oral administration; therefore, dosage adjustment of brexpiprazole is not necessary during concomitant use of such drugs.

● *Hypotensive Agents*

Because patients receiving brexpiprazole are at increased risk of orthostatic hypotension and syncope, monitoring of orthostatic vital signs is recommended in patients concomitantly receiving antihypertensive agents. (See Orthostatic Hypotension and Syncope under Cautions and also see Advice to Patients.)

● *Protein-bound Drugs*

Based on the results of in vitro studies, brexpiprazole protein binding does not appear to be affected by concurrent administration of other highly protein-bound drugs such as diazepam, digitoxin (no longer commercially available in the US), or warfarin. Therefore, clinically important drug interactions based on protein binding displacement appear to be unlikely with brexpiprazole.

● *Anticholinergic Agents*

Potential pharmacologic interaction (possible disruption of body temperature regulation); brexpiprazole should be used with caution in patients concurrently receiving drugs with anticholinergic activity. (See Body Temperature Dysregulation under Cautions.)

● *Fexofenadine*

Concomitant administration of brexpiprazole (2 mg daily for 11 days) with the P-gp substrate fexofenadine did not affect the pharmacokinetics of fexofenadine. No dosage adjustment is necessary when brexpiprazole is used concomitantly with fexofenadine.

● *Rosuvastatin*

Concomitant administration of brexpiprazole (2 mg daily for 11 days) with the BCRP substrate rosuvastatin did not affect the pharmacokinetics of rosuvastatin. No dosage adjustment is necessary when brexpiprazole is used concomitantly with rosuvastatin.

● *Ticlopidine*

Concomitant administration of brexpiprazole (single 2-mg dose) with the potent CYP2B6 inhibitor ticlopidine did not affect the pharmacokinetics of brexpiprazole. No dosage adjustment is necessary when brexpiprazole is used concomitantly with ticlopidine or other CYP2B6 inhibitors.

DESCRIPTION

Brexpiprazole is considered an atypical or second-generation antipsychotic agent; the drug is structurally similar to aripiprazole. The exact mechanism of action of brexpiprazole in major depressive disorder and schizophrenia has not been fully elucidated but is thought to be mediated through a combination of partial agonist activity at dopamine type 2 (D_2) and serotonin type 1A (5-HT_{1A}) receptors and antagonist activity at serotonin type 2A (5-HT_{2A}) receptors.

Brexpiprazole, like aripiprazole, differs from many other atypical antipsychotic agents (which primarily antagonize D_2 receptors) because it is a D_2 partial agonist; these drugs also are partial agonists at 5-HT_{1A} receptors and antagonists at 5-HT_{2A} receptors. Compared with aripiprazole, brexpiprazole appears to have lower intrinsic activity at D_2 receptors and higher activity at 5-HT_{1A} and 5-HT_{1B} receptors and demonstrates stronger antagonism at 5-HT_{2A} receptors. Brexpiprazole also is a partial agonist at D_3 receptors and an antagonist at 5-HT_{2B}, 5-HT_7, and α_{1A}-, α_{1B}-, α_{1D}-, and α_{2C}-adrenergic receptors. It has been suggested that the lower activity of brexpiprazole compared with aripiprazole at D_2 receptors may reduce the potential for certain D_2 partial agonist-mediated adverse effects (e.g., akathisia, insomnia, restlessness, nausea). In addition, brexpiprazole exhibits moderate affinity for histamine (H_1) receptors, which are associated with sedation, and very low affinity for muscarinic (M_1) receptors.

Following oral administration of brexpiprazole tablets, peak plasma concentrations of the drug occur within 4 hours. Administration of the tablets with a high-fat meal does not substantially affect peak plasma concentration or systemic exposure of brexpiprazole. The absolute oral bioavailability of brexpiprazole tablets is 95%. Steady-state plasma concentrations of the drug are achieved within 10–12 days. Higher concentrations of brexpiprazole have been observed in cytochrome P-450 (CYP) isoenzyme 2D6 poor metabolizers compared with CYP2D6 extensive metabolizers. (See Hepatic Microsomal Enzyme Considerations under Dosage and Administration: Special Populations.) Brexpiprazole has a large volume of distribution, which suggests extravascular distribution, and the drug is highly bound (greater than 99%) to plasma proteins (albumin and α_1-acid glycoprotein). The drug is extensively metabolized, principally by CYP3A4 and CYP2D6, to its principal metabolite, DM-3411. DM-3411 does not appear to contribute to the therapeutic effects of brexpiprazole. The elimination half-lives of brexpiprazole and DM-3411 are approximately 91 and 86 hours, respectively. Following administration of a single radiolabeled dose of brexpiprazole, approximately 46 and 25% of the dose is recovered in feces and urine (approximately 14% and less than 1% excreted unchanged), respectively.

ADVICE TO PATIENTS

Importance of advising patients and/or caregivers to read the patient information (medication guide).

Importance of advising patients that brexpiprazole tablets may be taken with or without food. Importance of also advising patients of the importance of following dosage escalation instructions.

Importance of advising patients and caregivers that geriatric patients with dementia-related psychosis treated with antipsychotic agents are at an increased risk of death. Patients and caregivers also should be informed that brexpiprazole is *not* approved for treating geriatric patients with dementia-related psychosis.

Risk of suicidal thoughts and behaviors; importance of patients, family, and caregivers being alert to and immediately reporting emergence of suicidality, especially during the first few months of therapy or during periods of dosage adjustment. (See Suicidal Thoughts and Behaviors in Children, Adolescents, and Young Adults under Cautions.)

Importance of informing patients and caregivers about the risk of neuroleptic malignant syndrome (NMS); importance of immediately contacting clinician or seeking emergency medical attention if signs and symptoms of this rare but potentially life-threatening syndrome develop (e.g., high fever, muscle stiffness, sweating, fast or irregular heart beat, change in blood pressure, confusion, kidney damage).

Importance of advising patients about the signs and symptoms of tardive dyskinesia. Importance of contacting a healthcare professional if abnormal muscle movements occur.

Importance of informing patients and caregivers about the risk of metabolic changes (e.g., hyperglycemia and diabetes mellitus, dyslipidemia, weight gain) with brexpiprazole and the need for specific monitoring for such changes during therapy. Importance of patients and caregivers being aware of the symptoms of hyperglycemia (e.g., increased thirst, increased urination, increased appetite, weakness) and monitoring all patients receiving brexpiprazole for these symptoms. Importance of informing patients who are diagnosed with diabetes or those with risk factors for diabetes (e.g., obesity, family history of diabetes) that they should have their blood glucose monitored at the beginning of and periodically during brexpiprazole therapy. Importance of informing patients that clinical monitoring of weight is recommended during brexpiprazole therapy.

Risk of pathological gambling and other compulsive behaviors. Importance of advising patients and caregivers of the possibility that they may experience compulsive urges to shop, intense urges to gamble, compulsive sexual urges, binge eating and/or other compulsive urges and the inability to control these urges during brexpiprazole therapy. In some cases, but not all, the urges reportedly stopped when the dosage was reduced or the drug was discontinued.

Risk of leukopenia, neutropenia, and agranulocytosis. Importance of advising patients with a preexisting low leukocyte count or a history of drug-induced leukopenia/neutropenia that they should have their complete blood cell (CBC) count monitored during brexpiprazole therapy.

Importance of informing patients about the risk of orthostatic hypotension and syncope, especially when initiating or reinitiating treatment or increasing the dosage.

Importance of avoiding overheating or dehydration.

Because somnolence and impairment of judgment, thinking, or motor skills may be associated with brexpiprazole, patients should be cautioned about performing activities requiring mental alertness, such as driving or operating hazardous machinery, while taking brexpiprazole until they gain experience with the drug's effects.

Importance of informing clinicians of existing or contemplated concomitant therapy, including prescription and OTC drugs or herbal supplements (see Drug Interactions), as well as any concomitant illnesses (e.g., cardiovascular disease, diabetes mellitus, seizures).

Importance of women informing clinicians if they are or plan to become pregnant or plan to breast-feed. Importance of clinicians informing patients about the benefits and risks of taking antipsychotics during pregnancy, and encouraging enrollment in the pregnancy registry (see Pregnancy under Cautions). Importance of advising patients not to stop taking brexpiprazole if they become pregnant without consulting their clinician; abruptly stopping antipsychotic agents may cause complications.

Importance of informing patients of other important precautionary information. (See Cautions.)

PREPARATIONS

Excipients in commercially available drug preparations may have clinically important effects in some individuals; consult specific product labeling for details.

Brexpiprazole

Oral		
Tablets	0.25 mg	**Rexulti®**, Otsuka (also promoted by Lundbeck)
	0.5 mg	**Rexulti®**, Otsuka (also promoted by Lundbeck)
	1 mg	**Rexulti®**, Otsuka (also promoted by Lundbeck)
	2 mg	**Rexulti®**, Otsuka (also promoted by Lundbeck)
	3 mg	**Rexulti®**, Otsuka (also promoted by Lundbeck)
	4 mg	**Rexulti®**, Otsuka (also promoted by Lundbeck)

Selected Revisions October 18, 2021, © Copyright, December 8, 2016, American Society of Health-System Pharmacists, Inc.

Cariprazine Hydrochloride

28:16.08.04 • ATYPICAL ANTIPSYCHOTICS

■ Cariprazine hydrochloride is considered an atypical or second-generation antipsychotic agent.

USES

● Schizophrenia

Cariprazine hydrochloride is used for the treatment of schizophrenia. Schizophrenia is a chronic major psychotic disorder that frequently has devastating effects on various aspects of the patient's life and is associated with an increased risk of suicide and increased overall mortality. The principal manifestations of schizophrenia usually are described in terms of positive, negative, and cognitive symptoms. Positive (i.e., psychotic) symptoms include hallucinations and delusions, while negative symptoms include decreases in emotional expression, initiation of goal-directed behavior (avolition), speech productivity (alogia), ability to experience pleasure from external stimuli (anhedonia), and apparent interest in social interactions (asociality). Cognitive symptoms include impairments in attention, concentration, and memory. Diagnostic criteria for schizophrenia also may include disorganized speech (e.g., frequent derailment or incoherence) or grossly disorganized or catatonic behavior.

Short-term efficacy of cariprazine monotherapy in the treatment of schizophrenia has been established in 3 randomized, multicenter, double-blind, placebo-controlled studies of 6 weeks' duration (studies 1, 2, and 3) in adults who met DSM-IV-TR criteria for schizophrenia and were experiencing an acute exacerbation of psychotic symptoms. The primary and secondary efficacy end points in these studies were the change from baseline to week 6 on the Positive and Negative Syndrome Scale (PANSS) total score and the Clinical Global Impressions-Severity (CGI-S) score, respectively. Studies 1 and 2 included an active control arm (risperidone and aripiprazole, respectively) to assess assay sensitivity. Study 1 evaluated 3 fixed dosages of cariprazine (1.5, 3, or 4.5 mg daily), study 2 evaluated 2 fixed dosages of cariprazine (3 or 6 mg daily), and study 3 evaluated flexible dosages of cariprazine in the range of 3–6 or 6–9 mg daily. In all 3 studies, cariprazine was found to be more effective than placebo in improving the PANSS total score and CGI-S score at week 6. Antipsychotic efficacy was demonstrated at cariprazine dosages ranging from 1.5–9 mg daily, and a modest dose-response relationship for efficacy was observed. However, there was a dose-related increase in certain adverse effects, particularly at dosages above 6 mg daily; therefore, the manufacturer states that the maximum recommended dosage of cariprazine for the treatment of schizophrenia is 6 mg daily. An examination of population subgroups did not reveal any clear evidence of differential responsiveness to the drug based on age (there were few patients over 55 years of age), gender, or race.

Efficacy and safety of cariprazine in the maintenance treatment of schizophrenia have been established in a randomized withdrawal study in adults with schizophrenia whose disease was clinically stable following 20 weeks of open-label cariprazine therapy at dosages of 3–9 mg daily. Patients were randomized to either continue cariprazine at their achieved stable dosage or to receive placebo for up to 72 weeks. The primary endpoint was time to relapse during the double-blind treatment phase. Patients continuing cariprazine therapy had a substantially longer time to relapse compared with those who were switched to placebo. Although efficacy of cariprazine was demonstrated at dosages ranging from 3 to 9 mg daily, dose-related increases in certain adverse effects were observed, particularly at dosages above 6 mg daily. Therefore, the maximum recommended dosage of cariprazine for the treatment of schizophrenia is 6 mg daily. (See Dosage under Dosage and Administration.)

Antipsychotic therapy is integral to the management of patients with schizophrenia, both for management of acute psychotic symptoms and for maintenance treatment to prevent symptom recurrence. The American Psychiatric Association (APA) and other experts consider antipsychotic agents (i.e., first- and second-generation antipsychotic agents) to be first-line drugs for the management of schizophrenia (including first psychotic episodes). The APA states that, with the possible exception of clozapine for the management of treatment-resistant symptoms, there currently is no definitive evidence that one antipsychotic agent will have superior efficacy compared with another agent, although meaningful differences

in response may be observed in individual patients. Therefore, initial choice of an antipsychotic agent should be individualized, and generally be made in the context of shared decision-making, taking into consideration multiple patient- and drug-related factors, including adverse effect profiles, concurrent medical conditions or risk factors, potential for drug interactions, and potential pharmacogenomic considerations, as well as the patient's preferences, prior responses to treatment, available formulations, and cost. Patient response and tolerance to antipsychotic agents are variable, and patients who do not respond to or tolerate one drug may be successfully treated with another drug with different receptor binding or adverse effect profile.

The APA recommends that patients with schizophrenia whose symptoms have improved with an antipsychotic agent continue to receive such therapy. The APA also suggests that patients whose symptoms have improved with an antipsychotic agent continue to be treated with the same antipsychotic agent; however, some circumstances (e.g., patient preferences, drug availability, adverse effects) may necessitate a change in antipsychotic agent. Drug therapy should be used as part of a comprehensive, patient-centered treatment plan that includes evidence-based nonpharmacologic and pharmacologic treatments for schizophrenia. Clinicians may consult APA's Practice Guideline for the Treatment of Patients with Schizophrenia (available at https://psychiatryonline.org/doi/book/10.1176/appi.books.9780890424841) for additional information on the treatment of schizophrenia.

For additional information on the symptomatic management of schizophrenia, including treatment recommendations, see Schizophrenia and Other Psychotic Disorders under Uses: Psychotic Disorders, in the Phenothiazines General Statement 28:16.08.24.

● Bipolar Disorder

Manic or Mixed Episodes associated with Bipolar Disorder

Cariprazine hydrochloride is used for the acute treatment of manic or mixed episodes associated with bipolar I disorder.

Efficacy of cariprazine in the acute treatment of bipolar mania was established in 3 double-blind, placebo-controlled studies of 3 weeks' duration (studies 1, 2, and 3) in adults who met DSM-IV-TR criteria for bipolar I disorder with manic or mixed episodes with or without psychotic features. The principal rating instrument used for assessing psychiatric signs and symptoms in these studies was the Young Mania Rating Scale (YMRS), an 11-item clinician-rated scale traditionally used to assess the degree of manic symptomatology in a range from 0 (no manic features) to 60 (maximum score). The main secondary rating instrument used in these trials was the CGI-S scale. The primary and secondary end points in these studies was the change from baseline to the end of week 3 on the YMRS and the CGI-S scores, respectively.

Study 1 evaluated flexible dosages of cariprazine in the ranges of 3–6 and 6–12 mg daily; studies 2 and 3 evaluated flexible dosages of cariprazine in the range of 3–12 mg daily. In all 3 studies, cariprazine was found to be more effective than placebo on the primary and secondary end points. Efficacy was demonstrated at daily cariprazine dosages ranging from 3–12 mg; however, no additional benefit was demonstrated at dosages above 6 mg daily and there was a dose-related increase in certain adverse effects. Therefore, the maximum recommended dosage of cariprazine in the acute treatment of manic or mixed episodes associated with bipolar I disorder is 6 mg daily. An examination of population subgroups did not reveal any clear evidence of differential responsiveness to the drug based on age (there were few patients over 55 years of age), gender, or race.

Depressive Episodes associated with Bipolar Disorder

Cariprazine hydrochloride is used for the treatment of depressive episodes associated with bipolar I disorder (bipolar depression).

Efficacy of cariprazine in the treatment of bipolar depression was established in 3 placebo-controlled studies of at least 6 weeks' duration (studies 7, 8, and 9) in adults with depressive episodes associated with bipolar I disorder according to DSM-IV-TR or DSM-5 criteria. The primary endpoint in each study was change from baseline in Montgomery-Asberg Depression Rating Scale (MADRS) total score at the end of week 6. The secondary endpoint was change from baseline to week 6 in CGI-S. In all 3 studies, cariprazine 1.5 mg daily was found to be superior to placebo in reduction of MADRS total scores at the end of week 6. In one of the studies, cariprazine 3 mg daily also was superior to placebo in reduction of MADRS total score at the end of week 6. In addition, cariprazine 1.5 mg daily substantially improved CGI-S at the end of week 6 compared with placebo in

2 of the studies. An examination of population subgroups did not reveal any clear evidence of differential responsiveness to the drug based on age (there were few patients over 55 years of age), gender, or race.

DOSAGE AND ADMINISTRATION

● Administration

Cariprazine hydrochloride is commercially available as capsules, which are administered orally once daily without regard to meals. (See Description.)

Patients receiving cariprazine should be monitored for possible worsening of depression and emergence of suicidal thoughts or behaviors, especially at the beginning of therapy or during periods of dosage adjustments. (See Suicidal Thoughts and Behaviors in Children, Adolescents, and Young Adults under Cautions.)

● Dosage

Dosage of cariprazine hydrochloride is expressed in terms of cariprazine.

Because of the long half-life of cariprazine and its active metabolites, changes in dosage will not be fully reflected in plasma concentrations for several weeks (see Description). Therefore, patients receiving the drug should be monitored for adverse effects and clinical response for several weeks after initiation of therapy and after each dosage change. In addition, plasma concentrations of cariprazine and its active metabolites may not be immediately reflected in patients' clinical symptoms following discontinuance of the drug. Plasma concentrations of cariprazine and its active metabolites will decrease by 50% in approximately 1 week.

There are no systematically collected data to specifically address switching patients from cariprazine to other antipsychotic agents or concerning concomitant administration of cariprazine with other antipsychotic agents.

Schizophrenia

For the management of schizophrenia in adults, the recommended dosage range of cariprazine is 1.5–6 mg orally once daily. Therapy should be initiated at 1.5 mg once daily and may be increased to 3 mg once daily on day 2. Based on clinical response and tolerability, further dosage adjustments can be made in increments of 1.5 or 3 mg once daily. The maximum recommended dosage of cariprazine is 6 mg daily. In short-term controlled studies, cariprazine dosages exceeding 6 mg daily did not provide increased efficacy sufficient to outweigh the risk of dose-related adverse effects.

In patients with schizophrenia whose symptoms have improved with an antipsychotic agent, continued treatment (i.e., maintenance therapy) with an antipsychotic agent is recommended to reduce the risk of relapse. The APA suggests that such patients continue to be treated with the same antipsychotic agent that was effective during acute treatment. Some experts have recommended maintenance antipsychotic therapy for at least 1–2 years after the first psychotic episode and for 2–5 years or longer following recurrent episodes. Indefinite maintenance antipsychotic treatment may be necessary in many cases; however, the benefits and risks of continued antipsychotic therapy should be assessed periodically in the context of shared decision-making, taking into consideration each patient's risk of relapse, drug-associated adverse effects, course of disease, and specific goals and needs.

Bipolar Disorder

Manic or Mixed Episodes associated with Bipolar Disorder

For the acute treatment of manic or mixed episodes associated with bipolar I disorder in adults, the recommended dosage range of cariprazine is 3–6 mg orally once daily. Therapy should be initiated at 1.5 mg once daily and increased to 3 mg once daily on day 2. Based on clinical response and tolerability, further dosage adjustments can be made in increments of 1.5 or 3 mg once daily. The maximum recommended dosage of cariprazine for the treatment of manic or mixed episodes associated with bipolar disorder is 6 mg daily. In short-term controlled studies, cariprazine dosages exceeding 6 mg daily did not provide increased efficacy sufficient to outweigh the risk of dose-related adverse effects.

Depressive Episodes associated with Bipolar Disorder

For the treatment of depressive episodes associated with bipolar I disorder (bipolar depression) in adults, the recommended dosage of cariprazine is 1.5 or 3 mg

orally once daily. Therapy should be initiated at 1.5 mg once daily and, depending on clinical response and tolerability, dosage may be increased to 3 mg once daily on day 15. The maximum recommended dosage of cariprazine for the treatment of bipolar depression is 3 mg daily.

● Special Populations

Dosage adjustment is not necessary in patients with mild to moderate renal impairment (creatinine clearance of 30 mL/minute or more). Cariprazine has not been studied in patients with severe renal impairment (creatinine clearance less than 30 mL/minute); use of the drug is not recommended in this patient population. (See Renal Impairment under Cautions.)

Dosage adjustment is not necessary in patients with mild to moderate hepatic impairment (Child-Pugh score 5–9). Cariprazine is not recommended in patients with severe hepatic impairment (Child-Pugh score 10–15); the drug has not been studied in this patient population. (See Hepatic Impairment under Cautions.)

In geriatric patients, the manufacturer states that dosage selection of cariprazine should be cautious, usually starting at the lower end of the recommended dosage range, reflecting the greater frequency of decreased hepatic, renal, and cardiac function; concomitant illnesses; and other drug therapy in this population. (See Geriatric Use under Cautions.)

Dosage adjustment is not required based on gender, race, or smoking status.

Drugs Affecting Hepatic Microsomal Enzymes

In patients receiving a stable dosage of cariprazine and in whom a potent inhibitor of cytochrome P-450 (CYP) isoenzyme 3A4 (e.g., itraconazole, ketoconazole) will be added to therapy, cariprazine dosage should be reduced to 50% of the current dosage. For patients taking 4.5 mg of cariprazine daily, the dosage should be reduced to 1.5 or 3 mg daily; for patients taking 1.5 mg daily, the dosing frequency should be reduced to every other day. Similarly, if cariprazine is initiated in patients already receiving a potent CYP3A4 inhibitor, the recommended initial dosage of cariprazine is 1.5 mg daily on days 1 and 3 (skipping day 2). From day 4 onward, the cariprazine dosage should be 1.5 mg daily; then, the dosage should be subsequently increased up to a maximum dosage of 3 mg daily. When the potent CYP3A4 inhibitor is withdrawn from combined therapy, the cariprazine dosage may need to be increased. (See Drugs Affecting Hepatic Microsomal Enzymes under Drug Interactions.)

Concomitant use of cariprazine and CYP3A4 inducers has not been evaluated and is not recommended. (See Drugs Affecting Hepatic Microsomal Enzymes under Drug Interactions.)

Pharmacogenomics and CYP2D6 Poor Metabolizer Phenotype

CYP2D6 poor metabolizer phenotype does not have a clinically important effect on the pharmacokinetics of cariprazine and its metabolites; therefore, dosage adjustment is unlikely to be necessary in patients who are CYP2D6 poor metabolizers.

CAUTIONS

● Contraindications

Known hypersensitivity to cariprazine. Hypersensitivity reactions, including rash, pruritus, urticaria, and manifestations of possible angioedema (e.g., swollen tongue, lip swelling, facial edema and swelling, pharyngeal edema), have been reported in patients receiving cariprazine.

● Warnings/Precautions

Warnings

Increased Mortality in Geriatric Patients with Dementia-related Psychosis

Geriatric patients with dementia-related psychosis treated with antipsychotic drugs are at an increased risk of death. Analyses of 17 placebo-controlled trials (modal duration of 10 weeks) revealed a 1.6- to 1.7-fold increase in mortality among geriatric patients who were mainly receiving atypical antipsychotic drugs (i.e., aripiprazole, olanzapine, quetiapine, risperidone) compared with that observed in patients receiving placebo. Over the course of a typical 10-week controlled trial, the rate of death in drug-treated patients was about 4.5% compared with a rate of about 2.6% in the placebo group. Although the causes of death were varied, most of the deaths appeared to be either cardiovascular (e.g., heart failure, sudden death) or infectious (e.g., pneumonia) in nature. The manufacturer states that cariprazine is *not* approved for the treatment of patients with dementia-related psychosis. (See Adverse Cerebrovascular Events, including Stroke, in Geriatric Patients with Dementia-related Psychosis and also see Geriatric Use under Cautions.)

Suicidal Thoughts and Behaviors in Children, Adolescents, and Young Adults

Antidepressants may increase the risk of suicidal thoughts and behaviors in children, adolescents, and young adults. Pooled analyses of short-term, placebo-controlled studies of antidepressants (i.e., selective serotonin-reuptake inhibitors [SSRIs] and other antidepressants) have shown an increased risk of suicidal thoughts and behaviors in children, adolescents, and young adults (24 years of age or younger) receiving antidepressants for major depressive disorder and other indications. Although the risk varied considerably between drugs, an increased risk was identified for most antidepressants studied. Differences in absolute risk of suicidal thoughts and behaviors were seen across the different indications, with the highest incidence in patients with major depressive disorder. An increased risk of suicidal thoughts and behaviors was not demonstrated with antidepressants compared with placebo in adults older than 24 years of age, and a reduced risk was observed in adults 65 years of age or older. Because the studies analyzed were short-term, it is not known whether the increased risk of suicidal thoughts or behaviors in such patients continues with longer-term antidepressant treatment (i.e., beyond 4 months). However, substantial evidence from placebo-controlled maintenance studies in adults with major depressive disorder indicates that antidepressants delay the recurrence of depression. Safety and efficacy of cariprazine have not been established in pediatric patients.

All patients being treated with antidepressants for any indication should be closely monitored for worsening of depression and emergence of suicidal thoughts and behaviors, particularly during initiation of therapy (i.e., the first few months) and during periods of dosage adjustments. Family members and caregivers of patients being treated with antidepressants also should be advised to monitor patients for changes in behavior and to alert a health-care provider if such changes occur. Consideration should be given to changing the therapeutic regimen or discontinuing therapy in patients whose depression is persistently worse or who are experiencing emergent suicidal thoughts or behaviors.

Other Warnings and Precautions

Adverse Cerebrovascular Events, including Stroke, in Geriatric Patients with Dementia-related Psychosis

An increased incidence of adverse cerebrovascular events (cerebrovascular accidents and transient ischemic attacks), including fatalities, has been observed in geriatric patients with dementia-related psychosis treated with certain atypical antipsychotic agents (aripiprazole, olanzapine, risperidone) in placebo-controlled studies. The manufacturer states that cariprazine is *not* approved for the treatment of patients with dementia-related psychosis. (See Increased Mortality in Geriatric Patients with Dementia-related Psychosis and also see Geriatric Use under Cautions.)

Neuroleptic Malignant Syndrome

Neuroleptic malignant syndrome (NMS), a potentially fatal syndrome characterized by hyperpyrexia, muscle rigidity, delirium, and autonomic instability, has been reported with antipsychotic agents. If NMS is suspected, antipsychotic therapy should be immediately discontinued and intensive symptomatic treatment and monitoring should be provided. (See Advice to Patients.) For additional information on NMS, see Neuroleptic Malignant Syndrome under Cautions: Nervous System Effects, in the Phenothiazines General Statement 28:16.08.24.

Tardive Dyskinesia

Because use of antipsychotic agents, including cariprazine, may be associated with tardive dyskinesia (a syndrome of potentially irreversible, involuntary, dyskinetic movements), cariprazine should be prescribed in a manner that is most likely to minimize the occurrence of this syndrome. Chronic antipsychotic treatment generally should be reserved for patients who suffer from a chronic illness that is known to respond to antipsychotic agents, and for whom alternative, equally effective, but potentially less harmful treatments are not available or appropriate. In patients who do require chronic treatment, the lowest dosage and the shortest duration of treatment producing a satisfactory clinical response should be sought, and the need for continued treatment should be reassessed periodically.

The American Psychiatric Association (APA) currently recommends that patients with schizophrenia who are receiving antipsychotic agents be assessed clinically for abnormal involuntary movements at baseline and at each follow-up visit and that assessment with a structured instrument (e.g., the Abnormal Involuntary Movement Scale [AIMS], Dyskinesia Identification System: Condensed User Scale [DISCUS]) occur at least every 6 months in patients considered at high risk for tardive dyskinesia (including patients older than 55 years of age; women; individuals with a mood disorder, substance use disorder, intellectual disability, or CNS injury; individuals with high cumulative exposure to antipsychotic medications, particularly high-potency dopamine type 2 [D_2] receptor antagonists; and patients who experience acute dystonic reactions, clinically significant parkinsonism, or akathisia) or at least every 12 months in other patients as well as if a new onset or exacerbation of preexisting movements is observed at any follow-up visit. In some jurisdictions, the frequency of monitoring for involuntary movements in individuals receiving antipsychotic agents may also be subject to local regulations.

If signs and symptoms of tardive dyskinesia appear in a cariprazine-treated patient, cariprazine discontinuance should be considered; however, some patients may require continued treatment with the drug despite the presence of the syndrome.

APA recommends that patients who have moderate to severe or disabling tardive dyskinesia associated with antipsychotic therapy be treated with a vesicular monoamine transporter 2 (VMAT2) inhibitor (e.g., deutetrabenazine, valbenazine, tetrabenazine); such treatment may also be considered for patients with mild tardive dyskinesia based on factors such as patient preference, associated impairment, and effect on psychosocial functioning. (See Deutetrabenazine 28:56, Tetrabenazine 28:56, and Valbenazine 28:56.)

For additional information on tardive dyskinesia, see Tardive Dyskinesia under Cautions: Nervous System Effects, in the Phenothiazines General Statement 28:16.08.24.

Late-occurring Adverse Effects

Adverse effects may first appear several weeks after initiation of cariprazine therapy, probably because plasma concentrations of cariprazine and its principal metabolites accumulate over time (see Description). Therefore, the incidence of adverse effects reported with cariprazine in short-term clinical trials may not reflect the incidence after longer-term exposure to the drug. Patients should therefore be monitored for adverse effects, including adverse extrapyramidal effects and akathisia, for several weeks after initiation of cariprazine therapy and after each dosage increase. (See Dosage under Dosage and Administration.)

Metabolic Changes

Atypical antipsychotic agents have been associated with metabolic changes, including hyperglycemia and diabetes mellitus, dyslipidemia, and body weight gain. While all of these drugs produce some metabolic changes, each drug has its own specific risk profile. (See Hyperglycemia and Diabetes Mellitus, see Dyslipidemia, and also see Weight Gain under Cautions.)

Hyperglycemia and Diabetes Mellitus

Hyperglycemia, sometimes severe and associated with ketoacidosis, hyperosmolar coma, or death, has been reported in patients receiving atypical antipsychotic agents. In short-term controlled trials in patients with schizophrenia or bipolar disorder, clinically important differences between cariprazine and placebo in the proportion of patients with shifts from normal or borderline to high fasting glucose concentrations were not observed. In longer-term, open-label studies, 4% of cariprazine-treated patients experienced a shift from normal to elevated (6.5% or higher) glycosylated hemoglobin (hemoglobin A_{1c}; HbA_{1c}) concentrations.

The manufacturer states that patients should undergo fasting blood glucose testing before or soon after initiation of cariprazine and periodically during long-term therapy.

Dyslipidemia

Undesirable changes in lipid parameters have been observed in patients treated with some atypical antipsychotic agents; however, cariprazine generally does not appear to adversely affect the lipid profile in patients receiving short-term therapy with the drug. In short-term, placebo-controlled studies in patients with schizophrenia or bipolar disorder, clinically important differences between cariprazine and placebo in the proportion of patients with shifts in fasting total cholesterol, low-density lipoprotein (LDL)-cholesterol, high-density lipoprotein (HDL)-cholesterol, and triglyceride concentrations were not observed.

The manufacturer recommends baseline and periodic follow-up lipid evaluations in patients receiving cariprazine therapy.

Weight Gain

Weight gain has been observed with atypical antipsychotic therapy, including cariprazine. Mean weight gain during short-term studies in patients receiving cariprazine for schizophrenia or bipolar mania was 0.5–1 kg compared with 0.2–0.3 kg in those receiving placebo. In the 6-week schizophrenia studies, 8 and 17% of patients receiving cariprazine daily dosages of 1.5–6 mg and 9–12 mg, respectively, gained 7% or more of their baseline body weight compared with 5% of placebo recipients. In longer-term, uncontrolled trials with cariprazine in schizophrenia, mean weight gain from baseline at 12, 24, and 48 weeks was 1.2, 1.7, and 2.5 kg, respectively.

The manufacturer recommends baseline and frequent monitoring of weight in patients receiving cariprazine.

Leukopenia, Neutropenia, and Agranulocytosis

Leukopenia and neutropenia have been reported with antipsychotic agents, including cariprazine. Agranulocytosis (including fatal cases) also has been reported with other antipsychotic agents.

Possible risk factors for leukopenia and neutropenia include preexisting low leukocyte or absolute neutrophil count (ANC) and a history of drug-induced leukopenia or neutropenia. Patients with a preexisting low leukocyte count or a history of drug-induced leukopenia or neutropenia should have their complete blood count monitored frequently during the first few months of therapy. Cariprazine should be discontinued at the first sign of a clinically important decline in leukocyte count in the absence of other causative factors.

Patients with neutropenia should be carefully monitored for fever or other signs or symptoms of infection and promptly treated if such signs and symptoms occur. In patients with severe neutropenia (ANC less than 1000/mm^3), cariprazine should be discontinued and the leukocyte count monitored until recovery occurs. Lithium reportedly has been used successfully in the treatment of several cases of leukopenia associated with aripiprazole, clozapine, and some other drugs; however, further clinical experience is needed to confirm these anecdotal findings.

Orthostatic Hypotension and Syncope

Atypical antipsychotic agents can cause orthostatic hypotension and syncope. The risk is usually the greatest during initial dosage titration and when dosage is increased. In clinical trials with cariprazine, the incidence of symptomatic orthostatic hypotension was infrequent and was not higher in cariprazine-treated patients compared with those receiving placebo; syncope was not observed in patients receiving the drug.

Orthostatic vital signs should be monitored in patients receiving cariprazine who are susceptible to hypotension (e.g., geriatric patients, patients with dehydration or hypovolemia, patients concomitantly receiving antihypertensive therapy), patients with cardiovascular disease (e.g., history of myocardial infarction, ischemic heart disease, heart failure, or conduction abnormalities), and patients with cerebrovascular disease.

Falls

Cariprazine therapy may cause somnolence, postural hypotension, and motor and sensory instability, which may lead to falls; as a consequence, fractures or other injuries may occur. For patients with diseases, conditions, or other drugs that could exacerbate these effects, fall risk assessments should be completed when initiating antipsychotic treatment and periodically during long-term antipsychotic therapy.

Seizures

As with other antipsychotic agents, cariprazine may cause seizures. The risk of seizures is greatest in patients with a history of seizures or with conditions that lower the seizure threshold; such conditions may be more prevalent in older patients.

Cognitive and Motor Impairment

Like other antipsychotic agents, cariprazine potentially may impair judgment, thinking, or motor skills. In short-term schizophrenia trials, somnolence (including hypersomnia and sedation) was reported in 7% of patients receiving cariprazine compared with 6% of patients receiving placebo. In short-term bipolar mania clinical trials, somnolence was reported in 8% of patients receiving cariprazine compared with 4% of placebo recipients. (See Advice to Patients.)

Body Temperature Dysregulation

Disruption of the body's ability to reduce core body temperature has been attributed to antipsychotic agents. The manufacturer recommends appropriate caution when cariprazine is used in patients who will be experiencing conditions that may contribute to an elevation in core body temperature (e.g., strenuous exercise, extreme heat, dehydration, concomitant use of agents with anticholinergic activity). (See Advice to Patients.)

Dysphagia

Esophageal dysmotility and aspiration have been associated with the use of antipsychotic agents. Dysphagia has been reported in patients receiving cariprazine. Cariprazine and other antipsychotic agents should be used with caution in patients at risk for aspiration.

Specific Populations

Pregnancy

There are no adequate and well-controlled studies to date of cariprazine use in pregnant women. The principal active metabolite of cariprazine, didesmethyl cariprazine (DDCAR), has been detected in adult patients up to 12 weeks following discontinuance of cariprazine. Based on animal findings, cariprazine may cause fetal harm. Fetal developmental toxicity (including reduced body weight, skeletal and external malformations, lower pup survival, and developmental delays) was observed when cariprazine was administered to pregnant rats at dosages 0.2–3.5 times the maximum recommended human dosage.

Neonates exposed to antipsychotic agents during the third trimester of pregnancy are at risk for extrapyramidal and/or withdrawal symptoms following delivery. Symptoms reported to date have included agitation, hypertonia, hypotonia, tardive dyskinetic-like symptoms, tremor, somnolence, respiratory distress, and feeding disorder. Neonates exhibiting such symptoms should be monitored. The complications have varied in severity; some neonates recovered within hours to days without specific treatment while others have required intensive care unit support and prolonged hospitalization.

National Pregnancy Registry for Atypical Antipsychotics: 866-961-2388 and http://womensmentalhealth.org/clinical-and-research-programs/pregnancyregistry/atypicalantipsychotic/.

Lactation

It is not known whether cariprazine is distributed into milk in humans. The drug is distributed into milk in rats. The effects of the drug on breastfed infants or on milk production are not known. The benefits of cariprazine therapy to the woman as well as the benefits of breast-feeding to the infant should be weighed against the potential risk of infant exposure to the drug or from the underlying maternal condition.

Pediatric Use

Safety and effectiveness of cariprazine in pediatric patients have not been established. The manufacturer states that pediatric clinical studies with cariprazine have not been conducted to date.

Antidepressants increased the risk of suicidal thoughts and behaviors in pediatric patients. (See Suicidal Thoughts and Behaviors in Children, Adolescents, and Young Adults under Cautions.)

Geriatric Use

Clinical trial experience with cariprazine in the treatment of schizophrenia and bipolar mania did not include sufficient numbers of patients 65 years of age and older to determine whether geriatric patients respond differently than younger adults.

Age did not have a clinically important effect on the pharmacokinetics of cariprazine and its principal metabolites (desmethyl cariprazine [DCAR] and didesmethyl cariprazine [DDCAR]). The manufacturer states that dosage selection in geriatric patients should be cautious, usually starting at the lower end of the dosage range, reflecting the greater incidence of decreased hepatic, renal, and cardiac function; concomitant illnesses; and other drug therapy in this population.

Geriatric patients with dementia-related psychosis treated with cariprazine are at an increased risk of death compared with those treated with placebo. In addition, an increased incidence of adverse cerebrovascular events (cerebrovascular accidents and transient ischemic attacks), including fatalities, has been observed in geriatric patients with dementia-related psychosis treated with certain atypical antipsychotic agents (aripiprazole, olanzapine, risperidone) in placebo-controlled studies. The manufacturer of cariprazine states that the drug is *not* approved for the treatment of patients with dementia-related psychosis (see Increased Mortality in Geriatric Patients with Dementia-related Psychosis under Cautions). For additional information on the use of antipsychotic agents in the management of dementia-related psychosis, see Geriatric Considerations under Uses: Psychotic Disorders, in the Phenothiazines General Statement 28:16.08.24.

Hepatic Impairment

Following multiple doses of cariprazine in individuals with mild or moderate hepatic impairment (Child-Pugh score 5–9), cariprazine exposure was approximately 25% higher and exposure to the drug's principal active metabolites, DCAR and DDCAR, was approximately 20–30% lower than in individuals with normal hepatic function. Dosage adjustment of cariprazine is not necessary in patients with mild to moderate hepatic impairment.

Cariprazine has not been studied in patients with severe hepatic impairment (Child-Pugh score 10–15), and use of the drug is not recommended in such patients.

Renal Impairment

Cariprazine and its principal active metabolites are minimally excreted in urine. Pharmacokinetic analyses indicate no substantial relationship between clearance of the drug and its metabolites and creatinine clearance. Dosage adjustment is not necessary for patients with mild to moderate renal impairment (creatinine clearance of 30 mL/minute or more). Cariprazine has not been studied in patients with severe renal impairment (creatinine clearance less than 30 mL/minute), and use of the drug is not recommended in such patients.

● Common Adverse Effects

Adverse effects occurring in 5% or more of patients receiving cariprazine for schizophrenia and at a frequency at least twice that reported with placebo in short-term clinical studies include extrapyramidal symptoms (e.g., parkinsonism, dystonia, dyskinesia, tardive dyskinesia) and akathisia.

Adverse effects occurring in 5% or more of patients receiving cariprazine for bipolar mania and at a frequency at least twice that reported with placebo in short-term clinical studies include extrapyramidal symptoms (e.g., parkinsonism, dystonia, dyskinesia, tardive dyskinesia), akathisia, dyspepsia, vomiting, somnolence, and restlessness.

Adverse effects occurring in 5% or more of patients receiving cariprazine for bipolar depression and at a frequency at least twice that reported with placebo in short-term clinical studies include nausea, akathisia, restlessness, and extrapyramidal symptoms.

DRUG INTERACTIONS

Cariprazine is metabolized primarily by cytochrome P-450 (CYP) isoenzyme 3A4 and, to a lesser extent, CYP2D6 to its major active metabolites, desmethyl cariprazine (DCAR) and didesmethyl cariprazine (DDCAR). (See Description.)

In vitro studies indicate that cariprazine and its major active metabolites are not substrates of P-glycoprotein (P-gp), organic anion transport proteins (OATP) 1B1 and 1B3, or breast cancer resistance protein (BCRP).

Based on in vitro studies, cariprazine is not expected to cause clinically important pharmacokinetic drug interactions with substrates of CYP isoenzymes 1A2, 2A6, 2C9, 2C19, 2D6, 2E, or 3A4; OATP1B1 and OATP1B3; BCRP; organic cation transporter (OCT) 2; or organic anion transporters (OAT) 1 and 3.

Cariprazine's major active metabolites possess little or no inhibitory effects on P-gp; however, cariprazine probably inhibits P-gp.

● Drugs Affecting Hepatic Microsomal Enzymes

Clinically important pharmacokinetic interactions with cariprazine and its active metabolites DCAR and DDCAR are possible with drugs that inhibit or induce CYP3A4. CYP2D6 inhibitors are not expected to substantially affect the pharmacokinetics of cariprazine or its active metabolites.

CYP3A4 Inhibitors

Concomitant use of cariprazine with a potent CYP3A4 inhibitor (e.g., itraconazole, ketoconazole) may result in increased systemic exposure to cariprazine and its major active metabolite, DDCAR. Cariprazine dosage should therefore be reduced when used concurrently with a potent CYP3A4 inhibitor. (See Special Populations under Dosage and Administration.)

The effect of moderate CYP3A4 inhibitors on the pharmacokinetics of cariprazine and its metabolites has not been studied to date.

Ketoconazole

Concomitant administration of ketoconazole (400 mg daily; a potent CYP3A4 inhibitor) and cariprazine (0.5 mg daily) increased peak plasma concentrations and AUC of cariprazine by approximately 3.5-fold and fourfold, respectively; increased peak concentrations and AUC of DDCAR by about 1.5-fold; and decreased peak concentrations and AUC of DCAR by about one-third.

CYP3A4 Inducers

CYP3A4 is responsible for the formation and elimination of the active metabolites of cariprazine (see Description). The effect of CYP3A4 inducers on the pharmacokinetics of cariprazine and its active metabolites has not been studied to date, and the net effect is not known. Therefore, concomitant use of cariprazine with a CYP3A4 inducer (e.g., carbamazepine, rifampin) is not recommended.

CYP2D6 Inhibitors

Based on observations in CYP2D6 poor metabolizers, CYP2D6 inhibitors are not likely to substantially affect the pharmacokinetics of cariprazine, DCAR, or DDCAR.

● Anticholinergic Agents

Potential pharmacologic interaction (possible disruption of body temperature regulation); use cariprazine with caution in patients concurrently receiving drugs with anticholinergic activity. (See Body Temperature Dysregulation under Cautions.)

● Hypotensive Agents

The manufacturer states that patients receiving cariprazine may be at increased risk of orthostatic hypotension and syncope. Therefore, monitoring of orthostatic vital signs is recommended in patients receiving cariprazine and antihypertensive agents concomitantly. (See Orthostatic Hypotension and Syncope under Cautions and see also Advice to Patients.)

● Pantoprazole

Concomitant administration of pantoprazole (40 mg daily) and cariprazine (6 mg daily) for 15 days in patients with schizophrenia did not substantially affect the exposure to cariprazine, DCAR, or DDCAR at steady state.

● Smoking

Cariprazine is not a substrate for CYP1A2; therefore, smoking should not alter the pharmacokinetics of the drug. Dosage adjustment of cariprazine in patients who smoke is not necessary.

DESCRIPTION

Cariprazine hydrochloride is considered an atypical or second-generation antipsychotic agent. The exact mechanism of action of cariprazine in schizophrenia and bipolar disorder has not been fully elucidated but may be mediated through a combination of partial agonist activity at central dopamine type 2 (D_2) and serotonin type 1 (5-hydroxytryptamine [5-HT_{1A}]) receptors and antagonist activity at serotonin type 2 (5-HT_{2A}) receptors.

Cariprazine acts as a partial agonist at D_2 and D_3 receptors with high binding affinity and at 5-HT_{1A} receptors in vitro. Cariprazine's partial agonist activity at D_2 receptors is similar to that of aripiprazole (another atypical antipsychotic agent with D_2 partial agonist activity) but cariprazine has shown approximately threefold to tenfold higher binding affinity at D_3 receptors compared with D_2 receptors; the clinical implications of the D_3-receptor selectivity are not known. In addition, cariprazine is a partial agonist at 5-HT_{1A} receptors; an antagonist at 5-HT_{2A} and 5-HT_{2B} receptors; and exhibits moderate to low binding affinity for histamine (H_1) receptors, lower binding affinity for 5-HT_{2C} and α_{1A}-adrenergic receptors than aripiprazole, and no appreciable affinity for muscarinic receptors.

The pharmacologic activity of cariprazine is thought to be mediated by cariprazine and its 2 principal active metabolites, desmethyl cariprazine (DCAR) and didesmethyl cariprazine (DDCAR). DCAR and DDCAR, which pharmacologically are as potent as cariprazine, are present in mean plasma concentrations that are approximately 30 and 400% of cariprazine plasma concentrations at the end of 12 weeks, respectively. Therefore, at steady state, DDCAR is the major active moiety circulating in plasma; in a pharmacokinetic study, DDCAR accounted for about 70% of the total activity after 27 days of dosing.

Following oral administration of cariprazine capsules, peak plasma concentrations of cariprazine occur in approximately 3–6 hours. Administration of a single dose of cariprazine with a high-fat meal does not substantially affect peak plasma concentration or systemic exposure of cariprazine or DCAR. Steady-state mean plasma concentrations of cariprazine and DCAR are achieved within 1–2 weeks. Steady-state plasma concentrations of DDCAR appear to approach steady state within about 4–8 weeks; however, the time varies and some patients did not reach steady-state DDCAR concentrations after 12 weeks of treatment. Cariprazine and its main metabolites are highly bound (91–97%) to plasma proteins. Cariprazine is extensively metabolized by cytochrome P-450 (CYP) isoenzyme 3A4 and, to a lesser extent, by CYP2D6 to DCAR and DDCAR. DCAR is further metabolized to DDCAR by CYP3A4 and CYP2D6; DDCAR is then metabolized by CYP3A4 to a hydroxylated metabolite. Following administration of cariprazine 12.5 mg daily for 27 days, approximately 21% of the daily dose is recovered in urine, with approximately 1.2% of the dose excreted in urine as unchanged cariprazine. The elimination half-lives of cariprazine and DDCAR are estimated to be 2–4 days and approximately 1–3 weeks, respectively. Following discontinuance of cariprazine, mean plasma concentrations of cariprazine and DCAR decrease by 50% in about 1 day and mean plasma concentrations of DDCAR decrease by about 50% in 1 week. CYP2D6 poor metabolizer status does not appear to affect the pharmacokinetics of cariprazine and its metabolites.

ADVICE TO PATIENTS

Importance of advising patients and/or caregivers to read the patient information (medication guide).

Importance of advising patients and caregivers that geriatric patients with dementia-related psychosis treated with antipsychotic agents are at an increased risk of death. Patients and caregivers also should be informed that cariprazine is *not* approved for treating geriatric patients with dementia-related psychosis.

Risk of suicidal thoughts and behaviors; importance of patients, family, and caregivers being alert to and reporting emergence of suicidality, especially during the first few months of therapy or during periods of dosage adjustment. (See Suicidal Thoughts and Behaviors in Children, Adolescents, and Young Adults under Cautions.)

Importance of advising patients that cariprazine hydrochloride capsules can be taken with or without food. Importance of advising patients to follow the dosage titration instructions for the drug.

Importance of informing patients and caregivers about the risk of neuroleptic malignant syndrome (NMS), a rare but potentially life-threatening syndrome that can cause high fever, stiff muscles, confusion, sweating, or changes in respiration, heart rate, or blood pressure. Importance of immediately contacting clinician or seeking emergency medical attention if signs and symptoms of this syndrome develop.

Importance of informing patients of the signs and symptoms of tardive dyskinesia. Importance of advising patients to report any abnormal movements to a healthcare professional.

Importance of informing patients that, because plasma concentrations of cariprazine and its metabolites accumulate over time, adverse effects may not appear until several weeks after the initiation of therapy.

Importance of informing patients and caregivers about the risk of metabolic changes (e.g., hyperglycemia and diabetes mellitus, dyslipidemia, weight gain) with cariprazine and the need for specific monitoring, including blood glucose, lipids, and weight, for such changes during therapy. Importance of patients and caregivers being aware of the symptoms of hyperglycemia and diabetes mellitus (e.g., increased thirst, increased urination, increased appetite, weakness).

Risk of leukopenia/neutropenia. Importance of advising patients with a pre-existing low leukocyte count or a history of drug-induced leukopenia/neutropenia that they should have their complete blood count (CBC) monitored during cariprazine therapy.

Importance of informing patients about the risk of orthostatic hypotension and syncope, especially when initiating or reinitiating treatment or increasing the dosage.

Because somnolence and impairment of judgment, thinking, or motor skills may be associated with cariprazine, patients should be cautioned about performing activities requiring mental alertness, such as driving or operating hazardous machinery, while taking the drug until they gain experience with the drug's effects.

Importance of avoiding overheating or dehydration.

Importance of informing clinicians of existing or contemplated concomitant therapy, including prescription (see Drug Interactions) and OTC drugs or herbal supplements, as well as any concomitant illnesses (e.g., cardiovascular disease, diabetes mellitus, seizures).

Importance of women informing clinicians if they are or plan to become pregnant or plan to breast-feed. Importance of clinicians informing patients about the benefits and risks of taking antipsychotics during pregnancy (see Pregnancy under Cautions). Importance of advising patients not to stop taking cariprazine if they become pregnant without consulting their clinician; abruptly stopping antipsychotic agents may cause complications.

Importance of informing patients of other important precautionary information. (See Cautions.)

PREPARATIONS

Excipients in commercially available drug preparations may have clinically important effects in some individuals; consult specific product labeling for details.

Cariprazine Hydrochloride

Oral			
Capsules		1.5 mg (of cariprazine)	**Vraylar®**, Allergan
		3 mg (of cariprazine)	**Vraylar®**, Allergan
		4.5 mg (of cariprazine)	**Vraylar®**, Allergan
		6 mg (of cariprazine)	**Vraylar®**, Allergan
Titration Pack		1 Capsule, 1.5 mg (of cariprazine) (Vraylar®)	**Vraylar® Titration Pack**, Allergan
		6 Capsules, 3 mg (of cariprazine) (Vraylar®)	

Selected Revisions October 18, 2021, © Copyright, June 12, 2017, American Society of Health-System Pharmacists, Inc.

cloZAPine

28:16.08.04 • ATYPICAL ANTIPSYCHOTICS

■ Clozapine has been referred to as an atypical or second-generation antipsychotic agent.

REMES

FDA approved a shared REMS for clozapine. The REMS may consist of the following: elements to assure safe use and implementation system. See the FDA REMS page (https://www.accessdata.fda.gov/scripts/cder/rems/index.cfm). (See General under Dosage and Administration.)

USES

● *Psychotic Disorders*

Clozapine is used for the symptomatic management of psychotic disorders (e.g., schizophrenia). Drug therapy is integral to the management of acute psychotic episodes in patients with schizophrenia and generally is required for long-term stabilization to sustain symptom remission or control and to minimize the risk of relapse. Antipsychotic agents are the principal class of drugs used for the management of all phases of schizophrenia. Patient response and tolerance to antipsychotic agents are variable, and patients who do not respond to or tolerate one drug may be successfully treated with an agent from a different class or with a different adverse effect profile.

Clozapine has been shown to be an effective, relatively rapid-acting, broad-spectrum antipsychotic agent in both uncontrolled and controlled studies of patients with schizophrenia. In these studies, improvement in manifestations of schizophrenia was based on the results of various psychiatric rating scales, principally the Brief Psychiatric Rating Scale (BPRS) that assesses factors such as anergy, thought disturbance, activation, hostility/suspiciousness, and anxiety/depression. In clinical studies, clozapine improved both positive (florid symptomatology such as hallucinations, conceptual disorganization, and suspiciousness) and negative ("deficit" symptomatology such as emotional withdrawal, motor retardation, blunted affect, and disorientation) manifestations of schizophrenia; conventional (typical) antipsychotic agents appear to have lesser effects on negative manifestations of the disorder. In comparative studies, clozapine was at least as effective as, or more effective than several conventional antipsychotic agents, including chlorpromazine, haloperidol, perphenazine, or trifluoperazine.

Unlike conventional antipsychotic agents, however, clozapine generally does not induce extrapyramidal effects and has not been clearly implicated as a causative agent in tardive dyskinesia.

While the risks of adverse neurologic effects with long-term clozapine therapy remain to be fully elucidated, other adverse effects, including some potentially serious effects (e.g., severe neutropenia, seizures), may occur more frequently with clozapine therapy. Consequently, the manufacturers and most clinicians state that use of clozapine should be reserved for patients with severe disease that fails to respond adequately to other antipsychotic therapy. The American Psychiatric Association (APA) recommends that a trial of clozapine be considered in patients with schizophrenia who fail to respond or experience a partial or suboptimal response to adequate trials of 2 antipsychotic agents (including at least one second-generation [atypical] antipsychotic), in patients with a history of chronic and persistent suicidal ideation and behavior that has not responded to other treatments, and in patients with persistent hostility and aggression.

Treatment-resistant Schizophrenia

Clozapine is used for the management of schizophrenia in severely ill patients who fail to respond adequately to standard antipsychotic therapy. Because of the risk of severe neutropenia and seizures associated with its use, clozapine should be used only in patients who have failed to respond adequately to standard antipsychotic treatment. (See Severe Neutropenia under Cautions: Hematologic Effects and also under Cautions: Precautions and Contraindications.)

Schizophrenia is a major psychotic disorder that frequently has devastating effects on various aspects of the patient's life and carries a high risk of suicide and other life-threatening behaviors. Manifestations of schizophrenia involve multiple psychologic processes, including perception (e.g., hallucinations), ideation, reality testing (e.g., delusions), emotion (e.g., flatness, inappropriate affect), thought processes (e.g., loose associations), behavior (e.g., catatonia, disorganization), attention, concentration, motivation (e.g., avolition, impaired intention and planning), and judgment. The principal manifestations of this disorder usually are described in terms of positive and negative (deficit) symptoms, and more recently, disorganized symptoms. Positive symptoms include hallucinations, delusions, bizarre behavior, hostility, uncooperativeness, and paranoid ideation, while negative symptoms include restricted range and intensity of emotional expression (affective flattening), reduced thought and speech productivity (alogia), anhedonia, apathy, and decreased initiation of goal-directed behavior (avolition). Disorganized symptoms include disorganized speech (thought disorder) and behavior and poor attention.

Evidence from both retrospective and controlled prospective studies indicates that clozapine is effective in many patients who fail to respond adequately to other antipsychotic therapy and/or in whom such therapy produces intolerable adverse effects. In a controlled, comparative study in patients with at least moderately severe schizophrenia whose disease was refractory to at least 3 antipsychotic agents from at least 2 different chemical classes during the past 5 years, an adequate clinical response (a 20% or greater decrease in total BPRS score and either a posttreatment Clinical Global Impressions [CGI] scale rating of mildly ill or a posttreatment BPRS score of 35 or less) was noted after 1–6 weeks of therapy in 30% of patients receiving clozapine (mean maximum dosage exceeding 600 mg daily) compared with 4% of patients receiving chlorpromazine (mean maximum dosage exceeding 1200 mg daily) plus benztropine. In addition, clozapine was substantially more effective than chlorpromazine plus benztropine in improving both positive and negative manifestations of schizophrenia. In this study, resistance to antipsychotic treatment prior to entry into the clozapine/chlorpromazine comparative phase was confirmed by a 6-week trial of haloperidol (mean dosage of 61 mg daily) combined with benztropine. This study provides evidence from both categorical and continuous measures not only of clozapine's efficacy as an antipsychotic agent but also of its superiority over conventional antipsychotic drug therapy in a well-defined group of antipsychotic-resistant patients. Similar 6-week response rates in treatment-resistant schizophrenia have been reported in other studies with the drug. Clinically important improvement in quality of life and social functioning, including deinstitutionalization, interpersonal relationships, and ability to hold a job or attend school, also have been reported following initiation of clozapine therapy in patients with antipsychotic-resistant schizophrenia.

For additional information on the symptomatic management of schizophrenia, including treatment recommendations, see Schizophrenia and Other Psychotic Disorders under Uses: Psychotic Disorders, in the Phenothiazines General Statement 28:16.08.24.

Pediatric Considerations

Although the manufacturers state that the safety and efficacy of clozapine in pediatric patients have not been established, the drug has been successfully used for the management of childhood-onset schizophrenia in a limited number of treatment-resistant children and adolescents†. While the lower risk of extrapyramidal adverse effects and tardive dyskinesia during treatment with atypical antipsychotic agents such as clozapine compared with conventional antipsychotic agents represents an advantage in the treatment of childhood-onset schizophrenia, concerns regarding serious adverse effects (e.g., neutropenia, seizures) associated with clozapine limit its use in clinical practice. (See Cautions: Pediatric Precautions.) Therefore, the American Academy of Child and Adolescent Psychiatry (AACAP) states that clozapine is not considered a first-line agent, and should be reserved for treatment-refractory patients who have failed to respond to adequate therapeutic trials (i.e., use of sufficient dosages over a period of 6 weeks) of at least 2 other first-line antipsychotic agents. For additional information on the symptomatic management of childhood-onset schizophrenia, see Pediatric Considerations under Psychotic Disorders: Schizophrenia, in Uses in the Phenothiazines General Statement 28:16.08.24.

In one randomized, double-blind, clinical study conducted by the National Institute of Mental Health (NIMH), a limited number of children and adolescents (mean: 14 years of age) with childhood-onset schizophrenia (i.e., development of the disorder by 12 years of age or younger) who were intolerant and/or nonresponsive to at least 2 different antipsychotic agents were treated with either clozapine (up to 525 mg daily; mean final dosage 176 mg daily) or haloperidol (up to 27 mg daily; mean final dosage 16 mg daily) for 6 weeks. In this study, children and adolescents receiving clozapine had substantially greater reductions in both positive and negative symptoms of schizophrenia than those receiving haloperidol. Additional follow-up of these patients over a 2-year period indicated that, as reported in adults, maximal antipsychotic effects in schizophrenic children and adolescents may not be evident until after 6–9 months of clozapine therapy. For most children and adolescents in the study, clozapine improved interpersonal functioning and enabled a return to a less restrictive setting. However, mild to moderate neutropenia occurred in 24% of the patients, and 29% required therapy with an anticonvulsant.

Suicide Risk Reduction in Schizophrenia and Schizoaffective Disorder

Clozapine is used to reduce the risk of recurrent suicidal behavior in patients with schizophrenia or schizoaffective disorder who are judged to be at chronic risk for such behavior, based on history and recent clinical state. Efficacy of clozapine for this indication has been established in a multicenter, randomized, open-label clinical study (the International Suicide Prevention Trial [InterSePT]) of 2 years' duration comparing clozapine and olanzapine in patients with schizophrenia (62%) or schizoaffective disorder (38%) who were judged to be at risk for recurrent suicidal behavior. These patients either had attempted suicide or had been hospitalized to prevent a suicide attempt within the 3 years prior to their baseline evaluation or had demonstrated moderate-to-severe suicidal ideation with a depressive component or command hallucinations to do self-harm within 1 week prior to their baseline evaluation. Treatment resistance (i.e., resistance to standard antipsychotic drug therapies) was not a requirement for inclusion in this study, and only 27% of the total patient population was identified as being treatment resistant at baseline.

In the InterSePT study, patients who received flexible dosages of clozapine (mean dosage: 274.2 mg daily) for approximately 2 years had a 26% reduction in their risk for suicide attempts or hospitalization to prevent suicide compared with those who received flexible dosages of olanzapine (mean dosage: 16.6 mg daily); the treatment-resistant status of patients was not predictive of response to clozapine or olanzapine. The cumulative probability of experiencing a suicide attempt, including a completed suicide, or hospitalization due to imminent suicide risk (including increased level of surveillance for suicidal behavior for patients already hospitalized) also was lower for patients receiving clozapine (24%) than for those receiving olanzapine (32%) at year 2. In addition, patients receiving clozapine had a statistically significant longer delay in the time to recurrent suicidal behavior than those receiving olanzapine. These results, however, may have been confounded by extensive use of other treatments to reduce the suicide risk, including concomitant psychotropic agents (84% with antipsychotics; 65% with anxiolytics; 53% with antidepressants; 28% with mood stabilizers), hospitalization, and psychotherapy, the contributions of which to clozapine's efficacy are unknown.

Some clinicians state that methodologic problems (e.g., lack of actively suicidal patients in the study, possible bias and unblinding of suicide monitoring board members during the study, use of concomitant psychotropic agents) associated with the InterSePT study limit definitive conclusions about the efficacy of clozapine for prevention of suicide in patients with schizophrenia or schizoaffective disorder. The FDA advises clinicians to interpret the results of the InterSePT study only as evidence of the efficacy of clozapine in delaying time to recurrent suicidal behavior, and not as efficacy of the drug for treatment of suicidal behaviors or as a demonstration of the superior efficacy of clozapine over olanzapine. However, the APA states that, based on the available evidence from the InterSePT study, clozapine should be preferentially considered for schizophrenia patients with a history of chronic and persistent suicidal ideation and behaviors. Decisions to initiate clozapine therapy or switch patients from other antipsychotics to clozapine, therefore, should be individualized. In addition, safety and efficacy of clozapine in actively suicidal patients have yet to be determined.

● *Parkinsonian Syndrome*

Clozapine has been used in a limited number of patients with advanced, idiopathic parkinsonian syndrome for the management of dopaminomimetic psychosis† associated with antiparkinsonian drug therapy, but adverse effects such as sedation, confusion, and increased parkinsonian manifestations may limit the benefit of clozapine therapy in these patients. Attempts to relieve antiparkinsonian drug-induced delusions, paranoia, and hallucinations by reduction of antiparkinsonian drug dosage or administration of typical antipsychotic agents often aggravate parkinsonian symptoms. Limited data suggest that administration of clozapine in dosages of 6.25–400 mg daily can improve psychotic symptoms within a few days, reportedly without exacerbating parkinsonian manifestations. However, in a controlled study in a limited number of patients receiving clozapine dosages up to 250 mg daily, exacerbation of parkinsonian manifestations and development of delirium occurred frequently despite prevention of antiparkinsonian-drug-induced deterioration of psychosis; it has been suggested that rapid clozapine dosage escalation may have contributed to the observed negative effect on parkinsonian manifestations and delirium. Clozapine dosages of 100–250 mg daily reportedly have been associated with hypersalivation, hypophonia, bradykinesia, and considerable sedation in patients with idiopathic parkinsonian syndrome, and withdrawal of clozapine therapy or a decrease in dosage also has exacerbated parkinsonian manifestations. Some clinicians suggest that the dosage of clozapine required to treat drug-induced dopaminomimetic psychosis may be substantially less than that required for treatment of psychosis in young, otherwise healthy individuals and that clozapine therapy should be initiated at low dosages (e.g., 6.25–50 mg daily) with cautious upward titration (e.g., to a maximum of 100–200 mg daily). Other clinicians have suggested that clozapine be used only as a last resort in patients with drug-induced dopaminomimetic psychosis.

DOSAGE AND ADMINISTRATION

● *General*

Pretreatment Screening

- Prior to initiating clozapine therapy, obtain a baseline complete blood cell (CBC) count, including absolute neutrophil count (ANC). In the general population, baseline ANC must be ≥1500/mm³ before clozapine therapy can be initiated. In patients with documented benign ethnic neutropenia (BEN), baseline ANC must be ≥1000/mm³ to be eligible for clozapine therapy.

Patient Monitoring

- Regular ANC monitoring is required during clozapine therapy because of the risk of severe neutropenia.

REMS

- Because of the risk of severe neutropenia, clozapine is available only through a restricted distribution program (Clozapine REMS program). As of October 12, 2015, all previous clozapine registries, which had been maintained individually by each manufacturer of clozapine, were replaced by a single, shared centralized system called the Clozapine REMS program. Under this shared program, only ANC is used to monitor patients for clozapine-induced neutropenia; white blood cell (WBC) count monitoring is no longer required. In addition, ANC thresholds for clozapine treatment interruption were lowered from the previous requirements to allow continued treatment for a greater number of patients, and patients with benign ethnic neutropenia (BEN) who were previously ineligible to receive clozapine are now eligible.

- Prescribers (who prescribe clozapine for outpatient use or initiate treatment for inpatients) must be certified with the Clozapine REMS program before they can prescribe clozapine; pharmacies must also certify with the program before they can receive and dispense the drug. Certified prescribers must enroll patients in the Clozapine REMS program and submit patients' ANC values to the program.

- On July 29, 2021, the Clozapine REMS program was modified to include changes to the authorization process for dispensing clozapine and changes to ANC reporting requirements. After November 15, 2021, pharmacists will no longer be able to use telecommunication verification (also known as the switch system) and will need to contact the REMS program by phone (888-586-0758) or online (www.clozapinerems.com) to verify safe use conditions and obtain authorization to dispense clozapine. In addition, prescribers will no longer need to submit ANC results according to the patient's monitoring frequency; the new process requires that ANC results be submitted monthly through a new Patient Status form, which will be used to document monitoring for all outpatients receiving the drug. Prescribers must re-enroll their existing patients, and pharmacies must recertify in the revised Clozapine REMS program by November 15, 2021 before they can prescribe and dispense clozapine.

● Administration

Clozapine is administered orally as conventional tablets, orally disintegrating tablets, or as an oral suspension without regard to meals; administration in divided doses may help minimize the risk of certain adverse effects. If daytime sleepiness occurs during therapy, bedtime administration may be helpful.

The orally disintegrating tablets and conventional tablets of clozapine are bioequivalent; the oral suspension and conventional tablets of the drug also are bioequivalent.

Clozapine also has been administered IM†, but a parenteral preparation currently is not commercially available in the US.

Orally Disintegrating Tablets

Patients receiving clozapine orally disintegrating tablets should be instructed not to remove a tablet from the blister until just prior to dosing. The tablet should not be pushed through the foil; instead, the foil blister backing should be peeled from the blister. The tablet should then be gently removed and immediately placed on the tongue, where it rapidly disintegrates in saliva, and then subsequently swallowed with or without liquid, or the tablet can be chewed as desired.

Oral Suspension

Clozapine oral suspension (Versacloz®) should be shaken for 10 seconds prior to each use. The bottle adapter and calibrated oral dosing syringe supplied by the manufacturer should be used to administer the suspension. After withdrawing the appropriate dose into the calibrated oral dosing syringe, the dose should be administered directly into the patient's mouth; clozapine oral suspension should not be stored in the syringe for later use.

● Dosage

Cautious dosage titration and administration of clozapine in divided doses are necessary to minimize the risk of certain adverse effects such as orthostatic hypotension, bradycardia, syncope, seizures, and sedation.

Treatment-resistant Schizophrenia

Adult Dosage

For the management of treatment-resistant schizophrenia, the usual initial adult dosage of clozapine is 12.5 mg given orally once or twice daily. If the drug is well tolerated, dosage may be increased in increments of 25–50 mg daily over a 2-week period until a target dosage of 300–450 mg daily (administered in divided doses) is achieved. Subsequent dosage increases can be made once or twice weekly in increments of up to 100 mg. The manufacturers state that use of a low initial daily dosage, a gradual titration schedule, and administration of the drug in divided doses are necessary to minimize the risks of orthostatic hypotension, bradycardia, syncope, seizures, and sedation.

Daily administration of clozapine in divided doses should continue until an effective and tolerable dosage is reached, usually within 2–5 weeks. Although many patients may respond adequately to dosages between 200–600 mg daily, a dosage of 600–900 mg daily may be required in some patients. In the multicenter study that provides the principal support for the effectiveness of clozapine in patients resistant to standard antipsychotic therapy, the maximum dosage of clozapine was 900 mg daily, which was given in 3 divided doses. The mean and median clozapine dosages in this study both were approximately 600 mg daily. Although some clinicians suggest that dosages exceeding 450–500 mg daily have not been shown to be associated with increased therapeutic benefit, others state that added response is observed at higher dosages in some patients and stress the need for individualized therapy. The manufacturers and most clinicians recommend that the maximum daily dosage of clozapine not exceed 900 mg. Because of the possibility that high dosages of clozapine may be associated with an increased risk of adverse reactions, particularly seizures, patients generally should be given adequate time to respond to a given dosage before dosage escalation is considered.

Pediatric Dosage

The dosage of clozapine for the management of schizophrenia in children and adolescents† has not been established. However, the National Institute of Mental Health (NIMH) protocol used an initial dosage of 6.25–25 mg given orally daily depending on the patient's weight. Dosages could be increased in this study every 3–4 days by 1–2 times the initial dose on an individual basis up to a maximum of 525 mg daily.

Duration of Therapy

While some clinicians state that clozapine therapy should be continued for longer than 6 weeks only in patients who exhibit substantial benefit within this period, others state that even less than substantial degrees of benefit may warrant continued therapy and that an adequate trial of clozapine may require at least 12 weeks (e.g., at daily dosages of 200–600 mg daily) or possibly 5–9 months or longer unless clinical deterioration or intolerable or potentially serious toxicity precludes it. The manufacturers state that patients who respond to clozapine therapy generally should continue to receive maintenance treatment with the drug at their effective dosage beyond the acute episode. Extended therapy in patients failing to show an acceptable response to clozapine generally should be avoided because of the substantial, continuing risks of neutropenia and seizures.

The American Psychiatric Association (APA) states that prudent long-term treatment options in patients with schizophrenia with remitted first or multiple episodes include either indefinite maintenance therapy or gradual discontinuance of the antipsychotic agent with close follow-up and a plan to reinstitute treatment upon symptom recurrence. Discontinuance of antipsychotic therapy should be considered only after a period of at least 1 year of symptom remission or optimal response while receiving the antipsychotic agent. In patients who have had multiple previous psychotic episodes or 2 psychotic episodes within 5 years, indefinite maintenance antipsychotic treatment is recommended.

Suicide Risk Reduction

For suicide risk reduction in schizophrenia and schizoaffective disorder, the usual initial adult dosage of clozapine is 12.5 mg given orally once or twice daily. If the drug is well tolerated, dosage may be increased in increments of 25–50 mg daily over a 2-week period until a target dosage of 300–450 mg daily (administered in divided doses) is achieved. Subsequent dosage increases can be made once or twice weekly in increments of up to 100 mg. The manufacturers state that use of a low initial daily dosage, a gradual titration schedule, and administration of the drug in divided doses are necessary to minimize the risks of orthostatic hypotension, bradycardia, syncope, seizures, and sedation. In the multicenter InterSePT study that provides the principal support for the effectiveness of clozapine for suicide risk reduction, mean dosage was about 300 mg daily (range: 12.5–900 mg daily).

The manufacturers state that patients who respond to clozapine therapy generally should continue to receive maintenance treatment with the drug at their effective dosage beyond the acute episode; efficacy of clozapine for this indication was demonstrated over a 2-year treatment period in the InterSePT study.

Discontinuance of Therapy

In the event of planned discontinuance of clozapine therapy, gradual reduction in dosage over a 1- to 2-week period is recommended if there is no evidence of moderate to severe neutropenia. However, if abrupt discontinuance of therapy is required because of moderate to severe neutropenia, ANC should be monitored according to the neutropenia monitoring recommendations. If abrupt discontinuance of clozapine is required for reasons unrelated to neutropenia, continuation of the existing ANC monitoring schedule is recommended; patients in the general population should be monitored until their ANC is in the normal range (i.e., ≥1500/mm³) while patients with BEN should be monitored until their ANC is ≥1000/mm³ or above their baseline. Additional ANC monitoring is necessary in any patient reporting onset of fever (temperature ≥38.5°C) during the 2 weeks after clozapine discontinuance. Patients should be observed carefully for recurrence of psychotic symptoms and symptoms related to cholinergic rebound such as profuse sweating, headache, nausea, vomiting, and diarrhea. Sudden withdrawal from clozapine therapy can lead to rapid decompensation and rebound psychosis.

Reinitiation of Therapy

If clozapine therapy is restarted in patients who have had even brief interruptions (i.e., 2 days or more since the last dose) in therapy, dosage generally should be titrated as with initial therapy (i.e., starting with 12.5 mg once or twice daily) to minimize the risk of hypotension, bradycardia, and syncope. If this dosage is well tolerated, dosage may be titrated back to the previous therapeutic dosage more quickly than recommended during initial treatment.

For clozapine treatment interruptions of less than 30 days in patients with normal ANC values, the same ANC monitoring schedule as before the treatment interruption may be continued. If clozapine treatment is interrupted for 30 days or more, the ANC monitoring schedule must be restarted as with initial therapy.

Patients who develop severe neutropenia (ANC <500/mm³) during clozapine therapy generally should not be restarted on the drug unless the clinician determines that the benefits of the drug outweigh the risks.

SPECIAL POPULATIONS

● Hepatic Impairment

Although the pharmacokinetics of clozapine have not been specifically studied in patients with hepatic impairment, increased plasma clozapine concentrations are possible in such patients since the drug is almost completely metabolized and then excreted. The manufacturers state that dosage reduction may be necessary in patients with substantial hepatic impairment.

● Renal Impairment

Although the pharmacokinetics of clozapine have not been specifically studied in patients with renal impairment, increased plasma clozapine concentrations are possible in such patients since the drug is almost completely metabolized and then excreted. The manufacturers state that dosage reduction may be necessary in patients with substantial renal impairment.

● Pharmacogenomics: Dosage in Poor CYP2D6 Metabolizers

The manufacturers state that dosage reduction of clozapine may be necessary in patients who are known poor metabolizers of cytochrome P-450 isoenzyme 2D6 (CYP2D6). (See Pharmacokinetics: Absorption.)

CAUTIONS

Although clozapine differs chemically from the phenothiazines, the drug may be capable of producing many of the toxic manifestations of phenothiazine derivatives. Not all adverse effects of the phenothiazines have been reported with clozapine, but the possibility that they may occur should be considered. Adverse effects of clozapine and the phenothiazines are numerous and may involve nearly all organ systems. Although these effects usually are reversible when dosage is reduced or the drug is discontinued, some effects may be irreversible and, rarely, fatal. In some patients, unexpected death associated with antipsychotic therapy has been attributed to cardiac arrest or asphyxia resulting from failure of the gag reflex. (See Cautions: Cardiovascular Effects.) In other cases, the cause of death could not be determined or definitely attributed to antipsychotic drug therapy. An increased risk of death has been observed in geriatric patients with dementia-related psychoses receiving antipsychotic agents. (See Cautions: Geriatric Precautions.)

The most frequent adverse effects of clozapine involve the central and autonomic nervous systems (e.g., drowsiness or sedation, hypersalivation) and the cardiovascular system (e.g., tachycardia, orthostatic hypotension, syncope). While the frequency and severity of some adverse effects (e.g., extrapyramidal reactions, tardive dyskinesia) appear to be less with clozapine than with other antipsychotic agents, other potentially serious adverse effects (e.g., severe neutropenia, seizures) may occur more frequently with clozapine therapy, and the potential risks and benefits should be evaluated carefully whenever therapy with the drug is considered. Because of the risk of severe clozapine-associated neutropenia, which may lead to serious and potentially fatal infections, clozapine is available only through a restricted distribution program that ensures appropriate monitoring of absolute neutrophil count (ANC). (See General under Dosage and Administration and also see Severe Neutropenia under Cautions: Hematologic Effects.)

● Hematologic Effects

Severe Neutropenia

Clozapine has been associated with neutropenia (i.e., a low absolute neutrophil count [ANC]) which can, when severe, increase the risk of serious and potentially fatal infections. Previously, the terms "severe leukopenia," "severe granulocytopenia," and "agranulocytosis" were used in the clozapine prescribing information (labeling) to describe this hematologic effect; however, to improve and standardize understanding, these terms have been replaced with "severe neutropenia" throughout the labeling for the drug. The ANC is usually available as a component of the complete blood count (CBC), including differential, and is considered more clinically relevant for drug-induced neutropenia than the white blood cell (WBC) count. Severe neutropenia is defined as an ANC value of less than 500/mm³ and occurs in a small percentage of patients receiving clozapine therapy.

Previously described agranulocytosis, which was defined as an ANC less than 500/mm³ and characterized by leukopenia (WBC count less than 2000/mm³) and relative lymphopenia, has been reported to have an estimated cumulative incidence of 1–2% after 1 year of clozapine therapy, as compared with an estimated incidence of 0.1–1% for phenothiazine-induced agranulocytosis. Some evidence has suggested that the incidence of clozapine-induced agranulocytosis is at least 10 times greater than the incidence associated with other antipsychotic agents, although it also has been suggested that the incidence of clozapine-induced agranulocytosis may be no higher than that associated with phenothiazines.

The precise mechanism by which clozapine induces neutropenia is not known and is not dose-dependent, but both immunologic and toxic mechanisms (including a direct myelotoxic effect of the drug and/or its metabolites) have been implicated. Some evidence suggests that granulocyte antibodies may be involved.

Identified risk factors for clozapine-induced neutropenia or agranulocytosis include advanced age, female gender, and African-American and Asian ethnicity; pediatric patients also are at an increased risk. Results of genetic typing indicate that genetic factors marked by a major histocompatibility complex haplotype (HLA-B38, DR4, DQw3) may be associated with the susceptibility of certain Jewish patients with schizophrenia to develop agranulocytosis when treated with clozapine; the incidence of some phenotypes common among Ashkenazi Jews has been found to be greatly increased in patients with clozapine-induced agranulocytosis.

The risk of clozapine-induced neutropenia appears to be greatest during the first 18 weeks of therapy and declines thereafter. However, rare cases of neutropenia or agranulocytosis have been reported after several years of treatment with the drug.

Benign ethnic neutropenia (BEN) is a condition observed in certain ethnic groups whose average ANC values are lower than standard laboratory ranges for neutrophils. BEN has an approximate prevalence of 25–50% in individuals of African descent and also is observed in some Middle Eastern ethnic groups and in other non-Caucasian ethnic groups with darker skin; the condition is more common in men than women. Patients with BEN have normal hematopoietic stem cell numbers and myeloid maturation, are healthy, and do not suffer from repeated or severe infections. Such patients are not at increased risk for developing clozapine-induced neutropenia. BEN may be diagnosed by repeated low ANC measurements (less than 1500/mm³ and usually 1000/mm³ or below) for several months without identifiable causes of the neutropenia. Additional evaluation may be necessary in some patients to determine whether their baseline neutropenia is caused by BEN. Consultation with a hematologist should be considered in patients with low baseline ANC values before initiating or during clozapine therapy, if necessary. Patients with documented BEN have different ANC monitoring and treatment recommendations during clozapine therapy than the general population because of their lower baseline ANC levels. (See Table 2.)

Because of the risk of severe neutropenia associated with clozapine use, patients must have a baseline CBC and ANC performed before initiation of therapy and regular ANC monitoring during treatment with the drug. Clozapine therapy should not be initiated if baseline ANC is less than 1500/mm³ (or less than 1000/mm³ in patients with documented BEN).

When initiating clozapine therapy, ANC must be monitored every week for the first 6 months of therapy and then every 2 weeks for the next 6 months if ANC values remain in the normal range. If ANC values continue to be maintained in the normal range after an additional 6 months (i.e., following 12 months of continuous treatment), the frequency of monitoring may be reduced to once every 4 weeks thereafter. If clozapine treatment is interrupted for 30 days or longer, the initial ANC monitoring schedule should be restarted beginning with once-weekly ANC monitoring.

See Tables 1 and 2 for clozapine treatment recommendations based on ANC monitoring in the general patient population and in patients with BEN, respectively.

For hospice patients (i.e., patients who are terminally ill with an estimated life expectancy of 6 months or less) receiving clozapine therapy, the ANC monitoring frequency may be reduced by the clinician to once every 6 months, after a discussion with the patient and caregiver. Treatment decisions in such individuals should weigh the importance of ANC monitoring in the context of the need to control psychiatric symptoms and the patient's terminal illness.

TABLE 1. Clozapine Treatment Recommendations based on ANC Monitoring in the General Patient Population

ANC Value	Treatment Recommendations	Frequency of ANC Monitoring
Normal range (ANC ≥1500/mm³)	Initiate treatment	Weekly from initiation to 6 months
	If treatment interrupted <30 days, continue monitoring as before	Every 2 weeks from 6–12 months
	If treatment interrupted ≥30 days, monitor as if new patient	Monthly after 12 months
Discontinuance for reasons other than neutropenia	(See Discontinuance of Therapy under Dosage and Administration.)	
Mild neutropenia (ANC 1000–1499/mm³) [a]	Continue treatment	3 times weekly until ANC ≥1500/mm³
		When ANC ≥1500/mm³, return to patient's last normal range ANC monitoring interval, if clinically appropriate
Moderate neutropenia (ANC 500–999/mm³) [a]	Recommend hematology consultation	Daily until ANC ≥1000/mm³
	Interrupt treatment for suspected clozapine-induced neutropenia	3 times weekly until ANC ≥1500/mm³
	Resume treatment once ANC ≥1000/mm³	When ANC ≥1500/mm³, monitor weekly for 4 weeks, then return to the patient's last normal range ANC monitoring interval, if clinically appropriate
Severe neutropenia (ANC <500/mm³) [a]	Recommend hematology consultation	Daily until ANC ≥1000/mm³
	Interrupt treatment for suspected clozapine-induced neutropenia	3 times weekly until ANC ≥1500/mm³
	Do not rechallenge unless prescriber determines benefits outweigh risks	If patient rechallenged, resume treatment and monitor as new patient under normal range monitoring once ANC ≥1500/mm³

[a] Confirm all *initial* reports of ANC <1500/mm³ with a repeat ANC measurement within 24 hours.

TABLE 2. Clozapine Treatment Recommendations based on ANC Monitoring in Patients with Benign Ethnic Neutropenia (BEN)

ANC Value	Treatment Recommendations	Frequency of ANC Monitoring
Normal BEN range (established ANC baseline ≥1000/mm³)	Obtain ≥2 baseline ANC values before initiating treatment	Weekly from initiation to 6 months
	If treatment interrupted <30 days, continue monitoring as before	Every 2 weeks from 6–12 months
	If treatment interrupted ≥30 days, monitor as if new patient	Monthly after 12 months
Discontinuance of treatment for reasons other than neutropenia	(See Discontinuance of Therapy and Dosage and Administration.)	
BEN neutropenia (ANC 500–999/mm³) [a]	Recommend hematology consultation	3 times weekly until ANC ≥1000/mm³ or at patient's known baseline
	Continue treatment	When ANC ≥1000/mm³ or at patient's known baseline, monitor weekly for 4 weeks, then return to the patient's last normal BEN range ANC monitoring interval, if clinically appropriate
BEN severe neutropenia (ANC <500/mm³) [a]	Recommend hematology consultation	Daily until ANC ≥500/mm³
	Interrupt treatment for suspected clozapine-induced neutropenia	3 times weekly until ANC at or above patient's baseline
	Do not rechallenge unless prescriber determines benefits outweigh risks	If patient rechallenged, resume treatment as a new patient under normal range monitoring once ANC ≥1000/mm³ or at patient's baseline

[a] Confirm all *initial* reports of ANC <1500/mm³ with a repeat ANC measurement within 24 hours.

If a patient develops fever (temperature of 38.5°C or higher) during therapy, clozapine should be interrupted and an ANC should be obtained. Fever is often the first sign of neutropenic infection. If fever occurs in any patient with an ANC value less than 1000/mm³, the patient should be appropriately evaluated (see Tables 1 and 2) and treated for infection. A hematology consultation should be considered in all clozapine-treated patients with fever or neutropenia.

Although some clinicians have suggested that body temperature be measured at least once daily for the first 18 weeks of clozapine therapy, others state that such monitoring is not an adequate means of assessing infection in clozapine-treated patients because of the drug's pharmacologic potential for causing temperature elevation (see Cautions: Fever). Patients receiving clozapine should be advised to immediately report the appearance of lethargy, weakness, fever, sore throat, or any other potential manifestations of infection.

Supportive therapy with biosynthetic hematopoietic agents, including filgrastim, a recombinant human granulocyte colony-stimulating factor (G-CSF), and sargramostim, a recombinant human granulocyte-macrophage colony-stimulating factor (GM-CSF), has been effective in a limited number of patients with clozapine-induced neutropenia and agranulocytosis. Consultation with a hematologist and infectious disease expert is recommended.

Lithium has been used successfully in the treatment of clozapine-induced neutropenia or to facilitate initiation of therapy or rechallenge† with the drug in a limited number of patients, including in some patients with BEN. However, lithium should be used concurrently with clozapine with caution because, in addition to the possible increased risk of NMS and seizures, the drug can mask the development or delay the detection of severe neutropenia and other blood dyscrasias. (See Drug Interactions: Other CNS-active Agents.)

When neutropenia is diagnosed and clozapine therapy is discontinued, patients usually recover in 7–28 days. Most of these patients require further antipsychotic therapy because of a recurrence of psychotic symptoms. (See Other Nervous System Effects under Cautions: Nervous System Effects.) Since there appears to be no cross-sensitivity between clozapine and other antipsychotics in terms of hematologic toxicity, other antipsychotic drugs generally may be used without causing further hematologic complications in patients who develop clozapine-induced neutropenia. Patients who develop severe clozapine-induced neutropenia generally should *not* be rechallenged with clozapine. However, for some patients who have no acceptable alternatives to clozapine, the risk of serious psychiatric illness from discontinuing treatment may outweigh the risk of severe neutropenia upon rechallenge; in such cases, consultation with a hematology specialist may be helpful in deciding whether to rechallenge a patient with clozapine.

Eosinophilia

Eosinophilia (defined as blood eosinophil count exceeding 700/mm^3) has been reported in approximately 1% of patients who received clozapine therapy in clinical trials. Clozapine-associated eosinophilia usually occurs during the first month of therapy and has been associated with myocarditis, pancreatitis, hepatitis, colitis, and/or nephritis in some patients. Such organ involvement could be consistent with drug reaction with eosinophilia and systemic symptoms (DRESS; also known as multiorgan hypersensitivity or drug-induced hypersensitivity syndrome).

The manufacturers state that if eosinophilia develops during clozapine therapy, the patient should be evaluated promptly for signs and symptoms of systemic reactions such as rash or other allergic symptoms, myocarditis, or other organ-specific disease associated with eosinophilia. If clozapine-associated systemic disease is suspected, the drug should be immediately discontinued. If a cause of eosinophilia unrelated to clozapine is identified (e.g., asthma, allergies, collagen vascular disease, parasitic infections, specific neoplasms), the underlying cause should be treated and clozapine therapy may be continued.

Clozapine-associated eosinophilia also has occurred without organ involvement and can resolve without intervention. In such cases, clozapine therapy may be continued with careful monitoring. If the patient's total eosinophil count continues to increase over several weeks in the absence of organ involvement, the decision whether to interrupt clozapine therapy and rechallenge after the eosinophil count decreases should be made based on the overall clinical assessment, in consultation with an internist or hematologist. There have been reports of successful rechallenge after discontinuance of clozapine without recurrence of eosinophilia.

Other Hematologic Effects

Other hematologic effects reported with clozapine therapy include leukopenia/decreased WBC count and neutropenia, which has been reported in 3% of patients. Other clozapine-induced hematologic effects reportedly include basophilia and a substantial reduction in B cells. Elevated hemoglobin/hematocrit, elevated erythrocyte sedimentation rate (ESR), sepsis, thrombocytosis, and thrombocytopenia have been reported in patients receiving clozapine during postmarketing surveillance; however, a causal relationship to the drug has not been established.

● *Nervous System Effects*

Seizures

Clozapine lowers the seizure threshold and can cause EEG changes, including the occurrence of spike and wave complexes. Seizures reportedly occurred in approximately 3.5% of patients exposed to the drug during clinical trials in the US (cumulative annual incidence of approximately 5%). In contrast, a seizure incidence of approximately 1% has been reported in patients treated with other antipsychotic agents. The risk of seizures with clozapine therapy is dose related, with a reported incidence of approximately 0.6–2% at dosages less than 300 mg daily, 1.4–5% at 300–600 mg daily, and 5–14% at high dosages (600–900 mg daily). Clozapine-induced seizures may be associated with rapid dosage escalations, particularly in patients receiving concomitant therapy with drugs that may cause increased plasma concentrations of clozapine. (See Seizures under Cautions: Precautions and Contraindications.)

One patient receiving clozapine experienced a generalized tonic-clonic (grand mal) seizure following accidental ingestion of an extra dose (total dose ingested within 24 hours: 1050 mg); the same patient had another seizure several weeks later, 2 hours after a usual 450-mg morning dose. Results of plasma clozapine determinations obtained at the time of the seizures revealed plasma clozapine concentrations of approximately 2000 ng/mL in each case. Another patient who had been taking clozapine for 27 months had a generalized tonic-clonic seizure following an apparent intentional overdosage (total dose ingested within 24 hours: approximately 3 g), after which the patient made an uneventful recovery. One hour after the seizure, the patient's plasma clozapine concentration was 1313 ng/mL.

Discontinuance of clozapine therapy, at least temporarily, should be seriously considered in patients who experience seizures while receiving the drug; however, some clinicians state that reduced clozapine dosage and/or, occasionally, addition of anticonvulsant therapy may adequately ameliorate this effect. If clozapine therapy is to be continued in such patients, many clinicians recommend obtaining additional informed consent from the patient. In patients in whom clozapine is withheld, it has been suggested that therapy with the drug can be reinitiated at one-half the previous dosage. Clozapine dosage may then be increased gradually, if clinically indicated, and the need for concomitant anticonvulsant therapy should be considered. Some clinicians recommend that patients who have experienced a clozapine-induced seizure *not* be given clozapine dosages exceeding 600 mg daily unless the results of an EEG performed prior to the anticipated dosage increase are normal; others suggest addition of anticonvulsant therapy and/or consultation with a neurologist in managing such patients. In patients with pre-existing seizure disorders who are treated concomitantly with certain anticonvulsants and clozapine, the anticonvulsant dosage may need to be increased. (See Drug Interactions: Drugs Affecting Hepatic Microsomal Enzymes.)

Extrapyramidal Reactions

In contrast to some other antipsychotic agents, clozapine has little or no potential for causing certain acute extrapyramidal effects (e.g., dystonias). Such effects, when they occur, have been limited principally to tremor, restlessness, rigidity, and akathisia. In addition, marked or total remission of such manifestations induced by other antipsychotics has occurred during treatment with clozapine in some patients.

One case of clozapine-associated tardive dystonia (blepharospasm) has been reported; the patient's symptoms in this case were alleviated by discontinuance of clozapine and initiation of clonazepam therapy.

Neuroleptic Malignant Syndrome

Neuroleptic malignant syndrome (NMS), a potentially fatal syndrome, has been reported in patients receiving antipsychotic agents, including clozapine. NMS attributable to clozapine therapy alone has been reported in some patients, and there also have been reports of NMS in patients treated concomitantly with clozapine and lithium or other CNS drugs; some clinicians suggest that NMS may be more likely to occur when clozapine or other antipsychotic agents are used concomitantly with lithium. Manifestations of NMS (e.g., muscle rigidity, hyperpyrexia, tachycardia, increased serum creatine kinase [CK, creatine phosphokinase, CPK], diaphoresis, somnolence), all of which may not occur in all patients with the condition, have occurred in a few patients treated with clozapine alone or combined with lithium or carbamazepine; resolution of the syndrome occurred following discontinuance of clozapine. However, clozapine also has been used successfully and apparently without recurrence of NMS in at least one patient who developed the syndrome while receiving chlorpromazine. Atypical presentations of NMS (e.g., absence of or lessened rigidity, absence of fever) also have been reported in some patients receiving clozapine.

The diagnostic evaluation of patients with NMS is complicated. In arriving at a diagnosis, serious medical illnesses (e.g., severe neutropenia, infection) and extrapyramidal symptoms must be excluded. Other important considerations in the differential diagnosis include central anticholinergic toxicity, heat stroke, drug fever, and primary CNS pathology.

The management of NMS should include immediate discontinuance of antipsychotic agents and other drugs not considered essential to concurrent therapy, intensive symptomatic treatment and medical monitoring, and treatment of any concomitant serious medical conditions for which specific treatments are available. There currently is no specific drug therapy for NMS, although dantrolene, bromocriptine, amantadine, and benzodiazepines have been used in a limited number of patients. If a patient requires antipsychotic therapy following recovery from NMS, the potential reintroduction of drug therapy should be carefully considered. In addition, such patients should be carefully monitored since NMS may recur. For additional information on NMS, including treatment, see Neuroleptic Malignant Syndrome under Cautions: Nervous System Effects, in the Phenothiazines General Statement 28:16.08.24.

Tardive Dyskinesia

Use of antipsychotic agents, including clozapine, may be associated with tardive dyskinesia, a syndrome of potentially irreversible, involuntary, dyskinetic movements. However, clozapine is considered less likely to cause tardive dyskinesia than many other antipsychotic agents, and dyskinetic movements in some patients have reportedly improved with clozapine therapy.

The risk of developing tardive dyskinesia and the likelihood that it will become irreversible are believed to increase as the duration of treatment and the total cumulative dose of antipsychotic drugs administered to the patient increase. However, the syndrome can develop following relatively brief treatment periods at low dosages. Management of tardive dyskinesia generally consists of gradual discontinuance of the precipitating antipsychotic agent when possible, reducing the dosage of the first-generation (conventional) antipsychotic agent or switching to a second-generation (atypical) antipsychotic agent, or switching to clozapine therapy. The syndrome may remit, partially or completely, if antipsychotic therapy is discontinued. However, antipsychotic therapy itself may suppress or partially suppress the signs and symptoms of the syndrome and thereby may possibly mask the underlying process. The effect that such symptomatic suppression has upon the long-term course of tardive dyskinesia is unknown. Vesicular monoamine transporter 2 (VMAT2) inhibitors (e.g., deutetrabenazine, valbenazine tosylate) have been shown to be effective in reducing symptoms of tardive dyskinesia in controlled clinical studies and may allow some patients to continue receiving antipsychotic therapy. (See Deutetrabenazine 28:56 and Valbenazine Tosylate 28:56.)

Clozapine should be prescribed in a manner that is most likely to minimize the occurrence of this syndrome. In patients who do require chronic treatment, the lowest dosage and the shortest duration of treatment producing a satisfactory clinical response should be sought, and the need for continued treatment should be reassessed periodically.

The American Psychiatric Association (APA) currently recommends that patients receiving atypical antipsychotic agents be assessed clinically for abnormal involuntary movements every 12 months and that patients considered to be at increased risk for tardive dyskinesia be assessed every 6 months. If signs and symptoms of tardive dyskinesia appear in a clozapine-treated patient, clozapine discontinuance should be considered; however, some patients may require continued treatment with the drug despite the presence of the syndrome.

For additional information on tardive dyskinesia, including manifestations and treatment, see Tardive Dyskinesia under Cautions: Nervous System Effects, in the Phenothiazines General Statement 28:16.08.24.

Other Nervous System Effects

Drowsiness and/or sedation occurs frequently in patients receiving clozapine. (See Effects on Sleep under Pharmacology: Nervous System Effects.) Somnolence reportedly occurred in 46% of patients receiving clozapine in the International Suicide Prevention Trial (InterSePT) compared with 25% of those receiving olanzapine. The sedative-hypnotic effect of clozapine is most pronounced initially, diminishes after 1–4 weeks, and then generally, but not always, disappears during continued therapy. Daytime sleepiness may be minimized by administration of clozapine at bedtime. (See Dosage and Administration and also see Cognitive and Motor Impairment under Cautions: Precautions and Contraindications.)

Dizziness and vertigo, headache, syncope, disturbed sleep (e.g., insomnia) or nightmares, hypokinesia or akinesia, and agitation have been reported with clozapine therapy. In the InterSePT study, dizziness (excluding vertigo) and insomnia reportedly occurred in 27 and 20% of patients receiving clozapine, respectively, compared with 12 and 33% of those receiving olanzapine, respectively. Clozapine also may cause confusion or delirium, which may be related to central anticholinergic effects and has been ameliorated in some cases by IV administration of physostigmine. Depression, fatigue, hyperkinesia, weakness or lethargy, and slurred speech also have been reported.

Delirium, abnormal EEG, myoclonus, paresthesia, possible cataplexy, status epilepticus, obsessive-compulsive symptoms, and post-discontinuation cholinergic rebound reactions have been reported in patients receiving clozapine during postmarketing surveillance; however, a causal relationship to the drug has not been established.

Abrupt discontinuance of clozapine (e.g., because of hematologic toxicity or other medical condition) may result in recurrence of psychotic symptoms or behavior, including autism, auditory hallucinations, suicide attempts, development of parkinsonian symptoms, anxiety, insomnia, delusions, and violent behavior. It has been suggested that this "rebound psychosis" may result, at least in part, from clozapine-induced supersensitivity of mesolimbic dopamine receptors (see Behavioral Effects in Animals under Pharmacology: Nervous System Effects) and that the essential feature of this phenomenon appears to be recurrence of positive symptoms of schizophrenia. Patients who develop rebound psychosis following discontinuance of clozapine may improve with initiation of other antipsychotic therapy; however, clozapine generally should *not* be reinstituted in patients in whom severe neutropenia has occurred. (See Cautions: Hematologic Effects.)

● Fever

Fever or transient temperature elevations exceeding 38°C generally have been reported in 5% or more of patients receiving clozapine. The peak incidence of fever occurs within the first 3 weeks of therapy, usually between days 5–20 of treatment. Fever generally is benign and self-limiting, responds to supportive measures, and usually diminishes within a few (4–8) days despite continued clozapine therapy; however, it may necessitate discontinuance of the drug. Fever occasionally may be associated with an increase or decrease in WBC count. Clozapine therapy should be interrupted as a precautionary measure; an ANC should be obtained in any patient who develops fever (38.5°C or higher) during treatment, and patients should be evaluated for severe neutropenia or infection. In addition, ANC should be monitored in any patient who develops fever within 2 weeks after discontinuance of clozapine. (See Cautions: Hematologic Effects.) Neuroleptic malignant syndrome also must be considered. (See Neuroleptic Malignant Syndrome under Cautions: Nervous System Effects.)

The mechanism of clozapine-induced fever (other than that occurring secondary to some other factor such as infection) is not yet known. It may result from the drug's pronounced anticholinergic activity (see Anticholinergic Effects under Pharmacology: Nervous System Effects) or a direct effect on the hypothalamic thermoregulatory center. Clozapine-induced hyperthermia may be a hypersensitivity reaction, a common mechanism underlying drug fevers. It has been suggested that decreasing the dosage of clozapine and then gradually increasing it to the previous level may reverse the hyperthermia and not be accompanied by a recurrence of elevated temperature; however, recurrence is possible despite such dosage adjustment.

● Cardiovascular Effects

Myocarditis, Cardiomyopathy, and Mitral Valve Incompetence

Myocarditis and cardiomyopathy, which are sometimes fatal, have been reported in patients receiving clozapine. Myocarditis most frequently presents within the first 2 months of clozapine treatment. Symptoms of clozapine-associated cardiomyopathy generally occur later than clozapine-associated myocarditis, usually after 8 weeks of treatment. However, myocarditis and cardiomyopathy can occur at any time during clozapine therapy. Overt manifestations of heart failure commonly are preceded by nonspecific flu-like symptoms (e.g., malaise, myalgia, pleuritic chest pain, low-grade fever). Typical laboratory findings include elevated troponin I or T concentrations, elevated CK-MB concentrations, peripheral eosinophilia, and elevated C-reactive protein (CRP) concentrations. Left ventricular dysfunction may be evident in cardiac imaging studies (e.g., electrocardiogram [ECG], radionucleotide studies, cardiac catheterization) and cardiac silhouette enlargement may be seen in chest radiographs.

The possibility of myocarditis or cardiomyopathy should be considered in patients receiving clozapine who present with chest pain, dyspnea, persistent tachycardia at rest, palpitations, fever, flu-like symptoms, hypotension, or other manifestations of heart failure or ECG changes associated with these conditions (e.g., low voltages, ST-T wave abnormalities, arrhythmias, right axis deviation, poor R wave progression). If myocarditis or cardiomyopathy is suspected, clozapine therapy should be discontinued and a cardiac evaluation should be obtained. Patients with a history of clozapine-associated myocarditis or cardiomyopathy generally should not be rechallenged with the drug. However, if the benefit of clozapine treatment is determined to outweigh the potential risks of recurrent myocarditis or cardiomyopathy, the clinician may consider rechallenge with the drug in consultation with a cardiologist, following a complete cardiac evaluation, and with close monitoring.

Mitral valve incompetence with mild or moderate mitral regurgitation has been reported in patients diagnosed with clozapine-associated cardiomyopathy. In patients with suspected cardiomyopathy, consideration should be given to performing a 2-dimensional Doppler echocardiogram to identify mitral valve incompetence.

Thromboembolic Effects

Deep-vein thrombosis and pulmonary embolism have been reported in patients receiving clozapine. Although a causal relationship between clozapine and these adverse effects has not been established, the possibility of pulmonary embolism should be considered in patients presenting with deep-vein thrombosis, acute dyspnea, chest pain, or respiratory symptomatology. (See Thromboembolic Events under Cautions: Precautions and Contraindications.)

Blood Pressure Effects

Hypotension and hypertension reportedly occur in less than 10% of patients receiving clozapine. When they occur, changes in blood pressure, principally reductions in systolic pressure, appear soon after initiation of clozapine therapy and may be associated with rapid dosage increases. A decrease in arterial blood pressure below 90 mm Hg was reported in 18% of male patients and 33% of female patients receiving clozapine in one retrospective study. Hypotension may result from clozapine's antiadrenergic effects (see Adrenergic Effects under Pharmacology: Nervous System Effects). However, tolerance to the hypotensive effects of clozapine often develops with continued therapy.

Orthostatic hypotension, bradycardia, syncope, and cardiac arrest have been reported, particularly during initial titration or rapid escalation of clozapine dosage. Rarely (approximately 1 case per 3000 patients), orthostatic hypotension has been accompanied by profound collapse and respiratory and/or cardiac arrest in patients receiving initial doses as low as 12.5 mg. Such reactions, which are sometimes fatal, are consistent with neurally-mediated reflex bradycardia. In some cases when collapse and cardiac and/or respiratory arrest developed during initial therapy, benzodiazepines or other psychotropic agents were used concomitantly, suggesting a possible adverse interaction between clozapine and these agents.

The risk of orthostatic hypotension may be reduced by initiating clozapine therapy at lower dosages, followed by gradual increases, and administration in divided doses. If hypotension occurs, dosage reduction of clozapine may be considered. In some cases, withholding the drug for 24 hours and then restarting at a lower dosage has been accomplished without recurrence of orthostatic hypotension. If clozapine therapy is temporarily interrupted (i.e., for 2 or more days), the manufacturers recommend that the drug be reinitiated at a lower dosage (12.5 mg once or twice daily).

Prolongation of QT Interval

Prolongation of the QT interval, torsades de pointes and other life-threatening ventricular arrhythmias, cardiac arrest, and sudden death have occurred in patients receiving clozapine. Patients at particular risk for these serious cardiovascular reactions include those with a history of QT-interval prolongation, long QT syndrome, family history of long QT syndrome or sudden cardiac death, significant cardiac arrhythmia, recent myocardial infarction, and uncompensated heart failure and those concurrently receiving other drugs that prolong the QT interval or inhibit the metabolism of clozapine. (See Drug Interactions: Drugs that Prolong the QT Interval and see also Drug Interactions: Drugs Affecting Hepatic Microsomal Enzymes.) Electrolyte abnormalities such as hypokalemia and hypomagnesemia also increase the risk of QT-interval prolongation.

Prior to initiating clozapine therapy, a careful physical examination should be performed and a medical and concomitant medication history should be obtained. A baseline ECG and serum chemistry panel should also be considered before initiating clozapine therapy. Clozapine should be discontinued if the corrected QT (QT$_c$) interval exceeds 500 msec. Clozapine should also be discontinued and a cardiac evaluation performed in patients who experience symptoms consistent with torsades de pointes or other arrhythmias (e.g., syncope, presyncope, dizziness, palpitations).

Baseline serum potassium and magnesium concentrations should be determined and electrolyte abnormalities, if present, should be corrected prior to initiating clozapine therapy. In addition, serum electrolytes should be periodically monitored during clozapine therapy.

Other Cardiovascular Effects

Tachycardia, which may persist throughout therapy in some cases, reportedly has been observed in up to 25% of patients receiving clozapine in clinical studies.

Postexercise decreases in left ventricular output, which may indicate left ventricular failure, have been reported in patients receiving clozapine. Although a causal relationship has not been established, atrial or ventricular fibrillation, ventricular tachycardia, palpitations, and myocardial infarction also have been reported during postmarketing surveillance in patients receiving the drug.

• *Autonomic Nervous System Effects*

Adverse autonomic nervous system effects occur in more than 5% of patients receiving clozapine. Dry mouth occurs frequently, but hypersalivation, an apparently paradoxical effect considering the drug's potent anticholinergic activity, is more common. (See Cautions: GI Effects.)

Other autonomic nervous system effects of clozapine include hyperhidrosis, decreased sweating, and visual disturbances. Increased salivation occurred in 31%, dry mouth and sweating in 6%, and visual disturbances in 5% of patients receiving clozapine in controlled clinical trials.

• *Hepatic Effects*

Transient increases in liver function test results, including serum aminotransferases (transaminases), LDH, and alkaline phosphatase, may occur with clozapine therapy. Clozapine-induced changes in liver function test results may be more pronounced than those with other tricyclic antipsychotic agents. Clozapine causes slight liver hyperplasia in rats; hyperplasia was reversible and no histologic changes were detectable. Clozapine also occasionally causes elevations of bilirubin concentration.

Cholestasis, hepatitis, jaundice, hepatotoxicity, hepatic steatosis, hepatic necrosis, hepatic fibrosis, hepatic cirrhosis, liver injury (hepatic, cholestatic, and mixed), and liver failure have been reported in patients receiving clozapine during postmarketing surveillance; however, a causal relationship to the drug has not been established.

Severe, life-threatening, and, in some cases, fatal hepatotoxicity, including hepatic failure, hepatic necrosis, and hepatitis, has been reported in postmarketing studies in clozapine-treated patients. (See Hepatotoxicity under Cautions: Precautions and Contraindications.)

• *Endocrine and Metabolic Effects*

Atypical antipsychotic agents have been associated with metabolic changes, including hyperglycemia, dyslipidemia, and weight gain. Such metabolic changes may be associated with increased cardiovascular and cerebrovascular risk.

Weight Gain

Weight gain has been observed with antipsychotic therapy. Clozapine may cause increased appetite, polyphagia, and weight gain in a substantial proportion (approximately one-third) of patients. Some clinicians suggest that the potential for weight gain with clozapine therapy may be similar to that with other antipsychotic agents; others state that they have observed greater weight gain with clozapine in some patients. In the 2-year InterSePT trial, weight gain reportedly occurred in 31% of patients receiving clozapine compared with 56% of those receiving olanzapine. Some clozapine-treated patients reportedly have gained up to 1 kg weekly for 6 weeks. Pooled data from 11 clinical studies in patients with schizophrenia indicate that 35% of clozapine-treated patients (median duration of exposure 609 days), 46% of olanzapine-treated patients (median duration of exposure 728 days), and 8% of chlorpromazine-treated patients (median duration of exposure 42 days) gained 7% or more of their baseline body weight.

Weight gain may result from the drug's serotonergic-, histaminergic-, and adrenergic-blocking properties. Weight gain has been reported to be a problem for some patients during long-term therapy with clozapine and may be a major cause of outpatient noncompliance. Some clinicians suggest using exercise and active measures (e.g., dietary counseling) to control dietary intake in clozapine-treated patients.

Hyperglycemia and Diabetes Mellitus

Hyperglycemia, sometimes severe and associated with ketoacidosis, hyperosmolar coma, or death, has been reported in patients receiving certain atypical antipsychotic agents, including clozapine. While confounding factors such as an increased background risk of diabetes mellitus in patients with schizophrenia and the increasing incidence of diabetes mellitus in the general population make it difficult to establish with certainty the relationship between use of agents in this drug class and glucose abnormalities, epidemiologic studies suggest an increased risk of treatment-emergent hyperglycemia-related adverse events in patients treated with the atypical antipsychotic agents included in the studies (e.g., clozapine, olanzapine, quetiapine, risperidone). (See Cautions: Precautions and Contraindications.)

Precise risk estimates for hyperglycemia-related adverse events in patients treated with atypical antipsychotics currently are not available. While some evidence suggests that the risk for diabetes may be greater with some atypical antipsychotics (e.g., clozapine, olanzapine) than with others (e.g., quetiapine, risperidone) in the class, available data are conflicting and insufficient to provide reliable estimates of relative risk associated with use of the various atypical antipsychotics.

In an analysis of 5 clinical studies in patients with schizophrenia (median treatment duration of 42 days), clozapine was associated with a greater average increase in fasting glucose concentrations compared with chlorpromazine (11 mg/dL versus 4 mg/dL, respectively). A greater proportion of patients receiving clozapine experienced shifts in fasting glucose concentrations from normal (less than 100 mg/dL) to high (126 mg/dL or higher) and from borderline (100–125 mg/dL) to high (126 mg/dL or higher) compared with those receiving chlorpromazine. Shifts in fasting glucose concentrations from normal to high were observed in 27 or 10%, and from borderline to high in 42 or 28% of patients receiving clozapine or chlorpromazine, respectively.

Dyslipidemia

Like some other antipsychotic agents, clozapine therapy has been associated with undesirable changes in lipid parameters, including elevations in serum cholesterol and triglyceride concentrations.

In a pooled analysis of 10 clinical studies in adults with schizophrenia, the mean increase in total cholesterol concentrations was 13 or 15 mg/dL in patients receiving clozapine or chlorpromazine, respectively, and in a pooled analysis of 2 studies in adults with schizophrenia, the mean increase in fasting triglyceride concentrations in clozapine-treated patients was 71 mg/dL (54%) compared with 39 mg/dL (35%) in chlorpromazine-treated patients. In these studies, the median duration of exposure was 45 or 38 days for clozapine or chlorpromazine, respectively; specific data on high-density lipoprotein (HDL)- or low-density lipoprotein (LDL)-cholesterol were not collected. An increase in serum total cholesterol concentrations (random or fasting) of 40 mg/dL or higher occurred in 33 or 25%, and increases in fasting serum triglyceride concentrations of 50 mg/dL or higher occurred in 50 or 43% of adults receiving clozapine or chlorpromazine, respectively. In addition, a greater proportion of patients receiving clozapine experienced an increase in serum total cholesterol concentrations from normal (below 200 mg/dL) to high (240 mg/dL or higher) or from borderline (200–239 mg/dL) to high (240 mg/dL or higher) compared with those receiving chlorpromazine.

The manufacturers recommend clinical monitoring, including baseline and periodic follow-up lipid evaluations, in patients receiving clozapine.

Hyperprolactinemia

Clozapine causes little or no elevation in serum prolactin concentrations. The drug has been reported to cause only a brief, transient elevation of prolactin concentration. (See Pharmacology: Neuroendocrine Effects.) Therefore, prolactin-dependent adverse effects such as galactorrhea and amenorrhea usually are not associated with clozapine therapy.

Other Endocrine and Metabolic Effects

Hyperuricemia, hyponatremia, weight loss, and pseudopheochromocytoma also have been reported in patients receiving clozapine during postmarketing surveillance, although a causal relationship to the drug has not been established.

Small decreases in protein-bound iodine or thyroxine concentrations have been reported in some patients receiving clozapine, but these values remained within normal limits.

● GI Effects

Increased salivation may occur in approximately one-third of patients receiving clozapine; in some studies, hypersalivation was reported in up to 75–85% of clozapine-treated patients. In the InterSePT trial, increased salivation reportedly occurred in 48% of patients receiving clozapine compared with 6% of those receiving olanzapine. Salivation may be profuse, very fluid, and particularly troublesome during sleep because of decreased swallowing. Since clozapine exhibits intrinsic anticholinergic properties, hypersalivation is an unexpected paradoxical effect. A muscle-relaxant effect of the drug may contribute to hypersalivation, but the cause has not been fully elucidated. Difficulty in swallowing has been reported in a few clozapine-treated patients, and it has been suggested that the drug may cause esophageal dysfunction, which may contribute to or exacerbate the nocturnal hypersalivation associated with clozapine therapy. Some clozapine-treated patients develop tolerance to increased salivation within a few weeks. Nonpharmacologic interventions such as the use of a towel on the pillow at night may help reduce the discomfort associated with clozapine-associated hypersalivation during sleep. Occasionally, hypersalivation may be ameliorated by reduction of clozapine dosage or cautious use of a peripherally acting anticholinergic drug; however, some clinicians generally advise against the use of anticholinergic therapy for this adverse effect because of possible potentiation of clozapine's anticholinergic activity. (See Anticholinergic Toxicity and see also GI Hypomotility with Severe Complications under Cautions: Precautions and Contraindications.)

Other GI effects associated with clozapine therapy include constipation, diarrhea, nausea and vomiting, dyspepsia or heartburn, and abdominal discomfort; some of these effects have been reported in more than 5% of patients. Constipation, nausea, vomiting, and dyspepsia reportedly occurred in 14–25% of patients receiving clozapine in the InterSePT trial compared with 8–10% of those receiving olanzapine. For additional information on clozapine-induced constipation and possible severe bowel complications, see GI Hypomotility with Severe Complications under Cautions: GI Effects and also under Cautions: Precautions and Contraindications. Although some clinicians advocate the use of metoclopramide (e.g., in doses less than 30 mg daily) for the treatment of clozapine-induced nausea, other clinicians suggest that metoclopramide or other dopamine antagonists not be used or be used with extreme caution for the treatment of clozapine-induced nausea because of their potential for causing parkinsonian manifestations and tardive dyskinesia.

Although a causal relationship to the drug has not been established, acute pancreatitis, dysphagia, salivary gland swelling, colitis, megacolon, and intestinal ischemia or infarction also have been reported in patients receiving clozapine during postmarketing surveillance.

GI Hypomotility with Severe Complications

Severe adverse GI effects have occurred with clozapine mainly due to its potent anticholinergic effects and resulting GI hypomotility. In postmarketing experience, these effects have ranged in severity from constipation to paralytic ileus. The increased frequency of constipation with clozapine and delayed diagnosis and treatment increased the risk of developing severe complications of GI hypomotility resulting in intestinal obstruction, fecal impaction, megacolon, and intestinal ischemia or infarction; these reactions have resulted in hospitalization, surgery, and death in some patients. The risk of severe adverse reactions in patients receiving clozapine is further increased with concomitant use of anticholinergic agents and other drugs that decrease GI peristalsis (including opiate analgesics); use of such drugs should therefore be avoided, if possible, during clozapine therapy.

Constipation is a frequent and well-established adverse effect associated with clozapine therapy; however, FDA states that serious and fatal bowel problems continue to be reported in patients receiving the drug. In January 2020, FDA therefore strengthened an existing warning in the clozapine prescribing information that constipation caused by the drug can, uncommonly, progress to serious bowel complications. FDA identified 10 cases of constipation that progressed to serious complications with clozapine use that were reported in the FDA Adverse Event Reporting System (FAERS) database from July 21, 2006 through July 20, 2016 and in the medical literature from July 21, 2006 through August 2, 2016. These cases resulted in hospitalization, surgery, and 5 deaths. Adverse events included necrotizing colitis (4 cases), intestinal ischemia or necrosis (5 cases), and volvulus

(1 case). The total daily dosage of clozapine in these patients ranged from 200–600 mg (median total daily dosage of 400 mg). The time to onset of serious bowel events ranged from 3 days to 6 months (median of 46 days). A preliminary review of additional FAERS data reported from July 21, 2016 through the end of 2019 identified similar findings. As a result of these findings, FDA is requiring a new warning and updates about this risk to be added to the prescribing information for all clozapine products.

The risk of constipation and severe bowel complications appears to be greater with clozapine than with other antipsychotic agents. Although clozapine can cause constipation and serious bowel complications when used alone, such serious complications of constipation have been reported with other antipsychotic agents (e.g., olanzapine) only when they were used in combination with other drugs with anticholinergic activity. The risk of such reactions is further increased at higher dosages of clozapine and when clozapine is used concurrently with drugs that have anticholinergic activity or other drugs that can cause constipation, including opiate analgesics.

Clozapine-induced GI hypomotility was objectively assessed and confirmed by measuring colonic transit time (CTT) using radiopaque markers in a study involving 37 patients. The study reviewed the effects of clozapine (monotherapy and combination antipsychotic therapy in 20 patients) and non-clozapine antipsychotic therapy (monotherapy and combination antipsychotic therapy in 17 patients) and concluded that nearly all patients receiving clozapine had increased CTTs. The median CTT in clozapine-treated patients was more than 4 times longer than in patients not receiving clozapine (105 hours versus 23 hours, respectively). Colonic hypomotility occurred in 80% of the patients receiving clozapine and in none of the patients receiving other antipsychotics (including aripiprazole, haloperidol, olanzapine, paliperidone, risperidone, and zuclopenthixol [not commercially available in the US]). An exposure-related increase in CTT was noted in this study (i.e., higher CTT observed with higher plasma clozapine concentrations). Patients receiving clozapine in this study did not report the hypomotility as subjective symptoms of constipation. (See GI Hypomotility with Severe Complications under Cautions: Precautions and Contraindications.)

● Genitourinary Effects

Genitourinary effects reported with clozapine therapy include polyuria, enuresis, and impotence. Acute interstitial nephritis, renal failure, nocturnal enuresis, priapism, and retrograde ejaculation also have been reported with clozapine therapy during postmarketing surveillance, although a causal relationship to the drug has not been established.

● Respiratory Effects

Although a causal relationship to the drug has not been established, aspiration, pleural effusion, sleep apnea, and pneumonia and lower respiratory tract infection have been reported with clozapine therapy during postmarketing surveillance.

Respiratory depression or failure, including arrest requiring resuscitation, also has been reported in patients receiving clozapine, usually at initiation of therapy and particularly in patients receiving concomitant benzodiazepine therapy or in those with a history of recent benzodiazepine use. Some evidence indicates that the incidence of respiratory arrest and vascular collapse is about 1–2% of patients receiving clozapine concomitantly with a benzodiazepine. For additional precautionary information about this potential effect, see Benzodiazepines under Drug Interactions: CNS Depressants.

● Dermatologic and Sensitivity Reactions

Rash has been reported in 2% of patients receiving clozapine.

Hypersensitivity reactions, including photosensitivity, vasculitis, erythema multiforme, skin pigmentation disorder, and Stevens-Johnson syndrome, have been reported with clozapine during postmarketing surveillance; however, a causal relationship to the drug has not been established.

● Other Adverse Effects

Myasthenic syndrome, rhabdomyolysis, systemic lupus erythematosus, angioedema, periorbital edema, leukocytoclastic vasculitis, and angle-closure (narrow angle) glaucoma have been reported with clozapine during postmarketing surveillance, although a causal relationship to the drug has not been established.

● Precautions and Contraindications

Clozapine shares many of the toxic potentials of other antipsychotic agents (e.g., phenothiazines), and the usual precautions associated with therapy with these agents should be observed. (See Cautions, in the Phenothiazines General Statement 28:16.08.24.)

Cognitive and Motor Impairment

Because of clozapine's sedative effects and because the drug potentially may impair cognitive and motor performance, clozapine-treated patients should be cautioned about operating hazardous machinery, including driving a motor vehicle, until they are reasonably certain that the drug does not adversely affect them. Because such effects may be dose-related, a reduction in clozapine dosage should be considered if they occur.

Hepatotoxicity

Severe, life-threatening, and sometimes fatal hepatotoxicity has been reported in clozapine-treated patients. Patients receiving clozapine should be monitored for possible signs and symptoms of liver injury such as fatigue, malaise, anorexia, nausea, jaundice, hyperbilirubinemia, coagulopathy, and hepatic encephalopathy. Liver function tests should also be monitored in patients receiving the drug. Permanent discontinuance of clozapine should be considered if hepatitis or elevated aminotransferase concentrations combined with other systemic symptoms are caused by the drug.

Fever

During clozapine therapy, patients may experience transient temperature elevations exceeding 38°C, with the peak incidence within the first 3 weeks of therapy. (See Cautions: Fever.) While this fever generally is benign and self-limiting, it may necessitate discontinuance of therapy. Occasionally, there may be an associated increase or decrease in leukocyte count.

Clozapine therapy should be interrupted as a precautionary measure and an ANC obtained in any patient who develops fever (38.5°C or higher) during treatment; patients should be carefully evaluated to rule out severe neutropenia or infection. In addition, ANC should be monitored in any patient who develops fever within 2 weeks after discontinuance of clozapine. In the presence of high fever, the possibility of neuroleptic malignant syndrome also must be considered. (See Neuroleptic Malignant Syndrome under Cautions: Nervous System Effects.)

Anticholinergic Toxicity

Clozapine has potent anticholinergic activity, and therapy with the drug may result in CNS and peripheral anticholinergic toxicity, particularly at higher dosages or in overdosage situations. (See Acute Toxicity.) Clozapine should therefore be used with caution in individuals whose condition may be aggravated by anticholinergic effects (e.g., patients with a current or previous history of constipation, clinically important prostatic hypertrophy, urinary retention, or angle-closure [narrow-angle] glaucoma).

Concomitant use of clozapine with other drugs that have anticholinergic activity should be avoided, if possible, because of the risk of anticholinergic toxicity and severe adverse GI reactions. (See Drug Interactions: Drugs with Anticholinergic Activity and Drugs that Decrease GI Peristalsis.)

Thromboembolic Events

Pulmonary embolism and deep-vein thrombosis have been reported with clozapine therapy. The possibility of pulmonary embolism should be considered in patients presenting with deep-vein thrombosis, acute dyspnea, chest pain, or other respiratory signs and symptoms.

Individuals with Phenylketonuria

Individuals with phenylketonuria (i.e., homozygous genetic deficiency of phenylalanine hydroxylase) and other individuals who must restrict their intake of phenylalanine should be warned that clozapine orally disintegrating tablets contain aspartame, which is metabolized in the GI tract to phenylalanine following oral administration; the respective manufacturer's labeling should be consulted for specific information regarding aspartame content of individual preparations and dosage strengths.

Neuroleptic Malignant Syndrome

Neuroleptic malignant syndrome (NMS), a potentially fatal syndrome requiring immediate discontinuance of the drug and intensive symptomatic treatment, has been reported in patients receiving antipsychotic agents, including clozapine. If a patient requires antipsychotic therapy following recovery from NMS, the potential reintroduction of drug therapy should be carefully considered. If antipsychotic therapy is reintroduced, the dosage generally should be increased gradually, and an antipsychotic agent other than the agent believed to have precipitated NMS generally should be chosen. In addition, such patients should be carefully monitored since recurrences of NMS have been reported. (See Neuroleptic Malignant Syndrome under Cautions: Nervous System Effects.) For additional information on NMS, see Neuroleptic Malignant Syndrome under Cautions: Nervous System Effects, in the Phenothiazines General Statement 28:16.08.24.

Metabolic Effects

Atypical antipsychotic agents are associated with metabolic changes that may increase cardiovascular and cerebrovascular risk (e.g., hyperglycemia, dyslipidemia, weight gain). While all atypical antipsychotics produce some metabolic changes, each drug has its own specific risk profile.

Hyperglycemia, sometimes severe and associated with ketoacidosis, hyperosmolar coma, or death, has been reported in patients receiving atypical antipsychotic agents, including clozapine. The manufacturers state that patients with preexisting diabetes mellitus in whom therapy with an atypical antipsychotic is initiated should be closely monitored for worsening glycemic control; those with risk factors for diabetes (e.g., obesity, family history of diabetes) should undergo fasting blood glucose testing upon therapy initiation and periodically throughout treatment. Any patient who develops manifestations of hyperglycemia (e.g., polydipsia, polyphagia, polyuria, weakness) during treatment with an atypical antipsychotic should undergo fasting blood glucose testing. In some cases, patients who developed hyperglycemia while receiving an atypical antipsychotic have required continuance of antidiabetic treatment despite discontinuance of the suspect drug; in other cases, hyperglycemia resolved with discontinuance of the antipsychotic.

Various experts have developed additional recommendations for the management of diabetes risks in patients receiving atypical antipsychotics; these include initial screening measures and regular monitoring (e.g., determination of diabetes risk factors; BMI determination using weight and height; waist circumference; blood pressure; fasting blood glucose; hemoglobin A_{1c} [HbA_{1c}]; fasting lipid profile), as well as provision of patient education and referral to clinicians experienced in the treatment of diabetes, when appropriate. Although some clinicians state that a switch from one atypical antipsychotic agent to another that has not been associated with substantial weight gain or diabetes should be considered in patients who experience weight gain (equal to or exceeding 5% of baseline body weight) or develop worsening glycemia or dyslipidemia at any time during therapy, such recommendations are controversial because differences in risk of developing diabetes associated with use of the different atypical antipsychotics remain to be fully established. Many clinicians consider antipsychotic efficacy the most important factor when making treatment decisions and suggest that detrimental effects of switching from a beneficial treatment regimen also should be considered in addition to any potential for exacerbation or development of medical conditions (e.g., diabetes). Decisions to alter drug therapy should be made on an individual basis, weighing the potential risks and benefits of the particular drug in each patient. (See Hyperglycemia and Diabetes Mellitus under Cautions: Endocrine and Metabolic Effects.)

Because undesirable changes in serum lipids have been observed with clozapine therapy, the manufacturers recommend appropriate clinical monitoring, including baseline and periodic follow-up lipid evaluations, in all patients receiving the drug. (See Dyslipidemia under Cautions: Endocrine and Metabolic Effects.)

Clozapine therapy may result in weight gain. Patients receiving the drug should be advised that weight gain has occurred during clozapine treatment. The manufacturers recommend clinical monitoring of weight in patients receiving the drug. (See Weight Gain under Cautions: Endocrine and Metabolic Effects.)

Falls

Clozapine therapy may cause somnolence, postural hypotension, and motor and sensory instability, which may lead to falls; as a consequence, fractures or other injuries may occur. For patients with diseases or conditions or receiving other drugs that could exacerbate these effects, fall risk assessments should be completed when initiating antipsychotic treatment and periodically during long-term therapy.

Orthostatic Hypotension, Bradycardia, and Syncope

Orthostatic hypotension, bradycardia, syncope, and cardiac arrest can occur with clozapine therapy; these effects are more likely to occur during initial titration of the drug, particularly with rapid dose escalation, but may even occur with the first dose at clozapine dosages as low as 12.5 mg. The risk of orthostatic hypotension may be reduced by initiating therapy at lower dosages, followed by gradual increases, and administration in divided doses. If hypotension occurs, dosage reduction of clozapine may be considered. Patients should be informed of the risk of orthostatic hypotension associated with use of clozapine, especially during the period of initial dosage titration. In addition, if clozapine therapy has been discontinued for more than 2 days, patients should be advised to contact their clinician for dosing instructions. .)

Clozapine should be used with particular caution in patients with known cardiovascular disease (history of myocardial infarction or ischemia, heart failure, or conduction abnormalities), cerebrovascular disease, or conditions that would predispose to hypotension (e.g., dehydration, hypovolemia, concomitant antihypertensive therapy).

GI Hypomotility with Severe Complications

Severe adverse GI reactions have occurred in patients receiving clozapine, primarily due to its potent anticholinergic effects and resulting GI hypomotility. In postmarketing experience, reported adverse effects ranged from constipation to paralytic ileus. Increased frequency of constipation and delayed diagnosis and treatment increased the risk of severe complications of GI hypomotility, resulting in intestinal obstruction, fecal impaction, megacolon, and intestinal ischemia or infarction. These reactions have resulted in hospitalization, surgery, and death. The risk of such severe adverse reactions is further increased with concomitant use of anticholinergic agents as well as with other drugs that decrease GI peristalsis (e.g., opiate agonists); therefore, concomitant use of clozapine with such drugs should be avoided whenever possible.

Prior to initiating clozapine therapy, patients should be screened for constipation and treated, if necessary. However, clinicians should keep in mind that subjective symptoms of constipation may not accurately reflect the degree of GI hypomotility in clozapine-treated patients. Therefore, clinicians should frequently reassess bowel function with careful attention to any changes in the frequency or character of bowel movements as well as possible signs and symptoms of hypomotility complications (e.g., nausea, vomiting, abdominal distension, abdominal pain). If constipation or GI hypomotility is identified, the patient should be closely monitored and treated promptly with appropriate laxatives, as needed, to prevent severe complications. In addition, the prophylactic use of laxatives in high-risk patients (e.g., those with a history of constipation or bowel obstruction) should be considered. Some clinicians recommend that laxatives should be prescribed prophylactically in all patients receiving clozapine.

Clinicians should educate patients and caregivers about the risks, prevention, and treatment of clozapine-induced constipation, including drugs to avoid when possible during therapy (e.g., drugs with anticholinergic activity). Appropriate hydration, physical activity, and fiber intake should be encouraged, and clinicians should emphasize that prompt attention to and treatment of developing constipation or other GI symptoms are essential in preventing severe complications. Patients and caregivers should be advised to contact their clinician if they experience symptoms of constipation (e.g., difficulty passing stools, incomplete passage of stool, decreased bowel movement frequency) or other symptoms associated with GI hypomotility (e.g., nausea, abdominal distension or pain, vomiting). (See GI Hypomotility with Severe Complications under Cautions: GI Effects.)

Geriatric Patients with Dementia-related Psychosis

Geriatric patients with dementia-related psychosis treated with antipsychotic drugs are at increased risk of death compared with patients receiving placebo.

An increased risk of adverse cerebrovascular events (e.g., stroke, transient ischemic attack), including fatalities, has been observed in geriatric patients with dementia-related psychosis treated with some atypical antipsychotic agents. Clozapine should therefore be used with caution in patients with risk factors for stroke.

The manufacturer states that clozapine is *not* approved for the treatment of patients with dementia-related psychosis.

Myocarditis, Cardiomyopathy, and Mitral Valve Incompetence

Because myocarditis and cardiomyopathy, which are sometimes fatal, have been reported in patients treated with clozapine, signs and symptoms suggestive of these reactions, including chest pain, dyspnea, persistent tachycardia at rest, palpitations, fever, flu-like symptoms, hypotension, other manifestations of heart failure, or ECG changes, should alert the clinician to perform further investigations. If the diagnosis of myocarditis or cardiomyopathy is confirmed, clozapine therapy should be discontinued and generally should *not* be reinitiated unless the benefit to the patient clearly outweighs the potential risk of recurrent myocarditis or cardiomyopathy.

Mitral valve incompetence with mild or moderate mitral regurgitation has been reported in patients diagnosed with cardiomyopathy during clozapine therapy. In patients with suspected cardiomyopathy, consideration should be given to performing a 2-dimensional Doppler echocardiogram to identify mitral valve incompetence.

Seizures

Generalized tonic-clonic (grand mal) seizures have occurred in patients receiving clozapine, particularly in patients receiving high dosages (greater than 600 mg daily) and/or in whom plasma clozapine concentrations were elevated. Clozapine should be used with caution in patients with a history of seizure disorders or other risk factors predisposing to seizures (e.g., history of head trauma or other preexisting CNS pathology, concomitant use of other drugs that lower the seizure threshold, history of alcohol abuse). Because of the substantial risk of seizures associated with clozapine use, patients should be advised not to engage in any activity where sudden loss of consciousness could cause serious risk to themselves or others (e.g., driving an automobile, operating complex machinery, swimming, climbing).

Severe Neutropenia

Because of the risk of severe neutropenia, which can lead to serious and potentially fatal infections, clozapine therapy should be reserved for use in patients who have failed to respond adequately to standard antipsychotic therapy. Patients should be warned of this risk and informed that clozapine is only available through the Clozapine REMS program that ensures baseline and periodic monitoring of neutrophil counts. (See General under Dosage and Administration and also see Cautions: Hematologic Effects.) In addition, patients receiving clozapine therapy should be advised to immediately report the development of flu-like symptoms, fever, lethargy, malaise, weakness, mucous membrane ulceration, skin, pharyngeal, vaginal, urinary, or pulmonary infection, or any other potential manifestation of infection. Patients who develop severe neutropenia (ANC less than 500/mm³) while receiving clozapine generally should *not* be rechallenged with the drug. However, for some patients who have no acceptable alternatives to clozapine, the risk of serious psychiatric illness from discontinuing treatment may outweigh the risk of severe neutropenia upon rechallenge; in such cases, consultation with a hematology specialist may be helpful in deciding whether to rechallenge a patient with clozapine.

It is not known whether concurrent use of other drugs known to cause neutropenia increases the risk or severity of clozapine-induced neutropenia. (See Drug Interactions: Other Drugs Associated with Neutropenia.)

Other Precautions and Contraindications

Clozapine is contraindicated in patients with a history of serious hypersensitivity to clozapine (e.g., photosensitivity, vasculitis, erythema multiforme, Stevens-Johnson syndrome) or any ingredient in the formulation. (See Cautions: Dermatologic and Sensitivity Reactions.)

● Pediatric Precautions

The manufacturers state that the safety and efficacy of clozapine in pediatric patients have not been established. However, clozapine has been used in a limited number of children and adolescents with treatment-refractory schizophrenia (see Pediatric Considerations under Psychotic Disorders: Treatment-resistant Schizophrenia, in Uses) and results of at least one randomized, double-blind clinical study indicate that adverse hematologic effects were a major concern for children and adolescents receiving clozapine†. Although no cases of agranulocytosis occurred in this study, 24% of these children and adolescents experienced mild to moderate neutropenia during 2 years of follow-up compared with an estimated cumulative risk of 1.5–2% of developing neutropenia in adults. The precise mechanism by which clozapine induces agranulocytosis is not known, but a higher concentration of the metabolite norclozapine, which has been associated with hematopoietic toxicity in children and adolescents receiving clozapine, has been suggested as a possible reason for the increased risk in this age group. As with adult patients, adjunctive lithium has been used successfully in the management of clozapine-induced neutropenia in pediatric patients with schizophrenia†.

In addition to adverse hematologic effects, clinically important seizure activity (e.g., epileptiform spikes, myoclonus, tonic-clonic seizures) also has been reported in children and adolescents with no previous history of epilepsy who received clozapine. In some cases, EEG abnormalities were associated with clinical deterioration (i.e., increased aggression, psychosis, irritability). Because some children and adolescents responded behaviorally to reduced dosages of clozapine and the addition of an anticonvulsant (e.g., valproate), it has been suggested that the EEG may be a sensitive indicator of clozapine toxicity in children as well as in adults.

● Geriatric Precautions

Clinical studies of clozapine did not include sufficient numbers of patients 65 years of age and older to determine whether geriatric patients respond differently than younger patients. Because geriatric patients may be at increased risk for certain cardiovascular (e.g., orthostatic hypotension, tachycardia) and anticholinergic effects of the drug (e.g., constipation, urinary retention in the presence of prostatic hypertrophy), clozapine should be used cautiously in this age group. In addition, geriatric patients generally are more sensitive than younger patients to drugs that affect the CNS. Data from clinical studies indicate that the incidence of tardive dyskinesia appears to be highest among geriatric patients, especially women. In general, dosage should be titrated carefully in geriatric patients, usually initiating therapy at the low end of the dosage range; the greater frequency of decreased hepatic, renal, and/or cardiac function and of concomitant disease and drug therapy observed in the elderly also should be considered.

Geriatric patients with dementia-related psychosis treated with antipsychotic drugs are at an increased risk of death compared with patients receiving placebo. Analyses of 17 placebo-controlled trials (modal duration of 10 weeks) revealed an approximate 1.6- to 1.7- fold increase in mortality among geriatric patients receiving atypical antipsychotic drugs (i.e., aripiprazole, olanzapine, quetiapine, risperidone) compared with that observed in patients receiving placebo. Over the course of a typical 10-week controlled trial, the rate of death in drug-treated patients was about 4.5% compared with a rate of about 2.6% in the placebo group. Although the causes of death were varied, most of the deaths appeared to be either cardiovascular (e.g., heart failure, sudden death) or infectious (e.g., pneumonia) in nature. Observational studies suggest that, similar to atypical antipsychotics, treatment with conventional (first-generation) antipsychotics may increase mortality; the extent to which the findings of increased mortality in observational studies may be attributed to the antipsychotic drug as opposed to some characteristic(s) of the patients remains unclear. Clozapine is not approved for the treatment of patients with dementia-related psychosis.

An increased risk of adverse cerebrovascular events has been observed in patients with dementia treated with some atypical antipsychotic agents. The mechanism for this increased risk is not known. The manufacturers state that an increased risk cannot be excluded for other antipsychotics, including clozapine, or other patient populations. Clozapine should therefore be used with caution in patients with risk factors for stroke.

● Mutagenicity and Carcinogenicity

Clozapine did not exhibit carcinogenic potential in long-term studies in mice and rats receiving dosages up to 0.3 and 0.4 times the maximum recommended human dosage on a mg/m² basis, respectively. Clozapine also did not exhibit genotoxic or mutagenic effects when assayed in appropriate bacterial and mammalian tests.

• Pregnancy, Fertility, and Lactation

Pregnancy

Reproduction studies in rats and rabbits using clozapine dosages up to 0.4 and 0.9 times the maximum recommended human dosage on a mg/m² basis, respectively, have not revealed evidence of harm to the fetus.

Neonates exposed to antipsychotic agents, including clozapine, during the third trimester of pregnancy are at risk for extrapyramidal and/or withdrawal symptoms following delivery. There have been reports of agitation, hypertonia, hypotonia, tardive dyskinetic-like symptoms, tremor, somnolence, respiratory distress, and feeding disorder in these neonates. The majority of cases were also confounded by other factors, including concomitant use of other drugs known to be associated with withdrawal symptoms, prematurity, congenital malformations, and obstetrical and perinatal complications; however, some cases suggested that neonatal extrapyramidal and withdrawal symptoms may occur with exposure to antipsychotic agents alone. Some of the cases described time of symptom onset, which ranged from birth to one month after birth. Any neonate exhibiting extrapyramidal or withdrawal symptoms following in utero exposure to antipsychotic agents should be monitored. Symptoms were self-limiting in some neonates but varied in severity; some infants required intensive care unit support and prolonged hospitalization. For further information on extrapyramidal and withdrawal symptoms in neonates, see Cautions: Pregnancy, Fertility, and Lactation, in the Phenothiazines General Statement 28:16.08.24.

The manufacturers state that there are no adequate and well-controlled studies to date using clozapine in pregnant women, and the drug should be used during pregnancy only when clearly needed. Women should be advised to notify their clinician if they become pregnant or plan to become pregnant during therapy with the drug. In addition, clinicians should advise women of childbearing potential about the benefits and risks of using antipsychotic agents during pregnancy. Patients should also be advised not to stop taking their antipsychotic agent if they become pregnant without first consulting with their clinician, since abruptly discontinuing the drugs can cause clinically important complications.

Fertility

Reproduction studies in rats using clozapine dosages up to 0.4 times the maximum recommended human dosage on a mg/m² basis have not revealed impaired fertility.

Lactation

Clozapine is distributed into milk in humans. Because of the potential for serious adverse reactions to clozapine in nursing infants, a decision should be made whether to discontinue nursing or the drug, taking into account the importance of the drug to the woman.

DRUG INTERACTIONS

• Drugs Affecting Hepatic Microsomal Enzymes

Clozapine is a substrate for many cytochrome P-450 (CYP) isoenzymes, in particular 1A2, 2D6, and 3A4. Concomitant use of clozapine with drugs that inhibit CYP1A2, CYP2D6, or CYP3A4 may result in increased plasma concentrations of clozapine. When used concomitantly with *potent* CYP1A2 inhibitors (e.g., ciprofloxacin, enoxacin [no longer commercially available in the US], fluvoxamine), clozapine dosage should be reduced to one-third of the original dosage. The dosage should be increased back to the original dosage when the potent CYP1A2 inhibitor is discontinued. When used concomitantly with moderate or weak CYP1A2 inhibitors (e.g., oral contraceptives, caffeine) or inhibitors of CYP2D6 or CYP3A4 (e.g., bupropion, cimetidine, duloxetine, erythromycin, escitalopram, fluoxetine, paroxetine, quinidine, sertraline, terbinafine), patients should be monitored for adverse effects and dosage reduction of clozapine should be considered, if necessary. If a moderate or weak CYP1A2 inhibitor or a CYP2D6 or CYP3A4 inhibitor is discontinued during clozapine therapy, patients should be monitored for decreased efficacy of clozapine and an increase in clozapine dosage may be necessary.

Conversely, concomitant use of clozapine with drugs or substances that induce CYP1A2 (e.g., tobacco smoke) or CYP3A4 (e.g., carbamazepine, phenytoin, rifampin, St. John's wort [*Hypericum perforatum*]) may result in decreased plasma concentrations of clozapine. The manufacturers state that concomitant use of a potent CYP3A4 inducer with clozapine is not recommended; however, if concomitant use cannot be avoided, patients should be monitored for decreased efficacy of clozapine and consideration should be given to increasing the dosage of clozapine, if necessary. If clozapine is used concomitantly with a moderate or weak CYP1A2 inducer (e.g., tobacco smoke), patients should be monitored for decreased efficacy of clozapine and an increase in clozapine dosage may be necessary. Likewise, if a CYP1A2 or CYP3A4 inducer is discontinued during clozapine therapy, patients should be monitored for possible adverse effects and dosage reduction of clozapine should be considered, if necessary.

Phenytoin

Substantial reductions in plasma clozapine concentrations and exacerbation of psychosis have been reported in patients receiving concomitant therapy with clozapine and phenytoin. In 2 patients stabilized for 1–2 weeks on a given dosage of clozapine, addition of phenytoin for prevention of clozapine-induced seizures resulted in a 65–85% decrease in steady-state plasma clozapine concentrations. Control of psychotic manifestations was regained in both patients by gradually increasing the clozapine dosage.

Because phenytoin is a potent inducer of CYP3A4, the manufacturers of clozapine state that concomitant use of these drugs generally is not recommended. However, if concomitant use of clozapine and phenytoin is necessary, patients should be monitored for decreased efficacy of clozapine and consideration should be given to increasing the dosage of clozapine, if necessary. Likewise, if phenytoin is discontinued during clozapine therapy, patients should be monitored for possible adverse effects and dosage reduction of clozapine should be considered, if necessary.

Carbamazepine

Concomitant use of clozapine and carbamazepine has been shown to decrease clozapine concentrations by about 40–50%. In addition, neuroleptic malignant syndrome has been reported rarely with clozapine therapy alone and during concomitant therapy with carbamazepine. (See Neuroleptic Malignant Syndrome under Cautions: Nervous System Effects.) Because carbamazepine is a potent inducer of CYP3A4, the manufacturers of clozapine state that concomitant use of these agents generally is not recommended. However, if concomitant use of clozapine and carbamazepine is necessary, patients should be monitored for decreased efficacy of clozapine and consideration should be given to increasing the dosage of clozapine if necessary. Likewise, if carbamazepine is discontinued during clozapine therapy, dosage reduction of clozapine should be considered.

Selective Serotonin-reuptake Inhibitors

Concomitant use of clozapine with certain selective serotonin-reuptake inhibitors (SSRIs), including escitalopram, fluoxetine, fluvoxamine, paroxetine, and sertraline, can increase plasma concentrations of clozapine due to inhibition of clozapine metabolism by SSRIs. Modest (less than twofold) elevations in plasma clozapine concentrations have been reported in patients receiving clozapine concomitantly with certain SSRIs (i.e., fluoxetine, paroxetine, sertraline).

Substantial (threefold) increases in trough plasma clozapine concentrations have occurred in patients receiving concomitant therapy with clozapine and the potent CYP1A2 inhibitor fluvoxamine. Clozapine dosage should be reduced to one-third of the usual dosage when used concomitantly with fluvoxamine and should be increased back to the original dosage if fluvoxamine is discontinued.

• Drugs Metabolized by Hepatic Microsomal Enzymes

Clozapine may increase systemic exposure of other drugs metabolized by CYP2D6 (e.g., some antidepressants, phenothiazines, carbamazepine, class Ic antiarrhythmics [e.g., encainide, flecainide, propafenone]). Caution should be exercised when such drugs are used concomitantly with clozapine. The manufacturers state that dosage reduction of the CYP2D6 substrate may be necessary.

• Other Drugs Associated with Neutropenia

It is not known whether concurrent use of other drugs known to cause neutropenia increases the risk or severity of clozapine-induced neutropenia. The manufacturers of clozapine currently state that there is no strong scientific rationale to avoid clozapine treatment in patients concurrently treated with such drugs. However, if clozapine is used in patients concurrently receiving other drugs known to cause neutropenia (e.g., some antineoplastic agents), the manufacturers state that closer monitoring than usually recommended should be considered and, in patients concomitantly receiving antineoplastic agents, the treating oncologist should be consulted.

Drugs Affecting the Seizure Threshold

Clozapine may lower the seizure threshold and is associated with dose-related increases in the risk of seizures (see Seizures under Cautions: Nervous System Effects). Therefore, the manufacturers state that clozapine should be used with caution in patients receiving concomitant therapy with other agents that lower the seizure threshold. In addition, caution is advised in patients in whom alcohol abuse is a concern.

CNS Depressants
Benzodiazepines

Severe hypotension (including absence of measurable blood pressure), respiratory or cardiac arrest, and loss of consciousness have been reported in several patients who received clozapine concomitantly with or following benzodiazepine (i.e., flurazepam, lorazepam, diazepam) therapy. Such effects occurred following administration of 12.5–150 mg of clozapine concurrently with or within 24 hours of the benzodiazepine, but patients generally have recovered within a few minutes to hours, usually spontaneously; the reactions usually developed on the first or second day of clozapine therapy. Although a causal relationship has not been established and such effects also have been observed in clozapine-treated patients who were not receiving a benzodiazepine concomitantly (see Cautions: Cardiovascular Effects), death resulting from respiratory arrest reportedly has occurred in at least one patient receiving clozapine concomitantly with a benzodiazepine. An increased incidence of dizziness and sedation and greater increases in liver enzyme test results also have been reported with this drug combination.

Other CNS-active Agents

Although a causal relationship has not been established, at least one death has been reported with concomitant clozapine and haloperidol therapy. A 31-year-old woman with schizophrenia developed respiratory arrest, became comatose, and died 4 days after receiving 10 mg of haloperidol orally and a single 100-mg dose of clozapine IM. The patient had been maintained on oral clozapine 200 mg daily for 2 years and also had received smaller doses of haloperidol concomitantly with clozapine therapy without unusual adverse effect.

Neuroleptic malignant syndrome has been reported rarely with clozapine therapy alone and during concomitant therapy with clozapine and carbamazepine, lithium, or other CNS-active agents. (See Neuroleptic Malignant Syndrome under Cautions: Nervous System Effects.)

Concomitant use of clozapine and lithium may also increase the risk of seizures.

Drugs that Prolong the QT Interval

Because of additive effects on QT-interval prolongation, clozapine should be used with caution in patients receiving other drugs known to prolong the QT interval, including class Ia antiarrhythmics (e.g., quinidine, procainamide), class III antiarrhythmics (e.g., amiodarone, sotalol), certain antipsychotic agents (e.g., chlorpromazine, haloperidol, iloperidone, mesoridazine [no longer commercially available in the US], pimozide, risperidone, thioridazine, ziprasidone), some anti-infective agents (e.g., erythromycin, gatifloxacin, moxifloxacin, sparfloxacin [no longer commercially available in the US]), and other drugs (e.g., dolasetron mesylate, droperidol, halofantrine [no longer commercially available in the US], levomethadyl acetate [no longer commercially available in the US], mefloquine, methadone, pentamidine, probucol [no longer commercially available in the US], tacrolimus). (See Prolongation of QT Interval under Cautions: Cardiovascular Effects.)

Drugs with Anticholinergic Activity and Drugs that Decrease GI Peristalsis

Clozapine has potent anticholinergic effects. Because of the risk of anticholinergic toxicity and severe GI adverse reactions related to hypomotility, concurrent use of clozapine and drugs with anticholinergic activity (e.g., benztropine, cyclobenzaprine, diphenhydramine) or drugs that decrease GI peristalsis (e.g., opiate analgesics) should be avoided whenever possible. (See GI Hypomotility with Severe

Complications and see also Anticholinergic Toxicity under Cautions: Precautions and Contraindications.)

Hypotensive Agents

Clozapine may be additive with or potentiate the actions of hypotensive agents; the drug should be used with particular caution in patients receiving concomitant antihypertensive therapy.

Smoking

Smoking tobacco products (e.g., cigarettes) moderately induces CYP1A2, and may substantially reduce plasma clozapine concentrations. Limited data indicate that plasma clozapine concentrations following a given dose in smokers average 60–82% of those in nonsmokers. The manufacturers state that if clozapine is used in smokers, patients should be monitored for decreased efficacy of clozapine and consideration should be given to increasing the dosage, if necessary. Likewise, if smoking is discontinued during clozapine therapy, patients should be monitored for possible adverse effects and dosage reduction of clozapine should be considered, if necessary.

ACUTE TOXICITY

Pathogenesis

Acute toxicity studies in animals revealed that the LD_{50}s for clozapine administered orally, IV, or intraperitoneally are approximately 145–325, 58–61, and 90 mg/kg, respectively.

Although the acute lethal dose of clozapine in humans remains to be established, fatal overdoses with the drug generally have been associated with doses exceeding 2.5 g. However, there also have been reports of patients surviving overdoses that substantially exceeded 4 g of the drug.

Manifestations

In general, overdosage of clozapine may be expected to produce effects that are extensions of the drug's pharmacologic and adverse effects. The most commonly reported signs and symptoms of clozapine overdosage have been altered states of consciousness and CNS depression (e.g., sedation, delirium, coma), tachycardia, hypotension, respiratory depression or failure, and hypersalivation. Seizures, cardiac arrhythmias, and aspiration pneumonia also have occurred with overdosage of clozapine in some patients. (See Seizures under Cautions: Nervous System Effects.)

A 24-year-old woman who ingested 2 g in excess of her prescribed daily dosage (i.e., total ingestion approximately 3 g within a 24-hour period) had a tonic-clonic (grand mal) seizure; her plasma clozapine concentration 1 hour after the seizure (1313 ng/mL) was 500 ng/mL higher than usual, but she recovered uneventfully. In a 50-year-old woman who ingested 1 g of clozapine, the only manifestations were confusion and hallucinations lasting about 48 hours. A 26-year-old man who ingested approximately 3 g of clozapine became drowsy, agitated, and disoriented; he also had visual hallucinations, dysarthria, tachycardia, and hypersalivation. The patient was treated with gastric lavage and also received diazepam, digitalis, and anti-infectives, but continued to exhibit manifestations of severe central anticholinergic toxicity. Administration of physostigmine salicylate 2 mg by slow IV injection resulted in improvement in the patient's mental status within minutes; however, symptoms recurred after approximately 1 hour. Symptoms finally remitted 18–24 hours later with no further treatment.

Treatment

Treatment of clozapine overdosage generally requires symptomatic and supportive care, including monitoring of cardiac and vital signs. There is no specific antidote for the management of clozapine overdosage.

The manufacturers recommend establishing and maintaining an airway and ensuring adequate ventilation and oxygenation. Electrolyte and acid-base balance should be monitored and adjusted accordingly. Peritoneal dialysis or hemodialysis is of limited value in the treatment of clozapine overdosage because the drug is almost totally bound to serum proteins. While physostigmine salicylate may be useful as adjunctive treatment if severe anticholinergic toxicity is present, the drug should *not* be used routinely because of its potential adverse effects.

In managing clozapine overdosage, the clinician should consider the possibility of multiple drug involvement.

CHRONIC TOXICITY

Chronic toxicity studies in mice, rats, dogs, and monkeys have revealed no specific organ toxicity. After 1 year of treatment with clozapine, a brown discoloration caused by increased lipopigment was observed in various organs in rats; this change normally appears with increasing age. Discoloration was noted in the thyroid, brain, liver, kidney, heart, spleen, and skeletal muscle of rats, but such increased pigmentation was not associated with deleterious changes. The liver did show slight, dose-dependent changes, including centrolobular vacuolation, hepatocyte swelling, and increased weight.

PHARMACOLOGY

Clozapine is a dibenzodiazepine-derivative antipsychotic agent. Clozapine shares some of the pharmacologic actions of other antipsychotic agents and has been described as an atypical or second-generation antipsychotic agent since many of its CNS effects differ from those of conventional (first-generation) agents (e.g., butyrophenones, phenothiazines). In fact, these apparent differences in actions on neostriatal dopaminergic receptors have led some investigators to question the importance of the dopaminergic system in mediating the therapeutic effects of neuroleptic drugs. The exact mechanism of antipsychotic action of clozapine has not been fully elucidated, but appears to be mediated through a combination of antagonist activity at dopamine type 2 (D_2) and serotonin type 2A (5-hydroxytryptamine [5-HT_{2A}]) receptors. Clozapine also acts as an antagonist at adrenergic, cholinergic, histaminergic, and other dopaminergic and serotonergic receptors.

● *Nervous System Effects*

Although the precise mechanism of action of antipsychotic drugs has not been fully elucidated, current data suggest that the therapeutic effects of atypical antipsychotic agents involve antagonism of dopaminergic and serotonergic systems in the CNS. In animals, classic neuroleptic agents increase muscle tone or induce postural abnormalities (catalepsy), antagonize stereotyped behaviors induced by the dopamine agonists apomorphine and amphetamine, accelerate dopamine turnover in various areas of the brain, increase serum prolactin concentrations, and produce dopamine receptor hypersensitivity on repeated administration. These effects, many of which have been attributed to blockade of dopamine receptors in the neostriatum, form the basis for the hypothesis that idiopathic psychoses result from overactivity of dopamine in neostriatal and mesolimbic systems.

Unlike typical antipsychotic agents, clozapine exerts relatively weak antidopaminergic action within the neostriatum and has a low propensity to produce extrapyramidal effects or stimulate prolactin secretion. While some studies have demonstrated that relatively high doses of clozapine suppress the conditioned avoidance response in animals, which is a characteristic of typical antipsychotic agents, this response is not completely blocked by clozapine, and tolerance to this effect develops rapidly with repeated dosing, suggesting that it is not specifically related to clozapine's antipsychotic action. Further research is needed to elucidate fully clozapine's antipsychotic action in terms of the drug's serotonergic, adrenergic, muscarinic, and peptidergic effects and their influences on functional alterations in dopamine receptor systems.

Antidopaminergic Effects

The therapeutic effects of antipsychotic drugs are thought to be mediated by dopaminergic blockade in the mesolimbic and mesocortical areas of the CNS, while antidopaminergic effects in the neostriatum appear to be associated with extrapyramidal effects. Several (at least 5) different types or subtypes of dopamine receptors have been identified in animals and humans. The relative densities of these receptors and their distribution and function vary for different neuroanatomical regions, and clozapine's unique effects may be secondary to regionally specific receptor interactions and/or other effects on dopaminergic neurons. Results obtained from receptor binding, behavioral, metabolic, and electrophysiologic studies of clozapine as well as the apparently low incidence of extrapyramidal effects associated with clozapine therapy suggest that the drug is more active in the mesolimbic than the neostriatal dopaminergic system. Results of some studies suggest that clozapine is more effective in increasing dopamine turnover and

release in the nucleus accumbens or olfactory tubercle than in the neostriatum with acute administration and that it reduces dopamine release in the accumbens but not in the neostriatum during prolonged administration, which suggests preferential effects on dopaminergic function in the limbic system. However, conflicting data (i.e., no preferential limbic effects) also have been reported with both acute and repeated administration of the drug, which may reflect differences in analytical techniques, regional differences in drug distribution or receptor affinity, or other variables.

Some evidence suggests that the effects of clozapine on dopamine metabolism in the neostriatum are dose related; unlike typical antipsychotic drugs, clozapine appears to increase striatal dopamine turnover only at supratherapeutic doses. Single high doses (80 mg/kg intraperitoneally) of clozapine in rats interfere with dopaminergic transmission by blocking postsynaptic dopamine receptors and causing a compensatory increase in dopaminergic neuronal firing, while lower doses retard dopamine release. Clozapine appears to increase striatal dopamine content when given either in single high doses or repeated low doses, and low doses of the drug reportedly decrease the degradation of dopamine to 3-methoxy-4-hydroxyphenylacetic acid (homovanillic acid, HVA) in the neostriatum. In a rodent model of tardive dyskinesia, single low doses (up to 1.2 mg/kg intraperitoneally) of clozapine suppressed ketamine-induced linguopharyngeal movements, which resemble symptoms of tardive dyskinesia (e.g., tongue protrusions, retrusions, and swallows), by 15–75% compared with baseline measures. At clozapine doses of 4.8 mg/kg or higher, clozapine caused total suppression of these movements, and duration of suppression became dose dependent. Since suppression of abnormal linguopharyngeal movements occurred at doses substantially lower than those reported to alter dopamine turnover, it has been suggested that doses of the drug lower than those required for antipsychotic activity may be useful for treating antipsychotic-induced tardive dyskinesia.

Current evidence suggests that the clinical potency and antipsychotic efficacy of both typical and atypical antipsychotic drugs generally are related to their affinity for and blockade of central dopamine D_2 receptors; however, antagonism at D_2 receptors does not appear to account fully for the antipsychotic effects of clozapine.

In in vitro studies, clozapine is a comparatively weak antagonist at D_2 receptors. Clozapine's affinity for the D_2 receptor on a weight basis reportedly is approximately one-third (33%) that of loxapine, one-tenth (10%) that of chlorpromazine, and one-fiftieth (2%) that of haloperidol. In oral dosages of 300 mg daily, clozapine produces a 40–65% occupancy of D_1 and D_2 receptors. During long-term clozapine therapy, the relative occupancy of D_1 receptors may become greater than that of D_2 receptors, or the long-term effects of the drug on D_2 receptors may be antagonized by its nondopaminergic properties. Although the in vitro affinity of clozapine for D_1 and D_2 receptors in brain tissue of animals appears to be similar, the drug's in vivo effects in many animals resemble those of D_1-receptor-specific antagonists. Compared with typical antipsychotic agents, clozapine shows greater affinity for and appears to produce greater blockade of neostriatal dopamine D_1 receptors; other data suggest that clozapine preferentially but not selectively antagonizes D_1 receptor-mediated functions. At clinically effective dosages, however, the drug produces comparable blockade of D_1 and D_2 receptors and less D_2 blockade than typical antipsychotic drugs. Long-term administration of clozapine leads to a 35–50% "up-regulation" of D_1 receptors, which is comparable to that observed with administration of selective D_1 antagonists; however, the number of D_2 receptors is not changed, possibly because the proportion of occupied receptors required to elicit a response is less for D_1 than for D_2 receptors. Limited evidence suggests that D_1 receptors may exist either coupled to adenylate cyclase or in uncoupled form. Clozapine appears to be a potent, competitive inhibitor of dopamine-stimulated adenylate cyclase in vitro, and the adenylate cyclase-coupled state of the D_1 receptor binds clozapine with high affinity; in contrast, typical antipsychotic agents bind preferentially to the uncoupled D_1 receptor.

Although their role in eliciting the pharmacologic effects of antipsychotic agents remains to be fully elucidated, dopamine D_3, D_4, and D_5 receptors also have been identified; clozapine appears to have a much higher affinity for the D_4 receptor than for D_2 or D_3 receptors. Current information on D_3-receptor affinity for antipsychotic drugs suggests that most antipsychotics probably bind to both D_2 and D_3 receptors, although with higher affinity to D_2 receptors; however, the magnitude of the difference in D_3- versus D_2-receptor binding is much less with atypical antipsychotics such as clozapine, suggesting that effects on D_3 receptors may play a more important role in the pharmacologic actions of atypical versus typical antipsychotic drugs. The high affinity of the D_4 receptor for clozapine and its preferential distribution in cortical and limbic areas in animals may explain, in part, the relative lack of tardive dyskinesia and extrapyramidal effects during clozapine therapy. The cloning of a gene for a neuron-specific dopamine D5 receptor, which binds antipsychotic drugs with similar affinity as the D1 receptor but has a tenfold higher affinity for dopamine, also has been reported.

Clozapine's clinical potency appears to be twice that of chlorpromazine on a weight basis, although the drug demonstrates considerably weaker D2-receptor binding affinity than chlorpromazine and appears to be much less potent in elevating dopamine metabolite concentrations in the brain. Clozapine produces a more potent blockade of central serotonergic, adrenergic, histamine H1, and muscarinic receptors than typical antipsychotic agents; also, long-term administration of clozapine enhances striatal D1-receptor function in animals and results in "down-regulation" of cortical, type 2 serotonergic (5-HT2) receptors, suggesting that an interaction between these central neurotransmitter systems may be important for the drug's antipsychotic efficacy. Antagonism at cholinergic and α1-adrenergic receptors in the mesolimbic system, compensating for dopaminergic blockade in the neostriatum, may explain the apparent selectivity and low incidence of extrapyramidal effects seen with clozapine. The amygdala also may be a site of action for clozapine, since repeated administration of the drug selectively induces supersensitivity to locally applied dopamine in the amygdala, and amygdaloid neurons are excited by clozapine but generally unresponsive to other antipsychotic agents (e.g., haloperidol).

Further studies are needed to elucidate the mechanism of clozapine's antipsychotic effects in various areas of the CNS.

Neurophysiologic Effects

In vitro and in vivo electrophysiologic studies in animals demonstrate different sensitivities of various brain areas to clozapine-mediated postsynaptic receptor blockade. While clozapine increases firing rates of both nigrostriatal (A9 pathway) and mesolimbic (A10 pathway) dopaminergic neurons after acute administration, only mesolimbic dopaminergic neurons exhibit prolonged depolarization blockade following repeated exposure to the drug. Repeated administration of typical antipsychotic agents (e.g., haloperidol) concomitantly with an anticholinergic agent (trihexyphenidyl) or an α1-adrenergic blocking drug (prazosin) mimicked these selective effects of clozapine on mesolimbic versus nigrostriatal dopaminergic neurons, suggesting that α1-adrenergic blocking and/or anticholinergic effects may be responsible, in part, for the differential effects of clozapine in these midbrain areas. Some evidence suggests that the nucleus accumbens has greater sensitivity for clozapine than do other regions, which may explain why the drug appears to produce depolarization blockade of dopaminergic neurons only in the mesolimbic area. However, some studies have shown that neurons in the neostriatum also may be responsive to clozapine. Clozapine reportedly produces an increase in dopamine metabolites in the neostriatum comparable to or even greater than that in the nucleus accumbens. Demonstrable dopamine-receptor supersensitivity in both striatal and limbic forebrain regions also has been reported with prolonged clozapine administration. Therefore, it has been suggested that there may be a dissociation between the effects of clozapine on synthesis and metabolism of dopamine within nigrostriatal neurons and the drug's effects on neuronal firing rate and dopamine release.

Adrenergic Effects

Clozapine has adrenergic-blocking activity, which may be partially responsible for the sedation, muscle relaxation, and cardiac effects observed in patients receiving the drug. (See Cautions: Cardiovascular Effects.) Although the drug appears to have relatively weak α-adrenergic blocking effects compared with typical antipsychotic drugs such as chlorpromazine, clozapine's in vitro affinity (relative to dopamine D2-receptor affinity) for α1- and α2-adrenergic receptors is much higher than that of conventional antipsychotics, including chlorpromazine, haloperidol, loxapine, and thioridazine. Clozapine increases the number and sensitivity of α1-adrenergic, but not dopamine D2, receptors. The turnover rate of epinephrine and norepinephrine also may be increased by clozapine, but to a lesser extent than that of dopamine. Substantial increases in plasma norepinephrine concentrations, which decreased following discontinuance of the drug but remained above basal levels, have been noted in both schizophrenic and healthy individuals receiving clozapine; such increases may be the result of feedback mechanisms activated by adrenergic blockade.

Clozapine's central α1-adrenergic blocking activity also may be responsible for the dose-related hypothermia observed in mice given the drug. Clozapine also

induces ataxia and blocks amphetamine-induced hyperactivity in mice, although repeated administration of the drug results in almost complete tolerance to these effects. It has been suggested that clozapine's α1-adrenergic blocking properties may, in part, mediate its differential effects on midbrain dopamine receptors and be responsible for its relative lack of extrapyramidal effects. However, the clinical importance of the drug's α1-adrenergic effects has not been fully elucidated.

Anticholinergic Effects

Clozapine possesses potent anticholinergic activity in vitro; the drug's affinity for muscarinic receptors substantially exceeds that of other antipsychotic agents (e.g., 39–50 times greater than that of chlorpromazine and 100 times that of loxapine) and may be similar to that of tricyclic antidepressants and antimuscarinic antiparkinsonian agents (e.g., benztropine, trihexyphenidyl). It has been suggested that clozapine's anticholinergic effects may be more potent centrally than peripherally and that adverse anticholinergic effects generally are not dose limiting; however, peripheral anticholinergic effects such as dry mouth are common and may be troublesome. Clozapine-induced delirium, which reportedly has occurred with rapid dosage escalation, has been reversed by physostigmine; this suggests that clozapine has central antimuscarinic activity. Some evidence also suggests that clozapine's anticholinergic properties may counteract the effects of dopamine receptor blockade in the neostriatum and thus prevent extrapyramidal reactions. Limited data suggest that the propensity of antipsychotic drugs to cause extrapyramidal effects varies inversely with anticholinergic potency and antimuscarinic activity; however, the relatively potent anticholinergic activity of clozapine does not appear to account adequately for its atypical actions.

Serotonergic Effects

It has been suggested that schizophrenia may involve a dysregulation of serotonin- and dopamine-mediated neurotransmission, and clozapine may at least partially restore a normal balance of neurotransmitter function, possibly through serotonergic regulation of dopaminergic tone. Clozapine blocks central type 2A serotonergic (5-HT2A) receptors; the drug also antagonizes central and peripheral type 3 serotonergic (5-HT3) receptors. Long-term and acute administration of clozapine has produced down-regulation of 5-HT2 receptors in the frontal cortex and neostriatum of male rats; single or repeated daily injections of clozapine also reduced the number of cortical 5-HT2 receptors but did not change receptor affinity. In contrast to effects caused by typical antipsychotic agents, an increase in brain tryptophan, serotonin, and 5-hydroxyindoleacetic acid (5-HIAA) concentrations generally has been reported with clozapine administration in animals. It has been suggested that these effects might contribute to the pronounced sedative effects of clozapine, although increases in blood serotonin concentrations occurring during clozapine treatment in humans have been inconsistent and variable. (See Effects on Sleep under Pharmacology: Nervous System Effects.) Clozapine's serotonergic effects also reportedly may contribute to the drug's efficacy against negative symptoms of schizophrenia and to the weight gain observed during clozapine therapy. (See Cautions: Endocrine and Metabolic Effects.)

Effects on Other Central Neurotransmitters

Clozapine appears to have important activity on the metabolism of γ-aminobutyric acid (GABA), which has inhibitory effects on dopaminergic neurons. In contrast to the effects of typical antipsychotic drugs, clozapine apparently augments GABA turnover in both the neostriatum and nucleus accumbens. Increases in neostriatal GABA turnover and release may attenuate extrapyramidal reactions, while a similar action in the nucleus accumbens may be related to antipsychotic efficacy.

Clozapine appears to have central histamine H1-receptor blocking activity; such activity reportedly may be associated with sedation, hypotension, and weight gain. The drug's affinity (relative to dopamine D2-receptor affinity) for histamine H1-receptors is approximately 30 times that of chlorpromazine and 4 times that of loxapine.

Behavioral Effects in Animals

Studies of the effects of clozapine on animal behavior routinely used to detect antipsychotic activity support its classification as an atypical antipsychotic drug. Such studies suggest that the neostriatum is relatively unresponsive to clozapine. Since the drug does not induce catalepsy or inhibit apomorphine-induced stereotypy, which are thought to be mediated principally by the nigrostriatal dopamine system, clozapine's antipsychotic activity appears to result from the drug's activity in other areas. Clozapine also does not block amphetamine-induced hyperactivity or apomorphine-induced emesis in animals as the typical antipsychotic agents do. Long-term administration of clozapine causes supersensitization of behaviors mediated by mesolimbic dopaminergic pathways (e.g., dopamine-induced locomotion) but not those mediated via neostriatal systems (e.g., dopamine-induced stereotypy). Long-term administration of clozapine in male rats caused a marked supersensitivity (of the same magnitude and duration as that of haloperidol) in the mesolimbic but not the nigrostriatal system. It has been suggested that supersensitivity of mesolimbic dopamine receptors may be associated with the apparent rebound psychosis that has been reported following clozapine therapy. (See Cautions: Other Nervous System Effects.)

EEG Effects

Clozapine may produce dose-related changes in the EEG, including increased discharge patterns similar to those associated with seizure disorders, and may lower the seizure threshold; seizures have occurred in patients receiving the drug, particularly with high dosages (greater than 600 mg daily), rapid dosage increases, and/or in the presence of high plasma concentrations. (See Seizures in Cautions: Nervous System Effects.) Some EEG changes associated with clozapine administration are atypical of those generally seen with other antipsychotic agents, resembling more closely those produced by antidepressants. Clozapine increases beta-, delta-, and theta-band amplitudes and slows dominant alpha frequencies in clinical EEG studies. However, in patients with severe, treatment-resistant schizophrenia, increases in delta and theta band frequencies are more pronounced with clozapine than with haloperidol or chlorpromazine therapy, a finding that appears to parallel the drugs' relative antiserotonergic, antihistaminic, and anticholinergic activities. Enhanced EEG synchronization, paroxysmal sharp-wave activity, and spike and wave complexes also may develop during clozapine therapy. Clozapine-induced EEG changes generally appear soon after initiation of the drug and return to baseline upon cessation of therapy. In one study, the EEG showed slight general changes or slight diffuse slowing in 75% of patients receiving clozapine; in another study, clozapine caused marked EEG changes, including a slowing of basal activity, in 5% of patients.

Effects on Sleep

Clozapine causes a shift in the sleep-wake pattern toward dozing in animals, with marked reductions in both slow-wave and paradoxical sleep times. However, tolerance to the drug's sedative effect usually occurs, although slowly in some patients, during continuous administration of clozapine. In a controlled study of short-term (3-day) administration in healthy young men, clozapine in dosages of 25 mg nightly substantially increased total sleep time on the first night of administration, but the duration of sleep returned to baseline by the third night. Clozapine did not substantially affect the time spent in stage 1, 2, 3, or slow-wave sleep, nor did it affect latency to the rapid eye movement (REM) period or the percentage of time spent in REM sleep. However, the percentage of time spent in stage 4 sleep was reduced substantially on the second and third nights of drug administration, while a variety of REM indices were increased on the third night of the study.

In a few patients receiving clozapine dosages of 150–800 mg daily, REM sleep increased to 85–100% of total sleep time after several days of drug therapy, with the onset of REM sleep occurring almost immediately after patients fell asleep. Intensification of dream activity also has been reported during clozapine therapy. Some clinicians have suggested that a correlation may exist between increases in body temperature and REM sleep and clozapine-induced improvement in psychosis. Cataplexy has been reported in some patients receiving clozapine.

Neuroendocrine Effects

In contrast to typical antipsychotic drugs, clozapine therapy in usual dosages generally produces little or no elevation of prolactin concentration in humans. Administration of clozapine to rats has produced a transient, dose-related increase in prolactin concentrations that is of much shorter duration than that caused by other antipsychotic agents. Prolactin normally is inhibited by dopamine released from tuberoinfundibular (TIDA) neurons into the pituitary portal circulation. In rats, clozapine acutely increases the activity of TIDA neurons, which inhibit the release of prolactin; activation of TIDA neurons may be mediated by an enhanced release of neurotensin. Clozapine's effect on prolactin appears to be transient, possibly because the drug appears to dissociate from dopamine receptors more rapidly than typical antipsychotic agents and is therefore eliminated from the brain more rapidly.

Clozapine has an effect on corticotropin (ACTH) and corticosterone, possibly through its effects on dopamine metabolism in the hypothalamus. Short-term administration of clozapine (cumulative dose: 200 mg) to a few patients with schizophrenia resulted in marked inhibition of apomorphine-induced somatotropin (growth hormone) response, suggesting that clozapine may block the dopamine receptors responsible for eliciting this response. In contrast to typical antipsychotic agents, clozapine decreases or has no effect on basal cortisol levels. Clozapine markedly increases corticosterone concentrations in a dose-dependent fashion; other antipsychotic agents appear to increase corticosterone concentrations only at doses producing substantial D_2-receptor blockade. Clozapine-induced stimulation of corticosterone secretion may result from stimulation, rather than blockade, of dopamine receptors, but the exact mechanism has not been fully elucidated.

Other Effects

Clozapine produced a dose-dependent delay in initiation of copulation in male rats, which may be related to blockade of mesolimbic dopamine receptors; however, the drug had no effect on copulatory behavior once the behavior had started. Fertility in male and female rats reportedly is not adversely affected by clozapine. (See Cautions: Pregnancy, Fertility, and Lactation.)

In animals, even small oral doses of clozapine cause ptosis, relaxation, and a reduction in spontaneous activity, effects that are consistent with the drug's sedative activity. Inhibition of locomotor activity induced by clozapine diminishes with repeated administration. With increasing doses of the drug, reactions to acoustic and tactile stimuli decline, and disturbances in equilibrium have been reported. Clozapine also inhibits isolation-induced aggression in mice at doses lower than those affecting motor function, suggesting a specific antiaggressive effect.

Studies in animals suggest that clozapine has a weak and variable diuretic effect; the clinical importance of this effect has not been established. In both rats and dogs, low doses of clozapine tend to increase the elimination of water and electrolytes, while higher doses are associated with increases in potassium excretion and sodium retention.

PHARMACOKINETICS

Absorption

Clozapine is rapidly and almost completely absorbed following oral administration. However, because of extensive hepatic first-pass metabolism, only about 27–50% of an orally administered dose reaches systemic circulation unchanged. Some, but not all, evidence suggests that clozapine may exhibit nonlinear, dose-dependent pharmacokinetics, with oral bioavailability being approximately 30% less following a single 75-mg dose than at steady state following multiple dosing. GI absorption appears to occur principally in the small intestine and is approximately 90–95% complete within 3.5 hours after an oral dose. Food does not appear to have a clinically important effect on the rate or extent of GI absorption of the drug when given as conventional tablets. Administration of clozapine orally disintegrating tablets or oral suspension with a high-fat meal decreases peak plasma concentrations of clozapine by about 20%, but does not affect area under the plasma concentration-time curve (AUC). The differences in peak plasma concentrations are not considered clinically important; therefore, the manufacturers state that clozapine (as conventional tablets, orally disintegrating tablets, or oral suspension) can be taken without regard to meals.

The relative oral bioavailability of clozapine has been shown to be equivalent following administration of 25-mg and 100-mg conventional tablets; commercially available clozapine oral suspension and conventional tablets and orally disintegrating tablets and conventional tablets also are bioequivalent.

Following oral administration of a single 25- or 100-mg oral dose of clozapine as tablets in healthy adults, the drug is detectable in plasma within 25 minutes, and peak plasma clozapine concentrations occur at about 1.5 hours. Peak plasma concentrations may be delayed with higher single doses and with multiple dosing of the drug. In a multiple-dose study, peak plasma clozapine concentrations at steady state averaged 319 ng/mL (range: 102–771 ng/mL) and occurred on average at 2.5 hours (range: 1–6 hours) after a dose with 100 mg twice daily as conventional tablets; minimum plasma concentrations at steady state averaged 122 ng/mL (range: 41–343 ng/mL). Steady-state plasma concentrations ranging from 200–600 ng/mL generally are achieved with oral dosages of 300 mg daily, and steady-state peak plasma concentrations generally occur within 2–4 hours after a dose. Steady-state plasma concentrations of clozapine are achieved after 7–10 days of continuous dosing.

Following multiple-dose administration of clozapine orally disintegrating tablets at a dosage of 100 mg twice daily in adults, peak plasma clozapine concentrations at steady state averaged 413 ng/mL (range: 132–854 ng/mL) and occurred on average at 2.3 hours (range: 1–6 hours). Minimum plasma concentrations at steady state in this study averaged 168 ng/mL (range: 45–574 ng/mL). Following multiple-dose administration of clozapine oral suspension at a dosage of 100–800 mg once daily, peak plasma clozapine concentrations at steady state averaged 275 ng/mL (range: 105–723 ng/mL) and occurred on average at 2.2 hours (range: 1–3.5 hours). Minimum plasma concentrations at steady state in this study averaged 75 ng/mL (range: 11–198 ng/mL).

Considerable interindividual variation in plasma clozapine concentrations has been observed in patients receiving the drug, and some patients may exhibit either extremely high or extremely low plasma concentrations with a given dosage. Such variability may be particularly likely at relatively high dosages (e.g., 400 mg daily) of the drug. In one study, a sixfold interindividual variation in steady-state plasma clozapine concentration was observed in patients receiving such dosages. In addition, considerable intraindividual variation, particularly from week to week, may occur in some patients. However, substantial intraindividual variations in pharmacokinetic parameters typically are not observed from day to day. Although the interindividual variability in plasma clozapine concentrations is consistent with that reported for other antipsychotic drugs and may be secondary to differences in absorption, distribution, metabolism, or clearance of the drug, further study is needed to clarify whether such variation results principally from variable pharmacokinetics or other variables.

There is some evidence that interindividual differences in pharmacokinetic parameters for clozapine may result, at least in part, from nonlinear, dose-dependent pharmacokinetics of the drug. However, a linear dose-concentration relationship also has been reported. Results of a study in patients with chronic schizophrenia revealed a correlation between oral clozapine dosages of 100–800 mg daily and steady-state plasma concentrations of the drug. In addition, linearly dose-proportional changes in area under the plasma concentration-time curve (AUC) and in peak and trough plasma concentrations have been observed with oral dosages of 37.5, 75, and 150 mg twice daily in other studies.

Because clozapine is a substrate for many cytochrome P-450 (CYP) isoenzymes, including CYP1A2, CYP2D6, and CYP3A4, patients with poor-metabolizer phenotypes of CYP2D6 may have higher plasma clozapine concentrations at usual dosages. In addition, smokers appear to achieve plasma clozapine concentrations that are approximately 60–80% of those achieved by nonsmokers following oral administration of the drug, due to induction of CYP1A2 activity by tobacco smoke. (See Drug Interactions: Smoking.) There also is limited evidence that gender may affect plasma clozapine concentrations, with concentrations being somewhat reduced, perhaps by as much as 20–30%, in males compared with females. In addition, smoking has a greater effect on clozapine plasma concentrations in men than in women, although this difference could result simply from gender differences in smoking behavior. Plasma concentrations may be increased in geriatric individuals compared with relatively young (e.g., 18–35 years old) individuals, possibly secondary to age-related decreases in hepatic elimination of clozapine.

Pharmacologic effects of clozapine (e.g., sedation) reportedly are apparent within 15 minutes and become clinically important within 1–6 hours. The duration of action of clozapine reportedly ranges from 4–12 hours following a single oral dose. In one study in patients with schizophrenia, the sedative effect was apparent within hours of the first dose of the drug and was maximal within 7 days. (See Effects on Sleep under Pharmacology: Nervous System Effects.) However, antipsychotic activity generally is delayed for one to several weeks after initiation of clozapine therapy, and maximal activity may require several months of therapy with the drug.

Correlations between steady-state plasma concentrations of clozapine and therapeutic efficacy have not been established, and some evidence suggests that the degree of clinical improvement is independent of plasma concentrations ranging from 100–800 ng/mL. However, it also has been suggested that serum clozapine concentrations less than 600 ng/mL may be adequate for therapeutic effect in most patients. Results of one study of 29 patients treated with clozapine 400 mg daily for 4 weeks showed that patients were most likely to respond to therapy when their plasma clozapine concentrations were at least 350 ng/mL and/

or when plasma concentrations of clozapine plus norclozapine (an active metabolite) totaled at least 450 ng/mL. Further study is needed to determine whether nonresponding patients with plasma clozapine concentrations less than 350 ng/mL will benefit from increasing their dosage in an attempt to achieve higher concentrations.

● Distribution

Distribution of clozapine into human body tissues is rapid and extensive; distribution of metabolites of the drug also appears to be extensive. In mice and rats, clozapine distributes principally into the lung, spleen, liver, kidney, gallbladder, and brain, achieving concentrations in these tissues up to 50 times those in blood. At 8 hours after IV injection, clozapine was still detectable in these organs but not in blood. There is limited evidence in animals that clozapine and its metabolites may be preferentially retained in the lungs by an energy-dependent, carrier-mediated process and by cellular binding. Evidence in animals also suggests that competition between clozapine and other drugs (e.g., chlorpromazine, imipramine, certain tetracycline antibiotics) for pulmonary binding sites may potentially affect plasma and tissue concentrations of clozapine, but the clinical importance, if any, of such an effect has not been established.

The volume of distribution of clozapine has been reported to be approximately 4.65 L/kg. In one study, the volume of distribution at steady state averaged 1.6 L/kg (range: 0.4–3.6 L/kg) in schizophrenic patients. Because the volume of distribution of clozapine is smaller than that of other antipsychotic agents, it has been suggested that clozapine is less sequestered in tissues than the other drugs. Clozapine is approximately 97% bound to serum proteins.

Results of receptor-binding studies in monkeys indicate that clozapine rapidly crosses the blood-brain barrier following IV injection. The highest brain uptake of the drug was in the striatum in these animals; lesser concentrations were achieved in the thalamus and mesencephalon, although they exceeded those in the cerebellum. The pharmacokinetic characteristics of the drug in the CNS paralleled those in plasma in these monkeys, with an elimination half-life from CNS of about 5 hours. Evidence from other animal studies indicates that CNS concentrations of the drug exceed those in blood. Distribution of the drug into the CNS in humans has not been characterized.

Clozapine reportedly is present in low concentrations in the placenta in animals; information on placental transfer of the drug in humans currently is unavailable. Clozapine distributes into human milk. (See Cautions: Pregnancy, Fertility, and Lactation.)

● Elimination

The decline of plasma clozapine concentrations in humans is biphasic. The elimination half-life of clozapine following a single 75-mg oral dose reportedly averages 8 hours (range: 4–12 hours); that after a 100-mg oral dose appears to be similar. The elimination half-life of clozapine at steady state following administration of 100 mg twice daily reportedly averages 12 hours (range: 4–66 hours). The rapid elimination phase may represent redistribution and is followed by a slower apparent mean terminal elimination half-life of 10.3–38 hours. Although a study comparing single and multiple dosing of clozapine demonstrated an increase in elimination half-life with multiple dosing, other evidence suggests this finding is not attributable to concentration-dependent pharmacokinetics.

Clozapine is almost completely metabolized in the liver prior to excretion by many CYP isoenzymes, particularly CYP1A2, CYP2D6, and CYP3A4. Clozapine may undergo N-demethylation, N-oxidation, 3′-carbon oxidation, epoxidation of the chlorine-containing aromatic ring, substitution of chlorine by hydroxyl or thiomethyl groups, and sulfur oxidation. A glucuronide metabolite, tentatively identified as a quaternary ammonium N-glucuronide of clozapine, also has been identified. Metabolism of clozapine may occur by one or more of these routes.

The rate of formation and biologic activity of clozapine metabolites have not been fully elucidated. The desmethyl metabolite of clozapine (norclozapine) has limited activity while the hydroxylated and N-oxide derivatives are inactive. The N-oxide and desmethyl derivatives are found in urine and plasma of humans in a proportion of 2:1.

Approximately 32% of a single oral dose of clozapine is found in plasma as the parent compound after 3 hours, 20% in 8 hours, and 10% up to 48 hours following the dose. Only limited amounts (approximately 2–5%) of unchanged drug are detected in urine and feces. Approximately 50% of an administered dose is excreted in urine and 30% in feces; maximum fecal excretion has been estimated at 38%. Approximately 46% of an oral dose of clozapine is excreted in urine within 120 hours.

Total plasma and blood clearance of clozapine reportedly average 217 and 250 mL/minute, respectively, but show considerable interindividual variation.

CHEMISTRY AND STABILITY

● Chemistry

Clozapine is a dibenzodiazepine-derivative antipsychotic agent. The drug is a piperazine-substituted tricyclic antipsychotic agent that is structurally similar to loxapine but that differs pharmacologically from this and other currently available antipsychotic agents (e.g., phenothiazines, butyrophenones). Because of these pharmacologic differences, clozapine is considered an atypical or second-generation antipsychotic agent.

While the structure-activity relationships of phenothiazine antipsychotic agents have been well described, these relationships for heterocyclic antipsychotic agents, including clozapine, have not been as fully characterized. Generally, the unsubstituted benzene ring seems to be important for interactions at dopamine receptors, while the chloro-substituted benzene ring seems more important for action at muscarinic receptors. In addition, an open carbon side chain replacing the piperazine moiety of clozapine generally leads to loss of activity.

Clozapine differs structurally from most currently available antipsychotic agents by the presence of a seven- rather than a six-membered central ring and the spatial relationship between the piperazine moiety and the chloro-substituted benzene ring. The core tricyclic ring system of clozapine is nonplanar and allows the piperazine moiety limited freedom of rotation.

Clozapine differs structurally from loxapine by the presence of a diazepine rather than an oxazepine central ring in the tricyclic nucleus and by the presence of a chlorine atom at position 8 rather than 2 of the tricyclic nucleus. The presence of a chlorine atom at position 8 of the tricyclic nucleus of clozapine appears to be associated with its distinct pharmacologic profile and may be responsible for the drug's antimuscarinic activity.

Clozapine occurs as a yellow, crystalline powder and is very slightly soluble in water.

● Stability

Commercially available conventional clozapine tablets should be stored in tight containers at a controlled room temperature of 20–25°C and not exceeding 30°C. Clozapine orally disintegrating tablets should be stored in their original package at a controlled room temperature of 20–25°C, but may be exposed to temperatures ranging from 15–30°C. The orally disintegrating tablets should be protected from

moisture. Clozapine oral suspension (e.g., Versacloz®) should be stored at a controlled room temperature of 20–25°C, but may be exposed to temperatures ranging from 15–30°C; the oral suspension should be protected from light and should not be refrigerated or frozen. The oral suspension is stable for 100 days after initial bottle opening.

PREPARATIONS

Clozapine is available only through a shared REMS program, the Clozapine REMS program, which ensures appropriate monitoring and management of patients with severe neutropenia. (See General under Dosage and Administration.)

Excipients in commercially available drug preparations may have clinically important effects in some individuals; consult specific product labeling for details.

cloZAPine

Oral		
Suspension	50 mg/mL	Versacloz® Jazz
Tablets	25 mg*	cloZAPine Tablets (scored)
		Clozaril® (scored), HLS
	50 mg*	cloZAPine Tablets (scored)
		Clozaril® (scored), HLS
	100 mg*	cloZAPine Tablets (scored)
		Clozaril® (scored), HLS
	200 mg*	cloZAPine Tablets (scored)
		Clozaril® (scored), HLS
Tablets, orally disintegrating	12.5 mg*	cloZAPine Orally Disintegrating Tablets
	25 mg*	cloZAPine Orally Disintegrating Tablets
	100 mg*	cloZAPine Orally Disintegrating Tablets
	150 mg*	cloZAPine Orally Disintegrating Tablets
	200 mg*	cloZAPine Orally Disintegrating Tablets

† Use is not currently included in the labeling approved by the US Food and Drug Administration.

* available from one or more manufacturer, distributor, and/or repackager by generic (nonproprietary) name

Selected Revisions September 29, 2021, © Copyright, September 1, 1991, American Society of Health-System Pharmacists, Inc.

Lurasidone Hydrochloride

28:16.08.04 • ATYPICAL ANTIPSYCHOTICS

■ Lurasidone hydrochloride is considered an atypical or second-generation antipsychotic agent.

USES

● Psychotic Disorders

Drug therapy is integral to the management of acute psychotic episodes in patients with schizophrenia and generally is required for long-term stabilization to sustain symptom remission or control and to minimize the risk of relapse. Antipsychotic agents are the principal class of drugs used for the management of all phases of schizophrenia. Patient response and tolerance to antipsychotic agents are variable, and patients who do not respond to or tolerate one drug may be successfully treated with an agent from a different class or with a different adverse effect profile.

Schizophrenia

Lurasidone hydrochloride is an atypical antipsychotic that is administered orally in the acute treatment of schizophrenia in adults. Schizophrenia is a major psychotic disorder that frequently has devastating effects on various aspects of the patient's life and carries a high risk of suicide and other life-threatening behaviors. Manifestations of schizophrenia involve multiple psychologic processes, including perception (e.g., hallucinations), ideation, reality testing (e.g., delusions), emotion (e.g., flatness, inappropriate affect), thought processes (e.g., loose associations), behavior (e.g., catatonia, disorganization), attention, concentration, motivation (e.g., avolition, impaired intention and planning), and judgment. The principal manifestations of this disorder usually are described in terms of positive and negative (deficit) symptoms and, more recently, disorganized symptoms. Positive symptoms include hallucinations, delusions, bizarre behavior, hostility, uncooperativeness, and paranoid ideation, while negative symptoms include restricted range and intensity of emotional expression (affective flattening), reduced thought and speech productivity (alogia), anhedonia, apathy, and decreased initiation of goal-directed behavior (avolition). Disorganized symptoms include disorganized speech (thought disorder) and behavior and poor attention.

The short-term efficacy of oral lurasidone in the acute management of schizophrenia was supported in 5 placebo-controlled, fixed-dose clinical trials of 6 weeks' duration in adults who met DSM-IV criteria for schizophrenia. Two of these studies included an active-control arm (olanzapine or extended-release quetiapine) to assess assay sensitivity. The studies used either the Positive and Negative Syndrome Scale (PANSS) or the Brief Psychiatric Rating Scale derived (BPRSd) and the Clinical Global Impression severity scale (CGI-S) to assess the effects of drug treatment in improving clinical manifestations of schizophrenia. Studies 1 and 3 both evaluated 2 fixed dosages of lurasidone hydrochloride (40 or 120 mg daily), study 2 evaluated a fixed dosage of 80 mg daily, study 4 evaluated 3 fixed dosages (40, 80, or 120 mg daily), and study 5 evaluated 2 fixed dosages of the drug (80 or 160 mg daily). In all 5 studies, lurasidone was found to be more effective than placebo; however, in study 4 only the 80-mg daily dosage of lurasidone hydrochloride was found to be more effective than placebo, and neither 40 mg nor 120 mg could be distinguished from placebo. Thus, the efficacy of 40-, 80-, 120-, and 160-mg daily dosages of lurasidone hydrochloride was established in these studies as assessed by the change from baseline in the PANSS or BPRSd total scores and the CGI-S. An examination of population subgroups did not reveal any clear evidence of differential responsiveness to the drug based on age, gender, or race.

The manufacturer states that if lurasidone is used for extended periods (i.e., longer than 6 weeks) in the treatment of schizophrenia, the long-term usefulness of the drug should be reassessed periodically on an individualized basis. (See Dosage and Administration: Dosage.)

The American Psychiatric Association (APA) considers most atypical antipsychotic agents first-line drugs for the management of the acute phase of schizophrenia (including first psychotic episodes), principally because of the decreased risk of adverse extrapyramidal effects and tardive dyskinesia, with the understanding that the relative advantages, disadvantages, and cost-effectiveness of conventional and atypical antipsychotic agents remain controversial. The APA states that, with the possible exception of clozapine for the management of treatment-resistant symptoms, there currently is no definitive evidence that one atypical antipsychotic agent will have superior efficacy compared with another agent in the class, although meaningful differences in response may be observed in individual patients. Conventional antipsychotic agents also may be an appropriate first-line option for some patients, including those who have been treated successfully in the past with or who prefer conventional agents. The choice of an antipsychotic agent should be individualized, considering past response to therapy, current symptomatology, concurrent medical conditions, other medications and treatments, adverse effect profile, and the patient's preference for a specific drug, including route of administration.

For additional information on the symptomatic management of schizophrenia, including treatment recommendations and results of the Clinical Antipsychotic Trials of Intervention Effectiveness (CATIE) research program, see Schizophrenia and Other Psychotic Disorders under Uses: Psychotic Disorders, in the Phenothiazines General Statement 28:16.08.24.

● Bipolar Disorder

Depressive Episodes Associated with Bipolar Disorder

Lurasidone hydrochloride is used orally as monotherapy or adjunctive therapy with lithium or valproate for the treatment of major depressive episodes associated with bipolar I disorder (bipolar depression) in adults.

The short-term efficacy of lurasidone monotherapy in the treatment of depressive episodes associated with bipolar I disorder was established in a randomized, double-blind, placebo-controlled, multicenter study of 6 weeks' duration in adults who met DSM-IV-TR criteria for major depressive episodes associated with bipolar I disorder, with or without rapid cycling and without psychotic features. The primary and key secondary end points were the change from baseline to week 6 on the Montgomery-Asberg Depression Rating Scale (MADRS) and the Clinical Global Impressions-Bipolar-Severity of Illness scale (CGI-BP-S) scores, respectively. Patients were randomized to receive lower-dose lurasidone hydrochloride (flexible dosage range of 20–60 mg daily), higher-dose lurasidone hydrochloride (flexible dosage range of 80–120 mg daily), or placebo. Lurasidone substantially reduced MADRS and CGI-BP-S scores at week 6 of therapy in both lurasidone dosage groups compared with placebo. The higher-dose range (80–120 mg daily) of lurasidone hydrochloride was not found to be more effective, on average, than the lower-dose regimen in this study.

The short-term efficacy of lurasidone as adjunctive therapy with lithium or valproate in the treatment of depressive episodes associated with bipolar I disorder was established in a randomized, double-blind, placebo-controlled, multicenter study of 6 weeks' duration in adults who met DSM-IV-TR criteria for major depressive episodes associated with bipolar I disorder, with or without rapid cycling and without psychotic features. Patients who remained symptomatic after lithium or valproate therapy were randomized to receive flexible-dose lurasidone hydrochloride (20–120 mg daily) or placebo. The primary end point was the change from baseline to week 6 in the MADRS score, and the secondary end point was the change from baseline to week 6 in the CGI-BP-S score. Lurasidone given as adjunctive therapy with lithium or valproate substantially reduced MADRS and CGI-BP-S scores at week 6 of therapy compared with placebo.

Clinical experience with lurasidone indicates that the drug is less likely to cause weight gain and to adversely affect metabolic parameters than some other atypical antipsychotic agents (e.g., olanzapine, quetiapine) that are used in the treatment of bipolar depression. Therefore, lurasidone may be a suitable alternative treatment for patients with bipolar depression who are at higher risk of metabolic abnormalities (e.g., those with diabetes mellitus or hyperlipidemia).

The manufacturer states that the efficacy of lurasidone for longer-term use (i.e., longer than 6 weeks) in bipolar depression has not been established in controlled studies. If lurasidone is used for extended periods, the long-term usefulness of the drug should be periodically reassessed on an individualized basis. (See Dosage and Administration: Dosage.)

The manufacturer states that the efficacy of lurasidone in the treatment of mania associated with bipolar disorder† has not been established.

For further information on the management of bipolar disorder, see Uses: Bipolar Disorder, in Lithium Salts 28:28.

DOSAGE AND ADMINISTRATION

● Administration

Lurasidone hydrochloride is commercially available as tablets, which are administered orally once daily, usually in the morning or evening, and should be taken with food (containing at least 350 calories) to increase absorption. Food increases peak concentrations and areas under the plasma concentration-time curve (AUC) of lurasidone threefold and twofold, respectively; however, lurasidone exposure was not affected as meal size was increased from 350 to 1000 calories and was independent of meal fat content. Lurasidone was administered with food in the controlled clinical studies.

Patients receiving lurasidone should be monitored for possible worsening of depression, suicidality, or unusual changes in behavior, especially at the beginning of therapy or during periods of dosage adjustments. (See Worsening of Depression and Suicidality Risk under Warnings/Precautions: Warnings, in Cautions.)

● Dosage

Dosage of lurasidone hydrochloride is expressed in terms of the hydrochloride salt.

Schizophrenia

For the acute management of schizophrenia in adults, the recommended initial dosage of lurasidone hydrochloride is 40 mg orally once daily. Initial dosage titration is not required. Dosages ranging from 40–160 mg daily were effective in 6-week controlled trials. The maximum recommended dosage of lurasidone hydrochloride for the treatment of schizophrenia is 160 mg daily.

The manufacturer states that efficacy of lurasidone in schizophrenia beyond 6 weeks has not been established in controlled studies. If lurasidone is used for an extended period, the long-term usefulness of the drug for the individual patient should be reassessed periodically.

The American Psychiatric Association (APA) states that prudent long-term treatment options in patients with schizophrenia with remitted first or multiple episodes include either indefinite maintenance therapy or gradual discontinuance of the antipsychotic agent with close follow-up and a plan to reinstitute treatment upon symptom recurrence. Discontinuance of antipsychotic therapy should be considered only after a period of at least 1 year of symptom remission or optimal response while receiving the antipsychotic agent. In patients who have had multiple previous psychotic episodes or 2 psychotic episodes within 5 years, indefinite maintenance antipsychotic treatment is recommended.

Depressive Episodes Associated with Bipolar Disorder

For the management of depressive episodes associated with bipolar I disorder in adults, either as monotherapy or as adjunctive therapy with lithium or valproate, the recommended initial dosage of lurasidone hydrochloride is 20 mg orally once daily. Initial dosage titration is not required. Dosages ranging from 20–120 mg daily as monotherapy or as adjunctive therapy with lithium or valproate were effective in 6-week controlled studies. In the monotherapy study, the higher dosage range (80–120 mg daily) did not provide additional efficacy, on average, over the lower dosage range (20–60 mg daily). The maximum recommended dosage of lurasidone hydrochloride for the treatment of bipolar depression, either as monotherapy or as adjunctive therapy with lithium or valproate, is 120 mg daily.

The manufacturer states that efficacy of lurasidone in bipolar depression beyond 6 weeks has not been established in controlled studies. If lurasidone is used for an extended period, the long-term usefulness of the drug for the individual patient should be reassessed periodically.

● Special Populations

The manufacturer recommends dosage adjustment in patients with moderate (creatinine clearance from 30 to less than 50 mL/minute) or severe renal impairment (creatinine clearance less than 30 mL/minute). The recommended initial lurasidone hydrochloride dosage in these patients is 20 mg daily. The maximum recommended dosage in patients with moderate or severe renal impairment is 80 mg daily. The manufacturer makes no specific dosage recommendations for patients with mild renal impairment. (See Renal Impairment under Warnings/Precautions: Specific Populations, in Cautions.)

The manufacturer recommends dosage adjustment in patients with moderate (Child-Pugh score 7–9) or severe hepatic impairment (Child-Pugh score 10–15). The recommended initial lurasidone hydrochloride dosage in these patients is

20 mg daily. The manufacturer states that lurasidone hydrochloride dosage in patients with moderate hepatic impairment should not exceed 80 mg daily and that dosage should not exceed 40 mg daily in patients with severe hepatic impairment. The manufacturer makes no specific dosage recommendations for patients with mild hepatic impairment. (See Hepatic Impairment under Warnings/Precautions: Specific Populations, in Cautions.)

In patients receiving lurasidone and in whom a moderate inhibitor of cytochrome P-450 (CYP) isoenzyme 3A4 (e.g., atazanavir, diltiazem, erythromycin, fluconazole, verapamil) will be added to therapy, the lurasidone dosage should be reduced to 50% of the original dosage. Similarly, in patients receiving a moderate CYP3A4 inhibitor in whom lurasidone hydrochloride is initiated, the recommended initial dosage of lurasidone hydrochloride is 20 mg daily and the maximum recommended dosage is 80 mg daily. If lurasidone is used concurrently with a moderate CYP3A4 inducer, it may be necessary to increase the lurasidone dosage after chronic therapy (i.e., 7 days or more) with the CYP3A4 inducer. Lurasidone should *not* be given concurrently with potent CYP3A4 inhibitors (e.g., clarithromycin, ketoconazole, ritonavir, voriconazole) or potent CYP3A4 inducers (e.g., carbamazepine, phenytoin, rifampin, St. John's wort [*Hypericum perforatum*]). (See Cautions: Contraindications and also see Drug Interactions.)

The manufacturer states that is not known whether dosage adjustment is necessary in geriatric patients on the basis of age alone. (See Geriatric Use under Warnings/Precautions: Specific Populations, in Cautions.)

Dosage adjustment is not recommended based on gender or race.

CAUTIONS

● Contraindications

Known hypersensitivity to lurasidone hydrochloride or any components in the formulation. Angioedema has been reported.

Concurrent use of potent cytochrome P-450 (CYP) isoenzyme 3A4 inhibitors (e.g., clarithromycin, ketoconazole, ritonavir, voriconazole) or potent CYP3A4 inducers (e.g., carbamazepine, phenytoin, rifampin, St. John's wort [*Hypericum perforatum*]). (See Drug Interactions.)

● Warnings/Precautions

Warnings

Increased Mortality in Geriatric Patients with Dementia-related Psychosis

Geriatric patients with dementia-related psychosis treated with antipsychotic drugs are at an increased risk of death. Analyses of 17 placebo-controlled trials (modal duration of 10 weeks) revealed a 1.6- to 1.7-fold increase in mortality among geriatric patients who were mainly receiving atypical antipsychotic drugs (i.e., aripiprazole, olanzapine, quetiapine, risperidone) compared with that observed in patients receiving placebo. Over the course of a typical 10-week controlled trial, the rate of death in drug-treated patients was about 4.5% compared with a rate of about 2.6% in the placebo group. Although the causes of death were varied, most of the deaths appeared to be either cardiovascular (e.g., heart failure, sudden death) or infectious (e.g., pneumonia) in nature. Observational studies suggest that, similar to atypical antipsychotics, treatment with conventional (first-generation) antipsychotics may increase mortality; the extent to which the findings of increased mortality in observational studies may be attributed to the antipsychotic drug as opposed to some characteristic(s) of the patients remains unclear. The manufacturer states that lurasidone is *not* approved for the treatment of patients with dementia-related psychosis. (See Adverse Cerebrovascular Events, including Stroke, in Geriatric Patients with Dementia-related Psychosis and see Dysphagia under Warnings/Precautions: Other Warnings and Precautions, in Cautions, and also see Geriatric Use under Warnings/Precautions: Specific Populations, in Cautions.)

Worsening of Depression and Suicidality Risk

Worsening of depression and/or the emergence of suicidal ideation and behavior (suicidality) or unusual changes in behavior may occur in both adult and pediatric (see Pediatric Use under Warnings/Precautions: Specific Populations, in Cautions) patients with major depressive disorder or other psychiatric disorders, whether or not they are taking antidepressants. This risk may persist until clinically important remission occurs. Suicide is a known risk of depression and certain other psychiatric disorders, and these disorders themselves are the strongest predictors of suicide. However, there has been a long-standing concern that antidepressants may have a role in inducing worsening of depression and the emergence of suicidality in certain patients during the early phases of treatment. Pooled analyses of short-term, placebo-controlled studies of antidepressants (i.e., selective serotonin-reuptake inhibitors [SSRIs] and other antidepressants) have shown an increased risk of suicidality in children, adolescents, and young adults (18–24 years of age) with major depressive disorder and other psychiatric disorders. An increased suicidality risk was not demonstrated with antidepressants compared with placebo in adults older than 24 years of age, and a reduced risk was observed in adults 65 years of age or older.

The US Food and Drug Administration (FDA) recommends that all patients being treated with antidepressants for any indication be appropriately monitored and closely observed for clinical worsening, suicidality, and unusual changes in behavior, particularly during initiation of therapy (i.e., the first few months) and during periods of dosage adjustments. Families and caregivers of patients being treated with antidepressants for major depressive disorder or other indications, both psychiatric and nonpsychiatric, also should be advised to monitor patients on a daily basis for the emergence of agitation, irritability, or unusual changes in behavior as well as the emergence of suicidality, and to report such symptoms immediately to a health-care provider.

Although a causal relationship between the emergence of symptoms such as anxiety, agitation, panic attacks, insomnia, irritability, hostility, aggressiveness, impulsivity, akathisia, hypomania, and/or mania and either the worsening of depression and/or the emergence of suicidal impulses has not been established, there is concern that such symptoms may represent precursors to emerging suicidality. Consequently, consideration should be given to changing the therapeutic regimen or discontinuing therapy in patients whose depression is persistently worse or in patients experiencing emergent suicidality or symptoms that might be precursors to worsening depression or suicidality, particularly if such manifestations are severe, abrupt in onset, or were not part of the patient's presenting symptoms. FDA also recommends that the drugs be prescribed in the smallest quantity consistent with good patient management, in order to reduce the risk of overdosage.

Sensitivity Reactions

Rash and pruritus have been reported frequently and angioedema has been reported rarely in patients receiving lurasidone. (See Contraindications under Cautions.)

Other Warnings and Precautions

Adverse Cerebrovascular Events, including Stroke, in Geriatric Patients with Dementia-related Psychosis

An increased incidence of adverse cerebrovascular events (cerebrovascular accidents and transient ischemic attacks), including fatalities, has been observed in geriatric patients with dementia-related psychosis treated with certain atypical antipsychotic agents (aripiprazole, olanzapine, risperidone) in placebo-controlled studies. The manufacturer states that lurasidone is *not* approved for the treatment of patients with dementia-related psychosis. (See Increased Mortality in Geriatric Patients with Dementia-related Psychosis under Warnings/Precautions: Warnings, and also see Geriatric Use under Warnings/Precautions: Specific Populations, in Cautions.)

Neuroleptic Malignant Syndrome

Neuroleptic malignant syndrome (NMS), a potentially fatal syndrome requiring immediate discontinuance of the drug and intensive symptomatic treatment, has been reported in patients receiving antipsychotic agents, including lurasidone. (See Advice to Patients.) For additional information on NMS, see Neuroleptic Malignant Syndrome under Cautions: Nervous System Effects, in the Phenothiazines General Statement 28:16.08.24.

Tardive Dyskinesia

Because use of antipsychotic agents, including lurasidone, may be associated with tardive dyskinesia (a syndrome of potentially irreversible, involuntary, dyskinetic movements), lurasidone should be prescribed in a manner that is most likely to minimize the occurrence of this syndrome. Chronic antipsychotic treatment generally should be reserved for patients who suffer from a chronic illness that is known to respond to antipsychotic agents, and for whom alternative, equally

effective, but potentially less harmful treatments are not available or appropriate. In patients who do require chronic treatment, the lowest dosage and the shortest duration of treatment producing a satisfactory clinical response should be sought, and the need for continued treatment should be reassessed periodically.

The American Psychiatric Association (APA) currently recommends that patients receiving atypical antipsychotic agents be assessed clinically for abnormal involuntary movements every 12 months and that patients considered to be at increased risk for tardive dyskinesia be assessed every 6 months. If signs and symptoms of tardive dyskinesia appear in a lurasidone-treated patient, lurasidone discontinuance should be considered; however, some patients may require continued treatment with the drug despite the presence of the syndrome. For additional information on tardive dyskinesia, see Tardive Dyskinesia under Cautions: Nervous System Effects, in the Phenothiazines General Statement 28:16.08.24.

Metabolic Changes

Atypical antipsychotic agents have been associated with metabolic changes that may increase cardiovascular and cerebrovascular risk, including hyperglycemia, dyslipidemia, and body weight gain. While all of these drugs produce some metabolic changes, each drug has its own specific risk profile. (See Hyperglycemia and Diabetes Mellitus, see Dyslipidemia, and also see Weight Gain under Warnings/Precautions: Other Warnings and Precautions, in Cautions.)

Hyperglycemia and Diabetes Mellitus

Hyperglycemia, sometimes severe and associated with ketoacidosis, hyperosmolar coma, or death, has been reported in patients receiving atypical antipsychotic agents. In short- and longer-term clinical trials in patients with schizophrenia or bipolar depression, clinically important differences between lurasidone and placebo in mean change from baseline to end point in serum glucose concentrations were not observed. While confounding factors such as an increased background risk of diabetes mellitus in patients with schizophrenia and the increasing incidence of diabetes mellitus in the general population make it difficult to establish with certainty the relationship between use of agents in this drug class and glucose abnormalities, epidemiologic studies (which did not include lurasidone) suggest an increased risk of treatment-emergent hyperglycemia-related adverse events in patients treated with the atypical antipsychotic agents included in the studies (e.g., clozapine, olanzapine, quetiapine, risperidone). It remains to be determined whether lurasidone also is associated with this increased risk.

Precise risk estimates for hyperglycemia-related adverse events in patients treated with atypical antipsychotics currently are not available. While some evidence suggests that the risk for diabetes may be greater with some atypical antipsychotics (e.g., clozapine, olanzapine) than with others (e.g., aripiprazole, asenapine, iloperidone, lurasidone, quetiapine, risperidone, ziprasidone) in the class, available data are conflicting and insufficient to provide reliable estimates of relative risk associated with use of the various atypical antipsychotics.

The manufacturers of atypical antipsychotic agents state that patients with preexisting diabetes mellitus in whom therapy with an atypical antipsychotic is initiated should be periodically monitored for worsening of glucose control; those with risk factors for diabetes (e.g., obesity, family history of diabetes) should undergo fasting blood glucose testing upon therapy initiation and periodically throughout treatment. Any patient who develops manifestations of hyperglycemia (including polydipsia, polyuria, polyphagia, and weakness) during treatment with an atypical antipsychotic should undergo fasting blood glucose testing. (See Advice to Patients.) In some cases, patients who developed hyperglycemia while receiving an atypical antipsychotic have required continuance of antidiabetic treatment despite discontinuance of the suspect drug; in other cases, hyperglycemia resolved with discontinuance of the antipsychotic.

For further information on managing the risk of hyperglycemia and diabetes mellitus associated with atypical antipsychotic agents, see Hyperglycemia and Diabetes Mellitus under Cautions: Precautions and Contraindications, in Clozapine 28:16.08.04.

Dyslipidemia

Undesirable changes in lipid parameters have been observed in patients treated with some atypical antipsychotic agents; however, lurasidone generally does not appear to adversely affect the lipid profile in patients receiving the drug. In a between-group comparison of pooled data from short-term, placebo-controlled studies, there were no clinically important changes in mean fasting total cholesterol and triglyceride concentrations from baseline to end point in the lurasidone-treated patients. In uncontrolled, longer-term schizophrenia studies, lurasidone was associated with decreases from baseline in mean total cholesterol and triglyceride concentrations of 3.8 and 15.1 mg/dL at week 24, 3.1 and 4.8 mg/dL at week 36, and 2.5 and 6.9 mg/dL at week 52, respectively. In an uncontrolled, longer-term bipolar depression study, lurasidone monotherapy was associated with decreases from baseline in mean total cholesterol and triglyceride concentrations of 0.5 and 1 mg/dL at week 24, respectively. In an uncontrolled, longer-term bipolar depression study of lurasidone given as adjunctive therapy with lithium or valproate, lurasidone was associated with a decrease in mean total cholesterol concentrations of 0.9 mg/dL and a mean increase in triglyceride concentrations of 5.3 mg/dL at week 24.

Weight Gain

Weight gain has been observed with atypical antipsychotic therapy. Although lurasidone generally appears to be associated with minimal weight gain and less weight gain than some other atypical antipsychotic agents (e.g., olanzapine, quetiapine, risperidone), the manufacturer recommends clinical monitoring of weight in patients receiving the drug.

Differences in mean weight gain between lurasidone-treated patients and placebo recipients were reported in short-term schizophrenia clinical studies. A mean weight gain of 0.43 kg was reported in lurasidone-treated patients compared with a loss of 0.02 kg in those receiving placebo; 4.8% of lurasidone-treated patients gained 7% or more of their baseline body weight compared with 3.3% of those receiving placebo. During uncontrolled, longer-term schizophrenia studies, lurasidone therapy was associated with a mean weight loss of 0.69 kg at week 24, 0.59 kg at week 36, and 0.73 kg at week 52.

The mean weight gain during a short-term study in patients receiving lurasidone as monotherapy for bipolar depression was 0.29 kg compared with a loss of 0.04 kg in those receiving placebo; 2.4% of lurasidone-treated patients gained 7% or more of their baseline body weight compared with 0.7% of those receiving placebo. During an uncontrolled, longer-term extension of this study, lurasidone monotherapy was associated with a mean weight loss of 0.02 kg at week 24. In the short-term studies of lurasidone as adjunctive therapy with lithium or valproate, lurasidone was associated with a mean weight gain of 0.11 kg compared with a gain of 0.16 kg in those receiving placebo. During an uncontrolled, longer-term bipolar depression study, lurasidone, given as adjunctive therapy with lithium or valproate, was associated with a mean weight gain of 1.28 kg at week 24.

For additional information on metabolic effects associated with atypical antipsychotic agents, see Hyperglycemia and Diabetes Mellitus under Warnings/Precautions: Other Warnings and Precautions, in Cautions.

Hyperprolactinemia

Similar to other antipsychotic agents and drugs with dopamine D_2 antagonistic activity, lurasidone can elevate serum prolactin concentrations.

In short-term schizophrenia clinical trials, the median change from baseline to end point in prolactin concentrations for lurasidone-treated patients was an increase of 0.4 ng/mL compared with a decrease of 1.9 ng/mL in the placebo group. The proportion of patients with prolactin elevations 5 or more times the upper limit of normal was 2.8% for lurasidone-treated patients compared with 1% for placebo recipients. In short-term bipolar depression trials, the median increase from baseline to end point in prolactin concentrations was 1.7 and 3.5 ng/mL in the lower- and higher-dosage lurasidone monotherapy groups, respectively, compared with an increase of 0.3 ng/mL in the placebo group. In the clinical study of lurasidone as adjunctive therapy with lithium or valproate, the median increase in prolactin was 2.8 ng/mL in the lurasidone-treated patients compared with no change in the placebo recipients. The increase in prolactin was generally greater in female patients than male patients. Clinical disturbances such as galactorrhea, amenorrhea, gynecomastia, and impotence have been associated with prolactin-elevating drugs. In addition, chronic hyperprolactinemia associated with hypogonadism may lead to decreased bone density in both female and male patients.

If lurasidone therapy is considered in a patient with previously detected breast cancer, clinicians should consider that approximately one-third of human breast cancers are prolactin-dependent in vitro.

Leukopenia, Neutropenia, and Agranulocytosis

In clinical trial and/or postmarketing experience, leukopenia and neutropenia have been temporally related to antipsychotic agents, including lurasidone. Agranulocytosis (including fatal cases) also has been reported with other antipsychotic agents.

Possible risk factors for leukopenia and neutropenia include preexisting low leukocyte count and a history of drug-induced leukopenia and neutropenia. Patients with a preexisting low leukocyte count or a history of drug-induced leukopenia or neutropenia should have their complete blood count monitored frequently during the first few months of therapy. Lurasidone should be discontinued at the first sign of a decline in leukocyte count in the absence of other causative factors.

Patients with neutropenia should be carefully monitored for fever or other signs or symptoms of infection and promptly treated if such signs and symptoms occur. In patients with severe neutropenia (absolute neutrophil count [ANC] less than 1000/mm³), lurasidone should be discontinued and the leukocyte count monitored until recovery occurs. Lithium reportedly has been used successfully in the treatment of several cases of leukopenia associated with aripiprazole, clozapine, and some other drugs; however, further clinical experience is needed to confirm these anecdotal findings.

Orthostatic Hypotension and Syncope

Orthostatic hypotension, dizziness, lightheadedness, tachycardia or bradycardia, and syncope may occur during lurasidone therapy in some patients, particularly early in treatment and when dosage is increased, perhaps because of the drug's α_1-adrenergic blocking activity. Patients at increased risk of these adverse reactions or of developing complications from hypotension include those with dehydration, hypovolemia, a history of cardiovascular disease (e.g., heart failure, myocardial infarction, ischemic heart disease, conduction abnormalities), or a history of cerebrovascular disease, as well as patients receiving concomitant antihypertensive therapy and those who are antipsychotic-naive.

In short-term schizophrenia trials, orthostatic hypotension was reported as an adverse event in 0.3% of patients receiving lurasidone compared with 0.1% of placebo recipients, and syncope was reported in 0.1% of patients receiving lurasidone compared with none of the placebo recipients. Orthostatic hypotension, as assessed by vital signs, was reported in 0.8, 2.1, 1.7, and 0.8% of patients receiving lurasidone hydrochloride 40, 80, 120, and 160 mg daily, respectively, compared with 0.7% of patients receiving placebo in short-term schizophrenia trials.

There were no reports of orthostatic hypotension or syncope as adverse events in short-term bipolar depression clinical trials. Orthostatic hypotension, as assessed by vital signs, occurred in 0.6–1.1% of lurasidone-treated patients compared with 0–0.9% of the placebo recipients in these trials.

The manufacturer recommends considering use of a lower initial lurasidone dosage and more gradual dosage titration in patients with a history of cardiovascular disease (e.g., heart failure, history of myocardial infarction, ischemic heart disease, conduction abnormalities) or cerebrovascular disease or with conditions that would predispose patients to hypotension (e.g., dehydration, hypovolemia, concomitant antihypertensive therapy) and in antipsychotic-naive patients. In addition, orthostatic vital signs should be monitored in such patients.

Seizures

In short-term schizophrenia trials, seizures occurred in 0.1% of patients receiving lurasidone compared with 0.1% of patients receiving placebo. There were no reports of seizures or convulsions in lurasidone-treated patients in short-term bipolar depression trials.

As with other antipsychotic agents, lurasidone should be used with caution in patients with a history of seizures or with conditions that lower the seizure threshold (e.g., dementia of the Alzheimer's type); conditions that lower the seizure threshold may be more prevalent in patients 65 years of age or older.

Cognitive and Motor Impairment

Like other antipsychotic agents, lurasidone potentially may impair judgment, thinking, or motor skills. In short-term, placebo-controlled schizophrenia trials, somnolence (including hypersomnia, hypersomnolence, and sedation) was reported in 17% of patients receiving lurasidone compared with 7.1% of placebo recipients. In a short-term bipolar depression trial, somnolence was reported in 7.3 and 13.8% of patients who received lower-dose (20–60 mg daily) and higher-dose (80–120 mg daily) lurasidone hydrochloride monotherapy, respectively, compared with 6.5% of placebo recipients. Frequency of somnolence was found to be dose related in the monotherapy study. (See Advice to Patients.)

Body Temperature Regulation

Disruption of the body's ability to reduce core body temperature has been attributed to antipsychotic agents. The manufacturer recommends appropriate caution when lurasidone is used in patients who will be experiencing conditions that may contribute to an elevation in core body temperature (e.g., strenuous exercise, extreme heat, concomitant use of agents with anticholinergic activity, dehydration). (See Advice to Patients.)

Suicide

There is an attendant risk of suicide in patients with psychotic illnesses; high-risk patients should be closely supervised. Lurasidone should be prescribed in the smallest quantity consistent with good patient management to reduce the risk of overdosage.

Activation of Mania/Hypomania

Antidepressants can increase the risk of developing manic or hypomanic episodes, particularly in patients with bipolar disorder. Manic or hypomanic episodes were reported in less than 1% of patients receiving lurasidone and in less than 1% of patients receiving placebo in the bipolar depression monotherapy and adjunctive therapy studies. Patients should be monitored for the emergence of manic or hypomanic episodes during lurasidone therapy.

Dysphagia

Esophageal dysmotility and aspiration have been associated with the use of antipsychotic agents. Aspiration pneumonia is a common cause of morbidity and mortality in geriatric patients, particularly in those with advanced Alzheimer's dementia. Lurasidone is *not* approved for the treatment of patients with dementia-related psychosis and should be used with caution in patients at risk for aspiration pneumonia. (See Increased Mortality in Geriatric Patients with Dementia-related Psychosis under Warnings/Precautions: Warnings, in Cautions.)

Neurologic Adverse Reactions in Patients with Parkinsonian Syndrome or Dementia with Lewy Bodies

Patients with parkinsonian syndrome or dementia with Lewy bodies reportedly have an increased sensitivity to antipsychotic agents. Clinical manifestations of this increased sensitivity have been reported to include confusion, obtundation, postural instability with frequent falls, extrapyramidal symptoms, and features consistent with NMS. For additional information on extrapyramidal adverse effects and NMS, see Cautions: Nervous System Effects, in the Phenothiazines General Statement 28:16.08.24.

Specific Populations

Pregnancy

Category B. (See Users Guide.)

Neonates exposed to antipsychotic agents during the third trimester of pregnancy are at risk for extrapyramidal and/or withdrawal symptoms following delivery. Symptoms reported to date have included agitation, hypertonia, hypotonia, tardive dyskinetic-like symptoms, tremor, somnolence, respiratory distress, and feeding disorder. Neonates exhibiting such symptoms should be monitored. The complications have varied in severity; some neonates recovered within hours to days without specific treatment while others have required intensive care unit support and prolonged hospitalization.

The effect of lurasidone on labor and delivery is unknown.

Lactation

Lurasidone is distributed into milk in rats. It is not known whether lurasidone and/or its metabolites are distributed into milk in humans. Because of the potential for serious adverse reactions to lurasidone in nursing infants, the manufacturer states that a decision should be made whether to discontinue nursing or lurasidone, taking into consideration the risk of drug discontinuance to the woman.

Pediatric Use

Safety and effectiveness of lurasidone in pediatric patients have not been established.

FDA warns that a greater risk of suicidal thinking or behavior (suicidality) occurred during the first few months of antidepressant treatment compared with placebo in children and adolescents with major depressive disorder, obsessive-compulsive disorder (OCD), or other psychiatric disorders based on pooled analyses of 24 short-term, placebo-controlled trials of 9 antidepressant drugs (SSRIs and other antidepressants). However, a later meta-analysis of 27 placebo-controlled trials of 9 antidepressants (SSRIs and others) in patients younger than 19 years of age with major depressive disorder, OCD, or non-OCD anxiety disorders suggests that the benefits of antidepressant therapy in treating these conditions may outweigh the risks of suicidal behavior or suicidal ideation. No suicides occurred in these pediatric trials. These findings should be carefully considered when assessing potential benefits and risks of lurasidone in a child or adolescent for any clinical use. (See Worsening of Depression and Suicidality Risk under Warnings/Precautions: Warnings, in Cautions.)

Geriatric Use

Clinical trial experience with lurasidone in patients with schizophrenia who are 65 years of age and older is insufficient to determine whether they respond differently than younger adults.

In geriatric patients (65–85 years of age) with psychosis, serum lurasidone concentrations were similar to those observed in younger adults. The manufacturer states that it is unknown whether dosage adjustment is necessary in geriatric patients on the basis of age alone.

Geriatric patients with dementia-related psychosis treated with lurasidone are at an increased risk of death compared with those treated with placebo. In addition, an increased incidence of adverse cerebrovascular events (cerebrovascular accidents and transient ischemic attacks), including fatalities, has been observed in geriatric patients with dementia-related psychosis treated with certain atypical antipsychotic agents (aripiprazole, olanzapine, risperidone) in placebo-controlled studies. The manufacturer states that lurasidone is *not* approved for the treatment of patients with dementia-related psychosis (see Increased Mortality in Geriatric Patients with Dementia-related Psychosis under Warnings/Precautions: Warnings, in Cautions and see also Adverse Cerebrovascular Events, including Stroke, in Geriatric Patients with Dementia-related Psychosis and see Dysphagia under Warnings/Precautions: Other Warnings and Precautions, in Cautions). For additional information on the use of antipsychotic agents in the management of dementia-related psychosis, see Geriatric Considerations under Uses: Psychotic Disorders, in the Phenothiazines General Statement 28:16.08.24.

In pooled data analyses, a *reduced* risk of suicidality was observed in adults 65 years of age or older with antidepressant therapy compared with placebo. (See Worsening of Depression and Suicidality Risk under Warnings/Precautions: Warnings, in Cautions.)

Hepatic Impairment

In a single-dose study, mean areas under the serum concentration-time curve (AUCs) of lurasidone were 1.5, 1.7, and 3 times higher in individuals with mild (Child-Pugh score 5–6), moderate (Child-Pugh score 7–9), and severe hepatic impairment (Child-Pugh score 10–15), respectively, compared with values in healthy matched individuals. Mean peak serum concentrations of lurasidone were 1.3, 1.2, and 1.3 times higher for patients with mild, moderate, and severe hepatic impairment, respectively, compared with values for healthy matched individuals. Dosage adjustment is recommended for patients with moderate or severe hepatic impairment. (See Dosage and Administration: Special Populations.)

Renal Impairment

After administration of a single 40-mg dose of lurasidone hydrochloride to patients with mild, moderate, or severe renal impairment, mean peak serum concentrations increased by 40, 92, and 54%, respectively, and mean AUCs increased by 53%, 91%, and twofold, respectively, compared with healthy matched individuals. Dosage adjustment is recommended for patients with moderate or severe renal impairment (creatinine clearance from 10 to less than 50 mL/minute). (See Dosage and Administration: Special Populations.)

• Common Adverse Effects

Adverse effects occurring in 5% or more of patients receiving lurasidone for schizophrenia and at a frequency at least twice that reported with placebo include somnolence (including hypersomnia, hypersomnolence, and sedation), akathisia, extrapyramidal symptoms (including parkinsonian symptoms and dyskinesia), and nausea. Akathisia and extrapyramidal symptoms were found to be dose related in these studies.

Adverse effects occurring in 5% or more of patients receiving lurasidone for bipolar depression as monotherapy or as adjunctive therapy with lithium or valproate and at a frequency at least twice that reported with placebo include somnolence (including hypersomnia, hypersomnolence, and sedation), akathisia, nausea, extrapyramidal symptoms (including parkinsonian symptoms and dyskinesia), vomiting, diarrhea, and anxiety. Nausea, somnolence, akathisia, and extrapyramidal symptoms were found to be dose related in the monotherapy study.

DRUG INTERACTIONS

● *Drugs Affecting or Metabolized by Hepatic Microsomal Enzymes*

CYP3A4 Inhibitors and Inducers

Lurasidone is predominantly metabolized by cytochrome P-450 (CYP) isoenzyme 3A4. Pharmacokinetic interactions of lurasidone with potent and moderate inhibitors or potent inducers of CYP3A4 have been observed.

Lurasidone should not be used in combination with potent inhibitors (e.g., clarithromycin, ketoconazole, ritonavir, voriconazole) or potent inducers (e.g., carbamazepine, phenytoin, rifampin, St. John's wort [*Hypericum perforatum*]) of CYP3A4. (See Contraindications and also see Drug Interactions: Ketoconazole and Drug Interactions: Rifampin.) Lurasidone dosage should be adjusted when used concurrently with moderate CYP3A4 inhibitors (e.g., atazanavir, diltiazem, erythromycin, fluconazole, verapamil). (See Dosage and Administration: Special Populations and also see Drug Interactions: Diltiazem.)

If lurasidone is used concurrently with a moderate CYP3A4 inducer, an increase in lurasidone dosage may be necessary after chronic therapy (i.e., 7 days or more) with the CYP3A4 inducer.

Inhibitors and Inducers of Other CYP Isoenzymes

Lurasidone is not a substrate of CYP isoenzymes 1A1, 1A2, 2A6, 4A11, 2B6, 2C8, 2C9, 2C19, 2D6, or 2E1; therefore, clinically important pharmacokinetic interactions between lurasidone and drugs that are either inhibitors or inducers of these enzymes are unlikely.

● *Anticholinergic Agents*

Potential pharmacologic interaction (possible disruption of body temperature regulation); use lurasidone with caution in patients concurrently receiving drugs with anticholinergic activity. (See Body Temperature Regulation under Warnings/Precautions: Other Warnings and Precautions, in Cautions.)

● *CNS Agents or Alcohol*

Potential pharmacologic interaction (additive CNS effects). Use with caution with other CNS agents and avoid use of alcohol during lurasidone therapy.

● *Digoxin*

Concomitant administration of lurasidone hydrochloride (120 mg daily at steady state) with a single 0.25-mg dose of digoxin, a P-glycoprotein substrate, increased peak plasma concentrations and areas under the serum concentration-time curve (AUCs) of digoxin by approximately 9 and 13%, respectively. Digoxin dosage adjustment is not required in patients receiving these drugs concurrently.

● *Diltiazem*

Concomitant administration of diltiazem (240 mg daily for 5 days), a moderate CYP3A4 inhibitor, and lurasidone hydrochloride (single 20-mg dose) increased peak serum lurasidone concentrations and AUCs by 2.1 and 2.2 times, respectively, compared with administration of lurasidone alone. If diltiazem is initiated in patients receiving lurasidone, the manufacturer states that lurasidone dosage should be reduced to 50% of the original dosage. If lurasidone is initiated in patients receiving diltiazem, the manufacturer recommends that lurasidone hydrochloride therapy be initiated at 20 mg daily and that dosage not exceed 80 mg daily.

● *Grapefruit*

Grapefruit and grapefruit juice should be avoided in patients receiving lurasidone since they may inhibit CYP3A4 and increase plasma concentrations of lurasidone. (See Advice to Patients.)

● *Hypotensive Agents*

Because of its α_1-adrenergic blocking activity, the manufacturer states that patients receiving lurasidone may be at increased risk of orthostatic hypotension and syncope and related adverse effects. A lower initial dosage of lurasidone and more gradual dosage titration should therefore be considered in patients concomitantly receiving antihypertensive agents; in addition, monitoring of orthostatic vital signs is recommended in such patients. (See Orthostatic Hypotension and Syncope under Warnings/Precautions: Other Warnings and Precautions, in Cautions and also see Advice to Patients.)

● *Ketoconazole*

Concomitant administration of ketoconazole (400 mg daily), a potent CYP3A4 inhibitor, and lurasidone hydrochloride (single 10-mg dose) increased peak serum concentrations and AUCs of lurasidone by 6.8 and 9.3 times, respectively, compared with administration of lurasidone alone. Ketoconazole should therefore not be used concurrently with lurasidone.

● *Lithium*

Concomitant administration of lithium (600 mg twice daily for 8 days) and lurasidone hydrochloride (120 mg daily for 8 days) decreased peak serum lurasidone concentrations by 8% and increased lurasidone AUC by 7% compared with lurasidone administration alone; these changes were not considered clinically important. In bipolar depression studies evaluating lurasidone and adjunctive lithium therapy, there was no evidence of additive CNS toxicity in patients receiving lurasidone and lithium in combination. Lurasidone dosage adjustment is not required in patients receiving lithium concurrently. In addition, lithium dosage adjustment is not necessary during concurrent use of lurasidone.

● *Midazolam*

Concomitant administration of lurasidone hydrochloride (120 mg daily at steady state) with a single 5-mg dose of midazolam, a CYP3A4 substrate, increased peak plasma concentrations and AUCs of midazolam by approximately 21 and 44%, respectively. Midazolam dosage adjustment is not required in patients receiving lurasidone concurrently.

● *Oral Contraceptives*

Concomitant administration of lurasidone hydrochloride (40 mg daily at steady state) with an oral contraceptive containing ethinyl estradiol and norgestimate resulted in equivalent peak plasma concentrations and AUCs of ethinyl estradiol and norgestimate relative to oral contraceptive administration alone. Sex hormone binding globulin concentrations also were not substantially affected by concurrent administration of the drugs. Oral contraceptive dosage adjustment is not required in patients receiving lurasidone concurrently.

● *Rifampin*

Concomitant administration of rifampin (600 mg daily for 8 days), a strong CYP3A4 inducer, and lurasidone hydrochloride (single 40-mg dose) decreased peak serum lurasidone concentrations and AUCs by approximately 85 and 82%, respectively. Rifampin should not be concurrently administered with lurasidone.

● *Smoking*

Lurasidone is not a substrate for CYP1A2 in vitro; therefore, smoking should not alter the pharmacokinetics of the drug.

● *St. John's Wort*

Lurasidone should not be used concurrently with St. John's wort (*Hypericum perforatum*), a potent inducer of CYP3A4.

● *Valproate*

The manufacturer states that a dedicated drug interaction study has not been conducted with lurasidone and valproate. However, pharmacokinetic data obtained from the bipolar depression studies indicate that valproate concentrations are not affected by concomitant use of lurasidone, and that lurasidone concentrations are not affected by concomitant use of valproate. Therefore, dosage adjustments are not required in patients receiving valproate and lurasidone concurrently.

DESCRIPTION

Lurasidone is a benzisothiazol-derivative antipsychotic agent and has been referred to as an atypical or second-generation antipsychotic agent. Lurasidone has also been described as an azapirone derivative. Although the exact mechanism of action of lurasidone in schizophrenia and bipolar depression is unknown, it has been suggested that the efficacy of lurasidone is mediated through a combination of antagonist activity at central dopamine type 2 (D_2) and serotonin type 2 (5-hydroxytryptamine [5-HT_{2A}]) receptors.

Lurasidone is an antagonist that exhibits high affinity for D_2, 5-HT_{2A}, and 5-HT_7 receptors and moderate affinity for α_{2C}-adrenergic receptors in vitro. The drug acts as a partial agonist at 5-HT_{1A} receptors and is an antagonist at α_{2A}-adrenergic receptors in vitro. Lurasidone exhibits weak affinity for α_1-adrenergic receptors and little or no affinity for histamine (H_1) receptors and muscarinic (M_1) receptors.

Lurasidone is rapidly absorbed following oral administration and reaches peak serum concentrations within about 1–3 hours. Approximately 9–19% of an administered dose is absorbed orally. Steady-state concentrations of the drug are achieved within 7 days. Lurasidone is highly bound (99.8%) to serum proteins, including albumin and α_1-acid glycoprotein. The drug is metabolized mainly via CYP3A4. The major biotransformation pathways are oxidative N-dealkylation, hydroxylation of the norbornane ring, and S-oxidation. Lurasidone is metabolized into 2 active metabolites (ID-14283 and ID-14326) and 2 major inactive metabolites (ID-20219 and ID-20220). Following administration of a single radiolabeled dose of lurasidone, approximately 80 and 9% of the dose is excreted in feces and urine, respectively.

ADVICE TO PATIENTS

Importance of providing a copy of written patient information (medication guide) each time lurasidone hydrochloride is dispensed. Importance of advising patients to read the patient information before taking lurasidone and each time the prescription is refilled.

Importance of advising patients and caregivers that geriatric patients with dementia-related psychosis treated with antipsychotic agents are at an increased risk of death. Patients and caregivers also should be informed that lurasidone is *not* approved for treating geriatric patients with dementia-related psychosis.

Risk of suicidality and activation of mania or hypomania; importance of patients, family, and caregivers being alert to and immediately reporting emergence of suicidality, worsening depression, manic or hypomanic symptoms, irritability, agitation, or unusual changes in behavior, especially during the first few months of therapy or during periods of dosage adjustment. (See Worsening of Depression and Suicidality Risk under Warnings/Precautions: Warnings, in Cautions.)

Importance of informing patients and caregivers about the risk of neuroleptic malignant syndrome (NMS), a rare but potentially life-threatening syndrome that can cause high fever, stiff muscles, sweating, fast or irregular heart beat, change in blood pressure, confusion, and kidney damage.

Importance of informing patients and caregivers about the risk of metabolic changes (e.g., hyperglycemia and diabetes mellitus, dyslipidemia, weight gain, cardiovascular reactions) with lurasidone and the need for specific monitoring for such changes during therapy. Importance of patients and caregivers being aware of the symptoms of hyperglycemia and diabetes mellitus (e.g., increased thirst, increased urination, increased appetite, weakness) and monitoring all patients receiving lurasidone for these symptoms. Importance of informing patients who are diagnosed with diabetes or those with risk factors for diabetes (e.g., obesity, family history of diabetes) that they should have their blood glucose monitored at the beginning of and periodically during lurasidone therapy; patients who develop symptoms of hyperglycemia during therapy should have their blood glucose assessed. Importance of informing patients that clinical monitoring of weight is recommended during lurasidone therapy.

Importance of informing patients about the risk of orthostatic hypotension, especially when initiating or reinitiating treatment or increasing the dosage.

Risk of leukopenia/neutropenia. Importance of advising patients with a preexisting low leukocyte count or a history of drug-induced leukopenia/neutropenia that they should have their complete blood cell (CBC) count monitored during lurasidone therapy.

Because somnolence (i.e., sleepiness, drowsiness) may be associated with lurasidone, patients should be cautioned about performing activities requiring mental alertness, such as driving or operating hazardous machinery, while taking lurasidone until they gain experience with the drug's effects.

Importance of avoiding eating grapefruit or drinking grapefruit juice during lurasidone therapy, since they can affect lurasidone concentrations in the blood.

Importance of avoiding alcohol during lurasidone therapy.

Importance of clinicians informing patients in whom chronic lurasidone use is contemplated about the risk of a movement problem called tardive dyskinesia. Importance of informing patients to report any muscle movements that cannot be stopped to a healthcare professional.

Importance of informing clinicians of existing or contemplated concomitant therapy, including prescription (see Drug Interactions) and OTC drugs or herbal supplements, as well as any concomitant illnesses (e.g., cardiovascular disease, diabetes mellitus, seizures).

Importance of women informing clinicians if they are or plan to become pregnant or plan to breast-feed. Importance of clinicians informing patients about the benefits and risks of taking antipsychotics during pregnancy (see Pregnancy under Warnings/Precautions: Specific Populations, in Cautions). Importance of advising patients not to stop taking lurasidone if they become pregnant without consulting their clinician; abruptly stopping antipsychotic agents may cause complications. Importance of advising patients not to breast-feed during lurasidone therapy.

Importance of avoiding overheating and dehydration.

Importance of informing patients of other important precautionary information. (See Cautions.)

PREPARATIONS

Excipients in commercially available drug preparations may have clinically important effects in some individuals; consult specific product labeling for details.

Lurasidone Hydrochloride

Oral

Tablets, film-coated		
	20 mg	Latuda®, Sunovion
	40 mg	Latuda®, Sunovion
	60 mg	Latuda®, Sunovion
	80 mg	Latuda®, Sunovion
	120 mg	Latuda®, Sunovion

† Use is not currently included in the labeling approved by the US Food and Drug Administration.

Selected Revisions March 2, 2015, © Copyright, September 27, 2011, American Society of Health-System Pharmacists, Inc.

OLANZapine

28:16.08.04 • ATYPICAL ANTIPSYCHOTICS

■ Olanzapine is considered an atypical or second-generation antipsychotic agent.

REMS

FDA approved a REMS for olanzapine to ensure that the benefits outweigh the risks. The REMS may apply to one or more preparations of olanzapine and consists of the following: medication guide, elements to assure safe use, communication plan, and implementation system. See the FDA REMS page (https://www.accessdata.fda.gov/scripts/cder/rems/index.cfm).

USES

Olanzapine is used orally for the symptomatic management of psychotic disorders (e.g., schizophrenia) in adults and adolescents 13–17 years of age. In addition, oral olanzapine is used alone in adults and adolescents 13–17 years of age or in conjunction with lithium or valproate in adults for the management of acute manic or mixed episodes associated with bipolar I disorder; the drug also is used for longer-term maintenance monotherapy in patients with this disorder. Short-acting olanzapine injection is used IM for the management of acute agitation in patients with bipolar disorder or schizophrenia. Long-acting olanzapine pamoate injection is used IM for the management of schizophrenia in adults.

Olanzapine is used orally in combination with fluoxetine for the treatment of acute depressive episodes associated with bipolar I disorder in adults and pediatric patients 10–17 years of age. The drug also is used orally in combination with fluoxetine for the acute and maintenance therapy of treatment-resistant depression.

Olanzapine has been used orally in combination with other antiemetic agents for the prevention of nausea and vomiting associated with highly emetogenic cancer chemotherapy†, including high-dose cisplatin therapy in adults. The drug also has been used as rescue antiemetic therapy in patients with breakthrough cancer chemotherapy-induced nausea and vomiting†.

● Psychotic Disorders

Olanzapine is used orally and parenterally for the symptomatic management of psychotic disorders (e.g., schizophrenia). Drug therapy is integral to the management of acute psychotic episodes in patients with schizophrenia and generally is required for long-term stabilization to sustain symptom remission or control and to minimize the risk of relapse. Antipsychotic agents are the principal class of drugs used for the management of all phases of schizophrenia. Patient response and tolerance to antipsychotic agents are variable, and patients who do not respond to or tolerate one drug may be successfully treated with an agent from a different class or with a different adverse effect profile.

Schizophrenia

Olanzapine is used orally for the management of schizophrenia in adults and adolescents from 13 to 17 years of age. The long-acting pamoate ester of olanzapine is used parenterally for the management of schizophrenia in adults. Schizophrenia is a major psychotic disorder that frequently has devastating effects on various aspects of the patient's life and carries a high risk of suicide and other life-threatening behaviors. Manifestations of schizophrenia involve multiple psychologic processes, including perception (e.g., hallucinations), ideation, reality testing (e.g., delusions), emotion (e.g., flatness, inappropriate affect), thought processes (e.g., loose associations), behavior (e.g., catatonia, disorganization), attention, concentration, motivation (e.g., avolition, impaired intention and planning), and judgment. The principal manifestations of this disorder usually are described in terms of positive and negative (deficit) symptoms, and more recently, disorganized symptoms. Positive symptoms include hallucinations, delusions, bizarre behavior, hostility, uncooperativeness, and paranoid ideation, while negative symptoms include restricted range and intensity of emotional expression (affective flattening), reduced thought and speech productivity (alogia), anhedonia, apathy, and decreased initiation of goal-directed behavior (avolition). Disorganized symptoms include disorganized speech (thought disorder) and behavior and poor attention.

The American Psychiatric Association (APA) considers most atypical antipsychotic agents (e.g., olanzapine, aripiprazole, quetiapine, risperidone, ziprasidone) first-line drugs for the management of the acute phase of schizophrenia (including first psychotic episodes), principally because of the decreased risk of adverse extrapyramidal effects and tardive dyskinesia, with the understanding that the relative advantages, disadvantages, and cost-effectiveness of conventional (first-generation) and atypical antipsychotic agents remain controversial. The APA states that, with the possible exception of clozapine for the management of treatment-resistant symptoms, there currently is no definitive evidence that one atypical antipsychotic agent will have superior efficacy compared with another agent in the class, although meaningful differences in response may be observed in individual patients. Conventional antipsychotic agents may be considered first-line in patients who have been treated successfully in the past with or who prefer conventional agents. The choice of an antipsychotic agent should be individualized, considering past response to therapy, adverse effect profile (including the patient's experience of subjective effects such as dysphoria), and the patient's preference for a specific drug, including route of administration.

To compare the long-term effectiveness and tolerability of older, first-generation antipsychotic agents (i.e., perphenazine) with those of newer, atypical antipsychotic agents (i.e., olanzapine, quetiapine, risperidone, ziprasidone), a double-blind, multicenter study (the first phase of Clinical Antipsychotic Trials of Intervention Effectiveness [CATIE]) was sponsored by the National Institute of Mental Health. More than 1400 patients with schizophrenia received one of these antipsychotics for up to 18 months or until therapy was discontinued for any reason. Patients with tardive dyskinesia could enroll in this trial; however, the randomization scheme prevented their assignment to the perphenazine group. The primary outcome measure in this study was the discontinuance of treatment for any cause; this measure was selected because discontinuing or switching an antipsychotic agent occurs frequently and is an important problem in the management of schizophrenia. In addition, this measure integrates the patient's and clinician's judgments concerning efficacy, safety, and tolerability into a more comprehensive measure of effectiveness reflecting therapeutic benefits in relation to adverse effects. Overall, 74% of patients in this study discontinued their medication before receiving the full 18 months of therapy because of inadequate efficacy, intolerable adverse effects, or for other reasons, suggesting substantial limitations in the long-term clinical effectiveness of currently available antipsychotic agents. Olanzapine appeared to be more effective than the other drugs evaluated in this study with a lower (64%) discontinuance rate and a lower rate of hospitalization for exacerbation of schizophrenia, while no significant differences between the effectiveness of the conventional agent, perphenazine, and the other second-generation agents studied were observed (discontinuance rates were 75, 82, 74, and 79% for perphenazine, quetiapine, risperidone, and ziprasidone, respectively). The time to discontinuance of therapy for any cause was found to be longer in the olanzapine group than in the quetiapine, risperidone, perphenazine, and ziprasidone groups in this study; however, the differences between the olanzapine and perphenazine groups and between the olanzapine and ziprasidone groups did not achieve statistical significance. Although there were no significant differences in the time until discontinuance of therapy because of drug intolerance among the drugs studied, the incidences of discontinuance for certain adverse effects differed among the drugs with olanzapine discontinued more frequently because of weight gain or metabolic effects (e.g., increases in glycosylated hemoglobin [hemoglobin A_{1c}; HbA_{1c}], cholesterol, and triglycerides) and perphenazine discontinued more frequently because of adverse extrapyramidal effects.

An open, multicenter, randomized, controlled trial comparing the relative long-term effectiveness (over a 1-year period) of a group of first-generation antipsychotic agents (e.g., chlorpromazine, flupentixol [not commercially available in the US], flupentixol decanoate [not commercially available in the US], fluphenazine decanoate, haloperidol, haloperidol decanoate, loxapine, methotrimeprazine [no longer commercially available in the US], pipothiazine palmitate [not commercially available in the US], sulpiride [not commercially available in the US], trifluoperazine, zuclopenthixol [not commercially available in the US], zuclopenthixol decanoate [not commercially available in the US]) with a group of second-generation antipsychotic agents other than clozapine (e.g., olanzapine, amisulpride [not commercially available in the US], quetiapine, risperidone, zotepine [not commercially available in the US]) in patients with schizophrenia was conducted throughout the United Kingdom by the National Health Service. In the Cost Utility of the Latest Antipsychotic Drugs in Schizophrenia Study (CUtLASS 1), the primary outcome measure was the Quality of Life Scale score, and secondary outcome measures included symptom improvement, adverse effects, patient satisfaction, and costs of health care. Patients in the first-generation antipsychotic group demonstrated a trend toward greater improvements in the Quality of Life Scale and symptom improvements scores in this study. In addition, the patients studied did not report a clear preference for either group of drugs and costs of health care in the 2 groups were found to be similar.

Emerging data from the first phase of the pivotal CATIE trial and the CUt-LASS 1 trial suggest that newer, atypical antipsychotics may not provide clinically important advantages over older, first-generation antipsychotics in patients with chronic schizophrenia and that several factors, including adequacy of symptom relief, tolerability of adverse effects, and cost of therapy, may influence a patient's ability and willingness to remain on long-term antipsychotic medication. In addition, these results suggest that it may often be necessary to try 2 or more different antipsychotic agents in an individual patient in order to provide optimal therapeutic benefit with an acceptable adverse effect profile.

In a randomized, double-blind, second phase trial, patients with schizophrenia who had discontinued an atypical antipsychotic agent during the first phase of the CATIE trial were reassigned to treatment with a different atypical antipsychotic agent (olanzapine, quetiapine, risperidone, or ziprasidone). Similarly to the first phase of the CATIE trial, efficacy and tolerability in this second phase study were principally measured by time until drug discontinuance for any reason. The time until antipsychotic treatment was discontinued was longer for patients receiving risperidone and olanzapine than for those receiving quetiapine and ziprasidone (median: 7, 6.3, 4, and 2.8 months, respectively). Among patients who discontinued their prior antipsychotic agent because of lack of efficacy, olanzapine was found to be more effective than quetiapine and ziprasidone, while risperidone was more effective than quetiapine.

In another study that was part of the second phase of the CATIE investigation, schizophrenic patients who had discontinued treatment with olanzapine, quetiapine, risperidone, or ziprasidone during the first phase of the CATIE investigation, principally because of inadequate efficacy, were randomized to receive open-label clozapine therapy or blinded treatment with another atypical antipsychotic agent not previously received in the trial. Clozapine was found to be more effective in this study than switching to another atypical antipsychotic agent. Patients receiving clozapine also were found to be less likely to discontinue treatment for any reason than patients receiving quetiapine or risperidone. In addition, the clozapine-treated patients were less likely to discontinue therapy because of an inadequate clinical response than were patients receiving the other atypical antipsychotic agents.

Pending further data clarifying the relative effectiveness and tolerability of first- and second-generation antipsychotics in the treatment of schizophrenia, many clinicians recommend that the choice of an antipsychotic agent be carefully individualized taking into consideration the clinical efficacy and adverse effect profile (including the risk for extrapyramidal effects, weight gain, and adverse metabolic effects) of the antipsychotic agent as well as the individual patient's risk factors; the patient's previous experience of subjective effects such as dysphoria; the patient's preference for and willingness to take (i.e., compliance) a specific drug, including route of administration; and the relative cost of therapy. Olanzapine and clozapine may be reasonable alternatives in any patient with schizophrenia who has not achieved a full clinical remission with other antipsychotic agents; however, the risk of adverse metabolic effects with both drugs necessitates dietary and exercise counseling before therapy is initiated, monitoring during drug therapy, and possible discontinuance of therapy if these effects become troublesome during therapy. Additional analyses from data generated by the CATIE trial addressing other schizophrenia treatment-related issues such as quality of life and predictors of response are ongoing.

Atypical antipsychotic agents, including olanzapine, generally appear less likely to induce adverse extrapyramidal effects and tardive dyskinesia than conventional, first-generation antipsychotic agents. In addition, stabilization of or improvement in tardive dyskinesia associated with conventional antipsychotic agents has been reported in some patients when they have been switched to second-generation antipsychotic therapy, including olanzapine. Therefore, the APA and some clinicians recommend that atypical antipsychotic agents be considered in patients with schizophrenia who have experienced tardive dyskinesia associated with conventional antipsychotic agents.

For additional information on the symptomatic management of schizophrenia, see Schizophrenia and Other Psychotic Disorders under Uses: Psychotic Disorders, in the Phenothiazines General Statement 28:16.08.24.

The efficacy of oral olanzapine for the management of psychotic disorders in adults has been established in hospital settings by 2 placebo-controlled studies of 6 weeks' duration in patients who met the DSM-III-R criteria for schizophrenia.

In these and several other studies, improvement in manifestations of schizophrenia was based principally on the results of various psychiatric rating scales, including the Brief Psychiatric Rating Scale (BPRS) that assesses factors such as anergy, thought disturbances, activation, hostility/suspiciousness, and anxiety/depression; the Scale for the Assessment of Negative Symptoms (SANS); the Positive and Negative Symptoms Scale (PANSS); and the Clinical Global Impression (CGI).

In the first 6-week, placebo-controlled study, olanzapine was given in a fixed dosage of 1 or 10 mg once daily. Results indicated that the 10-mg, but not the 1-mg, once-daily dosage was more effective than placebo in improving the scores on the PANSS total (also on the extracted BPRS total), the BPRS psychosis cluster, the PANSS Negative subscale, and the CGI Severity assessments. Results of the second 6-week, placebo-controlled study, which evaluated 3 fixed dosage ranges (5 ± 2.5 mg once daily, 10 ± 2.5 mg once daily, and 15 ± 2.5 mg once daily), found that the 2 highest dosages (actual mean dosages were 12 and 16 mg once daily, respectively) were more effective than placebo in reducing the BPRS total score, BPRS psychosis cluster, and CGI severity score; the highest dosage also was superior to placebo on the SANS. There appeared to be no therapeutic advantage for the higher dosage of olanzapine compared with the medium dosage in this study. No race- or gender-related differences in outcome were noted in either of these studies.

The efficacy of oral olanzapine for long-term use (i.e., longer than 6 weeks) in schizophrenia has been established in one controlled study in adults, and the drug has been used in some other patients for prolonged periods (e.g., reportedly up to 1 year) without apparent loss of clinical effect. In the long-term clinical trial, adult outpatients who predominantly met DSM-IV criteria for schizophrenia and who remained stable on olanzapine therapy during an open-label treatment phase lasting at least 8 weeks were randomized to continue receiving their current olanzapine dosage (ranging from 10–20 mg daily) or to receive placebo. Although the follow-up period to observe patients for relapse, which was defined in terms of increases in BPRS positive symptoms or hospitalization, initially was planned for 12 months, criteria were met for stopping the trial early because of an excess of placebo relapses compared with olanzapine relapses. In addition, olanzapine was found to be superior to placebo on prolonging time to relapse, which was the primary outcome measure in this study. Therefore, olanzapine was more effective than placebo at maintaining efficacy in schizophrenic patients stabilized for approximately 8 weeks and followed for an observation period of up to 8 months. If oral olanzapine is used for extended periods, the need for continued therapy should be reassessed periodically.

The short-term efficacy of long-acting IM olanzapine pamoate in schizophrenia has been established in a randomized, double-blind, placebo-controlled, multicenter study of 8 weeks' duration in 404 adults who were experiencing acute psychotic symptoms and met DSM-IV or DSM-IV-TR criteria for schizophrenia. Patients were randomized to receive IM injections of olanzapine pamoate (Zyprexa® Relprevv) in dosages of 210 mg (of olanzapine) every 2 weeks, 405 mg every 4 weeks, or 300 mg every 2 weeks or placebo every 2 weeks. Patients were discontinued from their previous antipsychotic regimen and underwent a washout period lasting 2–7 days. Supplementation with oral antipsychotics was not allowed throughout the study. The primary efficacy measure in this study was the change from baseline to end point in the total PANSS score (the mean baseline total PANSS score was 101). Total PANSS scores showed improvement from baseline to end point with each dosage of olanzapine pamoate compared with placebo. At week 8, PANSS total scores decreased by a mean of 22.5, 22.6, or 26.3 points in patients receiving IM olanzapine pamoate 210 mg every 2 weeks, 405 mg every 4 weeks, or 300 mg every 2 weeks, respectively, compared with a mean decrease of 8.5 points in patients receiving placebo. There were no substantial differences in efficacy among the 3 olanzapine pamoate dosage groups at the study end point. The onset of antipsychotic efficacy for the long-acting olanzapine pamoate injection was evident within the first week of treatment. The manufacturer states that the effectiveness of olanzapine pamoate injection in the treatment of schizophrenia also is supported by the established effectiveness of orally administered olanzapine.

Efficacy of long-acting IM olanzapine pamoate for long-term use (i.e., longer than 8 weeks) in the maintenance treatment of schizophrenia has been established in a randomized, double-blind, multicenter study in 1065 adults. Adult outpatients with schizophrenia who had remained stable on oral olanzapine therapy during an open-label treatment phase lasting 4–8 weeks were randomized to continue receiving their current olanzapine dosage orally (10, 15, or 20 mg daily) or to receive long-acting IM olanzapine pamoate (Zyprexa® Relprevv) in a low-dosage regimen (150 mg [of olanzapine] every 2 weeks), a medium-dosage regimen (405 mg every 4 weeks), or a high-dosage regimen (300 mg every 2 weeks), or a very low reference dosage regimen (45 mg every 4 weeks) for 24 weeks in the double-blind maintenance phase. No supplementation with oral antipsychotics was allowed throughout the study. The primary efficacy measure was time to exacerbation of symptoms of schizophrenia, which was defined as either increases in BPRS positive symptoms or hospitalization. IM olanzapine pamoate was found to be effective in the maintenance treatment of schizophrenia for up to 24 weeks and IM olanzapine pamoate dosage regimens of 150 mg every 2 weeks, 405 mg every 4 weeks, or 300 mg every 2 weeks were found to be superior to 45 mg every 4 weeks. Olanzapine pamoate generally demonstrated a similar safety profile to oral olanzapine with the exception of injection-related adverse effects. If IM olanzapine pamoate injection is used for extended periods, the need for continued therapy should be reassessed periodically.

Parenteral antipsychotic therapy with a long-acting IM preparation may be particularly useful in patients with schizophrenia and a history of poor compliance. In addition, long-acting antipsychotic preparations may be useful in patients with suspected GI malabsorption or variable GI absorption of the drug. The principal disadvantage of long-acting parenteral antipsychotics is the inability to terminate the drug's action when severe adverse reactions occur. The manufacturer of Zyprexa® Relprevv recommends that patients first receive oral olanzapine therapy to establish tolerability of the drug before long-acting IM olanzapine pamoate is used. Long-acting IM olanzapine pamoate may be most useful in schizophrenic patients who respond well to oral olanzapine therapy and for whom a depot antipsychotic can improve compliance.

Olanzapine has been shown to be an effective, relatively rapid-acting, broad-spectrum antipsychotic agent in both controlled and uncontrolled studies of patients with schizophrenia. Like other second-generation antipsychotic agents, olanzapine appears to improve both positive (florid symptomatology such as hallucinations, conceptual disorganization, and suspiciousness) and negative ("deficit" symptomatology such as emotional withdrawal, motor retardation, blunted affect, and disorientation) manifestations of schizophrenia; conventional antipsychotic agents may have lesser effects on negative manifestations of the disorder. Some evidence also suggests that atypical antipsychotic agents may be more effective in treating cognitive and mood symptoms as well as global psychopathology than conventional antipsychotic agents, but this is controversial and remains to be fully established. In addition, some patients with schizophrenia who have been stabilized on long-term conventional antipsychotic therapy have demonstrated further improvement following a switch to an atypical antipsychotic agent.

Results from one comparative study in adults suggest that oral olanzapine dosages of 7.5–17.5 mg daily may be as effective as oral haloperidol dosages of 10–20 mg daily in reducing positive symptoms of schizophrenia, while oral olanzapine dosages of 12.5–17.5 mg daily may be more effective than oral haloperidol dosages of 10–20 mg daily in reducing negative symptoms of schizophrenia. A randomized, controlled trial comparing the long-term (i.e., 1 year) effectiveness and cost of olanzapine and haloperidol therapy in patients with schizophrenia or schizoaffective disorder did not reveal any important advantage of olanzapine compared with haloperidol on measures of compliance, symptom improvement, adverse extrapyramidal effects, overall quality of life, and cost; olanzapine also was more frequently associated with weight gain. However, olanzapine therapy was associated with reduced akathisia, less tardive dyskinesia in a secondary analysis, and small but significant improvements in measures of memory and motor function compared with haloperidol. In other comparative studies, olanzapine usually was found to be at least as effective as or more effective than haloperidol and several other atypical antipsychotic agents, including quetiapine, risperidone, and ziprasidone. In a comparative, double-blind trial conducted in patients with schizophrenia or schizoaffective disorder, both olanzapine and risperidone were found to be effective and well tolerated, although greater reductions in the severity of positive and affective symptoms were noted in the risperidone-treated patients compared with those receiving olanzapine.

Olanzapine also has been studied in patients with treatment-refractory schizophrenia (i.e., patients who have demonstrated an inadequate response to prior antipsychotic therapy) in both open and comparative clinical trials. In an open trial of 6 weeks' duration, olanzapine (15–25 mg daily) was found to be effective and well tolerated in adult patients with treatment-refractory schizophrenia with 36% responding to the drug. In a double-blind trial of 8 weeks' duration, although olanzapine (25 mg daily) was found to be as effective as chlorpromazine (1.2 g daily with benztropine), the total amount of improvement with either drug was modest; olanzapine was better tolerated than chlorpromazine. In a double-blind trial of 14 weeks' duration comparing efficacy and safety of several atypical antipsychotics (olanzapine, clozapine, and risperidone) with each other and with haloperidol, olanzapine (mean dosage of approximately 30 mg daily) and

clozapine produced greater clinical improvement in global psychopathology and negative symptoms than haloperidol (mean dosage of approximately 26 mg daily) in patients with chronic schizophrenia or schizoaffective disorder, but the effects of atypical antipsychotic agents were considered small and of limited clinical importance. In another study using the manufacturer's clinical trial database to retrospectively identify treatment-resistant schizophrenic patients, olanzapine (mean dosage of approximately 11 mg daily) was found to be more effective than haloperidol therapy (mean dosage of approximately 10 mg daily) in improving positive, negative, and mood symptoms and produced fewer extrapyramidal effects. The results of clinical trials to date suggest that olanzapine may be somewhat less effective than or similarly effective to clozapine in the management of resistant schizophrenia patients. Clozapine generally appears to be more effective in the management of treatment-refractory schizophrenia than most first-generation and other second-generation antipsychotic agents and may produce greater improvement in negative symptoms of schizophrenia than other antipsychotic agents; however, tolerability concerns (e.g., hematologic toxicity, hypotension, dizziness, sedation) limit its use in many patients. Although higher olanzapine dosages (i.e., up to 60 mg daily) have been used in some patients with treatment-resistant schizophrenia, it remains to be established whether higher dosages of the drug result in improved efficacy in such patients, and higher dosages may increase the risk of extrapyramidal and other adverse effects.

Like some other atypical antipsychotic agents (e.g., clozapine, risperidone), olanzapine therapy appears to reduce the risk of violent behavior in patients with schizophrenia. Although the precise mechanism(s) for the antiaggressive effects are not known, improved compliance with atypical antipsychotic agents may play a role.

Olanzapine also has been used with a variety of adjunctive agents, including other antipsychotic agents, antidepressants (including selective serotonin-reuptake inhibitors such as fluoxetine and fluvoxamine), valproate (e.g., divalproex sodium, valproic acid, valproate sodium), and topiramate, in some patients with treatment-refractory schizophrenia, inadequate response to antipsychotic therapy, or acute exacerbations of schizophrenia in both controlled and uncontrolled trials. Further controlled trials of olanzapine combined with these agents are necessary to more clearly determine the potential risks and benefits of such combined therapy.

Pediatric Considerations

Olanzapine is used orally for the management of schizophrenia in adolescents 13 to 17 years of age. Clinicians treating pediatric patients with schizophrenia should be aware that pediatric schizophrenia is a serious mental disorder; however, its diagnosis can be challenging. Symptom profiles in such patients can be variable. Therefore, it is recommended that drug therapy for pediatric schizophrenia be initiated only after a thorough diagnostic evaluation has been performed and careful consideration given to the risks associated with medication treatment. Medication treatment should only be part of a total treatment program that often includes psychological, educational, and social interventions.

When deciding among the alternative treatments available for adolescents with schizophrenia, clinicians should consider the increased potential for weight gain and dyslipidemia in adolescents treated with olanzapine (as compared with adults). Clinicians also should consider the potential long-term risks when prescribing olanzapine to adolescents; in many cases, this may lead them to consider prescribing other drugs first in adolescent patients. (See Cautions: Endocrine and Metabolic Effects, Cautions: Precautions and Contraindications, and see also Cautions: Pediatric Precautions.)

The short-term efficacy and tolerability of oral olanzapine in 107 adolescent inpatients and outpatients 13–17 years of age with schizophrenia were established in a randomized, double-blind, placebo-controlled, multicenter trial of 6 weeks' duration in which olanzapine was given in a flexible dosage range of 2.5–20 mg once daily. The principal rating instrument used for assessing psychiatric signs and symptoms in this trial was the Anchored Version of the BPRS for Children (BPRS-C) total score. Olanzapine (mean modal dosage: 12.5 mg daily; mean dosage: 11.1 mg daily) was found to be more effective than placebo in treating adolescents with schizophrenia, since the olanzapine-treated adolescents had a substantially greater mean reduction in the BPRS-C total score compared with those receiving placebo. However, weight gain and hyperprolactinemia occurred more often in patients receiving olanzapine compared with those receiving placebo.

Olanzapine has been successfully used orally for the management of childhood-onset schizophrenia in a limited number of children† and other adolescents. However, the manufacturers state that the safety and effectiveness of the drug in children younger than 13 years of age have not been established.

Although there is no body of evidence available to determine how long adolescent patients treated with oral olanzapine should be maintained on the drug, the manufacturer states that such efficacy can be extrapolated from adult data in addition to comparisons of olanzapine pharmacokinetic parameters in adult and adolescent patients. If olanzapine is used for an extended period, the continued need for maintenance therapy should be reassessed periodically.

Based on the observed efficacy and tolerability of atypical antipsychotics in adults and the available clinical experience in pediatric patients, the American Academy of Child and Adolescent Psychiatry (AACAP) currently states that the use of atypical antipsychotic agents in children and adolescents with schizophrenia is justified, and many clinicians consider atypical antipsychotic agents, with the exception of clozapine, among the drugs of first choice in the management of childhood-onset schizophrenia. However, well-controlled studies are necessary to more clearly establish the efficacy and safety of atypical antipsychotics in pediatric patients, particularly during long-term therapy. For additional information on the symptomatic management of childhood-onset schizophrenia, see Pediatric Considerations under Psychotic Disorders: Schizophrenia, in Uses in the Phenothiazines General Statement 28:16.08.24.

Acute Agitation

Short-acting olanzapine injection (e.g., Zyprexa® IntraMuscular) is used IM for the management of acute agitation in adult patients with schizophrenia for whom treatment with olanzapine is appropriate and who require an IM antipsychotic agent for rapid control of behaviors that interfere with diagnosis and care (e.g., threatening behaviors, escalating or urgently distressing behavior, self-exhausting behavior). According to DSM-IV, psychomotor agitation is excessive motor activity associated with a feeling of inner tension. The efficacy of IM olanzapine for the management of acute agitation in patients with schizophrenia was established in 2 short-term (single-day), placebo-controlled trials in hospital settings; an active comparator treatment arm using haloperidol injection was included in both studies. The patients in this study exhibited a level of agitation that met or exceeded a threshold score of 14 on the 5 items comprising the Positive and Negative Syndrome Scale (PANSS) Excited Component (i.e., poor impulse control, tension, hostility, uncooperativeness, and excitement items) with at least one individual item score of 4 ("moderate") or greater using a 1–7 scoring system, where scores of 1 or 7 indicate absent or extreme agitation, respectively. The primary measure used for assessing efficacy in managing agitation in these trials was the change from baseline in the PANSS Excited Component at 2 hours post-injection. Patients could receive up to 3 injections of IM olanzapine; however, patients could not receive the second injection until after the initial 2-hour period when the primary efficacy measure was assessed.

In the first placebo-controlled trial, short-acting IM olanzapine was given in fixed single doses of 2.5, 5, 7.5, or 10 mg in agitated hospitalized patients with schizophrenia. All 4 IM olanzapine doses were found to be statistically superior to placebo in reducing the PANSS Excited Component score at 2 hours following injection; however, the effect was larger and more consistent for the 3 highest doses studied. There were no significant differences in efficacy noted for the 7.5- and 10-mg doses compared with the 5-mg dose in this study. In the second placebo-controlled trial in agitated patients with schizophrenia, a fixed, 10-mg dose of short-acting IM olanzapine was evaluated and found to be superior to placebo on the PANSS Excited Component at 2 hours following injection. An analysis of these 2 controlled studies as well as an additional controlled study conducted in agitated patients with bipolar mania for possible age-, race-, or gender-related effects on treatment outcome did not suggest any difference in efficacy based on these patient characteristics.

● Bipolar Disorder

Oral olanzapine is used alone in adults and adolescents 13–17 years of age or in conjunction with lithium or valproate in adults for the acute management of manic or mixed episodes associated with bipolar I disorder; the drug also is used orally for longer-term maintenance monotherapy in adults and adolescents 13–17 years of age with this disorder. In addition, oral olanzapine is used in combination with fluoxetine hydrochloride for the treatment of acute depressive episodes associated with bipolar I disorder in adults and pediatric patients 10–17 years of age. According to DSM-IV criteria, manic episodes are distinct periods lasting 1 week or longer (or less than 1 week if hospitalization is required) of abnormally and persistently elevated, expansive, or irritable mood accompanied by at least 3 (or 4 if the mood is only irritability) of the following 7 symptoms: grandiosity, reduced need for sleep, pressure of speech, flight of ideas, distractibility, increased goal-directed activity (either socially, at work or school, or sexually) or psychomotor

agitation, and engaging in high-risk behavior (e.g., unrestrained buying sprees, sexual indiscretions, foolish business investments).

For the initial management of less severe manic or mixed episodes in patients with bipolar disorder, current APA recommendations state that monotherapy with lithium, valproate (e.g., valproate sodium, valproic acid, divalproex), or an antipsychotic such as olanzapine may be adequate. For more severe manic or mixed episodes, combination therapy with an antipsychotic and lithium or valproate is recommended as first-line therapy. For further information on the management of bipolar disorder, see Uses: Bipolar Disorder, in Lithium Salts 28:28.

Acute Treatment of Manic or Mixed Episodes

Efficacy of oral olanzapine monotherapy in the acute treatment of manic or mixed episodes in adults has been demonstrated in 2 short-term (i.e., 3 or 4 weeks' duration), randomized, double-blind, placebo-controlled, parallel-group trials in patients who met DSM-IV criteria for bipolar I disorder (with or without a rapid-cycling course) and who met diagnostic criteria for an acute manic or mixed episode (with or without psychotic features). Olanzapine was given in an initial dosage of 10 mg once daily in the 3-week trial and 15 mg once daily in the 4-week trial; the dosage was subsequently adjusted within the range of 5–20 mg once daily in both of these trials. The principal rating instrument used for assessing manic symptoms in these trials was the Y-MRS score, an 11-item clinician-rated scale traditionally used to assess the degree of manic symptomatology (e.g., irritability, disruptive/aggressive behavior, sleep, elevated mood, speech, increased activity, sexual interest, language/thought disorder, thought content, appearance, insight) in a range from 0 (no manic features) to 60 (maximum score). All patients were hospitalized at the onset of these trials, but some patients were allowed to continue the studies on an outpatient basis after 1 week of hospitalization if their Clinical Global Impressions-Bipolar Version of severity of illness (CGI-BP) mania score was no greater than 3 (mild) and they had at least a 50% reduction in their Young Mania Rating Scale (Y-MRS) scores. In the 3- and 4-week placebo-controlled trials, approximately 49–65% of patients receiving 5–20 mg of olanzapine once daily achieved a 50% or greater improvement in Y-MRS total score from baseline compared with approximately 24–43% of those who received placebo. In addition, unlike therapy with typical antipsychotic agents, patients receiving olanzapine in these clinical studies did not experience a worsening in depressive symptoms (defined as an increase in the Hamilton Psychiatric Rating Scale for Depression-21 item [HAMD-21] score of at least 3 points) compared with those receiving placebo. In another 3-week, placebo-controlled trial that was designed identically to the first 3-week trial and was conducted simultaneously, olanzapine demonstrated a similar treatment difference in reduction of the Y-MRS total score but was not found to be superior to placebo on this outcome measure, possibly due to sample size and site variability.

Data from one limited comparative study suggest that oral olanzapine dosages of 10 mg daily may be as effective as lithium carbonate dosages of 400 mg twice daily in the treatment of manic episodes in adults with bipolar disorder. In a randomized, double-blind trial of 3 weeks' duration comparing olanzapine (5–20 mg daily) and divalproex sodium therapy in hospitalized adults with bipolar disorder experiencing acute manic or mixed episodes, olanzapine therapy was found to produce greater improvement in Y-MRS total scores, which was the primary efficacy measure in this trial. In addition, a substantially greater proportion of patients in the olanzapine group achieved remission compared with the divalproex group. In a randomized, double-blind study of 12 weeks' duration comparing olanzapine and divalproex sodium in patients with bipolar I disorder hospitalized for acute mania, the drugs were found to be equally effective although divalproex sodium was somewhat better tolerated than olanzapine.

Combined Therapy

Efficacy of oral olanzapine when used in combination with lithium or valproate in the short-term treatment of acute manic or mixed episodes has been demonstrated in 2 randomized, double-blind, placebo-controlled studies of 6 weeks' duration in adult patients who met the DSM-IV criteria for bipolar I disorder (with or without a rapid-cycling course) and who met diagnostic criteria for an acute manic or mixed episode (with or without psychotic features). In these studies, patients with bipolar disorder experiencing manic or mixed episodes (Y-MRS scores of 16 or greater) who had not responded to at least 2 weeks of lithium or divalproex sodium monotherapy despite adequate plasma drug concentrations (in a therapeutic range of 0.6–1.2 mEq/L for lithium or 50–125 mcg/mL of valproate for divalproex sodium) were randomized to receive either olanzapine (initial dosage of 10 mg once daily; range: 5–20 mg once daily) or placebo, in combination with their original therapy. Addition of olanzapine to lithium or divalproex sodium was shown to be superior to continued monotherapy with lithium or divalproex sodium in the reduction of Y-MRS total score in both of these studies.

The manufacturer states that efficacy of adjunctive therapy with olanzapine for longer-term use (i.e., longer than 6 weeks) in patients with bipolar I disorder has not been systematically evaluated in controlled trials.

Maintenance Monotherapy of Bipolar Disorder

Oral olanzapine is used for maintenance monotherapy in adults and adolescent patients 13–17 years of age with bipolar I disorder. The long-term efficacy of oral olanzapine as maintenance monotherapy in adults with bipolar disorder has been demonstrated in a double-blind, placebo-controlled trial and in double-blind comparative trials. In the placebo-controlled study, adult patients who met DSM-IV criteria for bipolar I disorder and experienced manic or mixed episodes and who had responded during an initial open-label treatment phase to oral olanzapine therapy (5–20 mg daily) for an average of about 2 weeks were randomized either to continue olanzapine at the same dosage or to receive placebo for up to 48 weeks and were observed for relapse. Response during the open-label phase was defined as a reduction in the Y-MRS total score of 12 or more and in the 21-item Hamilton Depression Rating Scale (HAM-D 21) of 8 or more; relapse during the double-blind phase of the study was defined as an increase in the Y-MRS or HAM-D 21 total score to 15 or more or being hospitalized for either mania or depression. Approximately 50% of the patients in the olanzapine group had discontinued therapy by day 59, and approximately 50% of the patients in the placebo group had discontinued placebo by day 23 of the double-blind phase. A longer time until relapse was observed in the patients receiving olanzapine compared with those receiving placebo (median of 174 and 22 days, respectively, for relapse into any mood episode) during the randomized phase of this study. The relapse rate also was significantly lower in the olanzapine group (approximately 47%) than in the placebo group (approximately 80%). If olanzapine is used for extended periods, the need for continued therapy should be reassessed periodically.

In a double-blind, 52-week trial comparing olanzapine and lithium maintenance therapy in adults with bipolar disorder, olanzapine was found to be significantly more effective than lithium in preventing relapses and recurrences of manic and mixed episodes following initial stabilization with combined olanzapine and lithium therapy. Olanzapine and lithium demonstrated comparable efficacy in preventing relapses and recurrences of depression in this study. In a retrospective analysis from this trial, patients were subcategorized into illness stage (early, intermediate, or later) based on the number of prior manic or mixed episodes they had experienced. The rates of relapse or recurrence of manic or mixed episodes were approximately 2 and 26%, 13 and 24%, and 24 and 33% for olanzapine and lithium in the early, intermediate, and later stage groups of bipolar patients, respectively; no substantial treatment effect for treatment or illness stage for depressive relapse or recurrence was observed. Because olanzapine was associated with a lower rate of relapse or recurrence of manic and mixed episodes in early-stage patients, it was suggested that the drug may be particularly effective early in the course of bipolar disorder.

In a double-blind, 47-week trial comparing monotherapy with olanzapine or divalproex sodium in adults with bipolar disorder experiencing manic or mixed episodes, mean improvement in Y-MRS scores was greater for olanzapine-treated patients. In addition, the median time to symptomatic mania remission was shorter for patients receiving olanzapine compared with those receiving divalproex sodium (14 days vs. 62 days, respectively). However, no significant differences in the rates of symptomatic mania remission and symptomatic relapse into mania or depression between the olanzapine- and divalproex-treated patients were observed in this study. In a double-blind, 18-month, relapse prevention trial comparing the efficacy of combined olanzapine plus lithium or valproate therapy with lithium or valproate therapy alone in patients with bipolar disorder, more sustained symptomatic remission (163 days vs 42 days, respectively) occurred in the group receiving combined olanzapine plus lithium or valproate therapy than in the group receiving lithium or valproate therapy alone.

Rapid-Cycling Bipolar Disorder

In an analysis of pooled data from several trials comparing the clinical response to olanzapine therapy in rapid-cycling and non-rapid-cycling adult patients with bipolar disorder, relative clinical response to olanzapine was found to be similar in the 2 groups, although earlier responses were observed in the rapid-cycling group of patients, and long-term outcomes were more favorable in the non-rapid-cycling group. Rapid-cycling patients were found to be less likely to achieve an initial symptomatic remission, more likely to experience recurrences, especially

of depression, and had more hospitalizations and suicide attempts than non-rapid-cycling patients in this study.

Depressive Episodes Associated with Bipolar Disorder

Oral olanzapine is used in combination with fluoxetine for the treatment of acute depressive episodes associated with bipolar I disorder in adults and pediatric patients 10–17 years of age. In 2 randomized, double-blind studies of 8 weeks' duration comparing a fixed combination of olanzapine and fluoxetine hydrochloride (Symbyax®) with olanzapine monotherapy and placebo in adults, the fixed combination (given in flexible daily dosages of 6 mg olanzapine with 25 or 50 mg of fluoxetine or 12 mg of olanzapine with 50 mg of fluoxetine) was more effective than olanzapine monotherapy (5–20 mg daily) or placebo in improvement in depressive symptoms as assessed by the Montgomery-Asberg Depression Rating Scale (MADRS). Although the manufacturer states that efficacy beyond 8 weeks' duration remains to be established, patients have received the fixed combination for up to 24 weeks in clinical trials. Clinicians who elect to extend therapy beyond 8 weeks should reevaluate the risks and benefits of continued therapy periodically.

The manufacturers state that olanzapine monotherapy is not indicated for the treatment of depressive episodes associated with bipolar I disorder.

Pediatric Considerations

Oral olanzapine is used as monotherapy in adolescents 13–17 years of age for the acute management of manic or mixed episodes associated with bipolar I disorder; the drug also is used orally for longer-term maintenance monotherapy in patients with this disorder. Oral olanzapine in combination with fluoxetine is used for the treatment of acute depressive episodes associated with bipolar I disorder in pediatric patients 10–17 years of age. When treating pediatric patients with bipolar I disorder, clinicians should be aware that pediatric bipolar I disorder is a serious mental disorder; however, its diagnosis can be challenging. Pediatric patients with bipolar disorder may have variable patterns of periodicity of manic or mixed symptoms. Therefore, it is recommended that drug therapy for pediatric bipolar disorder be initiated only after a thorough diagnostic evaluation has been performed and careful consideration given to the risks associated with medication treatment. Medication treatment should only be part of a total treatment program that often includes psychological, educational, and social interventions.

When deciding among the alternative treatments available for adolescents with bipolar disorder, clinicians should consider the increased potential for weight gain and dyslipidemia in adolescents receiving olanzapine (as compared with adults). Clinicians also should consider the potential long-term risks when prescribing olanzapine to adolescents; in many cases, this may lead them to consider prescribing other drugs first in adolescent patients. (See Cautions: Endocrine and Metabolic Effects, Cautions: Precautions and Contraindications, and see also Cautions: Pediatric Precautions.)

The short-term efficacy of oral olanzapine monotherapy in the acute treatment of bipolar I disorder in adolescents 13–17 years of age was established in a randomized, multicenter, double-blind, placebo-controlled trial of 3 weeks' duration in 161 patients who met DSM-IV-TR criteria for manic or mixed episodes associated with bipolar I disorder (with or without psychotic features). In this flexible-dosage trial, outpatients and inpatients were randomized to receive either olanzapine 2.5–20 mg daily (mean modal dosage of 10.7 mg daily; mean dosage of 8.9 mg daily) or placebo. Olanzapine was found to be more effective than placebo as demonstrated by substantially greater reduction in the total score on the Adolescent Structured Y-MRS, which was the primary efficacy measure in this study. However, the olanzapine-treated adolescents had substantially greater weight gain and elevations in serum transaminases, prolactin, fasting glucose, fasting total cholesterol, and uric acid compared with those receiving placebo.

The efficacy and safety of oral olanzapine in combination with fluoxetine hydrochloride for the acute treatment of depressive episodes associated with bipolar I disorder in pediatric patients 10–17 years of age were established in a randomized, double-blind, placebo-controlled trial of 8 weeks' duration in 255 patients who met the DSM-IV-TR criteria for bipolar I disorder, depressed episode. Patients randomized to receive olanzapine and fluoxetine were initially given 3 mg of olanzapine with 25 mg of fluoxetine and force-titrated to the maximum dosage of 12 mg of olanzapine with 50 mg of fluoxetine over 2 weeks; after 2 weeks, patients received flexible dosages of olanzapine 6–12 mg with fluoxetine 25–50 mg daily. At week 8, olanzapine in combination with fluoxetine was found to be substantially more effective than placebo in reducing the Children's Depression Rating Scale-Revised (CDRS-R) total score, which was the primary efficacy measure in this study. The average daily dosage was 7.7 mg of olanzapine and

37.6 mg of fluoxetine. The pediatric patients who received olanzapine in combination with fluoxetine had substantially greater weight gain and elevations in serum transaminases, serum lipids, and prolactin compared with those receiving placebo. The recommended initial dosage of the olanzapine/fluoxetine combination is lower in children and adolescents than in adults. In addition, the manufacturer states that flexible dosing is recommended in such patients instead of the forced-titration dosing initially used in this study. (See Bipolar Disorder under Dosage: Oral Dosage, in Dosage and Administration.)

Although there is no body of evidence available to determine how long adolescent patients with bipolar disorder treated with olanzapine should be maintained on the drug, the manufacturer states that such efficacy can be extrapolated from adult data in addition to comparisons of olanzapine pharmacokinetic parameters in adult and adolescent patients. If olanzapine is used for an extended period, the continued need for maintenance therapy should be reassessed periodically.

Based on the observed efficacy and tolerability of mood stabilizers and atypical antipsychotic agents in clinical trials in adults and the available clinical experience in pediatric patients, the American Academy of Child and Adolescent Psychiatry (AACAP) currently states that mood stabilizers (e.g., lithium, valproic acid, carbamazepine) and atypical antipsychotics (e.g., olanzapine, aripiprazole, risperidone, quetiapine, ziprasidone) are among drugs of first choice in the acute management of pediatric patients with bipolar I disorder experiencing manic or mixed episodes with or without psychosis. Additional controlled studies are necessary to more clearly establish the efficacy and safety of atypical antipsychotics in pediatric patients with bipolar disorder, particularly during long-term therapy.

Acute Agitation

Short-acting olanzapine injection (e.g., Zyprexa® IntraMuscular) is used IM for the management of acute agitation in patients with bipolar I disorder for whom treatment with olanzapine is appropriate and who require an IM antipsychotic agent for rapid control of behaviors that interfere with their diagnosis and care (e.g., threatening behaviors, escalating or urgently distressing behavior, self-exhausting behavior). According to DSM-IV, psychomotor agitation is excessive motor activity associated with a feeling of inner tension.

The efficacy of short-acting IM olanzapine for the management of acute agitation in adults with bipolar mania was established in a short-term (single-day), double-blind, placebo-controlled trial in agitated, hospitalized patients who met the DSM-IV criteria for bipolar I disorder and who displayed an acute manic or mixed episode with or without psychotic features. The patients in this study exhibited a level of agitation that met or exceeded a threshold score of 14 on the 5 items comprising the Positive and Negative Syndrome Scale (PANSS) Excited Component (i.e., poor impulse control, tension, hostility, uncooperativeness, and excitement items) with at least one individual item score of 4 ("moderate") or greater using a 1–7 scoring system where scores of 1 or 7 indicate absent or extreme agitation, respectively. An active comparator treatment arm using IM lorazepam was included in this study. The primary measure used for assessing efficacy in managing agitation in this trial was the change from baseline in the PANSS Excited Component at 2 hours post-injection of a fixed, 10-mg IM dose of olanzapine. Patients in this study could receive up to 3 injections of IM olanzapine; however, patients could not receive the second injection until after the initial 2-hour period when the efficacy was assessed. IM olanzapine was found to be statistically superior to placebo in reducing the PANSS Excited Component score at 2 hours and at 24 hours following the initial injection. An analysis of this study as well as 2 additional controlled studies conducted in agitated patients with schizophrenia for possible age-, race-, or gender-related effects on treatment outcome did not suggest any difference in efficacy based on these patient characteristics.

● Treatment-resistant Depression

Oral olanzapine is used in combination with fluoxetine hydrochloride for the acute and maintenance therapy of treatment-resistant depression (i.e., major depressive disorder in patients who do not respond to 2 separate trials of different antidepressants of adequate dosage and duration in the current episode).

The efficacy and safety of oral olanzapine in combination with fluoxetine for the acute treatment of treatment-resistant depression were demonstrated in 3 clinical studies conducted in 579 adults 18–85 years of age. Daily dosages evaluated in these studies ranged from 6–18 mg of olanzapine and 25–50 mg of fluoxetine. In the first study, efficacy of the fixed combination of olanzapine and fluoxetine (Symbyax®) was evaluated in 300 patients who met DSM-IV criteria for major depressive disorder and did not respond to 2 different antidepressants after at least 6 weeks at or above the minimally effective labeled dosage in their current episode. Patients enrolled in this study entered an open-label fluoxetine lead-in phase

in which the nonresponders were randomized to receive the fixed combination of olanzapine and fluoxetine, olanzapine alone, or fluoxetine alone for 8 weeks. The fixed combination of olanzapine and fluoxetine was flexibly dosed between 6–18 mg of olanzapine daily; all patients received 50 mg of fluoxetine daily. A substantially greater reduction in mean total MADRS scores from baseline to end point was observed in patients receiving olanzapine in fixed combination with fluoxetine compared with those receiving either fluoxetine or olanzapine alone. A second, smaller study with the same treatment-resistant depressed patient population also demonstrated a substantially greater reduction in MADRS scores in patients treated with the fixed combination compared with patients receiving fluoxetine or olanzapine monotherapy (when analyzed with change in MADRS score as the outcome measure). A third study demonstrated a substantially greater reduction in total MADRS scores in patients receiving the fixed combination of olanzapine and fluoxetine compared with those treated with fluoxetine or olanzapine alone, when data were analyzed in a subpopulation of 251 depressed patients who met the definition of treatment resistance (patients who had not responded to 2 antidepressants of adequate dosage and duration in the current episode).

The efficacy of oral olanzapine in combination with fluoxetine in the maintenance therapy of treatment-resistant depression was demonstrated in a 47-week study in 892 adults (18–65 years of age) who met DSM-IV criteria for major depressive disorder and did not respond to 2 different antidepressants after at least 6 weeks at or above the minimally effective labeled dosage in their current episode. Daily dosages evaluated in these studies ranged from 6–18 mg of olanzapine and 25–50 mg of fluoxetine. Patients were initially treated with open-label olanzapine and fluoxetine in fixed combination (Symbyax®). Patients who responded to and were stabilized on the fixed combination over approximately 20 weeks were randomized to continue receiving fixed-combination olanzapine and fluoxetine treatment or to receive fluoxetine alone for another 27 weeks. A total of 15.8% of patients receiving olanzapine and fluoxetine in fixed combination relapsed compared with 31.8% of patients receiving fluoxetine monotherapy; this difference was statistically significant. In addition, patients who continued to receive olanzapine and fluoxetine in fixed combination experienced a substantially longer time to relapse over the 27-week period compared with those receiving fluoxetine alone. If combined olanzapine and fluoxetine therapy is used for an extended period, the continued need for maintenance therapy should be reassessed periodically.

The manufacturer states that olanzapine monotherapy is not indicated for the treatment of treatment-resistant depression.

● Cancer Chemotherapy-induced Nausea and Vomiting

Olanzapine has been used orally in combination with other antiemetic agents for the prevention of acute and delayed nausea and vomiting associated with highly emetogenic cancer chemotherapy†, including high-dose cisplatin therapy. The drug also has been used as rescue therapy in patients with breakthrough cancer chemotherapy-induced nausea and vomiting†.

To prevent chemotherapy-induced nausea and vomiting associated with chemotherapy regimens with a high emetic risk (i.e., incidence of emesis exceeds 90% if no antiemetics are administered) in adults, the American Society of Clinical Oncology (ASCO) currently recommends a 4-drug antiemetic regimen consisting of a neurokinin 1 (NK$_1$) receptor antagonist (e.g., aprepitant, fosaprepitant, netupitant [in fixed combination with palonosetron], rolapitant), a type 3 serotonin (5-HT$_3$) receptor antagonist (e.g., dolasetron, granisetron, ondansetron, palonosetron, ramosetron [not commercially available in the US], tropisetron [not commercially available in the US]), dexamethasone, and olanzapine. If the fixed combination of netupitant and palonosetron is used as an NK$_1$ receptor antagonist, use of an additional 5-HT$_3$ receptor antagonist is not necessary. For adults receiving carboplatin with a target area under the plasma concentration-time curve (AUC) of 4 mg/mL per minute or more, ASCO recommends a 3-drug antiemetic regimen consisting of an NK$_1$ receptor antagonist, a 5-HT$_3$ receptor antagonist, and dexamethasone. For adults receiving other chemotherapy of moderate emetic risk (i.e., incidence of emesis without antiemetics exceeds 30% but does not exceed 90%), excluding carboplatin with a target AUC of 4 mg/mL per minute or more, ASCO recommends a 2-drug antiemetic regimen consisting of a 5-HT$_3$ receptor antagonist and dexamethasone. Because of the limited clinical experience with oral olanzapine in adults receiving moderately emetogenic chemotherapy, ASCO states that olanzapine is not recommended for routine prophylaxis in such patients. For adults receiving chemotherapy regimens with a low emetic risk (i.e., incidence of emesis without antiemetics exceeds 10% but does not exceed 30%), ASCO recommends a single dose of either a 5-HT$_3$ receptor antagonist or dexamethasone alone on the first day of chemotherapy. Routine antiemetic prophylaxis is not necessary in adults receiving chemotherapy with a minimal antiemetic risk (i.e., incidence of emesis is less than 10% without antiemetics).

For patients with breakthrough chemotherapy-induced nausea or vomiting, ASCO recommends that clinicians reevaluate emetic risk, disease status, concomitant medical conditions, and concurrent medications and determine whether the best antiemetic regimen is being provided for the emetic risk. Adults who experience nausea and vomiting despite optimal antiemetic prophylaxis and who have not received olanzapine prophylactically should be offered olanzapine in addition to continuing the standard antiemetic regimen. Adults who experience nausea or vomiting despite optimal antiemetic prophylaxis and who have already received olanzapine may be offered a drug from a different class such as an NK₁ receptor antagonist, lorazepam or alprazolam, a dopamine receptor antagonist (e.g., metoclopramide), dronabinol, or nabilone in addition to continuing the standard antiemetic regimen.

Clinical Experience

Efficacy of oral olanzapine for the prevention of nausea and vomiting associated with cancer chemotherapy was established in a randomized, double-blind, phase 3 study comparing olanzapine with placebo, in combination with an NK₁ receptor antagonist (either IV fosaprepitant or oral aprepitant), a 5-HT₃ receptor antagonist (e.g., oral or IV granisetron, oral or IV ondansetron, IV palonosetron), and oral dexamethasone, in 380 adults receiving highly emetogenic chemotherapy (cisplatin-containing regimens or anthracycline plus cyclophosphamide). Patients received olanzapine 10 mg or matching placebo orally once daily on days 1 through 4. The proportion of patients who experienced no chemotherapy-induced nausea was substantially higher with olanzapine than with placebo during the early assessment period (0–24 hours after chemotherapy; 74 versus 45%, respectively), the later assessment period (25–120 hours after chemotherapy; 42 versus 25%, respectively), and the overall period (0–120 hours after chemotherapy; 37 versus 22%, respectively). The proportion of patients with a complete response (no emetic episodes and no use of rescue medication) was also substantially higher in patients receiving olanzapine than in those receiving placebo in all 3 assessment periods (86 versus 65%, 67 versus 52%, and 64 versus 41% during the early, later, and overall assessment periods, respectively). Olanzapine was generally well tolerated and no serious adverse reactions to the drug were reported in this study; however, olanzapine-treated patients experienced more drowsiness on day 2 following chemotherapy than at baseline. The sedation generally resolved on days 3, 4, and 5 despite continued administration of olanzapine on days 3 and 4.

Efficacy of antiemetic prophylactic regimens including oral olanzapine and antiemetic regimens not including olanzapine was compared in a meta-analysis of 10 randomized controlled trials in patients receiving either highly or moderately emetogenic chemotherapy. Six of these studies included patients receiving only highly emetogenic chemotherapy and 4 studies included patients receiving either highly emetogenic or moderately emetogenic chemotherapy. Antiemetic regimens containing olanzapine were found to be statistically superior in 5 of 6 end points and clinically superior in 4 of 6 end points compared with antiemetic regimens not containing olanzapine in this meta-analysis.

In a randomized, multicenter, double-blind, phase 2, dose-finding study, efficacy and safety of 2 olanzapine dosage regimens (5 mg or 10 mg orally once daily on days 1 through 4) used in combination with standard antiemetic prophylaxis (e.g., aprepitant or fosaprepitant, palonosetron, and dexamethasone) for the prevention of nausea and vomiting associated with cancer chemotherapy were compared in 153 adults with malignant solid tumors who were receiving highly emetogenic chemotherapy with cisplatin. The primary end point in this study was complete response (no emesis and no use of rescue medications) in the delayed phase (24–120 hours after the start of cisplatin therapy). Both dosages of olanzapine produced a significant improvement in delayed emesis; complete response rates in the delayed phase were 85.7 and 77.6% in the 5- and 10-mg olanzapine dosage groups, respectively. Somnolence was the most commonly reported adverse effect in this study and occurred in 45.5 and 53.3% of patients in the 5- and 10-mg olanzapine dosage groups, respectively.

Olanzapine has been shown to be an effective rescue antiemetic in patients who develop breakthrough chemotherapy-induced nausea and vomiting despite having received optimal antiemetic prophylaxis. In a randomized, double-blind, phase 3 study, efficacy and safety of orally administered olanzapine and metoclopramide for the treatment of breakthrough chemotherapy-induced nausea and vomiting were compared in chemotherapy-naive adults receiving highly emetogenic chemotherapy (cisplatin or doxorubicin and cyclophosphamide)

who did not receive antiemetic prophylaxis with olanzapine. All patients had initially received guideline-directed antiemetic prophylaxis with fosaprepitant, palonosetron, and dexamethasone. Of 276 enrolled patients, 112 developed breakthrough nausea and vomiting and were randomized to receive olanzapine (10 mg orally once daily for 3 days) or metoclopramide (10 mg orally 3 times daily for 3 days); 108 of these patients were evaluable. Patients were monitored for emesis and nausea for 72 hours after receiving olanzapine or metoclopramide. During the 72-hour observation period after the breakthrough nausea and vomiting occurred, 70% of the olanzapine-treated patients had no emesis compared with 31% of the metoclopramide-treated patients and 68% of the olanzapine-treated patients had no nausea compared with 23% of the metoclopramide-treated patients. Olanzapine was found to be significantly better than metoclopramide in controlling breakthrough nausea and vomiting in patients receiving highly emetogenic chemotherapy. No grade 3 or 4 toxicities occurred with either olanzapine or metoclopramide.

DOSAGE AND ADMINISTRATION

● Reconstitution and Administration

Olanzapine is administered orally or by IM injection. Olanzapine pamoate is administered only by IM injection.

Restricted Distribution

Because of the risk of post-injection delirium/sedation syndrome (PDSS), extended-release olanzapine pamoate injection is available only under a restricted distribution program, the Zyprexa® Relprevv Patient Care Program. Zyprexa® Relprevv must not be dispensed directly to a patient. For a patient to receive treatment, the prescriber, healthcare facility, patient, and pharmacy must all be enrolled in the Patient Care Program. Clinicians may contact 877-772-9390 for additional information and to enroll in the Zyprexa® Relprevv Patient Care Program or consult the manufacturer's website (https://www.zyprexarelprevvprogram.com).

Oral Administration

Olanzapine conventional tablets, orally disintegrating tablets, and capsules (in fixed combination with fluoxetine hydrochloride) are administered orally. Since food does not appear to affect GI absorption of olanzapine, the drug generally can be administered as conventional tablets or orally disintegrating tablets without regard to meals. In patients who experience persistent or troublesome daytime sedation during oral olanzapine therapy for psychiatric indications (e.g., psychotic disorders, bipolar disorder, treatment-resistant depression), administration of the daily dosage in the evening at bedtime may be helpful.

Patients receiving olanzapine orally disintegrating tablets should be instructed not to remove a tablet from the blister until just prior to dosing. The tablet should not be pushed through the foil. With dry hands, the blister backing should be peeled completely off the blister. The tablet should then be gently removed and immediately placed on the tongue, where it rapidly disintegrates in saliva, and then subsequently swallowed with or without liquid.

The fixed combination capsules of olanzapine with fluoxetine hydrochloride (e.g., Symbyax®) are administered once daily in the evening. Although the manufacturer states that food has no appreciable effect on absorption of either drug when administered alone, absorption of the drugs when administered as the fixed combination with food has not been studied.

Dispensing and Administration Precautions

Because of similarities in spelling, dosage intervals (once daily), and tablet strengths (5 and 10 mg) of Zyprexa® (olanzapine) and Zyrtec® (cetirizine hydrochloride, an antihistamine), extra care should be exercised in ensuring the accuracy of prescriptions for these drugs. (See Cautions: Precautions and Contraindications.)

IM Administration

Clinicians should be aware that there are 2 IM formulations of olanzapine with different indications and dosing schedules; the short-acting, immediate-release formulation (e.g., Zyprexa IntraMuscular®; 10 mg per vial) is used for agitation associated with schizophrenia and bipolar mania and should not be confused with Zyprexa® Relprevv, a long-acting formulation (available in 210-, 300-, and 405-mg vial strengths) used for the treatment of schizophrenia.

Short-acting Olanzapine Injection for Acute Agitation associated with Bipolar Disorder or Schizophrenia

Commercially available short-acting olanzapine for injection (e.g., Zyprexa® IntraMuscular) must be reconstituted prior to administration by adding 2.1 mL of sterile water for injection to single-dose vials labeled as containing 10 mg of olanzapine to provide a solution containing approximately 5 mg/mL. Other solutions should not be used to reconstitute olanzapine for injection.

Following reconstitution, olanzapine for injection should be used immediately (within 1 hour). If necessary, the reconstituted solution may be stored for up to 1 hour at 20–25°C; after 1 hour, any unused portion should be discarded. Olanzapine for injection should be inspected visually for particulate matter and discoloration prior to administration whenever solution and container permit.

Olanzapine for injection is administered only by IM injection and should *not* be administered IV or subcutaneously. The drug should be injected slowly, deep into the muscle mass.

Extended-release Olanzapine Pamoate Injection for Schizophrenia

The manufacturer states that tolerability with oral olanzapine therapy should be established prior to initiating IM therapy with extended-release olanzapine pamoate (Zyprexa® Relprevv).

Because of the risk of post-injection delirium/sedation syndrome (PDSS), Zyprexa® Relprevv must be administered in a registered healthcare facility (e.g., hospital, clinic, residential treatment center, community healthcare center) with ready access to emergency response services. The medication guide should be provided to the patient or legal guardian prior to each injection. After each injection, patients should be continuously monitored at the healthcare facility for at least 3 hours by a healthcare professional. Patients should be alert, oriented, and absent of any signs and symptoms of PDSS prior to being released. All patients receiving an IM injection of olanzapine pamoate must be accompanied to their destination upon leaving the facility.

Patients should not drive or operate heavy machinery for the remainder of the day following the injection. Patients should be advised to be vigilant for the symptoms of PDSS and to obtain medical assistance if needed. Close medical supervision and monitoring should be instituted in a facility capable of resuscitation if PDSS is suspected in any patient. (See Post-injection Delirium/Sedation Syndrome under Cautions: Nervous System Effects and also under Cautions: Precautions and Contraindications and see also Acute Toxicity.)

Extended-release olanzapine pamoate injection is administered only by deep IM injection into the gluteal area and should *not* be administered IV or subcutaneously. The injection should be administered by a healthcare professional every 2–4 weeks.

Olanzapine pamoate is commercially available as the Zyprexa® Relprevv Convenience Kit, which contains 2 single-use vials, needles, and a syringe; one of the vials contains olanzapine pamoate powder for suspension and the other vial contains diluent. Olanzapine pamoate powder for suspension must be reconstituted using only the diluent provided in the convenience kit prior to IM administration; other diluents should not be substituted. Reconstitution and administration instructions included in the kit should be closely followed, and the suspension should be administered within 24 hours of mixing. Reconstituted olanzapine pamoate suspension remains stable for up to 24 hours in the vial. However, if the suspension is not used immediately, the vial should be shaken vigorously to resuspend the drug.

The manufacturer recommends that gloves are used while reconstituting olanzapine pamoate powder for suspension since it may be irritating to the skin. If contact is made with skin, the affected area should be flushed with water.

Following insertion of the needle into the gluteal muscle for the IM injection, the healthcare professional should aspirate for several seconds to ensure that no blood is drawn into the syringe. If blood appears in the syringe, the dose should not be injected; the needle should be withdrawn and the syringe and dose discarded. A new convenience kit should be used for the new dose of olanzapine pamoate with a new syringe and needle. Following IM administration, the injection site should not be massaged.

● *Dosage*

Olanzapine is commercially available as the base and as the pamoate salt; the dosage of olanzapine pamoate is expressed in terms of olanzapine.

Conventional olanzapine tablets and orally disintegrating tablets of the drug are bioequivalent. However, IM administration of a 5-mg dose of the commercially available short-acting olanzapine injection results in a maximum plasma olanzapine concentration that is about fivefold higher than that resulting from a 5-mg oral dose of the drug.

Dosage of olanzapine for psychiatric indications (e.g., psychotic disorders, bipolar disorder, treatment-resistant depression) must be adjusted carefully according to individual requirements and response, using the lowest possible effective dosage.

Oral Dosage
Schizophrenia

For the management of schizophrenia in adults, the recommended initial oral dosage of olanzapine is 5–10 mg daily, usually given as a single daily dose. Dosage may be increased by 5 mg daily within several days, to a target dosage of 10 mg daily. Because steady-state plasma concentrations of olanzapine may not be attained for approximately 7 days at a given dosage, subsequent dosage adjustments generally should be made at intervals of not less than 7 days, usually in increments or decrements of 5 mg once daily.

An initial adult olanzapine oral dosage of 5 mg daily is recommended in debilitated patients, in those predisposed to hypotension, in those who may be particularly sensitive to the effects of olanzapine, or in those who might metabolize olanzapine slowly (e.g., nonsmoking female patients who are 65 years of age or older). The manufacturers state that the presence of factors that might decrease the clearance or increase the pharmacodynamic response to olanzapine should lead to consideration of a lower initial dosage in all geriatric patients.

While a relationship between dosage and antipsychotic effect has not been established, the effective oral dosage of olanzapine in clinical studies in adults generally ranged from 10–15 mg daily. The manufacturers state that increasing olanzapine dosages beyond 10 mg daily usually does not result in additional therapeutic effect and recommend that such increases generally should occur only after the patient's clinical status has been assessed. In addition, the manufacturers state that olanzapine is not indicated for use in dosages exceeding 20 mg daily. However, olanzapine occasionally has been used in controlled and uncontrolled trials and in individual patients in dosages of up to 40 mg daily; dosages of up to 60 mg daily have been used in some patients with treatment-resistant schizophrenia. It remains to be established whether higher dosages of the drug are safe and result in improved efficacy in such patients. Some clinicians state that olanzapine dosages of up to 30 mg daily may produce further clinical improvement in schizophrenia patients who did not respond adequately to dosages of up to 20 mg daily; however, they recommend that caution be exercised when dosage of the drug exceeds 40 mg daily because of the potential for serious adverse effects (e.g., extrapyramidal reactions, excitement, metabolic changes, weight gain, cardiovascular complications).

For the management of schizophrenia in adolescents 13–17 years of age, the recommended initial oral dosage of olanzapine is 2.5 or 5 mg daily given as a single daily dose, and the recommended target dosage is 10 mg daily. When dosage adjustments are necessary, dosage increments or decrements of 2.5 or 5 mg daily are recommended. In clinical trials, efficacy of the drug in adolescents with schizophrenia was demonstrated based on a flexible dosage range of 2.5–20 mg daily, with a mean modal dosage of 12.5 mg daily (mean dosage of 11.1 mg daily). The manufacturer states that the safety and effectiveness of dosages exceeding 20 mg daily have not been evaluated in clinical trials.

The optimum duration of olanzapine therapy currently is not known, but maintenance therapy with antipsychotic agents is well established. The effectiveness of oral olanzapine given in a daily dosage of 10–20 mg in maintaining treatment response in adult schizophrenic patients who had been stable on olanzapine for approximately 8 weeks and were then followed for relapse has been demonstrated in a placebo-controlled study. If olanzapine is used for an extended period in adults, the long-term usefulness of the drug for the individual patient should be reassessed periodically.

Although there is no body of evidence available to determine how long adolescent patients treated with olanzapine should be maintained on the drug, the manufacturer states that such efficacy can be extrapolated from adult data in addition to comparisons of olanzapine pharmacokinetic parameters in adult and adolescent patients. Adolescent patients responding to olanzapine therapy should continue to receive the drug beyond the acute response, but at the lowest effective dosage, and the need for continued maintenance therapy with the drug should be reassessed periodically.

The American Psychiatric Association (APA) states that prudent long-term treatment options in adult patients with schizophrenia with remitted first episodes or multiple episodes include either indefinite maintenance therapy or gradual discontinuance of the antipsychotic agent with close follow-up and a plan to reinstitute treatment upon symptom recurrence. Discontinuance of antipsychotic therapy should be considered only after a period of at least 1 year of symptom remission or optimal response while receiving the antipsychotic agent. In patients who have had multiple previous psychotic episodes or 2 psychotic episodes within 5 years, indefinite maintenance antipsychotic treatment is recommended.

Bipolar Disorder

As monotherapy for the management of acute manic or mixed episodes associated with bipolar I disorder in adults, the usual initial oral dosage of olanzapine is 10 or 15 mg daily, given as a single dose. When dosage adjustments are necessary, the manufacturer recommends that dosage increments or decrements of 5 mg daily be made at intervals of not less than 24 hours, reflecting the procedures in the placebo-controlled trials. The effective dosage of olanzapine in short-term clinical studies generally has ranged from 5–20 mg daily. Safety of dosages exceeding 20 mg daily has not been established.

As monotherapy for the management of acute manic or mixed episodes associated with bipolar I disorder in adolescents 13–17 years of age, the recommended initial oral dosage of olanzapine is 2.5 or 5 mg daily, given as a single dose, with a target dosage of 10 mg daily. When dosage adjustments are necessary, the manufacturer recommends dosage increments or decrements of 2.5 or 5 mg daily. In short-term clinical trials, efficacy was demonstrated in a dosage range of 2.5–20 mg daily, with a mean modal dosage of 10.7 mg daily (average dosage of 8.9 mg daily). The manufacturer states that the safety and effectiveness of dosages exceeding 20 mg daily have not been evaluated in clinical trials.

When administered in conjunction with lithium or valproate for the management of acute manic or mixed episodes associated with bipolar I disorder in adults, the recommended initial oral dosage of olanzapine is 10 mg once daily. The effective dosage of olanzapine as adjunctive therapy for up to 6 weeks in clinical studies generally ranged from 5–20 mg daily. Safety of dosages exceeding 20 mg daily has not been established in clinical trials.

When used in fixed combination with fluoxetine hydrochloride (e.g., as the fixed combination Symbyax®) for acute depressive episodes in adults with bipolar disorder, olanzapine is administered once daily in the evening, usually initiating therapy with a dosage of 6 mg of olanzapine and 25 mg of fluoxetine. An initial dosage of 3 or 6 mg of olanzapine in fixed combination with 25 mg of fluoxetine should be used in patients with a predisposition to hypotensive reactions, patients with hepatic impairment, or those with factors that may slow metabolism of the drugs(s) (e.g., female gender, geriatric age, nonsmoking status); when indicated, dosage should be escalated with caution. In other patients, dosage can be increased according to patient response and tolerance as indicated. In clinical trials in adults, antidepressant efficacy was demonstrated at olanzapine dosages ranging from 6–12 mg daily and fluoxetine dosages ranging from 25–50 mg daily. Dosages exceeding 18 mg of olanzapine and 75 mg of fluoxetine daily have not been evaluated in clinical studies.

When used in conjunction with fluoxetine (as individual components of olanzapine and fluoxetine hydrochloride rather than the fixed-combination preparation) for acute depressive episodes in adults with bipolar disorder, olanzapine is administered once daily in the evening, usually initiating therapy with a dosage of 5 mg of olanzapine and 20 mg of fluoxetine. Dosage adjustments, if indicated, may be made based on efficacy and tolerability within the dosage ranges of olanzapine 5–12.5 mg daily and fluoxetine 20–50 mg daily. An initial dosage of 2.5–5 mg of olanzapine and 20 mg of fluoxetine should be used in patients with a predisposition to hypotensive reactions, patients with hepatic impairment, those with factors that may slow metabolism of the drugs(s) (e.g., female gender, geriatric age, nonsmoking status), or those who may be pharmacodynamically sensitive to olanzapine; when indicated, dosage adjustments should be made with caution in these patients. Dosages exceeding 18 mg of olanzapine and 75 mg of fluoxetine daily have not been evaluated in clinical studies.

The safety and efficacy of olanzapine and fluoxetine in combination (given as the individual components) were determined in clinical trials that supported the approval of Symbyax® (the fixed combination of olanzapine and fluoxetine). Dosage of the fixed-combination preparation ranges from olanzapine 3–12 mg and fluoxetine 25–50 mg daily. The following table provides the appropriate individual component dosages of olanzapine and fluoxetine compared with the fixed-combination preparation. If dosage adjustments are indicated, they should be made with the individual components according to efficacy and tolerability.

TABLE 1. Approximate Dosage Correspondence between Olanzapine in Fixed Combination with Fluoxetine (e.g., Symbyax®) and Combined Olanzapine (e.g., Zyprexa®) and Fluoxetine Therapy (Given Individually).

For fixed-combination dosages of:	Use in combination:	
	Olanzapine (mg/day)	Fluoxetine (mg/day)
3 mg olanzapine/25 mg fluoxetine	2.5	20
6 mg olanzapine/25 mg fluoxetine	5	20
12 mg olanzapine/25 mg fluoxetine	10 + 2.5	20
6 mg olanzapine/50 mg fluoxetine	5	40 + 10
12 mg olanzapine/50 mg fluoxetine	10 + 2.5	40 + 10

When used in fixed combination with fluoxetine hydrochloride (e.g., as the fixed combination Symbyax®) for acute depressive episodes in children and adolescents 10–17 years of age with bipolar disorder, olanzapine is administered once daily in the evening, usually initiating therapy with a dosage of 3 mg of olanzapine and 25 mg of fluoxetine. Dosage can then be adjusted to a target dosage within the FDA-labeled dosage range of olanzapine 6–12 mg daily and fluoxetine 25–50 mg daily. Concurrent administration of dosages exceeding 12 mg of olanzapine and 50 mg of fluoxetine daily has not been evaluated in pediatric clinical studies.

When used in conjunction with fluoxetine hydrochloride (as individual components of olanzapine and fluoxetine rather than the fixed-combination preparation) for acute depressive episodes in children and adolescents 10–17 years of age with bipolar disorder, olanzapine is administered once daily in the evening, usually initiating therapy with a dosage of 2.5 mg of olanzapine and 20 mg of fluoxetine. Dosage adjustments, if indicated, may be made based on efficacy and tolerability. Concurrent administration of dosages exceeding 12 mg of olanzapine and 50 mg of fluoxetine daily has not been evaluated in pediatric clinical studies.

The long-term efficacy of oral olanzapine (dosage range: 5–20 mg daily) for maintenance monotherapy in adults with bipolar disorder has been demonstrated in a double-blind, placebo-controlled trial of 52 weeks' duration and in comparative studies of 47–52 weeks' duration. The mean modal dosage of olanzapine in the placebo-controlled study was 12.5 mg daily. The manufacturer states that patients receiving oral olanzapine for extended periods should be reassessed periodically to determine the need for continued therapy.

Although the efficacy of oral olanzapine for maintenance treatment of adolescents with bipolar disorder has not been evaluated, the manufacturer states that such efficacy can be extrapolated from adult data in addition to comparisons of olanzapine pharmacokinetic parameters in adult and adolescent patients. If olanzapine is used for an extended period, the need for maintenance therapy should be reassessed periodically.

Although the manufacturer states that efficacy of the fixed combination of olanzapine and fluoxetine beyond 8 weeks' duration remains to be established, patients have received the fixed combination for up to 24 weeks in clinical trials. Clinicians who elect to use the fixed combination for extended periods should periodically reevaluate the long-term risks and benefits of the drug for the individual patient.

Treatment-resistant Depression

When used in fixed combination with fluoxetine hydrochloride (e.g., as the fixed combination Symbyax®) for the acute and maintenance treatment of treatment-resistant depression in adults, olanzapine is administered once daily in the evening, usually initiating therapy with a dosage of 6 mg of olanzapine and 25 mg of fluoxetine. An initial dosage of 3 or 6 mg of olanzapine in fixed combination with 25 mg of fluoxetine should be used in patients with a predisposition to hypotensive reactions, patients with hepatic impairment, or those with factors that may slow metabolism of the drugs(s) (e.g., female gender, geriatric age, nonsmoking status); when indicated, dosage should be escalated with caution. In other patients, dosage can be increased according to patient response and tolerance as indicated. In clinical trials in adults, antidepressant efficacy was demonstrated at olanzapine dosages ranging from 6–18 mg daily and fluoxetine dosages ranging from 25–50 mg daily. Dosages exceeding 18 mg of olanzapine and 75 mg of fluoxetine daily have not been evaluated in clinical studies. Clinicians who elect to use the fixed combination for extended periods should periodically reevaluate the long-term risks and benefits of the drug for the individual patient.

When used in conjunction with fluoxetine hydrochloride (as individual components of olanzapine and fluoxetine rather than the fixed-combination preparation) for the acute and maintenance treatment of treatment-resistant depression in adults, olanzapine is administered once daily in the evening, usually initiating therapy with a dosage of 5 mg of olanzapine and 20 mg of fluoxetine. Dosage adjustments, if indicated, may be made based on efficacy and tolerability within the dosage ranges of olanzapine 5–20 mg and fluoxetine 20–50 mg daily. An initial dosage of 2.5–5 mg of olanzapine and 20 mg of fluoxetine should be used in patients with a predisposition to hypotensive reactions, patients with hepatic impairment, those with factors that may slow metabolism of the drugs(s) (e.g., female gender, geriatric age, nonsmoking status), or those who may be pharmacodynamically sensitive to olanzapine; when indicated, dosage adjustment should be made with caution in these patients. Dosages exceeding 18 mg of olanzapine and 75 mg of fluoxetine daily have not been evaluated in clinical studies. Clinicians who elect to use the combination for extended periods should periodically reevaluate the long-term risks and benefits of the drug for the individual patient.

The safety and efficacy of olanzapine and fluoxetine in combination (given as the individual components) were determined in clinical trials that supported the approval of Symbyax® (the fixed combination of olanzapine and fluoxetine). Dosage of the fixed-combination preparation ranges from olanzapine 3–12 mg and fluoxetine 25–50 mg daily. Table 1 provides the appropriate individual component dosages of olanzapine and fluoxetine compared with the fixed-combination preparation. If dosage adjustments are indicated, they should be made with the individual components according to efficacy and tolerability.

Cancer Chemotherapy-induced Nausea and Vomiting

For the prevention of acute and delayed nausea and vomiting associated with highly emetogenic cancer chemotherapy† in adults, the American Society of Clinical Oncology (ASCO) currently recommends an oral olanzapine dosage of 10 mg once daily on the first day of chemotherapy (day 1) and then 10 mg once daily on days 2–4 of chemotherapy. Olanzapine usually has been administered as part of a 4-drug combination antiemetic regimen that includes a neurokinin 1 (NK_1) receptor antagonist, a 5-HT_3 receptor antagonist, and dexamethasone. This is the same dosage regimen that was used in the pivotal clinical study evaluating olanzapine as an antiemetic in patients receiving highly emetogenic chemotherapy. There is some evidence that 5-mg once-daily doses of olanzapine may be as effective as 10-mg once-daily doses in preventing chemotherapy-induced nausea and vomiting and reduce the risk of sedation observed with 10-mg once-daily doses; additional controlled studies are needed to determine the optimal dosing of olanzapine in prophylactic antiemetic regimens.

For the treatment of breakthrough nausea and vomiting† despite optimal antiemetic prophylaxis in adults receiving cancer chemotherapy, olanzapine has been given orally in a dosage of 10 mg orally once daily for 3 days in a pivotal clinical study. (See Uses: Cancer Chemotherapy-induced Nausea and Vomiting.)

IM Dosage

Immediate-release Olanzapine Injection for Acute Agitation associated with Bipolar Disorder or Schizophrenia

For the prompt control of acute agitation in patients with schizophrenia or bipolar mania, the recommended initial adult IM dose of olanzapine injection (e.g., Zyprexa® IntraMuscular) is 10 mg given as a single dose. A lower initial IM dose (2.5, 5, or 7.5 mg) may be considered when clinically warranted. In clinical trials, the efficacy of IM olanzapine for controlling agitation in patients with schizophrenia or bipolar mania has been demonstrated in a dosage range of 2.5–10 mg.

If agitation necessitating additional IM doses of olanzapine persists following the initial dose, subsequent single doses of up to 10 mg may be given. However, the manufacturer states that the efficacy of repeated doses of IM olanzapine in agitated patients has not been systematically evaluated in controlled clinical trials. In addition, the safety of IM dosages exceeding 30 mg daily or of 10-mg IM doses

given more frequently than 2 hours after the initial dose and 4 hours after the second dose has not been evaluated in clinical trials.

Maximal dosing of IM olanzapine (e.g., 3 doses of 10 mg administered 2–4 hours apart) may be associated with a substantial risk of clinically important orthostatic hypotension. Patients who experience drowsiness or dizziness after the IM injection should remain recumbent until an examination indicates that they are not experiencing orthostatic hypotension, bradycardia, and/or hypoventilation. (See Orthostatic Hypotension under Cautions: Precautions and Contraindications.)

If ongoing olanzapine therapy is clinically indicated, the manufacturer states that oral olanzapine may be initiated in a dosage range of 5–20 mg daily as soon as clinically appropriate. In one controlled study evaluating IM olanzapine in acutely agitated patients, patients initially received 1–3 IM injections of olanzapine 10 mg and were then switched to oral olanzapine therapy in dosages ranging from 5–20 mg daily for a period of 4 days.

A lower initial IM olanzapine dose of 5 mg may be considered for geriatric patients or when other clinical factors warrant. In addition, a lower IM dose of 2.5 mg per injection should be considered for patients who are debilitated, who may be predisposed to hypotensive reactions, or who may be more sensitive to the pharmacodynamic effects of olanzapine.

Extended-release Olanzapine Pamoate Injectable Suspension for Schizophrenia

The manufacturer recommends that patients first receive oral olanzapine to establish tolerability of the drug before the extended-release olanzapine pamoate injection is used IM.

The clinical efficacy of extended-release olanzapine pamoate injectable suspension (Zyprexa® Relprevv) in adults has been demonstrated within the dosage range of 150–300 mg administered every 2 weeks and with 405 mg administered every 4 weeks.

For the management of schizophrenia in *patients established on oral olanzapine 10 mg daily*, the recommended initial IM dosage of extended-release olanzapine pamoate is 210 mg administered every 2 weeks or 405 mg administered every 4 weeks during the first 8 weeks of therapy. Following the initial 8 weeks, the recommended maintenance dosage of olanzapine pamoate is 150 mg given every 2 weeks or 300 mg given every 4 weeks.

In *patients established on oral olanzapine 15 mg daily*, the recommended initial IM dosage of extended-release olanzapine pamoate is 300 mg administered every 2 weeks for the first 8 weeks of therapy. Following the initial 8 weeks, the recommended maintenance dosage of olanzapine pamoate is 210 mg given every 2 weeks or 405 mg given every 4 weeks.

In *patients established on oral olanzapine 20 mg daily*, the recommended initial and maintenance IM dosage of extended-release olanzapine pamoate is 300 mg administered every 2 weeks.

The manufacturer states that extended-release olanzapine pamoate IM dosages exceeding 405 mg every 4 weeks or 300 mg every 2 weeks have not been evaluated in clinical trials.

A lower initial IM olanzapine pamoate dosage of 150 mg every 4 weeks is recommended in patients who are debilitated, who may be predisposed to hypotensive reactions, who exhibit a combination of factors that may result in slower metabolism of olanzapine (e.g., nonsmoking female patients 65 years of age or older), or who may be more sensitive to the pharmacodynamic effects of the drug.

Although no controlled studies have been conducted to determine the optimum duration of extended-release olanzapine pamoate therapy in patients with stabilized schizophrenia, the long-term efficacy of the drug has been demonstrated over a 24-week period. In addition, long-term use of oral olanzapine has been shown to be effective in maintaining treatment response in patients with schizophrenia. If olanzapine pamoate is used for an extended period, the need for continued treatment should be reassessed periodically.

The manufacturer states that there are no systematically collected data to specifically address how to switch patients with schizophrenia receiving other antipsychotic agents to extended-release IM olanzapine pamoate therapy.

● Dosage in Renal and Hepatic Impairment

The manufacturer states that because only minimal amounts of olanzapine (about 7%) are excreted in urine and because the pharmacokinetics of olanzapine appear not to be altered in patients with renal or hepatic impairment, dosage adjustment is not necessary in such patients.

The manufacturer states that the extended-release IM formulation of olanzapine pamoate (Zyprexa® Relprevv) has not been specifically studied in patients with renal and/or hepatic impairment.

CAUTIONS

● Adverse Effects

The adverse effect profile of olanzapine generally is similar to that of other atypical (second-generation) antipsychotic agents (e.g., aripiprazole, clozapine, quetiapine, risperidone, ziprasidone). Although olanzapine differs chemically from the phenothiazines, the drug also may be capable of producing many of the toxic manifestations of phenothiazine derivatives. (See Cautions in the Phenothiazines General Statement 28:16.08.24.) Not all adverse effects of the phenothiazines have been reported with olanzapine, but the possibility that they may occur should be considered. Adverse effects of olanzapine, other atypical antipsychotics, and the phenothiazines are numerous and may involve nearly all body organ systems.

In controlled studies in adults, the most common adverse effects occurring more frequently in patients receiving oral olanzapine for schizophrenia or bipolar mania than in those receiving placebo included central and autonomic nervous system effects such as somnolence, asthenia, dry mouth, dizziness, tremor, personality disorder, and akathisia; cardiovascular system effects such as postural hypotension; GI effects such as constipation, dyspepsia, and increased appetite; and weight gain. There was no clear relationship between the incidence of adverse events and dosage in patients receiving oral olanzapine for schizophrenia in placebo-controlled trials except for certain extrapyramidal symptoms, asthenia or fatigue, dry mouth, nausea, somnolence, tremor, weight gain, and elevated prolactin concentrations. Discontinuance of olanzapine therapy was required in 5% of adult patients with schizophrenia compared with 6% for placebo in controlled trials; however, discontinuance because of increased serum ALT (SGPT) concentrations was required in 2% of the olanzapine-treated patients compared with none of those receiving placebo, and this adverse effect was considered to be drug related. Similar between olanzapine and placebo discontinuance rates were observed in the controlled trials for oral olanzapine for bipolar mania (2% for olanzapine and 2% for placebo) and IM olanzapine for acute agitation (0.4% for IM olanzapine and 0% for placebo).

Adverse effects occurring in 5% or more of adult patients with schizophrenia receiving oral olanzapine in short-term clinical studies and with an incidence of at least twice that of placebo included dizziness (11%), constipation (9%), personality disorder (i.e., nonaggressive objectionable behavior; 8%), weight gain (6%), postural hypotension (5%), and akathisia (5%).

Adverse effects occurring in 6% or more of adult patients with acute mania associated with bipolar disorder receiving oral olanzapine in clinical studies and with an incidence of at least twice that of placebo included somnolence (35%), dry mouth (22%), dizziness (18%), asthenia (15%), constipation (11%), dyspepsia (11%), increased appetite (6%), and tremor (6%).

When oral olanzapine was used in conjunction with lithium or divalproex sodium for treatment of acute mania associated with bipolar disorder in adults, adverse effects occurring in 5% or more of patients in clinical studies and with an incidence of at least twice that of placebo included dry mouth (32%), weight gain (26%), increased appetite (24%), dizziness (14%), back pain (8%), constipation (8%), speech disorder (7%), increased salivation (6%), amnesia (5%), and paresthesia (5%).

Adverse effects occurring in 5% or more of adolescents (13–17 years of age) with schizophrenia or bipolar disorder receiving oral olanzapine in short-term, placebo-controlled clinical studies and with an incidence of at least twice that of placebo included sedation (39–48%), weight gain (29–31%), headache (17%), increased appetite (17–29%), dizziness (7–8%), abdominal pain (6%), pain in extremities (5–6%), fatigue (3–14%), and dry mouth (4–7%).

When short-acting IM olanzapine was used for the management of acute agitation in short-term clinical studies, somnolence was the only adverse effect that occurred in 5% or more of patients with schizophrenia or bipolar mania and with an incidence at least twice that of placebo (6% and 3%, respectively).

When extended-release olanzapine pamoate injection was used IM in adults with schizophrenia in a short-term, placebo-controlled clinical study, adverse effects occurring in 5% or more of patients and more frequently than with placebo

included headache (13–18%), sedation (8–13%), weight gain (5–7%), cough (3–9%), diarrhea (2–7%), back pain (3–5%), nausea (4–5%), somnolence (1–6%), dry mouth (2–6%), nasopharyngitis (1–6%), increased appetite (1–6%), and vomiting (1–6%).

● Nervous System Effects

Seizures

Seizures occurred in about 0.9% of adult patients receiving oral olanzapine in controlled clinical trials during premarketing testing. During premarketing testing of extended-release olanzapine pamoate IM injection, seizures occurred in 0.15% of adult patients. Confounding factors that may have contributed to the occurrence of seizures were present in many of these cases.

Myoclonic status reportedly occurred shortly after initiation of olanzapine in one patient with probable dementia of the Alzheimer's type (Alzheimer's disease) who was concurrently receiving citalopram and donepezil; the myoclonic jerks in this patient coincided with EEG changes indicative of seizure activity (spikes and polyspike/wave complexes), and the seizures subsided following discontinuance of olanzapine. A new-onset seizure also reportedly occurred in an adult female patient upon the addition of quetiapine to maintenance therapy with olanzapine and following discontinuance of clonazepam therapy. In addition, an apparent lowering of seizure threshold occurred in at least 2 epileptic patients who experienced increased seizure activity following initiation of olanzapine therapy that resolved upon discontinuance of the drug. Fatal status epilepticus also has been reported in a patient who had been receiving olanzapine therapy for 5 months.

Olanzapine should be administered with caution to patients with a history of seizures or conditions known to lower the seizure threshold (e.g., dementia of the Alzheimer's type); conditions that lower the seizure threshold may be more prevalent in patients 65 years of age or older.

Extrapyramidal Reactions

Like other atypical antipsychotic agents, olanzapine has a low potential for causing certain adverse extrapyramidal effects (e.g., dystonias). Results from controlled clinical trials suggest that extrapyramidal reactions associated with olanzapine therapy are dose related.

Tremor was reported in about 4% of patients receiving oral olanzapine and in about 1% of patients receiving short-acting IM olanzapine in controlled clinical trials; the incidence of tremor appears to be dose related. In addition, akathisia occurred in about 3% of patients receiving oral olanzapine and in less than 1% of patients receiving short-acting IM olanzapine; hypertonia occurred in about 3% of patients receiving oral olanzapine in short-term controlled clinical trials. Oculogyric crisis also has been reported in a patient receiving olanzapine, lithium, and paroxetine concurrently. (See Drug Interactions: Other CNS-Active Agents and Alcohol.)

Neuroleptic Malignant Syndrome

Neuroleptic malignant syndrome (NMS), a potentially fatal symptom complex, has been reported in patients receiving antipsychotic agents, including olanzapine. Clinical manifestations of NMS generally include hyperpyrexia, muscle rigidity, altered mental status, and evidence of autonomic instability (irregular pulse or blood pressure, tachycardia, diaphoresis, and cardiac arrhythmias). Additional signs of NMS may include increased serum creatine kinase (CK, creatine phosphokinase, CPK), myoglobinuria (rhabdomyolysis), and acute renal failure. NMS attributable to olanzapine therapy alone has been reported in some patients, and there also have been reports of NMS in olanzapine-treated patients concomitantly receiving other drugs, including antipsychotic agents, antidepressants, lithium, or valproate. Extrapyramidal reactions were present in approximately two-thirds of the olanzapine-treated patients diagnosed with NMS. Atypical presentations of NMS (e.g., absence of or lessened rigidity, presenting as fever of unknown origin) and less severe presentations of NMS also have been reported in some patients receiving olanzapine or other atypical antipsychotic agents.

The diagnostic evaluation of patients with NMS is complicated. In arriving at a diagnosis, serious medical illnesses (e.g., pneumonia, systemic infection) and untreated or inadequately treated extrapyramidal signs and symptoms must be excluded. In addition, clinical features of NMS and serotonin syndrome sometimes overlap, and it has been suggested that these 2 syndromes may share certain underlying pathophysiologic mechanisms. Other important considerations in the differential diagnosis include central anticholinergic toxicity, heat stroke, drug fever, and primary CNS pathology.

The management of NMS should include immediate discontinuance of antipsychotic agents and other drugs not considered essential to concurrent therapy, intensive symptomatic treatment and medical monitoring, and treatment of any concomitant serious medical problems for which specific treatments are available. There currently is no specific drug therapy for NMS, although dantrolene, bromocriptine, amantadine, and benzodiazepines have been used in a limited number of patients. If a patient requires antipsychotic therapy following recovery from NMS, the potential reintroduction of drug therapy after several weeks should be carefully considered. If antipsychotic therapy is reintroduced, the dosage generally should be increased gradually and an antipsychotic agent other than the agent believed to have precipitated NMS generally is chosen. In addition, tolerability with oral olanzapine should be established prior to initiating treatment with extended-release IM olanzapine pamoate. Such patients should be carefully monitored since recurrences of NMS have been reported in some patients. For additional information on NMS, see Neuroleptic Malignant Syndrome under Cautions: Nervous System Effects, in the Phenothiazines General Statement 28:16.08.24.

Tardive Dyskinesia

Use of antipsychotic agents may be associated with tardive dyskinesia, a syndrome of potentially irreversible, involuntary, dyskinetic movements. Although the incidence of tardive dyskinesia appears to be highest among geriatric individuals, particularly geriatric females, it is not possible to reliably predict at the beginning of antipsychotic therapy which patients are likely to develop this syndrome. Tardive dyskinesia has been reported in less than 1% of patients receiving olanzapine therapy. Although the manufacturer states that it is not yet known whether antipsychotic agents differ in their potential to cause tardive dyskinesia, available evidence suggests that the risk appears to be substantially less with second-generation antipsychotic agents, including olanzapine, than with conventional, first-generation antipsychotic agents. Analyses from controlled, long-term trials have found an approximately 12-fold lower risk of tardive dyskinesia with olanzapine therapy compared with haloperidol therapy. In addition, stabilization of or improvement in tardive dyskinesia associated with conventional antipsychotic agents has been reported in some patients when they have been switched to second-generation antipsychotic therapy, including olanzapine. However, a transient increase in dyskinetic movements (sometimes referred to as withdrawal-emergent dyskinesia) occasionally may occur when a patient is switched from a first-generation to a second-generation antipsychotic agent or upon dosage reduction of an antipsychotic agent.

The risk of developing tardive dyskinesia and the likelihood that it will become irreversible are believed to increase as the duration of treatment and the total cumulative dose of antipsychotic drugs administered to the patient increase. However, the syndrome can develop, although much less commonly, following relatively brief treatment periods at low dosages or may even arise after discontinuance of treatment.

Management of tardive dyskinesia generally consists of gradual discontinuance of the precipitating antipsychotic agent when possible, reducing the dosage of the first-generation (conventional) antipsychotic agent or switching to a second-generation (atypical) antipsychotic agent, or switching to clozapine therapy. The syndrome may remit, partially or completely, if antipsychotic therapy is discontinued. However, antipsychotic therapy itself may suppress or partially suppress the signs and symptoms of the syndrome and thereby may possibly mask the underlying process. The effect that such symptomatic suppression has upon the long-term course of tardive dyskinesia is unknown. Vesicular monoamine transporter 2 (VMAT2) inhibitors (e.g., deutetrabenazine, valbenazine tosylate) have been shown to be effective in reducing symptoms of tardive dyskinesia in controlled clinical studies and may allow some patients to continue receiving antipsychotic therapy. (See Deutetrabenazine 28:56 and Valbenazine Tosylate 28:56.) There also is some evidence that vitamin E administration may reduce the risk of development of tardive dyskinesia; therefore, the American Psychiatric Association (APA) currently states that patients receiving antipsychotic agents may be advised to take 400–800 units of vitamin E daily for prophylaxis. (See Cautions in Vitamin E 88:20.)

Olanzapine should be prescribed in a manner that is most likely to minimize the occurrence of tardive dyskinesia. Chronic antipsychotic treatment generally should be reserved for patients who suffer from a chronic illness that is known to respond to antipsychotic agents, and for whom alternative, equally effective, but potentially less harmful treatments are not available or appropriate. In patients who do require chronic treatment, the smallest dosage and the shortest duration of treatment producing a satisfactory clinical response should be sought, and the need for continued treatment should be reassessed periodically.

The APA currently recommends that all patients receiving second-generation antipsychotic agents be assessed clinically for abnormal involuntary movements every 12 months and that patients considered to be at increased risk for tardive dyskinesia be assessed every 6 months. If signs and symptoms of tardive dyskinesia appear in a patient receiving olanzapine, drug discontinuance or a reduction in dosage should be considered. However, some patients may require treatment with olanzapine or another antipsychotic agent despite the presence of the syndrome.

For additional information on tardive dyskinesia, including manifestations and treatment, see Tardive Dyskinesia under Cautions: Nervous System Effects, in the Phenothiazines General Statement 28:16.08.24.

Post-injection Delirium/Sedation Syndrome

During premarketing studies of extended-release olanzapine pamoate (Zyprexa® Relprevv), adverse events that presented with signs and symptoms consistent with olanzapine overdosage, particularly sedation (ranging from mild in severity to coma) and/or delirium, were reported following injection of the drug. Such cases of post-injection delirium/sedation syndrome (PDSS) occurred in less than 0.1% of injections and in approximately 2% of patients who received injections for up to 46 months. These events were correlated with an unintentional rapid increase in serum olanzapine concentrations to supratherapeutic ranges in some cases. Although a rapid and greater than expected increase in serum olanzapine concentrations has been noted in some patients with these adverse events, the precise mechanism by which the drug was unintentionally introduced into the bloodstream in these cases is not known.

Clinical signs and symptoms of PDSS include dizziness, confusion, disorientation, malaise, slurred speech, altered gait, ambulation difficulties, weakness, agitation, extrapyramidal symptoms, hypertension, convulsions, and reduced levels of consciousness ranging from mild sedation to coma. The time after injection to PDSS in most reported cases ranged from soon after the injection to greater than 3 hours after the injection; patients had largely recovered by 72 hours. Because the risk of PDSS is the same at each injection, the risk per patient is cumulative (i.e., the risk increases with the number of injections). (See Post-injection Delirium/Sedation Syndrome under Cautions: Precautions and Contraindications and see also Acute Toxicity.)

Other Nervous System Effects

Somnolence or sedation, which usually appears to be moderate in severity compared with other antipsychotic agents and dose related, is among the most common adverse effects of olanzapine, occurring in approximately 29% of adults and 44% of adolescents receiving oral olanzapine in controlled clinical trials. In addition, sedation-related adverse events (defined as hypersomnia, lethargy, sedation, and somnolence) occurred more often in adolescents compared with adults. Sedation occurred in 8% of patients receiving extended-release olanzapine pamoate injection, and somnolence and sedation resulted in discontinuance of the drug in 0.6% of patients in the premarketing database. Somnolence associated with olanzapine and other antipsychotic agents generally is most pronounced during early therapy, since most patients develop some tolerance to the sedating effects with continued administration. Although sedation can have therapeutic benefits in some cases, persistent daytime drowsiness and increased sleep time can become troublesome in some patients and necessitate a lower dosage or evening administration of oral olanzapine. (See Reconstitution and Administration under Dosage and Administration, Cognitive and Motor Impairment under Cautions: Precautions and Contraindications, and see also Effects on Sleep under Pharmacology: Nervous System Effects.)

Insomnia occurred in about 12%, dizziness in about 11%, asthenia in about 10%, and abnormal gait in about 6% of adult patients receiving oral olanzapine in short-term controlled clinical trials. The incidence of asthenia appears to be dose related. In addition, articulation impairment was reported in about 2% of patients receiving oral olanzapine in short-term, controlled clinical trials.

Ataxia, decreased libido, dysarthria, stupor, and suicide attempt have been reported in 1% or less of patients receiving oral olanzapine in clinical trials.

In short-term (i.e., 24-hour), controlled clinical trials of short-acting IM olanzapine for acute agitation in adults, somnolence occurred in approximately 6%, dizziness in approximately 4%, and asthenia in about 2% of the patients.

● *Cardiovascular Effects*
Hemodynamic Effects

Oral olanzapine may produce orthostatic hypotension that may be associated with dizziness, tachycardia, bradycardia, and, in some patients, syncope, particularly during the initial period of dosage titration. These adverse hemodynamic effects probably are due to the drug's α_1-adrenergic blocking activity. In short-term, controlled clinical trials of oral olanzapine in adults, postural hypotension and tachycardia occurred in approximately 3% and hypertension occurred in approximately 2% of patients. In an analysis of vital sign data from 41 clinical trials conducted with oral olanzapine in adults, orthostatic hypotension was reported in 20% or more of patients. Vasodilatation has been reported in 1% or less of patients treated with oral olanzapine; this adverse effect has not been definitely attributed to the drug.

Hypotension, bradycardia with or without hypotension, tachycardia, and syncope also were reported during the clinical trials with short-acting IM olanzapine. In an open trial in nonagitated patients with schizophrenia designed to evaluate the safety and tolerability of a dosage regimen of three 10-mg IM doses of olanzapine administered 4 hours apart, approximately one-third of the patients experienced a substantial orthostatic decrease in systolic blood pressure (i.e., decrease of 30 mm Hg or more).

Syncope was reported in 0.6% of olanzapine-treated patients in phase 2 and 3 clinical trials of oral olanzapine, and in 0.3% of patients receiving short-acting IM olanzapine in the acute agitation clinical trials. In phase 1 trials of olanzapine, 3 healthy volunteers experienced hypotension, bradycardia, and sinus pauses of up to 6 seconds that spontaneously resolved; 2 of these cases occurred in association with short-acting IM olanzapine and one case involved oral olanzapine. In short-term, controlled clinical trials for short-acting IM olanzapine for acute agitation, hypotension occurred in approximately 2% and postural hypotension occurred in approximately 1% of patients. Syncope has been reported in 1% or less of patients receiving short-acting IM olanzapine in clinical trials. The manufacturer states that the risk for this sequence of hypotension, bradycardia, and sinus pause may be greater in nonpsychiatric patients compared with psychiatric patients, who may be more adapted to certain pharmacologic effects of psychotropic agents. Long-acting IM olanzapine pamoate also may cause orthostatic hypotension associated with dizziness, tachycardia, bradycardia, and syncope (in some cases). Syncope-related adverse effects have been reported in 0.1% of patients receiving long-acting IM olanzapine pamoate in clinical trials. (See Dosage and Administration and see also Orthostatic Hypotension, under Cautions: Precautions and Contraindications.)

ECG Effects

Pooled analyses from controlled clinical trials in adults as well as in adolescents did not reveal significant differences in the proportions of oral olanzapine-treated patients experiencing potentially important ECG changes, including QT, QT_c (Fridericia corrected), and PR intervals. Oral olanzapine was associated with a mean increase in heart rate of 2.4 beats/minute in adults and a mean increase of 6.3 beats/minute in adolescents compared with no change and a mean decrease of 5.1 beats/minute, respectively, among patients who received placebo in controlled trials. A comparison of extended-release IM olanzapine pamoate and oral olanzapine (in the 24-week study) did not reveal substantial differences in ECG changes between these formulations. The manufacturer states that the tendency to cause tachycardia may be related to olanzapine's potential for inducing orthostatic changes in blood pressure.

Like some other antipsychotic agents, olanzapine has been associated with prolongation of the QT_c interval in some patients and there is some evidence that higher dosages of the drug may increase the risk of QT_c-interval prolongation; however, the clinical relevance of these findings remains to be established.

Other Cardiovascular Effects

In short-term, controlled clinical trials for oral olanzapine, chest pain occurred in approximately 3% of patients. Cerebrovascular accident has been reported in 1% or less of patients.

Venous thromboembolic effects, including pulmonary embolism and deep venous thrombosis, have been reported in patients receiving olanzapine during postmarketing surveillance.

● Hepatic Effects

During premarketing clinical trials, oral olanzapine therapy was associated with asymptomatic elevations in serum aminotransferase (transaminase) concentrations, including elevations in serum concentrations of ALT (SGPT), AST (SGOT), and γ-glutamyltransferase (GGT). Clinically important ALT elevations 3 or more times the upper limit of the normal range were observed in 5% (77 of 1426) of adult patients exposed to olanzapine in placebo-controlled clinical studies; none of these patients experienced jaundice. ALT elevations 5 or more times the upper

limit of the normal range were observed in 2% (29 of 1438) of adult patients treated with olanzapine. ALT values returned to normal, or were decreasing, at last follow-up in the majority of patients who either continued olanzapine therapy or discontinued the drug. None of the patients with elevated ALT values experienced jaundice, liver failure, or met the criteria for Hy's rule. Within the larger premarketing database of about 2400 adult patients with baseline ALT values of 90 IU/L or less, the incidence of ALT elevation exceeding 200 IU/L was 2% (50 of 2381 patients). None of these patients experienced jaundice or other symptoms attributable to hepatic impairment, and most had transient changes that tended to normalize while olanzapine therapy was continued. (See Hepatic Effects under Cautions: Precautions and Contraindications.)

Changes in serum transaminase concentrations observed with extended-release IM olanzapine pamoate are similar to those reported with oral olanzapine. In placebo-controlled studies of the extended-release IM formulation, clinically important ALT elevations 3 or more times the upper limit of normal were observed in 2.7% (8 of 291) of adult patients exposed to the drug compared with 3.2% (3 of 94) of placebo recipients; none of these patients experienced jaundice. In 3 of the patients, transaminase concentrations returned to normal despite continuing IM olanzapine pamoate therapy; in the other 5 patients transaminase concentrations decreased but remained about the normal range at the end of therapy. Within the larger premarketing database of 1886 patients with baseline ALT values of 90 IU/L or less, the incidence of ALT elevation exceeding 200 IU/L was 0.8%. None of these patients experienced jaundice or other symptoms attributable to hepatic impairment, and most had transient changes that tended to normalize while olanzapine pamoate IM therapy was continued. (See Hepatic Effects under Cautions: Precautions and Contraindications.)

In clinical studies with oral olanzapine, adolescents were more likely to have greater increases in serum transaminase concentrations compared with adults. In placebo-controlled monotherapy studies, clinically important ALT elevations (3 or more times the upper limit of the normal range) were observed in 12% (22 of 192) of adolescent patients exposed to olanzapine. ALT elevations 5 or more times the upper limit of the normal range were observed in 4% (8 of 192) of adolescent patients treated with olanzapine. ALT values returned to normal, or were decreasing, at last follow-up in the majority of adolescent patients who either continued olanzapine therapy or discontinued the drug. None of the adolescents with elevated ALT values experienced jaundice, liver failure, or met the criteria for Hy's rule.

Hepatitis and jaundice have rarely been reported in patients receiving different formulations of olanzapine during postmarketing experience, as well as very rare cases of cholestatic or mixed hepatic injury. In addition, fatty deposit in the liver has been reported in less than 0.1% of patients receiving oral olanzapine in short-term clinical trials, although a causal relationship to the drug remains to be established.

● Endocrine and Metabolic Effects

Atypical antipsychotic agents have been associated with metabolic changes, including hyperglycemia, dyslipidemia, and weight gain. Such metabolic changes may be associated with increased cardiovascular and cerebrovascular risk.

Weight Gain

Like some conventional (first-generation) and atypical (second-generation) antipsychotic agents, olanzapine therapy may result in weight gain. In placebo-controlled studies of 6 weeks' duration in adults, weight gain occurred in approximately 6% of patients receiving oral olanzapine, and increased appetite occurred in 6% of patients receiving oral olanzapine in short-term controlled trials. In an analysis of 13 placebo-controlled monotherapy studies, adult patients receiving olanzapine gained an average of 2.6 kg compared with an average loss of 0.3 kg in those receiving placebo (with a median exposure of 6 weeks); 22.2% of the olanzapine-treated patients gained 7% or more of their baseline weight compared with 3% of placebo recipients (with a median exposure to event of 8 weeks). Dose group differences with regard to weight gain have been noted in a short-term, controlled study comparing fixed oral dosages of olanzapine in adults with schizophrenia or schizoaffective disorder; the mean baseline to end point increase in weight was 1.9 kg in patients receiving 10 mg of olanzapine daily, 2.3 kg in those receiving 20 mg daily, and 3 kg in those receiving 40 mg daily, with substantial differences between 10 and 40 mg daily. Discontinuance of olanzapine therapy because of weight gain occurred in 0.2% of olanzapine-treated patients compared with none of the placebo recipients. During long-term studies (at least 48 weeks' duration) with olanzapine in adults, mean weight gain was 5.6 kg (median exposure of 573 days); 64% of olanzapine-treated patients gained 7% or more of their baseline weight, 32% gained 15% or more of their baseline weight, and 12% gained 25% or more of their baseline weight.

In olanzapine-treated adolescent patients, both the magnitude of weight gain and the proportion of patients who had clinically significant weight gain were greater than in adult patients with comparable exposures. In short-term, placebo-controlled studies in adolescent patients with schizophrenia or bipolar disorder, weight gain occurred in approximately 30% of adolescents and increased appetite occurred in approximately 24% of adolescents receiving oral olanzapine. In 4 short-term, placebo-controlled monotherapy studies, adolescents receiving olanzapine gained an average of 4.6 kg compared with an average loss of 0.3 kg in those receiving placebo (with a median exposure of 3 weeks); 40.6% of the olanzapine-treated patients gained 7% or more of their baseline weight compared with 9.8% of placebo recipients (with median exposures to event of 4 and 8 weeks, respectively). Of the olanzapine-treated adolescents, 7.1% gained 15% or more of their baseline body weight compared with 2.7% of the placebo recipients (with median exposures to event of 19 and 8 weeks, respectively). In placebo-controlled studies of olanzapine therapy in adolescents, discontinuance due to weight gain occurred in 1% of olanzapine-treated patients compared with none of the placebo recipients. During long-term studies (at least 24 weeks' duration) in adolescents, the average weight gain was 11.2 kg (with a median exposure of 201 days). The percentages of adolescents who gained at least 7, 15, or 25% of their baseline body weight with long-term exposure were 89, 55, and 29%, respectively. Among adolescent patients, average weight gain according to baseline BMI category was 11.5, 12.1, and 12.7 kg for normal, overweight, and obese adolescents, respectively. Discontinuance because of weight gain occurred in 2.2% of olanzapine-treated adolescents following at least 24 weeks of olanzapine exposure.

In a 24-week, randomized, double-blind, fixed-dosage study that compared 3 different extended-release olanzapine pamoate IM dosage regimens in adult patients with schizophrenia, average weight gains of 0.7, 0.9, and 1.7 kg occurred in those receiving 150 mg of olanzapine every 2 weeks, 405 mg every 4 weeks, and 300 mg every 2 weeks, respectively.

Although the precise mechanism(s) remains to be clearly established, weight gain may result at least in part from the drug's serotonergic-, histaminergic-, and adrenergic-blocking properties. Weight gain has been reported to be troublesome for some patients during long-term therapy with atypical antipsychotics, particularly olanzapine and clozapine, and may be an important cause of outpatient noncompliance. Some clinicians suggest regular physical exercise and nutritional counseling in the prevention and treatment of weight gain associated with these drugs. There currently are no well established pharmacologic treatments for antipsychotic agent-induced weight gain; however, a number of drugs, including amantadine, bupropion, histamine H_2-receptor antagonists (e.g., nizatidine), orlistat, metformin, and topiramate, have been used with limited success to date. Because the potential risk of adverse effects in patients receiving these drugs may outweigh their possible weight-reducing effects in some cases, routine use of pharmacologic therapy currently is not recommended by most clinicians, although individual patients may benefit. Additional controlled studies are needed to more clearly determine the optimum management of antipsychotic-associated weight gain during long-term therapy with these drugs.

Hyperglycemia and Diabetes Mellitus

Hyperglycemia, sometimes severe and associated with ketoacidosis, hyperosmolar coma, or death, has been reported in patients receiving atypical antipsychotic agents, including olanzapine. While confounding factors such as an increased background risk of diabetes mellitus in patients with schizophrenia and the increasing incidence of diabetes mellitus in the general population make it difficult to establish with certainty the relationship between use of agents in this drug class and glucose abnormalities, epidemiologic studies suggest an increased risk of treatment-emergent hyperglycemia-related adverse events in patients treated with atypical antipsychotic agents. (See Hyperglycemia and Diabetes Mellitus under Cautions: Precautions and Contraindications.)

Precise risk estimates for hyperglycemia-related adverse events in patients treated with atypical antipsychotics currently are not available. While relative risk estimates are inconsistent, the association between atypical antipsychotics and increases in glucose concentrations appears to fall on a continuum, and olanzapine appears to have a greater association with hyperglycemia than some other atypical antipsychotic agents (e.g., quetiapine, risperidone).

In the first phase of Clinical Antipsychotic Trials of Intervention Effectiveness (CATIE), the mean increase in serum glucose concentration (fasting and nonfasting samples) from baseline to the average of the 2 highest serum concentrations was 15 mg/dL in olanzapine-treated adult patients (median exposure of about 9 months). In a study in healthy individuals, subjects who received olanzapine for 3 weeks had a mean increase in fasting blood glucose of 2.3 mg/dL compared with baseline; the subjects who received placebo had a mean increase in fasting blood glucose of 0.34 mg/dL compared with baseline.

In an analysis of 5 placebo-controlled monotherapy studies in adults with a median treatment duration of about 3 weeks, olanzapine was associated with a greater average increase in fasting glucose concentrations compared with placebo (2.76 mg/dL versus 0.17 mg/dL, respectively). The difference in mean changes between olanzapine and placebo was greater in patients with evidence of glucose dysregulation at baseline (e.g., patients diagnosed with diabetes mellitus or related adverse reactions, patients treated with antidiabetic agents, patients with a random baseline glucose concentration of 200 mg/dL or more and/or a baseline fasting glucose level of 126 mg/dL). Olanzapine-treated patients had a mean glycosylated hemoglobin (hemoglobin A_{1c} [HbA_{1c}]) concentration increase from baseline of 0.04% (median exposure: 21 days) compared with a mean HbA_{1c} decrease of 0.06% in placebo-treated individuals (median exposure of 17 days). In an analysis of 8 placebo-controlled studies (median treatment exposure of 4–5 weeks), 6.1% of olanzapine-treated subjects had treatment-emergent glycosuria compared with 2.8% of those receiving placebo. In adults receiving olanzapine monotherapy for at least 48 weeks, fasting glucose concentrations changed from normal (less than 100 mg/dL) to high (126 mg/dL or higher) and from borderline (between 100 and less than 126 mg/dL) to high (126 mg/dL or higher) in 12.8% and 26% of the patients, respectively. The mean change in fasting glucose for patients exposed to at least 48 weeks of olanzapine therapy was 4.2 mg/dL. In analyses of patients who completed 9–12 months of olanzapine therapy, the average change in fasting and nonfasting glucose concentrations continued to increase over time.

Although increases in fasting glucose concentrations were similar in adolescents and adults treated with olanzapine, the difference in these values between the olanzapine and placebo groups was greater in adolescents than in adults. In an analysis of 3 short-term, placebo-controlled olanzapine monotherapy studies of 3 or 6 weeks' duration in adolescent patients, olanzapine was associated with a greater mean change from baseline in fasting glucose concentrations compared with placebo (an increase of 2.68 mg/dL versus a decrease of 2.59 mg/dL, respectively). The average increase in fasting glucose concentrations for adolescents exposed to at least 24 weeks of olanzapine therapy was 3.1 mg/dL. In adolescents receiving olanzapine monotherapy for at least 24 weeks, fasting glucose concentrations changed from normal (less than 100 mg/dL) to high (126 mg/dL or higher) and from borderline (between 100 and less than 126 mg/dL) to high (126 mg/dL or higher) in 0.9% and 23.1% of the patients, respectively.

Diabetic coma and diabetic ketoacidosis have been reported in olanzapine-treated patients during postmarketing surveillance.

Dyslipidemia

Like some other antipsychotic agents, particularly clozapine, olanzapine therapy has been associated with undesirable changes in lipid parameters, including elevations in serum triglyceride and cholesterol concentrations. Clinically important, and sometimes very high (greater than 500 mg/dL), elevations in triglyceride concentrations have been observed with olanzapine therapy. Modest average increases in total cholesterol concentrations also have occurred with olanzapine use.

In an analysis of 5 placebo-controlled olanzapine monotherapy studies of up to 12 weeks' duration in adults, olanzapine-treated patients had increases from baseline in mean fasting serum total cholesterol, low-density lipoprotein (LDL)-cholesterol, and triglyceride concentrations of 5.3 mg/dL, 3 mg/dL, and 20.8 mg/dL, respectively, compared with decreases from baseline in mean fasting total cholesterol, LDL-cholesterol, and triglyceride concentrations of 6.1 mg/dL, 4.3 mg/dL, and 10.7 mg/dL for patients receiving placebo. For fasting high-density lipoprotein (HDL)-cholesterol, no clinically important differences were observed between olanzapine-treated patients and patients receiving placebo. Mean increases in fasting lipid values (total cholesterol, LDL-cholesterol, and triglycerides) were greater in patients without evidence of lipid dysregulation at baseline (defined as patients diagnosed with dyslipidemia or related adverse reactions, patients receiving antilipemic agents, or patients with high baseline lipid levels). In long-term studies (at least 48 weeks) in adults, patients had increases from baseline in mean fasting serum total cholesterol, LDL-cholesterol, and triglyceride concentrations of 5.6 mg/dL, 2.5 mg/dL, and 18.7 mg/dL, respectively, and a mean decrease in fasting HDL-cholesterol of 0.16 mg/dL. In an analysis of patients who completed 12 months of therapy, the mean nonfasting total cholesterol concentration did not increase further after approximately 4–6 months. In adult monotherapy studies, fasting serum triglyceride increases of 50 mg/dL or more occurred in approximately 61% of patients, fasting total cholesterol increases of 40 mg/dL or more occurred in approximately 33% of patients, and fasting LDL-cholesterol increases of 30 mg/dL or more occurred in approximately 40% of patients. In the first phase of the CATIE program, the mean increase in serum triglyceride concentrations in patients receiving olanzapine was 40.5 mg/dL (median exposure of about 9 months) and the mean increase in total cholesterol was 9.4 mg/dL.

In clinical studies, increases in fasting serum total cholesterol, LDL-cholesterol, and triglyceride concentrations were generally greater in adolescents than in adults treated with olanzapine. In an analysis of 3 placebo-controlled olanzapine monotherapy studies in adolescent patients, increases from baseline in mean fasting total cholesterol, LDL-cholesterol, and triglyceride concentrations of approximately 13 mg/dL, 7 mg/dL, and 28 mg/dL, respectively, occurred in adolescents receiving olanzapine compared with increases from baseline in mean fasting total cholesterol and LDL cholesterol of 1.3 mg/dL and 1 mg/dL and a decrease in triglycerides of 1.1 mg/dL in adolescents receiving placebo. For fasting HDL-cholesterol, no clinically important differences were observed between adolescents receiving olanzapine compared with adolescents receiving placebo. Adolescents receiving olanzapine monotherapy for at least 24 weeks had increases from baseline in mean fasting total cholesterol, LDL-cholesterol, and triglyceride concentrations of 5.5 mg/dL, 5.4 mg/dL, and 20.5 mg/dL, respectively, and a mean decrease in fasting HDL-cholesterol of 4.5 mg/dL. In adolescent monotherapy studies, fasting serum triglyceride increases of 50 mg/dL or more occurred in approximately 46% of adolescents, fasting total cholesterol increases of 40 mg/dL or more occurred in approximately 15% of patients, and fasting LDL-cholesterol increases of 30 mg/dL or more occurred in approximately 22% of patients.

Cholesterol concentrations of 240 mg/dL or higher and triglyceride concentrations of 1000 mg/dL or higher have been reported rarely during postmarketing surveillance.

The manufacturer recommends clinical monitoring, including baseline and periodic follow-up lipid evaluations, in all patients receiving olanzapine. In addition, some clinicians recommend that lipid profiles be monitored at baseline and periodically (e.g., every 3–6 months) in all patients receiving long-term therapy with atypical antipsychotic agents. There is some evidence from a study in individuals with developmental disabilities that the risk of dyslipidemia in patients receiving atypical antipsychotic agents may be minimized or avoided by careful monitoring, dietary management, and suitable physical activity. In patients who develop persistent and clinically important dyslipidemia during olanzapine therapy, nondrug therapies and measures (e.g., dietary management, weight control, an appropriate program of physical activity) and drug therapy (e.g., antilipemic agents) may be helpful. Consideration also may be given to switching to an alternative antipsychotic agent that is less frequently associated with dyslipidemia (such as aripiprazole, risperidone, or ziprasidone).

Hyperprolactinemia

As with other drugs that antagonize dopamine D_2 receptors, olanzapine can elevate serum prolactin concentrations, and the elevation may persist during chronic administration of the drug. However, in contrast to conventional (first-generation) antipsychotic agents and similar to many other atypical antipsychotic agents, olanzapine therapy in usual dosages generally produces transient elevations in serum prolactin concentrations in humans. It has been suggested that the more transient effect of atypical antipsychotic agents on prolactin may be because these drugs appear to dissociate from dopamine receptors more rapidly than conventional antipsychotic agents.

In placebo-controlled studies with olanzapine (up to 12 weeks) in adults, changes from normal to high serum prolactin concentrations were observed in 30% of olanzapine-treated adults compared with 10.5% of adults receiving placebo. In a pooled analysis from clinical studies involving 8136 adults treated with olanzapine, potentially associated clinical manifestations of hyperprolactinemia included menstrual-related events (2% of females), sexual function-related events (2% of females and males), and breast-related events (0.7% of females and 0.2% of males).

Adolescents treated with olanzapine had a higher incidence of elevated prolactin concentrations compared with adults; the incidence of galactorrhea and gynecomastia also was higher in adolescents compared with adults. In placebo-controlled olanzapine monotherapy studies of up to 6 weeks' duration in adolescent patients with schizophrenia or bipolar disorder, changes from normal to high serum

prolactin concentrations were observed in 47% of olanzapine-treated patients compared with 7% of those receiving placebo. In a pooled analysis from clinical trials that included 454 olanzapine-treated adolescents, potentially associated clinical manifestations included menstrual-related events (1% of females), sexual function-related events (0.7% of females and males), and breast-related events (2% of females and 2% of males).

In premarketing studies with extended-release IM olanzapine pamoate, substantial differences in prolactin concentrations have been observed in patients receiving different dosage regimens of the drug.

Olanzapine is considered by many experts to be relatively low to moderate among antipsychotic agents in its potential for inducing hyperprolactinemia in adults, and it has been recommended along with other prolactin-sparing atypical antipsychotics (e.g., aripiprazole, clozapine, quetiapine, ziprasidone) in patients with schizophrenia who are at risk of hyperprolactinemia. Although clinical disturbances such as galactorrhea, amenorrhea, gynecomastia, and impotence have been associated with prolactin-elevating drugs, the clinical importance of elevated prolactin concentrations is unknown for most patients.

Like other drugs that increase prolactin, an increase in mammary gland neoplasia was observed in olanzapine carcinogenicity studies conducted in mice and rats. However, neither clinical studies nor epidemiologic studies have demonstrated an association between chronic administration of dopamine antagonists and tumorigenesis in humans; the available evidence is considered too limited to be conclusive. (See Hyperprolactinemia under Cautions: Precautions and Contraindications and see also Cautions: Mutagenicity and Carcinogenicity.) In patients who develop elevated prolactin concentrations during antipsychotic therapy, some clinicians recommend reducing the dosage of the current antipsychotic agent or switching to a more prolactin-sparing antipsychotic agent (e.g., aripiprazole, clozapine, quetiapine, ziprasidone). Dopamine receptor agonists (e.g., bromocriptine) also may be helpful, and estrogen replacement therapy may be considered in hypoestrogenic female patients.

Other Endocrine and Metabolic Effects

Peripheral edema has been reported in approximately 3% of adult patients receiving oral olanzapine in short-term clinical trials; increased serum alkaline phosphatase concentrations have been reported in at least 1% of patients. Bilirubinemia and hypoproteinemia have been reported in 1% or less of patients receiving oral olanzapine in short-term trials.

Increased serum creatine phosphokinase concentrations have been reported in less than 1% of patients receiving IM olanzapine in short-term clinical trials; however, a causal relationship remains to be established.

● GI Effects

Dryness of the mouth and constipation both occurred in about 9%, dyspepsia in about 7%, vomiting in about 4%, and increased appetite in about 3% of adult patients receiving oral olanzapine in short-term controlled clinical trials.

Nausea (4–5%), vomiting (1–6%), dry mouth (2–6%), diarrhea (2–7%), and increased appetite (1–6%) occurred in adult patients receiving extended-release IM olanzapine pamoate therapy in a short-term controlled clinical trial.

Nausea has been reported in less than 1% of patients receiving short-acting IM olanzapine in clinical trials.

Tongue edema has been reported in 1% or less of oral olanzapine-treated patients. Ileus and intestinal obstruction have been reported in less than 0.1% of patients receiving oral olanzapine in short-term clinical trials.

● Respiratory Effects

Rhinitis occurred in about 7%, increased cough in about 6%, and pharyngitis in about 4% of adult patients receiving oral olanzapine in short-term controlled clinical trials. Dyspnea has been reported in at least 1% of patients receiving oral olanzapine in short-term clinical trials. Epistaxis has been reported in 1% or less of olanzapine-treated patients. In addition, dyspnea and hyperventilation, which appeared to be dose related, have been reported together in a patient treated with oral olanzapine.

Lung edema has been reported in less than 0.1% of adult patients receiving oral olanzapine; however, a causal relationship to the drug has not been clearly established. Respiratory failure developed in a geriatric individual with chronic lung disease who was receiving olanzapine therapy; although not clearly established, it was suggested that the respiratory failure was due at least in part to the sedative effect of the drug.

● Dermatologic and Sensitivity Reactions

Alopecia and photosensitivity reaction have been reported in 1% or less of olanzapine-treated adults. Allergic/hypersensitivity reactions (e.g., anaphylactoid reaction, angioedema, pruritus, urticaria, rash) also have been reported during postmarketing surveillance of olanzapine. In addition, a case of Guillain-Barré syndrome associated with an apparent hypersensitivity reaction to olanzapine (manifested as rash and hepatic impairment) has been reported in at least one olanzapine-treated patient; the symptoms of the reaction gradually improved in this patient following discontinuance of the drug and plasma exchange.

Eruptive xanthomas, which are associated with hyperlipidemia, have occurred in several patients receiving olanzapine therapy. Leukocytoclastic vasculitis also has been reported in a geriatric patient receiving olanzapine and warfarin concurrently; the vasculitis improved following discontinuance of olanzapine in this patient but recurred when the drug was subsequently reintroduced.

Drug Reaction with Eosinophilia and Systemic Symptoms

Drug reaction with eosinophilia and systemic symptoms (DRESS; also known as multiorgan hypersensitivity and hypersensitivity syndrome), a rare and serious dermatologic reaction, has been reported in patients receiving olanzapine. DRESS, which can be fatal in up to 10% of cases, consists of a combination of 3 or more of the following manifestations: cutaneous reaction (e.g., rash, exfoliative dermatitis), eosinophilia, fever, lymphadenopathy, and one or more systemic complications such as hepatitis, myocarditis, pericarditis, pancreatitis, nephritis, and pneumonitis. DRESS may start as a rash that can spread all over the body and include fever, lymphadenopathy, facial swelling, and injury to organs (including the liver, kidneys, lungs, heart, or pancreas) and possibly death.

FDA has identified 23 cases of DRESS, including one fatal case, associated with olanzapine use worldwide that were reported to its adverse event reporting system between 1996 and May 10, 2016. The median time to onset of symptoms in these cases was 19 days after initiation of olanzapine therapy and the median duration of olanzapine therapy was 2 months. The median reported olanzapine dosage was 20 mg daily; however, DRESS has been reported at olanzapine dosages as low as 5 mg daily. The 22 non-fatal cases all reported serious outcomes, including 18 that required hospitalization. Complete resolution of symptoms was reported in 9 cases after discontinuance of olanzapine. In one case, symptoms of DRESS recurred after reinitiation of the drug. In the fatal case, death was attributed to acute cardiac failure related to olanzapine; during hospitalization, the patient had an initial episode of DRESS, followed by a recurrence of DRESS. However, the patient in this case was taking multiple other drugs that may have contributed to death.

A published case report describes a severe and generalized pruritic eruption, fever, eosinophilia, and toxic hepatitis that developed in an adult male patient 60 days after beginning olanzapine therapy. The manifestations of DRESS/hypersensitivity syndrome in this patient improved following discontinuance of the drug, and skin and liver biopsy results suggested that the syndrome was caused by olanzapine. Another case of DRESS/hypersensitivity syndrome, which was manifested as rash, edema, generalized lymphadenopathy, hepatomegaly, eosinophilia, fever, and cough and confirmed by patch testing, was reported in an olanzapine-treated patient. (See Drug Reaction with Eosinophilia and Systemic Symptoms under Cautions: Precautions and Contraindications.)

● Local Effects

Pain at the injection site has been reported in at least 1% of patients receiving short-acting IM olanzapine in controlled clinical trials.

Injection site reactions were reported in 3.6% of patients receiving extended-release olanzapine pamoate IM in a short-term, placebo-controlled clinical trial, which included pain at the injection site, buttock pain, injection site mass, induration, and injection site induration. Pain at the injection site was reported most frequently (in 2.3% of patients). The injection site reactions were generally mild to moderate in severity, and none of the affected patients discontinued therapy because of the reactions.

● Genitourinary Effects

Urinary incontinence has been reported in approximately 2% of adult patients receiving oral olanzapine in short-term controlled clinical trials, although a causal relationship to the drug remains to be established. Amenorrhea, breast pain, decreased menstruation, increased menstruation, menorrhagia, metrorrhagia, lactation disorder, and gynecomastia have been reported in 1% or less of olanzapine-treated patients.

Impotence, polyuria, urinary frequency, urinary retention, urinary urgency, and impaired urination have been reported in 1% or less of adult patients receiving oral olanzapine in short-term clinical trials.

Priapism has been reported in several male patients and at least one case of clitoral priapism has been reported in a female patient. The α-adrenergic blocking effect of olanzapine appears to be responsible for this rare but potentially serious adverse effect requiring immediate medical attention to prevent long-term consequences such as erectile dysfunction.

● Musculoskeletal Effects

Joint pain, back pain, and extremity (other than joint) pain have been reported in 5% of adult patients receiving oral olanzapine in short-term controlled clinical trials. Osteoporosis has been reported in less than 0.1% of patients receiving oral olanzapine. Rhabdomyolysis also has been reported rarely in olanzapine-treated patients and may be seen as one of the clinical features of NMS. (See Neuroleptic Malignant Syndrome in Cautions: Nervous System Effects.)

● Ocular Effects

Amblyopia has been reported in 3% of adult patients receiving oral olanzapine in short-term clinical trials. Accommodation abnormality and dry eyes have been reported in 1% or less of oral olanzapine-treated patients. In addition, mydriasis has been reported in less than 0.1% of patients receiving oral olanzapine.

● Hematologic Effects

In clinical trial and/or postmarketing experience, leukopenia and neutropenia temporally related to antipsychotic agents, including olanzapine, have been reported. Agranulocytosis also has been reported.

Possible risk factors for leukopenia and neutropenia include a preexisting low leukocyte count and a history of drug-induced leukopenia or neutropenia. Therefore, patients with a history of clinically important low leukocyte count or drug-induced leukopenia and/or neutropenia should have their complete blood count monitored frequently during the first few months of olanzapine therapy. Discontinuance of olanzapine should be considered at the first sign of a clinically important decline in leukocyte count in the absence of other causative factors.

Patients with clinically significant neutropenia should be carefully monitored for fever or other signs or symptoms of infection and promptly treated if such signs or symptoms occur. In patients with severe neutropenia (absolute neutrophil count [ANC] less than 1000/mm^3), olanzapine should be discontinued and the leukocyte count monitored until recovery occurs.

Lithium reportedly has been used successfully in the treatment of several cases of leukopenia and neutropenia associated with aripiprazole, clozapine, olanzapine, and some other drugs; however, further clinical experience is needed to confirm these anecdotal findings.

Ecchymosis has been reported in 5% of adult patients receiving oral olanzapine in short-term clinical trials; however, a causal relationship to the drug remains to be established. Leukopenia and thrombocytopenia have been reported in less than 1% of patients receiving oral olanzapine. During premarketing clinical trials, asymptomatic elevation of the eosinophil count was reported in approximately 0.3% of patients receiving oral olanzapine.

● Other Adverse Effects

Accidental injury has been reported in approximately 12% of adult patients, and fever has been reported in approximately 6% of adult patients receiving oral olanzapine in short-term clinical trials. Chills and facial edema have been reported in 1% or less of oral olanzapine-treated patients. In addition, chills accompanied by fever, hangover effect, and sudden death have been reported in less than 0.1% of patients receiving oral olanzapine; however, a causal relationship to the drug has not been clearly established. Discontinuation reaction (diaphoresis, nausea, or vomiting) also has been reported during postmarketing surveillance of olanzapine.

Pancreatitis, which has been fatal in some cases, has occurred rarely in patients receiving atypical antipsychotic agents, including olanzapine, clozapine, and risperidone. In most of these cases, pancreatitis developed within 6 months of initiation of atypical antipsychotic therapy. Although the precise mechanism for this effect remains to be established, it has been suggested that it may be due at least in part to the adverse metabolic effects associated with these drugs.

● Precautions and Contraindications

Olanzapine shares many of the toxic potentials of other antipsychotic agents (e.g., other atypical antipsychotic agents, phenothiazines), and the usual precautions associated with therapy with these agents should be observed. (See Cautions in the Phenothiazines General Statement 28:16.08.24.)

When olanzapine is used in combination with fluoxetine, the usual cautions, precautions, and contraindications associated with fluoxetine must be considered in addition to those associated with olanzapine.

Laboratory Test Monitoring

The manufacturer recommends fasting blood glucose testing and lipid profile determinations at the beginning of olanzapine therapy and periodically during treatment with the drug. (See Cautions: Endocrine and Metabolic Effects and see also Dyslipidemia and Hyperglycemia and Diabetes Mellitus under Cautions: Precautions and Contraindications.)

Hyperprolactinemia

Similar to other antipsychotic agents, olanzapine can cause elevated serum prolactin concentrations, which may persist during chronic use of the drug. (See Hyperprolactinemia under Cautions: Endocrine and Metabolic Effects.) Clinical disturbances such as galactorrhea, amenorrhea, gynecomastia, and impotence have been associated with prolactin-elevating drugs. In addition, chronic hyperprolactinemia associated with hypogonadism may lead to decreased bone density.

If olanzapine therapy is considered in a patient with previously detected breast cancer, clinicians should consider that approximately one-third of human breast cancers are prolactin-dependent in vitro.

Cognitive and Motor Impairment

Dose-related somnolence occurred in 26% of patients receiving oral olanzapine compared with 15% of those receiving placebo, and resulted in discontinuance of the drug in 0.4% of the patients in the premarketing database. Sedation occurred in 8% of patients receiving extended-release olanzapine pamoate injection; somnolence and sedation resulted in discontinuance of the drug in 0.6% of patients in the premarketing database.

Because of olanzapine's sedative effects and because the drug potentially may impair judgment, thinking, and motor skills, olanzapine-treated patients should be cautioned about operating hazardous machinery, including driving a motor vehicle, until they are reasonably certain that the drug does not adversely affect them. In addition, because of the risk of post-injection delirium/sedation syndrome, patients receiving extended-release olanzapine pamoate injection should not drive or operate heavy machinery for the remainder of the day after each injection.

Seizures

Although seizures occurred in about 0.9% of patients receiving oral olanzapine in controlled clinical trials and in 0.15% of patients receiving extended-release olanzapine pamoate injection during premarketing testing, it should be noted that confounding factors that may have contributed to the occurrence of seizures were present in many of these cases. Olanzapine should be administered with caution to patients with a history of seizures, patients with conditions known to lower the seizure threshold (e.g., dementia of the Alzheimer's type), and during concurrent therapy with drugs that may lower the seizure threshold.

Body Temperature Regulation

Because disruption of the body's ability to reduce core body temperature has been associated with the use of antipsychotic agents, caution is advised when olanzapine is administered in patients exposed to conditions that may contribute to an elevation in core body temperature. Such conditions include strenuous exercise, exposure to extreme heat, concomitant use of drugs with anticholinergic activity, or dehydration. Patients receiving olanzapine should be advised regarding appropriate precautions to avoid overheating and dehydration. Patients also should be advised to contact their clinician immediately if they become severely ill and have some or all of the symptoms of dehydration, including sweating too much or not at all, dry mouth, feeling very hot or thirsty, and unable to produce urine.

Hepatic Effects

Because clinically important serum ALT elevations (3 or more times the upper limit of the normal range) were observed in adults and adolescents exposed to oral olanzapine and adults exposed to extended-release IM olanzapine pamoate in placebo-controlled clinical studies, the manufacturer states that olanzapine should be used with caution in patients with signs and symptoms of hepatic impairment, in patients with preexisting conditions associated with limited hepatic functional

reserve, and in patients who are being treated concurrently with potentially hepatotoxic drugs.

Drug Reaction with Eosinophilia and Systemic Symptoms

Drug reaction with eosinophilia and systemic symptoms (DRESS; also known as multiorgan hypersensitivity and hypersensitivity syndrome) has been reported in olanzapine-treated patients. (See Drug Reaction with Eosinophilia and Systemic Symptoms under Cautions: Dermatologic and Sensitivity Reactions.) Patients receiving olanzapine should be informed about the risk of DRESS and advised to seek immediate medical care if symptoms suggestive of DRESS, including rash, fever, facial swelling, and/or lymphadenopathy, occur. There currently is no specific treatment for DRESS. Management of the syndrome involves early recognition, immediate discontinuance of olanzapine if DRESS is suspected, and initiation of supportive care. Corticosteroid therapy also should be considered in cases of DRESS with extensive organ involvement.

Individuals with Phenylketonuria

Individuals with phenylketonuria (i.e., homozygous genetic deficiency of phenylalanine hydroxylase) and other individuals who must restrict their intake of phenylalanine should be warned that olanzapine orally disintegrating tablets contain aspartame (e.g., NutraSweet®), which is metabolized in the GI tract to provide phenylalanine following oral administration; the respective manufacturer's labeling should be consulted for specific information regarding phenylalanine content of individual preparations and dosage strengths.

Dysphagia

Esophageal dysmotility and aspiration have been associated with the use of antipsychotic agents. Aspiration pneumonia is a common cause of morbidity and mortality in patients with advanced Alzheimer's disease. The manufacturer states that olanzapine is *not* approved for the treatment of Alzheimer's disease.

Patients with Concomitant Illness

Clinical experience with olanzapine in patients with certain concurrent systemic diseases is limited. Olanzapine has demonstrated anticholinergic activity in vitro and constipation, dryness of the mouth, and tachycardia, possibly related to the drug's anticholinergic effects, have occurred in premarketing clinical trials. Although these adverse effects did not often result in drug discontinuance, the manufacturer states that olanzapine should be used with caution in patients with clinically important prostatic hypertrophy, angle-closure glaucoma, or a history of paralytic ileus or related conditions.

Olanzapine has not been adequately evaluated in patients with a recent history of myocardial infarction or unstable cardiovascular disease to date and patients with these conditions were excluded from premarketing clinical trials. Because of the risk of orthostatic hypotension associated with olanzapine, the manufacturer states that the drug should be used with caution in patients with cardiovascular disease. (See Cautions: Cardiovascular Effects and see also Orthostatic Hypotension under Cautions: Precautions and Contraindications.)

Concomitant Medication or Alcohol Use

Because of the potential for adverse drug interactions, the manufacturer recommends that patients receiving olanzapine be advised to notify their clinician if they are taking or plan to take other olanzapine-containing preparations (e.g., Symbyax® [an olanzapine/fluoxetine combination]). Patients receiving olanzapine should also be advised to inform their clinician if they are taking, plan to take, or have stopped taking any prescription or nonprescription (over-the-counter) medications, including herbal supplements. The manufacturer also recommends that patients be advised to avoid alcohol while receiving the drug. (See Drug Interactions.)

Tardive Dyskinesia

Because use of antipsychotic agents may be associated with tardive dyskinesia, a syndrome of potentially irreversible, involuntary, dyskinetic movements, olanzapine should be prescribed in a manner that is most likely to minimize the occurrence of this syndrome. Chronic antipsychotic treatment generally should be reserved for patients who suffer from a chronic illness that is known to respond to antipsychotic agents, and for whom alternative, equally effective, but potentially less harmful treatments are not available or appropriate. In patients who do require chronic treatment, the smallest dosage and the shortest duration of treatment producing a satisfactory clinical response should be sought, and the need for continued treatment should be reassessed periodically.

The APA currently recommends that patients receiving second-generation antipsychotic agents be assessed clinically for abnormal involuntary movements every 12 months and that patients considered to be at increased risk for tardive dyskinesia be assessed every 6 months. (See Tardive Dyskinesia under Cautions: Nervous System Effects.)

Falls

Olanzapine therapy may cause somnolence, postural hypotension, and motor and sensory instability, which may lead to falls; as a consequence, fractures or other injuries may occur. For patients with diseases or conditions or receiving other drugs that could exacerbate these effects, fall risk assessments should be completed when initiating antipsychotic treatment and periodically during long-term therapy.

Dispensing and Administration Precautions

Because of similarities in spelling, dosage intervals (once daily), and tablet strengths (5 and 10 mg) of Zyprexa® (the trade name for olanzapine) and Zyrtec® (the trade name for cetirizine hydrochloride, an antihistamine), several dispensing or prescribing errors have been reported to the manufacturer of Zyprexa®. These medication errors may result in unnecessary adverse events or a potential relapse in patients with schizophrenia or bipolar disorder. Therefore, the manufacturer of Zyprexa® cautions that extra care should be exercised in ensuring the accuracy of written prescriptions for Zyprexa® and Zyrtec® such as printing both the proprietary (brand) and nonproprietary (generic) names on all prescriptions for these drugs. The manufacturer also recommends that pharmacists assess various measures of avoiding dispensing errors and implement them as appropriate (e.g., placing drugs with similar names apart from one another on pharmacy shelves, patient counseling).

Leukopenia, Neutropenia, and Agranulocytosis

In clinical trial and/or postmarketing experience, leukopenia and neutropenia temporally related to antipsychotic agents, including olanzapine, have been reported; agranulocytosis also has been reported.

Because possible risk factors for leukopenia and neutropenia include a preexisting low leukocyte count and a history of drug-induced leukopenia and neutropenia, the manufacturer states that patients with a history of clinically important low leukocyte count or drug-induced leukopenia and/or neutropenia should have their complete blood count monitored frequently during the first few months of olanzapine therapy. Discontinuance of olanzapine should be considered at the first sign of a clinically important decline in leukocyte count in the absence of other causative factors.

Patients with clinically significant neutropenia should be carefully monitored for fever or other signs or symptoms of infection and promptly treated if such signs or symptoms occur. In patients with severe neutropenia (absolute neutrophil count [ANC] less than 1000/mm³), olanzapine should be discontinued and the leukocyte count monitored until recovery occurs. (See Cautions: Hematologic Effects.)

Orthostatic Hypotension

Orthostatic hypotension associated with dizziness, tachycardia, bradycardia, and/or syncope, particularly during the initial dosage titration period, has been reported in patients receiving oral olanzapine therapy. The risk of orthostatic hypotension and syncope may be minimized by initiating therapy with a dosage of 5 mg orally once daily. A more gradual titration to the target dosage should be considered if hypotension occurs. Patients should be cautioned about the risk of orthostatic hypotension, particularly during the initial dosage titration period and if the drug is given concurrently with drugs that may potentiate the orthostatic effect of olanzapine, including diazepam, or alcohol. Patients should be advised to change positions carefully to help prevent orthostatic hypotension and to lie down if they feel dizzy or faint until they feel better. Patients also should be advised to contact their clinician if they experience any of the following signs and symptoms associated with orthostatic hypotension: dizziness, fast or slow heart beat, or fainting.

Hypotension, bradycardia with or without hypotension, tachycardia, and syncope have been reported in patients receiving short-acting IM olanzapine. The use of maximum recommended dosages of IM olanzapine (i.e., 3 doses of 10 mg each given IM 2–4 hours apart) may be associated with a substantial risk of clinically important orthostatic hypotension. Patients who experience drowsiness or dizziness after the IM injection should remain recumbent until an examination indicates that they are not experiencing orthostatic hypotension, bradycardia, and/or hypoventilation. Patients requiring additional IM injections of olanzapine should be assessed for orthostatic hypotension prior to administration of any subsequent doses. Administration of additional IM doses to patients with clinically important postural change in blood pressure is not recommended.

Extended-release IM olanzapine pamoate therapy also may cause orthostatic hypotension associated with dizziness, tachycardia, bradycardia, and, in some cases, syncope.

The manufacturer states that olanzapine should be used with particular caution in patients with known cardiovascular disease (e.g., history of myocardial infarction or ischemia, heart failure, conduction abnormalities), cerebrovascular disease, and/or other conditions that would predispose patients to hypotension (e.g., dehydration, hypovolemia, concomitant antihypertensive therapy) where the occurrence of syncope, hypotension, and/or bradycardia might put the patient at increased risk. The manufacturer also states that the drug should be used with caution in patients receiving other drugs that can induce hypotension, bradycardia, or respiratory and CNS depression. (See Drug Interactions.) In such patients who have never taken oral olanzapine, tolerability should be established with oral olanzapine before initiating extended-release IM olanzapine pamoate therapy.

Concurrent administration of short-acting IM olanzapine and parenteral benzodiazepines is not recommended due to the potential for excessive sedation and cardiorespiratory depression. If use of short-acting IM olanzapine in combination with parenteral benzodiazepine therapy is considered, careful evaluation of the patient's clinical status for excessive sedation and cardiorespiratory depression is recommended.

Weight Gain

Olanzapine therapy may result in weight gain. In olanzapine-treated adolescent patients, both the magnitude of weight gain and the proportion of patients who had clinically important weight gain were greater compared with adult patients with comparable exposures. (See Endocrine and Metabolic Effects under Cautions and see also Cautions: Pediatric Precautions.)

The potential consequences of weight gain should be considered in adults and adolescents prior to starting olanzapine therapy. All patients receiving the drug should be advised that weight gain has occurred during olanzapine treatment and receive regular monitoring of their weight.

Dyslipidemia

Because undesirable changes in serum lipids have been observed with olanzapine therapy in both adults and adolescents, the manufacturer recommends appropriate clinical monitoring, including baseline and periodic follow-up lipid evaluations, in all patients receiving the drug. (See Endocrine and Metabolic Effects under Cautions and see also Cautions: Pediatric Precautions.)

Hyperglycemia and Diabetes Mellitus

Because hyperglycemia, sometimes severe and associated with ketoacidosis, hyperosmolar coma, or death, has been reported in patients receiving atypical antipsychotic agents, including olanzapine, the manufacturer states that clinicians should consider the risks and benefits when prescribing olanzapine to adult and adolescent patients with an established diagnosis of diabetes mellitus or in those having borderline increased blood glucose concentrations (i.e., fasting values of 100–126 mg/dL or nonfasting values of 140–200 mg/dL). The manufacturer recommends that all patients beginning olanzapine therapy undergo fasting blood glucose testing upon therapy initiation and periodically during treatment. The manufacturer also recommends that all patients receiving olanzapine be regularly monitored for worsening of glucose control. Any patient who develops manifestations of hyperglycemia (e.g., polydipsia, polyphagia, polyuria, weakness) during treatment with an atypical antipsychotic should undergo fasting blood glucose testing. In some cases, patients who developed hyperglycemia while receiving an atypical antipsychotic have required continuance of antidiabetic treatment despite discontinuance of the suspect drug; in other cases, hyperglycemia resolved with discontinuance of the antipsychotic or with continuance of both the suspect drug and initiation of antidiabetic treatment.

Various experts have developed additional recommendations for the management of diabetes risks in patients receiving atypical antipsychotics; these include initial screening measures and regular monitoring (e.g., determination of diabetes risk factors; BMI determination using weight and height; waist circumference; blood pressure; fasting blood glucose; HbA$_{1c}$; fasting lipid profile), as well as provision of patient education and referral to clinicians experienced in the treatment of diabetes, when appropriate. Although some clinicians state that a switch from one atypical antipsychotic agent to another that has not been associated with substantial weight gain or diabetes should be considered in patients who experience weight gain (equal to or exceeding 5% of baseline body weight) or develop worsening glycemia or dyslipidemia at any time during therapy, such recommendations are controversial because differences in risk of developing diabetes associated with use of the different atypical antipsychotics remain to be fully established. Many clinicians consider antipsychotic efficacy the most important factor when making treatment decisions and suggest that detrimental effects of switching from a beneficial treatment regimen also should be considered in addition to any potential for exacerbation or development of medical conditions (e.g., diabetes). Decisions to alter drug therapy should be made on an individual basis, weighing the potential risks and benefits of the particular drug in each patient.

Neuroleptic Malignant Syndrome

Neuroleptic malignant syndrome (NMS), a potentially fatal syndrome requiring immediate discontinuance of the drug and intensive symptomatic treatment, has been reported in patients receiving antipsychotic agents, including olanzapine. If a patient requires antipsychotic therapy following recovery from NMS, the potential reintroduction of drug therapy should be carefully considered. If antipsychotic therapy is reintroduced, the dosage generally should be increased gradually, and an antipsychotic agent other than the agent believed to have precipitated NMS generally should be chosen. In addition, such patients should be carefully monitored since recurrences of NMS have been reported in some patients. (See Neuroleptic Malignant Syndrome under Cautions: Nervous System Effects.)

Suicide

Because the possibility of a suicide attempt is inherent in patients with schizophrenia and bipolar disorder, close supervision of high-risk patients is recommended during olanzapine therapy. The manufacturer recommends that the drug be prescribed in the smallest quantity consistent with good patient management to reduce the risk of overdosage.

Geriatric Patients with Dementia-related Psychosis

Geriatric patients with dementia-related psychosis treated with antipsychotic drugs are at increased risk of death compared with patients receiving placebo. Analyses of 17 placebo-controlled trials (modal duration of 10 weeks) revealed an approximate 1.6- to 1.7-fold increase in mortality among geriatric patients receiving atypical antipsychotic drugs (i.e., aripiprazole, olanzapine, quetiapine, risperidone) compared with that observed in patients receiving placebo. Over the course of a typical 10-week controlled trial, the rate of death in drug-treated patients was about 4.5% compared with a rate of about 2.6% in the placebo group. Although the causes of death were varied, most of the deaths appeared to be either cardiovascular (e.g., heart failure, sudden death) or infectious (e.g., pneumonia) in nature. Observational studies suggest that, similar to atypical antipsychotics, treatment with conventional (first-generation) antipsychotics may increase mortality; the extent to which the findings of increased mortality in observational studies may be attributed to the antipsychotic drug as opposed to some characteristic(s) of the patients remains unclear. In placebo-controlled trials of geriatric patients with dementia-associated psychosis, the incidence of death was significantly greater in olanzapine-treated patients than in those receiving placebo (3.5 versus 1.5%, respectively).

Adverse cerebrovascular events (e.g., stroke, transient ischemic attack), including fatalities, have been reported in clinical trials of olanzapine in geriatric patients with dementia-related psychosis. In placebo-controlled studies, a significantly higher incidence of adverse cerebrovascular events was observed in olanzapine-treated patients compared with those receiving placebo.

The manufacturer states that olanzapine is *not* approved for the treatment of patients with dementia-related psychosis. (See Cautions: Geriatric Precautions.)

Post-injection Delirium/Sedation Syndrome

Clinicians should discuss the potential risk of post-injection delirium/sedation syndrome (PDSS) with patients each time they prescribe and administer extended-release olanzapine pamoate injection (Zyprexa® Relprevv). (See Post-injection Delirium/Sedation Syndrome under Cautions: Nervous System Effects.)

Patients should be advised not to drive or operate heavy machinery for the remainder of the day following each injection, and should be vigilant for symptoms of PDSS and able to obtain medical assistance if needed. If PDSS is suspected, close medical supervision and monitoring should be instituted in a facility capable of resuscitation. For additional information concerning the pathogenesis, clinical manifestations, and management of possible PDSS and other types of olanzapine overdosage, see Acute Toxicity.

In March 2015, FDA concluded a review of 2 unexplained deaths that occurred 3–4 days after the patients received an appropriate dose of long-acting olanzapine pamoate injection (Zyprexa® Relprevv), which is well beyond the 3-hour post-injection monitoring period required under the current REMS program. Both patients were found to have very high blood concentrations of olanzapine after death. High doses of olanzapine can cause delirium, cardiopulmonary arrest, cardiac arrhythmias, and reduced levels of consciousness, ranging from sedation to coma. The review suggested that much of the drug level increase could have occurred after death. It is unclear whether the patients in these 2 cases died from PDSS; FDA states that the results of their review were inconclusive, and that the possibility that the deaths were caused by rapid but delayed entry of the drug into the bloodstream following IM injection could not be excluded. In clinical trials, cases of PDSS were observed within 3 hours of administration of olanzapine pamoate; however, no deaths were reported. If therapy with extended-release olanzapine pamoate is initiated or continued in patients, the FDA recommends that clinicians continue to follow the REMS requirements as well as the recommendations in the prescribing information for Zyprexa® Relprevv. The FDA states that patients should not discontinue therapy with extended-release olanzapine pamoate injection without consulting their clinician. (See Extended-release Olanzapine Pamoate Injection for Schizophrenia under Dosage and Administration: Reconstitution and Administration.)

Contraindications

The manufacturer states that there are no contraindications associated with oral or short-acting IM olanzapine monotherapy.

When olanzapine is used in combination with fluoxetine, the usual contraindications associated with fluoxetine must be considered.

When olanzapine is used as adjunctive therapy with lithium or valproate, the manufacturer advises clinicians to refer to prescribing information for those other drugs.

The manufacturer states that there are no contraindications associated with use of the long-acting IM formulation of olanzapine pamoate.

● *Pediatric Precautions*

The safety and effectiveness of oral olanzapine in the treatment of schizophrenia and manic or mixed episodes associated with bipolar I disorder were established in short-term clinical trials in adolescents (13–17 years of age). Use of oral olanzapine in such adolescents is supported by evidence from adequate and well-controlled clinical trials in which 268 adolescents received olanzapine in a dosage range of 2.5–20 mg daily. The recommended initial dosage for adolescents is lower than that for adults (see Dosage and Administration: Dosage). Compared with adults in clinical trials, adolescents were likely to gain more weight, experience increased sedation, and have greater increases in serum concentrations of total cholesterol, triglycerides, LDL-cholesterol, prolactin, and hepatic transaminases. (See Pediatric Considerations under Psychotic Disorders: Schizophrenia in Uses, Pediatric Considerations under Bipolar Disorder in Uses, and Cautions.)

When deciding among the alternative treatments available for adolescents with schizophrenia or bipolar disorder, clinicians should consider the increased potential for weight gain and dyslipidemia with olanzapine in adolescents as compared with adults. Clinicians also should consider the potential long-term risks when prescribing olanzapine to adolescents; in many cases, this may lead them to consider prescribing other drugs first in such patients.

Adolescent patients and/or their caregivers should be advised that adolescent patients receiving olanzapine are likely to gain more weight and to develop sedation, dyslipidemia, higher prolactin elevations, and more elevated serum aminotransferase concentrations compared with adults. Adolescent patients and/or their caregivers also should be advised about the potential long-term risks associated with olanzapine therapy and that the risks may lead them to consider other drugs first.

Pediatric patients with schizophrenia or bipolar disorder should be advised that olanzapine is indicated as an integral part of a total treatment program that may include other measures (e.g., psychological, educational, social) for patients with the disorder. In addition, pediatric patients should be informed that atypical antipsychotic agents are not intended for use in pediatric patients who exhibit symptoms secondary to environmental factors and/or other primary psychiatric disorders. Appropriate educational placement is essential and psychosocial intervention is often helpful. The decision whether to prescribe atypical antipsychotic medication in pediatric patients with schizophrenia or bipolar disorder will depend upon the clinician's assessment of the chronicity and severity of the patient's symptoms.

Because adolescents receiving olanzapine are more likely to gain more weight and experience other metabolic problems compared with adults receiving the drug (see Cautions: Endocrine and Metabolic Effects), the American Academy of Child and Adolescent Psychiatry (AACAP) currently recommends that pediatric patients receiving atypical antipsychotic agents for the management of bipolar disorder have baseline body mass index (BMI), waist circumference, blood pressure, fasting glucose, and fasting lipid parameters determined at baseline. The AACAP also recommends that the BMI be followed monthly for the initial 3 months of therapy and then every 3 months thereafter. In addition, these experts recommend that blood pressure, fasting glucose, and lipid parameters be assessed after 3 months of therapy and then annually thereafter. (See Cautions: Precautions and Contraindications.)

The manufacturer states that safety and efficacy of oral olanzapine for the treatment of schizophrenia or manic or mixed episodes associated with bipolar I disorder in children and adolescents younger than 13 years of age have not been established. However, the drug has been used in a limited number of children and other adolescents with childhood-onset schizophrenia (see Pediatric Considerations under Psychotic Disorders: Schizophrenia, in Uses).

The safety and efficacy of oral olanzapine in combination with fluoxetine for the treatment of acute depressive episodes associated with bipolar I disorder were established in a short-term clinical trial in pediatric patients 10–17 years of age. Use of oral olanzapine and fluoxetine in such children and adolescents is supported by evidence from a well-controlled clinical trial in which 255 pediatric patients received olanzapine in a dosage range of 3–12 mg daily. The recommended initial dosage of olanzapine in combination with fluoxetine for adolescents is lower than that for adults (see Dosage and Administration: Dosage).

The manufacturer states that the safety and efficacy of oral olanzapine in combination with fluoxetine for the treatment of treatment-resistant depression have not been established in patients younger than 18 years of age.

The manufacturer states that the safety and efficacy of oral olanzapine in combination with fluoxetine have not been established in pediatric patients younger than 10 years of age.

Oral olanzapine also has been effective and well tolerated in a limited number of children† and adolescents with pervasive developmental disorder, including autistic disorder†. Additional controlled and longer-term studies are needed to confirm these initial findings and to evaluate the relative benefits and risks of olanzapine therapy in such patients.

The manufacturer states that the safety and efficacy of short-acting IM olanzapine have not been established in patients younger than 18 years of age.

The manufacturer states that the safety and efficacy of extended-release olanzapine pamoate IM injection in patients younger than 18 years of age have not been established.

● **Geriatric Precautions**

In premarketing clinical studies with oral olanzapine, 11% (263 of 2500) of the patients were 65 years of age or older. Clinical experience in patients with schizophrenia generally has not revealed differences in tolerability of oral olanzapine in geriatric patients compared with younger adults.

The first phase of the large-scale Clinical Antipsychotic Trials of Intervention Effectiveness—Alzheimer's Disease (CATIE-AD) trial was designed to evaluate the overall effectiveness of atypical antipsychotic agents in the treatment of psychosis, aggression, and agitation associated with Alzheimer's disease. Patients in this multicenter, double-blind, placebo-controlled trial were randomized to receive either olanzapine, quetiapine, risperidone, or placebo for up to 36 weeks; the principal outcomes were the time from initial treatment until discontinuance of treatment for any reason and the number of patients with at least minimum improvement on the Clinical Global Impression of Change (CGIC) Scale at 12 weeks. No statistically significant differences were found among the 4 groups with regard to the time until discontinuation of treatment for any reason; patients

remained on olanzapine, quetiapine, risperidone, and placebo for median times of approximately 8, 5, 7, and 8 weeks, respectively. In addition, no significant differences in CGIC Scale improvements were noted. However, patients receiving atypical antipsychotic therapy reportedly experienced more frequent adverse effects (e.g., drowsiness, weight gain, adverse extrapyramidal effects, confusion, and psychotic symptoms) compared with those receiving placebo. The authors stated that these results indicate that the overall therapeutic benefit of atypical antipsychotics in patients with Alzheimer's disease may be offset by the potential risk of adverse effects.

Studies in patients with dementia-related psychosis have suggested that oral olanzapine may have a different tolerability profile in patients 65 years of age or older with this condition compared with younger patients with schizophrenia. Geriatric patients with dementia-related psychosis receiving antipsychotic agents, including olanzapine, are at an increased risk of death compared with that among patients receiving placebo. Analyses of 17 placebo-controlled trials (average duration of 10 weeks) revealed an approximate 1.6- to 1.7-fold increase in mortality among geriatric patients receiving atypical antipsychotic drugs (i.e., olanzapine, aripiprazole, quetiapine, risperidone) compared with that in patients receiving placebo. Over the course of a typical 10-week controlled trial, the rate of death in drug-treated patients was about 4.5% compared with a rate of about 2.6% in the placebo group. Although the causes of death were varied, most of the deaths appeared to be either cardiovascular (e.g., heart failure, sudden death) or infectious (e.g., pneumonia) in nature.

In placebo-controlled trials with oral olanzapine in geriatric individuals with dementia-related psychosis, an increased incidence of death also was observed; the incidence of death in olanzapine-treated patients was significantly higher than in patients receiving placebo (3.5% and 1.5%, respectively). In addition, a significantly higher incidence of adverse cerebrovascular events (e.g., stroke, transient ischemic attack), including fatalities, was observed in patients receiving olanzapine compared with those receiving placebo in these trials. In 5 placebo-controlled studies of olanzapine in geriatric individuals with dementia-related psychosis, certain treatment-emergent adverse effects, including falls, somnolence, peripheral edema, abnormal gait, urinary incontinence, lethargy, increased weight, asthenia, pyrexia, pneumonia, dry mouth, and visual hallucinations, occurred in at least 2% of the patients and the incidence was significantly higher than in patients receiving placebo. Discontinuance of therapy because of adverse effects occurred in a significantly higher number of olanzapine-treated patients than in those receiving placebo (13% and 7%, respectively) in these studies.

The manufacturer states that olanzapine is *not* approved for the treatment of patients with dementia-related psychosis. Some clinicians recommend that the potential risks, therapeutic benefits, and individual needs of patients be carefully considered prior to prescribing olanzapine and other atypical antipsychotic agents for the management of behavioral problems associated with Alzheimer's disease. For additional information on the use of antipsychotic agents in the management of dementia-related psychosis, see Geriatric Considerations under Uses: Psychotic Disorders, in the Phenothiazines General Statement 28:16.08.24.

The manufacturer states that the presence of factors that might decrease the clearance of or increase the pharmacodynamic response to olanzapine should lead to consideration of a lower initial dosage of the drug in geriatric patients.

Clinical studies of olanzapine in combination with fluoxetine did not include sufficient numbers of patients 65 years of age or older to determine whether they respond differently than younger patients.

Clinical studies of extended-release IM olanzapine pamoate did not include sufficient numbers of patients 65 years of age or older to determine whether they respond differently than younger patients.

● **Mutagenicity and Carcinogenicity**

Olanzapine did not exhibit genotoxic potential in the Ames reverse mutation test, in vivo micronucleus mutation test in mice, the chromosomal aberration test in Chinese hamster ovary cells, unscheduled DNA synthesis test in rat hepatocytes, induction of forward mutation test in mouse lymphoma cells, or in vivo sister chromatid exchange test in bone marrow of Chinese hamsters.

In oral carcinogenicity studies conducted in mice, olanzapine was administered in 2 studies of 78-weeks' duration at dosages of 3, 10, and 30 mg/kg initially then reduced to 20 mg/kg daily (equivalent to 0.8–5 times the maximum recommended human daily oral dosage on a mg/m² basis) and 0.25, 2, and 8 mg/kg daily (equivalent to 0.06–2 times the maximum recommended human daily oral dosage on a mg/m² basis). In oral carcinogenicity studies conducted in rats, olanzapine was administered for 2 years at dosages of 0.25, 1, 2.5, and 4 mg/kg daily in males (equivalent to 0.13–2 times the maximum recommended human daily oral dosage on a mg/m² basis) and 0.25, 1, 4, and 8 mg/kg daily in females (equivalent to 0.13–4 times the maximum recommended human daily oral dosage on a mg/m² basis). An increased incidence of liver hemangiomas and hemangiosarcomas was observed in one mouse study in female mice receiving 8 mg/kg of the drug daily (equivalent to 2 times the maximum recommended human daily oral dosage on a mg/m² basis). The incidence of these tumors was not increased in another study in female mice receiving 10 or 30 mg/kg (later reduced to 20 mg/kg) of olanzapine daily (equivalent to 2–5 times the maximum recommended human daily dosage on a mg/m² basis); in this study, there was a high incidence of early mortalities in males in the 30 mg/kg (later reduced to 20 mg/kg) daily group. The incidence of mammary gland adenomas and adenocarcinomas was increased in female mice receiving 2 mg/kg or more of olanzapine daily and in female rats receiving 4 mg/kg or more of the drug daily (equivalent to 0.5 and 2 times the maximum recommended human daily oral dosage on a mg/m² basis, respectively).

Antipsychotic agents have been shown to chronically elevate prolactin concentrations in rodents. Serum prolactin concentrations were not measured during the olanzapine carcinogenicity studies; however, measurements during subchronic toxicity studies demonstrated that olanzapine administration produced up to a fourfold increase in serum prolactin concentrations in rats receiving the same dosages used in the carcinogenicity study. In addition, an increase in mammary gland neoplasms has been observed in rodents following chronic administration of other antipsychotic agents and generally is considered to be prolactin-mediated. However, the clinical importance in humans of this finding of prolactin-mediated endocrine tumors in rodents is unknown.

● Pregnancy, Fertility, and Lactation

Pregnancy

Limited experience to date with olanzapine administration during pregnancy has been encouraging and has not revealed evidence of any obvious teratogenic risks; however, additional cases of olanzapine exposure during pregnancy need to be evaluated to more fully determine the relative safety of olanzapine and other antipsychotic agents when administered during pregnancy. The manufacturer states that there have been 7 pregnancies reported during clinical trials with olanzapine, including 2 resulting in normal births, one resulting in neonatal death due to a cardiovascular defect, 3 therapeutic abortions, and one spontaneous abortion. In a separate compilation of pregnancy exposures to olanzapine reported to the manufacturer during clinical trials and from spontaneous reports worldwide, outcomes were available from 23 prospectively collected, olanzapine-exposed pregnancies. Spontaneous abortion occurred in 13% of these pregnancies, stillbirth in 5%, major malformations in 0%, and prematurity in 5%; these rates were all within the range of normal historical control rates. In 11 retrospectively collected, olanzapine-exposed pregnancies, there was one case of dysplastic kidney, one case of Down's syndrome, and one case of heart murmur and sudden infant death syndrome at 2 months of age. In another study, the majority of women with schizophrenia receiving atypical antipsychotic agents were found to be overweight and to have reduced folate intake and low serum folate concentrations, which may increase the potential risk of neural tube defects. In a prospective, comparative trial assessing pregnancy outcome in women receiving atypical antipsychotic agents (olanzapine, clozapine, risperidone, and quetiapine) during pregnancy, atypical antipsychotics did not appear to be associated with an increased risk of major congenital malformations. In addition, several case reports have described healthy infants born to women without complications despite prenatal exposure to olanzapine.

Neonates exposed to antipsychotic agents, including olanzapine, during the third trimester of pregnancy are at risk for extrapyramidal and/or withdrawal symptoms following delivery. There have been reports of agitation, hypertonia, hypotonia, tardive dyskinetic-like symptoms, tremor, somnolence, respiratory distress, and feeding disorder in these neonates. The majority of cases were also confounded by other factors, including concomitant use of other drugs known to be associated with withdrawal symptoms, prematurity, congenital malformations, and obstetrical and perinatal complications; however, some cases suggested that neonatal extrapyramidal and withdrawal symptoms may occur with exposure to antipsychotic agents alone. Some of the cases described time of symptom onset, which ranged from birth to one month after birth. Any neonate exhibiting extrapyramidal or withdrawal symptoms following in utero exposure to antipsychotic agents should be monitored. Symptoms were self-limiting in some neonates but varied in severity; some infants required intensive care unit support and prolonged hospitalization. For further information on extrapyramidal and

withdrawal symptoms in neonates, see Cautions: Pregnancy, Fertility, and Lactation, in the Phenothiazines General Statement 28:16.08.24.

The manufacturer and some clinicians state that there are no adequate and well-controlled studies to date using olanzapine in pregnant women, and the drug should be used during pregnancy only when the potential benefits justify the potential risks to the fetus. Women should be advised to notify their clinician if they become pregnant or plan to become pregnant during therapy with the drug. In addition, clinicians should advise women of childbearing potential about the benefits and risks of using antipsychotic agents during pregnancy. Patients should also be advised not to stop taking their antipsychotic agent if they become pregnant without first consulting with their clinician, since abruptly discontinuing the drugs can cause clinically important complications.

Parturition in rats was not affected by olanzapine. The effect of olanzapine on labor and delivery is unknown.

In oral reproduction studies in rats receiving dosages of up to 18 mg/kg daily and in rabbits at dosages of up to 30 mg/kg daily (equivalent to 9 and 30 times the maximum recommended human daily oral dosage on a mg/m² basis, respectively), no evidence of teratogenicity was observed. In an oral rat teratology study, early resorptions and increased numbers of nonviable fetuses were observed at a dosage of 18 mg/kg daily (9 times the maximum recommended human daily oral dosage on a mg/m² basis), and gestation was prolonged at a dosage of 10 mg/kg daily (equivalent to 5 times the maximum recommended human daily oral dosage on a mg/m² basis). In an oral rabbit teratology study, fetal toxicity, which was manifested as increased resorptions and decreased fetal weight, occurred at a maternally toxic dosage of 30 mg/kg daily (equivalent to 30 times the maximum recommended human daily oral dosage on a mg/m² basis).

Fertility

In an oral fertility and reproductive performance study in rats, male mating performance, but not fertility, was impaired at an olanzapine dosage of 22.4 mg/kg daily, and female fertility was decreased at a dosage of 3 mg/kg daily (equivalent to 11 and 1.5 times the maximum recommended human daily oral dosage on a mg/m² basis, respectively). Discontinuance of olanzapine administration reversed the effects on male mating performance. In a female rat fertility study, the precoital period was increased, and the mating index reduced at a dosage of 5 mg/kg daily (equivalent to 2.5 times the maximum recommended human daily oral dosage on a mg/m² basis). Diestrus was prolonged and estrus was delayed at a dosage of 1.1 mg/kg daily (equivalent to 0.6 times the maximum recommended human daily oral dosage on a mg/m² basis).

Lactation

Olanzapine is distributed into milk. The mean dosage received by an infant at steady state is estimated to be about 1.8% of the maternal dosage. The manufacturer recommends that women receiving olanzapine not breast-feed.

DRUG INTERACTIONS

● Drugs Affecting Hepatic Microsomal Enzymes

Olanzapine is a substrate for cytochrome P-450 (CYP) isoenzyme 1A2 and concomitant administration of drugs that induce CYP1A2 or glucuronyl transferase enzymes (e.g., carbamazepine, omeprazole, rifampin) may cause an increase in olanzapine clearance. Inhibitors of CYP1A2 (e.g., fluvoxamine) could potentially decrease olanzapine clearance. Although olanzapine is metabolized by multiple enzyme systems, induction or inhibition of a single enzyme may appreciably alter olanzapine clearance. Therefore, an increase or decrease in olanzapine dosage may be necessary during concomitant administration of olanzapine with specific drugs that induce or inhibit olanzapine metabolism, respectively.

Carbamazepine

Carbamazepine therapy (200 mg twice daily for 2 weeks) causes an approximately 50% increase in the clearance of a single, 10-mg dose of olanzapine. The manufacturer of olanzapine states that higher dosages of carbamazepine may cause an even greater increase in olanzapine clearance. Increased clearance of olanzapine probably is caused by carbamazepine-induced induction of CYP1A2 activity.

Selective Serotonin-reuptake Inhibitors

Concomitant administration of fluoxetine (60 mg as a single dose or 60 mg daily for 8 days) with a single 5-mg dose of oral olanzapine caused a small increase in peak plasma olanzapine concentrations (averaging 16%) and a small decrease (averaging 16%) in olanzapine clearance in one study; the elimination half-life was not substantially affected. A similar decrease in olanzapine clearance of 14% was observed in another study with concomitant administration of olanzapine doses of 6 or 12 mg and fluoxetine doses of 25 mg or more. Fluoxetine is an inhibitor of CYP2D6, and thereby may affect a minor metabolic pathway for olanzapine. Although the changes in pharmacokinetics are statistically significant when olanzapine and fluoxetine are given concurrently, the changes are unlikely to be clinically important in comparison to the overall variability observed between individuals; therefore, routine dosage adjustment is not recommended.

Fluvoxamine, a CYP1A2 inhibitor, has been shown to decrease the clearance of olanzapine, which is metabolized by CYP1A2; there is some evidence that fluvoxamine-induced CYP1A2 inhibition is dose dependent. In one pharmacokinetic study, peak plasma olanzapine concentrations increased by an average of 54 and 77% and area under the plasma concentration-time curve (AUC) increased by an average of 52 and 108% in female nonsmokers and male smokers, respectively, when fluvoxamine and olanzapine were administered concomitantly. Symptoms of olanzapine toxicity also have been reported in at least one patient during combined therapy. The manufacturer and some clinicians state that a lower olanzapine dosage should therefore be considered in patients receiving concomitant treatment with fluvoxamine. Preliminary data indicate that concurrent fluvoxamine administration may potentially be used to therapeutic advantage by reducing the daily dosage of olanzapine and thereby the cost of therapy; further controlled studies are needed to more fully evaluate this approach. Although combined therapy with olanzapine and fluvoxamine generally has been well tolerated and may be associated with clinical benefit, some clinicians recommend that caution be exercised and monitoring of plasma olanzapine concentrations be considered in patients receiving these drugs concurrently.

Preliminary results from a therapeutic drug monitoring service suggest that concurrent administration of sertraline and olanzapine does not substantially affect the pharmacokinetics of olanzapine.

Warfarin

Concomitant administration of a single 20-mg dose of warfarin (which has a potential CYP2C9 interaction) and a single oral 10-mg dose of olanzapine did not substantially alter the pharmacokinetics of olanzapine.

• Drugs Metabolized by Hepatic Microsomal Enzymes

In vitro studies utilizing human liver microsomes suggest that olanzapine has little potential to inhibit metabolism of CYP1A2, CYP2C9, CYP2C19, CYP2D6, and CYP3A substrates. Therefore, clinically important drug interactions between olanzapine and drugs metabolized by these isoenzymes are considered unlikely.

• Anticholinergic Agents

Because of the potential for disruption of body temperature regulation, olanzapine should be used with caution in patients concurrently receiving other drugs with anticholinergic activity. (See Body Temperature Regulation under Cautions: Precautions and Contraindications.)

• Levodopa and Dopamine Agonists

Olanzapine may antagonize the effects of levodopa and dopamine agonists.

• Lamotrigine

In a multiple-dose study in healthy individuals, the pharmacokinetics of olanzapine and lamotrigine were not substantially affected when the drugs were administered concomitantly. In another multiple-dose study conducted in healthy volunteers, olanzapine did not substantially alter lamotrigine pharmacokinetics when the drugs were administered concurrently. However, the time to reach maximal plasma concentrations of lamotrigine was substantially prolonged in this study, possibly because of olanzapine's anticholinergic activity. The tolerability of this combination was found to be similar to that of olanzapine alone, with mild sedative effects reported in some patients receiving the drugs concurrently. Although routine dosage adjustment does not appear to be necessary when olanzapine and lamotrigine are given concurrently, adjustment in lamotrigine dosage may be necessary in some patients for therapeutic reasons when olanzapine therapy is initiated or discontinued. In addition, careful monitoring of patients receiving high dosages of olanzapine and lamotrigine has been recommended by some clinicians.

• Other CNS-Active Agents and Alcohol

Because of the prominent CNS actions of olanzapine, the manufacturer states that caution should be exercised when olanzapine is administered concomitantly with other centrally acting drugs and alcohol. The manufacturer also states that concomitant use of olanzapine with CNS agents that are associated with hypotension (e.g., diazepam) may potentiate the orthostatic hypotension associated with olanzapine.

Benzodiazepines

Because of the prominent CNS actions of olanzapine, the manufacturer states that caution should be exercised when olanzapine is administered concomitantly with benzodiazepines. The manufacturer also states that concomitant use of olanzapine and diazepam or other benzodiazepines that are associated with hypotension may potentiate the orthostatic hypotension associated with olanzapine. However, administration of multiple doses of olanzapine did not substantially alter the pharmacokinetics of diazepam or its active metabolite N-desmethyldiazepam.

The pharmacokinetics of olanzapine, unconjugated lorazepam, and total lorazepam were not substantially affected when IM lorazepam (2 mg) was administered 1 hour after IM olanzapine (5 mg); however, increased somnolence was observed with this combination. Hypotension also has been reported when short-acting IM olanzapine and IM lorazepam have been administered concurrently. The manufacturer of olanzapine therefore states that concurrent use of short-acting IM olanzapine in conjunction with parenteral benzodiazepines is not recommended due to the potential for excessive sedation and cardiorespiratory depression.

Tricyclic Antidepressants

Administration of single doses of olanzapine did not substantially affect the pharmacokinetics of imipramine or its active metabolite desipramine.

Lithium

Multiple doses of oral olanzapine (10 mg for 8 days) did not affect the pharmacokinetics of a single dose of lithium. Although combined olanzapine and lithium therapy generally has been well tolerated in controlled clinical studies, rare cases of apparent lithium toxicity and adverse extrapyramidal effects, including oculogyric crisis, have been reported in patients receiving these drugs concurrently; the mechanism(s) for this potential drug interaction remains to be established. The manufacturer of olanzapine states that lithium dosage adjustment is not necessary during concurrent olanzapine administration.

Valproic Acid

In vitro studies using human liver microsomes indicated that olanzapine has little potential to inhibit the major metabolic pathway (glucuronidation) of valproic acid. In addition, valproic acid has little potential effect on the metabolism of olanzapine in vitro. In a pharmacokinetic study, olanzapine administration (10 mg daily for 2 weeks) did not affect the steady-state plasma concentrations of valproic acid. However, substantially decreased plasma olanzapine concentrations have been reported in several patients following initiation of valproate in patients already receiving oral olanzapine; it was suggested that induction of the hepatic enzymes responsible for olanzapine's metabolism by valproate may have been responsible for these findings. Further studies are needed to determine whether a pharmacokinetic interaction exists between olanzapine and valproic acid since these drugs are frequently used in combination in clinical practice. The manufacturer of olanzapine currently states that routine dosage adjustment of valproic acid is not necessary during concurrent olanzapine administration.

Alcohol

In a pharmacokinetic study, concomitant administration of a single dose of alcohol did not substantially alter the steady-state pharmacokinetics of olanzapine (given in dosages of up to 10 mg daily). However, concomitant use of olanzapine with alcohol potentiated the orthostatic hypotension associated with olanzapine. The manufacturer therefore states that alcohol should be avoided during olanzapine therapy.

• Hypotensive Agents

Olanzapine therapy potentially may enhance the effects of certain hypotensive agents during concurrent use. In addition, the administration of dopamine, epinephrine, and/or other sympathomimetic agents with β-agonist activity should be avoided in the treatment of olanzapine-induced hypotension, since such stimulation may worsen hypotension in the presence of olanzapine-induced α-blockade. (See Acute Toxicity: Treatment.)

• Antacids or Cimetidine

In pharmacokinetic studies, single doses of cimetidine (800 mg) or aluminum- and magnesium-containing antacids (30 mL) did not substantially affect the oral bioavailability of a single, 7.5-mg dose of olanzapine.

● Activated Charcoal

Concurrent administration of activated charcoal (1 g) reduced peak plasma concentrations and the AUC of a single, 7.5-mg oral dose of olanzapine by approximately 60%. Since peak plasma concentrations are not usually obtained until about 6 hours after oral administration, activated charcoal may be useful in the management of olanzapine intoxication. (See Acute Toxicity: Treatment.)

● Smoking

The manufacturer states that the clearance of olanzapine in smokers is approximately 40% higher than in nonsmokers. Therefore, plasma olanzapine concentrations generally are lower in smokers than in nonsmokers receiving the drug. Adverse extrapyramidal effects have been reported in one olanzapine-treated patient after a reduction in cigarette smoking, while worsened delusions, hostility, and aggressive behavior have been reported in another olanzapine-treated patient following a marked increase in smoking (i.e., an increase from 12 up to 80 cigarettes per day). Although the precise mechanism(s) for this interaction has not been clearly established, it has been suggested that induction of the CYP isoenzymes, particularly 1A2, by smoke constituents may be responsible at least in part for the reduced plasma olanzapine concentrations observed in smokers compared with nonsmokers.

Although the manufacturer states that routine dosage adjustment is not recommended in patients who smoke while receiving olanzapine, some clinicians recommend that patients treated with olanzapine should be monitored with regard to their smoking consumption and that dosage adjustment be considered in patients who have reduced or increased their smoking and/or who are not responding adequately or who are experiencing dose-related adverse reactions to the drug. In addition, monitoring of plasma olanzapine concentrations may be helpful in patients who smoke and have other factors associated with substantial alterations in metabolism of olanzapine (e.g., geriatric patients, women, concurrent fluvoxamine administration).

● Other Drugs

Multiple doses of olanzapine did not substantially alter the pharmacokinetics of theophylline or its metabolites.

Multiple doses of olanzapine did not substantially affect the pharmacokinetics of biperiden.

ACUTE TOXICITY

● Pathogenesis and Manifestations

The acute lethal dose of olanzapine in humans remains to be established. However, the toxic and lethal doses of olanzapine and other atypical antipsychotic agents appear to be highly variable and depend on concurrent administration of other drugs or toxic substances, patient age and habituation, and the time from exposure until treatment is initiated; pediatric and/or nonhabituated patients appear to be more sensitive to the toxic effects of these drugs.

During premarketing clinical studies of extended-release olanzapine pamoate (Zyprexa® Relprevv), adverse events that presented with signs and symptoms consistent with olanzapine overdosage, particularly sedation (ranging from mild in severity to coma) and/or delirium, were reported following IM injection of the drug. Such cases of post-injection delirium/sedation syndrome (PDSS) occurred in less than 0.1% of injections and in approximately 2% of patients who received injections for up to 46 months. These events were correlated with an unintentional rapid increase in serum olanzapine concentrations to supratherapeutic ranges in some cases. Although a rapid and greater than expected increase in serum olanzapine concentrations has been noted in some patients with these adverse events, the precise mechanism by which the drug was unintentionally introduced into the bloodstream in these cases is not known. Clinical signs and symptoms of PDSS include dizziness, confusion, disorientation, malaise, slurred speech, altered gait, ambulation difficulties, weakness, agitation, extrapyramidal symptoms, hypertension, convulsion, and reduced levels of consciousness ranging from mild sedation to coma. The time after injection to PDSS in the reported cases ranged from soon after the injection to greater than 3 hours after the injection. The majority of patients required hospitalization, and supportive care, including intubation, was necessary in several cases. All patients had largely recovered by 72 hours. Because the risk of PDSS is the same at each injection, the risk per patient is cumulative (i.e., the risk increases with the number of injections). (See Post-injection Delirium/Sedation Syndrome under Cautions: Nervous System Effects and also under Cautions: Precautions and Contraindications.)

In postmarketing reports of overdosage with oral olanzapine alone, symptoms have been reported in the majority of cases. Following acute overdosage of oral olanzapine or other atypical antipsychotic agents, toxic effects usually begin within 1–2 hours and maximal toxic effects usually are seen 4–6 hours following acute ingestion. In general, overdosage of olanzapine may be expected to produce effects that are extensions of its pharmacologic and adverse effects. The most commonly reported manifestations of olanzapine overdosage and those that have occurred in 10% or more of symptomatic patients following postmarketing overdosage reports with olanzapine alone are agitation and/or aggressiveness, dysarthria, tachycardia, anticholinergic syndrome, miosis, various extrapyramidal symptoms, jerking and myoclonus, hypersalivation, and reduced level of consciousness ranging in severity from sedation to coma. Less commonly reported but potentially medically serious events included aspiration, cardiopulmonary arrest, cardiac arrhythmias (e.g., supraventricular tachycardia), delirium, possible neuroleptic malignant syndrome, respiratory depression and/or arrest, convulsions, hypertension, and hypotension (including orthostatic hypotension); one patient experienced sinus pause with spontaneous resumption of normal rhythm. Fatalities in association with overdosage of oral olanzapine alone have been reported. In one such case, the amount of acutely ingested oral olanzapine was reported to be possibly as low as 450 mg of oral olanzapine; however, in another case, a patient reportedly survived an acute ingestion of approximately 2 g of oral olanzapine.

In some cases of acute olanzapine intoxication, rapid fluctuation in mental status (i.e., between sedation and agitation or agitation despite sedation) has been reported. In addition, olanzapine overdosage may resemble opiate overdosage because CNS depression and miosis sometimes are observed. Increased creatine kinase (CK, creatine phosphokinase, CPK) concentrations also have occurred following acute olanzapine overdosage. Cardiac arrhythmias, persistent choreoathetosis, nonconvulsive status epilepticus, hypersalivation, and coma occurred in an adult following an intentional ingestion estimated to be 750 mg of olanzapine; both coma and choreoathetosis persisted until the patient's death 8 weeks later.

The toxic effects of olanzapine and other atypical antipsychotic agents in pediatric patients appear to be similar to those seen in adults. In young children, marked CNS depression and anticholinergic delirium have occurred following ingestion of 7.5–15 mg of olanzapine (equivalent to 0.5–1 mg/kg). In an adolescent who ingested 275 mg of olanzapine and had an extremely high serum olanzapine concentration (1503 ng/mL), somnolence, agitation, and extrapyramidal symptoms developed initially, but the patient recovered without complications. A 400-mg olanzapine overdosage in another adolescent reportedly produced severe respiratory depression requiring intubation and mechanical ventilation; the patient recovered after 3 days. In addition, polyuria and other signs suggesting possible diabetes insipidus, including hypoosmolar urine, normoosmolar plasma, and increased serum sodium concentrations, have been reported in one adolescent following an overdosage of olanzapine and prazepam (a benzodiazepine; not commercially available in the US).

● Treatment

Clinicians should be aware that post-injection delirium/sedation syndrome (PDSS) may occur with any IM injection of extended-release olanzapine pamoate (Zyprexa® Relprevv). Signs and symptoms consistent with olanzapine overdosage have been observed in such cases, and access to emergency response services must be readily available for safe use.

Management of olanzapine overdosage generally involves symptomatic and supportive care, including continuous cardiovascular and respiratory monitoring and ensuring IV access. Cardiovascular monitoring should be initiated immediately and should include continuous ECG monitoring to detect possible arrhythmias. There is no specific antidote for olanzapine intoxication. In managing olanzapine overdosage, the clinician should consider the possibility of multiple drug intoxication.

The manufacturer and many clinicians recommend establishing and maintaining an airway and ensuring adequate ventilation and oxygenation, which may include intubation. Gastric lavage (following intubation, if the patient is unconscious) and/or activated charcoal, which may be used with sorbitol, should be considered. (See Drug Interactions: Activated Charcoal.) The possibility that obtundation, seizures, or dystonic reaction of the head and neck following olanzapine overdosage may create a risk of aspiration with induction of emesis should be considered.

Hypotension and circulatory collapse, if present, should be treated with appropriate measures, such as Trendelenburg's position, IV fluids, and/or sympathomimetic agents (e.g., norepinephrine, phenylephrine). However, dopamine, epinephrine, and/or other sympathomimetic agents with β-adrenergic agonist activity should be avoided, since such stimulation may worsen hypotension in the presence of olanzapine-induced α-adrenergic blockade. Tachycardia associated with olanzapine intoxication usually does not require specific therapy. Atrial and ventricular arrhythmias and conduction disturbances should be treated with appropriate measures; sodium bicarbonate may be helpful if QRS-interval prolongation is present. Seizures following olanzapine overdosage may be treated initially with a benzodiazepine followed by barbiturates, if necessary. Acute extrapyramidal reactions should be treated with anticholinergic agents (e.g., diphenhydramine, benztropine).

Physostigmine salicylate or benzodiazepine therapy may be useful in the management of severe agitation and delirium in patients with severe anticholinergic toxicity and a narrow QRS complex on their ECG. Physostigmine has been used successfully in the treatment of anticholinergic toxicity associated with overdosages of olanzapine or clozapine, another atypical antipsychotic agent. However, experience with physostigmine in the management of atypical antipsychotic overdosage is limited, and some clinicians recommend that the drug be used only by experienced clinicians and in cases in which the potential therapeutic benefit outweighs the potential risks.

Resolution of toxic effects following atypical antipsychotic intoxication generally occurs within 12–48 hours following acute overdosage, although it has taken up to 6 days. Patients should remain under close medical supervision and monitoring until fully recovered.

Hemodialysis has not been shown to be useful for enhancing elimination of olanzapine in acute overdosage. Clinical experience with other enhanced elimination techniques, including multiple-dose activated charcoal, hemoperfusion, forced diuresis, and urinary alkalinization, is lacking; however, these treatments also are unlikely to be beneficial following olanzapine overdosage because of the drug's large volume of distribution and extensive protein binding.

In animal studies prospectively designed to assess abuse and dependence potential, olanzapine was shown to produce acute CNS depressive effects but little or no potential for abuse or physical dependence in rats administered oral doses up to 15 times the maximum recommended human daily oral dosage (20 mg) and rhesus monkeys administered oral doses up to 8 times the maximum recommended human daily oral dosage on a mg/m² basis. Olanzapine has not been systematically evaluated in humans to date for its potential for abuse, tolerance, or physical dependence. While clinical trials did not reveal any tendency for drug-seeking behavior, these observations were not systematic, and it is not possible to predict on the basis of this limited experience the extent to which a CNS-active drug will be misused, diverted, and/or abused once marketed. Consequently, patients should be evaluated carefully for a history of drug abuse, and such patients should be observed closely for signs of misuse or abuse of olanzapine (e.g., development of tolerance, increases in dose, drug-seeking behavior).

PHARMACOLOGY

Olanzapine is a thienobenzodiazepine-derivative antipsychotic agent. The drug shares some of the pharmacologic actions of other antipsychotic agents and has been described as an atypical or second-generation antipsychotic agent. Like other atypical or second-generation antipsychotics (e.g., aripiprazole, asenapine, clozapine, quetiapine, risperidone, ziprasidone), olanzapine is less likely to cause adverse extrapyramidal effects and tardive dyskinesia than conventional (first-generation) antipsychotic agents, and is effective in the treatment of positive, negative, and depressive manifestations of schizophrenia.

● Nervous System Effects

The exact mechanism of antipsychotic action of olanzapine and other atypical antipsychotic agents has not been fully elucidated but appears to be more complex than that of conventional, first-generation antipsychotic agents and may involve central antagonism at serotonin type 2 (5-hydroxytryptamine [5-HT$_{2A}$, 5-HT$_{2C}$]), type 3 (5-HT$_3$), and type 6 (5-HT$_6$) and dopamine receptors.

The exact mechanism(s) of action of olanzapine in the treatment of acute manic or mixed episodes associated with bipolar disorder is not fully known. However, it has been suggested that the ability of olanzapine to block and downregulate 5-HT$_{2A}$ receptors may play a role in its antimanic activity. In addition, olanzapine's mood-stabilizing action may be caused at least in part by antagonism

of D$_2$ receptors. Further studies are needed to more clearly elucidate the potential mechanism(s) of the drug's antimanic activity.

Although not clearly established, the efficacy of IM olanzapine in the treatment of acute agitation appears to be due at least in part to its distinct calming effects rather than solely to nonspecific sedation.

Antidopaminergic Effects

The therapeutic effects of antipsychotic drugs are thought to be mediated by dopaminergic blockade in the mesolimbic and mesocortical areas of the CNS, while antidopaminergic effects in the neostriatum appear to be associated with extrapyramidal effects. The relatively low incidence of extrapyramidal effects associated with olanzapine therapy suggests that the drug is more active in the mesolimbic than the neostriatal dopaminergic system.

Several (at least 5) different types or subtypes of dopamine receptors have been identified in animals or humans. The relative densities of these receptors and their distribution and function vary for different neuroanatomical regions, and olanzapine's effects may be secondary to regionally specific receptor interactions and/or other effects on dopaminergic neurons. Current evidence suggests that the clinical potency and antipsychotic efficacy of both typical and atypical antipsychotic drugs generally are related at least in part to their affinity for and blockade of central dopamine D$_2$ receptors. Some studies suggest that clinically effective dosages of most antipsychotic agents result in occupation of between 60 and 80% of central dopamine D$_2$ receptors. However, antagonism at D$_2$ receptors does not appear to account fully for the antipsychotic effects of olanzapine. In vivo and in vitro studies have demonstrated that olanzapine is a comparatively weak antagonist at D$_2$ receptors. Although their role in eliciting the pharmacologic effects of antipsychotic agents remains to be fully elucidated, dopamine D$_3$, D$_4$, and D$_5$ receptors also have been identified. Olanzapine may have a higher affinity for D$_4$ receptors than for D$_2$ or D$_3$ receptors. K$_I$ values of olanzapine for dopamine D$_{1-4}$ receptors range from 11–31 nM.

Atypical antipsychotic agents generally have demonstrated relatively loose binding to dopamine D$_2$ receptors. Compared with typical antipsychotic agents, atypical antipsychotics appear to have faster dissociation rates from and lower affinity for dopamine D$_2$ receptors, which may result in fewer adverse extrapyramidal effects and less risk of elevated prolactin concentrations; however, further studies are needed to confirm these initial findings.

Serotonergic Effects

It has been suggested that schizophrenia may involve a dysregulation of serotonin- and/or dopamine-mediated neurotransmission, and olanzapine may at least partially restore a normal balance of neurotransmitter function, possibly through serotonergic modulation of dopaminergic tone. Olanzapine blocks serotonin type 2 (5-hydroxytryptamine [5-HT$_{2A}$ and 5-HT$_{2C}$; K$_I$ of 4 and 11 nM, respectively]), type 3 (5-HT$_3$; K$_I$ of 57 nM), and type 6 (5-HT$_6$; K$_I$ of 5 nM) receptors.

Anticholinergic Effects

Olanzapine blocks muscarinic cholinergic receptors and has demonstrated moderate affinity for all 5 muscarinic receptor subtypes (K$_I$ values for M$_{1-5}$ were 73, 96, 132, 32, and 48 nM, respectively). Anticholinergic activity in antipsychotic agents may contribute to certain adverse anticholinergic events associated with these drugs but also may help reduce the risk of adverse extrapyramidal reactions.

Effects on Other Central Neurotransmitters

Antagonism at receptors other than dopamine and 5-HT$_2$ receptors may produce some of the therapeutic and adverse effects associated with olanzapine. Olanzapine exhibits α$_1$-adrenergic blocking activity (K$_I$ of 19 nM), which may explain the occasional orthostatic hypotension associated with the drug. In addition, olanzapine blocks histamine H$_1$ receptors (K$_I$ of 7 nM), which may explain the sedative effects associated with the drug; affinity for H$_2$ and H$_3$ receptors appears to be low.

Olanzapine demonstrated weak binding affinity (K$_I$ exceeding 10 μM) for β-adrenergic, γ-aminobutyric acid (GABA), and benzodiazepine receptors; the drug also has little or no affinity for opiate receptors.

Neurophysiologic Effects

In vivo electrophysiologic studies demonstrate different sensitivities of various brain areas to antipsychotic-mediated postsynaptic receptor blockade. While conventional antipsychotics generally reduce spontaneous firing activity in both the mesolimbic (A10) and nigrostriatal regions (A9), chronic administration of atypical antipsychotics generally reduces the number of spontaneously active dopaminergic neurons in the mesolimbic region but not in the nigrostriatal region. Although not clearly established, it has been suggested that the ability to decrease A10 but not A9 neurons is associated clinically with a low potential to cause adverse extrapyramidal reactions and tardive dyskinesia. Olanzapine has demonstrated such mesolimbic selectivity in the in vivo studies conducted to date.

Cognitive Effects in Humans

Clinical experience suggests that second-generation antipsychotics, including olanzapine, improve cognition in patients with schizophrenia and that there may be differences between these drugs in their effects on neurocognitive functioning. In an initial clinical trial evaluating the short-term effects of atypical antipsychotic agents on cognitive function, olanzapine-treated schizophrenic patients demonstrated improved learning and memory, verbal fluency, and executive function. In a controlled clinical trial evaluating the neurocognitive effects of olanzapine, clozapine, risperidone, and haloperidol in patients with treatment-resistant schizophrenia or schizoaffective disorder, global neurocognitive function improved with olanzapine and risperidone treatment, and these improvements were found to be superior to those seen with haloperidol. Patients treated with olanzapine exhibited improvement in the general and attention domains but not more than that observed with the other antipsychotic agents. In another controlled trial, patients with schizophrenia receiving long-term (1 year) therapy with olanzapine demonstrated improved results on a general cognition index compared with those receiving haloperidol and risperidone. Neurocognition also improved in olanzapine- and risperidone-treated schizophrenic and schizoaffective patients receiving the drug for 1 year in another controlled study; improvements in executive function, learning and memory, processing speed, attention and vigilance, verbal working memory, and motor function were reported. The clinical relevance of these cognitive findings in the management of schizophrenia remains to be determined and requires further study.

EEG Effects

Olanzapine may cause EEG changes. In one study, olanzapine-induced EEG slowing to a lesser extent than clozapine in patients with schizophrenia and did not appear to substantially alter epileptiform activity in most of the patients studied; further studies are needed to determine whether olanzapine can affect the seizure threshold. Similarly, a comparative study found that epileptiform activity did not increase during olanzapine therapy; however, EEG slowing and other nonspecific EEG changes did occur more frequently in olanzapine-treated patients than in those receiving certain other antipsychotic agents. In another study that was retrospective in design, EEG changes occurred more frequently in patients receiving olanzapine or clozapine than in those receiving typical antipsychotic agents, quetiapine, or risperidone. In a study in patients with schizophrenia, olanzapine therapy was associated with increased rates of slow waves, sharp waves, and paroxysmal slow wave discharges on EEG recordings in the patients evaluated; however, spike- and sharp-slow-wave complexes that indicate seizure risk were not observed in this study.

Seizures have been reported rarely in olanzapine-treated patients but confounding factors were present in most of these cases. Further studies and postmarketing surveillance are needed to determine whether olanzapine can affect the seizure threshold and to evaluate the clinical relevance of the observed EEG findings in patients receiving the drug.

Effects on Sleep

The available evidence suggests that atypical antipsychotics, including olanzapine, clozapine, and risperidone, substantially increase total sleep time and stage 2 sleep; both olanzapine and risperidone also have been shown to enhance slow-wave sleep. Olanzapine's beneficial effects on sleep quality are thought to be mediated principally via type 2 serotonergic (5-HT_2) receptors.

In a controlled study, administration of single evening doses of olanzapine (5 or 10 mg orally) in healthy individuals significantly increased slow-wave sleep in a dose-related manner; sleep continuity measures and subjective sleep quality also increased significantly. Single 10-mg doses of the drug also suppressed rapid eye movement (REM) sleep and increased REM sleep latency in this study. In another study in healthy males and females, single 10-mg oral doses of olanzapine also were found to increase slow-wave sleep but preserved the normal structure of sleep; these effects were more prominent in females than in males.

During subchronic administration of olanzapine (15–20 mg) in patients with schizophrenia with predominantly negative symptoms in an uncontrolled study, parameters of sleep efficiency improved and delta sleep and REM sleep increased. Acute olanzapine administration (10 mg orally) in schizophrenic patients improved sleep continuity variables and total sleep time in another study; the principal changes observed in sleep architecture were a reduction in stage 1 sleep, a significant enhancement in stage 2 and delta sleep, and an increase in REM density. In a study comparing the effect of aging on the improvement of subjective sleep quality in patients with schizophrenia receiving atypical antipsychotic agents, including olanzapine, the proportion of patients experiencing improved subjective sleep quality was significantly higher in geriatric patients than in middle-aged patients.

● Neuroendocrine Effects

In contrast to conventional (first-generation) antipsychotic agents and similar to many other atypical antipsychotic agents, olanzapine therapy in usual dosages generally produces transient elevations in serum prolactin concentrations in humans. This prolactin-elevating effect appears to be mediated by dopamine blockade. The effect of atypical antipsychotic agents on prolactin generally appears to be transient, possibly because the drugs appear to dissociate from dopamine receptors more rapidly than conventional antipsychotic agents.

● Antiemetic Effects

Although the precise mechanism of olanzapine's antiemetic action has not been clearly established, its inhibitory activity at multiple dopaminergic and serotonergic receptors, particularly the D_2, 5-HT_{2C}, and 5-HT_3 receptors that may be involved in nausea and vomiting, may play a role in the drug's efficacy in both the prevention and rescue therapy of chemotherapy-induced nausea and vomiting†.

PHARMACOKINETICS

● Absorption

Olanzapine is well absorbed following oral administration. However, because of extensive first-pass metabolism, only about 60% of an orally administered dose reaches systemic circulation unchanged. Olanzapine exhibits linear and dose-proportional pharmacokinetics when given orally within the clinical dosage range. Food does not appear to affect the rate or the extent of GI absorption of the drug. The relative oral bioavailability of olanzapine has been shown to be equivalent following administration of the conventional and orally disintegrating tablets of the drug.

When olanzapine and fluoxetine hydrochloride are administered as the fixed-combination oral capsules, the pharmacokinetic characteristics of the drugs are expected to resemble those of the individual components; olanzapine pharmacokinetics are slightly altered when administered with fluoxetine, but the effects were not deemed to be clinically important. (See Selective Serotonin-reuptake Inhibitors under Drug Interactions: Drugs Affecting Hepatic Microsomal Enzymes.)

Following oral administration, peak plasma olanzapine concentrations occur in approximately 6 hours (range: 5–8 hours). Steady-state plasma concentrations of olanzapine are achieved after approximately 7 days of continuous dosing and are approximately twice those observed following single-dose administration.

Following IM administration of short-acting olanzapine injection (Zyprexa® IntraMuscular), olanzapine is rapidly absorbed with peak plasma olanzapine concentrations occurring within 15–45 minutes. In one pharmacokinetic study performed in healthy individuals, a single 5-mg IM dose of olanzapine produced peak plasma concentrations that were an average of approximately fivefold higher than the peak plasma concentrations produced following a single 5-mg oral dose of the drug. In this study, the areas under the plasma concentration-time curve (AUCs) achieved following IM and oral administration of the same dose of the drug were similar. Olanzapine exhibits linear pharmacokinetics when given IM within the clinical dosage range. Preliminary evidence suggests that the onset of antipsychotic action following IM administration of the drug is evident within 24 hours but may be observed as early as 2 hours after IM administration.

Following deep IM gluteal administration of extended-release olanzapine pamoate injection (Zyprexa® Relprevv), slow dissolution of the pamoate ester (which is practically insoluble) results in prolonged plasma olanzapine concentrations over a period of weeks to months. An IM injection every 2 or 4 weeks provides plasma olanzapine concentrations that are similar to those achieved with daily doses of oral olanzapine. Steady-state plasma concentrations achieved with extended-release olanzapine pamoate injection in IM dosages of 150–405 mg every 2 or 4 weeks are within the range achieved with oral olanzapine dosages of 5–20 mg daily. Plasma olanzapine concentrations generally reach a peak within the first week following each injection.

Plasma olanzapine concentrations may vary between individuals according to gender, smoking status, and age. There is limited evidence that gender may affect plasma olanzapine concentrations, with concentrations being somewhat higher, perhaps by as much as 30–40%, in females compared with males. Plasma concentrations of olanzapine also may be increased in geriatric individuals compared with younger individuals, possibly as a result of age-related decreases in hepatic elimination of the drug. Data from one limited study in children and adolescents 10–18 years of age with schizophrenia found that plasma olanzapine concentrations among adolescents were within the range reported in nonsmoking adult patients with schizophrenia. However, the manufacturer states that most adolescents (i.e., 13–17 years of age) in clinical studies were nonsmokers and had a lower average body weight, which resulted in higher average olanzapine exposure compared with adults. In vivo studies have shown that exposures to olanzapine are similar among Japanese, Chinese, and Caucasian individuals, particularly after normalization for body weight differences.

The therapeutic range for plasma olanzapine concentrations and the relationship of plasma concentration to clinical response and toxicity have not been clearly established; however, acutely ill schizophrenic patients with 24-hour post-dose plasma olanzapine concentrations of 9.3 ng/mL or higher in one study or 12-hour post-dose concentrations of 23.2 ng/mL or higher in another study appeared to have a better clinical response to therapy than patients with lower plasma concentrations.

● Distribution

Distribution of olanzapine, a highly lipophilic drug, into human body tissues is extensive.

The manufacturer states that the volume of distribution of olanzapine has been reported to be approximately 1000 L. In pharmacokinetic studies in healthy individuals, the apparent volume of distribution of the drug averaged 1150 L and ranged from 660 to 1790 L for the fifth to 95th percentiles. Olanzapine is 93% bound to plasma proteins over the concentration range of 7–1100 ng/mL, principally to albumin and α_1-acid glycoprotein.

Olanzapine and its glucuronide metabolite have been shown to cross the placenta in humans. Placental transfer of olanzapine also has been shown to occur in rat pups.

Olanzapine is distributed into milk. The manufacturer states that in a study in lactating, healthy women, the average infant dose of olanzapine at steady-state was estimated to be approximately 1.8% of the maternal olanzapine dose. In a separate study that evaluated the extent of infant exposure to olanzapine in 7 breastfeeding women who had been receiving 5–20 mg of olanzapine daily for periods ranging from 19–395 days, median and maximum relative infant doses of 1 and 1.2%, respectively, were observed. Olanzapine was not detected in the plasma of the breast-fed infants, and adverse effects possibly related to olanzapine exposure were not reported in the infants in this study. In addition, peak milk concentrations were achieved a median of 5.2 hours later than the corresponding maximal maternal plasma concentrations. In a case report, a relative infant dose of approximately 4% was estimated in one woman after 4 and 10 days (estimated to be at steady state) of olanzapine therapy at a dosage of 20 mg daily based on measurements of drug concentration in serum and in expressed breast milk. (See Cautions: Pregnancy, Fertility, and Lactation.)

● Elimination

Although the exact metabolic fate has not been clearly established, it appears that olanzapine is extensively metabolized. Following a single oral dose of radiolabeled olanzapine, 7% of the dose was recovered in urine as unchanged drug. Approximately 57 and 30% of the dose was recovered in the urine and feces, respectively.

In plasma, olanzapine accounted for only 12% of the AUC for total radioactivity, suggesting substantial exposure to metabolites. After multiple doses of olanzapine, the principal circulating metabolites are the 10-N-glucuronide, which is present at steady state at 44% of the plasma concentration of the parent drug, and 4′-N-desmethyl olanzapine, which is present at steady state at 31% of the plasma concentration of olanzapine. Both of these metabolites lack pharmacologic activity at the concentrations observed.

Direct glucuronidation and cytochrome P-450 (CYP)-mediated oxidation are the principal pathways for olanzapine metabolism. In vitro studies suggest that the CYP isoenzymes 1A2 and 2D6 and the flavin-containing monooxygenase system are involved in the oxidation of olanzapine. However, CYP2D6-mediated oxidation appears to be a minor metabolic pathway for olanzapine in vivo since the clearance of the drug is not reduced in individuals deficient in this enzyme.

Following oral administration, olanzapine has an elimination half-life ranging from 21 to 54 hours for the fifth to 95th percentiles of individual values with a mean of 30 hours. Following IM administration of short-acting olanzapine injection (Zyprexa® IntraMuscular), the half-life and metabolic profile of olanzapine were similar to those observed with oral administration. Following IM administration of extended-release olanzapine pamoate injection (Zyprexa® Relprevv), the elimination half-life is approximately 30 days. Therefore, exposure to olanzapine may persist for months after a single extended-release IM injection of the drug.

The apparent plasma clearance of olanzapine ranges from 12 to 47 L/hour (mean: 25 L/hour).

The clearance of olanzapine in smokers is approximately 40% higher than in nonsmokers. (See Drug Interactions: Smoking.)

The clearance of olanzapine in females may be reduced by approximately 30% compared with males.

In a single-dose pharmacokinetic study, the elimination half-life of orally administered olanzapine was 1.5 times longer in healthy geriatric individuals 65 years of age or older than in healthy younger adults. (See Dosage and Administration: Dosage and see also Cautions: Geriatric Precautions.)

In one pharmacokinetic study conducted in a limited number of children and adolescents 10–18 years of age with schizophrenia who were treated with oral olanzapine, the apparent plasma clearance at steady-state averaged 9.6 L/hr, which was approximately half of the clearance values reported in adult studies but similar to clearance values reported in nonsmoking male and female schizophrenic patients. The elimination half-life averaged 37.2 hours in this same study. (See Dosage and Administration: Dosage and see also Cautions: Pediatric Precautions.)

The combined effects of age, smoking, and gender could result in substantial pharmacokinetic differences in populations. The clearance in younger, smoking adult male patients may be 3 times higher than that in geriatric, nonsmoking females. Dosage adjustment may be necessary in patients who exhibit a combination of factors that may result in slower metabolism of olanzapine. (See Dosage and Administration: Dosage.)

Because olanzapine is extensively metabolized before excretion and only 7% of the drug is excreted unchanged, renal impairment alone is unlikely to substantially alter the pharmacokinetics of olanzapine. The pharmacokinetics of olanzapine were similar in patients with severe renal impairment and healthy individuals, suggesting that dosage adjustment based upon the degree of renal impairment is not necessary. The effect of renal impairment on the elimination of olanzapine's metabolites has not been evaluated to date.

Although the presence of hepatic impairment would be expected to reduce the clearance of olanzapine, a pharmacokinetic study evaluating the effect of impaired hepatic function in individuals with clinically important cirrhosis (Child-Pugh classification A and B) revealed little effect on the pharmacokinetics of olanzapine.

Olanzapine is not appreciably removed by hemodialysis, probably due to its large volume of distribution and extensive protein binding. Clinical experience with other enhanced elimination techniques, including multiple-dose activated charcoal, hemoperfusion, forced diuresis, and urinary alkalinization, is lacking; however, these treatments are unlikely to be beneficial following olanzapine overdosage because of the drug's large volume of distribution and extensive protein binding.

CHEMISTRY AND STABILITY

● Chemistry

Olanzapine is a thienobenzodiazepine-derivative antipsychotic agent. The drug is considered an atypical or second-generation antipsychotic agent. Olanzapine is structurally similar to clozapine.

Olanzapine occurs as a yellow crystalline solid that is practically insoluble in water.

Olanzapine for injection (short-acting) contains lactose monohydrate and tartaric acid; hydrochloric acid and/or sodium hydroxide may have been added to adjust pH. When olanzapine for injection is reconstituted as directed, the resulting solution should appear clear and yellow.

● Stability

Commercially available olanzapine conventional tablets, orally disintegrating tablets, and short-acting olanzapine for IM injection should be stored at a controlled room temperature of 20–25°C but may be exposed to temperatures ranging from 15–30°C. Olanzapine orally disintegrating tablets should be stored in their original sealed blister. The conventional and orally disintegrating tablets should be protected from light and moisture and olanzapine for injection should be protected from light and freezing. Extended-release olanzapine pamoate for IM injection should be stored at room temperature (not to exceed 30°C).

Following reconstitution, olanzapine for injection (short-acting) may be stored at a controlled room temperature of 20–25°C for up to 1 hour if necessary, but immediate use is preferred.

Following reconstitution, extended-release olanzapine pamoate injection suspension may be stored at room temperature for 24 hours. The vial should be agitated immediately prior to withdrawal of the suspension.

Olanzapine orally disintegrating tablets contain aspartame (e.g., NutraSweet®). (See Individuals with Phenylketonuria, under Cautions: Precautions and Contraindications.)

Olanzapine for IM injection (short-acting) should not be combined with diazepam injection in a syringe because precipitation occurs when these drugs are mixed. Olanzapine for IM injection also should not be combined in a syringe with haloperidol injection because the resulting pH has been shown to degrade olanzapine over time. In addition, lorazepam injection should not be used to reconstitute olanzapine for injection since this delays reconstitution time. Specialized references should be consulted for additional specific compatibility information.

PREPARATIONS

Long-acting IM olanzapine pamoate (Zyprexa® Relprevv) is available only through a restricted distribution program. (See Restricted Distribution under Dosage and Administration: Reconstitution and Administration.)

Excipients in commercially available drug preparations may have clinically important effects in some individuals; consult specific product labeling for details.

OLANZapine

Oral

Tablets, film-coated	2.5 mg*	ZyPREXA®, Lilly
	5 mg*	ZyPREXA®, Lilly
	7.5 mg*	ZyPREXA®, Lilly
	10 mg*	ZyPREXA®, Lilly
	15 mg*	ZyPREXA®, Lilly
	20 mg*	ZyPREXA®, Lilly
Tablets, orally disintegrating	5 mg*	ZyPREXA® Zydis®, Lilly
	10 mg*	ZyPREXA® Zydis®, Lilly
	15 mg*	ZyPREXA® Zydis®, Lilly
	20 mg*	ZyPREXA® Zydis®, Lilly

Parenteral

For injection, for IM use only	10 mg*	ZyPREXA® IntraMuscular, Lilly

* available from one or more manufacturer, distributor, and/or repackager by generic (nonproprietary) name

OLANZapine Combinations

Oral

Capsules	3 mg with Fluoxetine Hydrochloride 25 mg (of fluoxetine)*	Symbyax®, Lilly
	6 mg with Fluoxetine Hydrochloride 25 mg (of fluoxetine)*	Symbyax®, Lilly
	6 mg with Fluoxetine Hydrochloride 50 mg (of fluoxetine)*	Symbyax®, Lilly
	12 mg with Fluoxetine Hydrochloride 25 mg (of fluoxetine)*	Symbyax®, Lilly
	12 mg with Fluoxetine Hydrochloride 50 mg (of fluoxetine)*	Symbyax®, Lilly

* available from one or more manufacturer, distributor, and/or repackager by generic (nonproprietary) name

OLANZapine Pamoate

Parenteral

For injectable suspension, extended-release, for IM use only	210 mg (of olanzapine)	ZyPREXA® Relprevv (available as a convenience kit containing single-use vial, needles, syringe, and diluent), Lilly
	300 mg (of olanzapine)	ZyPREXA® Relprevv (available as a convenience kit containing single-use vial, needles, syringe, and diluent), Lilly
	405 mg (of olanzapine)	ZyPREXA® Relprevv (available as a convenience kit containing single-use vial, needles, syringe, and diluent), Lilly

† Use is not currently included in the labeling approved by the US Food and Drug Administration.

Selected Revisions November 12, 2018, © Copyright, June 1, 1997, American Society of Health-System Pharmacists, Inc.

Paliperidone

28:16.08.04 • ATYPICAL ANTIPSYCHOTICS

■ Paliperidone is considered an atypical or second-generation antipsychotic agent.

USES

● Psychotic Disorders

Paliperidone is used for the symptomatic management of psychotic disorders (e.g., schizophrenia). Drug therapy is integral to the management of acute psychotic episodes in patients with schizophrenia and generally is required for long-term stabilization to sustain symptom remission or control and to minimize the risk of relapse. Antipsychotic agents are the principal class of drugs used for the management of all phases of schizophrenia. Patient response and tolerance to antipsychotic agents are variable, and patients who do not respond to or tolerate one drug may be successfully treated with an agent from a different class or with a different adverse effect profile.

Schizophrenia

Paliperidone is used orally for the acute and maintenance treatment of schizophrenia in adults and adolescents 12–17 years of age. Schizophrenia is a major psychotic disorder that frequently has devastating effects on various aspects of the patient's life and carries a high risk of suicide and other life-threatening behaviors. Manifestations of schizophrenia involve multiple psychologic processes, including perception (e.g., hallucinations), ideation, reality testing (e.g., delusions), emotion (e.g., flatness, inappropriate affect), thought processes (e.g., loose associations), behavior (e.g., catatonia, disorganization), attention, concentration, motivation (e.g., avolition, impaired intention and planning), and judgment. The principal manifestations of this disorder usually are described in terms of positive and negative (deficit) symptoms, and more recently, disorganized symptoms. Positive symptoms include hallucinations, delusions, bizarre behavior, hostility, uncooperativeness, and paranoid ideation, while negative symptoms include restricted range and intensity of emotional expression (affective flattening), reduced thought and speech productivity (alogia), anhedonia, apathy, and decreased initiation of goal-directed behavior (avolition). Disorganized symptoms include disorganized speech (thought disorder) and behavior and poor attention.

The short-term efficacy of paliperidone in the acute treatment of schizophrenia in adults was established in 3 placebo-controlled and active comparator (olanzapine)-controlled, fixed-dose clinical trials of 6 weeks' duration in 1665 adult patients with schizophrenia. In these 3 studies, patients receiving paliperidone (3–15 mg daily as extended-release tablets) demonstrated substantially greater improvement in the Positive and Negative Syndrome Scale (PANSS) than did patients receiving placebo. The mean effects at all dosages (3, 6, 9, 12, and 15 mg daily) were fairly similar, although higher dosages produced numerically superior results. Paliperidone also was found to be superior to placebo in improving scores on the Personal and Social Performance (PSP) scale in these trials.

In a longer-term study, adult outpatients with schizophrenia who had clinically responded to oral paliperidone and who had received a stable fixed dosage of the drug for 2 weeks entered a 6-week, open-label, stabilization phase where they received a paliperidone dosage from 3–15 mg once daily as extended-release tablets. After the stabilization phase, patients were randomized in a double-blind manner to either continue receiving paliperidone at their stable dosage or to receive placebo until they experienced a relapse of schizophrenia symptoms. The median treatment exposure during this double-blind phase was 45 days for extended-release paliperidone and 29 days for placebo; the mean paliperidone dosage was approximately 11 mg daily throughout the phases of this trial. An interim analysis of the data showed a significantly longer time to relapse in the paliperidone-treated patients compared with those receiving placebo. In addition, 25% of the paliperidone-treated patients experienced a relapse of schizophrenia symptoms compared with 53% of those receiving placebo. The study was stopped early because maintenance of efficacy was demonstrated. If paliperidone is used for extended periods, the need for continued therapy should be reassessed periodically on an individualized basis. (See Dosage and Administration: Dosage.)

Short-term efficacy and safety of oral paliperidone in the acute treatment of schizophrenia in adolescents 12–17 years of age were established in a double-blind, placebo-controlled trial of 6 weeks' duration in 201 patients who met DSM-IV criteria for schizophrenia. The trial used a fixed-dosage, weight-based treatment group design over a dosage range of 1.5–12 mg once daily given as extended-release tablets. Patients were randomized to one of 4 treatment groups: a placebo group or a low-dosage (1.5 mg daily for all body weights), medium-dosage (3 or 6 mg daily depending on body weight), or high-dosage group (6 or 12 mg daily depending on body weight). Efficacy was evaluated using the PANSS. The study demonstrated the overall efficacy of paliperidone in adolescents with schizophrenia receiving dosages ranging from 3–12 mg once daily. However, no clear improvement in efficacy was observed at the higher dosages studied (i.e., 6 mg daily for adolescents weighing less than 51 kg and 12 mg daily for adolescents weighing 51 kg or more). Tolerability was adequate within the 3–12 mg daily dosage range; however, adverse effects were dose related. Longer-term efficacy and safety of extended-release paliperidone in adolescent patients with schizophrenia are currently being evaluated in clinical studies.

The American Psychiatric Association (APA) considers most atypical antipsychotic agents first-line drugs for the management of the acute phase of schizophrenia (including first psychotic episodes), principally because of the decreased risk of adverse extrapyramidal effects and tardive dyskinesia, with the understanding that the relative advantages, disadvantages, and cost-effectiveness of conventional and atypical antipsychotic agents remain controversial. The APA states that, with the possible exception of clozapine for the management of treatment-resistant symptoms, there currently is no definitive evidence that one atypical antipsychotic agent will have superior efficacy compared with another agent in the class, although meaningful differences in response may be observed in individual patients. Conventional antipsychotic agents may be considered first-line therapy in patients who have been treated successfully in the past with or who prefer conventional agents. The choice of an antipsychotic agent should be individualized, considering past response to therapy, adverse effect profile (including the patient's experience of subjective effects such as dysphoria), and the patient's preference for a specific drug, including route of administration.

For additional information on the symptomatic management of schizophrenia, including treatment recommendations and results of the Clinical Antipsychotic Trials of Intervention Effectiveness (CATIE) research program, see Schizophrenia and Other Psychotic Disorders under Uses: Psychotic Disorders, in the Phenothiazines General Statement 28:16.08.24.

● Schizoaffective Disorder

Paliperidone is used orally for the treatment of schizoaffective disorder as monotherapy and as an adjunct to mood stabilizers and/or antidepressant therapy in adults.

The acute efficacy of paliperidone in the treatment of schizoaffective disorder was principally established in 2 international, double-blind, placebo-controlled trials of 6 weeks' duration in nonelderly adults. Patients enrolled in these trials met DSM-IV criteria for schizoaffective disorder, had a PANSS total score of at least 60, and had prominent mood symptoms (confirmed by a score of at least 16 on the Young Mania Rating Scale [YMRS] and/or Hamilton Rating Scale for Depression [HRSD]). The patients in these trials included individuals with schizoaffective disorder bipolar and depressive types. In the first trial, efficacy was assessed in 211 patients who received flexible dosages of paliperidone (3–12 mg once daily as extended-release tablets). In the second trial, efficacy was assessed in 203 patients who were assigned to one of two different dosages of paliperidone: 6 mg with the option to reduce to 3 mg once daily or 12 mg with the option to reduce to 9 mg once daily. In both studies, patients received paliperidone either as monotherapy (55%) or as an adjunct to mood stabilizers and/or antidepressants (45%). The most commonly used mood stabilizers in the studies were valproic acid and lithium and the most commonly used antidepressants were selective serotonin-reuptake inhibitors and selective serotonin- and norepinephrine-reuptake inhibitors. Efficacy was principally evaluated using the PANSS; as secondary outcomes, mood symptoms were evaluated using the Hamilton Depression Rating Scale (HAM-D-21) and YMRS. The paliperidone-treated patients in the flexible-dose study (mean modal dosage of 8.6 mg daily) and the higher dosage group of paliperidone in the 2-dosage-level study were each found to be superior to placebo (as measured by the PANSS). The lower dosage group of paliperidone in the 2-dosage-level study (6 mg with option to reduce to 3 mg once daily) was not found to be substantially different from placebo (as measured by the PANSS). Improvements in mood symptoms (as measured by the HAM-D-21 and YMRS) also were observed in the studies.

In an analysis of both placebo-controlled studies in schizoaffective disorder, paliperidone improved the symptoms of schizoaffective disorder at the study end points when administered either as monotherapy or as an adjunct to mood stabilizers and/or antidepressants. An examination of population subgroups did not reveal evidence of differential responsiveness based on gender, age, or geographic region. There were insufficient data to explore differential effects based on race.

DOSAGE AND ADMINISTRATION

● *Administration*

Paliperidone extended-release tablets are administered orally once daily, usually in the morning, with or without food.

Paliperidone extended-release tablets should be swallowed whole with fluids and should *not* be chewed, divided, or crushed. Patients should be advised *not* to become concerned if they notice a tablet-like substance in their stools; this is normal since the tablet is designed to remain intact and slowly release the drug from a nonabsorbable shell during passage through the GI tract.

● *Dosage*

Schizophrenia

For the management of schizophrenia in adults, the usual recommended initial dosage of paliperidone is 6 mg orally once daily in the morning; initial dosage titration is not required. Although it remains to be systematically evaluated whether dosages exceeding 6 mg once daily provide additional clinical benefit, a general trend for greater clinical effects with higher dosages has been observed. However, the potential for increased clinical efficacy at higher dosages must be weighed against the potential for a dose-related increase in adverse effects. Some patients may benefit from higher dosages of up to 12 mg once daily, while a lower dosage of 3 mg once daily may be sufficient for other patients. The manufacturer states that increases beyond a dosage level of 6 mg once daily should be made only after clinical reassessment and generally should be made at intervals of more than 5 days. When dosage increases are necessary, increments of 3 mg daily are recommended. The maximum recommended dosage in adults is 12 mg once daily.

For the management of schizophrenia in adolescents 12–17 years of age, the usual recommended initial dosage of paliperidone is 3 mg (regardless of body weight) orally once daily in the morning; initial dosage titration is not required. The manufacturer states that dosage increases, if considered necessary, should be made only after clinical reassessment and should be made in increments of 3 mg daily at intervals of more than 5 days. The recommended adolescent dosage range for patients weighing less than 51 kg is 3–6 mg once daily and for those weighing 51 kg or more is 3–12 mg once daily. However, clinicians should consider that, in the adolescent schizophrenia study, there was no clear improvement in efficacy at the higher paliperidone dosage studied (i.e., 6 mg once daily for adolescents weighing less than 51 kg and 12 mg once daily for adolescents weighing 51 kg or more) while adverse effects were found to be dose related. The maximum recommended adolescent dosage is 6 mg once daily for adolescents weighing less than 51 kg and 12 mg once daily for adolescents weighing 51 kg or more.

The optimum duration of oral paliperidone therapy in patients with schizophrenia currently is not known, but maintenance therapy with paliperidone 3–15 mg daily as extended-release tablets has been shown to be effective in preventing relapse in adults. Patients responding to paliperidone therapy should continue to receive the drug as long as clinically necessary and tolerated but at the lowest possible effective dosage, and the need for continued therapy with the drug should be reassessed periodically. The American Psychiatric Association (APA) states that prudent long-term treatment options in patients with schizophrenia with remitted first- or multiple-episodes include either indefinite maintenance therapy or gradual discontinuance of the antipsychotic agent with close follow-up and a plan to reinstitute treatment upon symptom recurrence. Discontinuance of antipsychotic therapy should be considered only after a period of at least 1 year of symptom remission or optimal response while receiving the antipsychotic agent. In patients who have had multiple previous psychotic episodes or 2 psychotic episodes within 5 years, indefinite maintenance antipsychotic treatment is recommended.

Schizoaffective Disorder

The recommended initial and target dosage of paliperidone for the treatment of schizoaffective disorder in adults in 6 mg orally once daily. Initial dosage titration is not required. However, some patients may benefit from lower or higher dosages

within the recommended dosage range of 3–12 mg once daily. Although a general trend for greater clinical effects with higher dosages has been observed, the potential for increased clinical efficacy must be weighed against the potential for a dose-related increase in adverse effects. Dosage adjustment, if necessary, should occur only after clinical reassessment and generally should be made at intervals of more than 4 days. When dosage increases are necessary, increments of 3 mg daily are recommended. The maximum recommended adult dosage is 12 mg once daily.

● *Special Populations*

The manufacturer states that the dosage of paliperidone must be individualized according to the patient's renal function status. In patients with mild renal impairment (creatinine clearance of 50–79 mL/minute), the recommended initial oral dosage of paliperidone is 3 mg once daily. The dosage may then be increased up to a maximum of 6 mg once daily based on clinical response and tolerability. In patients with moderate to severe renal impairment (creatinine clearance of 10–49 mL/minute), the recommended initial dosage of paliperidone is 1.5 mg once daily, which may be increased up to a maximum of 3 mg once daily after clinical reassessment. Use in patients with a creatinine clearance below 10 mL/minute is not recommended since paliperidone has not been studied in such patients. (See Renal Impairment under Warnings/Precautions: Specific Populations, in Cautions.)

Dosage adjustment is not necessary in patients with mild to moderate hepatic impairment (Child-Pugh class A and B). Paliperidone has not been studied in patients with severe hepatic impairment. (See Hepatic Impairment under Warnings/Precautions: Specific Populations, in Cautions.)

Because geriatric patients may have reduced renal function, dosage adjustment may be required based on renal function status. Geriatric patients with normal renal function generally may receive the same dosage recommended for younger adults with normal renal function. In geriatric patients with moderate or severe renal impairment, the maximum recommended paliperidone dosage is 3 mg once daily. (See Renal Impairment under Warnings/Precautions: Specific Populations, in Cautions.)

No dosage adjustment is necessary based on race, gender, or smoking status (see Drug Interactions: Smoking).

CAUTIONS

● *Contraindications*

Hypersensitivity reactions, including anaphylactic reactions and angioedema, have been observed in patients receiving risperidone or paliperidone. Paliperidone is therefore contraindicated in patients with a known hypersensitivity to paliperidone, risperidone, or any ingredient in the paliperidone formulation.

● *Warnings/Precautions*

Warnings

Increased Mortality in Geriatric Patients with Dementia-related Psychosis

Geriatric patients with dementia-related psychosis treated with antipsychotic drugs appear to be at an increased risk of death. Analysis of 17 placebo-controlled trials (modal duration of 10 weeks) revealed an approximate 1.6- to 1.7-fold increase in mortality among geriatric patients receiving atypical antipsychotic drugs (i.e., aripiprazole, olanzapine, quetiapine, risperidone) compared with that observed in patients receiving placebo. Over the course of a typical 10-week controlled trial, the rate of death in drug-treated patients was about 4.5% compared with a rate of about 2.6% in the placebo group. Although the causes of death were varied, most of the deaths appeared to be either cardiovascular (e.g., heart failure, sudden death) or infectious (e.g., pneumonia) in nature. Observational studies suggest that, similar to atypical antipsychotics, treatment with conventional (first-generation) antipsychotics may increase mortality; the extent to which the findings of increased mortality in observational studies may be attributed to the antipsychotic drug as opposed to some characteristic(s) of the patients remains unclear. The manufacturer states that paliperidone is *not* approved for the treatment of patients with dementia-related psychosis. (See Adverse Cerebrovascular Events, including Stroke, in Geriatric Patients with Dementia-related Psychosis under Warnings/Precautions: Other Warnings and Precautions, in Cautions, Dysphagia under Warnings/Precautions: Other Warnings and Precautions, in Cautions, and also see Geriatric Use under Warnings/Precautions: Specific Populations, in Cautions.)

Sensitivity Reactions

Hypersensitivity reactions, including anaphylactic reactions and angioedema, have been observed in patients receiving risperidone or paliperidone. (See Contraindications under Cautions.)

Other Warnings and Precautions

Adverse Cerebrovascular Events, including Stroke, in Geriatric Patients with Dementia-related Psychosis

An increased incidence of adverse cerebrovascular events (cerebrovascular accidents and transient ischemic attacks), including fatalities, has been observed in geriatric patients with dementia-related psychosis treated with certain atypical antipsychotic agents (aripiprazole, olanzapine, risperidone) in placebo-controlled studies. The manufacturer states that paliperidone is *not* approved for the treatment of patients with dementia-related psychosis. (See Increased Mortality in Geriatric Patients with Dementia-related Psychosis under Warnings/Precautions: Warnings and also see Geriatric Use under Warnings/Precautions: Specific Populations, in Cautions.)

Neuroleptic Malignant Syndrome

Neuroleptic malignant syndrome (NMS), a potentially fatal syndrome requiring immediate discontinuance of the drug and intensive symptomatic treatment, has been reported in patients receiving antipsychotic agents, including paliperidone. (See Advice to Patients.) For additional information on NMS, see Neuroleptic Malignant Syndrome under Cautions: Nervous System Effects, in the Phenothiazines General Statement 28:16.08.24.

Prolongation of QT Interval

Paliperidone causes a modest increase in the corrected QT (QT_c) interval. The risk of torsades de pointes in association with drugs that prolong the QT_c interval may be increased in patients with bradycardia, hypokalemia, or hypomagnesemia; patients receiving other drugs that prolong the QT_c interval; and in those with congenital prolongation of the QT interval. Therefore, the manufacturer states that paliperidone should be avoided in patients concurrently receiving other drugs known to prolong the QT_c interval, patients with congenital long QT syndrome, and those with a history of cardiac arrhythmias. (See Drug Interactions: Drugs that Prolong QT Interval.)

Tardive Dyskinesia

Because use of antipsychotic agents may be associated with tardive dyskinesia (a syndrome of potentially irreversible, involuntary, dyskinetic movements), paliperidone should be prescribed in a manner that is most likely to minimize the occurrence of this syndrome. Chronic antipsychotic treatment generally should be reserved for patients who suffer from a chronic illness that is known to respond to antipsychotic agents, and for whom alternative, equally effective, but potentially less harmful treatments are not available or appropriate. In patients who do require chronic treatment, the lowest dosage and the shortest duration of treatment producing a satisfactory clinical response should be sought, and the need for continued treatment should be reassessed periodically.

The American Psychiatric Association (APA) currently recommends that patients receiving atypical antipsychotic agents be assessed clinically for abnormal involuntary movements every 12 months and that patients considered to be at increased risk for tardive dyskinesia be assessed every 6 months. If signs and symptoms of tardive dyskinesia appear in a paliperidone-treated patient, paliperidone discontinuance should be considered; however, some patients may require continued treatment with the drug despite the presence of the syndrome. For additional information on tardive dyskinesia, see Tardive Dyskinesia under Cautions: Nervous System Effects, in the Phenothiazines General Statement 28:16.08.24.

Metabolic Changes

Atypical antipsychotic agents have been associated with metabolic changes that may increase cardiovascular and cerebrovascular risk, including hyperglycemia, dyslipidemia, and body weight gain. While all of these drugs produce some metabolic changes, each drug has its own specific risk profile. (See Hyperglycemia and Diabetes Mellitus, see Dyslipidemia, and also see Weight Gain under Warnings/Precautions: Other Warnings and Precautions, in Cautions.)

Hyperglycemia and Diabetes Mellitus

Hyperglycemia and diabetes mellitus, sometimes severe and associated with ketoacidosis, hyperosmolar coma, or death, have been reported in patients treated with all atypical antipsychotic agents. These cases were mainly seen in postmarketing clinical use and epidemiologic studies, not in clinical trials, and there have been few reports of hyperglycemia or diabetes mellitus in paliperidone-treated patients to date. While confounding factors such as an increased background risk of diabetes mellitus in patients with schizophrenia and the increasing incidence of diabetes mellitus in the general population make it difficult to establish with certainty the relationship between use of agents in this drug class and glucose abnormalities, epidemiologic studies (which did not include paliperidone) suggest an increased risk of treatment-emergent hyperglycemia-related adverse events in patients treated with atypical antipsychotic agents. It remains to be determined whether paliperidone also is associated with this increased risk.

The manufacturers of atypical antipsychotic agents state that patients with preexisting diabetes mellitus in whom therapy with an atypical antipsychotic is initiated should be closely monitored for worsening of glucose control; those with risk factors for diabetes (e.g., obesity, family history of diabetes) should undergo fasting blood glucose testing upon therapy initiation and periodically throughout treatment. Any patient who develops manifestations of hyperglycemia (including polydipsia, polyuria, polyphagia, and weakness) during treatment with an atypical antipsychotic should undergo fasting blood glucose testing. (See Advice to Patients.) In some cases, patients who developed hyperglycemia while receiving an atypical antipsychotic have required continuance of antidiabetic treatment despite discontinuance of the suspect drug; in other cases, hyperglycemia resolved with discontinuance of the antipsychotic.

For further information on managing the risk of hyperglycemia and diabetes mellitus associated with atypical antipsychotic agents, see Hyperglycemia and Diabetes Mellitus under Cautions: Precautions and Contraindications, in Clozapine 28:16.08.04.

Dyslipidemia

Undesirable changes in lipid parameters have been observed in patients treated with some atypical antipsychotics. Data from short- and longer-term clinical studies suggest that the risk of developing clinically important dyslipidemia during paliperidone therapy is minimal.

Weight Gain

Weight gain has been observed with atypical antipsychotic therapy. Monitoring of weight is recommended in patients receiving paliperidone and other atypical antipsychotic agents. (See Pediatric Use under Warnings/Precautions: Specific Populations, in Cautions.)

Hyperprolactinemia

Similar to other antipsychotic agents and drugs with dopamine D_2 antagonistic activity, paliperidone can elevate serum prolactin concentrations. Paliperidone's prolactin-elevating effect is similar to that seen with risperidone, which appears to be associated with a higher level of prolactin elevation than other currently available antipsychotic agents. Clinical disturbances such as galactorrhea, amenorrhea, gynecomastia, and impotence have been associated with prolactin-elevating drugs. In addition, chronic hyperprolactinemia associated with hypogonadism may lead to decreased bone density in both female and male patients.

If paliperidone therapy is considered in a patient with previously detected breast cancer, clinicians should consider that approximately one-third of human breast cancers are prolactin-dependent in vitro.

Potential for GI Obstruction

As with other nondeformable material, extended-release paliperidone tablets do not appreciably change in shape in the GI tract. Therefore, extended-release tablets of the drug generally should not be administered to patients with severe, preexisting GI narrowing (either pathologic or iatrogenic). Rare cases of obstructive symptoms in patients with known strictures have been reported in association with the ingestion of drugs in nondeformable, controlled-release formulations. Because of the extended-release design of paliperidone tablets, the drug should only be used in patients who are able to swallow the tablet whole.

Decreased bioavailability of paliperidone extended-release tablets would be expected in patients with a decreased GI transit time (e.g., those with diarrhea) while an increased bioavailability would be expected in patients with an increased GI transit time (e.g., those with GI neuropathy, diabetic gastroparesis, or due to other causes). Such changes in bioavailability are more likely when changes in transit time occur in the upper GI tract.

Orthostatic Hypotension and Syncope

Orthostatic hypotension and syncope may occur during paliperidone therapy in some patients, particularly early in treatment, perhaps because of the drug's α_1-adrenergic blocking activity. Syncope occurred in about 0.8% of patients receiving paliperidone in controlled clinical trials.

Paliperidone should be used with caution in patients with known cardiovascular disease (e.g., heart failure, history of myocardial infarction, ischemic heart disease, conduction abnormalities), cerebrovascular disease, or conditions that would predispose patients to hypotension (e.g., dehydration, hypovolemia, concomitant antihypertensive therapy) and in antipsychotic-naive patients. Consideration should be given to monitoring orthostatic vital signs in paliperidone-treated patients who are susceptible to hypotension (e.g., geriatric patients).

Leukopenia, Neutropenia, and Agranulocytosis

In clinical trial and/or postmarketing experience, leukopenia and neutropenia have been temporally related to antipsychotic agents, including paliperidone. Agranulocytosis also has been reported with antipsychotic agents.

Possible risk factors for leukopenia and neutropenia include preexisting low leukocyte count and a history of drug-induced leukopenia and neutropenia. Patients with a preexisting low leukocyte count or a history of drug-induced leukopenia or neutropenia should have their complete blood count monitored frequently during the first few months of therapy. Paliperidone should be discontinued at the first sign of a decline in leukocyte count in the absence of other causative factors.

Patients with clinically important neutropenia should be carefully monitored for fever or other signs or symptoms of infection and promptly treated if such signs and symptoms occur. In patients with severe neutropenia (absolute neutrophil count [ANC] less than 1000/mm³), paliperidone should be discontinued and the leukocyte count monitored until recovery occurs. Lithium reportedly has been used successfully in the treatment of several cases of leukopenia associated with aripiprazole, clozapine, and some other drugs; however, further clinical experience is needed to confirm these anecdotal findings.

Cognitive and Motor Impairment

Like other antipsychotic agents, paliperidone potentially may impair judgment, thinking, or motor skills. In short-term, placebo-controlled trials in adults with schizophrenia, somnolence (including hypersomnia, hypersomnolence, and sedation) was reported in 6–11% of patients receiving the drug. The frequency of somnolence appears to be dose related. (See Advice to Patients.)

Seizures

Seizures have occurred in approximately 0.2% of patients with schizophrenia receiving paliperidone in premarketing clinical studies. As with other antipsychotic agents, paliperidone should be used with caution in patients with a history of seizures or with other conditions that may lower the seizure threshold (e.g., dementia of the Alzheimer's type); conditions that lower the seizure threshold may be more prevalent in patients 65 years of age or older.

Dysphagia

Esophageal dysmotility and aspiration have been associated with the use of antipsychotic agents. Aspiration pneumonia is a common cause of morbidity and mortality in geriatric patients, particularly in those with advanced Alzheimer's dementia. Paliperidone is *not* approved for the treatment of patients with dementia-related psychosis and should be used with caution in patients at risk for aspiration pneumonia. (See Increased Mortality in Geriatric Patients with Dementia-related Psychosis under Warnings/Precautions: Warnings, in Cautions.)

Suicide

There is an attendant risk of suicide in patients with psychotic illnesses; high-risk patients should be closely supervised. Paliperidone should be prescribed in the smallest quantity consistent with good patient management to reduce the risk of overdosage.

Priapism

Drugs possessing α-adrenergic blocking activity have been reported to cause priapism. Priapism has been reported in paliperidone-treated patients during postmarketing surveillance. Severe priapism may require surgical intervention.

Thrombotic Thrombocytopenic Purpura

Thrombotic thrombocytopenic purpura (TTP) has not been reported in clinical trials of paliperidone. TTP has been reported in association with risperidone therapy; however, the relationship of this adverse event to risperidone is unknown.

Body Temperature Regulation

Disruption of the body's ability to reduce core body temperature has been attributed to antipsychotic agents. The manufacturer recommends appropriate caution when paliperidone is used in patients who will be experiencing conditions that may contribute to an elevation in core body temperature (e.g., strenuous exercise, extreme heat, concomitant use of agents with anticholinergic activity, dehydration).

Antiemetic Effect

Antiemetic effects were observed in preclinical studies with paliperidone; these effects also may occur in humans and mask signs of overdosage of other drugs or obscure cause of vomiting in various disorders (e.g., intestinal obstruction, Reye's syndrome, brain tumor).

Concomitant Illnesses

Clinical experience with paliperidone in patients with certain concomitant illnesses is limited.

Patients with parkinsonian syndrome or dementia with Lewy bodies who receive antipsychotics reportedly have an increased sensitivity to antipsychotic agents. Clinical manifestations of this increased sensitivity have been reported to include confusion, obtundation, postural instability with frequent falls, extrapyramidal symptoms, and features consistent with NMS. For additional information on extrapyramidal adverse effects and NMS, see Cautions: Nervous System Effects, in the Phenothiazines General Statement 28:16.08.24.

Paliperidone has not been adequately evaluated in patients with a recent history of myocardial infarction or unstable cardiovascular disease to date and patients with these conditions were excluded from premarketing clinical trials. Because of the risk of orthostatic hypotension associated with paliperidone, the manufacturer states that the drug should be used with caution in patients with known cardiovascular disease. (See Orthostatic Hypotension and Syncope under Warnings/Precautions: Other Warnings and Precautions, in Cautions.)

Laboratory Test Monitoring

No specific laboratory tests are recommended in patients receiving paliperidone.

Specific Populations

Pregnancy

Category C. (See Users Guide.)

Neonates exposed to antipsychotic agents during the third trimester of pregnancy are at risk for extrapyramidal and/or withdrawal symptoms following delivery. Symptoms reported to date have included agitation, hypertonia, hypotonia, tardive dyskinetic-like symptoms, tremor, somnolence, respiratory distress, and feeding disorder. Neonates exhibiting such symptoms should be monitored. The complications have varied in severity; some neonates recovered within hours to days without specific treatment while others have required intensive care unit support and prolonged hospitalization. For further information on extrapyramidal and withdrawal symptoms in neonates, see Cautions: Pregnancy, Fertility, and Lactation, in the Phenothiazines General Statement 28:16.08.24.

Lactation

Paliperidone is distributed into milk in humans. The benefits of breastfeeding should be weighed against the unknown risks of infant exposure to the drug.

Pediatric Use

Safety and efficacy of oral paliperidone in the treatment of schizophrenia in adolescents 12–17 years of age have been established in a double-blind, placebo-controlled study of 6 weeks' duration.

Safety and efficacy of oral paliperidone in the treatment of schizophrenia have not been established in pediatric patients younger than 12 years of age.

Safety and efficacy of oral paliperidone in the treatment of schizoaffective disorder have not been established in pediatric patients younger than 18 years of age.

Weight gain has been associated with atypical antipsychotic use and monitoring of weight is recommended. However, in paliperidone-treated adolescents, weight gain should be assessed against that expected with normal growth. Weight gain in adolescents receiving paliperidone in an open-label, long-term study was not considered clinically substantial when compared with normative data.

The manufacturer states that the long-term effects of paliperidone on growth and sexual maturation have not been fully evaluated in children and adolescents.

Geriatric Use

In clinical studies, approximately 7% of nearly 1800 patients were 65 years of age or older. In addition, the short-term efficacy and safety of paliperidone have been demonstrated in a placebo-controlled trial of 6 weeks' duration in 114 geriatric patients with schizophrenia. While no substantial differences in efficacy or safety relative to younger adults were observed in these studies or in other clinical experience with the drug, increased sensitivity cannot be ruled out.

Because geriatric patients may have reduced renal function, dosage adjustment may be required based on renal function status; consider monitoring renal function. (See Dosage and Administration: Special Populations.)

Geriatric patients with dementia-related psychosis treated with atypical antipsychotic drugs appear to be at an increased risk of death compared with that among patients receiving placebo. Paliperidone is *not* approved for the treatment of dementia-related psychosis. (See Increased Mortality in Geriatric Patients with Dementia-related Psychosis under Warnings/Precautions: Warnings, in Cautions.)

Hepatic Impairment

Patients with moderate hepatic impairment (Child-Pugh class B) exhibited similar plasma concentrations of free paliperidone as healthy individuals, although total paliperidone exposure decreased because of decreased protein binding. Dosage adjustment is not necessary in patients with mild to moderate hepatic impairment (Child-Pugh class A and B). The effect of severe hepatic impairment on paliperidone pharmacokinetics is not known. (See Dosage and Administration: Special Populations.)

Renal Impairment

Clearance decreased by an average of 32, 64, and 71% in patients with mild, moderate, and severe renal impairment, respectively. Dosage adjustment is recommended in patients with renal impairment. (See Dosage and Administration: Special Populations.)

• Common Adverse Effects

Adverse effects reported in 5% or more of adults receiving paliperidone for schizophrenia and at a frequency at least twice that reported with placebo include extrapyramidal symptoms, tachycardia, and akathisia.

Adverse effects reported in 5% or more of adolescents receiving paliperidone for schizophrenia and at a frequency at least twice that reported with placebo include somnolence, extrapyramidal symptoms (e.g., akathisia, tremor, dystonia, cogwheel rigidity), anxiety, increased weight, and tachycardia.

Adverse effects reported in 5% or more of adults receiving paliperidone for schizoaffective disorder and at a frequency at least twice that reported with placebo include extrapyramidal symptoms, somnolence, dyspepsia, constipation, increased weight, and nasopharyngitis.

DRUG INTERACTIONS

• Drugs Affecting Hepatic Microsomal Enzymes

Inhibitors or inducers of cytochrome P-450 (CYP) isoenzymes 2D6, 3A4, 1A2, 2A6, 2C9, and 2C19: pharmacokinetic interaction unlikely.

• Drugs Metabolized by Hepatic Microsomal Enzymes

Substrates of CYP1A2, CYP2A6, CYP2C8/9/10, CYP2D6, CYP2E1, CYP3A4, or CYP3A5: pharmacokinetic interaction unlikely.

• Drugs Inhibiting P-glycoprotein Transport System

At therapeutic concentrations, paliperidone did not inhibit P-glycoprotein; clinically relevant interactions unlikely.

• Drugs that Prolong QT Interval

Potential pharmacologic interaction (additive effect on QT-interval prolongation); avoid concomitant use of other drugs known to prolong the QT interval (e.g., amiodarone, quinidine, procainamide, sotalol, other Class Ia and III antiarrhythmics, chlorpromazine, thioridazine, gatifloxacin, moxifloxacin). (See Prolongation of QT Interval under Warnings/Precautions: Other Warnings and Precautions, in Cautions.)

• Alcohol

Potential pharmacologic interaction (additive CNS effects). Avoid alcoholic beverages during paliperidone therapy.

• Other CNS Agents

Potential pharmacologic interaction (additive CNS effects). Use with caution.

• Anticholinergic Agents

Potential pharmacologic interaction (possible disruption of body temperature regulation); use paliperidone with caution in patients concurrently receiving drugs with anticholinergic activity. (See Body Temperature Regulation under Warnings/Precautions: Other Warnings and Precautions, in Cautions.)

• Carbamazepine

Concurrent administration of carbamazepine and paliperidone decreased mean steady-state peak plasma concentrations and area under the concentration-time curves (AUCs) of paliperidone by approximately 37%. The manufacturer recommends reevaluating the dosage of paliperidone upon initiation of carbamazepine and increasing it, if necessary, based on clinical assessment. Upon discontinuance of carbamazepine, the dosage of paliperidone should also be reevaluated and decreased, if necessary.

• Hypotensive Agents

Because of its α_1-adrenergic blocking activity and potential to cause hypotension, the manufacturer recommends that paliperidone be used with caution in patients receiving antihypertensive agents; monitoring of orthostatic vital signs should be considered in such patients. (See Orthostatic Hypotension and Syncope under Warnings/Precautions: Other Warnings and Precautions, in Cautions and also see Advice to Patients.)

• Levodopa and Dopamine Agonists

Potential pharmacologic interaction (antagonistic effects).

• Lithium

A pharmacokinetic interaction between paliperidone and lithium is unlikely.

• Paroxetine

Concomitant administration of paroxetine (20 mg daily) and a single dose of paliperidone (3 mg as extended-release tablets) caused a small, clinically insignificant increase in paliperidone AUCs compared with paliperidone administration alone. Therefore, dosage adjustment of paliperidone is not necessary.

• Protein-bound Drugs

Pharmacokinetic interaction unlikely.

• Risperidone

Concurrent use of paliperidone with risperidone has not been studied to date. However, because paliperidone is the principal active metabolite of risperidone, consideration should be given to additive paliperidone exposure if risperidone and paliperidone are concomitantly administered.

• Valproate

Concurrent administration of a single dose of paliperidone (12 mg) and divalproex sodium extended-release tablets (two 500-mg tablets once daily) resulted in an approximate 50% increase in peak plasma concentrations and AUCs of paliperidone. The manufacturer states that paliperidone dosage reduction should be considered when valproate is concomitantly administered with paliperidone.

• Smoking

Pharmacokinetic interaction unlikely. Dosage adjustment in patients who smoke is not necessary.

DESCRIPTION

Paliperidone is a benzisoxazole-derivative antipsychotic agent that differs chemically from other currently available first-generation (typical) antipsychotic agents (e.g., butyrophenones, phenothiazines) and has been referred to as an atypical or second-generation antipsychotic agent. The drug is the major active metabolite of risperidone, another atypical antipsychotic agent.

The exact mechanism of paliperidone's antipsychotic action, like that of other antipsychotic agents, has not been fully elucidated, but may involve antagonism of central dopamine type 2 (D_2) and serotonin type 2 (5-hydroxytryptamine [5-HT_{2A}]) receptors. Antagonism at α_1- and α_2-adrenergic and histamine (H_1) receptors may contribute to other therapeutic and adverse effects observed with the drug. Paliperidone possesses no affinity for cholinergic muscarinic and β_1- and β_2-adrenergic receptors.

In vitro studies have suggested a role for cytochrome P-450 (CYP) isoenzymes 2D6 and 3A4 in the metabolism of paliperidone; however, the results of in vivo studies indicate that these isoenzymes play a limited role in the overall elimination of the drug from the body.

Approximately 80% and 11% of a single 1-mg oral dose of radiolabeled, immediate-release paliperidone is recovered in urine and feces, respectively, within 1 week. About 59% of the administered dose is recovered as unchanged drug in urine and 32% is recovered as metabolites. Following single-dose oral administration as extended-release tablets, paliperidone appears to have a mean terminal elimination half-life of about 23 hours.

ADVICE TO PATIENTS

Importance of advising patients and caregivers that geriatric patients with dementia-related psychosis treated with antipsychotic agents are at an increased risk of death. Patients and caregivers also should be informed that paliperidone is *not* approved for treating geriatric patients with dementia-related psychosis.

Importance of informing patients about the risk of orthostatic hypotension, especially when initiating or reinitiating treatment or increasing the dosage. Importance of advising patients who experience dizziness or fainting during therapy to get up slowly when sitting or lying down.

Because somnolence and impairment of judgment, thinking, or motor skills may be associated with paliperidone, patients should be cautioned about driving, operating machinery, or performing hazardous tasks while taking paliperidone until they gain experience with the drug's effects. Importance of avoiding alcohol during paliperidone therapy.

Importance of patients being aware of the symptoms of hyperglycemia and diabetes mellitus (e.g., increased thirst, increased urination, increased appetite, weakness). Importance of informing patients who are diagnosed with diabetes, those with risk factors for diabetes, and those who develop hyperglycemic symptoms during treatment that they should have their blood glucose monitored at the beginning of and periodically during paliperidone therapy.

Risk of weight gain. Importance of patients being aware that they should have their weight monitored regularly during therapy.

Risk of leukopenia/neutropenia. Importance of advising patients with a preexisting low leukocyte count or a history of drug-induced leukopenia/neutropenia that they should have their complete blood cell (CBC) count monitored during paliperidone therapy.

Importance of informing patients and caregivers about the risk of neuroleptic malignant syndrome (NMS), a rare but potentially life-threatening syndrome that can cause high fever, stiff muscles, sweating, fast or irregular heart beat, change in blood pressure, confusion, and kidney damage.

Importance of clinicians informing patients in whom chronic paliperidone use is contemplated about the risk of tardive dyskinesia. Importance of informing patients to report any muscle movements that cannot be stopped to a healthcare professional.

Importance of informing clinicians of existing or contemplated concomitant therapy, including prescription (see Drug Interactions: Drugs that Prolong QT Interval) and OTC drugs, dietary supplements, and/or herbal products, as well as any concomitant illnesses (e.g., cardiovascular disease, diabetes mellitus, seizures).

Importance of women informing clinicians if they are or plan to become pregnant or plan to breast-feed. Importance of clinicians informing patients about the benefits and risks of taking antipsychotics during pregnancy (see Pregnancy under Warnings/Precautions: Specific Populations, in Cautions). Importance of advising patients not to stop taking paliperidone if they become pregnant without consulting their clinician; abruptly stopping antipsychotic agents may cause complications.

Importance of avoiding overheating or dehydration.

Importance of informing patients that paliperidone extended-release tablets should be swallowed whole with the aid of liquids, and should not be chewed, divided or crushed. Patients should not be concerned if they notice a tablet-like substance in their stool.

Importance of informing patients of other important precautionary information. (See Cautions.)

PREPARATIONS

Excipients in commercially available drug preparations may have clinically important effects in some individuals; consult specific product labeling for details.

Paliperidone

Oral		
Tablets, extended-release	1.5 mg	Invega®, Janssen
	3 mg	Invega®, Janssen
	6 mg	Invega®, Janssen
	9 mg	Invega®, Janssen

Selected Revisions February 16, 2017, © Copyright, December 1, 2007, American Society of Health-System Pharmacists, Inc.

QUEtiapine Fumarate

28:16.08.04 • ATYPICAL ANTIPSYCHOTICS

■ Quetiapine fumarate is considered an atypical or second-generation antipsychotic agent.

USES

● Psychotic Disorders

Quetiapine fumarate is used for the symptomatic management of psychotic disorders (e.g., schizophrenia). Drug therapy is integral to the management of acute psychotic episodes in patients with schizophrenia and generally is required for long-term stabilization to sustain symptom remission or control and to minimize the risk of relapse. Antipsychotic agents are the principal class of drugs used for the management of all phases of schizophrenia. Patient response and tolerance to antipsychotic agents are variable, and patients who do not respond to or tolerate one drug may be successfully treated with an agent from a different class or with a different adverse effect profile.

Schizophrenia

Short-term efficacy of quetiapine for the management of schizophrenia has been established by placebo-controlled studies of 6 weeks' duration principally in hospitalized patients with schizophrenia. Schizophrenia is a major psychotic disorder that frequently has devastating effects on various aspects of the patient's life and carries a high risk of suicide and other life-threatening behaviors. Manifestations of schizophrenia involve multiple psychologic processes, including perception (e.g., hallucinations), ideation, reality testing (e.g., delusions), emotion (e.g., flatness, inappropriate affect), thought processes (e.g., loose associations), behavior (e.g., catatonia, disorganization), attention, concentration, motivation (e.g., avolition, impaired intention and planning), and judgment. The principal manifestations of this disorder usually are described in terms of positive and negative (deficit) symptoms, and more recently, disorganized symptoms. Positive symptoms include hallucinations, delusions, bizarre behavior, hostility, uncooperativeness, and paranoid ideation, while negative symptoms include restricted range and intensity of emotional expression (affective flattening), reduced thought and speech productivity (alogia), anhedonia, apathy, and decreased initiation of goal-directed behavior (avolition). Disorganized symptoms include disorganized speech (thought disorder) and behavior and poor attention.

In clinical studies in patients with schizophrenia, quetiapine was more effective than placebo in reducing the severity of symptoms associated with this disorder. Quetiapine appears to improve both positive and negative manifestations of schizophrenia. Results from comparative clinical studies and meta-analyses suggest that quetiapine is at least as effective as chlorpromazine or haloperidol in reducing positive and negative symptoms of schizophrenia.

The American Psychiatric Association (APA) considers certain atypical antipsychotic agents (i.e., quetiapine, aripiprazole, olanzapine, risperidone, ziprasidone) first-line drugs for the management of the acute phase of schizophrenia (including first psychotic episodes), principally because of the decreased risk of adverse extrapyramidal effects and tardive dyskinesia, with the understanding that the relative advantages, disadvantages, and cost-effectiveness of conventional and atypical antipsychotic agents remain controversial. The APA states that, with the possible exception of clozapine for the management of treatment-resistant symptoms, there currently is no definitive evidence that one atypical antipsychotic agent will have superior efficacy compared with another agent in the class, although meaningful differences in response may be observed in individual patients. Conventional antipsychotic agents may be considered first-line therapy in patients who have been treated successfully in the past with or who prefer conventional agents. The choice of an antipsychotic agent should be individualized, considering past response to therapy, adverse effect profile (including the patient's experience of subjective effects such as dysphoria), and the patient's preference for a specific drug, including route of administration.

Although the efficacy of quetiapine for long-term use has not been established in controlled studies, the manufacturer states that beneficial effects of the drug were maintained for up to 4 years in some patients during an open-label extension study in patients who achieved an initial response to treatment during double-blind clinical studies. If quetiapine is used for extended periods, the need for continued therapy should be reassessed periodically on an individualized basis. (See Dosage and Administration: Dosage.)

For additional information on the symptomatic management of schizophrenia, including treatment recommendations and results of the Clinical Antipsychotic Trials of Intervention Effectiveness (CATIE) research program, see Schizophrenia and Other Psychotic Disorders under Uses: Psychotic Disorders, in the Phenothiazines General Statement 28:16.08.24.

● Bipolar Disorder

Quetiapine is used alone or in conjunction with lithium or divalproex sodium for the management of acute manic episodes associated with bipolar I disorder. Efficacy of quetiapine monotherapy in the treatment of acute manic episodes has been demonstrated in 2 placebo-controlled studies of 12 weeks' duration in patients who met the DSM-IV criteria for bipolar disorder and who met diagnostic criteria for an acute manic episode (with or without psychotic features). Patients with rapid cycling and mixed episodes were excluded from these studies. The principal rating instrument used for assessing manic symptoms in these studies was the Young Mania Rating Scale (YMRS) score, an 11-item clinician rated scale traditionally used to assess the degree of manic symptomatology in a range from 0 (no manic features) to 60 (maximum score). In these studies, quetiapine was shown to be superior to placebo in reduction of the YMRS total score after 3 and 12 weeks of treatment.

Efficacy of quetiapine when used in combination with lithium or divalproex sodium in the management of acute manic episodes has been demonstrated in a placebo-controlled study of 3 weeks' duration in patients who met the DSM-IV criteria for bipolar I disorder with acute manic episodes (with or without psychotic features). Patients with rapid cycling and mixed episodes were excluded from enrollment and patients included in the study may or may not have received an adequate course of therapy with lithium or divalproex sodium prior to randomization. Quetiapine was shown to be superior to placebo when added to lithium or divalproex sodium alone in the reduction of YMRS total score. However, in a similarly designed study, quetiapine was associated with an improvement of YMRS scores but did not demonstrate superiority to placebo.

For the initial management of less severe manic or mixed episodes in patients with bipolar disorder, current APA recommendations state that monotherapy with lithium, valproate (e.g., valproate sodium, valproic acid, divalproex), or an antipsychotic (e.g., olanzapine) may be adequate. For more severe manic or mixed episodes, combination therapy with an antipsychotic and lithium or valproate is recommended as first-line therapy. For further information on the management of bipolar disorder, see Uses: Bipolar Disorder, in Lithium Salts 28:28.

Quetiapine also is used for the treatment of depressive episodes associated with bipolar disorder. Efficacy of quetiapine in the treatment of depressive episodes has been demonstrated in 2 randomized, double-blind, placebo-controlled studies of 8 weeks' duration in patients with bipolar I or II disorder (with or without a rapid cycling course). Patients in these studies received fixed daily quetiapine dosages of 300 or 600 mg once daily. The principal rating instrument used for assessing depressive symptoms in these studies was the Montgomery-Asberg Depression Rating Scale (MADRS), a 10-item clinician-rated scale with scores ranging from 0 to 60. In both studies, quetiapine was found to be superior to placebo in reduction of MADRS scores at week 8, with improvements in scores evident within one week of treatment. In addition, patients receiving 300 mg of quetiapine daily demonstrated significant improvements compared to placebo recipients in overall quality of life and satisfaction related to various areas of functioning.

DOSAGE AND ADMINISTRATION

● Administration

Quetiapine fumarate is administered orally. While food reportedly can marginally increase the peak concentration and oral bioavailability of quetiapine, the drug generally can be administered without regard to meals.

Dispensing and Administration Precautions

Because of similarity in spelling between Seroquel® (the trade name for quetiapine fumarate) and Serzone® (the former trade name for nefazodone hydrochloride, an antidepressant agent; no longer commercially available in the US under this trade name), dispensing errors have been reported to the US Food and Drug Administration (FDA) and the manufacturer of Seroquel® (AstraZeneca). According to the medication error reports, the overlapping strengths (100 and 200 mg), dosage forms (tablets), and dosing intervals (twice daily) and the fact that these 2 drugs were stored closely together in pharmacies also were critical in causing these errors. Therefore, extra care should be exercised in ensuring the accuracy of both oral and written prescriptions for Seroquel® and Serzone®. Although the Serzone brand was discontinued in June 2004, clinicians may continue to refer to nefazodone by the former brand name in prescribing. Some experts recommend that pharmacists assess the measures of avoiding dispensing errors and implement them as appropriate (e.g., by verifying all orders for these agents by spelling both the trade and generic names to prescribers, using computerized name alerts, attaching reminders to drug containers and pharmacy shelves, separating the drugs on pharmacy shelves, counseling patients). (See Dispensing and Administration Precautions under Warnings/Precautions: General Precautions in Cautions.)

● Dosage

Dosage of quetiapine fumarate is expressed in terms of quetiapine and must be carefully adjusted according to individual requirements and response, using the lowest possible effective dosage.

Higher maintenance dosages of quetiapine may be required in patients receiving the antipsychotic drug concomitantly with phenytoin or other hepatic enzyme-inducing agents (e.g., carbamazepine, barbiturates, rifampin, glucocorticoids), and an increase in the maintenance dosage of quetiapine may be required to reestablish efficacy in patients receiving such concomitant therapy. (See Drug Interactions: Drugs Affecting Hepatic Microsomal Enzymes and also Phenytoin.)

Patients receiving quetiapine should be monitored for possible worsening of depression, suicidality, or unusual changes in behavior, especially at the beginning of therapy or during periods of dosage adjustments. (See Worsening of Depression and Suicidality Risk under Warnings/Precautions: Warnings, in Cautions.)

The manufacturer states that if quetiapine therapy is reinitiated after a drug-free period of less than 1 week, dosage titration is not necessary. However, if quetiapine therapy is reinitiated after a drug-free period exceeding 1 week, dosage generally should be titrated as with initial therapy.

Schizophrenia

For the management of schizophrenia, the recommended initial dosage of quetiapine in adults is 25 mg twice daily. Dosage may be increased in increments of 25–50 mg 2 or 3 times daily on the second or third day, as tolerated, to a target dosage of 300–400 mg daily in 2 or 3 divided doses by the fourth day. Because steady-state plasma concentrations of quetiapine may not be attained for 1–2 days at a given dosage, subsequent dosage adjustments generally should be made at intervals of not less than 2 days, usually in increments or decrements of 25–50 mg twice daily. Effective dosages of quetiapine in clinical trials generally ranged from 150–750 mg daily. While the manufacturer states that increasing quetiapine dosages beyond 300 mg daily usually does not result in additional therapeutic effect, dosages of 400–500 mg daily apparently have been required in some patients, and a dosage range of 300–800 mg daily has been recommended. Safety of quetiapine in dosages exceeding 800 mg daily has not been established.

The optimum duration of quetiapine therapy currently is not known, but the efficacy of maintenance therapy with antipsychotic agents used in the treatment of schizophrenia is well established. Patients responding to quetiapine therapy should continue to receive the drug as long as clinically necessary and tolerated but at the lowest possible effective dosage, and the need for continued therapy with the drug should be reassessed periodically. The American Psychiatric Association (APA) states that prudent long-term treatment options in patients with remitted first- or multiple-episodes include either indefinite maintenance therapy or gradual discontinuance of the antipsychotic agent with close follow-up and a plan to reinstitute treatment upon symptom recurrence. Discontinuance of antipsychotic therapy should be considered only after a period of at least 1 year of symptom remission or optimal response while receiving the antipsychotic agent. In patients who have had multiple previous psychotic episodes or 2 psychotic episodes within 5 years, indefinite maintenance antipsychotic treatment is recommended.

If antipsychotic therapy is to be discontinued in patients with schizophrenia, precautions should include slow, gradual dose reduction over many months, more frequent clinician visits, and use of early intervention strategies. Patients and their family and caregivers should be advised about early signs of relapse, and clinicians should collaborate with them to develop plans for action should they emerge. The

treatment program should be designed to respond quickly to evidence of prodromal symptoms or behaviors or exacerbations of schizophrenic symptoms.

Bipolar Disorder

For the management of depressive episodes associated with bipolar I or II disorder, the recommended dosage of quetiapine in adults is 50 mg administered once daily at bedtime on the first day of therapy. The dosage of quetiapine should then be increased to 100 mg once daily on the second day of therapy, 200 mg once daily on the third day of therapy, and 300 mg once daily on the fourth day of therapy. In clinical trials demonstrating clinical efficacy, quetiapine was given in a dosing schedule of 50, 100, 200, and 300 mg once daily on days 1–4, respectively; patients who received 600 mg daily received 400 mg daily on day 5 and 600 mg daily on day 8. Although antidepressant efficacy was demonstrated with quetiapine at dosages of 300 mg daily and 600 mg daily, no additional benefit was seen in the 600-mg daily group.

For the management of acute mania associated with bipolar I disorder (alone or in conjunction with lithium or divalproex sodium), the recommended initial dosage of quetiapine in adults is 100 mg daily, administered in 2 divided doses. The dosage of quetiapine should be increased in increments of up to 100 mg daily in 2 divided doses to 400 mg daily on the fourth day of therapy. Subsequent dosage adjustments up to 800 mg daily by the sixth day of therapy should be made in increments not exceeding 200 mg daily. Data indicate that most patients respond to 400–800 mg daily. The safety of quetiapine dosages exceeding 800 mg daily has not been established.

The APA states that for patients treated with an antipsychotic agent during an acute episode in bipolar disorder, the need for ongoing antipsychotic treatment should be reassessed upon entering the maintenance phase. The APA recommends that antipsychotics be slowly tapered and discontinued unless they are required to control persistent psychosis or provide prophylaxis against recurrence. While maintenance therapy with atypical antipsychotics may be considered, there currently is limited evidence regarding their efficacy in the maintenance phase compared with that of agents such as lithium or valproate. The manufacturer of quetiapine states that efficacy of the drug has not been systematically evaluated for more than 12 weeks as monotherapy of acute manic episodes associated with bipolar I disorder or for more than 3 weeks as combined therapy with divalproex or lithium. In addition, the manufacturer of quetiapine states that efficacy of the drug has not been systematically evaluated for more than 8 weeks in the management of depressive episodes in patients with bipolar I or II disorder. If quetiapine is used for extended periods, the need for continued therapy should be reassessed periodically on an individualized basis.

Switching to or Concomitant Use with Other Antipsychotic Agents

The manufacturer states that there are no systematically collected data that specifically address switching from other antipsychotic agents to quetiapine or concerning concomitant use of quetiapine with other antipsychotic agents. Although abrupt discontinuance of the previous antipsychotic agent may be acceptable for some patients with schizophrenia, gradual discontinuance may be most appropriate for others. In all cases, the period of overlapping antipsychotic administration should be minimized. In patients being switched from long-acting (depot) parenteral antipsychotic therapy to oral quetiapine therapy, the first oral dose of quetiapine should be administered in place of the next scheduled dose of the long-acting preparation. The need for continuing existing drugs used for the symptomatic relief of extrapyramidal manifestations should be reevaluated periodically.

● Special Populations

The manufacturer states that because quetiapine is substantially metabolized in the liver and because the pharmacokinetics of quetiapine appear to be altered in patients with hepatic impairment, an initial dosage of 25 mg daily should be used in adults with hepatic impairment. The dosage should be increased by 25–50 mg daily according to clinical response and tolerability until an effective dosage is reached.

Although elimination of quetiapine was reduced in patients with severe renal impairment (e.g., creatinine clearance of 10–30 mL/minute), the plasma quetiapine concentrations were similar to those in patients with normal renal function; therefore, the manufacturer states that dosage adjustment is not necessary in such patients.

Geriatric or debilitated patients and patients predisposed to hypotension or in whom hypotension would pose a risk (e.g., patients with dehydration or hypovolemia, those receiving antihypertensive drugs, patients with known cardiovascular or cerebrovascular disease) should have a slower rate of dosage titration and should receive lower target dosages of quetiapine. The risk of orthostatic hypotension can be minimized by limiting the initial dosage of quetiapine to 25 mg twice daily. If orthostatic hypotension occurs during titration to the target dosage, the manufacturer recommends a return to the previous dosage in the titration schedule

CAUTIONS

• Contraindications

The manufacturer states that there are no known contraindications to quetiapine use.

• Warnings/Precautions

Warnings

Increased Mortality in Geriatric Patients with Dementia-related Psychosis

Geriatric patients with dementia-related psychosis treated with atypical antipsychotic drugs appear to be at an increased risk of death compared with that among patients receiving placebo. Analyses of 17 placebo-controlled trials (average duration of 10 weeks) revealed an approximate 1.6- to 1.7-fold increase in mortality among geriatric patients receiving atypical antipsychotic drugs (i.e., quetiapine, aripiprazole, olanzapine, risperidone) compared with that in patients receiving placebo. Over the course of a typical 10-week controlled trial, the rate of death in drug-treated patients was about 4.5% compared with a rate of about 2.6% in the placebo group. Although the causes of death were varied, most of the deaths appeared to be either cardiovascular (e.g., heart failure, sudden death) or infectious (e.g., pneumonia) in nature. The manufacturer states that quetiapine is not approved for the treatment of dementia-related psychosis. (See Dosage and Administration: Special Populations and also see Geriatric Use under Warnings/Precautions: Specific Populations, in Cautions.)

Worsening of Depression and Suicidality Risk

Worsening of depression and/or the emergence of suicidal ideation and behavior (suicidality) or unusual changes in behavior may occur in both adult and pediatric (see Pediatric Use under Warnings/Precautions: Specific Populations, in Cautions) patients with major depressive disorder or other psychiatric disorders, whether or not they are taking antidepressants. This risk may persist until clinically important remission occurs with therapy. Suicide is a known risk of depression and certain other psychiatric disorders, and these disorders themselves are the strongest predictors of suicide. However, there has been a long-standing concern that antidepressants may have a role in inducing worsening of depression and the emergence of suicidality in certain patients during the early phases of treatment. Pooled analyses of short-term, placebo-controlled studies of antidepressants (i.e., selective serotonin-reuptake inhibitors and other antidepressants) have shown an increased risk of suicidality in children, adolescents, and young adults (18–24 years of age) with major depressive disorder and other psychiatric disorders. An increased suicidality risk was not demonstrated with antidepressants compared to placebo in adults older than 24 years of age and a reduced risk was observed in adults 65 years of age or older.

The US Food and Drug Administration (FDA) recommends that all patients being treated with antidepressants for any indication be appropriately monitored and closely observed for clinical worsening, suicidality, and unusual changes in behavior, particularly during initiation of therapy (i.e., the first few months) and during periods of dosage adjustments. Families and caregivers of patients being treated with antidepressants for major depressive disorder or other indications, both psychiatric and nonpsychiatric, also should be advised to monitor patients on a daily basis for the emergence of agitation, irritability, or unusual changes in behavior as well as the emergence of suicidality, and to report such symptoms immediately to a health-care provider.

Although a causal relationship between the emergence of symptoms such as anxiety, agitation, panic attacks, insomnia, irritability, hostility, aggressiveness, impulsivity, akathisia, hypomania, and/or mania and either the worsening of depression and/or the emergence of suicidal impulses has not been established, there is concern that such symptoms may represent precursors to emerging suicidality. Consequently, consideration should be given to changing the therapeutic regimen or discontinuing therapy in patients whose depression is persistently worse or

in patients experiencing emergent suicidality or symptoms that might be precursors to worsening depression or suicidality, particularly if such manifestations are severe, abrupt in onset, or were not part of the patient's presenting symptoms. FDA also recommends that the drugs be prescribed in the smallest quantity consistent with good patient management, in order to reduce the risk of overdosage.

Bipolar Disorder

It is generally believed (though not established in controlled trials) that treating a major depressive episode with an antidepressant alone may increase the likelihood of precipitating a mixed or manic episode in patients at risk for bipolar disorder. Therefore, patients should be adequately screened for bipolar disorder prior to initiating treatment with an antidepressant; such screening should include a detailed psychiatric history (e.g., family history of suicide, bipolar disorder, and depression). Quetiapine is approved for use in treating bipolar depression in adults. (See Bipolar Disorder under Uses.)

Neuroleptic Malignant Syndrome

Neuroleptic malignant syndrome (NMS), a potentially fatal syndrome requiring immediate discontinuance of the drug and intensive symptomatic treatment, has been reported in patients receiving antipsychotic agents, including quetiapine. (See Advice to Patients.) For additional information on NMS, see Neuroleptic Malignant Syndrome under Cautions: Nervous System Effects, in the Phenothiazines General Statement 28:16.08.24.

Tardive Dyskinesia

Use of antipsychotic agents, including quetiapine, may be associated with tardive dyskinesia, a syndrome of potentially irreversible, involuntary, dyskinetic movements. For additional information on tardive dyskinesia, see Tardive Dyskinesia under Cautions: Nervous System Effects, in the Phenothiazines General Statement 28:16.08.24.

Hyperglycemia and Diabetes Mellitus

Severe hyperglycemia, sometimes associated with ketoacidosis, hyperosmolar coma, or death, has been reported in patients receiving all atypical antipsychotic agents, including quetiapine. While confounding factors such as an increased background risk of diabetes mellitus in patients with schizophrenia and the increasing incidence of diabetes mellitus in the general population make it difficult to establish with certainty the relationship between use of agents in this drug class and glucose abnormalities, epidemiologic studies suggest an increased risk of treatment-emergent hyperglycemia-related adverse events in patients treated with the atypical antipsychotic agents included in the studies (e.g., quetiapine, clozapine, olanzapine, risperidone).

Precise risk estimates for hyperglycemia-related adverse events in patients treated with atypical antipsychotics currently are not available. While some evidence suggests that the risk for diabetes may be greater with some atypical antipsychotics (e.g., clozapine, olanzapine) than with others in the class (e.g., quetiapine, risperidone), available data are conflicting and insufficient to provide reliable estimates of relative risk associated with use of the various atypical antipsychotics.

The manufacturers of atypical antipsychotic agents state that patients with preexisting diabetes mellitus in whom therapy with an atypical antipsychotic is initiated should be closely monitored for worsening of glucose control; those with risk factors for diabetes (e.g., obesity, family history of diabetes) should undergo fasting blood glucose testing upon therapy initiation and periodically throughout treatment. Any patient who develops manifestations of hyperglycemia (e.g., polydipsia, polyphagia, polyuria, weakness) during treatment with an atypical antipsychotic should undergo fasting blood glucose testing. In some cases, patients who developed hyperglycemia while receiving an atypical antipsychotic have required continuance of antidiabetic treatment despite discontinuance of the suspect drug; in other cases, hyperglycemia resolved with discontinuance of the antipsychotic.

For further information on the risk of hyperglycemia and diabetes mellitus associated with atypical antipsychotic agents, see Cautions: Endocrine and Metabolic Effects and see also Hyperglycemia and Diabetes Mellitus under Cautions: Precautions and Contraindications, in Clozapine 28:16.08.04.

Sensitivity Reactions

Contact dermatitis, maculopapular rash, and photosensitivity reactions were reported infrequently during clinical trials. Anaphylaxis and Stevens-Johnson syndrome have been reported during postmarketing surveillance.

General Precautions
Cardiovascular Effects

Orthostatic hypotension with associated dizziness, tachycardia, and/or syncope, particularly during the initial dosage titration period, has been reported. The risk of orthostatic hypotension and syncope may be minimized by limiting initial dosage. (See Dosage and Administration: Special Populations.) Use with caution in patients with known cardiovascular (e.g., history of myocardial infarction or ischemia, heart failure, conduction abnormalities) or cerebrovascular disease and/or conditions that would predispose patients to hypotension (e.g., dehydration, hypovolemia, concomitant antihypertensive therapy).

● Ocular Effects

The development of cataracts in association with quetiapine was observed in animal studies. Lens changes also have been reported in some patients receiving long-term quetiapine therapy, although a causal relationship has not been established. Because the possibility of lens changes cannot be excluded, the manufacturer recommends ophthalmologic examination of the lens by methods adequate to detect cataract formation (e.g., slit lamp exam) be performed at the initiation of quetiapine therapy, or shortly thereafter, and at 6-month intervals during chronic quetiapine therapy.

● Nervous System Effects

Seizures occurred in 0.6% of patients receiving quetiapine in controlled clinical trials. Use with caution in patients with a history of seizures or with conditions known to lower the seizure threshold (e.g., dementia of the Alzheimer's type, geriatric patients).

Somnolence occurred in 16–18 or 34% of patients receiving quetiapine as monotherapy (for the treatment of schizophrenia or bipolar disorder) or in conjunction with lithium or divalproex sodium (for the treatment of bipolar disorder), respectively, during clinical studies compared with 4–11% of those receiving placebo.

● Endocrine Effects

Dose-related decreases in total and free thyroxine (T4) of approximately 20% were observed in patients receiving quetiapine dosages at the higher end of the therapeutic dosage range during clinical studies. These decreases were maximal during the first 2–4 weeks of therapy and were maintained without adaptation or progression during more chronic therapy. Generally, these changes were not considered clinically important and were reversible upon discontinuance of quetiapine, regardless of duration of therapy. Increases in TSH were observed in about 0.4 or 12% of patients receiving quetiapine alone or in conjunction with lithium or divalproex sodium, respectively. In patients receiving quetiapine monotherapy, thyroid replacement therapy was necessary in some patients who experienced increases in TSH.

Although not observed in patients receiving quetiapine during clinical trials, increases in prolactin concentrations and associated increases in mammary gland neoplasia were reported in animal studies.

● Metabolic Effects

During clinical studies, 23 or 21% of patients with schizophrenia or acute mania receiving quetiapine gained at least 7% of their baseline weight compared with 6–7% of those receiving placebo. In patients receiving quetiapine as adjunctive therapy for acute mania, 13% gained at least 7% of their baseline weight compared with 4% of those receiving placebo.

Increases from baseline in cholesterol and triglyceride concentrations of 11 and 17%, respectively, were reported in patients receiving quetiapine compared with slight decreases in patients receiving placebo in clinical studies in patients with schizophrenia. These changes were weakly related to increases in weight observed in patients receiving quetiapine. For additional information on metabolic effects, see Hyperglycemia and Diabetes Mellitus under Warnings/Precautions: Warnings, in Cautions.

● Hepatic Effects

Asymptomatic, transient, and reversible increases in serum transaminases, principally ALT, have been reported in patients receiving quetiapine; these changes usually occurred within the first 3 weeks and resolved despite continued quetiapine therapy.

● Priapism

Drugs possessing α-adrenergic blocking activity have been reported to cause priapism. One case of drug-induced priapism was reported in clinical studies of quetiapine. Severe priapism may require surgical intervention.

● Body Temperature Regulation

Although not reported in clinical studies with quetiapine, disruption of the body's ability to reduce core body temperature has been associated with use of antipsychotic agents. The manufacturer recommends appropriate caution when quetiapine is used in patients who will be experiencing conditions that may contribute to an elevation in core body temperature (e.g., strenuous exercise, extreme heat, concomitant use of agents with anticholinergic activity, dehydration).

● GI Effects

Esophageal dysmotility and aspiration have been associated with the use of antipsychotic agents. Use with caution in patients at risk for aspiration pneumonia (e.g., geriatric patients, those with advanced Alzheimer's dementia).

● Suicide

Attendant risk with bipolar disorder and psychotic illnesses; closely supervise high-risk patients. In clinical studies in patients with bipolar depression, the incidence of treatment-emergent suicidal ideation or suicide attempt in quetiapine-treated patients was low (1.7–2.6%) and similar to that observed with placebo (2%). Prescribe in the smallest quantity consistent with good patient management to reduce the risk of overdosage. (See Worsening of Depression and Suicidality Risk under Warnings/Precautions: Warnings, in Cautions.)

● Dispensing and Administration Precautions

Because of similarity in spelling between Seroquel® (the trade name for quetiapine fumarate) and Serzone® (the former trade name for nefazodone hydrochloride, an antidepressant agent; no longer commercially available in the US under this trade name), dispensing errors have been reported to the US Food and Drug Administration (FDA) and the manufacturer of Seroquel® (AstraZeneca). According to the medication error reports, the overlapping strengths (100 and 200 mg), dosage forms (tablets), and dosing intervals (twice daily) and the fact that these 2 drugs were stored closely together in pharmacies also were critical in causing these errors. These medication errors may be associated with adverse CNS (e.g., mental status deterioration, hallucination, paranoia, muscle weakness, lethargy, dizziness) and GI effects (e.g., nausea, vomiting, diarrhea). As of November 2001, 4 patients had required emergency room visits and 3 patients reportedly had been hospitalized because of dispensing errors involving these 2 agents. One female patient 25 years of age experienced fever and respiratory arrest after mistakenly taking Seroquel® for 3 days instead of taking Serzone®, and eventually died, although a causal relationship has not been established. FDA also is concerned that several patients unintentionally ingested Serzone® or Seroquel® for a prolonged period of time before the error was discovered. Therefore, extra care should be exercised in ensuring the accuracy of both oral and written prescriptions for Seroquel® and Serzone®. Although the Serzone brand was discontinued in June 2004, clinicians may continue to refer to nefazodone by the former brand name in prescribing. Some experts recommend that pharmacists assess the measures of avoiding dispensing errors and implement them as appropriate (e.g., by verifying all orders for these agents by spelling both the trade and generic names to prescribers, using computerized name alerts, attaching reminders to drug containers and pharmacy shelves, separating the drugs on pharmacy shelves, counseling patients).

Patients should be advised to question the dispensing pharmacist regarding any changes in the appearance of their prescription in terms of shape, color, or size of the tablets. Dispensing errors involving Seroquel® (quetiapine) and Serzone® (nefazodone) should be reported to the manufacturers or directly to the FDA MedWatch program by phone (800-FDA-1088), by fax (800-FDA-0178), by the Internet (http://www.fda.gov/Safety/MedWatch/default.htm), or by mail (FDA Safety Information and Adverse Event Reporting Program, FDA, 5600 Fishers Lane, Rockville, MD 20852-9787).

Specific Populations
Pregnancy

Category C. (See Users Guide.)

Neonates exposed to antipsychotic agents during the third trimester of pregnancy are at risk for extrapyramidal and/or withdrawal symptoms following delivery. Symptoms reported to date have included agitation, hypertonia, hypotonia, tardive dyskinetic-like symptoms, tremor, somnolence, respiratory distress, and feeding disorder. Neonates exhibiting such symptoms should be monitored. The complications have varied in severity; some neonates recovered within hours to days without specific treatment, while others have required intensive care unit support and prolonged hospitalization. For further information on extrapyramidal and withdrawal symptoms in neonates, see Cautions: Pregnancy, Fertility, and Lactation, in the Phenothiazines General Statement 28:16.08.24.

The effect of quetiapine on labor and delivery is unknown.

Lactation

Quetiapine appears to be distributed into human milk in relatively small amounts. The manufacturer recommends that women receiving quetiapine not breast-feed.

Pediatric Use

Safety and efficacy not established in children younger than 18 years of age.

FDA warns that a greater risk of suicidal thinking or behavior (suicidality) occurred during first few months of antidepressant treatment (4%) compared with placebo (2%) in children and adolescents with major depressive disorder, obsessive-compulsive disorder (OCD), or other psychiatric disorders based on pooled analyses of 24 short-term, placebo-controlled trials of 9 antidepressant drugs (selective serotonin-reuptake inhibitors [SSRIs] and other antidepressants). However, a more recent meta-analysis of 27 placebo-controlled trials of 9 antidepressants (SSRIs and others) in patients younger than 19 years of age with major depressive disorder, OCD, or non-OCD anxiety disorders suggests that the benefits of antidepressant therapy in treating these conditions may outweigh the risks of suicidal behavior or suicidal ideation. No suicides occurred in these pediatric trials.

Carefully consider these findings when assessing potential benefits and risks of quetiapine in a child or adolescent for any clinical use. (See Worsening of Depression and Suicidality Risk under Warnings/Precautions: Warnings, in Cautions.)

Geriatric Use

In clinical studies, approximately 7% of 3400 patients were 65 years of age or older. While no substantial differences in safety relative to younger adults were observed, factors that decrease pharmacokinetic clearance, increase the pharmacodynamic response, or cause poorer tolerance (e.g., orthostasis) may be present in geriatric patients. (See Dosage and Administration: Special Populations and also see Increased Mortality in Geriatric Patients with Dementia-related Psychosis under Warnings/Precautions: Warnings, in Cautions.)

In pooled data analyses, a *reduced* risk of suicidality was observed in adults 65 years of age or older with antidepressant therapy compared with placebo. (See Worsening of Depression and Suicidality Risk under Warnings/Precautions: Warnings, in Cautions.)

Hepatic Impairment

Increased plasma concentrations expected in patients with hepatic impairment; dosage adjustment may be necessary. (See Dosage and Administration: Special Populations.)

Renal Impairment

Clearance may be decreased in patients with severe renal impairment, but dosage adjustment is not necessary.

● Common Adverse Effects

The most common adverse effects reported in 5% or more of patients receiving quetiapine therapy for schizophrenia or bipolar disorder and at a frequency twice that reported among patients receiving placebo in clinical trials include somnolence, sedation, asthenia, lethargy, dizziness, dry mouth, constipation, increased ALT, weight gain, dyspepsia, abdominal pain, postural hypotension, and pharyngitis.

DRUG INTERACTIONS

● Drugs Affecting Hepatic Microsomal Enzymes

Inhibitors of cytochrome P-450 (CYP) isoenzyme 3A4 (e.g., erythromycin, fluconazole, itraconazole, ketoconazole): potential pharmacokinetic interaction (increased serum quetiapine concentrations). Use with caution.

Inducers of CYP3A4 (e.g., barbiturates, carbamazepine, glucocorticoids, phenytoin, rifampin): potential pharmacokinetic interaction (increased quetiapine metabolism and decreased serum quetiapine concentrations). Dosage adjustment may be necessary if these drugs are initiated or discontinued in patients receiving quetiapine. (See Drug Interactions: Phenytoin.)

● Drugs Metabolized by Hepatic Microsomal Enzymes

Substrates of CYP1A2, CYP3A4, CYP2C9, CYP2C19, or CYP2D6: pharmacokinetic interaction unlikely.

● Alcohol

Potential pharmacologic interaction (additive CNS effects). Avoid alcoholic beverages during quetiapine therapy.

● Anticholinergic Agents

Potential pharmacologic interaction (possible disruption of body temperature regulation); use quetiapine with caution in patients concurrently receiving drugs with anticholinergic activity. (See Body Temperature Regulation under Warnings/Precautions: General Precautions, in Cautions.)

● Cimetidine

Concomitant use of cimetidine (400 mg 3 times daily for 4 days) and quetiapine (150 mg 3 times daily) decreased mean clearance of quetiapine by 20%. However, dosage adjustment of quetiapine is not necessary.

● Divalproex

Potential pharmacokinetic interaction. Increased maximum plasma quetiapine concentrations, with no effect on extent of quetiapine absorption or mean clearance. Decreased maximum plasma valproic acid concentrations and extent of absorption (not clinically important).

● Fluoxetine, Haloperidol, Imipramine, Risperidone

No effect on steady-state pharmacokinetics of quetiapine observed.

● Hypotensive Agents

Potential pharmacologic interaction (additive hypotensive effects).

● Levodopa and Dopamine Agonists

Potential pharmacologic interaction (antagonistic effects).

● Lithium

No effect on steady-state lithium pharmacokinetics observed.

● Lorazepam

Potential pharmacokinetic interaction (decreased clearance of lorazepam). Concomitant use of quetiapine (250 mg 3 times daily) and lorazepam (single 2-mg dose) resulted in a 20% decrease in the mean clearance of lorazepam.

● Phenytoin

Concomitant use of quetiapine (250 mg 3 times daily) and phenytoin (100 mg 3 times daily) resulted in a fivefold increase in quetiapine clearance. An increase in quetiapine dosage may be required; caution advised if phenytoin is withdrawn and replaced with a noninducer of CYP3A4 (e.g., valproate).

● Thioridazine

Potential pharmacokinetic interaction (increased oral clearance of quetiapine).

● Other CNS Agents

Potential pharmacologic interaction (additive CNS effects). Use with caution.

● Smoking

Smoking does not affect the oral clearance of quetiapine.

DESCRIPTION

Quetiapine fumarate is a dibenzothiazepine-derivative antipsychotic agent. The drug is pharmacologically similar to clozapine, but differs pharmacologically from other currently available first-generation (typical) antipsychotic agents (e.g., phenothiazines, butyrophenones). Because of these pharmacologic differences, quetiapine is considered an atypical or second-generation antipsychotic agent.

The exact mechanism of quetiapine's antipsychotic action in schizophrenia and its mood stabilizing action in bipolar disorder has not been fully elucidated but may involve antagonism at serotonin type 1 (5-hydroxytryptamine [5-HT$_{1A}$]) and type 2 (5-HT$_{2A}$, 5-HT$_{2C}$) receptors, and at dopamine (D$_1$, D$_2$) receptors.

Current evidence suggests that the clinical potency and antipsychotic efficacy of both typical and atypical antipsychotic drugs generally are related to their affinity for and blockade of central dopamine D_2 receptors; however, antagonism at dopamine D_2 receptors does not appear to account fully for the antipsychotic effects of quetiapine. Results of in vivo and in vitro studies indicate that quetiapine is a comparatively weak antagonist at dopamine D_2 receptors. Receptor binding studies show quetiapine is a weak antagonist at D_1 receptors. Although their role in eliciting the pharmacologic effects of antipsychotic agents remains to be fully elucidated, dopamine D_3, D_4, and D_5 receptors also have been identified; quetiapine possesses no affinity for the dopamine D_4 receptor.

The therapeutic effects of antipsychotic drugs are thought to be mediated by dopaminergic blockade in the mesolimbic and mesocortical areas of the CNS, while antidopaminergic effects in the neostriatum appear to be associated with extrapyramidal effects. The apparently low incidence of extrapyramidal effects associated with quetiapine therapy suggests that the drug is more active in the mesolimbic than in the neostriatal dopaminergic system. In contrast to typical antipsychotic agents (e.g., chlorpromazine) but like other atypical antipsychotic drugs (e.g., clozapine), quetiapine does not cause sustained elevations in serum prolactin concentrations and therefore is unlikely to produce adverse effects such as amenorrhea, galactorrhea, and impotence.

Quetiapine exhibits α_1- and α_2-adrenergic blocking activity; blockade of α_1-adrenergic receptors may explain the occasional orthostatic hypotension associated with the drug. Quetiapine also blocks histamine H_1 receptors, which may explain the sedative effects associated with the drug. Quetiapine possesses little or no affinity for β-adrenergic, γ-aminobutyric acid (GABA), benzodiazepine, or muscarinic receptors.

Quetiapine is extensively metabolized in the liver principally via sulfoxidation and oxidation to inactive metabolites. In vitro studies suggest that the cytochrome P-450 (CYP) 3A4 isoenzyme is involved in the metabolism of quetiapine to the inactive sulfoxide metabolite, which is the principal metabolite. The mean terminal half-life of quetiapine is about 6 hours. Following oral administration of a single dose of quetiapine, approximately 73 and 20% of the dose is excreted in urine and feces, respectively; less than 1% of the dose is excreted unchanged. Based on in vitro studies, quetiapine and 9 of its metabolites do not appear likely to inhibit CYP isoenzymes 1A2, 3A4, 2C9, 2C19, or 2D6.

ADVICE TO PATIENTS

Risk of suicidality; importance of patients, family, and caregivers being alert to and immediately reporting emergence of suicidality, worsening depression, or unusual changes in behavior, especially during the first few months of therapy or during periods of dosage adjustment.

Importance of providing written patient information (medication guide) explaining risks of quetiapine each time the drug is dispensed.

Risk of orthostatic hypotension, especially during initial dosage titration and at times of reinitiation of therapy or increases in dosage.

Risk of somnolence and impairment of judgment, thinking, or motor skills; avoid driving, operating machinery, or performing hazardous tasks until effects on the individual are known.

Importance of avoiding alcohol during quetiapine therapy.

Importance of informing patients and caregivers about the risk of neuroleptic malignant syndrome (NMS), a rare but potentially life-threatening syndrome that can cause high fever, stiff muscles, sweating, fast or irregular heart beat, change in blood pressure, confusion, and kidney damage.

Importance of informing clinicians of existing or contemplated concomitant therapy, including prescription and OTC drugs, as well as any concomitant illnesses (e.g., diabetes mellitus).

Importance of women informing clinicians if they are or plan to become pregnant or plan to breast-feed. Importance of clinicians informing patients about the benefits and risks of taking antipsychotics during pregnancy (see Pregnancy under Warnings/Precautions: Specific Populations, in Cautions). Importance of advising patients not to stop taking quetiapine if they become pregnant without consulting their clinician; abruptly discontinuing antipsychotic agents may cause complications. Importance of advising patients not to breast-feed during quetiapine therapy.

Importance of avoiding overheating or dehydration.

Importance of informing patients of other important precautionary information. (See Cautions.)

PREPARATIONS

Excipients in commercially available drug preparations may have clinically important effects in some individuals; consult specific product labeling for details.

QUEtiapine Fumarate

Oral

Tablets, film-coated	25 mg (of quetiapine)	SEROquel®, AstraZeneca
	50 mg (of quetiapine)	SEROquel®, AstraZeneca
	100 mg (of quetiapine)	SEROquel®, AstraZeneca
	200 mg (of quetiapine)	SEROquel®, AstraZeneca
	300 mg (of quetiapine)	SEROquel®, AstraZeneca
	400 mg (of quetiapine)	SEROquel®, AstraZeneca

risperiDONE

28:16.08.04 • ATYPICAL ANTIPSYCHOTICS

■ Risperidone has been described as an atypical or second-generation antipsychotic agent.

USES

● Psychotic Disorders

Risperidone is used orally and parenterally for the symptomatic management of psychotic disorders (e.g., schizophrenia). Drug therapy is integral to the management of acute psychotic episodes in patients with schizophrenia and generally is required for long-term stabilization to sustain symptom remission or control and to minimize the risk of relapse. Antipsychotic agents are the principal class of drugs used for the management of all phases of schizophrenia.

The American Psychiatric Association (APA) considers most atypical antipsychotic agents first-line drugs for the management of the acute phase of schizophrenia (including first psychotic episodes), principally because of the decreased risk of adverse extrapyramidal effects and tardive dyskinesia, with the understanding that the relative advantages, disadvantages, and cost-effectiveness of conventional and atypical antipsychotic agents remain controversial. The APA states that, with the possible exception of clozapine for the management of treatment-resistant symptoms, there currently is no definitive evidence that one atypical antipsychotic agent will have superior efficacy compared with another agent in the class, although meaningful differences in response may be observed in individual patients. Conventional antipsychotic agents also may be an appropriate first-line option for some patients, including those who have been treated successfully in the past with or who prefer conventional agents. The choice of an antipsychotic agent should be individualized, considering past response to therapy, current symptomatology, concurrent medical conditions, other medications and treatments, adverse effect profile, and the patient's preference for a specific drug, including route of administration. Patient response and tolerance to antipsychotic agents are variable, and patients who do not respond to or tolerate one drug may be successfully treated with an agent from a different class or with a different adverse effect profile.

Schizophrenia

Risperidone is used orally for the treatment of schizophrenia in adults and adolescents 13–17 years of age and IM as an extended-release injection for the treatment of schizophrenia in adults. Schizophrenia is a major psychotic disorder that frequently has devastating effects on various aspects of the patient's life and carries a high risk of suicide and other life-threatening behaviors. Manifestations of schizophrenia involve multiple psychologic processes, including perception (e.g., hallucinations), ideation, reality testing (e.g., delusions), emotion (e.g., flatness, inappropriate affect), thought processes (e.g., loose associations), behavior (e.g., catatonia, disorganization), attention, concentration, motivation (e.g., avolition, impaired intention and planning), and judgment. The principal manifestations of this disorder usually are described in terms of positive and negative (deficit) symptoms, and more recently, disorganized symptoms. Positive symptoms include hallucinations, delusions, bizarre behavior, hostility, uncooperativeness, and paranoid ideation, while negative symptoms include restricted range and intensity of emotional expression (affective flattening), reduced thought and speech productivity (alogia), anhedonia, apathy, and decreased initiation of goal-directed behavior (avolition). Disorganized symptoms include disorganized speech (thought disorder) and behavior and poor attention.

Short-term efficacy of oral risperidone for the treatment of schizophrenia in adults was established in 4 controlled studies of 4–8 weeks' duration in patients who met DSM-III-R criteria for schizophrenia and who were hospitalized for psychotic symptoms. In these and other clinical studies conducted principally in patients with schizophrenia, oral risperidone was more effective than placebo and at least as effective as conventional (e.g., haloperidol, perphenazine) and certain atypical (e.g., olanzapine) antipsychotics in the treatment of schizophrenia. Data from limited clinical studies indicate that risperidone improves both positive and negative manifestations of schizophrenia, but that such improvements may not be substantially greater than those achieved by haloperidol, a conventional

antipsychotic. In these studies, improvement in manifestations of schizophrenia was based on the results of various psychiatric rating scales, including the Brief Psychiatric Rating Scale (BPRS) that assesses factors such as anergy, thought disturbances, activation, hostility/suspiciousness, and anxiety/depression; the BPRS psychosis cluster that assesses factors such as conceptual disorganization, hallucinatory behavior, suspiciousness, and unusual thought content in actively psychotic schizophrenic patients; the Scale for the Assessment of Negative Symptoms (SANS); the Positive and Negative Syndrome Scale (PANSS); and the Clinical Global Impression (CGI) scale.

Long-term efficacy of oral risperidone for the treatment of schizophrenia was established in a randomized, double-blind study in 365 adult outpatients who met DSM-IV criteria for schizophrenia or schizoaffective disorder. Patients were randomized to receive either flexible dosages of risperidone (2–8 mg daily) or haloperidol (5–20 mg daily) for 1–2 years and observed for relapse. Patients receiving risperidone experienced a substantially longer time to relapse than those who received haloperidol. In this study, approximately 25% of patients who received usual dosages of risperidone had relapsed by the end of the study compared with approximately 40% of those receiving usual dosages of haloperidol.

Efficacy of oral risperidone for the treatment of schizophrenia in adolescents was demonstrated in 2 short-term, double-blind clinical trials of 6–8 weeks' duration in adolescent patients 13–17 years of age who met DSM-IV criteria for schizophrenia and were experiencing an acute episode of schizophrenia at the time of enrollment. In the first study, patients were randomized to receive flexible dosages of risperidone of 1–3 mg daily or 4–6 mg daily or placebo. In the second study, patients were randomized to receive either risperidone target dosages of 0.15–0.6 mg daily or 1.5–6 mg daily. The primary efficacy measure in both studies was the change in total PANSS score from baseline. In these studies, risperidone in the target dosage groups from 1–6 mg daily was found to be more effective than placebo in substantially reducing the total PANSS score; however, dosages higher than 3 mg daily did not demonstrate additional efficacy.

Efficacy of the extended-release IM formulation of risperidone (Risperdal® Consta®) in the treatment of schizophrenia in adults was established, in part, based on extrapolation of efficacy data from oral risperidone. In addition, efficacy of extended-release IM risperidone was established in a multicenter, placebo-controlled study of 12 weeks' duration in adult inpatients and outpatients who met DSM-IV criteria for schizophrenia. During the 1-week run-in period of this study, other oral antipsychotic agents were discontinued and all patients received oral risperidone therapy (initially, 2 mg daily and titrated up to 4 mg daily for at least 3 days). During the 12-week, double-blind phase, patients were randomized to receive IM injections of 25, 50, or 75 mg of extended-release risperidone or placebo every 2 weeks. Patients receiving extended-release IM injections of risperidone were also given oral risperidone (2 mg daily in the 25-mg group, 4 mg in the 50-mg group, and 6 mg in the 75-mg group) for 3 weeks following the first injection to provide therapeutic plasma concentrations of the drug until the main release phase of risperidone from the IM injection site had begun; patients who received placebo injections were given placebo tablets. The primary efficacy measure in this study was the change in total PANSS score from baseline to end point. Total PANSS scores demonstrated substantially greater improvement in the patients treated with each of the 3 IM dosages of extended-release risperidone (25, 50, and 75 mg every 2 weeks) compared with patients receiving placebo. Although there were no significant differences in treatment effects between the 3 dosage groups, the effect size for the 75-mg group was numerically less than that of the 50-mg group. Subgroup analyses did not reveal any differences in treatment outcomes based on age, race, or gender.

Efficacy of extended-release IM risperidone in the treatment of schizophrenia has not been evaluated in controlled clinical trials for longer than 12 weeks; however, oral risperidone has been shown to be effective in delaying time to relapse with longer-term use. If the extended-release IM injection of risperidone is used for extended periods, the long-term risks and benefits of the drug should be reassessed periodically on an individualized basis.

Parenteral antipsychotic therapy with a long-acting IM preparation may be particularly useful in patients with schizophrenia and a history of poor compliance. In addition, long-acting antipsychotic preparations may be useful in patients with suspected GI malabsorption or variable GI absorption of the drug. The principal disadvantage of long-acting parenteral antipsychotics is the inability to terminate the drug's action when severe adverse reactions occur.

The manufacturer of extended-release IM risperidone recommends that patients should first receive oral risperidone therapy to establish tolerability of the drug before the long-acting IM preparation is used.

For additional information on the symptomatic management of schizophrenia, including treatment recommendations and results of the Clinical Antipsychotic Trials of Intervention Effectiveness (CATIE) research program, see Schizophrenia and Other Psychotic Disorders under Uses: Psychotic Disorders, in the Phenothiazines General Statement 28:16.08.24.

Geriatric Considerations

Although risperidone has been studied for use in the management of psychosis and aggression in institutionalized geriatric patients with moderate to severe dementia of the Alzheimer's type† (Alzheimer's disease, presenile or senile dementia), vascular dementia†, or a combination of the 2 types of dementia (i.e., mixed dementia†), use of the drug in geriatric patients with dementia-related psychosis is associated with an increased risk of adverse cerebrovascular events. In randomized, placebo-controlled studies in nursing home residents with dementia, oral risperidone at a dosage of approximately 1 mg daily was more effective than placebo in decreasing psychotic and behavioral symptoms (e.g., aggression, agitation) of dementia, as assessed by the Behavioral Pathology in Alzheimer's Disease scale (BEHAVE-AD) and the Cohen-Mansfield Agitation Inventory (CMAI). However, evidence from these studies showed a significantly higher incidence of adverse cerebrovascular events such as stroke and transient ischemic attacks (TIAs) associated with risperidone therapy relative to placebo. In addition, geriatric patients with dementia-related psychosis treated with atypical antipsychotic agents are at an increased risk of death compared with that among patients receiving placebo. (See Cautions: Geriatric Precautions.) Risperidone is not approved for the treatment of dementia-related psychosis.

● Bipolar Disorder

Risperidone is used orally as monotherapy for the treatment of acute manic and mixed episodes associated with bipolar I disorder in adults and adolescents 10–17 years of age, or in conjunction with lithium or valproate for the treatment of acute manic and mixed episodes associated with bipolar I disorder in adults. Risperidone as an extended-release injection is also used IM as monotherapy or adjunctive therapy with lithium or valproate for the maintenance treatment of bipolar I disorder in adults.

Efficacy of oral risperidone monotherapy in the treatment of acute manic and mixed episodes has been demonstrated in 2 placebo-controlled trials of 3 weeks' duration in adults who met the DSM-IV criteria for bipolar I disorder with acute manic or mixed episodes with or without psychotic features. The principal rating instrument used for assessing manic symptoms in these trials was the Young Mania Rating Scale (Y-MRS), an 11-item clinician-rated scale traditionally used to assess the degree of manic symptomatology in a range from 0 (no manic features) to 60 (maximum score). In the first 3-week, placebo-controlled trial, which was limited to patients with manic episodes, risperidone monotherapy was given at an initial dosage of 3 mg daily and subsequently in a flexible dosage ranging from 1–6 mg daily; the mean modal dosage was 4.1 mg daily. In the second 3-week, placebo-controlled trial, patients also were given an initial dosage of risperidone 3 mg daily and subsequently a flexible dosage ranging from 1–6 mg daily; the mean modal dosage was 5.6 mg daily. Risperidone was found to be superior to placebo in the reduction of the Y-MRS total score in both studies.

Efficacy of oral risperidone as monotherapy in the treatment of acute manic or mixed episodes associated with bipolar I disorder in children and adolescents 10–17 years of age was demonstrated in a 3-week, double-blind, placebo-controlled trial. The pediatric patients were randomized to receive 1 of 2 dosage ranges of risperidone or placebo. Risperidone was initiated at 0.25 mg daily and titrated to the maximum tolerated dosage within the target dosage ranges of 0.5–2.5 mg daily or 3–6 mg daily within 10 days. The principal rating instrument used for assessing manic symptoms in this trial was the Y-MRS. Both dosage ranges of risperidone were found to be substantially superior to placebo in reducing the Y-MRS total score; however, dosages exceeding 2.5 mg daily did not demonstrate greater efficacy than lower dosages of the drug (0.5–2.5 mg daily).

Efficacy of oral risperidone when used in conjunction with lithium or valproate in the treatment of acute manic or mixed episodes associated with bipolar I disorder has been demonstrated in one placebo-controlled trial of 3 weeks' duration in adults who met the DSM-IV criteria for bipolar I disorder (with or without a rapid cycling course) and who met diagnostic criteria for an acute manic or mixed episode (with or without psychotic features). In this study, inpatients and outpatients with bipolar disorder experiencing manic or mixed episodes who had not adequately responded to lithium or valproate monotherapy were randomized to receive risperidone, haloperidol, or placebo in conjunction with their original therapy. Risperidone therapy was given in an initial dosage of 2 mg daily and subsequently given in a flexible dosage ranging from 1–6 mg daily; the mean modal dosage was 3.8 mg daily. Lithium and valproate were given in conjunction with risperidone and plasma drug concentrations were maintained within therapeutic ranges of 0.6–1.4 mEq/L for lithium and 50–120 mcg/mL for valproate. Addition of risperidone to lithium or valproate was shown to be superior to continued monotherapy with lithium or valproate as assessed by reduction of Y-MRS total score.

In a second 3-week, placebo-controlled trial, inpatients and outpatients with bipolar mania receiving lithium, valproate (as divalproex), or carbamazepine therapy with inadequately controlled manic or mixed symptoms were randomized to receive oral risperidone or placebo in conjunction with their original therapy. Risperidone was given in a flexible dosage range of 1–6 mg daily, with an initial dosage of 2 mg daily; the mean modal dosage was 3.7 mg daily. Addition of risperidone to lithium, valproate, or carbamazepine therapy (with plasma drug concentrations maintained within therapeutic ranges of 0.6–1.4 mEq/L, 50–125 mcg/mL, or 4–12 mcg/mL, respectively) was not found to be superior to lithium, valproate, or carbamazepine given alone as assessed by reduction of the Y-MRS total score. A possible explanation for the failure of this trial was enzymatic induction of clearance of risperidone and its principal active metabolite, 9-hydroxyrisperidone, by carbamazepine in the subgroup of patients receiving combined therapy with these drugs, resulting in subtherapeutic plasma concentrations of risperidone and 9-hydroxyrisperidone.

Efficacy of the extended-release IM formulation of risperidone (Risperdal® Consta®) as monotherapy in the maintenance treatment of bipolar I disorder was established in a multicenter, placebo-controlled trial in adults who met the DSM-IV criteria for bipolar I disorder and who were either stable on their drug regimen or experiencing an acute manic or mixed episode. All patients in this study were treated with open-label extended-release IM risperidone therapy for 26 weeks. Patients received an initial risperidone dosage of 25 mg IM every 2 weeks; the dosage was increased to 37.5 or 50 mg or decreased to 12.5 mg every 2 weeks as clinically indicated; patients who maintained response at 26 weeks were randomized to double-blind treatment with either the same IM dosage of risperidone or placebo and then monitored for relapse. Time to relapse to any mood episode (the primary outcome variable) was substantially delayed in patients receiving extended-release IM risperidone therapy compared with placebo. The majority of relapses were caused by manic rather than depressive symptoms; based on patient history, patients enrolled in the study had more manic episodes than depressive episodes.

Efficacy of extended-release IM risperidone as adjunctive therapy with lithium or valproate in the maintenance treatment of bipolar I disorder was established in a multicenter, double-blind, placebo-controlled study in adults with bipolar I disorder treated with mood stabilizers (primarily lithium or valproate), antidepressants, and/or anxiolytics who had experienced at least 4 episodes of mood disorder requiring clinical intervention in the previous 12 months and at least 2 episodes in the previous 6 months. Following a 16-week, open-label treatment phase with extended-release IM risperidone (initial risperidone dosage of 25 mg every 2 weeks and increased to 37.5 or 50 mg or decreased to 12.5 mg, if necessary), patients who remained stable were randomized either to continue IM risperidone at the same dosage or to receive placebo for up to 52 weeks while continuing their usual treatment and were observed for relapse. Continuation of IM risperidone therapy in addition to mood stabilizers delayed time to relapse to any mood episode (depression, mania, hypomania, or mixed) compared with placebo; the relapses were approximately half depressive and half manic or mixed episodes in this study.

For the initial management of less severe manic or mixed episodes in patients with bipolar disorder, current APA recommendations state that monotherapy with lithium, valproate (e.g., valproate sodium, valproic acid, divalproex), or an antipsychotic such as olanzapine may be adequate. For more severe manic or mixed episodes, combined therapy with an antipsychotic and lithium or valproate is recommended as first-line therapy. For further information on the management of bipolar disorder, see Uses: Bipolar Disorder, in Lithium Salts 28:28.

The manufacturers state that clinicians who elect to use risperidone for extended periods should periodically reevaluate the long-term risks and benefits of the drug for the individual patient.

● Autistic Disorder

Risperidone is used orally for the management of irritability associated with autistic disorder in children and adolescents, including symptoms of aggression towards others, deliberate self-injuriousness, temper tantrums, and quickly changing moods.

Short-term efficacy of oral risperidone in children and adolescents with autistic disorder was established in 2 placebo-controlled trials of 8 weeks' duration in 156 children and adolescents (aged 5–16 years) who met the DSM-IV criteria for autistic disorder. Over 90% of the patients in these 2 trials were under 12 years of age and the majority weighed over 20 kg (weight range: 16–104.3 kg). The principal rating instruments used for assessing efficacy in these trials were the Aberrant Behavior Checklist (ABC) and the Clinical Global Impression-Change (CGI-C) scale. The primary outcome measure in both trials was the change from baseline to endpoint in the Irritability subscale of the ABC (ABC-I), which measures the emotional and behavioral symptoms of autism, including aggression toward others, deliberate self-injuriousness, temper tantrums, and rapidly changing moods. The CGI-C rating at endpoint was a co-primary outcome measure in one of the studies.

In the first 8-week, placebo-controlled trial, children and adolescents 5–16 years of age with autistic disorder received twice-daily placebo or risperidone 0.5–3.5 mg daily on a weight-adjusted basis, starting at 0.25 mg daily or 0.5 mg daily if baseline weight was less than 20 kg or 20 kg or greater, respectively; dosage was then titrated according to clinical response. Risperidone (mean modal dosage of 1.9 mg/day; equivalent to 0.06 mg/kg daily) was found to substantially improve scores on the ABC-I subscale and the CGI-C scale compared with placebo in this study.

In the second 8-week, placebo-controlled trial, children and adolescents 5–12 years of age with autistic disorder were given an initial risperidone dosage of 0.01 mg/kg daily, which was then titrated up to 0.02–0.06 mg/kg daily based on clinical response. Risperidone (mean modal dosage of 0.05 mg/kg daily; equivalent to 1.4 mg daily) substantially improved scores on the ABC-I subscale compared with placebo.

A third clinical trial conducted in children and adolescents 5–17 years of age who met DSM-IV criteria for autistic disorder and who had associated irritability and related behavioral symptoms compared 2 weight-based, fixed dosages of oral risperidone (high-dose and low-dose). Over 77% of the enrolled patients were younger than 12 years of age (mean age: 9 years) and 88% of the patients were male. In this 6-week, multicenter, double-blind study, patients were randomized to receive high-dose risperidone (1.25 mg daily for patients weighing from 20 to up to 45 kg and 1.75 mg daily for patients weighing 45 kg or more), low-dose risperidone (0.125 mg daily for those weighing from 20 to up to 45 kg and 0.175 mg daily for those weighing 45 kg or more), or placebo; the doses were administered once daily in the morning or evening (if sedation occurred). The primary outcome measure in this study was the change from baseline to end point in the ABC-I subscale. Treatment with risperidone substantially improved ABC-I scores in the high-dose risperidone group but not in the low-dose group, compared with placebo.

The efficacy of oral risperidone for long-term use (i.e., longer than 8 weeks) in children and adolescents with autistic disorder has been demonstrated in an open-label extension of the first 8-week, placebo-controlled trial in which 63 patients received risperidone for 4 or 6 months (depending on whether they received risperidone or placebo in the double-blind study). During the open-label treatment period, patients were maintained on a mean modal risperidone dosage of 1.8–2.1 mg daily (equivalent to 0.05–0.07 mg/kg daily).

Children and adolescents who maintained their positive response to risperidone (defined as at least a 25% improvement on the ABC-I subscale and a CGI-C rating of much improved or very much improved) during the 4–6 month, open-label treatment period (average duration of therapy was 140 days) were randomized to receive either risperidone or placebo during an 8-week, double-blind withdrawal trial. A substantially lower relapse rate was observed in the risperidone group compared with the placebo group during the pre-planned interim analysis of data from this trial. Based on the interim analysis results, the study was terminated since a statistically significant effect on relapse prevention was demonstrated. Relapse was defined as at least a 25% worsening on the most recent assessment of the ABC-I subscale (in relation to baseline for the randomized withdrawal phase).

The manufacturers state that clinicians who elect to use risperidone in children and adolescents with autistic disorder for extended periods should periodically re-evaluate the long-term risks and benefits of the drug for the individual patient.

Although not curative, pharmacologic agents, such as risperidone, generally are used in children and adolescents with autistic disorder to reduce behavioral disturbances associated with autism and to help facilitate the child's or adolescent's adjustment and engagement in intensive, targeted educational interventions. In clinical studies, risperidone was not found to improve certain core symptoms of autism (e.g., language deficits, impaired social relatedness). However, the drug was more effective than placebo in improving scores on subscales for sensory motor behaviors, affectual reactions, and sensory responses in a controlled study. The possible risks, including clinically important weight gain, tardive dyskinesia,

withdrawal dyskinesia, and other extrapyramidal reactions associated with the drug, should be considered. (See Cautions.)

Risperidone also has been used in a limited number of adults† for the treatment of autistic disorder and other pervasive developmental disorders.

DOSAGE AND ADMINISTRATION

● Administration

Risperidone is administered orally or by IM injection.

Oral Administration

Risperidone is administered orally, either in a once-daily dose or in 2 equally divided doses daily. Since food reportedly does not affect the rate or extent of GI absorption, the drug can be administered without regard to meals. Some experts state that once-daily administration of risperidone may be sufficient in most patients receiving maintenance therapy because of the extended half-life of the drug's principal active metabolite (9-hydroxyrisperidone).

Because risperidone can cause orthostatic hypotension and syncope, twice-daily oral administration of the drug may be preferable in geriatric patients and patients with renal or hepatic impairment to minimize the risk of these adverse effects.

In pediatric patients receiving risperidone for the management of schizophrenia or bipolar mania who experience persistent somnolence, twice-daily administration may be helpful.

In children and adolescents receiving risperidone for the management of irritability associated with autistic disorder who experience persistent somnolence, administering the drug once daily at bedtime, twice-daily administration, or a reduction in dosage may be helpful.

Risperidone oral solution may be administered directly from the calibrated pipette provided by the manufacturer or mixed in a beverage prior to administration. The oral solution is compatible in the following beverages: water, coffee, orange juice, and low-fat milk; risperidone oral solution is *not* compatible in cola or tea.

Patients receiving risperidone orally disintegrating tablets should be instructed not to remove a tablet from the blister until just prior to dosing. The tablet should not be pushed through the foil, since this may damage the tablet. With dry hands, the blister backing should be peeled back to expose the tablet. The tablet should then be gently removed and immediately placed on the tongue, where it rapidly disintegrates (i.e., within seconds) in saliva, and then subsequently swallowed with or without liquid. Risperidone orally disintegrating tablets should not be divided or chewed.

IM Administration

In patients who have never received oral risperidone, the manufacturer recommends that tolerability with oral risperidone therapy should be established prior to initiating IM therapy with extended-release risperidone (Risperdal® Consta®).

Risperidone extended-release injection is commercially available in a dose pack containing a vial of the drug in extended-release microspheres, a prefilled syringe containing 2 mL of diluent, a vial adapter device, and 2 safety needles for IM injection (one for deltoid and one for gluteal administration). Risperidone extended-release microspheres for injection must be reconstituted prior to administration using *only* the components of the dose pack supplied by the manufacturer. The dose pack should be allowed to sit at room temperature for at least 30 minutes before reconstitution; the dose pack should *not* be warmed any other way. Risperidone extended-release microspheres should be reconstituted using only the diluent in the prefilled syringe supplied by the manufacturer. The entire contents of the prefilled syringe should be injected into the vial, and the vial should be shaken vigorously while the plunger rod is held down with the thumb for at least 10 seconds to ensure a homogeneous suspension; the reconstituted suspension should appear uniform, thick, and milky. The manufacturer's prescribing information should be consulted for additional details on use of the components of the dose pack to reconstitute and administer risperidone injection. The manufacturer states that different dosage strengths of IM risperidone should not be combined in a single administration.

Following reconstitution, immediate use is necessary because the suspension will settle over time. Once the reconstituted suspension has been transferred to the syringe and the appropriate needle attached, the syringe should be vigorously shaken again to resuspend the drug just prior to the IM injection.

The entire contents of the vial should be administered by deep IM injection into either the deltoid muscle (using the 1-inch needle supplied by the manufacturer) or the upper outer quadrant of the gluteal area (using the 2-inch needle supplied by the manufacturer) every 2 weeks, alternating between the 2 arms or 2 buttocks, respectively. *Each injection should be administered by a health care professional.* IM injections at the same dosages into the deltoid and gluteal areas are bioequivalent and are, therefore, interchangeable. The injection should *not* be administered IV. In addition, care should be taken to avoid inadvertent injection into a blood vessel.

Dispensing and Administration Precautions

The US Food and Drug Administration (FDA) alerted healthcare professionals and patients of medication error reports in which patients were given risperidone (Risperdal®) instead of ropinirole hydrochloride (Requip®, a nonergot-derivative dopamine receptor agonist) and vice versa. As of June 2011, the FDA had evaluated 226 wrong drug medication errors associated with confusion between these 2 drugs; all of the reports involved tablet formulations of the drugs. Several of these cases resulted in adverse effects (including confusion, lethargy, ataxia, hallucinations, tiredness, dizziness, tingling, numbness, and altered mental status) and some of the patients who took the wrong drug required hospitalization. The FDA has determined that the factors contributing to the confusion between these 2 products include similarities in both the trade (brand) and generic (nonproprietary) names, similarities in the container labels and carton packaging, illegible handwriting on the prescriptions, and overlapping product characteristics (such as drug strengths, dosage forms, and dosing intervals). It is also possible that the 2 products may be stocked close to one another on pharmacy shelves whether they are alphabeticized by brand or generic name. In addition, some generic manufacturers make both products. Healthcare professionals are therefore reminded to clearly print out or spell out the drug name on prescriptions and to make sure their patients know the name of their prescribed drug and the reason they are taking it.

● *Dosage*

Schizophrenia

Oral Dosage

Risperidone has a bell-shaped dose-response curve, with therapeutic efficacy of oral dosages of 12–16 mg daily lower than that of dosages of 4–8 mg daily in adults. Because dosage information contained in the manufacturers' labeling principally is derived from early clinical studies of the drug in patients not typical of the general population of patients treated in the community (i.e., in hospitalized, chronically ill schizophrenic patients accustomed to high-dose antipsychotic therapies), dosage of risperidone should be individualized according to the patient's response and tolerance. Clinicians also may consider consulting published protocols for specific dosage information, particularly in geriatric or younger patients, and in those experiencing their first psychotic episode.

The manufacturers' labeling states that the initial oral dosage of risperidone for the treatment of schizophrenia in adults is 2 mg daily (given as either 2 mg once daily or 1 mg twice daily). The dosage may be increased in increments of 1–2 mg daily at intervals of 24 hours or greater, as tolerated, up to a target dosage of 4–8 mg daily (administered once daily or in 2 equally divided doses). The manufacturers state that slower dosage titration may be appropriate in certain patients.

Evidence from open-labeled studies and clinical experience with the drug indicate that an initial dosage of 1–2 mg daily, with dosage increases in increments of 0.5–1 mg daily titrated over 6–7 days, as tolerated, to a target dosage of 4 mg daily may be appropriate for the management of schizophrenia in most otherwise healthy adult patients. Lower initial dosages (e.g., 1 mg daily) and slower dosage titrations to an initial target dosage of 2 mg daily may be appropriate for younger patients and in those being treated for their first psychotic episode; dosage may then be titrated up to 4 mg daily depending on clinical response at the lower dosage and adverse neurologic effects. Such patients appear to benefit optimally from a risperidone dosage of 1–3 mg daily. A substantial number of patients being treated for their first psychotic episode start to develop extrapyramidal symptoms once dosages are increased above 2 mg daily. Dosage reductions should be considered in any patient who develops extrapyramidal symptoms.

While antipsychotic efficacy has been established in clinical trials at oral risperidone dosages ranging from 4–16 mg daily, the manufacturers and some clinicians state that dosages exceeding 6 mg daily, when given in 2 divided doses, did not result in further improvement but were associated with increases in some adverse effects, including extrapyramidal manifestations. Therefore, the

manufacturers state that dosages exceeding 6 mg (in 2 divided doses) daily generally are not recommended and those exceeding 16 mg daily have not been evaluated for safety. In a single study of once-daily dosing, efficacy results generally were stronger for 8 mg than for 4 mg.

For the treatment of schizophrenia in adolescents 13–17 years of age, the manufacturer recommends an initial oral risperidone dosage of 0.5 mg once daily in the morning or evening. Dosage adjustments may be made in increments of 0.5 or 1 mg daily at intervals of 24 hours or greater, as tolerated, up to the recommended dosage of 3 mg daily. While antipsychotic efficacy in adolescents has been demonstrated in clinical trials at oral dosages ranging from 1–6 mg daily, no additional benefit was observed with dosages exceeding 3 mg daily and higher dosages were associated with increased adverse effects. Dosages exceeding 6 mg daily in adolescents have not been evaluated in clinical studies. Pediatric patients who experience persistent somnolence may benefit from twice-daily administration of the drug in 2 equally divided doses.

The manufacturers state that there are no systematically collected data that specifically address switching from other antipsychotic agents to risperidone or concomitant administration with other antipsychotic agents. The first risperidone dose should be administered in place of the next scheduled parenteral antipsychotic dose in schizophrenic patients being switched from long-acting (depot) parenteral antipsychotic therapy to oral risperidone therapy.

The optimum duration of oral risperidone therapy currently is not known, but maintenance therapy with risperidone 2–8 mg daily has been shown to be effective in adults for up to 2 years. The manufacturers state that patients responding to risperidone therapy should generally continue to receive therapy at their effective dosage beyond the acute response. Patients should be reassessed periodically to determine the need for continued therapy with the drug. If risperidone therapy is reinitiated after a drug-free period, the manufacturers recommend that the appropriate recommended schedule of careful dosage titration be employed.

The American Psychiatric Association (APA) states that prudent long-term treatment options in adults with schizophrenia with remitted first episodes or multiple episodes include either indefinite maintenance therapy or gradual discontinuance of the antipsychotic agent with close follow-up and a plan to reinstitute treatment upon symptom recurrence. Discontinuance of antipsychotic therapy should be considered only after a period of at least 1 year of symptom remission or optimal response while receiving the antipsychotic agent. In patients who have had multiple previous psychotic episodes or 2 psychotic episodes within 5 years, indefinite maintenance antipsychotic treatment is recommended.

IM Dosage

For the management of schizophrenia in adults, the recommended dosage of extended-release risperidone injection is 25 mg administered by deep IM injection into the deltoid or gluteal area every 2 weeks. The manufacturer recommends that patients first receive oral risperidone to establish tolerability of the drug before the extended-release risperidone injection is used. To ensure that adequate plasma antipsychotic concentrations are maintained prior to the main release of risperidone from the injection site, therapy with oral risperidone or another oral antipsychotic agent (e.g., for patients being switched from other oral antipsychotic therapy to IM risperidone) should be given with the first IM injection of risperidone and continued for 3 weeks, then discontinued. The need for continuing any concomitant therapy for managing extrapyramidal manifestations should be periodically reevaluated.

Some patients not responding to the 25-mg dosage may benefit from increasing the IM dosage to 37.5 or 50 mg every 2 weeks. However, the dosage should not be increased more frequently than every 4 weeks, and clinical effects of the increased dosage should not be expected earlier than 3 weeks after the first injection of the higher dosage. The maximum IM dosage should not exceed 50 mg every 2 weeks since higher dosages were associated with an increased incidence of adverse effects, but no additional clinical benefit was observed.

In some patients, an initial risperidone dosage of 12.5 mg IM every 2 weeks and maintenance dosages as low as 12.5 mg every 2 weeks may be appropriate (e.g., patients with hepatic or renal impairment, patients who are receiving concurrent therapy with other drugs that increase plasma risperidone concentrations, patients with a history of poor tolerability to psychotropic drugs); however, efficacy of the 12.5 mg every 2 weeks dosage has not been evaluated in clinical trials.

Although no controlled studies have been conducted to establish the optimum duration of IM risperidone therapy in patients with schizophrenia, oral risperidone has been shown to be effective in delaying time to relapse with longer-term use. It is recommended that responding patients be continued on treatment with IM risperidone at the lowest dosage needed. Patients should periodically be reassessed to determine the need for continued treatment.

If therapy with IM risperidone is reinitiated after a drug-free period, oral risperidone (or another oral antipsychotic agent) should again be administered initially for supplementation.

Bipolar Disorder

Oral Dosage

For the management of acute manic or mixed episodes associated with bipolar I disorder in adults, either as monotherapy or as adjunctive therapy with lithium or valproate, the recommended initial oral dosage of risperidone is 2–3 mg given once daily. Dosage may be increased or decreased by 1 mg daily at intervals of not less than 24 hours, reflecting the procedures in the placebo-controlled trials. In these trials, the short-term (i.e., 3-week) antimanic efficacy of risperidone was demonstrated in a flexible dosage ranging from 1 to 6 mg daily. Safety of dosages exceeding 6 mg daily has not been established.

For the treatment of acute manic or mixed episodes associated with bipolar I disorder in children and adolescents 10–17 years of age, the recommended initial oral dosage of risperidone is 0.5 mg given once daily in the morning or evening. Dosage adjustments may be made in increments of 0.5–1 mg at intervals of not less than 24 hours, as tolerated, up to a target dosage of 1–2.5 mg daily. While efficacy in pediatric patients with bipolar mania has been demonstrated in clinical trials at oral dosages ranging from 0.5–6 mg daily, no additional benefit was observed with dosages exceeding 2.5 mg daily and higher dosages were associated with increased adverse effects. Safety and efficacy of oral dosages exceeding 6 mg daily in children and adolescents have not been evaluated in clinical studies. Pediatric patients who experience persistent somnolence may benefit from twice-daily administration of the drug in 2 equally divided doses.

The optimum duration of risperidone therapy for bipolar disorder currently is not known. While it is generally agreed that pharmacologic treatment beyond an acute response in mania is desirable, both for maintenance of the initial response and for prevention of new manic episodes, there are no systematically obtained data to support the use of oral risperidone beyond 3 weeks. Therefore, the manufacturers state that clinicians who elect to use risperidone for extended periods should periodically reevaluate the long-term risks and benefits of the drug for the individual patient.

IM Dosage

For the maintenance treatment of bipolar I disorder in adults, either as monotherapy or as adjunctive therapy with lithium or valproate, the recommended dosage of extended-release risperidone injection is 25 mg administered by deep IM injection in the deltoid or gluteal area every 2 weeks. The manufacturer recommends that patients first receive oral risperidone to establish tolerability of the drug before the extended-release risperidone injection is used. To ensure that adequate therapeutic plasma concentrations are maintained prior to the main release of risperidone from the injection site, therapy with oral risperidone or another oral antipsychotic agent (e.g., for patients being switched from other oral antipsychotic therapy to IM risperidone) should be given with the first IM injection of risperidone and continued for 3 weeks, then discontinued. The need for continuing any concomitant therapy for managing extrapyramidal manifestations should be periodically reevaluated.

Some patients not responding to an initial IM risperidone dosage of 25 mg every 2 weeks may benefit from increasing the dosage to 37.5 or 50 mg every 2 weeks. However, the dosage should not be increased more frequently than every 4 weeks, and clinical effects of the increased dosage should not be expected earlier than 3 weeks after the first injection of the higher dosage. Safety and efficacy of IM dosages exceeding 50 mg every 2 weeks have not been evaluated in clinical trials of risperidone in the maintenance treatment of bipolar disorder.

In some patients, an initial dosage of 12.5 mg IM every 2 weeks may be appropriate (e.g., patients with hepatic or renal impairment, patients concurrently receiving drugs that increase plasma concentrations of risperidone, or patients with a history of poor tolerability to psychotropic drugs); however, efficacy of the 12.5-mg IM dosage has not been evaluated in clinical trials.

If therapy with IM risperidone is reinitiated after a drug-free period, oral risperidone (or another oral antipsychotic agent) should again be administered initially for supplementation.

The manufacturer states that clinicians who elect to use extended-release IM risperidone for extended periods should periodically reevaluate the long-term risks and benefits of the drug for the individual patient.

Autistic Disorder

For the management of irritability associated with autistic disorder in children 5 years of age and older and adolescents, the recommended initial oral dosage of risperidone is 0.25 mg daily for patients weighing less than 20 kg and 0.5 mg daily for patients weighing 20 kg or more. The drug may be administered either once or twice daily. Patients experiencing persistent somnolence may benefit from a once-daily dosage administered at bedtime, administering half the daily dosage twice daily, or a reduction in dosage.

Dosage should be individualized according to clinical response and tolerability of the patient. After a minimum of 4 days following initiation of therapy, the dosage may be increased to the recommended dosage of 0.5 mg daily for patients weighing less than 20 kg and 1 mg daily for patients weighing 20 kg or more; this dosage should then be maintained for a minimum of 14 days. In patients not responding adequately, increases in dosage may be considered at intervals of 2 weeks or longer in increments of 0.25 mg daily for patients weighing less than 20 kg or 0.5 mg daily for patients weighing 20 kg or more. Dosages ranging from 0.5–3 mg daily were effective in clinical studies. Dosage data for children weighing less than 15 kg currently are lacking. In addition, safety and efficacy in pediatric patients younger than 5 years of age have not been established.

In the pivotal clinical trials, 90% of patients who responded to risperidone therapy (based on at least 25% improvement in the Irritability subscale of the Aberrant Behavior Checklist [ABC-I]) received dosages ranging from 0.5–2.5 mg daily. The maximum daily dosage in one of the trials, when the therapeutic effect reached a plateau, was 1 mg in patients weighing less than 20 kg, 2.5 mg in patients weighing 20 kg or more, and 3 mg in patients weighing more than 45 kg.

Once adequate clinical response has been achieved and maintained, a gradual reduction in dosage to achieve an optimal balance of efficacy and safety should be considered.

The manufacturers state that clinicians who elect to use risperidone in children and adolescents with autistic disorder for extended periods should periodically reevaluate the long-term risks and benefits of the drug for the individual patient.

Geriatric Patients and Others at Risk of Orthostatic Hypotension

Like other α-adrenergic blocking agents, risperidone can induce orthostatic hypotension (e.g., manifested as dizziness, tachycardia, and occasionally syncope), particularly during initiation of oral therapy with the drug. The manufacturers and some clinicians state that the risk of this effect can be minimized by limiting the initial oral dosage of risperidone to 2 mg daily, given as a single daily dose or 1 mg twice daily, in otherwise healthy adults and to 0.5 mg twice daily in geriatric patients or patients with renal or hepatic impairment. However, other clinicians recommend initiating risperidone therapy at a dosage of 0.25 mg daily in geriatric patients and gradually increasing the dosage as tolerated. (See Cautions: Geriatric Precautions.) Most geriatric patients should not be maintained at an oral dosage exceeding 3 mg daily.

For geriatric patients with schizophrenia or bipolar disorder, the recommended IM risperidone dosage of the extended-release injection is 25 mg every 2 weeks. Oral risperidone (or another oral antipsychotic agent) should be given with the first risperidone extended-release injection and should be continued for 3 weeks to ensure that adequate therapeutic plasma concentrations are maintained prior to the main release phase of risperidone from the injection site.

Geriatric patients and patients with a predisposition to hypotensive reactions or for whom such reactions would pose a particular risk should be instructed in nonpharmacologic interventions that help reduce the occurrence of orthostatic hypotension (e.g., sitting on the edge of the bed for several minutes before attempting to stand in the morning, slowly rising from a seated position). These patients should avoid sodium depletion or dehydration and circumstances that accentuate hypotension (e.g., alcohol intake, high ambient temperature). Monitoring of orthostatic vital signs also should be considered.

Particular caution also is warranted in patients with known cardiovascular disease (e.g., history of myocardial infarction or ischemia, heart failure, conduction abnormalities), cerebrovascular disease, or conditions that would predispose to hypotension (e.g., dehydration, hypovolemia, concomitant antihypertensive therapy) and in those for whom such reactions would pose a risk, and cautious dosage titration and careful monitoring are necessary in such patients. Dosage reduction should be considered in any patient in whom hypotension develops.

● Dosage in Renal and Hepatic Impairment

Because elimination of risperidone may be reduced and the risk of adverse effects, particularly hypotension, increased in patients with renal impairment, oral risperidone therapy should be initiated at a reduced dosage of 0.5 mg twice daily in adults with severe renal impairment (creatinine clearance less than 30 mL/minute) and increased as necessary and tolerated in increments of 0.5 mg or less, administered twice daily; increases beyond a dosage level of 1.5 mg twice daily should be made at intervals of at least 7 days. Likewise, this reduced oral dosage should be employed in patients with severe hepatic impairment (Child-Pugh score 10–15) because of the risk of an increased free fraction of risperidone in such patients.

If IM risperidone is used for management of schizophrenia or bipolar disorder in adults with renal or hepatic impairment, the patient should be treated with titrated doses of oral risperidone prior to initiating treatment with the extended-release injection. The recommended starting oral risperidone dosage is 0.5 mg twice daily during the first week, which can be increased to 1 mg twice daily or 2 mg once daily during the second week. If a dosage of at least 2 mg daily of oral risperidone is well tolerated, an IM dosage of 25 mg of the extended-release injection can be administered every 2 weeks. Alternatively, such patients may receive an initial dosage of 12.5 mg IM every 2 weeks; however, efficacy of the 12.5-mg dosage has not been evaluated in clinical trials. Oral supplementation should be continued for 3 weeks after the first injection until the main release of risperidone from the injection site has begun. In some patients, slower titration may be medically appropriate.

● Dosage Adjustments for Specific Drug Interactions

Adjustment of risperidone dosage may be necessary in patients receiving concomitant therapy with cytochrome P-450 (CYP) enzyme inducers (e.g., carbamazepine, phenobarbital, phenytoin, rifampin) or CYP2D6 inhibitors (e.g., fluoxetine, paroxetine). When risperidone is used concomitantly with a CYP enzyme inducer (e.g., carbamazepine), the manufacturers recommend that the dosage of oral risperidone be increased, up to double the patient's usual dosage.

In patients receiving IM risperidone, an increase in the IM dosage or addition of oral risperidone may be considered when used concomitantly with a CYP enzyme inducer.

A decrease in the dosage of oral or IM risperidone may be necessary when the CYP enzyme inducer is discontinued.

When oral risperidone is used concomitantly with fluoxetine or paroxetine (CYP2D6 inhibitors), the manufacturers recommend decreasing the dosage of risperidone and not exceeding 8 mg daily in adults. If oral risperidone is initiated in patients receiving fluoxetine or paroxetine, risperidone should be titrated slowly. When fluoxetine or paroxetine is discontinued, an increase in the dosage of risperidone may be necessary.

If fluoxetine or paroxetine is initiated in patients receiving IM risperidone, a dosage reduction may be considered; dosage of IM risperidone may be reduced 2–4 weeks before initiating fluoxetine or paroxetine. If fluoxetine or paroxetine is initiated in patients receiving IM risperidone 25 mg every 2 weeks, the manufacturer recommends continuing 25 mg every 2 weeks; dosage reduction to 12.5 mg every 2 weeks or interruption of therapy may be necessary based on clinical judgment. In patients already receiving fluoxetine or paroxetine, IM risperidone may be initiated at a dosage of 12.5 mg every 2 weeks; however, efficacy of the 12.5-mg dosage has not been evaluated in clinical trials.

CAUTIONS

Risperidone shares many of the toxic potentials of other antipsychotic agents (e.g., other atypical antipsychotic agents, phenothiazines), and the usual precautions associated with therapy with these agents should be observed. (See Cautions in the Phenothiazines General Statement 28:16.08.24.)

The most frequent adverse effects of oral risperidone reported in over 5% of patients who received the drug in clinical trials and with an incidence of at least twice that of those receiving placebo were parkinsonism, akathisia, dystonia, tremor, sedation, dizziness, anxiety, blurred vision, nausea, vomiting, upper abdominal pain, stomach discomfort, dyspepsia, diarrhea, salivary hypersecretion, constipation, dry mouth, increased appetite, weight gain, fatigue, rash, nasal congestion, upper respiratory tract infection, nasopharyngitis, and pharyngolaryngeal pain. Adverse effects associated with discontinuance of oral risperidone therapy in more than 1% of adults and/or more than 2% of pediatric patients were nausea, somnolence, sedation, vomiting, dizziness, and akathisia.

The most frequent adverse effects of oral risperidone reported in at least 5% of adult patients with schizophrenia who received the drug in 3 short-term (4–8

week) clinical studies and with an incidence of at least twice that of those who received placebo were nausea, parkinsonism, akathisia, sedation, and dizziness. Approximately 7% of adult patients receiving oral risperidone in placebo-controlled studies discontinued treatment because of adverse effects compared with 4% of those receiving placebo. Adverse effects associated with discontinuance of therapy in at least 2 risperidone-treated patients were dizziness, nausea, vomiting, parkinsonism, somnolence, dystonia, agitation, abdominal pain, orthostatic hypotension, and akathisia.

Adverse effects occurring in 5% or more of pediatric patients with schizophrenia receiving oral risperidone in a 6-week clinical study and with an incidence of at least twice that of those receiving placebo included salivary hypersecretion, sedation, parkinsonism, akathisia, dizziness, dystonia, and anxiety. Approximately 7% of pediatric patients receiving oral risperidone in the study discontinued treatment because of adverse effects compared with 4% of those receiving placebo. Adverse effects associated with discontinuance of therapy in more than one risperidone-treated patient included dizziness, somnolence, sedation, lethargy, anxiety, balance disorder, hypotension, and palpitation.

The most frequent adverse effects of oral risperidone reported in at least 5% of adult patients with bipolar mania who received the drug as monotherapy in placebo-controlled trials and with an incidence of at least twice that of those receiving placebo were nausea, parkinsonism, sedation, akathisia, tremor, and dystonia. In placebo-controlled trials of oral risperidone in conjunction with mood stabilizers, adverse effects reported in at least 5% of patients and with an incidence of at least twice that of those receiving placebo were parkinsonism, sedation, akathisia, dizziness, tremor, and pharyngolaryngeal pain. In placebo-controlled trials of risperidone monotherapy in adults, approximately 6% of patients receiving the drug discontinued therapy because of adverse effects compared with about 5% of those receiving placebo. Adverse effects associated with discontinuance of therapy in these studies included parkinsonism, lethargy, and dizziness.

Adverse effects reported in 5% or more of pediatric patients with bipolar mania receiving oral risperidone in a 3-week, placebo-controlled trial and with an incidence of at least twice that of those receiving placebo included blurred vision, upper abdominal pain, nausea, vomiting, diarrhea, dyspepsia, stomach discomfort, fatigue, increased appetite, sedation, dizziness, parkinsonism, dystonia, akathisia, anxiety, pharyngolaryngeal pain, and rash. In this study, 12% of pediatric patients receiving risperidone for bipolar mania discontinued treatment because of adverse effects compared with 7% of those receiving placebo. Adverse effects associated with discontinuance of therapy in at least one risperidone-treated patient were nausea, somnolence, sedation, and vomiting.

The most frequent adverse effects of oral risperidone reported in at least 5% of pediatric patients with irritability associated with autistic disorder who received the drug in 3 placebo-controlled trials and with an incidence of at least twice that of those receiving placebo were constipation, dry mouth, salivary hypersecretion, fatigue, nasopharyngitis, upper respiratory tract infection, weight gain, increased appetite, sedation, drooling, tremor, dizziness, parkinsonism, and nasal congestion. Sedation was the most frequent adverse effect in these trials, occurring in 63% of the risperidone-treated patients and in 15% of patients receiving placebo. (See Dosage and Administration: Administration and also see Cautions: Pediatric Precautions.)

The most frequent adverse effects associated with use of risperidone extended-release IM injection reported in at least 5% of adult patients with schizophrenia in clinical trials were headache, parkinsonism, dizziness, akathisia, fatigue, constipation, dyspepsia, sedation, weight gain, pain in extremity, and dry mouth. The most frequent adverse effects associated with the use of risperidone extended-release IM injection in adult patients with bipolar disorder were weight gain in the monotherapy study and tremor and parkinsonism in the adjunctive therapy study.

● Nervous System Effects
Tardive Dyskinesia

Use of antipsychotic agents may be associated with tardive dyskinesia, a syndrome of potentially irreversible, involuntary, dyskinetic movements. In one open-label study, an annual incidence of tardive dyskinesia of 0.3% was reported in patients with schizophrenia who received approximately 8–9 mg of oral risperidone daily for at least 1 year. The risk of developing tardive dyskinesia and the likelihood that it will become irreversible appear to increase with the duration of therapy and cumulative dose of antipsychotic agents administered; however, the syndrome may occur, although much less frequently, after relatively short periods of treatment with low dosages.

Management of tardive dyskinesia generally consists of gradual discontinuance of the precipitating antipsychotic agent when possible, reducing the dosage of the first-generation (conventional) antipsychotic agent or switching to a second-generation (atypical) antipsychotic agent, or switching to clozapine therapy. The syndrome may remit, partially or completely, if antipsychotic therapy is discontinued. However, antipsychotic therapy itself may suppress or partially suppress the signs and symptoms of the syndrome and thereby may possibly mask the underlying process. The effect that such symptomatic suppression has upon the long-term course of tardive dyskinesia is unknown. Vesicular monoamine transporter 2 (VMAT2) inhibitors (e.g., deutetrabenazine, valbenazine tosylate) have been shown to be effective in reducing symptoms of tardive dyskinesia in controlled clinical studies and may allow some patients to continue receiving antipsychotic therapy. (See Deutetrabenazine 28:56 and Valbenazine Tosylate 28:56.)

Risperidone should be prescribed in a manner that is most likely to minimize the occurrence of tardive dyskinesia. Chronic antipsychotic treatment generally should be reserved for patients who suffer from a chronic illness that is known to respond to antipsychotic agents, and for whom alternative, equally effective, but potentially less harmful treatments are not available or appropriate. In patients who do require chronic treatment, the smallest dosage and the shortest duration of treatment producing a satisfactory clinical response should be sought, and the need for continued treatment should be reassessed periodically.

The American Psychiatric Association (APA) currently recommends that patients receiving atypical antipsychotic agents be assessed clinically for abnormal involuntary movements every 12 months and that patients considered to be at increased risk for tardive dyskinesia be assessed every 6 months. If signs and symptoms of tardive dyskinesia appear in a risperidone-treated patient, risperidone discontinuance should be considered; however, some patients may require continued treatment with the drug despite the presence of the syndrome.

For additional information on tardive dyskinesia, including manifestations and treatment, see Tardive Dyskinesia under Cautions: Nervous System Effects, in the Phenothiazines General Statement 28:16.08.24.

Extrapyramidal Reactions

Extrapyramidal reactions occurred in 12–17% of adults with schizophrenia receiving oral risperidone dosages of 2–4 mg daily and in 20–35% of patients receiving dosages of 16 mg daily in clinical studies; these reactions appear to be dose related. At recommended therapeutic dosages of risperidone (4–8 mg daily) for schizophrenia, the severity of extrapyramidal reactions appears to be comparable to placebo and clozapine 400 mg daily, and substantially less than that associated with haloperidol 10 or 20 mg daily. Similarly, the severity of parkinsonian symptoms, as assessed on the parkinsonism subscale of the Extrapyramidal Symptom Rating Scale (ESRS), is also linearly related to risperidone dosages of 2–16 mg daily, with the incidence of parkinsonian symptoms at risperidone dosages of 6 mg daily or less comparable to that of placebo and substantially less than that seen with haloperidol dosages of 20 mg daily.

Neuroleptic Malignant Syndrome

Neuroleptic malignant syndrome (NMS), a potentially fatal syndrome requiring immediate discontinuance of therapy and intensive symptomatic treatment, has been reported in patients receiving antipsychotic agents, including risperidone. For additional information on NMS, see Neuroleptic Malignant Syndrome under Nervous System Effects: Extrapyramidal Reactions in Cautions, in the Phenothiazines General Statement 28:16.08.24.

Other Nervous System Effects

Dose-related somnolence is a commonly reported adverse effect associated with risperidone treatment. Approximately 41% of patients receiving 16 mg of oral risperidone daily and 16% of patients receiving placebo reported somnolence in a study utilizing a checklist to detect adverse events. Somnolence was reported in 5% of patients receiving extended-release IM risperidone in multiple-dose studies. (See Cautions: Pediatric Precautions.)

Insomnia and anxiety have been reported in 25–32 and 11–16%, respectively, of adult patients with schizophrenia receiving oral risperidone.

● Cardiovascular Effects

Orthostatic Hypotension

Orthostatic hypotension associated with dizziness, tachycardia, and in some patients, syncope, especially during the initial dose-titration period, has been reported in patients receiving risperidone, probably reflecting the drug's α-adrenergic antagonistic properties. Syncope was reported in 0.2% of patients receiving oral risperidone in phase 2 and 3 studies in adults with schizophrenia and in 0.8% of patients receiving extended-release IM risperidone in multiple-dose studies.

Risperidone should be used with particular caution in patients with known cardiovascular disease (history of myocardial infarction or ischemia, heart failure, or conduction abnormalities), cerebrovascular disease, or conditions that would predispose to hypotension (e.g., dehydration, hypovolemia). Clinically important hypotension has been observed with concomitant use of oral risperidone and antihypertensive drug therapy.

The risk of orthostatic hypotension and syncope may be minimized by limiting initial oral risperidone dosages to 2 mg daily (given as 2 mg once daily or as 1 mg twice daily) in otherwise healthy adults and to 0.5 mg twice daily in geriatric patients and patients with renal or hepatic impairment. (See Dosage and Administration.) Monitoring of orthostatic vital signs should be considered in patients for whom orthostatic hypotension is of concern. Dosage reduction of risperidone should be considered if hypotension occurs.

Other Cardiovascular Effects

Pooled analysis of results of placebo-controlled studies indicates that oral risperidone therapy generally is not associated with statistically significant changes in ECG parameters (e.g., PR, QT, or QT_c intervals) and heart rate. However, in short-term studies in adults with schizophrenia, higher oral dosages of risperidone (8–16 mg daily) were associated with a higher mean increase in heart rate of 4–6 beats per minute compared with placebo. In addition, sinus bradycardia, sinus tachycardia, atrioventricular (AV) block, and bundle branch block have been reported in patients receiving risperidone during clinical trials. Atrial fibrillation, cardiopulmonary arrest, QT interval prolongation, and sudden death also have been reported during postmarketing surveillance; however, a causal relationship to the drug has not been established.

● Endocrine and Metabolic Effects

Atypical antipsychotic agents have been associated with metabolic changes that may increase cardiovascular and cerebrovascular risk, including hyperglycemia, dyslipidemia, and body weight gain. While all of these drugs produce some metabolic changes, each drug has its own specific risk profile.

Hyperglycemia and Diabetes Mellitus

Severe hyperglycemia, sometimes associated with ketoacidosis, hyperosmolar coma, or death, has been reported in patients receiving certain atypical antipsychotic agents, including risperidone. While confounding factors such as an increased background risk of diabetes mellitus in patients with schizophrenia and the increasing incidence of diabetes mellitus in the general population make it difficult to establish with certainty the relationship between use of agents in this drug class and glucose abnormalities, epidemiologic studies suggest an increased risk of treatment-emergent, hyperglycemia-related adverse events in patients treated with the atypical antipsychotic agents included in the studies (e.g., risperidone, clozapine, olanzapine, quetiapine).

Precise risk estimates for hyperglycemia-related adverse events in patients treated with atypical antipsychotics currently are not available. While some evidence suggests that the risk for diabetes may be greater with some atypical antipsychotics (e.g., clozapine, olanzapine) than with others (e.g., risperidone, quetiapine) in the class, available data are conflicting and insufficient to provide reliable estimates of relative risk associated with use of the various atypical antipsychotics. (See Cautions: Precautions and Contraindications.)

In a pooled analysis of short-term, placebo-controlled studies of 3–8 weeks' duration in adults with schizophrenia or bipolar disorder, risperidone was associated with a mean increase in random serum glucose concentrations of 0.6–0.8 mg/dL compared with a decrease of 1.4 mg/dL for placebo. During longer-term studies in adults, risperidone was associated with a mean increase in serum glucose of 2.8 mg/dL at week 24 and 4.1 mg/dL at week 48.

In children and adolescents receiving risperidone 0.5–6 mg daily for schizophrenia, bipolar disorder, or autistic disorder in short-term studies, the proportion of patients experiencing an increase in fasting serum glucose from below 100 mg/dL to 126 mg/dL or higher was 0.8% for risperidone-treated patients compared with 0% for placebo recipients. During longer-term studies in children and adolescents, risperidone was associated with a mean increase in fasting glucose of 5.2 mg/dL at week 24.

Diabetic coma and diabetic ketoacidosis (in patients with impaired glucose metabolism) have been reported in risperidone-treated patients.

Dyslipidemia

Undesirable changes in lipid parameters have been observed in patients treated with atypical antipsychotics. In a pooled analysis of 7 short-term, placebo-controlled studies of 3–8 weeks' duration in adults receiving oral risperidone for schizophrenia or bipolar mania, random cholesterol concentrations increased from baseline by a mean of 6.9 and 1.8 mg/dL in patients receiving risperidone 1–8 mg and more than 8–16 mg daily, respectively, compared with 0.6 mg/dL in those receiving placebo. The proportion of patients with an increase in random cholesterol concentrations from below 200 mg/dL to 240 mg/dL or higher was 4.3% for those receiving risperidone 1–8 mg daily and 6.3% for those receiving more than 8–16 mg of risperidone daily compared with 2.7% for placebo recipients, and the proportion of risperidone-treated patients with an increase in triglyceride concentrations from below 500 mg/dL to 500 mg/dL or higher was 2.5–2.7% compared with 1.1% for placebo recipients. During longer-term studies of oral risperidone, therapy with the drug was associated with a mean increase in nonfasting cholesterol concentrations of 4.4 and 5.5 mg/dL at weeks 24 and 48, respectively, and a mean increase in nonfasting triglycerides of 19.9 mg/dL at week 24.

In children and adolescents receiving oral risperidone 0.5–6 mg daily for schizophrenia, bipolar mania, or autistic disorder in short-term studies, the proportion of risperidone-treated patients with an increase in fasting cholesterol concentrations from below 170 mg/dL to 200 mg/dL or higher was 3.8% compared with 2.4% for placebo recipients and the proportion of risperidone-treated patients with an increase in fasting triglyceride concentrations from below 150 mg/dL to 200 mg/dL or higher was 7.1% compared with 1.5% for placebo recipients. During longer-term studies in children and adolescents, oral risperidone was associated with a mean increase in fasting cholesterol and triglyceride concentrations of 2.1 and 6.8 mg/dL, respectively, at week 24.

Weight Gain

Weight gain has been observed with atypical antipsychotic therapy. The manufacturers recommend clinical monitoring of weight in patients receiving risperidone.

In short-term clinical studies in adults with schizophrenia or bipolar mania, a mean weight gain from baseline of 0.7 and 2.2 kg was reported in patients receiving oral risperidone 1–8 mg and more than 8–16 mg daily, respectively, compared with a weight loss of 0.3 kg in those receiving placebo. The proportion of patients experiencing a weight gain of 7% or more of their baseline body weight was 8.7% for those receiving risperidone 1–8 mg daily and 20.9% for those receiving more than 8–16 mg of risperidone daily compared with 2.9% for placebo recipients. During longer-term studies of risperidone in adults, risperidone was associated with a mean weight gain of 4.3 kg at week 24 and 5.3 kg at week 48.

Hyperprolactinemia

As with other drugs that antagonize dopamine D_2 receptors, risperidone can elevate serum prolactin concentrations, and the elevation may persist during chronic administration of the drug. Risperidone appears to be associated with a higher level of prolactin elevation than other antipsychotic agents. Elevated prolactin concentrations occur in children and adolescents as well as in adults receiving the drug. (See Cautions: Pediatric Precautions.) Clinical disturbances such as galactorrhea, amenorrhea, gynecomastia, and impotence have been associated with prolactin-elevating drugs. In addition, chronic hyperprolactinemia associated with hypogonadism may lead to decreased bone density in both female and male patients.

If risperidone therapy is considered in a patient with previously detected breast cancer, clinicians should consider that approximately one-third of human breast cancers are prolactin dependent in vitro.

Other Endocrine and Metabolic Effects

Increased serum creatine kinase (CK, creatine phosphokinase, CPK) concentrations, decreased appetite, polydipsia, and anorexia have been reported during clinical trials in patients receiving risperidone. Although a causal relationship has not been established, inappropriate antidiuretic hormone secretion and water intoxication have been reported in patients receiving risperidone during postmarketing surveillance. Precocious puberty and pituitary adenomas also have been reported during postmarketing surveillance; however, a causal relationship remains to be established.

● GI Effects

Adverse GI effects that have been reported in 5% or more of patients receiving oral or IM risperidone in clinical studies include nausea, vomiting, upper abdominal pain, stomach discomfort, dyspepsia, diarrhea, salivary hypersecretion, constipation, dry mouth, and increased appetite. In addition, abdominal discomfort has been reported in 1% or more of patients receiving oral risperidone in clinical studies.

Other adverse GI effects reported during clinical trials with oral risperidone include dysphagia, fecaloma, fecal incontinence, gastritis, lip swelling, cheilitis, and aptyalism. Toothache and tongue spasm have been reported in patients treated with extended-release IM risperidone. Although a causal relationship to risperidone has not been established, dysgeusia, ileus, pancreatitis, and intestinal obstruction have been reported during postmarketing surveillance.

● Respiratory Effects

Nasal congestion, upper respiratory tract infection, nasopharyngitis, and pharyngolaryngeal pain were the most common adverse respiratory effects reported in more than 5% of patients receiving oral risperidone during clinical studies. In addition, cough and dyspnea have been reported in up to 2% of patients receiving risperidone in clinical studies. Wheezing, aspiration pneumonia, sinus congestion, dysphonia, productive cough, pulmonary congestion, rales, hyperventilation, and nasal edema also have been reported in patients receiving risperidone in clinical studies. Although a causal relationship to the drug has not been established, sleep apnea and pulmonary embolism have been reported during postmarketing surveillance.

● Dermatologic Effects and Sensitivity Reactions

Rash and dry skin have been reported in at least 2% of patients with schizophrenia receiving oral risperidone in clinical studies. In addition, erythema, skin discoloration, skin lesion, pruritus, acne, hyperkeratosis, and seborrheic dermatitis have been reported in clinical trials.

Although a causal relationship has not been established, hypersensitivity reactions, including anaphylaxis and anaphylactic reactions, angioedema, and alopecia, have been reported in patients receiving risperidone during postmarketing surveillance. (See Cautions: Precautions and Contraindications.)

● Genitourinary Effects

Urinary tract infection has been reported in 1% or more of adult patients with schizophrenia receiving oral risperidone in clinical trials. Adverse genitourinary effects reported in adult and pediatric patients receiving oral risperidone in clinical trials include enuresis, dysuria, pollakiuria, urinary incontinence, cystitis, irregular menstruation, amenorrhea, vaginal discharge, menstrual disorder, erectile dysfunction, retrograde ejaculation, ejaculation disorder, sexual dysfunction, and breast enlargement. Although a causal relationship has not been established, urinary retention has been reported in patients receiving risperidone during postmarketing surveillance.

Rare cases of priapism have been reported in risperidone-treated patients during postmarketing surveillance. Severe priapism may require surgical intervention.

● Musculoskeletal Effects

Back or chest pain, arthralgia, and pain in extremities have been reported in 1–4% of patients with schizophrenia receiving oral risperidone in clinical studies. In addition, joint stiffness, joint swelling, musculoskeletal chest pain, abnormal posture, myalgia, neck pain, muscular weakness, and rhabdomyolysis have been reported in patients receiving oral risperidone in clinical trials.

● Hematologic Effects

In clinical trial and/or postmarketing experience, leukopenia and neutropenia temporally related to antipsychotic agents, including risperidone, have been reported. Agranulocytosis also has been reported.

Possible risk factors for leukopenia and neutropenia include a preexisting low leukocyte count and a history of drug-induced leukopenia or neutropenia. Therefore, patients with a history of clinically important low leukocyte count or drug-induced leukopenia and/or neutropenia should have their complete blood count monitored frequently during the first few months of risperidone therapy. Discontinuance of risperidone should be considered at the first sign of a clinically important decline in leukocyte count in the absence of other causative factors.

Patients with clinically important neutropenia should be carefully monitored for fever or other signs or symptoms of infection and promptly treated if such signs or symptoms occur. In patients with severe neutropenia (absolute neutrophil count [ANC] less than 1000/mm³), risperidone should be discontinued and the leukocyte count monitored until recovery occurs. (See Cautions: Precautions and Contraindications.)

Lithium reportedly has been used successfully in the treatment of several cases of leukopenia and neutropenia associated with aripiprazole, clozapine, olanzapine, and some other drugs; however, further clinical experience is needed to confirm these anecdotal findings.

Anemia, granulocytopenia, eosinophilia, and epistaxis have been reported in patients receiving risperidone in clinical studies.

Thrombotic thrombocytopenic purpura occurred in at least one patient (a 28 year-old female patient) receiving risperidone in a large, open-labeled study. This patient experienced jaundice, fever, and bruising but eventually recovered after receiving plasmapheresis. The relationship of this adverse event to risperidone therapy is unknown.

● Hepatic Effects

Elevated ALT or aminotransferase concentrations have been reported in patients receiving oral risperidone in clinical studies. Although a causal relationship to the drug has not been established, jaundice also has been reported during postmarketing surveillance.

● Ocular and Otic Effects

Blurred vision has been reported in 1–3% of adults with schizophrenia or bipolar mania and in 4–7% of pediatric patients with bipolar disorder receiving oral risperidone in clinical studies. Ocular hyperemia, eye discharge, conjunctivitis, eye rolling, eyelid edema, eye swelling, eyelid margin crusting, dry eye, increased lacrimation, photophobia, glaucoma, and reduced visual acuity have been reported in patients receiving risperidone in clinical studies. Ear pain and tinnitus also have been reported in clinical studies with the drug.

Retinal artery occlusion has been reported in a patient treated with extended-release IM risperidone during postmarketing surveillance. This case occurred in the presence of abnormal arteriovenous anastomosis.

● Precautions and Contraindications

Atypical antipsychotic agents are associated with metabolic changes that may increase cardiovascular and cerebrovascular risk (e.g., hyperglycemia, dyslipidemia, weight gain). While all atypical antipsychotics produce some metabolic changes, each drug has its own specific risk profile.

Because hyperglycemia, sometimes severe and associated with ketoacidosis, hyperosmolar coma, or death, has been reported in patients receiving certain atypical antipsychotic agents, including risperidone, the manufacturers of atypical antipsychotic agents state that patients with preexisting diabetes mellitus in whom therapy with an atypical antipsychotic is initiated should be closely monitored for worsening of glucose control; those with risk factors for diabetes (e.g., obesity, family history of diabetes) should undergo fasting blood glucose testing upon therapy initiation and periodically throughout treatment. (See Cautions: Endocrine and Metabolic Effects.) Any patient who develops manifestations of hyperglycemia during treatment with an atypical antipsychotic should undergo fasting blood glucose testing. In some cases, patients who developed hyperglycemia while receiving an atypical antipsychotic have required continuance of antidiabetic treatment despite discontinuance of the antipsychotic; in other cases, hyperglycemia resolved with discontinuance of the suspect drug. For further information on the management of diabetes risks in patients receiving atypical antipsychotics, see Hyperglycemia and Diabetes Mellitus under Cautions: Precautions and Contraindications, in Clozapine 28:16.08.04.

Because of the possibility of orthostatic hypotension, caution should be observed in patients with known cardiovascular disease (e.g., history of myocardial infarction or ischemia, heart failure, conduction abnormalities), cerebrovascular disease (see Cautions: Geriatric Precautions), conditions that would predispose patients to hypotension (e.g., dehydration, hypovolemia), and patients receiving antihypertensive agents. Since patients with a recent history of myocardial infarction or unstable heart disease were excluded from premarketing clinical studies, clinicians should be aware that risperidone has not been evaluated or used to any appreciable extent in such patients. Patients receiving risperidone should be advised of the risk of orthostatic hypotension, especially during the period of initial dosage titration. (See Geriatric Patients and Others at Risk of Orthostatic Hypotension under Dosage and Administration: Dosage and see Cautions: Cardiovascular Effects.)

Clinical experience with IM risperidone therapy in patients with certain concomitant diseases is limited. The manufacturer of extended-release IM risperidone advises using the drug with caution in patients with altered metabolism or hemodynamics.

Patients with parkinsonian syndrome or dementia with Lewy bodies reportedly have an increased sensitivity to antipsychotic agents, including risperidone. Clinical manifestations of this increased sensitivity have been reported to include confusion, obtundation, postural instability with more frequent falls, extrapyramidal adverse effects, and clinical features consistent with neuroleptic malignant syndrome. For additional information on extrapyramidal adverse effects and neuroleptic malignant syndrome, see Cautions: Nervous System Effects, in the Phenothiazines General Statement 28:16.08.24.

Clearance of risperidone and its principal active metabolite, 9-hydroxyrisperidone, are decreased by 60% in patients with moderate to severe renal impairment (creatinine clearance 15–59 mL/minute), and free fraction of risperidone is increased by about 35% in patients with hepatic impairment. Therefore, lower initial dosages of oral risperidone should be used in patients with severe renal or hepatic impairment. (See Dosage and Administration: Dosage in Renal and Hepatic Impairment.)

Patients with a history of clinically important low leukocyte count or drug-induced leukopenia and/or neutropenia should have their complete blood count monitored frequently during the first few months of risperidone therapy. Patients with clinically important neutropenia should be carefully monitored for fever or other signs or symptoms of infection and promptly treated if such signs or symptoms occur. (See Cautions: Hematologic Effects.)

Individuals with phenylketonuria (i.e., homozygous genetic deficiency of phenylalanine hydroxylase) and other individuals who must restrict their intake of phenylalanine should be warned that risperidone orally disintegrating tablets contain aspartame (e.g., NutraSweet®), which is metabolized in the GI tract to provide phenylalanine following oral administration; the respective manufacturer's labeling should be consulted for specific information regarding phenylalanine content of individual preparations and dosage strengths.

Because seizures have occurred in 0.3% of patients receiving risperidone orally or IM in clinical studies, the drug should be administered with caution to patients with a history of seizures.

Esophageal dysmotility and aspiration have been associated with the use of antipsychotic agents, including risperidone. Because aspiration pneumonia is a common cause of morbidity and mortality in patients with advanced dementia of the Alzheimer's type, risperidone and other antipsychotic drugs should be used with caution in patients at risk for aspiration pneumonia.

Because disruption of the body's ability to regulate body temperature has been associated with the use of antipsychotic agents and because both hypothermia and hyperthermia have been associated with oral and extended-release IM risperidone therapy, the drug should be administered with caution in patients who will be exposed to temperature extremes.

Because risperidone has the potential to impair judgment, thinking, or motor skills, patients should be cautioned about operating hazardous machinery, including driving automobiles, until they are reasonably certain that risperidone therapy does not adversely affect them.

Risperidone has an antiemetic effect in animals; this effect also may occur in humans, and may mask manifestations of overdosage with certain drugs or may obscure the cause of vomiting in various disorders such as intestinal obstruction, Reye's syndrome, or brain tumor.

Osteodystrophy, renal tubular tumors, and adrenomedullary pheochromocytomas have been observed in rats following IM administration of extended-release risperidone; these findings were not observed previously with oral risperidone. The clinical relevance of these findings to humans is not known.

Because the possibility of a suicide attempt is inherent in patients with schizophrenia or bipolar disorder, close supervision of high-risk patients is recommended during risperidone therapy. Because extended-release IM risperidone is administered by a health care professional, suicide due to an overdose is unlikely.

Patients should be advised to inform their clinician if they are taking, or plan to take, any prescription or nonprescription drugs, or have any concomitant illnesses (e.g., diabetes mellitus). Patients also should be advised to avoid alcohol while taking risperidone.

Risperidone is contraindicated in patients with known hypersensitivity to the drug. (See Cautions: Dermatologic Effects and Sensitivity Reactions.)

● Pediatric Precautions

The safety and efficacy of risperidone in children younger than 13 years of age with schizophrenia or younger than 10 years of age with bipolar I disorder have not been established. Safety and efficacy of oral risperidone for the treatment of schizophrenia in adolescents 13–17 years of age were demonstrated in 2 short-term clinical trials in 417 patients. (See Schizophrenia under Uses: Psychotic Disorders.)

Efficacy and safety of risperidone for the treatment of acute manic or mixed episodes associated with bipolar I disorder in children and adolescents 10–17 years of age were demonstrated in a 3-week, placebo-controlled study in 169 patients. (See Uses: Bipolar Disorder.)

Efficacy and safety of the drug in the treatment of irritability associated with autistic disorder have been evaluated in 3 placebo-controlled trials of 6–8 weeks' duration in 252 children and adolescents 5–17 years of age. (See Uses: Autistic Disorder.) Additional safety information also was assessed from long-term studies in patients with schizophrenia or autistic disorder and from short- and long-term studies in more than 1200 pediatric patients with other psychiatric disorders who were of similar age and weight and who received similar risperidone dosages as patients treated for irritability associated with autistic disorder.

In clinical trials in 1885 children and adolescents treated with risperidone, 2 patients (0.1%) reportedly developed tardive dyskinesia, which resolved upon discontinuance of therapy. In addition, approximately 15% of children and adolescents receiving 0.5–2.5 mg daily dosages of risperidone developed withdrawal dyskinesia during the discontinuance phase of one long-term (6 month), open-label study.

In children and adolescents receiving oral risperidone 0.5–6 mg daily for schizophrenia, bipolar mania, autistic disorder, or other psychiatric disorders in short-term studies, approximately 33% of the risperidone-treated patients gained 7% or more of their baseline body weight compared with 7% of those receiving placebo; mean weight gain was 2 and 0.6 kg in the risperidone and placebo groups, respectively. During longer-term, open-label studies of risperidone in children and adolescents, risperidone was associated with a mean weight gain of 5.5 kg at week 24 and 8 kg at week 48.

In long-term, open-label trials in patients with autistic disorder or other psychiatric disorders, a mean body weight gain of 7.5 kg after 12 months of risperidone therapy was reported, which was higher than the normal expected weight gain (i.e., 3–3.5 kg per year adjusted for age, based on the US Centers for Disease Control and Prevention normative data). The majority of the weight increase occurred within the first 6 months of drug exposure. When treating pediatric patients with risperidone, the manufacturers recommend that weight gain should be assessed against that expected with normal growth.

Somnolence frequently occurred in placebo-controlled trials of oral risperidone in pediatric patients with autistic disorder. Most cases were mild to moderate in severity, occurred early during therapy (peak incidence during the first 2 weeks of therapy), and were transient (median duration of 16 days). Somnolence also was the most common adverse effect in clinical trials in children and adolescents with bipolar disorder as well as in schizophrenia clinical trials in adolescents; as in the autistic disorder trials, somnolence usually occurred early during therapy and was transient. Pediatric patients experiencing persistent somnolence may benefit from a change in dosage regimen. (See Dosage and Administration: Administration.)

Risperidone has been shown to elevate prolactin concentrations in children and adolescents as well as adults. In double-blind, placebo-controlled trials of up to 8 weeks' duration in children and adolescents 5–17 years of age, 49% of oral risperidone-treated patients had elevated prolactin concentrations compared with 2% of those receiving placebo. Similarly, in placebo-controlled trials in children and adolescents 10–17 years of age with bipolar disorder or adolescents 13–17 years of age with schizophrenia, 82–87% of risperidone-treated patients had elevated prolactin concentrations compared with 3–7% of placebo recipients. Increases in prolactin concentrations were dose dependent and generally greater in female than male patients across indications.

In clinical trials conducted in 1885 children and adolescents, galactorrhea and gynecomastia reportedly occurred in 0.8 and 2.3%, respectively, of risperidone-treated patients.

The manufacturers state that the long-term effects of risperidone on growth and sexual maturation have not been fully evaluated in children and adolescents.

● Geriatric Precautions

Clinical studies of oral risperidone for the management of schizophrenia did not include sufficient numbers of patients 65 years of age and older to determine whether geriatric patients respond differently than younger patients. Other clinical experience with oral risperidone has not identified differences in responses between geriatric and younger patients. However, serious adverse effects, including an increased risk of death, have been reported in geriatric patients receiving risperidone or other atypical antipsychotic agents in clinical trials in patients with dementia-related psychosis. Risperidone is not approved for the treatment of dementia-related psychosis. (See Geriatric Considerations in Uses: Psychotic Disorders.)

Geriatric patients with dementia-related psychosis treated with antipsychotic drugs are at an increased risk of death. Analyses of 17 placebo-controlled trials (modal duration of 10 weeks) revealed an approximate 1.6- to 1.7-fold increase in mortality among geriatric patients receiving atypical antipsychotic drugs (i.e., risperidone, aripiprazole, olanzapine, quetiapine) compared with that in patients receiving placebo. Over the course of a typical 10-week controlled trial, the rate of death in drug-treated patients was about 4.5% compared with a rate of about 2.6% in the placebo group. Although the causes of death were varied, most of the deaths appeared to be either cardiovascular (e.g., heart failure, sudden death) or infectious (e.g., pneumonia) in nature. Observational studies suggest that, similar to atypical antipsychotics, treatment with conventional (first-generation) antipsychotics may increase mortality; the extent to which the findings of increased mortality in observational studies may be attributed to the antipsychotic drug as opposed to some characteristic(s) of the patients remains unclear.

A higher incidence of mortality also was observed in geriatric patients with dementia-related psychosis receiving oral risperidone and furosemide concurrently in 2 out of 4 placebo-controlled trials when compared with that in patients receiving risperidone alone or placebo and furosemide concurrently. The pathologic mechanism for this finding remains to be established and no consistent pattern for the cause of death was observed.

Adverse cerebrovascular events (e.g., stroke, transient ischemic attack), some of which resulted in fatalities, have been reported in clinical studies of risperidone in geriatric patients (mean age 85 years; range: 73–97) with dementia-related psychosis.

Because of the greater frequency of decreased hepatic, renal, and/or cardiac function and of concomitant disease and drug therapy observed in geriatric patients, oral risperidone generally should be initiated at lower dosages in such patients. Although geriatric patients exhibit a greater tendency to orthostatic hypotension, the manufacturers state that its risk may be minimized by limiting the initial oral dosage to 0.5 mg twice daily followed by careful titration and close monitoring of orthostatic vital signs in patients for whom this is of concern. However, there is some evidence that even lower initial dosages and slower dosage titration are better tolerated in these patients. Therefore, some clinicians recommend initiating oral risperidone therapy at 0.25 mg daily, and gradually increasing dosages, as tolerated, to a dosage of 2 mg daily in these patients. Higher oral dosages (e.g., 3 or 4 mg daily) may be required in some patients, but are usually associated with greater incidence of extrapyramidal reactions. Most geriatric patients should *not* be maintained at an oral risperidone dosage exceeding 3 mg daily. (See Geriatric Patients and Others at Risk of Orthostatic Hypotension under Dosage and Administration: Dosage.)

No differences in the tolerability of extended-release IM risperidone were observed in an open-label study in otherwise healthy geriatric patients and younger patients with schizophrenia or schizoaffective disorder. Therefore, the manufacturer states that extended-release IM risperidone dosage recommendations for otherwise healthy geriatric patients are the same as for younger adults.

● Mutagenicity and Carcinogenicity

Risperidone did not exhibit mutagenic or clastogenic potential in the Ames gene mutation test, mouse lymphoma assay, in vitro rat hepatocyte DNA-repair assay, in vivo micronucleus test in mice, the sex-linked recessive lethal test in Drosophila, or the chromosome aberration studies in human lymphocytes or Chinese hamster ovary cells.

Statistically significant increases in pituitary gland adenomas and mammary gland adenocarcinomas were observed in female mice receiving oral risperidone dosages of 0.63, 2.5, and 10 mg/kg (equivalent to approximately 2, 9, and 38 times the maximum recommended human dosage for schizophrenia on a mg/kg basis or 0.2, 0.75, and 3 times the maximum recommended human dosage on a mg/m² basis, respectively) for 18 months. In addition, statistically significant increases were observed in mammary gland adenocarcinomas in both male and female rats, and mammary gland neoplasms and endocrine pancreas adenomas in male rats receiving oral risperidone dosages of 0.63, 2.5, and 10 mg/kg (equivalent to approximately 2, 9, and 38 times the maximum recommended human dosage for schizophrenia on a mg/kg basis or 0.4, 1.5, and 6 times the maximum recommended human dosage on a mg/m² basis, respectively) for 25 months.

Although an increase in prolactin-mediated mammary, pituitary, and endocrine pancreas neoplasms has been found in rodents following long-term administration of other antipsychotic agents, no clinical or epidemiologic studies conducted to date have shown an association between long-term administration of antipsychotic drugs and tumorigenesis in humans; current evidence is considered too limited to be conclusive at this time. If risperidone therapy is considered in a patient with previously detected breast cancer, clinicians should consider that approximately one-third of human breast cancers are prolactin dependent in vitro.

● *Pregnancy, Fertility, and Lactation*
Pregnancy

Reproductive studies in rats and rabbits using risperidone dosages of 0.4–6 times the maximum recommended human dosage on a mg/m² basis have not revealed evidence of fetal malformation. However, risperidone has been shown to cross the placenta in rats, and an increased rate of stillborn rat pups occurred at dosages 1.5 times higher than the maximum recommended human dosage on a mg/m² basis. In 3 reproductive studies in rats, there was an increase in pup deaths during the first 4 days of lactation at dosages 0.1–3 times the human dosage on a mg/m² basis. It is not known whether these deaths resulted from a direct effect on the fetuses or pups or to effects on the dams. In a separate reproductive study in rats, an increased number of pup deaths (at birth or by the day after birth) and a decrease in birth weight were observed in pups of dams treated with risperidone. Risperidone also appeared to impair maternal behavior, as evidenced by reduced weight gain and decreased survival (from day 1–4 of lactation) in pups born to control dams but reared by risperidone-treated dams.

Although there are no adequate and controlled studies to date in humans, one case of agenesis of the corpus callosum has been reported in an infant exposed to risperidone in utero; however, a causal relationship to risperidone therapy is unknown.

Neonates exposed to antipsychotic agents, including risperidone, during the third trimester of pregnancy are at risk for extrapyramidal and/or withdrawal symptoms following delivery. There have been reports of agitation, hypertonia, hypotonia, tardive dyskinetic-like symptoms, tremor, somnolence, respiratory distress, and feeding disorder in these neonates. The majority of cases were also confounded by other factors, including concomitant use of other drugs known to be associated with withdrawal symptoms, prematurity, congenital malformations, and obstetrical and perinatal complications; however, some cases suggested that neonatal extrapyramidal symptoms and withdrawal may occur with exposure to antipsychotic agents alone. Some of the cases described time of symptom onset, which ranged from birth to one month after birth. Any neonate exhibiting extrapyramidal or withdrawal symptoms following in utero exposure to antipsychotic agents should be monitored. Symptoms were self-limiting in some neonates but varied in severity; some infants required intensive care unit support and prolonged hospitalization. For further information on extrapyramidal and withdrawal symptoms in neonates, see Cautions: Pregnancy, Fertility, and Lactation, in the Phenothiazines General Statement 28:16.08.24.

Risperidone should be used during pregnancy only if the potential benefit justifies the potential risk to the fetus.

The effect of risperidone on labor and delivery in humans is unknown.

Fertility

Oral risperidone (0.16–5 mg/kg) has been shown to impair mating, but not fertility, in Wistar rats in 3 reproductive studies at dosages 0.1–3 times the maximum recommended human dosage on a mg/m² basis. The effect appeared to be in females since impaired mating behavior was not noted in the mating and fertility study in which only males were treated. Sperm motility and concentration were decreased in beagles at dosages 0.6–10 times the maximum recommended human dosage on a mg/m² basis; dose-related decreases were also observed in serum testosterone concentrations at the same dosages. Serum testosterone and sperm parameters partially recovered but remained decreased after treatment was discontinued. A no-effect dosage was not found in these studies in either rats or dogs.

Lactation

Risperidone and its principal active metabolite, 9-hydroxyrisperidone, are distributed into milk. Because of the potential for serious adverse reactions to risperidone in nursing infants, the manufacturers of oral risperidone state that a decision should be made whether to discontinue nursing or risperidone, taking into consideration the importance of the drug to the woman. The manufacturer of the long-acting risperidone injection states that women receiving IM risperidone should not breast-feed during treatment and for at least 12 weeks after the last injection.

DESCRIPTION

Risperidone is a benzisoxazole-derivative antipsychotic agent. The drug has been described as an atypical or second-generation antipsychotic agent. The principal active metabolite of risperidone, 9-hydroxyrisperidone, has similar pharmacologic activity to the parent drug and is commercially available as paliperidone (another atypical antipsychotic agent); the clinical effects of risperidone result from combined concentrations of risperidone and 9-hydroxyrisperidone. The exact mechanism of antipsychotic action of risperidone has not been fully elucidated but, like that of clozapine, may involve antagonism of central type 2 serotonergic ($5\text{-}HT_2$) receptors and central dopamine D_2 receptors. Antagonism at other receptors (e.g., α_1- and α_2-adrenergic receptors, histamine H_1 receptors) may contribute to other therapeutic and adverse effects of risperidone (e.g., orthostatic hypotension, somnolence). Risperidone exhibits low to moderate affinity for other serotonin receptor subtypes (e.g., $5HT_{1C}$, $5HT_{1A}$, $5HT_{1D}$), and weak affinity for dopamine D_1 receptors and the haloperidol-sensitive sigma site. The drug possesses no affinity for cholinergic muscarinic or β_1- and β_2-adrenergic receptors.

PREPARATIONS

Excipients in commercially available drug preparations may have clinically important effects in some individuals; consult specific product labeling for details.

risperiDONE

Oral		
Solution	1 mg/mL*	RisperDAL®, Janssen
		risperiDONE Oral Solution
Tablets	0.25 mg*	RisperDAL®, Janssen
		risperiDONE Tablets
	0.5 mg*	RisperDAL®, Janssen
		risperiDONE Tablets
	1 mg*	RisperDAL®, Janssen
		risperiDONE Tablets
	2 mg*	RisperDAL®, Janssen
		risperiDONE Tablets
	3 mg*	RisperDAL®, Janssen
		risperiDONE Tablets
	4 mg*	RisperDAL®, Janssen
		risperiDONE Tablets
Tablets, orally disintegrating	0.25 mg*	risperiDONE Orally Disintegrating Tablets
	0.5 mg*	RisperDAL® M-TAB®, Janssen
		risperiDONE Orally Disintegrating Tablets

1 mg*	**RisperDAL® M-TAB®**, Janssen	
	risperiDONE Orally Disintegrating Tablets	
2 mg*	**RisperDAL® M-TAB®**, Janssen	
	risperiDONE Orally Disintegrating Tablets	
3 mg*	**RisperDAL® M-TAB®**, Janssen	
	risperiDONE Orally Disintegrating Tablets	
4 mg*	**RisperDAL® M-TAB®**, Janssen	
	risperiDONE Orally Disintegrating Tablets	

Parenteral

For injectable suspension, extended-release, for IM use	12.5 mg	**RisperDAL® Consta®** (available as dose pack containing a vial adapter device, 2 safety needles, and with 2-mL prefilled syringe diluent), Janssen
	25 mg	**RisperDAL® Consta®** (available as dose pack containing a vial adapter device, 2 safety needles, and with 2-mL prefilled syringe diluent), Janssen
	37.5 mg	**RisperDAL® Consta®** (available as dose pack containing a vial adapter device, 2 safety needles, and with 2-mL prefilled syringe diluent), Janssen
	50 mg	**RisperDAL® Consta®** (available as dose pack containing a vial adapter device, 2 safety needles, and with 2-mL prefilled syringe diluent), Janssen

* available from one or more manufacturer, distributor, and/or repackager by generic (nonproprietary) name

† Use is not currently included in the labeling approved by the US Food and Drug Administration.

Selected Revisions November 13, 2017, © Copyright, May 1, 1994, American Society of Health-System Pharmacists, Inc.

Haloperidol

28:16.08.08 · BUTYROPHENONES

■ Haloperidol is a butyrophenone-derivative antipsychotic agent. The drug is considered a conventional or first-generation antipsychotic agent.

USES

● Schizophrenia

Haloperidol is used orally and parenterally for the symptomatic management of psychotic disorders (i.e., schizophrenia). Drug therapy is integral to the management of acute psychotic episodes in patients with schizophrenia and generally is required for long-term stabilization to improve symptoms between episodes and to minimize the risk of recurrent acute episodes. Antipsychotic agents are the principal class of drugs used for the management of all phases of schizophrenia and generally are effective in all subtypes of the disorder and subgroups of patients. Conventional antipsychotic agents, such as haloperidol, generally are considered to exhibit similar efficacy in treating acute psychotic symptoms, although they vary in their potency and adverse effect profile. Haloperidol is a high-potency antipsychotic that has been shown to be effective in the management of acute and stable phases of schizophrenia, but is frequently associated with extrapyramidal reactions such as akathisia, dystonia, or parkinsonian symptoms, even at low dosages.

Results of short-term studies indicate that oral haloperidol is more effective than placebo and equally or less effective than atypical antipsychotics in the treatment of positive (e.g., delusions, hallucinations) and negative symptoms (e.g., withdrawal from social interaction, blunted emotional expression) of schizophrenia. However, in one clinical study, haloperidol was less effective than the atypical antipsychotic agent risperidone in preventing relapse in adult outpatients with clinically active schizophrenia or schizoaffective disorders who were assigned to receive either drug for a minimum of 1 year. In this study, approximately 40% of patients in the study who received usual dosages of haloperidol had relapsed by the end of the study compared with approximately 25% of those receiving usual dosages of risperidone.

Because atypical antipsychotics appear to be at least as effective in the treatment of positive symptoms and possibly more effective in the treatment of negative symptoms of schizophrenia and have fewer extrapyramidal reactions, some clinicians prefer use of atypical antipsychotics rather than conventional antipsychotics, such as haloperidol, for the management of schizophrenia, except in stable patients who have had good response to conventional antipsychotics without major adverse effects, in patients who require IM therapy, which is not yet available for some atypical antipsychotics, and for the acute management of aggression/violence in some patients, particularly those requiring long-acting (depot) parenteral preparations. However, patient response and tolerance to antipsychotic agents are variable, and patients who do not respond to or tolerate one drug may be successfully treated with an agent from a different class or with a different adverse effect profile.

The long-acting decanoate ester of haloperidol is used parenterally principally in patients requiring prolonged antipsychotic therapy (e.g., patients with chronic schizophrenic disorder). Parenteral antipsychotic therapy with a long-acting preparation may be particularly useful in patients with a history of poor compliance. In addition, long-acting antipsychotic preparations may be useful in patients with suspected GI malabsorption or variable GI absorption of the drug. The principal disadvantage of long-acting parenteral antipsychotics is the inability to terminate the drug's action when severe adverse reactions occur. Long-acting antipsychotic preparations should not be used in the acute management of severely agitated patients. Generally, patients should be stabilized on antipsychotic medication prior to conversion to haloperidol decanoate therapy and should have previously received and tolerated a shorter-acting haloperidol preparation so that the possibility of an unexpected adverse reaction that potentially could not be readily reversed following the decanoate can be minimized. For further information on the use of antipsychotic agents in the symptomatic treatment of schizophrenia, see Uses: Psychotic Disorders, in the Phenothiazines General Statement 28:16.08.24.

● Tourette's Syndrome

Haloperidol is used orally and parenterally for the control of tics and vocal utterances of Tourette's syndrome (Gilles de la Tourette's syndrome) in children and adults. Haloperidol generally has been considered the drug of choice for the management of Tourette's syndrome and pimozide has been an effective alternative in some patients who have an inadequate response to or do not tolerate haloperidol. Because limited data suggest that pimozide may be more effective than haloperidol in reducing tics and pimozide appears to be better tolerated than haloperidol, some clinicians and experts prefer the use of pimozide in patients with Tourette's syndrome.

In children with tic disorders (e.g., Tourette's syndrome) and comorbid attention deficit hyperactivity disorder† (ADHD) in whom stimulants alone cannot control tics, haloperidol may be used concomitantly with a stimulant.

● Delirium

Antipsychotic agents, mainly haloperidol, have been used in the management of delirium†.

General Considerations

Delirium is principally a disturbance of consciousness, attention, cognition, and perception but also may affect sleep, psychomotor activity, and emotions. It is a common psychiatric illness among medically compromised patients, particularly hospitalized patients, and may be a harbinger of substantial morbidity and mortality.

Prevalence and Course

The prevalence of delirium in hospitalized medically ill patients ranges from 10–30%; in those who are elderly, delirium ranges up to 40%. Up to 25% of hospitalized cancer patients and 30–40% of hospitalized patients with acquired immunodeficiency syndrome (AIDS) develop delirium. Up to about 50% of postoperative patients develop delirium, and up to 80% of terminally ill patients develop it near death. EEG abnormalities, mainly generalized slowing, have fairly good sensitivity for aiding in the diagnosis of delirium, but the absence of such changes does not rule out the diagnosis. Prodromal manifestations may progress to full-blown delirium over 1–3 days; the duration of delirium generally ranges from less than a week to more than 2 months, but typically does not exceed 10–12 days. Symptoms persist for up to 30 days or longer in up to 15% of patients, and frequently persist for longer than 1 month in geriatric patients. Although most patients recover fully, delirium may progress to stupor, coma, seizures, and death, particularly if untreated. Full recovery is less likely in geriatric patients and patients with AIDS, possibly because of underlying dementia in both populations.

Underlying general medical conditions associated with delirium include CNS disorders (e.g., head trauma, seizures, postictal state, vascular or degenerative disease), metabolic disorders (e.g., renal or hepatic failure, anemia, hypoxia, hypoglycemia, thiamine deficiency, endocrinopathy, fluid or electrolyte imbalance, acid-base imbalance), cardiopulmonary disorder (myocardial infarction, congestive heart failure, cardiac arrhythmia, shock, respiratory failure), and systemic illness (e.g., substance intoxication or withdrawal, infection, cancer, severe trauma, sensory deprivation, temperature dysregulation, postoperative state).

Management
Overview

Clinicians should undertake an essential array of psychiatric management tasks designed to provide immediate interventions for urgent general medical conditions, identify and treat the etiology of delirium, ensure safety of the patient and others in contact with the patient, and improve the patient's functioning. Environmental (e.g., varying light levels in intensive care units to heighten awareness about time of day and reduce the perception of timelessness) and supportive interventions (e.g., to deal with disorientation, to assure the patient that manifestations are temporary and reversible and do not reflect a persistent psychiatric disorder) also generally are offered to patients with delirium† and are designed to reduce factors that may exacerbate delirium, to reorient patients, and to provide support. Patients may have life-threatening medical conditions that require therapeutic intervention even before a specific or definitive cause of the delirium is determined. The goal of diagnosis is to identify potentially reversible causes of delirium and prevent complications through prompt treatment of these specific disorders. Psychiatric management is essential and should be undertaken for all patients with delirium. Somatic interventions principally consist of drug therapy. The choice of somatic intervention will depend on the specific features of the patient's clinical condition, the underlying etiology of the delirium, and any associated comorbid conditions.

Drug Therapy

Antipsychotic agents often are the drugs of choice for the management of delirium†. Although other drugs (e.g., phenothiazines, droperidol) have been used, haloperidol generally is considered the antipsychotic of choice for most patients with delirium because of its relatively low risk of anticholinergic activity and of sedative and hypotensive effects. In addition, haloperidol has been studied most extensively, although few studies have used standardized definitions of delirium or reliable and valid delirium symptom rating measures to assess symptom severity before and after initiation of treatment. For drugs other than haloperidol, there have been no large, prospective studies that included a control. Evidence of efficacy for such alternative therapies, including second-generation antipsychotic agents (e.g., olanzapine, quetiapine, risperidone, ziprasidone), is principally from small case series, case reports, or open-label studies. In addition, interpretation of findings from many such case presentations is difficult because of use of non-standardized delirium definitions and/or informal measures of delirium symptom severity. In general, evidence of the efficacy of antipsychotics, including haloperidol, in the management of delirium comes from numerous case reports and uncontrolled studies. However, evidence from a randomized, double-blind, comparator-drug controlled study (haloperidol, chlorpromazine, and lorazepam) in patients with AIDS that employed standardized clinical measures of delirium demonstrated clinical superiority of antipsychotic agents compared with benzodiazepines. Statistically significant improvement in the Delirium Rating Scale was evident after 2 days in patients receiving haloperidol or chlorpromazine but not in the lorazepam group (mean decreases in the score [i.e., improvement] were 8, 8.5, and 1, respectively). The symptomatic improvement in delirium occurred quickly among patients receiving antipsychotic therapy, usually before initiation of interventions directed at the medical etiologies of delirium.

Although various antipsychotic agents may be given orally, IM, or IV, IV administration is considered most effective in emergency situations or where oral access is limited. In addition, some evidence indicates that IV administration of antipsychotic agents may be associated with less severe extrapyramidal effects.

Special Precautions

Antipsychotic agents, particularly IV† haloperidol, used in the management of delirium have been associated with lengthening of the QT interval, possibly leading to atypical ventricular tachycardia (torsades de pointes), ventricular fibrillation, and sudden death. The manufacturer of Haldol® and the US Food and Drug Administration (FDA) state that although injectable haloperidol is approved *only* for IM injection and *not for IV administration*, there is considerable evidence from the medical literature that IV† administration of the drug is a relatively common, unlabeled ("off-label") clinical practice, principally for the treatment of severe agitation in intensive care units, and recommend ECG monitoring in any patient receiving the drug IV. Many clinicians also recommend that baseline and periodic or continuous ECG monitoring be performed with special attention paid to the length of the QT_c interval. Prolongation of the QT_c interval to greater than 450 msec or to greater than 15–25% over that in previous ECGs may warrant telemetry, a cardiology consultation, and dose reduction or discontinuance. Serum concentrations of magnesium and potassium also should be monitored at baseline and periodically in critically ill patients, especially those with baseline QT_c intervals of 440 msec or longer, those receiving other drugs known to increase the QT interval, and those who have electrolyte disorders. Limited evidence suggests that the incidence of torsades de pointes in patients receiving haloperidol IV is about 0.4–3.6%, but may increase to greater than 10% at relatively high IV doses (e.g., 35 mg or more over 24 hours). (See Cautions: Cardiovascular Effects and also see Cautions: Precautions and Contraindications.)

● Disruptive Behavior Disorder and Attention Deficit Hyperactivity Disorder

Haloperidol is used orally for the treatment of severe behavioral problems in children marked by combativeness and/or explosive hyperexcitable behavior (out of proportion to immediate provocations), and for the short-term treatment of hyperactive children who exhibit excessive motor activity with accompanying conduct disorders that are manifested as impulsive behavior, difficulty sustaining attention, aggression, mood lability, and/or poor frustration tolerance. However, the possible risks of tardive dyskinesia, withdrawal dyskinesia, and other extrapyramidal reactions should be considered. Some experts currently recommend use of haloperidol only for the treatment of comorbid tics in children with attention deficit hyperactivity disorder (ADHD). Some clinicians recommend routine administration of the Abnormal Involuntary Movement Scale (AIMS) to all children receiving antipsychotic agents.

● Nausea and Vomiting

Haloperidol also has been used in the prevention and control of severe nausea and vomiting† (e.g., cancer chemotherapy-induced emesis). Based on limited data, haloperidol appears to be as effective as phenothiazines in the prevention of

cancer chemotherapy-induced emesis. Additional studies are required to determine the efficacy of haloperidol in the prevention and control of severe nausea and vomiting.

DOSAGE AND ADMINISTRATION

● Administration

Haloperidol is administered orally. Haloperidol lactate is administered orally or by IM injection, and haloperidol decanoate is administered by IM injection. Pending accumulation of further data to establish safety and efficacy, IM administration of haloperidol lactate or decanoate in children is not recommended by the manufacturers. Haloperidol *lactate* also has been administered by IV injection† or infusion†. Haloperidol decanoate injection should *not* be administered IV.

Haloperidol decanoate should be administered by deep IM injection into the gluteal region using a 21-gauge needle. The manufacturers of haloperidol decanoate state that the maximum volume of haloperidol decanoate should not exceed 3 mL per IM injection site.

Haloperidol lactate and decanoate injections should be inspected visually for particulate matter and discoloration prior to administration whenever solution and container permit.

● Dosage

Dosage of haloperidol lactate and the decanoate is expressed in terms of haloperidol.

There is considerable interindividual variation in optimum dosage requirements of haloperidol, and dosage must be carefully adjusted according to individual requirements and response, using the lowest possible effective dosage. Dosage should be increased more gradually in children and in debilitated, emaciated, or geriatric patients. Because of the risk of adverse reactions associated with cumulative effects of butyrophenones, patients with a history of long-term therapy with haloperidol and/or other antipsychotic agents should be evaluated periodically to determine whether maintenance dosage could be decreased or drug therapy discontinued.

Oral Dosage

For the symptomatic management of psychotic disorders or Tourette's disorder in adults with *moderate symptomatology and in geriatric or debilitated patients*, the manufacturers state that the usual initial oral dosage of haloperidol is 0.5–2 mg administered 2 or 3 times daily. To achieve prompt control, higher initial dosages may be required in some patients. Subsequent dosage should be carefully adjusted according to the patient's tolerance and therapeutic response. Dosage during prolonged maintenance therapy should be kept at the lowest effective level.

For the symptomatic management of psychotic disorders or Tourette's disorder in adults with *severe symptomatology and/or chronic or resistant disorders*, the manufacturers state that the usual initial oral dosage of haloperidol is 3–5 mg administered 2 or 3 times daily. To achieve prompt control, higher initial dosages may be required in some patients. Subsequent dosage should be carefully adjusted according to the patient's tolerance and therapeutic response. Dosage during prolonged maintenance therapy should be kept at the lowest effective level.

Similarly, the American Psychiatric Association (APA) recommends oral haloperidol dosages ranging from 5–20 mg daily in the treatment of adults with schizophrenia. The APA states that determining the optimal dosage of antipsychotic agents during the acute phase of schizophrenia is complicated because there usually is a delay between initiation of therapy and full therapeutic response. An initial response to antipsychotic therapy may take 2–4 weeks and up to 6 months or longer may be needed for a full or optimal response.

Patients who remain severely disturbed or inadequately controlled despite receiving recommended dosages of haloperidol may require dosage adjustment. Some manufacturers state that oral haloperidol dosages up to 100 mg daily may be necessary in some cases to achieve an optimal response. In addition, these manufacturers further state that haloperidol has been used infrequently in dosages exceeding 100 mg daily in severely resistant disorders in adults, but that the limited use has not demonstrated the safety of prolonged administration of such high dosages of the drug. However, extensive clinical experience suggests that higher-dosage haloperidol regimens (i.e., those exceeding 20–40 mg daily) are unlikely to be more effective or result in a faster clinical response in the majority of patients with schizophrenia, including in those with refractory or chronic schizophrenia, and supports the use of more moderate dosage regimens (i.e., from 4 mg daily up to 15–20 mg daily) in such patients. In addition, high-dosage haloperidol regimens are more likely to be associated with unacceptable short- and long-term adverse effects (see Cautions).

The usual initial oral dosage of haloperidol in children 3–12 years of age and weighing 15–40 kg is 0.5 mg daily given in 2 or 3 divided doses. Subsequent dosage may be increased by 0.5 mg daily at 5- to 7-day intervals, depending on the patient's tolerance and therapeutic response.

For the symptomatic management of psychotic disorders in children 3–12 years of age, the usual oral dosage range is 0.05–0.15 mg/kg daily given in 2 or 3 divided doses; however, severely disturbed psychotic children may require higher dosages. Dosage during prolonged maintenance therapy should be kept at the lowest possible effective level; once an adequate response has been achieved, dosage should be gradually reduced and subsequently adjusted according to the patient's therapeutic response and tolerance.

For the management of non-psychotic behavioral problems and for the control of Tourette's disorder in children 3–12 years of age, the usual oral dosage range is 0.05–0.075 mg/kg daily given in 2 or 3 divided doses. Unlike psychotic disorders for which prolonged therapy is usually required, non-psychotic or hyperactive behavioral problems in children may be acute, and short-term administration of haloperidol may be adequate. A maximum effective dosage of haloperidol for the management of behavioral problems in children has not been established; however, the manufacturers state that there is little evidence that improvement in behavior is further enhanced at dosages greater than 6 mg daily.

IM Dosage
Haloperidol Lactate

For the prompt control of acutely agitated patients with moderately severe to very severe symptoms, the usual initial adult IM dose of haloperidol lactate is 2–5 mg (of haloperidol) given as a single dose. Depending on the response of the patient, this dose may be repeated as often as every hour; however, IM administration of haloperidol lactate every 4–8 hours may be adequate to control symptoms in some patients.

Oral therapy should replace short-acting parenteral therapy as soon as possible. Depending on the patient's clinical status, the first oral dose should be given within 12–24 hours following administration of the last parenteral dose of haloperidol lactate. Since bioavailability studies to establish bioequivalence between oral and parenteral dosage forms of haloperidol have not been conducted to date, the manufacturers suggest that the parenteral dosage administered during the preceding 24 hours be used for initial approximation of the total daily oral dosage required. Since this dosage is only an initial estimate, patients being switched from parenteral haloperidol lactate therapy to oral therapy should be closely monitored, particularly for clinical signs and symptoms of efficacy, sedation, and adverse effects, for the first several days following initiation of oral therapy. Subsequent dosage may be increased or decreased according to the patient's tolerance and therapeutic response, using the lowest possible effective dosage.

Haloperidol Decanoate

For patients requiring prolonged antipsychotic therapy (e.g., patients with chronic schizophrenic disorder), the long-acting haloperidol decanoate injection may be considered. If the decanoate is used, the patient's condition should initially be stabilized with an antipsychotic agent prior to attempting conversion to haloperidol decanoate. In addition, if the patient is receiving an antipsychotic agent other than haloperidol, it is recommended that the patient initially be converted to oral haloperidol therapy in order to minimize the risk of an unexpected adverse reaction to the drug, which might not be readily reversible following use of the decanoate.

The initial IM dose of haloperidol decanoate should be based on the patient's clinical history, physical condition, and response to previous antipsychotic therapy. To determine the minimum effective dosage, haloperidol decanoate therapy has been initiated at low initial doses and gradually titrated upward as necessary. A precise formula for converting from oral haloperidol to IM haloperidol decanoate dosage has not been established, but an initial adult dose 10–20 times the previous daily dose of oral haloperidol, not exceeding 100 mg (regardless of previous antipsychotic dosage requirements), is suggested, although limited clinical experience suggests that a lower initial dosage of the decanoate may be adequate. If conversion requires an initial dosage of haloperidol decanoate higher than 100 mg daily, such dosage should be administered in 2 injections (i.e., administering a maximum initial dose of 100 mg followed by the balance in 3–7 days). However, some clinicians have converted therapy to the decanoate using a higher initial dosage.

Lower initial IM dosages (e.g., 10–15 times the previous daily dose of oral haloperidol) and more gradual upward titration of haloperidol administered as the decanoate salt are recommended for patients who are geriatric, debilitated, or stabilized on low oral dosages (e.g., up to the equivalent of 10 mg daily of oral haloperidol). Higher initial IM dosages (e.g., 20 times the previous daily dosage of oral haloperidol) should be considered for patients who are stabilized on high oral dosages of antipsychotic agents, those who are at risk of relapse, and those who are tolerant to oral haloperidol, with downward titration on succeeding injections.

Haloperidol decanoate usually has been administered IM at monthly intervals (i.e., every 4 weeks), but individual response may dictate the need for adjusting the dosing interval as well as the dose.

The maintenance dosage of haloperidol decanoate must be individualized with upward or downward dosage titration based on clinical response. The usual adult maintenance IM dosage is 10–15 times the previous daily dosage of oral haloperidol for adult patients depending on the clinical response of the patient.

Close clinical observation is required during dosage titration in order to minimize the risk of overdosage and of emergence of psychotic manifestations prior to the next dose. If supplemental antipsychotic therapy is necessary during periods of dosage titration or for control of acute exacerbations of psychotic manifestations, a short-acting haloperidol preparation should be used. Experience with haloperidol decanoate dosages exceeding 450 mg (of haloperidol) monthly is limited.

IV Dosage
Haloperidol Lactate

The optimum dosage of haloperidol (administered as haloperidol lactate) for the treatment of delirium has not been established. However, initiation of IV† haloperidol with dosages of 1–2 mg every 2–4 hours in adults has been suggested. Lower IV dosages (e.g., 0.25–0.5 mg every 4 hours) have been suggested for geriatric patients with delirium; severely agitated adults may require titration to higher dosages. Although single IV doses up to 50 mg or total daily dosages of 500 mg have been reported in adults, the risk of adverse effects, particularly prolongation of the QT interval and torsades de pointes, must be considered. (See Uses: Delirium and also see Cautions: Cardiovascular Effects and Cautions: Precautions and Contraindications.) Some evidence suggests that the risk of torsades de pointes increases at total daily dosages of 35–50 mg or more. In patients requiring multiple IV injections of the drug to control delirium (e.g., more than eight 10-mg doses in 24 hours or more than 10 mg/hour for more than 5 consecutive hours), consideration can be given to continuous IV infusion† of haloperidol; in such patients, an initial 10-mg dose followed by an infusion of 5–10 mg/hour has been suggested. If agitation persists, repeat 10-mg IV doses at 30-minute intervals, accompanied by a 5 mg/hour increase in the infusion rate, can be considered. ECG should be determined at baseline and periodically or continuously thereafter, with special attention paid to possible prolongation of the QT interval, and dosage should be reduced or the drug discontinued if clinically important QT prolongation (e.g., 15–25% or more over baseline) occurs or the QT_c exceeds 450 msec.

CAUTIONS

Haloperidol shares the toxic potentials of phenothiazines, and the usual precautions of phenothiazine therapy should be observed. The overall incidence of adverse effects associated with haloperidol is similar to that associated with piperazine-derivative phenothiazines. (See Cautions in the Phenothiazines General Statement 28:16.08.24.)

Geriatric patients with dementia-related psychosis treated with antipsychotic agents are at an increased risk of mortality. (See Cautions: Geriatric Precautions.)

● Nervous System Effects

The most frequent adverse effects of haloperidol involve the CNS.

Extrapyramidal Reactions

Extrapyramidal reactions occur frequently with haloperidol, especially during the first few days of therapy. In most patients, these reactions consist of parkinsonian symptoms (e.g., marked drowsiness and lethargy, drooling or hypersalivation, fixed stare), which are mild to moderate in severity and are usually reversible following discontinuance of the drug. Other adverse neuromuscular reactions have been reported less frequently, but are often more severe, and include feelings of motor restlessness (i.e., akathisia), tardive dystonia, and dystonic reactions (e.g., hyperreflexia, opisthotonos, oculogyric crisis, torticollis, trismus). Generally, the occurrence and severity of most extrapyramidal reactions are dose related, since they occur at relatively high dosages and disappear or become less severe following a reduction in dosage; however, severe extrapyramidal reactions have reportedly occurred at relatively low dosages. Most patients respond rapidly to treatment with an anticholinergic antiparkinsonian drug (e.g., benztropine, trihexyphenidyl). If persistent extrapyramidal reactions occur, haloperidol therapy may have to be discontinued.

Neuroleptic malignant syndrome (NMS) may occur in patients receiving haloperidol or other antipsychotic therapy. NMS is potentially fatal and requires immediate discontinuance of the drug and initiation of intensive symptomatic and supportive care. For additional information on NMS, see Extrapyramidal Reactions in Cautions: Nervous System Effects, in the Phenothiazines General Statement 28:16.08.24.

Tardive Dyskinesia

Like other antipsychotic agents (e.g., phenothiazines), haloperidol has been associated with persistent dyskinesias. Tardive dyskinesia may occur in some patients during long-term administration of haloperidol or it may occur following discontinuance of the drug. The risk of developing tardive dyskinesia appears to be greater in geriatric patients receiving high dosages of the drug, especially females. The symptoms are persistent, and in some patients appear to be irreversible. Tardive dyskinesia is characterized by rhythmic involuntary movements of the tongue, face, mouth, or jaw (e.g., protrusion of the tongue, puffing of cheeks, chewing movements, puckering of the mouth), which sometimes may be accompanied by involuntary movements of the extremities and/or trunk. Although not clearly established, the risk of developing the syndrome and the likelihood that it will become irreversible may increase with the duration of therapy and total cumulative dose of antipsychotic agent(s) administered; however, the syndrome may occur, although much less frequently, after relatively short periods of treatment with low dosages.

Management of tardive dyskinesia generally consists of gradual discontinuance of the precipitating antipsychotic agent when possible, reducing the dosage of the first-generation (conventional) antipsychotic agent or switching to a second-generation (atypical) antipsychotic agent, or switching to clozapine therapy. The syndrome may partially or completely remit if antipsychotic agents are discontinued, although some patients may require many months for improvement. Tardive dyskinesia may be masked if antipsychotic therapy is reinstituted, dosage is increased, or therapy with another antipsychotic agent is initiated. The effect that masking of the symptoms may have on the long-term course of the syndrome is not known. Fine vermicular movement of the tongue may be an early sign of tardive dyskinesia; prompt discontinuance of haloperidol after this sign occurs may prevent development of the syndrome. Vesicular monoamine transporter 2 (VMAT2) inhibitors (e.g., deutetrabenazine, valbenazine tosylate) have been shown to be effective in reducing symptoms of tardive dyskinesia in controlled clinical studies and may allow some patients to continue receiving antipsychotic therapy. (See Deutetrabenazine 28:56 and Valbenazine Tosylate 28:56.) Antiparkinsonian agents do not alleviate and tend to exacerbate the symptoms of this syndrome.

In general, abrupt withdrawal of antipsychotic agents following short-term administration is not associated with adverse effects; however, transient dyskinetic signs have occurred following abrupt withdrawal in patients receiving prolonged maintenance therapy with haloperidol. In some patients, the dyskinetic movements are indistinguishable, except on the basis of their duration, from tardive dyskinesia. It is not known whether gradual withdrawal of antipsychotic agents reduces the incidence of withdrawal-emergent neurologic signs; however, if haloperidol therapy must be discontinued, gradual withdrawal of the drug is recommended, if possible, pending further accumulation of data.

For additional information on tardive dyskinesia, including manifestations and treatment, see Tardive Dyskinesia under Cautions: Nervous System Effects, in the Phenothiazines General Statement 28:16.08.24.

Other Nervous System Effects

Tardive dystonia, not associated with tardive dyskinesia, has occurred in patients receiving haloperidol. Tardive dystonia is characterized by delayed onset of choreic or dystonic movements, often is persistent, and potentially can become irreversible.

Other adverse nervous system effects of haloperidol include insomnia, restlessness, anxiety, euphoria, agitation, drowsiness, depression, lethargy, headache, confusion, vertigo, and tonic-clonic seizures. Exacerbation of psychotic symptoms (including hallucinations and catatonic-like behavior), which may subside following discontinuance of therapy or treatment with anticholinergic agents, has also been reported.

Adverse anticholinergic effects of haloperidol include dry mouth (xerostomia), blurred vision, constipation, urinary retention, and diaphoresis. Priapism has also occurred.

● Hematologic Effects

Mild and usually transient leukopenia/neutropenia and leukocytosis have been reported in patients receiving antipsychotic agents, including haloperidol.

Agranulocytosis (including fatal cases) has also been reported rarely in patients receiving haloperidol, but only when combined with other drugs. Possible risk factors for leukopenia and neutropenia include preexisting low leukocyte count and a history of drug-induced leukopenia or neutropenia. (See Cautions: Precautions and Contraindications.) Other adverse hematologic effects associated with haloperidol include anemia, minimal decreases in erythrocyte count, and a tendency toward lymphomonocytosis.

● Endocrine and Metabolic Effects

Moderate engorgement of the breast with lactation has occurred in some females receiving haloperidol. Galactorrhea, mastalgia, menstrual irregularities, gynecomastia, increased libido, impotence, hyperglycemia, hypoglycemia, and hyponatremia have also occurred in some patients. Antipsychotic agents increase serum prolactin concentrations. (See Cautions: Mutagenicity and Carcinogenicity.) Although not reported to date with haloperidol, the manufacturers caution that decreases in serum cholesterol concentration have occurred in patients receiving chemically related drugs.

● Cardiovascular Effects

Tachycardia, hypotension, hypertension, ECG changes (including those compatible with QT-interval prolongation and the polymorphous configuration of torsades de pointes), and sudden death have been reported in patients receiving haloperidol. The US Food and Drug Administration (FDA) states that there have been at least 28 case reports of QT-interval prolongation and torsades de pointes, including some that were fatal, in patients receiving the drug IV†. In addition, FDA states that case-control studies have demonstrated a dose-dependent relationship between IV haloperidol dosage and subsequent development of torsades de pointes. A postmarketing analysis of a worldwide safety database revealed 229 reports of QT-interval prolongation and torsades de pointes with oral or parenteral haloperidol; many of these cases were confounded by concomitant administration of drugs known to prolong the QT interval or medical conditions associated with QT-interval prolongation. The reports included 73 cases of torsades de pointes, 11 of which were fatal. In 8 out of 11 fatal cases, haloperidol was administered IV in various dosages. In another postmarketing analysis of adverse cardiovascular events associated with haloperidol decanoate, 13 cases of torsades de pointes, QT-interval prolongation, ventricular arrhythmias, and/or sudden death were identified.

FDA states that it is not possible to estimate the frequency with which QT-interval prolongation or torsades de pointes occurs following administration of haloperidol based on these case reports alone. However, use of higher than recommended doses of any haloperidol formulation and IV administration of the drug appear to be associated with an increased risk of these effects. Many of the reported cases of QT-interval prolongation and torsades de pointes have occurred in patients receiving relatively high dosages of IV haloperidol (e.g., exceeding 35 mg daily); however, such effects also have been reported in patients receiving lower IV dosages or oral therapy. Although cases of sudden death, torsades de pointes, and QT-interval prolongation have been reported even in the absence of predisposing factors, FDA, the manufacturer of Haldol®, and some clinicians state that particular caution is advised when using any formulation of haloperidol in patients who have other QT-interval prolonging conditions, including electrolyte imbalance (particularly hypokalemia and hypomagnesemia), underlying cardiac abnormalities, hypothyroidism, or familial long QT syndrome, or those who are concomitantly taking medications known to prolong the QT interval. (See Uses: Delirium, see Cautions: Precautions and Contraindications, and also see Acute Toxicity: Manifestations.) FDA states that clinicians should consider this cardiovascular risk information when making individual treatment decisions for their patients.

Cases of sudden and unexpected death have been reported in haloperidol-treated patients. The nature of the evidence makes it impossible to determine definitively what role, if any, haloperidol played in the outcome of the cases reported to date. Although the possibility that haloperidol played a causative role in these deaths cannot be excluded, it should be kept in mind that sudden and unexpected death may occur in psychotic patients when they remain untreated or when they are treated with other antipsychotic medications.

● Other Adverse Effects

Impaired liver function and/or jaundice, maculopapular and acneiform dermatologic reactions, photosensitivity, alopecia, anorexia, diarrhea, hypersalivation, dyspepsia, nausea, vomiting, cataracts, retinopathy, and visual disturbances have also been reported.

Hyperpyrexia and heat stroke, not associated with neuroleptic malignant syndrome (see Extrapyramidal Reactions in Cautions: Nervous System Effects), have been reported in some patients receiving haloperidol.

Laryngospasm, bronchospasm, and increased depth of respiration have occurred in patients receiving haloperidol. Bronchopneumonia, resulting in fatalities in some patients, has occurred following the use of antipsychotic agents, including haloperidol. It has been suggested that lethargy and decreased thirst, resulting from central inhibition, may cause dehydration, hemoconcentration, and reduced pulmonary ventilation.

Hyperammonemia following haloperidol treatment has been reported in at least one child with citrullinemia, an inherited disorder of ammonia excretion.

● Precautions and Contraindications

Haloperidol shares the toxic potentials of other antipsychotic agents (e.g., phenothiazines), and the usual precautions associated with therapy with these agents should be observed. (See Cautions in the Phenothiazines General Statement 28:16.08.24.)

Geriatric patients with dementia-related psychosis treated with antipsychotic agents are at an increased risk of mortality. (See Cautions: Geriatric Precautions.)

Patients should be warned that haloperidol may impair their ability to perform activities requiring mental alertness or physical coordination (e.g., operating machinery, driving a motor vehicle). Patients also should be warned that haloperidol may enhance their response to alcohol, barbiturates, or other CNS depressants.

Because of the possibility of transient hypotension and/or precipitation of angina, haloperidol should be used with caution in patients with severe cardiovascular disorders. If hypotension occurs, metaraminol, norepinephrine, or phenylephrine may be used; epinephrine should *not* be used since haloperidol causes a reversal of epinephrine's vasopressor effects and a further lowering of blood pressure.

Since haloperidol may lower the seizure threshold, the drug should be used with caution in patients receiving anticonvulsant agents and in those with a history of seizures or EEG abnormalities. Adequate anticonvulsant therapy should be maintained during administration of haloperidol.

The manufacturers state that haloperidol should be used with caution in patients with known allergies or with a history of allergic reactions to drugs.

When concomitant therapy with an antiparkinsonian drug is necessary to manage haloperidol-induced extrapyramidal symptoms, it may be necessary to continue the antiparkinsonian drug for a period of time after discontinuance of haloperidol in order to prevent emergence of these symptoms.

The manufacturers caution that when haloperidol is used to control mania in patients with bipolar disorder, there may be a rapid mood swing to depression.

Haloperidol should be used with caution in patients with thyrotoxicosis since severe neurotoxicity (e.g., rigidity, inability to walk or talk) may occur in these patients during therapy with an antipsychotic agent.

Cases of leukopenia and neutropenia have been reported in patients receiving antipsychotic agents, including haloperidol; agranulocytosis (including fatal cases) has also been reported. (See Cautions: Hematologic Effects.) Patients with a preexisting low leukocyte count or a history of drug-induced leukopenia or neutropenia should have their complete blood count monitored frequently during the first few months of therapy and haloperidol should be discontinued at the first sign of a decline in the leukocyte count in the absence of other causative factors. Haloperidol-treated patients with neutropenia should be carefully monitored for fever or other signs or symptoms of infection and be treated promptly should such signs and symptoms occur. Patients with severe neutropenia (absolute neutrophil count less than 1000/mm³) should discontinue haloperidol and have their leukocyte count followed until recovery.

Care should be taken to avoid skin contact with haloperidol lactate oral solution and injection, since contact dermatitis has occurred rarely.

Cases of sudden death, QT-interval prolongation, and torsades de pointes have been reported in patients receiving haloperidol. (See Uses: Delirium and also see Cautions: Cardiovascular Effects.) Use of higher than recommended doses of any haloperidol formulation and IV† administration of the drug appear to be associated with an increased risk of QT-interval prolongation and torsades de pointes. Although these effects have been reported in the absence of predisposing factors, haloperidol should be used with particular caution in patients with other conditions that prolong the QT interval, including electrolyte imbalance (particularly hypokalemia and hypomagnesemia), underlying cardiac abnormalities, hypothyroidism, and familial long QT syndrome, as well as in those concurrently receiving other drugs known to prolong the QT interval. In addition, ECG monitoring is recommended whenever haloperidol is administered IV. (See Uses: Delirium.)

Haloperidol is contraindicated in patients with severe toxic CNS depression or in those who are comatose from any cause. Haloperidol also is contraindicated in patients who are hypersensitive to the drug and in those with parkinsonian syndrome.

● Pediatric Precautions

Safety and efficacy of haloperidol decanoate or lactate injection in children have not been established, and safety and efficacy of other haloperidol preparations in children younger than 3 years of age have not been established. Hyperammonemia was reported during postmarketing surveillance in a 5.5-year-old child with citrullinemia, an inherited disorder of ammonia excretion, following haloperidol therapy.

● Geriatric Precautions

Clinical studies of haloperidol did not include sufficient numbers of geriatric patients 65 years of age and older to determine whether this age group responds differently from younger adults. Other reported clinical experience has not consistently identified differences in responses between geriatric and younger patients. However, the prevalence of tardive dyskinesia appears to be highest among geriatric patients, particularly elderly women. In addition, the pharmacokinetics of haloperidol generally warrant the use of reduced dosages in geriatric patients. (See Dosage and Administration: Dosage.)

Geriatric patients with dementia-related psychosis treated with either conventional or atypical antipsychotic agents are at an increased risk of mortality. Analyses of 17 placebo-controlled trials (modal duration of 10 weeks) in geriatric patients mainly receiving atypical antipsychotic agents revealed an approximate 1.6- to 1.7-fold increase in mortality compared with that in patients receiving placebo. Over the course of a typical 10-week controlled trial, the rate of death in drug-treated patients was about 4.5% compared with a rate of about 2.6% in those receiving placebo. Although the causes of death were varied in these trials, most of the deaths appeared to be either cardiovascular (e.g., heart failure, sudden death) or infectious (e.g., pneumonia) in nature. Subsequently, 2 observational, epidemiologic studies have indicated that, similar to atypical antipsychotic agents, treatment with conventional antipsychotic agents may increase mortality; the causes of death were not reported in the first study, and cancer and cardiac disease were the causes of death with the highest relative risk in the second study. However, the extent to which these findings of increased mortality in observational studies may be attributed to the antipsychotic agent as opposed to certain patient characteristics remains unclear.

The US Food and Drug Administration (FDA) currently advises clinicians that antipsychotic agents, including haloperidol, are *not* FDA labeled for the treatment of dementia-related psychosis. The FDA further advises clinicians that no drugs currently are approved for the treatment of dementia-associated psychosis and that other management options should be considered in patients with this disorder. The decision whether to prescribe antipsychotic agents "off-label" in the treatment of dementia symptoms is left to the discretion of the clinician. Clinicians who prescribe antipsychotic agents for geriatric patients with dementia-related psychosis should discuss the increased mortality risk with patients, their families, and their caregivers. In addition, patients currently receiving antipsychotic agents for dementia-associated symptoms should not abruptly stop taking the drugs; caregivers and patients should discuss any possible concerns with their clinician. For additional information on the use of antipsychotic agents for dementia-associated psychosis and other behavioral disturbances, see Geriatric Considerations under Psychotic Disorders: Schizophrenia, see Other Psychoneurologic Disorders, in Uses, and also see Cautions: Geriatric Precautions, in the Phenothiazines General Statement 28:16.08.24.

● Mutagenicity and Carcinogenicity

Haloperidol did not exhibit mutagenic potential in the Ames test. Negative or inconsistent positive findings have been reported in in vitro and in vivo studies on the effects of conventional preparations of haloperidol on chromosome structure and number. However, the available cytogenetic evidence is considered too inconsistent to be conclusive at this time.

Although an increase in mammary neoplasms has been found in rodents following long-term administration of prolactin-stimulating antipsychotic agents, no clinical or epidemiologic studies conducted to date have shown an association between long-term administration of these drugs and mammary tumorigenesis in humans. Current evidence is considered too limited to be conclusive, and further study is needed to determine the clinical importance in most patients of elevated serum prolactin concentrations associated with antipsychotic agents. Since in vitro tests indicate that approximately one-third of human breast cancers are prolactin dependent, haloperidol should be used with caution in patients with previously detected breast cancer.

● Pregnancy, Fertility, and Lactation

Pregnancy

Although there are no adequate and controlled studies to date in humans, 2 cases of limb malformations (e.g., phocomelia) have occurred in offspring of women who were given haloperidol concurrently with other potentially teratogenic drugs during the first trimester of pregnancy; these teratogenic effects have not been directly attributed to haloperidol. Haloperidol has been shown to be teratogenic and fetotoxic in animals at dosages 2–20 times the usual maximum human dosage.

Neonates exposed to antipsychotic agents, including haloperidol, during the third trimester of pregnancy are at risk for extrapyramidal and/or withdrawal symptoms following delivery. Symptoms reported in these neonates to date include agitation, hypertonia, hypotonia, tardive dyskinetic-like symptoms, tremor, somnolence, respiratory distress, and feeding disorder. Any neonate exhibiting extrapyramidal or withdrawal symptoms following in utero exposure to antipsychotic agents should be monitored. Symptoms were self-limiting in some neonates, but varied in severity; some infants required intensive care unit support and prolonged hospitalization. For further information on extrapyramidal and withdrawal symptoms in neonates, see Cautions: Pregnancy, Fertility, and Lactation, in the Phenothiazines General Statement 28:16.08.24.

Haloperidol should be used during pregnancy or in women likely to become pregnant only when the potential benefits justify the possible risks to the fetus.

Fertility

The effect of haloperidol on fertility in humans is not known. Impotence, increased libido, priapism, and menstrual irregularities have occurred in some individuals during haloperidol therapy.

Lactation

Haloperidol is distributed into milk. The manufacturers warn that nursing should not be undertaken by women receiving haloperidol.

DRUG INTERACTIONS

● CNS Depressants

Haloperidol may be additive with, or may potentiate the action of, other CNS depressants such as opiates or other analgesics, barbiturates or other sedatives, anesthetics, or alcohol. When haloperidol is used concomitantly with other CNS depressants, caution should be used to avoid excessive sedation.

● Lithium

Although most patients receiving lithium and an antipsychotic agent (e.g., haloperidol, phenothiazines) concurrently do not develop unusual adverse effects, an acute encephalopathic syndrome occasionally has occurred, especially when high serum lithium concentrations were present. Patients receiving such combined therapy should be observed for evidence of adverse neurologic effects; treatment should be promptly discontinued if such signs or symptoms appear. (See Drug Interactions: Antipsychotic Agents, in the monograph on Lithium Salts 28:28.)

● Anticoagulants

Haloperidol has been reported to antagonize the anticoagulant activity of phenindione in one patient. Further study is needed to determine the clinical importance of this interaction.

● Rifampin

Concomitant oral therapy with rifampin and haloperidol in schizophrenic patients resulted in a mean 70% decrease in plasma haloperidol concentrations and decreased antipsychotic efficacy. Following discontinuance of rifampin in other schizophrenic patients treated with oral haloperidol, mean haloperidol concentrations increased 3.3-fold. Careful monitoring of clinical status and appropriate dosage adjustment are warranted whenever rifampin is initiated or discontinued in patients stabilized on haloperidol.

● Drugs with Anticholinergic Effects

The manufacturers caution that increases in intraocular pressure may occur in patients receiving anticholinergic drugs, including antiparkinsonian agents, concurrently with haloperidol.

● Drugs that Prolong QT Interval

Cases of QT-interval prolongation and torsades de pointes have been reported in patients receiving haloperidol. Patients receiving higher than recommended dosages of any haloperidol preparation and those receiving the drug IV appear to be at a higher risk of developing these adverse effects. (See Uses: Delirium and see also Cautions: Cardiovascular Effects.) Particular caution is advised when oral or parenteral haloperidol is used in patients concurrently receiving other drugs that prolong the QT interval.

● Methyldopa

Dementia has reportedly occurred in several patients who received haloperidol and methyldopa concomitantly. Although the clinical importance of this possible interaction has not been determined, patients should be carefully observed for adverse psychiatric symptoms if the drugs are used concurrently.

ACUTE TOXICITY

● Manifestations

In general, overdosage of haloperidol may be expected to produce effects that are extensions of common adverse reactions; severe extrapyramidal reactions, hypotension, and sedation have been the principal effects reported. Coma with respiratory depression and hypotension (sometimes shock-like) may occur.

Substantial prolongation of the QT interval and atypical ventricular tachycardia (torsades de pointes) have occurred following haloperidol overdosage. The possibility of ECG changes associated with torsades de pointes should be considered following haloperidol overdosage, and ECG and vital signs should be monitored for signs of QT prolongation or dysrhythmias, continuing such monitoring until the ECG is normal.

Following accidental overdosage in a 2-year-old child, hypertension, rather than hypotension, reportedly occurred. Extrapyramidal reactions may consist of muscular weakness or rigidity and a generalized or localized tremor. Manifestations of overdosage with haloperidol decanoate injection may be prolonged.

● Treatment

Treatment of haloperidol overdosage generally involves symptomatic and supportive care. There is no specific antidote for haloperidol intoxication; however, anticholinergic or antiparkinsonian drugs may be useful in controlling extrapyramidal reactions associated with haloperidol overdosage.

Following acute ingestion of the drug, the stomach should be emptied by inducing emesis or by gastric lavage. If the patient is comatose, having seizures, or lacks the gag reflex, gastric lavage may be performed if an endotracheal tube with cuff inflated is in place to prevent aspiration of gastric contents. Activated charcoal should be administered after gastric lavage and/or emesis.

ECG and vital signs should be monitored, particularly for signs of QT prolongation or dysrhythmias. Severe arrhythmias should be treated with appropriate antiarrhythmic measures. Appropriate therapy should be instituted if hypotension or excessive sedation occurs; epinephrine should *not* be used (see Cautions: Precautions and Contraindications).

PHARMACOLOGY

The principal pharmacologic effects of haloperidol are similar to those of piperazine-derivative phenothiazines. The precise mechanism of antipsychotic action of haloperidol is unclear, but the drug appears to depress the CNS at the subcortical level of the brain, midbrain, and brain stem reticular formation. Haloperidol appears to inhibit the ascending reticular activating system of the brain stem (possibly through the caudate nucleus), thereby interrupting the impulse between the diencephalon and the cortex. The drug may antagonize the actions of glutamic acid within the extrapyramidal system. Inhibition of catecholamine receptors may also be important in the mode of action of haloperidol; the drug may also inhibit the reuptake of various neurotransmitters in the midbrain. Haloperidol appears to have strong central antidopaminergic and weak central anticholinergic activity. Like phenothiazines, haloperidol produces catalepsy and inhibits spontaneous motor activity and conditioned avoidance behaviors in animals. Haloperidol inhibits the central and peripheral effects of apomorphine, produces ganglionic blockade, and reduces affective responses. The precise mechanism of antiemetic action of haloperidol is unclear, but like some phenothiazines (e.g., chlorpromazine, prochlorperazine), haloperidol has been shown to directly affect the chemoreceptor trigger zone (CTZ), apparently by blocking dopamine receptors in the CTZ.

Like other dopamine receptor antagonists (e.g., phenothiazines), haloperidol may cause extrapyramidal reactions, and there appears to be a very narrow range between the effective therapeutic dosage for the management of acute psychotic disorders and that causing extrapyramidal symptoms.

Haloperidol produces less sedation, hypotension, and hypothermia than chlorpromazine.

PHARMACOKINETICS

● Absorption

Haloperidol is well absorbed from the GI tract following oral administration, but appears to undergo first-pass metabolism in the liver. Oral bioavailability of the drug has been reported to average 60%. The drug may undergo some enterohepatic circulation. Peak plasma concentrations of haloperidol occur within 2–6 hours following oral administration. Following IM administration of haloperidol lactate, peak plasma haloperidol concentrations occur within 10–20 minutes and peak pharmacologic action occurs within 30–45 minutes; in acutely agitated patients, control of psychotic manifestations may become apparent within 30–60 minutes, with substantial improvement often occurring within 2–3 hours. Haloperidol concentrations are detectable in plasma for several weeks following administration of a single dose of the drug.

Esterification of haloperidol results in slow and gradual release of haloperidol decanoate from fatty tissues, thus prolonging the duration of action; administration of the ester in a sesame oil vehicle further delays the rate of release. Following IM administration of haloperidol decanoate, plasma haloperidol concentrations are usually evident within 1 day and peak concentrations generally occur within about 6–7 days (range: 1–9 days). Steady-state plasma haloperidol concentrations are usually reached in approximately 3 months following once-monthly IM injection of the decanoate. In one group of patients receiving 20–400 mg monthly, data adjusted to 100-mg monthly doses suggested mean trough plasma haloperidol concentrations of 2 ng/mL after the first dose and of 4 ng/mL at steady state; accumulation during 24 months of therapy was not apparent. Within the usual dosage range, plasma haloperidol concentrations following IM administration of the decanoate are approximately proportional and linearly related to dosage; however, there is considerable interindividual and intraindividual variation in plasma concentrations attained with a given dosage.

● Distribution

Distribution of haloperidol into human body tissues and fluids has not been fully characterized. Following administration of haloperidol in animals, the drug is distributed mainly into the liver, with lower concentrations being distributed into the brain, lungs, kidneys, spleen, and heart.

Haloperidol is about 92% bound to plasma proteins.

Haloperidol is distributed into milk.

● Elimination

Although the exact metabolic fate has not been clearly established, it appears that haloperidol is principally metabolized in the liver. The drug appears to be metabolized principally by oxidative N-dealkylation of the piperidine nitrogen to form fluorophenylcarbonic acids and piperidine metabolites (which appear to be inactive), and by reduction of the butyrophenone carbonyl to the carbinol, forming hydroxyhaloperidol. Limited data suggest that the reduced metabolite, hydroxyhaloperidol, has some pharmacologic activity, although its activity appears to be less than that of haloperidol. Urinary metabolites in rats include p-fluorophenaceturic acid, β-p-fluorobenzoylpropionic acid, and several unidentified acids.

Haloperidol and its metabolites are excreted slowly in urine and feces. Approximately 40% of a single oral dose of haloperidol is excreted in urine within 5 days. About 15% of an oral dose of the drug is excreted in feces via biliary elimination. Small amounts of the drug are excreted for about 28 days following oral administration.

Following IM administration of haloperidol decanoate, the esterified compound is initially distributed into fatty tissue stores, from which the drug is then slowly and gradually released and subsequently undergoes hydrolysis by plasma and/or tissue esterases to form haloperidol and decanoic acid. Subsequent distribution, metabolism, and excretion of haloperidol appears to be similar to those of orally administered drug. Following IM administration of the decanoate, the drug has an apparent elimination half-life of approximately 3 weeks.

CHEMISTRY AND STABILITY

● Chemistry

Haloperidol is a butyrophenone-derivative antipsychotic agent. The drug is structurally similar to droperidol. Haloperidol is commercially available as the base, decanoic acid ester (decanoate), and lactate salt.

Haloperidol occurs as a white to faintly yellowish, amorphous or microcrystalline powder and has solubilities of less than 0.1 mg/mL in water and of approximately 16.7 mg/mL in alcohol at 25°C. The drug has a pK_a of 8.3.

Haloperidol decanoate occurs as a clear, light amber, oily liquid and is soluble in fixed oils (e.g., sesame oil) and in most organic solvents. The decanoate has a solubility of approximately 0.01 mg/mL in water. Haloperidol decanoate injection is commercially available as a sterile solution of the drug in sesame oil and contains benzyl alcohol as a preservative.

Haloperidol injection is prepared with the aid of lactic acid and contains the drug as the lactate salt; the injection is a sterile solution of the drug in water for injection. Commercially available injections are adjusted to pH 3–3.8 with lactic acid and also *may* contain parabens as preservatives. Haloperidol oral solution also is prepared with the aid of lactic acid and contains the drug as the lactate salt. The commercially available oral solution has a pH of 2.75–3.75.

● Stability

Commercially available haloperidol preparations should be stored in tight, light-resistant containers at controlled room temperature between 15–30°C; freezing of the oral solution and injections and refrigeration of the decanoate injection should be avoided.

Haloperidol lactate injection may be compatible with some drugs for a short period of time after mixing, but at least one manufacturer recommends that the lactate not be mixed with other drugs. Haloperidol decanoate injection is incompatible with sterile water for injection or sodium chloride injection and with other aqueous injections. Specialized references should be consulted for specific compatibility information.

PREPARATIONS

Excipients in commercially available drug preparations may have clinically important effects in some individuals; consult specific product labeling for details.

Haloperidol

Oral

Tablets	0.5 mg*	Haloperidol Tablets
	1 mg*	Haloperidol Tablets
	2 mg*	Haloperidol Tablets
	5 mg*	Haloperidol Tablets
	10 mg*	Haloperidol Tablets
	20 mg*	Haloperidol Tablets

* available from one or more manufacturer, distributor, and/or repackager by generic (nonproprietary) name

Haloperidol Decanoate

Parenteral

Injection, for IM use only	50 mg (of haloperidol) per mL*	Haldol® Decanoate, Ortho-McNeil-Janssen Haloperidol Decanoate Injection
	100 mg (of haloperidol) per mL*	Haldol® Decanoate, Ortho-McNeil-Janssen Haloperidol Decanoate Injection

* available from one or more manufacturer, distributor, and/or repackager by generic (nonproprietary) name

Haloperidol Lactate

Oral

Solution	2 mg (of haloperidol) per mL*	Haloperidol Lactate Oral Solution Concentrate

Parenteral

Injection	5 mg (of haloperidol) per mL*	Haldol®, Ortho-McNeil-Janssen Haloperidol Lactate Injection

* available from one or more manufacturer, distributor, and/or repackager by generic (nonproprietary) name

† Use is not currently included in the labeling approved by the US Food and Drug Administration.

Selected Revisions November 13, 2017, © Copyright, March 1, 1972, American Society of Health-System Pharmacists, Inc.

Benzodiazepines General Statement

28:24.08 · BENZODIAZEPINES

■ Benzodiazepines are used as anxiolytics, sedatives, hypnotics, anticonvulsants, and/or skeletal muscle relaxants.

USES

Benzodiazepines are used for preoperative relief of anxiety and provision of sedation, light anesthesia, and anterograde amnesia of perioperative events; for procedural sedation; for continuous sedation in intubated and mechanically ventilated patients undergoing treatment in a critical care setting (e.g., intensive care unit [ICU]); for induction and maintenance of anesthesia; as hypnotics in the treatment of insomnia; for the management of agitation associated with acute alcohol withdrawal; and for the management of anxiety (e.g., generalized anxiety disorder, panic disorder). Benzodiazepines also are used as anticonvulsants and skeletal muscle relaxants. In addition, benzodiazepines have been used alone and as adjuncts to antipsychotic agents in the management of schizophrenia† (e.g., in patients with akathisia associated with antipsychotic therapy).

All benzodiazepines have similar actions, and their use is more a reflection of the way in which the drugs have been studied and the way the manufacturers promote their use than real differences between the drugs. In general, there is no evidence that any one benzodiazepine is more effective than another if an adequate dosage is given. However, pharmacokinetic and pharmacodynamic differences have influenced the therapeutic application of these drugs.

● Anxiety and Insomnia

Benzodiazepines are used for the management of anxiety disorders and insomnia. These drugs appear to have a tranquilizing effect on the CNS with no appreciable effect on the respiratory or cardiovascular systems. Most clinicians prefer benzodiazepines to barbiturates or meprobamate for the management of anxiety and tension and to other hypnotics such as barbiturates in the management of insomnia, because benzodiazepines have a relatively low abuse potential, produce less sedation with effective anxiolytic doses, and produce less toxicity with acute overdosage. In addition, benzodiazepines generally do not induce hepatic microsomal enzymes or produce substantial changes in prothrombin time or in oral anticoagulant dosage requirements. (See Drug Interactions.) For the symptomatic treatment of anxiety or insomnia in geriatric patients and patients with liver disease, some clinicians prefer lorazepam, oxazepam, or triazolam to other benzodiazepines or barbiturates because they have a relatively short elimination half-life even in patients with liver disease, and they do not have active metabolites.

Anxiety Disorders

Benzodiazepines are used for the management of anxiety disorders, principally generalized anxiety disorder, and for the short-term relief of symptoms of anxiety or anxiety associated with depressive symptoms. Generalized anxiety disorder is characterized by unrealistic or excessive anxiety and worry (apprehensive expectation) about several life circumstances (e.g., misfortune of one's child; finances; academic, athletic, or social performance) for 6 months or longer, during which time such concerns are bothersome more often than not. When anxiety is present, it is accompanied by many signs of motor tension (e.g., trembling, twitching, shakiness, restlessness, easy fatigability), autonomic hyperactivity (e.g., shortness of breath, smothering sensation, tachycardia, palpitations, sweating, cold clammy hands, dry mouth, diarrhea, hot flushes), and vigilance and scanning (e.g., feeling keyed up or on edge, exaggerated startle response, trouble falling or staying asleep, difficulty concentrating or mind going blank because of anxiety). When such signs are associated with panic attacks, the patient may be suffering from panic disorder, which also can be treated effectively with benzodiazepines. Mild depressive symptoms commonly are associated with generalized anxiety disorder, and an associated and unrelated panic disorder or depressive disorder often is present.

In the management of anxiety disorders and anxiety symptoms, benzodiazepines are more effective than barbiturates or meprobamate. Anxiety or tension associated with the stress of everyday life usually does not require treatment with an anxiolytic. The efficacy of benzodiazepines for long-term use (i.e., longer than 4 months) as anxiolytics has not been evaluated. The need for continued therapy with benzodiazepines should be periodically reassessed.

Benzodiazepines (principally alprazolam and clonazepam, but also diazepam and lorazepam) have been used effectively in the management of panic disorder (an anxiety disorder), with or without agoraphobia. Panic disorder is characterized by recurrent, unexpected panic attacks (discrete periods of intense fear or discomfort), associated concern about having additional attacks, anxiety about the implications or consequences of the attacks, and/or a clinically important change in behavior related to the attacks. Panic attacks have a sudden onset, reach a peak effect rapidly (usually in 10 minutes or less), are associated with at least 4 characteristic symptoms, and often are accompanied by a feeling of imminent danger or impending doom and an urge to escape. Characteristic symptoms include palpitations, pounding heart, or tachycardia; sweating; trembling or shaking; dyspnea or smothering sensation; feeling of choking; chest pain or discomfort; nausea or abdominal distress; dizziness, unsteady feelings, lightheadedness, or faintness; derealization or depersonalization; fear of losing control or going crazy; fear of dying; paresthesias; and chills or hot flushes.

Efficacy of benzodiazepines in the management of panic disorder has been established mainly in short-term (for periods of 4–10 weeks) controlled studies, although the drugs have been used without apparent loss of efficacy for longer periods (e.g., 8–12 months or longer) in many patients. Benzodiazepines can reduce the number of spontaneous and situational panic attacks and associated anxiety, avoidance behavior, phobic fears, somatic manifestations, and secondary disability (e.g., interference with normal work or social activities). Although the drugs also can reduce depressive symptomatology in many patients with panic disorder, including those who are depressed or nondepressed, emergence of depressive symptomatology has occurred occasionally in such patients.

Following discontinuance of benzodiazepines, a relapse of the condition, including a rebound in panic attacks and anxiety, and/or the development of withdrawal frequently occurs. In one study despite gradual withdrawal over 4 weeks in patients receiving high-dose alprazolam therapy for 8 weeks, a rebound in panic attacks and anxiety occurred in 27 and 13% of patients, respectively, and a transient, mild to moderate withdrawal syndrome developed in 35% of patients, but both rebound effects and withdrawal manifestations subsided after 2 weeks. Additional study is needed to establish the optimum duration of benzodiazepine therapy in the management of panic disorder, and to determine the most appropriate method of tapered withdrawal of the drugs. The potential dependence liability of benzodiazepines should be considered in weighing the possible risks and benefits of therapy with the drugs in this condition.

Anxiety Associated with Myocardial Infarction

Benzodiazepines (e.g., diazepam) have been used to relieve anxiety associated with acute myocardial infarction (MI); however, evidence suggests that these drugs are no more effective than placebo in managing anxiety and ischemic-type pain in patients with MI. Experts state that routine use of anxiolytics is neither necessary nor recommended in patients with acute MI. Morphine sulfate is considered the drug of choice for relief of pain and associated anxiety following acute MI. (See Uses in the Opiate Agonists General Statement 28:08.08.)

Insomnia

Benzodiazepines have been used in the management of insomnia because of their established short- and intermediate-term efficacy and relative safety. However, non-benzodiazepine benzodiazepine receptor agonists (e.g., zaleplon, eszopiclone, zolpidem) may be preferred in some patients because of their relatively rapid onset of effect, short duration of action, and safety profile.

While experience to date in the management of insomnia principally has been with estazolam, flurazepam, quazepam, temazepam, and triazolam, other benzodiazepines also have been used for insomnia. Flurazepam was the first benzodiazepine approved by the FDA for use as a hypnotic.

The choice of a specific benzodiazepine must be individualized according to patient response and tolerance, taking into consideration pharmacokinetic and pharmacodynamic characteristics of the drug, patient age and other characteristics, and the underlying sleep disorder being treated. Benzodiazepines with a relatively short elimination half-life (e.g., triazolam) may be more likely to result in transient rebound insomnia after discontinuance and in pharmacodynamic tolerance and adaptation to the hypnotic effect after several weeks of therapy, with resultant diminished effectiveness during the end of each night's use (early morning insomnia) and, possibly, increased daytime anxiety. Benzodiazepines with a relatively long half-life (e.g., flurazepam, quazepam) may be more likely to result in residual daytime sedative effects and in impaired psychomotor and mental performance during continued therapy, although partial tolerance to these effects can occur. Differences in residual and cumulative CNS depressant effects may be particularly important in geriatric patients and in patients with potentially impaired elimination of the drugs and those whose job or lifestyle requires unimpaired intellectual or psychomotor function. Benzodiazepines with relatively slow GI absorption (e.g., temazepam) may be less effective in initial sleep induction; therefore, it has been suggested that the efficacy of such drugs may be diminished in patients whose principal symptom is initial difficulty in falling asleep (sleep-latency insomnia). Alterations in dosing (e.g., administering slowly absorbed drugs 1 or 2 hours before bedtime) may in part compensate for this delayed onset.

Treatment strategies for transient (insomnia of several days' duration related to minor situational stress), short-term (insomnia of several weeks' duration usually related to stress associated with work and/or family-life conditions such as job performance, job loss, bereavement, or illness), and long-term (insomnia of prolonged duration often associated with some underlying condition such as a psychiatric disorder, chronic drug and/or alcohol dependence, or other medical condition) insomnia will differ. For example, in the management of transient insomnia, use of relatively low-dose therapy with a relatively rapidly eliminated benzodiazepine for one to several nights may be preferred, unless sustained sedation is desired. For short-term insomnia, benzodiazepines are used as an adjunct to efforts aimed at improving sleep hygiene (e.g., avoidance of caffeine, alcohol, daytime naps, or retiring to bed too early), but therapy with the drugs generally should be limited to no more than several weeks, administering the drugs intermittently (e.g., skipping a nightly dose after one or two good nights' sleep) if possible; the choice of benzodiazepine should be individualized. Reevaluation of the patient's condition is recommended if continued hypnotic use exceeds 2–3 weeks, since sleep disturbance may be a presenting manifestation of an underlying physical and/or psychiatric disorder. Such underlying disorders also could result in worsening of insomnia or the emergence of new abnormalities of mentation or behavior; however, the possibility that such effects may be associated with benzodiazepine therapy itself also should be considered.

The management of long-term insomnia is more complex and depends in part on the presence of any identifiable underlying condition that is a contributing factor. The need for therapy with hypnotic drugs such as benzodiazepines may persist despite therapy aimed at treating the underlying condition; benzodiazepine therapy also may be useful in patients with no readily identifiable cause of the insomnia and usually is combined with psychological-behavioral therapies (e.g., relaxation techniques, sleep curtailment, stimulus control therapy) aimed at modifying negative conditioning related to sleep habits. If hypnotic drug therapy is employed, intermittent (e.g., every third night) therapy with a benzodiazepine having a relatively long elimination half-life has been suggested; efforts generally should be made to gradually discontinue such therapy after several months. Data from one study comparing the effects of triazolam and behavioral therapy on sleep latency in patients with persistent sleep-onset insomnia suggest that combined use of drug and behavioral therapies may offer both immediate relief and sustained effects upon drug discontinuance; however, behavioral therapy is a useful alternative to drug treatment and may be preferable, given its sustained effectiveness, particularly in individuals in whom use of hypnotic agents is problematic (e.g., individuals prone to drug abuse, pregnant or breast-feeding women). Referral to a sleep disorders clinic may be necessary for some patients.

Because of evidence from animal studies that the drugs can entrain circadian rhythms, benzodiazepines with a relatively short elimination half-life (e.g., triazolam) have been used for the prevention or short-term treatment of transient insomnia associated with sleep-wake schedule changes† (e.g., rapid travel across time zones ["jet lag"], rotating shift work). While such therapy may be useful in the management of sleep disorders associated with such schedule changes in some patients, the possibility that transient impairment of cognitive function (e.g., anterograde amnesia ["traveler's amnesia"]) may be induced by the drugs should be considered. (See Cautions: CNS Effects.)

Because benzodiazepines suppress stage 4 sleep, diazepam has been used effectively in some studies to prevent night terrors in adults.

● *Procedural Sedation*

Benzodiazepines (e.g., midazolam, diazepam) are used for procedural sedation, anxiolysis, and amnesia. Procedural sedation is a technique in which sedative and dissociative agents are administered with or without analgesics to allow patients to tolerate painful or unpleasant medical procedures; a depressed state of consciousness is intentionally induced while cardiorespiratory function is maintained. Because sedation is a continuum ranging from minimal sedation to general anesthesia, airway reflexes and cardiorespiratory function may be impaired if a deeper than intended level of sedation is produced. The appropriate level of sedation should be individualized according to the specific procedure and needs of the patient. Benzodiazepines are typically used to produce moderate to deep sedation for patients undergoing diagnostic or therapeutic procedures such as endoscopic procedures, radiologic procedures, coronary catheterization, coronary angiography, oncology procedures, and laceration repairs. Although these drugs can produce amnestic and sedative effects, they have no analgesic activity, and therefore, are usually administered in conjunction with an analgesic agent.

● *Preoperative Sedation, Anxiolysis, and Amnesia*

Benzodiazepines (e.g., lorazepam, midazolam, diazepam) are used preoperatively (prior to the induction of anesthesia) to relieve anxiety and produce sedation and anterograde amnesia. When used for this indication, benzodiazepines have been administered parenterally or orally. Benzodiazepines are particularly useful as a preoperative medication when relief of anxiety and diminished recall of events associated with the surgical procedure are desired. Studies have shown that diazepam, chlordiazepoxide hydrochloride (parenteral dosage form no longer commercially available in the US), or midazolam hydrochloride was as effective for preoperative sedation as opiate agonists or barbiturates and resulted in fewer undesirable effects, such as respiratory depression or hypotension. Because of midazolam's relatively rapid onset, short duration of effect, and improved local tolerance at the site of injection compared with other currently available parenteral benzodiazepines, some clinicians consider midazolam the benzodiazepine of choice for preoperative use associated with short surgical procedures.

● *Sedation in Critical Care Settings*

Benzodiazepines (e.g., lorazepam, midazolam, diazepam) are used for sedation of intubated and mechanically ventilated patients in a critical care setting (e.g., ICU). Midazolam has a quicker onset of action than lorazepam and is generally the preferred benzodiazepine for ICU sedation; lorazepam is used less frequently and diazepam is rarely used.

● *Alcohol Withdrawal*

Benzodiazepines (e.g., diazepam) are used in the management of acute alcohol withdrawal to relieve agitation and tremor and to prevent or to provide symptomatic relief of delirium tremens and hallucinations. It has not been proven that benzodiazepines prevent hallucinations or delirium tremens; however, some studies suggest that diazepam may shorten the duration and decrease the mortality of delirium tremens.

● *Seizure Disorders*

Status Epilepticus

Benzodiazepines (e.g., lorazepam, midazolam, diazepam) are considered the initial drugs of choice for the management of status epilepticus because of their rapid onset of action, demonstrated efficacy, safety, and tolerability.

Initial treatment of status epilepticus should include standard critical care and supportive therapy (e.g., blood pressure and respiratory support, oxygen, IV access, identification and correction of underlying causes), followed by administration of a benzodiazepine. Although IV lorazepam is generally preferred because of its longer duration of action, studies generally have not identified any substantial differences between IV lorazepam, IV diazepam, and IM midazolam in terms of seizure cessation, and experts consider these therapies to be equivalent first-line options. Selection of an appropriate benzodiazepine should be individualized based on local availability, route of administration, pharmacokinetics, cost, and other factors (e.g., treatment setting). To achieve a rapid therapeutic effect, IV administration of a benzodiazepine is preferred; however, administration via other routes (e.g., IM, rectal, intranasal, buccal) may be considered when IV administration is not possible (e.g., in the prehospital setting). If seizures continue after initial therapy with a benzodiazepine, a second-line anticonvulsant agent (e.g., IV fosphenytoin or phenytoin, IV valproate sodium, IV levetiracetam, IV phenobarbital) should be administered. If refractory status epilepticus occurs, continuous IV infusion of anticonvulsants, IV barbiturates, or general anesthetics may be necessary.

Other nonparenteral benzodiazepines that have been used for the treatment of status epilepticus include rectal diazepam, intranasal midazolam, and buccal midazolam; studies evaluating these benzodiazepines generally were conducted in the pediatric population. Potential limitations of these nonparenteral routes include difficulty with administration during an acute seizure episode, unpredictable absorption, and lack of commercially available dosage forms.

Other benzodiazepines such as clonazepam and chlordiazepoxide also have been evaluated for the treatment of status epilepticus, but are infrequently used due to the unavailability of a commercially available parenteral dosage form in the US.

Acute Repetitive Seizures or Seizure Clusters

Rectal diazepam and midazolam nasal spray also are used for the acute management of intermittent stereotypic episodes of increased seizure activity (also referred to as serial, cyclic, cluster, breakthrough, or crescendo seizures; acute repetitive seizures), especially for out-of-hospital management.

Midazolam also is administered intranasally for the acute management of seizures, including rescue therapy for prolonged, recurrent, or cyanotic seizures.

Adjunctive Therapy of Seizure Disorders

Benzodiazepines have been used orally as adjuncts to other anticonvulsants in the prophylactic management of partial seizures with elementary symptomatology, including those with motor symptoms (e.g., Jacksonian seizures), partial seizures with complex symptomatology (psychomotor seizures), absence (petit mal) seizures, seizures associated with Lennox-Gastaut syndrome (petit mal variant epilepsy), and akinetic or myoclonic seizures that are refractory to other drugs. Tolerance often develops to the anticonvulsant effects of benzodiazepines, which can limit their usefulness in the long-term management of seizure disorders.

● Skeletal Muscle Spasticity

Benzodiazepines may be useful adjuncts to rest, physical therapy, analgesics, and other measures for the relief of discomfort associated with acute, painful musculoskeletal conditions. There is no convincing evidence that oral benzodiazepines are more effective than barbiturates or meprobamate in these conditions. Most studies indicate that diazepam is superior to other skeletal muscle relaxants (e.g., methocarbamol, carisoprodol) for relief of musculoskeletal pain; however, there is some evidence that diazepam is no more effective than aspirin or placebo. The benzodiazepines are useful in the short- and long-term management of skeletal muscle spasticity such as reflex spasm secondary to local pathology (e.g., trauma, inflammation), spasticity caused by upper motor neuron disorders (e.g., cerebral palsy, paraplegia), athetosis, stiff-man syndrome, strychnine poisoning, or tetanus. Diazepam is generally as effective as dantrolene sodium or baclofen for spasticity in patients with various upper motor neuron disorders. For the management of moderate muscle spasm in tetanus, parenteral diazepam in large doses may be adequate; however, in severe tetanus, neuromuscular blocking agents may be the drugs of choice. The value of diazepam in neonatal tetanus has not been established.

● Cancer Chemotherapy-induced Nausea and Vomiting

Benzodiazepines (e.g., alprazolam, lorazepam) have been used in the management of nausea and vomiting associated with emetogenic cancer chemotherapy†. The antiemetic activity of benzodiazepines appears to be low, and their anxiolytic, sedative, and amnesic effects may account for beneficial effects in patients receiving emetogenic chemotherapy; the drugs appear to be most useful in reducing anticipatory and anxiety-related effects associated with administration of such chemotherapy. The American Society of Clinical Oncology (ASCO) guidelines on antiemetic therapy state that lorazepam is a useful adjunct to antiemetic drugs but is not recommended as a single-agent antiemetic.

● Delirium

Benzodiazepines, alone or combined with an antipsychotic agent, have been used in the management of delirium. However, the possibility that benzodiazepines may exacerbate symptoms of delirium in some patients and, when used alone, may be ineffective should be considered.

There are few controlled studies that evaluated the efficacy of benzodiazepines as monotherapy for the management of delirium. Limited data suggest that benzodiazepines alone may be ineffective or at least less effective than antipsychotic agents for general cases of delirium. While there appears to be little evidence to support the use of benzodiazepine monotherapy for general delirium, the drugs may have advantages and therefore would be preferred for certain types of delirium. For example, benzodiazepines are the drugs of choice for the management of delirium associated with alcohol or benzodiazepine withdrawal.

There is some evidence that combined use of a benzodiazepine and antipsychotic agent may decrease certain adverse effects and improve efficacy in certain patients with delirium (e.g., those with AIDS, those severely ill with cancer). If a benzodiazepine is used for the treatment of delirium, those with a short duration and no active metabolites (e.g., lorazepam) are preferred.

● Drug-induced Cardiovascular Emergencies

Benzodiazepines (e.g., diazepam, lorazepam) are used as adjuncts in the management of certain drug-induced cardiovascular emergencies†. If drug-induced cardiac arrest occurs, usual guidelines for advanced cardiovascular life support (ACLS) should be followed.

Cocaine-induced Acute Coronary Syndrome

Benzodiazepines have been used adjunctively in patients with severe cardiovascular toxicity associated with cocaine overdose†. Experts state that administration of a benzodiazepine may be beneficial for cocaine-induced hypertension or chest discomfort.

● Other Uses

Parenteral diazepam also has been used to relieve agitation in the management of neonatal opiate withdrawal†.

DOSAGE AND ADMINISTRATION

● Administration

Benzodiazepines are usually administered orally. When oral therapy is not feasible or when a rapid therapeutic effect is necessary, diazepam or lorazepam may be administered IV. Diazepam also may be given rectally. Midazolam hydrochloride is administered orally or by IM or IV injection and also has been administered intranasally† and intrabuccally†, and midazolam is administered intranasally. Although diazepam may also be given by deep IM injection, this route of administration is rarely justified because absorption of these drugs is slow and erratic. Chlordiazepoxide hydrochloride has also been given IV† and IM†; however, a parenteral dosage form of the drug is no longer commercially available in the US.

Concomitant oral administration of certain benzodiazepines (e.g., midazolam, triazolam) with grapefruit juice usually should be avoided since potentially clinically important increases in hemodynamic effects can result. (See Drug Interactions: Grapefruit Juice.)

● Dosage

Dosage of benzodiazepines must be carefully individualized, and the smallest effective dosage generally should be used (especially in geriatric or debilitated patients) to avoid oversedation. Sensitivity to the CNS depressant effects of the benzodiazepines differs among individual patients, and the patient's age, gender, physical or emotional status, and/or concurrent use of other drugs (including cigarette smoking) may alter the response.

Because of the episodic nature of anxiety, dosage may require frequent adjustments, and the drugs should generally be administered for a short period of time. The usefulness of the drug for each patient should be periodically reassessed. The effectiveness of benzodiazepines as anxiolytics for periods greater than 4 months or for panic disorder for periods greater than 4–10 weeks has not been established.

Because it is often difficult to predict how a patient will respond to a sedative agent, benzodiazepines used for procedural sedation should be titrated to effect.

The amount of time necessary for a particular benzodiazepine and its metabolites to reach steady-state plasma concentrations should be considered when dosage adjustments are made. (See Pharmacokinetics: Elimination.)

In patients who have received prolonged (e.g., for several months) benzodiazepine therapy, abrupt discontinuance of the drug should be avoided since manifestations of withdrawal, including rebound anxiety and insomnia, can be precipitated; if the drug is to be discontinued in such patients, it is recommended that dosage be gradually tapered. (See Chronic Toxicity.) It is particularly important that benzodiazepines *not* be discontinued abruptly in patients with a history of a seizure disorder to minimize the risk of precipitating seizures, seizure exacerbation, or status epilepticus. In addition, abrupt discontinuance of some benzodiazepines (e.g., those with a relatively short elimination half-life such as triazolam), even after relatively short periods of therapy (e.g., 1 week), can result in withdrawal effects such as rebound insomnia.

CAUTIONS

A boxed warning has been included in the prescribing information for all benzodiazepines describing the risks of abuse, misuse, addiction, physical dependence, and withdrawal reactions associated with all drugs in this class. Abuse and misuse can result in overdose or death, especially when benzodiazepines are combined with other medicines, such as opioid pain relievers, alcohol, or illicit drugs. Frequent follow-up with patients receiving benzodiazepines is important. Reassess patients regularly to manage their medical conditions and any withdrawal symptoms. Clinicians should assess a patient's risk of abuse, misuse, and addiction. Standardized screening tools are available (https://nida.nih.gov/nidamed-medical-health-professionals/screening-tools-resources/chart-screening-tools). To reduce the risk of acute withdrawal reactions, use a gradual dose taper when reducing the dosage or discontinuing benzodiazepines. Take precautions when benzodiazepines are used in combination with opioid medications.

• CNS Effects

Adverse CNS effects are an extension of the pharmacologic actions of benzodiazepines and include drowsiness, ataxia, fatigue, confusion, weakness, dizziness, vertigo, and syncope. Somnolence is the principal adverse effect associated with rectal diazepam administration, occurring in 13–33% of patients. Adverse CNS effects usually occur during the first few days of benzodiazepine therapy and may diminish with continued therapy or reduction in dosage. Geriatric or debilitated patients, children, and patients with liver disease or low serum albumin are most likely to experience these adverse CNS effects and generally should receive decreased initial dosages of the drugs. Benzodiazepines may produce prolonged CNS depression in neonates. Reversible dementia has been reported in geriatric patients after prolonged administration of benzodiazepines. Benzodiazepines with a relatively long elimination half-life may be more likely to cause residual daytime sedative effects and impaired psychomotor and mental performance during continued therapy, although partial tolerance to these effects can occur. Differences in residual and cumulative CNS depressant effects among benzodiazepines may be particularly important in geriatric patients and in patients with potentially impaired elimination of the drugs and those whose job or lifestyle requires unimpaired intellectual or psychomotor function. There is some evidence that ataxia and the risk of falling and associated hip fracture in geriatric patients is increased with use of benzodiazepines having a relatively long elimination half-life compared with use of those having a relatively short half-life. However, in several short-term studies in geriatric patients receiving quazepam, ataxia and morning hangover did not occur more frequently with the drug relative to placebo. Benzodiazepine therapy should be individualized and monitored closely in geriatric patients, and the need for continued therapy with the drugs should be determined periodically.

Amnesia

Benzodiazepines can cause amnesic effects, principally anterograde amnesia, and the magnitude and duration of these effects may vary depending on the patient (e.g., age), drug, dosage, and route of administration. Immediate recall usually does not appear to be affected substantially. Some evidence suggests that amnesic effects may be particularly likely with midazolam, triazolam, and lorazepam, although other benzodiazepines also have been reported to cause such effects. Anterograde amnesia may be particularly disturbing with triazolam, especially

when relatively high doses (e.g., 0.5 mg) are used. Anterograde amnesia ("traveler's amnesia") that occurred upon awakening and persisted for several hours has been reported in patients receiving triazolam for the prevention or treatment of insomnia associated with sleep-wake schedule changes (e.g., rapid travel across time zones ["jet lag"], rotating shift work); although behavior appeared normal in many of these patients (e.g., they performed what appeared to observers to be normal activities and they exhibited no apparent confusion or concern about memory at the time of amnesia), these patients subsequently had no recollection of the events that occurred during this period. Some of these patients consumed alcohol concomitantly, which also can cause anterograde amnesia. Similar anterograde amnesia has occurred in other patients receiving triazolam, and bizarre behavior has been associated with the period of amnesia in some patients. The risk of anterograde amnesia should be considered in patients receiving benzodiazepines, particularly when therapy with relatively high doses of triazolam is considered (e.g., for transient insomnia associated with sleep-wake schedule changes) or when the duration of drug effect is likely to exceed the intended period of sleep (e.g., when taken to induce sleep while traveling, such as during an airplane flight in which the patient will awake earlier than dissipation of hypnotic effects).

Behavioral Changes and Associated Effects

Potentially serious behavioral changes and abnormal mentation occasionally have been associated with benzodiazepine use. Such effects include confusion, bizarre or abnormal behavior, agitation, hyperexcitability, auditory and visual hallucinations, paranoid ideation, panic, delirium, depersonalization, agitation, sleepwalking, and disinhibition manifested as aggression, excessive extroversion, and/or antisocial acts; in some cases, amnesia about the behavior may occur. Decreased inhibition may be similar to that associated with use of alcohol or other CNS depressants. Emergence or worsening of mental depression, including suicidal ideation, also has been associated with benzodiazepine use, principally in patients with preexisting depression. It appears that some of these behavioral effects may be dose related. There also is some epidemiologic and other evidence that the risk of some such behavioral effects may be increased with triazolam; however, a precise causal relationship rarely can be established with certainty.

There also is a potential risk of complex sleep-related behaviors such as sleepdriving (i.e., driving while not fully awake after ingesting a sedative-hypnotic drug, with no memory of the event), making phone calls, or preparing and eating food while asleep in patients receiving benzodiazepines.

An analysis of spontaneous reports of adverse effects received by the FDA for triazolam and temazepam from the date of marketing through 1985 revealed that the reporting rates for confusion, amnesia, abnormal or bizarre behavior, agitation, and hallucinations were substantially higher for triazolam. An updated aggregate analysis of spontaneous reports in the US for the first 7 years of marketing for each drug confirmed the higher frequency associated with triazolam compared with temazepam. While it could not be completely ruled out that some selection factors may have contributed to the differences in reporting rates, analysis of these data with adjustment for various factors suggested that a higher occurrence of these reactions existed for triazolam; a large epidemiologic study that follows up new users for adverse reactions and includes adjustment for potentially contributing factors would be required to determine the risk factors for adverse behavioral effects associated with these and other benzodiazepines.

Data from a limited number of patients suggest that individuals with borderline personality disorder, a history of violent or aggressive behavior, or a history of alcohol or drug abuse may be at increased risk for adverse behavioral effects with benzodiazepine use. Irritability, hostility, and intrusive thoughts have been reported in patients with posttraumatic stress disorder during discontinuance of alprazolam. While emergence of abnormalities in behavior and mentation or worsening of preexisting abnormalities may be the consequence of an underlying, possibly unrecognized, physical and/or psychiatric condition, it rarely can be determined with certainty whether such effects are drug induced, spontaneous in origin, or secondary to such underlying causes. Therefore, the emergence of any new behavioral sign or symptom of concern during benzodiazepine therapy requires careful and immediate evaluation.

Seizures

When IV diazepam has been used to control absence status or Lennox-Gastaut syndrome status epilepticus, tonic status epilepticus has occurred. When oral benzodiazepines are used as adjuncts in the treatment of mixed epilepsy, increased frequency and/or severity of tonic-clonic seizures may occur, necessitating an increase in dosage of other anticonvulsants.

Abrupt withdrawal of diazepam therapy in patients with epilepsy may also result in a temporary increase in the frequency and/or severity of seizures. Changes in EEG patterns with characteristic low voltage, fast activity have been observed in some patients receiving benzodiazepines but are of no known importance. Withdrawal seizures also have been reported with alprazolam; in most cases, only a single seizure occurred, but multiple seizures and status epilepticus also have been reported. All anticonvulsants, including benzodiazepines, should be withdrawn gradually to minimize the risk of precipitating seizures, seizure exacerbation, or status epilepticus.

Other CNS Effects

Other adverse CNS effects of benzodiazepines include headache, vivid dreams, and dysarthria. Encephalopathy reportedly occurred in patients with renal failure receiving both diazepam and flurazepam. Extrapyramidal reactions, tremor, and oral buccal dyskinesia also have been reported. Abrupt withdrawal of benzodiazepines after use in the management of anxiety may lead to increased anxiety; rebound insomnia also has occurred following abrupt withdrawal of the drugs, particularly those with a relatively short elimination half-life. Withdrawal reactions also can be precipitated by dosage tapering and inadvertent dosage reduction (e.g., forgotten dose, admission to hospital). Such effects also can emerge in the early morning or between doses of benzodiazepines with a relatively short half-life.

Paradoxical CNS stimulation resulting in talkativeness, restlessness, anxiety, mania, euphoria, tremulousness, sleep disturbances, nightmares, excitement, hyperactivity, acute rage reactions, increased muscle spasticity, and hyperreflexia may occur, usually early in benzodiazepine therapy. Excitation is particularly likely to occur in psychiatric patients and in hyperactive aggressive children. Benzodiazepine therapy usually should be discontinued if CNS stimulation occurs.

The CNS depressant effect of benzodiazepines also can result in respiratory depression.

● *Respiratory and Cardiovascular Effects*

Parenteral administration of benzodiazepines may produce apnea, hypotension, bradycardia, or cardiac arrest, particularly in geriatric or severely ill patients and in patients with limited pulmonary reserve or unstable cardiovascular status or if the drug is administered too rapidly IV. IV diazepam has reportedly caused ventricular premature complexes and other arrhythmias when used prior to cardioversion. Death has occurred rarely shortly after initiation of alprazolam therapy in patients with severe pulmonary disease. Respiratory depression and apnea have been reported infrequently with benzodiazepines in patients with compromised respiratory function.

Decreased gag reflex has been reported when IV diazepam was used prior to endoscopy. During peroral endoscopic procedures, coughing, depressed respiration, dyspnea, hyperventilation, laryngospasm, and pain in the throat or chest have been reported. Although the risk of respiratory depression may be greatest with rapid IV administration or large doses of the drugs, such depression also has been reported with rectal administration. Respiratory and cardiovascular depressant effects may be caused in part by the propylene glycol present in diazepam injection, a formulation that also has been administered rectally. In clinical studies with diazepam rectal gel, respiratory depressant effects (e.g., hypoventilation) occurred rarely.

Palpitation, tachycardia, shortness of breath, diaphoresis, and flushing also have been reported in patients receiving benzodiazepines.

● *GI and Hepatic Effects*

Adverse GI effects reported in patients receiving benzodiazepines include nausea and other GI complaints, hiccups, constipation, increased appetite, anorexia, weight gain or loss, dry mouth, increased salivation and bronchial secretions, swollen tongue, and bitter or metallic taste. Animals have developed esophageal dilation after very high doses of lorazepam for prolonged periods, and patients receiving this drug should be observed for the development of GI disease. Benzodiazepines may cause elevated serum AST (SGOT), ALT (SGPT), LDH, and alkaline phosphatase and total and direct serum bilirubin; jaundice has been reported.

Hepatitis and hepatic failure have been reported during postmarketing experience with alprazolam; however, a causal relationship to the drug has not been established.

In addition to typical benzodiazepine-associated adverse effects, rectal administration of diazepam gel may result in diarrhea and rarely rectal burning/pain.

● *Dermatologic and Sensitivity Reactions*

There is a potential risk of anaphylaxis and angioedema in patients receiving benzodiazepines; such reactions may occur as early as with the first dose of the drug. Urticaria, rash, pruritus, photosensitivity, immediate hypersensitivity reactions, hypotension, nonthrombocytopenic purpura, and edema may occur in patients receiving benzodiazepines. Paresthesia, Stevens-Johnson syndrome, and a lupus-like syndrome have been reported.

● *Local Effects*

IM administration of parenteral benzodiazepines (e.g., diazepam, lorazepam, or midazolam) may result in pain. Redness, burning, induration, or muscle stiffness also has been reported with IM administration of some benzodiazepines (e.g., lorazepam). IV administration of benzodiazepines may result in pain or thrombophlebitis. Intra-arterial administration of diazepam and other parenteral benzodiazepines has resulted in tissue necrosis. Adverse local effects associated with IM or IV administration occur less frequently and generally are less severe with midazolam than with other currently available parenteral benzodiazepines (e.g., diazepam).

● *Genitourinary and Renal Effects*

Increased or decreased libido, menstrual irregularities, failure to ovulate, hyperprolactinemia, gynecomastia, and galactorrhea have been reported in patients receiving benzodiazepines. Genitourinary complaints such as urinary retention, difficulty in micturition, and urinary incontinence have occurred. Alprazolam exhibits weak uricosuric activity. Transient decreases in renal function have occurred after IV administration of diazepam or midazolam, and abnormal renal function test results have been reported after oral benzodiazepines.

● *Musculoskeletal Effects*

Serum creatine kinase (CK, creatine phosphokinase, CPK) concentrations increase after IM injection of diazepam. Body joint pains and muscle cramps also have been reported.

● *Hematologic Effects*

A few cases of leukopenia (including neutropenia and granulocytopenia), agranulocytosis, aplastic anemia, hemolytic anemia, decreased hematocrit, eosinophilia, and leukocytosis have been attributed to benzodiazepine administration.

● *Ocular Effects*

Conjunctivitis and visual disturbances such as diplopia, nystagmus, and blurred vision have occurred in patients receiving benzodiazepines.

● *Precautions and Contraindications*

In September of 2020, FDA announced that it is requiring that the boxed warning, FDA's most prominent warning, be updated by adding additional information to the prescribing information for all benzodiazepines. This information will describe the risks of abuse, misuse, addiction, physical dependence, and withdrawal reactions consistently across all the medicines in the class. FDA is also requiring updates to the existing patient medication guides for benzodiazepines to help educate patients and caregivers about these risks. Clinicians prescribing benzodiazepines should consider the patient's condition and the other drugs being taken, and assess the risk of abuse, misuse, and addiction. Clinicians should also limit the dosage and duration of therapy to the minimum needed to achieve the desired clinical effect when prescribing benzodiazepines either alone or in combination with other drugs. In addition, a gradual taper should be used when reducing the dosage of or discontinuing benzodiazepines to reduce the risk of acute withdrawal reactions. (See Dosage and Administration: Dosage, Drug Interactions: CNS Agents, and see also Chronic Toxicity.)

Concomitant use of benzodiazepines and opiate agonists or opiate partial agonists may result in profound sedation, respiratory depression, coma, and death.

Concomitant use of such drugs should be reserved for patients in whom alternative treatment options are inadequate; the lowest effective dosages and shortest possible duration of concomitant therapy should be used, and the patient should be monitored closely for respiratory depression and sedation. Patients receiving benzodiazepines and/or their caregivers should be apprised of the risks associated with concomitant therapeutic or illicit use of benzodiazepines and opiates. (See Opiate Agonists and Opiate Partial Agonists under Drug Interactions: CNS Agents.)

Patients should be warned that benzodiazepines may impair ability to perform hazardous activities requiring mental alertness or physical coordination (e.g., operating machinery, driving a motor vehicle). There also is a potential risk of complex sleep-related behaviors such as sleep-driving (i.e., driving while not fully awake after ingesting a sedative-hypnotic drug, with no memory of the event), making phone calls, or preparing and eating food while asleep in patients receiving benzodiazepines. Patients also should be warned about possible effects on memory (anterograde amnesia) and to report promptly to their physician any behavioral or mental change, including disturbing thoughts and unusual manners of conduct, that develops during benzodiazepine therapy. (See Cautions: CNS Effects.) Benzodiazepines should be used with caution and large quantities of the drugs should not be prescribed for patients with suicidal tendencies or whose history indicates that they may increase dosage on their own initiative.

Because benzodiazepines may produce psychologic and physical dependence, patients should be advised to consult their clinician before increasing the dose of, or abruptly discontinuing, benzodiazepine therapy. (See Chronic Toxicity.)

Liver and kidney function tests and blood cell counts should be performed regularly during long-term therapy, and benzodiazepines should be administered with caution to patients with hepatic or renal disease.

Benzodiazepines should be used with caution in patients with chronic pulmonary insufficiency or sleep apnea. Facilities and age- and size-appropriate equipment for respiratory or cardiovascular assistance should be readily available whenever benzodiazepines are administered IV. The drugs should not be administered IV to patients in whom the hypnotic or hypotensive effects may be prolonged or intensified such as those with shock or coma, to patients with depressed respiration, or to those who have recently received other respiratory depressant drugs. Diazepam rectal gel should be used with caution in patients with compromised respiratory function associated with a concurrent disease process (e.g., asthma, pneumonia) or neurologic damage.

Benzodiazepines generally should not be used in patients with depressive neuroses or psychotic reactions in which anxiety is not prominent. Many benzodiazepines are contraindicated in patients with known hypersensitivity to the drugs. Because the frequency of suicide appears to be increased in untreated patients with panic disorder, and because panic disorder may be associated with primary and secondary major depressive disorders, the usual precautions of psychotropic therapy in depressed patients or those at risk for concealed suicidal ideation should be exercised during benzodiazepine therapy for panic disorder. According to most manufacturers of benzodiazepines, the drugs are contraindicated in patients with acute angle-closure glaucoma but may be administered to patients receiving appropriate treatment for open-angle glaucoma. However, the clinical rationale for this contraindication has been questioned since benzodiazepines do not have anticholinergic effects and do not increase intraocular pressure; only one case of increased intraocular pressure after use of a benzodiazepine and other drugs has been reported.

● Pediatric Precautions

FDA warns that repeated or prolonged use of general anesthetics and sedation drugs, including benzodiazepines such as lorazepam and midazolam, in children younger than 3 years of age or during the third trimester of pregnancy may affect brain development. Animal studies in multiple species, including nonhuman primates, have demonstrated that use for longer than 3 hours of anesthetic and sedation drugs that block N-methyl-D-aspartic acid (NMDA) receptors and/or potentiate γ-aminobutyric acid (GABA) activity leads to widespread neuronal and oligodendrocyte cell loss and alterations in synaptic morphology and neurogenesis in the brain, resulting in long-term deficits in cognition and behavior. Across animal species, vulnerability to these neurodevelopmental changes occurs during the period of rapid brain growth or synaptogenesis; this period is thought to correlate with the third trimester of pregnancy through the first year of life in

humans, but may extend to approximately 3 years of age. The clinical relevance of these animal findings to humans is not known.

While some published evidence suggests that similar deficits in cognition and behavior may occur in children following repeated or prolonged exposure to anesthesia early in life, other studies have found no association between pediatric anesthesia exposure and long-term adverse neurodevelopmental outcomes. Most studies to date have had substantial limitations, and it is not clear whether the adverse neurodevelopmental outcomes observed in children were related to the drug or to other factors (e.g., surgery, underlying illness). There is some clinical evidence that a single, relatively brief exposure to general anesthesia in generally healthy children is unlikely to cause clinically detectable deficits in global cognitive function or serious behavioral disorders; however, further research is needed to fully characterize the effects of exposure to general anesthetics in early life, particularly for prolonged or repeated exposures and in more vulnerable populations (e.g., less healthy children).

Results from an observational study (the Pediatric Anesthesia Neurodevelopment Assessment [PANDA] study) and preliminary results from an ongoing multicenter, randomized trial (the General Anesthesia Compared to Spinal Anesthesia [GAS] trial) provide some evidence that a single, relatively brief exposure to general anesthesia in generally healthy children is unlikely to cause clinically detectable deficits in global cognitive function or serious behavioral disorders. The PANDA study compared global cognitive function (as measured by intelligence quotient [IQ] score) of children 8–15 years of age who had a single anesthesia exposure for elective inguinal hernia surgery before the age of 3 years with that of a biologically related sibling who had no anesthesia exposure before the age of 3 years. All of the children had a gestational age at birth of at least 36 weeks, and sibling pairs were within 3 years of being the same age. Children who underwent the elective procedure were mostly males (90%) and generally healthy. The mean duration of anesthesia was 84 minutes; 16% of those receiving anesthesia had exposures exceeding 2 hours. The study found no substantial difference in IQ score between children who had a single anesthesia exposure before the age of 3 years and their siblings who had not. The GAS trial was designed to compare neurodevelopmental outcomes in children who received general anesthesia with those in children who received awake regional (caudal and/or spinal) anesthesia for inguinal herniorrhaphy before they reached a postmenstrual age of 60 weeks (with a gestational age at birth of more than 26 weeks); the primary outcome was the Wechsler Preschool and Primary Scale of Intelligence Third Edition (WPPSI-III) Full Scale IQ at 5 years of age. In an interim analysis at the age of 2 years, no difference in composite cognitive score (as measured by the Bayley Scales of Infant and Toddler Development III) was detected between children who had received sevoflurane anesthesia of less than 1 hour's duration (median duration: 54 minutes) compared with those who had received awake regional anesthesia.

Anesthetic and sedation drugs are an essential component of care for children and pregnant women who require surgery or other procedures that cannot be delayed; no specific general anesthetic or sedation drug has been shown to be less likely to cause neurocognitive deficits than any other such drug. Pending further accumulation of data in humans from well-designed studies, decisions regarding the timing of elective procedures requiring anesthesia should take into consideration both the benefits of the procedure and the potential risks. When procedures requiring the use of general anesthetics or sedation drugs are considered for young children or pregnant women, clinicians should discuss with the patient, parent, or caregiver the benefits, risks (including potential risk of adverse neurodevelopmental effects), and appropriate timing and duration of the procedure. FDA states that procedures that are considered medically necessary should not be delayed or avoided.

● Pregnancy, Fertility, and Lactation

Pregnancy

Benzodiazepines can cause fetal harm when administered to pregnant women. Results of retrospective studies suggest an increased risk of congenital malformations in infants of mothers who received benzodiazepines (e.g., chlordiazepoxide, diazepam) during the first trimester of pregnancy. An increase in fetal heart rate has occurred after diazepam use during labor. Hypoactivity, hypotonia, hypothermia, apnea, feeding problems, impaired metabolic response to cold stress, hyperbilirubinemia, and kernicterus have been reported in neonates born to mothers who received large doses of diazepam (generally greater than 30 mg) shortly before delivery. Infants of mothers who chronically ingested benzodiazepines during pregnancy have been reported to have withdrawal symptoms.

Neonatal flaccidity, respiratory and feeding difficulties, and hypothermia have been reported in infants born to women who received benzodiazepines late in pregnancy. Since the use of anxiolytics is rarely urgent, their use during the first trimester of pregnancy should almost always be avoided. Benzodiazepines used solely as hypnotics (flurazepam, temazepam, triazolam) are contraindicated during pregnancy.

Although there is an association between anticonvulsant drug use in pregnant women with seizure disorders and an increased incidence of teratogenic effects in children born to such women, anticonvulsant therapy should not be discontinued in women in whom the drugs are administered to prevent seizures because of the strong possibility of precipitating status epilepticus and the attendant hypoxia and threat to life. In cases where the severity and frequency of the seizure disorder are such that removal of the anticonvulsant does not pose a serious threat to the patient, discontinuance of the drug may be considered prior to and during pregnancy. However, it cannot be said with confidence that even mild seizures do not pose some hazard to the developing embryo or fetus. In general, benzodiazepines should be considered for use as anticonvulsant therapy in women of childbearing potential, and more specifically during known pregnancy, only when the clinical situation warrants the risk to the fetus.

Based on animal data, repeated or prolonged use of general anesthetics and sedation drugs, including benzodiazepines such as lorazepam and midazolam, during the third trimester of pregnancy may result in adverse neurodevelopmental effects in the fetus. The clinical relevance of these animal findings to humans is not known; the potential risk of adverse neurodevelopmental effects should be considered and discussed with pregnant women undergoing procedures requiring general anesthetics and sedation drugs. (See Cautions: Pediatric Precautions.)

The possibility that a woman of childbearing potential may be pregnant at the time benzodiazepine therapy is initiated should be considered. Patients should be advised that if they become pregnant or intend to become pregnant during benzodiazepine therapy, they should communicate with their clinician about the desirability of discontinuing the drug.

Lactation

Since many benzodiazepines are distributed into milk and because of the potential for adverse reactions from the drugs in nursing infants, a decision should be made whether to discontinue nursing or the drug, taking into account the importance of the drug to the woman.

DRUG INTERACTIONS

• Drugs and Foods Affecting Hepatic Microsomal Enzymes

Some benzodiazepines (e.g., alprazolam, clobazam, diazepam, estazolam, midazolam, triazolam) are metabolized by cytochrome P-450 (CYP) isoenzymes, predominantly by CYP3A4 and/or CYP2C19. Clearance of these benzodiazepines may be reduced by drugs or foods that inhibit CYP3A4 (e.g., some azole antifungals, some macrolide antibiotics, HIV protease inhibitors, some calcium-channel blocking agents, some selective serotonin-reuptake inhibitors [SSRIs], nefazodone, grapefruit juice) or inhibit CYP2C19 (e.g., fluvoxamine, omeprazole, ticlopidine), possibly resulting in enhanced or prolonged benzodiazepine effects. Conversely, concomitant use of these benzodiazepines with drugs that induce CYP3A4 (e.g., carbamazepine, phenobarbital, phenytoin, rifampin) may decrease plasma concentrations of the benzodiazepines.

• Antihistamines

Concomitant administration of temazepam and diphenhydramine in a pregnant woman at the end of the third trimester has been associated with violent intrauterine fetal movements within several hours after maternal ingestion of the drugs; within 8 hours, the infant was delivered stillborn. Reproduction studies in rabbits have suggested that concomitant administration of these drugs markedly increases perinatal mortality; neonatal deaths were associated with increased irritability and seizures.

• Anti-infective Agents

Antifungal Agents

Concomitant use of some benzodiazepines (e.g., alprazolam, clobazam, estazolam, midazolam, triazolam) with some azole antifungal agents (e.g., fluconazole,

itraconazole, ketoconazole) may result in increased plasma concentrations and systemic exposure of these benzodiazepines. Following concomitant administration of oral midazolam with itraconazole or ketoconazole, large increases in the peak plasma concentration (up to 240 or 309%, respectively) and area under the serum concentration-time curve (AUC) (up to 980 or 1490%, respectively) of midazolam were observed. When alprazolam was given concomitantly with itraconazole or ketoconazole, increases of 2.7- or 4-fold, respectively, in the AUC of alprazolam were observed. In healthy adults receiving multiple doses of itraconazole (200 mg daily for 6 days), the elimination half-life of alprazolam was increased by 260% and AUC was increased by 270% following administration of a single 0.8-mg dose of alprazolam; substantial changes in psychomotor function (e.g., sleepiness) were also noted. Administration of a single 200-mg dose of itraconazole given 3, 12, or 24 hours prior to or simultaneously with a single 0.25-mg dose of triazolam increased the peak plasma concentration of triazolam by 140–180% and AUC of triazolam by 300–500%, depending on ingestion time of the dose, while the elimination half-life of triazolam was increased by 300%. When oral midazolam was administered concomitantly with fluconazole in healthy adults, the peak plasma concentration and AUC of midazolam were increased by 150 and 250%, respectively.

Alprazolam, estazolam, and triazolam are contraindicated in patients receiving concomitant therapy with potent CYP3A inhibitors such as ketoconazole and itraconazole; concomitant use of other azole antifungal agents that are considered potent CYP3A inhibitors is not recommended. Because of the potential for intense and prolonged sedation and respiratory depression, oral midazolam should be administered only when absolutely necessary and with extreme caution (e.g., with appropriate equipment and personnel available to respond to respiratory insufficiency) in patients receiving ketoconazole or itraconazole.

Antimycobacterial Agents

Isoniazid

Concomitant use of isoniazid with triazolam has been shown to increase the peak plasma concentration and half-life of triazolam by 20 and 31%, respectively, and decrease clearance of triazolam by 42%. Caution is advised when triazolam or other benzodiazepines that are metabolized by the CYP3A isoenzyme (e.g., alprazolam, estazolam) are used concomitantly with isoniazid.

Antiretroviral Agents

HIV Protease Inhibitors

Because of the potential for intense and prolonged sedation and respiratory depression, the manufacturers of HIV protease inhibitors (e.g., atazanavir, darunavir, fosamprenavir, indinavir, lopinavir/ritonavir, nelfinavir, ritonavir, saquinavir, tipranavir) state that concomitant use of these agents with midazolam or triazolam is contraindicated.

Concomitant use of HIV protease inhibitors (e.g., fosamprenavir, ritonavir, saquinavir) with certain other benzodiazepines (e.g., alprazolam, clorazepate, diazepam, flurazepam) also may result in increased concentrations of the benzodiazepine. While the clinical importance of the interaction is unknown, a reduction in dosage of the benzodiazepine may be needed.

Nonnucleoside Reverse Transcriptase Inhibitors

Concomitant use of efavirenz with midazolam or triazolam and of delavirdine with alprazolam, midazolam, or triazolam should be avoided because of the potential for the nonnucleoside reverse transcriptase inhibitor (NNRTI) to decrease metabolism of the benzodiazepine and result in intense or prolonged sedation or respiratory depression.

Macrolide Antibiotics

Concomitant use of erythromycin decreases clearance of midazolam and triazolam and could increase the pharmacologic effects of these benzodiazepines. Available data also suggest that some macrolide antibiotics (i.e., erythromycin, clarithromycin) might interact with alprazolam. In addition, it might be anticipated that erythromycin could interfere with the metabolism of estazolam.

Patients receiving benzodiazepines that are metabolized by the CYP3A isoenzyme concomitantly with some macrolide antibiotics (i.e., erythromycin, clarithromycin) should be monitored closely; reduction in the benzodiazepine dosage may be necessary.

● *Cardiovascular Agents*

Amiodarone

Although specific drug interaction studies are not available, concomitant use of amiodarone with some benzodiazepines (e.g., alprazolam, triazolam) may result in decreased metabolism of the benzodiazepine; caution is advised.

Calcium-channel Blocking Agents

Concomitant use of diltiazem or verapamil with oral midazolam results in increased plasma midazolam concentrations and may lead to increased and prolonged sedation and respiratory depression. If midazolam is used concomitantly with diltiazem or verapamil, caution is advised and dosage reduction of midazolam may be necessary.

Although specific drug interaction studies are not available, clinically important decreases in the metabolism and clearance of other benzodiazepines metabolized by the CYP3A isoenzyme (e.g., alprazolam, estazolam, triazolam) may occur when these benzodiazepines are used concomitantly with some calcium-channel blocking agents (e.g., diltiazem, verapamil); caution is advised. Drug interactions also are possible when some benzodiazepines (e.g., alprazolam, estazolam, triazolam) are used concomitantly with nicardipine or nifedipine.

Digoxin

Limited evidence suggests that diazepam may reduce the renal excretion of digoxin, resulting in an increased plasma half-life of the cardiac glycoside and possible digoxin toxicity. Digoxin toxicity has been reported in one geriatric patient who was receiving alprazolam and digoxin concurrently; serum digoxin concentrations increased threefold in this patient following initiation of alprazolam therapy, but returned to within normal limits following discontinuance of the benzodiazepine. Although the exact mechanism for the effect of benzodiazepines on the renal excretion of digoxin has not been clearly established, increased plasma protein binding of digoxin and/or an effect of benzodiazepines on the renal tubular transport of digoxin have been suggested. Pending further accumulation of data, serum digoxin concentrations should be monitored and patients should be carefully observed for signs and/or symptoms of digoxin toxicity during concomitant therapy with benzodiazepines and digoxin. Dosage reduction of digoxin may be necessary in some patients receiving concomitant therapy.

● *CNS Agents*

CNS Depressants

Additive CNS depression may occur when benzodiazepines are administered concomitantly with other CNS depressants, including other anticonvulsants, opiates, and alcohol. If benzodiazepines are used concomitantly with other depressant drugs, caution should be used to avoid overdosage. Patients receiving benzodiazepines should be advised to avoid alcohol.

Anticonvulsants

In patients receiving clonazepam and phenytoin concurrently, plasma concentrations of phenytoin may decrease; patients receiving these drugs concurrently should be closely observed.

Concurrent administration of carbamazepine with alprazolam or clonazepam has been shown to increase the rate of metabolism and decrease plasma concentrations of these benzodiazepines. In one study, administration of a single 0.8-mg dose of alprazolam after 10 days of low-dose carbamazepine (300 mg daily) resulted in a 2.4-fold increase in oral clearance of alprazolam and decreased the elimination half-life of alprazolam from 17.1 hours to 7.7 hours.

Concomitant administration of oral midazolam with phenytoin or carbamazepine has been shown to decrease the peak plasma concentration and AUC of midazolam by about 93–94%.

In a limited number of healthy men, concurrent use of valproate (250 mg twice daily orally, for 3 days) with a single 2-mg IV dose of lorazepam reportedly decreased total clearance of lorazepam by 40% and increased plasma concentration of the benzodiazepine approximately twofold (that persisted for at least 12 hours after dosing) compared with administration of lorazepam alone. The dosage of lorazepam should be reduced by approximately 50% when administered concomitantly with valproate.

Antidepressants

Nefazodone

Concomitant use of nefazodone with some benzodiazepines (e.g., alprazolam, triazolam) results in clinically important increases in plasma concentrations of the benzodiazepine. Concomitant use of triazolam and nefazodone should be avoided. If alprazolam is used concomitantly with nefazodone, caution is advised and reduction of the alprazolam dosage should be considered. Although specific drug interaction studies are not available, concomitant use of estazolam with nefazodone would be expected to increase plasma concentrations of estazolam.

Selective Serotonin-reuptake Inhibitors

Concomitant use of some SSRIs (e.g., fluoxetine, fluvoxamine) with alprazolam has been reported to decrease clearance and increase plasma concentrations of alprazolam and impair psychomotor performance. In one study, peak plasma concentrations of alprazolam were doubled, half-life of alprazolam was increased by 71%, and clearance of the drug was reduced by 49% when alprazolam was given concomitantly with fluvoxamine. When alprazolam was given concomitantly with fluoxetine, the peak plasma concentration and half-life of alprazolam were increased by 46 and 17%, respectively, and clearance of alprazolam was reduced by 21%. Caution is advised if fluvoxamine or fluoxetine is used concomitantly with alprazolam, midazolam, or triazolam. If fluvoxamine is used concomitantly with alprazolam, reduction of the alprazolam dosage also should be considered.

Although specific drug interaction studies are not available, concomitant use of estazolam with fluvoxamine would be expected to result in increased plasma concentrations of estazolam. In one study, concomitant use of estazolam (2 mg daily) and fluoxetine (20 mg twice daily) for 7 days did not appear to affect the peak plasma concentration or AUC of estazolam.

The clearance of diazepam was reduced by 65% and that of its active metabolite *N*-desmethyldiazepam could not be determined during concomitant administration with fluvoxamine in one study. Concomitant use of diazepam and fluvoxamine generally should be avoided.

The clearance of benzodiazepines that are metabolized by glucuronidation (e.g., lorazepam, oxazepam, temazepam) is unlikely to be affected by fluvoxamine.

In vitro studies suggest a possible interaction between triazolam and sertraline or paroxetine; caution is advised if these drugs are used concomitantly. Although in vitro data also suggest the possibility of an interaction between alprazolam and sertraline or paroxetine, no substantial changes in alprazolam pharmacokinetics were evident in one study involving multiple-dose administration of sertraline (50–150 mg daily) and single-dose administration of alprazolam (1 mg). Nonetheless, the manufacturers of alprazolam state that caution is advised when alprazolam is used concomitantly with sertraline or paroxetine.

Tricyclic Antidepressants

Although some studies showed no substantial alteration of tricyclic antidepressant plasma concentrations during simultaneous administration of benzodiazepines, one study indicated that the elimination half-life and steady-state plasma concentrations of amitriptyline may be increased in patients receiving diazepam. In addition, steady-state plasma concentrations of imipramine and desipramine reportedly were increased by 31 and 20%, respectively, in patients receiving these antidepressants concomitantly with alprazolam (up to 4 mg daily). The clinical importance of these possible interactions has not been determined. There have been reports of impaired motor function when tricyclic antidepressants were used with benzodiazepines, but these have not been confirmed and the drugs have often been administered concomitantly without adverse effects.

Antipsychotic Agents

Clozapine

Severe hypotension (including absence of measurable blood pressure), respiratory or cardiac arrest, and loss of consciousness have been reported in several patients who received benzodiazepines (i.e., diazepam, flurazepam, lorazepam) concomitantly with or before clozapine therapy. Such effects occurred following administration of 12.5–150 mg of clozapine concurrently with or within 24 hours of the benzodiazepine, but patients generally have recovered within a few minutes to hours, usually spontaneously; the reactions usually developed on the first or second day of clozapine therapy. Although a causal relationship has not definitely been established and such effects also have been observed in clozapine-treated patients who were not receiving a benzodiazepine concomitantly, death resulting from respiratory arrest reportedly has rarely occurred when a benzodiazepine (e.g., lorazepam) was used concomitantly with clozapine. An increased incidence of dizziness and sedation and greater increases in liver enzyme test results also have been reported when benzodiazepines and clozapine were used concomitantly.

The manufacturers of lorazepam and clozapine recommend caution when clozapine is initiated in patients receiving benzodiazepine therapy. However, some clinicians advise that, pending further accumulation of data, greater precaution should be exercised. These clinicians recommend that because initial titration of clozapine may cause respiratory arrest requiring resuscitation, which may be potentiated by recent benzodiazepine therapy, these latter drugs should be discontinued for at least 1 week prior to initiating clozapine therapy.

Other Antipsychotic Agents

Respiratory depression, stupor, and/or hypotension have been reported rarely in patients receiving lorazepam concomitantly with loxapine. In addition, apnea, coma, bradycardia, arrhythmia, cardiac arrest, and death have occurred in patients receiving lorazepam and haloperidol concomitantly. The manufacturer of lorazepam states that lorazepam should be used with caution in patients receiving haloperidol or loxapine because concomitant administration of these drugs has not been evaluated systematically.

Opiate Agonists and Opiate Partial Agonists

Concomitant use of benzodiazepines with opiate agonists or opiate partial agonists may result in profound sedation, respiratory depression, coma, and death. Epidemiologic studies have shown that a substantial proportion of fatal opiate overdoses involve the concurrent use of benzodiazepines.

Whenever possible, concomitant use of opiate agonists or partial agonists and benzodiazepines should be avoided. Opiate antitussive agents should be avoided in patients receiving benzodiazepines, and concomitant use of opiate analgesics and benzodiazepines should be reserved for patients in whom alternative treatment options are inadequate. (See Cautions: Precautions and Contraindications, in the Opiate Agonists General Statement 28:08.08.) If a decision is made to prescribe opiates and benzodiazepines concomitantly, the lowest effective dosages and shortest possible duration of concomitant therapy should be used, and the patient should be monitored closely for respiratory depression and sedation. If a benzodiazepine is required for any indication other than epilepsy in a patient receiving opiate therapy, the drug should be initiated at a lower dosage than indicated in the absence of opiate therapy and titrated based on clinical response. In patients receiving benzodiazepines, opiate analgesics should be initiated at a reduced dosage and titrated based on clinical response. Some experts state that consideration should be given to offering the opiate antagonist naloxone when opiates are prescribed for patients at increased risk of opiate overdosage, including those receiving benzodiazepines concomitantly.

● Cyclosporine

Although specific drug interaction studies are not available, concomitant use of cyclosporine with some benzodiazepines (e.g., alprazolam, triazolam) may result in decreased metabolism of the benzodiazepine; caution is advised.

● Disulfiram

Concurrent administration of disulfiram and benzodiazepines may result in inhibition of metabolism of some benzodiazepines. Disulfiram has reduced the plasma clearance and increased the plasma half-lives of chlordiazepoxide and diazepam during concomitant administration. It is likely that other benzodiazepines that undergo oxidative metabolism (e.g., alprazolam, clonazepam, clorazepate, estazolam, flurazepam, triazolam) would also interact with disulfiram. Benzodiazepines metabolized by glucuronide conjugation (e.g., lorazepam, oxazepam, temazepam) are probably not affected by disulfiram. Patients should be closely observed for evidence of enhanced benzodiazepine response during concomitant therapy with disulfiram; some patients may require reduction in benzodiazepine dosage.

● Ergot Alkaloids

Although specific drug interaction studies are not available, concomitant use of ergotamine with some benzodiazepines (e.g., alprazolam, triazolam) may result in decreased metabolism of the benzodiazepine; caution is advised.

● GI Drugs

Antacids

Concurrent administration of chlordiazepoxide or diazepam with antacids such as aluminum and magnesium hydroxides may decrease the rate, but not the extent, of GI absorption of chlordiazepoxide or diazepam. Concurrent administration of antacids and clorazepate may decrease the rate and extent of conversion of the latter drug to desmethyldiazepam, and these drugs should not be given concurrently.

Cimetidine

Concomitant administration of some benzodiazepines (e.g., alprazolam, chlordiazepoxide, clobazam, clorazepate, diazepam, midazolam, triazolam) and cimetidine may result in decreased benzodiazepine plasma clearance and increased plasma half-lives and concentrations of these benzodiazepines. Cimetidine reduces plasma clearance of benzodiazepines that undergo oxidative metabolism, apparently via inhibition of hepatic microsomal enzymes involved in oxidative metabolism. Consequently, the elimination of clonazepam, estazolam, and flurazepam may also be similarly affected by cimetidine. Benzodiazepines metabolized by conjugation with glucuronic acid (e.g., lorazepam, oxazepam, temazepam) do not appear to be affected by concomitant cimetidine therapy. Although an increased sedative effect has been observed in some patients receiving concomitant therapy with a benzodiazepine and cimetidine, the degree to which the pharmacologic response to the benzodiazepine may be increased is not well established. Benzodiazepine dosage reduction may be necessary in patients receiving concomitant therapy with cimetidine. Altered benzodiazepine response may occur following initiation or discontinuance of cimetidine therapy in patients receiving affected benzodiazepines.

Ranitidine

There have been reports of increased systemic availability of benzodiazepines (e.g., oral midazolam, triazolam) when these benzodiazepines were administered concomitantly with ranitidine. The mechanism has not been fully elucidated.

● Grapefruit Juice

Concomitant oral administration of grapefruit juice with midazolam or triazolam has been reported to increase bioavailability of the drugs. The interaction between grapefruit juice and benzodiazepine bioavailability appears to result from inhibition, probably prehepatic, of the cytochrome P-450 enzyme system by some constituent(s) in the juice. Following oral administration of these benzodiazepines, such prehepatic inhibition of drug metabolism by grapefruit juice appears mainly to involve the CYP3A4 isoenzyme, principally within the small intestinal wall (e.g., in the jejunum), thus increasing systemic availability of these drugs. (See Grapefruit Juice under Drug Interactions: Drugs and Foods Affecting Hepatic Microsomal Enzymes, in Cyclosporine 92:44.)

● Hormonal Contraceptives

In a limited number of healthy women, concurrent use of an oral estrogen-progestin contraceptive (1 mg of norethindrone acetate and 50 mcg of ethinyl estradiol daily for at least 6 months) with a single 2-mg IV dose of lorazepam decreased half-life of lorazepam by 55% and increased volume of distribution by 50%, resulting in an almost 3.7-fold increase in total clearance of lorazepam. Dosage of lorazepam may need to be increased when administered to women receiving oral contraceptives.

Concomitant use of oral contraceptives with alprazolam or triazolam has been shown to decrease clearance of these benzodiazepines. In one study, the peak plasma concentration and elimination half-life of alprazolam were increased by 18 and 29%, respectively, and clearance of alprazolam was decreased by 22% when oral contraceptives were given concomitantly. Similar results were observed in a study with triazolam; the peak plasma concentration and elimination half-life of triazolam were increased by 6 and 16%, respectively, and clearance of triazolam was decreased by 32% when oral contraceptives were given concomitantly.

Caution is advised when alprazolam or triazolam is used concomitantly with oral contraceptives.

Clobazam may reduce the efficacy of some hormonal contraceptives (e.g., oral or other hormonal contraceptives) that are metabolized by CYP3A4. Additional nonhormonal forms of contraception are recommended in women receiving hormonal contraceptives during clobazam therapy and for 28 days following discontinuance of the drug.

● Levodopa

A few levodopa-treated patients experienced decreased control of parkinsonian symptoms when chlordiazepoxide hydrochloride or diazepam was added to their therapeutic regimen. Therefore, benzodiazepines should be administered with caution to patients receiving levodopa.

● Probenecid

In a limited number of healthy adults, concurrent use of probenecid (500 mg every 6 hours) with a single 2-mg IV dose of lorazepam increased the half-life of lorazepam by 130% and decreased its clearance by 45%. Dosage of lorazepam should be reduced by 50% when administered concomitantly with probenecid.

● Scopolamine

An increased incidence of sedation, hallucinations, and irrational behavior has been reported in patients receiving lorazepam injection concomitantly with scopolamine. The manufacturer of lorazepam states that the benzodiazepine should be used with caution in patients receiving scopolamine, because concomitant administration of these drugs has not been evaluated systematically.

● Smoking

Cigarette smoking may decrease the sedative effects of usual doses of benzodiazepines. Clearance of benzodiazepines may be increased in smokers compared with nonsmokers. Plasma alprazolam concentrations reportedly are decreased by up to 50% in cigarette smokers compared with nonsmokers.

LABORATORY TEST INTERFERENCES

● Pregnancy Test

Chlordiazepoxide may cause a false-positive reaction in the Gravindex® pregnancy test.

● Tests for Urinary Steroids and Alkaloids

Chlordiazepoxide reportedly interferes with the Zimmerman reaction for urinary 17-ketosteroids, resulting in falsely elevated or decreased concentrations. Chlordiazepoxide and diazepam may interfere with urine alkaloids determined by the Frings thin layer chromatography procedure, resulting in falsely elevated readings.

● Tests for Urinary Glucose

False-negative reactions for glucose in the urine may occur in patients receiving diazepam when the test is performed with Clinistix® and Diastix®, but not with Tes-Tape®.

ACUTE TOXICITY

● Manifestations

Benzodiazepine overdosage may result in somnolence, impaired coordination, slurred speech, confusion, coma, and diminished reflexes. Hypotension, seizures, respiratory depression, and apnea also may occur. Although cardiac arrest has been reported, death from overdosage of benzodiazepines in the absence of concurrent ingestion of alcohol or other CNS depressants is rare. Most patients recover rapidly.

● Treatment

Treatment of benzodiazepine intoxication consists of general supportive therapy. Flumazenil, a benzodiazepine antagonist, can be used in the management of benzodiazepine overdosage, but the drug is an adjunct to, not a substitute for, appropriate supportive and symptomatic therapy. (See Flumazenil 28:92.) The possibility that the antagonist could precipitate withdrawal (e.g., seizures) in benzodiazepine-dependent individuals should be considered.

If ingestion of the benzodiazepine is recent and the patient is fully conscious, emesis should be induced. If the patient is comatose, gastric lavage may be done if an endotracheal tube with cuff inflated is in place to prevent aspiration of gastric contents. Activated charcoal and a saline cathartic may be administered after gastric lavage and/or emesis to remove any remaining drug. Pulse, respiration, and blood pressure should be monitored and the patient should be closely observed. IV fluids should be administered and an adequate airway maintained. Hypotension may be controlled, if necessary, by IV administration of norepinephrine or metaraminol. Although some manufacturers recommend use of caffeine and sodium benzoate to combat CNS depression, most authorities believe caffeine and other analeptic agents should *not* be used, because these drugs have questionable benefit and transient action. Instead, administration of flumazenil, if indicated, generally would be preferred. Hemodialysis is not useful in the treatment of benzodiazepine overdosage.

CHRONIC TOXICITY

Tolerance and psychologic and physical dependence may occur following prolonged use of benzodiazepines. The possibility that such effects also may occur following short-term use of benzodiazepines, particularly at high dosages, also should be considered. Symptoms of benzodiazepine dependence are similar to barbiturate dependence or chronic alcoholism and may include drowsiness, ataxia, slurred speech, and vertigo.

Sudden discontinuance of benzodiazepines in physically dependent patients (usually patients who have received excessive doses for an extended period of time but also occasionally with therapeutic dosages for relatively short periods) may produce severe withdrawal symptoms including anxiety, agitation, tension, dysphoria, anorexia, insomnia, sweating, vomiting, diarrhea, blurred vision, irritability, memory impairment, impaired concentrating ability, clouded sensorium, paresthesias, ataxia, tremors, muscle and abdominal cramps, heightened sensory perception, hallucinations, acute psychosis, decreased appetite/weight loss, and seizures which are clinically indistinguishable from tonic-clonic seizures. In addition, milder withdrawal symptoms such as dysphoria and insomnia have been reported following abrupt discontinuance of benzodiazepines in patients receiving therapeutic dosages for several months. It may be difficult to distinguish between withdrawal symptoms and those that are manifestations of illness return or rebound, although their management may differ. Because some benzodiazepines and their metabolites have long elimination half-lives, withdrawal symptoms may not occur until several days after the drugs have been discontinued.

Treatment of benzodiazepine physical dependence consists of cautious and gradual withdrawal of the drug using a dosage tapering schedule. Gradual dosage tapering is particularly important in patients with a seizure history. Occasionally, temporary reinstitution of benzodiazepine therapy at dosages adequate to suppress withdrawal symptoms may be necessary.

PHARMACOLOGY

The exact sites and mode of action of the benzodiazepines have not been fully elucidated, but the effects of the drugs appear to be mediated through the inhibitory neurotransmitter γ-aminobutyric acid (GABA). The drugs appear to act at the limbic, thalamic, and hypothalamic levels of the CNS, producing anxiolytic, sedative, hypnotic, skeletal muscle relaxant, and anticonvulsant effects. Benzodiazepines are capable of producing all levels of CNS depression—from mild sedation to hypnosis to coma.

Specific binding sites with high affinity for benzodiazepines have been detected in the CNS, and the affinity of these sites for the drugs is enhanced by both GABA and chloride. The sites and actions of benzodiazepines within the CNS appear to involve a macromolecular (oligomer or possibly a tetramer) complex (GABA$_A$-receptor-chloride ionophore complex) that includes GABA$_A$ receptors (GABA recognition sites), high-affinity benzodiazepine receptors, and chloride channels, although precise relationships between the sites of action of benzodiazepines and GABA-regulated (-gated) chloride channels remain to be more fully elucidated. Allosteric interactions of central benzodiazepine receptors with GABA$_A$ receptors and subsequent opening of chloride channels appear to be involved in eliciting the CNS effects of the drugs; the benzodiazepine receptors act as modulatory sites on the complex. Some evidence suggests that benzodiazepine receptor sites are heterogeneous, with at least 2 CNS subtypes (type 1 [BZ$_1$] and type 2 [BZ$_2$] benzodiazepine receptors) being described to date. While quazepam and 2-oxoquazepam (an active metabolite), like halazepam (another 1-*N*-trifluoroethyl derivative [no longer commercially available in the US]) but unlike other currently available benzodiazepines, exhibit relative selectivity for type 1 receptors (2-oxoquazepam is the most potent and selective of the three), the clinical importance, if any, of this finding remains to be established. Some evidence suggests that such selectivity may be responsible for the reduced ataxic effect of quazepam observed in animal studies; the possibility that the spectrum of other benzodiazepine-induced effects may be narrowed by such selectivity also has been suggested.

Clobazam, a 1,5-benzodiazepine, has been shown to have a broader spectrum of anticonvulsant activity and an improved adverse effect profile (e.g., less sedative effects) compared with the traditional 1,4-benzodiazepines (e.g., diazepam, lorazepam); these differences have been attributed to differences in binding affinity for the GABA$_A$ receptor. Because the active metabolite of clobazam, *N*-desmethylclobazam, is extensively metabolized by cytochrome P-450 (CYP) 2C19, genetic polymorphism of CYP2C19 can result in possible increased concentrations of the active metabolite. Systemic exposure to *N*-desmethylclobazam is approximately 3–5 and 2 times higher in poor (CYP2C19*2/*2) and intermediate (CYP2C19*1/*2) metabolizers of CYP2C19, respectively, than in extensive (CYP2C19*1/*1) metabolizers. The frequency of poor CYP2C19 metabolizers in the population varies widely depending on ethnic or racial background.

Anxiolytic and possibly paradoxical CNS stimulatory effects of benzodiazepines are postulated to result from release of previously suppressed responses (disinhibition). After usual doses of benzodiazepines for several days, the drugs cause a moderate decrease in rapid eye movement (REM) sleep. REM rebound does not occur when the drugs are withdrawn. Stage 3 and 4 sleep are markedly reduced by usual doses of the drugs; the clinical importance of these sleep stage alterations has not been established.

Benzodiazepines appear to produce skeletal muscle relaxation predominantly by inhibiting spinal polysynaptic afferent pathways, but the drugs may also inhibit monosynaptic afferent pathways. The drugs may inhibit monosynaptic and polysynaptic reflexes by acting as inhibitory neuronal transmitters or by blocking excitatory synaptic transmission. The drugs may also directly depress motor nerve and muscle function.

In animals, benzodiazepines protect against seizures induced by electrical stimulation and by pentylenetetrazol; benzodiazepines appear to act, at least partly, by augmenting presynaptic inhibition. The drugs suppress the spread of seizure activity but do not abolish the abnormal discharge from a focus in experimental models of epilepsy. In usual doses, benzodiazepines appear to have very little effect on the autonomic nervous system, respiration, or the cardiovascular system.

PHARMACOKINETICS

● *Absorption*

Benzodiazepines are generally well absorbed from the GI tract. Following IM administration of diazepam, absorption is slow and erratic. Absorption of lorazepam and midazolam hydrochloride after IM administration appears to be rapid and complete. Following oral administration of clorazepate dipotassium, it appears that most of the drug is rapidly decarboxylated in the GI tract and is absorbed as desmethyldiazepam (nordiazepam). The rate of decarboxylation of clorazepate decreases as gastric pH increases. Flurazepam undergoes first-pass metabolism in the liver, and plasma concentrations of the parent compound are minimal after oral administration. Plasma concentrations of the benzodiazepines

and their metabolites (which in general are active) exhibit considerable interpatient variation, and therapeutic plasma concentrations are difficult to define.

Following oral administration of usual doses of flurazepam, onset of hypnotic action is 15–45 minutes, and the duration of action is 7–8 hours. In general, orally administered benzodiazepines produce anxiolytic, skeletal muscle relaxant, and anticonvulsant effects after the first dose; however, these effects may increase until steady-state plasma concentrations are achieved. After IV administration of single doses of diazepam or lorazepam, the onset of anticonvulsant, anxiolytic, or sedative action occurs in 1–5 minutes; after usual doses of IV diazepam, the duration of action is 15 minutes–1 hour, and after IV lorazepam, the duration of action is 12–24 hours. Following repeated doses of IV diazepam, prolonged duration of sedative action may occur, because of the presence of its long-acting metabolites. Following IV administration of usual doses of midazolam hydrochloride, the onset of sedative, anxiolytic, and amnesic action usually occurs within 1–5 minutes. The duration of action following IV administration of midazolam is usually less than 2 hours; however, the pharmacologic effects may persist up to 6 hours in some patients and the duration of action appears to be dose related. After IM administration, the onset of action of lorazepam is 15–30 minutes, and the duration of action is 12–24 hours. Following IM administration of midazolam hydrochloride, onset of action occurs within 5–15 minutes but may not be maximal until 20–60 minutes; the duration of action usually is about 2 hours (range: 1–6 hours).

Midazolam appears to be rapidly and well absorbed transmucosally following intrabuccal administration. The drug also appears to be rapidly and well absorbed transmucosally following intranasal administration; however, the effect of increased nasal discharge and mucus production on intranasal midazolam absorption is unknown, and breathing may discharge drugs that are administered intranasally.

Diazepam is rapidly and well absorbed systemically following rectal administration as a gel or solution (e.g., using parenteral formulations). Peak plasma or serum concentrations generally are achieved within 5–90 minutes following rectal administration of these formulations, with bioavailabilities averaging 80–102%. Diazepam is less predictably absorbed systemically following rectal administration as suppositories (e.g., bioavailability of 67–84%), exhibiting slow and variable absorption. When a single 15-mg dose was administered rectally as a commercially available viscous gel (Diastat®) in healthy adults pretreated with an enema to ensure an empty rectum, plasma diazepam concentrations exceeded 200 ng/mL within 15 minutes and reached an initial peak of 373 ng/mL at 45 minutes and a second peak of 447 ng/mL at approximately 70 minutes. The manufacturer states that peak plasma concentrations of the drug are achieved within 1.5 hours following rectal administration of the gel in adults. In the healthy adults who received a single 15-mg rectal dose of diazepam following pretreatment with an enema, the absolute systemic bioavailability averaged about 90% (range: 71–110%). Peak plasma concentrations of the desmethyl metabolite in these adults averaged 62 ng/mL and were achieved 68 hours after rectal administration; areas under the plasma concentration-time curve (AUCs) and peak plasma concentrations for this metabolite were similar with rectal or IV administration. The elimination half-lives for diazepam and desmethyldiazepam averaged about 45–46 and 71–99 hours, respectively, following rectal administration of the gel in healthy adults. The pharmacokinetics of diazepam rectal gel in pediatric patients have not been determined, although some evidence suggests that more rapid absorption may be likely.

Clobazam is rapidly and almost completely absorbed following oral administration; peak plasma concentrations of the drug are achieved within 0.5–4 hours after single- or multiple-dose administration. The main circulating metabolite, *N*-desmethylclobazam, is pharmacologically active with potency estimates ranging from one-fifth to equal potency of the parent drug; therefore, the active metabolite may contribute to the efficacy and tolerability of the drug. At therapeutic dosages, plasma concentrations of *N*-desmethylclobazam are approximately 3–5 times higher than those of clobazam.

● *Distribution*

Benzodiazepines are widely distributed into body tissues and cross the blood-brain barrier. Following IV administration of diazepam, there is an early, rapid decline in plasma concentrations of the drug, principally associated with distribution into the tissues. After IV administration of lorazepam, plasma concentrations decline less rapidly. Generally, benzodiazepines and their metabolites cross the placenta; the concentration of diazepam in the fetal circulation has been reported to be equal to or greater than maternal plasma drug concentrations. The drugs and their metabolites are distributed into milk.

Benzodiazepines and their metabolites are highly bound to plasma proteins.

● **Elimination**

Elimination half-lives ($t_{1/2}$s) of benzodiazepines and their metabolites exhibit wide interpatient variation. (See Table 1.)

TABLE 1. The $t_{1/2}$s of benzodiazepines and their major active metabolites in healthy individuals

Drug ($t_{1/2}$ in hours)	Major Active Metabolites ($t_{1/2}$ in hours)
Alprazolam (11–15)	None
Chlordiazepoxide (5–30)	Demoxepam (14–95)
	Desmethylchlordiazepoxide (18)
	Desmethyldiazepam (30–200)
	Oxazepam (3–21)
Clobazam (36–42)	N-desmethylclobazam (71–82)
Clonazepam (18–50)	None
Clorazepate	Desmethyldiazepam (30–200)
	Oxazepam (3–21)
Diazepam (20–50)	Desmethyldiazepam (30–200)
	3-Hydroxydiazepam (5–20)
	Oxazepam (3–21)
Estazolam (10–24)	None
Flurazepam	Desalkylflurazepam (47–100)
	N-1-Hydroxyethylflurazepam (2–4)
Halazepam (14)	Desmethyldiazepam (30–200)
Lorazepam (10–20)	None
Midazolam (1–12.3)	1-Hydroxymethylmidazolam (1–1.3)
Oxazepam (3–21)	None
Quazepam (25–41)	2-Oxoquazepam (40)
	N-Desalkyl-2-oxoquazepam (70–75)
Temazepam (10–20)	None
Triazolam (1.6–5.4)	None

Geriatric patients and patients with liver disease may have prolonged elimination half-lives of all benzodiazepines and their metabolites, except possibly lorazepam, oxazepam, temazepam, and triazolam. However, limited data in healthy geriatric individuals (average age: 69 years) receiving single doses (0.125 or 0.25 mg) of triazolam indicate that values for peak plasma concentration and AUCs are increased and clearance decreased by an average of approximately 50% compared with values in younger adults (average age: 30 years). Evidence suggesting accumulation of triazolam (as determined by benzodiazepine receptor binding activity) with prolonged (i.e., 4 weeks) administration in geriatric individuals also has been reported. In premature and newborn infants, the half-lives of diazepam are longer than in adults and older children. Steady-state plasma concentrations of benzodiazepines and their metabolites are reached after administration of a fixed dosage for approximately 5 elimination half-lives. Plasma concentrations of metabolites with long half-lives may be greater than those of the unchanged drugs.

Benzodiazepines are metabolized in the liver. Lorazepam, oxazepam, temazepam, and the hydroxylated metabolites of chlordiazepoxide, clorazepate, diazepam, flurazepam, halazepam (no longer commercially available in the US), midazolam, quazepam, and triazolam are conjugated with glucuronic and/or sulfuric acid; these inactive conjugates are excreted principally in urine. Benzodiazepines are not appreciably removed by hemodialysis.

CHEMISTRY

Alprazolam, chlordiazepoxide, clobazam (see 28:12.08), clonazepam (see 28:12.08), clorazepate, diazepam, estazolam, flurazepam, lorazepam, midazolam, oxazepam, quazepam, temazepam, and triazolam are benzodiazepines that are used as anxiolytics, sedatives, hypnotics, anticonvulsants, and/or skeletal muscle relaxants. Benzodiazepines are subject to control under the Federal Controlled Substances Act of 1970.

Benzodiazepines contain a benzene ring structure fused to a 7-membered diazepine ring. The classic benzodiazepines (e.g., chlordiazepoxide, clonazepam, diazepam, lorazepam) are referred to as 1,4-benzodiazepines because they contain nitrogen atoms at positions 1 and 4 on the diazepine ring. Clobazam, a 1,5-benzodiazepine, differs structurally from 1,4-benzodiazepines in that its nitrogen atoms are at positions 1 and 5 and a keto group occupies the 4 position on the diazepine ring; clobazam is the only 1,5-benzodiazepine that is currently used in clinical practice. Commercially available 1,4-benzodiazepines, except alprazolam, chlordiazepoxide, estazolam, midazolam, quazepam, and triazolam, have the same characteristic structure but differ in the substitutions at the R^1, R^3, R^7, and $R^{2'}$ positions.

● **Comparative Structures of Benzodiazepines**

benzodiazepine nucleus

TABLE 2. Comparative structures of 1,4-benzodiazepines

	R^1	R^3	R^7	$R^{2'}$
Clonazepam	–H	–H	–NO$_2$	–Cl
Clorazepate dipotassium	–H	–COOK	–Cl	–H
Diazepam	–CH$_3$	–H	–Cl	–H
Flurazepam	–CH$_2$CH$_2$N(C$_2$H$_5$)$_2$	–H	–Cl	–F
Halazepam	–CH$_2$CF$_3$	–H	–Cl	–H
Lorazepam	–H	–OH	–Cl	–Cl
Oxazepam	–H	–OH	–Cl	–H
Quazepam	–CH$_2$CF$_3$	–H	–Cl	–F
Temazepam	–CH$_3$	–OH	–Cl	–H

In chlordiazepoxide, a 1,4-benzodiazepine-4-oxide, a methylamino group replaces the ketone at the 2 position, and a chlorine atom is at R^7. In alprazolam, estazolam, and triazolam, triazolobenzodiazepines, a triazolo ring is formed by the addition of a ring to the benzodiazepine nucleus at the 1 and 2 positions, and a chlorine atom is at R^7; triazolam also has a chlorine atom at $R^{2'}$. In midazolam, an imidazobenzodiazepine, an imidazole ring fused at positions 1 and

2 of the benzodiazepine nucleus replaces the ketone at position 2 of the nucleus; midazolam has a fluorine atom at $R^{2'}$ and a chlorine atom at R^7. Quazepam, a 1,4-benzodiazepine-2-thione, has a sulfur atom rather than a ketone at position 2 of the nucleus; the drug also has a trifluoroethyl group at R^1, a fluorine atom at $R^{2'}$, and a chlorine atom at R^7. The presence of the trifluoroethyl group (1-N-trifluoroethyl derivative) distinguishes halazepam (no longer commercially available in the US) and quazepam from other currently available benzodiazepines and results in relative selectivity for type 1 (BZ_1) benzodiazepine receptors. (See Pharmacology.)

For further information on chemistry and stability, uses, cautions, and dosage and administration of benzodiazepines, see the individual monographs in 28:24.08. See also the Anticonvulsants General Statement 28:12, Clobazam 28:12.08, and Clonazepam 28:12.08.

diazePAM

28:24.08 • BENZODIAZEPINES

■ Diazepam is a benzodiazepine. The drug has anticonvulsant, anxiolytic, sedative, and skeletal muscle relaxant properties.

USES

● Anxiety Disorders, Preoperative or Preprocedural Anxiolysis, Alcohol Withdrawal, and Musculoskeletal Conditions

Diazepam is used for preoperative sedation, anxiolysis, and anterograde amnesia; for relief of anxiety and stress in patients undergoing procedures (e.g., endoscopic procedures, cardioversion); for the management of agitation associated with acute alcohol withdrawal; as an adjunct for the relief of acute, painful musculoskeletal conditions; to manage skeletal muscle spasticity such as reflex spasm secondary to local pathology (e.g., trauma, inflammation), spasticity caused by upper motor neuron disorders (e.g., cerebral palsy, paraplegia), athetosis, stiff-man syndrome, or tetanus; and for the management of anxiety disorders or for the short-term relief of symptoms of anxiety.

The efficacy of diazepam for long-term use (i.e., longer than 4 months) has not been evaluated.

● Seizures

Diazepam is used parenterally (IV administration preferred) for the treatment of status epilepticus and severe recurrent convulsive seizures. Oral diazepam may be used for adjunctive therapy of seizure disorders; however, loss of response to the anticonvulsant effects of the drug often develops with prolonged use.

Diazepam also may be administered rectally either as a commercially available gel (e.g., Diastat®) or using parenteral† formulations for the management of seizure disorders and status epilepticus.

Status Epilepticus

Benzodiazepines are considered the initial drugs of choice for the management of status epilepticus because of their rapid onset of action, demonstrated efficacy, safety, and tolerability.

Status epilepticus is a medical emergency that must be treated promptly to reduce substantial morbidity and mortality. Initial treatment should include standard critical care and supportive therapy (e.g., blood pressure and respiratory support, oxygen, IV access, identification and correction of underlying causes), followed by administration of a benzodiazepine. Although IV lorazepam is generally preferred because of its longer duration of action, studies generally have not identified any substantial differences between IV lorazepam, IV diazepam, and IM midazolam in terms of seizure cessation, and experts consider these therapies to be equivalent first-line options. Selection of an appropriate benzodiazepine should be individualized based on local availability, route of administration, pharmacokinetics, cost, and other factors (e.g., treatment setting). To achieve a rapid therapeutic effect, IV administration of a benzodiazepine is preferred; however, administration via other routes (e.g., IM, rectal, intranasal, buccal) may be considered when IV administration is not possible (e.g., in the prehospital setting). If seizures continue after initial therapy with a benzodiazepine, a second-line anticonvulsant agent (e.g., IV fosphenytoin or phenytoin, IV valproate sodium, IV levetiracetam, IV phenobarbital) should be administered. If refractory status epilepticus occurs, continuous IV infusion of anticonvulsants, IV barbiturates, or general anesthetics may be necessary.

To achieve a rapid therapeutic effect, IV administration of a benzodiazepine generally is preferred for the management of status epilepticus; however, administration via other routes (e.g., rectal) may be considered when IV administration is not possible (e.g., in a prehospital setting). Rectal administration of diazepam may be particularly useful for out-of-hospital management of status attacks (e.g., at home or school, during transport to an emergency room).

Early treatment with benzodiazepines in the prehospital setting can improve outcomes in patients with status epilepticus. Results of a placebo-controlled study in adults with out-of-hospital status epilepticus indicated that IV administration

of benzodiazepines by paramedics was safe and effective in the management of this condition. Findings from this study indicated that both IV lorazepam and IV diazepam were more effective than placebo in controlling status epilepticus by the time of patient arrival in the emergency department. Because the need to establish IV access may delay administration of an IV benzodiazepine in the prehospital environment, use of other less invasive routes of administration may decrease the time to active treatment.

Acute Repetitive Seizures

Rectal diazepam also may be used for the management of acute repetitive seizures (also referred to as serial, cyclic, cluster, breakthrough, or crescendo seizures), especially for out-of-hospital management.

Acute repetitive seizures are exacerbations of an underlying seizure disorder that exhibit a pattern distinct from the patient's usual seizure pattern; the repetitive, periodic episodes often are predictable by the patient and caregivers according to a prodrome/aura, time of day when they originate, particular seizure type, and/or accompanying patient behavioral changes. Patients typically experience recovery between the repetitions; however, if untreated, acute repetitive seizures can evolve into more serious problems, including status epilepticus. The distinguishing features of these seizures are their predictability and pattern that differs from the underlying disorder rather than the actual seizure type; thus, while the pattern of presentation and patient and caregiver recognition are common features of the diagnosis, the actual seizure type can be different albeit definable for each individual patient.

In the 2 clinical studies establishing efficacy of rectal diazepam for the management of acute repetitive seizures in adults and children 2 years of age and older, the drug was more effective than placebo in reducing seizure frequency and improving global assessment of treatment outcome as judged by caregivers (e.g., frequency and severity of seizures and patient tolerance of therapy). In these studies, the time to next seizure was prolonged in diazepam-treated patients relative to placebo, and about 55–62% of patients were seizure-free during the 12-hour observation period versus 20–34% for placebo recipients. In these studies, patients with a history of acute repetitive seizures that typically progressed to status epilepticus were excluded from study entry. Similar efficacy has been reported in other placebo-controlled and open-label studies. Although formal economic analyses have not been performed to date, patients treated with rectal diazepam out of the hospital required emergency medical treatment less commonly than did placebo recipients.

● Sedation in Critical Care Settings

Diazepam has been used for the sedation of intubated and mechanically ventilated patients in critical care settings† (e.g., intensive care unit [ICU]). Because of some modest clinical benefits (e.g., reduced duration of mechanical ventilation, shorter time to extubation, reduced risk of delirium) and an overall favorable benefit-to-risk profile, nonbenzodiazepine sedatives (dexmedetomidine or propofol) are generally preferred to benzodiazepines (midazolam or lorazepam) in mechanically ventilated, critically ill adults. If a benzodiazepine is required, midazolam or lorazepam generally is used; diazepam is rarely used for this indication.

● Drug-induced Cardiovascular Emergencies

Diazepam has been used adjunctively in the management of certain drug-induced cardiovascular emergencies† and cocaine-induced acute coronary syndrome†.

● Other Uses

Diazepam has been used orally to prevent night terrors†. Although not recommended by the manufacturer, parenteral diazepam is used to reduce the requirements for opiate analgesics and produce anterograde amnesia during labor and delivery†. The drug has been used parenterally to manage neonatal opiate withdrawal†.

DOSAGE AND ADMINISTRATION

Diazepam is administered orally, by IV or IM injection, or rectally.

● Administration

Oral Administration

Diazepam is administered orally as tablets or oral solution.

When diazepam oral concentrate solution is used, the dose should be diluted (e.g., with water, juice, carbonated or soda-like beverages) or mixed with semi-solid foods (e.g., applesauce, pudding) using only the calibrated dropper provided by the manufacturer. The liquid or food mixture should be stirred gently for a few seconds and then consumed immediately; the mixture should not be stored for future use.

Parenteral Administration

When oral therapy is not feasible or when a rapid therapeutic effect is necessary, diazepam may be administered by slow IV injection at a rate not exceeding 5 mg/minute in adults and over a 3-minute period in children. When given IV, diazepam should be administered directly into a large vein to avoid thrombosis; if this is not feasible, the drug should be given into the tubing of a flowing IV solution as close as possible to the vein insertion. Small veins such as those of the wrist or the dorsum of the hand should not be used. Care should be taken to avoid intra-arterial administration or extravasation. Some clinicians have suggested IV administration of dilute solutions of the drug to avoid extravasation; however, the drug may precipitate when diluted and the manufacturers do not recommend this method of administration. (See Chemistry and Stability: Stability.)

Although diazepam may also be given by deep IM injection, this route of administration of the drug is rarely justified because absorption is slow and erratic.

Therapy with oral diazepam should replace parenteral administration as soon as possible.

Rectal Administration

When diazepam is administered rectally, the drug may be given as a commercially available rectal gel via the delivery device (a plastic applicator with a flexible molded tip) provided by the manufacturer. Diazepam also has been administered rectally as the parenteral solution† via a syringe and rectally inserted tubing or via a lubricated tuberculin syringe (*without* a needle) inserted 4–5 cm into the rectum.

Diazepam rectal gel is commercially available in prefilled syringe applicators containing 2.5, 10, or 20 mg of diazepam. The 2.5-mg Diastat® applicator delivers a dose of 2.5 mg of diazepam; the 10-mg Diastat® AcuDial® applicator can be set to deliver a dose of 5, 7.5, or 10 mg of the drug; and the 20-mg Diastat® AcuDial® applicator can be set to deliver a dose of 12.5, 15, 17.5, or 20 mg of the drug. Both the 2.5- and 10-mg applicators are fitted with a plastic applicator tip that is 4.4 cm in length; the 20-mg applicator is fitted with an applicator tip that is 6 cm in length. The 4.4-cm rectal tip applicator generally is used for pediatric patients. Although dosage of diazepam rectal gel is calculated on a mg/kg basis by age, the actual dose administered is approximate and determined by rounding upward to the next available dose (i.e., the next multiple of 2.5 mg).

Prior to dispensing the Diastat® AcuDial® preparation, the pharmacist must dial in and lock the correct dose to be administered. While holding the barrel of the applicator in one hand, the pharmacist turns the cap of the applicator to select the dose. After confirming that the dose visible in the display window is correct, the pharmacist locks the dose by grasping the locking ring and pushing upward to lock both sides of the ring. Once the dose-locking ring on the device is engaged, a green "ready" band becomes visible at the base of the applicator. The process should be repeated for each applicator to be dispensed. Upon receiving the drug from the pharmacy, the patient or caregiver should verify that the prescribed dose is visible in the display window and that the green "ready" band is visible.

Caregivers should be instructed carefully in the use of diazepam rectal gel and should be given a copy of the administration instructions provided by the manufacturer. As soon as an episode of acute repetitive seizures is recognized, the caregiver should place the patient on their side so they won't fall and administer the prescribed dose of rectal diazepam. Before the prescribed dose is administered, the expiration date of the appropriate applicator(s) should be checked to ensure that it is in date; with the AcuDial® applicators, the visibility of the green "ready" band and the dose displayed in the display window also should be checked. The applicator is prepared for use by removing the protective cap from the syringe and ensuring that the seal pin is removed with the cap. The rectal applicator tip should be lubricated with the water-soluble lubricant (jelly) provided by the manufacturer and the patient should be turned so that they are resting on their side facing the caregiver; the patient's upper leg should be bent forward and the buttocks separated to expose the rectum. The lubricated applicator tip should then be inserted rectally until the rim of the syringe is snug against the rectal opening; once inserted, the plunger should be pushed slowly (counting aloud slowly to 3) until it stops (i.e., until the entire dose of the applicator has been expelled into

the rectum). The caregiver should again count aloud slowly to 3 before removing the syringe from the rectum; to prevent leakage of the administered dose from the rectum, the buttocks should then be held together while again counting aloud slowly to 3. The patient should be left on their side facing the caregiver, the time the dose was given noted, and the patient observed. If bowel leakage occurs during rectal administration, it may be necessary to administer a supplemental dose. (See Dosage: Rectal Dosage, in Dosage and Administration.)

The rectal delivery system and all unused materials should be discarded in the garbage and *not* reused. Such disposal should be in a safe place away from children. Any diazepam rectal gel remaining in the AcuDial® applicator after use should be disposed of before the applicator is discarded. With the applicator tip pointed over the sink or toilet, the plunger should be pulled back and removed from the barrel of the syringe applicator and then replaced in the barrel and gently depressed until it stops, thereby forcing gel from the applicator tip into the sink or toilet. The toilet then should be flushed or the sink rinsed with water until gel is no longer visible. The applicator may then be discarded.

● Dosage

Dosage of diazepam must be individualized, and the smallest effective dosage should be used (especially in geriatric or debilitated patients or in those with liver disease or low serum albumin) to avoid oversedation. The doses recommended by the manufacturers for IM and IV administration are identical. When parenteral diazepam is used with an opiate analgesic, the dosage of the opiate should be reduced by at least one-third and administered in small increments. Because of the unpredictable response of children to CNS drugs, diazepam therapy should be initiated with the lowest dosage and increased as required. Since diazepam and its metabolites have long elimination half-lives, time to reach steady-state plasma concentrations should be considered when dosage adjustments are made.

In patients who have received prolonged (e.g., for several months) diazepam therapy, abrupt discontinuance of the drug should be avoided since manifestations of withdrawal can be precipitated; if the drug is to be discontinued in such patients, it is recommended that dosage be gradually tapered. It is particularly important that the drugs *not* be discontinued abruptly in patients with a history of a seizure disorder since seizures may be precipitated.

Oral Dosage
Adult Dosage

For the management of anxiety or for adjunctive treatment of seizure disorders, the usual adult oral dosage of diazepam is 2–10 mg 2–4 times daily as tablets or oral solution.

For adjunctive treatment of skeletal muscle spasticity, the usual adult oral dosage of diazepam is 2–10 mg 3 or 4 times daily as tablets or oral solution.

For the management of acute alcohol withdrawal, the usual adult oral dosage of diazepam is 10 mg 3 or 4 times as tablets or oral solution during the first 24 hours, followed by 5 mg 3 or 4 times daily as needed.

In adults with night terrors†, 5–20 mg of diazepam has been administered orally as tablets or oral solution at bedtime.

The initial oral dosage of diazepam for geriatric or debilitated patients should be 2–2.5 mg once or twice daily as tablets or oral solution. Dosage should be adjusted gradually according to response and tolerance.

Pediatric Dosage

The manufacturers state that children 6 months of age or older may receive an initial oral diazepam dosage of 1–2.5 mg 3 or 4 times daily as tablets or oral solution. When used as a sedative or muscle relaxant in children, some clinicians recommend an oral diazepam dosage of 0.12–0.8 mg/kg daily in 3 or 4 divided doses. Dosage should be adjusted gradually according to response and tolerance.

As an adjunct in the management of epilepsy in children, 6–15 mg daily (and occasionally up to 30 mg daily) in divided doses as tablets or oral solution has been used by some clinicians.

Parenteral Dosage
Adult Dosage

If diazepam injection is used for rapid relief of acute anxiety, the usual adult IV or IM dose is 2–5 mg for moderate anxiety or 5–10 mg for severe anxiety. The dose may be repeated in 3–4 hours if necessary. Some clinicians recommend that the adult dosage should not exceed 30 mg within an 8-hour period.

For the management of acute alcohol withdrawal, the manufacturer states that the usual adult dose of diazepam is 10 mg administered IM or IV initially; some clinicians recommend an initial dose of up to 20 mg. If necessary, the manufacturer states that an additional dose of 5–10 mg may be administered in 3–4 hours if necessary. For acute alcohol withdrawal, some clinicians recommend 10 mg of diazepam IV initially, followed by 10 mg at 20- to 30-minute intervals until the patient is calm.

To relieve anxiety and stress and produce amnesia in adults undergoing cardioversion, 5–15 mg of diazepam may be given IV within 5–10 minutes prior to the procedure.

To reduce anxiety prior to endoscopy, diazepam is administered slowly IV immediately before the procedure; dosage is titrated to obtain the desired sedative response, such as slurring of speech. Generally, IV administration of up to 10 mg is adequate in adults, but up to 20 mg may be required especially if opiates are not given concomitantly. If IV administration is not feasible, 5–10 mg of diazepam may be given IM approximately 30 minutes prior to endoscopy in adults.

For preoperative sedation in adults, 10 mg of diazepam may be administered parenterally 1–2 hours prior to surgery. IM administration is preferred. Some clinicians have recommended a dose of up to 20 mg preoperatively.

For the treatment of skeletal muscle spasticity in adults, 5–10 mg may be administered IM or IV initially, and 3–4 hours later if necessary. For tetanus in adults, larger doses may be required; up to 20 mg has been given every 2–8 hours.

For the treatment of status epilepticus or severe recurrent convulsive seizures, the usual initial adult dose of diazepam is 5–10 mg administered IV. The initial dose may be repeated at 10- to 15-minute intervals, if necessary, until a maximum total dose of 30 mg has been given. If necessary, therapy with diazepam may be repeated in 2–4 hours, with consideration that residual active metabolites may persist following readministration. Although IV administration is preferred, diazepam may be given IM if IV administration is not possible.

To reduce the requirements for opiate analgesics and produce anterograde amnesia during labor and delivery†, the usual parenteral dosage of diazepam is 10–20 mg.

If diazepam is used for sedation in intubated and mechanically ventilated adults in critical care settings†, an IV loading dose of 5–10 mg, followed by intermittent diazepam injections of 0.03–0.1 mg/kg every 0.5–6 hours as needed is recommended by some experts. Dosage should be titrated to the desired level of sedation; in most cases, a light rather than deep level of sedation is recommended in critically ill, mechanically ventilated adults. The depth and quality of sedation should be assessed frequently using a validated and reliable assessment tool.

In geriatric or debilitated patients or in patients receiving other sedative drugs, lower parenteral diazepam doses (usually 2–5 mg) should be used, and dosage should be slowly increased if needed.

Pediatric Dosage

In pediatric patients, IV diazepam should be given slowly over a 3-minute period. The manufacturers recommend that the initial dose not exceed 0.25 mg/kg. The dose may be repeated after 15–30 minutes; if relief of symptoms is not obtained after a third dose, adjunctive therapy appropriate to the condition being treated is recommended.

For the treatment of status epilepticus or severe recurrent convulsant seizures in children 30 days to less than 5 years of age, the usual initial dose of diazepam is 0.2–0.5 mg administered slowly IV; this dose may be repeated every 2–5 minutes up to a maximum total dose of 5 mg. In children 5 years of age or older, the initial dose for the management of seizures is 1 mg administered slowly IV; this dose may be repeated every 2–5 minutes up to a maximum total dose of 10 mg. If necessary, the initial dose of diazepam may be repeated in 2–4 hours. Although IV administration is preferred, diazepam may be given IM if IV administration is not possible. Some clinicians prefer IV lorazepam because of its more prolonged duration of effect. If seizures continue with either diazepam or lorazepam, an additional long-acting anticonvulsant (e.g., IV phenytoin or fosphenytoin) generally is initiated.

For tetanus in children, the manufacturers recommend 1–2 mg of diazepam for infants older than 30 days to 5 years of age and 5–10 mg for children older than 5 years of age administered slowly IV or by IM injection. This dose may be repeated every 3–4 hours as needed.

In painful musculoskeletal conditions and spasticity including tetanus in children, some clinicians recommend diazepam 0.04–0.3 mg/kg IV every 2–4 hours; however, dosage generally should not exceed 0.6 mg/kg in an 8-hour period.

Although the manufacturers have not established pediatric dosage recommendations for preoperative sedation, some clinicians have recommended IM administration of 0.4 mg/kg of diazepam in children older than 2 years of age 1–2 hours prior to surgery.

For acute anxiety reactions in children, some clinicians recommend 0.04–0.2 mg/kg of diazepam IV; this dose may be repeated in 3–4 hours, but dosage should not exceed 0.6 mg/kg in an 8-hour period.

Although the safety and efficacy of parenteral diazepam in infants 30 days of age or younger have not been established, neonates with agitation due to opiate withdrawal have received 0.5–2 mg IM every 8 hours followed by gradual reduction in dosage.

Rectal Dosage

When diazepam is administered rectally as the commercially available gel for the management of acute repetitive seizures, the dose should be individualized for maximum benefit. Children 2–5 years of age should receive 0.5 mg/kg and those 6–11 years of age should receive 0.3 mg/kg; adults and children 12 years of age and older should receive 0.2 mg/kg. These age-adjusted doses were based on the observation that diazepam clearance in children declines with age until about 12 years of age, at which time adult values are reached. The actual dose to be administered is determined by rounding up to the nearest commercially available dose (i.e., the next multiple of 2.5 mg). Using this method of rounded dosing, patients will receive 90–180% of the dose calculated on a weight and age basis. The safety of this dosing method has been established in clinical studies in adults and children 2 years of age and older. For geriatric or debilitated patients, the dose of the rectal gel should be adjusted downward to reduce the likelihood of ataxia and oversedation. The 2.5-mg applicator also may be used to provide a partial replacement dose (supplemental dose) for patients who partially expel the recommended dose within 5 minutes after administration.

If necessary for adequate seizure control, the usual age- and weight-adjusted dose of diazepam rectal gel may be repeated 4–12 hours after the initial dose. Although the usual dose was repeated a third time 8 hours after the second dose in adults in one clinical study, the additional dose resulted in increased sedation and appeared to negatively affect global caregiver assessment of treatment outcome; therefore, a third dose currently is not recommended by the manufacturer. Dosage should be adjusted periodically by the clinician to reflect changes in the patient's age and/or weight; the manufacturer recommends dosage reevaluation at 6-month intervals.

The manufacturer states that diazepam rectal gel is intended for use solely on an intermittent basis and therefore should be administered by caregivers outside the hospital no more frequently than one treatment course every 5 days nor more frequently than 5 treatment courses per month. In addition, chronic daily use of the rectal gel is not recommended because of the potential for development of tolerance to diazepam; chronic daily use may increase the frequency and/or severity of tonic-clonic seizures, requiring an increase in the dosage of concomitant chronic anticonvulsant therapy. In such cases, abrupt withdrawal of chronic diazepam also may be associated with a temporary increase in the frequency and/or severity of seizures.

Because caregivers will be responsible for recognizing seizure episodes suitable for treatment, making the decision to initiate treatment, administering the drug, monitoring the patient, and assessing the adequacy of response, a major component of the prescribing process is the careful instruction of these individuals. The clinician and caregiver must share a common explicit understanding of what constitutes a seizure episode (and/or the events, which may be nonconvulsive, presumed to herald their onset) that is appropriate for treatment, the timing of administration in relation to the onset of the episode, the mechanics of competently administering the drug, how and what to observe following administration, when to repeat a dose, and what would constitute an outcome requiring immediate and direct medical attention.

The caregiver should be instructed to contact the patient's clinician or seek other medical assistance if the seizure episode persists for longer than 15 minutes after administering the rectal gel (or as otherwise instructed), if the seizure behavior differs from other episodes, if the seizure frequency or severity or patient color or breathing is alarming, or if the patient is experiencing unusual or serious problems.

The patient's underlying seizure disorder should be stabilized with a standard chronic anticonvulsant drug regimen, and rectal diazepam should be used only as an adjunct to this regimen for characteristic breakthrough bouts of repetitive seizures.

When using the parenteral solution† of diazepam for rectal administration in the treatment of status epilepticus, a dose of 0.5 mg/kg (up to 20 mg) has been used in adults and children. Some clinicians state that a second dose of 0.25 mg/kg may be administered after 10 minutes if needed.

CAUTIONS

Drowsiness, fatigue, muscle weakness, and ataxia are the most common adverse effects of diazepam. With parenteral therapy, local reactions (venous thrombosis, phlebitis) at the injection site are the most common adverse effects of the drug. For further information on adverse effects reported with benzodiazepines, see Cautions in the Benzodiazepines General Statement 28:24.08

● Precautions and Contraindications

Diazepam shares the toxic potentials of the benzodiazepines, and the usual precautions of benzodiazepine administration should be observed. (See Cautions in the Benzodiazepines General Statement 28:24.08.)

A boxed warning has been included in the prescribing information for all benzodiazepines describing the risks of abuse, misuse, addiction, physical dependence, and withdrawal reactions associated with all drugs in this class. Abuse and misuse can result in overdose or death, especially when benzodiazepines are combined with other medicines, such as opioid pain relievers, alcohol, or illicit drugs. Frequent follow-up with patients receiving benzodiazepines is important. Reassess patients regularly to manage their medical conditions and any withdrawal symptoms. Clinicians should assess a patient's risk of abuse, misuse, and addiction. Standardized screening tools are available (https://nida.nih.gov/nidamed-medical-health-professionals/screening-tools-resources/chart-screening-tools). To reduce the risk of acute withdrawal reactions, use a gradual dose taper when reducing the dosage or discontinuing benzodiazepines. Take precautions when benzodiazepines are used in combination with opioid addiction medications.

Parenterally administered diazepam may cause hypotension and/or respiratory depression, particularly if the drug is administered too rapidly IV. The drug should be administered slowly IV at a rate not exceeding 5 mg/minute in adults and over a 3-minute period in children; facilities and equipment for respiratory or cardiovascular assistance should be readily available.

The possibility that respiratory depression could occur with rectal administration of diazepam also should be considered, although the risk of its development probably is less than that with IV administration. The drug should be used with caution in patients with compromised respiratory function secondary to an underlying disease (e.g., asthma, pneumonia) or neurologic damage. Repeated rectal therapy at relatively short intervals by out-of-hospital caregivers should be avoided because of the possibility of life-threatening respiratory depression; the manufacturer recommends that out-of-hospital rectal diazepam therapy be repeated no more frequently than once during a 5-day period or 5 times monthly and that dosing be limited to 2 doses per treatment course. (See Dosage: Rectal Dosage, in Dosage and Administration.)

Diazepam is contraindicated in patients with known hypersensitivity to the drug. The manufacturers state that the drug is contraindicated in patients with acute angle-closure glaucoma but may be used with caution in patients with open-angle glaucoma who are receiving appropriate therapy. However, the clinical rationale for this contraindication has been questioned.

● Pediatric Precautions

Safety and efficacy of oral diazepam in infants younger than 6 months of age have not been established. Safety and efficacy of parenteral diazepam in infants 30 days of age or younger have not been established. Safety and efficacy of rectal diazepam have not been established via clinical studies in children younger than 2 years of age, and the manufacturer states that the rectal gel is not recommended for use in infants younger than 6 months of age.

CHEMISTRY AND STABILITY

● Chemistry

Diazepam is a benzodiazepine. Diazepam occurs as an off-white to yellow, practically odorless, crystalline powder. The drug is sparingly soluble in propylene glycol and has solubilities of approximately 3 mg/mL in water and 62.5 mg/mL in alcohol at 25°C. Diazepam has a pK_a of 3.4. Sodium benzoate and benzoic acid are added to the commercially available injection to adjust the pH to 6.2–6.9.

Diazepam rectal gel is commercially available as a nonsterile viscous gel formulated in an aqueous base that contains propylene glycol, alcohol (10%), hydroxypropyl methylcellulose, sodium benzoate, benzyl alcohol (1.5%), and benzoic acid. The rectal gel is clear to slightly yellow and has a pH of 6.5–7.2.

● Stability

Diazepam injection should be protected from light and stored at 15–30°C; freezing should be avoided. Diazepam tablets and extended-release capsules should be stored in tight, light-resistant containers at 15–30°C. Diazepam oral solution and oral concentrate solution should be stored at 20–25°C.

The manufacturers state that diazepam injection should not be mixed with other drugs or IV fluids. Although some studies indicate that diazepam injection may be compatible with various drugs and IV fluids (e.g., diluted to a concentration of 5 mg/50 mL to 5 mg/100 mL with 0.9% sodium chloride, 5% dextrose, Ringer's, or lactated Ringer's injection), compatibility may depend on several factors (e.g., the concentration of the drugs, resulting pH, temperature). Specialized references should be consulted for more specific compatibility information. The addition of diazepam injection to an IV infusion solution or plastic syringes may result in adsorption of diazepam to the plastic container and tubing.

Diazepam rectal gel should be stored at a controlled room temperature of 25° but may be exposed to temperatures ranging from 15–30°C.

For further information on chemistry, pharmacology, pharmacokinetics, uses, cautions, chronic toxicity, acute toxicity, drug interactions, laboratory test interferences, and dosage and administration of diazepam, see the Benzodiazepines General Statement 28:24.08.

PREPARATIONS

Diazepam is subject to control under the Federal Controlled Substances Act of 1970 as a schedule IV (C-IV) drug.

Excipients in commercially available drug preparations may have clinically important effects in some individuals; consult specific product labeling for details.

diazePAM

Oral		
Solution	5 mg/5 mL*	diazePAM Solution (C-IV)
Solution, concentrate	5 mg/mL*	diazePAM Intensol® (C-IV), West-ward
		diazePAM Solution Concentrate (C-IV)
Tablets	2 mg*	diazePAM Tablets (C-IV)
		Valium® (C-IV; scored), Genentech
	5 mg*	diazePAM Tablets (C-IV)
		Valium® (C-IV; scored), Genentech
	10 mg*	diazePAM Tablets (C-IV)
		Valium® (C-IV; scored), Genentech

Parenteral		
Injection	5 mg/mL*	diazePAM Injection (C-IV)
Gel	5 mg/mL (2.5, 10, and 20 mg)*	Diastat® Rectal Delivery System (C-IV); in prefilled applicators with pediatric universal or adult applicator tips, Valeant
		diazePAM Gel Rectal Delivery System (C-IV); in prefilled applicators with pediatric universal or adult applicator tips

* available from one or more manufacturer, distributor, and/or repackager by generic (nonproprietary) name

† Use is not currently included in the labeling approved by the US Food and Drug Administration.

Selected Revisions September 28, 2022, © Copyright, March 01, 1980, American Society of Health-System Pharmacists, Inc.

LORazepam

28:24.08 • BENZODIAZEPINES

■ Lorazepam is a benzodiazepine. The drug has anticonvulsant, anxiolytic, and sedative properties.

USES

● Anxiety Disorders

Lorazepam is used for the management of anxiety disorders or for the short-term relief of symptoms of anxiety or anxiety associated with depressive symptoms. The efficacy of lorazepam for long-term use (i.e., longer than 4 months) has not been evaluated. The need for continued therapy with the drug should be periodically reassessed.

● Preoperative Sedation, Anxiolysis, and Amnesia

Lorazepam injection is used for preoperative sedation, anxiolysis, and anterograde amnesia. Administration of lorazepam is especially useful in patients with preoperative anxiety who prefer diminished recall of events associated with the day of surgery.

● Status Epilepticus

Lorazepam injection is used for the treatment of status epilepticus.

Efficacy of IV lorazepam was established in 2 multicenter controlled trials in patients (mostly 18–65 years of age) with tonic-clonic status epilepticus, simple partial and complex partial status epilepticus, or absence status. The first study was a double-blind, randomized, active-control study that compared lorazepam 2 mg (with an additional 2-mg IV dose given if necessary) with diazepam 5 mg (with an additional 5-mg IV dose given if necessary). In this study, 80 or 57% of patients receiving lorazepam or diazepam, respectively, were considered responders, defined as the percentage of patients in whom seizures were terminated within 10 minutes after administration of the drug and who continued to be seizure-free for at least an additional 30 minutes. When an additional dose of study drug was administered to nonresponders, the overall response rate increased to 93% with lorazepam and 86% with diazepam. The second study was a double-blind, dose comparison trial; in this study, 61, 57, and 76% of patients receiving 1, 2, and 4 mg of lorazepam, respectively, were responders (as defined above).

Clinical Perspective

Benzodiazepines are considered the initial drugs of choice for the management of status epilepticus because of their rapid onset of action, demonstrated efficacy, safety, and tolerability.

Status epilepticus is a medical emergency that must be treated promptly to reduce substantial morbidity and mortality. Initial treatment should include standard critical care and supportive therapy (e.g., blood pressure and respiratory support, oxygen, IV access, identification and correction of underlying causes), followed by administration of a benzodiazepine. Although IV lorazepam is generally preferred because of its longer duration of action, studies generally have not identified any substantial differences between IV lorazepam, IV diazepam, and IM midazolam in terms of seizure cessation, and experts consider these therapies to be equivalent first-line options. Selection of an appropriate benzodiazepine should be individualized based on local availability, route of administration, pharmacokinetics, cost, and other factors (e.g., treatment setting). To achieve a rapid therapeutic effect, IV administration of a benzodiazepine is preferred; however, administration via other routes (e.g., IM, rectal, intranasal, buccal) may be considered when IV administration is not possible (e.g., in the prehospital setting). If seizures continue after initial therapy with a benzodiazepine, a second-line anticonvulsant agent (e.g., IV fosphenytoin or phenytoin, IV valproate sodium, IV levetiracetam, IV phenobarbital) should be administered. If refractory status epilepticus occurs, continuous IV infusion of anticonvulsants, IV barbiturates, or general anesthetics may be necessary.

Early treatment with benzodiazepines in the prehospital setting can improve outcomes in patients with status epilepticus. Results of a placebo-controlled study in adults with out-of-hospital status epilepticus indicated that IV administration of benzodiazepines by paramedics was safe and effective in the management of this condition. Findings from this study indicated that both IV lorazepam and IV diazepam were more effective than placebo in controlling status epilepticus by the time of patient arrival in the emergency department. Because the need to establish IV access may delay administration of an IV benzodiazepine in the prehospital environment, use of other less invasive routes of administration may decrease the time to active treatment. Results of a randomized controlled study (RAMPART) indicate that IM administration of midazolam by paramedics in the prehospital setting may improve outcomes in patients with status epilepticus; in this study, 73% of patients who received IM midazolam achieved seizure resolution at the time of arrival in the emergency department compared with 63% of those who received IV lorazepam.

● Sedation in Critical Care Settings

Lorazepam, administered by intermittent injection or continuous IV infusion, has been used for sedation of intubated and mechanically ventilated adults and children in critical care settings† (e.g., intensive care unit [ICU]).

Clinical Perspective

Sedative agents are administered in critically ill patients to reduce agitation and anxiety and increase tolerance to invasive procedures (e.g., mechanical ventilation). The provision of adequate analgesia and other measures to ensure patient comfort is recommended before sedatives are administered. Sedative agents should be titrated to the desired level of sedation; in most cases, a light rather than deep level of sedation is recommended in critically ill, mechanically ventilated adults because of improved clinical outcomes that have been demonstrated (e.g., shortened duration of mechanical ventilation and reduced ICU length of stay). The depth and quality of sedation should be assessed using a validated and reliable assessment tool (e.g., Richmond Agitation-Sedation Scale [RASS], Sedation-Agitation Scale [SAS]). Common sedative agents used in the ICU include benzodiazepines (e.g., midazolam, lorazepam), propofol, and dexmedetomidine. These agents appear to be similarly effective in providing adequate sedation in critically ill, mechanically ventilated adults. However, modest benefits in terms of other clinical outcomes (e.g., reduced duration of mechanical ventilation, shorter time to extubation, reduced risk of delirium) have been observed with the nonbenzodiazepine sedatives (dexmedetomidine and propofol) compared with benzodiazepines.

Comparative studies have demonstrated a shorter time to light sedation and shorter time to extubation with propofol compared with benzodiazepines, and a shorter time to extubation and reduced risk of delirium with dexmedetomidine compared with benzodiazepines. In most of these studies, benzodiazepines were administered as a continuous IV infusion rather than as intermittent IV injections. Because of the apparent advantages and an overall favorable benefit-to-risk profile, experts state that nonbenzodiazepine sedatives (dexmedetomidine or propofol) may be preferred to benzodiazepines (midazolam or lorazepam) in mechanically ventilated, critically ill adults. This recommendation should be considered in the context of the specific clinical situation since benzodiazepines may still be preferred in certain situations (e.g., patients with anxiety, seizures, or alcohol or benzodiazepine withdrawal). When selecting an appropriate sedative agent, the patient's individual sedation goals should be considered in addition to specific drug-related (e.g., pharmacology, pharmacokinetics, adverse effects, availability, cost) and patient-related (e.g., comorbid conditions) factors.

Because of its greater potency and slower clearance, emergence from short-term sedation with lorazepam may be longer than with midazolam; however, comparative studies have suggested that midazolam is associated with greater variability and a longer time to awakening than lorazepam when used for prolonged sedation.

● Schizophrenia

Benzodiazepines have been used for augmentation of antipsychotic therapy or adjunctive therapy in patients with schizophrenia†.

The American Psychiatric Association (APA) suggests that a benzodiazepine may be used for the treatment of akathisia associated with antipsychotic therapy; however, the potential benefits of benzodiazepine therapy should be weighed against the potential adverse effects (e.g., somnolence, cognitive difficulties, problems with coordination, risk of misuse or development of a sedative use disorder, respiratory depression if used in high doses and particularly in combination with alcohol, other sedating medications, or opioids). Benzodiazepines (e.g., lorazepam) also have been used for augmentation treatment of catatonia.

● Cancer Chemotherapy-induced Nausea and Vomiting

Lorazepam also has been used in the management of nausea and vomiting associated with emetogenic cancer chemotherapy†. The American Society of Clinical Oncology (ASCO) guidelines on antiemetic therapy state that lorazepam is a useful adjunct to antiemetic drugs, but is not recommended as a single-agent antiemetic.

● Delirium

Lorazepam also has been used in the management of delirium.† Although there is little evidence to support the use of benzodiazepines alone for general cases of delirium, there may be certain types of delirium for which benzodiazepines may be useful (e.g., delirium related to alcohol or benzodiazepine withdrawal). If a benzodiazepine is used for the treatment of delirium, specific agents with a short duration and no active metabolites (e.g., lorazepam) are preferred.

● Drug-induced Cardiovascular Emergencies

Lorazepam has been used adjunctively in the management of certain drug-induced cardiovascular emergencies† and cocaine-induced acute coronary syndrome†.

DOSAGE AND ADMINISTRATION

● Administration

Lorazepam is administered orally, IM, or by IV injection or IV infusion. *The drug should not be administered by intra-arterial injection since arteriospasm can occur, which may cause gangrene and possibly require amputation.*

Oral Administration

Lorazepam is administered orally as tablets or oral solution.

Lorazepam oral concentrate solution should be mixed with a liquid (e.g., water, juices, carbonated or soda-like beverages) or semi-solid food (e.g., applesauce, pudding) just before administration using only the calibrated dropper provided by the manufacturer.

Parenteral Administration

IM administration: IM injections of lorazepam are administered as undiluted solutions; IM injections should be administered deep into the muscle mass.

IV injection: For direct IV administration, lorazepam injection must be diluted with an equal volume of compatible diluent, such as sterile water for injection, 0.9% sodium chloride injection, or 5% dextrose injection. Following dilution, the solution should be mixed thoroughly by gently inverting the container repeatedly until a homogenous solution is obtained; the solution should not be shaken vigorously. Solutions of lorazepam injection should *not* be used if they appear discolored or contain a precipitate. Following dilution, lorazepam may be injected directly into a vein or into the tubing of an existing IV infusion. Injections should be administered slowly at a rate not exceeding 2 mg/minute. Direct IV injection with the drug should be made with repeated aspiration to ensure that none of the drug is injected intra-arterially and that perivascular extravasation does not occur. Equipment necessary to maintain a patent airway and to support respiration and ventilation should be immediately available prior to administration of IV lorazepam. Vital signs should be monitored during IV infusion of the drug.

IV infusion: A standard concentration of 1 mg/mL has been recommended (see Standardize 4 Safety section below).

Standardize 4 Safety

Standardized concentrations for IV lorazepam have been established through Standardize 4 Safety (S4S), a national patient safety initiative to reduce medication errors, especially during transitions of care. Multidisciplinary expert panels were convened to determine recommended standard concentrations. Because recommendations from the S4S panels may differ from the manufacturer's prescribing

information, caution is advised when using concentrations that differ from labeling, particularly when using rate information from the label. For additional information on S4S (including updates that may be available), see https://www.ashp.org/pharmacy-practice/standardize-4-safety-initiative.

TABLE 1. Standardize 4 Safety Continuous IV Infusion Standard Concentration for Lorazepam

Patient Population	Concentration Standard	Dosing Units
Adults	1 mg/mL	mg/hour

● Dosage

Dosage of lorazepam must be individualized, and the smallest effective dosage should be used (especially in geriatric or debilitated patients, in those with low serum albumin, and in patients currently receiving other CNS depressants) to avoid oversedation.

Anxiety Disorders

The usual initial adult oral dosage of lorazepam for the symptomatic treatment of anxiety is 2–3 mg daily, divided in 2 or 3 doses; dosage should be adjusted if necessary and as tolerated. In geriatric or debilitated patients, lorazepam therapy should be initiated with 1–2 mg daily, divided in 2 or 3 doses; dosage should be adjusted if necessary and as tolerated. Dosage may range from 1–10 mg daily (usually 2–6 mg) in divided doses, with the largest single dose given at bedtime. For insomnia caused by anxiety or transient situational stress in adults, 2–4 mg of lorazepam is given as a single daily dose, usually at bedtime. In patients who have received prolonged (e.g., for several months) lorazepam therapy, abrupt discontinuance of the drug should be avoided since manifestations of withdrawal can be precipitated; if the drug is to be discontinued in such patients, it is recommended that dosage be gradually tapered.

Preoperative Sedation, Anxiolysis, and Amnesia

For preoperative IM use in adults, the usual dose of lorazepam is 0.05 mg/kg administered by deep IM injection at least 2 hours prior to surgery. The IM dose should be individualized, but should not exceed 4 mg.

Alternatively, lorazepam may be administered IV for preoperative use. For preoperative IV use, the usual initial dose of lorazepam for sedation and relief of anxiety is 0.044 mg/kg (or up to 2 mg total, whichever is smaller) administered 15–20 minutes prior to surgery; this dose is sufficient for sedating most adults and generally should not be exceeded in patients older than 50 years of age. For those patients in whom increased lack of recall about perioperative events is considered beneficial, lorazepam doses up to 0.05 mg/kg (maximum total dose of 4 mg) may be administered IV.

Status Epilepticus

For the management of status epilepticus, the usual dose of lorazepam in adults is 4 mg by slow IV injection (rate of 2 mg/minute); if seizures continue or recur after a 10- to 15-minute period of observation, an additional 4-mg dose of the drug may be administered. The manufacturer states that experience with administration of additional doses of lorazepam is limited. IM administration of lorazepam is not recommended for the treatment of status epilepticus because therapeutic plasma concentrations of the drug are not achieved as rapidly as with IV administration of the drug. However lorazepam may be given IM if IV access is not available.

For the management of status epilepticus in children†, IV doses of 0.05–0.1 mg/kg have been used.

Sedation in Critical Care Settings

Dosage of sedative agents should be titrated to the desired level of sedation; in most cases, a light rather than deep level of sedation is recommended in critically ill mechanically ventilated adults because of improved clinical outcomes that have been demonstrated (e.g., shortened duration of mechanical ventilation, reduced ICU length of stay). The depth and quality of sedation should be assessed frequently using a validated and reliable assessment tool (e.g., Richmond Agitation-Sedation Scale [RASS], Sedation-Agitation Scale [SAS]).

If lorazepam is used for sedation in intubated and mechanically ventilated adults in critical care settings†, some experts recommend an IV loading dose of 0.02–0.04 mg/kg (not to exceed 2 mg); the loading dose should be followed by intermittent injections of 0.02–0.06 mg/kg every 2–6 hours as needed or a continuous IV infusion at a rate of 0.01–0.1 mg/kg per hour (not to exceed 10 mg/hour). The infusion rate should be titrated to the lowest effective dosage to provide the desired level of sedation. Frequent assessment of the patient's sedation requirements and tapering of the infusion rate may prevent prolonged sedative effects.

Although there is limited information available on the use of lorazepam for sedation in intubated and mechanically ventilated children in critical care settings†, some clinicians have suggested lorazepam dosages of 0.025–0.05 mg/kg (maximum initial dose of 2 mg) given as intermittent IV infusions every 2–4 hours in children 2 months of age or older. Alternatively, in these pediatric patients, lorazepam may be administered by a continuous IV infusion, at a rate of 0.025 mg/kg per hour (up to 2 mg/hour) which may be titrated as necessary or supplemented with rapid ("bolus") injections of the drug to provide the desired level of sedation. Because of wide interpatient variations in dosage requirements and low hepatic metabolic function, the initial lorazepam dose should be reduced by 50% in infants younger than 2 months of age.

Cancer Chemotherapy-induced Nausea and Vomiting

For the management of nausea and vomiting associated with emetogenic cancer chemotherapy†, including that associated with cisplatin, adults have received 2.5 mg of lorazepam orally the evening before and just after initiation of chemotherapy. Alternatively, adults have received 1.5 mg/m² (usually up to a maximum dose of 3 mg) of lorazepam administered IV (usually over 5 minutes) 45 minutes before initiation of chemotherapy.

Delirium

For the management of delirium† in combination with haloperidol, combined therapy can be initiated in adults with an IV haloperidol dose of 3 mg followed immediately with an IV lorazepam dose of 0.5–1 mg. Dosage of the drugs should then be adjusted according to patient response and tolerance. ECG should be determined at baseline and periodically because of the risk of QT prolongation with haloperidol therapy. (See Uses: Delirium and also see Dosage: IV Dosage in Haloperidol 28:16.08.32.)

Dosage in Renal and Hepatic Impairment

The manufacturer states that a dosage adjustment is *not* required in patients with impaired renal function for single doses of lorazepam injection; however, caution should be exercised with administration of multiple doses of lorazepam injection over a short period of time.

Since the pharmacokinetics of parenteral lorazepam do not appear to be altered in patients with hepatic impairment, dosage adjustment is not necessary in such patients. However, because oral lorazepam may exacerbate hepatic encephalopathy, dosage of oral lorazepam should be adjusted carefully in patients with severe hepatic insufficiency and lower than recommended dosages may be sufficient in these patients.

CAUTIONS

Adverse effects reported with lorazepam are similar to those reported with other benzodiazepines. Changes in vital signs (e.g., respiratory rate, blood pressure) are the most frequent adverse effects associated with parenteral lorazepam administration. For further information on adverse effects reported with benzodiazepines, see Cautions in the Benzodiazepines General Statement 28:24.08. Flumazenil, a benzodiazepine antagonist, can be used in hospitalized patients as an adjunct, not a substitute for, proper management of lorazepam overdose.

● *Precautions and Contraindications*

Lorazepam shares the toxic potentials of the benzodiazepines, and the usual precautions of benzodiazepine administration should be observed. (See Cautions in the Benzodiazepines General Statement 28:24.08.)

A boxed warning has been included in the prescribing information for all benzodiazepines describing the risks of abuse, misuse, addiction, physical dependence, and withdrawal reactions associated with all drugs in this class. Abuse and misuse can result in overdose or death, especially when benzodiazepines are combined with other medicines, such as opioid pain relievers, alcohol, or illicit drugs. Frequent follow-up with patients receiving benzodiazepines is important. Reassess patients regularly to manage their medical conditions and any withdrawal symptoms. Clinicians should assess a patient's risk of abuse, misuse, and addiction. Standardized screening tools are available (https://nida.nih.gov/nidamed-medical-health-professionals/screening-tools-resources/chart-screening-tools). To reduce the risk of acute withdrawal reactions, use a gradual dose taper when reducing the dosage or discontinuing benzodiazepines. Take precautions when benzodiazepines are used in combination with opioid addiction medications.

Drugs that affect the CNS (e.g., phenothiazines, barbiturates, antidepressants, alcohol, scopolamine, monoamine oxidase inhibitors) may have additive CNS effects when used concomitantly with, or during the period of recovery from, lorazepam. Such combinations, or IV lorazepam used alone in higher than recommended doses, can produce excessive sedation which may result in partial airway obstruction. The manufacturer warns that scopolamine does *not* provide additional benefit when used concomitantly with lorazepam, but may increase sedation, hallucinations, and irrational behavior.

Concomitant use of benzodiazepines, including lorazepam, and opiate agonists or opiate partial agonists may result in profound sedation, respiratory depression, coma, and death. Patients receiving lorazepam and/or their caregivers should be apprised of the risks associated with concomitant therapeutic or illicit use of benzodiazepines and opiates. For further information on potential interactions with opiates, see Opiate Agonists and Opiate Partial Agonists under Drug Interactions: CNS Agents, in the Benzodiazepines General Statement 28:24.08.

When lorazepam is administered IV prior to regional or local anesthesia, especially at doses greater than 0.05 mg/kg or when opiate agonists or partial agonists are used concomitantly with recommended lorazepam doses, excessive sedation or drowsiness may occur; these effects may possibly interfere with patient cooperation in determining levels of anesthesia.

Lorazepam should be administered IV only in settings in which continuous monitoring of respiratory and cardiac function (i.e., pulse oximetry) is possible. Safety and efficacy of lorazepam may vary according to the dose administered and clinical status of the patient. Since lorazepam is capable of producing several levels of CNS depression—from mild to deep sedation, facilities, age- and size-appropriate equipment for bag/mask/valve ventilation and intubation, drugs, and skilled personnel necessary for ventilation and intubation, administration of oxygen, assisted or controlled respiration, airway management, and cardiovascular support should be immediately available whenever this drug is administered. Monitoring of vital signs also should continue during the recovery period. Lorazepam injection should be administered with extreme caution to geriatric or debilitated patients, and to patients with compromised pulmonary function (decreased reserve), since underventilation and/or hypoxic cardiac arrest may occur. For deeply sedated pediatric patients, a dedicated individual other than the clinician performing the procedure should monitor the patient throughout the procedure.

Lorazepam should only be used for the treatment of status epilepticus by clinicians experienced in the comprehensive management of the disease. Since these patients may be at increased risk of respiratory depression associated with administration of IV lorazepam, they require careful monitoring of respiratory rate and maintenance of an adequate, patent airway. Ventilatory support also may be needed in some patients. Because of the prolonged duration of action of lorazepam, it should be considered that the sedative effects of the drug (especially after multiple doses) may increase the impairment of consciousness observed in the postictal state.

The manufacturer warns that there is no evidence to date to support the use of lorazepam injection in patients with coma, shock, or acute alcohol intoxication. The manufacturer warns that there are insufficient data to support the use of lorazepam injection for outpatient endoscopic procedures; when these procedures are conducted in inpatients, adequate recovery room observation time is necessary and pharyngeal reflex activity should be minimized prior to the procedure by administering adequate topical or regional anesthesia.

Adverse effects associated with propylene glycol (e.g., lactic acidosis, hyperosmolality, hypotension) or polyethylene glycol (e.g., acute tubular necrosis) may occur in patients receiving lorazepam injection. Manifestations of toxicity are more likely to occur in patients with renal impairment and those receiving higher than recommended dosages, although total daily IV doses as low as 1 mg/kg also have been reported to cause propylene glycol toxicity.

Lorazepam injection is *not* recommended for use in patients with hepatic and/or renal failure, since the drug is most likely conjugated in the liver and since conjugated lorazepam is excreted via the kidneys. However, this does not preclude use of the drug in patients with mild to moderate hepatic or renal disease; in these patients, the lowest possible effective dose of lorazepam injection should be administered since the effects of the drug may be prolonged. The manufacturer states that administration of oral lorazepam may exacerbate hepatic encephalopathy and, therefore, the drug should be used with caution in patients with severe hepatic insufficiency and/or encephalopathy. Dosage of lorazepam should be adjusted carefully in patients with severe hepatic insufficiency; lower than recommended dosages may be sufficient in these patients. Because of the possibility of suicide in depressed patients, oral lorazepam should not be used in such patients without adequate antidepressant therapy.

Patients should be informed of the pharmacologic effects of lorazepam (e.g., sedation, relief of anxiety, lack of recall) and the duration of these effects (8 hours or longer) so that they may adequately perceive the risks and benefits of use of lorazepam injection. Patients should be warned that lorazepam injection may impair their ability to perform activities requiring mental alertness or physical coordination (e.g., operating machinery, driving a motor vehicle) for 24–48 hours following administration of the drug. Impaired performance may persist for longer periods in geriatric patients, in patients using other drugs concomitantly, and as a result of the stress of surgery or general condition of the patient. Patients also should be warned that premature ambulation (within 8 hours of receiving lorazepam injection) may result in injury from falling. Patients also should be warned that concomitant use of lorazepam with sedatives, opiate analgesics (opiate agonists or partial agonists), or tranquilizers may increase the extent and duration of impaired performance, may cause excessive sedation, and, rarely, may interfere with recall and recognition of events on the day of surgery and the following day. Patients should be advised to abstain from consumption of alcoholic beverages for 24–48 hours following administration of lorazepam injection.

Lorazepam is contraindicated in patients with known hypersensitivity to benzodiazepines or any ingredients in the formulation (i.e., polyethylene glycol, propylene glycol, or benzyl alcohol) and in patients with acute angle-closure glaucoma or sleep apnea syndrome. Lorazepam injection also is contraindicated in patients with severe respiratory insufficiency, except in those requiring relief of anxiety and/or diminished recall of events while being mechanically ventilated. In addition, the injection is contraindicated in premature infants because the formulation contains benzyl alcohol.

● **Pediatric Precautions**

Safety and efficacy of lorazepam tablets and oral concentrate solution in children younger than 12 years of age have not been established.

Safety and efficacy of lorazepam injection in pediatric patients younger than 18 years of age have not been established.

In several open label studies conducted in pediatric patients (neonates as young as a few hours up to adolescents 18 years of age), paradoxical excitation, characterized by tremors, agitation, euphoria, logorrhea, and brief episodes of visual hallucinations, was reported in 10–30% of children younger than 8 years of age. Seizures and myoclonus have been reported in pediatric patients (especially in very low birth-weight neonates) receiving lorazepam injection. Brief tonic-clonic seizures were reported in pediatric patients who received lorazepam for the management of atypical petit mal status epilepticus.

FDA warns that repeated or prolonged use of general anesthetics and sedation drugs, including lorazepam, in children younger than 3 years of age or during the third trimester of pregnancy may affect brain development. Animal studies in multiple species, including nonhuman primates, have demonstrated that use for longer than 3 hours of anesthetic and sedation drugs that block *N*-methyl-D-aspartic acid (NMDA) receptors and/or potentiate γ-aminobutyric acid (GABA) activity leads to widespread neuronal and oligodendrocyte cell loss and alterations in synaptic morphology and neurogenesis in the brain, resulting in long-term deficits in cognition and behavior. Across animal species, vulnerability to these neurodevelopmental changes occurs during the period of rapid brain growth or synaptogenesis; this period is thought to correlate with the third trimester of pregnancy through the first year of life in humans, but may extend to approximately 3 years of age. The clinical relevance of these animal findings to humans is not known. While some published evidence suggests that similar deficits in cognition and behavior may occur in children following repeated or prolonged exposure to anesthesia early in life, other studies have found no association between pediatric anesthesia exposure and long-term adverse neurodevelopmental outcomes. Most studies to date have had substantial limitations, and it is not clear whether the adverse neurodevelopmental outcomes observed in children were related to the drug or to other factors (e.g., surgery, underlying illness). There is some clinical evidence that a single, relatively brief exposure to general anesthesia in generally healthy children is unlikely to cause clinically detectable deficits in global cognitive function or serious behavioral disorders; however, further research is needed to fully characterize the effects of exposure to general anesthetics in early life, particularly for prolonged or repeated exposures and in more vulnerable populations (e.g., less healthy children).

Anesthetic and sedation drugs are an essential component of care for children and pregnant women who require surgery or other procedures that cannot be delayed; no specific general anesthetic or sedation drug has been shown to be less likely to cause neurocognitive deficits than any other such drug. Pending further accumulation of data in humans from well-designed studies, decisions regarding the timing of elective procedures requiring anesthesia should take into consideration both the benefits of the procedure and the potential risks. When procedures requiring the use of general anesthetics or sedation drugs are considered for young children or pregnant women, clinicians should discuss with the patient, parent, or caregiver the benefits, risks (including potential risk of adverse neurodevelopmental effects), and appropriate timing and duration of the procedure. FDA states that procedures that are considered medically necessary should not be delayed or avoided.

Lorazepam injection contains benzyl alcohol, polyethylene glycol, and propylene glycol and some pediatric patients (particularly premature and low-birth weight infants or those receiving high doses of the injection) may be susceptible to adverse effects associated with these ingredients. Although a causal relationship has not been established, administration of injections preserved with benzyl alcohol has been associated with toxicity in neonates. Toxicity appears to have resulted from administration of large amounts (i.e., 100–400 mg/kg daily) of benzyl alcohol in these neonates. Exposure to such excessive amounts of benzyl alcohol has been associated with CNS depression, metabolic acidosis, gasping respirations, gradual neurological deterioration, seizures, intracranial hemorrhage, hematologic abnormalities, skin breakdown, hepatic and renal failure, hypotension, bradycardia, and cardiovascular collapse. Although use of drugs preserved with benzyl alcohol should be avoided in neonates whenever possible, the American Academy of Pediatrics (AAP) states that the presence of small amounts of the preservative in a commercially available injection should not proscribe its use when indicated in neonates.

In pediatric patients, propylene glycol present in high doses of lorazepam injections, has been associated with adverse effects, including CNS toxicity, seizures, intraventricular hemorrhage, unresponsiveness, tachypnea, tachycardia, and diaphoresis.

● **Geriatric Precautions**

Clinical trials of lorazepam did not include sufficient numbers of patients ≥65 years of age to determine whether they respond differently than younger adults. However, unless enhanced suppression of recall is desired, patients >50 years of age generally should not be given an initial parenteral lorazepam dose greater than 2 mg since excessive and prolonged sedation may occur.

No age-related differences in the pharmacokinetics of lorazepam have been identified; however, because of greater sensitivity and increased frequency of impaired hepatic or renal function in geriatric patients, the manufacturer suggests that patients in this age group receive initial dosages of the drug in the lower end of the usual range. Geriatric patients should be warned that lorazepam injection may cause excessive sedation for 6–8 hours or longer after surgery.

● **Pregnancy, Fertility, and Lactation**

Pregnancy

Lorazepam may cause fetal toxicity when administered to pregnant women. An increased risk of congenital malformations associated with use of anxiolytic agents (i.e., chlordiazepoxide, diazepam, and/or meprobamate) during the first trimester of pregnancy has been suggested by several human studies. In humans, lorazepam and its glucuronide have been shown to cross the placenta (as determined from samples of umbilical cord blood). The drug has also been shown to cause various adverse fetal effects during reproduction studies in animals. Lorazepam injection should *not* be used during pregnancy. In addition, the manufacturer does *not* recommend preoperative use of the injection for obstetric procedures (e.g., cesarean section) or during labor and delivery, since safety of the injection has not been established in such procedures. Oral or injectable lorazepam should be used during pregnancy only in life-threatening situations or severe disease (e.g., status epilepticus) for which safer drugs cannot be used or are ineffective. The possibility that a woman of childbearing potential may be pregnant at the time lorazepam is initiated should be considered. When lorazepam is administered during pregnancy or if the patient becomes pregnant while receiving the drug, the patient should be advised of the potential hazard to the fetus and about the desirability of discontinuing lorazepam.

Based on animal data, repeated or prolonged use of general anesthetics and sedation drugs, including lorazepam, during the third trimester of pregnancy may result in adverse neurodevelopmental effects in the fetus. The clinical relevance of these animal findings to humans is not known; the potential risk of adverse neurodevelopmental effects should be considered and discussed with pregnant women undergoing procedures requiring general anesthetics and sedation drugs. (See Cautions: Pediatric Precautions.)

Fertility

It is not known whether lorazepam affects fertility in humans. No evidence of impaired fertility was observed in rats following oral administration of lorazepam doses of 20 mg/kg. At doses of 40 mg/kg or more, there was evidence of fetal resorption and increased fetal loss in rabbits.

Lactation

Lorazepam is distributed into milk. The potential exists that lorazepam can cause sedation or other adverse effects in nursing infants. The manufacturer of oral lorazepam states that the drug should not be administered to nursing women unless the potential benefits to the woman outweigh the possible risk to the infant. Nursing infants receiving oral lorazepam should be monitored for adverse effects (e.g., sedation, irritability). The manufacturer of lorazepam injection states that the drug should not be administered to nursing women because of possible adverse effects (e.g., sedation).

CHEMISTRY AND STABILITY

● Chemistry

Lorazepam is a benzodiazepine.

● Stability

Lorazepam oral concentrate solution and lorazepam injection should be stored at 2–8°C and protected from light. Lorazepam tablets should be stored in well-closed containers at 25°C, but may be exposed to temperatures of 15–30°C.

The manufacturer states that lorazepam injection should be diluted prior to IV administration with an equal volume of compatible diluent, including 0.9% sodium chloride injection or 5% dextrose injection. Solutions of lorazepam should not be used if they are discolored or contain a precipitate.

PREPARATIONS

Lorazepam is subject to control under the Federal Controlled Substances Act of 1970 as a schedule IV (C-IV) drug.

Excipients in commercially available drug preparations may have clinically important effects in some individuals; consult specific product labeling for details.

LORazepam

Oral		
For solution, concentrate	2 mg/mL*	LORazepam Solution Concentrate (C-IV)
Tablets	0.5 mg*	Ativan® (C-IV), Valeant LORazepam Tablets (C-IV),
	1 mg*	Ativan® (C-IV; scored), Valeant LORazepam Tablets (C-IV),
	2 mg*	Ativan® (C-IV; scored), Valeant LORazepam Tablets (C-IV),
Parenteral		
Injection	2 mg/mL*	Ativan® (C-IV), West-Ward LORazepam Injection (C-IV),
	4 mg/mL*	Ativan® (C-IV), West-Ward LORazepam Injection (C-IV),

* available from one or more manufacturer, distributor, and/or repackager by generic (nonproprietary) name

† Use is not currently included in the labeling approved by the US Food and Drug Administration.

Selected Revisions June 10, 2024, © Copyright, March 1, 1980, American Society of Health-System Pharmacists, Inc.

Midazolam, Midazolam Hydrochloride

28:24.08 • BENZODIAZEPINES

■ Midazolam is a benzodiazepine. The drug has anticonvulsant, anxiolytic, sedative/hypnotic, and amnestic properties.

USES

● Preoperative Sedation, Anxiolysis, and Amnesia

Midazolam hydrochloride is used parenterally (IM or IV) or orally for preoperative sedation, anxiolysis, and anterograde amnesia. The drug should be used only in monitored settings (i.e., hospital or ambulatory care setting).

Like other benzodiazepines (e.g., lorazepam, diazepam), midazolam is particularly useful as a premedication when relief of anxiety and diminished recall of events associated with the surgical procedure are desired. In studies using memory recall tests, IM midazolam produced anterograde amnesia in 40–73% of adults and up to 85% of pediatric patients. The degree and duration of anterograde amnesia appear to be dose related and can vary based on concomitantly administered drugs.

IM administration of midazolam usually results in less irritation at the site of injection than some other agents commonly used for preoperative sedation, including hydroxyzine or diazepam. In addition, IM midazolam appears to produce a more rapid onset of sedative effects, more pronounced anxiolytic effects during the first hour following administration, and more pronounced anterograde amnesia when compared with IM hydroxyzine. Because of midazolam's relatively rapid onset, short duration of effect, and improved local tolerance at the site of injection compared with other currently available parenteral benzodiazepines, some clinicians consider midazolam the benzodiazepine of choice for preoperative use associated with short surgical procedures. Midazolam also is used IV for preoperative sedation and anxiolysis with good results.

Oral midazolam is commonly used as a premedication to reduce anxiety in pediatric patients undergoing surgery. Studies have demonstrated that children may be separated from their parents as early as 10 minutes after receiving the drug. Efficacy of oral midazolam as a premedicant to sedate and calm pediatric patients prior to the induction of general anesthesia was evaluated in a randomized, double-blind study in patients 6 months to less than 16 years of age with ASA physical status I, II, or III. In this study, more than 90% of patients receiving midazolam achieved satisfactory sedation and anxiolysis within 30 minutes post-treatment. Similarly high proportions of patients exhibited satisfactory ease of separation from their parent or guardian and were cooperative at the time of mask induction with nitrous oxide and halothane administration.

● Procedural Sedation

Midazolam hydrochloride is used IV or orally for procedural sedation, anxiolysis, and amnesia, either alone or in combination with other CNS depressants. The drug should be used only in monitored settings (i.e., hospital or ambulatory care setting). Midazolam produces amnestic and sedative effects, but no analgesia; therefore, the drug is usually administered in conjunction with an analgesic agent.

Procedural sedation is a technique in which sedative or dissociative agents are administered with or without analgesics to allow patients to tolerate painful or unpleasant medical procedures; a depressed state of consciousness is intentionally induced while cardiorespiratory function is maintained. Because sedation is a continuum ranging from minimal sedation to general anesthesia, airway reflexes and cardiorespiratory function may be impaired if a deeper than intended level of sedation is produced. The appropriate level of sedation should be individualized according to the specific procedure and needs of the patient.

Procedures for which midazolam sedation has been used include dental or minor surgical procedures; diagnostic, therapeutic, or endoscopic procedures such as upper GI endoscopy, bronchoscopy, or cystoscopy; cardiac catheterization; coronary angiography; oncology procedures; radiologic procedures (e.g., computerized tomography); and suture of lacerations. Like other benzodiazepines, midazolam is particularly useful for sedation when relief of anxiety and diminished recall of events associated with such procedures are desired.

Anterograde amnesia occurs within 1–5 minutes following IV administration of midazolam and generally persists for 20–40 minutes after IV injection of a single dose. However, onset and duration of action depend on many factors, including the dose of midazolam, rate of administration, and concurrently administered drugs. IV midazolam produced amnestic effects (i.e., no recall of endoscope withdrawal) in 82% of adults in endoscopy studies. In pediatric patients, impaired or no recall of events related to lumbar puncture, bone marrow aspiration, or an oncology procedure was observed in 88–91% of those who received IV midazolam.

Midazolam generally produces less pain and venous irritation (e.g., thrombophlebitis) at the site of IV injection than diazepam. In addition, IV midazolam may have a slightly more rapid onset of action and more pronounced anterograde amnestic effects when compared with IV diazepam. Although data are conflicting, there is some evidence that midazolam's duration of action following IV administration may be slightly shorter than that of diazepam, but further comparative studies are needed; the duration of action of midazolam is substantially shorter than that of IV lorazepam. Because of the drug's relatively rapid onset and short duration of action, pronounced amnesic effect, and improved local tolerance at the site of injection compared with other currently available parenteral benzodiazepines, some clinicians consider midazolam the benzodiazepine of choice for moderate sedation (formerly known as conscious sedation) prior to short procedures.

● Induction and Maintenance of Anesthesia

Midazolam hydrochloride is used IV for induction of general anesthesia prior to administration of other anesthetic agents. Induction with IV midazolam results in anxiolysis, anterograde amnesia, and dose-related hypnotic effects (progressing from sedation to loss of consciousness), but not analgesia. Midazolam also is used as a component of balanced anesthesia (e.g., nitrous oxide and oxygen) for maintenance of anesthesia during short surgical procedures.

There is substantial interpatient variation in induction time and in the dose of midazolam required for induction of anesthesia, especially in young patients and/or patients who have not received premedication with an opiate agonist. Premedication with an opiate agonist results in more rapid and reliable induction of anesthesia within a narrower midazolam dosage range, and smaller doses of midazolam generally are required. Midazolam should not be used alone for maintenance of anesthesia; the drug usually is given in conjunction with inhalation anesthetic agents, balanced anesthesia (e.g., nitrous oxide and oxygen), and/or opiate agonists (e.g., fentanyl). Concurrent use of an opiate agonist usually is necessary to maintain adequate anesthesia.

The benefits of midazolam include its pronounced anterograde amnestic effects and good patient acceptability. The incidence of postoperative emergence delirium, nausea, and vomiting is relatively low following midazolam administration as compared with other anesthetic agents. Because midazolam does not appear to increase intraocular pressure, the drug appears to be safe for use in patients undergoing surgery for ocular trauma. Use of midazolam in patients without underlying ocular disease may result in moderate reduction of intraocular pressure. Midazolam generally has been well tolerated in patients with ischemic heart disease, although mild to moderate alterations in cardiovascular function may occur. Severe hypotension has occurred, however, when midazolam was used with high-dose fentanyl anesthesia in patients undergoing coronary artery bypass grafting procedures. Limited data suggest that midazolam attenuates both the postoperative emergence delirium and the cardiovascular stimulation associated with the use of ketamine during surgery.

IV midazolam has historically been compared with IV thiopental for induction and maintenance of anesthesia, and was considered to be more favorable than thiopental in certain characteristics (e.g., more pronounced anterograde amnesia, more gradual induction of anesthesia, less need for adjuvant anesthetic agents), but not in others (e.g., did not induce anesthesia as rapidly or consistently, required a longer recovery period). However, thiopental is no longer commercially available in the US and its use has been largely replaced by propofol.

● Sedation in Critical Care Settings

Midazolam is used as a continuous IV infusion for sedation of intubated and mechanically ventilated patients in critical care settings (e.g., intensive care unit [ICU]).

Clinical Perspective

Sedative agents are administered in critically ill patients to reduce agitation and anxiety and increase tolerance to invasive procedures (e.g., mechanical ventilation). The provision of adequate analgesia and other measures to ensure patient comfort is recommended before sedatives are administered. Sedative agents should be titrated to the desired level of sedation; in most cases, a light rather than deep level of sedation is recommended in critically ill, mechanically ventilated adults because of improved clinical outcomes that have been demonstrated (e.g., shortened duration of mechanical ventilation and reduced ICU length of stay). The depth and quality of sedation should be assessed using a validated and reliable assessment tool (e.g., Richmond Agitation-Sedation Scale [RASS], Sedation-Agitation Scale [SAS]). Common sedative agents used in the ICU include benzodiazepines (e.g., midazolam, lorazepam), propofol, and dexmedetomidine. These agents appear to be similarly effective in providing adequate sedation in critically ill, mechanically ventilated adults. However, modest benefits in terms of other clinical outcomes (e.g., reduced duration of mechanical ventilation, shorter time to extubation, reduced risk of delirium) have been observed with the nonbenzodiazepine sedatives (dexmedetomidine and propofol) compared with benzodiazepines.

Comparative studies have demonstrated a shorter time to light sedation and shorter time to extubation with propofol compared with benzodiazepines, and a shorter time to extubation and reduced risk of delirium with dexmedetomidine compared with benzodiazepines. In most of these studies, benzodiazepines were administered as a continuous IV infusion rather than as intermittent IV injections. Because of the apparent advantages and an overall favorable benefit-to-risk profile, experts state that nonbenzodiazepine sedatives (dexmedetomidine or propofol) may be preferred to benzodiazepines (midazolam or lorazepam) in mechanically ventilated, critically ill adults. This recommendation should be considered in the context of the specific clinical situation since benzodiazepines may still be preferred in certain situations (e.g., patients with anxiety, seizures, or alcohol or benzodiazepine withdrawal). When selecting an appropriate sedative agent, the patient's individual sedation goals should be considered in addition to specific drug-related (e.g., pharmacology, pharmacokinetics, adverse effects, availability, cost) and patient-related (e.g., comorbid conditions) factors.

Because of its greater potency and slower clearance, emergence from short-term sedation with lorazepam may be longer than with midazolam; however, comparative studies have suggested that midazolam is associated with greater variability and a longer time to awakening than lorazepam when used for prolonged sedation.

• Seizure Disorders

Status Epilepticus

Midazolam hydrochloride is used IM for the treatment of status epilepticus. While IM midazolam is FDA-labeled for use only in adults, the drug also has been used in pediatric patients† for the treatment of status epilepticus.

Midazolam also has been administered by intranasal† and buccal† routes for treatment of status epilepticus; limitations of these routes include unpredictable absorption, difficulty with administration during an acute seizure episode, and lack of commercial availability.

Clinical Perspective

Benzodiazepines are considered the initial drugs of choice for the management of status epilepticus because of their rapid onset of action, demonstrated efficacy, safety, and tolerability.

Status epilepticus is a medical emergency that must be treated promptly to reduce substantial morbidity and mortality. Initial treatment should include standard critical care and supportive therapy (e.g., blood pressure and respiratory support, oxygen, IV access, identification and correction of underlying causes), followed by administration of a benzodiazepine. Although IV lorazepam is generally preferred because of its longer duration of action, studies generally have not identified any substantial differences between IV lorazepam, IV diazepam, and IM midazolam in terms of seizure cessation, and experts consider these therapies to be equivalent first-line options. Selection of an appropriate benzodiazepine should be individualized based on local availability, route of administration, pharmacokinetics, cost, and other factors (e.g., treatment setting). If seizures continue after initial therapy with a benzodiazepine, a second-line anticonvulsant agent (e.g., IV fosphenytoin or phenytoin, IV valproate sodium, IV levetiracetam,

IV phenobarbital) should be administered. If refractory status epilepticus occurs, continuous IV infusion of anticonvulsants, IV barbiturates, or general anesthetics may be necessary.

Although IV administration of a benzodiazepine is the preferred method of treatment to achieve a rapid therapeutic effect in patients with status epilepticus, the need to establish IV access may delay administration of the drug in the prehospital environment. Results of a randomized controlled study (RAMPART) indicate that IM administration of midazolam by paramedics in the prehospital setting may improve outcomes in patients with status epilepticus; in this study, 73% of patients who received IM midazolam achieved seizure resolution at the time of arrival in the emergency department compared with 63% of those who received IV lorazepam.

Acute Repetitive Seizures or Seizure Clusters

Midazolam nasal spray is used for the acute treatment of intermittent, stereotypic episodes of frequent seizure activity (i.e., seizure clusters, acute repetitive seizures) that are distinct from the patient's usual seizure pattern.

Efficacy of intranasal midazolam for this use has been established in a randomized, double-blind, placebo-controlled study in epileptic patients 12 years of age or older who were receiving a stable anticonvulsant regimen, but were experiencing intermittent seizure activity distinct from their usual seizure pattern. The primary efficacy end point (i.e., termination of seizures within 10 minutes after administration of study drug and absence of recurrence within 6 hours) was achieved in substantially more patients receiving intranasal midazolam than those receiving placebo. Patients who received midazolam also experienced a longer time to the next seizure than those who received placebo.

• Other Uses

Parenterally administered midazolam has been used in the management of acute agitation†.

DOSAGE AND ADMINISTRATION

• Administration

Midazolam hydrochloride is administered orally, by IM or slow IV injection, or by IV infusion. Midazolam also has been used in IV patient-controlled analgesia (PCA). Midazolam is administered intranasally. Midazolam also has been orally administered as the maleate salt†; however, midazolam maleate currently is not commercially available in the US.

Because serious and life-threatening adverse cardiorespiratory effects can occur during therapy with midazolam, provision should be made for monitoring, detecting, and correcting such effects in every patient in whom the drug is administered, regardless of age or health status.

When IV or oral midazolam is used for sedation or anesthesia, the drug should be administered in a hospital or ambulatory care setting equipped to provide continuous monitoring of cardiorespiratory function. Resuscitative equipment, drugs, and personnel for airway and ventilation management should be immediately available. For deeply sedated pediatric patients, a dedicated individual other than the clinician performing the procedure should monitor the patient throughout the procedure.

When IM midazolam is used for status epilepticus, the drug should be administered in a monitored setting that allows for immediate access to resuscitative drugs, and the patient's cardiorespiratory function should be continuously monitored until stabilized.

When midazolam nasal spray is used, consideration should be given to administering the drug under the supervision of a healthcare professional.

Parenteral Administration

Midazolam Hydrochloride Injection for Sedation or Anesthesia

Midazolam hydrochloride injection is administered IV or IM for sedation or anesthesia; the parenteral preparation should not be administered by any other route (e.g., intrathecal, intra-arterial). Care should be taken to avoid intra-arterial injection or extravasation of the drug.

IM injection: IM injections of midazolam should be administered deep into a large muscle mass.

IV injection: IV injections of midazolam should be administered in incremental doses. The drug is a potent sedative that requires slow administration and individualized titration of dosage. The manufacturer states that the appropriate dose usually is injected over 2 or more minutes at intervals of at least 2 minutes for procedural sedation in healthy patients; incremental doses and the rate of IV injection should be reduced in patients ≥60 years of age, in debilitated patients, in patients with chronic disease states (e.g., congestive heart failure), and in patients with decreased pulmonary reserve, since such patients are at increased risk of underventilation, airway obstructions, and apnea, and the time to peak effect may be slower. For induction of anesthesia, the appropriate dose usually is injected over 20–30 seconds; supplemental doses may be given at 2-minute intervals. To facilitate dosage titration, the commercially available 1-mg/mL midazolam injection may be used, or the 1- or 5-mg/mL injection may be diluted with 0.9% sodium chloride injection or 5% dextrose injection. For procedural sedation, use of midazolam hydrochloride injection containing 1 mg/mL (of midazolam) is recommended to facilitate slow IV injection of the drug.

IV infusion: the manufacturer recommends that the 5-mg/mL midazolam injection should be diluted to a concentration of 0.5 mg/mL with 0.9% sodium chloride injection or 5% dextrose injection. Other standard concentrations for continuous IV infusion of midazolam have been recommended by ASHP's Standardize 4 Safety initiative in adults and pediatric patients (see Standardize 4 Safety section below).

Standardize 4 Safety

Standardize 4 safety (S4S) is a national patient safety initiative to standardize drug concentrations to reduce medication errors, especially during transitions of care. Multidisciplinary expert panels were convened to determine recommended standard concentrations. Because recommendations from the S4S panels may differ from the manufacturer's prescribing information, caution is advised when using concentrations that differ from labeling, particularly when using rate information from the label. For additional information on S4S (including updates that may be available), see https://www.ashp.org/pharmacy-practice/standardize-4-safety-initiative.

TABLE 1. Standardize 4 Safety Continuous IV Infusion Standard Concentrations for Midazolam

Patient Population	Concentration Standard	Dosing Units
Adults	1 mg/mL	mg/hr
	5 mg/mL	
Pediatric patients (<50 kg)	0.3 mg/mL (easier pump programming than 0.35 mg/mL less decimal)	mg/kg/hr
	1 mg/mL	
	5 mg/mL	

TABLE 2. Standardize 4 Safety PCA Standard Concentrations for Midazolam

Patient Population	Concentration Standard	Dosing Units
Adults	1 mg/mL	mg/kg/hr
	5 mg/mL	
Pediatric patients (<50 kg)	0.1 mg/mL	mg/kg/hr
	2 mg/mL	
	5 mg/mL	

Midazolam Hydrochloride Injection for Status Epilepticus

Midazolam hydrochloride injection (Seizalam®) should be administered by IM injection into the mid-outer thigh (vastus lateralis muscle). Administration of the injection by a clinician who has adequate training in the recognition and management of status epilepticus is recommended.

Oral Administration

Midazolam oral solution is intended for use in monitored settings (e.g., hospital or ambulatory care settings, including physician and dental offices) only, and is not intended for chronic or home use. For instruction on use of the special press-in bottle adapter and oral dispensers for administration of midazolam oral syrup, the manufacturer's labeling should be consulted. The drug should be administered from the individual oral dispenser directly into the child's mouth; the oral solution should *not* be mixed with any other liquid (e.g., grapefruit juice) prior to administration. Although the effect of food on absorption of the oral solution has not been determined, food intake generally is precluded prior to procedural sedation in pediatric patients.

Intranasal Administration

Midazolam nasal spray is administered intranasally using a single-dose nasal spray unit supplied by the manufacturer. Each nasal spray unit delivers 5 mg of midazolam in 0.1 mL of solution. The intranasal preparation is commercially available in boxes of 2 nasal spray units; each unit is contained within an individual blister pack that should not be opened until ready to use. The nasal spray unit should not be tested or primed before use. The manufacturer's instructions should be consulted for additional information on use of the midazolam nasal spray.

● Dosage

Midazolam is commercially available as midazolam or the hydrochloride salt; dosage is expressed in terms of midazolam. Midazolam is a potent sedative that requires individualized dosing.

When midazolam is used for sedation or anesthesia, dosage must be carefully adjusted according to individual requirements and response, age, body weight, physical and clinical status, underlying pathologic condition(s), type and amount of premedication or concomitant medication, and the nature and duration of the surgical or other procedure; however, individual response to the drug also may vary independent of these factors. Titration should be more gradual in patients 60 years of age and older for procedural sedation, in those 55 years of age and older for induction of anesthesia, and in patients with chronic debilitating diseases. Excessive doses or rapid or single large IV injections may result in respiratory depression and/or arrest, particularly in geriatric or debilitated patients and in patients receiving other cardio-respiratory depressants concomitantly. The smallest effective dose should be used, especially in geriatric and/or debilitated patients.

It should be recognized that the depth of sedation/anxiolysis needed for pediatric patients depends on the type of procedure performed. For example, simple light sedation in the preoperative period is different from the deeper sedation required for a therapeutic or diagnostic procedure (e.g., endoscopy); therefore, there is a broad dosage range. For all pediatric patients, regardless of the indications for sedation/anxiolysis, it is vital to titrate the midazolam dose and the dose of other concomitant drugs slowly for the desired clinical effect. Unlike adults, pediatric patients generally receive increments of midazolam on a mg/kg basis; drug dose in obese pediatric patients should be calculated on the basis of ideal body weight. Pediatric patients generally require higher dosages of midazolam on a mg/kg basis than adults, and pediatric patients younger than 6 years of age generally require higher dosages on a mg/kg basis than older pediatric patients and may require closer monitoring.

When midazolam is used for sedation in geriatric patients, the initial dose should be reduced, since some degree of organ impairment frequently is present. Dosage requirements in this age group generally appear to decrease with increasing age, and the possibility of profound and/or prolonged effects should be considered in older and/or debilitated patients. Low doses of midazolam usually are required in high-risk surgical patients, debilitated patients, and geriatric patients when the drug is administered with or without premedication.

Preoperative Sedation, Anxiolysis, and Amnesia

For preoperative sedation, anxiolysis, and amnesia in good-risk (e.g., ASA Physical Status I and II) *adults younger than 60 years of age*, the usual dose of midazolam is 0.07–0.08 mg/kg (about 5 mg) administered by IM injection approximately 30–60 minutes prior to surgery. The dosage must be individualized and reduced when IM midazolam is administered to patients with chronic obstructive pulmonary disease, other higher-risk surgical patients, patients 60 years of age or older, and patients who have received opiate agonists or other CNS depressants concomitantly. In a study in patients 60 years of age or older who did not receive concomitant opiate agonist therapy, IM doses of 2–3 mg (0.02–0.05 mg/kg) reportedly produced adequate sedation during the preoperative period; the manufacturer states that an IM midazolam dose of 1 mg may be sufficient in some geriatric patients if the anticipated intensity and duration of sedation are less critical. As with any potential respiratory depressant, such patients should be observed for signs of cardiorespiratory depression following administration of IM midazolam. Sedative effects usually are apparent within 15 minutes and peak at 30–60 minutes. Midazolam can be administered concomitantly with atropine sulfate, scopolamine hydrochloride, and/or reduced doses of opiate agonists.

If IM midazolam is used for preoperative sedation in *non-neonatal pediatric patients*, the usual dose is 0.1–0.15 mg/kg; doses in this range usually are effective and do not prolong emergence from general anesthesia. Sedation after IM administration of midazolam is age and dose dependent; higher doses may result in deeper and more prolonged sedation. For more anxious patients, IM doses of up to 0.5 mg/kg have been used. The manufacturer states that the total IM dose usually does not exceed 10 mg, although this has not been systematically studied. If midazolam is administered with an opiate, the initial dose of each drug must be reduced. IM midazolam may be used to initially sedate pediatric patients in order to facilitate less traumatic insertion of an IV catheter for further dosage titration.

If IV midazolam is used for preoperative sedation in *non-neonatal pediatric patients*, the usual dose (as an intermittent injection) is age dependent; prolonged sedation and risk of hypoventilation may be associated with the higher doses in each recommended range. IV injections of midazolam should be administered over 2–3 minutes. It is essential to wait 2–3 minutes to fully evaluate the sedative effect before starting the procedure or administering a repeat dose. In *pediatric patients 6 months to 5 years of age*, an initial IV dose of 0.05–0.1 mg/kg is recommended; a total dose of up to 0.6 mg/kg may be required to reach the desired end point, but usually does not exceed a total of 6 mg. In *pediatric patients 6–12 years of age*, an initial IV dose of 0.025–0.05 mg/kg is recommended; a total dose of up to 0.4 mg/kg may be required to reach the desired end point, but usually does not exceed a total of 10 mg. *Pediatric patients 12–16 years of age* should be dosed as adults; although some patients in this age range may require higher than recommended adult doses, the total dose usually does not exceed 10 mg. In nonintubated pediatric patients younger than 6 months of age, limited dosing information is available. The manufacturer states that because it is uncertain when a patient transfers from a neonatal to pediatric physiology, dosing recommendations are unclear in nonintubated pediatric patients younger than 6 months of age. However, because such patients are vulnerable to airway obstruction and hypoventilation, titration of drug dose in small increments to clinical effect and careful monitoring are essential.

If oral midazolam is used for preoperative sedation in *pediatric patients 6 months to 16 years of age*, a single dose of 0.25–0.5 mg/kg is recommended, depending on the status of the patient and the desired effect, up to a maximum of 20 mg. In general, it is recommended that the dose be individualized and modified based on patient age, level of anxiety, concomitantly administered drugs, and medical need. Younger pediatric patients (e.g., 6 months to younger than 6 years of age) and less cooperative patients may require a higher than usual oral dose of up to 1 mg/kg (up to a maximum of 20 mg). A dose of 0.25 mg/kg may be sufficient for older children 6–16 years of age or for cooperative patients, especially if the anticipated intensity and duration of sedation are less critical. For pediatric patients with cardiac or respiratory compromise, other higher-risk surgical pediatric patients, and pediatric patients who have received concomitant opiates or other CNS depressants, an oral dose of 0.25 mg/kg should be considered. Use of the oral solution in children younger than 6 months of age has not been established.

Procedural Sedation

For procedural sedation, midazolam may be administered by slow IV injection or as an oral solution before the procedure. In non-neonatal pediatric patients, IM midazolam may be used to initially sedate the patient in order to facilitate less traumatic insertion of an IV catheter for further dosage titration. The manufacturer of midazolam hydrochloride injection states that for peroral procedures (e.g., upper GI endoscopy, bronchoscopy), use of a topical anesthetic is generally recommended, and for bronchoscopy, use of an opiate analgesic for premedication also is generally recommended. For procedural sedation, premedication with an opiate agonist appears to produce less variable response to midazolam.

If IV midazolam is used for procedural sedation in healthy adults younger than 60 years of age, the manufacturer states that dosage should be titrated slowly to the desired effect (e.g., onset of slurred speech). The initial IV dose should not exceed 2.5 mg (administered over at least 2 minutes), although some patients may respond to as little as 1 mg of the drug. Patients 60 years of age or older and debilitated or chronically ill patients, and patients with decreased pulmonary reserve should receive 1–1.5 mg as an initial IV dose over a longer period of injection. The manufacturer recommends that not more than 1.5 mg over at least 2 minutes be administered as an initial dose in these patients. After waiting at least 2 minutes to fully evaluate the patient's clinical response, midazolam dosage may be further titrated in small increments if further sedative effect is required. Patients 60 years of age or older, chronically ill and/or debilitated patients, or patients with decreased pulmonary reserve should receive incremental doses of not more than 1 mg of midazolam. A total dose of up to 5 mg generally is adequate for procedural sedation in an average healthy adult younger than 60 years of age, and a total dose of up to 3.5 mg usually is adequate for patients 60 years of age or older, chronically ill and/or debilitated patients, and patients with decreased pulmonary reserve. If a thorough clinical evaluation clearly indicates a need for additional doses of midazolam to maintain the desired level of sedation, additional doses of the drug may be administered in increments of approximately 25% of the initial dose used to reach the first sedative end point. Some clinicians have recommended initiating dosing with 0.5–2 mg and repeating doses, as necessary, at 2- to 3-minute intervals up to a total dose of 0.1–0.15 mg/kg. In patients 60 years of age and older, these clinicians have recommended reducing midazolam dosage by 25% or more.

If IV midazolam is used concomitantly with an opiate agonist or other CNS depressant, dosage requirements of midazolam may be reduced by about 30% in healthy adults younger than 60 years of age and by at least 50% in patients 60 years of age or older, chronically ill and/or debilitated patients, and patients with decreased pulmonary reserve. Because the risk of underventilation or apnea is greatest in geriatric patients, patients with chronic debilitating disease, and patients with decreased pulmonary reserve, and because peak effect of the drug may occur later in these patients, increments in dose should be smaller, and the rate of injection should be slower.

If IM midazolam is used for procedural sedation in *non-neonatal pediatric patients*, the usual dose is 0.1–0.15 mg/kg. Sedation after IM administration of midazolam is age and dose dependent; higher doses may result in deeper and more prolonged sedation. For more anxious patients, IM doses of up to 0.5 mg/kg have been used. The manufacturer states that the total IM dose usually does not exceed 10 mg, although this has not been systematically studied. If midazolam is administered with an opiate, the initial dose of each must be reduced.

If IV midazolam is used for procedural sedation in *non-neonatal pediatric patients*, the usual IV dose (as an intermittent injection) is age dependent; prolonged sedation and risk of hypoventilation may be associated with the higher doses in each recommended range. IV injections of midazolam should be administered over 2–3 minutes. It is essential to wait 2–3 minutes to fully evaluate the sedative effect before starting the procedure or administering a repeat dose. In *pediatric patients 6 months to 5 years of age*, an initial IV dose of 0.05–0.1 mg/kg is recommended; a total dose of up to 0.6 mg/kg may be required to reach the desired end point, but usually does not exceed a total of 6 mg. In *pediatric patients 6–12 years of age*, an initial IV dose of 0.025–0.05 mg/kg is recommended; a total dose of up to 0.4 mg/kg may be required to reach the desired end point, but usually does not exceed a total of 10 mg. *Pediatric patients 12–16 years of age* should be dosed as adults; although some patients in this age range may require higher than recommended adult doses, the total dose usually does not exceed 10 mg. In nonintubated pediatric patients younger than 6 months of age, limited dosing information is available. The manufacturer states that because it is uncertain when a patient transfers from a neonatal to pediatric physiology, dosing recommendations are unclear in nonintubated pediatric patients younger than 6 months of age. However, because such patients are vulnerable to airway obstruction and hypoventilation, titration of drug dose in small increments to clinical effect and careful monitoring are essential.

If oral midazolam is used for procedural sedation in *pediatric patients 6 months to 16 years of age*, a single dose of 0.25–0.5 mg/kg is recommended, depending on the status of the patient and the desired effect, up to a maximum of 20 mg. In general, it is recommended that the dose be individualized and modified based on patient age, level of anxiety, concomitantly administered drugs, and medical need. Younger pediatric patients (e.g., 6 months to younger than 6 years of age) and less cooperative patients may require a higher than usual oral dose of up to 1 mg/kg (up to a maximum of 20 mg). A dose of 0.25 mg/kg may be sufficient for older children 6–16 years of age or for cooperative patients, especially if the anticipated intensity and duration of sedation are less critical. For pediatric patients with cardiac or respiratory compromise, other higher-risk surgical pediatric patients, and pediatric patients who have received concomitant opiates or other CNS depressants, an oral dose of 0.25 mg/kg should be considered. Use of the oral solution in children younger than 6 months of age has not been established.

Induction and Maintenance of Anesthesia

For induction of general anesthesia, midazolam should be administered prior to other anesthetic agents. Because individual response to midazolam is variable, especially when opiate agonist premedication is not used, dosage of midazolam should be titrated carefully to the desired clinical effect, taking into consideration the patient's age and clinical status. When midazolam is administered prior to other IV agents for induction of anesthesia, the initial dose of each of these agents may be substantially reduced, in some instances to as low as 25% of the usual initial dose of the individual agents.

For induction of general anesthesia prior to administration of other anesthetic agents, average adults younger than 55 years of age who have not received premedications usually require an initial midazolam dose of 0.3–0.35 mg/kg, administered IV over 20–30 seconds; approximately 2 minutes should be allowed for clinical effect. Some clinicians have suggested a lower initial dose (e.g., 0.2 mg/kg) in these adults. Supplemental doses of about 25% of the initial dose may be given as necessary to complete induction. Alternatively, induction of anesthesia may be completed with inhalation agents. Total IV induction doses of up to 0.6 mg/kg may be required in some resistant patients, but such doses may prolong recovery from anesthesia. Patients 55 years of age or older who have not been premedicated usually require lower induction doses of midazolam; the manufacturer recommends an initial IV induction dose of 0.3 mg/kg in these patients. Patients with severe systemic disease or other debilitation who have not been premedicated also usually require lower induction doses. Initial IV doses of 0.2–0.25 mg/kg usually are adequate in such patients, and doses as low as 0.15 mg/kg may be adequate for induction in some debilitated patients.

In premedicated patients, especially those who have received an opiate agonist, the usual IV induction dose of midazolam is 0.15–0.35 mg/kg. In premedicated adults younger than 55 years of age, the usual induction dose is 0.25 mg/kg administered IV over 20–30 seconds; about 2 minutes should be allowed for clinical effect. In premedicated, good-risk (e.g., ASA I and II) adults older than 55 years of age, an initial IV induction dose of 0.2 mg/kg is recommended by the manufacturer. In some premedicated patients with severe systemic disease or debilitation, an initial IV induction dose of 0.15 mg/kg may be sufficient.

For maintenance of anesthesia as a component of balanced anesthesia during surgical procedures, premedication with an opiate agonist is especially recommended. Midazolam may be administered in incremental IV doses of approximately 25% of the induction dose when lightening of anesthesia is evident and repeated, as necessary, to maintain the required level of anesthesia.

Sedation in Critical Care Settings

Dosage of sedative agents should be titrated to the desired level of sedation; in most cases, a light rather than deep level of sedation is recommended in critically ill mechanically ventilated adults because of improved clinical outcomes that have been demonstrated (e.g., shortened duration of mechanical ventilation, reduced ICU length of stay). The depth and quality of sedation should be assessed frequently using a validated and reliable assessment tool (e.g., Richmond Agitation-Sedation Scale [RASS], Sedation-Agitation Scale [SAS]).

For sedation in intubated and mechanically ventilated adult patients in critical care settings (e.g., ICU), midazolam is administered as a continuous IV infusion. In adults, if a loading dose is necessary to initiate sedation rapidly, 0.01–0.05 mg/kg (approximately 0.5–4 mg for a typical adult) may be given slowly or infused over several minutes. This dose may be repeated at 10- to 15-minute intervals until adequate sedation is achieved. For maintenance of sedation in adults, the usual initial infusion rate is 0.02–0.1 mg/kg per hour (approximately 1–7 mg per hour). Higher loading or maintenance infusion rates occasionally may be required in some patients. The lowest recommended doses should be used in patients with residual effects from anesthetic drugs, or in those currently receiving other sedatives or opiates. Individual response to midazolam is variable and the infusion rate should be titrated to the desired level of sedation, taking into account the patient's

age, clinical status, and current drugs. In general, midazolam should be infused at the lowest rate that produces the desired level of sedation. Assessment of sedation should be performed at regular intervals and the infusion rate adjusted up or down by 25–50% of the initial infusion rate to ensure adequate titration of the sedation level. Larger adjustments or even a small, incremental dose may be necessary if rapid changes in the level of sedation are required. In addition, the infusion rate should be decreased by 10–25% every few hours to find the minimum effective infusion rate. Finding the minimum effective infusion rate decreases the potential accumulation of midazolam and provides for the most rapid recovery once the infusion is terminated. Patients who exhibit agitation, hypertension, or tachycardia in response to noxious stimulation, but who are otherwise adequately sedated, may benefit from concomitant administration of an opioid analgesic; however, addition of an opiate generally will reduce the minimum effective midazolam infusion rate.

For sedation of intubated non-neonatal pediatric patients, midazolam generally is initiated with an IV loading dose of 0.05–0.2 mg/kg administered over at least 2–3 minutes; the drug should *not* be administered as a rapid IV injection. The loading dose may be followed by a continuous IV infusion to maintain the desired clinical effect. Based on pharmacokinetic parameters and clinical experience, continuous IV infusions of midazolam should be initiated at a rate of 0.06–0.12 mg/kg per hour (1–2 mcg/kg per minute). The infusion rate may be increased or decreased (generally by 25% of the initial or subsequent infusion rate) as required, or supplemental IV doses of midazolam may be administered to increase or maintain the desired effect. Frequent patient assessment at regular intervals using standard pain/sedation scales is recommended. Midazolam infusions have been used in pediatric patients whose trachea was intubated but who were allowed to breathe spontaneously; however, assisted ventilation is recommended for pediatric patients who are receiving other CNS depressants (e.g., opiates). Midazolam elimination may be delayed in patients receiving concomitant drugs (e.g., drugs interfering with midazolam metabolism), patients with hepatic dysfunction, patients with low cardiac output (especially those requiring inotropic support), and in neonates. Hypotension may be observed in patients who are critically ill, particularly those receiving opiates and/or if midazolam is administered rapidly. When initiating a midazolam infusion in pediatric patients who are hemodynamically compromised, the usual loading dose should be titrated in small increments and the patient monitored for hemodynamic instability (e.g., hypotension). These patients also are vulnerable to the respiratory depressant effects of midazolam and require careful monitoring of respiratory rate and oxygen saturation.

For sedation of intubated preterm neonates (i.e., born at less than 32 weeks' gestation) in critical care settings, midazolam generally is initiated as an IV infusion at a rate of 0.03 mg/kg per hour (0.5 mcg/kg per minute); for sedation of intubated neonates who were born after 32 weeks of gestation, midazolam is generally initiated as an IV infusion at a rate of 0.06 mg/kg per hour (1 mcg/kg per minute). IV loading doses should *not* be used in neonates; rather, the infusion may be administered more rapidly for the first several hours to establish therapeutic plasma drug concentrations. The infusion rate should be reassessed carefully and frequently, particularly after the first 24 hours, to administer the lowest possible effective dose and to reduce the potential for drug accumulation. This is particularly important because of the potential for adverse effects related to benzyl alcohol metabolism if not using the preservative-free formulation. Hypotension may be observed in critically ill neonates and in preterm and term neonates, especially in those receiving fentanyl and/or in patients in whom midazolam is administered rapidly. Because of an increased risk of apnea, extreme caution is advised when sedating a preterm or former preterm neonate whose trachea is not intubated.

Status Epilepticus

For the treatment of status epilepticus in adults, the manufacturer recommends a single midazolam dose of 10 mg by IM injection. The manufacturer states that safety and efficacy of midazolam for the treatment of status epilepticus have not been established in pediatric patients. However, the drug has been used in pediatric patients†. Some clinicians recommend an IM midazolam dose of 10 mg for the treatment of status epilepticus in patients weighing more than 40 kg and a dose of 5 mg for those weighing 13–40 kg. Other clinicians have recommended a usual weight-based dose of 0.15–0.3 mg/kg in both children and adults.

Acute Repetitive Seizures or Seizure Clusters

For the acute treatment of intermittent, stereotypic episodes of frequent seizure activity (e.g., seizure clusters, acute repetitive seizures), the recommended initial dose of intranasal midazolam in adults and pediatric patients 12 years of age or older is 1 spray (5 mg) into one nostril. An additional spray into the opposite nostril may be administered after 10 minutes if a response is not obtained with the first dose; however, a second dose should not be administered if the patient has difficulty breathing or excessive sedation that is uncharacteristic for the patient during a seizure cluster episode. No more than 2 doses should be used to treat a single seizure episode.

The manufacturer recommends that midazolam nasal spray be used to treat no more than one seizure episode every 3 days and no more than 5 seizure episodes a month.

CAUTIONS

Adverse effects reported with midazolam are similar to those reported with other benzodiazepines. Changes in vital signs (e.g., respiratory rate, blood pressure, pulse rate) are the most frequent adverse effects associated with parenteral midazolam administration. For further information on adverse effects reported with benzodiazepines, see Cautions in the Benzodiazepines General Statement 28:24.08.. The immediate availability of flumazenil, a specific benzodiazepine reversal agent, is highly recommended.

● Cardiorespiratory Effects

Midazolam can depress respiration. Relatively small doses, such as those used for preoperative sedation, usually do not substantially impair respiratory function; however, relatively large doses (e.g., more than 0.1–0.2 mg/kg) may substantially depress the ventilatory response to carbon dioxide (CO_2) stimulation. In addition, some patients (e.g., geriatric patients, patients with chronic obstructive pulmonary disease) may be predisposed to respiratory depression induced by midazolam.

Decreases in tidal volume and/or respiratory rate occur in about 23 or 11% of adults following IV or IM administration of midazolam, respectively. Apnea occurs in approximately 15% of adults receiving the drug parenterally. Desaturation or apnea has been reported in 4.6 or 2.8%, respectively, of pediatric patients receiving the drug IV. Hypoxia and laryngospasm were each reported in 2% of pediatric patients receiving the drug orally, and respiratory depression, rhonchi, airway obstruction, or upper airway obstruction was reported in 1% of these patients. Hypercarbia and stridor generally have been reported in less than 1% of patients receiving the drug orally. Serious, occasionally fatal, cardiorespiratory effects, including respiratory depression, apnea, respiratory arrest, and/or cardiac arrest, have occurred in patients receiving midazolam, particularly when the drug was used for procedural sedation. In some patients in whom midazolam-induced respiratory depression was not promptly recognized and effectively managed, hypoxic encephalopathy or death has resulted. Although many of the serious cardiorespiratory adverse effects reported to date have occurred in patients receiving excessive doses or rapid IV injection or infusion of midazolam, in geriatric or debilitated and/or higher-risk surgical patients, and in patients receiving other cardiorespiratory depressants concomitantly, some of these adverse reactions have occurred in younger, healthy patients, including those who did not receive concomitant drugs, and in patients receiving midazolam doses within the dosage range recommended by the manufacturer. Patients with chronic obstructive pulmonary disease appear to be particularly sensitive to the respiratory depressant effects of midazolam (e.g., impairment of the ventilatory response to CO_2), exhibiting more marked and prolonged depression than patients with healthy lungs.

Underventilation or apnea can result in potentially serious hypoxia and/or cardiac arrest unless effective countermeasures are initiated at the earliest sign of compromised respiration or ventilation. Early recognition and treatment of underventilation and apnea are necessary to avoid hypoxic cardiac arrest. Therefore, cardiorespiratory status should be monitored continuously during parenteral or oral midazolam use, dosage of the drug *must* be carefully individualized, and facilities and equipment for respiratory and ventilatory support should be readily available. Concomitant administration of CNS depressants may increase the risk of underventilation and apnea and may prolong and/or exacerbate the effects of midazolam. Use of supplemental oxygen should be considered when heavy sedation is anticipated or required.

Changes in systolic or diastolic blood pressure, principally decreases, and in heart rate are frequently associated with parenteral or oral administration of midazolam; however, in some cases, these effects may be associated with endotracheal intubation, changes in the depth of anesthesia, concomitantly administered drugs,

and/or surgical manipulation rather than with midazolam itself. Hypotensive episodes requiring treatment have been reported rarely during or following diagnostic or surgical manipulation in patients receiving midazolam. Concomitant administration of an opiate agonist (e.g., as premedication for moderate sedation [formerly known as conscious sedation]) appears to increase the risk of severe hypotension associated with midazolam administration. Severe hypotensive effects may be alleviated by the judicious administration of IV fluids, repositioning the patient, and/or the cautious use of vasopressors. Induction of anesthesia with midazolam in patients with a relatively slow baseline heart rate (less than 65 beats/minute) is associated with a slight increase in heart rate, especially in patients receiving a β-adrenergic blocking agent for angina. However, use of midazolam in patients with a relatively fast baseline heart rate (greater than 85 beats/minute) appears to result in slight slowing of the heart rate.

Other adverse respiratory effects of midazolam include hiccups and coughing, which occur in up to 4 and 1% of patients, respectively, receiving the drug IV. Laryngospasm, bronchospasm, dyspnea, hyperventilation, wheezing, shallow respiration, airway obstruction, and tachypnea occur in less than 1% of patients, principally those receiving the drug IV.

Other adverse cardiovascular effects of midazolam include decreases in systemic vascular resistance, cardiac index, and stroke index. Bradycardia has been reported in up to 1% of pediatric patients receiving midazolam oral solution. Bigeminy, ventricular premature complexes, vasovagal episodes, tachycardia, and nodal rhythms reportedly occur in less than 1% of patients. Trigeminy also has been reported in patients receiving midazolam.

● Nervous System Effects

Adverse nervous system effects of midazolam generally are extensions of the pharmacologic actions of the drug; however, some reactions (e.g., agitation, involuntary movements) may be paradoxical in nature, manifestations of an underlying iatrogenic disorder (e.g., cerebral hypoxia), and/or associated with the surgical or other procedures employed. Paradoxical reactions have been reported in 2% of pediatric patients receiving the drug IV.

Excessive sedation, headache, and drowsiness occur in 1–2% of patients following parenteral administration of midazolam. Agitation, involuntary movements (e.g., tonic/clonic movements, muscle tremor), hyperactivity, and combativeness also have been reported. Such reactions may have resulted from inadequate or excessive doses of midazolam, improper administration of the drug, or cerebral hypoxia, or may have been paradoxical. Agitation has been reported in 2% of pediatric patients receiving the drug orally. Seizure-like activity or nystagmus was reported in 1.1% of pediatric patients receiving the drug IV.

Other adverse nervous system effects that occur in less than 1% of patients receiving oral or IV midazolam include retrograde amnesia, euphoria, hallucinations, dysphoria, prolonged emergence from anesthesia, emergence delirium or agitation, dreaming during emergence, prolonged sedation, sleep disturbance, insomnia, nightmares, paresthesia, adverse behavior, mood swings, aggression, excitation, disinhibition, argumentativeness, nervousness, anxiety, restlessness, seizure-like activity, dysarthria, and athetoid movements. Confusion, grogginess, ataxia, dizziness, loss of balance or vertigo, lightheadedness, lethargy, yawning, faint feeling, weakness, slurred speech, blurred vision, strabismus, diplopia, and dysphonia have also been reported in less than 1% of patients.

Somnolence, headache, and dysarthria have been reported in 10, 4, and 2%, respectively, of patients receiving midazolam nasal spray.

Midazolam has reduced cerebral blood flow and oxygen consumption in animals and humans. In patients without intracranial pathology, induction of anesthesia with midazolam results in a moderate decrease in CSF pressure, similar to that occurring with thiopental (no longer commercially available in the US). There is some evidence that, in patients with normal intracranial pressure but decreased intracranial compliance who are undergoing intracranial surgery, induction of anesthesia with midazolam results in increased intracranial pressure during intubation similar to that occurring with thiopental.

● GI Effects

Nausea and/or vomiting occurs in 2–3% of adult patients receiving midazolam IV and in up to 4 or 8%, respectively, of pediatric patients receiving the drug orally. Acid taste, excessive salivation, gagging, drooling, and retching occur in less than 1% of patients. Other adverse GI effects include metallic taste, dry mouth, and constipation.

● Sensitivity Reactions

Hypersensitivity reactions reported in less than 1% of patients receiving midazolam include anaphylactoid reactions, urticaria, rash, and pruritus.

● Local Effects

Tenderness at the site of injection and pain during injection occur in 5–6% of patients receiving midazolam IV. Erythema and induration occur at the IV site in 2–3% of patients, and phlebitis occurs in less than 1%. Pain at the site of IM injection occurs in about 4% of patients, and local induration, erythema, and muscle stiffness occur in less than 1% of patients receiving midazolam IM. Adverse local effects associated with IM or IV administration occur less frequently and generally are less severe with midazolam than with other currently available parenteral benzodiazepines (e.g., diazepam).

Urticaria-like elevation at the injection site, swelling or feeling of burning, and warmth or coldness at the injection site occur in less than 1% of patients receiving midazolam parenterally, principally in those receiving the drug IV.

Nasal discomfort, throat irritation, rhinorrhea, and abnormal taste were reported in 9, 3, 3, and 2%, respectively, of patients receiving midazolam nasal spray.

● Ocular Effects

Adverse ocular effects occur in less than 1% of patients receiving parenteral midazolam, principally in those receiving the drug IV, and include blurred vision, diplopia, nystagmus, pinpoint pupils, cyclic movements of eyelids, visual disturbances, and focusing difficulty.

Increased lacrimation was reported in 2% of patients receiving midazolam nasal spray.

● Other Adverse Effects

Chills, toothache, blockage of ears, and hematoma occur in less than 1% of patients receiving midazolam parenterally, principally in those receiving the drug IV. Limited data suggest that administration of midazolam as an adjunct to anesthesia may result in transient decreases in renal blood flow and glomerular filtration rate.

● Precautions and Contraindications

Concomitant use of benzodiazepines, including midazolam, and opiate agonists or opiate partial agonists may result in profound sedation, respiratory depression, coma, and death. Patients receiving midazolam and/or their caregivers should be apprised of the risks associated with concomitant therapeutic or illicit use of benzodiazepines and opiates.

Agitation, involuntary movements, hyperactivity, and/or combativeness may be signs of inadequate or excessive dosing, improper administration, or cerebral hypoxia or may be paradoxical. If such adverse reactions occur during midazolam therapy, the patient's response to each dose of midazolam as well as to any concomitantly administered drug, including local anesthetics, should be evaluated before proceeding.

Midazolam should be used with caution and dosage individualized carefully in patients with renal impairment, since the pharmacokinetics of the drug may be altered in such patients. Induction of anesthesia may occur more rapidly in patients with renal impairment, and recovery may be prolonged.

Although the clinical importance has not been determined, some clinicians state that midazolam should be used with caution and dosage individualized carefully in patients with congestive heart failure. Pharmacokinetics of the drug may be substantially altered in such patients (e.g., prolonged elimination half-life, increased volume of distribution, delayed onset of action secondary to prolonged circulation time).

Patients should be informed of the potentially profound pharmacologic effects of midazolam (e.g., sedation, relief of anxiety, lack of recall) and that the duration of these effects varies considerably among individuals, so that they may adequately perceive the risks and benefits of use of the drug. Patients should also be warned that midazolam may impair their ability to perform activities requiring mental alertness or physical coordination (e.g., operating machinery, driving a motor vehicle). The decision regarding when patients who have received midazolam can safely perform such activities must be individualized, especially when

the patient received the drug as part of an outpatient procedure. Gross tests of recovery after awakening (e.g., orientation, ability to stand and walk, return to baseline Trieger competency) cannot be relied on alone to predict reaction time under stress. Patients should not operate a motor vehicle or hazardous machinery until the effects of the drug (e.g., drowsiness) have subsided or the day after anesthesia and surgery, whichever is longer. Impaired performance may persist for longer periods in geriatric patients, in patients using other drugs concomitantly, and secondary to the stress of surgery or general condition of the patient. For pediatric patients, particular care should be taken to ensure safe ambulation. Patients should be warned that concomitant use of midazolam with other CNS depressants may increase the extent and duration of impaired performance, cause excessive sedation, and interfere with recall and recognition of events on the day of surgery and the following day.

Some preparations of midazolam hydrochloride injection contain the preservative benzyl alcohol and should not be used in neonates and infants.

Midazolam is contraindicated in patients with known hypersensitivity to the drug. Midazolam oral solution also is contraindicated in patients allergic to cherries or to formulation excipients. Benzodiazepines can increase intraocular pressure in patients with glaucoma and some manufacturers state that the drug is contraindicated in patients with acute angle-closure glaucoma, but may be used in patients with open-angle glaucoma if they are receiving appropriate treatment. However, the clinical rationale for this contraindication has been questioned. The manufacturer of midazolam nasal spray states that patients with open-angle glaucoma may need an ophthalmologic evaluation following treatment with the drug.

Precautions Specific to the Use of Midazolam for Sedation or Anesthesia

Midazolam should be administered orally or IV only in hospital or ambulatory-care settings, including physicians' or dentists' offices, in which continuous monitoring of respiratory and cardiac function (i.e., pulse oximetry) is possible. Safety and efficacy of midazolam may vary in patients as functions of the dose administered and clinical status of the patient. Midazolam is a potent sedative and requires slow administration and individualized titration of dosage. Since the drug is capable of producing several levels of CNS depression—from mild to deep sedation, facilities, age- and size-appropriate equipment for bag/mask/valve ventilation and intubation, drugs, and skilled personnel necessary for ventilation and intubation, administration of oxygen, assisted or controlled respiration, airway management, and cardiovascular support should be immediately available whenever midazolam is administered. The immediate availability of specific benzodiazepine reversal agent (e.g., flumazenil) is highly recommended when the drug is administered IV or orally. Pediatric and adult patients undergoing procedures involving the upper airway, such as upper endoscopy or dental care, are particularly vulnerable to episodes of desaturation and hypoventilation due to partial airway obstruction. The incidence of such adverse events is higher in patients undergoing procedures involving the airway without the protective effect of an endotracheal tube. Patients receiving midazolam should be monitored continuously for early signs of underventilation or apnea since hypoxia and/or cardiac arrest can occur unless effective countermeasures are undertaken immediately. Monitoring of vital signs also should continue during the recovery period. Because midazolam can depress respiration and because opiate agonists or other sedatives can potentiate this effect, midazolam should be administered as an induction agent only by individuals who are experienced in the use of general anesthesia and should be used for procedural sedation only in the presence of personnel experienced in early detection of underventilation, maintenance of an adequate airway, and respiratory support. For deeply sedated pediatric patients, a dedicated individual other than the clinician performing the procedure should monitor the patient throughout the procedure. In addition, the possibility that the procedure may obscure early recognition of potential complications (e.g., performance of endoscopy in diminished light which can make visual observation of the patient difficult) or may interfere with effective countermeasures (e.g., patient positioning during colonoscopy) should be considered.

Careful monitoring and individualization of dosing are essential when parenteral midazolam is used for sedation or anesthesia; dosage individualization is particularly important in certain patient populations (e.g., geriatric patients, patients with various underlying disease states [e.g., chronic obstructive pulmonary disease, renal failure, congestive heart failure], and patients receiving other CNS depressants).

Midazolam should not be administered parenterally to patients with shock or who are comatose or to patients with acute alcohol intoxication and accompanying depression of vital signs. Caution should be exercised if midazolam is administered IV to patients with uncompensated acute illnesses, including severe fluid or electrolyte imbalances. Sedation guidelines recommend a careful presedation history to determine how a patient's underlying medical condition or concomitant drugs may affect the response to sedation/analgesia, as well as a physical examination including a focused examination of the airway for abnormalities. Further recommendations include appropriate presedation fasting.

There have been limited reports of intra-arterial injection of midazolam; adverse effects have included local reactions as well as isolated reports of seizure activity in which no clear causal relationship was established. Precautions against unintended intra-arterial injection should be taken, and drug extravasation should be avoided.

Midazolam does not fully prevent the increase in intracranial pressure or the cardiovascular effects (e.g., increase in blood pressure and/or heart rate) associated with endotracheal intubation under light general anesthesia. Midazolam also does not appear to prevent the usual cardiovascular stimulatory effects associated with administration of some neuromuscular blocking agents (e.g., succinylcholine, pancuronium) or the increase in intracranial pressure associated with succinylcholine.

Patients receiving continuous IV infusion of midazolam in critical care settings over an extended period of time may experience symptoms of withdrawal following discontinuance.

Precautions Specific to the Use of Midazolam Nasal Spray

If midazolam nasal spray is used in patients at risk of benzodiazepine-induced respiratory depression, it is recommended that the drug be administered under the supervision of a clinician.

The possibility of an increased risk of suicidality (suicidal behavior or ideation) should be considered in patients receiving midazolam nasal spray. An analysis of suicidality reports from 199 placebo-controlled studies found that patients receiving anticonvulsants for any indication had approximately twice the risk of suicidal behavior or ideation compared with those receiving placebo; the increased risk was observed as early as one week after beginning therapy and continued through 24 weeks. Although patients treated with an anticonvulsant for epilepsy, psychiatric disorders, and other conditions were all found to be at increased risk for suicidality when compared with those receiving placebo, the relative suicidality risk was higher for patients with epilepsy compared with those receiving anticonvulsants for other conditions. Clinicians should inform patients, their families, and caregivers of the potential for an increased risk of suicidality with anticonvulsant therapy; all patients currently receiving or beginning therapy with any anticonvulsant should be closely monitored for the emergence or worsening of suicidal thoughts or behavior or depression.

● Pediatric Precautions

The safety and efficacy of midazolam oral solution have not been established in pediatric patients younger than 6 months of age. Safety and efficacy of midazolam nasal spray have not been established in pediatric patients younger than 12 years of age.

Unlike adults, the dose of midazolam in pediatric patients is calculated on a mg/kg basis. As a group, pediatric patients require a higher parenteral dosage of midazolam on a mg/kg basis than do adults, and pediatric patients younger than 6 years of age generally require higher dosages on a mg/kg basis than do older pediatric patients and may require closer monitoring. In obese pediatric patients, the drug dose should be calculated on the basis of ideal body weight. When midazolam is administered in conjunction with opiates or other sedatives in the pediatric population, the potential for respiratory depression, airway obstruction, or hypoventilation is increased. Particular care should be taken to ensure safe ambulation of pediatric patients following sedation with midazolam. Clinicians who use this drug in pediatric patients should be aware of, and follow, accepted professional guidelines for pediatric sedation appropriate to the situation.

Higher-risk pediatric surgical patients may require lower midazolam doses, whether or not concomitant sedating drugs have been administered. Pediatric patients with cardiac or respiratory compromise may be unusually sensitive to the respiratory depressant effect of midazolam. Pediatric patients undergoing procedures involving the upper airway (e.g., upper endoscopy, dental care) are particularly vulnerable to episodes of desaturation and hypoventilation secondary to partial airway obstruction.

Because of reduced and/or immature organ function, neonates are vulnerable to profound and/or prolonged adverse respiratory effects of midazolam. The drug should not be administered by rapid IV injection in neonates. When administered as a rapid (i.e., over less than 2 minutes) IV injection in neonates, the drug has been associated with severe hypotension, particularly when coadministered with fentanyl. Likewise, severe hypotension has been observed in neonates receiving midazolam as a continuous infusion who then also received a rapid IV injection of fentanyl. Seizures also have been reported in neonates receiving midazolam as a rapid IV injection.

FDA warns that repeated or prolonged use of general anesthetics and sedation drugs, including midazolam, in children younger than 3 years of age or during the third trimester of pregnancy may affect brain development. Animal studies in multiple species, including nonhuman primates, have demonstrated that use for longer than 3 hours of anesthetic and sedation drugs that block N-methyl-ᴅ-aspartic acid (NMDA) receptors and/or potentiate γ-aminobutyric acid (GABA) activity leads to widespread neuronal and oligodendrocyte cell loss and alterations in synaptic morphology and neurogenesis in the brain, resulting in long-term deficits in cognition and behavior. Across animal species, vulnerability to these neurodevelopmental changes occurs during the period of rapid brain growth or synaptogenesis; this period is thought to correlate with the third trimester of pregnancy through the first year of life in humans, but may extend to approximately 3 years of age. The clinical relevance of these animal findings to humans is not known. While some published evidence suggests that similar deficits in cognition and behavior may occur in children following repeated or prolonged exposure to anesthesia early in life, other studies have found no association between pediatric anesthesia exposure and long-term adverse neurodevelopmental outcomes. Most studies to date have had substantial limitations, and it is not clear whether the adverse neurodevelopmental outcomes observed in children were related to the drug or to other factors (e.g., surgery, underlying illness). There is some clinical evidence that a single, relatively brief exposure to general anesthesia in generally healthy children is unlikely to cause clinically detectable deficits in global cognitive function or serious behavioral disorders; however, further research is needed to fully characterize the effects of exposure to general anesthetics in early life, particularly for prolonged or repeated exposures and in more vulnerable populations (e.g., less healthy children). For further information, see Cautions: Pediatric Precautions, in the Benzodiazepines General Statement 28:24.08.

Anesthetic and sedation drugs are an essential component of care for children and pregnant women who require surgery or other procedures that cannot be delayed; no specific general anesthetic or sedation drug has been shown to be less likely to cause neurocognitive deficits than any other such drug. Pending further accumulation of data in humans from well-designed studies, decisions regarding the timing of elective procedures requiring anesthesia should take into consideration both the benefits of the procedure and the potential risks. When procedures requiring the use of general anesthetics or sedation drugs are considered for young children or pregnant women, clinicians should discuss with the patient, parent, or caregiver the benefits, risks (including potential risk of adverse neurodevelopmental effects), and appropriate timing and duration of the procedure. FDA states that procedures that are considered medically necessary should not be delayed or avoided.

Midazolam hydrochloride injections containing benzyl alcohol should not be used in neonates or infants. Although a causal relationship has not been established, administration of injections preserved with benzyl alcohol has been associated with toxicity in neonates. Toxicity appears to have resulted from administration of large amounts (i.e., 100-400 mg/kg daily) of benzyl alcohol in these neonates. Exposure to such excessive amounts of benzyl alcohol has been associated with hypotension and metabolic acidosis in neonates, and an increased incidence of kernicterus, particularly in small, preterm infants. There have been reports of death, particularly in preterm infants, associated with exposure to excessive amounts of benzyl alcohol. Although use of drugs preserved with benzyl alcohol should be avoided in neonates whenever possible, the American Academy of Pediatrics (AAP) states that the presence of small amounts of the preservative in a commercially available injection should not proscribe its use when indicated in neonates. The amount of benzyl alcohol exposure from drugs usually is considered negligible compared with that from benzyl alcohol-containing flush solutions. Administration of high dosages of drugs containing this preservative, including midazolam hydrochloride, must take into account the total amount of benzyl alcohol administered. The recommended dosage range of midazolam for preterm and term infants includes amounts of benzyl alcohol well below that associated with toxicity; however, the amount of benzyl alcohol at which toxicity may occur is not known. If the patient requires more than the recommended midazolam dosages, or if other benzyl alcohol-containing preparations are to be used in the patient, the clinician must take into account the total daily metabolic load of benzyl alcohol from these sources.

● Geriatric Precautions

Because distribution of midazolam may be altered in geriatric patients and these patients may have decreased hepatic and/or renal function, the manufacturer of midazolam hydrochloride injection recommends that dosage of the drug be selected carefully in this age group. IV or IM dosage of midazolam should be reduced in geriatric or debilitated patients, particularly in those 70 years of age and older. When IV midazolam is used for induction of anesthesia, time to recovery may be delayed in this population. In addition, rare fatalities (possibly associated with cardiorespiratory depression) have been reported in geriatric and/or high-risk surgical patients receiving IV or IM midazolam (often in combination with other CNS depressants [e.g., opiates]).

The manufacturer of oral midazolam states that a safe dosing regimen has not been established in geriatric patients and that the drug should not be used in such patients until further information is available.

● Mutagenicity and Carcinogenicity

In vitro and in vivo microbial and mammalian test systems using midazolam have not revealed evidence of mutagenicity. No evidence of carcinogenic potential was seen in rats or mice receiving oral midazolam maleate dosages up to 9 mg/kg daily (about 25 times the recommended human dosage) for 24 months. However, an increased incidence of liver tumors was observed following oral administration of 80 mg/kg daily for 24 months in female mice, and an increased incidence of benign thyroid follicular cell tumors was observed following this dosage in male rats. The pathogenesis of induction of these tumors is not known. In addition, the relevance of these findings to usual use of midazolam in humans is not known, since these effects occurred after long-term administration of the drug in animals, whereas use in humans usually is short term.

● Pregnancy, Fertility, and Lactation

Pregnancy

An increased risk of congenital malformations associated with the use of benzodiazepines (e.g., chlordiazepoxide, diazepam) during pregnancy has been suggested by several retrospective studies in humans. Midazolam has been shown to cross the placenta in humans. Reproduction studies in rabbits and rats using IV midazolam in doses up to 1.85 times the human induction dose have not revealed evidence of fetal malformation. If the drug is administered during pregnancy, the patient should be informed of the potential hazard to the fetus. Use of midazolam injection for obstetric procedures or during labor and delivery is not recommended, since such use has not been evaluated and use of other benzodiazepines during the last weeks of pregnancy has caused CNS depression in the neonate.

Based on animal data, repeated or prolonged use of general anesthetics and sedation drugs, including midazolam, during the third trimester of pregnancy may result in adverse neurodevelopmental effects in the fetus. The clinical relevance of these animal findings to humans is not known; the potential risk of adverse neurodevelopmental effects should be considered and discussed with pregnant women undergoing procedures requiring general anesthetics and sedation drugs.

Fertility

No evidence of impaired fertility was observed in rats following oral administration of midazolam in doses producing exposures as high as 1.85 times the recommended human IV induction dose of 0.35 mg/kg.

Women who are pregnant while receiving midazolam nasal spray should be encouraged to enroll in the North American Antiepileptic Drug (NAAED) Pregnancy Registry at 888-233-2334 or https://www.aedpregnancyregistry.org.

Lactation

Midazolam is distributed into milk in humans, and caution should be exercised when midazolam is administered to nursing women.

DRUG INTERACTIONS

● Drugs Affecting Hepatic Microsomal Enzymes

Metabolism of midazolam is mediated by cytochrome P-450 (CYP) isoenzyme 3A4. Concomitant use of midazolam and drugs that inhibit CYP3A4 (e.g., erythromycin, diltiazem, verapamil, ketoconazole, fluconazole, itraconazole, HIV protease inhibitors) may result in clinically important increases in peak plasma concentrations and area under the plasma concentration-time curve (AUC) of midazolam; conversely, concomitant use of midazolam with drugs that induce CYP3A4 (e.g., rifampin, carbamazepine, phenytoin, phenobarbital) may result in clinically important decreases in peak plasma concentrations and AUC of midazolam. Caution should be observed if midazolam is administered concomitantly with these drugs and dosage adjustments may be necessary. The manufacturer states that oral midazolam should be used concomitantly with ketoconazole, itraconazole, or saquinavir only when absolutely necessary and with appropriate equipment and personnel available to respond to respiratory insufficiency.

Manufacturers of HIV protease inhibitors and the nonnucleoside reverse transcriptase inhibitors (NNRTIs) delavirdine and efavirenz state that concomitant use of midazolam with these antiretroviral agents is contraindicated; however, some experts state that a single midazolam dose can be used with caution for procedural sedation in monitored situations in patients receiving these antiretroviral agents.

● Commonly Used Drugs During Anesthesia or Surgery

Concomitant use of IV midazolam and IV fentanyl has resulted in severe hypotension in neonates. No adverse interactions have been observed when midazolam was administered concomitantly with other common premedications or drugs used during anesthesia or surgery (e.g., atropine, scopolamine, glycopyrrolate, diazepam, hydroxyzine, succinylcholine, nondepolarizing neuromuscular blocking agents, topical local anesthetics).

● Anesthetic Agents

Patients who have received midazolam as an induction agent may require reduced amounts of inhalation agents during maintenance of anesthesia.

The cardiovascular stimulatory effects and the postoperative emergence delirium usually associated with administration of ketamine appear to be antagonized, at least partially, by midazolam.

● Anticonvulsants

Concomitant administration of oral midazolam and phenytoin or carbamazepine has been shown to decrease peak plasma concentrations and AUC of midazolam by about 93–94%. Although not studied specifically, phenobarbital would be expected to have similar effects on the pharmacokinetics of midazolam.

● Antifungal Agents

Concomitant administration of oral midazolam in patients receiving ketoconazole or itraconazole has been shown to increase peak plasma concentrations of midazolam (by 309% or 80–240%, respectively) as a result of decreased plasma clearance. Because of the potential for intense and prolonged sedation and respiratory depression, midazolam oral solution should be coadministered with these drugs only if absolutely necessary and with appropriate equipment and personnel available to respond to respiratory insufficiency.

While fluconazole has been shown to increase peak plasma concentrations of midazolam by 150%, terbinafine does not appear to affect the pharmacokinetics of midazolam.

● Antimycobacterial Agents

Concomitant administration of oral midazolam and rifampin has been shown to decrease the peak plasma concentration of midazolam by 94% and the AUC of midazolam by 96%. Although not studied specifically, rifabutin would be expected to have similar effects on the pharmacokinetics of midazolam.

● Antiretroviral Agents

Large increases in peak plasma concentrations and AUC of midazolam (by about 235 and 514%, respectively) have been observed when saquinavir (1.2 g 3 times daily given as liquid-filled capsules [no longer commercially available in the US]) was administered concomitantly with oral midazolam. In one study, concomitant use of saquinavir (1.2 g 3 times daily for 5 days) with a single 0.05-mg/kg IV dose of midazolam decreased the clearance of midazolam by 56% and approximately doubled the half-life of the benzodiazepine. Because of the potential for intense and prolonged sedation and respiratory depression, the manufacturers of HIV protease inhibitors (e.g., atazanavir fosamprenavir, indinavir, lopinavir/ritonavir, nelfinavir, ritonavir, saquinavir, tipranavir) state that concomitant use of midazolam with HIV protease inhibitors is contraindicated. However, some experts state that a single midazolam dose can be used with caution for procedural sedation in a monitored situation in patients receiving HIV protease inhibitors.

The manufacturers of delavirdine and efavirenz state that concomitant use of these agents with midazolam should be avoided because of the potential for the NNRTI to decrease metabolism of midazolam and result in intense or prolonged sedation or respiratory depression. However, some clinicians state that a single midazolam dose can be used with caution for procedural sedation in a monitored situation in patients receiving delavirdine or efavirenz.

● Calcium-channel Blockers

Concomitant administration of oral midazolam and diltiazem or verapamil increased peak plasma concentrations of midazolam by 105 or 97%, respectively, and increased AUC of midazolam by 275 or 192%, respectively. In another study, half-life of midazolam was increased from 5 to 7 hours when the drug was administered in conjunction with diltiazem or verapamil.

Nifedipine does not appear to alter the pharmacokinetics of midazolam.

● CNS Depressants

Midazolam may potentiate the action of other CNS depressants, including opiate agonists or other analgesics, barbiturates or other sedatives, anesthetics, or alcohol, possibly resulting in respiratory depression and profound and/or prolonged underventilation or apnea. When midazolam is used concomitantly with a depressant drug, caution should be exercised and appropriate dosage adjustments should be made to avoid overdosage.

The sedative effect of IV midazolam is potentiated by premedication with CNS depressants, especially opiates, barbiturates, or combined fentanyl and droperidol. Midazolam dosage should be adjusted according to the type and amount of premedication administered.

Opiate Agonists and Opiate Partial Agonists

Concomitant use of benzodiazepines, including midazolam, and opiate agonists or opiate partial agonists may result in profound sedation, respiratory depression, coma, and death. Opiate agonists can impair the ventilatory response to carbon dioxide (CO_2), and appear to increase the risk of hypotension and prolong the recovery period compared with midazolam alone. Severe hypotension, possibly secondary to increased venous pooling, has occurred when midazolam was used concomitantly with high-dose fentanyl. When concomitant therapy is required, the lowest effective dosages and shortest possible duration of concomitant therapy should be used, and the patient should be monitored closely for respiratory depression and sedation. Opiate antitussive agents should be avoided in patients receiving benzodiazepines, and concomitant use of opiate analgesics and benzodiazepines should be reserved for patients in whom alternative treatment options are inadequate. For further information on potential interactions between benzodiazepines and opiates, see Opiate Agonists and Opiate Partial Agonists under Drug Interactions: CNS Agents, in the Benzodiazepines General Statement 28:24.08.

● Grapefruit Juice

Concomitant administration of grapefruit juice with oral midazolam has been reported to increase bioavailability of the drug. Grapefruit juice does not appear to interfere with metabolism following IV administration of the drug. The interaction between grapefruit juice and the benzodiazepine bioavailability appears to result from inhibition, probably prehepatic, of the cytochrome P-450 enzyme system by some constituent(s) in the juice. Following oral administration of midazolam, such prehepatic inhibition of drug metabolism by grapefruit juice appears mainly to involve the CYP3A4 isoenzyme, principally within the small intestinal wall (e.g., in the jejunum), thus increasing systemic availability of these drugs. The manufacturer states that oral midazolam should not be taken in conjunction with grapefruit juice.

● Histamine H₂-Receptor Antagonists

The effects of concomitant administration of midazolam and cimetidine or ranitidine have not been fully elucidated. Orally administered cimetidine or ranitidine did not substantially alter the pharmacokinetics of either IV or oral midazolam in one study in healthy adults. However, in another study, plasma midazolam concentrations were increased by about 30% following oral administration of cimetidine, but not ranitidine, in healthy adults receiving midazolam IV. Oral bioavailability of midazolam may be increased by up to about 30% when cimetidine or ranitidine is given concomitantly, possibly secondary to a pH-dependent enhancement of gastric absorption of midazolam and/or a reduction in hepatic clearance of the drug. In another study, concomitant administration of oral midazolam and cimetidine (800–1200 mg up to 4 times daily) increased peak plasma concentrations and AUC of midazolam by 6–138 and 10–102%, respectively; and concomitant administration of oral midazolam and ranitidine (150 mg 2 or 3 times daily or 300 mg once daily) increased peak plasma concentrations and AUC of midazolam by 15–67 and 9–66%, respectively. If changes in the pharmacokinetics of midazolam occur during concomitant use with one of these histamine H₂-receptor antagonists, enhanced pharmacologic effects of midazolam may result. Pending further accumulation of data, patients receiving midazolam and cimetidine or ranitidine concomitantly should be observed carefully for signs of midazolam-induced CNS and respiratory depression, and dosage of midazolam reduced if necessary.

● Macrolide Antibiotics

Concomitant administration of midazolam and erythromycin may affect the pharmacokinetics of midazolam. In one study, concomitant use of erythromycin (500 mg 3 times daily for 1 week) with a single 0.05-mg/kg IV dose of midazolam doubled the half-life of midazolam and reportedly decreased clearance of the benzodiazepine. In another study in healthy individuals, pretreatment with erythromycin (500 mg 3 times daily for 6 days) reportedly increased peak plasma concentrations and AUC of oral midazolam following a single 15-mg oral dose of the benzodiazepine. Because increased plasma concentrations of midazolam may be associated with excessive sedative effects, some clinicians state that erythromycin should not be given to patients receiving midazolam, or alternatively, the dose of midazolam should be reduced in patients receiving the anti-infective.

While erythromycin has been shown to increase peak plasma concentrations and AUC of oral midazolam by about 170 and 281–341%, respectively, azithromycin does not appear to affect the pharmacokinetics of midazolam.

● Neuromuscular Blocking Agents

Midazolam and pancuronium have been used concomitantly in adults without any clinically important changes in dosage, onset, or duration. Midazolam does not cause a clinically important change in dosage, onset, or duration of a single intubating dose of succinylcholine.

● Quinupristin and Dalfopristin

Concomitant use of midazolam and quinupristin/dalfopristin may affect the pharmacokinetics of midazolam. In healthy individuals, concomitant administration of a single IV dose of midazolam with IV quinupristin/dalfopristin increased mean peak plasma concentrations and AUC of midazolam by 14 and 33%, respectively.

ACUTE TOXICITY

● Pathogenesis

Limited information is available on the acute toxicity of midazolam in humans. The IV and oral LD₅₀s of midazolam have been reported to be about 86 and 760 mg/kg, respectively, in mice.

PHARMACOLOGY

Midazolam shares the actions of other benzodiazepines. Although initial data indicated that the sedative potency of midazolam was about 1.5–2.5 times that of diazepam, clinical experience with the drug suggests that potency may be 3–4 times that of diazepam.

For further information on the pharmacology of midazolam hydrochloride, see Acute Toxicity in the Benzodiazepines General Statement 28:24.08..

PHARMACOKINETICS

In studies described in the Pharmacokinetics section, midazolam was administered as the hydrochloride, maleate, or lactate salt; dosages and concentrations of the drug are expressed in terms of midazolam. Studies demonstrate that the pharmacokinetic properties of midazolam following administration of a single parenteral dose in pediatric patients aged 1 year and older are similar to those reported in adults.

● Absorption

Absorption of midazolam hydrochloride from IM injection sites is rapid and nearly complete (mean absolute bioavailability is greater than 90%). IM bioavailability of the lactate appears to be similar to or slightly less than that of the hydrochloride; however, any such difference does not appear to be clinically important. Pharmacologic effects of midazolam usually are apparent within 5–15 minutes but may not be maximal until 15–60 minutes following IM administration; the duration of action usually is about 2 hours (range: 1–6 hours). Peak plasma midazolam concentrations generally are attained within 30–45 minutes following IM administration. Following IM administration of a single 12.5-mg (of midazolam) dose of the hydrochloride in healthy adults, peak plasma midazolam concentrations of approximately 200 ng/mL (range: 88–269 ng/mL) are attained. Peak plasma concentrations of midazolam and 1-hydroxymethylmidazolam (an active metabolite) attained following IM injection are approximately 50% of those attained following IV injection of a dose.

Following IV administration of usual doses of midazolam hydrochloride, the onset of sedative, anxiolytic, and amnesic action usually occurs within 1–5 minutes. However, onset is affected by many factors, including total dose administered, rate of administration, patient age, serum albumin concentration, renal function, and the presence of other drugs. Induction of anesthesia usually occurs in about 1.5 minutes when opiate agonists are administered concurrently with midazolam and in 2–2.5 minutes when midazolam is administered without an opiate agonist or concurrently with other sedatives. Duration of action following IV administration is usually less than 2 hours; however, the pharmacologic effects may persist up to 6 hours in some patients, and the duration of action appears to be dose related. Limited data suggest that the onset may be more rapid and the duration prolonged in patients with chronic renal failure, probably secondary to decreased protein binding in these patients.

In one study in healthy adults who received a single 75-mcg/kg dose of midazolam IV over 1 minute, peak plasma concentrations of the drug averaged 323.8 ng/mL and plasma concentrations 0.25, 0.5, 1, 2, 4, 6, and 8 hours after the dose averaged 246.8, 206.8, 141.7, 84.2, 37.0, and 20.2 ng/mL, respectively. Following single IV doses, plasma concentrations of midazolam generally are 10–30 times higher than those of the principal metabolite, 1-hydroxymethylmidazolam.

Following intranasal administration of a single 5-mg dose of midazolam in healthy adults, peak plasma concentrations were obtained in approximately 17 minutes. Absolute bioavailability is approximately 44%. The onset of sedative and psychomotor impairment effects usually occurs within 10 minutes, while maximal effects are achieved within 30 minutes to 2 hours after a dose is administered.

Midazolam hydrochloride is absorbed rapidly from the GI tract, with maximum plasma concentrations usually occurring within 1–2 hours. Following oral administration, the drug undergoes substantial first-pass metabolism in the liver and intestine, with only about 40–50% (range: 28–72%) of an orally administered dose reaching systemic circulation unchanged. Pharmacologic effects of midazolam usually are apparent within 10–20 minutes following administration of midazolam oral solution in pediatric patients. In pharmacokinetic studies of pediatric patients (6 months to less than 16 years of age) receiving midazolam oral solution at doses of 250 mcg/kg, 500 mcg/kg, or 1 mg/kg, midazolam exhibited linear pharmacokinetics. The mean time to maximal plasma concentration in these patients ranged from 0.17–2.65 hours, and the absolute bioavailability of the drug was about 36%; bioavailability was not affected by pediatric age or weight. The effect of food on absorption of midazolam oral solution has not been studied; however, in adults receiving the drug as a 15-mg oral tablet, absorption was not affected by food.

A relationship between plasma midazolam concentrations and clinical effects has not been clearly established, and the manufacturer states that a direct relationship does not exist. However, some data suggest that sedation may be associated with plasma midazolam concentrations greater than 30–100 ng/mL. In one study, pronounced hypnotic effects (e.g., slurred speech, sleep with dreaming, nystagmus) were noted when plasma concentrations exceeded 100 ng/mL.

● Distribution

At physiologic pH, midazolam is highly lipophilic; however, the lipophilicity of the drug decreases with decreasing pH. Following IV administration in humans, midazolam is rapidly and apparently widely distributed. The apparent volume of distribution of the drug in healthy adults reportedly averages 0.8–2.5 L/kg (range: 0.6–6.6 L/kg). Volume of distribution of midazolam appears to be 1.5–2 times higher in adults with chronic renal failure and 2–3 times higher in adults with congestive heart failure compared with healthy adults. In pediatric patients (6 months to younger than 16 years of age) receiving IV midazolam 0.15 mg/kg, the mean steady-state volume of distribution ranged from 1.24–2.02 L/kg.

Following IV administration of midazolam hydrochloride in animals, the drug is widely distributed, with highest concentrations occurring in liver, kidneys, lungs, fat, and heart. The drug crosses the blood-brain barrier and distributes into CSF in humans and animals. In animals, equilibration of midazolam between plasma and CSF occurs within a few minutes following IV administration, and CSF:plasma ratios of the drug are highly correlated with unbound midazolam once equilibrium is reached. Distribution of the drug into human lumbar CSF may be slow and erratic. Distribution of midazolam may be altered in geriatric patients.

In both adult and pediatric patients older than 1 year of age, approximately 94–97% of midazolam hydrochloride is bound to plasma proteins, mainly to serum albumin; protein binding of the drug is decreased in patients with chronic renal failure. In healthy individuals, the drug's principal metabolite, 1-hydroxymethylmidazolam, is 89% protein bound. The degree of protein binding appears to be independent of the plasma concentration of the drug.

Midazolam crosses the placenta and is distributed into amniotic fluid in animals and humans; however, placental transfer of drug appears to occur more slowly than with diazepam. In humans, measurable midazolam concentrations were achieved in maternal venous serum, umbilical venous serum, umbilical arterial serum, and amniotic fluid following a single 15-mg (of midazolam) oral or 50-mcg/kg (of midazolam) IM dose of the maleate given 15–60 minutes prior to cesarean section; both umbilical venous and umbilical arterial midazolam concentrations were lower than maternal concentrations. Midazolam reportedly is distributed into milk in humans.

● Elimination

Plasma midazolam concentrations appear to decline in a biphasic manner following IV administration. Following a single IV dose in healthy adults, the half-life of midazolam in the initial distribution phase ($t_{1/2\alpha}$) averages 6–20 minutes, and the half-life in the terminal elimination phase ($t_{1/2\beta}$) averages 1–4 hours (range: 1–12.3 hours). Limited data suggest that the half-life of midazolam may be prolonged in obese patients (presumably secondary to an increased volume of distribution), geriatric individuals, and patients with impaired hepatic function or with congestive heart failure. The half-life of midazolam is also reportedly prolonged in patients receiving the drug for induction of anesthesia associated with major surgical procedures. Elimination half-life does not appear to be altered substantially in patients with chronic renal failure. Mean elimination half-life ranged from 2.2–6.8 hours following single oral doses of 250 mcg/kg, 500 mcg/kg, and 1 mg/kg of midazolam oral solution in pediatric patients (6 months to younger than 16 years of age). Mean elimination half-life ranged from 2.9–4.5 hours in pediatric patients (6 months to less than 16 years of age) receiving IV midazolam 150 mcg/kg. In seriously ill neonates, the terminal elimination half-life is substantially prolonged (i.e., 6.5–12 hours). Following IM administration of midazolam 10 mg, elimination half-life of the drug was approximately 4 hours. Following intranasal administration of midazolam nasal spray, elimination half-life of the drug ranged from 2.1 to 6.2 hours.

Midazolam is metabolized extensively in the liver and intestine by cytochrome P-450 CYP3A4. The drug rapidly undergoes hydroxylation via hepatic microsomal enzymes to form 1-hydroxymethylmidazolam (α-hydroxymidazolam), the principal metabolite, and 4-hydroxymidazolam; a small portion of

1-hydroxymethylmidazolam is further hydroxylated to 1-hydroxymethyl-4-hydroxymidazolam (α,4-dihydroxymidazolam). These metabolites undergo rapid conjugation with glucuronic acid in the liver. Although the elimination half-life of the principal metabolite, 1-hydroxymethylmidazolam, is not clearly established, it is estimated to be about 60–80 minutes. The 1-hydroxymethyl and 4-hydroxy metabolites are reportedly pharmacologically active; potency of 1-hydroxymethylmidazolam appears to be similar to that of midazolam. The 1-hydroxymethyl-4-hydroxy metabolite appears to have little, if any, pharmacologic activity.

Midazolam is excreted in urine almost entirely as conjugated metabolites. Approximately 45–57% of an IV dose is excreted in urine as conjugated 1-hydroxymethylmidazolam, small amounts as conjugates of 4-hydroxymidazolam and 1-hydroxymethyl-4-hydroxymidazolam, and less than 0.03% as unchanged drug. In healthy adults who received a single 10-mg oral dose of radiolabeled midazolam, about 90% of the radioactivity was excreted in urine within 24 hours, principally (about 60–70% of a dose) as conjugated 1-hydroxymethylmidazolam. Approximately 2–10% of an oral dose is excreted in feces.

It is not known whether midazolam is removed by hemodialysis or peritoneal dialysis.

Following IV administration in healthy individuals and pediatric patients, total apparent plasma clearance of midazolam averages 2.5–12.8 mL/minute per kg. In seriously ill neonates, the clearance is reduced to 0.07–0.12 L/hr per kg; it cannot be determined whether these differences are because of age, immature organ function or metabolism, underlying illness, or debility. Total apparent plasma clearance of the drug reportedly is decreased in geriatric individuals but, in one study, such clearance was decreased substantially only in geriatric males. Total plasma clearance and volume of distribution of total (bound and unbound) midazolam are 1.5–2 times higher in patients with chronic renal failure compared with individuals with normal renal function, but these alterations are attributable to changes in protein binding of the drug and are not apparent when these pharmacokinetic parameters are determined for unbound midazolam. Although the effects of hepatic impairment on the elimination of midazolam have not been fully evaluated, preliminary data suggest that total apparent plasma clearance of the drug may be decreased in some patients with chronic liver disease. In a limited number of patients with congestive heart failure, total body clearance of midazolam appeared to remain unchanged following a single 5-mg IV dose, although elimination half-life and volume of distribution were increased twofold to threefold.

CHEMISTRY AND STABILITY

● Chemistry

Midazolam is a benzodiazepine. The drug is an imidazobenzodiazepine, differing structurally from other benzodiazepines by the presence of an imidazole ring fused at positions 1 and 2 of the benzodiazepine nucleus, which replaces the ketone at position 2 of the nucleus. The imidazole ring results in the ability of midazolam to readily form salts, which have increased aqueous solubility and stability to hydrolysis compared with other benzodiazepines. Presence of a methyl group at position 1 of the imidazole ring may result in increased susceptibility to metabolism. In acidic solutions, such as in the commercially available oral solution (pH 2.8–3.6) or parenteral injections (pH 3–4 in the 1 mg/mL solutions and pH 3–3.6 in the 5 mg/mL solutions), a pH-dependent equilibrium exists between midazolam and a ring-opened structure (the corresponding benzophenone) at position 4 of the benzodiazepine nucleus, resulting in up to 40 or 25% ring-opened forms for the oral solution or parenteral injections, respectively. At physiologic pH (5–8), under which midazolam is absorbed into the systemic circulation, the drug is almost (at least 99%) completely ring-closed, resulting in increased lipophilicity.

Midazolam occurs as a white to light yellow, crystalline powder. Midazolam is commercially available as the hydrochloride salt, which is formed *in situ*. The aqueous solubility of midazolam hydrochloride is pH dependent; the drug has solubilities of approximately 0.24, 1.09, 3.67, 10.3, or greater than 22 mg (of midazolam) per mL in water at pH 6.2, 5.1, 3.8, 3.4, or 2.8, respectively, at 25°C. Midazolam has a pK$_a$ of 6.15. Midazolam also is commercially available as a solution for intranasal administration.

Midazolam hydrochloride injection is commercially available as a sterile solution for IM or IV administration. Hydrochloric acid and, if necessary, sodium hydroxide are added during manufacture of the injection to adjust the pH to about 3. The injection also contains disodium edetate and sodium chloride; some preparations also may contain benzyl alcohol. Commercially available midazolam hydrochloride oral solution is a red to purplish-red colored solution containing 2 mg/mL of the drug in a cherry-flavored vehicle. The pH of the oral solution has been adjusted to approximately 2.8–3.6 with hydrochloric acid. Commercially available midazolam nasal spray is a clear, colorless to yellowish colored solution; each 0.1 mL of solution contains 5 mg of midazolam.

● Stability

Midazolam hydrochloride injection should be stored at 20–25°C, but may be exposed to temperatures ranging from 15–30°C. The injection was physically stable when frozen for 3-day periods and allowed to thaw at room temperature. Preservative-free midazolam hydrochloride injection should be stored at 20–25°C. Midazolam oral solution should be stored at 20–25°C. Midazolam nasal spray should be stored at 20–25°C, but may be exposed to temperatures ranging from 15–30°C.

Midazolam hydrochloride injection is chemically and physically compatible with the following IV solutions: 5% dextrose, 0.9% sodium chloride, or lactated Ringer's. Midazolam hydrochloride injection that has been diluted to a final concentration of 0.5 mg or less per mL is stable for 24 hours in 5% dextrose or 0.9% sodium chloride injection and for 4 hours in lactated Ringer's injection when stored in glass or PVC containers at 25°C. When diluted and stored as recommended, it is not necessary to protect these solutions from light.

When admixed in the same syringe at room temperature, midazolam hydrochloride injection is reported to be physically compatible for at least 30 minutes with atropine sulfate, meperidine hydrochloride, morphine sulfate, or scopolamine hydrobromide, and for at least 8 hours with fentanyl citrate, glycopyrrolate, hydroxyzine hydrochloride, ketamine hydrochloride, nalbuphine hydrochloride, promethazine hydrochloride, or sufentanil citrate. Since the compatibility of these and other admixtures with midazolam hydrochloride injection depends on several factors (e.g., concentrations of the drugs, specific diluents used, resulting pH, temperature), specialized references should be consulted for specific information.

PREPARATIONS

Excipients in commercially available drug preparations may have clinically important effects in some individuals; consult specific product labeling for details.

Midazolam hydrochloride is subject to control under the Federal Controlled Substances Act of 1970 as a schedule IV (C-IV) drug.

Midazolam

Nasal

Solution	5 mg/0.1 mL	Nayzilam® Nasal Spray (C-IV), UCB

Midazolam Hydrochloride

Oral

Solution	2 mg (of midazolam) per mL*	Midazolam Hydrochloride Syrup (C-IV),

Parenteral

Injection	1 mg (of midazolam) per mL*	Midazolam Hydrochloride Injection (C-IV),
	5 mg (of midazolam) per mL*	Midazolam Hydrochloride Injection (C-IV),
		Seizalam® (C-IV), Meridian

* available from one or more manufacturer, distributor, and/or repackager by generic (nonproprietary) name

† Use is not currently included in the labeling approved by the US Food and Drug Administration

Eszopiclone

28:24.44 • NON-BENZODIAZEPINE HYPNOTICS

■ Eszopiclone, the S-enantiomer of zopiclone (not commercially available in the US), is a sedative and hypnotic agent structurally unrelated to the benzodiazepines.

USES

● Insomnia

Eszopiclone is used as a hypnotic agent in the management of transient and chronic insomnia. In controlled clinical studies, eszopiclone reportedly has been shown to have continued efficacy in decreasing sleep latency, improving sleep maintenance, and prolonging total sleep time when administered nightly for periods up to 6 months in duration.

Clinical Experience

Efficacy of eszopiclone for the management of transient insomnia was established in a controlled study in adults experiencing such insomnia during the first night in a sleep laboratory. In this study, 2- and 3-mg doses of eszopiclone were superior to placebo on the polysomnographic parameters of latency to persistent sleep (LPS) and wake time after sleep onset (WASO). Individuals receiving the 3-mg dose, but not those receiving the 2-mg dose, experienced substantially fewer awakenings than did individuals receiving placebo. Residual daytime psychomotor and/or cognitive impairment, as rated on a visual analog scale for morning sleepiness and assessed objectively using the Digit Symbol Substitution test (DSST), appeared to be minimal at eszopiclone doses of ≤3 mg. At such doses, sleep architecture (i.e., the percentage of time spent in each sleep stage) generally was preserved.

Efficacy of eszopiclone for the management of chronic insomnia was established in 5 controlled studies of up to 6 months' duration, including 3 studies in adults and 2 in geriatric patients. Results of these studies indicate that usual doses of eszopiclone (i.e., 2–3 mg in adults and 1–2 mg in geriatric patients) substantially decrease sleep latency; however, only the 3-mg dose in adults and the 2-mg dose in geriatric patients were superior to placebo on measures of sleep maintenance (e.g., WASO). Pharmacodynamic tolerance and adaptation to the hypnotic effect of eszopiclone were not observed during 6 months of therapy with the drug. Evidence to suggest, however, that such sleep improvements are maintained following discontinuance of eszopiclone is currently lacking.

Clinical Perspective

The American Academy of Sleep Medicine (AASM) and the American College of Physicians (ACP) have published clinical guidelines for the treatment of insomnia in adults. According to these guidelines, the goals of insomnia treatment are to improve sleep quality and quantity and to reduce insomnia-related daytime impairment, distress, and dysfunction. When possible, psychological and behavioral interventions are recommended as initial treatment. Pharmacologic therapy should be considered mainly in patients who are unable or unwilling to participate in cognitive behavioral therapy, are unresponsive to such therapy, or, in select cases, as a temporary adjunct to such therapy. When pharmacologic therapy is indicated, the choice of agent should be directed by symptoms, treatment goals, past treatment response, patient preference, drug cost and availability, comorbid conditions/contraindications, concomitant drug therapy/interactions, and potential adverse effects. Data on comparative efficacy of various sedative-hypnotic agents are limited, and an individualized and shared decision-making approach between patients and clinicians is advised.

Eszopiclone is among several agents recommended for the treatment of sleep onset and sleep maintenance insomnia. Pharmacologic therapy should be administered at the lowest effective dosage and should be short-term (e.g., 4–5 weeks) in duration; chronic use should be reserved for those individuals for whom cognitive behavioral therapy is either inaccessible or ineffective, who have been appropriately screened for contraindications to such treatment, who maintain long-term benefits with medication, and who are followed regularly. Patient monitoring should include ongoing assessment of effectiveness, monitoring for adverse effects, and evaluation for new onset or exacerbation of existing comorbid disorders.

DOSAGE AND ADMINISTRATION

● General

Pretreatment Screening

- Screen patients for diseases or conditions that may affect drug metabolism or hemodynamic responses.
- Consider the risk of respiratory depression prior to use of eszopiclone in patients with respiratory impairment.
- Screen patients for signs and symptoms of depression.
- Screen patients for a history of alcohol or drug abuse or psychiatric disorders.

Patient Monitoring

- Monitor for excess CNS depressant effects.
- Reevaluate patient if insomnia persists after 7–10 days of treatment.
- Carefully evaluate any new behavioral sign or symptom of concern.
- Closely monitor patients with a history of alcohol or drug abuse or psychiatric disorders.

● Administration

Eszopiclone is administered orally at bedtime. The drug should be taken immediately before retiring and only when the patient is able to get 7–8 hours of sleep before it is necessary to be active again.

Eszopiclone should not be administered with or immediately after a meal; administration with or immediately after a heavy, high-fat meal results in a decreased rate of absorption of eszopiclone and would be expected to decrease the drug's effect on sleep latency.

● Dosage

Dosage of eszopiclone should be individualized, and the lowest effective dosage should be used in all patient populations.

For the management of insomnia, the recommended initial adult dosage of eszopiclone is 1 mg immediately before bedtime. The recommended initial dosage is the same for women and men. If clinically indicated, dosage may be increased to 2 or 3 mg immediately before bedtime.

The dosage range of 2–3 mg has been shown to be effective in decreasing sleep latency and improving measures of sleep maintenance in adults <65 years of age. However, in some patients, the 2- or 3-mg dose may produce higher morning blood concentrations of eszopiclone, resulting in an increased risk of next-day impairment of driving and other activities that require full alertness. The adult dosage of eszopiclone should not exceed 3 mg immediately before bedtime.

● Special Populations

In geriatric or debilitated patients, the recommended initial dosage of eszopiclone is 1 mg immediately before bedtime. If clinically indicated, dosage may be increased to 2 mg immediately before bedtime. The dosage range of 1–2 mg has been shown to be effective in decreasing sleep latency and improving measures of sleep maintenance in geriatric patients. Dosage of eszopiclone in geriatric or debilitated patients should not exceed 2 mg immediately before bedtime.

In patients receiving a potent inhibitor of cytochrome P-450 (CYP) isoenzyme 3A4, dosage of eszopiclone should not exceed 2 mg immediately before bedtime.

Dosage adjustment is not necessary in patients with mild to moderate hepatic impairment. However, in patients with severe hepatic impairment, dosage of eszopiclone should not exceed 2 mg immediately before bedtime.

No eszopiclone dosage adjustment is necessary in patients with renal impairment.

CAUTIONS

● Contraindications

- History of a complex sleep behavior while taking eszopiclone, zaleplon, or zolpidem.

- Known hypersensitivity (e.g., anaphylaxis, angioedema) to eszopiclone or any ingredient in the formulation.

● Warnings/Precautions

Warnings

Complex Sleep Behaviors

Complex sleep behaviors such as sleepwalking, sleep driving (i.e., driving while not fully awake after ingesting a sedative-hypnotic drug, with no memory of the event), and engaging in other activities (e.g., making phone calls, preparing and eating food) while not fully awake have been reported in patients receiving sedative and hypnotic drugs. A boxed warning about the risk of complex sleep behaviors is included in the prescribing information for eszopiclone. Such complex sleep behaviors can result in serious injury and/or death. Complex sleep behaviors appear to be more common with eszopiclone, zaleplon, and zolpidem than other prescription medicines used for sleep. Patients usually have no memory of the events. These behaviors may occur when eszopiclone is used alone at recommended doses or when used concomitantly with alcohol or other CNS depressants. Serious injuries and fatalities from complex sleep behaviors have occurred in patients with and without a history of such behaviors and can occur even at the lowest recommended dosages and after just one dose of the hypnotic agent. Discontinue eszopiclone immediately in patients who experience a complex sleep behavior.

A total of 66 cases of complex sleep behaviors resulting in serious injuries or death in patients who took eszopiclone, zaleplon, or zolpidem were reported to the FDA Adverse Event Reporting System (FAERS) database and/or in published literature between December 1992 and March 2018. Of the 66 cases, 20 were reported as resulting in fatal outcomes and 46 reported serious nonfatal injuries; in the nonfatal cases, patients usually did not remember experiencing these complex sleep behaviors. These cases included falls with serious injuries such as intracranial hemorrhages, vertebral fractures, and hip fractures as well as fatal falls, self-injuries, accidental overdoses, hypothermia, suicide attempts and apparent completed suicides, fatal motor vehicle collisions, gunshot wounds, carbon monoxide poisoning, drowning or near drowning, burns, and homicide. Most of the patients in these cases reported using zolpidem (about 92%) when they experienced the complex sleep behavior; the remaining patients took eszopiclone (about 5%) or zaleplon (about 3%), reflecting the higher number of zolpidem prescriptions that were dispensed over this period compared with eszopiclone and zaleplon. The underlying mechanisms by which these drugs cause complex sleep behaviors are not fully understood.

Other Warnings and Precautions

Hypersensitivity Reactions

Angioedema involving the tongue, glottis, or larynx has occurred rarely following initial or subsequent doses of sedative and hypnotic drugs, including eszopiclone; airway obstruction may occur and may be fatal. Other symptoms suggestive of anaphylaxis (e.g., dyspnea, throat closing, nausea, vomiting) also have occurred. Medical therapy in the emergency department has been required in some patients.

Patients who develop angioedema following treatment with eszopiclone should not be rechallenged with the drug.

CNS Depressant Effects and Next-day Impairment

CNS depressant effects (i.e., memory impairment, confusion) have been reported in patients receiving higher doses of eszopiclone. In clinical studies evaluating CNS depressant effects of eszopiclone doses of 2–3 mg in adults, memory impairment was reported in 1–1.3% of patients receiving eszopiclone compared with 0% of those receiving placebo, and confusion was reported in 3% of patients receiving eszopiclone compared with 0% of those receiving placebo. In clinical studies evaluating CNS depressant effects of eszopiclone 2 mg in geriatric patients, memory impairment was reported in 1.5% of patients receiving eszopiclone compared with

0% of those receiving placebo, and confusion was reported in 2.5% of patients receiving eszopiclone compared with 0% of those receiving placebo.

Drowsiness and decreased levels of consciousness associated with eszopiclone may increase the risk of falls, particularly in geriatric patients.

Next-day impairment of psychomotor function has been reported in patients receiving the 3-mg dose of eszopiclone. In a study in 91 healthy individuals, treatment with eszopiclone 3 mg at bedtime was associated with next-morning impairment of psychomotor function (i.e., ability to maintain a motor vehicle in the driving lane, working memory, motor coordination); such impairment was most severe at 7.5 hours postdose but was still present and potentially clinically meaningful at 11.5 hours postdose. Patients often were unaware of these impairments.

The risk of next-day psychomotor impairment is increased if eszopiclone is administered with less than 7–8 hours of sleep time remaining. The risk of next-day impairment also is increased if a higher than recommended dose of eszopiclone is administered or when eszopiclone is used concomitantly with other CNS depressants or with drugs capable of increasing eszopiclone concentrations.

To reduce the potential risk of next-day impairment, the manufacturer and FDA have lowered the recommended initial dosage of eszopiclone from 2 mg to 1 mg immediately before bedtime. Women and men are equally susceptible to impairment from eszopiclone; therefore, the recommended initial dosage (1 mg immediately before bedtime) is the same for women and men. This lower initial dosage will result in less drug in the blood the next day. FDA states that patients currently receiving eszopiclone should continue therapy at the prescribed dosage and should contact their clinician to determine the most appropriate dosage. FDA is continuing to evaluate the risk of impaired mental alertness associated with other sedative and hypnotic drugs, including nonprescription (over-the-counter, OTC) preparations, and will update the public as new information becomes available. The agency states that nonprescription sedative and hypnotic drugs should not be considered safer than prescription drugs.

Patients receiving eszopiclone should be monitored for excessive CNS depressant effects; however, impairment may occur in the absence of symptoms and may not be reliably detected by ordinary clinical examination (i.e., formal psychomotor testing may be required). Patients receiving the 3-mg dose should be cautioned against driving or engaging in other activities that require complete mental alertness the day after use.

Concomitant use of eszopiclone with other CNS depressants (e.g., alcohol, benzodiazepines, opiates, tricyclic antidepressants) results in additive CNS depression. Concomitant use of eszopiclone with other sedative and hypnotic drugs, including OTC preparations used to treat insomnia (e.g., diphenhydramine, doxylamine succinate), at bedtime or in the middle of the night is not recommended.

Adequate Patient Evaluation

Because sleep disturbances may be a manifestation of a physical and/or psychiatric disorder, symptomatic treatment of insomnia should be initiated only after careful evaluation of the patient. Failure of insomnia to remit after 7–10 days of eszopiclone therapy, worsening of insomnia, or emergence of new abnormal thinking or behavior may indicate the presence of an underlying psychiatric, physical, and/or medical condition that requires evaluation; patients should be reevaluated if insomnia persists after 7–10 days of therapy.

Abnormal Thinking and Behavioral Changes

Abnormal thinking and behavioral changes have been reported in patients receiving sedative and hypnotic drugs. Some of these changes are similar to manifestations of alcohol intoxication or effects associated with other CNS depressants and include decreased inhibition (e.g., aggressiveness and extroversion that seem out of character), bizarre behavior, agitation, depersonalization, and hallucinations. Amnesia and other neuropsychiatric symptoms may occur unpredictably.

It can rarely be determined with certainty whether a particular instance of the abnormal behavior is drug induced, spontaneous, or results from an underlying psychiatric or physical disorder. Nevertheless, the emergence of any new behavioral sign or symptom of concern in patients receiving eszopiclone requires careful and immediate evaluation.

Withdrawal Effects

Manifestations of withdrawal have been reported following abrupt discontinuance or rapid reduction in dosage of sedative and hypnotic drugs. Clinical trials of eszopiclone did not reveal evidence of a serious withdrawal syndrome; however, anxiety, abnormal dreams, nausea, upset stomach, hyperesthesia, and neurosis were reported at an incidence of ≤2% after placebo substitution within 48 hours following the last dose of eszopiclone.

Rebound insomnia of 1 day's duration was noted in controlled trials of eszopiclone.

Abuse Potential

Studies using relatively high eszopiclone dosages (e.g., 2–4 times the maximum recommended hypnotic dosage) in individuals with a history of benzodiazepine abuse suggest that the abuse potential of eszopiclone is similar to that of benzodiazepines (e.g., diazepam); caution is advised in patients with a history of drug or alcohol abuse or a history of psychiatric disorders.

Tolerance

Pharmacodynamic tolerance and adaptation to the hypnotic effect of eszopiclone were not observed during studies of up to 6 months' duration.

Timing of Drug Doses

Ingesting eszopiclone while still up and about could result in adverse CNS effects such as short-term memory impairment, hallucinations, dizziness, and impaired coordination. Therefore, eszopiclone should be administered immediately before retiring.

Geriatric and/or Debilitated Patients

Geriatric and/or debilitated patients may be more sensitive to pharmacologic and adverse effects (e.g., impaired motor and/or cognitive performance) of sedative and hypnotic agents; reduction of the maximum dosage is recommended in such patients.

Concomitant Diseases

Experience in patients with concomitant disease is limited; eszopiclone should be used with caution in patients with diseases that may affect metabolism or hemodynamic responses.

Although respiratory depression was not reported in healthy individuals receiving doses 2.5-fold higher than the recommended dose, caution is advised in patients with impaired respiratory function.

Use in Patients with Depression

Worsening of depression and suicidal thoughts and actions (including completed suicides) have been reported in primarily depressed patients receiving sedative and hypnotic drugs.

As with other sedative and hypnotic agents, eszopiclone should be used with caution in patients with depression. Suicidal tendencies may be present, and protective measures may be required. Intentional overdosage is more common in this patient population, and the least amount of drug feasible should be prescribed and dispensed at any one time to avoid such intentional overdosage.

Specific Populations

Pregnancy

Available pharmacovigilance data on use of eszopiclone in pregnant women are insufficient to identify a drug-associated risk of major birth defects, miscarriage, or adverse maternal or fetal outcomes. There was no evidence of teratogenicity in animal reproduction studies in pregnant rats and rabbits administered eszopiclone throughout organogenesis. Administration of eszopiclone to rats throughout pregnancy and lactation resulted in offspring toxicities at all doses tested, with the lowest dose being approximately 200 times the maximum recommended human dose of 3 mg daily based on body surface area.

Lactation

It is not known whether eszopiclone is distributed into milk, affects the breast-fed infant, or affects milk production. Consider the developmental and health benefits of breast-feeding along with the mother's clinical need for eszopiclone and any potential adverse effects on the breast-fed infant from the drug or from the underlying maternal condition.

Pediatric Use

Safety and efficacy of eszopiclone have not been established in pediatric patients.

Eszopiclone has not been shown to be effective in the management of insomnia associated with attention deficit hyperactivity disorder (ADHD). In a 12-week controlled study in 483 pediatric patients (6–17 years of age) with insomnia associated with ADHD, eszopiclone (1, 2, or 3 mg at bedtime) did not decrease sleep latency as compared with placebo. In this study, the most frequent treatment-emergent adverse effects (compared with placebo) were psychiatric and nervous system effects, including dysgeusia (9 versus 1%), dizziness (6 versus 2%), hallucinations (2 versus 0%), and suicidal ideation (0.3 versus 0%). Discontinuance of therapy was required in 3% of patients receiving eszopiclone and in 2% of those receiving placebo.

Geriatric Use

In clinical studies, a total of 287 patients randomized to receive eszopiclone were 65 years of age or older (range: 65–86 years). The adverse effect profile of the 2-mg dose in geriatric patients (median age: 71 years) was similar to that observed in clinical trials of the drug in younger adults. However, patients ≥65 years of age had a longer elimination half-life and higher total systemic exposure to eszopiclone compared with younger adults. Reduction of the maximum dosage is recommended because of impaired motor and cognitive performance as well as increased sensitivity in geriatric patients.

Hepatic Impairment

Systemic exposure to eszopiclone is increased twofold in patients with severe hepatic impairment compared with healthy individuals.

Eszopiclone should be used with caution in patients with hepatic impairment. Dosage adjustment is not necessary in patients with mild to moderate hepatic impairment; however, reduction of the maximum dosage is recommended in those with severe hepatic impairment.

Renal Impairment

No dosage adjustment appears necessary in patients with renal impairment, since <10% of an oral dose of eszopiclone is excreted unchanged in urine.

● Common Adverse Effects

Adverse effects reported in ≥2% of patients receiving eszopiclone include unpleasant taste, headache, somnolence, respiratory infection, dizziness, dry mouth, rash, and viral infection.

DRUG INTERACTIONS

Eszopiclone is metabolized principally by cytochrome P-450 (CYP) isoenzymes 3A4 and 2E1; the drug does not appear to inhibit CYP isoenzymes 1A2, 2A6, 2C9, 2C19, 2D6, 2E1, or 3A4. Eszopiclone is not expected to alter the clearance of drugs that are metabolized by common CYP isoenzymes.

● Drugs Affecting Hepatic Microsomal Enzymes

Inhibitors of CYP3A4

Concomitant use of eszopiclone with inhibitors of CYP3A4 may result in increased systemic exposure to eszopiclone. When the potent CYP3A4 inhibitor ketoconazole (400 mg daily for 5 days) was administered concomitantly with eszopiclone (3 mg at bedtime), eszopiclone exposure, peak plasma concentration, and half-life were increased by 2.2-, 1.4-, and 1.3-fold, respectively.

If eszopiclone is used concomitantly with a potent CYP3A4 inhibitor (e.g., clarithromycin, itraconazole, ketoconazole, nefazodone, nelfinavir, ritonavir, troleandomycin), dosage of eszopiclone should not exceed 2 mg once daily immediately before bedtime.

Inducers of CYP3A4

Concomitant use of eszopiclone with inducers of CYP3A4 may result in decreased systemic exposure to and efficacy of eszopiclone. When zopiclone (not commercially available in the US) was administered concomitantly with the potent CYP3A4 inducer rifampin, exposure to zopiclone was decreased by 80%; a similar effect would be expected with eszopiclone.

● CNS-active Drugs

When eszopiclone was administered concomitantly with olanzapine, no alteration in the pharmacokinetics of either drug was observed; however, a pharmacodynamic interaction (effect on psychomotor function, as manifested by a decrease in Digit Symbol Substitution test [DSST] scores) was noted.

When eszopiclone (single dose) was administered concomitantly with paroxetine, no pharmacokinetic or pharmacodynamic interactions were observed; however, the possibility of a pharmacodynamic interaction between the drugs following long-term concomitant use cannot be ruled out.

● CNS Depressants

Concomitant use of eszopiclone with other CNS depressants (e.g., alcohol, benzodiazepines, opiates, sedatives and hypnotics, tricyclic antidepressants) may result in additive CNS depression. Concomitant use of alcohol with eszopiclone results in additive psychomotor impairment. Although no clinically important pharmacokinetic or pharmacodynamic interaction was observed following single-dose administration of eszopiclone with lorazepam, the possibility of a pharmacodynamic interaction between the drugs following long-term concomitant use cannot be ruled out.

Concomitant use of eszopiclone with alcohol should be avoided. Concurrent use of other sedative and hypnotic drugs used to treat insomnia (including OTC preparations such as diphenhydramine and doxylamine succinate) should also be avoided in patients receiving eszopiclone. When eszopiclone is used concomitantly with other CNS depressants, dosage reduction of eszopiclone and the CNS depressant may be necessary.

● Digoxin

The pharmacokinetics of digoxin were not affected following concomitant administration of eszopiclone (single 3-mg dose) with digoxin (0.5 mg twice daily for 1 day, followed by 0.25 mg daily for 6 days).

● Protein-bound Drugs

Because eszopiclone is not highly bound (52–59%) to plasma proteins, concomitant use of eszopiclone with highly protein-bound drugs is not expected to affect the free concentration of either drug.

● Warfarin

Concomitant administration of eszopiclone (3 mg daily for 5 days) with warfarin (single 25-mg dose) in healthy individuals did not affect the pharmacokinetics of *R*- or *S*-warfarin, nor were there any changes in the pharmacodynamic profile (prothrombin time).

DESCRIPTION

Eszopiclone, the *S*-enantiomer of zopiclone (not commercially available in the US), is a sedative and hypnotic agent that is structurally unrelated to benzodiazepines and other sedative and hypnotic agents that are commercially available in the US, including barbiturates, imidazopyridines (e.g., zolpidem), and pyrazolopyrimidines (e.g., zaleplon). Eszopiclone is pharmacologically similar to zaleplon and zolpidem; all of these agents have been shown to interact with the CNS γ-aminobutyric acid (GABA$_A$) receptor complex at binding domains located close to or allosterically coupled to benzodiazepine receptors. In vitro binding affinity of eszopiclone for benzodiazepine receptors is about 50 times that of the *R*-enantiomer of zopiclone. Preclinical data suggest that most, if not all, of the hypnotic effects of racemic zopiclone are attributable to the *S*-enantiomer. However, further studies are needed to determine whether these differences result in any clinical superiority of eszopiclone compared with zopiclone.

Eszopiclone is rapidly absorbed from the GI tract following oral administration. Eszopiclone has an intermediate duration of action (i.e., possesses a half-life of approximately 5–7 hours). Following oral administration, eszopiclone is extensively metabolized to several active and inactive metabolites via demethylation and oxidation by the cytochrome P-450 (CYP) 3A4 and 2E1 isoenzymes. Eszopiclone does not appear to have any inhibitory effect on CYP isoenzymes 1A2, 2A6, 2C9, 2C19, 2D6, 2E1, or 3A4.

ADVICE TO PATIENTS

- Provide patient with a copy of manufacturer's patient information. Advise patients to read the manufacturer's medication guide carefully prior to initiating therapy and each time the prescription is refilled.
- Instruct patients to administer the drug immediately before retiring.
- Instruct patients to take eszopiclone only when able to get a full night's sleep (i.e., 7–8 hours) before being active again.
- Advise patients to avoid taking eszopiclone with or immediately after a meal.
- Advise patients to take the drug only as prescribed; do not increase dosage or duration of therapy unless otherwise instructed by a clinician.
- Advise patients to contact their clinician if their insomnia worsens or does not improve within 7–10 days of treatment.
- Advise patients to avoid taking eszopiclone if alcohol has been consumed in the evening or before bedtime. Advise patients to avoid concurrent use of other sedative and hypnotic drugs used to treat insomnia (including OTC preparations such as diphenhydramine or doxylamine succinate) or CNS depressants during therapy, unless otherwise instructed by a clinician.
- Risk of serious injury and/or death resulting from complex sleep behaviors (e.g., sleep-walking, sleep-driving, preparing and eating food, making phone calls, or having sex while not being fully awake). Advise patients to discontinue eszopiclone and notify a clinician immediately if an episode of complex sleep behavior occurs during therapy, even if it did not result in a serious injury.
- Risk of next-day impairment, even when used as prescribed; impairment may be present despite feeling fully awake. Advise patients to exercise caution when operating machinery or performing hazardous tasks while using eszopiclone and to avoid these activities until they feel fully awake. Advise patients receiving the 3-mg dose to avoid driving or engaging in other activities that require complete mental alertness the day after use.
- Advise patients that drowsiness and decreased consciousness may increase the risk of falls in some patients.
- Risk of severe anaphylactic and anaphylactoid reactions; instruct patients to seek immediate medical attention if hypersensitivity reactions occur.
- Risk of abnormal thinking, behavioral changes, memory loss, and anxiety. Instruct patients to contact a clinician immediately if these adverse effects occur.
- Advise patients to immediately report any suicidal thoughts.
- Advise patients to inform clinicians of existing or contemplated concomitant therapy, including prescription and OTC drugs and herbal products, as well as concomitant or past illnesses (e.g., depression, substance abuse).
- Instruct women to inform their clinician if they are or plan to become pregnant or plan to breast-feed.
- Inform patients of other important precautionary information. (See Cautions.)

PREPARATIONS

Eszopiclone is subject to control under the Federal Controlled Substances Act of 1970 as a schedule IV (C-IV) drug.

Excipients in commercially available drug preparations may have clinically important effects in some individuals; consult specific product labeling for details.

Eszopiclone

Oral			
Tablets, film-coated	1 mg*	**Eszopiclone Tablets** (C-IV)	
		Lunesta® (C-IV), Sunovion	
	2 mg*	**Eszopiclone Tablets** (C-IV)	
		Lunesta® (C-IV), Sunovion	
	3 mg*	**Eszopiclone Tablets** (C-IV)	
		Lunesta® (C-IV), Sunovion	

* available from one or more manufacturer, distributor, and/or repackager by generic (nonproprietary) name

† Use is not currently included in the labeling approved by the US Food and Drug Administration.

Zaleplon

28:24.44 • NON-BENZODIAZEPINE HYPNOTICS

■ Zaleplon, a pyrazolopyrimidine derivative, is a sedative and hypnotic agent structurally unrelated to the benzodiazepines and other sedative-hypnotic agents.

USES

● Insomnia

Zaleplon is used in the short-term management of insomnia. Zaleplon has been shown to decrease sleep latency with repeated use for periods up to 30 days in duration. Because of the drug's short half-life, clinical studies have focused on decreasing sleep latency. Zaleplon has not been shown to substantially increase total sleep time or decrease the number of awakenings, and therefore appears to be most useful for sleep initiation disorders.

Clinical Experience

Efficacy of zaleplon for the treatment of transient insomnia was established in a controlled study in adults experiencing insomnia during the first night in a sleep laboratory; a 10-mg but not a 5-mg dose of zaleplon was superior to placebo in this patient population.

Efficacy for the treatment of chronic insomnia in adults was established in 9 controlled studies of 1–35 days' duration. The clinical efficacy trials ranged from a single night to 5 weeks in duration; the final formal assessments of sleep latency were performed at the end of treatment. The 10- and 20-mg doses of zaleplon were superior to placebo in decreasing sleep latency; some studies demonstrated efficacy versus placebo throughout the study, while others had a substantial number of placebo responders resulting in only 2 days' duration of superior efficacy for zaleplon. Although both the 10- and 20-mg doses were effective, the therapeutic effect was greater and more consistent with the 20-mg dose, and the 5-mg dose was less consistently effective. In one study, 10-mg doses of zaleplon were shown to have continued efficacy when administered for at least 30 consecutive nights. However, failure of insomnia to remit after 7–10 days of treatment may indicate the presence of a primary psychiatric and/or medical illness that should be evaluated. Insomnia may be the primary or first symptom of an unrecognized psychiatric and/or physical disorder.

Efficacy for the treatment of chronic initial insomnia in geriatric patients was established in 3 controlled studies of 2–14 days' duration in which 5- and 10-mg doses were shown to be superior to placebo in decreasing sleep latency.

Clinical Perspective

The American Academy of Sleep Medicine (AASM) and the American College of Physicians (ACP) have published clinical guidelines for the treatment of insomnia in adults. According to these guidelines, the goals of insomnia treatment are to improve sleep quality and quantity and to reduce insomnia-related daytime impairment, distress, and dysfunction. When possible, psychological and behavioral interventions are recommended as initial treatment. Pharmacologic therapy should be considered mainly in patients who are unable or unwilling to participate in cognitive behavioral therapy, are unresponsive to such therapy, or, in select cases, as a temporary adjunct to such therapy. When pharmacologic therapy is indicated, the choice of agent should be directed by symptoms, treatment goals, past treatment response, patient preference, drug cost and availability, comorbid conditions/contraindications, concomitant drug therapy/interactions, and potential adverse effects. Data on comparative efficacy of various sedative-hypnotic agents are limited, and an individualized and shared decision-making approach between patients and clinicians is advised.

Zaleplon is among several agents recommended for the treatment of sleep onset insomnia. Pharmacologic therapy should be administered at the lowest effective dosage and should be short-term (e.g., 4–5 weeks) in duration; chronic use should be reserved for those individuals for whom cognitive behavioral therapy is either inaccessible or ineffective, who have been appropriately screened for contraindications to such treatment, who maintain long-term benefits with medication, and who are followed regularly. Patient monitoring should include ongoing assessment of effectiveness, monitoring for adverse effects, and evaluation for new onset or exacerbation of existing comorbid disorders.

DOSAGE AND ADMINISTRATION

● General

Pretreatment Screening

● Screen patients for diseases or conditions that may affect drug metabolism or hemodynamic responses; use zaleplon with caution in such patients.

● Consider the risk of respiratory depression prior to use of zaleplon in patients with respiratory impairment, including those with sleep apnea or chronic obstructive pulmonary disease.

● Screen patients for a history of addiction to, or abuse of, drugs or alcohol.

Patient Monitoring

● Monitor for abnormal thinking and behavioral changes; carefully and immediately evaluate any new and concerning behavioral sign or symptom.

● Monitor geriatric and/or debilitated patients closely for adverse effects.

● Monitor patients with a history of addiction to, or abuse of, drugs or alcohol closely for zaleplon habituation and dependence.

● Administration

Zaleplon is administered orally without regard to meals, although administration with a high-fat meal should be avoided because of a potential decreased rate of drug absorption. Such delay in GI absorption could result in decreased efficacy on sleep latency.

Because of its rapid onset of action, zaleplon should be taken immediately before retiring when the patient is ready to go to sleep or after the patient has already gone to bed but has experienced difficulty falling asleep. Patients should be advised that zaleplon should only be used in circumstances where they are able to get a full night's sleep.

● Dosage

Dosage of zaleplon should be individualized. The lowest effective dosage of the drug should be used in all patient populations.

The recommended initial dosage of zaleplon for the management of insomnia in most adults <65 years of age is 10 mg immediately before bedtime or after unsuccessfully attempting to sleep. Although the risk of certain adverse effects appears to be dose dependent, 20-mg doses have been shown to be adequately tolerated and may be considered in most adults who do not respond adequately to lower doses. Doses >20 mg have not been adequately studied and are not recommended by the manufacturer.

● Special Populations

Hepatic Impairment

Patients with mild to moderate hepatic impairment should receive the 5-mg zaleplon dosage since drug clearance is reduced in these patients. Zaleplon is not recommended for use in patients with severe hepatic impairment.

Renal Impairment

No zaleplon dosage adjustment is necessary in patients with mild to moderate renal impairment; zaleplon has not been adequately studied in patients with severe renal impairment.

Geriatric and/or Debilitated Patients

For geriatric adults ≥65 years of age and debilitated patients, 5-mg doses of zaleplon are recommended. Doses >10 mg are not recommended in these populations.

Low-weight Patients

For certain low-weight nongeriatric adults, 5-mg doses of zaleplon may be sufficient.

Japanese Patients

Japanese adults demonstrated pharmacokinetic parameter differences that potentially could be explained by differences in body weight or hepatic enzyme activity.

Patients Receiving Cimetidine

Patients receiving cimetidine concomitantly should receive the 5-mg zaleplon dosage since drug clearance is reduced in these patients.

CAUTIONS

● *Contraindications*

● Hypersensitivity to zaleplon or any ingredient in the formulation.

● History of a complex sleep behavior while taking eszopiclone, zaleplon, or zolpidem.

● *Warnings/Precautions*

Warnings

Complex Sleep Behaviors

Complex sleep behaviors such as sleepwalking, sleep driving (i.e., driving while not fully awake after ingesting a sedative-hypnotic drug, with no memory of the event), and engaging in other activities (e.g., making phone calls, preparing and eating food) while not full awake have been reported in patients receiving sedative and hypnotic drugs. A boxed warning about the risk of complex sleep behaviors is included in the prescribing information for zaleplon. Such complex sleep behaviors can result in serious injury and/or death. Complex sleep behaviors appear to be more common with eszopiclone, zaleplon, and zolpidem than other prescription medicines used for sleep. Patients usually have no memory of the events. Serious injuries and fatalities from complex sleep behaviors have occurred in patients with and without a history of such behaviors and can occur even at the lowest recommended dosages and after just one dose of the hypnotic agent. These behaviors can occur when these drugs are taken alone or when taken with alcohol or other CNS depressants. Discontinue zaleplon immediately in patients who experience a complex sleep behavior.

A total of 66 cases of complex sleep behaviors resulting in serious injuries or death in patients who took eszopiclone, zaleplon, or zolpidem were reported to the FDA Adverse Event Reporting System (FAERS) database and/or in published literature between December 1992 and March 2018. Of the 66 cases, 20 were reported as resulting in fatal outcomes and 46 reported serious nonfatal injuries; in the nonfatal cases, patients usually did not remember experiencing these complex sleep behaviors. These cases included falls with serious injuries such as intracranial hemorrhages, vertebral fractures, and hip fractures as well as fatal falls, self-injuries, accidental overdoses, hypothermia, suicide attempts and apparent completed suicides, fatal motor vehicle collisions, gunshot wounds, carbon monoxide poisoning, drowning or near drowning, burns, and homicide. Most of the patients in these cases reported using zolpidem (about 92%) when they experienced the complex sleep behavior; the remaining patients took eszopiclone (about 5%) or zaleplon (about 3%), reflecting the higher number of zolpidem prescriptions that were dispensed over this period compared with eszopiclone and zaleplon. The underlying mechanisms by which these drugs cause complex sleep behaviors are not fully understood.

Other Warnings and Precautions

CNS Depression and Next-day Impairment

Like other sedative-hypnotic drugs, zaleplon has CNS-depressant effects. Because of its rapid onset of action, zaleplon should only be taken immediately prior to going to bed or after the patient has gone to bed and has experienced difficulty falling asleep. Drowsiness and decreased levels of consciousness associated with zaleplon may increase the risk of falls, particularly in geriatric patients.

Concomitant use of other CNS depressants (e.g., benzodiazepines, opiates, tricyclic antidepressants, alcohol) with zaleplon increases the risk of CNS depression. Because of the potential for additive effects, dosage adjustments of zaleplon and of concomitantly used CNS depressants may be necessary. The use of zaleplon with other sedative-hypnotic agents at bedtime or in the middle of the night is not recommended.

The risk of next-day psychomotor impairment, including impaired driving, is increased if zaleplon is taken with less than a full night of sleep (7–8 hours) remaining; if a higher than recommended dose is taken; if administered concomitantly with other CNS depressants, alcohol, or drugs that increase the blood levels of zaleplon. Warn patients against driving and engaging in other activities requiring complete mental alertness if zaleplon is taken in these circumstances.

Vehicle drivers and machine operators should be warned that, as with other sedative-hypnotic agents, there is a possible risk of adverse reactions (e.g., drowsiness, prolonged reaction time, dizziness, sleepiness, blurred/double vision, reduced alertness, and impaired driving) the morning after therapy. In order to minimize this risk, a full night of sleep (7–8 hours) is recommended.

Adequate Patient Evaluation

Since sleep disturbances may be a manifestation of a physical and/or psychiatric disorder, symptomatic treatment of insomnia should be initiated only after careful evaluation of the patient. The failure of insomnia to remit after 7–10 days of therapy may indicate the presence of an underlying psychiatric and/or medical condition requiring evaluation.

Worsening of insomnia or the emergence of new thinking or behavior abnormalities may be the consequence of an unrecognized psychiatric or physical disorder. Such findings have emerged during the course of treatment with sedative-hypnotic drugs, including zaleplon. Because some of the important adverse effects of zaleplon appear to be dose-related, it is important to use the lowest possible effective dose, especially in geriatric patients.

Sensitivity Reactions

Rare cases of angioedema involving the tongue, glottis, or larynx have been reported in patients receiving their first or subsequent doses of sedatives-hypnotics, including zaleplon. Some patients have experienced additional symptoms such as dyspnea, closing of the throat, or nausea and vomiting that suggest anaphylaxis. Some of these patients have required medical treatment in an emergency department. If angioedema involves the tongue, glottis, or larynx, airway obstruction may occur, which could be fatal. Patients who develop angioedema following treatment with zaleplon should not be rechallenged with the drug.

Some formulations of zaleplon contain the dye tartrazine (FD&C yellow No. 5), which may cause allergic reactions including bronchial asthma in susceptible individuals. Although the incidence of tartrazine sensitivity is low, it frequently occurs in patients who are sensitive to aspirin.

Abnormal Thinking and Behavioral Changes

Sedative-hypnotic agents are associated with numerous abnormal thought and behavioral processes (e.g., decreased inhibition, agitation, hallucinations, depersonalization, amnesia, depression/suicidal ideation); many are similar to manifestations of alcohol intoxication. Studies demonstrate short-term amnestic effects with zaleplon. Because of rapid clearance of the drug, amnestic effects peak at 1 hour after dosing, dissipate as early as 2 hours in some cases, and usually are gone within 3–4 hours; however, next-day memory impairment may occasionally occur and is dose dependent. As with other sedative-hypnotics, emergence of new psychiatric abnormalities during zaleplon therapy requires evaluation.

Abuse Potential

Studies using relatively high zaleplon doses (2.5–7.5 times the recommended hypnotic dose) suggest abuse potential similar to benzodiazepine and related hypnotics; the drug should be used with caution in patients with a history of drug or alcohol dependence or abuse.

Tolerance

No manifestations of tolerance for the therapeutic effects of zaleplon occurred during studies of 4 weeks' duration.

Dependence

Physical dependence results in the manifestation of withdrawal symptoms (e.g., rebound insomnia, anxiety) upon rapid dose decrease or abrupt discontinuance of many sedative-hypnotics, including zaleplon. Rebound insomnia of 1 day's duration was noted in controlled and open-label studies, principally in patients receiving the 20-mg dose of zaleplon. Although premarketing studies did not reveal evidence of a withdrawal syndrome other than such mild rebound insomnia, studies to date do not provide a reliable estimate of the incidence of dependence with zaleplon; in addition, at least 2 cases of seizure (one with a seizure history) have been reported.

Monitor patients closely during zaleplon discontinuance, as other sedative-hypnotics have manifested withdrawal symptoms such as seizures, vomiting, and abdominal cramps and experience with zaleplon to date is limited. Moreover, very short-acting hypnotics such as zaleplon may potentially demonstrate between-dose withdrawal symptoms, although no substantial clinical evidence of this phenomenon exists to date for zaleplon.

Timing of Drug Doses

Ingesting zaleplon while still up and about could result in adverse CNS effects such as short-term memory impairment, hallucinations, dizziness, and impaired coordination. Therefore, administer immediately before retiring or after experiencing difficulty falling asleep.

Geriatric or Debilitated Patients

Potential increased sensitivity to pharmacologic and adverse effects of hypnotic agents; use with caution and monitor such patients closely. To decrease the possibility of adverse effects, the recommended dosage of zaleplon in geriatric and/or debilitated patients is 5 mg.

Concomitant Illness

Experience is limited in patients with concomitant illnesses; zaleplon should be used with caution in patients with diseases or conditions that may affect metabolism or hemodynamic responses.

In general, sedative-hypnotic agents have the potential to depress respiration. Although no reports of respiratory depression have been noted with recommended zaleplon doses in studies to date (including in patients with moderate obstructive sleep apnea or mild to moderate chronic obstructive pulmonary disease [COPD]), patients with impaired respiratory function due to preexisting illness should be monitored carefully during zaleplon therapy.

Hepatic and Renal Disease

Reduce zaleplon dosage to 5 mg in patients with mild to moderate hepatic impairment. Use is not recommended in patients with severe hepatic impairment.

No adjustment of zaleplon dosage is necessary in patients with mild to moderate renal impairment. Zaleplon has not been adequately studied in patients with severe renal impairment.

Use in Patients with Depression

In primarily depressed patients treated with sedative-hypnotic agents, worsening of depression, including suicidal thoughts and actions (including completed suicides), have been reported. As with other sedative-hypnotic agents, zaleplon should be used with caution in patients with signs or symptoms of depression. Suicidal tendencies may be present in such patients and protective measures may be required. Intentional overdosage is more common in this patient population, and the least amount of drug that is feasible should be prescribed for the patient at any one time.

Specific Populations

Pregnancy

There are no studies of zaleplon in pregnant women to date. The manufacturer does not recommend use in this population, and there is no established use of the drug in labor and delivery.

Lactation

Zaleplon is distributed into milk. Since the effects of zaleplon on nursing infants are not known but even small amounts might be potentially important, the manufacturer does not recommend use in nursing women.

Pediatric Use

Safety and efficacy not established in pediatric patients <18 years of age.

Geriatric Use

Patients ≥65 years of age may be more sensitive to pharmacologic and adverse effects of sedative-hypnotic agents; initial and maximum dose reduction recommended.

Hepatic Impairment

Dosage reduction recommended for mild to moderate impairment; zaleplon use is not recommended in patients with severe impairment.

Renal Impairment

Dosage adjustment is not necessary in mild to moderate renal impairment; zaleplon has not been adequately studied in patients with severe renal impairment.

● Common Adverse Effects

Adverse effects occurring in ≥5% of patients receiving zaleplon include headache, asthenia, dizziness, nausea, abdominal pain, and somnolence.

DRUG INTERACTIONS

Zaleplon is metabolized principally by aldehyde oxidase, and to a lesser extent by CYP3A4; all metabolites of the drug are inactive.

● Drugs Affecting Hepatic Microsomal Enzymes

Cytochrome P-450 Isoenzyme 3A4 Inducers

Potential pharmacokinetic interaction with CYP3A4 inducers such as rifampin, phenytoin, carbamazepine, and phenobarbital: may result in decreased efficacy of zaleplon. Multiple-dose administration of rifampin (600 mg every 24 hours for 14 days) reduced zaleplon peak concentrations and AUC by approximately 80%. Consider an alternative sedative-hypnotic agent that is not a CYP3A4 substrate in patients receiving CYP3A4 inducers.

Cytochrome P-450 Isoenzyme 3A4 Inhibitors

Clinically important pharmacokinetic interaction is unlikely; routine adjustments of zaleplon dosage are not considered necessary when the drug is used concomitantly with CYP3A4 inhibitors. Concomitant administration of single, oral doses of zaleplon (10 mg) and erythromycin (800 mg), a strong, selective CYP3A4 inhibitor, resulted in increases in zaleplon peak plasma concentration and AUC of 34 and 20%, respectively. The effects of concomitant use of multiple doses of erythromycin on zaleplon pharmacokinetics are unknown. Other strong, selective CYP3A4 inhibitors (e.g., ketoconazole) also are expected to increase zaleplon exposure.

● Protein-bound Drugs

Zaleplon is not highly bound to plasma proteins; therefore, the disposition of zaleplon is not expected to be sensitive to alterations in protein binding. In addition, administration of zaleplon in patients receiving a highly protein-bound drug is not expected to cause a transient increase in free (unbound) concentration of the highly protein-bound drug.

● CNS Depressants

Potential pharmacodynamic interaction with other CNS depressants such as alcohol, imipramine, thioridazine, and diphenhydramine; anesthetics; anticonvulsants; antihistamines; sedatives and hypnotics; and opiates: may result in additive CNS effects. Concomitant administration of single doses of zaleplon 20 mg and imipramine 75 mg resulted in additive effects of decreased alertness and impaired psychomotor performance for 2–4 hours after administration; no alterations in the pharmacokinetics of either drug were observed. Concomitant administration of single doses of zaleplon 20 mg and thioridazine 50 mg resulted in additive effects of decreased alertness and impaired psychomotor performance for 2–4 hours after administration; no alterations in the pharmacokinetics of either drug were observed.

Concomitant use of sedative and hypnotic drugs used to treat insomnia should be avoided in patients receiving zaleplon.

Dosage adjustment of zaleplon and/or other CNS depressants may be necessary during concomitant use.

Alcohol

Potential pharmacodynamic interaction with alcohol: additive CNS effects. Administration of zaleplon 10 mg potentiated the CNS-impairing effects of ethanol 0.75 g/kg on balance testing and reaction time for 1 hour after ethanol administration and on the digit symbol substitution test (DSST), symbol copying test, and the variability component of the divided attention test for 2.5 hours after ethanol administration. Zaleplon did not affect the pharmacokinetics of ethanol. Alcohol should be avoided during zaleplon therapy.

● Cimetidine

Potential pharmacokinetic (CYP3A4 and aldehyde oxidase inhibition) interaction; initial zaleplon dose reduction to 5 mg recommended.

● Diphenhydramine

Pharmacokinetic (aldehyde oxidase inhibition) interaction unlikely; possible additive pharmacodynamic (CNS depressant) effect.

● Digoxin

Administration of zaleplon (10 mg) did not affect the pharmacokinetic or pharmacodynamic profile of digoxin (375 mcg once daily for 8 days).

● Ibuprofen

Pharmacokinetic interaction unlikely.

● Paroxetine

Concomitant administration of a single 20-mg dose of zaleplon and paroxetine 20 mg daily for 7 days did not result in any pharmacodynamic interaction related to psychomotor performance. In addition, the pharmacokinetics of zaleplon were not affected by paroxetine (a CYP2D6 inhibitor).

● Promethazine

Pharmacokinetic interaction unlikely; possible additive CNS effects. Concomitant administration of single doses of zaleplon 10 mg and promethazine 25 mg resulted in a 15% decrease in zaleplon peak plasma concentrations and no change in zaleplon AUC; however, the possible pharmacodynamic interaction between zaleplon and promethazine has not been evaluated. The manufacturer recommends using zaleplon and promethazine concomitantly with caution.

● Venlafaxine

Pharmacokinetic interaction unlikely. Concomitant administration of multiple doses of extended-release venlafaxine 150 mg and a single 10-mg dose of zaleplon did not result in a pharmacodynamic interaction and did not alter pharmacokinetics of either drug.

● Warfarin

Pharmacokinetic or pharmacodynamic (prothrombin time) interactions unlikely.

DESCRIPTION

Zaleplon, a pyrazolopyrimidine derivative, is a sedative and hypnotic agent structurally unrelated to the benzodiazepines and other sedative-hypnotic agents. Pharmacologically and pharmacokinetically, zaleplon is similar to zolpidem; both are hypnotic agents with short half-lives, and both have been shown to interact with the CNS γ-aminobutyric acid (GABA$_A$)-receptor-chloride ionophore complex at benzodiazepine (BZ) omega-1 (BZ$_1$, ω_1) receptors. In contrast, some benzodiazepines nonselectively activate central BZ$_1$ (ω_1) and BZ$_2$ (ω_2) receptors as well as peripheral BZ$_3$ (ω_3) receptors, resulting in nonspecific pharmacologic actions.

Zaleplon is extensively metabolized, principally by aldehyde oxidase, and to a lesser extent by the cytochrome P-450 (CYP) isoenzyme 3A4. Zaleplon generally appears to be absorbed and eliminated more rapidly than zolpidem.

ADVICE TO PATIENTS

- Provide patients with a copy of the manufacturer's medication guide.
- Advise patients to administer the drug immediately before retiring, or after attempting to fall asleep, and only when able to get a full night's sleep (7–8 hours) before it is necessary to be active again.
- Advise patients to avoid taking zaleplon with or immediately after a meal.
- Instruct patients to take zaleplon only as prescribed; do not increase the dose or duration of therapy unless otherwise instructed by a clinician.
- Advise patients to contact their clinician if their insomnia worsens or does not improve within 7–10 days of treatment.
- Risk of serious injury and/or death resulting from complex sleep behaviors (e.g., sleep-walking, sleep-driving, preparing and eating food, making phone calls, or having sex while not being fully awake). Advise patients to discontinue zaleplon and notify a clinician immediately if an episode of complex sleep behavior occurs during therapy, even if it did not result in a serious injury.
- Advise patients to exercise caution when operating machinery or performing hazardous tasks while using zaleplon and to avoid these activities until they feel fully awake. Inform patients that the risk of next-day psychomotor impairment, including impaired driving, is increased if zaleplon is taken with less than a full night of sleep (7–8 hours) remaining; if a higher than recommended dose is taken; if coadministered with other CNS depressants or alcohol; or if coadministered with other drugs that increase the blood levels of zaleplon; warn patients against driving and other activities requiring complete mental alertness if the drug is taken in these circumstances.
- Warn vehicle drivers and machine operators of the possible risk of adverse reactions including drowsiness, prolonged reaction time, dizziness, sleepiness, blurred/double vision, reduced alertness, and impaired driving the morning after therapy; in order to minimize this risk a full night of sleep (7-8 hours) is recommended.
- Advise patients to avoid alcohol and concurrent use of other sedative-hypnotic drugs used to treat insomnia (including OTC preparations such as diphenhydramine or doxylamine succinate) or CNS depressants during therapy unless otherwise instructed by a clinician.
- Advise patients that drowsiness and decreased consciousness may increase the risk of falls in some patients.
- Potential risk of severe hypersensitivity reactions; advise patients to immediately seek medical care if manifestations (e.g., angioedema, dyspnea, nausea, vomiting) of such reactions occur.
- Instruct patients to identify and report to clinicians any potential adverse effects, such as memory impairment, anxiety, or abnormal thinking or behavioral changes.
- Advise patient of possible rebound insomnia and withdrawal symptoms (e.g., unpleasant feelings, stomach and muscle cramps, vomiting, sweating, shakiness; seizures) for 1 or 2 nights after discontinuance.
- Advise patients to inform clinicians of existing or contemplated concomitant therapy, including prescription and OTC drugs and dietary or herbal supplements, as well as any concomitant illnesses (e.g., psychiatric disorders including depression or suicidality, history of drug or alcohol abuse or addiction, kidney or liver disease, lung disease or breathing difficulty).
- Advise women to inform clinicians if they are or plan to become pregnant or plan to breast-feed.
- Inform patients of other important precautionary information. (See Cautions.)

PREPARATIONS

Zaleplon is subject to control under the Federal Controlled Substances Act of 1970 as a schedule IV (C-IV) drug.

Excipients in commercially available drug preparations may have clinically important effects in some individuals; consult specific product labeling for details.

Zaleplon

Oral

Capsules	5 mg*	**Sonata®** (C-IV), Pfizer
		Zaleplon Capsules (C-IV)
	10 mg*	**Sonata®** (C-IV), Pfizer
		Zaleplon Capsules (C-IV)

* available from one or more manufacturer, distributor, and/or repackager by generic (nonproprietary) name

† Use is not currently included in the labeling approved by the US Food and Drug Administration.

Selected Revisions June 10, 2024, © Copyright, October 1, 1999, American Society of Health-System Pharmacists, Inc.

Zolpidem Tartrate

28:24.44 · NON-BENZODIAZEPINE HYPNOTICS

■ Zolpidem tartrate, a type A γ-aminobutyric acid (GABA$_A$)-receptor positive modulator of the imidazopyridine class, is a sedative and hypnotic agent structurally unrelated to the benzodiazepines and other sedative and hypnotic agents.

USES

● Insomnia

Zolpidem tartrate as conventional tablets or sublingual tablets (5 and 10 mg) is used as a hypnotic agent in the short-term management of insomnia characterized by difficulties with sleep initiation. Because zolpidem has a short half-life, the drug may be of particular benefit in the initiation of sleep (i.e., decreasing sleep latency). In controlled clinical studies, the drug reportedly has been effective in decreasing sleep latency for periods up to 35 days in duration.

Zolpidem tartrate as extended-release tablets is used for the short-term treatment of insomnia characterized by difficulty with sleep onset or sleep maintenance. However, the extended-release tablets may not be an appropriate treatment choice for patients with insomnia who need to drive or perform activities that require full alertness the next morning. In two 3-week, randomized, double-blind, placebo-controlled clinical trials in patients with chronic primary insomnia, zolpidem tartrate given as extended-release tablets improved sleep induction (as measured by latency to persistent sleep [LPS]) and sleep maintenance (as measured by wake time after sleep onset [WASO]). In one study in 212 adults 18–64 years of age, zolpidem tartrate 12.5 mg as extended-release tablets at bedtime decreased WASO for the first 7 hours during the first 2 nights of use and for the first 5 hours after 2 weeks of treatment. In a similarly designed study in 205 patients 65 years of age or older, a 6.25-mg dosage of the drug decreased WASO for the first 6 hours during the first 2 nights of use and for the first 4 hours after 2 weeks of treatment. In both studies, the drug decreased LPS during the first 2 nights of use and after 2 weeks of treatment and improved wakefulness at the end of the night (both measured by polysomnographic recordings) compared with placebo, and the drug was rated by patients as superior to placebo on a global impressions measure after 2 nights and after 3 weeks of use. In a 24-week, randomized, double-blind, placebo-controlled clinical trial in 1025 adults 18–64 years of age with chronic primary insomnia, zolpidem tartrate (12.5-mg administered as needed 3–7 nights per week as extended-release tablets) was superior to placebo on a patient-rated global impressions measure and on specific patient-reported parameters for sleep induction and maintenance; no substantial increase in frequency of drug use over time was observed.

Zolpidem tartrate as sublingual tablets (1.75 and 3.5 mg) is used as needed for the management of insomnia when middle-of-the-night awakening is followed by difficulty returning to sleep. The drug should be used in this manner *only* when 4 or more hours remain before the patient plans to awaken. In 2 randomized, double-blind, placebo-controlled clinical trials in patients with primary insomnia characterized by difficulty returning to sleep after a middle-of-the-night awakening, sublingual zolpidem tartrate improved sleep latency (as measured by polysomnography and patient-estimated reports) after middle-of-the-night awakening compared with placebo. In one crossover study, adults 19–64 years of age received each of 3 treatments (a 1.75- or 3.5-mg dose of zolpidem tartrate sublingual tablets or placebo) after a scheduled middle-of-the-night awakening on 2 consecutive nights in a sleep laboratory; the effect on sleep latency was similar for women receiving a 1.75-mg dose and men receiving a 3.5-mg dose. In the second study, adults 18–64 years of age received a 3.5-mg dose of zolpidem tartrate sublingual tablets or placebo on an as-needed basis over 4 weeks in an outpatient setting when the patient had difficulty returning to sleep after awakening in the middle of the night, provided at least 4 hours remained before the patient planned to awaken.

Hypnotics with a relatively short half-life may be more likely to result in transient rebound insomnia after discontinuance and in pharmacodynamic tolerance and adaptation to the hypnotic effect, with resultant diminished effectiveness during the end of each night's use (early morning insomnia) and, possibly, increased daytime anxiety. However, despite zolpidem's short half-life, the manufacturer states that increased wakefulness during the last third of the night and objective evidence of rebound insomnia following discontinuance of zolpidem tartrate as conventional tablets have not been observed in clinical trials to date, although there was subjective evidence of impaired sleep on the first posttreatment night in geriatric patients receiving zolpidem tartrate as conventional tablets in doses that exceeded the recommended geriatric dose of 5 mg. Rebound insomnia was observed in two 3-week clinical trials on the first night after abrupt discontinuance of zolpidem tartrate as extended-release tablets, but there was no worsening compared with baseline on the second night. In a 24-week clinical trial evaluating zolpidem tartrate extended-release tablets administered as needed 3–7 nights per week, a rebound effect was observed within the first month for total sleep time, but not for WASO, during the first night that the drug was not used; however, no further rebound insomnia was observed after the first month or after final treatment discontinuance.

In addition, hypnotics with relatively short half-lives may be less likely to result in residual daytime sedative effects and in impaired psychomotor and mental performance during continued therapy. Residual daytime sedative effects of zolpidem were evaluated in several placebo-controlled studies in healthy adults and in geriatric individuals. A small but statistically significant decrease in performance (determined by the Digit Symbol Substitution test [DSST]) was observed in some adults and geriatric individuals receiving zolpidem tartrate as conventional tablets compared with those receiving placebo. Several studies of zolpidem tartrate as conventional tablets in adults with insomnia found no evidence of residual daytime sedative effects, determined by DSST, the Multiple Sleep Latency Test (MSLT), and patient rating of alertness. In studies of zolpidem tartrate extended-release tablets (given at recommended doses) in adult and geriatric patients, neurocognitive tests performed 8 hours after a dose and patient reports of sedation revealed no evidence of decreased performance or next-day residual effects. However, during the 3-week clinical trials evaluating the extended-release tablets, next-day somnolence was reported by 15% or 2% of adults receiving zolpidem or placebo, respectively, and by 6% or 5% of geriatric patients receiving zolpidem or placebo, respectively. In the 24-week clinical trial, the overall incidence of next-day somnolence was 5.7% or 2% in patients receiving zolpidem tartrate as extended-release tablets or placebo, respectively. The minimal effect of zolpidem on sleep stages at usual hypnotic dosages may offer a therapeutic advantage. However, the fact that zolpidem has minimal anxiolytic and muscle relaxant properties at usual hypnotic doses also should be considered. Blood concentrations of zolpidem may be high enough in some patients on the morning after use to impair performance of activities that require alertness, including driving, and FDA states that all drugs used in the management of insomnia can impair driving and performance of activities that require alertness on the morning after use.

Clinical Perspective

The American Academy of Sleep Medicine (AASM) and the American College of Physicians (ACP) have published clinical guidelines for the treatment of insomnia in adults. According to these guidelines, the goals of insomnia treatment are to improve sleep quality and quantity and to reduce insomnia-related daytime impairment, distress, and dysfunction. When possible, psychological and behavioral interventions are recommended as initial treatment. Pharmacologic therapy should be considered mainly in patients who are unable or unwilling to participate in cognitive behavioral therapy, are unresponsive to such therapy, or, in select cases, as a temporary adjunct to such therapy. When pharmacologic therapy is indicated, the choice of agent should be directed by symptoms, treatment goals, past treatment response, patient preference, drug cost and availability, comorbid conditions/contraindications, concomitant drug therapy/interactions, and potential adverse effects. Data on comparative efficacy of various sedative hypnotic agents are limited, and an individualized and shared decision-making approach between patients and clinicians is advised.

Zolpidem is among several agents recommended for the treatment of sleep onset or sleep maintenance insomnia. Pharmacologic therapy should be used at the lowest effective dosage and should be short-term (e.g., 4–5 weeks) in duration; chronic use should be reserved for those individuals for whom cognitive behavioral therapy is either inaccessible or ineffective, who have been appropriately screened for contraindications to such treatment, who maintain long-term benefits with medication, and who are followed regularly. Patient monitoring should include ongoing assessment of effectiveness, monitoring for adverse effects, and evaluation for new onset or exacerbation of existing comorbid disorders.

DOSAGE AND ADMINISTRATION

● General

Pretreatment Screening

- Consider the risk of respiratory depression prior to use of zolpidem in patients with respiratory impairment, including those with sleep apnea or myasthenia gravis or in those receiving concomitant opiates or other CNS depressants.

Patient Monitoring

- Monitor for excessive CNS depression.

- Monitor for abnormal thinking and behavioral changes; carefully and immediately evaluate any new and concerning behavioral sign or symptom.

Other General Considerations

- Reevaluate patient if zolpidem is to be used for more than 2–3 weeks.

- Consider gradual dosage reduction (e.g., over several nights) when discontinuing therapy.

● Administration

Zolpidem tartrate is administered orally (as conventional tablets or extended-release tablets) or sublingually (as sublingual tablets).

Oral Administration

Zolpidem tartrate is administered orally at bedtime. Zolpidem tartrate should be taken only once per night immediately before bedtime and at least 7–8 hours before the planned time of awakening; patients should be advised of the importance of only taking the drug at such time. In addition, because food can reduce both the rate and extent of GI absorption of zolpidem tartrate, the drug should not be administered with or immediately after a meal in order to facilitate the onset of sleep.

Zolpidem tartrate extended-release tablets are commercially available as a coated bilayer formulation in which a portion of the labeled dose is contained in an immediate-release layer and the remaining portion is contained in a layer that slowly releases the drug. Following oral administration, the extended-release tablets exhibit biphasic absorption with a rapid initial absorption that is similar to that of immediate-release (conventional) tablets and extended absorption exceeding 3 hours after administration.

Zolpidem tartrate extended-release tablets should be swallowed whole and should *not* be divided, crushed, or chewed.

Sublingual Administration

Zolpidem tartrate 5- and 10-mg sublingual tablets should be taken only once per night immediately before bedtime and at least 7–8 hours before the planned time of awakening; patients should be advised of the importance of only taking the drug at such time. The tablet should be placed under the tongue, where it will disintegrate. The tablet should not be swallowed or administered with water. In addition, because food can reduce both the rate and extent of absorption of zolpidem tartrate, the drug should not be administered with or immediately after a meal in order to facilitate the onset of sleep.

Zolpidem tartrate 1.75- and 3.5-mg sublingual tablets should be taken in bed, only once per night as needed if a middle-of-the-night awakening is followed by difficulty returning to sleep, and only if at least 4 hours remain before the planned time of awakening; patients should be advised of the importance of only taking the drug at such time. The tablet should be placed under the tongue and allowed to disintegrate completely before swallowing. The tablet should not be swallowed whole. In addition, because food can reduce both the rate and extent of absorption of zolpidem tartrate, the drug should not be administered with or immediately after a meal for optimal effect. The tablet should be removed from the pouch just prior to administration.

● Dosage

The lowest effective dosage of zolpidem tartrate should be used. Long-term use of zolpidem is not recommended; treatment duration should be as short as possible.

Extended treatment should not take place without re-evaluation of the patient's status; risk of abuse and dependence increases with the duration of treatment.

The recommended initial doses of zolpidem tartrate for women and men differ because clearance of the drug is slower in women.

Because manifestations of withdrawal have been reported following abrupt discontinuance or rapid reduction in dosage of zolpidem, patients should be monitored for tolerance, abuse, and dependence. There also is evidence that abrupt discontinuance of sedative and hypnotic drugs, including zolpidem tartrate, may result in rebound insomnia, which usually persists for 1 or 2 nights; this effect may occur with some sedative and hypnotic drugs even after relatively short periods of therapy (e.g., 1 week). Therefore, some clinicians suggest that gradual dosage reduction (e.g., over several nights) be considered when discontinuing therapy, since the development of rebound insomnia can perpetuate continued use of hypnotics in patients with insomnia.

Oral Dosage

For the management of insomnia characterized by difficulties with sleep initiation, the recommended initial dose of zolpidem tartrate as an oral immediate-release preparation (conventional tablets) is a single dose of 5 mg in women and either 5 or 10 mg in men. If the 5-mg dose of immediate-release zolpidem tartrate is not effective in men or women, the dose may be increased to 10 mg.

For the management of insomnia characterized by difficulties with sleep initiation or sleep maintenance, the recommended initial dose of zolpidem tartrate as extended-release tablets is 6.25 mg in women and either 6.25 or 12.5 mg in men. If the 6.25-mg dose of extended-release zolpidem tartrate is not effective in men or women, the dose may be increased to 12.5 mg.

In some patients, higher morning blood concentrations following use of a 10-mg dose of immediate-release zolpidem tartrate or a 12.5-mg dose of extended-release zolpidem tartrate increase the risk of next-day impairment of driving and other activities that require full alertness. Total dosage should not exceed 10 mg of immediate-release zolpidem tartrate or 12.5 mg of extended-release zolpidem tartrate given once daily immediately before bedtime.

If zolpidem is used concomitantly with other CNS depressants, dosage adjustment of zolpidem and the concomitantly administered agent(s) may be necessary because of potentially additive effects.

Sublingual Dosage

For the short-term management of insomnia characterized by difficulties with sleep initiation, the recommended initial dose of zolpidem tartrate sublingual tablets is 5 mg for women and either 5 or 10 mg for men. If the 5-mg dose is not effective in men or women, the dose may be increased to 10 mg. In some patients, higher morning blood concentrations following use of a 10-mg dose increase the risk of next-day impairment of driving and other activities that require full alertness. Total dosage should not exceed 10 mg given once daily immediately before bedtime. If zolpidem is used concomitantly with other CNS depressants, dosage adjustment of zolpidem and the concomitantly administered agent(s) may be necessary because of potentially additive effects.

For as-needed use in the management of insomnia when middle-of-the-night awakening is followed by difficulty returning to sleep, the recommended and maximum dose of zolpidem tartrate sublingual tablets is 1.75 mg for women and 3.5 mg for men.

In patients receiving other CNS depressants concomitantly, the recommended sublingual dose of zolpidem tartrate for middle-of-the-night awakening is 1.75 mg; dosage adjustment of the concomitant CNS depressant may be necessary because of potentially additive effects.

● Special Populations

Hepatic Impairment

Zolpidem tartrate conventional tablets: For the management of insomnia characterized by difficulties with sleep initiation, the recommended dosage of zolpidem tartrate conventional tablets in patients with mild or moderate hepatic impairment is 5 mg once daily immediately before bedtime.

Zolpidem tartrate sublingual tablets: For the management of insomnia characterized by difficulties with sleep initiation, the recommended dosage of zolpidem tartrate sublingual tablets in patients with any degree of hepatic impairment is 5 mg once daily immediately before bedtime.

Zolpidem tartrate sublingual tablets: For use in the management of insomnia when middle-of-the-night awakening is followed by difficulty returning to sleep, the recommended sublingual dosage of zolpidem tartrate in patients with any degree of hepatic impairment is 1.75 mg once per night if needed.

Zolpidem tartrate extended-release tablets: For the management of insomnia characterized by difficulty with sleep initiation or sleep maintenance in patients with mild or moderate hepatic impairment, the recommended dosage of zolpidem tartrate as extended-release tablets is 6.25 mg once daily immediately before bedtime.

In patients with severe hepatic impairment, zolpidem may contribute to the occurrence of encephalopathy; the manufacturer of zolpidem conventional and extended-release tablets states that use should be avoided in such patients.

Renal Impairment

The manufacturers and some clinicians state that dosage adjustment is not necessary in patients with renal impairment. Other clinicians, however, state that the possibility that dosage reduction may be needed for patients with renal disease should be considered because of slower zolpidem elimination rates and other pharmacokinetic alterations observed in nondialyzed patients with chronic renal disease and in patients undergoing periodic dialysis.

Geriatric or Debilitated Patients

In geriatric or debilitated patients, the recommended bedtime dosage of zolpidem tartrate is 5 mg as an immediate-release preparation or 6.25 mg as extended-release tablets given once daily immediately before bedtime.

In geriatric or debilitated patients, the recommended sublingual dose of zolpidem tartrate for management of insomnia characterized by difficulties with sleep initiation is 5 mg once daily immediately before bedtime.

In patients >65 years of age, the recommended sublingual dosage of zolpidem tartrate for middle-of-the-night awakening is 1.75 mg taken only once per night if needed.

CAUTIONS

● *Contraindications*

- History of a complex sleep behavior while taking eszopiclone, zaleplon, or zolpidem.
- Known hypersensitivity to zolpidem.

● *Warnings/Precautions*

Warnings

Complex Sleep Behaviors

Complex sleep behaviors such as sleepwalking, sleep driving (i.e., driving while not fully awake after ingesting a sedative-hypnotic drug, with no memory of the event), and engaging in other activities (e.g., making phone calls, preparing and eating food) while not fully awake have been reported in patients receiving sedative and hypnotic drugs. A boxed warning about the risk of complex sleep behaviors is included in the prescribing information for zolpidem. Such complex sleep behaviors can result in serious injury and/or death. Complex sleep behaviors appear to be more common with eszopiclone, zaleplon, and zolpidem than other prescription medicines used for sleep. Patients usually have no memory of the events. These behaviors may occur when zolpidem is used alone at recommended doses or when used concomitantly with alcohol or other CNS depressants. Serious injuries and fatalities from complex sleep behaviors have occurred in patients with and without a history of such behaviors and can occur even at the lowest recommended dosages and after just one dose of the hypnotic agent. Discontinue zolpidem immediately in patients who experience a complex sleep behavior.

A total of 66 cases of complex sleep behaviors resulting in serious injuries or death in patients who took eszopiclone, zaleplon, or zolpidem were reported to the FDA Adverse Event Reporting System (FAERS) database and/or in published literature between December 1992 and March 2018. Of the 66 cases, 20 were reported as resulting in fatal outcomes and 46 reported serious nonfatal injuries; in the nonfatal cases, patients usually did not remember experiencing these complex sleep behaviors. These cases included falls with serious injuries such as

intracranial hemorrhages, vertebral fractures, and hip fractures as well as fatal falls, self-injuries, accidental overdoses, hypothermia, suicide attempts and apparent completed suicides, fatal motor vehicle collisions, gunshot wounds, carbon monoxide poisoning, drowning or near drowning, burns, and homicide. Most of the patients in these cases reported using zolpidem (about 92%) when they experienced the complex sleep behavior; the remaining patients took eszopiclone (about 5%) or zaleplon (about 3%), reflecting the higher number of zolpidem prescriptions that were dispensed over this period compared with eszopiclone and zaleplon. The underlying mechanisms by which these drugs cause complex sleep behaviors are not fully understood.

Other Warnings and Precautions

CNS Depression and Next-day Impairment

Like other sedative-hypnotic drugs, zolpidem has CNS-depressant effects and may impair daytime function in some patients even when used as prescribed. To decrease the potential risk of next-day impairment, clinicians should prescribe and patients should take the smallest effective dose. Bedtime dosages of zolpidem that currently are recommended by the manufacturers and FDA are lower than the original labeled dosages; such dosage reductions were prompted by concerns about excessively high concentrations of the drug in some patients on the morning after use and the attendant risks of next-day psychomotor impairment. Patients receiving zolpidem should be monitored for excessive CNS depressant effects; however, impairment may occur in the absence of symptoms and may not be reliably detected by ordinary clinical examination (i.e., formal psychomotor testing may be required). Drowsiness and decreased levels of consciousness associated with zolpidem may result in an increased risk of falls, particularly in geriatric patients. In order to minimize the risk of CNS effects, a full night of sleep (7–8 hours) is recommended.

Concomitant use of zolpidem with other CNS depressants (e.g., alcohol, benzodiazepines, opiates, tricyclic antidepressants) increases the risk of additive CNS depression, and reductions in dosage of zolpidem and any concomitant CNS depressants may be necessary. Patients taking zolpidem should be advised of the importance of not consuming alcohol in the evening or before bedtime. The use of zolpidem with other sedative and hypnotic drugs (including other zolpidem-containing preparations and OTC preparations used to treat insomnia at bedtime or in the middle of the night) also is not recommended.

All patients receiving zolpidem should be informed of the potential for next-day impairment, that the risk is increased if dosing instructions are not carefully followed, and that impairment may be present despite feeling fully awake. The risk of next-day psychomotor impairment, including impaired driving, is increased if zolpidem preparations intended for bedtime administration (e.g., conventional tablets, extended-release tablets, 5- or 10-mg sublingual tablets) are administered with less than 7–8 hours of sleep time remaining or if zolpidem preparations intended for middle-of-the-night administration (e.g., 1.75- or 3.5-mg sublingual tablets) are administered with less than 4 hours of sleep time remaining. Therefore, patients receiving zolpidem tartrate immediate-release preparations intended for bedtime administration (e.g., conventional tablets, 5- or 10-mg sublingual tablets) should be advised to wait at least 8 hours after administering zolpidem before driving or engaging in other activities requiring full mental alertness, and those receiving zolpidem tartrate preparations intended for middle-of-the-night administration (e.g., 1.75- or 3.5-mg sublingual tablets) should be advised to wait at least 4 hours and until they feel fully awake before engaging in such activities. Patients receiving zolpidem tartrate extended-release tablets should also be cautioned against driving a motor vehicle or performing other activities requiring complete mental alertness on the day after using the drug. Patients should be advised not to use zolpidem if they have consumed alcohol that evening or before bedtime.

Driving simulation and laboratory studies indicate that blood zolpidem concentrations exceeding approximately 50 ng/mL appear to be capable of impairing driving performance to a degree that increases the risk of a motor vehicle accident. The risk for next-morning impairment is highest for patients receiving extended-release preparations of the drug. Zolpidem tartrate extended-release tablets may not be an appropriate treatment choice for patients who need to drive or perform activities that require full alertness the next morning. While pharmacodynamic tolerance or adaptation to some adverse CNS depressant effects of extended-release zolpidem may develop, concentrations of the drug may remain high enough the next day to impair performance of these activities. In addition, women appear to be more susceptible than men to next-day psychomotor impairment because clearance of zolpidem is slower in women than in men. In pharmacokinetic studies evaluating 10-mg doses of immediate-release zolpidem tartrate (i.e., conventional tablet or bioequivalent preparations) in approximately 250 men and 250 women, zolpidem concentrations measured approximately 8 hours after a dose exceeded 50 ng/mL in 15% of women and 3% of men; results of 3 concentration measurements in women and 1 concentration measurement in men were at least 90 ng/mL. In pharmacokinetic studies evaluating 12.5-mg doses of extended-release zolpidem tartrate, zolpidem concentrations measured approximately 8 hours after a dose exceeded 50 ng/mL in 33% of women and 25% of men, and were at least 100 ng/mL in about 5% of patients. In studies evaluating 6.25-mg doses of extended-release zolpidem tartrate, zolpidem concentrations measured approximately 8 hours after a dose were 50 ng/mL or higher in about 15% of nongeriatric women, 5% of nongeriatric men, and 10% of both geriatric men and women.

The effect of middle-of-the-night sublingual administration of zolpidem tartrate on next-morning driving performance has been evaluated in a randomized, double-blind, placebo- and active-controlled crossover study in healthy individuals. In this study, individuals received a 3.5-mg sublingual dose of zolpidem tartrate 3 or 4 hours before driving, placebo, or an active control 9 hours before driving. When the driving test began 3 hours after the zolpidem dose, impairment (as measured by a standard test of road tracking precision ["weaving"]) was significantly worse than during the placebo test period, and testing was terminated for one individual (a 23-year-old woman) because of somnolence. When the driving test began 4 hours after the zolpidem dose, results were numerically worse than during the placebo period, but statistical significance was not established. Blood concentrations of zolpidem were not measured. However, the manufacturer states that the estimated zolpidem concentration in individuals with worse driving performance during the zolpidem test period is considered to present a risk for driving impairment. In some women, zolpidem concentrations remain at or sometimes considerably higher than this concentration for 4 or more hours after a 3.5-mg sublingual dose of the drug; therefore, the recommended dose of zolpidem tartrate for management of middle-of-the-night awakening in women is 1.75 mg. Because a small adverse effect on road tracking precision may remain 4 hours after a 1.75-mg dose in women or a 3.5-mg dose in men, potential impairment of driving performance at these recommended dosages cannot be completely excluded.

Adequate Patient Evaluation

Because sleep disturbances may be a manifestation of a physical and/or psychiatric disorder, symptomatic treatment of insomnia should be initiated only after careful evaluation of the patient. The failure of insomnia to remit after 7–10 days of zolpidem therapy may indicate the presence of an underlying psychiatric and/or medical condition that should be evaluated. Prolonged use of hypnotics (e.g., for longer than 2–3 weeks) usually is not indicated and should be undertaken only on further evaluation of the patient. Worsening of insomnia or emergence of new thinking or behavioral abnormalities during therapy with sedative and hypnotic drugs, including zolpidem, may be the consequence of an unrecognized psychiatric or physical disorder.

Severe Hypersensitivity Reactions

Angioedema involving the tongue, glottis, or larynx has been reported following initial or subsequent doses of sedative and hypnotic drugs, including zolpidem, and may result in airway obstruction and death. Anaphylaxis also has occurred. Patients who develop angioedema following treatment with zolpidem should not be rechallenged with the drug.

Abnormal Thinking and Behavioral Changes

Abnormal thinking and behavioral changes have been reported in patients receiving sedative and hypnotic drugs, including zolpidem. Some of these changes included decreased inhibition (e.g., aggressiveness and extroversion that seemed out of character), bizarre behavior, agitation, depersonalization, and visual and auditory hallucinations. Amnesia, anxiety, and other neuropsychiatric symptoms also may occur. Cases of delirium also have been reported.

The emergence of any new behavioral sign or symptom of concern in patients receiving zolpidem requires careful and immediate evaluation.

Use in Patients with Depression

In primarily depressed patients receiving treatment with sedative and hypnotic drugs, worsening of depression and suicidal thoughts and actions (including completed suicides) have been reported. Suicidal tendencies may be present in such patients, and protective measures may be required. Intentional overdosage is more common in this patient population; therefore, the least amount of zolpidem that is feasible should be prescribed for such patients at any one time. Patients should be advised to immediately inform their clinician if any suicidal thoughts occur.

Respiratory Depression

Although clinical studies did not reveal respiratory depressant effects following 10-mg doses of zolpidem tartrate in healthy individuals or in patients with mild-to-moderate chronic obstructive pulmonary disease (COPD), decreased oxygen saturation was observed in patients with mild-to-moderate sleep apnea. Respiratory insufficiency has been reported during postmarketing experience in patients receiving 10-mg doses of zolpidem tartrate, most of whom had preexisting respiratory impairment. Since sedative and hypnotic drugs have the capacity to depress respiratory drive, the drug should be used with caution in patients with compromised respiratory function and in patients receiving concomitant opiates or other CNS depressants. The risk of respiratory depression should be considered prior to use of zolpidem in patients with respiratory impairment, including those with sleep apnea or myasthenia gravis or in those receiving concomitant opiates or other CNS depressants.

Precipitation of Hepatic Encephalopathy

Precipitation of hepatic encephalopathy has been reported in patients with hepatic insufficiency receiving drugs affecting GABA receptors (e.g., zolpidem tartrate). In addition, zolpidem is eliminated more slowly in patients with hepatic insufficiency. Avoid use of zolpidem conventional or extended-release tablets in patients with severe hepatic impairment.

Tolerance, Dependence, and Abuse

Use of zolpidem may lead to the development of physical and/or psychological dependence. The risk of dependence increases with dose and duration of treatment and is greater in patients with a history of alcohol or drug abuse.

Because manifestations of withdrawal have been reported following abrupt discontinuance or rapid reduction in dosage of zolpidem, patients should be monitored for tolerance, abuse, and dependence. Withdrawal symptoms associated with sedative and hypnotic drugs range from mild dysphoria and insomnia to a withdrawal syndrome that may include abdominal and muscle cramps, vomiting, sweating, tremors, seizures, and delirium. In clinical trials with zolpidem in the US, manifestations of uncomplicated sedative and hypnotic withdrawal, including fatigue, nausea, flushing, lightheadedness, uncontrolled crying, emesis, stomach cramps, panic attack, nervousness, and abdominal discomfort, were reported after placebo substitution within 48 hours following the last dose of the drug. These adverse events occurred in 1% or less of patients. Available data cannot provide a reliable estimate of the frequency, if any, of dependency during therapy with recommended dosages of zolpidem. Studies of abuse potential in former drug abusers found that the effects of single 40-mg doses of zolpidem tartrate and 20-mg doses of diazepam were similar but not identical, while the effects of a 10-mg dose of zolpidem tartrate were difficult to distinguish from those of placebo. Because patients with a current or past history of addiction to or abuse of drugs or alcohol are at increased risk for misuse or abuse of or addiction to zolpidem, the drug should be used with extreme caution in such patients. Patients should be advised not to increase the dosage of zolpidem and to inform their clinician if the drug is not effective. Long-term use of zolpidem is not recommended; treatment duration should be as short as possible. Extended treatment should not take place without reevaluation of the patient's status; risk of abuse and dependence increases with the duration of treatment.

Specific Populations

Pregnancy

Published data from observational studies, birth registries, and case reports do not report a clear association between use of zolpidem and major birth defects. There are limited postmarketing reports of moderate to severe neonatal respiratory depression requiring artificial ventilation or intratracheal intubation when zolpidem was used late in the third trimester of pregnancy; the majority of neonates recovered within hours to a few weeks after birth once treated.

Zolpidem crosses the placenta and may cause respiratory depression and sedation in neonates. Neonates exposed to zolpidem during pregnancy and labor should be monitored for signs of excess sedation, hypotonia, and respiratory depression and treated as clinically appropriate.

Reproduction studies in animals were performed using zolpidem rather than zolpidem tartrate; dosages are expressed in terms of the base. Administration of zolpidem to pregnant rats and rabbits resulted in adverse effects on offspring development at dosages exceeding the maximum recommended human dosage (MRHD) of zolpidem tartrate as conventional tablets (10 mg daily); however, teratogenicity was not observed. When zolpidem was administered at oral dosages of 4, 20, and 100 mg/kg daily to pregnant rats during the period of organogenesis, delayed fetal development (incomplete fetal skull ossification) occurred at all but the lowest dosage (4 mg/kg daily, which is approximately 5 times the MRHD of zolpidem tartrate as conventional tablets on a mg/m^2 basis). In addition, administration of zolpidem to rats at oral dosages of 4, 20, and 100 mg/kg daily from day 15 of gestation through lactation delayed offspring growth and decreased survival at all but the lowest dosage. In rabbits receiving zolpidem during organogenesis at oral dosages of 1, 4, and 16 mg/kg daily, increased embryofetal death and incomplete fetal skeletal ossification occurred at the highest dosage studied. No risk of adverse effects on fetal development was observed following oral administration of zolpidem to pregnant rats and rabbits at clinically relevant doses.

Lactation

Zolpidem is distributed into milk in small amounts in humans. Excess sedation has been reported in nursing infants exposed to zolpidem through breast milk. The effects of zolpidem on milk production are not known.

Consider the developmental and health benefits of breast-feeding along with the mother's clinical need for zolpidem and any potential adverse effects on the breast-fed infant from the drug or from the underlying maternal condition. Infants exposed to zolpidem through breast milk should be monitored for excess sedation, hypotonia, and respiratory depression. Nursing women may consider interrupting breast-feeding and pumping and discarding breast milk during treatment and for 23 hours after administration of zolpidem to minimize drug exposure to a breast-fed infant.

Pediatric Use

Zolpidem tartrate is not recommended for use in pediatric patients. Safety and efficacy of the drug have not been established in pediatric patients younger than 18 years of age. In an 8-week clinical study in pediatric patients (6–17 years of age) with insomnia associated with attention deficit hyperactivity disorder (ADHD), zolpidem tartrate (0.25 mg/kg administered as an oral solution at bedtime) did not appear to decrease sleep latency as compared with placebo. In this study, the most frequent treatment-emergent adverse effects (compared with placebo) were nervous system effects, including dizziness (23.5 versus 1.5%), headache (12.5 versus 9.2%), and hallucinations (7 versus 0%).

Geriatric Use

Safety and efficacy of zolpidem for the treatment of insomnia in geriatric patients have been evaluated in controlled, double-blind studies. Geriatric or debilitated patients may be particularly sensitive to the effects of zolpidem. Adverse effects of the drug tend to be dose-related, particularly in geriatric patients. In addition, peak plasma zolpidem concentrations, elimination half-life, and AUC are increased substantially in geriatric patients compared with younger adults receiving zolpidem tartrate as conventional tablets.

In placebo-controlled clinical trials in geriatric patients receiving zolpidem tartrate doses of 10 mg or less (as conventional tablets), the most frequent adverse effects were dizziness, drowsiness, and diarrhea. In placebo-controlled trials in geriatric patients receiving zolpidem tartrate 6.25 mg as extended-release tablets, the most frequent adverse effects were headache, dizziness, and next-day somnolence. In clinical trials performed outside the US, involving approximately 2000 patients, falls were reported in about 1.5% of patients (93% of those being 70 years of age or older); 82% of the patients 70 years of age or older who experienced falls received zolpidem tartrate doses exceeding 10 mg (as conventional tablets). In these clinical trials, confusion was reported in 1.2% of patients (75% of those being 70 years of age or older); 78% of the patients 70 years of age or older who experienced confusion were receiving doses exceeding 10 mg (as conventional tablets).

The manufacturers recommend that zolpidem dosage be reduced in geriatric and/or debilitated patients to minimize adverse effects related to impaired motor and/or cognitive performance and unusual sensitivity to sedative and hypnotic drugs. Sedatives may cause confusion and oversedation in geriatric patients; geriatric patients should be observed closely. Geriatric patients are at a higher risk of falls related to drowsiness and CNS depression caused by zolpidem.

Hepatic Impairment

Elimination of zolpidem tartrate is prolonged in patients with hepatic impairment; dosage should be reduced in patients with mild or moderate hepatic impairment.

Avoid use of zolpidem conventional or extended-release tablets in patients with severe hepatic impairment since the drug may contribute to hepatic encephalopathy.

Renal Impairment

Pharmacokinetic alterations are possible in patients with renal impairment. Manufacturers state that dosage adjustment of zolpidem is not necessary; however, some clinicians recommend that dosage reduction be considered.

● Common Adverse Effects

Zolpidem tartrate conventional tablets generally are well tolerated at recommended doses (i.e., up to 10 mg). Adverse effects of the drug tend to be dose-related, particularly in geriatric patients and at doses exceeding those recommended. The most common adverse reactions with zolpidem conventional tablets when used in the short-term (<10 nights) include drowsiness, dizziness, and diarrhea; common adverse reactions reported with long-term use (28–35 nights) of the conventional tablets include dizziness and drugged feeling.

Adverse effects of zolpidem tartrate as extended-release tablets tend to be dose-related, particularly for certain adverse nervous system and GI effects. The most common adverse effects of zolpidem tartrate as extended-release tablets (occurring in >10% of adult patients) include headache, next-day somnolence, and dizziness.

The incidence of adverse effects in patients receiving zolpidem tartrate as 1.75- or 3.5-mg sublingual tablets were headache, fatigue, and nausea.

DRUG INTERACTIONS

Zolpidem is metabolized principally by cytochrome P-450 (CYP) isoenzyme 3A4 and, to a lesser extent, by CYP1A2 and CYP2D6.

● Drugs Affecting Hepatic Microsomal Enzymes

Some drugs that inhibit CYP3A may increase systemic exposure to zolpidem. Because of possible increased hypnotic effects, a lower dose of zolpidem should be considered when used concomitantly with a potent CYP3A4 inhibitor. The effect of inhibitors of other CYP isoenzymes on the pharmacokinetics (e.g., systemic exposure) of zolpidem is not known.

Some drugs that induce CYP3A may decrease systemic exposure to zolpidem. Concomitant use of zolpidem with potent CYP3A4 inducers is not recommended. The effect of other CYP inducers on the pharmacokinetics (e.g., systemic exposure) of zolpidem is not known.

● CNS Depressants

Concomitant use of zolpidem with other CNS depressants (e.g., alcohol, benzodiazepines, opiates, sedating antihistamines, tricyclic antidepressants) increases the risk of CNS depression. Concomitant use of zolpidem with these drugs may increase drowsiness and psychomotor impairment, including impaired driving ability.

Concomitant use of alcohol with zolpidem results in an additive adverse effect on psychomotor performance. Patients should be advised of the importance of not taking zolpidem after consuming alcohol in the evening or before bedtime.

Concomitant use of zolpidem with opiates may increase the risk of respiratory depression. Dosage and duration of concomitant use of zolpidem and opiates should be limited.

When zolpidem is used concomitantly with other CNS depressants, dosage adjustments of zolpidem and the concomitant CNS depressant may be necessary because of potentially additive effects. Concomitant use of zolpidem with other sedative and hypnotic drugs (including other zolpidem-containing preparations and OTC preparations used to treat insomnia [e.g., diphenhydramine, doxylamine succinate]) at bedtime or in the middle of the night is not recommended.

Chlorpromazine

Pharmacokinetic interactions have not been observed during concomitant use of zolpidem and chlorpromazine; however, additive effects in reducing alertness and psychomotor performance have been observed.

Cimetidine

Cimetidine does not appear to affect the pharmacokinetics or pharmacodynamics of zolpidem.

Ciprofloxacin

Concomitant use of ciprofloxacin (a strong inhibitor of CYP1A2 and a moderate inhibitor of CYP3A4) is likely to inhibit metabolism of zolpidem, potentially leading to an increase in zolpidem exposure.

Digoxin

Zolpidem had no effect on digoxin pharmacokinetics in healthy individuals.

Fluoxetine

Clinically important pharmacokinetic or pharmacodynamic interactions have not been observed when zolpidem was used concomitantly with fluoxetine in healthy individuals. In healthy men, concomitant use of fluoxetine (20 mg once daily for 17 days) with zolpidem tartrate (single 10-mg dose) resulted in no clinically important changes in the pharmacokinetics of zolpidem or fluoxetine, and no substantial changes in performance on psychomotor tests were observed. In healthy women, concomitant use of fluoxetine (20 mg once daily for 30 days) with zolpidem tartrate (10 mg once daily for 5 days) increased the half-life of zolpidem by 17%, but there was no evidence of additive effects on psychomotor function.

Fluvoxamine

Concomitant use of fluvoxamine (a strong inhibitor of CYP1A2 and a weak inhibitor of CYP3A4 and CYP2C9) is likely to inhibit metabolism of zolpidem, potentially leading to an increase in zolpidem exposure.

Haloperidol

Haloperidol does not appear to affect the pharmacokinetics or pharmacodynamics of zolpidem. However, the lack of an interaction following single-dose administration does not predict the absence of an effect following chronic administration.

Imipramine

Concomitant use of zolpidem and imipramine has been associated with a 20% decrease in peak plasma concentrations of imipramine; although other pharmacokinetic interactions have not been observed, an additive effect in reducing alertness has been observed during concomitant use.

Itraconazole

Concomitant use of the potent CYP3A4 inhibitor itraconazole (200 mg once daily for 4 days) with zolpidem tartrate (single 10-mg dose) in healthy individuals increased AUC of zolpidem by 34% but did not substantially alter patient ratings of drowsiness, performance on psychomotor tests, or postural sway compared with zolpidem alone.

Ketoconazole

Concomitant use of the potent CYP3A4 inhibitor ketoconazole (200 mg twice daily for 2 days) with zolpidem tartrate (single 5-mg dose) increased the peak plasma concentration, AUC, and elimination half-life of zolpidem by 30, 70, and 30%, respectively, and also increased pharmacodynamic effects of zolpidem. Because concomitant use may increase the hypnotic effects of zolpidem, a lower dose of zolpidem should be considered when the drug is used concomitantly with ketoconazole.

Ranitidine

Ranitidine does not appear to affect the pharmacokinetics or pharmacodynamics of zolpidem.

Rifampin

Rifampin, a potent CYP3A4 inducer, substantially reduces systemic exposure to and pharmacodynamic effects of zolpidem. Concomitant use with rifampin may decrease the hypnotic efficacy of zolpidem and is not recommended. In healthy women, concomitant use of zolpidem tartrate (single 20-mg dose) and rifampin (600 mg once daily for 5 days) reduced AUC, peak plasma concentration, and half-life of zolpidem by 73, 58, and 36%, respectively; substantial reductions in the effects of zolpidem on psychomotor performance also were observed.

Sertraline

Concomitant use of zolpidem and sertraline increases systemic exposure to zolpidem and may increase the pharmacodynamic effects of zolpidem, potentially resulting in earlier hypnotic onset and greater hypnotic effect. When zolpidem tartrate (10 mg daily at bedtime for 5 days) was used concomitantly with sertraline (50 mg daily in the morning for 17 days) in healthy women, peak plasma concentration of zolpidem was increased by 43% and time to peak plasma concentration of zolpidem was decreased by 53%. Zolpidem did not appear to have clinically important effects on the pharmacokinetics of sertraline or N-desmethylsertraline.

St. John's Wort

Concomitant use of St. John's wort (Hypericum perforatum), a CYP3A4 inducer, with zolpidem may decrease concentrations of zolpidem and is not recommended.

Warfarin

Zolpidem did not appear to affect prothrombin time (PT) when used concomitantly with warfarin in healthy individuals.

DESCRIPTION

Zolpidem tartrate, a type A γ-aminobutyric acid ($GABA_A$)-receptor positive modulator of the imidazopyridine class, is a sedative and hypnotic agent. Although zolpidem is structurally unrelated to the benzodiazepines and other sedative and hypnotic agents, it shares some of the pharmacologic properties of benzodiazepines and has been shown to interact with the CNS GABA-benzodiazepine-chloride ionophore receptor complex. Zolpidem is thought to exert its therapeutic effects in the short-term treatment of insomnia through binding to the benzodiazepine site of α_1 subunit containing GABA A receptors, increasing the frequency of chloride channel opening and resulting in the inhibition of neuronal excitation. Unlike some benzodiazepines, which nonselectively bind to and activate central type 1 (BZ_1) and 2 (BZ_2) benzodiazepine receptors, as well as peripheral type 3 (BZ_3) receptors, resulting in nonspecific pharmacologic actions, zolpidem binds preferentially to BZ_1 receptors with a greater affinity for the α_1 subunit relative to the α_2 and α_3 subunits; zolpidem has no appreciable binding affinity for the α_5 subunit. Such selectivity of zolpidem for the BZ_1 receptor is not absolute, but may account for the decreased muscle relaxant, anxiolytic, and anticonvulsant effects compared with benzodiazepines observed in certain animals and also may explain the preservation of deep (stages 3 and 4) sleep at hypnotic doses in humans. Such selectivity reportedly also may result in reduced abuse potential and tolerance development as well as in only minor effects on duration of sleep stages compared with benzodiazepines. However, some in vivo data from an animal (mouse) model have not confirmed such selectivity, and other data suggest that pharmacologic and toxicologic selectivity of zolpidem may be dose and species dependent. In addition, changes in sleep EEG observed with zolpidem are similar to those associated with benzodiazepines. Although some evidence suggests that the risk of residual daytime sedative effects and impairment of psychomotor and mental performance is minimal with zolpidem at usual dosages, blood concentrations of the drug may be high enough in some patients on the morning after use to impair performance of activities that require alertness, including driving. FDA states that all drugs used in the management of insomnia can impair driving and performance of activities that require alertness on the morning after use. Zolpidem has no appreciable binding affinity for dopaminergic D_2, serotonergic 5-HT_2, adrenergic, histaminergic or muscarinic receptors.

ADVICE TO PATIENTS

- Provide patients with a copy of the medication guide.
- Inform patients and their families of the benefits and risks of zolpidem therapy.
- Advise all patients of the potential for next-day impairment, that the risk is increased if dosing instructions are not carefully followed, and that impairment may be present despite feeling fully awake.
- Advise patients that drowsiness and decreased consciousness may increase the risk of falls in some patients.
- Advise patients to administer immediate-release zolpidem preparations intended for bedtime administration (conventional tablets, 5- and 10-mg sublingual tablets) immediately before getting into bed, at least 7–8 hours before being active again. Wait ≥8 hours after taking the drug before driving or engaging in other activities requiring full mental alertness.
- Advise patients to administer extended-release zolpidem immediately before getting into bed, at least 7–8 hours before being active again. Avoid driving or engaging in other activities requiring complete mental alertness the day after taking this preparation.
- Advise patients to administer the 1.75- or 3.5-mg sublingual tablets in bed, only once per night as needed, if middle-of-the-night awakening is followed by difficulty returning to sleep, and only if ≥4 hours remain before planned time of awakening. Wait ≥4 hours after taking this preparation and until feeling fully awake before driving or engaging in other activities requiring full mental alertness.
- Risk of serious injury and/or death resulting from complex sleep behaviors (e.g., sleep-walking, sleep-driving, preparing and eating food, making phone calls, or having sex while not being fully awake). Advise patients to discontinue zolpidem and notify a clinician immediately if an episode of complex sleep behavior occurs during therapy, even if it did not result in serious injury.
- Potential risk of abnormal thinking and behavioral changes; advise patients to immediately inform their clinician if any such changes occur.
- Advise patients to immediately inform their clinician of any suicidal thoughts or memory impairment.
- Potential risk of severe anaphylactic and anaphylactoid reactions; advise patients to immediately seek medical attention if manifestations of such reactions occur.
- Instruct patients to take zolpidem only as prescribed; do not increase dosage unless otherwise instructed by a clinician; inform clinician if the drug is not effective.
- Risk of withdrawal symptoms following abrupt discontinuance or rapid reduction in dosage. Advise patients to inform their clinician of any tolerance or dependence/withdrawal symptoms.
- Advise patients to not take zolpidem with or immediately after a meal.
- Instruct patients to take zolpidem sublingual tablet (5 or 10 mg) under the tongue and allow it to disintegrate; do not swallow or take with water.
- Instruct patients to place zolpidem sublingual tablet (1.75 or 3.5 mg) under the tongue and allow it to disintegrate completely before swallowing; do not swallow whole. Remove the tablet from the pouch just prior to dosing.
- Advise patients to inform their clinicians of existing or contemplated concomitant therapy, including prescription and OTC drugs, and any concomitant illnesses, particularly depression.
- Advise patients to not take zolpidem after consuming alcohol in the evening or before bedtime. Instruct patients to avoid concurrent use of other sedative and hypnotic drugs used to treat insomnia (including OTC preparations such as diphenhydramine or doxylamine succinate) or CNS depressants during therapy unless otherwise instructed by a clinician. Inform patients and caregivers that potentially serious additive effects may occur if zolpidem is used with opiates and not to use such drugs concomitantly with zolpidem unless supervised by a clinician.
- Advise women to inform their clinician if they are or plan to become pregnant or plan to breast-feed. Advise patients that use of zolpidem late in the third trimester may cause respiratory depression and sedation in neonates. Advise mothers who used zolpidem during the late third trimester of pregnancy to monitor neonates for signs of excess sleepiness, breathing difficulties, or limpness.
- Advise nursing women to monitor infants for increased sleepiness, breathing difficulties, or limpness and to seek immediate medical care if such signs occur. A lactating woman may consider pumping and discarding breast milk during treatment and for 23 hours after zolpidem administration to minimize drug exposure to a breast-fed infant.
- Inform patients of other important precautionary information. (See Cautions.)

PREPARATIONS

Zolpidem is subject to control under the Federal Controlled Substances Act of 1970 as a schedule IV (C-IV) drug.

Excipients in commercially available drug preparations may have clinically important effects in some individuals; consult specific product labeling for details.

Zolpidem Tartrate

Oral

Tablets, extended-release, film-coated	6.25 mg*	Ambien CR® (C-IV), Sanofi-Aventis
		Zolpidem Tartrate Extended-release Tablets (C-IV)
	12.5 mg*	Ambien CR® (C-IV), Sanofi-Aventis
		Zolpidem Tartrate Extended-release Tablets (C-IV)
Tablets, film-coated	5 mg*	Ambien® (C-IV), Sanofi-Aventis
		Zolpidem Tartrate Tablets (C-IV)
	10 mg*	Ambien® (C-IV), Sanofi-Aventis
		Zolpidem Tartrate Tablets (C-IV)

Sublingual

Tablets	1.75 mg*	Zolpidem Tartrate Sublingual Tablets (C-IV)
	3.5 mg*	Zolpidem Tartrate Sublingual Tablets (C-IV)
	5 mg*	Edluar® (C-IV), Meda
		Zolpidem Tartrate Sublingual Tablets (C-IV)
	10 mg*	Edluar® (C-IV), Meda
		Zolpidem Tartrate Sublingual Tablets (C-IV)

* available from one or more manufacturer, distributor, and/or repackager by generic (nonproprietary) name

† Use is not currently included in the labeling approved by the US Food and Drug Administration.

Selected Revisions June 10, 2024, © Copyright, September 1, 1993, American Society of Health-System Pharmacists, Inc.

hydrOXYzine Hydrochloride, hydrOXYzine Pamoate

28:24.92 · ANXIOLYTICS, SEDATIVES, AND HYPNOTICS, MISCELLANEOUS

■ Hydroxyzine is a piperazine-derivative antihistamine.

USES

Hydroxyzine is used for the symptomatic management of anxiety and tension associated with psychoneuroses and as an adjunct in patients with organic disease states who have associated anxiety; for the management of pruritus caused by allergic conditions such as chronic urticaria or atopic or contact dermatoses, and in histamine-mediated pruritus; and for its sedative effects before and after general anesthesia. The efficacy of hydroxyzine as an anxiolytic agent during long-term administration (i.e., longer than 4 months) has not been established; most clinicians believe that benzodiazepines, barbiturates, and meprobamate are more effective than hydroxyzine for anxiety. Patients with a history of long-term therapy with hydroxyzine should be evaluated periodically to determine the efficacy and need for further treatment. Hydroxyzine should not be used as the sole agent for the treatment of depression or psychoses.

Hydroxyzine has also been used for the management of agitation caused by acute alcohol withdrawal; to reduce opiate analgesic dosage; to control motion sickness; and to control nausea and vomiting of various etiologies (e.g., postoperative). Safe use of hydroxyzine for the prevention and treatment of nausea and vomiting of pregnancy has not been established, and the drug is contraindicated during early pregnancy.

DOSAGE AND ADMINISTRATION

● Administration

Hydroxyzine hydrochloride and hydroxyzine pamoate are administered orally; hydroxyzine hydrochloride may also be administered by IM injection. Because severe adverse effects may occur, the drug must *not* be administered by subcutaneous, intra-arterial, or IV injection. (See Cautions: Local Effects.) Oral therapy should replace IM therapy as soon as possible.

For IM administration, the commercially available hydroxyzine injection is used without further dilution. The Z-track technique of injection may be used to prevent subcutaneous infiltration. For IM administration in adults, injection should be made preferably deep into the upper outer quadrant of the gluteus maximus or the midlateral thigh. The deltoid area should be used with caution and only if well developed, in order to avoid radial nerve injury. IM injections should *not* be made into the lower and mid-third of the upper arm. For IM administration in children, injections should be made preferably into the midlateral muscles of the thigh; in infants and small children, the periphery of the upper outer quadrant of the gluteus maximus should be used only when necessary (e.g., burn patients), in order to minimize the possibility of damage to the sciatic nerve.

● Dosage

Dosage of hydroxyzine hydrochloride or pamoate is expressed in terms of the hydrochloride. Dosage must be carefully adjusted according to individual requirements and response, using the lowest possible effective dosage.

For the symptomatic management of anxiety and tension associated with psychoneuroses and as an adjunct in patients with organic disease states who have associated anxiety, the usual adult oral dosage of hydroxyzine is 50–100 mg 4 times daily. The usual oral dosage of hydroxyzine for the symptomatic management of anxiety and tension associated with psychoneuroses and as an adjunct in organic disease states in children 6 years of age or older is 50–100 mg daily given

in divided doses; for children younger than 6 years of age, the usual oral dosage is 50 mg daily given in divided doses.

For prompt control of acutely disturbed or hysterical patients and for the management of agitation caused by alcohol withdrawal, the usual adult IM dose of hydroxyzine is 50–100 mg. This dose may be repeated every 4–6 hours, as needed to control symptoms.

For the management of pruritus caused by allergic conditions such as chronic urticaria or atopic or contact dermatoses, and in histamine-mediated pruritus, the usual adult oral dosage of hydroxyzine is 25 mg 3 or 4 times daily. The usual oral dosage of hydroxyzine for the management of pruritus caused by allergic conditions in children 6 years of age or older is 50–100 mg daily given in divided doses; for children younger than 6 years of age, the usual oral dosage is 50 mg daily given in divided doses.

For sedation before and following general anesthesia, the usual adult dose of hydroxyzine is 50–100 mg orally or 25–100 mg IM. When used as a sedative before and following general anesthesia in children, the usual dose of hydroxyzine is 0.6 mg/kg orally or 1.1 mg/kg IM.

For control of nausea and vomiting (excluding nausea and vomiting of pregnancy), the usual initial IM dose of hydroxyzine is 25–100 mg in adults and 1.1 mg/kg in children. Subsequent dosage should be adjusted according to individual requirements and response.

For control of emesis, to permit reduction in opiate dosage, or to allay anxiety in prepartum and postpartum states, the usual initial adult IM dose of hydroxyzine is 25–100 mg. Subsequent dosage should be adjusted according to individual requirements and response.

CAUTIONS

Adverse reactions to hydroxyzine generally involve the CNS and are usually mild, transient, and reversible following discontinuance of the drug.

● Nervous System Effects

The most frequent adverse effects of hydroxyzine are drowsiness and dry mouth. Drowsiness usually diminishes with continued therapy or reduction in dosage. Other less frequent adverse nervous system effects of hydroxyzine include dizziness, ataxia, weakness, slurred speech, headache, agitation, and increased anxiety. Involuntary motor activity, including tremor and seizures, has occurred rarely, usually in patients receiving higher than recommended dosages of the drug.

● Local Effects

Marked local discomfort, sterile abcesses, erythema, local irritation, and tissue necrosis may occur at the site of IM injection, and marked localized subcutaneous tissue induration has been reported as a result of extravasation of the drug.

Following inadvertent intra-arterial injection of hydroxyzine hydrochloride, thrombosis and digital gangrene necessitating amputation have occurred. Phlebitis and hemolysis have been reported following IV administration of the drug. Following inadvertent subcutaneous administration of hydroxyzine hydrochloride, tissue necrosis, tissue slough, swelling, edema, petechial hemorrhage, and abscess have occurred.

● Other Adverse Effects

Other adverse effects that have been reported following administration of hydroxyzine include a bitter taste in the mouth, nausea, increased GI peristalsis, flushing, wheezing, and tightness of the chest.

● Precautions and Contraindications

Hydroxyzine shares the toxic potentials of the antihistamines, and the usual precautions of antihistamine therapy should be observed.

Because of the risk of adverse local effects, which may be severe (e.g., gangrene, thrombosis), IM administration of hydroxyzine should be performed with caution to avoid extravasation or inadvertent subcutaneous, IV, or intra-arterial injection.

Patients should be warned that hydroxyzine may impair their ability to perform activities requiring mental alertness or physical coordination (e.g., operating machinery, driving a motor vehicle). Patients also should be warned that hydroxyzine may enhance their response to alcohol, barbiturates, or other CNS depressants.

Hydroxyzine is contraindicated in patients who are hypersensitive to the drug.

● *Pregnancy, Fertility, and Lactation*

Pregnancy

Although there are no adequate and controlled studies to date in humans, hydroxyzine has been shown to be teratogenic in mice, rats, and rabbits when given at dosages substantially greater than the therapeutic human dosage. Pending accumulation of further data regarding safety in pregnant women, hydroxyzine is contraindicated during early pregnancy.

Lactation

It is not known whether hydroxyzine is distributed into milk. The manufacturers recommend that hydroxyzine not be given to nursing women.

DRUG INTERACTIONS

● *CNS Depressants*

Hydroxyzine may be additive with, or may potentiate the action of, other CNS depressants such as opiates or other analgesics, barbiturates or other sedatives, anesthetics, or alcohol. When hydroxyzine is used concomitantly with other CNS depressants, caution should be used to avoid excessive sedation, and the manufacturers recommend that dosage of the CNS depressant be reduced by up to 50%.

● *Anticholinergic Agents*

Additive anticholinergic effects may occur when hydroxyzine is administered concomitantly with other anticholinergic agents.

● *Epinephrine*

Hydroxyzine has been shown to inhibit and reverse the vasopressor effect of epinephrine. If a vasopressor agent is required in patients receiving hydroxyzine, norepinephrine or metaraminol should be used; epinephrine should *not* be used.

LABORATORY TEST INTERFERENCES

Hydroxyzine has been reported to cause falsely elevated urinary concentrations of 17-hydroxycorticosteroids when the Porter-Silber reaction or the Glenn-Nelson method is used.

ACUTE TOXICITY

Limited information is available on the acute toxicity of hydroxyzine. The acute lethal dose of hydroxyzine in humans is not known. In addition, there is no clearly defined relationship between plasma hydroxyzine concentration and severity of intoxication.

● *Manifestations*

In general, overdosage of hydroxyzine may be expected to produce effects that are extensions of common adverse reactions; excessive sedation has been the principal effect reported. Hypotension, although rare, may also occur.

● *Treatment*

Treatment of hydroxyzine overdosage generally involves symptomatic and supportive care; there is no specific antidote for hydroxyzine intoxication. Following acute ingestion of the drug, the stomach should be emptied immediately by inducing emesis or by gastric lavage. If the patient is comatose, having seizures, or lacks the gag reflex, gastric lavage may be performed if an endotracheal tube with cuff inflated is in place to prevent aspiration of gastric contents. Appropriate therapy

should be instituted if hypotension or excessive sedation occurs. If hypotension occurs, it may be controlled with IV fluids and norepinephrine or metaraminol; epinephrine should *not* be used. Although one manufacturer states that caffeine and sodium benzoate may be used to counteract CNS depressant effects of the drug, most authorities believe caffeine and other analeptics should *not* be used in overdosage resulting from CNS depressants. Although hemodialysis or peritoneal dialysis is probably *not* effective in enhancing elimination of hydroxyzine, if other agents (e.g., barbiturates) have been ingested concomitantly, dialysis may be indicated.

PHARMACOLOGY

The principal pharmacologic effects of hydroxyzine are similar to those of other antihistamines. (see Antihistamines General Statement 4:00)

● *Nervous System Effects*

Hydroxyzine has CNS depressant, anticholinergic, antispasmodic, and local anesthetic activity, in addition to antihistaminic effects. The drug also has sedative and antiemetic activity. The sedative and tranquilizing effects of hydroxyzine are thought to result principally from suppression of activity at subcortical levels of the CNS; the drug does not have cortical depressant activity. The precise mechanism of antiemetic and antimotion sickness actions of hydroxyzine are unclear, but appear to result, at least in part, from its central anticholinergic and CNS depressant properties.

Like many other centrally acting agents, hydroxyzine exhibits analgesic activity in a variety of analgesic test systems; this effect may be related to its sedative activity. Hydroxyzine also has primary skeletal muscle relaxant activity.

● *GI Effects*

Hydroxyzine does not appear to increase gastric secretions or acidity, and usually has mild antisecretory effects. The antispasmodic activity of hydroxyzine is apparently mediated through interference with the mechanism that responds to spasmogenic agents such as acetylcholine, histamine, and serotonin.

● *Cardiovascular Effects*

Although hydroxyzine does not appear to have clinically important antiarrhythmic properties, mild antiarrhythmic activity has been observed in some experimentally induced ventricular arrhythmias. Therapeutic dosages of hydroxyzine produce only minimal effects on blood pressure; however, hypotension may occur following overdosage.

● *Other Effects*

Hydroxyzine has been shown to produce bronchodilation in healthy individuals and in patients with chronic obstructive pulmonary disease.

PHARMACOKINETICS

● *Absorption*

Hydroxyzine is rapidly absorbed from the GI tract following oral administration.

The onset of sedative action of hydroxyzine is 15–30 minutes following oral administration. Sedative effects persist for 4–6 hours following administration of a single dose. Hydroxyzine suppresses the inflammatory response (wheal and flare reaction) and pruritus for up to 4 days after intradermal skin tests with allergens and histamine.

The therapeutic range for plasma hydroxyzine concentrations and the relationship of plasma concentration to clinical response or toxicity have not been established.

● *Distribution*

Distribution of hydroxyzine into human body tissues and fluids has not been fully characterized. Following administration of hydroxyzine in animals, the drug is widely distributed into most body tissues and fluids with highest concentrations in the liver, lungs, spleen, kidneys, and adipose tissue. The drug is also distributed into bile in animals.

It is not known if hydroxyzine crosses the placenta or is distributed into milk.

● **Elimination**

Although the exact metabolic fate of hydroxyzine is not clearly established, it appears that the drug is completely metabolized, principally in the liver. In animals, hydroxyzine and its metabolites are excreted in feces via biliary elimination. The carboxylic acid metabolite of hydroxyzine, cetirizine (Zyrtec®, Pfizer), is a long-acting antihistamine.

CHEMISTRY AND STABILITY

● **Chemistry**

Hydroxyzine is a piperazine-derivative antihistamine that is structurally similar to meclizine. Hydroxyzine is chemically unrelated to reserpine, meprobamate, benzodiazepines, or phenothiazines. Hydroxyzine is commercially available as the hydrochloride and pamoate salts.

Hydroxyzine hydrochloride occurs as a white, odorless powder and is very soluble in water and freely soluble in alcohol. The drug has pK_as of 2.6 and 7.0. Hydroxyzine hydrochloride injection is a sterile solution of the drug in water for injection. Sodium hydroxide is added during manufacture of the injection to adjust the pH to 3.5–6. The commercially available injection also contains benzyl alcohol as a preservative.

Hydroxyzine pamoate occurs as a light yellow, practically odorless powder and is practically insoluble in water and in alcohol. The commercially available hydroxyzine pamoate oral suspension has a pH of 4.5–7.

● **Stability**

Commercially available preparations of hydroxyzine should be stored in tight, light-resistant containers at a temperature less than 40°C, preferably at 15–30°C; freezing of the oral solution, oral suspension, or injection should be avoided.

Hydroxyzine hydrochloride injection is physically and/or chemically incompatible with some drugs, but the compatibility depends on several factors (e.g., concentrations of the drugs, specific diluents used, resulting pH, temperature). Specialized references should be consulted for specific compatibility information.

PREPARATIONS

Excipients in commercially available drug preparations may have clinically important effects in some individuals; consult specific product labeling for details.

hydrOXYzine Hydrochloride

Oral		
Solution	10 mg/5 mL*	Atarax® Syrup, Pfizer
		Hydroxyzine Hydrochloride Oral Solution
Tablets	10 mg*	Atarax®, Pfizer
		Hydroxyzine Hydrochloride Tablets
	25 mg*	Atarax®, Pfizer
		Hydroxyzine Hydrochloride Tablets
	50 mg*	Atarax®, Pfizer
		Hydroxyzine Hydrochloride Tablets
	100 mg	Atarax®, Pfizer
Tablets, film-coated	10 mg*	
	25 mg*	Anx® (scored), EconoMed
		Hydroxyzine Hydrochloride Film-coated Tablets
	50 mg*	
Parenteral		
Injection, for IM use only	25 mg/mL*	Vistaril®, Pfizer
		Hydroxyzine Hydrochloride Injection
	50 mg/mL*	Vistaril®, Pfizer
		Hydroxyzine Hydrochloride Injection

* available from one or more manufacturer, distributor, and/or repackager by generic (nonproprietary) name

hydrOXYzine Pamoate

Oral		
Capsules	equivalent to hydroxyzine hydrochloride 25 mg*	Vistaril®, Pfizer
		Hydroxyzine Pamoate Capsules
	equivalent to hydroxyzine hydrochloride 50 mg*	Vistaril®, Pfizer
		Hydroxyzine Pamoate Capsules
	equivalent to hydroxyzine hydrochloride 100 mg*	Vistaril®, Pfizer
		Hydroxyzine Pamoate Capsules
Suspension	equivalent to hydroxyzine hydrochloride 25 mg/5 mL	Vistaril® (with propylene glycol), Pfizer

* available from one or more manufacturer, distributor, and/or repackager by generic (nonproprietary) name

† Use is not currently included in the labeling approved by the US Food and Drug Administration.

Promethazine Hydrochloride

28:24.92 · ANXIOLYTICS, SEDATIVES, AND HYPNOTICS, MISCELLANEOUS

■ Promethazine hydrochloride is an ethylamino derivative of phenothiazine with potent sedative and antiemetic properties.

USES

Promethazine is used for its sedative and antiemetic effects in surgery and obstetrics (during labor). The drug reduces preoperative tension and anxiety, facilitates sleep, and reduces postoperative nausea and vomiting. As a preanesthetic medication, promethazine is used in conjunction with reduced doses of an opiate analgesic and an atropine-like drug. Promethazine also may be used as a routine sedative and as an adjunct to analgesics for control of pain.

For the use of promethazine as an antihistamine and for the management of motion sickness, see Promethazine Hydrochloride 4:04 and also see the Phenothiazines General Statement 28:16.08.24.

DOSAGE AND ADMINISTRATION

● Administration

Promethazine hydrochloride may be administered orally, rectally, or by deep IM injection. Promethazine hydrochloride also is administered by IV injection. However, because IV administration of the drug has been associated with severe tissue injury, including gangrene requiring amputation, the US Food and Drug Administration (FDA) states that deep IM injection is the preferred method for administration of promethazine hydrochloride injections. (See Cautions: Precautions and Contraindications.) If IV administration of promethazine hydrochloride is required, FDA states that the drug should be administered through the tubing of an IV infusion set that is known to be correctly functioning; FDA also states that the *maximum* rate of IV administration is 25 mg/minute, and the *maximum* concentration of the injection is 25 mg/mL. If the patient complains of pain at the injection site during presumed IV injection of the drug, the injection should immediately be stopped, and the possibility of intra-arterial placement of the needle or perivascular extravasation should be evaluated. Promethazine hydrochloride injection is commercially available in 2 strengths: 25 mg/mL and 50 mg/mL. FDA states that the preparation containing 50 mg/mL is for IM injection *only*; the preparation containing 25 mg/mL may be administered by IM or IV injection.

Because of the risk of severe tissue injury and amputations if promethazine hydrochloride is inadvertently administered intra-arterially or if extravasation were to occur, some medication safety experts (e.g., the Institute for Safe Medication Practices [ISMP]) recommend that parenteral administration of the drug be avoided and replaced by safer alternative therapies (e.g., a type 3 serotonin [5-HT₃] receptor antagonist such as ondansetron).

Subcutaneous or intra-arterial injection of promethazine hydrochloride is contraindicated.

Promethazine hydrochloride injections should be inspected visually for particulate matter and discoloration prior to administration whenever solution and container permit. The injection should be discarded if the solution is discolored or contains a precipitate.

● Dosage

Dosages of promethazine hydrochloride by the various routes of administration are identical.

For routine, preoperative or postoperative sedation or as an adjunct to analgesics for the control of pain, the usual adult dose of promethazine hydrochloride is 25–50 mg; children may receive 12.5–25 mg or 0.5–1.1 mg/kg. When promethazine is used as an adjunct to opiate analgesics, dosage of the analgesic should usually be reduced.

In obstetrics, 50 mg of promethazine hydrochloride may be given to provide sedation during the early stage of labor. When labor is established, 25–75 mg may

be given with a reduced therapeutic dose of an opiate agonist. Although additional doses are usually not required, the manufacturers state that 25- to 50-mg doses of promethazine may be repeated once or twice at 4-hour intervals if necessary. The maximum total dosage of promethazine during a 24-hour period of labor is 100 mg.

For the prevention and management of nausea and vomiting, the usual adult dose of promethazine hydrochloride is 12.5–25 mg; additional doses of 12.5–25 mg may be given every 4 hours if necessary. Children have been given 0.25–0.5 mg/kg or 7.5–15 mg/m² 4–6 times daily for the treatment of nausea and vomiting. (See Cautions: Pediatric Precautions.)

CAUTIONS

● Adverse Effects

Promethazine has adverse effects similar to those of other antihistamines and shares the toxic potentials of the phenothiazines; the usual precautions of antihistamine and phenothiazine therapy should be observed. (See Cautions in the Antihistamines General Statement 4:00 and in the Phenothiazines General Statement 28:16.08.24.) Although the risk of adverse reactions (e.g., blood dyscrasias, hepatotoxicity, reactivation of psychotic processes, tachycardia, cardiac arrest, endocrine disturbances, dermatologic disorders, ocular changes, hypersensitivity reactions) that have occurred during long-term administration of antipsychotic phenothiazines appears to be minimal, the possibility that such reactions could occur with prolonged administration of promethazine should be considered.

Adverse anticholinergic effects of promethazine include dryness of the mouth, blurring of vision and, rarely, dizziness. Confusion and disorientation also may occur. Extrapyramidal reactions may occur with high doses and usually subside with dosage reduction. Lassitude, fatigue, incoordination, tinnitus, diplopia, oculogyric crises, insomnia, excitation, nervousness, euphoria, hysteria, tremors, seizures, abnormal movements, nightmares, delirium, agitation, hallucinations, torticollis, tongue protrusion, oversedation, dystonic reactions, and catatonic-like states have been reported. Restlessness, akathisia, and, occasionally, marked irregular respiration have occurred. Neuroleptic malignant syndrome (NMS) also may occur. Patients with pain who have received inadequate or no analgesia have developed athetoid-like movements of the upper extremities following parenteral administration of promethazine. These symptoms usually disappeared when the pain was controlled.

Leukopenia, thrombocytopenia, thrombocytopenic purpura, and agranulocytosis have been reported in patients receiving promethazine.

Tachycardia, bradycardia, increased or decreased blood pressure, and faintness have occurred in patients receiving promethazine. Although rapid IV administration of promethazine may produce a transient fall in blood pressure, blood pressure usually is maintained or slightly elevated when the drug is given slowly. Venous thrombosis at the injection site also has been reported.

Promethazine has been associated with obstructive jaundice, which usually was reversible following discontinuance of the drug. Cholestatic jaundice, nausea, and vomiting have been reported in patients receiving promethazine. Photosensitivity has been reported and may be a contraindication to further promethazine therapy. Urticaria, dermatitis, asthma, dermatologic reactions, and angioedema also have occurred. Nasal stuffiness, respiratory depression (may be fatal), cardiac arrest, and apnea (may be fatal) also may occur.

Local Reactions Associated with Promethazine Hydrochloride Injection

Severe chemical irritation and damage to tissues (e.g., burning, pain, erythema, swelling, severe spasm of distal vessels, thrombophlebitis, venous thrombosis, phlebitis, abscesses, tissue necrosis, gangrene) may occur with administration of promethazine injection regardless of the route of administration. Such irritation and damage also may result from perivascular extravasation, unintentional intra-arterial injection, and intraneuronal or perineuronal infiltration. Parenteral administration of promethazine may produce nerve damage (ranging from temporary sensory loss to palsies and paralysis) while injection near or into a nerve may result in permanent tissue damage. In some cases, surgical intervention (e.g., fasciotomy, skin graft, amputation) may be needed. (See Dosage and Administration: Administration and see also Cautions: Precautions and Contraindications.)

● Precautions and Contraindications

Promethazine has adverse effects similar to those of other antihistamines and shares the toxic potentials of the phenothiazines; the usual precautions of antihistamine and phenothiazine therapy should be observed. (See Cautions: Precautions and Contraindications in the Antihistamines General Statement 4:00 and in the Phenothiazines General Statement 28:16.08.24.)

Ambulatory patients should be warned that promethazine may impair their ability to perform hazardous tasks requiring mental alertness or physical coordination such as operating machinery or driving a motor vehicle. It should be kept in mind that the antiemetic effect of promethazine may obscure signs of overdosage of other drugs or of symptoms of conditions such as intestinal obstruction or brain tumor, and thereby interfere with diagnosis.

Promethazine should be used with caution in patients with cardiovascular disease or impaired liver function or patients who are having an asthmatic attack. Some manufacturers state that promethazine should be used cautiously in individuals with peptic ulcer. Some manufacturers also state that the drug should be used with caution in patients with acute or chronic respiratory impairment, particularly children, because the cough reflex may be suppressed. Promethazine should be used with caution, if at all, in patients with sleep apnea. (See Cautions: Pediatric Precautions.)

Some commercially available formulations of promethazine hydrochloride contain sulfites that may cause allergic-type reactions, including anaphylaxis and life-threatening or less severe asthmatic episodes, in certain susceptible individuals. The overall prevalence of sulfite sensitivity in the general population is unknown but probably low; such sensitivity appears to occur more frequently in asthmatic than in nonasthmatic individuals.

Because IV administration of the drug has been associated with severe tissue injury, including gangrene requiring amputation, the US Food and Drug Administration (FDA) states that deep IM injection is the preferred method for administration of promethazine hydrochloride injections. If IV administration of promethazine hydrochloride is required, extreme care should be exercised to avoid extravasation or inadvertent intra-arterial injection. (See Dosage and Administration: Administration and see Local Reactions Associated with Promethazine Hydrochloride Injection under Cautions: Adverse Effects.) If the patient complains of pain at the injection site during presumed IV injection of the drug, the injection should immediately be stopped, and the possibility of intra-arterial placement of the needle or perivascular extravasation should be evaluated. Clinicians should be alert for signs and symptoms of potential tissue injury, including burning or pain at the site of injection, phlebitis, swelling, and blistering, and patients should be informed that adverse effects may occur immediately (i.e., while receiving the injection) or may develop hours to days after an injection of promethazine. Although there are no proven successful treatment regimens for the management of extravasation or inadvertent intra-arterial injection of promethazine, sympathetic block and administration of heparin are commonly employed during the acute management.

Because of the risk of severe tissue injury and amputations if promethazine hydrochloride is inadvertently administered intra-arterially or if extravasation were to occur, some medication safety experts (e.g., the Institute for Safe Medication Practices [ISMP]) recommend that parenteral administration of the drug be avoided and replaced by safer alternative therapies (e.g., a type 3 serotonin [5-HT$_3$] receptor antagonist such as ondansetron).

FDA states that subcutaneous or intra-arterial administration of promethazine hydrochloride is contraindicated. Promethazine hydrochloride should *not* be administered intra-arterially, because chemical irritation may be severe and cause severe arteriospasm, possibly resulting in impairment of circulation and gangrene requiring amputation. Since promethazine discolors blood on contact, aspiration of dark blood at the site of injection does *not* rule out the possibility of intra-arterial placement of the needle.

Promethazine is contraindicated in patients who have exhibited hypersensitivity or idiosyncrasy to promethazine or other phenothiazines. Promethazine also is contraindicated in pediatric patients younger than 2 years of age because of risk of developing potentially fatal respiratory depression. (See Cautions: Pediatric Precautions.) In addition, the drug is contraindicated in patients who have received large doses of other CNS depressants and/or who are comatose. The manufacturers state that the drug is contraindicated for use in the treatment of lower respiratory tract symptoms (e.g., asthma). There is some evidence that epileptic patients may experience increased severity of seizures if treated with promethazine, and the drug may be contraindicated in these patients. Since increases in blood pressure may occur, promethazine should be administered with extreme caution, if at all, to patients in hypertensive crisis. Some manufacturers state that promethazine also is contraindicated in patients with bone marrow depression, angle-closure glaucoma, prostatic hypertrophy, stenosing peptic ulcer, pyloroduodenal

obstruction, or bladder neck obstruction, although others state that the drug may be used with caution in such patients. Some experts do *not* recommend administering promethazine to pediatric patients who are vomiting, unless the vomiting is prolonged and there is a known cause. (See Cautions: Pediatric Precautions.)

● *Pediatric Precautions*

Because respiratory depression (sometimes fatal) has been reported in pediatric patients younger than 2 years of age receiving a wide range of weight-adjusted doses of promethazine during postmarketing surveillance, the drug is contraindicated in pediatric patients younger than 2 years of age.

Promethazine should be administered with caution in children 2 years of age and older because of possible respiratory depression and/or apnea that may be fatal. The lowest effective dose of the drug should be used. Concomitant use of promethazine with other respiratory depressant drugs should be avoided.

Children receiving promethazine should be supervised closely while performing hazardous activities such as bike riding. Adults responsible for the supervision of a child receiving promethazine should be warned that children may be at increased risk for experiencing CNS stimulant effects with antihistamines. Promethazine should not be used in vomiting of unknown etiology in children. The drug should not be used in acutely ill or dehydrated children or children with acute infections, since these patients have an increased susceptibility to dystonias. Use of promethazine also should be avoided in children with signs and symptoms that suggest Reye's syndrome, since the potential extrapyramidal effects produced by the drug may obscure the diagnosis of or be confused with the CNS signs and symptoms of this condition, and in children with signs and symptoms of other hepatic disease. Because promethazine may cause marked drowsiness that may be potentiated by other CNS depressants (e.g., sedatives, tranquilizers), promethazine should be used in children receiving one of these drugs only under the direction of a physician. Promethazine should not be used in children with asthma, liver disease, a seizure disorder, or glaucoma unless otherwise directed by a clinician.

Excessively high dosages of promethazine have caused sudden death in pediatric patients, although sleep apnea and sudden infant death syndrome (SIDS) have been reported in a number of infants and young children who were receiving usual dosages of promethazine or trimeprazine (no longer commercially available in the US). The relationship to the drugs and possible mechanism(s) of such effects have not been elucidated. In one study, the number but not the duration of central apneas during sleep was increased and obstructive apnea during sleep (accompanied by decreased heart rate and arterial oxygen pressure) developed in 4 healthy infants who were receiving 1 mg/kg of promethazine hydrochloride daily for 3 days. Promethazine should be used with caution in children with a history of sleep apnea, those with a family history of SIDS, and those who are less prone than usual to spontaneous arousal from sleep.

● *Geriatric Precautions*

Clinical studies of promethazine did not include sufficient numbers of patients 65 years of age and older to determine whether geriatric patients respond differently than younger patients. Although clinical experience generally has not revealed age-related differences in response to the drug, care should be taken in dosage selection of promethazine. Because of increased risk of sedative effects and confusion (associated with promethazine) and the greater frequency of decreased hepatic, renal, and/or cardiac function and of concomitant disease and drug therapy in geriatric patients, the manufacturers suggest that patients in this age group receive initial dosages of the drug in the lower end of the usual range.

● *Mutagenicity and Carcinogenicity*

Long-term animal studies to determine the carcinogenic potential of promethazine have not been performed to date. There was no evidence of promethazine-induced mutagenesis in the Ames microbial mutagen test. There are no human or other animal data concerning the carcinogenic or mutagenic potentials of the drug. For information on the carcinogenic potential of phenothiazines, see Cautions: Carcinogenicity, in the Phenothiazines General Statement 28:16.08.24.

● *Pregnancy, Fertility, and Lactation*
Pregnancy

Safe use of promethazine during pregnancy (except during labor) with respect to possible adverse effects on fetal development has not been established. Although there are no adequate and controlled studies to date in humans, promethazine has not been shown to be teratogenic in rats receiving oral dosages of 6.25–12.5

mg/kg daily (about 2.1–4.2 times the maximum recommended human dosage, depending on the use of the drug). The drug has been shown to produce fetal mortality in rats receiving intraperitoneal dosages of 25 mg/kg daily. Antihistamines, including promethazine, have been fetocidal in rodents, but the pharmacologic effects of histamine in rodents differ from those in humans. Promethazine should be used during pregnancy only when the potential benefits justify the possible risks to the fetus.

Fertility

There are no animal or human data concerning the effect of promethazine on fertility.

Lactation

It is not known whether promethazine is distributed into milk. Because many drugs are distributed in human milk and because of the potential for serious adverse reactions to promethazine in nursing infants if it were distributed, a decision should be made whether to discontinue nursing or the drug, taking into account the importance of the drug to the woman.

DRUG INTERACTIONS

● CNS Depressants

Promethazine hydrochloride is additive with or may potentiate the sedative action of opiates or other analgesics and other CNS depressants such as barbiturates or other sedatives, antihistamines, tranquilizers, or alcohol. When promethazine is used concomitantly with other depressant drugs, caution should be used to avoid overdosage. When promethazine is used concomitantly with barbiturates or narcotics, dosage of these drugs should be reduced by at least 50 or 25–50%, respectively.

● Epinephrine

Although reversal of the vasopressor effect of epinephrine has not been reported with promethazine, such possibility should be considered. If patients receiving promethazine require a vasopressor agent, norepinephrine or phenylephrine should be used; *epinephrine should not be used* because it may further decrease blood pressure in patients with partial adrenergic blockade.

● Anticholinergic Agents

Caution should be used during concomitant use of promethazine with drugs having anticholinergic properties.

● Monoamine Oxidase (MAO) Inhibitors

Increased incidence of extrapyramidal effects has been reported in patients receiving phenothiazines concomitantly with MAO inhibitors.

LABORATORY TEST INTERFERENCES

Promethazine may interfere with several immunologic urinary pregnancy tests. The drug may elicit a false-positive Gravindex® test and false-negative Prepurex® and Dap® test. Promethazine may interfere with blood grouping in the ABO system. The drug substantially alters the flare response in intradermal allergen tests.

ACUTE TOXICITY

● Manifestations

In adults, overdosage of promethazine may range from mild depression of the CNS and cardiovascular system to profound hypotension, respiratory depression, seizures, deep sleep, unconsciousness, and sudden death. Hyperreflexia, hypertonia, ataxia, athetosis, and extensor-plantar reflexes (Babinski reflex) also may occur. In children, a paradoxical reaction characterized by hyperexcitability, abnormal movements, nightmares, and respiratory depression may occur. A 12-year-old patient who had taken 200 mg of the drug exhibited numbness and pain in the left leg, tactile hallucinations, extreme hyperesthesia and hyperalgesia, and sinus tachycardia.

● Treatment

For information on the treatment of promethazine overdosage, see Acute Toxicity: Treatment in the Phenothiazines General Statement 28:16.08.24.

PHARMACOLOGY

Promethazine is a phenothiazine derivative with potent sedative properties. Although the drug can produce either CNS stimulation or CNS depression, CNS depression manifested by sedation is more common with therapeutic doses of promethazine. The precise mechanism of the CNS effects of the drug is not known.

Promethazine also has antihistaminic, antiemetic, antimotion sickness, anticholinergic, and local anesthetic effects. Although it has been reported that the drug has slight antitussive activity, this may result from its anticholinergic and CNS depressant effects. In therapeutic doses, promethazine appears to have no substantial effect on the cardiovascular system. Although rapid IV administration of promethazine may produce a transient fall in blood pressure, blood pressure usually is maintained or slightly elevated when the drug is given slowly.

PHARMACOKINETICS

● Absorption

Promethazine is well absorbed from the GI tract and from parenteral sites. Plasma concentrations of promethazine required for sedative effects are unknown. The onset of sedative effects occurs within 20 minutes following oral, rectal, or IM administration, and within 3–5 minutes following IV administration. The duration of sedative effects varies but may range from 2–8 hours depending on the dose and route of administration.

● Distribution

Promethazine is widely distributed in body tissues. Compared with other organs, lower concentrations of the drug are found in the brain, but this concentration is higher than the plasma concentration. Promethazine has been reported to be 93% protein bound when determined by gas chromatography and as 76–80% bound when determined by high-performance liquid chromatography. Promethazine readily crosses the placenta. It is not known whether the drug is distributed into milk.

● Elimination

Promethazine is metabolized in the liver. The drug is excreted slowly in urine (mainly) and feces principally as inactive promethazine sulfoxide and glucuronides.

CHEMISTRY AND STABILITY

● Chemistry

Promethazine hydrochloride is an ethylamino derivative of phenothiazine and occurs as a racemic mixture. The drug occurs as a white to faint yellow, practically odorless, crystalline powder that slowly oxidizes and turns blue on prolonged exposure to air. Promethazine hydrochloride is very soluble in water and in hot dehydrated alcohol. Commercially available promethazine hydrochloride injection has a pH of 4–5.5. The pK$_a$ of the drug is 9.1.

● Stability

Promethazine hydrochloride preparations should be protected from light. Promethazine hydrochloride oral solution and tablets should be stored in tight, light-resistant containers at 15–30 and 20–25°C, respectively, while the rectal suppositories should be stored in well-closed containers at 2–8°C. Freezing of the oral solution should be avoided. Following the date of manufacture, commercially available promethazine preparations have expiration dates of 2–5 years depending on the dosage form and manufacturer.

Promethazine hydrochloride injection should be stored in tight, light-resistant containers at 20–25°C, but may be exposed to temperatures ranging from 15–30°C. The injection should be discarded if the solution is discolored or contains a precipitate. Promethazine hydrochloride injection has been reported to be chemically incompatible with several drugs, especially those with an alkaline pH. However, the compatibility depends on several factors (e.g., concentration of the drugs, specific diluents used, resulting pH, temperature). Specialized references should be consulted for specific compatibility information.

PREPARATIONS

Excipients in commercially available drug preparations may have clinically important effects in some individuals; consult specific product labeling for details.

Promethazine Hydrochloride

Oral

Solution	6.25 mg/5 mL*	**Promethazine Hydrochloride Syrup**
Tablets	12.5 mg*	**Phenergan®** (scored), Wyeth
		Promethazine Hydrochloride Tablets
	25 mg*	**Phenergan®** (scored), Wyeth
		Promethazine Hydrochloride Tablets
	50 mg*	**Phenergan®**, Wyeth
		Promethazine Hydrochloride Tablets

Parenteral

Injection	25 mg/mL*	**Promethazine Hydrochloride Injection**
Injection, for IM use only	50 mg/mL*	**Promethazine Hydrochloride Injection**

Rectal

Suppositories	12.5 mg*	**Phenadoz®**, Paddock
		Phenergan®, Wyeth
		Promethazine Hydrochloride Suppositories
	25 mg*	**Phenadoz®**, Paddock
		Phenergan®, Wyeth
		Promethazine Hydrochloride Suppositories
	50 mg*	**Phenergan®**, Wyeth
		Promethazine Hydrochloride Suppositories
		Promethegan®, G&W

* available from one or more manufacturer, distributor, and/or repackager by generic (nonproprietary) name

Promethazine Hydrochloride Combinations

Oral

Solution	6.25 mg/ 5 mL with Phenylephrine Hydrochloride 5 mg/5 mL*	**Prometh® VC Syrup**, Actavis

* available from one or more manufacturer, distributor, and/or repackager by generic (nonproprietary) name

Selected Revisions September 24, 2018, © Copyright, May 1, 1976, American Society of Health-System Pharmacists, Inc.

Lithium Salts

28:28 • LITHIUM

■ Lithium salts are antimanic agents.

USES

Lithium salts are used in the treatment of a variety of psychiatric disorders but are most commonly used in the treatment of affective (mood) disorders. Currently, lithium salts are principally used in the treatment of bipolar disorder, particularly in the treatment of acute manic or mixed episodes in patients with bipolar 1 or bipolar 2 disorder. In addition, maintenance therapy with lithium salts has been shown to prevent or diminish the intensity of subsequent manic episodes in patients with bipolar disorder with a history of mania.

Lithium salts also are used in the prophylaxis and treatment of major depressive disorder† (unipolar depression).

● Bipolar Disorder

Diagnostic Considerations

Affective disorders currently are categorized as either bipolar (manic-depressive) or unipolar (depressive). A diagnosis of bipolar disorder is made if the patient has ever had a manic or hypomanic episode; otherwise, the criteria for bipolar depression and unipolar (major) depression are identical. According to DSM-IV-TR criteria, manic episodes are distinct periods lasting 1 week or longer (or less than 1 week if hospitalization is required) of abnormally and persistently elevated, expansive, or irritable mood accompanied by at least 3 (or 4 if the mood is only irritability) of the following 7 symptoms: inflated self-esteem or grandiosity, reduced need for sleep, pressure of speech, flight of ideas, distractibility, increased goal-directed activity (either socially, at work or school, or sexually) or psychomotor agitation, and engaging in high risk behavior (e.g., unrestrained buying sprees, sexual indiscretions, foolish business investments). In addition, to meet the criteria for manic episodes, the mood disturbances must be sufficiently severe that they cause marked impairment in occupational functioning, usual social activities, or relationships with others; they may necessitate hospitalization to prevent harm to self or others; and may be accompanied by psychotic features.

According to DSM-IV-TR criteria, bipolar disorder can be classified as bipolar 1 disorder, bipolar 2 disorder, cyclothymia, or bipolar disorder not otherwise specified. Bipolar 1 disorder is characterized by the occurrence of one or more manic episodes or mixed episodes. In addition, patients with bipolar I disorder often have had previous depressive episodes and most patients will have subsequent episodes that can be either manic or depressive. Hypomanic and mixed episodes also may occur in bipolar I disorder as well as substantial subthreshold mood lability between episodes. Bipolar 1 disorder is further characterized according to whether the patient is experiencing a first manic episode (which is classified as single manic episode) or whether the most recent episode is manic, hypomanic, depressive, mixed (concurrent or rapidly alternating manic and depressive features), or unspecified.

Patients meeting DSM-IV-TR criteria for bipolar 2 disorder have a history of one or more major depressive episodes accompanied by at least one hypomanic episode. However, patients with bipolar 2 disorder should not have had a previous manic or mixed episode.

Some patients with bipolar disorder may exhibit evidence of mood lability, hypomania, and depressive symptoms but fail to meet the diagnostic criteria for any specific bipolar disorder. This condition is called bipolar disorder not otherwise specified according to DSM-IV-TR criteria.

Cyclothymic disorder (cyclothymia) may be diagnosed in patients who have never experienced a manic, mixed, or major depressive episode but who have experienced numerous periods of depressive as well as hypomanic symptoms for at least 2 years in adults or 1 year in children, with no symptom-free period lasting longer than 2 months.

Bipolar 1 or 2 disorder may be diagnosed as rapid-cycling if the patient has 4 or more mood disturbances within a single year that meet DSM-IV-TR criteria for a major depressive, mixed, manic, or hypomanic episode. These episodes are demarcated either by a partial or full remission for at least 2 months or a switch to an episode of the opposite nature (e.g., from a major depressive to a manic episode). Rapid-cycling bipolar disorder is sometimes associated with certain medical conditions (e.g., hypothyroidism) or drug or substance abuse. Certain drugs, such as antidepressants, also may contribute to rapid cycling, particularly in patients who are not receiving a mood-stabilizing agent (e.g., lithium, carbamazepine, valproic acid).

Considerations in Choosing Therapy for Manic and Mixed Episodes

Although there presently is no cure for bipolar disorder, treatment may decrease the associated morbidity and mortality. The principal aim of acute treatment for patients with bipolar disorder experiencing a manic or mixed episode is to control the symptoms to allow a return to normal levels of psychosocial functioning. The rapid control of certain symptoms (e.g., agitation, aggression, impulsivity) may be particularly important for the safety of the patient and others.

A variety of drugs currently are available for the treatment of acute manic and mixed episodes, including mood-stabilizing agents, olanzapine and other antipsychotics, and benzodiazepines. In bipolar disorder, drugs generally are considered mood stabilizers if they provide relief from acute episodes of mania or depression or prevent such episodes from recurring and they do not worsen depression or mania or lead to increased cycling. Lithium salts, valproic acid or divalproex, carbamazepine, and some other anticonvulsants (e.g., oxcarbazepine, lamotrigine, gabapentin) have been used clinically as mood stabilizers in bipolar disorder. However, the American Psychiatric Association (APA) states that there is no consensus on the definitions of "mood stabilizers" and does not use this term in its most recent guidelines for the treatment of bipolar disorder.

For the initial management of less severe manic or mixed episodes in patients with bipolar disorder, monotherapy with lithium, valproate (e.g., sodium valproate, valproic acid, divalproex), or an antipsychotic agent such as olanzapine may be adequate. For more severe manic or mixed episodes, many experts recommend combination therapy involving lithium plus an antipsychotic or valproate plus an antipsychotic for first-line therapy. Some clinicians state that divalproex may be preferable to valproic acid in the treatment of bipolar disorder because of its more favorable adverse effect profile. Some experts recommend that carbamazepine or oxcarbazepine be used as alternatives to lithium or valproate therapy for patients who do not respond adequately to or who cannot tolerate other first-line therapies.

Bipolar patients experiencing manic or mixed episodes with psychotic features or psychosis often require therapy with an antipsychotic agent. Antipsychotic agents also are commonly used in the treatment of manic or mixed episodes in patients with bipolar disorder to control psychotic symptoms and for sedation. Some evidence indicates that certain atypical antipsychotic agents also possess mood-stabilizing properties and may therefore help to control depressive and manic episodes. When an antipsychotic agent is clinically indicated in patients with bipolar disorder, some experts recommend the use of atypical antipsychotics (e.g., olanzapine, risperidone) over conventional antipsychotic agents (e.g., chlorpromazine, haloperidol) because of their more favorable adverse effect profile and possible mood-stabilizing activity.

Short-term adjunctive therapy with a benzodiazepine (e.g., lorazepam, clonazepam) during manic episodes may be helpful for sedation and to help restore sleep in patients experiencing acute manic or mixed episodes. Some experts currently prefer high-potency benzodiazepines instead of antipsychotics in the management of acute manic episodes to avoid the risk of tardive dyskinesia and other adverse extrapyramidal effects associated with antipsychotic agents. However, benzodiazepines should be used with caution in bipolar patients with a history of substance abuse because of their addictive potential.

In bipolar patients who experience an acute manic or mixed episode while receiving antidepressant therapy, many experts recommend that the antidepressant be tapered and discontinued, if possible. If psychosocial therapy is used, this treatment should be combined with pharmacotherapy.

In patients with mixed episodes, many clinicians recommend valproate (valproic acid or divalproex) or carbamazepine rather than lithium as initial first-line therapy. In patients with dysphoric mania, combined divalproex and olanzapine currently is recommended by some clinicians.

In patients who experience a manic or mixed episode (i.e., a "breakthrough" episode) while receiving maintenance therapy, some experts recommend that the dosage(s) of the current medication be optimized as an initial approach (e.g., ensuring that plasma drug concentrations are within the therapeutic range). In addition, an antipsychotic agent may be added or reinitiated. Severely ill or agitated patients also may require short-term therapy with a benzodiazepine. When first-line therapy given at optimal dosages fails to control the symptoms, another first-line drug may be added to the regimen. Alternatively, carbamazepine or oxcarbazepine may be added instead of a first-line agent and an antipsychotic agent may be added in patients not already receiving one. In addition, changing to a different antipsychotic agent occasionally may be helpful.

In patients with refractory manic episodes, some experts recommend a trial of therapy with the antipsychotic clozapine. Electroconvulsive therapy (ECT) also may be considered in patients with particularly severe or treatment-resistant mania and in patients who prefer ECT in consultation with their clinician. ECT also has been recommended by some experts in patients experiencing mixed episodes or in patients who develop severe mania during pregnancy.

Lithium Therapy for Acute Manic and Mixed Episodes

Extensive clinical experience and data from randomized, controlled studies have shown lithium to be effective in the treatment of acute mania and the acute manic phase of mixed bipolar disorder. Based on data from 5 controlled clinical trials, lithium appears to be more effective than placebo in the treatment of acute manic and mixed episodes. Data from these studies indicate that about 70% of patients receiving lithium display at least a partial reduction of manic symptoms.

Based on data from several controlled clinical trials, lithium appears to be more effective than chlorpromazine in the treatment of acute mania. The percentage of patients achieving a complete or partial remission of a manic episode and the degree to which manic symptomatology is reduced are greater in patients treated with lithium than in those treated with chlorpromazine. Lithium is particularly effective in reducing affective and ideational signs and symptoms of mania, especially elation, grandiosity, feelings of persecution, flight of ideas, expansiveness, irritability, manipulativeness, anxiousness, and other manic behavior. Signs and symptoms of hyperactivity associated with mania, including sleep disturbances, pressured speech, increased motor activity, assaultive or threatening behavior, and distractability are reduced to a lesser extent. Because antipsychotic agents appear to be more effective than lithium in initially controlling the increased psychomotor activity of mania, many clinicians initiate treatment of acute mania with lithium or valproate (e.g., valproic acid, valproate sodium, divalproex) and an antipsychotic agent. Once psychomotor activity has been controlled (usually within 3–7 days), the antipsychotic agent usually is tapered and lithium or valproate therapy is continued to more specifically control disturbances of mood and ideation.

Considerations in Choosing Therapy for Depressive Episodes

In patients with bipolar disorder experiencing a depressive episode, many experts recommend that therapy with either lithium or lamotrigine be initiated as first-line therapy. Antidepressant monotherapy and therapy with tricyclic antidepressants generally should be avoided in such cases because of the possibility of inducing rapid cycling of symptoms. Alternatively, some clinicians recommend initiation of combination therapy with lithium and an antidepressant, particularly in patients with more severe depressive episodes. Psychotherapy (interpersonal therapy and cognitive behavior therapy) may be useful as an adjunct to pharmacotherapy. In patients with life-threatening inanition, suicidality, or psychosis, ECT may be considered. ECT may also be helpful for managing severe depressive episodes during pregnancy.

In bipolar patients who suffer from a breakthrough depressive episode despite maintenance therapy, many experts recommend optimizing the dosages of the current medication as an initial step. For acute depressive episodes in bipolar disorder patients not responding adequately to first-line interventions at optimal dosages, some experts recommend the addition of a selective serotonin-reuptake inhibitor (e.g., paroxetine), bupropion, venlafaxine, lamotrigine, or a monoamine oxidase (MAO) inhibitor. When an antidepressant is indicated in patients with bipolar depression, nonsedating antidepressants (i.e., bupropion, selective serotonin-reuptake inhibitors, MAO inhibitors) usually are preferred. ECT should be considered in bipolar patients with severe or treatment-resistant depression or in those with depression accompanied by psychotic or catatonic features.

Because the likelihood of antidepressant therapy precipitating a switch into a hypomanic or manic episode may be somewhat lower in patients with type 2 bipolar disorder than in patients with type 1 bipolar disorder, many clinicians choose to initiate antidepressant therapy earlier in patients with bipolar 2 disorder. Depressive episodes accompanied by psychotic features usually require adjunctive antipsychotic therapy.

Considerations in Choosing Therapy for Rapid Cycling

According to DSM-IV-TR criteria, rapid cycling refers to the occurrence of 4 or more mood-related disturbances within a single year that meet criteria for a major depressive, mixed, manic, or hypomanic episode. These episodes are demarcated either by partial or full remission for at least 2 months or a switch to an episode of the opposite nature (e.g., from a major depressive to a manic episode). Initially, many experts advise that any concurrent medical condition that may contribute to rapid cycling, such as hypothyroidism or drug or alcohol abuse, be identified and treated. Certain drugs, such as antidepressants, also may contribute to rapid cycling in bipolar disorder, particularly in patients not receiving other therapy such as lithium, carbamazepine, or valproic acid. Therefore, the need for continued antidepressant therapy should be reassessed in rapid-cycling patients and antidepressant therapy should be gradually discontinued, if possible.

The initial therapy in bipolar patients who experience rapid cycling usually includes lithium or valproate (e.g., valproate sodium, valproic acid, divalproex). Alternatively, lamotrigine may be used. In many patients, combination therapy (e.g., with 2 first-line agents or a combination of a first-line agent with an atypical antipsychotic) is required to adequately treat rapid cycling. Recent evidence suggests that atypical antipsychotic agents (e.g., olanzapine, clozapine) combined with mood stabilizers, such as valproic acid and/or lithium, may be effective in rapid cycling patients.

Considerations in Choosing Maintenance Therapy

Following treatment of an acute episode, patients with bipolar disorder remain at high risk of relapse. Therefore, following a single manic episode, maintenance therapy is recommended by many experts. The principal goals of maintenance therapy are relapse prevention, reduction of subthreshold symptoms, and reduction of suicide risk. Other aims of maintenance therapy include reduction in cycling frequency, reduction of mood instability, and improvement in overall functioning.

The choice of a maintenance regimen for initial therapy should be individualized and take into consideration illness severity, associated clinical features (e.g., rapid cycling, psychosis), and patient preference. Clinical experience to date indicates that either lithium or valproate (e.g., valproate sodium, valproic acid, divalproex) should be considered for first-line maintenance therapy in bipolar disorder; possible alternatives include lamotrigine, carbamazepine, or oxcarbazepine. If one of these agents was used to achieve remission from the most recent manic or depressive episode, many experts advise that it generally should be continued. Maintenance ECT therapy also should be considered in patients whose acute episode responded to ECT.

In patients who received an antipsychotic agent during the preceding acute episode, the need for continued antipsychotic therapy should be reassessed during the maintenance phase of therapy. Many experts recommend that antipsychotic therapy be tapered and discontinued unless needed for control of persisting psychotic symptoms or to prevent recurrence of such symptoms. Although maintenance therapy with atypical antipsychotic agents also may be considered, their efficacy as maintenance therapy compared with lithium or valproate has yet to be fully established. Patients with bipolar disorder are also likely to benefit from psychosocial interventions, including psychotherapy, during the maintenance phase.

Patients who continue to experience subthreshold symptoms or breakthrough episodes may require the addition of another mood-stabilizing maintenance agent (lithium or valproate), an atypical antipsychotic agent, or an antidepressant. Currently, data to support one combination over another are insufficient. Maintenance sessions of ECT also may be considered in patients whose acute episode responded to ECT.

Maintenance Therapy with Lithium

Lithium is effective in preventing or attenuating recurrences of bipolar episodes when used for long-term maintenance treatment of bipolar affective disorder. In patients with bipolar disorder, the drug is more effective at preventing signs and symptoms of mania than those of depression.

Approximately 65–90% of patients with bipolar disorder will have relapses if left untreated. During long-term lithium therapy, less than 40% of patients with bipolar disorder relapse during the first 2 years of therapy. The decision to initiate long-term prophylaxis with lithium in such patients is based on the history of recurrence of signs and symptoms.

Suicide Considerations

Patients with bipolar disorder are at high risk for suicide. Among the phases of bipolar disorder, depression is associated with the highest risk of suicide, followed by mixed episodes and the presence of psychotic symptoms, with episodes of mania being the least frequently associated with suicide. All patients with bipolar disorder should therefore be carefully evaluated to assess suicidal risk.

Long-term lithium therapy has been associated with a reduction in suicidal risk in patients with bipolar disorder. However, it has not been clearly established whether this reflects possible anti-impulsivity properties in addition to lithium's established mood-stabilizing activity. Lithium also may reduce the greater mortality risk observed among bipolar disorder patients from causes other than suicide. It remains to be established whether other drugs used as maintenance therapy such as valproic and carbamazepine also may prolong survival in patients with bipolar disorder.

● *Major Depression*

Lithium appears to be an effective antidepressant in some acutely depressed patients†. Depressive symptomatology, including feelings of hopelessness, worthlessness, and guilt; psychomotor retardation; weight loss; early awakening; and suicidal ideation, often improves during treatment with lithium. The acute antidepressant effect of lithium is more likely to occur in patients with bipolar disorder than in patients with major depression. In acutely depressed patients, complete or partial response occurs in 60–80% of patients treated with the drug. In controlled studies in acutely depressed patients, the antidepressant effect of lithium was about equal to that of tricyclic antidepressants; however, in one study imipramine was more effective than lithium. Because the effectiveness of other antidepressants (e.g., tricyclic antidepressants) in the treatment of acute depression is better established, and because lithium may worsen depressive symptoms in some patients, most clinicians reserve a trial of lithium therapy for those depressed patients who fail to respond to other antidepressants.

Based on data from several controlled studies, lithium appears to be more effective than placebo at reducing the rate of relapse in patients with recurrent depression† (recurrent unipolar affective disorder). Lithium also appears to be at least as effective as tricyclic antidepressants at reducing the number of depressive episodes in such patients. Although lithium appears to be effective in the prophylactic treatment of recurrent depression, only a small number of patients have been studied. Some clinicians believe that these studies justify the long-term use of lithium in recurrent depression; however, most clinicians believe that additional comparative studies are needed to determine the efficacy of lithium in the prophylactic treatment of recurrent depression.

● *Schizoaffective and Schizophrenic Disorders*

In patients with schizoaffective disorder† or schizophrenia†, lithium has been used with varying results. In patients with mildly active schizoaffective disorder in which the affective component predominates, lithium appears to be as effective as chlorpromazine. Such patients often show improvement in mannerisms, posturing, excitement, cooperation, and thought disorders during lithium therapy. In the treatment of patients with highly active schizoaffective disorder in which the schizophrenic component predominates, lithium appears to be less effective than chlorpromazine. In these patients, lithium alone generally fails to adequately control hostile, excited behavior. In patients with schizophrenia, lithium has demonstrated limited effectiveness when given as monotherapy and has caused worsening of the disorder in some cases.

Most clinicians consider antipsychotic agents to be the treatment of choice in patients with schizoaffective disorder or schizophrenia. The addition of lithium to a regimen containing an antipsychotic agent may be beneficial in some patients such as those with predominantly affective signs and symptoms who fail to respond to an antipsychotic agent alone, especially when acute episodes are of recent onset (e.g., less than 6 months). The American Psychiatric Association (APA) states that lithium has limited efficacy when used alone in the treatment of schizophrenia and is less effective than antipsychotic agents when used as monotherapy in patients with this condition. Earlier studies suggested that when added to antipsychotic agents in patients with schizophrenia, lithium increased overall efficacy and improved negative symptoms in particular. Other early studies indicated that lithium was beneficial in schizophrenic patients with prominent affective symptoms and in patients with schizoaffective disorder. However, more recent studies evaluating combined antipsychotic agent and lithium therapy have not confirmed those earlier findings and suggest that adjunctive therapy with lithium is not more effective than antipsychotics used alone in schizophrenia. The addition of relatively low doses of lithium over an 8-week period to an existing antipsychotic regimen improved anxiety but did not improve other symptoms in one placebo-controlled study. In another placebo-controlled study, the addition of lithium did not result in clinical improvement in schizophrenic patients who had not responded to 6 months of fluphenazine decanoate therapy. Although controlled studies of lithium combined with atypical antipsychotic agents are lacking, some of the newer antipsychotic agents have demonstrated antidepressant, anxiolytic, and mood stabilizing activity; therefore, the potential value of combined therapy with these agents and lithium may be limited.

When lithium and antipsychotic agents are used in combination, the APA states that lithium generally is added to the antipsychotic drug that the patient is already receiving after the patient has received an adequate trial but has reached a plateau in the level of clinical response and residual symptoms persist. The APA recommends that the dosage of lithium be adjusted so that serum lithium concentrations in the range of 0.8–1.2 mEq/L are achieved. Response to lithium therapy usually is evident soon after initiating therapy, and a trial of 3–4 weeks of lithium therapy usually is sufficient to determine effectiveness; however, clinical improvement may require 3 months or longer in some cases. In addition to monitoring for the usual adverse effects associated with lithium therapy, clinicians should carefully monitor patients for possible adverse drug interactions with the antipsychotic agent (e.g., adverse extrapyramidal effects, confusion, disorientation, and other signs of neuroleptic malignant syndrome), particularly during the early stage of combined therapy. For further information on the symptomatic management of schizophrenia, see Uses: Psychotic Disorders in the Phenothiazines General Statement 28:16.08.24.

● *Disorders of Impulse Control*

Lithium has been used successfully in the treatment of impulsive-aggressive behavior in a small number of adults with disorders of impulse control†. Lithium reduced temper outbursts, impulsive antisocial behavior, and the number of assaultive acts. Further studies are needed to confirm the usefulness of the drug in these patients.

● *Psychiatric Disorders in Children*

Lithium has been used to treat children with apparent mixed bipolar disorder symptomatology†, hyperactivity with psychotic or neurotic components†, or aggressive behavior† or aggressive outbursts† associated with attention-deficit hyperactivity disorder (ADHD). Although children with violent and aggressive behavior who do not have an underlying affective disorder may respond to lithium, children with a definite affective disorder are more likely to respond to the drug. Late-adolescent patients who have mixed bipolar disorder and a parent with a lithium-responsive mixed bipolar disorder are most likely to respond to lithium. Although lithium appears to be useful in children with mixed bipolar disorder†, emotionally unstable character disorder†, depression†, or aggressiveness†, data are too limited to support routine use of the drug in these children. When lithium is used in the treatment of these disorders after an adequate trial with more conservative therapy, the duration of lithium therapy should be short (i.e., not greater than 6 months) and continued only in the presence of unequivocal response to the drug.

● *Alcohol Dependence*

Although early studies reported limited evidence of improved outcomes in patients with or without depression who received lithium for the management of alcohol dependence†, evidence from a large, randomized, double-blind, placebo-controlled study sponsored by the Department of Veterans Affairs indicated that lithium was not an effective treatment for alcohol dependence in either depressed or nondepressed alcoholics. In this study, clinical outcome measurements such as abstinence rates, number of days of drinking, number of alcohol-related hospitalizations, change in severity of alcoholism, and change in severity of depression in alcoholics who received lithium were comparable to those of alcoholics who received placebo. Unlike previous studies, the Department of Veterans Affairs Cooperative Study was large enough to have sufficient statistical power to detect a medium-effect size difference between the efficacy of lithium and placebo. This study also was controlled for comorbidity; alcoholics with antisocial personality disorder and major psychiatric illnesses other than nonpsychotic depression were excluded from the study.

● *Neutropenia and Anemia*

Lithium has been used to treat neutropenia† or anemia† secondary to a variety of causes. Only in patients with antineoplastic drug-induced neutropenia have well-controlled studies of lithium therapy been reported.

In a limited number of patients with neutropenia secondary to myelosuppressive antineoplastic chemotherapy regimens, the addition of lithium to the regimen has decreased the number of days neutropenia is present, decreased the frequency of absolute neutrophil counts less than 500/mm³, and increased the neutrophil count at its nadir. The number of hospitalizations related to infection or fever and the number of infection-related deaths also have been reduced when lithium was added to a myelosuppressive antineoplastic chemotherapy regimen. There is no evidence to date that lithium increases the response of the underlying neoplastic disease to chemotherapy.

Patients receiving antineoplastic chemotherapy often are debilitated and generally are more susceptible to the adverse effects of lithium. Therefore, the benefit-to-risk ratio of lithium therapy in these patients remains to be established. Some clinicians recommend short-term lithium therapy when a patient has had severe neutropenic episodes during previous courses of chemotherapy or when a patient is undergoing treatment with combination chemotherapy known to be severely myelosuppressive.

Lithium has limited efficacy in the treatment of patients with congenital, idiopathic, or cyclic neutropenias†; Felty's syndrome†; or aplastic anemia†. In these patients, lithium has inconsistently increased leukocyte and/or erythrocyte counts. Most clinicians do not recommend routine use of lithium in these conditions since the efficacy of the drug has been limited and studies to date have not been adequately controlled.

● Other Uses

Lithium has been used in the treatment of hyperthyroidism†; however, because of its adverse effects, other treatments (e.g., radioactive iodine, surgery, propylthiouracil, methimazole) currently are preferred. Lithium also has been used to prolong the presence of radioactivity in the thyroid gland in patients receiving radioactive iodine†; however, use of the drug for this purpose requires further study.

Although lithium previously was considered one of the therapies of choice in the treatment of the syndrome of inappropriate secretion of antidiuretic hormone† (SIADH), it generally has been replaced with other more effective and/or less toxic therapies (e.g., demeclocycline).

DOSAGE AND ADMINISTRATION

● General Dosage and Administration

Lithium salts are administered orally, preferably with meals. Extended-release preparations should be swallowed intact and should *not* be chewed, crushed, or halved. Although there may be minor differences in bioavailability of commercially available lithium preparations, data do not support the use of one preparation over another. The choice of preparation usually is based on expense and patient preference. Lithium citrate oral solution may be useful in patients unable to swallow capsules or tablets; 5 mL of a commercially available solution contains about 8 mEq of lithium and is approximately equivalent to 300 mg of lithium carbonate.

Careful monitoring of serum lithium concentrations and clinical status of the patient is mandatory and patients should be carefully instructed in the safe use of the drug. The precautions and contraindications associated with lithium use should be reviewed carefully before initiating therapy. (See Cautions: Precautions and Contraindications.)

Serum lithium concentrations generally should be monitored twice weekly during initiation of the acute phase of therapy and until the serum concentration and clinical condition of the patient have been stabilized. Thereafter, serum concentrations should be monitored at least every 2 months in most patients. In patients whose affective disorder is not improving or in whom adverse effects are occurring, serum lithium concentrations should be monitored more frequently (e.g., weekly). There is wide interindividual variation in the dosage needed to achieve a given serum lithium concentration and in the serum lithium concentration needed to achieve therapeutic response. The established therapeutic range of serum lithium concentrations is based on correlations determined with monitoring of steady-state concentrations in the morning 12 hours after a dose in patients receiving a divided daily dosing regimen. Therefore, serum lithium concentrations should be determined at consistent times as close as possible to the twelfth hour after a dose. The manufacturers suggest that steady-state serum lithium concentrations be determined immediately before the next dose (i.e., 8–12 hours after the previous lithium dose). Total reliance must not be placed on serum lithium concentrations alone; accurate patient evaluation requires both careful clinical and laboratory evaluation. Dosage should be reduced and serum lithium concentration determined when a patient exhibits signs and symptoms of adverse nervous system, GI, or renal effects.

Although lithium has a long serum half-life and could be given in a single daily dose, the drug usually is given in divided doses because single daily doses often produce more frequent adverse effects (e.g., nausea, diarrhea). Several preliminary studies, however, indicate that the incidence of polyuria may be lower in patients receiving single daily doses rather than divided doses. Twice-daily dosing of conventional or extended-release preparations is sufficient for most patients. When adverse GI or nervous system effects occur, they may be minimized or prevented by giving the drug as conventional preparations in 3 or 4 divided doses.

When lithium is used during pregnancy (see Cautions: Pregnancy, Fertility, and Lactation), some clinicians recommend dividing the total daily dose of conventional preparations into 3–5 doses to avoid exposing the fetus to high peak serum concentrations of the drug.

● Dosage for Acute Episodes

Serum lithium concentrations of 1–1.2 mEq/L are usually required during acute affective episodes. Although higher serum lithium concentrations may be required in some patients, *the serum concentration should not exceed 1.5 mEq/L during the acute treatment phase.* If manifestations of lithium toxicity occur, the drug should be temporarily discontinued for 24–48 hours, then resumed at a lower dosage.

Adult Dosage

During acute episodes of an affective disorder, the manufacturers recommend an initial lithium dosage of 1.8 g daily as conventional capsules or tablets of lithium carbonate, given in 3 or 4 divided doses, or 30 mL (about 48 mEq of lithium) of lithium citrate oral solution daily, given in 3 divided doses. Alternatively, the usual initial dosage of lithium carbonate of 1.8 g daily may be administered as extended-release tablets of lithium carbonate, given in 2 or 3 divided doses. However, because long-term compliance may be affected by a patient's initial experience with the drug, some clinicians recommend that lower initial dosages of lithium be used (e.g., 900 mg of lithium carbonate daily or less), especially in geriatric patients, in an attempt to minimize initial adverse effects, and then dosage be titrated slowly to achieve therapeutic serum lithium concentrations. Dosage must be individualized according to serum lithium concentrations, patient tolerance, and clinical response. The manufacturers state that serum lithium concentrations should be determined twice weekly during the acute phase of therapy and until the serum concentration and clinical condition of the patient have been stabilized. However, some clinicians recommend more frequent monitoring of serum lithium concentrations (e.g., before and after each dosage increase), particularly if a rapid dosage increase is necessary (e.g., in the treatment of acute mania) or if toxicity is suspected. Following resolution of acute manic signs and symptoms, many patients will not tolerate serum lithium concentrations of 1–1.2 mEq/L, and dosage reduction with appropriate patient monitoring is usually necessary.

Pediatric Dosage

Although the usual dosage of lithium salts for acute episodes in children† has not been established, lithium carbonate dosages of 15–20 mg/kg (about 0.4–0.5 mEq/kg) daily or equivalent lithium citrate dosages have been given in 2 or 3 divided doses to children 11 years of age or younger. However, the usual adult dosage should not be exceeded. When lithium salts are used in children, dosage should be adjusted according to serum lithium concentrations, patient tolerance, and clinical response. Dosages for children 12 years of age and older usually are the same of those of adults.

● Maintenance Dosage

Maintenance dosage of lithium should be based on serum lithium concentrations noted during the acute phase of therapy and on steady-state serum lithium concentrations determined 12 hours after a dose. Manufacturers recommend maintaining steady-state serum lithium concentrations at 0.6–1.2 mEq/L, using the minimum effective dosage that produces serum concentrations in this range, while avoiding excessive adverse effects. Geriatric patients often can be maintained with dosages that produce serum concentrations at the lower end of this range. During maintenance therapy, serum lithium concentrations are generally determined at least every 2 months in patients whose disease is well controlled.

Adult Dosage

The usual adult maintenance dosage is 900 mg to 1.2 g daily of lithium carbonate as conventional tablets or capsules, given in 3 or 4 divided doses, or 15–20 mL of lithium citrate oral solution (about 24–32 mEq) daily, given in 3 or 4 divided doses. Alternatively, the usual maintenance dosage of lithium carbonate of 900 mg to 1.2 g daily may be administered as extended-release tablets, given in 2 or 3 divided doses. This dosage generally provides serum lithium concentrations of 0.6–1.2 mEq/L. Maintenance dosage usually should not exceed 2.4 g of lithium carbonate (65 mEq) daily.

Pediatric Dosage

The usual maintenance dosage of lithium salts in children† has not been established. When lithium salts are used in children†, dosage should be adjusted according to serum lithium concentrations, patient tolerance, and clinical response.

CAUTIONS

Adverse reactions to lithium generally involve the CNS, GI tract, and kidneys. These adverse reactions usually are dose-dependent and generally occur at 12-hour steady-state serum lithium concentrations greater than 1–1.3 mEq/L; however, adverse CNS effects have occurred at serum concentrations less than 1 mEq/L, especially in children and geriatric patients. Other adverse effects, particularly GI effects, have been related to high peak serum concentrations of lithium.

● Nervous System and Neuromuscular Effects

Mild adverse CNS and neuromuscular effects initially occur in about 40–50% of patients receiving lithium. Lethargy, fatigue, muscle weakness, and tremor occur most frequently. As many as 40% of patients receiving lithium initially complain of headache, minor memory impairment and mental confusion, and/or a slightly decreased ability to concentrate.

Hand tremor occurs in about 45–50% of patients during initiation of lithium therapy and is usually benign. The tremor is a fine, rapid intention tremor, which generally resolves during continued therapy with the drug. After 1 year of lithium therapy, less than 10% of patients exhibit tremor. A coarsening of the tremor or its spread to other parts of the body may indicate lithium intoxication. Although hand tremor usually occurs early in the course of therapy, it can occur at any time and may be aggravated by anxiety, caffeine, or thyrotoxicosis. Most patients do not find lithium-induced tremor particularly troublesome. For those who do, a reduction in lithium dosage or low doses of a β-adrenergic blocking agent (e.g., propranolol) may be beneficial. The tremor is not responsive to antimuscarinic or other antiparkinsonian drugs.

Transient muscle weakness occurs in about 30% of lithium-treated patients; after 1 year of lithium therapy, about 1% of lithium-treated patients complain of muscle weakness. Similarly, fatigue, lethargy, dulled senses, and ataxia occur early in therapy but seem to resolve after 2–3 weeks of therapy. Dysarthria and aphasia also have been reported.

Muscle hyperirritability (including fasciculations, twitching, clonic movements of limbs), hyperactive deep tendon reflexes, hypertonia (hypertonicity), and choreoathetoid movements occur in less than 15% of patients receiving lithium. Cogwheel rigidity occurs in about 5% of patients. In one study, cogwheel rigidity reportedly occurred in 75% of patients receiving lithium; however, persistent concentrations of antipsychotic agents may have accounted for the higher incidence of cogwheel rigidity noted in these patients. Lithium-induced cogwheel rigidity generally is mild to moderate. Although it rarely may be associated with other extrapyramidal signs, lithium-induced cogwheel rigidity does not respond to antiparkinsonian agents.

Blackout spells, giddiness, dizziness, vertigo, disturbances in accommodation, somnolence and tendency to sleep, stupor, coma, restlessness, psychomotor retardation, acute dystonia, down-beat nystagmus, centrally mediated incontinence of urine and feces, and worsening of organic brain syndrome have occurred during lithium therapy. In one study, vertigo and disturbances in accommodation occurred in 15 and 10% of patients receiving the drug, respectively. Asterixis has occurred in at least one patient.

Pseudotumor cerebri (with increased intracranial pressure and papilledema) has occurred in patients receiving lithium. If undetected, this condition may result in enlargement of the blind spot, constriction of visual fields, and/or eventual blindness resulting from optic atrophy. If pseudotumor cerebri occurs during lithium therapy, the drug should be discontinued, if clinically possible. Papilledema with no evidence of increased intracranial pressure has also been reported.

Seizures and localizing neurologic findings have occurred in patients receiving lithium. Seizures generally are associated with toxic serum lithium concentrations and/or other signs of lithium neurotoxicity, but seizures also have occurred when lithium concentrations were within the therapeutic range. In one study, there was an increased frequency of lithium-induced seizures in patients with temporal-lobe epilepsy. Various EEG changes, including diffuse slowing, widening of frequency spectrum, and potentiation and disorganization of background rhythm, also have been reported. (See Pharmacology: Nervous System Effects.)

● GI Effects

Adverse GI effects occur frequently during initiation of lithium therapy but tend to be mild and reversible. Nausea, anorexia, epigastric bloating, diarrhea, vomiting, or abdominal pain occur in about 10–30% of patients. These adverse GI effects usually resolve during continued therapy and are present in 1–10% of patients after 1–2 years of therapy. These effects often are related to high peak serum lithium concentrations and are alleviated by taking the drug with meals, dividing dosage, or using an extended-release preparation. Some patients report a reduction in adverse GI effects when switched from one conventional capsule or tablet preparation to another.

Dry mouth occurs in about 20–50% of patients receiving lithium and is related to lithium-induced polyuria. Dysgeusia and sialorrhea also have been reported. An increased frequency of dental caries has been reported in patients treated with lithium, but this effect is probably related to increased consumption of sugar-containing fluids by patients with lithium-induced polydipsia. Contact stomatitis has occurred in at least one patient and was attributed to the formulation of the preparation.

● Renal Effects

Nephrogenic diabetes insipidus manifested as polyuria and polydipsia occurs in about 30–50% of lithium-treated patients, usually develops shortly after starting lithium therapy, and persists in about 10–25% of treated patients after 1–2 years of therapy. Polydipsia is largely a consequence of polyuria; both usually are well tolerated in most patients. Polyuria rarely is associated with serum electrolyte abnormalities, weight loss, or other signs and symptoms of dehydration; however, these effects may occur in patients who develop severe diabetes insipidus during lithium therapy. Many patients actually respond to polyuria with weight gain, probably because of increased consumption of high-calorie fluids. Although polyuria is a persistent and sometimes progressive finding in patients treated with lithium, it usually is reversible within 1 year after discontinuance of the drug; irreversible diabetes insipidus occurs rarely. Polyuria has been treated with lithium dosage reduction and/or with thiazide diuretics or amiloride (See Drug Interactions: Diuretics.)

Nonspecific nephron atrophy characterized by glomerular sclerosis, tubular atrophy, interstitial fibrosis, and urinary casts has been observed in patients treated with lithium. The tubular lesions are limited mainly to the distal convoluted tubule and collecting ducts. Sclerosis of 10–20% of glomeruli has been noted in some patients. These nonspecific changes have not been associated with a decrease in renal function. Although available data do not support a causal relationship between these findings and lithium therapy, studies of large numbers of patients receiving the drug for many years have not been conducted. In several trials using appropriate controls, there was no difference in the frequency of abnormal renal findings in pretreatment and posttreatment patients. However, cellular pleomorphism in the distal renal tubule has been associated with a decrease in renal-concentrating ability. Albuminuria and glycosuria also have occurred.

Modest decreases in glomerular filtration rate occasionally occur in patients receiving long-term lithium therapy; however, a causal relationship has not yet been established. Oliguric renal failure, reported in a few intoxicated patients, probably is not a direct renal effect of lithium but is related to circulatory collapse that may accompany lithium intoxication. (See Chronic Toxicity: Manifestations.)

Distal renal tubular acidosis of the incomplete type has occurred in some patients receiving lithium, but it does not appear to be clinically important unless these patients are stressed by an acid load. Most patients receiving lithium show a normal urine acidification response.

● Endocrine Effects

In therapeutic concentrations, lithium causes clinically evident hypothyroidism in about 1–4% of patients receiving the drug. These patients may require supplemental thyroid therapy. Symptoms of hypothyroidism may vary from mild to severe myxedema and may occur within weeks to years after initiating lithium therapy; rarely, hypothyroidism may persist after discontinuance of the drug. In addition, about 5% of lithium-treated patients develop goiters, resulting from stimulation of the thyroid gland by an indirect lithium-induced increase in thyrotropin release. Goiters may develop even in the absence of hypothyroidism in some patients receiving lithium. Lithium-induced goiters usually are diffuse and nontender and often so small as to be noticed only on palpation. Many patients have only laboratory evidence of hypothyroidism, including decreased serum concentrations of thyroxine (T_4) and triiodothyronine (T_3) and increased radioactive iodine uptake. Even in patients whose baseline serum thyrotropin concentrations are within normal limits, an exaggerated thyrotropin response to IV protirelin often occurs. Geriatric patients and patients with antithyroglobulin antibody, a prior history of Graves' disease or Hashimoto's thyroiditis, or those receiving iodine may be more likely to develop hypothyroidism during lithium therapy. Paradoxically, a few cases of hyperthyroidism have been reported.

Mild asymptomatic primary hyperparathyroidism has occurred during long-term lithium therapy and, rarely, may persist after discontinuance of the drug. (See Pharmacology: Endocrine Effects.)

Transient hyperglycemia has occurred rarely in patients receiving lithium.

● Cardiovascular Effects

Benign, reversible ECG T-wave depression occurs in 20–30% of patients receiving lithium. Isoelectricity or inversion of T waves also may occur. Reversible sinus node dysfunction (e.g., sinus bradycardia, sinoatrial block), atrioventricular (AV) node dissociation with AV block and junctional rhythms, and ventricular premature depolarizations occur rarely at therapeutic and toxic serum lithium concentrations. Syncope has occurred in patients with lithium-induced nodal dysfunction. In contrast, lithium also has been found to reduce the frequency of preexisting atrial premature depolarizations and supraventricular tachycardia.

Mild to moderate pretibial edema has occurred in a few patients during lithium therapy and appears to be associated with high sodium intake (more than 170 mEq/day). The edema has responded to spironolactone. Edematous swelling of the wrists also has occurred.

Other cardiovascular effects, including hypotension and cardiovascular collapse, have been noted during severe lithium intoxication and probably are not direct effects of the drug. Peripheral circulatory collapse also has been reported. Cardiomyopathy with associated myocardial and thyroid fibrosis was reported in one patient receiving lithium, amitriptyline, and potassium iodide.

Signs and symptoms resembling Raynaud's disease, which included painful discoloration of fingers and toes and coldness of the extremities, occurred in some patients within 1 day after initiating lithium therapy. The mechanism of this effect is not known; recovery occurred following discontinuance of the drug.

● Dermatologic Effects

Adverse dermatologic effects occur in about 1% of patients receiving lithium and rarely necessitate discontinuance of the drug. Acneiform eruptions and folliculitis appear to occur most frequently. Lithium-induced acneiform eruptions usually involve the face, neck, axilla, groin, and breast. The papules may become confluent or may subside spontaneously. Temporary discontinuance of the drug usually results in resolution of the eruption. Lithium-induced folliculitis resembles keratosis pilaris, is asymptomatic and usually limited to the extensor surfaces of the extremities, and often remits spontaneously. Pruritic maculopapular rashes occur rarely and usually remit with dosage reduction or discontinuance of lithium.

Lithium-induced or -exacerbated psoriasis has occurred occasionally; it is unclear whether a causal relationship to the drug exists. Alopecia, drying and thinning of the hair, xerosis cutis, anesthesia of the skin, cutaneous ulcers, exfoliative dermatitis, and lupus erythematosus-like rash also have occurred.

● Hematologic Effects

Most patients receiving lithium develop a reversible leukocytosis, with leukocyte counts of 10,000–15,000/mm³. Increases in erythrocyte and platelet counts are less frequently observed.

Lithium has been associated with the development of leukemia (see Cautions: Mutagenicity and Carcinogenicity), but a causal relationship to the drug has not been established. Aplastic anemia has been reported in at least one patient receiving lithium. Positive serum titers for antinuclear antibodies (ANA) have occurred during lithium therapy, but patients with positive serum ANA titers usually were receiving other drugs in addition to lithium.

● Other Adverse Effects

Other adverse effects associated with lithium therapy include weight loss or excessive weight gain (which may be associated with polyuria, see Cautions: Renal Effects), transient scotomata, exophthalmos, and generalized discomfort.

● Precautions and Contraindications

Since lithium toxicity is closely related to serum lithium concentrations and may occur at doses closely associated with therapeutic serum concentrations, monitoring of serum lithium concentrations and the clinical status of the patient is necessary in all patients receiving the drug. Lithium dosing should be monitored carefully when a patient's initial manic symptoms begin to subside, since the patient's ability to tolerate high serum lithium concentrations decreases as these symptoms resolve. (See Dosage and Administration: Dosage for Acute Episodes.)

Patients receiving lithium should be carefully instructed to avoid dehydration and to report polyuria and any prolonged vomiting, diarrhea, or fever to their physician. Patients should maintain their usual fluid (2.5–3 L/day) and sodium intake, and supplement these in the event of fever (e.g., during infections), vomiting, or diarrhea. A temporary reduction in dosage or discontinuance of the drug also may be required in these patients. Lithium should be used cautiously in patients whose sodium intake is restricted; in these patients, sodium intake should be stabilized and lithium dosage carefully titrated to avoid increased serum lithium concentrations that may occur with sodium depletion.

Outpatients and their families should be warned that the patient must discontinue lithium therapy immediately and consult a physician if signs of lithium intoxication such as muscle twitching, tremor, mild ataxia, drowsiness, muscle weakness, diarrhea, or vomiting occur. Patients also should be warned that lithium may impair their ability to perform activities requiring mental alertness or physical coordination (e.g., operating machinery, driving a motor vehicle).

Because nonspecific nephron atrophy has occurred in patients receiving lithium, many clinicians recommend a thorough assessment of renal function before initiating therapy. Many clinicians recommend that measurement of 24-hour creatinine clearance, renal-concentrating ability, and a urinalysis should ideally be performed in all patients prior to initiating therapy. Many clinicians also recommend that renal function be evaluated every 2–3 months for the first 6 months, then every 6–12 months during therapy or whenever clinically indicated. If progressive or sudden changes in renal function, even within the normal range, occur during lithium therapy, the need for therapy with the drug should be reevaluated.

Lithium should be used cautiously in patients with preexisting cardiovascular or thyroid disease. Patients with underlying cardiovascular disease should be observed carefully for signs and symptoms of arrhythmia (including periodic ECG determinations), and serum lithium concentrations should be kept within the therapeutic range since nodal arrhythmias may occur. Patients with underlying hypothyroidism should have thyroid function (T_3, T_4, and TSH concentrations) evaluated yearly and be given supplemental thyroid therapy when needed.

Lithium should be used with caution in geriatric patients since they appear to be more susceptible to adverse effects of the drug (e.g., adverse nervous system and neuromuscular effects), even at therapeutic serum concentrations. Because geriatric patients are more prone than younger patients to developing lithium-induced goiter and clinical hypothyroidism, some clinicians recommend that thyroid function tests be performed every 6–12 months in these patients. In addition, because of decreased renal function, geriatric patients are more likely to develop lithium intoxication subsequent to accumulation of the drug.

Although most patients receiving lithium and an antipsychotic agent (e.g., haloperidol, phenothiazines) concurrently do not develop unusual adverse effects, an acute encephalopathic syndrome (consisting of confusion, disorientation, adverse extrapyramidal effects, and possibly neuroleptic malignant syndrome) occasionally has occurred, especially when high serum lithium concentrations were present and associated with dehydration. Patients receiving such combined therapy should be observed for evidence of adverse neurologic effects; treatment should be promptly discontinued if such signs or symptoms appear. (See Drug Interactions: Antipsychotic Agents.)

Lithium generally should not be used in patients with severe renal or cardiovascular disease or severe dehydration, sodium depletion, or debilitation since the risk of toxicity is increased in these patients. If the psychiatric indication is life-threatening and other forms of therapy are contraindicated or ineffective, lithium may be used with extreme caution in these patients; if lithium therapy is initiated in these patients, the patient should be hospitalized, serum lithium concentration should be monitored carefully, and dosage should be adjusted as necessary. Although the manufacturers caution against the concurrent use of lithium and a diuretic, when combined therapy is necessary, some clinicians recommend that the usual dosage of lithium initially be reduced by about 50%, the patient and serum lithium concentrations be monitored carefully, and lithium dosage be adjusted as necessary. (See Drug Interactions: Diuretics.)

● Pediatric Precautions

Safety and efficacy of lithium therapy in children younger than 12 years of age have not been established; however, the drug has been used in this age group when benefits were thought to outweigh risks. Transient acute dystonia and hyperreflexia occurred in a 15-kg child who ingested 300 mg of lithium carbonate.

● Geriatric Precautions

Clinical studies of lithium carbonate as extended-release tablets did not include sufficient numbers of patients 65 years of age and older to determine whether geriatric patients respond differently than younger patients. While clinical experience with lithium therapy generally has not revealed age-related differences in response to the drug, care should be taken in dosage selection of lithium. Because of the greater frequency of decreased hepatic, renal, and/or cardiac function and of concomitant disease and drug therapy in geriatric patients, patients in this age group should receive initial dosages of the drug in the lower end of the usual range. Lithium is substantially excreted by the kidneys and the risk of severe adverse reactions to the drug may be increased in patients with impaired renal function. Because geriatric patients may have decreased renal function, renal function should be monitored and dosage adjusted accordingly.

● Mutagenicity and Carcinogenicity

It is not known if lithium is mutagenic or carcinogenic.

An increased number of chromosomal breaks, gaps, and satellite associations, as well as a reduced percentage of replicating cells were found in one study of lithium-containing leukocyte cultures. Similar findings were not found in 2 other in vitro studies. Mice inoculated with viable sarcoma cells have shown an earlier incidence of tumor development but no change in tumor size when treated with lithium. The number and growth of induced mammary tumors in rats have not been increased by lithium.

There have been occasional reports of lithium-induced hematologic neoplasms (e.g., acute leukemia), but a causal relationship to the drug has not been established. Studies have shown no changes in blast and mature neutrophil counts in patients with various blood dyscrasias who were receiving lithium. One study found the incidence of leukemia not to be increased in a group of manic-depressive patients receiving chronic lithium therapy.

● Pregnancy, Fertility, and Lactation

Pregnancy

Lithium can cause fetal toxicity when administered to pregnant women, but potential benefits may be acceptable in certain conditions despite the possible risks to the fetus. Lithium should be used during pregnancy only in life-threatening situations or severe disease for which safer drugs cannot be used or are ineffective. When lithium is administered during pregnancy or if the patient becomes pregnant while receiving the drug, the patient should be informed of the potential hazard to the fetus. When possible, lithium should be withdrawn for at least the first trimester unless it is determined that this would seriously endanger the mother. Women of childbearing age receiving lithium should be counseled about methods of birth control.

When lithium is used during pregnancy, serum lithium concentrations should be carefully monitored and dosage adjusted if necessary since renal clearance of the drug and distribution of the drug into erythrocytes may be increased during pregnancy. Pregnant women receiving lithium may have subtherapeutic serum lithium concentrations if dosage of the drug is not increased during pregnancy. Immediately postpartum, renal clearance of lithium may decrease to pre-pregnancy levels; therefore, to decrease the risk of postpartum lithium intoxication, dosage of the drug should be reduced 1 week before parturition or when labor begins.

Lithium has caused various teratogenic effects in submammalian species and cleft palates in mice. Studies in rats, rabbits, and monkeys have shown no evidence of lithium-induced teratology.

Data from lithium birth registries suggest that the drug may increase the incidence of cardiac and other anomalies, especially Ebstein's anomaly (distorted tricuspid valve with secondary dilation of the right ventricular outflow tract). Atrial septal defect, patent foramen ovale, and right ventricular conduction delay also have occurred. Other reported fetal cardiovascular abnormalities included mitral atresia, coarctation of the aorta, ventricular septal defect, tricuspid atresia, patent ductus arteriosus, and dextrocardia. Down's syndrome, clubfoot, meningomyelocele, transient hypothyroidism with goiter, and transient nephrogenic diabetes insipidus also have been reported. Lithium-exposed neonates also have presented briefly with muscular hypotonia (floppy infant syndrome) and apneic spells. A 5-year follow-up study of children without apparent congenital abnormalities who were born to women treated with lithium found no increase in the frequency of physical or mental abnormalities in these children compared with matched controls (i.e., siblings during whose pregnancy the mother did not take lithium).

Fertility

The effect of lithium on fertility in humans is not known. Erective impotence has been noted by a few men receiving the drug. Lithium has had adverse effects on nidation in rats and on embryo viability in mice. In vitro metabolism of rat testes and human spermatozoa also have been observed.

Lactation

Lithium is distributed into milk. (See Pharmacokinetics: Distribution.) Because of the potential for serious adverse reactions from lithium in nursing infants, a decision generally should be made to discontinue nursing or the drug, taking into account the importance of the drug to the woman.

DRUG INTERACTIONS

● Diuretics

In general, the concomitant use of lithium and diuretics should be avoided. In those cases where concomitant use is necessary, extreme caution is advised because diuretic-induced sodium loss may reduce the renal clearance of lithium and increase the risk of lithium toxicity. When such combinations are used, the lithium dosage may need to be decreased and more frequent monitoring of serum lithium concentrations is recommended.

Thiazide diuretics, sometimes used in combination with lithium to reduce lithium-induced polyuria, will reduce renal lithium clearance within several days. The reduced lithium clearance has resulted in increased serum lithium concentrations and several cases of lithium intoxication. When thiazide diuretics are used to treat lithium-induced polyuria, most clinicians recommend reducing lithium dosage by about 50% and carefully monitoring serum lithium concentrations. Other diuretics that enhance sodium excretion (e.g., furosemide, spironolactone) also may reduce renal clearance of lithium; however, this effect does not occur consistently and lithium clearance often is increased initially. Urea also has increased renal clearance of lithium. Amiloride does not appear to substantially affect lithium pharmacokinetics in most patients. (See Drug Interactions: Lithium, in Amiloride Hydrochloride 40:28.10.)

● Antipsychotic Agents

Numerous pharmacokinetic and clinical interactions have been reported between phenothiazines and lithium. Phenothiazines have been shown to increase erythrocyte lithium concentrations and to increase renal clearance of lithium. Lithium has been reported to decrease serum chlorpromazine concentrations. The clinical result of these pharmacokinetic interactions is unpredictable; therefore, patients receiving lithium and a phenothiazine should be monitored for altered response to either drug. In addition, an acute encephalopathic syndrome (toxic-confusional state) consisting of confusion, disorientation, extrapyramidal adverse effects, and possibly neuroleptic malignant syndrome occasionally has been reported in patients receiving lithium and antipsychotic agents concurrently, particularly in dehydrated patients with high serum lithium concentrations. Therefore, patients receiving combined therapy should be observed for evidence of adverse neurologic effects (e.g., adverse extrapyramidal effects, confusion, disorientation, and other signs of neuroleptic malignant syndrome), particularly during the early stage of combined therapy. Nausea and vomiting, which are occasionally signs of lithium intoxication, may be masked by the antiemetic effect of some phenothiazines when used concurrently.

Occasionally, patients have developed acute encephalopathic syndromes or extrapyramidal reactions when concurrently using lithium and an antipsychotic agent (e.g., haloperidol, phenothiazines). Irreversible brain damage, parkinsonian movements, and dyskinesias have resulted. Although a causal relationship has not been established and most patients can receive the drugs concurrently without adverse effect, caution is advised. Patients receiving such combined therapy should be monitored for adverse neurologic effects, especially when large dosages of lithium and an antipsychotic agent are used; combined therapy should be promptly discontinued if such signs or symptoms appear.

● Nonsteroidal Anti-inflammatory Agents

Indomethacin, mefenamic acid, phenylbutazone, piroxicam, and ibuprofen have been reported to increase serum lithium concentrations by 30–60%, resulting in lithium toxicity in some cases. These nonsteroidal anti-inflammatory agents (NSAIAs) appear to decrease renal clearance of lithium. There is evidence that other NSAIAs, including selective inhibitors of cyclooxygenase-2 (COX-2), have the same effect. In one clinical study, mean steady-state plasma lithium concentrations increased approximately 17% in healthy individuals who received lithium (450 mg twice daily) in conjunction with celecoxib (200 mg twice daily) compared with those who received lithium alone. When these agents are started or discontinued in a patient receiving lithium, serum lithium concentrations should be closely monitored and the patient should be observed for signs and symptoms of lithium intoxication. Appropriate adjustment in lithium dosage may be required when therapy with the NSAIA is discontinued.

● Anticonvulsants

Adverse neurologic effects have occurred in patients receiving lithium concurrently with carbamazepine or phenytoin. Concurrent use of lithium and phenytoin also has resulted in increased serum lithium concentrations in at least one patient; however, the clinical importance of this effect has not been determined and further substantiation of this interaction is required.

● Angiotensin-converting Enzyme Inhibitors

Concomitant administration of lithium and an ACE inhibitor (e.g., captopril, enalapril, lisinopril) may result in elevated plasma lithium concentrations and has resulted in several cases of lithium intoxication. Consequently, at least one manufacturer of lithium and some clinicians recommend that such concomitant use of these agents be avoided, particularly in geriatric patients or in those with congestive heart failure, renal insufficiency, or volume depletion. The mechanism of this interaction is not known, but it has been postulated that dehydration and loss of sodium may decrease excretion of lithium. Moderate renal insufficiency (serum creatinine of 2.2 mg/dL or acute renal failure also has occurred in some patients receiving an ACE inhibitor concomitantly with lithium. (See Drug Interactions: Lithium, in Enalapril 24:32.04.) If lithium is used with an ACE inhibitor, the dosage of lithium may need to be reduced and serum lithium concentrations should be carefully monitored.

● Calcium-channel Blocking Agents

Serum lithium concentrations may decrease following initiation of verapamil in patients stabilized on lithium therapy. In a patient with bipolar disorder whose lithium dosage had been stabilized for several years, manic symptoms emerged and serum lithium concentrations decreased to subtherapeutic levels within 1 month after initiating 320 mg of verapamil hydrochloride daily, requiring an increase in lithium carbonate dosage from 900–1200 mg daily to 1800–2100 mg daily. Serum lithium concentrations also decreased in another patient and urinary excretion of the cation increased.

Although the mechanism of this interaction currently is not known, serum lithium concentrations and the patient should be monitored closely and lithium dosage adjusted accordingly when verapamil is initiated or discontinued in patients receiving lithium therapy.

There also is some evidence that calcium-channel blocking agents may potentiate the toxic effects of lithium; neurotoxicity (e.g., ataxia, choreoathetosis, tremors, tinnitus), adverse GI effects (e.g., nausea, vomiting, diarrhea), and bradycardia have been reported in patients receiving lithium concomitantly with a calcium-channel blocking agent. When 240 mg of verapamil hydrochloride daily was initiated for potential antimanic effects in a patient whose bipolar disorder was inadequately controlled with a therapeutic dosage of lithium, bipolar disorder was controlled within 1 week after initiating combined therapy, but manifestations of neurotoxicity occurred 2 days later despite therapeutic serum lithium concentrations. Neurotoxicity subsided within 2 days following discontinuance of verapamil but recurred when the patient was rechallenged with verapamil in an attempt to regain control of the bipolar disorder. Verapamil did not appear to affect the pharmacokinetics of lithium in this patient. The mechanism of this interaction is not known, but a similar interaction has been described in a patient receiving lithium and diltiazem concomitantly. Calcium-channel blocking agents appear to share some of the neuropharmacologic effects of lithium, and combined therapy with the drugs may potentiate neurotoxicity. Pending further accumulation of data, verapamil and possibly other calcium-channel blocking agents should be used concomitantly with lithium cautiously.

● Selective Serotonin-Reuptake Inhibitors

Adverse effects possibly associated with increased serum lithium concentrations, lithium toxicity, and/or serotonin syndrome (e.g., absence seizures, agitation, ataxia, confusion, diarrhea, dizziness, dysarthria, stiffness of the extremities, tremor) have been reported in patients receiving lithium concomitantly with selective serotonin-reuptake inhibitors (SSRIs). In addition, concomitant use of lithium and fluoxetine has resulted in both increased and decreased serum lithium concentrations; therefore, patients receiving such combined therapy should be monitored closely. Lithium appears to have some serotonergic activity and serotonin syndrome has been reported following initiation of lithium therapy in patients receiving SSRIs such as fluoxetine or paroxetine. For further information on serotonin syndrome, including manifestations and treatment, see Serotonin Syndrome under Drug Interactions: Drugs Associated with Serotonin Syndrome, in Fluoxetine Hydrochloride 28:16.04.20. The clinical importance of this potential interaction remains to be determined and further substantiation is required; however, caution should be exercised when lithium and serotonin reuptake-inhibitors are used concurrently.

● Neuromuscular Blocking Agents

Lithium has been reported to prolong the latency of neuromuscular blockade induced by succinylcholine or pancuronium. In limited clinical studies, however, no prolongation of neuromuscular blockade was noted in patients receiving electroconvulsive therapy, succinylcholine, and lithium concurrently. Patients receiving neuromuscular blocking agents should have lithium temporarily withdrawn during their use or should be carefully monitored if lithium is continued.

● Iodides

Concurrent use of lithium salts and iodides may result in an additive or synergistic hypothyroid effect. Lithium carbonate and potassium iodide have produced hypothyroidism in several patients when used concurrently. A lithium salt and potassium iodide generally should not be used concomitantly; when the drugs are used together, the patient should be monitored closely for signs and symptoms of hypothyroidism.

● Sodium

Changes in sodium intake in patients receiving lithium may alter the renal elimination of lithium. The renal clearance of lithium may be increased or decreased by as much as 30–50% by increased or decreased sodium intake, respectively. Patients should be advised to avoid substantial changes in their sodium intake. (See Cautions: Precautions and Contraindications.) When drugs with a high sodium content (e.g., antacids) are used concomitantly with lithium, serum lithium concentrations should be monitored.

● Electroconvulsive Therapy

Acute neurotoxicity with prominent delirium has occurred in patients receiving lithium and electroconvulsive therapy (ECT) concurrently. Some clinicians recommend decreasing lithium dosage or withdrawing the drug 2 days prior to ECT.

● Metronidazole

Initiation of short-term metronidazole therapy in patients stabilized on a relatively high dosage of lithium has been reported to increase serum lithium concentrations, resulting in signs of lithium toxicity in several patients; in some cases, signs of renal damage (e.g., persistent elevations in serum creatinine concentration, hypernatremia, abnormally dilute urine) were present. Pending further accumulation of data, caution should be exercised and frequent monitoring of serum lithium concentrations should be performed when metronidazole and lithium are administered concurrently.

● β-Adrenergic Blocking Agents

Although β-adrenergic blocking agents have been used to suppress lithium-induced tremor, the absence of tremor may make lithium intoxication more difficult to diagnose. Therefore, patients should be monitored for other signs and symptoms of lithium intoxication when the drugs are used concomitantly.

● Alkalinizing Agents

Urinary alkalinizing agents such as sodium bicarbonate may increase renal excretion of lithium, and a higher dosage of lithium may be required in patients receiving these agents concomitantly.

● Methyldopa

Symptoms of lithium intoxication, including confusion, disorientation, hand tremor, and slurred speech, have been reported occasionally when methyldopa was administered in patients already receiving lithium. Although plasma lithium concentrations were reported to be within the therapeutic range in some of the published cases, increased lithium concentrations have also been reported during concurrent administration of methyldopa. The possible mechanism for this interaction remains to be established. Pending further experience with this combination, some clinicians recommend that patients receiving lithium and methyldopa should be closely monitored for signs of lithium toxicity and that consideration should be given to the use of alternative antihypertensive agents in patients receiving lithium.

● Tetracycline

Tetracycline reportedly increased serum lithium concentrations when the 2 drugs were used concurrently in one patient; however, the clinical importance of this effect has not been determined.

● Diazepam

Profound hypothermia has been reported in one patient taking lithium and diazepam concurrently; however, widespread use of this combination without unusual adverse effects indicates that it is safe in most patients.

● Opiate Analgesics

Lithium reportedly interferes with opiate-induced euphoria and diminishes the analgesic effect of opiates (narcotic analgesics).

● Other Drugs

Decreased serum lithium concentrations as a result of increased urinary lithium excretion may occur when lithium is used concomitantly with acetazolamide or xanthine derivatives (e.g., aminophylline).

Hyperkinetic movements and tardive dyskinesia have been reported when lithium was used concomitantly with baclofen or a monoamine oxidase (MAO) inhibitor, respectively.

ACUTE TOXICITY

Since the pathophysiology, manifestations, and treatment of acute lithium intoxication are similar to those of chronic lithium intoxication, the Chronic Toxicity section should be consulted for additional information.

● Pathogenesis

Acute lithium intoxication occurs as the result of ingestion of a single toxic dose. The acute lethal dose of lithium varies but is generally associated with a dose that produces serum lithium concentrations greater than 3.5 mEq/L 12 hours after ingestion.

● Manifestations

In individuals not previously receiving the drug, acute ingestion of a single massive dose of lithium may produce only vomiting and diarrhea usually within 1 hour of ingestion. Manifestations associated with chronic lithium intoxication also may occur. A transient syndrome of acute dystonia and hyperreflexia has been reported in a 15-kg child following ingestion of 300 mg of lithium carbonate. Death has occurred in adults who ingested single 10- to 60-g doses of lithium. However, some patients who ingested a single 6-g dose of lithium have had no signs of lithium intoxication.

● Treatment

In acute overdosage, the stomach should be emptied immediately by inducing emesis or by gastric lavage. If the patient is comatose, having seizures, or lacks the gag reflex, gastric lavage may be performed if an endotracheal tube with cuff inflated is in place to prevent aspiration of gastric contents. Following induction of emesis or gastric lavage, the treatment described for chronic intoxication generally should be followed. (See Chronic Toxicity: Treatment.)

CHRONIC TOXICITY

● Pathogenesis

Chronic lithium intoxication, when it occurs, generally results from high dosages, prolonged therapy with high dosages, or changes in lithium pharmacokinetics. The main contributing factor to the development of chronic intoxication often is water loss, which may result from fever, decreased fluid or food intake during acute manic or depressive episodes, diuretics, abnormal GI conditions (e.g., nausea, diarrhea, vomiting), or pyelonephritis. Geriatric patients also are more prone to develop chronic lithium intoxication.

Although there is no clearly defined relationship between serum lithium concentration and severity of intoxication, the serum concentration 12 hours after the last dose may roughly predict severity of intoxication. Serum lithium concentrations of 1.5–2.5 mEq/L often indicate slight to moderate intoxication; concentrations of 2.5–3.5 mEq/L often indicate severe intoxication; and concentrations greater than 3.5 mEq/L often indicate potentially lethal intoxication. In addition to the serum lithium concentration, the severity of lithium intoxication depends on the length of time the serum concentration remains in the toxic range. *It is important to promptly recognize the signs and symptoms of lithium intoxication and to initiate treatment if necessary.*

● Manifestations

Initial manifestations of lithium intoxication often involve the nervous system and include drowsiness, confusion, giddiness, apathy, coarse hand tremor, and dysarthria. Occasionally, GI symptoms are seen (e.g., decreased appetite, nausea, vomiting, diarrhea). Muscle rigidity or fasciculations, slight ataxia, tinnitus, increased lethargy, increased deep tendon reflexes, blurred vision, and vertical nystagmus usually follow; photophobia also has occurred. Lithium intoxication can progress to impaired consciousness, increasing fasciculations and ataxia, coarse and irregular limb tremors, choreoathetoid movements, cogwheel rigidity, and other focal neurologic signs. Coma, twitching, coarse contractions of muscles, generalized tonic-clonic seizures, cardiovascular collapse with oliguria and anuria, and death may ensue. Arrhythmias, electrocardiographic widening of the QRS interval, inverted T waves, and myocardial infarction also have occurred. The clinical course of lithium intoxication is quite variable; patients may present with any of the above signs and symptoms.

Approximately 70–80% of lithium-intoxicated patients fully recover. Persistent sequelae, including dementia, ataxia, polyuria, dysarthria, spasticity, nystagmus, and tremor, have occurred in about 10% of intoxications. Death has occurred in 10–25% of reported lithium intoxications.

● Treatment

There is no specific antidote for lithium intoxication. Treatment of lithium intoxication is principally supportive and depends on the patient's clinical condition and serum lithium concentration. Early symptoms of milder lithium intoxication (e.g., diarrhea, vomiting, drowsiness, muscular weakness, lack of coordination) usually respond to dosage reduction or temporary discontinuance of the drug and correction of fluid and electrolyte abnormalities. When intoxication is more severe, the patient generally should be hospitalized and provided intensive, supportive care, including infection prophylaxis and regular chest X-rays. Discontinuance of lithium and any concurrently administered diuretic is essential.

IV infusion of 0.9% sodium chloride injection is begun when lithium intoxication is thought to be secondary to total body depletion of sodium. Rapid administration of large volumes of IV solutions, or IV administration of potassium or a diuretic apparently provides no additional benefit. Although diuretics (e.g., furosemide, mannitol, urea), carbonic anhydrase inhibitors, and xanthine derivatives (e.g., aminophylline) may increase lithium clearance. The increased clearance is insufficient to be useful in treating intoxication. Because dehydration resulting in sodium and lithium retention may also occur when these agents are used, these agents are not recommended for the treatment of lithium intoxication.

Hemodialysis is the only reliable method of rapidly removing excess lithium in patients who manifest lithium intoxication and/or who cannot excrete lithium. Because lithium is not metabolized and is only excreted renally, patients with chronic renal failure should undergo hemodialysis following potentially toxic exposures to lithium. In addition, patients with acute lithium intoxication who were not previously receiving the drug should undergo hemodialysis regardless of their clinical status if their serum lithium concentration equals or exceeds 4 mEq/L. These patients will not be able to excrete lithium in time to prevent a clinically important amount from entering the CNS and causing severe and potentially permanent neurologic toxicity. Because patients with an acute on chronic overdosage or chronic overdosage of lithium already have a body burden of the drug, a serum lithium concentration of 2.5 mEq/L or greater and moderate-to-severe neurologic toxicity are reasonable indications for hemodialysis. Hemodialysis for 8–12 hours is also recommended when fluid or electrolyte abnormalities are unresponsive to supportive treatment; when creatinine clearance or urine output decreases substantially; or when serum lithium concentration is not reduced by at least 20% in 6 hours. Serum lithium concentrations usually rebound within 5–8 hours after hemodialysis because of redistribution of the drug, often necessitating repeated courses of hemodialysis. The goal of hemodialysis is to produce a serum lithium concentration less than 1 mEq/L 8 hours after hemodialysis is completed. Although intermittent hemodialysis usually is performed in severe cases of lithium intoxication, continuous venovenous hemodialysis has also been successfully used in several patients in order to more slowly remove lithium from the body in hemodynamically unstable patients and to avoid postdialysis rebound elevations in lithium levels. Peritoneal dialysis is less effective at removing lithium and is used only when hemodialysis is not possible.

PHARMACOLOGY

Lithium has numerous pharmacologic effects. Although traces of lithium are found in animal tissues, lithium has no known physiologic function. Although the mechanisms of action have not been fully elucidated, lithium, as a monovalent cation, competes with other monovalent and divalent cations (potassium, sodium, calcium, magnesium) at cellular sites in body tissues, including the following: at cell membranes, where lithium passes readily through sodium channels and, at high concentrations, blocks potassium channels; at cellular binding sites sensitive to changes in cation concentration; at the level of cellular proteins sensitive to usual cation concentrations; and at cellular carrier-binding and transport sites for monovalent and divalent cations.

Lithium also interacts with a number of cyclic adenosine monophosphate (AMP) second-messenger cellular processes, including those regulated by polypeptide hormones. By inhibiting adenylate cyclase, lithium reduces intracellular concentrations of cyclic AMP. To a lesser extent, lithium also reduces plasma concentrations of cyclic guanosine monophosphate (cGMP).

● Nervous System Effects

Lithium has antimanic and antidepressant effects. Because of the complexity of the CNS, the exact mechanism(s) of these effects is unknown. Univalent and divalent cations appear to be critical to the synthesis, storage, release, and reuptake of central monoamine neurotransmitters, including indoleamines (e.g., serotonin) and catecholamines. These neurotransmitters appear to be involved in the pathogenesis of mania and depression.

Evidence suggests that dopamine and norepinephrine may be involved in the pathogenesis of mania. In animals, brain tissue lithium concentrations of 1–10 mEq/L inhibit depolarization-provoked and calcium-dependent release of norepinephrine, dopamine, and serotonin from nerve terminals and synapses. Lithium only minimally affects catecholamine-sensitive adenylate cyclase activity or the binding of ligands to adrenergic receptors in the CNS. Turnover of norepinephrine in the CNS is initially increased with lithium therapy, but the increased turnover does not persist with prolonged administration. Lithium may block the development of supersensitive dopamine receptors in the CNS of manic patients. Lithium blocks some of the behavioral manifestations of mania (e.g., euphoria, hyperactivity, talkativeness, decrease in sleep, increase in libido) induced by drugs (e.g., amphetamines, cocaine) that produce functional increases in CNS dopamine concentrations.

Serotonin may play a role in the pathogenesis of depressive episodes. Serotonin is present in low concentrations in the CNS of some patients with bipolar affective disorders. Animal studies have shown that lithium increases the concentrations of serotonin metabolites (e.g., 5-hydroxyindoleacetic acid) and decreases hemispheric asymmetry of serotonin and other indoleamines. Lithium is thought to increase neuronal tryptophan uptake and serotonin synthesis by decreasing the affinity of tryptophan hydroxylase for tryptophan at low tryptophan concentrations.

In healthy individuals, lithium has been shown to increase lethargy and lassitude, decrease clearheadedness, and cause deficits in cognitive motor tasks. Lithium also produces small but consistent delays in sleep-wake circadian rhythm and decreases rapid eye movement (REM) sleep, increases delta-wave sleep, and normalizes the sleep of some depressed patients. Lithium may cause benign EEG changes, including diffuse slowing and increased amplitude of alpha waves with an increase in beta-wave activity as alpha rhythm diminishes. In some patients, lithium has produced changes similar to those induced by electroconvulsive therapy (ECT), including marked epileptiform discharge; these effects generally are associated with toxic serum lithium concentrations and/or other signs of lithium neurotoxicity, but also have occurred when lithium concentrations were within the therapeutic range.

● Hematologic Effects

Lithium produces neutrophilia and may also increase erythrocyte and platelet counts and decrease lymphocyte counts; however, the latter 3 effects appear to occur less consistently than neutrophilia.

The hematologic effects of lithium appear to be related to its effect on the pluripotent stem cell of the myeloid series. Although there probably are many modifiers of stem-cell production, the monocyte appears to be the key modifier involved in the effect of lithium on the stem cell. Lithium stimulates the production of colony-stimulating factor by monocytes. Colony-stimulating factor in turn stimulates production of neutrophils by the pluripotent stem cell and, to a lesser extent, production of erythrocytes, platelets, and macrophages. The increase in colony-stimulating factor is related to the action of lithium on cyclic nucleotides.

Lithium causes a true increase in neutrophil production and survival time and in granulocyte marrow reserve; neutrophilia does not result from demargination. Neutrophilia is seen generally within 3–7 days after lithium therapy is initiated and occurs at serum lithium concentrations of 0.5–1 mEq/L; the effect rapidly reverses (within 1–2 weeks) when the drug is discontinued. Data from one in vitro study indicate that the effect of lithium on neutrophil production is apparently transient when stem cells are severely depleted, since increases in neutrophil counts were not seen after 4 weeks. Although some studies indicate that lithium produces neutrophilia at the expense of neutrophil function, most studies have shown no effect of the drug on phagocytosis, chemotaxis, adherence, or bactericidal activity of neutrophils. Although not clearly established, lithium may enhance lymphocyte activity.

● Renal Effects

Lithium causes alterations in renal function and often produces a mild nephrogenic diabetes insipidus manifested as polyuria. The drug decreases renal-concentrating ability and water reabsorption and initially increases sodium and potassium excretion. Some of these effects are overcome by counteracting physiologic mechanisms, while others may persist. Glomerular filtration rate may be slightly decreased in patients receiving prolonged lithium therapy.

A decrease in renal-concentrating ability occurs in 30–50% of patients shortly after starting lithium therapy and persists in about 25% of treated patients after 1–2 years of lithium therapy. The decrease in renal-concentrating ability is usually reversible following discontinuance of the drug; however, in one study, this effect persisted in more than 50% of patients 1 year after discontinuing lithium therapy. Lithium-induced polyuria results from a major disturbance in the water conservation system and a minor disturbance in the thirst regulatory system. Although a central mechanism for lithium-induced diabetes insipidus has been described in one patient, most evidence indicates that the impairment of renal-concentrating ability is nephrogenic, since lithium inhibits vasopressin-induced adenylate cyclase activity. In most patients with lithium-induced nephrogenic diabetes insipidus, plasma vasopressin concentrations usually are elevated and urine osmolality is reduced. Lithium-induced diabetes insipidus has been inhibited by increased urinary potassium or hydrogen ion concentrations, and by thiazide diuretics, triamterene, or amiloride.

The effects of lithium on serum and urinary electrolytes are variable and time and dose related. Lithium initially increases sodium and potassium excretion and urine volume; after 2–3 days, excretion of these electrolytes is reduced, probably because of a feedback increase in aldosterone. Sodium and potassium excretion return to pretreatment levels within 1 week of continuous therapy. Overall, lithium generally does not affect sodium reabsorption in the ascending limb of the loop of Henle or in the distal renal tubule; free water clearance is unchanged even in the presence of lithium-induced polyuria. However, high serum concentrations of lithium have been associated with increased renin release and resultant inhibition of sodium reabsorption in the proximal and distal renal tubules and collecting ducts.

● Endocrine Effects

Lithium has various effects on the thyroid gland, but its principal effect is to block the release of thyroxine (T_4) and triiodothyronine (T_3) mediated by thyrotropin. This results in a decrease in circulating T_4 and T_3 concentrations and a feedback increase in serum thyrotropin concentration. Lithium also inhibits thyrotropin-stimulated adenylate cyclase activity and thyrotropin-induced release of thyroidal iodine 131, decreases intrathyroidal iodothyronine-iodotyrosine ratios, and inhibits colloid droplet formation.

Long-term lithium therapy may alter calcium, magnesium, and parathyroid hormone homeostasis; these alterations may cause a mild asymptomatic primary hyperparathyroidism. Lithium may cause slight increases in serum calcium (total), magnesium, and parathyroid hormone concentrations and a decrease in serum phosphate concentration. Lithium may also cause slight alterations in bone mineral metabolism.

Lithium has varying effects on carbohydrate metabolism. Increased and decreased glucose tolerance and decreased sensitivity to insulin have been observed. It is unclear whether these are direct effects of lithium or are related to changes in the course of the underlying psychiatric disorder.

In animals, lithium decreases hepatic cholesterol and fatty acid synthesis.

● Cardiovascular Effects

In patients with therapeutic serum lithium concentrations, reversible ECG T-wave depression occurs frequently. T-wave inversion occurs rarely. Resting or exercise-induced ST-segment abnormalities have not been observed. Arrhythmias have occurred rarely. (See Cautions: Cardiovascular Effects.)

The cardiac effects of lithium may result partly from displacement of potassium from intracellular myocardial sites by lithium; this displacement may result in a slow, partial depletion of intracellular potassium.

● GI Effects

Lithium reduces intestinal absorption of glucose and water, probably by incompletely substituting for sodium in a sodium-dependent transport mechanism at the intestinal mucosa. These actions may be responsible for the osmotic diarrhea and other adverse GI effects that frequently occur during initiation of lithium therapy.

PHARMACOKINETICS

● Absorption

Lithium is readily absorbed from the GI tract. Food does not appear to affect the bioavailability of lithium. Although lithium carbonate capsules show a slightly longer dissolution time than do tablets, differences in the disintegration and dissolution properties of various preparations do not appear to be clinically important. Conventional lithium carbonate capsules and tablets are 95–100% absorbed. Extended-release lithium carbonate tablets are 60–90% absorbed, and lithium citrate oral solutions are essentially 100% absorbed.

Absorption from conventional lithium carbonate tablets and capsules is usually complete within 1–6 hours with peak serum lithium concentrations usually occurring within 0.5–3 hours. Following oral administration of a single 300-mg dose of lithium carbonate to fasting adults, peak serum lithium concentrations of 0.4–0.5 and 0.4–0.9 mEq/L have been reported for conventional tablets and capsules, respectively. Absorption of lithium carbonate from extended-release tablets is both delayed and prolonged, with peak serum lithium concentrations occurring within 4–12 hours. Oral solutions of lithium citrate are the most rapidly absorbed, with peak serum lithium concentrations usually occurring within 15–60 minutes. Following oral administration to fasting patients of single doses of lithium citrate solution equivalent in lithium content to 600 mg and 0.9–1 g of lithium carbonate, peak serum lithium concentrations of about 0.7 and 1 mEq/L, respectively, have been reported.

During the first 6–10 hours after dosing, serum lithium concentrations fluctuate depending on the absorption of the drug and tissue distribution. Therefore, the 12-hour steady-state serum lithium concentration is used by most clinicians for monitoring serum concentrations; this concentration shows a high intraindividual (but not interindividual) reproducibility. Steady-state serum lithium concentrations of 0.4–1.3 mEq/L are considered necessary for therapeutic effect in the treatment of affective and schizoaffective disorders. At 12- to 16-hour steady-state serum concentrations of less than 0.4 mEq/L, about 60% of lithium-responsive patients with bipolar disorder relapse, compared with about 15% relapse at concentrations of 0.4–0.59 mEq/L and about 20% relapse at concentrations of 0.6–1 mEq/L. Steady-state serum lithium concentrations of 1–1.4 mEq/L usually are required for an acute antimanic effect. Onset of the acute antimanic effect of lithium usually occurs within 5–7 days; full therapeutic effect often requires 10–21 days. The likelihood of toxicity increases substantially at steady-state serum lithium concentrations of 1.5 mEq/L or greater, but some patients who are sensitive to the effects of lithium may develop toxicity at serum concentrations less than 1 mEq/L. Salivary lithium concentrations have been used by some clinicians to monitor lithium therapy, but most clinicians have not found this method practical. (See Pharmacokinetics: Distribution.)

● Distribution

Lithium is widely distributed into most body tissues and fluids. Lithium is initially distributed into extracellular fluid and then gradually accumulates in varying degrees in tissues. The drug is rapidly distributed into thyroid, bone, and brain tissue; concentrations in these tissues often are 50% greater than simultaneous serum concentrations. Lithium is distributed more slowly and less completely into heart, lung, kidney, and muscle; concentrations in these tissues approximate those in serum. Lithium concentrations in CSF and liver usually are 30–50% of simultaneous serum concentrations.

Lithium also distributes into saliva. The ratio of serum-to-mixed saliva lithium concentrations shows considerable interindividual variation, but once steady-state is achieved there is little intraindividual variation. Steady-state mixed saliva lithium concentrations are generally 2- to 3-fold greater than concurrent serum concentrations.

Lithium distributes into erythrocytes against an electrochemical potential gradient, drawn by an oppositely directed sodium ion gradient. The ratio of the lithium concentration in erythrocytes to that in serum shows wide interindividual variation but less intraindividual variation. Steady-state lithium concentrations in erythrocytes may range from 30–90% of concurrent serum concentrations but usually are 50% or less. The ratio has been shown to be slightly higher in women (especially during pregnancy), in patients with bipolar illness compared with patients with unipolar illness, and in patients with affective illness in remission compared with those in acute stages; however, the clinical importance of these findings is unknown. Distribution of lithium into erythrocytes also may depend partially on genetic factors.

Lithium initially distributes into an apparent volume that is about 25–40% of body weight, and later into a volume that is equal to that of total body water. Steady-state and initial apparent distribution volumes of about 0.7–1 L/kg and 0.3–0.4 L/kg, respectively, have been reported. Geriatric patients may have slightly smaller volumes of distribution, while individuals younger than 30 years of age may have slightly larger volumes of distribution. Lithium is not bound to plasma proteins.

Lithium freely crosses the placenta; maternal and fetal serum concentrations are approximately equal. The milk of nursing women contains lithium concentrations that are approximately 33–50% of those in serum.

● Elimination

Serum concentrations of lithium appear to decline in a biphasic manner. In patients with normal renal function, an initial half-life ($t_{\frac{1}{2}\alpha}$) of 0.8–1.2 hours and a terminal half-life ($t_{\frac{1}{2}\beta}$) of 20–27 hours have been observed following single-dose administration of lithium. Patients receiving lithium for more than 1 year had terminal half-lives of 2.4 days in one study. In geriatric patients and patients with impaired renal function, serum half-lives of 36 and 40–50 hours, respectively, have been reported.

Lithium is not metabolized; it is excreted almost entirely in the urine. About 80% of the lithium that is filtered by the renal glomeruli is reabsorbed in the proximal renal tubules. Thus, renal plasma clearance of lithium is about 20% of the glomerular filtration rate or about 20–40 mL/minute. Geriatric patients may have lower, and younger patients and pregnant women may have higher, renal clearances. Proximal tubular reabsorption of lithium occurs against electrical and concentration gradients that do not distinguish between sodium and lithium. Lithium clearance can be increased or decreased by as much as 30–50% by sodium loading or depletion, respectively. Sodium depletion generally has a greater effect than does sodium loading. Several drugs (e.g., thiazide diuretics, aminophylline, urea) have been shown to increase or decrease renal clearance of lithium. Polyuria and potassium chloride administration do not increase renal clearance of lithium. Beyond the proximal tubule, lithium reabsorption is minimal. For this reason, most diuretics do not enhance renal lithium clearance. (See Drug Interactions: Diuretics.)

Approximately 95–99% of a single dose of lithium is excreted in urine. Small amounts may be excreted in feces as unabsorbed drug or in sweat. In patients with normal renal function, about 30–70% of a single dose is excreted in urine within 6–12 hours and 50–80% within 24 hours; the remainder is excreted slowly over 10–14 days. Lithium is readily removed by hemodialysis with reported clearances of about 50–90 mL/minute; however, the amount of lithium removed during hemodialysis depends of several factors (e.g., type of coil used, dialysis flow-rate). The drug is removed less readily by peritoneal dialysis, with reported clearances of 13–15 mL/minute. Because of slow equilibration between intracellular and extracellular fluid compartments, rebound increases in serum lithium concentration frequently occur 5–8 hours after dialysis.

CHEMISTRY AND STABILITY

● *Chemistry*

Lithium salts are antimanic agents. Lithium is a monovalent cation belonging to the group of alkali metals, but it also shares some of the chemical properties of calcium and magnesium. Lithium is commercially available as the carbonate and citrate salts.

Lithium Carbonate

Lithium carbonate occurs as a white, granular powder that has a slight saline taste. The drug is sparingly soluble in water, very slightly soluble in alcohol, and dissolves, with effervescence, in dilute mineral acids. Each gram of lithium carbonate contains 27 mEq of lithium.

Lithium Citrate

Lithium citrate occurs as a tetrahydrate, white, somewhat deliquescent, crystalline powder that has a slight saline taste. The drug is very soluble in water and practically insoluble in alcohol. Each gram of anhydrous lithium citrate contains approximately 14.3 mEq of lithium. Lithium citrate oral solution is prepared from lithium citrate or lithium hydroxide to which an excess of citric acid has been added. The oral solution has a pH of 4–5.

● *Stability*
Lithium Carbonate

Lithium carbonate conventional tablets, extended-release tablets, and capsules should be stored in well-closed containers at 15–30°C. When stored as directed, commercially available lithium carbonate extended-release tablets (Lithobid®) have an expiration date of 18 months following the date of manufacture.

Lithium Citrate

Lithium citrate oral solution should be stored in tight containers at 15–30°C.

PREPARATIONS

Excipients in commercially available drug preparations may have clinically important effects in some individuals; consult specific product labeling for details.

Lithium Carbonate

Oral		
Capsules	150 mg (4.06 mEq of lithium)*	Lithium Carbonate Capsules
	300 mg (8.12 mEq of lithium)*	Eskalith®, GlaxoSmithKline
		Lithium Carbonate Capsules
	600 mg (16.24 mEq of lithium)*	Lithium Carbonate Capsules, Roxane
Tablets	300 mg (8.12 mEq of lithium)	Lithium Carbonate Tablets (scored)
Tablets, extended-release	450 mg (12.18 mEq of lithium)*	Eskalith CR® (scored), GlaxoSmithKline
		Lithium Carbonate Extended-release Tablets
Tablets, extended-release, film-coated	300 mg (8.12 mEq of lithium)*	Lithobid® Slow-release, JDS Pharma
		Lithium Carbonate Extended-release Film-coated Tablets

* available from one or more manufacturer, distributor, and/or repackager by generic (nonproprietary) name

Lithium Citrate

Oral		
Solution	8 mEq (of lithium) per 5 mL	Lithium Citrate Syrup

† Use is not currently included in the labeling approved by the US Food and Drug Administration.

Selected Revisions January 1, 2006, © Copyright, July 1, 1983, American Society of Health-System Pharmacists, Inc.

Levodopa
Carbidopa

28:36.16 • DOPAMINE PRECURSORS

■ Levodopa is the levorotatory isomer of dihydroxyphenylalanine and the metabolic precursor of dopamine, and carbidopa is a decarboxylase inhibitor that inhibits the peripheral decarboxylation of levodopa to dopamine.

USES

● *Parkinsonian Syndrome*

Levodopa is used in the symptomatic treatment of parkinsonian syndrome, including parkinson disease (paralysis agitans) and parkinsonism resulting from encephalitis (postencephalitic parkinsonism), carbon monoxide intoxication, or manganese intoxication. Levodopa is commercially available in various fixed-combination preparations with carbidopa for this use.

Carbidopa is used to inhibit the decarboxylation of peripheral levodopa and increase the amount of levodopa available for transport to the brain. Concomitant administration of levodopa and carbidopa generally decreases levodopa dosage requirements by 70–80%, reduces the adverse peripheral effects of levodopa decarboxylation (e.g., nausea and vomiting), allows for more rapid dosage titration, and may provide a smoother response to levodopa. Certain patients who responded poorly to levodopa alone have improved when carbidopa was administered concomitantly; however, patients with markedly irregular "on-off" responses to levodopa (see Nervous System and Muscular Effects under Cautions) usually have not benefited from the addition of carbidopa. Carbidopa has no therapeutic effect when given alone to patients with parkinsonian syndrome and should be used only in conjunction with levodopa. A single-entity carbidopa preparation is commercially available for use in patients who are already receiving levodopa and carbidopa, but require additional carbidopa to reduce nausea and vomiting and/or facilitate more rapid dosage titration.

Levodopa (in combination with carbidopa) currently is the most effective drug for relieving the motor symptoms of parkinsonian syndrome and is considered by many clinicians to be the drug of choice for this use. Levodopa completely or partially relieves akinesia, rigidity, and tremor in about 80% of patients treated, and improves functional ability and other secondary motor manifestations such as those affecting gait, postural stability, facial expression, swallowing, speech, and handwriting. Levodopa also may be useful in the management of other symptoms of parkinsonian syndrome including dysphagia, sialorrhea, and seborrhea. Levodopa therapy often produces a general alerting response, increased vigor, and a sense of well-being. However, the effectiveness of levodopa decreases over time and most patients develop motor complications such as motor fluctuations (e.g., end-of-dose failure, "on-off" phenomenon, akinesia) and dyskinesias (drug-induced involuntary movements) with long-term use. Strategies for reducing the risk of motor complications include adjusting the dosage of levodopa or adding other antiparkinsonian agents such as a dopamine receptor agonist (e.g., pramipexole, ropinirole, rotigotine), selective monoamine oxidase (MAO)-B inhibitor (e.g., rasagiline, safinamide, selegiline), catechol-*O*-methyltransferase (COMT) inhibitor (e.g., entacapone), or amantadine. Alternatively, a levodopa-sparing strategy may be used in which other antiparkinsonian agents are initiated first and then levodopa is added when these other therapies no longer provide adequate symptom control. This delayed approach is often used in younger patients who have a higher risk of developing motor complications and a longer life expectancy. The appropriate treatment approach should be individualized based on the patient's age, symptoms, cognitive status, disease severity, adverse effects, and cost of therapy.

Motor complications associated with long-term use of standard oral formulations of levodopa are thought to result from fluctuating plasma concentrations of the drug due to its short half-life, delayed gastric emptying, and erratic absorption. Several non-oral preparations of levodopa have been developed to overcome these challenges and may be useful alternatives in patients with advanced parkinson disease whose motor symptoms are not effectively controlled with oral therapies. One such preparation is levodopa powder for oral inhalation, which is indicated for use as adjunctive therapy to levodopa-carbidopa for the intermittent treatment of "off" episodes in patients with parkinson disease. Inhaled levodopa has been shown to be effective only in patients who are already receiving levodopa-carbidopa therapy. Some clinicians state that this form of levodopa may be particularly useful in patients with severely delayed gastric emptying. Efficacy of levodopa oral inhalation powder has been established in a 12-week randomized, double-blind, placebo-controlled study in patients with parkinson disease who were experiencing at least 2 hours of "off" time per day while receiving levodopa-carbidopa therapy. Improvement in motor function (assessed by the change in Unified Parkinson Disease Rating Scale [UPDRS] motor score from predose to 30 minutes postdose) was substantially greater in patients receiving inhaled levodopa (84 mg) compared with those receiving placebo; in addition, 58% of levodopa-treated patients returned to an "on" state, which was sustained through 60 minutes postdose.

Another non-oral preparation of levodopa that may be used in advanced parkinson disease patients experiencing motor complications is carbidopa-levodopa enteral suspension. The enteral suspension is delivered continuously over a 16-hour period daily through a percutaneous endoscopic gastrojejunostomy (PEG-J) tube; this delivery method bypasses the stomach and eliminates the variability associated with gastric emptying, providing a more stable plasma concentration of levodopa. Efficacy of carbidopa-levodopa enteral infusion has been evaluated in several controlled prospective studies and observational studies. These studies have consistently demonstrated that treatment with the enteral suspension decreases total daily "off" time and increases "on" time without troublesome dyskinesia in patients with advanced parkinson disease; some studies also demonstrated improvements in nonmotor symptoms and quality of life measures. In a 12-week randomized, double-dummy, double-blind, active-controlled study, mean "off" time decreased by 4 hours following treatment with carbidopa-levodopa enteral suspension compared with a decrease of 2 hours with a standard oral immediate-release carbidopa-levodopa preparation. Results of longer-term studies suggest that the benefits of enterally administered continuous carbidopa-levodopa therapy are sustained over time; the longest reported duration of therapy is 16 years.

● *Other Uses*

Although levodopa is not effective in the management of extrapyramidal effects induced by antipsychotic agents and is not generally useful in the management of other neurologic diseases, the drug may be of some benefit in conditions in which marked akinesia is present. Levodopa is not useful in the treatment of psychiatric disorders.

DOSAGE AND ADMINISTRATION

● *Administration*

Levodopa and carbidopa are administered orally as fixed-combination or single-entity (carbidopa only) conventional tablets, orally disintegrating tablets, extended-release tablets, or extended-release capsules. Levodopa also is commercially available as a powder for oral inhalation. Carbidopa-levodopa enteral suspension is administered by direct intestinal infusion through a nasojejunal (NJ) tube or a percutaneous endoscopic gastrojejunostomy (PEG-J) tube.

In patients with moderate to severe motor fluctuations, better global improvement may be achieved in some patients when extended-release rather than conventional tablet preparations of carbidopa-levodopa are used. However, some studies have not found a substantial difference in "off" time between extended-release and immediate-release tablet preparations in such patients. In patients without motor fluctuations, the preparations were comparably effective but less frequent dosing was required with the extended-release preparation. Use of the extended-release capsule formulation of carbidopa-levodopa has been shown to improve "off" time compared with immediate-release preparations in patients with advanced parkinson disease. (See Absorption under Pharmacokinetics.)

Patients receiving other antiparkinsonian agents may continue taking these drugs while carbidopa-levodopa is administered; however, dosage adjustments of these drugs may be necessary.

Whenever a general anesthetic is required, levodopa may be continued as long as the patient is able to take fluids and medication orally. If therapy is interrupted, the patient should be observed for neuroleptic malignant syndrome and the usual daily dose may be given as soon as the patient can take oral medication.

Oral Administration

Fixed-combination carbidopa-levodopa oral dosage forms include conventional tablets, orally disintegrating tablets, extended-release tablets, and extended-release capsules. Carbidopa-levodopa conventional tablets and orally disintegrating tablets contain a 1:4 or 1:10 ratio of carbidopa to levodopa. Carbidopa-levodopa extended-release tablets and capsules contain a 1:4 ratio of carbidopa to levodopa. Carbidopa and levodopa also are commercially available in fixed combination with entacapone (Stalevo®) in a tablet preparation containing a 1:4 ratio of carbidopa to levodopa combined with 200 mg of entacapone. Carbidopa also is commercially available as single-entity conventional tablets.

Orally Disintegrating Carbidopa-Levodopa Tablets

Patients receiving carbidopa-levodopa orally disintegrating tablets should be instructed to gently remove a tablet from the bottle with dry hands just prior to administration. The tablet should then be immediately placed on the tongue to dissolve (usually within seconds) and swallowed with saliva; administration with liquid is not necessary.

Extended-release Carbidopa-Levodopa Tablets

Extended-release tablets of carbidopa-levodopa can be administered as whole or halved tablets; the tablets should be swallowed intact and not chewed or crushed. Patients should be advised that the extended-release tablets are designed to release the drugs over a 4- to 6-hour period and of the importance of taking the drug at regular intervals according to the prescribed schedule. Patients also should be advised that the onset of effect with the morning dose of extended-release tablets occasionally may be delayed up to 1 hour compared with that experienced with conventional tablets.

Extended-release Carbidopa-Levodopa Capsules

Extended-release carbidopa-levodopa capsules may be administered orally with or without food; however, administration with a high-fat, high-calorie meal may delay absorption of levodopa by about 2 hours. The capsules should be swallowed whole without chewing, dividing, or crushing. Patients with difficulty swallowing may open the capsules and sprinkle the entire contents on a small amount of applesauce (e.g., 1–2 tablespoons); the mixture should be administered immediately and not stored for later use.

Carbidopa, Levodopa, and Entacapone Fixed Combination (Stalevo®)

The fixed-combination preparation containing carbidopa, levodopa, and entacapone (Stalevo®) generally is used in patients receiving stable dosages of carbidopa, levodopa, and entacapone equivalent to those in the combination preparation. The fixed-combination preparation also may be used in certain patients receiving stable dosages of carbidopa and levodopa equivalent to those in the fixed-combination preparation when a decision has been made to add entacapone to the regimen. Stalevo® tablets should not be divided, and only one tablet should be administered per dosing interval.

Oral Inhalation

Levodopa powder is administered by oral inhalation using a special inhalation device (Inbrija® inhaler). The drug is commercially available as 42-mg capsules for oral inhalation; a total of 2 capsules should be administered (one at a time) to obtain the recommended dose. The capsules are for oral inhalation only and must not be swallowed as the intended effect will not be obtained. Inhaled levodopa is intended to be administered on an intermittent basis only in patients who are already receiving treatment with a carbidopa-levodopa combination.

The inhalers and capsules should be stored in a dry place at room temperature; capsules should not be stored in the inhalers. The capsules should not be removed from their foil-sealed blister packaging until immediately prior to use. To administer a dose, the first capsule should be loaded into the inhaler. Before inhaling the dose, the patient should exhale as completely as possible. While keeping the inhaler upright, the patient should place the mouthpiece of the inhaler between the lips and inhale deeply and slowly through the inhaler until a whirling sound is felt or heard; this is an indication that the inhaler is working. After inhaling the contents of a capsule, the patient should hold their breath for 5 seconds before exhaling. These steps should be repeated with the second capsule to complete the full dose. Patients should use a new inhaler with each new carton of levodopa inhalation powder. The manufacturer's prescribing information should be consulted for additional details on administration of levodopa powder for oral inhalation.

Enteral Administration

Carbidopa-levodopa enteral suspension is administered as a 16-hour continuous enteral infusion through a PEG-J tube using a portable infusion device (i.e., CADD® Legacy 1400 pump). Placement and removal of the PEG-J tube should be performed by a gastroenterologist or other experienced healthcare provider. A nasojejunal (NJ) tube may be used for short-term administration of the drug (e.g., as a trial to determine whether the patient responds to therapy and can manage the device) until a permanent PEG-J tube can be established. At the end of the daily 16-hour administration period, the patient's PEG-J tube should be disconnected from the pump and flushed with room temperature potable water.

The enteral suspension is commercially available in single-use cassettes containing 4.63 mg of carbidopa and 20 mg of levodopa per mL. Cassettes should be stored in the freezer (-20°C) and thawed in the refrigerator (2–8°C) prior to dispensing. Cassettes should be protected from light and kept in their cartons prior to use. Prior to administration, the cassette should be removed from the refrigerator and allowed to reach room temperature for 20 minutes; failure to administer the drug at room temperature may result in a subtherapeutic response. Cassettes are for single-use only and should not be used for longer than 16 hours; the cassette should be discarded after this time period even if some drug product remains.

The manufacturer's labeling should be consulted for more detailed information on administration of carbidopa-levodopa enteral suspension.

● *Dosage*

Parkinsonian Syndrome

Dosage of carbidopa-levodopa must be carefully adjusted according to individual requirements, response, and tolerance. Because patients receiving carbidopa dosages lower than 70–100 mg daily are likely to experience levodopa-induced nausea and vomiting, the minimum recommended daily dosage of carbidopa is 70–100 mg.

Because of the risk of precipitating a symptom complex resembling neuroleptic malignant syndrome (NMS), patients should be observed closely if levodopa dosage is reduced abruptly or the drug is discontinued; when discontinuing treatment, dosage should be reduced gradually. (See Precautions and Contraindications under Cautions.)

Immediate-release Oral Carbidopa-Levodopa Preparations

When immediate-release conventional tablets or orally disintegrating tablets of carbidopa and levodopa are used in patients with parkinsonian syndrome, therapy usually is initiated with a preparation containing 25 mg of carbidopa and 100 mg of levodopa; an initial dosage of 1 tablet (25 mg carbidopa/100 mg levodopa) 3 times daily is recommended. Dosage may be increased by 1 tablet every 1 or 2 days until a maximum dosage of 8 tablets daily (200 mg of carbidopa and 800 mg of levodopa) is reached. If an immediate-release combination preparation containing 10 mg of carbidopa and 100 mg of levodopa is used, therapy usually is initiated with 1 tablet 3 or 4 times daily; however, this dosage will not provide an adequate amount of carbidopa for many patients. Dosage may be increased by 1 tablet every 1 or 2 days until a maximum dosage of 8 tablets daily (80 mg of carbidopa and 800 mg of levodopa) is reached.

Maintenance therapy should be individualized and adjusted according to the desired therapeutic response. Patients should receive at least 70–100 mg of carbidopa daily during maintenance therapy, since peripheral aromatic l-amino acid decarboxylase is saturated at this dosage and patients receiving a lower daily dosage of carbidopa are likely to experience nausea and vomiting. Use of combination preparations containing a 1:10 ratio of carbidopa to levodopa may not provide an adequate amount of carbidopa. If a greater proportion of carbidopa is required in the combination, one tablet of an immediate-release preparation containing 25 mg of carbidopa and 100 mg of levodopa may be substituted for one tablet of the preparation containing 10 mg of carbidopa and 100 mg of levodopa. If additional carbidopa is still required, a 25-mg dose of carbidopa (as the single-entity tablet preparation) may be given with each first daily dose of carbidopa-levodopa, and additional 12.5-mg or 25-mg doses of carbidopa may be administered with each subsequent dose of carbidopa-levodopa as needed. If patients require higher dosages of levodopa while receiving an immediate-release combination preparation containing 100 mg of levodopa, patients should be switched to a combination preparation containing 250 mg of levodopa.

In general, the single-entity carbidopa preparation may be given with any dose of carbidopa-levodopa as required for optimum therapeutic response. Because experience with carbidopa daily dosages greater than 200 mg is limited, dosage of carbidopa should not exceed 200 mg daily.

Extended-release Carbidopa-Levodopa Tablets

Bioavailability of levodopa from the extended-release tablet formulation of carbidopa-levodopa is approximately 70–75% of immediate-release preparations; increased daily dosages may therefore be required to achieve the same level of symptomatic relief provided by immediate-release preparations. Dosage should be individualized based on patient tolerance and clinical response.

Patients being transferred from an immediate-release carbidopa-levodopa preparation should receive an initial dosage of the extended-release tablets that provides approximately 10% *more* levodopa daily than they previously were receiving with the immediate-release preparation. In some patients, up to 30% *more* levodopa daily may be required initially depending on clinical response.

For patients in whom levodopa therapy is initiated with extended-release carbidopa-levodopa tablets (i.e., those not being switched from existing levodopa therapy), an initial dosage of carbidopa 50 mg and levodopa 200 mg (as 1 extended-release tablet) twice daily is recommended. Initial dosage in such patients should not be given at intervals of less than 6 hours.

Following initiation of therapy, doses and/or dosing intervals can be increased or decreased according to patient tolerance and clinical response. Most patients are treated adequately with dosages providing 400–1600 mg of levodopa daily, administered in divided doses at intervals ranging from 4–8 hours while awake. Higher dosages (600 mg of carbidopa and 2400 mg or more of levodopa) and shorter intervals (less than 4 hours) have been used with the extended-release tablets but usually are not recommended. If the dosing interval is shorter than 4 hours and/or the divided doses are not equal, it is recommended that the smaller doses be given at the end of the day. Dosage of the extended-release tablets generally should be adjusted no more frequently than at 3-day intervals. Some patients with advanced disease may benefit from the addition of doses of a conventional preparation of carbidopa-levodopa during brief periods of the day when additional levodopa is needed for symptomatic control.

Extended-release Carbidopa-Levodopa Capsules

The extended-release capsule formulation of carbidopa-levodopa is less bioavailable than immediate-release preparations and increased daily dosages generally are required to achieve the same level of symptomatic relief provided by immediate-release preparations. Dosage should be individualized based on patient tolerance and clinical response.

In patients transferring from therapy with immediate-release carbidopa-levodopa preparations to the extended-release capsules, the patient's current total daily dosage of levodopa should be calculated and used to determine an appropriate starting dosage of the extended-release capsules (see Table 1).

TABLE 1. Conversion from Immediate-release Carbidopa-Levodopa Preparations to Extended-release Carbidopa-Levodopa Capsules (Rytary®)

Total Daily Dose of Levodopa in Immediate-release Carbidopa-Levodopa	Total Daily Dose of Levodopa in Extended-release Capsules
400–549 mg	855 mg (administered as 3 capsules [carbidopa 23.75 mg and levodopa 95 mg] 3 times daily)
550–749 mg	1140 mg (administered as 4 capsules [carbidopa 23.75 mg and levodopa 95 mg] 3 times daily)
750–949 mg	1305 mg (administered as 3 capsules [carbidopa 36.25 mg and levodopa 145 mg] 3 times daily)
950–1249 mg	1755 mg (administered as 3 capsules [carbidopa 48.75 mg and levodopa 195 mg] 3 times daily)
≥1250 mg	2340 mg (administered as 4 capsules [carbidopa 48.75 mg and levodopa 195 mg] 3 times daily) or 2205 mg (administered as 3 capsules [carbidopa 61.25 mg and levodopa 245 mg] 3 times daily)

Following conversion, the dose and/or dosing intervals can be increased or decreased as necessary based on patient tolerance and clinical response. In patients currently receiving carbidopa-levodopa in combination with a catechol-O-methyltransferase (COMT) inhibitor (e.g., entacapone), the total initial daily dose of levodopa in the extended-release capsule may need to be increased.

If extended-release capsules of carbidopa-levodopa are used in levodopa-naive patients (i.e., those not being switched from existing carbidopa-levodopa therapy), the recommended initial dosage is carbidopa 23.75 mg and levodopa 95 mg administered 3 times daily for the first 3 days. Dosage may be increased to carbidopa 36.25 mg and levodopa 145 mg 3 times daily on the fourth day of treatment. Thereafter, dosage may be increased based on patient tolerance and clinical response up to a maximum recommended dosage of carbidopa 97.5 mg and levodopa 390 mg 3 times daily; if needed, dosing frequency may be increased to a maximum of 5 times daily. Patients should be maintained on the lowest possible dosage necessary to achieve adequate symptom control while minimizing adverse effects.

The manufacturer recommends a maximum daily dose of carbidopa 612.5 mg and levodopa 2450 mg when using the extended-release capsules.

Carbidopa, Levodopa, and Entacapone Fixed Combination

For patients transferring from therapy with carbidopa-levodopa to the fixed-combination preparation containing carbidopa, levodopa, and entacapone (Stalevo®), recommendations are available for transferring patients currently receiving carbidopa-levodopa preparations containing a 1:4 ratio of carbidopa to levodopa.

Patients who are currently receiving entacapone 200 mg with each dose of carbidopa-levodopa (as a conventional tablet preparation) can be switched to the corresponding strength of the fixed-combination preparation containing the same amounts of carbidopa and levodopa. The manufacturer states that there is no experience to date in transitioning patients currently receiving extended-release preparations of carbidopa-levodopa or carbidopa-levodopa preparations not containing a 1:4 ratio to the fixed-combination preparation Stalevo®.

For patients initiating entacapone therapy, recommendations regarding use of the fixed-combination preparation Stalevo® should be individualized according to the current levodopa dosage and the presence of dyskinesias. Patients treated with carbidopa-levodopa conventional tablets who are receiving more than 600 mg of levodopa daily or have a history of moderate or severe dyskinesias before initiation of entacapone therapy are likely to require a reduction in levodopa dosage. In such patients, dosage should first be adjusted by administering carbidopa-levodopa (1:4 ratio) and entacapone as separate preparations. If it is determined that optimum maintenance dosages of levodopa, carbidopa, and entacapone correspond to the doses in the commercial combination product, the fixed-combination preparation containing carbidopa, levodopa, and entacapone (Stalevo®) may be used. For patients receiving levodopa dosages of 600 mg or less daily (conventional tablets, 1:4 ratio) and who do not have dyskinesias, an attempt can be made to initiate entacapone therapy with the fixed-combination preparation containing carbidopa, levodopa, and entacapone. The initial dosage of the fixed-combination preparation of carbidopa, levodopa and entacapone should provide the same dosage of carbidopa and levodopa that the patient currently is taking. However, a reduction in the dosage of carbidopa-levodopa or entacapone may be necessary. Because dosage of carbidopa, levodopa, or entacapone cannot be adjusted individually using the fixed-combination preparation, administration of carbidopa-levodopa and entacapone as separate preparations may be necessary.

Because there is limited clinical experience with entacapone dosages exceeding 1.6 g daily, the maximum recommended dosage of fixed-combination preparations containing carbidopa 12.5–37.5 mg, levodopa 50–150 mg, and entacapone 200 mg (Stalevo® 50, 75, 100, 125, and 150) is 8 tablets daily. Because there is limited clinical experience with carbidopa dosages exceeding 300 mg daily, the maximum recommended dosage of the fixed-combination preparation containing carbidopa 50 mg, levodopa 200 mg, and entacapone 200 mg (Stalevo® 200) is 6 tablets daily.

Levodopa Oral Inhalation

The recommended dosage of levodopa oral inhalation powder for the intermittent treatment of "off" episodes in adults with parkinson disease is 84 mg (contents of two 42-mg capsules) as needed, up to 5 times daily. The maximum recommended dose per "off" period is 84 mg and the maximum recommended daily dosage is 420 mg.

Carbidopa-Levodopa Enteral Suspension

Dosage of carbidopa-levodopa enteral suspension consists of 3 components: a morning dose (administered usually over 10–30 minutes), a continuous infusion (administered over 16 hours), and additional doses (i.e., extra doses) as needed for breakthrough symptoms. Prior to initiating treatment with the enteral suspension, patients should be converted from all forms of levodopa to oral immediate-release carbidopa-levodopa tablets (1:4 ratio). The initial dosage of the enteral suspension is based on the patient's previous daily dosage of oral levodopa (taken the day prior to initiation of enteral therapy).

The initial morning dose of carbidopa-levodopa enteral suspension (in mL) should be determined as follows. The total amount of levodopa (in mg) in the first dose of immediate-release carbidopa-levodopa taken the previous day should be calculated. This dose (in mg) should then be converted to mL by multiplying the dose by 0.8 and dividing by 20 mg/mL; an additional 3 mL should be added to account for priming volume.

The initial continuous dose of carbidopa-levodopa enteral suspension (in mL) should be determined as follows. The total amount of levodopa from oral immediate-release carbidopa-levodopa doses throughout the previous day (over 16 waking hours) should be calculated; doses taken at night should not be used in the calculation. The first oral levodopa dose taken the previous day (determined in the morning dose calculation) should be subtracted from the total oral levodopa dose taken over 16 hours; the resulting value should be divided by 20 mg/mL to obtain the continuous dose that should be administered over 16 hours. The hourly infusion rate (in mL/hour) is then calculated by dividing the continuous dose by 16 hours.

After the first day of treatment, the daily morning dose and continuous dose of carbidopa-levodopa should be titrated based on individual response and tolerability until a stable dosage is obtained. The maximum recommended daily dose is 2000 mg of levodopa (i.e., one cassette per day). If the patient experiences persistent or numerous "off" periods during the 16-hour infusion period, an increase in the continuous dose or extra doses may be given. In patients who require overnight treatment, an extended-release formulation of oral levodopa-carbidopa may be taken at bedtime after stopping the enteral infusion. If dyskinesias or other adverse effects occur, a decrease in the continuous dose or temporary interruption in therapy may be considered until adverse effects subside. The manufacturer's prescribing information should be consulted for recommendations on dosage adjustments.

Sudden discontinuance of therapy or rapid dose reduction should be avoided; when discontinuing therapy with the enteral suspension, dosage should be tapered or patients may be switched to oral immediate-release carbidopa-levodopa therapy.

CAUTIONS

Adverse effects occur in most patients who receive levodopa (with or without carbidopa). Adverse effects of levodopa are numerous and are usually dose dependent and reversible. The incidence of levodopa-induced nausea and vomiting is generally less when carbidopa is used in conjunction with the drug. However, concomitant administration of carbidopa does not decrease adverse reactions resulting from the central effects of levodopa; some CNS effects may occur at a lower dosage and more rapidly during therapy with levodopa-carbidopa combinations than with levodopa alone. The adverse effect profile of extended-release carbidopa-levodopa tablets is similar to conventional (immediate-release) preparations.

Whenever the fixed-combination preparation containing carbidopa, levodopa, and entacapone (Stalevo®) is used, consideration should be given to the possible adverse effects reported with the individual components.

● Nervous System and Muscular Effects

The most common adverse effects of levodopa are dyskinesias including choreiform, dystonic, dyskinetic, and other involuntary movements. Involuntary movements occur in about 50% of patients on long-term therapy and may consist of grimacing, bruxism, gnawing, chewing, twisting and protrusion of the tongue, rhythmic opening and closing of the mouth, bobbing and wave-like motions of the head with or without gesticulation, slow rhythmic movements of the neck, hands or feet, jerky movements of the shoulder or pelvic girdle, and opisthotonos or ballismus. Intermittent myoclonic body jerks during sleep, ataxia, increased hand tremor, and muscle twitching and blepharospasm (which may be an early sign of excessive dosage) may also occur. Dyskinesias usually are dose related and may require reduction of dosage. They do not usually occur in nonparkinsonian patients such as those with chronic manganese intoxication. Because carbidopa allows more levodopa to reach the brain, dyskinesias may occur at lower dosages and more rapidly when levodopa is used in conjunction with carbidopa than when levodopa is used alone.

Several types of motor fluctuations also may occur in patients receiving long-term levodopa therapy. In one form, a gradual return of parkinsonian symptoms may occur toward the end of an inter-dose period. This can be minimized by more frequent administration of the drug. In the "on-off" phenomenon, a sudden loss of effectiveness with an abrupt onset of akinesia ("off" effect) which may last from 1 minute to an hour followed by an equally sudden return of effectiveness ("on" effect) may occur many times daily. This occasionally can be minimized by increasing the number of doses per day. Akinesia paradoxica ("start hesitation"), a sudden hypotonic freezing in which the patient frequently falls because he becomes akinetic just as he starts to walk, may be relieved by reducing the dosage of levodopa. Although the cause of these episodes has not been precisely determined, it appears that they may result from a combination of progression of the disease and excessive levodopa dosage.

Numerous mild to severe CNS and psychiatric disturbances may be produced by levodopa and may include decreased attention span, memory loss, insouciance, nervousness, anxiety, agitation, restlessness, confusion, insomnia, vivid dreams, nightmares, daytime somnolence, euphoria, malaise, fatigue, pathologic gambling, increased libido (including hypersexuality), and symptoms related to impulse control. (See Precautions and Contraindications under Cautions.) Hallucinations and abnormal thoughts or behavior (e.g., paranoia, confusion, psychotic disorder, delusions, delirium, psychotic-like behavior, disorientation, aggressive behavior) have been reported in some patients receiving dopaminergic drugs. Hallucinations generally present soon after initiation of levodopa therapy and may be alleviated by reducing dosage of the drug. Serious psychiatric disturbances requiring reduction of dosage or complete withdrawal of levodopa have included severe depression with or without suicidal tendencies, dementia, toxic delirium, paranoid delusions, hallucinations, and hypomania with inappropriate or excessive sexual behavior. In clinical studies, depression was reported with increased frequency in patients receiving the enteral carbidopa-levodopa suspension compared with those receiving oral immediate-release preparations of the drug.

A symptom complex resembling neuroleptic malignant syndrome (NMS; characterized by elevated temperature, muscular rigidity, altered consciousness, autonomic instability) has been reported in association with rapid dosage reduction of, withdrawal of, or changes in dopaminergic therapy. (See Precautions and Contraindications under Cautions.)

Generalized neuropathy, most often characterized as sensory or sensorimotor, has been reported in patients receiving carbidopa-levodopa enteral suspension. Electrodiagnostic findings were most consistent with an axonal polyneuropathy.

● GI Effects

Nausea, vomiting, and anorexia (which may be accompanied by weight loss) occur frequently in patients receiving levodopa. Adverse GI effects of levodopa generally occur early in therapy while dosage is being increased and may be relieved by temporary reduction of dosage or administration of the drug with food. Other adverse GI effects which have been reported less frequently include duodenal ulcer, GI bleeding, constipation, diarrhea, epigastric and abdominal distress and pain, flatulence, hiccups, sialorrhea, dry mouth, dysphagia, change in taste sensation (including bitter taste), burning of the tongue, and trismus.

● Cardiovascular Effects

Orthostatic hypotension occurs frequently following therapeutic doses of levodopa; however, it is usually asymptomatic and tolerance usually develops within a few months.

Cardiac irregularities occur infrequently with levodopa and may include palpitation, sinus tachycardia, ventricular tachycardia or extrasystole, atrial flutter or fibrillation, or block of atrioventricular conduction. Other reported adverse cardiovascular effects of levodopa include flushing and hypertension.

Cardiac ischemic events have been reported with some preparations of levodopa-carbidopa (e.g., extended-release fixed-combination capsules).

● Respiratory Effects

Adverse respiratory effects of levodopa have included episodic hyperventilation, bizarre breathing patterns, hoarseness, and excessive nasal discharge.

Coughing is a frequent adverse effect of levodopa oral inhalation therapy. Temporary, asymptomatic reductions in forced expiratory volume in 1 second (FEV$_1$) have been reported in healthy individuals receiving this dosage form. In patients receiving levodopa oral inhalation therapy, spirometric testing did not reveal any clinically important changes in pulmonary function; however, patients with a recent history of chronic obstructive pulmonary disease (COPD), asthma, or other chronic respiratory conditions were not evaluated.

● Other Adverse Effects

Adverse reactions affecting the urinary tract include urinary frequency, retention, incontinence, and dark urine. Adverse ocular effects include blurred vision, diplopia, mydriasis or miosis, widening of the palpebral fissures, activation of latent Horner's syndrome, and oculogyric crises. However, levodopa has been reported to reduce the incidence and severity of oculogyric crises in some patients with postencephalitic parkinsonian syndrome. Rarely, phlebitis, leukopenia, hemolytic or nonhemolytic anemia, thrombocytopenia, agranulocytosis, and decreased hemoglobin and hematocrit have occurred. If leukopenia occurs during levodopa therapy, the drug should be discontinued, at least temporarily.

Other adverse effects reported to occur in patients receiving levodopa include muscle cramps, a sense of stimulation, headache, weakness, numbness, increased sweating, dark sweat or other body fluids (e.g., saliva), pigmentation of the skin and teeth, rash, hot flashes, postmenopausal bleeding, weight gain or loss, priapism, edema, and alopecia. The development or exacerbation of malignant melanoma has been reported rarely in patients receiving levodopa therapy; however, a causal relationship to the drug has not been fully established to date.

Transient elevations in serum alkaline phosphatase, AST, ALT, LDH, bilirubin, and BUN concentrations may occur in patients receiving levodopa therapy. Rarely, positive direct antiglobulin (Coombs') test results have been reported during prolonged therapy with levodopa. In controlled clinical trials, the incidence of patients experiencing increased BUN and CPK was increased with carbidopa-levodopa enteral suspension compared with oral immediate-release carbidopa-levodopa preparations.

● Precautions and Contraindications

Levodopa-carbidopa should be used with caution in patients with a history of myocardial infarction who have residual atrial, nodal, or ventricular arrhythmias; when initiating therapy in these patients, cardiac function should be monitored in an intensive coronary care facility. Levodopa also should be administered with caution to patients with severe cardiovascular, pulmonary (e.g., bronchial asthma), renal, hepatic, or endocrine disease.

Levodopa should be administered with caution to patients with a history of active peptic ulcer because there is a possibility that the drug may cause upper GI hemorrhage in such patients. Complications associated with the PEG-J procedure or device may occur in patients receiving carbidopa-levodopa enteral suspension and can sometimes result in serious outcomes including death and the need for surgery; these complications may include bezoar; ileus; implant site erosion/ulcer; intestinal hemorrhage, ischemia, obstruction, or perforation; intussusception; pancreatitis; peritonitis; pneumoperitoneum; and postoperative wound infection. Patients should be instructed to notify their clinician immediately if they experience abdominal pain, prolonged constipation, nausea, vomiting, fever, or melanotic stool while receiving the enteral suspension.

Patients receiving carbidopa-levodopa enteral suspension should be instructed on proper administration of the drug through the PEG-J tube and use of the ambulatory pump. Patients should be advised that if the pump is disconnected for short periods of time (e.g., less than 2 hours to swim, shower, or for a short medical procedure), no supplemental oral medication is needed, but an extra dose of the enteral suspension may be given before disconnecting. If the pump is disconnected for periods longer than 2 hours, the patient should contact their clinician and take oral carbidopa-levodopa until the enteral infusion can be resumed.

Patients receiving levodopa powder for oral inhalation should be instructed on proper use of the specific inhaler provided by the manufacturer. Patients should be instructed to take a dose when the return of their parkinsonian symptoms ("off" periods) first occurs. Patients should also be reminded that the contents of Inbrija® capsules are for oral inhalation only and must not be swallowed.

Since psychiatric changes have been reported with dopaminergic agents, levodopa and carbidopa generally should not be used in patients with major psychotic disorders. Because the incidence of depression was increased in patients receiving the enteral suspension of carbidopa-levodopa compared with those receiving oral immediate-release formulations, patients receiving the enteral suspension should be monitored for the development of depression and concomitant suicidal tendencies. Patients also should be cautioned about the possibility of developing hallucinations and instructed to notify a clinician promptly should these manifestations occur.

Because peripheral neuropathy has been reported in patients receiving the enteral suspension, such patients should be monitored for signs and symptoms of neuropathy prior to and during treatment, particularly in those with preexisting neuropathy or risk of neuropathy. Vitamin B supplementation has been reported to decrease the incidence of neuropathy.

Patients should be observed closely when levodopa dosage is reduced abruptly or the drug is discontinued, especially in patients receiving an antipsychotic agent concomitantly, since a symptom complex resembling NMS has occurred following abrupt withdrawal of antiparkinsonian agents. (See Nervous System and Muscular Effects under Cautions.) Sudden discontinuance or rapid dosage reduction of carbidopa-levodopa should be avoided, and dosage should be gradually reduced when treatment is being discontinued.

Patients receiving dopaminergic agents have reported falling asleep while engaged in activities of daily living, including operating a motor vehicle (which has sometimes resulted in accidents). Although many patients reported somnolence while receiving dopaminergic agents, some patients did not perceive warning signs, such as excessive drowsiness, and believed they were alert prior to the episode of falling asleep. Falling asleep while engaged in such activities usually occurs in a setting of preexisting somnolence, although some patients may not give such a history. Patients may not acknowledge drowsiness or sleepiness until directly questioned about these adverse effects during specific activities. Prior to initiating levodopa-carbidopa therapy, patients should be advised of the potential to develop drowsiness and specifically asked about any factors that may increase the risk of somnolence (e.g., concomitant use of sedating drugs, presence of sleep disorders). Patients should be continually reassessed for drowsiness or sleepiness during therapy, especially since some of the episodes of falling asleep occur well after starting treatment. Patients receiving therapy with dopaminergic agents, including levodopa, must be informed of this risk and advised to exercise caution when driving or operating machinery. Patients should be advised that they must refrain from these activities if they experience somnolence and/or an episode of sudden sleep onset. If a patient develops daytime sleepiness or episodes of falling asleep during activities that require active participation (e.g., driving a motor vehicle, conversations, eating), discontinuance of levodopa-carbidopa therapy should be considered. If a decision is made to continue therapy, the patient should be advised not to drive and to avoid other potentially dangerous activities. There is insufficient information to establish whether dosage reduction will eliminate this adverse event.

Data from epidemiologic studies indicate that patients with parkinsonian syndrome have a twofold to approximately sixfold greater risk of developing melanoma than the general population. It is unclear whether this increased risk is due to parkinsonian syndrome or other factors (e.g., drugs used to treat the disease). Because of these findings, patients should be monitored for melanoma on a frequent and regular basis. The manufacturer recommends that dermatologic examinations be performed periodically by qualified clinicians (e.g., dermatologists).

Intense urges (e.g., urge to gamble, increased sexual urges, other intense urges) and inability to control these urges have been reported in some patients receiving antiparkinsonian agents that increase central dopaminergic tone (including levodopa-carbidopa). These urges stopped in some cases when dosage was reduced or the drug was discontinued. Clinicians should ask patients whether they have developed new or increased gambling urges, sexual urges, or other urges while receiving levodopa-carbidopa and should advise them of the importance of reporting such urges. If a patient develops such urges while receiving levodopa-carbidopa, consideration should be given to reducing the dosage or discontinuing the drug.

Individuals with phenylketonuria (i.e., homozygous genetic deficiency of phenylalanine hydroxylase) and other individuals who must restrict their intake of phenylalanine should be warned that levodopa-carbidopa orally disintegrating tablets contain aspartame (NutraSweet®), which is metabolized in the GI tract to provide phenylalanine following oral administration.

Because of the risk of bronchospasm, use of levodopa powder for oral inhalation (Inbrija®) is not recommended in patients with asthma, COPD, or other chronic lung diseases.

When the fixed-combination preparation containing levodopa, carbidopa, and entacapone (Stalevo®) is used, the precautions and contraindications associated with all the drugs in the formulation must be considered.

Patients should be advised of the possibility that dark color (red, brown, black) may appear in saliva, urine, or sweat after ingestion of levodopa-carbidopa, and that garments may become discolored.

Periodic evaluations of hepatic, hematopoietic, cardiovascular, and renal function should be performed in all patients receiving prolonged levodopa therapy. Because some patients receiving levodopa have experienced abnormal bleeding episodes following prostatectomy, it has been recommended that hematologic studies be performed during the postoperative evaluation of all patients receiving the drug.

Levodopa and carbidopa are contraindicated in patients receiving nonselective monoamine oxidase inhibitors (e.g., phenelzine, tranylcypromine). Levodopa and carbidopa also are contraindicated in patients with known hypersensitivity to the drugs. Some manufacturers state that levodopa or levodopa-carbidopa products are contraindicated in patients with angle closure glaucoma, but patients with chronic wide-angle glaucoma may be treated cautiously with the drugs if intraocular pressure is monitored and remains well controlled.

● Pediatric Precautions

Safety and efficacy of levodopa and carbidopa preparations in patients <18 years of age have not been established.

● Geriatric Precautions

No overall differences in response have been observed between geriatric patients >65 years of age and younger adults receiving oral levodopa and carbidopa preparations, but greater sensitivity of some older individuals to adverse reactions such as hallucinations cannot be ruled out. In clinical studies evaluating levodopa powder for oral inhalation, cough, upper respiratory tract infection, nausea, vomiting, extremity pain, and discolored nasal discharge were reported with higher frequency in geriatric patients ≥65 years of age than in younger adults.

● Pregnancy, Fertility, and Lactation
Pregnancy

There are no adequate and well-controlled studies of levodopa and carbidopa in pregnant women. Reproduction studies in rodents using levodopa and carbidopa at dosages approximately 5 and 2 times greater than the maximum human dosage, respectively, have shown adverse effects on fetal and postnatal growth and viability, and studies in rabbits using the drug alone or in conjunction with carbidopa have shown visceral and skeletal malformations. Levodopa and carbidopa should be administered to pregnant women or women who might become pregnant only when the benefits to the mother outweigh the possible risks to the mother and fetus.

Levodopa is distributed into human milk. Carbidopa is distributed into milk in rats; it is not known whether carbidopa is distributed into human milk. Levodopa-carbidopa should be used with caution in nursing women. The known benefits of breast-feeding should be considered along with the mother's clinical need for the drug and any potential adverse effects on the infant from the drug or underlying maternal condition.

DRUG INTERACTIONS

● Anticholinergic Agents

Anticholinergic agents may act synergistically with levodopa to decrease tremor in the management of parkinsonian syndrome and this interaction is often used to therapeutic advantage; however, anticholinergic agents can exacerbate abnormal involuntary movements. In addition, these drugs (particularly in high dosage) may diminish the beneficial effects of levodopa by delaying its absorption thus increasing gastric metabolism of the drug. At least theoretically, this could result in levodopa toxicity when anticholinergic therapy is stopped.

● Benzodiazepines

A few levodopa-treated patients have experienced decreased control of parkinsonian symptoms when chlordiazepoxide or diazepam was added to their therapeutic regimen. For this reason, these drugs and probably other benzodiazepines should be administered with caution to patients receiving levodopa.

● Dopamine Antagonists

Dopamine antagonists (e.g., phenothiazines, butyrophenones, metoclopramide, risperidone) may reduce the therapeutic effects of levodopa; caution is advised if these drugs are used concomitantly and patients should be monitored for worsening parkinsonian symptoms.

Although metoclopramide-induced increases in gastric emptying may enhance the bioavailability of levodopa, metoclopramide can exacerbate parkinsonian symptoms secondary to its antagonistic effects on dopamine receptors.

● Dopamine-depleting Agents

Concomitant use of levodopa and dopamine-depleting agents (reserpine, tetrabenazine) or other drugs known to deplete monoamine stores is not recommended.

● Hypotensive Agents

Because of the risk of symptomatic orthostatic hypotension, levodopa should be used with caution in patients receiving hypotensive agents. If used concomitantly, dosage adjustment of the hypotensive agent may be necessary. In addition, methyldopa (like carbidopa) is a decarboxylase inhibitor and can cause toxic CNS effects such as psychosis if administered concomitantly with levodopa.

● Iron Salts

Iron salts can decrease absorption of levodopa-carbidopa; caution is advised if iron salts are used concomitantly with levodopa-carbidopa and patients should be monitored for worsening parkinsonian symptoms. Some clinicians recommend that iron supplements be taken at least 2 hours before or after administration of levodopa.

● Isoniazid

Isoniazid may antagonize the therapeutic effects of levodopa and should be used with caution during levodopa therapy; patients should be observed for loss of therapeutic response to levodopa.

● MAO Inhibitors

Concomitant use of nonselective monoamine oxidase (MAO) inhibitors (e.g., phenelzine, tranylcypromine) and levodopa-carbidopa is contraindicated because of the risk of hypertensive crises. Therapy with these MAO inhibitors must be discontinued at least 2 weeks prior to initiation of levodopa-carbidopa therapy.

Levodopa may be administered concomitantly with a selective MAO-B inhibitor (e.g., selegiline). However, concomitant use of levodopa-carbidopa and selegiline may be associated with severe orthostatic hypotension and patients should be monitored accordingly.

● Papaverine

Several patients have experienced decreased therapeutic response to levodopa when papaverine was added to their therapeutic regimen. Caution is advised if these drugs are used concomitantly and patients should be observed for loss of therapeutic response.

● Phenytoin

Phenytoin administration has substantially interfered with the therapeutic effects of levodopa in several patients receiving levodopa for the treatment of idiopathic parkinsonian syndrome or chronic manganese intoxication. Caution is advised if these drugs are used concomitantly and patients should be observed for loss of therapeutic response.

● *Pyridoxine*

Administration of 10–25 mg of pyridoxine hydrochloride (vitamin B₆) may cause a rapid reversal of antiparkinsonian effects of levodopa when levodopa is used alone. Concomitant administration of carbidopa with levodopa prevents the reversal of levodopa effects caused by pyridoxine.

● *Tricyclic Antidepressants*

Tricyclic antidepressants should be used with caution in patients receiving levodopa-carbidopa. Tricyclic antidepressants can augment postural hypotension and possibly interfere with absorption of levodopa by delaying gastric emptying and retarding delivery of levodopa to intestinal absorption sites. In addition, other adverse reactions, including hypertension and dyskinesia, have been reported rarely when the drugs were used concomitantly.

LABORATORY TEST INTERFERENCES

Elevated protein-bound iodine concentrations have been reported during levodopa therapy but were apparently caused by an iodine dye used to color the levodopa capsules used in the study. Elevation of serum and urinary uric acid concentrations have been noted during levodopa therapy when colorimetric test methods were used. Levodopa administration does not affect uric acid determinations utilizing uricase.

Levodopa can produce false-positive reactions for urinary glucose in tests based on cupric sulfate reagent (Benedict's reagent or Clinitest® tablets) and false-negative reactions in tests using glucose oxidase (Clinistix®, Tes-Tape®). An accurate measurement of urinary glucose may be obtained if the paper strip is only partially immersed in the urine so that the paper strip can act as an ascending chromatographic system; the top portion of the paper will give a true color change for glucose. False-positive reactions for urine ketones have been reported in patients receiving levodopa when the test was performed with sodium nitroprusside reagent (Acetest®, Ketostix®, Labstix®). In urine screening tests for phenylketonuria, the urine of patients receiving levodopa turned a black-brown color on addition of ferric chloride solution thus interfering with the test.

Patients receiving levodopa have also shown falsely elevated urinary catecholamine concentrations as measured by the Hingerty method. Although levodopa administration results in small increases in urinary VMA excretion, urinary VMA as measured by the Pisano method may be falsely decreased in patients receiving the drug.

ACUTE TOXICITY

Levodopa overdosage should be treated symptomatically. Immediate gastric lavage, maintenance of an adequate airway, and judicious administration of IV fluids is indicated. ECG monitoring and careful observation of the patient for development of cardiac arrhythmias are imperative. Antiarrhythmic therapy should be given if necessary. The value of hemodialysis in the management of levodopa overdosage is not known. Pyridoxine is not effective in reversing the actions of levodopa-carbidopa.

PHARMACOLOGY

Levodopa penetrates the CNS and is enzymatically converted to dopamine in the basal ganglia. There is considerable evidence that symptoms of parkinsonian syndrome, regardless of the cause of the syndrome, are related to depletion of dopamine in the corpus striatum, and levodopa is believed to act principally by increasing dopamine concentration in the brain. In addition, other metabolites of levodopa may contribute to the drug's antiparkinsonian activity. Dysregulation of brain serotonin activity may also occur.

Concurrent administration of a decarboxylase inhibitor such as carbidopa inhibits the peripheral decarboxylation of levodopa by aromatic l-amino acid decarboxylase without affecting the metabolism of the drug within the CNS. Thus, more levodopa is available for transport to the brain. Carbidopa, in doses that effectively inhibit peripheral decarboxylation of levodopa, has little effect on the CNS, cardiovascular system, or GI system.

PHARMACOKINETICS

● *Absorption*

Although substantial amounts of levodopa are metabolized in the lumen of the stomach and intestines, the drug is considered rapidly and well absorbed from the GI tract. GI absorption of levodopa from conventional preparations is slower and peak plasma concentrations are lower when the drug is ingested with food. Absorption of the drug may be particularly impaired in patients receiving a high-protein diet, since levodopa competes with certain amino acids for GI transport mechanisms. In one study in patients with parkinsonian syndrome receiving 3–8 g of levodopa daily as a conventional tablet preparation with food, average plasma concentrations of levodopa were approximately 1 mcg/mL with a range of 0.2–2.8 mcg/mL. However, considerable variation in plasma concentrations has been reported among patients and in the same patient on different occasions. The relationship of plasma levodopa concentrations to clinical effects has not been established.

Conventional (immediate-release) and orally disintegrating tablets of carbidopa-levodopa are formulated to begin releasing the drugs within 30 minutes of administration. Administration of levodopa and carbidopa as orally disintegrating tablets reportedly results in pharmacokinetic values similar to values observed with the conventional tablet preparation.

Oral bioavailability of levodopa from extended-release carbidopa-levodopa tablets is reduced and peak plasma concentrations are delayed compared with those from conventional tablet preparations; however, there is considerably less fluctuation in plasma levodopa concentrations between doses with the extended-release tablets. Food increases the extent of GI absorption and peak plasma levodopa concentrations by about 50 and 25%, respectively, following a single oral dose as extended-release tablets. In healthy geriatric individuals 56–67 years of age, the mean time to peak plasma levodopa concentration was 2 or 0.5 hours with single doses of extended-release or conventional tablet preparations of the combination, respectively, and the peak concentration achieved with the extended-release tablets was 35% of that achieved with conventional tablet preparations. Bioavailability of levodopa from the extended-release tablets was about 70–75% of that from conventional tablet preparations of the combination in this age group. Oral bioavailability and peak plasma levodopa concentrations are comparable following single doses and thrice-daily doses (at steady state) of extended-release tablets in geriatric individuals. In addition, mean trough plasma concentrations of levodopa at steady state with extended-release tablets were about twice those with conventional oral preparations.

The extended-release capsule formulation of carbidopa-levodopa consists of both immediate-release and extended-release components. The capsule formulation is designed to provide an initial rapid absorption of levodopa similar to immediate-release carbidopa-levodopa and then subsequently provide stable levodopa concentrations with reduced peak-to-trough fluctuations in plasma concentrations. Following oral administration of the extended-release capsules, an initial rapid increase in plasma levodopa concentrations is observed, followed by sustained plasma concentrations for about 4–5 hours; lower peak to trough fluctuation is observed at steady state with the extended-release capsules compared with immediate-release carbidopa-levodopa preparations. The bioavailability of levodopa from extended-release carbidopa-levodopa capsules is approximately 70% relative to immediate-release preparations. Peak levodopa concentrations achieved with the extended-release capsules is 30% of that achieved with immediate-release preparations when given in comparable doses.

Following oral inhalation of a single dose of levodopa inhalation powder, the median time to peak plasma concentration is about the same as that for immediate-release carbidopa-levodopa tablets (approximately 0.5 hours). Bioavailability of levodopa from inhaled levodopa is approximately 70% relative to immediate-release oral levodopa tablets. Time to peak plasma concentration of the drug following oral inhalation is approximately 15 minutes faster, but peak plasma concentrations and systemic exposure are substantially lower, compared with orally administered immediate-release carbidopa-levodopa.

Following initiation of the 16-hour infusion of carbidopa-levodopa enteral suspension, peak plasma concentrations of levodopa are obtained in 2.5 hours. Bioavailability of the enteral suspension is comparable to that of oral immediate-release carbidopa-levodopa. However, variability in plasma concentrations of carbidopa and levodopa is reduced with continuous enteral infusion compared with oral administration. Absorption of levodopa from the enteral suspension is not influenced by gastric emptying rate.

Therapeutic response to levodopa usually consists of short-duration improvement (occurring after each dose and disappearing within 5 hours) and long-duration improvement (occurring with prolonged therapy and not subsiding during the 10-hour period following the last dose at night and the first morning dose). The long-duration response usually does not disappear until 3–5 days after levodopa is discontinued.

About 40–70% of a dose of carbidopa is absorbed following oral administration. Although levodopa does not appear to enhance the absorption of carbidopa, carbidopa may enhance the absorption of levodopa by suppressing the metabolism of levodopa in the GI tract. Plasma levodopa concentrations are increased when carbidopa and levodopa are administered concomitantly, principally because of inhibition by carbidopa of the peripheral metabolism of levodopa. (See Elimination under Pharmacokinetics.)

● **Distribution**

Levodopa is widely distributed into most body tissues and the total volume of distribution is about 65% of body weight. There is considerable uptake of levodopa by the pancreas, liver, GI tract, salivary glands, kidneys, and skin. Probably less than 1% of absorbed levodopa penetrates the CNS and only a small amount enters the brain.

Levodopa is approximately 10–30% bound to plasma proteins.

Carbidopa is also widely distributed into most body tissues; however, it does not cross the blood-brain barrier. Carbidopa crosses the placenta and is distributed into milk.

At a concentration of 1 mcg/mL, about 36% of carbidopa is bound to plasma proteins.

● **Elimination**

The plasma half-life of levodopa is approximately 1 hour. The plasma half-life of carbidopa is 1–2 hours. When levodopa and carbidopa are administered concurrently, the plasma half-life of levodopa is increased to about 1.5–2 hours. When levodopa and carbidopa are administered with entacapone or tolcapone, (catechol-O-methyltransferase COMT inhibitors), the plasma half-life of levodopa is increased to 1.3–2 or 3.5 hours respectively. Because administration as extended-release tablets results in prolonged release and absorption of levodopa from the GI tract, the apparent half-life of levodopa may be prolonged with this formulation compared with conventional tablet formulations.

Substantial amounts of levodopa are metabolized in the lumen of the stomach and intestines and on first pass through the liver. There is some evidence that the metabolism of levodopa is accelerated during prolonged therapy, possibly secondary to enzyme induction. Most absorbed levodopa is decarboxylated to dopamine; more than 95% of the drug is decarboxylated peripherally by aromatic l-amino acid decarboxylase, a widely distributed enzyme. Carbidopa inhibits only the peripheral decarboxylation of levodopa since, like dopamine, carbidopa does not cross the blood-brain barrier. Peripheral aromatic l-amino acid decarboxylase is saturated by daily doses of 70–100 mg of carbidopa. Small amounts of levodopa are metabolized to norepinephrine, epinephrine, and 3-methoxytyramine. A small quantity of levodopa is methylated to 3-O-methyldopa; this metabolite is present in plasma and accumulates in the CNS because of its long half-life. The importance of these minor metabolites has not yet been determined, but 3-O-methyldopa does not appear to relieve parkinsonian symptoms. Dopamine is further metabolized to 3,4-dihydroxyphenylacetic acid (DOPAC) and 3-methoxy-4-hydroxyphenylacetic acid (homovanillic acid, HVA) and excreted in urine. HVA, DOPAC, and dopamine are the metabolites of levodopa present in CSF. Carbidopa is not extensively metabolized; about 30% of an oral dose of carbidopa is excreted in urine unchanged within 24 hours.

About 80–85% of a dose of radiolabeled levodopa is excreted in urine within 24 hours. DOPAC and HVA account for about 50% and HVA has been reported to account for 13–42% of an ingested dose. Small amounts of the drug are excreted in urine as vanillylmandelic acid (VMA), 3-O-methyldopa, and norepinephrine. Less than 1% of a dose of levodopa is excreted in urine unchanged. When carbidopa and levodopa are administered concurrently, the urinary excretion of

dopamine, DOPAC, and HVA is substantially diminished, and the amount of unchanged levodopa excreted in urine has been reported to be increased to 6%.

CHEMISTRY AND STABILITY

● **Chemistry**

Levodopa

Levodopa is the levorotatory isomer of dihydroxyphenylalanine and the metabolic precursor of dopamine. Levodopa is commercially available in combination with carbidopa. Levodopa also is commercially available as a fixed-combination preparation containing levodopa, carbidopa, and entacapone (Stalevo®). Levodopa occurs as a white to off-white, odorless, crystalline powder and is slightly soluble in water and insoluble in alcohol.

Extended-release tablets of levodopa and carbidopa (Sinemet® CR) contain the drugs in a polymeric-based delivery system that controls the release of the drugs over an approximately 4- to 6-hour period by slowly eroding in the GI tract.

The extended-release capsule formulation of carbidopa-levodopa (Rytary®) consists of both immediate-release and extended-release components.

Carbidopa

Carbidopa is a decarboxylase inhibitor that inhibits decarboxylation of levodopa to dopamine. Carbidopa is commercially available in combination with levodopa and is also available as a single entity. Carbidopa occurs as a white to creamy white, odorless or practically odorless powder and is slightly soluble in water and practically insoluble in alcohol. Although carbidopa is commercially available as the monohydrate, potency is described in terms of anhydrous carbidopa.

● **Stability**

Levodopa is rapidly oxidized and darkens in the presence of moisture; the color change indicates loss of potency. Commercially available preparations containing levodopa and carbidopa should be protected from exposure to light, moisture, and excessive heat. Tablets containing levodopa and carbidopa should be stored at a temperature of 25°C but may be exposed briefly to temperatures ranging from 15–30°C. Extended-release capsules of levodopa and carbidopa should be stored at 25°C, but may be exposed to temperatures ranging from 15–30°C.

The Inbrija® inhaler and capsules should be stored in a dry place at 20–25°C, but may be exposed to temperatures of 15–30°C. The capsules should be kept in their blister pack until ready to use and should not be stored in inhalers.

Cassettes containing carbidopa-levodopa enteral suspension should be stored in the freezer at -20°C. Prior to dispensing, the cassettes should be thawed in the refrigerator at 2–8°C. The cassettes should be protected from light and kept in the carton prior to use.

PREPARATIONS

Excipients in commercially available drug preparations may have clinically important effects in some individuals; consult specific product labeling for details.

Carbidopa

Oral

Tablets	25 mg (of anhydrous carbidopa)*	Carbidopa Tablets Lodosyn® (scored), Valeant

* available from one or more manufacturer, distributor, and/or repackager by generic (nonproprietary) name

Levodopa

Oral-Inhalation

Powder for inhalation (contained in capsules)	42 mg	Inbrija®, Acorda

* available from one or more manufacturer, distributor, and/or repackager by generic (nonproprietary) name

Carbidopa-Levodopa

Oral

Capsules, extended-release	Carbidopa 23.75 mg (of anhydrous carbidopa) and Levodopa 95 mg	**Rytary®**, Amneal
	Carbidopa 36.25 mg (of anhydrous carbidopa) and Levodopa 145 mg	**Rytary®**, Amneal
	Carbidopa 48.75 mg (of anhydrous carbidopa) and Levodopa 195 mg	**Rytary®**, Amneal
	Carbidopa 61.25 mg (of anhydrous carbidopa) and Levodopa 245 mg	**Rytary®**, Amneal
Suspension, enteral	4.63 mg (of anhydrous carbidopa) per mL and 20 mg (of levodopa) per mL	**Duopa®** (available as single-use 100-mL cassettes), AbbVie
Tablets	Carbidopa 10 mg (of anhydrous carbidopa) and Levodopa 100 mg*	**Carbidopa and Levodopa Tablets** **Sinemet®**, Merck
	Carbidopa 25 mg (of anhydrous carbidopa) and Levodopa 100 mg*	**Carbidopa and Levodopa Tablets** **Sinemet®**, Merck
	Carbidopa 25 mg (of anhydrous carbidopa) and Levodopa 250 mg*	**Carbidopa and Levodopa Tablets** **Sinemet®**, Merck
Tablets, extended-release	Carbidopa 50 mg (of anhydrous carbidopa) and Levodopa 200 mg*	**Carbidopa and Levodopa Extended-release Tablets** **Sinemet® CR**, Merck
	Carbidopa 25 mg (of anhydrous carbidopa) and Levodopa 100 mg*	**Carbidopa and Levodopa Extended-release Tablets** **Sinemet® CR**, Merck

Tablets, orally disintegrating	Carbidopa 10 mg (of anhydrous carbidopa) and Levodopa 100 mg*	**Carbidopa and Levodopa Orally-disintegrating Tablets**
	Carbidopa 25 mg (of anhydrous carbidopa) and Levodopa 100 mg*	**Carbidopa and Levodopa Orally-disintegrating Tablets**
	Carbidopa 25 mg (of anhydrous carbidopa) and Levodopa 250 mg*	**Carbidopa and Levodopa Orally-disintegrating Tablets**

* available from one or more manufacturer, distributor, and/or repackager by generic (nonproprietary) name

Other Carbidopa Combinations

Oral

Tablets, film-coated	Carbidopa 12.5 mg (of anhydrous carbidopa) Entacapone 200 mg and Levodopa 50 mg	**Stalevo®**, Novartis
	Carbidopa 18.75 mg (of anhydrous carbidopa) Entacapone 200 mg and Levodopa 75 mg	**Stalevo®**, Novartis
	Carbidopa 25 mg (of anhydrous carbidopa) Entacapone 200 mg and Levodopa 100 mg	**Stalevo®**, Novartis
	Carbidopa 31.25 mg (of anhydrous carbidopa) Entacapone 200 mg and Levodopa 125 mg	**Stalevo®**, Novartis
	Carbidopa 37.5 mg (of anhydrous carbidopa) Entacapone 200 mg and Levodopa 150 mg	**Stalevo®**, Novartis
	Carbidopa 50 mg (of anhydrous carbidopa) Entacapone 200 mg and Levodopa 200 mg	**Stalevo®**, Novartis

* available from one or more manufacturer, distributor, and/or repackager by generic (nonproprietary) name

Selected Revisions October 18, 2021, © Copyright, September 1, 1976, American Society of Health-System Pharmacists, Inc.

Memantine Hydrochloride

28:92 • CENTRAL NERVOUS SYSTEM AGENTS, MISCELLANEOUS

■ Memantine hydrochloride is an N-methyl-D-aspartate (NMDA) receptor antagonist.

USES

● Alzheimer's Disease

Memantine hydrochloride is used for the management of moderate to severe dementia of the Alzheimer's type (Alzheimer's disease).

Short-term use of memantine in patients with moderate to severe Alzheimer's disease has been associated with improvements in cognitive function, behavior, and activities of daily living; however, the benefits have been modest. Because memantine may provide some beneficial effects and has a favorable safety profile, experts state that the drug may be considered (alone or in combination with a cholinesterase inhibitor) in patients with moderate to severe Alzheimer's disease. Although memantine also has been used in patients with mild Alzheimer's disease†, clinical trials have shown that the drug is no more effective than placebo when used for milder forms of the disease. The long-term efficacy of memantine (e.g., beyond 6 months) has not been established, and additional studies are needed to determine whether benefits of the drug are sustained.

Efficacy of conventional preparations of memantine hydrochloride (tablets and oral solution) has been established in 2 short-term (24 or 28 weeks), randomized, controlled clinical studies in adults (50–93 years of age) with moderate to severe Alzheimer's disease. In both studies, patients treated with memantine hydrochloride received an initial dosage of 5 mg once daily, with weekly increases in increments of 5 mg daily until a dosage of 10 mg twice daily was reached. Patients enrolled in the 24-week study were receiving donepezil hydrochloride (a cholinesterase inhibitor) at a stable dosage prior to randomization and continued to receive such therapy in addition to either memantine or placebo during the study period. In both studies, changes from baseline in cognitive performance were assessed using the Severe Impairment Battery (SIB) scale. Changes from baseline in overall daily function and overall clinical effects (including information from caregivers) were assessed using the modified Alzheimer's disease Cooperative Study Activities of Daily Living inventory (ADCS-ADL) and the Clinician's Interview Based Impression of Change (CIBIC plus) scales, respectively. In both studies, patients receiving memantine experienced less deterioration in cognitive and daily function than patients receiving placebo. In the 24-week study, patients receiving memantine experienced less decline in CIBIC plus scores than patients receiving placebo; however, while improvements in CIBIC plus scores were observed in patients receiving memantine in the 28-week study, the difference from placebo (intent-to-treat analysis) was not statistically significant. In an unpublished 24-week, open-label extension of the 28-week trial, improvement relative to the projected rate of continued decline in cognition, daily function, and overall clinical impression of change was observed in patients who were switched from placebo to memantine.

A third randomized, controlled clinical study of 12 weeks' duration was conducted in nursing home patients with severe dementia (Alzheimer's disease or vascular dementia) using conventional preparations of memantine (e.g., Namenda®). In this study, memantine hydrochloride was initiated at a dosage of 5 mg once daily and increased to 10 mg once daily after 1 week. Daily function was assessed using the care dependency subscale of the Behavioral Rating Scale for Geriatric Patients (BGP), and overall clinical effects were assessed using the Clinical Global Impression of Change scale (CGI-C); cognitive function was not evaluated. In a subset of patients diagnosed as having Alzheimer's disease, memantine was more effective than placebo, as assessed by changes from baseline in both the BGP and CGI-C scales.

Efficacy of memantine hydrochloride extended-release capsules (e.g., Namenda XR®) has been established in a randomized, double-blind study in patients with moderate to severe Alzheimer's disease receiving a cholinesterase inhibitor (e.g., donepezil, galantamine, rivastigmine). Patients were randomized to receive add-on therapy with memantine hydrochloride extended-release capsules (28 mg once daily) or placebo. At 24 weeks, patients who received memantine had statistically significant improvements in cognitive function (as assessed by the SIB scale) and overall clinical effect (as assessed by the CIBIC plus scale). However, a wide range of responses was observed in the cognitive performance measure.

Memantine may be used in combination with a cholinesterase inhibitor. A fixed-combination preparation containing memantine hydrochloride and donepezil hydrochloride (Namzaric®) is commercially available for the treatment of moderate to severe dementia of the Alzheimer's type in patients receiving a stable donepezil hydrochloride dosage of 10 mg once daily. There is some evidence indicating that the addition of memantine to established therapy with a cholinesterase inhibitor may result in less clinical deterioration than therapy with a cholinesterase inhibitor alone in patients with moderate to severe Alzheimer's disease, but the effect size appears to be small and of uncertain clinical importance.

● Autism Spectrum Disorders

Because glutamatergic neurotransmission has been implicated in the pathophysiology of autism spectrum disorders (ASD)†, drugs that modulate glutamate such as memantine have been investigated as potential treatments. However, efficacy of memantine has not been established for this use, and clinical studies generally have found no difference with the drug compared with placebo on primary efficacy measures in patients with autism. In 2 randomized controlled studies in children 6–12 years of age with ASD, no statistically significant difference in scores on the Social Responsiveness Scale (SRS), a rating instrument evaluating core symptoms of autism (i.e., social awareness, information processing, capacity for reciprocal response, anxiety/avoidance, and autistic preoccupations and traits), was observed in patients receiving memantine and those receiving placebo. In these studies, memantine hydrochloride was administered as extended-release capsules in dosages ranging from 3–15 mg daily based on weight.

DOSAGE AND ADMINISTRATION

● Administration

Memantine hydrochloride is administered orally (as tablets, extended-release capsules, or oral solution) without regard to meals. Memantine hydrochloride tablets and oral solution are equivalent on a mg-per-mg basis.

The oral solution should be administered using the oral dosing syringe provided by the manufacturer, referring to the accompanying patient information for instructions. Memantine hydrochloride oral solution should not be mixed with any other liquid.

The extended-release capsules should be swallowed intact and not divided, chewed, or crushed; alternatively, the capsules may be opened, sprinkled on applesauce, and swallowed without chewing.

The fixed-combination preparation containing memantine hydrochloride and donepezil hydrochloride (Namzaric®) may be used in patients currently receiving a stable dosage of donepezil hydrochloride 10 mg daily. The fixed-combination capsules should be swallowed intact (and not divided, chewed, or crushed); alternatively, the capsules may be opened, sprinkled on applesauce, and swallowed without chewing. The entire contents of each capsule should be consumed; the dose should not be divided.

If a dose of memantine is missed, the next dose should be taken as scheduled; the dose should not be doubled to make up for a missed dose. If treatment is interrupted for several days, the drug may need to be restarted with a lower dosage and retitrated.

● Dosage

Memantine is commercially available as memantine hydrochloride; dosage is expressed in terms of the hydrochloride salt.

Tablets and Oral Solution

The recommended initial adult dosage of memantine hydrochloride (as tablets or oral solution) for the treatment of moderate to severe dementia of the Alzheimer's type is 5 mg once daily. Dosage should be increased to the recommended maintenance dosage of 10 mg twice daily (effective dosage in clinical trials) in increments of 5 mg daily at minimum intervals of 1 week. The manufacturer states that dosage should be increased as follows: first to 10 mg daily (5 mg twice daily), then to 15 mg daily (5 mg and 10 mg as separate doses), and then to 20 mg daily (10 mg twice daily).

Extended-release Capsules

The recommended initial adult dosage of memantine hydrochloride (as extended-release capsules) for the treatment of moderate to severe dementia of the Alzheimer's type is 7 mg once daily. If the drug is well tolerated, dosage should be increased to the recommended maintenance dosage of 28 mg once daily (effective dosage in clinical trials) by increments of 7 mg daily at minimum intervals of 1 week.

Patients currently receiving memantine hydrochloride conventional tablets or oral solution at a dosage of 10 mg twice daily may be switched to the extended-release capsules at a dosage of 28 mg once daily; the transition should occur on the day following the last dose of the conventional preparation.

Fixed Combination of Memantine and Donepezil (Namzaric®)

Patients receiving a stable donepezil hydrochloride dosage of 10 mg daily and not currently receiving memantine who are switching to the fixed-combination preparation: The recommended initial dosage of the fixed-combination preparation is 7 mg of memantine hydrochloride and 10 mg of donepezil hydrochloride once daily in the evening. Dosage may be increased in increments of 7 mg of the memantine hydrochloride component at minimum intervals of at least 1 week up to the maximum recommended maintenance dosage of 28 mg of memantine hydrochloride and 10 mg of donepezil hydrochloride once daily in the evening.

Patients who are switching from separate memantine and donepezil preparations (i.e., donepezil hydrochloride 10 mg daily; memantine hydrochloride 10 mg twice daily or 28 mg once daily as the extended-release preparation) to the fixed-combination preparation: Initial dosage of the fixed-combination preparation is 28 mg of memantine hydrochloride and 10 mg of donepezil hydrochloride once daily in the evening. Therapy with the fixed-combination preparation should be initiated on the day following the last dose of the individual preparations.

● Special Populations

No dosage adjustment is needed in patients with mild to moderate hepatic impairment. Memantine should be used with caution in patients with severe hepatic impairment.

No dosage adjustment is needed in patients with mild to moderate renal impairment. In patients with severe renal impairment (i.e., creatinine clearance of 5–29 mL/minute), the recommended maintenance dosage of memantine hydrochloride is 5 mg twice daily (as conventional tablets or oral solution) or 14 mg once daily (as extended-release capsules).

CAUTIONS

● Contraindications

Known hypersensitivity to memantine hydrochloride or any ingredient in the formulation.

● Warnings/Precautions

General Precautions

Urinary Excretion

Conditions that increase urinary pH (e.g., dietary changes [e.g., from a high-protein to a vegetarian diet], concomitant use of drugs that alkalinize urine [e.g., carbonic anhydrase inhibitors, sodium bicarbonate], renal tubular acidosis, severe urinary tract infections) may decrease elimination of memantine, resulting in increased plasma memantine concentrations; the drug should be used with caution under such conditions.

Specific Populations

Pregnancy

There are no adequate data to inform the developmental risks associated with the use of memantine in pregnant women. In animal reproduction studies, adverse developmental effects (e.g., decreased body weight, decreased skeletal ossification) were observed when the drug was administered to pregnant rats during the period of organogenesis or from late gestation throughout lactation to weaning at doses higher than those used clinically.

Lactation

It is not known whether memantine is distributed into human milk or if the drug has any effects on the nursing infant or milk production. The known benefits of breast-feeding should be considered along with the mother's clinical need for memantine and any potential adverse effects on the breast-fed infant from the drug or underlying maternal condition.

Pediatric Use

Safety and efficacy of memantine have not been established in pediatric patients.

Memantine has been evaluated in children 6–12 years of age with autism spectrum disorders (ASD)†; however, efficacy has not been demonstrated. (See Uses: Autism Spectrum Disorders.)

Geriatric Use

Clinical studies have been conducted principally in older patients since dementia of the Alzheimer's type occurs mainly in patients 65 years of age or older. Memantine pharmacokinetics were similar in elderly patients and younger adults.

Hepatic Impairment

In patients with moderate hepatic impairment (Child-Pugh class B), no change in exposure of memantine was observed compared with individuals with normal hepatic function; however, terminal half-life was increased by about 16% in patients with moderate hepatic impairment. No dosage adjustment is necessary in patients with mild or moderate hepatic impairment. Memantine has not been evaluated in patients with severe hepatic impairment and should be used with caution in such patients.

Renal Impairment

The area under the plasma concentration-time curve (AUC) was increased by 4, 60, or 115% in individuals with mild (creatinine clearance exceeding 50–80 mL/minute), moderate (creatinine clearance 30–49 mL/minute), or severe (creatinine clearance 5–29 mL/minute) renal impairment, respectively. Terminal elimination half-life was increased by 18, 41, or 95% in those with mild, moderate, or severe renal impairment, respectively. Dosage adjustment is recommended in patients with severe renal impairment, but not in those with mild or moderate renal impairment. (See Dosage and Administration: Special Populations.)

● Common Adverse Effects

Common adverse effects reported with conventional preparations of memantine include dizziness, confusion, headache, and constipation.

Common adverse effects reported with the extended-release capsule formulation of the drug include headache, diarrhea, and dizziness.

DRUG INTERACTIONS

● Drugs Affecting or Metabolized by Hepatic Microsomal Enzymes

Memantine is minimally metabolized by cytochrome P-450 (CYP) isoenzymes. Drugs that inhibit or induce these enzymes are not likely to alter the pharmacokinetics of memantine.

Memantine produces minimal inhibition of CYP1A2, 2A6, 2C9, 2D6, 2E1, and 3A4 in vitro. No induction of CYP1A2, 2C9, 2E1, or 3A4/5 has been observed in vitro at concentrations exceeding those associated with therapeutic efficacy.

● Protein-bound Drugs

Because plasma protein binding of memantine is low (45%), a pharmacokinetic interaction with drugs that are highly protein bound (e.g., digoxin, warfarin) is unlikely.

● Drugs Secreted by Renal Tubular Cationic Transport

When memantine is used with drugs secreted by the same renal cationic system (e.g., cimetidine, hydrochlorothiazide, metformin, nicotine, quinidine, ranitidine, triamterene), altered plasma concentrations of the drugs are possible. However, concomitant use of memantine with a fixed combination of hydrochlorothiazide and triamterene did not affect bioavailability of either memantine or triamterene, and maximum plasma concentrations and area under the plasma concentration-time curve (AUC) of hydrochlorothiazide decreased by only 20%. In addition, concomitant use of memantine with a fixed combination of glyburide and metformin hydrochloride did not affect the pharmacokinetics of memantine, metformin, or glyburide, and the hypoglycemic effects of the glyburide-metformin combination were not affected.

● Alkalinizing Agents

There is a potential for decreased memantine clearance with resulting increases in adverse effects when the drug is used concomitantly with agents that increase urine pH (e.g., carbonic anhydrase inhibitors, sodium bicarbonate). Caution is advised. Memantine clearance was decreased by approximately 80% at alkaline urine conditions (i.e., pH 8).

● *Bupropion*

Results of a pharmacokinetic study showed that memantine did not affect the pharmacokinetics of bupropion or its hydroxy-bupropion metabolite.

● *Cholinesterase Inhibitors*

Concomitant use of memantine with the cholinesterase inhibitor donepezil did not affect the pharmacokinetics of either drug or substantially alter acetylcholinesterase inhibition by donepezil. In a 24-week clinical study in patients with moderate to severe Alzheimer's disease, adverse effects observed with combination therapy with memantine and donepezil were similar to those observed with donepezil alone. In vitro and animal studies indicate that memantine does not affect the reversible inhibition of acetylcholinesterase produced by donepezil or galantamine.

● *N-Methyl-D-aspartate (NMDA) Antagonists*

Concomitant use of memantine with other NMDA antagonists (e.g., amantadine, ketamine, dextromethorphan) has not been systematically evaluated. Caution is advised if these drugs are used concomitantly.

● *Warfarin*

Memantine did not affect the pharmacokinetics or pharmacodynamics of warfarin (as assessed by the INR).

DESCRIPTION

Memantine hydrochloride is a low- to moderate-affinity, noncompetitive *N*-methyl-D-aspartate (NMDA) receptor antagonist that binds preferentially to NMDA receptor-operated cation channels. The drug differs structurally and pharmacologically from other currently available agents used for the palliative treatment of Alzheimer's disease.

Memantine is thought to act by blocking the actions of glutamate, the principal excitatory neurotransmitter in the CNS. The effects of glutamate are mediated by different receptor types, including NMDA receptors, which play a role in physiologic processes such as learning and memory formation. Persistent activation of NMDA receptors by glutamate has been implicated as a possible cause of neurodegeneration in various types of dementia, including dementia of the Alzheimer's type (Alzheimer's disease), and is thought to contribute to the symptomatology of Alzheimer's disease. In vitro studies have shown that β-amyloid, which accumulates to form amyloid plaques in patients with Alzheimer's disease, increases the release of glutamate upon neuronal depolarization, supporting a role for pathologic NMDA receptor activation in the disease. It has been postulated that low- to moderate-affinity NMDA receptor antagonists may prevent glutamate-induced neurotoxicity without interfering with the physiologic processes mediated by the activation of NMDA receptors. However, there currently is no evidence that memantine prevents or slows neurodegeneration in patients with Alzheimer's disease.

In addition to exhibiting antagonist activity at the NMDA receptor, memantine exhibits antagonist activity at the type 3 serotonergic (5-HT$_3$) receptor with a potency that appears to be similar to that at the NMDA receptor. Memantine also blocks the nicotinic acetylcholine receptor with a potency of about one-sixth to one-tenth that at the NMDA receptor. Memantine exhibits little or no affinity for γ-aminobutyric acid (GABA), benzodiazepine, dopamine, adrenergic, histamine, or glycine receptors or for voltage-dependent calcium, sodium, or potassium channels.

Memantine hydrochloride is well absorbed following oral administration of conventional preparations, with peak plasma concentrations achieved in about 3–7 hours. Following multiple-dose administration of extended-release capsules of the drug, peak plasma concentrations are achieved in about 9–12 hours. Memantine is eliminated principally in urine, with approximately 48% of an administered dose excreted as unchanged drug; the remainder of the dose is converted to metabolites that exhibit minimal NMDA receptor antagonist activity. The hepatic microsomal cytochrome P-450 (CYP) isoenzyme system does not play a substantial role in the metabolism of memantine. The terminal elimination half-life of memantine is approximately 60–80 hours.

ADVICE TO PATIENTS

Importance of instructing patients and caregivers regarding proper dosing and administration of memantine.

Importance of instructing patients and/or caregivers in proper use of the oral dosing syringe if the oral solution is used. Ensure that patients and/or caregivers are aware of the patient instruction sheet that is enclosed with the solution. Oral solution should not be mixed with any other liquids. Advise patients that questions about administration should be directed to their pharmacist or clinician.

Importance of informing clinician of existing or contemplated concomitant therapy, including prescription and OTC drugs, as well as any concomitant illnesses.

Importance of women informing clinicians if they are or plan to become pregnant or plan to breast-feed.

Importance of informing patients of other important precautionary information. (See Cautions.)

PREPARATIONS

Excipients in commercially available drug preparations may have clinically important effects in some individuals; consult specific product labeling for details.

Memantine Hydrochloride

Oral		
Capsules, extended-release	7 mg*	Memantine Hydrochloride Extended-release Capsules
		Namenda XR®, Allergan
	14 mg*	Memantine Hydrochloride Extended-release Capsules
		Namenda XR®, Allergan
	21 mg*	Memantine Hydrochloride Extended-release Capsules
		Namenda XR®, Allergan
	28 mg*	Memantine Hydrochloride Extended-release Capsules
		Namenda XR®, Allergan
Solution	10 mg/5 mL*	Memantine Hydrochloride Solution
Tablets, film-coated	5 mg*	Memantine Hydrochloride Tablets
		Namenda®, Allergan
	10 mg*	Memantine Hydrochloride Tablets
		Namenda®, Allergan
	5 mg (28 tablets) and 10 mg (21 tablets)	Namenda® Titration Pak, Allergan

* available from one or more manufacturer, distributor, and/or repackager by generic (nonproprietary) name

Memantine Hydrochloride Combinations

Oral		
Capsules, extended-release	7 mg with Donepezil Hydrochloride 10 mg	Namzaric®, Allergan
	14 mg with Donepezil Hydrochloride 10 mg	Namzaric®, Allergan
	21 mg with Donepezil Hydrochloride 10 mg	Namzaric®, Allergan
	28 mg with Donepezil Hydrochloride 10 mg	Namzaric®, Allergan

† Use is not currently included in the labeling approved by the US Food and Drug Administration.

Table of Contents

§ Omitted from the print version of *AHFS Drug Information*® because of space limitations. This monograph is available on the *AHFS Drug Information*® website, http://www.ahfsdruginformation.com.

Table of Contents

40:00 ELECTROLYTIC, CALORIC, AND WATER BALANCE

§ Omitted from the print version of *AHFS Drug Information* because of space limitations. This monograph is available on the *AHFS Drug Information* web site, http://www.ahfsdruginformation.com.

Citrates

40:08 • ALKALINIZING AGENTS

■ Citrates (i.e., potassium citrate and citric acid, sodium citrate, sodium citrate and citric acid, tricitrates) are alkalinizing agents.

USES

● Alkalinizing Alternatives to Sodium Bicarbonate

Administration of sodium citrate and other citrate preparations appears to be associated with formation of bicarbonate; therefore, the drugs are used as alkalinizing agents.

Oral citrate solutions, including potassium citrate and citric acid, sodium citrate and citric acid, and tricitrates, are used as alkalinizing agents in conditions where long-term maintenance of an alkaline urine is desirable and in the management of chronic metabolic acidosis associated with conditions such as chronic renal insufficiency or renal tubular acidosis.

Selection of a specific preparation may in part be determined by the potassium and sodium contents. Preparations containing sodium citrate and citric acid are especially useful when administration of potassium salts is undesirable or contraindicated, while those containing potassium citrate and citric acid are used when administration of sodium salts is undesirable or contraindicated. Unlike sodium bicarbonate solution, these preparations are generally considered highly palatable and pleasant tasting, and may be particularly useful as an alkalinizing agent in patients who do not tolerate the taste of sodium bicarbonate oral solution.

● Adjuvant in Gout Therapy

Potassium citrate and citric acid oral solution and tricitrates oral solution are used as adjuvant therapy to uricosuric agents in gout therapy.

● Prevention of Milk Curdling

Sodium citrate has been used to alter cow's milk so that large hard curds are not formed in the stomach of feeding infants†.

DOSAGE AND ADMINISTRATION

● Administration

Citrate preparations (i.e., potassium citrate and citric acid, sodium citrate, sodium citrate and citric acid, tricitrates) are administered orally. Oral citrate solutions should be diluted with adequate amounts of water prior to administration to minimize the risk of GI complications, and followed by additional water after administration; palatability may be enhanced by chilling the solution before administration. For reconstitution of potassium citrate and citric acid for oral solution in single-dose packets, the contents of one packet should be mixed thoroughly with at least 180 mL of cool water or juice prior to administration and followed by additional water or juice after administration. Oral citrate solutions should preferably be taken after meals to avoid the saline laxative effect of the drug.

● Dosage

Potassium Citrate and Citric Acid

The usual adult dosage of potassium citrate and citric acid solution is 15–30 mL after meals and at bedtime. The usual dosage of potassium citrate and citric acid solution in children is 5–15 mL after meals and at bedtime. The usual adult dosage of potassium citrate and citric acid for oral solution is one single-dose packet (containing 3300 mg of potassium citrate monohydrate and 1002 mg of citric acid monohydrate), reconstituted as directed 4 times daily, after meals and at bedtime. The single-dose packets of potassium citrate and citric acid for oral solution are not recommended for pediatric use, since dosage for these patients can be more easily regulated with the commercially available oral solution. Dosage should be individualized according to the patient's tolerance and response.

Sodium Citrate

The usual adult dosage of sodium citrate as an alkalinizing agent is 1–2 g every 2–4 hours as necessary.

To prevent formation of large curds in the stomach of feeding infants, 100 mg of sodium citrate has been added to each 30 mL of cow's milk.

Sodium Citrate and Citric Acid

The usual adult dosage of sodium citrate and citric acid solution is 10–30 mL, diluted in 30–90 mL of water, after meals and at bedtime. The usual dosage of sodium citrate and citric acid solution in children 2 years of age or older is 5–15 mL of solution, diluted in 30–90 mL of water, after meals and at bedtime. A clinician should be consulted for use of the drug in children younger than 2 years of age. Dosage should be individualized according to the patient's tolerance and response.

Sodium citrate and citric acid may be used as a buffer to maintain an approximate pH in various extemporaneous formulations. Addition of the following concentration of the drugs should generally produce a solution buffered to the approximate pH listed:

TABLE 1. Citrate Buffer

pH	Citric Acid Monohydrate g/L	Sodium Citrate Dihydrate g/L
2.5	64.4	7.8
3.0	57.4	17.6
3.5	47.6	31.4
4.0	40.6	41.2
4.5	30.8	54.9
5.0	19.6	70.6
5.5	9.8	84.3
6.0	4.2	92.1
6.5	1.8	95.6

Adapted from Schumacher GE. Buffer formulations. *Am J Hosp Pharm*. 1966; 23:628-9.

Tricitrates

The usual adult dosage of tricitrates solution is 15–30 mL diluted in water 4 times daily, after meals and at bedtime. The usual dosage of tricitrates solution in children is 5–15 mL 4 times daily, after meals and at bedtime. Dosage should be individualized according to the patient's tolerance and response.

CAUTIONS

● Adverse Effects

Oral citrate preparations generally are well tolerated when given in the usual dosages to patients with normal renal function and urine output. Excessive doses of sodium-containing formulations may cause metabolic alkalosis, especially in patients with renal dysfunction or hypocalcemia. Large doses also may cause tetany or depression of the heart associated with decreasing ionized calcium concentrations. Large doses of potassium-containing formulations may cause hyperkalemia and alkalosis, particularly in patients with impaired renal function. Listlessness, weakness, mental confusion, and paresthesia of the extremities may be associated with hyperkalemia. Oral citrate preparations may have a saline laxative effect when administered orally.

● Precautions and Contraindications

To avoid complications, the clinical condition of the patient should be evaluated and laboratory determinations (e.g., serum electrolytes, acid-base balance) obtained periodically during therapy with oral citrate preparations, especially in patients with renal disorders. Patients with renal impairment are at risk of developing hypernatremia or alkalosis in the presence of hypocalcemia.

Sodium-containing citrate preparations should be used with caution in patients with low urine output unless the patient is closely supervised during therapy. Citrate preparations containing sodium should be used with extreme caution in patients with congestive heart failure, hypertension, renal dysfunction, peripheral or pulmonary edema, or toxemia of pregnancy. Citrate preparations containing potassium should be used with extreme caution in patients in whom excessive potassium may have a deleterious effect.

Sodium citrate and citric acid oral solution (Cytra-2, Bicitra®) is contraindicated in patients receiving a sodium-restricted diet and in those with severe renal impairment. Tricitrates oral solution is contraindicated in patients with severe renal impairment with azotemia or oliguria, untreated Addison's disease, or severe myocardial damage. Sodium citrate and citric acid (Oracit®) is contraindicated in patients with severe renal impairment, oliguria or azotemia, untreated Addison's disease, adynamia episodica hereditaria, acute dehydration, heat cramps, anuria, severe myocardial damage, and hyperkalemia. Potassium citrate and citric acid oral solution and potassium citrate and citric acid for oral solution are also contraindicated in patients with adynamia episodica hereditaria, acute dehydration, heat cramps, anuria, severe myocardial damage, or hyperkalemia (from any cause).

● Pregnancy, Fertility, and Lactation

Pregnancy

Controlled studies to date in pregnant women receiving potassium citrate have not shown a risk to the fetus in the first trimester of pregnancy and there is no evidence of risk in subsequent trimesters.

Lactation

It is not known whether potassium citrate is distributed into milk. Because potassium freely distributes into and out of milk, use of potassium citrate by a nursing woman with normal plasma potassium concentrations should have no adverse effect on the nursing infant; milk potassium concentrations may be increased in hyperkalemic women.

DRUG INTERACTIONS

● Antacids

Concomitant use of citrate preparations and aluminum-containing antacids may increase GI absorption of aluminum. In patients with chronic kidney disease who require aluminum-containing phosphate binders, concomitant use of citrate preparations should be avoided because of the risk of aluminum absorption and potential toxicity with concomitant use. Sodium bicarbonate may be an alternative to citrates if aluminum-containing phosphate binders are required.

● Cardiac Glycosides

The potential for toxicity exists in patients receiving cardiac glycosides concomitantly with citrate preparations.

● Drugs Affecting the Renin-Angiotensin-Aldosterone System

Concomitant use of potassium-containing citrate preparations with an angiotensin converting-enzyme (ACE) inhibitor or mineralocorticoid (aldosterone) receptor antagonist (e.g., eplerenone, spironolactone) may increase serum potassium concentrations and increase the risk of hyperkalemia and associated toxicity.

● Drugs Increasing Serum Potassium Concentrations

Concomitant administration of potassium-containing citrate preparations with potassium-sparing diuretics (e.g., amiloride, triamterene) or potassium-containing agents may increase serum potassium concentrations and increase the risk of hyperkalemia and associated toxicity.

● Drugs with pH-dependent Urinary Excretion

Alkalinization of the urine with citrates may enhance urinary excretion and decrease therapeutic and toxic effects of salicylates. (For further information on the effects of alkalinizing agents on salicylate pharmacokinetics, see Drug Interactions: Acidifying and Alkalinizing Agents and also see Pharmacokinetics: Elimination, in the Salicylates General Statement 28:08.04.24.) Alkalinization of the urine with citrates also may enhance urinary excretion of chlorpropamide and lithium.

Alkalinization of the urine with citrates may decrease urinary excretion of amphetamines, pseudoephedrine, and quinidine and increase serum concentrations of these drugs. Dosage reduction of pseudoephedrine may be necessary. Concomitant use of amphetamines and citrates should be avoided, especially in patients with amphetamine overdosage, since toxicity will be prolonged. If citrate therapy is initiated or discontinued in a patient receiving a stable quinidine dosage regimen, ECGs and serum quinidine concentrations should be monitored.

PHARMACOLOGY

Citrates (i.e., potassium citrate and citric acid, sodium citrate, sodium citrate and citric acid, tricitrates) are alkalinizing agents. Metabolism of these drugs appears to be associated with formation of bicarbonate. Citrates are extensively metabolized, and less than 5% of an oral dose is excreted in urine unchanged.

Sodium citrate has anticoagulant activity. Sodium citrate prevents the clotting of blood by forming an undissociated calcium citrate complex, making calcium unavailable to the clotting mechanism. Anticoagulant sodium citrate solution, when added to blood, prevents the clotting of blood and the crenation or swelling of cells. The sterile solution is used as an anticoagulant for banked blood for transfusion and to prepare citrated human plasma and blood for fractionation.

Sodium citrate prevents the curdling of milk by rennin, and has been used for this purpose to alter cow's milk so that large hard curds are not formed in the stomach of feeding infants.

CHEMISTRY AND STABILITY

● Chemistry

Citrates (i.e., potassium citrate and citric acid, sodium citrate, sodium citrate and citric acid, tricitrates) are alkalinizing agents.

Citric Acid

Citric acid occurs as colorless, translucent crystals or as a white, granular to fine, crystalline powder. The drug is odorless or practically odorless and has a strongly acidic taste. Citric acid may occur as the anhydrous form or may contain 1 molecule of water; concentration is expressed in terms of anhydrous citric acid. Citric acid is very soluble in water and freely soluble in alcohol.

Potassium Citrate

Potassium citrate occurs as transparent crystals or as a white, granular powder. The drug is odorless and has a cooling, saline taste. Potassium citrate may occur as the anhydrous form or may contain 1 molecule of water; concentration is expressed in terms of anhydrous potassium citrate. The drug is freely soluble in water and almost insoluble in alcohol.

Potassium Citrate and Citric Acid for Oral Solution

Potassium citrate and citric acid for oral solution contains potassium citrate and citric acid in a sugar-free base. Each single-dose packet contains 3300 mg of potassium citrate monohydrate and 1002 mg of citric acid monohydrate and when reconstituted as directed, each single-dose packet provides 2 mEq of potassium, which is equivalent to 2 mEq of bicarbonate. Each packet of potassium citrate and citric acid for oral solution is equivalent to 15 mL of the potassium citrate and citric acid oral solution.

Potassium Citrate and Citric Acid Oral Solution

Potassium citrate and citric acid oral solution is a solution of potassium citrate and citric acid in a suitable aqueous medium. Each 100 mL of potassium citrate and citric acid oral solution contains 7.55–8.35 g of potassium, 12.18–13.46 g of citrate (equivalent to 20.9–23.1 g of potassium citrate monohydrate), and 6.34–7.02 g of citric acid monohydrate. Each mL of potassium citrate and citric acid oral solution contains about 2 mEq of potassium and provides approximately 2 mEq of bicarbonate. Potassium citrate and citric acid oral solution has a pH of 4.9–5.4.

Sodium Citrate

Sodium citrate occurs as colorless crystals or as a white, crystalline powder. Sodium citrate may occur as the anhydrous form or may contain 2 molecules of hydration; concentration is expressed in terms of anhydrous sodium citrate. The hydrous form of the drug is freely soluble in water, very soluble in boiling water, and insoluble in alcohol.

Sodium Citrate and Citric Acid Oral Solution

Sodium citrate and citric acid oral solution is a solution of sodium citrate and citric acid in a suitable aqueous medium and occurs as a clear solution having the color of any added preservative or flavoring agent. Each 100 mL of sodium citrate and citric acid oral solution contains 2.23–2.46 g of sodium, 6.11–6.75 g of citrate (equivalent to 9.5–10.5 g of sodium citrate dihydrate), and 6.34–7.02 g of citric acid monohydrate. Each mL of sodium citrate and citric acid oral solution contains about 1 mEq of sodium and provides approximately 1 mEq of bicarbonate. Sodium citrate and citric acid oral solution has a pH of 4–4.4.

Tricitrates Oral Solution

Tricitrates oral solution is a solution of citric acid, potassium citrate, and sodium citrate in a suitable aqueous medium. Each 100 mL of tricitrates oral solution contains 6.34–7.02 g of citric acid monohydrate, 12.20–13.48 g of citrate as potassium citrate and sodium citrate, 3.78–4.18 g of potassium (equivalent to 10.45–11.55 g of potassium citrate monohydrate), and 2.23–2.46 g of sodium (equivalent to 9.5–10.5 g of sodium citrate dihydrate). Each mL of tricitrates oral solution contains about 1 mEq each of potassium and sodium and provides approximately 2 mEq of bicarbonate. Tricitrates oral solution has a pH of 4.9–5.4.

● Stability

Citric Acid

The hydrous form of citric acid is efflorescent in dry air.

Potassium Citrate

Potassium citrate is deliquescent when exposed to moist air.

Potassium Citrate and Citric Acid for Oral Solution

Potassium citrate and citric acid for oral solution should be protected from excessive heat and freezing.

Potassium Citrate and Citric Acid Oral Solution

Potassium citrate and citric acid oral solution should be stored in tight, light-resistant container at 20–25°C and protected from excessive heat and freezing.

Sodium Citrate and Citric Acid Oral Solution

Sodium citrate and citric acid oral solution generally should be stored in tight containers and protected from freezing or excessive heat. The manufacturer's labeling should be consulted for specific storage recommendations.

Tricitrates Oral Solution

Tricitrates oral solution should be stored in tight container at 20–25°C and protected from excessive heat and freezing.

PREPARATIONS

Excipients in commercially available drug preparations may have clinically important effects in some individuals; consult specific product labeling for details.

Potassium Citrate and Citric Acid

Oral		
For solution	Potassium Citrate Monohydrate 3300 mg and Citric Acid Monohydrate 1002 mg per packet	Cytra-K Crystals, Cypress
Solution	Potassium Citrate Monohydrate 1100 mg/5 mL and Citric Acid Monohydrate 334 mg/5 mL*	Cytra-K, Cypress Potassium Citrate Monohydrate and Citric Acid Monohydrate Solution

* available from one or more manufacturer, distributor, and/or repackager by generic (nonproprietary) name

Sodium Citrate

Powder

Sodium Citrate and Citric Acid

Oral		
Solution (Shohl's Solution)	Hydrous Sodium Citrate 490 mg/5 mL and Citric Acid 640 mg/5 mL	Oracit®, Carolina Medical
	Sodium Citrate Dihydrate 500 mg (321.5 mg of citrate) per 5 mL and Citric Acid Monohydrate 334 mg/5 mL	Bicitra®, Ortho-McNeil Cytra-2, Cypress

Tricitrates

Oral		
Solution	Citric Acid Monohydrate 334 mg/5 mL, Potassium Citrate Monohydrate 550 mg/5 mL, and Sodium Citrate Dihydrate 500 mg (321.5 mg of citrate) per 5 mL*	Citric Acid Monohydrate, Potassium Citrate Monohydrate, and Sodium Citrate Dihydrate Solution Cytra-3 Syrup, Cypress

* available from one or more manufacturer, distributor, and/or repackager by generic (nonproprietary) name

† Use is not currently included in the labeling approved by the US Food and Drug Administration.

Sodium Bicarbonate

40:08 · ALKALINIZING AGENTS

■ Sodium bicarbonate is an alkalinizing agent.

USES

● Overview

Sodium bicarbonate is used as an alkalinizing agent in the treatment of metabolic acidosis. Sodium bicarbonate also is used to increase urinary pH in order to increase the solubility of certain weak acids (e.g., cystine, sulfonamides, uric acid) or in the treatment of hemolytic reactions requiring alkalinization of the urine to diminish the nephrotoxic effects of blood pigments. In addition, the drug is used in the treatment of severe diarrhea accompanied by substantial GI bicarbonate loss.

● Acidosis

Sodium bicarbonate is used in the treatment of metabolic acidosis associated with many conditions including severe renal disease (e.g., renal tubular acidosis), uncontrolled diabetes (ketoacidosis), extracorporeal circulation of the blood, cardiac arrest, circulatory insufficiency caused by shock or severe dehydration, ureterosigmoidostomy, lactic acidosis, alcoholic ketoacidosis, use of carbonic anhydrase inhibitors, and ammonium chloride administration. In metabolic acidosis, the principal disturbance is a loss of proton acceptors (e.g., loss of bicarbonate during severe diarrhea) or accumulation of an acid load (e.g., ketoacidosis, lactic acidosis, renal tubular acidosis).

Mild acidosis may have minimal clinical importance and require no corrective therapy; physiologic compensatory mechanisms may be adequate to correct the disorder. When the underlying cause can be treated effectively in more severe acidosis, there is often no need to specifically treat the acid-base disorder. Generally, administration of sodium bicarbonate is not necessary unless the acidosis is severe (e.g., arterial pH less than 7.1–7.2 or plasma bicarbonate concentration of 8 mEq/L or less) or the underlying cause of the acidosis cannot be determined and/or corrected.

When specific alkalinizing therapy is necessary, complete correction of the acidosis with an alkalinizing agent is usually not necessary, and may be hazardous, since metabolic alkalosis can be precipitated. Generally, the goal of alkalinizing therapy is to correct the acid-base disturbance toward normal and allow physiologic compensatory mechanisms to complete the correction, if possible. Sodium bicarbonate is generally considered the alkalinizing agent of choice for oral or parenteral therapy. When sodium bicarbonate is used in the treatment of metabolic acidosis, the acid-base status of the patient must be monitored frequently and dosage modified according to response; the bicarbonate deficit can only be estimated, and no more than 50% of the calculated deficit should be replaced initially in patients whose compensatory mechanisms are expected to contribute to correction of the acidosis.

● Diabetic Ketoacidosis

The specific role of sodium bicarbonate therapy in the treatment of diabetic ketoacidosis has not been established. Because correction of the underlying metabolic disorder generally results in correction of acid-base abnormalities and because of the potential risks of sodium bicarbonate therapy in the treatment of this disorder, administration of sodium bicarbonate is generally reserved for the treatment of severe acidosis (e.g., arterial pH less than 7–7.15 or serum bicarbonate concentration of 8 mEq/L or less). Rapid correction of acidosis with sodium bicarbonate in patients with diabetic ketoacidosis may cause hypokalemia, paradoxical acidosis in CSF since carbon dioxide diffuses more rapidly into CSF than does bicarbonate, and lactic acidosis since increased pH increases hemoglobin-oxygen affinity which, when combined with erythrocyte 2,3-diphosphoglycerate (2,3-DPG) deficiency in these patients, results in peripheral tissue hypoxia. However, the benefits and risks of sodium bicarbonate therapy in ketoacidosis have not been fully determined, and additional controlled studies of the safety and efficacy of the drug are necessary. Generally, when sodium bicarbonate is used in the treatment of diabetic ketoacidosis, the acidosis should only be partially corrected (e.g., to an arterial pH of about 7.2) to avoid rebound metabolic alkalosis as ketones are metabolized.

● Advanced Cardiovascular Life Support

The American Heart Association (AHA) guidelines for cardiopulmonary resuscitation (CPR) and emergency cardiovascular care state that IV sodium bicarbonate is not recommended for *routine* use during cardiac arrest. There are only limited data that support therapy with buffers during cardiac arrest, and routine administration of sodium bicarbonate has not been reported to improve outcomes of resuscitation. There is no evidence indicating that sodium bicarbonate improves the likelihood of defibrillation or survival rates in animals with ventricular fibrillation and cardiac arrest. In addition, the drug potentially may have detrimental effects (e.g., compromised coronary perfusion pressure [CPP] caused by reduction of systemic vascular resistance; paradoxical intracellular acidosis caused by production of carbon dioxide that freely diffuses into myocardial and cerebral cells and may depress function, especially in ischemic myocardium; shift in the oxyhemoglobin saturation curve, inhibiting release of oxygen; induction of hyperosmolarity and hypernatremia; adverse effects secondary to extracellular alkalosis; exacerbation of central venous acidosis; inactivation of concomitantly administered catecholamines).

Restoration of oxygen content with appropriate ventilation with oxygen, support of some tissue perfusion and cardiac output with good chest compressions, then rapid return of spontaneous circulation (ROSC), are the mainstays of restoring acid-base balance during cardiac arrest. By ensuring adequate alveolar ventilation, a major component of depressed pH (respiratory acidosis) during cardiac arrest generally can be managed without sodium bicarbonate. Sodium bicarbonate may be useful in some resuscitation situations (e.g., preexisting metabolic acidosis, hyperkalemia, tricyclic antidepressant overdosage). In addition, some experts state that sodium bicarbonate may be considered in the treatment of ventricular arrhythmias associated with cocaine toxicity in addition to standard treatments.

It must be kept in mind that administration of sodium bicarbonate is followed by release of carbon dioxide, which requires adequate alveolar ventilation to assure continued excretion of this source of potential acid. Thus, the importance of adequate alveolar ventilation in the control of pH must be emphasized, as well as the need for repeated arterial determination of blood pH and $Paco_2$, if possible. Whenever possible, sodium bicarbonate therapy should be guided by the bicarbonate concentration or calculated base deficit obtained from blood gas analysis or laboratory measurement. To minimize the risk of iatrogenically induced alkalosis, complete correction of the base deficit should not be attempted. Some experts state that other non-carbon dioxide generating buffers (e.g., tromethamine) have shown a potential to minimize some adverse effects of sodium bicarbonate (e.g., carbon dioxide generation, hyperosmolarity, hypernatremia, hypoglycemia, intracellular acidosis, myocardial acidosis, overshoot alkalosis) when used in certain resuscitation situations; however, clinical experience is limited and outcome studies are lacking.

● Antacid Therapy

For the use of sodium bicarbonate as an antacid, see Antacids 56:04.

DOSAGE AND ADMINISTRATION

● Administration

Sodium bicarbonate is administered by IV infusion. Sodium bicarbonate may be administered by rapid IV injection when initial immediate administration of the drug is considered necessary (e.g., during cardiac arrest). The drug also may be administered orally in the treatment of mild to moderately severe acidosis, in conditions (e.g., chronic renal failure) requiring prolonged therapy with an alkalinizing agent, and in conditions in which IV administration of the drug is not necessary (e.g., alkalinization of the urine). The drug has also been administered by subcutaneous injection if diluted to isotonicity (1.5% sodium bicarbonate solution). Extravasation of hypertonic sodium bicarbonate injections must be avoided. (See Cautions: Adverse Effects.) Sodium bicarbonate also has been administered by intraosseous (IO) injection† in the setting of pediatric advanced life support (PALS); onset of action and systemic concentrations are comparable to those achieved with venous administration. However, acid-base balance analysis may be inaccurate after administration of sodium bicarbonate via the IO cannula.

In neonates and children younger than 2 years of age, hypertonic sodium bicarbonate injections generally should be administered by slow IV infusion of a 4.2% solution up to 8 mEq/kg daily. (See Cautions: Pediatric Precautions.)

IV Administration

Standardize 4 Safety

Standardized concentrations for sodium bicarbonate have been established through Standardize 4 Safety (S4S), a national patient safety initiative to reduce medication errors, especially during transitions of care. Multidisciplinary expert panels were convened to determine recommended standard concentrations. Because recommendations from the S4S panels may differ from the manufacturer's prescribing information, caution is advised when using concentrations that differ from labeling, particularly when using rate information from the label. For additional information on S4S (including updates that may be available), see https://www.ashp.org/pharmacy-practice/standardize-4-safety-initiative.

TABLE 1. Standardize 4 Safety Continuous IV Infusion Standard Concentrations for Sodium Bicarbonate

Patient Population	Concentration Standards	Dosing Units
Pediatric patients (<50 kg)	0.5 mEq/mL	mEq/kg/hour
	1 mEq/mL	

● Dosage

Dosage of sodium bicarbonate injection is determined by severity of the acidosis, appropriate laboratory determinations, and the patient's age, weight, and clinical condition. Frequent laboratory determinations and clinical evaluation of the patient are essential during therapy with sodium bicarbonate, especially during prolonged therapy, to monitor changes in fluid and electrolyte and acid-base balance.

Generally, full correction of bicarbonate deficit should not be attempted during the first 24 hours of sodium bicarbonate therapy, since this may result in precipitation of metabolic alkalosis because of delayed physiologic compensatory mechanisms. When total carbon dioxide content is returned to normal or beyond within the first day of therapy, substantially alkaline values for blood pH and subsequent adverse effects are likely to occur. When initial, rapid administration of the drug is considered necessary, it is generally recommended that no more than 33–50% of the calculated bicarbonate requirements be administered initially. Several methods for estimating bicarbonate requirements in patients with metabolic acidosis have been suggested; specialized references on fluid and electrolyte and acid-base balance should be consulted for specific recommendations.

Sodium bicarbonate is not recommended for *routine* use in advanced cardiovascular life support (ACLS) during cardiac arrest (see Uses: Advanced Cardiovascular Life Support); however, if the drug is used in certain resuscitation situations (e.g., preexisting metabolic acidosis, hyperkalemia, tricyclic antidepressant overdosage), an IV dose of 1 mEq/kg is usually given initially in adults. Whenever possible, dosage of sodium bicarbonate should be guided by the bicarbonate concentration or by the calculated base deficit obtained from blood gas analysis or laboratory measurement. Complete correction of the base deficit is not recommended to minimize the risk of alkalosis. For the management of cardiac arrest due to hyperkalemia in adults, 50 mEq of sodium bicarbonate has been administered IV over 5 minutes as adjunctive therapy to other standard ACLS measures.

If sodium bicarbonate is used for pediatric resuscitation, the guidelines for pediatric advanced life support (PALS) recommend a pediatric dose of 1 mEq/kg, administered slowly by IV or IO† injection. If blood gas tensions and pH measurements are available, subsequent doses should be determined by the following equation:

$$mEq\ NaHCO_3 = 0.3 \times bodyweight\ (in\ kg) \times base\ deficit\ (in\ mEq/L)$$

In less urgent forms of metabolic acidosis, a 2–5 mEq/kg dose of sodium bicarbonate may be administered to older children or adults as a 4- to 8-hour IV infusion. Subsequent doses should be determined by the response of the patient

and appropriate laboratory determinations. Sodium bicarbonate therapy should be planned in a stepwise manner, since the degree of response following a given dose is not always predictable. Generally, the dose and frequency of administration should be reduced after severe symptoms have improved.

For the treatment of ventricular arrhythmias associated with cocaine toxicity in pediatric patients, 1–2 mEq/kg of IV sodium bicarbonate has been administered.

Although the specific role of sodium bicarbonate therapy in the treatment of diabetic ketoacidosis has not been established (see Uses: Diabetic Ketoacidosis), when IV sodium bicarbonate is administered, the acidosis should only partially be corrected, generally to an arterial pH of about 7.2, in order to avoid rebound alkalosis.

For the treatment of acidosis associated with chronic renal failure, oral sodium bicarbonate therapy is generally initiated when plasma bicarbonate concentration is less than 15 mEq/L. Therapy is usually initiated in adults with an oral sodium bicarbonate dosage of 20–36 mEq daily, given in divided doses. Dosage is then titrated to provide a plasma bicarbonate concentration of about 18–20 mEq/L. Because of the sodium content of sodium bicarbonate, the fluid and electrolyte balance of the patient must be carefully monitored during therapy with the drug. To relieve symptoms and prevent or stabilize renal failure and osteomalacia in patients with renal tubular acidosis, higher dosages of sodium bicarbonate are necessary. In adults with distal (type 1) renal tubular acidosis, an initial oral dosage of 0.5–2 mEq/kg daily, given in 4 or 5 divided doses, has been suggested. Dosage is titrated until hypercalciuria and acidosis are controlled, and according to the response and tolerance of the patient. Alternatively, an adult dosage of 48–72 mEq (about 4–6 g) daily has been suggested. Higher dosages are generally required in patients with proximal (type 2) renal tubular acidosis; oral dosages of 4–10 mEq/kg daily, given in divided doses, have been suggested.

The usual oral dosage of sodium bicarbonate for alkalinization of urine in adults is 48 mEq (4 g) initially, followed by 12–24 mEq (1–2 g) every 4 hours. Dosages of 30–48 mEq (2.5–4 g) every 4 hours, up to 192 mEq (16 g) daily, may be required in some patients. Dosage should be individually titrated to maintain the desired urinary pH. For alkalinization of urine in children, an oral dosage of 1–10 mEq (84–840 mg) per kg daily, adjusted according to response, has been suggested.

CAUTIONS

● Adverse Effects

Gastric distention and flatulence may occur when sodium bicarbonate is administered orally. Inadvertent extravasation of hypertonic solutions of sodium bicarbonate has reportedly caused chemical cellulitis because of their alkalinity, subsequently resulting in tissue necrosis, ulceration, and/or sloughing at the site of injection. One manufacturer recommends that extravasation be treated by elevating the affected area, applying warm compresses to the site, and locally injecting lidocaine or hyaluronidase.

Sodium bicarbonate, when given in large doses or to patients with renal insufficiency, may cause metabolic alkalosis. Metabolic alkalosis may be accompanied by hyperirritability or tetany. The manufacturers recommend that severe bicarbonate-induced alkalosis be treated with a parenteral calcium salt (e.g., calcium gluconate) and/or an acidifying agent (e.g., ammonium chloride). In patients with ketoacidosis, rapid alkalinization with sodium bicarbonate may reportedly result in clouding of consciousness, cerebral dysfunction, obtundation, seizures, and peripheral tissue hypoxia and lactic acidosis.

Sodium and water retention and edema may occur during sodium bicarbonate therapy, especially when the drug is given in large doses or to patients with renal insufficiency, congestive heart failure, or those predisposed to sodium retention and edema. Sodium and water overload may result in hypernatremia and hyperosmolality. Severe hyperosmolal states may develop during cardiopulmonary resuscitation when excessive doses of sodium bicarbonate are administered. (See Pharmacology.)

● Precautions and Contraindications

Generally, the goal of alkalinizing therapy is to correct the acid-base disturbance while avoiding overdosage and resultant metabolic alkalosis.

Sodium bicarbonate should be used with extreme caution in patients with congestive heart failure or other edematous or sodium-retaining conditions; in patients with renal insufficiency, especially those with severe insufficiency such as oliguria or anuria; and in patients receiving corticosteroids or corticotropin, since each gram of sodium bicarbonate contains about 12 mEq of sodium. (For the sodium content of commercially available injections, see Chemistry and Stability: Chemistry.) IV administration of sodium bicarbonate may cause fluid and/or solute overload resulting in dilution of serum electrolytes, overhydration, congestive conditions, or pulmonary edema. The risk of dilutional conditions is inversely proportional to the electrolyte concentration administered, and the risk of solute overload and resultant congestive conditions with peripheral and/or pulmonary edema is directly proportional to the electrolyte concentration administered.

Potassium depletion may predispose to metabolic alkalosis and coexistent hypocalcemia may result in tetany and carpopedal spasm as the plasma pH increases. To minimize the risks of preexisting hypokalemia and/or hypocalcemia, these electrolyte disturbances should be corrected prior to initiation of, or concomitantly with, sodium bicarbonate therapy.

Sodium bicarbonate is generally contraindicated in patients with metabolic or respiratory alkalosis, in patients with hypocalcemia in whom alkalosis may induce tetany, in patients with excessive chloride loss from vomiting or continuous GI suctioning, and in patients at risk of developing diuretic-induced hypochloremic alkalosis. Sodium bicarbonate should not be used orally as an antidote in the treatment of acute ingestion of strong mineral acids, since carbon dioxide gas forms during neutralization and may cause gastric distention and possible rupture. Some experts state that non-lipid soluble drugs (e.g., sodium bicarbonate) may injure the airway and should not be administered via the endotracheal route.

● Pediatric Precautions

One manufacturer cautions that rapid injection (10 mL/minute) of hypertonic sodium bicarbonate solutions in neonates and children younger than 2 years of age may produce hypernatremia, decreased CSF pressure, and possible intracranial hemorrhage. It is recommended that the rate of IV administration in these children not exceed 8 mEq/kg daily and that slow IV administration of a 4.2% solution may be preferred. In emergencies such as cardiac arrest, the risk of rapid infusion of the drug in these children must be weighed against the potential for death from acidosis.

● Pregnancy, Fertility, and Lactation

Pregnancy

Animal reproduction studies have not been performed with sodium bicarbonate. It is also not known whether sodium bicarbonate can cause fetal harm when administered to pregnant women. Sodium bicarbonate should be used during pregnancy only when clearly needed.

PHARMACOLOGY

Sodium bicarbonate is an alkalinizing agent which dissociates to provide bicarbonate ion.

Bicarbonate is the conjugate base component of the principal extracellular buffer in the body, the bicarbonate:carbonic acid buffer. Various metabolic processes in the body either generate or consume hydrogen ions. Despite the dynamic nature of these processes, the hydrogen ion concentration in plasma and interstitial fluid is maintained at an almost constant level between 38–42 nmole/L (pH 7.37–7.42). The acid-base balance is maintained by 3 interacting mechanisms: buffers, regulation of carbonic acid concentration by the pulmonary system, and renal excretion of acid or base.

In body fluids, there are many buffers, including hemoglobin, proteins, and phosphates; however, the principal extracellular buffer is the bicarbonate:carbonic acid buffer. At a given pH, the ratio of bicarbonate:carbonic acid is constant. At pH 7.4, the bicarbonate:carbonic acid ratio is 20:1. Although buffers are most efficient when the ratio is 1, the unique characteristics of the bicarbonate:carbonic acid buffer make it highly effective even at a ratio of 20:1. In a solution such as plasma, all buffers are in equilibrium with the same hydrogen ion concentration and with each other. Thus, assessment of any one of these buffers (e.g., bicarbonate:carbonic acid) is reflective of the hydrogen ion concentration of the entire solution and the ratios of conjugate base to undissociated acid for all buffers. The bicarbonate:carbonic acid buffer is the only buffer in the body whose component concentrations can be varied independently by physiologic regulatory mechanisms. The bicarbonate buffer is extremely effective in buffering fixed acids and bases since changes in its components can be compensated by physiologic mechanisms such as formation and excretion of high concentrations of carbon dioxide, regulation by the pulmonary system of carbon dioxide concentration in body fluids, and generation or excretion by the kidney of substantial amounts of bicarbonate. Since carbonic acid is readily converted to or from carbon dioxide gas, its concentration is responsive to changes in alveolar Pco_2 and can be readily altered by changes in pulmonary ventilation.

Carbonic acid and dissolved carbon dioxide constitute the weak acid component and bicarbonate is the conjugate base component in the bicarbonate:carbonic acid buffer. The bicarbonate:carbonic acid buffer can be expressed as the following form of the Henderson-Hasselbalch equation:

$$pH = 6.1 + \log (HCO_3^- / (H_2CO_3 + \text{dissolved } CO_2))$$

At equilibrium, the amount of dissolved carbon dioxide in plasma greatly exceeds that of carbonic acid. Thus, measurement of carbon dioxide is used to determine the concentration of the weak acid component of the buffer. Since the concentration of dissolved carbon dioxide in plasma (liquid phase) is in equilibrium with alveolar carbon dioxide (gas phase), the concentration of carbon dioxide in plasma can be calculated from the partial pressure of carbon dioxide using the following equation:

$$CO_2 \text{ (mmol/L)} = 0.03 \times Pco_2 \text{ (mm Hg)}$$

and the Henderson-Hasselbalch equation can be expressed as follows:

$$pH = 6.1 + \log (HCO_3^- / (0.03 \times Pco_2))$$

Changes in the concentration of either component of the buffer can cause a decrease or increase in pH. Administration of sodium bicarbonate will increase the plasma bicarbonate concentration and possibly increase plasma pH; however, pH is usually maintained within the normal range, since compensatory mechanisms such as increased glomerular filtration and decreased tubular reabsorption of bicarbonate in the kidneys will rapidly decrease the plasma concentration of bicarbonate and restore the bicarbonate:carbonic acid ratio. Although metabolic alkalosis may result from IV infusion or ingestion of large amounts of sodium bicarbonate, renal mechanisms for increasing bicarbonate excretion are usually adequate to compensate for the acid-base imbalance. Primary acid-base disturbances (i.e., respiratory acidosis or alkalosis and metabolic acidosis or alkalosis) result from an initial change in one of the components of the bicarbonate:carbonic acid buffer. Generally, compensatory physiologic mechanisms and correction of the underlying cause of the disturbance are sufficient to restore acid-base balance. Occasionally, when acidemia is severe or plasma bicarbonate concentration is severely depleted, administration of sodium bicarbonate may be necessary to restore acid-base balance in patients with metabolic or respiratory acidosis. However, administration of sodium bicarbonate in these patients may result in metabolic alkalosis.

Changes in acid-base balance also stimulate compensatory ion-exchange mechanisms. Cations such as potassium and sodium can exchange for extracellular hydrogen ions. When the extracellular hydrogen ion concentration increases, as in acidosis, there is a redistribution of potassium ions from intracellular to extracellular fluid. Administration of sodium bicarbonate, by decreasing pH, can cause a redistribution of potassium ions into cells in patients with acidosis.

Since sodium bicarbonate provides bicarbonate which is readily excreted in urine, administration of the drug will increase urinary pH in patients with normal renal function. Alkalinizing the urine can increase the solubility of certain weak acids (e.g., cystine, uric acid) and can increase the ionization and urinary excretion of lipid-soluble organic acids (e.g., phenobarbital, salicylates) that are reabsorbed in the kidney via diffusion of the un-ionized species.

Sodium bicarbonate has a potent antacid action. Each gram of sodium bicarbonate has an in vitro neutralizing capacity of about 12 mEq of acid. For a discussion on sodium bicarbonate's antacid action, see Antacids 56:04.

CHEMISTRY AND STABILITY

● *Chemistry*

Sodium bicarbonate is an alkalinizing agent. Sodium bicarbonate occurs as a white, crystalline powder which has a saline and slightly alkaline taste. The drug is soluble in water and insoluble in alcohol. Aqueous solutions of sodium bicarbonate, when freshly prepared, are alkaline to litmus; alkalinity increases as the solutions stand, are agitated, or are heated. Each 84 mg or 1 g of sodium bicarbonate contains 1 or about 12 mEq, respectively, each of sodium and bicarbonate ions.

Sodium bicarbonate injections are sterile solutions of the drug in water for injection. Carbon dioxide may be added during the manufacture of the injection to adjust the pH to 7–8.5. An 8.4% solution contains 1 mEq each of sodium and bicarbonate ions per mL and has a calculated osmolarity of 2000 mOsm/L. A 7.5% solution contains 0.892 mEq/mL each of sodium and bicarbonate ions and has a calculated osmolarity of 1786 mOsm/L. A 5% solution contains 0.595 mEq each of sodium and bicarbonate ions per mL and has a calculated osmolarity of 1190–1203 mOsm/L. A 4.2% solution contains 0.5 mEq each of sodium and bicarbonate ions per mL and has a calculated osmolarity of 1000 mOsm/L. Sodium bicarbonate is also available as a 4% small volume parenteral additive solution (Neut®) which provides 2.4 mEq each of sodium and bicarbonate ions per 5 mL and is used to increase the pH of acidic infusion solutions.

A 1.5% solution of sodium bicarbonate is isotonic. A 1.5% sodium bicarbonate solution can be prepared by diluting each mL of an 8.4, 7.5, or 4.2% solution of the drug with 4.6, 4, or 1.8 mL of sterile water for injection, respectively.

● *Stability*

Sodium bicarbonate tablets and effervescent tablets should be stored in tightly closed containers at a temperature less than 40°C, preferably between 15–30°C. Sodium bicarbonate injection should be stored at a temperature less than 40°C, preferably between 15–30°C; freezing should be avoided.

Sodium bicarbonate is stable in dry air, but slowly decomposes into sodium carbonate, carbon dioxide, and water in moist air. When heated, sodium bicarbonate loses water and carbon dioxide and is converted into sodium carbonate. Solutions of sodium carbonate are much more alkaline than sodium bicarbonate; since sodium carbonate may be formed when the dry salt or its solutions are sterilized with heat, the pH of heat-sterilized solutions or of solutions prepared from heat-sterilized powder should be determined prior to use. When sodium bicarbonate is combined with acids in aqueous solutions, a vigorous evolution of carbon dioxide gas occurs; the liberated carbon dioxide bubbles through the solution resulting in effervescence. In the dry state, sodium bicarbonate and acids do not react.

Sodium bicarbonate is physically and/or chemically incompatible with many drugs including acids, acidic salts, and many alkaloidal salts, but the compatibility depends on several factors (e.g., concentrations of the drugs, specific diluent used, resulting pH, temperature). Sodium bicarbonate injection should not be admixed with solutions containing calcium salts, except where compatibility has been specifically established, since haze formation or precipitation may result from such combinations. Also, sodium bicarbonate should not be admixed with or administered in the same IV line as catecholamines (e.g., epinephrine) because sodium bicarbonate may inactivate simultaneously administered catecholamines. Specialized references should be consulted for specific compatibility information.

PREPARATIONS

Excipients in commercially available drug preparations may have clinically important effects in some individuals; consult specific product labeling for details.

Sodium Bicarbonate

Oral		
Powder	325 mg*	**Arm & Hammer® Baking Soda**, Church & Dwight
Tablets	650 mg*	**Soda Mint**, CMC
		Sodium Bicarbonate Tablets
Parenteral		
Injection	4.2% (0.5 mEq/mL) (2.5 or 5 mEq)*	**Sodium Bicarbonate Injection**
	5% (0.595 mEq/mL) (297.5 mEq)*	**Sodium Bicarbonate Injection**
	7.5% (0.892 mEq/mL) (8.92 or 44.6 mEq)*	**Sodium Bicarbonate Injection**
	8.4% (1 mEq/mL) (10 or 50 mEq)*	**Sodium Bicarbonate Injection**
Injection, for preparation of IV admixtures	7.5% (0.892 mEq/mL) (178.4 mEq) pharmacy bulk package	**Sodium Bicarbonate Injection MaxiVial®**, Abraxis
Solution, sterile, to adjust pH of injections	4% (0.48 mEq/mL) (2.4 mEq)	**Neut®**, Hospira
	4.2% (0.5 mEq/mL) (2.5 mEq)*	**Sodium Bicarbonate Additive Solution**

* available from one or more manufacturer, distributor, and/or repackager by generic (nonproprietary) name

† Use is not currently included in the labeling approved by the US Food and Drug Administration.

Selected Revisions June 10, 2024, © Copyright, January 1, 1959, American Society of Health-System Pharmacists, Inc.

Lactulose

40:10 • AMMONIA DETOXICANTS

■ Lactulose, a synthetic derivative of lactose, is an ammonia detoxicant.

USES

● Portal-Systemic Encephalopathy

Lactulose is used as an adjunct to protein restriction and supportive therapy for the prevention and treatment of portal-systemic encephalopathy (PSE) including hepatic pre-coma and coma. Lactulose has been useful in the management of PSE resulting from surgical portacaval shunts or from chronic hepatic diseases such as cirrhosis. In patients with PSE, lactulose therapy reduces the blood ammonia concentration and this is usually accompanied by substantial improvement in the mental state of the patient and improved EEG tracings. Many patients are able to tolerate increased dietary protein during lactulose therapy. The drug does not, however, alter the course of the underlying liver disease. Therefore, use of lactulose in the treatment of PSE does not obviate treatment of underlying liver disease, nor preclude other measures used in the treatment of PSE.

A good clinical response has been achieved in 75–85% of PSE patients receiving lactulose therapy. Because lactulose is relatively nontoxic, it is a valuable alternative to antibiotics such as neomycin, especially when prolonged therapy is required or when neomycin is contraindicated. Some well-controlled comparative studies have shown that the efficacy of lactulose is superior to that of laxative controls (such as magnesium sulfate or sorbitol) and about equal to that of neomycin in the treatment of acute and chronic PSE. Some patients who had previously failed to respond to neomycin and dietary protein restriction responded to lactulose therapy. Conversely, other patients responded better to neomycin than to lactulose.

Since neomycin destroys bacteria and lactulose requires bacterial degradation for its effectiveness, concomitant therapy with these agents is theoretically counterproductive. (See Drug Interactions: Anti-infective Agents.) It appears, however, that lactulose remains active when administered with neomycin and, in fact, there is some evidence that concomitant therapy with lactulose and neomycin may be more effective than either drug alone. Some clinicians recommend neomycin for acute episodes of PSE and lactulose for the long-term management of chronic PSE.

Lactulose is not useful in the management of non-nitrogenous types of encephalopathy such as those induced by drugs or metabolic or electrolyte disturbances. Lactulose therapy is not effective in the treatment of coma associated with infectious hepatitis or other acute disorders of the liver. In a case of hyperammonemia, which was apparently caused by an inborn error of metabolism, lactulose therapy was ineffective.

● Constipation

Lactulose is useful as a laxative in the treatment of chronic constipation in adults and geriatric patients. The drug has been used in the treatment of chronic constipation in children†; however, the manufacturers state that safety and efficacy of lactulose for the treatment of chronic constipation in children have not been established. Lactulose has also been used to restore regular bowel movements in hemorrhoidectomy patients†. Following a barium meal examination, the drug has been used to induce bowel evacuation in geriatric patients with colonic retention of barium and severe constipation†. Although lactulose is effective in the treatment of chronic constipation, its superiority to conventional laxatives has not been established.

DOSAGE AND ADMINISTRATION

● Reconstitution and Administration

Lactulose is usually administered orally. The sweet taste of lactulose solution, which may be unpleasant to some patients, can be minimized by diluting the solution with water, fruit juice, or milk or administering it in food such as desserts. When lactulose solution is administered via a gastric tube, it should be well diluted to prevent induction of vomiting and the possibility of aspiration pneumonia.

Lactulose may also be administered rectally to adults with portal-systemic encephalopathy (PSE) during stages of hepatic pre-coma or coma when the possibility of aspiration exists, or when necessary endoscopic or intubation procedures interfere with oral administration.

For oral administration, lactulose powder should be reconstituted by dissolving the contents of a packet labeled as containing 10 or 20 g of the drug in approximately 120 mL of water.

● Dosage

Each 15 mL of commercially available lactulose solution provides approximately 10 g of the drug; corresponding doses provided by 2.5, 5, 7.5, 10, 30, 40, 45, 90, 150, and 300 mL of the commercial solution are approximately 1.67, 3.3, 5, 6.67, 20, 27, 30, 60, 100, and 200 g, respectively. Following reconstitution of the oral powder as directed, a 10 or 20 g dose is provided by the total volume.

Portal-Systemic Encephalopathy

For the prevention and treatment of PSE in adults, the usual initial oral dosage of lactulose is 20–30 g 3 or 4 times daily. Dosage is then adjusted every 1–2 days as necessary to produce 2 or 3 soft stools daily. Some clinicians recommend that dosage be adjusted according to the acidity of the colonic contents by measuring stool pH (with indicator paper) at the start of therapy and adjusting the dosage until stool pH is about 5. This pH is usually achieved when the patient has 2 or 3 soft stools daily during lactulose therapy. For most adults, lactulose dosage is usually 60–100 g daily, although some patients may require higher dosage.

In the management of acute episodes of PSE in adults, 20–30 g may be given orally at 1- to 2-hour intervals to induce rapid laxation. When the laxative effect has been achieved, the dose of lactulose is reduced to the amount required to produce 2 or 3 soft stools daily. When lactulose is administered in the treatment of PSE, improvement in the clinical condition of the patient usually occurs within 1–3 days. Continuous long-term therapy with lactulose may decrease the severity and prevent the recurrence of PSE.

Based on limited information, the initial oral dosage of lactulose for the prevention and treatment of PSE in infants is 1.67–6.67 g daily given in divided doses. In older children and adolescents, the total daily dose of lactulose suggested by the manufacturers is 27–60 g. Dosage is adjusted every 1–2 days as necessary to produce 2–3 soft stools daily. If the initial dose of lactulose produces diarrhea, the dose should be reduced immediately; if diarrhea persists, the drug should be discontinued.

When lactulose is used rectally in the treatment of PSE to reverse hepatic coma in adults, 200 g is diluted with 700 mL of water or 0.9% sodium chloride solution; the diluted solution is administered rectally via a rectal balloon catheter and retained for 30–60 minutes. Lactulose retention enemas may be administered every 4–6 hours; if the enema is retained for less than 30 minutes, it may be repeated immediately. In some patients, reversal of hepatic coma may occur within 2 hours of the first enema. Before discontinuance of lactulose retention enemas, recommended oral dosages of the drug should be started. Cleansing enemas containing soapsuds or other alkaline agents should not be used concomitantly with lactulose enemas.

Constipation

For the treatment of chronic constipation in adults, the usual initial dosage of lactulose is 10–20 g daily. Dosage may be increased to 40 g daily if necessary. Following oral lactulose administration, 24–48 hours may be required to restore normal bowel movements.

For the treatment of chronic constipation in children†, lactulose dosages of at least 5 g daily, usually given as a single dose after breakfast, have been used. When lactulose was used to restore bowel movements in hemorrhoidectomy patients†, a 10-g dose was given twice during the day before surgery and twice daily for 5 days postoperatively. To induce bowel evacuation in geriatric patients with colonic retention of barium and severe constipation following a barium meal examination†, lactulose dosages of 3.3–6.7 g twice daily for 1–4 weeks have been used.

CAUTIONS

● Adverse Effects

During the first few days of therapy, lactulose frequently produces gaseous distention, belching, flatulence, borborygmi, and/or abdominal discomfort such as cramping. These adverse effects usually subside with continued therapy, but dosage reduction may be required. Diarrhea indicates overdosage and responds to dosage reduction. Potential complications of diarrhea include fluid loss, hypokalemia, and hypernatremia. Infants receiving lactulose may develop dehydration and hyponatremia. Nausea and vomiting have been reported infrequently in patients receiving the drug.

● Precautions and Contraindications

In the treatment of PSE, it is important to remember that the serious underlying liver disease may produce complications such as electrolyte disturbances (e.g., hypokalemia) which require additional therapy. In addition, if diarrhea occurs it may severely deplete fluids and potassium and may intensify symptoms of PSE. For these reasons, some clinicians recommend periodic determinations of serum potassium concentrations during long-term treatment with lactulose.

Lactulose solution should be administered with caution to patients who may require electrocautery procedures during proctoscopy or colonoscopy, since the drug can cause accumulation of hydrogen gas in high concentrations which in the presence of an electrical spark may theoretically result in an explosive reaction. Although this reaction has not been reported to date, patients receiving lactulose therapy should have a thorough bowel cleansing with a nonfermentable solution prior to these procedures. In addition, insufflation of carbon dioxide may be used but is probably an unnecessary measure.

If an unusual diarrheal condition occurs during lactulose therapy, patients should contact their physician. Geriatric, debilitated patients who receive lactulose for more than 6 months should have serum electrolytes (e.g., potassium, chloride, carbon dioxide) measured periodically during therapy.

Since lactulose solution contains some free lactose and galactose, the drug should be used with caution in patients with diabetes mellitus and is contraindicated in patients who require a low-galactose diet.

Laxatives should not be administered with lactulose. (See Drug Interactions: Laxatives.)

● Pediatric Precautions

Limited information on the use of lactulose for prevention and treatment of PSE in young children and adolescents is available. Safety and efficacy of the drug for the treatment of chronic constipation in children have not been established.

● Mutagenicity and Carcinogenicity

Data on the long-term mutagenic potential of lactulose in animals or humans and on the long-term carcinogenic potential in humans are not available. Administration of lactulose solution in concentrations of 3 and 10% v/w in the diet of mice for 18 months did not produce evidence of carcinogenicity.

● Pregnancy, Fertility, and Lactation
Pregnancy

Use of lactulose during pregnancy has not been studied in humans. Reproduction studies in rats, mice, and rabbits receiving oral lactulose doses up to 6 times the usual human oral dose have not revealed evidence of harm to the fetus. Lactulose should be used during pregnancy only when clearly needed.

Fertility

Reproduction studies in rats, mice, and rabbits using oral lactulose dosages of up to 4 or 8 g/kg (6 or 12 mL/kg) daily did not reveal evidence of impaired fertility.

Lactation

It is not known if lactulose is distributed into milk. The drug should be used with caution in nursing women.

DRUG INTERACTIONS

● Laxatives

Additional laxatives should not be administered with lactulose solution, especially when lactulose therapy is initiated, because the loose stools produced may be falsely interpreted as an indication that adequate dosage of lactulose has been achieved.

● Anti-infective Agents

Theoretically, orally administered neomycin and possibly other anti-infective agents, when administered concurrently with lactulose, could eliminate colonic bacteria that are necessary to metabolize lactulose and thereby prevent acidification of the contents of the colon. Limited data obtained from experiments in healthy individuals tend to support the theoretical incompatibility of these agents.

There is, however, evidence that lactulose remains active when administered with neomycin to patients with PSE. In addition, there have been reports that concomitant therapy with lactulose and neomycin may be more effective than either drug alone in the treatment of PSE. Therefore, until there is conclusive evidence that concurrent administration of lactulose and neomycin or other oral anti-infective agents is efficacious, patients receiving lactulose and an oral anti-infective agent should be closely monitored for possible inadequate response to lactulose.

● Antacids

Results of limited studies in rats and humans suggest that nonabsorbable antacids administered concomitantly with lactulose may inhibit the desired decrease in fecal pH in the colon. The potential lack of desired effect of lactulose should be considered before a nonabsorbable antacid is administered concomitantly with lactulose.

ACUTE TOXICITY

No information is available on the acute overdosage of lactulose in humans. The oral LD_{50} of the drug is 48.8 mL/kg in mice and greater than 30 mL/kg in rats. Overdosage of lactulose presumably would be manifested by abdominal cramps and diarrhea (which could result in severe fluid and electrolyte depletion), and treatment would consist of fluid and electrolyte replacement, as required.

PHARMACOLOGY

In patients with portal-systemic encephalopathy (PSE), lactulose causes a decrease in blood ammonia concentration and reduces the degree of PSE. Although the mechanism of action of lactulose has not been clearly defined, it appears to be associated primarily with the metabolism of the sugar in the lower intestinal tract. The breakdown of lactulose to organic acids (i.e., lactic acid and small amounts of formic and acetic acids) by the saccharolytic bacteria in the colon acidifies the contents of the colon. In patients with PSE who respond to lactulose, a decrease in fecal pH occurs. Acidification of colon contents inhibits the nonionic diffusion of ammonia from the colon into the blood. In addition, since the contents of the colon are more acidic than is blood, ammonia (NH_3) can diffuse from the blood into the colon. In the acidic colon, ammonia is converted to ammonium ions (NH_4^+) thereby preventing its absorption. In a similar manner, the absorption of amines (which may also contribute to the development of PSE) may also be reduced. Finally the cathartic action of lactulose (which is probably caused by the osmotic effect of the organic acid metabolites of the drug) expels the trapped ammonium ions and possibly other nitrogenous substances from the colon. The osmotic effect of the organic acid metabolites of lactulose causes an increase in water content of the stool and a softening of the stool; this effect on the stool may not be seen for 24–48 hours after administration of the drug. In patients with chronic constipation, the drug increases the number of bowel movements per day and the number of days when bowel movements occur.

PHARMACOKINETICS

Following oral administration, less than 3% of a dose of lactulose is absorbed from the small intestine. Absorbed lactulose is not metabolized and is excreted in the urine unchanged within 24 hours. Unabsorbed lactulose reaches the colon unchanged where it is metabolized by bacteria to form lactic acid and small amounts of acetic and formic acids. The bacteria normally present in the colon which are capable of metabolizing lactulose include *Lactobacilli, Bacteroides, Escherichia coli,* and *Clostridia,* but not *Proteus mirabilis, Enterococcus faecalis* (formerly *Streptococcus faecalis*), *Salmonella,* or *Shigella.* Only negligible amounts of lactulose or its metabolites are absorbed from the colon.

CHEMISTRY AND STABILITY

● Chemistry

Lactulose, a disaccharide sugar containing one molecule of galactose and one molecule of fructose, is a synthetic derivative of lactose. Lactulose occurs as a white powder or crystals and is very soluble in water and very slightly soluble in alcohol.

Each 10 g of lactulose powder for oral solution also contains a combined total of 0.3 g of galactose and lactose. Following reconstitution of the powder as directed, resultant solutions are colorless to slightly pale yellow and have a pH of 3–7. Commercially available lactulose solutions (which also contain galactose,

lactose, and other sugars) are pale yellow to yellow, sweet, viscous liquids. Sodium hydroxide is added to the commercially available solutions to adjust pH when necessary; the pH of the solutions is 2.5–6.5.

● *Stability*

Lactulose powder and solutions should be stored at 15–30°C; freezing of the solutions should be avoided. Although heat causes cloudiness, and heat and light cause darkening of the solutions, the manufacturers state that these changes do not indicate loss of potency. Prolonged exposure to freezing temperatures may cause lactulose solutions to become semisolid and too viscous to pour; viscosity returns to normal following warming to room temperature. Lactulose solutions have an expiration date of 2 years following the date of manufacture.

PREPARATIONS

Excipients in commercially available drug preparations may have clinically important effects in some individuals; consult specific product labeling for details.

Lactulose

Oral

For solution	10 g/packet*	Kristalose®, Mylan (also promoted by Cumberland)
		Lactulose for Oral Solution
	20 g/packet*	Kristalose®, Mylan (also promoted by Cumberland)
		Lactulose for Oral Solution
Solution	3.33 g/5 mL*	Constilac® Syrup, Alra
		Constulose®, Actavis
		Evalose® Syrup, Teva
		Lactulose Oral Solution

Oral or Rectal

Solution	3.33 g/5 mL*	Cholac® Syrup, Alra
		Enulose®, Actavis
		Generlac®, Morton Grove
		Heptalac®, Teva
		Lactulose Oral or Rectal Solution

* available from one or more manufacturer, distributor, and/or repackager by generic (nonproprietary) name

† Use is not currently included in the labeling approved by the US Food and Drug Administration.

Selected Revisions January 1, 2009, © Copyright, March 1, 1977, American Society of Health-System Pharmacists, Inc.

Calcium Salts

40:12 · REPLACEMENT PREPARATIONS

■ Calcium salts are used as a source of calcium, an essential nutrient cation.

USES

Calcium salts are used as a source of calcium cation for the treatment or prevention of calcium depletion in patients in whom dietary measures are inadequate. Conditions that may be associated with calcium deficiency include hypoparathyroidism, achlorhydria, chronic diarrhea, vitamin D deficiency, steatorrhea, sprue, pregnancy and lactation, menopause, pancreatitis, renal failure, alkalosis, and hyperphosphatemia. Administration of certain drugs (e.g., some diuretics, anticonvulsants) may sometimes result in hypocalcemia which may warrant calcium replacement therapy. Calcium should be administered in long-term electrolyte replacement regimens and is also recommended for the routine prophylaxis of hypocalcemia during transfusions with citrated blood. Administration of calcium salts should not preclude the use of other measures intended to correct the underlying cause of calcium depletion.

● Dietary Requirements

Since 1941, the Institute of Medicine's (IOM) Food and Nutrition Board of the National Academy of Sciences (NAS) has developed guidelines for adequate dietary intake of essential nutrients. Nutrient recommendations are issued through Dietary Reference Intakes (DRIs), which are a set of reference values that can be used for planning and assessing diets for healthy populations and for many other purposes. DRIs for calcium include the Estimated Average Requirement (EAR), Recommended Dietary Allowance (RDA), Adequate Intake (AI), and Tolerable Upper Intake Level (UL). DRIs apply to the healthy general population and consider nutrient levels needed to prevent deficiency as well as those associated with disease risk reduction. The current methods for establishing DRIs differ from those used in the past and incorporate increased understanding of both population and individual nutrient needs. The EAR is the nutrient intake value that is estimated to meet the nutrient needs of 50% of individuals in a particular life-stage and gender group. The RDA, which is derived from the EAR, currently is defined as the estimated daily dietary intake level that is sufficient to meet the nutrient requirements of 97.5% of the population's requirements. The RDA for a given nutrient, in a prescriptive sense, is the *goal* for dietary intake in individuals. If data are insufficient to establish an RDA for a given life-stage group, the AI may be used instead. AIs are based on observed or experimentally determined approximations of the average nutrient intake, by a defined population or subgroup, that appears to sustain a defined nutritional state (e.g., usual circulating nutrient levels, nutrient levels for normal growth).

The previous NAS report from 1997 was unable to establish EARs and RDAs for calcium because of inadequate data attributed in part to uncertainties in the methods used in calcium balance studies, the lack of concordance between observational and experimental data, and the lack of longitudinal data to verify the association between calcium intake, calcium retention, and bone loss. Since then, emerging data from large-scale randomized controlled studies and more recent calcium balance studies have allowed for estimation of EARs and RDAs in all life stage groups except for infants.

The principal goal of maintaining an adequate intake of calcium in the US and Canada is to support the development and preservation of bone mass at a level sufficient to prevent fractures associated with osteopenia or osteoporosis in later life and of other calcified tissues (e.g., teeth), although other biologic roles for calcium and related nutrients (e.g., fluoride, magnesium, phosphorus) have been considered in establishing DRIs. Lifelong intake of adequate calcium is necessary for good bone health at any age. Although some evidence indicates an inverse relationship between calcium intake and blood pressure and that increased calcium intake can reduce blood pressure in certain healthy individuals and some hypertensive patients, there currently is no rationale for recommending calcium supplementation solely to reduce blood pressure; the importance of maintaining adequate calcium intake should be emphasized though, since potential secondary benefits on blood pressure may result.

Adequate intakes of calcium can be accomplished through changes in food consumption behaviors, consumption of nutrient-fortified foodstuffs, use of dietary supplements, or a combination of these. In the US and Canada, calcium principally is obtained from dairy products. Other principal sources include fruits, vegetables, and grain products. In addition, many healthy individuals take dietary supplements containing calcium.

For specific information on currently recommended dietary reference intakes for calcium, see Dosage and Administration: Dosage.

● Parenteral Preparations

Calcium salts are administered IV to treat acute hypocalcemic tetany secondary to renal failure, hypoparathyroidism, premature delivery, and/or maternal diabetes mellitus in infants, and poisoning with magnesium, oxalic acid, radiophosphorus, carbon tetrachloride, fluoride, phosphate, strontium, or radium. Some experts state that administration of calcium also may be useful in the treatment of β-adrenergic blocking agent toxicity in patients with shock refractory to other treatment measures.

IV calcium gluconate is considered by most clinicians to be the salt of choice for the treatment of acute hypocalcemia. In some situations (e.g., critically ill children with hypocalcemia), calcium chloride may be preferred because it can provide a greater increase in ionized calcium concentrations. Some clinicians believe that calcium chloride is the calcium salt of choice for the prevention of hypocalcemia during transfusions with citrated blood. In addition to being irritating, however, the chloride salt is acidifying and generally should not be used when acidosis coincides with hypocalcemia (e.g., renal failure).

Calcium salts have been used IV as adjunctive therapy to reduce spasms in renal†, biliary†, intestinal†, or lead colic. Calcium salts also have been used IV as adjuncts to relieve muscle cramps in the treatment of insect bites or stings (e.g., black widow spider) or to decrease capillary permeability in sensitivity reactions characterized by urticaria or angioedema† and in allergic conditions, including nonthrombocytopenic purpura, dermatitis herpetiformis, drug-induced pruritus, hay fever†, and asthma†.

The calcium glycerophosphate and calcium lactate fixed-combination injection is used IM to increase serum calcium concentrations.

Calcium infusions ("calcium challenge") are used to diagnose the Zollinger-Ellison syndrome† and medullary thyroid carcinoma†. In addition, calcium salt injections are used to antagonize neuromuscular blockade† resulting from the use of aminoglycoside antibiotics (e.g., gentamicin, kanamycin, neomycin) with or without agents possessing neuromuscular blocking properties (e.g., gallamine triethiodide).

Advanced Cardiovascular Life Support

Because of the lack of demonstrated benefit and potential for detrimental effects, the American Heart Association (AHA) guidelines for cardiopulmonary resuscitation (CPR) and emergency cardiovascular care currently state that calcium should not be used routinely for advanced cardiovascular life support (ACLS) during cardiac arrest in adults and pediatric patients unless there is documented hypocalcemia, calcium-channel blocker toxicity, hypermagnesemia, or hyperkalemia. When used in this setting, experts state that either calcium chloride or calcium gluconate may be administered.

● Oral Preparations

Oral calcium therapy may be used for the treatment of osteoporosis, osteomalacia, chronic hypoparathyroidism, rickets, latent tetany, and hypocalcemia secondary to the administration of anticonvulsant drugs. Calcium salts are also used orally in the adjunctive treatment of myasthenia gravis and the Eaton-Lambert syndrome, and as supplemental therapy for pregnant, postmenopausal, or nursing women. In general, any of the oral calcium salts may be used for chronic replacement therapy.

Although some evidence from early trials suggested a beneficial effect of calcium supplementation on preeclampsia, a more recent, large, well-designed study did *not* confirm a beneficial effect of calcium supplementation in preventing preeclampsia during pregnancy. In this study, supplemental administration of calcium (2 g of elemental calcium daily) beginning during the 13th–21st week and continued for the remainder of pregnancy did not prevent preeclampsia, pregnancy-associated hypertension, or adverse perinatal outcomes in healthy nulliparous women. However, these findings do not obviate adequate dietary calcium intake during pregnancy nor do they address whether adequate or increased calcium intake can affect blood pressure favorably in pregnant women.

Calcium acetate or carbonate is considered to be the salt of choice in patients with chronic renal failure. In addition to providing a source of calcium, calcium acetate or carbonate sequesters phosphate in the intestine by forming insoluble phosphates that are excreted fecally, thus reducing serum phosphate concentrations and secondary hyperparathyroidism; calcium carbonate also partially corrects metabolic acidosis which may occur in patients with chronic renal failure. Because of the risk of aluminum accumulation and resultant neurotoxic and osteomalacic effects, most clinicians no longer use aluminum hydroxide to inhibit phosphorus absorption; instead calcium acetate or carbonate and/or non-calcium-, non-aluminum-, non-magnesium-containing phosphate binders (e.g., lanthanum carbonate, sevelamer hydrochloride) currently are used. Therapeutic measures to control hyperphosphatemia in patients with chronic renal disease include reduction in dietary intake of phosphates, inhibition of intestinal phosphate absorption, and removal via dialysis. In individuals with moderate to severe renal impairment (i.e., glomerular filtration rate of 15–59 mL/minute per 1.73 m²), calcium carbonate or acetate may be used to sequester phosphates in the intestine if serum phosphorus or parathyroid hormone (PTH) concentrations are not controlled through dietary restrictions and/or vitamin D therapy. In patients with chronic renal failure, reductions in serum phosphate through dietary restrictions and dialysis generally are insufficient, and inhibition of intestinal phosphate absorption usually is necessary. In these individuals, either a calcium-containing phosphate binder or a non-calcium-, non-aluminum-, non-magnesium-containing phosphate binder may be used as primary therapy. Some experts state that dialysis patients who remain hyperphosphatemic despite treatment with either calcium-based phosphate binders or non-calcium-, non-aluminum-, non-magnesium-containing phosphate binders should receive both types of phosphate binders in combination. Non-calcium-containing phosphate binders are preferred in dialysis patients with severe vascular and/or other soft-tissue calcification. Calcium-containing phosphate binders should not be used in dialysis patients who are hypercalcemic or whose plasma PTH concentrations are less than 150 pg/mL on 2 consecutive measurements. Use of aluminum-containing phosphate binders should be limited to short periods of time (e.g., a single 4-week course) in patients with difficult-to-control serum phosphorus concentrations (e.g., concentrations exceeding 7 mg/dL).

When taken with meals, calcium acetate or carbonate can contribute to controlling hyperphosphatemia in patients with chronic renal failure by binding to and inhibiting absorption of phosphates in the GI tract. Caution should be observed in patients undergoing chronic hemodialysis to prevent hypophosphatemia. Patients with end-stage renal failure may develop hypercalcemia when calcium is administered with meals; therefore, other calcium supplementation should not be given concomitantly when calcium salts are used to control hyperphosphatemia in such patients. Progressive hypercalcemia secondary to overdose of calcium salts in patients with chronic renal disease can occur and may require emergency treatment measures. Chronic hypercalcemia also may lead to vascular and other soft-tissue calcification. Therefore, periodic (e.g., twice weekly) monitoring of calcium concentrations is recommended during the initial dose adjustment period in patients with chronic renal failure. One manufacturer recommends that the serum calcium times phosphate (Ca×P) product should not exceed 66. Radiographic evaluation of a suspected anatomic region for early soft-tissue calcification may be useful.

Vitamin D analogs may be administered concomitantly with oral calcium salts for the treatment of chronic hypocalcemia, especially when caused by vitamin D deficiency.

Calcium chloride, an acid-forming salt, has been used to promote diuresis but, because it is irritating and loses effectiveness after a few days, it is rarely used for this effect.

For the use of calcium carbonate as an antacid, see Antacids 56:04.

Osteoporosis

Calcium salts (e.g., calcium carbonate, calcium citrate) are used as supplements for the prevention and treatment of osteoporosis in patients whose dietary intake of calcium is insufficient.

A principal long-term consequence of inadequate calcium intake is osteoporosis, which is characterized by reduced bone mass, increased bone fragility, and increased fracture risk. Reduced absorption of calcium causes declines in circulating ionized calcium concentrations, which induce increased parathyroid hormone (PTH) synthesis and release. PTH then acts to restore circulating calcium concentrations to normal levels by promoting the reabsorption of calcium in the distal renal tubule, by indirectly increasing intestinal absorption secondary to stimulation of activated vitamin D synthesis, and by inducing bone resorption. Thus, while circulating calcium concentrations can be maintained at normal levels during calcium deprivation, it is at the expense of skeletal mass.

Adequate intake of calcium and vitamin D (which increases absorption of calcium) is universally recommended for all individuals to diminish age-related bone loss and prevent osteoporosis. Controlled clinical studies have demonstrated that the combination of calcium and vitamin D can reduce fracture

risk. In addition to lifestyle modifications (e.g., regular weight-bearing exercise, avoidance of excessive alcohol and tobacco use), the National Osteoporosis Foundation recommends a calcium intake of 1 g daily in men 50–70 years of age, and an intake of 1.2 g daily in women 51 years of age or older and men 71 years of age or older. There is no evidence to suggest that increasing intake above these amounts will provide any additional benefit on bone strength; excess calcium intake has been linked to increased risks of kidney stones, cardiovascular disease, and stroke. It is important to also ensure sufficient calcium and vitamin D intake in children and younger adults to prevent the development of osteoporosis. (See Uses: Dietary Requirements.) If adequate calcium cannot be obtained from diet, calcium supplements are recommended.

Glucocorticoid-induced Osteoporosis

The American College of Rheumatology (ACR) recommends optimizing dietary intake of calcium (1–1.2 g daily) and vitamin D (600–800 units daily) for the prevention of glucocorticoid-induced osteoporosis in all patients receiving long-term glucocorticoid therapy (defined as a daily dosage equivalent to 2.5 mg of prednisone or greater for at least 3 months). Because of concerns about potential harms (e.g., adverse cardiovascular effects), ACR states that additional study is needed to determine the potential benefits versus risks of calcium and vitamin D supplementation in patients receiving glucocorticoids. For additional information on the prevention and treatment of glucocorticoid-induced osteoporosis, see Cautions: Musculoskeletal Effects, in the Corticosteroids General Statement 68:04.

DOSAGE AND ADMINISTRATION

• Administration

The acetate, carbonate, citrate, gluconate, lactate, and phosphate salts of calcium are administered orally. It has been recommended that most oral calcium supplements be administered 1–1.5 hours after meals or with a demulcent (e.g., milk). However, calcium carbonate powder (i.e., CAL CARB-HD®) should generally be administered with meals, since the manufacturer recommends mixing the powder with food for administration. Calcium salts used to bind dietary phosphate in patients with end-stage renal disease should be administered with meals (e.g., 10–15 minutes before, or during, the meal).

Calcium chloride and calcium gluconate may be administered IV. Calcium chloride also may be administered by intraosseous (IO) injection† in the setting of pediatric resuscitation; onset of action and systemic concentrations are comparable to those achieved with venous administration. Parenteral calcium salts may be administered in large volume IV infusion fluids.

IV calcium injections must be administered slowly at a rate not exceeding 0.7–1.8 mEq/minute, and the injection should be stopped if the patient complains of discomfort. Following IV injection, the patient should remain recumbent for a short time. Close monitoring of serum calcium concentrations is essential during IV administration of calcium. Calcium chloride should not be injected IM or into subcutaneous or perivascular tissue, since severe necrosis and sloughing may occur. Although other calcium salts may cause mild to severe local reactions, they are generally less irritating than calcium chloride. (See Cautions.) The fixed combination of calcium glycerophosphate and calcium lactate is injected IM. Although some manufacturers previously stated that calcium gluconate could be injected IM when IV administration was not possible, manufacturers of calcium gluconate currently state that the drug should not be injected IM or into subcutaneous tissue because of the potential for severe local reactions. In children, calcium salts should not be administered through scalp veins. Oral administration of calcium supplements or calcium-rich foods should replace parenteral calcium therapy as soon as possible.

The interaction of calcium and phosphate in parenteral nutrition solutions is a complex phenomenon; various factors have been identified as playing a role in the solubility or precipitation of a given combination. Calcium salts are conditionally compatible with phosphate in parenteral nutrition solutions; incompatibility is dependent on a solubility and concentration phenomenon and is not entirely predictable. Precipitation may occur during compounding or at some time after compounding is completed. Specialized references should be consulted for specific compatibility information.

• Dosage

Dosage of the oral calcium supplements is usually expressed in grams or mg of elemental calcium and depends on the requirements of the individual patient. Dosage of parenteral calcium replacements is usually expressed as mEq of calcium and depends on individual patient requirements. One mEq of elemental calcium is equivalent to 20 mg. See Table 1 for the approximate calcium content of the various calcium salts.

TABLE 1.

Calcium Salt	Calcium Content
calcium acetate	253 mg (12.7 mEq) per g
calcium carbonate	400 mg (20 mEq) per g
calcium chloride	270 mg (13.5 mEq) per g
calcium citrate	211 mg (10.6 mEq) per g
calcium gluceptate	82 mg (4.1 mEq) per g
calcium gluconate	90 mg (4.5 mEq) per g
calcium glycerophosphate	191 mg (9.6 mEq) per g
calcium lactate	130 mg (6.5 mEq) per g
calcium phosphate dibasic anhydrous	290 mg (14.5 mEq) per g
calcium phosphate dibasic dihydrate	230 mg (11.5 mEq) per g
calcium phosphate tribasic	400 mg (20 mEq) per g

Oral calcium supplements usually are administered in 3 or 4 divided doses daily. Optimum calcium absorption may require supplemental vitamin D in individuals with inadequate vitamin D intake, those with impaired renal activation of the vitamin, or those not receiving adequate exposure to sunlight.

Dietary and Replacement Requirements

Because of insufficient data to establish estimated average requirements (EARs) in infants younger than 1 year of age, the National Academy of Sciences (NAS) has developed adequate intakes (AIs) for calcium in this population (see Uses: Dietary Requirements). Calcium requirements in infants are presumed to be met by human milk; thus, AIs developed for this age group are principally based on mean intake data from infants receiving human milk. The AI recommended for healthy **infants up to 6 months of age** is 200 mg daily and for **infants 6–12 months of age** is 260 mg daily (taking into account additional intake of calcium from food).

In **children and adolescents 1–18 years of age**, the recommended dietary reference intake values for calcium are determined based on levels required to support bone accretion and calcium retention. Using this approach, the EAR of elemental calcium currently recommended by the NAS for healthy children 1–3, 4–8, or 9–18 years of age is 500, 800, or 1100 mg daily, respectively, and the Recommended Dietary Allowance (RDA) for these respective age groups is 700, 1000, and 1300 mg daily. Many chronic illnesses that affect children are associated with abnormalities in calcium metabolism and bone mineralization, and special consideration should be given for different calcium requirements in such children; some such diseases include juvenile rheumatologic conditions, renal disease, liver failure, and certain endocrine disorders, including type 1 (insulin-dependent) diabetes mellitus.

The goal of calcium intake in **adults 19–50 years of age** is to promote bone maintenance and neutral calcium balance. Based on a series of controlled calcium balance studies in this age group, NAS recommends an EAR of 800 mg daily and an RDA of 1 g daily.

Calcium intake in **adults 51–70 years of age** is principally focused on lessening the degree of bone loss that manifests during later stages of adulthood. Because of menopause, the natural process of bone loss occurs earlier for women than for men. Findings from the Women's Health Initiative (WHI) study revealed modest improvements in BMD and risk of fractures in women 50–79 years of age who received daily supplementation with 1 g calcium plus 400 units vitamin D; however, these results should be interpreted cautiously because of possible confounding factors (e.g., concomitant use of hormone replacement therapy). While considering these limitations, NAS states that the emerging evidence indicates that a somewhat higher intake of calcium may be justified in postmenopausal women 51–70 years of age compared with similarly aged men. In men 51–70 years of age, the recommended EAR for calcium is 800 mg daily and the RDA is

1 g daily; in women 51–70 years of age, the recommended EAR for calcium is 1 g daily and the recommended RDA is 1.2 g daily.

Bone loss and resulting risk of fractures are the predominant concerns when developing calcium intake recommendations in **adults older than 70 years of age**. However, a dose-response relationship for calcium and fracture risk has not been established and calcium balance studies are lacking in this age group. Given these limitations, NAS recommends the same calcium requirements in adults older than 70 years of age as for those recommended in postmenopausal women (EAR of 1 g daily and RDA of 1.2 g daily).

Because of adaptive maternal responses to fetal calcium needs (e.g., changes in calciotropic hormones and resultant enhanced calcium absorption) and the fact that the maternal skeleton does not appear to act as a reservoir for fetal calcium needs, calcium requirements are not increased during pregnancy. Randomized controlled studies have not demonstrated any additional benefits to the mother or fetus from increased intake of calcium during pregnancy. Therefore, the usual calcium recommendations that are appropriate for age in nonpregnant women should be used in pregnant women. Likewise, there is no evidence that calcium requirements are increased during lactation and the same calcium intake recommendations are given for lactating as for nonlactating women. Physiologic changes occur naturally in maternal bone during and after lactation to provide the infant with calcium without impairing maternal bone mass, and increased calcium intake does not appear to alter this process.

Calcium replacement requirements can be estimated by clinical condition and/or serum calcium determinations. Prophylactic administration of calcium supplements may be necessary in some patients in order to maintain serum calcium above 9 mg/dL. The average adult oral dosage of elemental calcium for prevention of hypocalcemia is about 1 g daily, and the usual oral dosage for treatment of calcium depletion is 1–2 g or more daily. In children, the usual supplemental dosage of elemental calcium is 45–65 mg/kg daily. In neonatal hypocalcemia, the daily dosage of elemental calcium is 50–150 mg/kg and should not exceed 1 g.

Calcium gluconate is usually administered IV as a 10% solution and calcium chloride as a 2–10% solution. The manufacturers state that the usual initial IV dose of calcium for prompt elevation of serum calcium is 2.3–14 mEq for adults, 0.93–2.3 mEq for children, and less than 0.93 mEq for infants. It has been recommended that these doses be repeated every 1–3 days depending on the patient's response. Alternatively, one manufacturer recommends a pediatric IV dose of 0.272 mEq of calcium per kg, up to a maximum total daily dosage of 1.36–13.6 mEq, in the treatment of hypocalcemic disorders. For the treatment of hypocalcemic tetany, 4.5–16 mEq doses of calcium may be administered IV to adults until therapeutic response occurs. In children with hypocalcemic tetany, 0.5–0.7 mEq/kg may be administered IV 3 or 4 times daily or until tetany is controlled. Neonatal tetany may be treated with divided doses totaling about 2.4 mEq/kg daily.

The usual adult IM dosage of the calcium glycerophosphate and calcium lactate fixed-combination preparation given to increase serum calcium concentrations is 0.8 mEq of calcium 1–4 times weekly or as directed by a clinician.

Advanced Cardiovascular Life Support
Adult Dosage

If calcium administration is necessary during cardiac arrest, an IV dose of 0.109–0.218 mEq/kg (repeated as necessary) using calcium chloride has been recommended. Alternatively, adults have been given IV calcium doses of 7–14 mEq using calcium chloride. However, routine administration of calcium in patients with cardiac arrest is not recommended. (See Advanced Cardiovascular Life Support under Uses: Parenteral Preparations.)

Pediatric Dosage

If administration of calcium is indicated for the treatment of hypocalcemia, calcium-channel blocker overdosage, hypermagnesemia, or hyperkalemia during pediatric resuscitation, experts recommend a pediatric IV or IO† calcium dose of 0.272 mEq/kg using calcium chloride. In critically ill children, calcium chloride may provide a greater increase in ionized calcium than calcium gluconate. The appropriate dose should be administered by slow IV or IO† injection.

Other Dosages

When calcium acetate is used orally to control hyperphosphatemia in adults with chronic renal failure, the recommended initial dosage is 1.334 g of calcium acetate (338 mg of calcium) with each meal. Dosage may be increased gradually according to serum phosphate concentrations, provided hypercalcemia does not occur. The manufacturer states that most patients require about 2–2.67 g (about 500–680 mg of calcium) with each meal. However, some experts state that the dosage of calcium provided by calcium-containing phosphate binders should not exceed 1.5 g daily and that the total calcium intake (including dietary calcium) should not exceed 2 g daily. These experts state that dialysis patients who remain hyperphosphatemic despite such therapy should receive a calcium-containing phosphate binder in combination with a non-calcium-, non-aluminum-, non-magnesium-containing phosphate binder. The manufacturer recommends that serum calcium concentrations be monitored twice weekly during initiation of calcium acetate therapy and subsequent dosage adjustment; serum phosphorus concentrations also should be monitored periodically. If hypercalcemia occurs, dosage should be reduced or the salt should be withheld. If severe hypercalcemia occurs, specific measures (e.g., hemodialysis) for the management of overdosage may be necessary. Patients should be advised of the importance of dosage compliance, adherence to instructions about diet, and avoidance of concomitant use of antacids or other preparations containing clinically important concentrations of calcium. Patients also should be advised of potential manifestations of hypercalcemia.

For the treatment of hyperkalemia with secondary cardiac toxicity, 2.25–14 mEq of calcium may be administered IV while monitoring the ECG. Doses may be repeated after 1–2 minutes if necessary.

Magnesium intoxication in adults is treated initially with 7 mEq of IV calcium; subsequent doses should be adjusted according to patient response. Alternatively, for the treatment of hypermagnesemia in adults, an IV calcium dose of 6.8–13.6 mEq using 10% calcium chloride (5–10 mL) has been administered, and repeated as necessary.

For the treatment of drug-induced cardiovascular emergencies associated with calcium-channel blocking agent toxicity in pediatric patients, an IV calcium dose of 0.272 mEq/kg using 10% calcium chloride (0.2 mL/kg) has been administered over 5–10 minutes; if a beneficial effect was observed, an IV calcium infusion of 0.27–0.68 mEq/kg per hour using calcium chloride has been administered. Ionized calcium concentrations should be monitored to prevent hypercalcemia.

Calcium is also administered IV during exchange transfusions in neonates in a dosage of 0.45 mEq of calcium after every 100 mL of citrated blood exchanged. In adults receiving transfusions of citrated blood, about 1.35 mEq of calcium should be administered IV concurrently with each 100 mL of citrated blood.

In the calcium infusion test†, calcium is given IV in a dosage of 0.25 mEq/kg per hour for a 3-hour period; serum gastrin concentrations are determined 30 minutes before the infusion, at the start of the infusion, and at 30-minute intervals thereafter for 4 hours. In most patients with Zollinger-Ellison syndrome, pre-infusion serum gastrin concentrations increase by more than 50% or by greater than 500 pg/mL during the infusion. In the diagnosis of medullary thyroid carcinoma†, about 7 mEq of calcium is given IV over 5–10 minutes. In patients with medullary thyroid carcinoma, plasma calcitonin concentrations are elevated above normal basal concentrations.

CAUTIONS

● Local Effects

Calcium salts are irritating to tissue when administered by IM or subcutaneous injection and cause mild to severe local reactions including burning, necrosis and sloughing of tissue, cellulitis, and soft tissue calcification; venous irritation may occur with IV administration. When injected IV, calcium salts should be administered slowly through a small needle into a large vein to avoid too rapid an increase in serum calcium and extravasation of calcium solution into the surrounding tissue with resultant necrosis. Patients may complain of tingling sensations, a sense of oppression or heat waves, and a calcium or chalky taste following IV administration of calcium salts.

● Cardiovascular Effects

Rapid IV injection of calcium salts may cause vasodilation, decreased blood pressure, bradycardia, cardiac arrhythmias, syncope, and cardiac arrest.

● GI Effects

Orally administered calcium salts may be irritating to the GI tract. Calcium salts also may cause constipation. Calcium chloride, by any route of administration, produces more irritation than the other calcium salts and has been reported to cause GI hemorrhage when taken orally.

● Hypercalcemia

Hypercalcemia is rarely produced by administration of calcium alone, but may occur when large doses are given to patients with chronic renal failure. Since hypercalcemia may be more dangerous than hypocalcemia, overtreatment of hypocalcemia should be avoided. Mild hypercalcemia may be asymptomatic or manifest as constipation, anorexia, nausea, and vomiting, with mental changes such as confusion, delirium, stupor, and coma becoming evident as the degree of hypercalcemia increases. Mild hypercalcemia usually is readily controlled by reducing calcium intake (e.g., decreasing the dose of or avoiding supplemental calcium); more severe hypercalcemia may require specific management (e.g., hemodialysis). In dialysis patients with chronic renal failure receiving calcium salts, adjustments in calcium concentrations in the dialysate may be necessary to reduce the risk of hypercalcemia. The long-term effect of chronic calcium administration (e.g., in patients with chronic renal failure receiving calcium salts to control hyperphosphatemia) on progression of vascular or soft-tissue calcification is not known.

● Renal Calculi

Because the principal constituents of most renal calculi (kidney stones) are calcium salts, a high dietary intake of calcium has long been suspected as contributing to the risk of renal calculi, and restriction of calcium intake (i.e., low-calcium diets) had long been considered a reasonable measure in an attempt to prevent calculi formation in patients with idiopathic hypocalciuria. However, recent evidence from studies in men 40–75 years of age with no history of kidney stones and in women 34–59 years of age participating in the Nurses'; Health Study I indicates that high dietary intake of calcium actually decreases the risk of symptomatic renal calculi, while intake of supplemental calcium may increase the risk of symptomatic stones. High calcium intake can reduce urinary oxalate excretion, which is thought to lower the risk of renal calculi. In addition, dietary calcium can reduce the GI absorption of oxalate. Therefore, differences in calculi risk between high dietary calcium intake and calcium supplementation may be associated in part with differences in the timing of calcium ingestion relative to oxalate consumption or with other factors present in dairy products (the principal source of dietary calcium) that are not present in supplements.

● Precautions and Contraindications

Frequent determinations of serum calcium concentrations should be performed, and serum calcium concentrations should be maintained at 9–10.4 mg/dL (4.5–5.2 mEq/L). Some clinicians prefer to maintain serum calcium at slightly lower concentrations. Serum calcium concentrations usually should not be allowed to exceed 12 mg/dL. Administration of calcium in patients who have received transfusions of citrated blood may result in higher than normal total serum calcium concentrations. In these patients, however, most of the excess calcium is bound to citrate and is inactive; therefore, serious toxicity usually does not result. Although determinations of urine calcium have been advised, they are generally unreliable and hypercalciuria can occur in the presence of hypocalcemia. Some clinicians recommend forcing fluids to produce increased urine volume and thus prevent the formation of renal stones in patients with hypercalciuria. When hypercalcemia occurs, discontinuance of the drug is usually sufficient to return serum calcium concentrations to normal.

Calcium salts should be used cautiously, if at all, in patients with sarcoidosis, renal or cardiac disease, and in patients receiving cardiac glycosides. (See Drug Interactions: Cardiac Glycosides.) Calcium salts are contraindicated in patients with ventricular fibrillation or hypercalcemia. IV administration of calcium is contraindicated when serum calcium concentrations are above normal.

DRUG INTERACTIONS

● Bisphosphonates

Concomitant administration of calcium salts with bisphosphonates (e.g., alendronate, etidronate, ibandronate, risedronate) may reduce absorption of the bisphosphonate from the GI tract. To minimize this effect, the drugs should be administered at separate times.

● Cardiac Glycosides

The inotropic and toxic effects of cardiac glycosides and calcium are synergistic and arrhythmias may occur if these drugs are given together (particularly when calcium is given IV). IV administration of calcium should be avoided in patients receiving cardiac glycosides, particularly if digoxin toxicity is suspected; if necessary, calcium should be given slowly in small amounts.

● **Iron Preparations**

Concomitant administration of calcium salts and oral iron preparations may result in reduced absorption of iron. Patients should be advised to take the drugs at different times, whenever possible.

● **Levothyroxine**

Calcium carbonate may form an insoluble chelate with levothyroxine, resulting in decreased levothyroxine absorption and increased serum thyrotropin concentrations. To minimize or prevent this interaction, oral levothyroxine sodium should be administered at least 4 hours apart from calcium carbonate.

● **Quinolones**

Concomitant administration of calcium salts and some fluoroquinolones (e.g., ciprofloxacin) may reduce oral bioavailability of the fluoroquinolone. For further information, including any specific instructions regarding timing of drug administration when concomitant use is necessary, see the individual monographs for quinolones in 8:12.18.

● **Tetracyclines**

Calcium complexes tetracycline antibiotics rendering them inactive; the 2 drugs should not be given at the same time orally nor should they be mixed for parenteral administration.

For further information on drug interactions with calcium salts, see Drug Interactions in Antacids 56:04.

LABORATORY TEST INTERFERENCES

Transient elevations of plasma 11-hydroxycorticosteroid concentrations (Glenn-Nelson technique) may occur when IV calcium is administered, but concentrations return to control values after 1 hour. In addition, IV calcium salts can produce false-negative values for serum and urinary magnesium as measured by the Titan yellow method.

PHARMACOLOGY

Calcium is essential for maintenance of the functional integrity of nervous, muscular, and skeletal systems and cell-membrane and capillary permeability. The cation is an important activator in many enzymatic reactions and is essential to a number of physiologic processes including transmission of nerve impulses; contraction of cardiac, smooth, and skeletal muscles; renal function; respiration; and blood coagulation. Calcium also plays regulatory roles in the release and storage of neurotransmitters and hormones, in the uptake and binding of amino acids, and in cyanocobalamin (vitamin B_{12}) absorption and gastrin secretion. There is evidence indicating an inverse relationship between calcium intake and blood pressure and that calcium supplementation may be associated with a reduction in blood pressure in healthy young adults and healthy pregnant women and in some patients with hypertension; however, further study is needed to evaluate further the role of calcium in blood pressure regulation.

Calcium accounts for 1–2% of adult body weight, and more than 99% of total body calcium is found in bone and teeth. Calcium also is present in blood, extracellular fluid, muscle, and other tissues where it has roles in mediating vascular contraction and vasodilation, muscle contraction, nerve transmission, and glandular secretion. Calcium is present in bone mainly as hydroxyapatite, with bone mineral content representing about 40% of bone weight. Bone is a dynamic tissue that constantly undergoes osteoclastic bone resorption and osteoblastic bone formation, with a portion of bone being remodeled (reabsorbed and replaced with new bone) each year. Formation exceeds resorption in growing children, is balanced with resorption in healthy adults, and lags behind resorption after menopause and with aging in both genders. The rate of cortical (compact) bone remodeling can be as high as 50% annually in young children and is about 5% annually in adults; trabecular (cancellous) bone remodeling is about fivefold that of cortical remodeling in adults. In addition to serving as a structural support for the body, the skeleton also serves as a reservoir for calcium. Although both exercise and calcium intake influence bone mass, it currently is unclear whether calcium intake influences the degree of benefit on bone derived from exercise.

Conditions associated with reduced concentrations of circulating estrogen alter calcium homeostasis. Exercise-induced amenorrhea results in reduced calcium retention and lower bone mass, and anorexia-induced amenorrhea results in reduced net calcium absorption, increased urinary calcium excretion, and a reduced rate of bone formation, when compared with eumenorrheic women. Decreased estrogen production at menopause is associated with accelerated bone loss, particularly from the lumbar spine, for about 5 years, during which time skeletal mass loss averages about 3% per year. Reduced estrogen concentrations are associated with reduced calcium absorption efficiency and increased bone turnover rates. While it is unclear whether the principal effect of estrogens on calcium is at the skeletal or intestinal level, examination of the skeletal response to calcium supplementation in premenopausal and early postmenopausal women indicates that increased calcium intake will not prevent the rapid trabecular bone loss that occurs during the first 5 years after menopause and that the calcium intake requirement for women does not appear to change acutely with menopause. Calcium responsiveness of cortical bone appears to depend less on menopausal status than does that of trabecular bone. Calcium requirements in vegetarians may be increased because of the negative effects of oxalate and phytate (present in high concentrations in vegetarian diets) on calcium bioavailability. Because lactose-intolerant individuals often avoid consumption of dairy products, the principal source of calcium in the US and Canada, they may be calcium deficient; however, there is no evidence to indicate that lactose intolerance influences the calcium requirement per se, although it may negatively influence calcium intake.

PHARMACOKINETICS

● **Absorption**

Calcium is absorbed from the GI tract by active transport and passive diffusion. Calcium is actively absorbed in the duodenum and proximal jejunum and, to a lesser extent, in the more distal segments of the small intestine. The degree of absorption depends on a number of factors; calcium is never completely absorbed from the intestine. For absorption to occur, calcium must be in a soluble, ionized form. The efficiency of intestinal calcium absorption may be increased when calcium intake is reduced and during pregnancy and lactation when calcium requirements are higher than normal. However, when hypocalcemia is caused by deficiency of either parathyroid hormone or vitamin D, calcium absorption decreases. As serum calcium concentration rises, negative feedback control by parathyroid hormone results in decreased calcium absorption. Vitamin D, in its activated forms, is required for calcium absorption and increases the capability of the absorptive mechanisms. Active transport of calcium into enterocytes and out on the serosal side of the intestinal mucosa depends on the action of activated vitamin D (1,25-dihydroxyvitamin D) and its intestinal receptors; this mechanism accounts for most of the calcium absorption from the GI tract at low and moderate intake levels. Calcium also diffuses passively between intestinal mucosal cells, depending on the luminal:serosal concentration gradient of the ion; the importance of passive diffusion increases with high calcium intakes. An acidic intestinal pH is necessary for ionization of calcium; thus an alkaline pH impedes absorption.

Oral bioavailability of calcium from nonfood sources and supplements depends on intestinal pH, the presence or absence of a meal, and the dose. When a 250-mg dose of calcium is administered with a standardized breakfast, average oral bioavailability in adults ranges from 25–35% with various salts; under the same conditions, absorption from milk was about 29%. Calcium absorption is decreased in the absence of a meal. The extent of calcium absorption from supplements is greatest when calcium is taken in doses of 500 mg or less.

Fractional calcium absorption varies with age, being highest during infancy (about 60%), declining to about 28% in prepubertal children, and rising again during early puberty (about 34%); fractional absorption remains at about 25% in young adults, although it increases during the last 2 trimesters of pregnancy. With aging, fractional absorption declines, decreasing on average by 0.21% annually in postmenopausal women. Similar declines also appear to occur with aging in men.

Absorption is retarded by certain anions (e.g., oxalates, phytates, sulfates) and by fatty acids which precipitate or complex calcium ions; however, an intestinal pH of 5–7 facilitates maximal dissolution and dissociation of these complexes. As a result, calcium may be poorly absorbed from foods rich in oxalic acid (e.g., spinach, sweet potatoes, rhubarb, beans) or phytic acid (e.g., unleavened bread, raw beans, seeds, nuts, grains, soy isolates). Although soybeans contain high concentrations of phytic acid, calcium absorption is relatively high from this food. Glucocorticoids and low serum concentrations of calcitonin may depress the absorption of calcium. Calcium absorption is decreased in patients with certain disease states such as achlorhydria, renal osteodystrophy, steatorrhea, or uremia.

IM or IV administered calcium salts are absorbed directly into the blood stream. Following IV injection of calcium salts, serum calcium concentrations increase almost immediately and may return to previous values in 30 minutes to 2 hours.

● **Distribution**

Following absorption, calcium first enters the extracellular fluid and is then rapidly incorporated into skeletal tissue. Bone formation, however, is not stimulated by administration of calcium. Bone contains 99% of the body's calcium; the remaining 1% is distributed equally between the intracellular and extracellular fluids.

Normal total serum calcium concentrations range from 9–10.4 mg/dL (4.5–5.2 mEq/L), but only ionized calcium is physiologically active. Serum calcium concentrations are not necessarily accurate indications of total body calcium; total body calcium may be decreased in the presence of hypercalcemia, and hypocalcemia can occur even though total body calcium is increased. Of the total serum calcium concentration, 50% is in the ionic form and 5% is complexed by phosphates, citrates, and other anions. Approximately 45% of the serum calcium is bound to plasma proteins; for a change in serum albumin of 1 g/dL, the serum calcium concentration may change about 0.8 mg/dL (0.04 mEq/dL). Hyperproteinemia is associated with increased total serum calcium concentrations; in hypoproteinemia, total serum calcium concentrations decrease. Acidosis results in increased concentrations of ionic calcium, while alkalosis promotes a decrease in the ionic serum calcium concentration.

CSF concentrations of calcium are about 50% of serum calcium concentrations and tend to reflect ionized serum calcium concentrations. Calcium crosses the placenta and reaches higher concentrations in fetal blood than in maternal blood. Calcium is distributed into milk.

● **Elimination**

Calcium is excreted mainly in the feces and consists of unabsorbed calcium and that secreted via bile and pancreatic juice into the lumen of the GI tract. Most of the calcium filtered by renal glomeruli is reabsorbed in the ascending limb of the loop of Henle and proximal and distal convoluted tubules. Only small amounts of the cation are excreted in urine. Parathyroid hormone, vitamin D, and thiazide diuretics decrease urinary excretion of calcium, whereas other diuretics, calcitonin, and growth hormone promote renal excretion of the cation. Urinary excretion of calcium decreases with reduction of ionic serum calcium concentrations but is proportionately increased as serum ionized calcium concentrations increase. In healthy adults on a regular diet, urinary excretion of calcium may be as high as 250–300 mg daily. With low calcium diets, urinary excretion usually does not exceed 150 mg daily. Urinary excretion of calcium decreases during pregnancy and in the early stages of renal failure. Urinary excretion of calcium decreases with aging, possibly because of age-related decreases in intestinal calcium absorption efficiency and an associated decrease in filtered calcium load. Endogenous fecal calcium excretion does not change appreciably with aging. Calcium is also excreted by the sweat glands.

CHEMISTRY AND STABILITY

● Chemistry

Calcium is an essential nutrient cation, and calcium salts are used for the prevention or treatment of calcium depletion. For oral administration, the acetate, carbonate, citrate, gluconate, lactate, and phosphate salts of calcium are available as single ingredients and/or as components of combination products. The chloride, gluconate, and a combination of the glycerophosphate and lactate salts are available as injections.

Calcium chloride is freely soluble, and calcium lactate and calcium acetate are soluble in water. Calcium gluconate and calcium glycerophosphate are sparingly soluble, and the carbonate and phosphate salts of calcium are insoluble in water. Calcium chloride is deliquescent, and calcium lactate is somewhat efflorescent. Calcium gluconate injection may contain small amounts of calcium d-saccharate or other calcium salts as stabilizers and has a pH of 6–8.2. Calcium chloride injection has a pH of 5.5–7.5 and calcium glycerophosphate-calcium lactate injection has a pH of about 7.

● Stability

The interaction of calcium and phosphate in parenteral nutrition solutions is a well-documented, but complex, phenomenon (see Dosage and Administration: Administration). Calcium injections have been reported to be incompatible with IV solutions containing various drugs. Published data are too varied and/or limited to permit generalizations, and specialized references should be consulted for specific compatibility information.

PREPARATIONS

Excipients in commercially available drug preparations may have clinically important effects in some individuals; consult specific product labeling for details.

Calcium Acetate

Powder		
		Calcium Acetate Powder
Oral		
Capsules	667 mg (169 mg calcium; 8.45 mEq of Ca++)*	Calcium Acetate Capsules
		PhosLo® GelCaps, Fresenius

* available from one or more manufacturer, distributor, and/or repackager by generic (nonproprietary) name

Calcium Carbonate, Precipitated

Powder		
		Calcium Carbonate, Precipitated Powder
Oral		
Capsules	1.25 g (500 mg calcium)	Calci-Mix®, Watson
Capsules, liquid-filled	600 mg (240 mg of calcium)	Liqui-Cal® Softgels®, Advanced Nutritional Technology
Suspension	1.25 g (500 mg calcium) per 5 mL*	Calcium Carbonate Suspension
Tablets	650 mg (260 mg calcium)*	Calcium Carbonate Tablets
	1.25 g (500 mg calcium)*	Calcium Carbonate Tablets (scored)
		Os-Cal® 500, GlaxoSmithKline
Tablets, chewable	420 mg (168 mg calcium)	Titralac®, 3M
	500 mg (200 mg calcium)	Chooz®, Insight
	750 mg (300 mg calcium)	Tums E-X® 750, GlaxoSmithKline
	850 mg (340 mg calcium)	Alka-Mints®, Bayer
	1 g (400 mg calcium)	Tums® Ultra 1000, GlaxoSmithKline
	1.25 g (500 mg calcium)*	Calci-Chew®, Watson
		Calcium Carbonate Chewable Tablets
		Os-Cal® 500, GlaxoSmithKline
Tablets, film-coated	1.5 g (600 mg calcium)*	Calcium Carbonate Tablets
		Caltrate® 600, Wyeth

* available from one or more manufacturer, distributor, and/or repackager by generic (nonproprietary) name

Calcium Carbonate, Precipitated, Combinations

Oral		
Pieces, chewable	1.25 g (500 mg calcium) with Cholecalciferol 100 units and Phytonadione 40 mcg	Viactiv® Soft Calcium Chews, McNeil
Tablets	Calcium Carbonate 240 mg with Calcium Gluconate 240 mg, Calcium Lactate 240 mg, (152.8 mg calcium) and Cholecalciferol 100 units	Calcet®, Mission
	1.25 g (500 mg calcium) with Cholecalciferol 200 units	Os-Cal® 500+D, GlaxoSmithKline
	1.5 g (600 mg calcium) with Cholecalciferol 125 units*	Calcium Carbonate, Precipitated, and Cholecalciferol Tablets

Tablets, film-coated	1.5 g (600 mg calcium) with Cholecalciferol 280 units*	**Calcium Carbonate, Precipitated, and Cholecalciterol Tablets**
		Healthy Woman® (scored), Personal Products
Tablets, film-coated	1.5 g (600 mg calcium) with Cholecalciferol 400 units	**Caltrate® 600 + Vitamin D,** Wyeth

* available from one or more manufacturer, distributor, and/or repackager by generic (nonproprietary) name

Calcium Chloride

Powder

| | | **Calcium Chloride Powder** |

Parenteral

| Injection | 10% (1.36–1.4 mEq of Ca⁺⁺ and Cl⁻ per mL)* | **Calcium Chloride Injection** |

* available from one or more manufacturer, distributor, and/or repackager by generic (nonproprietary) name

Calcium Citrate

Oral

| Tablets | 950 mg (200 mg calcium) | **Citracal®,** Bayer |

Calcium Citrate Combinations

Oral

| Tablets | 1.5 g (315 mg calcium) with Cholecalciferol 250 units | **Citracal® + D Caplets®,** Bayer |

Calcium Gluceptate

Powder

| | | **Calcium Gluceptate Powder** |

Calcium Gluconate

Powder

| | | **Calcium Gluconate Powder** |

Oral

Tablets	500 mg (45 mg calcium)*	**Calcium Gluconate Tablets**
	650 mg (58.5 mg calcium)*	**Calcium Gluconate Tablets**
	1 g (90 mg calcium)*	**Calcium Gluconate Tablets**

Parenteral

| Injection | 10% (0.45–0.48 mEq of Ca⁺⁺ per mL provided by calcium gluconate and other calcium salt stabilizers)* | **Calcium Gluconate Injection** |
| **Injection, for preparation of IV admixtures** | 10% (0.45–0.48 mEq of Ca⁺⁺ per mL provided by calcium gluconate and calcium saccharate or other calcium salts stabilizers) pharmacy bulk package* | **Calcium Gluconate Injection** |

* available from one or more manufacturer, distributor, and/or repackager by generic (nonproprietary) name

Calcium Glycerophosphate

Powder

| | | **Calcium Glycerophosphate Powder** |

Calcium Glycerophosphate and Calcium Lactate

Parenteral

| Injection | 0.08 mEq of Ca⁺⁺ (provided by calcium glycerophosphate 5 mg and calcium lactate 5 mg) per mL | **Calphosan®,** Glenwood |

Calcium Lactate

Powder

| | | **Calcium Lactate Powder** |

Oral

| Tablets | 325 mg (42.25 mg calcium)* | **Calcium Lactate Tablets** |
| | 650 mg (84.5 mg calcium)* | **Calcium Lactate Tablets** |

* available from one or more manufacturer, distributor, and/or repackager by generic (nonproprietary) name

Calcium Phosphate Dibasic

Powder

| | | **Calcium Phosphate Dibasic Powder** |

Calcium Phosphate Tribasic

Powder

| | | **Calcium Phosphate Tribasic Powder** |

Oral

| Tablets, film-coated | 1.5652 g (600 mg calcium) | **Posture®** (scored), Inverness |

Calcium Phosphate Tribasic Combinations

Oral

| Tablets, film-coated | 1.5652 g (600 mg calcium) with Cholecalciferol 125 units | **Posture-D®** (scored), Inverness |

Calcium salts are also commercially available in combination with vitamins, minerals, electrolytes, and antacids.

† Use is not currently included in the labeling approved by the US Food and Drug Administration.

Selected Revisions January 7, 2019, © Copyright, September 1, 1979, American Society of Health-System Pharmacists, Inc.

Hetastarch

40:12 • REPLACEMENT PREPARATIONS

■ Hetastarch, a nonprotein synthetic colloid, is a plasma volume expander.

USES

● Hypovolemia

Hetastarch solutions are used for plasma volume expansion in the treatment of hypovolemia associated with elective surgery; safety of hetastarch in the treatment of hypovolemia in situations other than elective surgery has not been established. Hetastarch should not be used as a substitute for whole blood or plasma.

Plasma volume expansion produced by hetastarch solutions is comparable to that of albumin. For additional information on use of colloids in the treatment of hypovolemia, see Uses in Albumin Human 16:00.

● Leukapheresis

Solutions containing 6% hetastarch in 0.9% sodium chloride injection are used as an adjunct in leukapheresis to enhance the yield of granulocytes by centrifugal means. The solution containing 6% hetastarch in lactated electrolyte injection, however, is *not* indicated for such use.

● Other Uses

Hetastarch has been used as a cryoprotective agent for the long-term storage of whole blood†.

DOSAGE AND ADMINISTRATION

● Administration

Hetastarch solutions are administered by IV infusion.

When used as an adjunct in leukapheresis, 6% hetastarch in 0.9% sodium chloride injection should be thoroughly mixed with a citrate anticoagulant prior to IV infusion. (See Dosage and Administration: Dosage.) Hetastarch volumes of 500–560 mL are compatible with citrate concentrations up to 2.5% for 24 hours at room temperature. The safety and compatibility of additives other than citrate have not been established.

Because 6% hetastarch in lactated electrolyte injection contains calcium, it should not be administered simultaneously with blood through the same administration set due to the potential risk of coagulation.

Hetastarch solutions contain no preservatives and are intended for single use only; partially used containers of the drug should be discarded.

Hetastarch solutions should be stored at room temperature (25°C); brief exposure to temperatures up to 40°C does not adversely affect the preparation. Hetastarch solutions should not be frozen or exposed to excessive heat.

● Dosage

When hetastarch is used for the treatment of hypovolemia, total dosage and rate of infusion depend on the amount of blood or plasma lost, the resultant hemoconcentration, and the patient's age, weight, and clinical condition. The usual adult dose of hetastarch is 30–60 g (500–1000 mL of 6% hetastarch in 0.9% sodium chloride injection or 6% hetastarch in lactated electrolyte injection). Hetastarch doses up to 90 g (1500 mL) have been used during surgery, generally without a need for blood or blood products. The manufacturers state that daily dosages exceeding 1.2 g/kg (20 mL/kg) or 90 g (1500 mL) usually are not required; however, such dosages have been used when severe blood loss has occurred (e.g., in postoperative or trauma patients), although generally only in conjunction with the administration of blood and blood products.

When used as an adjunct in leukapheresis, a citrate anticoagulant should be added to 250–700 mL of 6% hetastarch in 0.9% sodium chloride injection and mixed thoroughly. The resultant solution should be aseptically added to the input line of the centrifugation apparatus and infused at a ratio of 1:8 to 1:13 to venous whole blood.

● Special Populations

There are no specific dosage recommendations for geriatric patients; however, because of the greater frequency of decreased renal function in these patients, dosage should be selected with caution. (See Geriatric Use and also see Renal Impairment under Warnings/Precautions: Specific Populations, in Cautions.)

CAUTIONS

● Contraindications

Hydroxyethyl starch (HES) preparations, including hetastarch, are contraindicated in critically ill adult patients, including those with sepsis, because of the increased risk of mortality and renal replacement therapy in such patients. (See Increased Mortality and Severe Renal Injury under Warnings/Precautions: Warnings, in Cautions.) HES preparations also are contraindicated in patients with severe liver disease, preexisting coagulation or bleeding disorders, and/or clinical conditions that may be exacerbated by volume overload (e.g., congestive heart failure, renal disease with oliguria or anuria not related to hypovolemia). The drug also is contraindicated in patients with known hypersensitivity to HES.

Because 6% hetastarch in lactated electrolyte injection contains lactate, the solution is contraindicated in the treatment of lactic acidosis.

● Warnings/Precautions

Warnings

Increased Mortality and Severe Renal Injury

Increased mortality and/or severe renal injury requiring renal replacement therapy have been reported in critically ill adults, including patients with sepsis, receiving various preparations of HES. Data from randomized controlled trials in critically ill adults receiving lower-molecular-weight HES preparations (e.g., 6% hydroxyethyl starch 130/0.4) indicate that increased mortality and/or severe renal injury occurred within the recommended dosage range for HES (30–90 g [500–1500 mL] daily). Although the increased risks were reported principally with lower-molecular-weight HES preparations, such safety results may be applicable to higher-molecular-weight HES (e.g., 6% hydroxyethyl starch 450/0.7) because of similarities in chemical structure and mechanism of action, and also because lower- and higher-molecular-weight HES preparations are both metabolized by α-amylase into similar smaller fragments that may be associated with renal toxicity. Data from several meta-analyses and observational studies evaluating various preparations of HES confirmed the increased risk of mortality and/or severe renal injury in critically ill adults. Based on the reported evidence, the US Food and Drug Administration (FDA) considers the increased risk of mortality and renal injury requiring renal replacement therapy in critically ill adults, including those with sepsis, to be class effects of HES.

No evidence of renal injury was noted in a review of randomized controlled trials in which HES preparations were administered in the operating room to adult and pediatric patients who were undergoing surgery and were monitored for a short period of time (less than 7 days). Possible explanations for the lack of observed toxicity in these surgical populations include low exposure to HES in a relatively healthier population, requirement for post-administration follow-up monitoring, and/or other unknown factors.

Because of the increased risk of mortality and severe renal injury, HES solutions are contraindicated in critically ill adults, including those with sepsis. HES solutions should be avoided in patients with preexisting renal dysfunction. Use of HES should be discontinued at the first sign of renal injury. Because the need for renal replacement therapy has been reported up to 90 days after administration of HES, renal function should be monitored for at least 90 days in hospitalized patients receiving HES. (See Advice to Patients.)

Sensitivity Reactions

Hypersensitivity Reactions

Life-threatening anaphylactic or anaphylactoid reactions (e.g., rash, erythema multiforme, urticaria, pruritus, angioedema, facial and periorbital edema, chills, flushing, severe hypotension, tachycardia, bradycardia, ventricular fibrillation, cardiac arrest, wheezing, shortness of breath, stridor, tachypnea, cough, chest pain, noncardiac pulmonary edema, laryngeal edema, bronchospasm, restlessness, fever, sneezing) have been reported rarely in patients receiving hetastarch; death has occurred, but a causal relationship to the drug has not been established. Hypersensitivity reactions can occur after discontinuance of hetastarch.

Hetastarch is made from corn starch; the drug should be used with caution in patients with known allergy to corn because such patients may also exhibit sensitivity to hetastarch.

If a hypersensitivity reaction occurs, hetastarch should be discontinued immediately and appropriate treatment and supportive measures should be initiated and continued until symptoms have resolved.

Other Warnings and Precautions

Hemodilution and Circulatory Overload

Substantial hemodilution may occur following administration of hetastarch volumes exceeding 25% of blood volume in less than 24 hours. Slight decreases in platelet counts and hemoglobin concentrations have occurred as a result of the volume-expanding effects of hetastarch and the collection of platelets and erythrocytes in donors undergoing repeated leukapheresis procedures. Hemoglobin concentration usually returns to normal within 24 hours. Hemodilution by hetastarch may also result in 24-hour reductions in concentrations of total protein, albumin, calcium, and fibrinogen; these reductions are not considered clinically relevant.

The risk of circulatory overload is largely dependent on clinical circumstances; however, use of hetastarch doses exceeding 1.2 g/kg (20 mL/kg) within 24 hours may substantially increase such risk.

Excessive hemodilution and circulatory overload should be avoided, particularly in patients at risk of congestive heart failure or pulmonary edema. If excessive hemodilution occurs, administration of blood or blood products (e.g., packed red blood cells, platelets, fresh frozen plasma) should be considered.

Hematologic Effects and Coagulopathy

Administration of large volumes of hetastarch may transiently alter the coagulation mechanism (due to hemodilution and direct inhibition of factor VIII). Transient prolongation of prothrombin time (PT), activated partial thromboplastin time (aPTT), clotting time, and bleeding time may occur. Large volumes of hetastarch solution may decrease hematocrit and dilute plasma proteins. Bleeding, anemia (secondary to hemodilution and/or factor VIII deficiency), and coagulopathy (including rare cases of disseminated intravascular coagulation and hemolysis) have been reported. Increased risk of coagulation abnormalities and bleeding is associated with higher hetastarch doses. (See Patient Evaluation and Laboratory Monitoring under Warnings/Precautions: Other Warnings and Precautions, in Cautions.)

The safety of prolonged use (i.e., over several days) of hetastarch has not been established in situations other than leukapheresis. Prolonged use of the drug has been associated with coagulation abnormalities in conjunction with an acquired, reversible von Willebrand-like syndrome and/or factor VIII deficiency. Replacement therapy should be considered if severe factor VIII deficiency or von Willebrand disease occurs. Coagulopathy may take several days to resolve. Certain conditions appear to be associated with substantial risk during chronic use of hetastarch. Clinically important bleeding may occur in patients with subarachnoid hemorrhage receiving hetastarch repeatedly over a number of days for the prevention of cerebral vasospasm; severe intracranial bleeding resulting in cerebral herniation and death has been reported in at least one patient receiving 6% hetastarch in 0.9% sodium chloride injection. Therefore, it currently is recommended that hetastarch *not* be used for the management of cerebral vasospasm associated with subarachnoid hemorrhage or for conditions other than leukapheresis that necessitate repeated use of the drug over several days. In addition, some clinicians suggest that use of hetastarch be avoided in all neurosurgical patients, since prevention of intracranial hemorrhage in such patients is critical.

Increased bleeding has been reported in patients undergoing open heart surgery in association with cardiopulmonary bypass receiving HES solutions; such excess bleeding occurred irrespective of the molecular weight or molar substitution of the HES preparation and, therefore, is considered by FDA to be a class effect of HES. The coagulation status of patients undergoing open heart surgery in association with cardiopulmonary bypass should be monitored. 6% Hetastarch in 0.9% sodium chloride injection should not be used as a cardiac bypass pump prime, during cardiopulmonary bypass, or in the immediate period after discontinuance of the pump. Use of HES should be discontinued at the first sign of coagulopathy.

Hepatic Effects

Elevated indirect serum bilirubin concentrations have been reported in 2 of 20 healthy individuals who received multiple infusions of 6% hetastarch in 0.9% sodium chloride injection; however, total bilirubin concentrations remained within normal limits. Indirect bilirubin concentrations returned to normal within 96 hours after the final infusion. The importance of these elevations is not known; however, hetastarch should be used with caution in patients with a history of liver disease.

Liver function should be monitored in patients receiving HES preparations, including hetastarch.

Hetastarch and other HES preparations are contraindicated in patients with severe liver disease.

Pancreatic Effects

Transient increases in amylase concentrations may occur following administration of hetastarch; elevated serum amylase concentrations may persist for longer periods in patients with renal impairment. There is no association of the increased amylase concentration with pancreatitis, but this effect limits the use of serum amylase concentrations as an aid in the diagnosis of pancreatitis for up to 3–5 days after hetastarch administration.

Hetastarch has not been shown to increase serum lipase concentrations.

Electrolyte and Other Components of Hetastarch Preparations

Solutions containing 6% hetastarch in 0.9% sodium chloride injection contain sodium; at least one manufacturer states that preparations containing sodium should be used with caution in patients receiving concomitant therapy with drugs affecting electrolyte balance (e.g., corticosteroids, corticotropin). Such preparations should be used with extreme caution, if at all, in patients with edema with sodium retention.

The solution containing 6% hetastarch in lactated electrolyte injection contains dextrose and various electrolytes (e.g., lactate, potassium, sodium). Therefore, the preparation should be used with caution in patients with known subclinical or overt diabetes mellitus, patients with cardiac disease (particularly those receiving digoxin), and patients receiving concomitant therapy with drugs affecting electrolyte balance (e.g., corticosteroids, corticotropin). The preparation should be used with extreme caution in patients with metabolic or respiratory alkalosis and in patients with conditions that result in increased concentrations or impaired utilization of lactate ions (e.g., severe hepatic impairment). The solution containing 6% hetastarch in lactated electrolyte injection also should be used with extreme caution, if at all, in patients with hyperkalemia, potassium retention, or edema with sodium retention.

Patient Evaluation and Laboratory Monitoring

When used for treatment of hypovolemia, the patient's vital signs, fluid balance, electrolyte concentrations, acid-base balance, hemoglobin, hematocrit, platelet count, PT, and aPTT should be closely monitored.

When used as an adjunct in leukapheresis, regular and frequent clinical evaluation and complete blood cell counts (CBCs) are necessary. Additional laboratory determinations (i.e., total leukocyte and platelet counts, leukocyte differential count, hemoglobin, hematocrit, PT, and aPTT) should be considered if the frequency of leukapheresis exceeds the guidelines for whole blood donation.

Specific Populations

Pregnancy

Category C. (See Users Guide.)

Lactation

It is not known whether hetastarch is distributed into milk in humans. Caution is advised if the drug is administered to nursing women.

Pediatric Use

Safety and efficacy of hetastarch have not been established in pediatric patients. However, in a small double-blind study in which a limited number of pediatric patients (1–15.5 years of age) were randomized to receive either hetastarch (i.e., 6% hetastarch in 0.9% sodium chloride injection) or albumin as a postoperative volume expander during the first 24 hours after surgery for repair of congenital heart disease, no differences in coagulation parameters or amount of required replacement fluids were found between pediatric patients receiving 1.2 g/kg (20 mL/kg) or less of hetastarch compared with those receiving albumin. However, an increase in PT was observed among patients receiving more than 1.2 g/kg of hetastarch.

Geriatric Use

In clinical trials of 6% hetastarch in lactated electrolyte injection, 30% of patients were 65 years of age or older, and 12% were 70 years of age or older. Experience with 6% hetastarch in 0.9% sodium chloride injection has not revealed overall differences in response relative to younger adults, but increased sensitivity in some older individuals cannot be ruled out.

Because hetastarch is primarily excreted by the kidneys and geriatric patients are more likely to have decreased renal function, caution should be exercised in dosage selection, and renal function should be monitored for at least 90 days in hospitalized patients receiving HES. (See Increased Mortality and Severe Renal Injury under Warnings/Precautions: Warnings and also see Renal Impairment under Warnings/Precautions: Specific Populations, in Cautions.)

Hepatic Impairment

Hetastarch should be used with caution in patients with a history of liver disease. (See Hepatic Effects under Warnings/Precautions: Other Warnings and Precautions, in Cautions.) Liver function should be monitored in patients receiving HES preparations, including hetastarch. (See Hepatic Effects under Warnings/Precautions: Other Warnings and Precautions, in Cautions.)

Hetastarch and other HES preparations are contraindicated in patients with severe liver disease.

Because of the lactate component in 6% hetastarch in lactated electrolyte injection, the preparation should be used with extreme caution in patients with severe hepatic impairment. (See Electrolyte and Other Components of Hetastarch Preparations under Warnings/Precautions: Other Warnings and Precautions, in Cautions.)

Renal Impairment

The manufacturers and FDA state that HES solutions, including hetastarch, should be avoided in patients with preexisting renal impairment. (See Increased Mortality and Severe Renal Injury under Warnings/Precautions: Warnings, in Cautions.) Hetastarch is contraindicated in patients with renal disease with oliguria or anuria not related to hypovolemia. (See Cautions: Contraindications.)

Limited data suggest that in the presence of renal glomerular damage, larger molecules of hetastarch can leak into urine and elevate the specific gravity, which can obscure the diagnosis of renal failure.

● Common Adverse Effects

Adverse effects reported in patients receiving hetastarch include hypersensitivity reactions, coagulopathy, hemodilution, circulatory overload, metabolic acidosis, congestive heart failure, pulmonary edema, bleeding, vomiting, peripheral edema, submaxillary and parotid glandular enlargement, mild influenza-like symptoms, headache, and muscle pain.

DRUG INTERACTIONS

● Drugs Affecting Coagulation

Because hetastarch may alter the coagulation mechanism, the drug should be used with caution in patients receiving drugs that affect the coagulation system.

● Drugs Affecting Electrolyte Balance

Because of the electrolyte components in hetastarch preparations, at least one manufacturer states that hetastarch should be used with caution in patients receiving concomitant therapy with drugs that affect electrolyte balance (e.g., corticosteroids, corticotropin).

DESCRIPTION

Hetastarch, a hydroxyethyl starch (HES), is a synthetic colloid derived from a waxy starch composed mainly of amylopectin. Hydroxyethyl ether groups are introduced into glucose units of the starch, and the resultant material is hydrolyzed to yield a product with a molecular weight suitable for use as a plasma volume expander and for use in leukapheresis to promote erythrocyte sedimentation and thereby enhance granulocyte yield. Hetastarch resembles glycogen, and the polymerized D-glucose units in the hetastarch polymer are primarily joined by α-1-4-glycosidic linkages with occasional α-1-6 linkages. Hetastarch is characterized by its molecular weight and molar substitution. The average molecular weight of hetastarch is approximately 600 (6% hetastarch in 0.9% sodium chloride injection [Hespan®]) or 670 (6% hetastarch in lactated electrolyte injection [Hextend®]); while the average molecular weight of hetastarch ranges from 450–800, at least 80% of the polymers have molecular weights ranging from 200–2600. The molar substitution of hetastarch is approximately 0.75 (i.e., there are 75 hydroxyethyl groups per 100 glucose units). Hetastarch is commercially available as premixed solutions containing 6 g of hetastarch per 100 mL of 0.9% sodium chloride injection (e.g., Hespan®) or lactated electrolyte injection (Hextend®). Hespan® and Hextend® are designated as 6% HES 450/0.7.

Hetastarch exhibits colloidal oncotic effects. The drug retains intravascular fluid, resulting in plasma volume expansion. The degree of plasma volume expansion and improvement in hemodynamic state depend on the intravascular status of the patient. Plasma volume expansion produced by hetastarch is comparable to that of albumin human 5% solution. Maximum plasma volume expansion in hypovolemic patients is reached within a few minutes after the end of infusion; the extent and duration of the expansion in plasma volume vary with the volume of solution infused and depend on the preadministration plasma volume, the distribution of hetastarch through body water, and the rate of renal clearance of the drug. Following IV infusion, plasma volume expansion diminishes over 24–36 hours. In hypovolemic patients, hetastarch causes a temporary increase in arterial and venous pressures, cardiac index, stroke work index, and pulmonary wedge pressure. When added to whole blood, 6% hetastarch in 0.9% sodium chloride injection increases the erythrocyte sedimentation rate.

Hetastarch is not completely metabolized. The hydroxyethyl group is not cleaved during metabolism but remains intact and attached to glucose units when excreted; therefore, metabolism of hetastarch does not produce substantial amounts of glucose. Hetastarch is primarily excreted by the kidneys; molecules with a molecular weight of less than 50 are rapidly excreted, while larger molecules are retained for varying periods depending on their size and ease of breakdown. Following IV infusion of a single 30-g (500-mL) dose of 6% hetastarch in 0.9% sodium chloride injection, about 33% of the dose is excreted in urine within 24 hours. Although excretion of hetastarch is variable, intravascular concentration of the drug decreases to less than 10% of the total administered dose within 2 weeks following IV infusion. Biliary excretion of hetastarch accounts for less than 1% of the dose. Hetastarch is not removed by hemodialysis; it is not known whether hetastarch is removed by other extracorporeal elimination techniques.

Each liter of 6% hetastarch in 0.9% sodium chloride injection provides 154 mEq each of sodium and chloride. Each liter of 6% hetastarch in lactated electrolyte injection provides 143 mEq of sodium, 124 mEq of chloride, 28 mEq of lactate, 5 mEq of calcium, 3 mEq of potassium, and 0.9 mEq of magnesium; the electrolyte content of 6% hetastarch in lactated electrolyte injection resembles that of the principal ionic constituents of normal plasma. Commercially available hetastarch solutions have a pH of approximately 5.9 and a calculated osmolarity of approximately 307–309 mOsm/L.

ADVICE TO PATIENTS

Risk of severe kidney damage. Importance of immediately reporting signs and symptoms suggestive of kidney damage (e.g., change in frequency, volume, or color of urine; blood in urine; difficulty in urinating; swelling of the legs, ankles, feet, face, or hands; unusual weakness or fatigue; nausea and vomiting; shortness of breath).

Importance of informing clinicians of existing or contemplated concomitant therapy, including prescription and OTC drugs and herbal supplements, as well as any concomitant illnesses (e.g., congestive heart failure, liver disease, renal impairment).

Importance of women informing clinicians if they are or plan to become pregnant or plan to breast-feed.

Importance of informing patients of other important precautionary information. (See Cautions.)

PREPARATIONS

Excipients in commercially available drug preparations may have clinically important effects in some individuals; consult specific product labeling for details.

Hetastarch in Sodium Chloride

Parenteral

Injection, for IV infusion only	6% Hetastarch in 0.9% Sodium Chloride*	**Hespan®**, Braun
		6% Hetastarch in 0.9% Sodium Chloride Injection

* available from one or more manufacturer, distributor, and/or repackager by generic (nonproprietary) name

Hetastarch in Lactated Electrolyte Injection

Parenteral

Injection, for IV infusion only	6% Hetastarch in Lactated Electrolyte Injection	**Hextend®**, Hospira

† Use is not currently included in the labeling approved by the US Food and Drug Administration.

Selected Revisions April 29, 2014, © Copyright, July 1, 1973, American Society of Health-System Pharmacists, Inc.

Potassium Supplements

40:12 • REPLACEMENT PREPARATIONS

■ Potassium supplements are used as a source of potassium, an essential nutrient cation.

USES

● Potassium Depletion

Potassium supplements are used as a source of potassium cation for treatment or prevention of potassium depletion in patients in whom dietary measures are inadequate. Conditions which may indicate or result in potassium deficiency include vomiting, diarrhea, drainage of GI fluids, hyperadrenalism, malnutrition, debilitation, prolonged negative nitrogen balance, prolonged parenteral alimentation without addition of potassium, dialysis, metabolic alkalosis, metabolic or diabetic acidosis, GI tract abnormalities which result in poor absorption, certain renal diseases, and familial periodic paralysis characterized by hypokalemia. Potassium should be included in long-term electrolyte replacement regimens and has been recommended for routine prophylactic administration following surgery after adequate urine flow has been established. Administration of certain drugs including thiazide diuretics, carbonic anhydrase inhibitors, furosemide, ethacrynic acid, some corticosteroids, corticotropin, aminosalicylic acid, and amphotericin B may sometimes result in potassium depletion which may warrant potassium replacement therapy. Ingestion of potassium-rich foods and/or use of potassium-containing salt substitutes may prevent potassium depletion in patients receiving potassium-depleting drugs; however, judicious prophylactic administration of potassium may be advisable in selected patients during prolonged diuretic or corticosteroid therapy, especially if they are digitalized.

Potassium chloride is usually the salt of choice in the treatment of potassium depletion, since the chloride ion is required to correct hypochloremia which frequently accompanies potassium deficiency. In addition, hypochloremia may develop if the citrate, bicarbonate, gluconate, or another alkalinizing salt of potassium is administered, particularly in conjunction with chloride-restricted diets. In the rare instances in which metabolic acidosis exists concurrently with potassium depletion (e.g., renal tubular acidosis), alkalinizing salts of potassium are preferred.

● Hypertension

Inadequate dietary intake of potassium may play an important role in the development of hypertension, and high dietary intake of potassium (e.g., with supplementation) may protect against the development of high blood pressure and improve blood pressure control in patients with hypertension. Epidemiologic studies have suggested that a lower sodium-potassium ratio may result in a lower risk of cardiovascular disease as compared with that observed with a reduction of sodium or increase in potassium alone. Most experts currently recommend enhanced intake of potassium (3.5–5 g daily) as part of lifestyle modifications for hypertensive patients, unless contraindicated by chronic kidney disease (CKD) or use of drugs that reduce potassium excretion. (See Cautions: Precautions and Contraindications.) Potassium supplementation is recommended particularly in those unable to adequately reduce their sodium intake. Adequate intake of potassium also should be considered as a means of preventing the development of hypertension. Food sources high in potassium such as fruits and vegetables preferably should be used instead of potassium supplements. In pooled analysis of data from 33 randomized controlled trials in which potassium supplementation was the only difference between intervention and control groups, such supplementation was associated with a reduction in mean systolic blood pressure of 3.11 mm Hg and a reduction in mean diastolic blood pressure of 1.97 mm Hg. The effects of potassium supplementation appeared to be particularly evident in patients exposed to high sodium intake.

● Other Uses

Potassium salts may be used cautiously to abolish arrhythmias of cardiac glycoside toxicity precipitated by a loss of potassium. It has been reported that elevation of plasma potassium concentrations by 0.5–1.5 mEq/L or to the upper limits of normal may be useful in the management of tachyarrhythmias following cardiac surgery. This regimen should not be used in patients with atrioventricular block, however, since potassium may further impair nodal conduction.

Limited data suggest that potassium may be useful in the treatment of thallium poisoning; however, such treatment is limited by the amount of thallium that can be released into the blood without worsening cerebral symptoms.

DOSAGE AND ADMINISTRATION

● Administration

The acetate, bicarbonate, chloride, citrate, and gluconate salts of potassium are administered orally. Potassium chloride, potassium acetate, and potassium phosphate may be administered by slow IV infusion. Rarely, potassium-containing injections are given by hypodermoclysis, in which case potassium concentrations should not exceed 10 mEq/L in order to avoid local pain. Whenever possible, potassium supplements should be given orally since the relatively slow absorption from the GI tract prevents sudden, large increases in plasma potassium concentrations. Oral potassium supplements should preferably be administered as liquid with or after meals with a full glass of water or fruit juice to minimize the possibility of GI irritation and a saline cathartic effect. Enteric-coated (no longer commercially available in the US) and wax matrix tablets must be swallowed and not allowed to dissolve in the mouth. Other commercially available oral dosage forms of potassium should be dissolved and/or diluted and administered according to the instructions of the manufacturer.

Potassium for injection concentrates must be diluted with a compatible IV solution prior to administration. Diluted solutions of potassium acetate, potassium chloride, and potassium phosphate for injection concentrates *must* be administered slowly. Potassium injections should generally be administered only in patients with adequate urine flow. In dehydrated patients, 1 liter of potassium-free fluid should be administered prior to initiating potassium therapy. Generally, potassium concentrations in IV fluids should not exceed 40 mEq/L and the rate of administration should not exceed 20 mEq/hour. However, higher potassium concentrations (e.g., 60–80 mEq/L) administered more rapidly occasionally may be needed initially in cases of severe hypokalemia and associated cardiac arrhythmias or for the management of diabetic ketoacidosis or the diuretic phase of acute renal failure. Local vascular intolerance may limit the ability to administer such concentrated solutions. In such cases, use of a large vein with a relatively high blood flow (e.g., femoral vein) or splitting and administering the dose in less concentrated solutions via 2 veins simultaneously can be considered. Administration of such concentrated potassium solutions via a subclavian, jugular, or right atrial catheter should be *avoided* since local potassium concentrations achieved in the heart may be high and potentially cardiotoxic. The ECG should be monitored closely when the rate of IV potassium administration exceeds 20 mEq/hour. Peaking of the T wave or other ECG changes associated with hyperkalemia (see Cautions: Hyperkalemia) indicate that the rate of potassium infusion is excessive and should be reduced.

Viaflex® Plus containers of potassium chloride injections should be checked for minute leaks by firmly squeezing the bag. The injection should be discarded if the container seal is not intact or leaks are found or if the solution is cloudy or contains a precipitate. The injection in plastic containers should not be used in series connections with other plastic containers, since such use could result in air embolism from residual air being drawn from the primary container before administration of fluid from the secondary container is complete.

Oral administration of potassium supplements or ingestion of potassium-rich foods should replace IV potassium therapy as soon as possible.

● Dosage

Dosage of potassium supplements is usually expressed as mEq of potassium and depends on the requirements of the individual patient. The normal adult daily requirement and the usual dietary intake of potassium is 40–80 mEq; infants may require 2–3 mEq/kg or 40 mEq/m^2 daily. Potassium replacement requirements can be estimated only by initial clinical condition and response, ECG monitoring, and/or plasma potassium determinations. Prophylactic administration of potassium supplements may be necessary in some patients in order to maintain plasma potassium concentration above 3.0 mEq/L. The average oral dosage of potassium supplements for the prevention of hypokalemia is about 20 mEq daily, and the usual oral dosage of potassium for the treatment of potassium depletion is 40–100 mEq or more daily. However, it is important to remember that dosage must be individualized for each patient. Forty mEq of potassium is provided by approximately:

3.9 g of potassium acetate
4.0 g of potassium bicarbonate
3.0 g of potassium chloride
4.3 g of potassium citrate
9.4 g of potassium gluconate
5.4 g of monobasic potassium phosphate
3.5 g of dibasic potassium phosphate

Oral potassium supplements are usually administered in 2–4 doses daily. To avoid serious hyperkalemia, replacement of potassium deficits must be undertaken gradually usually over a 3- to 7-day period depending on the severity of the deficit. Potassium dosage for adults should usually not exceed 150 mEq daily, and the dosage for young children should not exceed 3 mEq/kg daily. Close monitoring of the ECG and plasma potassium concentrations is essential during IV administration of potassium.

CAUTIONS

● GI and Other Local Effects

Adverse effects of potassium salts may include nausea, vomiting, diarrhea, flatulence, and abdominal pain or discomfort. Small bowel ulcerations have been reported following administration of enteric-coated potassium chloride tablets (no longer commercially available in the US). Ulcerations have been accompanied by stenosis, hemorrhage, obstruction, and perforation; surgery is frequently required and deaths have been reported. A few cases of small bowel ulceration, stricture, and perforation have been associated with wax matrix formulations of potassium chloride. Esophageal ulceration and stricture have occurred in patients with esophageal compression associated with an enlarged left atrium, and mouth ulceration occurred when a patient sucked rather than swallowed the wax matrix tablets. Following release of the drug from wax matrix tablets, the expended wax matrix is not absorbed systemically and may be detected in feces. Numerous wax matrices accumulated in a patient with partial obstruction of the lower bowel causing an impaction. To date, the incidence of GI lesions (ulceration, stricture, and perforation) with wax matrix tablets appears to be much lower than with enteric-coated (no longer commercially available in the US) tablets (less than 1 per 100,000 patient-years vs 40–50 per 100,000 patient-years). Extended-release tablets containing coated potassium chloride crystals are also formulated to minimize the likelihood of the drug causing GI lesions, but the frequency of GI lesions with these tablets currently is not known. Like enteric-coated tablets (no longer commercially available in the US), the wax matrix tablets and extended-release tablets containing coated crystals of the drug should be administered with caution and should be discontinued immediately if abdominal pain, distention, severe vomiting, or GI bleeding occurs. (See Cautions: Precautions and Contraindications.) Some authorities question the use of any potassium tablet, since use of dilute liquid preparations of potassium minimizes the risk of GI complications.

Pain at the site of injection and phlebitis may occur during IV administration of solutions containing 30 mEq or more potassium per liter.

● Hyperkalemia

Hyperkalemia is the most common and serious hazard of potassium therapy. Since an exact measurement of potassium deficiency is not usually possible, potassium supplements should be administered slowly and with caution. The presence of adequate renal function must be confirmed, and frequent observations of the clinical status of the patient and periodic ECGs and/or determinations of plasma potassium concentrations should be made. ECG changes are probably the most important indicator of potassium toxicity and include tall, peaked T waves, depression of the ST segment, disappearance of the P wave, prolongation of the QT interval, and widening and slurring of the QRS complex. Clinical signs and symptoms of potassium overdosage include paresthesia of the extremities, listlessness, mental confusion, weakness or heaviness of the legs, flaccid paralysis, cold skin, gray pallor, peripheral vascular collapse with fall in blood pressure, cardiac arrhythmias, and heart block. Extremely high plasma potassium concentrations (8–11 mEq/L) may cause death from cardiac depression, arrhythmias, or arrest. It has been suggested that hyperkalemia may decrease the excitability of the myocardium to electrical stimulation resulting in the possibility that the myocardium may not respond to implanted pacemakers.

Except in the presence of severe renal impairment, hyperkalemia is not likely to result from oral administration or from slow IV administration of dilute solutions of potassium. Nonetheless, hyperkalemia can occur from therapeutic doses of potassium salts and, when detected, must be treated immediately since lethal

plasma potassium concentrations can be reached within a few hours. Hyperkalemia may result from rapid IV administration of potassium solutions. Hyperkalemia has occurred following addition of concentrated potassium chloride solutions to infusions from a hanging flexible plastic container, apparently as a result of pooling of the concentrated potassium solution at the base of the container and infusion of undiluted solution. Squeezing the container did not facilitate mixing but tended to pump the concentrated solution into the infusion chamber. Mixing of the solutions can be achieved if the plastic container is inverted during the addition of potassium solutions and subsequently agitated and/or kneaded.

Treatment of hyperkalemia depends on its severity and various regimens have been recommended. It must be kept in mind that rapid lowering of plasma potassium concentrations in digitalized patients can cause cardiac glycoside toxicity. Administration of potassium-rich foods and drugs and potassium-sparing diuretics must be discontinued. In patients with severe hyperkalemia, measures which facilitate shift of potassium into cells, such as administration of sodium bicarbonate, a calcium salt, and/or dextrose with or without insulin, have been recommended. In patients with plasma potassium concentrations greater than 6.5 mEq/L, IV infusion of 40–160 mEq of sodium bicarbonate over a 5-minute period has been recommended. This dose may be repeated after 10–15 minutes if ECG abnormalities persist. Dextrose therapy usually consists of IV infusion of 300–500 mL of 10–25% dextrose injection containing 5–10 units of insulin per 20 grams of dextrose over a 1-hour period. Some clinicians report that dextrose is less reliable and does not produce effects as rapidly as does sodium bicarbonate. In addition, studies indicate that the addition of insulin to an infusion solution results in adsorption of insulin to the glass and tubing. For this reason, it has been recommended that insulin be given as a separate injection. Patients whose ECGs show absent P waves or a broad QRS complex and who are *not* receiving cardiac glycosides should immediately be given 0.5–1 g (5–10 mL of a 10% solution) of calcium gluconate or another calcium salt IV over a 2-minute period (with continuous ECG monitoring) to antagonize the cardiotoxic effects of potassium. If ECG abnormalities persist, repeated doses of the calcium salt may be given, allowing 1–2 minutes between doses. When hyperkalemia is associated with water loss, administration of potassium-free fluids may be useful to decrease plasma potassium concentrations.

When the ECG approaches normal, efforts should be directed toward removal of excess potassium from the body. Some adsorption and/or exchange of potassium may be accomplished by administration of sodium polystyrene sulfonate orally or as a retention enema. Hemodialysis or peritoneal dialysis will reduce plasma potassium concentrations and may be required in patients with renal insufficiency. Administration of large doses of sodium chloride has been recommended to increase urinary excretion of potassium in patients with functional kidneys. Other drugs which have been used in an effort to reduce plasma potassium concentrations include testosterone to promote anabolism, and desoxycorticosterone acetate in patients with adrenal insufficiency who have adequate renal function.

● Precautions and Contraindications

Potassium supplements should be administered with caution in patients with cardiac disease. These drugs may intensify symptoms of myotonia congenita. Potassium supplements should not be administered to patients receiving potassium-sparing drugs such as amiloride, spironolactone, and triamterene. Potassium should generally not be given in the immediate postoperative period until urine flow is established. In patients with renal impairment, its use must be carefully controlled by frequent determinations of plasma potassium concentrations.

Because intestinal and gastric ulceration and bleeding have occurred with extended-release potassium chloride preparations, these dosage forms of the drug should be reserved for patients who cannot tolerate or refuse to take liquid or effervescent potassium preparations or for those in whom there is a problem of compliance with these latter dosage forms. If abdominal pain, distension, severe vomiting, or GI bleeding occurs in patients receiving an extended-release preparation, the drug should be discontinued immediately and the possibility of intestinal obstruction or perforation considered. Because Micro-K® LS contains docusate sodium as a dispersing agent, minor changes in consistency of feces may commonly occur; these changes are generally well tolerated. However, rarely, patients may experience diarrhea and cramping or abdominal pain. Patients with severe or chronic diarrhea or who are dehydrated generally should not receive supplemental potassium therapy using Micro-K® LS.

Some preparations of potassium contain the dye tartrazine (FD&C yellow No. 5), which may cause allergic reactions including bronchial asthma in susceptible individuals. Although the incidence of tartrazine sensitivity is low, it frequently occurs in patients who are sensitive to aspirin.

Potassium supplements are contraindicated in patients with severe renal impairment with oliguria, anuria, or azotemia; untreated chronic adrenocortical insufficiency (Addison's disease); the hyperkalemic form of familial periodic paralysis or other hyperkalemias; acute dehydration; heat cramps; or extensive tissue breakdown such as severe burns. Wax matrix formulations of potassium chloride should not be administered to patients with esophageal compression caused by an enlarged left atrium; a liquid preparation of potassium should be used in these patients. Solid oral dosage forms of potassium supplements are contraindicated in patients in whom there is a structural, pathological (e.g., diabetic gastroparesis), and/or pharmacologic (e.g., induced by anticholinergic agents) cause for arrest or delay in passage of the dosage form through the GI tract; an oral liquid preparation of potassium should be used in these patients.

PHARMACOLOGY

Potassium is the major cation of intracellular fluid and is essential for maintenance of acid-base balance, isotonicity, and electrodynamic characteristics of the cell. Potassium is an important activator in many enzymatic reactions and is essential to a number of physiologic processes including transmission of nerve impulses; contraction of cardiac, smooth, and skeletal muscles; gastric secretion; renal function; tissue synthesis; and carbohydrate metabolism.

PHARMACOKINETICS

● Absorption

Potassium salts are well absorbed from the GI tract. Enteric-coated potassium chloride tablets (no longer commercially available in the US) pass through the stomach releasing the drug in the small intestine and may produce dangerously high, localized concentrations of potassium chloride. Ingestion of sugar-coated tablets containing potassium chloride imbedded in a wax matrix (e.g., Kaon-Cl®, Slow-K®) produces a slow release of the drug. The wax matrix and potassium chloride crystals are blended so that the salt can be slowly leached from the tablet by GI fluids, and thus the potassium chloride is gradually released over a large segment of the intestine. Compared to liquid preparations, absorption of potassium from a single dose in these wax matrix formulations is somewhat delayed, probably because of the time required for dissolution of the drug. However, when potassium chloride is administered chronically, the bioavailability of potassium from the wax matrix preparations appears to be similar to that of liquid preparations of the drug. Dangerously high, localized concentrations of potassium chloride are not likely to occur with this dosage form unless blockage of passage of the tablet through the GI tract occurs. Similarly, extended-release granules for suspension and tablets containing coated potassium chloride crystals produce a slow release of the drug and minimize the likelihood of high, localized concentrations in the GI tract.

● Distribution

Potassium first enters the extracellular fluid and is then actively transported into the cells where its concentration is up to 40 times that outside the cell. Dextrose, insulin, and oxygen facilitate movement of potassium into cells. In healthy adults, plasma potassium concentrations generally range from 3.5–5 mEq/L. Plasma concentrations up to 7.7 mEq/L may be normal in neonates. Plasma potassium concentrations, however, are not necessarily accurate indications of cellular potassium concentrations; cellular deficits can occur without decreases in plasma potassium concentrations and hypokalemia may occur without substantial depletion of cellular potassium. Changes in extracellular fluid pH produce reciprocal effects on plasma potassium concentrations. A change of 0.1 unit in plasma pH has been reported to produce an inverse change of 0.6 mEq/L in plasma potassium concentration. Potassium concentrations in gastric and intestinal secretions are higher than plasma concentrations, and diarrheal fluid may contain up to 60 mEq/L.

● Elimination

Potassium is excreted mainly by the kidneys. The cation is filtered by the glomeruli, reabsorbed in the proximal tubule, and secreted in the distal tubule, the site of sodium-potassium exchange. Tubular secretion of potassium is also influenced by chloride ion concentration, hydrogen ion exchange, acid-base equilibrium, and adrenal hormones. Healthy patients on potassium-free diets usually excrete 40–50 mEq of potassium daily. Surgery and/or tissue injury result in increased urinary excretion of potassium which may continue for several days. Postoperative

patients or patients under stress of disease with normal kidneys may excrete up to 80–90 mEq of potassium daily, even though they are not receiving any potassium. Small amounts of potassium may be excreted via the skin and intestinal tract, but most of the potassium excreted into the intestine is later reabsorbed.

CHEMISTRY AND STABILITY

● Chemistry

Potassium supplements are used in the prevention or treatment of potassium depletion. For oral administration, the acetate, bicarbonate, chloride, citrate, and gluconate salts of potassium are available as single ingredients and/or components of combination products. Potassium acetate, potassium chloride, and potassium phosphate are available as concentrates for injection that must be diluted prior to IV administration (for injection concentrate). In addition, potassium chloride is a component of several multiple electrolyte IV infusion fluids. The salts used as potassium supplements are very soluble or freely soluble in water. Potassium chloride for injection concentrate has a pH of 4–8, potassium acetate for injection concentrate has a pH of 7.1–7.7, and potassium phosphates for injection concentrate has a pH of 7–7.8.

● Stability

Some commercially available injections of potassium chloride are provided in Viaflex® Plus containers. Viaflex® Plus plastic containers are fabricated from specially formulated polyvinyl chloride (PL 146® plastic). The amount of water that can permeate from inside the container into the overwrap is insufficient to substantially affect the solution. Solutions in contact with the plastic can leach out some of its chemical components in very small amounts (e.g., bis(2-ethylhexyl)phthalate [BEHP, DEHP] in up to 5 ppm) within the expiration period of the injection; however, safety of the plastic has been confirmed in tests in animals according to USP biological tests for plastic containers as well as by tissue culture toxicity studies.

Potassium chloride, potassium acetate, and potassium phosphates concentrates for injection have been reported to be physically incompatible with IV solutions containing various drugs. Published data are too varied and/or limited to permit generalizations, and specialized references should be consulted for specific compatibility information.

PREPARATIONS

Excipients in commercially available drug preparations may have clinically important effects in some individuals; consult specific product labeling for details.

Potassium Acetate

Parenteral		
For injection concentrate	2 mEq of K⁺/mL and CH₃COO⁻/mL*	**Potassium Acetate Injection**
	2 mEq of K⁺/mL and CH₃COO⁻/mL pharmacy bulk package*	**Potassium Acetate Injection** **Potassium Acetate Injection MaxiVial®**, Abraxis
	4 mEq of K⁺/mL and CH₃COO⁻/mL*	**Potassium Acetate Injection**

* available from one or more manufacturer, distributor, and/or repackager by generic (nonproprietary) name

Potassium Bicarbonate

Oral		
Tablets, for solution	6.5 mEq of K⁺	**Quic-K®**, Western Research
	25 mEq of K⁺*	**K⁺ Care® Effervescent Tablets**, Alra
		K-Lyte® Effervescent Tablets, Bristol-Myers Squibb
		Klor-Con®/EF, Upsher-Smith
		Potassium Bicarbonate Effervescent Tablets

* available from one or more manufacturer, distributor, and/or repackager by generic (nonproprietary) name

Potassium Chloride

Oral		
Capsules, extended-release	8 mEq of K$^+$ and Cl$^-$*	**Micro-K®**, Ther-Rx **Potassium Chloride Extended-Release Capsules**
	10 mEq of K$^+$ and Cl$^-$*	**Micro-K®**, Ther-Rx **Potassium Chloride Extended-Release Capsules**
For solution	20 mEq of K$^+$ and Cl$^-$ per packet*	**K+ Care®**, Alra **K-Lor®**, Abbott **Kay Ciel®**, Forest **Klor-Con® Powder**, Upsher-Smith **Potassium Chloride for Oral Solution**
	25 mEq of K$^+$ and Cl$^-$ per packet	**Klor-Con®/25 Powder**, Upsher-Smith
Solution	6.7 mEq of K$^+$/5 mL and Cl$^-$/5 mL*	**Kaochlor® 10%**, Savage **Kay Ciel®**, Forest **Potassium Chloride Oral Solution**
	10 mEq of K$^+$/5 mL and Cl$^-$/5 mL*	**Potassium Chloride Oral Solution** **Rum-K®**, Fleming
	13.3 mEq of K$^+$/5 mL and Cl$^-$/5 mL*	**Kaon-Cl® 20% Elixir**, Savage **Potassium Chloride Oral Solution**
Tablets, extended-release	8 mEq of K$^+$ and Cl$^-$*	**Potassium Chloride Extended-Release Tablets** **Slow-K®**, Novartis
	10 mEq of K$^+$ and Cl$^-$*	**Kaon-Cl-10®**, Savage
Tablets, extended-release (containing coated potassium chloride crystals)	10 mEq of K$^+$ and Cl$^-$	**K-Dur® 10**, Key
	20 mEq of K$^+$ and Cl$^-$	**K-Dur® 20** (scored), Key
Tablets, extended-release, film-coated	8 mEq of K$^+$ and Cl$^-$*	**K+ 8®**, Alra **Klor-Con® 8**, Upsher-Smith **Potassium Chloride Extended-Release Tablets**
	10 mEq of K$^+$ and Cl$^-$*	**K+ 10®**, Alra **Klor-Con® 10**, Upsher-Smith **Klotrix®**, Bristol-Myers Squibb **K-Tab® Filmtab®**, Abbott **Potassium Chloride Extended-Release Tablets**
Tablets, film-coated	2.5 mEq of K$^+$ and Cl$^-$*	**Potassium Chloride Tablets**
	10 mEq K$^+$ and Cl$^-$*	**Potassium Chloride Tablets**
Parenteral		
For injection concentrate	1.5 mEq of K$^+$ and Cl$^-$ per mL*	**Potassium Chloride for Injection Concentrate**
	2 mEq of K$^+$ and Cl$^-$ per mL*	**Potassium Chloride for Injection Concentrate**
	2 mEq of K$^+$ and Cl$^-$ per mL pharmacy bulk package*	**Potassium Chloride for Injection Concentrate**
For injection concentrate, for IV infusion	0.1 mEq of K$^+$ and Cl$^-$ per mL (10 mEq)*	**Potassium Chloride for Injection Concentrate** **Potassium Chloride Injection Highly Concentrated (Viaflex®)**, Baxter
	0.2 mEq of K$^+$ and Cl$^-$ per mL (10 and 20 mEq)*	**Potassium Chloride Injection Highly Concentrated (Viaflex®)**, Baxter
	0.3 mEq of K$^+$ and Cl$^-$ per mL (30 mEq)*	**Potassium Chloride Injection Highly Concentrated (Viaflex®)**, Baxter
	0.4 mEq of K$^+$ and Cl$^-$ per mL (20 and 40 mEq)*	**Potassium Chloride Injection Highly Concentrated (Viaflex®)**, Baxter

* available from one or more manufacturer, distributor, and/or repackager by generic (nonproprietary) name

Potassium Chloride in Dextrose Injection

Parenteral		
Injection, for IV infusion only	10 mEq of K$^+$ per L in 5% Dextrose*	**10 mEq/L Potassium Chloride in 5% Dextrose Injection (Viaflex®)**, Baxter
	20 mEq of K$^+$ per L in 5% Dextrose*	**20 mEq/L Potassium Chloride in 5% Dextrose Injection (Viaflex®)**, Baxter **20 mEq/L 0.15% Potassium Chloride in 5% Dextrose Injection**
	30 mEq of K$^+$ per L in 5% Dextrose*	**30 mEq/L Potassium Chloride in 5% Dextrose Injection (Viaflex®)**, Baxter **30 mEq/L 0.224% Potassium Chloride in 5% Dextrose Injection**
	40 mEq of K$^+$ per L in 5% Dextrose*	**40 mEq/L Potassium Chloride in 5% Dextrose Injection (Viaflex®)**, Baxter **40 mEq/L 0.3% Potassium Chloride in 5% Dextrose Injection**

* available from one or more manufacturer, distributor, and/or repackager by generic (nonproprietary) name

Potassium Chloride in Sodium Chloride Injection

Parenteral		
Injection, for IV infusion only	20 mEq of K$^+$ per L in 0.9% Sodium Chloride*	**20 mEq/L Potassium Chloride in 0.9% Sodium Chloride Injection (Viaflex®)**, Baxter **20 mEq/L 0.15% Potassium Chloride in 0.9% Sodium Chloride Injection**
	40 mEq of K$^+$ per L in 0.9% Sodium Chloride*	**40 mEq/L Potassium Chloride in 0.9% Sodium Chloride Injection (Viaflex®)**, Baxter **40 mEq/L 0.3% Potassium Chloride in 0.9% Sodium Chloride Injection**

* available from one or more manufacturer, distributor, and/or repackager by generic (nonproprietary) name

Potassium Chloride in Dextrose and Lactated Ringer's Injection

Parenteral

Injection, for IV infusion only	20 mEq of K⁺ per L in 5% Dextrose and Lactated Ringer's*	20 mEq/L Potassium Chloride in 5% Dextrose and Lactated Ringer's Injection (Viaflex®), Baxter
		20 mEq/L 0.15% Potassium Chloride in 5% Dextrose and Lactated Ringer's Injection
	40 mEq of K⁺ per L in 5% Dextrose and Lactated Ringer's*	40 mEq/L Potassium Chloride in 5% Dextrose and Lactated Ringer's Injection (Viaflex®), Baxter
		40 mEq/L 0.3% Potassium Chloride in 5% Dextrose and Lactated Ringer's Injection

* available from one or more manufacturer, distributor, and/or repackager by generic (nonproprietary) name

Potassium Chloride in Dextrose and Sodium Chloride Injection

Parenteral

Injection, for IV infusion only	10 mEq of K⁺ per L in 5% Dextrose and 0.2–0.225% Sodium Chloride*	10 mEq/L Potassium Chloride in 5% Dextrose and 0.2% Sodium Chloride Injection (Viaflex®), Baxter
		10 mEq/L 0.075% Potassium Chloride in 5% Dextrose and 0.2% Sodium Chloride Injection
		10 mEq/L 0.075% Potassium Chloride in 5% Dextrose and 0.225% Sodium Chloride Injection
	10 mEq of K⁺ per L in 5% Dextrose and 0.3–0.33% Sodium Chloride*	10 mEq/L (0.075%) Potassium Chloride in 5% Dextrose and 0.3% Sodium Chloride Injection
		10 mEq/L Potassium Chloride in 5% Dextrose and 0.33% Sodium Chloride Injection (Viaflex®), Baxter
	10 mEq of K⁺ per L in 5% Dextrose and 0.45% Sodium Chloride*	10 mEq/L Potassium Chloride in 5% Dextrose and 0.45% Sodium Chloride Injection (Viaflex®), Baxter
		10 mEq/L 0.075% Potassium Chloride in 5% Dextrose and 0.45% Sodium Chloride Injection
	20 mEq of K⁺ per L in 5% Dextrose and 0.2–0.225% Sodium Chloride*	20 mEq/L Potassium Chloride in 5% Dextrose and 0.2% Sodium Chloride Injection (Viaflex®), Baxter
		20 mEq/L 0.15% Potassium Chloride in 5% Dextrose and 0.225% Sodium Chloride Injection
		0.15% 20 mEq/L Potassium Chloride in 5% Dextrose and 0.2% Sodium Chloride Injection
	20 mEq K⁺ per L in 5% Dextrose and 0.3–0.33% Sodium Chloride*	20 mEq/L Potassium Chloride in 5% Dextrose and 0.33% Sodium Chloride Injection (Viaflex®), Baxter
		20 mEq/L 0.15% Potassium Chloride in 5% Dextrose and 0.3% Sodium Chloride Injection
	20 mEq of K⁺ per L in 5% Dextrose and 0.45% Sodium Chloride*	20 mEq Potassium Chloride in 5% Dextrose and 0.45% Sodium Chloride Injection (Viaflex®), Baxter
		20 mEq/L 0.15% Potassium Chloride in 5% Dextrose and 0.45% Sodium Chloride Injection
	20 mEq of K⁺ per L in 5% Dextrose and 0.9% Sodium Chloride*	20 mEq/L Potassium Chloride in 5% Dextrose and 0.9% Sodium Chloride Injection (Viaflex®), Baxter
		20 mEq 0.15% Potassium Chloride in 5% Dextrose and 0.9% Sodium Chloride Injection
	20 mEq of K⁺ per L in 10% Dextrose and 0.2% Sodium Chloride*	0.15% 20 mEq/L Potassium Chloride in 10% Dextrose and 0.2% Sodium Chloride Injection
	30 mEq of K⁺ per L in 5% Dextrose and 0.2–0.225% Sodium Chloride*	30 mEq/L Potassium Chloride in 5% Dextrose and 0.2% Sodium Chloride Injection (Viaflex®), Baxter
		30 mEq/L 0.224% Potassium Chloride in 5% Dextrose and 0.225% Sodium Chloride Injection
		0.22% 30 mEq/L Potassium Chloride in 5% Dextrose and 0.2% Sodium Chloride Injection
	30 mEq of K⁺ per L in 5% Dextrose and 0.3–0.33% Sodium Chloride*	30 mEq/L Potassium Chloride in 5% Dextrose and 0.33% Sodium Chloride Injection (Viaflex®), Baxter
		30 mEq/L 0.224% Potassium Chloride in 5% Dextrose and 0.3% Sodium Chloride Injection
	30 mEq of K⁺ per L in 5% Dextrose and 0.45% Sodium Chloride*	30 mEq/L Potassium Chloride in 5% Dextrose and 0.45% Sodium Chloride Injection (Viaflex®), Baxter
		30 mEq/L 0.224% Potassium Chloride in 5% Dextrose and 0.45% Sodium Chloride Injection
		0.22% 30 mEq/L Potassium Chloride in 5% Dextrose and 0.45% Sodium Chloride Injection
	40 mEq of K⁺ per L in 5% Dextrose and 0.2–0.225% Sodium Chloride*	40 mEq/L Potassium Chloride in 5% Dextrose and 0.2% Sodium Chloride Injection (Viaflex®), Baxter
		40 mEq/L 0.3% Potassium Chloride in 5% Dextrose and 0.225% Sodium Chloride Injection
		0.3% 40 mEq/L Potassium Chloride in 5% Dextrose and 0.2% Sodium Chloride Injection

	40 mEq of K⁺ per L in 5% Dextrose and 0.3–0.33% Sodium Chloride*	40 mEq/L Potassium Chloride in 5% Dextrose and 0.33% Sodium Chloride Injection
		40 mEq/L 0.3% Potassium Chloride in 5% Dextrose and 0.3% Sodium Chloride Injection
	40 mEq of K⁺ per L in 5% Dextrose and 0.45% Sodium Chloride*	40 mEq/L Potassium Chloride in 5% Dextrose and 0.45% Sodium Chloride Injection (Viaflex®), Baxter
		40 mEq/L 0.3% Potassium Chloride in 5% Dextrose and 0.45% Sodium Chloride Injection
	40 mEq of K⁺ per L in 5% Dextrose and 0.9% Sodium Chloride*	40 mEq/L Potassium Chloride in 5% Dextrose and 0.9% Sodium Chloride Injection (Viaflex®), Baxter

* available from one or more manufacturer, distributor, and/or repackager by generic (nonproprietary) name

Potassium Chloride in Water

Parenteral		
Injection, for IV infusion only	0.1 mEq per mL (10 mEq)*	**Potassium Chloride in Water for Injection (Premixed)** (LifeCare®), Hospira
	0.2 mEq per mL (10 and 20 mEq)*	**Potassium Chloride in Water for Injection (Premixed)** (LifeCare®), Hospira
	0.3 mEq per mL (30 mEq)*	**Chloride in Water for Injection (Premixed)** (LifeCare®), Hospira
	0.4 mEq per mL (20 and 40 mEq)*	**Potassium Chloride in Water for Injection (Premixed)** (LifeCare®), Hospira

* available from one or more manufacturer, distributor, and/or repackager by generic (nonproprietary) name

Potassium Gluconate

Oral		
Elixir	6.7 mEq of K⁺ per 5 mL*	**Kaon® Elixir**, Savage
		Potassium Gluconate Elixir
Tablets	2 mEq of K⁺*	**Glu-K®**, Western Research
		Potassium Gluconate Tablets

* available from one or more manufacturer, distributor, and/or repackager by generic (nonproprietary) name

Potassium Acetate, Potassium Bicarbonate, and Potassium Citrate

| **Oral** | | |
| **Solution** | 15 mEq of K⁺ (provided by potassium acetate 500 mg, potassium bicarbonate 500 mg, and potassium citrate 500 mg) per 5 mL | **Tri-K®**, Century |

Potassium Bicarbonate and Potassium Chloride

Oral		
Tablets, for solution	25 mEq of K⁺ and Cl⁻ (provided by potassium bicarbonate 0.5 g and potassium chloride 1.5 g)*	**Potassium Bicarbonate and Potassium Chloride Effervescent Tablets**
	25 mEq of K⁺ and Cl⁻ (provided by potassium bicarbonate 0.5 g, potassium chloride 1.5 g, and lysine hydrochloride 0.91 g)	**K-Lyte/CL® Effervescent Tablets**, Bristol-Myers Squibb
		Potassium Bicarbonate and Potassium Chloride Effervescent Tablets
	50 mEq of K⁺ and Cl⁻ (provided by potassium bicarbonate 2 g, potassium chloride 2.24 g, and lysine hydrochloride 3.65 g)	**K-Lyte/CL® 50 Effervescent Tablets**, Bristol-Myers Squibb
		Potassium Bicarbonate and Potassium Chloride Effervescent Tablets

* available from one or more manufacturer, distributor, and/or repackager by generic (nonproprietary) name

Potassium Bicarbonate and Potassium Citrate

| **Oral** | | |
| **Tablets, for solution** | 50 mEq of K⁺ (provided by potassium bicarbonate 2.5 g and potassium citrate 2.7 g) | **K-Lyte® DS Effervescent Tablets**, Bristol-Myers Squibb |

Potassium Citrate and Potassium Gluconate

| **Oral** | | |
| **Solution** | 6.7 mEq of K⁺ (provided by potassium citrate 0.17 g and potassium gluconate 1.17 g) per 5 mL | **Twin-K®**, Boots |

Potassium Phosphates

Parenteral		
For injection concentrate	4.4 mEq of K⁺ and 3 mM of P (provided by potassium phosphate dibasic 236 mg and potassium phosphate monobasic 224 mg) per mL*	**Potassium Phosphates Injection**
	4.4 mEq of K⁺ and 3 mM of P (provided by potassium phosphate dibasic 236 mg and potassium phosphate monobasic 224 mg) per mL pharmacy bulk package*	**Potassium Phosphates Injection**

* available from one or more manufacturer, distributor, and/or repackager by generic (nonproprietary) name

Selected Revisions March 25, 2019, © Copyright, September 1, 1976, American Society of Health-System Pharmacists, Inc.

Patiromer Sorbitex Calcium

40:18.18 • POTASSIUM-REMOVING AGENTS

■ Patiromer sorbitex calcium, which consists of patiromer, a nonabsorbed cation-exchange polymer, and a calcium-sorbitol counterion, is used for the removal of excess potassium.

USES

● Hyperkalemia

Patiromer sorbitex calcium is used in the treatment of hyperkalemia. Patiromer has been shown to decrease elevated serum potassium concentrations and to reduce the recurrence of hyperkalemia in patients with chronic kidney disease who are receiving drugs that inhibit the renin-angiotensin-aldosterone system. Because of the delayed onset of action of patiromer, the drug is not used as an emergency treatment for life-threatening hyperkalemia.

Efficacy of patiromer was established in a 2-part single-blind study that consisted of a 4-week single-group treatment phase followed by an 8-week, randomized, placebo-controlled withdrawal phase. Patients with stage 3 or 4 chronic kidney disease who were hyperkalemic with serum potassium concentrations of 5.1 to less than 6.5 mEq/L and who were receiving stable dosages of at least one drug that inhibits the renin-angiotensin-aldosterone system (i.e., angiotensin-converting enzyme [ACE] inhibitor, angiotensin II receptor antagonist, aldosterone antagonist) were included in the study. The mean patient age was 64 years and most patients were male (58%) and Caucasian (98%); approximately 97% of patients had hypertension, 57% had type 2 diabetes mellitus, and 42% had heart failure.

In the initial phase of the study, 243 patients received patiromer. Initial dosage of the drug was based on baseline serum potassium concentration; patients with mild or moderate-to-severe hyperkalemia (baseline serum potassium concentration of 5.1 to less than 5.5 mEq/L or 5.5 to less than 6.5 mEq/L, respectively) received an initial patiromer dosage of 8.4 or 16.8 g daily, respectively, in 2 divided doses. Dosage was adjusted based on serum potassium concentration on day 3 and at weeks 1, 2, and 3 to achieve and maintain concentrations in the target range of 3.8 to less than 5.1 mEq/L. The mean patiromer dosage was 13 or 21 g daily in patients with mild or moderate-to-severe hyperkalemia, respectively. The mean reduction in serum potassium concentration from baseline to week 4 was 1.01 mEq/L; 76% of patients had serum potassium concentrations within the target range at week 4.

The randomized placebo-controlled withdrawal phase included 107 patients with moderate-to-severe hyperkalemia at study entry whose serum potassium concentration was in the target range at the end of the initial study phase, and who were still receiving drugs that inhibit the renin-angiotensin-aldosterone system. Patients randomized to continue patiromer therapy received the same dosage they were receiving at the end of the initial study phase. For those who received patiromer, the mean dosage was 21 g daily at the beginning of and during the withdrawal phase. The primary end point of the randomized withdrawal phase was change in serum potassium concentration from the start of the withdrawal phase to the earliest visit at which the patient's serum potassium concentration was outside the range of 3.8 to less than 5.5 mEq/L, or to week 4 of the withdrawal phase if the patient's serum potassium concentration remained in range. Serum potassium concentration increased by a median of 0.72 mEq/L in patients who were switched to placebo but was unchanged in patients who continued receiving patiromer. A greater proportion of patients who received placebo had a serum potassium concentration of 5.1 mEq/L or greater (91 versus 43%) or 5.5 mEq/L or greater (60 versus 15%) at any time during the withdrawal phase compared with those who received patiromer.

Efficacy of patiromer in reducing serum potassium concentration is maintained with continued use. In a phase 2, open-label, dose-ranging study in 304 hyperkalemic patients with chronic kidney disease and type 2 diabetes mellitus who were receiving drugs that inhibit the renin-angiotensin-aldosterone system, the effect of patiromer on serum potassium concentration was maintained during continued therapy for periods of up to 52 weeks. The mean patiromer dosage during the study was 14 g daily in patients with a baseline serum potassium concentration of greater than 5 to 5.5 mEq/L who received an initial dosage of 8.4 g daily in 2 divided doses and was 20 g daily in those with a baseline serum potassium concentration of greater than 5.5 to 6 mEq/L who received an initial dosage of 16.8 g daily in 2 divided doses.

DOSAGE AND ADMINISTRATION

● Administration

Patiromer sorbitex calcium should be administered at least 3 hours before or 3 hours after other oral drugs. (See Drug Interactions: Effects on GI Absorption of Drugs.)

Patiromer is administered orally without regard to food. Patiromer should not be heated (e.g., in a microwave) or added to heated foods or liquids.

Patiromer should not be taken in its dry form. The powder should be mixed with water immediately prior to administration to form an oral suspension. The entire contents of the packet(s) containing patiromer should be emptied into a glass or cup containing 40 mL of water. The mixture should be stirred and then an additional 40 mL of water should be added to the suspension. The suspension should again be stirred thoroughly and more water may be added to achieve the desired consistency. The suspension should be administered immediately after preparation. If powder remains in the glass after initial administration, more water should be added and the mixture should be stirred and then administered immediately; this should be repeated, as needed, until the entire dose is administered.

● Dosage

Dosage of patiromer sorbitex calcium is expressed in terms of patiromer.

The recommended initial adult dosage of patiromer is 8.4 g once daily. Serum potassium concentration should be monitored, and the dosage of patiromer may be increased (in 8.4-g increments at intervals of 1 week or longer, up to a maximum dosage of 25.2 g once daily) or reduced based on the serum potassium concentration and desired target range.

● Special Populations

Dosage adjustments are not necessary in patients with renal impairment.

CAUTIONS

● Contraindications

Patiromer is contraindicated in patients with known hypersensitivity to the drug or to any ingredient in the formulation.

● Warnings/Precautions

Worsening of GI Motility Disorders

Patients with a history of bowel obstruction or major GI surgery, severe GI disorders, or swallowing disorders were excluded from clinical studies evaluating patiromer. Use of patiromer should be avoided in patients with severe constipation, bowel obstruction, or fecal impaction, including abnormal postoperative bowel motility disorders, because the drug may not be effective and may worsen GI conditions.

Hypomagnesemia

Hypomagnesemia was reported in 5.3% of patients receiving patiromer in clinical studies. Patiromer binds to magnesium in the colon, which can lead to hypomagnesemia. Serum magnesium concentrations should be monitored in patients receiving patiromer, and magnesium supplementation should be considered in those with low serum magnesium concentrations.

Specific Populations

Pregnancy

Patiromer is not expected to cause fetal harm when administered to pregnant women because the drug is not absorbed systemically following oral administration.

Lactation

Breast-feeding is not expected to result in risk to infants of patiromer-treated women because the drug is not absorbed systemically following oral administration.

Pediatric Use

Safety and efficacy of patiromer have not been established in pediatric patients.

Geriatric Use

In clinical studies of patiromer, 60% of patients receiving the drug were 65 years of age or older, while 20% were 75 years of age or older. No overall differences in efficacy were observed between geriatric patients and younger adults. However, adverse GI effects were reported more frequently in those 65 years of age or older compared with younger patients.

Renal Impairment

In clinical studies of patiromer, 93% of patients receiving the drug had chronic kidney disease. No dosage adjustments are necessary in patients with renal impairment.

● Common Adverse Effects

Adverse effects reported in 2% or more of patients receiving patiromer include constipation, hypomagnesemia, diarrhea, nausea, abdominal discomfort, and flatulence.

DRUG INTERACTIONS

● Effects on GI Absorption of Drugs

In vitro binding studies have shown that patiromer binds to approximately 50% of the oral drugs tested; in clinical interaction studies, concomitant oral administration with patiromer altered the bioavailability of some of these drugs. Clinically meaningful in vitro binding (i.e., 30% or more) was not observed between patiromer and allopurinol, amoxicillin, apixaban, aspirin, atorvastatin, cephalexin, digoxin, glipizide, lisinopril, phenytoin, riboflavin, rivaroxaban, spironolactone, or valsartan. Although clinically meaningful in vitro binding was observed between patiromer and amlodipine, cinacalcet, clopidogrel, furosemide, lithium, metoprolol, trimethoprim, verapamil, and warfarin, studies in healthy individuals indicated that systemic exposure to these drugs was not affected by concomitant oral administration with patiromer. Decreased systemic exposure to ciprofloxacin, levothyroxine, and metformin was observed when these oral drugs were administered concomitantly with patiromer but not when the administration times were separated by 3 hours. Since binding of patiromer to other concomitantly administered oral drugs could reduce GI absorption of the drugs and result in loss of efficacy when administration times are close to those of patiromer, other oral agents should be administered at least 3 hours before or 3 hours following administration of patiromer.

DESCRIPTION

Patiromer sorbitex calcium, which consists of patiromer, a nonabsorbed cation-exchange polymer, and a calcium-sorbitol counterion, is used for the removal of excess potassium. The drug increases fecal potassium excretion via binding of potassium in the lumen of the GI tract, which decreases the concentration of free potassium in the GI lumen and, consequently, reduces serum potassium concentrations. Animal studies indicate that orally administered patiromer is not absorbed systemically and is excreted in feces.

In an open-label study in patients with chronic kidney disease and hyperkalemia (mean baseline serum potassium concentration of 5.9 mEq/L), serum potassium concentrations were reduced by 0.2 and 0.8 mEq/L at 7 and 48 hours, respectively, following initiation of therapy with patiromer (16.8 g daily in divided doses for 2 days); potassium concentrations remained stable for 24 hours after the last dose and then began to increase. Following twice-daily dosing, maximum (steady-state) effects on serum potassium concentration are attained in approximately 7–14 days.

In healthy individuals, patiromer produced a dose-dependent increase in fecal potassium excretion with a corresponding dose-dependent decrease in urinary potassium excretion, resulting in no change in serum potassium concentrations, when administered at dosages up to 50.4 g daily in 3 divided doses for 8 days. Substantial increases in mean daily fecal potassium excretion with concomitant decreases in mean daily urinary potassium excretion also were observed in healthy individuals receiving patiromer 25.2 g daily for 6 days; fecal and urinary potassium excretion were similar whether the drug was administered as a single daily dose or in 2 or 3 divided doses daily. Mean patiromer dosage and effects of the drug on serum potassium concentration are similar whether patiromer is administered with or without food.

ADVICE TO PATIENTS

Importance of informing patients who are taking other oral drugs to administer these drugs at least 3 hours before or 3 hours after administration of patiromer.

Importance of informing patients that patiromer may be administered without regard to food and that patients should adhere to their prescribed diets.

Importance of preparing each dose immediately before administration according to the manufacturer's instructions. Importance of advising patients that patiromer should not be heated (e.g., in a microwave) or added to heated foods or liquids and that the drug should not be taken in its dry form.

Importance of women informing clinicians if they are or plan to become pregnant or plan to breast-feed.

Importance of informing clinicians of existing or contemplated concomitant therapy, including prescription and OTC drugs, as well as any concomitant illnesses.

Importance of informing patients of other important precautionary information. (See Cautions.)

PREPARATIONS

Excipients in commercially available drug preparations may have clinically important effects in some individuals; consult specific product labeling for details.

Patiromer Sorbitex Calcium

Oral		
For suspension	8.4 g (of patiromer) per packet	**Veltassa®**, Relypsa
	16.8 g (of patiromer) per packet	**Veltassa®**, Relypsa
	25.2 g (of patiromer) per packet	**Veltassa®**, Relypsa

Selected Revisions November 12, 2018, © Copyright, September 13, 2016, American Society of Health-System Pharmacists, Inc.

Sodium Polystyrene Sulfonate

40:18.18 • POTASSIUM-REMOVING AGENTS

■ Sodium polystyrene sulfonate is a sulfonated cation-exchange resin that is used for the removal of excess potassium.

USES

● Hyperkalemia

Sodium polystyrene sulfonate is used in the treatment of hyperkalemia. The drug aids in the removal of excess potassium from the body and should be considered an adjunct to other measures such as restriction of electrolyte intake, control of acidosis, and a high caloric diet. Before therapy is instituted, the cause of hyperkalemia should be determined and eliminated if possible. Because the action of the resin is slow, sodium polystyrene sulfonate alone may be insufficient (effective lowering of serum potassium may occur within hours to days) to rapidly correct severe hyperkalemia, including that associated with states of rapid tissue breakdown (e.g., burns, renal failure). Treatments that facilitate shift of potassium into cells, such as administration of sodium bicarbonate and/or dextrose (with or without insulin), and/or other treatments (e.g., a calcium salt) are indicated in patients with hyperkalemia evidenced by conduction defects (widening of the QRS complex) or arrhythmias. If hyperkalemia is severe, other definitive measures, including dialysis, should be considered. Sodium polystyrene sulfonate is most useful when hyperkalemia is not life-threatening or when other measures have reduced the dangers of hyperkalemia. The drug should not be used as an emergency treatment for life-threatening hyperkalemia.

DOSAGE AND ADMINISTRATION

● Reconstitution and Administration

Sodium polystyrene sulfonate is administered orally or rectally.

Oral Administration

Oral administration of sodium polystyrene sulfonate should be separated from oral administration of other drugs by at least 3 hours, and the separation time should be increased to 6 hours for patients with gastroparesis. (See Drug Interactions: Effects on GI Absorption of Drugs.)

When sodium polystyrene sulfonate is administered orally, each 1 g of the powdered resin should be reconstituted in 3–4 mL of water or a syrup and given as a suspension; usually 20–100 mL of fluid is used. Alternatively, the resin may be administered orally as a commercially available suspension. The suspension should be shaken well prior to administration. Sodium polystyrene sulfonate suspension also may be introduced into the stomach via a tube or the powdered resin or suspension may be mixed with the patient's food. The drug should *not* be mixed with foods or liquids that contain a large amount of potassium such as bananas or orange juice. Full precautions to prevent aspiration (e.g., placing and keeping the patient in an upright position during administration) should be observed.

Rectal Administration

When sodium polystyrene sulfonate is administered rectally as a retention enema, each dose of the powdered resin is administered in 100–200 mL of an aqueous vehicle, such as 1% methylcellulose, 10% dextrose, or water, which has been warmed to body temperature. Although a somewhat thicker suspension may be used, care should be taken that a paste, which would greatly reduce the exchange surface and be particularly ineffective if deposited in the rectal ampulla, is not formed. Alternatively, 120–200 mL of a commercially available suspension may be administered as a retention enema, after the suspension has been warmed to body temperature. The suspension should be shaken well prior to administration. After an initial cleansing enema, a soft, large (French 28) rubber tube should be inserted about 20 cm into the rectum, with the tip well into the sigmoid colon, and taped in place. The extemporaneously prepared suspension of the resin, kept in suspension by stirring, or the commercially available suspension is then administered rectally by gravity feed. The tube may then be flushed with 50–100 mL of fluid,

clamped, and left in place. If back leakage occurs, the hips should be elevated on pillows or a knee-chest position assumed. The suspension is retained in the colon for at least 30–60 minutes or for several hours if possible, after which the colon is irrigated with a non-sodium-containing solution at body temperature to remove the resin. Returns should be drained constantly through a Y-tube connection. Care should be taken to ensure that adequate volumes of non-sodium-containing cleansing enemas are administered. Approximately 2 L of irrigating solution may be needed to adequately flush out the resin. Proper removal of the resin is particularly important if sorbitol is used (administration of sorbitol is not recommended). Some clinicians believe that the preferred method of rectal administration is to place the resin in a sealed dialysis bag and insert the bag into the rectum.

● Dosage

Hyperkalemia

The dosage and duration of sodium polystyrene sulfonate therapy must be individualized and depend on daily assessment of total body potassium. (See Cautions: Precautions and Contraindications.)

The usual adult oral dosage of sodium polystyrene sulfonate is 15 g (approximately 4 level teaspoonfuls of the powder or 60 mL of the commercially available suspension) 1–4 times daily (average 15–60 g daily).

Sodium polystyrene sulfonate may also be given rectally as a retention enema (see Rectal Administration, in Dosage and Administration: Reconstitution and Administration) in adult doses of 30–50 g (120–200 mL of the commercially available suspension) every 6 hours.

Reduced dosage is recommended in infants and small children. Pediatric dosage may be based on the fact that 1 g of the resin binds approximately 1 mEq of potassium. Oral administration is contraindicated in neonates. Some manufacturers also state that rectal administration is contraindicated in neonates and premature infants. (See Cautions: Pediatric Precautions.)

CAUTIONS

● GI Effects

Sodium polystyrene sulfonate may cause some degree of gastric irritation. Anorexia, nausea, vomiting, and constipation may occur, especially if large doses are given. Large doses of the drug may cause fecal impaction, especially in geriatric patients. If clinically important constipation occurs, therapy with sodium polystyrene sulfonate should be discontinued until normal bowel movements resume; administration of magnesium hydroxide laxatives or sorbitol is not recommended. (See Drug Interactions.) Occasionally, the resin causes diarrhea.

Intestinal necrosis, which may be fatal, and other serious adverse GI events (bleeding, ischemic colitis, perforation) have been reported in patients receiving sodium polystyrene sulfonate. Most cases have occurred in patients receiving sorbitol concomitantly; many of the patients had risk factors for adverse GI events (e.g., prematurity, history of intestinal disease or surgery, hypovolemia, renal insufficiency or failure). (See Cautions: Precautions and Contraindications.) Although a causal relationship to the resin and/or sorbitol has not been established, some clinicians have suggested that studies in uremic rats implicate sorbitol rather than sodium polystyrene sulfonate as being principally responsible for intestinal necrosis. However, the occurrence of GI injury in patients receiving sodium polystyrene sulfonate without sorbitol and the presence of sodium polystyrene sulfonate crystals in injured segments of the GI tract have led others to suggest that the resin itself may be pathogenic.

In a systematic review of 58 cases of adverse GI events associated with sodium polystyrene sulfonate use, 71% of patients received the resin in combination with sorbitol, and 77% received the resin orally; 71% of patients had a history of chronic kidney disease or end-stage renal disease requiring dialysis, 16% had undergone prior solid organ transplantation, and 28% had undergone a recent surgical procedure. The colon was the most common site of injury (76% of patients); injuries in more proximal segments of the GI tract often were accompanied by colonic injury. Histolopathologic examination of GI specimens revealed transmural necrosis in 62% and ulceration in 48% of patients; sodium polystyrene sulfonate crystals were detected in injured segments of the GI tract in 90% of patients. Common presenting symptoms included abdominal pain and distension, GI bleeding, nausea and vomiting, and diarrhea; the median time from initiation of therapy to onset of symptoms was 2 days. The mortality rate in this series of patients was 33%, with 94% of the deaths occurring in patients with evidence of colonic necrosis.

● Electrolyte Effects

Hypokalemia and clinically important sodium retention may occur in patients receiving sodium polystyrene sulfonate therapy. Since the cation-exchange action of sodium polystyrene sulfonate is not totally selective for potassium, increased excretion of other cations occurs. (See Pharmacology.) Hypocalcemia and other electrolyte disturbances may occur.

● Pulmonary Effects

Acute bronchitis and bronchopneumonia following aspiration of sodium polystyrene sulfonate particles have been reported.

● Precautions and Contraindications

Patients receiving sodium polystyrene sulfonate should be monitored for electrolyte (e.g., calcium, magnesium, potassium) abnormalities. Serum potassium concentrations should be determined frequently within each 24-hour period during therapy; the duration of treatment with the resin must be determined individually for each patient. Because intracellular potassium deficiency is not always reflected by serum potassium concentrations, electrocardiograms and the clinical condition of the patient also should be closely monitored. ECG abnormalities seen with hypokalemia include lengthened QT intervals; widened, flat, or inverted T waves; and prominent U waves. Cardiac abnormalities, including premature atrial, nodal, or ventricular contractions and supraventricular and ventricular tachycardias, may also occur. Early signs of severe hypokalemia include a pattern of irritable confusion, delayed thought processes, and muscle cramps. Marked hypokalemia can also be manifested by severe muscle weakness and occasionally frank paralysis. The risk of precipitating hypokalemia-induced cardiotoxic effects of cardiac glycosides should be considered when sodium polystyrene sulfonate is administered to patients receiving these glycosides.

Because of the potential for intestinal necrosis and other serious adverse GI events (bleeding, ischemic colitis, perforation), sodium polystyrene sulfonate should be used only in patients with normal bowel function. Use of the drug should be avoided in patients at risk for developing constipation or impaction (e.g., those with a history of fecal impaction, chronic constipation, inflammatory bowel disease, ischemic colitis, vascular intestinal atherosclerosis, previous bowel resection, or bowel obstruction) and in postoperative patients who have not had a bowel movement following surgery. Because most of the reported cases of intestinal necrosis or other serious adverse GI events occurred in patients who received sorbitol concomitantly with sodium polystyrene sulfonate, concomitant administration of sorbitol is not recommended. Most commercially available suspensions of sodium polystyrene sulfonate have been reformulated without sorbitol; however, preparations in a 33% sorbitol vehicle remain commercially available. Therapy with sodium polystyrene sulfonate should be discontinued if constipation occurs.

Precautions (e.g., placing and keeping the patient in an upright position during oral administration) should be taken to prevent aspiration. Patients with an impaired gag reflex, altered level of consciousness, or predisposition to regurgitation may be at an increased risk of aspirating sodium polystyrene sulfonate following oral administration.

Because administration of sodium polystyrene sulfonate may represent a clinically important sodium load (see Chemistry and Stability: Chemistry), the resin should be administered cautiously to patients whose sodium intake must be restricted, such as those with heart failure, hypertension, or edema. In these patients, compensatory restriction of sodium intake from other sources may be indicated.

In vitro studies have shown that sodium polystyrene sulfonate can bind to other drugs, which may decrease the extent of absorption of these drugs following concomitant oral administration. Other oral drugs should be administered at least 3 hours before or 3 hours after oral administration of sodium polystyrene sulfonate, and the separation time should be increased to 6 hours for patients with gastroparesis. (See Drug Interactions: Effects on GI Absorption of Drugs.)

Sodium polystyrene sulfonate is contraindicated in patients with hypokalemia, those with obstructive bowel disease, and those with known hypersensitivity to sodium polystyrene sulfonate resins. The drug also is contraindicated in neonates with decreased gut motility. Oral administration of sodium polystyrene sulfonate is contraindicated in neonates; some manufacturers state that use of the drug (oral or rectal administration) is contraindicated in neonates and premature infants. (See Cautions: Pediatric Precautions.)

● Pediatric Precautions

Efficacy of sodium polystyrene sulfonate in pediatric patients has not been established.

Sodium polystyrene sulfonate is contraindicated in neonates with reduced gut motility. Premature or low-birthweight infants may have an increased risk of adverse GI effects (e.g., intestinal necrosis) with sodium polystyrene sulfonate use. Some manufacturers state that use of the drug is contraindicated in premature infants.

Oral administration of sodium polystyrene sulfonate is contraindicated in neonates. The drug should be administered rectally in children and neonates with particular caution, since excessive dosages or inadequate dilution may result in impaction of the resin; care should be taken to ensure an adequate volume of non-sodium-containing cleansing enemas after rectal administration. Some manufacturers state that rectal administration is contraindicated in neonates.

● Geriatric Precautions

Large doses of sodium polystyrene sulfonate may cause fecal impaction in geriatric patients.

● Pregnancy, Fertility, and Lactation

Animal reproduction studies have not been performed with sodium polystyrene sulfonate. Sodium polystyrene sulfonate is not absorbed systemically following oral or rectal administration, and use in pregnant women is not expected to result in fetal risk.

Breast-feeding is not expected to result in risk to infants of sodium polystyrene sulfonate-treated women because the drug is not absorbed systemically.

DRUG INTERACTIONS

● Effects on GI Absorption of Drugs

In vitro studies have shown that sodium polystyrene sulfonate may bind to other drugs (e.g., amlodipine, amoxicillin, furosemide, metoprolol, phenytoin, warfarin). Binding of sodium polystyrene sulfonate to other oral drugs could reduce GI absorption of the concomitantly administered agents and result in loss of efficacy when administration times are close to those of sodium polystyrene sulfonate. Therefore, other oral drugs should be administered at least 3 hours before or 3 hours after oral administration of sodium polystyrene sulfonate. Patients with gastroparesis or other conditions resulting in delayed gastric emptying may require a 6-hour separation. FDA states that the recommended spacing interval is based on the expected time for either sodium polystyrene sulfonate or the other drug to pass through the stomach. Clinical response and/or blood concentrations of the drugs should be monitored whenever possible. The manufacturers state that sodium polystyrene sulfonate may decrease absorption of lithium and thyroxine.

● Antacids and Laxatives

Sodium polystyrene sulfonate, when given orally with cation-donating antacids and laxatives such as magnesium hydroxide or calcium carbonate, has been reported to cause metabolic alkalosis in patients with renal disease. Magnesium hydroxide and calcium carbonate neutralize gastric hydrochloric acid and form the ionizable compounds magnesium chloride and calcium chloride. Upon entry into the small intestine, the magnesium and calcium ions react with bicarbonate and form magnesium carbonate and calcium carbonate, both of which are insoluble. However, sodium polystyrene sulfonate prevents this reaction by binding with the magnesium and calcium before they react with bicarbonate. This results in a loss of hydrogen ions from the stomach without a loss of bicarbonate ions from the intestine and, subsequently, in metabolic alkalosis. Rectal use of sodium polystyrene sulfonate may avoid this reaction.

In one study in patients with renal impairment (i.e., creatinine clearance ranging from 10–60 mL/minute), increases in plasma CO_2 concentration and in plasma and urinary pH were reported following concomitant use of sodium polystyrene sulfonate and calcium- or magnesium-containing antacids. Severe systemic alkalosis and a tonic-clonic seizure reportedly occurred in one patient with chronic hypocalcemia secondary to renal failure who received magnesium hydroxide and sodium polystyrene sulfonate concomitantly. In one patient with impaired renal function and chronic metabolic acidosis, the systemic alkalosis produced by concomitant use of sodium polystyrene sulfonate and magnesium hydroxide was used to therapeutic advantage.

Simultaneous oral administration of cation-donating antacids and laxatives with sodium polystyrene sulfonate may also reduce the resin's potassium exchange capability. Although there are no controlled studies to date, some clinicians have observed resistance to the potassium-lowering effect of sodium polystyrene sulfonate in hyperkalemic patients receiving magnesium hydroxide; response to sodium polystyrene sulfonate was reportedly restored when magnesium hydroxide was discontinued.

One case of small bowel obstruction resulting from aluminum hydroxide concretion has been reported to be associated with concurrent sodium polystyrene sulfonate therapy. However, the patient was receiving 720–1440 mL of aluminum hydroxide gel per day, and intestinal obstruction has been reported to occur with doses of aluminum hydroxide gel as low as 120 mL per day without concurrent administration of the resin.

Sodium polystyrene sulfonate and calcium- or magnesium-containing antacids or laxatives should be used with caution, especially in patients with renal impairment. The manufacturer warns that magnesium hydroxide should not be used as a laxative for the treatment of sodium polystyrene sulfonate-induced constipation.

● Sorbitol

Concomitant use of sorbitol with sodium polystyrene sulfonate may result in intestinal necrosis and is not recommended. (See Cautions: GI Effects and Cautions: Precautions and Contraindications.)

● Cardiac Glycosides

Sodium polystyrene sulfonate-induced hypokalemia may increase toxic effects of cardiac glycosides on the heart (e.g., ventricular arrhythmias, AV nodal dissociation).

PHARMACOLOGY

Sodium polystyrene sulfonate is a cation-exchange resin that releases sodium in exchange for other cations. Following oral administration, sodium is released from the resin in exchange for hydrogen ions in the acidic environment of the stomach. As the resin passes through the intestines, hydrogen cations exchange with those cations that are in greater concentrations and the cationically modified resin is excreted in the feces. Because of the relatively high concentration of potassium present in the large intestine, conversion of the resin to the potassium form occurs principally at this site. Following rectal administration of sodium polystyrene sulfonate, sodium ions are partially released from the resin in exchange for other cations present. In clinical use, much of the exchange capacity of sodium polystyrene sulfonate is utilized for cations other than potassium such as calcium, magnesium, iron, organic cations, lipids, steroids, and proteins. Thus, although 1 g of the resin has an in vitro exchange capacity of about 3.1 mEq of potassium, an in vivo exchange capacity greater than 1 mEq of potassium per g of resin is not likely.

CHEMISTRY AND STABILITY

● Chemistry

Sodium polystyrene sulfonate is a sulfonated cation-exchange resin prepared in the sodium phase and used for the removal of excess potassium. Each gram of the resin has an in vitro exchange capacity of about 3.1 mEq (range: 2.81–3.45 mEq) of potassium. Sodium polystyrene sulfonate occurs as a cream to light brown, fine

powder that is odorless and tasteless and is insoluble in water. Each gram of the powdered resin contains approximately 4.1 mEq of sodium.

Sodium polystyrene sulfonate is commercially available as the powder or as a suspension. The commercially available suspension is an amber-colored, cherry-flavored suspension of the resin; the vehicle contains purified water, propylene glycol, magnesium aluminum silicate, sucralose, citric acid, flavoring agent, and parabens as a preservative. Each 100 mL of the commercially available suspension contains 25 g of sodium polystyrene sulfonate and 114 mEq of sodium. The drug also remains available as a light brown, cherry-flavored suspension in a 33% sorbitol vehicle that contains alcohol, purified water, propylene glycol, magnesium aluminum silicate, sodium saccharin, flavoring agent, and parabens as a preservative. (See Drug Interactions: Sorbitol.)

● Stability

Sodium polystyrene sulfonate powder and commercially available suspensions should be stored in well-closed containers at a temperature of 20–25°C, but some preparations may be exposed to temperatures ranging from 15–30°C. If repackaged, the commercially available suspensions should be refrigerated and used within 14 days of repackaging.

Sodium polystyrene sulfonate should not be heated because changes in the exchange properties of the resin may occur. The manufacturers of the powdered resin state that extemporaneous suspensions of the resin should be freshly prepared and should not be stored for more than 24 hours. However, an extemporaneously prepared 25% suspension of the powdered resin in water using a combination of 0.5% carboxymethylcellulose and 0.3% magnesium aluminum silicate as suspending agents was reportedly stable (i.e., easily redispersed, minimal sedimentation) for at least 30 days.

PREPARATIONS

Excipients in commercially available drug preparations may have clinically important effects in some individuals; consult specific product labeling for details.

Sodium Polystyrene Sulfonate

Oral or Rectal		
Powder, for suspension		Kionex®, Perrigo
		Sodium Polystyrene Sulfonate Powder
Suspension	1.25 g/5 mL*	Kionex®, Perrigo
		Sodium Polystyrene Sulfonate Suspension
		SPS®, CMP

* available from one or more manufacturer, distributor, and/or repackager by generic (nonproprietary) name

Selected Revisions November 12, 2018, © Copyright, January 1, 1984, American Society of Health-System Pharmacists, Inc.

Bumetanide

40:28.08 • LOOP DIURETICS

■ Bumetanide is a sulfonamide loop-type diuretic and antihypertensive agent.

USES

● Edema

Bumetanide is used for the management of edema associated with heart failure or hepatic or renal disease (including nephrotic syndrome). The drug may be effective in some patients whose condition is unresponsive or refractory to other diuretics. In a limited number of patients, approximately 60% of those with edema refractory to other diuretic therapy showed an improved diuretic response with bumetanide. Patients who had received 80–160 mg of furosemide daily with little or no diuretic response showed a marked diuresis with 2–6 mg of bumetanide daily; however, in some of these patients, improvement observed during initial therapy did not continue during maintenance therapy with bumetanide. Further study is needed to determine the role of bumetanide in the management of edema refractory to other diuretics.

Careful etiologic diagnosis should precede the use of any diuretic. Because the potent diuretic effect of loop diuretics may result in severe electrolyte imbalance and excessive fluid loss, hospitalization of the patient during initiation of therapy is advisable, especially for patients with hepatic cirrhosis and ascites or chronic renal failure. In prolonged diuretic therapy, intermittent use of the loop diuretics for only a few days each week may be advisable.

Heart Failure

Bumetanide is effective for the short- and long-term management of edema associated with heart failure. In addition to decreasing edema, the drug relieves other signs and symptoms of heart failure such as dyspnea, rales, and hepatomegaly. Bumetanide appears to be as effective as furosemide in reducing edema, body weight, abdominal girth, rales, hepatomegaly, blood pressure, and heart rate in patients with heart failure.

Most experts state that all patients with symptomatic heart failure who have evidence for, or a history of, fluid retention generally should receive diuretic therapy in conjunction with moderate sodium restriction, an agent to inhibit the renin-angiotensin-aldosterone-aldosterone (RAA) system (e.g., angiotensin-converting enzyme [ACE] inhibitor, angiotensin II receptor antagonist, angiotensin receptor-neprilysin inhibitor [ARNI]), a β-adrenergic blocking agent (β-blocker), and in selected patients, an aldosterone antagonist. Some experts state that because of limited and inconsistent data, it is difficult to make precise recommendations regarding daily sodium intake and whether it should vary with respect to the type of heart failure (e.g., reduced versus preserved ejection fraction), disease severity (e.g., New York Heart Association [NYHA] class), heart failure-related comorbidities (e.g., renal dysfunction), or other patient characteristics (e.g., age, race). The American College of Cardiology Foundation (ACCF) and American Heart Association (AHA) state that limiting sodium intake to 1.5 g daily in patients with ACCF/AHA stage A or B heart failure may be reasonable. While data currently are lacking to support recommendation of a specific level of sodium intake in patients with ACCF/AHA stage C or D heart failure, ACCF and AHA state that limiting sodium intake to some degree (e.g., less than 3 g daily) in such patients may be considered for symptom improvement. Diuretics play a key role in the management of heart failure because they produce symptomatic benefits more rapidly than any other drugs, relieving pulmonary and peripheral edema within hours or days compared with weeks or months for cardiac glycosides, ACE inhibitors, or β-blockers. However, since there are no long-term studies of diuretic therapy in patients with heart failure, the effects of diuretics on morbidity and mortality in such patients are not known. Although there are patients with heart failure who do not exhibit fluid retention in the absence of diuretic therapy and even may develop severe volume depletion with low doses of diuretics, such patients are rare and the unique pathophysiologic mechanisms regulating their fluid and electrolyte balance have not been elucidated.

Most experts state that loop diuretics (e.g., bumetanide, ethacrynic acid, furosemide, torsemide) are the diuretics of choice for most patients with heart failure. However, thiazides may be preferred in some patients with concomitant hypertension because of their sustained antihypertensive effects. If resistance to diuretics occurs, IV administration of a diuretic or concomitant use of 2 or more diuretics (e.g., a loop diuretic and metolazone, a loop diuretic and a thiazide diuretic) may be necessary; alternatively, short-term administration of a drug that increases blood flow (e.g., a positive inotropic agent such as dopamine) may be necessary. ACCF and AHA state that IV loop diuretics should be administered promptly to all hospitalized heart failure patients with substantial fluid overload to reduce morbidity. In addition, ACCF and AHA state that low-dose dopamine infusions may be considered in combination with loop diuretics to augment diuresis and preserve renal function and renal blood flow in patients with acute decompensated heart failure, although data are conflicting and additional study and experience are needed. For additional information, see Heart Failure under Uses: Edema, in the Thiazides General Statement 40:28.20.

Hepatic Disease

Bumetanide is used for the short- and long-term management of edema and ascites associated with hepatic disease (e.g., cirrhosis). Short-term administration of 2–4 mg of bumetanide daily or long-term administration of up to 6 mg daily has produced appreciable diuretic and natriuretic effects without substantial serum electrolyte disturbance in some patients with this condition. Patients with hepatic ascites reportedly have responded to an initial bumetanide dosage of 1 mg daily with weight loss averaging about 0.6 kg daily and a marked increase in urinary volume and natriuresis. The major complications observed during bumetanide therapy in these patients included hypokalemia and hyponatremia; however, electrolyte disturbances are commonly observed in patients with severe hepatic disease who are receiving diuretic therapy. Some patients developed encephalopathy during bumetanide administration.

Bumetanide appears to be as effective as furosemide in reducing body weight and in causing diuresis and increased urinary excretion of sodium, potassium, and chloride in patients with hepatic cirrhosis and ascites. Following IV administration, single 0.5-mg doses of bumetanide were as effective as 20-mg doses of furosemide in patients with refractory ascites.

In most clinical studies in patients with hepatic cirrhosis and ascites, patients received concomitant therapy with bumetanide and potassium salts or potassium-sparing diuretics to prevent hypokalemia.

Renal Disease

Bumetanide is used for the management of edema in patients with impaired renal function. In patients with severe renal impairment (i.e., GFR less than 10 mL/minute), high dosages of the drug may be needed to produce an adequate diuretic response.

Bumetanide (1–10 mg orally daily) appears to be as effective as furosemide (40–400 mg orally daily) in reducing edema, body weight, and abdominal girth in patients with edema secondary to renal disease. However, in one study, substantial reductions in body weight, edema, and mean arterial pressure were observed in patients with severe renal impairment who received oral bumetanide dosages of 1–18 mg daily but not in those who received oral furosemide dosages of 20–480 mg daily.

Oral bumetanide dosages of 2–6 mg daily appear to be as effective as oral furosemide dosages of 40–160 mg daily in reducing edema in patients with nephrotic syndrome; however, in some patients with nephrotic syndrome and moderately impaired renal function (i.e., creatinine clearance of 4–34 mL/minute), a decreased response compared with that of patients with nephrotic syndrome and normal renal function has been reported.

Other Edematous Conditions

Bumetanide has been used for the management of postoperative† or premenstrual edema† and edema associated with disseminated carcinoma†.

● Hypertension

Bumetanide has been used alone or in combination with other classes of antihypertensive agents for the management of hypertension†, especially when complicated by heart failure, acute pulmonary edema, or renal disease. Because of established clinical benefits (e.g., reductions in overall mortality and in adverse cardiovascular, cerebrovascular, and renal outcomes), current evidence-based practice guidelines for the management of hypertension in adults generally recommend the use of drugs from 4 classes of antihypertensive agents (ACE inhibitors, angiotensin II receptor antagonists, calcium-channel blockers, and thiazide diuretics). (See Uses: Hypertension in Adults, in the Thiazides General Statement 40:28.20.) However, some experts state that loop diuretics (e.g., furosemide, bumetanide, torsemide) are preferred over thiazides in patients with moderate to severe chronic kidney disease (CKD) or symptomatic heart failure. Loop diuretics may be particularly useful in patients with heart failure and reduced left ventricular ejection fraction (LVEF) who have evidence of fluid retention; however, some experts state that thiazide diuretics my be considered in hypertensive patients with heart failure and mild fluid retention because of their more persistent antihypertensive effect.

For further information on the role of diuretics in antihypertensive drug therapy and information on overall principles and expert recommendations for treatment of hypertension, see Uses: Hypertension in Adults and also see Uses: Hypertension in Pediatric Patients, in the Thiazides General Statement 40:28.20.

Other Uses

Bumetanide has been used to enhance the elimination of drugs or toxic substances following intoxication. Like furosemide, bumetanide has been used as an adjunct in forced alkaline diuresis to enhance salicylate elimination following acute aspirin intoxication. (See Measures to Enhance Salicylate Elimination in Acute Toxicity: Treatment, in the Salicylates General Statement 28:08.04.24.) IV bumetanide and IV sodium bicarbonate have reportedly produced a more rapid decrease in blood salicylate concentration compared with parenteral fluid therapy alone.

DOSAGE AND ADMINISTRATION

Administration

Oral Administration

Bumetanide is usually administered orally as a single daily dose in the morning. Bumetanide may also be given by intermittent administration on alternate days or on 3 or 4 consecutive days alternating with drug-free periods of 1 or 2 days. For optimum therapeutic effect in some patients, it may be necessary to administer bumetanide in 2 divided doses in the morning and evening. Administration of bumetanide in 2 divided doses daily has been reported to be more effective in increasing urinary sodium output and urinary volume than administration of the drug as a single daily dose, and the evening dose appeared to have a greater diuretic effect than the morning dose. Therefore, some clinicians suggest that, when the drug is administered once daily, it may be preferable to administer the dose in the evening. Further study is needed to determine the optimum dosage schedule for oral bumetanide administration.

IV Administration

When the patient is unable to take oral medication or GI absorption is impaired, bumetanide may be administered by IM or IV injection or by IV infusion. Parenteral administration of bumetanide should be replaced by oral therapy as soon as possible. Bumetanide injection should be inspected visually for particulate matter and discoloration prior to administration.

For IV injection, bumetanide should be given slowly over a period of 1–2 minutes. For IV infusion, bumetanide injection should be diluted in 5% dextrose, 0.9% sodium chloride, or lactated Ringer's injection. IV infusions should be freshly prepared and used within 24 hours.

Standardize 4 Safety

Standardized concentrations for IV bumetanide have been established through Standardize 4 Safety (S4S), a national patient safety initiative to reduce medication errors, especially during transitions of care. Multidisciplinary expert panels were convened to determine recommended standard concentrations. Because recommendations from the S4S panels may differ from the manufacturer's prescribing information, caution is advised when using concentrations that differ from labeling, particularly when using rate information from the label. For additional information on S4S (including updates that may be available), see https://www.ashp.org/ pharmacy-practice/standardize-4-safety-initiative.

TABLE 1. Standardize 4 Safety Continuous IV Infusion Standard Concentrations for Bumetanide

Patient Population	Concentration Standards	Dosing Units
Adults	0.25 mg/mL	mg/hour
Pediatric patients (<50 kg)	0.04 mg/mL	mcg/kg/hour[a]
	0.25 mg/mL	

[a] dosing units differ from concentration units

Dosage

Dosage of bumetanide should be adjusted according to individual requirements and response. Since the diuretic response following oral or parenteral administration is similar, bumetanide dosage is identical for oral, IV, or IM administration. For the management of fluid retention (e.g., edema) associated with heart failure, experts state that diuretics should be administered at a dosage sufficient to achieve optimal volume status and relieve congestion without inducing an excessively rapid reduction in intravascular volume, which could result in hypotension, renal dysfunction, or both. The manufacturer states that, in furosemide-allergic patients, bumetanide may be substituted for furosemide at approximately a 1:40 ratio since cross-sensitivity between the drugs does not appear to occur; however, some clinicians question the safety of bumetanide administration in furosemide-sensitive patients.

Edema

Oral Dosage

For the management of edema, the usual initial adult oral dosage of bumetanide recommended by the manufacturers is 0.5–2 mg daily. If the diuretic response to an initial dose of the drug is inadequate, repeated doses may be given at 4- to 5-hour intervals until the desired response is obtained or a maximum dosage of 10 mg daily is reached. For maintenance therapy, the effective dose of bumetanide may be administered intermittently. For the management of fluid retention (e.g., edema) associated with heart failure, some experts recommend initiating bumetanide at a low dosage (e.g., 0.5–1 mg once or twice daily) and increasing the dosage (maximum of 10 mg daily) until urine output increases and weight decreases, generally by 0.5–1 kg daily. (See Dosage and Administration: Administration.)

Parenteral Dosage

The usual initial adult IV or IM dose of bumetanide for the management of edema is 0.5–1 mg. In patients with inadequate response to the initial parenteral dose of bumetanide, repeated doses may be given at 2- to 3-hour intervals until the desired diuretic response is obtained or a maximum dosage of 10 mg daily is reached.

Hypertension

Oral Dosage

For the management of hypertension† in adults, the usual oral dosage of bumetanide is 0.5–2 mg daily, administered in 2 divided doses.

Monitoring and Blood Pressure Treatment Goals

The patient's renal function and electrolytes should be assessed 2–4 weeks after initiation of diuretic therapy. Blood pressure should be monitored regularly (i.e., monthly) during therapy and dosage of the antihypertensive drug adjusted until blood pressure is controlled. If an adequate blood pressure response is not achieved, the dosage may be increased or another antihypertensive agent with demonstrated benefit and preferably with a complementary mechanism of action (e.g., angiotensin-converting enzyme [ACE] inhibitor, angiotensin II receptor antagonist, calcium-channel blocker) may be added; if target blood pressure is still not achieved, a third drug may be added. (See Uses: Hypertension in Adults, in the Thiazides General Statement 40:28.20.) In patients who develop unacceptable adverse effects with bumetanide, the drug should be discontinued and another antihypertensive agent from a different pharmacologic class should be initiated.

The goal of hypertension management and prevention is to achieve and maintain optimal control of blood pressure. However, the optimum blood pressure threshold for initiating antihypertensive drug therapy and specific treatment goals remain controversial. A 2017 multidisciplinary hypertension guideline from the American College of Cardiology (ACC), American Heart Association (AHA), and a number of other professional organizations generally recommends a blood pressure goal of less than 130/80 mm Hg in all adults, regardless of comorbidities or level of atherosclerotic cardiovascular disease (ASCVD) risk. Many patients will require at least 2 drugs from different pharmacologic classes to achieve this blood pressure goal; the potential benefits of hypertension management and drug cost, adverse effects, and risks associated with the use of multiple antihypertensive drugs also should be considered when deciding a patient's blood pressure treatment goal.

For additional information on target levels of blood pressure and on monitoring therapy in the management of hypertension, see Blood Pressure Monitoring and Treatment Goals under Dosage: Hypertension, in Dosage and Administration in the Thiazides General Statement 40:28.20.

Pediatric Dosage

Although the manufacturer states that safety and efficacy have not been established, dosages of 0.015 mg/kg on alternate days to 0.1 mg/kg daily have been used safely and effectively in a limited number of children with heart failure†. For information on overall principles for treatment of hypertension and overall expert recommendations for such disease in pediatric patients, see Uses: Hypertension in Pediatric Patients, in the Thiazides General Statement 40:28.20.

● Dosage in Renal and Hepatic Impairment

Although the manufacturer recommends that maximum oral or parenteral dosage of bumetanide not exceed 10 mg daily, oral or IV dosages up to 20 mg daily have been administered to patients with impaired renal function for the management of edema. Single-dose studies have shown that IV doses greater than 2 mg are needed to achieve a diuretic response in patients with creatinine clearances less than 5 mL/minute.

In patients with impaired hepatic function, bumetanide dosage should be kept to a minimum; if bumetanide dosage must be increased in these patients, it should be adjusted carefully.

CAUTIONS

Adverse effects occurring frequently during bumetanide therapy include muscle cramps, dizziness, hypotension, headache, nausea, and encephalopathy; these adverse effects may be related to bumetanide. The manufacturer states that one or more of these adverse effects occurs in 4.1% of bumetanide-treated patients. Laboratory test alterations, including electrolyte, hematologic, renal, and hepatic abnormalities, occur in approximately 49% of patients receiving the drug. Many of the adverse effects associated with bumetanide therapy may be caused by diuresis or the underlying disease being treated.

● Fluid, Electrolyte, Cardiovascular, and Renal Effects

Bumetanide may produce profound diuresis resulting in fluid and electrolyte depletion. Fluid and electrolyte depletion is more likely to occur with excessive doses or too frequent administration of the drug or in those with restricted sodium intake.

Too vigorous diuresis may result in profound water loss and dehydration, especially in geriatric patients. The resultant hypovolemia may lead to circulatory collapse or thromboembolic episodes such as vascular thromboses and/or emboli. Pronounced reductions in plasma volume associated with rapid or excessive diuresis may also result in an abrupt fall in glomerular filtration rate, as evidenced by increased BUN and serum creatinine concentration. Hypotension reportedly occurs in less than 1% of patients receiving bumetanide. Orthostatic hypotension has occurred during concomitant therapy with other hypotensive agents.

Hypokalemia and hypochloremia reportedly occur in about 15% of patients receiving bumetanide and hyponatremia occurs in about 10% of patients. Hypophosphatemia and hypocalcemia have been reported less frequently. Potassium depletion is particularly likely to occur in patients with hyperaldosteronism with normal renal function, hepatic cirrhosis and ascites, potassium-losing renal diseases, or certain diarrheal conditions and may require particular attention in patients with heart failure receiving cardiac glycosides and diuretics, those with a history of ventricular arrhythmias, and those with other conditions in which hypokalemia is considered to represent a risk. Prevention of hypokalemia is particularly important in these patients. Diuretic-induced hypokalemia and hypochloremia may result in metabolic alkalosis, especially in patients with other losses of potassium and chloride secondary to vomiting, diarrhea, GI drainage, excessive sweating, paracentesis, or potassium-losing renal diseases. Metabolic alkalosis, with increased serum bicarbonate concentration and changes in total CO_2 content, has been reported in patients receiving bumetanide. Sudden changes in electrolyte balance may precipitate hepatic encephalopathy and coma in patients with hepatic cirrhosis and ascites. Supplemental therapy with potassium chloride or potassium-sparing diuretics (e.g., spironolactone) may be necessary for the prevention of hypokalemia and/or metabolic alkalosis in some patients. Diuretics also have shown to increase urinary excretion of magnesium, which may result in hypomagnesemia.

Other adverse cardiovascular effects of bumetanide include ECG changes and chest pain.

Hyperuricemia has been reported in about 20% of patients receiving bumetanide; however, most reported cases to date have been asymptomatic. Gouty arthritis has occurred in at least one patient receiving the drug. Serum uric acid concentrations have returned to pretreatment levels in some patients during continued therapy with the drug. Serum uric acid concentrations have increased to more than 12 mg/dL in a few patients receiving bumetanide but have returned to within normal limits following discontinuance of the drug.

Reversible azotemia and increased serum creatinine concentration have been reported in 10% or less of bumetanide-treated patients. These adverse renal effects are especially likely to occur in patients with impaired renal function and appear to be associated with dehydration. Decreased creatinine clearance reportedly has been observed in less than 1% of patients receiving the drug. Bumetanide-induced renal failure has occurred rarely. Although acute interstitial nephritis has been reported rarely with furosemide, there are no reports to date of this adverse renal effect with bumetanide.

● Otic Effects

Ototoxicity has been reported in cats, dogs, and guinea pigs receiving bumetanide. On a weight basis, the ototoxic potential of bumetanide in these animals was 5–6 times greater than that of furosemide; however, the relative ototoxic potential of bumetanide at equivalent diuretic dosages was 0.11–0.16 times that of furosemide, since bumetanide has about 40–60 times the diuretic potency of furosemide. The likelihood of serum bumetanide concentrations achieving a level necessary to produce ototoxicity in humans is small; however, the possibility of bumetanide-induced ototoxicity must be considered following IV administration of the drug, especially at high dosages, after too rapid administration, in patients with impaired renal function, and/or in patients receiving other ototoxic drugs (e.g., aminoglycosides). Impaired hearing and otic discomfort have reportedly occurred rarely in patients receiving bumetanide. Combined data from comparative studies indicate that the frequency of drug-related hearing loss based on audiometric testing was 1.1% in patients receiving oral bumetanide dosages of 0.5–18 mg daily and 6.4% in patients receiving oral furosemide dosages of 20–640 mg daily. In addition, there are reports of furosemide-induced ototoxicity that improved following substitution of bumetanide therapy.

● Metabolic Effects

Although changes in plasma insulin, glucagon, or growth hormone concentration or in glucose tolerance generally have not been observed to date in patients receiving bumetanide, the possibility that the drug may adversely affect glucose metabolism should be considered. Hyperglycemia has reportedly occurred in about 7% of patients receiving the drug. Although comparative differences have not been fully determined, the frequency of bumetanide-induced hyperglycemia has been reported to be lower than that of furosemide. Bumetanide has also been associated with glycosuria and proteinuria in less than 1% of patients. The drug has been associated with decreased glucose tolerance without glycosuria in at least one patient. In general, diabetic control has not been adversely affected in patients with diabetes mellitus who were receiving bumetanide for the management of edema.

Diuretics, including bumetanide, can increase serum total cholesterol concentrations in some patients; increases in low-density lipoprotein cholesterol and/or very low-density lipoprotein cholesterol subfractions appear to be principally responsible for these increases.

● Musculoskeletal Effects

Adverse musculoskeletal effects reportedly occurring in about 1% or less of patients receiving bumetanide include muscle cramps, arthritic pain, musculoskeletal pain, muscle stiffness and tenderness, and asterixis. Musculoskeletal pain (sometimes severe) generally develops about 4 hours following oral administration or 1–2 hours following IV administration of the drug and persists for about 6–12 hours. In most patients, musculoskeletal pain is more severe in the extremities. The development of musculoskeletal pain appears to be a dose-related effect but varies among individuals. Some clinicians suggest that bumetanide-induced musculoskeletal pain may be related to electrolyte disturbances.

● Nervous System Effects

Adverse nervous system effects occurring in 1% or less of patients receiving bumetanide include dizziness, headache, weakness, vertigo, and fatigue.

● Hepatic Effects

Adverse hepatic effects of bumetanide include alteration of liver function test results and encephalopathy (in patients with preexisting hepatic disease). Increased total serum bilirubin, serum LDH, AST (SGOT), ALT (SGPT), or alkaline phosphatase concentration and increased or decreased cholesterol concentration have occurred in 1% or less of patients receiving bumetanide. Although these adverse hepatic effects have been associated with bumetanide, a causal relationship to the drug has not been established.

● Hematologic Effects

Adverse hematologic effects of bumetanide reportedly occurring in less than 1% of patients include increased or decreased hemoglobin concentration, prothrombin time, or hematocrit. Thrombocytopenia, increased or decreased leukocyte count, and changes in the differential leukocyte count, including eosinophilia, have occurred rarely. Bumetanide-induced leukopenia and thrombocytopenia have usually been transient and not associated with serious adverse systemic effects; however, one patient developed purpura alone and another developed purpura, epistaxis, and intestinal hemorrhage which proved fatal. Although the development of blood dyscrasias has been associated with bumetanide, a causal relationship to the drug has not been established.

● GI Effects

Adverse GI effects reportedly occurring in less than 1% of patients receiving bumetanide include nausea, abdominal pain, vomiting, xerostomia, dyspepsia, diarrhea, and stomach cramps.

● Dermatologic Effects

Adverse dermatologic effects reportedly occurring rarely in patients receiving bumetanide include pruritus, urticaria, and rash. The drug has been associated with Stevens-Johnson syndrome in at least one patient; a causal relationship to bumetanide has been suggested since the condition resolved following discontinuance of the drug.

● Other Adverse Effects

Premature ejaculation, erectile impotence, and nipple tenderness have occurred rarely in patients receiving bumetanide. Bumetanide has been associated with the development of mammary tenderness or gynecomastia in a few patients; however, a causal relationship to the drug has not been established and some of these patients were receiving concomitant therapy with spironolactone.

Other adverse effects of bumetanide include sweating, hyperventilation, and increased or decreased serum protein concentrations.

● Precautions and Contraindications

Bumetanide is a potent diuretic that may produce profound diuresis with fluid and electrolyte depletion, especially when administered at high dosages or for prolonged periods. Patients receiving bumetanide should be carefully observed for signs of electrolyte depletion, especially hypokalemia. Patients should be informed of the signs and symptoms of electrolyte imbalance and instructed to report to their physician if weakness, dizziness, fatigue, faintness, mental confusion, lassitude, muscle cramps, headache, paresthesia, thirst, anorexia, nausea, and/or vomiting occur. Excessive fluid and electrolyte loss may be minimized by monitoring the patient carefully and by initiating therapy with small doses, adjusting dosage carefully, and using an intermittent dosage schedule if possible. Careful monitoring, including hospitalization during initiation of therapy, and dosage adjustment are especially important in patients with hepatic cirrhosis and ascites.

Serum potassium concentration should be measured periodically during therapy with bumetanide. Supplemental therapy with potassium chloride or potassium-sparing diuretics may be used if necessary to prevent or treat hypokalemia and/or metabolic alkalosis. Prevention of hypokalemia is particularly important for patients with heart failure receiving cardiac glycosides and diuretics or for those with hepatic cirrhosis and ascites, hyperaldosteronism with normal renal function, potassium-losing renal diseases, certain diarrheal conditions, or other conditions (e.g., history of ventricular arrhythmias) in which hypokalemia is considered to represent a risk. Periodic determination of other serum electrolyte concentrations is recommended for patients receiving therapy at high dosages or for prolonged periods, especially in those with restricted sodium intake. Administration of bumetanide at high dosages or for prolonged periods may cause profound water loss, electrolyte depletion, dehydration, or hypovolemia and circulatory collapse with the possibility of vascular thrombosis and embolism, especially in geriatric patients. If excessive diuresis and/or electrolyte abnormalities occur, the drug should be withdrawn or dosage reduced until homeostasis is restored. Electrolyte abnormalities should be corrected by appropriate measures.

Bumetanide should be used with caution in patients with hepatic cirrhosis and ascites, since sudden alterations in fluid and electrolyte balance may precipitate hepatic encephalopathy and/or coma. Bumetanide administration in these patients should be initiated at low dosages in a hospital setting with careful monitoring of the patient's fluid and electrolyte balance and clinical status. Supplemental therapy with potassium chloride or potassium-sparing diuretics may be used to prevent hypokalemia and metabolic alkalosis in these patients.

Although changes in plasma insulin, glucagon, or growth hormone concentration or in glucose tolerance generally have not been observed during therapy with bumetanide, the possibility of an adverse effect on glucose metabolism cannot be excluded. Blood glucose concentration should be determined periodically, especially in patients with known or suspected (e.g., marginally impaired glucose tolerance) diabetes mellitus.

Patients receiving bumetanide should be observed carefully for the development of blood dyscrasias (especially thrombocytopenia), liver damage, or idiosyncratic reactions which have been reported occasionally during therapy with the drug.

Although bumetanide's potential for producing ototoxicity is small compared with furosemide, the possibility of bumetanide-induced ototoxicity must be considered following IV administration of the drug, especially at high dosages, after too rapid administration, in patients with impaired renal function, and/or in patients receiving other ototoxic drugs.

Bumetanide should be used with extreme caution, if at all, in patients who are allergic to sulfonamides, since these patients may show hypersensitivity to bumetanide. Although the manufacturer states that bumetanide does not appear to exhibit cross-sensitivity in patients allergic to furosemide, the drugs are structurally similar and some clinicians believe that there is insufficient evidence to support a lack of cross-sensitivity. Bumetanide is contraindicated in patients with known hypersensitivity to the drug.

Bumetanide is contraindicated in patients with anuria. Although bumetanide may be used to produce diuresis in patients with impaired renal function, the drug is contraindicated for further use when marked increases in BUN or serum creatinine concentration or oliguria occur during treatment of progressive renal disease. In patients with hepatic coma or severe electrolyte depletion, bumetanide therapy should not be instituted until the basic condition is improved or corrected.

● Pediatric Precautions

Safety and efficacy of bumetanide in children younger than 18 years of age have not been established. Bumetanide has been used effectively as a diuretic for up to 40 weeks in a limited number of infants ranging from 2 weeks to 7 months of age who had congenital heart disease and heart failure†. However, in vitro studies using pooled serum from critically ill neonates have shown substantial displacement of bilirubin from albumin by bumetanide. Therefore, bumetanide should be used with caution in critically ill or jaundiced neonates who are at risk for kernicterus. In addition, the elimination of bumetanide appears to be slower in neonates than in adults, possibly because of immature renal and hepatobiliary functions. For information on overall principles and expert recommendations for treatment of hypertension in pediatric patients, see Uses: Hypertension in Pediatric Patients, in the Thiazides General Statement 40:28.20.

● *Mutagenicity and Carcinogenicity*

It is not known whether bumetanide is mutagenic or carcinogenic in humans. Bumetanide did not produce mutagenic activity in various strains of *Salmonella typhimurium* when tested with or without metabolic activation. Following oral administration of bumetanide, an increased number of mammary tumors was observed in female rats receiving 2000 times the maximum recommended human dosage for 18 months; however, these findings could not be duplicated when the study was repeated with the same dosage.

● *Pregnancy, Fertility, and Lactation*

Pregnancy

Limited clinical experience with bumetanide in pregnant women to date has not revealed evidence of harm to the fetus; however, the possibility of adverse fetal effects cannot be excluded. Bumetanide should be used during pregnancy only when the potential benefits justify the possible risks to the fetus.

Although there are no adequate and controlled studies to date in humans, bumetanide has been shown to have a slight embryocidal effect in rats when given at a dosage 3400 times the maximum recommended human dosage; evidence of moderate growth retardation and delayed ossification of sternebrae in fetal offspring and maternal weight loss also occurred. Fetotoxic effects were not observed in rats when bumetanide was administered at 1000–2000 times the maximum recommended human dosage. Reproduction studies in mice using dosages up to 3400 times the maximum recommended human dosage have not revealed evidence of teratogenic or embryocidal effects. Bumetanide was not teratogenic in hamsters following oral administration of 0.5 mg/kg daily (17 times the maximum recommended human dosage) or in mice or rats at IV dosages up to 140 times the maximum recommended human dosage. A dose-related decrease in litter size and increase in fetal resorption rate occurred in rabbits receiving oral dosages of 0.1 and 0.3 mg/kg daily (3.4 and 10 times the maximum recommended human dosage, respectively); a slight embryocidal effect occurred in those receiving 0.1 mg/kg daily, and an increased frequency of delayed ossification of the sternebrae also occurred in those receiving 0.3 mg/kg daily. Adverse fetal effects were not observed in rabbits receiving 0.03 mg/kg daily.

Fertility

The effect of bumetanide on fertility in humans is not known. Reproduction studies in rats using bumetanide dosages of 10, 30, 60, or 100 mg/kg daily showed a slightly decreased rate of pregnancy; however, the differences were small and not statistically significant.

Lactation

Since it is not known if bumetanide is distributed into milk, the manufacturer cautions that nursing should not be undertaken in women receiving the drug.

DRUG INTERACTIONS

● *Diuretics*

Concomitant administration of bumetanide and most other diuretics results in enhanced diuretic and natriuretic effects. Spironolactone, triamterene, or amiloride hydrochloride may reduce the potassium loss resulting from bumetanide therapy; this effect has been used to therapeutic advantage.

● *Drugs Affected by or Causing Potassium Depletion*

In patients receiving a cardiac glycoside (e.g., digoxin), electrolyte disturbances produced by bumetanide (principally hypokalemia but also hypomagnesemia)

predispose the patient to digitalis toxicity; possibly fatal cardiac arrhythmias may result. Therefore, it is particularly important that hypokalemia be prevented in patients receiving bumetanide and a cardiac glycoside concomitantly. Periodic electrolyte determinations should be performed in patients receiving a cardiac glycoside and bumetanide, and correction of hypokalemia undertaken if warranted. Bumetanide does not affect serum digoxin concentrations or renal excretion of digoxin when the drugs are used concomitantly.

Like furosemide, bumetanide potentially can cause prolonged neuromuscular blockade in patients receiving nondepolarizing neuromuscular blocking agents (e.g., tubocurarine chloride, gallamine triethiodide [no longer commercially available in the US]), presumably because of potassium depletion or decreased urinary excretion of the muscle relaxant. Although there are no reports to date of prolonged neuromuscular blockade during concomitant administration of bumetanide and nondepolarizing neuromuscular blocking agents, the possibility of this drug interaction should be considered.

Some drugs such as corticosteroids, corticotropin, and amphotericin B also cause potassium loss, and severe potassium depletion may occur when one of these drugs is administered during bumetanide therapy.

● *Lithium*

Renal clearance of lithium is apparently decreased in patients receiving diuretics, and lithium toxicity may result. Bumetanide and lithium should generally not be given together. If concomitant therapy is necessary, serum lithium concentrations should be monitored carefully and dosage adjusted accordingly.

● *Hypotensive Agents*

The antihypertensive effect of hypotensive agents may be enhanced during concomitant bumetanide administration. This effect is usually used to therapeutic advantage; however, orthostatic hypotension may result. Dosage of the hypotensive agent, and possibly both drugs, should be reduced when bumetanide is added to an existing antihypertensive regimen.

● *Indomethacin*

Indomethacin may reduce the diuretic and natriuretic effects of bumetanide. The mechanism(s) of these interactions has not been established but has been attributed to indomethacin-induced inhibition of prostaglandin synthesis which may result in fluid retention and/or changes in vascular resistance. Indomethacin also inhibits the bumetanide-induced increase in plasma renin activity. Although the clinical importance of these interactions has not been determined, the manufacturer states that concomitant therapy with bumetanide and indomethacin is not recommended. However, some clinicians suggest that, if concomitant therapy is necessary, an increase in bumetanide dosage may overcome an indomethacin-induced decrease in diuretic activity.

● *Probenecid*

Probenecid may reduce the diuretic and natriuretic effects of bumetanide. Probenecid may also inhibit the bumetanide-induced increase in plasma renin activity. The mechanism(s) of these interactions does not appear to result from direct inhibition of sodium excretion but probably involves inhibition by probenecid of the renal tubular secretion of bumetanide. Although the clinical importance of these interactions has not been determined, the manufacturer recommends that probenecid not be administered concomitantly with bumetanide.

● *Ototoxic Drugs*

Concomitant parenteral administration of bumetanide and aminoglycoside antibiotics or other ototoxic drugs (e.g., cisplatin) may result in increased risk of ototoxicity, especially in patients with impaired renal function. Although potentiation of aminoglycoside-induced ototoxicity with bumetanide has not been reported to date in humans, permanent changes in cochlear activity have occurred following administration of bumetanide in animals pretreated with kanamycin. Concomitant parenteral administration of bumetanide and aminoglycoside antibiotics should be avoided, except in life-threatening conditions.

● *Nephrotoxic Drugs*

Although there is no clinical experience to date with concomitant administration of bumetanide and nephrotoxic agents, concomitant use of these drugs should be avoided since bumetanide may enhance the nephrotoxic effects.

● Anticoagulants

Bumetanide does not appear to affect the plasma prothrombin activity or the metabolism of oral anticoagulants (e.g., warfarin). In 2 studies in healthy individuals, no substantial differences in prothrombin time or in plasma concentration or half-life of warfarin were observed when a single dose of warfarin (40–65 mg) was administered alone or concomitantly with 1 or 2 mg of bumetanide daily.

ACUTE TOXICITY

● Pathogenesis

The LD_{50} of bumetanide following IV administration has been reported to be 330 mg/kg in mice and 70 mg/kg in rabbits. The oral LD_{50} of the drug in rabbits has been reported to be 350 mg/kg. However, mice and rats have survived oral doses of 2000 mg/kg in one study and 6000 mg/kg in another study.

● Manifestations

Overdosage of bumetanide may result in acute, profound water loss, volume and electrolyte depletion, and hypovolemia and circulatory collapse with a possibility of vascular thrombosis and embolism. Electrolyte depletion may be manifested as weakness, dizziness, mental confusion, anorexia, lethargy, vomiting, and cramps.

Following intraperitoneal administration of 300 mg/kg of bumetanide to mice, ataxia, reduced muscle tone, tremors, and seizures occurred and persisted for 1 day. In dogs receiving 0.5 mg/kg of the drug IV, leg muscle fasciculations, opisthotonos, and trismus occurred and were present from 10 seconds to 2 minutes followed by complete recovery.

● Treatment

In acute bumetanide overdose, supportive and symptomatic treatment consisting of fluid and electrolyte replacement should be initiated. Urinary output and serum and urinary electrolyte concentrations should be carefully monitored.

PHARMACOLOGY

The pharmacologic effects of bumetanide are similar to those of furosemide.

● Renal Effects

Bumetanide acts directly on the ascending limb of the loop of Henle to inhibit sodium and chloride reabsorption. Although the exact mechanism(s) of action has not been established, bumetanide decreases electrolyte reabsorption by inhibiting the active chloride and, possibly, sodium transport systems in the ascending limb of the loop of Henle. Bumetanide may interfere with renal cyclic 3′,5′-adenosine monophosphate (cAMP) activity or with binding of cAMP to renal tissue. Inhibition of cAMP-dependent protein kinase or sodium-potassium adenosine triphosphatase (ATPase), an enzyme with high activity in the ascending limb of the loop of Henle, may be involved. Unlike ethacrynic acid, bumetanide does not bind sulfhydryl groups of renal cellular proteins. Bumetanide also appears to inhibit electrolyte reabsorption in the proximal renal tubule. Since phosphate and bicarbonate reabsorption occur mainly in the proximal tubule, phosphaturia and increased bicarbonate excretion during bumetanide-induced diuresis are indicative of this additional effect. Inhibition of electrolyte reabsorption in the proximal tubule may result from inhibition of sodium phosphate-linked transport, but is apparently not related to inhibition of carbonic anhydrase activity. Bumetanide indirectly increases potassium secretion in the distal renal tubule secondary to an increased sodium load in the tubule; the drug does not appear to have a direct effect on electrolyte reabsorption in the distal tubule. The drug is not an aldosterone antagonist. Although bumetanide reportedly has about 40 times the diuretic activity of furosemide on a weight basis, the relative potency may vary when different dosages and/or routes of administration are compared.

Bumetanide increases urinary excretion of sodium, chloride, potassium, hydrogen, calcium, magnesium, and ammonium; excretion of phosphate and bicarbonate may also be increased. The chloruretic effect of the drug is greater than its natriuretic effect and its effect on urinary calcium and magnesium excretion is less than that on sodium excretion. Although urinary excretion of calcium and magnesium is initially (4–6 hours after administration) increased, retention

of these electrolytes subsequently occurs and no substantial net loss of calcium or magnesium is observed over a 24-hour period. Bumetanide-induced increases in urinary excretion of hydrogen and ammonium ions are generally associated with little or no effect on urinary pH; however, in one study, urinary pH decreased from 6.1 to 5.1 following administration of the drug. The drug decreases free water clearance in humans during hydration and tubular free water reabsorption during hydropenia. The decrease in free water clearance results from inhibition of electrolyte reabsorption and active transport at the ascending limb of the loop of Henle.

Bumetanide decreases uric acid excretion and increases serum uric acid concentration. Hyperuricemia has been reported in some patients receiving the drug. (See Cautions: Renal Effects.) The overall decrease in uric acid excretion appears to be less than that attributed to therapeutically equivalent doses of furosemide.

Bumetanide produces renal vascular dilation and substantially increases renal blood flow. Maximum increases in renal blood flow have ranged from 30–40% during bumetanide therapy. In animals, the drug causes redistribution of renal blood flow to the midcortical and juxtamedullary regions of the kidney. Increased urinary prostaglandin E concentrations have been observed in bumetanide-treated animals. It has been suggested that the drug's effect on renal prostaglandin activity may result in changes in renal hemodynamics. Although the effect of bumetanide on prostaglandin activity in humans has not been determined, the drug's effects on renal blood flow and renal cortical redistribution in animals are inhibited by prior treatment with a prostaglandin synthetase inhibitor (e.g., indomethacin). Bumetanide has a variable effect on glomerular filtration rate (GFR) in humans.

Bumetanide produces variable but substantial increases in plasma renin activity (PRA). In one study in healthy adults, increased PRA was observed 1 hour after bumetanide administration and persisted for up to 12 hours.

● Cardiovascular Effects

Bumetanide may produce hypotensive effects resulting from decreased plasma volume. Substantial reductions in blood pressure and in body weight have been observed in patients with hypertensive cardiovascular disease and heart failure who received the drug. Reductions in mean pulmonary venous pressure, left ventricular end-diastolic pressure (LVEDP), mean pulmonary artery pressure, and mean right atrial pressure have also been observed in patients with valvular heart disease receiving bumetanide; pulmonary and systemic arteriolar resistance were slightly reduced. Following administration of the drug in patients with coronary artery disease, reductions in cardiac output, cardiac index, stroke volume, stroke index, and in diastolic pressures (beginning, mean, and end) have occurred.

● Metabolic Effects

There is conflicting evidence to date on bumetanide's effect on carbohydrate metabolism. In healthy individuals receiving the drug, changes in plasma insulin, glucagon, or growth hormone concentration or in glucose tolerance generally have not been observed. However, hyperglycemia reportedly has occurred in some patients receiving the drug. Diuretic-induced hyperglycemia may result from potassium depletion which has been associated with impaired insulin secretion. In one study in healthy individuals, a single 1-mg IV dose of bumetanide did not alter insulin response to IV glucose or the rate of decrease in blood glucose concentration. In individuals with impaired glucose tolerance (chemical, latent, or borderline diabetes mellitus), 1 mg of the drug daily for 10 days did not impair glucose tolerance further. When the effects of bumetanide and furosemide on oral glucose tolerance and insulin response to glucose were compared in another study, similar effects on carbohydrate metabolism were observed in bumetanide- and in furosemide-treated patients. Further study is needed to fully characterize the effects of bumetanide on carbohydrate metabolism; however, the drug does not appear to be associated with consistent or clinically important changes in blood glucose concentration.

PHARMACOKINETICS

● Absorption

Bumetanide is rapidly and almost completely absorbed from the GI tract. In several studies in healthy individuals, at least 85–95% of a single oral dose of the drug was absorbed; however, in one study, the bioavailability of bumetanide tablets reportedly was only 72%. The oral bioavailability of the drug in patients with impaired renal or hepatic function does not appear to differ substantially from that in healthy individuals. Limited data suggest that food may delay the absorption of oral bumetanide. The drug appears to be completely absorbed following IM administration.

Following oral administration, bumetanide appears in plasma within 15–20 minutes and peak plasma concentrations of the drug generally occur within 0.5–2 hours. Following oral administration of a single 1-mg dose of the drug in healthy adults, peak plasma or serum bumetanide concentrations have reportedly averaged 31–48 ng/mL; after a single 2-mg dose in one study, the peak plasma concentration averaged 73 ng/mL.

Bumetanide-induced diuresis begins within 30–60 minutes following oral administration, about 40 minutes following IM administration, and within a few minutes following IV administration; peak diuretic activity generally occurs within 1–2 hours following oral or IM administration and within 15–30 minutes after IV administration. Diuresis is generally complete within 4 hours following oral or IM administration of 1–2 mg of the drug; however, diuretic activity may persist for up to 5–6 hours, particularly when doses greater than 2 mg are used. Following IV administration, diuresis generally persists for 2–3 hours.

● **Distribution**

Distribution of bumetanide into human body tissues and fluids has not been fully characterized. Following IV administration of bumetanide in dogs, highest concentrations of the drug were observed in kidney, liver, and plasma, with lowest concentrations in heart, lung, muscle, and adipose tissue; bumetanide showed 3 times the affinity for renal tissue compared with that of furosemide. Following IV administration of bumetanide in healthy adults, the steady-state volume of distribution (V_{ss}) has been reported to range from 9.45–19.7 L and the volume of distribution of the central compartment (V_c) has been reported to range from 3.26–5.84 L. Following IV administration of bumetanide in neonates, the mean volume of distribution has been reported to range from 0.26–0.38 L/kg. V_{ss} may be decreased in patients with hepatic impairment. V_{ss} may be increased in patients with renal impairment. In one study in patients with varying degrees of renal dysfunction, V_{ss}, but not V_c, was increased compared with that of individuals with normal renal function (V_{ss}: 22 versus 17 L).

Approximately 94–97% of bumetanide is bound to plasma proteins in vitro. In vivo, approximately 92.6 or 96% of the drug is bound to plasma proteins based on Sephadex batch or ultrafiltration method, respectively. Protein binding may be decreased in patients with renal impairment; binding appears to be correlated with plasma albumin concentration in these patients. In one study, when bumetanide or furosemide was added to pooled human serum (adult or neonatal) in equimolar concentrations, bumetanide's displacement of bilirubin from albumin-binding sites was equivalent to that of furosemide in adult serum but less than that of furosemide in neonatal cord serum. In addition, results of an vitro study of pooled serum from critically ill neonates indicate that serum concentrations of free (unbound) bilirubin increased in a linear manner at bumetanide concentrations of 0.5–50 mcg/mL; however, such a correlation was not observed at bumetanide concentrations of 0.25 mcg/mL. Bumetanide does not appear to bind to erythrocytes.

Bumetanide and its metabolites are distributed into bile. Following oral administration of radiolabeled bumetanide in one patient with a biliary T tube in place, 1.8% of the dose was distributed into bile as unchanged drug and 12.6% as metabolites.

It is not known whether bumetanide crosses the blood-brain barrier or the placenta or is distributed into milk.

● **Elimination**

Plasma concentrations of bumetanide have generally been reported to decline in a monophasic or biphasic manner; however, studies using sensitive assay methods indicate that plasma concentrations may decline in a triphasic manner following IV administration.

Following oral administration, the terminal elimination half-life of bumetanide reportedly ranges from 1–1.5 hours in healthy adults. Following IV administration in adults with normal renal and hepatic function, the half-life in the initial phase ($t_{\frac{1}{2}\alpha}$) averages 5–6.9 minutes, the half-life in the secondary phase ($t_{\frac{1}{2}\beta}$) averages 46–47 minutes, and the half-life in the terminal phase ($t_{\frac{1}{2}\gamma}$) averages 3.1–3.4 hours. Serum concentrations of bumetanide may be higher and the terminal elimination half-life prolonged in patients with impaired renal and/or hepatic function. In neonates and infants, the elimination of bumetanide appears to be slower than in older pediatric patients and adults, possibly because of immature renal and hepatobiliary functions. The mean serum elimination half-life of bumetanide reportedly is 2.5 and 1.5 hours in infants younger than 2 months of age and in those 2–6 months of age, respectively. In addition, limited data indicate that the apparent half-life of the drug may be prolonged to about 6 hours (with a range up to 15 hours) in premature or full-term neonates with respiratory disorders receiving IV bumetanide.

Total body clearance of bumetanide from plasma reportedly averages 120–250 mL/minute in adults with normal renal and hepatic function; renal clearance of the drug is about 50–65% of the total body clearance. Total body clearance of bumetanide is decreased in patients with impaired renal function, with or without concomitant hepatic impairment; in patients with only renal impairment, nonrenal clearance of the drug is about 90% or more of the total body clearance. Clearance also may be decreased in neonates and infants possibly, because of immature renal and hepatobiliary functions. In neonates with volume overload, mean serum clearance of bumetanide reportedly was about 2.2 and 3.8 mL/minute per kg in those younger than 2 months of age and 2–6 months of age, respectively. In addition, limited data indicate that serum clearance of the drug may be decreased to about 0.2–1.1 mL/minute per kg in premature or full-term neonates with respiratory disorders receiving IV bumetanide.

Bumetanide is partially metabolized in the liver to at least 5 metabolites. Metabolism apparently occurs only by oxidation of the N-butyl side chain of the bumetanide molecule; the phenyl ring structures do not appear to be metabolized. Hydroxylation occurs at each carbon of the N-butyl side chain. The major urinary metabolite is the 3′-alcohol derivative. The major metabolite excreted in bile and/or feces is the 2′-alcohol derivative. Minor metabolites include the 4′-alcohol, N-desbutyl, and 3′-acid derivatives. Bumetanide metabolites in urine and bile are present as conjugates, principally glucuronide conjugates. Conjugates of the drug and its metabolites do not appear in feces.

Bumetanide and its metabolites are excreted principally in urine. Renal excretion of the drug appears to occur mainly via glomerular filtration; tubular secretion may also occur. Following oral or IV administration in healthy adults, about 80% of a dose is excreted in urine and 10–20% in feces within 48 hours; about 50% of a dose is excreted unchanged in urine. Bumetanide is excreted in feces almost completely as metabolites, apparently via biliary elimination; less than 2% of a dose is excreted unchanged in feces within 48 hours. Following IV administration of radiolabeled bumetanide in one study in patients with varying degrees of renal dysfunction, about 25% of a dose was excreted in urine within 48 hours and about 40% (range: 4–94%) was excreted in feces within 7 days.

CHEMISTRY AND STABILITY

● **Chemistry**

Bumetanide is a sulfonamide-type, loop diuretic. The drug is a derivative of metanilamide and is structurally related to furosemide. Bumetanide differs structurally from furosemide by the presence of 4-phenoxy and 5-butylamino substituents.

Bumetanide occurs as a practically white, crystalline powder with a slightly bitter taste. The drug has solubilities of 0.1 mg/mL in water and 30.6 mg/mL in alcohol at 25°C. Bumetanide has pK_as of 0.3, 4, and 10. Commercially available bumetanide injection is a sterile solution of the drug containing 0.85% sodium chloride and 0.4% ammonium acetate as buffers, 1% benzyl alcohol as a preservative, and 0.01% disodium edetate. Sodium hydroxide is added during the manufacture of the injection to adjust the pH to 6.8–7.8.

● **Stability**

Bumetanide is photosensitive and will discolor when exposed to light. Commercially available preparations of bumetanide should be protected from light and stored at 15–30°C. Bumetanide tablets should be stored in tight, light-resistant containers. The commercially available tablets are stable for 5 years and the injection is stable for 3 years after the date of manufacture.

Bumetanide injection is reportedly stable at a pH of 4–10. Substantial adsorption of the drug to glass or PVC containers reportedly does not occur. Bumetanide injection is physically and chemically compatible in glass and PVC containers with the following IV solutions: 5% dextrose, 0.9% sodium chloride, or lactated Ringer's injection. Bumetanide injection that has been diluted with one of these compatible IV solutions should be used within 24 hours after preparation.

PREPARATIONS

Excipients in commercially available drug preparations may have clinically important effects in some individuals; consult specific product labeling for details.

Bumetanide

Oral		
Tablets	0.5 mg*	Bumetanide Tablets
	1 mg*	Bumetanide Tablets
	2 mg*	Bumetanide Tablets
Parenteral		
Injection	0.25 mg/mL*	Bumetanide Injection

* available from one or more manufacturer, distributor, and/or repackager by generic (nonproprietary) name

† Use is not currently included in the labeling approved by the US Food and Drug Administration.

Selected Revisions June 10, 2024, © Copyright, July 1, 1984, American Society of Health-System Pharmacists, Inc.

Furosemide

40:28.08 • LOOP DIURETICS

■ Furosemide is a sulfonamide, loop-type diuretic and antihypertensive agent.

USES

● Edema

Furosemide is used in the management of edema associated with heart failure, nephrotic syndrome, and hepatic cirrhosis. IV furosemide also may be used as an adjunct in the treatment of acute pulmonary edema.

Careful etiologic diagnosis should precede the use of any diuretic. Because the potent diuretic effect of furosemide may result in severe electrolyte imbalance and excessive fluid loss, hospitalization of the patient during initiation of therapy is advisable, especially for patients with hepatic cirrhosis and ascites or chronic renal failure. In prolonged diuretic therapy, intermittent use of the drug for only a few days each week may be advisable. Furosemide may be administered cautiously for additive effect with most other diuretics; however, since furosemide and other loop diuretics (e.g., ethacrynic acid) act in a similar manner, there is no rationale for using these drugs together.

Heart Failure

Furosemide is used in the management of edema associated with heart failure. Most experts state that all patients with symptomatic heart failure who have evidence for, or a history of, fluid retention generally should receive diuretic therapy in conjunction with moderate sodium restriction, an agent to inhibit the renin-angiotensin-aldosterone (RAA) system (e.g., angiotensin-converting enzyme [ACE] inhibitor, angiotensin II receptor antagonist, angiotensin receptor-neprilysin inhibitor [ARNI]), a β-adrenergic blocking agent (β-blocker), and in selected patients, an aldosterone antagonist. Some experts state that because of limited and inconsistent data, it is difficult to make precise recommendations regarding daily sodium intake and whether it should vary with respect to the type of heart failure (e.g., reduced versus preserved ejection fraction), disease severity (e.g., New York Heart Association [NYHA] class), heart failure-related comorbidities (e.g., renal dysfunction), or other patient characteristics (e.g., age, race). The American College of Cardiology Foundation (ACCF) and American Heart Association (AHA) state that limiting sodium intake to 1.5 g daily in patients with ACCF/AHA stage A or B heart failure may be reasonable. While data currently are lacking to support recommendation of a specific level of sodium intake in patients with ACCF/AHA stage C or D heart failure, ACCF and AHA state that limiting sodium intake to some degree (e.g., less than 3 g daily) in such patients may be considered for symptom improvement.

Diuretics play a key role in the management of heart failure because they produce symptomatic benefits more rapidly than any other drugs, relieving pulmonary and peripheral edema within hours or days compared with weeks or months for cardiac glycosides, ACE inhibitors, or β-blockers. However, since there are no long-term studies of diuretic therapy in patients with heart failure, the effects of diuretics on morbidity and mortality in such patients are not known. Although there are patients with heart failure who do not exhibit fluid retention in the absence of diuretic therapy and even may develop severe volume depletion with low doses of diuretics, such patients are rare and the unique pathophysiologic mechanisms regulating their fluid and electrolyte balance have not been elucidated.

Most experts state that loop diuretics (e.g., bumetanide, ethacrynic acid, furosemide, torsemide) are the diuretics of choice for most patients with heart failure. If resistance to diuretics occurs, IV administration of a diuretic or concomitant use of 2 or more diuretics (e.g., a loop diuretic and metolazone, a loop diuretic and a thiazide diuretic) may be necessary; alternatively, short-term administration of a drug that increases blood flow (e.g., a positive inotropic agent such as dopamine) may be necessary. ACCF and AHA state that IV loop diuretics should be administered promptly to all hospitalized heart failure patients with substantial fluid overload to reduce morbidity. In addition, ACCF and AHA state that

low-dose dopamine infusions may be considered in combination with loop diuretics to augment diuresis and preserve renal function and renal blood flow in patients with acute decompensated heart failure, although data are conflicting and additional study and experience are needed. For additional information, see Heart Failure under Uses: Edema, in the Thiazides General Statement 40:28.20.

Pulmonary Disease

Furosemide may be administered IV as an adjunct in the treatment of acute pulmonary edema; however, the drug should be used cautiously when pulmonary edema is a complication of cardiogenic shock associated with acute myocardial infarction because diuretic-induced hypovolemia may reduce cardiac output.

Hepatic and Renal Disease

Furosemide also may be used cautiously in the management of edema associated with the nephrotic syndrome and in patients with hepatic cirrhosis, but such edema is frequently refractory to treatment. When metabolic alkalosis may be anticipated, a potassium-rich diet, potassium supplements, or potassium-sparing diuretics may be necessary before and during furosemide therapy to mitigate or prevent hypokalemia in cirrhotic, nephrotic, or digitalized patients. (See Cautions: Fluid, Electrolyte, Cardiovascular, and Renal Effects.)

Large oral or IV doses of furosemide have been employed as an adjunct to other therapy, including peritoneal dialysis or hemodialysis, in patients with acute or chronic renal failure. In some patients, the use of furosemide may delay the need for dialysis, increase the intervals between dialyses, shorten the period of hospitalization, or permit a slightly more liberal fluid intake.

● Hypertension

Furosemide may be used alone or in combination with other classes of antihypertensive agents for the management of hypertension, especially when complicated by heart failure or renal disease. Because of established clinical benefits (e.g., reductions in overall mortality and in adverse cardiovascular, cerebrovascular, and renal outcomes), current evidence-based practice guidelines for the management of hypertension in adults generally recommend the use of drugs from 4 classes of antihypertensive agents (ACE inhibitors, angiotensin II receptor antagonists, calcium-channel blockers, and thiazide diuretics). (See Uses: Hypertension in Adults, in the Thiazides General Statement 40:28.20) However, some experts state that loop diuretics (e.g., bumetanide, furosemide, torsemide) are preferred over thiazides in patients with moderate to severe chronic kidney disease (CKD) or symptomatic heart failure. Loop diuretics may be particularly useful in patients with heart failure and reduced left ventricular ejection fraction (LVEF) who have evidence of fluid retention; however, some experts state that thiazide diuretics may be considered in hypertensive patients with heart failure and mild fluid retention because of their more persistent antihypertensive effect.

In most patients, hypertension not controllable by thiazides alone probably will not respond adequately to furosemide alone.

For information on antihypertensive therapy for patients with chronic kidney disease or heart failure, see Chronic Kidney Disease and also see Heart Failure under Hypertension in Adults: Considerations for Drug Therapy in Patients with Underlying Cardiovascular and Other Risk Factors, in Uses in the Thiazides General Statement 40:28.20.

For further information on the role of diuretics in antihypertensive therapy and information on overall principles and expert recommendations for treatment of hypertension, see Uses: Hypertension in Adults and also see Uses: Hypertension in Pediatric Patients, in the Thiazides General Statement 40:28.20.

Hypertensive Crises

IV furosemide has been found useful as an adjunct to hypotensive agents in the treatment of hypertensive crises†, especially when associated with acute pulmonary edema or renal failure. In addition to producing a rapid diuresis, furosemide enhances the effects of other hypotensive drugs and counteracts the sodium retention caused by some of these agents.

● Other Uses

Furosemide has been used IV alone or with 0.9% sodium chloride injection or sodium sulfate to increase renal excretion of calcium in patients with hypercalcemia†. Oral furosemide has been suggested for maintenance.

DOSAGE AND ADMINISTRATION

● Administration

Furosemide is administered orally; the drug can also be administered by IM or IV injection.

IV Administration

IV injections of furosemide should be given slowly over 1–2 minutes. Parenteral administration of furosemide should be replaced by oral therapy as soon as possible. If high-dose parenteral furosemide therapy is necessary, the manufacturer recommends that the drug be administered as a controlled infusion at a rate not exceeding 4 mg/minute in adults. For IV infusion, furosemide should be diluted with an infusion solution of 0.9% sodium chloride, lactated Ringer's, or 5% dextrose, adjusting the pH to greater than 5.5 when necessary.

Standardize 4 Safety

Standardized concentrations for IV furosemide have been established through Standardize 4 Safety (S4S), a national patient safety initiative to reduce medication errors, especially during transitions of care. Multidisciplinary expert panels were convened to determine recommended standard concentrations. Because recommendations from the S4S panels may differ from the manufacturer's prescribing information, caution is advised when using concentrations that differ from labeling, particularly when using rate information from the label. For additional information on S4S (including updates that may be available), see https://www.ashp.org/pharmacy-practice/standardize-4-safety-initiative.

TABLE 1. Standardize 4 Safety Continuous IV Infusion Standard Concentrations for Furosemide

Patient Population	Concentration Standards	Dosing Units
Adults	2 mg/mL	mg/hour
	10 mg/mL	
Pediatric patients (<50 kg)	2 mg/mL	mg/kg/hour
	10 mg/mL	

● Dosage

Dosage of furosemide injection, in which the drug is present as the sodium salt (see Chemistry and Stability: Chemistry), is expressed in terms of furosemide. Furosemide dosage must be adjusted according to the patient's requirements and response. If furosemide is added to the regimen of a patient stabilized on a potent hypotensive agent, the dosage of the hypotensive agent and possibly both drugs should initially be reduced in order to avoid severe hypotension.

For the management of fluid retention (e.g., edema) associated with heart failure, experts state that diuretics should be administered at a dosage sufficient to achieve optimal volume status and relieve congestion without inducing an excessively rapid reduction in intravascular volume, which could result in hypotension, renal dysfunction, or both.

When high-dose furosemide infusions are used, dosage should be individualized according to patient response, titrating the dosage to gain maximum therapeutic effect while using the lowest possible effective dosage; the patient should be closely observed during therapy.

Edema

Oral Dosage

The usual initial adult oral dose of furosemide for the management of edema is 20–80 mg given as a single dose, preferably in the morning. In adults who do not respond, the second and each succeeding oral dose may be increased in 20- to 40-mg increments every 6–8 hours until the desired diuretic response (including weight loss) is obtained. The effective dose may be given once or twice daily thereafter, or, in some cases, by intermittent administration on 2–4 consecutive days each week. For maintenance, dosage may be reduced in some patients. Adult oral dosage of furosemide may be carefully titrated up to 600 mg daily in severely edematous patients.

For the management of fluid retention (e.g., edema) associated with heart failure, some experts recommend initiating furosemide at a low dosage (e.g., 20–40 mg once or twice daily) and increasing the dosage (maximum of 600 mg daily) until urine output increases and weight decreases, generally by 0.5–1 kg daily.

For infants and children, the usual initial oral dose of furosemide for the management of edema is 2 mg/kg administered as a single dose. If necessary, dosage may be increased in increments of 1 or 2 mg/kg every 6–8 hours to maximum individual doses of 6 mg/kg; however, it usually is not necessary to exceed individual doses of 4 mg/kg or a dosing frequency of once or twice daily. For maintenance, the minimum effective dosage should be employed.

Parenteral Dosage

As a diuretic, the usual adult IM or IV dose is 20–40 mg given as a single injection. In adults who do not respond to the initial parenteral dose of furosemide, the second and each succeeding dose may be increased in 20-mg increments and given not more often than every 2 hours until the desired diuretic response is obtained. The effective single dose may then be given once or twice daily.

For the management of acute pulmonary edema in adults, 40 mg of furosemide may be slowly injected IV over 1–2 minutes. If the initial adult dose does not produce a satisfactory response within 1 hour, the dose may be increased to 80 mg IV given over 1–2 minutes. In adults with hypertensive crises†, who have normal renal function, 40–80 mg of furosemide (administered concomitantly with other hypotensive agents) may be given IV over 1–2 minutes; in patients with reduced renal function higher does may be required.

For infants and children, the usual initial IV or IM dose of furosemide for the management of acute pulmonary edema or edema associated with heart failure or renal disease† is 1 mg/kg. If necessary for resistant forms of edema, the initial dose may be increased by 1 mg/kg no more often than every 2 hours until the desired effect has been obtained. Adequate response usually is obtained with individual parenteral doses of 1 mg/kg, but occasionally individual doses of 2 mg/kg may be required. Maximum individual parenteral doses recommended by the manufacturer for infants and children are 6 mg/kg; however, the potential risks associated with large parenteral doses of the drug should be considered and the patient should be monitored closely.

Literature reports suggest that the recommended maximum dosage of furosemide injection for respiratory distress syndrome (RDS) in premature neonates less than 31 weeks postconception age (gestational age at birth plus postnatal age) should not exceed 1 mg/kg in 24 hours.(See Cautions: Pediatric Precautions.)

Large doses of furosemide have been administered orally or IV to adults with acute or chronic renal failure. One investigator recommends beginning therapy in adults with 80 mg of furosemide orally daily and increasing dosage in increments of 80–120 mg daily until the desired effect is achieved. When immediate diuresis is needed, an initial adult dose of 320–400 mg orally daily has been suggested. Some patients have received as much as 4 g orally daily†. Initial IV doses have ranged from 100 mg to 2 g in adults. In some studies, the initial IV doses were doubled at 2- to 24-hour intervals until the desired effect was attained. The highest IV dosage of furosemide was 6 g daily.

Hypertension

Adult Dosage

The manufacturer states that the usual adult oral dosage of furosemide for the management of hypertension is 40 mg twice daily initially and for maintenance. If a satisfactory lowering of blood pressure does not occur, dosage can be increased gradually. Careful monitoring of blood pressure is essential when furosemide is used alone or in combination with other hypotensive agents, especially during initial therapy. If a satisfactory lowering of blood pressure does not occur when 40 mg is administered orally twice daily, the manufacturer recommends adding other antihypertensive agents rather than increasing the dosage of furosemide. Some experts state that the usual oral antihypertensive dosage of furosemide for adults is 20–80 mg daily given in 2 divided doses.

Monitoring and Blood Pressure Treatment Goals

The patient's renal function and electrolytes should be assessed 2–4 weeks after initiation of diuretic therapy. Blood pressure should be monitored regularly (i.e., monthly) during therapy and dosage of the antihypertensive drug adjusted until blood pressure is controlled. If an adequate blood pressure response is not achieved, the dosage may be increased or another antihypertensive agent with demonstrated benefit and preferably with a complementary mechanism of action (e.g., angiotensin-converting enzyme [ACE] inhibitor, angiotensin II receptor antagonist, calcium-channel blocker) may be added; if target blood pressure is still not achieved, a third drug may be added.(See Uses: Hypertension in Adults, in the Thiazides General Statement 40:28.20.) In patients who develop unacceptable adverse effects with furosemide, the drug should be discontinued and another antihypertensive agent from a different pharmacologic class should be initiated.

The goal of hypertension management and prevention is to achieve and maintain optimal control of blood pressure. However, the optimum blood pressure threshold for initiating antihypertensive drug therapy and specific treatment goals remain controversial. A 2017 multidisciplinary hypertension guideline from the American College of Cardiology (ACC), American Heart Association (AHA), and a number of other professional organizations generally recommends a blood pressure goal of less than 130/80 mm Hg in all adults, regardless of comorbidities or level of atherosclerotic cardiovascular disease (ASCVD) risk. Many patients will require at least 2 drugs from different pharmacologic classes to achieve this blood pressure goal; the potential benefits of hypertension management and drug cost, adverse effects, and risks associated with the use of multiple antihypertensive drugs also should be considered when deciding a patient's blood pressure treatment goal.

For additional information on target levels of blood pressure and on monitoring therapy in the management of hypertension, see Blood Pressure Monitoring and Treatment Goals under Dosage: Hypertension, in Dosage and Administration in the Thiazides General Statement 40:28.20.

Pediatric Dosage

For the management of hypertension in children†, some experts have recommended an initial oral dosage of 0.5–2 mg/kg administered once or twice daily. Such experts have suggested that dosage may be increased as necessary up to 6 mg/kg daily. For information on overall principles and expert recommendations for treatment of hypertension in pediatric patients, see Uses: Hypertension in Pediatric Patients in the Thiazides General Statement 40:28.20.

Other

In the treatment of hypercalcemia†, adults have been given 80–100 mg of furosemide IV at intervals of 1–2 hours. In one study, total IV dosage ranged from 160 mg to 3.2 g. Slight elevations of blood calcium concentration have been treated with 120 mg of oral furosemide daily.

Dosage in Renal Impairment

Large doses of furosemide have been administered orally or IV to adults with acute or chronic renal failure. One investigator recommends beginning therapy in adults with 80 mg of furosemide orally daily and increasing dosage in increments of 80–120 mg daily until the desired effect is achieved. When immediate diuresis is needed, an initial adult dose of 320–400 mg orally daily has been suggested. Some patients have received as much as 4 g orally daily†. Initial IV doses have ranged from 100 mg to 2 g in adults. In some studies, the initial IV doses were doubled at 2- to 24-hour intervals until the desired effect was attained. The highest IV dosage of furosemide was 6 g daily.

CAUTIONS

● Fluid, Electrolyte, Cardiovascular, and Renal Effects

Furosemide may produce profound diuresis resulting in fluid and electrolyte depletion. Fluid and electrolyte depletion are especially likely to occur when large doses are given and/or in patients with restricted sodium intake.

Too vigorous diuresis, as evidenced by rapid and excessive weight loss, may induce orthostatic hypotension or acute hypotensive episodes, and the patient's blood pressure should be closely monitored. Excessive dehydration is most likely to occur in geriatric patients and/or patients with chronic cardiac disease treated with prolonged sodium restriction or those receiving sympatholytic agents. The resultant hypovolemia may cause hemoconcentration, which could lead to circulatory collapse or thromboembolic episodes such as possibly fatal vascular thromboses and/or emboli. Pronounced reductions in plasma volume associated with

rapid or excessive diuresis may also result in an abrupt fall in glomerular filtration rate and renal blood flow, which may be restored by replacement of fluid loss. Rarely, sudden death from cardiac arrest has been reported following IV or IM administration of furosemide.

Potassium depletion occurs frequently in patients with secondary hyperaldosteronism which may be associated with cirrhosis or nephrosis and is particularly important in cirrhotic, nephrotic, or digitalized patients. Hypokalemia and hypochloremia may result in metabolic alkalosis, especially in patients with other losses of potassium and chloride due to vomiting, diarrhea, GI drainage, excessive sweating, paracentesis, or potassium-losing renal diseases. In patients with cor pulmonale, alkalosis may cause compensatory respiratory depression. Intermittent administration of furosemide and/or ingestion of potassium-rich foods or administration of a potassium-sparing diuretic may reduce or prevent potassium depletion. However, potassium supplements may be necessary in patients whose serum potassium concentration is less than approximately 3 mEq/L or those receiving digitalis glycosides. To prevent hypokalemic and hypochloremic alkalosis, potassium chloride supplementation should be used. Furosemide increases calcium excretion; rarely, tetany has been reported. Magnesium depletion may also occur.

Furosemide may cause a transient rise in BUN which is usually readily reversible upon withdrawal of the drug. Elevated BUN is especially likely to occur in patients with chronic renal disease. Hyperuricemia may result from furosemide administration and rarely gout has been precipitated; patients with a history of gout or elevated serum uric acid concentrations should be observed closely during therapy. However, large IV doses of furosemide may cause temporary uricosuria. Elevations of BUN and uric acid concentrations may be associated with dehydration, which should be avoided, particularly in patients with renal insufficiency. Allergic interstitial nephritis leading to reversible renal failure has been attributed to furosemide. Blood ammonia concentrations may be increased, especially in patients with preexisting elevations of blood ammonia.

Chronic administration of furosemide 50 mg/kg in rats has caused renal tubular degeneration. Calcification and scarring of the renal parenchyma has occurred in dogs receiving 10 mg/kg for 6 months.

● Otic Effects

Tinnitus, reversible or permanent hearing impairment, or reversible deafness have occurred, usually following rapid IV or IM administration of furosemide in doses greatly exceeding the usual therapeutic dose of 20–40 mg. Otic effects are most likely to occur in patients with severe impairment of renal function and/or in patients receiving other ototoxic drugs (e.g., aminoglycosides). (See Drug Interactions: Other Drugs.) It has been postulated that administering furosemide by slow IV infusion rather than as a bolus may reduce the ototoxic effects of the drug by preventing high peak plasma concentrations; if high-dose parenteral furosemide therapy is necessary in patients with severely impaired renal function, the manufacturers recommend that the drug be infused in adults at a rate not exceeding 4 mg/minute.

● GI Effects

Adverse GI effects of furosemide include nausea, anorexia, oral and gastric irritation, vomiting, cramping, diarrhea, and constipation. Because furosemide oral solutions contain sorbitol, they may cause diarrhea, especially in children, when high dosages are administered. In children, mild to moderate abdominal pain has been reported after furosemide was administered IV. In addition, rare occurrences of sweet taste have been reported, but a causal relationship to the drug has not been established.

● Metabolic Effects

Furosemide may produce hyperglycemia and glycosuria, possibly as a result of hypokalemia, in patients with predisposition to diabetes. Rarely, precipitation of diabetes mellitus has been reported.

Diuretics, including furosemide, can increase serum total cholesterol concentrations in some patients; increases in low-density lipoprotein (LDL)-cholesterol and/or very low-density lipoprotein (VLDL)-cholesterol subfractions appear to be principally responsible for these increases. In addition, the ratio of serum total cholesterol to high-density lipoprotein (HDL)-cholesterol has been increased in some patients in whom total serum cholesterol did not appear to be elevated. Increases in serum triglyceride concentrations also can occur.

Nervous System Effects

Adverse nervous system effects of furosemide include dizziness, lightheadedness, vertigo, headache, xanthopsia, blurred vision, and paresthesias.

Hematologic Effects

Anemia, hemolytic anemia, leukopenia, neutropenia, and thrombocytopenia have occurred in patients receiving furosemide. In addition, rare cases of agranulocytosis and aplastic anemia have been reported.

Dermatologic and Sensitivity Reactions

Adverse dermatologic and/or hypersensitivity reactions to furosemide include purpura, photosensitivity, rash, urticaria, pruritus, exfoliative dermatitis, erythema multiforme, interstitial nephritis, and necrotizing angiitis (vasculitis, cutaneous vasculitis). Patients with known sulfonamide sensitivity may show allergic reactions to furosemide. Anaphylaxis, manifested as urticaria, angioedema, and hypotension, occurred within 5 minutes after IV administration of furosemide in at least one patient; subsequent intradermal skin testing showed sensitivity to furosemide and other sulfonamides.

Local Effects

Transient pain at the injection site has been reported after IM administration of furosemide. Thrombophlebitis has occurred with IV administration.

Other Adverse Effects

Other adverse effects of furosemide include increased perspiration, weakness, fever, restlessness, muscle spasm, urinary bladder spasm, and urinary frequency. A few cases of flank and loin pain have been reported in adults receiving oral furosemide, possibly resulting from calyceal dilation, increased bladder pressure, or spasms caused by formation of calcium-containing crystals in the urine. Intrahepatic cholestatic jaundice and pancreatitis have also occurred in patients receiving furosemide. Furosemide may possibly exacerbate or activate systemic lupus erythematosus.

Precautions and Contraindications

Patients receiving furosemide must be carefully observed for signs of hypovolemia, hyponatremia, hypokalemia, hypocalcemia, hypochloremia, and hypomagnesemia. Patients should be informed of the signs and symptoms of electrolyte imbalance and instructed to report to their physicians if weakness, dizziness, fatigue, faintness, mental confusion, lassitude, muscle cramps, headache, paresthesia, thirst, anorexia, nausea, and/or vomiting occur. Excessive fluid and electrolyte loss may be minimized by initiating therapy with small doses, careful dosage adjustment, using an intermittent dosage schedule if possible, and monitoring the patient's weight. To prevent hyponatremia and hypochloremia, intake of sodium may be liberalized in most patients; however, patients with cirrhosis usually require at least moderate sodium restriction while on diuretic therapy. Determinations of serum electrolytes, BUN, and carbon dioxide should be performed early in therapy with furosemide and periodically thereafter. If excessive diuresis and/or electrolyte abnormalities occur, the drug should be withdrawn or dosage reduced until homeostasis is restored. Electrolyte abnormalities should be corrected by appropriate measures.

Furosemide should be used with caution in patients with hepatic cirrhosis because rapid alterations in fluid and electrolyte balance may precipitate hepatic precoma or coma.

Periodic blood studies and liver function tests should be performed in patients receiving furosemide, especially in those on prolonged therapy.

Urine and blood glucose concentration determinations should be made periodically in diabetics and suspected latent diabetics receiving furosemide.

Furosemide therapy during the first few weeks of life in premature neonates reportedly may increase the risk of persistent patent ductus arteriosus (PDA), possibly through a prostaglandin E (PGE)-mediated process.

Furosemide is contraindicated in patients with anuria. The drug is contraindicated for further use if increasing azotemia and/or oliguria occur during the treatment of severe, progressive renal disease. In patients with hepatic coma or electrolyte depletion, therapy should not be instituted until the basic condition is improved or corrected. Furosemide is also contraindicated in patients with a history of hypersensitivity to the drug.

Pediatric Precautions

In premature neonates with respiratory distress syndrome (RDS), diuretic therapy with furosemide during the first weeks of life may increase the risk of persistent patent ductus arteriosus (PDA), an effect that may be mediated by prostaglandins, presumably of the E series. Hearing loss has been reported in neonates receiving furosemide. Ototoxicity may be associated with elevated plasma concentrations of furosemide secondary to renal immaturity in these patients. Therefore, the manufacturers state that parenteral furosemide dosages should not exceed 1 mg/kg per 24 hours in premature neonates with less than 31 weeks postconception age (gestational age at birth plus postnatal age), because higher dosages may be associated with potentially toxic plasma concentrations of the drug.

Pregnancy, Fertility, and Lactation

Pregnancy

In reproduction studies in mice, rats, and rabbits, administration of furosemide caused unexplained abortions and maternal and fetal deaths. In addition, an increased incidence of hydronephrosis occurred in fetuses of animals treated with the drug. There are no adequate and well controlled studies in pregnant women. Furosemide should be used during pregnancy only when the potential benefits justify the possible risks to the fetus.

Fertility

Reproduction studies in male and female rats using furosemide dosages of 100 mg/kg daily (the maximum effective diuretic dosage in rats and 8 times the maximum human dosage of 600 mg daily) have not revealed evidence of impaired fertility.

Lactation

Since furosemide is distributed into milk, the manufacturers recommend that nursing be discontinued if administration of the drug is necessary.

DRUG INTERACTIONS

Diuretics

Concomitant administration of furosemide and most other diuretics results in enhanced effects, and furosemide should be administered in reduced dosage when the drug is added to an existing diuretic regimen. Spironolactone, triamterene, or amiloride hydrochloride may reduce the potassium loss resulting from furosemide therapy; this effect has been used to therapeutic advantage.

Drugs Affected by or Causing Potassium Depletion

In patients receiving cardiac glycosides, electrolyte disturbances produced by furosemide (principally hypokalemia but also hypomagnesemia) predispose the patient to glycoside toxicity. Possibly fatal cardiac arrhythmias may result. Periodic electrolyte determinations should be performed in patients receiving a cardiac glycoside and furosemide, and correction of hypokalemia undertaken if warranted. (See Cautions: Fluid, Electrolyte, Cardiovascular, and Renal Effects.)

Furosemide reportedly causes prolonged neuromuscular blockade in patients receiving nondepolarizing neuromuscular blocking agents (e.g., tubocurarine chloride, gallamine triethiodide [no longer commercially available in the US]), presumably because of potassium depletion or decreased urinary excretion of the muscle relaxant. Furosemide may also cause decreased arterial responsiveness to pressor amines. Orally administered furosemide should be discontinued 1 week, and parenterally administered furosemide 2 days, prior to elective surgery.

Some drugs such as corticosteroids, corticotropin, and amphotericin B also cause potassium loss, and severe potassium depletion may occur when one of these drugs is administered during furosemide therapy.

Lithium

Renal clearance of lithium is apparently decreased in patients receiving diuretics, and lithium toxicity may result. Furosemide and lithium should generally not be given together. If concomitant therapy is necessary, the patient should be hospitalized. Serum lithium concentrations should be monitored carefully and dosage adjusted accordingly.

• Antidiabetic Agents

Administration of furosemide to diabetic patients may interfere with the hypo-glycemic effect of insulin or oral antidiabetic agents, possibly as a result of hypo-kalemia. Patients should be observed for possible decrease of diabetic control. If correction of the potassium deficit does not restore control, dosage adjustments of the antidiabetic agent may be needed.

• Hypotensive Agents

The antihypertensive effect of hypotensive agents may be enhanced when given concomitantly with furosemide. This effect is usually used to therapeutic advan-tage; however, orthostatic hypotension may result. Dosage of the hypotensive agent, and possibly both drugs, should be reduced when furosemide is added to an existing regimen.

• Indomethacin

In some patients, indomethacin may reduce the natriuretic and hypotensive effects of furosemide. The mechanism(s) of these interactions is uncertain but has been attributed to indomethacin-induced inhibition of prostaglandin synthe-sis which may result in fluid retention and/or changes in vascular resistance. The clinical importance of these interactions has not been established; however, when indomethacin and furosemide are administered concurrently, patients should be observed closely to determine if the desired diuretic and/or hypotensive effect is obtained. When evaluating plasma renin activity in hypertensive patients, it should be kept in mind that indomethacin blocks the furosemide-induced increase in plasma renin activity.

• Ototoxic Drugs

Concomitant administration of furosemide and aminoglycoside antibiotics or other ototoxic drugs may result in increased incidence of ototoxicity and con-comitant use of these drugs should be avoided. In addition, the possibility that IV furosemide may increase aminoglycoside toxicity by altering serum and tis-sue concentrations of the antibiotic should be considered. It has been proposed, but not proven, that furosemide may enhance the nephrotoxicity of neomycin.

• Nonsteroidal Anti-inflammatory Agents

Furosemide and salicylates reportedly have competitive renal excretory sites and, therefore, patients receiving high doses of salicylates with furosemide may experience salicylate toxicity at lower dosage than usual. Concomitant admin-istration of furosemide and aspirin reportedly has been associated with a tran-sient reduction in creatinine clearance in a few patients with chronic renal insufficiency. Weight gain and increases in BUN, serum creatinine, and serum potassium concentrations also have been reported in patients receiving furo-semide in combination with other nonsteroidal anti-inflammatory agents (NSAIAs).

• Anticonvulsants

In one study, epileptic patients receiving chronic anticonvulsant therapy had a reduced diuretic response to furosemide as compared to controls. All of the epi-leptic patients were receiving phenytoin sodium and phenobarbital and some were also receiving other anticonvulsants. It has been postulated that renal sensi-tivity to furosemide is diminished by these drugs.

• Chloral Hydrate

A reaction characterized by diaphoresis, flushes, variable blood pressure includ-ing hypertension, and uneasiness has been reported in some patients with acute myocardial infarction and heart failure who received furosemide IV within 24 hours after administration of an oral hypnotic dose of chloral hydrate (no longer commercially available in the US). Therefore, it may be preferable to use an alternate hypnotic drug (e.g., a benzodiazepine) in patients who require IV furosemide.

• Probenecid or Sulfinpyrazone

It has been suggested that furosemide, by increasing serum uric acid concentra-tions, may interfere with the uricosuric effects of probenecid or sulfinpyrazone. Serum uric acid concentrations should be monitored in patients receiving both drugs, and dosage of the uricosuric drug should be increased if necessary.

PHARMACOLOGY

The pharmacologic effects of furosemide are similar to those of ethacrynic acid. The exact mode of action of furosemide has not been clearly defined; in contrast to ethacrynic acid, it does not bind sulfhydryl groups of renal cellular proteins. Furosemide inhibits the reabsorption of electrolytes in the ascending limb of the loop of Henle. The drug also decreases reabsorption of sodium and chloride and increases potassium excretion in the distal renal tubule and exerts a direct effect on electrolyte transport at the proximal tubule. Furosemide does not inhibit car-bonic anhydrase and is not an aldosterone antagonist.

Furosemide diuresis results in enhanced excretion of sodium, chloride, potas-sium, hydrogen, calcium, magnesium, ammonium, bicarbonate, and possi-bly phosphate. Chloride excretion exceeds that of sodium. In studies in patients with normal renal function, the diuretic response was similar following oral or IV administration of equal doses of furosemide. In one study in uremic patients, however, diuresis and urinary excretion of sodium and potassium were greater after IV administration of furosemide than after equal oral doses. Excessive losses of potassium, hydrogen, and chloride may result in metabolic alkalosis. Urinary pH usually falls after administration of furosemide; however, increased bicarbon-ate excretion in some patients may temporarily raise urinary pH. Low doses of furosemide promote uric acid retention while large IV doses may cause tempo-rary uricosuria. Maximum diuresis and electrolyte loss is greater with furosemide than with the thiazides or most other diuretics except ethacrynic acid. Like the thiazide diuretics and ethacrynic acid, the effectiveness of furosemide is indepen-dent of the acid-base balance of the patient.

Furosemide has some renal vasodilator effect; renal vascular resistance decreases and renal blood flow increases following administration of the drug. A temporary but substantial increase in glomerular filtration rate, as well as decreased peripheral vascular resistance and increased peripheral venous capac-itance, has been reported following IV administration of furosemide in patients with heart failure associated with acute myocardial infarction. The renal and peripheral vascular effects may contribute toward the beneficial effects of the drug in these patients, as a decrease in left ventricular filling pressure occurs before the onset of substantial diuresis. In addition, IV administration of furosemide in patients with heart failure results in a decrease in plasma volume, increased hema-tocrit, and a fall in mean arterial pressure associated with increased cardiac output and decreased peripheral resistance. When large doses of furosemide are adminis-tered to patients with chronic renal insufficiency, glomerular filtration rate may be increased temporarily. A fall in renal blood flow and glomerular filtration rate may occur if excessive drug-induced diuresis results in a reduction in plasma volume.

As with other diuretics, a hypotensive effect may result from decreased plasma volume in patients receiving furosemide. However, the drug has been reported to produce only mild decreases in the supine systolic blood pressure and in the erect systolic and diastolic blood pressures when administered alone in the rec-ommended oral dosage.

Furosemide appears to have less effect on carbohydrate metabolism and blood glucose concentrations than do the thiazides; however, the drug may cause eleva-tions of blood glucose, glycosuria, and alterations in glucose tolerance possibly as a result of hypokalemia.

PHARMACOKINETICS

• Absorption

In one study in patients with normal renal function, approximately 60% of a sin-gle 80-mg oral dose of furosemide was absorbed from the GI tract. When admin-istered to fasting adults in this dosage, the drug appeared in the serum within 10 minutes, reached a peak concentration of 2.3 mcg/mL in 60–70 minutes, and was almost completely cleared from the serum in 4 hours. When the same dose was given after a meal, the serum concentration of furosemide increased slowly to a peak of about 1 mcg/mL after 2 hours and similar concentrations were present 4 hours after ingestion. However, a similar diuretic response occurred regardless of whether the drug was given with food or to fasting patients. In another study, the rate and extent of absorption varied considerably when 1 g of furosemide was given orally to uremic patients. An average of 76% of a dose was absorbed, and peak plasma concentrations were achieved within 2–9 hours (average 4.4 hours).

Serum concentrations required to produce maximum diuresis are not known, and it has been reported that the magnitude of response does not correlate with either the peak or the mean serum concentrations.

The diuretic effect of orally administered furosemide is apparent within 30 minutes to 1 hour and is maximal in the first or second hour. The duration of action is usually 6–8 hours. The maximum hypotensive effect may not be apparent until several days after furosemide therapy is begun. After IV administration of furosemide, diuresis occurs within 5 minutes, reaches a maximum within 20–60 minutes, and persists for approximately 2 hours. After IM administration, peak plasma concentrations are attained within 30 minutes; onset of diuresis occurs somewhat later than after IV administration. In patients with severely impaired renal function, the diuretic response may be prolonged.

● Distribution

Only limited information is available on the distribution of furosemide. The drug crosses the placenta and is distributed into milk.

Furosemide is approximately 95% bound to plasma proteins in both normal and azotemic patients.

● Elimination

Plasma concentrations of furosemide decline in a biphasic manner. Various investigators have reported a wide range of elimination half-lives for furosemide. In one study, the elimination half-life averaged about 30 minutes in healthy patients who received 20–120 mg of the drug IV. In another study, the elimination half-life averaged 9.7 hours in patients with advanced renal failure who received 1 g of furosemide IV. The elimination half-life was more prolonged in 1 patient with concomitant liver disease.

In patients with normal renal function, a small amount of furosemide is metabolized in the liver to the defurfurylated derivative, 4-chloro-5-sulfamoylanthranilic acid. Furosemide and its metabolite are rapidly excreted in urine by glomerular filtration and by secretion from the proximal tubule. In patients with normal renal function, approximately 50% of an oral dose and 80% of an IV or IM dose are excreted in urine within 24 hours; 69–97% of these amounts is excreted in the first 4 hours. The remainder of the drug is eliminated by nonrenal mechanisms including degradation in the liver and excretion of unchanged drug in the feces. In patients with marked renal impairment without liver disease, nonrenal clearance of furosemide is increased so that up to 98% of the drug is removed from the plasma within 24 hours. One patient with uremia and hepatic cirrhosis eliminated only 58% of an IV dose in 24 hours. Furosemide is not removed by hemodialysis.

CHEMISTRY AND STABILITY

● Chemistry

Furosemide is a sulfonamide-type, loop diuretic. The drug occurs as a white to slightly yellow, odorless, crystalline powder with a pK_a of 3.9. Furosemide is insoluble in dilute acids, practically insoluble in water, sparingly soluble in alcohol, and freely soluble in alkali hydroxides.

Furosemide injection, a nonpyrogenic, sterile solution of the drug, contains the sodium salt of furosemide which is formed *in situ* by the addition of sodium hydroxide during the manufacturing process. The injection contains 0.162 mEq of sodium per mL and has a pH of 8–9.3.

● Stability

Furosemide injection should be stored at a temperature of 15–30°C and protected from light; injections having a yellow color should not be used. Exposure of furosemide tablets to light may cause discoloration; discolored tablets should not be dispensed. Furosemide tablets should be stored and dispensed in well-closed, light-resistant containers at a controlled room temperature of 15–30°C. Commercially available 40-mg furosemide tablets have an expiration date of 5 years and the commercially available injection has an expiration date 42 months following the date of manufacture. The 20-mg tablets do not have a specific expiration dating period. Furosemide oral solutions should be stored at 15–30°C and protected from light and freezing; once opened, unused portions of the oral solution should be discarded after the time period recommended by the manufacturer.

Furosemide injection usually can be mixed with weakly alkaline and neutral solutions having a pH of 7–10, such as 0.9% sodium chloride injection or Ringer's injection, and with some weakly acidic solutions having a low buffer capacity. The injection should *not* be mixed with strongly acidic solutions (i.e., pH less than 5.5), such as those containing ascorbic acid, tetracycline, epinephrine, or norepinephrine, because furosemide may be precipitated. In addition, furosemide may precipitate at pH less than 7 and should not be used with certain drugs (e.g., amrinone, ciprofloxacin, labetalol, milrinone). Other drugs which should not be mixed with furosemide injection include most salts of organic bases including local anesthetics, alkaloids, antihistamines, hypnotics, meperidine, and morphine. Specialized references should be consulted for specific compatibility information.

PREPARATIONS

Excipients in commercially available drug preparations may have clinically important effects in some individuals; consult specific product labeling for details.

Furosemide

Oral		
Solution	40 mg/5 mL*	Furosemide Solution
	10 mg/mL*	Furosemide Solution
Tablets	20 mg*	Furosemide Tablets
		Lasix®, Sanofi-Aventis
	40 mg*	Furosemide Tablets
		Lasix® (scored), Sanofi-Aventis
	80 mg*	Furosemide Tablets
		Lasix®, Sanofi-Aventis

Parenteral		
Injection	10 mg/mL*	Furosemide Injection

* available from one or more manufacturer, distributor, and/or repackager by generic (nonproprietary) name

† Use is not currently included in the labeling approved by the US Food and Drug Administration.

Selected Revisions June 10, 2024. © Copyright, January 1, 1976, American Society of Health-System Pharmacists, Inc.

Torsemide

40:28.08 • LOOP DIURETICS

■ Torsemide is a sulfonamide, loop-type diuretic and antihypertensive agent.

USES

● Edema

Torsemide is used for the management of edema associated with heart failure or hepatic or renal disease. Most experts state that all patients with symptomatic heart failure who have evidence for, or a history of, fluid retention generally should receive diuretic therapy in conjunction with moderate sodium restriction, an agent to inhibit the renin-angiotensin-aldosterone (RAA) system (e.g., angiotensin-converting enzyme [ACE] inhibitor, angiotensin II receptor antagonist, angiotensin receptor-neprilysin inhibitor [ARNI]), a β-adrenergic blocking agent (β-blocker), and in selected patients, an aldosterone antagonist. For additional information on the use of loop diuretics in the management of edema associated with heart failure, see Heart Failure under Uses: Edema, in Bumetanide, Ethacrynic Acid, and Furosemide 40:28.08.

● Hypertension

Torsemide is used alone or in combination with other classes of antihypertensive agents for the management of hypertension. Because of established clinical benefits (e.g., reductions in overall mortality and in adverse cardiovascular, cerebrovascular, and renal outcomes), current evidence-based practice guidelines for the management of hypertension in adults generally recommend the use of drugs from 4 classes of antihypertensive agents (ACE inhibitors, angiotensin II receptor antagonists, calcium-channel blockers, and thiazide diuretics). (See Uses: Hypertension in Adults, in the Thiazides General Statement 40:28.20.) However, some experts state that loop diuretics (e.g., bumetanide, furosemide, torsemide) are preferred over thiazides in patients with moderate to severe chronic kidney disease (CKD) or symptomatic heart failure. Loop diuretics may be particularly useful in patients with heart failure and reduced left ventricular ejection fraction (LVEF) who have evidence of fluid retention; however, some experts state that thiazide diuretics may be considered in hypertensive patients with heart failure and mild fluid retention because of their more persistent antihypertensive effect.

For further information on the role of diuretics in antihypertensive drug therapy and information on overall principles and expert recommendations for treatment of hypertension, see Uses: Hypertension in Adults, and also see Uses: Hypertension in Pediatric Patients, in the Thiazides General Statement 40:28.20.

DOSAGE AND ADMINISTRATION

● Administration

Torsemide usually is administered orally. Food decreases the rate but not the extent of GI absorption, and the manufacturers state that the drug may be administered without regard to meals.

Torsemide also may be given by IV injection when a rapid onset of diuresis is desired or when oral therapy is not practical. IV injections of torsemide should be administered slowly over 2 minutes ("bolus"); alternatively, the drug may be administered as a continuous IV infusion.

If torsemide injection is administered through an IV line, it is recommended that the IV line be flushed with 0.9% sodium chloride injection before and after the drug is administered. Because the pH of torsemide injection exceeds 8.3, flushing is necessary to avoid potential incompatibilities that may result from differences in pH.

For administration of torsemide as a continuous IV infusion, 200 mg of the drug may be diluted in 250 mL of 5% dextrose or 0.9% sodium chloride injection or in 500 mL of 0.45% sodium chloride injection; alternatively, 50 mg of torsemide may be diluted in 500 mL of 5% dextrose, 0.9% sodium chloride injection, or 0.45% sodium chloride injection. Following dilution in these solutions in plastic containers, the drug is stable for up to 24 hours at room temperature.

● Dosage

The manufacturers state that since oral and IV doses of torsemide are therapeutically equivalent, torsemide dosage is identical for oral or IV administration.

For the management of fluid retention (e.g., edema) associated with heart failure, experts state that diuretics should be administered at a dosage sufficient to achieve optimal volume status and relieve congestion without inducing an excessively rapid reduction in intravascular volume, which could result in hypotension, renal dysfunction, or both.

Safety and efficacy of torsemide in children have not been established.

Edema

For the management of edema associated with heart failure, the usual initial adult oral or IV dosage of torsemide is 10–20 mg daily, given as a single dose. If the diuretic response is inadequate, dosage can be titrated upward by approximately doubling the daily dose until the desired response is attained. The manufacturers state that single doses exceeding 200 mg have not been adequately studied. Some experts recommend initiating torsemide at a low dosage (10–20 mg once daily) and increasing the dosage (maximum of 200 mg daily) until urine output increases and weight decreases, generally by 0.5–1 kg daily.

Hypertension

For the management of hypertension, the usual initial adult dosage of torsemide recommended by the manufacturers is 5 mg once daily. If a satisfactory lowering of blood pressure does not occur within 4–6 weeks, dosage of torsemide may be increased to 10 mg once daily. Some experts state that the usual dosage of torsemide is 5–10 mg once daily. If a satisfactory lowering of blood pressure does not occur when 10 mg is administered daily, other antihypertensive agents should be added to the regimen.

Monitoring and Blood Pressure Treatment Goals

The patient's renal function and electrolytes should be assessed 2–4 weeks after initiation of diuretic therapy. Blood pressure should be monitored regularly (i.e., monthly) during therapy and dosage of the antihypertensive drug adjusted until blood pressure is controlled. If an adequate blood pressure response is not achieved, the dosage may be increased or another antihypertensive agent with demonstrated benefit and preferably with a complementary mechanism of action (e.g., angiotensin-converting enzyme [ACE] inhibitor, angiotensin II receptor antagonist, calcium-channel blocker) may be added; if target blood pressure is still not achieved, a third drug may be added. (See Uses: Hypertension in Adults, in the Thiazides General Statement 40:28.20.) In patients who develop unacceptable adverse effects with torsemide, the drug should be discontinued and another antihypertensive agent from a different pharmacologic class should be initiated.

The goal of hypertension management and prevention is to achieve and maintain optimal control of blood pressure. However, the optimum blood pressure threshold for initiating antihypertensive drug therapy and specific treatment goals remain controversial. A 2017 multidisciplinary hypertension guideline from the American College of Cardiology (ACC), American Heart Association (AHA), and a number of other professional organizations generally recommends a blood pressure goal of less than 130/80 mm Hg in all adults, regardless of comorbidities or level of atherosclerotic cardiovascular disease (ASCVD) risk. Many patients will require at least 2 drugs from different pharmacologic classes to achieve this blood pressure goal; the potential benefits of hypertension management and drug cost, adverse effects, and risks associated with the use of multiple antihypertensive drugs also should be considered when deciding a patient's blood pressure treatment goal.

For additional information on target levels of blood pressure and on monitoring therapy, see Blood Pressure Monitoring and Treatment Goals under Dosage: Hypertension, in Dosage and Administration in the Thiazides General Statement 40:28.20.

● Dosage in Renal and Hepatic Impairment

For the management of edema in patients with chronic renal failure, the usual initial adult oral or IV dosage of torsemide is 20 mg daily, given as a single dose. If the diuretic response is inadequate, dosage may be titrated upward by doubling the dose until desired response is attained. However, the manufacturers state that single doses exceeding 200 mg or chronic use in patients with renal impairment have not been adequately studied.

For the management of edema in patients with hepatic cirrhosis, torsemide is administered concomitantly with an aldosterone antagonist or a potassium-sparing diuretic; the usual initial adult oral or IV dosage of torsemide is 5–10 mg daily, given as a single dose. If the diuretic response to this initial dosage is inadequate, dosage may be titrated upward by doubling the dose until the desired response is attained. Single doses exceeding 40 mg have not been adequately studied in patients with hepatic cirrhosis.

DESCRIPTION

Torsemide is a sulfonamide-type, loop diuretic.

PREPARATIONS

Excipients in commercially available drug preparations may have clinically important effects in some individuals; consult specific product labeling for details.

Torsemide

Oral			
Tablets	5 mg*	**Demadex®**, Roche	
		Torsemide Tablets	
	10 mg*	**Demadex®** (scored), Roche	
		Torsemide Tablets	
	20 mg*	**Demadex®** (scored), Roche	
		Torsemide Tablets	
	100 mg*	**Demadex®** (scored), Roche	
		Torsemide Tablets	
Parenteral			
Injection, for IV use	10 mg/mL*	**Torsemide Injection**	

* available from one or more manufacturer, distributor, and/or repackager by generic (nonproprietary) name

† Use is not currently included in the labeling approved by the US Food and Drug Administration.

Selected Revisions September 10, 2024, © Copyright, May 1, 1994, American Society of Health-System Pharmacists, Inc.

Mannitol

40:28.12 · OSMOTIC DIURETICS

■ Mannitol is an osmotic diuretic.

USES

● Oliguric Acute Renal Failure

In conjunction with adequate replacement of water and electrolytes and maintenance of normal blood pressure, mannitol is used to promote diuresis for the prevention and/or treatment of the oliguric phase of acute renal failure which may occur after massive hemorrhage, trauma, shock, burns, transfusion reactions caused by mismatched blood, or major surgery. The drug may prevent or reverse acute functional renal failure before there is evidence of tubular necrosis or multiple vascular thrombosis; however, mannitol has no effect and may be harmful if used after tubular necrosis and irreversible renal failure become established.

Mannitol has been used during cardiovascular surgical procedures, including open heart surgery and surgery to correct aortic aneurysms. Use of the drug may prevent hemoglobin buildup during cardiopulmonary bypass procedures. Mannitol has been used to protect renal function in patients with poor renal function undergoing various surgical procedures such as nephrolithotomy or renal artery surgery; however, the drug does not permit prolonging the time of occlusion and renal ischemia during renovascular reconstructive surgery. The drug has also been recommended for use during abdominal surgery or other major surgery, especially in jaundiced patients who appear to be particularly susceptible to postoperative renal failure. In one study, mannitol prevented azotemia, but not systemic acidosis, caused by amphotericin B in 4 patients being treated for systemic fungal infections following kidney transplantation.

● Reduction of Intracranial Pressure

Mannitol is used prior to and during neurosurgery to reduce greatly increased intracranial pressure and for the treatment of cerebral edema. The drug is especially indicated when there is evidence of herniation and developing brainstem compression. A rebound increase in intracranial pressure may occur approximately 12 hours after osmotic diuresis is employed; however, this occurs less frequently with mannitol than with urea. Mannitol is also useful for the early treatment of cerebral edema in patients with diabetic ketoacidosis or in patients in hypoglycemic coma who fail to respond to increases in blood glucose concentrations. Mannitol has also been used to reduce edema in the traumatized area of the spinal cord prior to corrective surgery.

● Reduction of Intraocular Pressure

Mannitol is used to reduce elevated intraocular pressure when the pressure cannot be lowered by other means. The drug is especially useful for treating acute episodes of angle-closure, absolute, or secondary glaucoma and for lowering intraocular pressure prior to intraocular surgery. Mannitol may be of value in those cases of cataract extraction in which vitreous loss is likely. Unlike urea, mannitol does not penetrate the eye and may be used when irritation is present.

● Other Uses

Mannitol is used alone or with other diuretics such as furosemide or ethacrynic acid to promote the urinary excretion of toxins such as aspirin or other salicylates, some barbiturates, bromides, or imipramine as an adjunct to usual treatment regimens in patients with severe intoxications. Continuous infusion of mannitol in some cases of drug poisoning has reduced the period of unconsciousness and maintained urine flow. Renal lesions caused by inhalation or ingestion of carbon tetrachloride may possibly be prevented by early treatment with mannitol. Unlike many other diuretics, mannitol increases the urinary excretion of lithium and may be useful for the treatment of lithium intoxication. The drug has also been used to promote excretion of uric acid and prevent hyperuricemia and/or uric acid nephropathy in patients who develop uricemia following chemotherapy or radiation therapy for leukemia or lymphoma. Concomitant administration of sodium bicarbonate may be needed to alkalinize the urine in the treatment of salicylate or barbiturate poisonings or uricemia. Mannitol has also been found useful in treating carbon monoxide poisoning and ethylene glycol intoxication.

There is limited evidence that mannitol may be useful in the management of ciguatera fish poisoning, but additional study and experience are necessary.

Although the mechanism(s) of action is not known, the drug appeared to reverse neurologic and neurosensory manifestations of such poisoning as well as GI manifestations in a limited number of patients. No specific antidote for ciguatera fish poisoning has been identified to date, and treatment remains supportive and symptomatic; therefore, pending further accumulation of data, some clinicians suggest that use of mannitol (e.g., 1 g/kg by IV infusion) be considered for initial therapy, combined with other supportive therapy as necessary, in patients with clinically important manifestations of such poisoning.

Mannitol has been used alone or in conjunction with other diuretics to promote diuresis for the supportive treatment of edema and ascites of nephrotic, cirrhotic, or cardiac origin. The drug may also be useful to relieve the symptoms and congestion of pulmonary edema caused by bronchopneumonia. Mannitol may be indicated when thiazides or other diuretics that act by inhibiting transport mechanisms fail because of decreased glomerular filtration rate caused by shock, dehydration, or trauma or when further depression of renal function produced by other diuretics is contraindicated. However, mannitol diuresis offers only symptomatic relief of edema and is independent of and has no effect on the underlying disease process. IV therapy with mannitol is impractical for the treatment of chronic edema. Use of the drug requires larger volumes of fluid to be administered than do other osmotic diuretics; however, unlike dextrose, it is not contraindicated for use in diabetic patients and it causes less local irritation and necrosis than does urea.

Mannitol is also used as an irrigating solution in transurethral prostatic resection. Use of the drug minimizes the hemolytic effects of water, the entrance of hemolyzed blood into the circulation, and the resulting hemoglobinemia which is considered a major factor in producing serious renal complications. In addition, mannitol has been administered IV before, during and after transurethral prostatectomy to maintain urine output, promote rapid excretion of absorbed irrigants, and reduce the need for postoperative irrigation.

Mannitol has been administered by intra-amniotic instillation in attempts to terminate pregnancy; however, the drug has been reported to have a high failure rate and therefore to be unreliable for this purpose.

For the use of mannitol to measure glomerular filtration rate, see Mannitol 36:40.

DOSAGE AND ADMINISTRATION

● Administration

Mannitol injections are administered by IV infusion. An administration set with a filter should be used for infusion of injections containing 20% or more, since mannitol crystals may be present. For transurethral prostatic resection, mannitol irrigation solutions are instilled into the bladder via an indwelling urethral catheter.

● Dosage

The dosage, concentration of solution, and rate of administration of mannitol vary with the condition being treated and the patient's fluid requirements, urinary output, and response to the drug.

Test Dose

Patients with marked oliguria or suspected inadequate renal function should receive a dose of about 0.2 g/kg or 12.5 g as a 15 or 20% solution infused over a period of 3–5 minutes to test renal response before mannitol therapy is initiated. A response is considered adequate if at least 30–50 mL of urine per hour is excreted over the next 2–3 hours. If an adequate response is not attained, a second test dose may be given. If a satisfactory response is not obtained after the second test dose, the patient should be reevaluated and mannitol should not be used.

Oliguric Acute Renal Failure

For the prevention of oliguria or acute renal failure, 50–100 g of mannitol may be given. Generally, a concentrated solution of the drug is given initially followed by a 5 or 10% solution. When used prophylactically in surgical procedures, administration of the drug may be initiated before or immediately following surgery and may be continued postoperatively. When mannitol was used to reduce nephrotoxicity caused by amphotericin B, 12.5 g of mannitol was administered immediately before and after each dose of amphotericin B. For the treatment of oliguria, 100 g of mannitol is usually given as a 15 or 20% solution over 90 minutes to several hours.

Reduction of Intracranial or Intraocular Pressure

To reduce intracranial pressure and brain mass, and to lower elevated intraocular pressure, the usual dose of mannitol is 1.5–2 g/kg administered as a 15, 20, or 25%

solution over a period of 30–60 minutes. Some clinicians have recommended as little as 1 g or as much as 3.2 g/kg to lower intraocular pressure. When used preoperatively, the drug should be administered 1–1.5 hours prior to surgery in order to achieve maximum reduction of pressure before surgery.

Other Parenteral Uses

To promote diuresis in the adjunctive treatment of severe drug intoxications, various mannitol regimens have been used. In general, a urinary output of at least 100 mL/hour, but preferably 500 mL/hour, and a positive fluid balance of 1–2 L should be maintained. Some clinicians recommend an initial loading dose of 25 g, followed by infusion of a solution at a rate that will maintain a urinary output of at least 100 mL/hour. In barbiturate poisoning, an initial dose of 0.5 g/kg, followed by administration of a 5 or 10% solution at a rate to maintain the desired urine output, has been recommended. Alternatively, it has been recommended that 1 L of a 10% solution be given during the first hour. Urine volume and pH should be measured and cumulative fluid balance calculated at the end of the first hour and subsequent 2-hour periods. If positive fluid balance remains at 1–2 L, another liter of 10% mannitol may be given over the next 2 hours. If positive fluid balance falls below 1 L, mannitol should be replaced with 1 L of (1/6) M sodium lactate over the next 2 hours (if urine pH is less than 7) or 1 L of 0.9% sodium chloride over 2 hours (if urine pH is greater than 7). If the positive fluid balance is more than 2 L, 10% mannitol may be given at the slowest possible rate. IV administration of furosemide was recommended if the positive fluid balance exceeded 2.5 L. For the treatment of uricemia, 50 g/m² has been given in 24 hours.

As a diuretic for the adjunctive treatment of edema and ascites, 100 g of mannitol may be infused as a 10–20% solution over a period of 2–6 hours.

Transurethral Prostatic Resection

Solutions containing 2.5–5% mannitol are used as irrigating solutions in transurethral prostatic resection. One limited study indicates that mannitol concentrations of at least 3.5% are necessary to prevent hemolysis.

Pediatric Dosage

Mannitol dosage requirements for patients 12 years of age and younger have not been established. However, some clinicians have suggested the following dosages for pediatric patients. In oliguria or anuria, a test dose of 0.2 g/kg or 6 g/m² may be given as a single dose over 3–5 minutes. For therapeutic purposes, 2 g/kg or 60 g/m² may be given. For the treatment of edema and ascites, this dose may be given as a 15 or 20% solution over 2–6 hours. To reduce cerebral or ocular edema, the dose may be given as a 15 or 20% solution over 30–60 minutes. For the treatment of intoxications, the drug may be given as a 5 or 10% solution as needed.

CAUTIONS

● Effects on Fluids and Electrolytes

The most severe adverse effects encountered during mannitol therapy are fluid and electrolyte imbalance. Accumulation of mannitol caused by inadequate urinary output or to rapid administration of large doses may result in overexpansion of extracellular fluid. The resulting circulatory overload may result in pulmonary edema, signs and symptoms of water intoxication, and fulminating congestive heart failure, especially in patients with diminished cardiac reserve. Overhydration may be corrected by hemodialysis or administration of a potent diuretic (e.g., furosemide).

Electrolyte imbalance, in some cases severe enough to alter acid-base balance or depress respiration, may result from mannitol-induced diuresis. Hyponatremia or hypernatremia and hypokalemia or hyperkalemia may occur. The shift of sodium-free intracellular fluid into extracellular spaces may result in dilutional lowering of serum sodium concentrations and may cause hyponatremia or aggravate preexisting hyponatremia. Hyponatremia may be accompanied by tremor or seizures and may result in death. Loss of water in excess of sodium, as may occur during prolonged therapy with mannitol, may result in hypernatremia and hyperosmolality. A natriuretic agent such as a thiazide may be administered concomitantly if this occurs.

● Nervous System Effects

Symptoms of CNS toxicity have occurred in 3 patients with acute renal failure who received 25 g of mannitol every 12 hours for at least 36 hours. When large doses of mannitol are administered, especially in the presence of acidosis, the drug may cross the blood-brain barrier and interfere with the ability of the brain to maintain CSF pH. Cerebral dessication may also occur, and the mechanisms that protect the brain from the effects of systemic acidosis may be disrupted. CNS damage may result, and death has occurred in patients with organic CNS disease who received mannitol.

● Other Adverse Effects

Other adverse effects that have occurred during mannitol therapy include acidosis, dryness of the mouth, thirst, urinary retention, headache, blurred vision, uricosuria, nausea, vomiting, rhinitis, arm pain, backache, thrombophlebitis, chills, dizziness, urticaria, hypotension, hypertension, tachycardia, fever, transient muscle rigidity, and angina-like chest pain.

Vacuolar nephrosis, possibly irreversible, has occurred during administration of mannitol. Reversible, acute oligoanuric renal failure has occurred in several patients with normal pretreatment renal function who received large IV dosages (400–900 g daily) of mannitol for the reduction of intracranial or intraocular pressure; the mechanism of this effect has not been fully elucidated. Urine output and glomerular filtration rate declined abruptly in these patients but returned toward or exceeded normal within several days after discontinuance of mannitol; one patient underwent ultrafiltration and hemodialysis.

Extravasation of mannitol should be avoided, since local edema and skin necrosis may result. In a patient with a history of allergies, mannitol caused a severe allergic reaction and anaphylaxis which responded to treatment with epinephrine hydrochloride. Intraocular hemorrhage has also occurred but could not be definitely attributed to mannitol.

● Precautions and Contraindications

Mannitol should not be administered until the adequacy of the patient's renal function and urine flow has been established. A test dose may be employed for this purpose. (See Dosage and Administration: Dosage.) In patients with shock with oliguria and rising BUN, mannitol should not be administered until fluids, plasma, blood, and electrolytes have been replaced. The cardiovascular status of the patient should also be carefully evaluated prior to mannitol administration.

Renal function, urine output, fluid balance, serum sodium and potassium concentrations, and central venous pressure should be monitored during mannitol administration. If urine output continues to decline, the patient's clinical status should be reviewed and mannitol discontinued if necessary. If central venous pressure rises or there is any other evidence of circulatory overload, the infusion should be slowed or stopped. Fluid administration should not exceed 1 L/day in excess of urinary output. The sustained diuresis caused by mannitol may obscure and intensify inadequate hydration or hypovolemia. Tissue dehydration may occur, especially when urine output is less than 40 mL/minute, and may lead to coma. Hypovolemia reduces glomerular filtration rate and enhances the reabsorption of sodium and water, thus promoting oliguria. In addition, preexisting hemoconcentration may be intensified.

Mannitol is not a substitute for fluid and electrolyte therapy, and homeostasis should be maintained by hydration and electrolyte therapy. Volume and electrolyte depletion may be prevented or treated by administering dilute mannitol solutions with sodium chloride added or by alternating each liter of mannitol solution with a liter of sodium chloride injection to which 40 mEq of potassium chloride has been added. If the threat of renal shutdown exists, potassium supplementation should be administered subsequent to, but not concomitantly with, mannitol.

Mannitol is contraindicated in patients with well established anuria caused by severe renal disease or impaired renal function who do not respond to a test dose. (See Dosage and Administration: Dosage.) The drug is also contraindicated in patients with severe pulmonary congestion, frank pulmonary edema, severe congestive heart disease, severe dehydration, metabolic edema associated with capillary fragility or membrane permeability and not due to renal, cardiac or hepatic disease, or active intracranial bleeding except during craniotomy. Mannitol is contraindicated for further use when progressive renal disease or dysfunction, including increasing oliguria and azotemia, or progressive heart failure or pulmonary congestion occur after institution of mannitol therapy. Electrolyte-free mannitol solutions should not be given concomitantly with blood. If blood must be given simultaneously with mannitol, at least 20 mEq of sodium chloride should be added to each liter of mannitol solution to avoid pseudoagglutination.

● Pregnancy, Fertility, and Lactation
Pregnancy

Animal reproduction studies have not been performed with mannitol. It is also not known whether mannitol can caused fetal harm when administered to pregnant women. Mannitol should be used during pregnancy only when clearly needed.

Fertility

It is not known whether mannitol affects fertility in humans.

DRUG INTERACTIONS

Because mannitol increases urinary excretion of lithium, patients being treated with lithium should be observed for possible impairment of response to that drug if they receive mannitol.

LABORATORY TEST INTERFERENCES

In addition to alterations in laboratory test values resulting from mannitol-induced electrolyte changes, the drug may affect the results of other tests. Determinations of inorganic phosphorus blood concentrations are interfered with by use of the drug; values may be increased or decreased. Mannitol will also interfere with laboratory determinations of blood ethylene glycol concentrations, because both substances are oxidized to an aldehyde during the test procedure.

PHARMACOLOGY

IV administration of mannitol induces diuresis mainly by elevating the osmotic pressure of the glomerular filtrate to such an extent that the tubular reabsorption of water and solutes is hindered. For mannitol to be effective, enough renal blood flow and glomerular filtration must exist to enable the drug to reach the tubules. Increased renal blood flow resulting from dilation of vascular segments between the renal artery and glomeruli, lowered renal vascular resistance, and reduced blood viscosity may also contribute to the diuretic effect of the drug. Mannitol promotes the excretion of sodium; however, proportionately more water than sodium is excreted. Excretion of potassium, chloride, calcium, phosphorus, lithium, magnesium, urea, and uric acid is also increased during mannitol-induced diuresis. The drug protects the kidneys from nephrotoxins by preventing toxins from becoming concentrated in the tubular fluid.

Mannitol may prevent or reverse acute functional renal failure by reversing the acute reductions in renal blood flow, glomerular filtration rate, urine flow, and sodium excretion which may occur after trauma. However, the drug must exert its effect before decreases in filtration rate and renal blood flow produce tubular damage, interstitial edema, and/or diffuse ischemia.

The osmotic effect of mannitol causes water to be drawn from cells to extracellular fluid and from erythrocytes cells to plasma. As a result, extracellular fluid volume, plasma volume, and circulation time are increased and extracellular stores of sodium are diluted. Cellular dehydration may result. Plasma pH is decreased. Erythrocyte volume becomes more concentrated and hematocrit is decreased. The fluid shifts caused by the drug result in reduction of cerebral edema by a reduction in brain mass and in the lowering of elevated CSF pressure. However, a rebound increase in intracranial pressure may occur approximately 12 hours after the administration of mannitol. Fluids are also withdrawn from the anterior chamber of the eye, resulting in a reduction of elevated intraocular pressure.

When administered orally, mannitol causes profound osmotic diarrhea, resulting in a loss of fluid, sodium, and potassium. Serum sodium concentrations are increased, but serum potassium and blood urea concentrations are reduced.

PHARMACOKINETICS

● Absorption

Although mannitol has been thought not to be absorbed when administered orally, one study revealed that about 17% of an oral dose of radiolabeled drug was excreted unchanged in urine.

Diuresis may occur within 1–3 hours after IV administration of mannitol. Lowering of elevated intraocular pressure occurs within 30–60 minutes and persists for 4–6 hours. Elevated CSF pressure may be reduced within 15 minutes after starting an infusion of mannitol, and the effect may last for 3–8 hours after the infusion is stopped.

● Distribution

When administered IV, mannitol remains confined to the extracellular compartment. The drug does not cross the blood-brain barrier unless very high concentrations are present in the plasma or the patient has acidosis. Unlike urea, mannitol does not penetrate the eye.

● Elimination

Mannitol is metabolized only very slightly, if at all, to glycogen in the liver. The drug is freely filtered by the glomeruli, with less than 10% tubular reabsorption; it is not secreted by tubular cells. The elimination half-life in adults is about 100 minutes.

Approximately 80% of a 100-g dose is excreted unchanged in urine within 3 hours. When large dose are given as in forced diuresis, retention of the drug may occur. In the presence of renal disease in which glomerular function is impaired or in conditions that impair small vessel circulation, such as congestive heart failure, cirrhosis with ascitic accumulation, shock, or dehydration, mannitol clearance is lower than normal.

CHEMISTRY AND STABILITY

● Chemistry

Mannitol, a hexahydroxy alcohol chemically related to mannose, is an osmotic diuretic. Mannitol occurs as a white, crystalline powder or free-flowing granules with a sweet taste. The drug is very slightly soluble in alcohol and has a solubility of approximately 182 mg/mL in water at 25°C. Commercially available mannitol injections have a pH of 4.5–7.

The approximate osmolarities of mannitol solutions are as follows:

% Mannitol	mOsm/L
5	275
10	550
15	825
20	1100
25	1375

● Stability

Mannitol solutions should be stored at 15–30°C and protected from freezing. Solutions of mannitol are chemically stable but, in concentrations of 15% and more, mannitol may crystallize when exposed to low temperatures. If crystallization occurs, the solution should be autoclaved or warmed by immersing the container in hot water (approximately 60°C) and periodically shaking vigorously. The solution should be cooled to body temperature before administration. If all crystals cannot be completely dissolved, the solution should not be used. The addition of potassium or sodium chloride to mannitol solutions of 20% concentration or greater may cause precipitation of mannitol. Mannitol should not be added to whole blood for transfusion.

PREPARATIONS

Excipients in commercially available drug preparations may have clinically important effects in some individuals; consult specific product labeling for details.

Mannitol

Powder
Parenteral

Injection	5%*	Mannitol Injection
		Osmitrol®, Baxter
	10%*	Mannitol Injection
		Osmitrol®, Baxter
	15%*	Mannitol Injection
		Osmitrol®, Baxter
	20%*	Mannitol Injection
		Osmitrol®, Baxter
	25%*	Mannitol Injection

* available from one or more manufacturer, distributor, and/or repackager by generic (nonproprietary) name

Mannitol Combinations

Urogenital

Solution	0.54% with Sorbitol 2.7%*	Sorbitol-Mannitol Irrigating Solution

* available from one or more manufacturer, distributor, and/or repackager by generic (nonproprietary) name

Triamterene

40:28.16 • POTASSIUM-SPARING DIURETICS

■ Triamterene is a potassium-sparing diuretic.

USES

● Edema

Triamterene is used in the management of edema associated with heart failure, cirrhosis of the liver, or the nephrotic syndrome, as well as in the management of steroid-induced edema, idiopathic edema, and edema caused by secondary hyperaldosteronism. Careful etiologic diagnosis should precede the use of any diuretic. Triamterene should not be used alone as initial therapy in severe heart failure since its maximum therapeutic effect may occur slowly. However, it may be used in combined initial therapy with more effective, rapidly acting diuretics such as thiazides, chlorthalidone, furosemide, or ethacrynic acid or after rapid initial diuresis has been achieved by other means. Triamterene may be particularly useful in patients excreting excessive amounts of potassium (especially those who cannot tolerate potassium supplements) and for those in whom potassium loss could be detrimental, such as digitalized patients or those with myasthenia gravis. Triamterene promotes increased diuresis when patients prove resistant or only partially responsive to thiazides or other diuretics because of secondary hyperaldosteronism. Unlike spironolactone, the effectiveness of triamterene is independent of aldosterone concentrations; therefore, triamterene may be effective in some patients unresponsive to spironolactone. Although triamterene is effective alone, its chief value lies in combined therapy with other diuretics that act at different sites in the nephron. Some patients resistant to triamterene alone may respond to combined therapy with a thiazide diuretic, furosemide, ethacrynic acid, or chlorthalidone. Triamterene decreases potassium excretion caused by kaliuretic diuretics.

Heart Failure

Triamterene generally is used concomitantly with other more effective, rapidly acting diuretics (e.g., thiazides, chlorthalidone, loop diuretics) in the management of edema associated with heart failure. Most experts state that all patients with symptomatic heart failure who have evidence for, or a history of, fluid retention generally should receive diuretic therapy in conjunction with moderate sodium restriction, an agent to inhibit the renin-angiotensin-aldosterone (RAA) system (e.g., angiotensin-converting enzyme [ACE] inhibitor, angiotensin II receptor antagonist, angiotensin receptor-neprilysin inhibitor [ARNI]), a β-adrenergic blocking agent (β-blocker) and in selected patients, an aldosterone antagonist. Some experts state that because of limited and inconsistent data, it is difficult to make precise recommendations regarding daily sodium intake and whether it should vary with respect to the type of heart failure (e.g., reduced versus preserved ejection fraction), disease severity (e.g., New York Heart Association [NYHA] class), heart failure-related comorbidities (e.g., renal dysfunction), or other patient characteristics (e.g., age, race). The American College of Cardiology Foundation (ACCF) and American Heart Association (AHA) state that limiting sodium intake to 1.5 g daily in patients with ACCF/AHA stage A or B heart failure may be reasonable. While data currently are lacking to support recommendation of a specific level of sodium intake in patients with ACCF/AHA stage C or D heart failure, ACCF and AHA state that limiting sodium intake to some degree (e.g., less than 3 g daily) in such patients may be considered for symptom improvement.

Diuretics play a key role in the management of heart failure because they produce symptomatic benefits more rapidly than any other drugs, relieving pulmonary and peripheral edema within hours or days compared with weeks or months for cardiac glycosides, ACE inhibitors, or β-blockers. However, since there are no long-term studies of diuretic therapy in patients with heart failure, the effects of diuretics on morbidity and mortality in such patients are not known. Although there are patients with heart failure who do not exhibit fluid retention in the absence of diuretic therapy and even may develop severe volume depletion with low doses of diuretics, such patients are rare and the unique pathophysiologic mechanisms regulating their fluid and electrolyte balance have not been elucidated.

Most experts state that loop diuretics (e.g., bumetanide, ethacrynic acid, furosemide, torsemide) are the diuretics of choice for most patients with heart failure. However, thiazides may be preferred in some patients with concomitant

hypertension because of their sustained antihypertensive effects. For additional information, see Heart Failure under Uses: Edema in the Thiazides General Statement 40:28.20.

● Hypertension

Triamterene has been used in the management of hypertension†. However, because of established clinical benefits (e.g., reductions in overall mortality and in adverse cardiovascular, cerebrovascular, and renal outcomes), current evidence-based practice guidelines for the management of hypertension in adults generally recommend the use of drugs from 4 classes of antihypertensive agents (ACE inhibitors, angiotensin II receptor antagonists, calcium-channel blockers, and thiazide diuretics). (See Uses: Hypertension in Adults, in the Thiazides General Statement 40:28.20.) Triamterene alone has little if any hypotensive effect; however, it may be used with another diuretic (e.g., hydrochlorothiazide) or a hypotensive agent in the management of mild to moderate hypertension. In the management of hypertension, triamterene is used principally in patients with diuretic-induced hypokalemia or to prevent hypokalemia in patients receiving diuretics and at risk of this adverse effect. Potassium-sparing diuretics should be avoided in patients with substantial renal insufficiency.

For additional information on overall principles and expert recommendations for treatment of hypertension, see Uses: Hypertension in Adults and also see Uses: Hypertension in Pediatric Patients, in the Thiazides General Statement 40:28.20.

DOSAGE AND ADMINISTRATION

● Administration

Triamterene is administered orally. Triamterene has been administered IV†, but the poor solubility of the drug and acidity of the solutions make administration by this route extremely difficult and a parenteral dosage form currently is not available in the US.

● Dosage

Dosage of triamterene should be individualized according to the patient's requirements and response. It has been theorized that abrupt withdrawal of triamterene may result in rebound kaliuresis; therefore, the drug should be withdrawn gradually. Experts state that diuretics should be administered at a dosage sufficient to achieve optimal volume status and relieve congestion without inducing an excessively rapid reduction in intravascular volume, which could result in hypotension, renal dysfunction, or both.

Triamterene Therapy
Edema

The usual initial adult dosage of triamterene in the management of edema is 100 mg twice daily after meals. Once edema is controlled, most patients can be maintained on 100 mg daily or every other day. Dosage should not exceed 300 mg daily. When triamterene is used in combination with other diuretics, the initial dosage of each drug should be lowered and adjusted to individual requirements and tolerance.

For the management of fluid retention (e.g., edema) associated with heart failure, some experts recommend initiating triamterene at a low dosage (e.g., 50–75 mg twice daily) and increasing the dosage (maximum of 200 mg daily) until urine output increases and weight decreases, generally by 0.5–1 kg daily.

Hypertension

When triamterene is used in the management of hypertension† in adults (usually in combination with a kaliuretic diuretic), some experts state that the usual dosage range is 50–100 mg daily given as a single dose or in 2 divided doses.

The patient's renal function and electrolytes should be assessed 2–4 weeks after initiation of diuretic therapy. Blood pressure should be monitored regularly (i.e., monthly) during therapy and dosage of the antihypertensive drug adjusted until blood pressure is controlled. If an adequate blood pressure response is not achieved, the dosage may be increased or another antihypertensive agent with demonstrated benefit and preferably with a complementary mechanism of action (e.g., angiotensin-converting enzyme [ACE] inhibitor, angiotensin II receptor antagonist, calcium-channel blocker) may be added; if target blood pressure is still not achieved, a third drug may be added. (See Uses: Hypertension.) In patients who develop unacceptable adverse effects with triamterene, the drug should be discontinued and another antihypertensive agent from a different pharmacologic class should be initiated.

The goal of hypertension management and prevention is to achieve and maintain optimal control of blood pressure. However, the optimum blood pressure threshold for initiating antihypertensive drug therapy and specific treatment goals remain controversial. A 2017 multidisciplinary hypertension guideline from the American College of Cardiology (ACC), American Heart Association (AHA), and a number of other professional organizations generally recommends a blood pressure goal of less than 130/80 mm Hg in all adults, regardless of comorbidities or level of atherosclerotic cardiovascular disease (ASCVD) risk. Many patients will require at least 2 drugs from different pharmacologic classes to achieve this blood pressure goal; the potential benefits of hypertension management and drug cost, adverse effects, and risks associated with the use of multiple antihypertensive drugs also should be considered when deciding a patient's blood pressure treatment goal.

For additional information on target levels of blood pressure and on monitoring therapy in the management of hypertension, see Blood Pressure Monitoring and Treatment Goals under Dosage: Hypertension, in Dosage and Administration in the Thiazides General Statement 40:28.20.

Triamterene/Hydrochlorothiazide Fixed-combination Therapy

Commercially available preparations containing triamterene and hydrochlorothiazide in fixed combination generally should not be used as initial therapy, except in patients in whom the clinical consequences of potential thiazide-induced hypokalemia represent an important risk (e.g., patients receiving cardiac glycosides or patients with cardiac arrhythmias).

When Dyazide®, Maxzide® or Maxzide®-25 mg, or therapeutically equivalent formulations of the combination are used, the manufacturers state that the usual adult dosage in terms of triamterene is 37.5–75 mg once daily with appropriate monitoring of serum potassium concentrations. Patients who become hypokalemic while receiving hydrochlorothiazide 25 or 50 mg daily may be switched to a fixed-combination preparation containing triamterene in combination with the equivalent hydrochlorothiazide dosage. In patients who require hydrochlorothiazide and in whom hypokalemia cannot be risked, therapy with the fixed combination may be initiated at a triamterene dosage of 37.5 mg daily (with hydrochlorothiazide 25 mg daily). The manufacturers state that clinical experience with the fixed-combination tablets suggests that the risk of electrolyte imbalance and renal dysfunction may be increased when triamterene 75 mg daily (with hydrochlorothiazide 50 mg daily) is administered in 2 divided doses rather than as a single daily dose. The manufacturers also state that there is no clinical experience to date with dosages of these more bioavailable formulations exceeding 75 mg of triamterene and 50 mg of hydrochlorothiazide daily. (See Pharmacokinetics: Absorption.)

Pediatric Dosage

The safety and efficacy of triamterene in children† have not been established; however, some clinicians suggest an initial dosage of 4 mg/kg daily or 115 mg/m² daily, given in two divided doses after meals. If necessary, dosage may be increased to 6 mg/kg daily; however, pediatric dosage should not exceed 300 mg daily. Dosage should be reduced if triamterene is used with other diuretics.

If triamterene is used for the management of hypertension in children†, some experts have recommended an initial triamterene dosage of 1–2 mg/kg daily given in 2 divided doses. Such experts have suggested that dosage may be increased as necessary up to 3–4 mg/kg (maximum 300 mg) daily given in 2 divided doses. For information on overall principles and expert recommendations for treatment of hypertension in pediatric patients, see Uses: Hypertension in Pediatric Patients, in the Thiazides General Statement 40:28.20.

CAUTIONS

● Adverse Effects

In general, adverse effects of triamterene are mild and respond to withdrawal of the drug. The most serious adverse effect of triamterene therapy is electrolyte imbalance, mainly hyperkalemia (serum potassium concentrations may exceed 5.5 mEq/L), especially in patients with renal insufficiency or diabetes, geriatric or severely ill patients, or those receiving prolonged therapy with large doses. Hyperkalemia may be associated with cardiac irregularities. At least 3 fatal cases of hyperkalemia have been reported in patients receiving triamterene and a thiazide

diuretic; however, 2 of these patients were also receiving spironolactone which may have contributed to the hyperkalemia.

Potassium loss has been reported during triamterene therapy in some patients with hepatic cirrhosis and may result in signs and symptoms of hepatic coma or precoma. Serum potassium concentrations should be closely monitored in patients with hepatic cirrhosis and potassium supplementation administered if required.

Diuretics increase urinary sodium excretion and decrease physical signs of fluid retention in patients with heart failure. Results of short-term studies in patients with heart failure indicate that diuretic therapy is associated with a reduction in jugular venous pressures, pulmonary congestion, ascites, peripheral edema, and body weight within a few days of initiating such therapy. In addition, diuretics may improve cardiac function, symptoms, and exercise tolerance in these patients. However, since there are no long-term studies of diuretic therapy in patients with heart failure, the effects of diuretics on morbidity and mortality are not known. Nevertheless, most long-term studies of therapeutic interventions for heart failure have been in patients receiving diuretic therapy. Diuretics should *not* be used as monotherapy in patients with heart failure even if symptoms of fluid overload (e.g., peripheral edema, pulmonary congestion) are well controlled, because diuretics alone do not prevent progression of heart failure.

Depending on the dosage employed, diuretics may alter the efficacy and safety of concomitantly used drugs in heart failure, and therefore diuretic dosage should be selected carefully. Excessive diuretic dosages may lead to volume depletion, which can increase the risk of hypotension in patients receiving angiotensin-converting enzyme (ACE) inhibitors or vasodilators and renal insufficiency in patients receiving ACE inhibitors or angiotensin II receptor antagonists. Inadequate diuretic dosages may lead to fluid retention, which can decrease the response to ACE inhibitors and increase the risk of β-adrenergic blocking agent (β-blocker) therapy. Patients with mild heart failure may respond favorably to low doses of diuretics, since absorption of diuretics from the GI tract is rapid and the drugs are distributed rapidly to the renal tubules in such patients; however, as heart failure advances, absorption of the drugs may be delayed because of bowel edema or intestinal hypoperfusion, and distribution may be impaired because of decreases in renal perfusion and function. Therefore, dosage of diuretics usually needs to be increased with progression of heart failure; eventually, patients may become resistant to even high dosages of diuretic therapy. If resistance to diuretics occurs, IV administration of a diuretic or concomitant use of 2 or more diuretics (e.g., a loop diuretic and metolazone, a loop diuretic and a thiazide diuretic) may be necessary, or alternatively, short-term administration of a drug that increases blood flow (e.g., a positive inotropic agent such as dopamine) may be necessary. ACCF and AHA state that IV loop diuretics should be administered promptly to all hospitalized heart failure patients with substantial fluid overload to reduce morbidity. ACCF and AHA state that low-dose dopamine infusions may be considered in combination with loop diuretics to augment diuresis and preserve renal function and renal blood flow in patients with acute decompensated heart failure, although data are conflicting and additional study and experience are needed.

Most experts state that the diuretics of choice for most patients with heart failure usually are loop diuretics (e.g., bumetanide, ethacrynic acid, furosemide, torsemide), especially in those with renal impairment or substantial fluid retention, since loop diuretics increase sodium excretion to 20–25% of the filtered load of sodium, enhance free water clearance, and maintain their efficacy unless renal function is severely impaired (e.g., creatinine clearance less than 5 mL/minute). In contrast, thiazide diuretics increase fractional sodium excretion to only 5–10% of the filtered load, tend to decrease free water clearance, and lose their efficacy in patients with moderate renal impairment (e.g., creatinine clearance less than 30 mL/minute). Thiazides may be preferred in some patients with concomitant hypertension because of their sustained effects. If electrolyte imbalance(s) occurs during diuretic therapy for heart failure, the patient should be treated aggressively (preferably with low doses of a potassium-sparing diuretic instead of potassium or magnesium supplements) and diuresis should be continued. In patients who develop azotemia or hypotension before therapeutic goals are achieved, consideration to decreasing the rate of diuresis may be made, but diuretic therapy should continue until fluid retention is eliminated, provided that decreases in blood pressure remain asymptomatic; excessive concern about hypotension and azotemia may result in suboptimal diuretic therapy leading to refractory edema.

Once fluid retention has resolved in patients with heart failure, diuretic therapy should be maintained to prevent recurrence of fluid retention. Ideally, diuretic therapy should be adjusted according to changes in body weight (as an indicator of fluid retention) rather than maintained at a fixed dose.

Sodium depletion may occur when triamterene is administered to markedly edematous patients whose sodium chloride intake is restricted. Magnesium depletion may also occur, especially if triamterene is used concomitantly with another diuretic such as a thiazide which also increases excretion of magnesium. Serum chloride may be increased and serum bicarbonate decreased during triamterene therapy, resulting in decreased alkali reserve with the possibility of metabolic acidosis. Slight alkalinization of the urine may occur.

Increased BUN concentration caused by decreased glomerular filtration rate has been reported during therapy with triamterene. However, a rise in BUN concentration seldom occurs with intermittent (every other day) therapy and is reversible upon withdrawal of the drug. Serum creatinine concentration may be moderately increased during administration of triamterene but returns to pretreatment levels in 7–14 days after the drug is discontinued. Serum uric acid concentrations may be increased, especially in patients with gouty arthritis.

Megaloblastic anemia has occurred in patients with alcoholic cirrhosis receiving triamterene.

Renal colic occurred in one patient receiving triamterene and hydrochlorothiazide who had a previously asymptomatic partial urinary tract obstruction. Triamterene has occasionally caused nephrolithiasis. Renal calculi have been composed of triamterene and/or its metabolites (i.e., 6-p-hydroxytriamterene and its sulfate) alone, but apparently in a protein matrix, or combined with other usual calculus components (e.g., calcium oxalate monohydrate and dihydrate, uric acid, hydroxylapatite). Triamterene usually appears as the nucleus of the calculus as a central amorphous deposit around which calcium oxalate monohydrate or dihydrate or uric acid is deposited. Triamterene has reportedly caused acute interstitial nephritis in one patient.

Other adverse effects of triamterene include nausea, vomiting, diarrhea, or other GI disturbances. Nausea may be minimized by giving the drug after meals; however, nausea and vomiting may also be symptoms of electrolyte imbalance. Dizziness, hypotension, weakness, headache, muscle cramps, dry mouth, anaphylaxis, photosensitivity, rash, and blood dyscrasias such as granulocytopenia and eosinophilia have also been attributed to use of the drug.

● Precautions and Contraindications

When triamterene is used as a fixed-combination preparation that includes hydrochlorothiazide, the cautions, precautions, and contraindications associated with thiazide diuretics must be considered in addition to those associated with triamterene.

Patients receiving prolonged triamterene therapy should be monitored for signs of electrolyte imbalance, especially those with heart failure, renal disease, or cirrhosis of the liver. It is particularly important that serum potassium concentrations be checked periodically, especially in geriatric, cirrhotic, or diabetic patients; in patients with impaired renal function; or when there is a change in dosage of triamterene. If hyperkalemia occurs, the drug should be discontinued. Periodic BUN and serum creatinine determinations should be performed, especially in patients with suspected or confirmed renal insufficiency.

Potassium supplementation in the form of potassium salts, a high potassium diet, or salt substitutes should not be given to patients receiving triamterene alone. When triamterene is added to other diuretic therapy or when patients are switched to triamterene from other diuretics, potassium supplementation should be discontinued. Patients receiving triamterene concomitantly with a thiazide or other diuretic that promotes potassium excretion (kaliuretic diuretic) should receive dietary potassium supplements only if they develop hypokalemia or their dietary intake of potassium is markedly impaired. It has been theorized that abrupt withdrawal of triamterene after intense or prolonged therapy may result in a rebound kaliuresis; therefore, the drug should be discontinued gradually.

Although a causal relationship has not been established between the drug and megaloblastic anemia, triamterene should be used with caution in pregnant women and in patients with alcohol dependence since these patients may have reduced stores of folate. Periodic blood studies should be performed in cirrhotic patients with splenomegaly as they are subject to marked hematologic variations; such patients also should be observed for exacerbation of underlying hepatic disease.

Triamterene should be used with caution in patients with impaired hepatic function. Diuretic therapy in such patients should be initiated while the patient is hospitalized, because rapid alterations in fluid and electrolyte balance may precipitate hepatic coma. Patients receiving the drug should be observed for signs of liver damage, blood dyscrasias, or other idiosyncratic reactions. Triamterene should be administered cautiously to patients with impaired renal function. Although the manufacturer states that triamterene should be used with caution in patients with a history of renal calculi, some clinicians recommend that the drug not be used in these patients because of the risk of triamterene nephrolithiasis. If a patient passes a urinary calculus during triamterene therapy, the drug should be discontinued and the calculus analyzed for the presence of triamterene and/or its metabolites. (See Cautions: Adverse Effects.)

Triamterene should be administered with caution to patients with diabetes mellitus and should be given only to those diabetic patients whose blood glucose concentration is well controlled. The drug does not appear to be diabetogenic or to alter carbohydrate metabolism; however, diabetic patients appear to be more sensitive to changes in serum potassium concentrations than are nondiabetics. Elevations of serum potassium concentrations are exacerbated by administration of large quantities of glucose; therefore, comatose diabetic patients receiving triamterene therapy should not be tested for hypoglycemia by IV administration of dextrose.

Potassium-conserving therapy should generally be avoided in severely ill patients in whom respiratory or metabolic acidosis may occur; acidosis may result in rapid increases in serum potassium concentrations. If potassium-conserving therapy (e.g., triamterene) is used, frequent assessment of acid-base balance and serum electrolytes should be performed.

Triamterene is contraindicated in patients with severe or progressive kidney disease, severe hepatic disease, preexisting or drug-induced hyperkalemia, or hypersensitivity to the drug. Triamterene should also not be used in patients who develop hyperkalemia while receiving the drug.

● Pediatric Precautions

Safety and efficacy of triamterene in children have not been established. For information on overall principles and expert recommendations for treatment of hypertension in pediatric patients, see Uses: Hypertension in Pediatric Patients, in the Thiazides General Statement 40:28.20.

● Mutagenicity and Carcinogenicity

Studies to determine the mutagenic and carcinogenic potentials of triamterene currently are not available.

● Pregnancy, Fertility, and Lactation

Pregnancy

There are no adequate and well-controlled studies using triamterene in pregnant women, and the drug should be used during pregnancy only when the potential benefits justify the possible risks (these include adverse effects reported in adults) to the fetus.

Fertility

Reproduction studies in rats using triamterene doses up to 30 times the human dose have not revealed evidence of harm to the fetus or impaired fertility. The drug has been shown to cross the placental barrier and appear in the cord blood of ewes; similar distribution may occur in humans.

Lactation

Since triamterene has been shown to distribute into milk in animals and may distribute into human milk, the drug should not be used in nursing women. If use of triamterene is deemed essential, nursing should be discontinued.

DRUG INTERACTIONS

● Potassium-sparing Agents

Triamterene should not be used concurrently with another potassium-sparing agent (e.g., amiloride, spironolactone), since concomitant therapy with these drugs may increase the risk of hyperkalemia compared with triamterene alone. At least 2 deaths have been reported in patients receiving triamterene and spironolactone concurrently; in one patient, recommended dosages were exceeded and, in the other patient, serum electrolytes were not closely monitored.

Potassium-sparing diuretics should be used with caution and serum potassium should be determined frequently in patients receiving an angiotensin-converting enzyme (ACE) inhibitor (e.g., captopril, enalapril), since concomitant administration with an ACE inhibitor may increase the risk of hyperkalemia. Dosage of triamterene should be reduced or the drug should be discontinued as necessary. Patients with renal impairment may be at increased risk of hyperkalemia.

● Potassium-containing Preparations

Concurrent administration of triamterene with potassium supplements, potassium-containing medications (e.g., parenteral penicillin G potassium), or other substances containing potassium (e.g., salt substitutes, low-salt milk) may increase the risk of hyperkalemia as compared with triamterene alone, and such combined use is contraindicated.

● Nonsteroidal Anti-inflammatory Agents

Concomitant use of triamterene and indomethacin has adversely affected renal function. In one study, concomitant administration of indomethacin and triamterene to 4 healthy adults resulted in a 60–70% decrease in creatinine clearance in 2 individuals; renal function returned to normal within 2 weeks after both drugs were discontinued. When the drugs were given separately, triamterene caused no consistent change in renal function; indomethacin induced an average 10% decrease in creatinine clearance. Acute anuric renal failure occurred within 2 days after concomitant use of indomethacin and triamterene in a 79-year-old woman with compensated heart failure. BUN and serum creatinine concentrations increased to 102 and 10.2 mg/dL, respectively, 5 days after discontinuance of the drugs in this woman, and subsequently returned toward normal over 2 months; anuria persisted for 11 days after discontinuance of the drugs. Although the mechanism of this interaction was not determined, it has been postulated that indomethacin may inhibit triamterene-stimulated synthesis of renal prostaglandins that mediate an adaptive mechanism for renal blood flow preservation in response to triamterene-mediated renal vasoconstriction. The manufacturer of indomethacin recommends that the combination of indomethacin and triamterene not be used. Triamterene should be used with caution in patients receiving other nonsteroidal anti-inflammatory agents.

● Angiotensin-converting Enzyme Inhibitors

Potassium-sparing diuretics (e.g., triamterene) should be used with caution and serum potassium should be determined frequently in patients receiving an ACE inhibitor (e.g., enalapril), since hyperkalemia may occur. Potassium-sparing diuretics should be used with great caution, if at all, in patients receiving an ACE inhibitor (e.g., enalapril) for heart failure. Potassium-sparing diuretics should be discontinued or their dosage reduced as necessary in patients receiving an ACE inhibitor. (See Drug Interactions: Drugs Increasing Serum Potassium Concentration in Enalapril 24:32.04.)

● Other Drugs

Although triamterene alone does not consistently cause hypotension, lowering of blood pressure may occur, especially when it is used with hypotensive agents.

Diuretics including triamterene, generally should not be used concurrently with lithium since diuretics reduce renal lithium clearance and may increase the risk of lithium toxicity. (See Lithium Salts 28:28.)

LABORATORY TEST INTERFERENCES

A pale blue fluorescence may be produced in urine of patients receiving triamterene which may interfere with methods of enzyme assay that depend on fluorometry, such as determinations of lactic dehydrogenase activity. Triamterene interferes with the fluorometric assay of quinidine as the two drugs have similar fluorescence spectra.

ACUTE TOXICITY

● Pathogenesis

The amount of triamterene ingested as a single dose that would usually be associated with symptoms of overdosage or would likely be life-threatening is not known. The oral LD_{50} of the drug in mice is 380 mg/kg.

● Manifestations

Overdosage of triamterene may cause electrolyte imbalance, especially hyperkalemia. Nausea, vomiting, other GI disturbances, and weakness may also occur. Hypotension may also result, especially when the drug is used concomitantly with hydrochlorothiazide or other diuretics or hypotensive agents.

● Treatment

Severe hypotension may be alleviated by administration of pressor agents such as norepinephrine. Immediate gastric lavage or emesis should be induced in conscious patients. Careful evaluation of the electrolyte pattern and fluid balance should be made and corrective therapy initiated if indicated. Although triamterene is relatively highly protein bound, dialysis may be of some benefit.

PHARMACOLOGY

Like amiloride, triamterene acts directly on the distal renal tubule of the nephron to depress reabsorption of sodium and excretion of potassium and hydrogen which are stimulated at that site by aldosterone. Triamterene is a potassium-sparing diuretic that does not competitively inhibit aldosterone, and its activity is independent of aldosterone concentrations. Triamterene does not inhibit carbonic anhydrase.

Administration of triamterene increases excretion of sodium, calcium, magnesium, and bicarbonate. Excretion of chloride is increased but not always in proportion to sodium excretion; slightly more sodium than chloride is excreted. Excretion of potassium is usually reduced; however, slight potassium loss was reported in one study in some patients with cirrhosis and ascites. Serum concentrations of potassium and chloride are usually increased, and serum bicarbonate is consistently decreased during triamterene therapy. Triamterene may cause decreased alkali reserve with the possibility of metabolic acidosis. Urinary pH is increased slightly.

Glomerular filtration rate is reduced during daily but not during intermittent administration of the drug, suggesting a reversible effect on renal blood flow. Cardiac output is decreased. In contrast to other diuretics, triamterene does not appear to inhibit excretion of uric acid; however, serum uric acid concentrations may be elevated in some patients, especially those predisposed to gouty arthritis. Triamterene has been reported to inhibit dehydrofolate reductase in vitro; however, in vivo interference with folic acid utilization has not been demonstrated.

Triamterene alone has little if any hypotensive effect. The drug does not appear to be diabetogenic or to alter carbohydrate metabolism.

PHARMACOKINETICS

● Absorption

Triamterene is rapidly absorbed from the GI tract; however, the degree of absorption varies in different individuals. Diuresis usually occurs within 2–4 hours and diminishes in approximately 7–9 hours after oral administration of the drug, although the total duration of action may be 24 hours or longer. The maximum therapeutic effect may not occur until after several days of therapy. Peak plasma concentrations of 0.05–0.28 mcg/mL are achieved within 2–4 hours following administration of a 100- to 200-mg single oral dose.

Oral bioavailability of hydrochlorothiazide from the original formulation (no longer commercially available) of Dyazide® capsules was about 50–65% that from Maxzide® tablets or single-entity tablets or solutions of the drug. In one crossover study in a limited number of healthy adults receiving single doses of the drug, the mean hydrochlorothiazide dose recovered in urine within 72 hours was about 30% for the original formulation of Dyazide® capsules and about 60% for Maxzide® or single-entity tablets of the drug. In 1995, Dyazide® capsules were reformulated to improve the oral bioavailability of triamterene and hydrochlorothiazide. The oral bioavailabilities of triamterene and hydrochlorothiazide from the reformulated Dyazide® capsules now are comparable to those of aqueous suspensions of the individual drugs, averaging 85 and 82%, respectively, for the new formulation and 100 and 100%, respectively, for the suspensions. In addition, intraindividual variation in bioavailability from the reformulated Dyazide® capsules was reduced by about 40% compared with the original formulation. The manufacturer states that the reformulated Dyazide® capsules also are bioequivalent to single-entity 25-mg hydrochlorothiazide tablets and 37.5-mg triamterene capsules. Administration of reformulated Dyazide® with a high-fat meal in healthy adults increased the average bioavailabilities of triamterene by about 67%, 6-p-hydroxytriamterene by about 50%, and hydrochlorothiazide by about 17% and the peak concentrations of triamterene and its p-hydroxy metabolite and delayed the absorption of the active drugs by up to 2 hours.

Distribution

In animals, triamterene has been detected in the brain, heart, ocular fluid, fat, liver, and skeletal muscles. The drug is distributed into bile. Approximately 67% of the drug in the plasma is bound to proteins. Triamterene crosses the placenta in animals. No human data are available indicating whether triamterene appears in the milk of nursing women; however, animal studies have demonstrated the presence of very small amounts of the drug in breast milk.

Elimination

The plasma half-life of triamterene is 100–150 minutes. The metabolic and excretory fate of triamterene has not been fully determined. The drug is reportedly metabolized to 6-*p*-hydroxytriamterene and its sulfate conjugate. Triamterene is excreted in urine as unchanged drug and metabolites. In one study in healthy males, the urinary excretion of 6-*p*-hydroxytriamterene was up to 3 times that of unchanged drug. Limited data indicate that the renal clearances of triamterene, hydroxytriamterene sulfate, and hydrochlorothiazide are reduced in geriatric patients receiving combined triamterene and hydrochlorothiazide therapy, principally as a result of age-related reductions in renal function.

CHEMISTRY AND STABILITY

Chemistry

Triamterene is a pteridine derivative, potassium-sparing diuretic that is structurally related to folic acid. Triamterene occurs as a yellow, odorless, crystalline powder and is practically insoluble in water and very slightly soluble in alcohol. The drug has a pK$_a$ of 6.2.

Stability

Triamterene capsules should be stored in tight, light-resistant containers at a temperature less than 40°C, preferably between 15–30°C.

PREPARATIONS

Excipients in commercially available drug preparations may have clinically important effects in some individuals; consult specific product labeling for details.

Triamterene

Oral		
Capsules	50 mg	**Dyrenium®**, WellSpring
	100 mg	**Dyrenium®**, WellSpring

Triamterene and Hydrochlorothiazide (Co-triamterzide)

Oral		
Capsules	37.5 mg Triamterene and Hydrochlorothiazide 25 mg*	**Dyazide®**, GlaxoSmithKline
		Triamterene and Hydrochlorothiazide Capsules
Tablets	37.5 mg Triamterene and Hydrochlorothiazide 25 mg*	**Maxzide®-25** (scored), Mylan
		Triamterene and Hydrochlorothiazide Tablets
	75 mg Triamterene and Hydrochlorothiazide 50 mg*	**Maxzide®** (scored), Mylan
		Triamterene and Hydrochlorothiazide Tablets

* available from one or more manufacturer, distributor, and/or repackager by generic (nonproprietary) name

† Use is not currently included in the labeling approved by the US Food and Drug Administration.

Selected Revisions April 29, 2019, © Copyright, January 1, 1976, American Society of Health-System Pharmacists, Inc.

Thiazides General Statement

40:28.20 · THIAZIDE DIURETICS

■ Thiazides are diuretics and antihypertensive agents.

USES

● Edema

Thiazide diuretics are used in the management of edema resulting from a number of causes; however, careful etiologic diagnosis should precede the use of any diuretic. There are no substantial differences in the clinical effects or toxicity of comparable dosages of the thiazides or thiazide-like diuretics except that metolazone may be more effective than other thiazide-like diuretics in the management of edema in patients with impaired renal function. Determination of the specific agent to be used is, therefore, usually determined by factors such as cost and patient convenience.

Heart Failure

Clinical Role

Thiazides are used in the management of edema associated with heart failure. Most experts state that all patients with symptomatic heart failure who have evidence for, or a history of, fluid retention generally should receive diuretic therapy in conjunction with moderate sodium restriction, an agent to inhibit the renin-angiotensin-aldosterone (RAA) system (e.g., angiotensin-converting enzyme [ACE] inhibitor, angiotensin II receptor antagonist, angiotensin receptor-neprilysin inhibitor [ARNI]), a β-adrenergic blocking agent (β-blocker), and in selected patients, an aldosterone antagonist. Some experts state that because of limited and inconsistent data, it is difficult to make precise recommendations regarding daily sodium intake and whether it should vary with respect to the type of heart failure (e.g., reduced versus preserved ejection fraction), disease severity (e.g., New York Heart Association [NYHA] class), heart failure-related comorbidities (e.g., renal dysfunction), or other patient characteristics (e.g., age, race). The American College of Cardiology Foundation (ACCF) and American Heart Association (AHA) state that limiting sodium intake to 1.5 g daily in patients with ACCF/AHA stage A or B heart failure may be reasonable. While data currently are lacking to support recommendation of a specific level of sodium intake in patients with ACCF/AHA stage C or D heart failure, ACCF and AHA state that limiting sodium intake to some degree (e.g., less than 3 g daily) in such patients may be considered for symptom improvement.

Diuretics play a key role in the management of heart failure because they produce symptomatic benefits more rapidly than any other drugs, relieving pulmonary and peripheral edema within hours or days compared with weeks or months for cardiac glycosides, ACE inhibitors, or β-blockers. However, since there are no long-term studies of diuretic therapy in patients with heart failure, the effects of diuretics on morbidity and mortality in such patients are not known. Although there are patients with heart failure who do not exhibit fluid retention in the absence of diuretic therapy and even may develop severe volume depletion with low doses of diuretics, such patients are rare and the unique pathophysiologic mechanisms regulating their fluid and electrolyte balance have not been elucidated.

Most experts state that loop diuretics (e.g., bumetanide, ethacrynic acid, furosemide, torsemide) are the diuretics of choice for most patients with heart failure, especially in those with renal impairment or substantial fluid retention, since loop diuretics increase sodium excretion to 20–25% of the filtered load of sodium, enhance free water clearance, and maintain their efficacy unless renal function is severely impaired (e.g., creatinine clearance less than 5 mL/minute). In contrast, thiazide diuretics increase fractional sodium excretion to only 5–10% of the filtered load, tend to decrease free water clearance, and lose their efficacy in patients with moderate renal impairment (e.g., creatinine clearance less than 30 mL/minute). However, thiazides may be preferred in some patients with concomitant hypertension because of their sustained antihypertensive effects. In patients who develop azotemia or hypotension before therapeutic goals are achieved, consideration to decreasing the rate of diuresis may be made, but diuretic therapy should continue until fluid retention is eliminated, provided that decreases in blood pressure remain asymptomatic; excessive concern about hypotension and azotemia may result in suboptimal diuretic therapy leading to refractory edema.

Efficacy

Diuretics increase urinary sodium excretion and decrease physical signs of fluid retention in patients with heart failure. Results of short-term studies in patients with heart failure indicate that diuretic therapy is associated with a reduction in jugular venous pressures, pulmonary congestion, ascites, peripheral edema, and body weight within a few days of initiating such therapy. In addition, diuretics may improve cardiac function, symptoms, and exercise tolerance in these patients. However, since there are no long-term studies of diuretic therapy in patients with heart failure, the effects of diuretics on morbidity and mortality are not known. Nevertheless, most long-term studies of therapeutic interventions for heart failure have been in patients receiving diuretic therapy. Diuretics should *not* be used as monotherapy in patients with heart failure even if symptoms of fluid overload (e.g., peripheral edema, pulmonary congestion) are well controlled, because diuretics alone do not prevent progression of heart failure.

Dosing Considerations

Depending on the dosage employed, diuretics may alter the efficacy and safety of concomitantly used drugs in heart failure, and therefore diuretic dosage should be selected carefully. Excessive diuretic dosages may lead to volume depletion, which can increase the risk of hypotension in patients receiving ACE inhibitors or vasodilators and renal insufficiency in patients receiving ACE inhibitors or angiotensin II receptor antagonists. Inadequate diuretic dosages may lead to fluid retention, which can decrease the response to ACE inhibitors and increase the risk of β-blocker therapy. Patients with mild heart failure may respond favorably to low doses of diuretics, since absorption of diuretics from the GI tract is rapid and the drugs are distributed rapidly to the renal tubules in such patients; however, as heart failure advances, absorption of the drugs may be delayed because of bowel edema or intestinal hypoperfusion, and distribution may be impaired because of decreases in renal perfusion and function. Therefore, dosage of diuretics usually needs to be increased with progression of heart failure; eventually, patients may become resistant to even high dosages of diuretics. If resistance to diuretics occurs, IV administration of a diuretic or concomitant use of 2 or more diuretics (e.g., a loop diuretic and metolazone, a loop diuretic and a thiazide diuretic) may be necessary, or alternatively, short-term administration of a drug that increases blood flow (e.g., a positive inotropic agent such as dopamine) may be necessary. ACCF and AHA state that IV loop diuretics should be administered promptly to all hospitalized heart failure patients with substantial fluid overload to reduce morbidity. In addition, ACCF and AHA state that low-dose dopamine infusions may be considered in combination with loop diuretics to augment diuresis and preserve renal function and renal blood flow in patients with acute decompensated heart failure, although data are conflicting and additional study and experience are needed.

Maintenance Therapy

Once fluid retention has resolved in patients with heart failure, diuretic therapy should be maintained to prevent recurrence of fluid retention. Ideally, diuretic therapy should be adjusted according to changes in body weight (as an indicator of fluid retention) rather than maintained at a fixed dosage. Diuretics also should be continued in patients with comorbid conditions (e.g., hypertension) where ongoing therapy with the drugs is indicated.

Other Edematous Conditions

In edema secondary to nephrotic syndrome, thiazides may be useful if the patient fails to respond to corticosteroid therapy. Edema secondary to nephrotic syndrome is more likely to become refractory to therapy than edema associated with heart failure, and more potent diuretics may be required. Other forms of edema caused by renal disease and edema caused by corticosteroids and estrogens also may be relatively resistant to treatment with the thiazides. Thiazides and thiazide-like diuretics (with the exception of metolazone) are ineffective in patients with serum creatinine or BUN concentrations greater than about twice normal. Some clinicians state that thiazides are ineffective in patients with a glomerular filtration rate (GFR) of less than 15–25 mL/minute, whereas others suggest that use of a more potent diuretic should be considered whenever the GFR is less than 50 mL/minute.

Edema associated with pregnancy generally responds well to thiazides except when caused by renal disease. Hypertension during pregnancy also responds well, but preeclampsia and eclampsia may require more potent diuretics. The routine use of thiazides is contraindicated in pregnant women with mild edema who are otherwise healthy.

• *Hypertension in Adults*

Thiazide diuretics are used alone or in combination with other classes of antihypertensive agents in the management of all stages of hypertension.

Current evidence-based practice guidelines for the management of hypertension in adults generally recommend the use of drugs from 4 classes of antihypertensive agents (ACE inhibitors, angiotensin II receptor antagonists, calcium-channel blockers, and thiazide diuretics); data from clinical outcome trials indicate that lowering blood pressure with any of these drug classes can reduce the complications of hypertension and provide similar cardiovascular protection. However, recommendations for initial drug selection and use in specific patient populations may vary across these expert guidelines. This variability is due, in part, to differences in the guideline development process and the types of studies (e.g., randomized controlled studies only versus a range of studies with different study designs) included in the evidence reviews. Ultimately, choice of antihypertensive therapy should be individualized, considering the clinical characteristics of the patient (e.g., age, ethnicity/race, comorbid conditions, cardiovascular risk factors) as well as drug-related factors (e.g., ease of administration, availability, adverse effects, costs).

Thiazide diuretics historically have been considered the drugs of choice for most patients with uncomplicated hypertension because of their established benefits, cost, and favorable adverse effects profile. However, current evidence indicates no overall differences in clinical outcomes between thiazide diuretics and other classes of antihypertensive drugs, including calcium-channel blockers, ACE inhibitors, and angiotensin II receptor antagonists. While there may be individual differences with respect to specific outcomes, these antihypertensive drug classes all generally produce comparable effects on overall mortality and cardiovascular, cerebrovascular, and renal outcomes. Because many patients eventually will need drugs from 2 or more antihypertensive classes, experts generally state that the emphasis should be placed on achieving appropriate blood pressure control rather than on identifying a preferred drug to achieve that control.

Disease Overview

Worldwide, hypertension is the most common modifiable risk factor for cardiovascular events and mortality. The lifetime risk of developing hypertension in the US exceeds 80%, with higher rates observed among African Americans and Hispanics compared with whites or Asians. The systolic blood pressure (SBP) and diastolic blood pressure (DBP) values defined as hypertension (see Blood Pressure Classification under Uses: Hypertension in Adults) in a 2017 multidisciplinary guideline of the American College of Cardiology (ACC), AHA, and a number of other professional organizations (subsequently referred to as the 2017 ACC/AHA hypertension guideline in this monograph) are lower than those defined in the Seventh Report of the Joint National Committee on Prevention, Detection, Evaluation, and Treatment of High Blood Pressure (JNC 7) guidelines, which results in an increase of approximately 14% in the prevalence of hypertension in the US. However, this change in definition results in only a 2% increase in the percentage of patients requiring antihypertensive drug therapy because nonpharmacologic treatment is recommended for most adults now classified by the 2017 ACC/AHA hypertension guideline as hypertensive who would *not* meet the JNC 7 definition of hypertension. Among US adults receiving antihypertensive drugs, approximately 53% have inadequately controlled blood pressure according to current ACC/AHA treatment goals.

Cardiovascular and Renal Sequelae

The principal goal of preventing and treating hypertension is to reduce the risk of cardiovascular and renal morbidity and mortality, including target organ damage. The relationship between blood pressure and cardiovascular disease is continuous, consistent, and independent of other risk factors. It is important that very high blood pressure be managed promptly to reduce the risk of target organ damage. The higher the blood pressure, the more likely the development of myocardial infarction (MI), heart failure, stroke, and renal disease. For adults 40–70 years of age, each 20-mm Hg increment in SBP or 10-mm Hg increment in DBP doubles the risk of developing cardiovascular disease across the entire blood pressure range of 115/75 to 185/115 mm Hg. For those older than 50 years of age, SBP is a much more important risk factor for developing cardiovascular disease than is DBP. The rapidity with which treatment is required depends on the patient's clinical presentation (presence of new or worsening target organ damage) and the presence or absence of cardiovascular complications; the 2017 ACC/AHA hypertension guideline states that treatment of very high blood pressure should be initiated within 1 week.

Blood Pressure Classification

Accurate blood pressure measurement is essential for the proper diagnosis and management of hypertension. Error in measuring blood pressure is a major cause of inadequate blood pressure control and may lead to overtreatment. Because a patient's blood pressure may vary in an unpredictable fashion, a single blood pressure measurement is not sufficient for clinical decision-making. An average of 2 or 3 blood pressure measurements obtained on 2–3 separate occasions using proper technique should be used to minimize random error and provide a more accurate blood pressure reading. Out-of-office blood pressure measurements may be useful for confirming and managing hypertension. The 2017 ACC/AHA hypertension guideline document (available on the ACC and AHA websites) should be consulted for key steps on properly measuring blood pressure.

According to the 2017 ACC/AHA hypertension guideline, blood pressure in adults is classified into 4 categories: normal, elevated, stage 1 hypertension, and stage 2 hypertension. (See Table 1.) The 2017 ACC/AHA hypertension guideline lowers the blood pressure threshold used to define hypertension in the US; previous hypertension guidelines (JNC 7) considered adults with SBP of 120–139 mm Hg or DBP of 80–89 mm Hg to have prehypertension, those with SBP of 140–159 mm Hg or DBP of 90–99 mm Hg to have stage 1 hypertension, and those with SBP of 160 mm Hg or higher or DBP of 100 mm Hg or higher to have stage 2 hypertension. The blood pressure definitions in the 2017 ACC/AHA hypertension guideline are based upon data from studies evaluating the association between SBP/DBP and cardiovascular risk and the benefits of blood pressure reduction. Individuals with SBP and DBP in 2 different categories should be designated as being in the higher blood pressure category.

TABLE 1. ACC/AHA Blood Pressure Classification in Adults [a][b]

Category	SBP (mm Hg)		DBP (mm Hg)
Normal	<120	and	<80
Elevated	120–129	and	<80
Hypertension, Stage 1	130–139	or	80–89
Hypertension, Stage 2	≥140	or	≥90

[a] Source: Whelton PK, Carey RM, Aronow WS et al. 2017 ACC/AHA/AAPA/ABC/ACPM/AGS/APhA/ASH/ASPC/NMA/PCNA guideline for the prevention, detection, evaluation, and management of high blood pressure in adults: a report of the American College of Cardiology/American Heart Association Task Force on Clinical Practice Guidelines. *Hypertension.* 2018;71:e13-115.

[b] Individuals with SBP and DBP in 2 different categories (e.g., elevated SBP and normal DBP) should be designated as being in the higher blood pressure category (i.e., elevated BP).

The blood pressure thresholds used to define hypertension, when to initiate drug therapy, and the ideal target blood pressure values remain controversial. The 2017 ACC/AHA hypertension guideline recommends a blood pressure goal of less than 130/80 mm Hg in all adults who have confirmed hypertension and known cardiovascular disease or a 10-year atherosclerotic cardiovascular disease (ASCVD) event risk of 10% or higher; the ACC/AHA guideline also states that this blood pressure goal is reasonable to attempt to achieve in adults with confirmed hypertension who do *not* have increased cardiovascular risk. The lower blood pressure values used to define hypertension and the lower target blood pressure goals outlined in the 2017 ACC/AHA hypertension guideline are based on clinical studies demonstrating a substantial reduction in the composite end point of major cardiovascular disease events and the combination of fatal and nonfatal stroke when a lower SBP/DBP value (i.e., 130/80 mm Hg) was used to define hypertension. These lower target blood pressure goals also are based upon clinical studies demonstrating continuing reduction of cardiovascular risk at progressively lower levels of SBP. A linear relationship has been demonstrated between cardiovascular risk and blood pressure even at low blood pressures (e.g., 120–124 mm Hg SBP). The 2017 ACC/AHA hypertension guideline recommends estimating a patient's ASCVD risk using the ACC/AHA Pooled Cohort equations (available online at http://tools.acc.org/ASCVD-Risk-Estimator), which are based on a variety of factors including age, race, gender, cholesterol levels, statin use, blood pressure, treatment for hypertension, history of diabetes mellitus, smoking status, and aspirin use. While the 2017 ACC/AHA hypertension guideline has lowered the threshold for *diagnosing* hypertension in adults, the threshold for *initiating drug therapy* has only been lowered for those patients who are at high risk of cardiovascular disease. Clinicians who support the 2017 ACC/AHA hypertension guideline believe that these recommendations have the potential to increase hypertension awareness, encourage lifestyle modification, and focus antihypertensive drug initiation and intensification in those adults at high risk for cardiovascular disease.

The lower blood pressure goals advocated in the 2017 ACC/AHA hypertension guideline have been questioned by some clinicians who have concerns regarding the guideline's use of extrapolated observational data, the lack of generalizability of some of the randomized trials (e.g., SPRINT) used to support the guideline, the difficulty of establishing accurate representative blood pressure values in typical clinical practice settings, and the accuracy of the cardiovascular risk calculator used in the guideline. Some clinicians state the lower blood pressure threshold used to define hypertension in the 2017 ACC/AHA hypertension guideline is not fully supported by clinical data, and these clinicians have expressed concerns about the possible harms (e.g., adverse effects of antihypertensive therapy) associated with classifying more patients as being hypertensive. Some clinicians also state that using this guideline, a large number of young, low-risk patients would need to be treated in order to observe a clinical benefit, while other clinicians state that the estimated gains in life expectancy attributable to long-term use of blood pressure-lowering drugs are correspondingly greater in this patient population.

Treatment Benefits

In clinical trials, antihypertensive therapy has been found to reduce the risk of developing stroke by about 34–40%, MI by about 20–25%, and heart failure by more than 50%. In a randomized, controlled study (SPRINT) that included hypertensive patients without diabetes mellitus who had a high risk of cardiovascular disease, intensive SBP lowering of approximately 15 mm Hg was associated with a 25% reduction in cardiovascular disease events and a 27% reduction in all-cause mortality. However, the exclusion of patients with diabetes mellitus, prior stroke, and those younger than 50 years of age may decrease the generalizability of these findings. Some experts estimate that if the SBP goals of the 2017 ACC/AHA hypertension guideline are achieved, major cardiovascular disease events may be reduced by an additional 340,000 and total deaths by an additional 156,000 compared with implementation of the JNC 8 expert panel guideline goals but these benefits may be accompanied by an increase in the frequency of adverse events. While there was no overall difference in the occurrence of serious adverse events in patients receiving intensive therapy for blood pressure control (SBP target of less than 120 mm Hg) compared with those receiving less intense control (SBP target of less than 140 mm Hg) in the SPRINT study, hypotension, syncope, electrolyte abnormalities, and acute kidney injury or acute renal failure occurred in substantially more patients receiving intensive therapy.

Clinical Benefits of Thiazides in Hypertension

The Antihypertensive and Lipid-Lowering Treatment to Prevent Heart Attack Trial (ALLHAT), which compared the long-term cardiovascular morbidity and mortality benefit of chlorthalidone (a thiazide-like diuretic), amlodipine (a long-acting dihydropyridine calcium-channel blocker), and lisinopril (an ACE inhibitor), supports the clinical benefits of thiazides in the management of hypertension.

ALLHAT provides strong evidence that usual dosages of chlorthalidone, amlodipine, and lisinopril are comparably effective in providing important cardiovascular benefit in a broad population of patients with stage 1 or 2 hypertension at risk for coronary heart disease, but apparent differences in certain secondary outcomes were observed. After a mean follow-up of 4.9 years, an intent-to-treat analysis revealed no difference in the primary outcome of combined fatal coronary heart disease or nonfatal myocardial infarction among the treatments. Compared with chlorthalidone, the relative risks for the primary outcome were 0.98 for amlodipine and 0.99 for lisinopril. In addition, all-cause mortality, a secondary outcome, did not differ among the treatments.

Chlorthalidone was superior to amlodipine (by 25%) in preventing heart failure overall and also for hospitalized or fatal cases, although the drugs were comparably effective in preventing overall cardiovascular disease. Subgroup analysis (age [younger than 65 years vs 65 years or older], race [black vs nonblack], gender, underlying diabetes mellitus status) revealed no subgroup differences in outcomes between amlodipine and chlorthalidone therapy. Unlike some previously reported evidence with short-acting calcium-channel blockers (see Cautions: Precautions and Contraindications, in Diltiazem 24:28.92 and Cautions in Nifedipine 24:28.08), ALLHAT revealed no evidence of excess coronary heart disease associated with long-acting calcium-channel blocker therapy.

Chlorthalidone also was superior to lisinopril in preventing aggregate cardiovascular events, principally stroke, heart failure, angina, and the need for coronary revascularization. Much of the superiority in reducing these events may be attributable to the greater antihypertensive effect of chlorthalidone (i.e., an overall difference of 2–4 mm Hg in SBP) compared with that of lisinopril. In addition, chlorthalidone was better tolerated than lisinopril.

In ALLHAT, an α-blocker (doxazosin) treatment arm was terminated prematurely after an interim analysis indicated that use of doxazosin in high-risk (at least 2 risk factors for coronary heart disease) hypertensive patients 55 years of age and older was associated with a higher risk of stroke and incidence of combined cardiovascular disease events. (See Uses: Hypertension, in Doxazosin 24:20.)

Post hoc analysis of ALLHAT directly comparing cardiovascular and other outcomes in patients receiving amlodipine versus those receiving lisinopril revealed no difference in the primary outcome of combined fatal coronary heart disease or nonfatal MI between patients receiving the ACE inhibitor and those receiving the calcium-channel blocker. However, patients receiving lisinopril were at higher risk for stroke, combined cardiovascular disease, GI bleeding, and angioedema, while those receiving amlodipine were at higher risk of developing heart failure. ALLHAT investigators suggested that the observed differences in cardiovascular outcome may be attributable, at least in part, to the greater antihypertensive effect of amlodipine compared with that of lisinopril, especially in women and black patients.

Subgroup analysis for race-related effects revealed no difference in the primary outcome of combined fatal coronary heart disease or nonfatal MI among the treatments in both black and nonblack patients. However, substantial race-related effects were observed in the incidence of secondary outcomes (e.g., stroke, combined cardiovascular disease events, heart failure). Compared with chlorthalidone, the relative risk for lisinopril was 1.4 or 1 (in black or nonblack patients, respectively) for stroke and 1.19 or 1.06 (in black or nonblack patients, respectively) for combined cardiovascular disease events. When amlodipine was compared with chlorthalidone, the only race-related difference observed was in the incidence of heart failure; the relative risk was 1.46 or 1.32 (in black or nonblack patients, respectively). The relative risk for heart failure in black patients versus nonblack patients receiving lisinopril was not considered to be statistically significant, and the overall relative risk for both groups was 1.19. In addition, after 4 years, in each treatment group, blood pressure reductions were greater in nonblack than in black patients; about 68 or 60% of nonblack or black patients, respectively, achieved a SBP/DBP of less than 140/90 mm Hg. In nonblack patients receiving chlorthalidone, amlodipine, or lisinopril 69, 69, or 67% achieved the mentioned blood pressure, respectively, while in black patients receiving chlorthalidone, amlodipine, or lisinopril 63, 60, or 54% achieved such blood pressure, respectively.

Based on cost and other considerations (e.g., differences in secondary outcomes, differences in patient tolerance), ALLHAT provides compelling evidence that thiazides, in particular the long-acting drug chlorthalidone, should be considered as one of the initial drugs of choice in most patients with hypertension. ALLHAT did not include a first-line β-blocker treatment arm.

General Considerations for Initial and Maintenance Antihypertensive Therapy
Nonpharmacologic Therapy

Nonpharmacologic measures (i.e., lifestyle/behavioral modifications) that are effective in lowering blood pressure include weight reduction (for those who are overweight or obese), dietary changes to include foods such as fruits, vegetables, whole grains, and low-fat dairy products that are rich in potassium, calcium, magnesium, and fiber (i.e., adoption of the Dietary Approaches to Stop Hypertension [DASH] eating plan), sodium reduction, increased physical activity, and moderation of alcohol intake. Such lifestyle/behavioral modifications, including smoking cessation, enhance antihypertensive drug efficacy and decrease cardiovascular risk and remain an indispensable part of the management of hypertension. Lifestyle/behavioral modifications without antihypertensive drug therapy are recommended for individuals classified by the 2017 ACC/AHA hypertension guideline as having elevated blood pressure (SBP 120–129 mm Hg and DBP less than 80 mm Hg) and in those with stage 1 hypertension (SBP 130–139 mm Hg or DBP 80–89 mm Hg) who do *not* have preexisting cardiovascular disease or an estimated 10-year ASCVD risk of 10% or greater.

Initiation of Drug Therapy

Drug therapy in the management of hypertension must be individualized and adjusted based on the degree of blood pressure elevation while also considering cardiovascular risk factors. Drug therapy generally is reserved for patients who respond inadequately to nondrug therapies or in whom the degree of blood pressure elevation or coexisting risk factors, especially increased cardiovascular risk, require more prompt or aggressive therapy; however, the optimum blood pressure threshold for initiating antihypertensive drug therapy and specific treatment goals remain controversial. Recommendations generally are based on specific blood pressure levels shown in clinical studies to produce clinical benefits and can therefore vary depending on the studies selected for review.

The 2017 ACC/AHA hypertension guideline and many experts currently state that the treatment of hypertension should be based not only on blood pressure values but also on patients' cardiovascular risk factors. For *secondary prevention* of recurrent cardiovascular disease events in adults with clinical cardiovascular disease or for *primary prevention* in adults with an estimated 10-year ASCVD risk of 10% or higher, the 2017 ACC/AHA hypertension guideline recommends initiation of antihypertensive drug therapy in conjunction with lifestyle/behavioral modifications at an average SBP of 130 mm Hg or an average DBP of 80 mm Hg or higher. For *primary prevention* of cardiovascular disease events in adults with a low (less than 10%) estimated 10-year risk of ASCVD, the 2017 ACC/AHA hypertension guideline recommends initiation of antihypertensive drug therapy in conjunction with lifestyle/behavioral modifications at an SBP of 140 mm Hg or higher or a DBP of 90 mm Hg or higher. After initiation of antihypertensive drug therapy, regardless of the ASCVD risk, the 2017 ACC/AHA hypertension guideline generally recommends a blood pressure goal of less than 130/80 mm Hg in all adults. In addition, an SBP goal of less than 130 mm Hg also is recommended for non-institutionalized ambulatory patients 65 years of age or older. While these blood pressure goals are lower than those recommended for most patients in previous guidelines, they are based upon clinical studies demonstrating continuing reduction of cardiovascular risk at progressively lower levels of SBP.

Most data indicate that patients with a higher cardiovascular risk will benefit the most from tighter blood pressure control; however, some experts state this treatment goal also may be beneficial in those at lower cardiovascular risk. Other clinicians believe that the benefits of such blood pressure lowering do not outweigh the risks in those patients considered to be at lower risk of cardiovascular disease and that reclassifying individuals formerly considered to have prehypertension as having hypertension may potentially lead to use of drug therapy in such patients without consideration of cardiovascular risk. Previous hypertension guidelines, such as those from the JNC 8 expert panel, generally recommended initiation of antihypertensive treatment in patients with an SBP of at least 140 mm Hg or DBP of at least 90 mm Hg, targeted a blood pressure goal of less than 140/90 mm Hg regardless of cardiovascular risk, and used higher SBP thresholds and targets in geriatric patients. Some clinicians continue to support the target blood pressures recommended by the JNC 8 expert panel because of concerns that such recommendations in the 2017 ACC/AHA hypertension guideline are based on extrapolation of data from the high-risk population in the SPRINT study to a lower-risk population. Also, because more than 90% of patients in SPRINT were already receiving antihypertensive drugs at baseline, data are lacking on the effects of *initiating* drug therapy at a lower blood pressure threshold (130/80 mm Hg) in patients at high risk of cardiovascular disease. The potential benefits of hypertension management and drug cost, adverse effects, and risks associated with the use of multiple antihypertensive drugs should be considered when deciding a patient's blood pressure treatment goal.

The 2017 ACC/AHA hypertension guideline recommends an ASCVD risk assessment for all adults with hypertension; however, experts state that it can be assumed that patients with hypertension and diabetes mellitus or chronic kidney disease (CKD) are at high risk for cardiovascular disease and that antihypertensive drug therapy should be initiated in these patients at a blood pressure of 130/80 mm Hg or higher. The 2017 ACC/AHA hypertension guideline also recommends a blood pressure goal of less than 130/80 mm Hg in patients with hypertension and diabetes mellitus or CKD. These recommendations are based on a systematic review of high-quality evidence from randomized controlled trials, meta-analyses, and post hoc analyses that have demonstrated substantial reductions in the risk of important clinical outcomes (e.g., cardiovascular events) regardless of comorbid conditions or age when SBP is lowered to less than 130 mm Hg. However, some clinicians have questioned the generalizability of findings from some of the trials (e.g., SPRINT) used to support the 2017 ACC/AHA hypertension guideline. For example, SPRINT included adults (mean age: 68 years) *without* diabetes mellitus who were at high risk of cardiovascular disease. While benefits of intensive blood pressure control were observed in this patient population, some clinicians have questioned whether these findings apply to younger patients who have a low risk of cardiovascular disease. In patients with CKD in the SPRINT trial,

intensive blood pressure management (achieving a mean SBP of approximately 122 mm Hg compared with 136 mm Hg with standard treatment) provided a similar beneficial reduction in the composite cardiovascular disease primary outcome and all-cause mortality as in the full patient cohort. Because most patients with CKD die from cardiovascular complications, the findings of this study further support a lower blood pressure target of less than 130/80 mm Hg.

Data are lacking to determine the ideal blood pressure goal in patients with hypertension and diabetes mellitus; also, studies evaluating the benefits of intensive blood pressure control in patients with diabetes mellitus have provided conflicting results. Clinical studies reviewed for the 2017 ACC/AHA hypertension guideline have shown similar quantitative benefits from blood pressure lowering in hypertensive patients with or without diabetes mellitus. In a randomized, controlled study (ACCORD-BP) that compared a higher (SBP less than 140 mm Hg) versus lower (SBP less than 120 mm Hg) blood pressure goal in patients with diabetes mellitus, there was no difference in the incidence of cardiovascular outcomes (e.g., composite outcome of cardiovascular death, nonfatal MI, and nonfatal stroke). However, some experts state that this study was underpowered to detect a difference between the 2 treatment groups and that the factorial design of the study complicated interpretation of the results. Although SPRINT did not include patients with diabetes mellitus, patients in this study with prediabetes demonstrated a similar cardiovascular benefit from intensive treatment of blood pressure as normoglycemic patients. A meta-analysis of data from ACCORD and SPRINT suggests that the findings of both studies are consistent and that patients with diabetes mellitus benefit from more intensive blood pressure control. These data support the 2017 ACC/AHA hypertension guideline recommendation of a blood pressure treatment goal of less than 130/80 mm Hg in patients with hypertension and diabetes mellitus. Alternatively, the American Diabetes Association (ADA) recommends a blood pressure goal of less than 140/90 mm Hg in patients with diabetes mellitus. The ADA states that a lower blood pressure goal (e.g., less than 130/80 mm Hg) may be appropriate for patients with a high risk of cardiovascular disease and diabetes mellitus if it can be achieved without undue treatment burden.

Further study is needed to more clearly define optimum blood pressure goals in patients with hypertension, particularly in high-risk groups (e.g., patients with diabetes mellitus, cardiovascular disease, or cerebrovascular disease; black patients); when determining appropriate blood pressure goals, individual risks and benefits should be considered in addition to the evidence from clinical studies.

Choice of Initial Drug Therapy

In current hypertension management guidelines, thiazide diuretics are recommended as one of several preferred drugs for the initial treatment of hypertension. Results of clinical trials (e.g., ALLHAT) indicate that thiazide diuretics appear to prevent cardiovascular complications associated with hypertension as effectively as ACE inhibitors or calcium-channel blockers and better than β-blockers. (See Clinical Benefits of Thiazides in Hypertension under Hypertension in Adults: Treatment Benefits, in Uses.) These findings, in addition to cost and other considerations, have prompted some experts in the past to recommend thiazides as the initial drugs of choice in most patients with hypertension. ACC/AHA and most experts currently recommend selection of the initial antihypertensive agent from among several preferred drug classes that have been shown to reduce clinical events. The 2017 ACC/AHA hypertension guideline states that a thiazide or thiazide-like diuretic (preferably chlorthalidone), ACE inhibitor, angiotensin II receptor antagonist, or calcium-channel blocker are all acceptable choices for initial antihypertensive drug therapy in the general population of nonblack patients, including those with diabetes mellitus; drugs from any of these classes generally produce similar benefits in terms of overall mortality and cardiovascular, cerebrovascular, and renal outcomes. In black patients, including those with diabetes mellitus, the initial drug choice should include a thiazide diuretic or calcium-channel blocker. Because many patients eventually will need more than one antihypertensive drug to achieve blood pressure control, any of the recommended drug classes may be considered for add-on therapy.

In patients with hypertension and compelling indications (e.g., CKD with albuminuria [urine albumin 300 mg/day or greater, or urine albumin:creatinine ratio of 300 mg/g or equivalent in the first morning void]), angiotensin II receptor antagonists are usually considered an alternative for ACE inhibitor-intolerant patients. (See Chronic Kidney Disease under Hypertension in Adults: Considerations for Drug Therapy in Patients with Underlying Cardiovascular and Other Risk Factors, in Uses.) However, data indicate no difference in efficacy between ACE inhibitors and angiotensin II receptor antagonists with regard to blood pressure lowering and clinical outcomes (i.e., all-cause mortality, cardiovascular mortality, MI, heart failure, stroke, and end-stage renal disease). Adverse events (e.g., cough, angioedema) leading to drug discontinuance occur more frequently with ACE inhibitor therapy than with angiotensin II receptor antagonist therapy. Because of similar efficacy and a lower frequency of adverse effects, some experts believe that angiotensin II receptor antagonists should be used instead of an ACE inhibitor for the treatment of hypertension or hypertension with certain compelling indications.

Most guidelines no longer recommend β-blockers as first-line therapy for hypertension because of the lack of established superiority over other recommended drug classes and evidence from at least one study demonstrating that they may be less effective than angiotensin II receptor antagonists in preventing cardiovascular death, MI, or stroke. However, therapy with a β-blocker may still be considered in some patients with a compelling indication such as ischemic heart disease, history of MI, or heart failure.

Experts state that in patients with stage 1 hypertension (especially the elderly, those with a history of hypotension, or those who have experienced adverse drug effects), it is reasonable to initiate drug therapy using the stepped-care approach in which one drug is initiated and titrated and other drugs are added sequentially to achieve the target blood pressure. Although some patients can begin treatment with a single antihypertensive agent, starting with 2 drugs in different pharmacologic classes (either as separate agents or in a fixed-dose combination) is recommended in patients with stage 2 hypertension and an average blood pressure more than 20/10 mm Hg above their target blood pressure. Such combined therapy may increase the likelihood of achieving goal blood pressure in a more timely fashion, but also may increase the risk of adverse effects (e.g., orthostatic hypotension) in some patients (e.g., elderly). Drug regimens with complementary activity, where a second antihypertensive agent is used to block compensatory responses to the first agent or affect a different pressor mechanism, can result in additive blood pressure lowering and are preferred. Drug combinations that have similar mechanisms of action or clinical effects (e.g., the combination of an ACE inhibitor and an angiotensin II receptor antagonist) generally should be avoided. Many patients who begin therapy with a single antihypertensive agent will subsequently require at least 2 drugs from different pharmacologic classes to achieve their blood pressure goal. Experts state that other patient-specific factors, such as age, concurrent medications, drug adherence, drug interactions, the overall treatment regimen, cost, and comorbidities, also should be considered when deciding on an antihypertensive drug regimen. For any stage of hypertension, antihypertensive drug dosages should be adjusted and/or other agents substituted or added until goal blood pressure is achieved. (See Follow-up and Maintenance Drug Therapy under Hypertension in Adults: General Considerations for Initial and Maintenance Antihypertensive Therapy, in Uses.)

Follow-up and Maintenance Drug Therapy

Several strategies are used for the titration and combination of antihypertensive drugs; these strategies, which are generally based on those used in randomized controlled studies, include maximizing the dosage of the first drug before adding a second drug, adding a second drug before achieving maximum dosage of the initial drug, or initiating therapy with 2 drugs simultaneously (either as separate preparations or as a fixed-dose combination). Combined use of an ACE inhibitor and angiotensin II receptor antagonist should be avoided because of the potential risk of adverse renal effects. After initiating a new or adjusted antihypertensive drug regimen, patients should have their blood pressure reevaluated monthly until adequate blood pressure control is achieved. Effective blood pressure control can be achieved in most hypertensive patients, but many will ultimately require therapy with 2 or more antihypertensive drugs. In addition to measuring blood pressure, clinicians should evaluate patients for orthostatic hypotension, adverse drug effects, adherence to drug therapy and lifestyle modifications, and the need for drug dosage adjustments. Laboratory testing such as electrolytes and renal function status and other assessments of target organ damage also should be performed.

Considerations for Drug Therapy in Patients with Underlying Cardiovascular and Other Risk Factors

Drug therapy in patients with hypertension and underlying cardiovascular or other risk factors should be carefully individualized based on the underlying disease(s), concomitant drugs, tolerance to drug-induced adverse effects, and blood pressure goal.

The following table lists compelling indications for which certain antihypertensive drug classes are recommended. The drug selections recommended for these compelling indications are based on favorable outcome data from clinical trials and existing expert guidelines; the specific drug classes that are included in the table are meant to be considered, but not necessarily all administered at the same time in an individual patient. For additional information on the management of hypertension in patients with compelling indications, individual expert clinical guidelines should be consulted.

TABLE 2. Compelling Indications for Drug Classes based on Comorbid Conditions

Compelling Indication [a]	Recommended Drugs					
	Diuretics	β-Blockers	ACE Inhibitors	Angiotensin II Receptor Antagonists	Calcium-channel Blockers	Aldosterone Antagonists [b]
Heart failure	x	x	x	x		x
Post-MI		x	x	x		x
Ischemic heart disease		x	x	x	x	
Diabetes mellitus [c]			x	x		
Chronic kidney disease [d]			x	x		
Recurrent stroke prevention	x		x	x		

[a] Compelling indications for antihypertensive drugs are based on benefits from outcome studies or existing clinical guidelines; the compelling indication is managed in parallel with hypertension.

[b] e.g., eplerenone, spironolactone

[c] The 2017 ACC/AHA hypertension guideline states that in adults with diabetes mellitus and hypertension who do not have albuminuria, all first-line classes of antihypertensive agents (i.e., thiazide diuretics, ACE inhibitors, angiotensin II receptor antagonists, calcium-channel blockers) are useful and effective; ACE inhibitors (or angiotensin II receptor antagonists if intolerant of ACE inhibitors) are preferred in patients with albuminuria.

[d] The 2017 ACC/AHA hypertension guideline states that adults with hypertension and stage 1 or 2 CKD without albuminuria can be treated with any of the first-line classes of antihypertensive agents (i.e., thiazide diuretics, ACE inhibitors, angiotensin II antagonists, and calcium-channel blockers); use of ACE inhibitor or angiotensin II receptor antagonist may be reasonable in those with hypertension and stage 1 or 2 CKD with albuminuria or stage 3 CKD.

Ischemic Heart Disease

Adequate control of blood pressure in patients with ischemic heart disease substantially reduces cardiovascular morbidity and mortality (e.g., stroke, coronary events, death). The 2017 ACC/AHA hypertension guideline recommends initiating antihypertensive drug therapy in patients with stable ischemic heart disease who have a blood pressure of 130/80 mm Hg or higher; alternatively, other experts recommend initiating antihypertensive drug therapy in patients with coronary artery disease who have a blood pressure of 140/90 mm Hg or higher, including in those with stable ischemic heart disease. The selection of an appropriate antihypertensive agent should be based on individual patient characteristics, but may include ACE inhibitors and/or β-blockers, with the addition of other drugs such as thiazide diuretics or calcium-channel blockers as necessary to achieve blood pressure goals. Many experts recommend the use of ACE inhibitors in hypertensive patients with stable ischemic heart disease because of the cardioprotective benefits of these drugs; angiotensin II receptor antagonists are recommended as an alternative if ACE inhibitors are not tolerated or are contraindicated. Because of the demonstrated mortality benefit of β-blockers following MI, these drugs should be administered in all patients who have survived an MI. Aldosterone receptor antagonists are also recommended to reduce morbidity and mortality following an acute MI in patients with reduced left ventricular ejection fraction (LVEF) (40% or less) who develop symptoms of heart failure or have a history of diabetes mellitus.

Heart Failure

Thiazide diuretics may be considered in hypertensive patients with heart failure and mild fluid retention. ACCF, AHA, and the Heart Failure Society of America (HFSA) also recommend the addition of an aldosterone antagonist (i.e., spironolactone or eplerenone) in selected patients with chronic heart failure and reduced LVEF who are already receiving an agent to inhibit the renin-angiotensin system (e.g., ACE inhibitor, angiotensin II receptor antagonist) and a β-blocker. The 2017 ACC/AHA hypertension guideline states that diuretics should be used to control hypertension in patients with heart failure with preserved ejection fraction who have symptoms of volume overload.

Diabetes Mellitus

The presence of diabetes mellitus increases the risk of coronary events by twofold in men and fourfold in women, and observational studies suggest that the risk of cardiovascular disease is approximately twice as high in hypertensive patients with diabetes mellitus as in nondiabetic hypertensive patients. Epidemiologic data indicate that SBP and DBP exceeding 115 and 75 mm Hg, respectively, are associated with increased cardiovascular event rates and mortality in patients with diabetes mellitus. Data are lacking to determine the ideal blood pressure goal in patients with hypertension and diabetes mellitus. Some randomized clinical studies have shown benefit from lowering SBP to less than 140 mm Hg and DBP to less than 80 mm Hg in patients with diabetes mellitus and hypertension, while other data indicate that lower blood pressure targets (e.g., less than 130/80 mm Hg) provide additional benefits. (See General Considerations for Initial and Maintenance Antihypertensive Therapy under Uses: Hypertension in Adults.) Results of several studies indicate that adequate control of blood pressure in patients with type 2 diabetes mellitus reduces the development or progression of complications of diabetes (e.g., diabetes-related death, stroke, heart failure, microvascular disease).

The ADA recommends lifestyle/behavioral modification in adults with diabetes mellitus who have elevated blood pressure (i.e., higher than 120/80 mm Hg); if blood pressure is higher than 140/90 mm Hg, the ADA recommends prompt initiation of drug therapy in addition to these nondrug interventions. However, other experts recommend initiating drug therapy at a blood pressure of 130/80 mm Hg or higher in addition to nondrug interventions in such patients.

Experts state that initial treatment of hypertension in adults with diabetes mellitus and hypertension should include any of the usual first-line agents (thiazide diuretics, ACE inhibitors, angiotensin II receptor antagonists, calcium-channel blockers). In adults with diabetes mellitus, hypertension, and albuminuria, treatment with an ACE inhibitor or angiotensin II receptor antagonist may be considered to reduce the progression of kidney disease. In the absence of albuminuria, the risk of progressive kidney disease is low, and ACE inhibitors and angiotensin II receptor antagonists have not demonstrated superior cardioprotection when compared with other first-line agents. Most patients with diabetes mellitus will require 2 or more antihypertensive agents to achieve blood pressure control.

Chronic Kidney Disease

Hypertensive patients with CKD (GFR less than 60 mL/minute per 1.73 m² or kidney damage for 3 or more months) usually will require more than one antihypertensive agent to reach target blood pressure. Use of ACE inhibitors or angiotensin II receptor antagonists may be reasonable in patients with diabetic or nondiabetic CKD (stage 1 or 2 with albuminuria or stage 3 or higher); these drugs have been shown to slow the progression of kidney disease. Evidence of a renoprotective benefit is strongest in those with higher levels of albuminuria. Increases in serum creatinine (up to 30%) may be observed as a result of a decrease in intraglomerular pressure and concurrent reduction in GFR. The 2017 ACC/AHA hypertension guideline states that in patients with less severe kidney disease (i.e., stage 1 or 2 CKD without albuminuria), any of the first-line antihypertensive agents (e.g., thiazide diuretics, ACE inhibitors, angiotensin II receptor antagonists, calcium-channel blockers) can be used for the initial treatment of hypertension. Diuretics also may be useful in the management of CKD, and may potentiate the effects of ACE inhibitors, angiotensin II receptor antagonists, and other antihypertensive agents when used in combination. Thiazides are not effective in patients with advanced renal impairment (e.g., GFR less than 30 mL/minute per 1.73 m², serum creatinine 1.5 mg/dL or greater); loop diuretics should be used instead in such patients.

Cerebrovascular Disease

Some experts recommend a blood pressure goal of less than 140/90 mm Hg in patients with ischemic stroke or transient ischemic attack (TIA), while others state that a blood pressure goal of less than 130/80 mm Hg may be reasonable. The 2017 ACC/AHA hypertension guideline states that adults not previously treated for hypertension who experience a stroke or TIA and who have an established blood pressure of 140/90 mm Hg or higher should receive antihypertensive therapy a few days after the event to reduce the risk of recurrent stroke or other vascular events. In patients with a recent lacunar stroke, experts suggest that an SBP goal of 130 mm Hg may be reasonable based on results of a randomized open-label study (the Secondary Prevention of Small Subcortical Strokes [SPS3] trial). Although experts state that the optimal choice of drug for the management of hypertension in patients with a previous TIA or ischemic stroke is uncertain, available data indicate that a thiazide diuretic, ACE inhibitor, angiotensin II receptor antagonist, or the combination of a thiazide diuretic and an ACE inhibitor may be effective. Administration of an ACE inhibitor in combination with a thiazide diuretic has been shown to lower rates of recurrent stroke.

Other Special Considerations for Antihypertensive Drug Therapy

Race

Most patients with hypertension, especially black patients, will require at least 2 antihypertensive drugs to achieve adequate blood pressure control. In general, black hypertensive patients tend to respond better to monotherapy with thiazide diuretics or calcium-channel blockers than to monotherapy with ACE inhibitors, angiotensin II receptor antagonists, or β-blockers. In a prespecified subgroup analysis of the ALLHAT study, a thiazide-like diuretic was more effective than an ACE inhibitor in improving cerebrovascular and cardiovascular outcomes in black patients; when compared with a calcium-channel blocker, the ACE inhibitor was less effective in reducing blood pressure and was associated with a 51% higher rate of stroke. However, the combination of an ACE inhibitor or an angiotensin II receptor antagonist with a calcium-channel blocker or thiazide diuretic produces similar blood pressure lowering in black patients as in other racial groups. In addition, some experts state that when use of ACE inhibitors, angiotensin II receptor antagonists, or β-blockers is indicated in hypertensive patients with underlying cardiovascular or other risk factors, these indications should be applied equally to black hypertensive patients. (See Considerations for Drug Therapy in Patients with Underlying Cardiovascular and Other Risk Factors under Uses: Hypertension in Adults.)

Advanced Age

Antihypertensive drugs recommended for initial therapy in geriatric patients, including those with isolated systolic hypertension, generally are the same as those recommended for younger patients. US guidelines have provided inconsistent recommendations regarding the optimal target SBP in geriatric patients. While some experts have recommended a higher blood pressure threshold for initiating treatment (e.g., 150/90 mm Hg) and a higher target blood pressure (less than 150/90 mm Hg) for older patients, the 2017 ACC/AHA hypertension guideline generally recommends the same blood pressure treatment lowering goal in patients regardless of age. The recommendation of higher blood pressure goals in geriatric patients was based on studies providing moderate to strong evidence that lowering blood pressure to less than 150/90 mm Hg in individuals 60 years of age or older was associated with clinical benefits (i.e., reduction in incidence of stroke, heart failure, and coronary heart disease) and some evidence, albeit less compelling, that an SBP goal of less than 140 mm Hg provided no additional benefit over a higher SBP goal (e.g., 140–160 mm Hg) in this age group. The 2017 ACC/AHA hypertension guideline recommendation that patients 65 years of age and older generally should have the same target SBP goal of younger adults (less than 130 mm Hg) is supported by data from several large, randomized, controlled studies demonstrating that more intensive blood pressure control results in lower rates of cardiovascular disease in patients older than 65, 75, and 80 years of age and does not exacerbate orthostatic hypotension or increase the risk of injurious falls. However, elderly patients should be carefully monitored for orthostatic hypotension while they are receiving antihypertensive drugs, especially when 2 agents are initiated simultaneously. Some experts state that it can be assumed that most adults 65 years of age or older with hypertension have a 10-year ASCVD risk of at least 10%, which places these individuals in the higher-risk category that requires initiation of antihypertensive drugs at an SBP of 130 mm Hg or higher. In geriatric patients with hypertension, multiple comorbidities, and a limited life expectancy, clinical judgment and patient preference should be used to determine the intensity of blood pressure lowering and the choice of antihypertensive drugs.

In several controlled studies, thiazide diuretics alone or in combination with other antihypertensive agents have been shown to reduce morbidity and mortality effectively in patients 50 years of age or older, including those with isolated systolic hypertension. Antihypertensive therapy initiated with a calcium-channel blocker also has been shown to reduce cardiovascular morbidity in older patients with isolated systolic hypertension. Although some experts state that diuretics or calcium-channel blockers may be preferred in geriatric patients, ACE inhibitors and angiotensin II receptor antagonists also have shown beneficial effects and may be considered in this population. Results of a prospective, randomized, open-label study in about 6000 hypertensive patients 65–84 years of age (the Second Australian National Blood Pressure trial) have demonstrated that initiation of therapy with ACE inhibitors may result in slightly better outcomes (concerning cardiovascular events), particularly in men, than those associated with diuretics.

Thiazides may be preferred in patients with osteoporosis. Limited data suggest that thiazide therapy may have a secondary beneficial effect in geriatric patients of reducing the risk of osteoporosis secondary to the drugs' effect on calcium homeostasis and bone mineralization.

Elevated Uric Acid and Gout

Hyperuricemia is common in patients with untreated hypertension and thiazides can increase serum uric acid concentrations. Thiazides generally should be avoided or used with caution in patients with a history of gout unless the patient is on uric acid-lowering therapy. (See Cautions: Electrolyte, Fluid, and Renal Effects.)

● Hypertension in Pediatric Patients

Disease Overview

Clinical studies have shown that elevated blood pressure during childhood increases the risk of adult hypertension and metabolic syndrome. Additionally, children with hypertension are likely to experience accelerated vascular aging. Because the long-term health risks in hypertensive children and adolescents may be substantial, it is important that clinical measures be taken to reduce such risks and optimize health outcomes.

Primary hypertension is now the predominant form of hypertension seen in children and adolescents in the US. The general characteristics of a child with primary hypertension include older age (6 years of age or older), family history of hypertension, and excess body weight (overweight or obese). An extensive evaluation for secondary causes of hypertension is not needed in such patients or in those without physical examination findings suggestive of a secondary cause.

Secondary hypertension is more common in children than in adults. The most common secondary causes of hypertension in children are renal and renovascular diseases. Hypertension secondary to a renal cause should be strongly considered in hypertensive children, particularly in those younger than 6 years of age.

Obesity and other Risk Factors

Pediatric patients with primary hypertension frequently are overweight; the rate of hypertension increases with increasing body mass index (BMI) percentile. In addition, obesity in children with hypertension may be accompanied by other cardiometabolic risk factors (e.g., dyslipidemia, disordered glucose metabolism) that may affect blood pressure. Poor diet, inactivity, and obesity contribute to pediatric hypertension and lipid disorders. Children with other chronic conditions such as sleep-disordered breathing, CKD, and those born preterm also are more likely to have hypertension.

Blood Pressure Classification

The current definition of hypertension in children and adolescents is based on the normative distribution of blood pressure (auscultatory measurements) in healthy, normal-weight children. According to a 2017 clinical practice guideline of the American Academy of Pediatrics (AAP), normal blood pressure in patients 1 to less than 13 years of age is defined as an SBP and DBP that are less than in the 90th percentile for gender, age, and height, and hypertension is defined as an average SBP and/or DBP that is at least in the 95th percentile on at least 3 separate occasions. An ambulatory blood pressure monitor should be used to confirm a diagnosis of hypertension; however, for technical reasons, ambulatory monitoring may need to be limited to those who can tolerate the procedure and those for whom reference data are available. In patients 1 to less than 13 years of age, elevated blood pressure is defined as blood pressure levels that range from the 90th percentile or 120/80 mm Hg (whichever is lower) to less than the 95th percentile, stage 1 hypertension is defined as blood pressure levels that range from the 95th percentile to less than 12 mm Hg above 95th percentile (or 130/80–139/89

mm Hg, whichever is lower), and stage 2 hypertension is defined as blood pressure levels of at least 12 mm Hg above the 95th percentile (or at least 140/90 mm Hg, whichever is lower). For patients 13 years of age or older, hypertension is defined using the same blood pressure values as those recommended by ACC and AHA for adults (see Table 1). Using data from the 2001–2016 National Health and Nutrition Examination Survey (NHANES), the US Centers for Disease Control and Prevention (CDC) has estimated that approximately 800,000 individuals 12–19 years of age would be newly classified as having hypertension according to the 2017 ACC/AHA hypertension guidelines.

Considerations for Initial and Maintenance Antihypertensive Therapy

The overall goals for the treatment of pediatric hypertension include achieving a blood pressure that reduces both the risk of childhood target organ damage and the risk of hypertension and cardiovascular disease in adulthood. Lifestyle/behavioral modifications that include weight reduction (for those who are overweight or obese), dietary changes, and increased physical activity are strongly encouraged in pediatric patients to limit or prevent future or excess increases in blood pressure. Data from clinical studies suggest that the relationship between diet, physical activity, and blood pressure in childhood is similar to that observed in adults.

When a pediatric patient has been diagnosed with hypertension (blood pressure being in the 95th percentile or greater), management decisions should be determined by the degree or severity of hypertension. The treatment goal for most children and adolescents treated with antihypertensive drugs and lifestyle/behavior modifications is a reduction in blood pressure to less than in the 90th percentile or less than 130/80 mm Hg. While previous guidelines have recommended a goal blood pressure less than in the 95th percentile, some evidence suggests that markers of target organ damage can be detected among children with blood pressure greater than in the 90th percentile (or greater than 120/80 mm Hg). Because hypertension is a known risk factor for the progression of CKD, a target 24-hour mean arterial pressure (MAP) less than the 50th percentile by ambulatory blood pressure monitoring is recommended in children and adolescents with hypertension and CKD to reduce the rate of decline in kidney function.

Choice of Initial Drug Therapy

Drug therapy in the management of hypertension must be individualized and adjusted based on the degree of blood pressure elevation and other patient- and drug-related factors. Drug therapy generally is reserved for pediatric patients who inadequately respond to nondrug therapies or in whom the degree of blood pressure elevation or coexisting risk factors require more prompt or aggressive therapy. Some experts recommend antihypertensive drug therapy in all pediatric patients with symptomatic hypertension, those with secondary hypertension without a clearly modifiable factor (e.g., obesity), those with persistent hypertension who fail to respond to lifestyle/behavioral modifications (especially those with an abnormal echocardiogram), and those with diabetes mellitus or CKD.

For initial drug therapy, many experts recommend use of a single antihypertensive drug (e.g., an ACE inhibitor, an angiotensin II receptor antagonist, a long-acting calcium-channel blocker, a thiazide diuretic) given at the low end of the dosing range. Because black patients may not have a robust response to an ACE inhibitor, a higher initial dosage of an ACE inhibitor may be considered in such patients; alternatively, therapy may be initiated with a thiazide diuretic or long-acting calcium-channel blocker. Clinical studies comparing the effectiveness of different antihypertensive agents in children are lacking; however, a few studies have demonstrated no clinically important differences in the degree of blood pressure lowering among drugs. It is recommended that hypertensive pediatric patients with underlying or concurrent medical conditions receive specific classes of hypotensive agents (e.g., use of ACE inhibitors or angiotensin II receptor antagonists in children with diabetes, proteinuria, or CKD). For further information on drug therapy in patients with underlying or concurrent medical conditions, see Considerations for Drug Therapy in Patients with Underlying Cardiovascular and Other Risk Factors under Uses: Hypertension in Adults.

For additional information on the management of hypertension in children, the AAP Clinical Practice Guideline for Screening and Management of High Blood Pressure in Children and Adolescents may be consulted at https://www.aap.org.

Follow-up and Maintenance Drug Therapy

In pediatric patients who fail to respond adequately to initial therapy with a single drug (i.e., a thiazide diuretic, an ACE inhibitor, an angiotensin II receptor antagonist, a long-acting calcium-channel blocker), dosage of the initial drug therapy may be increased every 2–4 weeks until the desired blood pressure goal is achieved or the maximum recommended dosage is attained or tolerated; an antihypertensive agent from another class (preferably an agent having complementary mechanism of action with the initial drug) may then be added.

Although the dosage of antihypertensive drugs may be increased every 2–4 weeks based on home blood pressure measurements, the patient should be evaluated every 4–6 weeks by a clinician until blood pressure has normalized. After the patient's blood pressure is at goal, the patient may be evaluated less frequently (i.e., every 3–4 months). Pediatric hypertensive patients also should be periodically monitored for target organ damage and adverse effects while emphasizing nonpharmacologic measures and the importance of drug therapy adherence.

● Diabetes Insipidus

Thiazides have been widely used in the treatment of diabetes insipidus†. The drugs are effective in both the neurohypophyseal and nephrogenic forms of the disease, decreasing urine volume by up to 50%. Thiazides are particularly useful in nephrogenic diabetes insipidus, since this form of the disease is unresponsive to vasopressin or lypressin and chlorpropamide. Thiazides are also useful in patients who are allergic or refractory to vasopressin or lypressin and have been used in combination with one of these hormones and a low-salt diet in patients who excrete an exceptionally large volume of urine.

● Other Uses

Thiazide diuretics have been used with success in the prophylaxis of renal calculus formation associated with hypercalciuria† and in the treatment of the electrolyte disturbances associated with renal tubular acidosis†.

DOSAGE AND ADMINISTRATION

● Administration

Thiazides are administered orally. Chlorothiazide sodium is administered IV; however, the IV route should be reserved for emergency situations or when patients are unable to take the drug orally.

● Dosage

Dosage of the thiazides should be adjusted according to the patient's requirements and response. The response of the patient depends on factors such as the nature and degree of the disease, state of hydration, cardiac output, physical activity, diet, and concurrent administration of other drugs. Therapy should be adjusted to attain the maximum therapeutic effect at minimum dosage. Dosage among the individual thiazides varies greatly; however, the maximum diuretic response is approximately equal with all agents.

Maintenance therapy with thiazides may be intermittent, such as administration of the drug on alternate days or once daily 3–5 days a week to minimize electrolyte imbalances. In hypertensive patients, however, a decrease in hypotensive effect often occurs during intermittent therapy, except when agents with a very long duration of action (e.g., chlorthalidone, a thiazide-like diuretic) are used. If the response is reduced when intermittent therapy is instituted, the drug should be given more frequently and alternate measures should be used to minimize electrolyte disturbances.

Edema

In the management of severe edema, a large thiazide dosage may be administered until fluid retention is resolved, then a lower maintenance dosage may be instituted. Large initial dosages generally are not necessary in other conditions.

For the management of fluid retention (e.g., edema) associated with heart failure, experts state that diuretics should be administered at a dosage sufficient to achieve optimal volume status and relieve congestion without inducing an excessively rapid reduction in intravascular volume, which could result in hypotension, renal dysfunction, or both.

Hypertension

Chlorthalidone dosages of 12.5–25 mg once daily or hydrochlorothiazide dosages of 25–50 mg once daily have been shown to provide optimal benefit in patients with hypertension; the effectiveness of lower dosages is unknown or has been shown to be less effective in clinical studies. The usual dosages of other thiazide or thiazide-like diuretics for the treatment of hypertension include indapamide 1.25–2.5 mg once daily and metolazone 2.5–5 mg once daily.

The patient's renal function and electrolytes should be assessed 2–4 weeks after initiation of diuretic therapy. Blood pressure should be monitored regularly

(i.e., monthly) during therapy and dosage of the antihypertensive drug adjusted until blood pressure is controlled. If an adequate blood pressure response is not achieved with thiazide monotherapy, the dosage may be increased or another antihypertensive agent with demonstrated benefit (e.g., angiotensin-converting enzyme [ACE] inhibitor, angiotensin II receptor antagonist, calcium-channel blocking agent) and preferably with a complementary mechanism of action may be added; if target blood pressure is still not achieved, a third drug may be added. (See Uses: Hypertension in Adults.) In patients who develop unacceptable adverse effects with a thiazide, the drug should be discontinued and another antihypertensive agent from a different pharmacologic class should be initiated.

Blood Pressure Monitoring and Treatment Goals

Blood pressure monitoring using an out-of-office (home [self-monitored]) or ambulatory method (using a device that measures blood pressure over a 24-hour period) as an adjunct to in-office monitoring generally is recommended to provide a more reliable assessment of blood pressure; studies suggest that out-of-office blood pressure may be a better predictor of hypertension-induced organ damage and cardiovascular risk than office blood pressure. Periodic determination of blood pressure in both the morning and evening (before taking the morning or evening dose) is useful in monitoring daytime control and ensuring that the surge in blood pressure that occurs with arising has been modulated adequately. Occasionally, particularly in geriatric patients and those with orthostatic symptoms, monitoring should include blood pressure determinations in both the seated position and, to recognize possible postural hypotension, after standing quietly for 2–5 minutes.

Once antihypertensive drug therapy has been initiated, dosage generally is adjusted at approximately monthly intervals if blood pressure control is inadequate at a given dosage; additional drugs may need to be added to an antihypertensive drug regimen to achieve adequate blood pressure control. Once blood pressure has been stabilized, follow-up visits generally can be scheduled at 3- to 6-month intervals, depending on patient status.

The goal of hypertension management and prevention is to achieve and maintain optimal control of blood pressure. However, the optimum blood pressure threshold for initiating antihypertensive drug therapy and specific treatment goals remain controversial. While other hypertension guidelines have based target blood pressure goals on age and comorbidities, the 2017 ACC/AHA hypertension guideline incorporates underlying cardiovascular risk into decision making regarding treatment and generally recommends the same target blood pressure (i.e., less than 130/80 mm Hg) for all adults. Many patients will require at least 2 drugs from different pharmacologic classes to achieve this blood pressure goal; the potential benefits of hypertension management and drug cost, adverse effects, and risks associated with the use of multiple antihypertensive drugs also should be considered when deciding a patient's blood pressure treatment goal. (See General Considerations for Initial and Maintenance Antihypertensive Therapy under Uses: Hypertension in Adults.)

In children with hypertension with or without diabetes mellitus, blood pressure should be reduced to less than the corresponding age-adjusted 90th percentile value and to less than 130/80 mm Hg in adolescents at least 13 years of age. In children and adolescents with hypertension and CKD, the 24-hour mean arterial pressure (MAP) as determined by ambulatory blood pressure monitoring should be decreased to a value less than the 50th percentile.

Long-term Regimen Adjustments

A reduction in the dosage or number of antihypertensive drugs in the regimen may be possible in some patients after hypertension has been controlled effectively for an extended period. Such step-down therapy is more often successful in patients who are making lifestyle modifications. The reduction should be gradual and accompanied by frequent monitoring, since blood pressure often rises again to hypertensive levels.

Combination Therapy

When combination therapy is required in the management of hypertension, dosage of each agent can be adjusted first by administering each drug separately. If it is determined that the optimum maintenance dosage of both drugs corresponds to the ratio in a commercial combination preparation, a fixed combination may be used. Alternatively, therapy can be initiated with a fixed combination of 2 antihypertensive agents. Use of fixed-combination preparations may result in increased patient compliance. However, fixed-combination preparations containing 3 different antihypertensive agents may contain a thiazide diuretic dosage that is lower than recommended for the treatment of hypertension.

Whenever dosage adjustment is necessary, the drugs then can be administered separately again or increased with certain fixed combinations according to the manufacturer's recommendations. Initiating therapy and adjusting dosage with separate administration of each drug are particularly important with combination preparations containing antihypertensive agents that have wide ranges in their effective dosages and may require frequent dosage alterations (e.g., methyldopa, guanethidine).

For information on commercially available preparations containing hydrochlorothiazide in fixed combination with a potassium-sparing diuretic, see the individual monographs in 40:28.10.

● *Dosage in Renal Impairment*

For information on dosage of thiazide and thiazide-like diuretics in patient with renal impairment, see the individual monographs in 40:28.10.

CAUTIONS

Adverse effects associated with some thiazides (e.g., hydrochlorothiazide) may be dose-related.

● *Electrolyte, Fluid, and Renal Effects*

One of the most common adverse effects of the thiazides is potassium depletion which occurs in most patients. Potassium depletion may cause cardiac arrhythmias and is particularly important in patients receiving cardiac glycosides because hypokalemia potentiates the cardiac toxicity (e.g., increased ventricular irritability) of these agents. Potassium concentrations may be especially low in patients with primary or secondary aldosteronism, in patients with a low potassium intake, in those receiving other potassium-depleting drugs, and in patients with other losses of potassium, as in vomiting and diarrhea. Intermittent rather than continuous administration of the thiazides and/or ingestion of potassium-rich foods may reduce or prevent potassium depletion; however, prophylactic administration of a potassium supplement such as potassium chloride solution or a potassium-sparing diuretic may be necessary in patients whose serum potassium concentration is less than about 3 mEq/L. Enteric-coated potassium-containing tablets should not be used because of the possibility of GI ulceration.

Rarely, sudden death from cardiac arrest has been associated with thiazide monotherapy, and this effect may be dose related. Since the risk of sudden cardiac death with thiazide therapy appears to be reduced by the addition of a potassium-sparing diuretic, it has been suggested that changes in serum concentrations of potassium or magnesium may contribute to the risk of sudden cardiac death; however, possible reductions in thiazide dosage that may have accompanied the addition of a potassium-sparing diuretic also may have contributed to the risk reduction with combined therapy.

Hypochloremic alkalosis may occur with hypokalemia, especially in patients with other losses of potassium and chloride such as those with vomiting, diarrhea, GI drainage, excessive sweating, paracentesis, or potassium-losing renal diseases. Patients with hepatic cirrhosis who are receiving thiazides are also very susceptible to hypokalemic hypochloremic alkalosis with the thiazides. Blood ammonia concentrations may be further increased in patients with previously elevated concentrations. The diuretic may induce hepatic encephalopathy secondary to electrolyte imbalances.

Dilutional hyponatremia may occasionally occur or be aggravated during thiazide therapy and can be life-threatening. Such hyponatremia usually develops insidiously during chronic therapy and is asymptomatic and of modest degree, and in such cases, serum sodium concentrations return rapidly to within the normal range following withdrawal of the diuretic, water restriction, and potassium and/or magnesium supplementation. However, severe hyponatremia (serum sodium concentration less than 120 mEq/L) can occur rarely. Dilutional hyponatremia most commonly occurs in hot weather in patients with chronic heart failure or hepatic disease, is usually present before diuretic therapy, and is manifested by signs of edema associated with hyponatremia. Geriatric patients, especially females who are underweight, have poor oral intake of fluid and electrolytes, and/ or excessive intake of low-sodium nutritional supplements, may be at increased risk of dilutional hyponatremia induced by the drugs. Dilutional hyponatremia usually is treated by restriction of fluid intake to about 500 mL per day and withdrawal of the diuretic. Sodium chloride should not be administered unless the hyponatremia is life threatening. If sodium chloride is administered to correct severe, symptomatic hyponatremia, care should be taken to avoid early overcorrection to normonatremia or hypernatremia since resultant rapid osmolar changes may be associated with the development of central pontine myelinolysis.

Therefore, although prognosis appears to depend on rapid correction of severe hyponatremia during the first 1 or 2 days, such correction initially should only be to a state of mild hyponatremia; it is recommended that serum sodium concentration be corrected by no more than 20 mEq/L during the first 24 hours. Avoidance of hypernatremia during subsequent days also is important. Patients with severe, symptomatic hyponatremia generally should be managed in an intensive care facility with frequent monitoring of fluid and electrolyte balance.

Hypercalcemia may also occur infrequently in patients receiving thiazides, especially in patients receiving vitamin D or having mild hyperparathyroidism. Hypomagnesemia may also occur.

Hyperuricemia occurs in many patients receiving a thiazide or related diuretic. Hyperuricemia is usually asymptomatic and rarely leads to clinical gout except in patients with a history of gout, familial predisposition to gout, or chronic renal failure. If therapy is required, hyperuricemia and gout may be treated with a uricosuric agent.

Impairment of renal function, interstitial nephritis (which may be allergic), and reversible renal failure have been reported mainly in patients with preexisting renal disease (proliferative glomerulonephritis or nephrotic syndrome) who were receiving thiazides; however, a direct causative relationship has not been demonstrated.

● *Metabolic and Endocrine Effects*

Pathologic changes in the parathyroid gland with hypercalcemia and hypophosphatemia have occurred occasionally during prolonged thiazide therapy. (See Cautions: Precautions and Contraindications.) Common complications of hyperparathyroidism such as nephrolithiasis, bone resorption, and peptic ulceration have not been reported.

Thiazides and related diuretics can produce hyperglycemia and glycosuria in diabetics. Insulin or oral antidiabetic agent requirements of diabetics may be altered by the thiazides and, in addition, diabetes mellitus has been precipitated in prediabetic patients receiving thiazides. However, results of a large, prospective, cohort study found that the increased risk of developing type 2 diabetes mellitus in patients receiving antihypertensive drug therapy (e.g., thiazide diuretics) appears to be related to the presence of hypertension. In this study, development of type 2 diabetes mellitus was shown to be almost 2.5 times more likely in hypertensive patients than in normotensive patients. In addition, once the study investigators accounted for the presence of hypertension, the risk of developing diabetes mellitus among hypertensive patients receiving thiazide diuretics was shown to be no greater than that among those receiving no drug therapy. Abnormal glucose tolerance usually does not develop in patients receiving thiazides who previously exhibited normal glucose tolerance. Hyperglycemia and impairment of glucose tolerance are almost always reversible by discontinuance of the drugs, and correction of hypokalemia may improve glucose tolerance.

Thiazides and related diuretics can slightly increase serum total cholesterol concentrations; increases in the low-density lipoprotein cholesterol and/or very low-density lipoprotein cholesterol subfractions appear to be principally responsible for these increases. The effect of these diuretics on high-density lipoprotein cholesterol concentrations has not been fully elucidated but appears to be variable. Increases in serum triglyceride concentrations also can occur in thiazide-treated patients. Whether changes in serum lipid and lipoprotein concentrations are dose-related and whether such changes persist during long-term diuretic therapy has not been established. In addition, the clinical importance of these effects is not known and further evaluation is needed. The diuretic-induced increase in serum cholesterol concentration can generally be counteracted by concomitant use of a diet low in saturated fat and cholesterol.

● *Uncommon Adverse Effects*

Adverse effects of thiazides other than electrolyte and metabolic disturbances are rare.

Dermatologic and Sensitivity Reactions

Dermatologic reactions are uncommon with thiazides but purpura, photosensitivity, rash, alopecia, urticaria, erythema multiforme including Stevens-Johnson syndrome, exfoliative dermatitis including toxic epidermal necrolysis, and polyarteritis nodosa may occur. Cross-photosensitivity has been reported in a patient who received quinethazone after previously having photosensitivity reactions with 2 thiazides. Allergic reactions are most likely to occur in patients with a history of allergy or bronchial asthma, and the possibility of exacerbation or activation of systemic lupus erythematosus has been reported.

Most information reporting cross-reactivity among sulfonamide derivatives is based on case reports. The mechanism of sulfonamide sensitivity is poorly understood, and the contribution of allergens, haptens, and/or other immune mechanisms remains to be established. Although there is an association between hypersensitivity to sulfonamide anti-infectives and subsequent sensitivity reactions to non-anti-infective sulfonamides such as thiazides and thiazide manufacturers state that use of the diuretics is contraindicated in patients who are allergic to any sulfonamide derivative, this association appears to result from a predisposition to allergic reactions in general rather than to cross-reactivity to the sulfa moiety per se. In fact, a retrospective cohort study using the UK General Practice Research Database found that the risk of associated allergic reactions in sulfonamide anti-infective-sensitive patients was even greater following exposure to penicillins than following exposure to non-anti-infective sulfonamides such as thiazides. In addition, the risk of an allergic reaction following administration of a non-anti-infective sulfonamide (e.g., thiazides, sulfonylurea antidiabetic agents, furosemide, dapsone, probenecid) was lower in patients with a history of sensitivity to sulfonamide anti-infectives than in those with a history of penicillin sensitivity. There also is other evidence, including a pooled analysis of data from clinical trials with celecoxib (an arylsulfonamide) and a cohort study of the risk of cross-sensitivity between co-trimoxazole and dapsone (a sulfone), to support the apparent lack of chemical cross-reactivity among sulfa derivatives. Therefore, based on current evidence from cohort studies and pooled analyses, some researchers suggest that clinicians should understand that patients with a history of any allergic reaction to sulfonamides or penicillins may be at increased risk for reactions to other drugs in general, and a history of sensitivity to sulfonamide anti-infectives should not be considered an absolute contraindication to subsequent use of non-anti-infective sulfonamides.

Cardiovascular Effects

Orthostatic hypotension may occur rarely, and hypotensive episodes have occurred during surgery in patients receiving thiazides. The hypotensive effect of the drugs may be enhanced in postsympathectomy patients. Transient cerebral ischemic attacks related to thiazide-induced hypotension have been reported.

GI Effects

GI adverse effects reported with the thiazides include anorexia, gastric irritation, nausea, vomiting, sialadenitis, cramping, diarrhea, constipation, intrahepatic cholestatic jaundice, and pancreatitis.

CNS Effects

CNS reactions associated with thiazides include dizziness, vertigo, paresthesia, headache, and xanthopsia.

Hematologic Effects

Infrequently, hematologic reactions including leukopenia, hemolytic anemia, thrombocytopenic purpura, agranulocytosis, and aplastic anemia have been reported with some of the thiazides.

Other Adverse Effects

Muscle spasms, impotence, renal failure, renal dysfunction, interstitial nephritis, weakness, restlessness, transient blurred vision, fever, respiratory distress, necrotizing angiitis (vasculitis and cutaneous vasculitis), and anaphylactic reactions have also been reported with thiazides.

Rarely, pulmonary edema and allergic pneumonitis have been reported with hydrochlorothiazide. Hematuria has been reported in at least one patient receiving IV chlorothiazide.

● Precautions and Contraindications

Electrolyte disturbances may occur during thiazide therapy, and patients should be observed for signs of electrolyte imbalance such as dryness of mouth, thirst, weakness, lethargy, drowsiness, restlessness, confusion, seizures, oliguria, or muscle pains or cramps, muscular fatigue, hypotension, tachycardia, or GI disturbances such as nausea and vomiting. Periodic determination of serum electrolyte concentrations (particularly potassium, sodium, chloride, and bicarbonate) should be performed and measures to maintain normal serum concentrations should be instituted if necessary. Serum and urinary electrolyte measurements are especially important in diabetic patients and in patients who are vomiting,

have diarrhea, are receiving parenteral fluids, or are expected to undergo excessive diuresis. It has been recommended that electrolytes be measured weekly or more frequently early in the course of therapy. Once the electrolyte response has stabilized, it may be possible to extend the interval between electrolyte determinations to 3 months or longer.

Thiazides should be used with caution in patients with severe renal disease because the drugs decrease the glomerular filtration rate (GFR) and may precipitate azotemia. The effects of thiazides may be cumulative in patients with impaired renal function. If progressive renal impairment becomes evident as indicated by rising nonprotein nitrogen, BUN, or serum creatinine concentrations, careful reappraisal of therapy is necessary with consideration given to interrupting or discontinuing thiazide therapy. The drugs should also be used with caution in patients with impaired hepatic function or progressive liver disease, particularly when potassium deficiency exists, because they may precipitate hepatic coma as a result of alterations in electrolyte balance. Thiazides should be discontinued immediately if signs of impending hepatic coma appear.

Thiazides are contraindicated in patients with anuria and in those who are allergic to any of the thiazides. The manufacturers state that thiazides are contraindicated in patients who are allergic to other sulfonamide derivatives. However, there currently is limited evidence to support this latter contraindication, and some suggest that a history of sensitivity to sulfonamide anti-infectives ("sulfa sensitivity") should not be considered an absolute contraindication to non-anti-infective sulfonamides such as thiazides. (See Uncommon Adverse Effects: Dermatologic and Sensitivity Reactions, in Cautions.)

● Pregnancy, Fertility, and Lactation

Pregnancy

The routine use of thiazides is contraindicated in pregnant women with mild edema who are otherwise healthy. Thiazides cross the placenta and appear in cord blood. Thrombocytopenia has been reported in newborn infants of women receiving thiazides; however, this appears to be an unpredictable idiosyncratic reaction. Amniotic fluid concentrations of uric acid and creatinine are elevated in women receiving thiazides near term. Jaundice may also occur in the fetus or neonate. These risks and the possibility that other effects of the thiazides may occur in the fetus or neonate must be weighed against the potential benefits of therapy.

Although some evidence suggests that thiazide use during pregnancy may be associated with an increased risk of fetal abnormalities, other data do not support such an association. Some experts have considered thiazide diuretics to be contraindicated during pregnancy, except in patients with heart disease or chronic hypertension, because of the theoretical fetal risk associated with plasma volume reduction. The American College of Obstetricians and Gynecologists (ACOG) states that thiazide diuretics may be used as second-line antihypertensive agents and may be particularly useful in women who are sodium sensitive. The goal of antihypertensive treatment in pregnant women with hypertension is to minimize the acute complications of maternal hypertension while avoiding therapy that could compromise fetal well-being. Antihypertensive therapy is recommended in pregnant women with chronic hypertension who have persistent, severely elevated blood pressure (e.g., systolic blood pressure [SBP] of 160 mm Hg or higher or diastolic blood pressure [DBP] of 105 mm Hg or higher); it is less clear whether antihypertensive therapy should be initiated in women with mild to moderate chronic hypertension. If initiation of antihypertensive therapy is necessary in a pregnant woman, use of labetalol, nifedipine, or methyldopa is recommended. Angiotensin-converting enzyme (ACE) inhibitors, angiotensin II receptor antagonists, and aldosterone antagonists should not be used in pregnant women. In women who are already receiving antihypertensive therapy prior to pregnancy, ACOG states there are insufficient data to make recommendations regarding the continuance or discontinuance of such therapy; treatment decisions should be individualized in these situations. Thiazide diuretics are not recommended for the prevention or management of gestational hypertension or preeclampsia.

Lactation

Thiazides are distributed into the milk of nursing women in low concentrations; however, the drug is considered to be compatible with breastfeeding. The potential for idiosyncratic or allergic reactions in the infant should be considered, however, and some manufacturers state that women receiving thiazides should not nurse their infants.

DRUG INTERACTIONS

● *Drugs Affected by or Causing Potassium Depletion*

In patients receiving digitalis glycosides, electrolyte disturbances produced by the thiazides (principally hypokalemia, but also hypomagnesemia and hypercalcemia) predispose the patient to digitalis toxicity. Periodic electrolyte determinations should be performed in patients receiving a thiazide and a digitalis glycoside, and correction of hypokalemia should be undertaken if warranted. (See Cautions: Electrolyte, Fluid, and Renal Effects.)

It has been stated that the thiazides and related diuretics may cause prolonged neuromuscular blockade in patients receiving nondepolarizing neuromuscular blocking agents, such as tubocurarine chloride or gallamine triethiodide (no longer commercially available in the US), presumably because of potassium depletion. Actual case reports are lacking, however.

Some drugs such as corticosteroids, corticotropin, and amphotericin B also cause potassium loss, and severe potassium depletion may occur when one of these drugs is administered during thiazide therapy.

● *Lithium*

Thiazides, sometimes used in combination with lithium to reduce lithium-induced polyuria, will reduce renal lithium clearance within several days. The reduced lithium clearance has resulted in increased serum lithium concentrations and several cases of lithium intoxication. When thiazide diuretics are used to treat lithium-induced polyuria, most clinicians recommend reducing lithium dosage by about 50% and carefully monitoring serum lithium concentrations. Thiazides and lithium should generally not be used concomitantly because of the increased risk of lithium toxicity.

● *Antidiabetic Agents*

The hyperglycemic effect of the thiazides may exacerbate diabetes mellitus, resulting in increased requirements of insulin or sulfonylurea antidiabetic agents, temporary loss of diabetic control, or secondary failure to the antidiabetic agent.

● *Hypotensive Agents*

The hypotensive effects of most other hypotensive agents are increased by the thiazide diuretics. This effect is usually used to therapeutic advantage in antihypertensive therapy, but severe postural hypotension may result if a thiazide is added to the regimen of a patient stabilized on a potent hypotensive agent such as guanethidine sulfate, methyldopa, or a ganglionic blocking agent. The hyperglycemic, hypotensive, and hyperuricemic effects of diazoxide may be potentiated by the thiazide diuretics. Caution should be used in administering the thiazides with diazoxide.

● *Probenecid*

Probenecid blocks thiazide-induced uric acid retention when administered concomitantly with the thiazides. It appears that probenecid enhances excretion of calcium, magnesium, and citrate during thiazide therapy, but urinary calcium concentrations remain below normal. The excretion of sodium, potassium, ammonia, chloride, bicarbonate, phosphate, and titratable acid during thiazide therapy do not seem to be affected by concomitant probenecid therapy. Probenecid also blocks the renal tubular secretion of the thiazides, but its effect on the duration of action of the thiazides has apparently not been studied.

● *Nonsteroidal Anti-inflammatory Agents*

Diuretics may increase the risk of nonsteroidal anti-inflammatory agent (NSAIA)-induced renal failure. Such NSAIA-induced renal failure appears to be secondary to decreased renal blood flow resulting from prostaglandin inhibition by the drugs. In addition, NSAIAs may interfere with the natriuretic, diuretic, and antihypertensive response to diuretics. Therefore, patients receiving the drugs concomitantly should be observed closely for possible adverse effects and/or attenuation of diuretic-induced therapeutic effects.

● *Other Drugs*

Since the pH of the urine becomes slightly more alkaline during thiazide therapy, the urinary excretion of some amines such as amphetamine and quinidine may be decreased somewhat when given concurrently with the thiazides; however, since the change in urine pH is not great during thiazide therapy, toxic blood concentrations of these drugs usually do not occur. Patients receiving amines (e.g., amphetamine, quinidine) should be monitored for signs of toxicity following initiation of thiazide therapy. Urinary alkalinization may decrease the effectiveness of methenamine compounds which require a urinary pH of 5.5 or less for optimal activity. The pH of the urine should be monitored during concurrent therapy with a thiazide and a methenamine compound.

Alcohol, barbiturates, and opiates are reported to increase the postural hypotensive effect of the thiazides.

It has been proposed that the thiazides may antagonize the effects of oral anticoagulants; however, studies which demonstrate this effect are lacking.

Cholestyramine or colestipol resin may bind thiazides and reduce their absorption from the GI tract, with cholestyramine reportedly producing greater binding in vitro. Thiazides should be administered at least 2 hours before cholestyramine or colestipol when these drugs are used concomitantly.

A decrease in arterial responsiveness to vasopressors has been reported during thiazide therapy; however, the clinical importance of this interaction has not been established.

LABORATORY TEST INTERFERENCES

In addition to alterations in laboratory test values resulting from the metabolic changes caused by the thiazides, the drugs may affect the results of a number of other tests. Thiazides may cause false-negative results in both the tyramine and phentolamine tests and probably the histamine test for pheochromocytoma. Protein-bound iodine values may be decreased during thiazide therapy, although usually not to subnormal levels. Triiodothyronine resin uptake may be decreased slightly, but the 24-hour I 131 uptake is not affected. Thyroid function is not affected by the thiazides.

Since thiazides may cause elevations in serum calcium in the absence of known disorders of calcium metabolism, the drugs should be discontinued prior to performing tests of parathyroid function.

It has been reported that hydrochlorothiazide causes falsely decreased values in the spectrophotometric assay of total urinary estrogen by interfering with formation of the Kober chromogen, and with the assay of estriol by degrading estriol at the acid hydrolytic stage of the assay. These interferences apparently do not occur with chlorothiazide.

Serum amylase values may be increased substantially in both asymptomatic patients and in patients developing acute pancreatitis who are receiving thiazides. Thiazides have been reported to decrease urinary corticosteroid values by interfering in vitro with the absorbance in the modified Glenn-Nelson technique for urinary 17-hydroxycorticosteroids. The drugs may also decrease urinary excretion of cortisol. The importance of the effect of thiazides on urinary corticosteroids is not clear.

Thiazides compete with phenolsulfonphthalein (PSP) for secretion by the proximal renal tubules, but the importance of this effect on PSP excretion is unknown.

ACUTE TOXICITY

● *Manifestations*

In addition to diuresis and resultant dehydration, overdosage of thiazides may produce lethargy, nausea, weakness, and electrolyte imbalance; lethargy may progress to coma within a few hours with minimal depression of respiratory and cardiovascular function and without evidence of dehydration or serum electrolyte changes. The mechanism of thiazide-induced CNS depression is unknown. GI irritation and hypermotility may occur, and temporary elevation of the BUN has been reported. Serum electrolyte changes (e.g., hypokalemia, hypochloremia, hyponatremia) may occur, especially in patients with impaired renal function.

● *Treatment*

In the treatment of thiazide overdosage, gastric contents may be evacuated taking caution to avoid aspiration, especially in unconscious patients. If the patient is conscious, induction of vomiting with ipecac syrup is effective in removing the drug from the stomach. Cathartics should *not* be administered because they tend to promote loss of fluid and electrolytes. Treatment is generally supportive. Serum electrolytes and renal function should be monitored, and replacement of fluid and electrolytes may be indicated. Measures may be required to maintain respiratory, cardiovascular, and renal function. GI irritation is usually of short duration, but may be treated symptomatically.

PHARMACOLOGY

Thiazides and related diuretics enhance excretion of sodium, chloride, and water by interfering with the transport of sodium ions across the renal tubular epithelium. Their primary site of action appears to be the cortical diluting segment of the nephron. The exact mechanism of action of the thiazides is unclear; however, they may act by altering metabolism of the tubular cells.

Thiazides decrease the glomerular filtration rate (GFR), but whether this results from a direct effect on renal vasculature or is secondary to the decrease in intravascular fluid volume or an increase in tubular pressure caused by the inhibition of sodium and water reabsorption is unclear. The fall in GFR is not important in the mechanism of action of the drugs, but contributes to their decreased efficacy in patients with impaired renal function. Thiazides also exhibit a carbonic anhydrase inhibiting effect which varies considerably among the various agents.

In addition to increasing sodium and chloride excretion, thiazides affect excretion of other electrolytes. Potassium excretion is substantially increased because of the increased amount of sodium reaching the distal tubular site of sodium-potassium exchange. The ratio of potassium to sodium excreted may vary among the thiazides and related diuretics and at different dosages of the drugs; however, the differences in excretion are generally clinically insignificant. Long-term thiazide therapy can cause mild metabolic alkalosis associated with hypokalemia and hypochloremia.

Thiazides increase bicarbonate excretion (although to a lesser extent than chloride excretion) but change in urinary pH is usually minimal. The diuretic efficacy of the thiazides is not affected by the acid-base balance of the patient. Magnesium, phosphate, bromide, and iodide excretion are also increased. Excretion of ammonia may decrease slightly, and blood ammonia concentrations may be increased. Urinary calcium excretion may increase transiently when therapy is initiated; however, during long-term administration, it is substantially decreased. The hypocalciuric effect is thought to result from a decrease in extracellular fluid (ECF) volume, although calcium reabsorption in the nephron may be increased. Thiazides also have been reported to cause slight or intermittent elevations in serum calcium concentration. The rate of excretion of uric acid is decreased, probably because of competitive inhibition of uric acid secretion or a decrease in ECF volume and a secondary increase in uric acid reabsorption. Lithium excretion may also be decreased.

Thiazides have hypotensive activity in hypertensive patients, and they augment the action of other hypotensive agents. The precise mechanism of hypotensive action has not been determined, but it has been postulated that part of this effect is caused by direct arteriolar dilation. Initially, thiazides cause appreciable decreases in ECF volume, plasma volume, and cardiac output which may account for the decrease in blood pressure. After several weeks of therapy, however, plasma and ECF volumes approach, but remain slightly below, normal. Cardiac output returns to normal or slightly above, and peripheral vascular resistance remains decreased. Total body sodium also remains slightly below pretreatment values, which may be due to chronic depletion of sodium. Slight decreases in plasma and ECF volumes and total body sodium during prolonged thiazide therapy are not sufficient to explain the long-term decrease in blood pressure, but may explain the efficacy of thiazides in combination with most other hypotensive agents which tend to increase sodium retention and plasma volume.

Plasma renin activity is considerably elevated during thiazide therapy, probably because of plasma volume changes. The aldosterone secretion rate is slightly but substantially increased and contributes to the hypokalemia caused by thiazides.

Paradoxically, thiazides decrease urine volume in patients with diabetes insipidus. The urine becomes less hypotonic, but not hypertonic, and thirst and water consumption are decreased. This effect is thought to result mainly from the decrease in plasma volume and from sodium depletion with a resultant increase in renal water and sodium reabsorption, although other factors may play a role.

Thiazides can induce hyperglycemia, exacerbate preexisting diabetes mellitus, or precipitate diabetes in prediabetic patients. The mechanism of this action of the thiazides is not known, but there is evidence that the drugs act at both pancreatic and peripheral sites and that potassium depletion may decrease glucose tolerance.

PHARMACOKINETICS

● Absorption

Thiazides are absorbed from the GI tract in varying degrees. The onset of diuretic action of the thiazides following oral administration occurs within 2 hours, and the peak effect occurs 3–6 hours after administration. Following IV administration, chlorothiazide sodium has an onset of action within 15 minutes and a peak effect in 30 minutes. The duration of diuretic action of the individual agent is determined by the rate of its excretion. The approximate duration of diuretic action of a single dose of the thiazides and related diuretics is as follows:

TABLE 3. Duration of Diuretic Action

Drug	Duration of Diuretic Action (hours)
Chlorothiazide (IV)	2
Chlorothiazide (oral)	6–12
Hydrochlorothiazide	6–12
Metolazone	12–24
Hydroflumethiazide	12–24
Bendroflumethiazide	18–24
Methyclothiazide	24
Trichlormethiazide	24
Chlorthalidone	24–72

The onset of hypotensive action is generally 3 or 4 days, and the hypotensive action dissipates during the first week after discontinuing chronic therapy.

● Distribution

Thiazides are distributed in the extracellular space and cross the placenta. Thiazides also are distributed into milk.

● Elimination

Most thiazides are excreted in urine, principally unchanged. The drugs are excreted by glomerular filtration and active secretion in the proximal tubule. The renal clearance of the thiazides varies; those with the lowest renal clearance generally require the lowest dosage for therapeutic effect. In patients with uncompensated heart failure or impaired renal function, excretion of the drugs may be delayed.

CHEMISTRY

Thiazide (benzothiadiazine) diuretics are derivatives of 1,2,4-benzothiadiazine-7-sulfonamide 1,1-dioxide. Substitution in the R^2 and R^3 positions of the thiazide nucleus increases the activity of the compound. In most thiazides, the 3-4 bond is saturated and all presently marketed compounds have a chloride or CF_3 substituent at the 6 position of the thiazide nucleus. Quinethazone and metolazone, which are pharmacologically similar to the thiazides, are quinazoline derivatives and differ from the thiazides in having a carbonyl group rather than a sulfoxide group at the 1 position. Chlorthalidone is also pharmacologically and structurally similar to the thiazides, but is a phthalimidine derivative of benzenesulfonamide. Diazoxide, a nondiuretic hypotensive agent, is structurally related to the thiazides, but lacks the 7-sulfamyl group common to the thiazide diuretics.

In general, thiazides occur as white or nearly white, crystalline powders and are very slightly soluble or practically insoluble in water.

For further information on chemistry and stability, pharmacology, pharmacokinetics, and dosage and administration of thiazides, see the individual monographs in 40:28.

† Use is not currently included in the labeling approved by the US Food and Drug Administration.

hydroCHLOROthiazide

40:28.20 • THIAZIDE DIURETICS

■ Hydrochlorothiazide is a thiazide diuretic and antihypertensive agent.

DOSAGE AND ADMINISTRATION

● Administration

Hydrochlorothiazide is administered orally.

Extemporaneously Compounded Oral Liquid

Extemporaneously compounded oral liquid formulations of hydrochlorothiazide containing 5 mg/mL have been prepared.

Standardize 4 Safety

Standardized concentrations for an extemporaneously prepared oral liquid formulation of hydrochlorothiazide have been established through Standardize 4 Safety (S4S), a national patient safety initiative to reduce medication errors, especially during transitions of care. Because recommendations from the S4S panels may differ from the manufacturer's prescribing information, caution is advised when using concentrations that differ from labeling, particularly when using rate information from the label. For additional information on S4S (including updates that may be available), see https://www.ashp.org/pharmacy-practice/standardize-4-safety-initiative.

TABLE 1. Standardize 4 Safety Compounded Oral Liquid Standards for Hydrochlorothiazide

Concentration Standards
5 mg/mL

● Dosage

Dosage of hydrochlorothiazide should be individualized according to the patient's requirements and response. The lowest dosage necessary to produce the desired clinical effect should be used. If hydrochlorothiazide is added to the regimen of a patient stabilized on a potent hypotensive agent, dosage of the hypotensive agent should initially be reduced to avoid the possibility of severe hypotension.

Edema

For the management of edema, the usual adult dosage of hydrochlorothiazide is 25–100 mg daily in 1–3 divided doses. Many patients also may respond to intermittent therapy (e.g., on alternate days or on 3–5 days weekly). Excessive diuretic response and the resulting undesirable electrolyte imbalance are less likely to occur with such intermittent administration of the drug.

For the management of fluid retention (e.g., edema) associated with heart failure, some experts recommend initiating hydrochlorothiazide at a low dosage (e.g., 25 mg once or twice daily) and increasing the dosage (maximum of 200 mg daily) until urine output increases and weight decreases, generally by 0.5–1 kg daily. When hydrochlorothiazide is used for sequential nephron blockade in the management of fluid retention in heart failure, some experts recommend an initial dosage of 25–100 mg once or twice daily in combination with a loop diuretic. Experts state that diuretics should be administered at a dosage sufficient to achieve optimal volume status and relieve congestion without inducing an excessively rapid reduction in intravascular volume, which could result in hypotension, renal dysfunction, or both.

Hypertension

Usual Dosage

For the management of hypertension in adults, the manufacturers recommend an initial hydrochlorothiazide dosage of 12.5–25 mg once daily and a usual maximum dosage of 50 mg daily (in 1 or 2 divided doses). Dosages of 25–100 mg daily (in 1 or 2 divided doses) have been used in randomized controlled studies; experts recommend a dosage of 25–50 mg daily for optimal balance between efficacy and safety in the management of hypertension in adults. Dosages exceeding 50 mg daily usually are associated with marked hypokalemia; some manufacturers state that such dosages are not recommended.

Fixed-combination Therapy

When combination therapy is required in the management of hypertension, dosage can first be adjusted by administering each drug separately. If it is determined that the optimum maintenance dosage corresponds to the ratio in the commercial combination preparation, the fixed combination may be used. Alternatively, therapy can be initiated with a fixed combination of 2 antihypertensive agents. Use of fixed-combination preparations may increase patient compliance.

For information on commercially available preparations containing hydrochlorothiazide in fixed combination with a potassium-sparing diuretic, see the individual monographs in 40:28.10.

Monitoring and Blood Pressure Treatment Goals

The patient's renal function and electrolytes should be assessed 2–4 weeks after initiation of diuretic therapy. Blood pressure should be monitored regularly (i.e., monthly) during therapy and dosage of the antihypertensive drug adjusted until blood pressure is controlled. If an adequate blood pressure response is not achieved with hydrochlorothiazide monotherapy, another antihypertensive agent with demonstrated benefit and preferably with a complementary mechanism of action (e.g., angiotensin-converting enzyme [ACE] inhibitor, angiotensin II receptor antagonist, calcium-channel blocker) may be added; if goal blood pressure is still not achieved, a third drug may be added. (See Uses: Hypertension in Adults, in the Thiazides General Statement 40:28.20.) In patients who develop unacceptable adverse effects with hydrochlorothiazide, the drug should be discontinued and another antihypertensive agent from a different pharmacologic class should be initiated.

The goal of hypertension management and prevention is to achieve and maintain optimal control of blood pressure. However, the optimum blood pressure threshold for initiating antihypertensive drug therapy and specific treatment goals remain controversial. A 2017 multidisciplinary hypertension guideline from the American College of Cardiology (ACC), American Heart Association (AHA), and a number of other professional organizations generally recommends a blood pressure goal of less than 130/80 mm Hg in all adults regardless of comorbidities or level of atherosclerotic cardiovascular disease (ASCVD) risk. Many patients will require at least 2 drugs from different pharmacologic classes to achieve this blood pressure goal; the potential benefits of hypertension management and drug cost, adverse effects, and risks associated with the use of multiple antihypertensive drugs also should be considered when deciding a patient's blood pressure treatment goal.

For additional information on target levels of blood pressure and on monitoring therapy in the management of hypertension, see Blood Pressure Monitoring and Treatment Goals under Dosage: Hypertension, in Dosage and Administration in the Thiazides General Statement 40:28.20.

Pediatric Dosage

In children 6 months to 12 years of age, the usual dosage of hydrochlorothiazide for the management of hypertension or for diuresis is 1–2 mg/kg daily given as a single dose or in 2 divided doses. Infants younger than 6 months of age may require up to 3 mg/kg daily in 2 divided doses. The total daily dosage should not exceed 37.5 mg for children up to 2 years of age or 100 mg for children 2–12 years of age. Experts recommend initiation of the drug at the low end of the dosage range; the dosage may be increased every 2–4 weeks until blood pressure is controlled, the maximum dosage is reached, or adverse effects occur. For information on overall principles and expert recommendations for treatment of hypertension in pediatric patients, see Uses: Hypertension in Pediatric Patients, in the Thiazides General Statement 40:28.20.

Geriatric Dosage

Because an increased incidence of adverse effects to hydrochlorothiazide and excessive reduction in blood pressure may occur in geriatric patients (older than 65 years of age), hydrochlorothiazide should be initiated at the lowest dosage (12.5 mg daily); dosage may be adjusted in increments of 12.5 mg if needed.

CAUTIONS

Hydrochlorothiazide shares the pharmacologic actions, uses, and toxic potentials of the thiazides, and the usual precautions of thiazide administration should be observed. (See Cautions in the Thiazides General Statement 40:28.20.)

When hydrochlorothiazide is used in fixed combination with other drugs, the cautions, precautions, contraindications, and interactions associated with the concomitant agent(s) should be considered in addition to those associated with hydrochlorothiazide.

Some commercially available formulations of hydrochlorothiazide contain sulfites that may cause allergic-type reactions, including anaphylaxis and life-threatening or less severe asthmatic episodes, in certain susceptible individuals. The overall prevalence of sulfite sensitivity in the general population is unknown but probably low; such sensitivity appears to occur more frequently in asthmatic than in nonasthmatic individuals.

PHARMACOKINETICS

Hydrochlorothiazide is well absorbed from the GI tract, with an oral bioavailability of approximately 65–75%. Although the rate and extent of absorption have been reported to vary depending on the formulation administered, no studies have been performed to determine the clinical importance (if any) of variations in absorption in patients receiving chronic hydrochlorothiazide therapy. Following oral administration of hydrochlorothiazide at doses of 12.5–100 mg, peak plasma concentrations of 70–490 ng/mL are observed within 1–5 hours of dosing. Food decreases the rate and extent of absorption of hydrochlorothiazide capsules (Microzide®). Bioavailability and peak plasma concentrations of the drug were decreased by about 10 and 20%, respectively, when hydrochlorothiazide capsules (Microzide®) were administered with food. Times to peak plasma concentration for such capsules were delayed by 1.3 hours (from 1.6 to 2.9 hours). Absorption of hydrochlorothiazide is reduced in patients with heart failure.

Approximately 40–68% of the drug is bound to plasma proteins.

Hydrochlorothiazide exhibits linear pharmacokinetics. Based on determination of plasma drug concentrations over a period of at least 24 hours, the plasma half-life of hydrochlorothiazide reportedly ranges from 5.6–15 hours. Hydrochlorothiazide apparently is not metabolized and is excreted unchanged in urine. At least 61% of the drug is reportedly eliminated from the body within 24 hours. Increased hydrochlorothiazide plasma concentrations and a prolonged elimination half-life have been reported in patients with renal impairment. The effect of hemodialysis on the elimination of the drug has not been determined.

CHEMISTRY AND STABILITY

● Chemistry

Hydrochlorothiazide is a thiazide diuretic. Hydrochlorothiazide occurs as a white or practically white, practically odorless, crystalline powder and has a slightly bitter taste. The drug is slightly soluble in water and soluble in alcohol and has pK_as of 7.9 and 9.2.

● Stability

Hydrochlorothiazide tablets and capsules should be stored in tightly closed containers at a controlled room temperature of 15–30°C and protected from light, moisture, and freezing. Hydrochlorothiazide oral solution should be stored in well-closed containers at a temperature less than 40°C, preferably at 15–30°C. Freezing of the oral solution should be avoided. Commercially available hydrochlorothiazide tablets have an expiration date of 3 or 5 years following the date of manufacture depending on the packaging.

For further information on chemistry and stability, pharmacology, pharmacokinetics, uses, cautions, acute toxicity, drug interactions, laboratory test interferences, and dosage and administration of hydrochlorothiazide, see the Thiazides General Statement 40:28.20.

PREPARATIONS

Excipients in commercially available drug preparations may have clinically important effects in some individuals; consult specific product labeling for details.

hydroCHLOROthiazide

Oral

Capsules	12.5 mg*	hydroCHLOROthiazide Capsules
		Microzide®, Watson
Tablets	12.5 mg*	hydroCHLOROthiazide Tablets
	25 mg*	hydroCHLOROthiazide Tablets
	50 mg*	hydroCHLOROthiazide Tablets

* available from one or more manufacturer, distributor, and/or repackager by generic (nonproprietary) name

Amiloride Hydrochloride and hydroCHLOROthiazide

Oral

Tablets	5 mg of Anhydrous Amiloride Hydrochloride and Hydrochlorothiazide 50 mg*	Amiloride Hydrochloride and hydroCHLOROthiazide Tablets

* available from one or more manufacturer, distributor, and/or repackager by generic (nonproprietary) name

Captopril and hydroCHLOROthiazide

Oral

Tablets	25 mg Captopril and Hydrochlorothiazide 15 mg*	Captopril and hydroCHLOROthiazide Tablets
	25 mg Captopril and Hydrochlorothiazide 25 mg*	Captopril and hydroCHLOROthiazide Tablets
	50 mg Captopril and Hydrochlorothiazide 15 mg*	Captopril and hydroCHLOROthiazide Tablets
	50 mg Captopril and Hydrochlorothiazide 25 mg*	Captopril and hydroCHLOROthiazide Tablets

* available from one or more manufacturer, distributor, and/or repackager by generic (nonproprietary) name

Enalapril Maleate and hydroCHLOROthiazide

Oral

Tablets	5 mg Enalapril Maleate and Hydrochlorothiazide 12.5 mg*	Enalapril Maleate and hydroCHLOROthiazide Tablets
	10 mg Enalapril Maleate and Hydrochlorothiazide 25 mg*	Enalapril Maleate and hydroCHLOROthiazide Tablets
		Vaseretic®, Valeant

* available from one or more manufacturer, distributor, and/or repackager by generic (nonproprietary) name

Methyldopa and hydroCHLOROthiazide

Oral

Tablets, film-coated	250 mg Methyldopa and Hydrochlorothiazide 15 mg*	Methyldopa and hydroCHLOROthiazide Tablets
	250 mg Methyldopa and Hydrochlorothiazide 25 mg*	Methyldopa and hydroCHLOROthiazide Tablets

* available from one or more manufacturer, distributor, and/or repackager by generic (nonproprietary) name

Metoprolol Tartrate and hydroCHLOROthiazide

Oral

Tablets

	50 mg Metoprolol Tartrate and Hydrochlorothiazide 25 mg*	**Lopressor® HCT** (scored), Validus
		Metoprolol Tartrate and hydroCHLOROthiazide Tablets
	100 mg Metoprolol Tartrate and Hydrochlorothiazide 25 mg*	**Lopressor® HCT** (scored), Validus
		Metoprolol Tartrate and hydroCHLOROthiazide Tablets
	100 mg Metoprolol Tartrate and Hydrochlorothiazide 50 mg*	**Lopressor® HCT** (scored), Validus
		Metoprolol Tartrate and hydroCHLOROthiazide Tablets

* available from one or more manufacturer, distributor, and/or repackager by generic (nonproprietary) name

Propranolol Hydrochloride and hydroCHLOROthiazide

Oral

Tablets

	40 mg Propranolol Hydrochloride and Hydrochlorothiazide 25 mg*	**Propranolol Hydrochloride and hydroCHLOROthiazide Tablets**
	80 mg Propranolol Hydrochloride and Hydrochlorothiazide 25 mg*	**Propranolol Hydrochloride and hydroCHLOROthiazide Tablets**

* available from one or more manufacturer, distributor, and/or repackager by generic (nonproprietary) name

Spironolactone and hydroCHLOROthiazide

Oral

Tablets, film-coated

	25 mg Spironolactone and Hydrochlorothiazide 25 mg*	**Aldactazide®**, Pfizer
		Spironolactone and hydroCHLOROthiazide Tablets
	50 mg Spironolactone and Hydrochlorothiazide 50 mg	**Aldactazide®** (scored), Pfizer

* available from one or more manufacturer, distributor, and/or repackager by generic (nonproprietary) name

Triamterene and hydroCHLOROthiazide (Co-triamterzide)

Oral

Capsules

	37.5 mg Triamterene and Hydrochlorothiazide 25 mg*	**Dyazide®**, GlaxoSmithKline
		Triamterene and hydroCHLOROthiazide Capsules

Tablets

	37.5 mg Triamterene and Hydrochlorothiazide 25 mg*	**Maxzide®** (scored), Mylan
		Triamterene and hydroCHLOROthiazide Tablets
	75 mg Triamterene and Hydrochlorothiazide 50 mg*	**Maxzide®** (scored), Mylan
		Triamterene and hydroCHLOROthiazide Tablets

* available from one or more manufacturer, distributor, and/or repackager by generic (nonproprietary) name

Other hydroCHLOROthiazide Combinations

Oral

Tablets

	12.5 mg with Candesartan 16 mg	**Atacand® HCT**, AstraZeneca
	12.5 mg with Candesartan 32 mg	**Atacand® HCT**, AstraZeneca
	12.5 mg with Fosinopril Sodium 10 mg*	**Fosinopril Sodium and hydroCHLOROthiazide Tablets**
	12.5 mg with Fosinopril Sodium 20 mg*	**Fosinopril Sodium and hydroCHLOROthiazide Tablets**
	12.5 mg with Irbesartan 150 mg	**Avalide®**, Bristol-Myers Squibb (also promoted by Sanofi-Synthelabo)
	12.5 mg with Irbesartan 300 mg	**Avalide®**, Bristol-Myers Squibb (also promoted by Sanofi-Synthelabo)
	12.5 mg with Lisinopril 10 mg*	**Lisinopril and hydroCHLOROthiazide Tablets**
		Prinzide®, Merck
		Zestoretic®, AstraZeneca
	12.5 mg with Lisinopril 20 mg*	**Lisinopril and hydroCHLOROthiazide Tablets**
		Prinzide®, Merck
		Zestoretic®, AstraZeneca
	12.5 mg with Telmisartan 40 mg*	**Micardis® HCT**, Boehringer Ingelheim
		Telmisartan and hydroCHLOROthiazide Tablets
	12.5 mg with Telmisartan 80 mg*	**Micardis® HCT**, Boehringer Ingelheim
		Telmisartan and hydroCHLOROthiazide Tablets
	25 mg with Irbesartan 300 mg	**Avalide®**, Bristol-Myers Squibb (also promoted by Sanofi-Synthelabo)
	25 mg with Lisinopril 20 mg*	**Lisinopril and hydroCHLOROthiazide Tablets**
		Prinzide®, Merck
		Zestoretic®, AstraZeneca
	25 mg with Telmisartan 80 mg*	**Micardis® HCT**, Boehringer Ingelheim
		Telmisartan and hydroCHLOROthiazide Tablets

Tablets, film-coated

	6.25 mg with Benazepril Hydrochloride 5 mg*	**Benazepril Hydrochloride and hydroCHLOROthiazide Tablets**
		Lotensin® HCT (scored), Novartis
	6.25 mg with Bisoprolol Fumarate 2.5 mg*	**Bisoprolol Fumarate and hydroCHLOROthiazide Tablets**
		Ziac®, Duramed
	6.25 mg with Bisoprolol Fumarate 5 mg*	**Bisoprolol Fumarate and hydroCHLOROthiazide Tablets**
		Ziac®, Duramed
	6.25 mg with Bisoprolol Fumarate 10 mg*	**Bisoprolol Fumarate and hydroCHLOROthiazide Tablets**
		Ziac®, Duramed
	12.5 mg with Aliskiren Hemifumarate 150 mg (of aliskiren)	**Tekturna® HCT**, Noden
	12.5 mg with Aliskiren Hemifumarate 300 mg (of aliskiren)	**Tekturna® HCT**, Noden
	12.5 mg with Amlodipine Besylate 5 mg (of amlodipine) and Olmesartan Medoxomil 20 mg	**Tribenzor®**, Daiichi Sankyo
	12.5 mg with Amlodipine Besylate 5 mg (of amlodipine) and Olmesartan Medoxomil 40 mg	**Tribenzor®**, Daiichi Sankyo
	12.5 mg with Amlodipine Besylate 5 mg (of amlodipine) and Valsartan 160 mg*	**Amlodipine Besylate, Valsartan, and hydroCHLOROthiazide Tablets**
		Exforge HCT®, Novartis
	12.5 mg with Amlodipine Besylate 10 mg (of amlodipine) and Olmesartan Medoxomil 40 mg	**Tribenzor®**, Daiichi Sankyo
	12.5 mg with Amlodipine Besylate 10 mg (of amlodipine) and Valsartan 160 mg*	**Amlodipine Besylate, Valsartan, and hydroCHLOROthiazide Tablets**
		Exforge HCT®, Novartis
	12.5 mg with Benazepril Hydrochloride 10 mg*	**Benazepril Hydrochloride and hydroCHLOROthiazide Tablets**
		Lotensin® HCT (scored), Novartis

12.5 mg with Benazepril Hydrochloride 20 mg*	**Benazepril Hydrochloride and Hydrochlorothiazide Tablets** **Lotensin® HCT** (scored), Novartis	25 mg with Amlodipine Besylate 5 mg (of amlodipine) and Valsartan 160 mg*	**Amlodipine Besylate, Valsartan, and hydroCHLOROthiazide Tablets** **Exforge HCT®**, Novartis
12.5 mg with Eprosartan Mesylate 600 mg (of eprosartan)	**Teveten® HCT**, Abbott	25 mg with Amlodipine Besylate 10 mg (of amlodipine) and Olmesartan Medoxomil 40 mg	**Tribenzor®**, Daiichi Sankyo
12.5 mg with Losartan Potassium 50 mg	**Hyzaar®**, Merck	25 mg with Amlodipine Besylate 10 mg (of amlodipine) and Valsartan 160 mg*	**Amlodipine Besylate, Valsartan, and hydroCHLOROthiazide Tablets** **Exforge HCT®**, Novartis
12.5 mg with Losartan Potassium 100 mg	**Hyzaar®**, Merck	25 mg with Amlodipine Besylate 10 mg (of amlodipine) and Valsartan 320 mg*	**Amlodipine Besylate, Valsartan, and hydroCHLOROthiazide Tablets** **Exforge HCT®**, Novartis
12.5 mg with Moexipril Hydrochloride 7.5 mg*	**Moexipril Hydrochloride and hydroCHLOROthiazide Tablets** **Uniretic®** (scored), UCB	25 mg with Benazepril Hydrochloride 20 mg*	**Benazepril Hydrochloride and hydroCHLOROthiazide Tablets** **Lotensin® HCT** (scored), Novartis
12.5 mg with Moexipril 15 mg*	**Moexipril Hydrochloride and hydroCHLOROthiazide Tablets** **Uniretic®** (scored), UCB	25 mg with Eprosartan Mesylate 600 mg (of eprosartan)	**Teveten® HCT**, Abbott
12.5 mg with Olmesartan Medoxomil 20 mg	**Benicar® HCT**, Daiichi-Sankyo	25 mg with Losartan Potassium 100 mg	**Hyzaar®**, Merck
12.5 mg with Olmesartan Medoxomil 40 mg	**Benicar® HCT**, Daiichi-Sankyo	25 mg with Moexipril Hydrochloride 15 mg*	**Moexipril Hydrochloride and hydroCHLOROthiazide Tablets** **Uniretic®** (scored), UCB
12.5 mg with Quinapril Hydrochloride 10 mg (of quinapril)*	**Accuretic®** (scored), Pfizer **Quinapril Hydrochloride and hydroCHLOROthiazide Tablets**	25 mg with Olmesartan Medoxomil 40 mg	**Benicar® HCT**, Daiichi-Sankyo
12.5 mg with Quinapril Hydrochloride 20 mg (of quinapril)*	**Accuretic®** (scored), Pfizer **Quinapril Hydrochloride and hydroCHLOROthiazide Tablets**	25 mg with Quinapril Hydrochloride 20 mg (of quinapril)*	**Accuretic®** (scored), Pfizer **Quinapril Hydrochloride and hydroCHLOROthiazide Tablets**
12.5 mg with Valsartan 80 mg*	**Diovan® HCT**, Novartis **Valsartan and hydroCHLOROthiazide Tablets**	25 mg with Valsartan 160 mg*	**Diovan® HCT**, Novartis **Valsartan and hydroCHLOROthiazide Tablets**
12.5 mg with Valsartan 160 mg*	**Diovan® HCT**, Novartis **Valsartan and hydroCHLOROthiazide Tablets**	25 mg with Valsartan 320 mg*	**Diovan® HCT**, Novartis **Valsartan and hydro-CHLOROthiazide Tablets**
12.5 mg with Valsartan 320 mg*	**Diovan® HCT**, Novartis **Valsartan and hydroCHLOROthiazide Tablets**		
25 mg with Aliskiren Hemifumarate 150 mg (of aliskiren)	**Tekturna® HCT**, Noden		
25 mg with Aliskiren Hemifumarate 300 mg (of aliskiren)	**Tekturna® HCT**, Noden		
25 mg with Amlodipine Besylate 5 mg (of amlodipine) and Olmesartan Medoxomil 40 mg	**Tribenzor®**, Daiichi Sankyo		

* available from one or more manufacturer, distributor, and/or repackager by generic (nonproprietary) name

† Use is not currently included in the labeling approved by the US Food and Drug Administration.

Selected Revisions June 10, 2024, © Copyright, May 1, 1975, American Society of Health-System Pharmacists, Inc.

Chlorthalidone

40:28.24 • THIAZIDE-LIKE DIURETICS

■ Chlorthalidone, which is structurally and pharmacologically similar to the thiazides, is a diuretic and antihypertensive agent.

DOSAGE AND ADMINISTRATION

● Administration

Chlorthalidone is administered orally.

● Dosage

Dosage of chlorthalidone should be individualized according to the patient's requirements and response. If chlorthalidone is added to the regimen of a patient stabilized on a potent hypotensive agent, the dosage of the hypotensive agent should initially be reduced to avoid the possibility of severe hypotension.

Edema

For the management of edema in adults, the usual initial dosage of chlorthalidone is 50–100 mg daily in a single dose after breakfast. Alternatively, therapy may be initiated at a dosage of 100 mg every other day or 3 times a week. Some patients require dosages of 150–200 mg daily or every other day. Dosages greater than 200 mg daily do not produce a greater response. In edematous patients, reduction of dosage to a lower maintenance level may be possible after several days or when nonedematous weight is attained.

For the management of fluid retention (e.g., edema) associated with heart failure, some experts recommend initiating chlorthalidone at a low dosage (e.g., 12.5–25 mg once daily) and increasing the dosage (maximum of 100 mg daily) until urine output increases and weight decreases, generally by 0.5–1 kg daily. Experts state that diuretics should be administered at a dosage sufficient to achieve optimal volume status and relieve congestion without inducing an excessively rapid reduction in intravascular volume, which could result in hypotension, renal dysfunction, or both.

Hypertension

The usual manufacturer-recommended initial dosage of chlorthalidone for the management of hypertension in adults is 25 mg once daily. If blood pressure remains uncontrolled, the dosage may be increased to 50 mg once daily. Some experts recommend a chlorthalidone dosage of 12.5–25 mg once daily based on efficacy and tolerance demonstrated in clinical studies. Dosages of chlorthalidone exceeding 100 mg daily usually do not increase efficacy.

Fixed-combination Therapy

When combination therapy is required in the management of hypertension, dosage can be adjusted first by administering each drug separately. If it is determined that the optimum maintenance dosage corresponds to the ratio in a commercial combination preparation, the fixed combination may be used. The manufacturer states that commercially available preparations containing chlorthalidone in fixed combination with atenolol should not be used for initial antihypertensive therapy; however, some experts state that initiation of therapy with a fixed-combination preparation may increase patient compliance.

Monitoring and Blood Pressure Treatment Goals

The patient's renal function and electrolytes should be assessed 2–4 weeks after initiation of diuretic therapy. Blood pressure should be monitored regularly (i.e., monthly) during therapy and dosage of the antihypertensive drug adjusted until blood pressure is controlled. If an adequate blood pressure response is not achieved with chlorthalidone monotherapy, another antihypertensive agent with demonstrated benefit and preferably with a complementary mechanism of action (e.g., angiotensin-converting enzyme [ACE] inhibitor, angiotensin II receptor antagonist, calcium-channel blocker) may be added; if goal blood pressure is still not achieved, a third drug may be added. (See Uses: Hypertension in Adults, in the Thiazides General Statement 40:28.20.) In patients who develop unacceptable adverse effects with chlorthalidone, the drug should be discontinued and another antihypertensive agent from a different pharmacologic class should be initiated.

The goal of hypertension management and prevention is to achieve and maintain optimal control of blood pressure. However, the optimum blood pressure threshold for initiating antihypertensive drug therapy and specific treatment goals remain controversial. A 2017 multidisciplinary hypertension guideline from the American College of Cardiology (ACC), American Heart Association (AHA), and a number of other professional organizations generally recommends a blood pressure goal of less than 130/80 mm Hg in all adults, regardless of comorbidities or level of atherosclerotic cardiovascular disease (ASCVD) risk. Many patients will require at least 2 drugs from different pharmacologic classes to achieve this blood pressure goal; the potential benefits of hypertension management and drug cost, adverse effects, and risks associated with the use of multiple antihypertensive drugs also should be considered when deciding a patient's blood pressure treatment goal.

For additional information on target levels of blood pressure and on monitoring therapy in the management of hypertension, see Blood Pressure Monitoring and Treatment Goals under Dosage: Hypertension, in Dosage and Administration in the Thiazides General Statement 40:28.20.

Pediatric Dosage

For the management of hypertension in children†, some experts recommend an initial dosage of 0.3 mg/kg once daily. Experts state that the dosage should be increased every 2–4 weeks until blood pressure is controlled, the maximum dosage is reached (2 mg/kg [up to 50 mg] daily), or adverse effects occur. For information on overall principles and expert recommendations for treatment of hypertension in pediatric patients, see Uses: Hypertension in Pediatric Patients, in the Thiazides General Statement 40:28.20.

CAUTIONS

Chlorthalidone shares the pharmacologic actions, uses, and toxic potentials of the thiazides, and the usual precautions of thiazide administration should be observed. (See Cautions in the Thiazides General Statement 40:28.20.)

PHARMACOKINETICS

Chlorthalidone is absorbed from the GI tract. Little information is available on the extent of absorption of the drug.

About 90% of chlorthalidone is bound in the body, principally to or in red blood cells. The high degree of binding accounts for the long half-life of the drug which is reported to be 54 hours. During long-term oral administration, 30–60% of the daily dose is excreted unchanged in urine.

CHEMISTRY AND STABILITY

● Chemistry

Chlorthalidone is a phthalimidine derivative of benzenesulfonamide that is structurally and pharmacologically similar to the thiazide diuretics. The drug occurs as a white to yellowish-white, crystalline powder. The drug is practically insoluble in water and slightly soluble in alcohol and has a pK_a of 9.4.

● Stability

Chlorthalidone tablets should be stored in tight, light-resistant containers at 20–25°C.

For further information on chemistry, pharmacology, pharmacokinetics, cautions, acute toxicity, uses, drug interactions, laboratory test interferences, and dosage and administration of chlorthalidone, see the Thiazides General Statement 40:28.20.

PREPARATIONS

Excipients in commercially available drug preparations may have clinically important effects in some individuals; consult specific product labeling for details.

Chlorthalidone

Oral		
Tablets	25 mg*	Chlorthalidone Tablets
	50 mg*	Chlorthalidone Tablets

* available from one or more manufacturer, distributor, and/or repackager by generic (nonproprietary) name

Atenolol and Chlorthalidone

Oral		
Tablets	Atenolol 50 mg and Chlorthalidone 25 mg*	Atenolol and Chlorthalidone Tablets
		Tenoretic®, AstraZeneca
	Atenolol 100 mg and Chlorthalidone 25 mg*	Atenolol and Chlorthalidone Tablets
		Tenoretic®, AstraZeneca

* available from one or more manufacturer, distributor, and/or repackager by generic (nonproprietary) name

† Use is not currently included in the labeling approved by the US Food and Drug Administration.

Table of Contents

44:00 ENZYMES

44:04 Enzyme Inhibitors

44:08 Enzyme Cofactor/Chaperones

§ Omitted from the print version of *AHFS Drug Information*® because of space limitations. This monograph is available on the *AHFS Drug Information*® website, http://ahfsdruginformation.com.

Table of Contents

§ Omitted from the print version of *AHFS Drug Information* because of space limitations. This monograph is available on the *AHFS Drug Information* web site, http://www.ahfsdruginformation.com.

Codeine Phosphate
Codeine Sulfate

48:08 · ANTITUSSIVES

■ Codeine is a phenanthrene-derivative opiate agonist antitussive agent.

USES

● Cough

Codeine is used, alone or in combination with other antitussives or expectorants, in the symptomatic relief of nonproductive cough. Since the cough reflex may be a useful physiologic mechanism which clears the respiratory passages of foreign material and excess secretions and may aid in preventing or reversing atelectasis, cough suppressants should not be used indiscriminately.

Antitussives containing codeine should *not* be used in patients younger than 18 years of age. (See Cautions: Pediatric Precautions.)

● Pain

For use of codeine as an analgesic, see 28:08.08.

DOSAGE AND ADMINISTRATION

● Administration

Codeine sulfate and codeine phosphate are administered orally as antitussives.

● Dosage
Cough

Codeine preparations should be given in the smallest effective dose and as infrequently as possible to minimize the development of tolerance and physical dependence. Reduced dosage is indicated in poor-risk patients and in very old patients.

The usual oral antitussive dosage of codeine phosphate or codeine sulfate conventional (immediate-release) preparations in adults is 10–20 mg every 4–6 hours, not to exceed 120 mg daily.

CAUTIONS

● Adverse Effects

Adverse reactions occur infrequently with usual oral antitussive doses of codeine. Nausea, vomiting, constipation with repeated doses, dizziness, sedation, palpitation, pruritus, and, rarely, excessive perspiration and agitation have been reported. Although equianalgesic doses of codeine and morphine produce similar degrees of respiratory depression, respiratory depression seldom occurs with oral antitussive doses of codeine.

● Precautions and Contraindications

Codeine is *contraindicated* in children younger than 12 years of age for the management of cough and cold. In addition, FDA states that use of antitussives containing codeine is *not* recommended in pediatric patients younger than 18 years of age. (See Cautions: Pediatric Precautions.)

Individuals who are ultrarapid metabolizers of cytochrome P-450 (CYP) 2D6 substrates are likely to have higher than expected serum concentrations of morphine, the active metabolite of codeine; therefore, FDA states that codeine should *not* be used in such patients. (See Pharmacokinetics: Pharmacogenomics.)

Because concomitant use of opiate agonists and benzodiazepines or other CNS depressants may result in profound sedation, respiratory depression, coma, and death, opiate antitussives should be *avoided* in patients receiving CNS depressants. (See Drug Interactions.) Patients receiving codeine and/or their caregivers should be apprised of the risks associated with concomitant therapeutic or illicit use of benzodiazepines, alcohol, or other CNS depressants.

When preparations containing codeine in fixed combination with other drugs are used, the cautions, precautions, and contraindications applicable to each ingredient must be considered.

In patients with asthma or pulmonary emphysema, the indiscriminate use of antitussives may precipitate respiratory insufficiency resulting from increased viscosity of bronchial secretions and suppression of the cough reflex.

Tolerance and physical dependence may occur following prolonged administration of codeine. Patients should be warned that codeine may impair their ability to perform activities requiring mental alertness or physical coordination (e.g., operating machinery, driving a motor vehicle). Codeine should be used with caution in debilitated patients. The drug should also be used with caution in patients who have undergone thoracotomies or laparotomies, since suppression of the cough reflex may lead to retention of secretions postoperatively in these patients.

FDA states that use of codeine is *not* recommended in nursing women, especially those who have evidence of ultrarapid metabolism of CYP2D6 substrates. Serious adverse events (i.e., excessive sedation, difficulty nursing, respiratory depression), including death, have been reported in nursing infants exposed to codeine. One case of opiate toxicity resulting in neonatal death has been reported in the nursing infant of a woman receiving codeine; genetic testing of the woman indicated that she was an ultrarapid metabolizer of codeine. (See Pharmacokinetics: Pharmacogenomics.) Higher than expected concentrations of morphine were found in breast milk and in the blood of the infant. Somnolence also has been reported more frequently in nursing infants whose mothers received codeine in combination with acetaminophen compared with those whose mothers received acetaminophen alone; evidence of ultrarapid metabolism of CYP2D6 substrates was identified in some of these women. Concentrations of morphine in breast milk are low and dose dependent in women who are normal metabolizers of codeine. Although not routinely used in clinical practice, FDA-approved tests (e.g., AmpliChip® CYP450 Test) are available to identify an individual's CYP2D6 genotype. However, testing alone may not adequately predict the risk of adverse reactions. Infants exposed to codeine through breast milk should be monitored closely for clinical manifestations of opiate toxicity (e.g., sedation, difficulty breast-feeding or breathing, hypotonia). If such manifestations occur, caregivers should seek immediate medical treatment for the infant.

Codeine is contraindicated in patients with known hypersensitivity to the drug.

For additional information on the usual precautions of opiate agonist therapy, see Cautions in the Opiate Agonists General Statement 28:08.08.

● Pediatric Precautions

Pediatric patients receiving codeine for the management of cough and cold, especially those who are obese, have obstructive sleep apnea or severe lung disease, or have evidence of ultrarapid metabolism of CYP2D6 substrates, are at increased risk of respiratory depression. Between January 1969 and May 2015, the FDA Adverse Event Reporting System (AERS) received 64 reports of respiratory depression, including 24 reports of death, worldwide that were associated with codeine use in pediatric patients younger than 18 years of age; in all 10 of the reports that provided information about CYP2D6 metabolizer status, the patients were ultrarapid or extensive metabolizers of CYP2D6 substrates. (See Pharmacokinetics: Pharmacogenomics.) Most of the cases of respiratory depression, including most of the deaths, occurred in children younger than 12 years of age. Respiratory depression may occur despite serum concentrations of codeine or morphine being within the therapeutic range; one patient who had concentrations within the therapeutic range died following use of codeine for management of pain after tonsillectomy and adenoidectomy. In addition, a review initiated by the European Medicines Agency (EMA) in 2014 identified 14 cases of morphine toxicity, including 4 deaths, in children 17 days to 6 years of age receiving codeine for relief of symptoms of upper respiratory tract infection (e.g., cough).

Because the risks of respiratory depression, misuse, abuse, addiction, overdosage, and death outweigh the potential benefit in pediatric patients, FDA states that antitussive agents containing opiates, including codeine, should *not* be used in pediatric patients younger than 18 years of age. In addition, use of codeine for the management of cough is *contraindicated* in children younger than 12 years of age. FDA is requiring inclusion of this warning against antitussive use of codeine in pediatric patients younger than 18 years of age and this contraindication to antitussive use of codeine in children younger than 12 years of age in the labeling of codeine-containing cough and cold preparations available by prescription; FDA also is considering additional regulatory action for fixed-combination codeine-containing cough and cold preparations available without a prescription in some states. FDA and EMA consider that cough and cold generally are self-limiting conditions and that evidence of codeine's efficacy in the management of these conditions in children is limited.

Serious adverse events, including deaths, also have been reported in children receiving codeine for management of pain. For additional information on precautions and contraindications associated with the use of codeine as an analgesic in pediatric patients, see Cautions: Pediatric Precautions in Codeine 28:08.08.

DRUG INTERACTIONS

Concomitant use of opiate agonists and benzodiazepines or other CNS depressants (e.g., anxiolytics, sedatives, hypnotics, tranquilizers, muscle relaxants, general anesthetics, antipsychotics, other opiate agonists, alcohol) may result in profound sedation, respiratory depression, coma, and death. Opiate agonist antitussives should be avoided in patients taking benzodiazepines, other CNS depressants, or alcohol. Concomitant use of opiate agonists with serotonergic drugs can cause serotonin syndrome. (See Drug Interactions in the Opiate Agonists General Statement 28:08.08.)

ACUTE TOXICITY

Toxic doses of codeine may produce exhilaration, excitement, seizures, delirium, hypotension, miosis, slow pulse, tachycardia, narcosis, flushed facies, tinnitus, lassitude, muscular weakness, and circulatory collapse or respiratory paralysis. Codeine should be discontinued if any of the aforementioned effects occur. Respiratory arrest, coma, and death have occurred in young children receiving oral codeine doses of 5–12 mg/kg. Severe respiratory depression resulting from acute toxicity may be reversed by administration of an opiate antagonist (i.e., naloxone hydrochloride).

PHARMACOLOGY

Codeine causes suppression of the cough reflex by a direct effect on the cough center in the medulla of the brain and appears to exert a drying effect on respiratory tract mucosa and to increase viscosity of bronchial secretions. On a weight basis, antitussive activity of codeine is less than that of morphine. Codeine also has mild analgesic and sedative effects.

PHARMACOKINETICS

Codeine is well absorbed from the GI tract. Following oral administration, peak antitussive effects usually occur within 1–2 hours and antitussive activity may persist for 4 hours. Codeine is distributed into milk.

Like other phenanthrene derivatives, codeine is metabolized in the liver. The drug undergoes O-demethylation (by cytochrome P-450 [CYP] isoenzyme 2D6), N-demethylation (by CYP3A4), and partial conjugation with glucuronic acid and is excreted in the urine as norcodeine and morphine in the free and conjugated forms. Negligible amounts of codeine and its metabolites are found in the feces.

Codeine is metabolized by the CYP microsomal enzyme system, principally by CYP3A4, and to a lesser extent by CYP2D6 (debrisoquine hydroxylase). Although the CYP2D6 isoenzyme accounts for only 10% of the metabolism of codeine, it plays an essential role in converting the drug to its active O-demethylated metabolite, morphine.

Pharmacogenomics: Metabolism of certain drugs, including codeine, is influenced by CYP2D6 polymorphism. Individuals who lack functional alleles of the CYP2D6 gene are described as poor metabolizers, those with one or two functional alleles are described as extensive metabolizers, and those who carry a duplicate or amplified gene are described as ultrarapid metabolizers. Genetically determined differences in drug metabolism can affect an individual's response to a drug or risk of having an adverse event. Individuals who are poor metabolizers experience no analgesic effects of codeine; individuals who are ultrarapid metabolizers are likely to have higher than expected serum concentrations of morphine.

Variations in CYP2D6 polymorphism occur at different frequencies among subpopulations of different ethnic or racial origin. Approximately 1–7% of Caucasians and 10–30% of Ethiopians and Saudi Arabians carry the genotype associated with ultra-rapid metabolism of CYP2D6 substrates.

CHEMISTRY AND STABILITY

● Chemistry

Codeine is a phenanthrene-derivative opiate agonist antitussive agent. Codeine occurs as colorless or white crystals or as a white, crystalline powder and is slightly soluble in water and freely soluble in alcohol. The phosphate and sulfate salts of codeine occur as white, needle-shaped crystals or white, crystalline powders. Codeine phosphate is freely soluble in water and slightly soluble in alcohol. Codeine sulfate is soluble in water and very slightly soluble in alcohol. Because of its greater water solubility, codeine phosphate is most frequently used for extemporaneous compounding.

● Stability

Codeine sulfate tablets should be stored in well-closed, light-resistant containers at a temperature less than 40°C, preferably between 15–30°C.

For further information on chemistry and stability, pharmacology, pharmacokinetics, uses, cautions, and dosage and administration of codeine, see 28:08.08. See also the Opiate Agonists General Statement 28:08.08.

PREPARATIONS

Codeine preparations are subject to control under the Federal Controlled Substances Act of 1970.

Excipients in commercially available drug preparations may have clinically important effects in some individuals; consult specific product labeling for details.

Codeine Phosphate

Crystal	
Powder	

Guaifenesin and Codeine Phosphate

Oral		
Solution	100 mg/5 mL Guaifenesin and Codeine Phosphate 6.3 mg/5 mL	RelCof-C® (C-V), Burel
		M-Clear® WC (C-V), R.A. McNeil
	100 mg/5 mL Guaifenesin and Codeine Phosphate 10 mg/5 mL*	Cheratussin® AC (C-V), Qualitest
		Guaiatussin® AC (C-V), Hi-Tech
		Guaifenesin AC Cough Syrup (C-V)
		Guaifenesin and Codeine Phosphate Oral Solution (C-V)
		Robafen® AC (C-V), Major
	200 mg/5 mL Guaifenesin and Codeine Phosphate 8 mg/5 mL	Codar® GF (C-V), Respa
	200 mg/5 mL Guaifenesin and Codeine Phosphate 10 mg/5 mL	Coditussin® AC (C-V), Glendale
	225 mg/5 mL Guaifenesin and Codeine Phosphate 7.5 mg/5 mL	Mar-Cof® CG (C-V), Marnel

Codeine phosphate is also commercially available in combination with other antihistamines, decongestants, and expectorants.

* available from one or more manufacturer, distributor, and/or repackager by generic (nonproprietary) name

Codeine Sulfate

Powder	

Oral		
Solution	30 mg/5 mL*	Codeine Sulfate Oral Solution (C-II)
Tablets	15 mg*	Codeine Sulfate Tablets (C-II)
	30 mg*	Codeine Sulfate Tablets (C-II)
	60 mg*	Codeine Sulfate Tablets (C-II)

* available from one or more manufacturer, distributor, and/or repackager by generic (nonproprietary) name

Selected Revisions November 5, 2018, © Copyright, January 1, 1973, American Society of Health-System Pharmacists, Inc.

Dextromethorphan
Dextromethorphan Hydrobromide

48:08 • ANTITUSSIVES

■ Dextromethorphan, a derivative of levorphanol, is an antitussive agent.

USES

Dextromethorphan is used for the temporary relief of coughs caused by minor throat and bronchial irritation such as may occur with common colds or with inhaled irritants. Dextromethorphan is most effective in the treatment of chronic, nonproductive cough. The drug is a common ingredient in commercial cough mixtures available without prescription.

Although cough and cold preparations that contain cough suppressants (including dextromethorphan), nasal decongestants, antihistamines, and/or expectorants commonly are used in pediatric patients younger than 2 years of age, systematic reviews of controlled trials have concluded that nonprescription (over-the-counter, OTC) cough and cold preparations are *not* more effective than placebo in reducing acute cough and other symptoms of upper respiratory tract infection in these patients. Furthermore, adverse events, including deaths, have been (and continue to be) reported in pediatric patients younger than 2 years of age receiving these preparations. (See Cautions: Pediatric Precautions and see Acute Toxicity: Manifestations.)

For information on abuse of dextromethorphan, see Cautions.

For use of dextromethorphan hydrobromide in fixed combination with quinidine sulfate in the treatment of pseudobulbar affect (PBA), see Dextromethorphan Hydrobromide and Quinidine Sulfate 28:92.

DOSAGE AND ADMINISTRATION

● Administration

Dextromethorphan preparations are administered orally. Lozenges containing dextromethorphan hydrobromide should not be used in children younger than 6 years of age and liquid-filled capsules containing the drug should not be used in children younger than 12 years of age, unless otherwise directed by a clinician.

● Dosage

Dosages of dextromethorphan hydrobromide and dextromethorphan polistirex are expressed in terms of dextromethorphan hydrobromide.

The usual dosage of dextromethorphan hydrobromide for adults and children 12 years of age or older is 10–20 mg every 4 hours or 30 mg every 6–8 hours, not to exceed 120 mg daily, or as directed by a clinician. The usual dosage for children 6 to younger than 12 years of age is 5–10 mg every 4 hours or 15 mg every 6–8 hours, not to exceed 60 mg daily, or as directed by a clinician. Children 2 to younger than 6 years of age may receive 2.5–5 mg every 4 hours or 7.5 mg every 6–8 hours, not to exceed 30 mg daily, or as directed by a clinician. Dosage in children younger than 2 years of age must be individualized. Suggested dosages for children younger than 2 years of age† for some cough and cold preparations have been published in various references for prescribing and parenting. Using recommended dosages for adults and older children, some clinicians have extrapolated dosages for these preparations based on the weight or age of children younger than 2 years of age. However, these extrapolations were based on assumptions that pathology of the disease and pharmacology of the drugs are similar in adults and pediatric patients. There currently are *no* specific dosage recommendations (i.e., approved by the US Food and Drug Administration [FDA]) for cough and cold preparations for this patient population. (See Cautions: Pediatric Precautions.)

The usual dosage of dextromethorphan hydrobromide as the extended-release oral suspension containing the polistirex for adults and children 12 years of age or

older is 60 mg twice daily. The usual dosage as the extended-release oral suspension for children 6 to younger than 12 years of age is 30 mg twice daily; children 2 to younger than 6 years of age may receive 15 mg twice daily.

CAUTIONS

Adverse effects with dextromethorphan are rare, but nausea and/or other GI disturbances, slight drowsiness, and dizziness sometimes occur. The drug produces no analgesia or addiction and little or no CNS depression.

● Abuse

Abuse and recreational use of dextromethorphan have been reported with nonprescription (over-the-counter [OTC]) dextromethorphan-containing preparations and with dextromethorphan powder sold illicitly. Dextromethorphan is a safe and effective cough suppressant with minimal adverse effects when used at recommended dosages; however, the drug can have euphoric, stimulant, and dissociative effects at higher dosages. Abuse of the drug for its euphoric and dissociative effects occurs mainly in adolescents.

While dextromethorphan abuse is not a new phenomenon, a more recent trend involving illicit sale of pure dextromethorphan powder that has been encapsulated and sold as a street drug has caused concern. There also has been an increasing trend in abuse of dextromethorphan-containing OTC preparations. One study that analyzed the trend in dextromethorphan abuse in California identified Coricidin® HBP® Cough and Cold tablets as the most commonly abused OTC product. Abuse of dextromethorphan can result in serious adverse events, including death. (See Acute Toxicity.) Fatalities have been reported in adolescents that were possibly associated with consumption of powdered dextromethorphan sold illicitly in capsules.

● Precautions and Contraindications

Administration of dextromethorphan may be associated with histamine release, and the drug should be used with caution in atopic children. Dextromethorphan also should be used with caution in sedated or debilitated patients and in patients confined to the supine position. Dextromethorphan should not be taken for persistent or chronic cough (e.g., with smoking, emphysema, asthma) or when coughing is accompanied by excessive secretions, unless directed by a clinician. If cough persists for longer than 1 week, tends to recur, or is accompanied by high fever, rash, or persistent headache, a clinician should be consulted.

Individuals with phenylketonuria (i.e., homozygous deficiency of phenylalanine hydroxylase) and other individuals who must restrict their intake of phenylalanine should be warned that some commercially available preparations of dextromethorphan contain aspartame (NutraSweet®), which is metabolized in the GI tract to phenylalanine following oral administration.

Because cases of apparent serotonin syndrome, including 2 fatalities, have been reported in patients receiving dextromethorphan and monoamine oxidase (MAO) inhibitors concomitantly, dextromethorphan preparations should not be used in patients receiving these drugs or for 2 weeks after discontinuing them. For detailed information on serotonin syndrome, including its management, see Drug Interactions: Drugs Associated with Serotonin Syndrome, in the Monoamine Oxidase Inhibitors General Statement 28:16.04.12.

● Pediatric Precautions

Despite the lack of efficacy in children younger than 2 years of age, dextromethorphan use in such children has continued, in some cases with other prescription and/or nonprescription (over-the-counter, OTC) cough and cold preparations containing other agents (e.g., antihistamines, expectorants, nasal decongestants). In a report published by the US Centers for Disease Control and Prevention (CDC), cough and cold preparations containing dextromethorphan, acetaminophen, carbinoxamine, doxylamine, and/or pseudoephedrine were determined by medical examiners or coroners to be the underlying cause of death in 3 infants 6 months of age or younger during 2005. The actual cause of death might have been overdosage of one drug, interaction of different drugs, an underlying medical condition, or a combination of drugs and underlying medical conditions. In addition, an estimated 1519 children younger than 2 years of age were treated in emergency departments in the US during 2004–2005 for adverse events, including overdoses, associated with cold and cough preparations. (See Acute Toxicity:

Manifestations; also see Cautions: Pediatric Precautions in Pseudoephedrine Hydrochloride 12:12.12.)

The dosages at which cough and cold preparations can cause illness or death in pediatric patients younger than 2 years of age are not known, and there are no specific dosage recommendations (i.e., approved by the US Food and Drug Administration [FDA]) for patients in this age group. (See Dosage and Administration: Dosage.) Because of the absence of dosage recommendations, limited published evidence of effectiveness, and risks for toxicity (including fatal overdosage), FDA stated that nonprescription cough and cold preparations should not be used in children younger than 2 years of age; the agency continues to assess safety and efficacy of these preparations in older children. Meanwhile, because children 2–3 years of age also are at increased risk of overdosage and toxicity, some manufacturers of oral nonprescription cough and cold preparations agreed to voluntarily revise the product labeling to state that such preparations should not be used in children younger than 4 years of age. FDA recommends that parents and caregivers adhere to the dosage instructions and warnings on the product labeling that accompanies the preparation if administering to children and consult with their clinician about any concerns. Clinicians should ask caregivers about use of nonprescription cough and cold preparations to avoid overdosage.

ACUTE TOXICITY

Dextromethorphan has a low order of toxicity, with the potential for toxic effects following acute overdosage being low. Although a few cases of toxicity and death have been reported, doses in excess of 100 times the usual adult dose have not been fatal.

● Manifestations

Manifestations following acute overdosage of dextromethorphan have included nausea, vomiting, drowsiness, dizziness, blurred vision, nystagmus, ataxia, shallow respiration, urinary retention, stupor, toxic psychosis, seizures, and coma. However, the presentation of dextromethorphan intoxication depends on the ingested dose. Manifestations of minimal intoxication include tachycardia, hypertension, vomiting, mydriasis, diaphoresis, nystagmus, euphoria, loss of motor coordination, and giggling/laughing. Manifestations of moderate intoxication include those associated with minimal intoxication, hallucinations, and a plodding ataxic gait ("zombie-like" walking). Severely intoxicated individuals may be agitated or somnolent.

From 1969–1981, the US Food and Drug Administration received 15 case reports of adverse reactions to dextromethorphan in children 1–10 years of age; these reactions included hallucinations, urticaria, nausea, insomnia, and hysteria, but no fatalities. Deaths that were possibly associated with consumption of powdered dextromethorphan (sold illicitly in capsules) have been reported in adolescents. Ataxia, facial edema, and urticaria occurred following acute ingestion of 225 mg of dextromethorphan in a 2-year-old child, and lateral nystagmus, ataxia, unstable gait, and excitability occurred in a 22-month-old child who ingested 360 mg of the drug. Lethargy, somnolence, ataxia, and nystagmus occurred in a 3-year-old who ingested 270 mg of the drug.

● Treatment

Treatment of dextromethorphan overdosage includes symptomatic and supportive measures. In one child, ataxia resolved rapidly following IV naloxone, and other neurologic manifestations resolved within 8 hours. In another child, manifestations of toxicity resolved following IV naloxone and oral administration of activated charcoal.

PHARMACOLOGY

Dextromethorphan retains only the antitussive activity of other morphinan derivatives. The drug is about equal to codeine in depressing the cough reflex and has no expectorant action. In therapeutic dosages, dextromethorphan does not inhibit ciliary activity.

PHARMACOKINETICS

Dextromethorphan is rapidly absorbed from the GI tract and exerts its antitussive effect in 15–30 minutes after oral administration. The duration of action is approximately 3–6 hours with conventional dosage forms.

CHEMISTRY AND STABILITY

● Chemistry

Dextromethorphan is an antitussive agent. Dextromethorphan is the methyl ether of the dextrorotatory form of levorphanol, an opiate analgesic. Dextromethorphan hydrobromide occurs as practically white crystals or crystalline powder and is sparingly soluble in water and freely soluble in alcohol.

● Stability

Dextromethorphan preparations should be stored in tight containers, and solutions and liquid-filled capsules containing dextromethorphan should be stored in tight, light-resistant containers.

Dextromethorphan is incompatible with penicillins, tetracyclines, salicylates, phenobarbital sodium, hydriodic acid, and high concentrations of sodium or potassium iodide.

PREPARATIONS

Excipients in commercially available drug preparations may have clinically important effects in some individuals; consult specific product labeling for details.

Dextromethorphan Hydrobromide

Oral

Capsules, liquid-filled	15 mg	Robitussin® Long-Acting CoughGels®, Pfizer
Lozenges	5 mg	Hold® DM, Ascher
	10 mg	Sucrets® DM Cough Formula, Insight
Solution	7.5 mg/5 mL*	Dextromethorphan Hydrobromide Solution
	10 mg/5 mL*	Dextromethorphan Hydrobromide Solution
		Vicks® 44 Custom Care Dry Cough, Procter & Gamble
	15 mg/5 mL*	Dextromethorphan Hydrobromide Solution

* available from one or more manufacturer, distributor, and/or repackager by generic (nonproprietary) name

Dextromethorphan Hydrobromide Combinations

Oral

Capsules, liquid-filled	10 mg with Acetaminophen 325 mg, Chlorpheniramine Maleate 2 mg, and Phenylephrine Hydrochloride 5 mg	Alka-Seltzer Plus® Cold & Cough Formula Liquid Gels®, Bayer Tylenol® Cold Multi-Symptom Nighttime Rapid Release Gels®, McNeil
	10 mg with Acetaminophen 325 mg, Doxylamine Succinate 6.25 mg, and Phenylephrine Hydrochloride 5 mg	Alka-Seltzer Plus® Night Cold Formula Liquid Gels®, Bayer
	10 mg with Acetaminophen 325 mg and Phenylephrine Hydrochloride 5 mg	Alka-Seltzer® Plus Day Cold Formula Liquid Gels®, Bayer Vicks® DayQuil® Cold & Flu Relief LiquiCaps®, Procter & Gamble
	15 mg with Acetaminophen 325 mg and Doxylamine Succinate 6.25 mg	Vicks® NyQuil® Cold & Flu Relief LiquiCaps®, Procter & Gamble
For solution	30 mg with Acetaminophen 1 g, Guaifenesin 400 mg, and Pseudoephedrine Hydrochloride 60 mg per packet	Theraflu® Max-D Severe Cold & Flu, Novartis

Kit	12 Tablets, film-coated, Acetaminophen 325 mg with Dextromethorphan Hydrobromide 10 mg and Phenylephrine Hydrochloride 5 mg (Comtrex® Daytime Caplets®)	**Comtrex® Cold & Cough Day-Night Maximum Strength Caplets®**, Novartis
	12 Tablets, film-coated, Acetaminophen 325 mg with Chlorpheniramine Maleate 2 mg, Dextromethorphan Hydrobromide 10 mg, and Phenylephrine Hydrochloride 5 mg (Comtrex® Nighttime Caplets®)	
Solution	3.3 mg/5 mL with Acetaminophen 108.3 mg/5 mL, Doxylamine Succinate 1.25 mg/5 mL, and Phenylephrine Hydrochloride 1.6 mg/5 mL	**Tylenol® Cold Multi-Symptom Nighttime**, McNeil
	3.3 mg/5 mL with Acetaminophen 108.3 mg/5 mL, Guaifenesin 66.6 mg/5 mL, and Phenylephrine Hydrochloride 1.6 mg/5 mL	**Tylenol® Cold Multi-Symptom Severe**, McNeil **Tylenol® Cold & Flu Severe**, McNeil
	3.3 mg/5 mL with Acetaminophen 108.3 mg/5 mL and Phenylephrine Hydrochloride 1.6 mg/5 mL	**Tylenol® Cold Multi-Symptom Daytime**, McNeil **Vicks® DayQuil® Cold & Flu Relief**, Procter & Gamble
	5 mg/5 mL with Acetaminophen 108.3 mg/5 mL and Doxylamine Succinate 2.08 mg/5 mL	**Vicks® NyQuil® Cold & Flu Relief**, Procter & Gamble
	5 mg/5 mL with Acetaminophen 160 mg/5 mL	**Children's Tylenol® Plus Cough & Sore Throat**, Prestige Brands **Triaminic® Cough and Sore Throat**, Novartis
	5 mg/5 mL with Acetaminophen 160 mg/5 mL and Chlorpheniramine Maleate 1 mg/5 mL	**Children's Tylenol® Plus Cough & Runny Nose**, McNeil
	5 mg/5 mL with Acetaminophen 160 mg/5 mL, Chlorpheniramine Maleate 1 mg/5 mL, and Phenylephrine Hydrochloride 2.5 mg/5 mL	**Children's Dimetapp® Multi-Symptom Cold & Flu**, Pfizer **Children's Tylenol® Plus Flu**, McNeil
	5 mg/5 mL with Acetaminophen 166.6 mg/5 mL	**Tylenol® Cold & Cough Daytime**, McNeil
	5 mg/5 mL with Acetaminophen 166.6 mg/5 mL and Doxylamine Succinate 2.08 mg/5 mL	**Tylenol® Cold & Cough Nighttime**, McNeil
	5 mg/5 mL with Brompheniramine Maleate 1 mg/5 mL and Phenylephrine Hydrochloride 2.5 mg/5 mL	**Children's Dimetapp® Cold & Cough**, Pfizer
	5 mg/5 mL with Chlorpheniramine Maleate 0.67 mg/5 mL	**Children's Vicks® NyQuil® Cold/Cough**, Procter & Gamble
	5 mg/5 mL with Chlorpheniramine Maleate 1 mg/5 mL and Pseudoephedrine Hydrochloride 15 mg/5 mL	**Kidkare® Cough & Cold Liquid**, Watson
	5 mg/5 mL with Doxylamine Succinate 2.08 mg/5 mL	**Vicks® NyQuil® Cough**, Procter & Gamble
	5 mg/5 mL with Guaifenesin 50 mg/5 mL and Phenylephrine Hydrochloride 2.5 mg/5 mL	**Robitussin® Children's Cough & Cold CF**, Pfizer
	5 mg/5 mL with Guaifenesin 100 mg/5 mL	**Pediacare® Cough & Congestion**, Prestige Brands

	5 mg/5 mL with Phenylephrine Hydrochloride 2.5 mg/5 mL	**Children's Sudafed PE® Cold & Cough**, McNeil **Pediacare® Multi-Symptom Cold**, Prestige Brands **Triaminic® Daytime Cold & Cough**, Novartis
	6.7 mg/5 mL with Guaifenesin 66.7 mg/5 mL	**Vicks® Formula 44® Custom Care Chesty Cough**, Procter & Gamble
	7.5 mg/5 mL with Acetaminophen 160 mg/5 mL and Chlorpheniramine Maleate 1 mg/5 mL	**Triaminic® Multi-Symptom Fever**, Novartis
	10 mg/5 mL with Acetaminophen 216.7 mg/5 mL and Chlorpheniramine Maleate 1.3 mg/5 mL	**Vicks® Formula 44® Custom Care Cough & Cold PM**, Procter & Gamble
	10 mg/5 mL with Guaifenesin 100 mg/5 mL*	**Cheracol D® Cough Formula**, Lee **Dextromethorphan Hydrobromide with Guaifenesin Syrup** **Diabetic Tussin® DM**, Health Care Products **Guiatuss DM®**, Goldline **Robitussin® Peak Cold Cough + Chest Congestion DM**, Pfizer **Robitussin® Sugar-Free Cough + Chest Congestion DM**, Pfizer
	10 mg/5 mL with Guaifenesin 100 mg/5 mL and Phenylephrine Hydrochloride 5 mg/5 mL*	**Robitussin® Peak Cold Multi-Symptom Cold®**, Pfizer
	10 mg/5 mL with Guaifenesin 200 mg/5 mL	**Diabetic Tussin® DM Maximum Strength**, Health Care Products **Robitussin® Maximum Strength Cough + Chest Congestion**, Pfizer **Robitussin® Peak Cold Maximum Strength Cough + Chest Congestion**, Pfizer
	15 mg/5 mL with Guaifenesin 100 mg/5 mL*	**Safe Tussin®**, Kramer
	15 mg/5 mL with Promethazine Hydrochloride 6.25 mg/5 mL*	**Promethazine Hydrochloride with Dextromethorphan Hydrobromide Cough Syrup**
	5 mg/mL with Guaifenesin 50 mg/mL and Phenylephrine Hydrochloride 2.5 mg/mL	**Suppress® DX Pediatric Drops**, Kramer Novis
Suspension	5 mg/5 mL with Acetaminophen 160 mg/5 mL	**Pediacare® Fever Reducer Plus Cough & Sore Throat**, Prestige Brands
	5 mg/5 mL with Acetaminophen 160 mg/5 mL and Chlorpheniramine Maleate 1 mg/5 mL	**Pediacare® Fever Reducer Plus Cough & Runny Nose**, Prestige Brands
	5 mg/5 mL with Acetaminophen 160 mg/5 mL, Chlorpheniramine Maleate 1 mg/5 mL, and Phenylephrine Hydrochloride 2.5 mg/5 mL	**Children's Tylenol® Plus Multi-Symptom Cold**, McNeil **Pediacare® Fever Reducer Plus Multi-Symptom Cold**, Prestige Brands **Pediacare® Fever Reducer Plus Flu**, Prestige Brands

	5 mg/5 mL with Acetaminophen 160 mg/5 mL and Phenylephrine Hydrochloride 2.5 mg/5 mL	**Pediacare® Fever Reducer Plus Cold & Cough**, Prestige Brands
Tablets	10 mg with Acetaminophen 325 mg, Guaifenesin 200 mg, and Phenylephrine Hydrochloride 5 mg	**Tylenol® Cold & Flu Severe**, McNeil
		Tylenol® Cold Head Congestion Severe, McNeil
	10 mg with Acetaminophen 325 mg and Phenylephrine Hydrochloride 5 mg	**Tylenol® Cold Multi-Symptom Daytime**, McNeil
	10 mg with Acetaminophen 325 mg and Phenylephrine Hydrochloride 15 mg	**Comtrex® Cold & Cough Multi-Symptom Relief Maximum Strength Tablets**, Novartis
	30 mg with Chlorpheniramine Maleate 4 mg	**Coricidin® HBP® Cough & Cold**, Schering-Plough
Tablets, chewable	10 mg with Chlorpheniramine Maleate 2 mg and Pseudoephedrine Hydrochloride 30 mg	**Dicel® DM**, Centrix
Tablets, extended-release	15 mg with Acetaminophen 500 mg and Chlorpheniramine Maleate 2 mg	**Coricidin® HBP® Flu Maximum Strength**, Schering-Plough
	30 mg with Guaifenesin 600 mg	**Mucinex® DM**, Reckitt Benckiser
	60 mg with Guaifenesin 1200 mg	**Maximum Strength Mucinex® DM**, Reckitt Benckiser

Tablets, film-coated	10 mg with Acetaminophen 325 mg, Chlorpheniramine Maleate 2 mg, and Phenylephrine Hydrochloride 5 mg	**Theraflu® Warming Relief Nighttime Multi-Symptom Cold**, Novartis
	10 mg with Acetaminophen 325 mg and Phenylephrine Hydrochloride 5 mg	**Comtrex® Non-Drowsy Maximum Strength Caplets®**, Novartis
		Theraflu® Warming Relief Daytime Multi-Symptom Cold, Novartis
		Tylenol® Cold Multi-Symptom Daytime, McNeil
	15 mg with Acetaminophen 325 mg, Guaifenesin 200 mg, and Phenylephrine Hydrochloride 5 mg	**Tylenol® Cold Head Congestion Severe**, McNeil

Dextromethorphan hydrobromide is also commercially available in combination with analgesic-antipyretics, antihistamines, and decongestants.

* available from one or more manufacturer, distributor, and/or repackager by generic (nonproprietary) name

Dextromethorphan Polistirex

Oral

| **Suspension, extended-release** | equivalent to Dextromethorphan Hydrobromide 30 mg/5 mL | **Delsym®**, Reckitt Benckiser |

† Use is not currently included in the labeling approved by the US Food and Drug Administration.

Selected Revisions February 1, 2016, © Copyright, April 1, 1961, American Society of Health-System Pharmacists, Inc.

HYDROcodone Bitartrate

48:08 • ANTITUSSIVES

■ Hydrocodone bitartrate is a phenanthrene-derivative opiate agonist antitussive and analgesic agent.

REMS

FDA approved a REMS for hydrocodone to ensure that the benefits outweigh the risks. The REMS may apply to one or more preparations of hydrocodone and consists of the following: medication guide and elements to assure safe use. See the FDA REMS page (https://www.accessdata.fda.gov/scripts/cder/rems/index.cfm).

USES

● Cough

Hydrocodone bitartrate and hydrocodone polistirex are used in combination with other antitussives or expectorants for the symptomatic relief of nonproductive cough. Since the cough reflex may be a useful physiologic mechanism that clears the respiratory passages of foreign material and excess secretions and may aid in preventing or reversing atelectasis, cough suppressants should not be used indiscriminately.

Antitussives containing hydrocodone should *not* be used in patients younger than 18 years of age. (See Cautions: Pediatric Precautions.)

● Pain

For use of hydrocodone as an analgesic agent, see 28:08.08.

DOSAGE AND ADMINISTRATION

● Administration

Hydrocodone bitartrate and hydrocodone polistirex are administered orally.

When the extended-release oral suspension containing hydrocodone polistirex and chlorpheniramine polistirex (e.g., Tussionex® Pennkinetic®) is used, patients and caregivers should be strongly advised to use an accurate, calibrated dosing device to measure doses of the suspension. Use of a household teaspoon as a measuring device could result in overdosage. The extended-release oral suspension should not be diluted with other liquids or mixed with other drugs, since this may alter resin binding, thereby altering the rate of hydrocodone absorption and possibly resulting in toxicity. The extended-release oral suspension should not be given more frequently than every 12 hours; if cough is not controlled, the clinician should be contacted. The extended-release oral suspension should be shaken well before each use.

● Dosage

Cough

Hydrocodone bitartrate and hydrocodone polistirex are currently commercially available only in combination products. Dosage of hydrocodone polistirex is expressed in terms of hydrocodone bitartrate.

Hydrocodone preparations should be given in the smallest effective dose and as infrequently as possible to minimize the development of tolerance and physical dependence. Reduced dosage is indicated in debilitated or poor-risk patients and in very old patients.

The recommended adult antitussive dosage of hydrocodone bitartrate conventional (immediate-release) preparations is 5 mg every 4–6 hours as needed, not to exceed 30 mg in a 24-hour period. However, recommended and maximum dosages of other drugs included in the combination preparations must be considered and may further limit the maximum hydrocodone bitartrate dosage given in a 24-hour period.

In adults, the usual antitussive dosage of hydrocodone bitartrate using the extended-release oral suspension containing hydrocodone polistirex and chlorpheniramine polistirex (e.g., Tussionex® Pennkinetic®) is 10 mg (5 mL) every 12 hours; the dosage should not exceed 20 mg (10 mL) daily.

CAUTIONS

● Adverse Effects

Adverse reactions occur infrequently with usual oral antitussive doses of hydrocodone. The most common adverse effects of hydrocodone are lightheadedness, dizziness, sedation, nausea, and vomiting. These adverse effects appear to be more prominent in ambulatory patients than in nonambulatory patients, and some of these effects may be alleviated if the patient lies down. Other adverse effects include constipation, rash, pruritus, euphoria, and dysphoria.

● Precautions and Contraindications

Hydrocodone shares the toxic potentials of the opiate agonists, and the usual precautions of opiate agonist therapy should be observed. (See Cautions in the Opiate Agonists General Statement 28:08.08.)

Because concomitant use of opiate agonists and benzodiazepines or other CNS depressants may result in profound sedation, respiratory depression, coma, and death, opiate antitussives should be *avoided* in patients receiving CNS depressants. (See Drug Interactions.) Patients receiving hydrocodone should be apprised of the risks associated with concomitant therapeutic or illicit use of benzodiazepines, alcohol, or other CNS depressants.

In patients with asthma or pulmonary emphysema, indiscriminate use of antitussives may precipitate respiratory insufficiency resulting from increased viscosity of bronchial secretions and suppression of the cough reflex. Tolerance and physical dependence may occur following prolonged administration of hydrocodone preparations.

Patients should be warned that hydrocodone may impair their ability to perform activities requiring mental alertness or physical coordination (e.g., operating machinery, driving a motor vehicle).

As with other opiate agonist antitussives, hydrocodone may cause respiratory depression in large doses, when given more frequently than recommended, or in sensitive patients; this effect seldom occurs with usual oral doses. Overdosage and toxicity (including fatal respiratory depression) have been reported in adults and children receiving hydrocodone. (See Cautions: Pediatric Precautions.) Patients should be advised to immediately seek medical attention if they have trouble breathing, slow heartbeat, severe sleepiness, dizziness, confusion, or cold, clammy skin. Severe respiratory depression resulting from acute toxicity may be reversed by administration of an opiate antagonist (e.g., naloxone hydrochloride).

Hydrocodone should be used with caution in geriatric or debilitated patients and in those with hypothyroidism, Addison's disease, prostatic hypertrophy, urethral stricture, pulmonary disease, or severe renal or hepatic impairment. Hydrocodone also should be used with caution in patients with head injury, other intracranial lesions, or preexisting increased intracranial pressure, since opiate agonists may increase CSF pressure and markedly exaggerate these conditions; in addition, adverse CNS effects of the drug may obscure the clinical course of the underlying condition. The drug should also be used with caution in patients who have undergone thoracotomies or laparotomies, since suppression of the cough reflex may lead to retention of secretions postoperatively in these patients.

Hydrocodone may obscure the diagnosis or clinical course in patients with acute abdominal conditions.

Long-term use of hydrocodone may result in obstructive bowel disease, especially in patients with an underlying intestinal motility disorder.

Hydrocodone is contraindicated in patients who are hypersensitive to the drug or any ingredient in the formulation.

● Pediatric Precautions

Because the risks of respiratory depression, misuse, abuse, addiction, overdosage, and death outweigh the potential benefit in pediatric patients, FDA states that antitussive agents containing opiates, including hydrocodone, should *not* be used in pediatric patients younger than 18 years of age. In addition, use of hydrocodone for the management of cough and cold is *contraindicated* in children younger than 6 years of age.

● Geriatric Precautions

Clinical studies of hydrocodone polistirex and chlorpheniramine polistirex extended-release suspension did not include sufficient numbers of patients 65 years of age and older to determine whether they respond differently than younger adults.

While other clinical experience generally has not revealed age-related differences in safety or response to the drug, care should be taken in dosage selection in geriatric patients. Because of the greater frequency of decreased hepatic, renal, and/or cardiac function and of concomitant disease and drug therapy in geriatric patients, the manufacturer suggests that patients in this age group receive initial dosages of this preparation in the lower end of the usual range.

Hydrocodone is substantially eliminated in urine and the risk of toxicity may be increased in patients with impaired renal function. Because geriatric patients are more likely to have decreased renal function, caution should be used when selecting dosages for such patients and monitoring of renal function should be considered.

● Pregnancy, Fertility, and Lactation

Pregnancy

Safe use of hydrocodone during pregnancy has not been established; therefore, the drug should not be administered to pregnant women unless the possible benefits outweigh the potential risks.

Lactation

It is not known whether hydrocodone is distributed into human milk. A decision should be made to discontinue nursing or the drug, taking into account the importance of the drug to the woman.

DRUG INTERACTIONS

Concomitant use of opiate agonists and benzodiazepines or other CNS depressants (e.g., anxiolytics, sedatives, hypnotics, tranquilizers, muscle relaxants, general anesthetics, antipsychotics, other opiate agonists, alcohol) may result in profound sedation, respiratory depression, coma, and death. Opiate agonist antitussives should be avoided in patients taking benzodiazepines, other CNS depressants, or alcohol. Concurrent use of anticholinergic agents with hydrocodone may produce paralytic ileus. Concomitant use of opiate agonists with serotonergic drugs can cause serotonin syndrome. (See Drug Interactions in the Opiate Agonists General Statement 28:08.08.)

PHARMACOLOGY

Hydrocodone causes suppression of the cough reflex by a direct effect on the cough center in the medulla of the brain. The drug also appears to exert a drying effect on respiratory tract mucosa and to increase viscosity of bronchial secretions. On a weight basis, antitussive activity of hydrocodone is slightly greater than that of codeine. At equivalent therapeutic doses, hydrocodone is more sedating than codeine. The constipating effect of hydrocodone is less than that of morphine and not greater than that of codeine.

PHARMACOKINETICS

Hydrocodone is well absorbed from the GI tract. Following oral administration of a single 10-mg dose of hydrocodone to adult males in one study, a mean peak serum hydrocodone concentration of 23.6 ng/mL occurred after 1.3 hours. Following oral administration, antitussive action is maintained for 4–6 hours. Following multiple doses of the extended-release oral suspension containing hydrocodone polistirex and chlorpheniramine polistirex (Tussionex® Pennkinetic®), a mean peak plasma hydrocodone concentration of 22.8 ng/mL occurred after 3.4 hours.

The elimination half-life of hydrocodone is reportedly about 3.8 hours in healthy adults. Like other phenanthrene derivatives, hydrocodone is probably metabolized in the liver and excreted mainly in urine. Metabolism of hydrocodone includes O-demethylation, N-demethylation, and 6-keto reduction.

CHEMISTRY AND STABILITY

● Chemistry

Hydrocodone bitartrate is a phenanthrene-derivative opiate agonist that is used as an antitussive and analgesic agent. Hydrocodone is a hydrogenated ketone derivative of codeine. Hydrocodone bitartrate occurs as fine, white crystals or crystalline

powder and is soluble in water and slightly soluble in alcohol. Hydrocodone polistirex consists of hydrocodone with a cation-exchange resin copolymer complex of sulfonated styrene-divinylbenzene. Hydrocodone bitartrate and hydrocodone polistirex are currently commercially available only in combination products.

● Stability

Hydrocodone bitartrate is affected by light. Hydrocodone bitartrate preparations should be stored in tight, light-resistant containers at 15–30°C.

For further information on the chemistry, pharmacology, pharmacokinetics, uses, cautions, chronic toxicity, acute toxicity, and dosage and administration of hydrocodone bitartrate, see the Opiate Agonists General Statement 28:08.08 and Hydrocodone Bitartrate 28:08.08.

PREPARATIONS

Fixed-combination preparations containing hydrocodone in a concentration of 15 mg or less per dosage unit or 5 mL combined with a therapeutic amount of one or more nonopiate drugs or with a fourfold or greater quantity of isoquinolone opium alkaloid previously were subject to control under the Federal Controlled Substances Act of 1970 as schedule III (C-III) drugs. However, because of increasing concerns about misuse, abuse, and diversion, these preparations have been rescheduled and, effective October 6, 2014, are subject to control as schedule II (C-II) drugs. For additional information on the rescheduling of hydrocodone preparations, see Cautions: Misuse and Abuse, in Hydrocodone Bitartrate 28:08.08.

Excipients in commercially available drug preparations may have clinically important effects in some individuals; consult specific product labeling for details.

HYDROcodone Bitartrate Combinations

Oral		
Solution	5 mg/5 mL with Chlorpheniramine Maleate 4 mg/5 mL	Vituz® (C-II), Hawthorn
	5 mg/5 mL with Chlorpheniramine Maleate 4 mg/5 mL and Pseudoephedrine Hydrochloride 60 mg/5 mL*	HYDROcodone Bitartrate, Chlorpheniramine Maleate, and Pseudoephedrine Hydrochloride Oral Solution (C-II)
		Zutripro® (C-II), Hawthorn
	5 mg/5 mL with Homatropine Methylbromide 1.5 mg/5 mL*	HYDROcodone Bitartrate and Homatropine Methylbromide Syrup (C-II)
		Hydromet® Syrup (C-II), Actavis
	5 mg/5 mL with Pseudoephedrine Hydrochloride 60 mg/5 mL*	HYDROcodone Bitartrate and Pseudoephedrine Hydrochloride Oral Solution (C-II)
		Rezira® (C-II), Hawthorn
Tablets	5 mg with Homatropine Methylbromide 1.5 mg*	HYDROcodone Bitartrate and Homatropine Methylbromide Tablets (C-II)
		Tussigon® (C-II; scored), Pfizer

* available from one or more manufacturer, distributor, and/or repackager by generic (nonproprietary) name

HYDROcodone Polistirex Combinations

Oral		
Suspension, extended-release	equivalent to HYDROcodone Bitartrate 10 mg/5 mL with Chlorpheniramine Polistirex equivalent to Chlorpheniramine Maleate 8 mg/5 mL*	HYDROcodone Polistirex and Chlorpheniramine Polistirex Extended-Release Suspension (C-II)
		Tussionex® Pennkinetic® (C-II), UCB

* available from one or more manufacturer, distributor, and/or repackager by generic (nonproprietary) name

Selected Revisions November 19, 2018, © Copyright, January 1, 1973, American Society of Health-System Pharmacists, Inc.

Canakinumab

48:10.20 • INTERLEUKIN ANTAGONISTS

■ Canakinumab, a recombinant human anti-human interleukin-1 beta (IL-1β) monoclonal antibody, is an IL-1β blocker.

USES

● Periodic Fever Syndromes

Canakinumab is used for the management of periodic fever syndromes including cryopyrin-associated periodic syndromes (CAPS), such as familial cold autoinflammatory syndrome (FCAS) and Muckle-Wells syndrome (MWS), in adults and children ≥4 years of age.

Canakinumab is also used for the following periodic fever syndromes: tumor necrosis factor receptor associated periodic syndrome (TRAPS), hyperimmunoglobulin D syndrome (HIDS)/mevalonate kinase deficiency (MKD), and familial Mediterranean fever (FMF), in adult and pediatric patients.

Canakinumab is designated an orphan drug by the US FDA for use in these conditions.

Clinical Experience

Cryopyrin-associated Periodic Syndromes

Safety and efficacy of canakinumab in the treatment of CAPS have been evaluated in a randomized, double-blind, placebo-controlled study with 3 parts conducted sequentially in 35 adults and children with MWS. Patients in this study were 9–74 years of age, had genetic evidence of NLRP-3 (nucleotide-binding domain, leucine rich family [NLR], pyrin domain containing 3; also known as cold-induced autoinflammatory syndrome-1 [CIAS1]) gene mutation, and had the MWS phenotype of CAPS. Part 1 of the study was an 8-week open-label period during which all 35 patients received a single dose of canakinumab. Patients who achieved a complete clinical response during part 1 and did not relapse by week 8 were randomized into part 2 of the study, a 24-week randomized, double-blind, placebo-controlled withdrawal period. Patients who completed part 2 or experienced a disease flare entered part 3 of the study, a 16-week open-label active treatment phase.

Complete response to treatment was defined as ratings of minimal or better for physician's assessment of global disease activity and assessment of skin disease and serum concentrations of C-reactive protein (CRP) and serum amyloid A (SAA) <10 mg/L. Disease flare was defined as CRP and/or SAA concentrations exceeding 30 mg/L and either a score of mild or worse for physician's assessment of disease activity or a score of minimal or worse for physician's assessment of disease activity and assessment of skin disease.

The rate of complete clinical response in part 1 of the study, with all patients receiving a single dose of canakinumab, was 71% at 1 week and 97% by week 8. Serum CRP and SAA concentrations normalized within 8 days of treatment initiation in most patients. During part 2 of the study, the randomized withdrawal period, disease flare occurred in 81% of the 16 patients receiving placebo and in none of the 15 patients receiving canakinumab. All 15 patients receiving canakinumab (compared with 25% of patients receiving placebo) had absent or minimal disease activity at the end of part 2 of the study.

During part 2 of the study, serum CRP and SAA concentrations returned to abnormal values in patients receiving placebo and returned to normal after reintroduction of canakinumab in part 3; normal values for these markers were sustained throughout the study in patients who received uninterrupted treatment with canakinumab. Clinical and biochemical remission of CAPS was sustained in 97% of the 29 patients who completed part 3 of the study. Safety and efficacy of canakinumab in the treatment of CAPS also were evaluated in an open-label study in patients 4–74 years of age with MWS or FCAS. Treatment with canakinumab was associated with clinically important improvement in signs and symptoms of CAPS and normalization of serum CRP and SAA concentrations in most patients within 1 week.

Tumor Necrosis Factor Receptor Associated Periodic Syndrome, Hyperimmunoglobulin D Syndrome/Mevalonate Kinase Deficiency, and Familial Mediterranean Fever

Canakinumab was studied for the treatment of TRAPS, HIDS/MKD, and FMF in a multi-part study that consisted of the 3 disease cohorts with a total of 185 patients (CLUSTER). Part 1 of the study was a 12-week screening period to determine the disease-flare onset. Patients were 2–76 years of age and were randomized into a double-blind, placebo-controlled treatment over 16 weeks. Patients received either canakinumab 150 mg (in patients weighing >40 kg) or 2 mg/kg (in patients weighing ≤40 kg) subcutaneously or placebo every 4 weeks. An additional dose of canakinumab 150 mg (in patients weighing >40 kg) or 2 mg/kg (in patients weighing ≤40 kg) was provided to patients with a persistent flare (Physician's Global Assessment [PGA] ≥2 or C-reactive protein [CRP] >10 mg/L with <40% reduction from baseline) or those who did not experience resolution of their disease flare from day 8–14. Another dose of canakinumab 150 mg (in patients weighing >40 kg) or 2 mg/kg (in patients weighing ≤40 kg) was provided to patients with persistent disease activity or for those who did not experience resolution of their disease flare from day 15–28, defined as PGA ≥2 or CRP ≥10 mg/L and no reduction by at least 70% from baseline. Patients with PGA ≥2 or CRP ≥30 mg/L on or after day 29 were also up-titrated; patients who were up-titrated remained at the higher dose of 300 mg (>40 kg) or 4 mg/kg (≤40 kg).

The primary endpoint was the proportion of complete responders, defined as the patients who experienced resolution of index disease flare at day 15 without a new disease flare during the rest of the study period. Resolution was defined as a PGA Disease Activity score <2 and CRP ≤10 mg/L or a reduction ≥70% from baseline. A PGA score ≥2 and CRP ≥30 mg/L was considered a new flare. Patients who required a dose escalation, who changed from placebo to canakinumab, or who discontinued were classified as nonresponders. The efficacy of canakinumab was evaluated in 3 separate cohorts described below.

In the TRAPS cohort of the CLUSTER trial (N=46), median age was 15.5 years (range, 2–76 years), 57.8% did not have fever at baseline, and patients had 6 flares per year (median, 9 flares) with a PGA ≥2 and CRP >10 mg/L (median, 112.5 mg/L). Half of patients randomized to canakinumab 150 mg every 4 weeks were up-titrated to 300 mg every 4 weeks; 87.5% (21 of 24) of patients were crossed over from placebo to canakinumab. The proportion of patients who resolved their index disease flare at day 15 without a new flare over the 16-week treatment period was higher with canakinumab compared to placebo in the TRAPS cohort (45.5 vs 8.3%).

In the HIDS/MKD cohort of the CLUSTER trial (N=72), median age was 11 years (range, 2–47 years), 41.7% did not have fever at baseline and had a history of ≥3 febrile acute flares within 6 months (median per year, 12), with a PGA ≥2 and CRP >10 mg/L (median 113.5 mg/L). Of the patients who were randomized to canakinumab 150 mg every 4 weeks, 51.4% were up-titrated to 300 mg every 4 weeks; in addition, 88.6% of patients were crossed over from placebo to canakinumab. The proportion of patients who resolved their index disease flare at day 15 without a new flare was higher with canakinumab compared to placebo in the HIDS/MKD cohort (35.1 vs 5.7%) over the 16-week treatment period. Long-term studies found canakinumab effective for patients with HIDS/MKD over an additional 72 weeks.

In the FMF cohort of the CLUSTER trial (N=63), median age was 18 years (range, 2–69 years), 76.2% did not have fever at baseline, and patients had active disease despite colchicine treatment or were intolerant to colchicine treatment. Active disease was defined as at least 1 flare per month (median per year, 18) and CRP >10 mg/L (median, 94 mg/L). Colchicine could be continued without changes and 55 of 63 patients continued colchicine after randomization. Of the patients who were randomized to canakinumab 150 mg every 4 weeks, 32.3% were up-titrated to 300 mg every 4 weeks; 84.4% of placebo recipients were crossed over to canakinumab. The proportion of patients who resolved their index disease flare at day 15 without a new flare over the 16-week treatment period was higher with canakinumab compared to placebo for FMF (61.3 vs 6.2%). Long-term studies found canakinumab effective for patients with FMF over an additional 72 weeks.

Clinical Perspective

An American Academy of Allergy, Asthma, and Immunology (AAAAI) and American College of Allergy, Asthma, and Immunology (ACAAI) practice parameter includes recommendations for the management of CAPS, FMF,

TRAPS, and HIDS/MKD. This practice parameter recommends use of interleukin (IL)-1 inhibitors, including anakinra, rilonacept, and canakinumab, for patients with CAPS. Colchicine is the recommended mainstay of therapy for FMF; however, IL-1 inhibitors have been successful in patients who are unresponsive to colchicine therapy. Recommended therapies for TRAPS include corticosteroids, TNF-blocking agents, and IL-1 inhibitors. For the management of HIDS/MKD, therapeutic trials of corticosteroids and inflammatory cytokine inhibitors should be undertaken; most reports indicate a significant beneficial effect from TNF-α and IL-1ß inhibitors.

● Still's Disease

Canakinumab is used for the treatment of active Still's disease, including adult-onset Still's disease (AOSD) and systemic juvenile idiopathic arthritis (SJIA), in patients ≥2 years of age. Canakinumab is designated an orphan drug by the FDA for use in these conditions.

Clinical Experience

Canakinumab was studied for the treatment of active SJIA in two phase 3 studies (SJIA study 1 and SJIA study 2). These studies included patients between 2–19 years of age with a confirmed diagnosis of SJIA at least 2 months prior to study enrollment. Active disease was defined as ≥2 joints with active arthritis, intermittent spiking fever (body temperature >38°C), and CRP >30 mg/L. Stable doses of methotrexate, corticosteroids, and/or nonsteroid anti-inflammatory agents (NSAIAs) were continued; only corticosteroids could be tapered. At baseline, patients had a mean age of 8.5 years, mean disease duration of 3.5 years, mean number of active joints of 15.4, and mean CRP of 200.5 mg/L.

The SJIA study 1 was a randomized, double-blind, single-dose study in 84 patients evaluating the efficacy of canakinumab 4 mg/kg subcutaneously (n=43) compared to placebo (n=41). The primary endpoint was the proportion of patients who achieved at least 30% improvement in American College of Rheumatology (ACR30) response and absence of fever (defined as ≥38°C) in the previous 7 days at day 15. The ACR30 responses with canakinumab and placebo were 84% and 10% at day 15, respectively, and 81% and 10% at day 29. Results were consistent for both ACR50 and ACR70 responses each at day 15 and day 29. The patient pain score (0–100 mm visual analogue scale) decreased 50 mm with canakinumab and increased by 4.5 mm with placebo at day 15, which was consistent at day 29. No patients treated with canakinumab experienced fever at day 3, compared to 87% of patients treated with placebo.

The SJIA study 2 was a randomized, double-blind, placebo-controlled, withdrawal study evaluating the prevention of flare with canakinumab. Flare was defined as worsening of ≥30% in at least 3 of 6 Pediatric ACR response variables, plus improvement of ≥30% in no more than 1 of 6 variables, or reappearance of fever (not due to infection) over at least 2 consecutive days. In part 1, 177 patients received canakinumab 4 mg/kg subcutaneously every 4 weeks; 100 patients continued to part 2 to receive canakinumab 4 mg/kg or placebo subcutaneously every 4 weeks. Corticosteroid tapering was permitted from week 9 through week 28 if there was at least an adapted JIA ACR 50 response (indicating the absence of fever and an improvement of ≥50% in at least 3 of the 6 core criteria for JIA, with a worsening of >30% in no more than one of the criteria) Of 92 patients who attempted corticosteroid tapering, 62% successfully tapered the dose and 46% discontinued the corticosteroid. In part 2 of the study, the probability of a flare was lower with canakinumab compared to placebo. Canakinumab was also effective for up to 5 years in the long-term extension study. Tapering canakinumab after clinical remission was possible in 33% of 75 patients, all of whom maintained clinical remission for at least 24 weeks.

The efficacy of canakinumab in patients with AOSD was based on pharmacokinetic exposure and extrapolation of efficacy data in patients with SJIA. In addition, a randomized, double-blind, placebo-controlled study of 36 patients (22–70 years of age) found consistent efficacy data compared to the pooled efficacy analysis of SJIA patients.

Clinical Perspective

The American College of Rheumatology published a guideline for the treatment of juvenile idiopathic arthritis. In patients without macrophage activation syndrome, the guideline conditionally recommends NSAIAs, IL-1 inhibitors, and IL-6 inhibitors as initial therapy. The guideline also strongly recommends IL-1 inhibitors and IL-6 inhibitors over conventional synthetic disease-modifying antirheumatic drugs in those without a response or with intolerance to NSAIAs or glucocorticoids. In patients with macrophage activation syndrome, IL-1 inhibitors and IL-6 inhibitors are conditionally recommended over calcineurin inhibitors alone; glucocorticoids are also conditionally recommended as initial treatment. For treatment of AOSD, some experts state that corticosteroids are considered first-line treatment, and refractory disease may be treated with IL-1 inhibitors (e.g., anakinra, canakinumab, rilonacept), IL-6 inhibitors (e.g., tocilizumab), and TNF-blocking agents (e.g., infliximab, etanercept, adalimumab).

● Gout Flares

Canakinumab is used for the symptomatic treatment of adults with gout flares in whom NSAIAs and colchicine are contraindicated, not tolerated, or do not provide an adequate response, and in whom repeated courses of corticosteroids are inappropriate.

Clinical Experience

Canakinumab was initially evaluated for the treatment of gout flares in two 12-week, randomized, double-blind, active-controlled studies enrolling patients for whom NSAIAs and/or colchicine were contraindicated, ineffective, or intolerable, and who experienced ≥3 gout flares in the prior year (studies 1 and 2). These initial studies were continued via active-control and open-label extensions, up to a maximum of 36 months where all patients were treated with canakinumab upon occurrence of a new gout flare. In study 1, 230 patients were randomly assigned to canakinumab 150 mg subcutaneously or triamcinolone acetonide 40 mg intramuscularly at baseline for subsequent treatment of a new gout flare. In study 2, 226 patients were similarly randomized to canakinumab or triamcinolone acetonide (same dosage regimen) at baseline for subsequent treatment of a new flare. In both study 1 and 2, the co-primary endpoints were patient's assessment of gout flare pain intensity at the most affected joint at 72 hours post-dose measured on a 0-100 mm visual analogue scale (VAS) and the time to first new gout flare.

Most patients (73%) in studies 1 and 2 reported between 3-6 flares in the year prior to study entry; the remaining patients reported ≥7 flares during that time period. Approximately 33% of enrolled patients had contraindications, intolerance, or an inadequate response to both NSAIAs and colchicine; the remainder had contraindications, intolerance, or an inadequate response to either NSAIAs or colchicine. At least 1 comorbidity was reported in the majority (>85%) of enrolled patients. These included hypertension (60%), obesity (53%), chronic kidney disease (stage ≥3; 25%), diabetes (15%), and ischemic heart disease (12%). Results revealed that pain intensity of the most affected joint at 72 hours post-dose was consistently improved for patients randomized to canakinumab as compared to those administered triamcinolone acetonide. Additionally, the time to new gout flare over 12 weeks from randomization showed a reduction in the risk of a new flare among patients treated with canakinumab as compared to those treated with triamcinolone acetonide.

Another 12-week, randomized, double-blind, active-controlled study (study 3) randomly assigned 397 patients to canakinumab 150 mg subcutaneously or triamcinolone acetonide 40 mg intramuscularly for management of subsequent gout flares. In study 3, approximately 44% of enrolled patients had contraindications, intolerance, or an inadequate response to NSAIAs and colchicine. The primary endpoint was pain intensity at the most affected joint, assessed on a 0-100 mm VAS at 72 hours post-dose; time to first new gout flare was a secondary endpoint. Similar to studies 1 and 2, treatment with canakinumab resulted in an improvement in pain intensity and time to new gout flare in the subpopulation of patients unable to use NSAIAs and colchicine.

Clinical Perspective

The American College of Rheumatology released guidelines for the management of gout in 2020, including optimal use of urate lowering therapy, treatment of gout flares, and lifestyle and other medication recommendations. For gout flare management, the guidelines strongly recommend colchicine, NSAIAs, or glucocorticoids (oral, intraarticular, or intramuscular) as first-line treatments over IL-1 inhibitors (e.g., canakinumab) or adrenocorticotropic hormone (ACTH). This recommendation is based on the availability of substantial data demonstrating efficacy, tolerability, and the relatively low cost of these agents, particularly when given early after symptom onset. The administration of an IL-1 inhibitor was conditionally recommended over no therapy for patients experiencing a gout flare who are unable to tolerate, had an ineffective response, or had contraindications to first-line treatments.

DOSAGE AND ADMINISTRATION

● General

Pretreatment Screening

● Confirm absence of active infection. Evaluate for and, if necessary, treat latent tuberculosis infection before initiating treatment.

● Ensure that patients receive all recommended vaccinations, including pneumococcal and inactivated influenza vaccines, before initiating treatment with canakinumab.

Patient Monitoring

● Monitor patients with Still's disease for worsening of underlying symptoms and symptoms of infection as these are known triggers for macrophage activation syndrome.

● Monitor all patients for signs and symptoms of infection suggestive of tuberculosis.

● Administration

Canakinumab is administered by subcutaneous injection *only*. Injection of canakinumab should be performed by a clinician; the drug should *not* be self-administered. Do not inject into scar tissue since this may result in insufficient exposure to the drug. Do not inject into areas where skin is swollen or erythematous.

Store unopened vials at 2–8°C; protect from light; the vials should be stored in the original carton until time of use.

Administration

Commercially available canakinumab solution has a concentration of 150 mg/mL. Do not shake. The solution should be clear to opalescent, colorless to slightly brownish-yellow, and essentially free from particulates. Do not use if the solution has a distinctly brown discoloration, is highly opalescent, or contains visible particles.

Using a sterile 1-mL syringe and 18-gauge, 2-inch needle, withdraw the required volume for administration. Use a 27-gauge, ½-inch needle for the subcutaneous injection. Discard unused portions of the solution since the solution contains no preservatives.

● Dosage

Pediatric Patients

Cryopyrin-Associated Periodic Syndromes

Children ≥4 years of age with body weight >40 kg: recommended dosage is 150 mg once every 8 weeks.

Children ≥4 years with body weight 15 to ≤40 kg: recommended dosage is 2 mg/kg once every 8 weeks. The dosage can be increased to 3 mg/kg once every 8 weeks if the clinical response is not adequate.

Tumor Necrosis Factor Receptor Associated Periodic Syndrome, Hyperimmunoglobulin D Syndrome/Mevalonate Kinase Deficiency, Familial Mediterranean Fever

Body weight ≤40 kg: recommended dosage is 2 mg/kg every 4 weeks. The dosage can be increased to 4 mg/kg every 4 weeks if the clinical response is not adequate.

Body weight >40 kg: recommended dosage is 150 mg every 4 weeks. The dosage can be increased to 300 mg every 4 weeks if the clinical response is not adequate.

Still's Disease

Children ≥2 years of age with body weight ≥7.5 kg: recommended dosage is 4 mg/kg (maximum of 300 mg) every 4 weeks.

Adults

Cryopyrin-Associated Periodic Syndromes

Body weight >40 kg: recommended dosage is 150 mg once every 8 weeks.

Body weight 15 to ≤40 kg: recommended dosage is 2 mg/kg once every 8 weeks.

Tumor Necrosis Factor Receptor Associated Periodic Syndrome, Hyperimmunoglobulin D Syndrome/Mevalonate Kinase Deficiency, Familial Mediterranean Fever

Body weight ≤40 kg: recommended dosage is 2 mg/kg every 4 weeks. The dosage can be increased to 4 mg/kg every 4 weeks if the clinical response is not adequate.

Body weight >40 kg: recommended dosage is 150 mg every 4 weeks. The dosage can be increased to 300 mg every 4 weeks if the clinical response is not adequate.

Still's Disease

Recommended dosage is 4 mg/kg (maximum of 300 mg) every 4 weeks.

Gout Flares

Recommended dose: 150 mg. If retreatment is required, there should be an interval of at least 12 weeks before a new dose may be administered.

Hepatic Impairment

The manufacturer makes no specific dosage recommendations for patients with hepatic impairment.

Renal Impairment

The manufacturer makes no specific dosage recommendations for patients with renal impairment.

Geriatric Patients

The manufacturer makes no specific dosage recommendations for geriatric patients.

CAUTIONS

● Contraindications

● Confirmed hypersensitivity to canakinumab or any ingredient in the formulation.

● Warnings/Precautions

Serious Infections

Canakinumab has been associated with an increased risk of serious infections. In a clinical trial in patients with cryopyrin-associated periodic syndromes (CAPS), canakinumab therapy was associated with an increased incidence of suspected infections compared with placebo. Infections, predominantly involving the upper respiratory tract and in some cases serious, have been reported in patients receiving canakinumab in clinical trials; these infections generally responded to standard therapy. Isolated cases of unusual or opportunistic infections (e.g., aspergillosis, atypical mycobacterial infections, cytomegalovirus, herpes zoster) were reported during canakinumab treatment. Do not initiate canakinumab in patients with an active infection requiring medical treatment or a chronic infection (including infection with human immunodeficiency virus [HIV], hepatitis B virus [HBV], or hepatitis C virus [HCV]), and discontinue the drug in patients who develop a serious infection. Use canakinumab with caution in patients with infections, a history of recurring infections, or underlying conditions that may predispose them to infections.

Drugs that affect the immune system by blocking tumor necrosis factor (TNF, TNF-α) have been associated with an increased risk of new tuberculosis and reactivation of latent tuberculosis. Canakinumab, which blocks IL-1, may increase the risk of reactivation of tuberculosis or opportunistic infections. Evaluate patients using appropriate screening tests for active and latent tuberculosis prior to initiation of canakinumab therapy. Canakinumab has not been studied in patients with latent tuberculosis infection, and the safety of canakinumab in such individuals is not known. When indicated, initiate an appropriate antimycobacterial regimen for the treatment of latent tuberculosis infection prior to canakinumab therapy. Instruct patients to seek medical advice if signs, symptoms, or high risk exposure suggestive of tuberculosis (e.g., persistent cough, weight loss, subfebrile temperature) appear during or after canakinumab treatment.

Immunosuppression

The effect of canakinumab on the development of malignancies is not known. However, treatment with immunosuppressive agents, including canakinumab, may result in an increased risk of malignancies.

Hypersensitivity

Hypersensitivity reactions have been reported with canakinumab. Symptoms of the underlying disease may be similar to symptoms of hypersensitivity. If hypersensitivity reactions occur, discontinue canakinumab and initiate appropriate therapy.

Immunizations

IL-1 blockade may interfere with the immune response to vaccines. When use of canakinumab is being considered, review the vaccination status of all adult and pediatric patients and administer all age-appropriate vaccines, including pneumococcal vaccine and influenza virus vaccine inactivated, prior to initiation of canakinumab therapy.

No data are available on the efficacy or on the risks of secondary transmission of infection by live vaccines in patients receiving canakinumab Safety and/or efficacy of concomitant administration of live or inactivated vaccines in patients receiving canakinumab have not been established. Do not administer live vaccines to patients receiving canakinumab.

Macrophage Activation Syndrome

Macrophage activation syndrome (MAS), a life-threatening disorder, may develop in patients with rheumatic conditions, particularly Still's disease; if MAS develops, it should be aggressively treated. Eleven of 201 patients with systemic juvenile idiopathic arthritis (SJIA) treated with canakinumab developed MAS. No definitive conclusions can be made as to whether canakinumab increases the incidence of MAS. Monitor patients with Still's disease for worsening of underlying symptoms and symptoms of infection because these are known triggers for MAS.

Immunogenicity

In clinical studies, antibodies against canakinumab were observed in 1.4, 1.2, and 3.5% of patients treated with canakinumab for CAPS, SJIA, and gout flares, respectively. Neutralizing antibodies were detected in <1% of patients with gout flares and no correlation of antibody development to clinical response or adverse events was observed. No patients in clinical studies evaluating use of 150 mg and 300 mg doses of canakinumab over 16 weeks for TRAPS, HIDS/MKD, FMF, SJIA, or AOSD tested positive for anti-canakinumab antibodies.

Specific Populations

Pregnancy

There are limited available data regarding use of canakinumab in pregnant women to inform a drug-associated risk of major birth defects, miscarriage, or adverse maternal or fetal outcomes. In animal embryofetal development studies, no evidence of embryotoxicity or fetal malformations was observed with canakinumab during the period of organogenesis and later in gestation at doses that produced exposures approximately 11 times the exposure at the maximum recommended human dose (MRHD) and greater. Delays in fetal skeletal development were observed in animal studies following prenatal exposure to canakinumab at concentrations approximately 11 times the MRHD and greater and during the period of organogenesis.

Because IL-1 blockade may interfere with immune response to infections, consider risks and benefits of administering live vaccines to infants who were exposed to canakinumab in utero for at least 4-12 months following the mother's last dose of canakinumab.

Lactation

The presence of canakinumab in human milk or its effects on milk production is not known. A small number of case reports do not establish an association between maternal canakinumab use during lactation and adverse effects on breast-fed infants. Consider the developmental and health benefits of breast-feeding along with the mother's clinical need for canakinumab and adverse effects on the breast-fed infant from canakinumab and from the underlying maternal condition.

Pediatric Use

Canakinumab has been evaluated in 23 pediatric patients 4–17 years of age with CAPS. Most patients demonstrated improvement from baseline in clinical symptoms and objective markers of inflammation (e.g., serum amyloid A [SAA], C-reactive protein [CRP]). Overall efficacy and safety were similar to those observed in adults; the most frequently reported infections involved the upper respiratory tract.

The manufacturer states that safety and efficacy of canakinumab in patients with CAPS <4 years of age have not been established.

The TRAPS, HIDS/MKD, and FMF trials evaluated 102 pediatric patients between 2–17 years of age. Clinical symptoms and objective markers of inflammation were improved in a majority of pediatric patients and no meaningful differences in efficacy, safety, and tolerability were observed between pediatric and adult patients.

The safety and efficacy of canakinumab in patients with SJIA <2 years of age have not been established.

The safety and efficacy of canakinumab for the treatment of gout flares in pediatric patients have not been established.

Avoid use of live virus vaccines in pediatric patients receiving canakinumab and in infants exposed in utero following maternal administration. Administer all recommended vaccinations to pediatric patients prior to initiating canakinumab treatment.

Geriatric Use

Experience in those ≥65 years of age with CAPS, TRAPS, HIDS/MKD, FMF, and Still's disease is insufficient to determine whether they respond differently than younger adults.

In clinical studies of canakinumab for treatment of gout flares, 85 (17.3%) patients were ≥65 years of age and 16 (3.3%) patients were ≥75 years of age. The efficacy profile was similar between patients 65 to 75 years of age and those <65 years of age. Studies did not include sufficient numbers of patients ≥75 years of age to determine whether they respond differently than younger patients. No new safety findings were reported in these age groups.

Hepatic Impairment

The pharmacokinetics of canakinumab have not been formally studied in patients with hepatic impairment.

Renal Impairment

The pharmacokinetics of canakinumab have not been formally studied in patients with renal impairment.

● Common Adverse Effects

Adverse effects reported in >10% of patients receiving canakinumab for CAPS include nasopharyngitis, diarrhea, influenza, rhinitis, headache, nausea, bronchitis, gastroenteritis, musculoskeletal pain, pharyngitis, vertigo, and weight gain.

Adverse effects reported in ≥10% of patients receiving canakinumab for TRAPS, HIDS/MKD, and FMF include injection site reactions and nasopharyngitis.

Adverse effects reported in ≥10% of patients receiving canakinumab for Still's disease include infections (nasopharyngitis and upper respiratory tract infections), abdominal pain, and injection site reactions.

Adverse effects reported in ≥2% of patients receiving canakinumab for gout flares include nasopharyngitis, upper respiratory tract infections, urinary tract infections, hypertriglyceridemia, and back pain.

DRUG INTERACTIONS

Formal drug interaction studies have not been conducted to date.

● Drugs Metabolized by Hepatic Microsomal Enzymes

Increased levels of cytokines (e.g., interleukin-1 [IL-1]) during chronic inflammation suppress the formation of cytochrome P-450 (CYP) enzymes; drugs that bind to IL-1, including canakinumab, are expected to normalize CYP enzyme formation. If canakinumab is initiated in a patient already receiving a CYP isoenzyme substrate that has a narrow therapeutic index (e.g., warfarin), monitor efficacy or concentrations of the concomitant drug, and adjust dosage of the concomitant drug as needed.

● IL-1 Blocking Agents

Concomitant use of canakinumab with other IL-1 antagonists has not been evaluated. Because of the potential for pharmacologic interactions between canakinumab and a recombinant IL-1 receptor antagonist (IL-1Ra), concomitant use of canakinumab with other agents that block IL-1 or its receptors (e.g., anakinra, rilonacept) is not recommended.

● TNF Blocking Agents

Canakinumab has not been used concomitantly with agents that block tumor necrosis factor (TNF, TNF-α) in clinical studies. However, an increased risk of serious infections and an increased risk of neutropenia were observed when anakinra (an IL-1 receptor antagonist) and etanercept (an agent that blocks TNF) were used concomitantly in patients with active rheumatoid arthritis. Similar toxicities would be expected with concomitant use of canakinumab and TNF blocking agents. Therefore, concomitant use of canakinumab and TNF blocking agents is not recommended.

● Immunizations

Information is not available regarding the efficacy of live vaccines or the risk of secondary transmission of infection following administration of live vaccines in patients receiving canakinumab. Therefore, live vaccines should not be administered to patients receiving canakinumab. The manufacturer makes no specific recommendations regarding the length of time to wait between discontinuance of canakinumab and administration of a live vaccine or the length of time to wait between administration of a live vaccine and initiation of canakinumab therapy.

Information is not available regarding the efficacy of inactivated vaccines in patients receiving canakinumab. Because canakinumab may interfere with normal immune response to new antigens, vaccinations may not be effective in patients receiving canakinumab.

DESCRIPTION

Canakinumab is a recombinant human immunoglobulin G₁ (IgG₁) kappa monoclonal antibody. The drug is an anti-human interleukin-1 beta (IL-1β) antibody.

Cryopyrin-associated periodic syndromes (CAPS) are rare genetic syndromes generally caused by mutations in the NLRP-3 gene. Inflammation in CAPS is usually associated with mutations in the NLRP-3 gene that encodes the protein cryopyrin, which is an important component of the inflammasome. Cryopyrin regulates the protease caspase-1 and controls the activation of IL-1β. Mutations in the NLRP-3 gene result in an overactive inflammasome, which causes excessive release of activated IL-1β. Still's disease is a severe autoinflammatory disease, driven by innate immunity by means of proinflammatory cytokines such as IL-1β. Gout flares are characterized by activation of resident macrophages and infiltrating neutrophils in the joint, with concomitant overproduction of IL-1β resulting in an acute painful inflammatory response. Canakinumab binds to IL-1β and neutralizes its activity by blocking its interaction with IL-1 receptors. The drug does not bind interleukin-1 alpha (IL-1α) or interleukin-1 receptor antagonist (IL-1Ra).

Concentrations of serum amyloid A (SAA) and C-reactive protein (CRP), indicators of inflammatory disease activity, are elevated in patients with CAPS and gout flares. Elevated SAA concentrations have been associated with the development of systemic amyloidosis in patients with CAPS; treatment with canakinumab resulted in a normalization of CRP and SAA within 8 days. In patients with gout flares, CRP and SAA were rapidly reduced following canakinumab therapy, and reductions were sustained throughout the 24-week observation period. In SJIA, the median percent reduction in CRP from baseline to day 15 was 91%.

The pharmacokinetics of canakinumab are typical for an IgG-type antibody and are comparable in different disease states, but influenced by body weight. The absolute bioavailability of canakinumab following subcutaneous injection is estimated to be 66%. Peak plasma concentrations were achieved approximately 7 days following subcutaneous administration of a single 150-mg dose in adults with CAPS and approximately 2–7 days following subcutaneous administration of a single dose of 150 mg or 2 mg/kg in pediatric patients with CAPS. The mean terminal half-life of the drug is approximately 26 days in adults. Pharmacokinetic properties in the pediatric populations are similar in patients with CAPS, TRAPS, HIDS/MKD, FMF, and SJIA.

ADVICE TO PATIENTS

- Provide a copy of the manufacturer's patient information to all patients and advise of the importance of reading the information.

- Inform patients of the risk of injection site reactions (e.g., pain, erythema, swelling, pruritus, bruising, mass, inflammation, dermatitis, edema, urticaria, vesicles, warmth, hemorrhage). Instruct patients to inform their clinician of any persistent injection site reaction.

- Inform patients of the risk of serious infection. Instruct patients to inform their clinicians immediately if any signs or symptoms of infection (e.g., fever, cough, redness in one part of the body, warmth or swelling of the skin) occur.

- Instruct patients to inform their clinician if they have an active infection, have a history of recurrent infection, or have had human immunodeficiency virus (HIV), hepatitis B, or hepatitis C.

- Advise patients that they should not take canakinumab if they have an active or chronic infection.

- Instruct patients to contact their clinician immediately if they develop signs of an allergic reaction, such as difficulty breathing or swallowing, nausea, dizziness, skin rash, itching, hives, palpitations, or low blood pressure.

- Advise patients to review their vaccination status with their clinician and receive all age-appropriate vaccines prior to initiation of canakinumab therapy.

- Advise patients to inform clinicians of existing or contemplated concomitant therapy, including prescription (e.g., IL-1 antagonists such as anakinra, rilonacept; TNF-blocking agents such as etanercept, infliximab, certolizumab, golimumab, or adalimumab; immunizations; corticosteroids) and OTC drugs, dietary supplements, and/or herbal products, as well as any concomitant illnesses (e.g., active or chronic infections).

- Advise women to inform clinicians if they are or plan to become pregnant or plan to breast-feed.

- Inform patients of other important precautionary information.

PREPARATIONS

Canakinumab can only be obtained through designated specialty pharmacies and distributors. Contact the manufacturer for additional information regarding enrollment.

Excipients in commercially available drug preparations may have clinically important effects in some individuals; consult specific product labeling for details.

Canakinumab

Parenteral		
Injection, for subcutaneous use	150 mg/mL	Ilaris®, Novartis

† Use is not currently included in the labeling approved by the US Food and Drug Administration.

Tezepelumab-ekko

48:10.20 • INTERLEUKIN ANTAGONISTS

■ Tezepelumab, a human immunoglobulin (IgG_2) lamda monoclonal antibody, is a thymic stromal lymphopoietin (TSLP) blocker.

USES

● Asthma

Tezepelumab-ekko is used for the add-on maintenance treatment of adults and adolescents ≥12 years of age with severe asthma. The drug is *not* indicated for relief of acute bronchospasm or status asthmaticus. In clinical trials, tezepelumab-ekko was shown to be more effective than placebo for reducing annual asthma exacerbation rate and improving lung function.

Clinical Experience

Safety and efficacy of tezepelumab-ekko were evaluated in 2 multicenter, randomized, double-blind, placebo-controlled studies (PATHWAY and NAVIGATOR) in patients ≥12 years of age with severe asthma. In both trials, patients were required to have an Asthma Control Questionnaire 6 (ACQ-6) score of 1.5 or more at screening and reduced lung function at baseline. Reduced lung function was defined as pre-bronchodilator forced expiratory volume in 1 second (FEV1) below 80% predicted in adults and below 90% predicted in adolescents. Treatment with a medium or high-dose inhaled corticosteroid (ICS) and at least 1 additional asthma controller, with or without oral corticosteroids (OCS) was required. Patients continued background asthma therapy throughout the trials. In both trials, patients were enrolled without requiring a minimum baseline level of blood eosinophils or fraction of expired nitrous oxide (FeNO). Both trials had the same primary outcome of clinically significant asthma exacerbation rate over 52 weeks. A clinically significant exacerbation was defined as worsening of asthma requiring the use of or increased use of OCS or ICS for at least 3 days, a single depo-injection of corticosteroids, and/or emergency room visits requiring use of OCS or ICS, and/or hospitalization.

In the phase 2b dose-ranging PATHWAY trial, 550 adults with a history of at least 2 asthma exacerbations that required oral or injectable corticosteroid treatment or 1 asthma exacerbation that resulted in hospitalization in the past 12 months were included. Patients were randomly assigned to either subcutaneous placebo or tezepelumab-ekko (70 mg every 4 weeks, 210 mg every 4 weeks, or 280 mg every 2 weeks). The annualized asthma exacerbation rate was 0.20 with tezepelumab and 0.72 in the placebo group with a rate ratio of 0.29. Exacerbation rates requiring an emergency room visit or hospitalization were 0.03 per year with tezepelumab and 0.18 per year with placebo (rate ratio: 0.15). Exacerbation rates requiring hospitalization were 0.02 and 0.14 per year with tezepelumab and placebo, respectively (rate ratio 0.14). The least squares mean change from baseline in FEV1 demonstrated an increase of 0.08 L with tezepelumab and a decrease of 0.06 L with placebo (difference from placebo: 0.13). Measures of patient-reported symptoms and quality of life demonstrated improvement with tezepelumab compared to placebo. In a post-hoc analysis, outcomes were compared between patients with and without perennial allergy. Compared to placebo, tezepelumab reduced the annual asthma exacerbation rate to a similar extent in both populations. A reduction in eosinophil counts and FeNO and improvement in lung function was observed with tezepelumab in patients with and without perennial allergy.

In the phase 3 NAVIGATOR trial, 1061 patients ≥12 years of age with a history of at least 2 asthma exacerbations that required oral or injectable corticosteroid treatment or resulted in hospitalization in the past 12 months were included. Patients were randomly assigned to either subcutaneous placebo or tezepelumab-ekko 210 mg every 4 weeks. The annualized asthma exacerbation rate was 0.93 with tezepelumab and 2.10 in the placebo group with a rate ratio of 0.44. Exacerbation rates requiring an emergency room visit or hospitalization were 0.06 with tezepelumab and 0.28 with placebo (rate ratio: 0.21). Exacerbation rates requiring hospitalization were 0.03 and 0.19 per year with tezepelumab and placebo, respectively (rate ratio: 0.15). Fewer exacerbations were demonstrated regardless of baseline levels of blood eosinophils or FeNO. The time to an exacerbation was significantly longer with tezepelumab compared to placebo. The least squares mean change from baseline in FEV1 demonstrated an increase of 0.23 L with tezepelumab versus 0.10 with placebo (difference from placebo 0.13). Measures of patient-reported symptoms and quality of life demonstrated improvement with tezepelumab compared to placebo.

Reduction in the use of maintenance OCS with tezepelumab was compared to placebo in a randomized, double-blind clinical trial (SOURCE). The trial included 150 adults with severe asthma who required daily OCS (7.5–30 mg daily of prednisone or prednisolone) treatment in addition to regular use of high-dose ICS and a long-acting beta-agonist with or without an additional controller. A statistically significant reduction in maintenance OCS dose while maintaining asthma control was not observed with tezepelumab compared to placebo after 48 weeks of treatment.

Clinical Perspective

Several clinical practice guidelines are available for asthma management including the Global Initiative for Asthma (GINA) guidelines, which are published annually. The GINA guideline provides evidence-based recommendations for the management of asthma in adults, adolescents, and children ≥6 years of age. The guideline states that all patients with asthma should be evaluated for symptom control, risk of future exacerbations, treatment issues (e.g., inhaler technique and adherence), and comorbidities. A stepwise approach to treatment is recommended where specific drugs are added or adjusted up or down through a series of steps (1 through 5) to achieve symptom control while keeping the patient on the lowest effective treatment. Drugs used in the management of asthma include inhaled corticosteroids (ICS)-formoterol, long-acting beta agonists (LABA), short-acting beta agonists (SABA), long-acting muscarinic agonists (LAMA), leukotriene receptor antagonists, theophylline, oral corticosteroids, and biologic agents. Biologic agents such as tezepelumab are generally recommended as add-on therapy for severe asthma. Higher blood eosinophils and higher FeNO levels are associated with a greater risk of severe exacerbations and are predictive markers for Type 2 inflammation, which is found in the majority of individuals with severe asthma. The GINA guideline states that tezepelumab can be considered as add-on therapy in patients ≥12 years of age with severe asthma. High blood eosinophils and high FeNO levels are strongly predictive of a good response with the drug. The use of tezepelumab can also be considered in patients without elevation in type 2 inflammatory markers.

DOSAGE AND ADMINISTRATION

● General

Pretreatment Screening

- Treat preexisting helminth infections prior to initiating therapy.

Patient Monitoring

- Monitor patients for signs and symptoms of hypersensitivity reactions.

Other General Considerations

- Concomitant oral or inhaled corticosteroids should not be discontinued abruptly. If appropriate, reduction in corticosteroid dosage should be done gradually and under the direct supervision of a physician.

● Administration

Tezepelumab-ekko is commercially available as a single-dose vial, single-dose prefilled syringe, or single-dose prefilled pen.

Store refrigerated at 2–8°C; do not freeze. Protect from light. If needed, the drug may be stored at room temperature between 20–25°C for no longer than 30 days. Do not refrigerate once the drug has been stored at room temperature.

Allow the product to reach room temperature before administration. This takes about 60 minutes once removed from refrigeration. Do not shake the drug or expose to heat.

Visually inspect the contents of the vial or prefilled syringe or pen for particulate matter and discoloration prior to administration. Tezepelumab is a clear to opalescent, colorless to light yellow solution; do not use if the liquid is cloudy, discolored, or if it contains large particles or foreign particulate matter.

The manufacturer states that tezepelumab-ekko vials and prefilled syringes are intended for administration by a healthcare provider. Tezepelumab-ekko prefilled pens may be administered by a healthcare provider or by patients/caregivers after proper training in subcutaneous injection technique and after the healthcare provider determines it is appropriate. Inject the entire contents of the vial, prefilled syringe, or pen subcutaneously into the thigh or abdomen, except for the 2 inches around the navel. The upper arm can also be used if a healthcare provider or caregiver administers the injection. Rotate injection sites. Do not inject into tender, bruised, erythematous, or hardened skin areas.

If a dose is missed, administer the dose as soon as possible. Resume regular dosing on the usual day of administration. If the next dose is already due, administer as planned.

Administration of the Prefilled Syringe

Pinch the skin gently and administer the prefilled syringe subcutaneously at an approximately 45° angle into the recommended injection site (upper arm, thigh, or abdomen, except for the 2 inches around the navel). Inject all of the drug by pushing the plunger all the way until it is completely between the needle guard activation clips. This is necessary to activate the needle guard. After the injection, maintain pressure on the plunger head and remove the needle from the skin. Release pressure on the plunger head to allow the needle guard to cover the needle.

Administration of the Prefilled Pen

Pinch the skin gently or give the injection without pinching the skin. Position the pen by placing the orange needle guard flat against the skin at a 90° angle. Press down firmly until the orange needle guard is not visible. The first clicking sound will signal that the injection has started. The orange plunger will move down in the viewing window during the injection. Hold down firmly for about 15 seconds. A second clicking sound will indicate that the injection has finished. The orange plunger will fill the viewing window. After the injection is complete, lift the pen straight up. The orange needle guard will slide down and lock into place over the needle.

● Dosage

Asthma

The recommended dosage of tezepelumab-ekko in adults and adolescents ≥12 years of age with severe asthma is 210 mg given subcutaneously once every 4 weeks.

Hepatic Impairment

The manufacturer makes no specific dosage recommendations for patients with hepatic impairment.

Renal Impairment

The manufacturer makes no specific dosage recommendations for patients with renal impairment.

Geriatric Patients

The manufacturer makes no specific dosage recommendations for geriatric patients.

CAUTIONS

● Contraindications

- Known history of hypersensitivity to the drug or any ingredient in the formulation.

● Warnings/Precautions

Hypersensitivity Reactions

Hypersensitivity reactions (e.g., rash, allergic conjunctivitis, anaphylaxis) can occur following administration of tezepelumab-ekko. These reactions can occur within hours of administration, but in some instances have a delayed onset

(i.e., days). In the event of a hypersensitivity reaction, consider the benefits and risks for the individual patient to determine whether to continue or discontinue treatment with tezepelumab.

Acute Asthma Symptoms or Deteriorating Disease

Tezepelumab-ekko should not be used to treat acute asthma symptoms such as bronchospasm or acute exacerbations, including status asthmaticus. Patients should seek medical advice if their asthma remains uncontrolled or worsens after initiation of treatment with tezepelumab.

Risk Associated with Abrupt Reduction of Corticosteroid Dosage

Do not discontinue systemic or inhaled corticosteroids abruptly upon initiation of therapy with tezepelumab. Reductions in corticosteroid dosage, if appropriate, should be gradual and performed under the direct supervision of a physician. Reduction in corticosteroid dosage may be associated with systemic withdrawal symptoms and/or unmask conditions previously suppressed by systemic corticosteroid therapy.

Parasitic (Helminth) Infection

Thymic stromal lymphopoietin (TSLP) may be involved in the immunologic response to some helminth infections. Patients with known helminth infections were excluded from participation in clinical trials of tezepelumab-ekko. It is unknown if tezepelumab will influence a patient's response against helminth infections.

Treat patients with pre-existing helminth infections before initiating therapy with tezepelumab. If patients become infected while receiving treatment with tezepelumab and do not respond to antihelmintic treatment, discontinue treatment with tezepelumab until infection resolves.

Live Attenuated Vaccines

The concomitant use of tezepelumab-ekko and live attenuated vaccines has not been evaluated. The use of live attenuated vaccines should be avoided in patients receiving the drug.

Specific Populations

Pregnancy

There are no available data on tezepelumab-ekko use in pregnant women to evaluate for any drug-associated risk of major birth defects, miscarriage, or other adverse maternal or fetal outcomes. Placental transfer of monoclonal antibodies such as tezepelumab is greater during the third trimester of pregnancy; therefore, potential effects on a fetus are likely to be greater during the third trimester of pregnancy.

In an enhanced pre- and post-natal development study conducted in cynomolgus monkeys, placental transport of tezepelumab was observed but there was no evidence of fetal harm following IV administration of tezepelumab throughout pregnancy at doses that produced maternal exposures up to 168 times the exposure at the maximum recommended human dose (MRHD) of 210 mg administered subcutaneously.

Lactation

There is no information regarding the presence of tezepelumab in human milk, its effects on the breast-fed infant, or its effects on milk production. However, tezepelumab is a human monoclonal antibody immunoglobulin G2λ (IgG2λ), and immunoglobulin G (IgG) is present in human milk in small amounts. Tezepelumab was present in the milk of cynomolgus monkeys postpartum following dosing during pregnancy.

The developmental and health benefits of breast-feeding should be considered along with the mother's clinical need for tezepelumab and any potential adverse effects on the breast-fed infant from tezepelumab or from the underlying maternal condition.

Pediatric Use

The safety and effectiveness of tezepelumab-ekko for the add-on maintenance treatment of severe asthma have been established in pediatric patients ≥12 years of age. Use of tezepelumab for this indication is supported by evidence from a total of 82 pediatric patients 12–17 years of age enrolled in the NAVIGATOR study.

Compared with placebo, improvements in annualized asthma exacerbation and FEV1 were observed in pediatric patients treated with tezepelumab-ekko. The safety profile and pharmacodynamic responses in pediatric patients were generally similar to the overall study population.

The safety and effectiveness of tezepelumab-ekko in patients <12 years of age have not been established.

Geriatric Use

Of the 665 patients with asthma treated with tezepelumab-ekko in clinical trials (PATHWAY and NAVIGATOR) for severe asthma, 119 patients (18%) were ≥65 years of age. No overall differences in safety or effectiveness of tezepelumab have been observed between these geriatric patients and younger patients.

Hepatic Impairment

Pharmacokinetic studies of tezepelumab have not been conducted in patients with hepatic impairment, and the manufacturer makes no specific dosage recommendations for such patients. Since tezepelumab is not metabolized by hepatic-specific enzymes, changes in hepatic function are not expected to influence the drug's clearance.

Renal Impairment

The clearance of tezepelumab was similar in patients with normal renal function (creatinine clearance [Cl_{cr}] ≥90 mL/minute) and those with mild (Cl_{cr} 60–89 mL/minute) and moderate (Cl_{cr} 30–59 mL/minute) renal impairment. Pharmacokinetic studies of tezepelumab-ekko have not been conducted in patients with severe (Cl_{cr} <30 mL/minute) renal impairment.

• Common Adverse Effects

Adverse effects reported in ≥3% of patients with severe asthma receiving tezepelumab in controlled clinical studies include pharyngitis, arthralgia, and back pain.

DRUG INTERACTIONS

No formal drug interaction studies have been performed with tezepelumab.

Tezepelumab-ekko is not metabolized by hepatic enzymes.

• Leukotriene Receptor Antagonists

Based on population pharmacokinetic analysis, co-administered asthma medications, including leukotriene receptor antagonists, did not have a clinically meaningful effect on tezepelumab clearance.

• Theophylline/Aminophylline

Based on population pharmacokinetic analysis, co-administered asthma medications, including theophylline/aminophylline, did not have a clinically meaningful effect on tezepelumab clearance.

• Oral and Inhaled Corticosteroids

Based on population pharmacokinetic analysis, co-administered asthma medications, including oral and inhaled corticosteroids, did not have a clinically meaningful effect on tezepelumab clearance.

• Live Attenuated Vaccines

The concomitant use of tezepelumab-ekko and live attenuated vaccines has not been evaluated. The use of live attenuated vaccines should be avoided in patients receiving tezepelumab.

DESCRIPTION

Tezepelumab is a thymic stromal lymphopoietin (TSLP) blocker; the drug is a human monoclonal antibody immunoglobulin G_2 (IgG_2) lambda that binds to human TSLP and blocks its interaction with the heterodimeric TSLP receptor. TSLP is a cytokine mainly derived from epithelial cells that occupies an upstream position in the asthma inflammatory cascade.

Airway inflammation is an important component in the pathogenesis of asthma. Multiple cell types (e.g., mast cells, eosinophils, neutrophils, macrophages, lymphocytes, group 2 innate lymphoid [ILC2] cells) and mediators (e.g., histamine, eicosanoids, leukotrienes, cytokines) are involved in airway inflammation. Blocking TSLP with tezepelumab reduces biomarkers and cytokines associated with inflammation including blood eosinophils, airway submucosal eosinophils, IgE, fraction of expired nitrous oxide (FeNO), IL-5, and IL-13. However, the mechanism of tezepelumab action in asthma has not been definitively established.

Following administration of a single subcutaneous dose of tezepelumab-ekko over a dose range from 2.1–420 mg, the pharmacokinetics of tezepelumab were found to be dose-proportional. When administered every 4 weeks, the drug achieves steady-state after 12 weeks. The maximum serum concentration was reached in 3–10 days. Bioavailability is approximately 77% with no clinically relevant differences when administered to different injection sites. Administration every 4 weeks reduced blood eosinophil counts, FeNO, and concentrations of IL-5 and IL-13 from baseline with an onset of 2 weeks after initiation. Tezepelumab is degraded by proteolytic enzymes that are widely distributed in the body, is not metabolized by hepatic enzymes, and is eliminated by intracellular catabolism. The elimination half-life is approximately 26 days.

Age (12 to 80 years), sex, and race did not demonstrate meaningful effects on tezepelumab pharmacokinetics. Although higher body weight was associated with lower exposure, no meaningful impact on efficacy or safety was observed.

ADVICE TO PATIENTS

- Advise the patient to read the FDA-approved patient labeling (patient information).

- Inform patients that hypersensitivity reactions (e.g., rash, allergic conjunctivitis, anaphylaxis) can occur following administration of tezepelumab. These reactions can occur within hours of administration, but in some instances have a delayed onset (i.e., days). Instruct patients to contact their healthcare provider if they experience symptoms of an allergic reaction.

- Inform patients that tezepelumab does not treat acute asthma symptoms or acute exacerbations. Instruct patients to seek medical advice if their asthma remains uncontrolled or worsens after initiation of treatment with tezepelumab.

- Inform patients to not discontinue systemic or inhaled corticosteroids except under the direct supervision of a healthcare provider. Inform patients that reduction in corticosteroid dose may be associated with systemic withdrawal symptoms and/or unmask conditions previously suppressed by systemic corticosteroid therapy.

- Instruct patients to inform the healthcare provider that they are taking tezepelumab prior to a potential vaccination.

- Advise patients to refrigerate tezepelumab at 2-8°C. Tezepelumab may be kept at room temperature between 20-25°C for a maximum of 30 days. Inform patients and caregivers of the need for proper disposal of the prefilled pen after use, including the use of a sharps disposal container.

- Advise women to inform their clinician if they are or plan to become pregnant or plan to breast-feed.

- Advise patients to inform their clinician of existing or contemplated concomitant therapy, including prescription and OTC drugs and dietary or herbal supplements, as well as any concomitant illnesses.

- Advise patients of other important precautionary information.

PREPARATIONS

Tezepelumab-ekko can only be obtained through designated specialty pharmacies. Contact the manufacturer for specific availability information.

Excipients in commercially available drug preparations may have clinically important effects in some individuals; consult specific product labeling for details.

Tezepelumab-ekko

Parenteral

Injection, for subcutaneous use	110 mg/mL	Tezspire® (available as single-dose prefilled syringes, prefilled pens, and single-dose vials), Amgen and AstraZeneca

† Use is not currently included in the labeling approved by the US Food and Drug Administration.

Selected Revisions September 10, 2024, © Copyright, December 22, 2021, American Society of Health-System Pharmacists, Inc.

Montelukast Sodium

Montelukast Sodium

48:10.24 • LEUKOTRIENE MODIFIERS

■ Montelukast sodium, a synthetic leukotriene-receptor antagonist, is an antiasthmatic agent.

USES

Montelukast is used in the management of asthma and for the prevention of exercise-induced bronchospasm. Montelukast is also used for the symptomatic treatment of seasonal or perennial allergic rhinitis and has been evaluated for the management of urticaria†.

● Bronchospasm

Asthma

Montelukast is used for the prevention and long-term symptomatic management of asthma.

Montelukast is not a bronchodilator and should *not* be used to relieve symptoms of acute asthma, including status asthmaticus; however, therapy with the drug can be continued during acute asthmatic attacks. All patients receiving montelukast should be provided with a short-acting, orally inhaled β_2-adrenergic agonist (e.g., albuterol) to use as supplemental therapy for acute symptoms that may occur despite montelukast therapy. Patients receiving montelukast should be cautioned not to decrease the dose of, or discontinue therapy with, other antiasthmatic agents unless instructed to do so by a clinician.

Because of the risk of neuropsychiatric effects, the benefits and risks of montelukast treatment should be considered before prescribing the drug for patients with asthma. (See Cautions: Precautions and Contraindications.)

Mild Persistent Asthma

Drugs for asthma may be categorized as relievers (e.g., bronchodilators taken as needed for acute symptoms) or controllers (principally inhaled corticosteroids or other anti-inflammatory agents taken regularly to achieve long-term control of asthma). When control of symptoms deteriorates in patients with intermittent asthma and symptoms become persistent (e.g., daytime symptoms of asthma more than twice weekly but less than once daily, and nocturnal symptoms of asthma 3–4 times per month), current asthma management guidelines and most clinicians recommend initiation of an anti-inflammatory agent, preferably with a low-dose orally inhaled corticosteroid (e.g., 88–264, 88–176, or 176 mcg of fluticasone propionate [or its equivalent] daily via a metered-dose inhaler in adolescents and adults, children 5–11 years of age, or children 4 years of age or younger, respectively) as first-line therapy for persistent asthma, supplemented by as-needed use of a short-acting, inhaled β_2-agonist. Alternatives to low-dose inhaled corticosteroids for mild persistent asthma include certain leukotriene modifiers (i.e., montelukast, zafirlukast), extended-release theophylline (in adults and children 5 years of age or older), or mast-cell stabilizers (e.g., cromolyn, nedocromil [preparation for oral inhalation no longer commercially available in the US]), but these agents are less effective and generally not preferred as initial therapy. Limited evidence suggests that montelukast may be considered for maintenance therapy in young children with mild persistent asthma when inhaled corticosteroid delivery is suboptimal as a result of poor technique or adherence.

Moderate Persistent Asthma

According to current asthma medication guidelines, therapy with a long-acting inhaled β_2-agonist such as salmeterol or formoterol generally is recommended in adults and adolescents who have moderate persistent asthma and daily asthmatic symptoms that are inadequately controlled following addition of low-dose inhaled corticosteroids to as-needed inhaled β_2-agonist treatment. However, the National Asthma Education and Prevention Program recommends that the beneficial effects of long-acting inhaled β_2-agonists should be weighed carefully against the increased risk (although uncommon) of severe asthma exacerbations and asthma-related deaths associated with daily use of such agents. (See Asthma-related Death and Life-threatening Events under Cautions: Respiratory Effects, in Salmeterol 12:12.08.12.)

Current asthma management guidelines also state that an alternative, but equally preferred option for management of moderate persistent asthma that is not adequately controlled with a low dosage of inhaled corticosteroid is to increase the maintenance dosage to a medium dosage (e.g., exceeding 264 but not more than 440 mcg of fluticasone propionate [or its equivalent] daily via a metered-dose inhaler in adults and adolescents). Alternative less effective therapies that may be added to a low dosage of an inhaled corticosteroid include oral extended-release theophylline or certain leukotriene modifiers (i.e., montelukast, zafirlukast). Considerations favoring these leukotriene modifiers in combination with orally inhaled corticosteroids include intolerance to long-acting β_2-adrenergic agonists, marked preference for oral therapy, and demonstration of superior responsiveness to these leukotriene modifiers. Limited data are available in infants and children 11 years of age or younger with moderate persistent asthma, and recommendations of care are based on expert opinion and extrapolation from studies in adults. According to current asthma management guidelines, a long-acting inhaled β_2-agonist (e.g., salmeterol, formoterol), a leukotriene modifier (i.e., montelukast, zafirlukast), or extended-release theophylline (with appropriate monitoring) may be added to low-dose inhaled corticosteroid therapy in children 5–11 years of age. Because comparative data establishing relative efficacy of these agents in this age group are lacking, there is no clearly preferred agent for use as adjunctive therapy with a low-dose inhaled corticosteroid for treatment of asthma in these children.

Severe Persistent Asthma

Maintenance therapy with an inhaled corticosteroid at medium (e.g., exceeding 264 but not more than 440 mcg of fluticasone propionate in adults and adolescents or 176 but not more than 352 mcg of the drug [or its equivalent] in children 5–11 years of age daily via a metered-dose inhaler) or high dosages (e.g., exceeding 440 mcg of fluticasone propionate in adults and adolescents or 352 mcg of the drug [or its equivalent] in children 5–11 years of age daily via a metered-dose inhaler) and adjunctive therapy with a long-acting inhaled β_2-agonist is the preferred treatment according to current asthma management guidelines in adults and children 5 years of age or older with severe persistent asthma (i.e., continuous daytime asthma symptoms, nighttime symptoms 7 times per week). Such recommendations in children 5–11 years of age are based on expert opinion and extrapolation from studies in older children and adults. Alternatives to a long-acting inhaled β_2-agonist for severe persistent asthma in adults and children 5 years of age or older receiving medium-dose inhaled corticosteroids include certain leukotriene modifiers (i.e., montelukast, zafirlukast) or extended-release theophylline, but these therapies are generally not preferred. Omalizumab may be considered in adults and adolescents with severe persistent asthma with an allergic component who are inadequately controlled with high-dose inhaled corticosteroids and a long-acting β_2-agonist. In infants and children 4 years of age or younger with severe asthma, maintenance therapy with an inhaled corticosteroid at medium (e.g., exceeding 176 but not more than 352 mcg of fluticasone propionate [or its equivalent] daily via a metered-dose inhaler) or high dosages (e.g., exceeding 352 mcg of fluticasone propionate [or its equivalent] daily via a metered-dose inhaler) and adjunctive therapy with either a long-acting inhaled β_2-agonist or montelukast is the only preferred treatment according to current asthma management guidelines. Recommendations for care of infants and children with severe asthma are based on expert opinion and extrapolation from studies in adolescents and adults. For additional details on the stepped-care approach to drug therapy in asthma, see Asthma under Uses: Bronchospasm, in Albuterol 12:12.08.12 and see Asthma under Uses: Respiratory Diseases, in the Corticosteroids General Statement 68:04.

Clinical Experience with Leukotriene Modifiers

While efficacy of montelukast in the management of asthma has not been directly compared with that of zafirlukast or zileuton, improvements in forced expiratory volume in 1 second (FEV_1) and asthma symptoms reported with montelukast generally have been similar to those reported with zafirlukast or zileuton. For the management of mild persistent asthma, advantages of leukotriene modifiers relative to orally inhaled corticosteroids include ease of administration of an oral dosage form (and presumably improved compliance) and rapid onset of action (1 day versus a week or longer). The effects of montelukast appear to be additive with those of orally inhaled corticosteroids, and such combination therapy may improve asthma control in patients with moderate to severe asthma. In addition, montelukast therapy reduces the requirements for long-term inhaled corticosteroids in stable patients. Leukotriene modifiers may be especially useful in children and adults in whom disadvantages of using, continuing, or increasing the dose of orally inhaled corticosteroids have been identified. Additional clinical settings where therapy with a leukotriene modifier may be especially useful include patients with aspirin-induced asthma, exercise-induced bronchospasm (e.g., children who want to exercise at school without having to use an orally inhaled β_2-adrenergic agonist, those whose jobs require exercise under atmospheric conditions likely to induce an asthmatic episode), nocturnal asthma, acute allergen-induced asthma, or coexisting allergic rhinitis. Conversely, because leukotrienes do not play a major role in asthma pathology in patients with naturally occurring mutations in the 5-lipoxygenase gene, such patients are unlikely to respond to therapy with leukotriene modifiers.

Current data indicate that leukotriene modifiers such as montelukast generally produce modest improvements in lung function, diminish asthma symptoms, and decrease the need for supplemental, short-acting β_2-adrenergic agonist therapy in patients with mild to moderate persistent asthma. However, not all patients receiving leukotriene modifiers have substantial clinical improvement. While patients with aspirin-sensitive asthma generally respond to leukotriene modifiers, it currently is not possible to identify patients most likely to benefit from such therapy.

Clinical Efficacy of Montelukast

Efficacy of montelukast has been established in 2 clinical trials in adults and adolescents 15 years of age or older with mild to moderate intermittent or persistent asthma (i.e., a baseline FEV_1 averaging 66% of the predicted normal value and an inhaled, short-acting β_2-adrenergic agonist requirement averaging 5 puffs daily) who generally received montelukast for 12 weeks. Efficacy of montelukast also has been established in a clinical trial in children 6–14 years of age with mild to moderate intermittent or persistent asthma (i.e., a baseline FEV_1 averaging 72% of the predicted normal value and an inhaled, short-acting β_2-adrenergic agonist requirement averaging 3 or 4 puffs daily) who generally received montelukast for 8 weeks. Approximately 77–95% of children, adolescents, and adults enrolled in these studies had a history of exercise-induced bronchospasm, and 61–96% had a history of allergic rhinitis. In these clinical trials, adults and pediatric patients received montelukast once daily in the evening; evening administration was selected to provide high montelukast plasma concentrations in the early morning, the time of maximal airway narrowing. In these trials, montelukast was more effective than placebo in alleviating respiratory symptoms (i.e., daytime asthma symptoms, nighttime awakenings), improving pulmonary function (as measured by FEV_1 and peak expiratory flow rate [PEFR]), and reducing the need for supplemental therapy with an orally inhaled β_2-adrenergic agonist. The therapeutic effects of montelukast are evident after the first dose and persist for at least 24 hours.

Studies to date indicate that tolerance to montelukast does not occur and the therapeutic effect has been maintained for over 2.5 years in patients 15 years of age or older and at least 1.5 years in children 6–14 years of age. Discontinuance of long-term (i.e., 12 weeks) montelukast therapy is not associated with rebound deterioration in asthma symptoms. Efficacy of montelukast in the management of asthma in children 2–5 years of age is supported by evidence from studies in adults, adolescents, and children 6–14 years of age, the similar pathophysiology of asthma and the drug's effect in these populations, and data regarding the pharmacokinetics of montelukast in these patients.

Montelukast has been evaluated for the management of asthma in 2 randomized, controlled studies (the US study, the multinational study) that included 1576 patients 15 years of age or older with mild to moderate asthma who were allowed to receive an orally inhaled β_2-adrenergic agonist on an as-needed basis. Patients in the US study were randomized to receive montelukast 10 mg daily or placebo; about 23% of these patients also received an orally inhaled corticosteroid on a routine basis. Patients in the multinational study were randomized to receive montelukast 10 mg daily, placebo, or active control (i.e., orally inhaled beclomethasone dipropionate 200 mcg [dose expressed as amount of drug released during actuation from the valve stem] twice daily). In these studies, therapy with montelukast was associated with greater improvement than placebo in daytime asthma symptom scores, fewer nighttime awakenings per week, and improvement in other asthma-related outcomes. Compared with baseline values, reductions in asthma symptom scores (on a scale of 0–6) averaged 0.45 or 0.22 for montelukast or placebo, respectively; nighttime awakenings per week were reduced by 1.84 or 0.79, respectively. Montelukast produced modest improvements in pulmonary function compared with baseline values in this study, with increases in FEV_1, morning PEFR, and evening PEFR averaging 0.32 L, 24.5 L/minute, and 17.9 L/minute, respectively. In the US study, montelukast produced improvements in FEV_1 of 13.1% versus 4.2% with placebo. Montelukast therapy also enabled a reduction averaging about 1.56 puffs/day in the use of supplemental orally inhaled β_2-adrenergic agonist.

Therapy with montelukast in these studies was associated with a reduction in the number of patients experiencing an acute asthma episode (11.6% versus 18.4%), number of patients requiring oral corticosteroid rescue (10.7% versus 17.5%), fewer days with exacerbations (12.8% versus 20.5%), more days without symptoms (38.5% versus 27.2%), and greater improvement in physician and patient global evaluation scores than placebo. In the US study, the clinical effects of montelukast were not affected by gender, age, race, history of exercise-induced bronchoconstriction, history of allergic rhinitis, or concomitant use of orally inhaled corticosteroids. In patients 15 years of age and older, montelukast dosages exceeding 10 mg daily are not associated with additional clinical benefit.

In the multinational study, orally inhaled beclomethasone dipropionate 200 mcg (dose expressed as amount of drug released during actuation from the valve stem) twice daily was more effective in the management of asthma than montelukast. In patients 15 years of age or older, improvements in FEV_1 reported with inhaled beclomethasone (13.3% versus 7.49%) and decreases in asthma symptom scores (0.7 versus 0.49) generally have been greater than those reported with montelukast.

In a randomized, placebo-controlled study in 336 children 6–14 years of age or older with mild to moderate asthma who were allowed to receive an orally inhaled β_2-adrenergic agonist on an as-needed basis (36% also received an orally inhaled corticosteroid on a routine basis), therapy with montelukast 5 mg (chewable tablet) daily produced modest improvements in pulmonary function compared with baseline values, with increases in FEV_1 and morning PEFR (determined in clinic setting) averaging 0.16 L and 27.85 L/minute, respectively. Montelukast produced improvements in FEV_1 of 8.7% versus 8.2% with placebo. Montelukast therapy also enabled a reduction averaging about 0.56 puffs daily in the use of supplemental orally inhaled β_2-adrenergic agonists. Therapy with montelukast and intermittent use of an orally inhaled β_2-adrenergic agonist (with or without an orally inhaled corticosteroid) was associated with fewer days with asthma exacerbations (20.6% versus 25.7%) and greater improvement in clinician and parent global evaluation scores than intermittent use of a β_2-adrenergic agonist (with or without an orally inhaled corticosteroid). Subgroup analysis indicates that improvement in FEV_1 in children 6–11 years of age (7.7%) was essentially the same as in children 12–14 years of age (9.8%). In this study, the effects of montelukast on FEV_1 and as-needed inhaled β_2-adrenergic agonist use were not affected by gender, race, Tanner stage, history of allergic rhinitis, history of exercise-induced bronchospasm, or use of orally inhaled corticosteroids.

Montelukast has been evaluated for the management of asthma in children 2–5 years of age with mild persistent asthma. In a randomized, double-blind, placebo-controlled study, children received either montelukast 4 mg (as a chewable tablet) or placebo daily; about 27–29% of these patients also were receiving an orally inhaled corticosteroid on a routine basis. Patients were allowed to receive an orally inhaled β_2-adrenergic agonist on an as-needed basis. The primary end point was determination of the safety profile of montelukast, and secondary end points evaluated asthma control. In this study, therapy with montelukast was associated with improvement in daytime asthma symptom scores, days without symptoms, and days requiring β-adrenergic agonist use. Therapy with montelukast also was associated with a reduction in the number of patients requiring oral corticosteroid rescue.

Concomitant Corticosteroid Therapy

The role of montelukast as a corticosteroid-sparing agent in patients receiving orally inhaled corticosteroids has been evaluated in asthmatic adults. In one study in adults with stable asthma (a baseline FEV_1 averaging 84% of the predicted normal value), addition of montelukast to therapy with orally inhaled corticosteroids allowed a reduction in inhaled corticosteroid use while maintaining adequate asthma control. In this study, inhaled corticosteroids (i.e., metered-dose aerosol or dry powder for oral inhalation) used and their mean baseline requirement (dosage may not be expressed as dosage delivered from the mouthpiece) include beclomethasone dipropionate (1203 mcg/day), triamcinolone acetonide (2004 mcg/day), fluticasone propionate (1083 mcg/day), and budesonide (1192 mcg/day). Prior to study initiation, the dosage of orally inhaled corticosteroid was reduced to the lowest effective dosage, a reduction of 37%. An additional 47 or 30% reduction in corticosteroid dosage was reported in patients receiving montelukast or placebo for 12 weeks. In addition, about 40 or 29% of patients receiving montelukast or placebo reportedly were no longer receiving orally inhaled corticosteroids at study conclusion. Whether results of this study are applicable to patients who are maintained on higher doses of orally inhaled corticosteroids or systemic corticosteroid therapy remains to be determined.

Montelukast has been evaluated for use in combination with orally inhaled corticosteroids in asthmatic adults whose symptoms were not controlled by 336 mcg/day of beclomethasone dipropionate. Patients were randomized to receive combined therapy with beclomethasone and montelukast, beclomethasone alone, montelukast alone (beclomethasone withdrawn), or placebo (beclomethasone withdrawn). Treatment with beclomethasone and montelukast was more effective in improving pulmonary function (as measured by FEV_1) than therapy with beclomethasone alone, montelukast alone, or placebo. In addition, beclomethasone alone was more effective than montelukast alone in alleviating respiratory symptoms (i.e., daytime asthma symptoms, nighttime awakenings), improving pulmonary function (as measured by FEV_1 and PEFR), and reducing the need for supplemental therapy with an orally inhaled β_2-adrenergic agonist. While combined therapy with orally inhaled corticosteroids and montelukast may improve asthma control in patients not adequately controlled with orally inhaled corticosteroids alone, substitution of montelukast for orally inhaled corticosteroids is not likely to result in improved asthma control in these patients. The relative merits of adding montelukast to a regimen of orally inhaled corticosteroids in patients whose symptoms are inadequately controlled versus doubling the dose of the orally inhaled corticosteroid remain to be determined.

In adults with documented aspirin sensitivity who were receiving orally inhaled and/or systemic corticosteroids, addition of montelukast improved asthma control compared with placebo. The magnitude of the effect of montelukast in aspirin-sensitive patients was similar to that observed in the general population of asthma patients enrolled in clinical trials. Montelukast-treated patients with aspirin sensitivity should avoid aspirin or nonsteroidal anti-inflammatory agents (NSAIAs) since montelukast has not been shown to truncate the bronchoconstrictor response to aspirin or other NSAIAs in aspirin-sensitive patients.

Exercise-induced Bronchospasm

Montelukast is used for the prevention of exercise-induced bronchospasm. In adults and adolescents 15 years of age or older with a FEV_1 averaging 83% of the predicted normal value and exercise-induced exacerbation of asthma, montelukast (10 mg daily 20–24 hours prior to exercise) reduced the mean maximal fall in FEV_1 and time to recovery compared with placebo. In this study, the response to montelukast was similar after 4, 8, and 12 weeks; however, not all patients responded to montelukast. Montelukast did not prevent clinically important deterioration in the maximal fall in FEV_1 after exercise (i.e., a 20% or greater decrease from baseline [before exercise]) in 52% of patients. While about 23% of patients experienced complete protection (i.e., a decrease in FEV_1 of less than 10% after exercise), 25% had little or no response (i.e., decrease in FEV_1 of more than 30% after exercise).

In one multinational, randomized, double-blind, placebo-controlled crossover study, efficacy of montelukast was evaluated in 64 pediatric patients 6–14 years of age with exercise-induced bronchospasm who received a single dose of montelukast 5 mg as a chewable tablet or placebo administered 2 hours before exercise. Exercise challenge testing was conducted at 2 and 24 hours in these patients following administration of montelukast or placebo. In this study, the primary end point was the mean maximum percent fall in FEV_1 following the post-dose exercise challenge at 2 hours. Results of the study showed that montelukast 5 mg demonstrated a substantial protective effect against exercise-induced bronchospasm in these patients compared with placebo. Similar results were shown for the secondary end point of mean maximum percent fall in FEV_1 following the post-dose exercise challenge at 24 hours. However, the protective effect of montelukast for prevention of exercise-induced bronchospasm did not persist for all patients 24 hours following administration of the drug.

Results of 2 randomized, controlled studies in adults (15–46 years of age) with exercise-induced bronchospasm indicate that the bronchoprotective effect of montelukast is similar to that of salmeterol. Efficacy of montelukast in exercise-induced bronchoconstriction versus other therapies (e.g., orally inhaled albuterol, cromolyn sodium, or nedocromil [preparation for oral inhalation no longer commercially available in the US]) has not been established.

Advantages of montelukast for the management of exercise-induced bronchospasm compared with some other therapies (e.g., orally inhaled albuterol, cromolyn sodium, nedocromil [no longer commercially available in the US]) include oral administration and a protective effect that persists for 20–24 hours. While leukotriene modifiers are not included as first-line agents or as alternative agents to orally inhaled β_2-adrenergic agonists for the prevention or treatment of exercise-induced bronchoconstriction in current guidelines, current evidence supports their bronchoprotective efficacy, and the addition of montelukast may provide an additional measure of control in patients currently maintained on long-term controller therapy. The National Collegiate Athletic Association, the US Olympic Committee, and the International Olympic Committee allow competitors to use leukotriene modifiers without prior approval. The manufacturer states that patients who experience exacerbations of asthma after exercise should have a short-acting orally inhaled β_2-adrenergic agonist available for rescue. Daily administration of montelukast for the chronic treatment of asthma has not been established to prevent acute episodes of exercise-induced bronchospasm.

Because of the risk of neuropsychiatric effects, the benefits and risks of montelukast treatment should be considered before prescribing the drug for patients with exercise-induced bronchospasm. (See Cautions: Precautions and Contraindications.)

• Allergic Rhinitis

Montelukast is used for the symptomatic treatment of seasonal or perennial allergic rhinitis. Montelukast has been evaluated in a number of placebo-controlled or comparative trials with loratadine or cetirizine for the treatment of seasonal or perennial allergic rhinitis in patients 15–82 years of age. Therapy with montelukast generally has been associated with modest improvement in rhinitis end points (scores evaluating nasal congestion, nasal itching, rhinorrhea, nasal pruritus, sneezing) compared with placebo. Therapy with montelukast alone or in combination with loratadine has been associated with improved ocular manifestations, daytime nasal symptoms, nighttime symptoms, global evaluations, and quality of life compared with placebo.

Because the benefits of montelukast treatment may not outweigh the risks of neuropsychiatric effects in patients with allergic rhinitis, use of the drug in such patients should be reserved for those who have an inadequate response or intolerance to alternative therapies. (See Cautions: Precautions and Contraindications.)

• Urticaria

Montelukast (5–20 mg daily) has been used successfully in a limited number of patients with chronic idiopathic urticaria†; one retrospective analysis involving 18 patients indicated that many patients may benefit from the addition of a leukotriene modifier to existing therapy. Additional study is needed to elucidate further the role of leukotriene modifiers in the treatment of urticaria.

DOSAGE AND ADMINISTRATION

• Administration

In patients with asthma with or without coexisting allergic rhinitis, montelukast is administered orally as a single daily dose in the evening. Safety and efficacy of montelukast in the management of asthma were established in clinical trials in which the drug was administered in the evening without regard to meals in adults, adolescents, and children 2–14 years of age. Evening dosing has been employed so that achievement of peak plasma concentrations of the drug might coincide with peak airway reactivity in the morning. In patients with allergic rhinitis, the time of administration may be individualized to suit patient needs. Efficacy was demonstrated in patients with seasonal allergic rhinitis when montelukast was administered in the morning or evening without regard to food intake.

Pharmacokinetic and clinical data support use of the 10-mg film-coated tablet of montelukast in adults and adolescents 15 years of age or older, use of the 5-mg chewable tablet in children 6–14 years of age, use of the 4-mg chewable tablet or 4-mg oral granules formulation in children 2–5 years of age, and use of the 4-mg oral granules formulation in infants and children 12–23 months of age for the treatment of asthma and in infants and children 6–23 months of age for the treatment of perennial allergic rhinitis.

Oral granules may be administered orally alone (directly in the mouth) or mixed with 1 teaspoonful (5 mL) of cold or room temperature baby formula or breast milk, or a spoonful of cold or room temperature soft food (applesauce, carrots, rice, or ice cream only); the stability of the drug when mixed with other foods has not been determined. Oral granules are not intended to be dissolved in any liquid other than baby formula or breast milk prior to administration. However, liquids may be taken subsequent to administration, and oral granules can be administered without regard to meals. The packet should not be opened until ready to use. After opening the packet of granules, patients should receive the full dose within 15 minutes; do not store the opened packet or mixtures of the drug with food, breast milk, or baby formula. Any unused portions should be discarded.

• Dosage

Dosage of montelukast sodium is expressed in terms of montelukast.

Asthma

Patients should be advised that montelukast must be taken at regular intervals (i.e., daily) to be therapeutically effective. In addition, patients should be advised that the drug will *not* provide immediate symptomatic relief and should *not* be used for relief of acute bronchospasm; however, montelukast therapy can be continued during acute exacerbations of asthma. Patients should *not* discontinue or reduce the dosage of other antiasthmatic agents, even if they feel better as a result of initiation of montelukast therapy, unless instructed to do so by their clinician.

No additional dosage is needed for the treatment of allergic rhinitis in patients already receiving chronic therapy for asthma.

Adult Dosage

For the prevention and long-term symptomatic control of asthma with or without allergic rhinitis, the usual dosage of montelukast for adults and adolescents 15 years of age or older is 10 mg once daily as film-coated tablets. The pharmacokinetic profile of montelukast in geriatric adults generally is similar to that in younger adults, and the manufacturer states that dosage of the drug in geriatric patients does not need to be modified based solely on age.

Pediatric Dosage

Adolescents 15 years of age or older may receive the usual adult dosage of montelukast of 10 mg once daily as film-coated tablets.

For the prevention and long-term symptomatic control of asthma with or without allergic rhinitis, the usual dosage of montelukast for children 6–14 years of age is 5 mg once daily as chewable tablets. The usual dosage of montelukast for the prevention and long-term symptomatic control of asthma with or without allergic rhinitis in children 2–5 years of age is 4 mg once daily as chewable tablets or oral granules. The usual dosage of montelukast for the prevention and long-term symptomatic control of asthma with or without allergic rhinitis in pediatric patients 12–23 months of age is 4 mg once daily as oral granules.

Exercise-induced Bronchospasm

For the prevention of exercise-induced bronchospasm, montelukast should be administered at least 2 hours before exercise. Patients already taking montelukast for another indication, including chronic asthma, should not take an additional dose of the drug to prevent exercise-induced bronchospasm. All patients should have a short-acting β_2-adrenergic agonist available for exacerbations of asthma that may occur after exercise despite montelukast therapy.

Adult Dosage

For the prevention of exercise-induced bronchospasm, the usual dosage of montelukast for adults and adolescents 15 years of age or older not already taking the drug for another indication is 10 mg as a film-coated tablet administered at least 2 hours prior to exercise; an additional dose should not be taken within 24 hours of the previous dose. The pharmacokinetic profile of montelukast in geriatric adults generally is similar to that in younger adults, and the manufacturer states that dosage of the drug in geriatric patients does not need to be modified based solely on age.

Pediatric Dosage

For prevention of exercise-induced bronchospasm in children 6–14 years of age not already taking the drug for another indication, the usual dosage is 5 mg as a chewable tablet administered at least 2 hours prior to exercise; an additional dose should not be taken within 24 hours of the previous dose. Safety and efficacy of montelukast for exercise-induced bronchospasm in patients younger than 6 years of age have not been established.

Allergic Rhinitis
Adult Dosage

For symptomatic control of seasonal or perennial allergic rhinitis with or without asthma, the usual dosage of montelukast is 10 mg once daily as film-coated tablets.

Pediatric Dosage

Adolescents 15 years of age or older with allergic rhinitis with or without asthma may be given 10 mg once daily as film-coated tablets.

For the symptomatic control of seasonal or perennial allergic rhinitis with or without asthma, the usual dosage of montelukast for children 6–14 years of age is 5 mg once daily as chewable tablets. In children 2–5 years of age with seasonal or perennial allergic rhinitis with or without asthma, the usual dosage is 4 mg once daily as chewable tablets or oral granules. In infants and children 12–23 months of age or older with allergic rhinitis and asthma, the usual dosage of montelukast is 4 mg once daily as oral granules. The usual dosage of montelukast in pediatric patients 6–23 months of age with perennial allergic rhinitis is 4 mg once daily as oral granules.

● Dosage in Renal and Hepatic Impairment

Limited evidence in patients with mild to moderate hepatic impairment and clinical evidence of cirrhosis indicate that area under the plasma concentration-time curve (AUC) of montelukast is increased 41% and plasma montelukast

elimination half-life is prolonged in these patients relative to patients with normal hepatic function. However, the manufacturer makes no specific recommendations for adjustment of montelukast dosage in patients with mild to moderate hepatic impairment. The pharmacokinetics of montelukast in patients with severe hepatic impairment or with hepatitis have not been evaluated.

The manufacturer makes no specific recommendations for dosage adjustment in patients with renal impairment. The drug is extensively metabolized and excreted principally in feces.

CAUTIONS

Montelukast generally is well tolerated. Safety of montelukast has been evaluated in adults and adolescents 15 years of age or older with asthma or allergic rhinitis, in children 2–14 years of age with allergic rhinitis, in children 12 months of age or older with asthma, and in infants 6–23 months with perennial allergic rhinitis. While most adults and children 2 years of age or older with asthma received montelukast in clinical trials of 12 weeks' duration, safety data also have been collected from long-term studies lasting up to 2 years. The types of adverse effects reported in long-term studies were comparable to those reported in short-term, controlled studies.

A causal relationship between many adverse effects and montelukast has not been established. In clinical studies in adults and adolescents 15 years of age or older with asthma, adverse effects occurring in at least 1% of patients receiving montelukast and more frequently than with placebo included headache, influenza, abdominal pain, cough, increased serum ALT or AST concentration, dyspepsia, dizziness, asthenia/fatigue, dental pain, nasal congestion, rash, fever, infectious gastroenteritis, trauma, and pyuria, and the safety profile did not change substantially over time. In studies in asthmatic children 6–14 years of age, influenza, fever, dyspepsia, diarrhea, laryngitis, pharyngitis, nausea, otitis, sinusitis, and viral infection occurred in at least 2% of patients and more frequently in those receiving montelukast than in those receiving placebo; the safety profile in these children generally was similar to that in adults and did not change substantially over time. In clinical studies in asthmatic children 2–5 years of age, adverse effects occurring in at least 2% of patients receiving montelukast and more frequently than with placebo included fever, cough, abdominal pain, diarrhea, headache, rhinorrhea, sinusitis, otitis, influenza, rash, otic pain, gastroenteritis, eczema, urticaria, varicella, pneumonia, dermatitis, and conjunctivitis. In clinical studies in asthmatic children 6–23 months of age, upper respiratory tract infection, wheezing, otitis media, pharyngitis, tonsillitis, cough, and rhinitis occurred in at least 2% of patients receiving montelukast and more frequently than with placebo.

Discontinuance of montelukast therapy was required in about 2% of adolescents and adults and 4% of children 6–14 years of age in clinical studies, principally because of exacerbation of asthma.

● Nervous System Effects

Headache is the most frequently reported adverse effect with montelukast, occurring in 18–19% of children 6 years of age or older, adolescents, and adults. Headache has been reported in at least 2% of children 2–8 years of age with asthma receiving montelukast and in at least 1% (and more frequently than with placebo) of adults and adolescents 15 years of age or older with asthma. Sinus headache has been reported in at least 1% of adult and adolescent patients 15 years of age or older with perennial allergic rhinitis receiving montelukast and more frequently than in those receiving placebo. Dizziness or asthenia/fatigue has occurred in about 1.8–1.9% of patients 15 years of age or older receiving the drug in clinical studies. Dream abnormalities, hallucinations, agitation including aggressive behavior or hostility, anxiousness, paresthesia/hypoesthesia, seizures, drowsiness, insomnia, somnambulism, irritability, depression, suicidal thinking and behavior (including suicide), tremor, and restlessness also have been reported. (See Cautions: Precautions and Contraindications.)

● GI Effects

Abdominal pain has occurred in 2.9% of patients 15 years of age or older receiving montelukast. Dyspepsia, infectious gastroenteritis, and dental pain have been reported in 2.1, 1.5, and 1.7% of patients in this age group, respectively. Diarrhea or nausea has been reported in at least 2% of children 6–14 years of age receiving montelukast. Abdominal pain, diarrhea, and gastroenteritis have been reported in at least 2% of children 2–5 years of age with asthma and more frequently than in those receiving placebo. Gastroenteritis has been reported in at least 2% of children 6–8 years of age with asthma and more frequently than in those receiving placebo. Nausea, vomiting, dyspepsia, pancreatitis (rarely), and diarrhea also have been reported with montelukast therapy during postmarketing experience.

● Hepatic Effects

Elevations in the results of one or more liver function tests have occurred in patients receiving montelukast in clinical studies. Increases in serum ALT (SGPT) or AST (SGOT) concentrations occurred in 2.1 or 1.6%, respectively, of patients 15 years of age or older with asthma receiving montelukast in clinical studies. Increases in ALT occurred in at least 1% of adult and adolescent patients 15 years of age or older with perennial allergic rhinitis receiving montelukast in clinical studies and more frequently than in those receiving placebo. Changes in laboratory values returned to normal despite continuing montelukast therapy or were not directly attributable to drug therapy. Elevations in serum aminotransferase (transaminase) concentrations also have been reported in children 2–14 years of age receiving montelukast, but the incidence of these elevations was similar to that in children receiving placebo. Hepatic eosinophilic infiltration has been reported very rarely through postmarketing experience with montelukast. (See Dermatologic and Sensitivity Reactions.) Hepatocellular injury, cholestatic hepatitis, or mixed-pattern liver injury also has been reported rarely through postmarketing experience with montelukast. Confounding factors were present in most of these patients, such as the concomitant use of other drugs or alcohol or in the presence of coexisting conditions (e.g., other forms of hepatitis).

● Dermatologic and Sensitivity Reactions

Rash has occurred in 1.6% of adults and adolescents 15 years of age or older receiving montelukast. Rash, eczema, dermatitis, or urticaria has been reported in at least 2% of children 2–5 years of age receiving the drug. Atopic dermatitis, varicella, and skin infection have been reported in at least 2% of children 6–8 years of age with asthma receiving montelukast and more frequently than in those receiving placebo. Hypersensitivity reactions, including anaphylaxis, angioedema, pruritus, urticaria, and rarely hepatic eosinophilic infiltration, have been reported in patients receiving montelukast.

Eosinophilia and Churg-Strauss Syndrome

Although montelukast therapy generally is associated with a decrease in peripheral blood eosinophil counts in asthmatic patients (see Pharmacology: Effects on Eosinophils), systemic eosinophilia, sometimes presenting with clinical features of vasculitis consistent with Churg-Strauss syndrome, has been reported rarely in patients receiving leukotriene modifiers (e.g., montelukast, pranlukast, zafirlukast); in almost all cases, these events were associated with a reduction (tapered dosage) or withdrawal of oral or high-dose inhaled corticosteroid therapy.

Churg-Strauss syndrome (allergic granulomatosis and angiitis) is an uncommon vasculitis of unknown etiology that is potentially fatal and characterized by at least 4 of the following 6 features: moderate to severe asthma, peripheral blood eosinophilia (greater than 10% on differential leukocyte count), mononeuropathy or polyneuropathy, nonfixed pulmonary infiltrates on radiograph, paranasal sinus abnormality, and blood vessel biopsy with extravascular eosinophils. The incidence of this syndrome in patients receiving leukotriene modifiers (e.g., zafirlukast) has been estimated to be approximately 60 cases/million patient-years of exposures; this is similar to the estimated incidence of this syndrome reported in patients receiving other antiasthmatic drugs (bambuterol, salmeterol, nedocromil [preparation for oral inhalation no longer commercially available in the US]). The onset of Churg-Strauss syndrome has been reported to range from 2 days to 10 months after initiation of leukotriene modifier therapy, and in most cases corticosteroid therapy had been withdrawn or dosage tapered within 3 months of the development of the syndrome.

Although the exact mechanism of Churg-Strauss syndrome has not been determined, it is unlikely that its development during therapy with leukotriene modifiers is directly attributable to these drugs. Instead, the occurrence of Churg-Strauss syndrome in patients receiving leukotriene modifiers is believed to result from unmasking of an underlying vasculitic syndrome that initially was diagnosed as moderate to severe asthma. In such patients, it has been postulated that corticosteroid therapy had suppressed or delayed the development of overt Churg-Strauss syndrome, and initiation of therapy with leukotriene modifiers resulted in decreased steroid requirements, with a subsequent unmasking of the syndrome as corticosteroid therapy was tapered or withdrawn. Remission of the syndrome usually can be induced with systemic corticosteroid therapy alone, although other immunodulating agents (e.g., cyclophosphamide, methotrexate) may be necessary in some patients.

● Respiratory Effects

Influenza, cough, and nasal congestion have been reported in 4.2, 2.7, and 1.6%, respectively, of montelukast-treated patients with asthma 15 years of age or older. Upper respiratory tract infection occurred in 1.9 or at least 2% of patients

15 years of age or older or 2–14 years of age, respectively, with seasonal allergic rhinitis. Upper respiratory tract infection, wheezing, pharyngitis, tonsillitis, cough, and rhinitis occurred in at least 2% of patients 12–23 months of age with asthma. Pharyngitis occurred in at least 2% of patients 2–14 years of age with seasonal allergic rhinitis. Laryngitis, pharyngitis, sinusitis, and viral infection have occurred in at least 2% of children 6–14 years of age with asthma receiving montelukast and more frequently than in those receiving placebo. Rhinorrhea, cough, sinusitis, influenza, and pneumonia have been reported in at least 2% of montelukast-treated children 2–5 years of age with asthma and more frequently than in those receiving placebo. Sinusitis, upper respiratory tract infection, or cough occurred in at least 1% of adult and adolescent patients 15 years of age or older with perennial allergic rhinitis receiving montelukast and more frequently than in those receiving placebo. Infective rhinitis and acute bronchitis occurred in at least 2% of montelukast-treated children 6–8 years of age with asthma and more frequently than in those receiving placebo.

● Other Adverse Effects

Fever or trauma occurred in 1.5 or 1% of patients 15 years of age or older receiving montelukast. Fever also has been reported in children 2–14 years of age. Fever, otic pain, or otitis occurred in at least 2% of children 2–5 years of age with asthma and more frequently than in those receiving placebo. Otitis has occurred in at least 2% of the children 6–14 years of age with asthma and more frequently than in those receiving placebo. Otitis media has occurred in at least 2% of montelukast-treated patients 12–23 months of age with asthma or 2–14 years of age with seasonal allergic rhinitis and more frequently than in those receiving placebo. Pyuria has occurred in 1% of patients 15 years of age or older and more frequently than with placebo. At least 2% of montelukast-treated children 2–5 years of age experienced conjunctivitis, varicella, leg pain, or thirst, each occurring more frequently than with placebo. Tooth infection and myopia have been reported in at least 2% of montelukast-treated children 6–8 years of age with asthma and more frequently than in those receiving placebo. Epistaxis occurred in at least 1% of adult and adolescent patients 15 years of age or older with perennial allergic rhinitis receiving montelukast and more frequently than in those receiving placebo. Edema has been reported through postmarketing experience with montelukast. Myalgia (including muscle cramps) arthralgia, palpitations, bruising, edema, and an increased tendency for bleeding also has occurred in montelukast-treated patients.

● Precautions and Contraindications

Patients should be advised that montelukast must be taken at regular intervals to be therapeutically effective. In addition, patients should be advised that the drug will not provide immediate symptomatic relief and should *not* be used for the relief of acute bronchospasm; however, montelukast therapy can be continued during acute exacerbations of asthma. Patients receiving montelukast should be provided with and instructed in the use of a short-acting, inhaled β_2-adrenergic bronchodilator as supplemental therapy for acute asthma symptoms. Patients should not discontinue or reduce the dosage of other antiasthmatic agents, even if they feel better as a result of initiation of montelukast therapy, unless instructed to do so by their clinician.

The manufacturer states that patients who experience exacerbations of asthma after exercise should have a short-acting orally inhaled β_2-adrenergic agonist available for rescue. (See Exercise-induced Bronchospasm under Uses: Bronchospasm.)

Patients in whom asthma is precipitated by aspirin or other nonsteroidal anti-inflammatory agents (NSAIAs) should continue to avoid aspirin and NSAIAs while receiving montelukast. While montelukast can improve airway function in asthmatic patients with documented aspirin sensitivity, the drug has *not* been shown to truncate the bronchoconstrictor response to aspirin or other NSAIAs in such patients.

Although orally inhaled corticosteroid requirements in patients with stable asthma may be reduced during montelukast therapy, only gradual (e.g., at 2-week intervals) reduction of the steroid dosage should be undertaken. Montelukast should not be abruptly substituted for oral or inhaled corticosteroids.

Serious neuropsychiatric effects have been reported during postmarketing experience with montelukast. These postmarketing reports have been highly variable and included, but were not limited to, agitation, aggressive behavior or hostility, anxiousness, depression, disorientation, disturbance in attention, dream abnormalities, dysphemia (stuttering), hallucinations, insomnia, irritability, memory impairment, obsessive-compulsive symptoms, restlessness, somnambulism, suicidal thoughts and behavior (including completed suicides), tic, and tremor in adults, adolescents, and pediatric patients with or without a history of psychiatric disorders. Neuropsychiatric effects have been reported mainly during montelukast treatment and resolved after the drug was discontinued; however, some of these effects developed or continued following discontinuance of the drug. Based on available data, it is difficult to identify risk factors for or to quantify the risk of neuropsychiatric effects with use of montelukast. The mechanisms underlying neuropsychiatric effects associated with use of montelukast are not well understood; however, it is known that montelukast distributes into the brain in rats. FDA evaluated reports for all neuropsychiatric adverse effects (including completed suicides) associated with use of montelukast from February 1998 (date of drug approval) through May 2019. A total of 82 cases of completed suicide associated with montelukast use were identified; many of these cases reported the development of concomitant neuropsychiatric symptoms prior to the event. Most of these reports did not contain sufficient information (e.g., time to onset of event, use of concomitant medications, presence of comorbidities or other risk factors) to determine the exact relationship between montelukast and these neuropsychiatric events. Following extensive review of the postmarketing reports and analysis of available clinical data, FDA convened a panel of outside experts to reevaluate the benefits and risks of montelukast and concluded that there was a need to strengthen existing warnings in the labeling for the drug, including restrictions for use in patients with allergic rhinitis. (See Uses: Allergic Rhinitis.) The manufacturer of montelukast states that patients receiving the drug and their caregivers and/or clinicians should be alert to the potential for neuropsychiatric effects, including changes in behavior or new neuropsychiatric symptoms. The benefits and risks of using montelukast should be considered when deciding to prescribe or continue therapy with the drug. Prior to initiation of therapy, patients should be asked about any history of psychiatric illness. Patients should be advised to discontinue montelukast and to contact their clinician immediately if changes in behavior, new neuropsychiatric symptoms, or suicidal thoughts and/or behavior occur during therapy with montelukast. Clinicians should provide patient monitoring and supportive care until such symptoms resolve, and should carefully evaluate the risks and benefits of reinitiating treatment with montelukast if such effects occur.

Eosinophilia, vasculitic rash, worsening pulmonary symptoms, cardiac complications, and/or neuropathy consistent with Churg-Strauss syndrome, a systemic eosinophilic vasculitis, have been reported rarely in patients receiving leukotriene modifiers (e.g., montelukast, pranlukast, zafirlukast). While a causal relationship between this syndrome and leukotriene modifiers has not been established, clinicians should be alert to the development of such manifestations in patients receiving leukotriene modifiers. Patients should inform their clinician immediately if symptoms of Churg-Strauss syndrome (e.g., feeling of pins and needles or numbness of extremities, flu-like symptoms, rash, sinusitis) occur. (See Eosinophilia and Churg-Strauss Syndrome under Cautions: Dermatologic and Sensitivity Reactions.)

Patients should be advised that an increase in frequency of administration of short-acting inhaled bronchodilators or inadequate control of symptoms while receiving the maximum prescribed dosage of an inhaled bronchodilator may indicate substantial worsening of asthma that requires evaluation.

Montelukast is contraindicated in patients hypersensitive to the drug or any ingredient in the formulation. Individuals with phenylketonuria (i.e., homozygous genetic deficiency of phenylalanine hydroxylase) and other individuals who must restrict their intake of phenylalanine should be advised that montelukast chewable tablets contain aspartame (Nutrasweet®), which is metabolized in the GI tract to provide 0.674 mg of phenylalanine for each 4-mg chewable tablet or 0.842 mg of phenylalanine for each 5-mg chewable tablet of montelukast.

● *Pediatric Precautions*

Safety and efficacy of montelukast for the treatment of asthma in children younger than 12 months of age have not been established. Safety and efficacy of montelukast for the prevention of exercise-induced bronchospasm in children younger than 6 years of age have not been established.

Safety and efficacy of montelukast in infants younger than 6 months of age with perennial allergic rhinitis have not been established. Safety and efficacy of montelukast in pediatric patients younger than 2 years of age with seasonal allergic rhinitis have not been established.

Safety of montelukast oral granules in pediatric patients 12–23 months with asthma has been demonstrated in a placebo-controlled trial and other clinical experience. Efficacy of montelukast in this age group was explored as a secondary end point in a safety study and is extrapolated from demonstrated efficacy in patients 6 years of age or older based on similar mean systemic exposure to montelukast and the substantial similarity of the disease course, pathophysiology, and effects of the drug among these populations.

Safety and efficacy of montelukast have been established in adequate and well-controlled studies in children 6–14 years of age with asthma and are similar

to those reported in adults. Safety of the drug in children 2–5 years of age with asthma is extrapolated from demonstrated efficacy in asthmatic adults, adolescents, and children 6 years of age or older based on similar mean systemic exposure to montelukast and the substantial similarity of the disease course, pathophysiology, and effects of the drug among these populations. Efficacy of montelukast in children 2–5 years of age is supported by exploratory efficacy assessments from a large, well-controlled safety study.

Efficacy of montelukast in pediatric patients 2–14 years or 6 months to 14 years of age with seasonal or perennial allergic rhinitis, respectively, is supported by extrapolation from demonstrated efficacy in patients 15 years of age and older with allergic rhinitis and the assumption that the disease course, pathophysiology, and drug's effect are substantially similar among these populations. Safety of the montelukast in pediatric patients aged 2–14 years of age with allergic rhinitis is supported by data from studies in pediatric patients 2–14 years of age with asthma. Data from a safety study of montelukast therapy in pediatric patients 2–14 years of age with seasonal allergic rhinitis demonstrated a safety profile similar to that of placebo. Safety of montelukast in pediatric patients 6–23 months with perennial allergic rhinitis is supported by data from studies in pediatric patients 6–23 months of age with asthma and by pharmacokinetic data comparing systemic exposure in such pediatric patients with that in adults.

The effect of long-term therapy with montelukast on linear growth in pediatric patients has been assessed in a 56-week, multicenter, double-blind, randomized study with an active control (beclomethasone dipropionate) and placebo control in 360 children 6–8 years of age with mild asthma. Montelukast (5 mg once daily) did not affect growth rate in children compared with placebo; however, growth rate was slowed in children taking orally inhaled beclomethasone dipropionate (168 mcg twice daily) with chlorofluorocarbon propellants (no longer commercially available in the US) compared with placebo.

● *Geriatric Precautions*

When the total number of patients studied in clinical trials of montelukast is considered, 3.5% were 65 years of age or older, while 0.4% were 75 years of age or older. Although no overall differences in safety or efficacy were observed between geriatric and younger patients, and other clinical experience revealed no evidence of age-related differences, the possibility that some older patients may exhibit increased sensitivity to the drug cannot be ruled out.

Changes in the plasma elimination half-life of montelukast occur in geriatric individuals but do not affect the dosing regimen.

● *Mutagenicity and Carcinogenicity*

Montelukast was not mutagenic or clastogenic in the microbial mutagenesis assay, the V-79 mammalian cell mutagenesis assay, the alkaline elution assay in rat hepatocytes, the chromosomal aberration assay in Chinese hamster ovary cells, or the in vivo mouse bone marrow chromosomal aberration assay.

Montelukast was not tumorigenic in a 2-year carcinogenicity study in rats at oral (gavage) dosages up to 200 mg/kg daily (estimated exposure approximately 120 and 75 times the area under the plasma concentration-time curve [AUC] for adults and children, respectively, at the maximum recommended daily oral dose) or in a 92-week carcinogenicity study in mice at oral (gavage) dosages up to 100 mg/kg daily (estimated exposure approximately 45 and 25 times the AUC for adults and children, respectively, at the maximum recommended daily oral dose).

● *Pregnancy, Fertility, and Lactation*
Pregnancy

Montelukast crosses the placenta following oral dosing in rats and rabbits. Reproduction studies in rats using oral dosages up to 400 mg/kg daily (estimated exposure approximately 100 times the AUC for adults at the maximum recommended daily oral dose) and in rabbits using oral dosages up to 300 mg/kg daily (estimated exposure approximately 110 times the AUC for adults at the maximum recommended daily oral dose) have not revealed evidence of harm to the fetus.

There are no adequate and well-controlled studies to date using montelukast in pregnant women, and the manufacturer states that montelukast should be used during pregnancy only when clearly needed. The American College of Obstetricians and Gynecologists (ACOG) generally recommends use of leukotriene modifiers as an alternative to a long-acting β₂-agonist in pregnant women with moderate persistent asthma who are inadequately controlled with low to medium dosages of an inhaled corticosteroid. (See Uses: Asthma.)

During postmarketing experience with montelukast, congenital limb defects have been reported rarely in the children of women treated with the drug;

however, most of these women were receiving other antiasthmatic agents during their pregnancies. A causal relationship between montelukast use and the development of these congenital anomalies has not been established. The manufacturer maintains a registry to monitor pregnancy outcomes in women exposed to montelukast during pregnancy. Patients may be enrolled by calling 800-986-8999.

Fertility

While reproduction studies in female rats using oral montelukast doses up to 100 mg/kg (estimated exposure approximately 20 times the AUC for adults at the maximum recommended daily oral dose) have not revealed evidence of impaired fertility, oral doses of 200 mg/kg (estimated exposure approximately 70 times the AUC for adults at the maximum recommended daily oral dose) have been associated with reduced fertility and fecundity indices. Reproduction studies in male rats using oral montelukast doses up to 800 mg/kg (estimated exposure approximately 160 times the AUC for adults at the maximum recommended daily oral dose) have not revealed evidence of impaired fertility.

Lactation

Montelukast is distributed into milk in rats. Since it is not known whether montelukast is distributed in human milk, the drug should be used with caution in nursing women.

DRUG INTERACTIONS

Montelukast has been used concomitantly in clinical studies with other drugs used routinely for the prevention and long-term symptomatic management of asthma without an apparent increase in adverse effects. In addition, montelukast has been used concomitantly with benzodiazepines, decongestants, nonsteroidal anti-inflammatory agents (NSAIAs), sedative-hypnotics, or thyroid hormones without evidence of an increase in adverse effects.

In drug-interaction studies, usual dosages of montelukast did not have clinically important effects on the pharmacokinetics of theophylline, warfarin, terfenadine (no longer commercially available in the US), digoxin, oral contraceptives (ethinyl estradiol with norethindrone), prednisone, or prednisolone.

● Nonsteroidal Anti-inflammatory Agents

Montelukast-treated patients with known aspirin sensitivity should continue to avoid aspirin and other NSAIAs. Although montelukast can improve airway function in asthmatics with aspirin sensitivity, the drug has *not* been shown to truncate the bronchoconstrictor response to aspirin or other NSAIAs in such patients, and an anaphylactic reaction has been reported following exposure to a NSAIA (e.g., diclofenac) in at least one aspirin-sensitive individual receiving montelukast.

● Drugs Affecting Hepatic Microsomal Enzymes

Metabolism of montelukast is mediated in part by the cytochrome P-450 (CYP) isoenzymes 3A4 and 2C9, and the possibility exists that drugs that induce or inhibit these isoenzymes may alter the plasma concentrations of montelukast. Montelukast does not appear to have any inhibitory effect on CYP3A4, CYP2C9, CYP1A2, CYP2A6, CYP2C19, or CYP2D6. Data from in vitro studies indicate that montelukast is a potent inhibitor of CYP2C8. However, data from several clinical drug interaction studies evaluating montelukast and rosiglitazone or repaglinide, substrates for the CYP2C8 isoenzyme, indicate that montelukast does not inhibit CYP2C8 in vivo. Therefore, clinical drug interactions involving montelukast and CYP2C8 substrates (e.g., paclitaxel, rosiglitazone, repaglinide) are not anticipated.

The effect of drugs that inhibit CYP3A4 (e.g., erythromycin, ketoconazole) or CYP2C9 (e.g., fluconazole) on the pharmacokinetics of montelukast remains to be determined.

Phenobarbital

Administration of phenobarbital, which induces cytochrome P-450 isoenzymes, and a single 10-mg dose of montelukast resulted in a reduction of 40% in area under the plasma montelukast concentration-time curve (AUC). The manufacturer of montelukast states that the drug can be administered without dosage adjustment in patients also receiving phenobarbital. However, patients receiving montelukast with drugs that are potent inducers of cytochrome P-450 isoenzymes (e.g., phenobarbital) should be monitored for alterations in clinical response and/or adverse effects.

Theophylline

Although theophylline may be metabolized to some extent via the CYP3A4 isoenzyme, drug interaction studies did not reveal evidence of a pharmacokinetic interaction with usual dosages of montelukast; however, the potential for an interaction exists with higher than recommended montelukast dosages. Following IV administration of a single theophylline dose (4.65 mg/kg of anhydrous drug) in healthy adults who had achieved steady-state plasma montelukast concentrations while receiving montelukast 10 mg daily, clinically important changes in the pharmacokinetics of theophylline were not observed.

At daily montelukast dosages that were 20-fold higher (200 mg once daily) than the currently recommended dosage, montelukast decreased the peak concentration achieved with a single oral (250 mg) or IV (5 mg/kg) theophylline dose by 12 or 10% respectively, the AUC by 43 or 44%, respectively, and the elimination half-life by 44 or 39%, respectively. At a montelukast dosage that was 60-fold higher (200 mg 3 times daily) than recommended, the drug decreased the peak concentration of a single 250-mg oral dose of theophylline by 25%, AUC by 66%, and elimination half-life by 63%.

Warfarin

Although warfarin is eliminated principally via CYP-dependent hepatic metabolism (see Pharmacokinetics: Elimination, in Warfarin 20:12.04.08) and montelukast is highly (99%) protein bound, drug interaction studies did not identify clinically important pharmacokinetic interactions between the drugs. Concomitant administration of montelukast and warfarin does not appear to affect the pharmacokinetics of warfarin. The effect of a single 30-mg dose of warfarin on prothrombin time (PT) or international normalized ratio (INR) was not altered in healthy adults who had achieved steady-state plasma montelukast concentrations while receiving montelukast 10 mg daily. Montelukast did not exhibit a clinically important effect on AUCs or peak plasma concentrations of R- or S-warfarin, although slight but statistically significant decreases in the time to peak for both warfarin enantiomers and in elimination half-life of the less potent R-enantiomer were observed; the latter changes were not considered clinically important.

Rifampin

Although specific drug interaction studies have not been performed to date, the manufacturer states that it is reasonable to employ appropriate clinical monitoring when a potent cytochrome P-450 enzyme inducer such as rifampin is used concomitantly with montelukast.

Antihistamines

Administration of terfenadine (60 mg twice daily; no longer commercially available in the US) following achievement of steady-state plasma montelukast concentrations in adults receiving montelukast 10 mg daily did not alter the plasma concentration profile of terfenadine or fexofenadine, the active carboxylated metabolite, and did not affect ECG parameters (i.e., QT_c interval).

● Digoxin

Administration of digoxin in adults who had achieved steady-state plasma montelukast concentrations while receiving montelukast 10 mg daily did not alter the pharmacokinetic profile or urinary excretion of digoxin.

● Estrogen-Progestin Combinations

Administration of an oral contraceptive (a fixed combination of ethinyl estradiol 35 mcg with norethindrone 1 mg) following achievement of steady-state plasma montelukast concentrations in women receiving montelukast 100 mg or more daily did not alter the plasma concentrations of either the estrogen or the progestin.

● Corticosteroids

Administration of oral prednisone or IV prednisolone in patients who had achieved steady-state plasma montelukast concentrations while receiving montelukast 100 mg or more daily did not result in clinically important changes in the plasma profiles of the corticosteroids.

ACUTE TOXICITY

Limited information is available on the acute toxicity of montelukast. Single oral doses of up to 5 g/kg in mice (estimated exposure approximately 335 and 210 times the area under the plasma concentration-time curve [AUC] for adults and children, respectively, at the maximum recommended daily oral dose) and rats (estimated exposure approximately 230 and 145 times the AUC for adults and children, respectively, at the maximum recommended daily oral dose) were not lethal.

● Manifestations

Montelukast has been administered to adults with asthma in dosages up to 200 mg daily for 22 weeks, and in dosages up to 900 mg daily for approximately 1 week without clinically important adverse experiences.

There have been reports of acute overdosage with montelukast doses of up to 1 g in adults and children. While adverse effects were not reported in most incidents of overdosage, the most frequently reported adverse experiences that were reported included abdominal pain, somnolence, thirst, headache, vomiting, and psychomotor hyperactivity. Clinical and laboratory findings associated with these reports were consistent with the safety profile of the drug in adults and pediatric patients. In one 43-month-old child who ingested 65 mg of the drug and complained only of thirst, most of the ingested tablets were recovered via saline gastric lavage.

● Treatment

If acute overdosage of montelukast occurs, supportive and symptomatic treatment should be initiated and the patient closely observed. If indicated, unabsorbed material should be removed from the GI tract. Whether peritoneal dialysis or hemodialysis removes montelukast is unknown.

PHARMACOLOGY

● Anti-inflammatory Effects

Asthma and Allergic Rhinitis

Montelukast sodium, a selective, competitive leukotriene-receptor antagonist, affects inflammatory processes involved in asthma and allergic rhinitis. Current evidence indicates that asthma is a chronic inflammatory disorder of the airways involving the production and activity of several endogenous inflammatory mediators, including leukotrienes. Montelukast exerts beneficial effects in patients with asthma by inhibiting the action of leukotrienes at specific receptor sites (i.e., the cysteinyl leukotrienes C_4 [LTC_4], D_4 [LTD_4], and E_4 [LTE_4]) on airway smooth muscle and nasal mucosa. Cysteinyl leukotrienes are released from the nasal mucosa after allergen exposure and are associated with manifestations of allergic rhinitis (e.g., increased nasal airway resistance, nasal obstruction). Leukotriene modifiers (e.g., montelukast, zafirlukast, zileuton) have actions consistent with those of anti-inflammatory agents in that an expert panel of the National Asthma Education and Prevention Program has defined anti-inflammatory agents as those that reduce the markers of airway inflammation (e.g., eosinophils, mast cells, activated lymphocytes, macrophages, cytokines) in airway tissue or airway secretions and thereby reduce the intensity of airway hyperresponsiveness. However, the precise anti-inflammatory actions responsible for the therapeutic effects of drugs in asthma (e.g., symptom reduction, improvement in expiratory flow, reduction in airway hyperresponsiveness, prevention of exacerbations, prevention of airway wall remodeling) remain to be fully elucidated.

Effects on Leukotrienes

Leukotrienes are products of arachidonic acid metabolism via the 5-lipoxygenase pathway; the contribution of this pathway to the inflammatory process is complemented by the cyclooxygenase pathway, which converts arachidonic acid into other biologic mediators (e.g., prostaglandins, thromboxanes). Arachidonic acid is liberated by cell membranes in response to various factors, such as antigen-antibody interactions, IgE-receptor activation, microorganisms, and physical stimuli (e.g., cold, altered ionic conditions). The cysteinyl leukotrienes (LTC_4, LTD_4, LTE_4) and leukotriene B_4 (LTB_4, a potent chemotactic mediator) are derived from the initial unstable product of arachidonic acid metabolism, leukotriene A_4 (LTA_4). Cysteinyl leukotrienes are produced by a number of cell types, including eosinophils, basophils, mast cells, macrophages, and monocytes; however, the physiologic effects of these leukotrienes appear to be mediated through binding to a common receptor, CysLT. While several other mediators (e.g., histamine, prostaglandins) also act on target cells within airways to induce manifestations typical of asthma, the cysteinyl leukotrienes (formerly referred to as "slow-reacting substance of anaphylaxis" [SRSA]) are especially important in the pathogenesis of this disease, causing increased mucus secretion and vascular permeability, airway edema, bronchoconstriction, and altered cellular activity associated with the inflammatory process.

The involvement of leukotrienes in asthma is supported by evidence of increased concentrations of leukotrienes in biologic fluids (i.e., urine, bronchoalveolar lavage fluid, nasal fluid, plasma) of some patients with asthma compared with healthy individuals; increased urinary leukotriene concentrations also have been observed in patients following allergen challenge, episodes of asthma, and exercise or aspirin challenge. Compared with histamine or prostaglandins, cysteinyl leukotrienes are 100–1000 times more potent as bronchoconstrictors. In addition, patients with asthma are substantially more responsive to the effects of leukotrienes than are healthy individuals. In one study, patients with asthma were 25–100 times more sensitive to the bronchoconstrictor effects of inhaled LTD_4 than nonasthmatic individuals. However, there is substantial interindividual variability in airway sensitivity to the contractile effects of leukotrienes among both healthy individuals and patients with asthma.

Because of the role of leukotrienes in the pathogenesis of asthma, modification of leukotriene activity may be used to reduce airway symptoms, decrease bronchial smooth muscle tone, and improve asthma control. Inhibition of leukotriene-mediated effects may be achieved by drugs that interrupt 5-lipoxygenase activity and prevent formation of leukotrienes (e.g., zileuton) or by antagonism of leukotriene activity at specific receptor sites in the airway (e.g., montelukast, zafirlukast). The antagonist activity of montelukast is selective, competitive, and reversible. Montelukast competitively inhibits the action of LTD_4 at a subgroup of CysLT receptors ($CysLT_1$) in airway smooth muscle. In vitro, montelukast possesses affinity for the $CysLT_1$ receptor that is similar to that of LTD_4. In in vitro studies, montelukast antagonized contraction of isolated animal smooth muscle produced by LTD_4, but did not antagonize contraction produced by LTC_4. In animal studies, montelukast antagonized contraction of airway smooth muscle produced by LTD_4 or antigen.

Inhibition of Bronchoconstriction

In patients with asthma, oral montelukast inhibits bronchoconstriction induced by exposure to known precipitating factors (e.g., allergens, cold and/or dry air, exercise); in addition, both the acute bronchoconstrictor response (immediate/early asthmatic response [IAR, EAR]) and the delayed inflammatory response (late asthmatic response [LAR]) to inhaled antigen are inhibited. Montelukast reduces sensitivity to inhaled LTD_4 in patients with asthma. In studies evaluating the in vivo potency of montelukast, oral administration of a single 5-mg dose of montelukast attenuated LTD_4-induced bronchoconstriction. The effect of montelukast on LTD_4-induced bronchoconstriction is evident within 4 hours of drug administration and persists for 24 hours or longer. Montelukast is associated with a longer duration of inhibition of LTD_4-induced bronchoconstriction than oral zafirlukast. In addition, montelukast inhibits both the acute bronchoconstrictor response and the delayed inflammatory response to inhaled antigen. In one crossover, placebo-controlled study, montelukast inhibited the acute bronchoconstrictor and delayed inflammatory response to antigen by 75 and 57%, respectively. Following IV administration of montelukast 7 mg (not commercially available in the US) in patients with asthma, forced expiratory volume in 1 second (FEV_1) increased 15% over baseline at 15 minutes and 18.43% at 60 minutes; following administration of a single oral dose of montelukast 10 mg in patients with asthma, FEV_1 increased 4.67% at 15 minutes and 12.9% at 60 minutes.

In a limited number of patients with asthma, single oral doses of montelukast 100 or 250 mg increased the FEV_1 regardless of concomitant use of inhaled corticosteroids. In addition, data from one clinical study indicate the bronchodilatory effects of inhaled corticosteroids and montelukast are additive.

● Effects on Eosinophils

Montelukast therapy decreased mean peripheral blood eosinophil count 9–15% from baseline in pediatric (at least 2 years of age) and adult patients with asthma. While a decrease in peripheral blood eosinophil count may indicate that montelukast has important effects on parameters of asthmatic inflammation, the clinical importance of changes in eosinophil counts in asthmatic patients remains to be determined.

Similarly, therapy with montelukast in patients with seasonal allergic rhinitis (15 years of age or older) either prevented the rise in mean peripheral blood eosinophil counts observed with placebo or actually decreased mean peripheral blood eosinophil counts compared with placebo.

● Other Effects

Montelukast has essentially no affinity for prostanoid, cholinergic, or β-adrenergic receptors.

PHARMACOKINETICS

While safety and efficacy of montelukast (10 or 5 mg daily) have been established in clinical studies in which the drug was administered in the evening without regard to meals, pharmacokinetics have been studied principally in healthy nonasthmatic adults and in asthmatic children who received the drug in the morning. Pharmacokinetic studies have not revealed diurnal or gender-related differences in the pharmacokinetics of the drug; further study is needed to determine if there are race-related differences.

The plasma concentration profile following oral administration of montelukast 10 mg in adolescents 15 years of age or older is similar to that in young adults. In addition, the plasma concentration profile following oral administration of montelukast 4 or 5 mg chewable tablets in children 2–5 or 6–14 years of age, respectively, is similar to the profile in adults receiving montelukast 10 mg (as the commercially available film-coated tablet). In children 6–11 months of age, systemic exposure to montelukast and variability in plasma drug concentrations are greater than those observed in adults. Based on population analyses, the mean area under the plasma concentration-time curve (AUC) and the mean peak plasma drug concentration were 60 and 89% higher, respectively, than those observed in adults. Systemic exposure following administration of 4-mg granules in infants 12–23 months of age is less variable than that with the same formulation in younger children, but the mean AUC and mean peak plasma concentration were 33 and 60% higher, respectively, than that following administration of 10-mg film-coated tablets in adults. Changes in disposition kinetics of montelukast occur in geriatric individuals but do not affect the dosing regimen. Pharmacokinetics of montelukast are linear for oral doses up to 50 mg.

Bioequivalence of the 10-mg film-coated tablet versus the 5-mg chewable tablet (2 tablets) has not been evaluated; however, limited data indicate that absorption of montelukast administered as a 10-mg chewable tablet (not commercially available) is more rapid and more complete than when the drug is administered as the commercially available film-coated tablet. The 4-mg oral granule formulation is bioequivalent to the 4-mg chewable tablet when administered to fasting adults, and the oral granules can be used as an alternative to the chewable tablets in patients 2–5 years of age.

● Absorption

Montelukast is rapidly absorbed from the GI tract, and peak plasma concentrations are attained within 3–4, 2–2.5, or 2 hours following oral administration in the fasted state of a single 10-mg film-coated (in adults), 5-mg chewable (in adults), or 4-mg chewable (in children 2–5 years of age) tablet, respectively. Oral bioavailability of montelukast administered as a 10-mg tablet in adults is 58–66%; presence of food in the GI tract does not affect bioavailability when the 10-mg film-coated tablet is administered with a standard meal in the morning. Oral bioavailability of the drug administered as a 5-mg chewable tablet in adults is 73% when the drug is administered in fasting individuals and 63% when the drug is administered with a standard meal in the morning. Ingestion of a high-fat meal in the morning with the 4-mg oral granules formulation had no effect on the AUC of montelukast; however, the time to peak plasma concentrations was prolonged from 2.3 hours to 6.4 hours and peak plasma concentrations were reduced by 35%. Administration of montelukast granules with applesauce does not appear to have a clinically important effect on the pharmacokinetics of montelukast.

Following oral administration of montelukast 10 mg daily for 7 days in fasting young adults, peak plasma concentrations averaged 541 ng/mL on day 1 and 602.8 ng/mL on day 7. Trough concentrations on days 3–7 were essentially constant and ranged from 18–24 ng/mL. In this study, values for area under the plasma concentration-time curve (AUC) at steady-state were about 14–15% higher than those achieved with a single dose, and were reached within 2 days.

The therapeutic effects of montelukast (e.g., as determined by improvements in asthma symptoms and/or lung function test results, decreased use of β-agonist bronchodilators) are evident after the first dose and persist for at least 24 hours.

In patients receiving montelukast 10 mg daily with mild to moderate hepatic impairment and clinical evidence of cirrhosis, the AUC of the drug was increased by 41% compared with the AUC in healthy individuals receiving montelukast.

● Distribution

Distribution of montelukast in body tissues and fluids has not been fully characterized. The steady-state volume of distribution of montelukast is 8–11 L.

Studies in rats indicate that only minimal amounts of radiolabeled material are detected in all tissues at 24 hours after administration of radiolabeled montelukast. Minimal amounts of radiolabeled montelukast cross the blood-brain barrier in rats.

Montelukast is more than 99% bound to plasma proteins.

It is not known whether montelukast crosses the placenta in humans; the drug crosses the placenta following oral administration in rats and rabbits. While it is not known whether montelukast is distributed in human milk, the drug is distributed into milk in rats.

● Elimination

The metabolic fate of montelukast has not been fully determined, but the drug is extensively metabolized in the GI tract and/or liver and excreted in bile. Several metabolic pathways have been identified including acyl glucuronidation, and oxidation catalyzed by several cytochrome P-450 (CYP) isoenzymes. In vitro studies indicate that the microsomal P-450 isoenzyme CYP3A4 is the major enzyme involved in formation of the 21-hydroxy metabolite (M5) and a sulfoxide metabolite (M2), and CYP2C9 is the major isoenzyme involved in the formation of the 36-hydroxy metabolite (M6). Other identified metabolites include an acyl glucuronide (M1) and a 25-hydroxy (a phenol, M3) analog.

Following oral administration of 54.8 mg of radiolabeled montelukast, metabolites of the drug represented less than 2% of circulating radioactivity. Montelukast metabolites that have been identified in plasma in radiolabeled studies include the 21-hydroxy (diastereomers of a benzylic acid, M5a and M5b) and the 36-hydroxy (diastereomers of a methyl alcohol, M6a and M6b) metabolites. Following oral administration of therapeutic doses of montelukast, plasma concentrations of metabolites at steady-state in adults and children were below the level of detection.

The mean plasma elimination half-life of montelukast in adults 19–48 years of age is 2.7–5.5 hours, and plasma clearance averages 45 mL/minute. A plasma elimination half-life of 3.4–4.2 hours has been reported in children 6–14 years of age. Limited data indicate that the plasma elimination half-life of montelukast is prolonged slightly in geriatric adults and in patients with mild to moderate hepatic impairment, although dosage adjustment is not required. A plasma elimination half-life of 6.6 or 7.4 hours has been reported in geriatric adults 65–73 years of age or patients with mild to moderate hepatic impairment, respectively.

Pharmacokinetics of montelukast have not been evaluated in patients with renal impairment. It is not known whether montelukast is removed from the body by hemodialysis or peritoneal dialysis.

Following oral administration, montelukast is excreted principally in bile as unchanged drug and metabolites. Following oral administration of radiolabeled montelukast, 86% of administered radioactivity was recovered in feces and less than 2% was recovered in urine over a 5-day collection period.

CHEMISTRY AND STABILITY

● Chemistry

Montelukast sodium, a synthetic leukotriene-receptor antagonist, is an antiasthmatic agent. Montelukast is a cysteinyl leukotriene analog that was developed based on a quinoline-containing compound that was modified with leukotriene structural elements. Structural modifications resulted in improved potency, oral bioavailability, clinical efficacy, and/or safety profile relative to early leukotriene antagonists (e.g., MK-571, verlukast). Montelukast consists of a 7-chloro-2-quinolinyl ethenylphenyl connected to a {[(1-hydroxy-1-methylethyl)phenyl]propyl} thiomethyl cyclopropaneacetic acid. Because montelukast contains polar and nonpolar groups at opposite ends of the molecule, the drug has amphophilic physicochemical properties.

Montelukast is pharmacologically but not structurally related to zafirlukast. Montelukast, like zafirlukast, differs chemically and pharmacologically from other currently available antiasthmatic agents (e.g., corticosteroids, mast-cell stabilizers, β-adrenergic agonist bronchodilators, theophylline, zileuton).

Montelukast sodium occurs as a hygroscopic, white to off-white powder. Montelukast sodium has solubilities of 0.2–0.5 mcg/mL in water at 25°C; the drug is freely soluble in alcohol. The apparent pK_as of the drug in water are 2.8 and 5.7.

Montelukast sodium chewable tablets contain aspartame (Nutrasweet®). Following metabolism of aspartame in the GI tract, each 4- or 5-mg chewable tablet of montelukast provides 0.674 or 0.824 mg of phenylalanine, respectively.

● *Stability*

Commercially available montelukast sodium film-coated and chewable tablets and oral granules should be stored at 25°C and protected from light and moisture with exposure for short periods to temperatures of 15–30°C permitted. When stored as directed, montelukast sodium film-coated and chewable tablets have an expiration date of 2 years after the date of manufacture.

PREPARATIONS

Excipients in commercially available drug preparations may have clinically important effects in some individuals; consult specific product labeling for details.

Montelukast Sodium

Oral		
Granules	4 mg (of montelukast)	**Singulair®**, Merck
Tablets, chewable	4 mg (of montelukast)*	**Singulair®**, Merck
	5 mg (of montelukast)*	**Singulair®**, Merck
Tablets, film-coated	10 mg (of montelukast)*	**Singulair®**, Merck

† Use is not currently included in the labeling approved by the US Food and Drug Administration.

Selected Revisions December 21, 2020, © Copyright, July 1, 2000, American Society of Health-System Pharmacists, Inc.

guaiFENesin

48:16 • EXPECTORANTS

■ Guaifenesin is an expectorant.

USES

● Cough

Guaifenesin is used as an expectorant in the symptomatic management of coughs associated with the common cold, bronchitis, laryngitis, pharyngitis, pertussis, influenza, and measles, and coughs provoked by chronic paranasal sinusitis. While there is clinical evidence that guaifenesin is an effective expectorant (i.e., increasing expectorated sputum volume over the first 4–6 days of a productive cough, decreasing sputum viscosity and difficulty in expectoration, and improving associated symptoms), there currently is insufficient evidence to support efficacy of the drug as an antitussive (cough suppressant). Therefore, guaifenesin's principal benefit in the symptomatic treatment of coughs results from the drug's ability to loosen and thin sputum and bronchial secretions and ease expectoration. Although such facilitation of evacuation of secretions may indirectly diminish the tendency to cough, the mechanism of this effect differs from that of antitussives, which inhibit or suppress cough. In addition to usefulness in the management of productive cough, guaifenesin's effects on sputum production and viscosity and on ease of expectoration suggest that the drug may prove useful in the management of irritative nonproductive cough and coughs productive of scanty amounts of thick, viscous secretions.

Although cough and cold preparations that contain cough suppressants, nasal decongestants, antihistamines, and/or expectorants commonly are used in pediatric patients younger than 2 years of age, systematic reviews of controlled trials have concluded that over-the-counter cough and cold preparations are *not* more effective than placebo in reducing acute cough and other symptoms of upper respiratory tract infection in these patients. Furthermore, adverse events, including deaths, have been (and continue to be) reported in pediatric patients younger than 2 years of age receiving these preparations. (See Cautions: Pediatric Precautions.)

Guaifenesin is combined with bronchodilators, decongestants, antihistamines, or opiate antitussives in numerous commercial liquid cough preparations.

DOSAGE AND ADMINISTRATION

● Administration

Guaifenesin is administered orally.

Mucinex® 600-mg extended-release tablets should not be broken, crushed, or chewed and should not be used in children younger than 12 years of age; the tablets should be kept out of reach of young children to avoid accidental swallowing and choking.

● Dosage

Cough

The usual dosage of guaifenesin as an expectorant in adults and children 12 years of age and older is 200–400 mg as conventional preparations every 4 hours, not to exceed 2.4 g daily. The usual dosage of guaifenesin 600-mg extended-release tablets as an expectorant in adults and children 12 years of age and older is 600 mg or 1.2 g every 12 hours, not to exceed 2.4 g daily. The usual dosage of guaifenesin as an expectorant for children 6 to younger than 12 years of age is 100–200 mg as conventional preparations every 4 hours, not to exceed 1.2 g daily. Alternatively, children 6–12 years of age may receive 600 mg as an appropriate extended-release preparation every 12 hours, not to exceed 1.2 g daily. Children 2 to younger than 6 years of age may receive 50–100 mg as conventional preparations every 4 hours, not to exceed 600 mg daily. Alternatively, children 2–6 years of age may receive 300 mg as an appropriate extended-release preparation every 12 hours, not to exceed 600 mg daily. Dosage of guaifenesin in children younger than 2 years of age must be individualized. Suggested dosages for children younger than 2 years of age† for some cough and cold preparations have been published in various references for prescribing and parenting. Using recommended dosages for adults

and older children, some clinicians have extrapolated dosages for these preparations based on the weight or age of children younger than 2 years of age. However, these extrapolations were based on assumptions that pathology of the disease and pharmacology of the drugs are similar in adults and pediatric patients. There currently are *no* specific dosage recommendations (i.e., approved by the US Food and Drug Administration [FDA]) for cough and cold preparations for this patient population. (See Cautions: Pediatric Precautions.)

CAUTIONS

Doses of guaifenesin larger than those required for expectorant action may produce emesis, but GI upset at ordinary dosage levels is rare.

For *self-medication*, unless directed by a physician, guaifenesin should not be used for persistent or chronic cough such as that occurring with smoking, asthma, chronic bronchitis, or emphysema, or for cough accompanied by excessive phlegm. A persistent cough may be indicative of a serious condition. If cough persists for more than one week, is recurrent, or is accompanied by fever, rash, or persistent headache, a physician should be consulted.

When preparations containing guaifenesin in fixed combination with other agents (e.g., acetaminophen, chlorpheniramine, codeine, dextromethorphan, ephedrine, phenylephrine, pseudoephedrine) are used, the cautions, precautions, and contraindications applicable to each ingredient should be considered.

● Pediatric Precautions

Overdosage and toxicity (including death) have been reported in children younger than 2 years of age receiving nonprescription (over-the-counter, OTC) preparations containing antihistamines, cough suppressants, expectorants, and nasal decongestants alone or in combination for relief of symptoms of upper respiratory tract infection. There is limited evidence of efficacy for these preparations in this age group, and appropriate dosages (i.e., approved by the US Food and Drug Administration [FDA]) for the symptomatic treatment of cold and cough have not been established. Therefore, FDA stated that nonprescription cough and cold preparations should not be used in children younger than 2 years of age; the agency continues to assess safety and efficacy of these preparations in older children. Meanwhile, because children 2–3 years of age also are at increased risk of overdosage and toxicity, some manufacturers of oral nonprescription cough and cold preparations agreed to voluntarily revise the product labeling to state that such preparations should not be used in children younger than 4 years of age. FDA recommends that parents and caregivers adhere to the dosage instructions and warnings on the product labeling that accompanies the preparation if administering to children and consult with their clinician about any concerns. Clinicians should ask caregivers about use of nonprescription cough and cold preparations to avoid overdosage. For additional information on precautions associated with the use of cough and cold preparations in pediatric patients, see Cautions: Pediatric Precautions in Dextromethorphan 48:08.

PHARMACOLOGY

By increasing respiratory tract fluid, guaifenesin reduces the viscosity of tenacious secretions and acts as an expectorant.

CHEMISTRY AND STABILITY

● Chemistry

Guaifenesin is an expectorant. Guaifenesin occurs as a white to slightly gray, crystalline powder, having a bitter taste. Guaifenesin may have a slight characteristic odor. Guaifenesin is soluble in alcohol and in water.

● Stability

Guaifenesin powder tends to become lumpy on storage. Guaifenesin preparations should be stored in tight containers.

PREPARATIONS

Excipients in commercially available drug preparations may have clinically important effects in some individuals; consult specific product labeling for details.

guaiFENesin

Oral

Granules	50 mg per packet	**Mucinex® Mini Melts®**, Reckitt Benckiser
	100 mg per packet	**Mucinex® Mini Melts®**, Reckitt Benckiser
Solution	100 mg/5 mL*	**Children's Mucinex® Chest Congestion**, Reckitt Benckiser
		Diabetic Tussin® Expectorant, Health Care Products
		Guaifenesin Oral Solution
		Guiatuss® Syrup, Goldline
	200 mg/5 mL	**Diabetic Tussin® Mucus Relief**, Health Care Products
Tablets	200 mg*	**Guaifenesin Tablets**
Tablets, extended-release	600 mg	**Mucinex®**, Reckitt Benckiser
	1.2 g	**Mucinex® Maximum Strength**, Reckitt Benckiser

* available from one or more manufacturer, distributor, and/or repackager by generic (nonproprietary) name

guaiFENesin and Codeine Phosphate

Oral

Solution	100 mg/5 mL Guaifenesin and Codeine Phosphate 10 mg/5 mL*	**Cheratussin® AC** (C-V), Qualitest
		Guaiatussin® AC (C-V), Hi-Tech
		Guaifenesin AC Cough Syrup (C-V)
		Guaifenesin and Codeine Phosphate Oral Solution (C-V)
		Robafen® AC (C-V), Major
	200 mg/5 mL Guaifenesin and Codeine Phosphate 8 mg/5 mL	**Codar® GF** (C-V), Respa

* available from one or more manufacturer, distributor, and/or repackager by generic (nonproprietary) name

Other guaiFENesin Combinations

Oral

For Solution	400 mg/packet with Acetaminophen 1 g/packet	**Theraflu® Flu & Chest Congestion**, Novartis
	400 mg/packet with Acetaminophen 1 g/packet, Dextromethorphan Hydrobromide 30 mg/packet, and Pseudoephedrine Hydrochloride 60 mg/packet	**Theraflu® Max-D® Severe Cold & Flu**, Novartis
Granules	50 mg per packet with Dextromethorphan Hydrobromide 5 mg/packet	**Mucinex® Cough Mini Melts®**, Reckitt Benckiser
Solution	33.3 mg/5 mL with Dextromethorphan Hydrobromide 3.3 mg/5 mL	**Vicks® Nature Fusion® Cough and Chest Congestion**, Procter & Gamble
	50 mg/5 mL with Dextromethorphan Hydrobromide 5 mg/5 mL and Phenylephrine Hydrochloride 2.5 mg/5 mL	**Children's Robitussin® Cold & Cough CF**, Pfizer
	50 mg/5 mL with Phenylephrine Hydrochloride 2.5 mg/5 mL	**Triaminic® Chest and Nasal Congestion**, Novartis
	66.6 mg/5 mL with Acetaminophen 108.3 mg/5 mL, Dextromethorphan Hydrobromide 3.3 mg/5 mL, and Phenylephrine Hydrochloride 1.6 mg/5 mL	**Tylenol® Cold Multi-Symptom Severe**, McNeil **Tylenol® Cold & Flu Severe**, McNeil
	66.6 mg/5 mL with Acetaminophen 108.3 mg/5 mL, and Phenylephrine Hydrochloride 1.6 mg/5 mL	**Theraflu Warming Relief® Cold & Chest Congestion**, Novartis
	66.6 mg/5 mL with Dextromethorphan Hydrobromide 3.3 mg/5 mL	**Vicks® DayQuil® Mucus Control DM**, Procter & Gamble
	66.6 mg/5 mL with Dextromethorphan Hydrobromide 6.6 mg/5 mL	**Vicks® Formula 44® Custom Care Chesty Cough**, Procter & Gamble
	100 mg/5mL with Acetaminophen 162.5 mg/5 mL, Dextromethorphan Hydrobromide 5 mg/5 mL, and Phenylephrine Hydrochloride 2.5 mg/5 mL	**Children's Mucinex® Cold, Cough, and Sore Throat**, Reckitt Benckiser
	100 mg/5 mL with Dextromethorphan Hydrobromide 5 mg/5 mL	**Children's Mucinex® Multi-symptom Cold & Fever**, Reckitt Benckiser
		Children's Mucinex® Cough, Reckitt Benckiser
	100 mg/5 mL with Dextromethorphan Hydrobromide 5 mg/5 mL and Phenylephrine Hydrochloride 2.5 mg/5 mL	**Pediacare® Children's Cough & Congestion**, Prestige Brands **Children's Mucinex® Multi-symptom Cold**, Reckitt Benckiser
	100 mg/5 mL with Dextromethorphan Hydrobromide 10 mg/5 mL	**Robitussin® Peak Cold Cough + Chest Congestion DM**, Pfizer
	100 mg/5 mL with Dextromethorphan Hydrobromide 10 mg/5 mL and Phenylephrine Hydrochloride 5 mg/5 mL	**Robitussin® Peak Cold Multi-Symptom Cold®**, Pfizer
	100 mg/5 mL with Phenylephrine Hydrochloride 2.5 mg/5 mL	**Children's Mucinex® Stuffy Nose & Cold**, Reckitt Benckiser
	100 mg/5 mL with Phenylephrine Hydrochloride 5 mg/5 mL	**Rescon®-GG**, Capellon
	200 mg/5 mL with Dextromethorphan Hydrobromide 10 mg/5 mL	**Robitussin® Peak Cold Maximum Strength Cough + Chest Congestion DM**, Pfizer
	200 mg/5 mL with Dextromethorphan Hydrobromide 10 mg/5 mL and Phenylephrine Hydrochloride 5 mg/5 mL	**Robitussin® Peak Cold Maximum Strength Multi-Symptom Cold®**, Pfizer
Tablets	200 mg with Acetaminophen 325 mg, Dextromethorphan 10 mg, and Phenylephrine Hydrochloride 5 mg	**Tylenol® Cold Multi-symptom Severe**, McNeil **Tylenol® Cold & Flu Severe**, McNeil
	200 mg with Ephedrine Hydrochloride 12.5 mg	**Primatene®**, Pfizer
	400 mg with Ephedrine Sulfate 25 mg	**Bronkaid® Dual Action Caplets®**, Bayer
	400 mg with Pseudoephedrine Hydrochloride 60 mg	**Congestac® Caplets®**, Ascher
Tablets, extended-release	600 mg with Dextromethorphan Hydrobromide 30 mg	**Mucinex® DM**, Reckitt Benckiser
	600 mg with Pseudoephedrine Hydrochloride 60 mg	**Mucinex® D**, Reckitt Benckiser
	1.2 g with Dextromethorphan Hydrobromide 60 mg	**Mucinex® DM Maximum Strength**, Reckitt Benckiser
	1.2 g with Pseudoephedrine Hydrochloride 120 mg	**Mucinex® D Maximum Strength**, Reckitt Benckiser

Guaifenesin also is commercially available in combination with antihistamines, antitussives, bronchodilators, decongestants, and expectorants.

† Use is not currently included in the labeling approved by the US Food and Drug Administration.

Selected Revisions February 1, 2016, © Copyright, November 1, 1963, American Society of Health-System Pharmacists, Inc.

Table of Contents

52:00 EYE, EAR, NOSE, AND THROAT PREPARATIONS

§ Omitted from the print version of *AHFS Drug Information*® because of space limitations. This monograph is available on the *AHFS Drug Information*® website, http://ahfsdruginformation.com

Table of Contents

56:00 GASTROINTESTINAL DRUGS

§ Omitted from the print version of *AHFS Drug Information* because of space limitations. This monograph is available on the *AHFS Drug Information* website, http://www.ahfsdruginformation.com.

Antacids

56:04 · ANTACIDS AND ADSORBENTS

■ Antacids are inorganic salts that dissolve in acid gastric secretions releasing anions that partially neutralize gastric hydrochloric acid.

USES

Antacids are used as an adjunct to other drugs for the relief of peptic ulcer pain and to promote the healing of peptic ulcers. Antacids also are used for the relief of esophageal reflux, acid indigestion, heartburn, dyspepsia, and sour stomach; for the prevention of stress ulceration and GI bleeding; to reduce the risk associated with gastric aspiration; and for the management of hyperphosphatemia.

● Considerations in Choosing an Antacid

The choice of a specific antacid preparation depends on palatability, cost, adverse effects, acid neutralizing capacity, the sodium content of the antacid, and the patient's renal and cardiovascular function. Because of its high sodium content, sodium bicarbonate generally is used only for occasional heartburn or indigestion and not for chronic high-dose management of peptic ulcer disease. The role of calcium carbonate in the management of peptic ulcers is controversial because this antacid may cause acid rebound, which is especially important when the drug is administered at bedtime. Most clinicians believe that calcium carbonate should not be used in the management of peptic ulcers. However, some clinicians postulate that frequent administration of calcium carbonate may ameliorate acid rebound and reduce the clinical importance of gastric hypersecretion and believe that calcium carbonate is useful because it has a rapid onset of action, high acid neutralizing capacity, and a prolonged effect and is relatively inexpensive. Magnesium and/or aluminum antacids are the most commonly used and are often administered concurrently or in commercially available combinations to control the frequency and consistency of bowel movements. In any antacid combination product, each active antacid ingredient must contribute at least 25% of the in vitro acid neutralizing capacity. With administration of fixed combinations, ideal regulation of bowel function is seldom achieved, and patients should be taught to supplement their antacid therapy with appropriate doses of magnesium, calcium, or aluminum antacids to regulate bowel function.

Fixed combinations of antacids and histamine H$_2$-receptor antagonists can be used for relief of *occasional* symptoms of heartburn (pyrosis) associated with acid indigestion (hyperchlorhydria) and sour stomach, with the antacid providing intital rapid relief and the histamine H$_2$-receptor antagonist providing more prolonged relief.

Fixed combinations of antacids with nonantacid laxatives are rational only if the laxative is used to counteract the constipating effect of the antacid. Antacid combinations containing analgesics or simethicone should be administered only when concurrent symptoms require the effects of both an antacid and the nonantacid drug. However, fixed combinations of antacids and analgesics are not indicated for the management of peptic ulcers. Antacid combinations containing an anticholinergic, sedative-hypnotic, antiemetic, antipepsin, or proteolytic agents, bile, or bile salts are irrational, unsafe, and ineffective. Optimal use of antacids and anticholinergics or sedative-hypnotics requires that the dosage of each drug be adjusted by administering each drug separately. Bismuth salts and milk have no appreciable acid neutralizing activity.

● Peptic Ulcers

Few well-designed clinical studies are available demonstrating the efficacy or inefficacy of antacids in the healing of peptic ulcers or for the relief of peptic ulcer pain. However, most clinicians believe that based upon the ability of antacids to increase gastric pH these drugs are useful in the management of peptic ulcers. In one well-controlled 4-week trial in outpatients, placebo was compared with 1- and 3-hour postprandial and bedtime administration of a suspension containing magnesium and aluminum hydroxides and simethicone (about 144 mEq of acid neutralizing capacity per dose); the antacid regimen was more effective than placebo in healing duodenal ulcer craters (endoscopically proven), but the antacid was no more effective than placebo in relieving ulcer pain.

In another study in outpatients with gastric or duodenal ulcers, calcium carbonate (about 8.2 mEq of acid neutralizing capacity) in tablet form administered every hour while the patient was awake and as necessary for abdominal discomfort produced a greater incidence of radiologically confirmed healing and pain relief in patients with gastric ulcers but not in those with duodenal ulcers after 30 days as compared with placebo. In a third well-controlled 3-week trial in hospitalized gastric ulcer patients, placebo was compared to administration of 30 mL of a suspension containing magnesium and aluminum hydroxides and simethicone (acid neutralizing capacity not specified) every 2 hours while the patient was awake; gastric ulcer healing and pain relief were not different in antacid-treated and placebo-treated patients. In a 5-day clinical study, 15 mL of an antacid (30 mEq of acid neutralizing capacity per dose) was alternately administered every 30 minutes with placebo as needed to relieve duodenal ulcer pain; antacid was not different from placebo. In the same study, a single 30-mL dose of the antacid was not more effective than placebo in relieving duodenal ulcer pain.

In one well-controlled study, 4 weeks of oral therapy with 1.2 g of cimetidine daily was compared to that with 1- and 3-hour postprandial and bedtime administration of magnesium and aluminum hydroxides antacid suspension (about 123 mEq of acid neutralizing capacity per dose); cimetidine and antacid did not differ significantly (64 *vs* 52%) in healing of duodenal ulcer craters and erosions or pain relief. Well-controlled clinical studies are not available comparing the efficacy of anticholinergic agents to antacids in the management of peptic ulcers.

Current epidemiologic and clinical evidence supports a strong association between gastric infection with *Helicobacter pylori* and the pathogenesis of duodenal and gastric ulcers; long-term *H. pylori* infection also has been implicated as a risk factor for gastric cancer. For additional information on the association of this infection with these and other GI conditions, see Helicobacter pylori infection, under Uses, in Clarithromycin 8:12.12.92.

Conventional antiulcer therapy with antacids, H$_2$-receptor antagonists, proton-pump inhibitors, and/or sucralfate heals ulcers but generally is ineffective in eradicating *H. pylori*, and such therapy is associated with a high rate of ulcer recurrence (e.g., 60–100% per year). The American College of Gastroenterology (ACG), the National Institutes of Health (NIH), and most clinicians currently recommend that *all* patients with initial or recurrent duodenal or gastric ulcer and documented *H. pylori* infection receive anti-infective therapy for treatment of the infection. Although 3-drug regimens consisting of a bismuth salt (e.g., bismuth subsalicylate) and 2 anti-infective agents (e.g., tetracycline or amoxicillin plus metronidazole) administered for 10–14 days have been effective in eradicating the infection, resolving associated gastritis, healing peptic ulcer, and preventing ulcer recurrence in many patients with *H. pylori*-associated peptic ulcer disease, current evidence principally from studies in Europe suggests that 1 week of such therapy provides comparable *H. pylori* eradication rates. Other regimens that combine one or more anti-infective agents (e.g., clarithromycin, amoxicillin) with a bismuth salt and/or an antisecretory agent (e.g., omeprazole, lansoprazole, H$_2$-receptor antagonist) also have been used successfully for *H. pylori* eradication, and the choice of a particular regimen should be based on the rapidly evolving data on optimal therapy, including consideration of the patient's prior exposure to anti-infective agents, the local prevalence of resistance, patient compliance, and cost of therapy.

Current evidence suggests that inclusion of a proton-pump inhibitor (e.g., omeprazole, lansoprazole) in anti-*H. pylori* regimens containing 2 anti-infectives enhances effectiveness, and limited data suggest that such regimens retain good efficacy despite imidazole (e.g., metronidazole) resistance. Therefore, the ACG and many clinicians currently recommend 1 week of therapy with a proton-pump inhibitor and 2 anti-infective agents (usually clarithromycin and amoxicillin or metronidazole), or a 3-drug, bismuth-based regimen (e.g., bismuth-metronidazole-tetracycline) concomitantly with a proton-pump inhibitor, for treatment of *H. pylori* infection. For a more complete discussion of *H. pylori* infection, including details about the efficacy of various regimens and rationale for drug selection, see Helicobacter pylori Infection, under Uses, in Clarithromycin 8:12.12.92.

● Acid Indigestion

Although the efficacy of antacids for the relief of acid indigestion, heartburn, sour stomach, and pressure and/or bloating (commonly referred as gas), generally has not been established systematically by well-designed studies, most experts believe that, since these symptoms may be caused by gastric acid, antacids are probably useful.

● Gastroesophageal Reflux

Antacids also may be useful to increase gastric pH and to increase lower esophageal sphincter pressure in the management of esophageal reflux. The ACG states that antacids and antirefluxants such as alginic acid are more effective than placebo in relieving symptoms of heartburn induced by a meal, and are useful for *self-medication* as initial therapy for milder forms of gastroesophageal reflux disease (GERD). However, suppression of gastric acid secretion with a proton-pump inhibitor or histamine H$_2$- receptor antagonist to control symptoms and prevent complications of the disease is considered by the ACG to be the principal therapeutic goal in the management of GERD. Other measures such as avoidance of constrictive clothing, treatment of obesity, reducing meal size and dietary fat intake, avoidance of foods that increase reflux, avoiding recumbency after meals, and elevating the head of the bed should be initiated and continued throughout the course of treatment. For further information on the treatment of GERD, see Uses: Gastroesophageal Reflux, in Omeprazole 56:28.36.

● Upper GI Bleeding

Antacids may be effective in the prevention of stress ulceration and GI bleeding. In one randomized controlled study in critically ill patients, antacids administered prophylactically to maintain gastric pH above 3.5 decreased the incidence of acute GI bleeding.

● Gastric Aspirations

Antacids have been administered prophylactically as an adjunct to reduce the risk of gastric acid aspiration in patients undergoing cesarean section or emergency surgery.

● Hyperphosphatemia

The hypophosphatemic effect of aluminum-containing antacids (except aluminum phosphate) has been used in conjunction with a low phosphate diet in the management of calcinosis universalis, in hyperparathyroidism secondary to chronic hemodialysis, and to prevent recurrent phosphatic renal calculi. Since aluminum carbonate reportedly binds phosphate more than does aluminum hydroxide, aluminum carbonate is generally preferred.

● Calcium Replacement

For the use of calcium carbonate as replacement therapy, see Calcium Salts 40:12. For the use of magnesium preparations as laxatives, see the Cathartics and Laxatives General Statement 56:12. For the use of sodium bicarbonate as an alkalinizing agent, see Sodium Bicarbonate 40:08.

DOSAGE AND ADMINISTRATION

Antacids are administered orally. The dose of antacids should be expressed in terms of mEq of acid neutralizing capacity. Dose and frequency of administration depend on the acid secretory rate of the stomach, gastric emptying time, and the disorder being treated. The duration of action of antacids is determined principally by gastric emptying time. In fasting subjects, antacids have a duration of action of 20–60 minutes. However, if the drugs are administered 1 hour after meals, acid neutralizing effects may persist up to 3 hours. Sodium bicarbonate generally has a shorter duration of action than other antacids. Antacids should be used for longer than 2-week periods only under the management of a physician and as part of a carefully planned therapeutic regimen.

There is considerable variation in in vivo acid neutralizing capacity of equal volumes of different antacids and antacid products. Since suspensions are more rapidly and effectively solubilized than powders or tablets, antacid suspensions have a greater ability to react with and neutralize gastric acid. Antacid suspensions have a smaller particle size than do tablets and drying of antacid suspensions to prepare powders and tablets causes substantial loss of ability to neutralize acid. In general, an antacid suspension is preferable to a tablet or powder; tablets should be reserved for chronic use in patients who refuse suspensions because they are inconvenient or unpalatable. Tablets should be thoroughly chewed before swallowing.

The US Food and Drug Administration (FDA) requires that antacids have a minimum in vitro acid neutralizing capacity of 5 mEq per dose and that antacid labeling contain the in vitro acid neutralizing capacity; however, this FDA in vitro test does not correlate with in vivo acid neutralizing capacity.

For peptic ulcer disease, dosages of antacids are empirical and various antacid dosages have been used. In patients with uncomplicated duodenal ulcers or gastric ulcers, an antacid is administered 1 and 3 hours postprandially and at bedtime. In patients with duodenal ulcers, antacids are usually given for 4–6 weeks, and in patients with gastric ulcers, antacids are administered until healing is complete. If symptoms of duodenal ulcer recur, some clinicians recommend that

antacids be administered 1 and 3 hours postprandially and at bedtime for 1 week and, if pain is relieved, less frequently for an additional 1–2 weeks; these patients should consult their physicians if pain worsens or is not relieved after the first week of therapy. Additional doses of antacids may be administered to relieve ulcer pain which occurs between regularly scheduled doses.

For the acute management of moderate or severe esophageal reflux, an antacid suspension is administered every hour; if symptoms persist, antacids may be given every 30 minutes. For long-term therapy of esophageal reflux, antacids are administered 1 and 3 hours postprandially and at bedtime and whenever symptoms recur.

In the management of GI bleeding and stress ulceration, antacids are usually administered every hour and, for GI bleeding, the antacid dosage should be titrated to maintain the nasogastric aspirate above pH 3.5. For severe symptoms, antacid suspensions may be diluted with water or milk and given by continuous intragastric infusion.

To reduce the risk of anesthesia-induced gastric acid aspiration, an antacid suspension has been given 30 minutes before anesthesia.

In conjunction with dietary phosphate restriction in the management of hyperphosphatemia, 30–40 mL of aluminum hydroxide or aluminum carbonate suspension is administered 3 or 4 times daily.

CAUTIONS

● Precautions and Contraindications

Most antacids contain sodium as an impurity, and antacid products must be labeled with their sodium content if they contain more than 0.2 mEq of sodium per dose. Sodium bicarbonate is contraindicated and use of other sodium-containing antacids should be restricted in patients on low-sodium diets and in those with congestive heart failure, renal failure, edema, or cirrhosis. Antacid products containing more than 25 mEq of potassium in the recommended daily dosage should be used cautiously in patients with renal disease and only under the supervision of a physician.

Since antacids may alter the absorption of certain concomitantly administered oral drugs, patients taking oral drugs should be advised to consult their physician or other health professional before taking concomitant antacids. (See Drug Interactions.)

The most common adverse effects associated with prolonged administration of antacids are constipation and diarrhea. Although fixed-combination antacid products are frequently administered to balance the laxative and cathartic effects of each, bowel function must often be regulated by administering supplemental doses of an antacid with constipating (i.e., aluminum salt) or laxative (i.e., magnesium salt) action.

Some commercially available antacids contain the dye tartrazine (FD&C yellow No. 5), which may cause allergic reactions including bronchial asthma in susceptible individuals. Although the incidence of tartrazine sensitivity is low, it frequently occurs in patients who are sensitive to aspirin. Individuals with phenylketonuria (i.e., homozygous genetic deficiency of phenylalanine hydroxylase) and other individuals who must restrict their intake of phenylalanine should be warned that some antacids may contain aspartame, which is metabolized in the GI tract to phenylalanine following oral administration.

Serious medication errors have been reported to the US Food and Drug Administration (FDA) in which consumers used Maalox® Total Relief (bismuth subsalicylate) when they intended to use traditional Maalox® liquid antacid products containing aluminum hydroxide, magnesium hydroxide, and simethicone (e.g., Maalox® Advanced Regular Strength, Maalox® Advanced Maximum Strength). Because of the potential for serious adverse effects associated with accidental use of bismuth subsalicylate (which is chemically related to aspirin), the manufacturer of Maalox® Total Relief initially agreed to change the trade name of the product to one that did not include "Maalox"; however, the manufacturer instead discontinued the bismuth subsalicylate preparation in the summer of 2010.

Aluminum Antacids

The most frequent adverse effect of aluminum antacids is constipation. Decreased bowel motility, dehydration, or fluid restriction may predispose patients to intestinal obstruction. Hemorrhoids and fissures or fecal impaction may occur.

Long-term administration of aluminum antacids in patients with renal failure or chronic renal failure may result in hyperaluminemia since small amounts of aluminum are absorbed from the GI tract and excretion of aluminum is decreased in patients with renal failure. Absorbed aluminum becomes bound to serum proteins (e.g., albumin, transferrin) and therefore is not easily dialyzed; aluminum may then accumulate in bones, lungs, and nerve tissue. Aluminum accumulation in the CNS may be the cause of dialysis encephalopathy, while aluminum accumulation in the bones may result in or worsen dialysis osteomalacia. Dialysis dementia also may occur in patients with renal failure receiving long-term aluminum antacid therapy for hyperphosphatemia. Several cases of dialysis encephalopathy have been associated with increased aluminum concentrations in the dialysate water. Aluminum intoxication with severe osteomalacia and extensive aluminum deposition at the junction between calcified and noncalcified bone has been reported in several young children who were receiving large dosages of aluminum hydroxide for the management of hyperphosphatemia associated with azotemia; the children were not undergoing hemodialysis during aluminum hydroxide therapy.

Aluminum salts may cause phosphorus depletion which is generally negligible. However, with prolonged administration or large doses, hypophosphatemia may occur, especially in patients with inadequate dietary intake of phosphorus; hypercalciuria secondary to bone resorption and increased intestinal absorption of calcium results. This phosphorus depletion syndrome is characterized by anorexia, malaise, and muscle weakness, and prolonged aluminum antacid therapy may cause urinary calculi, osteomalacia, and osteoporosis. A low-phosphorus diet, diarrhea, excessive phosphorus losses from malabsorption, and restoration of renal function after a kidney transplant increase the likelihood of the syndrome. Serum phosphate concentrations should be monitored at monthly or bimonthly intervals in patients on maintenance hemodialysis who are receiving chronic aluminum antacid therapy.

Calcium Carbonate

The major limiting factor to the chronic use of calcium carbonate is gastric hypersecretion and acid rebound. Increased gastric acid secretion begins within 2 hours after administration of the drug and has occurred following a single 500-mg dose of calcium carbonate. In one study in peptic ulcer patients receiving large doses of calcium carbonate (500 mg/kg daily), hypercalcemia occurred in 14% of patients within 3 days of initiating therapy. Calcium carbonate may cause the milk-alkali syndrome which is characterized by hypercalcemia, metabolic alkalosis and, rarely, renal insufficiency; hypercalcemia may cause nausea, vomiting, anorexia, weakness, headache, dizziness, and change in mental status. Patients with renal impairment or dehydration and electrolyte imbalance are predisposed to developing the milk-alkali syndrome. Hypercalcemia has also been reported in chronic hemodialysis patients receiving calcium carbonate. Serum calcium concentrations should be monitored weekly and whenever symptoms of hypercalcemia occur in patients receiving large doses of calcium carbonate. Calcium carbonate reportedly causes constipation. Belching and flatulence may occur. When dietary phosphate is low, hypophosphatemia may occur.

Magnesium Antacids

Magnesium-containing antacids commonly cause a laxative effect and frequent administration of these antacids alone often cannot be tolerated; repeated doses cause diarrhea which may cause fluid and electrolyte imbalances. Chronic administration of magnesium trisilicate infrequently produces silica renal stones.

In patients with severe renal impairment, hypermagnesemia characterized by hypotension, nausea, vomiting, ECG changes, respiratory or mental depression, and coma has occurred after administration of magnesium-containing antacids. Magnesium-containing antacids should not be administered in patients with renal failure, and antacid products containing more than 50 mEq of magnesium in the recommended daily dosage should be used cautiously and only under the supervision of a physician who should monitor electrolytes in patients with renal disease.

Sodium Bicarbonate

Gastric distension and flatulence may occur with sodium bicarbonate preparations. Sodium bicarbonate, when given in large doses or in patients with renal insufficiency, may cause metabolic alkalosis. Chronic administration of bicarbonate with milk or calcium may cause the milk-alkali syndrome which is characterized by hypercalcemia, renal insufficiency, metabolic alkalosis, nausea, vomiting, headache, mental confusion, and anorexia. During the acute phase of the milk-alkali syndrome, the condition is reversible when the calcium and alkali are withdrawn. However, in patients with chronic milk-alkali syndrome, reduced renal function may persist even after calcium and alkali are discontinued. Patients with a salt-losing nephropathy have an increased risk of developing the milk-alkali syndrome.

The maximum daily dosage of sodium or bicarbonate is 200 mEq in patients younger than 60 years of age and 100 mEq in patients older than 60 years of age. Sodium bicarbonate is contraindicated for prolonged therapy because it may cause metabolic alkalosis or sodium overload.

DRUG INTERACTIONS

All antacids potentially may increase or decrease the rate and/or extent of absorption of concomitantly administered oral drugs by changing GI transit time or by binding or chelating the drug. In vitro studies indicate that magnesium hydroxide or trisilicate has the greatest potential for drug binding and aluminum hydroxide and calcium carbonate are intermediate. Antacid-induced increases in GI pH may affect the disintegration, dissolution, solubility, or ionization of enteric-coated preparations and weakly acidic or basic drugs.

Simultaneous administration of aluminum-, calcium-, or magnesium-containing antacids with orally administered tetracyclines reduces the absorption of the tetracycline, probably because of chelation of these antacids by the tetracycline. Therefore, doses of tetracyclines should be spaced 1–2 hours from doses of antacids.

Concurrent administration of antacids and orally administered digoxin, indomethacin, or iron salts may decrease the absorption of these drugs. Doses of these drugs should be spaced as far apart as possible from doses of antacids. Concurrent administration of isoniazid and aluminum hydroxide gel may decrease the absorption of isoniazid; therefore, isoniazid should be administered at least 1 hour before aluminum-containing antacids. Absorption of buffered or enteric-coated aspirin is increased by simultaneous administration of antacids. Antacid-induced changes in urine pH increase urinary excretion and decrease blood concentrations of salicylates. Concurrent administration of dicumarol and an aluminum and magnesium hydroxides preparation reportedly increases the absorption of dicumarol; patients receiving antacids and oral anticoagulants should probably use warfarin rather than dicumarol. Concurrent administration of aluminum hydroxide and pseudoephedrine or diazepam increases the rate of absorption of the latter drugs. Administration of a magnesium and aluminum hydroxide preparation with chlordiazepoxide decreases the rate of chlordiazepoxide absorption. Administration of sodium bicarbonate with naproxen increases the rate of naproxen absorption, while concurrent administration of magnesium oxide or aluminum hydroxide with naproxen decreases the rate of naproxen absorption.

Antacid-induced increases in urine pH may decrease excretion of weakly basic drugs and increase excretion of weakly acidic drugs. Urinary excretion of amphetamines and quinidine are markedly decreased in patients whose urine is alkalinized with sodium bicarbonate and patients receiving these drugs concomitantly may have increased amphetamine or quinidine effects.

PHARMACOLOGY

The clinical use of antacids is based on their ability to increase the pH of gastric secretions. With usual doses, antacids generally do not increase and maintain gastric pH above 4–5. Although antacids do not neutralize all gastric acid, increasing gastric pH from 1.3 to 2.3 neutralizes 90% and increasing pH to 3.3 neutralizes 99% of gastric acid. Consequently, the amount of gastric acid back-diffusing through the gastric mucosa and the amount of acid reaching the duodenum is decreased. It is not known how much or for how long neutralization is required for optimal healing of peptic ulcers, but most clinicians believe that gastric pH should be maintained at about 3–3.5 for as many of the 24 hours as is possible. Antacids, in decreasing order of their ability to neutralize a given amount of acid, are calcium carbonate, sodium bicarbonate, magnesium salts, and aluminum salts. Magnesium hydroxide and aluminum hydroxide are the most potent magnesium and aluminum salts. Magnesium oxide has essentially the same acid neutralizing effect as magnesium hydroxide. Because magnesium trisilicate is slowly solubilized, it is a less effective buffer than magnesium hydroxide, carbonate, or phosphate.

Sodium bicarbonate rapidly reacts with hydrochloric acid to form sodium chloride, carbon dioxide, and water; excess bicarbonate that does not neutralize gastric acid rapidly empties into the small intestine and is absorbed. When sodium bicarbonate is given orally, gastric acid is neutralized by exogenous bicarbonate instead of intestinal bicarbonate. The net effect of administering sodium bicarbonate whether it reacts with gastric acid or reaches the small intestine is that all of a dose reaches the extracellular fluid. Mild metabolic alkalosis occurs; in patients with normal renal function, the kidneys excrete the excess sodium and bicarbonate ions and the urine becomes alkaline.

Antacids other than sodium bicarbonate neutralize gastric secretions but generally do not cause metabolic alkalosis, because the cation formed in the stomach is minimally absorbed and regains a basic anion in the small intestine. However, to the extent that the cation is absorbed and does not react with intestinal bicarbonate, the extracellular fluid receives a bicarbonate load; urinary pH is usually increased.

Calcium carbonate is slowly solubilized in the stomach and reacts with hydrochloric acid to form calcium chloride, carbon dioxide, and water. About 90% of the calcium chloride formed is converted to insoluble calcium salts (mainly calcium carbonate and to a lesser extent calcium phosphate) and calcium soaps in the small intestine and is not absorbed. When calcium carbonate is administered orally, a limited amount of calcium and intestinal bicarbonate are absorbed and hypercalcemia may occur. In some patients, metabolic alkalosis and the milk-alkali syndrome may occur. Calcium is excreted by the kidneys and hypercalciuria frequently occurs in patients receiving calcium carbonate.

Aluminum hydroxide or oxide is slowly solubilized in the stomach and reacts with hydrochloric acid to form aluminum chloride and water. In addition to forming aluminum chloride, dihydroxyaluminum sodium carbonate and aluminum carbonate form carbon dioxide, and aluminum phosphate forms phosphoric acid. About 17–30% of the aluminum chloride formed is absorbed and is rapidly excreted by the kidneys in patients with normal renal function. In the small intestine, aluminum chloride is rapidly converted to insoluble, poorly absorbed basic aluminum salts which are probably a mixture of hydrated aluminum oxide, oxyaluminum hydroxide, various basic aluminum carbonates, and aluminum soaps. Aluminum-containing antacids (except aluminum phosphate) also combine with dietary phosphate in the intestine forming insoluble, nonabsorbable aluminum phosphate which is excreted in the feces. If phosphate intake is limited in patients with normal renal function, aluminum antacids (except aluminum phosphate) decrease phosphate absorption and hypophosphatemia and hypophosphaturia occur; calcium absorption is increased. In vitro studies indicate that aluminum hydroxide binds bile salts with an affinity and capacity similar to that of cholestyramine; aluminum phosphate binds bile salts, but to a much lesser degree than does aluminum hydroxide.

Magnesium hydroxide rapidly reacts with hydrochloric acid to form magnesium chloride and water. In addition, magnesium carbonate forms carbon dioxide. Magnesium trisilicate is slowly solubilized and reacts with hydrochloric acid to form magnesium chloride, silicon dioxide, and water. About 15–30% of the magnesium chloride formed is absorbed and is rapidly excreted by the kidneys in patients with normal renal function. Any magnesium hydroxide that is not converted to magnesium chloride in the stomach is presumably subsequently changed in the small intestine to soluble but poorly absorbed salts. Magnesium hydroxide binds bile salts in vitro, but to a much lesser extent than does aluminum hydroxide. Magnesium-containing antacids have a laxative action. (See Saline Laxatives 56:12.)

Antacid-induced increases in gastric pH inhibit the proteolytic action of pepsin, an effect which is particularly important in patients with peptic ulcer disease. The optimum pH for pepsin activity is 1.5–2.5 and progressive inhibition occurs as gastric pH increases; above pH 4, the proteolytic activity of pepsin is minimal. Although some investigators have reported that aluminum- or calcium-containing antacids adsorb pepsin and thus have direct antipepsin effects, one study in which pH was controlled indicates that the antipepsin effects of antacids are due entirely to increased pH. Antacids do not coat the lining of peptic ulcers or the GI mucosa. Although some antacids, such as aluminum hydroxide, have astringent and demulcent actions, these effects are probably not important in the treatment of peptic ulcers.

In patients with peptic ulcers, antacids increase serum gastrin concentrations probably by increasing gastric pH. Single dose studies indicate that calcium carbonate causes gastric acid hypersecretion and acid rebound probably as a result of a local effect of calcium on gastrin-producing cells. Other antacids also increase secretion of gastric acid but do not cause acid rebound after the antacid has left the stomach. Aluminum-containing antacids delay gastric emptying time, an effect that is related to the concentration of aluminum in the stomach.

CHEMISTRY AND STABILITY

● Chemistry

Antacids are inorganic salts that dissolve in acid gastric secretions releasing anions that partially neutralize gastric hydrochloric acid.

Aluminum Antacids
Aluminum Carbonate

Dried basic aluminum carbonate gel occurs as a white powder and is insoluble in water and in alcohol. Aluminum carbonate suspension is a white, creamy,

thixotropic gel and contains the equivalent of 4.9–5.3% aluminum oxide and not less than 2.4% carbon dioxide.

Aluminum Hydroxide

Dried aluminum hydroxide gel occurs as a white, odorless, tasteless, amorphous powder and is insoluble in water and in alcohol. The powder contains 50–57.5% aluminum oxide as the hydrated oxide and may contain varying amounts of aluminum carbonate and bicarbonate. Tablets of dried aluminum hydroxide gel contain 62–72% of the labeled amount of aluminum hydroxide as aluminum oxide. Aluminum hydroxide gel is a white, viscous suspension. The suspension contains the equivalent of 3.6–4.4% w/w aluminum oxide in the form of aluminum hydroxide and hydrated oxide. The suspension also may contain basic aluminum carbonate and bicarbonate, flavoring agents, sweeteners and antimicrobial agents. Aluminum hydroxide gel suspension should not be frozen.

Aluminum Phosphate

Aluminum phosphate gel is a white, viscous suspension. The suspension contains 4–5% w/w aluminum phosphate and may contain preservatives.

Dihydroxyaluminum Aminoacetate

Dihydroxyaluminum aminoacetate occurs as a white, odorless powder that has a faintly sweet taste and is insoluble in water. The powder contains 35.5–38.5% aluminum oxide calculated on a dried basis and may contain small amounts of aluminum oxide or aminoacetic acid.

Calcium Carbonate

Precipitated calcium carbonate occurs as a fine, white, odorless, tasteless, microcrystalline powder and is practically insoluble in water and insoluble in alcohol.

Magnesium Antacids
Magnesium Carbonate

Magnesium carbonate occurs as light, white, friable masses (heavy magnesium carbonate) or as a bulky, white powder (light magnesium carbonate). The drug is odorless and is practically insoluble in water and insoluble in alcohol. Magnesium carbonate contains the equivalent of 40–43.5% magnesium oxide.

Magnesium Hydroxide

Magnesium hydroxide occurs as a bulky, white powder which is practically insoluble in water and in alcohol. Milk of Magnesia, Double-strength Milk of Magnesia, and Triple-strength Milk of Magnesia are suspensions containing 80, 160, and 240 mg of magnesium hydroxide per mL, respectively. Milk of Magnesia USP occurs as a white, opaque, more or less viscous suspension.

Magnesium Oxide

Magnesium oxide occurs as a very bulky, white, powder (light magnesium oxide) or as a relatively dense, white powder (heavy magnesium oxide). Magnesium oxide is practically insoluble in water and insoluble in alcohol. Light magnesium oxide suspends more readily in liquids than does heavy magnesium oxide.

Magnesium Trisilicate

Magnesium trisilicate, a compound of magnesium oxide and silicon dioxide, occurs as a fine, white, odorless, tasteless powder free from grittiness. The powder is insoluble in water and in alcohol. The powder contains not less than 20% magnesium oxide and not less than 45% silicon dioxide.

Miscellaneous Antacids
Dihydroxyaluminum Sodium Carbonate

Dihydroxyaluminum sodium carbonate is a single molecule that reportedly combines the antacid properties of aluminum hydroxide and sodium bicarbonate. Dihydroxyaluminum sodium carbonate occurs as a fine, white, odorless powder that is slightly hygroscopic at room temperature. The powder is practically insoluble in water and contains the equivalent of 34.8–38.2% aluminum oxide.

Sodium Bicarbonate

Sodium bicarbonate occurs as a white, crystalline powder with a saline and slightly alkaline taste. The drug is soluble in water and insoluble in alcohol. Aqueous solutions of sodium bicarbonate, when freshly prepared, are alkaline to litmus; alkalinity increases as the solutions stand, are agitated, or are heated.

Magaldrate

Magaldrate, a chemical combination of aluminum and magnesium hydroxides and sulfate, occurs as a white, odorless, crystalline powder and is insoluble in water and in alcohol. The powder contains the equivalent of 34–46% magnesium oxide, the equivalent of 21–30% aluminum oxide, and 13.3–17.5% sulfur trioxide, calculated on the dried basis. Each gram of magaldrate in the oral suspension and tablets contains the equivalent of 340–460 mg of magnesium oxide and 210–300 mg of aluminum oxide.

● *Stability*

Aluminum Antacids

Aluminum Hydroxide

Aluminum hydroxide gel suspension should not be frozen. On standing, small amounts of clear liquid may separate from aluminum hydroxide gel suspension.

Aluminum Phosphate

On standing, small amounts of water may separate from aluminum phosphate gel suspension.

Magnesium Antacids

Magnesium Hydroxide

Milk of Magnesia USP should preferably be stored at less than 35°C; however, freezing should be avoided. On standing, varying proportions of water usually separate from Milk of Magnesia USP suspension.

Magnesium Oxide

Magnesium oxide readily absorbs water and carbon dioxide when exposed to air and, in the presence of a limited amount of water, forms a cement-like mass. In water, magnesium oxide is converted to magnesium hydroxide.

PREPARATIONS

Excipients in commercially available drug preparations may have clinically important effects in some individuals; consult specific product labeling for details.

Aluminum Carbonate, Basic

Oral

Capsules	equivalent to dried aluminum hydroxide gel 608 mg or aluminum hydroxide 500 mg	**Basaljel®**, Wyeth
Tablets	equivalent to dried aluminum hydroxide gel 608 mg or aluminum hydroxide 500 mg	**Basaljel®** (scored), Wyeth

Aluminum Hydroxide

Oral

Capsules	475 mg	**Alu-Cap®**, 3M
Suspension	320 mg/5 mL*	**Aluminum Hydroxide Suspension**
		Amphojel®, Wyeth
	600 mg/5 mL	**ALternaGEL®**, J&J-Merck
Tablets	300 mg	**Amphojel®**, Wyeth
Tablets, film-coated	600 mg	**Alu-Tab®**, 3M

* available from one or more manufacturer, distributor, and/or repackager by generic (nonproprietary) name

Calcium Carbonate, Precipitated (Precipitated Chalk)

Powder
Oral

Pieces, chewing gum	500 mg	**Chooz®**, Insight
Suspension	400 mg/5 mL	**Mylanta® Children's Upset Stomach Relief**, J&J-Merck
	1.25 g/5 mL*	**Calcium Carbonate Suspension**

Tablets	1.25 g*	**Calcium Carbonate Tablets** (scored)
Tablets, chewable	400 mg	**Mylanta® Children's Upset Stomach Relief**, J&J-Merck
	420 mg	**Titralac® Regular**, 3M
	500 mg	**Tums® Antacid/Calcium Supplement**, GlaxoSmithKline
	650 mg*	**Calcium Carbonate Chewable Tablets**
	750 mg	**Titralac® Extra Strength**, 3M
	850 mg	**Tums® E-X Antacid/Calcium Supplement**, GlaxoSmithKline
	850 mg	**Alka-Mints®**, Bayer
	1 g	**Tums® Ultra Antacid/Calcium Supplement**, GlaxoSmithKline
Tablets, chewable, rapidly disintegrating	600 mg	**Maalox® Quick Dissolve® Chewables**, Novartis
	1 g	**Maalox® Quick Dissolve® Chewables Maximum Strength**, Novartis

* available from one or more manufacturer, distributor, and/or repackager by generic (nonproprietary) name

Dihydroxyaluminum Sodium Carbonate

Powder

Magaldrate (Aluminum Magnesium Hydroxide)

Oral

Suspension	540 mg/5 mL	**Lowsium®**, Rugby

Magaldrate Combinations

Oral

Suspension	540 mg/5 mL with Simethicone 40 mg/5 mL	**Lowsium® Plus**, Rugby
		Riopan Plus®, Wyeth
	1080 mg/5 mL with Simethicone 40 mg/5mL	**Riopan Plus® Double Strength**, Wyeth

Magnesium Carbonate

Powder

Magnesium Hydroxide

Powder
Oral

Suspension	400 mg/5 mL*	**Milk of Magnesia**
		Phillips'® Milk of Magnesia, Bayer
	800 mg/5 mL	**Phillips'® Milk of Magnesia Concentrate**, Bayer
	1.2 g/5 mL*	**Milk of Magnesia Concentrate**, Roxane
Tablets	300 mg*	**Phillips'® Milk of Magnesia**, Bayer

* available from one or more manufacturer, distributor, and/or repackager by generic (nonproprietary) name

Magnesium Oxide

Powder
Oral

Capsules	140 mg	**Uro-Mag®**, Blaine
Tablets	400 mg*	**Magnesium Oxide Tablets**
		Mag-Ox® 400, Blaine
	420 mg*	**Magnesium Oxide Tablets**

* available from one or more manufacturer, distributor, and/or repackager by generic (nonproprietary) name

Magnesium Trisilicate

Powder

Sodium Bicarbonate (Baking Soda)

Powder
Oral

For solution	0.78 g/3.9 g	**Citrocarbonate®** Granules, Lee
Tablets	325 mg*	**Sodium Bicarbonate Tablets**
	650 mg*	**Sodium Bicarbonate Tablets**

* available from one or more manufacturer, distributor, and/or repackager by generic (nonproprietary) name

Aluminum Hydroxide and Magnesium Carbonate

Oral

Suspension	Aluminum Hydroxide 31.7 mg/5 mL and Magnesium Carbonate 119.3 mg/5 mL	**Gaviscon® Liquid**, GlaxoSmithKline **Genaton® Liquid**, Teva
	Aluminum Hydroxide 254 mg/5 mL and Magnesium Carbonate 237.5 mg/5 mL	**Gaviscon® Extra Strength**, GlaxoSmithKline
Tablets, chewable	Aluminum Hydroxide 160 mg and Magnesium Carbonate 105 mg	**Gaviscon® Extra Strength**, GlaxoSmithKline

Aluminum Hydroxide and Magnesium Hydroxide

Oral

Suspension	Aluminum Hydroxide 200 mg/5 mL and Magnesium Hydroxide 200 mg/5 mL	**Mag-Al®**, Pharmaceutical Associates
	Aluminum Hydroxide 225 mg/5 mL and Magnesium Hydroxide 200 mg/5 mL	**Alamag®**, Teva, URL **Maalox®**, Novartis **Rulox®**, Rugby
	Aluminum Hydroxide 600 mg/5 mL and Magnesium Hydroxide 300 mg/5 mL	**Maalox® TC**, Novartis
Tablets, chewable	Aluminum Hydroxide 200 mg and Magnesium Hydroxide 200 mg	**Rulox® #1**, Rugby

Aluminum Hydroxide and Magnesium Hydroxide Combinations

Oral

Suspension	Aluminum Hydroxide 200 mg/5 mL, Magnesium Hydroxide 200 mg/5 mL, and Simethicone 20 mg/5 mL	**Almacone®**, Rugby **Di-Gel®**, Schering-Plough **Maalox Advanced Regular Strength®**, Novartis **Mag-Al® Plus**, Pharmaceutical Associates **Mygel®**, Sandoz **Mylanta® Fast-Acting**, J&J-Merck
	Aluminum Hydroxide 225 mg/5 mL, Magnesium Hydroxide 200 mg/5 mL, and Simethicone 25 mg/5 mL	**Alamag® Plus**, Teva
	Aluminum Hydroxide 400 mg/5 mL, Magnesium Hydroxide 400 mg/5 mL, and Simethicone 40 mg/5 mL	**Almacone® II Hi-Potency**, Rugby **Antacid Double Strength®**, Teva **Maalox Advanced Maximum Strength®**, Novartis **Mag-Al® XS**, Pharmaceutical Associates **Mygel® II**, Sandoz **Mylanta® Fast-Acting Double Strength**, J&J-Merck

Tablets, chewable	Aluminum Hydroxide 500 mg/5 mL, Magnesium Hydroxide 450 mg/5 mL, and Simethicone 40 mg/5 mL	**Kudrox®**, Schwarz **Maalox® Antacid/Anti-Gas Maximum Strength**, Novartis
	Aluminum Hydroxide 200 mg, Magnesium Hydroxide 200 mg, and Simethicone 20 mg	**Almacone®**, Rugby
	Aluminum Hydroxide 200 mg, Magnesium Hydroxide 200 mg, and Simethicone 25 mg	**Tempo®**, Blairex

Aluminum Hydroxide and Magnesium Trisilicate

Oral

Tablets, chewable	Aluminum Hydroxide 80 mg and Magnesium Trisilicate 20 mg	**Gaviscon®**, GlaxoSmithKline **Genaton®**, Teva

Calcium Carbonate and Magnesium Carbonate

Oral

Suspension	Calcium Carbonate 520 mg/5 mL and Magnesium Carbonate 400 mg/5 mL	**Marblen®**, Fleming

Calcium Carbonate and Magnesium Hydroxide

Oral

Suspension	Calcium Carbonate 400 mg/5 mL and Magnesium Hydroxide 135 mg/5 mL	**Mylanta® Supreme Fast Acting**, J&J-Merck
Tablets	Calcium Carbonate 550 mg and Magnesium Hydroxide 125 mg	**Mylanta® Gelcaps®**, J&J-Merck
Tablets, chewable	Calcium Carbonate 350 mg and Magnesium Hydroxide 150 mg	**Mylanta® Fast-Acting**, J&J-Merck
	Calcium Carbonate 500 mg and Magnesium Hydroxide 110 mg	**Rolaids® Antacid**, Pfizer
	Calcium Carbonate 700 mg and Magnesium Hydroxide 300 mg	**Mylanta® Fast-Acting Maximum Strength**, J&J-Merck

Calcium Carbonate and Magnesium Hydroxide Combinations

Oral

Tablets	Calcium Carbonate 280 mg, Magnesium Hydroxide 128 mg, and Simethicone 20 mg	**Di-Gel®**, Schering-Plough
Tablets, chewable	Calicum Carbonate 800 mg, Magnesium Hydroxide 165 mg, and Famotidine 10 mg	**Pepcid® Complete**, J&J-Merck

Other Calcium Carbonate Combinations

Oral

Tablets	420 mg with Simethicone 21 mg	**Titralac® Plus**, 3M
Tablets, chewable, rapidly disintegrating	1 g with Simethicone 60 mg	**Maalox® Max® Quick Dissolve Chewables Antacid/Antigas Maximum Strength**, Novartis

Potassium Bicarbonate and Sodium Bicarbonate

Oral

Tablets, for solution	Potassium Bicarbonate 312 mg and Sodium Bicarbonate 958 mg	**Alka-Seltzer® Gold Effervescent Antacid**, Bayer

Selected Revisions February 1, 2011, © Copyright, March 1, 1979, American Society of Health-System Pharmacists, Inc.

Bismuth Salts

56:08 · ANTIDIARRHEA AGENTS

■ Bismuth subsalicylate is an antidiarrheal agent and antidyspepsia agent; bismuth subgallate is an internal deodorant.

Bismuth subcitrate potassium and bismuth subsalicylate are antiulcer agents (used as part of multiple-drug regimens for Helicobacter pylori infection).

USES

● Diarrhea

Bismuth subsalicylate is used as *self-medication* in children and adults for symptomatic control of acute nonspecific diarrhea and travelers' diarrhea.

Bismuth subsalicylate has been used in adults for prevention of travelers' diarrhea†; however, the drug is less effective than anti-infective agents.

● Helicobacter pylori Infection and Duodenal Ulcer Disease

Bismuth subsalicylate or bismuth subcitrate potassium is used for treatment of *Helicobacter pylori* infection and duodenal ulcer disease (active disease or history of duodenal ulcer); eradication of *H. pylori* has been shown to reduce the risk of duodenal ulcer recurrence.

Bismuth subsalicylate or bismuth subcitrate potassium is used in multiple-drug regimens that also include metronidazole, tetracycline hydrochloride, and a histamine H_2-receptor antagonist or proton-pump inhibitor (quadruple therapy); such drug combinations are recommended by the American College of Gastroenterology (ACG) as a first-line treatment option for eradication of *H. pylori* infection. ACG recommends consideration of such quadruple-drug regimens in penicillin-allergic patients and those who have previously received a macrolide antibiotic. If the initial 14-day regimen does not eradicate *H. pylori*, retreat with a multiple-drug regimen that does not include metronidazole to avoid possible development of metronidazole resistance.

Multiple-drug regimens including bismuth subsalicylate, metronidazole, tetracycline hydrochloride, and a proton-pump inhibitor (instead of a histamine H_2-receptor antagonist) may be more effective against metronidazole-resistant strains of *H. pylori*; such regimens are recommended by ACG as an acceptable treatment option for persistent *H. pylori* infection ("salvage" treatment).

The fixed combination containing bismuth subcitrate potassium, metronidazole, and tetracycline hydrochloride (Pylera®) is used in conjunction with omeprazole for the treatment of *H. pylori* infection and duodenal ulcer disease (active ulcer or history of duodenal ulcer within past 5 years).

● Flatulence or Stool Odor

Bismuth subgallate is used as *self-medication* in children and adults for the reduction of flatulence or stool odor from a colostomy or ileostomy.

Bismuth subgallate has been used as *self-medication* for the reduction of odor from fecal incontinence†, irritable bowel syndrome†, or bariatric surgery†.

Bismuth subgallate is *not* expected to be effective for the reduction of odor from faulty personal hygiene†.

● Dyspepsia (Upset Stomach)

Bismuth subsalicylate is used as *self-medication* in children and adults for the symptomatic relief of dyspepsia (e.g., upset stomach, nausea, heartburn, fullness, belching, gas) secondary to overindulgence in food and drink.

The effectiveness of bismuth salts in the treatment of nonulcer dyspepsia† is uncertain. The drugs are not recommended as first-line therapy because of the potential risk of neurotoxicity with long-term use; they may be useful as second-line agents.

DOSAGE AND ADMINISTRATION

● Administration

Oral Administration

Capsules

Bismuth subgallate: Administer orally up to 4 times daily with meals. Swallow the capsule whole.

Bismuth subcitrate potassium in fixed combination with metronidazole and tetracycline hydrochloride (Pylera®): Administer orally 4 times daily after meals and at bedtime; give omeprazole concomitantly as part of the regimen. (See Fixed Combination Containing Bismuth Subcitrate Potassium, Metronidazole, and Tetracycline Hydrochloride [Pylera®] under Dosage: Helicobacter pylori Infection and Duodenal Ulcer Disease, in Dosage and Administration.) Swallow the capsule whole. Administer with a full glass (240 mL) of water, particularly with bedtime doses, to reduce the risk of esophageal irritation and ulceration by the tetracycline hydrochloride component. If a dose of Pylera® is missed, take the next dose at the regularly scheduled time; do not double the dose. Contact a clinician if more than 4 doses are missed.

Suspension

Bismuth subsalicylate: Shake the suspension well prior to administration. Use the dose cup provided by the manufacturer for accurate dosing. For Diotame®, twist off the lid and dispense the appropriate dose by squeezing the tube.

Chewable Tablets

Bismuth subgallate: Administer orally up to 4 times daily with meals. Chew or swallow whole.

Bismuth subsalicylate: Chew or dissolve in the mouth and swallow.

Bismuth subsalicylate (with metronidazole and tetracycline hydrochloride in the Helidac® Therapy kit): Administer each component orally 4 times daily with meals and at bedtime. Chew and swallow the bismuth subsalicylate tablets. Administer the tetracycline hydrochloride and metronidazole components with a full glass (240 mL) of water, particularly with bedtime doses, to reduce the risk of esophageal irritation and ulceration by the tetracycline hydrochloride component. If a dose of Helidac® Therapy is missed, take the next dose at the regularly scheduled time; do not double the dose. If more than 4 doses are missed, contact a clinician.

Conventional Tablets

Bismuth subsalicylate (e.g., Pepto-Bismol® Easy-to-Swallow Caplets): Swallow with water; do not chew.

● Dosage

Bismuth salts are available as bismuth subgallate, bismuth subcitrate potassium, and bismuth subsalicylate; dosages are expressed in terms of the salts.

Bismuth subcitrate potassium is available in fixed combination with metronidazole and tetracycline hydrochloride (Pylera®); dosage of Pylera® is expressed as number of capsules.

Acute Nonspecific Diarrhea and Travelers' Diarrhea

Bismuth Subsalicylate

Adults and children 12 years of age or older: 525 mg every 30–60 minutes or 1.05 g every hour as needed, not to exceed 4.2 g in a 24-hour period. Use until diarrhea stops, but not for more than 2 days. Alternatively, administer 1.05 g every 30 minutes† to every hour as needed, not to exceed 4.2 g in a 24-hour period. *Self-medication* should not exceed 2 days.

Prevention of Travelers' Diarrhea

Bismuth Subsalicylate

Adults: For prevention of travelers' diarrhea†, 525 mg 4 times daily has been recommended.

Helicobacter pylori Infection and Duodenal Ulcer Disease

Bismuth Subsalicylate, Metronidazole, and Tetracycline Hydrochloride Regimen

Adults: Administer 525 mg of bismuth subsalicylate in conjunction with metronidazole (250 mg) and tetracycline hydrochloride (500 mg) 4 times daily for 10–14 days; give concomitantly with ranitidine (150 mg) twice daily or the usual dosage of a proton-pump inhibitor once or twice daily.

Salvage therapy for persistent *H. pylori* infection: Administer for 7–14 days.

Bismuth Subsalicylate (with Metronidazole and Tetracycline Hydrochloride) in Helidac® Therapy Kit

Adults: Administer 525 mg of bismuth subsalicylate in conjunction with metronidazole (250 mg) and tetracycline hydrochloride (500 mg) 4 times daily (at meals and at bedtime) for 14 days; give concomitantly with usual dosage of H$_2$-receptor antagonist.

Fixed Combination Containing Bismuth Subcitrate Potassium, Metronidazole, and Tetracycline Hydrochloride (Pylera®)

Adults: Administer 3 capsules 4 times daily (after meals and at bedtime) for 10 days; give concomitantly with omeprazole 20 mg twice daily (after morning and evening meal) for 10 days.

Flatulence or Stool Odor
Bismuth Subgallate

Adults and children 12 years of age or older: Administer 200–400 mg up to 4 times daily.

Dyspepsia (Upset Stomach)
Bismuth Subsalicylate

Adults and children 12 years of age or older: Administer 525 mg every 30–60 minutes as needed, not to exceed 4.2 g in a 24-hour period. Do not use for more than 2 days. Alternatively, administer 1.05 g every 30–60 minutes† as needed, not to exceed 4.2 g in a 24-hour period. *Self-medication* should not exceed 2 days.

● Special Populations

No special population dosage recommendations at this time. (See Cautions: Geriatric Use and also see Cautions: Renal Impairment.)

CAUTIONS

● Contraindications

Helidac® Therapy (kit containing bismuth subsalicylate, metronidazole, tetracycline hydrochloride) is contraindicated in pregnant or nursing women, pediatric patients, patients with hepatic or renal impairment, patients with known allergy to aspirin or salicylates, and those with known hypersensitivity to any component of the kit.

Pylera® (fixed-combination capsule containing bismuth subcitrate potassium, metronidazole, tetracycline hydrochloride) is contraindicated in pregnant or nursing women, pediatric patients, patients with hepatic or renal impairment, and those with known hypersensitivity to any ingredient in the capsule.

● Warnings/Precautions
Warnings
GI Disorders

Bismuth subsalicylate should not be used for *self-medication* in patients with an ulcer, bleeding disorder, or bloody or black stools.

Reye's Syndrome

A risk of Reye's syndrome exists with bismuth subsalicylate in children or adolescents who have or are recovering from varicella or influenza-like symptoms. (See Pediatric Use under Warnings/Precautions: Specific Populations, in Cautions.)

Neurotoxicity

Neurotoxicity associated with excessive doses of bismuth salts has been reported rarely; this effect is reversible following discontinuance of the drug.

Discoloration of Tongue and/or Stool

A transient and harmless darkening of the tongue and/or black stool is possible with bismuth treatment; do not confuse stool darkening with melena.

Lead Content

Bismuth mined from the ground, and commercially available Pepto-Bismol® preparations, may contain small amounts of naturally occurring lead. Amounts of lead in Pepto-Bismol® preparations are low compared with average daily lead exposure. Pepto-Bismol® preparations are *not* intended for chronic use.

Sensitivity Reactions
Hypersensitivity

Bismuth subsalicylate contains salicylate; do not use in patients allergic to salicylates (including aspirin).

General Precautions
Selection and Use of Anti-infectives in H. pylori Regimens

To reduce the development of drug-resistant bacteria and maintain effectiveness of Helidac® Therapy, Pylera®, and other anti-infective agents, use only for the treatment or prevention of infections proven or strongly suspected to be caused by susceptible bacteria.

When selecting or modifying anti-infective therapy, use results of culture and in vitro susceptibility testing. In the absence of such data, consider local epidemiology and susceptibility patterns when selecting anti-infectives for empiric therapy.

Phenylketonuria

Diotame® chewable tablets contain aspartame (NutraSweet®), which is metabolized in the GI tract to phenylalanine following oral administration.

Medication Errors

Serious medication errors have been reported to the US Food and Drug Administration (FDA) in which consumers used Maalox® Total Relief (bismuth subsalicylate) when they intended to use traditional Maalox® liquid antacid products containing aluminum hydroxide, magnesium hydroxide, and simethicone (e.g., Maalox® Advanced Regular Strength, Maalox® Advanced Maximum Strength). Because of the potential for serious adverse effects associated with accidental use of bismuth subsalicylate (which is chemically related to aspirin), the manufacturer of Maalox® Total Relief initially agreed to change the trade name of the product to one that did not include "Maalox"; however, the manufacturer instead discontinued the bismuth subsalicylate preparation in the summer of 2010.

Use of Fixed Combinations or Multiple-Drug Kits

When the fixed-combination preparation containing bismuth subcitrate potassium, metronidazole, and tetracycline hydrochloride (Pylera®) or the kit containing bismuth subsalicylate, metronidazole, and tetracycline hydrochloride (Helidac® Therapy) is used for the treatment of *H. pylori* infection and duodenal ulcer disease, the cautions, precautions, and contraindications associated with metronidazole and tetracycline hydrochloride must be considered in addition to those associated with bismuth subcitrate potassium or bismuth subsalicylate.

Laboratory Test Interferences

Bismuth absorbs x-rays; may interfere with radiographic diagnostic procedures of the GI tract.

Darkening of stool from bismuth salts does not interfere with any tests for occult blood.

Specific Populations
Pregnancy

Bismuth subsalicylate: Category C (Category D in third trimester). (See Users Guide.)

Helidac® Therapy, Pylera®: Category D. (See Users Guide.)

Helidac® Therapy, Pylera®: Effect on labor and delivery unknown.

Lactation

Bismuth subsalicylate: Use with caution.

Helidac® Therapy, Pylera®: Discontinue nursing or the drug.

Pediatric Use

Do *not* use bismuth subsalicylate in children or adolescents who have or are recovering from varicella or influenza-like symptoms. Changes in behavior accompanied by nausea and vomiting in children or adolescents taking the drug may be an early sign of Reye's syndrome.

Safety and efficacy of the commercially available Helidac® Therapy kit or the fixed-combination preparation Pylera® in pediatric patients infected with *H. pylori* have not been established. Pylera® or the Helidac® Therapy kit should not be used in children younger than 8 years of age. (See Contraindications under Cautions.)

Geriatric Use

There is insufficient experience in patients 65 years of age or older to determine whether they respond differently than younger adults to the commercially available Helidac® Therapy kit or the fixed-combination preparation Pylera® for treatment of *H. pylori* infection and duodenal ulcer disease.

Consider age-related decreases in hepatic, renal, and/or cardiac function and concomitant disease and drug therapy.

Hepatic Impairment

Accumulation of bismuth salts may occur in patients with severe hepatic disease, presumably because of biliary excretion of bismuth from the body. The commercially available Helidac® Therapy kit and the fixed-combination preparation Pylera® are contraindicated in patients with hepatic impairment. (See Cautions: Contraindications.)

Renal Impairment

Use bismuth subsalicylate with caution, if at all, in patients with renal impairment. The commercially available Helidac® Therapy kit and the fixed-combination preparation Pylera® are contraindicated in patients with renal impairment. (See Contraindications under Cautions.)

● Common Adverse Effects

Bismuth: Transient and harmless darkening of the tongue and/or black stools, decreased peristalsis (with bismuth subgallate).

Helidac® Therapy: Nausea, diarrhea, abdominal pain, melena, upper respiratory infection.

Pylera®: Stool abnormality, diarrhea, dyspepsia, abdominal pain, nausea, headache, flu syndrome, taste perversion, asthenia, vaginitis, dizziness.

DRUG INTERACTIONS

● Anticoagulants

Salicylate salts (e.g., bismuth subsalicylate) may increase the risk of bleeding with concomitant anticoagulant therapy. Monitor anticoagulant therapy and adjust anticoagulant dosage as needed.

● Antidiabetic Agents

Possibly enhanced hypoglycemic effects with concomitant salicylate salt therapy. Use with caution.

● Aspirin

Use with caution.

● Ciprofloxacin

Bismuth subsalicylate slightly decreases peak plasma concentrations and area under the concentration-time curve (AUC) of ciprofloxacin. This effect is not considered clinically important.

● Doxycycline

Bismuth subsalicylate may decrease absorption of doxycycline. Avoid using bismuth subsalicylate for *self-medication* in travelers taking doxycycline for malaria prophylaxis.

● Methotrexate

Avoid using bismuth subsalicylate for *self-medication* concomitantly with methotrexate.

● Omeprazole

Omeprazole increases the extent of absorption of bismuth from Pylera® capsules following concomitant administration.

● Probenecid

Use concomitantly with caution, if at all.

● Salicylates

Do not use bismuth subsalicylate for *self-medication* concomitantly with other salicylate drugs.

● Sulfinpyrazone

Use concomitantly with caution.

● Tetracycline

Bismuth and/or calcium carbonate (excipient of bismuth subsalicylate tablets) reduces systemic absorption of tetracycline; the clinical importance is unknown

since relative contribution of systemic versus local antimicrobial activity against *H. pylori* has not been determined.

PHARMACOKINETICS

● Absorption

Bioavailability

Bismuth subsalicylate: Hydrolyzed in GI tract to bismuth and salicylic acid following oral administration.

Bismuth: <1% absorbed from GI tract into systemic circulation following oral administration of bismuth subsalicylate.

Salicylic acid: >80% absorbed following oral administration of bismuth subsalicylate chewable tablets.

Food

Food reduces systemic absorption of all three components of fixed-combination preparation containing bismuth subcitrate potassium, metronidazole, and tetracycline hydrochloride (Pylera®); effect not considered clinically important. (See Administration under Dosage and Administration.)

● Distribution

Extent

Bismuth: Distributed throughout body.

Plasma Protein Binding

Bismuth: >90%.

Salicylic acid: About 90%.

● Elimination

Metabolism

Salicylic acid: Extensively metabolized.

Elimination Route

Bismuth: Excreted principally via urine and biliary routes.

Salicylic acid: About 10% excreted in urine as unchanged drug.

Half-life

Bismuth: Multiple disposition half-lives; intermediate and terminal half-lives of 5–11 and 21–72 days, respectively.

Metabolic clearance of salicylic acid is saturable.

Salicylic acid: Terminal half-life of 2–5 hours following a single oral 525-mg dose of bismuth subsalicylate.

Special Populations

Severe liver disease may be associated with accumulation of bismuth because of suggested biliary excretion of bismuth from the body.

Metabolic clearance of salicylic acid lower in women than in men.

DESCRIPTION

Bismuth subsalicylate may protect gastric mucosa, bind to ulcer base and mucosa, bind bile acids, and decrease endogenous prostaglandin and bicarbonate secretion.

Bismuth subsalicylate reduces number of bowel movements, aids in firming stool, normalizes fluid movement via antisecretory mechanisms, binds bacterial toxins, and exhibits antimicrobial activity in patients with diarrhea.

Mechanism of antibacterial action of bismuth salts not fully elucidated.

Bismuth salts may exert bactericidal action by complexing in bacterial wall and periplasmic space, inhibiting urease, catalase and lipase/phospholipase, ATP synthesis, and *H. pylori* adherence.

Multiple-drug regimen of bismuth subsalicylate, metronidazole, and tetracycline hydrochloride and the fixed-combination preparation containing bismuth subcitrate potassium, metronidazole, and tetracycline hydrochloride (Pylera®) active against most strains of *H. pylori* in vitro and in clinical infections.

Bismuth subgallate may reduce number of odor-producing anaerobic intestinal microbes and/or directly interact with sulfur-containing compounds; reduces flatulence odor but not flatulence itself.

Each 262.4-mg tablet of bismuth subsalicylate contains an amount of salicylate comparable to that in approximately 130 mg of aspirin.

ADVICE TO PATIENTS

Importance of advising patients of the cautions, precautions, and contraindications associated with metronidazole and tetracycline hydrochloride when using Helidac® Therapy or Pylera®.

Importance of informing patient that temporary and harmless darkening of the tongue and/or black stool may occur with bismuth salts, and that stool darkening should not be confused with blood in the stool.

Do not use bismuth subsalicylate for *self-medication* in presence of peptic ulcers, bleeding disorders, bloody or black stool, known allergy to salicylates (including aspirin), or if taking other salicylates; consult clinician before use if diarrhea is accompanied by fever, mucus in stools, or if patient is on a sodium-restricted diet or currently taking drugs for anticoagulation, diabetes, gout, or arthritis.

Importance of instructing patients to discontinue bismuth subsalicylate for *self-medication* and inform clinician if symptoms worsen, ringing in the ears or loss of hearing occurs, or if diarrhea or other symptoms do not improve after 2 days of therapy.

Importance of advising patients *not* to use bismuth subsalicylate in children or adolescents who have or are recovering from chickenpox or flu-like symptoms. Importance of informing clinician if changes in behavior accompanied by nausea and vomiting occur while using bismuth subsalicylate, because these symptoms may be an early sign of Reye's syndrome.

Importance of adequate hydration (with clear fluids) to help prevent dehydration caused by diarrhea.

Importance of informing patients with phenylketonuria that Diotame® chewable tablets contain aspartame.

Importance of instructing patients about correct administration of Helidac® Therapy or Pylera® capsules, including administration of each dose after meals and at bedtime and with a full glass of water (particularly at bedtime to reduce risk of esophageal irritation and ulceration), swallowing Pylera® capsules whole, chewing and swallowing bismuth subsalicylate tablets, and about duration of therapy.

Importance of informing patients that Helidac® Therapy contains salicylates, and to contact a clinician if ringing in the ears occurs with concomitant aspirin therapy.

Importance of advising patient that if a dose of Helidac® Therapy or Pylera® is missed, the next dose should be taken at the regularly scheduled time; the dose should not be doubled. Importance of informing clinicians if more than 4 doses of Helidac® Therapy or Pylera® are missed.

Importance of advising patients that antibacterials (including Helidac® Therapy and Pylera®) should only be used to treat bacterial infections and not used to treat viral infections (e.g., the common cold).

Importance of completing full course of therapy, even if feeling better after a few days.

Advise patients that skipping doses or not completing the full course of therapy may decrease effectiveness and increase the likelihood that bacteria will develop resistance and will not be treatable with Helidac® Therapy or other anti-infective agents in the future.

Advise patients that Helidac® Therapy or the Pylera® fixed combination may reduce the effectiveness of oral contraceptives and that alternative nonhormonal contraceptive measures should be used.

Importance of informing clinician of existing or contemplated concomitant therapy, including prescription and OTC drugs and dietary or herbal products, as well as any concomitant illnesses.

Importance of women informing clinicians if they are or plan to become pregnant or plan to breast-feed.

Importance of advising patients of other important precautionary information. (See Cautions.)

PREPARATIONS

Excipients in commercially available drug preparations may have clinically important effects in some individuals; consult specific product labeling for details.

Bismuth Subcitrate Potassium Combinations

Oral

Capsules	140 mg with Metronidazole 125 mg and Tetracycline Hydrochloride 125 mg	Pylera®, Axcan Pharma

Bismuth Subgallate

Oral

Capsules	200 mg	Devrom®, Parthenon
Tablets, chewable	200 mg	Devrom®, Parthenon

Bismuth Subsalicylate

Oral

Suspension	87.3 mg/5 mL*	Bismatrol®, Major
		Bismuth Subsalicylate Oral Suspension
		Diotame® Instydose, Medique
		Kaopectate®, Chattem
		Kao-Tin®, Major
		Peptic Relief®, Rugby
		Pepto-Bismol®, Procter & Gamble
		Pink Bismuth Suspension
	175 mg/5 mL*	Bismatrol® Maximum Strength, Major
		Bismuth Subsalicylate Oral Suspension
		Kaopectate® Extra Strength, Chattem
		Pepto-Bismol® Maximum Strength, Procter & Gamble
		Pink Bismuth Maximum Strength Suspension
Tablets	262 mg*	Bismuth Subsalicylate Tablets
		Pepto-Bismol® Easy-to-Swallow Caplets, Procter & Gamble
		Pink Bismuth Caplets
Tablets, chewable	262 mg*	Bismatrol®, Major
		Bismuth Subsalicylate Chewable Tablets
		Diotame®, Medique
		Peptic Relief®, Rugby
		Pepto-Bismol® Chewables, Procter & Gamble
		Pink Bismuth Chewable Tablets

* available from one or more manufacturer, distributor, and/or repackager by generic (nonproprietary) name

Bismuth Subsalicylate Combinations

Oral

Kit	8 Tablets, chewable, Bismuth Subsalicylate 262.4 mg	Helidac® Therapy (available as 14 blister cards), Prometheus
	4 Tablets, Metronidazole 250 mg	
	4 Capsules, Tetracycline Hydrochloride 500 mg	

† Use is not currently included in the labeling approved by the US Food and Drug Administration.

Loperamide Hydrochloride

56:08 • ANTIDIARRHEA AGENTS

■ Loperamide hydrochloride, a synthetic piperidine-derivative, is an antiperistaltic antidiarrhea agent.

USES

● Diarrhea

Loperamide hydrochloride is used in the control and symptomatic relief of acute, nonspecific diarrhea and in the control and symptomatic relief of chronic diarrhea associated with inflammatory bowel disease. The drug has also been effective in controlling chronic functional (idiopathic) diarrhea† and chronic diarrhea caused by bowel resection or organic lesions†.

For self-medication, loperamide hydrochloride is used for symptomatic control of diarrhea, including travelers' diarrhea. The fixed combination containing loperamide hydrochloride and simethicone is used for self-medication for symptomatic control of diarrhea and symptomatic control of gas (gastric bloating, pressure, cramps).

Double-blind clinical studies have shown that loperamide is at least as effective as diphenoxylate for control of acute diarrhea and more effective than diphenoxylate in decreasing daily stool frequency, improving fecal consistency, and controlling chronic diarrhea.

Loperamide should not be used as primary therapy in patients with acute dysentery (characterized by blood in stools and high fever), acute ulcerative colitis, bacterial enterocolitis caused by invasive organisms (e.g., Salmonella, Shigella, Campylobacter), or pseudomembranous colitis associated with the use of anti-infectives. Fluid and electrolyte depletion may occur in patients who have diarrhea, and the use of loperamide does not preclude administration of appropriate fluid and electrolyte therapy.

Travelers' Diarrhea

Antiperistaltic agents (e.g., loperamide, diphenoxylate) are used for symptomatic treatment of mild or uncomplicated travelers' diarrhea, including that occurring in adult travelers with human immunodeficiency virus (HIV) infection, and also have been used for adjunctive therapy when anti-infectives are indicated for the treatment of moderate to severe travelers' diarrhea.

The most common cause of travelers' diarrhea (80–90% of cases) is bacteria (e.g., enterotoxigenic Escherichia coli, Campylobacter jejuni, Shigella, Salmonella, Aeromonas, Plesiomonas). Travelers' diarrhea caused by bacteria often is self-limited and resolves within 3–7 days without treatment. In travelers with only mild diarrhea (without fever or bloody stools), use of loperamide may provide symptomatic relief in less that 24 hours. If diarrhea is moderate to severe, associated with fever or bloody stools, or extremely disruptive to travel plans, short-term (1–3 days) empiric treatment with an appropriate anti-infective (e.g., ciprofloxacin or levofloxacin, azithromycin, rifaximin) is recommended. Adjunctive therapy with an antiperistaltic agent during the first few days may shorten the duration of illness or reduce the frequency of bowel movements so that travelers can continue with travel plans while waiting for the beneficial effects of anti-infective treatment. However, loperamide and diphenoxylate are not usually recommended in travelers with high fever or bloody diarrhea or in young children. (See Cautions.)

For additional information on treatment of travelers' diarrhea, see Travelers' Diarrhea under Uses: GI Infections, in Ciprofloxacin 8:12.18.

● Ileostomy Discharge

Loperamide hydrochloride is used to reduce the volume of discharge from ileostomies. Although not statistically significant, in one study loperamide appeared to have a greater effect on ileostomy discharge than did diphenoxylate with atropine. The greater the initial ileostomy discharge, the more benefit obtained by the patient from loperamide therapy.

DOSAGE AND ADMINISTRATION

● Administration

Loperamide hydrochloride is administered orally.

The oral solution or suspension should be administered using only the calibrated measuring cup provided by the manufacturer; the suspension should be shaken well prior to each dose.

Patients should receive appropriate fluid and electrolyte replacement as needed. Patients using the drug for self-medication should be advised to drink plenty of clear fluids to help prevent dehydration caused by diarrhea.

● Dosage

Dosage of loperamide hydrochloride is expressed in terms of the salt.

Adult Dosage

Acute Diarrhea

For control and symptomatic relief of acute, nonspecific diarrhea in adults, the initial dosage of loperamide hydrochloride is 4 mg, followed by 2 mg after each unformed stool. The maximum recommended dosage of loperamide hydrochloride for adults is 16 mg daily.

For self-medication to control symptoms of diarrhea, including travelers' diarrhea, in adults, the initial dosage of loperamide hydrochloride (alone or in fixed combination with simethicone) is 4 mg, followed by 2 mg after each subsequent unformed stool. The maximum recommended dosage of loperamide hydrochloride for self-medication in adults is 8 mg in a 24-hour period; the duration of therapy should not exceed 2 days unless directed by a clinician.

Clinical improvement of acute diarrhea usually occurs within 48 hours after initiation of loperamide. The drug should be discontinued and a clinician consulted if there is no improvement after 48 hours of therapy.

Chronic Diarrhea

For control and symptomatic relief of chronic diarrhea associated with inflammatory bowel disease in adults, the initial dosage of loperamide hydrochloride is 4 mg, followed by 2 mg after each unformed stool until symptoms are controlled; dosage should then be reduced for maintenance as required. When the optimal dosage for maintenance therapy has been established, the daily dosage may then be administered as a single dose or in divided doses. In clinical trials, the average adult maintenance dosage was 4–8 mg daily and only rarely exceeded 16 mg daily. If improvement does not occur in patients with chronic diarrhea after treatment with loperamide hydrochloride given in a dosage of 16 mg daily for at least 10 days, symptoms are unlikely to be controlled by further administration of the drug. Loperamide therapy may be continued if diarrhea cannot be adequately controlled with diet or specific treatment.

Pediatric Dosage

Acute Diarrhea

For control and symptomatic relief of acute, nonspecific diarrhea in children 2–12 years of age, dosage of loperamide hydrochloride is based on age and body weight. (See Table 1 for initial pediatric dosage for the first day of therapy.) On the second and subsequent days of therapy, children 2–12 years of age should receive a dosage of 0.1 mg/kg only after each unformed stool. Dosage on the second and subsequent days should not exceed the age-appropriate dosages recommended for the initial 24 hours of therapy.

TABLE 1. Initial Dosage of Loperamide Hydrochloride in Children 2–12 Years of Age

Age (weight)	Dosage (initial 24 hours)
2–5 years (13–20 kg)	1 mg 3 times daily
6–8 years (20–30 kg)	2 mg twice daily
8–12 years (>30 kg)	2 mg 3 times daily

For self-medication in children 12 years of age or older to control symptoms of diarrhea, including travelers' diarrhea, the initial dosage of loperamide hydrochloride (alone or in fixed combination with simethicone) is 4 mg, followed by 2 mg after each subsequent unformed stool. The maximum recommended dosage of loperamide hydrochloride for self-medication in children 12 years of age or older is 8 mg in a 24-hour period; the duration of therapy should not exceed 2 days unless directed by a clinician.

For *self-medication* in children 9–11 years of age (27.3–43.2 kg) to control symptoms of diarrhea, including travelers' diarrhea, the usual dosage of loperamide hydrochloride (alone or in fixed combination with simethicone) is 2 mg after the first unformed stool, followed by 1 mg after each subsequent unformed stool. The maximum recommended dosage of loperamide hydrochloride for *self-medication* in children 9–11 years of age is 6 mg daily in a 24-hour period; the duration of therapy should not exceed 2 days unless directed by a clinician.

For *self-medication* in children 6–8 years of age (21.8–26.8 kg) to control symptoms of diarrhea, including travelers' diarrhea, the usual dosage of loperamide hydrochloride (alone or in fixed combination with simethicone) is 2 mg after the first unformed stool, followed by 1 mg after each subsequent unformed stool. The maximum recommended dosage of loperamide hydrochloride for *self-medication* in children 6–8 years of age is 4 mg in a 24-hour period; the duration of therapy should not exceed 2 days unless directed by a clinician.

Loperamide hydrochloride (alone or in fixed combination with simethicone) should *not* be used for *self-medication* in children younger than 6 years of age unless directed by a clinician.

Clinical improvement of acute diarrhea usually occurs within 48 hours after initiation of loperamide. The drug should be discontinued and a clinician consulted if there is no improvement after 48 hours of therapy.

Chronic Diarrhea

A therapeutic dosage of loperamide hydrochloride for the treatment of chronic diarrhea in pediatric patients has not been established. A dosage of 0.08–0.24 mg/kg daily in 2 or 3 divided doses† has been used in a limited number of children for the management of chronic diarrhea and has been recommended by some clinicians.

● Dosage in Renal and Hepatic Impairment

Dosage adjustments are not necessary when loperamide hydrochloride is used in patients with renal impairment.

Loperamide hydrochloride should be used with caution in patients with hepatic impairment since first-pass metabolism may be decreased in such patients. (See Cautions: Precautions and Contraindications.)

CAUTIONS

● Adverse Effects

In clinical trials evaluating loperamide hydrochloride for the treatment of diarrhea, adverse effects generally were minor and self-limiting and were reported more frequently in patients receiving the drug for treatment of chronic diarrhea than in those receiving the drug for treatment of acute diarrhea. Some adverse effects reported with loperamide during clinical trials and postmarketing experience are difficult to distinguish from symptoms of the underlying diarrheal syndrome.

The most frequently reported adverse effects in patients receiving recommended dosages of the drug are nausea, constipation, abdominal cramps, and dizziness. Dry mouth, abdominal pain, abdominal distention or discomfort, vomiting, flatulence, dyspepsia, drowsiness, fatigue, and urinary retention also have been reported. Children may be more sensitive to adverse CNS effects of the drug than adults.

Paralytic ileus and megacolon (including toxic megacolon) have been reported in patients receiving loperamide. There have been rare reports of toxic megacolon in patients with human immunodeficiency virus (HIV) infection who had infectious colitis associated with viral or bacterial pathogens and received loperamide. (See Cautions: Precautions and Contraindications.)

Hypersensitivity reactions, including rash, pruritus, urticaria, and angioedema, have been reported in patients receiving loperamide. There have been rare reports of severe hypersensitivity reactions (e.g., anaphylactic shock, anaphylactoid reactions) and bullous eruptions (e.g., erythema multiforme, Stevens-Johnson syndrome, toxic epidermal necrolysis).

Potentially fatal, serious cardiovascular effects (e.g., QT interval prolongation, torsades de pointes or other ventricular arrhythmias, syncope, cardiac arrest) have been reported in patients taking loperamide. Cardiovascular effects have been reported rarely in patients receiving recommended dosages of loperamide hydrochloride; the majority of reported cases involved higher than recommended dosages, usually in individuals misusing or abusing the drug. (See Misuse and Abuse Potential under Cautions: Precautions and Contraindications.)

● Precautions and Contraindications

Loperamide is contraindicated in patients with known hypersensitivity to the drug or any ingredient in the formulation.

Loperamide is contraindicated in patients with abdominal pain in the absence of diarrhea.

The drug is used only for control and symptomatic relief of diarrhea. Whenever an underlying etiology for the diarrhea can be determined, specific treatment should be given if indicated or appropriate.

Loperamide is contraindicated in patients with acute dysentery (characterized by blood in stools and high fever), acute ulcerative colitis, bacterial enterocolitis caused by invasive organisms (e.g., *Salmonella, Shigella, Campylobacter*), or pseudomembranous colitis associated with anti-infective therapy.

Because of the possible risk of serious sequelae, including ileus, megacolon, and toxic megacolon, loperamide should *not* be used when inhibition of peristalsis should be avoided. The drug *must* be discontinued promptly if constipation, abdominal distention, or ileus occurs. Based on rare reports of toxic megacolon in HIV-infected patients with infectious colitis associated with viral or bacterial pathogens, loperamide should be discontinued in HIV-infected patients at the earliest signs of abdominal distention.

Fluid and electrolyte depletion often occurs in patients with diarrhea, and administration of appropriate fluid and electrolytes is important in such cases. Loperamide therapy does not preclude administration of appropriate fluid and electrolyte therapy. When loperamide is used for *self-medication*, patients should be advised to drink plenty of clear fluids to help prevent dehydration caused by diarrhea.

Because tiredness, dizziness, or drowsiness may occur in the setting of diarrheal syndromes treated with loperamide, patients should be advised to use caution when driving a car or operating machinery.

Loperamide should be used with caution in patients with hepatic impairment. Such patients should be monitored closely for signs and symptoms of CNS toxicity during loperamide therapy, since first-pass metabolism of the drug may be decreased in patients with hepatic impairment.

Patients receiving loperamide should be advised to consult a clinician if diarrhea persists for longer than 2 days, if blood is present in stools, or if fever or abdominal distention develops.

Loperamide should be used with caution in patients predisposed to QT interval prolongation, torsades de pointes, or other serious arrhythmias. The drug also should be used with caution in patients who are receiving drugs that inhibit loperamide metabolism or transport (i.e., inhibitors of hepatic cytochrome P-450 [CYP] isoenzymes 3A4 and 2C8, inhibitors of P-glycoprotein [P-gp]) since increased plasma concentrations of loperamide may increase the risk of serious cardiovascular effects. (See Misuse and Abuse Potential under Cautions: Precautions and Contraindications and see Drug Interactions.)

Precautions Related to *Self-medication*

For *self-medication*, loperamide should not be used for longer than 2 days unless directed by a clinician. Loperamide also should not be used for *self-medication* if diarrhea is accompanied by fever, if mucus or blood is present in the stool, or if rash or other allergic reaction to the drug has occurred previously.

If a patient is receiving an anti-infective or has a history of liver disease, a clinician should be consulted before the drug is used for *self-medication*.

When loperamide is used for *self-medication*, patients should be advised to discontinue the drug and contact a clinician if diarrhea symptoms worsen or last longer than 2 days or if abdominal swelling or bulging develops.

Precautions Related to Use of Fixed Combinations

When the fixed combination containing loperamide and simethicone is used, the cautions, precautions, contraindications, and drug interactions associated with both drugs should be considered. Cautionary information applicable to specific populations (e.g., pregnant or nursing women, individuals with hepatic or renal impairment, geriatric patients) should be considered for both loperamide and simethicone.

Misuse and Abuse Potential

FDA has warned clinicians to consider the potential for misuse and abuse of loperamide hydrochloride.

Serious cardiovascular effects, including fatalities, have occurred when loperamide hydrochloride was used at dosages higher than recommended. The majority of serious cardiovascular effects reported with loperamide have occurred in individuals who were intentionally misusing and abusing high dosages of the drug in an attempt to self-treat opiate withdrawal symptoms or to achieve a feeling of euphoria. The maximum recommended adult dosage of loperamide hydrochloride is 8 mg daily for *self-medication* or 16 mg daily for prescription use; in some cases of misuse and abuse, individuals ingested loperamide hydrochloride dosages of 70–1600 mg daily.

FDA recommends that clinicians consider loperamide as a possible cause of unexplained cardiac events (e.g., QT interval prolongation, torsades de pointes or other ventricular arrhythmias, syncope, cardiac arrest).

If loperamide-induced cardiotoxicity is suspected, loperamide should be promptly discontinued and appropriate therapy initiated to manage and prevent cardiac arrhythmias and severe outcomes. In some cases of torsades de pointes, drug treatment may be ineffective and electrical pacing or cardioversion may be required. Patients with opiate use disorders should be referred for treatment. When excessive loperamide ingestion is suspected, specific testing may be required to measure blood levels of the drug; standard drug screens for opiates may not include an assay for loperamide and may yield negative results even in the presence of loperamide.

Individuals abusing loperamide often take other drugs with the antidiarrheal agent in an attempt to increase loperamide absorption and penetration across the blood-brain barrier, inhibit loperamide metabolism, and enhance its euphoric effects. FDA warns that the risk of serious cardiac problems (e.g., abnormal heart rhythms) may be increased if high loperamide dosages are taken with drugs that interact with loperamide (e.g., cimetidine, clarithromycin, erythromycin, gemfibrozil, itraconazole, ketoconazole, quinidine, quinine, ranitidine, ritonavir). (See Drug Interactions.)

FDA states that patients and consumers should be advised to take loperamide *only* in the dosage prescribed by their clinician or stated on the label of the over-the-counter (OTC, nonprescription) product and should be warned that taking larger doses of loperamide (either intentionally or unintentionally) may lead to abnormal heart rhythms and serious cardiac events that can be fatal. In addition, patients and consumers should be warned that taking loperamide with some commonly used drugs also may increase the risk of serious cardiac adverse events. To help deter misuse and abuse of OTC loperamide products, FDA has approved packaging changes for several tablet and capsule formulations of the drug (including Imodium® brandname products) that limit the total loperamide hydrochloride content of the package to 48 mg and require use of single-dose (e.g., blister) packaging. FDA continues to work with manufacturers, including manufacturers of OTC generic and liquid formulations of the drug, to institute appropriate packaging changes.

Patients and consumers should be advised to immediately seek medical attention if they or someone else taking loperamide experiences fainting, rapid heartbeat or irregular heart rhythm, or are unresponsive (i.e., can't be wakened or is not answering or reacting normally).

● **Pediatric Precautions**

Loperamide is contraindicated in children younger than 2 years of age because of the risks of respiratory depression and serious adverse cardiac reactions.

There have been rare reports of paralytic ileus associated with abdominal distention in patients receiving loperamide; most cases occurred in the setting of acute dysentery, overdosage, and with infants younger than 2 years of age.

Loperamide should not be used for *self-medication* in children younger than 6 years of age unless directed by a clinician.

Loperamide should be used with particular caution in young children because of the greater variability of response in this age group. The presence of dehydration, especially in younger children, may further influence the variability of response to the drug.

● **Geriatric Precautions**

Formal studies have not been conducted to evaluate loperamide in geriatric patients. There are no apparent differences in disposition of the drug in elderly patients with diarrhea relative to younger adults.

● **Mutagenicity and Carcinogenicity**

In a study in rats using loperamide hydrochloride dosages up to 40 mg/kg daily (21 times the maximum human dose of 16 mg daily based on body surface area comparison) for 18 months, there was no evidence of carcinogenicity.

Loperamide was not genotoxic in the Ames test, the SOS chromotest in *Escherichia coli*, the dominant lethal test in female mice, or the mouse embryo cell transformation assay.

● **Pregnancy, Fertility, and Lactation**

Pregnancy

There are no adequate and well-controlled studies using loperamide in pregnant women, and the drug should be used during pregnancy only if potential benefits to the woman justify potential risks to the fetus.

Reproduction studies in rats and rabbits using loperamide hydrochloride dosages up to 40 mg/kg daily (43 times the human dosage based on body surface comparison) did not reveal evidence of teratogenicity; however, a dosage of 40 mg/kg daily in rats produced impaired growth and survival of offspring.

Fertility

Although reproduction studies in female and male rats using loperamide hydrochloride dosages up to 10 mg/kg daily (5 times the human dosage based on body surface area comparison) did not reveal evidence of impaired fertility, a dosage of 20 or 40 mg/kg daily resulted in marked impairment of fertility in females and a dosage of 40 mg/kg daily resulted in impairment of fertility in males.

Lactation

Because loperamide is distributed into milk in low concentrations, the drug is not recommended in nursing women.

DRUG INTERACTIONS

● **Drugs Affecting Hepatic Microsomal Enzymes**

Loperamide hydrochloride is metabolized principally by hepatic cytochrome P-450 (CYP) isoenzymes 3A4 and 2C8.

Concomitant use of loperamide with drugs that are CYP3A4 inhibitors (e.g., clarithromycin, erythromycin, itraconazole, ketoconazole) or CYP2C8 inhibitors (e.g., gemfibrozil) may increase plasma loperamide concentrations and may increase the risk of serious cardiovascular effects. Caution is advised if loperamide is used in patients receiving a CYP3A4 or CYP2C8 inhibitor.

● **Drugs Affecting P-glycoprotein Transport**

Loperamide hydrochloride is a P-glycoprotein (P-gp) substrate.

Concomitant use of loperamide with drugs that are P-gp inhibitors (e.g., quinidine, quinine, ritonavir) may increase plasma loperamide concentrations and may increase the risk of enhanced central effects or serious cardiovascular effects. Caution is advised if loperamide is used in patients receiving a P-gp inhibitor.

● **GI Drugs**

Cimetidine or ranitidine can potentially interact with loperamide if the drugs are used concomitantly.

● **Antiretroviral Agents**

Concomitant use of loperamide hydrochloride (single 16-mg dose) and ritonavir (single 600-mg dose) resulted in up to a threefold increase in plasma loperamide concentrations. Loperamide should be used concomitantly with ritonavir with caution since increased plasma loperamide concentrations may result in enhanced central effects of the drug.

Concomitant use of loperamide hydrochloride (single 16-mg dose) and saquinavir (single 600-mg dose) resulted in a 54% decrease in saquinavir exposure, which may result in decreased efficacy of the antiretroviral agent. If loperamide and saquinavir are used concomitantly, therapeutic efficacy of saquinavir should be closely monitored.

● **Quinidine**

Concomitant use of loperamide hydrochloride (single 16-mg dose) and quinidine (single 600-mg dose) resulted in up to a threefold increase in plasma loperamide concentrations. Loperamide should be used concomitantly with quinidine with caution since increased plasma loperamide concentrations may result in enhanced central effects of the drug and may increase the risk of serious cardiovascular effects.

ACUTE TOXICITY

● **Manifestations**

Overdosage of loperamide hydrochloride (including relative overdosage due to hepatic dysfunction) may be manifested by urinary retention, paralytic ileus, CNS depression, and GI effects (e.g., vomiting, abdominal pain or burning). Children may be more sensitive to CNS effects than adults. An adult who took three 20-mg doses of loperamide hydrochloride within 24 hours was nauseated after the second dose and vomited after the third dose. In studies designed to evaluate the potential for adverse effects, intentional ingestion of single doses of up to 60 mg did not result in any clinically important adverse effects.

Intentional or unintentional overdosage of loperamide (intentional misuse or abuse in an attempt to self-treat opioid withdrawal symptoms or to achieve a feeling of euphoria, suspected suicide attempt) or long-term use of high loperamide dosages has resulted in serious cardiovascular effects, including fatalities. Use of excessive loperamide dosage also has resulted in severe CNS effects (e.g., catatonia). In some cases of misuse and abuse, individuals ingested loperamide hydrochloride dosages of 70–1600 mg daily. (See Misuse and Abuse Potential under Cautions: Precautions and Contraindications.)

● **Treatment**

In the treatment of loperamide overdosage, gastric lavage is recommended, followed by administration of 100 g of activated charcoal slurry through the gastric tube. If vomiting has occurred spontaneously, 100 g of activated charcoal slurry should be administered orally as soon as fluids can be retained. Patients should be monitored for signs of CNS depression for at least 24 hours. Naloxone may be administered if CNS depression occurs. Because the duration of action of loperamide is greater than that of naloxone, the patient must be closely watched and additional doses of naloxone administered as necessary. Vital signs should be monitored for recurrence of symptoms of drug overdose for at least 24 hours after the last dose of naloxone. Forced diuresis would not be expected to be effective in loperamide overdosage, since relatively little drug is excreted in urine.

PHARMACOLOGY

Loperamide hydrochloride slows intestinal motility through a direct effect on the nerve endings and/or intramural ganglia of the intestinal wall. The drug is generally believed to act by interfering with the cholinergic and noncholinergic mechanisms involved in the peristaltic reflex, decreasing the activity of circular and longitudinal muscles in the intestinal wall. However, some data indicate that the drug may act, like diphenoxylate and morphine, by enhancing contractions of intestinal circular musculature, thus increasing segmentation and retarding forward motion through the intestine.

Loperamide prolongs the transit time of intestinal contents and therefore reduces fecal volume, increases fecal viscosity and bulk density, and diminishes loss of fluid and electrolytes. As an antidiarrhea agent, loperamide is reported to be more specific, longer acting, and 2–3 times more potent on a weight basis than diphenoxylate. Tolerance to the antidiarrheal effect of loperamide has not been reported.

In animals, loperamide has no analgesic activity even in extremely high doses. Although loperamide binds to opiate receptors in the brain and myenteric plexus, the drug has not produced opiate-like CNS effects in rats, even in large doses. Studies in monkeys, however, have demonstrated that high doses of loperamide can produce morphine-like symptoms of physical dependence and prevent signs of morphine withdrawal in morphine-dependent animals. In humans, the naloxone challenge pupil test, which when positive indicates opiate-like effects, was negative when performed after a single 16-mg dose of loperamide, and after more than 2 years of therapeutic use of the drug. Physical dependence on loperamide has not been reported in humans.

PHARMACOKINETICS

● **Absorption**

Peak plasma concentrations of loperamide occur about 5 or 2.5 hours following administration of loperamide hydrochloride capsules or oral solution, respectively. After a 2-mg oral dose of loperamide hydrochloride capsules, peak plasma concentrations of 2 ng/mL have been reported. The oral bioavailability of capsules and solution of the drug, as determined by area under the plasma concentration-time curve (AUC), is reportedly similar. Peak plasma concentrations of loperamide metabolites are reached 8 hours following oral administration of capsules of the drug.

● **Distribution**

It is not known whether loperamide crosses the placenta. The drug is distributed into milk in low concentrations.

● **Elimination**

Loperamide undergoes oxidative metabolism, principally by hepatic cytochrome P-450 (CYP) isoenzymes 2C8 and 3A4; CYP2B6 and CYP2D6 may also be involved.

The unchanged drug and metabolites are excreted principally in feces. A manufacturer reports that after oral administration of 4 mg of loperamide hydrochloride, less than 2% of the dose is excreted in urine and 30% of the dose is excreted in feces as intact drug. In animals, loperamide has been shown to undergo enterohepatic circulation.

The apparent elimination half-life of loperamide in healthy adults receiving recommended dosages of the drug is 10.8 hours (range 9.1–14.4 hours). Half-lives as high as 41 hours have been reported in individuals who ingested higher than recommended dosages of the drug.

CHEMISTRY AND STABILITY

● **Chemistry**

Loperamide hydrochloride is a synthetic piperidine-derivative antidiarrhea agent. The drug occurs as a white to slightly yellow powder and is slightly soluble in water and freely soluble in alcohol. Loperamide hydrochloride oral solution has a pH of about 5. The drug has a pK_a of 8.6.

● **Stability**

Loperamide hydrochloride capsules should be stored at 20–25°C in a well-closed container.

Loperamide hydrochloride solutions, suspensions, film-coated tablets, and chewable tablets commercially available for *self-administration* should be stored at 20–25°C.

Tablets containing a fixed combination of loperamide hydrochloride and simethicone commercially available for *self-administration* should be stored at 20–25°C and protected from light.

PREPARATIONS

Excipients in commercially available drug preparations may have clinically important effects in some individuals; consult specific product labeling for details.

Loperamide Hydrochloride

Oral		
Capsules	2 mg*	Loperamide Hydrochloride Capsules
Solution	1 mg/5 mL*	Imodium® A-D, McNeil
		Loperamide Hydrochloride Oral Solution
Suspension	1 mg/7.5 mL*	Imodium® A-D, McNeil
		Loperamide Hydrochloride Oral Suspension
Tablets, film-coated	2 mg*	Imodium® A-D Caplets®, McNeil
		Loperamide Hydrochloride Tablets
Tablets, chewable	2 mg	Imodium® A-D EZ Chews, McNeil

* available from one or more manufacturer, distributor, and/or repackager by generic (nonproprietary) name

Loperamide Hydrochloride Combinations

Oral		
Tablets	2 mg with Simethicone 125 mg*	Imodium® Multi-Symptom Relief Caplets®, McNeil
		Loperamide Hydrochloride and Simethicone Tablets
Tablets, chewable	2 mg with Simethicone 125 mg*	Imodium® Multi-Symptom Relief Chewable Tablets, McNeil
		Loperamide Hydrochloride and Simethicone Chewable Tablets

* available from one or more manufacturer, distributor, and/or repackager by generic (nonproprietary) name

† Use is not currently included in the labeling approved by the US Food and Drug Administration.

Selected Revisions January 27, 2020, © Copyright, November 1, 1977, American Society of Health-System Pharmacists, Inc.

Cathartics and Laxatives General Statement

56:12 · CATHARTICS AND LAXATIVES

■ Cathartic, laxative, and purgative are terms describing drugs that promote evacuation of the intestine; the difference between the terms is largely one of degree.

GENERAL

Cathartic, laxative, and purgative are terms describing drugs that promote evacuation of the intestine; the difference between the terms is largely one of degree. Cathartic and purgative are interchangeable terms describing drugs that promote rapid evacuation of the intestine and noticeable alteration of stool consistency. The evacuant action of a laxative is less pronounced, but large doses of a laxative may produce catharsis or purgation. Cathartic, laxative, and purgative drugs will be referred to as laxatives.

Laxatives are usually subdivided into several categories, including the bulk-forming, hyperosmotic, lubricant, saline, and stimulant laxatives and the stool softeners. The bulk-forming laxatives include cellulose derivatives, karaya, malt soup extract, psyllium preparations, and dietary bran. Glycerin, sorbitol, and polyethylene glycol are commonly termed hyperosmotic laxatives. Mineral oil is a lubricant laxative. Laxatives containing magnesium cations or phosphate anions are commonly termed saline laxatives. Anthraquinone laxatives (aloe [preparations containing aloe are no longer commercially available in the US], cascara sagrada [preparations containing cascara sagrada are no longer commercially available in the US], senna), the diphenylmethane derivatives (bisacodyl, phenolphthalein [preparations containing phenolphthalein are no longer commercially available in the US]), castor oil, and dehydrocholic acid are stimulant laxatives. The stool softeners include the calcium, potassium, and sodium salts of docusate.

PHARMACOLOGY

The precise mechanisms of action of the laxatives are not known. Recent evidence indicates that the actions of the various laxatives may be pharmacologically similar but dose dependent and that most laxatives promote defecation by altering intestinal fluid and electrolyte transport. Active ion secretion stimulated by most laxatives may be the driving force for intestinal fluid accumulation and subsequent defecation.

● Bulk-forming Laxatives

Bulk-forming laxatives dissolve or swell in water to form an emollient gel or viscous solution. It is thought that the resulting bulk in the feces promotes peristalsis and reduces transit time. Reductions in fecal pH and in serum cholesterol, and altered composition of fecal bile acids have been observed following administration of some bulk-forming laxatives; some pharmacologists believe these actions may also contribute to the laxative effect of some of these drugs.

● Hyperosmotic Laxatives

When administered rectally, glycerin and sorbitol exert a hygroscopic and/or local irritant action, drawing water from the tissues into the feces and reflexly stimulating evacuation. The extent to which the simple physical distention of the rectum and the hygroscopic and/or local irritant actions are responsible for the laxative effects of some of these drugs is not known. Only extremely high oral doses of sorbitol (25 g daily) or glycerin exert laxative action.

Polyethylene glycol 3350 electrolyte solution is a nonabsorbable solution that passes through the bowel without net absorption or secretion; therefore, substantial fluid and electrolyte shifts are avoided. Polyethylene glycol 3350 electrolyte solution osmotically increases intraluminal fluids to induce diarrhea and rapidly cleanse the bowel.

● Mineral Oil

Oral mineral oil appears to lubricate fecal material and the intestinal mucosa by retarding reabsorption of water from the intestinal tract. Increased water retention may secondarily increase the bulk of the stool and hasten evacuation. Mineral oil emulsion reportedly has better wetting properties than does nonemulsified mineral oil and penetration of the feces thus may be enhanced. Rectal enemas of heavy or light mineral oil exert laxative action via a lubricant effect and/or simple physical distention of the rectum.

● Saline Laxatives

It is commonly believed that the action of the saline laxatives results from the hyperosmotic effect of poorly absorbed magnesium or phosphate ions within the small intestine and from the retention of water which indirectly stimulates stretch receptors and increases peristalsis. These mechanisms of action are unproven, and conversely, it has been noted that isosmolarity is present at the ligament of Treitz following ingestion of hyperosmolar meals. The laxative action of magnesium also may be the result of cholecystokinin release or decreased transit time. The effectiveness of phosphate enemas may simply reflect the volume of liquid introduced rectally.

Orally administered saline laxatives act mainly on the small intestine. Saline suppositories or enemas generally promote evacuation of the colon only.

The amount of sodium biphosphate in rectal suppositories containing sodium acid pyrophosphate, sodium bicarbonate, and sodium biphosphate is probably insufficient to exert an effect as a saline laxative, but it is included to facilitate the chemical reaction that produces carbon dioxide (CO_2). Rectal suppositories containing potassium bitartrate and sodium bicarbonate also produce CO_2. The expanding CO_2 promotes laxation by exerting pressure in the rectum.

● Stimulant Laxatives

It has commonly been thought that the stimulant laxatives induce defecation by stimulating propulsive peristaltic activity of the intestine through local irritation of the mucosa or through a more selective action on the intramural nerve plexus of intestinal smooth muscle, thus increasing motility. However, recent studies show that these drugs alter fluid and electrolyte absorption, producing net intestinal fluid accumulation and laxation. Some of these drugs may directly stimulate active intestinal ion secretion. Increased concentrations of cyclic 3',5'-adenosine monophosphate (cAMP), occurring in colonic mucosal cells following administration of stimulant laxatives, may alter the permeability of these cells and mediate active ion secretion thereby producing net fluid accumulation and laxative action.

Stimulant laxatives mainly promote evacuation of the colon; however, castor oil and phenolphthalein (laxatives containing phenolphthalein are no longer commercially available in the US) also directly or reflexly increase activity of the small intestine. Rectal suppositories of some stimulant laxatives reportedly promote laxation by physical distention of the rectum.

With the exception of aloe (preparations containing aloe extract or aloe flower extract are no longer commercially available in the US) and aloin which are reportedly very irritating, the anthraquinone laxatives are considered to be the mild laxatives in the stimulant category. The laxative action of dehydrocholic acid also appears to be relatively mild. The diphenylmethanes have a more pronounced laxative effect. Castor oil produces violent purgation in therapeutic doses.

● Stool Softeners

In vitro studies suggest that the stool softeners soften fecal material and ease defecation by lowering surface tension at the oil-water interface of fecal material, permitting water and lipids to penetrate. Recent in vivo evidence suggests that the laxative properties of these drugs may result from stimulation of electrolyte and water secretion in the colon. Increased concentrations of cAMP, occurring in colonic mucosal cells following administration of these drugs, may alter the permeability of these cells and mediate active ion secretion thereby producing net fluid accumulation and laxative action.

USES

● GI Conditions

Although there are few valid indications for laxatives, these drugs are self-prescribed and overused by a large portion of the population. Constipation usually is best avoided or relieved with proper diet (high fiber content such as bran), adequate fluid intake, prompt response to the defecation reflex, and exercise. The normal frequency of bowel movements varies from once daily to 1–2 times weekly. If constipation (i.e., decreased frequency of bowel movements with prolonged and difficult passage of stools) occurs, the cause should be identified carefully before initiating laxative use. Use of laxatives in infants and children should be avoided; childhood constipation is best treated by counseling the parents regarding acceptable variations in the frequency of bowel movements.

When laxatives are indicated, the *mildest* effective laxative should be used. Rectal suppositories or enemas are routinely used to empty the colon prior to surgery or radiologic or colonoscopic procedures but, except for these uses, should not be used when oral laxatives are effective. Single-ingredient laxative products facilitate necessary dosage adjustment and usually are as effective as and safer than combination products. Combinations of two different types of laxatives may be desirable in some patients such as those with both painful and infrequent bowel movements, but there is no rationale for combinations containing more than 2 laxatives. Most clinicians consider fixed combinations of laxatives with other drugs (e.g., belladonna alkaloids, other antimuscarinics, bismuth salts, vitamins, minerals, trace elements) unsafe and irrational.

Most clinicians consider bulk-forming laxatives to be the laxatives of choice for the initial treatment of most cases of simple constipation which is usually caused by a low-fiber and/or low-fluid diet; use of saline or stimulant laxatives for simple constipation is seldom necessary or desirable. If a stimulant laxative is used, most clinicians prefer senna or cascara (preparations containing cascara sagrada are no longer commercially available in the US) derivatives or dehydrocholic acid to the other stimulant laxatives. Aloin, aloe (preparations containing aloe extract or aloe flower extract are no longer commercially available in the US), and castor oil are avoided because they reportedly produce violent purgation, and phenolphthalein (laxatives containing phenolphthalein are no longer commercially available in the US) is avoided because it causes fixed skin eruptions.

Bulk-forming laxatives, stool softeners, or mineral oil are preferred to other laxatives in patients with conditions in which straining at defecation should be avoided (e.g., myocardial infarction, vascular diseases, diseases of the anus or rectum, hernias, recent rectal surgery). Oral stool softeners or mineral oil are preferred to bulk-forming laxatives to ease evacuation of feces in patients with constipation associated with hard, dry stools. Many clinicians consider the stool softeners to be the treatment of choice in childhood constipation associated with hard, dry stools and to be safer and more efficacious than mineral oil for conditions in which straining at defecation is to be avoided.

Bulk-forming and stimulant laxatives have been used to treat constipation that occurs following prolonged bed rest or hospitalization. These laxatives have also been used to treat constipation resulting from diminished colonic motor response in geriatric patients but, because this type of constipation is frequently due to psychological or physical laxative dependence, the bulk-forming laxatives are preferred.

Bulk-forming, hyperosmotic, stimulant, and mild saline laxatives (e.g., oral magnesium hydroxide or milk of magnesia) and stool softeners have been used to treat constipation occurring during pregnancy or the puerperium, but bulk-forming laxatives or stool softeners are usually preferred. Because the anthraquinone and diphenylmethane stimulant laxatives may be distributed into milk, other laxatives usually are used for postpartum constipation.

Mineral oil or stool softeners may be administered orally or rectally for the treatment of constipation associated with stricture of the colon or to soften fecal impactions. Some clinicians consider stool softeners to be safer and more efficacious than mineral oil for these purposes. After softening impacted feces with a stool softener or mineral oil, stimulant or saline laxatives may be administered rectally to evacuate the impacted colon. Alternatively, phosphate-containing saline enemas may be administered rectally to promote evacuation of fecal impactions after manual disimpaction.

Stimulant laxatives are used to treat constipation occurring secondary to idiopathic slowing of transit time, to constipating drugs, or to irritable bowel or spastic colon syndrome. They have also been used to treat constipation in patients with neurologic constipation.

Saline laxatives have been used to eliminate parasites and toxic anthelmintics prior to and/or after therapy with some anthelmintics (e.g., quinacrine hydrochloride). Because oral or rectal preparations of sodium phosphate and sodium biphosphate apparently do not destroy osmotically sensitive trophozoites of *Entamoeba histolytica* or *Giardia lamblia*, these preparations have been used to facilitate collection of stool samples for parasitic examination. However, most clinicians agree that with the newer anthelmintics use of laxatives to eliminate parasites or the anthelmintic is not necessary, may complicate identification of the parasite, and may be harmful to the patient.

Oral saline (usually magnesium citrate or sodium phosphates) and/or oral stimulant laxatives (usually castor oil, bisacodyl, or standardized senna fruit extract) are used to empty the bowel prior to surgery or radiologic, proctoscopic, or sigmoidoscopic procedures. These laxatives are usually supplemented with administration of rectal evacuants, such as saline, stimulant, or soapsuds enemas, immediately before radiologic procedures. Polyethylene glycol 3350 electrolyte solutions also are used to empty the bowel prior to colonoscopy and barium enema radiologic examinations. The American Society of Colon and Rectal Surgeons (ASCRS), American Society for Gastrointestinal Endoscopy (ASGE), and Society of American Gastrointestinal and Endoscopic Surgeons (SAGES) recommend the use of polyethylene glycol 3350 electrolyte solutions in patients with electrolyte or fluid imbalances (e.g., those with renal or liver insufficiency, congestive heart failure, liver failure, or advanced liver disease with ascites). These experts also recommend use of polyethylene glycol 3350 electrolyte solutions for colonic cleansing in infants and children. Glycerin and sorbitol also have been used before these procedures, but these laxatives do not always entirely empty the colon. Bisacodyl tannex has been added to barium sulfate enemas to aid in coating the intestinal mucosa and enhance colonic evacuation prior to radiologic examination of the colon. Bisacodyl and mineral oil enemas are used to cleanse the colon postoperatively. Bisacodyl suppositories may be used to cleanse the colon in pregnant women prior to delivery if they are given at least 2 hours before onset of the second stage of labor.

Sorbitol is used orally or rectally to facilitate the passage of sodium polystyrene sulfonate through the intestinal tract, to prevent constipation caused by the resin, and, by acting as a hyperosmotic laxative, to aid in potassium removal; sorbitol also improves the palatability of the resin.

Bisacodyl has been used to facilitate flushing of colostomies, but the value and safety of the drug as compared to irrigations have not been established.

Semisynthetic celluloses and psyllium bulk-forming laxatives have been used to increase the bulk of stools in patients with chronic, watery diarrhea; subjective improvement has been noted in these patients but the total water content of the stool has been unchanged. Bulk-forming laxatives and dietary bran have also been used, with some success, to reduce intraluminal and rectosigmoid pressure, and pain in patients with diverticular disease. One manufacturer suggests that stool softeners may be useful in the treatment of ulcerative colitis or diverticulitis.

Malt soup extract, in conjunction with other therapy such as proper diet and hygiene, has been used in the treatment of pruritus ani; however, evidence that the drug is effective for this condition is lacking. Bulk-forming laxatives have also been used in the management of obesity but their effectiveness in this condition is questionable.

● *Other Uses*

Saline laxatives are also used, after inducing emesis or performing gastric lavage, to hasten removal of some poisons from the GI tract, but should not be used after poisonings with ingested acids or alkalies. Magnesium laxatives should not be used to remove poisons producing CNS depression or renal function impairment.

Some manufacturers have suggested that oral phosphate saline laxatives may be useful for the symptomatic relief of gallbladder disorders, but their effectiveness in these conditions has not been proven.

When used as an adjunct to dietary therapy, oral psyllium hydrophilic mucilloid (3.4 g 3 times daily before meals as a sugar-free preparation) has produced modest reductions in serum total cholesterol, low-density lipoprotein (LDL)-cholesterol, and apolipoprotein B concentrations and the ratio of LDL cholesterol to high-density lipoprotein (HDL)-cholesterol in adults with mild to moderate hypercholesterolemia†.

CAUTIONS

When used in appropriate dosages for a limited period of time (one week or less), most laxatives are relatively free from adverse effects such as diarrhea, GI irritation, and fluid and electrolyte depletion. Stimulant laxatives are the laxatives most likely to produce these adverse effects. Chronic use or overdosage of laxatives may produce persistent diarrhea, hypokalemia, loss of essential nutritional factors, and dehydration.

Because magnesium, potassium, or sodium accumulation may occur in patients with renal disease, laxative products containing more than 50 mEq of magnesium, 25 mEq of potassium, or 1 mEq of sodium per dose should be used by these patients only under the supervision of a physician who should monitor electrolytes. Although no information is available on the amount of sodium absorbed following ingestion of carboxymethylcellulose sodium, this drug usually contains 2.7–4 mEq of sodium per gram. Congestive heart failure has occurred following indiscriminate use of saline laxatives containing sodium. Use of carboxymethylcellulose sodium and sodium-containing saline laxatives should be restricted in patients on low-sodium diets. Use of sodium-containing saline laxatives should also be restricted in those with congestive heart failure, edema, or cirrhosis.

Because standardized senna fruit extract and some psyllium preparations contain large amounts of sugar, the caloric value of these preparations should be considered in patients with diabetes mellitus.

All laxatives are contraindicated in patients with acute abdominal pain, nausea, vomiting, or other symptoms of appendicitis or undiagnosed abdominal pain. Stimulant laxatives are contraindicated in patients with intestinal obstruction. Bulk-forming laxatives are *not* useful when prompt or thorough bowel evacuation is necessary (e.g., poisonings, radiologic examination, bowel surgery) and are contraindicated in patients with partial obstruction of the bowel or dysphagia. Patients should consult their clinicians if sudden changes in bowel habits persist for longer than 2 weeks or if use of a laxative for one week has no effect. Polyethylene glycol 3350 electrolyte solutions are contraindicated in patients with GI obstruction, gastric retention, bowel perforation, toxic colitis, toxic megacolon, or ileus. Sodium phosphates are contraindicated in patients with biopsy-proven acute phosphate nephropathy, GI obstruction, gastric bypass or stapling surgery, bowel perforation, toxic colitis, toxic megacolon, congestive heart failure, history of kidney disease or clinically important renal function impairment, paralytic ileus, active inflammatory bowel disease, imperforate anus, decreased intravascular volume or dehydration, uncorrected electrolyte abnormalities, or known hypersensitivity to sodium phosphate salts or any ingredient in the formulation. (See Sodium Phosphates Preparations under Cautions: Saline Laxatives.)

● Bulk-forming Laxatives

Adverse effects occur rarely with the use of bulk-forming laxatives. Rare cases of allergic reactions and urticaria have been associated with the use of karaya. Bowel and/or esophageal obstruction, swelling or blockage of the throat, choking, or asphyxiation has occurred when insufficient liquid was administered with some of these laxatives; some of these effects probably result from formation of a viscous, semi-solid mass rather than the emollient gel or viscous solution that results when sufficient fluid is added to these laxatives. Therefore, at least one full glass (250 mL) of liquid should be administered with each dose of bulk-forming laxatives. Patients should be informed of the symptoms of esophageal obstruction and instructed to contact their physician if chest pain and/or pressure, regurgitation, vomiting, or difficulty in swallowing and/or breathing occur. Bulk-forming laxatives should not be used in individuals with esophageal obstruction, problems of the throat, or those who have difficulty in swallowing.

Potentially severe hypersensitivity reactions, including rhinoconjunctivitis, acute bronchospasm, and anaphylaxis, can occur in susceptible individuals (e.g., those with psyllium sensitivity or suffering from respiratory disorders) following inhalation of psyllium dust particles. Therefore, inhalation of psyllium hydrophilic mucilloid particles should be avoided. To minimize exposure and, therefore, sensitization to airborne particles of psyllium, one manufacturer suggests that health-care personnel dispense powdered psyllium preparations with a spoon rather than pouring them directly from the container into the glass for administration. In some cases, reassignment of health-care personnel to areas (e.g., nongeriatric units) where use of bulk powder formulations of psyllium was minimal has been necessary.

● Hyperosmotic Laxatives

Adverse effects occur rarely following rectal administration of glycerin or sorbitol. Glycerin may produce rectal discomfort, irritation, burning or griping, cramping pain and tenesmus. Hyperemia of the rectal mucosa with minimal amounts of hemorrhage and mucus discharge may also occur. These adverse effects occur less frequently following rectal administration of sorbitol. Diarrhea frequently occurs with the dosages of sorbitol used as adjuncts to sodium polystyrene sulfonate therapy.

Polyethylene glycol 3350 electrolyte solutions (oral or nasogastric) may produce malaise, nausea, abdominal distention, abdominal fullness and/or bloating, abdominal cramps, vomiting, anal irritation, and thirst. Generalized tonic-clonic seizures associated with electrolyte abnormalities (e.g., hyponatremia, hypokalemia) have been reported following use of polyethylene glycol 3350 electrolyte solutions for bowel cleansing in patients without a history of seizures. Such neurologic effects resolved with correction of fluid and electrolyte abnormalities. Polyethylene glycol 3350 electrolyte solutions (Golytely®, Colyte®, MoviPrep®) should be used with caution in patients with severe ulcerative colitis. In addition, polyethylene glycol 3350 electrolyte solutions should be used with caution in patients

receiving drugs that increase the risk of electrolyte abnormalities (e.g., diuretics, angiotensin-converting enzyme [ACE] inhibitors). Consideration should be given to measuring electrolyte, BUN, and creatinine concentrations before and after colonoscopy in patients receiving such drugs and in those with known or suspected hyponatremia. Since MoviPrep® contains sodium ascorbate and ascorbic acid, the drug should be used with caution in patients with glucose-6-phosphate dehydrogenase (G-6-PD) deficiency, especially those with an active infection, with a history of hemolysis, or those taking concomitant drugs known to precipitate hemolytic reactions. If severe bloating, distention, or abdominal pain occurs in patients receiving therapy with polyethylene glycol 3350 electrolyte solutions, administration should be slowed or temporarily discontinued until symptoms subside. If GI obstruction or perforation is suspected, appropriate tests should be performed to rule out these conditions before administration of polyethylene glycol 3350 electrolyte solution.

If rectal bleeding, nausea, bloating, cramping, or abdominal pain worsens, or the patient experiences diarrhea or requires more than 7 days of use of polyethylene glycol 3350 solution (MiraLAX®) for the treatment of constipation, the drug should be discontinued and a clinician notified.

● Mineral Oil

Adverse effects associated with the proper use of mineral oil are few. Seepage of mineral oil from the rectum may occur following oral or rectal administration, particularly when high doses are given. Seepage may cause soiling of the skin and clothing, anal irritation, and pruritus ani; impair normal rectal reflex mechanisms; and increase infection of anorectal lesions and interfere with their healing. Seepage of mineral oil may be minimized by reducing dosage.

Infrequently, aspiration of orally administered mineral oil may occur, particularly in young children and geriatric or debilitated patients, causing lipid pneumonitis.

Rarely, and only with chronic, oral use of plain mineral oil, absorption of fat-soluble vitamins, including provitamin A and vitamins A, D, and K, may be impaired. Hypoprothrombinemia and hemorrhagic disease of the newborn has occurred when mineral oil was chronically administered orally to pregnant women. Clinically important malabsorption of fat-soluble vitamins can be minimized by administering mineral oil on an empty stomach and limiting use of the drug to periods of less than 1 week.

Systemic absorption of mineral oil has caused foreign-body granulomatous reactions or paraffinomas, particularly in mesenteric lymph nodes and in the liver and spleen. Tissue depositions of mineral oil have simulated neoplasms and, in rare instances, carcinomas have been associated with industrial exposure to unrefined mineral oils or injection of refined mineral oil in animals and humans.

Oral administration of mineral oil is contraindicated in children younger than 6 years of age; in bedridden, geriatric, debilitated, or pregnant patients; and in patients with esophageal or gastric retention, dysphagia, or hiatal hernia.

● Saline Laxatives

Saline laxatives generally do not produce serious adverse effects except when used for prolonged periods or when overdoses are administered. The bitter taste of magnesium sulfate, which may cause nausea, can be masked by mixing the drug with lemon juice. Common adverse effects associated with sodium phosphates preparations include dehydration, abdominal pain, bloating, nausea, vomiting, headache, and dizziness. Rectal discomfort and burning sensations have occurred occasionally in patients receiving carbon dioxide-releasing suppositories, because of inadequate moistening of the suppository prior to insertion and/or the sudden stretch reflex caused by expanding gas.

Dehydration may result from repeated administration of hypertonic solutions of saline laxatives but can be avoided by administering the laxatives with sufficient fluid. Serious, potentially life-threatening electrolyte disturbances may occur with long-term use or overdosage of saline laxatives.

Magnesium Sulfate Preparations

Symptoms of hypermagnesemia, including muscle weakness, ECG changes, sedation, and confusion, may occur when plasma magnesium concentrations exceed 1.5–2.2 mEq/L. When plasma magnesium concentrations exceed 4 mEq/L, deep tendon reflexes become depressed and at 12–15 mEq/L, respiratory paralysis may occur. Complete heart block occasionally occurs when plasma magnesium concentrations are elevated. In patients with impaired renal function, oral or rectal administration of 30 g (243 mEq magnesium) or greater of magnesium sulfate has been fatal. If hypermagnesemia occurs, urinary excretion of magnesium may be increased by administration of diuretics (e.g., furosemide, ethacrynic acid, ammonium chloride).

Sodium Phosphates Preparations

Overdosage

Overdosage has been reported in adults and pediatric patients receiving non-prescription (over-the-counter, OTC) sodium phosphates preparations (i.e., oral solution, enema) for *self-medication* of occasional constipation.

In 1998, following reports of inadvertent overdosage and death associated with the use of large-size containers of sodium phosphates oral solution, FDA limited the container size of the drugs to no more than 90 mL when used as a nonprescription laxative. In addition, FDA required that the product information of nonprescription oral and rectal sodium phosphates preparations contain warning and direction statements to inform patients that exceeding the recommended dosages in a 24-hour period can be harmful. According to a subsequent FDA review of the safety of oral sodium phosphates preparations, use of more than 45 mL (usually 90 mL or more) of sodium phosphates oral solution in a 24-hour period and/or use in patients at increased risk for electrolyte abnormalities has been associated with severe electrolyte abnormalities, dehydration, metabolic acidosis, renal failure, tetany, and death.

Between 1957 and August 2013, a total of 54 cases of serious adverse effects associated with oral or rectal sodium phosphate laxative preparations, including severe dehydration, electrolyte abnormalities (e.g., hypernatremia, hyperphosphatemia, hypocalcemia), acute kidney injury, cardiac arrhythmias, and/or death, have been identified in the FDA Adverse Event Reporting System (AERS) and the medical literature. Nearly half (12/25) of adult cases and 3% (1/29) of pediatric cases resulted in a fatal outcome. The remaining nonfatal cases were life-threatening in more than two-thirds of affected adults and in all of the affected children; these included acute deterioration in respiratory status, mental status, and heart function; dialysis; suspected bowel perforation requiring surgery; abdominal distention requiring surgery; and residual neurologic defects. The severity of reported adverse events was similar regardless of whether the drugs were administered orally or rectally.

In the 50 cases (27 pediatric, 23 adult) for which the administered dose was reported, the majority of adverse events occurred in patients who received higher than recommended dosages in a 24-hour period (i.e., a single dose that was larger than recommended or more than one dose in a day) or in patients at increased risk of developing sodium phosphate-induced toxicity (e.g., those with dehydration, kidney disease, acute colitis, or delayed bowel emptying or receiving concomitant therapy with drugs that affect renal function [e.g., diuretics, angiotensin converting-enzyme [ACE] inhibitors, angiotensin II receptor antagonists, nonsteroidal anti-inflammatory agents [NSAIAs]). Forty percent (11/27) of the pediatric cases for which the dose was reported occurred in young children for whom FDA has not proposed a safe and effective dose (9 cases in children younger than 2 years of age receiving a rectal preparation, and 2 cases in children younger than 5 years of age receiving an oral preparation); these children received doses comparable to those recommended on the label for use in adults or older children. The duration of sodium phosphates use in the majority of the overdose cases was 1–2 days.

In light of these findings, FDA issued a drug safety communication in 2014, warning patients of possible harm from exceeding the recommended dosages of nonprescription sodium phosphates preparations. The agency stated that the maximum recommended oral or rectal dosage of nonprescription sodium phosphates preparations should not be exceeded, and that additional doses are not recommended within 24 hours, even in patients who do not have a bowel movement after receiving a dose. FDA also stated that clinicians should be cautious in recommending use of nonprescription sodium phosphates preparations in patients older than 55 years of age; patients with hypovolemia, decreased intravascular volume, kidney disease, decreased bowel transit time, or active colitis; and patients receiving drugs that affect renal perfusion or function (e.g., diuretics, ACE inhibitors, angiotensin II receptor antagonists, NSAIAs). FDA recommended that serum electrolytes and renal function be assessed in patients who may be at increased risk of serious adverse effects, including those who have retained a rectal dose for more than 30 minutes, who are vomiting, or who may have signs of dehydration. Nonprescription sodium phosphates preparations should not be used concomitantly with other laxatives containing sodium phosphate. Patients should be advised to discontinue sodium phosphates therapy and to immediately seek medical attention if symptoms of kidney injury (e.g., drowsiness; sluggishness; decreased urine; swelling of the ankles, feet, or legs) occur.

Nonprescription sodium phosphates oral solution should not be used for *self-medication* of occasional constipation in children 5 years of age or younger, and nonprescription sodium phosphates enema should not be used for such *self-medication* in children 2 years of age or younger. Sodium phosphates preparations should not be used for *self-medication* of occasional constipation for longer than 3 days.

Serious Adverse Effects Associated with Oral Sodium Phosphates

Electrolyte abnormalities (e.g., hyperphosphatemia, hypernatremia, hypocalcemia, hypokalemia) resulting in prolongation of the QT interval, generalized tonic-clonic seizures, and/or loss of consciousness have been reported rarely with sodium phosphates preparations. Renal failure, acute phosphate nephropathy, and nephrocalcinosis, often resulting in *permanent* renal impairment and sometimes requiring long-term dialysis, also have been reported rarely in patients receiving oral sodium phosphates preparations (i.e., oral solution, OsmoPrep® tablets) for bowel cleansing prior to colonoscopy or other procedures. Onset of kidney injury occurred from several days to several months after use of the oral sodium phosphates preparation. Although certain patients (e.g., patients older than 55 years of age; patients with hypovolemia, increased bowel transit time, bowel obstruction, active colitis, or kidney disease; patients receiving drugs that affect renal perfusion or function, such as diuretics, ACE inhibitors, angiotensin II receptor antagonists, and possibly NSAIAs) appear to be at increased risk of developing acute phosphate nephropathy, this adverse effect has occurred in patients *without* identifiable risk factors; however, FDA states that the possibility that some of these patients were dehydrated prior to or did not drink sufficient fluids after ingestion of oral sodium phosphates preparations cannot be ruled out. Death secondary to substantial fluid shifts, severe electrolyte abnormalities, and cardiac arrhythmias also has occurred in patients with renal impairment, patients with bowel perforation, and patients who misused or administered overdosages of sodium phosphates preparations prior to colonoscopy. Prolonged use or overdosage of phosphate laxatives may result in inorganic phosphate poisoning, which reduces plasma calcium concentrations; acidosis also may occur.

Regulatory Actions in 2008 Involving Oral Sodium Phosphates

Because of continued reports of acute renal injury in patients receiving oral sodium phosphates preparations for bowel cleansing, in 2008 FDA required the manufacturer to add a boxed warning to the labeling of OsmoPrep®, an oral sodium phosphates preparation available by prescription only.

Because acute phosphate nephropathy also had been reported following use of nonprescription oral sodium phosphates preparations (i.e., oral solutions) as bowel cleansing regimens (i.e., at dosages higher than those used for relief of constipation), FDA stated that these preparations should be used for bowel cleansing *only* when a prescription for such use has been issued by a clinician. In response to FDA's announcement, at least one manufacturer (i.e., Fleet Laboratories) ceased distribution and initiated a voluntary recall of some of its nonprescription oral sodium phosphates preparations used for bowel cleansing (i.e., Fleet® Phospho-soda® Oral Saline Laxative, Fleet® Phospho-soda® EZ-PREP® Bowel Cleansing System) effective December 12, 2008. Health-care professionals were advised to cease recommending oral sodium phosphates preparations for bowel cleansing and to remove them from pharmacy shelves; patients requesting a nonprescription oral sodium phosphates preparation for bowel cleansing should be advised to consult their clinician for an alternative bowel cleansing preparation (i.e., one available by prescription only).

Because nonprescription oral sodium phosphates preparations had not been associated with acute kidney injury when used as laxatives (i.e., for relief of constipation), FDA concluded that these preparations should continue to be available over-the-counter for such use.

Subsequent Regulatory Actions Involving Oral Sodium Phosphates

Despite efforts to inform healthcare professionals and consumers about the risks associated with the use of sodium phosphates oral solution for bowel cleansing, FDA reported in 2011 that the agency continued to receive reports of acute kidney injury following administration of usual recommended dosages of the drugs for *self-medication* (i.e., approximately 60 g of sodium phosphates [dibasic sodium phosphate and monobasic sodium phosphate salts] administered as two 45-mL doses given 12 hours apart, or approximately 50 g of sodium phosphates administered as a 45-mL dose initially, followed by a 30-mL dose 12 hours later).

A review of reports received from 1969–2005 revealed 33 reports of acute kidney injury (i.e., chronic kidney failure requiring hospitalization or dialysis, end-stage kidney disease requiring transplantation) associated with the use of nonprescription sodium phosphates oral solution for bowel cleansing; in most cases, acute kidney injury occurred within the recommended dosages for *self-medication* for bowel cleansing, including the lower-dose regimen (i.e., approximately 50 g of sodium phosphates administered as a 45-mL dose initially, followed by a 30-mL dose 10–12 hours later). Seizures, serious cardiac events, and death also have been reported with nonprescription sodium phosphates oral solution, although most of these cases occurred following use of dosages higher than those recommended for *self-medication* for bowel cleansing.

As a result of these findings, FDA has tentatively concluded that the usual recommended dosage of nonprescription oral sodium phosphates *for self-medication* for bowel cleansing based on professional labeling in an OTC monograph poses an unacceptable risk of serious adverse events. Therefore, in February 2011, the agency issued a proposed rule amending the tentative final monograph on nonprescription laxative drug products to classify the individual sodium phosphate salts (i.e., dibasic sodium phosphate, monobasic sodium phosphate) as *not* generally recognized as safe (GRAS) for bowel cleansing. In the proposed rule, FDA also suggested that the professional labeling for sodium phosphates (which discusses use of the drugs as part of a bowel cleansing regimen) be removed from the 1985 tentative final monograph for over-the-counter laxative drug products. In response to FDA's proposed rule, some manufacturers have removed the indication for bowel cleansing from labeling of nonprescription sodium phosphates preparations.

Precautions and Contraindications Involving Use of Oral Sodium Phosphates for Bowel Cleansing

FDA states that use of prescription-only oral sodium phosphates preparations as bowel cleansing regimens should be *avoided* in patients younger than 18 years of age; these agents should be used with caution as bowel cleansing regimens in patients older than 55 years of age; patients with dehydration, kidney disease, delayed bowel emptying, or acute colitis; and patients receiving drugs that may affect renal perfusion or function (e.g., diuretics, ACE inhibitors, angiotensin II receptor antagonists, possibly NSAIAs).

Furthermore, the manufacturer of sodium phosphates tablets (OsmoPrep®) states that these preparations (which are intended for use in cleansing the bowel prior to colonoscopy) should be used with caution in patients with renal disease or renal impairment (creatinine clearance less than 30 mL/minute), congestive heart failure, ascites, unstable angina, gastric retention, ileus, pseudo-obstruction of the bowel, severe chronic constipation, severe active ulcerative colitis, acute exacerbation of chronic inflammatory bowel disease, or hypomotility syndrome. Sodium phosphates tablets also should be used with caution in patients with a history of acute phosphate nephropathy or inflammatory bowel disease, known or suspected electrolyte disturbances (e.g., dehydration), an increased risk of arrhythmias (i.e., history of cardiomyopathy or uncontrolled arrhythmias, recent history of myocardial infarction, evidence of prolonged QT interval), or a history or an increased risk of seizures (e.g., those receiving drugs that lower the seizure threshold [e.g., tricyclic antidepressants], those in alcohol or benzodiazepine withdrawal, those with known or suspected hyponatremia). Electrolyte abnormalities (e.g., hypernatremia, hyperphosphatemia, hypokalemia, hypocalcemia) should be corrected prior to initiation of oral sodium phosphates therapy for bowel cleansing.

Patients receiving oral sodium phosphates preparations for bowel cleansing should receive instructions on preparation for the procedure and be informed of symptoms of acute phosphate nephropathy (e.g., malaise; lethargy; drowsiness; decreased amount of urine; swelling of the ankles, feet, and legs). Patients should be advised not to exceed recommended dosages and to *avoid* use of additional laxatives, particularly sodium phosphate-based preparations. Patients also should be advised to drink sufficient quantities of clear fluids before, during, and after bowel cleansing.

IV hydration in a hospital setting may be used to support frail patients who are unable to drink an appropriate volume of fluid or who do not have adequate assistance at home. The fluid intake volume necessary to minimize electrolyte abnormalities and to lower the risk of acute phosphate nephropathy is not known; furthermore, it is not known whether fluid intake should be individualized based on weight, age, gender, concomitant drug therapy, or medical conditions. However, some data indicate that use of an electrolyte or carbohydrate-electrolyte replacement solution may help minimize electrolyte abnormalities and hypovolemia associated with bowel cleansing with oral sodium phosphates preparations.

The manufacturer states that sodium phosphates tablets are contraindicated in patients with biopsy-proven acute phosphate nephropathy, GI obstruction, gastric bypass or stapling surgery, bowel perforation, toxic colitis, toxic megacolon, or known hypersensitivity to sodium phosphate salts or any ingredient in the formulation.

FDA recommends that baseline and postprocedural (e.g., postcolonoscopy) laboratory measurements, including serum concentrations of electrolytes (e.g., potassium, sodium), phosphate, calcium, creatinine, and BUN, be obtained in patients who may be at increased risk of acute phosphate nephropathy, including those with vomiting and/or manifestations of dehydration. FDA

also recommends monitoring of the glomerular filtration rate in smaller, frail patients. In addition, the manufacturers of sodium phosphates tablets recommend that baseline and postprocedural laboratory measurements also be considered in patients with a history of renal impairment, history of acute phosphate nephropathy, known or suspected electrolyte disorders, seizures, arrhythmias, cardiomyopathy, prolonged QT interval, recent history of myocardial infarction, or known or suspected hyperphosphatemia, hypocalcemia, hypokalemia, or hypernatremia. In addition, baseline and postprocedural ECGs should be considered in patients at high risk of serious cardiac arrhythmias.

Precautions and Contraindications Involving Use of Oral Sodium Phosphates for Occasional Constipation

When oral sodium phosphates solution is used for *self-medication* for the relief of occasional constipation, patients should be advised to drink sufficient quantities of fluids and should be advised not to exceed recommended dosages. The manufacturer states that use of oral sodium phosphates solution for *self-medication* of occasional constipation should be avoided in patients with a history of kidney disease or clinically important renal function impairment, congestive heart failure, decreased intravascular volume, dehydration, or uncorrected electrolyte abnormalities and in children younger than 5 years of age. Patients should be advised to consult their clinician before initiating *self-medication* with oral sodium phosphates solution if they are under a clinician's care for any medical condition, if their dietary sodium intake is restricted, or if they are receiving therapy with other prescription or nonprescription drugs.

Precautions and Contraindications Involving Sodium Phosphates Enemas

Because dehydration, hypocalcemia, hyperphosphatemia, hypernatremia, hypokalemia, and acidosis may occur following administration of sodium phosphates rectal solutions, these preparations should be used with caution in patients with cardiac disease, colostomy, or preexisting electrolyte disturbances (e.g., patients receiving diuretics) and in those receiving drugs that may affect serum electrolyte concentrations (e.g., diuretics). If fluid or electrolyte disturbances occur or if sodium phosphates rectal solutions are retained, fluid and electrolyte balance should be restored promptly as necessary; serum concentrations of calcium, phosphorus, chloride, and sodium should be monitored. Children with anatomic abnormalities of the colon or with abnormal colonic motility (e.g., megacolon) appear to be at particular risk of developing marked, potentially life-threatening fluid and electrolyte disturbances and altered acid-base balance during therapy with phosphate laxatives.

Sodium phosphates rectal solutions are contraindicated in patients with congestive heart failure, clinically important renal function impairment, known or suspected GI obstruction, congenital or acquired megacolon, paralytic ileus, perforation, active inflammatory bowel disease, imperforate anus, dehydration, or increased absorption capacity or decreased elimination capacity; sodium phosphates rectal solutions also are contraindicated in children younger than 2 years of age and patients with known hypersensitivity to sodium phosphate salts or any ingredient in the formulation.

The manufacturer states that patients should be advised to consult their clinician before initiating *self-medication* with sodium phosphates rectal solutions for the relief of occasional constipation if they have kidney disease or if their dietary sodium intake is restricted. Recommended dosages of sodium phosphates rectal solutions should not be exceeded.

● Stimulant Laxatives

In therapeutic oral doses, all stimulant laxatives may produce some degree of abdominal discomfort, nausea, mild cramps, griping, and/or faintness. Rectal administration of bisacodyl suspensions or suppositories may cause irritation and a sensation of burning of the rectal mucosa and mild proctitis. Some clinicians state that stimulant laxative suppositories or enemas should not be used in patients with abdominal cramps, anal or rectal fissures, or ulcerated hemorrhoids. Aloe (preparations containing aloe extract or aloe flower extract are no longer commercially available in the US), aloin, and castor oil reportedly cause excessive irritation of the colon, and violent purgation usually accompanies administration of therapeutic doses. Castor oil may rarely cause pelvic congestion.

With long-term use or overdosage of stimulant laxatives, electrolyte disturbances including hypokalemia, hypocalcemia, metabolic acidosis or alkalosis, abdominal pain, diarrhea, malabsorption, weight loss, and protein-losing enteropathy may occur. Electrolyte disturbances may produce vomiting and muscle weakness; rarely, osteomalacia, secondary aldosteronism, and tetany may occur. Pathologic changes including structural damage to the myenteric plexus, severe and permanent interference with colonic motility, and hypertrophy of the muscularis mucosae may occur with chronic use. "Cathartic colon" with atony and dilation of the colon, especially of the right side, has occurred with habitual use (often for several years) and often resembles ulcerative colitis.

Anthraquinone laxatives may discolor colonic mucosa (melanosis coli), but this adverse effect is usually innocuous and reversible. Anthraquinones also produce a pink to red or brown to black discoloration of the urine; phenolphthalein (laxatives containing phenolphthalein are no longer commercially available in the US) colors alkaline urine pink to red. The diphenylmethane and anthraquinone laxatives may be distributed into the milk of nursing women but usually in amounts insufficient to produce a laxative effect. Although specific evidence of carcinogenic potential in humans is not available, danthron-containing preparations were withdrawn from the US market in 1987 because mice and rats developed intestinal and hepatic tumors following chronic administration of high dosages of the laxative. In addition, danthron and other anthraquinone laxatives have been shown to be mutagenic in some in vitro studies.

Phenolphthalein and dehydrocholic acid rarely have produced hypersensitivity reactions. Phenolphthalein allergy often has been manifested by dermal reactions including polychromatic, fixed skin eruptions with macules and nonspecific rashes, itching, burning, and pigmentation that may last for several months. Phenolphthalein allergy also has produced renal irritation, encephalitis, cardiac arrest, respiratory disturbances, and, rarely, death.

Current evidence indicates that phenolphthalein is potentially genotoxic and carcinogenic in humans. FDA reached this conclusion after reviewing animal data demonstrating carcinogenic activity of the drug in rodents and subsequent data indicating that the mechanism of this activity probably was secondary to a genotoxic effect. Drug exposures used in the in vivo and in vitro studies showing the carcinogenic and genotoxic effects of phenolphthalein were in the range of those that could occur with human laxative use. These findings indicate that chronic use of the drug could result in damage to the human genome (including p53, which is known to be a tumor suppressor gene) and could increase the risk of malignancy; some human cancers have been associated with alterations of the p53 gene. As a result, all preparations containing phenolphthalein for *self-medication* (over-the-counter [OTC] use) are no longer generally recognized as safe and effective. Therefore, US manufacturers have reformulated phenolphthalein-containing preparations to include other laxatives.

As part of its ongoing review of OTC drug products, the FDA has determined that existing data are insufficient to establish safety and efficacy of aloe and cascara sagrada as stimulant laxatives. This determination was made after no comments or data were submitted in response to the FDA's request for mutagenicity, genotoxicity, and carcinogenicity data on these agents. Therefore, any OTC drug product containing laxative ingredients derived from aloe (i.e., aloe extract, aloe flower extract) or cascara sagrada (i.e., casanthranol, cascara fluidextract aromatic, or cascara sagrada bark, extract, or fluidextract) is considered by the FDA to be misbranded. Effective November 5, 2002, any such OTC drug product introduced or initially delivered for introduction into interstate commerce is considered to be misbranded, and manufacturers are required to reformulate preparations containing aloe or cascara sagrada to delete and/or replace these ingredients. In addition, previously marketed OTC products containing aloe or cascara sagrada may not be repackaged or relabeled after this date.

Hepatotoxicity may result if sufficient tannic acid is absorbed from bisacodyl tannex laxatives. Bisacodyl tannex should be used with caution, if at all, in patients receiving multiple enemas or in those with extensive ulceration of the colon since increased tannic acid absorption may occur.

In general, use of stimulant laxatives should be avoided in children younger than 6–10 years of age. Because the possibility of tannic acid absorption has not been studied adequately in children younger than 10 years of age, bisacodyl tannex is contraindicated in these patients. Castor oil is contraindicated in pregnant or menstruating women. Safe use of bisacodyl tannex during pregnancy has not been established.

● *Stool Softeners*

Adverse effects associated with the use of stool softeners are rare. Occasionally, mild, transitory GI cramping pains or rashes may occur. Irritation of the throat has occurred following oral administration of docusate sodium solutions. In one study, docusate sodium was found to be toxic to hepatic cells in vitro.

DRUG INTERACTIONS

By increasing intestinal motility, all laxatives may potentially decrease transit time of concomitantly administered oral drugs and thereby decrease their absorption.

Mineral oil may impair absorption of many orally administered drugs including fat-soluble vitamins (i.e., vitamins A, D, E, and K), carotene, oral contraceptives, and coumarin and indandione derivative anticoagulants. By mixing with nonabsorbable sulfonamides (e.g., phthalylsulfathiazole) in the feces, mineral oil may interfere with antibacterial activity of these drugs. Patients receiving any of these drugs should be discouraged from ingesting more than therapeutic amounts of mineral oil and from taking these drugs concurrently with mineral oil.

Stool softeners (i.e., docusate salts) theoretically may enhance the absorption of many orally administered drugs. Docusate sodium increases the extent of mineral oil absorption and the rate of phenolphthalein (laxatives containing phenolphthalein are no longer commercially available in the US) absorption. Greater intestinal mucosal damage has reportedly occurred following concomitant administration of aspirin and docusate sodium than occurs with aspirin alone. Oral stool softeners should not be administered concurrently with oral mineral oil, and some clinicians recommend that stool softeners not be administered concurrently with any oral drugs having low therapeutic indices.

Magnesium hydroxide, in antacid preparations also containing aluminum hydroxide, has been shown to decrease the rate and extent of chlordiazepoxide, chlorpromazine, dicumarol, digoxin, and isoniazid absorption. The effect of magnesium hydroxide laxative preparations on drug bioavailability is not known.

Cellulose binds orally administered digitalis, nitrofurantoin, and salicylates in the GI tract. Although the clinical importance of these interactions has not been determined for other cellulose derivatives such as methylcellulose, patients taking bulk-forming laxatives concurrently with digitalis, nitrofurantoin, or salicylates should consult their physician or pharmacist before initiating or discontinuing use of these laxatives. Some clinicians recommend that bulk-forming laxatives be administered at least 3 hours after or before administration of these drugs.

Several manufacturers of polyethylene glycol 3350 electrolyte solution suggest that other oral drugs should be administered at least 1 hour before polyethylene glycol 3350 electrolyte solutions.

LABORATORY TEST INTERFERENCES

By discoloring the urine, anthraquinone laxatives and phenolphthalein (laxatives containing phenolphthalein are no longer commercially available in the US) may produce an apparent increase in the urinary excretion of phenolsulfonphthalein (PSP). These laxatives may also give false-positive test results for urinary urobilinogen and for estrogens when measured by the Kober procedure.

DOSAGE AND ADMINISTRATION

● *Administration*

Laxatives are usually administered orally and in conjunction with adequate fluid intake. Rectal suppositories or enemas may be used when oral laxatives are not effective or to prepare for surgery, or radiologic or colonoscopic procedures.

Suppositories should be moistened with lukewarm water before being inserted high into the rectum and retained in the rectum for as long as possible. Before administering laxative enemas, the patient should lie on his left side with knees bent or should kneel on the bed with the head and chest lowered and forward until the left side of the face is resting on the surface of the bed. With steady pressure, the enema nozzle should be inserted into the rectum, with the nozzle toward the navel, and the container squeezed until the entire dose is expelled. Enema fluids, if properly introduced, usually provide adequate evacuation if retained until definite lower abdominal cramping is felt.

● *Dosage*

Laxatives should be used as infrequently as possible, at the lowest effective dosage level, and usually for periods not exceeding one week; laxatives should be used for longer periods only under the management of a physician and as part of a carefully planned therapeutic regimen.

For further information on chemistry, pharmacology, pharmacokinetics, uses, and dosage and administration of the Cathartics and Laxatives, see the individual monographs in 56:12.

† Use is not currently included in the labeling approved by the US Food and Drug Administration.

Naldemedine Tosylate

56:18.04 • OPIOID ANTAGONISTS

■ Naldemedine tosylate is a peripherally acting μ-opiate receptor antagonist.

USES

● Opiate-induced Constipation

Naldemedine tosylate is used for the management of opiate-induced constipation in patients with chronic non-cancer-related pain, including those with chronic pain related to prior cancer or its treatment who do not require frequent (e.g., weekly) increases in opiate dosage.

Safety and efficacy of naldemedine were established in 2 identical, randomized, double-blind, placebo-controlled studies (COMPOSE-1 and COMPOSE-2) in 1100 patients (mean age of 54 years, 59% women, 80% white) with chronic non-cancer-related pain and active opiate-induced constipation who had received a stable opiate dosage (equivalent to 30 mg or more of oral morphine sulfate daily) for at least 4 weeks prior to study enrollment. Opiate-induced constipation was defined as no more than 4 spontaneous bowel movements over 14 consecutive days and fewer than 3 spontaneous bowel movements per week with at least 25% of spontaneous bowel movements associated with straining, hard or lumpy stools, a sensation of incomplete evacuation, and/or a sensation of anorectal obstruction or blockage. Patients with evidence of substantial structural abnormalities of the GI tract, those with no bowel movements during a 3-week period (the 2-week qualifying period and the preceding 7 days), and patients who had never received laxatives for the management of opiate-induced constipation were excluded from these studies. Patients in these studies received naldemedine 0.2 mg once daily or placebo without regard to food for 12 weeks. No laxatives other than a "rescue" laxative regimen (bisacodyl for an episode of no bowel movements for 72 hours, followed by one-time use of an enema if no bowel movement occurred within 24 hours following bisacodyl administration) were permitted during the studies.

Patients enrolled in the studies had received their current opiate analgesic for an average of approximately 5 years; the mean baseline opiate dosage was equivalent to morphine sulfate 121–132 mg daily. Back or neck pain (61%) was the most common indication for opiate analgesia. The mean baseline number of spontaneous bowel movements was 1.2–1.3 per week.

The primary end point of the studies was response, defined as 3 or more spontaneous bowel movements per week and a change from baseline of 1 or more spontaneous bowel movements per week for at least 9 of the 12 study weeks and at least 3 of the final 4 weeks of the study. Response to naldemedine was superior to the placebo response in both studies; response rates for naldemedine and placebo were 48 and 35%, respectively, in COMPOSE-1 and 53 and 34%, respectively, in COMPOSE-2.

Secondary end points included the change in frequency of spontaneous bowel movements, spontaneous bowel movements without straining, and complete spontaneous bowel movements per week from baseline to the final 2 weeks of treatment, as well as the change in frequency of spontaneous bowel movements per week from baseline to week 1 of treatment. On each of these secondary end points, naldemedine was superior to placebo. From baseline to the final 2 weeks of treatment, spontaneous bowel movements, spontaneous bowel movements without straining, and complete spontaneous bowel movements in naldemedine-treated patients versus placebo recipients increased in frequency by a mean of 3.1 versus 2, 1.3 versus 0.7, and 2.3 versus 1.5 bowel movements per week, respectively, in COMPOSE-1 and by 3.3 versus 2.1, 1.8 versus 1.1, and 2.6 versus 1.6 bowel movements per week, respectively, in COMPOSE-2. From baseline to week 1 of treatment, spontaneous bowel movements in naldemedine-treated patients versus placebo recipients increased in frequency by a mean of 3.3 versus 1.3 and by 3.7 versus 1.6 bowel movements per week in these respective studies.

DOSAGE AND ADMINISTRATION

● General

Changes in the analgesic dosing regimen are not required prior to initiation of naldemedine therapy. Patients receiving opiates for less than 4 weeks may be less responsive to naldemedine therapy. Naldemedine should be discontinued if therapy with opiate analgesics is discontinued.

● Administration

Naldemedine tosylate is administered orally without regard to food.

● Dosage

Dosage of naldemedine tosylate is expressed in terms of naldemedine.

The recommended adult dosage of naldemedine for the management of opiate-induced constipation in patients with chronic non-cancer-related pain is 0.2 mg once daily.

● Special Populations

No dosage adjustment of naldemedine is required in patients with mild or moderate hepatic impairment. Use of naldemedine should be avoided in patients with severe hepatic impairment. The manufacturer makes no specific dosage recommendations for geriatric patients or patients with renal impairment. (See Specific Populations under Cautions: Warnings/Precautions.)

CAUTIONS

● Contraindications

Because of the potential for GI perforation, naldemedine is contraindicated in patients with known or suspected GI obstruction and in patients at increased risk for recurrent GI obstruction. (See GI Perforation under Cautions: Warnings/Precautions.)

Naldemedine also is contraindicated in patients with known hypersensitivity to the drug.

● Warnings/Precautions

GI Perforation

GI perforation has been reported with use of methylnaltrexone, another peripherally acting opiate antagonist, in patients with underlying conditions that may be associated with localized or diffuse reduction of structural integrity in the GI tract wall (e.g., peptic ulcer disease, Ogilvie's syndrome, diverticular disease, infiltrative GI tract malignancies or peritoneal metastases). Risks and benefits of naldemedine therapy should be carefully considered in patients with these conditions or with other conditions that might result in impaired integrity of the GI tract wall (e.g., Crohn's disease). Patients receiving naldemedine should be monitored for the development of severe, persistent, or worsening abdominal pain. Naldemedine should be discontinued if such symptoms occur.

Opiate Withdrawal

Manifestations consistent with opiate withdrawal, including hyperhidrosis, chills, increased lacrimation, hot flush/flushing, pyrexia, sneezing, feeling cold, abdominal pain, diarrhea, nausea, and vomiting, have been reported in patients receiving naldemedine.

Pooled data from the COMPOSE-1 and COMPOSE-2 studies indicated that the incidence of opiate-withdrawal manifestations (defined as same-day or consecutive-day occurrence of 3 or more adverse effects potentially related to opiate withdrawal) over 12 weeks of treatment was similar (1%) in patients receiving naldemedine and those receiving placebo. In a long-term (52-week) safety study, opiate-withdrawal manifestations occurred in 3 or 1% of patients receiving naldemedine or placebo, respectively. In most naldemedine-treated patients, the incidence of withdrawal manifestations confined solely to the GI tract was approximately equivalent to that of combined GI and non-GI manifestations.

Patients with disruptions in the blood-brain barrier may be at increased risk for opiate withdrawal or reduced analgesia; risks and benefits of naldemedine therapy should be carefully considered in such patients, and these patients should be monitored for symptoms of opiate withdrawal.

Sensitivity Reactions

Hypersensitivity reactions, including bronchospasm and rash, have been reported in patients receiving naldemedine.

Specific Populations

Pregnancy

Naldemedine should be used in pregnant women only if the potential benefits justify the potential risk to the fetus. There are no adequate and well-controlled studies of naldemedine in pregnant women. Naldemedine crosses the placenta; because of the immature fetal blood-brain barrier, use of naldemedine during pregnancy may precipitate opiate withdrawal in the fetus. No adverse effects of the drug on embryofetal development have been observed in animal reproduction studies.

Lactation

It is not known whether naldemedine is distributed into human milk, affects milk production, or affects the breast-fed infant. Naldemedine is distributed into milk in rats. Because of the potential for serious adverse effects, including opiate withdrawal, in nursing infants, a decision should be made whether to discontinue nursing or the drug, taking into account the importance of the drug to the woman. If naldemedine is discontinued, nursing may be resumed 3 days after the final dose of the drug.

Pediatric Use

Safety and efficacy of naldemedine have not been established in pediatric patients.

Geriatric Use

In clinical studies, 16% of patients who received naldemedine were 65 years of age and older, while 3% were 75 years of age and older. Although no overall differences in safety and efficacy were observed between geriatric patients and younger adults, the possibility that some older patients may exhibit increased sensitivity to the drug cannot be ruled out. A population pharmacokinetic analysis revealed no age-related differences in the pharmacokinetics of naldemedine.

Hepatic Impairment

The pharmacokinetic profile of naldemedine in patients with mild or moderate (Child-Pugh class A or B) hepatic impairment is similar to that in individuals with normal hepatic function. The effect of severe (Child-Pugh class C) hepatic impairment on the pharmacokinetics of naldemedine has not been established. Use of naldemedine should be avoided in patients with severe hepatic impairment.

Renal Impairment

The pharmacokinetic profile of naldemedine in patients with renal impairment (mild, moderate, or severe renal impairment or end-stage renal disease requiring hemodialysis) is similar to that in individuals with normal renal function. Naldemedine is not removed by hemodialysis.

● Common Adverse Effects

Adverse effects reported in 2% or more of patients receiving naldemedine and at a greater incidence than that observed with placebo include abdominal pain, diarrhea, nausea, vomiting, and gastroenteritis.

DRUG INTERACTIONS

Naldemedine is metabolized principally by cytochrome P-450 (CYP) isoenzyme 3A4 (CYP3A4), with minimal contribution from uridine diphosphate-glucuronosyltransferase (UGT) 1A3; naldemedine also is a substrate of P-glycoprotein (P-gp). Naldemedine did not inhibit CYP isoenzyme 1A2, 2A6, 2B6, 2C8, 2C9, 2C19, 2D6, 2E1, 3A4/5, or 4A11 in vitro at clinically relevant concentrations. The drug also did not substantially induce CYP isoenzyme 1A2, 2B6, or 3A4 or UGT 1A2, 1A6, or 2B7.

Naldemedine does not inhibit organic anion transport protein (OATP) 1B1 or 1B3, organic cation transporter (OCT) 1 or 2, organic anion transporter (OAT) 1 or 3, breast cancer resistance protein (BCRP), or P-gp.

● Drugs Affecting Hepatic Microsomal Enzymes

Concomitant use of naldemedine with moderate (e.g., aprepitant, atazanavir, diltiazem, erythromycin, fluconazole) or potent (e.g., clarithromycin, itraconazole, ketoconazole, ritonavir, saquinavir) CYP3A inhibitors may result in increased plasma concentrations of naldemedine. Patients receiving naldemedine concomitantly with moderate or potent CYP3A inhibitors should be monitored for naldemedine-related adverse effects.

Potent CYP3A inducers (e.g., carbamazepine, phenytoin, rifampin, St. John's wort [Hypericum perforatum]) can substantially reduce plasma naldemedine concentrations and may decrease efficacy of the drug. Use of naldemedine with potent CYP3A inducers should be avoided.

● Drugs that Inhibit P-glycoprotein

Concomitant use of naldemedine and inhibitors of P-gp (e.g., amiodarone, captopril, cyclosporine, quercetin, quinidine, verapamil) may result in increased plasma concentrations of naldemedine. Patients receiving such concomitant therapy should be monitored for naldemedine-related adverse effects.

● Cyclosporine

Concomitant administration of naldemedine (single 0.4-mg dose) and the combined P-gp and weak CYP3A inhibitor cyclosporine (single 600-mg dose) increased the peak plasma concentration and area under the plasma concentration-time curve (AUC) of naldemedine by 45 and 78%, respectively. Patients receiving concomitant therapy with naldemedine and cyclosporine should be monitored for naldemedine-related adverse effects.

● Efavirenz

Pharmacokinetic simulations suggest that concomitant use of efavirenz, a moderate CYP3A inducer, decreases exposure to naldemedine by 43%. The clinical importance of this reduced exposure is unknown.

● Fluconazole

Concomitant administration of naldemedine (single 0.2-mg dose) and the combined P-gp and moderate CYP3A inhibitor fluconazole (400 mg on day 1, then 200 mg daily for 6 days) increased peak plasma concentration and AUC of naldemedine by 38 and 90%, respectively. Patients receiving concomitant therapy with naldemedine and fluconazole should be monitored for naldemedine-related adverse effects.

● Itraconazole

Concomitant administration of naldemedine (single 0.2-mg dose) and the combined P-gp and potent CYP3A inhibitor itraconazole (200 mg twice daily on day 1, then 200 mg once daily for 6 days) increased the peak plasma concentration and AUC of naldemedine by 12% and 2.91-fold, respectively. Patients receiving concomitant therapy with naldemedine and itraconazole should be monitored for naldemedine-related adverse effects.

● Opiate Antagonists

Concomitant use of naldemedine and other opiate antagonists should be avoided because of the potential for additive opiate receptor antagonism and an increased risk of opiate withdrawal.

● Rifampin

Concomitant administration of naldemedine (single 0.2-mg dose) and the combined P-gp and potent CYP3A inducer rifampin (600 mg once daily for 17 days) reduced the peak plasma concentration and AUC of naldemedine by approximately 38 and 83%, respectively. Concomitant use of rifampin and naldemedine may decrease the efficacy of naldemedine and should be avoided.

DESCRIPTION

Naldemedine tosylate, a derivative of naltrexone, is a peripherally acting μ-opiate receptor antagonist that also binds to and exhibits antagonistic activity at δ- and κ-opiate receptors. The mechanism of action of naldemedine in the management of opiate-induced constipation stems from the drug's ability to block μ-opiate receptors in the GI tract, thereby reversing opiate-induced constipating effects (e.g., slowing of GI transit). Naldemedine differs structurally from naltrexone by the addition of a large polar side chain that decreases the ability of the drug to cross the blood-brain barrier. In addition, naldemedine is a substrate of the P-glycoprotein (P-gp) efflux transporter. Because of these properties, CNS penetration of naldemedine is expected to be negligible at the recommended dosage, limiting the potential for interference with centrally mediated opiate analgesia.

Following oral administration in the fasted state, peak plasma concentrations of naldemedine are attained in approximately 45 minutes. Peak plasma concentration and area under the plasma concentration-time curve (AUC) increase in a dose-proportional or almost dose-proportional manner. Administration of naldemedine with a high-fat meal decreases the peak plasma concentration by approximately 35% and delays the time to peak plasma concentration by approximately 1.75 hours, but does not affect the extent of absorption. Naldemedine is 93–94% bound to plasma proteins and has a terminal elimination half-life of 11 hours. Naldemedine is metabolized principally by cytochrome P-450 isoenzyme 3A4 (CYP3A4), with minor contribution by uridine diphosphate-glucuronosyltransferase (UGT) isoenzyme 1A3 (UGT1A3), to form metabolites (nornaldemedine and naldemedine 3-glucuronide, respectively) that are less-potent opiate receptor antagonists. At usual clinical concentrations, these metabolites are not expected to contribute to the drug's pharmacologic effects. Naldemedine also is cleaved in the GI tract to form benzamidine and naldemedine carboxylic acid. Following oral administration of a radiolabeled dose of naldemedine, 57% of the dose was excreted in urine and 35% in feces, with 16–18% of the administered dose excreted as unchanged drug in urine. Benzamidine was the principal metabolite excreted in urine and feces, accounting for 32 and 20%, respectively, of the administered dose.

ADVICE TO PATIENTS

Importance of advising patients to read the manufacturer's medication guide.

Importance of discontinuing naldemedine following discontinuance of opiate analgesic therapy.

Possible risk of GI perforation. Importance of discontinuing naldemedine and promptly seeking medical attention if unusually severe, persistent, or worsening abdominal pain occurs.

Importance of advising patients that manifestations consistent with opiate withdrawal may occur and that they should inform their clinician if such manifestations occur.

Importance of women informing clinicians if they are or plan to become pregnant or plan to breast-feed. Women of child-bearing potential should be informed that naldemedine use during pregnancy may precipitate opiate withdrawal in the fetus because the fetal blood-brain barrier is immature. Women also should be advised *not* to breast-feed while receiving naldemedine and for 3 days following the final dose of the drug because of the potential for opiate withdrawal in nursing infants.

Importance of informing clinicians of existing or contemplated concomitant therapy, including prescription and OTC drugs and dietary supplements (especially those that alter activity of cytochrome P-450 isoenzyme 3A4 [CYP3A4]), as well as any concomitant illnesses.

Importance of informing patients of other important precautionary information. (See Cautions.)

PREPARATIONS

Excipients in commercially available drug preparations may have clinically important effects in some individuals; consult specific product labeling for details.

Naldemedine Tosylate

Oral

| Tablets, film-coated | 0.2 mg (of naldemedine) | Symproic®, Purdue |

† Use is not currently included in the labeling approved by the US Food and Drug Administration.

Selected Revisions May 10, 2024, © Copyright, April 12, 2017, American Society of Health-System Pharmacists, Inc.

Naloxegol Oxalate

56:18.04 • OPIOID ANTAGONISTS

■ Naloxegol is a peripherally acting μ-opiate receptor antagonist.

USES

● Opiate-induced Constipation

Naloxegol oxalate is used for the management of opiate-induced constipation in patients with chronic non-cancer-related pain, including those with chronic pain related to prior cancer or its treatment who do not require frequent (e.g., weekly) increases in opiate dosage.

Safety and efficacy of naloxegol were established in 2 identical randomized, double-blind, placebo-controlled, phase 3 studies (KODIAC-04 and KODIAC-05) in 1352 patients (mean age of 52 years) with non-cancer-related pain and active opiate-induced constipation who had received an oral opiate analgesic (at a stable dosage equivalent to 30 mg to 1 g of morphine sulfate daily) for at least 4 weeks prior to study enrollment. Opiate-induced constipation was defined as fewer than 3 spontaneous bowel movements per week during the 4 weeks prior to screening, with at least 25% of spontaneous bowel movements associated with straining, hard or lumpy stools, and/or a sensation of incomplete evacuation or anorectal obstruction. Patients with suspected clinically important disruptions of the blood-brain barrier were not enrolled in the studies. Patients in the studies were randomized to receive naloxegol 12.5 or 25 mg once daily or placebo for 12 weeks. No laxatives or bowel-therapy regimens other than a "rescue" laxative regimen (up to three 10- to 15-mg doses of bisacodyl followed, if necessary, by one-time use of an enema for an episode of no bowel movements for 72 hours) were permitted during the studies. Back pain (56–57%) and arthritis (10%) were the most common indications for opiate analgesia in the 2 studies. Patients enrolled in the studies had received their current opiate analgesic for an average of 3.6–3.7 years. The mean baseline opiate dosage was equivalent to 136–140 mg of morphine sulfate daily.

Laxative use on at least one occasion within 2 weeks prior to study enrollment was reported by 71% of patients. Approximately 53–55% of patients enrolled in the studies had an inadequate response to laxatives prior to study enrollment. Inadequate response to laxatives was defined as laxative use on at least 4 of the previous 14 days with at least 1 of the following symptoms of moderate, severe, or very severe intensity: incomplete bowel movements, hard stool, straining, or sensation of needing to pass a bowel movement but being unable to do so. In the subgroup of patients with inadequate response to laxatives, 42–50% of patients reported daily use of laxatives, most frequently stool softeners (18–24%), stimulants (16–18%), and polyethylene glycol (5–6%), prior to enrollment. Combined use of 2 laxative classes was reported by 27–31% of these patients at any time during the 14 days prior to enrollment; the most commonly reported combination was stimulants and stool softeners (8–10%).

The primary end point of the studies was response, defined as 3 or more spontaneous bowel movements per week and a change from baseline of 1 or more spontaneous bowel movements per week for at least 9 of the 12 study weeks and at least 3 of the final 4 study weeks. Response to naloxegol 25 mg daily was superior to the placebo response in both studies; however, response to naloxegol 12.5 mg daily was superior to the placebo response in only one of the studies. Response rates for naloxegol 25 mg, naloxegol 12.5 mg, and placebo were 44, 41, and 29%, respectively, in KODIAC-04 and 40, 35, and 29%, respectively, in KODIAC-05.

Key secondary end points of the studies included time to first postdose spontaneous bowel movement, change from baseline in the mean number of days per week with 1–3 spontaneous bowel movements, and response rate in patients with an inadequate response to laxatives prior to study enrollment. On each of these 3 key secondary end points, naloxegol 25 mg daily was superior to placebo in both studies and naloxegol 12.5 mg daily was superior to placebo in KODIAC-04; statistical significance for secondary end points could not be established for the 12.5-mg dosage in KODIAC-05 since this study failed to established efficacy of the 12.5-mg dosage for the primary efficacy end point. In the subgroup of patients with an inadequate response to laxatives, response rates were 49, 43, and 29% in KODIAC-04 for naloxegol 25 mg, naloxegol 12.5 mg, and placebo, respectively, and 47 and 31% in KODIAC-05 for naloxegol 25 mg and placebo, respectively. In KODIAC-04, median times to first postdose spontaneous bowel movement were 6, 20, and 36 hours with naloxegol 25 mg, naloxegol 12.5 mg, and placebo, respectively. In KODIAC-05, median times to first postdose spontaneous bowel movement were 12 and 37 hours with naloxegol 25 mg and placebo, respectively. A spontaneous bowel movement occurred within 24 hours of the first dose in 61–70 or 58% of patients receiving naloxegol 25 or 12.5 mg, respectively.

Mean daily opiate dosages remained stable during the studies, and mean changes from baseline in pain intensity (as measured on a scale of 0–10) were small and not clinically important.

DOSAGE AND ADMINISTRATION

● General

All maintenance laxative therapy should be discontinued prior to initiating naloxegol; laxatives may be used as needed if the patient's response to naloxegol is suboptimal after 3 days of therapy.

Changes in the analgesic dosing regimen are not required prior to initiation of naloxegol therapy. Patients receiving opiates for less than 4 weeks may be less responsive to naloxegol therapy.

● Administration

Naloxegol oxalate is administered orally on an empty stomach at least 1 hour before or 2 hours after the first meal of the day. For patients who have cannot swallow naloxegol oxalate tablets whole, the tablet may be crushed to a powder and mixed with 120 mL of water in a glass; the resulting mixture should be stirred and then swallowed immediately. To ensure consumption of the entire dose, the glass should be rinsed with 120 mL of water; the resulting mixture should be stirred and then swallowed immediately.

For administration through a nasogastric tube, the nasogastric tube should first be flushed with 30 mL of water using a 60-mL syringe. The tablet should then be crushed to a powder and mixed with approximately 60 mL of water in a container. The resulting mixture should be drawn up into the 60-mL syringe and administered through the nasogastric tube. To facilitate delivery of the entire dose, the container should be rinsed with approximately 60 mL of water, the mixture should be drawn up into the same syringe, and the entire contents of the syringe should be used to flush the nasogastric tube.

Plasma concentrations of naloxegol attained when a crushed naloxegol oxalate tablet is mixed in water and administered either orally or through a nasogastric tube are comparable to those attained following oral administration of an intact tablet of the drug.

● Dosage

Dosage of naloxegol oxalate is expressed in terms of naloxegol.

The recommended adult dosage of naloxegol for the management of opiate-induced constipation in patients with chronic non-cancer-related pain is 25 mg once daily in the morning. If patients cannot tolerate the 25-mg daily dosage, dosage of naloxegol may be reduced to 12.5 mg once daily in the morning.

If concomitant use of moderate cytochrome P-450 (CYP) 3A4 inhibitors (e.g., diltiazem, erythromycin, verapamil) is unavoidable, dosage of naloxegol should be reduced to 12.5 mg once daily, and the patient should be monitored for adverse effects. (See Drug Interactions.)

● Special Populations

The recommended initial dosage of naloxegol in patients with moderate or severe renal impairment (i.e., creatinine clearance less than 60 mL/minute), including those with end-stage renal disease, is 12.5 mg once daily. If the initial naloxegol dosage is well tolerated but symptoms of opiate-induced constipation persist, dosage may be increased to 25 mg once daily, taking into consideration the potential for markedly increased systemic exposure to the drug in some patients with renal impairment and the associated increased risk of adverse effects. (See Renal Impairment under Warnings/Precautions: Specific Populations, in Cautions.)

No dosage adjustment is needed in patients with mild (Child-Pugh class A) or moderate (Child-Pugh class B) hepatic impairment. Use of naloxegol should be avoided in patients with severe (Child-Pugh class C) hepatic impairment; an appropriate dosage has not been established. (See Hepatic Impairment under Warnings/Precautions: Specific Populations, in Cautions.)

No dosage adjustment is required in geriatric patients based solely on age.

CAUTIONS

● Contraindications

Because of the potential for GI perforation, naloxegol is contraindicated in patients with known or suspected GI obstruction and in patients at increased risk for recurrent GI obstruction (see GI Perforation under Cautions: Warnings/Precautions).

Naloxegol is contraindicated in patients receiving potent inhibitors of cytochrome P-450 (CYP) isoenzyme 3A4 (CYP3A4) (e.g., clarithromycin, ketoconazole) because of the potential for increased exposure to naloxegol and precipitation of opiate withdrawal (see Drug Interactions).

Naloxegol also is contraindicated in patients with known serious or severe hypersensitivity reactions to the drug or any ingredient in the formulation.

● Warnings/Precautions

Opiate Withdrawal

In 2 controlled clinical trials of naloxegol in patients with opiate-induced constipation, possible opiate withdrawal (defined as the same-day occurrence of at least 3 adverse effects, not all related to the GI tract, that are potential manifestations of opiate withdrawal [e.g., hyperhidrosis, chills, diarrhea, abdominal pain, anxiety, irritability, yawning]) occurred in 1% of patients receiving naloxegol 12.5 mg daily, 3% of patients receiving naloxegol 25 mg daily, and less than 1% of those receiving placebo. In both trials, the incidence of adverse GI effects potentially related to opiate withdrawal was higher in patients receiving methadone compared with those receiving other opiate analgesics (39 versus 26% of those receiving naloxegol 12.5 mg daily and 75 versus 34% of those receiving naloxegol 25 mg daily).

Patients with disruptions in the blood-brain barrier may be at increased risk for opiate withdrawal or reduced analgesia; risks and benefits of naloxegol therapy should be carefully considered in such patients, and these patients should be monitored for symptoms of opiate withdrawal.

Severe Abdominal Pain and Diarrhea

Severe abdominal pain and/or diarrhea, sometimes resulting in hospitalization, have been reported in patients receiving naloxegol. Most cases of severe abdominal pain have been reported in patients receiving a naloxegol dosage of 25 mg daily. Symptoms generally have occurred within a few days following initiation of therapy. Patients receiving naloxegol should be monitored for the development of abdominal pain and/or diarrhea. Naloxegol should be discontinued if severe symptoms occur. If appropriate, consideration can be given to reinitiating naloxegol therapy at a dosage of 12.5 mg once daily.

GI Perforation

GI perforation has been reported with use of methylnaltrexone, another peripherally acting opiate antagonist, in patients with underlying conditions that may be associated with localized or diffuse reduction of structural integrity in the GI tract wall (e.g., peptic ulcer disease, Ogilvie's syndrome, diverticular disease, infiltrative GI tract malignancies or peritoneal metastases). Risks and benefits of naloxegol therapy should be carefully considered in patients with these conditions or with other conditions that might result in impaired integrity of the GI tract wall (e.g., Crohn's disease). Patients receiving naloxegol should be monitored for the development of severe, persistent, or worsening abdominal pain. Naloxegol should be discontinued if such symptoms occur.

Specific Populations

Pregnancy

Category C. (See Users Guide.)

Naloxegol should be used in pregnant women only if the potential benefits justify the potential risk to the fetus. There are no adequate and well-controlled studies of naloxegol in pregnant women. Because of the immature fetal blood-brain barrier, use of naloxegol during pregnancy may precipitate opiate withdrawal in the fetus. No adverse effects of the drug on embryofetal development have been observed in animal reproduction studies.

Lactation

It is not known whether naloxegol is distributed into human milk; however, naloxegol is distributed into milk in rats and is absorbed in nursing rat pups. Because of the potential for serious adverse effects, including opiate withdrawal, in nursing infants, a decision should be made whether to discontinue nursing or the drug, taking into account the importance of the drug to the woman.

Pediatric Use

Safety and efficacy of naloxegol have not been established in pediatric patients.

Geriatric Use

In clinical studies of naloxegol, 11% of patients were 65 years of age and older, while 2% were 75 years of age and older. Although no overall differences in efficacy or safety were observed between geriatric patients and younger adults, and other clinical experience revealed no evidence of age-related differences in response, the possibility that some older patients may exhibit increased sensitivity to the drug cannot be ruled out.

Naloxegol exposure was higher in healthy geriatric Japanese individuals compared with younger individuals; however, no dosage adjustment is required in geriatric patients.

Hepatic Impairment

Following oral administration of a single 25-mg dose of naloxegol, slight decreases in area under the concentration-time curve (AUC) of the drug were observed in patients with mild (Child-Pugh class A) or moderate (Child-Pugh class B) hepatic impairment compared with those with normal hepatic function. No dosage adjustment is required in patients with mild or moderate hepatic impairment. The effect of severe hepatic impairment (Child-Pugh class C) on the pharmacokinetics of naloxegol has not been established. Use of naloxegol in patients with severe hepatic impairment should be avoided, as appropriate dosage in these patients has not been determined.

Renal Impairment

Following oral administration of a single 25-mg dose of naloxegol in patients with moderate or severe renal impairment or end-stage renal disease not yet requiring dialysis (i.e., creatinine clearance less than 60 mL/minute), the pharmacokinetic profile of naloxegol in most patients was similar to that observed in healthy individuals. However, some patients with renal impairment (including patients with moderate, severe, or end-stage renal disease) had markedly increased systemic exposure to the drug (e.g., up to tenfold higher than that observed in healthy individuals). Some patients with end-stage renal disease requiring dialysis also were included in the pharmacokinetic study. Plasma concentrations of naloxegol in these patients were similar to concentrations observed in healthy individuals whether the drug was administered before or after hemodialysis.

The reason for the high exposures observed in some patients with renal impairment is unknown; however, because the risk of adverse effects increases as systemic exposure increases, a reduced initial dosage of naloxegol is recommended in patients with creatinine clearances of less than 60 mL/minute. (See Dosage and Administration: Special Populations.) No dosage adjustment is required in patients with mild renal impairment.

● Common Adverse Effects

Adverse effects reported in 3% or more of patients receiving naloxegol 12.5 or 25 mg daily and at an incidence greater than that observed with placebo include abdominal pain, diarrhea, nausea, flatulence, vomiting, headache, and hyperhidrosis.

DRUG INTERACTIONS

Naloxegol is metabolized principally by cytochrome P-450 (CYP) 3A isoenzymes and is a substrate, but not a clinically important inhibitor, of P-glycoprotein

(P-gp). Naloxegol did not inhibit CYP 1A2, 2C9, 2C19, 2D6, or 3A4 nor substantially induce CYP 1A2, 2B6, or 3A4 in vitro at clinically relevant concentrations, and is not expected to alter metabolic clearance of drugs metabolized by these enzymes.

Naloxegol does not substantially inhibit breast cancer resistance protein (BCRP), organic anion transporter (OAT) 1 or 3, organic cation transporter (OCT) 2, or organic anion transport protein (OATP) 1B1 or 1B3.

Drugs Affecting Hepatic Microsomal Enzymes

Concomitant use of naloxegol with potent CYP3A4 inhibitors (e.g., clarithromycin, itraconazole, ketoconazole) or moderate CYP3A4 inhibitors (e.g., diltiazem, erythromycin, verapamil) may result in increased plasma concentrations of naloxegol and increased risk of adverse effects. Use of naloxegol with potent CYP3A4 inhibitors is contraindicated. Use of naloxegol with moderate CYP3A4 inhibitors should be avoided; if concomitant use is unavoidable, dosage of naloxegol should be reduced to 12.5 mg once daily and the patient should be monitored for adverse effects. When naloxegol is used concomitantly with weak CYP3A4 inhibitors (e.g., cimetidine, quinidine), clinically important increases in naloxegol concentrations are not expected and dosage adjustments are not required.

Potent CYP3A4 inducers (e.g., carbamazepine, rifampin, St. John's wort [*Hypericum perforatum*]) can substantially decrease plasma naloxegol concentrations and may decrease the efficacy of naloxegol. Use of naloxegol with potent CYP3A4 inducers is not recommended.

Diltiazem

Concomitant administration of naloxegol (single 25-mg dose) and the combined P-gp and moderate CYP3A4 inhibitor diltiazem (240 mg of extended-release diltiazem hydrochloride once daily) increased peak plasma concentration and area under the concentration-time curve (AUC) of naloxegol by 2.9- and 3.4-fold, respectively. Concomitant use of naloxegol with diltiazem should be avoided; if concomitant use cannot be avoided, dosage of naloxegol should be reduced to 12.5 mg once daily and the patient should be monitored for adverse effects.

Efavirenz

Pharmacokinetic simulations suggested that concomitant administration of a single 25-mg dose of naloxegol with the moderate CYP3A inducer efavirenz (400 mg once daily) results in naloxegol exposures similar to those achieved with administration of naloxegol 12.5 mg alone (i.e., a 50% reduction in exposure).

Grapefruit or Grapefruit Juice

When consumed concomitantly with naloxegol, grapefruit or grapefruit juice can increase plasma naloxegol concentrations. Consumption of grapefruit or grapefruit juice should be avoided by patients receiving naloxegol. The manufacturer states that the effect of grapefruit juice varies widely among brands and is dependent on the concentration, dose, and preparation. Studies have demonstrated that some preparations of grapefruit juice (e.g., high dose, double strength) are potent CYP3A inhibitors, while other preparations (e.g., low dose, single strength) are moderate CYP3A inhibitors.

Ketoconazole

Concomitant administration of naloxegol (single 25-mg dose) and the combined P-gp and potent CYP3A4 inhibitor ketoconazole (400 mg once daily) increased peak plasma concentration and AUC of naloxegol by 9.6- and 12.9-fold, respectively. Concomitant use of naloxegol with ketoconazole is contraindicated.

Morphine

In healthy individuals receiving IV morphine sulfate (5 mg per 70 kg), single doses of naloxegol (8 mg to 1 g) had no meaningful effect on systemic exposure to morphine or its major circulating metabolites. With increasing naloxegol dose, there was no trend toward increasing or decreasing morphine exposure compared with morphine administered alone.

Opiate Antagonists

When naloxegol is used concomitantly with other opiate antagonists, the potential exists for additive opiate receptor antagonism and an increased risk of opiate withdrawal. Concomitant use of naloxegol with other opiate antagonists should be avoided.

Quinidine

Because of its inhibitory effect on P-gp, the combined potent P-gp and weak CPY3A4 inhibitor quinidine sulfate (single 600-mg dose) increased peak plasma concentration and AUC of naloxegol (given as a single 25-mg dose) by 2.5- and 1.4-fold, respectively. However, no dosage adjustment is necessary.

Rifampin

Concomitant administration of naloxegol (single 25-mg dose) and the combined P-gp and potent CYP3A4 inducer rifampin (600 mg once daily) decreased peak plasma concentration and AUC of naloxegol by 76 and 89%, respectively. Concomitant use of naloxegol with rifampin is not recommended.

DESCRIPTION

Naloxegol, a covalent conjugate of naloxone and polyethylene glycol (PEG), is a peripherally acting μ-opiate receptor antagonist. Naloxegol exhibits antagonist effects at the μ- and δ-opiate receptors and weak partial agonist activity at κ-opiate receptors, but has highest affinity for μ-opiate receptors; affinity of naloxegol for μ-opiate receptors is approximately 20-fold lower than that of naloxone. The mechanism of action of naloxegol in the management of opiate-induced constipation stems from the drug's ability to block μ-opiate receptors in the GI tract, thereby reversing opiate-induced constipating effects (e.g., slowing of GI motility and transit). Conjugation with PEG results in reduced passive permeability of the drug across the blood-brain barrier and renders naloxegol a substrate for P-glycoprotein, which results in increased efflux of the drug across the blood-brain barrier. CNS penetration of naloxegol is expected to be negligible at recommended dosages, limiting the potential for interference with centrally mediated opiate analgesia.

Naloxegol is rapidly absorbed from the GI tract, with peak plasma concentrations attained in less than 2 hours following oral administration. The presence of a secondary peak concentration has been observed approximately 0.4–3 hours after the first peak concentration in most individuals, suggesting that the drug undergoes enterohepatic circulation. Peak plasma concentration and area under the concentration time-curve (AUC) increase in a dose-proportional or almost dose-proportional manner. Administration with a high-fat meal increases the extent and rate of absorption of naloxegol; peak plasma concentration and AUC were increased by approximately 30 and 45%, respectively, when the drug was administered with a high-fat meal. Naloxegol is minimally bound to plasma proteins (approximately 4%) and has a half-life of 6–11 hours. Naloxegol is extensively metabolized, principally via cytochrome P-450 (CYP) 3A isoenzymes; the drug undergoes N-dealkylation, O-demethylation, oxidation, and shortening of the PEG chain. Approximately 68% of an oral dose is eliminated in feces (approximately 16% of which is unchanged drug) and 16% is eliminated in urine.

ADVICE TO PATIENTS

Importance of advising patients to read the manufacturer's medication guide before initiating therapy and each time the prescription is refilled.

Importance of discontinuing all maintenance laxative therapy prior to initiation of naloxegol therapy. Laxatives may be used as needed if the response to naloxegol is suboptimal after 3 days.

Importance of taking naloxegol on an empty stomach at least 1 hour before or 2 hours after the first meal of the day. If the patient cannot swallow the tablets intact or the drug must be administered through a nasogastric tube, the tablets may be crushed, mixed with water, and administered according to the manufacturer's instructions.

Importance of informing clinician if naloxegol therapy is not tolerated, as dosage adjustment may be appropriate.

Importance of informing clinician if opiate analgesics are discontinued, since naloxegol should be discontinued if opiate analgesics are discontinued.

Importance of advising patients that symptoms consistent with opiate withdrawal (e.g., sweating, chills, diarrhea, abdominal pain, anxiety, irritability, yawning) may occur. Importance of informing patients who are receiving methadone that they may be more likely than patients receiving other opiates to experience adverse GI effects that may be related to opiate withdrawal.

Importance of advising patients that severe abdominal pain and/or diarrhea may occur following initiation of naloxegol therapy; patients should be advised to discontinue therapy with the drug and contact their clinician if they experience such severe symptoms.

Possible risk of GI perforation. Importance of discontinuing naloxegol and promptly seeking medical attention if unusually severe, persistent, or worsening abdominal pain occurs.

Importance of women informing clinicians if they are or plan to become pregnant or plan to breast-feed. Women should be informed that naloxegol use during pregnancy may precipitate opiate withdrawal in the fetus because the fetal blood-brain barrier is immature. Women also should be advised *not* to breast-feed while receiving naloxegol because of the potential for opiate withdrawal in nursing infants.

Importance of informing clinicians of existing or contemplated concomitant therapy, including prescription and OTC drugs (especially those that alter activity of cytochrome P-450 isoenzyme 3A4 [CYP3A4]), as well as any concomitant illnesses. Patients receiving naloxegol should be advised to avoid consumption of grapefruit or grapefruit juice and to inform their clinician when they initiate or discontinue any concomitant drug therapy.

Importance of informing patients of other important precautionary information. (See Cautions.)

PREPARATIONS

Excipients in commercially available drug preparations may have clinically important effects in some individuals; consult specific product labeling for details.

Naloxegol Oxalate

Oral		
Tablets, film-coated	12.5 mg (of naloxegol)	**Movantik®**, AstraZeneca
	25 mg (of naloxegol)	**Movantik®**, AstraZeneca

† Use is not currently included in the labeling approved by the US Food and Drug Administration.

Selected Revisions May 10, 2024, © Copyright, February 25, 2016, American Society of Health-System Pharmacists, Inc.

Lubiprostone

56:18.08 • CHLORIDE CHANNEL ACTIVATORS

■ Lubiprostone, a bicyclic fatty acid that selectively activates intestinal ClC-2 chloride channels, increases intestinal fluid secretion.

USES

● Chronic Idiopathic Constipation

Lubiprostone is used for the management of chronic idiopathic constipation in adults.

Safety and efficacy of lubiprostone have been evaluated in 2 randomized, double-blind, placebo-controlled studies in a total of 479 adults (mean age: about 47 years, range: 20–81 years; 89% female; 80.8% white; 9.6% black; 7.3% Hispanic; 1.5% Asian) with chronic idiopathic constipation. In these studies, constipation was characterized by an average of less than 3 spontaneous bowel movements per week and the presence of one or more of 3 symptoms (very hard stools, sensation of incomplete evacuation, straining at defecation) occurring at least 25% of the time over a 6-month period prior to randomization. In these trials, patients receiving lubiprostone (24 mcg twice daily) had a higher frequency of spontaneous bowel movements, a decrease in signs and symptoms of constipation (including abdominal bloating, abdominal discomfort, stool consistency, and straining), and a decrease in constipation severity ratings compared with those receiving placebo. 57–63% of patients receiving lubiprostone (24 mcg twice daily) experienced spontaneous bowel movements within 24 hours after administration of treatment compared with 32–37% of those receiving placebo. In addition, the time to first spontaneous bowel movement was shorter in patients receiving the drug than in those receiving placebo. A rebound effect was not observed upon withdrawal of the drug following 4 weeks of treatment.

In 3 long-term, open-label safety trials in a total of 871 patients with chronic idiopathic constipation, lubiprostone (24 mcg twice daily for 6–12 months) was associated with decreases in abdominal bloating, abdominal discomfort, and severity of constipation throughout the treatment period.

● Irritable Bowel Syndrome with Constipation in Women

Lubiprostone is used for the treatment of irritable bowel syndrome (IBS) with constipation in women 18 years of age or older.

Safety and efficacy of lubiprostone have been evaluated in 2 double-blind, placebo-controlled studies in a total of 1154 adults (mean age: about 47 years, range: 18–85 years; 91.6% female; 77.4% white; 13.2% black; 8.5% Hispanic; 0.4% Asian) with IBS with constipation. In these studies, IBS was defined as abdominal pain or discomfort occurring over at least 6 months with 2 or more of 3 characteristics (relief with defecation, onset associated with change in stool frequency, or onset associated with change in stool form). The subtype of IBS with constipation was defined by the presence of 2 of 3 symptoms (less than 3 spontaneous bowel movements per week, more than 25% hard stools, more than 25% of spontaneous bowel movements associated with straining). Patients were randomized to receive lubiprostone 8 mcg twice daily (16 mcg daily) or placebo twice daily for 12 weeks. The primary end point was the number of "overall responders" as determined by patients' response (frequency of IBS) to a questionnaire. The percentage of patients qualifying as overall responders was 13.8 and 12.1% in study 1 and 2, respectively, while percentages of overall responders were 7.8 and 5.7% in those receiving placebo in study 1 and 2, respectively. In study 1, a rebound effect was not observed upon withdrawal of the drug following 12 weeks of treatment. Results of an open-label extension of these studies found that lubiprostone remained safe and effective for an additional 36 weeks.

DOSAGE AND ADMINISTRATION

● General

Lubiprostone is administered orally twice daily with food and water. Food may decrease peak plasma concentrations of the drug by 55%; however, the clinical importance of this effect has not been elucidated and the manufacturer states that lubiprostone should be taken with food and water to reduce symptoms of nausea.

● Dosage

Clinicians and patients (with chronic idiopathic constipation or irritable bowel syndrome with constipation) should periodically assess the need for continued therapy.

Chronic Idiopathic Constipation

The recommended adult dosage of lubiprostone for the treatment of chronic idiopathic constipation is 24 mcg twice daily.

Because dose-dependent nausea (sometimes severe) occurred frequently in patients receiving lubiprostone 24 mcg twice daily, dosage reduction to 24 mcg daily was allowed in such patients in the open-label, long-term studies.

Irritable Bowel Syndrome with Constipation in Women

The recommended adult dosage of lubiprostone for the treatment of irritable bowel syndrome with constipation in women is 8 mcg twice daily.

● Special Populations

No special population recommendations at this time.

CAUTIONS

● Contraindications

Known hypersensitivity to lubiprostone or any ingredient in the formulation. Known or suspected mechanical GI obstruction.

● Warnings/Precautions

Warnings

GI Obstruction

Patients with symptoms suggestive of mechanical GI obstruction should be evaluated thoroughly to confirm absence of such obstruction prior to initiating lubiprostone therapy. (See Cautions: Contraindications.)

Fetal/Neonatal Morbidity and Mortality

Women of childbearing potential should have a negative pregnancy test prior to receiving lubiprostone and should use an effective method of contraception during therapy with the drug.

General Precautions

GI Effects

Dose-dependent nausea may occur. Symptoms may be reduced by coadministration with food and water.

Possible diarrhea (may be severe). Lubiprostone should not be prescribed to patients experiencing severe diarrhea.

Respiratory Effects

Possible dyspnea (may result in discontinuance of drug). Acute onset of symptoms (e.g., sensation of chest tightness, difficulty in breathing) may occur, generally within 30–60 minutes after taking first dose. Symptoms usually resolve within a few hours; however, they frequently recur with subsequent doses.

Specific Populations

Pregnancy

Category C. (See Users Guide.) (Also see Fetal/Neonatal Morbidity and Mortality under Warnings/Precautions: Warnings, in Cautions.)

Lactation

Not known whether lubiprostone is distributed into human milk; discontinue nursing or the drug, taking into account the importance of the drug to the woman.

Pediatric Use

Safety and efficacy not established in patients younger than 18 years of age.

Geriatric Use

Efficacy of lubiprostone in geriatric patients (65 years of age and older) with chronic idiopathic constipation was consistent with efficacy of the drug in the overall study population. Geriatric patients experienced a lower incidence (18 versus 29%) of associated nausea than the overall study population.

Experience in those 65 years of age or older with irritable bowel syndrome (IBS) with constipation was insufficient to determine whether they respond differently from younger adults. Safety profile of lubiprostone in these patients was consistent with the safety profile in the overall study population.

Hepatic or Renal Impairment

Lubiprostone has not been studied in patients with renal or hepatic impairment.

● Common Adverse Effects

Adverse effects reported in about 2% or more of patients receiving lubiprostone for the management of chronic idiopathic constipation include nausea, diarrhea, headache, abdominal distention, abdominal pain, flatulence, vomiting, dizziness, edema, loose stools, abdominal discomfort (abdominal tenderness, abdominal rigidity, GI discomfort), dyspepsia, chest discomfort/pain, dyspnea, and fatigue.

Adverse effects reported in about 3% or more of women receiving lubiprostone for the treatment of IBS with constipation include nausea, diarrhea, abdominal pain, and abdominal distention.

DRUG INTERACTIONS

● Drugs Affecting or Metabolized by Hepatic Microsomal Enzymes

Pharmacokinetic interactions unlikely. In vitro, lubiprostone does not inhibit cytochrome P-450 (CYP) isoenzymes 1A2, 2A6, 2B6, 2C9, 2C19, 2D6, 2E1, or 3A4 or induce isoenzymes 1A2, 2B6, 2C9, or 3A4. Lubiprostone is not metabolized by CYP isoenzymes.

● Highly Protein-bound Drugs

Pharmacokinetic interaction unlikely.

DESCRIPTION

Lubiprostone, a bicyclic fatty acid that selectively activates intestinal ClC-2 chloride channels, increases intestinal chloride and fluid secretion without affecting serum sodium and potassium concentrations. Lubiprostone activates the ClC-2 chloride channel which is located on the apical (luminal) membrane of the human intestinal epithelium, independent of the actions of protein kinase A.

Decreased intestinal motility is a possible cause of chronic idiopathic constipation. Lubiprostone increases intestinal motility by increasing intestinal fluid secretion, consequently increasing the passage of stool and alleviating symptoms of chronic idiopathic constipation. Activation of ClC-2 by lubiprostone also may stimulate recovery of mucosal barrier function by restoring tight junction protein complexes in the intestine.

The drug also delays gastric emptying, which may cause nausea (the most common adverse effect associated with lubiprostone therapy).

Lubiprostone has low systemic bioavailability following oral administration, and plasma concentrations of the drug are below the limit of quantitation (10 pg/mL).

Lubiprostone is rapidly and extensively metabolized, probably in the stomach and jejunum, by processes mediated by carbonyl reductase; hepatic cytochrome P-450 enzymes are not involved in the metabolism of the drug. About 60% of an orally administered dose is excreted in the urine within 24 hours, while about 30% of such dose is excreted in feces within 168 hours.

ADVICE TO PATIENTS

Advise patients to take the drug twice daily (morning and evening) with food and water.

Importance of advising patients to swallow capsules whole without chewing or breaking apart.

Importance of advising patients that nausea may occur. Administration of the drug with food and water may reduce symptoms of nausea. Advise patients to contact a clinician if nausea becomes severe.

Clinicians and patients should periodically assess the need for continued treatment.

Importance of advising patients that diarrhea may occur. Advise patients to notify a clinician and not to take lubiprostone if they experience severe diarrhea.

Advise patients that dyspnea may occur; notify clinician if dyspnea becomes severe.

Importance of women informing clinicians if they are or plan to become pregnant or plan to breast-feed. Advise pregnant women of risk to the fetus. Importance of using effective method of contraception.

Importance of informing clinicians of existing or contemplated concomitant therapy, including prescription and OTC drugs, as well as any concomitant illnesses.

Importance of informing patients of other important precautionary information. (See Cautions.)

PREPARATIONS

Excipients in commercially available drug preparations may have clinically important effects in some individuals; consult specific product labeling for details.

Lubiprostone

Oral		
Capsules	8 mcg	Amitiza®, Sucampo
	24 mcg	Amitiza®, Sucampo

† Use is not currently included in the labeling approved by the US Food and Drug Administration.

Linaclotide

56:18.12 • GUANYLATE CYCLASE C (GC-C) RECEPTOR AGONISTS

■ Linaclotide, a guanylate cyclase-C (GC-C) agonist, stimulates secretion of chloride and bicarbonate into the intestinal lumen, which increases intestinal fluid and accelerates intestinal transit.

USES

● Irritable Bowel Syndrome with Constipation

Linaclotide is used in adults for the symptomatic treatment of irritable bowel syndrome (IBS) with constipation.

Efficacy and safety of linaclotide for the symptomatic treatment of IBS with constipation have been evaluated in 2 randomized, double-blind, placebo-controlled studies (trial 31 and trial 302) in adults (mean age 44 years; 90% female; 77% white, 19% black, and 12% Hispanic) who met Rome II criteria for IBS. Eligible patients also were required to meet the following criteria during the 14-day baseline period: a mean abdominal pain score of at least 3 (on a scale of 0–10), fewer than 3 complete spontaneous bowel movements (CSBMs) per week, and 5 or fewer spontaneous bowel movements (SBMs) per week. In both studies, patients were randomized to receive linaclotide 290 mcg once daily or placebo. In trial 31, the assigned treatment was continued for 12 weeks; patients who completed 12 weeks of linaclotide therapy then were rerandomized to receive linaclotide 290 mcg once daily or placebo for 4 additional weeks, while those who had received placebo for 12 weeks were reassigned to receive linaclotide 290 mg once daily for 4 weeks. In trial 302, the originally assigned treatment was continued for 26 weeks. In both studies, the primary end point was efficacy over the first 12 weeks. Data on patients' symptoms were collected via daily patient reports.

In the first study (trial 31), 34% of patients receiving linaclotide and 21% of patients receiving placebo achieved the combined efficacy end point (defined as at least 30% improvement in mean abdominal pain score and an increase of one or more CSBMs per week compared with baseline) in the same week for at least 6 out of 12 weeks of treatment. The individual components of this end point were achieved by 50 and 49%, respectively, of patients receiving linaclotide and 37 and 30%, respectively, of those receiving placebo. In patients who switched to placebo after completing 12 weeks of linaclotide therapy, abdominal pain scores and CSBM frequency returned toward baseline values within 1 week following drug discontinuance; those who continued receiving linaclotide maintained their response over 4 additional weeks of treatment.

In the second study (trial 302), 34% of patients receiving linaclotide and 14% of those receiving placebo achieved the combined efficacy end point (at least 30% improvement in mean abdominal pain score and an increase of one or more CSBMs per week compared with baseline) in the same week for at least 6 out of the first 12 weeks of treatment. The individual components of this end point were achieved by 49 and 48%, respectively, of patients receiving linaclotide and 34 and 23%, respectively, of those receiving placebo. Results for the entire 26-week treatment period were consistent with those for the first 12 weeks, with 32% of linaclotide-treated patients and 13% of placebo recipients achieving the combined end point for at least 13 out of 26 weeks.

In both studies, assessments of changes in individual symptoms of IBS, measures of bowel function (frequency of SBMs, stool consistency, amount of straining with bowel movements), and patient ratings of the adequacy and degree of relief also favored linaclotide over placebo. Improvements in abdominal pain scores were apparent within the first week of linaclotide therapy and were maximal in 6–9 weeks; maximal effects on CSBM frequency were achieved within the first week of therapy.

A post-hoc analysis of data from trials 31 and 302 indicated that linaclotide improved abdominal symptoms in subsets of patients with severe symptoms at baseline (defined as any baseline abdominal pain, discomfort, bloating, fullness, or cramping rated 7 or greater on a scale of 0–10). At 12 weeks, the mean change in abdominal symptom scores from baseline in these subsets of patients was substantially greater in patients receiving linaclotide compared with those receiving placebo.

● Chronic Idiopathic Constipation

Linaclotide is used in adults for the symptomatic treatment of chronic idiopathic constipation.

Efficacy and safety of linaclotide (145 or 290 mcg daily) for the symptomatic treatment of chronic idiopathic constipation have been evaluated in 2 randomized, double-blind, placebo-controlled studies (trial 01 and trial 303) in adults who reported having had fewer than 3 SBMs per week and having experienced straining, lumpy or hard stools, and/or a sensation of incomplete evacuation during more than 25% of bowel movements for at least 12 weeks out of the previous 12 months. Patients were excluded if they met Rome II criteria for IBS. In the 2 studies combined, the mean age of patients was 48 years, and most patients were female (89%) and white (76%; 22% black, 10% Hispanic). In each study, patients were randomized to receive linaclotide 290 mcg, linaclotide 145 mcg, or placebo once daily for 12 weeks. In trial 303, patients who completed 12 weeks of linaclotide therapy were rerandomized to receive linaclotide (at the originally assigned dosage) or placebo for 4 additional weeks, while those who had received placebo for 12 weeks were reassigned to receive linaclotide 290 mcg daily for 4 weeks. Data on bowel function and patients' symptoms were collected via daily patient reports. The combined primary efficacy end point was defined as 3 or more CSBMs per week *and* an increase of at least 1 CSBM per week compared with baseline for at least 9 weeks during the 12-week treatment period.

Results from trial 303 showed that 19, 20, or 3% of patients receiving linaclotide 290 mcg, linaclotide 145 mcg, or placebo, respectively, achieved the combined efficacy end point. In patients who switched to placebo after receiving 12 weeks of linaclotide therapy, CSBM and SBM frequency returned toward baseline values within 1 week following drug discontinuance; those who continued receiving linaclotide maintained their response over 4 additional weeks of treatment.

Results from trial 01 showed that 20, 15, or 6% of patients receiving linaclotide 290 mcg, linaclotide 145 mcg, or placebo, respectively, achieved the combined efficacy end point.

Although both dosages of linaclotide were effective, the studies provided no consistent evidence indicating that the 290-mcg daily dosage confers additional clinical benefit beyond that produced by the 145-mcg daily dosage.

In both studies, assessments of changes in individual symptoms of constipation, measures of bowel function (frequency of SBMs, stool consistency, amount of straining with bowel movements), and overall severity of constipation also favored linaclotide over placebo. Maximal effects on CSBM frequency were achieved within the first week of therapy and were sustained throughout the treatment period.

Efficacy of linaclotide at a dosage of 72 mcg daily was established in a third randomized, double-blind, placebo-controlled study in adults who met modified Rome III criteria for functional constipation. The study design through week 12 was the same as that in trial 01 and trial 303. The mean age of patients was 46 years, and most patients were female (77%) and white (71%). The combined efficacy end point (3 or more CSBMs in a given week and an increase of at least 1 CSBM from baseline in the same week for a minimum of 9 weeks out of the 12-week treatment period) was achieved by 13% of patients receiving linaclotide 72 mcg daily compared with 5% of those receiving placebo. In a separate analysis using an alternate definition of response (3 or more CSBMs in a given week and an increase of at least 1 CSBM from baseline in the same week for a minimum of 9 weeks out of the 12-week treatment period and for at least 3 of the last 4 weeks of the treatment period), response rates were 12% for patients receiving linaclotide 72 mcg daily and 5% for those receiving placebo.

DOSAGE AND ADMINISTRATION

● Administration

Linaclotide is administered orally on an empty stomach, at least 30 minutes prior to the first meal of the day. Administration immediately after a high-fat breakfast resulted in looser stools and increased frequency of stools when compared with administration in the fasted state. In clinical trials, linaclotide was administered at least 30 minutes before breakfast.

Linaclotide capsules should be swallowed whole. Alternatively, for patients who are unable to swallow whole capsules, linaclotide capsules may be opened and the contents (beads) may be sprinkled on applesauce and administered orally or dispersed in water and administered orally or via a nasogastric or gastrostomy tube. The manufacturer states that sprinkling the capsule contents of linaclotide capsules on soft foods other than applesauce or dispersing the contents in liquids other than water has not been studied. The capsules or capsule contents should not be crushed or chewed.

For administration in applesauce, the entire contents of one capsule of linaclotide should be sprinkled on one teaspoonful of room-temperature applesauce in a clean container. The entire mixture should be consumed (without chewing) immediately and should not be stored for later use.

For oral administration mixed in water, the entire contents of one capsule of linaclotide should be added to a clean cup containing approximately 30 mL of room-temperature bottled water, the mixture should be gently swirled for at least 20 seconds, and then the entire contents should be consumed immediately. Any beads remaining in the cup should be dispersed in an additional 30 mL of water, gently swirled again for at least 20 seconds, and then consumed immediately. The mixture should not be stored for later use. The manufacturer states that linaclotide is coated on the surface of the beads and will dissolve off the beads into the water. Thus, consumption of all the beads is not necessary to deliver a complete dose of the drug.

For administration via nasogastric or gastrostomy feeding tube, the entire contents of one linaclotide capsule should be added to a clean cup containing 30 mL of room-temperature bottled water, the mixture should be gently swirled for at least 20 seconds, and then the entire contents should be drawn up into an appropriately sized catheter-tipped syringe and administered into the nasogastric or gastrostomy tube rapidly (10 mL per 10 seconds) using steady pressure. Any beads remaining in the cup should be dispersed in an additional 30 mL of water and the process should be repeated. Following administration of the dose, the nasogastric or gastrostomy tube should be flushed with at least 10 mL of water. Because linaclotide is coated on the surface of the beads and will dissolve off the beads into the water, the manufacturer states that it is not necessary to administer all the beads to deliver a complete dose of the drug.

● **Dosage**

Adult Dosage

Irritable Bowel Syndrome with Constipation

The recommended adult dosage of linaclotide for the symptomatic treatment of irritable bowel syndrome (IBS) with constipation is 290 mcg once daily.

Chronic Idiopathic Constipation

The recommended adult dosage of linaclotide for the symptomatic treatment of chronic idiopathic constipation is 145 mcg once daily. A dosage of 72 mcg once daily may be used based on individual presentation and tolerability.

● **Special Populations**

Dosage adjustments are not needed in patients with renal or hepatic impairment.

The manufacturer makes no specific dosage recommendations for geriatric patients.

CAUTIONS

● **Contraindications**

Linaclotide is contraindicated in infants and children younger than 6 years of age. (See Pediatric Use under Warnings/Precautions: Specific Populations, in Cautions.) The drug also is contraindicated in any patient with known or suspected mechanical GI obstruction.

● **Warnings/Precautions**

Warnings

Pediatric Risk

In toxicology studies, linaclotide caused deaths due to dehydration in neonatal mice when administered in single, clinically relevant, adult oral doses. Linaclotide is contraindicated in infants and children younger than 6 years of age and should be avoided in children and adolescents 6 years to younger than 18 years of age. (See Pediatric Use under Warnings/Precautions: Specific Populations, in Cautions.)

Other Warnings and Precautions

Diarrhea

Diarrhea may occur, generally during the first 2 weeks of linaclotide therapy. The incidence of diarrhea is similar in patients with either irritable bowel syndrome (IBS) with constipation or chronic idiopathic constipation. In clinical trials in patients with these conditions, severe diarrhea was reported in 2% of patients receiving a linaclotide dosage of 145 or 290 mcg daily and in less than 1% of those receiving a dosage of 72 mcg daily. Cases of severe diarrhea that were associated with dizziness, syncope, hypotension, and electrolyte abnormalities (hypokalemia and hyponatremia) and that required hospitalization or administration of IV fluids have been reported during postmarketing experience with the drug. If severe diarrhea occurs, linaclotide therapy should be interrupted and the patient should be rehydrated.

Specific Populations

Pregnancy

Since systemic absorption of linaclotide and its active metabolite is negligible following oral administration, the drug is not expected to result in fetal exposure if administered to pregnant women. However, available data on use of linaclotide in pregnant women are insufficient to inform fetal risk.

No adverse effects on embryofetal development were observed in rats or rabbits when linaclotide was administered orally during organogenesis at dosages of up to 100,000 or 40,000 mcg/kg daily, respectively. Severe maternal toxicity and associated effects on fetal morphology were observed in mice at dosages of at least 40,000 mcg/kg daily. No developmental abnormalities and no effects on growth, learning and memory, or fertility were observed in the offspring of rats that received linaclotide orally at dosages up to 100,000 mcg/kg daily during the period of organogenesis through lactation. Limited systemic exposure to linaclotide was achieved in rats, rabbits, and mice during the period of organogenesis. Animal and human doses should not be compared directly for evaluating relative exposure.

Lactation

It is not known whether linaclotide is distributed into human milk, affects milk production, or affects the breast-fed infant.

Systemic absorption of linaclotide and its active metabolite is negligible following oral administration. It is not known whether the negligible systemic absorption observed in adults will result in clinically important exposure in breast-fed infants. The benefits of breast-feeding and the importance of linaclotide to the woman should be considered along with potential adverse effects on the breast-fed infant from the drug or from the underlying maternal condition. Exposure of infants to linaclotide could result in serious adverse effects. (See Pediatric Use under Warnings/Precautions: Specific Populations, in Cautions.)

Pediatric Use

Linaclotide is contraindicated in infants and children younger than 6 years of age and should be avoided in children and adolescents 6 years to younger than 18 years of age.

Safety and efficacy of linaclotide in pediatric patients younger than 18 years of age have not been established, and the drug has caused deaths within 24 hours of administration in toxicology studies in neonatal mice (age approximately equivalent to a human age of 0–28 days). In neonatal mice, administration of linaclotide 10 mcg/kg daily caused deaths on postnatal day 7. Tolerability to linaclotide increased with age in juvenile mice. In 2-week-old mice, linaclotide was well tolerated at a dosage of 50 mcg/kg daily, but deaths occurred after a single oral dose of 100 mcg/kg. In 3-week-old mice, linaclotide was well tolerated at a dosage of 100 mcg/kg daily, but deaths occurred after a single oral dose of 600 mcg/kg. The deaths in neonatal mice were due to rapid and severe dehydration resulting from increased fluid secretion into the intestine as a consequence of guanylate cyclase-C (GC-C) stimulation. Because of increased intestinal expression of GC-C, infants and children younger than 6 years of age may be at greater risk of developing diarrhea and its potentially serious consequences compared with individuals 6 years of age and older. Although no deaths occurred in older juvenile mice, use of the drug in children and adolescents 6 years to younger than

18 years of age should be avoided because of the deaths reported in younger mice and the lack of safety and efficacy data in pediatric patients.

Geriatric Use

Clinical studies of linaclotide did not include sufficient numbers of patients 65 years of age and older to determine whether geriatric patients respond differently than younger adults. In clinical trials in patients with IBS with constipation, 5% of patients were 65 years of age or older, while 1% were 75 years of age and older; in clinical trials in patients with chronic idiopathic constipation, 11% were 65 years of age or older, while 2% were 75 years of age and older. In general, dosage should be selected with caution in geriatric patients because of the greater frequency of decreased hepatic, renal, and/or cardiac function and of concomitant disease and/or drug therapy.

Hepatic Impairment

Linaclotide has not been studied in patients with hepatic impairment. However, because linaclotide is metabolized within the GI tract and has negligible systemic bioavailability following oral administration, hepatic impairment is not expected to affect metabolism or clearance of the drug or its metabolite.

Renal Impairment

Linaclotide has not been studied in patients with renal impairment. However, because linaclotide is metabolized within the GI tract and has negligible systemic bioavailability following oral administration, renal impairment is not expected to affect clearance of the drug or its metabolite.

● Common Adverse Effects

Adverse effects reported in 2% or more of patients receiving linaclotide 290 mcg daily for the treatment of IBS with constipation, and more frequently with the drug than with placebo, include diarrhea, abdominal pain, flatulence, abdominal distension, viral gastroenteritis, and headache.

Adverse effects reported in 2% or more of patients receiving linaclotide 145 mcg daily for the treatment of chronic idiopathic constipation, and more frequently with the drug than with placebo, include diarrhea, abdominal pain, flatulence, abdominal distension, upper respiratory tract infection, and sinusitis.

Adverse effects reported in 2% or more of patients receiving linaclotide 72 mcg daily for the treatment of chronic idiopathic constipation, and more frequently with the drug than with placebo, include diarrhea and abdominal distension.

DRUG INTERACTIONS

No formal drug interaction studies have been conducted with linaclotide to date. However, systemic exposure to linaclotide and its active metabolite is negligible following oral administration at recommended dosages, and in vitro studies indicate that linaclotide does not interact with cytochrome P-450 (CYP) isoenzymes or with common efflux and uptake transporters, including the P-glycoprotein (P-gp) efflux transporter. Thus, no interactions mediated by CYP enzymes or common transporters are anticipated.

DESCRIPTION

Linaclotide, a guanylate cyclase-C (GC-C) agonist, is a 14-amino acid peptide structurally related to endogenous guanylin peptide hormones that regulate fluid and electrolyte balance in the intestine. The parent drug and its active metabolite bind to GC-C receptors on the luminal surface of the intestinal epithelium, which increases intracellular and extracellular concentrations of cyclic guanosine monophosphate (cGMP). In turn, increased intracellular concentrations of cGMP trigger a signal-transduction cascade activating the cystic fibrosis transmembrane conductance regulator (CFTR) ion channel. This results in secretion of chloride and bicarbonate into the intestinal lumen causing increased intestinal fluid and accelerated intestinal transit. Linaclotide has been shown to change stool consistency and increase stool frequency.

In animal models, linaclotide also decreased visceral hyperalgesia and abdominal pain. This effect in animals is thought to be mediated by activation of GC-C leading to increased extracellular concentrations of cGMP, which inhibits colonic nociceptors. Further research is needed to determine the precise mechanism(s) by which linaclotide relieves abdominal pain in patients with irritable bowel syndrome (IBS) with constipation.

After oral administration, linaclotide is minimally absorbed with negligible systemic bioavailability. Linaclotide is metabolized by carboxypeptidase A within the GI tract to an active metabolite; both the parent drug and active metabolite are further degraded within the intestinal lumen to smaller peptides and amino acids. Following multiple-dose oral administration, about 3–5% of the drug is recovered in feces as active peptide, principally as active metabolite.

ADVICE TO PATIENTS

Importance of reading the manufacturer's patient information (medication guide) prior to initiation of therapy and each time the prescription is refilled.

Importance of advising patients that accidental ingestion of linaclotide by a child, especially a child younger than 6 years of age, may result in severe diarrhea and dehydration; importance of keeping linaclotide out of reach of children and of properly disposing of any unused drug. (See Pediatric Use under Warnings/Precautions: Specific Populations, in Cautions.)

Importance of advising patients that abdominal pain or diarrhea may occur and that they should discontinue linaclotide and contact their clinician if severe diarrhea or unusual or severe abdominal pain occurs, especially if associated with hematochezia or melena.

Importance of taking linaclotide once daily on an empty stomach; the capsule should be swallowed whole, and the capsule or capsule contents should not be crushed or chewed. Importance of advising patient of alternative forms of administration if patient is unable to swallow whole capsule.

Importance of storing linaclotide in the original container, with the lid tightly closed and the contents protected from moisture; importance of not removing the desiccant from the container and of not repackaging the capsules.

If a dose is missed, the missed dose should be omitted and the next dose taken at the regularly scheduled time. Two doses should not be taken at the same time to make up for a missed dose.

Importance of informing clinicians of existing or contemplated concomitant therapy, including prescription and OTC drugs, as well as any concomitant illnesses.

Importance of women informing clinicians if they are or plan to become pregnant or plan to breast-feed.

Importance of informing patients of other important precautionary information. (See Cautions.)

PREPARATIONS

Excipients in commercially available drug preparations may have clinically important effects in some individuals; consult specific product labeling for details.

Linaclotide

Oral			
Capsules	72 mcg		Linzess®, Allergan
	145 mcg		Linzess®, Allergan
	290 mcg		Linzess®, Allergan

† Use is not currently included in the labeling approved by the US Food and Drug Administration.

Plecanatide

56:18.12 • GUANYLATE CYCLASE C (GC-C) RECEPTOR AGONISTS

■ Plecanatide, a guanylate cyclase-C (GC-C) agonist, stimulates secretion of chloride and bicarbonate into the intestinal lumen, which increases intestinal fluid and accelerates intestinal transit.

USES

● Chronic Idiopathic Constipation

Plecanatide is used in adults for the symptomatic treatment of chronic idiopathic constipation.

Efficacy and safety of plecanatide for the symptomatic treatment of chronic idiopathic constipation have been evaluated in 2 randomized, double-blind, placebo-controlled studies in adults who met modified Rome III criteria for functional constipation for a minimum of 3 months prior to screening, with symptom onset at least 6 months prior to diagnosis. The modified Rome III criteria specified fewer than 3 defecations per week, rare occurrence of loose stool in the absence of laxative use, no use of manual maneuvers to facilitate defecation, failure to meet criteria for irritable bowel syndrome with constipation, and presence of 2 or more of the following symptoms for at least 25% of defecations: straining, lumpy or hard stool, sensation of incomplete evacuation, or sensation of anorectal obstruction/blockage. Patients also were required to meet the following 3 criteria during the last 2 weeks of the screening period: fewer than 3 complete spontaneous bowel movements (CSBMs) in each of the 2 weeks, a score of 6 or 7 on the Bristol Stool Form Scale for fewer than 25% of spontaneous bowel movements (SBMs), and one of the following criteria: a score of 1 or 2 on the Bristol Stool Form Scale for 25% or more of defecations, a straining value recorded on at least 25% of days when a bowel movement was reported, or a sense of incomplete evacuation following at least 25% of bowel movements. In the 2 studies combined, the mean age of patients was 45 years, and most patients were female (80%) and white (72%). Eligible patients were randomized to receive plecanatide 3 or 6 mg once daily or placebo for 12 weeks and then were followed for an additional 2 weeks. In the 2 studies combined, the intention-to-treat population included 2656 patients.

On a daily basis, patients recorded information on bowel function and symptoms in an electronic diary. The primary efficacy end point of both studies was the proportion of patients who achieved a response, defined as 3 or more CSBMs in a given week and an increase of 1 or more CSBMs from baseline in the same week for a minimum of 9 weeks out of the 12-week treatment period and for at least 3 of the last 4 weeks of the study. In both studies, a greater proportion of patients receiving plecanatide 3 mg daily compared with those receiving placebo (21 versus 10–13%, respectively) achieved a response. An increase in CSBM frequency (i.e., number of CSBMs per week) was observed within the first week of therapy and was sustained through week 12. The difference between patients receiving plecanatide 3 mg daily and those receiving placebo in the mean change in CSBM frequency from baseline to week 12 was approximately 1.1 CSBMs per week.

Over the 12-week treatment period, improvements were observed in stool frequency (number of CSBMs and SBMs per week), stool consistency (as measured by the Bristol Stool Form Scale), and/or amount of straining with bowel movements in patients receiving plecanatide 3 mg daily compared with those receiving placebo. During the 2-week period following discontinuance of treatment, patients' diary entries generally reverted to baseline status.

Plecanatide 6 mg once daily did not provide additional clinical benefit beyond that provided by the 3-mg daily dosage and was associated with an increased incidence of adverse effects. A response was achieved by 20% of patients receiving the 6-mg daily dosage.

DOSAGE AND ADMINISTRATION

● Administration

Plecanatide is administered orally without regard to food. Although administration with a meal resulted in looser stools when compared with administration in the fasted state, plecanatide was administered with or without food in clinical trials.

Plecanatide tablets should be swallowed whole. Alternatively, for patients who are unable to swallow whole tablets, plecanatide tablets may be crushed and administered orally mixed in applesauce or dispersed in water and administered orally or via a nasogastric or gastric feeding tube. The manufacturer states that mixing crushed plecanatide tablets in soft foods other than applesauce or dispersing the tablets in liquids other than water has not been studied.

If a dose of plecanatide is missed, a double dose should not be administered to make up for the missed dose. The next dose should be taken at the regularly scheduled time.

For administration in applesauce, a plecanatide 3-mg tablet should be crushed to a powder and mixed with one teaspoonful of room-temperature applesauce in a clean container. The entire mixture should be consumed immediately and should not be stored for later use.

For oral administration as an aqueous dispersion, a plecanatide 3-mg tablet should be placed in a clean cup, approximately 30 mL of room-temperature water should then be added to the cup, and the mixture should be gently swirled for at least 10 seconds to disperse the disintegrating tablet. The entire mixture should be consumed immediately. Any residue remaining in the cup should be dispersed in an additional 30 mL of water, gently swirled again for at least 10 seconds, and then consumed immediately. The mixture should not be stored for later use.

For administration via nasogastric or gastric feeding tube, a plecanatide 3-mg tablet should be placed in a clean cup, approximately 30 mL of room-temperature water should be added to the cup, and the mixture should be gently swirled for at least 15 seconds to disperse the disintegrating tablet. The nasogastric or gastric feeding tube should be flushed with 30 mL of water and then the entire contents of the mixture should be drawn up into a syringe and administered immediately. Any residue remaining in the cup should be dispersed in an additional 30 mL of water, gently swirled again for at least 15 seconds, and then administered via the nasogastric or gastric feeding tube using the same syringe. Following administration of the dose, the nasogastric or gastric feeding tube should be flushed with at least 10 mL of water using either the same syringe or a new syringe. The mixture should not be stored for later use.

● Dosage

The recommended adult dosage of plecanatide for the symptomatic treatment of chronic idiopathic constipation is 3 mg once daily. A dosage of 6 mg daily is not recommended; in clinical trials, the 6-mg daily dosage did not provide additional clinical benefit beyond that provided by the 3-mg daily dosage and was associated with an increased incidence of adverse effects.

● Special Populations

The manufacturer makes no specific dosage recommendations for geriatric patients or for patients with renal or hepatic impairment. (See Specific Populations under Cautions: Warnings/Precautions.)

CAUTIONS

● Contraindications

Plecanatide is contraindicated in infants and children younger than 6 years of age. (See Pediatric Use under Warnings/Precautions: Specific Populations, in Cautions.) The drug also is contraindicated in any patient with known or suspected mechanical GI obstruction.

● Warnings/Precautions

Warnings

Pediatric Risk

In toxicology studies, plecanatide caused deaths due to dehydration in young juvenile mice within 24 hours following single-dose oral administration. Plecanatide is contraindicated in infants and children younger than 6 years of age and should be avoided in children and adolescents 6 years to younger than 18 years of age. (See Pediatric Use under Warnings/Precautions: Specific Populations, in Cautions.)

Other Warnings and Precautions
Diarrhea

In clinical trials in patients with chronic idiopathic constipation, diarrhea resulting in drug discontinuance occurred in 2% of patients receiving plecanatide 3 mg daily compared with 0.5% of patients receiving placebo, while severe diarrhea was reported in 0.6 or 0.3% of patients receiving plecanatide 3 mg daily or placebo, respectively. Most reported cases of diarrhea occurred within 4 weeks of drug initiation, and severe diarrhea occurred within the first 3 days of treatment. Plecanatide therapy should be interrupted and the patient should be rehydrated if severe diarrhea develops.

Specific Populations
Pregnancy

Since systemic absorption of plecanatide and its active metabolite is negligible following oral administration, the drug is not expected to result in fetal exposure if administered to pregnant women. However, available data on use of plecanatide in pregnant women are insufficient to inform fetal risk.

No adverse effects on embryofetal development were observed in mice or rabbits when plecanatide was administered orally during organogenesis at dosages up to 800 or 250 mg/kg daily, respectively. In addition, no developmental abnormalities and no effects on growth, learning and memory, or fertility were observed in the offspring of mice that received plecanatide orally at dosages up to 600 mg/kg daily during the period of organogenesis through lactation. Limited systemic exposure to plecanatide was achieved in rabbits during the period of organogenesis. Animal and human doses should not be compared directly for evaluating relative exposure.

Lactation

It is not known whether plecanatide is distributed into human milk, affects milk production, or affects the breast-fed infant.

Systemic absorption of plecanatide and its active metabolite is negligible following oral administration. It is not known whether the negligible systemic absorption observed in adults will result in clinically important exposure in breast-fed infants. The benefits of breast-feeding and the importance of plecanatide to the woman should be considered along with potential adverse effects on the breast-fed infant from the drug or from the underlying maternal condition. Exposure of infants to plecanatide could result in serious adverse effects. (See Pediatric Use under Warnings/Precautions: Specific Populations, in Cautions.)

Pediatric Use

Plecanatide is contraindicated in infants and children younger than 6 years of age and should be avoided in children and adolescents 6 years to younger than 18 years of age.

Safety and efficacy of plecanatide in pediatric patients younger than 18 years of age have not been established, and the drug has caused deaths within 24 hours of administration in toxicology studies in juvenile mice (age approximately equivalent to a human age of 1 month to younger than 2 years). The deaths in young juvenile mice occurred following single oral doses of plecanatide 0.5 and 10 mg/kg administered on postnatal days 7 and 14, respectively. The deaths apparently were due to dehydration resulting from increased fluid secretion into the intestine as a consequence of guanylate cyclase-C (GC-C) stimulation. Because of increased intestinal expression of GC-C, infants and children younger than 6 years of age may be at greater risk of developing diarrhea and its potentially serious consequences compared with individuals 6 years of age and older. Although no deaths were observed in older juvenile mice, use of plecanatide should be avoided in children and adolescents 6 years to younger than 18 years of age because of the deaths reported in younger mice and the lack of safety and efficacy data in pediatric patients. Although administration of the recommended plecanatide dosage (approximately 0.05 mg/kg daily in a 60-kg individual) in adults does not result in measurable plasma concentrations of the drug, systemic absorption was observed in juvenile animal toxicology studies; animal and human doses should not be compared directly for evaluating relative exposure.

Geriatric Use

Clinical trials of plecanatide did not include sufficient numbers of patients 65 years of age and older to determine whether geriatric patients respond differently than younger adults. In clinical trials in patients with chronic idiopathic constipation, 10% of patients were 65 years of age and older, while 2% were 75 years of age and older. Because of the greater frequency of decreased hepatic, renal, and/or cardiac function and of concomitant disease and drug therapy observed in the elderly, dosage selection for geriatric patients should be cautious.

Hepatic Impairment

The pharmacokinetics of plecanatide have not been formally studied in patients with hepatic impairment since the drug is not appreciably absorbed after oral administration.

Renal Impairment

The pharmacokinetics of plecanatide have not been formally studied in patients with renal impairment since the drug is not appreciably absorbed after oral administration.

● Common Adverse Effects

Diarrhea was reported in 5% of patients with chronic idiopathic constipation receiving plecanatide 3 mg daily and more frequently with the drug than with placebo.

DRUG INTERACTIONS

Because plasma concentrations of plecanatide and its active metabolite are not measurable in adults following oral administration at the recommended dosage, only enzyme and transporter systems that are expressed in the GI tract have been evaluated for interaction potential. In vitro studies indicate that plecanatide and its active metabolite do not inhibit cytochrome P-450 (CYP) isoenzyme 2C9 or 3A4, do not induce CYP3A4, and are not substrates or inhibitors of P-glycoprotein (P-gp) or breast cancer resistance protein (BCRP).

DESCRIPTION

Plecanatide, a guanylate cyclase-C (GC-C) agonist, is a 16-amino acid peptide structurally related to endogenous uroguanylin peptide hormone. The parent drug and its active metabolite bind to GC-C receptors on the luminal surface of the intestinal epithelium, which increases intracellular and extracellular concentrations of cyclic guanosine monophosphate (cGMP). In turn, increased intracellular concentrations of cGMP trigger a signal-transduction cascade activating the cystic fibrosis transmembrane conductance regulator (CFTR) ion channel. This results in secretion of chloride and bicarbonate into the intestinal lumen causing increased intestinal fluid and accelerated intestinal transit.

In animal models, plecanatide has been shown to reduce abdominal muscle contractions (a measure of intestinal pain), increase fluid secretion into the GI tract, accelerate intestinal transit, and change stool consistency. Further research is needed to determine the precise mechanism(s) by which plecanatide relieves intestinal pain.

After oral administration, plecanatide is minimally absorbed with negligible systemic bioavailability. Administration of a single 9-mg dose of plecanatide with either a low-fat, low-calorie or a high-fat, high-calorie meal resulted in looser stools compared with administration in the fasting state. Plecanatide is metabolized in the GI tract to an active metabolite via lysis of the terminal leucine moiety. Plecanatide and its metabolite are proteolytically degraded within the intestinal lumen to smaller peptides and naturally occurring amino acids.

ADVICE TO PATIENTS

Importance of reading the manufacturer's patient information (medication guide) prior to initiation of therapy and each time the prescription is refilled.

Importance of advising patients that accidental ingestion of plecanatide by a child, especially a child younger than 6 years of age, may result in severe diarrhea and dehydration; importance of keeping plecanatide out of reach of children and of properly disposing of any unused drug. (See Pediatric Use under Warnings/Precautions: Specific Populations, in Cautions.)

Importance of advising patients that diarrhea may occur and that they should discontinue plecanatide and notify their clinician if diarrhea becomes severe.

Importance of advising patient of alternative forms of administration if patient is unable to swallow whole tablets.

Importance of storing plecanatide in the original container, with the lid tightly closed and the contents protected from moisture; importance of removing the polyester coil after opening the container, of not removing the desiccant from the container, and of not repackaging the tablets.

If a dose is missed, the missed dose should be omitted and the next dose taken at the regularly scheduled time. Two doses should not be taken at the same time to make up for a missed dose.

Importance of informing clinicians of existing or contemplated concomitant therapy, including prescription and OTC drugs, as well as any concomitant illnesses.

Importance of women informing clinicians if they are or plan to become pregnant or plan to breast-feed.

Importance of informing patients of other important precautionary information. (See Cautions.)

PREPARATIONS

Excipients in commercially available drug preparations may have clinically important effects in some individuals; consult specific product labeling for details.

Plecanatide

Oral

Tablets	3 mg	Trulance®, Synergy

† Use is not currently included in the labeling approved by the US Food and Drug Administration.

Selected Revisions May 10, 2024, © Copyright, March 8, 2017, American Society of Health-System Pharmacists, Inc.

dimenhyDRINATE

56:22.08 • ANTIHISTAMINES

- Dimenhydrinate, an ethanolamine-derivative antihistamine containing a diphenhydramine moiety, is an antiemetic.

USES

● Motion Sickness

Dimenhydrinate is used principally in the prevention and treatment of nausea, vomiting, and/or vertigo associated with motion sickness, although scopolamine, promethazine, or meclizine may be more effective. Dimenhydrinate is most effective against motion sickness when given prophylactically, although susceptibility to motion sickness may vary with the patient's age, previous exposure to motion, and the type, severity, and duration of motion.

● Other Uses

Dimenhydrinate has been used for symptomatic treatment of Ménière's disease† and other vestibular disturbances†. Like other antihistamines, dimenhydrinate may be less effective than the phenothiazines in controlling nausea and vomiting not related to vestibular stimulation.

Although dimenhydrinate is a histamine antagonist, its use in allergic states has not been evaluated.

DOSAGE AND ADMINISTRATION

● Administration

Dimenhydrinate may be administered orally or by IM or IV injection. For IV injection, each 50 mg of dimenhydrinate must be diluted with 10 mL of 0.9% sodium chloride injection and administered slowly over a period of 2 minutes.

● Dosage

For the prevention of motion sickness, dimenhydrinate should be taken orally 30 minutes before exposure to motion. For the prevention and treatment of nausea, vomiting, and/or vertigo associated with motion sickness, the usual oral dosage of dimenhydrinate for *self-medication* in adults and children 12 years of age or older is 50–100 mg every 4–6 hours, not to exceed 400 mg in 24 hours, or as directed by a clinician. The same dosage can be given parenterally in adults to treat motion sickness. Children 6 to younger than 12 years of age may receive 25–50 mg orally every 6–8 hours, not to exceed 150 mg in 24 hours, or as directed by a clinician. Children 2 to younger than 6 years of age may receive 12.5–25 mg orally every 6–8 hours, not to exceed 75 mg in 24 hours, or as directed by a clinician. Alternatively, children may be given 1.25 mg/kg or 37.5 mg/m², orally or IM 4 times daily, up to a maximum of 300 mg daily. Children younger than 2 years of age should receive oral dimenhydrinate only under the direction of a clinician. IV dosage has not been established for children.

For symptomatic relief of Ménière's disease, 25–50 mg of dimenhydrinate has been given orally 3 times daily for maintenance, or 50 mg has been given IM for acute attacks.

CAUTIONS

● Adverse Effects

Drowsiness commonly occurs after administration of dimenhydrinate. Paradoxical CNS stimulation may occur in children and occasionally in adults.

Other adverse effects include headache, blurred vision, tinnitus, dryness of the mouth and respiratory passages, incoordination, palpitation, dizziness, and hypotension. Anorexia, constipation or diarrhea, urinary frequency, and dysuria are less common. Pain may occur at the site of IM injection. Because dimenhydrinate contains diphenhydramine, the possibility of other diphenhydramine-related adverse effects should also be considered. (See the Antihistamines General Statement 4:00 and Diphenhydramine Hydrochloride 4:04.)

● Precautions and Contraindications

Patients should be warned that dimenhydrinate may impair their ability to perform hazardous activities requiring mental alertness or physical coordination (e.g., operating machinery or driving a motor vehicle). Sedation may be enhanced by other CNS depressants. (See Drug Interactions: CNS Depressants.)

Dramamine® chewable tablets contain the dye tartrazine (FD&C yellow No. 5), which may cause allergic reactions including bronchial asthma in certain susceptible individuals. Although the incidence of tartrazine sensitivity is low, it frequently occurs in individuals who are sensitive to aspirin.

Dimenhydrinate should be used with caution in patients with seizure disorders. The anticholinergic effects of the drug should be considered when administering dimenhydrinate to patients with conditions that might be aggravated by anticholinergic therapy (e.g., angle-closure glaucoma, enlargement of the prostate gland). The drug may mask symptoms of ototoxicity and therefore should be administered with caution to patients receiving known ototoxic drugs. These patients should be closely monitored during therapy with dimenhydrinate.

● Pregnancy, Fertility, and Lactation

Pregnancy

Reproduction studies in rats and rabbits using dimenhydrinate doses up to 20 and 25 times the human dose (on a mg/kg basis), respectively, have not revealed evidence of harm to the fetus. There are no adequate and well-controlled studies using dimenhydrinate in pregnant women. Clinical studies to date in pregnant women receiving the drug have not indicated an increased risk of abnormalities when administered during any trimester. Although the possibility of harm to the fetus appears remote, dimenhydrinate should be used during pregnancy only when clearly needed.

Fertility

Reproduction studies in rats and rabbits using dimenhydrinate doses up to 20 and 25 times the human dose (on a mg/kg basis), respectively, have not revealed evidence of impaired fertility.

Lactation

Small amounts of dimenhydrinate are distributed into milk. Because of the potential for adverse reactions to dimenhydrinate in nursing infants, a decision should be made whether to discontinue nursing or the drug, taking into account the importance of the drug to the woman.

DRUG INTERACTIONS

● CNS Depressants

Dimenhydrinate may enhance the effects of other CNS depressants such as alcohol and barbiturates. If dimenhydrinate is used concomitantly with other CNS depressants, caution should be used to avoid overdosage.

● Drugs with Anticholinergic Effects

Because dimenhydrinate also has anticholinergic activity, it may potentiate the effects of other drugs with anticholinergic activity including tricyclic antidepressants.

● Ototoxic Drugs

When given concurrently with aminoglycoside antibiotics or other ototoxic drugs, dimenhydrinate may mask the early symptoms of ototoxicity. (See Cautions: Precautions and Contraindications.)

● Other Drugs

Although dimenhydrinate has been reported to induce hepatic microsomal enzymes in animals, there is no clinical evidence that dimenhydrinate influences the metabolism of other drugs in humans.

ACUTE TOXICITY

● Manifestations

Accidental antihistamine overdose occurs frequently in infants and children. Symptoms of dimenhydrinate toxicity in children may resemble atropine overdosage and include dilated pupils, flushed face, excitation, hallucinations, confusion, ataxia, intermittent clonic convulsions, coma, cardiorespiratory collapse, and death. Symptoms may be delayed for up to 2 hours after ingestion; death may occur within 18 hours.

In adults, 500 mg or more of dimenhydrinate may cause extreme difficulty in speech and swallowing, and produces a psychosis indistinguishable from that of atropine poisoning. CNS excitation may be preceded by sedation, leading to a cycle of CNS excitation, seizures, and postictal depression.

● Treatment

Treatment of dimenhydrinate toxicity is symptomatic and supportive. Emetics are usually ineffective, but in the absence of seizures, early gastric lavage (with an endotracheal tube with cuff inflated in place to prevent aspiration of gastric contents) may be beneficial. Patients should be kept quiet to minimize CNS stimulation; seizures may be treated with diazepam in adults and phenobarbital in children. Mechanical respiratory assistance may be required.

PHARMACOLOGY

The pharmacologic effects of dimenhydrinate are believed to result principally from its diphenhydramine moiety. Like diphenhydramine, dimenhydrinate has CNS depressant, anticholinergic, antiemetic, antihistaminic, and local anesthetic effects. Although its exact mechanism of antiemetic action is unknown, dimenhydrinate has been shown to inhibit vestibular stimulation, acting first on the otolith system, and in larger doses on the semicircular canals. Dimenhydrinate inhibits acetylcholine; some investigators believe this is its primary mechanism of action, since cholinergic stimulation in the vestibular and reticular systems may be responsible for the nausea and vomiting of motion sickness. Tolerance to CNS depressant effects usually occurs after a few days of treatment, and some decrease in antiemetic effectiveness may be noted after prolonged use.

PHARMACOKINETICS

● Absorption

Dimenhydrinate is well absorbed after oral or parenteral administration. Antiemetic effects occur almost immediately after IV administration, within 15–30 minutes after oral administration, and 20–30 minutes after IM administration. The duration of action is 3–6 hours.

● Distribution and Elimination

Little information is available on the distribution and metabolic fate of dimenhydrinate. Like other antihistamines, the drug probably is widely distributed into body tissues, crosses the placenta, is metabolized by the liver, and is excreted in urine. Small amounts of dimenhydrinate are distributed into milk.

CHEMISTRY AND STABILITY

● Chemistry

Dimenhydrinate is an ethanolamine-derivative antihistamine that is used as an antiemetic. The drug contains 53–55.5% diphenhydramine and 44–47% 8-chlorotheophylline. Dimenhydrinate occurs as a white, odorless, crystalline powder with a bitter, numbing taste, and is slightly soluble in water and freely soluble in alcohol and in propylene glycol. Dimenhydrinate injection is a sterile solution of the drug in a mixture of propylene glycol and water and has a pH of 6.4–7.2.

● Stability

Dimenhydrinate preparations should be stored at room temperature; freezing of the oral solution and injection should be avoided. Dimenhydrinate tablets should be stored in well-closed containers and the oral solution in tight containers.

Dimenhydrinate injection has been reported to be incompatible with many drugs, but the compatibility depends on several factors (e.g., concentrations of the drugs, specific diluents used, resulting pH, temperature). Specialized references should be consulted for specific compatibility information.

PREPARATIONS

Excipients in commercially available drug preparations may have clinically important effects in some individuals; consult specific product labeling for details.

dimenhyDRINATE

Oral		
Solution	12.5 mg/5 mL*	**DMH®** Syrup, Alra
		Dramamine® Children's (with methylparaben), Pfizer
Tablets	50 mg*	**Dramamine®** (scored), Pfizer
Tablets, chewable	50 mg	**Dramamine® Children's** (with sorbitol and tartrazine; scored), Pfizer
Tablets, film-coated	50 mg	**TripTone® Caplets®** (scored), Del
Parenteral		
Injection	50 mg/mL*	**dimenhyDRINATE Injection** (with propylene glycol and benzyl alcohol), Abraxis

* available from one or more manufacturer, distributor, and/or repackager by generic (nonproprietary) name

† Use is not currently included in the labeling approved by the US Food and Drug Administration.

Selected Revisions July 1, 2006, © Copyright, May 1, 1977, American Society of Health-System Pharmacists, Inc.

Meclizine Hydrochloride

56:22.08 • ANTIHISTAMINES

■ Meclizine, a piperazine-derivative antihistamine, is an antiemetic.

USES

● Motion Sickness

Meclizine hydrochloride is used in the prevention and treatment of nausea, vomiting, and/or vertigo associated with motion sickness. Meclizine is most effective against motion sickness when given prophylactically, although susceptibility to motion sickness may vary with the patient's age, previous exposure to motion, and the type, severity, and duration of motion. Although scopolamine generally is considered to be the most effective drug for the treatment of motion sickness, most clinicians prefer an antihistamine such as meclizine because it produces fewer adverse anticholinergic effects than does scopolamine. Meclizine and dimenhydrinate generally are considered to be equally effective in the treatment of motion sickness, but dimenhydrinate causes drowsiness more frequently. Meclizine has a longer duration of action than scopolamine and most other antihistamines. Promethazine may be more effective than other antihistamines in the treatment of motion sickness.

● Other Uses

Meclizine has been used in the symptomatic treatment of vertigo associated with diseases affecting the vestibular system (e.g., labyrinthitis, Ménière's disease), but the value of the drug in these conditions has not been established. Like other antihistamines, meclizine is less effective than the phenothiazines in controlling nausea and vomiting not related to vestibular stimulation.

Although meclizine is a histamine H_1-receptor antagonist, its use in allergic states has not been evaluated.

DOSAGE AND ADMINISTRATION

● Administration

Meclizine hydrochloride is administered orally.

● Dosage

For the prevention and treatment of nausea, vomiting, and/or vertigo associated with motion sickness, the usual oral dosage of meclizine hydrochloride in adults and children 12 years of age or older is 25–50 mg once daily or as directed by a physician. For the prevention of motion sickness, 25–50 mg of the drug may be given 1 hour before exposure to motion.

For the control of vertigo associated with diseases affecting the vestibular system, the usual adult dosage is 25–100 mg daily, administered in divided doses.

For further information on pharmacology, cautions, and acute toxicity in therapy with meclizine, see the Antihistamines General Statement 4:00.

CAUTIONS

● Adverse Effects

Drowsiness, fatigue, dry mouth, and, rarely, blurred vision have occurred after administration of meclizine.

● Precautions and Contraindications

Patients should be warned that meclizine may impair their ability to perform hazardous activities requiring mental alertness or physical coordination (e.g., operating machinery, driving a motor vehicle). In addition, additive CNS depression may occur when antihistamines, such as meclizine, are administered concomitantly with other CNS depressants including barbiturates, tranquilizers, and alcohol. If meclizine is used concomitantly with other depressant drugs, caution should be used to avoid overdosage. The anticholinergic effects of the drug should be considered when administering meclizine to patients with angle-closure glaucoma or prostatic hypertrophy.

Meclizine is contraindicated in patients who are hypersensitive to it.

● Pediatric Precautions

Safety and efficacy of meclizine in children younger than 12 years of age have not been established; therefore, the manufacturers state that use of the drug in this age group is not recommended. If the drug is used in this age group (e.g., for the prevention and treatment of nausea, vomiting, and/or vertigo associated with motion sickness), it should be only under the advice and supervision of a physician.

● Pregnancy, Fertility, and Lactation

Pregnancy

Meclizine is teratogenic in animals. Although retrospective studies in humans suggest that the use of meclizine during pregnancy is probably not associated with teratogenic effects, the manufacturers state that the drug is contraindicated in women who are or may become pregnant.

PHARMACOLOGY

Meclizine has CNS depressant, anticholinergic, antiemetic, antispasmodic, and local anesthetic effects in addition to antihistaminic activity. The drug depresses labyrinth excitability and conduction in vestibular-cerebellar pathways. The antiemetic and antimotion-sickness actions of meclizine result, at least in part, from its central anticholinergic and CNS depressant properties.

PHARMACOKINETICS

The onset of action of meclizine hydrochloride is about 1 hour and the drug has a prolonged duration of action, with effects persisting 8–24 hours following administration of a single oral dose. The drug has a plasma half-life of 6 hours. The metabolic fate of meclizine in humans is unknown. In rats, meclizine is metabolized (probably in the liver) to norchlorcyclizine. This metabolite is distributed throughout most body tissues and crosses the placenta. The drug is excreted in feces unchanged and in urine as norchlorcyclizine.

CHEMISTRY AND STABILITY

● Chemistry

Meclizine is a piperazine-derivative antihistamine that is used as an antiemetic. Meclizine hydrochloride occurs as a white or slightly yellowish, crystalline powder, has a slight odor and is tasteless, and is practically insoluble in water and slightly soluble in alcohol.

● Stability

Meclizine hydrochloride preparations should be stored at a temperature less than 40°C, preferably between 15–30°C; the conventional tablets should be stored in well-closed containers.

PREPARATIONS

Excipients in commercially available drug preparations may have clinically important effects in some individuals; consult specific product labeling for details.

Meclizine Hydrochloride

Oral		
Capsules	25 mg	**Meni-D**®, Seatrace
Tablets	12.5 mg*	**Antivert**®, Pfizer
	25 mg*	**Antivert**®, Pfizer
		Dramamine® Less Drowsy, Pfizer
	50 mg*	**Antivert**® (scored), Pfizer
Tablets, chewable	25 mg*	**Bonine**® (scored), Insight

* available from one or more manufacturer, distributor, and/or repackager by generic (nonproprietary) name

Selected Revisions January 1, 2006, © Copyright, January 1, 1979, American Society of Health-System Pharmacists, Inc.

Prochlorperazine, Prochlorperazine Edisylate, Prochlorperazine Maleate

56:22.08 • ANTIHISTAMINES

■ Prochlorperazine, a phenothiazine derivative, is an antiemetic.

USES

Prochlorperazine is used for the control of severe nausea and vomiting of various etiologies. The drug is effective for the management of postoperative nausea and vomiting, and that caused by toxins, radiation, or cytotoxic drugs. Prochlorperazine also is effective for the relief of acute migraine attacks and associated nausea and vomiting. (For further information on management and classification of migraine headache, see Vascular Headaches: General Principles in Migraine Therapy, under Uses in Sumatriptan 28:32.28.) Prochlorperazine is not effective in preventing vertigo or motion sickness, or for the management of emesis caused by the action of drugs on the nodose ganglion or locally on the GI tract. Because safety of prochlorperazine for the prevention and treatment of nausea and vomiting associated with pregnancy has not been established, use of the drug is not recommended during pregnancy except in cases of severe nausea and vomiting so serious and intractable that, in the judgment of the clinician, pharmacologic intervention is required and the potential benefits justify the possible risks to the fetus. (See Cautions: Pregnancy, Fertility, and Lactation in the Phenothiazines General Statement 28:16.08.24.)

For the use of prochlorperazine as an antipsychotic agent, see 28:16.08.24.

DOSAGE AND ADMINISTRATION

● Administration

Prochlorperazine edisylate is administered orally, by deep IM injection, or by direct IV injection or by IV infusion. When administered by direct IV injection, prochlorperazine is administered at a rate not exceeding 5 mg/minute; the drug should not be given as a bolus injection. Subcutaneous administration of the drug is not recommended because of local irritation. Prochlorperazine maleate is administered orally. Prochlorperazine is administered rectally.

For IV infusion, 20 mg (4 mL) of prochlorperazine injection should be diluted in 1 L of a compatible IV infusion solution (e.g., 0.9% sodium chloride).

● Dosage

Dosage of prochlorperazine and its salts is expressed in terms of prochlorperazine. Dosage must be carefully adjusted according to individual requirements and response, using the lowest possible effective dosage. Dosage should be increased more gradually in debilitated, emaciated, or geriatric patients. Since geriatric patients may be more susceptible to hypotension and neuromuscular reactions, these patients should be observed closely; in general, dosages in the lower end of the range are sufficient for most geriatric patients. Since children appear to be more prone to extrapyramidal reactions, even at moderate dosages, they should receive the lowest possible effective dosage and parents should be instructed not to exceed the prescribed dosage.

For the control of severe nausea and vomiting in patients who can tolerate oral administration of the drug, the usual adult oral dosage of prochlorperazine is 5 or 10 mg 3 or 4 times daily. Alternatively, a dosage of 15 mg (as the extended-release Spansule®) once daily upon arising or 10 mg (as the extended-release Spansule®) every 12 hours may be used; some patients subsequently may require a dosage of 30 mg (using the appropriate number of 10- or 15-mg extended-release Spansules®) once daily in the morning. Oral dosages exceeding 40 mg daily should be used only in resistant cases. The usual adult rectal dosage of prochlorperazine for the control of severe nausea and vomiting is 25 mg twice daily. The usual initial adult IM dose of prochlorperazine for the control of severe nausea and vomiting

is 5–10 mg. If necessary, the initial IM dose may be repeated every 3 or 4 hours, but total IM dosage should not exceed 40 mg daily. For the control of severe nausea and vomiting, the usual adult IV dose of prochlorperazine is 2.5–10 mg; single IV doses of the drug should not exceed 10 mg and total IV dosage should not exceed 40 mg daily. For the control of severe nausea and vomiting in children older than 2 years of age and weighing more than 9 kg, the usual oral or rectal dosage of prochlorperazine is 0.4 mg/kg or 10 mg/m² daily given in 3 or 4 divided doses. Alternatively, the oral or rectal dosage of prochlorperazine for the control of severe nausea and vomiting in children older than 2 years of age and weighing 9.1–13.2 kg is 2.5 mg once or twice daily, but not exceeding 7.5 mg daily; children weighing 13.6–17.7 kg may receive 2.5 mg 2 or 3 times daily, but no more than 10 mg daily; and children weighing 18.2–38.6 kg may receive 2.5 mg 3 times daily or 5 mg twice daily, but no more than 15 mg daily. Generally, it is not necessary to continue oral or rectal therapy for longer than 24 hours in most pediatric patients. The usual IM dose of prochlorperazine for the control of severe nausea and vomiting in children 2 years of age or older and weighing more than 9 kg is 0.13 mg/kg. Generally, a single IM dose is sufficient to control nausea and vomiting in most pediatric patients.

For the control of severe nausea and vomiting during surgery, the usual initial adult IM dose of prochlorperazine is 5–10 mg given 1–2 hours before induction of anesthesia. If necessary, the initial IM dose may be repeated once, 30 minutes after the initial dose. To control acute symptoms during or after surgery, the usual adult IM dose is 5–10 mg, repeated once in 30 minutes, if necessary. For the control of severe nausea and vomiting during surgery, the usual adult IV dose of prochlorperazine is 5–10 mg given 15–30 minutes before induction of anesthesia. If necessary, the initial IV dose may be repeated once before surgery. To control acute symptoms during or after surgery, the usual adult IV dose is 5–10 mg, repeated once, if necessary; however, single IV doses of the drug should not exceed 10 mg. For the control of severe nausea and vomiting during surgery, prochlorperazine also may be given by IV infusion. For IV infusion, an infusion containing prochlorperazine 20 mg/L is begun 15–30 minutes before induction of anesthesia. Prochlorperazine is not recommended for the control of severe nausea and vomiting during surgery in children.

For further information on chemistry and stability, pharmacology, pharmacokinetics, uses, cautions, acute toxicity, drug interactions, laboratory test interferences, and dosage and administration of prochlorperazine, see the Phenothiazines General Statement 28:16.08.24. For information on the use of prochlorperazine in psychiatric disorders, see 28:16.08.24.

CAUTIONS

● Precautions

Prochlorperazine shares the toxic potentials of other phenothiazines, and the usual precautions of phenothiazine therapy should be observed. (See Cautions in the Phenothiazines General Statement 28:16.08.24.) The incidence of extrapyramidal reactions associated with prochlorperazine therapy appears to be relatively high in hospitalized psychiatric patients and in children.

Care should be taken to avoid skin contact with prochlorperazine edisylate oral solution or injection, since contact dermatitis has occurred rarely.

● Pediatric Precautions

Safety and efficacy of prochlorperazine in children younger than 2 years of age or those weighing less than 9 kg have not been established.

Use of prochlorperazine should be avoided in children and adolescents with suspected Reye's syndrome, since the antiemetic and potential extrapyramidal effects produced by the drug may obscure the diagnosis of or be confused with the CNS signs of this condition; the drug also is hepatotoxic.

Prochlorperazine should not be used in children during surgery or in conditions for which pediatric dosage has not been established.

PHARMACOLOGY

The precise mechanism of antiemetic action of prochlorperazine is unclear, but the drug inhibits apomorphine-induced vomiting and has been shown to directly affect the medullary chemoreceptor trigger zone (CTZ), apparently by blocking dopamine receptors in the CTZ.

PHARMACOKINETICS

Following oral administration of prochlorperazine maleate in a tablet formulation, the drug has an onset of action of approximately 30–40 minutes and a duration of action of 3–4 hours. The onset of action following oral administration of prochlorperazine maleate in an extended-release formulation is approximately 30–40 minutes; the duration of action is 10–12 hours. Rectally administered prochlorperazine in a suppository has an onset of action of approximately 60 minutes and a duration of action of approximately 3–4 hours. Following IM administration of prochlorperazine edisylate, the drug has an onset of action within 10–20 minutes and a duration of action of 3–4 hours.

CHEMISTRY AND STABILITY

● Chemistry

Prochlorperazine is a phenothiazine antiemetic. The drug is a propylpiperazine derivative of phenothiazine. Prochlorperazine is commercially available as the base, edisylate salt, and maleate salt. Each 7.5 mg of prochlorperazine edisylate or 8 mg of prochlorperazine maleate is approximately equivalent to 5 mg of prochlorperazine.

Prochlorperazine occurs as a clear, pale yellow, viscous liquid and is very slightly soluble in water and freely soluble in alcohol. Prochlorperazine edisylate occurs as a white to very light yellow, odorless, crystalline powder and has approximate solubilities of 500 mg/mL in water and 0.67 mg/mL in alcohol at 25°C. Prochlorperazine maleate occurs as a white to pale yellow, practically odorless, crystalline powder and is practically insoluble in water and has a solubility of approximately 0.83 mg/mL in alcohol at 25°C. Prochlorperazine edisylate injection is a sterile solution of the drug in water for injection. The commercially available injection has a pH of 4.2–6.2 and may contain benzyl alcohol as a preservative and other excipients. The commercially available prochlorperazine edisylate oral solution has a pH of 4.5–5.

● Stability

Commercially available preparations of prochlorperazine should be stored in tight, light-resistant containers. Prochlorperazine edisylate oral solutions and injection, and prochlorperazine maleate tablets and extended-release capsules should be stored at a temperature less than 40°C, preferably between 15–30°C; freezing of the oral solutions and injection should be avoided. Prochlorperazine suppositories should be stored at a temperature less than 37°C. Slight yellowish discoloration of the oral solutions or injection will not affect potency or efficacy, but they should not be used if markedly discolored or if a precipitate is present. Prochlorperazine edisylate injection is physically and/or chemically incompatible with some drugs, but the compatibility depends on several factors (e.g., concentrations of the drugs, specific diluents used, resulting pH, temperature). Specialized references should be consulted for specific compatibility information.

PREPARATIONS

Excipients in commercially available drug preparations may have clinically important effects in some individuals; consult specific product labeling for details.

Prochlorperazine

Rectal			
Suppositories	2.5 mg		**Compazine®**, GlaxoSmithKline
	5 mg		**Compazine®**, GlaxoSmithKline
	25 mg		**Compazine®**, GlaxoSmithKline
			Compro®, Paddock
			Prochlorperazine Suppositories

Prochlorperazine Edisylate

Oral			
Solution	5 mg (of prochlorperazine) per 5 mL		**Compazine® Syrup,** GlaxoSmithKline
Parenteral			
Injection	5 mg (of prochlorperazine) per mL*		**Compazine®**, GlaxoSmithKline

* available from one or more manufacturer, distributor, and/or repackager by generic (nonproprietary) name

Prochlorperazine Maleate

Oral			
Capsules, extended-release	10 mg (of prochlorperazine)		**Compazine Spansule®,** GlaxoSmithKline
	15 mg (of prochlorperazine)		**Compazine® Spansule®,** GlaxoSmithKline
Tablets, film-coated	5 mg (of prochlorperazine)*		**Compazine®**, GlaxoSmithKline
			Prochlorperazine Film-coated Tablets
	10 mg (of prochlorperazine)*		**Compazine®**, GlaxoSmithKline
			Prochlorperazine Film-coated Tablets

* available from one or more manufacturer, distributor, and/or repackager by generic (nonproprietary) name

† Use is not currently included in the labeling approved by the US Food and Drug Administration.

Ondansetron Hydrochloride

56:22.20 · 5-HT₃ RECEPTOR ANTAGONISTS

■ Ondansetron hydrochloride, a selective, first-generation inhibitor of type 3 serotonin (5-HT₃) receptors, is an antiemetic.

USES

● Cancer Chemotherapy-induced Nausea and Vomiting

Ondansetron is used orally or IV for the prevention of nausea and vomiting associated with emetogenic cancer chemotherapy. The drug is used IV with initial and repeat courses of emetogenic cancer chemotherapy, including high-dose cisplatin therapy. Ondansetron is used orally with highly emetogenic cancer chemotherapy (including cisplatin at a dosage of 50 mg/m² or greater). Ondansetron also is used orally with initial and repeat courses of moderately emetogenic cancer chemotherapy. The drug has been used effectively for the prevention of chemotherapy-induced emesis in patients receiving cisplatin alone or in combination with other antineoplastic agents and in those receiving other antineoplastic regimens (e.g., cyclophosphamide plus fluorouracil, doxorubicin, methotrexate, and/or vincristine) that did not include cisplatin.

To prevent chemotherapy-induced nausea and vomiting associated with *highly emetogenic* chemotherapy regimens (including an anthracycline plus cyclophosphamide), the American Society of Clinical Oncology (ASCO) currently recommends a 3-drug antiemetic regimen consisting of a neurokinin-1 (NK₁) receptor antagonist (e.g., either oral aprepitant or IV fosaprepitant dimeglumine), a type 3 serotonin (5-HT₃) receptor antagonist (e.g., dolasetron, granisetron, ondansetron, palonosetron, ramosetron [not commercially available in the US], tropisetron [not commercially available in the US]), and dexamethasone. ASCO states that the oral, fixed-combination of netupitant and palonosetron plus dexamethasone is an additional antiemetic treatment option in this setting.

For patients receiving *moderately emetogenic* chemotherapy regimens, ASCO recommends a 2-drug antiemetic regimen preferably consisting of palonosetron and dexamethasone. If palonosetron is not available, a first-generation 5-HT₃ receptor antagonist (preferably granisetron or ondansetron) may be substituted. Limited evidence suggests that aprepitant may be added to this regimen; in such cases, ASCO states that any of the 5-HT₃ receptor antagonists is appropriate.

For patients receiving chemotherapy regimens with a *low emetogenic risk*, ASCO recommends administration of a single dose of dexamethasone prior to chemotherapy.

In patients receiving chemotherapy regimens with a *minimal emetogenic risk*, antiemetics should not be routinely administered prior to or following chemotherapy.

● Postoperative Nausea and Vomiting

Ondansetron is used orally or IV for the prevention of postoperative nausea and vomiting. Oral or IV ondansetron has been used effectively to prevent nausea and vomiting in surgical patients where nausea and vomiting must be avoided postoperatively; IV ondansetron also has been used effectively to prevent further episodes of nausea and vomiting in patients who did not receive prophylactic antiemetic therapy and developed postoperative nausea and/or vomiting. Studies of oral ondansetron for the prevention of postoperative nausea and vomiting to date have included only women undergoing inpatient surgical procedures; no studies have been performed in males. Controlled studies comparing oral versus IV administration of ondansetron have not been performed to date. The manufacturer states that as with other antiemetics, routine prophylaxis with ondansetron is not recommended in patients in whom there is little expectation that nausea and/or vomiting will occur postoperatively. However, use of the drug is recommended for patients in whom nausea and/or vomiting must be avoided postoperatively, even when the anticipated incidence of such nausea and/or vomiting is low.

● Radiation-induced Nausea and Vomiting

Ondansetron is used orally for the prevention of radiation-induced nausea and vomiting. The drug has been used effectively to prevent nausea and vomiting in patients receiving total body irradiation or single high-dose fraction or daily fractionated radiation to the abdomen.

DOSAGE AND ADMINISTRATION

● Reconstitution and Administration

Ondansetron hydrochloride generally is administered orally or IV; the manufacturer states that, alternatively, the drug may be administered *undiluted* by IM injection in adults for prevention of postoperative nausea and vomiting. (See Dosage: Postoperative Nausea and Vomiting.) For prevention of cancer chemotherapy-induced nausea and vomiting, ondansetron hydrochloride injection should be diluted in 50 mL of 5% dextrose injection or 0.9% sodium chloride injection and infused IV over 15 minutes.

For prevention of postoperative nausea and vomiting, ondansetron hydrochloride injection in single- or multiple-dose vials does *not* require dilution. The undiluted drug is administered by IV injection over a period of at least 30 seconds and, preferably, over a period of 2–5 minutes.

Ondansetron hydrochloride occasionally precipitates at the stopper/vial interface in vials that are stored upright; the manufacturer states that potency and safety of the drug are not affected. If a precipitate is found, the drug may be resolubilized by vigorous shaking of the vial.

Patients receiving ondansetron orally disintegrating tablets should be instructed not to remove a tablet from the blister until just prior to dosing. The tablet should not be pushed through the foil. With dry hands, the blister backing should be peeled completely off the blister. The tablet should then be gently removed and immediately placed on the tongue to dissolve and be swallowed with the saliva; administration with liquid is not necessary.

● Dosage

Dosage of ondansetron, which is available for oral or IV use as the hydrochloride dihydrate and also for oral use as ondansetron base (orally disintegrating tablets), is expressed in terms of ondansetron.

Cancer Chemotherapy-induced Nausea and Vomiting
Oral Dosage

For the prevention of nausea and vomiting associated with moderately emetogenic cancer chemotherapy in adults and children 12 years of age and older, an initial ondansetron dose of 8 mg is given 30 minutes before administration of an emetogenic drug and the dose is repeated 8 hours after the initial dose. An 8-mg dose should be administered at 12-hour intervals for 1–2 days following completion of the emetogenic chemotherapy.

For children 4–11 years of age, an initial ondansetron dose of 4 mg is given 30 minutes before administration of a moderately emetogenic cancer chemotherapy drug, with subsequent doses 4 and 8 hours after the initial dose. A 4-mg dose should then be administered at 8-hour intervals for 1–2 days following completion of emetogenic cancer chemotherapy. Little information currently is available regarding dosages for children younger than 4 years of age.

For the prevention of nausea and vomiting associated with highly emetogenic cancer chemotherapy in adults, a single oral 24-mg dose of ondansetron is given 30 minutes before administration of single-day chemotherapy. The manufacturer states that multiple-day, single-daily-dose oral administration of ondansetron 24 mg has not been studied to date. In addition, safety and efficacy of single-daily-dose oral administration of the 24-mg dose have not been established in pediatric patients.

The manufacturer states that dosage modification is not necessary in geriatric patients.

IV Dosage

For the prevention of cancer chemotherapy-induced nausea and vomiting in adults and pediatric patients 6 months of age and older, an initial IV ondansetron dose of 0.15 mg/kg (up to a maximum of 16 mg per dose) is given as a 15-minute infusion beginning 30 minutes before administration of an emetogenic drug and is repeated twice at 4-hour intervals following the initial dose. Because of the risk of QT interval prolongation (see Cautions: Cardiovascular Effects), an antiemetic regimen consisting of a single IV ondansetron dose of 32 mg no longer is recommended for prevention of cancer chemotherapy-induced nausea and vomiting. Efficacy and safety of alternative single-dose IV ondansetron regimens for prevention of cancer chemotherapy-induced nausea and vomiting have not been established.

The manufacturer states that dosage modification is not necessary in geriatric patients. Little information currently is available regarding dosages for pediatric patients younger than 6 months of age.

Postoperative Nausea and Vomiting

For the prevention of postoperative nausea and vomiting in adults, a single ondansetron IV dose of 4 mg is given immediately before induction of anesthesia or postoperatively if the patient experiences nausea and/or vomiting shortly after surgery. In pediatric patients 1 month to 12 years of age, the recommended dosage of ondansetron is a single IV dose of 4 mg in patients weighing more than 40 kg or a single IV dose of 0.1 mg/kg in patients weighing 40 kg or less; the dose should be given immediately before or after induction of anesthesia or postoperatively if the patient experiences nausea and/or vomiting shortly after surgery. Little information is available regarding dosages for patients weighing more than 80 kg. The manufacturer states that adults who do not achieve adequate control of postoperative nausea and vomiting with a single 4-mg IV dose of ondansetron given prior to induction of anesthesia will not obtain additional benefit from administration of a second 4-mg dose of the drug postoperatively. Efficacy of a second dose of ondansetron in pediatric patients who did not achieve adequate control of postoperative nausea and vomiting following a single prophylactic dose of the drug has not been evaluated.

If ondansetron is used orally for the prevention of postoperative nausea and vomiting in adults, a single 16-mg dose is given 1 hour before induction of anesthesia. The manufacturer states that oral or IV dosage modification is not necessary in geriatric patients and that there is no experience with the use of oral ondansetron for the prevention of postoperative nausea and vomiting in children.

As an alternative to IV administration for the prevention of postoperative nausea and vomiting in adults, an ondansetron dose of 4 mg may be given IM *undiluted* as a single injection.

Radiation-induced Nausea and Vomiting

For prevention of radiation-induced nausea and vomiting in adults undergoing total body irradiation or single high-dose fraction or daily fractionated radiation to the abdomen, the usual oral dosage of ondansetron is 8 mg 3 times daily. Patients undergoing total body irradiation should receive one 8-mg dose 1–2 hours before each fraction of radiation therapy each day. Patients undergoing single high-dose fraction radiation therapy to the abdomen should receive one 8-mg dose 1–2 hours before radiation, with subsequent doses administered every 8 hours for 1–2 days after completion of radiation therapy. For patients undergoing daily fractionated radiation to the abdomen, one 8-mg dose should be given 1–2 hours before radiation therapy and then every 8 hours, with this regimen repeated for each day radiation therapy is given. The manufacturer states that dosage modification is not necessary in geriatric patients and that there is no experience with use of the drug for the prevention of radiation-induced nausea and vomiting in children.

● *Dosage in Renal and Hepatic Impairment*

The manufacturer states that patients with renal impairment do not require ondansetron dosage adjustment, but there is no experience with continuing ondansetron beyond the first day of therapy in such patients. Although only about 5% of the drug is eliminated by the kidneys and renal impairment was not expected to substantially alter elimination of ondansetron, mean plasma clearance has been decreased by about 41–50% in patients with severe renal impairment (creatinine clearances less than 30 mL/minute). However, the decrease in clearance was variable and not consistent with an increase in plasma half-life of the drug. In patients with severe hepatic impairment (Child-Pugh score of 10 or greater) clearance is decreased and apparent volume of distribution of ondansetron is increased with a resultant increase in plasma half-life; therefore, the manufacturer recommends that the total daily dose not exceed 8 mg in such patients.

CAUTIONS

Ondansetron generally is well tolerated. Most adverse effects reported in clinical trials have been mild to moderate in severity. Adverse effects rarely have resulted in discontinuance of the drug. The most frequent adverse effects of ondansetron in patients receiving the drug for the prevention of chemotherapy-induced nausea and vomiting involve the nervous system (e.g., headache) and GI tract (e.g., diarrhea, constipation). Because most patients receiving ondansetron in clinical trials for chemotherapy-induced nausea and vomiting had serious underlying disease (e.g., cancer) and were receiving toxic drugs (e.g., cisplatin), diuretics, and IV fluids concomitantly, it may be difficult to attribute various adverse effects to ondansetron. In trials comparing ondansetron and metoclopramide, adverse effects occurring substantially more frequently for one drug compared with the other included headache and constipation for ondansetron and diarrhea and

extrapyramidal/dystonic manifestations for metoclopramide; adverse effects resulting in drug discontinuance were less common with ondansetron.

The adverse effect profile of ondansetron in patients receiving the drug for the prevention of radiation-induced nausea and vomiting is similar to that in patients receiving the drug for the prevention of chemotherapy-induced nausea and vomiting, although specific incidences of effects may vary; the most common adverse effects of the drug in patients undergoing radiation were headache, constipation, and diarrhea.

In clinical trials in patients receiving ondansetron for the prevention of postoperative nausea and vomiting, the incidences of adverse effects associated with ondansetron, with the exception of headache, did not differ substantially from those associated with placebo. Most such patients were receiving concomitantly multiple preoperative and postoperative drugs. Studies of oral ondansetron for the prevention of postoperative nausea and vomiting to date have included only women undergoing inpatient surgical procedures; no studies have been performed in males.

● *Nervous System Effects*

Headache is the most common adverse nervous system effect of ondansetron, occurring in 11–24% of patients receiving the drug orally or IV in recommended dosages for prevention of chemotherapy-induced nausea and vomiting and in 9–17% of those receiving the drug for postoperative nausea and vomiting in controlled clinical trials; headache occurred in 5% of patients receiving ondansetron for radiation-induced nausea and vomiting. Preliminary observations in a small number of patients suggest that headache occurs more frequently when ondansetron orally disintegrating tablets are taken with water as compared to ingestion without water. Headache generally is mild to moderate in severity and generally responds to mild analgesics. While some evidence suggests that the incidence of headache may be dose related, other evidence failed to establish a clear relationship, particularly regarding severity. Migraine headache has been reported rarely with oral or IV ondansetron.

Dizziness has been reported in 7% of patients receiving ondansetron orally in recommended dosages for prevention of postoperative nausea and vomiting in controlled clinical trials. Dizziness has occurred occasionally in patients receiving the drug IV (mainly during or shortly after IV infusion) and in 4–5% of patients receiving ondansetron orally for prevention of chemotherapy-induced nausea and vomiting; however, a direct causal relationship to the drug has not been established. Although not directly attributed to the drug, other adverse nervous system effects reported include drowsiness or sedation, which occurred in 8%, and paresthesia, which occurred in 2%, of patients receiving the drug IV in the recommended dosage for prevention of postoperative nausea and vomiting; these effects also occurred occasionally in patients receiving the drug orally or IV for prevention of chemotherapy-induced nausea and vomiting. Drowsiness/sedation occurred in 20%, and anxiety/agitation in 6%, of patients receiving oral ondansetron for prevention of postoperative nausea and vomiting in clinical trials. Anxiety or agitation also has occurred in patients receiving the drug IV for prevention of postoperative nausea and vomiting.

Although extrapyramidal reactions were not reported with ondansetron in clinical trials comparing the drug with metoclopramide, manifestations consistent with, but not necessarily diagnostic of, such reactions have been reported rarely in patients receiving ondansetron. Oculogyric crisis, appearing alone, as well as other dystonic reactions, have been reported during postmarketing experience in patients receiving IV ondansetron.

Restlessness, akathisia, ataxia, lightheadedness, and insomnia have been reported rarely with IV ondansetron. Lightheadedness was reported mainly during IV infusion of ondansetron and resolved rapidly. Panic attacks also have been reported rarely.

Seizures (including tonic-clonic seizures) have been reported rarely in patients receiving ondansetron.

● *GI Effects*

Diarrhea is the most common adverse GI effect of ondansetron, occurring in 16% of patients receiving the drug IV in recommended dosages for prevention of chemotherapy-induced nausea and vomiting in controlled clinical trials and in 4–6% of patients receiving the drug orally in recommended dosages. Because most patients receiving ondansetron IV for chemotherapy-induced nausea and vomiting were receiving cisplatin concomitantly, which can cause diarrhea, a causal relationship to ondansetron has not been established. Constipation occurred in 3% of ondansetron-treated patients receiving single-day IV therapy, but is more common in patients receiving multiple-day therapy, occurring in 11% of patients receiving multiple-day IV therapy and in 6–9% of patients receiving multiple-day oral therapy in the recommended dosage for chemotherapy-induced nausea and vomiting. The incidence of constipation may be dose related. Dyspepsia or heartburn, thirst, flatulence, abdominal cramps, abdominal pain, abnormal taste, anorexia, xerostomia, and intestinal obstruction also have been reported with oral or IV ondansetron for prevention of chemotherapy-induced nausea and vomiting.

● Hepatic Effects

Increased serum concentrations of ALT (SGPT) and AST (SGOT) exceeding twice the upper limit of normal have been reported in approximately 1–2% of patients receiving ondansetron orally for prevention of chemotherapy-induced nausea and vomiting, in approximately 5% of patients receiving the drug IV for prevention of chemotherapy-induced nausea and vomiting, and in approximately 1% of patients receiving the drug IV for prevention of postoperative nausea and vomiting. The increases were transient and appeared to be unrelated to dose or duration of ondansetron therapy; however, similar transient increases recurred in some courses of therapy with repeat exposure to the drug, but symptomatic hepatic disease did not occur. In patients with cancer, the role of cancer chemotherapy in these increases cannot be clearly determined. Hepatosplenomegaly, jaundice, and increased serum concentrations of bilirubin and γ-glutamyltransferase (GGT, γ-glutamyltranspeptidase, GGTP) also have been reported rarely.

Liver failure and death have been reported rarely in patients with cancer receiving ondansetron concomitantly with other drugs, including potentially hepatotoxic cytotoxic chemotherapy and antibiotics; the etiology of the liver failure is unclear.

● Dermatologic and Sensitivity Reactions

Pruritus has been reported in 2% of patients receiving ondansetron IV and in 5% of those receiving the drug orally for prevention of postoperative nausea and vomiting in controlled clinical trials. Rash, which may be maculopapular and/or accompanied by pruritus, has occurred in approximately 1% of patients receiving the drug orally or IV for prevention of chemotherapy-induced nausea and vomiting in controlled clinical trials. Rarely, rash may be followed by desquamation and hyperpigmentation.

Serious hypersensitivity reactions have occurred in patients receiving ondansetron orally or IV. In patients with cancer, these reactions have been reported to occur mainly following the first dose during the second or third course of cancer chemotherapy. These reactions may include anaphylaxis/anaphylactoid reactions, angioedema, bronchospasm, cardiopulmonary arrest, hypotension, laryngeal edema, laryngospasm, shock, shortness of breath, stridor, wheezing, facial edema, and urticaria. Sensitivity reactions also have been reported in patients who have exhibited sensitivity to other selective 5-HT₃-receptor antagonists. If a hypersensitivity reaction occurs during ondansetron therapy, the drug should be discontinued, and severe acute hypersensitivity reactions should be treated with appropriate therapy (e.g., epinephrine, corticosteroids, maintenance of an adequate airway, oxygen, IV fluids, antihistamines, maintenance of blood pressure) as indicated.

● Cardiovascular Effects

Prolongation of the QT interval and cases of torsades de pointes have been reported in patients receiving ondansetron. Preliminary results of a randomized, double-blind, placebo- and active-controlled crossover study conducted in healthy adults to assess the drug's effects on the QT interval indicate that ondansetron prolongs the QT interval in a dose-dependent manner. Following IV infusion of ondansetron 8 or 32 mg over 15 minutes, the maximum mean baseline-corrected increase in the QT_c interval (QT interval corrected for heart rate using Fridericia's formula) relative to placebo was 5.8 or 19.6 milliseconds, respectively. Other studies in postoperative patients or healthy individuals also suggest that ondansetron can prolong the QT interval. Based on these findings, an antiemetic regimen consisting of a single IV ondansetron dose of 32 mg given prior to emetogenic cancer chemotherapy no longer is recommended. Individual IV doses of the drug should *not* exceed 16 mg. (See Cautions: Precautions and Contraindications.)

Hypotension has occurred in 5% of patients receiving oral ondansetron for prevention of postoperative nausea and vomiting. Unspecified chest pain and hypotension have been reported in patients receiving ondansetron IV for prevention of postoperative nausea and vomiting in controlled clinical trials, but these effects have not been directly attributed to the drug.

Angina (chest pain), hypotension, flushing, tachycardia, ECG alterations (including arrhythmias and prolongation of PR, QRS, and QT intervals), and

vascular occlusive events (e.g., myocardial infarction, cerebrovascular accident, pulmonary embolism, deep-vein thrombosis) have been reported rarely during clinical trials or postmarketing experience in patients receiving ondansetron orally or IV for prevention of chemotherapy-induced nausea and vomiting; a definite causal relationship to the drug has not been established. Arrhythmias (including ventricular and supraventricular tachycardia, premature ventricular complexes, and atrial fibrillation), bradycardia, ECG alterations (including second-degree heart block and ST-segment depression), hypertension, syncope, and palpitations have been reported in patients receiving IV ondansetron, although these effects have not been directly attributed to the drug. Transient ECG alterations including QT-interval prolongation have been reported rarely, mainly in patients receiving the drug IV; cases of torsades de pointes have been reported during postmarketing experience in patients receiving ondansetron. Bradycardia also was reported in 6% of patients receiving oral ondansetron in clinical trials for prevention of postoperative nausea and vomiting.

● Ocular Effects

Transient blurred vision, occasionally associated with abnormalities of accommodation, has been reported rarely in patients during or shortly after IV infusion of ondansetron. This adverse effect may be ameliorated with a slower infusion rate or following discontinuance of the infusion. Transient blindness, which resolved within a few minutes to 48 hours, also has been reported, generally during IV administration of the drug.

● Other Adverse Effects

Fever occurred in 8% of patients receiving ondansetron IV for prevention of chemotherapy-induced nausea and vomiting and in 2% of patients receiving the drug IV for prevention of postoperative nausea and vomiting in controlled clinical trials. Malaise or fatigue was reported in 9–13% and weakness was reported in up to 2% of patients receiving ondansetron orally for prevention of chemotherapy-induced nausea and vomiting. Pyrexia was reported in 8% of patients receiving oral ondansetron for prevention of postoperative nausea and vomiting in controlled trials. Shivers have been reported in 5% of patients receiving ondansetron orally for prevention of postoperative nausea and vomiting in controlled clinical trials, and occasionally in patients receiving the drug orally for prevention of chemotherapy-induced nausea and vomiting. However, these effects have not been directly attributed to the drug. Sweating also has been reported rarely with IV ondansetron.

Injection site reactions (including pain, erythema, swelling, and burning) occurred in 4% of patients receiving ondansetron IV for prevention of postoperative nausea and vomiting and occasionally in patients receiving the drug IV for prevention of chemotherapy-induced nausea and vomiting in controlled clinical trials. Wound problems were reported in 28% of patients receiving ondansetron orally for postoperative nausea and vomiting in controlled trials. Throat problems and hemorrhage also have been reported in patients receiving ondansetron orally or IV for prevention of postoperative nausea and vomiting.

Cold sensation occurred in 2% of patients receiving ondansetron IV for prevention of postoperative nausea and vomiting in controlled clinical trials, although a causal relationship has not been established. Urinary retention has occurred in 5%, and gynecologic disorder in 7%, of patients receiving oral ondansetron for prevention of postoperative nausea and vomiting. Sensation of cold has been reported in patients receiving ondansetron IV for prevention of chemotherapy-induced nausea and vomiting; sensation of warmth also has been reported rarely with IV ondansetron therapy. Musculoskeletal pain has been reported in patients receiving IV ondansetron. Hypoxia has been reported in 9% of those receiving the drug orally for postoperative nausea and vomiting. Dyspnea, hypoxia, and hiccups also have been reported with ondansetron.

Although a definite causal relationship to ondansetron has not been established, hypokalemia has been reported rarely in patients receiving the drug orally or IV for prevention of cancer chemotherapy-induced nausea and vomiting.

● Precautions and Contraindications

Because of the risk of QT-interval prolongation, ondansetron should be avoided in patients with congenital long QT syndrome. ECG monitoring is recommended in patients with electrolyte abnormalities such as hypokalemia or hypomagnesemia, congestive heart failure, or bradyarrhythmias and in those receiving other drugs known to prolong the QT interval. Electrolyte abnormalities should be corrected prior to IV administration of ondansetron. Because effects of ondansetron on the QT interval are dose related, use of single IV doses exceeding 16 mg should be avoided. Patients receiving ondansetron should be advised to seek immediate medical care if feelings of faintness, lightheadedness, irregular heartbeat, shortness of breath, or dizziness occur.

Like other antiemetics, ondansetron may mask a progressive ileus and/or gastric distention in patients undergoing abdominal surgery or in patients with chemotherapy-induced nausea and vomiting.

Because ondansetron does not stimulate gastric or intestinal peristalsis, it should not be used as a substitute for nasogastric suction.

Because clearance of ondansetron is decreased and apparent volume of distribution and plasma half-life are increased in patients with severe hepatic impairment, the drug should be used with caution and at reduced dosage in such patients. (See Dosage and Administration: Dosage in Renal and Hepatic Impairment.)

Ondansetron rarely may cause serious hypersensitivity reactions, and patients should be advised of this possibility and instructed to discontinue the drug and contact their clinician at the first sign of rash or any other sign of hypersensitivity. (See Cautions: Dermatologic and Sensitivity Reactions.) Ondansetron is contraindicated in patients with known hypersensitivity to the drug or any ingredient in the formulation.

Because profound hypotension and loss of consciousness have been reported when ondansetron was administered concomitantly with apomorphine, concomitant use of these drugs is contraindicated.

Individuals with phenylketonuria (i.e., homozygous genetic deficiency of phenylalanine hydroxylase) and other individuals who must restrict their intake of phenylalanine should be warned that each 4- and 8-mg Zofran® ODT® orally disintegrating tablet contains aspartame (NutraSweet®), which is metabolized in the GI tract to provide less than 0.03 mg of phenylalanine following oral administration.

● Pediatric Precautions

The manufacturer states that little information is available on IV use of ondansetron for the prevention of postoperative nausea and vomiting in pediatric patients younger than 1 month of age or for the prevention of cancer chemotherapy-induced nausea and vomiting in pediatric patients younger than 6 months of age. Little information is available on oral dosage of ondansetron in pediatric patients 4 years of age or younger. Efficacy of the single 24-mg oral dose of ondansetron for the prevention of nausea and vomiting induced by highly emetogenic cancer chemotherapy in pediatric patients younger than 18 years of age has not been established. Efficacy of oral ondansetron for prevention of radiation-induced and postoperative nausea and vomiting in pediatric patients younger than 18 years of age has not been established. In prevention of cancer chemotherapy-induced emesis, safety and efficacy of the drug orally and IV generally are comparable to that observed in older children and adults.

In placebo-controlled trials evaluating IV ondansetron for prevention of postoperative nausea and vomiting in pediatric patients, adverse effects occurred at similar frequencies in pediatric patients receiving recommended dosages of ondansetron and those receiving placebo; however, among pediatric patients 1–24 months of age, diarrhea occurred more frequently in those receiving ondansetron compared with those receiving placebo (2 versus less than 1%).

Pediatric cancer or surgical patients younger than 18 years of age generally tend to have higher clearances and shorter half-lives of ondansetron compared with adults. However, in infants 1–4 months of age, clearance of the drug is reduced and half-life is prolonged (by approximately 2.5-fold relative to values in infants older than 4 months up to 24 months of age); thus, the manufacturer recommends that infants younger than 4 months of age receiving ondansetron therapy be closely monitored.

● Geriatric Precautions

While safety and efficacy of ondansetron have not been established specifically in geriatric patients, a large proportion of patients treated with the drug for chemotherapy-induced nausea and vomiting and prevention of postoperative nausea and/or vomiting have been 65 years of age or older. Plasma clearance of ondansetron may be decreased and elimination half-life increased in patients older than 75 years of age. In clinical studies with ondansetron that included patients 65 years of age and older, no overall differences in efficacy or safety were observed between patients in this age group and younger patients. However, the possibility that some older patients may exhibit increased sensitivity to the drug cannot be ruled out.

● Mutagenicity and Carcinogenicity

Ondansetron was not mutagenic in standard tests performed for mutagenicity. In rats and mice receiving oral dosages up to 10 and 30 mg/kg daily, respectively (approximately 3.6 and 5.4 times, respectively, the recommended human IV dosage of 0.15 mg/kg given 3 times daily [calculated on the basis of body surface area]), ondansetron did not produce evidence of carcinogenicity.

● Pregnancy, Fertility, and Lactation
Pregnancy

Reproduction studies in rats and rabbits receiving oral ondansetron dosages up to 15 and 30 mg/kg daily, respectively, and IV ondansetron dosages up to 4 mg/kg daily (approximately 1.4 and 2.9 times, respectively, the recommended human IV dosage of 0.15 mg/kg given 3 times daily [calculated on the basis of body surface area]) have not revealed evidence of harm to the fetus. There are no adequate and controlled studies to date using ondansetron in pregnant women, and the drug should be used during pregnancy only when clearly needed.

Fertility

Reproduction studies in male and female rats using oral ondansetron dosages up to 15 mg/kg daily (approximately 3.8 times the recommended human IV dosage based on body surface area) have not revealed evidence of impaired fertility.

Lactation

It is not known whether ondansetron is distributed into human milk; however, the drug is distributed into the milk of lactating rats. Because many drugs are distributed in human milk, ondansetron should be used with caution in nursing women.

DESCRIPTION

Ondansetron hydrochloride, a selective inhibitor of type 3 serotonin (5-HT₃) receptors, is an antiemetic. The antiemetic activity of ondansetron appears to be mediated both centrally and peripherally via inhibition of 5-HT₃ receptors. Current evidence indicates that 5-HT₃ receptors play a major role in acute emesis, but only a minor role in delayed nausea and vomiting.

The role of serotonin as a mediator of acute chemotherapy (e.g., cisplatin) induced emesis has been strongly suggested by the temporal relationship between the emetogenic action of such drugs and the release (e.g., from GI enterochromaffin cells) of serotonin (e.g., as reflected by increases in plasma and urine concentrations of the serotonin metabolite 5-hydroxyindoleacetic acid [5-HIAA]) as well as by the clinical efficacy of antiemetic agents that act as inhibitors of 5-HT₃ receptors (e.g., ondansetron, metoclopramide, granisetron). Studies in animals have shown that such chemotherapy-induced emesis can be prevented completely by ablation of the area postrema (the locus of the chemoreceptor trigger zone [CTZ]) or depletion of serotonin from this area; in addition, high levels of 5-HT₃ receptors have been demonstrated in this area, and direct injection of 5-HT₃ receptor antagonists into the area postrema also can prevent such chemotherapy-induced emesis. Therefore, current evidence suggests that the emetogenic action of such chemotherapy may be initiated by degenerative changes in the GI tract (e.g., small intestine) induced by these drugs and associated increases in endogenous serotonin release; serotonin then stimulates vagal and splanchnic nerve receptors that project to the medullary vomiting (emetic) center of the brain and also appears to stimulate 5-HT₃ receptors in the area postrema. Thus, 5-HT₃ receptor antagonists appear to prevent or ameliorate acute chemotherapy-induced emesis by inhibiting visceral (from the GI tract) afferent stimulation of the emetic center probably indirectly at the level of the area postrema and by directly inhibiting serotonin activity within the area postrema and CTZ.

Alternative mechanisms appear to be principally responsible for delayed nausea and vomiting induced by such chemotherapy (e.g., cisplatin), since similar temporal relationships between serotonin and emesis beyond the first day after a dose have not been established, and inhibitors of 5-HT₃ receptors do not appear to be effective alone in preventing or ameliorating delayed effects.

PREPARATIONS

Excipients in commercially available drug preparations may have clinically important effects in some individuals; consult specific product labeling for details.

Ondansetron

Oral

Tablets, orally disintegrating	4 mg*	**Ondansetron Orally Disintegrating Tablets**
		Zofran® ODT®, GlaxoSmithKline
	8 mg*	**Ondansetron Orally Disintegrating Tablets**
		Zofran® ODT®, GlaxoSmithKline

* available from one or more manufacturer, distributor, and/or repackager by generic (nonproprietary) name

Ondansetron Hydrochloride

Oral

Solution	4 mg (of ondansetron) per 5 mL*	**Ondansetron Hydrochloride Oral Solution**
		Zofran®, GlaxoSmithKline
Tablets, film-coated	4 mg (of ondansetron)*	**Ondansetron Hydrochloride Tablets**
		Zofran®, GlaxoSmithKline
	8 mg (of ondansetron)*	**Ondansetron Hydrochloride Tablets**
		Zofran®, GlaxoSmithKline

Parenteral

| Injection, for IV use | 2 mg (of ondansetron) per mL* | **Ondansetron Hydrochloride Injection** |
| | | Zofran®, GlaxoSmithKline |

* available from one or more manufacturer, distributor, and/or repackager by generic (nonproprietary) name

Selected Revisions December 6, 2016, © Copyright, May 1, 1992, American Society of Health-System Pharmacists, Inc.

Aprepitant
Fosaprepitant
Dimeglumine

56:22.32 • NEUROKININ-1 RECEPTOR ANTAGONISTS

■ Fosaprepitant dimeglumine, a prodrug of aprepitant, and aprepitant, a selective, high-affinity antagonist at substance P/neurokinin-1 (NK_1) receptors, are antiemetics.

USES

● Cancer Chemotherapy-induced Nausea and Vomiting

Aprepitant and fosaprepitant dimeglumine are used in combination with other antiemetic agents for the prevention of acute and delayed nausea and vomiting associated with initial and repeat courses of moderately to highly emetogenic cancer chemotherapy, including high-dose cisplatin therapy in adults.

To prevent chemotherapy-induced nausea and vomiting associated with *highly emetogenic* chemotherapy regimens (including an anthracycline plus cyclophosphamide), the American Society of Clinical Oncology (ASCO) currently recommends a 3-drug antiemetic regimen consisting of a neurokinin-1 (NK_1) receptor antagonist (e.g., either oral aprepitant or IV fosaprepitant dimeglumine), a type 3 serotonin (5-HT_3) receptor antagonist (e.g., dolasetron, granisetron, ondansetron, palonosetron, ramosetron [not commercially available in the US], tropisetron [not commercially available in the US]), and dexamethasone. ASCO states that the oral, fixed-combination of netupitant and palonosetron plus dexamethasone is an additional antiemetic treatment option in this setting.

For patients receiving *moderately emetogenic* chemotherapy regimens, ASCO recommends a 2-drug antiemetic regimen preferably consisting of palonosetron and dexamethasone. If palonosetron is not available, a first-generation 5-HT_3 receptor antagonist (preferably granisetron or ondansetron) may be substituted. Limited evidence suggests that aprepitant may be added to this regimen; in such cases, ASCO states that any of the 5-HT_3 receptor antagonists is appropriate.

For patients receiving chemotherapy regimens with a *low emetogenic risk*, ASCO recommends administration of a single dose of dexamethasone prior to chemotherapy.

In patients receiving chemotherapy regimens with a *minimal emetogenic risk*, antiemetics should not be routinely administered prior to or following chemotherapy.

Safety and efficacy of aprepitant for chronic use or for treatment of established nausea and vomiting have not been established.

Clinical Experience

Pivotal clinical efficacy studies for the prevention of acute and delayed nausea and vomiting associated with chemotherapy were conducted with oral aprepitant. Efficacy of aprepitant in patients receiving highly emetogenic chemotherapy was established in 2 controlled clinical studies comparing a regimen containing aprepitant in combination with a 5-HT_3 receptor antagonist (ondansetron) and a corticosteroid (dexamethasone) with a standard regimen containing ondansetron and dexamethasone alone. In these studies, 63–73% of those receiving the regimen with oral aprepitant or 43–52% of those receiving the standard regimen experienced a complete response (i.e., no emetic episodes and no use of rescue therapy) from 0–120 hours after treatment with cisplatin. In the acute phase (0–24 hours) after cisplatin treatment, 83–89% of patients receiving the aprepitant regimen or 68–78% of those receiving the standard regimen experienced a complete response. In the delayed phase (25–120 hours) after cisplatin treatment, 68–75% of patients receiving the aprepitant regimen or 47–56% of those receiving the standard regimen experienced complete response. In addition, antiemetic efficacy of the regimen containing aprepitant was maintained through up to 5 additional chemotherapy cycles in patients who continued into a multiple-cycle extension phase of these 2 studies.

Efficacy of aprepitant in patients receiving moderately emetogenic chemotherapy was established in a double-blind clinical study comparing a regimen containing aprepitant in combination with a 5-HT_3 receptor antagonist (ondansetron) and a corticosteroid (dexamethasone) with a standard regimen containing ondansetron and dexamethasone alone. In this study, a significantly higher proportion of patients with breast cancer receiving the aprepitant regimen (51%) had a complete response (i.e., no emetic episodes and no use of rescue therapy) compared with those receiving the standard regimen (42%) from 0–120 hours after treatment with cyclophosphamide and doxorubicin or epirubicin. In addition, more patients in the aprepitant group than in the standard regimen group reported minimal or no impact of chemotherapy-induced nausea and vomiting on daily living overall (64 versus 56%, respectively). Antiemetic efficacy of the regimen containing aprepitant was maintained through up to 3 additional chemotherapy cycles in patients who continued into a multiple-cycle extension phase of this study.

● Postoperative Nausea and Vomiting

Aprepitant is used for the prevention of postoperative nausea and vomiting in adults. Efficacy of aprepitant was established in 2 randomized, double-blind, active-comparator (ondansetron) clinical studies of similar design in 1658 patients. Patients were randomized to receive an oral aprepitant dose of 40 or 125 mg given 1–3 hours prior to anesthesia, or an IV ondansetron dose of 4 mg immediately before anesthesia induction. Aprepitant doses of 125 mg did not appear to provide additional benefit compared with 40-mg aprepitant doses. In the first study, significantly more patients receiving aprepitant 40-mg doses experienced no emesis (i.e., no emetic episodes regardless of use of rescue therapy) compared with patients receiving IV ondansetron (84 versus 71%, respectively) in the initial 24-hour period following surgery. Complete response (i.e., no emetic episodes and no use of rescue therapy) was reported in about 64 or 55% of those receiving aprepitant or ondansetron, respectively. Similar results were observed for up to 48 hours following surgery; no emesis was reported in about 82 or 66% of patients receiving aprepitant or ondansetron, respectively. Although aprepitant delayed the time to first emetic episode, it did not affect time to first use of rescue therapy compared with ondansetron.

The second study failed to support the primary hypothesis that a 40-mg oral aprepitant dose is superior to a 4-mg IV ondansetron dose in the prevention of postoperative nausea and vomiting as measured by the proportion of patients with complete response in the 24 hours following end of surgery. A similar percentage of patients who received 40 mg of aprepitant orally or 4 mg of IV ondansetron (45 versus 42%, respectively) achieved a complete response, and did not require rescue therapy for established emesis or nausea in the initial 24-hour period following surgery. A higher proportion of patients receiving aprepitant had a clinically meaningful effect compared with those receiving IV ondansetron (about 90 versus 74%, respectively) in the initial 24-hour period following surgery.

A combined analysis of the 2 pivotal studies showed that both aprepitant doses (40 and 125 mg) improved protection against nausea and vomiting and reduced the need for rescue therapy, compared with ondansetron. The 40-mg aprepitant dose also was found to be superior to ondansetron on the 3 measures of efficacy (accounting for any nausea, any vomiting, and any use of rescue therapy in the same patient).

Aprepitant capsules and fosaprepitant dimeglumine for injection have not been studied for chronic use or treatment of established nausea and vomiting.

DOSAGE AND ADMINISTRATION

● Administration

Dispensing and Administration Precautions

Because of similarities in spelling and/or pronunciation between Emend® (the trade name for aprepitant) and Amen® (a former trade name for medroxyprogesterone acetate; no longer commercially available under this trade name in the US) or Vfend® (the trade name for voriconazole), extra care should be exercised in ensuring the accuracy of prescriptions for these drugs. (See Dispensing and Administration Precautions under Warnings/Precautions: General Precautions, in Cautions.)

Oral Administration

Aprepitant is administered orally without regard to meals.

IV Administration

Fosaprepitant dimeglumine is administered by IV infusion over a period of 15 minutes. Fosaprepitant should not be mixed or reconstituted with solutions containing divalent cations (e.g., lactated Ringer's injection, Hartmann's solution).

For the prevention of cancer chemotherapy-induced nausea and vomiting, fosaprepitant dimeglumine injection should be reconstituted with 5 mL of 0.9% sodium chloride injection. The solution should be gently swirled; shaking and jetting saline into the vial should be avoided. The entire volume from the vial should be withdrawn aseptically and transferred into an infusion bag containing 110 mL of 0.9% sodium chloride injection, yielding a total volume of 115 mL and a final concentration of 1 mg/mL. The solution should be mixed by gentle inversion of the bag 2–3 times.

● Dosage

Dosage of fosaprepitant dimeglumine is expressed in terms of fosaprepitant.

● Cancer Chemotherapy-induced Nausea and Vomiting

Aprepitant is administered orally for 3 days as part of a regimen that includes a 5-HT$_3$ receptor antagonist and a corticosteroid.

The recommended oral adult dosage of aprepitant for moderately to highly emetogenic cancer chemotherapy is 125 mg administered 1 hour before chemotherapy on day 1, followed by 80 mg once daily in the morning on days 2 and 3 of the treatment regimen.

Alternatively, a 115-mg dose of fosaprepitant, infused over 15 minutes and administered 30 minutes prior to chemotherapy, may be substituted for aprepitant 125 mg on day 1 *only* of the 3-day regimen.

In clinical studies, the aprepitant regimen included 1 or 4 days of ondansetron and dexamethasone for moderately or highly emetogenic chemotherapy, respectively. For moderately emetogenic chemotherapy, ondansetron 8 mg was administered orally 30–60 minutes before chemotherapy and repeated 8 hours later on day 1 and dexamethasone 12 mg was administered orally 30 minutes prior to chemotherapy on day 1. For highly emetogenic chemotherapy, ondansetron 32 mg was administered IV 30 minutes before chemotherapy on day 1. Dexamethasone was given orally as 12 mg administered 30 minutes before chemotherapy on day 1, followed by 8 mg once daily in the morning on days 2–4. These are reduced dexamethasone dosages relative to the dosages often used to prevent cancer chemotherapy-induced nausea and vomiting to account for decreased dexamethasone metabolism when aprepitant is used concomitantly.

● Postoperative Nausea and Vomiting

The recommended oral adult dosage of aprepitant for the prevention of postoperative nausea and vomiting is 40 mg administered once within 3 hours before anesthesia induction.

● Special Populations

No special population dosage recommendations at this time.

CAUTIONS

● Contraindications

Concomitant use of aprepitant or fosaprepitant dimeglumine with astemizole (no longer commercially available in the US), cisapride (currently commercially available in the US only under a limited-access protocol), pimozide, or terfenadine (no longer commercially available in the US). (See Drug Interactions: Drugs Metabolized by Hepatic Microsomal Enzymes.)

Known hypersensitivity to aprepitant, fosaprepitant dimeglumine, polysorbate 80, or any ingredient in the formulations.

● Warnings/Precautions

Sensitivity Reactions

Stevens-Johnson syndrome has been reported in one patient receiving aprepitant with antineoplastic agents. Hypersensitivity reactions, including anaphylaxis, hives, rash, itching, and urticaria, which may be serious and can cause difficulty in breathing or swallowing, have been reported in patients receiving aprepitant or fosaprepitant. Angioedema was reported in one patient receiving aprepitant.

General Precautions

Dispensing and Administration Precautions

A potential dispensing error exists because of the similarity in spelling and/or pronunciation of Emend® (the trade name for aprepitant and fosaprepitant dimeglumine) and Amen® (a former trade name for medroxyprogesterone acetate; no longer commercially available under this trade name in the US) or Vfend® (the trade name for voriconazole). The manufacturer advises precautionary measures,

including removal of Amen® from the drug database, alerting pharmacy personnel about the potential for error, verifying verbal or telephone orders by spelling the drug name to the prescriber, and confirmation of the patient's understanding of the prescribed drug's purpose and use during patient counseling.

Specific Populations

Pregnancy

Category B. (See Users Guide.)

Lactation

Aprepitant is distributed into milk in rats; it is not known whether the drug is distributed into milk in humans. Discontinue nursing or the drug, taking into account the importance of the drug to the woman.

Gender

In women, peak plasma concentrations of oral aprepitant are 16% higher, and plasma half-life is decreased compared with those reported in men. Not considered to be clinically important, and no dosage adjustment is necessary.

Pediatric Use

Safety and efficacy of fosaprepitant dimeglumine and aprepitant not established in children younger than 18 years of age.

Geriatric Use

No substantial differences in safety, efficacy, or pharmacokinetics of oral aprepitant relative to younger adults; no dosage adjustment necessary.

Hepatic Impairment

Oral aprepitant has not been adequately studied in patients with severe hepatic impairment (Child-Pugh score exceeding 9). No specific dosage adjustment is recommended by the manufacturer, but caution is advised in such patients. Area under the plasma concentration-time curve (AUC) decreased in patients with mild hepatic impairment, but increased in those with moderate hepatic impairment. However, these changes were not considered clinically important, and no dosage adjustment is necessary.

Fosaprepitant is metabolized by extrahepatic tissue; therefore hepatic insufficiency not expected to alter conversion of fosaprepitant to aprepitant.

Renal Impairment

Total (protein bound and unbound) aprepitant AUCs and peak plasma concentrations are decreased in patients with severe renal impairment or end-stage renal disease requiring hemodialysis, but AUC of active unbound drug is unaffected. No dosage adjustment necessary in such patients. Hemodialysis had no substantial effect on pharmacokinetics of aprepitant.

● Common Adverse Effects

Adverse effects occurring in 3% or more of patients receiving oral aprepitant capsules and more frequently than in those receiving standard therapy include asthenia and/or fatigue, dizziness, hypoesthesia, disorientation, nausea, anorexia, constipation, diarrhea, dyspepsia, heartburn, abdominal pain, epigastric discomfort, stomatitis, gastritis, hiccups, perforating duodenal ulcer, enterocolitis, neutropenia, alopecia, bradycardia, hypotension, hypertension, sinus tachycardia, hot flush, pharyngolaryngeal pain, neutropenic sepsis, pneumonia, pruritus, and dehydration.

Since fosaprepitant dimeglumine for injection is converted into aprepitant, adverse effects associated with aprepitant also may be expected to occur with the injection. Adverse effects occurring with IV fosaprepitant dimeglumine include infusion site reactions (e.g., pain, induration) and headache.

DRUG INTERACTIONS

Because fosaprepitant is rapidly metabolized to aprepitant in vivo, interactions reported with aprepitant are expected to occur with fosaprepitant.

● Drugs Metabolized by Hepatic Microsomal Enzymes

Substrates of cytochrome P-450 (CYP) 3A4 (CYP3A4) isoenzyme: Potential pharmacokinetic interaction (altered metabolism of CYP3A4 substrates). Aprepitant is an inhibitor and inducer of CYP3A4 and an inducer of CYP2C9. There is evidence that aprepitant-induced CYP3A4 inhibition is dose dependent. A single 40-mg dose of aprepitant is a weak inhibitor of CYP3A4 and is not expected to have a clinically important effect on plasma concentrations of concomitantly administered drugs that are primarily metabolized by this enzyme. However, when given at higher dosages (i.e., in a regimen consisting of 125 mg on day 1 followed by 80 mg on days 2 and 3) or in repeated doses at any dose level, aprepitant is a moderate inhibitor of CYP3A4, and concomitant administration with drugs metabolized primarily by this enzyme may result in a clinically important effect. Aprepitant (at a dosage level of 125 mg on day 1 followed by 80 mg on days 2 and 3) may increase plasma concentrations of a CYP3A4 substrate to a lesser extent when the substrate is given IV rather than orally. Use with caution; dosage adjustment of concomitantly administered drugs (e.g., dexamethasone) may be necessary. (See Dosage and Administration: Cancer Chemotherapy-induced Nausea and Vomiting and see Drug Interactions: Corticosteroids.) Serious or life-threatening reactions may occur if aprepitant is used concomitantly with astemizole (no longer commercially available in the US), cisapride (currently commercially available in the US only under a limited-access protocol), pimozide, or terfenadine (no longer commercially available in the US).

Substrates of CYP2C9: Potential pharmacokinetic interaction (increased metabolism of CYP2C9 substrates [e.g., phenytoin, tolbutamide, S-warfarin] resulting in decreased plasma concentrations).

Drugs Affecting Hepatic Microsomal Enzymes

Inhibitors of CYP3A4 (e.g., clarithromycin, diltiazem, itraconazole, ketoconazole, nefazodone, nelfinavir, ritonavir, troleandomycin): Potential pharmacokinetic interaction (decreased aprepitant metabolism, resulting in increased plasma aprepitant concentrations). Use with caution.

Inducers of CYP3A4 (e.g., carbamazepine, phenytoin, rifampin): Potential pharmacokinetic interaction (increased aprepitant metabolism). Decreased efficacy possible with strong CYP3A4 inducers (e.g., rifampin).

Antineoplastic Agents

Potential pharmacokinetic interaction (increased plasma antineoplastic concentrations) with antineoplastic agents that are metabolized by CYP3A4. Use with caution and careful monitoring.

5-HT$_3$ Receptor Antagonists

Pharmacokinetic interaction unlikely.

Corticosteroids

Potential pharmacokinetic interaction (increased plasma corticosteroid concentrations) with corticosteroids that are metabolized by CYP3A4 (e.g., dexamethasone, methylprednisolone), particularly when given concomitantly with the 3-day aprepitant regimen (consisting of 125 mg on day 1 followed by 80 mg on days 2 and 3) or with fosaprepitant followed by aprepitant. Decreased dosage of oral and IV corticosteroids may be necessary. The manufacturer of fosaprepitant dimeglumine and aprepitant recommends that dosages of oral dexamethasone and methylprednisolone be reduced by 50% and IV dosage of methylprednisolone be reduced by 25% when these drugs are used concomitantly with fosaprepitant dimeglumine followed by aprepitant, or the 3-day oral aprepitant regimen. Because of weak inhibition of CYP3A4 associated with single 40-mg doses of aprepitant, dosage adjustments of corticosteroids are not required when used concomitantly with this aprepitant regimen.

Digoxin

Pharmacokinetic interaction unlikely.

Diltiazem

Potential pharmacokinetic interaction (increased plasma aprepitant and diltiazem concentrations), but no clinically important changes in ECG, heart rate, or blood pressure were observed in one study with oral aprepitant. The manufacturer recommends caution when aprepitant is used concomitantly with diltiazem.

In studies with fosaprepitant dimeglumine, a small but clinically meaningful decrease in diastolic blood pressure and a small but possibly clinically meaningful decrease in systolic blood pressure were reported. However, no clinically important changes in heart rate or PR interval beyond those induced by diltiazem were reported.

Docetaxel

Pharmacokinetic interaction unlikely when administered with the 3-day aprepitant regimen (consisting of 125 mg on day 1 followed by 80 mg on days 2 and 3).

Midazolam

Potential pharmacokinetic interaction (altered plasma midazolam concentrations). Dosage adjustment for IV midazolam may be necessary when administered concomitantly with the 3-day oral aprepitant regimen. Consider the potential effect of increased benzodiazepine plasma concentrations when midazolam is used concomitantly with the 3-day regimen of aprepitant or fosaprepitant followed by aprepitant.

Increase in plasma midazolam concentrations not considered clinically important when concomitantly administered with a single dose of fosaprepitant 100 mg or aprepitant 40 mg.

Oral Contraceptives

Potential pharmacokinetic interaction (decreased plasma steroid concentrations). Use alternative or additional contraceptive methods during fosaprepitant and aprepitant treatment and for 1 month following the last dose.

Paroxetine

Potential pharmacokinetic interaction (decreased plasma aprepitant and paroxetine concentrations.

Vinorelbine

Pharmacokinetic interaction unlikely when administered with the 3-day aprepitant regimen (consisting of 125 mg on day 1 followed by 80 mg on days 2 and 3).

Warfarin

Potential pharmacokinetic interaction (decreased plasma S-warfarin concentrations). Monitor prothrombin time closely for 2 weeks (particularly 7–10 days) after initiation of fosaprepitant followed by aprepitant, the 3-day oral aprepitant regimen, or aprepitant 40 mg as a single dose.

DESCRIPTION

Fosaprepitant dimeglumine, a prodrug of aprepitant, is rapidly (within 30 minutes of infusion completion) converted in hepatic and extrahepatic tissues to aprepitant, a selective, high-affinity antagonist at substance P/neurokinin 1 (NK$_1$) receptors. Aprepitant crosses the blood-brain barrier and occupies NK$_1$ receptors in the brain. The drug acts in the CNS to inhibit emesis induced by cytotoxic chemotherapy, including both the acute and delayed emesis induced by cisplatin therapy. Studies indicate that aprepitant augments the antiemetic activity of ondansetron and dexamethasone and inhibits both the acute and delayed phases of cisplatin-induced emesis.

Aprepitant is extensively metabolized to weakly active metabolites by the cytochrome P-450 (CYP) enzyme system, principally by CYP3A4, and to a lesser extent by CYP1A2 and CYP2C19. Aprepitant is both a moderate inhibitor and an inducer of CYP3A4; the drug also is an inducer of CYP2C9.

ADVICE TO PATIENTS

Importance of reading the fosaprepitant and aprepitant patient information provided by the manufacturer before beginning therapy and rereading each time the prescription is renewed.

Importance of using fosaprepitant and aprepitant only as directed by the clinician.

Advise patients that aprepitant may be taken with or without food.

Importance of taking first oral aprepitant (125-mg) dose 1 hour before initiation of antineoplastic chemotherapy.

Importance of taking aprepitant (40-mg) dose within 3 hours prior to induction of anesthesia for prevention of postoperative nausea and vomiting.

Importance of discontinuing aprepitant and promptly contacting a clinician if symptoms of an allergic reaction occur.

Importance of women informing clinicians if they are or plan to become pregnant or plan to breast-feed. Importance of women using alternative or additional contraceptive methods during fosaprepitant or aprepitant use (and for 1 month after last dose) if oral contraceptives are being taken.

Importance of informing clinician of existing or contemplated concomitant therapy, including prescription and OTC drugs and herbal products. Importance of closely monitoring prothrombin time in patients receiving chronic warfarin therapy during the 2 weeks (particularly 7–10 days) after initiation of the 3-day regimen of fosaprepitant followed by aprepitant or the 3-day oral aprepitant regimen for each antineoplastic chemotherapy cycle, or administration of aprepitant for prevention of postoperative emesis.

Importance of informing patients of other important precautionary information. (See Cautions.)

PREPARATIONS

Excipients in commercially available drug preparations may have clinically important effects in some individuals; consult specific product labeling for details.

Aprepitant

Oral		
Capsules	40 mg	Emend®, Merck
	80 mg	Emend®, Merck
	125 mg	Emend®, Merck

Fosaprepitant Dimeglumine

Parenteral		
For injection, for IV infusion only	115 mg (of fosaprepitant)	Emend®, Merck

Selected Revisions December 5, 2016, © Copyright, November 1, 2003, American Society of Health-System Pharmacists, Inc.

Netupitant and Palonosetron Hydrochloride

56:22.32 • NEUROKININ-1 RECEPTOR ANTAGONISTS

■ Netupitant and palonosetron hydrochloride (netupitant/palonosetron) is a fixed combination of 2 antiemetic agents; netupitant is a selective antagonist at substance P/neurokinin-1 (NK_1) receptors and palonosetron is a selective, second-generation inhibitor of type 3 serotonergic ($5\text{-}HT_3$) receptors.

USES

● Cancer Chemotherapy-induced Nausea and Vomiting

Netupitant and palonosetron hydrochloride are used orally in fixed combination (Akynzeo®) for the prevention of acute and delayed nausea and vomiting associated with initial and repeat courses of cancer chemotherapy, including, but not limited to, highly emetogenic chemotherapy. Palonosetron prevents nausea and vomiting during the acute phase and netupitant prevents nausea and vomiting during both the acute and delayed phase after cancer chemotherapy. Fixed-combination netupitant and palonosetron is used in an antiemetic regimen that also includes dexamethasone.

To prevent chemotherapy-induced nausea and vomiting associated with *highly emetogenic* chemotherapy regimens (including an anthracycline plus cyclophosphamide), the American Society of Clinical Oncology (ASCO) currently recommends a 3-drug antiemetic regimen consisting of a neurokinin-1 (NK_1) receptor antagonist (e.g., either oral aprepitant or IV fosaprepitant dimeglumine), a type 3 serotonin ($5\text{-}HT_3$) receptor antagonist (e.g., dolasetron, granisetron, ondansetron, palonosetron, ramosetron [not commercially available in the US], tropisetron [not commercially available in the US]), and dexamethasone. ASCO states that oral, fixed-combination netupitant and palonosetron plus dexamethasone is an additional antiemetic treatment option in this setting.

For patients receiving *moderately emetogenic* chemotherapy regimens, ASCO recommends a 2-drug antiemetic regimen preferably consisting of palonosetron and dexamethasone. If palonosetron is not available, a first-generation $5\text{-}HT_3$ receptor antagonist (preferably granisetron or ondansetron) may be substituted. Limited evidence suggests that aprepitant may be added to this regimen; in such cases, ASCO states that any of the $5\text{-}HT_3$ receptor antagonists is appropriate.

For patients receiving chemotherapy regimens with a *low emetogenic risk*, ASCO recommends administration of a single dose of dexamethasone prior to chemotherapy.

In patients receiving chemotherapy regimens with a minimal emetogenic risk, antiemetics should not be routinely administered prior to or following chemotherapy.

Clinical Experience

Efficacy and safety of fixed-combination netupitant and palonosetron in combination with dexamethasone in the prevention of acute and delayed nausea and vomiting associated with initial and repeat courses of chemotherapy have been established in 2 randomized, double-blind, multicenter, controlled clinical studies. One of the trials was conducted in patients receiving highly emetogenic chemotherapy and the other trial was conducted in patients receiving moderately emetogenic chemotherapy. In both trials, complete response rates (i.e., no emetic episodes and no use of rescue therapy) were substantially higher with fixed-combination netupitant and palonosetron than with palonosetron alone.

In study 1, which was dose-finding in design, efficacy and safety of a single oral dose of netupitant (300 mg) in combination with oral palonosetron (0.5 mg), administered with oral dexamethasone (12 mg on day 1 and 8 mg once daily on days 2–4), were compared with a single oral dose of palonosetron (0.5 mg), administered with oral dexamethasone (20 mg on day 1 and 8 mg twice daily on days 2–4), in 694 chemotherapy-naive, adult cancer patients receiving a highly emetogenic, cisplatin-based chemotherapy regimen (median cisplatin dose was 75 mg/m²). In this study, 86% of the patients who received netupitant in combination with palonosetron concomitantly received an antineoplastic agent in addition to protocol-mandated cisplatin. The most common antineoplastic agents and the percentage of patients exposed were cyclophosphamide (34%), fluorouracil (24%), etoposide (21%), and doxorubicin (16%). Primary efficacy endpoints were complete responses (i.e., no emetic episodes and no use of rescue therapy) in the delayed phase (25–120 hours), complete responses in the acute phase (0–24 hours), and complete responses in the overall phase (0–120 hours) after the initiation of treatment with cisplatin. A substantially greater proportion of patients in the netupitant and palonosetron treatment arm attained complete responses (90.4% [delayed phase], 98.5% [acute phase], and 89.6% [overall phase]) compared with those who received palonosetron alone (80.1% [delayed phase], 89.7% [acute phase], and 76.5% [overall phase]).

In study 2, efficacy and safety of a single oral dose of netupitant (300 mg) in combination with oral palonosetron (0.5 mg) were compared with a single dose of oral palonosetron (0.5 mg) in 1455 chemotherapy-naive, adult cancer patients scheduled to receive their first cycle of a moderately emetogenic chemotherapy regimen containing an anthracycline and cyclophosphamide for treatment of a solid malignant tumor. All patients also received a single oral dose of dexamethasone (12 or 20 mg on day 1 in patients who received netupitant in combination with palonosetron or palonosetron alone, respectively). After completion of cycle 1, patients had the option to enter a multiple-cycle extension phase and receive the same treatment assigned in cycle 1. Of the 1450 patients who received either netupitant in combination with palonosetron or palonosetron alone, 1438 patients (99%) completed cycle 1; 1286 patients (88%) continued treatment in the multiple-cycle extension phase, and 907 patients (62%) completed the multiple-cycle extension phase up to a maximum of 8 treatment cycles. The majority of patients who received netupitant in combination with palonosetron were treated with cyclophosphamide, and all patients also received either doxorubicin (68%) or epirubicin (32%). During the first cycle, 32% of patients treated with fixed-combination netupitant and palonosetron received a concomitant chemotherapeutic agent in addition to protocol-mandated regimens; the most common chemotherapeutic agents administered were fluorouracil (28%) and docetaxel (3%).

The primary efficacy endpoint in study 2 was the complete response rate in the delayed phase (25–120 hours) following initiation of the chemotherapy regimen; secondary endpoints included complete response in the acute phase (0–24 hours) and overall phase (0–120 hours). Patients continued into the multiple-cycle extension phase for up to 7 additional cycles of chemotherapy; however, only a limited number of patients received treatment beyond cycle 6. In cycle 1, a greater proportion of patients in the fixed-combination netupitant and palonosetron treatment arm attained a complete response (77% [delayed phase], 88% [acute phase], and 74% [overall phase]) compared with those who received palonosetron alone (70% [delayed phase], 85% [acute phase], and 67% [overall phase]). During all subsequent cycles, the complete response rate in the delayed phase was higher in patients who received netupitant in combination with palonosetron compared with those who received palonosetron alone. In addition, the antiemetic activity of netupitant in combination with palonosetron was maintained throughout repeat cycles in those patients who continued to receive the fixed combination in each of the multiple cycles.

Two additional clinical trials were conducted to support the efficacy of netupitant and palonosetron in fixed combination. In study 3, which was multinational, randomized, and double-blind in design, efficacy of a single oral dose of netupitant (300 mg) in fixed combination with palonosetron (0.5 mg) given on day 1 with oral dexamethasone was maintained throughout all cycles in 309 chemotherapy-naive, adult cancer patients undergoing initial and repeat cycles of moderately or highly emetogenic chemotherapy (including carboplatin, cisplatin, oxaliplatin, and doxorubicin-containing regimens). The fixed-dose combination of netupitant and palonosetron also was found to be well tolerated when given over multiple chemotherapy cycles in this study.

In a multinational, randomized, active-controlled, double-blind, clinical noninferiority study (study 4), efficacy and safety of a single oral dose of palonosetron (0.5 mg) were compared with IV palonosetron (0.25 mg) in 739 cancer patients scheduled to receive highly emetogenic cisplatin-based chemotherapy (70 mg/m² or more). The intent of this study was to demonstrate that oral palonosetron (0.5 mg) contributes to the efficacy of fixed-combination netupitant and palonosetron during the acute phase (i.e., the first 24 hours after cancer chemotherapy) in the setting of cisplatin-based chemotherapy. The primary efficacy endpoint was complete response (defined as no emetic episode and no use of rescue medication) within 24 hours (acute phase) following initiation of cisplatin-based chemotherapy. In patients who received oral palonosetron, 89.4% attained a complete response in the acute phase compared with 86.2% of those who received IV palonosetron; noninferiority of oral versus IV palonosetron was demonstrated in a statistical analysis of the complete response results.

For IV use of palonosetron hydrochloride as an antiemetic, see Palonosetron Hydrochloride 56:22.20.

DOSAGE AND ADMINISTRATION

• Administration

The fixed-combination capsules containing netupitant and palonosetron hydrochloride (netupitant/palonosetron; Akynzeo®) are administered orally approximately one hour before the start of chemotherapy without regard to meals.

The manufacturer states that the antiemetic regimen also should include oral dexamethasone administered 30 minutes prior to chemotherapy on days 1–4 for highly emetogenic chemotherapy (including cisplatin-based chemotherapy), or on day 1 only for anthracycline- and cyclophosphamide-based chemotherapy and chemotherapy not considered highly emetogenic.

• Dosage

Netupitant and palonosetron hydrochloride is a fixed combination preparation containing 300 mg of netupitant and 0.5 mg of palonosetron.

The netupitant component is provided as netupitant; the palonosetron component is provided as palonosetron hydrochloride (dosage of this component is expressed in terms of palonosetron).

Cancer Chemotherapy-induced Nausea and Vomiting

For the prevention of acute and delayed nausea and vomiting associated with initial and repeat courses of *highly emetogenic cancer chemotherapy, including cisplatin-based chemotherapy*, in adults, the recommended dosage of fixed-combination netupitant and palonosetron is 1 capsule (300 mg of netupitant and 0.5 mg of palonosetron) administered approximately 1 hour prior to the start of chemotherapy; dexamethasone 12 mg should be administered orally 30 minutes prior to chemotherapy on day 1, followed by 8 mg orally once daily on days 2–4 of the treatment regimen. (See Drug Interactions: Dexamethasone.)

For the prevention of acute and delayed nausea and vomiting associated with initial and repeat courses of *anthracycline- and cyclophosphamide-based chemotherapy and chemotherapy not considered highly emetogenic* in adults, the recommended dosage of fixed-combination netupitant and palonosetron is 1 capsule (300 mg of netupitant and 0.5 mg of palonosetron) administered approximately 1 hour prior to the start of chemotherapy; dexamethasone 12 mg should be administered orally 30 minutes prior to chemotherapy on day 1 of the treatment regimen. The manufacturer states that administration of dexamethasone on days 2–4 is not necessary. (See Drug Interactions: Dexamethasone.)

• Special Populations

Dosage adjustments are not necessary when fixed-combination netupitant and palonosetron is used in patients with mild or moderate hepatic impairment (Child-Pugh score of 5–8). However, fixed-combination netupitant and palonosetron should *not* be used in patients with severe hepatic impairment (Child-Pugh score exceeding 9) because the fixed combination has not been adequately studied in such patients.

Dosage adjustments are not necessary when fixed-combination netupitant and palonosetron is used in patients with mild to moderate renal impairment. However, fixed-combination netupitant and palonosetron should not be used in patients with severe renal impairment or end-stage renal disease.

Caution generally should be used when dosing fixed-combination netupitant and palonosetron in geriatric patients because of the greater frequency of decreased hepatic, renal, and/or cardiac function and concomitant diseases and other drug therapy in such patients.

CAUTIONS

• Contraindications

The manufacturer states there are no known contraindications to the use of the fixed combination of netupitant and palonosetron hydrochloride.

• Warnings/Precautions

Sensitivity Reactions

Hypersensitivity reactions, including anaphylaxis, have been reported in patients receiving palonosetron; the reactions have occurred in patients with or without

known hypersensitivity to other type 3 serotonergic (5-HT₃) receptor antagonists. (See Advice to Patients.)

Other Warnings and Precautions

Serotonin Syndrome

Development of serotonin syndrome has been reported in patients receiving 5-HT₃ receptor antagonists. Most of the cases have been associated with concomitant use of other serotonergic drugs (e.g., selective serotonin-reuptake inhibitors [SSRIs], serotonin- and norepinephrine-reuptake inhibitors [SNRIs], monoamine oxidase [MAO] inhibitors, mirtazapine, fentanyl, lithium, tramadol, IV methylene blue). Some of the reported cases of serotonin syndrome were fatal. Serotonin syndrome occurring with overdosage of another 5-HT₃ receptor antagonist alone (ondansetron) also has been reported. The majority of reports of serotonin syndrome related to 5-HT₃ receptor antagonist use have occurred in a post-anesthesia care unit or an infusion center.

Manifestations associated with serotonin syndrome may include mental status changes (e.g., agitation, hallucinations, delirium, coma), autonomic instability (e.g., tachycardia, labile blood pressure, dizziness, diaphoresis, flushing, hyperthermia), neuromuscular symptoms (e.g., tremor, rigidity, myoclonus, hyperreflexia, incoordination), and seizures with or without GI symptoms (e.g., nausea, vomiting, diarrhea).

Patients receiving 5-HT₃ receptor antagonists, including fixed-combination netupitant and palonosetron, should be monitored for the emergence of serotonin syndrome, particularly with concomitant use of other serotonergic drugs. If symptoms of serotonin syndrome occur, fixed-combination netupitant and palonosetron should be discontinued, and supportive treatment should be initiated. (See Drug Interactions: Serotonergic Agents and also see Advice to Patients.)

For further information on serotonin syndrome, including manifestations and treatment, see Drug Interactions: Serotonergic Drugs, in Fluoxetine Hydrochloride 28:16.04.20.

Specific Populations

Pregnancy

Category C. (See Users Guide.)

Lactation

It is not known whether netupitant or palonosetron is distributed into human milk. Because many drugs are excreted in milk and because of the potential tumorigenicity palonosetron demonstrated in an animal carcinogenicity study, a decision should be made whether to discontinue nursing or the fixed combination of netupitant and palonosetron, taking into account the importance of the drugs to the woman.

Pediatric Use

The manufacturer states that the safety and efficacy of netupitant and palonosetron hydrochloride have not been established in pediatric patients younger than 18 years of age.

Geriatric Use

In the main clinical studies with the fixed combination of netupitant and palonosetron, 18% of adult cancer patients were 65 years of age or older and 2% were 75 years of age or older. No overall differences in safety were observed in these geriatric patients compared with younger adults in these studies. Exploratory analyses of the effect of age on efficacy were performed in 2 clinical studies comparing the fixed combination of netupitant and palonosetron with palonosetron. In study 1 in patients receiving cisplatin chemotherapy, the difference in complete response rates between fixed-combination netupitant and palonosetron and palonosetron alone was similar between patients 65 years of age or older and those younger than 65 years of age in both the acute and delayed phases. In study 2 in patients receiving anthracycline plus cyclophosphamide chemotherapy, the difference in complete response rates between fixed-combination netupitant and palonosetron and palonosetron alone also was similar between patients 65 years of age or older and those younger than 65 years of age in the acute phase. In the delayed phase, the difference in complete response rates between fixed-combination netupitant and palonosetron and palonosetron alone was higher in patients younger than 65 years of age; this difference may be explained, at least in part, by a higher complete response rate in the delayed phase with palonosetron alone in geriatric patients (81%) compared with younger patients treated with palonosetron alone (67%).

In a population pharmacokinetic analysis, age (within the range of 29–75 years of age) did not affect the pharmacokinetics of netupitant or palonosetron in cancer patients receiving the fixed combination of the 2 drugs. In healthy individuals older than 65 years of age, mean systemic exposure and peak plasma concentrations were 25 and 36% higher for netupitant, respectively, and 37 and 10% higher for palonosetron, respectively, compared with those in healthy younger adults (22–45 years of age).

Caution is advised when dosing fixed-combination netupitant and palonosetron in geriatric patients because of the greater frequency of decreased hepatic, renal, and/or cardiac function and of concomitant diseases and other drug therapy in such patients.

Hepatic Impairment

The effects of hepatic impairment on the pharmacokinetics of netupitant and palonosetron were studied following administration of a single oral dose of the fixed combination to patients with mild (Child-Pugh score of 5–6), moderate (Child-Pugh score of 7–9), or severe (Child-Pugh score exceeding 9) hepatic impairment. In patients with mild or moderate hepatic impairment, mean exposure of netupitant was 67 and 86% higher, respectively, than in healthy individuals and mean peak plasma concentration for netupitant was approximately 40 and 41% higher, respectively, than in healthy individuals. In patients with mild or moderate hepatic impairment, mean exposure of palonosetron was 33 and 62% higher, respectively, than in healthy individuals and mean peak plasma concentration for palonosetron was approximately 14% higher and unchanged, respectively, compared with healthy individuals. The manufacturer states that no dosage adjustment is necessary in patients with mild to moderate hepatic impairment.

The pharmacokinetics of netupitant and palonosetron were available from only 2 patients with severe hepatic impairment, and the manufacturer states that the data are too limited to draw a conclusion. Use of fixed-combination netupitant and palonosetron should therefore be avoided in patients with severe hepatic impairment.

Renal Impairment

In a population pharmacokinetic analysis, mild and moderate renal impairment did not substantially affect the pharmacokinetics of netupitant in cancer patients. The manufacturer states that no dosage adjustment of fixed-combination netupitant and palonosetron is necessary in patients with mild to moderate renal impairment.

The pharmacokinetics and safety of netupitant have not been studied in patients with severe renal impairment; however, severe renal impairment did not substantially affect the pharmacokinetics of palonosetron. In a study with IV palonosetron, total systemic exposure to palonosetron increased by approximately 28% in patients with severe renal impairment, compared with healthy individuals. The pharmacokinetics of netupitant and palonosetron have not been studied in patients with end-stage renal disease requiring hemodialysis. The manufacturer states that use of fixed-combination netupitant and palonosetron should be avoided in patients with severe renal impairment or end-stage renal disease.

● Common Adverse Effects

Adverse effects reported in 3% or more of patients receiving the oral fixed combination of netupitant and palonosetron concomitantly with highly emetogenic, cisplatin-based chemotherapy and that occurred more frequently than in those receiving palonosetron alone include dyspepsia, fatigue, constipation, and erythema.

Adverse effects reported in 3% or more of patients receiving fixed-combination netupitant with palonosetron concomitantly with anthracycline- and cyclophosphamide-based chemotherapy (cycle 1) and that occurred at a rate that exceeded palonosetron alone include headache, asthenia, and fatigue.

DRUG INTERACTIONS

Metabolism of netupitant is primarily mediated by cytochrome P-450 (CYP) isoenzyme 3A4 and, to a lesser extent, by CYP2C9 and CYP2D6.

Based on in vitro studies and confirmed in an in vivo study, netupitant is a moderate inhibitor of CYP3A4; its M1 metabolite also is an inhibitor of CYP3A4 based on in vitro studies. Based on in vitro studies, netupitant and its metabolites are unlikely to have clinically important pharmacokinetic drug interactions via inhibition of CYP isoenzymes 1A2, 2B6, 2C8, 2C9, 2C19, and 2D6 at the usual clinical dose of 300 mg.

Netupitant and its metabolites (M1, M2, and M3) do not induce CYP isoenzymes 1A2, 2B6, 2C9, 2C19, and 3A4.

Based on in vitro studies, netupitant inhibits P-glycoprotein (P-gp) and breast cancer resistance protein (BCRP) transporters. Netupitant is not a substrate for P-gp, but its M2 metabolite is a P-gp substrate.

In vitro studies indicate that netupitant and its 3 major metabolites are unlikely to have clinically important drug interactions with human efflux transporters bile salt export pump (BSEP), multidrug resistance protein (MRP) 2, and human uptake transporters organic anion transport protein (OATP) 1B1 or 1B3, organic anion transporter (OAT) 1 or 3, and organic cation transporter (OCT) 1 or 2 at the usual clinical dose of 300 mg.

In vitro studies suggest that CYP2D6 and, to a lesser extent, CYP3A4 and CYP1A2 are involved in the metabolism of palonosetron. Palonosetron does not inhibit CYP isoenzymes 1A2, 2A6, 2B6, 2C9, 2D6, 2E1, and 3A4/5 or induce CYP isoenzymes 1A2, 2D6, or 3A4/5 based on in vitro studies; CYP2C19 was not studied.

● Drugs Affecting or Metabolized by Hepatic Microsomal Enzymes

Concomitant use of fixed-combination netupitant and palonosetron with potent CYP3A4 inhibitors (e.g., ketoconazole) can substantially increase systemic exposure to the netupitant component of the fixed combination. (See Drug Interactions: Ketoconazole.) However, the manufacturer states that dosage adjustment is not necessary for single-dose administration of fixed-combination netupitant and palonosetron during concomitant use of potent CYP3A4 inhibitors.

Plasma concentrations of CYP3A4 substrates may increase when used concomitantly with fixed-combination netupitant and palonosetron. The inhibitory effect of netupitant on CYP3A4 can last for multiple days. Therefore, fixed-combination netupitant and palonosetron should be used with caution in patients concomitantly receiving drugs that are principally metabolized by CYP3A4.

Potent CYP3A inducers can decrease the efficacy of fixed-combination netupitant and palonosetron by substantially reducing plasma concentrations of the netupitant component. The manufacturer therefore states that concomitant use of fixed-combination netupitant and palonosetron should be avoided in patients who are receiving long-term therapy with a potent CYP3A4 inducer (e.g., rifampin). (See Drug Interactions: Rifampin.)

● Antineoplastic Agents

Systemic exposure to antineoplastic agents that are metabolized by CYP3A4 (e.g., docetaxel, paclitaxel, etoposide, irinotecan, cyclophosphamide, ifosfamide, imatinib, vinorelbine, vinblastine, vincristine) can increase when administered concomitantly with the fixed combination of netupitant and palonosetron. Systemic exposure to IV docetaxel, etoposide, and cyclophosphamide was increased when administered with fixed-combination netupitant with palonosetron. Systemic exposure to IV docetaxel, etoposide, and cyclophosphamide was increased when administered with fixed-combination netupitant with palonosetron compared with palonosetron administration alone in patients with cancer.

Concurrent administration of fixed-combination netupitant and palonosetron increased the mean peak plasma concentration and area under the concentration-time curve (AUC) of docetaxel by 49 and 35%, respectively, and increased the mean peak plasma concentration and AUC of etoposide by 10 and 28%, respectively, compared with palonosetron administration alone.

Following concomitant administration of fixed-combination netupitant and palonosetron, mean peak plasma concentration and AUC of cyclophosphamide were 27 and 20% higher, respectively, compared with concomitant administration of palonosetron alone.

The mean AUC of palonosetron was approximately 65% higher when fixed-combination netupitant and palonosetron was concomitantly administered with docetaxel than with etoposide or cyclophosphamide; the mean AUC of netupitant was similar among groups that received docetaxel, etoposide, or cyclophosphamide.

Caution and monitoring for chemotherapy-related adverse effects are advised in patients concomitantly receiving antineoplastic agents that are principally metabolized by CYP3A4.

● Serotonergic Agents

Serotonin syndrome (including altered mental status, autonomic instability, and neuromuscular symptoms) has been reported following the concomitant use of type 3 serotonin (5-HT$_3$) receptor antagonists and other serotonergic drugs, including selective serotonin-reuptake inhibitors (SSRIs), serotonin- and norepinephrine-reuptake inhibitors (SNRIs), monoamine oxidase (MAO) inhibitors, mirtazapine, fentanyl, lithium, tramadol, and IV methylene blue. Patients should be monitored for the emergence of serotonin syndrome, particularly during concomitant use of fixed-combination netupitant and palonosetron and other serotonergic drugs. If symptoms of serotonin syndrome occur, fixed-combination netupitant and palonosetron should be discontinued, and supportive treatment should be initiated. (See Serotonin Syndrome under Warnings/Precautions: Other Warnings and Precautions, in Cautions and also see Advice to Patients.)

● Netupitant and Palonosetron

The pharmacokinetics of netupitant and palonosetron were not substantially affected when oral netupitant (450 mg) and oral palonosetron (0.75 mg) were concurrently administered.

● Dexamethasone

Concomitant administration of a single dose of netupitant (300 mg on day 1) and a dexamethasone regimen (20 mg on day 1, followed by 8 mg twice daily on days 2–4) increased systemic exposure to dexamethasone approximately twofold. The mean AUC of dexamethasone increased by 1.7-fold on day 1 and up to 2.4-fold on days 2 and 4; the duration of this effect was not studied beyond 4 days. Therefore, the manufacturer states that a reduced dose of dexamethasone (i.e., 8 or 12 mg orally) should be administered when used with fixed-combination netupitant and palonosetron. (See Dosage and Administration: Dosage.)

● Digoxin

Concurrent administration of netupitant (450 mg) did not substantially affect systemic exposure and urinary excretion of digoxin, a P-gp substrate, at steady state. Therefore, concurrent administration of fixed-combination netupitant and palonosetron and digoxin is not expected to affect systemic exposure of digoxin.

● Erythromycin

Systemic exposure of erythromycin was highly variable and the mean peak concentration and AUC of erythromycin were increased by 92 and 56%, respectively, when erythromycin (500 mg) was concurrently administered with netupitant (300 mg). The pharmacokinetics of netupitant were not affected by concurrent administration of erythromycin.

● Ketoconazole

A single dose of fixed-combination netupitant and palonosetron was administered with ketoconazole (a potent CYP3A4 inhibitor) following once-daily administration of ketoconazole 400 mg for 12 days. Concurrent administration of ketoconazole increased the mean peak plasma concentrations and AUC of netupitant by 25 and 140%, respectively, and increased mean AUC and peak plasma concentrations of palonosetron by 10 and 15%, respectively, compared with administration of fixed-combination netupitant and palonosetron alone. Although ketoconazole can substantially increase systemic exposure to the netupitant component of the fixed combination, the manufacturer states that dosage adjustment is not necessary for single-dose administration of fixed-combination netupitant and palonosetron.

● Midazolam

Systemic exposure of midazolam was substantially higher when administered with netupitant. Following concomitant administration of netupitant (300 mg) and a single oral dose of midazolam (7.5 mg), the mean peak plasma concentration and AUC of midazolam were 36 and 126% higher, respectively. The pharmacokinetics of netupitant were unaffected by concomitant administration of midazolam. The manufacturer states that the potential effects of increased plasma concentrations of midazolam or other benzodiazepines metabolized by CYP3A4 (e.g., alprazolam, triazolam) should be considered when administering these drugs with fixed-combination netupitant and palonosetron.

● Oral Contraceptives

Single-dose netupitant in fixed combination with palonosetron, when given with a single oral dose of ethinyl estradiol 60 mcg and levonorgestrel 300 mcg, increased the AUC of levonorgestrel by 46%. However, fixed-combination netupitant and palonosetron did not substantially affect the AUC of ethinyl estradiol. A clinically important effect of fixed-combination netupitant and palonosetron on the efficacy of oral contraceptives containing levonorgestrel and ethinyl estradiol is therefore considered unlikely, and dosage adjustments are not necessary during concomitant use of these drugs.

● Rifampin

Single-dose, fixed-combination netupitant and palonosetron was administered with rifampin, a potent CYP3A4 inducer, following once-daily administration of rifampin (600 mg for 17 days). Concurrent administration of rifampin decreased the mean peak plasma concentration and exposure of netupitant by 62 and 82%, respectively, compared with those following administration of fixed-combination netupitant and palonosetron alone. Concurrent administration of rifampin decreased the mean peak plasma concentration and AUC of palonosetron by 15 and 19%, respectively.

Because potent CYP3A4 inducers can decrease the efficacy of fixed-combination netupitant and palonosetron by substantially reducing plasma concentrations of the netupitant component, use of fixed-combination netupitant and palonosetron should be avoided in patients receiving long-term therapy with potent CYP3A4 inducers such as rifampin.

DESCRIPTION

Netupitant and palonosetron hydrochloride is a fixed oral combination of 2 antiemetic agents: netupitant, a highly selective antagonist at substance P/neurokinin-1 (NK$_1$) receptors, and palonosetron, a selective, second-generation inhibitor of type 3 serotonergic (5-HT$_3$) receptors.

Palonosetron is pharmacologically related to first-generation 5-HT$_3$ receptor antagonists (e.g., dolasetron, granisetron, ondansetron). However, palonosetron has a higher potency, higher binding affinity for 5-HT$_3$ receptors, a longer elimination half-life, and a different molecular interaction with 5-HT$_3$ receptors than other commercially available 5-HT$_3$ receptor antagonists and exhibits little or no affinity for other receptors.

Current evidence suggests that chemotherapeutic agents produce acute nausea and vomiting by inducing degenerative changes in the GI tract (e.g., small intestine), thereby increasing endogenous serotonin release from the enterochromaffin cells of the small intestine. Serotonin then stimulates 5-HT$_3$ receptors on vagal and splanchnic nerves that project to the medullary vomiting (emetic) center of the brain and also appears to stimulate 5-HT$_3$ receptors in the area postrema. Thus, 5-HT$_3$ receptor antagonists appear to prevent or ameliorate acute chemotherapy-induced emesis by inhibiting visceral (from the GI tract) afferent stimulation of the emetic center probably indirectly at the level of the area postrema and by directly inhibiting serotonin activity within the area postrema and chemoreceptor trigger zone (CTZ).

Delayed emesis has been mainly associated with the activation of tachykinin family NK$_1$ receptors, which are widely distributed in the central and peripheral nervous systems, by substance P. Netupitant has been shown to inhibit substance P-mediated responses in in vitro and in vivo studies. Netupitant crosses the blood-brain barrier and occupies NK$_1$ receptors in the brain. In addition, the combination of palonosetron and netupitant may inhibit the action of substance P synergistically.

Following single-dose, oral administration of fixed-combination netupitant and palonosetron hydrochloride in healthy individuals, peak plasma concentrations of netupitant and palonosetron are achieved within approximately 5 hours.

In a pooled analysis, peak plasma concentration of netupitant was 35% higher in females than in males, while AUC was similar between males and females. In females, mean AUC and peak plasma concentration of palonosetron were 35 and 26% higher, respectively, compared with males.

Plasma protein binding of netupitant is greater than 99.5% at drug concentrations ranging from 10–1300 ng/mL and protein binding of its principal metabolites is greater than 97% at drug concentrations ranging from 100–2000 ng/mL. Approximately 62% of palonosetron is bound to plasma proteins. Netupitant is extensively metabolized to form 3 principal metabolites: a desmethyl derivative (M1), an N-oxide derivative (M2), and a OH-methyl derivative (M3). Following a single oral dose of netupitant, the apparent elimination half-life in cancer patients is 80 hours. The elimination half-life of palonosetron in cancer patients is 48 hours. Approximately 50% of a single, oral radiolabeled dose of netupitant was recovered in urine and feces within 120 hours following oral administration. A total of approximately 4 and 71% of a radiolabeled dose of netupitant was recovered in urine and feces collected over 336 hours, respectively; less than 1% of the dose was recovered in urine as unchanged drug. Following oral administration of a single dose of radiolabeled palonosetron in healthy individuals, 85–93% of the dose was excreted in urine and 5–8% was excreted in feces; approximately 40% of the dose was recovered in urine as unchanged drug.

ADVICE TO PATIENTS

Importance of reading patient information provided by the manufacturer before beginning therapy and rereading it each time the fixed-combination netupitant and palonosetron hydrochloride is taken.

Importance of informing patients to take fixed-combination netupitant and palonosetron hydrochloride with or without food approximately 1 hour before initiation of antineoplastic chemotherapy.

Importance of informing patients that hypersensitivity reactions, including anaphylaxis, have been reported in patients receiving palonosetron. Clinicians should advise patients to seek immediate medical attention if any signs or symptoms of a hypersensitivity reaction occur while receiving netupitant and palonosetron in fixed combination.

Importance of informing patients of the possibility of serotonin syndrome, particularly with concomitant use of fixed-combination netupitant and palonosetron and another serotonergic agent such as antidepressants and antimigraine agents. Clinicians should advise patients to seek immediate medical attention should they experience any of the following serotonin syndrome symptoms: changes in mental status, autonomic instability, or neuromuscular symptoms, either with or without GI symptoms.

Importance of women informing their clinician if they are or plan to become pregnant or plan to breast-feed.

Importance of informing clinicians of existing or contemplated concomitant therapy, including prescription and OTC drugs and dietary or herbal supplements, as well as any concomitant illnesses.

Importance of informing patients of other precautionary information. (See Cautions.)

PREPARATIONS

Excipients in commercially available drug preparations may have clinically important effects in some individuals; consult specific product labeling for details.

Netupitant and Palonosetron Hydrochloride

Oral

Capsules	Netupitant 300 mg and Palonosetron Hydrochloride 0.5 mg (of palonosetron)	Akynzeo®, Helsinn

Selected Revisions March 4, 2019, © Copyright, December 5, 2016, American Society of Health-System Pharmacists, Inc.

Rolapitant Hydrochloride

56:22.32 • NEUROKININ-1 RECEPTOR ANTAGONISTS

■ Rolapitant hydrochloride, a highly selective and competitive antagonist at substance P/neurokinin-1 (NK$_1$) receptors, is an antiemetic.

USES

● Cancer Chemotherapy-induced Nausea and Vomiting

Rolapitant is used in combination with other antiemetic agents in adults for the prevention of delayed nausea and vomiting associated with initial and repeat courses of emetogenic cancer chemotherapy, including, but not limited to, highly emetogenic chemotherapy.

Safety and efficacy of rolapitant for this use are based on the results of several randomized controlled trials.

Clinical Experience

Safety and efficacy of rolapitant in patients receiving *highly emetogenic chemotherapy* were established in 2 multicenter, randomized, double-blind, parallel group, active-controlled studies. In Study 1, 526 adults 20–90 years of age (mean age 57 years) were randomized 1:1 to receive either rolapitant or placebo in addition to cisplatin protocol-mandated chemotherapy. The mean cisplatin dose was 77 mg/m^2 and 82% of patients received a concomitant chemotherapeutic agent in addition to protocol-mandated cisplatin therapy. The most common concomitant chemotherapeutic agents administered during cycle 1 were gemcitabine (17%), paclitaxel (12%), fluorouracil (11%), etoposide (10%), vinorelbine (9%), docetaxel (9%), pemetrexed (7%), doxorubicin (6%), and cyclophosphamide (5%). Those assigned to the rolapitant regimen received oral rolapitant 180 mg, oral dexamethasone 20 mg, and IV granisetron 10 mcg/kg on day 1, and oral dexamethasone 8 mg twice daily on days 2–4. Patients assigned to the control regimen received placebo plus oral dexamethasone 20 mg, and IV granisetron 10 mcg/kg on day 1, and oral dexamethasone 8 mg twice daily on days 2–4. Rolapitant or placebo was administered 1–2 hours prior to chemotherapy on day 1. Dexamethasone and granisetron were administered 30 minutes prior to chemotherapy on day 1. The primary endpoint of the study was complete response, defined as no emetic episodes and no use of rescue medication, in the delayed phase (25–120 hours) of chemotherapy-induced nausea and vomiting in cycle 1. In Study 1, a greater proportion of patients who received rolapitant therapy achieved a complete response in the delayed phase, compared with those who received the control regimen (72.7 versus 58.4%).

In Study 2, 544 adults 18–83 years of age (mean age 58 years) were randomized 1:1 to receive either rolapitant or placebo in addition to their cisplatin protocol-mandated chemotherapy. The mean cisplatin dose was 76 mg/m^2 and 85% of patients received a concomitant chemotherapeutic agent in addition to protocol-mandated cisplatin therapy. The most common concomitant chemotherapeutic agents administered during cycle 1 were vinorelbine (16%), gemcitabine (15%), fluorouracil (12%), etoposide (11%), pemetrexed (9%), docetaxel (7%), paclitaxel (7%), epirubicin (5%), and capecitabine (4%). Those assigned to the rolapitant regimen received oral rolapitant 180 mg, oral dexamethasone 20 mg, and IV granisetron 10 mcg/kg on day 1, and oral dexamethasone 8 mg twice daily on days 2–4. Patients assigned to the control regimen received placebo plus oral dexamethasone 20 mg and IV granisetron 10 mcg/kg on day 1, and oral dexamethasone 8 mg twice daily on days 2–4. Rolapitant or placebo was administered 1–2 hours prior to chemotherapy on day 1. Dexamethasone and granisetron were administered 30 minutes prior to chemotherapy on day 1. The primary endpoint of Study 2 was complete response, defined as no emetic episodes and no use of rescue medication, in the delayed phase (25–120 hours) of chemotherapy-induced nausea and vomiting in cycle 1. A greater proportion of patients who received rolapitant therapy in Study 2 achieved a complete response in the delayed phase, compared with those who received the control regimen (70.1 versus 61.9%).

Safety and efficacy of rolapitant in patients receiving *moderately emetogenic chemotherapy* were established in a multicenter, randomized, double-blind, parallel group, active-controlled study (Study 3) in 1332 adults 22–88 years of age

(mean age 57 years) who were receiving such chemotherapy; at least 50% of the patients were receiving a combination of anthracycline and cyclophosphamide. Thirty percent of patients also received carboplatin in cycle 1. Patients were randomized 1:1 to either the rolapitant or control treatment arm. Those assigned to the rolapitant regimen received oral rolapitant 180 mg, oral dexamethasone 20 mg, and oral granisetron 2 mg on day 1, and oral granisetron 2 mg once daily on days 2–3. Patients assigned to the control regimen received placebo plus oral dexamethasone 20 mg and oral granisetron 2 mg on day 1, and oral granisetron 2 mg once daily on days 2–3. Rolapitant was administered 1–2 hours prior to chemotherapy on day 1. Dexamethasone and granisetron were administered 30 minutes prior to chemotherapy on day 1. The primary endpoint of Study 3 was complete response, defined as no emetic episodes and no rescue drug therapy, in the delayed phase (25–120 hours) of chemotherapy-induced nausea and vomiting. A greater proportion of patients who received rolapitant therapy (71.3%) achieved a complete response, compared with those who received the control regimen (61.6%).

Patients enrolled in Studies 1, 2, and 3 could enter a multiple-cycle extension study for up to 5 additional cycles of chemotherapy receiving the same treatment as assigned in cycle 1. At days 6–8 following initiation of chemotherapy, patients were asked to recall whether they had any episode of vomiting or retching or nausea that interfered with normal daily life. In nearly all cycles, a greater proportion of patients receiving rolapitant reported no emesis and no nausea interfering with daily life for the remaining chemotherapy cycles (cycles 2–6), compared with those who received control therapy.

Clinical Perspective

The American Society of Clinical Oncology (ASCO) issued updated antiemetic guidelines in 2020 for the use of prophylactic antiemetic therapy prior to emetogenic antineoplastic therapy. The guidelines state that all patients should receive the most active antiemetic regimen appropriate for the antineoplastic agents being administered. Patients treated with combinations of antineoplastic agents should be offered antiemetic therapy appropriate for the agent of greatest emetic risk. The ASCO guidelines generally support the use of a neurokinin-1 (NK$_1$) receptor antagonist such as rolapitant in combination regimens to prevent delayed nausea and vomiting in patients receiving high- or moderate-risk emetogenic antineoplastic therapy. Unlike other currently available NK$_1$ antagonists, rolapitant is not approved for prevention of acute nausea and vomiting associated with cancer chemotherapy.

To prevent chemotherapy-induced nausea and vomiting associated with *highly emetogenic antineoplastic regimens* that include cisplatin and other high-emetic-risk single agents, ASCO currently recommends a 4-drug antiemetic regimen consisting of an NK$_1$ receptor antagonist, a serotonin (5-HT$_3$) receptor antagonist, dexamethasone, and olanzapine on day 1 followed by continued dexamethasone and olanzapine therapy on days 2–4. To prevent chemotherapy-induced nausea and vomiting associated with a *highly emetogenic antineoplastic regimen* that includes an anthracycline plus cyclophosphamide, ASCO currently recommends a 4-drug antiemetic regimen consisting of an NK$_1$ receptor antagonist, a 5-HT$_3$ receptor antagonist, dexamethasone, and olanzapine on day 1 followed by continued olanzapine therapy on days 2–4.

To prevent chemotherapy-induced nausea and vomiting associated with *moderately emetogenic antineoplastic regimens* that include carboplatin AUC ≥4 mg/mL/min, patients should be offered a 3-drug combination of an NK$_1$ receptor antagonist, a 5-HT$_3$ receptor antagonist, and dexamethasone on day 1. Adults treated with *moderately emetogenic antineoplastic regimens* that do not include carboplatin AUC ≥4 mg/mL/min should be offered a 2-drug combination consisting of a 5-HT$_3$ receptor antagonist and dexamethasone on day 1; those receiving cyclophosphamide, doxorubicin, oxaliplatin, and other moderate-emetic-risk antineoplastic agents known to cause delayed nausea and vomiting may be offered dexamethasone on days 2 to 3.

ASCO recommends that patients receiving antineoplastic regimens with a *low emetogenic risk* should be offered a single dose of a 5-HT$_3$ receptor antagonist or a single dose of dexamethasone 8 mg prior to the antineoplastic treatment.

In adults receiving antineoplastic regimens with a *minimal emetogenic risk*, ASCO states that antiemetics should not be routinely administered.

For patients with breakthrough nausea or vomiting, clinicians should re-evaluate emetic risk, disease status, concurrent illnesses, and medications to determine whether the best regimen is being administered for the emetic risk.

DOSAGE AND ADMINISTRATION

● Administration

Rolapitant is administered prior to initiation of each chemotherapy cycle, but at intervals of no less than 2 weeks. Rolapitant should be administered within 2 hours prior to initiation of chemotherapy.

Rolapitant is administered orally without regard to meals.

● Dosage

Rolapitant is administered orally on day 1 as part of a 4-day regimen that includes a 5-HT₃ receptor antagonist and dexamethasone.

Rolapitant is commercially available as the hydrochloride salt; dosage is expressed in terms of rolapitant.

Prevention of Nausea and Vomiting Associated with Cisplatin-Based Highly Emetogenic Cancer Chemotherapy

When used with a 5-HT₃ receptor antagonist and dexamethasone for the prevention of nausea and vomiting associated with cisplatin-based highly emetogenic cancer chemotherapy in adults, rolapitant 180 mg should be administered as a single oral dose within 2 hours prior to initiation of chemotherapy on day 1. Dexamethasone 20 mg should be administered 30 minutes prior to initiation of chemotherapy on day 1, and the 5-HT₃ receptor antagonist should be administered on day 1 according to the prescribing information for the specific 5-HT₃ receptor antagonist. Dexamethasone should be continued on days 2–4 at a dosage of 8 mg twice daily.

In clinical studies, the rolapitant regimen for prevention of nausea and vomiting associated with cisplatin-based highly emetogenic chemotherapy included oral dexamethasone 20 mg and IV granisetron 10 mcg/kg on day 1, and oral dexamethasone 8 mg twice daily on days 2–4. In all studies, rolapitant was administered 1–2 hours prior to chemotherapy, and dexamethasone and granisetron were administered 30 minutes prior to chemotherapy on day 1.

Prevention of Nausea and Vomiting Associated with Moderately Emetogenic Cancer Chemotherapy and Combinations of Anthracycline and Cyclophosphamide

When used with a 5-HT₃ receptor antagonist and dexamethasone for the prevention of nausea and vomiting associated with moderately emetogenic cancer chemotherapy and combinations of anthracycline and cyclophosphamide in adults, rolapitant 180 mg should be administered as a single oral dose within 2 hours prior to initiation of chemotherapy on day 1. Dexamethasone 20 mg should be administered 30 minutes prior to initiation of chemotherapy on day 1. The 5-HT₃ receptor antagonist should be administered on days 1–4 according to the prescribing information for the specific 5-HT₃ receptor antagonist.

In clinical studies, the rolapitant regimen for prevention of delayed nausea and vomiting associated with moderately emetogenic cancer chemotherapy and combinations of anthracycline and cyclophosphamide included oral dexamethasone 20 mg and oral granisetron 2 mg on day 1, and oral granisetron 2 mg on days 2–3. In all studies, rolapitant was administered 1–2 hours prior to chemotherapy, and dexamethasone and granisetron were administered 30 minutes prior to chemotherapy on day 1.

● Special Populations

Hepatic Impairment

No dosage adjustment is necessary in patients with mild or moderate (Child-Pugh class A or B) hepatic impairment. Use of rolapitant should be avoided in patients with severe (Child-Pugh class C) hepatic impairment.

Renal Impairment

The manufacturer makes no special dosage recommendations at this time.

Geriatric Patients

The manufacturer makes no special dosage recommendations at this time.

CAUTIONS

● Contraindications

● Concurrent therapy with CYP2D6 substrates with a narrow therapeutic index such as pimozide or thioridazine.

● Pediatric patients <2 years of age.

● Warnings/Precautions

Interactions with CYP2D6 Substrates

Rolapitant is a moderate inhibitor of the CYP2D6 isoenzyme; the inhibitory effect of the drug is expected to persist beyond 28 days. Concomitant use of rolapitant and CYP2D6 substrates with a narrow therapeutic index such as pimozide or thioridazine is contraindicated. The resulting increase in plasma concentrations of pimozide or thioridazine may cause serious and/or life-threatening events of QT prolongation and torsades de pointes. If these drugs are required, use an alternative antiemetic to rolapitant or an alternative to thioridazine or pimozide.

Before starting treatment with rolapitant in patients receiving other CYP2D6 substrates, consult the manufacturer's prescribing information for the CYP2D6 substrate to obtain additional information about interactions.

Specific Populations

Pregnancy

Data are insufficient to inform a drug-associated risk of adverse developmental outcomes when rolapitant is used in pregnant women. Animal reproduction studies revealed no teratogenic or embryofetal effects when the drug was administered to pregnant rats and rabbits during the period of organogenesis; however, maternal toxicity, including reduced body weight gain and/or body weight loss and a concomitant reduction in food consumption during the first week of dosing in rats, was observed.

Lactation

It is not known whether rolapitant is distributed in human milk or whether the drug has any effects on the breastfed infant or on milk production. Rolapitant was found to distribute into the milk of lactating rats.

Consider the developmental and health benefits of breastfeeding along with the mother's clinical need for rolapitant and any potential adverse effects on the breastfed infant from the drug or underlying maternal condition or the use of concomitant chemotherapy.

Females and Males of Reproductive Potential

In animal fertility studies, rolapitant impaired the fertility of female rats in a reversible fashion. A transient decrease in maternal body weight gain, increases in the incidence of pre- and post-implantation loss, and slight decreases in number of corpora lutea and implantation sites were observed in these studies.

Rolapitant did not affect the fertility or general reproductive performance of male rats in animal fertility studies.

Pediatric Use

Safety and efficacy of rolapitant have not been established in pediatric patients. Rolapitant is contraindicated in pediatric patients <2 years of age.

Administration of rolapitant to juvenile rats at the human age equivalent of birth to 2 years resulted in abnormal ovarian and uterine development, early sexual development in female rats, delayed sexual development in male rats, and impaired fertility.

Geriatric Use

Of the 1294 patients who received rolapitant in clinical studies, 25% were ≥65 years of age, and 5% were ≥75 years of age. No overall differences in safety and efficacy were observed between geriatric patients and younger adults. However, the possibility of greater sensitivity of some older patients cannot be ruled out.

Hepatic Impairment

Following administration of a single oral dose of rolapitant 180 mg to patients with mild hepatic impairment (Child-Pugh class A), the pharmacokinetics of rolapitant were comparable with those of healthy individuals. In patients with moderate hepatic impairment (Child-Pugh class B), the mean peak plasma concentration of rolapitant was reduced by 25%, while the mean AUC was similar to those of healthy individuals. Median time to peak plasma concentration of a metabolite of rolapitant (M19) was 204 hours in patients with mild or moderate hepatic impairment, compared to 168 hours in healthy individuals. Pharmacokinetics of rolapitant were not studied in patients with severe hepatic impairment (Child-Pugh class C).

Use of rolapitant should be avoided in patients with severe hepatic impairment. If use is unavoidable, patients should be monitored for adverse effects.

Renal Impairment

In population pharmacokinetic analyses, rolapitant pharmacokinetics in cancer patients with mild (creatinine clearance of 60–90 mL/minute) or moderate (creatinine clearance of 30–60 mL/minute) renal impairment were comparable to cancer patients with normal renal function. Insufficient data are available regarding the effect of rolapitant in patients with severe renal impairment. Pharmacokinetics of rolapitant were not studied in patients with end-stage renal disease requiring hemodialysis.

● Common Adverse Effects

Cisplatin-based highly emetogenic chemotherapy: Adverse effects reported in ≥3% of patients include neutropenia, hiccups, and abdominal pain.

Moderately emetogenic chemotherapy and combinations of anthracycline and cyclophosphamide: Adverse effects reported in ≥3% of patients include decreased appetite, neutropenia, dizziness, dyspepsia, urinary tract infection, stomatitis, and anemia.

DRUG INTERACTIONS

Rolapitant is metabolized by cytochrome P-450 (CYP) 3A4 isoenzyme. The drug does not inhibit or induce CYP3A4 when given as a single oral dose. Rolapitant is a moderate inhibitor of CYP2D6, an inhibitor of P-glycoprotein (P-gp), and an inhibitor of breast cancer resistance protein (BCRP).

In vitro studies suggest that rolapitant is not an inhibitor of CYP1A2 or CYP2E1. Rolapitant inhibits CYP2A6; however, clinically meaningful interaction via inhibition of CYP2A6 is unlikely.

Oral rolapitant is unlikely to inhibit organic anion transporting polypeptides (OATP) 1B1 and 1B3, organic anion transporters (OAT1 and OAT3), organic cation transporter (OCT) 2, and multidrug and toxin extrusion proteins (MATE1 and MATE2K).

● Drugs Affecting or Affected by Hepatic Microsomal Enzymes

CYP2D6 Substrates

Concomitant administration of rolapitant and CYP2D6 substrates can increase plasma concentrations and adverse effects of the CYP2D6 substrate. The inhibitory effect of rolapitant on CYP2D6 substrates can persist beyond 28 days for an unknown duration following administration of the drug.

Concomitant administration of rolapitant and CYP2D6 substrates with a narrow therapeutic index such as pimozide or thioridazine increases plasma concentrations of the substrate, which can cause serious and/or life-threatening events including QT prolongation and torsades de pointes. Concomitant use is contraindicated. If patients require these drugs, use an alternative antiemetic to rolapitant or an alternative to pimozide or thioridazine that is not metabolized by CYP2D6.

Consider the possibility of a clinically relevant interaction with other CYP2D6 substrates. Before starting treatment with rolapitant in patients taking other CYP2D6 substrates, consult the prescribing information of the CYP2D6 substrate to obtain further information about interactions with CYP2D6 inhibitors.

CYP3A4 Inducers

Coadministration of rolapitant with rifampin, a strong CYP3A4 inducer, can significantly reduce the plasma concentrations of rolapitant and decrease the drug's efficacy. Avoid use of rolapitant in patients who require chronic administration of strong CYP3A4 inducers.

● BCRP Substrates with Narrow Therapeutic Index

Concomitant administration of rolapitant and BCRP substrates with a narrow therapeutic index (e.g., methotrexate, topotecan, or irinotecan) may increase the plasma concentration of the BCRP substrate, which could potentially result in adverse effects. If concomitant use of a BCRP substrate with a narrow therapeutic index cannot be avoided, patients should be monitored for adverse effects related to the concomitant drug.

● P-gp Substrates with Narrow Therapeutic Index

Concomitant administration of rolapitant and P-gp substrates with a narrow therapeutic index (e.g., digoxin) increases the plasma concentration of the P-gp substrate, which could potentially result in adverse effects. If digoxin is used concomitantly with rolapitant, monitor digoxin concentrations and adjust the dosage as necessary to maintain therapeutic concentrations. If concomitant use of other P-gp substrates with a narrow therapeutic index cannot be avoided, patients should be monitored for adverse effects.

● Dexamethasone

Rolapitant has no substantial effects on the pharmacokinetics of dexamethasone (a CYP3A4 substrate). No dosage adjustment for dexamethasone is needed when co-administered with rolapitant.

● Dextromethorphan

A 3-fold increase in the systemic exposure of dextromethorphan, a CYP2D6 substrate, was observed 7 days following coadministration of dextromethorphan 30 mg and a single dose of rolapitant 180 mg. Inhibition of CYP2D6 persisted on day 28 with a 2.3-fold increase in dextromethorphan concentrations. The increase in plasma concentrations of dextromethorphan may result in potential adverse reactions.

● Digoxin

Concomitant administration of a single dose of rolapitant 180 mg and digoxin 0.5 mg increases peak plasma concentration and AUC of digoxin by 70 and 30%, respectively. Monitor digoxin concentrations and adjust the dosage as needed to maintain therapeutic concentrations.

● Efavirenz

No clinically important interaction was observed on the pharmacokinetics of efavirenz, a CYP2B6 substrate, when the drug was administered with rolapitant.

● Ketoconazole

Concomitant administration of the strong CYP3A4 inhibitor ketoconazole 400 mg once daily for 21 days and a single dose of rolapitant 90 mg did not substantially affect the peak plasma concentration of rolapitant, while the AUC of rolapitant was increased by 21%.

● Midazolam

Concomitant administration of rolapitant had no substantial effects on the pharmacokinetics of oral midazolam (a CYP3A4 substrate) when the drugs were coadministered.

● Omeprazole

No clinically important interaction was observed on the pharmacokinetics of omeprazole, a CYP2C19 substrate, when the drug was administered with rolapitant.

● Ondansetron

Concomitant administration of a single dose of rolapitant 180 mg and IV ondansetron (a CYP3A4 substrate) had no substantial effects on the pharmacokinetics of ondansetron.

● Repaglinide

No clinically important interaction was observed on the pharmacokinetics of repaglinide, a CYP2C8 substrate, when the drug was administered with rolapitant.

● Rifampin

Plasma concentrations and AUC of rolapitant were decreased by 30 and 85%, respectively, when rifampin, a strong CYP3A4 inducer, was administered concomitantly with rolapitant. The mean half-life of rolapitant decreased from 176 hours without concomitant rifampin administration to 41 hours with concomitant rifampin administration. Avoid concomitant use of rolapitant in patients who require chronic administration of rifampin.

• Sulfasalazine

Concomitant administration of rolapitant and sulfasalazine (a BCRP substrate) increased peak plasma concentrations and AUC of sulfasalazine by 140 and 130%, respectively, on day 1. Peak plasma concentrations and AUC of sulfasalazine were increased by 17 and 32%, respectively, on day 8 when a second dose of sulfasalazine was given without rolapitant administration.

• Tolbutamide

No clinically important interaction was observed on the pharmacokinetics of tolbutamide, a CYP2C9 substrate, when the drug was administered with rolapitant.

• Warfarin

Coadministration of a single dose of IV rolapitant (unapproved route of administration with a higher peak plasma concentration than the oral route) with warfarin increased peak plasma concentrations and AUC of S-warfarin by 3% and 18%, respectively, on day 1. On day 8, the increases were 3% for peak plasma concentrations and 21% for AUC. The effects on INR and prothrombin time were not studied.

Monitor INR and prothrombin time and adjust the dosage of warfarin as needed with concomitant use of rolapitant.

DESCRIPTION

Rolapitant is a selective and competitive antagonist of human substance P/neurokinin-1 (NK_1) receptors. Rolapitant does not have substantial affinity for the NK_2 or NK_3 receptors or for a battery of other receptors, transporters, enzymes, and ion channels. Rolapitant crosses the blood-brain barrier and occupies NK_1 receptors in the brain. The drug demonstrates a dose-dependent increase in mean NK_1 receptor occupancy in the dose range of 4.5–180 mg. At a rolapitant dose of 180 mg, the mean NK_1 receptor occupancy was 73% in the striatum at 120 hours after the dose was administered to healthy individuals. However, the relationship between NK_1 receptor occupancy and clinical efficacy of rolapitant is yet to be determined.

Rolapitant has a high bioavailability (greater than 90%) and is highly bound to plasma proteins (99.8%). Peak plasma concentrations are attained in approximately 4 hours following administration of a single oral dose of 180 mg under fasting conditions in healthy individuals. Accumulation of rolapitant is approximately 5-fold following multiple oral doses of 9–45 mg once daily. Systemic exposure of rolapitant increases in a dose-proportional manner over the dose range of 4.5 to 180 mg. Following single oral doses of rolapitant, the mean terminal half-life ranges from 169 to 183 hours (approximately 7 days) and is independent of dose. Rolapitant is metabolized principally by cytochrome P-450 (CYP) 3A4 to a major active metabolite (M19). Formation of M19 is relatively slow resulting in a delayed median time to peak plasma concentration of 120 hours (range: 24–168 hours); mean half-life of M19 is 158 hours. Exposure ratio of M19 to rolapitant is approximately 50% in plasma. Following administration of a single oral 180-mg radiolabeled dose of rolapitant, 14.2% (range 9–20%) and 73% (range 52–89%) of the dose is recovered in the urine and feces, respectively, over 6 weeks. In pooled samples collected over 2 weeks, 8.3% of the dose is recovered in the urine principally as metabolites, and 37.8% of the dose is recovered in the feces principally as unchanged drug. Unchanged rolapitant or M19 was not found in the pooled urine sample. Age, sex, and race have no substantial effect on the pharmacokinetics of rolapitant.

ADVICE TO PATIENTS

- Advise patients to read the FDA-approved patient labeling (Patient Information).

- Advise patients to tell their healthcare provider when they start or stop taking any concomitant medications. Rolapitant is a moderate CYP2D6 inhibitor and can increase plasma concentrations of CYP2D6 substrates.

- Advise females of reproductive potential that rolapitant may impair fertility. Importance of women informing clinicians if they are or plan to become pregnant or plan to breast-feed.

- Advise patients to inform their clinicians of existing or contemplated concomitant therapy, including prescription and OTC drugs, as well as any concomitant illnesses.

- Advise patients of other important precautionary information. (See Cautions.)

PREPARATIONS

Excipients in commercially available drug preparations may have clinically important effects in some individuals; consult specific product labeling for details.

Rolapitant Hydrochloride

Oral		
Tablets, film-coated	90 mg (of rolapitant)	Varubi®, TerSera Therapeutics

Selected Revisions January 16, 2023, © Copyright, September 14, 2016, American Society of Health-System Pharmacists, Inc.

Famotidine

56:28.12 • HISTAMINE H₂-ANTAGONISTS

■ Famotidine is a histamine H_2-receptor antagonist.

USES

Famotidine is used orally for the treatment of active duodenal or gastric ulcer, gastroesophageal reflux disease, endoscopically diagnosed erosive esophagitis, and as maintenance therapy for duodenal ulcer. Oral famotidine also is used for the management of pathological GI hypersecretory conditions. IV famotidine is used in hospitalized individuals with pathological GI hypersecretory conditions or intractable ulcers, or when oral therapy is not feasible.

● Duodenal Ulcer

Acute Therapy

Famotidine is used for the short-term treatment of endoscopically or radiographically confirmed active duodenal ulcer. Antacids may be used concomitantly as needed for relief of pain. In controlled studies in patients with endoscopically confirmed duodenal ulcers, reported rates of ulcer healing for famotidine were substantially higher than those for placebo. In a multicenter, double-blind study in patients with endoscopically confirmed duodenal ulcer, reported rates of ulcer healing for oral famotidine dosages of 40 mg at bedtime daily, 20 mg twice daily, or 40 mg twice daily vs placebo were 32, 38, or 34%, respectively, vs 17%, at 2 weeks; 70, 67, or 75%, respectively, vs 31%, at 4 weeks; and 82–83% for these famotidine dosage regimens vs 45% for placebo, at 8 weeks. Famotidine also produced greater reductions in daytime and nocturnal pain and antacid consumption than did placebo, with complete relief of pain in most patients usually occurring within 2 weeks after initiation of famotidine therapy.

Famotidine appears to be at least as effective as cimetidine or ranitidine for the short-term treatment of active duodenal ulcer. An oral famotidine dosage of 40 mg at bedtime daily generally appears to be more effective than an oral cimetidine dosage of 800 mg daily and as effective as an oral ranitidine dosage of 300 mg daily (as a single or divided dose) in this condition. In a multicenter, double-blind study in patients with endoscopically confirmed duodenal ulcers, 68–81 or 76% of ulcers were healed following administration of famotidine (20 mg twice daily, 40 mg at bedtime daily, or 40 mg twice daily) or ranitidine (150 mg twice daily), respectively, for 4 weeks and 87–92 or 90%, respectively, were healed following therapy for 8 weeks. In geriatric patients, famotidine and ranitidine, in dosages of 40 mg at bedtime daily and 150 mg twice daily, respectively, were equally effective in healing active duodenal ulcers and providing symptomatic relief; 57 and 51% of ulcers were healed following administration of famotidine and ranitidine, respectively, for 8 weeks. In several studies, there appeared to be little difference between famotidine and ranitidine in reductions of daytime and nocturnal pain and antacid consumption.

Daily bedtime doses of famotidine generally appear to be as effective as a twice-daily regimen of the drug in healing active duodenal ulcer, although the bedtime regimen may be slightly less effective than twice-daily regimens at 4 but not 8 weeks. Ulcer healing rates averaged 32, 34, or 38% at 2 weeks; 68–70, 75–81, or 67–77% at 4 weeks; and 83–87, 82–92, or 82–92 at 8 weeks following oral famotidine dosages of 40 mg at bedtime daily, 40 mg twice daily, or 20 mg twice daily, respectively. Antacid consumption appeared to be similar with the various famotidine dosage regimens employed. Evidence from a multicenter, controlled study indicates that healing rates for duodenal ulcers in patients receiving famotidine may not be affected substantially by cigarette smoking or alcohol consumption, although healing rates were slightly higher in nonsmokers than in smokers.

Safety and efficacy of long-term famotidine therapy for active duodenal ulcer have not been determined. Studies to date have been limited to short-term treatment of active duodenal ulcer, and the safety and efficacy of treatment for active disease beyond 8 weeks have not been determined. Most patients with duodenal ulcer respond to famotidine therapy during the initial 4-week course of therapy; an additional 4 weeks of therapy may contribute to healing in some patients. However, short-term famotidine therapy (i.e., up to 8 weeks) for the treatment of active duodenal disease will not prevent recurrence following acute healing and discontinuance of the drug. Current epidemiologic and clinical evidence supports a strong association between gastric infection with Helicobacter pylori and the pathogenesis of duodenal and gastric ulcers; long-term H. pylori infection also

has been implicated as a risk factor for gastric cancer. For additional information on the association of this infection with these and other GI conditions, see Helicobacter pylori Infection, under Uses, in Clarithromycin 8:12.12.92.

Conventional antiulcer therapy with H_2-receptor antagonists, proton-pump inhibitors, sucralfate, and/or antacids heals ulcers but generally is ineffective in eradicating H. pylori, and such therapy is associated with a high rate of ulcer recurrence (e.g., 60–100% per year). Duodenal ulcers have recurred within 6 months in 52–73% of patients following discontinuance of famotidine therapy. The American College of Gastroenterology (ACG), the National Institutes of Health (NIH), and most clinicians currently recommend that all patients with initial or recurrent duodenal or gastric ulcer and documented H. pylori infection receive anti-infective therapy for treatment of the infection. Although 3-drug regimens consisting of a bismuth salt (e.g., bismuth subsalicylate) and 2 anti-infective agents (e.g., tetracycline or amoxicillin plus metronidazole) administered for 10–14 days have been effective in eradicating the infection, resolving associated gastritis, healing peptic ulcer, and preventing ulcer recurrence in many patients with H. pylori-associated peptic ulcer disease, current evidence principally from studies in Europe suggests that 1 week of such therapy provides comparable H. pylori eradication rates. Other regimens that combine one or more anti-infective agents (e.g., clarithromycin, amoxicillin) with a bismuth salt and/ or an antisecretory agent (e.g., omeprazole, lansoprazole, H_2-receptor antagonist) also have been used successfully for H. pylori eradication, and the choice of a particular regimen should be based on the rapidly evolving data on optimal therapy, including consideration of the patient's prior exposure to anti-infective agents, the local prevalence of resistance, patient compliance, and costs of therapy.

Current evidence suggests that inclusion of a proton-pump inhibitor (e.g., omeprazole, lansoprazole) in anti-H. pylori regimens containing 2 anti-infectives enhances effectiveness, and limited data suggest that such regimens retain good efficacy despite imidazole (e.g., metronidazole) resistance. Therefore, the ACG and many clinicians currently recommend 1 week of therapy with a proton-pump inhibitor and 2 anti-infective agents (usually clarithromycin and amoxicillin or metronidazole), or a 3-drug, bismuth-based regimen (e.g., bismuth-metronidazole-tetracycline) concomitantly with a proton-pump inhibitor, for treatment of H. pylori infection. For a more complete discussion of H. pylori infection, including details about the efficacy of various regimens and rationale for drug selection, see Helicobacter pylori Infection, under Uses, in Clarithromycin 8:12.12.92.

Maintenance Therapy

Famotidine is used in reduced dosage as maintenance therapy following healing of active duodenal ulcer to reduce ulcer recurrence. In placebo-controlled studies, duodenal ulcer recurrence rates after 3, 6, and 12 months ranged from 9–14, 16–30, and 23–38%, respectively, for 20 or 40 mg of famotidine at bedtime daily vs 39, 52–73, and 57–77%, respectively, for placebo. Because the efficacy of H_2-receptor antagonists in preventing duodenal ulcer recurrence appears to be substantially reduced in patients who are cigarette smokers compared with nonsmokers, patients who are cigarette smokers should be advised of the importance of discontinuing smoking in the prevention of ulcer recurrence. Maintenance therapy with famotidine has not been studied for longer than 1 year in placebo-controlled studies, and the effect of maintenance therapy with the drug in patients with previously healed duodenal ulcers remains to be more fully evaluated.

● Pathologic GI Hypersecretory Conditions

Famotidine is used for the treatment of pathologic GI hypersecretory conditions (e.g., Zollinger-Ellison syndrome, multiple endocrine adenomas). Famotidine reduces gastric acid secretion and associated symptoms (including diarrhea, nausea, and epigastric burning and pain) in patients with these conditions. Antimuscarinics (e.g., isopropamide iodide) have been used concomitantly with famotidine to augment famotidine-induced inhibition of gastric acid secretion in some patients with GI hypersecretory conditions.

In a limited number of patients with GI hypersecretory conditions, famotidine has effectively inhibited gastric acid hypersecretion and produced inhibition of longer duration than cimetidine and somewhat longer than that of ranitidine. However, these drugs appear to be comparably effective for the treatment of hypersecretion when adequate, equipotent dosages are used and patient compliance is optimal. In one study, patients with GI hypersecretory conditions who were successfully treated with 1.2–9 or 0.6–5.4 g of cimetidine or ranitidine, respectively, alone daily subsequently were treated successfully with 50–800 mg of famotidine alone daily. Although famotidine, cimetidine, and ranitidine were equally effective in controlling gastric hypersecretion, substantially lower doses of famotidine were required and with less frequency than with cimetidine or ranitidine. Famotidine therapy alone or in combination with an antimuscarinic agent has been continued in a few patients for up to 34 months.

● Gastric Ulcer

Famotidine is used for short-term treatment of active, benign gastric ulcer. The efficacy of famotidine in the treatment of gastric ulcer appears to be similar to that of cimetidine or ranitidine, with 40–47, 36–71, or 40–76% of ulcers healed at 4 weeks; 65–68, 66–95, or 68–90% healed at 6 weeks; and 64–80, 67–86, or 79–91% healed at 8 weeks following therapy with famotidine, cimetidine, or ranitidine, respectively. In several other studies in patients with gastric ulcer, famotidine promoted healing of ulcers in about 42–65, 60–95, and 78 to greater than 91% of patients after 4, 6, and 8 weeks of treatment, respectively. Response of gastric ulcers to famotidine therapy does not appear to be affected by patient age or gender, cigarette smoking, alcohol consumption, or duration of disease. Patients with a history of chronic gastric ulcers (history of disease of 10 years or longer) appear to respond as well to famotidine therapy as patients with a brief history of disease. Famotidine also generally produced greater reductions in pain (fasting, postprandial, nocturnal) and other symptoms (including belching, nausea, anorexia) and in antacid consumption than did placebo. Safety and efficacy of famotidine in the treatment of gastric ulcer have not been established for periods exceeding 8 weeks; therefore, use of the drug for more prolonged treatment of active disease or for maintenance therapy of previously healed gastric ulcer remains to be more fully evaluated. If famotidine is used in the treatment of gastric ulcer, it should be kept in mind that symptomatic response does not preclude the presence of gastric malignancy.

Current epidemiologic and clinical evidence supports a strong association between gastric infection with *H. pylori* and the pathogenesis of gastric ulcers, and the ACG, NIH, and most clinicians currently recommend that *all* patients with initial or recurrent gastric ulcer and documented *H. pylori* infection receive anti-infective therapy for treatment of the infection. The choice of a particular regimen should be based on the rapidly evolving data on optimal therapy, including consideration of the patient's prior exposure to anti-infective agents, the local prevalence of resistance, patient compliance, and costs of therapy (See Duodenal Ulcer: Acute Therapy, in Uses.) For a more complete discussion of *H. pylori* infection, including details about the efficacy of various regimens and rationale for drug selection,see Helicobacter pylori Infection, under Uses, in Clarithromycin 8:12.12.92.

● Gastroesophageal Reflux Disease

Famotidine is used to provide short-term symptomatic relief of gastroesophageal reflux disease (GERD). Famotidine also is used for short-term treatment of esophagitis associated with gastroesophageal reflux, including endoscopically proven erosive or ulcerative disease. By increasing gastric pH, H₂-receptor antagonists have relieved heartburn and other symptoms of reflux and have been associated with somewhat higher healing rates of endoscopically proven esophagitis when compared with placebo and have reduced antacid consumption.

Suppression of gastric acid secretion is considered by the ACG to be the mainstay of treatment for GERD, and a proton-pump inhibitor or histamine H₂- receptor antagonist is used to achieve acid suppression, control symptoms, and prevent complications of the disease. The ACG states that a histamine H₂- receptor antagonist administered daily in divided doses is effective in many patients with less severe GERD, and over-the-counter (OTC) antacids and histamine H₂- receptor antagonists are appropriate for *self*-medication as initial therapy in such individuals. A histamine H₂-receptor antagonist is particularly useful when taken before certain activities (e.g., heavy meal, exercise) that may result in acid reflux symptoms in some patients. The ACG states that H₂-receptor antagonists generally may be used interchangeably, although the drugs may differ in potency and in their onset and duration of action. However, proton-pump inhibitors are more effective (i.e., provide more frequent and more rapid symptomatic relief and healing of esophagitis) than histamine H₂-receptor antagonists in the treatment of GERD. Although higher doses and more frequent administration of histamine H₂-receptor antagonists appear to increase their efficacy, such dosages are less effective and more expensive than proton-pump inhibitor therapy. Once-daily administration of a histamine H₂-receptor antagonist at full dosage is *not* considered to be appropriate therapy for GERD.

Based on data from a limited number of patients, famotidine 20 mg administered twice daily appears to be at least as effective as famotidine 40 mg administered at bedtime and more effective than placebo in improving symptoms of gastroesophageal reflux in patients who had no evidence of endoscopically proven erosive or ulcerative disease. Within 2 weeks of therapy, symptomatic relief was reported in a higher percentage of patients receiving famotidine compared with those receiving placebo; symptoms improved in 82, 69, and 62% of these patients at 6 weeks

for famotidine 20 mg twice daily, famotidine 40 mg at bedtime, or placebo, respectively. In controlled studies in patients with endoscopically evaluated gastroesophageal reflux disease, reported rates of ulcer healing for famotidine were higher than those for placebo. Healing rates from controlled studies employing various dosage regimens were approximately 48, 32–34, 29, and 7–18% at 6 weeks and 69, 50–54, 43, and 26–29% at 12 weeks for famotidine 40 mg twice daily, 20 mg twice daily, 40 mg at bedtime, and placebo, respectively. Patients receiving famotidine reported faster relief of daytime and nocturnal heartburn and greater reduction in antacid consumption than those receiving placebo. Nocturnal heartburn relief was reported in a higher percentage of patients receiving famotidine than those receiving placebo; nocturnal heartburn relief occurred in about 58, 50, and 49% of patients receiving famotidine 20 mg twice daily, 40 mg at bedtime, and placebo, respectively, while daytime heartburn relief occurred in approximately 56, 42, and 46% of such patients, respectively. In a study in patients with gastroesophageal reflux who had endoscopically evaluated erosive or ulcerative disease, reported rates of ulcer or erosion healing at 6 weeks were 48 and 42% in patients receiving famotidine 40 mg twice daily or ranitidine 150 mg twice daily, respectively, while at 12 weeks rates of healing were 71 or 60% in patients receiving famotidine 40 mg twice daily or ranitidine 150 mg twice daily, respectively. However, ranitidine was as effective as famotidine in improving symptoms of gastroesophageal reflux.

H₂-receptor antagonists also have been used in combination with metoclopramide in a limited number of patients who failed to respond to an H₂-receptor antagonist alone, but the ACG states that frequent and potentially severe adverse CNS effects of metoclopramide have appropriately decreased regular use of the drug for GERD. Although some clinicians have suggested that a histamine H₂- receptor antagonist also may be used in combination with bethanechol† in patients who fail to respond to a histamine H₂-receptor antagonist alone, the ACG states that bethanechol has limited efficacy in the treatment of GERD.

Short-term therapy (i.e., up to 12 weeks) with H₂-receptor antagonists for the treatment of GERD will not prevent recurrence following ulcer healing and discontinuance of such therapy. Esophagitis has recurred within 6 months in up to 80% of patients following discontinuance of H₂-receptor antagonist therapy. Because GERD is considered a chronic disease, many patients with GERD require long-term, even lifelong, treatment. The ACG states that proton-pump inhibitors are effective and appropriate as maintenance therapy in many patients with the disease. Maintenance therapy† with an H₂-receptor antagonist also has been used to reduce recurrence of GERD. However, many patients initially responding to proton-pump inhibitors experience symptomatic relapse and failure of esophageal healing with subsequent use of a histamine H₂-receptor antagonist.

For further information on the treatment of GERD, see Uses: Gastroesophageal Reflux, in Omeprazole 56:28.36.

● Other Uses

Famotidine may be used for *self-medication* for relief of symptoms of *occasional* heartburn (pyrosis), acid indigestion (hyperchlorhydria), or sour stomach and for prevention of such symptoms caused by consumption of food or beverages. Famotidine also may be used in fixed combination with calcium carbonate and magnesium hydroxide (Pepcid® Complete) for *self-medication* for relief of symptoms of *occasional* heartburn (pyrosis) associated with acid indigestion (hyperchlorhydria) or sour stomach.

Famotidine also has been used in a limited number of patients to control intragastric pH and/or stress-induced GI bleeding in critically ill patients (e.g., traumatized or postoperative patients, patients in shock or with respiratory insufficiency)†. In patients with GI bleeding† secondary to duodenal or stress ulcers or gastritis, the drug may control GI bleeding and reduce the need for emergency surgery, but may not prevent bleeding recurrence. Additional study to further evaluate the effect of famotidine on morbidity and mortality in patients with these conditions is necessary.

DOSAGE AND ADMINISTRATION

● Reconstitution and Administration

Famotidine is usually administered orally. The drug may also be given by slow IV injection or by slow IV infusion in hospitalized patients with pathologic hypersecretory conditions or intractable duodenal ulcers, or when oral therapy is not feasible. Antacids may be administered concomitantly as necessary for relief of pain. (See Drug Interactions: Food and Antacids.)

Parenteral solutions of famotidine should be inspected visually for particulate matter and discoloration prior to administration whenever solution and container permit.

Oral Suspension

For oral administration, famotidine oral suspension may be substituted for famotidine tablets in patients who are unable to swallow tablets. The powder for suspension should be reconstituted at the time of dispensing by adding 46 mL of water to a bottle containing 400 mg of famotidine to provide a suspension containing 40 mg/5 mL. The suspension should be agitated well for 5–10 seconds after adding the water for reconstitution and again immediately prior to administration of each dose.

Orally Disintegrating Tablets

Patients receiving famotidine orally disintegrating tablets should be instructed not to remove a tablet from the blister until just prior to dosing. The tablet should *not* be pushed through the foil. With dry hands, the blister package should be peeled completely off the blister. The tablet should then be gently removed and immediately placed on the tongue to dissolve and be swallowed with the saliva; administration with liquid is not necessary.

IV Injection

Famotidine concentrate for injection must be diluted prior to IV administration. For IV injection, 20 mg of famotidine is diluted to a total of 5 or 10 mL with 0.9% sodium chloride injection or another comparable IV solution (see Chemistry and Stability: Stability) to provide a solution containing approximately 4 or 2 mg/mL, respectively. The appropriate dose is injected IV at a rate no faster than 10 mg/minute.

IV Infusion

For intermittent IV infusion, 20 mg of famotidine as the concentrate is added to 100 mL of 5% dextrose injection or another compatible IV solution (see Chemistry and Stability: Stability) to provide a solution containing approximately 0.2 mg/mL. This solution is infused IV over 15–30 minutes.

Alternatively, famotidine that is commercially available as a diluted solution (0.4 mg of famotidine per mL) in 0.9% sodium chloride may be used for intermittent IV infusion. The commercially available diluted solution should only be administered by IV infusion over 15–30 minutes. The container should be checked for minute leaks by firmly squeezing the bag. The injection should be discarded if the seal is not intact or leaks are found or if the solution is cloudy or contains a precipitate. Additives should not be introduced into the injection container. The injection should not be used in series connections with other plastic containers, since such use could result in air embolism from residual air being drawn from the primary container before administration of fluid from the secondary container is complete.

• Dosage

Duodenal Ulcer

For the treatment of active duodenal ulcer, the usual adult oral dosage of famotidine is 40 mg at bedtime daily. Alternatively, 20 mg twice daily may be administered orally in adults. The advantage of one oral regimen over another for particular patients with active duodenal ulcer has not been determined, although a once-daily bedtime dosage may be used for patients in whom dosing convenience is considered important for patient compliance. Healing may occur within 2 weeks in some patients and within 4 weeks in most patients. Some patients may benefit from an additional 4 weeks of therapy. It occasionally may be necessary to continue full-dose famotidine therapy for longer than 6–8 weeks; however, the safety and efficacy of continuing full-dose therapy beyond 8 weeks have not been determined. In hospitalized adults with intractable duodenal ulcers or when oral therapy is not feasible, the manufacturer states that famotidine may be administered IV in a dosage of 20 mg every 12 hours.

For maintenance therapy following healing of acute duodenal ulcer to reduce ulcer recurrence, the usual adult oral dosage of famotidine is 20 mg at bedtime daily.

For the treatment of duodenal ulcer in children 1–16 years of age, the manufacturer recommends an oral famotidine dosage of 0.5 mg/kg daily given at bedtime or in 2 divided doses, up to a total daily dosage of 40 mg. In hospitalized children 1–16 years of age with intractable ulcers or when oral therapy is not feasible, the manufacturer states that a famotidine dosage of 0.25 mg/kg may be administered IV (over not less than 2 minutes or as a 15-minute infusion) every

12 hours, up to a total daily dosage of 40 mg. Data from uncontrolled studies in pediatric patients suggest that famotidine is effective for gastric acid suppression when given in dosages of up to 1 mg/kg daily; however, data are insufficient to establish the percentage of these patients who respond to a given dose and duration of therapy. (See Cautions: Pediatric Precautions.) Therefore, treatment duration (initially based on recommendations in adults) and dosage in such patients should be individualized based on clinical response and/or gastric or esophageal pH determination and endoscopy.

Pathologic GI Hypersecretory Conditions

For the treatment of pathologic GI hypersecretory conditions (e.g., Zollinger-Ellison syndrome, multiple endocrine adenomas), dosages of famotidine should be individualized according to patient response and tolerance. The usual initial adult dosage is 20 mg orally every 6 hours; however, higher initial dosages may be necessary in some patients. Subsequent famotidine dosage should be adjusted according to the patient's requirements and response, and therapy continued as long as clinically necessary. Periodic (e.g., once to several times yearly) increases in famotidine dosage may be necessary during long-term therapy. Oral dosages ranging from 20–160 mg every 6 hours generally have been necessary to maintain basal gastric acid secretion at less than 10 mEq/hour; determination of gastric acid secretion during the hour prior to a dose may be useful in establishing optimum dosage. Dosages up to 800 mg daily in divided doses have been administered to individuals with severe disease, although the manufacturer recommends dosages only up to 160 mg every 6 hours (640 mg daily). In hospitalized patients with pathologic GI hypersecretory conditions or when oral therapy is not feasible, the manufacturer states that famotidine may be administered IV in a dosage of 20 mg every 6 hours in adults; however, higher initial doses may be necessary in some patients. Subsequent IV dosage should be adjusted according to the patient's requirements and response.

The famotidine dosage necessary in patients who have previously received therapy with cimetidine or ranitidine is directly related to the severity of the GI hypersecretory condition and the dosage regimen of cimetidine or ranitidine. Patients who require low or high dosages of cimetidine or ranitidine will also require low or high dosages, respectively, of famotidine.

Gastric Ulcer

For the short-term treatment of active, benign gastric ulcer, the usual adult oral dosage of famotidine is 40 mg daily at bedtime. Most patients demonstrate complete healing of gastric ulcers within 8 weeks; the safety and efficacy of continuing famotidine therapy beyond 8 weeks have not been determined.

For the treatment of gastric ulcer in children 1–16 years of age, the manufacturer recommends an oral famotidine dosage of 0.5 mg/kg daily given at bedtime or in 2 divided doses, up to a total daily dosage of 40 mg. In hospitalized children 1–16 years of age with intractable ulcers or when oral therapy is not feasible, the manufacturer states that a famotidine dosage of 0.25 mg/kg may be administered IV (over not less than 2 minutes or as a 15-minute infusion) every 12 hours, up to a total daily dosage of 40 mg. Data from uncontrolled studies in pediatric patients suggest that famotidine is effective for gastric acid suppression when given in dosages of up to 1 mg/kg daily; however, data are insufficient to establish the percentage of these patients who respond to a given dose and duration of therapy. (See Cautions: Pediatric Precautions.) Therefore, treatment duration (initially based on recommendations in adults) and dosage in such patients should be individualized based on clinical response and/or gastric or esophageal pH determination and endoscopy.

Gastroesophageal Reflux

For the symptomatic relief of gastroesophageal reflux, the usual adult oral dosage of famotidine is 20 mg twice daily for up to 6 weeks. Famotidine dosages of 40 mg at bedtime also have been used for the symptomatic relief of gastroesophageal reflux; however, famotidine administered twice daily appears to be more effective in improving symptoms of gastroesophageal reflux than famotidine administered just at bedtime. In addition, the American College of Gastroenterology (ACG) states that once-daily administration of a histamine H₂-receptor antagonist at full dosage is *not* considered to be appropriate therapy for gastroesophageal reflux disease (GERD). For the symptomatic relief of esophagitis associated with gastroesophageal reflux, including endoscopically proven erosive or ulcerative disease, the usual adult oral dosage of famotidine is 20 or 40 mg twice daily for up to 12 weeks.

For the symptomatic relief of gastroesophageal reflux with or without esophagitis including erosions and ulcerations in children 1–16 years of age, the manufacturer recommends an initial oral famotidine dosage of 1 mg/kg daily in 2 divided doses, up to 40 mg twice daily. Data from uncontrolled studies in pediatric patients suggest that famotidine is effective in the management of gastroesophageal reflux with or without esophagitis including erosions and ulcerations when given in oral dosages of up to 2 mg/kg daily; however, data are insufficient to establish the percentage of these patients who respond to a given dose and duration of therapy. (See Cautions: Pediatric Precautions.) Therefore, treatment duration (initially based on recommendations in adults) and dosage in such patients should be individualized based on clinical response and/or gastric or esophageal pH determination and endoscopy.

The manufacturer states that dosages and dosage regimens for parenteral famotidine in patients with gastroesophageal reflux disease have not been established.

Self-medication

For *self-medication* in relieving symptoms of occasional heartburn, acid indigestion, or sour stomach or in preventing such symptoms caused by consumption of food or beverages in patients 12 years of age or older, a famotidine dosage of 10 or 20 mg once or twice daily is recommended; when used prophylactically, the dose should be taken 10 minutes to 1 hour before eating or drinking. When the fixed combination of famotidine, calcium carbonate, and magnesium hydroxide (Pepcid® Complete) is used for *self-medication* for relief of occasional heartburn associated with acid indigestion or sour stomach, the usual dosage in adults and children 12 years of age or older is 1 tablet (10 mg of famotidine) once or twice daily. When famotidine chewable tablets are used for *self-medication*, the tablets should be chewed thoroughly before swallowing. When the 10-mg tablets are used for *self-medication*, the manufacturer recommends that the dosage of famotidine not exceed 20 mg in 24 hours. Alternatively, when the 20-mg tablets are used for *self-medication*, the manufacturer recommends that dosage of famotidine not exceed 40 mg in 24 hours. Famotidine for *self-medication* should not exceed 2 weeks of *continuous* therapy unless otherwise directed by a clinician. Persistent symptoms should be reported to a clinician.

● Dosage in Renal Impairment

In patients with renal impairment, doses and/or frequency of administration of famotidine can be modified in response to the degree of renal impairment. Adverse CNS effects have been reported in patients with moderate or severe renal insufficiency receiving famotidine, and modification of dosage and/or dosing interval may be used to avoid excess accumulation of the drug in such patients. In adults with moderate (creatinine clearances less than 50 mL/minute) or severe (creatinine clearances less than 10 mL/minute) renal impairment, the manufacturer states that dosage of famotidine may be reduced to half the usual dosage or the dosing interval may be prolonged to 36–48 hours as necessary according to the patient's clinical response. Some clinicians have recommended that one-half the usual adult dosage be administered in adults with creatinine clearances of 30–60 mL/minute per 1.48 m² and that one-fourth the usual adult dosage be administered in those with creatinine clearances less than 30 mL/minute per 1.48 m².

Based on the comparison of pharmacokinetic parameters of famotidine in adults and children, dosage adjustment also should be considered in children with moderate or severe renal impairment.

CAUTIONS

Famotidine generally is well tolerated. A causal relationship between many adverse reactions and the drug has not been established but cannot be excluded. In some studies, the incidence of reported adverse effects was similar in patients receiving famotidine or placebo. The frequency of adverse effects of the drug does not appear to be affected by patient age in adults.

Overall, the frequency of adverse effects produced by famotidine is similar to that produced by ranitidine. Famotidine does not appear to exhibit substantial antiandrogenic activity nor to substantially affect serum prolactin concentrations, and the drug also does not appear to affect hepatic clearance of other drugs. Adverse nervous system effects (e.g., headache, dizziness) and GI effects (e.g., constipation, diarrhea) occur most frequently during famotidine therapy. Although adverse effects of the drug generally are not severe, discontinuance of famotidine therapy has been necessary in up to 14% of patients. Adverse effects generally are similar when famotidine is administered orally or IV.

● Nervous System Effects

Headache and dizziness occur in about 5 and 1% of patients, respectively, receiving famotidine. Weakness (asthenia), fatigue, paresthesia, tonic-clonic (grand

mal) seizure, insomnia, drowsiness, and reversible psychic disturbances such as depression, disorientation, confusion, anxiety, agitation, decreased libido, and hallucinations have been reported in 1% or less of patients receiving famotidine but have not been directly attributed to the drug in many cases. The risk of adverse CNS effects of famotidine may be greater in patients with impaired renal function.

● GI Effects

Constipation and diarrhea occur in 1–2% of patients receiving famotidine. Nausea, vomiting, abdominal discomfort, flatulence, belching, anorexia, dry mouth, heartburn, and dysgeusia have been reported in 1% or less of patients receiving famotidine but have not been directly attributed to the drug in many cases.

● Dermatologic and Sensitivity Reactions

Adverse dermatologic effects occur in 1% or less of patients receiving famotidine, but a causal relationship to the drug has not been established. Dermatologic effects include acne, pruritus, urticaria, and dry skin. Rash also has been reported and occasionally has required discontinuance of the drug. Some of these adverse dermatologic effects appear to be hypersensitivity reactions. Anaphylaxis, angioedema, bronchospasm, orbital or facial edema, and conjunctival congestion also have been reported. Alopecia has occurred during famotidine therapy but was attributed to removal of the antiandrogenic effects of the previously administered high-dose cimetidine therapy. Toxic epidermal necrolysis has been reported very rarely with famotidine therapy. Transient irritation at the site of injection may occur following IV administration of famotidine.

● Renal Effects

Increases in BUN or serum creatinine concentrations and proteinuria have been reported occasionally during famotidine therapy. There is limited evidence that, unlike cimetidine, famotidine does not substantially inhibit renal tubular secretion of creatinine.

● Hepatic Effects

Increases in total serum bilirubin, and cholestatic jaundice have been reported rarely during famotidine therapy and have required discontinuance of the drug in some patients. Increases in serum aminotransferase (transaminase) (AST [SGOT] and ALT [SGPT]) and alkaline phosphatase concentrations also have occurred, occasionally requiring discontinuance of the drug. Hepatomegaly was reported in one patient during famotidine therapy.

● Respiratory Effects

Community-acquired Pneumonia

Administration of gastric antisecretory agents (e.g., H₂-receptor antagonists, proton-pump inhibitors) has been associated with an increased risk for developing certain infections (e.g., community-acquired pneumonia). A possible association between chronic administration of gastric acid-suppressive drugs and occurrence of community-acquired pneumonia has been evaluated using a large Dutch database (Integrated Primary Care Information [IPCI]) containing information on approximately 500,000 patients, 364,683 of whom (average follow-up: 2.7 years) were selected for evaluating any such association. During the 8-year population-based, case-control study, gastric acid suppressants were first prescribed in 19,459 individuals (10,177 received H₂-receptor antagonists [mean duration of use: 2.8 months] and 12,337 received proton-pump inhibitors [mean duration of use: 5 months]; some individuals received both drugs). Most patients did not undergo endoscopy and were treated empirically for upper GI symptoms. In this study, first occurrence of pneumonia (confirmed by radiography or microbiologic testing in 18% of patients) was reported in 5551 individuals; development of pneumonia occurred in 185 individuals while receiving gastric acid suppressants and in 292 individuals who had discontinued such use.

The adjusted relative risk for development of pneumonia (or the incidence rate) was 0.6, 2.3 and 2.5 per 100 person-years for individuals not receiving acid-suppressive drugs, for those receiving H₂-receptor antagonists, and for those receiving proton-pump inhibitors, respectively. Patients using gastric acid suppressants developed community-acquired pneumonia 4.5 (95% confidence interval of 3.8–5.1) times more often than those who never used such drugs. When evaluating use of all gastric acid suppressants, current use of the drugs was associated with a small (27%) overall increase in the risk of pneumonia (adjusted odds ratio 1.27 and 95% confidence interval of 1.06–1.54). Higher risks were observed for current users of H₂-receptor antagonists and proton-pump inhibitors; the adjusted relative risk for developing community-acquired pneumonia was 1.63 (95% confidence interval of 1.07–2.48) or 1.89 (95% confidence interval of

1.36–2.62), respectively, for these classes of drugs compared with those who discontinued using these agents. Estimates for developing pneumonia were higher (1.7 [95% confidence interval of 0.8–2.9] for H_2-receptor antagonists) and 2.2 [95% confidence interval of 1.4–3.5] for proton-pump inhibitors) when only laboratory-confirmed cases of pneumonia were considered for analysis.

Although there was variation among individual H_2-receptor antagonists and individual proton-pump inhibitors, the numbers were small and the heterogeneity was not considered significant. For patients currrently receiving proton-pump inhibitors, a dose-response relationship for developing pneumonia was observed; individuals using more than one defined daily dose of these drugs had a 2.3-fold increased risk for developing pneumonia compared with those who discontinued gastric acid suppressants. Such a dose-response relationship for developing pneumonia was not observed in patients receiving H_2-receptor antagonists; however, dose variation of these drugs was limited. Among current users of H_2-receptor antagonists or proton-pump inhibitors, the risk for developing pneumonia was most pronounced among those who initiated such therapies within the past 30 days.

Although the exact mechanism for development of community-acquired pneumonia in patients receiving gastric acid suppressants has not been fully elucidated, it has been suggested that reduction of gastric acid secretion by acid suppressive therapy and consequent increases of gastric pH may result in a favorable environment for the development of infection. Intragastric acidity constitutes a major nonspecific defense mechanism of the stomach to ingested pathogens; when gastric pH is less than 4, most pathogens are killed, while at higher gastric pH, pathogens may survive. Since for the effective management of upper GI symptoms, intragastric pH should be maintained above 4 for several hours, acid suppressive therapy may lead to insufficient elimination or, even, increased colonization of ingested pathogens. Some evidence indicates that acid-supressive therapy may result in nosocomial infections.

It should be considered that certain patients (e.g., those with pleuritic chest pain, hypothermia, systolic hypotension, tachypnea, diabetes mellitus, neoplastic disease, neurologic disease, bacteremia, leukopenia, multilobar pulmonary infiltrate) are at increased risk for developing infections and in these individuals community-acquired pneumonia may be associated with increased mortality. Some clinicians state that gastric acid-suppressive drugs should be used in patients in whom community-acquired pneumonia may be severe (e.g., those with asthma or chronic obstructive lung disease, immunocompromised patients, pediatric or geriatric individuals) only when clearly needed and the lowest effective dose should be employed.

● Other Adverse Effects

Fever, hypertension, flushing, musculoskeletal pain (including muscle cramps), arthralgia, and tinnitus have been reported in 1% or less of patients receiving famotidine, but a causal relationship to the drug has not been established in many cases. An acute episode of gout occurred in one patient during therapy with the drug.

Leukocytosis, leukopenia, neutropenia, pancytopenia, agranulocytosis, eosinophilia, prolonged erythrocyte sedimentation rate (ESR), and thrombocytopenia have occurred rarely in patients receiving famotidine. Changes in serum protein or cholesterol concentrations also have occurred.

Unlike cimetidine, famotidine does not appear to exhibit substantial antiandrogenic activity. (See Pharmacology: Endocrine and Gonadal Effects.) Famotidine did not produce gynecomastia, impotence, or decreased libido in one study in males with GI hypersecretory conditions who were receiving dosages of 80–640 mg daily for periods longer than 12 months, but such effects occasionally have been associated with therapy with the drug. The manufacturer states that in controlled studies the incidence of impotence in patients receiving famotidine was not greater than that in patients receiving placebo. Impotence and gynecomastia, which developed in one male during cimetidine therapy, continued during subsequent therapy with ranitidine and then with famotidine, but did not resolve following discontinuance of famotidine. In at least one patient, androgenic activity that had been inhibited by cimetidine appeared to become disinhibited (as evidenced by worsening of pre-existing alopecia) when famotidine was substituted. Menstrual abnormalities have occurred in at least one woman receiving famotidine.

Cardiac arrhythmias, palpitations, and AV block have been reported in 1% or less of patients receiving famotidine. There is limited evidence suggesting that famotidine may have a negative inotropic effect, but further study is necessary to confirm these preliminary findings.

● Precautions and Contraindications

Symptomatic response to famotidine should *not* be interpreted as precluding the presence of gastric malignancy.

The possibility that gastric acid-suppressive therapy may increase the risk of community-acquired pneumonia should be considered. (See Respiratory Effects: Community-acquired Pneumonia, in Cautions.)

Adverse CNS effects have been reported in patients with moderate (i.e., creatinine clearance less than 50 mL/minute) or severe (i.e., creatinine clearance less than 10 mL/minute) renal impairment receiving famotidine, and the drug should be used with caution and dosage and/or frequency of administration reduced in such patients, since the drug is excreted principally by the kidneys. (See Dosage and Administration: Dosage in Renal Impairment.)

Unless otherwise directed by a clinician, patients receiving famotidine for *self-medication* should be advised to discontinue the drug and consult a clinician if symptoms of heartburn (pyrosis), acid indigestion (hyperchlorhydria), or sour stomach persist after 2 weeks of continuous use of the drug.

Individuals with phenylketonuria (i.e., homozygous genetic deficiency of phenylalanine hydroxylase) and other individuals who must restrict their intake of phenylalnine should be warned that Pepcid AC® chewable tablets and Pepcid RPD® orally disintegrating tablets contain aspartame (NutraSweet®), which is metabolized in the GI tract to phenylalanine following oral administration.

Famotidine is contraindicated in patients with known hypersensitivity to the drug or any ingredient in the formulation. Since cross-sensitivity has been observed among H_2-receptor antagonists, famotidine should not be administered to patients with a history of hypersensitivity to other drugs in this class.

● Pediatric Precautions

Safety and efficacy of famotidine in children 1–16 years of age is supported by evidence from adequate and well-controlled studies in adults and by a limited number of studies in pediatric patients. In studies in a limited number of pediatric patients 1–15 years of age, clearance and area under the curve (AUC) were similar to those values reported in adults. Limited evidence also suggests that the relationship between serum concentration and acid suppression is similar in children 1–15 years of age as compared with adults. While uncontrolled studies suggest efficacy of famotidine in the treatment of gastroesophageal reflux disease and peptic ulcer, data in pediatric patients are insufficient to establish percent response with dose and duration of therapy. Therefore, treatment duration (initially based on adult duration recommendations) and dose should be individualized based on clinical response and/or pH determination (gastric or esophageal) and endoscopy. In uncontrolled clinical studies in pediatric patients, dosages of up to 1 mg/kg daily for peptic ulcer and 2 mg/kg daily for gastroesophageal reflux disease with or without esophagitis including erosions and ulcerations have been used. The manufacturer states that no pharmacokinetic or pharmacodynamic data for famotidine are available in children younger than 1 year of age. Famotidine should not be used for *self-medication* in children younger than 12 years of age unless directed by a clinician.

● Geriatric Precautions

Of almost 5000 patients in clinical studies of famotidine, 9.8% were 65 years of age or older, while 1.7% were older than 75 years of age. Although no overall differences in efficacy and safety were observed between geriatric and younger patients, the possibility that some older patients may exhibit increased sensitivity to the drug cannot be ruled out. Clinically important changes in the pharmacokinetics of famotidine have not been observed in geriatric individuals, and dosage of the drug does not need to be modified based on age alone. However, famotidine dosage should be selected carefully in geriatric patients because these individuals may have decreased renal function, and patients with renal impairment may be at increased risk of famotidine-induced toxicity. Monitoring of renal function may be useful for patients in this age group. Doses and/or frequency of administration of famotidine should be modified in geriatric patients with moderate (creatinine clearance less than 50 mL/minute) or severe (creatinine clearance less than 10 mL/minute) renal impairment. (See Dosage and Administration: Dosage in Renal Impairment)

● Mutagenicity and Carcinogenicity

No evidence of mutagenicity was observed in in vitro studies using famotidine concentrations up to 10 mg per plate in the Ames microbial mutagen test with or without metabolic activation and in in vivo studies in mice using a micronucleus test and a chromosomal aberration test.

No evidence of carcinogenicity was seen in long-term studies in mice or rats receiving oral famotidine dosages up to 2 g/kg daily (approximately 2500 times the usual human dosage). Although famotidine did not produce changes in gastric mucosal cells in animals, long-term effects of the drug on human gastric mucosal morphology are not known, and the risk, if any, of gastric neoplasms and long-term therapy with an H$_2$-receptor antagonist remains controversial.

● Pregnancy, Fertility, and Lactation

Pregnancy

Reproduction studies in rats and rabbits using oral famotidine dosages up to 2 (approximately 2500 times the maximum human dosage) and 0.5 g/kg daily, respectively, or IV dosages up to 0.2 (approximately 250 times the maximum human dosage) and 0.1 g/kg daily, respectively, have not revealed evidence of harm to the fetus. Oral dosages of 2 g/kg daily inhibited weight gain in pregnant rats, and those of 0.5 and/or 2 g/kg daily on days 7–17 of gestation decreased fetal weight and delayed sternal ossification in the offspring. Decreased food intake and decreased weight gain also occurred in offspring of rats receiving these dosages from days 10–28 post partum. Death and locomotor dysfunction were observed in pregnant rats receiving IV famotidine dosages of 100 or 200 mg/kg daily. IV dosages of 100 or 200 mg/kg daily in rats have decreased pup body weight during the post-weaning period. Although no direct fetotoxic effects have been observed, sporadic abortions and decreases in fetal weight occurred secondary to substantial decreases in food intake in pregnant rabbits receiving oral dosages of 200 mg/kg (250 times the usual human dosage) or more daily. Decreased number of sacrocaudal vertebrae and delayed ossification have occurred in rabbits receiving oral famotidine dosages of 0.5 g/kg daily. There are no adequate and controlled studies to date using famotidine in pregnant women, and the drug should be used during pregnancy only when clearly needed. Women who are pregnant or nursing should seek the advice of a health professional before using famotidine for *self-medication*.

Fertility

Reproduction studies in rats and rabbits using oral famotidine dosages up to 2 (approximately 2500 times the maximum human dosage) and 0.5 g/kg daily, respectively, or IV dosages up to 0.2 (approximately 250 times the maximum human dosage) and 0.1 g/kg daily, respectively, have not revealed evidence of impaired fertility.

Lactation

Famotidine is distributed into milk in humans and in animals. The drug has produced transient growth depression in the offspring of lactating rats receiving dosages at least 600 times the usual human dosage. Because of the potential for serious adverse reactions to famotidine in nursing infants, a decision should be made whether to discontinue nursing or the drug, taking into account the importance of the drug to the woman.

DRUG INTERACTIONS

● Food and Antacids

Food appears to slightly enhance, and antacids appear to slightly decrease, the bioavailability of famotidine, but these effects do not appear to be clinically important. Famotidine can be administered concomitantly with antacids.

In one study following concomitant administration of food and a single oral 40-mg dose of famotidine, mean peak plasma concentration, fraction of the dose excreted in urine, bioavailability, and renal clearance of famotidine increased slightly; however, area under the plasma concentration-time curve (AUC) and time to reach the peak were decreased slightly. In the same study following concomitant administration of 10 mL of an aluminum and magnesium hydroxides antacid (Mylanta-II®) and 40 mg of famotidine orally, the mean peak plasma concentration decreased from 81 to 60 ng/mL, and the mean AUC decreased from 443 to 355 mcg/hour per L. The time to reach the peak and the fraction of the dose excreted in urine also decreased slightly, and renal clearance increased slightly.

● Effects on Hepatic Clearance of Drugs

Unlike cimetidine or ranitidine, famotidine does not appear to inhibit the metabolism of drugs, including warfarin, theophylline, phenytoin, diazepam, or procainamide, by the hepatic cytochrome P-450 (microsomal) enzyme system. Metabolism of aminopyrine or antipyrine and clearance and/or half-life of the drugs also do not appear to be affected substantially by famotidine therapy. However, minimal effects of the drug on cytochrome P-450 enzymes have been suggested, and additional experience with long-term therapy and with relatively high dosages is necessary to determine the potential, if any, for clinically important effects. Famotidine does not appear to affect elimination of indocyanine green.

ACUTE TOXICITY

There has been no experience to date with acute overdosage of famotidine.

● Pathogenesis

The oral and IV LD$_{50}$s of famotidine have been reported to be greater than 3000 and 254–563 mg/kg, respectively, in both mice and rats, and the intraperitoneal and subcutaneous LD$_{50}$s have been reported to be greater than 778 and greater than 800 mg/kg, respectively, in these animals. The minimum acute oral and IV lethal doses have been reported to be greater than 2000 and about 300 mg/kg, respectively, in dogs. In rabbits, oral famotidine dosages of 200 mg/kg or more daily produce substantial anorexia and growth retardation; however, no evidence of toxicity was observed following high oral dosages in dogs and rats. In dogs, IV dosages of 5–200 mg/kg daily produce vomiting; restlessness; pallor of the mucous membranes or redness of the mouth and ears; and cardiovascular effects, including hypotension, tachycardia, and collapse.

Oral dosages up to 800 mg of famotidine daily produced no evidence of serious toxicity when the drug was used in patients with pathologic GI hypersecretory conditions.

● Treatment

In acute famotidine overdose, usual measures to remove unabsorbed drug from the GI tract and clinical monitoring should be employed. Supportive and symptomatic treatment should be initiated.

PHARMACOLOGY

● GI Effects

Famotidine competitively inhibits the action of histamine on the H$_2$ receptors of parietal cells, reducing gastric acid secretion and concentration under daytime and nocturnal basal conditions and also when stimulated by food, histamine, or pentagastrin. The H$_2$-receptor antagonist activity of famotidine reportedly is slowly reversible, since the drug dissociates slowly from the H$_2$ receptor. Famotidine has been shown to be 20–150 or 3–20 times as potent on a molar basis as cimetidine or ranitidine, respectively, in inhibiting stimulated gastric acid secretion.

The degree of inhibition of gastric acid secretion by famotidine is similar to that observed following equipotent doses of cimetidine or ranitidine. A 5-mg dose of famotidine appears to produce inhibition of gastric acid secretion similar in degree to that produced by a 300-mg dose of cimetidine. The degree of inhibition of gastric acid secretion (especially nocturnal or food-stimulated) by famotidine is directly related to the dose and the time of administration of the drug. In one study in healthy individuals who were hypersecretors of gastric acid (basal gastric acid output of 5 or more mEq/hour), the total volume of gastric acid secretion was decreased 55–65% following single 20-mg oral or 10- or 20-mg IV doses of the drug, but the largest decrease was observed following the 20-mg IV dose. In another study in healthy individuals, a single 40-mg evening dose of famotidine inhibited 95 and 32% of nocturnal and daytime gastric acid secretion, respectively; 24-hour gastric acid secretion was inhibited about 70%.

Evening (bedtime) doses produce maximal inhibitory effects on nocturnal or breakfast-stimulated gastric acid secretion, but produce minimal inhibition of lunch- or dinner-stimulated secretion; administration of famotidine twice daily before meals produces substantial inhibition of meal-stimulated gastric acid secretion.

Basal and nocturnal gastric acid secretion appear to be inhibited to a greater extent than are food- or pentagastrin-stimulated gastric acid secretion following a given dose of famotidine in both healthy individuals and patients with duodenal ulcer or GI hypersecretory conditions. Following oral administration of a single 20- or 40-mg evening dose of famotidine, 86 or 94% of nocturnal gastric acid secretion, respectively, is inhibited for at least 10 hours. Following oral administration of a single 20- or 40-mg morning dose, 76 or 84% of food-stimulated gastric acid secretion, respectively, is inhibited for up to 3–5 hours and 25 or 30%, respectively, for up to 8–10 hours. However, inhibition of food-stimulated gastric acid secretion disappeared within 6–8 hours following administration of a 20-mg dose in some individuals. Following oral administration of a single 40-mg bedtime dose of the drug, basal or pentagastrin-stimulated gastric acid secretion is inhibited by 70 or 30%, respectively, for 12 hours and by 55 or 9%, respectively, for 20 hours.

The inhibitory effects of famotidine on gastric acid secretion do not appear to be cumulative following repeated administration of the drug, and tolerance to the drug's effects does not develop rapidly.

The increases in gastric pH that occur secondary to inhibition of gastric acid secretion by famotidine also are dose dependent. Nocturnal gastric pH increased to a mean of 5 or 6.4 following oral administration of a single 20- or 40-mg evening dose of famotidine, respectively, and basal gastric pH increased to about 5 for 3–8 hours after a single 20- or 40-mg morning (after breakfast) dose of the drug. Following administration of a single evening dose of 20 mg orally, 10 mg IV, 20 mg IV, or placebo, nocturnal gastric pH averaged 4.4, 5.5, 6.2, or 1.7, respectively, 2 hours after the dose; nocturnal gastric pH averaged 6, 5.4, and 4.4 at 7, 8, and 10 hours after the 20-mg IV dose or 4, 3.3, and 3 at 7, 8, and 10 hours after the 10-mg IV dose. Gastric pH for a 24-hour period (measured every 5 seconds) was greater than 6 about half the time during continuous IV infusion of famotidine dosages of 3.2 or 4 mg/hour in patients with duodenal ulcer; however, during postprandial periods of the day, pH exceeded 6 only 10% of the time.

Famotidine indirectly causes a dose-dependent reduction in pepsin secretion by decreasing the volume of gastric acid secretion. The drug appears to have minimal effects on fasting and postprandial serum gastrin concentrations. Serum gastrin concentrations have increased in some patients during famotidine therapy but remained within the normal range. Famotidine may protect the gastric mucosa from the irritant effects caused by certain drugs (e.g., aspirin, nonsteroidal anti-inflammatory agents).

Famotidine does not appear to affect gastric emptying, lower esophageal sphincter pressure, or biliary secretion.

Famotidine concentrations ranging from 128–1024 mcg/mL are necessary to inhibit growth of various strains of *Helicobacter pylori* (formerly *Campylobacter pylori* or *C. pyloridis*), an organism possibly contributing to the etiology of duodenal and gastric ulcers. The MIC$_{50}$ and MIC$_{90}$ of famotidine for susceptible strains of *H. pylori* are reportedly 512 and greater than 1024 mcg/mL, respectively.

● *Endocrine and Gonadal Effects*

Famotidine has been shown to have little, if any, effect on serum prolactin concentrations. Although changes in serum prolactin concentrations occurred following a 20-mg IV dose of the drug in some healthy individuals and patients with duodenal ulcer, these changes were considered within normal physiologic variations. Serum prolactin concentrations remained unchanged following single IV doses of 20 mg or following oral dosages of 80–640 mg daily for periods longer than 12 months.

Famotidine does not appear to have substantial antiandrogenic effects. Unlike cimetidine but like ranitidine, famotidine has been shown to have little, if any, effect on serum concentrations of testosterone, luteinizing hormone (LH), follicle-stimulating hormone (FSH), estradiol, parathyroid hormone (PTH), cortisol, insulin, glucagon, thyrotropin (TSH), thyroxine (T$_4$), triiodothyronine (T$_3$), or thyroxine-binding globulin (TBG).

● *Other Effects*

Famotidine has been shown to produce few, if any, CNS, cardiovascular, or respiratory effects. The drug does not appear to affect hepatic or portal blood flow in healthy individuals or patients with chronic liver disease. Unlike cimetidine, famotidine does not inhibit hepatic metabolism of antipyrine. Famotidine does not appear to affect the volume or bicarbonate or amylase content of exocrine pancreatic secretions.

In animals, famotidine did not inhibit immediate hypersensitivity reactions involving antigen-induced mediator release from mast cells or cellular and humoral immune responses.

PHARMACOKINETICS

● *Absorption*

Famotidine is incompletely absorbed from the GI tract following oral administration, and the drug reportedly undergoes minimal first-pass metabolism. The oral bioavailability of famotidine in adults is about 40–50%. Studies in a limited number of children 11–15 years of age indicate a similar oral bioavailability of famotidine (mean bioavailability: 50%). The film-coated tablets, oral suspension, and orally disintegrating tablets of famotidine reportedly are bioequivalent. Food may slightly enhance and antacids may slightly decrease the bioavailability of famotidine, but these alterations do not appear to be clinically important. (See Drug Interactions: Food and Antacids.)

Following IV injection of a single 20-mg dose of famotidine, peak plasma concentrations of 272 ng/mL occur within 20 minutes and decrease to 163, 98, 64, 25, and 11 ng/mL 1, 2, 4, 8, and 12 hours, respectively, after the dose. Following oral administration of a 5-, 10-, 20-, or 40-mg dose of famotidine, peak plasma concentrations of 17–22, 29–39, 40–71, or 78–132 ng/mL, respectively, occur within 1–4 hours.

Plasma famotidine concentrations necessary to inhibit 50% of tetragastrin-stimulated gastric acid secretion (IC$_{50}$) are estimated to be 13 ng/mL. Plasma famotidine concentrations greater than 50 ng/mL result in inhibition of more than 80% of gastric acid secretion; however, inhibition generally appears to diminish at lower concentrations. Data are conflicting regarding the relationship between plasma famotidine concentrations and a given therapeutic effect of acid inhibition. However, in one study, the decline in the degree of inhibition of gastric acid secretion appeared to be proportional to decreases in plasma famotidine concentrations.

Inhibition of gastric acid secretion is apparent within 1 hour following IV or oral administration of famotidine. Peak inhibition occurs within 0.5–3 or 1–4 hours following IV or oral administration, respectively. The duration of inhibition of gastric acid secretion and maximal inhibition produced by famotidine are dose dependent. The duration of inhibition of basal and nocturnal secretion following a single 20- or 40-mg oral dose of the drug reportedly is 10–12 hours. Inhibition of food-stimulated secretion generally persists for 8–10 hours when these doses are administered in the morning, but this inhibition may dissipate within 6–8 hours after a 20-mg oral dose in some patients. Following equipotent doses of famotidine (60 mg), cimetidine (1.9 g), or ranitidine (530 mg) in one study in patients with GI hypersecretory conditions, gastric acid secretion 12 hours after discontinuance of the drugs was reduced by 58, 27, or 38%, respectively, compared with basal secretion, and the time required for secretion to return to 20 mEq/hour averaged 12, 9, or 10 hours, respectively, following discontinuance of the drugs. The duration of inhibition of nocturnal gastric acid secretion is 10–15 hours following a single 10- or 20-mg IV famotidine dose. In one study in healthy individuals who were hypersecretors of gastric acid (basal gastric acid output of 5 or more mEq/hour), maximal inhibition of gastric acid secretion was 97.4, 99.7, or 99.4% 2–4 hours and 73.8, 77.2, or 83.3% 12 hours following a single famotidine dose of 10 or 20 mg IV or 20 mg orally, respectively.

● *Distribution*

Distribution of famotidine into human body tissues and fluids has not been fully characterized. The apparent volume of distribution of the drug is reported to be 1.1–1.4 L/kg in adults and does not appear to be altered substantially in patients with renal dysfunction. In children 1–15 years of age, a volume of distribution of 1.5–2.07 L/kg has been reported. Following oral or IV administration in rats, famotidine is widely distributed, appearing in highest concentrations in the kidney, liver, pancreas, and submandibular gland. The drug is 15–20% protein bound.

In rats, famotidine appears to distribute only minimally into the CNS, and does not cross the placenta. It is not known whether the drug crosses the placenta in humans. Famotidine is distributed into milk in rats; however, it is not known whether the drug is distributed into milk in humans.

● *Elimination*

The elimination half-life of famotidine averages 2.5–4 hours in adults with normal renal function. An elimination half-life of 2.3–3.38 hours has been reported in children 1–15 years of age. The elimination of famotidine does not appear to be affected substantially by age in adults, but is prolonged in patients with renal impairment; adjustment of dosage or dosing interval may be necessary to avoid excess accumulation of the drug in patients with moderate or severe renal impairment. (See Dosage and Administration: Dosage in Renal Impairment.) In adults with creatinine clearances of 10 mL or less per minute, the elimination half-life of the drug may exceed 20 hours, with an elimination half-life of about 24 hours in anuric patients. There is some evidence that plasma concentrations of famotidine decline in a biphasic manner. In adults with normal renal function and those with creatinine clearances of 60–90, 30–60, or less than 30 mL/minute per 1.48 m², the plasma half-life in the distribution phase (t$_{\frac{1}{2}\alpha}$) was not affected substantially by renal function, averaging 0.18, 0.23, 0.25, or 0.24 hours, respectively; the half-life in the terminal elimination phase (t$_{\frac{1}{2}\beta}$) averaged 2.6, 2.9, 4.7, or 12 hours, respectively.

Famotidine is metabolized in the liver to famotidine S-oxide (S-famotidine). The metabolite does not appear to inhibit gastric acid secretion. Orally administered famotidine undergoes minimal metabolism on first pass through the liver.

Famotidine is excreted principally in urine via glomerular filtration and tubular secretion. Approximately 25–30 or 65–80% of a dose is excreted unchanged in urine within 24 hours following oral or IV administration, respectively, and approximately 13–49 or 52–82% of a single 40-mg oral or IV dose, respectively, is excreted within 72 hours. The cumulative renal excretion of famotidine is decreased in patients with renal dysfunction, with 72, 69, 65, or 21% of an administered dose excreted in individuals with normal renal function or those with creatinine clearances of 60–90, 30–60, or less than 30 mL/minute per 1.48 m², respectively. A small fraction of an orally administered dose is excreted in urine as famotidine S-oxide. The remainder of an orally administered dose is eliminated in feces. Nonrenal excretion of famotidine did not show a compensatory increase in patients with severe renal impairment, but rather decreased by about 40% in these patients. Interindividual variation in the metabolism and excretion of famotidine has been reported. Following oral administration of a 20-mg dose, 24–56 or 28–79% of the administered dose reportedly was excreted in urine or feces, respectively.

Total body clearance of famotidine from plasma averages 381–483 mL/minute, and renal clearance of the drug averages 250–450 mL/minute. Total body and renal clearances are decreased in patients with renal dysfunction. In patients with creatinine clearances of 30–60 or less than 30 mL/minute per 1.48 m², total body clearance from plasma averaged 241 or 71–83 mL/minute, respectively, and renal clearance averaged 157 or 9.5–21 mL/minute, respectively.

Famotidine does not appear to be removed by hemodialysis.

CHEMISTRY AND STABILITY

● Chemistry

Famotidine is a histamine H₂-receptor antagonist. Unlike the earlier histamine H₂-receptor antagonists, burimamide and metiamide, which are not commercially available, and cimetidine and ranitidine, famotidine contains a guanidine-substituted thiazole ring rather than an imidazole or furan ring.

Famotidine occurs as a white to pale yellow, odorless, crystalline powder having a moderately bitter taste. Famotidine has solubilities of 740 mcg/mL in water and 360 mcg/mL in alcohol at 20°C. The drug has a pK$_a$ of 7.1 in water at 25°C.

Famotidine is commercially available for oral administration as film-coated, chewable, gelatin-coated, or orally disintegrating tablets and as a powder for oral suspension. Some famotidine chewable tablet preparations (Pepcid® AC) and famotidine orally disintegrating tablets (Pepcid RPD®) contain aspartame (Nutrasweet®). (See Cautions: Precautions and Contraindications.) Following metabolism of aspartame in the GI tract, each 20- or 40-mg orally disintegrating tablet provides 1.05 or 2.1 mg, respectively, of phenylalanine.

Famotidine powder for suspension occurs as a white to off-white powder. When reconstituted as directed, oral suspensions of the drug occur as smooth, mobile, off-white homogenous suspensions and have a pH of 6.5–7.5.

Famotidine concentrate for injection is a clear, colorless, sterile solution of the drug in water for injection. The concentrate also contains mannitol; multiple-dose vials also contain benzyl alcohol as a preservative. Famotidine concentrate for injection has a pH of 5–5.6. The preservative-free injection has an osmolarity of 217 mOsm/L, and the injection preserved with benzyl alcohol has an osmolarity of 290 mOsm/L. Famotidine injection that is commercially available as a diluted solution in 0.9% sodium chloride is iso-osmotic and has a pH of 5.7–6.4. This injection contains approximately 7.8 mEq of sodium per 50 mL.

● Stability

Commercially available famotidine film-coated tablets (Pepcid®) should be stored in well-closed, light-resistant containers at 25°C, but may be exposed to temperatures ranging from 15–30°C. These tablets have an expiration date of 30 months following the date of manufacture when stored under these conditions. Famotidine orally disintegrating tablets (Pepcid RPD®) should be stored at 25°C, but may be exposed to temperatures ranging from 15–30°C. Famotidine tablets and chewable tablets for self-medication (Pepcid® AC, Pepcid® Complete) should be stored at a temperature between 25–30°C and protected from moisture.

Commercially available famotidine powder for oral suspension should be stored in tight containers at 25°C, but may be exposed to temperatures ranging from 15–30°C. The powder for oral suspension has an expiration date of 18 months following the date of manufacture when stored at a temperature less than 40°C. Following reconstitution, oral suspensions of the drug should be stored at a temperature less than 30°C and, although not necessary, may be refrigerated; freezing should be avoided. Any unused suspension should be discarded after 30 days.

Commercially available famotidine concentrate for injection should be refrigerated at 2–8°C and has an expiration date of 24 months following the date of manufacture when stored at this temperature. If freezing occurs, the injection should be thawed at room temperature or by warming it in a water bath or under running hot tap water, allowing sufficient time for dissolution of all ingredients. The injection should not be thawed by exposure to microwave radiation because of the potential hazard of rapidly increased temperature and vapor pressure in a closed system. When diluted with most commonly used IV solutions (e.g., 0.9% sodium chloride injection, 5 or 10% dextrose injection, lactated Ringer's, water for injection), famotidine solutions are stable for 7 days at room temperature. However, the manufacturer states that data on the maintenance of sterility of these solutions after dilution are unavailable. Therefore, the manufacturer recommends that solutions prepared by dilution of famotidine concentrate for injection, if not used immediately after dilution, should be refrigerated and used within 48 hours.

Famotidine injection that is commercially available as a diluted solution in 0.9% sodium chloride should be stored at room temperature (25°C) and is stable for 15 months when stored as recommended. Brief exposure to temperatures up to 35°C will not adversely affect the stability of the solution, but the solution should be protected from exposure to excessive heat. The commercially available injection of famotidine in 0.9% sodium chloride is provided in a plastic container fabricated from specially designed multilayered plastic PL 2501 (Galaxy® container). Solutions in contact with the plastic can leach out some of its chemical components in very small amounts within the expiration period of the injection; however, safety of the plastic has been confirmed in tests in animals according to USP biological tests for plastic containers as well as by tissue culture toxicity studies.

PREPARATIONS

Excipients in commercially available drug preparations may have clinically important effects in some individuals; consult specific product labeling for details.

Famotidine

Oral		
For suspension	40 mg/5 mL	Pepcid®, Merck
Tablets	10 mg	Pepcid® AC Gelcaps, J&J-Merck
Tablets, chewable	10 mg	Pepcid® AC, J&J-Merck
Tablets, film-coated	10 mg	Pepcid® AC, J&J-Merck
	20 mg*	Pepcid®, Merck
		Pepcid® AC Maximum Strength, J&J-Merck
	40 mg	Pepcid®, Merck
Tablets, orally disintegrating	20 mg	Pepcid® RPD, Merck
	40 mg	Pepcid® RPD, Merck
Parenteral		
For injection, concentrate	10 mg/mL (pharmacy bulk package)	Famotidine for Injection
For injection concentrate, for IV use	10 mg/mL	Famotidine for Injection Pepcid® I.V., Merck

* available from one or more manufacturer, distributor, and/or repackager by generic (nonproprietary) name

Famotidine in Sodium Chloride.

Parenteral		
Injection, for IV use only	0.4 mg/mL (20 mg) in 0.9% Sodium Chloride	Pepcid® Premixed in Iso-osmotic Sodium Chloride Injection (Galaxy® [Baxter]), Merck

Famotidine Combinations

Oral		
Tablets, chewable	10 mg with calcium carbonate 800 mg and magnesium hydroxide 165 mg	Pepcid® Complete, J&J-Merck

† Use is not currently included in the labeling approved by the US Food and Drug Administration.

Misoprostol

56:28.28 • PROSTAGLANDINS

■ Misoprostol, a synthetic analog of prostaglandin E₁ (alprostadil), is a gastric antisecretory agent with protective effects on the gastroduodenal mucosa; the drug also increases the amplitude and frequency of uterine contractions and stimulates uterine bleeding and total or partial expulsion of uterine contents in pregnant women.

USES

Misoprostol is used for reducing the risk of nonsteroidal anti-inflammatory agent (NSAIA)-induced gastric ulcer in patients at high risk of developing complications from these ulcers and in patients at high risk of developing gastric ulceration. Misoprostol has been used for the short-term treatment of active duodenal ulcer† and for the short-term treatment of active, benign gastric ulcer†. Misoprostol also has been used as maintenance therapy following healing of gastric ulcer to reduce ulcer recurrence†.

Misoprostol is used as an adjunct to mifepristone for the medical termination of intrauterine pregnancy (i.e., medical abortion). The drug has been used for induction of labor† and for treatment of serious postpartum hemorrhage† in the presence of uterine atony.

For information on the use of misoprostol in fixed combination with diclofenac, a NSAIA, see Diclofenac 28:08.04.92.

● Prevention of NSAIA-induced Ulcers

Misoprostol is used for reducing the risk of NSAIA-induced gastric ulcers in patients at high risk of developing complications (e.g., bleeding, perforation, death) from these ulcers, such as patients with a concomitant debilitating disease and geriatric patients, and in patients at high risk of developing gastric ulceration, such as those with a history of upper GI ulcer. While the drug also has been used for the prevention of NSAIA-induced duodenal ulcers† in a limited number of patients, current evidence is insufficient to establish efficacy in these patients.

Serious adverse GI effects (e.g., bleeding, ulceration, perforation) can occur at any time in patients receiving chronic NSAIA therapy, and such effects may *not* be preceded by warning signs or symptoms. Results of studies to date are inconclusive concerning the relative risk of various NSAIAs in causing serious GI effects. In patients receiving prototypical NSAIAs and observed in clinical studies of several months' to 2-years' duration, symptomatic upper GI ulcers, gross bleeding, or perforation appeared to occur in approximately 1% of patients treated for 3–6 months and in about 2–4% of those treated for 1 year. These trends continue with long-term therapy and increase the likelihood of a serious GI event occurring at some time during the course of therapy. Studies have shown that patients with a history of peptic ulcer disease and/or GI bleeding who are receiving NSAIAs have a greater than tenfold higher risk for developing GI bleeding than patients without these risk factors. In addition, several comorbid conditions and concomitant therapies have been shown to increase the risk for GI bleeding, including concomitant use of oral corticosteroids or anticoagulants, longer duration of NSAIA therapy, smoking, alcoholism, older age, and poor general health status. In addition, geriatric or debilitated patients appear to tolerate GI ulceration and bleeding less well than other individuals, and most spontaneous reports of fatal NSAIA-induced GI effects have been in such patients. Therefore, consideration can be given to concomitant preventive therapy with misoprostol in these and other patients deemed at high risk of developing complications resulting from NSAIA-induced gastric ulcer or at high risk of developing such ulcers.

Clinical Experience

Efficacy of misoprostol for the prevention of NSAIA-induced gastric ulcer has been established principally in short-term studies (up to 3 months' duration). Therefore, although continuous misoprostol therapy for the duration of NSAIA use currently is recommended by the manufacturer, the long-term safety and efficacy and optimum duration of misoprostol therapy in patients receiving NSAIAs chronically remain to be established. In addition, although NSAIA-induced

gastric injury is asymptomatic in most patients, most studies conducted to date have included only patients with symptomatic injury. It also should be recognized that while misoprostol is intended for use in the prevention of NSAIA-induced gastric injury in patients at high risk of complications from such injury, efficacy of the drug in most high-risk patient groups has not been specifically established. Despite the lack of such data, however, high-risk patients are thought to be most likely to benefit from prophylactic therapy with misoprostol.

Misoprostol has reduced the rate of endoscopically documented NSAIA-induced gastroduodenal mucosal injury in healthy individuals. The drug also has reduced the rate of gastroduodenal ulcer formation in osteoarthritic patients with GI symptoms but no evidence of ulcer prior to initiation of misoprostol. Gastroduodenal mucosal injury also has been reduced and healing of gastroduodenal ulcer promoted in patients with rheumatoid arthritis who had GI symptoms and evidence of mucosal injury and/or ulcer when misoprostol was initiated. However, misoprostol does not appear to be effective in reducing associated GI symptoms (e.g., pain).

In several short-term (about 1-week duration) studies in a limited number of healthy individuals receiving a NSAIA (e.g., aspirin, ibuprofen, naproxen, tolmetin), reported rates of endoscopically documented gastric or duodenal mucosal injury were 10–30% in those receiving oral misoprostol dosages of 100 or 200 mcg 4 times daily and 70–75% in those receiving placebo. In a limited number of healthy individuals, misoprostol also has been more effective than sucralfate in preventing aspirin-induced gastroduodenal mucosal injury and more effective than cimetidine in preventing tolmetin-induced gastric but not duodenal mucosal injury.

In a multicenter controlled study in patients with osteoarthritis who were receiving chronic NSAIA therapy (e.g., 3 months or longer with ibuprofen, naproxen, or piroxicam) and had GI symptoms but no endoscopic evidence of gastric ulcer, 100 or 200 mcg of misoprostol 4 times daily reduced the rate of NSAIA-induced gastric ulcer formation; at 12 weeks, 21–30% of patients receiving placebo developed gastric ulcers while only 1.4–3 or 6–8% of patients receiving the 200- or 100-mcg regimen, respectively, developed such ulcers. However, the 100-mcg regimen was less effective than the 200-mcg regimen, producing a significant reduction in gastric ulcer formation compared with placebo in only one of the study groups. In addition, misoprostol was not effective in relieving associated GI symptoms (e.g., daytime or nocturnal abdominal pain, nausea, vomiting, anorexia) with either regimen.

In a study in patients with rheumatoid arthritis who were receiving aspirin therapy for at least 4 weeks and had GI symptoms and endoscopically confirmed gastric and/or duodenal injury, 8 weeks of concomitant misoprostol (200 mcg 4 times daily) therapy promoted gastroduodenal healing, including healing of ulcers. Healing of gastric or duodenal mucosal injury occurred at 8 weeks in 70 or 86%, respectively, of patients receiving misoprostol compared with 25 or 53%, respectively, of those receiving placebo, and healing of gastroduodenal ulcers occurred in 67% of patients receiving the drug compared with 26% of those receiving placebo. There was similar evidence of misoprostol-induced healing at 4 weeks. Misoprostol also appeared to prevent formation of new ulcers and did not interfere with the efficacy of aspirin as determined by relief of pain and stiffness, reduction of swelling, improvement of mobility and grip strength, or erythrocyte sedimentation rate (ESR).

Clinical Perspective

The American College of Gastroenterology (ACG) has published guidelines for the prevention of NSAIA-related ulcer complications. The guidelines state that misoprostol (administered in full doses of 800 mcg daily) is very effective in preventing ulcers and ulcer complications in patients taking NSAIDs; however, the drug's usefulness is limited by its adverse GI effects. There is evidence that lower doses (400–600 mcg daily) may also confer significant protection with a similar adverse effect profile to placebo.

● Gastric Ulcer

Acute Therapy

Misoprostol has been used in the short-term treatment of active, benign, gastric ulcer†. However, the drug does not appear to offer any superiority over H₂-receptor antagonists and is less effective than these agents in relieving ulcer pain. Because misoprostol is associated with severe adverse effects (e.g., fetal mortality, premature birth, birth defects), it is not considered a drug of choice for the treatment of peptic ulcer disease (e.g., gastric ulcer) and is not included in the current American College of Gastroenterology (ACG) guidelines for the treatment of this condition.

Epidemiologic and clinical evidence supports a strong association between gastric infection with *H. pylori* and the pathogenesis of gastric ulcers. The ACG, National Institutes of Health (NIH), and most clinicians currently recommend that *all* patients with initial or recurrent gastric ulcer and documented *H. pylori* infection receive anti-infective therapy for treatment of the infection. The choice of a particular regimen should be based on the rapidly evolving data on optimal therapy, including consideration of the patient's prior exposure to anti-infective agents, the local prevalence of resistance, patient compliance, and costs of therapy. (See Duodenal Ulcer: Acute Therapy, in Uses.)

Maintenance Therapy

Misoprostol has been used in reduced dosage for up to 14 months in a limited number of patients as maintenance therapy following healing of active gastric ulcer to reduce ulcer recurrence†. However, additional studies are needed to evaluate the safety and efficacy of maintenance therapy with the drug.

● *Duodenal Ulcer*

Acute Therapy

Misoprostol has been used for the short-term treatment of endoscopically or radiographically confirmed active duodenal ulcer†. Limited data suggest that misoprostol also may be effective in some patients with duodenal ulcer refractory to H$_2$-antagonist therapy. However, misoprostol does not appear to be effective in reducing daytime and nocturnal pain or antacid consumption in patients with duodenal ulcers; aluminum-containing antacids have been used concomitantly with the drug as needed for relief of pain.

Some clinicians state that misoprostol does not appear to offer any superiority over other existing antiulcer therapies for active duodenal ulcers in terms of healing efficacy, dosing schedule, or recurrence after treatment, but is less effective in relieving associated GI pain. Because misoprostol may represent a risk of uterine bleeding and/or abortion when inadvertently used by pregnant women, it is not considered a drug of choice for the treatment of peptic ulcer disease (e.g., duodenal ulcer) and is not included in the current ACG guidelines for the treatment of this condition.

Current epidemiologic and clinical evidence supports a strong association between gastric infection with *Helicobacter pylori* and the pathogenesis of duodenal and gastric ulcers; long-term *H. pylori* infection also has been implicated as a risk factor for gastric cancer. The ACG, NIH, and most clinicians currently recommend that *all* patients with initial or recurrent duodenal or gastric ulcer and documented *H. pylori* infection receive anti-infective therapy for treatment of the infection. Anti-*H. pylori* regimens that combine one or more anti-infective agents (e.g., clarithromycin, amoxicillin) with a bismuth salt and/or an antisecretory agent (e.g., omeprazole, lansoprazole, H$_2$-receptor antagonist) have been used successfully for *H. pylori* eradication. The choice of a particular regimen should be based on the rapidly evolving data on optimal therapy, including consideration of the patient's prior exposure to anti-infective agents, the local prevalence of resistance, patient compliance, and costs of therapy.

● *Termination of Pregnancy*

Misoprostol is used in conjunction with mifepristone for medical termination of an intrauterine pregnancy. Although the manufacturer of misoprostol states that it has not conducted and does not intend to conduct research to support such usage, mifepristone is labeled by FDA for use with misoprostol for termination of pregnancy and the American College of Obstetricians and Gynecologists (ACOG) states that the medication abortion regimen supported by major medical organizations nationally and internationally includes mifepristone and misoprostol; if mifepristone is unavailable, then a misoprostol-only regimen is an acceptable alternative. For additional information on the use of misoprostol with mifepristone for this indication, see Mifepristone 76:00.

● *Other Obstetric Uses*

ACOG states that misoprostol has been used effectively (e.g., 25 mcg every 3–6 hours intravaginally† using tablets formulated for oral administration) to improve cervical inducibility (cervical "ripening") in pregnant women with a medical or obstetric need for labor induction†. Although the manufacturer of misoprostol states that it has not conducted and does not intend to conduct research to support use in pregnancy (e.g., labor induction), some experts state that vaginal administration of misoprostol appears to be safe and effective for induction of labor in appropriately selected women with unfavorable cervices. However, such use in women with prior uterine surgery or cesarean section should be avoided because of the risk of possible uterine rupture.

Misoprostol also has been used for prevention or treatment of serious postpartum hemorrhage† in the presence of uterine atony.

● *Other Uses*

Misoprostol has been used in a limited number of patients for the management of fat malabsorption† associated with cystic fibrosis, and for the management of hemorrhagic gastritis†, reflux esophagitis†, alcohol-induced gastritis†, and NSAIA-induced nephropathy†. The drug has been effective in some patients with these conditions, but further studies are needed.

DOSAGE AND ADMINISTRATION

● *Administration*

Misoprostol usually is administered orally.

When used to reduce the risk of nonsteroidal anti-inflammatory agent (NSAIA)-induced gastric ulcers, the incidence of misoprostol-induced diarrhea may be minimized by administering the drug in divided doses after meals and at bedtime and by avoiding concomitant administration with a magnesium-containing or other laxative antacid.

When used in conjunction with mifepristone for the medical termination of pregnancy, misoprostol is administered intrabuccally 24–48 hours following mifepristone administration; patients should be instructed to place 2 misoprostol tablets in each side of the mouth between the cheek and gums for 30 minutes, then swallow any remnants with water or another liquid. Misoprostol should be administered in an appropriate setting for the patient, taking into account that expulsion of uterine contents could begin within 2 hours of misoprostol administration.

Misoprostol also has been administered intravaginally† using tablets formulated for oral administration.

● *Dosage*

Prevention of NSAIA-Induced Ulcers

For reducing the risk of NSAIA-induced gastric ulcer, the usual adult dosage of misoprostol is 200 mcg 4 times daily. Dosage can be reduced to 100 mcg 4 times daily in patients who do not tolerate the usual dosage; however, this reduced dosage may be somewhat less effective in preventing NSAIA-induced gastric ulcers. Misoprostol dosages of 200 mcg twice daily also have been used for reducing the risk of NSAIA-induced gastric ulcer. The optimum duration of misoprostol therapy has not been elucidated and safety and efficacy have been established in controlled studies only for periods up to 3 months' duration; however, the manufacturer currently recommends that the drug be continued for the duration of NSAIA therapy.

Termination of Pregnancy

When misoprostol is used in conjunction with mifepristone for the medical termination of an intrauterine pregnancy, 800 mcg of misoprostol is administered intrabuccally (two 200-mcg tablets placed in each cheek pouch) 24–48 hours following mifepristone administration. Efficacy of the combined regimen may be reduced if misoprostol is administered less than 24 hours or more than 48 hours after mifepristone.

If mifepristone is unavailable, ACOG states that misoprostol administration alone† may be an acceptable alternative. The recommended dose of misoprostol (when used alone) is 800 mcg administered vaginally, sublingually, or buccally. This dose may be repeated every 3 hours for up to 3 doses. Of note, although studies have typically used no more than 3 doses for the initial treatment regimen, the World Health Organization (WHO) does not specify a maximum number of misoprostol doses for this medication abortion regimen.

Gastric Ulcer

For the short-term treatment of active, benign gastric ulcer†, a misoprostol dosage of 100 or 200 mcg 4 times daily for 8 weeks has been used in adults.

Duodenal Ulcer

For the short-term treatment of active duodenal ulcer†, misoprostol dosages of 100 or 200 mcg 4 times daily or 400 mcg twice daily for 4–8 weeks have been used in adults.

Induction of Labor

Although the optimal misoprostol dosage regimen for cervical ripening and induction of labor† remains to be determined, the American College of Obstetricians and Gynecologists (ACOG) states that misoprostol 25 mcg (¼ of a 100-mcg oral tablet) given intravaginally† can be considered for the initial dose. Subsequent 25-mcg doses have been administered every 3–6 hours.

● Dosage in Renal Impairment and in Geriatric Patients

Routine reduction of misoprostol dosage in patients with renal impairment or in geriatric patients does not appear to be necessary; however, if patients are unable to tolerate the usual adult dosage, dosage can be reduced.

CAUTIONS

Misoprostol generally is well tolerated. The frequency of adverse effects does not appear to be affected by patient age in adults. The most frequent adverse effects associated with misoprostol therapy involve the GI tract (e.g., diarrhea, nausea, abdominal pain).

● GI Effects

Diarrhea is the most common adverse effect of misoprostol. In controlled clinical studies in patients receiving NSAIAs, the incidence of diarrhea associated with a misoprostol dosage of 800 mcg daily was 14–40%. In all studies (including those in which the drug was being studied for the treatment of acute duodenal or gastric ulcers), the incidence of diarrhea averaged 13% with dosages of 400–800 mcg daily. Diarrhea, which appears to be dose related, usually is apparent after about 2 weeks of misoprostol therapy, and generally is self-limiting, often resolving within about a week after onset. However, diarrhea has been severe enough to require discontinuance of misoprostol therapy in about 2% of patients receiving the drug for the prevention of NSAIA-induced ulcer. Profound diarrhea (e.g., voluminous, watery diarrhea) and resultant severe dehydration has been reported rarely in patients receiving misoprostol therapy; such diarrhea also has resulted in severe metabolic acidosis and can be life-threatening. Patients with inflammatory bowel disease may be at increased risk of developing such diarrhea during misoprostol therapy (e.g., secondary to an unmasking or exacerbation of a previously quiescent GI inflammatory condition). Misoprostol-induced diarrhea may be minimized by administering the drug in divided doses after meals and at bedtime and by avoiding concomitant administration with a magnesium-containing or other laxative antacid.

Abdominal pain occurred in about 13–20% of patients receiving misoprostol concomitantly with NSAIAs and in about 7% overall in studies with the drug, but the incidence of this effect did not differ consistently from that reported with placebo. Nausea, flatulence, dyspepsia, vomiting, and constipation occur in about 1–4% of patients receiving misoprostol, but the incidences of these effects were similar to those reported with placebo. Pancreatitis has been reported rarely in patients receiving the drug.

GI bleeding, GI inflammation and/or infection, rectal disorder, gingivitis, dysgeusia, reflux, changes in appetite, and dysphagia also have been reported, but a causal relationship to misoprostol has not been established. The possibility that preexisting NSAIA-induced gastropathy can progress following initiation of misoprostol therapy should be considered.

● Nervous System Effects

Headache occurs in about 2% of patients receiving misoprostol. Asthenia, fatigue, anxiety, depression, drowsiness, dizziness, peripheral neuropathy, confusion, and neurosis also have been reported, but a causal relationship to misoprostol has not been established. Vertigo and lethargy have been reported rarely in patients receiving the drug.

● Genitourinary and Renal Effects

Menstrual irregularities (e.g., cramps, dysmenorrhea, hypermenorrhea, spotting) have occurred in 0.1–0.7% of women receiving misoprostol in clinical studies. Postmenopausal vaginal bleeding may also occur in some women receiving the drug; if such bleeding occurs, the possibility of an underlying gynecologic abnormality should be ruled out. Spontaneous abortions have occurred in pregnant women receiving the drug. Uterine rupture has been reported in pregnant women following administration of misoprostol to induce labor or to induce abortion beyond the eighth week of pregnancy; death of the fetus has occurred in some cases.

Polyuria, dysuria, hematuria, and urinary tract infection have been reported in patients receiving misoprostol, but a causal relationship to the drug has not been established.

● Hematologic Effects

Anemia, abnormal differential blood cell count, thrombocytopenia, and increased erythrocyte sedimentation rate (ESR) have been reported in patients receiving misoprostol, although these effects have not been directly attributed to the drug.

● Ocular and Otic Effects

Visual abnormalities, conjunctivitis, deafness, tinnitus, and earache have been reported in patients receiving misoprostol, but a causal relationship to the drug has not been established.

● Dermatologic and Sensitivity Reactions

Rash, dermatitis, alopecia, pallor, purpura, and diaphoresis have been reported in patients receiving misoprostol, although these effects have not been directly attributed to the drug. Anaphylaxis has been reported in patients receiving misoprostol.

● Cardiovascular Effects

Chest pain, edema, diaphoresis, hypotension, hypertension, arrhythmia, phlebitis, increased serum concentrations of cardiac enzymes, syncope, myocardial infarction (some fatal), and thromboembolic events (e.g., pulmonary embolism, arterial thrombosis, cerebrovascular accident) have been reported in patients receiving misoprostol, but a causal relationship to the drug has not been established.

● Hepatic Effects

Abnormal hepatobiliary function and increased serum alkaline phosphatase or aminotransferase concentrations have been reported in patients receiving misoprostol, but these effects have not been directly attributed to the drug.

● Respiratory Effects

Upper respiratory tract infection, bronchitis, bronchospasm, dyspnea, pneumonia, and epistaxis have been reported in patients receiving misoprostol, but a causal relationship to the drug has not been established.

● Other Adverse Effects

Fever, rigors, weight change, thirst, breast pain, impotence, loss of libido, arthralgia, myalgia, muscle cramps, stiffness, and back pain have been reported in patients receiving misoprostol, but these effects have not been directly attributed to the drug.

● Precautions and Contraindications

Patients receiving misoprostol for reducing the risk of NSAIA-induced gastric ulcer should be advised about such use and that the drug should be used only as directed. A copy of the patient information provided by the manufacturer should be given to each patient receiving the drug, and the latest version should be issued with each prescription refill. Patients should be instructed to read the patient information before initiation of misoprostol therapy and every time the prescription is refilled, since the information may have been revised. It is particularly important that all patients understand misoprostol's abortifacient properties and attendant risks (See Cautions: Pregnancy, Fertility, and Lactation), and that the drug is intended only for their use for the specific condition for which it was prescribed. Sharing the drug with another individual, particularly a woman of childbearing potential, could be hazardous. Patients should be advised to contact their clinician promptly if they have problems with or questions about misoprostol.

Because severe adverse cardiovascular effects have been reported with misoprostol, the manufacturer states that the drug should be used with caution in patients with preexisting cardiovascular disease.

Because misoprostol may exacerbate intestinal inflammation and produce severe diarrhea in patients with inflammatory bowel disease, the drug should be used with extreme caution in these patients and their condition monitored carefully. Because dehydration rarely may occur secondary to misoprostol-induced diarrhea, the drug also should be used with careful monitoring in patients prone to dehydration or in whom its consequences would be dangerous.

Misoprostol should not be used in pregnant women for reducing the risk of NSAIA-induced gastric ulcers. Misoprostol also should not be used for reducing the risk of NSAIA-induced gastric ulcers in women of childbearing potential unless the woman is at high risk of developing gastric ulcers or of complications resulting from NSAIA-induced gastric ulcers. Misoprostol therapy should *not* be initiated in such women until the possibility of pregnancy has been excluded and an effective method of contraception has been started.

Misoprostol is contraindicated in patients with known hypersensitivity to prostaglandins.

● Pediatric Precautions

Safety and efficacy of misoprostol in children <18 years of age have not been established.

● Pregnancy, Fertility, and Lactation

Pregnancy

Misoprostol exhibits abortifacient activity and therefore can cause serious fetal harm when administered to pregnant women. A boxed warning about this risk is included in the prescribing information for the drug. Misoprostol should not be used in pregnant women for reducing the risk of NSAIA-induced gastric ulcers. The drug also should not be used for reducing the risk of NSAIA-induced gastric ulcers in women of childbearing potential unless the woman is at high risk of developing gastric ulcers or of complications resulting from NSAIA-induced gastric ulcers; such women should not receive misoprostol until pregnancy is excluded and other necessary precautions are ensured.

Misoprostol has been reported to produce uterine contractions and to stimulate uterine bleeding and total or partial expulsion of the products of conception in pregnant women. Spontaneous abortions induced by the drug may be incomplete, may require hospitalization and/or surgery, and can result in dangerous uterine bleeding, premature birth, or birth defects.

Intravaginal use of misoprostol may result in hyperstimulation of the uterus, which may progress to uterine tetany with marked impairment of uteroplacental blood flow, uterine rupture (requiring surgical repair, hysterectomy, and/or salpingo-oophorectomy), or amniotic fluid embolism. Pelvic pain, retained placenta, severe genital bleeding, shock, fetal bradycardia, and fetal and maternal death have been reported. Use of intravaginal misoprostol dosages exceeding 25 mcg may be associated with an increased risk of uterine tachysystole, uterine rupture, meconium passage, meconium staining of amniotic fluid, and cesarean delivery resulting from uterine hyperstimulation. The risk of uterine rupture increases with advancing gestational age, prior uterine surgery (including cesarean delivery), and grand multiparity; the American College of Obstetricians and Gynecologists (ACOG) states that intravaginal use of misoprostol for cervical ripening or labor induction is not recommended in patients with a previous cesarean delivery or prior major uterine surgery.

Serious, sometimes fatal, bacterial (e.g., *Clostridium sordellii*) infection and sepsis or prolonged heavy vaginal bleeding have been reported following spontaneous, surgical, and medical abortions, including in patients receiving mifepristone and misoprostol for termination of pregnancy; a causal relationship to the regimen has not been established.

Congenital abnormalities, sometimes associated with fetal death, have been reported subsequent to the unsuccessful use of misoprostol as an abortifacient. Some data indicate that use of misoprostol during the first trimester of pregnancy has been associated with skull defects, cranial nerve palsies, facial malformations, and limb defects; however, the precise mechanism(s) for these teratogenic effects has not been fully elucidated. Effects of misoprostol on later growth, development, and functional maturation of the child whose mother received the drug for cervical ripening or labor induction have not been established. The effects of misoprostol on the need for forceps delivery or other intervention are not known.

Currently, it is recommended that misoprostol be used for reducing the risk of NSAIA-induced gastric ulcers in women of childbearing potential *only* if they are at high risk of complications resulting from NSAIA-induced gastric ulceration or are at high risk of developing gastric ulceration. Such therapy should be initiated in such women *only* after determining that they are reliable and able to comply with effective contraceptive measures and ensuring that they have received both oral and written warnings concerning the hazards associated with misoprostol therapy, the risk of possible contraceptive failure, and the danger to other women of childbearing potential should the drug be taken by them. In addition, a reliable, blood pregnancy test must be performed within 2 weeks prior to beginning misoprostol therapy and the drug should *not* be provided to the patient until the pregnancy test is reported as negative, initiating therapy on the second or third day of the next normal menstrual cycle.

If misoprostol is inadvertently administered during pregnancy or if the patient becomes pregnant while receiving the drug for reducing the risk of NSAIA-induced gastric ulcer, misoprostol should be discontinued and the patient informed of the potential hazard to the fetus.

Reproduction studies in rats and rabbits using oral misoprostol dosages up to 10 and 1 mg/kg (625 and 63 times the usual human dosage), respectively, have not revealed evidence of fetotoxicity or teratogenicity. However, increased fetal resorption occurred in rabbits, suggesting possible embryotoxicity.

Fertility

Reproduction studies in male and female rats using oral misoprostol dosages of 0.1–10 mg/kg daily (6.25–625 times the usual human dosage) have revealed dose-related pre- and post-implantation losses and a decrease in the number of live offspring at the highest dosage administered. These effects suggest that the drug may impair fertility in both males and females.

Lactation

It is not known whether misoprostol and/or misoprostol acid cross the placenta. The drug is metabolized rapidly to the free acid following oral administration, which is biologically active and distributed into breast milk. There are no published reports of adverse effects associated with misoprostol in breast-fed infants. Caution is advised if the drug is used during breast-feeding.

DRUG INTERACTIONS

● Food and Antacids

Food and antacids decrease the rate of absorption of misoprostol, resulting in delayed and decreased peak plasma concentrations of misoprostol acid, the active metabolite of the drug. Antacids and possibly food also appear to decrease the oral bioavailability of misoprostol; however, it has been suggested that such decreases may not be clinically important since misoprostol's activity in protecting the GI mucosa appears to be local rather than systemic. Magnesium-containing antacids also may increase the incidence of misoprostol-induced diarrhea. Therefore, if concomitant administration of an antacid is necessary, a magnesium-containing or other laxative antacid should be avoided and a constipating (e.g., aluminum-containing) antacid used instead.

● Drugs Metabolized by Hepatic Microsomal Enzymes

Misoprostol does not appear to interfere with the metabolism of drugs, including diazepam or propranolol, by the hepatic cytochrome P-450 (CYP) enzyme system.

● Nonsteroidal Anti-inflammatory Agents

No substantial pharmacokinetic interactions between misoprostol and ibuprofen, piroxicam, or diclofenac have been observed to date.

Absorption or peak plasma concentrations of misoprostol or aspirin do not appear to be affected substantially by concomitant administration, although AUC of aspirin may be decreased by about 20% when the drugs are administered concomitantly. This interaction does not appear to be clinically important since misoprostol did not interfere with the efficacy of aspirin as determined by relief of pain and stiffness, reduction of swelling, improvement of mobility and grip strength, or erythrocyte sedimentation rate (ESR) in patients with rheumatoid arthritis who received usual dosages of the drugs concomitantly.

In a study in a limited number of healthy individuals receiving oral indomethacin 75 mg twice daily concomitantly with oral misoprostol 400 mcg twice daily, steady-state plasma indomethacin concentrations reportedly were decreased by 20–60%. However, reanalysis of data from this study using different statistical methods suggested that oral bioavailability of indomethacin was not affected substantially by concomitant misoprostol. Further studies are needed to determine whether a potential pharmacokinetic interaction exists between the drugs.

PHARMACOLOGY

• GI Effects

Misoprostol, a synthetic prostaglandin E_1 analog, is a gastric antisecretory agent with protective effects on the gastroduodenal mucosa. The drug inhibits gastric acid secretion and protects the mucosa from the irritant and/or other (e.g., pharmacologic) effects of certain drugs (e.g., nonsteroidal anti-inflammatory agents [NSAIAs]) and may have similar antisecretory and mucosal effects in patients with gastric or duodenal ulcer.

The role of endogenous prostaglandins in the GI tract is complex. Endogenous prostaglandins decrease acid secretion from parietal cells and may have a cytoprotective effect on the gastric mucosa by increasing mucus and bicarbonate secretion, preventing disruption of the gastric mucosal barrier, inhibiting or reducing back diffusion of hydrogen ions, regulating mucosal blood flow, preventing microvascular stasis, and preserving mucosal capacity to regenerate cells. Enhancement of transmucosal diffusion potential and cellular bicarbonate and chloride exchange, stabilization of lysosomal membranes with a resultant reduction in enzyme release, and modulation of endogenous sulfhydryl concentrations also may contribute to the GI cytoprotective effect of endogenous prostaglandins.

Inhibition of the synthesis of prostaglandins (e.g., prostaglandins of the E series, prostacyclin) that are believed to exhibit cytoprotective effects on the gastric mucosa has been suggested as a possible mechanism for gastric mucosal damage induced by NSAIAs. However, the exact relationship between NSAIA-induced GI mucosal damage and prostaglandins has not been fully elucidated. NSAIAs may decrease bicarbonate and mucus secretion by inhibiting prostaglandin synthesis and decreasing mucosal prostaglandin concentrations. NSAIAs also may reduce gastric transmucosal potential difference, decrease gastric blood flow, cause capillary stasis, and selectively increase permeability of the gastric mucosa to cations and thus enhance back diffusion of hydrogen ions into the mucosa. Increased entry of acid into the gastric mucosa causes cellular damage, which leads to additional alterations in mucosal permeability. Gastric mucosal damage induced by NSAIAs can result in ulceration and/or bleeding. Mucosal prostaglandin synthesis also appears to be reduced in some patients with gastric or duodenal ulceration compared with that in healthy individuals.

The exact mechanisms of the protective effect of misoprostol on the gastroduodenal mucosa have not been fully elucidated, but it appears that several actions may contribute to the drug's activity in the prevention and/or healing of gastroduodenal ulcers. In addition, it appears that the drug's protective effect on the gastroduodenal mucosa is local rather than systemic. However, because the therapeutic GI effects of the drug have been observed principally at antisecretory dosages, which are higher than cytoprotective dosages in animals, the extent to which the antisecretory and mucosal protective activities contribute to misoprostol's effect in preventing and/or healing gastroduodenal ulcers in humans currently is not known.

Inhibition of Gastric Acid Secretion

Misoprostol reduces gastric acid secretion via a direct action at the parietal cells. Secretion is inhibited under basal conditions and also when stimulated by food, histamine, pentagastrin, betazole, tetragastrin, NSAIAs, alcohol, or caffeine. Misoprostol also inhibits nocturnal gastric acid secretion but does not appear to reduce the volume of such secretion.

In vitro receptor-binding studies have shown that animal parietal cells contain prostaglandin receptors in proximity to histamine H_2 receptors. It has been postulated that stimulation of prostaglandin receptors may inhibit the activation of the histamine-sensitive enzyme adenylate cyclase, and that such inhibition may depend on guanosine-5′-triphosphate (GTP), a regulator in several adenylate cyclase receptor systems. Binding to prostaglandin receptors appears to be a saturable, reversible, and stereospecific process. These receptors have high affinity for prostaglandins of the E series, including misoprostol and misoprostol acid (an active metabolite of the drug), but not for prostaglandins of the F or I series or for compounds such as histamine or histamine H_2-receptor antagonists (e.g., cimetidine). Limited data have shown that the antisecretory activity of misoprostol may be positively correlated with its receptor-site affinity. High affinity for these receptors may allow misoprostol to be effective locally when taken with food despite the lower serum concentrations of the drug that may be attained compared with those attained in the fasted state.

The degree of inhibition of gastric acid secretion by misoprostol is directly related to dose. The inhibitory effect of a 50-mcg oral dose of misoprostol generally is considered modest and is relatively short in duration, whereas oral 200-mcg doses are required for substantial inhibitory effects on basal, nocturnal, and food- or histamine-stimulated gastric acid secretion and reportedly are similar in degree although not in duration to those produced by 300-mg oral doses of cimetidine. However, other evidence suggests that misoprostol may not be as effective as histamine H_2-antagonists in decreasing gastric acid secretion, particularly nocturnal secretion. Following oral administration of 100- or 200-mcg of misoprostol in healthy individuals, gastric acid secretion is decreased by 83 or 85–98%, respectively. Following oral administration of 200 mcg of the drug, 85 or 75% of meal-stimulated gastric acid secretion is inhibited within 60 or 90 minutes, respectively; inhibition persists for at least 3 hours. Following oral administration of a single 200-, 400-, or 800-mcg dose of misoprostol, pentagastrin-stimulated gastric acid secretion is inhibited by 45, 60, or 65%, respectively, for at least 1–2 hours. Following oral administration of a single 100- or 200-mcg dose of misoprostol, histamine-stimulated gastric acid secretion is inhibited by 98 or 100%, respectively, for at least 2 hours.

Mucosal Protective Effects

The mucosal protective effects of misoprostol may contribute to the drug's effect in preventing and/or healing gastroduodenal ulceration and bleeding. The exact mechanisms have not been established, but it appears that several actions may contribute to the protective effects of misoprostol on the gastric mucosa. Misoprostol may increase mucus secretion, increase bicarbonate secretion from nonparietal cells, enhance or maintain blood flow of the mucosa (possibly via direct vasodilation), protect submucosal cell proliferation, stabilize mucosal membrane systems, prevent mucosal barrier disruption, enhance transmucosal diffusion potential, and inhibit or reduce back diffusion of hydrogen ions into the mucosa. However, the exact relationship between these effects and the mucosal protective activity of misoprostol has not been clearly established. Limited data indicate that inhibition of adenyl cyclase does not contribute to the drug's mucosal protective effects.

In animals, doses smaller than those necessary for inhibition of gastric acid secretion have provided protection of the gastric mucosa. However, a mucosal protective dose has not been established in humans. In addition, because antisecretory dosages generally appear to be necessary for optimal therapeutic GI effects in humans, it is difficult to determine whether prevention of mucosal injury results from misoprostol-induced gastric acid inhibition, mucosal protection, or both. While it has been suggested that the protective effects of misoprostol on the gastroduodenal mucosa may not depend on inhibition of gastric acid secretion, current evidence is insufficient to substantiate this suggestion, and further studies are needed to determine the mechanisms and possible therapeutic contribution of the drug's mucosal protective activity.

It appears that the extent of increased mucus and bicarbonate secretion induced by misoprostol is directly related to dose. Following oral administration of single 200-, 400-, or 800-mcg doses in healthy individuals, basal gastric mucus secretion increased by 37, 82, or 95%, respectively. In one study, following oral administration of 50 mcg of misoprostol 4 times daily for 2 days in healthy individuals who also were receiving aspirin dosages of 975 mg 4 times daily, no appreciable changes in mucus secretion were observed.

Following oral administration of 100–400 mcg of misoprostol in healthy individuals, dose-related stimulation of basal bicarbonate secretion has been reported; lower doses do not appear to produce appreciable effects on bicarbonate secretion. Results from studies on the effects of misoprostol on blood flow in the gastric mucosa have been conflicting and species dependent. In a study in dogs, IV misoprostol produced vasodilation and increased the ratio of gastric mucosal blood flow to the rate of acid secretion; however, in other animals, the drug had no effect on basal or stimulated mucosal blood flow following intragastric or IV administration. Further studies are needed to evaluate the relationship, if any, between gastric mucosal blood flow and mucus secretion and the mucosal protective effect of misoprostol.

Misoprostol has protected the gastroduodenal mucosa from the irritant and/or other (e.g., pharmacologic) effects of various NSAIAs, including aspirin, and those of alcohol, and from stress-induced effects, as determined by reduction or prevention of fecal blood loss or by endoscopy. Misoprostol's activity against the irritant effects of taurocholate has been equivocal, and limited evidence suggests that the drug may not protect the gastric mucosa from the effects of systemically administered cytotoxic agents.

Other GI Effects

Equivocal effects on pepsin secretion have been observed in animals and humans receiving misoprostol. The drug has produced a moderate reduction in pepsin concentration in gastric juice under basal conditions but not when stimulated by histamine. In healthy individuals, misoprostol also has inhibited tetragastrin-stimulated and nocturnal pepsin secretion. However, in at least one study in animals, misoprostol increased pepsin volume and secretion. Misoprostol does not appear to have a substantial effect on intrinsic factor secretion or serum concentrations of polypeptide hormones, including gastrin (basal or meal-stimulated), somatostatin, vasoactive intestinal peptide, or motilin.

At usual dosages, misoprostol can produce diarrhea, probably via stimulation of intestinal fluid secretion and effects on motility. Following IV administration of the drug in animals, initial (for 1–2 hours after dosing) inhibition of intestinal motility was observed together with stimulation of intestinal fluid secretion, which was followed by the development of organized propulsive spike-burst patterns of motility similar to those associated with other forms of diarrhea. Limited evidence suggests that the drug does not affect gastric emptying or lower esophageal sphincter tone, but additional study is necessary.

● Genitourinary and Renal Effects

Misoprostol has been reported to increase the amplitude and frequency of uterine contractions and to stimulate uterine bleeding and total or partial expulsion of uterine contents in pregnant women. Other prostaglandins of the E series (e.g., prostaglandin E_2) are known abortifacients. In addition, menstrual irregularities have been reported occasionally in nonpregnant women receiving the drug. Because of the potential abortifacient effect of misoprostol, the drug should not be used in pregnant women for reducing the risk of NSAIA-induced gastric ulcers.

Misoprostol does not appear to have clinically important effects on serum creatinine or uric acid concentrations.

● Endocrine and Gonadal Effects

Misoprostol does not appear to have clinically important effects on serum concentrations of prolactin (although reductions have been reported in men), thyrotropin (TSH), somatotropin (growth hormone), thyroxine (T_4), follicle-stimulating hormone (FSH, follitropin), luteinizing hormone (lutropin), sex-hormone binding globulin, progesterone (in women, although reductions have been reported), testosterone (in men), estradiol (in women), or gonadotropin. Although serum cortisol concentrations have been reported to increase in some women receiving misoprostol, they remained within the normal range.

● Other Effects

In healthy individuals, misoprostol did not inhibit cellular or humoral immune responses. The drug also does not appear to affect platelet aggregation or to produce clinically important cardiovascular or respiratory effects.

PHARMACOKINETICS

● Absorption

Misoprostol is rapidly and almost completely absorbed from the GI tract; however, the drug undergoes extensive and rapid first-pass metabolism (de-esterification) to form misoprostol acid (the free acid), the principal and active metabolite of the drug. There is evidence from animal studies that such metabolism may occur at least in part in the GI tract (e.g., in parietal cells). An average of 88% of a dose of misoprostol reportedly is absorbed following oral administration in healthy individuals, but only negligible amounts of unchanged drug are attained in plasma.

Food and antacids decrease the rate of absorption of misoprostol, resulting in delayed and decreased peak plasma concentrations of misoprostol acid. Following oral administration of single 400-mcg doses of misoprostol, average peak plasma misoprostol acid concentrations occur within about 14 minutes in the fasted state compared with about 20 minutes when administered with antacids and about 1 hour when taken with food. The extent of absorption also appears to be decreased by antacids and possibly by food, but it has been suggested that such decreases may not be clinically important since the GI effects of misoprostol appear to be local rather than systemic.

There is considerable interindividual variation in plasma concentrations attained with a given dose of misoprostol; however, it appears that plasma concentrations of the free acid increase linearly with single misoprostol doses of 200–400 mcg. Following oral administration of a single 200- or 400-mcg dose of misoprostol in fasting, healthy individuals, average peak plasma misoprostol acid concentrations occur within 14–20 minutes.

Steady-state plasma concentrations of misoprostol acid generally are reached within 48 hours following continuous dosing. Accumulation of misoprostol acid does not appear to occur during chronic administration of misoprostol.

Peak plasma misoprostol acid concentrations and AUC in patients with renal impairment (creatinine clearance of 0.5–37 mL/minute) were about twofold those observed in patients with normal renal function; however, no clear correlation was established between AUCs achieved and degree of renal impairment. AUC of misoprostol acid also may be increased in geriatric patients (older than 64 years of age) compared with those in younger adults, probably secondary to decreased volume of distribution (V_d) in geriatric patients; however, peak plasma concentrations do not appear to be affected.

Following single 50- to 200-mcg oral doses of misoprostol, inhibition of gastric acid secretion under basal and nocturnal conditions and also when stimulated by food, histamine, pentagastrin, or caffeine is apparent within 30 minutes, reaches a maximum within 60–90 minutes, and persists for at least 3 hours. The degree and duration of inhibition of gastric acid secretion produced by misoprostol are directly related to the dose with single misoprostol doses of 200–400 mcg. It appears that misoprostol doses exceeding 400 mcg do not produce further increases in inhibition of gastric acid secretion. In animals, doses lower than those necessary for inhibition of gastric acid secretion have provided protection of the gastric mucosa. In humans, however, a relationship between dose and mucosal protective activity has not been established since therapeutic effects (e.g., prevention of injury) on the gastroduodenal mucosa have been observed principally with antisecretory doses.

● Distribution

Distribution of misoprostol into human body tissues and fluids has not been fully characterized. Following oral administration of misoprostol in rats, the drug is widely distributed, achieving concentrations in stomach, intestines, liver, blood, and kidneys that are 6–73 times that in plasma.

Misoprostol acid is approximately 80–90% bound to serum proteins. Protein binding of the drug does not appear to be affected by plasma concentrations of misoprostol acid or misoprostol in the therapeutic range, age of the patient, or concomitant administration of other highly protein-bound drugs.

It is not known whether misoprostol and/or the free acid cross the placenta. Misoprostol is metabolized rapidly to the free acid following oral administration, which is distributed into breast milk.

● Elimination

Misoprostol is rapidly metabolized to misoprostol acid (the free acid) following oral administration. The parent drug reportedly has a half-life of 6 minutes in vitro. Plasma concentrations of the free acid and other metabolites of the drug appear to decline in a biphasic manner. Following oral administration of misoprostol in healthy adults, the elimination half-life of the free acid is about 20–40 minutes. Following oral administration of radiolabeled drug in healthy adults, the half-life of misoprostol metabolites averages about 1.5 hours in the initial distribution phase, corresponding principally to organic metabolites of the drug, and about 144–177 hours in the terminal elimination phase, corresponding principally to radiolabeled water.

In patients with renal impairment (creatinine clearance of 0.5–37 mL/minute), half-life may be increased twofold compared with that in patients with normal renal function. It appears that half-life of misoprostol is not increased in geriatric patients.

The exact metabolic fate of misoprostol has not been clearly established, but the drug is rapidly and extensively metabolized, principally via de-esterification to form misoprostol acid, which is pharmacologically active. Animal evidence suggests that de-esterification of the drug may occur at least in part in the GI tract (e.g., in parietal cells). Misoprostol acid undergoes extensive, rapid β-oxidation of the α side chain to form the tetranor metabolite of misoprostol acid, and *omega*-oxidation of the β side chain with subsequent ketone reduction to form prostaglandin F analogs. Studies in animals indicate that misoprostol acid is approximately as potent as misoprostol in inhibiting gastric acid secretion; the dinor and tetranor metabolites of misoprostol acid appear to be pharmacologically inactive.

Following oral or IV administration of misoprostol, the free acid and other metabolites of the drug are excreted mainly in urine; smaller amounts of metabolites are excreted in feces, probably via biliary elimination. Only negligible amounts of unchanged drug are excreted in urine following oral or IV administration. Following a single oral 200-mcg dose of misoprostol in healthy adults, about 73% of the dose is excreted in urine and about 15% in feces within 7 days; most urinary excretion occurs within 8–24 hours. The principal urinary metabolites are the dinor and tetranor of misoprostol acid. In healthy adults, less than 1% of a single oral dose of misoprostol is excreted in urine as unchanged drug and misoprostol acid. Approximately 5% of a single oral dose is excreted in feces within 24 hours as the dinor and tetranor of misoprostol acid.

CHEMISTRY AND STABILITY

● Chemistry

Misoprostol is a synthetic analog of prostaglandin E$_1$ (alprostadil). Misoprostol differs structurally from prostaglandin E$_1$ by the presence of a methyl ester at C-1, a methyl group at C-16, and a hydroxy group at C-16 rather than at C-15. These structural differences appear to increase the antisecretory potency, prolong the duration of action, and improve the safety profile of misoprostol compared with prostaglandin E$_1$.

● Stability

Commercially available misoprostol tablets should be stored in a dry place at a temperature of 25°C or less.

PREPARATIONS

Excipients in commercially available drug preparations may have clinically important effects in some individuals; consult specific product labeling for details.

Misoprostol

Oral

Tablets	100 mcg*	Cytotec®, Pfizer
		Misoprostol Tablets
	200 mcg*	Cytotec®, Pfizer
		Misoprostol Tablets

Misoprostol Combinations

Oral

| Tablets, enteric-coated core, film-coated | 200 mcg Misoprostol outer layer with 50 mg Diclofenac Sodium enteric-coated core | Arthrotec®, Pfizer |
| | 200 mcg Misoprostol outer layer with 75 mg Diclofenac Sodium enteric-coated core | Arthrotec®, Pfizer |

* available from one or more manufacturer, distributor, and/or repackager by generic (nonproprietary) name

† Use is not currently included in the labeling approved by the US Food and Drug Administration.

Selected Revisions March 28, 2023, © Copyright, October 01, 1989, American Society of Health-System Pharmacists, Inc.

Dexlansoprazole

56:28.36 • PROTON-PUMP INHIBITORS

■ Dexlansoprazole, commonly referred to as an acid- or proton-pump inhibitor, is a gastric antisecretory agent. Dexlansoprazole is the *R*-isomer of lansoprazole.

USES

● Gastroesophageal Reflux

Dexlansoprazole is used for short-term (up to 8 weeks) treatment of all grades of erosive esophagitis, as maintenance therapy (for up to 6 months) following healing of erosive esophagitis to reduce recurrence of the disease, and for short-term (up to 4 weeks) management of symptoms (e.g., heartburn) of gastroesophageal reflux disease (GERD) in patients without erosive esophagitis.

Suppression of gastric acid secretion is considered by the American College of Gastroenterology (ACG) to be the mainstay of treatment for GERD, and a proton-pump inhibitor or histamine H_2-receptor antagonist is used to achieve acid suppression, control symptoms, and prevent complications of the disease. Because GERD is a chronic condition, the ACG states that continuous therapy to control symptoms and prevent complications is appropriate, and chronic, even lifelong, use of a proton-pump inhibitor is effective and appropriate as maintenance therapy in many patients with GERD. The ACG states that proton-pump inhibitors are more effective (i.e., provide more frequent and more rapid symptomatic relief and healing of esophagitis) than histamine H_2-receptor antagonists in the treatment of GERD. Proton-pump inhibitors also provide greater control of acid reflux than do prokinetic agents (e.g., cisapride [no longer commercially available in the US], metoclopramide) without the risk of severe adverse effects associated with these agents.

Efficacy of dexlansoprazole in the treatment of endoscopically diagnosed erosive esophagitis was established in 2 controlled studies in patients receiving dexlansoprazole 60 or 90 mg daily or lansoprazole 30 mg daily for 8 weeks. Healing rates at 4 weeks were similar for dexlansoprazole 60 mg daily and lansoprazole 30 mg daily (66–70 and 65%, respectively). Findings of one study showed higher rates of healing (85 versus 79%) for dexlansoprazole 60 mg daily versus lansoprazole 30 mg daily at 8 weeks; however, in the other study, healing rates at 8 weeks for these 2 regimens did not differ significantly (87 versus 85%, respectively). No additional benefit of the 90-mg dosage over the 60-mg dosage of dexlansoprazole was reported.

Efficacy of dexlansoprazole as maintenance therapy following healing of erosive esophagitis was established in a controlled study in patients with endoscopically confirmed healing of erosive esophagitis who received dexlansoprazole 30 or 60 mg daily or placebo for 6 months. Healing was maintained in 66% of patients receiving dexlansoprazole 30 mg daily compared with 14% of patients receiving placebo. In addition, patients receiving dexlansoprazole 30 mg daily reported a higher percentage of heartburn-free 24-hour periods over 6 months of maintenance therapy than did patients receiving placebo. Most patients receiving placebo discontinued such treatment between months 2 and 6 because of recurrent erosive esophagitis. No additional clinical benefit of the 60-mg dosage over the 30-mg dosage was reported.

Efficacy in patients with symptomatic nonerosive GERD was established in a controlled study in patients with a 6-month or longer history of heartburn episodes, no endoscopic evidence of erosive esophagitis, and heartburn for at least 4 of the 7 days immediately prior to randomization; patients received dexlansoprazole 30 or 60 mg daily or placebo for 4 weeks. The median percentage of days (24-hour periods) without heartburn was 55 or 19% during 4 weeks of therapy with dexlansoprazole or placebo, respectively; no additional benefit of the 60-mg dosage over the 30-mg dosage was reported.

For further information on the treatment of GERD, see Uses: Gastroesophageal Reflux, in Omeprazole 56:28.36.

● Crohn's Disease-associated Ulcers

Although evidence currently is limited, proton-pump inhibitors have been used for gastric acid-suppressive therapy as an adjunct in the symptomatic treatment of upper GI Crohn's disease†, including esophageal, gastroduodenal, and jejunoileal disease. Most evidence of efficacy to date has been from case studies in patients with Crohn's-associated peptic ulcer disease unresponsive to other therapies (e.g., histamine H_2-receptor antagonists, cytoprotective agents,

antacids, and/or sucralfate). (See Uses: Crohn's Disease-associated Ulcers in Omeprazole 56:28.36.)

For further information on the management of Crohn's disease, see Uses: Crohn's Disease, in Mesalamine 56:36.

DOSAGE AND ADMINISTRATION

● Administration

Dexlansoprazole is administered orally once daily. The drug may be taken without regard to food; however, because the effect on gastric pH during the initial 4 hours after a dose may be decreased slightly when dexlansoprazole is taken after a meal, patients with postprandial symptoms that do not respond adequately to postprandial administration may benefit from preprandial administration of the drug. Dexlansoprazole capsules should be swallowed whole; alternatively, the contents of a capsule may be sprinkled on a tablespoonful of applesauce and swallowed immediately without chewing.

Dispensing and Administration Precautions

Dispensing errors have occurred because of similarity in spelling between Kapidex® (the former trade name for dexlansoprazole) and Casodex® (the trade name for bicalutamide, a nonsteroidal antiandrogenic antineoplastic agent) or Kadian® (a trade name for an extended-release capsule preparation of morphine sulfate, an opiate agonist analgesic). Therefore, in April 2010, the manufacturer of Kapidex® changed the trade name for dexlansoprazole from Kapidex® to Dexilant® to avoid future dispensing errors. (See Dispensing and Administration Precautions under Cautions: Warnings/Precautions.)

● Dosage

Gastroesophageal Reflux

For short-term treatment of erosive esophagitis, the recommended adult dosage of dexlansoprazole is 60 mg once daily for up to 8 weeks. For maintenance therapy following healing of erosive esophagitis, the recommended adult dosage of dexlansoprazole is 30 mg once daily for up to 6 months. The manufacturer states that controlled studies of dexlansoprazole maintenance therapy beyond 6 months have not been performed. For short-term management of symptomatic gastroesophageal reflux disease (GERD) in patients without erosive esophagitis, the recommended adult dosage of dexlansoprazole is 30 mg once daily for 4 weeks. However, the American College of Gastroenterology (ACG) states that chronic, even lifelong, therapy with a proton-pump inhibitor is appropriate in many patients with GERD.

● Special Populations

No adjustment of dexlansoprazole dosage is necessary in geriatric patients, patients with renal impairment, or patients with mild hepatic impairment (Child-Pugh class A). The manufacturer states that a maximum dosage of 30 mg daily should be considered in patients with moderate hepatic impairment (Child-Pugh class B). The drug has not been studied in patients with severe hepatic impairment (Child-Pugh class C).

CAUTIONS

● Contraindications

Known hypersensitivity to dexlansoprazole or any ingredient in the formulation.

● Warnings/Precautions

Sensitivity Reactions

Hypersensitivity Reactions

Hypersensitivity reactions (e.g., anaphylaxis, toxic epidermal necrolysis, Stevens-Johnson syndrome) have been reported with dexlansoprazole.

Gastric Malignancy

Symptomatic response to therapy with dexlansoprazole does not preclude the presence of gastric malignancy.

Clostridium difficile Infection

Available data suggest a possible association between use of proton-pump inhibitors and risk of *Clostridium difficile* infection, including *C. difficile*-associated diarrhea and colitis (CDAD; also known as antibiotic-associated diarrhea and colitis or pseudomembranous colitis). In most observational studies to date, the risk of *C. difficile* infection in patients exposed to proton-pump inhibitors has ranged from 1.4–2.75 times that in patients not exposed to proton-pump inhibitors; however, some observational studies have found no increase in risk. Although many of the cases occurred in patients who had other risk factors for CDAD, including advanced age, comorbid conditions, and/or use of broad-spectrum anti-infectives, the US Food and Drug Administration (FDA) concluded that a contributory role for proton-pump inhibitors could not be definitively ruled out. The mechanism by which proton-pump inhibitors might increase the risk of CDAD has not been elucidated. Although it has been suggested that reduction of gastric acidity by gastric antisecretory agents might facilitate colonization with *C. difficile*, some studies have raised questions about this proposed mechanism or have suggested that the observed association is the result of confounding with other risk factors for CDAD. FDA also is reviewing the risk of CDAD in patients exposed to histamine H_2-receptor antagonists.

CDAD can be serious in patients who have one or more risk factors for *C. difficile* infection and are receiving concomitant therapy with a proton-pump inhibitor; colectomy and, rarely, death have been reported. FDA recommends that patients receive proton-pump inhibitors at the lowest effective dosage and for the shortest possible time appropriate for their clinical condition. Patients experiencing persistent diarrhea should be evaluated for CDAD and should be managed with appropriate supportive therapy (e.g., fluid and electrolyte management), anti-infective therapy directed against *C. difficile* (e.g., metronidazole, vancomycin), and surgical evaluation as clinically indicated.

Musculoskeletal Effects

Findings from several observational studies suggest that therapy with proton-pump inhibitors, particularly in high dosages (i.e., multiple daily doses) and/or for prolonged periods of time (i.e., one year or longer), may be associated with an increased risk of osteoporosis-related fractures of the hip, wrist, or spine. The magnitude of risk is unclear; causality has not been established. (See Cautions: Musculoskeletal Effects, in Omeprazole 56:28.36.) FDA is continuing to evaluate this safety concern. Although controlled studies are required to confirm these findings, patients should receive proton-pump inhibitors at the lowest effective dosage and for the shortest possible time appropriate for their clinical condition. Individuals who are at risk for osteoporosis-related fractures should receive an adequate intake of calcium and vitamin D and should have their bone health assessed and managed according to current standards of care.

Hypomagnesemia

Hypomagnesemia, symptomatic and asymptomatic, has been reported rarely in patients receiving long-term therapy (for at least 3 months or, in most cases, for longer than one year) with proton-pump inhibitors, including dexlansoprazole. Clinically serious adverse effects associated with hypomagnesemia, which are similar to manifestations of hypocalcemia, include tetany, seizures, tremors, carpopedal spasm, arrhythmias (e.g., atrial fibrillation, supraventricular tachycardia), and abnormal QT interval. Other reported adverse effects include paresthesia, muscle weakness, muscle cramps, lethargy, fatigue, and unsteadiness. In most patients, treatment of hypomagnesemia required magnesium replacement and discontinuance of the proton-pump inhibitor. Following discontinuance of the proton-pump inhibitor, hypomagnesemia resolved within a median of one week; upon rechallenge, hypomagnesemia recurred within a median of 2 weeks.

In patients expected to receive long-term therapy with a proton-pump inhibitor or in those receiving a proton-pump inhibitor concomitantly with digoxin or drugs that may cause hypomagnesemia (e.g., diuretics), clinicians should consider measurement of serum magnesium concentrations prior to initiation of prescription proton-pump inhibitor therapy and periodically thereafter. (See Cautions: Hypomagnesemia and also Cautions: Precautions and Contraindications, in Omeprazole 56:28.36.)

Respiratory Effects

Administration of proton-pump inhibitors has been associated with an increased risk for developing certain infections (e.g., community-acquired pneumonia). For further precautionary information about this adverse effect, see Community-acquired Pneumonia under Cautions: Respiratory Effects, in Omeprazole 56:28.36.

Dispensing and Administration Precautions

Because of similarity in spelling between Kapidex® (the former trade name for dexlansoprazole) and Casodex® (the trade name for bicalutamide, a nonsteroidal antiandrogenic antineoplastic agent) or Kadian® (a trade name for morphine

sulfate, an opiate agonist), dispensing errors have been reported. Therefore, in April 2010, the manufacturer of Kapidex® changed the trade name for dexlansoprazole from Kapidex® to Dexilant® to avoid future dispensing errors. The potential exists for serious adverse effects to occur if patients receive the incorrect drug. Bicalutamide may cause fetal harm if used during pregnancy, and use of this drug is contraindicated in women. Kadian® is an extended-release morphine sulfate preparation intended for use in managing moderate to severe pain when a continuous around-the-clock opiate analgesic is needed for an extended period of time; ingestion of 100- or 200-mg Kadian® capsules by patients who are not opiate tolerant can cause fatal respiratory depression. In addition, there is a potential for the trade name Kapidex® to be confused with Capadex® (a trade name for a fixed-combination preparation containing propoxyphene and acetaminophen that is available via the Internet and marketed in certain other countries [e.g., Australia]). Some experts recommend that pharmacists assess measures of avoiding dispensing errors and implement them as appropriate (e.g., by using computerized name alerts, matching the prescribed drug with the patient's medical history, verifying orders for these drugs) and that clinicians consider including the intended use of the drug on the prescription.

Specific Populations

Pregnancy

Category B. (See Users Guide.)

Lactation

It is unknown whether dexlansoprazole is distributed into milk. However, lansoprazole and its metabolites are distributed into milk in rats; the manufacturer states that a decision should be made whether to discontinue nursing or the drug, taking into account the importance of the drug to the woman.

Pediatric Use

Safety and efficacy have not been established in pediatric patients younger than 18 years of age.

Geriatric Use

No substantial differences in safety and efficacy relative to younger adults, but increased sensitivity of some older patients cannot be ruled out.

Hepatic Impairment

Systemic exposure to dexlansoprazole is increased approximately twofold in individuals with moderate hepatic impairment. The drug has not been studied in severe hepatic impairment. (See Dosage and Administration: Special Populations.)

Renal Impairment

Because dexlansoprazole is extensively metabolized in the liver to inactive metabolites, and unchanged drug is not recovered in urine following administration of an oral dose, renal impairment is not expected to affect the pharmacokinetics of the drug.

● Common Adverse Effects

Adverse effects reported in 2% or more of patients receiving dexlansoprazole and more frequently than with placebo include diarrhea, abdominal pain, nausea, upper respiratory infection, vomiting, and flatulence.

DRUG INTERACTIONS

● Drugs Affecting or Metabolized by Hepatic Microsomal Enzymes

Dexlansoprazole is metabolized by cytochrome P-450 (CYP) isoenzymes 2C19 and 3A4. In vitro studies indicate that dexlansoprazole is unlikely to inhibit CYP isoenzymes 1A1, 1A2, 2A6, 2B6, 2C8, 2C9, 2C19, 2D6, 2E1, or 3A4; therefore, interactions with drugs metabolized by these isoenzymes are considered unlikely. Dexlansoprazole did not alter the pharmacokinetics of diazepam (a CYP2C19 substrate) in healthy individuals (mainly extensive or intermediate metabolizers of CYP2C19 substrates), nor did dexlansoprazole alter the pharmacokinetics of phenytoin (a CYP2C9 substrate) or theophylline (a CYP1A2 substrate) in healthy individuals; CYP1A2 genotypes were not determined.

● Drugs that Cause Hypomagnesemia

Potential pharmacologic interaction (possible increased risk of hypomagnesemia). In patients receiving diuretics (i.e., loop or thiazide diuretics) or other drugs that may cause hypomagnesemia, monitoring of magnesium concentrations should be considered prior to initiation of prescription proton-pump inhibitor therapy and periodically thereafter. (See Hypomagnesemia under Warnings/Precautions: General Precautions, in Cautions.)

● Gastric pH-dependent Drugs

Pharmacokinetic interaction is possible when dexlansoprazole is used concomitantly with gastric pH-dependent drugs (e.g., ketoconazole, iron salts, digoxin, ampicillin esters); altered absorption at increased gastric pH values.

● Antiretroviral Agents

Atazanavir

Potential pharmacokinetic interaction with atazanavir (possible altered oral absorption of atazanavir at increased gastric pH, resulting in decreased plasma atazanavir concentrations). Concomitant use of omeprazole 40 mg once daily and atazanavir (with or without low-dose ritonavir) results in a substantial decrease in plasma concentrations of atazanavir and possible loss of the therapeutic effect of the antiretroviral agent. The manufacturer of dexlansoprazole states that concomitant administration with atazanavir is not recommended. If atazanavir is administered in a treatment-naive patient receiving a proton-pump inhibitor, a *ritonavir-boosted* regimen of 300 mg of atazanavir once daily with ritonavir 100 mg once daily with food is recommended. The dose of the proton-pump inhibitor should be administered approximately 12 hours before *ritonavir-boosted* atazanavir; the dose of the proton-pump inhibitor should not exceed omeprazole 20 mg daily (or equivalent). Concomitant use of proton-pump inhibitors with atazanavir is not recommended in treatment-experienced patients.

Fosamprenavir

Concomitant use of esomeprazole with fosamprenavir (with or without ritonavir) did not substantially affect concentrations of amprenavir (active metabolite of fosamprenavir). No dosage adjustment is required when proton-pump inhibitors are used concomitantly with fosamprenavir (with or without ritonavir).

Lopinavir

Concomitant use of omeprazole with the fixed combination of lopinavir and ritonavir (lopinavir/ritonavir) did not have a clinically important effect on plasma concentrations or area under the concentration-time curve (AUC) of lopinavir. No dosage adjustment is required when proton-pump inhibitors are used concomitantly with lopinavir/ritonavir.

Raltegravir

Pharmacokinetic interaction with omeprazole (substantially increased peak plasma concentration and AUC of raltegravir); however, no dosage adjustment is recommended when proton-pump inhibitors are used concomitantly with raltegravir.

Rilpivirine

Pharmacokinetic interaction with omeprazole (decreased plasma concentrations and AUC of rilpivirine). Concomitant use of other proton-pump inhibitors also may result in decreased plasma concentrations of rilpivirine. Concomitant use of rilpivirine and proton-pump inhibitors is contraindicated.

Saquinavir

Potential pharmacokinetic interaction (increased peak plasma concentration and AUC of saquinavir). Concomitant use of omeprazole 40 mg once daily and *ritonavir-boosted* saquinavir (saquinavir 1 g twice daily and ritonavir 100 mg twice daily) increased the peak plasma concentration and AUC of saquinavir by 75 and 82%, respectively. Caution is advised if proton-pump inhibitors are used concomitantly with *ritonavir-boosted* saquinavir, and patients should be monitored for saquinavir toxicity.

● Clopidogrel

Potential pharmacokinetic interaction (decreased plasma concentration of the active metabolite of clopidogrel) and pharmacodynamic interaction (reduced antiplatelet effects) between proton-pump inhibitors and clopidogrel. Clopidogrel is metabolized to its active metabolite by CYP2C19. Concurrent use of omeprazole or esomeprazole, which inhibit CYP2C19, with clopidogrel reduces exposure to the active metabolite of clopidogrel and decreases platelet inhibitory eff

ects. Although the clinical importance has not been fully elucidated, a reduction in the effectiveness of clopidogrel in preventing cardiovascular events is possible. Proton-pump inhibitors vary in their potency for inhibiting CYP2C19. The change in inhibition of adenosine diphosphate (ADP)-induced platelet aggregation associated with concomitant use of proton-pump inhibitors is related to the change in exposure to the active metabolite of clopidogrel. In pharmacokinetic and pharmacodynamic studies in healthy individuals, concomitant use of dexlansoprazole, lansoprazole, or pantoprazole had less effect on the antiplatelet activity of clopidogrel than did concomitant use of omeprazole or esomeprazole. In individuals who were extensive metabolizers of CYP2C19 substrates, use of dexlansoprazole (60 mg once daily) concomitantly with clopidogrel (75 mg once daily) for 9 days reduced exposure to the active metabolite of clopidogrel by about 9% compared with use of clopidogrel alone. The observed effects of dexlansoprazole on metabolite exposure and clopidogrel-induced platelet inhibition were not considered clinically important, and the manufacturer of dexlansoprazole states that no adjustment of clopidogrel dosage is necessary if clopidogrel is used concomitantly with recommended dosages of dexlansoprazole.

The decision to use a proton-pump inhibitor concomitantly with clopidogrel should be based on the assessed risks and benefits in individual patients. The American College of Cardiology Foundation/American College of Gastroenterology/American Heart Association (ACCF/ACG/AHA) states that the reduction in GI bleeding risk with proton-pump inhibitors is substantial in patients with risk factors for GI bleeding (e.g., advanced age; concomitant use of warfarin, corticosteroids, or nonsteroidal anti-inflammatory agents [NSAIAs]; H. pylori infection) and may outweigh any potential reduction in the cardiovascular efficacy of antiplatelet treatment associated with a drug-drug interaction. In contrast, ACCF/ACG/AHA states that patients without such risk factors receive little if any absolute risk reduction from proton-pump inhibitor therapy, and the risk/benefit balance may favor use of antiplatelet therapy without a proton-pump inhibitor in these patients.

If concomitant therapy with a proton-pump inhibitor and clopidogrel is considered necessary, use of an agent with little or no CYP2C19-inhibitory activity should be considered. Alternatively, treatment with a histamine H$_2$-receptor antagonist (ranitidine, famotidine, nizatidine) may be considered, although such agents may not be as effective as a proton-pump inhibitor in providing gastric protection; cimetidine should *not* be used since it also is a potent CYP2C19 inhibitor. There currently is no evidence that histamine H$_2$-receptor antagonists (other than cimetidine) or other drugs that reduce gastric acid (e.g., antacids) interfere with the antiplatelet effects of clopidogrel. For further information on interactions between proton-pump inhibitors and clopidogrel, see Drug Interactions: Proton-Pump Inhibitors, in Clopidogrel Bisulfate 20:12.18.

● Digoxin

Hypomagnesemia (e.g., resulting from long-term use of proton-pump inhibitors) sensitizes the myocardium to digoxin and, thus, may increase the risk of digoxin-induced cardiotoxic effects. In patients receiving digoxin, monitoring of magnesium concentrations should be considered prior to initiation of prescription proton-pump inhibitor therapy and periodically thereafter.

● Methotrexate

Potential pharmacokinetic interaction (increased serum methotrexate concentrations, possibly resulting in toxicity) when proton-pump inhibitors, including dexlansoprazole, are used concomitantly with methotrexate. Increased serum concentrations and delayed clearance of methotrexate and/or its metabolite hydroxymethotrexate, with or without symptoms of methotrexate toxicity, have been reported in patients receiving methotrexate (usually at doses of 300 mg/m^2 to 12 g/m^2) concomitantly with a proton-pump inhibitor. Although most of the reported cases occurred in patients receiving high doses of methotrexate, toxicity also has been reported in patients receiving low dosages of methotrexate (e.g., 15 mg per week) concomitantly with a proton-pump inhibitor. No formal studies of interactions between high-dose methotrexate and proton-pump inhibitors have been conducted to date.

The manufacturer of dexlansoprazole states that temporary discontinuance of proton-pump inhibitor therapy may be considered in some patients receiving high-dose methotrexate therapy. Some clinicians recommend either withholding proton-pump inhibitor therapy for several days before and after methotrexate administration or substituting a histamine H$_2$-receptor antagonist for the proton-pump inhibitor when acid suppressive therapy is indicated during methotrexate therapy. Pending further evaluation, some clinicians state that these recommendations should extend to patients receiving low-dose methotrexate.

● *Tacrolimus*

Potential pharmacokinetic interaction (increased whole blood concentrations of tacrolimus, particularly in transplant patients who are intermediate or poor metabolizers of CYP2C19 substrates).

● *Warfarin*

When warfarin 25 mg was administered orally on day 6 of an 11-day course of dexlansoprazole 90 mg once daily in healthy individuals, the pharmacokinetics of warfarin and the international normalized ratio (INR) were not altered; however, increased INR and prothrombin time have been reported in patients receiving warfarin concomitantly with proton-pump inhibitors. The INR and prothrombin time may need to be monitored when dexlansoprazole is used concomitantly with warfarin.

DESCRIPTION

Dexlansoprazole, a proton-pump inhibitor, is a gastric antisecretory agent that is structurally and pharmacologically related to esomeprazole, lansoprazole, omeprazole, pantoprazole, and rabeprazole. The drugs are substituted benzimidazoles and are chemically and pharmacologically unrelated to H_2-receptor antagonists or antimuscarinics. Dexlansoprazole is the *R*-isomer of lansoprazole, which is a racemic mixture of *R*- and *S*-isomers. Both isomers inhibit hydrogen-potassium ATPase, but plasma clearance of dexlansoprazole is slower than that of *S*-lansoprazole.

Dexlansoprazole binds to hydrogen-potassium ATPase in gastric parietal cells; inactivation of this enzyme system (also known as the proton, hydrogen, or acid pump) blocks the final step in the secretion of hydrochloric acid by these cells, resulting in potent, long-lasting inhibition of gastric acid secretion.

The commercially available delayed-release capsules of dexlansoprazole contain 2 types of enteric-coated granules of the drug that dissolve at different pH values. Following oral administration of this formulation, an initial (smaller) peak plasma concentration of the drug occurs at 1–2 hours followed by a second (larger) peak concentration at 4–5 hours. Following once-daily administration for 5 days, gastric pH exceeds 4 for 17 hours per day with dexlansoprazole 60 mg versus 14 hours per day with lansoprazole 30 mg. Dexlansoprazole is extensively metabolized in the liver by oxidation, reduction, and subsequent formation of inactive sulfate, glucuronide, and glutathione conjugates. Cytochrome P-450 (CYP) isoenzymes 2C19 and 3A4 are involved in the metabolism of dexlansoprazole. The drug is eliminated in urine (51%) and feces (48%); unchanged drug is not recovered in urine. Because the CYP2C19 isoenzyme is polymorphically expressed, systemic exposure to the drug generally is increased in individuals who are intermediate or poor metabolizers of CYP2C19 substrates. In one small study in Japanese men, systemic exposure (as measured by area under the serum concentration-time curve [AUC]) was increased twofold in intermediate metabolizers and up to 12-fold in poor metabolizers compared with extensive metabolizers.

Increased gastric pH during dexlansoprazole therapy stimulates gastrin secretion via a negative feedback mechanism. Enterochromaffin-like (ECL) cell hyperplasia has been reported during proton-pump inhibitor therapy. Gastric biopsy specimens obtained from 653 patients receiving dexlansoprazole 30–90 mg daily for up to one year revealed no instances of ECL cell hyperplasia.

Although rats have demonstrated carcinoid lesions, no adenomatoid, dysplastic, or neoplastic changes have occurred to date in patients receiving long-term proton-pump inhibitor therapy.

Therapy with proton-pump inhibitors, particularly in high dosages and/or for prolonged periods of time, may be associated with an increased risk of osteoporosis-related fractures of the hip, wrist, or spine. (See Cautions: Musculoskeletal Effects.) The mechanism by which these drugs may increase risk of such fractures has not been elucidated but may involve decreased insoluble calcium absorption secondary to increased gastric pH.

ADVICE TO PATIENTS

Necessity of swallowing dexlansoprazole capsules whole or, alternatively, of sprinkling the capsule contents on a tablespoonful of applesauce and swallowing immediately without chewing.

Dexlansoprazole may be administered without regard to food.

Importance of continuing therapy for the entire treatment course, unless directed otherwise.

Importance of advising patients that use of multiple daily doses of the drug for an extended period of time may increase the risk of fractures of the hip, wrist, or spine.

Risk of hypomagnesemia; importance of advising patients to immediately report and seek care for any cardiovascular or neurologic manifestations (e.g., palpitations, dizziness, seizures, tetany).

Possible increased risk of *Clostridium difficile* infection; importance of contacting a clinician if persistent watery stools, abdominal pain, and fever occur.

Importance of informing clinicians of existing or contemplated concomitant therapy, including prescription and OTC drugs and herbal supplements, as well as any concomitant illnesses.

Importance of informing clinicians of any symptoms suggestive of an allergic reaction (e.g., facial swelling, rash).

Importance of women informing clinicians if they are or plan to become pregnant or plan to breast-feed.

Importance of informing patients of other important precautionary information. (See Cautions.)

PREPARATIONS

Excipients in commercially available drug preparations may have clinically important effects in some individuals; consult specific product labeling for details.

Dexlansoprazole

Oral

Capsules, delayed-release (containing enteric-coated granules)	30 mg	**Dexilant®**, Takeda
	60 mg	**Dexilant®**, Takeda

† Use is not currently included in the labeling approved by the US Food and Drug Administration.

Esomeprazole Magnesium
Esomeprazole Sodium

56:28.36 • PROTON-PUMP INHIBITORS

■ Esomeprazole, commonly referred to as an acid- or proton-pump inhibitor, is a gastric antisecretory agent. Esomeprazole is the *S*-isomer of omeprazole.

USES

● Gastroesophageal Reflux

Esomeprazole magnesium is used for short-term (4–8 weeks) treatment of diagnostically confirmed erosive esophagitis in patients with gastroesophageal reflux disease (GERD). The drug also is used as maintenance therapy following healing of erosive esophagitis to reduce recurrence of the disease. In addition, esomeprazole is used for short-term (4–8 weeks) treatment of symptoms (e.g., heartburn) of GERD in patients without erosive esophagitis. In infants, esomeprazole is used for short-term (up to 6 weeks) treatment of erosive esophagitis due to acid-mediated GERD. Potential benefits of proton-pump inhibitors in gastroesophageal reflux and esophagitis are thought to result principally from reduced acidity of gastric contents induced by the drugs and resultant reduced irritation of esophageal mucosa; the drugs can effectively relieve symptoms of esophagitis (e.g., heartburn) and promote healing of ulcerative and erosive lesions. Because esomeprazole (*S*-omeprazole) is not eliminated as rapidly as *R*-omeprazole, more drug reaches and blocks the proton pump, providing greater control of intragastric pH than racemic omeprazole.

Suppression of gastric acid secretion is considered by the American College of Gastroenterology (ACG) to be the mainstay of treatment for GERD, and a proton-pump inhibitor or histamine H_2-receptor antagonist is used to achieve acid suppression, control symptoms, and prevent complications of the disease. Because GERD is considered to be a chronic disease, the ACG states that many patients with GERD will require long-term, even lifelong, treatment. The ACG states that proton-pump inhibitors are more effective (i.e., provide more frequent and more rapid symptomatic relief and healing of esophagitis) than histamine H_2-receptor antagonists for treatment of GERD, and are effective and appropriate as maintenance therapy in many patients with the disease. Proton-pump inhibitors also provide greater control of acid reflux than do prokinetic agents (e.g., cisapride [no longer commercially available in the US], metoclopramide) without the risk of severe adverse effects associated with these agents.

Efficacy of esomeprazole in the treatment of endoscopically diagnosed erosive esophagitis was established in 4 controlled studies in patients receiving esomeprazole 20 or 40 mg daily or omeprazole 20 mg daily for 8 weeks. Rates of healing and sustained resolution of heartburn achieved with esomeprazole were similar to or exceeded those achieved with omeprazole.

Efficacy in the long-term maintenance of healing was established in 2 controlled studies in patients with endoscopically confirmed healing of erosive esophagitis receiving esomeprazole 10, 20, or 40 mg daily or placebo for 6 months. Patients receiving esomeprazole remained in remission longer and experienced fewer recurrences than patients receiving placebo; although esomeprazole 10 mg daily provided less benefit than esomeprazole 20 or 40 mg daily, no additional benefit of the 40-mg daily dosage over the 20-mg daily dosage was reported.

Efficacy in patients with symptomatic GERD was established in 2 controlled studies in patients with a 6-month or longer history of heartburn episodes, no endoscopic evidence of erosive esophagitis, and heartburn for at least 4 of the 7 days immediately prior to randomization; patients received esomeprazole 20 or 40 mg daily or placebo for 4 weeks. The percentage of patients who were symptom-free was substantially higher in the group receiving esomeprazole than in the group receiving placebo; no additional benefit of the 40-mg dosage over the 20-mg dosage was reported.

In patients with erosive esophagitis who are unable to take esomeprazole orally, esomeprazole sodium may be used IV for short-term treatment of GERD. In several open-label crossover studies in patients with symptoms of GERD with or without erosive esophagitis, IV administration of esomeprazole 20 or 40 mg as either a 3-minute injection or a 15-minute infusion once daily for 10 days inhibited gastric acid secretion to a similar extent as the corresponding (20 or 40 mg) oral dosage of the drug.

For further information on the treatment of GERD, see Uses: Gastroesophageal Reflux, in Omeprazole 56:28.36.

● Duodenal Ulcer

Esomeprazole magnesium is used in combination with amoxicillin and clarithromycin (triple therapy) for short-term (10 days) treatment of patients with *H. pylori* infection and duodenal ulcer disease (active duodenal ulcer or a history of duodenal ulcer within the preceding 5 years).

Efficacy of esomeprazole-based triple therapy for *H. pylori* eradication was established in 2 controlled studies in patients with documented *H. pylori* infection and at least one endoscopically verified duodenal ulcer (or documented history of duodenal ulcer disease in the preceding 5 years). At 4 weeks after treatment, *H. pylori* eradication rates were substantially higher in patients receiving triple therapy (esomeprazole 40 mg once daily, amoxicillin 1 g twice daily, and clarithromycin 500 mg twice daily) for 10 days than in those receiving dual therapy (esomeprazole 40 mg daily and clarithromycin 500 mg twice daily) or monotherapy with esomeprazole 40 mg daily for 10 days.

● Prevention of Nonsteroidal Anti-inflammatory Agent-induced Ulcers

Esomeprazole magnesium is used for reducing the occurrence of gastric ulcers associated with chronic nonsteroidal anti-inflammatory agent (NSAIA) therapy in patients at risk for developing these ulcers, including individuals 60 years of age or older and/or those with a documented history of gastric ulcers. Efficacy for this indication was established in two 6-month randomized, controlled studies in patients receiving chronic therapy with either a prototypical NSAIA or a selective cyclooxygenase-2 (COX-2) inhibitor; individuals enrolled in these studies were considered to be at risk for developing NSAIA-associated ulcers because of their age (60 years or older) and/or a history of documented gastric or duodenal ulcer within the previous 5 years, but they had no evidence of gastric or duodenal ulcers on endoscopic examination at the start of the studies. Results of the studies indicated that esomeprazole 20 or 40 mg daily was more effective than placebo in preventing gastric ulcer occurrence during 6 months of treatment; however, no additional benefit was observed with the 40-mg daily dosage compared with the 20-mg daily dosage. In these studies, 94.7–95.4% of patients receiving esomeprazole 20 mg daily, 95.3–96.7% of those receiving esomeprazole 40 mg daily, and 83.3–88.2% of those receiving placebo remained free of gastric ulcers, as determined by serial endoscopic examinations, throughout the 6-month study. The occurrence rate of duodenal ulcers was too low to determine the effect of esomeprazole therapy on duodenal ulcer occurrence.

In 2 other randomized studies, combined therapy with esomeprazole and naproxen was associated with a lower cumulative incidence of gastric ulcer compared with naproxen therapy alone over 6 months of treatment (4.1–7.1 versus 23.1–24.3%). Patients in these studies were randomized to receive either esomeprazole in fixed combination with naproxen (as immediate-release esomeprazole 20 mg and delayed-release naproxen 500 mg twice daily) or delayed-release naproxen (500 mg twice daily) alone. In both studies, patients receiving combined therapy with esomeprazole and naproxen were less likely than patients receiving naproxen alone to discontinue therapy because of adverse upper GI effects, including duodenal ulcers (4 versus 12%). Most patients (83%) in these studies were 50–69 years of age; those younger than 50 years of age were required to have a history of documented gastric or duodenal ulcer within the previous 5 years. About one-fourth of patients also received low-dose aspirin. Efficacy in patients receiving concomitant aspirin therapy was similar to that in the overall study population.

● Pathologic GI Hypersecretory Conditions

Esomeprazole magnesium is used for the long-term treatment of pathologic GI hypersecretory conditions. Efficacy for this indication was established in an open-label study in a limited number of patients with previously diagnosed pathologic GI hypersecretory conditions (e.g., Zollinger-Ellison syndrome, idiopathic gastric acid hypersecretion); patients received total daily dosages of esomeprazole ranging from 80 mg–240 mg. The drug generally was well tolerated at these dosages for the duration of the study (12 months). At 12 months of therapy, 90% of patients treated with esomeprazole had controlled basal acid output (BAO) levels, defined as BAO of less than 5 or 10 mEq/hour in patients who had or had not previously undergone gastric acid-reducing surgery, respectively.

● Crohn's Disease-associated Ulcers

Although evidence currently is limited, proton-pump inhibitors have been used for gastric acid-suppressive therapy as an adjunct in the symptomatic treatment of upper GI Crohn's disease†, including esophageal, gastroduodenal, and jejunoileal disease. Most evidence of efficacy to date has been from case studies in patients with Crohn's-associated peptic ulcer disease unresponsive to other therapies (e.g., H₂-receptor antagonists, cytoprotective agents, antacids, and/or sucralfate). (See Uses: Crohn's Disease-associated Ulcers in Omeprazole 56:28.36.)

For further information on the management of Crohn's disease, see Uses: Crohn's Disease, in Mesalamine 56:36.

DOSAGE AND ADMINISTRATION

• Administration

Oral Administration

Esomeprazole magnesium is administered orally once or twice daily. Because the area under the plasma concentration-time curve (AUC) of a single 40-mg dose of esomeprazole administered after the intake of food is decreased by 43–53%, the manufacturer states that esomeprazole magnesium delayed-release capsules and delayed-release oral suspension should be taken at least 1 hour before a meal. The manufacturer states that tablets containing immediate-release esomeprazole magnesium in fixed combination with delayed-release naproxen should taken at least 30 minutes before a meal.

Esomeprazole Oral Capsules

Esomeprazole magnesium delayed-release capsules should be swallowed whole and the contents should not be crushed or chewed. Alternatively, for patients with difficulty swallowing, the contents of a capsule may be mixed with a tablespoon of applesauce and swallowed immediately. The applesauce should not be hot and should be soft enough to be swallowed without chewing. The applesauce and esomeprazole enteric-coated granule mixture should *not* be stored for future use.

For patients with a nasogastric tube, the contents of a capsule can be mixed with 50 mL of water in a 60-mL catheter-tipped syringe. The syringe should be shaken vigorously for 15 seconds and then held with the tip pointed up and inspected for dissolved or disintegrated granules and granules remaining in the tip. The mixture should not be used if dissolved or disintegrated granules are observed. The mixture should be administered immediately and the tube should be flushed with additional water.

Esomeprazole Oral Suspension

For reconstitution of esomeprazole magnesium for delayed-release oral suspension in single-dose packets, the contents of a 2.5- or 5-mg packet should be mixed thoroughly with 5 mL of water and the contents of a 10-, 20-, or 40-mg packet should be mixed thoroughly with 15 mL of water; the mixture should be allowed to thicken for 2–3 minutes. If a single dose requires 2 packets, the oral suspension may be reconstituted with twice the amount of water needed for 1 packet. Within 30 minutes of preparation, the mixture should be stirred and consumed. If any material remains after the mixture is ingested, additional water should be added, mixed, and ingested immediately.

For patients with a nasogastric or gastric tube, the contents of a 2.5- or 5-mg packet should be mixed with 5 mL of water and the contents of a 10-, 20-, or 40-mg packet should be mixed with 15 mL of water in a catheter-tipped syringe and then shaken immediately. The mixture should be allowed to thicken for 2–3 minutes. The mixture should be administered within 30 minutes of reconstitution; prior to administration, the syringe should be shaken again and the mixture injected into the stomach through the nasogastric or gastric tube (French size 6 or larger). The syringe should be refilled with additional water (5 or 15 mL, respectively), shaken, and used to flush any remaining drug mixture from the nasogastric or gastric tube into the stomach.

Esomeprazole and Naproxen Fixed-combination Tablets

Tablets containing immediate-release esomeprazole magnesium in fixed combination with delayed-release naproxen should be swallowed whole with liquid, and should not be split, chewed, crushed, or dissolved.

IV Administration

Esomeprazole sodium is administered by IV injection over no less than 3 minutes or by IV infusion over 10–30 minutes.

For direct IV injection of a 20- or 40-mg dose in adults, esomeprazole sodium powder for injection is reconstituted by adding 5 mL of 0.9% sodium chloride injection to a vial labeled as containing 20 or 40 mg of esomeprazole. A volume of 5 mL

of reconstituted solution (20 or 40 mg, respectively) should be withdrawn from the vial and injected over a period of no less than 3 minutes. Reconstituted solutions should be stored at room temperature (up to 30°C) and used within 12 hours of reconstitution. Each vial of esomeprazole sodium is intended for single use only.

For IV infusion of a 20- or 40-mg dose in adults, esomeprazole sodium powder for injection is reconstituted by adding 5 mL of 0.9% sodium chloride injection, lactated Ringer's injection, or 5% dextrose injection to a vial labeled as containing 20 or 40 mg of esomeprazole. The reconstituted solution should be further diluted with 0.9% sodium chloride injection, lactated Ringer's injection, or 5% dextrose injection to a final volume of 50 mL prior to IV infusion over 10–30 minutes. Esomeprazole sodium infusion solutions prepared using 0.9% sodium chloride injection or lactated Ringer's injection should be stored at room temperature (up to 30°C) and used within 12 hours of preparation; infusion solutions prepared using 5% dextrose injection should be stored at room temperature (up to 30°C) and used within 6 hours.

For IV infusion in pediatric patients 1 month to 17 years of age, esomeprazole sodium powder for injection is reconstituted by adding 5 mL of 0.9% sodium chloride injection to a vial labeled as containing 20 or 40 mg of esomeprazole to provide a solution containing 4 or 8 mg/mL, respectively. The reconstituted 4- or 8-mg/mL solution should be further diluted with 0.9% sodium chloride injection to a final volume of 50 mL to yield a final concentration of 0.4 or 0.8 mg/mL, respectively. The appropriate dose of esomeprazole should be withdrawn from the diluted solution and administered as an IV infusion over 10–30 minutes.

Parenteral esomeprazole sodium solutions should be inspected visually for particulate matter and discoloration prior to administration whenever solution and container permit.

The manufacturer states that esomeprazole sodium should not be administered simultaneously through the same IV line with other drugs. The IV line should be flushed with 0.9% sodium chloride injection, lactated Ringer's injection, or 5% dextrose injection before and after esomeprazole administration.

• Dosage

Dosage of esomeprazole magnesium or esomeprazole sodium is expressed in terms of esomeprazole.

Duration of therapy with a proton-pump inhibitor should be based on safety and efficacy data associated with a specific indication, dosing frequency as described by the manufacturer, and the needs of individual patients. The potential benefits versus possible risks of initiating or continuing proton-pump inhibitor therapy should be weighed carefully.

Adult Dosage

Gastroesophageal Reflux

The recommended oral dosage of esomeprazole for short-term treatment of erosive esophagitis in adults with GERD is 20 or 40 mg once daily for 4–8 weeks; an additional 4- to 8-week course of treatment may be considered if esophageal healing is incomplete after the first course of treatment. For maintenance therapy following healing of erosive esophagitis, the recommended adult oral dosage of esomeprazole is 20 mg once daily; the manufacturer states that controlled studies of esomeprazole maintenance therapy beyond 6 months have not been performed. The recommended oral dosage for the short-term treatment of symptomatic GERD in adults without erosive esophagitis is 20 mg once daily for 4 weeks; the manufacturer states that an additional 4-week course of therapy may be considered in patients whose symptoms have not completely resolved after the first course of treatment. However, the American College of Gastroenterology (ACG) states that chronic, even lifelong, therapy with a proton-pump inhibitor is appropriate in many patients with GERD.

In adults with erosive esophagitis who are unable to take esomeprazole orally, the usual dosage of IV esomeprazole for treatment of GERD is 20 or 40 mg administered by IV injection (over no less than 3 minutes) or by IV infusion (over 10–30 minutes) once daily; safety and efficacy of IV use beyond 10 days have not been established. Treatment with IV esomeprazole should be discontinued as soon as the patient is able to take the drug orally.

Duodenal Ulcer

When esomeprazole is used in combination with amoxicillin and clarithromycin (triple therapy) for eradication of *H. pylori* infection in patients with duodenal ulcer disease (active duodenal ulcer or a history of duodenal ulcer in the preceding 5 years), the recommended adult oral dosage is 40 mg once daily for 10 days.

Prevention of Nonsteroidal Anti-inflammatory Agent-induced Ulcers

For reducing the risk of nonsteroidal anti-inflammatory agent (NSAIA)-induced gastric ulcer, the usual adult oral dosage of esomeprazole is 20 or 40 mg once daily for up to 6 months; the manufacturer states that controlled studies of esomeprazole therapy in patients considered to be at risk for NSAIA-induced gastric ulcers did not extend beyond 6 months. When esomeprazole is administered in fixed combination with naproxen, the recommended adult dosage of esomeprazole is 20 mg (with naproxen 375 or 500 mg) twice daily. The fixed-combination preparation should not be used in patients requiring a total daily esomeprazole dosage of less than 40 mg.

Pathologic GI Hypersecretory Conditions

The recommended adult oral dosage of esomeprazole for the treatment of pathologic GI hypersecretory conditions (e.g., Zollinger-Ellison syndrome) is 40 mg twice daily. The manufacturer states that the dosage should be adjusted to individual patient needs; dosages up to 240 mg daily for up to 12 months have been administered.

Pediatric Dosage

Oral dosage of esomeprazole for short-term (up to 6 weeks) treatment of erosive esophagitis due to acid-mediated GERD in infants 1 month to less than 1 year of age is based on weight. Infants weighing 3–5 kg may receive an oral esomeprazole dosage of 2.5 mg once daily, those weighing more than 5 kg but not more than 7.5 kg may receive 5 mg once daily, and those weighing more than 7.5 kg but not more than 12 kg may receive 10 mg once daily. The manufacturer states that dosages exceeding 1.33 mg/kg daily have not been studied in infants 1 month to less than 1 year of age.

The recommended oral dosage for the short-term treatment of symptomatic GERD in children 1–11 years of age without erosive esophagitis is 10 mg once daily for up to 8 weeks. The recommended oral dosage of esomeprazole for the short-term treatment of erosive esophagitis in children 1–11 years of age weighing less than 20 kg is 10 mg once daily for 8 weeks; 10 or 20 mg once daily for 8 weeks is recommended in children 1–11 years of age weighing 20 kg or more. The manufacturer states that dosages exceeding 1 mg/kg daily have not been studied in children 1–11 years of age.

The recommended oral dosage of esomeprazole for the short-term treatment of GERD in adolescents 12–17 years of age is 20 or 40 mg once daily for up to 8 weeks.

Pediatric patients who are unable to take esomeprazole orally for the treatment of GERD with erosive esophagitis may receive the drug IV. Infants 1 month to less than 1 year of age may receive an IV esomeprazole dosage of 0.5 mg/kg once daily; children and adolescents 1–17 years of age may receive an IV dosage of 10 mg once daily if they weigh less than 55 kg or 20 mg once daily in they weigh 55 kg or more. Esomeprazole should be administered by IV infusion (over 10–30 minutes) in infants, children, and adolescents. Treatment with IV esomeprazole should be discontinued as soon as the patient is able to take the drug orally.

● Special Populations

The oral or IV dosage of esomeprazole in patients with severe hepatic impairment (Child-Pugh class C) should *not* exceed 20 mg daily because AUCs of esomeprazole in such patients are 2–3 times greater than those in patients with normal hepatic function. Dosage adjustment is not necessary in patients with mild to moderate (Child-Pugh class A or B) hepatic impairment, patients with renal impairment, or geriatric patients. However, the commercially available tablets containing esomeprazole magnesium in fixed combination with naproxen are not recommended for use in patients with severe hepatic impairment or moderate to severe renal impairment (creatinine clearance less than 30 mL/minute).

CAUTIONS

● Contraindications

Known hypersensitivity to esomeprazole or other substituted benzimidazoles (e.g., lansoprazole, omeprazole, pantoprazole, rabeprazole) or any ingredient in the formulation.

● Warnings/Precautions

Sensitivity Reactions

Hypersensitivity Reactions

Hypersensitivity reactions (e.g., angioedema, anaphylactic shock) have been reported with esomeprazole.

Gastric Malignancy

Symptomatic response to therapy with esomeprazole does not preclude the presence of gastric malignancy.

Atrophic Gastritis

Atrophic gastritis has been noted occasionally in patients receiving long-term treatment with omeprazole.

Clostridium difficile Infection

Available data suggest a possible association between use of proton-pump inhibitors and risk of *Clostridium difficile* infection, including *C. difficile*-associated diarrhea and colitis (CDAD; also known as antibiotic-associated diarrhea and colitis or pseudomembranous colitis). In most observational studies to date, the risk of *C. difficile* infection in patients exposed to proton-pump inhibitors has ranged from 1.4–2.75 times that in patients not exposed to proton-pump inhibitors; however, some observational studies have found no increase in risk. Although many of the cases occurred in patients who had other risk factors for CDAD, including advanced age, comorbid conditions, and/or use of broad-spectrum anti-infectives, the US Food and Drug Administration (FDA) concluded that a contributory role for proton-pump inhibitors could not be definitively ruled out. The mechanism by which proton-pump inhibitors might increase the risk of CDAD has not been elucidated. Although it has been suggested that reduction of gastric acidity by gastric antisecretory agents might facilitate colonization with *C. difficile*, some studies have raised questions about this proposed mechanism or have suggested that the observed association is the result of confounding with other risk factors for CDAD. FDA also is reviewing the risk of CDAD in patients exposed to histamine H₂-receptor antagonists.

CDAD can be serious in patients who have one or more risk factors for *C. difficile* infection and are receiving concomitant therapy with a proton-pump inhibitor; colectomy and, rarely, death have been reported. FDA recommends that patients receive proton-pump inhibitors at the lowest effective dosage and for the shortest possible time appropriate for their clinical condition. Patients experiencing persistent diarrhea should be evaluated for CDAD and should be managed with appropriate supportive therapy (e.g., fluid and electrolyte management), anti-infective therapy directed against *C. difficile* (e.g., metronidazole, vancomycin), and surgical evaluation as clinically indicated.

Musculoskeletal Effects

Findings from several observational studies suggest that therapy with proton-pump inhibitors, particularly in high dosages (i.e., multiple daily doses) and/or for prolonged periods of time (i.e., one year or longer), may be associated with an increased risk of osteoporosis-related fractures of the hip, wrist, or spine. The magnitude of risk is unclear; causality has not been established. (See Cautions: Musculoskeletal Effects, in Omeprazole 56:28.36.) FDA is continuing to evaluate this safety concern. Although controlled studies are required to confirm these findings, patients should receive proton-pump inhibitors at the lowest effective dosage and for the shortest possible time appropriate for their clinical condition. Individuals who are at risk for osteoporosis-related fractures should receive an adequate intake of calcium and vitamin D and should have their bone health assessed and managed according to current standards of care.

Hypomagnesemia

Hypomagnesemia, symptomatic and asymptomatic, has been reported rarely in patients receiving long-term therapy (for at least 3 months or, in most cases, for longer than one year) with proton-pump inhibitors, including esomeprazole. Clinically serious adverse effects associated with hypomagnesemia, which are similar to manifestations of hypocalcemia, include tetany, seizures, tremors, carpopedal spasm, arrhythmias (e.g., atrial fibrillation, supraventricular tachycardia), and abnormal QT interval. Other reported adverse effects include paresthesia, muscle weakness, muscle cramps, lethargy, fatigue, and unsteadiness. In most patients, treatment of hypomagnesemia required magnesium replacement and discontinuance of the proton-pump inhibitor. Following discontinuance of the proton-pump inhibitor, hypomagnesemia resolved within a median of one week; upon rechallenge, hypomagnesemia recurred within a median of 2 weeks.

In patients expected to receive long-term therapy with a proton-pump inhibitor or in those receiving a proton-pump inhibitor concomitantly with digoxin or drugs that may cause hypomagnesemia (e.g., diuretics), clinicians should consider measurement of serum magnesium concentrations prior to initiation of prescription proton-pump inhibitor therapy and periodically thereafter. (See Cautions: Hypomagnesemia and also Cautions: Precautions and Contraindications, in Omeprazole 56:28.36.)

Interactions with Diagnostic Tests for Neuroendocrine Tumors

Increases in intragastric pH may result in hypergastrinemia, enterochromaffin-like cell hyperplasia, and increased serum chromogranin A (CgA) concentrations. Increased CgA concentrations may produce false-positive results for diagnostic tests for neuroendocrine tumors. Clinicians should temporarily discontinue esomeprazole therapy before assessing CgA concentrations and consider repeating the test if initial CgA concentrations are high.

Cardiac Effects

Although preliminary safety data from 2 long-term clinical trials comparing esomeprazole or omeprazole with antireflux surgery in patients with severe gastroesophageal reflux disease (GERD) raised concerns about a potential increased risk of cardiac events (myocardial infarction, heart failure, and sudden death) in patients receiving these drugs, the US Food and Drug Administration (FDA) has reviewed safety data from these and other studies of the drugs and has concluded that long-term use of esomeprazole or omeprazole is not likely to be associated with an increased risk of such cardiac events. FDA has concluded that the apparent increase in cardiac events observed in the early analyses is not a true effect of the drugs and recommends that clinicians continue to prescribe and patients continue to use these drugs in the manner described in the manufacturers' labelings. (See Cautions: Cardiovascular Effects, in Omeprazole 56:28.36.)

Respiratory Effects

Administration of proton-pump inhibitors has been associated with an increased risk for developing certain infections (e.g., community-acquired pneumonia). (For further precautionary information about this adverse effect, see Community-acquired Pneumonia under Cautions: Respiratory Effects, in Omeprazole 56:28.36.)

Use of Fixed Combinations

When esomeprazole is used in fixed combination with naproxen, the usual cautions, precautions, and contraindications associated with naproxen must be considered in addition to those associated with esomeprazole.

Specific Populations

Pregnancy

Category B. (See Users Guide.)

Lactation

It is unknown whether esomeprazole is distributed into milk. However, omeprazole is distributed into human milk; discontinue nursing or drug because of potential risk in nursing infants.

Pediatric Use

Safety and efficacy of oral esomeprazole for short-term (4–8 weeks) treatment of GERD in pediatric patients 1–17 years of age are supported by evidence from controlled clinical trials in adults and by safety and pharmacokinetic studies in children and adolescents. Safety and tolerability of oral esomeprazole 5, 10, or 20 mg daily for up to 8 weeks were evaluated in children 1–11 years of age with endoscopically diagnosed GERD; the presence or absence of erosive esophagitis was confirmed endoscopically in this study. Safety and tolerability of oral esomeprazole 20 or 40 mg daily for up to 8 weeks were evaluated in adolescents 12–17 years of age with clinically diagnosed GERD; the presence or absence of erosive esophagitis was not confirmed endoscopically in this study. Adverse effects reported in children and adolescents were similar to those reported during clinical trials in adults; however, a higher incidence of somnolence was reported in children.

Safety and efficacy of oral esomeprazole for short-term (up to 6 weeks) treatment of erosive esophagitis due to acid-mediated GERD in infants 1 month to less than 1 year of age are supported by controlled clinical trials in adults and by safety, pharmacokinetic, and pharmacodynamic studies in pediatric patients. The most commonly reported adverse effects in infants 1–11 months of age receiving oral esomeprazole include irritability and vomiting.

Safety and efficacy of oral esomeprazole for other uses in pediatric patients have not been established. In a randomized, controlled, treatment-withdrawal study in infants 1–11 months of age with symptomatic GERD (diagnosed clinically

in most patients), the proportion of patients discontinuing treatment because of worsening symptoms was similar in the esomeprazole and placebo groups.

Safety and efficacy of IV esomeprazole for short-term treatment of GERD with erosive esophagitis in pediatric patients 1 month to 17 years of age are supported by pharmacokinetic studies of IV esomeprazole in pediatric patients and adults and by pharmacodynamic studies of oral esomeprazole in pediatric patients and of IV esomeprazole in adults. Adverse effects of IV esomeprazole in pediatric patients 1 month to 17 years of age were consistent with the known safety profile of the drug.

Safety and efficacy of IV esomeprazole in neonates younger than 1 month of age have not been established.

Geriatric Use

No substantial differences in safety and efficacy relative to younger adults, but increased sensitivity of some older patients cannot be ruled out.

Severe Hepatic Impairment

Use with caution. (See Dosage and Administration: Special Populations.)

● Common Adverse Effects

Adverse effects occurring in 1% or more of patients receiving oral esomeprazole include headache, diarrhea, nausea, flatulence, abdominal pain, constipation, and dry mouth. Common adverse effects of IV esomeprazole generally are similar to those reported with oral esomeprazole, although injection site reaction, dizziness/vertigo, and pruritus also occur commonly with IV administration.

DRUG INTERACTIONS

● Drugs Affecting or Metabolized by Hepatic Microsomal Enzymes

Esomeprazole is extensively metabolized by the cytochrome P-450 (CYP) 2C19 isoenzyme and to a lesser extent by CYP3A4. Esomeprazole also may interfere with CYP2C19 activity.

Potential pharmacokinetic interaction with drugs metabolized by CYP2C19 (esomeprazole-induced inhibition of metabolism). Concomitant administration of esomeprazole and diazepam (a CYP2C19 substrate) decreased diazepam clearance by 45%.

Concomitant use of esomeprazole and cilostazol, a substrate of CYP3A4 and CYP2C19, is expected to result in increased concentrations of cilostazol and its active metabolite; therefore, reduction of cilostazol dosage (from 100 mg twice daily to 50 mg twice daily) should be considered during such concomitant use.

Pharmacokinetic interaction with drugs metabolized by CYP isoenzymes 3A4, 1A2, 2A6, 2C9, 2D6, or 2E1 is considered unlikely.

Potential pharmacokinetic interaction (esomeprazole exposure may increase more than twofold) with combined inhibitors of CYP2C19 and CYP3A4 (e.g., voriconazole); dosage adjustment of esomeprazole usually is not required but may be considered in patients receiving high dosages (up to 240 mg daily), such as those with Zollinger-Ellison syndrome.

Potential pharmacokinetic interaction (decreased esomeprazole concentrations) with drugs that induce CYP2C19 and/or CYP3A4 (e.g., St. John's wort [Hypericum perforatum], rifampin). Concomitant use of omeprazole, of which esomeprazole is an enantiomer, and St. John's wort (300 mg 3 times daily for 14 days) in healthy men resulted in decreased systemic exposure to omeprazole; peak plasma concentrations and area under the plasma concentration-time curve (AUC) of omeprazole were decreased by 37.5 and 37.9%, respectively, in poor CYP2C19 metabolizers and by 49.6 and 43.9%, respectively, in extensive metabolizers. Concomitant use of esomeprazole with St. John's wort or rifampin should be avoided.

● Drugs that Cause Hypomagnesemia

Potential pharmacologic interaction (possible increased risk of hypomagnesemia). In patients receiving diuretics (i.e., loop or thiazide diuretics) or other drugs that may cause hypomagnesemia, monitoring of magnesium concentrations should be considered prior to initiation of prescription proton-pump inhibitor therapy and periodically thereafter. (See Hypomagnesemia under Cautions: Warnings/Precautions.)

● Gastric pH-dependent Drugs

Potential pharmacokinetic interaction (altered absorption at increased gastric pH) with gastric pH-dependent drugs (e.g., ketoconazole, iron salts, digoxin, atazanavir, erlotinib).

Concomitant use of omeprazole 20 mg once daily and digoxin in healthy individuals increased digoxin bioavailability by 10% (up to 30% in some individuals). Because esomeprazole is an enantiomer of omeprazole, concomitant use of esomeprazole with digoxin is expected to increase systemic exposure to digoxin; therefore, monitoring for manifestations of digoxin toxicity may be required during such concomitant use.

Absorption of ketoconazole, iron salts, atazanavir, or erlotinib may be decreased in patients receiving esomeprazole concomitantly.

• *Antiretroviral Agents*

Atazanavir

Potential pharmacokinetic interaction (possible altered oral absorption of atazanavir at increased gastric pH, resulting in decreased plasma atazanavir concentrations). Concomitant use of omeprazole 40 mg once daily and atazanavir (with or without low-dose ritonavir) results in a substantial decrease in plasma concentrations of atazanavir and possible loss of the therapeutic effect of the antiretroviral agent or development of drug resistance. Concomitant use of omeprazole 40 mg once daily (administered 2 hours before atazanavir) and atazanavir 400 mg once daily decreased the AUC and peak plasma concentration of atazanavir by 94 and 96%, respectively. The manufacturer of esomeprazole states that concomitant administration with atazanavir is not recommended. If atazanavir is administered in an antiretroviral treatment-naive patient receiving a proton-pump inhibitor, a *ritonavir-boosted* regimen of 300 mg of atazanavir once daily with ritonavir 100 mg once daily with food is recommended. The dose of the proton-pump inhibitor should be administered approximately 12 hours before *ritonavir-boosted* atazanavir; the dose of the proton-pump inhibitor should not exceed omeprazole 20 mg daily (or equivalent). Concomitant use of proton-pump inhibitors with atazanavir is not recommended in antiretroviral treatment-experienced patients.

Fosamprenavir

Concomitant use of esomeprazole and fosamprenavir increased the AUC of esomeprazole by about 55% but did not substantially alter plasma concentrations of amprenavir (active metabolite of fosamprenavir). Concomitant use of esomeprazole and *ritonavir-boosted* fosamprenavir did not substantially affect concentrations of either amprenavir or esomeprazole. No dosage adjustment is required when proton-pump inhibitors are used concomitantly with fosamprenavir (with or without ritonavir).

Lopinavir

Concomitant use of omeprazole with the fixed combination of lopinavir and ritonavir (lopinavir/ritonavir) did not have a clinically important effect on plasma concentrations or AUC of lopinavir. No dosage adjustment is required when proton-pump inhibitors are used concomitantly with lopinavir/ritonavir.

Nelfinavir

Potential pharmacokinetic interaction (decreased plasma nelfinavir concentrations). Concomitant use of omeprazole 40 mg once daily (given 30 minutes before a nelfinavir dose) and nelfinavir 1.25 g twice daily decreased peak plasma concentrations and AUCs of nelfinavir by 37 and 36%, respectively, and of its major active metabolite M8 by 89 and 92%, respectively. The manufacturer of esomeprazole states that concomitant administration with nelfinavir is not recommended.

Raltegravir

Pharmacokinetic interaction with omeprazole (substantially increased peak plasma concentration and AUC of raltegravir); however, no dosage adjustment is recommended when proton-pump inhibitors are used concomitantly with raltegravir.

Rilpivirine

Pharmacokinetic interaction with omeprazole (decreased plasma concentrations and AUC of rilpivirine). Concomitant use of other proton-pump inhibitors also may result in decreased plasma concentration of rilpivirine. Concomitant use of rilpivirine and proton-pump inhibitors is contraindicated.

Saquinavir

Potential pharmacokinetic interaction (increased peak plasma concentration and AUC of saquinavir). Concomitant use of omeprazole 40 mg once daily and *ritonavir-boosted* saquinavir (saquinavir 1 g twice daily and ritonavir 100 mg twice daily) increased the peak plasma concentration and AUC of saquinavir by 75 and 82%, respectively. Caution is advised if proton-pump inhibitors are used concomitantly with *ritonavir-boosted* saquinavir, and patients should be monitored for saquinavir toxicity. The manufacturer of esomeprazole states that dosage reduction of saquinavir may be considered on an individual basis.

• *Clopidogrel*

Potential pharmacokinetic interaction (decreased plasma concentration of the active metabolite of clopidogrel) and pharmacodynamic interaction (reduced antiplatelet effects) between proton-pump inhibitors and clopidogrel. Clopidogrel is metabolized to its active metabolite by CYP2C19. Concurrent use of omeprazole or esomeprazole, which inhibit CYP2C19, with clopidogrel reduces exposure to the active metabolite of clopidogrel and decreases platelet inhibitory effects. Although the clinical importance has not been fully elucidated, a reduction in the effectiveness of clopidogrel in preventing cardiovascular events is possible. Proton-pump inhibitors vary in their potency for inhibiting CYP2C19. The change in inhibition of adenosine diphosphate (ADP)-induced platelet aggregation associated with concomitant use of proton-pump inhibitors is related to the change in exposure to the active metabolite of clopidogrel. In pharmacokinetic and pharmacodynamic studies in healthy individuals, concomitant use of dexlansoprazole, lansoprazole, or pantoprazole had less effect on the antiplatelet activity of clopidogrel than did concomitant use of omeprazole or esomeprazole. In individuals who were extensive metabolizers of CYP2C19 substrates, use of esomeprazole (40 mg once daily) concomitantly with clopidogrel (75 mg once daily) for 9 days reduced exposure to the active metabolite of clopidogrel by about 16% compared with use of clopidogrel alone. The manufacturer of clopidogrel states that concomitant use of esomeprazole and clopidogrel should be avoided.

The decision to use a proton-pump inhibitor concomitantly with clopidogrel should be based on the assessed risks and benefits in individual patients. The American College of Cardiology Foundation/American College of Gastroenterology/American Heart Association (ACCF/ACG/AHA) states that the reduction in GI bleeding risk with proton-pump inhibitors is substantial in patients with risk factors for GI bleeding (e.g., advanced age; concomitant use of warfarin, corticosteroids, or nonsteroidal anti-inflammatory agents [NSAIAs]; *H. pylori* infection) and may outweigh any potential reduction in the cardiovascular efficacy of antiplatelet treatment associated with a drug-drug interaction. In contrast, ACCF/ACG/AHA states that patients without such risk factors receive little if any absolute risk reduction from proton-pump inhibitor therapy, and the risk/benefit balance may favor use of antiplatelet therapy without a proton-pump inhibitor in these patients.

If concomitant therapy with a proton-pump inhibitor and clopidogrel is considered necessary, use of an agent with little or no CYP2C19-inhibitory activity should be considered. Alternatively, treatment with a histamine H_2-receptor antagonist (ranitidine, famotidine, nizatidine) may be considered, although such agents may not be as effective as a proton-pump inhibitor in providing gastric protection; cimetidine should *not* be used since it also is a potent CYP2C19 inhibitor. There currently is no evidence that histamine H_2-receptor antagonists (other than cimetidine) or other drugs that reduce gastric acid (e.g., antacids) interfere with the antiplatelet effects of clopidogrel. For further information on interactions between proton-pump inhibitors and clopidogrel, see Drug Interactions: Proton-Pump Inhibitors, in Clopidogrel Bisulfate 20:12.18.

• *Digoxin*

Hypomagnesemia (e.g., resulting from long-term use of proton-pump inhibitors) sensitizes the myocardium to digoxin and, thus, may increase the risk of digoxin-induced cardiotoxic effects. In patients receiving digoxin, monitoring of magnesium concentrations should be considered prior to initiation of prescription proton-pump inhibitor therapy and periodically thereafter.

• *Methotrexate*

Potential pharmacokinetic interaction (increased serum methotrexate concentrations, possibly resulting in toxicity) when proton-pump inhibitors, including esomeprazole, are used concomitantly with methotrexate. Increased serum concentrations and delayed clearance of methotrexate and/or its metabolite hydroxymethotrexate, with or without symptoms of methotrexate toxicity, have been reported in patients receiving methotrexate (usually at doses of 300 mg/m^2 to 12 g/m^2) concomitantly with a proton-pump inhibitor. Although most of the reported cases occurred in patients receiving high doses of methotrexate, toxicity also has been reported in patients receiving low dosages of methotrexate (e.g., 15 mg per week) concomitantly with a proton-pump inhibitor. No formal studies of interactions between high-dose methotrexate and proton-pump inhibitors have been conducted to date.

The manufacturer of esomeprazole states that temporary discontinuance of proton-pump inhibitor therapy may be considered in some patients receiving high-dose methotrexate therapy. Some clinicians recommend either withholding proton-pump inhibitor therapy for several days before and after methotrexate administration or substituting a histamine H_2-receptor antagonist for the proton-pump inhibitor when acid suppressive therapy is indicated during methotrexate therapy. Pending further evaluation, some clinicians state that these recommendations should extend to patients receiving low-dose methotrexate.

● *Nonsteroidal Anti-inflammatory Agents*

Pharmacokinetic interactions with naproxen or rofecoxib (no longer commercially available in the US) are unlikely.

● *Sucralfate*

In a single-dose study, concomitant administration of omeprazole 20 mg and sucralfate 1 g resulted in delayed absorption of omeprazole and decreased omeprazole bioavailability by 16%. Proton-pump inhibitors should be administered at least 30 minutes before sucralfate.

● *Tacrolimus*

Potential pharmacokinetic interaction (increased serum concentrations of tacrolimus).

● *Warfarin*

Potential increased international normalized ratio (INR) and prothrombin time when warfarin is used concomitantly with proton-pump inhibitors, including esomeprazole. Potential for abnormal bleeding and death; monitor for INR and prothrombin time increases when esomeprazole is used concomitantly with warfarin.

DESCRIPTION

Esomeprazole, a proton-pump inhibitor, is a gastric antisecretory agent that is structurally and pharmacologically related to lansoprazole, omeprazole, pantoprazole, and rabeprazole. The drugs are substituted benzimidazoles and are chemically and pharmacologically unrelated to H_2-receptor antagonists, antimuscarinics, or prostaglandin analogs. Esomeprazole is the *S*-isomer of omeprazole, which is a racemic mixture of *R*- and *S*-isomers.

Esomeprazole binds to hydrogen-potassium ATPase in gastric parietal cells; inactivation of this enzyme system (also known as the proton, hydrogen, or acid pump) blocks the final step in the secretion of hydrochloric acid by these cells, resulting in potent, long-lasting inhibition of gastric acid secretion.

Because the esomeprazole molecule is acid labile, the commercially available delayed-release capsules and packets for delayed-release oral suspension containing enteric-coated granules of the drug increase oral bioavailability. Esomeprazole is extensively metabolized, principally by the hepatic cytochrome P-450 (CYP) 2C19 isoenzyme and to a lesser extent by CYP3A4, to form metabolites lacking antisecretory activity. The CYP2C19 isoenzyme is polymorphically expressed; poor metabolizers (about 3% of Caucasians and 15–20% of Asians) lack the isoenzyme, and the metabolism of esomeprazole and omeprazole is decreased in such individuals compared with the rest of the population (i.e., extensive or rapid metabolizers). However, esomeprazole undergoes less metabolic transformation by CYP2C19 and may exhibit less variation in plasma concentrations between slow and rapid metabolizers than omeprazole. At steady state, the ratio of the area under the plasma concentration-time curve (AUC) of esomeprazole in poor metabolizers to the AUC of the drug in rapid metabolizers is about 2:1.

A proton-pump inhibitor (e.g., esomeprazole, omeprazole) can suppress but not eradicate gastric *Helicobacter pylori* in patients with duodenal ulcer and/or reflux esophagitis infected with the organism. Therapy with esomeprazole in combination with clarithromycin and amoxicillin can effectively eradicate *H. pylori* gastric infection.

Increased gastric pH during esomeprazole therapy stimulates gastrin secretion via a negative feedback mechanism and results in enterochromaffin-like cell (ECL) hyperplasia. Although rats have demonstrated carcinoid lesions, no adenomatoid, dysplastic, or neoplastic changes have occurred to date in patients receiving esomeprazole or other proton-pump inhibitors for up to 1 year.

Therapy with proton-pump inhibitors, particularly in high dosages and/or for prolonged periods of time, may be associated with an increased risk of osteoporosis-related fractures of the hip, wrist, or spine. (See Musculoskeletal Effects under Cautions: Warnings/Precautions.) The mechanism by which these drugs may increase risk of such fractures has not been elucidated but may involve decreased insoluble calcium absorption secondary to increased gastric pH.

ADVICE TO PATIENTS

Importance of taking oral esomeprazole at least 1 hour before a meal.

Necessity of swallowing capsules whole, without crushing or chewing the delayed-release granules. For patients with difficulty swallowing, necessity of mixing capsule contents with cool, soft applesauce and swallowing immediately without chewing. Importance of *not* storing mixture of applesauce and capsule contents for future use.

If using oral suspension, necessity of mixing packet contents with an appropriate amount of water, allowing suspension to thicken for 2–3 minutes, and stirring and drinking mixture within 30 minutes of preparation. Importance of swallowing suspension without crushing or chewing granules.

Antacid administration is permissible during esomeprazole therapy.

Importance of advising patients that use of multiple daily doses of the drug for an extended period of time may increase the risk of fractures of the hip, wrist, or spine.

Risk of hypomagnesemia; importance of advising patients to immediately report and seek care for any cardiovascular or neurologic manifestations (e.g., palpitations, dizziness, seizures, tetany).

Possible increased risk of *Clostridium difficile* infection; importance of contacting a clinician if persistent watery stools, abdominal pain, and fever occur.

Importance of informing clinicians of existing or contemplated concomitant therapy, including prescription and OTC drugs, as well as concomitant illnesses.

Importance of continuing therapy for the entire treatment course, unless directed otherwise.

Importance of women informing clinicians if they are or plan to become pregnant or plan to breast-feed.

Importance of informing patients of other important precautionary information. (See Cautions.)

PREPARATIONS

Excipients in commercially available drug preparations may have clinically important effects in some individuals; consult specific product labeling for details.

Esomeprazole Magnesium

Oral

Capsules, delayed-release (containing enteric-coated granules)	20 mg (of esomeprazole)	NexIUM®, AstraZeneca
	40 mg (of esomeprazole)	NexIUM®, AstraZeneca
For Suspension, delayed-release (containing enteric-coated granules)	2.5 mg (of esomeprazole) per packet	NexIUM®, AstraZeneca
	5 mg (of esomeprazole) per packet	NexIUM®, AstraZeneca
	10 mg (of esomeprazole) per packet	NexIUM®, AstraZeneca
	20 mg (of esomeprazole) per packet	NexIUM®, AstraZeneca
	40 mg (of esomeprazole) per packet	NexIUM®, AstraZeneca

Esomeprazole Magnesium Combinations

Oral

Tablets, delayed-release core (naproxen only)	20 mg (of esomeprazole) with Naproxen 375 mg	Vimovo®, AstraZeneca
	20 mg (of esomeprazole) with Naproxen 500 mg	Vimovo®, AstraZeneca

Esomeprazole Sodium

Parenteral

For injection, for IV use	20 mg (of esomeprazole)	NexIUM® IV, AstraZeneca
	40 mg (of esomeprazole)	NexIUM® IV, AstraZeneca

† Use is not currently included in the labeling approved by the US Food and Drug Administration.

Selected Revisions December 8, 2012, © Copyright, August 1, 2001, American Society of Health-System Pharmacists, Inc.

Lansoprazole

56:28.36 • PROTON-PUMP INHIBITORS

- Lansoprazole, commonly referred to as an acid- or proton-pump inhibitor, is a gastric antisecretory agent.

USES

Lansoprazole is used orally for the short-term treatment and symptomatic relief of active duodenal and benign gastric ulcer and as maintenance therapy following healing of duodenal ulcers. Lansoprazole also is used orally in combination with amoxicillin (dual therapy) or with clarithromycin and amoxicillin (triple therapy) for the treatment of *Helicobacter pylori* infection and duodenal ulcer disease. Lansoprazole also has been used in other multiple-drug regimens† for the treatment of *H. pylori* infection associated with peptic ulcer disease. Lansoprazole also is used orally for the treatment of nonsteroidal anti-inflammatory agent (NSAIA)-induced gastric ulcers in patients who continue NSAIA use, and for the prevention of NSAIA-induced gastric ulcers in patients with a documented history of gastric ulcer who require the use of an NSAIA. Oral lansoprazole also is used for short-term treatment and symptomatic relief of gastroesophageal reflux disease (e.g., erosive esophagitis), as maintenance therapy following healing of erosive esophagitis to reduce its recurrence and in the long-term treatment of pathologic GI hypersecretory conditions. Lansoprazole is used orally as *self-medication* for short-term treatment of frequent heartburn.

● Gastroesophageal Reflux

Acute Therapy

Lansoprazole is used orally to provide short-term (up to 8 weeks) treatment and symptomatic relief of all grades of erosive esophagitis in patients with gastroesophageal reflux disease (GERD). Oral lansoprazole also is used for the short-term (up to 8 weeks) treatment of symptomatic GERD (e.g., heartburn). Potential benefits of lansoprazole in gastroesophageal reflux and esophagitis result principally from reduced acidity of gastric contents induced by the drug and resultant reduced irritation of esophageal mucosa; the drug can effectively relieve symptoms of esophagitis (e.g., heartburn) and promote healing of ulcerative and erosive lesions.

Suppression of gastric acid secretion is considered by the American College of Gastroenterology (ACG) to be the mainstay of treatment for GERD, and a proton-pump inhibitor or histamine H_2-receptor antagonist is used to achieve acid suppression, control symptoms, and prevent complications of the disease. The ACG states that proton-pump inhibitors are more effective (i.e., provide more frequent and more rapid symptomatic relief and healing of esophagitis) than histamine H_2-receptor antagonists in the treatment of GERD. Proton-pump inhibitors also provide greater control of acid reflux than do prokinetic agents (e.g., cisapride [no longer commercially available in the US], metoclopramide) without the risk of severe adverse effects associated with these agents.

In a controlled study in patients with manifestations of GERD (e.g., heartburn) and the absence of erosive esophageal lesions, symptomatic improvement (reduction in frequency and severity of heartburn) with lansoprazole was greater than that with placebo. In this study in patients with endoscopically confirmed GERD, the median percentage of days without heartburn was 84, 82, or 13% at week 8 of therapy with lansoprazole 15 mg daily, lansoprazole 30 mg daily, or placebo, respectively; the median percentage of nights without heartburn in these respective treatment groups was 92, 80, or 36% at week 8. Administration of 30 mg of lansoprazole daily did not provide improved relief compared with 15 mg daily in this study.

In controlled studies in patients with endoscopically evaluated GERD, reported rates of healing with lansoprazole were higher than those with placebo or an H_2-receptor antagonist and at least as high as those with omeprazole. Generally, antacids were used concomitantly for pain relief. In a controlled study in patients with esophagitis, reported rates of healing were 91, 95, 94, or 53% at 8 weeks in patients receiving lansoprazole 15 mg daily, 30 mg daily, 60 mg daily, or placebo, respectively. Healing rates from controlled studies were 80–84 or 39–52%

at 4 weeks and 91–92 or 53–70% at 8 weeks for lansoprazole 30 mg daily or ranitidine 150 mg twice daily, respectively. Patients receiving lansoprazole reported faster relief of daytime and nocturnal heartburn and self-administered less antacid than those receiving placebo or an H_2-receptor antagonist; however, since the recommended dosage of ranitidine for esophagitis is 150 mg four times daily and patients treated with ranitidine received only 150 mg twice daily, further study is needed to evaluate relative efficacy. Lansoprazole also has been shown to be effective in promoting healing and providing symptomatic relief in a substantial proportion of patients failing to respond to usual or relatively high dosages of H_2-receptor antagonists.

Although lansoprazole has been used IV for short-term (up to 7 days) treatment of erosive esophagitis in patients who are unable to take the drug orally, a parenteral dosage form no longer is commercially available in the US. In one controlled study in patients with erosive esophagitis receiving oral lansoprazole, the degree of inhibition of gastric acid secretion following IV administration of lansoprazole 30 mg daily for 7 days was similar to that achieved following repeated oral administration of the drug.

Short-term lansoprazole therapy for the treatment of erosive esophagitis will not prevent recurrence of the disease following discontinuance of the drug. Most patients with erosive esophagitis respond to lansoprazole during an initial 8-week course of therapy; however, an additional 8 weeks of therapy may contribute to healing and symptomatic improvement in some patients (i.e., patients experiencing a recurrence of erosive esophagitis or patients who fail to heal after the initial course of therapy). If symptomatic GERD or severe esophagitis recur, the manufacturer states that additional 8-week courses of lansoprazole may be given. However, the ACG states that chronic, even lifelong, therapy with a proton-pump inhibitor is appropriate in many patients with GERD.

Maintenance Therapy

Lansoprazole is used as maintenance therapy following healing of erosive esophagitis to reduce recurrence of the disease. In a multicenter, double-blind study, endoscopically documented remission of esophagitis was maintained at 6 months in 81, 93, or 27% of patients receiving lansoprazole 15 mg daily, 30 mg daily, or placebo, respectively, and such remission was maintained at 12 months in 79, 90, or 24% of patients, respectively. In another multicenter, double-blind study in patients with endoscopically confirmed healed esophagitis, remission of esophagitis was maintained at 6 months in 72, 72, or 13% of patients receiving lansoprazole 15 mg daily, 30 mg daily, or placebo, respectively, and at 12 months in 67, 55, or 13% of patients, respectively. Remission rates of esophagitis were independent of the patient's initial grade of erosive esophagitis and the daily dosage of lansoprazole (15 or 30 mg).

Because GERD is a chronic condition, the ACG states that continuous therapy to control symptoms and prevent complications is appropriate, and chronic, even lifelong, use of a proton-pump inhibitor is effective and appropriate as maintenance therapy in many patients with GERD. The frequent marked improvement in symptoms associated with full dosage of a proton-pump inhibitor generally is followed by rapid recurrence of symptoms once the drug is discontinued, and reduced-dosage regimens (e.g., every other day, "weekend" dosage) have not been shown to be consistently effective for maintenance therapy.

For further information on the treatment of GERD, see Uses: Gastroesophageal Reflux, in Omeprazole 56:28.36.

Self-medication

Lansoprazole is used orally in adults 18 years of age or older as *self-medication* for short-term (14 days) treatment of frequent (2 or more days per week) heartburn. Because 1–4 days may be required for complete relief of symptoms, lansoprazole for *self-medication* is not intended for the immediate relief of heartburn. However, some individuals may experience complete relief of symptoms within 24 hours of taking the first dose of lansoprazole. In 2 controlled studies in adults with frequent (2 or more days per week) heartburn, the percentage of days (24-hour periods) without heartburn during 14 days of treatment was greater with lansoprazole 15 mg daily than with placebo (59.9–64.7 versus 45–45.7%). The percentage of heartburn-free nights during the 14-day treatment period was 79.5–81.6% with lansoprazole therapy compared with 76.3–77% with placebo. On day 1 of treatment, 50.4–50.7% of lansoprazole-treated patients experienced no heartburn compared with 33–37.9% of those receiving placebo. In a controlled study in adults with frequent nocturnal heartburn, the percentage of heartburn-free nights during 14 days of treatment was greater with lansoprazole 15 or 30 mg (61.3–61.7%) compared with placebo (47.8%). The percentage of days (24-hour periods) without heartburn and the percentage of patients without heartburn on day 1 of treatment also were greater with lansoprazole therapy than with placebo.

● Gastric Ulcer

Acute Therapy

Lansoprazole is used for the short-term treatment and symptomatic relief of active benign gastric ulcer. Antacids may be used concomitantly as needed for pain relief. In controlled studies in patients with endoscopically confirmed gastric ulcers, reported rates of ulcer healing for lansoprazole were substantially higher than those for placebo. In a multicenter, double-blind study in patients with endoscopically confirmed gastric ulcer, reported rates of ulcer healing in patients receiving lansoprazole 15 or 30 mg each morning or placebo were 65, 58, or 38%, respectively, at 4 weeks and 92, 97, or 77%, respectively, at 8 weeks. Lansoprazole also produced greater reductions in daytime and nocturnal pain and antacid consumption than did placebo.

Current epidemiologic and clinical evidence supports a strong association between gastric infection with *H. pylori* and the pathogenesis of gastric ulcers, and the ACG, NIH, and most clinicians currently recommend that *all* patients with initial or recurrent gastric ulcer and documented *H. pylori* infection receive anti-infective therapy for treatment of the infection. The choice of a particular regimen should be based on current data on optimal therapy, including consideration of the patient's prior exposure to anti-infective agents, the local prevalence of resistance, patient compliance, and costs of therapy. (See Duodenal Ulcer: Acute Therapy, in Uses.) For a more complete discussion of *H. pylori* infection, including details about the efficacy of various regimens and rationale for drug selection, see Uses: *Helicobacter pylori* Infection, in Clarithromycin 8:12.12.92.

● NSAIA-induced Ulcers

Treatment

Lansoprazole is used for the treatment of NSAIA-induced gastric ulcers in patients who continue NSAIA use. In 2 controlled studies in patients with endoscopically confirmed NSAIA-associated gastric ulcer who continued their NSAIA use, substantially more patients receiving lansoprazole 30 mg daily experienced ulcer healing at 8 weeks compared with those receiving an active control drug. In one study, healing of gastric ulcers occurred in 60 and 79% of patients receiving lansoprazole, compared with 28 and 55% of those receiving an active control drug at 4 and 8 weeks, respectively. In the second study, ulcer healing occurred in 77% of patients receiving lansoprazole or in 50% of those receiving an active control drug at 4 and 8 weeks. However, there was no substantial difference in the number of patients experiencing symptomatic (e.g., abdominal pain) relief between those receiving lansoprazole and those receiving the active control.

For treatment of NSAIA-induced ulcers, it is preferable to discontinue NSAIA therapy and initiate therapy with a drug (e.g., proton-pump inhibitor, histamine H_2-receptor antagonist) indicated for the treatment of ulcers. When NSAIA therapy must be continued, a proton-pump inhibitor is considered the drug of choice for treatment of ulcers since the efficacy of H_2-receptor antagonists is substantially decreased by continued use of NSAIAs. Treatment of *H. pylori* infection is recommended in patients receiving NSAIAs who have ulcers and are infected with this organism. For further information on *H. pylori* infection, including details about the efficacy of various regimens and rationale for drug selection, see Uses: *Helicobacter pylori* Infection, in Clarithromycin 8:12.12.92.

Prevention

Lansoprazole is used for the prevention of NSAIA-induced gastric ulcers in patients with a documented history of gastric ulcer who require the use of an NSAIA. In a controlled study in patients with a history of gastric ulcer who required NSAIA therapy, lansoprazole 15 or 30 mg daily was more effective than placebo but less effective than misoprostol 200 mcg 4 times daily in preventing gastric ulcer recurrence at 4, 8, and 12 weeks of therapy. About one-half of the patients also had a history of duodenal ulcer. About 51, 93, 80, or 82% of those receiving placebo, misoprostol, or lansoprazole 15 or 30 mg, respectively, remained free of gastric ulcers at 12 weeks. In a subsequent subset analysis of patients receiving only naproxen or naproxen and aspirin (up to 325 mg daily), lansoprazole 15 or 30 mg daily was more effective than placebo and as effective as

misoprostol in preventing gastric ulcer recurrence at 4, 8, and 12 weeks of therapy; about 33, 83, 89, or 83% of those receiving placebo, misoprostol, or lansoprazole 15 or 30 mg, respectively, remained free of gastric ulcers at 12 weeks. Serious NSAIA-related GI complications (e.g., bleeding, perforation, obstruction) were not reported during the study; however, the study was not designed to assess the effect of lansoprazole on the risk of such complications or on the risk of duodenal ulcers.

Serious adverse GI effects (e.g., bleeding, ulceration, perforation) can occur at any time in patients receiving chronic NSAIA therapy, and such effects may *not* be preceded by warning signs or symptoms. Results of studies to date are inconclusive concerning the relative risk of various NSAIAs in causing serious GI effects. In patients receiving prototypical NSAIAs and observed in clinical studies of several months' to 2-years' duration, symptomatic upper GI ulcers, gross bleeding, or perforation appeared to occur in approximately 1% of patients treated for 3–6 months and in about 2–4% of those treated for 1 year. These trends continue with long-term therapy and increase the likelihood of a serious GI event occurring at some time during the course of therapy. Studies have shown that patients with a history of peptic ulcer disease and/or GI bleeding who are receiving NSAIAs have a greater than tenfold higher risk for developing GI bleeding than patients without these risk factors. In addition to a history of ulcer disease, pharmacoepidemiologic studies have identified several comorbid conditions and concomitant therapies that may increase the risk for GI bleeding, including concomitant use of oral corticosteroids or anticoagulants, longer duration of NSAIA therapy, high NSAIA dosage, smoking, alcoholism, older age, and poor general health status. In addition, geriatric or debilitated patients appear to tolerate GI ulceration and bleeding less well than other individuals, and most spontaneous reports of fatal NSAIA-induced GI effects have been in such patients.

For patients at high risk for complications from NSAIA-induced GI ulceration (e.g., bleeding, perforation), concomitant use of misoprostol can be considered for preventive therapy. (See Misoprostol 56:28.28.) Alternatively, use of a proton-pump inhibitor (e.g., lansoprazole) may be used concomitantly to decrease the incidence of serious GI toxicity associated with NSAIA therapy. Another approach in high-risk patients who would benefit from NSAIA therapy is use of an NSAIA that is a selective inhibitor of cyclooxygenase-2 (COX-2), since these agents are associated with a lower incidence of serious GI bleeding than are prototypical NSAIAs. However, while celecoxib (200 mg twice daily) was comparably effective to diclofenac sodium (75 mg twice daily) plus omeprazole (20 mg daily) in preventing recurrent ulcer bleeding (recurrent ulcer bleeding probabilities of 4.9 versus 6.4%, respectively, during the 6-month study) in *H. pylori*-negative arthritis (principally osteoarthritis) patients with a recent history of ulcer bleeding, the protective efficacy was unexpectedly low for both regimens and it appeared that neither could completely protect patients at high risk. Additional study is necessary to elucidate optimal therapy for preventing GI complications associated with NSAIA therapy in high-risk patients.

● Duodenal Ulcer

Acute Therapy

Lansoprazole is used for the short-term treatment of endoscopically or radiographically confirmed active duodenal ulcer. Antacids may be used concomitantly as needed for pain relief. In controlled studies in patients with endoscopically confirmed duodenal ulcers, reported rates of ulcer healing for lansoprazole were substantially higher than those for placebo. In a multicenter, double-blind study in patients with endoscopically confirmed duodenal ulcer, reported rates of ulcer healing for an oral lansoprazole dosage of 15 mg daily or placebo were 42 or 11%, respectively, at 2 weeks and 89 or 46%, respectively, at 4 weeks. A similar response was observed in patients receiving 30 or 60 mg of lansoprazole daily. Lansoprazole also produced greater reductions in daytime and nocturnal abdominal pain and antacid consumption than did placebo. Clinically important differences in the rates of ulcer healing between men and women receiving lansoprazole therapy do not appear to exist.

Lansoprazole appears to be at least as effective as H_2-receptor antagonists or other proton-pump inhibitors (e.g., omeprazole) for short-term treatment of active duodenal ulcer. In a multicenter, controlled study in patients with endoscopically confirmed duodenal ulcers, 35 or 31% of ulcers were healed following 2 weeks of oral therapy with lansoprazole 20 mg daily or ranitidine 300 mg twice daily, respectively, and 92 or 71%, respectively, were healed after 4 weeks of therapy. A lansoprazole dosage of 30 mg daily was similarly effective. In another multicenter, controlled study in patients with endoscopically confirmed duodenal ulcers, 88 or 82% of ulcers were healed following 2 weeks of oral therapy with lansoprazole 30 mg daily or omeprazole 20 mg daily, respectively, and 98 or 97%, respectively, were healed after 4 weeks of therapy.

Most patients with duodenal ulcer respond to lansoprazole therapy during the usual 4-week course of therapy. However, short-term lansoprazole therapy for the treatment of active duodenal disease will not prevent recurrence of the disease following acute healing and discontinuance of the drug.

Lansoprazole is used in combination with amoxicillin and clarithromycin for the treatment of *H. pylori* infection and duodenal ulcer disease. Lansoprazole also is used in combination with amoxicillin for the treatment of *H. pylori* infection and duodenal ulcer disease in patients who are either allergic to or intolerant of clarithromycin or in whom clarithromycin resistance is known or suspected. Lansoprazole also has been used in other multiple-drug regimens† for the treatment of *H. pylori* infection and peptic ulcer disease. Current epidemiologic and clinical evidence supports a strong association between gastric infection with *H. pylori* and the pathogenesis of duodenal and gastric ulcers; long-term *H. pylori* infection also has been implicated as a risk factor for gastric cancer. For additional information on the association of this infection with these and other GI conditions, see Helicobacter pylori Infection, under Uses, in Clarithromycin 8:12.12.92. Conventional antiulcer therapy with H_2-receptor antagonists, proton-pump inhibitors, sucralfate, and/or antacids heals ulcers but generally is ineffective in eradicating *H. pylori*, and such therapy is associated with a high rate of ulcer recurrence (e.g., 60–100% per year). The American College of Gastroenterology (ACG), the National Institutes of Health (NIH), and most clinicians currently recommend that *all* patients with initial or recurrent duodenal or gastric ulcer and documented *H. pylori* infection receive anti-infective therapy for treatment of the infection. Although 3-drug regimens consisting of a bismuth salt (e.g., bismuth subsalicylate) and 2 anti-infective agents (e.g., tetracycline or amoxicillin plus metronidazole) administered for 10–14 days have been effective in eradicating the infection, resolving associated gastritis, healing peptic ulcer, and preventing ulcer recurrence in many patients with *H. pylori*-associated peptic ulcer disease, current evidence principally from studies in Europe suggests that 1 week of such therapy provides comparable *H. pylori* eradication rates. Other regimens that combine one or more anti-infective agents (e.g., clarithromycin, amoxicillin) with a bismuth salt and/or an antisecretory agent (e.g., omeprazole, lansoprazole, H_2-receptor antagonist) also have been used successfully for *H. pylori* eradication, and the choice of a particular regimen should be based on current data on optimal therapy, including consideration of the patient's prior exposure to anti-infective agents, the local prevalence of resistance, patient compliance, and costs of therapy.

Current evidence suggests that inclusion of a proton-pump inhibitor (e.g., lansoprazole, omeprazole) in anti-*H. pylori* regimens containing 2 anti-infectives enhances effectiveness, and limited data suggest that such regimens retain good efficacy despite imidazole (e.g., metronidazole) resistance. Therefore, the ACG and many clinicians currently recommend 1 week of therapy with a proton-pump inhibitor and 2 anti-infective agents (usually clarithromycin and amoxicillin or metronidazole), or a 3-drug, bismuth-based regimen (e.g., bismuth-metronidazole-tetracycline) concomitantly with a proton-pump inhibitor, for treatment of *H. pylori* infection.

Therapy with an antisecretory drug and a single anti-infective agent (i.e., "dual therapy") also has been used successfully for treatment of *H. pylori* infection. However, while some studies demonstrate that certain 2-drug anti-*H. pylori* regimens (e.g., clarithromycin-omeprazole, ranitidine bismuth citrate-omeprazole, amoxicillin-omeprazole) can successfully eradicate *H. pylori* infection and prevent recurrence of duodenal ulcer at least in the short term (e.g., at 6 months following completion of anti-*H. pylori* therapy), the ACG and some clinicians currently state that anti-*H. pylori* regimens consisting of at least 3 drugs (e.g., 2 anti-infective agents plus a proton-pump inhibitor) are recommended because of enhanced *H. pylori* eradication rates, decreased failures due to resistance, and shorter treatment periods compared with those apparently required with 2-drug regimens. Additional randomized, controlled studies comparing various anti-*H. pylori* regimens are needed to clarify optimum drug combinations, dosages, and durations of treatment for *H. pylori* infection. For a more complete discussion of *H. pylori* infection, including details about the efficacy of various regimens and rationale for drug selection, see Uses: Helicobacter pylori Infection, in Clarithromycin 8:12.12.92.

Maintenance Therapy

Lansoprazole is used as maintenance therapy following healing of duodenal ulcers to reduce ulcer recurrence. In 2 controlled studies of patients with endoscopically documented healed duodenal ulcers, those receiving lansoprazole 15 or 30 mg daily remained healed substantially longer, and experienced substantially fewer recurrences than those receiving placebo over a 12 month period. In one study, 90, 87, and 84% of patients receiving lansoprazole 15 mg daily, and 49, 41, and 39% of patients receiving placebo, remained in endoscopically documented remission over 3, 6, and 12 months, respectively. In another study, 94, 94, and 85% of patients receiving lansoprazole 30 mg daily and 87, 79, and 70% of those receiving lansoprazole 15 mg daily were still in endoscopically documented remission at 3, 6, and 12 months, respectively. In comparison, only 33% of those receiving placebo remained in endoscopically documented remission over 3 months, and none were in remission at 6 or 12 months. There was no substantial difference between lansoprazole 15 or 30 mg daily in maintaining remission.

● Pathologic GI Hypersecretory Conditions

Lansoprazole is used for the long-term treatment of pathologic GI hypersecretory conditions (e.g., Zollinger-Ellison syndrome, multiple endocrine adenomas, systemic mastocytosis). The drug reduces gastric acid secretion and associated symptoms (including diarrhea, anorexia, and pain) in patients with these conditions. In dosages ranging from 15 mg every other day to 180 mg daily, lansoprazole can maintain basal acid secretion below 5 or 10 mEq/hour in patients who have or have not undergone gastric surgery, respectively. Lansoprazole therapy has been continued in some patients for longer than 4 years.

● Crohn's Disease-associated Ulcers

Although evidence currently is limited, proton-pump inhibitors have been used for gastric acid-suppressive therapy as an adjunct in the symptomatic treatment of upper GI Crohn's disease†, including esophageal, gastroduodenal, and jejunoileal disease. Most evidence of efficacy to date has been from case studies in patients with Crohn's-associated peptic ulcer disease unresponsive to other therapies (e.g., H_2-receptor antagonists, cytoprotective agents, antacids, and/or sucralfate). (See Uses: Crohn's Disease-associated Ulcers in Omeprazole 56:28.36.)

For further information on the management of Crohn's Disease, see Uses: Crohn's Disease, in Mesalamine 56:36.

DOSAGE AND ADMINISTRATION

● Administration

Lansoprazole is administered orally. Lansoprazole also has been administered by IV infusion; however, a parenteral dosage form no longer is commercially available in the US.

If a dose of lansoprazole is missed, the dose should be taken as soon as possible. However, if the next scheduled dose is due, the missed dose should be omitted, and the next dose taken at the regularly scheduled time. A double dose should not be administered to make up for a missed dose.

Oral Administration

Lansoprazole is administered orally as capsules or orally disintegrating tablets. To avoid decomposition of lansoprazole in the acidic pH of the stomach, the commercially available delayed-release capsules contain enteric-coated granules of the drug, and the orally disintegrating tablets contain enteric-coated microgranules of the drug. The contents of the capsules should *not* be chewed or crushed, nor should the orally disintegrating tablets be broken, cut, or chewed.

Lansoprazole usually is administered once daily, generally in the morning; however, the manufacturer states that administration of the drug in 2 equally divided doses in the morning and evening may improve efficacy in patients receiving more than 120 mg daily. When lansoprazole is used in combination with amoxicillin or with clarithromycin and amoxicillin for the treatment of *Helicobacter pylori* infection associated with duodenal ulcer, lansoprazole is given in 2 or 3 divided doses daily.

Following administration of lansoprazole with meals, the rate and extent of GI absorption are reduced. Therefore, lansoprazole should be taken before meals.

Since an acidic environment in the parietal cell canaliculi is required for conversion of proton-pump inhibitors (e.g., lansoprazole) to their active sulfenamide metabolites, the American College of Gastroenterology suggests that proton-pump inhibitors are most effective when given about 30 minutes prior to meals and that effectiveness may be compromised if these drugs are administered during the basal state (e.g., to fasting patients at bedtime) or concomitantly with other antisecretory agents (e.g., anticholinergics, histamine H_2-receptor antagonists, somatostatin analogs, misoprostol). Lansoprazole may be administered concomitantly with antacids but should be administered at least 30 minutes before sucralfate (see Drug Interactions).

Extemporaneously Compounded Oral Suspension

An extemporaneously compounded 3 mg/mL oral suspension of lansoprazole has been prepared using the commercially available capsules and an 8.4% sodium bicarbonate vehicle. An extemporaneous suspension also has been prepared by pulverizing one 30-mg enteric-coated microgranule tablet in 10 mL of Ora-Blend to provide a suspension containing 3 mg/mL.

Standardize 4 Safety

Standardized concentrations for an extemporaneously prepared oral suspension of lansoprazole have been established through Standardize 4 Safety (S4S), a national patient safety initiative to reduce medication errors, especially during transitions of care. Multidisciplinary expert panels were convened to determine recommended standard concentrations. Because recommendations from the S4S panels may differ from the manufacturer's prescribing information, caution is advised when using concentrations that differ from labeling, particularly when using rate information from the label. For additional information on S4S (including updates that may be available), see https://www.ashp.org/pharmacy-practice/standardize-4-safety-initiative.

TABLE 1. Standardize 4 Safety Compounded Oral Liquid Standards for Lansoprazole

Concentration Standards
3 mg/mL

Oral Capsules

Lansoprazole capsules may be swallowed whole. Alternatively, the contents of a capsule may be sprinkled on a tablespoonful of a suitable soft food and swallowed without chewing; mixed with apple, orange, or tomato juice and consumed; or mixed with apple juice and given via a nasogastric tube.

In patients who have difficulty swallowing capsules, the contents of a capsule may be sprinkled on a tablespoonful of applesauce, liquid dietary supplement (e.g., Ensure®) pudding, cottage cheese, yogurt, or strained pears and ingested immediately without a clinically important effect on the drug's bioavailability. The granules should not be chewed or crushed. The manufacturer states that administration of lansoprazole mixed in other foods has not been evaluated clinically and is not recommended.

Alternatively, the contents of a capsule may be emptied into a small volume (i.e., 60 mL, about 2 ounces) of apple, orange, or tomato juice, mixed briefly, and swallowed immediately. To ensure complete consumption of the dose, the glass should be rinsed with 120 mL or more of juice, and the contents swallowed immediately. The manufacturer states that administration of lansoprazole mixed in other beverages has not been evaluated clinically and is not recommended.

For patients with a nasogastric tube, the contents of a capsule can be mixed with 40 mL of apple juice in a syringe and administered immediately (i.e., within 3–5 minutes) without any clinically important effect on the drug's bioavailability; the manufacturer states that other liquids should not be used. To facilitate delivery of the entire dose and to maintain patency of the nasogastric tube, the syringe and tube should be flushed with additional apple juice.

The manufacturer states that lansoprazole capsules for *self-medication* should be swallowed whole with a glass of water; the capsules should not be crushed or chewed.

Orally Disintegrating Tablets

Lansoprazole orally disintegrating tablets containing enteric-coated microgranules of the drug may be allowed to disintegrate on the tongue and then swallowed without chewing; alternatively, a tablet may be dispersed in a compatible liquid and administered orally using an oral syringe or given via a nasogastric tube. The orally disintegrating tablets should not be broken or cut.

For oral administration, the orally disintegrating tablet should be placed on the tongue and allowed to disintegrate (usually in less than 1 minute) with or without water, and the particles swallowed without chewing.

For administration using an oral syringe, a 15- or 30-mg orally disintegrating tablet should be placed in an oral syringe, about 4 or 10 mL, respectively, of water should be drawn into the syringe, and the syringe should be shaken gently to ensure rapid dispersal of the particles. The contents of the syringe should be administered within 15 minutes of preparation. An additional 2 mL (for a 15-mg dose) or 5 mL (for a 30-mg dose) of water should be drawn into the syringe, mixed gently, and the entire contents ingested to ensure complete consumption of the dose.

For administration via a nasogastric tube, a 15- or 30-mg orally disintegrating tablet should be placed in a syringe, about 4 or 10 mL, respectively, of water should be drawn into the syringe, and the syringe should be shaken gently to ensure rapid dispersal of the particles. The contents of the syringe should be administered through a nasogastric tube (8 French or larger) within 15 minutes of preparation. An additional 5 mL of water should be drawn into the syringe, mixed gently, and used to flush the nasogastric tube.

● Dosage
Adult Dosage
Gastroesophageal Reflux

For the short-term treatment of symptomatic gastroesophageal reflux disease (GERD), the usual adult dosage of lansoprazole is 15 mg once daily for up to 8 weeks.

For the short-term symptomatic treatment of all grades of erosive esophagitis, the usual adult dosage of lansoprazole is 30 mg once daily. Therapy is continued until healing occurs, usually within 8 weeks; an additional 8 weeks of therapy (up to 16 weeks for a single course) may contribute to healing and symptomatic improvement in some patients. If the erosive esophagitis recurs, the manufacturer states that an additional 8-week course of lansoprazole may be given. However, the American College of Gastroenterology (ACG) states that chronic, even lifelong, therapy with a proton-pump inhibitor is appropriate in many patients with GERD.

For maintenance therapy following healing of erosive esophagitis to reduce recurrence, the usual adult dosage of lansoprazole is 15 mg daily. Safety and efficacy of lansoprazole maintenance therapy for longer than 1 year have not been established.

For *self-medication* to relieve symptoms of frequent heartburn in adults 18 years of age or older, a lansoprazole dosage of 15 mg once daily in the morning for 14 days is recommended. For *self-medication*, the manufacturer recommends that the dosage of lansoprazole not exceed 15 mg in 24 hours. In addition, the drug should not be used for *self-medication* for longer than 14 days of *continuous* use and individuals should not exceed one course of therapy every 4 months unless otherwise directed by a clinician.

Gastric Ulcer

For the short-term treatment of active benign gastric ulcer, the usual adult dosage of lansoprazole is 30 mg daily for up to 8 weeks.

Nonsteroidal Anti-inflammatory Agent (NSAIA)-induced Ulcers

For the treatment of nonsteroidal anti-inflammatory agent (NSAIA)-associated gastric ulcers in patients continuing NSAIA use, the usual adult dosage of lansoprazole is 30 mg once daily for 8 weeks.

For prevention of NSAIA-associated gastric ulcers in patients with a documented history of gastric ulcer who require the use of an NSAIA, the usual adult dosage of lansoprazole is 15 mg once daily for up to 12 weeks. Efficacy of lansoprazole for periods exceeding 12 weeks in preventing of NSAIA-induced gastric ulcers has not been studied.

Duodenal Ulcer

For the short-term treatment of active duodenal ulcer, the usual adult dosage of lansoprazole is 15 mg once daily. Although an oral dosage of 30 mg daily often was administered in clinical studies, the manufacturer states that dosages of 30 or even 60 mg daily were no more effective at healing active duodenal ulcers than 15 mg daily. Therapy should be continued up to 4 weeks or until healing occurs.

When lansoprazole is used in combination with amoxicillin and clarithromycin (triple therapy) for the treatment of *H. pylori* infection in patients with active duodenal ulcer, the usual adult dosage is 30 mg every 12 hours (morning and evening) for 10 or 14 days. When lansoprazole is used in combination with amoxicillin (dual therapy) for the treatment of *H. pylori* infection in patients with active duodenal ulcer, the usual adult dosage is 30 mg every 8 hours for 14 days.

For maintenance therapy following healing of duodenal ulcer to reduce recurrence, the usual adult dosage of lansoprazole is 15 mg daily. Safety and efficacy of lansoprazole maintenance therapy for longer than 1 year have not been established.

Pathologic GI Hypersecretory Conditions

For the long-term treatment of pathologic GI hypersecretory conditions (e.g., Zollinger-Ellison syndrome, multiple endocrine adenomas, systemic mastocytosis), dosages of lansoprazole should be individualized according to patient response and tolerance. The usual initial adult dosage is 60 mg once daily. Subsequent lansoprazole dosage should be adjusted as tolerated and necessary to adequately suppress gastric acid secretion, and therapy continued as long as clinically necessary.

Oral dosages ranging from 15 mg every other day to 180 mg daily have been necessary to maintain basal gastric acid secretion at less than 10 mEq/hour in patients without a history of gastric surgery and less than 5 mEq/hour in those who have undergone gastric surgery; generally, determination of gastric acid secretion during the hour prior to a dose is useful in establishing optimum dosage. The manufacturer recommends that daily dosages exceeding 120 mg be administered in 2 equally divided doses in the morning and evening. Lansoprazole has been given continuously for longer than 4 years in some patients with Zollinger-Ellison syndrome.

Pediatric Dosage

Gastroesophageal Reflux

For the short-term treatment of symptomatic GERD or erosive esophagitis in children 1–11 years of age, the usual oral dosage of lansoprazole for children weighing 30 kg or less is 15 mg once daily for up to 12 weeks; dosage for children weighing more than 30 kg is 30 mg once daily for up to 12 weeks. Dosage in children 1–11 years of age has been increased to up to 30 mg twice daily in patients remaining symptomatic after 2 or more weeks of treatment.

For children 12–17 years of age, the usual oral dosage of lansoprazole for treatment of nonerosive GERD is 15 mg daily for up to 8 weeks, and that for erosive esophagitis is 30 mg daily for up to 8 weeks.

● *Special Populations*

The manufacturer states that lansoprazole dosage adjustment is not necessary in geriatric patients. Although pharmacokinetics of lansoprazole may be altered slightly in patients with renal impairment, dosage adjustment is not necessary. However, the commercially available daily administration pack containing lansoprazole, amoxicillin, and clarithromycin (Prevpac®) is not recommended for use in patients with creatinine clearance values less than 30 mL/minute. In patients with severe hepatic impairment, lansoprazole dosage reduction should be considered. (See Specific Populations under Cautions: Warnings/Precautions.)

CAUTIONS

● *Contraindications*

Known severe hypersensitivity to lansoprazole or any ingredient in the formulation.

● *Warnings/Precautions*

Gastric Malignancy

Symptomatic response to therapy with lansoprazole does not preclude the presence of gastric malignancy.

Clostridium difficile Infection

Available data suggest a possible association between use of proton-pump inhibitors and risk of *Clostridium difficile* infection, including *C. difficile*-associated diarrhea and colitis (CDAD; also known as antibiotic-associated diarrhea and colitis or pseudomembranous colitis). In most observational studies to date, the risk of *C. difficile* infection in patients exposed to proton-pump inhibitors has ranged from 1.4–2.75 times that in patients not exposed to proton-pump inhibitors; however, some observational studies have found no increase in risk. Although many of the cases occurred in patients who had other risk factors for CDAD, including advanced age, comorbid conditions, and/or use of broad-spectrum anti-infectives, the US Food and Drug Administration (FDA) concluded that a contributory role for proton-pump inhibitors could not be definitively ruled out. The mechanism by which proton-pump inhibitors might increase the risk of CDAD has not been elucidated. Although it has been suggested that reduction of gastric acidity by gastric antisecretory agents might facilitate colonization with *C. difficile*, some studies have raised questions about this proposed mechanism or have suggested that the observed association is the result of confounding with other risk factors for CDAD. FDA also is reviewing the risk of CDAD in patients exposed to histamine H_2-receptor antagonists.

CDAD can be serious in patients who have one or more risk factors for *C. difficile* infection and are receiving concomitant therapy with a proton-pump inhibitor; colectomy and, rarely, death have been reported. FDA recommends that patients receive proton-pump inhibitors at the lowest effective dosage and for the shortest possible time appropriate for their clinical condition. Patients experiencing persistent diarrhea should be evaluated for CDAD and should be managed with appropriate supportive therapy (e.g., fluid and electrolyte management), anti-infective therapy directed against *C. difficile* (e.g., metronidazole, vancomycin), and surgical evaluation as clinically indicated.

Respiratory Effects

Administration of proton-pump inhibitors has been associated with an increased risk for developing certain infections (e.g., community-acquired pneumonia). For further precautionary information about this adverse effect, see Community-acquired Pneumonia under Cautions: Respiratory Effects, in Omeprazole 56:28.36.

Musculoskeletal Effects

Findings from several observational studies suggest that therapy with proton-pump inhibitors, particularly in high dosages (i.e., multiple daily doses) and/or for prolonged periods of time (i.e., one year or longer), may be associated with an increased risk of osteoporosis-related fractures of the hip, wrist, or spine. The magnitude of risk is unclear; causality has not been established. (See Cautions: Musculoskeletal Effects, in Omeprazole 56:28.36.) FDA is continuing to evaluate this safety concern. Although controlled studies are required to confirm these findings, patients should receive proton-pump inhibitors at the lowest effective dosage and for the shortest possible time appropriate for their clinical condition. Individuals who are at risk for osteoporosis-related fractures should receive an adequate intake of calcium and vitamin D and should have their bone health assessed and managed according to current standards of care.

Hypomagnesemia

Hypomagnesemia, symptomatic and asymptomatic, has been reported rarely in patients receiving long-term therapy (for at least 3 months or, in most cases, for longer than one year) with proton-pump inhibitors, including lansoprazole. Clinically serious adverse effects associated with hypomagnesemia, which are similar to manifestations of hypocalcemia, include tetany, seizures, tremors, carpopedal spasm, arrhythmias (e.g., atrial fibrillation, supraventricular tachycardia), and abnormal QT interval. Other reported adverse effects include paresthesia, muscle weakness, muscle cramps, lethargy, fatigue, and unsteadiness. In most patients, treatment of hypomagnesemia required magnesium replacement and discontinuance of the proton-pump inhibitor. Following discontinuance of the proton-pump inhibitor, hypomagnesemia resolved within a median of one week; upon rechallenge, hypomagnesemia recurred within a median of 2 weeks.

In patients expected to receive long-term therapy with a proton-pump inhibitor or in those receiving a proton-pump inhibitor concomitantly with digoxin or drugs that may cause hypomagnesemia (e.g., diuretics), clinicians should consider measurement of serum magnesium concentrations prior to initiation of prescription proton-pump inhibitor therapy and periodically thereafter. (See Cautions: Hypomagnesemia and also Cautions: Precautions and Contraindications, in Omeprazole 56:28.36.)

Phenylketonuria

Individuals with phenylketonuria (i.e., homozygous genetic deficiency of phenylalanine hydroxylase) and other individuals who must restrict their intake of phenylalanine should be warned that each 15- or 30-mg Prevacid® SoluTab® orally disintegrating tablet contains aspartame (NutraSweet®), which is metabolized in the GI tract to provide about 2.5 or 5.1 mg, respectively, of phenylalanine following oral administration.

Specific Populations

Pregnancy

Category B. (See Users Guide.)

Lactation

Lansoprazole or its metabolites are distributed into milk in rats; it is not known whether lansoprazole is distributed into human milk. The manufacturer states that a decision should be made whether to discontinue nursing or the drug, taking into account the importance of the drug to the woman.

Pediatric Use

Safety and efficacy of oral lansoprazole in pediatric patients 1–17 years of age have been established for short-term treatment of symptomatic gastroesophageal reflux disease (GERD) and erosive esophagitis. In an open-label study in children 1–11 years of age, symptomatic improvement occurred following 8–12 weeks of lansoprazole therapy in 76% of children with symptomatic GERD; in a limited subset of children with endoscopically documented erosive esophagitis, rates of symptomatic improvement and healing were 81 and 100%, respectively. Lansoprazole was initiated at a dosage of 15 mg daily in children weighing 30 kg or less and a dosage of 30 mg daily in those weighing more than 30 kg; dosage could be increased up to 30 mg twice daily in children who continued to experience symptoms 2 or more weeks after initiating therapy with the drug. In an open-label study in adolescents 12–17 years of age with GERD, symptomatic improvement occurred following 8 weeks of therapy with lansoprazole 15 mg daily in 71% of those with nonerosive disease; in a smaller group of adolescents with erosive esophagitis, rates of symptomatic improvement and healing were 78 and 96%, respectively, following 8–12 weeks of therapy with lansoprazole 30 mg daily. The most commonly reported adverse effects in pediatric patients receiving lansoprazole include headache, abdominal pain, constipation, nausea, and dizziness.

Efficacy of oral lansoprazole has not been established in infants younger than 1 year of age. In a controlled study in infants 1 month to younger than 1 year of age with symptomatic GERD, lansoprazole was no more effective than placebo in reducing feeding-associated episodes of crying, fussing, or irritability; in both the placebo and lansoprazole groups, the response rate was 54%.

Safety and efficacy of lansoprazole for *self-medication* of frequent heartburn have not been established in children younger than 18 years of age.

Geriatric Use

The frequency of adverse effects in geriatric patients appears to be similar to that in younger patients. Clearance of lansoprazole may be decreased in geriatric patients, but accumulation of the drug does not occur with once-daily dosing and dosage adjustment is not necessary.

Hepatic Impairment

Systemic exposure to lansoprazole, as measured by area under the serum concentration-time curve (AUC), may be increased by up to 500% in patients with chronic hepatic impairment. Dosage reduction should be considered in patients with severe hepatic impairment.

Renal Impairment

Although the pharmacokinetics of lansoprazole may be altered slightly in patients with renal impairment, dosage adjustment is not necessary.

● Common Adverse Effects

Adverse effects occurring in 1% or more of patients receiving oral lansoprazole and more frequently than with placebo include abdominal pain, diarrhea, nausea, and constipation.

DRUG INTERACTIONS

● Drugs Metabolized by Hepatic Microsomal Enzymes

Lansoprazole is metabolized by cytochrome P-450 (CYP) isoenzymes 2C19 and 3A. In studies in healthy individuals, clinically important interactions were not observed between lansoprazole and other drugs (e.g., antipyrine, clarithromycin, diazepam, ibuprofen, indomethacin, phenytoin, prednisone, propranolol, warfarin) metabolized by CYP isoenzymes, including the 1A2, 2C9, 2C19, 2D6, and 3A isoenzymes.

● Drugs that Cause Hypomagnesemia

Potential pharmacologic interaction (possible increased risk of hypomagnesemia). In patients receiving diuretics (i.e., loop or thiazide diuretics) or other drugs that may cause hypomagnesemia, monitoring of magnesium concentrations should be considered prior to initiation of prescription proton-pump inhibitor therapy and periodically thereafter. (See Hypomagnesemia under Cautions: Warnings/Precautions.)

● Gastric pH-dependent Drugs

Pharmacokinetic interaction is theoretically possible when lansoprazole is used concomitantly with gastric pH-dependent drugs (e.g., ampicillin esters, digoxin, iron salts, ketoconazole); altered drug absorption at increased gastric pH values.

● Amoxicillin

Clinically important interaction is unlikely.

● Antacids

Efficacy of lansoprazole is not altered by concomitant administration of antacids.

● Antiretroviral Agents

Atazanavir

Potential pharmacokinetic interaction with atazanavir (possible altered oral absorption of atazanavir at increased gastric pH, resulting in decreased plasma atazanavir concentrations). Concomitant use of omeprazole 40 mg once daily and atazanavir (with or without low-dose ritonavir) results in a substantial decrease in plasma concentrations of atazanavir and possible loss of the therapeutic effect of the antiretroviral agent. The manufacturer of lansoprazole states that concomitant administration with atazanavir is not recommended. If atazanavir is administered in an antiretroviral treatment-naive patient receiving a proton-pump inhibitor, a *ritonavir-boosted* regimen of 300 mg of atazanavir once daily with ritonavir 100 mg once daily with food is recommended. The dose of the proton-pump inhibitor should be administered approximately 12 hours before *ritonavir-boosted* atazanavir; the dose of the proton-pump inhibitor should not exceed omeprazole 20 mg daily (or equivalent). Concomitant use of proton-pump inhibitors with atazanavir is not recommended in antiretroviral treatment-experienced patients.

Fosamprenavir

Concomitant use of esomeprazole with fosamprenavir (with or without ritonavir) did not substantially affect concentrations of amprenavir (active metabolite of fosamprenavir). No dosage adjustment is required when proton-pump inhibitors are used concomitantly with fosamprenavir (with or without ritonavir).

Lopinavir

Concomitant use of omeprazole with the fixed combination of lopinavir and ritonavir (lopinavir/ritonavir) did not have a clinically important effect on plasma concentrations or area under the concentration-time curve (AUC) of lopinavir. No dosage adjustment is required when proton-pump inhibitors are used concomitantly with lopinavir/ritonavir.

Raltegravir

Pharmacokinetic interaction with omeprazole (substantially increased peak plasma concentration and AUC of raltegravir); however, no dosage adjustment is recommended when proton-pump inhibitors are used concomitantly with raltegravir.

Rilpivirine

Pharmacokinetic interaction with omeprazole (decreased plasma concentrations and AUC of rilpivirine). Concomitant use of other proton-pump inhibitors also may result in decreased plasma concentrations of rilpivirine. Concomitant use of rilpivirine and proton-pump inhibitors is contraindicated.

Saquinavir

Potential pharmacokinetic interaction (increased peak plasma concentration and AUC of saquinavir). Concomitant use of omeprazole 40 mg once daily and *ritonavir-boosted* saquinavir (saquinavir 1 g twice daily and ritonavir 100 mg twice daily) increased the peak plasma concentration and AUC of saquinavir by 75 and 82%, respectively. Caution is advised if proton-pump inhibitors are used concomitantly with *ritonavir-boosted* saquinavir, and patients should be monitored for saquinavir toxicity.

● Clopidogrel

Potential pharmacokinetic interaction (decreased plasma concentration of the active metabolite of clopidogrel) and pharmacodynamic interaction (reduced antiplatelet effects) between proton-pump inhibitors and clopidogrel. Clopidogrel is metabolized to its active metabolite by CYP2C19. Concurrent use of omeprazole or esomeprazole, which inhibit CYP2C19, with clopidogrel reduces exposure to the active metabolite of clopidogrel and decreases platelet inhibitory effects. Although the clinical importance has not been fully elucidated, a reduction in the effectiveness of clopidogrel in preventing cardiovascular events is possible. Proton-pump inhibitors vary in their potency for inhibiting CYP2C19. The change in inhibition of adenosine diphosphate (ADP)-induced platelet aggregation associated with concomitant use of proton-pump inhibitors is related to the change in exposure to the active metabolite of clopidogrel. In pharmacokinetic and pharmacodynamic studies in healthy individuals, concomitant use of dexlansoprazole, lansoprazole, or pantoprazole had less effect on the antiplatelet activity of clopidogrel than did concomitant use of omeprazole or esomeprazole. In individuals who were extensive metabolizers of CYP2C19 substrates, use of lansoprazole (30 mg once daily) concomitantly with clopidogrel (75 mg once daily) for 9 days reduced exposure to the active metabolite of clopidogrel by about 14% compared with use of clopidogrel alone. The observed effects of lansoprazole on metabolite exposure and clopidogrel-induced platelet inhibition were not considered clinically important, and the manufacturer of lansoprazole states that no adjustment of clopidogrel dosage is necessary if clopidogrel is used concomitantly with recommended dosages of lansoprazole.

The decision to use a proton-pump inhibitor concomitantly with clopidogrel should be based on the assessed risks and benefits in individual patients. The American College of Cardiology Foundation/American College of Gastroenterology/American Heart Association (ACCF/ACG/AHA) states that the reduction in GI bleeding risk with proton-pump inhibitors is substantial in patients with risk factors for GI bleeding (e.g., advanced age; concomitant use of warfarin, corticosteroids, or nonsteroidal anti-inflammatory agents [NSAIAs]; *H. pylori* infection) and may outweigh any potential reduction in the cardiovascular efficacy of antiplatelet treatment associated with a drug-drug interaction. In contrast, ACCF/ACG/AHA states that patients without such risk factors receive little if any absolute risk reduction from proton-pump inhibitor therapy, and the risk/benefit balance may favor use of antiplatelet therapy without a proton-pump inhibitor in these patients.

If concomitant therapy with a proton-pump inhibitor and clopidogrel is considered necessary, use of an agent with little or no CYP2C19-inhibitory activity

should be considered. Alternatively, treatment with a histamine H_2-receptor antagonist (ranitidine, famotidine, nizatidine) may be considered, although such agents may not be as effective as a proton-pump inhibitor in providing gastric protection; cimetidine should *not* be used since it also is a potent CYP2C19 inhibitor. There currently is no evidence that histamine H_2-receptor antagonists (other than cimetidine) or other drugs that reduce gastric acid (e.g., antacids) interfere with the antiplatelet effects of clopidogrel. For further information on interactions between proton-pump inhibitors and clopidogrel, see Drug Interactions: Proton-Pump Inhibitors, in Clopidogrel Bisulfate 20:12.18.

● Digoxin

Hypomagnesemia (e.g., resulting from long-term use of proton-pump inhibitors) sensitizes the myocardium to digoxin and, thus, may increase the risk of digoxin-induced cardiotoxic effects. In patients receiving digoxin, monitoring of magnesium concentrations should be considered prior to initiation of prescription proton-pump inhibitor therapy and periodically thereafter.

● Methotrexate

Potential pharmacokinetic interaction (increased serum methotrexate concentrations, possibly resulting in toxicity) when proton-pump inhibitors, including lansoprazole, are used concomitantly with methotrexate. Increased serum concentrations and delayed clearance of methotrexate and/or its metabolite hydroxymethotrexate, with or without symptoms of methotrexate toxicity, have been reported in patients receiving methotrexate (usually at doses of 300 mg/m^2 to 12 g/m^2) concomitantly with a proton-pump inhibitor. Although most of the reported cases occurred in patients receiving high doses of methotrexate, toxicity also has been reported in patients receiving low dosages of methotrexate (e.g., 15 mg per week) concomitantly with a proton-pump inhibitor. In patients with rheumatoid arthritis receiving low-dose methotrexate (7.5–15 mg weekly), concomitant use of lansoprazole (30 mg daily) and naproxen (500 mg twice daily) for 7 days had no effect on the pharmacokinetics of methotrexate or 7-hydroxymethotrexate. However, no formal studies of interactions between high-dose methotrexate and proton-pump inhibitors have been conducted to date.

The manufacturer of lansoprazole states that temporary discontinuance of proton-pump inhibitor therapy may be considered in some patients receiving high-dose methotrexate therapy. Some clinicians recommend either withholding proton-pump inhibitor therapy for several days before and after methotrexate administration or substituting a histamine H_2-receptor antagonist for the proton-pump inhibitor when acid suppressive therapy is indicated during methotrexate therapy. Pending further evaluation, some clinicians state that these recommendations should extend to patients receiving low-dose methotrexate.

● Sucralfate

Potential pharmacokinetic interaction. Concomitant administration of lansoprazole with sucralfate resulted in delayed absorption and decreased (by 17%) bioavailability of lansoprazole. Lansoprazole should be administered at least 30 minutes before sucralfate.

● Tacrolimus

Potential pharmacokinetic interaction (increased whole blood concentrations of tacrolimus), particularly in transplant patients who are intermediate or poor metabolizers of CYP2C19 substrates.

● Theophylline

Potential pharmacokinetic interaction. Concomitant administration of theophylline and lansoprazole may result in a slight (10%) increase in theophylline clearance. The interaction is unlikely to be clinically important, although some patients may require adjustment of theophylline dosage when lansoprazole therapy is initiated or discontinued.

● Warfarin

When warfarin was administered concomitantly with single or multiple doses of lansoprazole 60 mg in healthy individuals, the pharmacokinetics of warfarin and the prothrombin time were not altered; however, increased international normalized ratio (INR) and prothrombin time have been reported in patients receiving warfarin concomitantly with proton-pump inhibitors, including lansoprazole.

The INR and prothrombin time may need to be monitored when lansoprazole is used concomitantly with warfarin.

DESCRIPTION

Lansoprazole is a substituted benzimidazole gastric antisecretory agent. Lansoprazole is structurally and pharmacologically related to dexlansoprazole, esomeprazole, omeprazole, pantoprazole, and rabeprazole; lansoprazole differs structurally from omeprazole by the presence of a trifluoroethoxy group in position 4 of the pyridine ring and the absence of methyl and methoxy groups on the pyridine and benzimidazole rings, respectively. The drugs are chemically and pharmacologically unrelated to H_2-receptor antagonists, antimuscarinics, or prostaglandin analogs. Lansoprazole is a racemic mixture of R- and S-isomers. Both isomers inhibit hydrogen/potassium adenosine triphosphatase (H^+K^+-exchanging ATPase), but plasma clearance of the R-isomer (dexlansoprazole) is slower than that of the S-isomer; following oral administration of racemic lansoprazole, plasma concentrations of the R-isomer are markedly higher than those of the S-isomer.

Lansoprazole binds to H^+K^+-exchanging ATPase in gastric parietal cells; inactivation of this enzyme system (also known as the proton, hydrogen, or acid pump) blocks the final step in the secretion of hydrochloric acid by these cells. Therefore, gastric antisecretory agents such as lansoprazole are commonly referred to as acid- or proton-pump inhibitors. Lansoprazole, a weak base, does not directly inhibit this enzyme system, but instead, it concentrates under the acid conditions of the parietal cell secretory canaliculi, where the drug undergoes rearrangement to active sulfenamide metabolites; these active metabolites then react with the sulfhydryl groups of H^+K^+-exchanging ATPase inactivating the proton pump. Because the sulfenamide metabolites form an irreversible covalent bond to H^+K^+-exchanging ATPase, acid secretion is inhibited until additional enzyme is synthesized, resulting in a prolonged duration of action.

Lansoprazole inhibits basal and stimulated gastric acid secretion; in addition, because the drug inhibits the final step in the secretory pathway, it inhibits such secretion regardless of the stimulus. The degree of inhibition of gastric acid secretion is related to the dose and duration of therapy, but lansoprazole is a more potent inhibitor of such secretion than are H_2-receptor antagonists. Following oral administration of 15 or 30 mg of lansoprazole, inhibition of gastric acid secretion is apparent within 2–3 or 1–2 hours, respectively. After multiple daily doses, increased gastric pH is apparent within 1 hour of administration of 30 mg of lansoprazole and within 1–2 hours after administration of 15 mg of the drug.

Although lansoprazole has a short terminal plasma half-life, the drug has a long duration of action (secondary to the prolonged presence of active lansoprazole metabolites within the parietal cell where they bind to H^+K^+-exchanging ATPase). Following continuous oral administration of 15 or 30 mg of lansoprazole, the percent of time during a 24-hour period that the gastric pH exceeds 4 is 49 or 66%, respectively. Inhibition of basal gastric secretion is 71% after an initial oral dose of 30 mg and 80% or greater after 7 days of oral administration of 30 mg of lansoprazole daily. Stimulated gastric secretion initially is reduced 81% after an oral dose of 30 mg of lansoprazole and gastric secretion is reduced 88% after 7 days of oral administration of 30 mg of lansoprazole daily. Oral administration of lansoprazole 60 mg produced almost complete inhibition of gastric acid secretion in some patients. Following discontinuance of lansoprazole therapy, gastric acid secretion returns to baseline over a 2- to 4-day period, without rebound gastric acidity.

The degree of inhibition of gastric acid secretion is similar following oral or IV administration (a parenteral formulation no longer is commercially available in the US) of lansoprazole 30 mg daily for 7 days in healthy individuals. Following oral or IV administration of the drug, the percent of time during a 24-hour period that the gastric pH exceeds 4 is about 67 or 71%, respectively, after an initial dose of 30 mg and about 78 or 80%, respectively, after 5 days of administration of lansoprazole 30 mg daily in healthy individuals.

Lansoprazole increases plasma gastrin concentrations; this increase occurs in response to a negative feedback mechanism resulting from decreased gastric acid secretion. Although a single oral dose of 30 mg of lansoprazole did not affect serum gastrin levels in healthy adults, patients with gastric ulcer receiving 30–60 mg of lansoprazole once daily for 2 months developed a 50–100% increase from baseline in median fasting serum gastrin concentration; however, median serum gastrin levels remained within the normal range. Serum gastrin concentrations reach a plateau within 2 months of lansoprazole therapy and return to pretreatment values within 1–12 weeks after discontinuing therapy with the drug. Although marked hypergastrinemia with subsequent enterochromaffin-like (ECL) cell proliferation and carcinoid lesions have been observed in animal studies, no evidence of similar ECL cell effects were observed in patients receiving the drug for periods of at least one year. Longer-term study and experience are needed to rule out the possibility of an increased risk of gastric tumors in patients receiving prolonged lansoprazole therapy.

Lansoprazole also decreases pepsin secretion and activity and increases serum pepsinogen; however, these effects are not as pronounced as the drug's inhibition of gastric acid secretion. Suppression of pepsin activity appears to be secondary to increased gastric pH, as conversion of the inactive precursor pepsinogen to pepsin requires an acidic gastric milieu. Pepsin output is inhibited in healthy adults receiving 30 mg of lansoprazole daily for 7 days in the morning or evening by 42–58 or 67–88%, respectively. When the dose is increased to 60 mg daily, no additional inhibition of pepsin secretion is observed. Pepsin activity also is inhibited by lansoprazole 30 mg daily administered in the morning or evening by 23 or 35%, respectively. Lansoprazole also substantially prolongs gastric emptying of digestible solids, but does not appear to affect lower esophageal sphincter pressure.

Lansoprazole can suppress *Helicobacter pylori* (formerly *Campylobacter pylori* or *C. pyloridis*) in patients with gastric or duodenal ulcers infected with the organism. Combined therapy with lansoprazole and one or more appropriate anti-infectives (e.g., amoxicillin, clarithromycin) can effectively eradicate *H. pylori* gastric infection. (See Duodenal Ulcer: Acute Therapy, in Uses.)

Lansoprazole is extensively metabolized in the liver. Cytochrome P-450 (CYP) isoenzymes 2C19 and 3A4 are involved in the metabolism of the drug. Following single-dose oral administration of lansoprazole, approximately one-third of the administered dose is eliminated in urine and two-thirds in feces; unchanged drug is not recovered in urine.

Therapy with proton-pump inhibitors, particularly in high dosages and/or for prolonged periods of time, may be associated with an increased risk of osteoporosis-related fractures of the hip, wrist, or spine. (See Musculoskeletal Effects under Cautions: Warnings/Precautions.) The mechanism by which these drugs may increase risk of such fractures has not been elucidated but may involve decreased insoluble calcium absorption secondary to increased gastric pH.

ADVICE TO PATIENTS

Importance of instructing patients regarding proper administration of delayed-release oral preparations (see Oral Administration under Dosage and Administration: Administration). Necessity of swallowing the preparation without crushing or chewing the delayed-release granules. Importance of administering lansoprazole delayed-release oral preparations before eating.

Importance of advising patients that use of multiple daily doses of the drug for an extended period of time may increase the risk of fractures of the hip, wrist, or spine.

Risk of hypomagnesemia; importance of advising patients to immediately report and seek care for any cardiovascular or neurologic manifestations (e.g., palpitations, dizziness, seizures, tetany).

Advise patients that *self-medication* with lansoprazole is not intended for immediate relief of heartburn; the drug may relieve symptoms within 24 hours, but 1–4 days may be required for complete relief.

Importance of not using lansoprazole for *self-medication* for longer than 14 days of *continuous* use and of not exceeding one course of therapy every 4 months unless otherwise directed by a clinician. Advise patients to discontinue use of lansoprazole as *self-medication* and to consult a clinician if their heartburn persists or worsens or if they need to use the drug for longer than 14 days or require more than one course of therapy every 4 months.

Advise patients to consult a clinician before using lansoprazole for *self-medication* if they have liver disease, have had heartburn for longer than 3 months, or are experiencing heartburn with lightheadedness, dizziness, or sweating; chest or shoulder pain with shortness of breath, sweating, lightheadedness, or pain spreading to the arms, neck, or shoulders; frequent chest pain; frequent wheezing (especially with heartburn); unexplained weight loss; nausea or vomiting; or stomach pain. Advise patients with difficulty or pain with swallowing, those vomiting blood, and those with bloody or blackened stools that they should not use lansoprazole for *self-medication* and should consult a clinician.

Possible increased risk of *Clostridium difficile* infection; importance of contacting a clinician if persistent watery stools, abdominal pain, and fever occur.

Importance of informing clinicians of existing or contemplated concomitant therapy, including prescription and OTC drugs, as well as any concomitant illnesses. Antacid administration is permissible with lansoprazole delayed-release preparations.

Importance of informing patients with phenylketonuria that lansoprazole delayed-release orally disintegrating tablets contain aspartame.

Importance of women informing clinicians if they are or plan to become pregnant or plan to breast-feed.

Importance of informing patients of other important precautionary information. (See Cautions.)

PREPARATIONS

Excipients in commercially available drug preparations may have clinically important effects in some individuals; consult specific product labeling for details.

Lansoprazole

Oral		
Capsules, delayed-release (containing enteric-coated granules)	15 mg*	Lansoprazole Delayed-Release Capsules
		Prevacid®, Takeda
		Prevacid® 24HR, Novartis
	30 mg*	Lansoprazole Delayed-Release Capsules
		Prevacid®, Takeda
Tablets, delayed-release (containing enteric-coated microgranules), orally disintegrating	15 mg	Prevacid® SoluTab®, Takeda
	30 mg	Prevacid® SoluTab®, Takeda

* available from one or more manufacturer, distributor, and/or repackager by generic (nonproprietary) name

Lansoprazole Combinations

Oral		
Kit	4 Capsules, Amoxicillin (trihydrate) 500 mg (of amoxicillin)	Prevpac®, Takeda
	2 Capsules, delayed-release (containing enteric-coated granules), Lansoprazole, 30 mg (Prevacid®)	
	2 Tablets, film-coated, Clarithromycin, 500 mg (Biaxin® Filmtab®)	

† Use is not currently included in the labeling approved by the US Food and Drug Administration.

Omeprazole
Omeprazole Magnesium

56:28.36 • PROTON-PUMP INHIBITORS

■ Omeprazole, commonly referred to as an acid- or proton-pump inhibitor, is a gastric antisecretory agent.

USES

Omeprazole is used in adults for the short-term treatment of active duodenal and benign gastric ulcer. Omeprazole also is used in combination with clarithromycin (dual therapy) or with amoxicillin and clarithromycin (triple therapy) for the treatment of *Helicobacter pylori* infection and duodenal ulcer disease in adults. Omeprazole also has been used in other multiple-drug regimens (with or without clarithromycin)† for the treatment of *H. pylori* infection associated with peptic ulcer disease. Omeprazole is used in adults and children 1 year of age and older for short-term treatment and symptomatic relief of gastroesophageal reflux disease (e.g., erosive esophagitis, heartburn) and as maintenance therapy following healing of erosive esophagitis to reduce its recurrence. The drug also is used as *self-medication* for short-term treatment and symptomatic relief of frequent heartburn in adults. Omeprazole is used for the long-term treatment of pathologic GI hypersecretory conditions in adults. Omeprazole also is used to decrease the risk of upper GI bleeding in critically ill adults.

● Duodenal Ulcer
Acute Therapy

Omeprazole immediate- and delayed-release capsules, omeprazole immediate-release oral suspension, and omeprazole magnesium delayed-release oral suspension are used in adults for the short-term treatment of endoscopically or radiographically confirmed active duodenal ulcer. Antacids may be used concomitantly as needed for pain relief. In controlled studies in patients with endoscopically confirmed duodenal ulcers, reported rates of ulcer healing for omeprazole were substantially higher than those for placebo. In a multicenter, double-blind study in patients with endoscopically confirmed duodenal ulcer, reported rates of ulcer healing for an oral omeprazole dosage of 20 mg each morning or placebo were 41 or 13%, respectively, at 2 weeks and 75 or 27%, respectively, at 4 weeks. Omeprazole also produced greater reductions in daytime and nocturnal pain and antacid consumption than did placebo, with complete relief of pain in most patients usually occurring within 4 weeks after initiation of omeprazole therapy.

Omeprazole appears to be at least as effective as histamine H_2-receptor antagonists for short-term treatment of active duodenal ulcer. In a multicenter, controlled study in patients with endoscopically confirmed duodenal ulcers, 42 or 34% of ulcers were healed following oral administration of omeprazole 20 mg each morning or ranitidine 150 mg twice daily, respectively, for 2 weeks and 82 or 63%, respectively, were healed after 4 weeks of therapy. In another multicenter, controlled study in patients with endoscopically confirmed duodenal ulcers, ulcer healing occurred faster in patients given omeprazole 20 or 40 mg daily compared with patients given ranitidine 150 mg twice daily. Ulcer healing rates averaged 83 or 53% at 2 weeks, 97–100 or 82% at 4 weeks, and 100 or 94% at 8 weeks with the omeprazole regimens or ranitidine 150 mg twice daily, respectively. In several studies, ulcer healing was less likely in patients who were smokers and in those with large ulcers than in other patients.

Most patients with duodenal ulcer respond to omeprazole therapy during the initial 4-week course of therapy; an additional 4 weeks of therapy may contribute to healing in some patients.

Omeprazole delayed-release capsules and omeprazole magnesium delayed-release oral suspension are used in combination with clarithromycin and amoxicillin (triple therapy) for the treatment of *H. pylori* infection and duodenal ulcer disease in adults. Omeprazole delayed-release capsules and omeprazole magnesium delayed-release oral suspension also are used in combination with clarithromycin (dual therapy) in adults for the treatment of *H. pylori* infection and duodenal ulcer disease. Omeprazole also has been used in other multiple-drug regimens† for the treatment of *H. pylori* infection associated with peptic ulcer disease. Current epidemiologic and clinical evidence supports a strong association

between gastric infection with *H. pylori* and the pathogenesis of duodenal and gastric ulcers; long-term *H. pylori* infection also has been implicated as a risk factor for gastric cancer. For additional information on the association of this infection with these and other GI conditions, see Helicobacter pylori Infection, under Uses, in Clarithromycin 8:12.12.92. Conventional antiulcer therapy with histamine H_2-receptor antagonists, proton-pump inhibitors, sucralfate, and/or antacids heals ulcers but generally is ineffective in eradicating *H. pylori*, and such therapy is associated with a high rate of ulcer recurrence (e.g., 60–100% per year). The American College of Gastroenterology (ACG), the National Institutes of Health (NIH), and most clinicians currently recommend that *all* patients with initial or recurrent duodenal or gastric ulcer and documented *H. pylori* infection receive anti-infective therapy for treatment of the infection. Although 3-drug regimens consisting of a bismuth salt (e.g., bismuth subsalicylate) and 2 anti-infective agents (e.g., tetracycline or amoxicillin plus metronidazole) administered for 10–14 days have been effective in eradicating the infection, resolving associated gastritis, healing peptic ulcer, and preventing ulcer recurrence in many patients with *H. pylori*-associated peptic ulcer disease, current evidence principally from studies in Europe suggests that 1 week of such therapy provides comparable *H. pylori* eradication rates. Other regimens that combine one or more anti-infective agents (e.g., clarithromycin, amoxicillin) with a bismuth salt and/or an antisecretory agent (e.g., omeprazole, lansoprazole, histamine H_2-receptor antagonist) also have been used successfully for *H. pylori* eradication, and the choice of a particular regimen should be based on the rapidly evolving data on optimal therapy, including consideration of the patient's prior exposure to anti-infective agents, the local prevalence of resistance, patient compliance, and costs of therapy.

Current evidence suggests that inclusion of a proton-pump inhibitor (e.g., omeprazole, lansoprazole) in anti-*H. pylori* regimens containing 2 anti-infectives enhances effectiveness, and limited data suggest that such regimens retain good efficacy despite imidazole (e.g., metronidazole) resistance. Therefore, the ACG and many clinicians currently recommend 1 week of therapy with a proton-pump inhibitor and 2 anti-infective agents (usually clarithromycin and amoxicillin or metronidazole), or a 3-drug, bismuth-based regimen (e.g., bismuth-metronidazole-tetracycline) concomitantly with a proton-pump inhibitor, for treatment of *H. pylori* infection.

Therapy with an antisecretory drug and a single anti-infective agent (i.e., "dual therapy") also has been used successfully for treatment of *H. pylori* infection. However, while some studies demonstrate that certain 2-drug anti-*H. pylori* regimens (e.g., clarithromycin-omeprazole, ranitidine bismuth citrate-omeprazole, amoxicillin-omeprazole) can successfully eradicate *H. pylori* infection and prevent recurrence of duodenal ulcer at least in the short term (e.g., at 6 months following completion of anti-*H. pylori* therapy), the ACG and some clinicians currently state that anti-*H. pylori* regimens consisting of at least 3 drugs (e.g., 2 anti-infective agents plus a proton-pump inhibitor) are recommended because of enhanced *H. pylori* eradication rates, decreased failures due to resistance, and shorter treatment periods compared with those apparently required with 2-drug regimens. Additional randomized, controlled studies comparing various anti-*H. pylori* regimens are needed to clarify optimum drug combinations, dosages, and durations of treatment for *H. pylori* infection. For a more complete discussion of *H. pylori* infection, including details about the efficacy of various regimens and rationale for drug selection, see Uses: Helicobacter pylori Infection, in Clarithromycin 8:12.12.92.

● Gastric Ulcer
Acute Therapy

Omeprazole immediate- and delayed-release capsules, omeprazole immediate-release oral suspension, and omeprazole magnesium delayed-release oral suspension are used in adults for the short-term treatment and symptomatic relief of active benign gastric ulcer. In controlled studies in patients with endoscopically confirmed gastric ulcers, reported rates of ulcer healing with omeprazole therapy were substantially higher than those with placebo. In a multicenter, double-blind study in patients with endoscopically confirmed gastric ulcer, reported rates of ulcer healing with omeprazole 20 or 40 mg daily or placebo were 48, 56, or 31%, respectively, at 4 weeks and 75, 83, or 48%, respectively, at 8 weeks. In patients with an ulcer larger than 1 cm in size, the percentage of patients with healed ulcers at 8 weeks was greater with the 40-mg dosage than with the 20-mg dosage of omeprazole. Otherwise, for patients with smaller ulcers, no difference in ulcer healing rates between the 40- and 20-mg dosages was observed.

In a multicenter, comparative study in patients with endoscopically confirmed gastric ulcer, ulcer healing occurred at 4 weeks in 64 or 78% of patients receiving omeprazole 20 or 40 mg daily, respectively, compared with 56% of those receiving ranitidine 150 mg twice daily; at 8 weeks, 82, 91, or 78% of patients receiving omeprazole 20 mg daily, omeprazole 40 mg daily, or ranitidine 150 mg twice daily, respectively, had healed ulcers.

● *Crohn's Disease-associated Ulcers*

Although evidence currently is limited, proton-pump inhibitors have been used for gastric acid-suppressive therapy as an adjunct in the symptomatic treatment of upper GI Crohn's disease†, including esophageal, gastroduodenal, and jejunoileal disease. The drugs have been used for symptomatic relief of upper GI symptoms and to promote healing of Crohn's disease-associated peptic ulcer disease. Most evidence of efficacy to date has been from case studies in patients with Crohn's-associated peptic ulcer disease unresponsive to other therapies (e.g., histamine H_2-receptor antagonists, cytoprotective agents, antacids, and/or sucralfate). Omeprazole (20 or 40 mg daily) was associated with resolution of symptoms and ulcer healing within about 2 and 4 weeks, respectively, in some patients, while others required several months of acid-suppressive therapy. Subsequent symptomatic relief may be maintained with prolonged acid-suppressive therapy with a proton-pump inhibitor or H_2-receptor antagonist, with or without an immunosuppressive agent (e.g., azathioprine). Adjunctive inhibition of gastric acid secretion is likely to be more effective in promoting ulcer healing in Crohn's disease than corticosteroid therapy. Pending accumulation of more definitive evidence, some experts and clinicians state that therapy with a proton-pump inhibitor may be a useful adjunct to provide symptomatic relief and promote ulcer healing in patients with upper GI Crohn's disease.

For further information on the management of Crohn's Disease, see Uses: Crohn's Disease, in Mesalamine 56:36.

● *Gastroesophageal Reflux*

Omeprazole delayed-release capsules and omeprazole magnesium delayed-release oral suspension are used in adults and children 1 year of age and older, and omeprazole immediate-release capsules and immediate-release oral suspension are used in adults for the short-term treatment and symptomatic relief of gastroesophageal reflux disease (GERD) (e.g., erosive esophagitis, heartburn) and as maintenance therapy following healing of erosive esophagitis to prevent its recurrence. Safety and efficacy of omeprazole immediate-release capsules and immediate-release oral suspension have not been established in pediatric patients. Omeprazole magnesium delayed-release capsules are used in adults as *self-medication* for the short-term treatment and symptomatic relief of frequent heartburn.

GERD is considered to be a chronic disease, and many patients with GERD require long-term, even lifelong, treatment. Typical GERD symptoms include heartburn and/or regurgitation, often occurring after meals, especially large and/or fatty meals. The symptoms often are aggravated by recumbency or bending, and are relieved by antacids. GERD symptoms generally are controlled by appropriate medical therapy. Suppression of gastric acid secretion is considered by the ACG to be the mainstay of treatment for GERD, and a proton-pump inhibitor or histamine H_2-receptor antagonist is used to achieve acid suppression, control symptoms, and prevent complications of the disease. The ACG states that proton-pump inhibitors are more effective than histamine H_2-receptor antagonists for acute therapy of GERD and also are appropriate as maintenance therapy in many patients with the disease. Lifestyle modifications (e.g., elevation of the head of the bed, decreased dietary fat intake, smoking cessation, avoidance of recumbency for 3 hours after a meal, avoidance of foods that increase reflux, weight loss) should be initiated and continued throughout the course of treatment.

Acute Therapy

Omeprazole delayed-release capsules and omeprazole magnesium delayed-release oral suspension are used in adults and children 1 year of age and older, and omeprazole immediate-release capsules and immediate-release oral suspension are used in adults for the short-term (4–8 weeks) treatment of endoscopically diagnosed erosive esophagitis in patients with GERD. Omeprazole delayed-release capsules and omeprazole magnesium delayed-release oral suspension are used in adults and children 1 year of age and older, and omeprazole immediate-release capsules and immediate-release oral suspension are used in adults for the short-term (4–8 weeks) treatment of symptomatic GERD (e.g., heartburn). Potential benefits of omeprazole in gastroesophageal reflux and esophagitis are thought to result principally from reduced acidity of gastric contents induced by the drug and resultant reduced irritation of esophageal mucosa; the drug can effectively relieve symptoms of esophagitis (e.g., heartburn) and promote healing of ulcerative and erosive lesions.

Drug Selection Considerations

The ACG states that proton-pump inhibitors are more effective (i.e., provide more frequent and more rapid symptomatic relief and healing of esophagitis) than histamine H_2-receptor antagonists in the treatment of GERD. Although higher doses and more frequent administration of histamine H_2-receptor antagonists appear to increase their efficacy, such dosages are less effective than proton-pump inhibitor therapy. In addition, the ACG states that proton-pump inhibitors provide greater control of acid reflux than do prokinetic agents (e.g., cisapride [no longer commercially available in the US], metoclopramide) without the risk of severe adverse effects associated with these agents. Correction of esophageal and gastric motility defects that cause GERD might theoretically control the disease and make suppression of normal gastric acid secretion unnecessary, and prokinetic agents have been used in the treatment of GERD. However, cisapride was withdrawn from the US market because of its association with serious cardiac arrhythmias and death (see Cisapride 56:32), and metoclopramide frequently is associated with adverse CNS effects (e.g., restlessness, drowsiness, fatigue, lassitude). The ACG states that the frequent occurrence of adverse CNS effects has appropriately decreased regular use of metoclopramide for treatment of GERD. Cisapride or metoclopramide therapy appears to provide symptomatic relief and esophageal healing as effectively as a standard dosage of a histamine H_2-receptor antagonist, and improved efficacy has been reported when a prokinetic agent has been used in combination with a histamine H_2-receptor antagonist. Bethanechol, a cholinergic drug that increases GI motility, may increase lower esophageal sphincter pressure to a small degree, but the ACG states that the drug has limited efficacy in the treatment of GERD.

The ACG states that a histamine H_2-receptor antagonist administered daily in divided doses is effective in many patients with less severe GERD, and over-the-counter (OTC) antacids and histamine H_2-receptor antagonists are appropriate for *self-medication* as initial therapy in such individuals. A histamine H_2-receptor antagonist is particularly useful when taken before certain activities (e.g., heavy meal, exercise) that may result in acid reflux symptoms in some patients.

Other Considerations

The ACG states that initial empiric therapy including suppression of gastric acid secretion and lifestyle modification is appropriate for patients with typical symptoms of uncomplicated GERD, and a diagnosis of GERD is reasonably assumed in those who respond to such therapy. Diagnostic testing (e.g., endoscopy, endoscopic biopsy, ambulatory pH testing, esophageal manometry) may be indicated when empiric drug therapy is unsuccessful, continuous medical therapy is required for symptomatic relief, chronic symptoms occur in patients at risk for esophageal metaplasia (e.g., Barrett's epithelium), or manifestations suggestive of complicated disease (e.g., dysphagia, bleeding, weight loss, choking [acid causing cough, shortness of breath, or hoarseness], chest pain) occur. In patients with symptoms refractory to empiric drug therapy, the diagnosis of GERD should be carefully confirmed with diagnostic testing before chronic, high-dose acid-suppression therapy or antireflux surgery is undertaken. Higher dosage and a longer therapeutic trial of a gastric antisecretory agent may be required in patients with atypical or extraesophageal symptoms (e.g., chronic chest pain, cough, hoarseness, asthma, dental erosions).

Clinical Trials

In a controlled study in patients with manifestations of GERD (e.g., heartburn) and the absence of erosive esophageal lesions, symptomatic improvement with omeprazole was better than that with placebo. Complete resolution of heartburn was reported in 56, 36, or 14% of patients with endoscopically confirmed GERD and in 46, 31, or 13% of all enrolled patients after up to 4 weeks of therapy with omeprazole 20 mg daily, omeprazole 10 mg daily, or placebo, respectively.

In an uncontrolled, open-label study of 113 pediatric patients 2–16 years of age with a history of symptoms suggestive of nonerosive GERD, patients received an omeprazole dosage of 10 or 20 mg once daily (based on body weight) either as an intact capsule or as an open capsule in applesauce. The number and intensity of either pain-related symptoms or vomiting/regurgitation episodes was successfully reduced in 60 or 59% of those receiving omeprazole 10 or 20 mg, respectively. In another uncontrolled study in 12 children 1–2 years of age with a history of clinically diagnosed GERD, administration of omeprazole (0.5–1.5 mg/kg as an opened capsule in 8.4% sodium bicarbonate solution) for 8 weeks reduced episodes of vomiting/regurgitation from baseline by at least 50% in 9 patients (75%).

In controlled studies in patients with endoscopically diagnosed erosive esophagitis and symptoms of GERD, reported rates of healing with omeprazole were higher than those with placebo or an H_2-receptor antagonist. Healing rates from a controlled study were 39, 45, or 7% at 4 weeks and 74, 75, or 14% at 8 weeks for omeprazole 20 mg daily, 40 mg daily, or placebo, respectively. In controlled studies in patients with esophagitis, reported rates of healing were 57–74 or 27–43% at 4 weeks and 78–87 or 28–56% at 8 weeks in patients given omeprazole or ranitidine, respectively. Patients receiving omeprazole reported faster relief of daytime and nocturnal heartburn than those receiving placebo or an H_2-receptor antagonist. Omeprazole also has been shown to be effective in promoting healing and providing symptomatic relief in a substantial proportion of patients who failed to respond to an adequate course of relatively high dosages of an H_2-receptor antagonist.

In an uncontrolled, open-label dose-titration study in 57 pediatric patients aged 1–16 years of age with erosive esophagitis, omeprazole dosages of 0.7–3.5 mg/kg daily were required to promote healing. Dosages were initiated at 0.7 mg/kg daily and if therapeutic goals (intraesophageal pH below 4 for less than 6% of a 24-hour period) were not achieved after 5–14 days of treatment, the dosage was increased to 1.4 mg/kg daily. Based on additional measurements of intraesophageal pH and/ or presence of pathologic acid reflux, the dosages were increased up to a maximum dosage of 3.5 mg/kg or 80 mg daily. After titration of omeprazole dosage, patients remained on treatment for 3 months (healing phase); patients with persistent erosive esophagitis after 3 months received a discretionary dosage increase and treatment for an additional 3 months. Erosive esophagitis was healed in 90% of children completing the first course of treatment in the healing phase of the study; 5% received a second treatment course. Healing occurred in 44% of the patients receiving omeprazole 0.7 mg/kg daily, and an additional 28% were healed with 1.4 mg/kg daily. After 3 months of treatment, 33% of the children had no overall symptoms, 57% had mild reflux symptoms, and 40% had less frequent regurgitation or vomiting.

Most patients with GERD respond to omeprazole therapy during an initial 8-week course of therapy; however, an additional 4 weeks of therapy may contribute to healing and symptomatic improvement in some patients. Short-term omeprazole therapy for the treatment of GERD will not prevent recurrence following discontinuance of the drug. If symptomatic GERD or erosive esophagitis recur, the manufacturers state that additional 4- to 8-week courses of omeprazole may be given. However, the ACG states that chronic therapy with a proton-pump inhibitor is appropriate in many patients with GERD.

Maintenance Therapy

Omeprazole delayed-release capsules and omeprazole magnesium delayed-release oral suspension are used in adults and children 1 year of age and older, and omeprazole immediate-release capsules and immediate-release oral suspension are used in adults as maintenance therapy following healing of erosive esophagitis to reduce recurrence of the disease. In a multicenter, double-blind study, endoscopically documented remission of esophagitis was maintained at 6 months in 70, 34, or 11% of patients receiving omeprazole 20 mg daily, 20 mg on 3 consecutive days each week, or placebo, respectively. In another multicenter, double-blind study in patients with endoscopically confirmed healed esophagitis, endoscopic remission of esophagitis was maintained at 12 months in 77, 58, or 46% of patients receiving omeprazole 20 mg daily, 10 mg daily, or ranitidine 150 mg twice daily, respectively. However, patients with initial grade 3 or 4 erosive esophagitis required 20 mg of omeprazole daily for maintenance of healing.

In an uncontrolled, open-label study in 46 pediatric patients, maintenance dosages were half the dosages that were required for promotion of healing in 54% of the children studied. The remaining patients required a dosage increase (0.7 to a maximum of 2.8 mg/kg daily) for all or part of the maintenance period. There was no relapse of erosive esophagitis in 41% of the patients, and no symptoms occurred in 63% of the pediatric patients receiving omeprazole maintenance therapy.

Because GERD is a chronic condition, the ACG states that continuous therapy to control symptoms and prevent complications of the disease is appropriate, and chronic, even lifelong, use of a proton-pump inhibitor is effective and appropriate as maintenance therapy in many patients with GERD. Although neither medical nor surgical therapy of GERD appears to result in regression of Barrett's epithelium in the esophagus, chronic use of a proton-pump inhibitor at full dosage decreases the recurrence of esophageal strictures, increases the interval between symptomatic relapses, and may improve esophageal motility. In a double-blind, controlled study, antisecretory therapy had no clinically important effect on Barrett's mucosa in 106 patients receiving omeprazole (40 mg twice daily for 12 months, followed by 20 mg twice daily for 12 months) or ranitidine (300 mg twice daily for 24 months). Although neosquamous epithelium developed during antisecretory therapy, complete elimination of Barrett's mucosa was not achieved.

The frequent marked improvement in symptoms associated with full dosage of a proton-pump inhibitor generally is followed by rapid recurrence of symptoms

once the drug is discontinued, and reduced-dosage regimens (e.g., every other day, "weekend" dosage) have not been shown to be consistently effective for maintenance therapy. In addition, many patients initially responding to proton-pump inhibitors experience symptomatic relapse and failure of esophageal healing when switched subsequently to a histamine H_2-receptor antagonist or prokinetic agent (e.g., cisapride, metoclopramide). Furthermore, prokinetic agents have been associated with severe adverse effects. Cisapride has been withdrawn from the US market because of its association with serious cardiac arrhythmias and death (see Cisapride 56:32), and metoclopramide frequently is associated with CNS adverse effects (e.g., restlessness, drowsiness, fatigue, lassitude) and may cause irreversible tardive dyskinesia with prolonged use. Once-daily administration of a histamine H_2-receptor antagonist at full dosage is *not* considered to be appropriate therapy for GERD. Although antacids and lifestyle modifications may provide long-term symptomatic control in up to 20% of patients with GERD, frequent symptomatic relapses may occur despite appropriate therapy in up to 50% of patients with chronic gastroesophageal reflux.

Self-Medication

Omeprazole magnesium delayed-release capsules are used in adults 18 years of age or older as *self-medication* for short-term (14 days) treatment and symptomatic relief of frequent (e.g., 2 or more days a week) heartburn. Because 1–4 days may be required for complete relief of symptoms, omeprazole for *self-medication* is not intended for the immediate relief of heartburn, and other agents (e.g., antacids, histamine H_2-receptor antagonists) may be needed for initial relief. However, some individuals may experience complete relief of symptoms within 24 hours of taking the first dose of omeprazole. In 2 controlled studies, 50% of patients receiving omeprazole 20 mg daily experienced no heartburn during the first day of therapy, and the percentage of patients experiencing complete relief continued to increase in subsequent days; 30% of those receiving placebo experienced no heartburn during the first day of therapy. Omeprazole should not be used for *self-medication* of occasional heartburn (i.e., heartburn that occurs once weekly or less frequently) or for prevention of occasional meal- or beverage-induced heartburn.

● Pathologic GI Hypersecretory Conditions

Omeprazole delayed-release capsules and omeprazole magnesium delayed-release oral suspension are used in adults for the long-term treatment of pathologic GI hypersecretory conditions (e.g., Zollinger-Ellison syndrome, multiple endocrine adenomas, systemic mastocytosis). The drug reduces gastric acid secretion and associated symptoms (including diarrhea, anorexia, and pain) in patients with these conditions. In dosages ranging from 20 mg every other day to 360 mg daily, omeprazole can maintain basal acid secretion below 5 or 10 mEq/hour in patients who have or have not undergone gastric surgery, respectively. In addition, dosages ranging from 20–360 mg daily have been effective in resolving acid-related pathology in most patients with Zollinger-Ellison syndrome, including those whose symptoms were unresponsive to H_2-receptor antagonist therapy.

● Upper GI Bleeding

Omeprazole immediate-release oral suspension is used to decrease the risk of upper GI bleeding in critically ill adults. Efficacy of omeprazole was evaluated in a controlled, double-blind randomized clinical trial in critically ill patients who were randomized to receive either omeprazole immediate-release oral suspension (2 doses of 40 mg 6–8 hours apart on the first day, then 40 mg daily) via a gastric tube or IV cimetidine (300 mg loading dose, then 50–100 mg/hour continuously) for up to 14 days. The primary efficacy end point of the study was clinically important upper GI bleeding (defined as bright red blood that did not clear after tube adjustment and 5–10 minutes of lavage or positive test for occult blood in gastric aspirate ["coffee ground material"] for 8 consecutive hours on days 1 and 2, or for 2–4 hours on days 3–14 that did not clear with 100 mL of lavage). Omeprazole was at least as effective as IV cimetidine in preventing clinically important upper GI bleeding. In the intent-to-treat population, clinically important gastric bleeding occurred in 3.9% of patients receiving omeprazole and in 5.5% of those receiving IV cimetidine.

DOSAGE AND ADMINISTRATION

● Administration

Omeprazole immediate-release and delayed-release capsules and omeprazole magnesium delayed-release tablets for *self-administration* are administered orally; oral suspensions of the drug are administered orally or through a gastric tube. To avoid decomposition of omeprazole in the acidic pH of the stomach, the commercially available delayed-release capsules and delayed-release oral suspension contain enteric-coated granules of the drug, and the immediate-release capsules and immediate-release oral suspension contain sodium bicarbonate.

Omeprazole immediate-release capsules (Zegerid®) are administered orally and must be swallowed intact with water; other liquids should not be used. The capsules should not be opened and mixed with food. Both the 20- and 40-mg capsules contain the same amount of sodium bicarbonate (1100 mg). Therefore, two 20-mg capsules are not equivalent to and should not be substituted for one 40-mg capsule.

Patients should be advised that the delayed-release capsules must be swallowed intact and *not* chewed or crushed. However, for adult and pediatric patients with difficulty swallowing, the delayed-release capsule may be opened, the contents carefully emptied on and mixed with a tablespoon of applesauce in a bowl, and the mixture swallowed immediately with a glass of cool water to ensure complete swallowing of the pellets. The applesauce should not be hot and should be soft enough to be swallowed without chewing. The applesauce and omeprazole enteric-coated pellet mixture should *not* be stored for future use. The manufacturer states that the 40-mg capsule, but not the 20-mg capsule, is bioequivalent when administered with or without applesauce. When the contents of a 20-mg capsule were administered with applesauce, the peak plasma omeprazole concentration decreased by 25%, but the area under the concentration-time curve (AUC) was not substantially changed. However, the clinical importance of this is unknown.

Tablets used for *self-medication* must be swallowed intact with a glass of water; the tablets should *not* be chewed or crushed and should *not* be crushed in food.

Omeprazole magnesium powder for delayed-release oral suspension (Prilosec®) should be reconstituted prior to administration by pouring the contents of a single-dose packet containing 2.5 or 10 mg of the drug into a small cup containing 5 or 15 mL, respectively, of water. The suspension should be stirred well and allowed to thicken for 2–3 minutes. Within 30 minutes of preparation, the mixture should be stirred and consumed. If any material remains in the cup after the mixture is ingested, additional water should be added, mixed, and ingested immediately. If the delayed-release oral suspension is to be administered through a nasogastric or gastric tube, the contents of a 2.5- or 10-mg packet should be mixed with 5 or 15 mL of water, respectively, in a catheter-tipped syringe and then shaken immediately. The mixture should be allowed to thicken for 2–3 minutes. The mixture should be administered within 30 minutes of reconstitution; prior to administration, the syringe should be shaken again and the mixture injected into the stomach through the nasogastric or gastric tube (French size 6 or larger). The syringe should be refilled with additional water (5 or 15 mL, respectively), shaken, and used to flush any remaining drug mixture from the nasogastric or gastric tube into the stomach.

Omeprazole powder for immediate-release oral suspension (Zegerid®) should be reconstituted prior to administration by pouring the contents of a single-dose packet containing 20 or 40 mg of the drug into a small cup containing 15–30 mL of water. The 20- and 40-mg powder for oral suspension packets contain the same amount of sodium bicarbonate (1680 mg). Therefore, two 20-mg packets are not equivalent to and should not be substituted for one 40-mg packet. The suspension should be stirred well and ingested immediately. The cup should be refilled with water and the contents ingested to ensure complete consumption of the dose. The manufacturer states that omeprazole powder for immediate-release oral suspension should not be mixed with any liquids (other than water) or foods. If the oral suspension is to be administered through a nasogastric or orogastric tube, the contents of each packet should be reconstituted with approximately 20 mL of water, stirred well and administered immediately. An appropriate-sized syringe should be used to instill the suspension into the tube. The suspension should then be flushed through the tube with 20 mL of water.

Following administration of delayed-release capsules of omeprazole with meals, the rate of GI absorption is reduced. Therefore, omeprazole should be taken before meals; administration up to 2 minutes prior to a meal reportedly has no adverse effect on oral bioavailability. However, since an acidic environment in the parietal cell canaliculi is required for conversion of proton-pump inhibitors (e.g., omeprazole) to their active sulfenamide metabolites, the American College of Gastroenterology suggests that proton-pump inhibitors are most effective when given about 30 minutes prior to meals; effectiveness may be compromised if these drugs are administered during the basal state (e.g., to fasting patients at bedtime) or concomitantly with other antisecretory agents (e.g., anticholinergics, histamine H₂-receptor antagonists, somatostatin analogs, misoprostol). The manufacturer states that delayed-release preparations of omeprazole should be administered at least 1 hour before a meal. Antacids may be administered concomitantly with the delayed-release preparations of omeprazole.

The manufacturer states that immediate-release preparations of omeprazole (Zegerid®) should be administered on an empty stomach at least 1 hour prior to a meal. For patients receiving continuous feedings via a nasogastric or orogastric tube, enteral feeding should be stopped temporarily for 3 hours before, and for 1 hour after administration of omeprazole immediate-release oral suspension. Also, the manufacturer states that antacids, antacid/alginic acid combinations, histamine H₂-receptor antagonists, or histamine H₂-receptor antagonist and antacid combinations may be used for "breakthrough" symptoms; however, efficacy of these agents for this use has not been established.

Omeprazole usually is administered once daily in the morning; however, administering the drug in divided doses (e.g., every 12 hours) has been reported to improve efficacy in patients receiving more than 80 mg daily.

● Dosage

The manufacturer states that omeprazole dosage adjustments based on age are not necessary in geriatric patients. However, since the bioavailability of omeprazole appears to be increased substantially in Asians, the manufacturer states that dosage adjustment should be considered in Asian patients, especially when such patients are receiving long-term omeprazole therapy for maintenance of healing of erosive esophagitis. There is no evidence from the omeprazole prescription safety database that Asians experience excess risk from omeprazole, or that accumulation of omeprazole in the blood is harmful when used over a short period of time (e.g., 14 days of *self-medication*) in Asian patients.

Dosage of omeprazole magnesium is expressed in terms of omeprazole.

Duodenal Ulcer

For the short-term treatment of active duodenal ulcer, the usual adult dosage of omeprazole is 20 mg once daily. Therapy should be continued until healing occurs, usually within 2–4 weeks; some patients may benefit from an additional 4 weeks of therapy. Occasionally, dosages up to 40 mg daily may be necessary in patients who have been poorly responsive to therapy with H₂-receptor antagonists.

When omeprazole is used in combination with clarithromycin (dual therapy) for the treatment of *Helicobacter pylori* infection in patients with active duodenal ulcer, the usual adult dosage of omeprazole is 40 mg once daily (in the morning) for 14 days. In patients who have an active ulcer present at the time anti-*H. pylori* therapy is initiated, an additional 14 days of therapy with omeprazole 20 mg once daily is recommended for ulcer healing and symptom relief. When omeprazole is used in combination with clarithromycin and amoxicillin (triple therapy) for the treatment of *H. pylori* infection in patients with active duodenal ulcer, the usual adult dosage of omeprazole is 20 mg *twice* daily (morning and evening) for 10 days. In patients who have an active ulcer present at the time anti-*H. pylori* therapy is initiated, an additional 18 days of therapy with omeprazole 20 mg *once* daily is recommended for ulcer healing and symptom relief. Multiple-drug regimens currently recommended by the American College of Gastroenterology (ACG) and many clinicians for the treatment of *H. pylori* infection consist of a proton-pump inhibitor (e.g., omeprazole) and 2 anti-infective agents (e.g., clarithromycin and amoxicillin or metronidazole) or a 3-drug, bismuth-based regimen (e.g., bismuth-metronidazole-tetracycline) concomitantly with a proton-pump inhibitor; when omeprazole has been used in these regimens, dosages of 20 mg once daily to 80 mg twice daily (generally 20 mg twice daily) for 7–28 days have been used. While the minimum duration of therapy required to eradicate *H. pylori* infection with these 3- or 4-drug regimens has not been fully elucidated, the ACG and many clinicians state that treatment for longer than 1 week probably is not necessary. However, more prolonged therapy is recommended for patients with complicated, large, or refractory ulcers; therapy in such patients should be continued at least until successful eradication of *H. pylori* has been confirmed. (See Uses: Helicobacter pylori Infection, in Clarithromycin 8:12.12.92.)

Gastric Ulcer

For the short-term treatment of active benign gastric ulcer, the usual adult dosage of omeprazole is 40 mg once daily for 4–8 weeks.

Gastroesophageal Reflux

For the short-term, symptomatic treatment of gastroesophageal reflux disease (GERD) without erosive esophageal lesions, the usual adult dosage of omeprazole is 20 mg once daily for 4 weeks. For the short-term treatment of erosive esophagitis, the usual adult dosage of omeprazole is 20 mg once daily for 4–8 weeks. Occasionally, dosages up to 40 mg daily may be necessary in some patients. Therapy is continued until healing occurs, usually within 4–8 weeks; an additional 4 weeks of therapy (up to 12 weeks for a single course) may contribute to healing and symptomatic improvement in some patients. If erosive esophagitis or symptomatic

GERD (heartburn) recurs, the manufacturer states that additional 4- to 8-week courses of omeprazole may be considered. However, the American College of Gastroenterology (ACG) states that chronic, even lifelong, therapy with a proton-pump inhibitor is appropriate in many patients with GERD.

For maintenance therapy following healing of erosive esophagitis to reduce recurrence, the usual adult dosage of omeprazole is 20 mg daily. Safety and efficacy of omeprazole maintenance therapy for longer than 1 year have not been established.

For the treatment of symptomatic GERD or erosive esophagitis and for maintenance of healing of erosive esophagitis in pediatric patients 1–16 years of age, a dosage of 5 mg of omeprazole daily is recommended for pediatric patients weighing at least 5 kg but less than 10 kg, 10 mg daily is recommended for those weighing at least 10 kg but less than 20 kg, and 20 mg daily is recommended for those weighing 20 kg or more. Omeprazole was administered as a single daily dose for 4 weeks in one study of children with symptomatic nonerosive GERD. On a mg/kg basis, the dosage of omeprazole required to heal erosive esophagitis in pediatric patients is greater than that required in adults. In an uncontrolled open-label study, dosages of 0.7–3.5 mg/kg daily (up to a maximum dosage of 80 mg daily) for 3–6 months were required for healing in children 1–16 years of age; a dosage of 0.7 mg/kg daily resulted in healing of erosive esophagitis in 44% of children, but a dosage of 1.4 mg/kg daily was required for healing to occur in an additional 28% of the children. In an uncontrolled open-label study of 46 pediatric patients, dosages of omeprazole for maintenance therapy following healing of erosive esophagitis were half those required for initial healing in 54% of children, but the remainder required an increased dosage (0.7 to a maximum of 2.8 mg/kg daily) for all or part of the maintenance period; maintenance therapy was continued for about 2 years.

Self-Medication

For *self-medication* to relieve symptoms of frequent heartburn in adults 18 years of age or older, an omeprazole dosage of 20 mg once daily in the morning for 14 days is recommended. For *self-medication*, the manufacturer recommends that the dosage of omeprazole not exceed 20 mg in 24 hours. In addition, the drug should not be used for *self-medication* for longer than 14 days of *continuous* use and individuals should not exceed one course of therapy every 4 months unless otherwise directed by a clinician.

Pathologic GI Hypersecretory Conditions

For the treatment of pathologic GI hypersecretory conditions (e.g., Zollinger-Ellison syndrome, multiple endocrine adenomas, systemic mastocytosis), dosages of omeprazole should be individualized according to patient response and tolerance. The usual initial adult dosage is 60 mg (as delayed-release capsules or delayed-release oral suspension) once daily. Subsequent omeprazole dosage should be adjusted as tolerated and necessary to adequately suppress gastric acid secretion, and therapy continued as long as clinically necessary. Daily dosages exceeding 80 mg should be administered in divided doses.

Oral dosages ranging from 20 mg every other day to 360 mg daily (given in 3 divided doses) have been necessary to maintain basal gastric acid secretion at less than 10 mEq/hour in patients without a history of gastric surgery and less than 5 mEq/hour in those who have undergone gastric surgery; determination of gastric acid secretion during the hour prior to a dose may be useful in establishing optimum dosage. Omeprazole has been given continuously for more than 5 years in some patients with Zollinger-Ellison syndrome.

Upper GI Bleeding

For reduction of risk of upper GI bleeding in critically ill adults, the initial loading dose of omeprazole is 40 mg (as immediate-release oral suspension) followed by another 40-mg dose after 6–8 hours on the first day; thereafter, 40 mg (as immediate-release oral suspension) is administered once daily for up to 14 days. Safety and efficacy of omeprazole immediate-release oral suspension in critically ill patients for longer than 14 days have not been established.

● *Dosage in Renal and Hepatic Impairment*

Although pharmacokinetics may be altered in patients with renal impairment, dosage adjustment does not appear necessary in patients with such impairment. However, the manufacturers state that dosage adjustment should be considered in patients with hepatic impairment, particularly in such patients receiving long-term omeprazole therapy for maintenance of healing of erosive esophagitis. Some clinicians recommend that such patients with hepatic dysfunction receiving dosages exceeding 20 mg daily should be monitored closely for possible adverse effects.

CAUTIONS

Omeprazole generally is well tolerated. The most frequent adverse effects associated with omeprazole therapy involve the GI tract (e.g., diarrhea, nausea, constipation, abdominal pain, vomiting, flatulence) and the CNS (e.g., headache, dizziness). In short-term studies, the incidence of reported adverse effects was similar in patients receiving omeprazole or placebo. In addition, while the most common effects have been reported in 1–7% of patients receiving omeprazole, they were considered by investigators as being possibly, probably, or definitely related to the drug in only 0.2–2.4% of patients. Overall, the frequency and type of adverse effects produced by omeprazole appear to be similar to those produced by ranitidine, and the frequency of omeprazole-induced effects does not appear to be affected by age in adults. In dose-ranging studies, a relationship between doses ranging from 10–60 mg and the frequency of adverse effects was not observed. Adverse effects were severe enough to result in discontinuance of omeprazole therapy in less than 2% of patients in clinical studies. The manufacturer states that the adverse event profile of omeprazole in pediatric patients is similar to that in adults. However, the most frequently reported adverse effects in pediatric patients were respiratory effects, which were reported in about 75 or 18% of those 1–2 or 2–16 years of age, respectively; fever was frequently reported (33%) in children 1–2 years of age, and accidental injuries were frequently reported (about 4%) in those 2–16 years of age.

In controlled clinical trials with combined omeprazole-clarithromycin or omeprazole-clarithromycin-amoxicillin therapy, no adverse drug experiences peculiar to these combinations were noted.

In a controlled clinical trial, the adverse event profile was similar for critically ill patients receiving either omeprazole immediate-release suspension or IV cimetidine for up to 14 days. The most frequent adverse effects reported in patients receiving omeprazole were pyrexia (20.2%), hypokalemia (12.4%), nosocomial pneumonia (11.2%), hyperglycemia (10.7%), thrombocytopenia (10.1%), hypomagnesemia (10.1%), and hypotension (9.6%).

● GI Effects

Diarrhea, abdominal pain, nausea, vomiting, constipation, flatulence, and acid regurgitation are the most frequent adverse GI effects reported with omeprazole therapy, occurring in about 1–5% of patients. Constipation, diarrhea, and gastric hypomotility occurred in 4.5, 3.9, and 1.7%, respectively, of critically ill patients receiving omeprazole immediate-release oral suspension or in 4.4, 8.3, and 3.3%, respectively, of those receiving IV cimetidine in a controlled clinical trial. Dysphagia, abdominal swelling, anorexia, irritable colon, fecal discoloration, pancreatitis (sometimes fatal), esophageal candidiasis, mucosal atrophy of the tongue, taste perversion, dry mouth, stomatitis, and microscopic colitis have been reported during postmarketing surveillance in patients receiving omeprazole; a causal relationship to the drug was not established in many cases. Benign gastric fundic polyps have been reported rarely and appear to resolve upon discontinuation of omeprazole therapy. Long-term administration of omeprazole has produced dose-related increases in gastric carcinoid tumors and enterochromaffin-like (ECL) cell hyperplasia in rats. Carcinoid tumors also have been observed in rats subjected to fundectomy or long-term treatment with other proton-pump inhibitors or high dosages of H_2-receptor antagonists. Gastric biopsy specimens obtained from patients in long-term studies with omeprazole have demonstrated an increased frequency of ECL cell hyperplasia. However, no cases of ECL cell carcinoid tumor, dysplasia, or neoplasia were found. (See Cautions: Mutagenicity and Carcinogenicity.)

Adverse GI effects observed in controlled trials with combined omeprazole and clarithromycin therapy that were not reported with omeprazole monotherapy include taste perversion in 15% of such patients and tongue discoloration in 2%.

As with other agents that elevate intragastric pH, administration of omeprazole for 14 days in healthy individuals increased the intragastric concentration of viable bacteria. The pattern of bacteria isolated was similar to that of saliva. Alterations in the intragastric bacterial flora were reversible following discontinuance of omeprazole. Treatment with proton-pump inhibitors may result in a slight increase in the risk of GI infections caused by such organisms as *Salmonella* and *Campylobacter* species.

Available data suggest a possible association between use of proton-pump inhibitors and risk of *Clostridium difficile* infection, including *C. difficile*-associated diarrhea and colitis (CDAD; also known as antibiotic-associated diarrhea and colitis or pseudomembranous colitis). In most observational studies to date, the risk of *C. difficile* infection in patients exposed to proton-pump inhibitors has ranged from 1.4–2.75 times that in patients not exposed to proton-pump inhibitors; however, some observational studies have found no increase in risk. Although many of the cases occurred in patients who had other risk factors for CDAD, including advanced age, comorbid conditions, and/or use of broad-spectrum anti-infectives, the US Food and Drug Administration (FDA) concluded that a contributory role for proton-pump inhibitors could not be definitively ruled out. The mechanism by which proton-pump inhibitors might increase the risk of CDAD has not been elucidated. Although it has been suggested that reduction of gastric acidity by gastric antisecretory agents might facilitate colonization with *C. difficile*, some studies have raised questions about this proposed mechanism or have suggested that the observed association is the result of confounding with other risk factors for CDAD. FDA also is reviewing the risk of CDAD in patients exposed to histamine H_2-receptor antagonists.

CDAD can be serious in patients who have one or more risk factors for *C. difficile* infection and are receiving concomitant therapy with a proton-pump inhibitor; colectomy and, rarely, death have been reported. FDA recommends that patients receive proton-pump inhibitors at the lowest effective dosage and for the shortest possible time appropriate for their clinical condition. Patients experiencing persistent diarrhea should be evaluated for CDAD and should be managed with appropriate supportive therapy (e.g., fluid and electrolyte management), anti-infective therapy directed against *C. difficile* (e.g., metronidazole, vancomycin), and surgical evaluation as clinically indicated.

● *Nervous System Effects*

Headache and dizziness are the most common adverse nervous system effects of omeprazole, occurring in 6.9 and 1.5%, respectively, of patients in US clinical studies. In a controlled clinical trial in critically ill patients, agitation occurred in 3.4 or 8.8% of patients receiving omeprazole immediate-release oral suspension or IV cimetidine, respectively. Asthenia has been reported in 1.1–1.3% of patients receiving omeprazole; in controlled studies, the incidence of this effect was similar in patients receiving omeprazole, ranitidine, or placebo. Psychic and sleep disturbances, including depression, agitation, aggression, hallucinations, confusion, insomnia, nervousness, tremors, apathy, somnolence, anxiety, and dream abnormalities, have been reported during postmarketing surveillance in patients receiving omeprazole; a causal relationship to the drug was not established in many cases. Other infrequent nervous system effects for which a causal relationship may not have been established include pain, fatigue, malaise, vertigo, paresthesia, and hemifacial dysesthesia.

● *Respiratory Effects*

Upper respiratory tract infections and cough have occurred in 1.9 and 1.1%, respectively, of patients receiving omeprazole; in controlled studies, the incidence of these effects was similar in patients receiving omeprazole, ranitidine, or placebo. Acute respiratory distress syndrome, respiratory failure, and pneumothorax occurred in 3.4, 1.7, and 0.6%, respectively, of critically ill patients receiving omeprazole immediate-release oral suspension or in 3.9, 3.3, and 4.4%, respectively, of those receiving IV cimetidine in a controlled clinical trial. Epistaxis and pharyngeal pain have been reported during postmarketing surveillance in patients receiving omeprazole; a causal relationship to the drug was not established. Adverse respiratory effects have been reported in about 75% of children 1–2 years of age and in about 18% of those 2–16 years of age.

Other adverse respiratory effects observed in controlled trials with combined omeprazole and clarithromycin therapy that were not reported with omeprazole monotherapy were rhinitis in 2% of patients, pharyngitis in 1%, and flu syndrome in 1%.

Community-acquired Pneumonia

Administration of gastric antisecretory agents (e.g., proton-pump inhibitors, H_2-receptor antagonists) has been associated with an increased risk for developing certain infections (e.g., community-acquired pneumonia). A possible association between chronic administration of gastric acid-suppressive drugs and occurrence of community-acquired pneumonia has been evaluated using a large Dutch database (Integrated Primary Care Information [IPCI]) containing information on approximately 500,000 patients, 364,683 of whom (average follow-up: 2.7 years) were selected for evaluating any such association. During the 8-year population-based, case-control study, gastric acid suppressants were first prescribed in 19,459 individuals (12,337 received proton-pump inhibitors [mean duration of use: 5 months] and 10,177 received H_2-receptor antagonists [mean duration of use: 2.8 months]; some individuals received both drugs). Most patients did not

undergo endoscopy and were treated empirically for upper GI symptoms. In this study, first occurrence of pneumonia (confirmed by radiography or microbiologic testing in 18% of patients) was reported in 5551 individuals; development of pneumonia occurred in 185 individuals while receiving gastric acid suppressants and in 292 individuals who had discontinued such use.

The adjusted relative risk for development of pneumonia (or the incidence rate) was 0.6, 2.3 and 2.5 per 100 person-years for individuals not receiving acid-suppressive drugs, for those receiving H_2-receptor antagonists, and for those receiving proton-pump inhibitors, respectively. Patients using gastric acid suppressants developed community-acquired pneumonia 4.5 (95% confidence interval of 3.8–5.1) times more often than those who never used such drugs. When evaluating use of all gastric acid suppressants, current use of the drugs was associated with a small (27%) overall increase in the risk of pneumonia (adjusted odds ratio 1.27 and 95% confidence interval of 1.06–1.54). Higher risks were observed for current users of proton-pump inhibitors and H_2-receptor antagonists; the adjusted relative risk for developing community-acquired pneumonia was 1.89 (95% confidence interval of 1.36–2.62) or 1.63 (95% confidence interval of 1.07–2.48), respectively, for these classes of drugs compared with those who discontinued using these agents. Estimates for developing pneumonia were higher (2.2 [95% confidence interval of 1.4–3.5] for proton-pump inhibitors and 1.7 [95% confidence interval of 0.8–2.9] for H_2-receptor antagonists) when only laboratory-confirmed cases of pneumonia were considered for analysis.

Although there was variation among individual proton-pump inhibitors and individual H_2-receptor antagonists, the numbers were small and the heterogeneity was not considered significant. For patients currently receiving proton-pump inhibitors, a dose-response relationship for developing pneumonia was observed; individuals using more than one defined daily dose of these drugs had a 2.3-fold increased risk for developing pneumonia compared with those who discontinued gastric acid suppressants. Such a dose-response relationship for developing pneumonia was not observed in patients receiving H_2-receptor antagonists; however, dose variation of these drugs was limited. Among current users of proton-pump inhibitors or H_2-receptor antagonists, the risk for developing pneumonia was most pronounced among those who initiated such therapies within the past 30 days.

Although the exact mechanism for development of community-acquired pneumonia in patients receiving gastric acid suppressants has not been fully elucidated, it has been suggested that reduction of gastric acid secretion by acid suppressive therapy and consequent increases of gastric pH may result in a favorable environment for the development of infection. Intragastric acidity constitutes a major nonspecific defense mechanism of the stomach to ingested pathogens; when gastric pH is less than 4, most pathogens are killed, while at higher gastric pH, pathogens may survive. Since intragastric pH should be maintained above 4 for several hours for the effective management of upper GI symptoms, acid suppressive therapy may lead to insufficient elimination or even increased colonization of ingested pathogens. Some evidence indicates that acid-suppressive therapy may result in nosocomial infections.

It should be considered that certain patients (e.g., those with pleuritic chest pain, hypothermia, systolic hypotension, tachypnea, diabetes mellitus, neoplastic disease, neurologic disease, bacteremia, leukopenia, multilobar pulmonary infiltrate) are at increased risk for developing infections and in these individuals community-acquired pneumonia may be associated with increased mortality. Some clinicians state that gastric acid-suppressive drugs should be used in patients in whom community-acquired pneumonia may be severe (e.g., those with asthma or chronic obstructive lung disease, immunocompromised patients, pediatric or geriatric individuals) only when clearly needed and the lowest effective dose should be employed.

● *Musculoskeletal Effects*

Back pain has been reported in about 1% of patients receiving omeprazole. Other musculoskeletal effects have been reported during postmarketing surveillance; a causal relationship to the drug was not established in many cases. Such effects include muscle cramps, myalgia, muscle weakness, joint pain, and leg pain. Bone fracture also has been reported during postmarketing surveillance in patients receiving omeprazole.

Findings from several observational studies suggest that therapy with proton-pump inhibitors, particularly in high dosages (i.e., multiple daily doses) and/or for prolonged periods of time (i.e., one year or longer), may be associated with an increased risk of osteoporosis-related fractures of the hip, wrist, or spine. The magnitude of the risk is not clear. To date, most of the observational studies assessing fracture risk in patients receiving proton-pump inhibitor therapy have limited the study population to individuals at least 50 years of age or older. Some of the studies found that the risk of hip fracture was increased with use of higher dosages of the drugs (e.g., average dosage of at least 1.5 "pills" daily) or with long-term use of the drugs, particularly long-term use of high dosages (e.g., dosages exceeding 1.75 times the average daily dosage for more than one year). Study results relating duration of proton-pump inhibitor use to emergence of increased fracture risk have been variable; one study found an increased risk of hip fracture after more than one year of use, whereas another study found an increased risk of hip fracture or osteoporosis-related fracture after 5 or 7 years of use, respectively. In yet another study, an increased risk of hip or spinal fracture was observed when the drugs were last used within the previous year but not when last use was more distant. One study that excluded patients with major risk factors for hip fracture found no relationship between proton-pump inhibitor use and hip fracture occurrence. Because these observational studies relied extensively on claims data from computerized administrative databases, the clinical relevance of reported findings is difficult to determine. FDA states that a causal relationship between proton-pump inhibitor use and fracture occurrence has not been established. To further evaluate this safety issue, FDA intends to analyze data obtained from several large, long-term, placebo-controlled trials of bisphosphonates in women at risk for osteoporosis-related fractures to assess risk of fractures based on use or nonuse of proton-pump inhibitors.

The mechanism by which proton-pump inhibitors may increase risk of fractures has not been elucidated, but it has been suggested that the mechanism may involve decreased insoluble calcium absorption secondary to increased gastric pH. Results of 3 observational studies showed no consistent relationship between proton-pump inhibitor use and bone mineral density. Additional studies evaluating effects of these drugs on bone homeostasis, including effects on biomarkers of bone formation and resorption, are ongoing.

Hypomagnesemia

Hypomagnesemia, symptomatic and asymptomatic, has been reported rarely in patients receiving long-term therapy (for at least 3 months or, in most cases, for longer than one year) with proton-pump inhibitors, including omeprazole. (See Cautions: Precautions and Contraindications.) On March 2, 2011, after reviewing reports of hypomagnesemia in patients receiving proton-pump inhibitors (i.e., 38 cases from the Adverse Event Reporting System [AERS] database, 23 cases from the medical literature [at least 8 of which have been identified in AERS]), FDA confirmed that long-term use (in most cases, longer than one year) of proton-pump inhibitors may be associated with an increased risk of hypomagnesemia; the incidence of this adverse effect could not be quantified because hypomagnesemia is likely underrecognized and underreported. The mechanism responsible for hypomagnesemia associated with long-term use of proton-pump inhibitors is unknown; however, long-term use of these agents may be associated with changes in intestinal absorption of magnesium.

Clinically serious adverse effects associated with hypomagnesemia, which are similar to manifestations of hypocalcemia, include tetany, seizures, tremors, carpopedal spasm, arrhythmias (e.g., atrial fibrillation, supraventricular tachycardia), and abnormal QT interval. Other reported adverse effects include paresthesia, muscle weakness, muscle cramps, lethargy, fatigue, and unsteadiness. Manifestations of hypomagnesemia secondary to proton-pump inhibitor therapy may not be present in all patients. Hypomagnesemia also produces impaired parathyroid hormone secretion, which may lead to hypocalcemia. In most patients, treatment of hypomagnesemia required magnesium replacement and discontinuance of the proton-pump inhibitor. Following discontinuance of the proton-pump inhibitor, hypomagnesemia resolved within a median of one week; upon rechallenge, hypomagnesemia recurred within a median of 2 weeks. In a few patients in whom reinitiation of proton-pump inhibitor therapy was necessary, use of pantoprazole, the least potent proton-pump inhibitor, in combination with oral magnesium supplements resulted in acceptable control of GI discomfort (e.g., dyspepsia, reflux symptoms) without causing recurrent hypomagnesemia; further study is needed to establish the role, if any, of pantoprazole in patients with proton-pump inhibitor-induced hypomagnesemia.

Because nonprescription (over-the-counter, OTC) proton-pump inhibitors are marketed at low dosages and are only intended for a 14-day course of treatment up to 3 times per year, FDA states that there is very little risk of hypomagnesemia when these preparations are used in accordance with the directions on the labeling.

Hepatic Effects

Mild and, rarely, marked increases in serum ALT (SGPT), AST (SGOT), γ-glutamyltransferase (GGT, γ-glutamyltranspeptidase, GGTP), alkaline phosphatase, and bilirubin concentrations have been reported during postmarketing surveillance in patients receiving omeprazole, but in many cases a causal relationship has not been established. In a controlled clinical trial in critically ill patients, abnormal liver function test results (not otherwise specified) occurred in 1.7 or 3.3% of patients receiving omeprazole immediate-release oral suspension or IV cimetidine, respectively. Rare occurrences of symptomatic liver disease have been reported, including hepatocellular, cholestatic, or mixed hepatitis, jaundice, liver necrosis, hepatic failure, and hepatic encephalopathy. Fatalities have been reported in some patients with hepatic failure or liver necrosis.

Dermatologic and Sensitivity Reactions

In a controlled clinical trial in critically ill patients, rash and decubitus ulcer occurred in 5.6 and 3.4%, respectively, of patients receiving omeprazole immediate-release oral suspension or in 6.1 and 2.8%, respectively, of those receiving IV cimetidine.

Rash has been reported during postmarketing surveillance in patients receiving omeprazole; severe generalized reactions such as toxic epidermal necrolysis (some fatal), Stevens-Johnson syndrome, erythema multiforme, exfoliative dermatitis, and lichenoid eruptions have been reported. Other adverse dermatologic effects reported during postmarketing surveillance include skin inflammation, urticaria, purpura and/or petechiae (some cases with rechallenge) angioedema, pruritus, photosensitivity, alopecia, dry skin, and hyperhidrosis. Hypersensitivity reactions, including anaphylaxis, anaphylactic shock, angioedema, bronchospasm, interstitial nephritis, and urticaria, have been reported with omeprazole therapy. In many cases, a causal relationship to omeprazole has not been established.

Hematologic Effects

Short-term use of omeprazole does not appear to be associated with substantial changes in hematologic parameters. However, in a controlled clinical trial of critically ill patients, thrombocytopenia, anemia, and aggravated anemia occurred in 10.1, 7.9 and 2.2%, respectively, of those receiving omeprazole immediate-release oral suspension, or in 6.1, 7.7, and 3.9%, respectively, of those receiving IV cimetidine. Agranulocytosis (occasionally fatal) has been reported rarely with omeprazole therapy, but a causal relationship to the drug is uncertain. Other adverse hematologic effects reported during postmarketing surveillance include pancytopenia, thrombocytopenia, neutropenia, leukopenia, anemia, and leukocytosis. Hemolytic anemia has been reported rarely in patients receiving omeprazole. In many cases, a causal relationship with omeprazole has not been established.

Genitourinary Effects

Acute interstitial nephritis (some cases with positive rechallenge), urinary tract infection, microscopic pyuria, urinary frequency, elevated serum creatinine concentration, proteinuria, hematuria, glycosuria, testicular pain, and gynecomastia have been reported during postmarketing surveillance in patients receiving omeprazole; in many cases a causal relationship to the drug has not been established. Sexual disturbances (e.g., priapism) have been reported occasionally in patients receiving omeprazole.

Cardiovascular Effects

In a controlled clinical trial of critically ill patients, hypotension and hypertension occurred in 9.6 and 7.9%, respectively, of patients receiving omeprazole immediate-release oral suspension, or in 6.6 and 3.3%, respectively, of those receiving IV cimetidine. Atrial fibrillation, ventricular tachycardia, bradycardia, supraventricular tachycardia and tachycardia (not otherwise specified) occurred in 6.2, 4.5, 3.9, 3.4, and 3.4%, respectively, of patients receiving omeprazole or in 3.9, 3.3, 2.8, 1.1, and 3.3%, respectively, of patients receiving IV cimetidine.

Chest pain, angina pectoris, tachycardia, bradycardia, palpitation, elevated blood pressure, and peripheral edema have been reported during postmarketing surveillance in patients receiving omeprazole; a causal relationship to the drug has not been established in many cases.

Although preliminary safety data from 2 long-term clinical trials comparing omeprazole or esomeprazole with antireflux surgery in patients with severe gastroesophageal reflux disease (GERD) raised concerns about a potential increased risk of cardiac events (myocardial infarction, heart failure, and sudden death) in patients receiving these drugs, FDA has reviewed safety data from these and other studies of the drugs and has concluded that long-term use of omeprazole or esomeprazole is not likely to be associated with an increased risk of such cardiac events. FDA has concluded that the apparent increase in cardiac events observed in the early analyses is not a true effect of the drugs.

In one study (a 14-year study comparing omeprazole with antireflux surgery in 298 patients), death from cardiac causes (heart failure, sudden death) or nonfatal myocardial infarction occurred in 8 or 9 patients, respectively, randomized to receive omeprazole and in 2 or 2 patients, respectively, randomized to undergo surgery. However, the findings may have been biased by baseline differences between the 2 groups, since patients in the surgery group tended to be younger and healthier and were less likely to have a history of myocardial infarction than those receiving omeprazole. In addition, some patients withdrew from the study prior to undergoing surgery, and several underwent surgery and also received drug therapy. Fewer than half of the patients remained in the study until its completion. Preliminary data from the second study (an ongoing study comparing esomeprazole with antireflux surgery in 554 patients) also suggested a difference in occurrence of cardiac events between treatment groups; however, after 5 years of follow-up, a similar number of patients in each treatment group had experienced cardiac-related events. FDA reviewed safety data from 14 additional comparative studies of omeprazole (including 4 placebo-controlled studies) and indicated that these studies do not suggest that omeprazole is associated with an increased risk of cardiac events. None of the studies were designed to assess cardiac risk, and patient follow-up in the studies was incomplete.

● Ocular Effects

Blurred vision, ocular irritation, dry eye syndrome, optic atrophy, anterior ischemic optic neuropathy, optic neuritis, and double vision have been reported during postmarketing surveillance in patients receiving omeprazole; in many cases a causal relationship to the drug has not been established.

● Other Adverse Effects

In a controlled clinical trial of critically ill patients, hypophosphatemia, hypocalcemia, fluid overload, and hyponatremia occurred in 6.2, 6.2, 5.1, and 3.9%, respectively, of patients receiving omeprazole immediate-release oral suspension or in 3.9, 5.5, 7.7, and 2.8%, respectively, of patients receiving IV cimetidine. Hypoglycemia, hyperkalemia, and hypernatremia occurred in 3.4, 2.2, and 1.7%, respectively, of those receiving omeprazole or in 4.4, 3.3, and 5%, respectively, of patients receiving IV cimetidine. Hyperpyrexia and edema occurred in 4.5 and 2.8%, respectively, of patients receiving omeprazole or in 1.7 and 6.1%, respectively, of patients receiving IV cimetidine. Sepsis (not otherwise specified), oral candidiasis, urinary tract infection, and candidal infection (not otherwise specified) occurred in 5.1, 3.9, 2.2, and 1.7%, respectively, of patients receiving omeprazole or in 5, 0.6, 3.3, and 3.9%, respectively, of patients receiving IV cimetidine.

Hyponatremia, hypoglycemia, weight gain, fever, and tinnitus have been reported during postmarketing surveillance in patients receiving omeprazole, but in many cases were not attributed to the drug. Acute gout also has been reported during omeprazole therapy.

Accidental injury occurred in about 4% of pediatric patients 2–16 years of age receiving omeprazole in clinical studies.

Limited evidence suggests that omeprazole therapy may cause a dose-dependent reduction in cyanocobalamin absorption, although conflicting data also exist. In one study, absorption of protein-bound cyanocobalamin decreased from a median value of 2.2 or 2.3% at baseline to 0.8 or 0.5% in healthy men receiving 20 or 40 mg, respectively, of omeprazole daily for 2 weeks. (See Cautions: Precautions and Contraindications.)

● Precautions and Contraindications

Symptomatic response to omeprazole should not be interpreted as precluding the presence of gastric malignancy.

While available endoscopic and histologic examinations of gastric biopsy specimens from humans exposed short-term to omeprazole have failed to reveal any associated risk, a dose-related increase in gastric carcinoid tumors has been observed during long-term exposure in animals, and further data from humans are needed to rule out the possibility of an increased risk of tumors during long-term exposure to the drug. (See Cautions: Mutagenicity and Carcinogenicity.)

Atrophic gastritis occasionally has been noted in gastric corpus biopsies from patients receiving long-term treatment with omeprazole.

The possibility that gastric acid-suppressive therapy may increase the risk of community-acquired pneumonia should be considered. (See Respiratory Effects: Community-acquired Pneumonia, in Cautions.)

Findings from several observational studies suggest that therapy with proton-pump inhibitors, particularly in high dosages and/or for prolonged periods of time, may be associated with an increased risk of osteoporosis-related fractures of the hip, wrist, or spine. (See Cautions: Musculoskeletal Effects.) Although controlled studies are required to confirm these findings, patients should receive proton-pump inhibitors at the lowest effective dosage and for the shortest possible time

appropriate for their clinical condition. Individuals using omeprazole for *self-medication* should be advised that they should use the drug only as directed for no longer than 14 days of *continuous* use and that they should not exceed one course of therapy every 4 months. Patients who are at risk for osteoporosis-related fractures should receive an adequate intake of calcium and vitamin D and should have their bone health assessed and managed according to current standards of care.

Long-term use (in most cases, longer than one year) of proton-pump inhibitors may be associated with an increased risk of hypomagnesemia. In patients expected to receive long-term therapy with a proton-pump inhibitor or in those receiving a proton-pump inhibitor concomitantly with digoxin or drugs that may cause hypomagnesemia (e.g., diuretics), clinicians should consider measurement of serum magnesium concentrations prior to initiation of prescription proton-pump inhibitor therapy and periodically thereafter. Patients receiving proton-pump inhibitors should be advised to seek immediate care if manifestations of hypomagnesemia (e.g., arrhythmias, tetany, tremor, seizures) occur; in children, abnormal heart rates may cause fatigue, upset stomach, dizziness, and lightheadedness. Patients receiving nonprescription proton-pump inhibitors should be advised to follow the manufacturer's directions on the package carefully; if therapy with a nonprescription proton-pump inhibitor is continued for longer than the maximum recommended duration (an unlabeled [off-label] use), patients should be informed of the potential increased risk of hypomagnesemia.

Although preliminary safety data from 2 long-term clinical trials comparing omeprazole or esomeprazole with antireflux surgery in patients with severe gastroesophageal reflux disease (GERD) raised concerns about a potential increased risk of cardiac events (myocardial infarction, heart failure, and sudden death) in patients receiving these drugs, FDA has reviewed safety data from these and other studies of the drugs and has concluded that long-term use of omeprazole or esomeprazole is not likely to be associated with an increased risk of such cardiac events. FDA has concluded that the apparent increase in cardiac events observed in the early analyses is not a true effect of the drugs and recommends that clinicians continue to prescribe and patients continue to use these drugs in the manner described in the manufacturers' labelings. (See Cautions: Cardiovascular Effects.)

Because available data suggest a possible association between use of proton-pump inhibitors and risk of *Clostridium difficile* infection, patients should be advised to contact a clinician if persistent watery stools, abdominal pain, and fever occur.

Limited data suggest that omeprazole therapy may cause a dose-dependent reduction in cyanocobalamin absorption. (See Cautions: Other Adverse Effects.) Whether such a reduction in cyanocobalamin absorption can result in a deficiency of the vitamin has not been determined, although it has been suggested that pending further study, serum cyanocobalamin concentrations should be monitored in patients receiving long-term therapy with omeprazole.

Increases in intragastric pH may result in hypergastrinemia, enterochromaffin-like cell hyperplasia, and increased serum chromogranin A (CgA) concentrations. Increased CgA concentrations may produce false-positive results for diagnostic tests for neuroendocrine tumors. Clinicians should temporarily discontinue omeprazole therapy before assessing CgA concentrations and consider repeating the test if initial CgA concentrations are high.

Each 20- or 40-mg packet of omeprazole powder for immediate-release oral suspension (Zegerid®) contains 1680 mg of sodium bicarbonate (460 mg [20 mEq] of sodium). Each 20- or 40-mg immediate-release capsule of omeprazole (Zegerid®) contains 1100 mg of sodium bicarbonate (304 mg [13 mEq] of sodium). The sodium content of these preparations should be taken into consideration in patients whose sodium intake must be restricted; increased sodium intake may produce edema and weight increase. Sodium bicarbonate may cause metabolic alkalosis, seizures, and tetany, and chronic use with calcium or milk may cause milk-alkali syndrome. Acute toxicity associated with sodium bicarbonate overdose may include hypocalcemia, hypokalemia, hypernatremia, and seizures. Sodium bicarbonate should be used with caution in patients with Bartter's syndrome, hypokalemia, respiratory alkalosis, or acid-base abnormalities. Sodium bicarbonate is contraindicated in patients with metabolic alkalosis or hypocalcemia.

In clinical trials in patients who received combined clarithromycin-omeprazole therapy for *H. pylori* infection, some *H. pylori* isolates demonstrated an increase in clarithromycin MICs over time, indicating decreased susceptibility and increasing resistance to the drug. Susceptibility testing should be performed if possible in patients with *H. pylori* infection in whom therapy with combined clarithromycin-omeprazole fails (i.e., as determined in clinical trials by a positive result for *H. pylori* on culture or histologic testing 4 weeks following completion of therapy); if resistance to clarithromycin is demonstrated or susceptibility testing is not possible, alternative anti-infective therapy should be instituted. The American College of

Gastroenterology (ACG) states that clarithromycin or metronidazole should not be used subsequently in patients with *H. pylori* infection who fail therapy that includes these drugs since resistance consistently emerges during such unsuccessful therapy. (See Uses: *Helicobacter pylori* Infection, in Clarithromycin 8:12.12.92.)

Patients should be advised to consult their clinician before using omeprazole for *self-medication* if they are taking warfarin, an antifungal agent (e.g., ketoconazole), diazepam, or digoxin. Patients with heartburn that has persisted for more than 3 months or heartburn in conjunction with lightheadedness, sweating, or dizziness should consult their clinician before using omeprazole for *self-medication*. Patients should be advised to consult their clinician before using omeprazole for *self-medication* if they are experiencing chest or shoulder pain with lightheadedness, shortness of breath, sweating, or pain spreading to arms, neck, or shoulders. Those with frequent chest pain, unexplained weight loss, nausea and vomiting, stomach pain, or frequent wheezing (especially with heartburn) also should consult their clinician before using omeprazole for *self-medication*. Patients should discontinue taking omeprazole for *self-medication* and consult their clinician if heartburn persists, or worsens after 14 days of therapy, or a course of treatment is needed more frequently than every 4 months. Patients with difficulty or pain with swallowing, vomiting with blood, or bloody or blackened stools should not use omeprazole for *self-medication*; such manifestations should be reported promptly to a clinician, since they may be indicative of a serious condition requiring alternative treatment. Women who are pregnant or breast feeding should consult their clinician before using omeprazole for *self-medication*.

Omeprazole is contraindicated in patients with known hypersensitivity to the drug, esomeprazole, or other substituted benzimidazoles (e.g., lansoprazole, pantoprazole, rabeprazole), or any ingredient in the formulation.

● **Pediatric Precautions**

Safety and efficacy of omeprazole (omeprazole delayed-release capsules and omeprazole magnesium delayed-release oral suspension) have been established for the treatment of symptomatic gastroesophageal reflux disease (GERD), erosive esophagitis, and maintenance of healing of erosive esophagitis in pediatric patients 1–16 years of age. Use in pediatric patients is supported by adequate and well-controlled studies in adults and additional pharmacokinetic data and clinical and safety studies in children. (See Gastroesophageal Reflux: Clinical Trials and see Gastroesophageal Reflux: Maintenance Therapy, in Uses.)

Safety and efficacy of omeprazole in pediatric patients younger than 1 year of age have not been established. Safety and efficacy of omeprazole for *self-medication* in those younger than 18 years of age have not been established. Safety and efficacy of omeprazole immediate-release capsules and oral suspension (Zegerid®) have not been established in pediatric patients younger than 18 years of age.

● **Geriatric Precautions**

In US and European clinical trials, more than 2000 patients treated with omeprazole were 65 years of age or older. Although no overall differences in efficacy or safety were observed between geriatric and younger patients, and other clinical experience revealed no evidence of age-related differences, the possibility that some older patients may exhibit increased sensitivity to the drug cannot be ruled out.

Although elimination of omeprazole may be somewhat delayed and oral bioavailability increased in the elderly, clinically important differences in the pharmacokinetic profile of omeprazole between geriatric individuals and younger adults generally do not appear to exist. Therefore, dosage adjustment solely on the basis of age generally is not required for geriatric patients.

The adverse effect profile of omeprazole is similar in geriatric patients and those 65 years of age and younger.

● **Mutagenicity and Carcinogenicity**

No evidence of mutagenicity was observed in vivo in the rat liver DNA damage assay or in some in vitro test systems, including the microbial (Ames test) and mammalian (mouse lymphoma) assays. Omeprazole was positive for clastogenic effects in an in vitro human lymphocyte chromosome aberration assay, in 1 of 2 in vivo mouse micronucleus tests, and in an in vivo bone marrow cell chromosomal aberration assay.

In animals, long-term administration of relatively high dosages of omeprazole results in morphologic changes in the gastric mucosa. Such changes observed in rats during long-term (24-month) administration of the drug include dose-related increases in gastric carcinoid tumors and enterochromaffin-like (ECL) cell hyperplasia, which are thought to represent exaggerated physiologic responses occurring secondary to profound inhibition of gastric acid secretion and subsequent hypergastrinemia and reversible hypertrophy of oxyntic mucosa. While

such changes have not been observed following short-term administration of the drug in humans, additional long-term data are needed to rule out the possibility of an increased risk of gastric tumors in patients receiving long-term omeprazole therapy. In two 24-month studies in rats given omeprazole dosages of 1.7, 3.4, 13.8, 44, and 140.8 mg/kg daily (about 0.7–57 times the human dosage of 20 mg daily based on body surface area), the drug caused a dose-related increase in gastric ECL cell carcinoids in both male and female rats; the increase in carcinoids occurred more frequently in female rats. In addition, ECL cell hyperplasia was observed in both male and female rats receiving omeprazole. In female rats given omeprazole dosages of 13.8 mg/kg daily (about 6 times the human dosage of 20 mg daily based on body surface area) for 1 year and then observed for another year without the drug, carcinoids were not detected but ECL hyperplasia occurred in 94% of rats given omeprazole versus 10% of controls at the end of 1 year; at the end of the second year, hyperplasia was observed in 46% of rats given omeprazole versus 26% of controls. Gastric adenocarcinoma was reported in one rat; similar tumors were not seen in male or female rats treated for 2 years. For this strain of rat no similar tumor had been noted historically, but the finding of this tumor in only one rat is difficult to interpret. In a 1-year toxicity study in Sprague-Dawley rats, brain astrocytomas were found in a small number of males (but not in females) given omeprazole at dosage levels of 0.4, 2, and 16 mg/kg daily (about 0.2–6.5 times the human dosage of 20 mg daily based on body surface area). In a 2-year carcinogenicity study in Sprague-Dawley rats, no astrocytomas were found in males or females at 140.8 mg/kg daily (about 57 times the human dosage of 20 mg daily based on body surface area). Long-term carcinogenicity studies (78 weeks) in mice did not demonstrate increased tumor occurrence; however, the manufacturer states that the study was inconclusive. The drug was not carcinogenic in a 26-week p53± transgenic mouse study.

A number of patients with Zollinger-Ellison syndrome receiving long-term therapy with omeprazole have developed gastric carcinoids; however, Zollinger-Ellison syndrome is known to be associated with such tumors, and these findings are believed to be related to the underlying disease rather than to omeprazole therapy. Gastric corpus biopsy specimens obtained from more than 3000 patients in long-term studies with omeprazole have demonstrated an increased frequency of ECL cell hyperplasia (including micronodular hyperplasia of argyrophil cells) in association with increased plasma gastrin concentrations and progression to subatrophic or atrophic gastritis. However, no evidence of ECL cell carcinoids, dysplasia, or neoplasia has been observed in these patients, and it has been suggested that the development of mucosal cell hyperplasia may be related to the severity and natural progression of gastritis rather than to hypergastrinemia.

● **Pregnancy, Fertility, and Lactation**

Pregnancy

Omeprazole crosses the placenta in animals and in humans. Reproductive studies in rats or rabbits using omeprazole dosages up to 138 or 69 mg/kg daily (about 56 times the human dosage of 20 mg daily based on body surface area), respectively, have not revealed evidence of teratogenicity. However, in rabbits given omeprazole dosages of 6.9–69.1 mg/kg daily (about 5.6–56 times the human dosage of 20 mg daily based on body surface area), dose-related increases in embryolethality, fetal resorptions, and pregnancy loss occurred. In rats, dose-related embryo/fetal toxicity and postnatal developmental toxicity were observed in offspring resulting from administration of omeprazole in dosages of 13.8–138 mg/kg daily (about 5.6–56 times the human dosage of 20 mg daily based on body surface area) to parents.

There are no adequate and controlled studies using omeprazole in pregnant women. Most reported experience with omeprazole during human pregnancy has been first trimester exposure; duration of use (i.e., intermittent, long-term) rarely has been specified. A review of published data (considered fair in quality and quantity) by the Teratogen Information System (TERIS) concluded that therapeutic dosages of omeprazole during pregnancy are unlikely to pose a substantial teratogenic risk. Data from cohort studies have not demonstrated that omeprazole exposure is associated with a statistically significant increase in the rate of major birth defects; however, the studies lacked the power to detect small increases in birth defects or in rare malformations. Therefore, additional study is needed.

A population-based retrospective cohort epidemiologic study using data from the Swedish Medical Birth Registry reported on outcomes in infants whose mothers used omeprazole during pregnancy; most (about 86%) were exposed to omeprazole during the first trimester, 4% during and beyond the first trimester, and about 10% were exposed only after the first trimester of pregnancy. Exposure to omeprazole was not associated with increased risk of any malformation (odds ratio 0.82 and 95% confidence interval of 0.50–1.34), low birth weight, or low Apgar score. The number of infants born with ventricular septal defects and the number of stillborn infants was slightly higher in the omeprazole-exposed infants than the expected number in the normal population, but both effects may be random. In an earlier study using data from the Swedish Medical Birth Registry, exposure to proton-pump inhibitors was not associated with increased risk of congenital malformation.

In a retrospective cohort study, the incidence of congenital malformations in women who received omeprazole or histamine H_2-antagonists (cimetidine or ranitidine) in the first trimester of pregnancy was compared with a control group of women who were not exposed to acid-suppressant drugs. The overall malformation rate was 4.4% (95% confidence interval of 3.6–5.3), the malformation rate for nonexposed women was 3.8% (95% confidence interval of 3–4.9), and the malformation rate associated with omeprazole exposure was 3.6% (95% confidence interval of 1.5–8.1). The relative risk of malformations associated with first-trimester exposure to omeprazole (compared with nonexposed women) was 0.9 (95% confidence interval of 0.3–2.2). The study could effectively rule out a relative risk greater than 2.5 for all malformations. Rates of preterm delivery or growth retardation did not differ between the groups.

A controlled prospective observational study followed women exposed to omeprazole, disease-paired controls exposed to histamine H_2-receptor antagonists, and controls exposed to nonteratogenic agents (e.g., acetaminophen, dental radiation) during pregnancy; major congenital malformations occurred in 4, 2.8, and 2%, respectively, of live births, or in 5.1%, 3.1%, and 3%, respectively, of live births when exposure occurred during the first trimester of pregnancy. Rates of spontaneous and elective abortions, preterm deliveries, gestational age at delivery, and mean birth weight did not differ between the groups. The study lacked statistical power to detect a small increase in major malformations; the sample size had 80% power to detect a fivefold increase in the major malformation rate.

The manufacturers state that several studies reported that adverse short-term effects were not observed in infants when a single oral or IV dose of omeprazole was administered to pregnant women as premedication for cesarean section under general anesthesia.

Omeprazole immediate-release capsules and oral suspension contain sodium bicarbonate; chronic use of sodium bicarbonate may lead to systemic alkalosis, and increased sodium intake may produce edema and weight increase.

Because there are no adequate and controlled studies using omeprazole in pregnant women, and because studies to date in animals and pregnant women cannot rule out the possibility of harm, the drug should be used during pregnancy only when clearly needed and only when the potential benefits justify the possible risk to the fetus.

Fertility

Reproductive studies in rats using omeprazole dosages of up to 138 mg/kg daily (about 56 times the human dose of 20 mg daily based on body surface area) have not revealed evidence of impaired fertility.

Lactation

Omeprazole is distributed into human milk; following oral administration of omeprazole 20 mg in one lactating woman, the peak concentration of the drug in breast milk was less than 7% of the peak serum concentration. Because of the potential for serious adverse reactions to omeprazole in nursing infants, and because of the potential for tumorigenicity shown in animal studies, a decision should be made whether to discontinue nursing or the drug, taking account the importance of the drug to the woman. In addition, omeprazole immediate-release capsules and oral suspension contain sodium bicarbonate, which should be used with caution in nursing mothers.

DRUG INTERACTIONS

• Drugs Affecting or Metabolized by Hepatic Microsomal Enzymes

Omeprazole can prolong the elimination of diazepam, warfarin (the *R*-isomer), phenytoin, cyclosporine, disulfiram, and benzodiazepines, and the possibility that dosages of these and other drugs that are metabolized by cytochrome P-450 (CYP)-mediated oxidation in the liver may require adjustment should be considered when concomitant omeprazole therapy is initiated or discontinued.

Omeprazole is extensively metabolized by the CYP enzyme system. Drugs that induce CYP2C19 or CYP3A4 (e.g., rifampin, St. John's wort [*Hypericum perforatum*]) can substantially decrease omeprazole concentrations. In a crossover study, concomitant use of omeprazole and St. John's wort (300 mg 3 times daily for 14 days) in healthy men resulted in decreased exposure to omeprazole; peak plasma concentrations and area under the concentration-time curve (AUC) of omeprazole were decreased by

37.5 and 37.9%, respectively, in poor CYP2C19 metabolizers and by 49.6 and 43.9%, respectively, in extensive metabolizers. Concomitant use of omeprazole with St. John's wort or rifampin should be avoided.

• Drugs that Cause Hypomagnesemia

In patients receiving diuretics (i.e., loop or thiazide diuretics) or other drugs that may cause hypomagnesemia, monitoring of magnesium concentrations should be considered prior to initiation of prescription proton-pump inhibitor therapy and periodically thereafter. (See Cautions: Hypomagnesemia.)

• Gastric pH-dependent Drugs

The possibility that omeprazole-induced increases in gastric pH may affect the bioavailability of drugs such as ketoconazole, ampicillin esters, iron salts, erlotinib, or digoxin (where gastric acidity is an important determinant in oral absorption) should be considered. Concomitant use of omeprazole 20 mg once daily and digoxin in healthy individuals increased digoxin bioavailability by 10% (up to 30% in some individuals); monitoring for manifestations of digoxin toxicity may be required when omeprazole is used concomitantly.

• Antiretroviral Agents

Atazanavir

Concomitant use of omeprazole 40 mg once daily and atazanavir (with or without low-dose ritonavir) results in a substantial decrease in plasma concentrations of atazanavir and possible loss of the therapeutic effect of the antiretroviral agent. The manufacturers of omeprazole state that concomitant use of omeprazole with atazanavir is not recommended. If atazanavir is administered in an antiretroviral treatment-naive patient receiving a proton-pump inhibitor, a *ritonavir-boosted* regimen of 300 mg of atazanavir once daily with ritonavir 100 mg once daily with food is recommended. The dose of the proton-pump inhibitor should be administered approximately 12 hours before *ritonavir-boosted* atazanavir; the dose of the proton-pump inhibitor should not exceed omeprazole 20 mg daily (or equivalent). Concomitant use of proton-pump inhibitors with atazanavir is not recommended in antiretroviral treatment-experienced patients.

Darunavir

Concomitant use of omeprazole with *ritonavir-boosted* darunavir resulted in decreased plasma concentrations of omeprazole; plasma concentrations of darunavir were not affected. However, no dosage adjustment of either drug is required when omeprazole is used concomitantly with *ritonavir-boosted* darunavir.

Fosamprenavir

Concomitant use of esomeprazole and fosamprenavir increased the AUC of esomeprazole by about 55% but did not substantially alter plasma concentrations of amprenavir (active metabolite of fosamprenavir). Concomitant use of esomeprazole and *ritonavir-boosted* fosamprenavir did not substantially affect concentrations of either amprenavir or esomeprazole. No dosage adjustment is required when proton-pump inhibitors are used concomitantly with fosamprenavir (with or without ritonavir).

Lopinavir

Concomitant use of omeprazole with the fixed combination of lopinavir and ritonavir (lopinavir/ritonavir) did not have a clinically important effect on plasma concentrations or AUC of lopinavir. No dosage adjustment is required when proton-pump inhibitors are used concomitantly with lopinavir/ritonavir.

Nelfinavir

Concomitant use of omeprazole 40 mg once daily (given 30 minutes before a nelfinavir dose) and nelfinavir 1.25 g twice daily decreased peak plasma concentrations and AUCs of nelfinavir by 37 and 36%, respectively, and of its major active metabolite M8 by 89 and 92%, respectively. The manufacturers of omeprazole state that concomitant use with nelfinavir is not recommended.

Raltegravir

Concomitant use of omeprazole with raltegravir resulted in substantially increased peak plasma concentration and AUC of raltegravir; however, no dosage adjustment is recommended when proton-pump inhibitors are used concomitantly with raltegravir.

Rilpivirine

Concomitant use of omeprazole with rilpivirine resulted in decreased plasma concentrations and AUC of rilpivirine. Concomitant use of rilpivirine and proton-pump inhibitors is contraindicated.

Saquinavir

Concomitant use of omeprazole 40 mg once daily and saquinavir 1 g twice daily (with ritonavir 100 mg twice daily) increased peak serum concentrations and AUC of saquinavir by 75 and 82%, respectively. If omeprazole is used concomitantly with *ritonavir-boosted* saquinavir, clinical and laboratory monitoring for saquinavir toxicity is recommended, and reduction of saquinavir dosage should be considered.

Tipranavir

Concomitant use of omeprazole with *ritonavir-boosted* tipranavir resulted in decreased plasma concentrations of omeprazole; plasma concentrations of tipranavir were not affected. An increase in omeprazole dosage may be required when omeprazole is used concomitantly with *ritonavir-boosted* tipranavir.

● Cilostazol

Concomitant use of omeprazole (40 mg daily for one week) and cilostazol in healthy individuals resulted in increased peak plasma concentrations and AUC of cilostazol (by 18 and 16%, respectively) and one of its active metabolites (by 29 and 69%, respectively). Therefore, reduction of cilostazol dosage (from 100 mg twice daily to 50 mg twice daily) should be considered during such concomitant use.

● Clarithromycin

Concomitant administration of clarithromycin (500 mg 3 times daily) and omeprazole (40 mg daily) in healthy men resulted in increases of 30, 89, and 34% in the peak plasma concentration, AUC, and elimination half-life, respectively, of omeprazole. Increases in omeprazole AUC and half-life had a modest effect on gastric pH; mean 24-hour gastric pH was 5.2 when omeprazole was administered alone versus 5.7 with concomitant administration of clarithromycin. Acid suppression resulting from omeprazole appears to enhance the activity of anti-infective therapy against *H. pylori*. Serum concentrations and AUCs of clarithromycin and 14-hydroxyclarithromycin also are increased by concomitant administration of omeprazole. (See Pharmacokinetics: Absorption, in Clarithromycin 8:12.12.92.)

● Clopidogrel

Because omeprazole inhibits CYP2C19, concurrent use of omeprazole with clopidogrel, which is metabolized to its active metabolite by CYP2C19, reduces plasma concentrations of clopidogrel's active metabolite and potentially may reduce clopidogrel's clinical efficacy.

In a crossover clinical trial in healthy individuals who received clopidogrel (a 300-mg loading dose, followed by 75 mg daily) alone or with omeprazole (80 mg administered at the same time as the clopidogrel dose) for 5 days, exposure to the active metabolite of clopidogrel was decreased by 46% and 42% on days 1 and 5, respectively, when the drugs were administered simultaneously. In addition, mean inhibition of platelet aggregation was reduced by 47% at 24 hours and by 30% on day 5. When administration of the 2 drugs (at the same dosages) was separated by 12 hours in another study, results were similar. Concomitant use of clopidogrel and omeprazole also has been associated with decreased antiplatelet effects as determined by vasodilator-stimulated phosphoprotein (VASP) phosphorylation.

The clinical importance of these effects has not yet been established but reduction in clopidogrel's effectiveness in preventing cardiovascular events is possible. Several observational studies involving large numbers of patients suggest that proton-pump inhibitors reduce the effectiveness of clopidogrel in preventing cardiovascular events (e.g., recurrent myocardial infarction, rehospitalization for acute coronary syndromes, urgent target vessel revascularization, death). However, data discounting the clinical importance of an interaction between clopidogrel and proton-pump inhibitors also have been reported. Some experts, including the American College of Cardiology (ACC) and the American Heart Association (AHA), state that additional data from large, prospective trials are needed to fully elucidate the clinical consequences, if any, of the observed interaction between clopidogrel and certain proton-pump inhibitors, including omeprazole.

Proton-pump inhibitors vary in their potency for inhibiting CYP2C19. The change in inhibition of adenosine diphosphate (ADP)-induced platelet aggregation associated with concomitant use of proton-pump inhibitors with clopidogrel is related to the change in exposure to the active metabolite of clopidogrel. In pharmacokinetic and pharmacodynamic studies in healthy individuals, concomitant use of dexlansoprazole, lansoprazole, or pantoprazole had less effect on the antiplatelet activity of clopidogrel than did concomitant use of omeprazole or esomeprazole. For further information on interactions between proton-pump inhibitors and clopidogrel, see Drug Interactions: Proton-Pump Inhibitors, in Clopidogrel Bisulfate 20:12.18. Concomitant use of clopidogrel and either omeprazole or esomeprazole should be avoided. Administration of the drugs at separate times will not prevent the interaction.

The decision to use a proton-pump inhibitor concomitantly with clopidogrel should be based on the assessed risks and benefits in individual patients. The American College of Cardiology Foundation/American College of Gastroenterology/American Heart Association (ACCF/ACG/AHA) states that the reduction in GI bleeding risk with proton-pump inhibitors is substantial in patients with risk factors for GI bleeding (e.g., advanced age; concomitant use of warfarin, corticosteroids, or nonsteroidal anti-inflammatory agents [NSAIAs]; *H. pylori* infection) and may outweigh any potential reduction in the cardiovascular efficacy of antiplatelet treatment associated with a drug-drug interaction. In contrast, ACCF/ACG/AHA states that patients without such risk factors receive little if any absolute risk reduction from proton-pump inhibitor therapy, and the risk/benefit balance may favor use of antiplatelet therapy without a proton-pump inhibitor in these patients. (See Drug Interactions: Proton Pump Inhibitors, in Clopidogrel Bisulfate 20:12.18.)

If concomitant proton-pump inhibitor use is considered necessary, use of an agent with little or no CYP2C19-inhibitory activity should be considered. Alternatively, treatment with a histamine H_2-receptor antagonist (ranitidine, famotidine, nizatidine) may be considered, although such agents may not be as effective as a proton-pump inhibitor in providing gastric protection; cimetidine should *not* be used since it also is a potent CYP2C19 inhibitor. There currently is no evidence that histamine H_2-receptor antagonists (other than cimetidine) or other drugs that reduce gastric acid (e.g., antacids) interfere with the antiplatelet effects of clopidogrel.

● Digoxin

Hypomagnesemia (e.g., resulting from long-term use of proton-pump inhibitors) sensitizes the myocardium to digoxin and, thus, may increase the risk of digoxin-induced cardiotoxic effects. In patients receiving digoxin, monitoring of magnesium concentrations should be considered prior to initiation of prescription proton-pump inhibitor therapy and periodically thereafter.

● Methotrexate

Data from case reports, population pharmacokinetic studies, and retrospective analyses suggest that concomitant use of proton-pump inhibitors, including omeprazole, with methotrexate may result in increased serum methotrexate concentrations and possibly result in toxicity. Increased serum concentrations and delayed clearance of methotrexate and/or its metabolite hydroxymethotrexate, with or without symptoms of methotrexate toxicity, have been reported in patients receiving methotrexate (usually at doses of 300 mg/m^2 to 12 g/m^2) concomitantly with a proton-pump inhibitor. Although most of the reported cases occurred in patients receiving high doses of methotrexate, toxicity also has been reported in patients receiving low dosages of methotrexate (e.g., 15 mg per week) concomitantly with a proton-pump inhibitor. No formal studies of interactions between high-dose methotrexate and proton-pump inhibitors have been conducted to date.

The manufacturer of omeprazole states that temporary discontinuance of proton-pump inhibitor therapy may be considered in some patients receiving high-dose methotrexate therapy. Some clinicians recommend either withholding proton-pump inhibitor therapy for several days before and after methotrexate administration or substituting a histamine H_2-receptor antagonist for the proton-pump inhibitor when acid suppressive therapy is indicated during methotrexate therapy. Pending further evaluation, some clinicians state that these recommendations should extend to patients receiving low-dose methotrexate.

● Tacrolimus

Concomitant use of omeprazole with tacrolimus may result in increased serum concentrations of tacrolimus.

● Voriconazole

Concomitant use of omeprazole (40 mg daily for 7 days) with voriconazole (a combined inhibitor of CYP2C19 and CYP3A4; 400 mg every 12 hours for one day, then 200 mg for 6 days) in healthy individuals increased peak plasma concentrations and AUC of omeprazole by an average of twofold and fourfold, respectively. Dosage adjustment of omeprazole usually is not required but may be considered in patients receiving high dosages (up to 240 mg daily), such as those with Zollinger-Ellison syndrome.

● Warfarin

Increases in international normalized ratio (INR) and prothrombin time have been reported in patients receiving warfarin concomitantly with a proton-pump inhibitor, including omeprazole. Because such increases may lead to abnormal bleeding and death, monitoring of INR and prothrombin time may be necessary in patients receiving warfarin and a proton-pump inhibitor concomitantly.

DESCRIPTION

Omeprazole is a substituted benzimidazole gastric antisecretory agent. Omeprazole is structurally and pharmacologically related to esomeprazole, lansoprazole, pantoprazole, and rabeprazole. Omeprazole is a racemic mixture of *R*- and *S*-isomers; esomeprazole is the *S*-isomer of omeprazole. The drugs are chemically and pharmacologically unrelated to H_2-receptor antagonists, antimuscarinics, or prostaglandin analogs.

Because the omeprazole molecule is acid labile, the drug is administered orally as a delayed-release capsule, tablet, or oral suspension or as a buffered immediate-release capsule or oral suspension. The commercially available omeprazole delayed-release capsules increase oral bioavailability by delaying absorption until after the capsule leaves the stomach; peak plasma concentrations of omeprazole occur 30 minutes to 3.5 hours after administration. Following administration of omeprazole magnesium delayed-release oral suspension, the peak plasma concentration and area under the concentration-time curve (AUC) of the drug are 88 and 87%, respectively, of the values achieved following oral administration of omeprazole delayed-release capsules. Omeprazole immediate-release capsules and oral suspension are rapidly absorbed immediate-release formulations that contain sodium bicarbonate to neutralize gastric acid; mean peak plasma concentrations of omeprazole occur at about 30 minutes (range 10–90 minutes) after oral administration of a single dose or repeated doses of the immediate-release capsule or oral suspension on an empty stomach (1 hour prior to a meal).

Omeprazole binds to hydrogen/potassium adenosine triphosphatase (H^+K^+-exchanging ATPase) in gastric parietal cells; inactivation of this enzyme system (also known as the proton, hydrogen, or acid pump) blocks the final step in the secretion of hydrochloric acid by these cells. Therefore, gastric antisecretory agents such as omeprazole and lansoprazole are commonly referred to as acid- or proton-pump inhibitors. Omeprazole, a weak base, does not directly inhibit this enzyme system, but instead, it concentrates under the acid conditions of the parietal cell secretory canaliculi, where the drug undergoes rearrangement to its active sulfenamide metabolite; this metabolite then reacts with sulfhydryl groups of H^+K^+-exchanging ATPase, inactivating the proton pump. Because the sulfenamide metabolite forms an irreversible covalent bond to H^+K^+-exchanging ATPase, acid secretion is inhibited until additional enzyme is synthesized, resulting in a prolonged duration of action. In an animal model, the pharmacologic effect of the drug at this enzyme was shown to correlate directly with sulfenamide formation.

Omeprazole inhibits basal and stimulated gastric acid secretion; in addition, because the drug inhibits the final step in the secretory pathway, it inhibits such secretion regardless of the stimulus. The degree of inhibition of gastric acid secretion is related to the dose and duration of therapy, but omeprazole is a more potent inhibitor of such secretion than are H_2-receptor antagonists. Following oral administration of omeprazole, inhibition of gastric acid secretion is apparent within 1 hour, peaks within 2 hours, and persists for up to 72 hours. Inhibition of gastric acid secretion increases with continuous drug administration and reaches a plateau after about 4 days of omeprazole therapy. Although omeprazole has a short terminal plasma half-life, the drug has a long duration of action (presumably secondary to prolonged binding of the drug to H^+K^+-exchanging ATPase). Following continuous oral administration of omeprazole, 78 and 58–80% of basal gastric acid secretion is inhibited 2–6 and 24 hours, respectively, after a 20-mg dose, and 94 and 80–93% of basal gastric acid secretion is inhibited, respectively, after a 40-mg dose. Following continuous oral administration, 79 and 50–59% of peak gastric acid output is inhibited 2–6 and 24 hours, respectively, after a 20-mg dose, and 88 and 62–68% of peak gastric acid output is inhibited, respectively, after a 40-mg dose. Oral administration of omeprazole 10–40 mg daily has reduced 24-hour intragastric acidity by 100% in some patients. Following discontinuance of omeprazole therapy, gastric acid secretion returns to baseline over a 3–5 day period.

Following oral administration of omeprazole 20 or 40 mg daily (as the immediate-release oral suspension) in healthy individuals, the median decrease in 24-hour integrated gastric acidity from baseline was 82 or 84%, respectively, the percent of time during a 24-hour period that the gastric pH exceeded 4 was 51 or 77%, respectively, and the median 24-hour gastric pH was 4.2 or 5.2, respectively. In critically ill patients receiving omeprazole 40 mg daily as the immediate-release oral suspension via nasogastric or orogastric tube, the median daily gastric pH was above 4 in at least 95% of patients over the course of a 14-day trial. Gastric pH was above 4 in 99% of patients 1–2.5 hours after the first dose, and in 92% of patients 6 hours after the first dose.

Omeprazole increases plasma gastrin concentrations; this increase occurs via a negative feedback mechanism resulting from decreased gastric acid secretion. Because of omeprazole's greater potency as an inhibitor of gastric acid secretion,

the drug also causes secondary increases in plasma gastrin concentrations that exceed those produced by H_2-receptor antagonists. For example, administration of omeprazole 20 mg once daily for 1–2 weeks results in a 1.3- to 3.6-fold increase in plasma gastrin concentration, whereas administration of an H_2-receptor antagonist usually results in only a 1.1- to 1.8-fold increase. Plasma gastrin concentrations return to pretreatment values with 1–4 weeks after discontinuing omeprazole therapy. Despite omeprazole-induced reductions in gastric acid secretion, the drug does not contribute appreciably to increased plasma gastrin concentrations in most patients with Zollinger-Ellison syndrome, since gastrin is produced principally by the tumor rather than in response to achlorhydria in such patients. Omeprazole also indirectly causes a dose-dependent reduction in pepsin secretion by decreasing the volume of gastric acid secretion. A systematic dose-dependent effect on basal or stimulated pepsin secretion has not been observed in humans; basal pepsin output is low and pepsin activity is decreased when intragastric pH is maintained above 4. The drug does not appear to affect intrinsic factor secretion.

Omeprazole can suppress gastric *Helicobacter pylori* (formerly *Campylobacter pylori* or *C. pyloridis*) in patients with duodenal ulcer and/or reflux esophagitis infected with the organism. Combined therapy with omeprazole and one or more appropriate anti-infectives (e.g., clarithromycin, amoxicillin), can effectively eradicate *H. pylori* gastric infection. (See Duodenal Ulcer: Acute Therapy, in Uses.) Omeprazole does not appear to affect gastric emptying or lower esophageal sphincter pressure.

Short-term administration (2–4 weeks) of omeprazole dosages of 30–40 mg daily does not appear to affect thyroid function, carbohydrate metabolism, or plasma/serum concentrations of parathyroid hormone (parathormone), cortisol, estradiol, testosterone, prolactin, cholecystokinin, or secretin. However, the drug may decrease antral somatostatin concentrations.

Therapy with proton-pump inhibitors, particularly in high dosages and/or for prolonged periods of time, may be associated with an increased risk of osteoporosis-related fractures of the hip, wrist, or spine. (See Cautions: Musculoskeletal Effects.) The mechanism by which these drugs may increase risk of such fractures has not been elucidated but may involve decreased insoluble calcium absorption secondary to increased gastric pH.

PREPARATIONS

Excipients in commercially available drug preparations may have clinically important effects in some individuals; consult specific product labeling for details.

Omeprazole

Oral		
Capsules	20 mg	Zegerid®, Santarus
	40 mg	Zegerid®, Santarus
Capsules, delayed-release (containing enteric- coated granules)	10 mg*	**Omeprazole Delayed-release Capsules**
		PriLOSEC®, AstraZeneca
	20 mg*	**Omeprazole Delayed-release Capsules**
		PriLOSEC®, AstraZeneca
	40 mg*	**Omeprazole Delayed-release Capsules**
		PriLOSEC®, AstraZeneca
For suspension, powder	20 mg/packet	Zegerid®, Santarus
	40 mg/packet	Zegerid®, Santarus

* available from one or more manufacturer, distributor, and/or repackager by generic (nonproprietary) name

Omeprazole Magnesium

Oral		
For suspension, delayed-release (containing enteric-coated granules)	2.5 mg (of omeprazole) per packet	PriLOSEC®, AstraZeneca
	10 mg (of omeprazole) per packet	PriLOSEC®, AstraZeneca
Tablets, delayed-release	20 mg (of omeprazole)	PriLOSEC® OTC, Procter & Gamble

† Use is not currently included in the labeling approved by the US Food and Drug Administration.

Selected Revisions December 8, 2012, © Copyright, January 1, 1994, American Society of Health-System Pharmacists, Inc.

Pantoprazole Sodium

56:28.36 • PROTON-PUMP INHIBITORS

■ Pantoprazole sodium, commonly referred to as an acid- or proton-pump inhibitor, is a gastric antisecretory agent that can suppress gastric *Helicobacter pylori* in patients with duodenal ulcer and/or reflux esophagitis infected with the organism.

USES

● Gastroesophageal Reflux

Pantoprazole sodium is used orally for the short-term (up to 8 weeks) treatment and symptomatic relief of erosive esophagitis in patients with gastroesophageal reflux disease (GERD). Pantoprazole sodium also is used orally as maintenance therapy following healing of erosive esophagitis to reduce recurrence of the disease. Pantoprazole sodium is used IV for up to 7–10 days in the treatment of GERD in patients with a history of erosive esophagitis. IV pantoprazole should be discontinued as soon as the patient is able to initiate or resume treatment with oral pantoprazole. Potential benefits in gastroesophageal reflux and esophagitis result principally from reduced acidity of gastric contents induced by the drug and resultant reduced irritation of esophageal mucosa; the drug can effectively relieve symptoms of esophagitis (e.g., heartburn, regurgitation) and promote healing of ulcerative and erosive lesions.

Suppression of gastric acid secretion is considered by the American College of Gastroenterology (ACG) to be the mainstay of treatment for GERD, and a proton-pump inhibitor or histamine H_2-receptor antagonist is used to achieve acid suppression, control symptoms, and prevent complications of the disease. Because GERD is considered to be a chronic disease, the ACG states that many patients with GERD require long-term, even lifelong, treatment. The ACG states that proton-pump inhibitors are more effective (i.e., provide more frequent and more rapid symptomatic relief and healing of esophagitis) than histamine H_2-receptor antagonists in the treatment of GERD, and are effective and appropriate as maintenance therapy in many patients with the disease. Proton-pump inhibitors also provide greater control of acid reflux than do prokinetic agents (e.g., cisapride [no longer commercially available in the US], metoclopramide) without the risk of severe adverse effects associated with these agents.

Safety and efficacy of oral pantoprazole for treating GERD and erosive esophagitis (grade 2 or greater on the Hetzel-Dent scale) were established in 2 short-term (up to 8 weeks), controlled studies in adults; pantoprazole was more effective than placebo or nizatidine in healing lesions and providing symptomatic relief. In other studies, pantoprazole was more effective than famotidine or ranitidine and at least as effective as omeprazole.

Safety and efficacy of oral pantoprazole as maintenance therapy following healing of erosive esophagitis were established in two 12-month controlled studies in adults. Pantoprazole (40 mg daily) was more effective than ranitidine (150 mg twice daily) in maintaining healing and decreasing the number of daytime and nocturnal heartburn episodes.

Safety and efficacy of IV pantoprazole for short-term (up to 7–10 days) use in the treatment of GERD in patients with a history of erosive esophagitis have been established in several studies. In a controlled study in adults receiving oral pantoprazole prior to study entry, the degree of inhibition of gastric acid secretion following substitution of IV pantoprazole (40 mg once daily for 7 days) was similar to that achieved following oral administration of the drug at the same daily dosage. In 2 controlled studies evaluating short-term (up to 7 days) use of IV pantoprazole as initial treatment for GERD in adults, the degree of inhibition of gastric acid secretion following IV administration of pantoprazole 40 mg once daily was similar to that achieved following oral administration of pantoprazole at the same daily dosage. In addition, relief of GERD symptoms and healing of esophageal lesions were comparable for IV and oral administration of pantoprazole.

Safety and efficacy of IV pantoprazole use for more than 10 days have not been established.

For further information on the treatment of GERD, see Uses: Gastroesophageal Reflux, in Omeprazole 56:28.36.

● Pathologic GI Hypersecretory Conditions

Pantoprazole sodium is used orally or IV for the treatment of pathologic GI hypersecretory conditions associated with Zollinger-Ellison syndrome or other neoplastic conditions. The drug reduces the volume of gastric acid output and hydrogen ion concentration of gastric secretions in patients with these conditions.

In an uncontrolled study in a limited number of patients with pathologic GI hypersecretory conditions (e.g., Zollinger-Ellison syndrome with or without multiple endocrine neoplasia type I), oral administration of pantoprazole at dosages of 80–240 mg daily maintained gastric acid secretion below 5 or 10 mEq/hour in patients who had or had not undergone gastric acid-reducing surgery, respectively. The drug was well tolerated at these dosages for more than 2 years in some patients.

Administration of IV pantoprazole in a limited number of patients with Zollinger-Ellison syndrome (with or without multiple endocrine neoplasia type I) resulted in control of gastric acid secretion to 10 mEq/hour or less with substantial reductions in hydrogen ion concentration and volume of gastric secretions within 45 minutes of drug administration. In another study, control of gastric acid secretion was maintained or improved in a limited number of patients switched from an oral proton-pump inhibitor to IV pantoprazole. In both studies, IV pantoprazole 160 or 240 mg daily in divided doses for up to 6 days maintained basal gastric acid secretion below target levels (10 mEq/hour in patients without or 5 mEq/hour in those with prior gastric acid-reducing surgery) for at least 24 hours in all patients and through the end of treatment (3–7 days) in nearly all patients. Dosage was individualized in both studies, but a regimen of 80 mg every 12 hours controlled gastric acid secretion in more than 80% of patients. There was no evidence of tolerance once acid secretion was controlled.

● Crohn's Disease-associated Ulcers

Although evidence currently is limited, proton-pump inhibitors have been used for gastric acid-suppressive therapy as an adjunct in the symptomatic treatment of upper GI Crohn's disease, including esophageal, gastroduodenal, and jejunoileal disease. Most evidence of efficacy to date has been from case studies in patients with Crohn's-associated peptic ulcer disease unresponsive to other therapies (e.g., H_2-receptor antagonists, cytoprotective agents, antacids, and/or sucralfate). (See Uses: Crohn's Disease-associated Ulcers in Omeprazole 56:28.36.)

For further information on the management of Crohn's Disease, see Uses: Crohn's Disease, in Mesalamine 56:36.

● Other Uses

Pantoprazole also has been used orally for treatment of gastric† or duodenal ulcers†. The recommended dosage of IV pantoprazole does *not* raise gastric pH sufficiently to contribute to the treatment of some conditions (e.g., life-threatening GI bleeding), and the drug's safety and efficacy in the treatment of conditions other than GERD or pathologic GI hypersecretory conditions associated with Zollinger-Ellison syndrome or other neoplastic conditions have not been established.

DOSAGE AND ADMINISTRATION

● Reconstitution and Administration

Pantoprazole sodium is administered orally or IV; the drug is *not* intended for other parenteral routes of administration. Pantoprazole is administered once daily in the management of gastroesophageal reflux disease (GERD) and erosive esophagitis; in the management of pathologic GI hypersecretory conditions, pantoprazole generally is given twice daily, although the drug may be given IV every 8 hours if necessary.

Oral Administration

Pantoprazole sodium delayed-release tablets should be swallowed intact and not split, crushed, or chewed. For patients unable to swallow the 40-mg tablets, a 40-mg dose may be administered using two 20-mg tablets. Food may delay the rate but does not affect the extent of GI absorption of the tablets; therefore, pantoprazole delayed-release tablets may be administered without regard to meals. Antacids do not affect the absorption of pantoprazole and may be administered concomitantly with the delayed-release tablets.

Pantoprazole delayed-release oral suspension should be administered 30 minutes before a meal. Pantoprazole sodium delayed-release granules for oral suspension should be mixed with applesauce or apple juice prior to administration; the granules should *not* be mixed with any other foods or liquids (including water). The delayed-release granules in the suspension should be swallowed intact and not crushed or chewed. The contents of a single-dose packet of pantoprazole sodium delayed-release granules for oral suspension should be sprinkled onto one teaspoonful of applesauce and administered within 10 minutes of preparation. After swallowing the pantoprazole and applesauce mixture, the patient should take sips of water, repeated as necessary, to ensure complete delivery of the dose. Alternatively, the contents of a single-dose packet may be sprinkled into 5 mL of apple juice; the resulting suspension should be stirred for 5 seconds and then swallowed immediately. The granules will not dissolve. The container should be rinsed once or twice with apple juice and the rinsings swallowed immediately to ensure complete delivery of the dose. The contents of a packet of delayed-release granules for oral suspension should not be divided to prepare a dose that is smaller than the full labeled dose (e.g., a 40-mg packet should not be used to prepare a 20-mg dose for a pediatric patient who is unable to swallow the delayed-release tablets).

Pantoprazole delayed-release oral suspension also can be administered via a nasogastric or gastrostomy tube (16 French or larger). The plunger should be removed from a 60-mL syringe and the catheter tip of the syringe attached to the nasogastric or gastrostomy tube; then, the contents of a single-dose packet of pantoprazole sodium delayed-release granules for oral suspension should be emptied into the barrel of the syringe while the syringe is held as high as possible to prevent bending of the tubing. A volume of 10 mL of apple juice should be added to the syringe and the syringe gently tapped or shaken to facilitate emptying; the syringe and tubing should be rinsed with 10 mL of apple juice at least 2 more times (until no granules remain).

IV Administration

For the treatment of GERD, one vial of pantoprazole sodium for injection should be reconstituted with 10 mL of 0.9% sodium chloride injection to provide a solution containing about 4 mg/mL of pantoprazole; the reconstituted solution may be stored for up to 24 hours at room temperature and does not need to be protected from light prior to IV injection over not less than 2 minutes. Alternatively, the reconstituted solution may be stored for up to 6 hours at room temperature prior to further dilution with 100 mL of 0.9% sodium chloride injection, 5% dextrose injection, or lactated Ringer's injection to provide a final concentration of about 0.4 mg/mL. The diluted solution may be stored at room temperature but must be used within 24 hours after initial reconstitution. Neither the reconstituted nor diluted solution needs to be protected from light. The diluted solution may be infused IV over a period of about 15 minutes (about 2.7 mg of the drug or 7 mL of solution per minute).

For the treatment of hypersecretory conditions, each of two 40-mg (of pantoprazole) vials of pantoprazole sodium for injection should be reconstituted with 10 mL of 0.9% sodium chloride injection; the total volume (approximately 20 mL) of reconstituted solution may be stored for up to 24 hours at room temperature and does not need to be protected from light prior to IV injection over not less than 2 minutes. Alternatively, the contents of both vials may be combined and stored for up to 6 hours at room temperature prior to further dilution with 80 mL of 0.9% sodium chloride injection, 5% dextrose injection, or lactated Ringer's injection to a final volume of about 100 mL, providing a final concentration of about 0.8 mg/mL. The diluted solution may be stored at room temperature but must be used within 24 hours after initial reconstitution. Neither the reconstituted nor diluted solution needs to be protected from light. The diluted solution may be infused IV over a period of about 15 minutes (about 5.3 mg of the drug or 7 mL of solution per minute).

For the treatment of pathologic hypersecretory conditions associated with Zollinger-Ellison syndrome or other neoplastic conditions, pantoprazole sodium for injection is administered IV every 8 or 12 hours. The frequency of administration may be individualized based on acid output measurements. Patients with Zollinger-Ellison syndrome may be vulnerable to serious complications of increased gastric acid secretion, even after a brief loss of gastric acid suppression. Therefore, transition from oral to IV and IV to oral formulations of gastric acid inhibitors should be performed in such a manner to ensure continuity of gastric acid suppression effects.

Health-care personnel (e.g., pharmacists, nurses) preparing reconstituted solutions using spiked IV system adapters should use caution because of the potential for breakage of the glass vial.

Pantoprazole sodium should be administered IV through a dedicated IV line or via a Y-site. Parenteral pantoprazole sodium solutions should be inspected visually for particulate matter and discoloration prior to and during administration whenever solution and container permit. Pantoprazole sodium for injection is incompatible by Y-site administration with midazolam hydrochloride injection and may be incompatible with solutions containing zinc. Y-site administration of IV pantoprazole should be discontinued immediately if precipitation or discoloration occurs.

Standardize 4 Safety

Standardized concentrations for pantoprazole have been established through Standardize 4 Safety (S4S), a national patient safety initiative to reduce medication errors, especially during transitions of care. Multidisciplinary expert panels were convened to determine recommended standard concentrations. Because recommendations from the S4S panels may differ from the manufacturer's prescribing information, caution is advised when using concentrations that differ from labeling, particularly when using rate information from the label. For additional information on S4S (including updates that may be available), see https://www.ashp.org/ pharmacy-practice/standardize-4-safety-initiative.

TABLE 1. Standardize 4 Safety Continuous IV Infusion Standard Concentrations for Pantoprazole

Patient Population	Concentration Standards	Dosing Units
Pediatric patients (<50 kg)	0.8 mg/mL	mg/kg/hour

● Dosage

Dosage of pantoprazole sodium is expressed in terms of pantoprazole.

Gastroesophageal Reflux

For the treatment of erosive esophagitis associated with GERD, the recommended adult oral dosage of pantoprazole is 40 mg daily. The duration of therapy is 8 weeks, and therapy may be extended for an additional 8 weeks if esophageal healing is incomplete. For maintenance therapy following healing of erosive esophagitis, the recommended adult oral dosage of pantoprazole is 40 mg once daily. Although the American College of Gastroenterology (ACG) states that chronic, even lifelong, therapy with a proton-pump inhibitor is appropriate in many patients with GERD, the manufacturer states that the safety and efficacy of continuing pantoprazole maintenance therapy for more than 1 year has not been established.

For the treatment of GERD associated with a history of erosive esophagitis, the recommended adult IV dosage of pantoprazole is 40 mg once daily. Treatment with IV pantoprazole should be discontinued as soon as the patient is able to initiate or resume treatment with the oral drug; safety and efficacy of IV pantoprazole use for more than 10 days have not been established.

For the treatment of erosive esophagitis associated with GERD in children 5 years of age or older, the recommended oral dosage of pantoprazole is 20 mg once daily in children weighing at least 15 kg but less than 40 kg and 40 mg once daily in children weighing 40 kg or more. Treatment may be continued for up to 8 weeks; safety beyond 8 weeks has not been established in pediatric patients.

Pathologic GI Hypersecretory Conditions

For the treatment of pathologic GI hypersecretory conditions (e.g., Zollinger-Ellison syndrome, multiple endocrine neoplasia type I), the recommended adult oral dosage of pantoprazole is 40 mg twice daily. Dosages should be individualized and continued for as long as clinically necessary. Oral dosages up to 240 mg daily have been administered, and some patients have received the drug for more than 2 years.

The recommended adult IV dosage of pantoprazole for the treatment of pathologic GI hypersecretory conditions is 80 mg administered IV every 12 hours. In patients requiring a higher daily dosage, 80 mg administered IV every

8 hours is expected to maintain acid output below 10 mEq/hour. Safety and efficacy of dosages exceeding 240 mg daily, and use of IV pantoprazole for longer than 6 days have not been established.

● Special Populations

Dosage adjustment is not necessary in patients with renal impairment, patients undergoing hemodialysis, patients with hepatic impairment, or in geriatric patients. However, dosages exceeding 40 mg daily have not been studied in patients with hepatic impairment.

Reduction of pantoprazole dosage should be considered in pediatric patients who are poor metabolizers of cytochrome P-450 (CYP) 2C19 substrates, since exposure to the drug is increased by more than sixfold compared with that in extensive or moderate metabolizers. However, no dosage adjustment is required in adults who are poor metabolizers of CYP2C19 substrates, since minimal (23% or less) accumulation of the drug occurs with once-daily dosing.

CAUTIONS

● Contraindications

Known hypersensitivity to pantoprazole, any other ingredient in the formulation, or other substituted benzimidazoles (e.g., esomeprazole, lansoprazole, omeprazole, rabeprazole).

● Warnings/Precautions

Sensitivity Reactions

Anaphylaxis has been reported with the use of IV pantoprazole sodium. Immediate medical intervention and drug discontinuance are required if anaphylaxis or other severe hypersensitivity reaction occurs.

Gastric Malignancy

Symptomatic response to therapy with pantoprazole does not preclude the presence of gastric neoplasm. Because of the chronic nature of the disease, there may be a potential for prolonged administration of pantoprazole in patients with gastroesophageal reflux disease (GERD); in long-term animal studies, pantoprazole caused rare types of GI tumors, although the relevance of these findings to humans is unknown.

Atrophic Gastritis

Atrophic gastritis occasionally has been noted in gastric corpus biopsy specimens from patients receiving long-term treatment with pantoprazole, especially those infected with *Helicobacter pylori*.

Clostridium difficile Infection

Available data suggest a possible association between use of proton-pump inhibitors and risk of *Clostridium difficile* infection, including *C. difficile*-associated diarrhea and colitis (CDAD; also known as antibiotic-associated diarrhea and colitis or pseudomembranous colitis). In most observational studies to date, the risk of *C. difficile* infection in patients exposed to proton-pump inhibitors has ranged from 1.4–2.75 times that in patients not exposed to proton-pump inhibitors; however, some observational studies have found no increase in risk. Although many of the cases occurred in patients who had other risk factors for CDAD, including advanced age, comorbid conditions, and/or use of broad-spectrum anti-infectives, the US Food and Drug Administration (FDA) concluded that a contributory role for proton-pump inhibitors could not be definitively ruled out. The mechanism by which proton-pump inhibitors might increase the risk of CDAD has not been elucidated. Although it has been suggested that reduction of gastric acidity by gastric antisecretory agents might facilitate colonization with *C. difficile*, some studies have raised questions about this proposed mechanism or have suggested that the observed association is the result of confounding with other risk factors for CDAD. FDA also is reviewing the risk of CDAD in patients exposed to histamine H$_2$-receptor antagonists.

CDAD can be serious in patients who have one or more risk factors for *C. difficile* infection and are receiving concomitant therapy with a proton-pump inhibitor; colectomy and, rarely, death have been reported. FDA recommends that patients receive proton-pump inhibitors at the lowest effective dosage and for the shortest possible time appropriate for their clinical condition. Patients experiencing persistent diarrhea should be evaluated for CDAD and should be managed with appropriate supportive therapy (e.g., fluid and electrolyte management), anti-infective therapy directed against *C. difficile* (e.g., metronidazole, vancomycin), and surgical evaluation as clinically indicated.

Musculoskeletal Effects

Findings from several observational studies suggest that therapy with proton-pump inhibitors, particularly in high dosages (i.e., multiple daily doses) and/or for prolonged periods of time (i.e., one year or longer), may be associated with an increased risk of osteoporosis-related fractures of the hip, wrist, or spine. The magnitude of risk is unclear; causality has not been established. (See Cautions: Musculoskeletal Effects, in Omeprazole 56:28.36.) FDA is continuing to evaluate this safety concern. Although controlled studies are required to confirm these findings, patients should receive proton-pump inhibitors at the lowest effective dosage and for the shortest possible time appropriate for their clinical condition. Individuals who are at risk for osteoporosis-related fractures should receive an adequate intake of calcium and vitamin D and should have their bone health assessed and managed according to current standards of care.

Hypomagnesemia

Hypomagnesemia, symptomatic and asymptomatic, has been reported rarely in patients receiving long-term therapy (for at least 3 months or, in most cases, for longer than one year) with proton-pump inhibitors, including pantoprazole. Clinically serious adverse effects associated with hypomagnesemia, which are similar to manifestations of hypocalcemia, include tetany, seizures, tremors, carpopedal spasm, arrhythmias (e.g., atrial fibrillation, supraventricular tachycardia), and abnormal QT interval. Other reported adverse effects include paresthesia, muscle weakness, muscle cramps, lethargy, fatigue, and unsteadiness. In most patients, treatment of hypomagnesemia required magnesium replacement and discontinuance of the proton-pump inhibitor. Following discontinuance of the proton-pump inhibitor, hypomagnesemia resolved within a median of one week; upon rechallenge, hypomagnesemia recurred within a median of 2 weeks.

In patients expected to receive long-term therapy with a proton-pump inhibitor or in those receiving a proton-pump inhibitor concomitantly with digoxin or drugs that may cause hypomagnesemia (e.g., diuretics), clinicians should consider measurement of serum magnesium concentrations prior to initiation of prescription proton-pump inhibitor therapy and periodically thereafter. (See Cautions: Hypomagnesemia and also Cautions: Precautions and Contraindications, in Omeprazole 56:28.36.)

Cyanocobalamin Malabsorption

Hypochlorhydria or achlorhydria resulting from daily treatment with acid-suppressive drugs over a long period (e.g., longer than 3 years) may lead to malabsorption of cyanocobalamin. Cyanocobalamin deficiency has been reported rarely. The possibility of such malabsorption should be considered if manifestations of cyanocobalamin deficiency occur.

Injection Site Reactions

Injection site reactions, including thrombophlebitis and abscess, have been associated with IV administration of pantoprazole.

Edetate Disodium Content

Pantoprazole sodium for injection contains edetate disodium (disodium EDTA), which is a potent metal ion (e.g., zinc) chelator. Zinc supplementation should be considered during IV pantoprazole therapy in patients who are prone to zinc deficiency and caution should be exercised when IV pantoprazole is used concomitantly with other IV preparations that contain edetate disodium.

Laboratory Test Interferences

Cannabinoid Tests

False-positive results for urine screening tests for tetrahydrocannabinol (THC) have been reported in patients receiving proton-pump inhibitors, including pantoprazole. An alternative confirmatory test should be considered to verify positive urine THC screening results in these patients.

Respiratory Effects

Administration of proton-pump inhibitors has been associated with an increased risk for developing certain infections (e.g., community-acquired pneumonia). For further precautionary information about this adverse effect, see Community-acquired Pneumonia under Cautions: Respiratory Effects, in Omeprazole 56:28.36.

Glass Vial Breakage

The manufacturer and the US Food and Drug Administration (FDA) have received reports of glass vial breakage during attempts to connect pantoprazole sodium vials to spiked IV system adapters. Such breakage may be a safety issue for health-care personnel (e.g., pharmacists, nurses) attempting to connect these system components either manually or with mechanical assistance, but is not considered by the manufacturer to be a quality issue for pantoprazole sodium for injection. Although the manufacturer is reviewing the use of pantoprazole sodium vials with such systems in order to understand the problem, the manufacturer has not performed studies with these systems to date and currently does not recommend use of spiked IV system adapters with pantoprazole sodium vials. The manufacturer of pantoprazole sodium states that if a decision is made to use spiked adapters, the manufacturer of the adapters should be contacted to provide assistance.

Specific Populations

Pregnancy

Category B. (See Users Guide.)

Lactation

Pantoprazole is distributed into milk; discontinue nursing or the drug because of potential risk in nursing infants.

Pediatric Use

Efficacy and safety of oral pantoprazole for short-term treatment of erosive esophagitis associated with GERD in pediatric patients 1–16 years of age are supported by controlled clinical trials in adults and additional safety, efficacy, and pharmacokinetic studies in pediatric patients. However, because an appropriate dosage formulation is not available for children younger than 5 years of age, oral pantoprazole is labeled for use only in children 5 years of age or older. Safety and efficacy of oral pantoprazole for uses other than treatment of erosive esophagitis have not been established in pediatric patients.

Oral pantoprazole was evaluated in several clinical trials in pediatric patients 1–16 years of age with endoscopically diagnosed or symptomatic GERD, including a limited number of patients with endoscopically diagnosed erosive esophagitis. Because these clinical trials had no placebo or active comparator group and provided no evidence of a dose-related response to the pantoprazole dosages studied, the results were inconclusive regarding efficacy of pantoprazole for the treatment of symptomatic GERD in pediatric patients. Adverse effects reported in more than 4% of patients included upper respiratory tract infection, headache, fever, diarrhea, vomiting, rash, and abdominal pain. Following oral administration of a single 40-mg dose of pantoprazole, exposure to the drug was about 39% higher in children 6–11 years of age and about 10% higher in adolescents 12–16 years of age compared with adults.

Efficacy of oral pantoprazole in infants younger than 1 year of age has not been established. In a treatment-withdrawal study in infants 1–11 months of age with symptomatic GERD, pantoprazole was not more effective than placebo.

Safety and efficacy of IV pantoprazole in pediatric patients have not been established.

Geriatric Use

There are no substantial differences in safety and efficacy relative to younger adults. No dosage adjustment is necessary in geriatric patients.

● Common Adverse Effects

Adverse effects occurring in more than 2% of patients receiving oral pantoprazole and reported more frequently with pantoprazole than with placebo include headache, diarrhea, abdominal pain, vomiting, flatulence, dizziness, and arthralgia.

Adverse effects occurring in more than 1% of patients receiving IV pantoprazole and that generally had an unclear relationship to the drug include headache, injection site reaction (including thrombophlebitis and abscess), abdominal pain, constipation, dyspepsia, nausea, diarrhea, insomnia, dizziness, and rhinitis.

DRUG INTERACTIONS

● Drugs Affecting Hepatic Microsomal Isoenzymes

Pharmacokinetic interaction unlikely. Pantoprazole is extensively metabolized, mainly via hepatic cytochrome P-450 (CYP) 2C19 isoenzyme; CYP3A4, CYP2D6, and CYP2C9 isoenzymes metabolize the drug to a much lesser extent. However, no clinically important drug interactions between pantoprazole and other drugs metabolized by the same isoenzymes were identified in clinical studies. Pantoprazole may have a lower potential for drug interactions than lansoprazole, omeprazole, and rabeprazole.

● Drugs that Cause Hypomagnesemia

Potential pharmacologic interaction (possible increased risk of hypomagnesemia). In patients receiving diuretics (i.e., loop or thiazide diuretics) or other drugs that may cause hypomagnesemia, monitoring of magnesium concentrations should be considered prior to initiation of prescription proton-pump inhibitor therapy and periodically thereafter. (See Hypomagnesemia under Cautions: Warnings/Precautions.)

● Gastric pH-Dependent Drugs

Pharmacokinetic interaction theoretically possible when pantoprazole is used concomitantly with gastric pH-dependent drugs (e.g., ampicillin esters, iron salts, ketoconazole); increased or decreased drug absorption at increased gastric pH values.

● Antiretroviral Agents

Atazanavir

Potential pharmacokinetic interaction with atazanavir (possible altered oral absorption of atazanavir at increased gastric pH, resulting in decreased plasma atazanavir concentrations). Concomitant use of omeprazole 40 mg once daily and atazanavir (with or without low-dose ritonavir) results in a substantial decrease in plasma concentrations of atazanavir and possible loss of the therapeutic effect of the antiretroviral agent or development of drug resistance. The manufacturer of pantoprazole states that concomitant use with atazanavir is not recommended. If atazanavir is administered in a treatment-naive patient receiving a proton-pump inhibitor, a *ritonavir-boosted* regimen of 300 mg of atazanavir once daily with ritonavir 100 mg once daily with food is recommended. The dose of the proton-pump inhibitor should be administered approximately 12 hours before *ritonavir-boosted* atazanavir; the dose of the proton-pump inhibitor should not exceed omeprazole 20 mg daily (or equivalent). Concomitant use of proton-pump inhibitors with atazanavir is not recommended in treatment-experienced patients.

Fosamprenavir

Concomitant use of esomeprazole with fosamprenavir (with or without ritonavir) did not substantially affect concentrations of amprenavir (active metabolite of fosamprenavir). No dosage adjustment is required when proton-pump inhibitors are used concomitantly with fosamprenavir (with or without ritonavir).

Lopinavir

Concomitant use of omeprazole with the fixed combination of lopinavir and ritonavir (lopinavir/ritonavir) did not have a clinically important effect on plasma concentrations or area under the concentration-time curve (AUC) of lopinavir. No dosage adjustment is required when proton-pump inhibitors are used concomitantly with lopinavir/ritonavir.

Nelfinavir

Potential pharmacokinetic interaction (decreased plasma nelfinavir concentrations). Concomitant use of omeprazole 40 mg once daily (given 30 minutes before a nelfinavir dose) and nelfinavir 1.25 g twice daily decreased peak plasma concentrations and AUCs of nelfinavir by 37 and 36%, respectively, and of its major active metabolite M8 by 89 and 92%, respectively. The manufacturer of pantoprazole states that concomitant use of proton-pump inhibitors with nelfinavir is not recommended.

Raltegravir

Pharmacokinetic interaction with omeprazole (substantially increased peak plasma concentration and AUC of raltegravir); however, no dosage adjustment is recommended when proton-pump inhibitors are used concomitantly with raltegravir.

Rilpivirine

Pharmacokinetic interaction with omeprazole (decreased plasma concentrations and AUC of rilpivirine). Concomitant use of other proton-pump inhibitors also may result in decreased plasma concentrations of rilpivirine. Concomitant use of rilpivirine and proton-pump inhibitors is contraindicated.

Saquinavir

Potential pharmacokinetic interaction (increased peak plasma concentration and AUC of saquinavir). Concomitant use of omeprazole 40 mg once daily and *ritonavir-boosted* saquinavir (saquinavir 1 g twice daily and ritonavir 100 mg twice daily) increased the peak plasma concentration and AUC of saquinavir by 75 and 82%, respectively. Caution is advised if proton-pump inhibitors are used concomitantly with *ritonavir-boosted* saquinavir, and patients should be monitored for saquinavir toxicity.

● Clopidogrel

Potential pharmacokinetic interaction (decreased plasma concentration of the active metabolite of clopidogrel) and pharmacodynamic interaction (reduced antiplatelet effects) between proton-pump inhibitors and clopidogrel. Clopidogrel is metabolized to its active metabolite by cytochrome P-450 (CYP) isoenzyme 2C19 (CYP2C19). Concurrent use of omeprazole or esomeprazole, which inhibit CYP2C19, with clopidogrel reduces exposure to the active metabolite of clopidogrel and decreases platelet inhibitory effects. Although the clinical importance has not been fully elucidated, a reduction in the effectiveness of clopidogrel in preventing cardiovascular events is possible. Proton-pump inhibitors vary in their potency for inhibiting CYP2C19. The change in inhibition of adenosine diphosphate (ADP)-induced platelet aggregation associated with concomitant use of proton-pump inhibitors is related to the change in exposure to the active metabolite of clopidogrel. In pharmacokinetic and pharmacodynamic studies in healthy individuals, concomitant use of dexlansoprazole, lansoprazole, or pantoprazole had less effect on the antiplatelet activity of clopidogrel than did concomitant use of omeprazole or esomeprazole. Use of pantoprazole (80 mg daily, administered at the same time as clopidogrel) concomitantly with clopidogrel (300-mg loading dose followed by 75 mg daily) for 5 days reduced exposure to the active metabolite of clopidogrel by about 14% compared with use of clopidogrel alone. The observed effects of pantoprazole on metabolite exposure and clopidogrel-induced platelet inhibition were not considered clinically important, and the manufacturer of pantoprazole states that no adjustment of clopidogrel dosage is necessary if clopidogrel is used concomitantly with recommended dosages of pantoprazole.

The decision to use a proton-pump inhibitor concomitantly with clopidogrel should be based on the assessed risks and benefits in individual patients. The American College of Cardiology Foundation/American College of Gastroenterology/American Heart Association (ACCF/ACG/AHA) states that the reduction in GI bleeding risk with proton-pump inhibitors is substantial in patients with risk factors for GI bleeding (e.g., advanced age; concomitant use of warfarin, corticosteroids, or nonsteroidal anti-inflammatory agents [NSAIAs]; *H. pylori* infection) and may outweigh any potential reduction in the cardiovascular efficacy of antiplatelet treatment associated with a drug-drug interaction. In contrast, ACCF/ACG/AHA states that patients without such risk factors receive little if any absolute risk reduction from proton-pump inhibitor therapy, and the risk/benefit balance may favor use of antiplatelet therapy without a proton-pump inhibitor in these patients.

If concomitant therapy with a proton-pump inhibitor and clopidogrel is considered necessary, use of an agent with little or no CYP2C19-inhibitory activity should be considered. Alternatively, treatment with a histamine H_2-receptor antagonist (ranitidine, famotidine, nizatidine) may be considered, although such agents may not be as effective as a proton-pump inhibitor in providing gastric

protection; cimetidine should *not* be used since it also is a potent CYP2C19 inhibitor. There currently is no evidence that histamine H_2-receptor antagonists (other than cimetidine) or other drugs that reduce gastric acid (e.g., antacids) interfere with the antiplatelet effects of clopidogrel. For further information on interactions between proton-pump inhibitors and clopidogrel, see Drug Interactions: Proton-Pump Inhibitors, in Clopidogrel Bisulfate 20:12.18.

● Digoxin

Hypomagnesemia (e.g., resulting from long-term use of proton-pump inhibitors) sensitizes the myocardium to digoxin and, thus, may increase the risk of digoxin-induced cardiotoxic effects. In patients receiving digoxin, monitoring of magnesium concentrations should be considered prior to initiation of prescription proton-pump inhibitor therapy and periodically thereafter.

● Methotrexate

Potential pharmacokinetic interaction (increased serum methotrexate concentrations, possibly resulting in toxicity) when proton-pump inhibitors, including pantoprazole, are used concomitantly with methotrexate. Increased serum concentrations and delayed clearance of methotrexate and/or its metabolite hydroxymethotrexate, with or without symptoms of methotrexate toxicity, have been reported in patients receiving methotrexate (usually at doses of 300 mg/m² to 12 g/m²) concomitantly with a proton-pump inhibitor. Although most of the reported cases occurred in patients receiving high doses of methotrexate, toxicity also has been reported in patients receiving low dosages of methotrexate (e.g., 15 mg per week) concomitantly with a proton-pump inhibitor. No formal studies of interactions between high-dose methotrexate and proton-pump inhibitors have been conducted to date.

The manufacturer of pantoprazole states that temporary discontinuance of proton-pump inhibitor therapy may be considered in some patients receiving high-dose methotrexate therapy. Some clinicians recommend either withholding proton-pump inhibitor therapy for several days before and after methotrexate administration or substituting a histamine H_2-receptor antagonist for the proton-pump inhibitor when acid suppressive therapy is indicated during methotrexate therapy. Pending further evaluation, some clinicians state that these recommendations should extend to patients receiving low-dose methotrexate.

● Sucralfate

Potential delayed absorption and decreased bioavailability of proton-pump inhibitor (e.g., lansoprazole, omeprazole); administer proton-pump inhibitor at least 30 minutes before sucralfate.

● Warfarin

Potential increased international normalized ratio (INR) and prothrombin time when warfarin is used concomitantly with proton-pump inhibitors, including pantoprazole. Potential for abnormal bleeding and death; monitor for INR and prothrombin time increases when pantoprazole is used concomitantly with warfarin.

DESCRIPTION

Pantoprazole sodium, a proton-pump inhibitor, is a gastric antisecretory agent that is structurally and pharmacologically related to esomeprazole, lansoprazole, omeprazole, and rabeprazole. The drugs are substituted benzimidazoles and are chemically and pharmacologically unrelated to H_2-receptor antagonists, antimuscarinics, or prostaglandin analogs.

Pantoprazole, a weak base, concentrates under the acidic conditions of the parietal cell secretory canaliculi, where it is activated by rearrangement to a cationic cyclic sulfenamide. The activated form covalently binds to 2 sites of the hydrogen/potassium ATPase in the gastric parietal cells; inactivation of this enzyme system (also known as the proton, hydrogen, or acid pump) blocks the final step in the secretion of hydrochloric acid by these cells, resulting in potent, long-lasting inhibition of gastric acid secretion.

The duration of antisecretory effect of orally administered pantoprazole continues for more than 24 hours. Within 2.5 hours of administration of a 40-mg oral dose to healthy individuals, gastric acid secretion was inhibited by a mean of 51%, which increased to a mean of 85% following administration of 40 mg orally once daily for 7 days. Gastric acid secretion returned to normal within a week after pantoprazole discontinuance, and there was no evidence of rebound hypersecretion. Because the pantoprazole molecule is acid labile, the drug is commercially available for oral administration as delayed-release, enteric-coated formulations (tablets, granules for oral suspension) that increase oral bioavailability by delaying absorption until after the preparation leaves the stomach. The duration of antisecretory effect of IV pantoprazole was 24 hours. Following IV administration of a single 20- to 120-mg dose of pantoprazole to healthy individuals, onset of gastric acid suppression occurred within 15–30 minutes, and suppression of cumulative 24-hour acid output was dose dependent for doses of 20–80 mg. Within 2 hours of IV administration of pantoprazole 80 mg, complete suppression of acid output was achieved; no substantial additional suppression was observed following a 120-mg dose of the drug.

Pantoprazole is extensively metabolized, mainly via hepatic cytochrome P-450 (CYP) 2C19 isoenzyme; CYP3A4, CYP2D6, and CYP2C9 isoenzymes metabolize the drug to a much lesser extent. (See Dosage and Administration: Special Populations.)

Pantoprazole can suppress gastric *Helicobacter pylori* in patients with duodenal ulcer and/or reflux esophagitis infected with the organism. Combined therapy with pantoprazole and one or more anti-infectives (e.g., amoxicillin, clarithromycin) can effectively eradicate *H. pylori* gastric infection.

A moderate increase in enterochromaffin-like cell (ECL) density, which began after the first year of therapy and appeared to plateau after 4 years, occurred in patients receiving pantoprazole dosages of 40–240 mg daily for up to 5 years. Dose-related increases in ECL-cell proliferation and gastric neuroendocrine-cell tumors were observed in animal studies.

Therapy with proton-pump inhibitors, particularly in high dosages and/or for prolonged periods of time, may be associated with an increased risk of osteoporosis-related fractures of the hip, wrist, or spine. (See Musculoskeletal Effects under Cautions: Warnings/Precautions.) The mechanism by which these drugs may increase risk of such fractures has not been elucidated but may involve decreased insoluble calcium absorption secondary to increased gastric pH.

ADVICE TO PATIENTS

Importance of informing clinicians of existing or contemplated concomitant therapy, including prescription and OTC drugs, as well as concomitant illnesses. Antacid administration is permissible with pantoprazole delayed-release tablets.

Importance of women informing clinicians if they are or plan to become pregnant or plan to breast-feed.

Importance of instructing patients regarding proper administration of delayed-release oral preparations. Necessity of swallowing delayed-release tablets whole, without crushing or chewing. Importance of preparing the delayed-release

suspension according to the manufacturer's directions and of administering the suspension 30 minutes before a meal. Importance of not dividing the contents of a packet of delayed-release granules for oral suspension to prepare a dose that is smaller than the full labeled dose.

Importance of advising patients that use of multiple daily doses of the drug for an extended period of time may increase the risk of fractures of the hip, wrist, or spine.

Risk of hypomagnesemia; importance of advising patients to immediately report and seek care for any cardiovascular or neurologic manifestations (e.g., palpitations, dizziness, seizures, tetany).

Possible increased risk of *Clostridium difficile* infection; importance of contacting a clinician if persistent watery stools, abdominal pain, and fever occur.

Importance of continuing therapy for the entire treatment course, unless directed otherwise.

Importance of informing patients of other important precautionary information. (See Cautions.)

PREPARATIONS

Excipients in commercially available drug preparations may have clinically important effects in some individuals; consult specific product labeling for details.

Pantoprazole Sodium

Oral

For suspension, delayed-release (containing enteric-coated granules)	40 mg (of pantoprazole) per packet	**Protonix®**, Pfizer
Tablets, delayed-release (enteric-coated)	20 mg (of pantoprazole)*	**Pantoprazole Sodium Delayed-release Tablets**
		Protonix®, Pfizer
	40 mg (of pantoprazole)*	**Pantoprazole Sodium Delayed-release Tablets**
		Protonix®, Pfizer

Parenteral

For injection, for IV infusion	40 mg (of pantoprazole)	**Protonix® I.V.**, Pfizer

* available from one or more manufacturer, distributor, and/or repackager by generic (nonproprietary) name

† Use is not currently included in the labeling approved by the US Food and Drug Administration.

Selected Revisions June 10, 2024, © Copyright, January 1, 2001, American Society of Health-System Pharmacists, Inc.

Metoclopramide Hydrochloride

56:32 • PROKINETIC AGENTS

■ Metoclopramide hydrochloride is a dopamine-receptor antagonist, an antiemetic, and a stimulant of upper GI motility (prokinetic agent).

USES

Metoclopramide is used in a variety of GI disorders, but principally for the management of GI motility disorders, especially gastric stasis, for the management of gastroesophageal reflux, for the prevention of cancer chemotherapy-induced nausea and vomiting, and for the prevention of postoperative nausea and vomiting when nasogastric suction is considered undesirable. The drug is also used to facilitate intubation of the small intestine and as an adjunct during radiographic examination of the upper GI tract.

Therapy with metoclopramide, including all dosage forms and routes of administration, should not exceed 12 weeks' duration because of the risk for developing tardive dyskinesia with longer-term use. (See Tardive Dyskinesia under Cautions: Nervous System Effects.) Oral and nasal formulations of the drug are recommended for use in adults *only*. (See Cautions: Pediatric Precautions.)

● *Diabetic Gastric Stasis*

Metoclopramide is used for the symptomatic treatment of acute and recurrent diabetic gastric stasis (gastroparesis). Treatment of diabetic gastric stasis with metoclopramide is not curative.

Symptomatic treatment of diabetic gastric stasis may include dietary modifications, optimization of glycemic control, avoidance of drugs that adversely affect GI motility, antiemetics for relief of associated nausea and vomiting, and, in more severe cases, prokinetic agents to improve gastric emptying. Current prokinetic treatment options are limited, and the risks and benefits of such therapy must be considered. The American Diabetes Association states that metoclopramide should be reserved for use in patients with severe diabetic gastric stasis that is unresponsive to other therapies, since evidence of benefit in the management of diabetic gastric stasis is weak and the drug is associated with serious adverse effects (see Cautions: Nervous System Effects).

The motility of the stomach is abnormal in patients with diabetic gastric stasis; fundic and antral contractility are markedly diminished and gastric emptying of liquids and solids is delayed. Although a correlation between gastric stasis and autonomic neuropathy has not been shown in diabetics, these patients may have signs of vagal nerve damage.

In patients with diabetic gastric stasis, metoclopramide increases the rate of gastric emptying and decreases usual symptoms of gastric stasis including nausea, vomiting, heartburn, anorexia, persistent postprandial fullness, abdominal pain and distention, and early satiety. Symptoms of delayed gastric emptying appear to respond to metoclopramide within different time intervals. Relief of nausea usually occurs soon after initiating metoclopramide therapy and continues to improve over a 3-week period. Subsequently, relief of vomiting and anorexia may precede relief of abdominal fullness by 1 week or longer.

In most patients with diabetic gastric stasis, metoclopramide-induced reduction of symptoms does not correlate well with improvement in gastric emptying. In some patients, complete relief of symptoms occurs despite minimal increases in the rate of gastric emptying, while in others, symptoms of gastric stasis persist despite a normalization in gastric emptying.

● *Postsurgical Gastric Stasis*

Metoclopramide has been used for the symptomatic treatment of acute and chronic postsurgical gastric stasis† following vagotomy and gastric resection or vagotomy and pyloroplasty. The drug has improved gastric emptying and decreased the usual symptoms of gastric stasis in patients with these conditions.

● *Prevention of Cancer Chemotherapy-induced Emesis*

Metoclopramide is used parenterally in high doses for the prevention of nausea and vomiting associated with emetogenic cancer chemotherapy. The drug also has been administered orally† for the prevention of chemotherapy-induced nausea and vomiting.

To prevent chemotherapy-induced nausea and vomiting associated with chemotherapy regimens with a high emetic risk (i.e., incidence of emesis exceeds 90% if no antiemetics are administered), the American Society of Clinical Oncology (ASCO) currently recommends a 3-drug antiemetic regimen consisting of a type 3 serotonin (5-HT$_3$) receptor antagonist (e.g., dolasetron, granisetron, ondansetron, palonosetron, tropisetron [not commercially available in the US]), dexamethasone, and aprepitant.

Antiemetic agents with a lower therapeutic index (i.e., less efficacious and generally associated with more frequent adverse effects), including metoclopramide, cannabinoids (e.g., dronabinol, nabilone), butyrophenones, and phenothiazines are *not* considered by ASCO to be appropriate first-line antiemetics for any group of patients receiving chemotherapy of high emetic risk; ASCO states that these drugs should be reserved for patients unable to tolerate or refractory to first-line agents.

The antiemetic combination of a 5-HT$_3$ receptor antagonist, dexamethasone, and aprepitant also is preferred in patients receiving combination chemotherapy with an anthracycline and cyclophosphamide.

For patients receiving other chemotherapy of moderate emetic risk (i.e., incidence of emesis without antiemetics exceeds 30% but does not exceed 90%), ASCO recommends a 2-drug antiemetic regimen consisting of a 5-HT$_3$ receptor antagonist and dexamethasone.

For patients receiving chemotherapy regimens with a low emetic risk (i.e., incidence of emesis without antiemetics exceeds 10% but does not exceed 30%), ASCO recommends dexamethasone alone on the first day of chemotherapy.

Antiemetics can be prescribed on an as-needed basis in patients receiving chemotherapy with a minimal emetic risk (incidence of emesis is less than 10% without antiemetics).

In patients experiencing vomiting and nausea despite recommended prophylaxis regimens, ASCO recommends that clinicians consider adding a benzodiazepine (e.g., alprazolam, lorazepam) to the regimen, substituting high-dose intravenous metoclopramide for the 5-HT$_3$ receptor antagonist in the regimen, or adding a butyrophenone or phenothiazine to the regimen.

For the prevention of *delayed* emesis in patients receiving cisplatin or other chemotherapy associated with a high emetic risk, these authorities currently recommend a 2-drug combination of dexamethasone and aprepitant.

Although antihistamines (e.g., diphenhydramine) and benzodiazepines (e.g., alprazolam, lorazepam) may be useful as adjunctive antiemetic agents, they currently are not recommended as monotherapy as antiemetic agents. However, many clinicians find benzodiazepines useful in the management of anticipatory emesis.

Cisplatin

Metoclopramide is used parenterally for the prevention of cisplatin-induced nausea and vomiting. The drug has been used effectively for the prevention of chemotherapy-induced emesis in patients receiving cisplatin alone or in combination with other antineoplastic agents. In patients receiving cisplatin, high-dose metoclopramide (2 mg/kg) reduces the number and duration of vomiting episodes and the volume of emesis. In some patients, cisplatin-induced nausea and vomiting are completely prevented with metoclopramide therapy. Clinical evaluations of metoclopramide in the prevention of cisplatin-induced emesis have shown that the antiemetic effect of metoclopramide is greater than that of placebo, prochlorperazine, or tetrahydrocannabinol (THC). However, it appears that type 3 serotonergic (5-HT$_3$) receptor antagonists (e.g., dolasetron, granisetron, ondansetron, palonosetron, tropisetron [not commercially available in the US]) and aprepitant generally are more effective and better tolerated than metoclopramide, which reportedly is pharmacologically less selective, and therefore, these 5-HT$_3$ receptor antagonists given in combination with dexamethasone and aprepitant may be preferred for the initial prophylaxis of acute emetic effects in many patients; in some cases, these drugs may be effective in treating nausea and emesis that develop despite metoclopramide prophylaxis. Currently available 5-HT$_3$ receptor antagonists (i.e., dolasetron, granisetron, ondansetron, palonosetron, tropisetron [not commercially available in the US]) appear to be comparably effective in preventing acute cisplatin- and other chemotherapy-induced nausea and vomiting. The addition of dexamethasone to monotherapy with a 5-HT$_3$ receptor antagonist or metoclopramide increases the antiemetic efficacy of either drug alone, and such combined therapy may be useful in patients whose nausea and vomiting are refractory to monotherapy. Although addition of diphenhydramine to metoclopramide and dexamethasone therapy may increase the antiemetic efficacy further and decrease metoclopramide-induced adverse effects, combined therapy with a selective 5-HT$_3$ receptor antagonist and dexamethasone appears to be more effective than this triple-drug combination. In addition, some evidence suggests that such combined therapy may be more effective, albeit not optimally, than monotherapy for the prevention and treatment of delayed emesis. Various combinations of antiemetic agents have been used, and comparative efficacy is continually being evaluated.

Remaining most problematic is the management of *delayed* and *anticipatory* nausea and vomiting; pending further elucidation of optimal regimens, some clinicians suggest combined regimens of 2 or 3 drugs that include a 5-HT$_3$ receptor antagonist (e.g., dolasetron, granisetron, ondansetron, palonosetron, tropisetron [not commercially available in the US]), aprepitant, a corticosteroid (e.g., dexamethasone), metoclopramide, and/or benzodiazepine (e.g., lorazepam for anxiolytic, amnesic, and possibly antiemetic effects). In several clinical trials, oral† metoclopramide has been effective when given in combination with dexamethasone for the prevention of delayed emesis in patients receiving chemotherapy.

Based on limited published data, maximum efficacy of metoclopramide appears to depend greatly on the use of the appropriate dose, route, and schedule during administration of the drug. (See Prevention of Cancer Chemotherapy-induced Emesis, in Dosage and Administration: Dosage.) The efficacy of lower than currently recommended doses and/or alternate administration schedules for metoclopramide in the prevention of cisplatin-induced emesis remains to be clearly established. In one study in patients receiving cisplatin, optimum antiemetic effect was generally associated with serum metoclopramide concentrations greater than 850 ng/mL.

Metoclopramide is more likely to be effective in patients who were not previously exposed to cancer chemotherapy than in patients whose symptoms are refractory to conventional antiemetic agents. The antiemetic efficacy of metoclopramide appears to be maintained during subsequent doses of cisplatin.

Other Antineoplastic Agents

Metoclopramide is used for prevention of nausea and vomiting associated with other antineoplastic agents (e.g., cyclophosphamide, dacarbazine, doxorubicin, methotrexate) and with cancer chemotherapy regimens that do not include cisplatin. Since various antineoplastic agents may induce emesis by different mechanisms, the efficacy of metoclopramide depends on their relative potential and specific pharmacologic pathways for inducing emesis. In patients receiving dacarbazine, high-dose metoclopramide (2 mg/kg) appears to be an effective antiemetic. When oral metoclopramide (10 mg 1–2 hours before chemotherapy and then every 8 hours for a week) was combined with IV dexamethasone (10 mg immediately before initiation of IV chemotherapy) in patients receiving cyclophosphamide, methotrexate, and fluorouracil for breast cancer (a moderately emetogenic regimen), this antiemetic combination appeared to be comparably effective overall to oral ondansetron (8 mg 1–2 hours before chemotherapy and then every 8 hours for a week) in preventing emesis during the 7-day treatment period but was more effective than ondansetron in reducing the frequency of nausea during the first day of chemotherapy. Additional study is needed to further evaluate the role of metoclopramide alone or combined with other antiemetics in the prevention of nausea and vomiting associated with the many different regimens used for cancer chemotherapy.

● Intubation of the Small Intestine

Metoclopramide is used parenterally to facilitate intubation of the small intestine in adults and children in whom the tube (e.g., endoscope, biopsy tube) does not pass through the pylorus with conventional maneuvers. The beneficial effect of metoclopramide on intubation of the small intestine is principally related to the pharmacologic action of the drug on GI motility and contractility. (See Pharmacology: GI Effects.) Metoclopramide has little influence on the time required for biopsy capsules to reach the pylorus, but substantially reduces the time required for the capsules to pass through the pylorus.

In several controlled trials in patients with or without GI disease (e.g., inflammatory bowel disease, chronic diarrhea, malabsorption, celiac disease, peptic ulcer) undergoing intubation of the small intestine, IV metoclopramide (10 mg) reduced the time required for intubation and facilitated performance of the procedure; however, administration of the drug generally did not influence patient tolerance of the procedure.

● Radiographic Examination of the Upper GI Tract

Metoclopramide is used parenterally to stimulate gastric emptying and intestinal transit of barium in patients in whom delayed emptying interferes with radiographic examination of the stomach and/or small intestine. In patients receiving oral barium, IV metoclopramide increases the rate of gastric emptying and reduces transit time of the barium in the small intestine. Metoclopramide markedly reduces the time required for radiographic examination of the small intestine and is effective in preventing nausea or regurgitation of barium that occurs in some patients with gastric atonia, pylorospasm, or spasm of the duodenal bulb.

● Gastroesophageal Reflux

Metoclopramide is used orally for the short-term (4–12 weeks) relief of symptomatic, documented gastroesophageal reflux in adults who are unresponsive to conventional therapy, including changes in lifestyle, habits, and/or diet (which may be contributing or precipitating factors); weight reduction in obese patients; and acid-suppressive therapy (e.g., proton-pump inhibitors, histamine H$_2$-receptor antagonists, antacids). Agents that suppress gastric acid secretion (e.g., proton-pump inhibitors, histamine H$_2$-receptor antagonists) currently are considered to be the mainstay of treatment for gastroesophageal reflux disease (GERD).

Metoclopramide produces a dose-related increase in the resting tone of the lower esophageal sphincter in healthy adults and in patients with gastroesophageal reflux. There reportedly is substantial interindividual variation in the effect of metoclopramide on lower esophageal sphincter pressure. In patients with gastroesophageal reflux, metoclopramide increases gastric emptying rate both in those with normal or delayed gastric emptying, and reduces daytime and nocturnal heartburn and regurgitation; however, metoclopramide therapy produces greater reductions in severity and occurrence of daytime and postprandial heartburn and regurgitation than in nocturnal symptoms associated with gastroesophageal reflux. If symptoms are associated with particular situations or precipitating factors (e.g., following the evening meal), administration of a single dose of metoclopramide prior to the provocative situation rather than daily administration of multiple doses of the drug should be considered.

Based on data from a limited number of patients, metoclopramide appears to be more effective than an aluminum hydroxide antacid or placebo and about as effective as cimetidine in improving the symptoms of gastroesophageal reflux. Objective parameters (i.e., endoscopy, lower esophageal sphincter pressure, esophageal contraction amplitude) for response were not consistently improved in these patients following short-term (4–8 weeks) administration of metoclopramide; however, in one unpublished study, endoscopic evidence of healing was observed following administration of metoclopramide (15 mg 4 times daily) for 12 weeks. Since there is no documented correlation between symptoms and healing of esophageal lesions in patients with gastroesophageal reflux, therapy in patients with documented lesions should be accompanied by appropriate endoscopic evaluation. In a study comparing single oral doses of metoclopramide (15 mg) with an aluminum hydroxide antacid (30 mL) or placebo in patients with reflux esophagitis, metoclopramide was reportedly more effective than antacid in reducing the symptoms associated with reflux. Metoclopramide increased the resting tone of the lower esophageal sphincter in all patients for at least 1 hour and prevented gastroesophageal reflux following administration of an intragastric acid load. Although metoclopramide may be effective for the short-term relief of gastroesophageal reflux, safety and efficacy of metoclopramide therapy beyond 12 weeks have not been evaluated and such prolonged use is not recommended.

The potential risks (e.g., severe and potentially irreversible adverse CNS effects) and benefits of metoclopramide relative to other effective therapies must be considered. The American Gastroenterological Association (AGA) recommends against use of metoclopramide for treatment of GERD because of the drug's adverse effect profile and a lack of high-quality data supporting its use. Both the AGA and the American College of Gastroenterology (ACG) state that proton-pump inhibitors provide greater control of acid reflux and heartburn than do other currently available agents, including prokinetic agents (e.g., cisapride [no longer commercially available in the US], metoclopramide). Suppression of gastric acid secretion is considered by these experts to be the mainstay of treatment for GERD, and a proton-pump inhibitor or histamine H$_2$-receptor antagonist is used to achieve acid suppression, control symptoms, and prevent complications of the disease. For further information on the treatment of GERD, see Uses: Gastroesophageal Reflux, in Omeprazole 56:28.36.

● Other Uses

Metoclopramide is used parenterally for the prevention of postoperative nausea and vomiting when nasogastric suction is considered undesirable.

Metoclopramide has been used for the management of migraine†. Some experts state that metoclopramide may be considered as adjunctive therapy for control of nausea in patients with acute migraine attacks and that the IV drug may be considered for relief of migraine pain. For further information on management and classification of migraine headache, see Vascular Headaches: General Principles in Migraine Therapy, under Uses in Sumatriptan 28:32.28.

Metoclopramide has been used as an antiemetic for the prevention of nausea and vomiting associated with drugs other than antineoplastic agents†, radiation therapy†, and other causes†. The drug also has been used for the management of intractable hiccups†, to promote postpartum lactation†, and to empty the stomach of blood prior to endoscopy in patients with upper GI hemorrhage†. The safety and efficacy of metoclopramide in these conditions have not been established.

DOSAGE AND ADMINISTRATION

● Administration

Metoclopramide is administered orally, intranasally, by IM or direct IV injection, or by IV infusion.

Therapy with the drug, including all dosage forms and routes of administration, should not exceed 12 weeks' duration because of the risk for developing tardive dyskinesia with longer-term use. (See Tardive Dyskinesia under Cautions: Nervous System Effects.) Oral and intranasal preparations of metoclopramide are recommended for adults *only*.

Oral Administration

Metoclopramide is administered orally on an empty stomach as conventional tablets, an oral solution, or orally disintegrating tablets. At least one manufacturer states that the dose should not be repeated if inadvertently administered with food.

Because metoclopramide orally disintegrating tablets rapidly absorb moisture, each dose should be removed from the blister packaging with dry hands and immediately placed on the tongue. The tablet should disintegrate on the tongue in approximately one minute (range: 10 seconds to 14 minutes). The orally disintegrating tablets are intended to be taken without liquid; it is unknown whether administration with liquid affects the pharmacokinetics of the drug. Any orally disintegrating tablet that breaks or crumbles during handling should be discarded.

Intranasal Administration

Metoclopramide nasal spray is administered by nasal inhalation using a metered-dose spray pump. Patients should be instructed carefully in the use of the nasal spray pump, including the need to prime the pump prior to first use or after a period of nonuse (i.e., 2 weeks or more). To obtain optimum results, patients also should be given a copy of the patient instructions provided by the manufacturer. The manufacturer's instructions for use should be consulted for complete information on administration technique for the metered-dose spray pump.

An extra dose or a double dose should not be administered to make up for a missed dose, and a dose should not be repeated if the patient is uncertain whether the spray entered the nostril; instead, the next dose should be administered at the regularly scheduled time.

IM or IV Administration

For IM or direct IV injection, the commercially available metoclopramide injection is used without further dilution. For direct IV injection, each 10 mg of the drug should be administered slowly over 1–2 minutes, since a transient but intense feeling of anxiety and restlessness, followed by drowsiness, may occur with rapid IV injection.

For doses exceeding 10 mg, metoclopramide injection should be diluted in 50 mL of a compatible IV solution.

For IV infusion, metoclopramide hydrochloride injection should be diluted in 50 mL of one of the following IV solutions: 5% dextrose, 0.9% sodium chloride, 5% dextrose and 0.45% sodium chloride, Ringer's, or lactated Ringer's. Because the drug is most stable when diluted in 0.9% sodium chloride injection, the manufacturers state that this is the preferred solution for preparing IV infusions. IV infusions should be given slowly over at least 15 minutes. Other IV solutions flowing through a common administration tubing or site generally should be discontinued while metoclopramide is being infused unless the solutions are known to be compatible and the flow rate is adequately controlled.

Metoclopramide injection and diluted solutions of the drug should be inspected for particulate matter and discoloration prior to administration

whenever solution and container permit; the solution should be discarded if particulate matter or discoloration is observed.

● Dosage

Although USP currently states that potency of metoclopramide hydrochloride preparations should be expressed both in terms of the salt and the base ("active moiety"), dosage currently is expressed in terms of the base. (See Chemistry and Stability: Chemistry.)

Metoclopramide nasal spray delivers 15 mg of metoclopramide per 70-µL metered spray. Each bottle contains 9.8 mL of solution, which is sufficient for administration 4 times daily over a period of 4 weeks.

Diabetic Gastric Stasis

For relief of symptoms associated with acute and recurrent diabetic gastric stasis, the usual adult oral dosage of metoclopramide is 10 mg 4 times daily, given 30 minutes before meals and at bedtime. The maximum recommended dosage is 40 mg daily. In patients who have severe symptoms or when oral administration of metoclopramide is not feasible, the drug may be given by IM or IV injection. The usual adult IM or IV dosage of metoclopramide for symptomatic relief of diabetic gastric stasis is 10 mg 4 times daily, given 30 minutes before meals and at bedtime; parenteral administration of metoclopramide for up 10 days may be required until symptoms subside sufficiently to allow oral administration of the drug. However, a thorough assessment of the risks and benefits should be made prior to continuing further metoclopramide therapy.

The recommended adult dosage of intranasal metoclopramide for relief of symptoms associated with acute and recurrent diabetic gastric stasis is 15 mg (one spray in one nostril) administered 30 minutes before meals and at bedtime (maximum of 4 times daily).

Therapy with metoclopramide is usually continued for 2–8 weeks, depending on patient response. The lowest effective dosage should be used to reduce the risk of adverse effects. Therapy with metoclopramide, including all dosage forms and routes of administration, should not exceed 12 weeks' duration.

Dosage adjustment is required in patients receiving concomitant therapy with potent inhibitors of cytochrome P-450 isoenzyme 2D6 (CYP2D6). (See CYP2D6 Inhibitors under Drug Interactions: Drugs Affecting or Metabolized by Hepatic Microsomal Enzymes.)

Prevention of Cancer Chemotherapy-induced Emesis

For the prevention of cancer chemotherapy-induced emesis, the manufacturer states that metoclopramide is usually given by IV infusion 30 minutes before administration of cancer chemotherapy, and repeated every 2 hours for 2 additional doses, then every 3 hours for 3 additional doses. For adults, the manufacturer states that the initial 2 doses of metoclopramide should be 2 mg/kg if highly emetogenic drugs (e.g., cisplatin, dacarbazine, dactinomycin) are used alone or in combination, while a metoclopramide dose of 1 mg/kg may be sufficient for less emetogenic drugs or chemotherapy regimens. However, combinations of other antiemetic agents generally are preferred as first-line antiemetic regimens in patients receiving chemotherapy of moderate or high emetic risk (see Uses: Prevention of Cancer Chemotherapy-induced Emesis). If extrapyramidal symptoms occur during these IV metoclopramide dosage regimens, diphenhydramine hydrochloride (e.g., 25–50 mg given IV or IM) may be administered.

Metoclopramide has been administered orally† for the prevention of delayed emesis in patients receiving chemotherapy (i.e., vomiting occurring 24 or more hours after chemotherapy). When given in combination with dexamethasone in clinical trials, oral metoclopramide dosages of 20–40 mg (or 0.5 mg/kg) given 2–4 times daily for 3 or 4 days have been used.

Prevention of Postoperative Nausea and Vomiting

For the prevention of postoperative nausea and vomiting when nasogastric suction is considered undesirable, the manufacturer states that the usual adult IM dose of metoclopramide is 10 mg administered near the end of the surgical procedure, although a 20-mg dose also may be used.

Intubation of the Small Intestine

For patients undergoing intubation of the small intestine in whom the tube has not passed through the pylorus during 10 minutes of conventional maneuvers, the usual dose of metoclopramide to facilitate intubation in adults and children older than 14 years of age is 10 mg, given as a single, direct IV injection. To facilitate intubation in children, the usual single IV dose of metoclopramide is 0.1 mg/kg in children younger than 6 years of age or 2.5–5 mg in children 6–14 years of age.

Radiographic Examination of the Upper GI Tract

For patients in whom delayed gastric emptying interferes with radiographic examination of the stomach and/or small intestine, the usual adult dose of metoclopramide to stimulate gastric emptying and intestinal transit of barium is 10 mg, given as a single, direct IV injection.

Gastroesophageal Reflux

For the symptomatic treatment of gastroesophageal reflux in patients who have not responded to conventional therapy, the usual adult oral dosage of metoclopramide in those who require continuous dosing is 10–15 mg 4 times daily, given 30 minutes before meals and at bedtime, for 4–12 weeks; treatment duration should be based on endoscopic evaluation of response, but the duration should not exceed 12 weeks. The maximum recommended dosage is 60 mg daily. (See Uses: Gastroesophageal Reflux.) If symptoms occur only intermittently or at specific times of the day, single oral doses of up to 20 mg given prior to the provocative situation may be preferred to daily administration of multiple doses of the drug.

Dosage adjustment is required in patients receiving concomitant therapy with potent CYP2D6 inhibitors. (See CYP2D6 Inhibitors under Drug Interactions: Drugs Affecting or Metabolized by Hepatic Microsomal Enzymes.)

● Dosage in Renal and Hepatic Impairment

Renal Impairment

Because metoclopramide is eliminated principally via renal excretion, doses and/or frequency of administration of the drug should be modified in response to the degree of impairment in patients with impaired renal function. The manufacturers recommend that patients with creatinine clearances less than 40 mL/minute receive initial parenteral dosages that are approximately 50% of the usual recommended dosages. Dosage subsequently should be increased or decreased according to the patient's clinical response and tolerance.

Diabetic Gastric Stasis

In adults with moderate or severe renal impairment (creatinine clearance less than 60 mL/minute), the recommended oral dosage of metoclopramide for the relief of symptoms associated with diabetic gastric stasis is 5 mg 4 times daily, given 30 minutes before meals and at bedtime; the maximum recommended dosage is 20 mg daily. In adults with end-stage renal disease, including those undergoing hemodialysis or continuous ambulatory peritoneal dialysis, the recommended oral dosage for the relief of symptoms associated with diabetic gastric stasis is 5 mg twice daily and the maximum recommended oral dosage is 10 mg daily.

Metoclopramide nasal spray is not recommended for use in patients with moderate or severe renal impairment (creatinine clearance less than 60 mL/minute) because dosage of the drug cannot be adjusted to reduce systemic exposure. Adults with mild renal impairment may receive the usual recommended intranasal dosage.

Gastroesophageal Reflux

In adults with moderate or severe renal impairment (creatinine clearance of 60 mL/minute or less), the recommended oral dosage of metoclopramide for the symptomatic treatment of gastroesophageal reflux is 5 mg 4 times daily, given 30 minutes before meals and at bedtime, or 10 mg 3 times daily; the maximum recommended oral dosage is 30 mg daily. In adults with end-stage renal disease, including those undergoing hemodialysis or continuous ambulatory peritoneal dialysis, the recommended oral dosage for the symptomatic treatment of gastroesophageal reflux is 5 mg 4 times daily, given 30 minutes before meals and at bedtime, or 10 mg twice daily; the maximum recommended oral dosage is 20 mg daily.

Hepatic Impairment

Diabetic Gastric Stasis

In adults with moderate or severe hepatic impairment (Child-Pugh class B or C), the recommended oral dosage of metoclopramide for the relief of symptoms associated with diabetic gastric stasis is 5 mg 4 times daily, given 30 minutes before meals and at bedtime; the maximum recommended oral dosage is 20 mg daily. Adults with mild hepatic impairment (Child-Pugh class A) may receive the usual recommended oral dosage.

Metoclopramide nasal spray is not recommended for use in patients with moderate or severe hepatic impairment because dosage of the drug cannot be adjusted to reduce systemic exposure. Adults with mild hepatic impairment may receive the usual recommended intranasal dosage.

Gastroesophageal Reflux

In adults with moderate or severe hepatic impairment, the recommended oral dosage of metoclopramide for the symptomatic treatment of gastroesophageal reflux is 5 mg 4 times daily, given 30 minutes before meals and at bedtime, or 10 mg 3 times daily; the maximum recommended oral dosage is 30 mg daily. Adults with mild hepatic impairment may receive the usual recommended oral dosage.

● Dosage in Geriatric Patients

Because geriatric adults may be more sensitive to the therapeutic or adverse effects of metoclopramide, a reduced initial dosage of the drug is recommended. (See Cautions: Geriatric Precautions.)

Diabetic Gastric Stasis

For relief of symptoms associated with diabetic gastric stasis in geriatric patients, a reduced initial oral metoclopramide dosage of 5 mg 4 times daily, given 30 minutes before meals and at bedtime, should be considered. Dosage may be titrated to a dosage of 10 mg 4 times daily based on response and tolerability. The maximum recommended oral dosage is 40 mg daily.

Metoclopramide nasal spray is not recommended as initial therapy for relief of acute and recurrent diabetic gastric stasis in geriatric patients 65 years of age or older. Geriatric patients may be switched from an alternative metoclopramide preparation administered at a stable dosage of 10 mg 4 times daily to the nasal formulation administered at a dosage of 15 mg (one spray in one nostril) given 30 minutes before meals and at bedtime (maximum 4 times daily).

Gastroesophageal Reflux

For the symptomatic treatment of gastroesophageal reflux in geriatric patients, a reduced initial oral metoclopramide dosage of 5 mg 4 times daily, given 30 minutes before meals and at bedtime, should be considered. Dosage may be titrated to a dosage of 10–15 mg 4 times daily based on response and tolerability. The maximum recommended oral dosage is 60 mg daily.

● Pharmacogenomic Dosage Considerations

The manufacturers make no specific recommendations for parenteral metoclopramide dosage in patients who are poor metabolizers of CYP2D6 substrates.

Diabetic Gastric Stasis

In adults who are poor CYP2D6 metabolizers, the recommended oral dosage of metoclopramide for the relief of symptoms associated with diabetic gastric stasis is 5 mg 4 times daily, given 30 minutes before meals and at bedtime. The maximum recommended oral dosage is 20 mg daily.

Metoclopramide nasal spray is not recommended for use in poor CYP2D6 metabolizers because dosage of the drug cannot be adjusted to reduce systemic exposure.

Gastroesophageal Reflux

In adults who are poor CYP2D6 metabolizers, the recommended oral dosage of metoclopramide for the symptomatic treatment of gastroesophageal reflux is 5 mg 4 times daily, given 30 minutes before meals and at bedtime, or 10 mg 3 times daily. The maximum recommended oral dosage is 30 mg daily.

CAUTIONS

Adverse reactions to metoclopramide generally involve the CNS and GI tract. In general, the incidence of metoclopramide-induced adverse effects is related to dosage and duration of therapy. Adverse effects reported in patients receiving metoclopramide orally disintegrating tablets are similar to those reported with the conventional tablets. In patients receiving intranasal metoclopramide, dysgeusia is the most commonly reported adverse effect; other adverse effects have been similar to those reported with oral administration.

● Nervous System Effects

The most frequent adverse effects of metoclopramide involve the CNS. Restlessness, drowsiness, fatigue, and lassitude have been reported in patients receiving the drug; these effects occur in about 10% of patients receiving a dosage of 10 mg 4 times daily. Insomnia, headache, confusion, dizziness, or depression with suicidal ideation occurs less frequently. The risk of drowsiness is increased at higher doses, occurring in about 70% of patients receiving doses of 1–2 mg/kg. Seizures and hallucinations have been reported. Feelings of anxiety or agitation also may occur, especially following rapid IV injection of the drug. Delirium, severe dysphoria, obsessive rumination, and mania have been reported occasionally.

Extrapyramidal Reactions

Extrapyramidal reactions (e.g., acute dystonic reactions, akathisia) may occur in patients receiving metoclopramide and apparently are mediated via blockade of central dopaminergic receptors involved in motor function. Although extrapyramidal reactions may occur in all age groups and at any dose, they occur more frequently in pediatric patients and adults younger than 30 years of age and following IV administration of high doses of the drug (e.g., those used in prophylaxis of cancer chemotherapy-induced vomiting). Extrapyramidal reactions generally occur within 24–48 hours after starting therapy and usually subside within 24 hours following discontinuance of the drug. Most patients respond rapidly to treatment with diazepam or an agent with central anticholinergic activity such as diphenhydramine or benztropine.

Acute dystonic reactions, which resemble the acute dyskinesias produced by antipsychotic drugs (e.g., phenothiazines, butyrophenones), reportedly occur in less than 1% of adults receiving usual dosages of metoclopramide (e.g., 30–40 mg daily). However, dystonic reactions occur in approximately 25% of young adults (i.e., 18–30 years of age) receiving high dosages of metoclopramide (e.g., 2 mg/kg per dose) during cancer chemotherapy; in adults older than 30 years of age who are receiving similar dosages of metoclopramide, the incidence of dystonic reactions is only about 1.8%. Dystonic reactions associated with metoclopramide therapy include involuntary movements of limbs, trismus, torticollis, facial spasms, rhythmic protrusions of the tongue, bulbar type of speech, opisthotonos, oculogyric crisis, and dystonic reactions resembling tetanus. Dystonic reactions rarely may present as upper airway obstruction with stridor and dyspnea, possibly secondary to laryngospasm or supraglottic dystonia; cardiorespiratory arrest, which was fatal, also has occurred in at least one patient with an acute dystonic reaction. An acute dystonic reaction combined with myoclonus and asterixis also has been reported.

Akathisia combined with severe dysphoria, anxiety, agitation, feelings of jitteriness, and insomnia has been reported. Akathisia appears to be related to the peak plasma metoclopramide concentration. If symptoms resolve, reinitiation of therapy at a lower dosage may be considered.

Tardive Dyskinesia

Treatment with metoclopramide may result in tardive dyskinesia, a potentially irreversible disorder manifested by involuntary movements of the tongue, face, mouth, or jaw, and sometimes by involuntary movements of the trunk and/or extremities; movements may be choreoathetotic in appearance. The risk that patients receiving metoclopramide will develop tardive dyskinesia and the likelihood that it will become irreversible increase with duration of therapy and total cumulative dose; an analysis of drug utilization patterns indicated that the syndrome occurs in about 20% of patients receiving the drug for longer than 12 weeks. In addition, the risk of developing tardive dyskinesia is increased in geriatric patients, especially older women, and patients with diabetes mellitus. Treatment with metoclopramide, including all dosage forms and routes of administration, for longer than 12 weeks should be avoided, and dosage should be reduced in geriatric patients.

Metoclopramide should be discontinued immediately in patients who develop signs or symptoms of tardive dyskinesia. The syndrome may remit, either partially or completely, in some patients within several weeks to months after metoclopramide is discontinued. Metoclopramide itself may suppress or partially suppress the manifestations of tardive dyskinesia, thereby masking the underlying disease process. Whether this symptomatic suppression affects the long-term course of tardive dyskinesia is unknown. Therefore, metoclopramide should not be used for symptomatic control of tardive dyskinesia. Vesicular monoamine transporter 2 (VMAT2) inhibitors (e.g., deutetrabenazine, valbenazine tosylate) have been shown to be effective in reducing symptoms of tardive dyskinesia in controlled clinical studies. (See Deutetrabenazine 28:56 and Valbenazine Tosylate 28:56.)

For additional information on tardive dyskinesia, including manifestations and treatment, see Tardive Dyskinesia under Cautions: Nervous System Effects, in the Phenothiazines General Statement 28:16.08.24.

Neuroleptic Malignant Syndrome

Neuroleptic malignant syndrome (NMS), a potentially fatal symptom complex characterized by hyperpyrexia, muscular rigidity, altered mental status, and autonomic dysfunction, has been reported with dopamine antagonists. NMS has occurred following metoclopramide overdosage in patients receiving concomitant therapy with other drugs known to be associated with NMS. In patients with clinical manifestations consistent with NMS, it is important to determine whether untreated or inadequately treated extrapyramidal reactions and serious medical illness (e.g., pneumonia, systemic infection) may coexist. Other important considerations in the differential diagnosis of NMS include the possibility of central anticholinergic toxicity, heat stroke, malignant hyperthermia, drug fever, serotonin syndrome, and primary CNS pathology. Treatment of NMS includes immediate discontinuance of metoclopramide therapy and other drugs not considered essential to concurrent therapy, intensive symptomatic treatment and medical monitoring, and treatment of any concomitant serious medical condition for which specific therapies are available. (For additional information on NMS, see Neuroleptic Malignant Syndrome under Cautions: Nervous System Effects, in the Phenothiazines General Statement 28:16.08.24.)

Parkinsonian Effects

Parkinsonian symptoms, including tremor, rigidity, bradykinesia, akinesia, and mask-like facies, have occurred in patients receiving metoclopramide. Such symptoms develop more commonly during the first 6 months of metoclopramide therapy but also may occur after longer periods; following discontinuance of the drug, parkinsonian symptoms generally subside within 2–3 months.

Depression

Depression has been reported in patients receiving metoclopramide, including patients with or without a history of an underlying depressive disorder. In some patients, depression has been severe and included unprovoked episodes of uncontrollable crying, suicidal ideation, and suicide. In most patients, signs of depression resolved following discontinuance of the drug.

● GI Effects

Nausea and bowel disturbances, principally diarrhea but also constipation, have occurred in patients receiving metoclopramide. Xerostomia also has occurred. In a placebo-controlled trial evaluating intranasal metoclopramide, dysgeusia was reported in 15% of patients receiving intranasal metoclopramide (14 mg 4 times daily) and 4% of those receiving placebo.

● Sensitivity Reactions

Hypersensitivity reactions, including bronchospasm (especially in patients with a history of asthma), urticaria, and rash (e.g., maculopapular rash), have been reported in patients receiving metoclopramide. Angioedema, including laryngeal, glossal, or periorbital edema, also has been reported.

● Hematologic Effects

Agranulocytosis, neutropenia, and leukopenia have been reported in patients receiving metoclopramide. Methemoglobinemia and sulfhemoglobinemia also have been reported in patients receiving the drug; individuals with deficient or reduced cytochrome-b_5 reductase activity are at an increased risk of developing methemoglobinemia and/or sulfhemoglobinemia. (See Cautions: Precautions and Contraindications and also see Cautions: Pediatric Precautions.) One child reportedly developed symptoms of acute intermittent porphyria immediately following IM administration of metoclopramide; the patient had a known history of acute intermittent porphyria exacerbated by various drugs.

● Genitourinary Effects

Metoclopramide is a potent stimulator of prolactin secretion in both genders; however, the clinical importance of the drug's effect on prolactin has not been fully determined. (See Cautions: Mutagenicity and Carcinogenicity.) Galactorrhea, gynecomastia, and menstrual disorders (e.g., amenorrhea) may occur in some patients during administration of metoclopramide. Impotence secondary to hyperprolactinemia can occur. Serum prolactin concentration usually returns to normal within 1 week following discontinuance of metoclopramide; adverse effects associated with increased serum prolactin concentration usually subside within a few weeks to months following discontinuance of the drug. Urinary frequency and incontinence also have been reported.

● **Cardiovascular Effects**

Metoclopramide may elevate blood pressure; IV administration of the drug in hypertensive patients has been shown to result in catecholamine release. AV block, hypotension, acute congestive heart failure, and hypertension have been reported. In addition, the drug may cause hypertensive crisis in patients with pheochromocytoma, apparently by causing release of catecholamines from the tumor. Metoclopramide-induced hypertensive crisis in patients with pheochromocytoma may be controlled with phentolamine. Metoclopramide should be discontinued in any patient who experiences a rapid increase in blood pressure. Supraventricular tachycardia has been reported following parenteral administration of the drug. Transient flushing of the face and upper body have occurred with large IV doses of the drug. Severe bradycardia has reportedly occurred in one patient immediately following IV administration of 15–17 mg of metoclopramide.

● **Other Adverse Effects**

Visual disturbances have been reported in patients receiving metoclopramide. Fluid retention secondary to transient metoclopramide-induced elevations in serum aldosterone concentration also can occur. Hepatotoxicity, manifested as jaundice and alterations in liver function test results, has occurred in patients receiving metoclopramide concomitantly with other drugs with hepatotoxic potential.

● **Precautions and Contraindications**

The manufacturer's medication guide should be provided to the patient or caregiver each time metoclopramide is dispensed. The patient or caregiver should be instructed to read the medication guide before initiating therapy and each time the prescription is refilled. Patients and/or caregivers should be informed that metoclopramide can cause serious adverse effects, including tardive dyskinesia, extrapyramidal reactions, NMS, and depression and/or suicidality, and should be instructed to discontinue metoclopramide therapy and contact a clinician immediately if such adverse effects occur. Because numerous other medications can precipitate or worsen these adverse reactions, patients and caregivers should be advised to ensure that all prescribing clinicians are aware that the patient is receiving metoclopramide. In addition, patients and caregivers should be informed that oral and intranasal formulations of metoclopramide are recommended for use in adults *only*.

Patients should be warned that metoclopramide may impair their ability to perform activities requiring mental alertness or physical coordination (e.g., operating machinery, driving a motor vehicle). Patients also should be warned that concomitant use of metoclopramide with CNS depressants (e.g., alcohol, sedatives, hypnotics, opiate analgesics, anxiolytics) or drugs known to cause extrapyramidal reactions may increase mental and/or physical impairment; such concomitant use should be avoided.

Extrapyramidal reactions may occur during metoclopramide therapy, especially in pediatric patients and adults younger than 30 years of age, or when high doses such as those used for prophylaxis of cancer chemotherapy-induced nausea and vomiting are administered. Because use of metoclopramide may result in tardive dyskinesia, a syndrome of potentially irreversible, involuntary, dyskinetic movements, therapy with metoclopramide, including all dosage forms and routes of administration, for longer than 12 weeks should be avoided. Metoclopramide should be discontinued immediately in patients who develop signs or symptoms of tardive dyskinesia. Because metoclopramide can exacerbate parkinsonian symptoms, the drug should be avoided in patients with parkinsonian syndrome and in other patients receiving antiparkinsonian drugs. NMS, a potentially fatal syndrome requiring immediate discontinuance of the drug and intensive symptomatic treatment, has been reported in patients receiving metoclopramide. (See Cautions: Nervous System Effects.) Use of metoclopramide should be avoided in patients receiving drugs that are associated with NMS or that are likely to cause tardive dyskinesia or extrapyramidal reactions (e.g., antipsychotic agents).

Metoclopramide should be avoided in patients with a history of mental depression.

Because metoclopramide can stimulate GI motility, the drug theoretically could produce increased pressure on suture lines following GI anastomosis

or closure. This possibility should be considered and weighed when deciding whether to use metoclopramide or nasogastric suction for the prevention of postoperative nausea and vomiting.

In patients with moderate to severe renal impairment, clearance of metoclopramide is decreased, resulting in increased systemic exposure to the drug and the potential for increased adverse effects. (See Pharmacokinetics: Elimination.) Therefore, patients with moderate to severe renal impairment, including those undergoing hemodialysis or continuous ambulatory peritoneal dialysis, should receive reduced dosages of the drug. (See Dosage and Administration: Dosage in Renal and Hepatic Impairment.)

In patients with severe hepatic impairment, clearance of metoclopramide is decreased by approximately 50%, resulting in increased systemic exposure to the drug and the potential for increased adverse effects. Pharmacokinetic data are lacking in patients with moderate hepatic impairment. Therefore, patients with moderate or severe hepatic impairment should receive reduced dosages of the drug. (See Dosage and Administration: Dosage in Renal and Hepatic Impairment.)

Because of the potential for transient increases in plasma aldosterone concentrations and sodium retention, the manufacturer and some clinicians state that certain patients (e.g., those with hepatic impairment, cirrhosis, or congestive heart failure) may be at risk of developing fluid retention and volume overload or hypokalemia and should be closely monitored while receiving the drug. The manufacturer states that if fluid retention or volume overload occurs at any time during metoclopramide therapy, the drug should be discontinued.

Because metoclopramide may increase blood pressure and there is some evidence in hypertensive patients that the drug may increase circulating catecholamines, metoclopramide should be avoided in patients with hypertension and in those receiving monoamine oxidase (MAO) inhibitors. Hypertensive crisis has been reported in patients with undiagnosed pheochromocytoma, and metoclopramide should be discontinued in any patient who experiences a rapid increase in blood pressure.

Adverse reactions, particularly those involving the CNS (including dizziness, nervousness, and/or headaches), may occur following discontinuance of metoclopramide therapy.

Because metoclopramide is metabolized by cytochrome P-450 isoenzyme 2D6 (CYP2D6), patients who are CYP2D6 poor metabolizers may eliminate metoclopramide more slowly than individuals who are CYP2D6 intermediate, extensive, or ultra-rapid metabolizers. Poor metabolizers may be at increased risk of dystonic and other adverse reactions to the drug. Therefore, reduced dosage is recommended in patients who are CYP2D6 poor metabolizers. (See Dosage and Administration: Pharmacogenomic Dosage Considerations.)

Patients with cytochrome-b_5 reductase deficiency have an increased risk of methemoglobinemia and/or sulfhemoglobinemia when metoclopramide is administered. In patients with glucose-6-phosphate dehydrogenase (G-6-PD) deficiency who experience metoclopramide-induced methemoglobinemia, methylene blue treatment is not recommended. (See Acute Toxicity: Treatment.)

Individuals who must restrict their intake of phenylalanine should be advised that each 5- or 10-mg orally disintegrating tablet of metoclopramide contains aspartame, which is metabolized in the GI tract to provide 4.7 mg of phenylalanine per tablet.

Some formulations of metoclopramide oral solution may contain the dye tartrazine (FD&C yellow No. 5), which may cause allergic reactions including bronchial asthma in susceptible individuals. Although the incidence of tartrazine sensitivity is low, it frequently occurs in patients who are sensitive to aspirin.

Metoclopramide is contraindicated in patients with a history of tardive dyskinesia or a dystonic reaction to the drug.

Metoclopramide is contraindicated in patients with known hypersensitivity to the drug. Although there are no reports to date, patients allergic to procainamide theoretically may exhibit cross-sensitivity to metoclopramide, since the drugs are structurally similar.

Metoclopramide is contraindicated in patients in whom stimulation of GI motility might be dangerous (e.g., in the presence of mechanical obstruction or perforation). Although the manufacturers state that metoclopramide also is contraindicated in patients with GI hemorrhage, the drug has been used by some clinicians to empty the stomach of blood prior to endoscopy in patients with acute upper GI hemorrhage.

Metoclopramide is contraindicated in patients with pheochromocytoma or other catecholamine-releasing paragangliomas, since the drug may cause hypertensive/pheochromocytoma crisis in these patients.

Metoclopramide is contraindicated in patients with a history of seizure disorders since the frequency and severity of seizures may be increased by the drug.

Pediatric Precautions

The safety profile of metoclopramide in adults cannot be extrapolated to pediatric patients. Dystonias and other extrapyramidal reactions to metoclopramide are more common in pediatric patients than in adults.

Safety and efficacy of oral and intranasal formulations of metoclopramide have not been established in pediatric patients, and these formulations are *not* recommended for use in pediatric patients because of the risk of tardive dyskinesia and other extrapyramidal reactions, as well as the risk of methemoglobinemia in neonates.

Safety and efficacy of metoclopramide injection in pediatric patients have been established *only* for use to facilitate intubation of the small intestine. Metoclopramide injection should be used with caution in pediatric patients, since the incidence of extrapyramidal reactions is increased in these patients. In addition, metoclopramide injection should be administered with caution to neonates because decreased clearance may result in increased serum concentrations of the drug. (See Pharmacokinetics: Elimination.) In addition, since neonates have reduced concentrations of cytochrome-b_5 reductase, they may be more susceptible to methemoglobinemia.

Following oral or IV administration of metoclopramide in infants and children, pharmacodynamics of the drug are highly variable, and a relationship between drug plasma concentrations and pharmacodynamic effects has not been established. Data are insufficient to determine whether the pharmacokinetics of the drug in children are similar to those in adults.

Geriatric Precautions

Geriatric patients are more likely to have decreased renal function and may be more sensitive to therapeutic or adverse effects of metoclopramide. Geriatric patients, especially older women, are at increased risk for tardive dyskinesia. In addition, the risk of developing parkinsonian symptoms increases with increasing dosage. Therefore, geriatric patients should receive the lowest effective dosage of metoclopramide. If parkinsonian symptoms develop in a geriatric patient receiving metoclopramide, metoclopramide generally should be discontinued before any specific antiparkinsonian therapy is considered. Sedation has been reported in patients receiving metoclopramide and may be manifested as confusion and oversedation in geriatric patients.

Metoclopramide is known to be substantially eliminated by the kidneys, and the risk of adverse reactions to the drug, including tardive dyskinesia, may be increased in patients with impaired renal function. Reduced dosage should be considered in geriatric patients. In general, dosage should be selected carefully, usually initiating therapy at the low end of the dosage range; the greater frequency of decreased renal function and of concomitant disease and drug therapy observed in geriatric patients also should be considered. (See Dosage and Administration: Dosage in Geriatric Patients.)

Mutagenicity and Carcinogenicity

No evidence of metoclopramide-induced mutagenicity was observed in the Ames microbial mutagen test, the unscheduled DNA synthesis assay in rat and human hepatocytes, or the rat micronucleus assay. However, mutagenic effects were observed in the Chinese hamster lung cell assay measuring forward mutations of the HGPRT locus, and clastogenic effects were observed in the human lymphocyte chromosome aberration assay.

Hyperprolactinemia may potentially stimulate prolactin-dependent breast cancer; however, some clinical and epidemiologic studies have not shown an association between administration of dopamine D_2-receptor antagonists and tumorigenesis in humans. In a 77-week study in rats receiving metoclopramide at dosages of approximately 6 times the maximum recommended human dosage (MRHD), persistent elevation of prolactin concentrations and an increase in mammary neoplasms were observed following long-term administration. In a rat model assessing tumor promotion potential, administration of metoclopramide at a dosage of approximately 35 times the MRHD for 2 weeks enhanced the tumorigenic effect of *N*-nitrosodiethylamine.

Pregnancy, Fertility, and Lactation

Pregnancy

Published studies, including retrospective cohort studies, national registry studies, and meta-analyses, have not revealed an increased risk of adverse pregnancy-related outcomes with metoclopramide use during pregnancy. However, metoclopramide crosses the placenta and may cause extrapyramidal reactions and methemoglobinemia in neonates whose mothers received the drug during delivery; these neonates should be monitored for extrapyramidal effects. (See Extrapyramidal Reactions under Cautions: Nervous System Effects.)

Reproduction studies in pregnant rats and rabbits using metoclopramide dosages of approximately 6 and 12 times, respectively, the MRHD have not revealed evidence of adverse developmental effects.

Fertility

Reproduction studies in male and female rats using metoclopramide dosages of up to approximately 3 times the MRHD have not revealed evidence of impaired fertility or altered reproductive performance. Menstrual disturbances and impotence have occurred in some individuals during metoclopramide therapy. (See Cautions: Genitourinary Effects.)

Lactation

Limited published data indicate that metoclopramide is distributed into milk; the estimated dose received by breast-fed infants is less than 10% of the maternal weight-adjusted dose. In one study, the estimated dose received by infants from breast milk ranged from 6–24 mcg/kg daily at 3–9 days postpartum and from 1–13 mcg/kg daily at 8–12 weeks postpartum. Exposure is expected to be similar following maternal doses of 10 mg administered orally or 15 mg administered intranasally. Adverse GI effects, including intestinal discomfort and increased intestinal gas formation, have been reported in breast-fed infants who were exposed to metoclopramide. Although metoclopramide increases prolactin concentrations, data are not adequate to support drug-related effects on milk production.

The developmental and health benefits of breast-feeding should be considered along with the mother's clinical need for metoclopramide and any potential adverse effects on the breast-fed child from the drug or from the underlying maternal condition. Nursing neonates should be monitored for extrapyramidal effects (dystonias) and methemoglobinemia. (See Extrapyramidal Reactions under Cautions: Nervous System Effects and also see Acute Toxicity.)

DRUG INTERACTIONS

Metoclopramide undergoes metabolism via cytochrome P-450 isoenzyme 2D6 (CYP2D6), as well as conjugation with glucuronic acid and sulfuric acid.

Effects on GI Absorption of Drugs

Because of its pharmacologic effects on transit time in the stomach and small intestine, metoclopramide may alter the absorption of certain drugs. The extent of absorption of drugs that disintegrate, dissolve, and/or are absorbed mainly in the stomach (e.g., digoxin) may be diminished by metoclopramide, whereas the rate and extent of absorption of drugs that are mainly absorbed in the small intestine (e.g., acetaminophen, aspirin, cyclosporine, diazepam, ethanol, levodopa, lithium, tetracycline) may be enhanced. Absorption of atovaquone, fosfomycin, and posaconazole oral suspension (but not posaconazole delayed-release tablets) also may be diminished by metoclopramide. Patients receiving drugs with possible diminished GI absorption should be monitored for reduced efficacy. In patients receiving digoxin concomitantly with metoclopramide, digoxin concentrations should be monitored and digoxin dosage should be increased as needed. Because absorption of orally administered cyclosporine, sirolimus, or tacrolimus may be increased by metoclopramide, concentrations of these drugs should be monitored and dosage of the immunosuppressive agent should be adjusted as needed.

Drugs Affecting GI Motility

The effects of metoclopramide on GI motility are antagonized by anticholinergic agents (e.g., atropine) and opiate analgesics.

Drugs that impair GI motility (e.g., antiperistaltic antidiarrheal agents, anticholinergic drugs, opiates) may reduce oral absorption of metoclopramide;

patients requiring such concomitant therapy should be monitored for reduced efficacy of metoclopramide.

● Drugs Affecting or Metabolized by Hepatic Microsomal Enzymes

CYP2D6 Inhibitors

Concomitant administration of metoclopramide (20-mg oral dose) and the potent CYP2D6 inhibitor fluoxetine (60 mg orally daily) in healthy individuals increased peak plasma concentration and area under the concentration-time curve (AUC) of metoclopramide by 40 and 90%, respectively, compared with administration of metoclopramide alone. Such increases in plasma concentrations of metoclopramide may be associated with exacerbation of extrapyramidal symptoms.

If metoclopramide is used concomitantly with a potent CYP2D6 inhibitor (e.g, bupropion, fluoxetine, paroxetine, quinidine), metoclopramide dosage should be reduced. In adults receiving potent CYP2D6 inhibitors, the recommended oral dosage of metoclopramide for the relief of symptoms associated with diabetic gastric stasis is 5 mg given 4 times daily (maximum 20 mg daily) and the recommended oral dosage for the symptomatic treatment of gastroesophageal reflux is 5 mg given 4 times daily or 10 mg given 3 times daily (maximum 30 mg daily). The manufacturers make no specific recommendations for parenteral metoclopramide dosage in patients receiving potent CYP2D6 inhibitors. Concomitant use of intranasal metoclopramide and potent CYP2D6 inhibitors is not recommended since dosage of the intranasal preparation cannot be adjusted to reduce exposure.

CYP2D6 Substrates

Although in vitro studies suggest that metoclopramide can inhibit CYP2D6, metoclopramide is unlikely to interact with CYP2D6 substrates in vivo at clinically relevant concentrations.

● Drugs with Similar Adverse Effect Profiles

Because of the potential for additive adverse effects, metoclopramide should be avoided in patients receiving drugs that are likely to cause extrapyramidal reactions or drugs that are associated with tardive dyskinesia or neuroleptic malignant syndrome (NMS). (See Cautions: Precautions and Contraindications.)

● Anesthetic Agents

Acute hypotension reportedly occurred in some patients receiving IV metoclopramide during neurosurgical procedures in which hypotensive anesthetic agents were used; various anesthetic agents, with or without concomitant administration of ganglionic blocking agents, were used. The mechanism and clinical importance of this adverse reaction are not known.

● Antipsychotic Agents

Concomitant use of metoclopramide and antipsychotic agents may result in additive adverse effects, including increased frequency and severity of tardive dyskinesia, parkinsonian or other extrapyramidal symptoms, and NMS. Such concomitant use should be avoided.

● CNS Depressants

Metoclopramide may be additive with, or may potentiate the action of, other CNS depressants such as opiates or other analgesics, sedatives or hypnotics, anxiolytic agents, anesthetics, or alcohol. Such concomitant use should be avoided.

● Dopaminergic Agents

Concomitant use of metoclopramide and dopamine receptor agonists (e.g., apomorphine, bromocriptine, cabergoline, pramipexole, ropinirole, rotigotine) or other drugs that increase dopamine concentrations (e.g., levodopa) may result in reduced efficacy of metoclopramide and possible exacerbation of parkinsonian symptoms because of the opposing effects of the drugs on dopamine. Because of the potential for exacerbation of parkinsonian symptoms, such concomitant use should be avoided. However, if such concomitant therapy is required, therapeutic effects of the drugs should be monitored.

● Insulin

Gastric stasis may be responsible for poor diabetic control in some patients; exogenously administered insulin may begin to act before food has left the stomach,

potentially resulting in hypoglycemia. Increases in blood glucose concentrations may occur secondary to metoclopramide-induced increases in GI motility and increased delivery of food to the intestines. Monitoring of blood glucose concentrations and adjustment of insulin dosage or timing of administration may be necessary in patients with insulin-controlled diabetes mellitus.

● Monoamine Oxidase Inhibitors

Metoclopramide has been shown to cause release of catecholamines in patients with essential hypertension. Because concomitant use of metoclopramide and monoamine oxidase (MAO) inhibitors increases the risk of hypertension, concomitant use of these drugs should be avoided.

● Neuromuscular Blocking Agents

Metoclopramide inhibits plasma cholinesterase leading to enhanced neuromuscular blockade by neuromuscular blocking agents (e.g., mivacurium [no longer commercially available in the US], succinylcholine). Patients receiving such concomitant therapy should be monitored for prolonged neuromuscular blockade.

ACUTE TOXICITY

Limited information is available on the acute toxicity of metoclopramide.

● Pathogenesis

The acute lethal dose of metoclopramide in humans is not known. In addition, there is no clearly defined relationship between plasma metoclopramide concentration and severity of intoxication. The oral LD_{50} of metoclopramide is 465 mg/kg in mice, 760 mg/kg in rats, and 870 mg/kg in rabbits. In animals, lethal doses produced dyspnea, excessive lacrimation, decreased activity, ataxia, miosis, tachycardia, tremors, and tonic seizures. Oral metoclopramide dosages up to 1 g daily have been used for several weeks in some patients receiving the drug for the management of psychiatric disorders.

● Manifestations

One patient who intentionally ingested 360 mg of metoclopramide experienced only drowsiness and disorientation. Although the patient was not lucid at the time of hospitalization, no focal neurologic abnormalities or cardiovascular symptoms were present, and gastric lavage was performed. Another patient had an uneventful recovery after ingesting 800 mg of metoclopramide; the patient had no abnormal neurologic, autonomic, or cardiovascular signs or symptoms. There have been numerous reports of overdosage in children; most of these children were younger than 1 year of age and were inadvertently given excessive amounts (1–11.6 mg/kg) orally over a 2- to 3-day period. One 5-month-old infant who weighed 7 kg was given a single 5-mg IM dose of metoclopramide; symptoms of overdose appeared within 30 minutes following administration and subsided within 12 hours. Manifestations of overdosage in these children included drowsiness, ataxia, agitation, hyperexcitability, dystonic extrapyramidal reactions, attacks of muscular contractions of the face or neck, oculogyric crisis, opisthotonos, and seizures. None of these patients lost consciousness, and all recovered spontaneously within 12–48 hours.

Methemoglobinemia, which responded to methylene blue therapy, and reduced oxyhemoglobin saturation occurred in a neonate who inadvertently received 1 mg/kg of metoclopramide orally every 6 hours for 36 hours. The neonate presented with manifestations of cyanosis, lethargy, poor feeding, diarrhea, and respiratory distress. Methemoglobinemia also has developed in several other infants following overdosage with the drug, and this age group may be predisposed to developing this toxicity.

In general, overdosage of metoclopramide may be expected to produce effects that are extensions of common adverse reactions; drowsiness, disorientation, and extrapyramidal reactions have been the principal effects reported. Other reported effects associated with metoclopramide overdosage have included feelings of anxiety or restlessness, headache, vertigo, nausea, vomiting, constipation, weakness, hypotension, and xerostomia; in addition, generalized seizures and methemoglobinemia have occurred. Deaths have been reported. Neuroleptic malignant syndrome (NMS) has been reported following metoclopramide overdosage in patients receiving concomitant therapy with other drugs associated with NMS.

• Treatment

Treatment of metoclopramide overdosage generally involves symptomatic and supportive care. There is no specific antidote for metoclopramide intoxication; however, agents with central anticholinergic activity (e.g., diphenhydramine, benztropine) may be useful in controlling extrapyramidal reactions. Following acute ingestion of the drug, the stomach should be emptied immediately. If the patient is comatose, having seizures, or lacks the gag reflex, gastric lavage may be performed if an endotracheal tube with cuff inflated is in place to prevent aspiration of gastric contents. Symptoms of metoclopramide overdosage are generally self-limiting and usually subside within 24 hours. Appropriate therapy should be instituted if hypotension or excessive sedation occurs. Methemoglobinemia should be treated with methylene blue. However, in patients with glucose-6-phosphate dehydrogenase (G-6-PD) deficiency, methylene blue can induce hemolytic anemia, which may be fatal. Hemodialysis or peritoneal dialysis does not substantially enhance the elimination of metoclopramide.

PHARMACOLOGY

The pharmacology of metoclopramide is complex and its mechanism(s) of action has not been fully elucidated. The principal pharmacologic effects of metoclopramide involve the GI tract and CNS.

• GI Effects

Metoclopramide has several effects on mechanical activity of GI smooth muscle. At low concentrations in vitro, metoclopramide increases the resting tone and phasic contractile activity of GI smooth muscle, while at high concentrations, the drug inhibits mechanical activity. Metoclopramide increases lower esophageal sphincter pressure in patients with hiatal hernia with or without associated gastroesophageal reflux and in healthy individuals. Following oral or IV administration of the drug, lower esophageal sphincter pressure generally increases to a greater extent in healthy individuals than in patients with reflux; there appears to be substantial interindividual variation in the effect of metoclopramide on lower esophageal sphincter pressure.

Metoclopramide accelerates gastric emptying and intestinal transit from the duodenum to the ileocecal valve by increasing the amplitude and duration of esophageal contractions, the resting tone of the lower esophageal sphincter, and the amplitude and tone of gastric (especially antral) contractions and by relaxing the pyloric sphincter and the duodenal bulb, while increasing peristalsis of the duodenum and jejunum. Unlike nonspecific cholinergic-like stimulation of upper GI smooth muscle, the stimulant effects of metoclopramide on GI smooth muscle coordinate gastric, pyloric, and duodenal motor activity. Metoclopramide is most effective in patients with reduced antral tone and duodenal activity. Metoclopramide lowers the pressure threshold for occurrence of the peristaltic reflex and enhances the frequency and amplitude of longitudinal muscle contractions. In addition to its ability to enhance motor activity of upper GI smooth muscle, metoclopramide may also increase gastric emptying by inhibiting receptive relaxation of the gastric fundus.

Although metoclopramide has been reported to have little, if any, effect on motility of the colon in several studies, there is some evidence that the drug may increase colonic motility. The effect of metoclopramide on motility of the gallbladder has been variable.

The pharmacologic actions of metoclopramide on the upper GI tract are similar to those of cholinergic drugs (e.g., bethanechol); however, unlike cholinergic drugs, metoclopramide does not stimulate gastric, biliary, or pancreatic secretions and does not affect serum gastrin concentration.

Although the exact mechanism of action of metoclopramide is unclear, the effects of metoclopramide on GI motility may be mediated via enhancement of cholinergic excitatory processes at the postganglionic neuromuscular junction; antagonism of nonadrenergic, noncholinergic inhibitory motor nerves (i.e., dopaminergic); and/or a direct effect on smooth muscle.

The effects of metoclopramide on GI motility do not depend on intact vagal innervation but are reduced or abolished by anticholinergic drugs (e.g., atropine) and potentiated by cholinergic drugs (e.g., carbachol, methacholine). These findings suggest that metoclopramide's effects on GI motility may depend in part on intramural cholinergic neurons of smooth muscle that are intact after vagal denervation. Unlike cholinergic drugs, metoclopramide requires intrinsic neuronal storage sites of acetylcholine to exert its pharmacologic effects. Postsynaptic

activity results from metoclopramide's ability to enhance release of acetylcholine from postganglionic cholinergic neurons in the GI tract and to sensitize muscarinic receptors of GI smooth muscle to the actions of acetylcholine.

Metoclopramide does *not* exhibit anticholinesterase activity and its GI stimulant actions are not affected by ganglionic blocking drugs; however, the sensitization to acetylcholine may be prevented by ganglionic blocking drugs (e.g., hexamethonium).

Metoclopramide is a potent dopamine-receptor antagonist, and some of the actions of metoclopramide on GI smooth muscle may be mediated via antagonism of dopaminergic neurotransmission. Specific dopamine receptors in the esophagus and stomach have been identified; however, it is not known if there is a dopaminergic control system for smooth muscle function in the upper GI tract. In the GI tract, dopamine is principally an inhibitory neurotransmitter. Dopamine decreases the intensity of esophageal contractions, relaxes the proximal stomach, and reduces gastric secretion. Although metoclopramide blocks these inhibitory effects of dopamine, the actual role of dopamine in the peripheral control of GI motility has not been fully elucidated. Since cholinergic mechanisms are responsible for most excitatory motor activity in the GI tract, it appears that metoclopramide's therapeutic effects are principally caused by the drug's cholinergic-like activity; however, antagonism of GI dopaminergic activity may augment metoclopramide's cholinergic-like activity.

• Nervous System Effects

Metoclopramide is a potent central dopamine-receptor antagonist. The drug has antiemetic and sedative activity.

Antiemetic Effect

The precise mechanism of antiemetic action of metoclopramide is unclear, but the drug has been shown to directly affect the medullary chemoreceptor trigger zone (CTZ) in the area postrema, apparently by blocking dopamine (e.g., D_2) receptors in the CTZ. Metoclopramide increases the CTZ threshold and decreases the sensitivity of visceral nerves that transmit afferent impulses from the GI tract to the vomiting center in the lateral reticular formation. The drug also enhances gastric emptying, which is believed to minimize stasis that precedes vomiting. It also has been suggested that inhibition of serotonin (i.e., 5-HT₃) receptors, at least when relatively high doses of metoclopramide are used, may contribute to the antiemetic action of the drug. Metoclopramide inhibits the central and peripheral emetic effects of apomorphine, hydergine, and levodopa.

Other Nervous System Effects

In animals, metoclopramide exhibits neuroleptic effects similar to those of antipsychotic agents (e.g., phenothiazines); metoclopramide produces catalepsy and reverses behavioral effects mediated by amphetamine and apomorphine. Following administration of usual dosages (e.g., 40 mg daily), metoclopramide exhibits little, if any, antipsychotic or tranquilizing activity in psychiatric patients; however, antipsychotic effects have been observed in a limited number of patients with chronic schizophrenic disorder receiving oral metoclopramide dosages of 520–1000 mg daily for up to 24 days.

Metoclopramide produces varying degrees of sedation and lethargy in healthy adults. The drug may cause EEG changes, including increased slow-wave activity. Based on limited data in animals, usual IV doses of metoclopramide do not appear to lower the seizure threshold.

Like other dopamine-receptor antagonists (e.g., phenothiazines), metoclopramide may cause extrapyramidal reactions. (See Cautions: Nervous System Effects.) Metoclopramide may worsen symptoms in patients with parkinsonian syndrome.

• Cardiovascular and Renal Effects

Although metoclopramide does *not* appear to have clinically important antiarrhythmic activity, transient antiarrhythmic effects have been observed in animals and humans following administration of large IV doses. Following IV administration of a single 20-mg dose to patients with valvular heart disease (e.g., mitral stenosis) in one study, metoclopramide did *not* produce ECG changes nor did it exert a clinically important effect on hemodynamic parameters, including cardiac output, left ventricular end-diastolic pressure, or pulmonary arterial pressure. In a controlled ECG study in healthy individuals, a single 80-mg intranasal dose of metoclopramide had no effect on the corrected QT (QT_c) interval. At doses greater than 40 mg/kg in animals, metoclopramide produces only minimal

ECG changes, including enhancement of R and T waves and a transient decrease in heart rate.

In healthy adults in one study, metoclopramide potentiated the vasopressor response to dopamine; however, in animals, metoclopramide reportedly blocks the hypertensive effect of dopamine. Potentiation of the vasopressor response to dopamine in humans may result from inhibition of a central homeostatic reflex by metoclopramide.

Limited data suggest that metoclopramide decreases renal plasma flow, at least at high doses given IV. The mechanism of this effect and its clinical importance remain to be established.

● Metabolic and Endocrine Effects

Metoclopramide indirectly stimulates secretion of prolactin from the anterior pituitary gland by inhibiting dopamine receptors in the pituitary and hypothalamus. Hyperprolactinemia may suppress hypothalamic gonadotropin-releasing hormone secretion, resulting in reduced pituitary gonadotropin secretion, which may inhibit reproductive function by impairing gonadal steroidogenesis in males and females. The elevated prolactin concentrations persist during long-term administration and, like other prolactin-stimulating drugs, may be associated with galactorrhea, amenorrhea, gynecomastia, and impotence.

Metoclopramide does *not* appear to substantially alter the secretion of growth hormone, corticotropin, luteinizing hormone (LH), or follicle-stimulating hormone (FSH); however, following oral administration of a single 10-mg dose in one study in healthy adults, metoclopramide caused a small decrease in serum growth hormone, LH, and FSH concentrations. In another study in hypogonadal males, metoclopramide caused an increase in serum growth hormone concentration following IV administration of 10 mg of the drug. Serum thyrotropin concentrations may be increased by metoclopramide; however, serum thyrotropin concentrations usually remain within normal limits, and the clinical importance of this alteration has not been determined.

Metoclopramide produces a transient increase in plasma aldosterone concentrations. Although the exact mechanism has not been fully determined, metoclopramide appears to increase plasma aldosterone concentrations by stimulating the secretion of aldosterone via a direct effect on adrenal tissue; metoclopramide does not affect the metabolic clearance of aldosterone. There is no correlation between the changes in aldosterone and prolactin concentrations, suggesting that the effect on plasma aldosterone is not mediated via prolactin secretion. Metoclopramide does *not* alter plasma renin activity or plasma potassium or cortisol concentrations. Although the possibility of sodium retention and hypokalemia exists, especially in patients with edema (e.g., those with cirrhosis or congestive heart failure), plasma aldosterone concentrations reportedly return to pretreatment levels during prolonged administration of metoclopramide.

PHARMACOKINETICS

In all studies described in the Pharmacokinetics section, metoclopramide was administered as the monohydrochloride monohydrate salt; dosages and concentrations of the drug are expressed in terms of metoclopramide.

● Absorption

Metoclopramide is rapidly and almost completely absorbed from the GI tract following oral administration; however, absorption may be delayed or diminished in patients with gastric stasis. Considerable interindividual variations (up to five-fold) in peak plasma concentration have been reported with the same oral dose of metoclopramide. This variability apparently results from interindividual differences in first-pass metabolism of the drug. Bioavailability of metoclopramide appears to correlate with the ratio of free:conjugated metoclopramide concentrations in urine. The absolute bioavailability of orally administered metoclopramide has not been clearly established in humans, but limited data indicate that 30–100% of an oral dose of the drug reaches systemic circulation as unchanged metoclopramide. Following IM administration, the absolute bioavailability of metoclopramide is 74–96%.

Following oral administration of a single 10-mg dose of the drug in healthy, fasting adults in one study, peak plasma metoclopramide concentrations of 32–44 ng/mL occurred at 1–2 hours; following oral administration of a single 20-mg dose, peak plasma metoclopramide concentrations of 72–87 ng/mL occurred at an average of 2 hours. In a study in infants (3.5 weeks–5.4 months of age) with gastroesophageal reflux who received 0.15-mg/kg oral doses of metoclopramide every 6 hours for 10 doses as an oral solution, the mean peak plasma concentration (56.8 ng/mL) of the drug after the 10th dose was twofold higher compared with that after the first dose (29 ng/mL), suggesting that metoclopramide accumulates in plasma following multiple oral dosing in this age group.

When administered under fasting conditions in adults, metoclopramide orally disintegrating tablets are bioequivalent to metoclopramide conventional tablets. Administration of the orally disintegrating tablets immediately after a high-fat meal did not affect the extent of absorption, but decreased the peak blood concentration by 17%; the time to peak concentration was increased from approximately 1.75 hours when administered under fasting conditions to 3 hours when administered immediately after a high-fat meal. The clinical importance of the decrease in peak blood concentration if the orally disintegrating tablets are inadvertently administered with food is unknown.

Following intranasal or IV administration of metoclopramide 10 mg, bioavailability of intranasally administered metoclopramide was 47% that of IV metoclopramide. Absorption of the drug is reduced following intranasal administration compared with oral administration; systemic exposure (peak concentration and area under the concentration-time curve [AUC]) and time to reach peak concentration are similar following a 15-mg intranasal dose or a 10-mg oral dose. Over an intranasal dose range of 10–80 mg, exposure to the drug is proportional to dose. Metoclopramide AUC and peak concentration following intranasal administration are increased by 34 and 42%, respectively, in females compared with males. Lean body weight (range: 34–94 kg) also appears to affect the pharmacokinetics of the intranasally administered drug, with lower systemic exposure expected in individuals with higher lean body weight. The clinical relevance of these findings is unknown.

The onset of the principal pharmacologic actions of metoclopramide on the GI tract is 1–3 minutes following IV administration, 10–15 minutes following IM administration, and 30–60 minutes following oral administration. Pharmacologic effects persist for 1–2 hours following administration of a single dose.

The therapeutic range for plasma metoclopramide concentrations and the relationship of plasma concentration to clinical response and toxicity have not been clearly established. In one study, a maximum change in lower esophageal sphincter pressure correlated poorly with peak plasma metoclopramide concentration. Data from patients receiving large IV doses of metoclopramide (8 mg/kg in 4 divided doses) for the prevention of cisplatin-induced nausea and vomiting indicate that serum metoclopramide concentrations greater than 850 ng/mL may be required for optimum antiemetic effect in patients receiving cisplatin. Metoclopramide-induced akathisia is reportedly associated with peak plasma metoclopramide concentrations greater than 120 ng/mL.

● Distribution

Distribution of metoclopramide into human body tissues and fluids has not been fully characterized. The apparent volume of distribution of metoclopramide is reportedly 2.2–3.5 L/kg in adults and 1.93–4.4 L/kg in children. Following IM administration of metoclopramide in mice, the drug is rapidly distributed into most body tissues and fluids with high concentrations in the GI mucosa, liver, biliary tract, and salivary glands, and lower concentrations in brain, heart, thymus, adrenals, adipose tissue, and bone marrow. Metoclopramide crosses the blood-brain barrier and enters the CNS in animals, with high concentrations in the area postrema, which contains the chemoreceptor trigger zone (CTZ).

Metoclopramide is weakly bound to plasma proteins; in vitro, metoclopramide is 13–30% protein bound, principally to albumin.

Metoclopramide crosses the placenta and is distributed into milk; concentrations of the drug in milk are higher than those in plasma 2 hours after oral administration. (See Cautions: Pregnancy, Fertility, and Lactation.)

● Elimination

Plasma concentrations of metoclopramide decline in a biphasic manner.

Although limited data from single-dose studies have suggested that elimination of metoclopramide is dose dependent, other studies using oral doses up to 100 mg have *not* shown a dose-dependent pharmacokinetic profile. In addition, one pharmacokinetic study using high doses of metoclopramide did *not* demonstrate dose-dependent elimination. In adults, the half-life of metoclopramide in the initial phase ($t_{\frac{1}{2}\alpha}$) is about 5 minutes, and the half-life in the terminal phase ($t_{\frac{1}{2}\beta}$) ranges from 2.5–6 hours. A half-life of 8.1 hours has been reported following intranasal administration. In children receiving oral or IV metoclopramide, the elimination half-life of the drug reportedly is 4.1–4.5 hours. Following oral administration of 0.15-mg/kg doses of metoclopramide every 6 hours for 10 doses in an infant (3.5 weeks of age), elimination half-lives of 23.1 and 10.3 hours were observed after the first and 10th dose, respectively, which were substantially longer than those reported in older infants, suggesting a reduced clearance in the neonate possibly being associated with immature renal and hepatic functions present at birth. Total body clearance of metoclopramide is reportedly 10.9–11.7 mL/minute per kg in adults with normal renal function. In children receiving oral or IV metoclopramide, clearance of the drug reportedly is 6.16–11.1 mL/minute per kg.

Metoclopramide undergoes enzymatic metabolism via oxidation as well as conjugation with glucuronic acid and sulfuric acid in the liver. Monodeethyl-metoclopramide, a major oxidative metabolite, is formed mainly by cytochrome P-450 isoenzyme 2D6 (CYP2D6), an enzyme subject to genetic variability.

Metoclopramide and its metabolites are excreted in urine and feces. In a limited number of adults with normal renal function, approximately 85% of an oral dose of radiolabeled metoclopramide was excreted in urine within 72 hours of administration, principally as unchanged drug and glucuronide or sulfate conjugates of metoclopramide. About 18–20% of an oral dose of metoclopramide is excreted in urine as unchanged drug within 36 hours. Approximately 5% of an oral dose of the drug is excreted in feces via biliary elimination.

Plasma metoclopramide concentrations may be higher and the half-life prolonged in patients with impaired renal function. In patients with moderate or severe renal impairment, systemic exposure to metoclopramide, as measured by AUC, following oral administration is approximately twice that observed in individuals with normal renal function; in those with end-stage renal disease requiring dialysis, systemic exposure is approximately 3.5 times that observed in individuals with normal renal function. Metoclopramide is only minimally removed by hemodialysis or peritoneal dialysis.

In a limited number of patients with severe hepatic impairment (Child-Pugh class C), average clearance of metoclopramide following oral administration was reduced by approximately 50% compared with patients with normal hepatic function.

CHEMISTRY AND STABILITY

● Chemistry

Metoclopramide hydrochloride, a synthetic substituted benzamide, is a dopamine-receptor antagonist, an antiemetic, and a stimulant of upper GI motility. The drug is a derivative of p-aminobenzoic acid and is structurally related to procainamide, but lacks local anesthetic and antiarrhythmic properties. Metoclopramide differs structurally from procainamide by the presence of 5-chloro and 2-methoxy aryl substituents.

Metoclopramide hydrochloride occurs as a monohydrate, white, odorless, crystalline powder. The drug has solubilities of approximately 1.43 g/mL in water and 333 mg/mL in alcohol. Metoclopramide hydrochloride has pK_as of 0.6 and 9.3.

Commercially available metoclopramide hydrochloride oral solution occurs as an orange-colored, palatable, aromatic, sugar-free liquid. The oral solution contains parabens as preservatives. Metoclopramide hydrochloride nasal solution is an aqueous solution of the drug; the nasal solution has a pH of 5.5 and contains benzalkonium chloride as a preservative. Each actuation of the metered-spray pump delivers 15 mg of metoclopramide per 70-μL spray.

Metoclopramide hydrochloride injection is a clear, colorless, sterile, nonpyrogenic solution of the drug in water for injection. The injection also contains sodium chloride. The injection has a pH of 2.5–6.5.

USP currently states that potency of metoclopramide hydrochloride preparations should be expressed both in terms of the salt and the base ("active moiety"). Previously, potency was expressed only in terms of metoclopramide base. Dosage currently continues to be expressed in terms of the base. Therefore, care should be taken to avoid confusion between labeled potencies as the salt and base and dosage of metoclopramide hydrochloride.

● Stability

Metoclopramide hydrochloride is photosensitive and will degrade when exposed to light. Commercially available preparations of metoclopramide hydrochloride should be protected from light.

Metoclopramide hydrochloride tablets, orally disintegrating tablets, injection, and oral solution should be stored at controlled room temperature between 20–25°C. The orally disintegrating tablets should be protected from moisture, and the oral solution should be protected from freezing. Metoclopramide hydrochloride tablets and metoclopramide hydrochloride oral solution should be stored in tight, light-resistant containers (i.e., amber glass bottles). The commercially available tablets are stable for 3 years and the oral solution and injection are stable for 5 years after manufacture.

Metoclopramide hydrochloride nasal solution should be stored at 20–25°C, but may be exposed to temperatures ranging from 15–30°C. The nasal solution should be discarded 4 weeks after opening.

Metoclopramide hydrochloride injection is reportedly stable at pH 2–9. Metoclopramide hydrochloride injection is physically and chemically compatible with the following IV solutions: 5% dextrose, 0.9% sodium chloride, 5% dextrose and 0.45% sodium chloride, Ringer's, and lactated Ringer's. Solutions of metoclopramide hydrochloride that have been prepared by dilution of the injection with 50 mL of one of these compatible IV solutions are stable for up to 48 hours when stored at 4–30°C and protected from light or for up to 24 hours when stored at these temperatures and exposed to normal light conditions. Solutions prepared by dilution of the injection with 0.9% sodium chloride injection may be frozen in PVC bags immediately after preparation and are stable for up to 4 weeks at –20°C. Solutions prepared by dilution of the injection with 5% dextrose injection should *not* be frozen in PVC bags since loss of potency of up to about 40% occurs within 4 weeks. Any unused portion remaining in the vial should be discarded and not stored for later use. The manufacturer's prescribing information and specialized references should be consulted for specific information on compatibility with other drugs.

PREPARATIONS

Excipients in commercially available drug preparations may have clinically important effects in some individuals; consult specific product labeling for details.

Metoclopramide Hydrochloride

Nasal		
Solution	15 mg (of metoclopramide) per metered spray	**Gimoti®**, Evoke
Oral		
Solution	5 mg (of metoclopramide) per 5 mL*	Metoclopramide Hydrochloride Oral Solution
Tablets	5 mg (of metoclopramide)*	Metoclopramide Hydrochloride Tablets
		Reglan®, ANI
	10 mg (of metoclopramide)*	Metoclopramide Hydrochloride Tablets
		Reglan®, scoredANI
Tablets, orally disintegrating	5 mg (of metoclopramide)*	Metoclopramide Hydrochloride Orally Disintegrating Tablets
	10 mg (of metoclopramide)*	Metoclopramide Hydrochloride Orally Disintegrating Tablets
Parenteral		
Injection	5 mg (of metoclopramide) per mL*	Metoclopramide Hydrochloride Injection

* available from one or more manufacturer, distributor, and/or repackager by generic (nonproprietary) name

† Use is not currently included in the labeling approved by the US Food and Drug Administration

Prucalopride Succinate

56:32 • PROKINETIC AGENTS

■ Prucalopride succinate, a selective type 4 serotonin (5-HT₄) receptor agonist, is a GI prokinetic agent.

USES

● Chronic Idiopathic Constipation

Prucalopride succinate is used for the symptomatic treatment of chronic idiopathic constipation.

Efficacy and safety of prucalopride for the symptomatic treatment of chronic idiopathic constipation have been evaluated in 6 similarly designed, phase 3 or 4, randomized, double-blind, placebo-controlled studies in a total of 2484 adults (mean age: 47 years, 76% female, 76% Caucasian, mean duration of constipation: 16 years) with chronic constipation not considered to be drug induced or caused by other medical conditions. An integrated analysis of data from the 6 studies indicated that prucalopride increases the frequency of complete spontaneous bowel movements (CSBMs) in patients with chronic idiopathic constipation.

Although there were minor variations among the studies in inclusion criteria, chronic constipation generally was defined as fewer than 3 CSBMs per week for at least 6 months *and* the presence of one of 3 symptoms (hard or very hard stools, a sensation of incomplete evacuation, straining during defecation) during at least 25% of bowel movements. Most of the patients randomized to receive prucalopride in these studies received a dosage of 2 mg daily. A prucalopride dosage of 4 mg daily also was evaluated in 3 studies. In 2 studies, geriatric patients received an initial dosage of 1 mg daily, with dosage increased to 2 mg daily if response was insufficient; dosage was increased in 81% of patients receiving the lower initial dosage. Treatment was continued for 12 weeks in 5 studies and for 24 weeks in one study. The prespecified primary end point in all 6 studies defined response as a mean of 3 or more CSBMs per week evaluated over 12 or 24 weeks of treatment. In a post hoc analysis, an alternative definition of response, based on FDA's efficacy standard for chronic idiopathic constipation, was utilized: 3 or more CSBMs per week *and* an increase of at least 1 CSBM per week compared with baseline for at least 9 weeks during a 12-week treatment period and for at least 3 of the last 4 weeks of the 12-week treatment period. On a daily basis, patients recorded information on bowel function and symptoms in an electronic diary.

In 5 of the 6 studies, both the prespecified primary end point and the alternative (post hoc) end point were achieved in greater proportions of patients receiving prucalopride 1 or 2 mg daily for 12 weeks compared with those receiving placebo (33, 38, 19, 29, and 24% versus 10, 18, 10, 13, and 12%, respectively, for the prespecified end point; 26, 32, 13, 19, and 16% versus 9, 14, 5, 8, and 5%, respectively, for the alternative end point). In the sixth study (24-week study), response rates for prucalopride-treated patients and placebo recipients did not differ significantly (25 versus 20%, respectively, for the prespecified end point; 17 versus 13%, respectively, for the alternative end point). In all studies, an increase in the frequency of CSBMs (i.e., number of CSBMs per week) was observed as early as the first week of therapy and was sustained through week 12. The median time to first spontaneous bowel movement or first CSBM following initiation of therapy was 0.1–0.4 or 1.4–4.7 days, respectively, for patients receiving prucalopride 1 or 2 mg daily compared with 1–1.6 or 9.1–20.6 days, respectively, for placebo recipients.

The 4-mg daily dosage of prucalopride was not found to provide any additional benefit over the 2-mg dosage.

DOSAGE AND ADMINISTRATION

● Administration

Prucalopride succinate is administered orally once daily without regard to food.

● Dosage

Dosage of prucalopride succinate is expressed in terms of prucalopride.

For the symptomatic treatment of chronic idiopathic constipation, the recommended adult dosage of prucalopride is 2 mg once daily. In clinical trials, a dosage of 4 mg daily was not found to provide any additional benefit over the 2-mg

dosage. In addition, most patients (81%) who received an initial dosage of 1 mg daily required an increase in dosage to 2 mg daily. (See Uses: Chronic Idiopathic Constipation.)

● Special Populations

No dosage adjustment is required in patients with hepatic impairment or those with mild or moderate renal impairment (creatinine clearance of 30 mL/minute or greater). For patients with severe renal impairment (creatinine clearance less than 30 mL/minute), dosage of prucalopride should be reduced to 1 mg once daily. Use of the drug should be avoided in patients with end-stage renal disease requiring dialysis. Dosage in geriatric patients should be based on renal function. (See Specific Populations under Cautions: Warnings/Precautions.)

CAUTIONS

● Contraindications

Prucalopride is contraindicated in patients with intestinal perforation or obstruction due to a structural or functional disorder of the gut wall, obstructive ileus, or severe inflammatory conditions of the intestinal tract including Crohn's disease, ulcerative colitis, and toxic megacolon/megarectum. Prucalopride also is contraindicated in patients with known hypersensitivity to the drug.

● Warnings/Precautions

Sensitivity Reactions

Hypersensitivity reactions including dyspnea, rash, pruritus, urticaria, and facial edema have been reported in patients receiving prucalopride.

Suicidal Ideation and Behavior

In clinical trials, suicides, suicide attempts, and suicidal ideation have been reported in patients receiving prucalopride. However, a causal relationship to the drug has not been established. In double-blind trials, suicide attempt was reported in one patient 7 days after discontinuance of prucalopride therapy (2 mg daily) and by no patients receiving placebo. In open-label trials, suicide attempt was reported in 2 patients receiving the drug and suicidal ideation was reported in one additional patient. Completed suicide was reported in 2 patients who had discontinued prucalopride therapy (2 or 4 mg daily) at least one month prior to the event.

Patients receiving prucalopride should be monitored for persistent worsening of depression and for emergence of suicidal thoughts and behaviors. Families and caregivers of patients receiving the drug should be advised to monitor patients for unusual changes in mood or behavior and to report such changes to a clinician. Patients should be instructed to discontinue prucalopride therapy immediately and to contact their clinician if they experience persistent worsening of depression or emerging suicidal thoughts or behaviors.

Cardiovascular Safety

Although certain nonselective type 4 serotonin (5-HT₄) receptor agonists (i.e., cisapride, tegaserod) have been associated with adverse cardiovascular events, results of a retrospective, observational, population-based cohort study revealed no increase in the risk of major adverse cardiovascular events (i.e., myocardial infarction, stroke, cardiovascular death) in patients receiving prucalopride, a selective 5-HT₄ receptor agonist. (See Description.) The observational study utilized data from European healthcare databases to estimate the risk of major adverse cardiovascular events with prucalopride versus polyethylene glycol 3350 therapy in patients with chronic constipation. The incidence estimates (6.57 or 10.24 per 1000 patient-years of exposure to prucalopride or polyethylene glycol 3350, respectively) excluded an increase in risk above the prespecified safety margin of a threefold increase in risk for prucalopride compared with polyethylene glycol use.

In double-blind clinical trials of prucalopride, the incidence of major adverse cardiovascular events was 3.5 per 1000 patient-years of prucalopride exposure compared with 5.2 per 1000 patient-years of placebo exposure; the incidence was 3.3 per 1000 patient-years of prucalopride exposure in double-blind and open-label trials combined. In healthy individuals, prucalopride did not cause clinically important prolongation of the QT interval at doses of 5 times the recommended dose.

Specific Populations

Pregnancy

Available data from case reports of prucalopride use in pregnant women are insufficient to identify any drug-associated risks of spontaneous abortion, major birth defects, or adverse maternal or fetal outcomes. In animal reproduction studies in rats and rabbits, no adverse embryofetal developmental effects were observed at dosages up to approximately 390 and 780 times, respectively, the recommended human dosage. The highest dosage in rats was maternally toxic; a slight decrease in pup survival was observed at this dosage.

Lactation

Prucalopride is distributed into human milk. It is not known whether prucalopride affects the breast-fed child or affects milk production. The benefits of breast-feeding should be considered along with the importance of the drug to the woman and any potential adverse effects on the breast-fed child from the drug or underlying maternal condition.

During weaning, prucalopride was distributed into human breast milk with a milk-to-plasma ratio of 2.65:1 (based on area under the concentration-time curve [AUC]); mean infant exposure was estimated to be 1.74 mcg/kg daily (about 6% of the maternal dose) adjusted for body weight. However, the manufacturer states that the prucalopride concentration in breast milk during weaning may not reflect the concentration attained during full milk production.

Pediatric Use

Safety and efficacy of prucalopride have not been established in pediatric patients.

Geriatric Use

In controlled trials of at least 12-weeks' duration in patients with chronic idiopathic constipation, 15% of patients receiving prucalopride 1 or 2 mg daily were 65 years of age or older, while 5% were 75 years of age or older. No overall differences in safety and efficacy were observed in these studies between geriatric patients and younger adults, and no unanticipated safety concerns were identified in an additional 4-week double-blind, placebo-controlled, dose-escalation study in 89 geriatric nursing home patients with chronic idiopathic constipation. Geriatric patients had higher prucalopride exposure (26–28% higher AUC and peak plasma concentrations) compared with younger adults; however, the effect of age on the pharmacokinetics of prucalopride appears to be related to decreased renal function. Therefore, dosage of the drug in geriatric patients should be based on renal function.

Hepatic Impairment

Following oral administration of a single 2-mg dose of prucalopride, peak plasma concentration and AUC averaged 10–20% higher in patients with moderate or severe (Child-Pugh class B or C) hepatic impairment compared with individuals with normal hepatic function, but these increases in exposure were not considered to be clinically important.

Renal Impairment

Prucalopride is eliminated mainly by the kidneys, and the risk of adverse effects may be increased in patients with renal impairment. Following oral administration of a single 2-mg dose of prucalopride, AUC in patients with mild, moderate, or severe renal impairment (creatinine clearances of 60–89, 30–59, or 15–29 mL/minute, respectively) was increased by 1.23-, 1.4-, or 2.38-fold, respectively, compared with that in individuals with normal renal function. No dosage adjustment of prucalopride is necessary in patients with mild to moderate renal impairment; however, reduced dosage is recommended in patients with severe renal impairment. (See Dosage and Administration: Special Populations.) The pharmacokinetic profile of prucalopride in patients with end-stage renal disease or requiring dialysis has not been fully established, and the manufacturer states that use of the drug should be avoided in patients with end-stage renal disease requiring dialysis.

● Common Adverse Effects

Adverse effects reported in clinical trials in 2% or more of patients with chronic idiopathic constipation receiving prucalopride and at an incidence greater than that reported with placebo include headache, abdominal pain, nausea, diarrhea, abdominal distension, dizziness, vomiting, flatulence, and fatigue.

DRUG INTERACTIONS

● Drugs Affecting or Metabolized by Hepatic Microsomal Enzymes

In vitro, prucalopride is a substrate of cytochrome P-450 (CYP) isoenzyme 3A4. In vitro studies indicate that prucalopride has limited potential to inhibit CYP isoenzymes 1A2, 2A6, 2B6, 2C8, 2C9, 2C19, 2D6, 2E1, and 3A4 or to induce CYP isoenzymes 1A2, 2B6, and 3A4 at clinically relevant concentrations.

● Drugs Affecting or Affected by Transport Systems

In vitro, prucalopride is a substrate of P-glycoprotein (P-gp) and breast cancer resistance protein (BCRP). In vitro studies indicate that prucalopride has limited potential to inhibit P-gp, BCRP, organic anion transport protein (OATP) 1B1 or 1B3, organic anion transporter (OAT) 1 or 3, organic cation transporter (OCT) 1 or 2, multidrug and toxin extrusion (MATE) 1 or 2-K transporters, bile salt export pump (BSEP), or multidrug resistance protein (MRP) 2 at clinically relevant concentrations.

● Cimetidine

No clinically important effect on the pharmacokinetics of prucalopride was observed when cimetidine, an inhibitor of multiple CYP isoenzymes and transport systems, was administered concomitantly with prucalopride.

● Digoxin

No clinically important effect on the pharmacokinetics of digoxin, a P-gp substrate, was observed when digoxin was administered concomitantly with prucalopride.

● Erythromycin

When prucalopride was administered with erythromycin (500 mg orally 4 times daily), a substrate and moderate inhibitor of CYP3A4 and an inhibitor of P-gp and OATP 1B1 and 1B3, the mean peak plasma concentration and area under the concentration-time curve (AUC) of erythromycin were increased by 40 and 28%, respectively. The mechanism for this interaction is not clear, but the increased exposure to erythromycin is unlikely to be clinically important. No clinically important effect on the pharmacokinetics of prucalopride was observed.

● Estrogens and Progestins

When a combination oral contraceptive containing ethinyl estradiol and norethisterone was administered concomitantly with prucalopride, no clinically important effect on the pharmacokinetics of either the estrogen or progestin was observed.

● Ketoconazole

When prucalopride was administered with ketoconazole (200 mg twice daily), a potent CYP3A4 inhibitor and an inhibitor of P-gp and BCRP, the peak plasma concentration and AUC of prucalopride were increased by approximately 40%. However, the manufacturer states that this effect is unlikely to be clinically important.

● Paroxetine

When paroxetine, a substrate and potent inhibitor of CYP2D6, was administered concomitantly with prucalopride, no clinically important effect on the pharmacokinetics of either drug was observed.

● Probenecid

No clinically important effect on the pharmacokinetics of prucalopride was observed when probenecid, an OAT1 and OAT3 inhibitor, was administered concomitantly with prucalopride.

● Warfarin

No clinically important effect on the pharmacokinetics of warfarin, a CYP2C9 substrate, was observed when warfarin was administered concomitantly with prucalopride.

DESCRIPTION

Prucalopride, a selective type 4 serotonin (5-HT$_4$) receptor agonist, is a GI prokinetic agent. The drug increases bowel motility by binding with high affinity to 5-HT$_4$ receptors, facilitating release of acetylcholine to enhance the amplitude of contractions and stimulate colonic peristalsis. In animal studies, prucalopride has been shown to induce contractions starting from the proximal colon to the anal sphincter. Following oral administration of a single 2-mg dose of prucalopride in patients with chronic idiopathic constipation, the number of high-amplitude propagating contractions was increased during the first 12 hours; with once-daily administration, mean colonic transit time was reduced by 12 hours from a baseline of 65 hours.

Prucalopride is devoid of effects mediated via type 2A, 2B, or 3 serotonin (5-HT$_{2A}$, 5-HT$_{2B}$, or 5-HT$_3$), motilin, or cholecystokinin A receptors in vitro at concentrations exceeding the 5-HT$_4$ receptor affinity by 150-fold or greater. In animal pharmacology studies, prucalopride had no clinically relevant effects on cardiovascular and cardiac electrophysiologic parameters at concentrations of at least 50 times the therapeutic peak plasma concentration in humans. Certain nonselective 5-HT$_4$ receptor agonists (i.e., cisapride, tegaserod) have been associated with adverse cardiovascular events; while cardiac arrhythmias associated with cisapride use have been attributed to the drug's lack of selectivity for the 5-HT$_4$ receptor (i.e., affinity for the human ether-a-go-go gene [hERG]-encoded cardiac potassium channel), the precise mechanism by which tegaserod use may be associated with ischemic cardiovascular events has not been fully established. (See Cardiovascular Safety under Cautions: Warnings/Precautions.)

Following oral administration, bioavailability of prucalopride exceeds 90% and peak plasma concentrations are achieved within 2–3 hours. Administration with a high-fat meal does not alter oral bioavailability. Pharmacokinetics of prucalopride are dose proportional and time independent during continued use. The elimination half-life is approximately 1 day. The parent drug accounts for 92–94% of plasma exposure. Prucalopride is eliminated mainly by the kidneys by passive filtration and active secretion and to a lesser extent (up to 35%) by nonrenal mechanisms. Approximately 84.2% of an orally administered dose is excreted in urine, with 60–65% of the dose excreted in urine as unchanged drug; 13.3% of an administered dose is excreted in feces, with 5% of the dose excreted in feces as unchanged drug. Prucalopride is a substrate of cytochrome P-450 (CYP) isoenzyme 3A4 in vitro. Seven minor metabolites have been identified; the most common metabolite (O-desmethylprucalopride acid) accounts for only 3.2 or 3.1% of the dose recovered in urine or feces, respectively. Age, sex, race, and body weight (after adjustment for renal function) do not appear to affect the pharmacokinetics of prucalopride.

ADVICE TO PATIENTS

Importance of advising patients to read the manufacturer's patient information.

Importance of advising patients and their caregivers and families that suicidal thoughts and behavior have been reported in patients receiving prucalopride. Importance of being alert for persistent worsening of symptoms of depression, unusual changes in mood or behavior, and emergence of suicidal thoughts or behavior. Importance of immediately discontinuing prucalopride and contacting a clinician if such symptoms occur.

Importance of women informing clinicians if they are or plan to become pregnant or plan to breast-feed.

Importance of patients informing clinicians of existing or contemplated concomitant therapy, including prescription and OTC drugs, as well as any concomitant illnesses.

Importance of informing patients of other important precautionary information. (See Cautions.)

PREPARATIONS

Excipients in commercially available drug preparations may have clinically important effects in some individuals; consult specific product labeling for details.

Prucalopride Succinate

Oral

| Tablets, film-coated | 1 mg (of prucalopride) | Motegrity®, Shire |
| | 2 mg (of prucalopride) | Motegrity®, Shire |

Selected Revisions October 28, 2019, © Copyright, January 14, 2019, American Society of Health-System Pharmacists, Inc.

Table of Contents

§ Omitted from the print version of *AHFS Drug Information®* because of space limitations. This monograph is available on the *AHFS Drug Information®* website, http://ahfsdruginformation.com.

Corticosteroids General Statement

68:04 · ADRENALS

■ Corticosteroids are hormones secreted by the adrenal cortex or synthetic analogs of these hormones. They exhibit glucocorticoid and/or mineralocorticoid activity and affect almost all body systems, but are used principally for their potent anti-inflammatory and immunosuppressant effects and for replacement.

USES

In physiologic dosages, corticosteroids are used to replace deficient endogenous hormones. In pharmacologic dosages, the drugs have both therapeutic and diagnostic applications based on their ability to suppress secretion of normal adrenal hormones. Glucocorticoids are also used in pharmacologic dosages for their anti-inflammatory and immunosuppressant properties and their effects on blood and lymphatic systems in the palliative treatment of various diseases.

When glucocorticoids are used for their anti-inflammatory and immunosuppressant properties, synthetic glucocorticoids that have minimal mineralocorticoid activity are preferred to cortisone or hydrocortisone. *Glucocorticoid therapy is not curative and is rarely indicated as the primary method of treatment, but rather as supportive therapy to be used adjunctively with other indicated therapies.* If prolonged oral administration of glucocorticoids is required, alternate-day therapy should be used whenever possible to minimize adverse reactions, and continual attempts should be made to reduce the dosage or, preferably, to withdraw glucocorticoid therapy completely. (See General Dosage under Dosage and Administration: Dosage.)

● Adrenocortical Insufficiency

Corticosteroids are administered in physiologic dosages to replace deficient endogenous hormones in patients with adrenocortical insufficiency. Because production of both mineralocorticoids and glucocorticoids is deficient in these patients, hydrocortisone or cortisone (in conjunction with liberal salt intake) is usually the corticosteroid of choice for replacement therapy. Concomitant administration of a more potent mineralocorticoid (fludrocortisone) may be required in some patients, particularly in infants. If synthetic glucocorticoids are used instead of hydrocortisone or cortisone, a mineralocorticoid must also be given. In suspected or known adrenal insufficiency, parenteral therapy may be used preoperatively or during serious trauma, illness, or shock unresponsive to conventional therapy. In shock caused by acute adrenocortical insufficiency, IV administration of hydrocortisone (or a synthetic glucocorticoid) in conjunction with other therapy for shock is essential.

● Adrenogenital Syndrome

In salt-losing forms of congenital adrenogenital syndrome, cortisone or hydrocortisone is administered in conjunction with liberal salt intake. Because of the risk of growth retardation with excessive dosage (see Cautions: Pediatric Precautions), the minimum dosage of the corticosteroid required to suppress adrenocortical hyperfunction should be used. If sodium loss and hypotension are not adequately controlled by cortisone or hydrocortisone, an additional mineralocorticoid drug should be given. Mineralocorticoid replacement can usually be discontinued in children 5–7 years of age, but a glucocorticoid must be continued throughout life. Patients with the hypertensive form of congenital adrenogenital syndrome (who secrete excessive amounts of desoxycorticosterone) should be treated with a "short-acting" glucocorticoid with minimal mineralocorticoid activity (e.g., prednisone). Longer acting glucocorticoids (e.g., dexamethasone) should not be used in such patients because there is a tendency toward overdosage and growth may be retarded.

● Hypercalcemia

Glucocorticoids promote a reduction in serum calcium concentrations and are effective as hypocalcemic agents in patients with steroid-sensitive malignancies (e.g., multiple myeloma, lymphoma) and in patients with hypercalcemia due to sarcoidosis or vitamin D intoxication. Glucocorticoids are not effective in hypercalcemia caused by hyperparathyroidism.

● Thyroiditis

The anti-inflammatory action of glucocorticoids dramatically relieves symptoms such as fever and acute thyroid pain and swelling in granulomatous (subacute, nonsuppurative) thyroiditis. The drugs are indicated in moderate to high dosages for palliative therapy in severely ill patients unresponsive to salicylates and thyroid hormones. Glucocorticoids may also be effective in reducing orbital edema in endocrine exophthalmos (thyroid ophthalmopathy). Changes in thyroid status may necessitate adjustment of glucocorticoid dosage.

● Rheumatic Disorders and Collagen Diseases

In rheumatic disorders and collagen diseases, glucocorticoids relieve inflammation and suppress symptoms, but do not affect progression of the disease. The drugs are rarely indicated except for palliative, short-term treatment of acute exacerbations and systemic complications in patients refractory to more conservative therapy. Dosage in life-threatening situations is often high and is reduced rapidly after the crisis is past. Maintenance therapy with glucocorticoids is rarely indicated in rheumatoid arthritis, acute gouty arthritis, or systemic lupus erythematosus, but may be used as part of a total treatment program in selected patients when more conservative therapies have proven ineffective. Glucocorticoid withdrawal is extremely difficult in patients with these conditions, as relapses or rebounds usually occur upon discontinuance of the drugs.

In the symptomatic treatment of rheumatoid arthritis that involves only a few persistently inflamed joints or in the treatment of inflammation of tendons or bursae, local injections of slightly soluble glucocorticoids may be beneficial. Patients usually experience dramatic relief initially. Although inflammation tends to recur and sometimes it is more intense after cessation of therapy, the drugs can prevent invalidism by facilitating movement of joints that might otherwise become immobile.

Systemically administered glucocorticoids control acute manifestations of rheumatic carditis more rapidly than salicylates and may be life-saving in certain conditions, but glucocorticoids, like salicylates, cannot prevent valvular damage and are no better than salicylates for long-term treatment. Salicylates used concomitantly with glucocorticoids may decrease inflammatory rebound when the steroids are withdrawn. (See Drug Interactions: Nonsteroidal Anti-Inflammatory Agents.) Cytotoxic therapy is the treatment of choice in Wegener's granulomatosis, but glucocorticoids may be used adjunctively for severe systemic complications.

Glucocorticoids remain the primary treatment to control symptoms and prevent severe, often life-threatening complications in patients with dermatomyositis and polymyositis, polyarteritis nodosa, relapsing polychondritis, polymyalgia rheumatica and giant-cell (temporal) arteritis, or mixed connective tissue disease syndrome. High dosage may be required for acute situations; after a response has been obtained, glucocorticoids must often be continued for long periods at low dosage. Polymyositis associated with malignancy and childhood dermatomyositis may not respond well to glucocorticoids.

Systemic glucocorticoids are rarely indicated in psoriatic arthritis, diffuse scleroderma (progressive systemic sclerosis), acute and subacute bursitis, and osteoarthritis. Risks outweigh benefits received, and more conservative therapy should be used. In osteoarthritis, intra-articular injections of glucocorticoids may be beneficial but should be limited in number as joint damage may occur.

● Dermatologic Diseases

In dermatologic diseases such as pemphigus and pemphigoid, exfoliative dermatitis, bullous dermatitis herpetiformis, severe erythema multiforme (Stevens-Johnson syndrome), uncontrollable eczema, cutaneous sarcoidosis, mycosis fungoides, and lichen planus, systemic glucocorticoids should generally be reserved for acute exacerbations unresponsive to conservative therapy. In all these dermatologic diseases, high dosage of glucocorticoids may be required. Early initiation of systemic glucocorticoid therapy may be life-saving in pemphigus vulgaris and pemphigoid, and high or massive doses may be required. Dosage should be reduced gradually to the lowest effective level, but discontinuance may not be possible; alternate-day therapy may often be used beneficially.

Although chronic skin disorders are seldom an indication for systemic glucocorticoids, intralesional or sublesional injections may occasionally be indicated for localized chronic disorders (including keloids, psoriatic plaques, alopecia areata, discoid lupus erythematosus, and granuloma annulare) unresponsive to topical therapy. Systemic glucocorticoids are rarely indicated for psoriasis or alopecia (areata, totalis, or universalis). When systemic corticosteroids are used in the treatment of psoriasis, exacerbation of the disease may occur when the drugs are withdrawn or dosage is decreased. Although glucocorticoids may stimulate hair growth in patients with alopecia, hair loss returns when the drugs are discontinued.

● Allergic Conditions

Systemic glucocorticoids are used for control of severe or incapacitating allergic conditions that do not respond to adequate trials of conventional therapy in patients with bronchial asthma, seasonal or perennial allergic rhinitis, atopic dermatitis, urticaria associated with transfusion, or acute noninfectious laryngeal edema (although epinephrine is the drug of choice). Systemic glucocorticoids also may be used in acute manifestations of angioedema, serum sickness, contact dermatitis, drug hypersensitivity, and allergic symptoms of trichinosis. In acute conditions, the drugs may be used for short periods in high dosage with other therapy such as antihistamines and sympathomimetics.

In the symptomatic treatment of chronic allergic conditions, systemic glucocorticoids generally should be reserved for acute conditions and severe exacerbations. Prolonged treatment of chronic allergic conditions should be reserved for patients with disabling conditions unresponsive to more conservative therapy and for whom the risks of long-term glucocorticoid therapy are justified.

● Ocular Disorders

Optic Neuritis

Systemic glucocorticoids have been used for the treatment of acute optic neuritis†. Interest in the use of IV methylprednisolone in the management of acute relapses of multiple sclerosis has been heightened as a result of the Optic Neuritis Treatment Trial. In this trial in which short-term glucocorticoid therapy (IV methylprednisolone 1 g daily for 3 days followed by oral prednisone 1 mg/kg daily for 11 days versus oral prednisone alone at this dosage for 14 days) was compared with placebo for the treatment of initial episodes of acute optic neuritis, the rate of vision recovery was faster with the methylprednisolone regimen, with the greatest benefit being observed in patients with visual acuity of 20/50 or worse at entry; however, there were no substantial differences in visual outcomes between the groups at 6 months. Use of oral prednisone alone did not improve the rate of vision recovery compared with placebo and was associated with an increased risk of new episodes of optic neuritis in either eye.

At 2-year follow-up, patients who had received the methylprednisolone regimen had a lower rate of progression to clinically definite multiple sclerosis than those who received placebo. This beneficial effect was most evident in patients at the highest risk for multiple sclerosis (i.e., those with multicentric brain lesions on magnetic resonance imaging [MRI] at study entry). However, after 3 years, differences between the treatment groups were no longer significant, suggesting that IV methylprednisolone delayed but did not arrest the development of multiple sclerosis after optic neuritis. At 5-year follow-up, most patients who had received the methylprednisolone regimen retained good to excellent vision, even if there had been single or multiple recurrences of optic neuritis during the 5-year period. The cumulative probability of having a new episode of optic neuritis over the 5-year follow-up period was 19% for affected eyes, 17% for fellow eyes, and 30% for either eye.

Patients who developed clinically diagnosed multiple sclerosis over the follow-up period were more likely to have recurrences of optic neuritis in the affected or fellow eye and also were more likely to have slight worsening of vision between the 6-month and 5-year follow-up examinations than patients without clinically diagnosed multiple sclerosis.

Other Ocular Disorders

Systemic glucocorticoids may be used to suppress a variety of allergic and nonpyogenic ocular inflammations and to reduce scarring in ocular injuries. Glucocorticoids have been used for the treatment of severe acute and chronic allergic and inflammatory processes involving the eye that are intractable to adequate trials of conventional treatment (e.g., allergic conjunctivitis, keratitis, allergic corneal marginal ulcers, herpes zoster ophthalmicus, iritis and iridocyclitis, chorioretinitis, diffuse posterior uveitis and choroiditis, anterior segment inflammation, temporal arteritis, sympathetic ophthalmia). Moderate dosage is used initially and is quickly discontinued after the acute condition is controlled. Some disorders may relapse upon discontinuance of therapy and low-dose maintenance therapy may be required. Glucocorticoids are of no value in the treatment of degenerative ocular diseases such as cataracts.

Topically applied glucocorticoids appear to be as effective as systemic steroids for the treatment of most anterior ocular inflammations. Systemic glucocorticoid therapy may be required, however, in stubborn cases of anterior segment eye disease and is necessary when deeper ocular structures are involved.

● Respiratory Diseases

Asthma

Corticosteroids are used as adjunctive treatment of asthma. The Global Initiative for Asthma (GINA) guidelines provide evidence-based recommendations for the management of asthma in adults, adolescents, and children ≥6 years of age. The guideline states that all patients with asthma should be evaluated for symptom control, risk of future exacerbations, treatment issues (e.g., inhaler technique and adherence), and comorbidities. A stepwise approach to treatment is recommended where specific drugs are added or adjusted up or down through a series of steps (1 through 5) to achieve symptom control while keeping the patient on the lowest effective treatment. Drugs used in the management of asthma include inhaled corticosteroids (ICS)-formoterol, long-acting beta agonists (LABA), short-acting β_2-adrenergic agonists (SABA), long-acting muscarinic agonists (LAMA), leukotriene receptor antagonists, theophylline, oral corticosteroids, and biologic agents.

Chronic Obstructive Pulmonary Disease

Oral and inhaled corticosteroids have been used in the management of chronic obstructive pulmonary disease (COPD). The Global Initiative for Chronic Obstructive Lung Disease (GOLD) guideline states that oral glucocorticoids play a role in the acute management of COPD exacerbations, but have no role in the chronic daily treatment of COPD because of the lack of benefit and high rate of systemic complications.

Sarcoidosis

In the management of sarcoidosis, systemic glucocorticoids are indicated for ocular, CNS, glandular, myocardial, or severe pulmonary involvement or for hypercalcemia or severe skin lesions unresponsive to intralesional or sublesional injections of glucocorticoids. Long-term therapy may be required.

Advanced Pulmonary and Extrapulmonary Tuberculosis

Systemic glucocorticoids have been used as adjunctive therapy in some patients with severe pulmonary or extrapulmonary tuberculosis in an attempt to suppress manifestations related to the host's inflammatory response to the *Mycobacterium tuberculosis* bacillus and ameliorate complications of the disease. While evidence from studies of *M. tuberculosis* infection in both animals and humans indicates that glucocorticoids can have deleterious effects (e.g., increased virulence of the organism) in the absence of adequate antituberculosis therapy, such effects generally appear to be prevented by coadministration of effective antimycobacterial agents (e.g., streptomycin, isoniazid). Data from randomized, controlled trials are limited and principally consist of studies conducted before the use of current 4-drug, short-course antituberculosis regimens; however, an analysis of available evidence suggests that adjunctive glucocorticoid therapy may enhance short-term resolution of disease manifestations (e.g., clinical and radiographic abnormalities) in patients with advanced pulmonary tuberculosis and also may reduce mortality associated with certain forms of extrapulmonary disease (e.g., meningitis, pericarditis). Additional randomized, controlled studies in patients receiving current short-course antituberculosis regimens are needed to fully elucidate the potential benefits and risks of adjunctive glucocorticoid therapy in pulmonary or extrapulmonary tuberculosis. Dosage of adjunctive corticosteroids may need to be adjusted upward in patients receiving rifampin-containing antituberculosis regimens as a result of rifampin-induced increases in corticosteroid metabolism.

Advanced Pulmonary Tuberculosis

Adjunctive systemic glucocorticoid therapy has been used to treat severe systemic and respiratory manifestations in patients with advanced pulmonary tuberculosis. Although benefit to the patient is unclear, radiographically evident abnormalities (other than cavities) usually resolve more rapidly with glucocorticoid therapy. No improvement in long-term outcomes (chronic respiratory disease or death) has been observed. In patients receiving adequate antituberculosis therapy (2 or more effective agents), glucocorticoid use does not appear to delay the time to conversion of sputum culture to negative or affect long-term cure rates.

Tuberculous Meningitis

Use of systemic adjunctive glucocorticoids (e.g., dexamethasone, prednisone) in patients with moderate to severe tuberculous meningitis appears to reduce sequelae (e.g., intellectual impairment) and/or improve survival. In a randomized, controlled study in young children (mean age younger than 36 months) with tuberculous meningitis, therapy with prednisone (2–4 mg/kg daily) reduced mortality in patients with stage III disease from 17% to 4% but did not reduce the incidence of permanent motor deficits (hemiparesis and quadriparesis). Results from a prospective, randomized, placebo-controlled study in adults and adolescents older than 14 years of age with tuberculous meningitis (with or without HIV infection) also showed reduced mortality (relative risk of death of 0.69; 95% confidence interval of 0.52–0.92) in patients receiving dexamethasone (IV therapy tapered over 2–4 weeks, depending on disease severity, followed by oral therapy tapered over 4 weeks), but dexamethasone therapy was not associated with a substantial reduction in the proportion of severely disabled patients among survivors or in the proportion of patients who had either died or were severely disabled after 9 months. A faster resolution of abnormal CSF parameters (e.g., elevated intracranial pressure, basal exudate, CNS tuberculomas) occurs with glucocorticoids use, which may aid in patient management. Available data suggest that response is most favorable in patients with disease of intermediate severity (as opposed to early or late disease) and that continuation of glucocorticoid therapy for at least 4 weeks may be associated with better outcomes than with shorter regimens.

Tuberculous Pericarditis

Limited data suggest that adjunctive systemic glucocorticoid therapy is effective in the management of acute tuberculous pericarditis, rapidly reducing the size of pericardial effusions and the need for drainage procedures and decreasing mortality (probably through control of hemodynamically threatening effusion). However, glucocorticoid therapy does not appear to alter the incidence of progression to constrictive disease when used for treatment of either the acute or intermediate stage of pericarditis.

Tuberculous Pleurisy

While most studies of adjunctive systemic glucocorticoid therapy in patients with tuberculous pleurisy have not been randomized or controlled, limited evidence suggests that such therapy hastens the resolution of pain, dyspnea, and fever associated with this form of the disease. However, glucocorticoids appear to have little efficacy in preventing fibrotic changes and resultant constrictive lung disease, and some clinicians advise against their routine use.

Other Tuberculosis Complications

Limited data suggest that intrathoracic adenopathy associated with primary tuberculosis may resolve more rapidly with the use of adjunctive systemic glucocorticoids. While a few studies have reported a reduced frequency of complications (e.g., recurrent abdominal pain, intestinal obstruction) with adjunctive glucocorticoid therapy in patients with peritoneal tuberculosis, data from randomized trials are lacking, and rapid improvement in symptoms occurred in these patients with antituberculosis therapy alone. Although it has been suggested that atelectasis associated with endobronchial tuberculosis may benefit from glucocorticoid therapy, results of a randomized, controlled trial in a limited number of patients with this form of the disease suggested no important benefit of glucocorticoid therapy over antituberculosis therapy alone with regard to healing rates and changes in pulmonary function. Inadequate data are available regarding the safety and efficacy of adjunctive glucocorticoid therapy in patients with tuberculous lymphadenitis, miliary or laryngeal tuberculosis, or HIV-associated tuberculosis.

Lipid Pneumonitis

In lipid pneumonitis, glucocorticoids appear to promote the breakdown or dissolution of pulmonary lesions and eliminate lipids in the sputum. Although high doses of glucocorticoids are commonly used in hydrocarbon pneumonitis to prevent pulmonary edema and fibrosis, there is no evidence that they prevent any complications or improve the recovery rate.

Pneumocystis jirovecii Pneumonia

The use of systemic glucocorticoids as an adjunct to anti-infective therapy for the treatment of moderate to severe pneumonia caused by *Pneumocystis jirovecii*† (formerly *Pneumocystis carinii*) in patients with human immunodeficiency virus (HIV) infection, including acquired immunodeficiency syndrome (AIDS), can decrease the likelihood of deterioration of oxygenation, respiratory failure, and/or death in those with moderate to severe pneumonia. Based on the results of controlled, randomized studies, experts recommend that adults and adolescents older than 13 years of age with documented or suspected HIV infection and documented or suspected pneumocystis pneumonia be given systemic glucocorticoid therapy in addition to anti-infective treatment if they have moderate to severe pulmonary dysfunction, defined as an arterial oxygen pressure of less than 70 mm Hg or an arterial-alveolar gradient of 35 mm Hg or greater on room air. It is not known whether patients with mild pneumocystis pneumonia (arterial oxygen pressure exceeding 70 mm Hg or arterial-alveolar gradient less than 35 mm Hg on room air) might have clinically important benefit with adjunctive glucocorticoid therapy, and such benefit may be difficult to demonstrate in clinical studies because of the generally good clinical outcome of this group.

It is recommended that adjunctive glucocorticoid therapy be initiated as early as possible, preferably within the first 24–72 hours after initiation of specific anti-infective therapy. Benefit in controlled studies has not been demonstrated with initiation of glucocorticoid therapy more than 72 hours after initiation of specific antipneumocystis therapy; however, most clinicians would initiate such therapy in those with moderate to severe pneumocystis pneumonia even if it has been more than 72 hours after initiation of anti-infective therapy. Glucocorticoid therapy can be started in patients with presumed AIDS-associated pneumocystis pneumonia if these patients meet the recommended oxygenation criteria. The diagnosis of HIV infection and pneumocystis pneumonia should be confirmed promptly to minimize the likelihood of masking and/or exacerbating other treatable diseases (e.g., tuberculosis) and to avoid adverse effects of unnecessary drugs. Pending the availability of specific efficacy or safety data, it may be reasonable to consider adjunctive systemic glucocorticoid therapy for pneumocystis pneumonia in immunosuppressed patients *without* HIV infection or in pregnant women with HIV infection according to the same criteria as for nonpregnant adults with HIV infection.

When glucocorticoid therapy is used as an adjunct to anti-infective therapy in HIV-infected patients with moderate to severe pneumocystis pneumonia, experts recommend specific regimens of prednisone or, if parenteral therapy is required, methylprednisolone. (See Dosage and Administration, in Prednisone 68:04 and Methylprednisolone 68:04.) Higher dosages for patients whose condition is not improving on glucocorticoids, or newly initiated glucocorticoid therapy for those patients in whom standard treatment alone is failing, may or may not be beneficial; available evidence is inadequate to provide specific recommendations.

Coronavirus Disease 2019 (COVID-19)

Corticosteroid therapy (e.g., dexamethasone, hydrocortisone, methylprednisolone, prednisone) has been used as adjunctive therapy in the treatment of serious complications from coronavirus disease 2019 (COVID-19)†. Patients with severe COVID-19 may develop a systemic inflammatory response that can result in lung injury and multisystem organ dysfunction. The potent anti-inflammatory effects of corticosteroids may prevent or mitigate these deleterious effects.

The National Institutes of Health (NIH) COVID-19 Treatment Guidelines Panel issued guidelines for the treatment of COVID-19, including recommendations for use of corticosteroids in patients with COVID-19. For the treatment of COVID-19 in nonhospitalized adults and hospitalized adults who do not require supplemental oxygen, the NIH guidelines panel recommends against the use of dexamethasone or other corticosteroids. However, the NIH panel recommends use of dexamethasone (6 mg daily orally or IV for up to 10 days or until hospital discharge, whichever comes first) in hospitalized adults with COVID-19 who require supplemental oxygen or are receiving mechanical ventilation or extracorporeal membrane oxygenation (ECMO). The NIH panel states that it is not known at this time whether other corticosteroids will have a similar benefit as dexamethasone. However, if dexamethasone is not available, the panel recommends using alternative corticosteroids (e.g., hydrocortisone, methylprednisolone, prednisone).

Data regarding potential adverse effects of dexamethasone in patients with COVID-19, efficacy in combination with other treatments (e.g., remdesivir, tocilizumab, baricitinib), and efficacy in other patient populations (e.g., pediatric patients, pregnant women) are insufficient to date. Although efficacy of concomitant use of dexamethasone and remdesivir has not been rigorously studied, the NIH panel states there is a theoretical rationale for using dexamethasone plus remdesivir in some patients with severe COVID-19 and clinically important drug interactions are not expected. Specifically, the NIH guideline panel recommends concomitant use of dexamethasone and remdesivir in hospitalized patients requiring increasing amounts of supplemental oxygen or use of dexamethasone alone when combined therapy with remdesivir cannot be used or is unavailable in such patients. Similarly, the NIH panel recommends the use of dexamethasone alone or in combination with remdesivir in hospitalized patients requiring high-flow oxygen or noninvasive ventilation. For such patients who were recently hospitalized with rapidly increasing oxygen needs and systemic inflammation, the panel also recommends the addition of baricitinib or tocilizumab to either monotherapy with dexamethasone or combination therapy with dexamethasone and remdesivir. For hospitalized COVID-19 patients requiring invasive mechanical ventilation or ECMO, the NIH panel recommends therapy with dexamethasone alone, although dexamethasone in combination with remdesivir may be considered in patients who were recently intubated. For those receiving invasive mechanical ventilation or ECMO who are within 24 hours of ICU admission with rapid respiratory decompensation, the NIH panel recommends dexamethasone in combination with tocilizumab. Clinicians should consult the most recent NIH COVID-19 treatment guidelines for additional information on use of corticosteroids in patients with COVID-19.

The World Health Organization (WHO) Guideline Development Group also issued guidelines for the use of systemic corticosteroids in patients with COVID-19. For the treatment of patients with nonsevere COVID-19, the WHO Guideline Development Group suggests not using systemic corticosteroids, regardless of hospitalization status; however, if the clinical condition of such patients worsens (e.g., increased respiratory rate, signs of respiratory distress, or hypoxemia), systemic corticosteroids are recommended for treatment. The WHO Guideline Development Group strongly recommends the use of systemic corticosteroids (e.g., dexamethasone 6 mg orally or IV once daily or hydrocortisone 50 mg IV every 8 hours for 7-10 days) over no systemic corticosteroid therapy for the treatment of patients with severe and/or critical COVID-19, regardless of hospitalization status. This treatment recommendation includes critically ill patients with COVID-19 who could not be hospitalized or receive oxygen supplementation because of resource limitations. The WHO Guideline Development Group also recommends the concomitant use of systemic corticosteroids with an interleukin (IL-6) inhibitor (e.g., sarilumab, tocilizumab) for patients with severe or critical COVID-19. These experts recommend against discontinuing systemic corticosteroids in patients with nonsevere COVID-19 who are receiving systemic corticosteroids for chronic conditions (e.g., COPD, autoimmune diseases). Clinicians should consult the most recent WHO COVID-19 treatment guidelines for additional information.

In one randomized, controlled, open-label study (NCT04381936; RECOVERY), the effect of potential treatments (including low-dose dexamethasone) on all-cause mortality in hospitalized patients with COVID-19 was evaluated. Patients were randomized to receive dexamethasone (6 mg once daily orally or IV for up to 10 days) plus standard care or standard care alone. Preliminary data analysis indicated that overall 28-day mortality was reduced in patients who received dexamethasone compared with those who received standard care alone, and the greatest benefit was observed in patients receiving invasive mechanical ventilation or those receiving supplemental oxygen without mechanical ventilation. However, no survival benefit was observed with dexamethasone and there was a possibility of harm in patients who did not require respiratory support at study enrollment. (See Uses: Coronavirus Disease 2019 [COVID-19] in Dexamethasone 68:04.)

In another randomized, controlled, open-label, multicenter study (NCT04327401; CoDEX), the effect of dexamethasone on the number of ventilator-free days was evaluated in patients with COVID-19-associated moderate or severe acute respiratory distress syndrome (ARDS) who were receiving mechanical ventilation. Patients were randomized to receive dexamethasone (20 mg IV once daily for 5 days followed by 10 mg IV once daily for another 5 days or until ICU discharge) plus standard care or standard care alone. Preliminary data analysis indicated that use of dexamethasone plus standard care was associated with a higher mean number of ventilator-free days (6.6 days) compared with those receiving standard care alone (4 days). This trial was terminated early after results of the RECOVERY trial became available and, therefore, was likely underpowered to determine secondary outcomes such as mortality. (See Uses: Coronavirus Disease 2019 [COVID-19] in Dexamethasone 68:04.)

In one randomized, double-blind sequential trial (NCT02517489; CAPE COVID), the effect of low-dose hydrocortisone on treatment failure was evaluated in critically ill patients with COVID-19-related acute respiratory failure compared with placebo. In the hydrocortisone treatment group, 76 patients received a continuous IV infusion of hydrocortisone at an initial dosage of 200 mg daily for 7 days followed by 100 mg daily for 4 days, and then 50 mg daily for 3 days (total of 14 days; some patients received a shorter regimen); 73 patients received placebo. The primary study end point was treatment failure (defined as death or persistent dependency on mechanical ventilation or high-flow oxygen therapy) on day 21. Treatment failure on day 21 occurred in 42.1% of patients receiving hydrocortisone compared with 50.7% of patients receiving placebo. No substantial difference was observed between the treatment groups; however, the study was discontinued early after results of the RECOVERY trial became available and, therefore, was likely underpowered to determine a statistically and clinically important difference in the primary outcome.

In another randomized, open-label, multicenter study (NCT02735707; REMAP-CAP), an embedded multifactorial adaptive platform was used to evaluate patients receiving multiple interventions within multiple domains. In the COVID-19 corticosteroid domain, adults with suspected or confirmed COVID-19 following ICU admission for respiratory or cardiovascular organ support were randomized to receive a fixed 7-day regimen of IV hydrocortisone (50 or 100 mg every 6 hours), a shock-dependent regimen of IV hydrocortisone (50 mg every 6 hours when shock was clinically evident), or no hydrocortisone or other corticosteroid. The primary study end point was organ support-free days (defined as days alive and free of ICU-based respiratory or cardiovascular support) within 21 days. The 7-day fixed regimen and the shock-dependent regimen of hydrocortisone were associated with a 93 and 80% probability of benefit in terms of organ support-free days compared with no hydrocortisone. However, the trial was discontinued early after results of the RECOVERY trial were available and no treatment strategy met the prespecified criteria for statistical superiority, precluding definitive conclusions. In addition, serious adverse effects were reported in 2.6% of patients in the study (4 patients receiving the fixed-dosage regimen and 5 patients receiving the shock-dependent regimen compared with 1 patient receiving no hydrocortisone).

In one randomized, parallel, double-blind, placebo-controlled, phase 2b trial (NCT04343729; Metcovid), the effect of a short course of IV methylprednisolone was evaluated compared with placebo in hospitalized adults with suspected COVID-19 from a single center in Brazil. Patients were enrolled prior to laboratory confirmation of COVID-19 to avoid treatment delays and the presence of COVID-19 was later confirmed based on RT-PCR testing in 81.3% of these patients. At time of enrollment, 34% of patients in each treatment group required invasive mechanical ventilation. Supplemental oxygen was required in 51% of patients receiving methylprednisolone and in 45% of those receiving placebo. In the methylprednisolone treatment group, 194 patients received IV methylprednisolone at a dosage of 0.5 mg/kg twice daily for 5 days; 199 patients received placebo. A modified intent-to-treat analysis was conducted; the primary study end point was 28-day mortality. Overall, the 28-day mortality rate was 37.1 or 38.2% in patients who received methylprednisolone or placebo, respectively, showing no substantial difference in overall mortality between the treatment groups. However, a subgroup analysis found a lower mortality rate in patients older than 60 years of age who received methylprednisolone compared with placebo (46.6 vs 61.9%, respectively). Patients older than 60 years of age reportedly had a higher degree of systemic inflammatory disease as manifested by increased median concentrations of C-reactive protein (CRP) compared with patients 60 years of age or younger. In those 60 years of age or younger, there was a higher incidence of fatal outcomes in the methylprednisolone group. The authors concluded that caution is needed when using systemic corticosteroids in patients with less severe COVID-19 since a trend toward more harm was noted in the younger age group.

In another multicenter, observational, longitudinal study (NCT04323592), the association between use of prolonged, low-dose methylprednisolone treatment and ICU admission, intubation, or all-cause death within 28 days (composite primary end point) was evaluated in patients with severe COVID-19 pneumonia admitted to 14 respiratory high-dependency units in Italy. A total of 173 patients were enrolled in the study with 83 patients receiving methylprednisolone plus standard care and 90 patients receiving standard care alone. In the methylprednisolone treatment group, patients received a loading dose of IV methylprednisolone 80 mg at study entry followed by IV infusion of the drug at a dosage of 80 mg daily at a rate of 10 mL/hr for at least 8 days until achievement of either a PaO2/FiO2 (P/F ratio) greater than 350 mm Hg or CRP concentrations less than 20 mg/L. Subsequently, twice-daily administration of either oral methylprednisolone 16 mg or IV methylprednisolone 20 mg was given until achievement of a P/F ratio greater than 400 mm Hg or CRP concentrations reached less than 20% of the normal range. The composite primary end point was reached by 22.9 or 44.4% of patients in the group receiving methylprednisolone or standard care alone, respectively. Therefore, use of methylprednisolone was associated with a reduction in the risk of ICU admission, invasive mechanical ventilation, or death within 28 days (adjusted hazard ratio: 0.41). Specifically, 18.1 or 30% of patients required ICU admission and 16.9 or 28.9% of patients required invasive mechanical ventilation in those receiving methylprednisolone or standard care alone, respectively. In addition, use of methylprednisolone was associated with a 28-day lower risk of all-cause mortality than use of standard care alone (7.2 vs 23.3%, respectively) with an adjusted hazard ratio of 0.29. Overall, there was no difference in adverse effects between treatment groups with the exception of increased reports of hyperglycemia and mild agitation in the methylprednisolone-treated patients; no adverse effects resulted in drug discontinuation. The authors concluded that early, low-dose, prolonged therapy with methylprednisolone resulted in decreased ICU burden, reduced need for invasive mechanical ventilation, and lower mortality along with improvement in systemic inflammation and oxygenation markers in hospitalized patients with severe COVID-19 pneumonia at high risk of progression to acute respiratory failure.

In one multicenter quasi-experimental study with single pretest and posttest (NCT04374071), the efficacy of early, short-term therapy with systemic methylprednisolone was evaluated in hospitalized adults with confirmed moderate to severe COVID-19 from a multicenter health system in Michigan. A total of 213 patients were enrolled with 132 patients receiving early therapy with IV methylprednisolone at dosages of 0.5–1 mg/kg daily in 2 divided doses for 3 days plus standard care and 81 patients receiving early therapy with standard care alone. The primary end point was a composite based on the need for ICU transfer, progression to respiratory failure requiring mechanical ventilation, or in-hospital all-cause mortality. The primary composite end point occurred at a substantially lower rate in the group receiving early corticosteroid therapy (34.9%) compared with the group receiving early therapy with standard care alone (54.3%). The early corticosteroid group had a median time to initiation of methylprednisolone of 2 days compared with 5 days for the standard care group. The median hospital length of stay was substantially reduced from 8 to 5 days in patients receiving early corticosteroid therapy compared with those receiving early therapy with standard care alone. ARDS occurred in 26.6% of patients receiving early corticosteroid therapy compared with 38.3% of those in the standard care group. The authors concluded that early, short-term therapy with methylprednisolone in patients with moderate to severe COVID-19 may prevent disease progression and improve clinical outcomes.

In a prospective meta-analysis of studies using systemic corticosteroids (i.e., dexamethasone, hydrocortisone, or methylprednisolone) from the WHO Rapid Evidence Appraisal for COVID-19 Therapies (REACT) Working Group, data were pooled from 7 randomized clinical trials in 12 countries that evaluated the efficacy of corticosteroids in 1703 critically ill patients with COVID-19. The primary outcome was all-cause mortality up to 30 days after randomization to treatment. Administration of systemic corticosteroids was associated with lower all-cause mortality at 28 days compared with usual care or placebo (222 deaths among 678 patients who received corticosteroids and 425 deaths among 1025 patients who received usual care or placebo). The effect of corticosteroids on reduced mortality was observed in critically ill patients who were and were not receiving mechanical ventilation at randomization and also in patients from the RECOVERY trial who required supplemental oxygen with or without non-invasive ventilation, but who were not receiving invasive mechanical ventilation at the time of randomization. The odds ratios for the association between corticosteroids and mortality were similar for dexamethasone and hydrocortisone. The optimal dosage and duration of corticosteroid treatment could not be determined from this analysis; however, there was no evidence suggesting that a higher dosage of corticosteroids was associated with greater benefit than a lower dosage. The authors also concluded that there was no suggestion of an increased risk of serious adverse effects associated with corticosteroid use.

In a retrospective, case-control study, the efficacy of early, low-dose, short-term therapy with systemic methylprednisolone or prednisone was evaluated in hospitalized adults with nonsevere COVID-19 pneumonia from a single center in China. A total of 475 patients were enrolled with 55 of these patients receiving early, low-dose corticosteroids. Methylprednisolone 20 or 40 mg IV daily was administered to 50 of these patients for 3–5 days, and oral prednisone 20 mg daily (equivalent dosage to methylprednisolone) was administered to 5 such patients for 3 days. Systemic corticosteroid therapy was initiated within a median of 2 days following hospital admission. A total of 420 patients received standard therapy (no corticosteroids); using propensity score matching, 55 of these patients were selected as matched controls. The primary outcome was the rate of patients who developed severe disease and mortality. In the corticosteroid treatment group, 12.7% of patients developed severe disease compared with 1.8% of patients in the control group. There was one death in the group receiving methylprednisolone and none in the control group. Regarding secondary outcomes, duration of fever, virus clearance time, and length of hospital stay were all substantially longer in patients receiving corticosteroids compared with no corticosteroid therapy. Because of the finding that early, low-dose, short-term systemic corticosteroid therapy was associated with worse clinical outcomes in hospitalized adult patients with nonsevere COVID-19 pneumonia, the authors concluded that the study results do not support the use of corticosteroids in this population. However, it is difficult to interpret these results because of potential confounding factors inherent in the nonrandomized study design. It is unclear if the results of this study apply to corticosteroids other than methylprednisolone or prednisone.

Other Respiratory Diseases

Systemic glucocorticoids may be used for symptomatic relief of acute manifestations of respiratory diseases including symptomatic idiopathic eosinophilic pneumonias (e.g., Löffler's syndrome) not manageable by other means, idiopathic pulmonary fibrosis, allergic bronchopulmonary aspergillosis, idiopathic bronchiolitis obliterans with organizing pneumonia, aspiration pneumonitis, hypersensitivity pneumonitis, and berylliosis. Glucocorticoids also are used in fulminating or disseminated tuberculosis (see Advanced Pulmonary and Extrapulmonary Tuberculosis under Uses: Respiratory Diseases) in conjunction with appropriate antituberculosis therapy. High dosage may be required for several days. Glucocorticoids are not indicated for uncomplicated chronic respiratory diseases.

● Complications of Prematurity
Antenatal Use in Preterm Labor

Short-course IM therapy with glucocorticoids (e.g., dexamethasone, betamethasone) is used in selected women with preterm labor to hasten fetal maturation (e.g., lungs, cerebral blood vessels), including women with preterm premature rupture of membranes, preeclampsia, or third-trimester hemorrhage. Antenatal administration of glucocorticoids generally appears to reduce the incidence and/or severity of neonatal respiratory distress syndrome (RDS) as indicated by a reduction in requirements for neonatal ventilatory support or surfactant therapy, and the beneficial effects are additive with those of surfactant.

Antenatal glucocorticoid therapy also can improve neonatal circulatory stability and reduce the incidence or severity of intraventricular hemorrhage. The incidence of necrotizing enterocolitis also is reduced by the use of antenatal glucocorticoids. The combined effects on multiple organ maturation during glucocorticoid therapy reduces the incidence of neonatal mortality, and the beneficial effects extend to a broad range of gestational ages (i.e., 24–34 weeks) and are not limited by gender or race.

Data are conflicting concerning the effects of antenatal glucocorticoids on the incidence of bronchopulmonary dysplasia, and patent ductus arteriosus in neonates, and the efficacy and safety of antenatal therapy with the drugs before 24 weeks or after 34 weeks of gestation have not been established. Short-term adverse effects of antenatal glucocorticoid administration include transient neonatal and maternal adrenal suppression and increased risk of infection. No long-term sequelae were noted in children up to 12 years of age who had been exposed to short-term antenatal glucocorticoids.

Antenatal use of glucocorticoids to reduce infant morbidity and mortality in women with preterm premature rupture of membranes is somewhat controversial, since the magnitude of neonatal benefit on RDS appears to be less and the risk of neonatal infection is greater than those in women with intact membranes. However, even in the presence of preterm premature rupture of membranes, the incidence of neonatal mortality and intraventricular hemorrhage is reduced with antenatal glucocorticoid therapy. In addition, the magnitude of increased risk of neonatal infection associated with such therapy appears to be small. Therefore, because of the benefit on mortality and hemorrhage in fetuses younger than 30–32 weeks' gestation and the apparently small risk, antenatal maternal glucocorticoid therapy is considered appropriate in the absence of clinically important chorioamnionitis.

Antenatal therapy with IM dexamethasone phosphate (6 mg every 12 hours for 2 days) or IM betamethasone sodium phosphate in fixed combination with betamethasone acetate (12 mg once daily for 2 days) has been studied most extensively, and some experts state that these drugs generally have been preferred for use in preterm labor because of similarities in potency and efficacy and their ability to readily cross the placenta, as well as the relative absence of mineralocorticoid activity and relatively weak immunosuppressive effects. These glucocorticoids also have been preferred because of their longer duration of action compared with hydrocortisone or methylprednisone.

Beneficial effects of IM glucocorticoids on fetal maturation are greatest more than 24 hours after initiating therapy and extend up to at least 7 days; however, clinically important improvement in neonatal outcomes also has been observed in women receiving an incomplete course of glucocorticoid therapy (i.e., less than 24 hours), and antenatal administration of even a partial course of glucocorticoids should be attempted unless immediate delivery is anticipated. Some experts recommend a single course of treatment for all pregnant women between 24–34 weeks' gestation who are at risk of preterm delivery within 7 days and state that repeat courses of antenatal glucocorticoids should not be used routinely because data evaluating the risks and benefits of such therapy are insufficient. A recent clinical study evaluated the overall effect on neonatal morbidity of repeated weekly courses of antenatal glucocorticoid therapy compared with a single course of treatment in pregnant women at risk of preterm delivery. The incidence of neonatal morbidity (defined as the presence of severe RDS, bronchopulmonary dysplasia, severe intraventricular hemorrhage [IVH], periventricular leukomalacia, necrotizing enterocolitis, proven sepsis, or death between randomization and nursery discharge) observed with weekly treatment courses (22.5%) was similar to that observed with single courses of therapy (28%). Other clinical studies are in progress to determine if a specific number of exposures to antenatal corticosteroids or an increased interval between treatment courses will improve neonatal outcomes in women at risk of preterm delivery.

Maternal use of tocolytic agents in conjunction with glucocorticoids may delay delivery in patients with preterm labor long enough for the fetus to derive benefit from glucocorticoid-induced accelerated fetal maturation. Combined use of the drugs has been shown to reduce the risk of neonatal RDS, and women between 24–34 weeks' gestation at risk of preterm delivery are candidates for antenatal glucocorticoid therapy regardless of fetal race, gender, or availability of surfactant. Because β-adrenergic tocolytic monotherapy may be associated with an increased risk of intraventricular hemorrhage, the addition of antenatal glucocorticoid therapy could have a secondary benefit of reducing this risk.

Antenatal glucocorticoid therapy appears to have an additive effect with postnatal prophylactic lung surfactant therapy in reducing the incidence of RDS and neonatal mortality. In addition, antenatal glucocorticoids can reduce the incidence and/or severity of intraventricular hemorrhage, which surfactant therapy alone does not appear to benefit. However, data are limited concerning the prophylactic use of combination therapy for respiratory distress syndrome in women less than 28 weeks' gestation.

Postnatal Use for Bronchopulmonary Dysplasia

Although some evidence indicates that postnatal IV glucocorticoids (e.g., dexamethasone) may be useful in preventing or treating bronchopulmonary dysplasia in preterm neonates with very low birth weight (i.e., less than 1.5 kg) who require mechanical ventilation, other evidence suggests that such therapy may be associated with an increased risk of serious adverse effects. Glucocorticoid therapy may provide short-term pulmonary benefits (e.g., reduced incidence of bronchopulmonary dysplasia, facilitation of weaning from mechanical ventilation) but does not reduce overall mortality and may be associated with both short-term adverse effects (e.g., hyperglycemia, hypertension, GI bleeding or intestinal perforation, hypertrophic obstructive cardiomyopathy, poor weight gain, poor growth of head circumference) and long-term sequelae. Long-term follow-up of preterm infants receiving IV glucocorticoids within 12 hours after birth indicates that postnatal glucocorticoid therapy is associated with an increased incidence of neurodevelopmental delay, cerebral palsy, impaired cognitive function, and stunted growth at or before school age. Therefore, the American Academy of Pediatrics (AAP) currently states that routine use of systemic glucocorticoids for prevention or treatment of bronchopulmonary dysplasia in very low birth weight infants is *not* recommended.

● *Hematologic Disorders*

Glucocorticoids are used in the management of acquired (autoimmune) hemolytic anemia, idiopathic thrombocytopenic purpura (ITP), secondary thrombocytopenia, erythroblastopenia, congenital (erythroid) hypoplastic anemia (Diamond-Blackfan syndrome), and pure red cell aplasia.

Although there is no evidence that glucocorticoids affect the course or duration of hematologic disorders, high or even massive dosage of the drugs is often used to decrease bleeding tendencies and normalize blood counts. When treatment is indicated in adults or children with moderate to severe idiopathic thrombocytopenic purpura (ITP), glucocorticoids, immune globulin IV (IGIV), or splenectomy are considered first-line therapies depending on the extent of bleeding involved. Other methods of treatment, such as splenectomy, should be considered if glucocorticoids must be continued for prolonged periods (exceeding several months), especially in patients with idiopathic or secondary thrombocytopenia, acquired (autoimmune) hemolytic anemia, erythroblastopenia (RBC anemia), or congenital (erythroid) hypoplastic anemia. Cytotoxic drugs produce better results in erythroblastopenia, but glucocorticoids may enhance response.

Glucocorticoids may not affect or prevent renal complications in Henoch-Schoenlein purpura. Glucocorticoids have been widely used in aplastic anemia in children, but there is no evidence to prove their effectiveness.

● *GI Diseases*

In ulcerative colitis, regional enteritis, and celiac disease, moderate to high dosage glucocorticoids may be useful as short-term palliative therapy for acute exacerbations and systemic complications of these chronic conditions. Glucocorticoids should not be used if there is a probability of impending perforation, abscess, or other pyogenic infection. Systemic and topical (rectal enema) glucocorticoids may be useful in acute ulcerative colitis. Sulfasalazine is the drug of choice for chronic ulcerative colitis, and a gluten-free diet is the primary method of therapy for celiac disease.

Glucocorticoids are rarely indicated for maintenance therapy in chronic GI diseases (ulcerative colitis, celiac disease) as they do not prevent relapses and may produce severe adverse reactions with long-term administration. Gastric hemorrhage and malignant hypertension are especially frequent. Occasionally, however, low dosages of glucocorticoids, in conjunction with other supportive therapy, may be useful for patients unresponsive to the usual therapy indicated for chronic conditions.

Crohn's Disease

Conventional systemic glucocorticoids (e.g., prednisone, prednisolone, methylprednisolone) have been used for the management of mildly to moderately active and moderately to severely active Crohn's disease†, while budesonide (a more recently approved glucocorticoid) is used orally as delayed-release capsules for the management of mildly-to-moderately active Crohn's disease involving the ileum and/or ascending colon. Conventional glucocorticoids are at least as effective as sulfasalazine, mesalamine, budesonide, or azathioprine in patients with Crohn's disease; however, many clinicians and experts state that conventional glucocorticoids should not be used for the management of mildly to moderately active disease, because of their high incidence of adverse effects and, therefore, their use should be reserved for patients with moderately to severely active disease.

Although no appropriate dose-ranging studies have been performed to evaluate conventional glucocorticoid dosing or dosage schedules for Crohn's disease, comparable clinical effects have been reported in placebo-controlled and active comparator clinical trials in which 50–70% of patients received glucocorticoid dosages equivalent to prednisone (40 mg daily; tapered after clinical response). In these patients, resolution of certain symptoms and resumption of weight gain usually occurred after 1–4 weeks of therapy, while clinical remission was achieved over 8–12 weeks. Parenteral glucocorticoids (dosages equivalent to prednisone 40–60 mg, given as divided doses or as a continuous infusion) are recommended for patients with severe fulminant Crohn's disease†; individuals with inflammatory abdominal mass should receive broad-spectrum anti-infective agents in conjunction with glucocorticoids. Once patients respond to parenteral therapy, they should gradually be switched to an equivalent regimen of an oral glucocorticoid. About 50% of patients with active Crohn's disease, who are receiving systemic glucocorticoids, become glucocorticoid-dependent or glucocorticoid-resistant; such patients should receive drugs with steroid-sparing effects (e.g., azathioprine, mercaptopurine) or, alternatively, infliximab. Glucocorticoids should not be used for maintenance therapy of Crohn's disease, because both conventional glucocorticoids and budesonide usually do not prevent relapses and the drugs (especially conventional glucocorticoids) may produce severe adverse reactions with long-term administration.

Systemic conventional glucocorticoids (e.g., prednisone 1–2 mg/kg daily up to 60 mg daily) have been used in pediatric patients with mild esophageal or gastroduodenal Crohn's disease†. In addition, glucocorticoids (e.g., prednisone or methylprednisolone 1–2 mg/kg daily up to 60 mg daily) are recommended for the management of moderately to severely active Crohn's disease, in children. Results of a 12-week comparator-drug (prednisone versus budesonide) controlled study in pediatric patients 8–18 years of age (weighing more than 20 kg) with mildly to moderately active Crohn's disease (Pediatric Crohn's Disease Activity Index [PCDI] score of 12.5–40) indicate that remission rates in children receiving prednisone (40 mg daily for 2 weeks and then tapered until discontinuance) were similar (50% for prednisone versus 47% for budesonide) to those receiving budesonide (9 mg daily for 8 weeks, tapered until discontinuance). Incidence of adverse effects was substantially lower (about 32% for budesonide versus 71% for prednisone) and less severe in pediatric patients receiving budesonide than in those receiving prednisone.

Trichinosis

Glucocorticoids are used in the treatment of trichinosis with neurologic or myocardial involvement.

● Neoplastic Diseases

Glucocorticoids in high dosage are used alone or as a component of various chemotherapeutic regimens in the palliative treatment of neoplastic diseases of the lymphatic system (e.g., leukemias and lymphomas in adults and acute leukemias in children). Massive dosage of glucocorticoids has occasionally been used in the treatment of neoplastic diseases but rarely offers any additional benefit and greatly increases adverse effects. Beneficial results are enhanced, however, when glucocorticoids are used as part of a total treatment regimen in combination with cytotoxic and immunosuppressive drugs; such a regimen should be administered only by an experienced oncologist.

In adults, acute lymphocytic (lymphoblastic) leukemia, chronic lymphocytic leukemia, and Hodgkin's disease respond well to combination regimens that include a glucocorticoid (usually prednisone or prednisolone). Acute myeloblastic leukemia, lymphosarcoma, and the blast crisis of chronic myelocytic leukemia may fail to respond or may relapse upon discontinuance of therapy.

In moderate dosage, glucocorticoids induce tumor remission in approximately 15% of patients with breast cancer. Because glucocorticoids used alone are not as effective as other agents (e.g., cytotoxic agents, hormones, antiestrogens) in the treatment of breast cancer, their use should be reserved for patients unresponsive to other therapy.

Glucocorticoids (e.g., prednisone) also have been used alone or as a component of various combination chemotherapeutic regimens in the treatment of advanced, symptomatic (i.e., painful) hormone-refractory prostate cancer. Use of glucocorticoids and/or chemotherapeutic agents in the treatment of advanced, hormone-resistant prostate cancer is palliative, with patients having median survival durations of less than 1 year; no therapy has been shown to improve survival to date, and therefore the principal goal of therapy in such cancer currently is improvement in quality of life, particularly pain. Randomized studies have shown that the addition of an antineoplastic agent (e.g., mitoxantrone) to glucocorticoid therapy results in a greater proportion of patients achieving a palliative response (i.e., pain reduction) and a longer duration of such response compared with glucocorticoid treatment alone. Improvement in certain quality-of-life measures, including indicators related to pain, physical activity or function, constipation, and mood, also may favor combination therapy.

Glucocorticoids (e.g., dexamethasone, prednisone) also have been used as a component of various combination chemotherapeutic regimens in the treatment of multiple myeloma. Dexamethasone has been used in combination chemotherapeutic regimens in various doses (20–40 mg) and schedules. Although high-dose dexamethasone has been associated with increased adverse effects (e.g., hyperglycemia, psychiatric effects, insomnia, hyperactivity, infectious complications), high-dose dexamethasone is an effective component of combination chemotherapeutic regimens for the treatment of multiple myeloma.

● Cancer Chemotherapy-induced Nausea and Vomiting

Corticosteroids (e.g., dexamethasone, methylprednisolone) have been used for the prevention of nausea and vomiting associated with emetogenic cancer chemotherapy† including that associated with cisplatin. Most clinical experience to date has been with dexamethasone.

● Liver Diseases

Glucocorticoids may be beneficial or harmful in patients with liver disease. Although evidence is conflicting, the drugs probably are of no value in patients with acute hepatitis and massive necrosis. In patients with subacute hepatic necrosis and chronic active hepatitis, administration of glucocorticoids in high dosage can decrease serum bilirubin, ascites, and mortality rate. Prolonged low-dosage maintenance therapy may be necessary. In nonalcoholic cirrhosis in women, glucocorticoids increase survival rate in the absence of ascites, but not when ascites is present. The drugs are ineffective in men with nonalcoholic cirrhosis. Glucocorticoids may decrease mortality rate in patients with alcoholic cirrhosis with hepatic encephalopathy, but they should not be used in less seriously ill patients. Acute viral hepatitis is usually benign and self-limited, and glucocorticoids are rarely indicated.

● Cerebral Edema

Glucocorticoids administered parenterally, in high dosage, may be useful to decrease cerebral edema associated with brain tumors and neurosurgery. Some patients with cerebral edema associated with pseudotumor cerebri may also benefit from use of glucocorticoids, but the efficacy of the drugs is controversial and remains to be established. Edema resulting from brain abscesses is less responsive than that resulting from brain tumors.

The use of glucocorticoids in the management of cerebral edema is not a substitute for careful neurosurgical evaluation and definitive management such as neurosurgery or other specific therapy. Effects of glucocorticoids are not apparent for several hours and in acute situations the drugs should only be used adjunctively with other indicated therapy. Although any glucocorticoid may be effective, those having minimal mineralocorticoid activity are preferable. Glucocorticoids do not appear to be beneficial in cerebral edema associated with cerebral infarction.

Head Injury

Pooled analyses of small controlled studies of glucocorticoids in patients with head injury have failed to clearly establish the efficacy of glucocorticoid therapy in this patient population. Because of a lack of evidence of efficacy, some experts have recommended against the use of glucocorticoids for improving outcomes or reducing intracranial pressure in patients with head injury. More recent evidence from a large, international, randomized, placebo-controlled study (Corticosteroid Randomization after Significant Head Injury [CRASH]) indicates that use of glucocorticoids in patients with head injuries may be detrimental. Results from this study in more than 10,000 patients with head injury and a Glasgow coma score not exceeding 14 within 8 hours of injury indicate that glucocorticoid therapy (e.g., methylprednisolone 2 g administered by IV infusion over 1 hour, followed by methylprednisolone 0.4 g/hour by IV infusion for 48 hours) is associated with a substantial increase in risk of death (21.1% with methylprednisolone versus 17.9% with placebo) within 2 weeks after head injury; the relative risk of death from all causes within 2 weeks in patients receiving methylprednisolone compared with placebo in this study was 1.18 (95% confidence interval of 1.09–1.27). The cause of the observed increase in mortality in patients receiving glucocorticoids is unclear because cause of death was not documented. Recruitment of patients for this study was halted after results from interim analyses were reported. Results regarding effects of glucocorticoid therapy on disability 6 months after head injury are pending.

● Acute Spinal Cord Injury

Some evidence indicates that therapy with large IV doses of glucocorticoids (i.e., methylprednisolone) can improve motor and sensory function in patients with acute spinal cord injury† when treatment is initiated promptly following injury. However, benefit in controlled studies in humans has been demonstrated to date only in patients receiving high-dose IV methylprednisolone within 8 hours after spinal cord injury, and whether improvement in neurologic function with such therapy will routinely lead to specific improvements in disability has not been established.

In a multicenter, comparative study, patients with acute spinal cord injuries† who received an initial 30-mg/kg dose of methylprednisolone (as the sodium succinate salt) by rapid IV injection (over 15 minutes) within 8 hours of injury, followed by infusion of the drug at 5.4 mg/kg per hour for an additional 23 hours, had substantial improvement in motor function and pinprick and touch sensation at 6 weeks and 6 months compared with those who received IV naloxone hydrochloride (5.4 mg/kg by rapid IV injection followed by 4 mg/kg per hour for an additional 23 hours) or placebo. The benefits of methylprednisolone therapy were observed in patients with complete as well as incomplete loss of motor and sensory function, and neurologic improvement observed at 6 weeks in methylprednisolone-treated patients was still evident at 6 months. Patients receiving naloxone or placebo and those in whom therapy with high-dose methylprednisolone was initiated later than 8 hours (but usually within 14 hours) after injury did not have substantial improvement in motor function or touch sensation. Mortality at 6 months was similar among treatment groups, and overall mortality was low (6%) compared with that of previous studies. Although the use of glucocorticoids in patients with spinal cord injuries has been associated with increased morbidity in some studies, clinically important differences in the incidence of wound infections, GI bleeding, and other complications among treatment groups in this study were not observed.

Limited evidence in animals suggests that the ameliorative effects of glucocorticoids in spinal cord injury† are related to dose and time of initiation of therapy; these effects appear to be characterized by a biphasic, bell-shaped response curve. In one study in animals with experimentally induced spinal cord injury, posttraumatic spinal cord ischemia was effectively minimized by a 30-mg/kg dose of methylprednisolone administered 30 minutes but not several hours after injury; at 30 minutes, a 15-mg/kg dose produced little benefit, while a dose of 60 mg/kg was ineffective or deleterious. Such studies suggest that the lack of appreciable benefit observed in an earlier controlled study of patients with acute spinal cord injury who were treated up to 48 hours after injury using a methylprednisolone dose of 100 mg or 1 g (approximately 15 mg/kg) daily for 10 days may have been related in part to delayed administration of the drug or administration of an insufficient dose. Additional studies are needed to determine the optimal timing, dosage, and duration of therapy with methylprednisolone or other glucocorticoids in patients with acute spinal cord injury and to elucidate further the potential benefits of glucocorticoid therapy on functional status in such patients.

● Low Back Pain

Glucocorticoids (alone or combined with a local anesthetic and/or an opiate analgesic) have been used epidurally† for symptomatic relief of low back pain†. Although this use remains controversial and convincing evidence of efficacy remains to be established, most experts state that this invasive form of therapy

is an option for short-term relief of acute, subacute, or chronic radicular pain in patients with low back pain and radiculopathy associated with disk disease or herniation or spinal stenosis when more conservative therapies (e.g., rest, analgesics, physical therapy) fail and as a means of potentially avoiding surgery. The effect of epidural glucocorticoid injections on long-term outcomes of unremitting low back pain remains unclear. Epidural therapy for low back pain and radiculopathy involves injection of the drug(s) into the epidural space near the site where the nerve roots pass before entering the intervertebral foramen. Such therapy theoretically allows a concentrated amount of drug(s) to be deposited and retained locally, exposing nerves to the drug(s) for prolonged periods in an attempt to reduce inflammation, swelling, and pain. Epidural injections may be performed by caudal, interlaminar, or transforaminal approaches; the transforaminal approach requires the smallest injection volume and appears to be the most specific and possibly most effective route.

Because of the potential for complications related to improper needle placement or drug administration, many experts state that epidural injections should be performed by an experienced clinician using fluoroscopic guidance and contrast control to ensure that the needle is correctly positioned and that the injection is not performed intravascularly, intrathecally, or into tissues other than the epidural space. While some clinicians suggest that fluoroscopic guidance may not be necessary in patients who have not undergone previous surgery and whose spinal anatomy is normal, and for whom there are no other factors making the procedure technically difficult (e.g., obesity), serious adverse neurologic effects have been reported following epidural glucocorticoid injection both with and without fluoroscopic guidance. (See Cautions: Nervous System Effects.) Long-acting injectable suspension formulations of methylprednisolone, triamcinolone, and betamethasone are the most commonly used preparations for epidural injections. Optimal technique, dosage, timing of initial injection, and injection frequency, as well as maximum number of epidural glucocorticoid injections, remain to be established.

Water-soluble glucocorticoid preparations typically have not been used for epidural injection because they are cleared rapidly from the spinal canal and have been associated with adverse neurologic effects (e.g., seizures, segmental hyperalgesia) when injected intrathecally in animals. Limited evidence suggests that large particles (e.g., exceeding 50 μm) in glucocorticoid suspension preparations potentially may cause embolic vascular occlusion during inadvertent intra-arterial injection; it appears that some particulate suspensions (e.g., methylprednisolone acetate, triamcinolone hexacetonide) may contain substantial amounts of these large particles, and some clinicians have suggested that a glucocorticoid solution preparation (e.g., dexamethasone sodium phosphate) or a suspension with an overall smaller size of particulate matter (e.g., fixed combination of betamethasone sodium phosphate and betamethasone acetate) may be preferred for epidural injections. Long-acting injectable suspension preparations of glucocorticoids (e.g., Aristospan®, Celestone® Soluspan®, Depo-Medrol®, Kenalog®) also contain preservatives and/or suspending agents (e.g., benzalkonium chloride, benzyl alcohol, myristyl-γ-picolinium chloride, polyethylene glycol) that have been associated with neurotoxic effects in animals or humans. While most reports of neurotoxicity with intraspinal glucocorticoid therapy in humans have involved intrathecal administration, the safety of epidural injections using preserved glucocorticoid formulations is controversial, and epidural administration of these formulations is not recommended by the manufacturers. Currently there are no studies supporting the use of any one formulation over any other in terms of safety.

The principal risk of epidural injection therapy for low back pain and radiculopathy is rare epidural abscess. However, other serious adverse effects, including infectious complications (e.g., meningitis), neurologic effects (e.g., arachnoiditis, spinal cord trauma, increased intracranial pressure, nerve injury, seizures, bladder or bowel dysfunction, paraparesis or paralysis, brain damage), ocular effects, embolic vascular complications, and death may occur following attempted epidural injection (see Cautions). Systemic glucocorticoid effects (e.g., hypothalamic-pituitary-adrenal [HPA] axis suppression, hypercorticism, Cushing's syndrome, osteoporosis, fluid retention, hyperglycemia) also may occur after epidural glucocorticoid administration.

Data from the American Society of Anesthesiologists (ASA) Closed Claims Project database, which includes closed anesthesia malpractice claims arising from chronic pain management, suggest that serious injuries (e.g., brain damage, death) can occur when glucocorticoids are combined with local anesthetics and/or opiate analgesics for epidural injection and that patient safety may be improved by excluding typical epidural doses (volumes in excess of intrathecal test doses) of local anesthetics and/or opiate analgesics from epidural glucocorticoid injections.

Limited evidence suggests that therapeutic facet joint† and intradiscal glucocorticoid injections† are minimally effective or ineffective in the treatment of low back pain, although some clinicians report that facet joint injections may be useful in some patients with facet arthropathy. Inclusion of a glucocorticoid in trigger point injections also does not appear to be beneficial. Sacroiliac joint injections performed using fluoroscopic guidance may provide temporary pain relief in some patients when the principal source of spinal pain is the sacroiliac joint.

Although oral glucocorticoids have been used by some clinicians in the treatment of low back pain†, they do not appear to be effective and evidence supporting such use is lacking.

Bacterial Meningitis

Glucocorticosteroids have been used as adjunctive therapy in patients with bacterial meningitis†; however, results of many studies evaluating this use have been inconclusive or conflicting. Most trials were conducted with dexamethasone. In a Cochrane review which included 25 randomized controlled studies of corticosteroid use in acute bacterial meningitis, corticosteroids were found to reduce hearing loss and neurological sequelae, but did not improve overall mortality. Subgroup analysis showed that the benefits were limited to high-income countries; there was no beneficial effect of corticosteroid therapy in low-income countries. In most of the studies, the corticosteroid used was dexamethasone; hydrocortisone or prednisone were used in a few studies.

Multiple Sclerosis

Glucocorticoids currently are considered the drugs of choice for the management of acute relapses of multiple sclerosis. The anti-inflammatory and immunomodulating effects of the drugs can accelerate neurologic recovery by restoring the blood-brain barrier, reducing edema, and possibly improving axonal conduction.

For moderate to severe relapses, methylprednisolone has been administered IV in a dosage of 1 g daily for 3–5 days, followed by 60 mg of oral prednisone daily, tapering the dosage over 12 days. Alternative regimens have included 1 g or 15 mg/kg of IV methylprednisolone tapered over 15 days to 1 mg/kg and followed by oral prednisone or prednisolone in gradually decreasing dosages over several weeks to months.

Interest in the use of IV methylprednisolone in the management of acute relapses of multiple sclerosis heightened as a result of the Optic Neuritis Treatment Trial in which the rate of recovery in vision was faster in those receiving the drug and the risk of development of clinically definite multiple sclerosis was reduced during the first 2 years of follow-up. (See Uses: Ocular Disorders.) The beneficial effect of the methylprednisolone regimen on disease progression was transient since results at 3- and 5-year follow-up indicate that there were not clinically important differences among treatment groups in the rate of development of clinically definite multiple sclerosis or the degree of neurologic disability among those who developed the disease during the 5-year follow-up period. Additional study is needed and under way to determine whether pulsed doses of glucocorticoids given every other month can slow progression of the disease in patients with moderate disability and secondary progressive multiple sclerosis.

Myasthenia Gravis

Glucocorticoids (e.g., prednisone) are used in the management of myasthenia gravis, usually in patients who have had an inadequate response to anticholinesterase therapy. Glucocorticoids also have been administered parenterally in the treatment of myasthenic crisis.

Organ Transplants

In massive dosage, glucocorticoids may be used concomitantly with other immunosuppressive drugs to prevent rejection of transplanted organs. Because the incidence of secondary infections is high in patients receiving these drugs, such therapy should be administered by physicians experienced in its use.

Nephrotic Syndrome

Glucocorticoids can induce diuresis and remission of proteinuria in children and adults with nephrotic syndrome secondary to primary renal disease, especially when there is minimal renal histologic change. Lupus nephritis may also respond to glucocorticoids. High dosage may be required for prolonged periods, and alternate-day therapy should be used to decrease adverse effects. Nephrotic syndrome secondary to diabetes mellitus, renal amyloidosis, glomerulonephritis, or other diseases is generally refractory to glucocorticoids.

Diagnostic Uses

Dexamethasone inhibits pituitary adrenocorticotropic hormone (ACTH) release and decreases output of endogenous corticosteroids when given in an amount which does not itself appreciably affect concentrations of urinary 17-hydroxycorticosteroids. This effect is utilized in the dexamethasone suppression test for the diagnosis of Cushing's syndrome and the differential diagnosis of adrenocortical tumors. (See Dexamethasone 68:04.)

The dexamethasone suppression test (DST) has been used for the detection, diagnosis, and management of mental depression; however, considerable controversy currently exists regarding the clinical utility of the test. The sensitivity of the DST in patients with major depression is relatively modest (about 40–50%), and a positive test result (nonsuppression) does not appear to reliably predict response to antidepressant therapy and a negative test result (suppression) is not an indication for withholding antidepressant therapy. Therefore, the American Psychiatric Association, American College of Physicians, and other experts currently state that, pending further studies and evaluation, the DST should not be used *routinely* for the diagnosis and management of depression, although judicious use of the DST may be a useful adjunct in clinical decision making in selected situations and as a research tool.

Duchenne Muscular Dystrophy

The current standard of care for patients with Duchenne muscular dystrophy includes the use of corticosteroids (e.g., prednisone, deflazacort) for improving muscle function and strength. The American Academy of Neurology recommends the use of prednisone or deflazacort to improve muscle strength, pulmonary function, and possibly also slow the development of scoliosis and need for surgery in patients with Duchenne muscular dystrophy. Results of direct comparative studies suggest that prednisone and deflazacort are similarly effective in improving motor function, but differ in their adverse effect profiles (e.g., prednisone may be associated with more weight gain while deflazacort may be associated with a greater risk of cataracts).

Cardiovascular Disorders
Shock

Use of corticosteroids in the treatment of septic shock has been controversial. Although some controlled studies have shown beneficial effects of high-dose regimens on morbidity and mortality in septic shock, many studies have not. Results of one prospective, controlled study suggest that glucocorticoids do not improve overall survival in patients with severe, late septic shock but may be beneficial early in the course of septic shock and in certain subgroups of patients. However, 2 subsequent, prospective, controlled studies failed to show a benefit of high-dose glucocorticoid therapy that was initiated *early* (i.e., within 2.8 hours of diagnosis) in patients with presumed sepsis or septic shock. In addition, there was some evidence that such therapy may be associated with an increased risk of mortality in certain patients (i.e., those with serum creatinine concentrations exceeding 2 mg/dL at diagnosis and those who developed secondary infection). More recent meta-analyses found that systemic corticosteroid use accelerated the resolution of shock and increased vasopressor-free days; however, corticosteroids increased neuromuscular weakness without a clear effect on short- or long-term mortality. The Surviving Sepsis Campaign guidelines suggest the use of IV corticosteroids for adults with septic shock and an ongoing requirement for vasopressor therapy; this recommendation is based on a moderate quality of evidence. The optimal dose, timing of initiation, and duration of corticosteroids remain uncertain. The typical corticosteroid used in adults with septic shock is IV hydrocortisone at a dose of 200 mg daily given as 50 mg IV every 6 hours or as a continuous infusion. The guidelines suggest that this is commenced at a dose of norepinephrine or epinephrine ≥0.25 mcg/kg/min at least 4 hours after initiation.

Pericarditis

Systemic corticosteroids (e.g. prednisone) have been used in the treatment of pericarditis†, but is generally considered a second- or third-line treatment. Corticosteroid use (mostly with high dosages) in this setting has been associated with recurrence and a prolonged disease course. In a nonrandomized observational study, use of higher doses of corticosteroids (i.e., prednisone 1 mg/kg/day) for recurrent pericarditis was associated with increased risk of adverse effects, recurrence, and hospitalizations compared with low-dose corticosteroid therapy (i.e., prednisone 0.2 to 0.5 mg/kg).

● Chronic Fatigue Syndrome

Because of evidence that chronic fatigue syndrome† is associated with subnormal cortisol secretion secondary to impaired activation of the hypothalamic-pituitary-adrenal (HPA) axis, glucocorticoid supplementation has been studied in patients with this condition. In a study in patients 18–55 years of age who met the US Centers for Disease Control and Prevention (CDC) case criteria for chronic fatigue syndrome, low-dose oral glucocorticoid therapy (approximately 13 mg/m^2 [20–30 mg] of hydrocortisone every morning and 3 mg/m^2 [5 mg] every afternoon for about 12 weeks) produced some symptomatic improvement as determined by a global self-rating wellness scale; however, there was no evidence of improvement in several other self-rating scales, including mood, depression, and activity scales. Because the modest symptomatic improvement with glucocorticoid therapy was associated with clinically important adrenal suppression, such therapy is not practical nor advisable for the chronic management of chronic fatigue syndrome.

● Other Uses

In miscellaneous inflammatory reactions, such as those resulting from dental procedures, short-term glucocorticoid therapy can decrease edema and may alleviate pain associated with such inflammations.

Local injection of glucocorticoids (e.g., methylprednisolone, betamethasone) into the tissue near the carpal tunnel has been used in a limited number of patients to relieve symptoms (e.g., pain, edema, sensory deficit) of carpal tunnel syndrome. In clinical studies, short-term response was noted in most patients, but the improvement in symptoms waned during the following 11–24 months. Limited evidence suggests that injection technique may influence the duration of effect.

Glucocorticoids (e.g., betamethasone, dexamethasone, methylprednisolone) have been used by local injection for the management of cystic tumors of an aponeurosis or tendon (ganglia).

For EENT and topical uses of the corticosteroids, see 52:08.08 and 84:06.08.

DOSAGE AND ADMINISTRATION

● Administration

Glucocorticoids, in appropriate forms, may be administered orally, by oral inhalation, and by IV, IM, subcutaneous, intra-articular, intrabursal, intradermal, intrasynovial, intralesional, or soft tissue injection. Long-acting injectable suspension formulations of some glucocorticoids (e.g., betamethasone, methylprednisolone, triamcinolone) have been administered by epidural injection, although the safety of epidural injections using preserved glucocorticoid formulations is controversial and epidural administration of these formulations is not recommended by the manufacturers. (See Uses: Low Back Pain and see Cautions: Nervous System Effects.) The manufacturer of Depo-Medrol® (sterile methylprednisolone acetate suspension) states that this formulation of methylprednisolone acetate contains benzyl alcohol, which is potentially toxic when administered locally to neural tissue, and that this formulation should not be administered intrathecally because of reports of severe adverse events with such use. (See Cautions: Nervous System Effects.) Whenever possible, topical corticosteroid therapy (see 52:08.08 and 84:06.08) is preferable to systemic therapy.

Because injections of slightly soluble glucocorticoids may produce atrophy at the site of injection, IM injections of these products should be made deeply into gluteal muscle; repeated IM injections at the same site should be avoided, and these products should not be administered subcutaneously. Knee, ankle, wrist, elbow, shoulder, phalangeal, and hip joints are suitable sites for intra-articular injections of glucocorticoids; spinal joints and joints without synovial spaces are not suitable for intra-articular injection. For intra-articular injections, a 20- to 24-gauge needle should be used; needle placement should be verified by aspirating a few drops of synovial fluid prior to drug administration with a second syringe. Joints should be injected where the synovial cavity is most superficial and free from large vessels and nerves. Joint fluid should be examined to exclude sepsis, and injection into an infected site should be avoided; if joint sepsis is evident, appropriate antibacterial therapy should be instituted. Symptoms of septic arthritis include local swelling, further restriction of joint motion, fever, or malaise. Glucocorticoids should not be injected into unstable joints and patients should be cautioned not to overuse joints in which the inflammatory process is still active despite symptomatic improvement.

For management of tenosynovitis and tendinitis, glucocorticoids should be injected into affected tendon sheaths rather than into tendons.

For disorders of the foot (bursitis, tenosynovitis, acute gouty arthritis), a tuberculin syringe with a 25-gauge, ¾-inch needle should be used for intra-articular or soft-tissue administration.

For dermatologic conditions, a tuberculin syringe with a 25-gauge, ½-inch needle should be used for intralesional administration.

In treatment of intercostal neuritis or neuralgia, local injections of glucocorticoids should be made cautiously to avoid penetration of the pleura, which may be indicated by appearance of sudden sharp pain during the injection.

● Dosage

General Dosage

In the management of acute disorders, glucocorticoid dosage should be sufficient to ensure that symptoms are controlled quickly, and treatment should be discontinued as soon as possible. Acute disorders respond most rapidly to divided daily doses. In life-threatening situations where adrenal insufficiency may be the precipitating cause, glucocorticoids can be administered in any dosage required without serious complications, even before a definite diagnosis has been made.

Dosage ranges for glucocorticoids are extremely wide, and patient responses are quite variable. The amount of drug each patient receives should be individualized according to the diagnosis, severity, prognosis and probable duration of the disease, and patient response and tolerance. Occasionally, patients may respond better to one glucocorticoid than another but this is unpredictable.

Types of dosages generally used in various disease states are: *physiologic* or *replacement* (amount of glucocorticoid normally secreted by the adrenal cortex each day—approximately 20 mg of hydrocortisone), *pharmacologic* (any dosage greater than a physiologic dosage) which includes *maintenance* or *low* (dosage slightly in excess of physiologic amounts—e.g., 5–15 mg of prednisone daily), *moderate* (approximately 0.5 mg of prednisone/kg daily), *high* (approximately 1–3 mg of prednisone/kg daily), and *massive* (approximately 15–30 mg of prednisolone/kg daily). The *approximate* equivalent oral glucocorticoid dosages established by various laboratory assays are as follows:

TABLE 1. Equivalent Oral Dosages of Glucocorticoids

Drug	Equivalent Dosage
Cortisone	25 mg
Hydrocortisone	20 mg
Prednisolone	5 mg
Prednisone	5 mg
Methylprednisolone	4 mg
Triamcinolone	4 mg
Dexamethasone	0.75 mg
Betamethasone	0.6 mg

"Equivalent dosages" are general approximations and may not apply to all diseases or routes of administration (especially oral inhalation, IM or intrasynovial injections). In addition, duration of HPA-axis suppression and degree of mineralocorticoid activities must be considered separately. (See Pharmacology.)

Estimated equivalent daily dosages of inhaled glucocorticoids for the treatment of asthma for adults and adolescents 12 years of age or older are as follows:

TABLE 2. Equivalent Daily Dosages of Inhaled Glucocorticoids for Adults and Adolescents

Drug	Low Daily Dosage (mcg)	Medium Daily Dosage (mcg)	High Daily Dosage (mcg)
Beclomethasone with Fluoroethane Propellant	80–240	>240–480	>480
Budesonide Powder for Oral Inhalation	180–600	>600–1200	>1200
Flunisolide with Hydro-fluoroalkane (HFA) Propellant	320	>320–640	>640
Fluticasone with Fluoroethane Propellant	88–264	>264–440	>440
Fluticasone Powder for Oral Inhalation	100–300	>300–500	>500
Mometasone Powder for Oral Inhalation	200	400	>400
Triamcinolone Acetonide with Dichlorodifluoromethane Propellant	300–750	>750–1500	>1500

Estimated equivalent daily dosages of inhaled glucocorticoids for the treatment of asthma for infants and children are as follows (Table 3):

TABLE 3. Equivalent Daily Dosages of Inhaled Glucocorticoids for Infants and Children

Drug	Low Daily Dosage		Medium Daily Dosage		High Daily Dosage	
	Infants and Children 0–4 years of age[a]	Children 5–11 years of age	Infants and Children 0–4 years of age[a]	Children 5–11 years of age	Infants and Children 0–4 years of age[a]	Children 5–11 years of age
Beclomethasone with Fluoroethane Propellant	NA[b]	80–160 mcg	NA	>160–320 mcg	NA	>320 mcg
Budesonide Powder for Oral Inhalation	NA	180–400 mcg	NA	>400–800 mcg	NA	>800 mcg
Budesonide Suspension for Nebulization	0.25–0.5 mg	0.5 mg	>0.5–1 mg	1 mg	>1 mg	2 mg
Flunisolide with Hydrofluoroalkane (HFA) Propellant	NA	160 mcg[c]	NA	320 mcg[c]	NA	≥640 mcg[c]

TABLE 3. Continued

Drug	Low Daily Dosage		Medium Daily Dosage		High Daily Dosage	
	Infants and Children 0–4 years of age[a]	Children 5–11 years of age	Infants and Children 0–4 years of age[a]	Children 5–11 years of age	Infants and Children 0–4 years of age[a]	Children 5–11 years of age
Fluticasone with Fluoroethane Propellant	176 mcg	88–176 mcg	>176–352 mcg	>176–352 mcg	>352 mcg	>352 mcg
Fluticasone Powder for Oral Inhalation	NA	100–200 mcg	NA	>200–400 mcg	NA	>400 mcg
Triamcinolone Acetonide with Dichlorodifluoromethane Propellant	NA	300–600 mcg	NA	>600–900 mcg	NA	>900 mcg

[a] Safety and efficacy of inhaled corticosteroids in children younger than 1 year of age have not been established.

[b] NA: not applicable.

[c] Safety and efficacy of flunisolide inhalation aerosol in children younger than 6 years of age have not been established.

Long-term glucocorticoid therapy should not be initiated without due consideration of its risks. Other less dangerous drugs should be used if possible. If glucocorticoids are clearly necessary, the drugs should be administered in the smallest dosage possible and should generally be used only as adjuncts to other treatments. Patients should be continually monitored for signs that indicate dosage adjustment is necessary, such as remission or exacerbations of the disease and stress (surgery, infection, trauma). Periodic attempts should be made to decrease dosage or, preferably, to withdraw the drugs completely. Prescription refills should always be limited so that periodic evaluations can be made of the patient's condition.

Coronavirus Disease 2019 (COVID-19)

When used for adjunctive treatment in adults with coronavirus disease 2019 (COVID-19)†, dexamethasone has been used IV or orally in a dosage of 6 mg daily for up to 10 days or until hospital discharge, whichever comes first. If dexamethasone is not available, use of other systemic corticosteroids is recommended. It is not known at this time whether other corticosteroids (e.g., hydrocortisone, methylprednisolone, prednisone) will have a similar benefit as dexamethasone. For equivalent daily dosages of these alternative corticosteroids to dexamethasone, see Table 4.

TABLE 4. Equivalent IV or Oral Total Daily Dosages of Corticosteroids[a]

Drug	Equivalent Daily Dosage	Frequency of Administration
Dexamethasone	6 mg	Once daily
Methylprednisolone	32 mg	Once daily or in 2 divided doses daily
Prednisone	40 mg	Once daily or in 2 divided doses daily
Hydrocortisone	160 mg	2–4 divided doses daily

[a] Dosages recommended by the National Institutes of Health (NIH) COVID-19 Treatment Guidelines Panel.

When used for adjunctive treatment in pediatric patients with COVID-19†, the NIH COVID-19 Treatment Guidelines Panel recommends dexamethasone 0.15 mg/kg (maximum dosage 6 mg) given IV or orally for up to 10 days. If dexamethasone is not available, equivalent dosages of alternative corticosteroids may be considered.

Clinicians should consult the most recent NIH COVID-19 treatment guidelines for additional information on use of corticosteroids in patients with COVID-19.

Alternate-Day Therapy

Alternate-day therapy is the dosage regimen of choice for long-term oral glucocorticoid treatment of most conditions. In alternate-day therapy, a single dose is administered every other morning. The drug is administered in the morning to simulate the natural circadian rhythm of corticosteroid secretion which is high in the morning and low in the evening. This regimen provides relief of symptoms while minimizing adrenal suppression, protein catabolism, and other adverse effects. However, some patients, especially those with rheumatoid arthritis or ulcerative colitis, require daily glucocorticoid therapy because symptoms of the underlying disease cannot be controlled by alternate-day therapy. Only "short-acting" steroids (e.g., prednisone, prednisolone, methylprednisolone) that suppress the HPA axis for less than 1.5 days after a single oral dose should be used for alternate-day therapy.

Several methods of transferring patients from initial divided-dose oral therapy to alternate-day therapy have been described. Twice the total daily dose that has been found to be effective may be administered as a single dose every other morning; this dose may then be gradually decreased to maintenance levels. Alternatively, the daily dose may be decreased to maintenance levels prior to initiation of alternate-day therapy; then twice the daily dose is given every other day. A third method is to establish a maintenance dose that is administered every morning as a single dose; alternate-day therapy is then introduced by gradual increases of this dose on alternate mornings with corresponding decreases in the dose administered on intervening mornings until twice the daily dose is being taken on alternate mornings.

Because an intact HPA axis is necessary for alternate-day therapy to be effective, it may be difficult to transfer a patient who has been maintained on divided-dose therapy for prolonged periods to alternate-day therapy, but continual attempts should be made to do so. Symptomatic treatment with other drugs on the "off day" or a trial of more than double the daily dose every other day may be helpful. When alternate-day therapy is not possible, the entire daily dose of glucocorticoid can usually be administered as a single morning dose; however, some patients will require divided daily doses of glucocorticoids.

Discontinuance of Therapy

Although high-dose glucocorticoid therapy used for only brief periods in emergency situations may be reduced and discontinued quite rapidly, withdrawal following long-term therapy with pharmacologic dosages of systemic glucocorticoids should be very gradual until recovery of HPA-axis function occurs. (See Cautions: Adrenocortical Insufficiency.) These precautions also apply when a patient is transferred from a systemic glucocorticoid to oral or nasal inhalation therapy with beclomethasone dipropionate, budesonide, fluticasone propionate, or flunisolide.

For certain acute allergic conditions (e.g., contact dermatitis such as poison ivy), glucocorticoids may be administered short term (e.g., for 6 days), giving an initially high dose (e.g., 30 mg of prednisone in divided doses) on the first day of therapy, and then withdrawing therapy by tapering the dose over several days (e.g., by 5 mg of prednisone daily). (See Dosage and Administration: Dosage, in Methylprednisolone 68:04 and also Prednisone 68:04.)

Many methods of slow withdrawal or "tapering" have been described. In one suggested regimen, glucocorticoid dosage is decreased by the equivalent of 2.5–5 mg of prednisone every 3–7 days until the physiologic dose (e.g., 5 mg of prednisone or prednisolone, 0.75 mg of dexamethasone, or 20 mg of hydrocortisone) is reached. Other recommendations state that decrements usually should not exceed 2.5 mg of prednisone (or its equivalent) every 1–2 weeks except in patients on alternate-day therapy in whom it may be possible to decrease dosage in decrements of 5 mg of prednisone (or its equivalent) at 1- to 2-week intervals. If the disease flares up during withdrawal, dosage may need to be increased and followed by a more gradual withdrawal. In addition, increased dosage will be required during periods of stress. When a physiologic dosage has been reached, it has been suggested that single 20-mg oral morning doses of hydrocortisone be substituted for whatever glucocorticoid the patient has been receiving. After 2–4 weeks, the dosage of hydrocortisone may be decreased by 2.5 mg every week until a single morning dosage of 10 mg daily is reached.

The time required for complete HPA function recovery following discontinuance of glucocorticoid therapy is variable. Tests of adrenal function may be used to measure recovery of adrenocortical function. Normal morning plasma cortisol concentrations (exceeding 10 mcg/dL) indicate that basal pituitary-adrenal function is adequate and that maintenance therapy can be discontinued. However, this does not assure that adrenal function has recovered sufficiently to adequately increase cortisol production in response to stress and, therefore, supplemental glucocorticoids may still be required during stress. Complete recovery of HPA function generally can be assumed and supplementary therapy during stress can usually be discontinued when response to a corticotropin or cosyntropin test is normal.

CAUTIONS

Short-term administration of glucocorticoids, even in massive dosages, is unlikely to produce harmful effects. When the drugs are used for longer than brief periods, however, they can produce a variety of devastating effects, including adrenocortical atrophy and generalized protein depletion.

● Adrenocortical Insufficiency

When given in supraphysiologic doses for prolonged periods, glucocorticoids may cause decreased secretion of endogenous corticosteroids by suppressing pituitary release of corticotropin (secondary adrenocortical insufficiency). The degree and duration of adrenocortical insufficiency produced by the drugs is highly variable among patients and depends on the dose, frequency and time of administration, and duration of glucocorticoid therapy. This effect may be minimized by use of alternate-day therapy. (See Alternate-Day Therapy under Dosage and Administration: Dosage.)

As in patients with primary adrenocortical insufficiency maintained on corticosteroids, patients who develop secondary adrenocortical insufficiency require higher corticosteroid dosage when they are subjected to stress (e.g., infection, surgery, trauma). In addition, acute adrenal insufficiency (even death) may occur if the drugs are withdrawn abruptly or if patients are transferred from systemic glucocorticoid therapy to oral inhalation therapy. Therefore, the drugs should be withdrawn very gradually following long-term therapy with pharmacologic dosages. (See Discontinuance of Therapy under Dosage and Administration: Dosage.) Adrenal suppression may persist up to 12 months in patients who receive large dosages for prolonged periods. Until recovery occurs, patients may show signs and symptoms of adrenal insufficiency when they are subjected to stress and replacement therapy may be required. Since mineralocorticoid secretion may be impaired, sodium chloride and/or a mineralocorticoid should also be administered.

● Musculoskeletal Effects

Muscle wasting, muscle pain or weakness, delayed wound healing, and atrophy of the protein matrix of the bone resulting in osteoporosis, vertebral compression fractures, aseptic necrosis of femoral or humeral heads, or pathologic fractures of long bones are manifestations of protein catabolism which may occur during prolonged therapy with glucocorticoids. These adverse effects may be especially serious in geriatric or debilitated patients. Before initiating glucocorticoid therapy in postmenopausal women, the fact that they are especially prone to osteoporosis should be considered. Glucocorticoids should be withdrawn if osteoporosis develops, unless their use is life-saving. A high-protein diet may help to prevent adverse effects associated with protein catabolism.

An acute myopathy has been observed with the use of high doses of glucocorticoids, particularly in patients with disorders of neuromuscular transmission (e.g., myasthenia gravis) or in patients receiving concomitant therapy with neuromuscular blocking agents (e.g., pancuronium). This acute myopathy is generalized, may involve ocular and respiratory muscles, and may result in quadriparesis. Myopathy may be accompanied by elevated serum creatine kinase [CK, creatine phosphokinase, CPK] concentrations. Resolution or clinical improvement of the myopathy may occur weeks to years after discontinuance of glucocorticoid therapy.

Tendon rupture, particularly of the Achilles tendon, has occurred in patients receiving glucocorticoids.

Osteoporosis

Osteoporosis and related fractures are some of the most serious adverse effects of long-term glucocorticoid therapy. More than 10% of patients are diagnosed with a fracture and 30–40% have radiographic evidence of vertebral fractures during long-term glucocorticoid use. Glucocorticoid-induced bone loss and osteoporosis result from increased osteoclast-mediated bone resorption and decreased osteoblast-mediated bone formation. Contributing mechanisms include: 1) effects on calcium homeostasis (e.g., decreased intestinal absorption of calcium and phosphate, increased urinary calcium excretion possibly secondary to a direct effect on tubular reabsorption, resultant secondary hyperparathyroidism leading to increased bone resorption if persistent), 2) effects on sex hormones (e.g., decreased sex hormone production both indirectly by reducing endogenous pituitary hormone concentrations and adrenal androgen production and directly through effects on gonadal hormone release, decreased pituitary secretion of luteinizing hormone with resultant decreased ovarian estrogen and testicular androgen production), 3) inhibition of bone formation (e.g., inhibition of osteoblast proliferation and attachment to matrix, inhibition of the synthesis of type I collagen and noncollagenous proteins by osteoblasts, and dose-related decreases in circulating osteocalcin, possibly mediated by effects on oncogene expression, prostaglandin E production, and the production of insulin-like growth factors and transforming growth factor), and 4) other effects (e.g., effects on the normal forces of muscle contraction on bone resulting from glucocorticoid-induced myopathy and muscle weakness, contribution of the underlying inflammatory condition being treated). Bone loss is most rapid during the first 3–6 months following initiation of glucocorticoid therapy and continues at a slower, steadier rate with prolonged use.

Patients with such bone loss are predisposed to fractures (particularly vertebral fractures because of greater effects of glucocorticoids on trabecular than cortical bone). The risk of fractures is both dose and duration dependent, with higher daily or cumulative doses of glucocorticoids and longer durations of use associated with greater risk. A high glucocorticoid dosage generally is considered a daily dosage equivalent to more than 7.5 mg of prednisone. However, some studies have reported an increased risk of fracture with daily dosages as low as 2.5–7.5 mg of prednisolone or equivalent, while others have found no appreciable decline in bone density with prednisone dosages averaging 8 mg daily or dosages of less than 5 mg daily. Alternate-day regimens have not been shown to be associated with less risk of bone loss than daily regimens. Bone loss has even been associated with oral inhalation of glucocorticoids. However, risk of osteoporosis is uncertain in patients receiving recommended doses of inhaled glucocorticoids.

Glucocorticoid-induced bone loss can be both prevented and treated; however, many patients receiving long-term glucocorticoid therapy do not receive appropriate therapies to prevent bone loss or are treated only after a fracture has occurred. The American College of Rheumatology (ACR) recommends that preventive therapy be considered for patients in whom the benefits of such therapy outweigh the potential harms. ACR recommendations are based on a risk-stratification approach in which an individual's risk level for developing a fracture (low, moderate, or high) is determined based on predisposing factors including the individual's preexisting or anticipated glucocorticoid dosage. An initial clinical fracture risk assessment is recommended as soon as possible, but at least within 6 months of initiating long-term glucocorticoid therapy and reassessments are recommended every 12 months during continued treatment. ACR states that the available data on fracture risk and risk reduction are more limited in children and adults younger than 40 years of age; nevertheless such patients also should be assessed for their fracture risk and managed accordingly.

To minimize the risk of glucocorticoid-induced bone loss, the smallest possible effective dosage and duration should be used. Topical and inhaled preparations should be used whenever possible. Lifestyle modifications to reduce the risk of osteoporosis (e.g., cigarette smoking cessation, limitation of alcohol consumption, participation in a weight-bearing exercise for 30–60 minutes daily) should be encouraged in all patients. In addition, patients should receive adequate calcium and vitamin D supplementation to preserve bone mass and limit the extent of glucocorticoid-induced bone loss. Patients who are considered

to be at moderate-to-high risk of fracture generally should receive additional pharmacologic therapy. Bisphosphonates generally are preferred and have been shown to reduce the incidence of radiographic vertebral fractures in patients with glucocorticoid-induced osteoporosis.

The ACR guideline for the prevention and treatment of glucocorticoid-induced osteoporosis recommends calcium and vitamin D supplementation in addition to lifestyle modification in any patient receiving long-term (at least 3 months) glucocorticoid therapy at a daily dosage equivalent to at least 2.5 mg of prednisone. No further preventive measure is generally recommended in patients who are considered to be at low risk of fracture; however, such patients should be monitored closely during continued glucocorticoid therapy, with fracture risk assessments and bone mineral density (BMD) measurements performed at regular intervals. ACR recommends an additional pharmacologic agent in patients who are considered to be at moderate-to-high risk of fracture. Oral bisphosphonates generally are preferred in most situations because of their demonstrated benefits in reducing fracture risk as well as their safety and low cost; other suggested options include IV bisphosphonates, teriparatide, denosumab, and raloxifene (for postmenopausal women if no other therapy is appropriate). Because of some uncertainty regarding the relative benefits versus harms of these interventions, ACR states that most of their recommendations are conditional and that treatment decisions should be individualized based on patient preferences, values, and comorbidities.

● *Increased Susceptibility to Infection*

Glucocorticoids, especially in large doses, increase susceptibility to and mask symptoms of infection. Infections with any pathogen, including viral, bacterial, fungal, protozoan, or helminthic infections in any organ system, may be associated with glucocorticoids alone or in combination with other immunosuppressive agents. These infections may be mild, but they can be severe or fatal, and localized infections may disseminate.

Patients who become immunosuppressed while receiving glucocorticoids have increased susceptibility to infections compared with healthy individuals. Some infections such as varicella (chickenpox) and measles can have a more serious or even fatal outcome in such patients, particularly in children.

Immunosuppression is most likely to occur in patients receiving high-dose (e.g., equivalent to at least 1 mg/kg of prednisone daily), systemic glucocorticoid therapy for any period of time, particularly in conjunction with glucocorticoid-sparing drugs (e.g., troleandomycin) and/or concomitant immunosuppressant agents; however, patients receiving moderate dosages of systemic glucocorticoids for short periods or low dosages for prolonged periods also may be at risk.

FDA states that the possibility of orally inhaled glucocorticoid therapy causing sufficient immunosuppression to place a patient at risk of infection also should be considered. However, the risk of such therapy, including any possible contribution of local pulmonary immunosuppressant effects of inhaled drug to the development of serious pulmonary infections (e.g., varicella pneumonia), remains to be more fully elucidated.

Glucocorticoid-dependent children should undergo anti-varicella-zoster virus antibody testing. Vaccination should be considered for those who have absent or inadequate antibody concentrations. In addition, such children and any adult who are not likely to have been exposed to varicella or measles should avoid exposure to these infections while receiving glucocorticoids. If exposure to varicella or measles occurs in such individuals, administration of varicella zoster immune globulin (VZIG) or immune globulin, respectively, may be indicated. If varicella develops, treatment with an antiviral agent (e.g., acyclovir) may be considered, although fatal outcome (e.g., in those developing hemorrhagic varicella) may not always be avoided even if such therapy is initiated aggressively.

The immunosuppressive effects of glucocorticoids may result in activation of latent infection or exacerbation of intercurrent infections, including those caused by *Candida*, *Mycobacterium*, *Toxoplasma*, *Strongyloides*, *Pneumocystis*, *Cryptococcus*, *Nocardia*, or *Ameba*. Glucocorticoids should be used with great care in patients with known or suspected *Strongyloides* (threadworm) infection. In such patients, glucocorticoid-induced immunosuppression may lead to *Strongyloides* hyperinfection and dissemination with widespread larval migration, often accompanied by severe enterocolitis and potentially fatal gram-negative septicemia.

The National Institutes of Health (NIH) COVID-19 Treatment Guidelines panel states that prolonged use of systemic corticosteroids in patients with COVID-19† may increase the risk of reactivation of latent infections (e.g., hepatitis B virus [HBV], herpesvirus, strongyloidiasis, tuberculosis). The risk of reactivation of latent infections following a 10-day course of dexamethasone (6 mg once daily) is not well established. When initiating dexamethasone in patients with COVID-19, appropriate screening and treatment to reduce the risk of *Strongyloides* hyperinfection in those at high risk of strongyloidiasis (e.g., patients from tropical, subtropical, or warm, temperate regions or those engaged in agricultural activities) and reduce the risk of fulminant reactivation of HBV should be considered.

Some experts advise that the need to continue at least physiologic replacement dosages of glucocorticoids in glucocorticoid-dependent patients developing serious infection should be considered since discontinuance of the drugs before or after the development of varicella may have contributed to fatal outcome in some reported cases. Additional insight is needed regarding the dosages, routes, and types of glucocorticoids as well as immunologic characteristics likely to place patients at substantial risk of immunosuppression and serious infection.

The most common adverse effect of oral inhalation therapy with glucocorticoids is *Candida albicans* or *Aspergillus niger* infections of the mouth, pharynx, and occasionally the larynx. Oral candidiasis also is one of the most frequent adverse effects of therapy with long-term oral glucocorticoids. The occurrence of these fungal infections appears to be dose dependent; they also occur more frequently in women than in men. Some clinicians recommend that patients rinse their mouths with water and swallow after each oral inhalation dose to prevent *Candida* infection. Usually, *Candida* or *Aspergillus* infections are of little clinical importance, but occasionally they may require antifungal therapy or discontinuance of the oral inhalation.

The principal risk of epidural injection therapy for low back pain and radiculopathy is rare epidural abscess. Infectious complications (including bacterial meningitis) have been reported following epidural injection. Fungal and bacterial infections (including meningitis) have been reported in patients who received epidural or intra-articular therapy with contaminated glucocorticoid injections prepared by compounding pharmacies.

● Fluid and Electrolyte Disturbances

Sodium retention with resultant edema, potassium loss, hypokalemic alkalosis, and hypertension may occur in patients receiving glucocorticoids. Congestive heart failure may occur in susceptible patients. These mineralocorticoid effects are less frequent with synthetic glucocorticoids (except fludrocortisone) than with hydrocortisone or cortisone, but may occur, especially when synthetic glucocorticoids are given in high dosage for prolonged periods. Dietary salt restriction is advisable and potassium supplementation may be necessary in patients receiving glucocorticoids for anti-inflammatory or immunosuppressant effects. When glucocorticoids with substantial mineralocorticoid activity are administered, patients should be instructed to notify their physicians if edema develops. All glucocorticoids increase calcium excretion and may cause hypocalcemia.

● Ocular Effects

Prolonged use of glucocorticoids may result in posterior subcapsular and nuclear cataracts (particularly in children), exophthalmos, or increased intraocular pressure which may result in glaucoma or may occasionally damage the optic nerve. However, data from several studies indicate that the risk of subcapsular and nuclear cataracts associated with inhaled glucocorticoid use is negligible in young asthmatic patients, but the risk of such cataracts may be elevated in older patients. Data from a case-control study indicate that the risk of ocular hypertension or open-angle glaucoma was increased in patients receiving high dosages of orally inhaled glucocorticoids (at least 1600 mcg of beclomethasone dipropionate, budesonide, or triamcinolone acetonide) daily for at least 3 months. Patients receiving lower dosages of orally inhaled or intranasal glucocorticoids were not at increased risk for these adverse ocular effects. Results from a population-based study indicate that use of orally inhaled corticosteroids is associated with development of posterior subcapsular and nuclear cataracts. Establishment of secondary fungal and viral infections of the eye may also be enhanced in patients receiving glucocorticoids. Blindness has occurred rarely following intralesional injection of

glucocorticoids around the face and head. Ocular effects (e.g., transient blindness, amblyopia, acute retinal necrosis syndrome, intraocular hemorrhage, cortical blindness) also have occurred following epidural injection. Eye irritation and eyelid edema have been reported in patients receiving glucocorticoids in clinical trials.

● Endocrine Effects

When glucocorticoids are administered over a prolonged period, they may produce various endocrine disorders including hypercorticism (cushingoid state) and amenorrhea or other menstrual difficulties. Corticosteroids may decrease glucose tolerance, produce hyperglycemia, and aggravate or precipitate diabetes mellitus especially in patients predisposed to diabetes mellitus. If steroid therapy is required in patients with diabetes mellitus, changes in insulin or oral antidiabetic agent dosage or diet may be necessary. Corticosteroids have also been reported to increase or decrease motility and number of sperm in some men.

● GI Effects

Adverse GI effects of corticosteroids include nausea, vomiting, anorexia which may result in weight loss, increased appetite which may result in weight gain, diarrhea or constipation, abdominal distention, pancreatitis, gastric irritation, and ulcerative esophagitis. Indigestion is one of the most frequently occurring adverse effects in patients receiving long-term therapy with oral corticosteroids. Blood in the stool has been reported in patients receiving prednisolone orally disintegrating tablets in clinical trials. Corticosteroids have been implicated in the development, reactivation, perforation, hemorrhage, and delayed healing of peptic ulcers. Although concomitant administration of antacids or other antiulcer agents (e.g., cimetidine) has been suggested to prevent peptic ulcer formation in patients receiving high dosages of corticosteroids, routine concomitant use of these agents does not appear to be warranted since corticosteroid-induced ulcers occur infrequently (in 2% or less of patients receiving corticosteroids) and the efficacy of antiulcer therapy in preventing these ulcers has not been established. However, selective use of preventive antiulcer therapy may be considered in patients receiving corticosteroids who are at increased risk of peptic ulcer formation (e.g., those receiving other ulcerogenic drugs). Gastric irritation may be reduced if oral corticosteroids are taken immediately before, during, or immediately after meals, or with food or milk.

● Nervous System Effects

Adverse neurologic effects of glucocorticoids have included headache, vertigo, insomnia, restlessness and increased motor activity, ischemic neuropathy, electroencephalogram (EEG) abnormalities, and seizures. Glucocorticoids may precipitate mental disturbances ranging from euphoria, mood swings, depression and anxiety, and personality changes to frank psychoses. Emotional instability or psychotic tendencies may be aggravated by the drugs. Increased intracranial pressure with papilledema (i.e., pseudotumor cerebri) has been reported, generally in association with withdrawal of glucocorticoid therapy.

Aseptic meningitis, arachnoiditis, exacerbation of pain, spinal cord trauma, subdural injection, intracranial air injection, increased intracranial pressure, nerve injury, seizures, bladder or bowel dysfunction, paraparesis or paralysis, sensory disturbances, and brain damage have been reported following epidural injection and/or intrathecal administration. It is unclear whether reports of neurologic effects associated with epidural glucocorticoid administration involved improper needle placement or were related to administration of the drug and/or preservatives.

Serious, potentially permanent, adverse neurologic events (e.g., spinal cord infarction, paraplegia, quadriplegia, cortical blindness, stroke, seizures, nerve injury, brain edema), including death, have been reported rarely following epidural glucocorticoid injection both with and without fluoroscopic guidance. In addition to potential direct needle trauma to the spinal cord, such adverse events also may be the result of inadvertent intra-arterial injection of the particulate glucocorticoid suspension with subsequent embolization. Many of the events occurred within minutes to 48 hours after epidural injection of the glucocorticoid. In some cases, diagnoses of adverse neurologic events were confirmed by magnetic resonance imagining or computed tomography. Patients should be advised to immediately seek emergency medical attention for unusual symptoms (e.g., loss of or changes in vision, tingling in extremities, sudden weakness or numbness affecting the face or occurring unilaterally or bilaterally in the arms or legs, dizziness, severe headache, seizures) occurring after epidural glucocorticoid injection.

● Dermatologic Effects

Various adverse dermatologic effects are associated with systemic glucocorticoid administration and include impaired wound healing, skin atrophy and thinning, acne, increased sweating, hirsutism, facial erythema, striae, petechiae, ecchymoses, and easy bruising. Long-term therapy with high dosages of inhaled corticosteroids is associated with skin thinning and easy bruising, particularly among women. Dermatologic manifestations of hypersensitivity to the corticosteroids include hives and/or allergic dermatitis, urticaria, and angioedema. Burning or tingling of the perineal area may occur after IV injection of the drugs. Parenteral corticosteroid therapy has also produced hypopigmentation or hyperpigmentation, scarring, induration, delayed pain or soreness, subcutaneous and cutaneous atrophy, and sterile abscesses. Kaposi's sarcoma has been reported to occur in patients receiving glucocorticoid therapy; discontinuance of such therapy may result in remission of the disease.

Dermal and/or subdermal changes forming depressions in the skin at the injection site have been reported with use of methylprednisolone acetate injectable suspension (Depo-Medrol®). Caution should be used to minimize the incidence of dermal and subdermal atrophy.

● Other Adverse Effects

A steroid withdrawal syndrome seemingly unrelated to adrenocortical insufficiency and consisting of anorexia, nausea and vomiting, lethargy, headache, fever, joint pain, desquamation, easy bruising, myalgia, weight loss, and/or hypotension has been reported following abrupt withdrawal of glucocorticoids. Symptoms often occurred while plasma glucocorticoid concentrations were still high but were falling rapidly; apparently the abrupt change in glucocorticoid concentration rather than a low concentration per se was responsible for the phenomenon. Bradycardia has occurred during or after IV administration of large doses of methylprednisolone sodium succinate but did not appear to be related to the rate or duration of infusion.

A few patients have experienced hoarseness, dry mouth, and sore throat during oral inhalation therapy with glucocorticoids; these adverse effects have also occurred in patients receiving only the aerosol vehicle and may be minimized by rinsing the mouth and swallowing after using the aerosol. Pharyngolaryngeal pain has been reported in patients receiving glucocorticoids in clinical trials. Dysphonia also has been reported following epidural glucocorticoid injection.

Injections of slightly soluble glucocorticoids may produce atrophy at the site of injection. (See Dosage and Administration: Administration.) Intra-articularly administered corticosteroids have caused postinjection flare and Charcot-like arthropathy. Epidural lipomatosis has been reported with repeated epidural glucocorticoid injections but appears to resolve following discontinuance of such therapy. Cerebral or pulmonary embolism, hematoma formation, pneumothorax, intravascular injection, and vascular injury also have been reported following epidural injection therapy.

Minor transient complications of epidural glucocorticoid therapy include headache, nausea, facial flushing, fever, and inadvertent spinal tap. Headache appears to occur commonly with epidural injection of glucocorticoids presumably secondary to pressure changes in the epidural space or accidental puncture of the dura.

Intranasal administration of these drugs has been associated with allergic reactions and rhinitis. Temporary or permanent visual impairment, including blindness, has been reported with glucocorticoid administration by intranasal, ophthalmic, and other routes of administration. Increased intraocular pressure, infection, residue or slough at the injection site, and ocular and periocular inflammation, including allergic reactions, have been reported with ophthalmic administration of glucocorticoids.

Hypercholesterolemia, atherosclerosis, thrombosis, thromboembolism, fat embolism, and thrombophlebitis have also been associated with corticosteroid therapy, particularly with cortisone. Hypertrophic cardiomyopathy has been reported in premature infants receiving glucocorticoids (e.g., prednisolone). Thrombocytopenia has been observed in a few patients following prolonged,

high-dose glucocorticoid therapy. Palpitation, tachycardia, swelling of mouth and tongue, frequency and urgency of urination, and enuresis have been reported rarely. Anaphylactic reactions also have been reported rarely with parenteral glucocorticoid therapy. Glucocorticoids may decrease serum concentrations of ascorbic acid (vitamin C) and vitamin A; symptoms of vitamin A or C deficiency may occur rarely.

Transient, mild, asymptomatic elevations in ALT (SGPT), AST (SGOT), and alkaline phosphatase concentrations have been reported in patients receiving glucocorticoids; these effects are not associated with any clinical syndrome and generally resolve upon discontinuance of glucocorticoid therapy.

● Precautions and Contraindications

Prior to initiation of long-term glucocorticoid therapy, baseline ECGs, blood pressures, chest and spinal radiographs, glucose tolerance tests, and evaluations of HPA-axis function should be performed on all patients. Upper GI radiographs should be performed in patients predisposed to GI disorders, including those with known or suspected peptic ulcer disease. During long-term therapy, periodic height, weight, chest and spinal radiographs, hematopoietic, electrolyte, glucose tolerance, and ocular and blood pressure evaluations should be performed.

Patients receiving glucocorticoids should be instructed to notify their physicians of any infections, signs of infections (e.g., fever, sore throat, pain during urination, muscle aches), or injuries that develop during therapy or within 12 months after therapy is discontinued, so that adjustments in dosage can be made or glucocorticoid therapy reintroduced if necessary. In addition, when surgery is required, patients should be advised to inform the attending physician, dentist, or anesthesiologist that they are receiving or have recently (within 12 months) received glucocorticoids. Patients should carry identification cards listing the diseases for which they are being treated, the glucocorticoid they are receiving and its dosage, and the name and telephone number of their physician. Patients being transferred from systemic corticosteroid to oral inhalation therapy should carry special identification (e.g., card, bracelet) indicating the need for supplementary systemic corticosteroids during periods of stress. Patients receiving orally inhaled glucocorticoid therapy who are currently being withdrawn or who have been withdrawn from systemic corticosteroids should be advised to immediately resume full therapeutic dosages of systemic corticosteroids and to contact their clinician for further instructions during stressful periods (e.g., severe infection, severe asthmatic attack).

Because anaphylactoid reactions have occurred in patients receiving glucocorticoids parenterally, precautionary measures should be taken prior to parenteral administration of the drugs, particularly in patients with history of a drug allergy. Some patients who appear to be hypersensitive to parenteral glucocorticoids may actually be hypersensitive to the paraben preservatives present in some injectable formulations.

Because an apparent association has been suggested between use of corticosteroids and left ventricular free-wall rupture after a recent myocardial infarction, corticosteroids should be used with extreme caution in these patients.

Some commercially available oral preparations of prednisolone, and triamcinolone contain the dye tartrazine (FD&C yellow No. 5), which may cause allergic reactions including bronchial asthma in susceptible individuals. Although the incidence of tartrazine sensitivity is low, it frequently occurs in patients who are sensitive to aspirin.

Some commercially available formulations of dexamethasone, hydrocortisone, and prednisolone contain sulfites that may cause allergic-type reactions, including anaphylaxis and life-threatening or less severe asthmatic episodes, in certain susceptible individuals. The overall prevalence of sulfite sensitivity in the general population is unknown but probably low; such sensitivity appears to occur more frequently in asthmatic than in nonasthmatic individuals.

Glucocorticoids should be used with caution in patients with hypothyroidism or cirrhosis, because such patients often show exaggerated response to the drugs. Glucocorticoids should be used with caution in psychotic patients or patients with hypertension or congestive heart failure.

Corticosteroids should be used with caution in patients with active or latent peptic ulcer, diverticulitis, nonspecific ulcerative colitis (if there is a probability of impending perforation, abscess, or other pyogenic infection), and in those with recent intestinal anastomoses. Manifestations of peritoneal irritation following GI perforation may be minimal or absent in patients receiving glucocorticoids.

Glucocorticoids should be used cautiously in patients with myasthenia gravis, particularly in those receiving anticholinesterase therapy. If possible, anticholinesterase agents should be withdrawn at least 24 hours prior to initiating glucocorticoid therapy. Because cortisone has been reported rarely to increase blood coagulability and to precipitate intravascular thrombosis, thromboembolism, and thrombophlebitis, corticosteroids should be used with caution in patients with thromboembolic disorders. Glucocorticoids should be used with caution in patients with seizure disorders, renal insufficiency, osteoporosis, or herpes simplex infections of the eye; some manufacturers state that glucocorticoids should not be used in patients with active ocular herpes simplex infections. Corneal perforation may occur in patients with ocular herpes simplex infections who are receiving glucocorticoids. Glucocorticoids are not recommended for use in the treatment of optic neuritis as such use may increase the risk of new episodes.

Because glucocorticoids increase susceptibility to and mask symptoms of infection, the drugs should not be used, except in life-threatening situations, in patients with viral infections or bacterial infections not controlled by anti-infectives. Manufacturers state that glucocorticoid oral inhalation therapy should be used with caution, if at all, in patients with untreated systemic fungal, bacterial, viral, or parasitic infections. Patients whose susceptibility to infection is high, such as those receiving glucocorticoids as immunosuppressive therapy, are especially likely to develop secondary infections. Patients receiving glucocorticoids who are potentially immunosuppressed should be warned of the risk of exposure to certain infections (e.g., chickenpox, measles) and of the importance of obtaining medical advice if such exposure occurs. Since glucocorticoid therapy can reactivate tuberculosis, treatment of latent tuberculosis infection should be included in the regimen of patients with a history of active tuberculosis undergoing prolonged glucocorticoid therapy. If glucocorticoids are indicated in patients with latent tuberculosis or tuberculin reactivity, close observation is necessary. Use of glucocorticoids in patients with active tuberculosis should be restricted to those with fulminating or disseminated tuberculosis in which glucocorticoids are used in conjunction with appropriate antimycobacterial chemotherapy. Manufacturers state that glucocorticoid oral inhalation therapy should be used with caution, if at all, in patients with clinical or asymptomatic *Mycobacterium tuberculosis* infections of the respiratory tract. Since glucocorticoids can reactivate latent amebiasis, any patient who has been in the tropics or who has unexplained diarrhea should be evaluated for amebiasis to exclude these patients prior to initiating therapy. In the treatment of acute or disseminated tuberculosis, glucocorticoids should only be used as part of a total antituberculosis regimen. Corticosteroids should not be used in patients with cerebral malaria. The manufacturers of methylprednisolone warn that the efficacy of glucocorticoids in the treatment of sepsis syndrome and septic shock has not been established, and that at least one study suggested that such use in certain patients (e.g., those with serum creatinine concentrations exceeding 2 mg/dL at diagnosis and those who develop secondary infections) may be associated with an increased risk of mortality.

Some clinicians state that glucocorticoid oral inhalation therapy probably should be avoided when the risk of activating bronchopulmonary mycoses appears high, as in patients with bronchiectasis or inadequate immunologic responses. Although manufacturers state that glucocorticoids are contraindicated in patients with systemic fungal infections, most authorities believe that glucocorticoid therapy may be initiated in patients with known infections (including those from fungi) if effective specific chemotherapy is administered concomitantly. The manufacturers of methylprednisolone acetate state that although the drug is contraindicated in patients with systemic fungal infections, it may be used as an intra-articular injection for localized joint conditions. In patients with acute infection, methylprednisolone acetate should not be administered intra-articularly, bursally, or into a tendon for local effects.

FDA states that the efficacy and safety of epidural administration of glucocorticoids have not been established, and glucocorticoids are not FDA-labeled for such use. Prior to initiating such therapy, healthcare providers should discuss with patients the potential benefits and risks of epidural glucocorticoid injections and alternative treatments. Epidural administration of glucocorticoids is contraindicated in patients with local or systemic infection; individuals with bleeding disorders or receiving concurrent anticoagulant therapy (e.g., warfarin, heparin, antiplatelet agents); patients with known hypersensitivity to local anesthetic agents, contrast agents, or glucocorticoids; and patients who experienced complications with prior glucocorticoid injections. Epidural glucocorticoid therapy should be used with caution in patients with congestive heart failure or diabetes mellitus. Fluoroscopy (recommended for ensuring proper needle placement) is contraindicated in pregnant women.

IM administration of corticosteroids is contraindicated in patients with idiopathic thrombocytopenic purpura.

● *Pediatric Precautions*

The effects of glucocorticoids on the pathophysiology and course of diseases are considered to be similar in adults and children. Evidence of safety and efficacy for prednisolone in pediatric patients has been provided through studies using the drug in pediatric patients for the treatment of nephrotic syndrome (in patients older than 2 years of age) and aggressive leukemias and lymphomas (in patients older than 1 month of age). However, some of the conclusions of these studies, and evidence of safety and efficacy for other pediatric indications (e.g., severe asthma and wheezing), are based on controlled trials in adults.

The adverse effects of prednisolone in pediatric patients are similar to those in adults. As in adults, periodic evaluations of height, weight, ocular pressure, and blood pressure should be performed in children receiving glucocorticoids. Children, like adults, also should undergo clinical evaluation for the presence of infection, psychosocial disturbances, thromboembolism, peptic ulcers, cataracts, and osteoporosis.

Long-term administration of pharmacologic dosages of glucocorticoids to children should be avoided if possible, since the drugs may retard bone growth when administered by any route. If prolonged therapy is necessary, the growth and development of infants and children should be closely monitored, and the potential effects on growth should be weighed against clinical benefits and the availability of alternative therapy. Most children receiving recommended dosages of inhaled glucocorticoids achieved their predicted adult heights but at a later than normal age, and the potential but small risk of delayed growth is well balanced by the improved health outcomes associated with inhaled glucocorticoid therapy for mild or moderate persistent asthma in such children. Therapy with low-to-medium dose inhaled glucocorticoids is associated with a short-term (first year of treatment) decrease in growth rates (approximately 1 cm), but such effects appear to be temporary and do not predict final adult height. Effects on growth are not likely with inhaled glucocorticoid dosages of up to 200 mcg daily, and HPA-axis suppression is unlikely at dosages of less than 200 mcg daily of budesonide [or its equivalent] daily dosage. Results of controlled longitudinal studies and several cross-sectional studies in children with asthma receiving long-term inhaled glucocorticoid (2–5 years) therapy indicate that bone mineral density was not affected by use of inhaled glucocorticoids. High dosages of inhaled glucocorticoids for prolonged periods of time (e.g., exceeding 1 year), particularly in combination with frequent courses of systemic glucocorticoid therapy may be associated with adverse growth effects and/or reduced bone mineral density. Retardation of bone growth has been observed at low systemic doses of glucocorticoids and in the absence of hypothalamic-pituitary-adrenal (HPA) axis suppression (e.g., as determined by tests of HPA axis function such as cosyntropin stimulation and basal plasma cortisol concentrations). Growth velocity may therefore be a more sensitive indicator of systemic glucocorticoid exposure than some commonly used tests of HPA axis function. In order to minimize the potential effects of glucocorticoids on growth, dosage in children should be titrated to the lowest effective level. Alternate-day therapy minimizes growth suppression and should be instituted if growth suppression occurs.

Glucocorticoid-induced osteoporosis and associated fractures are common in children and adolescents receiving long-term systemic therapy with the drugs since bone turnover is high and the rates of bone formation required to maintain adequate mineralization of the rapidly growing skeleton also are high in this age group. In addition, glucocorticoids by inhibiting bone formation may prevent achievement of peak bone mass during adolescence. The underlying pediatric condition for which glucocorticoids are prescribed also may be associated independently with an increased risk of osteoporosis. Methods for monitoring bone mineralization (e.g., dual-energy x-ray absorptiometry [DXA]) in children and adolescents are similar to those in adults. However, the roles of various preventive or corrective therapies for glucocorticoid-induced bone loss in children currently are not well defined. At this time, the most prudent approach to minimizing the negative effects of glucocorticoids on BMD in children and adolescents is by ensuring that the patients consistently ingest adequate calcium and vitamin D, either through diet or supplementation. (See Uses: Corticosteroid-induced Osteoporosis, in the Vitamin D Analogs General Statement 88:16.)

High dosages of glucocorticoids in children may cause acute pancreatitis leading to pancreatic destruction. Children have developed increases in intracranial pressure (pseudotumor cerebri), causing papilledema, oculomotor or abducens nerve paralysis, visual loss, and headache. Pseudotumor cerebri has occurred most frequently following reduction of dosage or a change in the steroid administered.

Some commercially available injections of dexamethasone, hydrocortisone, methylprednisolone, and triamcinolone contain benzyl alcohol as a preservative. Although a causal relationship has not been established, administration of injections preserved with benzyl alcohol has been associated with toxicity in neonates. Toxicity appears to have resulted from administration of large amounts (i.e., 100–400 mg/kg daily) of benzyl alcohol in these neonates. Although manufacturers of some benzyl alcohol-containing injectable glucocorticoids state that these drugs are contraindicated in premature infants and use of drugs preserved with benzyl alcohol should be avoided in neonates whenever possible, the American Academy of Pediatrics states that the presence of small amounts of the preservative in a commercially available injection should not proscribe its use when the medication is indicated in neonates and comparable benzyl alcohol-free preparations are not available.

The safety and efficacy of dexamethasone or other corticosteroids for COVID-19† treatment have not been fully evaluated in pediatric patients. Therefore, caution should be used when extrapolating recommendations for adults with COVID-19 to patients younger than 18 years of age. The NIH COVID-19 Treatment Guidelines Panel recommends use of dexamethasone (see Coronavirus Disease 2019 [COVID-19] under Dosage and Administration: Dosage) for hospitalized pediatric patients with COVID-19 who are receiving high-flow oxygen, noninvasive ventilation, invasive mechanical ventilation, or extracorporeal membrane oxygenation (ECMO); dexamethasone is not routinely recommended for pediatric patients who require only low levels of oxygen support (i.e., nasal cannula only). If dexamethasone is not available, the NIH panel states that alternative corticosteroids such as hydrocortisone, methylprednisolone, or prednisone may be considered. Use of corticosteroids for treatment of severe COVID-19 in pediatric patients who are profoundly immunocompromised has not been evaluated to date and may be harmful; therefore, the NIH panel states that such use should be considered only on a case-by-case basis. IV corticosteroids have been used as first-line therapy in pediatric patients with multisystem inflammatory syndrome in children (MIS-C); however, the NIH panel recommends consultation with a multidisciplinary team when considering and managing immunomodulating therapy for children with this condition. The optimal choice and combination of immunomodulating therapies for children with MIS-C have not been definitely established. Clinicians should consult the most recent NIH COVID-19 treatment guidelines for additional information on the use of corticosteroids in pediatric patients with COVID-19.

● Pregnancy, Fertility, and Lactation

Pregnancy

Glucocorticoids may cause fetal damage when administered to pregnant women. One retrospective study of 260 women who received pharmacologic dosages of glucocorticoids during pregnancy revealed 2 instances of cleft palate, 8 stillbirths, 1 spontaneous abortion, and 15 premature births. Another study reported 2 cases of cleft palate in 86 births. Occurrence of cleft palate in these studies is higher than in the general population but could have resulted from the underlying diseases as well as from the steroids. Other fetal abnormalities that have been reported following glucocorticoid administration in pregnant women include hydrocephalus and gastroschisis. Women should be instructed to inform their physicians if they become or wish to become pregnant while receiving glucocorticoids. If glucocorticoids must be used during pregnancy or if the patient becomes pregnant while taking one of these drugs, the potential risks should be carefully considered.

In a retrospective study of 260 women, administration of glucocorticoids throughout pregnancy has been reported to precipitate adrenal crisis in one neonate, but in other studies there was no evidence of this. Infants born to women who receive glucocorticoids during pregnancy should be carefully monitored for symptoms of adrenal insufficiency and appropriate therapy begun immediately if such symptoms appear.

Lactation

Corticosteroids may be distributed into milk and could suppress growth, interfere with endogenous glucocorticoid production, or cause other adverse effects in nursing infants. Since adequate reproductive studies have not been performed in humans with glucocorticoids, these drugs should be administered to nursing mothers only if the benefits of therapy are judged to outweigh the potential risks to the infant.

DRUG INTERACTIONS

● Drugs Affecting Hepatic Microsomal Enzymes

Metabolism of certain glucocorticoids is mediated by the cytochrome P-450 (CYP) isoenzyme 3A4, and the possibility exists that drugs that induce, inhibit, or compete for this isoenzyme may alter metabolism and clearance of glucocorticoids. Conversely, some glucocorticoids (e.g. betamethasone) inhibit the action of CYP3A4, and some glucocorticoids (e.g., dexamethasone) induce CYP3A4. These glucocorticoids may alter the metabolism of drugs metabolized by CYP3A4.

Cyclosporine

Concomitant administration of prednisolone and cyclosporine may result in decreased plasma clearance of prednisolone, and plasma concentrations of cyclosporine may be increased during concomitant therapy with methylprednisolone. In addition, seizures reportedly have occurred in adult and pediatric patients receiving high-dose glucocorticoid therapy concurrently with cyclosporine. The mechanism of this interaction may involve competitive inhibition of hepatic microsomal enzymes. The potential drug interaction between cyclosporine and prednisolone or methylprednisolone and the possibility of exacerbated toxicity, as well as the need for appropriate dosage adjustment, should be considered when these drugs are administered concomitantly.

Other Drugs

Drugs that induce cytochrome P-450 (CYP) isoenzyme 3A4 (e. g., barbiturates, phenytoin, rifampin, ephedrine, carbamazepine) may enhance metabolism of, and reduce, glucocorticoid concentrations. Dosage of glucocorticoids given in combination with such cytochrome P-450 inducers may need to be increased to achieve the desired response. Conversely, concomitant administration of certain glucocorticoids with drugs that inhibit CYP3A4 (e.g., macrolide antibiotics, ketoconazole) may decrease glucocorticoid clearance; dosage of glucocorticoids given in combination with cytochrome P-450 inhibitors may need to be decreased to avoid potential adverse effects.

● Antidiabetic Therapy

Because glucocorticoids may increase blood glucose concentrations, patients with diabetes mellitus receiving concurrent insulin and/or oral hypoglycemic agents may require adjustments in the dosage of such therapy.

● Estrogens

Estrogens may potentiate effects of hydrocortisone, possibly by increasing the concentration of transcortin and thus decreasing the amount of hydrocortisone available to be metabolized. Effects of other glucocorticoids that bind to transcortin could be similarly potentiated and dosage adjustments may be required if estrogens are added to or withdrawn from a stable dosage regimen.

● Nonsteroidal Anti-inflammatory Agents

Concomitant administration of ulcerogenic drugs such as indomethacin during corticosteroid therapy may increase the risk of GI ulceration. Aspirin should be used cautiously in conjunction with glucocorticoids in patients with hypoprothrombinemia. Although concomitant therapy with salicylates and corticosteroids does not appear to increase the incidence or severity of GI ulceration, the possibility of this effect should be considered.

Serum salicylate concentrations may decrease when corticosteroids are administered concomitantly. Likewise, when corticosteroids are discontinued in patients receiving salicylates, serum salicylate concentration may increase; salicylate intoxication has been precipitated rarely. Several mechanisms may be involved in this interaction. In one study in healthy individuals and in patients with polyarthritis who received both drugs concomitantly, corticosteroids increased the renal clearance of salicylate, possibly by increasing glomerular filtration rate. Corticosteroids may also induce the metabolism of salicylate. Salicylates and corticosteroids should be used concurrently with caution. Patients receiving both drugs should be observed closely for adverse effects of either drug. It may be necessary to increase salicylate dosage when corticosteroids are administered concurrently or decrease salicylate dosage when corticosteroids are discontinued in patients receiving salicylates.

In one study in patients with rheumatoid arthritis, concomitant administration of indomethacin and prednisolone resulted in increased plasma concentrations of free prednisolone; total plasma prednisolone concentrations were unchanged. It was suggested that indomethacin may have a steroid-sparing effect.

● Potassium-depleting Drugs

Potassium-depleting diuretics (e.g., thiazides, furosemide, ethacrynic acid) and other drugs that deplete potassium, such as amphotericin B, may enhance the potassium-wasting effect of glucocorticoids. Serum potassium should be closely monitored in patients receiving glucocorticoids and potassium-depleting drugs.

● Vaccines and Toxoids

Because corticosteroids inhibit antibody response, the drugs may cause a diminished response to toxoids and live or inactivated vaccines. In addition, corticosteroids may potentiate replication of some organisms contained in live, attenuated vaccines and supraphysiologic dosages of the drugs can aggravate neurologic reactions to some vaccines. Routine administration of vaccines or toxoids should generally be deferred until corticosteroid therapy is discontinued. Administration of live virus or live, attenuated vaccines, including smallpox vaccine, is contraindicated in patients receiving immunosuppressive dosages of glucocorticoids. In addition, if inactivated vaccines are administered to such patients, expected serum antibody response may not be obtained. The Advisory Committee on Immunization Practices (ACIP) states that administration of live virus vaccines usually is not contraindicated in patients receiving corticosteroid therapy as short-term (less than 2 weeks) treatment, in low to moderate dosages, as long-term alternate-day treatment with short-acting preparations, in maintenance physiologic dosages (replacement therapy), or if corticosteroids are administered topically, ophthalmically, intra-articularly, bursally, or into a tendon. If immunization is necessary in a patient receiving corticosteroid therapy, serologic testing may be needed to ensure adequate antibody response and additional doses of the vaccine or toxoid may be necessary. Immunization procedures may be undertaken in patients receiving nonimmunosuppressive doses of glucocorticoids or in patients receiving glucocorticoids as replacement therapy (e.g., Addison's disease). For specific information on administration of vaccines or toxoids in patients receiving corticosteroids, see the individual monographs in 80:00.

● Oral Anticoagulants

The effect of glucocorticoids on oral anticoagulant therapy is variable, and the efficacy of oral anticoagulants has been reported to be enhanced or diminished with concomitant glucocorticoid administration. Patients receiving glucocorticoids and oral anticoagulants concomitantly should be monitored (e.g., using coagulation indices) in order to maintain desired anticoagulant effect.

LABORATORY TEST INTERFERENCES

Glucocorticoids may decrease iodine 131 uptake and protein-bound iodine concentrations, making it difficult to monitor the therapeutic response of patients receiving the drugs for thyroiditis. Glucocorticoids may produce false-negative results in the nitroblue tetrazolium test for systemic bacterial infection. Glucocorticoids may suppress reactions to skin tests. Phenytoin interferes with dexamethasone suppression tests.

PHARMACOLOGY

Pharmacology of the corticosteroids is complex and the drugs affect almost all body systems. Maximum pharmacologic activity lags behind peak blood concentrations, suggesting that most effects of the drugs result from modification of enzyme activity rather than from direct actions by the drugs.

Aldosterone is a naturally occurring mineralocorticoid, and it affects electrolyte and fluid balance by acting on the distal renal tubule to promote sodium reabsorption and potassium and hydrogen excretion. Although glomerular filtration rate is also increased which promotes sodium excretion, the net effect is almost always sodium retention with resultant edema and hypertension. The naturally occurring glucocorticoids, hydrocortisone (cortisol) and cortisone, have some mineralocorticoid activity in addition to their glucocorticoid activity. Synthetic glucocorticoids also exhibit some degree of mineralocorticoid activity, especially with prolonged, high-dose therapy. Fludrocortisone has extremely potent mineralocorticoid properties and is only used for this purpose; prednisone and prednisolone have approximately half the mineralocorticoid activity of hydrocortisone and cortisone; and betamethasone, dexamethasone, meprednisone (no longer commercially available in the US), methylprednisolone, and triamcinolone have relatively little mineralocorticoid activity.

In physiologic doses (see General Dosage under Dosage and Administration: Dosage), corticosteroids are administered to replace deficient endogenous hormones. In larger (pharmacologic) doses, glucocorticoids decrease inflammation by stabilizing leukocyte lysosomal membranes, preventing release of destructive acid hydrolases from leukocytes; inhibiting macrophage accumulation in inflamed areas; reducing leukocyte adhesion to capillary endothelium; reducing capillary wall permeability and edema formation; decreasing complement components; antagonizing histamine activity and release of kinin from substrates; reducing fibroblast proliferation, collagen deposition, and subsequent scar tissue formation; and possibly by other mechanisms as yet unknown. The drugs suppress the immune response by reducing activity and volume of the lymphatic system, producing lymphocytopenia, decreasing immunoglobulin and complement concentrations, decreasing passage of immune complexes through basement membranes, and possibly by depressing reactivity of tissue to antigen-antibody interactions. Glucocorticoids stimulate erythroid cells of bone marrow, prolong survival time of erythrocytes and platelets, and produce neutrophilia and eosinopenia. Glucocorticoids promote gluconeogenesis, redistribution of fat from peripheral to central areas of the body, and protein catabolism, which results in negative nitrogen balance. They reduce intestinal absorption and increase renal excretion of calcium.

In pharmacologic doses, systemically administered glucocorticoids suppress release of corticotropin (adrenocorticotropic hormone, ACTH) from the pituitary; thus the adrenal cortex ceases secretion of endogenous corticosteroids (secondary adrenocortical insufficiency). The degree and duration of hypothalamic-pituitary-adrenal (HPA) axis suppression produced by the drugs is highly variable among patients and depends on the dose, frequency and time of administration, and duration of glucocorticoid therapy. If suppressive doses of glucocorticoids are administered for prolonged periods, the adrenal cortex atrophies and patients develop cushingoid (hypercorticism) features and respond to stress like patients with primary adrenocortical insufficiency (Addison's disease, hypocorticism). (See Cautions: Adrenocortical Insufficiency.)

The duration of anti-inflammatory activity of glucocorticoids approximately equals the duration of HPA-axis suppression. In one study, the duration of HPA-axis suppression after a single oral dose of glucocorticoids was as follows:

TABLE 4. Duration of HPA-Axis Suppression After Single-Dose Oral Glucocorticoids

Drug	Duration of Suppression
Hydrocortisone 250 mg	1.25–1.5 days
Cortisone 250 mg	1.25–1.5 days
Methylprednisolone 40 mg	1.25–1.5 days
Prednisone 50 mg	1.25–1.5 days
Prednisolone 50 mg	1.25–1.5 days
Triamcinolone 40 mg	2.25 days
Dexamethasone 5 mg	2.75 days
Betamethasone 6 mg	3.25 days

Following IM administration of a single dose of 40–80 mg of triamcinolone acetonide, 50 mg of triamcinolone diacetate, 9 mg of betamethasone sodium phosphate and betamethasone acetate suspension, or 40–80 mg of methylprednisolone, the duration of HPA suppression is 2–4 weeks, 1 week, 1 week, and 4–8 days, respectively. Suppression of the HPA axis below the normal clinical range did not occur when beclomethasone dipropionate was administered by oral inhalation in dosages up to and including 640 mcg daily; however, a dose-dependent reduction of adrenal cortisol production was observed. Since inhaled beclomethasone dipropionate is absorbed into circulation and can be systemically active, HPA axis suppression could occur when recommended dosages are exceeded or in particularly sensitive individuals. With recommended dosages of triamcinolone acetonide administered by oral inhalation, suppression of the HPA axis has occurred within 6–12 weeks in some patients.

In a comparative pharmacodynamic study in healthy geriatric individuals (65–89 years of age) and in younger adults (23–34 years of age), geriatric individuals receiving a single dose of IV prednisolone (0.8 mg/kg, no longer commercially available in the US) or oral prednisone (0.8 mg/kg) exhibited a higher area under the concentration-time curve (AUC) for cortisol than that observed in younger adults. Increased cortisol concentrations in geriatric patients may be the result of attenuated suppression of endogenous cortisol or decreased hepatic clearance of cortisol compared with younger adults.

The mechanism of antiemetic action of corticosteroids remains to be established.

PHARMACOKINETICS

● Absorption

Most glucocorticoids appear to be readily absorbed when administered orally as free alcohols, ketones, cypionates, or acetates. Following IM administration, absorption of the water-soluble sodium phosphate and sodium succinate salts is rapid; the rate of absorption of the lipid-soluble acetate and acetonide esters is much slower. Following intra-articular administration of betamethasone sodium phosphate and betamethasone acetate injectable suspension, systemic absorption of the soluble portion (betamethasone sodium phosphate) is rapid. When the most rapid onset of action is desired, a water-soluble glucocorticoid ester should be administered IV. Systemic absorption occurs slowly following intra-articular, intrabursal, intrasynovial, intradermal, or soft tissue injection of most glucocorticoids.

Following oral inhalation, glucocorticoids are absorbed from the GI and respiratory tracts. After oral inhalation of beclomethasone dipropionate given via metered-dose aerosol with a tetrafluoroethane (non-CFC) propellant, most of the dose (e.g., 51–60% is deposited in the respiratory tract; approximately 27–33% of a dose is deposited in the oropharynx. Systemic bioavailability of fluticasone propionate is about 30 or 13.5% following oral inhalation of the aerosol (via metered spray) or of the powder (via the Diskhaler® device, no longer commercially available in the US), respectively. Systemic bioavailability of budesonide is about 39% in healthy individuals following oral inhalation of the powder (via the Turbuhaler® device) and about 6% in asthmatic children (4–6 years of age) following administration of the micronized suspension for nebulization (via jet nebulizer). Following oral inhalation of 320 mcg of flunisolide, the oral bioavailability is less than 7%. Absolute (compared with IV administration) bioavailability of orally inhaled mometasone furoate as a powder averaged less than 1%. Bioavailability following oral administration of fluticasone propionate is negligible (less than 1%), principally because of incomplete absorption and presystemic metabolism of the drug. Systemic bioavailability of a single orally ingested dose of budesonide is higher in patients with Crohn's disease (21%) than in healthy individuals (about 9%); however, bioavailabilities approach those of healthy individuals following multiple dosing.

Prednisolone sodium phosphate orally disintegrating tablets and solution are bioequivalent based on comparison of area under the plasma concentration-time curves (AUCs) and peak plasma concentrations of the 2 formulations.

Results of a pharmacokinetic study in healthy geriatric adults and younger adults (23–34 years of age) receiving a single IV dose of prednisolone (0.8 mg/kg, no longer commercially available in the US) or oral dose of prednisone (0.8 mg/kg) indicate that the plasma prednisolone concentrations and AUCs of total and unbound prednisolone in geriatric adults are higher than that reported in younger adults. (See Pharmacokinetics: Elimination.)

Normal endogenous plasma concentrations of cortisol and cortisone are 4–30 mcg/dL and 1–2 mcg/dL, respectively.

● Distribution

Animal studies indicate that most glucocorticoids are rapidly removed from the blood and distributed to muscles, liver, skin, intestines, and kidneys.

Glucocorticoids vary in the extent to which they are bound to plasma proteins. Cortisol (hydrocortisone) is extensively bound to corticosteroid-binding globulin (transcortin) and albumin, which are plasma proteins. With physiologic concentrations, cortisol is bound primarily to transcortin and only 5–10% of cortisol in plasma is unbound and is biologically active. Prednisolone (unlike other synthetic glucocorticoids such as betamethasone, dexamethasone, or triamcinolone) has a high affinity for transcortin and competes with cortisol for this binding protein. Results of a pharmacokinetic study in healthy geriatric adults and younger adults (23-34 years of age) receiving a single IV dose of prednisolone (0.8 mg/kg, no longer commercially available in the US) or oral dose of prednisone (0.8 mg/kg) indicate that the mean unbound fraction of prednisolone was higher, and the steady-state volume of distribution of unbound prednisolone was reduced in geriatric adults compared with younger adults. Because only unbound drug is pharmacologically active, patients with low serum albumin concentrations may be more susceptible to effects of glucocorticoids than patients with normal serum albumin concentrations.

Glucocorticoids cross the placenta and may be distributed into milk.

● Elimination

Glucocorticoids having a ketone group at C-11 (e.g., cortisone, prednisone) must be reduced (primarily in the liver) to their corresponding 11-hydroxy analogs (hydrocortisone, prednisolone, and meprednisolone) in order to be pharmacologically active. Prednisone is rapidly converted to prednisolone, but much of cortisone is inactivated before it can be converted to hydrocortisone.

Pharmacologically active glucocorticoids are metabolized in most tissues, but primarily in the liver, to biologically inactive compounds. The metabolic clearance of hydrocortisone may be decreased in patients with hypothyroidism and increased in those with hyperthyroidism. Changes in thyroid status may necessitate adjustment of glucocorticoid dosage. The metabolic clearance of prednisolone is impaired in geriatric patients (as evidenced by a reduced fractional urinary clearance of 6β-hydroxyprednisolone) compared with younger adults. Inactive metabolites are excreted by the kidneys, primarily as glucuronides and sulfates, but also as unconjugated products. Small amounts of unmetabolized drugs are also excreted in urine. Negligible amounts of most of the drugs are excreted in bile; enterohepatic circulation does not occur.

CHEMISTRY

Corticosteroids are hormones secreted by the adrenal cortex or synthetic analogs of these hormones. Traditionally, corticosteroids have been classified as mineralocorticoids or glucocorticoids based on their primary pharmacologic activity; however, separation of the drugs into these classes is not absolute. (See Pharmacology.) Of the corticosteroids that are used clinically, beclomethasone, betamethasone, budesonide, cortisone, dexamethasone, flunisolide, fluticasone, hydrocortisone, methylprednisolone, prednisolone, prednisone, and triamcinolone are classified as glucocorticoids. Although fludrocortisone is also a glucocorticoid, it has very potent mineralocorticoid properties and is used for its mineralocorticoid effects.

For further information on chemistry and stability, uses, cautions, and dosage and administration of corticosteroids, see the individual monographs in 68:04.

---

† Use is not currently included in the labeling approved by the US Food and Drug Administration.

Budesonide

68:04 • ADRENALS

■ Budesonide is a synthetic, nonhalogenated corticosteroid that has potent glucocorticoid and weak mineralocorticoid activity.

USES

Budesonide is used orally for the management of mild to moderate Crohn's disease. Budesonide is used by oral inhalation for the management of bronchial asthma. Budesonide in fixed combination with formoterol fumarate is used by oral inhalation for the treatment of asthma and also for maintenance treatment of airflow obstruction in patients with chronic obstructive pulmonary disease (COPD), including chronic bronchitis and emphysema.

● Crohn's Disease

Budesonide is used orally as delayed-release capsules for the management of mildly to moderately active Crohn's disease involving the ileum and/or ascending colon and for maintenance of clinical remission for up to 3 months in this condition.

Safety and efficacy of delayed-release budesonide capsules in the management of active Crohn's disease were evaluated in 5 randomized, double-blind (2 placebo-controlled and 3 comparative) studies that included 994 adults (17–85 years of age [mean age: 35 years]; 40% male; 97% white) with mild to moderately active Crohn's disease involving the ileum and/or the ascending colon. For clinical assessment, the Crohn's Disease Activity Index (CDAI) was used. The CDAI score is based on subjective observations by the patient (e.g., the daily number of liquid or very soft stools, severity of abdominal pain, general well-being) and objective evidence (e.g., number of extraintestinal manifestations, presence of an abdominal mass, use or nonuse of antidiarrheal drugs, the hematocrit, body weight). Clinical improvement, defined as a CDAI score of 150 or less, assessed after 8 weeks of treatment, was the primary efficacy parameter in these studies. In the 2 placebo-controlled studies, patients were randomized to receive placebo or budesonide dosages of 3, 9, or 15 mg daily. In one of these studies (patients having a median CDAI score of 290), a statistically significant difference in clinical improvement was observed in patients receiving 9-mg (4.5 mg twice daily) daily dosages of budesonide (as the delayed-release capsules) when compared with those receiving placebo (51% for budesonide versus 20% for placebo). Improvements in the quality of life, as measured by the patients' responses to the inflammatory bowel disease questionnaire, highly correlated with CDAI scores. In this study, no additional benefit in the management of active Crohn's disease was observed when budesonide dosages were increased to 15 mg daily (7.5 mg twice daily). Clinical improvement was similar in patients receiving 3-mg (1.5 mg twice daily) daily dosages of budesonide to those receiving placebo. In the other placebo-controlled study (patients having a median CDAI score of 263), no statistically significant difference in clinical improvement was observed in patients receiving 9-mg (9 mg once daily or 4.5 mg twice daily) daily dosages of budesonide delayed-release capsules when compared with those receiving placebo (48–53% for budesonide versus 33% for placebo).

Results of a comparator-drug (budesonide versus mesalamine) controlled study (patients having a median CDAI score of 272) indicate that clinical improvement was substantially higher in adults receiving 9-mg daily dosages of budesonide delayed-release capsules than in those receiving 2-g twice daily dosages of mesalamine delayed-release tablets (69% for budesonide versus 45% for mesalamine). In addition to a higher clinical improvement rate, quality-of-life scores (e.g., anxiety, depressed mood, sense of well-being, self-control, general health, vitality) were improved to a greater extent in patients receiving budesonide than in those receiving mesalamine. Similar or lower clinical improvement rates were observed (although the difference was not statistically significant) in 2 comparative clinical trials (patients having a median CDAI score of 277) when oral budesonide delayed-release capsules were compared with oral prednisolone (40 mg daily initially and then tapered). In one 12-week study, clinical improvement was observed in 42–60% of patients receiving budesonide (42% in patients receiving 4.5 mg twice daily and 60% in those receiving 9 mg once daily for 8 weeks; dosage was tapered thereafter) compared with 60% of those receiving prednisolone (40 mg daily for 2 weeks and tapered thereafter). In the second trial (10 weeks' duration), clinical improvement was observed in 52 or 65% of patients receiving budesonide (9 mg daily for 8 weeks followed by 6 mg daily for 2 weeks) or prednisolone (40 mg daily for 2 weeks, 30 mg for 2 weeks, 25 mg for 2 weeks; daily dosage was then decreased by 5 mg each week for the last 4 weeks), respectively.

Results of a pooled analysis of randomized clinical trials have shown that adults with an active episode of mildly to moderately active Crohn's disease receiving budesonide are 82 or 73% more likely to achieve remission than those receiving placebo (relative risk of 1.82) or mesalamine (relative risk of 1.73), respectively. In addition, results of the pooled analysis indicate that budesonide (using preparations other than Entocort® EC) and conventional corticosteroids (e.g., prednisolone) were associated with similar remission rates in patients with mildly to moderately active Crohn's disease (CDAI scores of 200–300), although conventional corticosteroids were more likely to induce remission than oral budesonide when the patient population included individuals with severely active Crohn's disease.

Safety and efficacy of oral budesonide delayed-release capsules for maintenance therapy of Crohn's disease has been established in 4 randomized, double-blind, placebo-controlled studies of 12 months' duration in patients 18–73 (mean: 37) years of age, 60% of whom were female and 99% of whom were Caucasian. The mean CDAI score at study entry was 96 and approximately 75% had exclusively ileal disease. Budesonide has been effective in prolonging time to relapse defined as an increase in CDAI score of at least 60 units to a total score exceeding 150 or withdrawal secondary to disease deterioration. The median time to relapse in pooled analysis was 268 or 154 days for budesonide (6 mg daily) or placebo, respectively, and budesonide reduced the portion of patients with loss of symptom control relative to placebo at 3 months (28 versus 45%, respectively).

The potential benefits of corticosteroids for maintenance therapy of Crohn's disease should be considered carefully, because both conventional corticosteroids and budesonide do not prevent relapses and the drugs (especially conventional corticosteroids) may produce severe adverse reactions with long-term administration. (See Uses: GI Diseases, in Corticosteroids General Statement 68:04.)

Crohn's Disease in Pediatric Patients

Although safety and efficacy of budesonide delayed-release capsules in pediatric patients have not been established, budesonide (using preparations other than Entocort® EC) has been used for the management of mildly to moderately active Crohn's disease† in a limited number of children 9.5–18 years of age. In one retrospective study in pediatric patients 9.5–18 years of age with mild to moderately active Crohn's disease (Pediatric Crohn's Disease Activity Index [PCDI] score of 12.5–40), budesonide pH-dependent-release preparations (0.45 mg/kg daily up to a maximum dosage of 9 mg daily) were compared with prednisone (2 mg/kg daily up to a maximum dosage of 40 mg daily). Remission was defined as the absence of clinical symptoms and a PCDI score of 10 or less, assessed after 8 weeks of treatment. Results of this study showed that 48 or 77% of pediatric patients achieved remission with budesonide or prednisone, respectively. In addition, 59% of pediatric patients who had shown no improvement with previous mesalamine therapy achieved remission with budesonide.

In addition, results of a 12-week comparator-drug (prednisone versus budesonide) controlled study in pediatric patients† 8–18 years of age (weighing more than 20 kg) with mildly to moderately active Crohn's disease (Pediatric Crohn's Disease Activity Index [PCDI] score of 12.5–40), indicate that remission rates in children receiving prednisone (40 mg daily for 2 weeks and then tapered to discontinuance) were similar (50% for prednisone versus 47% for budesonide) to those receiving budesonide pH- dependent-release preparations (9 mg daily for 8 weeks and then tapered to discontinuance). Total incidence of adverse effects was substantially lower (about 32% for budesonide versus 71% for prednisone) and less severe in pediatric patients receiving budesonide than those receiving prednisone.

For further information on the management of Crohn's disease, see Uses: Crohn's Disease, in Mesalamine 56:36.

● Asthma

Budesonide powder is used by oral inhalation, via the Flexhaler®, for the treatment of bronchial asthma in adults and pediatric patients 6 years of age or older who require chronic administration of corticosteroids to control symptoms. Budesonide inhalation suspension (administered via nebulization) is used by oral inhalation for the treatment of bronchial asthma in children 1–8 years of age. The inhalation aerosol containing budesonide in fixed combination with formoterol fumarate (Symbicort®) is used by oral inhalation for the treatment of asthma in adults and children 6 years of age or older. The fixed combination of budesonide and formoterol fumarate is used only in patients with asthma who have not responded adequately to long-term asthma controller therapy, such as inhaled corticosteroids, or whose disease severity clearly warrants initiation of treatment with both an inhaled corticosteroid and a long-acting β_2-adrenergic agonist. Once asthma control is achieved and maintained, the patient should be assessed at regular intervals and therapy should be stepped down (e.g., discontinuance of budesonide in fixed combination with formoterol fumarate), if possible without loss of asthma control, and the patient should be maintained on long-term asthma controller therapy, such as inhaled corticosteroids. Budesonide in fixed combination with formoterol fumarate should not be used in patients whose asthma is adequately controlled on low or medium dosage of inhaled corticosteroids. (See Serious Asthma-related Events under Warnings/Precautions: Warnings, in Cautions.) Orally inhaled budesonide, alone or in fixed combination with formoterol fumarate, should not be used in the management of acute bronchospasm.

Well-controlled clinical studies have shown that oral inhalation of budesonide improves pulmonary function and relieves symptoms of bronchial asthma. Following continuous use of the oral inhalation of budesonide powder (administered via a Flexhaler®) or the micronized suspension (administered via nebulization), improvement may occur within 1 or 2–8 days of therapy, respectively; however, maximum symptomatic relief may require at least 1–2 or 4–6 weeks, respectively. In corticosteroid-dependent patients, use of budesonide oral inhalation therapy may permit a reduction in the daily maintenance dosage of the systemic corticosteroid and gradual discontinuance of corticosteroid maintenance dosages. In 2 randomized, double-blind, placebo-controlled clinical studies in patients with mild to severe asthma, orally inhaled budesonide (160 or 320 mcg twice daily) in fixed combination with formoterol fumarate (9 mcg twice daily) produced greater improvement in most indices of pulmonary function (e.g., mean percent change from baseline in forced expiratory volume in 1 second [FEV_1] or morning and evening peak expiratory flow rate [PEFR]) than either drug alone and similar efficacy as concurrent therapy with both agents given separately. For information on the stepped-care approach to drug therapy in asthma, see Asthma under Uses: Respiratory Diseases, in the Corticosteroids General Statement 68:04.

● Chronic Obstructive Pulmonary Disease

The inhalation aerosol containing budesonide in fixed combination with formoterol fumarate is used by oral inhalation for maintenance treatment of airflow obstruction in patients with chronic obstructive pulmonary disease (COPD), including chronic bronchitis and emphysema. Orally inhaled budesonide in fixed combination with formoterol fumarate is *not* indicated for the relief of acute bronchospasm.

In 2 randomized, double-blind, placebo-controlled studies of 6 or 12 months' duration in patients with COPD, orally inhaled budesonide (320 mcg twice daily) in fixed combination with formoterol fumarate (9 mcg twice daily) produced greater improvements in the mean percent change from baseline in predose FEV_1 than formoterol alone or placebo and in 1-hour postdose FEV_1 than budesonide alone or placebo. The fixed combination containing 160 mcg of budesonide and 9 mcg of formoterol fumarate twice daily did not produce greater improvements from baseline in predose FEV_1 than formoterol alone or placebo. Therefore, the fixed combination containing 320 mcg of budesonide and 9 mcg of formoterol fumarate twice daily is the only recommended dosage for the treatment of airflow obstruction in COPD. For information on the stepped-care approach to drug therapy in COPD, see Chronic Obstructive Pulmonary Disease under Uses: Bronchospasm, in Ipratropium Bromide 12:08.08.

DOSAGE AND ADMINISTRATION

● Administration

Budesonide is administered orally as delayed-release capsules. For oral inhalation, budesonide is available as an inhalation powder administered via an inhaler device (Flexhaler®), as a micronized suspension administered via nebulization, and as an inhalation aerosol containing budesonide in fixed combination with formoterol fumarate (Symbicort®) administered via an oral aerosol inhaler with hydrofluoroalkane (HFA) propellant. Patients receiving orally inhaled budesonide should rinse their mouth with water after each dose to remove residual drug in the oropharyngeal area and to minimize the development of fungal overgrowth and/or infection.

Oral Administration

Budesonide is administered orally once daily as delayed-release capsules containing enteric-coated granules. The capsules should be swallowed intact; they should not be chewed or broken. However, limited data indicate that the release characteristics of the delayed-release capsules were not affected when the unencapsulated granules were added to applesauce for 30 minutes. Because grapefruit juice has been shown to inhibit cytochrome P-450 (CYP) isoenzyme 3A4, an enzyme involved in the metabolism of budesonide, concomitant use of budesonide

capsules with grapefruit juice should be avoided. (See Drug Interactions: Drugs or Foods Affecting Hepatic Microsomal Enzymes.) Although administration with a high-fat meal delays time to reach peak plasma concentrations of budesonide by about 2.5 hours, the manufacturer makes no specific recommendation regarding administration of budesonide capsules with food.

Oral Inhalation via Powder Inhaler

Budesonide oral inhalation powder (Pulmicort®) is administered by oral inhalation using an inhaler device (Flexhaler®). Budesonide inhalation powder should only be used with the inhaler supplied with the product. Before initial use, the inhaler must be primed; the priming procedure does not have to be repeated even if the inhaler is not used for a long period of time. The inhaler device should not be shaken. Before inhaling the dose, the patient should exhale fully, being careful not to blow into the mouthpiece. The patient should place the mouthpiece between the lips and inhale deeply and forcefully. The patient should not use another dose even if they did not sense the presence of the drug entering their lungs from the Flexhaler® device. Rinsing the mouth after inhalation of budesonide inhalation powder and spitting out the water are advised. The outside of the mouthpiece of the inhaler should be wiped clean with a dry tissue every 7 days. The inhaler should be discarded when the dose indicator reads zero. The canister should never be immersed in water to determine if the canister is empty.

Each actuation of the oral powder inhaler containing budesonide delivers 80 mcg of budesonide from the inhaler labeled as containing 90 mcg or 160 mcg of budesonide from the inhaler labeled as containing 180 mcg (based on testing at 60 L/minute for 2 seconds). Dose delivery for the oral powder inhaler is dependent on airflow through the device. The commercially available inhalation powder contains 60 actuations per 90-mcg inhaler device and 120 actuations per 180-mcg inhaler device.

Oral Inhalation via Nebulization

Commercially available budesonide suspension for oral inhalation is administered via nebulization. *The oral inhalation suspension should not be administered parenterally or used with ultrasonic nebulizers.* Budesonide inhalation suspension should be administered using a jet nebulizer (with face mask or mouthpiece) connected to a compressor that has an adequate air flow. The face mask should be properly adjusted to optimize delivery and to avoid exposure of the eyes to nebulized drug. When a face mask is used for nebulization of budesonide suspension, the face should be washed after each use to avoid dermatologic corticosteroid effects (e.g., rash, contact dermatitis). In clinical trials, a Pari-LC-Jet Plus® Nebulizer was used to deliver budesonide inhalation suspension (Pulmicort® Respules®). The manufacturer states that safety and efficacy of budesonide inhalation suspension administered by a nebulizer other than the Pari-LC-Jet Plus® Nebulizer or a compressor other than the Pari Master compressor have not been established. Since stability and safety of budesonide suspension mixed with other drugs in a nebulizer have not been established, budesonide oral inhalation suspension for nebulization should not be mixed with other drugs. When the commercially available Pulmicort® Respules® are used, the amount of drug delivered to the lungs depends on the type of jet nebulizers used, performance of the compressor, and on factors such the patient's inspiratory flow. Using standardized in vitro testing at a flow rate of 5.5 L per minute, the mean delivered dose at the mouthpiece of the commercially available budesonide suspension (Pulmicort® Respules®) is 17% of the nominal dose.

Oral Inhalation via Aerosol Inhaler

Budesonide in fixed combination with formoterol fumarate (Symbicort®) is administered by oral inhalation using an oral aerosol inhaler with hydrofluoroalkane (HFA) propellant. Budesonide/formoterol fumarate inhalation aerosol should only be used with the actuator supplied with the product. Before each inhalation, the inhaler must be shaken well for 5 seconds. The aerosol inhaler should be test sprayed twice into the air (away from the face) before initial use, and shaken well for 5 seconds before each spray. If the inhaler has not been used for more than 7 days or if the inhaler was dropped, the inhaler should be test sprayed twice into the air (away from the face) and shaken well for 5 seconds before each spray. Rinsing the mouth after inhalation of budesonide/formoterol fumarate inhalation aerosol and spitting out the water are advised. The mouthpiece of the inhaler should be wiped clean with a dry cloth every 7 days. The inhaler should be discarded when the labeled number of inhalations have been used or within 3 months after removal from the foil pouch. The canister should never be immersed in water to determine the amount of drug remaining in the canister ("float test").

Each actuation of the oral aerosol inhaler containing the fixed combination of budesonide and formoterol fumarate delivers 91 or 181 mcg of budesonide and 5.1

mcg of formoterol fumarate from the valve. Dosages of budesonide and formoterol fumarate in the fixed-combination inhalation aerosol are expressed in terms of drug delivered from the mouthpiece; each actuation of the inhaler delivers 80 or 160 mcg of budesonide and 4.5 mcg of formoterol fumarate from the actuator per metered spray. The amount of drug delivered to the lungs depends on factors such as the patient's coordination between the actuation of the inhaler and inspiration through the delivery system. The commercially available inhalation aerosol containing budesonide in fixed combination with formoterol fumarate delivers 60 metered sprays per 6- or 6.9-g canister and 120 metered sprays per 10.2-g canister.

● Dosage

Crohn's Disease

For the management of mild to moderately active Crohn's disease involving the ileum and/or the ascending colon, the recommended adult oral dosage of delayed-release budesonide capsules is 9 mg administered daily in the morning for 8 weeks. Results of a double-blind, multicenter study indicate that in patients who have not experienced remission during the initial 8-week course of budesonide, a second 8-week (16 weeks of continuous therapy) course with the drug may be beneficial in some patients. The manufacturer states that for recurrent episodes of active Crohn's disease, a repeated 8-week course of oral budesonide may be given.

For maintenance of clinical remission following 8 weeks of active treatment once symptoms have been controlled (CDAI score of less than 150), the recommended adult oral dosage of delayed-release budesonide capsules is 6 mg once daily for up to 3 months. If symptom control is maintained at 3 months, an attempt to taper dosage to complete cessation is recommended. The manufacturer states that continued therapy beyond 3 months has not been shown to provide substantial clinical benefit.

Reduction of budesonide dosage should be considered in patients receiving a known inhibitor of the CYP3A4 isoenzyme concomitantly. (See Drugs and Foods that Inhibit CYP3A4 under Drug Interactions: Drugs or Foods Affecting Hepatic Microsomal Enzymes.)

No episodes of adrenal insufficiency have been reported in patients with mild to moderately active Crohn's disease (involving the ileum and/or the ascending colon) who have been switched from oral prednisolone to oral budesonide therapy. It should be considered, however, that abrupt discontinuance of prednisolone is not recommended and, therefore, dosage of prednisolone should be tapered when initiating budesonide therapy. (See Withdrawal of Systemic Corticosteroid Therapy under Warnings/Precautions: Warnings, in Cautions.)

Asthma

The recommended initial and maximum dosages of budesonide suspension for oral inhalation are based on previous asthma therapy. The recommended initial dosage of the oral inhalation aerosol containing budesonide in fixed combination with formoterol fumarate is based on the patient's asthma severity. Safety and efficacy of dosages exceeding those recommended by the manufacturer have not been established. The manufacturer suggests that in patients who were receiving prior oral corticosteroid therapy, reduction of alternate-day or daily dosing should be initiated approximately 1 week after starting budesonide oral inhalation, followed by further reductions after an interval of 1 or 2 weeks; decrements usually should not exceed 2.5 mg or 25% of prednisone (or its equivalent) in patients receiving budesonide inhalation suspension administered via nebulization. The manufacturer of budesonide oral inhalation powder states that patients who were receiving prior oral corticosteroid therapy should be withdrawn slowly from systemic corticosteroid use after transferring to oral inhalation therapy by reducing the prednisone daily dosage by 2.5 mg (or its equivalent) on a weekly basis. The manufacturer of the oral inhalation aerosol containing budesonide in fixed combination with formoterol fumarate states that patients requiring oral corticosteroids should be withdrawn slowly from systemic corticosteroid use after transferring to budesonide in fixed combination with formoterol fumarate. The manufacturer also states that prednisone dosage reduction may be accomplished by reducing the daily dosage by 2.5 mg on a weekly basis during therapy with the oral inhalation aerosol containing budesonide in fixed combination with formoterol fumarate. Once oral corticosteroids are discontinued and symptoms of asthma have been controlled, the dosage of budesonide should be titrated to the lowest effective level. (See Withdrawal of Systemic Corticosteroid Therapy under Warnings/Precautions: Warnings, in Cautions and also see Advice to Patients.)

Oral Inhalation via Powder Inhaler

In asthmatic adults 18 years of age or older, the recommended initial dosage of budesonide oral inhalation powder is 320 mcg (labeled 360 mcg) twice daily. In some patients, an initial dosage of 160 mcg (labeled 180 mcg) twice daily may be adequate. If required, the dosage of budesonide may be increased to a maximum of 640 mcg (labeled 720 mcg) twice daily.

In asthmatic children and adolescents 6–17 years of age, the recommended initial dosage of budesonide oral inhalation powder is 160 mcg (labeled 180 mcg) twice daily. In some patients, an initial dosage of 320 mcg (labeled 360 mcg) twice daily may be appropriate. If required, the dosage may be increased to a maximum of 320 mcg (labeled 360 mcg) twice daily.

For all patients, the dosage of budesonide oral inhalation powder should be titrated to the lowest effective dosage after adequate asthma stability is achieved.

Oral Inhalation via Nebulization in Children (1–8 years of age)

When budesonide suspension is administered via a nebulizer in children who previously were receiving bronchodilators alone, the recommended initial dosage of budesonide is 0.5 mg, given in 1 or 2 divided daily doses; the recommended maximum dosage is 0.5 mg daily. In children who were previously receiving inhaled corticosteroids, the recommended initial dosage of budesonide suspension, given via a nebulizer, is 0.5 mg, given in 1 or 2 divided daily doses; the recommended maximum dosage is 1 mg daily. In children who previously were receiving oral corticosteroids, the recommended initial dosage of budesonide inhalation suspension, given via a nebulizer, is 1 mg, given in 1 or 2 divided daily doses; the recommended maximum dosage is 1 mg daily. In children who are not receiving oral corticosteroids and who do not respond adequately to the initial once-daily administration of budesonide suspension, increasing the dosage or giving the drug in 2 divided doses daily should be considered.

In children with asthma symptoms who do not respond to nonsteroidal (e.g., bronchodilator, mast-cell stabilizer) therapy, an initial 0.25-mg daily dosage of budesonide inhalation suspension, given via a nebulizer, may be considered. However, if the once-daily dosage does not provide adequate control of asthma symptoms, the total daily dosage should be increased and/or administered in divided doses.

Budesonide/Formoterol Fumarate Fixed-combination Therapy

In asthmatic adults and adolescents 12 years of age or older, the recommended initial dosage of the oral inhalation aerosol containing budesonide in fixed combination with formoterol fumarate is based on the patient's asthma severity, level of control of asthma symptoms, and/or risk of asthma exacerbations during current therapy with inhaled corticosteroids. The dosage of the inhalation aerosol fixed-combination preparation is 160 or 320 mcg of budesonide and 9 mcg of formoterol fumarate (2 inhalations) twice daily, given approximately 12 hours apart (morning and evening). The maximum recommended dosage of budesonide in fixed combination with formoterol fumarate is 320 mcg of budesonide with 9 mcg of formoterol fumarate (2 inhalations) twice daily. The manufacturer states that administration of the inhalation aerosol containing budesonide in fixed combination with formoterol fumarate more frequently than twice daily or in excess of 2 inhalations twice daily is not recommended. Patients receiving the fixed combination of budesonide and formoterol fumarate should not use additional long-acting β_2-agonists for any reason.

In asthmatic children 6 to less than 12 years of age, the recommended dosage of the oral inhalation aerosol containing budesonide in fixed combination with formoterol fumarate is 160 mcg of budesonide and 9 mcg of formoterol fumarate (2 inhalations) twice daily, given approximately 12 hours apart (morning and evening).

Improvement in asthma control following inhalation of budesonide in fixed combination with formoterol fumarate may occur within 15 minutes of initiating treatment, although maximum benefit may not be achieved for 2 weeks or longer after therapy initiation. Individual patients will experience a variable time to onset and degree of symptom relief. If control of asthma is inadequate after 1–2 weeks of therapy at the lower dosage, increasing the strength of the fixed combination (higher strengths contain higher dosages of budesonide only) may provide additional asthma control. If acute asthmatic symptoms arise despite therapy with budesonide in fixed combination with formoterol fumarate, a short-acting inhaled β_2-adrenergic agonist should be administered for immediate relief. Patients should be advised not to discontinue budesonide in fixed combination with formoterol fumarate without medical supervision, as symptoms may recur after treatment discontinuation. If a previously effective dosage of budesonide in fixed combination with formoterol fumarate fails to provide adequate asthma control, the therapeutic regimen should be reevaluated and additional therapeutic options should be considered (e.g., increasing the strength of the fixed combination [higher strengths contain higher dosages of budesonide only], adding additional inhaled corticosteroids, initiating systemic corticosteroids). The manufacturer warns that therapy with the fixed combination of budesonide and formoterol fumarate should *not* be initiated in patients during rapidly deteriorating or potentially life-threatening episodes of asthma.

Chronic Obstructive Pulmonary Disease
Budesonide/Formoterol Fumarate Fixed-combination Therapy

For maintenance therapy of airflow obstruction in patients with chronic obstructive pulmonary disease (COPD), the recommended dosage of the oral inhalation aerosol containing budesonide in fixed combination with formoterol fumarate in adults is 320 mcg of budesonide and 9 mcg of formoterol fumarate (2 inhalations) twice daily (morning and evening). In clinical studies, the fixed combination containing 160 mcg of budesonide and 9 mcg of formoterol fumarate (2 inhalations) twice daily did not produce greater improvements from baseline in predose FEV_1 than formoterol alone or placebo; therefore, the fixed combination containing 320 mcg of budesonide and 9 mcg of formoterol fumarate (2 inhalations) twice daily is the only recommended dosage for the treatment of airflow obstruction in COPD. If shortness of breath occurs despite therapy with budesonide in fixed combination with formoterol fumarate, a short-acting inhaled β_2-adrenergic agonist should be taken for immediate relief. Patients should be advised not to discontinue budesonide in fixed combination with formoterol fumarate without medical supervision, as symptoms may recur after treatment discontinuance. The manufacturer warns that therapy with the fixed combination of budesonide and formoterol fumarate should *not* be initiated in patients during rapidly deteriorating or potentially life-threatening episodes of COPD. The manufacturer states that administration of the inhalation aerosol containing budesonide in fixed combination with formoterol fumarate more frequently than twice daily or in excess of 2 inhalations twice daily is not recommended. Patients receiving the fixed combination of budesonide and formoterol fumarate should not use additional long-acting β_2-agonists for any reason.

● Special Populations

Patients with Crohn's disease and moderate to severe hepatic impairment should be monitored for increased signs and symptoms of hypercorticism; reduction of budesonide oral dosage is recommended in these patients.

When budesonide is used in fixed combination with formoterol fumarate, dosage requirements for formoterol fumarate should be considered.

The manufacturer of budesonide in fixed combination with formoterol fumarate states that dosage adjustment is not required in geriatric patients. The manufacturer of budesonide in fixed combination with formoterol fumarate makes no specific dosage recommendations for patients with hepatic or renal impairment at this time. However, since budesonide and formoterol fumarate are cleared predominantly by the liver, impaired liver function theoretically may lead to accumulation of the drugs in plasma. Therefore, the manufacturer of budesonide in fixed combination with formoterol fumarate states that patients with hepatic disease should be closely monitored.

CAUTIONS

● Contraindications

Known hypersensitivity to budesonide or any ingredient in the formulation.

Orally inhaled budesonide is contraindicated as primary treatment of acute asthmatic attacks or status asthmaticus when intensive measures (e.g., an orally inhaled β_2-adrenergic agonist, an orally inhaled anticholinergic agent, subcutaneous epinephrine, IV aminophylline, and/or an oral/IV glucocorticoid) are required.

Orally inhaled budesonide powder (Pulmicort® Flexhaler®) is contraindicated in patients with severe hypersensitivity to milk proteins.

Budesonide in fixed combination with formoterol fumarate (Symbicort®) is contraindicated as primary treatment of status asthmaticus or other acute episodes of asthma or chronic obstructive pulmonary disease (COPD) when intensive measures are required.

When budesonide is used in fixed combination with formoterol fumarate, contraindications associated with formoterol fumarate should be considered.

● Warnings/Precautions
Warnings
Use of Fixed Combinations

When budesonide is used in fixed combination with formoterol fumarate, the usual cautions, precautions, contraindications, and interactions associated with formoterol fumarate should be considered. Cautionary information applicable to specific populations (e.g., pregnant or nursing women, individuals with hepatic or renal impairment, geriatric patients) should be considered for each drug in the fixed combination.

Serious Asthma-related Events

Monotherapy with long-acting β_2-adrenergic agonists, such as formoterol, a component of Symbicort®, increases the risk of asthma-related death. Data from a large (approximately 26,000 patients), placebo-controlled study (Salmeterol Multi-center Asthma Research Trial [SMART]) evaluating the safety of another long-acting β_2-adrenergic agonist, salmeterol, in patients with asthma showed an increase in asthma-related deaths in patients receiving salmeterol. (See Asthma-related Death and Life-threatening Events under Cautions: Respiratory Effects, in Salmeterol 12:12.08.12.) In addition, available data from controlled clinical trials suggest that monotherapy with long-acting β_2-adrenergic agonists increases the risk of asthma-related hospitalization in pediatric and adolescent patients.

However, FDA has concluded that there is no clinically important increased risk of serious asthma-related events, including hospitalization, intubation, or death, associated with concomitant use of long-acting β_2-adrenergic agonists (e.g., formoterol) and inhaled corticosteroids (e.g., budesonide) compared with inhaled corticosteroids alone based on the results of several large clinical studies. In addition, these studies showed that combination therapy with long-acting β_2-adrenergic agonists and inhaled corticosteroids was more effective in reducing the incidence of asthma exacerbations (i.e., events requiring use of systemic corticosteroids for at least 3 outpatient days or an asthma-related hospitalization or emergency department visit requiring use of systemic corticosteroids) compared with use of inhaled corticosteroids alone. (See Asthma-related Death and Serious Asthma-related Events under Warnings/Precautions: Warnings, in Cautions, in Formoterol 12:12.08.12.)

In the treatment of asthma, the fixed combination of budesonide and formoterol fumarate is used only in patients who have not responded adequately to long-term asthma controller therapy, such as inhaled corticosteroids, or whose disease severity warrants initiation of treatment with both an inhaled corticosteroid and a long-acting β_2-adrenergic agonist. (See Uses: Asthma.)

Withdrawal of Systemic Corticosteroid Therapy

In patients being switched from systemic corticosteroids to oral or orally inhaled budesonide, systemic corticosteroid therapy should be withdrawn gradually because life-threatening adrenal insufficiency may occur. Patients who have been maintained on 20 mg or more of prednisone (or its equivalent) daily may be most susceptible to such adverse events, particularly when their systemic corticosteroid therapy has been almost completely withdrawn. *In most patients, following withdrawal of systemic corticosteroid therapy, several months are required for total recovery of HPA function.* These patients should be carefully monitored during and for a number of months after withdrawal of systemic corticosteroids because of the risk of corticosteroid withdrawal symptoms (e.g., joint pain, muscular pain, lassitude, depression); acute adrenal insufficiency during exposure to trauma, surgery, or infection (particularly gastroenteritis) or other conditions associated with acute electrolyte loss; or symptomatic exacerbation of allergic conditions previously controlled by systemic corticosteroid therapy (e.g., rhinitis, conjunctivitis, eczema, arthritis, eosinophilic conditions). Clinicians should be alert for the potential for eosinophilia, vasculitic rash, worsening of pulmonary symptoms, cardiac complications, and/or neuropathy consistent with Churg-Strauss syndrome. In asthmatic patients, death, possibly resulting from acute adrenal insufficiency, has occurred rarely during and after transfer from a systemic corticosteroid to budesonide oral inhalation therapy. Systemic corticosteroid dosage should be carefully tapered and patients should be monitored during dosage reduction for objective signs of adrenal insufficiency and for benign intracranial hypertension. In general, the greater the dosage and duration of systemic corticosteroid therapy, the greater the time required for withdrawal of systemic corticosteroids and replacement by orally inhaled corticosteroids.

Immunosuppressed Patients

Patients who are taking immunosuppressant drugs have increased susceptibility to infections compared with healthy individuals, and certain infections (e.g., varicella [chickenpox], measles) can have a more serious or even fatal outcome in such patients, particularly in children. In patients who have not had these diseases or been properly vaccinated, particular care should be taken to avoid exposure. If exposure to varicella occurs in such individuals, administration of varicella zoster immune globulin (VZIG) or pooled IV immunoglobulin (IVIG) may be indicated; if exposure to measles occurs, pooled IM immune globulin (IG) may be indicated.

If varicella (chickenpox) develops, treatment with an antiviral agent may be considered. It is not known how the dosage, route and duration of administration of a corticosteroid, or the contribution of the underlying disease and/or prior corticosteroid therapy affect the risk of developing a disseminated infection. For additional information, see Cautions: Increased Susceptibility to Infection and also see Precautions and Contraindications, in the Corticosteroids General Statement 68:04.

Hypothalamic-Pituitary-Adrenal (HPA) Axis Suppression

Since glucocorticoids can reduce HPA-axis response to stress (e.g., surgery), supplementation with a systemic corticosteroid in patients undergoing such stress is recommended.

Bronchospasm

As with other inhaled drugs for asthma, bronchospasm may occur, resulting in an immediate increase in wheezing following oral inhalation of budesonide. If bronchospasm occurs, appropriate treatment (e.g., use of a short-acting β-adrenergic agonist) should be initiated immediately, and budesonide therapy should be discontinued and alternate therapy instituted.

General Precautions
Infections

Localized candidal infections of the mouth and/or pharynx have been reported in patients receiving orally inhaled budesonide therapy. When infection occurs, appropriate local or systemic antifungal treatment may be necessary while still continuing with inhaled budesonide therapy, although discontinuance of such therapy (under close medical supervision) may be required in some patients. Inhaled corticosteroid therapy should be used with extreme caution, if at all, in patients with clinical or asymptomatic *Mycobacterium tuberculosis* infections of the respiratory tract; untreated systemic fungal, bacterial, viral, or parasitic infections; or ocular herpes simplex. Clinicians should remain vigilant for the possible development of pneumonia in patients with COPD who are receiving budesonide in fixed combination with formoterol fumarate, since the clinical features of pneumonia and COPD exacerbations frequently overlap. Lower respiratory tract infections, including pneumonia, have been reported in patients with COPD following the administration of inhaled corticosteroids.

Ophthalmic Effects

Glaucoma, increased intraocular pressure (IOP), and cataracts have been reported rarely in patients receiving orally inhaled corticosteroids.

Concomitant Disease States

The manufacturer states that budesonide delayed-release capsules should be used with caution in patients with tuberculosis, hypertension, diabetes mellitus, osteoporosis, peptic ulcer, glaucoma or cataracts, a family history of diabetes or glaucoma, or any other condition in which glucocorticoids may be associated with adverse effects.

Systemic Corticosteroid Effects

Administration of higher than recommended dosages of orally inhaled budesonide or prolonged oral administration of budesonide capsules may result in manifestations of hypercorticism and suppression of HPA function.

Long-Term Administration

The long-term local and systemic effects of budesonide in humans, particularly local effects on developmental or immunologic processes in the mouth, pharynx, trachea, and lung, are unknown.

Musculoskeletal Effects

Long-term use of orally inhaled corticosteroids may affect normal bone metabolism, resulting in a loss of bone mineral density. (See Osteoporosis under Cautions: Musculoskeletal Effects, in the Corticosteroids General Statement 68:04.) The manufacturer of budesonide in fixed combination with formoterol states that patients with major risk factors for decreased bone mineral density, such as prolonged immobilization, family history of osteoporosis, postmenopausal status, tobacco use, advanced age, poor nutrition, or chronic use of drugs that can reduce bone mass (e.g., anticonvulsants, oral corticosteroids) should be monitored and treated using established standards of care. Since patients with COPD often have multiple risk factors for reduced bone mineral density, assessment of bone mineral density is recommended prior to initiation of therapy with budesonide in fixed combination with

formoterol fumarate and periodically thereafter. If appreciable reductions in bone mineral density are seen and use of budesonide in fixed combination with formoterol fumarate is considered to be important for the patient's COPD therapy, use of agents to treat or prevent osteoporosis should be strongly considered.

Specific Populations
Pregnancy

Category B (orally inhaled powder and inhalation suspension); category C (oral capsules and the fixed combination of budesonide and formoterol fumarate oral inhalation aerosol). (See Users Guide.) Hypoadrenalism may occur in infants of women receiving corticosteroid therapy during pregnancy. These infants should be carefully monitored.

Lactation

Like other corticosteroids, budesonide is distributed into milk; however, data are not available on the effects of the drug on the breast-fed child or on milk production. The benefits of breast-feeding and the importance of budesonide to the woman should be considered along with any potential adverse effects on the breast-fed infant from the drug or underlying maternal condition. The manufacturer of budesonide oral inhalation powder (Pulmicort® Flexhaler®) states that the drug should be used in nursing women only if clinically appropriate and that therapy should be titrated to the lowest effective dosage. In addition, budesonide powder inhaler should be used immediately after nursing to minimize infant exposure to the drug.

Pediatric Use

Safety and efficacy of oral budesonide delayed-release capsules have not been established in pediatric patients younger than 18 years of age with Crohn's disease. Oral budesonide (using preparations other than Entecort® EC) has been used for the management of mild to moderately active Crohn's disease in a limited number of pediatric patients without unusual adverse effects. Benign intracranial hypertension has been reported in at least one pediatric patient with Crohn's disease receiving the drug.

Safety and efficacy of budesonide inhalation powder have not been established in children younger than 6 years of age. Efficacy of budesonide inhalation suspension has not been established in children younger than 1 year of age, while safety of the suspension has not been established in children younger than 6 months of age. Safety and efficacy of budesonide in fixed combination with formoterol fumarate (Symbicort®) inhalation aerosol in patients 12 years of age or older with asthma have been established in studies of up to 12 months' duration; in addition, safety and efficacy of the fixed-combination preparation in children 6 to less than 12 years of age with asthma have been established in studies of up to 12 weeks' duration. The manufacturer states that safety and efficacy of the fixed-combination preparation in children younger than 6 years of age with asthma have not been established. Use of corticosteroids may lead to suppression of growth in children and adolescents. Therefore, children receiving prolonged therapy with orally inhaled budesonide should be monitored periodically for possible adverse effects on growth and development. (See Cautions: Pediatric Precautions, in the Corticosteroids General Statement 68:04.)

Geriatric Use

Clinical studies of oral budesonide delayed-release capsules or budesonide oral inhalation powder did not include sufficient numbers of patients 65 years of age or older to determine whether geriatric patients respond differently than younger patients. While other clinical experience with budesonide inhalation powder or inhalation suspension or with the inhalation aerosol containing budesonide in fixed combination with formoterol fumarate has not revealed age-related differences in response, oral drug dosage generally should be titrated carefully in geriatric patients, usually initiating therapy at the low end of the dosage range. Safety of budesonide inhalation powder in patients 65 years of age or older was similar to that observed in younger adults. No substantial differences in safety and efficacy of budesonide in fixed combination with formoterol fumarate were observed in geriatric patients relative to younger adults. The greater frequency of decreased hepatic, renal, and/or cardiac function and of concomitant disease and drug therapy observed in the elderly also should be considered. (See Dosage and Administration: Special Populations.)

Hepatic Impairment

May affect elimination of corticosteroids; increased systemic availability of oral budesonide capsules has been reported in patients with liver cirrhosis. Patients with mild hepatic impairment are minimally affected. Pharmacokinetics were not studied in patients with severe hepatic impairment. The manufacturer states that patients with hepatic disease receiving budesonide in fixed combination with formoterol fumarate should be closely monitored. (See Dosage and Administration: Special Populations.)

Renal Impairment

Pharmacokinetics of budesonide have not been studied in patients with renal impairment. However, since only the metabolites (having negligible glucocorticoid activity), and not the unchanged drug, are excreted by the kidneys, increased adverse effects are not expected in such patients receiving the drug.

● Common Adverse Effects

Adverse effects occurring in at least 5% of patients receiving budesonide oral capsules include headache, dizziness, nausea, vomiting, dyspepsia, diarrhea, abdominal pain, flatulence, sinusitis, respiratory infection, viral infection, pain (including back pain), arthralgia, and fatigue. Adverse effect profile in long-term treatment was similar to that of short-term treatment.

Adverse effects occurring in 1% or more of patients receiving budesonide by oral inhalation (as a powder using a Flexhaler® or a Turbuhaler® [no longer commercially available in the US] or as an inhalation suspension, administered via nebulization) include infections (e.g., respiratory infection, ocular infection), nasopharyngitis, pharyngitis, nasal congestion, allergic rhinitis, sinusitis, viral infection (e.g., herpes simplex), cough, voice alteration, stridor, earache, otitis (media or externa), viral infection, flu-like syndrome, moniliasis, oral candidiasis, flu syndrome, fever, headache, migraine, insomnia, dysphonia, hyperkinesia, asthenia, fatigue, emotional lability, pain (e.g., back pain), arthralgia, myalgia, hypertonia, fractures, dyspepsia, gastroenteritis, nausea, vomiting, diarrhea, abdominal pain, dry mouth, taste perversion, weight gain, anorexia, epistaxis, ecchymosis, purpura, cervical lymphadenopathy, conjunctivitis, rash (may be pustular), pruritus, allergic reaction, contact dermatitis, syncope, and chest pain.

DRUG INTERACTIONS

The following information addresses potential interactions with budesonide. When budesonide is used in fixed combination with formoterol fumarate, interactions associated with formoterol fumarate should be considered. No formal drug interaction studies have been performed to date with the fixed-combination preparation containing budesonide and formoterol fumarate.

● Drugs or Foods Affecting Hepatic Microsomal Enzymes

Drugs and Foods that Inhibit Isoenzyme CYP3A4

Since budesonide is metabolized in the liver by the cytochrome P-450 (CYP) 3A4 isoenzyme, concomitant use with drugs that are potent inhibitors of the CYP3A4 isoenzyme may result in increased plasma budesonide concentrations. Concomitant use of oral budesonide with oral ketoconazole resulted in an eightfold increase in budesonide systemic exposure. Patients in whom concomitant use of a known inhibitor of the CYP3A4 isoenzyme (e.g., erythromycin, itraconazole, clarithromycin, ketoconazole, indinavir, ritonavir, saquinavir) with oral budesonide capsules is indicated should be carefully monitored for increased signs and symptoms of hypercorticism and reduction of budesonide dosage should be considered.

Oral contraceptives containing ethinyl estradiol (also metabolized by CYP3A4 isoenzyme) do not appear to affect the pharmacokinetics of budesonide; in addition, budesonide does not appear to affect plasma concentrations of these oral contraceptives.

Concomitant use of oral budesonide delayed-release capsules with grapefruit juice resulted in a twofold increase in budesonide systemic exposure; therefore, such concomitant use should be avoided.

Drugs that Induce Isoenzyme CYP3A4

Concomitant administration of budesonide with drugs that induce CYP3A4 isoenzyme may result in decreased budesonide plasma concentrations.

● Drugs Affecting GI pH

Because budesonide delayed-release oral capsules containing enteric-coated granules are formulated to dissolve at a relatively nonacidic pH (exceeding 5.5) (see Description), concomitant use of drugs that affect GI pH may affect release properties and systemic uptake of oral budesonide delayed-release capsules. Although administration of gastric antisecretory agents (e.g., omeprazole, cimetidine) did not

appear to affect the pharmacokinetic parameters (e.g., absorption) of the commercially available budesonide delayed-release capsules, slightly increased peak plasma concentrations and rate of absorption of budesonide have been reported following concomitant use of cimetidine (1 g daily) with a nonenteric-coated formulation of budesonide, resulting in substantial suppression of the hypothalamic-pituitary-adrenal (HPA) axis.

DESCRIPTION

Budesonide is a synthetic, nonhalogenated corticosteroid. Budesonide has potent glucocorticoid and weak mineralocorticoid activity. The exact mechanism of action of budesonide in the management of Crohn's disease is not known. The drug appears to have immunosuppressant and substantial topical anti-inflammatory activity and lower systemic availability than conventional corticosteroids. Budesonide oral delayed-release capsules have been formulated to release the drug at the site of inflammation (usually in the terminal ileum and ascending colon). For further information on the pharmacology of corticosteroids, see Pharmacology in the Corticosteroids General Statement 68:04.

Budesonide is commercially available as oral delayed-release capsules, oral inhalation powder, oral micronized suspension for nebulization, and an oral inhalation aerosol containing budesonide in fixed combination with formoterol fumarate.

Budesonide oral delayed-release capsules contain enteric-coated granules in an extended-release matrix. The enteric coating of the granules is formulated to dissolve at a relatively nonacidic pH (exceeding 5.5; i.e., in the small intestine); thereafter, budesonide is released slowly (in a time-dependent manner) from the matrix of ethylcellulose within the intestinal lumen. Budesonide powder for inhalation is administered by an inhaler (Flexhaler®), micronized sterile budesonide inhalation suspension for oral inhalation is administered by a jet nebulizer (with face mask or mouthpiece) connected to a compressor that has an adequate air flow, and budesonide in fixed combination with formoterol fumarate (Symbicort®) for oral inhalation is administered via an oral aerosol inhaler with hydrofluoroalkane (HFA) propellant. (See Dosage and Administration: Administration.)

In healthy individuals, following oral administration of 9 mg of budesonide as delayed-release capsules, the drug appears to be completely absorbed; peak plasma concentrations of 2.2 ng/mL are achieved within 0.5–10 hours. Systemic bioavailability of a single orally ingested dose of budesonide is higher (21%) in patients with Crohn's disease than in healthy individuals (about 9–15%); however, bioavailabilities approach those of healthy individuals following multiple dosing.

In healthy individuals, systemic bioavailability of budesonide inhalation powder (administered via a metered-dose inhaler [no longer commercially available in the US]), has been about 39%. The absolute bioavailability of budesonide inhalation suspension administered via a jet nebulizer in asthmatic children (4–6 years of age) has been reported to be 6%. Following oral inhalation of 1 mg of budesonide inhalation suspension for nebulization in asthmatic children (4–6 years of age), peak plasma concentrations of 1.1 ng/mL occurred about 20 minutes after nebulization. Following oral inhalation of budesonide powder, peak plasma concentrations in adults with asthma occur within about 10 minutes. The therapeutic effects of orally inhaled budesonide are thought to result from local actions of the deposited inhaled dose on the respiratory tract rather than from the systemic actions of the swallowed portion of the dose.

Budesonide undergoes extensive (about 80–95%) metabolism on first pass through the liver via the cytochrome P-450 enzyme system, mainly by the isoenzyme 3A4 (CYP3A4) to 2 metabolites with negligible (less than 1%) glucocorticoid activity when compared with the parent compound. Following oral or IV administration, the drug is excreted in urine (60%) and feces as metabolites; unchanged budesonide has not been detected in urine.

Race, gender, or advanced age does not appear to affect pharmacokinetics of budesonide.

ADVICE TO PATIENTS

When budesonide is used in fixed combination with formoterol fumarate, importance of informing patients of important cautionary information about formoterol fumarate.

Importance of informing patients receiving the fixed combination of budesonide and formoterol fumarate that monotherapy with long-acting β_2-adrenergic agonists, including formoterol, a component of Symbicort®, increases the risk of asthma-related death and may increase the risk of asthma-related hospitalization in pediatric and adolescent patients.

Necessity of swallowing budesonide capsules whole, without chewing or breaking. Patients should be advised that concomitant use of budesonide capsules with grapefruit juice should be avoided.

Advise that oral inhalation of budesonide must be used at regular intervals to be therapeutically effective. Importance of adherence to prescribed budesonide dosage, unless otherwise instructed by a clinician.

Advise that although improvement may occur within 1 or 2–8 days of therapy with budesonide oral inhalation powder or inhalation suspension, respectively; at least 1–2 or 4–6 weeks, respectively, of continuous therapy may be required for optimum effects to be achieved. Advise that although improvement in asthma control following administration of the oral inhalation aerosol containing budesonide in fixed combination with formoterol fumarate may occur within 15 minutes of initiating treatment, maximum benefit may not be achieved for 2 weeks or longer.

Patients should be carefully instructed in the use of the oral aerosol inhaler containing budesonide alone or in fixed combination with formoterol fumarate. Provide copy of manufacturer's patient information and medication guide.

Advise that orally inhaled budesonide alone or in fixed combination with formoterol fumarate should not be used as a bronchodilator and that the drug is not indicated for emergency use (e.g., relief of acute bronchospasm).

Importance of all patients being provided with a short-acting, inhaled β_2-adrenergic agonist as supplemental therapy for acute asthma symptoms. Importance of informing a clinician if a short-acting β_2-adrenergic agonist is not available for use.

Importance of discontinuing *regular* use of a short-acting, inhaled β_2-adrenergic agonist when initiating therapy with the fixed combination of budesonide and formoterol fumarate.

Advise patients being transferred from systemic corticosteroid to budesonide oral inhalation therapy to carry special identification (e.g., card) indicating the need for supplementary systemic corticosteroids during periods of stress or severe exacerbation of asthma. Such patients should immediately resume therapy with large doses of systemic corticosteroids and contact their clinician for further instructions during stressful periods (e.g., stress, severe asthmatic attack).

Importance of not exceeding the recommended dosage and of contacting a clinician immediately if asthma symptoms do not improve or worsen.

Importance of contacting a clinician if decreased effectiveness of a short-acting, inhaled β_2-adrenergic agonist (requiring more inhalations than usual) for acute symptoms occurs.

Importance of not using additional formoterol or other long-acting inhaled β_2-adrenergic agonists for any reason when the fixed combination of budesonide and formoterol fumarate is used.

In immunosuppressed patients, importance of avoiding exposure to chickenpox or measles, and, if exposed, of immediately consulting their clinician.

Importance of informing patients that corticosteroids may decrease bone mineral density.

Importance of informing patients that long-term use of inhaled corticosteroids may increase the risk for development of some ocular disorders (cataracts or glaucoma); regular eye examinations should be considered.

Importance of informing patients that orally inhaled corticosteroids may cause a reduction in growth velocity when administered to pediatric patients.

Importance of adequate understanding of proper storage and inhalation techniques, including use of the inhalation delivery systems.

Advise patients receiving orally inhaled budesonide to rinse their mouth with water after each dose to remove residual drug in the oropharyngeal area and to minimize the development of fungal overgrowth and/or infection.

Importance of informing patients with COPD receiving budesonide in fixed combination with formoterol fumarate that they have a higher risk of pneumonia and to contact their clinician if they develop symptoms of pneumonia.

Importance of women informing clinicians if they are or plan to become pregnant or plan to breast-feed.

Importance of informing clinicians of existing or contemplated concomitant therapy, including prescription and OTC drugs, as well as any concomitant illnesses.

Importance of informing patients of other important precautionary information. (See Cautions.)

PREPARATIONS

Excipients in commercially available drug preparations may have clinically important effects in some individuals; consult specific product labeling for details.

Budesonide

Oral

Capsules, delayed-release (containing enteric-coated granules)	3 mg	Entocort® EC, AstraZeneca

Oral Inhalation

Powder, for oral inhalation only	90 mcg (delivers 80 mcg per inhalation)	Pulmicort® Flexhaler®, AstraZeneca
	180 mcg (delivers 160 mcg per inhalation)	Pulmicort® Flexhaler®, AstraZeneca
Suspension, for nebulization	0.25 mg/2 mL	Pulmicort® Respules® (available in flexible ampuls), AstraZeneca
	0.5 mg/2 mL	Pulmicort® Respules® (available in flexible ampuls), AstraZeneca

Budesonide Combinations

Oral Inhalation

Aerosol	80 mcg with Formoterol Fumarate Dihydrate 4.5 mcg per metered spray	Symbicort® (with hydrofluoroalkane propellant), AstraZeneca
	160 mcg with Formoterol Fumarate Dihydrate 4.5 mcg per metered spray	Symbicort® (with hydrofluoroalkane propellant), AstraZeneca

† Use is not currently included in the labeling approved by the US Food and Drug Administration.

Fluticasone Propionate

68:04 • ADRENALS

■ Fluticasone propionate is a synthetic trifluorinated glucocorticoid.

USES

● Bronchospasm

Asthma

Fluticasone propionate is used for the long-term prevention of bronchospasm in patients with asthma. The fixed combination of fluticasone propionate and salmeterol xinafoate is used only in patients with asthma who have not responded adequately to long-term asthma controller therapy, such as inhaled corticosteroids, or whose disease severity clearly warrants initiation of treatment with both an inhaled corticosteroid and a long-acting β_2-adrenergic agonist. Once asthma control is achieved and maintained, the patient should be assessed at regular intervals and therapy should be stepped down (e.g., discontinuance of fluticasone propionate in fixed combination with salmeterol xinafoate), if possible without loss of asthma control, and the patient should be maintained on long-term asthma controller therapy, such as inhaled corticosteroids. Fluticasone propionate in fixed combination with salmeterol xinafoate should not be used in patients whose asthma is adequately controlled on low or medium dosage of inhaled corticosteroids. (See Serious Asthma-related Events under Warnings/Precautions: Warnings, in Cautions.)

Orally inhaled fluticasone propionate alone or combined with salmeterol xinafoate should not be used for the primary treatment of severe acute asthmatic attacks or status asthmaticus when intensive measures (e.g., oxygen, parenteral bronchodilators, IV corticosteroids) are required. Fluticasone propionate oral inhalation is not a bronchodilator, and patients should be warned that the drug alone or in fixed combination with salmeterol xinafoate should not be used for rapid relief of bronchospasm.

Mild Persistent Asthma

Drugs for asthma may be categorized as relievers (e.g., bronchodilators taken as needed for acute symptoms) or controllers (principally inhaled corticosteroids or other anti-inflammatory agents taken regularly to achieve long-term control of asthma). In the stepped-care approach to antiasthmatic drug therapy, current asthma management guidelines and most clinicians recommend initiation of a controller drug such as an anti-inflammatory agent, preferably a low-dose orally inhaled corticosteroid (e.g., 88–264, 88–176, or 176 mcg of fluticasone propionate [or its equivalent] daily via a metered-dose inhaler in adolescents and adults, children 5–11 years of age, or children 4 years of age or younger, respectively) as first-line therapy for persistent asthma (e.g., patients with daytime symptoms of asthma more than twice per week, but less than once daily, and nocturnal symptoms of asthma 3–4 times per month), supplemented by as-needed use of a short-acting, inhaled β_2-agonist.

Moderate Persistent Asthma

According to current asthma management guidelines, therapy with a long-acting β_2-agonist such as salmeterol or formoterol generally is recommended in adults and adolescents who have moderate persistent asthma and daily asthma symptoms that are inadequately controlled following addition of low-dose inhaled corticosteroids to as-needed inhaled β_2-agonist treatment. However, the National Asthma Education and Prevention Program (NAEPP) recommends that the beneficial effects of long-acting inhaled β_2-agonists should be weighed carefully against the increased risk (although uncommon) of severe asthma exacerbations and asthma-related deaths associated with daily use of such agents. (See Asthma-related Death and Life-threatening Events under Cautions: Respiratory Effects, in Salmeterol 12:12.08.12.) Current asthma management guidelines also state that an alternative, but equally preferred option for management of moderate persistent asthma that is not adequately controlled with a low dosage of inhaled corticosteroid is to increase the maintenance dosage to a medium dosage (e.g., exceeding 264 but not more than 440 mcg of fluticasone propionate [or its equivalent] daily via a metered-dose inhaler in adults and adolescents).

In children 5–11 years of age with moderate persistent asthma that is not controlled with a low dosage of an inhaled corticosteroid, a long-acting inhaled β_2-agonist (i.e., salmeterol, formoterol), a leukotriene modifier (i.e., montelukast, zafirlukast), or extended-release theophylline (with appropriate monitoring) may be added to low-dose inhaled corticosteroid therapy; another preferred option according to current asthma management guidelines is to increase the maintenance dosage of the inhaled corticosteroid to a medium dosage (e.g., exceeding 176 but not more than 352 mcg of fluticasone propionate [or its equivalent] daily via a metered-dose inhaler). In infants and children 4 years of age or younger with moderate persistent asthma that is not controlled by a low dosage of an inhaled corticosteroid, the only preferred option is to increase the maintenance dosage of the inhaled corticosteroid to a medium dosage (e.g., exceeding 176 but not more than 352 mcg of fluticasone propionate [or its equivalent] daily via a metered-dose inhaler).

Severe Persistent Asthma

Maintenance therapy with an inhaled corticosteroid at medium or high dosages (e.g., exceeding 440 mcg of fluticasone propionate [or its equivalent] daily in adults and adolescents or 352 mcg of the drug daily in children 5–11 years of age via a metered-dose inhaler) and adjunctive therapy with a long-acting inhaled β_2-agonist is the preferred treatment according to current asthma management guidelines for adults and children 5 years of age or older with severe persistent asthma (i.e., continuous daytime asthma symptoms, nighttime symptoms 7 times per week). In infants and children 4 years of age or younger with severe asthma, maintenance therapy with an inhaled corticosteroid at medium or high dosages (e.g., exceeding 352 mcg of fluticasone propionate or its equivalent daily via a metered-dose inhaler) and adjunctive therapy with either a long-acting inhaled β_2-agonist or montelukast is the only preferred treatment according to current asthma management guidelines.

Poorly Controlled Asthma

If asthma symptoms in patients with moderate to severe asthma are very poorly controlled (i.e., at least 2–3 exacerbations per year requiring oral corticosteroids), a short course of an oral corticosteroid (3–10 days) may be added to gain prompt control of asthma. Regular use of oral corticosteroids as add-on therapy in adults and children 5 years of age or older with severe asthma who are inadequately controlled with high-dose inhaled corticosteroid, intermittent oral corticosteroid therapy, and a long-acting inhaled β_2-agonist bronchodilator is suggested, based on consensus and clinical experience. A short (2-week) course of oral corticosteroids may be considered to confirm clinical response prior to implementing long-term therapy with these agents. Once long-term oral corticosteroid therapy is initiated, the lowest possible effective dosage (i.e., alternate-day or once-daily administration) should be used, and the patient should be monitored carefully for adverse effects. Once asthma is well-controlled, repeated attempts should be made to reduce the oral corticosteroid dosage. (See Asthma under Uses: Respiratory Diseases, in the Corticosteroids General Statement 68:04.) Use of orally inhaled fluticasone propionate as adjunctive therapy in patients who require chronic administration of systemic corticosteroids to control asthma symptoms may permit a reduction in dosage or discontinuance of systemic corticosteroids. When used in recommended dosages in responsive patients, fluticasone propionate oral inhalation may permit control of asthmatic symptoms with less suppression of hypothalamic-pituitary-adrenal (HPA) function than therapeutically equivalent oral dosages of prednisone. For additional details on the stepped-care approach to drug therapy in asthma, see Asthma under Uses: Bronchospasm, in Albuterol 12:12.08.12 and see Asthma under Uses: Respiratory Diseases, in the Corticosteroids General Statement 68:04.

Clinical Experience with Fluticasone Propionate

Well-controlled clinical studies have shown that oral inhalation of fluticasone propionate relieves symptoms of bronchial asthma (cough, dyspnea, wheezing) and improves pulmonary function. Although substantial improvement may occur within the first day of therapy, optimum symptomatic relief may require at least 1–2 weeks of continuous fluticasone propionate oral inhalation therapy. In corticosteroid-dependent patients, use of fluticasone propionate oral inhalation therapy may permit a substantial reduction in the daily maintenance dosage of the systemic corticosteroid and gradual discontinuance of corticosteroid maintenance dosages.

In several randomized, double-blind, placebo-controlled clinical trials in adults or children with mild to severe persistent asthma, fluticasone propionate (50, 100, 250, 500, or 1000 mcg twice daily) powder for oral inhalation produced greater improvement in pulmonary function (e.g., mean percent change from baseline in forced expiratory volume in 1 second [FEV_1] or morning or evening peak expiratory flow [PEF]) than placebo. Data from an open-label extension study in pediatric patients (4–11 years of age) with mild to moderate persistent asthma indicate that fluticasone propionate (100 mcg twice daily or 200 mcg once daily) maintained improvement in lung function for up to 1 year.

In several randomized, double-blind, placebo-controlled clinical trials in patients with mild to severe asthma, fluticasone propionate (100, 250, or 500 mcg) in fixed combination with salmeterol xinafoate (50 mcg as salmeterol) for oral inhalation produced greater improvement in most indices of pulmonary function (e.g., mean percent change from baseline in FEV_1, morning FEV_1, or PEF) than either drug alone and similar efficacy as concurrent therapy with both agents given separately. Additional randomized, double-blind, comparative trials in patients with mild to moderate persistent asthma who were not optimally controlled with their current antiasthma therapy, the fixed combination of fluticasone propionate 90, 230, or 460 mcg twice daily and salmeterol (42 mcg twice daily) with a hydrofluoroalkane propellant (HFA) for oral inhalation via a metered-dose inhaler (Advair® HFA) produced greater improvement in indices of pulmonary function (e.g., mean percent change from baseline in FEV_1 or morning and evening PEF) than either drug alone.

Chronic Obstructive Pulmonary Disease

Fluticasone propionate in fixed combination with salmeterol xinafoate as the inhalation powder (Advair® Diskus®) is used for the maintenance treatment of airflow obstruction in patients with chronic obstructive pulmonary disease (COPD), including chronic bronchitis and/or emphysema. Fluticasone propionate in fixed combination with salmeterol xinafoate as the inhalation powder (Advair® Diskus®) also is used to reduce exacerbations of COPD in patients with a history of such exacerbations. Fluticasone propionate in fixed combination with salmeterol xinafoate is *not* indicated for the relief of acute bronchospasm.

In several randomized, double-blind, placebo-controlled studies of 6 or 12 months' duration in patients with COPD, orally inhaled fluticasone propionate (250 or 500 mcg twice daily) in fixed combination with salmeterol (50 mcg twice daily) as the inhalation powder produced greater improvement in lung function (defined as predose and postdose FEV_1) than either drug alone or placebo. The improvement in lung function with fluticasone propionate 500 mcg and salmeterol 50 mcg in fixed combination was similar to that observed with fluticasone propionate 250 mcg and salmeterol 50 mcg in fixed combination. In two randomized, double-blind studies of 12 months' duration in patients with COPD, orally inhaled fluticasone propionate (250 mcg twice daily) in fixed combination with salmeterol (50 mcg twice daily) as the inhalation powder produced a greater reduction in the annual incidence of moderate/severe COPD exacerbations and exacerbations requiring treatment with oral corticosteroids compared with salmeterol alone. No studies have been conducted to directly compare the efficacy of fluticasone propionate 250 mcg and salmeterol 50 mcg in fixed combination with fluticasone propionate 500 mcg and salmeterol 50 mcg in fixed combination in reducing exacerbations; however, in clinical studies, the reduction in exacerbations observed with fluticasone propionate 500 mcg and salmeterol 50 mcg in fixed combination was not greater than the reduction in exacerbations observed with fluticasone propionate 250 mcg and salmeterol 50 mcg in fixed combination. In a double-blind, placebo-controlled study of 3 years' duration in patients with COPD, orally inhaled fluticasone propionate (500 mcg) in fixed combination with salmeterol (50 mcg) as the inhalation powder did not improve all-cause mortality compared with either drug alone or placebo. Fluticasone propionate 250 mcg and salmeterol 50 mcg in fixed combination twice daily is the only recommended dosage for the treatment of COPD; an efficacy advantage of the higher dosage of the fixed combination (500 mcg of fluticasone propionate and 50 mcg of salmeterol) over the lower dosage (250 mcg of fluticasone propionate and 50 mcg of salmeterol) has not been established.

● Other Uses

Fluticasone also has been administered as oral tablets (formulation currently not commercially available in the US) in the management of ulcerative colitis†, Crohn's disease†, and celiac sprue†.

DOSAGE AND ADMINISTRATION

● General

Dosage of fluticasone propionate alone or in fixed combination with salmeterol xinafoate should be adjusted carefully according to individual requirements and response. The recommended initial and maximum dosages of fluticasone propionate for oral inhalation are based on previous asthma therapy. The recommended initial dosage of the inhalation powder preparation containing fluticasone propionate in fixed combination with salmeterol (Advair® Diskus®) is based on the patient's asthma severity, and the recommended initial dosage of the inhalation aerosol containing fluticasone propionate in fixed combination with salmeterol

(Advair® HFA) is based on the patient's current asthma therapy. The lowest effective dosage of fluticasone should be achieved, particularly in children, since inhaled corticosteroids have the potential to affect growth.

● Administration

Fluticasone propionate alone and in fixed combination with salmeterol is administered as a microcrystalline suspension by oral inhalation using an oral aerosol inhaler with hydrofluoroalkane (HFA; non-chlorofluorocarbon) propellant or as the inhalation powder using the Diskus® device that delivers the drug from foil-wrapped blisters. Fluticasone propionate in fixed combination with salmeterol xinafoate is also administered as an inhalation powder using the Diskus® device that delivers the drugs from foil-wrapped blisters.

Oral Inhalation via Aerosol Inhaler

The fluticasone propionate HFA inhalation aerosol canister should be shaken well for 5 seconds immediately prior to use. The fluticasone propionate HFA aerosol canister should be used only with the supplied actuator (inhaler). The aerosol inhaler should be actuated 4 times prior to the initial use of fluticasone propionate. In addition, the inhaler should be shaken well for 5 seconds and actuated once prior to use if it has not been used for longer than 1 week or if the inhaler has been dropped. Patients should exhale slowly and completely and place the mouthpiece of the inhaler well into the mouth with lips closed around it. Patients should inhale slowly and deeply through the mouth while actuating the inhaler. Patients should hold their breath for up to 10 seconds, withdraw the mouthpiece from the mouth, and then exhale slowly. Subsequent actuations of the aerosol inhaler should be performed 30 seconds after the previous inhalation. Following each treatment, the patient should rinse the mouth thoroughly. The inhaler should be cleaned at least once a week after the evening dose by removing the mouthpiece cap from the inhaler and washing the mouthpiece with moistened cotton; the actuator should be allowed to air-dry overnight. When the dose counter on the inhaler reads "020", the patient should contact the pharmacy for a refill or consult their clinician to determine whether a refill is needed. The inhaler should be discarded when the dose counter reads "000". The canister should never be immersed in water to determine the amount of drug remaining in the canister ("float test").

Fluticasone propionate/salmeterol inhalation aerosol (Advair® HFA) should only be used with the actuator provided with the product. Before each inhalation, the inhaler must be shaken well for 5 seconds. The aerosol inhaler should be test sprayed 4 times into the air (away from the face) before initial use, and shaken well for 5 seconds before each spray. If the inhaler has not been used for more than 4 weeks or if the inhaler was dropped, the inhaler should be test sprayed twice into the air (away from the face) and shaken well for 5 seconds before each spray.

The cap covering the mouthpiece should be removed; the strap on the cap will stay attached to the actuator. The patient should look for foreign objects inside the inhaler prior to use and verify that the canister is fully inserted into the actuator. After exhaling as completely as possible, the patient should place the mouthpiece of the inhaler well into the mouth and close the lips firmly around it. Then the patient should inhale slowly and deeply through the mouth while actuating the inhaler. The patient should remove the mouthpiece from the mouth and hold the breath for as long as possible, up to 10 seconds, and then exhale normally. It is recommended that 30 seconds should elapse between inhalations. Rinsing the mouth thoroughly after inhalation of fluticasone propionate/salmeterol inhalation aerosol and spitting out the water are advised. The opening for the spray of the metal canister should be wiped dry with a dry cotton swab and the mouthpiece should be wiped clean with a dampened tissue at least once a week after the evening dose. The actuator should be allowed to air-dry overnight. When the dose counter on the inhaler reads "020," the patient should contact the pharmacy for a refill or consult their clinician to determine whether a refill is needed. The inhaler should be discarded when the dose counter reads "000." The counter should never be altered or removed from the canister.

Oral Inhalation via Dry Powder Inhaler

The oral inhalation powder of fluticasone propionate alone or in fixed combination with salmeterol xinafoate is administered using a special preloaded oral inhaler (Diskus®). To obtain optimal benefit, the patient should be given a copy of the patient instructions or medication guide provided by the manufacturer with Flovent® Diskus® or Advair® Diskus®, respectively. Children should use Flovent® Diskus® or Advair® Diskus® under adult supervision as instructed by a clinician. The patient should hold the Diskus® device in one hand, put the thumb of the other hand on the thumbgrip, and push the thumbgrip until the mouthpiece appears and snaps into position. The lever on the Diskus® should then be depressed in a direction away from the patient while the inhaler is held in a level, horizontal position until a click is heard; the lever pierces the foil blister and releases the powdered drug into an exit port. To avoid releasing and wasting additional doses of the drug, the patient should not tilt or close the Diskus® device, play with the lever, or advance the lever more than once at this point. A dose counter will advance each time the lever is depressed.

Before inhaling the dose, the patient should exhale as completely as possible; the patient should *not* exhale into the Diskus® device because pressure from the exhalation will interfere with proper inhaler operation. The patient should then place the mouthpiece of the inhaler between the lips and inhale deeply and quickly through the inhaler with a steady, even breath; pressure from the inhalation will disperse drug from the exit port into the air stream created by the patient's inhalation. The patient should remove the inhaler from the mouth, hold his or her breath for a few seconds (i.e., 10 seconds), and then exhale slowly. While patients may or may not taste or feel a dose of drug delivered from the Diskus® device, they should be instructed not to use an extra dose even if they do not perceive that the dose has been delivered. Rinsing the mouth after inhalation of fluticasone propionate alone or in fixed combination with salmeterol is advised. The Diskus® device may be closed and reset for the next dose by sliding the thumbgrip towards the patient as far as it will go. The inhaler should not be washed but should be stored in a dry place away from direct heat or sunlight. The Flovent® Diskus® inhaler should be discarded when every blister has been used (when the dose indicator reads "0") or 6 weeks after removal from its foil overwrap pouch. The Advair® Diskus® inhaler should be discarded when every blister has been used or 1 month after removal from its foil overwrap pouch, whichever comes first. The inhaler should not be taken apart.

● *Dosage*

Unless otherwise stated, the dose of fluticasone propionate administered as an aerosol via metered-dose inhaler with a hydrofluoroalkane (HFA) propellant is expressed as the amount of drug delivered from the actuator of the inhaler per metered spray; the dose of fluticasone propionate (and of salmeterol in the combination preparation Advair®) administered as an oral inhalation powder is expressed as the nominal (labeled) dose contained in each foil-wrapped blister. The manufacturer states that spacer devices should not be used with Advair® or Flovent® Diskus®.

Each actuation of the commercially available fluticasone propionate HFA oral inhalation aerosol labeled as containing 44, 110, or 220 mcg of fluticasone propionate per metered spray delivers 50, 125, or 250 mcg from the valve, respectively, and 44, 110, or 220 mcg from the actuator, respectively. The 10.6-g (labeled as containing 44 mcg of fluticasone propionate) or 12-g canister (labeled as containing 110 or 220 mcg of fluticasone propionate) delivers 120 metered sprays of fluticasone propionate.

Each actuation of the oral aerosol inhaler containing the fixed combination of fluticasone propionate and salmeterol xinafoate delivers 50, 125, or 250 mcg of fluticasone propionate and 25 mcg of salmeterol from the valve. Dosages of fluticasone propionate and salmeterol in the fixed-combination inhalation aerosol are expressed in terms of drug delivered from the mouthpiece; each actuation of the inhaler delivers 45, 115, or 230 mcg of fluticasone propionate and 21 mcg of salmeterol from the mouthpiece. The commercially available inhalation aerosol of fluticasone propionate in fixed combination with salmeterol delivers 60 or 120 metered sprays per 8- or 12-g canister, respectively.

With commercially available fluticasone propionate inhalation powder (Flovent® Diskus®, Advair® Diskus®) delivered via the Diskus® device, the amount of drug delivered to the lungs depends on factors such as the patient's inspiratory flow. Using standardized in vitro testing at a flow rate of 60 L per minute for 2 seconds, the Flovent® Diskus® labeled as containing 50, 100, or 250 mcg of fluticasone propionate delivers 46, 94, or 235 mcg of fluticasone propionate, respectively. In adults with obstructive lung disease and severely compromised lung function (FEV₁ 20–30% of predicted), mean peak inspiratory flow through the Diskus® device was 82.4 L/minute. In children 4 and 8 years of age with asthma, mean peak inspiratory flow through the Diskus® device was 70 and 104 L/minute, respectively. Using standardized in vitro testing at a flow rate of 60 L per minute for 2 seconds, the Advair® Diskus® device delivered 93, 233, and 465 mcg of fluticasone propionate and 45 mcg of salmeterol per activation from a Diskus® labeled as containing 100, 250, or 500 mcg of fluticasone propionate and 50 mcg of salmeterol, respectively. In adults with obstructive lung disease and severely compromised lung function (FEV₁ 20–30% of predicted), mean peak inspiratory flow through

the Diskus® device was 82.4 L/minute for Advair®. In adults and adolescents with asthma, mean peak inspiratory flow through the Diskus® device was 122.2 L/minute. In a group of children 4 years of age, mean peak inspiratory flow through the Advair® Diskus® device averaged 75.5 L/minute; in children 8 years of age, mean peak inspiratory flow averaged 107.3 L/minute.

Asthma
Fluticasone Propionate

When the fluticasone propionate HFA oral inhalation aerosol is used, the initial, maintenance, and maximum dosage in children 4–11 years of age is 88 mcg twice daily. The recommended initial dosage of fluticasone propionate for adults and adolescents 12 years of age or older who previously were receiving bronchodilators alone is 88 mcg twice daily; the maximum recommended dosage is 440 mcg twice daily. In adults and adolescents 12 years of age or older who previously were receiving inhaled corticosteroids, the recommended initial dosages of fluticasone propionate, using the HFA oral inhalation aerosol, are 88–220 mcg twice daily; the maximum recommended dosage is 440 mcg twice daily. Initial dosages exceeding 88 mcg twice daily should be considered in patients with poorer asthma control or in those who were receiving inhaled corticosteroids at the higher end of the dosing range. In adults and adolescents 12 years of age or older who previously were receiving oral corticosteroids, the recommended initial and maximum dosage of fluticasone propionate, using the HFA oral inhalation aerosol, is 440 and 880 mcg twice daily, respectively. If control of asthma is inadequate after 2 weeks of therapy at the initial dosage, replacing the current strength with a higher strength may provide additional asthma control.

When fluticasone propionate inhalation powder is administered via the Diskus® device, the recommended initial dosage of fluticasone propionate in adults and adolescents 12 years of age or older who previously were receiving bronchodilators alone is 100 mcg twice daily; the maximum recommended dosage is 500 mcg twice daily. In adults and adolescents 12 years of age or older who previously were receiving inhaled corticosteroids, the recommended initial dosage of fluticasone propionate using the inhalation powder (administered via a Diskus®) is 100–250 mcg twice daily; the maximum recommended dosage is 500 mcg twice daily. Initial dosages exceeding 100 mcg twice daily should be considered in patients with poorer asthma control or in those who were receiving inhaled corticosteroids at the higher end of the dosing range. In adults and adolescents 12 years of age or older who previously were receiving oral corticosteroids, the recommended initial dosage of fluticasone propionate using the powdered drug is 500–1000 mcg twice daily (administered via the Diskus® device); the maximum recommended dosage for the Diskus® device is 1000 mcg twice daily.

When the fluticasone propionate inhalation powder is administered via the Diskus® device in children 4 to younger than 12 years of age who previously were receiving bronchodilators alone or with inhaled corticosteroids, the recommended initial dosage of fluticasone propionate is 50 mcg twice daily; the recommended maximum dosage is 100 mcg twice daily. Initial dosages exceeding 50 mcg twice daily should be considered in children with poorer asthma control or in those who were receiving inhaled corticosteroids at the higher end of the dosing range. Because patient responses may vary, pediatric patients previously maintained on fluticasone propionate inhalation powder administered via the Diskhaler® (50 or 100 mcg twice daily) may require dosage adjustments upon transfer to the drug administered via the Diskus® device.

Conversion to Orally Inhaled Therapy in Patients Receiving Systemic Corticosteroids

When orally inhaled corticosteroids are administered to patients receiving systemic corticosteroids, the patient's asthma should be reasonably stable before treatment with the oral inhalation begins. Initially, fluticasone propionate inhalation powder is given concurrently with the maintenance dosage of the systemic corticosteroid. The manufacturer suggests that in patients who were receiving prior oral corticosteroid therapy, reduction of oral corticosteroid dosage should be initiated at least 1 week after starting fluticasone propionate oral inhalation and decrements usually should not exceed 2.5–5 mg of prednisone (or its equivalent) each week. Once oral corticosteroids are discontinued and symptoms of asthma have been controlled, the dosage of fluticasone propionate should be titrated to the lowest effective level. The inability to decrease the dosage of oral corticosteroids during systemic corticosteroid withdrawal may indicate the need to increase the dosage of fluticasone propionate up to a maximum of 1000 mcg twice daily. The manufacturer of the oral inhalation powder containing fluticasone propionate in fixed combination with salmeterol (Advair® Diskus®) states that patients requiring oral corticosteroids should be withdrawn slowly from systemic corticosteroid use after transferring to fluticasone propionate in fixed combination with salmeterol inhalation powder. The manufacturer also states that prednisone dosage reduction may be accomplished by reducing the daily dosage of prednisone by 2.5 mg on a weekly basis during therapy with the oral inhalation powder containing fluticasone propionate in fixed combination with salmeterol. The oral inhalation aerosol containing fluticasone propionate in fixed combination with salmeterol (Advair® HFA) should *not* be used to transfer patients from systemic corticosteroid therapy. (See Dosage and Administration in the Corticosteroids General Statement 68:04.) *Particular care is needed in gradually withdrawing systemic corticosteroids following long-term therapy, since death has occurred in some individuals in whom systemic corticosteroids were withdrawn too rapidly.* (See Withdrawal of Systemic Corticosteroid Therapy under Warnings/Precautions: Warnings, in Cautions.)

Fluticasone Propionate/Salmeterol Fixed-combination Therapy

In asthmatic patients 4–11 years of age who are inadequately controlled on an inhaled corticosteroid, the recommended dosage of the commercially available inhalation powder preparation containing fluticasone propionate in fixed combination with salmeterol (Advair® Diskus®) is 100 mcg of fluticasone propionate and 50 mcg of salmeterol (1 inhalation) twice daily, given approximately 12 hours apart (morning and evening).

In asthmatic patients 12 years of age or older, the recommended initial dosage of the commercially available inhalation powder preparation containing fluticasone propionate in fixed combination with salmeterol (Advair® Diskus®) is based on the patient's asthma severity. The dosage of the inhalation powder fixed-combination preparation is 100, 250, or 500 mcg of fluticasone propionate and 50 mcg of salmeterol (1 inhalation) twice daily, given approximately 12 hours apart (morning and evening). The maximum recommended dosage of fluticasone propionate in fixed combination with salmeterol is 500 mcg of fluticasone propionate and 50 mcg of salmeterol twice daily. The manufacturer states that administration of the inhalation powder containing fluticasone propionate in fixed combination with salmeterol more frequently than twice daily or exceeding 1 inhalation twice daily is not recommended.

In asthmatic patients 12 years of age or older, the recommended initial dosage of the inhalation aerosol containing fluticasone propionate in fixed combination with salmeterol (Advair® HFA) is based on the patient's current asthma therapy. The dosage of the inhalation aerosol fixed-combination preparation is 90, 230, or 460 mcg of fluticasone propionate and 42 mcg of salmeterol (2 inhalations) twice daily, given approximately 12 hours apart (morning and evening). The maximum recommended dosage of fluticasone propionate is 460 mcg in fixed combination with 42 mcg of salmeterol (2 inhalations) twice daily. The manufacturer states that administration of the inhalation aerosol containing fluticasone propionate in fixed combination with salmeterol more frequently than twice daily or exceeding 2 inhalations twice daily is not recommended.

If control of asthma is inadequate after 2 weeks of therapy at the initial dosage, replacing the current strength of the fixed combination with a higher strength (higher strengths contain higher dosages of fluticasone propionate only) may provide additional asthma control. Patients receiving the fixed combination of fluticasone propionate and salmeterol twice daily should not use additional salmeterol or other long-acting β_2-adrenergic agonists (e.g., formoterol) for any reason, including the treatment of asthma or prevention of exercise-induced bronchospasm. Patients also should be advised not to discontinue fluticasone propionate in fixed combination with salmeterol without medical supervision, as symptoms may recur after treatment discontinuance. If a previously effective dosage of fluticasone propionate in fixed combination with salmeterol fails to provide adequate improvement in asthma control, the therapeutic regimen should be reevaluated and additional therapeutic options should be considered (e.g., increasing the strength of the fixed combination [higher strengths contain higher dosages of fluticasone propionate only], adding additional inhaled corticosteroids, initiating systemic corticosteroids). The manufacturer warns that therapy with the fixed combination of fluticasone propionate and salmeterol should *not* be initiated in patients during rapidly deteriorating or potentially life-threatening episodes of asthma. (See Respiratory Effects under Cautions: Warnings/Precautions and also see Cautions: Precautions and Contraindications, in Salmeterol 12:12.08.12.)

Chronic Obstructive Pulmonary Disease
Fluticasone Propionate/Salmeterol Fixed-combination Therapy

For maintenance therapy of COPD, the recommended dosage of fluticasone propionate in fixed combination with salmeterol (Advair® Diskus®) in adults

is 250 mcg of fluticasone propionate and 50 mcg of salmeterol (1 inhalation) twice daily, given approximately every 12 hours (morning and evening). If shortness of breath occurs between doses, an inhaled, short-acting β_2-agonist should be used for immediate relief. Higher dosages of salmeterol in fixed combination with fluticasone propionate (e.g., 500 mcg of fluticasone propionate and 50 mcg of salmeterol twice daily) do not result in additional benefit and are not recommended. Patients receiving fluticasone propionate in fixed combination with salmeterol should not use additional salmeterol or other long-acting β_2-agonists (e.g., arformoterol, formoterol) for any reason, including the treatment of COPD.

● Special Populations

The following information addresses dosage of fluticasone propionate in special populations. When fluticasone propionate is used in fixed combination with salmeterol, dosage requirements for salmeterol should be considered.

Dosage of fluticasone propionate HFA inhalation aerosol in geriatric patients should be selected with caution, reflecting the greater frequency of decreased hepatic function, presence of coexisting conditions, or other drug therapies in such patients. Dosage adjustments based solely on age are not recommended in geriatric patients receiving fluticasone propionate inhalation powder alone or fluticasone propionate inhalation powder or aerosol in fixed combination with salmeterol.

CAUTIONS

● Contraindications

Primary treatment of severe acute asthmatic attacks or status asthmaticus when intensive measures (e.g., oxygen, parenteral bronchodilators, IV corticosteroids) are required.

Fluticasone propionate in fixed combination with salmeterol is contraindicated as primary treatment of status asthmaticus or other acute episodes of asthma or chronic obstructive pulmonary disease (COPD) when intensive measures are required.

Known hypersensitivity to fluticasone propionate or any ingredient (e.g., milk protein) in the formulation.

When fluticasone propionate is used in fixed combination with salmeterol, contraindications associated with salmeterol should be considered.

● Warnings/Precautions
Warnings
Use of Fixed Combinations

When preparations containing fluticasone propionate in fixed combination with salmeterol are used, the usual cautions, precautions, and contraindications associated with salmeterol should be considered. Cautionary information applicable to specific populations (e.g., pregnant or nursing women, individuals with hepatic or renal impairment, geriatric patients) should be considered for each drug in the fixed combination.

Serious Asthma-related Events

Monotherapy with long-acting β_2-adrenergic agonists, such as salmeterol, a component of Advair® Diskus® and Advair® HFA, increases the risk of asthma-related death. Data from a large (approximately 26,000 patients), placebo-controlled study (Salmeterol Multi-center Asthma Research Trial [SMART]) evaluating the safety of salmeterol in patients with asthma showed an increase in asthma-related deaths in those receiving the drug. Results of a post hoc analysis revealed a statistically significant greater risk of asthma-related deaths or life-threatening experiences with salmeterol therapy in African-American patients and in patients not receiving concomitant inhaled corticosteroid therapy (53% of study patients) compared with placebo. In addition, available data from controlled clinical trials suggest that monotherapy with long-acting β_2-adrenergic agonists increases the risk of asthma-related hospitalization in pediatric and adolescent patients. (See Asthma-related Death and Life-threatening Events under Cautions: Respiratory Effects, in Salmeterol 12:12.08.12.)

However, FDA has concluded that there is no clinically important increased risk of serious asthma-related events, including hospitalization, intubation, or death, associated with concomitant use of long-acting β_2-adrenergic agonists (e.g., salmeterol) and inhaled corticosteroids (e.g., fluticasone) compared with inhaled corticosteroids alone based on the results of several large clinical studies. In addition, these studies showed that combination therapy with long-acting β_2-adrenergic agonists and inhaled corticosteroids was more effective in reducing the incidence of asthma exacerbations (i.e., events requiring use of systemic corticosteroids for at least 3 outpatient days or an asthma-related hospitalization or emergency department visit requiring use of systemic corticosteroids) compared with use of inhaled corticosteroids alone. (See Asthma-related Death and Life-Threatening Events under Cautions: Respiratory Effects, in Salmeterol 12:12.08.12.)

In the treatment of asthma, the fixed combination of fluticasone propionate and salmeterol xinafoate is used only in patients who have not responded adequately to long-term asthma controller therapy, such as inhaled corticosteroids, or whose disease severity clearly warrants initiation of treatment with both an inhaled corticosteroid and a long-acting β_2-adrenergic agonist. (See Asthma under Uses: Bronchospasm.)

Withdrawal of Systemic Corticosteroid Therapy

The fixed combination of fluticasone propionate and salmeterol xinafoate as the inhalation aerosol (Advair® HFA) should not be used for transferring patients from systemic corticosteroid therapy. In patients being switched from systemic corticosteroids to orally inhaled fluticasone propionate, systemic corticosteroid therapy should be withdrawn gradually and patients should be monitored during dosage reduction for objective signs of adrenal insufficiency (e.g., hypotension, fatigue, lassitude, weakness, nausea, vomiting) since a life-threatening exacerbation of asthma or adrenal insufficiency could occur. Lung function (FEV$_1$ or morning PEF), adjunctive β_2-adrenergic agonist use, and asthma symptoms should be carefully monitored during withdrawal of systemic corticosteroid therapy. *In most patients, several months are required for total recovery of HPA function following withdrawal of systemic corticosteroid therapy.* Patients who have been previously maintained on a corticosteroid dosage equivalent to 20 mg or more of prednisone daily may be most susceptible to adrenal insufficiency, particularly when systemic corticosteroids have been almost completely withdrawn. Corticosteroid withdrawal symptoms (e.g., joint pain, muscular pain, fatigue, lassitude, depression) may occur. Acute adrenal insufficiency may occur during exposure to trauma, surgery, or infection (particularly gastroenteritis or other conditions associated with acute electrolyte loss). Clinicians should be alert for the potential for eosinophilia, vasculitic rash, worsening of pulmonary symptoms, cardiac complications, and/or neuropathy consistent with Churg-Strauss syndrome; or unmasking of conditions previously controlled by systemic corticosteroid therapy (e.g., rhinitis, conjunctivitis, eczema, arthritis, eosinophilic conditions).

Immunosuppressed Patients

Patients who become immunosuppressed while receiving corticosteroids have increased susceptibility to infections compared with healthy individuals, and certain infections (e.g., varicella [chickenpox], measles) can have a more serious or even fatal outcome in such patients, particularly in children. Patients receiving corticosteroids who are potentially immunosuppressed should be warned of the risk of exposure to certain infections (e.g., chickenpox, measles) and of the importance of obtaining medical advice if such exposure occurs. Such patients should take particular care to avoid exposure to these infections. If exposure to varicella (chickenpox) or measles occurs in susceptible patients, administration of varicella zoster immune globulin (VZIG) or pooled immune globulin (IG), respectively, should be considered. If chickenpox develops, treatment with an antiviral agent should be considered. For additional information, see Cautions: Increased Susceptibility to Infection and also see Cautions: Precautions and Contraindications, in the Corticosteroids General Statement 68:04.

Bronchospasm

As with other inhaled drugs for asthma, bronchospasm may occur, resulting in an immediate increase in wheezing following oral inhalation of fluticasone propionate. If bronchospasm occurs, appropriate treatment (e.g., use of a short-acting β_2-adrenergic agonist) should be instituted immediately and fluticasone propionate therapy should be discontinued.

Acute Exacerbations of Asthma or Chronic Obstructive Pulmonary Disease

Therapy with the fixed combination of fluticasone propionate and salmeterol xinafoate should not be initiated in patients with substantially worsening or acutely deteriorating asthma or acute symptoms of chronic obstructive pulmonary disease (COPD). Failure to respond to a previously effective dosage of fluticasone propionate in fixed combination with salmeterol xinafoate may indicate substantially worsening asthma or COPD that requires reevaluation. If inadequate control of symptoms

persists with supplemental β_2-agonist bronchodilator therapy (i.e., if there is a need to increase the dose or frequency of administration of the short-acting bronchodilator) or an appreciable decrease in lung function (e.g., peak expiratory flow [PEF]) occurs, prompt reevaluation of asthma therapy is required; however, extra/increased doses of salmeterol or other long-acting inhaled β_2-agonists (e.g., formoterol) should not be used in such situations or for any indication. Such reevaluation may include increasing the strength of the fixed combination (higher strengths contain higher dosages of fluticasone propionate only), adding additional inhaled corticosteroid, or initiating systemic corticosteroids. Patients should not increase the frequency of administration of the fixed combination. (See Cautions: Precautions and Contraindications, in Salmeterol 12:12.08.12.)

Sensitivity Reactions

Immediate hypersensitivity reactions, including urticaria, angioedema, rash, bronchospasm, hypotension, and anaphylaxis, may occur following oral inhalation of fluticasone in fixed combination with salmeterol.

Anaphylactic reactions, including reactions in patients with severe milk protein allergy, have been reported following oral inhalation of powder products containing lactose, such as fluticasone in fixed combination with salmeterol (Advair® Diskus®). (See Cautions: Contraindications.)

General Precautions
Infections

Localized candidal infections of the pharynx have been reported in patients receiving orally inhaled fluticasone propionate therapy. When infection occurs, appropriate local or systemic treatment of the infection may be necessary and/or discontinuance of orally inhaled fluticasone propionate therapy may be required. Inhaled corticosteroid therapy should be used with extreme caution, if at all, in patients with clinical or asymptomatic *Mycobacterium tuberculosis* infections of the respiratory tract; untreated fungal, bacterial, or parasitic infections; or ocular herpes simplex or untreated systemic viral infections. Clinicians should remain vigilant for the possible development of pneumonia in patients with COPD who are receiving the inhalation powder preparation containing fluticasone propionate in fixed combination with salmeterol (Advair® Diskus®), since the clinical features of pneumonia and COPD exacerbations frequently overlap. Lower respiratory tract infections, including pneumonia, have been reported in patients with COPD following the administration of inhaled corticosteroids, including fluticasone propionate and the inhalation powder preparation containing fluticasone propionate in fixed combination with salmeterol (Advair® Diskus®).

Ophthalmic Effects

Glaucoma, increased intraocular pressure, and cataracts rarely have been reported in patients receiving orally inhaled corticosteroids, including fluticasone propionate; regular eye examinations should be considered.

Systemic Corticosteroid Effects

Administration of higher than recommended dosages of orally inhaled fluticasone propionate may result in manifestations of hypercorticism and suppression of HPA function. If such changes occur, the dosage of fluticasone propionate should be reduced slowly, consistent with accepted procedures for reducing corticosteroid dosage and management of asthma symptoms. Particular care should be taken in monitoring patients postoperatively or during periods of stress for evidence of inadequate adrenal response.

Musculoskeletal Effects

Long-term use of orally inhaled corticosteroids may affect normal bone metabolism, resulting in a loss of bone mineral density. (See Osteoporosis under Cautions: Musculoskeletal Effects, in the Corticosteroids General Statement 68:04.) In a 2-year study in adults with asthma, orally inhaled fluticasone propionate was not associated with appreciable changes in lumbar spine bone mineral density. The manufacturer of fluticasone propionate in fixed combination with salmeterol states that use of this preparation can pose additional risks in patients with major risk factors for decreased bone mineral density, such as tobacco use, advanced age, sedentary lifestyle, poor nutrition, family history of osteoporosis, or chronic use of drugs that can reduce bone mass (e.g., anticonvulsants, corticosteroids). Since patients with chronic obstructive pulmonary disease (COPD) often have multiple risk factors for reduced bone mineral density, assessment of bone mineral density is recommended prior to initiation of therapy and periodically thereafter. If appreciable reductions in bone mineral density are seen and use of fluticasone propionate and salmeterol in fixed combination is considered to be important for the patient's COPD therapy, use of agents to treat or prevent osteoporosis should be strongly considered.

Specific Populations

Pregnancy

Category C. (See Users Guide.)

Lactation

While it is not known whether fluticasone propionate is distributed into milk in humans, the drug is distributed into milk in rats. In addition, other corticosteroids are distributed into milk. Data also are not available on the effects of the drug on the breast-fed child or on milk production. Since data are not available on the use of fluticasone propionate oral inhalation aerosol in nursing women, caution is advised if the drug is administered in nursing women. The benefits of breast-feeding should be considered along with the woman's clinical need for fluticasone propionate oral inhalation and any potential adverse effects on the breast-fed child from the drug or underlying maternal condition.

Pediatric Use

Safety and efficacy of fluticasone propionate inhalation aerosol or powder alone in children younger than 4 years of age have not been established. Safety and efficacy of the inhalation powder containing fluticasone propionate in fixed combination with salmeterol (Advair® Diskus®) in children younger than 4 years of age have not been established. Safety and efficacy of the inhalation aerosol containing fluticasone propionate in fixed combination with salmeterol (Advair® HFA) in children younger than 12 years of age have not been established. Use of the inhalation powder containing fluticasone propionate in children 4–11 years of age is supported by data from several clinical trials. Use of fluticasone propionate inhalation aerosol or the inhalation powder containing fluticasone propionate in fixed combination with salmeterol (Advair® Diskus®) in children 4–11 years of age is supported by data from several clinical trials and by extrapolation of efficacy data from older patients. The adverse effect profile of Flovent® HFA in pediatric patients (4–11 years of age) generally is similar to that observed in adolescents and adults.

Use of corticosteroids or inadequate control of chronic diseases (e.g., asthma) may lead to suppression of growth in children and adolescents. Therefore, children receiving prolonged therapy with orally inhaled fluticasone propionate should be monitored periodically (e.g., via stadiometry) for possible adverse effects on growth and development. The benefits of corticosteroid therapy should be weighed against the possibility of growth suppression and the risks associated with alternative therapies. Children should be maintained on the lowest possible dosage of fluticasone propionate that controls asthma symptoms. (See Cautions: Pediatric Precautions, in the Corticosteroids General Statement 68:04.)

Geriatric Use

Although no overall differences in safety and efficacy of orally inhaled fluticasone propionate alone or fluticasone propionate in fixed combination with salmeterol as the inhalation aerosol (Advair® HFA) were observed relative to younger adults, the possibility that some older patients may exhibit increased sensitivity to the drug cannot be ruled out. Experience with the inhalation powder containing fluticasone propionate in fixed combination with salmeterol (Advair® Diskus®) in those 65 years of age or older with asthma is insufficient to determine whether geriatric patients respond differently than younger patients. In clinical studies evaluating the inhalation powder containing fluticasone propionate in fixed combination with salmeterol for COPD, patients 65 years of age or older experienced a higher incidence of serious adverse effects compared with those younger than 65 years of age, although the distribution of adverse effects was similar in the two groups. Dosage of fluticasone propionate HFA inhalation aerosol in geriatric patients should be selected with caution, reflecting the greater frequency of decreased hepatic function, presence of coexisting conditions, or other drug therapies in such patients. Dosage adjustments based solely on age are not recommended in geriatric patients receiving fluticasone propionate inhalation powder alone or fluticasone propionate inhalation powder or aerosol in fixed combination with salmeterol.

● Common Adverse Effects

Adverse effects occurring in more than 3% of patients older than 12 years of age receiving fluticasone propionate HFA oral inhalation aerosol in controlled clinical trials include upper respiratory tract infection, headache, throat irritation, upper respiratory inflammation, sinusitis/sinus infection, candidiasis (including oral candidiasis), cough, hoarseness/dysphonia, and bronchitis. Adverse effects

reported in clinical trials with fluticasone propionate HFA inhalation aerosol in pediatric patients (4–11 years of age) generally were similar to those observed in adolescents and adults.

Adverse effects occurring in more than 3% of patients receiving fluticasone propionate oral inhalation powder in controlled clinical trials include upper respiratory tract infection, throat irritation, sinusitis/sinus infection, upper respiratory inflammation, rhinitis, viral respiratory infection, cough, bronchitis, oral candidiasis, nausea and vomiting, GI discomfort and pain, viral GI infection, musculoskeletal pain, muscle injury, headache, fever, and viral infection.

DRUG INTERACTIONS

The following information addresses potential interactions with fluticasone propionate. When fluticasone propionate is used in fixed combination with salmeterol, interactions associated with salmeterol should be considered. No formal drug interaction studies have been performed to date with the fixed-combination preparations containing fluticasone propionate and salmeterol.

● Drugs Affecting Hepatic Microsomal Enzymes

Since fluticasone propionate is metabolized in the liver by the cytochrome P-450 (CYP) 3A4 isoenzyme, concomitant use of drugs that affect cytochrome P-450 hepatic microsomal enzymes could alter the metabolism of fluticasone.

Cushing's syndrome and adrenal suppression have been reported during postmarketing experience in patients receiving concomitant therapy with fluticasone propionate and ritonavir, a highly potent CYP3A4 inhibitor. Concomitant use of ritonavir and fluticasone propionate is not recommended unless the potential benefit is considered to outweigh the risk of systemic corticosteroid adverse effects.

Administration of a single 1-mg dose of orally inhaled fluticasone propionate in healthy individuals receiving ketoconazole (200 mg once daily to steady state) increased mean plasma fluticasone concentrations, resulting in a depression of certain indices of HPA-axis function (as determined by a reduction in area under the plasma cortisol concentration-time curve [AUC]). Care should be exercised when fluticasone propionate is used concomitantly with long-term ketoconazole or other potent isoenzyme CYP3A4 inhibitors.

Concomitant use of fluticasone propionate (500 mcg twice daily) and erythromycin (333 mg 3 times daily) did not affect fluticasone propionate pharmacokinetics.

DESCRIPTION

Fluticasone propionate is a synthetic trifluorinated glucocorticoid. For a discussion of the pharmacology of fluticasone propionate, see Pharmacology in the Corticosteroids General Statement 68:04 and in Fluticasone Propionate 52:08.08.

Bioavailability following oral administration of fluticasone propionate is negligible (less than 1%), principally because of incomplete absorption and presystemic metabolism of the drug. Following oral inhalation, fluticasone propionate is absorbed into systemic circulation from the surface of the lungs; in healthy adults, the systemic bioavailability of the drug was about 18% following oral inhalation of the powder for inhalation (via the Diskus® device). However, results of comparative studies using fluticasone propionate administered orally or by inhalation indicate that the clinical efficacy of the orally inhaled drug appears to result from local action rather than from systemic absorption.

Fluticasone propionate is metabolized in the liver by the cytochrome P-450 (CYP) isoenzyme 3A4; the only identified metabolite is the inactive 17 β-carboxylic acid derivative. Fluticasone propionate is excreted principally in the feces, both as unchanged drug and metabolites. Following oral administration of radiolabeled fluticasone propionate, less than 5% of the administered dose was excreted in urine as metabolites.

ADVICE TO PATIENTS

When fluticasone propionate is used in fixed combination with salmeterol xinafoate, importance of informing patients of important cautionary information about salmeterol xinafoate.

A copy of the manufacturer's patient information (medication guide) for fluticasone propionate in fixed combination with salmeterol (Advair® Diskus® and Advair® HFA) must be provided to all patients with each prescription of the drug. Importance of instructing patients to read the medication guide prior to initiation of therapy and each time the prescription is refilled.

Importance of informing patients receiving the fixed combination of fluticasone propionate and salmeterol xinafoate that monotherapy with long-acting β_2-adrenergic agonists, including salmeterol, a component of Advair® Diskus® and Advair® HFA, increases the risk of asthma-related death and may increase the risk of asthma-related hospitalization in pediatric and adolescent patients.

Importance of instructing patients in the use of oral inhaler and Diskus® devices and providing a copy of the manufacturer's instructions for patients.

Importance of pediatric patients receiving therapy under adult supervision.

Importance of adequate understanding of proper storage, preparation, and inhalation techniques, including use of the inhalation delivery systems.

Importance of rinsing the mouth after oral inhalation.

Importance of advising patients that fluticasone propionate oral inhalation must be used at regular intervals to be therapeutically effective.

Importance of not exceeding the recommended dosage and of contacting a clinician immediately if symptoms of asthma or chronic obstructive pulmonary disease (COPD) occur that are not responsive to bronchodilators.

Importance of advising patients that if a dose of fluticasone propionate alone or in fixed combination with salmeterol is missed, the next dose should be taken at the regularly scheduled time; the dose should not be doubled.

Importance of not discontinuing therapy with fluticasone propionate, alone or in fixed combination with salmeterol, without clinician guidance, as symptoms may recur.

Importance of discontinuing *regular* use of oral or inhaled, short-acting β_2-adrenergic agonists and using inhaled, short-acting β_2-adrenergic agonists only for relief of acute symptoms (e.g., shortness of breath) after initiation of therapy with the fixed combination of fluticasone propionate and salmeterol.

Importance of availability of a short-acting, inhaled β_2-adrenergic agonist for acute asthma symptoms. Importance of informing a clinician if a short-acting, inhaled β_2-adrenergic agonist is not available for use.

Importance of contacting a clinician if decreased effectiveness of a short-acting β_2-adrenergic agonist (exceeding 4 inhalations for greater than 2 consecutive days or 1 canister in an 8-week period) for acute symptoms occurs.

Importance of advising patients that although substantial improvement may occur within the first day of therapy with fluticasone propionate, at least 1–2 weeks or more of continuous therapy may be required for optimum effects.

Importance of advising patients using fluticasone in fixed combination with salmeterol that at least 1 week of therapy may be required for optimum effects to be achieved. Importance of contacting a clinician if asthma symptoms do not improve after 1 week of therapy with the fixed-combination preparation.

Importance of informing patients receiving therapy with the fixed combination of fluticasone propionate and salmeterol regarding common adverse effects associated with β_2-adrenergic agonists such as palpitations, chest pain, rapid heart rate, tremor, or nervousness.

Importance of informing patients that corticosteroids may decrease bone mineral density.

Importance of informing patients that long-term use of inhaled corticosteroids may increase the risk for development of some eye problems (cataracts or glaucoma).

Importance of informing a clinician of heart problems, high blood pressure, seizures, thyroid disorders, diabetes mellitus, liver disorders, osteoporosis, or immune disorders prior to initiation of therapy.

Importance of advising patients that orally inhaled fluticasone propionate should not be used as a bronchodilator and that the drug is not indicated for emergency use (e.g., relief of acute bronchospasm).

Importance of advising patients that additional salmeterol or other long-acting inhaled β_2-adrenergic agonists should not be used for prevention of exercise-induced bronchospasm, treatment of asthma or COPD, or any other reason when the fixed combination of fluticasone propionate and salmeterol xinafoate is used.

Importance of advising patients being transferred from systemic corticosteroid to fluticasone propionate oral inhalation therapy to carry special identification (e.g., card, bracelet) indicating the need for supplementary systemic corticosteroids during periods of stress. Importance of advising such patients that they should immediately resume full therapeutic dosages of systemic corticosteroids and contact their clinician for further instructions during stressful periods (e.g., severe infection, severe asthmatic attack).

Importance of patients avoiding exposure to chickenpox or measles, and, if exposed, of immediately consulting their clinician.

Importance of informing patients with COPD receiving the inhalation powder preparation containing fluticasone propionate in fixed combination with salmeterol (Advair® Diskus®) that they have a higher risk of pneumonia and to contact their clinician if they develop symptoms of pneumonia.

Importance of informing clinicians of existing or contemplated concomitant therapy, including therapy with prescription drugs, particularly ritonavir, other orally inhaled bronchodilators or corticosteroids, OTC drugs, vitamins, or herbal supplements.

Importance of informing clinicians of allergies to fluticasone, salmeterol (in fixed combination), other drugs, or foods.

Importance of women informing clinicians if they are or plan to become pregnant or plan to breast-feed.

Importance of informing patients of other important precautionary information. (See Cautions.)

PREPARATIONS

Excipients in commercially available drug preparations may have clinically important effects in some individuals; consult specific product labeling for details.

Fluticasone Propionate

Oral Inhalation

Aerosol	44 mcg/metered spray	**Flovent® HFA** (with tetrafluoroethane propellant), GlaxoSmithKline
	110 mcg/metered spray	**Flovent® HFA** (with tetrafluoroethane propellant), GlaxoSmithKline
	220 mcg/metered spray	**Flovent® HFA** (with tetrafluoroethane propellant), GlaxoSmithKline
Powder for inhalation	50 mcg/inhalation	**Flovent® Diskus®**, GlaxoSmithKline
	100 mcg/inhalation	**Flovent® Diskus®**, GlaxoSmithKline
	250 mcg/inhalation	**Flovent® Diskus®**, GlaxoSmithKline

Fluticasone Propionate Combinations

Oral Inhalation

Aerosol	45 mcg with salmeterol xinafoate 21 mcg (of salmeterol) per metered spray (from the actuator)	**Advair® HFA** (with hydrofluoroalkane propellant), GlaxoSmithKline
	115 mcg with salmeterol xinafoate 21 mcg (of salmeterol) per metered spray (from the actuator)	**Advair® HFA** (with hydrofluoroalkane propellant), GlaxoSmithKline
	230 mcg with salmeterol xinafoate 21 mcg (of salmeterol) per metered spray (from the actuator)	**Advair® HFA** (with hydrofluoroalkane propellant), GlaxoSmithKline
Powder for inhalation	100 mcg with salmeterol xinafoate 50 mcg (of salmeterol) per inhalation	**Advair® Diskus®**, GlaxoSmithKline
	250 mcg with salmeterol xinafoate 50 mcg (of salmeterol) per inhalation	**Advair® Diskus®**, GlaxoSmithKline
	500 mcg with salmeterol xinafoate 50 mcg (of salmeterol) per inhalation	**Advair® Diskus®**, GlaxoSmithKline

† Use is not currently included in the labeling approved by the US Food and Drug Administration.

Selected Revisions November 19, 2018, © Copyright, September 1, 2001, American Society of Health-System Pharmacists, Inc.

Mometasone Furoate

68:04 • ADRENALS

■ Mometasone furoate is a synthetic glucocorticoid.

USES

● Bronchospasm

Asthma

Mometasone furoate is used for the maintenance treatment of asthma as prophylactic therapy.

The fixed combination of mometasone furoate and formoterol fumarate (mometasone/formoterol) is used for the treatment of asthma in patients not responding adequately to long-term asthma controller therapy (e.g., inhaled corticosteroids) or whose asthma severity warrants initiation of treatment with both an inhaled corticosteroid and a long-acting β_2-adrenergic agonist.

Orally inhaled mometasone furoate alone or in fixed combination with formoterol fumarate should *not* be used for the primary treatment of severe acute asthmatic attacks or status asthmaticus when intensive measures (e.g., oxygen, parenteral bronchodilators, IV corticosteroids) are required. Mometasone furoate alone or in fixed combination with formoterol fumarate should *not* be used as a bronchodilator or for the rapid relief of bronchospasm.

National Asthma Education and Prevention Program (NAEPP) guidelines include recommendations for assessing asthma severity and asthma control as principal components for effective management of asthma. Assessment of asthma severity is used principally to determine initial therapy; once therapy is initiated, asthma control is assessed to guide decisions about adjusting or maintaining therapy using a stepped-care approach.

In the stepped-care approach to antiasthmatic drug therapy, asthma management guidelines and most clinicians recommend initiation of a controller drug such as an anti-inflammatory agent, preferably a low-dose orally inhaled corticosteroid (e.g., 88–264, 88–176, or 176 mcg of fluticasone propionate [or its equivalent] daily via a metered-dose inhaler in adolescents and adults, children 5–11 years of age, or children 4 years of age or younger, respectively) as first-line therapy for persistent asthma (i.e., patients with daytime symptoms of asthma more than twice per week, but less than once daily, and nocturnal symptoms of asthma 3 or 4 times per month), supplemented by as-needed use of a short-acting, inhaled β_2-agonist. For equivalent orally inhaled dosages of corticosteroids, see General Dosage under Dosage and Administration: Dosage, in the Corticosteroids General Statement 68:04.

According to asthma management guidelines, therapy with a long-acting β_2-agonist (e.g., formoterol, salmeterol) generally is recommended in adults and adolescents who have moderate persistent asthma and daily asthmatic symptoms that are inadequately controlled following addition of low-dose inhaled corticosteroids to as-needed short-acting inhaled β_2-agonist treatment. However, NAEPP recommends that the beneficial effects of long-acting β_2-agonists should be weighed carefully against the increased risk (although uncommon) of severe asthma exacerbations and asthma-related deaths associated with daily use of such agents. (See Asthma-Related Death and Life-Threatening Events under Cautions: Respiratory Effects, in Salmeterol 12:12.08.12.) Asthma management guidelines also state that an alternative, but equally preferred option for management of moderate persistent asthma that is not adequately controlled with a low dosage of inhaled corticosteroid is to increase the maintenance dosage to a medium dosage (e.g., exceeding 264 but not more than 440 mcg of fluticasone propionate [or its equivalent] daily via a metered-dose inhaler in adults and adolescents).

Maintenance therapy with an inhaled corticosteroid at medium or high dosages (e.g., exceeding 440 mcg of fluticasone propionate in adults and adolescents or 352 mcg of the drug in children 5–11 years of age [or its equivalent] daily via a metered-dose inhaler) and adjunctive therapy with a long-acting inhaled β_2-agonist is the preferred treatment according to current asthma management guidelines for adults and children 5 years of age or older with severe persistent asthma (i.e., continuous daytime asthma symptoms, nighttime symptoms 7 times per week).

If asthma symptoms in patients with moderate to severe asthma are very poorly controlled (i.e., at least 2–3 exacerbations per year requiring oral corticosteroids), a short course of an oral corticosteroid (3–10 days) may be added to gain prompt control of asthma. Regular use of oral corticosteroids as add-on therapy in adults and children 5 years of age or older with severe asthma who are inadequately controlled with a high-dose inhaled corticosteroid, intermittent oral corticosteroid therapy, and a long-acting inhaled β_2-agonist bronchodilator is suggested, based on consensus and clinical experience. A short (2-week) course of oral corticosteroids may be considered to confirm clinical response prior to implementing long-term oral corticosteroid therapy. Once long-term oral corticosteroid therapy is initiated, the lowest possible effective dosage (i.e., alternate-day or once-daily administration) should be used, and the patient should be monitored carefully for adverse effects. Once asthma is well controlled, repeated attempts should be made to reduce the oral corticosteroid dosage. (See Dosage: Discontinuance of Therapy, under Dosage and Administration in the Corticosteroids General Statement 68:04.)

Well-controlled clinical studies have shown that oral inhalation of mometasone relieves symptoms of bronchial asthma and improves pulmonary function. Optimum symptomatic relief may require at least 1–2 weeks of continuous mometasone oral inhalation therapy. In corticosteroid-dependent patients, use of mometasone oral inhalation therapy may permit a substantial reduction in the daily maintenance dosage, or discontinuance, of the systemic corticosteroid.

Clinical Experience with Mometasone Furoate

In several studies in patients with mild to moderate asthma who were receiving short-acting β_2-adrenergic agonists alone, orally inhaled mometasone furoate (220 mcg once or twice daily or 440 mcg once daily) produced greater improvements in pulmonary function (e.g., morning predose forced expiratory volume in 1 second [FEV_1], morning or evening peak expiratory flow rate [PEFR]) than placebo. In adolescents and adults with mild to moderate asthma who were receiving inhaled corticosteroids, substitution of mometasone furoate (220 or 440 mcg once daily; 110, 220, or 440 mcg twice daily) for the previous inhaled corticosteroid (at existing or reduced dosage) maintained or improved pulmonary function (e.g., as assessed by morning predose FEV_1). In pediatric patients 4–11 years of age with mild to moderate asthma who were receiving inhaled corticosteroids, substitution of mometasone furoate (110 mcg once or twice daily) for the previous inhaled corticosteroid improved pulmonary function (e.g., change in percentage of predicted FEV_1 from baseline to end point).

In a 12-week, double-blind, placebo-controlled study in patients with severe persistent asthma who were receiving chronic oral therapy with prednisone (approximately 12 mg daily) usually in conjunction with inhaled corticosteroids, discontinuance of oral prednisone therapy was achieved in 40 or 0% of patients receiving orally inhaled mometasone furoate 440 mcg twice daily or placebo, respectively, following discontinuance of any previous inhaled corticosteroid therapy. At the study end point, oral prednisone dosage was decreased by 46% in patients receiving orally inhaled mometasone furoate 440 mcg twice daily and increased by 164% in those receiving placebo.

Clinical Experience with Fixed Combination of Mometasone Furoate and Formoterol Fumarate

In one randomized, double-blind, placebo-controlled, 26-week study in patients with asthma 12 years of age or older, orally inhaled mometasone/formoterol (2 inhalations of a preparation containing mometasone furoate 100 mcg/formoterol fumarate dihydrate 5 mcg administered twice daily) was compared with either orally inhaled mometasone furoate 100 mcg, formoterol fumarate dihydrate 5 mcg, or placebo (2 inhalations administered twice daily). A co-primary efficacy end point in this study was the change from baseline in FEV_1 AUC from 0–12 hours. In this study, patients receiving the mometasone/formoterol fixed combination had substantially greater increases in FEV_1 AUC 0–12 hours at 12 weeks compared with those receiving single-entity mometasone furoate or placebo; such improvements were maintained over the 26-week study period. Another primary end point in this study was deterioration in asthma or reduction in lung function. Patients who received the mometasone/formoterol fixed combination had fewer reports of asthma deterioration compared with patients receiving single-entity formoterol fumarate.

In a randomized, double-blind, 12-week study in patients with asthma 12 years of age or older, orally inhaled mometasone/formoterol (2 inhalations of a preparation containing mometasone furoate 100 or 200 mcg/formoterol fumarate dihydrate 5 mcg administered twice daily) was compared with orally inhaled mometasone furoate 200 mcg (2 inhalations administered twice daily). Patients with asthma who received either dosage of the mometasone/formoterol fixed combination had substantially greater increases in FEV_1 from baseline and over 12 weeks compared with those receiving single-entity mometasone furoate.

For EENT and topical uses of mometasone furoate, see 52:08.08 and 84:06.08, respectively.

DOSAGE AND ADMINISTRATION

● *Administration*

Oral Inhalation

Mometasone furoate (Asmanex® Twisthaler®) is administered by oral inhalation as an oral inhalation powder using the Twisthaler® breath-actuated dry powder inhalation device.

Mometasone furoate (Asmanex® HFA) is administered by oral inhalation as an oral inhalation suspension using a metered-dose aerosol inhaler with a hydrofluoroalkane (HFA; non-chlorofluorocarbon) propellant.

Mometasone furoate in fixed combination with formoterol fumarate (mometasone/formoterol; Dulera®) is administered by oral inhalation as an oral inhalation suspension using a metered-dose aerosol inhaler with an HFA propellant.

Following each mometasone furoate or mometasone/formoterol oral inhalation treatment, the mouth should be rinsed thoroughly with water without swallowing.

Children should only use the oral inhalation devices under adult supervision as instructed by a clinician.

Oral Inhalation via Dry-Powder Inhaler

Mometasone furoate (Asmanex® Twisthaler®) is administered by oral inhalation as an oral inhalation powder. This preparation should be administered as a single inhalation once or twice daily. When administered once daily, it should be used at the same time each day, preferably in the evening for optimal efficacy.

Removal of the cap from the Twisthaler® device (by twisting in a counterclockwise direction) loads a single dose of drug from the drug storage unit into the inhalation channel, making the dose available for administration via oral inhalation through the mouthpiece. The dose counter will decrease by 1 each time the cap is removed. Before inhaling the dose, the patient should exhale as completely as possible; the patient should *not* exhale into the Twisthaler® device. The patient should then place the mouthpiece of the inhaler between the lips and inhale quickly and deeply through the inhaler. Patients should not cover the ventilation holes on either side of the inhaler while inhaling the dose. The patient should remove the inhaler from the mouth, hold the breath for about 10 seconds, then exhale slowly.

The Twisthaler® device should be closed and reloaded for the next dose by twisting the cap in a clockwise direction until a click is heard. Patients should wipe the mouthpiece dry with a dry cloth or tissue and store the device in a dry place. The inhaler should not be washed. The inhaler should be discarded when every inhalation has been used (when the dose indicator reads "00") or 45 days after removal from its foil pouch, whichever comes first.

Oral Inhalation via Aerosol

Mometasone furoate (Asmanex® HFA) is administered by oral inhalation using an oral aerosol inhaler with HFA propellant. This preparation should be administered as 2 inhalations twice daily (morning and evening). The aerosol inhaler should be primed by releasing 4 test sprays into the air (away from the face) before initial use and shaken well before each spray. If the inhaler has not been used for more than 5 days, the inhaler should be primed again by releasing 4 test sprays into the air (away from the face) and shaken well before each spray. The cap from the mouthpiece of the actuator should be removed before use. The mouthpiece should be cleaned using a dry wipe after every 7 days of use; water should not be used to clean the inhaler. Mometasone oral inhalation aerosol should only be used with the actuator supplied with the product.

Mometasone/formoterol fixed combination (Dulera®) is administered by oral inhalation using an aerosol inhaler with HFA propellant. The fixed combination should be administered as 2 inhalations twice daily (morning and evening). Mometasone/formoterol should only be used with the actuator supplied with the product. The aerosol inhaler should be primed by releasing 4 test sprays into the air (away from the face) before initial use and shaken well before each spray. If the inhaler has not been used for more than 5 days, it should be primed again by releasing 4 test sprays into the air (away from the face) and shaken well before each spray. Before each inhalation, the inhaler must be shaken well. The mouthpiece of the inhaler should be wiped clean with a dry cloth every 7 days; water should not be used to clean the inhaler.

● *Dosage*

Dosage of mometasone furoate is expressed in terms of the salt.

Mometasone/formoterol is a fixed combination of mometasone furoate and formoterol fumarate dihydrate; dosage of the mometasone component is expressed in terms of the salt and dosage of the formoterol component is expressed in terms of the hydrated salt.

The strength and dosage of mometasone furoate administered as an oral inhalation powder (Asmanex® Twisthaler®) is expressed as the nominal (labeled) dose contained in the Twisthaler® device. The actual amount of drug delivered to the lungs depends on factors such as the patient's inspiratory flow. Based on standardized in vitro testing at a flow rate of 30 and 60 L/minute at a constant volume of 2 L, each actuation of the Twisthaler® inhaler labeled as containing 220 or 110 mcg of mometasone furoate delivers 200 or 100 mcg of mometasone furoate, respectively, from the mouthpiece. In adults and adolescents 12 years of age or older with asthma of varying severity, mean peak inspiratory flow through the Twisthaler® device was 69 L/minute. Mean peak inspiratory flow through the Twisthaler® device in pediatric patients 5–8 or 9–12 years of age exceeded 50 or 60 L/minute, respectively.

Each actuation of the mometasone furoate oral aerosol metered-dose inhaler (Asmanex® HFA) delivers 115 or 225 mcg of mometasone furoate from the valve and 100 or 200 mcg of mometasone furoate from the actuator, depending on the preparation used. The strength and dosage of these mometasone preparations are expressed in terms of drug delivered from the mouthpiece of the actuator. The actual amount of drug delivered to the lungs may depend on factors such as the patient's coordination between actuation of the device and inspiration through the delivery system. Commercially available Asmanex® HFA aerosol inhaler delivers 120 actuations per 13-g canister.

Each actuation of the oral aerosol inhaler containing the fixed combination of mometasone furoate and formoterol fumarate (Dulera®) delivers 115 or 225 mcg of mometasone furoate and 5.5 mcg of formoterol fumarate dihydrate from the valve and delivers 100 or 200 mcg of mometasone furoate and 5 mcg of formoterol fumarate dihydrate from the actuator per metered spray, depending on the preparation used. The strength and dosage of mometasone/formoterol preparations are expressed in terms of drug delivered from the mouthpiece of the actuator. The actual amount of drug delivered to the lungs may depend on factors such as the patient's coordination between actuation of the device and inspiration through the delivery system. Commercially available mometasone/formoterol aerosol inhaler delivers 60 or 120 metered sprays per 8.8- or 13-g canister, respectively.

Asthma

Dosage of mometasone furoate alone or in fixed combination with formoterol fumarate should be adjusted carefully according to individual requirements and response. The recommended initial and maximum dosages of mometasone furoate are based on previous asthma therapy. The lowest effective dosage of mometasone furoate should be used, particularly in children and adolescents, since inhaled corticosteroids have the potential to affect growth. (See Pediatric Use under Warnings/Precautions: Specific Populations, in Cautions.) Safety and efficacy of mometasone furoate dosages exceeding those recommended by the manufacturer have not been established.

Mometasone Furoate

When mometasone furoate oral inhalation powder (Asmanex® Twisthaler®) is used, the initial and maximum dosage in children 4–11 years of age is 110 mcg once daily in the evening, regardless of previous therapy. The recommended initial dosage of mometasone furoate for adults and adolescents 12 years of age or older who were previously receiving bronchodilators alone or inhaled corticosteroids is 220 mcg once daily in the evening. If control of asthma is inadequate in patients 12 years of age or older after 2 weeks of mometasone furoate therapy at the initial dosage, a higher dosage of the drug may provide additional asthma control. If required, the dosage may be increased to a maximum of 440 mcg daily (given as 440 mcg once daily or 220 mcg twice daily). The recommended initial and maximum dosage of mometasone furoate in adults and adolescents 12 years of age or older who were previously receiving oral corticosteroids is 440 mcg twice daily.

When mometasone furoate oral inhalation aerosol (Asmanex® HFA) is used, the initial dosage is based on previous asthma therapy. The initial dosage in adults and adolescents 12 years of age or older previously receiving inhaled medium-dose corticosteroids is 200 mcg (2 inhalations of preparation containing 100 mcg) twice daily. The initial dosage in adolescents 12 years of age or older previously receiving inhaled high-dose corticosteroids or oral corticosteroids is 400 mcg (2 inhalations of preparation containing 200 mcg) twice daily. If control of asthma is inadequate after 2 weeks of mometasone furoate therapy at the lower dosage, switching to a higher strength preparation of the drug, initiating therapy with an oral corticosteroid, or initiating oral inhalation therapy with a fixed-combination preparation containing a corticosteroid and a long-acting β_2-agonist should be considered.

Fixed Combination of Mometasone Furoate and Formoterol Fumarate

When the mometasone/formoterol fixed-combination oral inhalation aerosol (Dulera®) is used in patients with asthma, the recommended initial dosage is based on the patient's asthma severity, previous asthma therapy (including previous inhaled corticosteroid dosage), current control of asthma symptoms, and risk of future asthma exacerbations.

In adults and adolescents 12 years of age or older, the dosage of orally inhaled mometasone/formoterol fixed combination is 200 or 400 mcg of mometasone furoate and 10 mcg of formoterol fumarate dihydrate (2 inhalations of preparation containing 100 or 200 mcg of mometasone furoate and 5 mcg of formoterol fumarate dihydrate) twice daily. If control of asthma is inadequate after 2 weeks of mometasone/formoterol therapy at the lower dosage, switching to a higher strength preparation of the fixed combination (higher strengths contain higher dosages of mometasone only) may provide additional asthma control. The maximum recommended daily dosage of the mometasone/formoterol fixed combination in asthmatic adults and adolescents 12 years of age or older is 800 mcg of mometasone and 20 mcg of formoterol fumarate dihydrate (maximum of 2 inhalations of preparation containing mometasone furoate 200 mcg and formoterol fumarate 5 mcg dihydrate twice daily).

Conversion to Orally Inhaled Therapy in Patients Receiving Systemic Corticosteroids

When switching to an orally inhaled corticosteroid in patients receiving systemic corticosteroids, the patient's asthma should be reasonably stable before oral inhalation therapy begins. Initially, mometasone furoate inhalation powder is given concurrently with the maintenance dosage of the systemic corticosteroid. Reduction of the systemic corticosteroid dosage should be initiated at least 1 week after starting mometasone furoate oral inhalation, and dosage reductions should not exceed 2.5 mg daily of prednisone (or its equivalent) each week. *Particular care is needed in gradually withdrawing systemic corticosteroids following long-term therapy with these drugs, since death due to adrenal insufficiency has occurred in some individuals in whom systemic corticosteroids were withdrawn too rapidly.* (See Withdrawal of Systemic Corticosteroids under Cautions: Warnings/Precautions.)

● Special Populations

Patients with hepatic impairment should be closely monitored for signs of increased drug exposure during mometasone therapy.

In patients with renal impairment, there are no specific dosage recommendations for mometasone at this time.

When the mometasone/formoterol fixed combination is used, dosage requirements for formoterol fumarate should be considered.

CAUTIONS

● Contraindications

Mometasone furoate and the fixed combination containing mometasone furoate and formoterol fumarate (mometasone/formoterol) are contraindicated for primary treatment of severe acute asthmatic attacks or status asthmaticus when intensive measures (e.g., oxygen, parenteral bronchodilators, IV corticosteroids) are required.

Mometasone furoate is contraindicated in patients hypersensitive to the drug or any ingredient (e.g., milk proteins) in the formulation. Mometasone oral inhalation powder contains small amounts of lactose, which has trace amounts of milk proteins. Anaphylactic reactions in patients with milk protein allergy have been reported; therefore, patients with known milk protein allergy should not receive mometasone oral inhalation powder.

Mometasone/formoterol fixed combination is contraindicated in patients hypersensitive to mometasone, formoterol, or any ingredient in the formulation.

● Warnings/Precautions

Use of Fixed Combinations

When mometasone furoate is used in fixed combination with formoterol fumarate, cautions, precautions, contraindications, and interactions associated with formoterol fumarate should be considered. (See Risk of Serious Asthma-related Events under Cautions: Warnings/Precautions.)

Cautionary information applicable to specific populations (e.g., pregnant or nursing women, individuals with hepatic or renal impairment, geriatric patients) should be considered for each drug in the fixed combination.

Acute Exacerbations of Asthma

Orally inhaled mometasone furoate alone or in fixed combination with formoterol fumarate should *not* be used as a bronchodilator and is not indicated for emergency use (e.g., status asthmaticus) or relief of acute bronchospasm. Acute asthma symptoms should be treated with a short-acting β_2-agonist bronchodilator. If inadequate control of symptoms persists with supplemental β_2-agonist bronchodilator therapy, prompt reevaluation of asthma therapy is required. Such reevaluation may include dosage adjustment of inhaled corticosteroids or initiation of systemic corticosteroids.

Localized Candidal Infections

Candidal infections of the mouth and pharynx have been reported in patients receiving orally inhaled mometasone therapy. If such infections occur, appropriate local or systemic antifungal treatment of the infection may be necessary while still continuing orally inhaled mometasone therapy, although interruption of mometasone therapy may be required in some patients. Patients receiving mometasone or mometasone/formoterol should be instructed to rinse their mouths with water (without swallowing) after each dose to help reduce the risk of oropharyngeal candidiasis.

Immunosuppressed Patients

Patients who are taking immunosuppressant drugs have increased susceptibility to infections compared with healthy individuals, and certain infections (e.g., varicella [chickenpox], measles) can have a more serious or even fatal outcome in such patients. Patients receiving corticosteroids who are potentially immunosuppressed and who have not had these diseases or have not been properly vaccinated against these diseases should be warned of the risk of exposure to certain infections (e.g., chickenpox, measles) and take particular care to avoid exposure. If exposure to chickenpox or measles occurs in susceptible individuals, administration of varicella zoster immune globulin (VZIG) or immune globulin IM (IGIM), respectively, may be indicated. If chickenpox develops, treatment with an antiviral agent may be considered.

It is not known how the dosage, route, and duration of administration of a corticosteroid, or the contribution of the underlying disease and/or prior corticosteroid therapy, affect the risk of developing a disseminated infection. Inhaled corticosteroid therapy should be used with caution, if at all, in patients with clinical or asymptomatic *Mycobacterium tuberculosis* infections of the respiratory tract; untreated systemic fungal, bacterial, parasitic, or viral infections; or ocular herpes simplex. For additional information, see Cautions: Increased Susceptibility to Infection and also see Precautions and Contraindications, in the Corticosteroids General Statement 68:04.

Withdrawal of Systemic Corticosteroids

Systemic corticosteroid therapy should be withdrawn gradually in patients being switched from systemic corticosteroids to less systemically available orally inhaled corticosteroids. Patients should be monitored during dosage reduction for objective signs and symptoms of adrenal insufficiency (e.g., fatigue, lassitude, weakness, nausea, vomiting, hypotension) since life-threatening adrenal insufficiency could occur. Lung function (forced expiratory volume in 1 second [FEV$_1$] or peak expiratory flow rate [PEFR]), adjunctive β_2-adrenergic agonist use, and asthma symptoms should be carefully monitored during withdrawal of systemic corticosteroid therapy. *In most patients, several months are required for total recovery of hypothalamic-pituitary-adrenal (HPA) function following withdrawal of systemic corticosteroid therapy.* Patients who have been maintained on a systemic corticosteroid dosage equivalent to 20 mg or more of prednisone daily may be most susceptible to adrenal insufficiency, particularly when systemic corticosteroids have been almost completely withdrawn. These patients should be carefully monitored during and for a number of months after withdrawal of systemic corticosteroids for corticosteroid withdrawal symptoms (e.g., joint pain, muscular pain, lassitude, depression); acute adrenal insufficiency during exposure to trauma, surgery, or infection (particularly gastroenteritis) or other conditions associated with acute electrolyte loss; or symptomatic exacerbation of allergic conditions previously controlled by systemic corticosteroid therapy (e.g., rhinitis, conjunctivitis, eczema, arthritis, eosinophilic conditions).

In patients who have been withdrawn from systemic corticosteroids, reinitiation of systemic corticosteroid therapy will likely be necessary during periods of stress or severe asthmatic attack. Since glucocorticoids can reduce HPA-axis response to stress, supplementation with a systemic corticosteroid in patients undergoing such stress is recommended.

Systemic Corticosteroid Effects

Although minimal absorption of mometasone furoate into systemic circulation occurs following oral inhalation of the drug at recommended dosages, manifestations of hypercorticism and HPA-axis suppression could occur if recommended dosages are exceeded over prolonged periods of time or in particularly sensitive individuals. If such changes occur, the dosage of mometasone furoate should be reduced slowly, consistent with accepted procedures for reducing systemic corticosteroid dosage and management of asthma symptoms. Particular care should be taken in monitoring patients postoperatively or during periods of stress for evidence of inadequate adrenal response.

Musculoskeletal Effects

Long-term use of orally inhaled corticosteroids, including mometasone furoate, may affect normal bone metabolism, resulting in a loss of bone mineral density. (See Osteoporosis under Cautions: Musculoskeletal Effects, in the Corticosteroids General Statement 68:04.) Although appreciable reduction in lumbar spine bone mineral density was noted in a 2-year study in adults receiving 220 mcg of mometasone furoate twice daily, this adverse effect was not confirmed in another 2-year study in adults receiving 440 mcg of the drug twice daily.

Patients with major risk factors for decreased bone mineral density, such as family history of osteoporosis, prolonged immobilization, or chronic use of drugs that can reduce bone mass (e.g., anticonvulsants, corticosteroids), should be monitored and treated using established standards of care.

Ophthalmic Effects

Glaucoma, increased intraocular pressure (IOP), and cataracts have been reported in patients receiving long-term therapy with orally inhaled corticosteroids. Referral to an ophthalmologist should be considered in patients who develop ophthalmic symptoms or in those receiving long-term therapy with mometasone furoate.

Bronchospasm

As with other inhaled drugs for asthma, paradoxical bronchospasm may occur, resulting in an immediate increase in wheezing following oral inhalation of mometasone furoate.

If paradoxical bronchospasm occurs, appropriate treatment (e.g., use of a short-acting inhaled β_2-adrenergic agonist) should be instituted immediately, and mometasone therapy should be discontinued.

Sensitivity Reactions

Cases of anaphylaxis, rash, pruritus, angioedema, urticaria, flushing, allergic dermatitis, and bronchospasm have been reported with mometasone furoate oral inhalation therapy in clinical trials and during postmarketing experience. Orally inhaled mometasone furoate should be discontinued if such reactions occur.

Mometasone furoate oral inhalation powder contains small amounts of lactose with trace amounts of milk proteins. Anaphylactic reactions in patients with milk protein allergy have been reported; therefore, patients with known milk protein allergy should not receive this preparation of mometasone furoate. (See Cautions: Contraindications.)

Risk of Serious Asthma-related Events

Monotherapy with long-acting β_2-adrenergic agonists, such as formoterol, a component of the mometasone/formoterol fixed combination, increases the risk of asthma-related death. Data from a large placebo-controlled safety study (Salmeterol Multi-center Asthma Research Trial [SMART]) evaluating the safety of another long-acting β_2-adrenergic agonist, salmeterol, in patients with asthma showed an increase in asthma-related deaths in patients receiving salmeterol. (See Asthma-related Death and Life-threatening Events under Cautions: Respiratory Effects, in Salmeterol 12:12.08.12.) In addition, available data from controlled clinical trials suggest that monotherapy with long-acting β_2-adrenergic agonists increases the risk of asthma-related hospitalization in pediatric and adolescent patients.

However, FDA has concluded that there is no clinically important increased risk of serious asthma-related events, including hospitalization, intubation, or death, associated with concomitant use of long-acting β_2-adrenergic agonists (e.g., formoterol) and inhaled corticosteroids (e.g., mometasone) compared with inhaled corticosteroids alone based on the results of several large clinical studies. In addition, these studies showed that combination therapy with long-acting β_2-adrenergic agonists and inhaled corticosteroids was more effective in reducing the incidence of asthma exacerbations (i.e., events requiring use of systemic corticosteroids for at least 3 outpatient days or an asthma-related hospitalization or emergency department visit requiring use of systemic corticosteroids) compared with use of inhaled corticosteroids alone. (See Asthma-related Death and Serious Asthma-related Events under Warnings/Precautions: Warnings, in Cautions, in Formoterol Fumarate 12:12.08.12.)

In the treatment of asthma, the mometasone/formoterol fixed combination should be used only in patients who have not responded adequately to long-term asthma controller therapy, such as inhaled corticosteroids, or whose disease severity warrants initiation of treatment with both an inhaled corticosteroid and a long-acting β_2-adrenergic agonist.

Specific Populations

Pregnancy

Category C. (See Users Guide.)

There are no adequate and well-controlled studies with mometasone furoate in pregnant women. The drug should be used during pregnancy only if potential benefits justify potential risks to the fetus.

There is an increased risk of adverse perinatal outcomes (e.g., preeclampsia, premature birth, low birth weight, neonates small for gestational age) in women with poorly or moderately controlled asthma. Pregnant women with asthma should be closely monitored and therapy adjusted as necessary to maintain optimal asthma control.

The effects of mometasone furoate in fixed combination with formoterol fumarate during labor and delivery are not known. Because of the potential for β-agonist interference with uterine contractility, use of the mometasone/formoterol fixed combination during labor should be restricted to those patients in whom the benefits clearly outweigh the risks.

Hypoadrenalism may occur in infants of women who have received substantial oral corticosteroid dosages during pregnancy. These infants should be carefully monitored.

Lactation

It is not known whether mometasone furoate is distributed into milk; however, other corticosteroids are distributed into milk. Data are not available on the effects of the drug on the breast-fed child or milk production. The benefits of breast-feeding and the importance of mometasone to the woman should be considered along with any potential adverse effects on the breast-fed infant from the drug or underlying maternal condition. The manufacturer of mometasone oral inhalation powder (Asmanex® Twisthaler®) states that caution is advised if mometasone furoate is administered in nursing women.

The manufacturer of the mometasone/formoterol fixed combination states that a decision should be made whether to discontinue nursing or the drug, taking into account the importance of the drug to the woman.

Pediatric Use

Safety and efficacy of mometasone furoate oral inhalation powder have not been established in children younger than 4 years of age.

Safety and efficacy of mometasone furoate oral inhalation aerosol have not been established in children younger than 12 years of age.

Safety and efficacy of the mometasone/formoterol fixed combination have not been established in children younger than 12 years of age.

Use of corticosteroids may lead to suppression of growth in children and adolescents. Therefore, pediatric patients receiving prolonged therapy with orally inhaled mometasone should be monitored periodically (e.g., via stadiometry) for possible adverse effects on growth and development. The benefits of corticosteroid therapy should be weighed against the possibility of growth suppression and the availability of safe and effective alternative therapies. Pediatric patients should be maintained on the lowest possible dosage of mometasone that controls asthma symptoms. (See Cautions: Pediatric Precautions, in the Corticosteroids General Statement 68:04.)

Geriatric Use

Although no overall differences in safety and efficacy of orally inhaled mometasone furoate were observed in geriatric patients relative to younger adults, the possibility that some older patients may exhibit increased sensitivity to the drug cannot be ruled out.

● Common Adverse Effects

Adverse effects occurring in 5% or more of patients receiving mometasone furoate oral inhalation powder for the treatment of asthma include headache, allergic rhinitis, pharyngitis, upper respiratory tract infection, sinusitis, oral candidiasis, dysmenorrhea, musculoskeletal pain, back pain, and dyspepsia.

Adverse effects occurring in 3% or more of patients receiving mometasone furoate oral inhalation aerosol for the treatment of asthma include nasopharyngitis, headache, sinusitis, bronchitis, and influenza.

Adverse effects occurring in 3% or more of patients receiving the mometasone/formoterol fixed combination for the treatment of asthma and more frequently than in those receiving placebo include nasopharyngitis, sinusitis, and headache.

DRUG INTERACTIONS

The following information addresses potential interactions with mometasone furoate. When mometasone furoate is used in fixed combination with formoterol fumarate (mometasone/formoterol), interactions associated with formoterol also should be considered. No formal drug interaction studies have been performed to date with the mometasone/formoterol fixed combination.

● Drugs Affecting Hepatic Microsomal Enzymes

Drugs that Inhibit Isoenzyme CYP3A4

Since mometasone furoate is principally metabolized in the liver by the cytochrome P-450 (CYP) 3A4 isoenzyme, concomitant use with drugs that are potent inhibitors of the CYP3A4 isoenzyme (e.g., atazanavir, clarithromycin, cobicistat-containing preparations, indinavir, itraconazole, ketoconazole, nefazodone, nelfinavir, ritonavir, saquinavir) may result in increased plasma mometasone concentrations.

Caution should be exercised when considering concomitant use of mometasone furoate with ketoconazole and other known inhibitors of the CYP3A4 isoenzyme. The benefits of such concomitant use should be weighed against the risk of systemic corticosteroid effects. If concomitant use is necessary, patients should be monitored for adverse systemic corticosteroid effects related to increased systemic exposure to mometasone furoate.

DESCRIPTION

Mometasone furoate is a synthetic nonfluorinated glucocorticoid. For a discussion of the pharmacology of mometasone, see Pharmacology in the Corticosteroids General Statement 68:04.

Systemic bioavailability of mometasone furoate following oral inhalation of a single 400-mcg dose is reported to be less than 1%. Most of an orally inhaled dose of the drug is swallowed and excreted unchanged in feces. Any systemically absorbed drug is extensively metabolized in the liver, principally by the cytochrome P-450 (CYP) 3A4 isoenzyme, and is excreted principally in feces and to a lesser extent in urine.

ADVICE TO PATIENTS

When mometasone furoate is used in fixed combination with formoterol fumarate, importance of informing patients of important cautionary information about formoterol fumarate.

Importance of instructing patients to read manufacturer's patient instructions prior to initiation of therapy.

Importance of pediatric patients receiving therapy under adult supervision.

Importance of adequate understanding of proper storage, preparation, and inhalation techniques, including use of the oral inhalation delivery systems.

Importance of informing clinician of any history of hypersensitivity reactions to mometasone or other ingredients in the formulations or of known allergy to milk proteins.

Importance of rinsing the mouth with water without swallowing after oral inhalation.

Importance of advising patients that mometasone furoate oral inhalation must be used at regular intervals to be therapeutically effective. Importance of adherence to prescribed dosage regimen; do not increase the frequency of administration without consulting a clinician.

Importance of advising patients that if a dose of mometasone furoate alone or in fixed combination with formoterol fumarate is missed, the next dose should be taken at the regularly scheduled time; the dose should not be doubled.

Importance of advising patients that at least 1–2 weeks of continuous therapy may be required for optimum effects to be achieved. Importance of contacting a clinician if asthma symptoms do not improve in such a time frame.

Importance of advising patients that orally inhaled mometasone furoate should not be used as a bronchodilator and that the drug is not indicated for emergency use (e.g., relief of acute bronchospasm).

Importance of availability and use of a short-acting β_2-adrenergic agonist for relief of acute asthma symptoms.

Importance of contacting a clinician immediately when asthmatic attacks are not controlled by current bronchodilator therapy.

Importance of gradual withdrawal from systemic corticosteroids during transfer to orally inhaled mometasone furoate and of monitoring by a clinician during such transfer of therapy. (See Conversion to Orally Inhaled Therapy in Patients Receiving Systemic Corticosteroids under Dosage: Asthma, in Dosage and Administration.)

Importance of advising patients being transferred from systemic corticosteroid to mometasone furoate oral inhalation therapy to carry special identification (e.g., card) indicating the need for supplementary systemic corticosteroids during periods of stress or severe exacerbation of asthma. Importance of advising patients to immediately resume therapy with large doses of systemic corticosteroids and contact their clinician for further instructions during stressful periods (e.g., stress, severe asthmatic attack, surgery, trauma, infection).

Importance of informing patients that corticosteroids may decrease bone mineral density. (See Musculoskeletal Effects under Cautions: Warnings/Precautions.)

Risk of localized candidal infections of mouth and pharynx. (See Localized Candidal Infections under Cautions: Warnings/Precautions.)

Risk for development of cataracts or glaucoma associated with long-term use of inhaled corticosteroids (e.g., mometasone). Importance of reporting any vision changes to a clinician. (See Ophthalmic Effects under Cautions: Warnings/Precautions.)

Risk of systemic corticosteroid effects (e.g., hypercorticism, potentially life-threatening adrenal suppression). Importance of informing a clinician of fatigue, weakness, nausea, vomiting, dizziness, or fainting. (See Systemic Corticosteroid Effects under Cautions: Warnings/Precautions.)

Risk of reduction in growth velocity in children and adolescents with orally inhaled corticosteroids. (See Pediatric Use under Warnings/Precautions: Specific Populations, in Cautions.)

Importance of immunosuppressed patients avoiding exposure to chickenpox or measles, and, if exposed, of immediately consulting a clinician. (See Immunosuppressed Patients under Cautions: Warnings/Precautions.)

Importance of advising immunosuppressed patients of potential worsening of existing tuberculosis; fungal, bacterial, parasitic, or viral infections; or ocular herpes simplex. Importance of immunosuppressed patients informing clinician of a history of infections.

Importance of women informing clinicians if they are or plan to become pregnant or plan to breast-feed.

Importance of informing clinicians of existing or contemplated concomitant therapy, including prescription (e.g., anticonvulsants, systemic corticosteroids) and OTC drugs, as well as any concomitant illnesses (e.g., infections).

Importance of informing patients of other important precautionary information. (See Cautions.)

PREPARATIONS

Excipients in commercially available drug preparations may have clinically important effects in some individuals; consult specific product labeling for details.

Mometasone Furoate

Oral Inhalation

Aerosol	100 mcg per metered spray	**Asmanex® HFA** (with hydrofluoroalkane propellant), Merck
	200 mcg per metered spray	**Asmanex® HFA** (with hydrofluoroalkane propellant), Merck
Powder, for oral inhalation	110 mcg (delivers 100 mcg per inhalation)	**Asmanex® Twisthaler®**, Teva
	220 mcg (delivers 200 mcg per inhalation)	**Asmanex® Twisthaler®**, Teva

Mometasone Furoate Combinations

Oral Inhalation

Aerosol	100 mcg with Formoterol Fumarate Dihydrate 5 mcg per metered spray	**Dulera®** (with hydrofluoroalkane propellant), Merck
	200 mcg with Formoterol Fumarate Dihydrate 5 mcg per metered spray	**Dulera®** (with hydrofluoroalkane propellant), Merck

Selected Revisions November 11, 2019, © Copyright, June 1, 2008, American Society of Health-System Pharmacists, Inc.

Triamcinolone

68:04 · ADRENALS

■ Triamcinolone is a synthetic glucocorticoid.

USES

Triamcinolone is used principally as an anti-inflammatory or immunosuppressant agent. Because it has virtually no mineralocorticoid properties, the drug is inadequate alone for the management of adrenocortical insufficiency. If triamcinolone is used in the treatment of this condition, concomitant therapy with a mineralocorticoid is also required.

● Asthma

Triamcinolone acetonide is used by oral inhalation for the long-term prevention of bronchospasm in patients with asthma.

Orally inhaled triamcinolone acetonide should not be used for the primary treatment of severe acute asthmatic attacks or status asthmaticus when intensive measures (e.g., oxygen, parenteral bronchodilators, IV corticosteroids) are required. Triamcinolone acetonide oral inhaler is not a bronchodilator, and patients should be warned that the drug should not be used for rapid relief of bronchospasm.

Mild Persistent Asthma

Drugs for asthma may be categorized as relievers (e.g., bronchodilators taken as needed for acute symptoms) or controllers (principally inhaled corticosteroids or other anti-inflammatory agents taken regularly to achieve long-term control of asthma). In the stepped-care approach to antiasthmatic drug therapy, current asthma management guidelines and most clinicians recommend initiation of a controller drug such as an anti-inflammatory agent, preferably a low-dose orally inhaled corticosteroid (e.g., 88–264, 88–176, or 176 mcg of fluticasone propionate [or its equivalent] daily via a metered-dose inhaler in adolescents and adults, children 5–11 years of age, or children 4 years of age or younger, respectively) as first-line therapy for persistent asthma (i.e., patients with daytime symptoms of asthma more than twice per week, but less than once daily, and nocturnal symptoms of asthma 3–4 times per month), supplemented by as-needed use of a short-acting, inhaled β₂-agonist. For equivalent orally inhaled dosages of corticosteroids, see General Dosage under Dosage and Administration: Dosage, in the Corticosteroids General Statement 68:04.

Moderate Persistent Asthma

According to current asthma management guidelines, therapy with a long-acting β₂-agonist such as salmeterol or formoterol generally is recommended in adults and adolescents who have moderate persistent asthma and daily asthmatic symptoms that are inadequately controlled following addition of low-dose inhaled corticosteroids to as-needed inhaled β₂-agonist treatment. However, the National Asthma Education and Prevention Program (NAEPP) recommends that the beneficial effects of long-acting inhaled β₂-agonists should be weighed carefully against the increased risk (although uncommon) of severe asthma exacerbations and asthma-related deaths associated with daily use of such agents. (See Asthma-related Death and Life-threatening Events under Cautions: Respiratory Effects, in Salmeterol 12:12.08.12.) Current asthma management guidelines also state that an alternative, but equally preferred option for management of moderate persistent asthma that is not adequately controlled with a low dosage of inhaled corticosteroid is to increase the maintenance dosage to a medium dosage (e.g., exceeding 264 but not more than 440 mcg of fluticasone propionate [or its equivalent] daily via a metered-dose inhaler in adults and adolescents).

In children 5–11 years of age with moderate persistent asthma that is not controlled with a low dosage of an inhaled corticosteroid, a long-acting inhaled β₂-agonist (e.g., salmeterol, formoterol), a leukotriene modifier (i.e., montelukast, zafirlukast), or extended-release theophylline (with appropriate monitoring) may be added to low-dose inhaled corticosteroid therapy according to current asthma management guidelines; another preferred option is to increase the maintenance dosage of the inhaled corticosteroid to a medium dosage (e.g., exceeding 176 but not more than 352 mcg of fluticasone propionate [or its equivalent] daily via a metered-dose inhaler). In infants and children 4 years of age or younger with moderate persistent asthma that is not controlled by a low dosage of an inhaled corticosteroid, the only preferred option is to increase the maintenance dosage of the inhaled corticosteroid to a medium dosage (e.g., exceeding 176 but not more than 352 mcg of fluticasone propionate [or its equivalent] daily via a metered-dose inhaler).

Severe Persistent Asthma

Maintenance therapy with an inhaled corticosteroid at medium or high dosages (e.g., exceeding 440 mcg of fluticasone propionate or its equivalent daily in adults and adolescents or 352 mcg of the drug in children 5–11 years of age or its equivalent via a metered-dose inhaler) and adjunctive therapy with a long-acting inhaled β₂-agonist is the preferred treatment according to current asthma management guidelines for adults and children 5 years of age or older with severe persistent asthma (i.e., continuous daytime asthma symptoms, nighttime symptoms 7 times per week). In infants and children 4 years of age or younger with severe asthma, maintenance therapy with an inhaled corticosteroid at medium or high dosages (e.g., exceeding 352 mcg of fluticasone propionate daily or its equivalent via a metered-dose inhaler) and adjunctive therapy with either a long-acting inhaled β₂-agonist or montelukast is recommended in current asthma management guidelines as the only preferred treatment.

Poorly Controlled Asthma

If asthma symptoms in patients with moderate to severe asthma are very poorly controlled (i.e., at least 2–3 exacerbations per year requiring oral corticosteroids), a short course of an oral corticosteroid (3–10 days) may be added to gain prompt control of asthma. Regular use of oral corticosteroids as add-on therapy in adults and children 5 years of age or older with severe asthma who are inadequately controlled with high-dose inhaled corticosteroid, intermittent oral corticosteroid therapy, and a long-acting inhaled β₂-agonist bronchodilator is suggested, based on consensus and clinical experience. A short (2-week) course of oral corticosteroids may be considered to confirm clinical response prior to implementing long-term therapy with these agents. Once long-term oral corticosteroid therapy is initiated, the lowest possible effective dosage (i.e., alternate-day or once-daily administration) should be used, and the patient should be monitored carefully for adverse effects. Once asthma is well-controlled, repeated attempts should be made to reduce the oral corticosteroid dosage. Use of orally inhaled triamcinolone acetonide as adjunctive therapy in patients who require chronic administration of systemic corticosteroids to control asthma symptoms may permit a reduction in dosage or discontinuance of systemic corticosteroids. When used in recommended dosages in responsive patients, triamcinolone acetonide oral inhalation may permit control of asthmatic symptoms with less suppression of hypothalamic-pituitary-adrenal (HPA) function than therapeutically equivalent oral dosages of prednisone. For additional details on the stepped-care approach to drug therapy in asthma, see Asthma under Uses: Bronchospasm, in Albuterol 12:12.08.12 and see Asthma under Uses: Respiratory Diseases, in the Corticosteroids General Statement 68:04.

DOSAGE AND ADMINISTRATION

The route of administration and dosage of triamcinolone and its derivatives depend on the condition being treated and the response of the patient. IM therapy is generally reserved for patients who are not able to take the drug orally. Dosage for infants and children should be based on the severity of the disease and the response of the patient rather than on strict adherence to dosage indicated by age, body weight, or body surface area. After a satisfactory response is obtained, dosage should be decreased in small decrements to the lowest level that maintains an adequate clinical response, and the drug should be discontinued as soon as possible. Patients should be continually monitored for signs that indicate dosage adjustment is necessary, such as remissions or exacerbations of the disease and stress (surgery, infection, trauma). One manufacturer recommends that an alternate-day dosage regimen be considered when long-term oral triamcinolone therapy is necessary. However, most authorities state that only methylprednisolone, prednisolone, and prednisone have been proven to be suitable for alternate-day glucocorticoid therapy. Following long-term therapy, triamcinolone should be withdrawn gradually. (See Discontinuance of Therapy under Dosage and Administration: Dosage, in the Corticosteroids General Statement 68:04.)

● Triamcinolone

Triamcinolone is administered orally. The initial adult dosage of triamcinolone may range from 4–48 mg daily depending on the disease being treated and is usually administered in 1–4 doses. Some clinicians state that children may be given a dosage of 0.117–1.66 mg/kg daily or 3.3–50 mg/m² daily, administered in 4 divided doses.

● *Triamcinolone Acetonide*

Triamcinolone acetonide may be administered by IM, intra-articular, intrasynovial, intralesional (intradermal) or sublesional, and soft-tissue injection or by oral inhalation. Because it is slowly absorbed and its effects may persist for several weeks, IM administration of triamcinolone acetonide is not indicated when an immediate effect of short duration is required.

The usual IM dose for adults and children older than 12 years of age is 60 mg (using the 40-mg/mL sterile suspension). Additional IM doses of 20–100 mg (usually 40–80 mg) may be given when signs and symptoms recur. Some clinicians recommend that triamcinolone acetonide be administered IM at 6-week intervals, if possible, to minimize HPA suppression. Some clinicians state that children 6–12 years of age may receive 0.03–0.2 mg/kg or 1–6.25 mg/m² IM at 1- to 7-day intervals. IM dosage for children younger than 6 years of age has not been established, and triamcinolone acetonide should not be administered IM to children in this age group.

For intralesional (or sublesional) injections, the 10-mg/mL sterile suspension of triamcinolone acetonide is used. The usual intralesional or sublesional dose of triamcinolone acetonide is 1 mg per injection site and may be repeated 1 or more times a week depending on the response of the patient. A tuberculin syringe should be used to facilitate intralesional or sublesional dosage measurement. Multiple sites may be injected if they are at least 1 cm apart, but the total amount of triamcinolone acetonide administered intralesionally at any one time should not exceed 30 mg.

For intra-articular, intrasynovial, and soft-tissue injection, the usual dose of triamcinolone acetonide (using either the 10-mg/mL or 40-mg/mL sterile suspension) is 2.5–40 mg depending on the location of the affected area and the degree of inflammation; the dose may be repeated when signs and symptoms recur. Anti-inflammatory effects may be maintained for several weeks following intra-articular administration of the drug. A local anesthetic, such as procaine hydrochloride, may be infiltrated into the soft tissue surrounding the joint and/or injected into the joint before administration of triamcinolone acetonide. For large joints such as the knee, 15–40 mg of triamcinolone acetonide may be used. For smaller joints, 2.5–10 mg may be adequate. For soft-tissue injection in the treatment of tendon sheath inflammation, the usual dose is 2.5–10 mg.

For oral inhalation use, the triamcinolone acetonide oral aerosol inhaler delivers about 200 mcg of drug from the valve and 75 mcg from the spacer mouthpiece per metered spray under defined in vitro test conditions. The commercially available aerosol delivers at least 240 metered sprays; however, since reliable dosage delivery cannot be assured after 240 metered sprays, the aerosol inhaler should not be used after 240 actuations and patients should be cautioned against longer use of an individual inhaler. Patients should be carefully instructed in the use of the oral inhaler. To obtain optimum results, patients should also be given a copy of the patient instructions provided by the manufacturer. The inhaler should be shaken well immediately prior to use and inverted prior to actuation. After exhaling as completely as possible, the mouthpiece of the inhaler should be placed well into the mouth and the lips closed firmly around it. The patient should then inhale slowly and deeply through the mouth while pressing the metal canister down with the forefinger. After holding the breath for as long as possible (about 5–10 seconds), the mouthpiece should be removed and the patient should exhale slowly. If additional inhalations are required, the patient should wait 1 minute between inhalations, shake the inhaler again, and repeat the procedure. Following each treatment, the patient should rinse the mouth thoroughly with water or mouthwash to remove drug deposited in the oropharyngeal area.

Dosage of triamcinolone acetonide oral inhalation must be carefully adjusted according to individual requirements and response. The usual initial adult dosage by oral inhalation is 150 mcg (2 sprays) 3 or 4 times daily or 300 mcg (4 sprays) twice daily (450 or 600 mcg total). In adults with severe asthma, it may be advisable to start with 12–16 sprays daily (900–1200 mcg total), and then reduce the dosage to the lowest effective level. While the manufacturer states that a triamcinolone acetonide dosage of 1200 mcg (16 sprays) daily in adults should not be exceeded, some experts state that higher dosages may be used in adults with severe persistent asthma.

In children 6–12 years of age, the usual initial dosage is 75 or 150 mcg (1 or 2 sprays) 3 or 4 times daily (225–600 mcg total) or 150 or 300 mcg (2–4 sprays) twice daily (300–600 mcg total); dosage is adjusted according to patient response. While the manufacturer states that dosage for children 6–12 years of age should not exceed 900 mcg (12 sprays) daily, some experts state that higher dosages may be used in children with severe persistent asthma. The manufacturer states that

the drug is not recommended for use in children younger than 6 years of age. When orally inhaled triamcinolone acetonide is administered to patients receiving systemic corticosteroids, the patient's asthma should be reasonably stable before treatment with the oral inhalation begins. Initially, the aerosol is given concurrently with the maintenance dosage of the systemic corticosteroid. After about 1 week, the systemic corticosteroid is gradually withdrawn. (See Discontinuance of Therapy under Dosage and Administration: Dosage, in the Corticosteroids General Statement 68:04.) *Gradual withdrawal of systemic corticosteroids following long-term therapy is strongly recommended, since death has occurred in some individuals in whom systemic corticosteroids were withdrawn too rapidly.* After systemic corticosteroids have been withdrawn, if exacerbations of asthma occur during triamcinolone acetonide oral inhalation therapy, short courses of systemic corticosteroids should be given, then tapered as symptoms subside.

● *Triamcinolone Hexacetonide*

Triamcinolone hexacetonide may be administered by intra-articular, intralesional, or sublesional injection. Sterile suspensions of triamcinolone hexacetonide may be diluted with a local anesthetic such as 1% or 2% lidocaine hydrochloride prior to intra-articular or intralesional injection or with sterile water for injection, 0.9% sodium chloride injection, or 5% or 10% dextrose in 0.9% sodium chloride injection prior to intralesional administration. Diluents containing preservatives such as parabens or phenols should be avoided. (See Chemistry and Stability: Stability.) For intralesional (or sublesional) injection, the 5-mg/mL sterile suspension of triamcinolone hexacetonide is used.

The usual dosage for intralesional (or sublesional) injection is up to 0.5 mg per square inch of affected skin. Additional injections should be administered according to the response of the patient. For intra-articular injections, the usual dosage of triamcinolone hexacetonide (using the 20-mg/mL sterile suspension) is 2–20 mg depending on the size of the joint, degree of inflammation and amount of fluid present; doses may be repeated at intervals of 3–4 weeks. For large joints such as the knee, 10–20 mg may be used. For smaller joints such as in the fingers, 2–6 mg may be adequate.

CHEMISTRY AND STABILITY

● *Chemistry*

Triamcinolone is a synthetic glucocorticoid. The free alcohol occurs as a white or practically white, odorless, crystalline powder and is very slightly soluble in water and slightly soluble in alcohol. Triamcinolone acetonide occurs as a white to cream-colored, crystalline powder having not more than a slight odor and is practically insoluble in water and very soluble in dehydrated alcohol. The diacetate ester of triamcinolone occurs as a white to off-white, fine crystalline powder with not more than a slight odor and is practically insoluble in water and sparingly soluble in alcohol. Triamcinolone hexacetonide occurs as a white to cream-colored powder and is practically insoluble in water and very slightly soluble in alcohol.

Commercially available sterile suspensions of triamcinolone acetonide and triamcinolone hexacetonide have a pH of 5–7.5 and 4–8, respectively.

For oral inhalation, triamcinolone acetonide is commercially available as an aerosol containing a microcrystalline suspension of the drug in a vehicle of a fluorocarbon propellant (dichlorodifluoromethane) and dehydrated alcohol. Although triamcinolone acetonide is administered by an oral inhaler that produces metered sprays containing 200 mcg of triamcinolone acetonide per spray, each actuation of the inhaler delivers a dose equivalent to 100 mcg of triamcinolone acetonide, since a portion of each spray is retained within the delivery device.

● *Stability*

Commercially available oral and parenteral preparations of triamcinolone should be stored at a temperature less than 40 °C, preferably between 15–30 °C; freezing of the sterile suspensions should be avoided. Exposure of sterile suspensions of the drug to freezing temperatures can result in irreversible clumping or agglomeration (granular appearance); such suspensions should *not* be used. Triamcinolone tablets should be stored in well-closed containers. Triamcinolone acetonide sterile suspension should be protected from light. Triamcinolone acetonide oral inhaler should be stored at controlled room temperature (20–25 °C). Because the contents of the oral inhaler are under pressure, the aerosol container should *not* be punctured, used or stored near heat or an open flame, exposed to temperatures exceeding 49 °C, or placed into a fire or incinerator for disposal.

Sterile suspensions of triamcinolone hexacetonide should not be mixed with diluents or local anesthetics containing preservatives (such as parabens or phenols) because flocculation of the suspension may result. Unused diluted suspensions of the hexacetonide esters of triamcinolone should be discarded after 7 days.

For further information on chemistry, pharmacology, pharmacokinetics, uses, cautions, drug interactions, laboratory test interferences, and dosage and administration of triamcinolone, see the Corticosteroids General Statement 68:04. For EENT and topical uses, see 52:08.08 and 84:06.08, respectively.

PREPARATIONS

Abbott discontinued the manufacture of triamcinolone acetonide oral inhalation aerosol (Azmacort®) effective December 31, 2009. The US Food and Drug Administration (FDA) states that triamcinolone acetonide oral inhalation aerosol with chlorofluorocarbon (CFC) propellants will not be manufactured, sold, or dispensed in the US after December 31, 2010.

Excipients in commercially available drug preparations may have clinically important effects in some individuals; consult specific product labeling for details.

Triamcinolone

Oral		
Tablets	4 mg	**Aristocort®** (scored), Astellas

Triamcinolone Acetonide

Parenteral		
Injectable suspension	10 mg/mL	**Kenalog®**, Bristol-Myers Squibb
	40 mg/mL	**Kenalog®**, Bristol-Myers Squibb

Triamcinolone Acetonide (Microcrystalline)

Oral Inhalation		
Aerosol	75 mcg/metered spray	**Azmacort®** Oral Inhaler, Abbott

Triamcinolone Hexacetonide (Microcrystalline)

Parenteral		
Injectable suspension	5 mg/mL	**Aristospan®** Intralesional, Sandoz
	20 mg/mL	**Aristospan®** Intra-articular, Sandoz

Selected Revisions January 29, 2018, © Copyright, May 1, 1978, American Society of Health-System Pharmacists, Inc.

methylTESTOSTERone

68:08 · ANDROGENS

■ Methyltestosterone is a synthetic androgenic anabolic steroid hormone.

USES

Methyltestosterone is used mainly for replacement or substitution of diminished or absent endogenous testicular hormone.

● Uses in Males

In males, methyltestosterone is used for the management of congenital or acquired primary hypogonadism such as that resulting from orchiectomy or from testicular failure caused by cryptorchidism, bilateral torsion, orchitis, or vanishing testis syndrome. Methyltestosterone also is used in males for the management of congenital or acquired hypogonadotropic hypogonadism such as that resulting from idiopathic gonadotropin or gonadotropin releasing hormone (luteinizing hormone releasing hormone) deficiency or from pituitary-hypothalamic injury caused by tumors, trauma, or radiation. If any of these conditions occur before puberty, androgen replacement therapy will be necessary during adolescence for the development of secondary sexual characteristics and prolonged therapy will be required to maintain these characteristics. Prolonged androgen therapy also is required to maintain sexual characteristics in other males who develop testosterone deficiency after puberty.

When the diagnosis is well established, methyltestosterone may be used to stimulate puberty in carefully selected males with delayed puberty. These males usually have a family history of delayed puberty that is not caused by a pathologic disorder. Brief treatment with conservative doses of an androgen may occasionally be justified in these males if they do not respond to psychologic support. Because androgens may adversely affect bone maturation in these prepubertal males, this potential risk should be fully discussed with the patient and his parents prior to initiation of androgen therapy. (See Cautions: Pediatric Precautions.) If androgen therapy is initiated in these prepubertal males, radiographs of the hand and wrist should be obtained at 6-month intervals to determine the effect of therapy on the epiphyseal centers.

The safety and efficacy of methyltestosterone in patients with low testosterone concentrations related to aging (i.e., late-onset hypogonadism) have not been established. Although endogenous testosterone concentrations decline with aging and manifestations of hypogonadism such as decreased libido, impotence, decreased body hair growth, decreased muscle mass, increased risk of cardiovascular disease, and decreased bone mass and resultant osteoporosis may occur, it is unclear whether these symptoms are related to such decreased concentrations or to normal aging; therefore, the need to replace testosterone in aging men is unclear. For further information on management of low testosterone concentrations related to aging, see Late-onset Hypogonadism under Uses: Uses in Males, in Testosterone 68:08.

For additional information on the management of male hypogonadism, see Uses: Uses in Males in Testosterone 68:08.

● Other Uses

In females, methyltestosterone is used for the palliative treatment of androgen-responsive, advanced, inoperable, metastatic (skeletal) carcinoma of the breast in women who are 1–5 years postmenopausal. Primary goals of therapy in these women include ablation of the ovaries. Other methods of counteracting estrogen activity include adrenalectomy, hypophysectomy, and/or antiestrogen therapy (e.g., tamoxifen). Androgen therapy also has been used in premenopausal women with carcinoma of the breast who have benefited from oophorectomy and are considered to have a hormone-responsive tumor. The decision to use androgen therapy in women with carcinoma of the breast should be made by an oncologist with expertise in the treatment of this carcinoma.

Methyltestosterone also has been used for the prevention of postpartum breast pain and engorgement; however, the drug does not appear to prevent or suppress lactation.

In females, methyltestosterone is used in combination with estrogens for the management of moderate to severe vasomotor symptoms† associated with menopause in patients who do not respond adequately to estrogens alone. While estrogen/androgen combinations were found to be effective for the management of vasomotor symptoms associated with menopause under a determination made by the FDA in 1976, formal administrative proceedings were initiated by the

FDA in April 2003 to examine the effectiveness of estrogen/androgen combinations for this indication. FDA is undertaking this action because the agency does not believe there is substantial evidence available to establish the contribution of androgens to the effectiveness of estrogen/androgen combinations for the management of vasomotor symptoms in menopausal women who do not respond to estrogens alone. The FDA will allow continued marketing of combination estrogen/androgen products while the matter is under study.

Although methyltestosterone has been used in other conditions (e.g., fractures, surgery, convalescence, functional uterine bleeding), there is a lack of substantial evidence that androgens are effective in these conditions. In addition, the FDA states that there currently is no evidence to support the safety and efficacy of methyltestosterone as an aphrodisiac (i.e., to arouse or increase sexual desire or to improve sexual performance).

● Misuse, Abuse, and Dependence

Because of their anabolic and androgenic effects on performance (ergogenic potential) and physique, androgens have been misused and abused by athletes, bodybuilders, weight lifters, and others, including high school- and college-aged individuals engaged in sports. Following review of data from published literature and case reports in October 2016, the FDA concluded that misuse and abuse of androgens are associated with serious adverse cardiovascular, hepatic, endocrine, and mental health effects. (See Cautions; also see Uses: Misuse, Abuse, and Dependence, in Testosterone 68:08.)

Serum testosterone concentrations should be evaluated in patients who may be misusing or abusing androgens (e.g., patients experiencing serious adverse cardiovascular or psychiatric effects); however, serum testosterone concentrations may be below or within the normal range in patients abusing synthetic derivatives of testosterone.

DOSAGE AND ADMINISTRATION

Diagnosis of male hypogonadism must be confirmed by laboratory testing prior to initiation of methyltestosterone therapy. To confirm this diagnosis, serum testosterone concentrations should be measured in the morning on at least 2 separate days and must be consistently below the normal range. Serum testosterone concentrations may be low later in the day in men with or without hypogonadism; therefore, measuring testosterone concentrations later in the day should be avoided.

● Administration

Methyltestosterone is administered orally; the drug usually is given in divided daily doses. Methyltestosterone also has been administered intrabuccally.

● Dosage

Dosage of methyltestosterone is variable and should be individualized according to the condition being treated, the severity of symptoms, and the patient's age, gender, and history of prior androgenic therapy.

Male Hypogonadism

For replacement of endogenous testicular hormone in androgen-deficient males, the usual oral dosage of methyltestosterone is 10–50 mg daily as capsules. Alternatively, buccal tablets have been administered in a dosage of 5–25 mg daily. For the management of postpubertal cryptorchidism in patients with evidence of hypogonadism, several manufacturers recommend an oral methyltestosterone dosage of 30 mg daily as capsules. Alternatively, buccal tablets have been administered in a dosage of 15 mg daily.

Various dosage regimens have been used to induce pubertal changes in hypogonadal males. Some clinicians recommend that lower dosages be used initially, followed by gradual increases in dosage as puberty progresses; subsequently, the dosage may be decreased to maintenance levels. Other clinicians state that higher dosages are required initially to induce pubertal changes and lower dosages can then be used for maintenance therapy after puberty. The chronologic and skeletal ages of the patient must be considered when determining the initial dosage and subsequent dosage adjustment. In general, short-term administration (e.g., 4–6 months) of methyltestosterone and dosages in the lower end of the usual range for replacement (i.e., 10 mg daily) are used for the treatment of delayed puberty in males.

Inoperable Carcinoma of the Breast

For the palliative treatment of advanced, inoperable, metastatic carcinoma of the breast in women, the usual oral dosage of methyltestosterone is 50–200 mg daily as capsules. Alternatively, buccal tablets have been administered in a dosage of 25–100 mg daily.

Postpartum Breast Pain and Engorgement

For the prevention of postpartum breast pain and engorgement, the usual oral dosage of methyltestosterone is 80 mg daily as capsules for 3–5 days after parturition. Alternatively, buccal tablets have been administered in a dosage of 40 mg daily for 3–5 days after parturition.

Vasomotor Symptoms Associated with Menopause

When methyltestosterone is used in combination with an estrogen (i.e., conjugated estrogens or esterified estrogens) for the short-term management of moderate to severe vasomotor symptoms† associated with menopause, the lowest possible effective dosage should be used and therapy should be discontinued as soon as possible. Attempts to reduce dosage or discontinue the drugs should be made at 3- to 6-month intervals. The combined drugs are administered for 21 consecutive days, followed by 7 days without the drugs, and then this regimen is repeated as necessary. The manufacturers' labeling for the respective drugs or drug combinations should be consulted for usual recommended dosages for combination therapy. Women with an intact uterus receiving combination therapy should be closely monitored for signs of endometrial carcinoma, and appropriate diagnostic measures should be employed if persistent or recurring abnormal vaginal bleeding occurs during therapy with the drugs.

CAUTIONS

● Adverse Effects

Cardiovascular events (e.g., myocardial infarction [MI], stroke) have been reported with methyltestosterone therapy. Long-term clinical safety studies have not been conducted to date to determine the cardiovascular effects of testosterone replacement therapy in men. Epidemiologic data and results from randomized, controlled clinical trials have been inconclusive for determining the risk of serious adverse cardiovascular events (i.e., nonfatal MI, nonfatal stroke, death) with testosterone use compared with nonuse.

Because the current evidence regarding the cardiovascular risk associated with testosterone replacement therapy is weak because of the limited scope, quality, design, and size of the clinical trials, the FDA has requested additional evidence from well-designed studies to further elucidate the cardiovascular risk associated with testosterone use. Following review of data from several observational studies and meta-analyses in March 2015, the FDA concluded that use of testosterone is associated with a possible increased risk of serious adverse cardiovascular events. Clinicians should inform patients of this potential increased risk when deciding whether to use or continue to use testosterone replacement therapy. For further precautionary information about adverse cardiovascular effects, see Cautions: Cardiovascular Effects, in Testosterone 68:08.

Venous thromboembolic events, including deep-vein thrombosis (DVT) and pulmonary embolism (PE), have been reported during postmarketing experience with testosterone preparations, including methyltestosterone. Patients reporting symptoms of pain, edema, warmth, and erythema in a lower extremity or presenting with acute shortness of breath should be evaluated for possible DVT or PE, respectively. If venous thromboembolism is suspected, methyltestosterone therapy should be discontinued and appropriate evaluation and management should be initiated.

Adverse effects associated with methyltestosterone are similar to those of other synthetic or natural androgens and include acne, gynecomastia, and edema. If edema is present before or develops during therapy, administration of diuretics may be required. Gynecomastia frequently develops and occasionally persists in patients being treated for hypogonadism.

Oligospermia and decreased ejaculatory volume may occur in males receiving excessive dosage or prolonged administration of the drug. Priapism or excessive sexual stimulation in males, especially geriatric patients, also may occur. If priapism or excessive sexual stimulation develops during methyltestosterone therapy, the drug should be discontinued temporarily, since these are signs of excessive dosage; if therapy with methyltestosterone is reinstituted, a lower dosage should be used. Male pattern of baldness also may occur.

Amenorrhea and other menstrual irregularities and inhibition of gonadotropin secretion occur commonly in females. Virilization, including deepening of the voice, hirsutism, and clitoral enlargement, also occur commonly in females; these changes may not be reversible following discontinuance of the drug.

Hypersensitivity reactions, including skin manifestations and anaphylactoid reactions, have occurred rarely with methyltestosterone.

Hypercalcemia resulting from osteolysis, especially in immobile patients and those with metastatic carcinoma of the breast, has been reported in patients receiving methyltestosterone. The drug should be discontinued if hypercalcemia occurs in patients with cancer since this may indicate progression of metastases to the bone. Retention of water, sodium, chloride, potassium, and inorganic phosphates also has occurred in patients receiving the drug.

Cholestatic hepatitis and jaundice and abnormal liver function test results may occur in patients receiving 17-α-alkylandrogens such as methyltestosterone. These adverse hepatic effects may occur at relatively low doses of the drug. Drug-induced jaundice usually is reversible following discontinuance of the drug. Methyltestosterone should be discontinued if cholestatic jaundice or hepatitis occurs, or if liver function test results become abnormal during therapy with the drug, and the etiology of these disorders should be determined. Peliosis of the liver and hepatic neoplasms, including hepatocellular carcinoma, have been reported rarely in patients receiving long-term administration of androgenic anabolic steroids. Peliosis of the liver can be a life-threatening or fatal complication of androgen therapy.

Serious adverse effects (e.g., increased aggression, antisocial behavior, manic episode, hostility, depression, changes in libido, increased risk of cardiovascular events, hepatotoxicity, testicular atrophy, sperm abnormalities) are associated with misuse and abuse of androgens (see Uses: Misuse, Abuse, and Dependence). Methyltestosterone preparations currently are subject to control under the Federal Controlled Substances Act of 1970, as amended by the Anabolic Steroids Control Act of 1990 and 2004, as schedule III (C-III) drugs.

Manifestations of withdrawal (e.g., depressed mood, major depression, fatigue, cravings, restlessness, irritability, anorexia, insomnia, decreased libido, hypogonadotropic hypogonadism) may occur if androgens are discontinued abruptly or dosage is substantially reduced in physically dependent patients or in those taking supratherapeutic dosages of such drugs; withdrawal symptoms may persist for weeks or months.

Other adverse effects associated with methyltestosterone therapy include nausea, polycythemia, headache, anxiety, mental depression, generalized paresthesia, and suppression of clotting factors II, V, VII, and X. Serum cholesterol concentration may increase during androgen therapy.

● Precautions and Contraindications

Methyltestosterone shares the toxic potentials of other androgens, and the usual precautions of androgen therapy should be observed. When methyltestosterone is used in combination with estrogens, the usual precautions associated with estrogen therapy also should be observed. (See Cautions in Conjugated Estrogens 68:16.04.) Clinicians prescribing estrogens should be aware of the risks associated with these drugs, and the manufacturers' labeling should be consulted for further discussion of these risks and associated precautions.

Methyltestosterone should be used with caution in patients with cardiac, renal, or hepatic dysfunction since edema, with or without congestive heart failure, may occur as a result of sodium and water retention. If edema occurs during methyltestosterone therapy and it is considered a serious complication, the drug should be discontinued; diuretic therapy also may be necessary. Liver function should be evaluated periodically during use of methyltestosterone.

Some experts recommend that methyltestosterone be used with caution in patients at high risk for cardiovascular disease, such as older men or those with diabetes mellitus or obesity, since serious adverse cardiovascular events (i.e., MI, stroke, death) may occur. (See Cautions: Adverse Effects.)

Females should be carefully monitored for signs of virilization (e.g., deepening of the voice, hirsutism, clitoromegaly, menstrual irregularities) during methyltestosterone therapy. The drug should generally be discontinued when mild virilization is evident, since some adverse androgenic effects (e.g., voice changes) may not subside following discontinuance of the drug. The woman and physician may decide that some virilization is acceptable during treatment for carcinoma of the breast.

Males should be carefully monitored for the development of priapism or excessive sexual stimulation since these are signs of excessive dosage. Males, especially geriatric patients, may become overly stimulated. Stimulation to the point of increasing the nervous, mental, and physical activities beyond the patient's cardiovascular capacity should be avoided when methyltestosterone is used to treat climacteric in males. (See also Cautions: Adverse Effects.) Geriatric males may be at increased risk of developing prostatic hypertrophy and carcinoma during androgen therapy.

Adult or adolescent males should be advised to report too frequent or persistent penile erections to their physician. Females should be advised to report hoarseness, acne, menstrual changes, or the growth of facial hair to their physician. All patients should be advised to report nausea, vomiting, changes in skin color, or ankle swelling to their physician.

Patients receiving high dosages of methyltestosterone should have periodic hemoglobin and hematocrit determinations, since polycythemia may occur.

Methyltestosterone is contraindicated in males with carcinoma of the breast or known or suspected carcinoma of the prostate. Some manufacturers state that the drug also is contraindicated in patients with cardiac, renal, or hepatic decompensation; hypercalcemia; impaired liver function; and in patients who are easily sexually stimulated. Because of the potential risk of serious adverse health effects, methyltestosterone should not be used for enhancement of athletic performance or physique. (See Uses: Misuse, Abuse and Dependence, in Testosterone 68:08.) Patients should be informed of the serious adverse effects associated with misuse and abuse of androgens.

● **Pediatric Precautions**

Androgens should be used with extreme caution in children and only by specialists who are aware of the adverse effects of these drugs on bone maturation. Methyltestosterone should be used cautiously to stimulate puberty, and only in carefully selected males with delayed puberty. (See Uses: Uses in Males.) In children, methyltestosterone may accelerate bone maturation without producing compensatory gain in linear growth. This adverse effect may result in compromised adult stature. The younger the child, the greater the risk of methyltestosterone compromising final mature stature. If methyltestosterone is administered to prepubertal children (e.g., to stimulate puberty in males), the drug should be used with extreme caution, and radiographic examination of the hand and wrist should be performed every 6 months to determine the rate of bone maturation and to assess the effect of treatment on the epiphyseal centers. If methyltestosterone is to be used to stimulate puberty in a male with delayed puberty, the potential risk of therapy should be fully discussed with the patient and his parents prior to initiation of the drug.

● **Mutagenicity and Carcinogenicity**

Hepatocellular carcinoma reportedly has occurred in patients receiving long-term therapy with high dosages of androgens. Regression of the tumor does not always occur following discontinuance of androgen therapy. Geriatric patients may be at increased risk of developing prostatic hypertrophy and carcinoma during androgen therapy.

Following implantation of testosterone in mice, cervical-uterine tumors developed and occasionally metastasized. There is some evidence to suggest that injection of testosterone into some strains of female mice increases their susceptibility to hepatomas. Testosterone also has been shown to increase the number of tumors and decrease the degree of differentiation of chemically induced tumors in rats. It is not known whether androgens, including methyltestosterone, are mutagenic.

● **Pregnancy, Fertility, and Lactation**

Pregnancy

Methyltestosterone may cause fetal harm when administered to pregnant women. Androgenic effects including clitoral hypertrophy, labial fusion of the external genital fold to form a scrotal-like structure, abnormal vaginal development, and persistence of a urogenital sinus have occurred in the female offspring of women who were given androgens during pregnancy. The degree of masculinization is related to the amount of drug given to the woman and the age of the fetus; masculinization is most likely to occur in a female fetus when exposure to androgens occurs during the first trimester. Since the risks clearly outweigh the possible benefits in women who are or may become pregnant, methyltestosterone is contraindicated in such women. Women who become pregnant while receiving the drug should be informed of the potential hazard to the fetus.

Fertility

Although the effect of methyltestosterone on fertility in humans has not been conclusively determined, the drug produces oligospermia and decreased ejaculatory volume in males. Priapism and excessive sexual stimulation also have occurred

in males receiving the drug. (See Cautions: Adverse Effects and Precautions and Contraindications.) Increased or decreased libido also has been reported.

Lactation

It is not known whether methyltestosterone is distributed into milk. Because of the potential for serious adverse reactions to androgens in nursing infants, a decision should be made whether to discontinue nursing or to not use methyltestosterone, taking into account the importance of the drug to the woman.

DRUG INTERACTIONS

Methyltestosterone may potentiate the action of oral anticoagulants, causing bleeding in some patients. When methyltestosterone therapy is initiated in patients receiving oral anticoagulants, dosage reduction of the anticoagulant may be required to prevent an excessive hypoprothrombinemic response. Patients receiving oral anticoagulants also should be closely monitored when androgen therapy is discontinued.

The metabolic effects of androgens may decrease blood glucose concentrations and insulin requirements in patients with diabetes.

LABORATORY TEST INTERFERENCES

Protein bound iodine (PBI) concentrations may be decreased in some patients during methyltestosterone therapy; however, this does not appear to be clinically important. Androgens may decrease thyroxine-binding globulin concentrations, resulting in decreased total serum thyroxine (T_4) concentrations and increased resin uptake of triiodothyronine (T_3) and T_4. Free thyroid hormone concentrations remain unchanged, and there is no clinical evidence of thyroid dysfunction.

PHARMACOLOGY

Endogenous androgens are essential hormones that are responsible for the normal growth and development of the male sex organs and for maintenance of secondary sex characteristics, including the growth and maturation of the prostate, seminal vesicles, penis, and scrotum; development of male hair distribution, such as beard, pubic, chest, and axillary hair; laryngeal enlargement and thickening of the vocal cords; and alterations in body musculature and fat distribution.

Like testosterone and other androgenic anabolic hormones, methyltestosterone also produces retention of nitrogen, potassium, sodium, and phosphorus; increases protein anabolism; and decreases amino acid catabolism and urinary calcium concentrations. Nitrogen balance is improved only when there is sufficient intake of calories and protein.

Androgens are responsible for the growth spurt that occurs during adolescence and for the eventual termination of linear growth that results from fusion of the epiphyseal growth centers. Although exogenous androgens accelerate linear growth rates in children, the drugs may cause a disproportionate advancement in bone maturation, and long-term administration of the drugs in prepubertal children may result in fusion of the epiphyseal growth centers and premature termination of the growth process.

Exogenous administration of androgens inhibits the release of endogenous testosterone via feedback inhibition of pituitary luteinizing hormone (LH). Following administration of large doses of exogenous androgens, spermatogenesis also may be suppressed as a result of feedback inhibition of pituitary follicle-stimulating hormone (FSH).

Androgens reportedly stimulate the production of erythrocytes, apparently by enhancing the production of erythropoietic stimulating factor.

CHEMISTRY AND STABILITY

● **Chemistry**

Methyltestosterone is a synthetic androgenic anabolic steroid hormone. The drug is structurally similar to testosterone, but is methylated at the 17 position of the steroid nucleus. Methylation at the 17 position is associated with less hepatic metabolism and enhanced pharmacologic activity following oral administration compared with testosterone.

Methyltestosterone occurs as white or creamy white, odorless, slightly hygroscopic crystals or a crystalline powder and is practically insoluble in water and soluble in alcohol.

● Stability

Commercially available preparations of methyltestosterone should be protected from light and stored in well-closed containers at a temperature less than 40°C, preferably between 2–30°C, unless otherwise specified by the manufacturer.

PREPARATIONS

Most methyltestosterone-containing preparations are subject to control under the Federal Controlled Substances Act of 1970, as amended by the Anabolic Steroids Control Act of 1990 and 2004, as schedule III (C-III) drugs. However, manufacturers of certain preparations containing androgenic anabolic steroids (principally combinations that also include estrogens) have applied for and obtained for their product(s) an exemption from the record-keeping and other regulatory requirements of the Federal Controlled Substances Act. (See the introductory paragraph under Preparations, in Testosterone 68:08.) Because regulatory requirements for a given preparation containing an androgenic

anabolic steroid may be subject to change under the provisions of the Act, the manufacturer should be contacted when specific clarification about a preparation's status is required.

Excipients in commercially available drug preparations may have clinically important effects in some individuals; consult specific product labeling for details.

methylTESTOSTERone

Oral

Capsules	10 mg*	**Android®** (C-III), Valeant
		methylTESTOSTERone Capsules (C-III)
		Testred® (C-III), Valeant
Tablets	10 mg*	**Methitest®** (C-III; scored), Global
		methylTESTOSTERone Tablets (C-III)

* available from one or more manufacturer, distributor, and/or repackager by generic (nonproprietary) name

† Use is not currently included in the labeling approved by the US Food and Drug Administration.

Selected Revisions November 27, 2017, © Copyright, January 1, 1959, American Society of Health-System Pharmacists, Inc.

Testosterone

68:08 • ANDROGENS

■ Testosterone, the principal endogenous androgen, is a naturally occurring androgenic anabolic steroid hormone.

REMS

FDA approved a REMS for testosterone to ensure that the benefits outweigh the risks. The REMS may apply to one or more preparations of testosterone. See the FDA REMS page (https://www.accessdata.fda.gov/scripts/cder/rems/index.cfm).

USES

Testosterone is used for replacement or substitution of diminished or absent endogenous testicular hormone caused by certain medical conditions.

Diagnosis of hypogonadism must be confirmed by laboratory testing prior to initiation of testosterone therapy. (See Dosage and Administration.)

The safety and efficacy of testosterone replacement therapy in men with low testosterone concentrations related to aging have not been established. (See Late-onset Hypogonadism under Uses: Uses in Males.)

● Uses in Males

Hypogonadism

In males, testosterone is used for the management of congenital or acquired primary hypogonadism such as that resulting from orchiectomy or from testicular failure caused by cryptorchidism, bilateral torsion, orchitis, or vanishing testis syndrome. Testosterone also is used in males for the management of congenital or acquired hypogonadotropic hypogonadism such as that resulting from idiopathic gonadotropin or gonadotropin-releasing hormone (luteinizing hormone releasing hormone) deficiency or from pituitary-hypothalamic injury caused by tumors, trauma, or radiation. If any of these conditions occur before puberty, androgen replacement therapy will be necessary during adolescence for the development of secondary sexual characteristics and prolonged therapy will be required to maintain these characteristics. Prolonged androgen therapy also is required to maintain sexual characteristics in other males who develop testosterone deficiency after puberty.

Manifestations

Hypogonadism in males may manifest with signs and symptoms of testosterone deficiency and/or infertility, with manifestations depending principally on the age of the patient at the time of development. Hypogonadism seldom is recognized before the age of puberty unless it is associated with growth retardation or other anatomic and/or endocrine abnormalities. When hypogonadism develops before puberty onset, manifestations include small testes, phallus, and prostate; minimal pubic and axillary hair; disproportionately long arms and legs (secondary to delayed epiphyseal closure); reduced male musculature; gynecomastia; and a persistently high-pitched voice. Postpubertal loss of testicular function results in slowly evolving subtle clinical manifestations, which may be difficult to appreciate in aging men because they often are attributed to growing old. Growth of body hair usually slows, while the voice and size of the phallus and prostate remain unchanged. Patients with postpubertal hypogonadism may manifest a progressive decrease in muscle mass, libido loss, impotence, oligospermia or azoospermia, and/or occasionally menopause-type hot flushes (with acute onset of hypogonadism). Hypogonadism also is associated with a risk of osteoporosis and resultant fractures. Many cases of postpubertal hypogonadism are initially detected during fertility evaluations.

Hypogonadism Associated with HIV Infection

Hypogonadism occurs commonly in human immunodeficiency virus (HIV)-infected men, particularly as their disease progresses to acquired immunodeficiency syndrome (AIDS). Hypogonadism has been reported in up to 50% of HIV-infected men, being most likely in those with AIDS; however, the incidence may now be lower as a result of highly active antiretroviral therapy (HAART) and resultant improved overall health in HIV-infected patients. Such patients generally exhibit low serum testosterone concentrations and usually low (indicating hypothalamic-pituitary involvement) or occasionally high (indicating testicular involvement) gonadotropin concentrations. In addition to typical manifestations of hypogonadism (e.g., impaired sexual mood and functioning, loss of body hair, gynecomastia, bone loss, impaired sense of well-being), hypogonadal HIV-infected men may exhibit a disproportionate loss of lean body mass and muscle wasting. The etiology of hypotestosteronism in HIV-infected men likely is multifactorial and may show interindividual variation and may include primary testicular problems, changes in the hypothalamic-pituitary-gonadal axis, and/or changes caused by chronic illness, poor nutrition, or medications; approximately 25% of hypogonadism cases in HIV-infected men are primary. Testosterone replacement therapy is considered the androgen of choice for the treatment of androgen deficiency (e.g., hypogonadism) and AIDS wasting in HIV-infected men.

Late-onset Hypogonadism

The safety and efficacy of testosterone replacement therapy for men with late-onset hypogonadism (i.e., low testosterone concentrations related to aging) have not been established. Although endogenous testosterone concentrations decline with aging and manifestations of hypogonadism such as decreased libido, impotence, decreased body hair growth, decreased muscle mass, increased risk of cardiovascular disease, and decreased bone mass and resultant osteoporosis may occur, it is unclear whether these symptoms are related to such decreased concentrations or to normal aging; therefore, the need to replace testosterone in aging men is unclear.

There currently is a paucity of information from well-designed studies on the use of testosterone in middle-aged or older men who do not meet the clinical diagnostic criteria for established hypogonadism but who may have testosterone levels in the low range for young adults and/or who show one or more manifestations common to both aging and hypogonadism. In addition, studies that have been conducted generally have been of short duration, involved small numbers of patients, and often lacked adequate controls. Therefore, assessments of risks and benefits have been limited to date, and uncertainties remain about the value of testosterone therapy in older men without a clinical diagnosis of hypogonadism. In most studies to date, it appears that older men were given testosterone dosages that increased testosterone levels to the normal physiologic range for young adult males. Because of the potential risks of testosterone therapy and the availability of other safe and effective intervention options for some of the diseases and conditions it is intended to prevent or treat (e.g., bisphosphonates for osteoporosis), testosterone should be considered a therapeutic rather than a preventative measure in aging men. Although endogenous testosterone levels clearly decline with aging, it currently is unclear whether such decreased levels affect health outcomes in older men. Much remains unknown about how physiologic pathways are affected by changes in endogenous testosterone concentrations or by the administration of exogenous testosterone in aging men.

Current limited evidence suggests that testosterone therapy in aging men may produce beneficial effects on body composition, strength, bone density, frailty, cognitive function, mood, sexual function, and quality of life. However, additional evidence from well-designed studies is needed to further elucidate the role of testosterone therapy in men with low testosterone concentrations related to aging.

Testosterone Replacement Therapy for Hypogonadism

Men with symptomatic hypogonadism and clearly low testosterone concentrations (free or total, considering SHBG) are potential candidates for testosterone replacement therapy; however, the potential prostatic risk must be considered. Serum total (bound and free) testosterone concentrations less than 300 ng/dL generally are considered indicative of hypogonadism in men, and the biochemical goal of hormone replacement therapy with testosterone generally is to increase serum total testosterone concentrations to within the normal physiologic range of 300–1200 ng/mL. The principal goals of testosterone replacement are to restore sexual function, libido, well-being, and behavior; to stimulate and maintain virilization (e.g., secondary sex characteristics such as muscle mass, body hair, phallus growth); to optimize bone density and prevent osteoporosis; to possibly normalize somatotropin (growth hormone) concentrations in geriatric men; to potentially improve cardiovascular risk; and to restore fertility in cases of hypogonadotropic hypogonadism. In HIV-infected men, additional goals include improvement in mood (e.g., depression), energy level (fatigue), quality of life, and lean body mass (wasting syndrome); however, clinical response to testosterone therapy in HIV-infected men is not necessarily correlated to baseline serum testosterone concentrations, and eugonadal HIV-infected men may benefit from such therapy.

Delayed Puberty

When the diagnosis is well established, testosterone may be used to stimulate puberty in carefully selected males with delayed puberty. These males usually have a family history of delayed puberty that is not caused by a pathologic disorder. Brief treatment with conservative doses of an androgen may occasionally be justified in these males if they do not respond to psychologic support. Because androgens may adversely affect bone maturation in these prepubertal males, this potential risk should be fully discussed with the patient and his parents prior to initiation of androgen therapy. (See Cautions: Pediatric Precautions.) If androgen therapy is initiated in these prepubertal males, radiographs of the hand and wrist should be obtained at 6-month intervals to determine the effect of therapy on the epiphyseal centers. Testosterone is designated an orphan drug by the FDA for use in this condition.

Corticosteroid-induced Hypogonadism and Osteoporosis

Patients receiving long-term corticosteroid therapy may develop hypogonadism secondary to inhibition of secretion of luteinizing hormone (LH) and follicle-stimulating hormone (FSH) from the pituitary as well as secondary to direct effects on the testes and ovaries, and such hypogonadism may be associated with bone loss. Therefore, all patients receiving prolonged corticosteroid therapy should be assessed for possible hypogonadism, which should be corrected if present. Unlike experience with hormone replacement therapy (HRT, combined estrogen and progestin therapy) in postmenopausal women receiving chronic prednisone therapy, there currently is only limited information on the effect of androgen (e.g., testosterone) replacement therapy in men with hypogonadism secondary to long-term corticosteroid therapy. In a small study in men with corticosteroid-treated asthma and low serum testosterone concentrations, lumbar spine bone mass density (BMD) was increased nearly 4% after 12 months of monthly testosterone injections; lean body mass also was increased and fat mass was reduced. Therefore, men who develop low serum testosterone concentrations while receiving long-term corticosteroid therapy should be offered testosterone replacement therapy in an attempt to treat hypogonadism and possibly reduce the risk of corticosteroid-induced osteoporosis† when contraindications to androgen therapy are not present. Some experts (e.g., the American College of Rheumatology) recommend that such men with serum testosterone concentrations below the physiologic range (i.e., less than 300 ng/mL) receive replacement therapy. The goal of testosterone replacement therapy in men receiving long-term corticosteroid therapy is to provide serum testosterone concentrations within the therapeutic range. It is important that the possibility of prostate cancer be ruled out in any man being considered for such replacement therapy. For additional information on the management of corticosteroid-induced osteoporosis, see Cautions: Musculoskeletal Effects in the Corticosteroids General Statement 68:04.

Erectile Dysfunction

Although testosterone replacement therapy may restore sexual function in hypogonadal men (see Uses in Males: Hypogonadism, in Uses), the American Urological Association (AUA) states that the drug is not indicated for the treatment of erectile dysfunction in men with normal serum testosterone concentrations†. Outcome measures in studies to date are inadequate to evaluate testosterone's efficacy in eugonadal men. In men with borderline testosterone concentrations, a clinical trial of replacement therapy may be warranted in the management of erectile dysfunction; however, the risks of hormone replacement must be weighed carefully.

● Uses in Females

Inoperable Carcinoma of the Breast

In females, testosterone has been used for the palliative treatment of androgen-responsive, advanced, inoperable, metastatic (skeletal) carcinoma of the breast in women who are 1–5 years postmenopausal. Primary goals of therapy in these women include ablation of the ovaries. Other methods of counteracting estrogen activity include adrenalectomy, hypophysectomy, and/or antiestrogen therapy (e.g., tamoxifen). Androgen therapy also has been used in premenopausal women with carcinoma of the breast who have benefited from oophorectomy and

are considered to have a hormone-responsive tumor. The decision to use androgen therapy in women with carcinoma of the breast should be made by an oncologist with expertise in the treatment of this carcinoma.

Postpartum Breast Pain and Engorgement

Testosterone formerly was used for the prevention of postpartum breast pain and engorgement†; however, the drug does not appear to prevent or suppress lactation. Testosterone esters also have been used in combination with estrogens for the prevention of postpartum breast pain and engorgement; however, the FDA has withdrawn approval of estrogen-containing drugs for this indication. Data from controlled studies indicate that the incidence of substantial painful engorgement is low in untreated women, and the condition usually responds to analgesic or other supportive therapy.

Menopause

In females, testosterone esters also are used in combination with estrogens for the management of moderate to severe vasomotor symptoms† associated with menopause in patients who do not respond adequately to estrogens alone. While estrogen/androgen combinations were found to be effective for the management of vasomotor symptoms associated with menopause under a determination made by the FDA in 1976, formal administrative proceedings were initiated by the FDA in April 2003 to examine the effectiveness of estrogen/androgen combinations for this indication. FDA is undertaking this action because the agency does not believe there is substantial evidence available to establish the contribution of androgens to the effectiveness of estrogen/androgen combinations for the management of vasomotor symptoms in menopausal women who do not respond to estrogens alone. The FDA will allow continued marketing of combination estrogen/androgen products while the matter is under study.

● Misuse, Abuse, and Dependence

Because of their anabolic and androgenic effects on performance (ergogenic potential) and physique, androgens have been misused and abused by athletes, bodybuilders, weight lifters, and others, including high school- and college-aged individuals engaged in sports. The drugs also have been misused and abused for cosmetic purposes by noncompetitors attempting to achieve bodies with lean muscle mass. Although historically the drugs have been regarded as ineffective for anabolic and androgenic uses in athletes, limited evidence suggests that androgens may increase skeletal muscle mass and strength when used in conjunction with proper (e.g., high-protein, high calorie) diet and training but that their use is not associated with increased power or capacity for aerobic work. There continues to be a lack of evidence of long-term beneficial effects, and the drugs have been associated with substantial adverse health effects and toxicity. When used to improve athletic performance and physique, dosages employed often substantially (e.g., 10- to 1000-fold) exceed usual therapeutic dosages of the drugs. In addition, several androgens often are taken concomitantly ("stacking") for extended periods. The extent of misuse and abuse of androgens has not been fully determined, but nonmedical use is believed to be widespread. Estimates for the rate of misuse and abuse by weight lifters and body builders have ranged up to 50–80%. However, in terms of actual numbers, it has been suggested that most misuse and abuse of androgens are by individuals who never compete in sports. Evidence from one study indicates that about 7% of male high school seniors use or have used the drugs. Although the likelihood of use was increased in males intending to participate in school-sponsored sports (particularly football and wrestling), 35% of users had no intention of participating in school-sponsored sports. About 40% of these high school students admitted initiating use of the drugs at 15 years of age or younger. In studies of college students, androgen use among athletes ranged up to about 20%.

Following review of data from published literature and case reports in October 2016, the FDA concluded that misuse and abuse of androgens are associated with serious adverse effects. Serious adverse effects including increased aggression, hostility, and antisocial behavior ("roid rage"); psychotic manifestations and affective disorders (e.g., manic episode, depression, paranoia, psychosis, delusions, hallucinations); changes in libido; cardiovascular events (e.g., cardiac arrest, myocardial infarction [MI], hypertrophic cardiomyopathy, congestive heart failure [CHF], cerebrovascular accident); and hepatotoxicity (e.g., abnormal liver function test results, liver tumors [hepatic adenomas, hepatocellular carcinoma], peliosis hepatis, jaundice) have been reported in individuals who misuse and abuse androgens. Other potential adverse effects of androgens in adolescents or younger children include premature bone maturation and epiphyseal closure with resultant irreversible short stature, precocious puberty, possible increased risk of ruptured tendons and ligaments and of tendinitis, and acne. Other potential adverse effects of androgens in males include transient ischemic attacks, convulsions, hypomania, irritability, dyslipidemias, gynecomastia, hair loss, testicular atrophy and sperm abnormalities (oligospermia, decreased motility, abnormal morphology, azoospermia), impotence, subfertility, infertility, and prostatic enlargement with resultant difficulty in urinating. Other potential adverse effects in females include clitoral enlargement (which may be irreversible), menstrual irregularities, hirsutism, androgenetic alopecia, deepened voice, breast atrophy, and virilization. Manifestations of withdrawal (e.g., depressed mood, major depression, fatigue, cravings, restlessness, irritability, anorexia, insomnia, decreased libido, hypogonadotropic hypogonadism) may occur if androgens, such as testosterone, are discontinued abruptly or the dosage is substantially reduced in patients who are physically dependent or receiving supratherapeutic doses of the drug; withdrawal symptoms may persist for weeks or months.

Serum testosterone concentrations should be evaluated in patients who may be misusing or abusing androgens (e.g., patients experiencing serious adverse cardiovascular or psychiatric effects); however, serum testosterone concentrations may be below or within the normal range in patients abusing synthetic derivatives of testosterone. Because of the potential for serious adverse effects associated with misuse and abuse of androgens, preventive measures have been initiated, including educational programs, interdiction of black market supplies, drug screening of athletes with associated penalties for use, and other control measures. The prescription, dispensing, distribution, and use of most androgens currently are restricted as controlled substances. In addition, medical and sports experts, including the American College of Sports Medicine, American Medical Association, American Academy of Pediatrics, American College Health Association, National Strength and Conditioning Association, National Collegiate Athletic Association, National Football League, US Olympic Committee, and the International Olympic Committee, consider the use of androgens to enhance athletic performance or physique inappropriate and unacceptable because of known adverse effects, lack of data regarding long-term gains in size and strength, and potential long-term adverse sequelae and because their use by athletes is contrary to the rules and ethical principles of athletic competition.

DOSAGE AND ADMINISTRATION

Diagnosis of hypogonadism must be confirmed by laboratory testing prior to initiation of testosterone therapy. To confirm this diagnosis, serum testosterone concentrations should be measured in the morning on at least 2 separate days and must be consistently below the normal range. Serum testosterone concentrations may be low later in the day in men with or without hypogonadism; therefore, measuring testosterone concentrations later in the day should be avoided.

● Administration

Testosterone is administered by IM injection; percutaneously by topical application of a transdermal system, solution, or gel to the skin; intranasally; subcutaneously as a biodegradable implant; and intrabuccally (transmucosally) as a buccal tablet.

IM Injection

Testosterone cypionate (Depo®-testosterone), testosterone enanthate (Delatestryl®), and testosterone undecanoate (Aveed®) are administered by deep IM injection into the gluteal muscle; the usual precautions for IM administration should be followed.

Because of the risk of serious pulmonary oil microembolism reactions and anaphylaxis following IM administration of testosterone undecanoate, patients should be observed for 30 minutes in a healthcare setting following each IM injection of the drug.

Restricted Distribution Program

Because of the potential for serious pulmonary oil microembolism reactions and anaphylaxis in patients receiving IM testosterone undecanoate (Aveed®) (see Cautions: Sensitivity Reactions and also Other Adverse Effects), testosterone undecanoate must be obtained through a restricted distribution program, the Aveed® Risk Evaluation and Mitigation Strategy (REMS) Program, designed to minimize

the risk of pulmonary oil microembolism reactions and anaphylaxis. Clinicians and institutions that prescribe and/or dispense testosterone undecanoate must enroll in and comply with all requirements of the Aveed® REMS Program. Institutions are required to have appropriate equipment for the treatment of serious pulmonary oil microembolism and anaphylactic reactions for immediate use in patients receiving the drug. For additional information or to enroll in the Aveed® REMS program, clinicians may contact 855-755-0494 or visit www.AveedREMS.com.

Subcutaneous Administration

Testosterone pellets are administered as a biodegradable implant subcutaneously into the hip or other fatty area by a clinician; the usual precautions for subcutaneous implantation should be followed.

Transdermal Administration

Patients receiving transdermal testosterone therapy (Androderm®) should be carefully instructed in the proper use and disposal of the transdermal system. To obtain optimum results, patients should be given a copy of the patient instructions provided by the manufacturer. To expose the adhesive surface of the system, the protective liner should be peeled and discarded prior to administration.

The transdermal system should then be applied topically to a clean, dry area of skin on the back, abdomen, upper arm, or thigh by firmly pressing the system with the adhesive side touching the skin; the system should *not* be applied to the scrotum. The system should be applied immediately after removal from its protective pouch and removal of the protective liner. The system should be pressed firmly in place, ensuring good contact, particularly around the edges. The application site should not be oily, damaged, or irritated. Application of transdermal systems over bony prominences or on a part of the body that may be subject to prolonged pressure during sleep or sitting (e.g., the deltoid region of the upper arm, the greater trochanter of the femur, the ischial tuberosity) should be avoided, because burn-like blisters may occur. If the transdermal system becomes loose, the system should be smoothed down by firmly rubbing around the edges. If the system should inadvertently come off before noon following application the previous evening, a new system may be applied until the next scheduled application that evening. If the transdermal system comes off later in the day, the system should not be replaced until the next scheduled application that evening. If a system comes off, it should not be reapplied with tape.

To minimize and/or prevent potential skin irritation, each testosterone transdermal system should be applied at a different site, with an interval of at least 1 week allowed between applications to a particular site. Mild skin irritation may be ameliorated by application of over-the-counter topical hydrocortisone *cream* after system removal; alternatively, a small amount of triamcinolone acetonide *cream* 0.1% may be applied to the skin under the drug reservoir to minimize irritation (ointment formulations should *not* be used because they may reduce testosterone absorption).

Testosterone transdermal systems are applied once daily; to produce serum testosterone concentrations that mimic endogenous profiles, the system should be applied at night (e.g., 10 p.m.). The system should be left in place for approximately 24 hours; after this period, the system should be removed and discarded and a new system applied.

The transdermal system does not need to be removed during sexual intercourse nor while showering or bathing; however, patients should avoid swimming, showering, or washing the administration site for at least 3 hours following application.

Topical Administration

Patients receiving testosterone topical gel (AndroGel®, Fortesta®, Testim®, Vogelxo®) or solution (Axiron®) should be instructed on use of the gel or solution and given a copy of the patient instructions provided by the manufacturer.

AndroGel® is commercially available as unit-dose packets or as a metered-dose pump. AndroGel® should be applied topically once daily, preferably in the morning, to clean, dry, intact skin only; testosterone topical gel 1% (AndroGel® 1%) should be applied on the shoulders, upper arms, and/or abdomen and testosterone topical gel 1.62% (AndroGel® 1.62%) should be applied only on the shoulders and upper arms. The gel should *not* be applied to other parts of the body (e.g., genitals, chest, axillae, knees, back). To apply a dose from the unit-dose packet, the entire contents of the packet should be squeezed into the palm of the hand

and immediately applied to the application site; alternatively, a portion of the contents should be squeezed into the palm of the hand and applied to the application site and the procedure repeated until the entire contents of the packet has been applied. Alternatively, the gel can be applied directly to the application site. Patients using the metered-dose pump should be instructed to prime the pump prior to initial use by depressing the pump 3 times; this gel should be discarded by rinsing down the sink or placing in household trash in a manner that avoids accidental exposure or ingestion by household members or pets. To apply a dose from the metered-dose pump, the gel may be collected in the palm of the hand by pressing the pump firmly and fully; the gel is applied to the application site. Patients should immediately wash their hands with soap and water following application of the gel. Before dressing, the patient should allow the application site to dry; after the gel has dried, the application site should be covered with clothing (e.g., a shirt) to prevent transfer of testosterone to another individual. Following application of AndroGel® 1 or 1.62%, patients should avoid swimming, showering, or washing the application site for at least 5 or 2 hours, respectively.

Testim® is commercially available as unit-dose tubes. Testim® should be applied topically once daily, preferably in the morning, to clean, dry, intact skin only on the shoulders and/or upper arms; the gel should *not* be applied to the abdomen or genitals. Upon opening the tube, the entire contents should be squeezed into the palm of the hand and immediately applied to the application site. Patients should immediately wash their hands with soap and water following application of the gel. Before dressing, the patient should allow the application site to dry; after the gel has dried, the application site should be covered with clothing (e.g., a shirt) to prevent transfer of testosterone to another individual. Patients should avoid swimming, showering, or washing the administration site for at least 2 hours following application.

Vogelxo® is commercially available as unit-dose tubes or packets and as a metered-dose pump. Vogelxo® should be applied topically once daily to clean, dry, intact skin only on the shoulders and/or upper arms; the gel should *not* be applied to the abdomen or genitals. To apply a dose from the unit-dose tube or packet, the entire contents of the tube or packet should be squeezed into the palm of the hand and immediately applied to the application site. Patients using the metered-dose pump should be instructed to prime the pump prior to initial use by pressing the pump 3 times; this gel should be discarded by rinsing down the sink to avoid accidental exposure or ingestion by others. To apply a dose from the metered-dose pump, the gel may be collected in the palm of the hand by pressing the pump firmly and fully; the gel is applied to the application site. Patients should immediately wash their hands with soap and water following application of the gel. Before dressing, the patient should allow the application site to dry; after the gel has dried, the application site should be covered with clothing (e.g., a shirt) to prevent transfer of testosterone to another individual. Patients should avoid swimming, showering, or washing the application site for at least 2 hours following administration.

Fortesta® is commercially available as a metered-dose pump. Fortesta® should be applied topically once daily, in the morning, to clean, dry, intact skin only on the front and inner thighs; the gel should *not* be applied to the genitals or other parts of the body. Patients should be instructed to prime the pump prior to initial use by pressing the pump 8 times; this gel should be discarded by rinsing down the sink or placing in household trash in a manner that avoids accidental exposure or ingestion by others. To apply a dose from the metered-dose pump, the gel should be applied directly to the application site; the area of the thigh adjacent to the scrotum should be avoided. Patients should use one finger to gently and evenly rub the gel into the application site. Patients should immediately wash their hands with soap and water following application of the gel. Before dressing, the patient should allow the application site to dry; after the gel has dried, the application site should be covered with clothing (e.g., pants, shorts) to prevent transfer of testosterone to another individual. Patients should avoid swimming, showering, or washing the application site for at least 2 hours following administration.

Axiron® is commercially available as a metered-dose pump. Axiron® should be applied topically once daily to clean, dry, intact skin only on the axilla; the solution should *not* be applied to the genitals or other parts of the body (i.e., abdomen, shoulders, upper arms). Patients should be instructed to prime the pump prior to initial use by pressing the pump 3 times; this solution should be discarded by rinsing down a basin, sink, or toilet. To dispense a dose from the metered-dose pump, the solution should be dispensed into the applicator cup. To apply a dose from the applicator cup, the applicator cup should be held upright and placed onto the

application site and then wiped steadily up and down. If the solution drips or runs, excess solution should be collected using the applicator cup; the solution should *not* be rubbed in with fingers or hands. Application sites should be allowed to dry completely prior to another application. Deodorants and antiperspirants should not affect the efficacy of Axiron®; however, application of a deodorant or antiperspirant (stick or roll-on) should occur prior to application of Axiron® to avoid contamination of the deodorant or antiperspirant product. Patients should immediately wash their hands with soap and water following application of the solution. Before dressing, the patient should allow the application site to dry; after the solution has dried, the application site should be covered with clothing (e.g., shirt) to prevent transfer of testosterone to another individual. Patients should avoid swimming, showering, or washing the application site for at least 2 hours following administration.

Prior to any situation in which skin-to-skin contact with other individuals at the site of testosterone gel or solution application is anticipated, patients should wash the application site(s) thoroughly with soap and water to remove any testosterone residue. If unwashed or unclothed skin at the site of testosterone gel or solution application comes in contact with the skin of another individual, the general area of contact should be washed with soap and water as soon as possible. Studies show that residual testosterone is removed from the skin surface by washing with soap and water. Signs of virilization in children (e.g., changes in genital size, libido, or development of pubic hair) and women (e.g., changes in body hair distribution, substantial increases in acne) and the possibility of secondary exposure to topical testosterone products (AndroGel®, Axiron®, Fortesta®, Testim®, Vogelxo®) should be brought to the attention of a clinician. (See Cautions: Precautions and Contraindications.)

Buccal Administration

Patients receiving testosterone extended-release buccal (transmucosal) tablets (Striant®) should be instructed on use of the buccal system and given a copy of the patient instructions provided by the manufacturer. Testosterone extended-release buccal (transmucosal) tablets are applied to the gum region twice daily, morning and evening (approximately 12 hours apart). Upon opening the packet, the rounded-side surface of the buccal tablet should be placed against the gum and held in place with a finger over the lip and against the buccal tablet for 30 seconds. The buccal tablet should be placed just above the incisor tooth; the application site should be alternated between the left and right upper incisors. The buccal tablet is designed to stay in place until removed. Care should be taken not to dislodge the buccal tablet; placement of the tablet should be verified after tooth brushing, use of mouthwash, and eating or drinking liquids. The buccal tablet should not be chewed or swallowed. If the buccal tablet fails to properly adhere to the gum or falls off, the buccal tablet should be removed and a new tablet applied. If the buccal tablet must be replaced within 8 hours after application, the new tablet can remain in place until the next regularly scheduled dose (i.e., the application schedule employed should be continued). If the tablet must be replaced more than 8 hours after application, the replacement tablet can remain in place for the remainder of the current dosing interval as well as the next full dosing interval. To remove the buccal tablet, the tablet should be slid downward from the gum toward the tooth.

Intranasal Administration

Testosterone nasal gel (Natesto®) is administered intranasally using a metered-dose nasal pump. Patients should be instructed carefully in the use of the nasal pump. To obtain optimum results, patients also should be given a copy of the patient instructions provided by the manufacturer. Testosterone nasal gel should be administered intranasally 3 times daily; the nasal gel should *not* be applied to other parts of the body. Patients should be instructed to prime the pump prior to initial use by depressing the pump 10 times; this gel should be discarded by rinsing down a sink with warm water. Prior to administration of testosterone nasal gel, patients should clear their nasal passages. Patients should place their right index finger on the pump of the actuator and slowly insert the actuator into the left nostril until the finger reaches the base of the nose. To ensure adequate application of the gel, the tip of the actuator should be in contact with the lateral wall of the nostril. To dispense a dose from the metered-dose pump, the pump should be slowly pressed until it stops and the tip of the actuator should be wiped along the inside of the lateral nostril wall upon removal from the nose. This procedure is then repeated using the patient's left index finger for administration to the right nostril. Patients should lightly massage the application site by pressing on the nostrils just below the nasal bridge. Patients should avoid blowing their nose or sniffing for 1 hour following application. If testosterone nasal gel gets on the hands, patients should wash their hands with soap and warm water.

● Dosage

Dosage of testosterone is variable and should be individualized according to the condition being treated; the severity of symptoms; the patient's age, gender, and history of prior androgenic therapy; and the specific testosterone preparation being used.

Various dosage regimens have been used to induce pubertal changes in hypogonadal males. Some clinicians recommend that lower dosages be used initially, followed by gradual increases in dosage as puberty progresses; subsequently, the dosage may be decreased to maintenance levels. Other clinicians state that higher dosages are required initially to induce pubertal changes and lower dosages can then be used for maintenance therapy after puberty. The chronologic and skeletal ages of the patient must be considered when determining the initial dosage and subsequent dosage adjustment.

IM Dosage

Male Hypogonadism

For replacement of endogenous testicular hormone in androgen-deficient males, the usual IM dosage of testosterone cypionate or testosterone enanthate is 50–400 mg every 2–4 weeks. The recommended initial dosage of testosterone undecanoate is 750 mg every 4 weeks for the first 2 doses, then 750 mg every 10 weeks thereafter. In general, testosterone therapy is initiated with full therapeutic doses; subsequent dosage adjustment should be made according to the patient's tolerance and therapeutic response.

Alternatively, some clinicians state that complete androgen replacement in hypogonadal men generally can be achieved with 50–100 mg of testosterone cypionate or testosterone enanthate administered IM every 7–10 days. This regimen generally will achieve relatively physiologic testosterone concentrations throughout the time interval between doses. Longer time intervals between IM doses are more convenient but are associated with greater fluctuations in testosterone concentrations. Higher dosages produce longer-term effects but higher peak concentrations and wider swings between peak and nadir testosterone concentrations and resultant symptom fluctuation in many patients. If less frequent injection is desired, 100–150 mg IM every 2 weeks may be considered. While 300 mg IM every 3 weeks also may be considered for convenience, such dosing is associated with wider testosterone fluctuations and generally is inadequate to ensure a consistent clinical response. For men who develop pronounced symptoms in the week prior to the next dose with such prolonged dosing intervals, a smaller dose at a shorter dosing interval should be tried; in general, serum total testosterone concentrations should exceed 250–300 ng/dL just before the next dose.

If full androgen replacement is not required, lower testosterone dosages are used. For example, in adult males with prepubertal onset of hypogonadism who are going through puberty for the first time with IM testosterone replacement, testosterone therapy may be initiated at 50 mg every 3–4 weeks, gradually increasing the dose in subsequent months as tolerated up to full replacement within 1 year.

Attainment of full virilization in men with hypogonadism may require up to 3–4 years of IM testosterone replacement. Patients generally should be monitored at 4–6 months to assess clinical progress, review compliance, and determine whether any complications or psychologic adjustment problems are present.

For delayed puberty, the usual IM dosage of testosterone enanthate is 50–200 mg every 2–4 weeks for a limited period of time (e.g., 4–6 months).

Inoperable Carcinoma of the Breast

For the palliative treatment of advanced, inoperable, metastatic carcinoma of the breast in women, the usual IM dosage of testosterone enanthate is 200–400 mg every 2–4 weeks.

Subcutaneous Dosage

For replacement of endogenous testicular hormone in androgen-deficient males, the usual dosage of testosterone pellets is 150–450 mg implanted subcutaneously every 3–6 months. Dosage adjustment should be made according to the patient's tolerance and therapeutic response.

For delayed puberty, the dosage of testosterone pellets is generally less than the dosage used for male hypogonadism and for a limited period of time (e.g., 4–6 months).

Transdermal Dosage

Transdermal testosterone (Androderm®) is commercially available as a system delivering 2 mg/24 hours or 4 mg/24 hours. Dosage should be adjusted according to determinations of serum testosterone concentrations.

When Androderm® is used for the treatment of male hypogonadism, the usual initial transdermal dosage is 4 mg once daily administered nightly as one system delivering 4 mg/24 hours. Dosage should be adjusted according to morning serum testosterone concentrations approximately 2 weeks following initiation of therapy. Depending on requirements, dosage can be increased to 6 mg once daily administered nightly as one system delivering 4 mg/24 hours plus one delivering 2 mg/24 hours or can be decreased to 2 mg once daily administered nightly as one system delivering 2 mg/24 hours.

Patients currently maintained on a transdermal dosage of 2.5 mg once daily may be switched to one system delivering 2 mg/24 hours at the next scheduled dose. Patients currently maintained on a transdermal dosage of 5 mg once daily may be switched to one system delivering 4 mg/24 hours at the next scheduled dose. Patients currently maintained on a transdermal dosage of 7.5 mg once daily may be switched to 6 mg once daily with one system delivering 4 mg/24 hours plus one delivering 2 mg/24 hours.

Approximately 2 weeks after switching therapy, the early morning serum testosterone concentrations should be measured in patients following system application the previous evening to ensure proper dosing.

Topical Gel Dosage

Topical testosterone is commercially available as a 1% gel in unit-dose packets containing a 25-mg dose of testosterone (2.5 g of gel) (AndroGel®) or a 50-mg dose of testosterone (5 g of gel) (AndroGel®, Vogelxo®); as a 1.62% gel in unit-dose packets (AndroGel®) containing a 20.25- or 40.5-mg dose of testosterone (1.25 or 2.5 g of gel, respectively); as a nonaerosol metered-dose pump (AndroGel® [each actuation of the pump delivers 1.25 g of gel containing 20.25 mg of testosterone after priming], Fortesta® [each actuation of the pump delivers 0.5 g of gel containing 10 mg of testosterone after priming], Vogelxo® [each actuation of the pump delivers 1.25 g of gel containing 12.5 mg of testosterone after priming]); or in unit-dose tubes (Testim®, Vogelxo®) containing a 50-mg dose (5 g of gel).

For the treatment of male hypogonadism, the usual initial dosage of testosterone gel 1% (AndroGel® 1%, Testim®, Vogelxo®) is the entire contents of a packet or tube containing 50 mg of testosterone, the entire contents of 2 packets containing 25 mg of testosterone, or 4 actuations of the pump (5 g of gel) applied topically once daily, preferably in the morning; this dose delivers about 5 mg of testosterone systemically. The usual initial dosage of testosterone gel 1.62% (AndroGel® 1.62%) is the entire contents of a packet containing 40.5 mg of testosterone or 2 actuations of the pump (2.5 g of gel) applied topically once daily in the morning. The usual initial dosage of Fortesta® is 40 mg of testosterone or 4 actuations of the pump (2 g of gel) applied topically once daily in the morning. Dosage should be adjusted according to serum testosterone concentrations obtained at regular intervals following initiation of AndroGel® 1% therapy, approximately 14 days after initiating daily application of Testim® or Vogelxo®, approximately 14 and 28 days after initiating daily application or dosage adjustment of AndroGel® 1.62%, and approximately 14 and 35 days after initiating daily application or dosage adjustment of Fortesta®.

If serum testosterone concentrations are below the normal range in a patient receiving AndroGel® 1%, the dosage can be increased initially to 75 mg of testosterone (7.5 g of gel) and, if necessary, subsequently to 100 mg of testosterone (10 g of gel). If serum testosterone concentrations exceed the normal range in a patient receiving AndroGel® 1% therapy, the daily dosage may be decreased. AndroGel® 1% should be discontinued if the serum testosterone concentrations consistently exceed the normal range at a daily dosage of 50 mg of testosterone (5 g of gel).

If serum testosterone concentrations are below the normal range in a patient receiving Testim® or Vogelxo®, the dosage can be increased to 100 mg of testosterone (10 g of gel, 8 actuations of the pump).

If serum testosterone concentrations exceed 750 ng/dL in a patient receiving AndroGel® 1.62%, the dosage should be decreased to 20.25 mg of testosterone (1.25 g of gel, 1 actuation of the pump). If serum testosterone concentrations are below 350 ng/dL in a patient receiving AndroGel® 1.62%, the dosage should be increased initially to 60.75 mg of testosterone (3.75 g of gel, 3 actuations of the pump) and, if necessary, subsequently to 81 mg of testosterone (5 g of gel, 4 actuations of the pump).

In patients receiving Fortesta®, the dosage should be decreased by 20 mg of testosterone (2 actuations of the pump) if serum testosterone concentrations reach or exceed 2500 ng/dL or by 10 mg of testosterone (1 actuation of the pump) if serum testosterone concentrations are 1250 ng/dL or greater, but less than 2500 ng/dL; however, if a 10-mg dosage of testosterone requires further reduction, Fortesta® should be discontinued. If serum testosterone concentrations are below 500 ng/dL in a patient receiving Fortesta®, the dosage of testosterone can be adjusted in 10-mg increments (1 actuation of the pump); however, the daily dosage should not exceed 70 mg of testosterone (7 actuations of the pump).

Topical Solution Dosage

Topical testosterone is commercially available as a solution in a metered-dose pump (Axiron®; each actuation of the pump delivers 1.5 mL of solution containing 30 mg of testosterone after priming). For the treatment of male hypogonadism, the recommended initial dosage of testosterone solution is 60 mg (2 actuations of the pump) applied topically once daily. Dosage should be adjusted according to serum testosterone concentrations obtained following initiation of therapy and at least 14 days after initiating daily application or dosage adjustment of testosterone solution. If serum testosterone concentrations exceed 1050 ng/dL in a patient receiving testosterone topical solution, the dosage should be decreased from 60 mg (2 actuations of the pump) to 30 mg (1 actuation of the pump); however, if a 30-mg dosage of testosterone requires further reduction, testosterone topical solution should be discontinued. If serum testosterone concentrations are below 300 ng/dL in a patient receiving testosterone topical solution, the dosage of testosterone can be adjusted in 30-mg increments (1 actuation of the pump); however, the daily dosage should not exceed 120 mg of testosterone (4 actuations of the pump).

Buccal (Transmucosal) Dosage

When testosterone buccal (transmucosal) tablets (Striant®) are used for the treatment of male hypogonadism, the usual dosage is 30 mg (one extended-release tablet) twice daily, morning and evening (about 12 hours apart). Serum testosterone concentrations should be obtained just prior to the morning dose 4–12 weeks after initiation of therapy with testosterone buccal tablets. If total serum testosterone concentrations are consistently outside of the normal range, testosterone buccal tablets should be discontinued.

Intranasal Dosage

Intranasal testosterone is commercially available as a gel in a metered-dose nasal pump (Natesto®; each actuation of the pump delivers 0.122 g of gel containing 5.5 mg of testosterone after priming). For the treatment of male hypogonadism, the recommended initial dosage of testosterone nasal gel is 1 actuation of the pump per nostril for a total dosage of 11 mg 3 times daily. Dosage should be adjusted according to serum testosterone concentrations obtained at least 1 month after initiating therapy and periodically thereafter. If serum testosterone concentrations consistently exceed 1050 ng/dL, testosterone nasal gel should be discontinued. If serum testosterone concentrations are consistently below 300 ng/dL, testosterone nasal gel should be discontinued and alternative therapy considered. If severe rhinitis occurs, testosterone nasal gel should be temporarily interrupted until resolution of symptoms; however, if severe rhinitis persists, testosterone nasal gel should be discontinued and alternative therapy considered.

● Dosage in Renal and Hepatic Impairment

The manufacturers of testosterone enanthate injection, testosterone undecanoate injection, and testosterone transdermal system, topical gel, topical solution, nasal gel, and buccal tablets state that clinical studies involving patients with renal or hepatic impairment have not been conducted. Therefore, there are no special population dosage recommendations at this time.

CAUTIONS

Adverse effects associated with testosterone are similar to those of other synthetic or natural androgens and include acne, flushing of the skin, gynecomastia, increased or decreased libido, habituation, and edema. In addition, gynecomastia frequently develops and occasionally persists in patients being treated for hypogonadism.

● Cardiovascular Effects

Long-term clinical safety studies have not been conducted to date to determine the cardiovascular effects of testosterone replacement therapy in men. Epidemiologic data and results from randomized, controlled clinical trials have been inconclusive for determining the risk of serious adverse cardiovascular events (i.e., nonfatal myocardial infarction [MI], nonfatal stroke, death) with testosterone use compared with nonuse.

In 2 observational studies, the risk of serious adverse cardiovascular events was increased in patients receiving testosterone replacement therapy compared with those not receiving such therapy; however, 2 other observational studies found a mortality benefit with use of testosterone replacement therapy and one observational study was inconclusive. In addition, findings from 2 meta-analyses of data from published, randomized, controlled clinical trials show conflicting results. Because the current evidence regarding the cardiovascular risk associated with testosterone replacement therapy is weak because of the limited scope, quality, design, and size of the clinical trials, the FDA has requested additional evidence from well-designed studies to further elucidate the cardiovascular risk associated with testosterone use.

Following review of the data from several observational studies and meta-analyses in March 2015, the FDA concluded that use of testosterone is associated with a possible increased risk of serious adverse cardiovascular events. Clinicians should inform patients of this potential increased risk when deciding whether to use or continue to use testosterone replacement therapy. Although the FDA Bone, Reproductive and Urologic Drugs Advisory Committee (BRUDAC) and the Drug Safety and Risk Management Advisory Committee (DSaRM) concluded that there was insufficient evidence to suggest that the potential cardiovascular risk was confined to a certain subset of patients, some experts state that testosterone replacement therapy should be used with caution in patients at high risk for cardiovascular disease, such as older men or those with diabetes mellitus or obesity.

● Local Effects

IM administration of anabolic steroids has been associated with urticaria and inflammation at the injection site, postinjection induration, and furunculosis.

Pellet extrusion at or near the implantation site, generally during the first month following subcutaneous implantation of testosterone pellets (Testopel®), has been reported in postmarketing surveillance; infection also may occur at the implantation site. Infection and/or extrusion at the implantation site may be manifested with induration, inflammation, fibrosis, bleeding, contusions, wound drainage, pain, and pruritus.

The most common adverse effect associated with transdermal testosterone is local irritation at the site of application. In clinical studies with Androderm® transdermal systems, most patients developed mild to moderate erythema at the site of application at some time during therapy; 37% of patients receiving this preparation experienced pruritus at the application site, 12% experienced burn-like blisters (manifesting with bullae, epidermal necrosis, or ulceration) on the skin immediately under the system, and 6, 3, and 3% developed vesicles, burning, and induration, respectively, at the application site. In patients who developed burn-like blisters, most such lesions were associated with application of the system over bony prominences or on body parts that may have been subject to prolonged pressure during sleep or sitting (e.g., over the deltoid region of the upper arm, the greater trochanter of the femur, or the ischial tuberosity), and such administration should be avoided; the more severe lesions healed over several weeks with occasional scarring, and such lesions should be treated as burns. Application site reactions occurring in less than 3% of patients receiving Androderm® include bullae, mechanical irritation, and contamination.

In one comparative study, the incidence of application site reactions was substantially less with Testoderm® TTS (no longer commercially available in the US) than with Androderm®, possibly because of the lower amount of delivered alcohol (a permeation-enhancer excipient in the transdermal systems) per unit area of skin with Testoderm® TTS. The possibility exists that excipients other than alcohol also may play a role in application site reactions. Mild skin irritation may be ameliorated with topical application of over-the-counter hydrocortisone *cream;* alternatively, application of triamcinolone acetonide 0.1% *cream* under the central drug reservoir of the transdermal system may decrease the incidence and severity of application site reactions.

Application site reactions were reported in 5, 3, or 4% of patients who received 50, 75, or 100 mg, respectively, of testosterone gel 1% (as AndroGel® 1%) topically for up to 6 months in a clinical trial, but none of these patients required treatment or discontinued the drug because of these reactions. Application site reactions were reported in 2.14% of patients who received testosterone gel 1.62% (as Andro-Gel® 1.62%), but none of these patients discontinued the drug because of these reactions. In a long-term (up to 3 years) follow-up study, application site reactions were reported in 5.6% of patients. Application site reactions were reported in 2 or 4% of patients receiving 50- or 100-mg doses, respectively, of another testosterone gel formulation (Testim®, Vogelxo®) compared with placebo (3%). Application site reactions were reported in 16.1% of patients receiving another testosterone gel formulation (Fortesta®). AndroGel® 1% appears to have minimal potential for inducing phototoxic reactions. Other application site reactions reported with AndroGel® 1% during postmarketing surveillance include pruritus, dry skin, erythema, rash, discolored hair, and paresthesia. The possibility that testosterone transfer to another individual (including women and children) could occur when skin-to-skin contact is made with the application site should be considered. (See Cautions: Precautions and Contraindications.) In vitro studies have shown that 96% of residual testosterone is removed from the skin by washing with soap and water.

In clinical studies with a testosterone topical solution (Axiron®), irritation (5–7% of patients) or erythema (7–8% of patients) developed at the application site following 120 or 180 days of therapy, respectively.

The most common adverse effects associated with testosterone nasal gel are nasal discomfort, nasal scabbing, rhinorrhea, epistaxis, nasopharyngitis, bronchitis, upper respiratory tract infection, and sinusitis. In a clinical study with Natesto® nasal gel, most patients developed mild to moderate adverse effects; however, long-term effects of testosterone nasal gel are unknown because of limited data.

Gum or mouth irritation, bitter taste, and gum pain or tenderness have been reported in 9.2, 4.1, and 3.1%, respectively, of patients receiving testosterone buccal tablets (Striant®) in one controlled study. Gum edema or taste perversion occurred in 2% of patients receiving the drug in this study. Most gum-related adverse effects were transient; gum irritation generally resolved in 1–8 days and tenderness resolved in 1–14 days.

● Genitourinary Effects

Oligospermia and decreased ejaculatory volume may occur in males receiving excessive dosage or prolonged administration of testosterone. Priapism or excessive sexual stimulation in males, especially geriatric patients, may also occur. If priapism or excessive sexual stimulation develops during testosterone therapy, the drug should be discontinued temporarily, since these are signs of excessive dosage; if therapy with testosterone is reinstituted, a lower dosage should be used. Male pattern of baldness may also occur.

Amenorrhea and other menstrual irregularities and inhibition of gonadotropin secretion occur commonly in females.

Gynecomastia can occur in males receiving testosterone replacement therapy as a result of aromatization of testosterone to estradiol and changes in sex hormone binding globulin (SHBG). Surgery can be considered for such patients.

Testosterone, especially its active metabolite dihydrotestosterone (DHT), stimulates growth of the prostate and seminal vesicles. In hypogonadal men receiving testosterone replacement, such growth did not exceed the volumes expected in normal men. Testosterone therapy was associated with an overall mean increase in serum prostate-specific antigen (PSA) concentrations of 0.11–0.14, 0.13, 0.1–0.2, or 0.5 ng/mL in studies evaluating the effect of topical testosterone gel (AndroGel®), topical testosterone solution (Axiron®), testosterone nasal gel (Natesto®), or testosterone undecanoate injection (Aveed®), respectively, on serum PSA concentrations in men with hypogonadism. In one study, PSA was reduced in 21%, unchanged in 22%, and increased in 57% of patients receiving testosterone replacement therapy for 1 year. Increased serum PSA concentrations also were observed in 18% of hypogonadal men receiving AndroGel® 1% for up to 42 months; most of these increases occurred within the first year of therapy. No clear relationship between testosterone replacement therapy and prostate cancer has been established to date, although anecdotal reports have been published;

additional long-term studies are needed to clarify the potential risk. (See Cautions: Mutagenicity and Carcinogenicity.)

Other adverse genitourinary effects of testosterone include epididymitis and bladder irritability. Impaired urination, prostatic enlargement, prostate cancer, testicular atrophy, oligospermia, priapism, gynecomastia, and mastodynia have been reported during postmarketing experience with topical testosterone gel (AndroGel® 1%).

● Endocrine and Metabolic Effects

Virilization, including deepening of the voice, hirsutism, and clitoral enlargement, occur commonly in females; these changes may not be reversible following discontinuance of the drug.

Secondary exposure to testosterone resulting in virilization of children has been reported with use of topical testosterone gel during postmarketing surveillance. (See Cautions: Precautions and Contraindications.) The FDA has fully reviewed 8 reports of secondary exposure to testosterone from testosterone gel products in children 9 months to 5 years of age. Additional cases in children have been reported and currently are under FDA review. Signs and symptoms have included enlargement of the penis or clitoris, development of pubic hair, increased erections and libido, aggressive behavior, and advanced bone age. In most cases, these signs and symptoms resolved with removal of the testosterone exposure. However, in a few cases, enlarged genitalia did not fully return to age-appropriate normal size, and bone age remained modestly greater than chronologic age. In some of these children, invasive diagnostic procedures were performed as a result of the delay in recognizing the underlying cause of the signs and symptoms. Direct contact of the child with application sites on the skin of men using testosterone gel was reported in most of the cases. The possibility of secondary exposure from contact with items such as shirts and bed linens of men receiving testosterone gel also may be considered.

Because of the aromatization of testosterone to estradiol, lipid abnormalities usually do not develop secondary to testosterone replacement, and the ratio of HDL to total cholesterol generally remains constant. However, the possibility that lipid abnormalities may develop should be considered. (See Cautions: Precautions and Contraindications.) Anabolic steroids that do not undergo aromatization increase LDL-cholesterol and lower HDL-cholesterol, which could increase cardiovascular risk.

Hypercalcemia resulting from osteolysis, especially in immobile patients and those with metastatic carcinoma of the breast, has been reported in patients receiving testosterone. (See Cautions: Precautions and Contraindications.) The drug should be discontinued if hypercalcemia occurs in patients with cancer, since this may indicate progression of metastases to the bone. Retention of water, sodium, chloride, potassium, and inorganic phosphates has also occurred in patients receiving the drug. If edema is present before or develops during therapy, administration of diuretics may be required.

● Nervous System Effects

Sleep apnea has occurred occasionally in men receiving testosterone replacement. Although the mechanism of testosterone-induced apnea remains to be elucidated, a relationship between sex hormones and sleep apnea has been suggested since untreated males are more likely than females to develop this disorder and disordered breathing during sleep is more common among healthy males than among premenopausal women. In addition, loud snoring is more common in untreated men than in women, and physiologic mechanisms for snoring and obstructive sleep apnea are similar. Therefore, it has been postulated that abnormal relaxation of pharyngeal muscles seen in both snoring and obstructive sleep apnea is affected by circulating concentrations of hormones, including testosterone. If manifestations of sleep apnea occur or worsen in testosterone-treated patients, sleep studies should be performed and testosterone replacement dosage should be decreased or the drug discontinued if sleep apnea is confirmed. In addition, patients receiving testosterone replacement should be advised to report any sleep-associated changes such as snoring, daytime somnolence, and emotional disturbances.

Sleeplessness, headache, anxiety, mental depression, and generalized paresthesia also have occurred in patients receiving testosterone. Headache, dizziness, sleep apnea, insomnia, depression, emotional lability, nervousness, hostility, amnesia, and anxiety have been reported during postmarketing experience with topical testosterone (AndroGel® 1%).

● Sensitivity Reactions

Hypersensitivity reactions, including skin manifestations and anaphylactoid reactions, have occurred rarely with testosterone. Allergic contact dermatitis has been reported with topical administration (e.g., as transdermal systems) of testosterone. (See Cautions: Local Effects.)

● Hematologic Effects

Supraphysiologic concentrations of testosterone can stimulate erythropoiesis. Increased hemoglobin and hematocrit and possibly adverse effects secondary to hyperviscosity may result. In addition, leukopenia, polycythemia, and suppression of clotting factors II, V, VII, and X also have occurred in patients receiving testosterone.

● Hepatic Effects

Cholestatic hepatitis, peliosis hepatis, hepatic neoplasms, jaundice and abnormal liver function test results have occurred in patients receiving androgens, principally 17-α-alkylandrogens such as fluoxymesterone or methyltestosterone. (See Cautions in Fluoxymesterone 68:08 and in Methyltestosterone 68:08.) Multiple hepatic adenomas have been reported with long-term use of testosterone enanthate injection. Abnormal liver function tests (e.g., ALT, AST, gamma-glutamyltranspeptidase [GGTP], bilirubin) also have been reported during postmarketing surveillance with topical testosterone (AndroGel® 1%).

● Other Adverse Effects

Other adverse effects associated with testosterone therapy include nausea, chills, and excitation. Nausea, asthenia, edema, malaise, dyspnea, acne, alopecia, sweating, weight gain, hypertension, and vasodilation (hot flushes) have been reported during postmarketing experience with topical testosterone (AndroGel® 1%).

Serious pulmonary oil microembolism reactions, including cough, urge to cough, dyspnea, hyperhidrosis, throat tightness, angina, dizziness, and syncope, have occurred rarely with IM testosterone undecanoate. In clinical trials, pulmonary oil microembolism reactions have occurred during or immediately following IM administration of 750 mg or 1 g of testosterone undecanoate; these reactions have been reported following administration of the third and tenth injection of the drug. Although these reactions generally lasted a few minutes and resolved following initiation of supportive measures, some reactions persisted for several hours and required emergency care and/or hospitalization. (See Dosage and Administration: Administration.)

● Precautions and Contraindications

Testosterone shares the toxic potentials of other androgens, and the usual precautions of androgen therapy should be observed. When testosterone esters are used in combination with estrogens, the usual precautions associated with estrogen therapy should also be observed. (See Cautions in Conjugated Estrogens 68:16.04.) Clinicians prescribing estrogens should be aware of the risks associated with use of these drugs and the manufacturers' labeling should be consulted for further discussion of these risks and associated precautions.

Patients receiving testosterone replacement therapy should be monitored periodically for response and tolerance. Some clinicians recommend that patients be monitored every 3–4 months during the first year of testosterone replacement, and periodically thereafter. Patients with benign prostatic hyperplasia (BPH) receiving androgen therapy are at increased risk for worsening of signs and symptoms of BPH. Patients treated with androgens also may be at increased risk for development of BPH and/or prostate cancer. (See Cautions: Mutagenicity and Carcinogenicity.) The manufacturers of testosterone transdermal system, nasal gel, and topical solution state that evaluation of patients for prostate cancer is appropriate prior to initiation of therapy, 3–6 months after initiation of therapy, and then in accordance with current standards of care. The manufacturers of testosterone topical gel, testosterone buccal tablets, and testosterone undecanoate injection state that evaluation of patients for prostate cancer is appropriate prior to initiating and during androgen therapy. Some clinicians recommend that rectal prostate examination be performed routinely along with assessment of prostate-related symptoms every 6–12 months. Additionally, determination of PSA should be performed annually in older men.

Increases in hematocrit may occur during testosterone therapy as a manifestation of increased red blood cell (RBC) mass, and may require dosage reduction or discontinuance of testosterone. Increased RBC mass also may increase the risk for a thromboembolic event. Annual determination of hematocrit is recommended by some clinicians during testosterone replacement therapy because of the hormone's erythropoietic potential. Determination of hematocrit should occur prior to initiation of therapy, and is appropriate 3–6 months after initiation of therapy, and then annually thereafter. Patients receiving high dosages of testosterone should have periodic hemoglobin and hematocrit determinations, since polycythemia may occur. Some clinicians state that hyperviscosity states are relative contraindications to testosterone therapy.

Changes in serum lipid profiles may require dosage adjustment or discontinuance of testosterone therapy. Some clinicians recommend that patients receiving testosterone replacement have a lipid profile performed at baseline, 6–12 months after initiation of therapy, and then annually thereafter. Androgen therapy should be used with caution in cancer patients at risk of hypercalcemia (and associated hypercalciuria). Regular monitoring of serum calcium concentrations is recommended in these patients.

Cardiovascular events, including MI or stroke, have been reported during postmarketing experience with testosterone preparations. Testosterone should be used with caution in patients at high risk for cardiovascular disease (e.g., older men, those with diabetes mellitus or obesity). Patients should be advised to immediately report symptoms suggestive of MI or stroke (e.g., chest pain, shortness of breath, unilateral weakness, difficulty talking) to their clinician.

Venous thromboembolic events, including deep-vein thrombosis (DVT) and pulmonary embolism (PE), have been reported during postmarketing experience with testosterone preparations. Patients reporting symptoms of pain, edema, warmth, and erythema in a lower extremity or presenting with acute shortness of breath should be evaluated for possible DVT or PE, respectively. If venous thromboembolism is suspected, testosterone therapy should be discontinued and appropriate evaluation and management should be initiated.

Testosterone should be used with caution in patients with cardiac, renal, and/or hepatic dysfunction since edema may occur as a result of sodium and water retention. Edema, with or without congestive heart failure, may be a serious complication in patients with preexisting cardiac, renal, and/or hepatic disease. If edema occurs during testosterone therapy and it is considered a serious complication, the drug should be discontinued; diuretic therapy may also be necessary. Testosterone cypionate (Depo®-testosterone) is contraindicated in patients with serious cardiac, hepatic, or renal disease.

Females should be carefully monitored for signs of virilization (e.g., deepening of the voice, hirsutism, clitoromegaly, menstrual irregularities) during testosterone therapy. The drug should generally be discontinued when mild virilization is evident, since some adverse androgenic effects (e.g., voice changes) may not subside following discontinuation of the drug. The woman and physician may decide that some virilization is acceptable during treatment for carcinoma of the breast.

Males should be carefully monitored for the development of priapism or excessive sexual stimulation since these are signs of excessive dosage. Males, especially geriatric patients, may become overly stimulated. Stimulation to the point of increasing the nervous, mental, and physical activities beyond the patient's cardiovascular capacity should be avoided when testosterone is used to treat decreased testosterone concentrations related to aging. Geriatric males may be at increased risk of developing prostatic hypertrophy and carcinoma during androgen therapy.

Adult or adolescent males should be advised to report too frequent or persistent penile erections to their physician. Females should be advised to report hoarseness, acne, menstrual changes, or the growth of facial hair to their physician. All patients should be advised to report nausea, vomiting, changes in skin color, or ankle swelling to their physician.

Treatment of hypogonadal men with testosterone products may potentiate sleep apnea in some patients, especially those with risk factors such as obesity or chronic lung diseases. Some clinicians also state that a history of sleep apnea is a relative contraindication to testosterone therapy. (See Cautions: Systemic Effects.)

Testosterone topical gels and topical solution contain a flammable vehicle (alcohol), and should not be exposed to an open flame or ignited materials (e.g., a lighted cigarette). The topical gel or topical solution is no longer flammable once the gel or solution has dried.

Virilization in children and women can occur following secondary exposure to testosterone in topical testosterone preparations, including gels or solution.

Cases of secondary exposure resulting in virilization of children have been reported during postmarketing surveillance of topical testosterone preparations. (See Cautions: Endocrine and Metabolic Effects.) Signs and symptoms of virilization in children have included enlargement of the penis or clitoris, development of pubic hair, increased erections and libido, aggressive behavior, and advanced bone age. In most cases, these signs and symptoms regressed with removal of the testosterone exposure. However, in a few cases, enlarged genitalia did not fully return to age-appropriate normal size, and bone age remained modestly greater than chronologic age.

The risk of testosterone transfer in some of these reported cases was increased by lack of adherence to precautions for the appropriate use of the topical testosterone preparations. Men using topical testosterone gel or solution should strictly adhere to the recommended instructions for use and appropriate precautions from the manufacturers to minimize the potential for secondary exposure to testosterone in other individuals. (See Dosage and Administration: Administration.) Children and women should avoid contact with application sites on the skin of men using topical testosterone products.

Inappropriate changes in genital size or development of pubic hair or libido in children, changes in body hair distribution, substantial increase in acne, or other signs of virilization in adult women, and the possibility of secondary exposure to testosterone topical gel should be brought to the attention of a clinician. Testosterone topical gel should be promptly discontinued at least until the cause of virilization in such children and women has been identified.

Testosterone transdermal system (Androderm®) should be removed before undergoing magnetic resonance imaging (MRI), since the transdermal system contains aluminum and may cause skin burns at the application site.

Serious pulmonary oil microembolism reactions and anaphylaxis have been reported following IM administration of testosterone undecanoate. Patients should be monitored for 30 minutes following each dose of IM testosterone undecanoate.

Adverse nasal reactions have been reported with testosterone nasal gel. Because of limited data in patients with a history of nasal disorders (e.g., nasal or sinus surgery, nasal fracture within the previous 6 months, nasal fracture resulting in a deviated anterior nasal septum), mucosal inflammatory disorders (e.g., Sjogren's syndrome), and/or sinus disease, testosterone nasal gel is not recommended in such patients. Patients should be advised to report nasal symptoms to their clinician to determine if further evaluation by an ear, nose, and throat (ENT) specialist or discontinuance of testosterone nasal gel is necessary.

Testosterone topical gel, topical solution, nasal gel, transdermal system, and buccal tablets and testosterone undecanoate injection (Aveed®) are not indicated for use in women, have not been evaluated in women, and should not be used in women.

Testosterone is contraindicated in males with carcinoma of the breast or known or suspected carcinoma of the prostate. Testosterone also is contraindicated in women who are or may become pregnant or who are breastfeeding. (See Cautions: Pregnancy, Fertility, and Lactation.) Testosterone cypionate injection, testosterone enanthate injection, and testosterone undecanoate injection are contraindicated in patients with known hypersensitivity to the drug or any ingredient in the respective formulation. Because of the potential risk of serious adverse health effects, testosterone should not be used for enhancement of athletic performance or physique. (See Uses: Misuse, Abuse, and Dependence.) Patients should be informed of the serious adverse effects associated with misuse and abuse of androgens.

● Pediatric Precautions

Androgens should be used with extreme caution in children and only by specialists who are aware of the adverse effects of these drugs on bone maturation. Testosterone should be used cautiously to stimulate puberty, and only in carefully selected males with delayed puberty. (See Uses: Uses in Males.) In children, testosterone may accelerate bone maturation without producing compensatory gain in linear growth. This adverse effect may result in compromised adult stature. The younger the child, the greater the risk of testosterone compromising final mature stature. If testosterone is administered to prepubertal children (e.g., to stimulate puberty in males), the drug should be used with extreme caution, and radiographic examination of the hand and wrist should be performed every 6 months to determine the rate of bone maturation and to assess the effect of treatment on the epiphyseal centers. If testosterone is to be used to stimulate puberty in a male with delayed puberty, the potential risk of therapy should be fully discussed with the patient and his parents prior to initiation of the drug.

Safety and efficacy of testosterone topical gel, topical solution, nasal gel, transdermal system, and buccal tablets and testosterone undecanoate injection (Aveed®) in pediatric patients younger than 18 years of age have not been established. Safety and efficacy of testosterone cypionate injection (Depo®-testosterone) in pediatric patients younger than 12 years of age have not been established. Secondary exposure to testosterone in children can occur with the use of topical testosterone preparations, including gels or solution, in other individuals. (See Cautions: Precautions and Contraindications.)

● Geriatric Precautions

Clinical studies evaluating testosterone enanthate injection (Delatestryl®), testosterone undecanoate injection (Aveed®), and testosterone topical gel (AndroGel®, Fortesta®), topical solution, nasal gel, and transdermal system have not included sufficient numbers of adults 65 years of age or older to determine whether geriatric patients respond differently than younger adults. There also are insufficient long-term safety data with testosterone enanthate injection, testosterone undecanoate injection, and testosterone topical gel (AndroGel®, Fortesta®, Testim®, Vogelxo®). topical solution, nasal gel, and transdermal system to determine the potential risks of cardiovascular disease, prostate cancer, and prostatic hyperplasia in geriatric adults. The manufacturer of testosterone buccal tablets (Striant®) states that no substantial differences in safety and efficacy were observed in clinical studies in patients 65 years of age or older relative to younger adults. Differences in pharmacokinetics were observed between geriatric and younger adults in studies with Striant®, but it is not known whether these differences are clinically important.

● Mutagenicity and Carcinogenicity

Hepatocellular carcinoma has reportedly occurred in patients receiving long-term therapy with high dosages of androgens. Regression of the tumor does not always occur following discontinuance of androgen therapy. Geriatric patients may be at increased risk of developing prostatic hypertrophy and carcinoma during androgen therapy, although the manufacturers state that conclusive evidence to support this risk is lacking. Testosterone replacement is contraindicated in men with known or suspected prostate cancer or male breast cancer since the drug can stimulate tumor growth in androgen-dependent neoplasms. The prostate and breasts should be examined carefully prior to initiating testosterone therapy in men and at follow-up visits. Baseline and follow-up determinations of PSA also should be performed in older men (e.g., older than 50 years of age) at increased risk for prostate cancer.

Following implantation of testosterone in mice, cervical-uterine tumors developed which occasionally metastasized. There is some evidence to suggest that injection of testosterone into some strains of female mice increases their susceptibility to hepatomas. Testosterone has also been shown to increase the number of tumors and decrease the degree of differentiation of chemically induced tumors in rats. It is not known whether androgens, including testosterone, are mutagenic.

● Pregnancy, Fertility, and Lactation

Pregnancy

Testosterone may cause fetal harm when administered to pregnant women due to the potential for virilization of a female fetus. Androgenic effects including clitoral hypertrophy, labial fusion of the external genital fold to form a scrotal-like structure, abnormal vaginal development, and persistence of a urogenital sinus have occurred in the female offspring of women who were given androgens during pregnancy. The degree of masculinization is related to the amount of drug given to the woman and the age of the fetus; masculinization is most likely to occur in a female fetus when exposure to androgens occurs during the first trimester. Since the risks clearly outweigh the possible benefits in women who are or may become pregnant, testosterone is contraindicated in such women. Women who become pregnant while receiving the drug should be informed of the potential hazard to the fetus.

Pregnant women or those who may become pregnant should be aware of the possibility that testosterone could be transferred from patients treated with topical preparations of the drug such as their sexual partners or other individuals in close physical contact. (See Cautions: Precautions and Contraindications.) Testosterone transdermal system (Androderm®) has an occlusive backing that prevents the partner from coming in contact with active ingredient in the system. Transdermal systems that inadvertently are transferred to a sexual partner should be removed immediately and the contacted skin washed. Pregnant women should avoid skin contact with testosterone topical gel application sites in men. (See Cautions: Precautions and Contraindications.) If unwashed or unclothed skin to which testosterone topical gel has been applied comes in direct contact with the skin of a pregnant woman, the general area of contact by the woman should be washed with soap and water immediately. In vitro studies show that residual testosterone is removed by such washing.

Fertility

Although the effect of testosterone on fertility in humans has not been conclusively determined, the drug produces oligospermia and decreased ejaculatory volume in males. With high dosages of androgen therapy, spermatogenesis may be suppressed through feedback inhibition of pituitary follicle-stimulating hormone possibly leading to adverse effects on semen parameters including sperm count. Priapism and excessive sexual stimulation also have occurred in males receiving the drug. (See Cautions: Precautions and Contraindications.) Increased or decreased libido also has been reported.

Lactation

It is not known whether testosterone is distributed into milk. The manufacturers of testosterone enanthate injection (Delatestryl®) and testosterone pellets (Testopel®) state that because of the potential for serious adverse reactions to androgens in nursing infants, a decision should be made whether to discontinue nursing or the drug, taking into account the importance of the drug to the woman. The manufacturer of testosterone cypionate injection (Depo®-testosterone) states that use in nursing women is not recommended. Testosterone topical gel, topical solution, nasal gel, transdermal system, and buccal tablets and testosterone undecanoate injection (Aveed®) are not indicated for use in women. Testosterone topical gel, topical solution, nasal gel, and buccal tablets and testosterone undecanoate injection also are contraindicated in nursing women because of the potential for serious adverse reactions in nursing infants. Exposure of a female nursing infant to androgens may result in varying degrees of virilization. Testosterone and other androgens also may adversely affect lactation.

DRUG INTERACTIONS

Testosterone may potentiate the action of oral anticoagulants, causing bleeding in some patients. When testosterone therapy is initiated in patients receiving oral anticoagulants, dosage reduction of the anticoagulant may be required to prevent an excessive hypoprothrombinemic response. In patients receiving concomitant therapy with testosterone and anticoagulants, more frequent monitoring of INR and prothrombin time is recommended, especially during initiation or discontinuance of therapy.

Increased serum oxyphenbutazone concentrations have reportedly occurred in patients receiving androgens concurrently with oxyphenbutazone.

Changes in insulin sensitivity or glycemic control may occur in patients receiving androgen therapy. The metabolic effects of androgens may decrease blood glucose concentrations and insulin requirements in patients with diabetes.

Concomitant administration of testosterone with ACTH or corticosteroids may result in increased fluid retention and edema formation. Therefore, testosterone should be administered with caution in patients with cardiac, renal, and/or hepatic disease. Patients should be monitored for fluid retention and edema formation.

Administration of IM testosterone cypionate resulted in increased clearance of propranolol in one study. It is not known whether there is a potential for this interaction with topically administered testosterone gel.

Topical administration of 0.1% triamcinolone cream prior to application of a testosterone transdermal system did not alter absorption of testosterone; however, pretreatment with topical administration of triamcinolone ointment substantially reduced absorption of testosterone.

Administration of intranasal oxymetazoline, a sympathomimetic nasal decongestant, prior to administration of testosterone nasal gel (Natesto®) did not alter absorption of testosterone. Concomitant administration of testosterone nasal gel with other drugs administered intranasally has not been studied. The manufacturer does not recommend concomitant use with such drugs.

LABORATORY TEST INTERFERENCES

Protein bound iodine (PBI) concentrations may be decreased in some patients during testosterone therapy; however, this does not appear to be clinically important. Androgens may decrease thyroxine-binding globulin concentrations, resulting in decreased total serum thyroxine (T_4) concentrations and increased resin uptake of triiodothyronine (T_3) and T_4. Free thyroid hormone concentrations remain unchanged, and there is no clinical evidence of thyroid dysfunction.

Testosterone may cause a decrease in creatinine and creatine excretion and increase the excretion of 17-ketosteroids.

Electrolyte changes (e.g., nitrogen, calcium, potassium, phosphorus, sodium), changes in serum lipids (e.g., hyperlipidemia, elevated triglycerides, decreased high-density lipoprotein [HDL]-cholesterol), impaired glucose tolerance, and fluctuating testosterone concentrations have been reported during postmarketing surveillance with a topical testosterone gel (AndroGel®).

PHARMACOLOGY

Testosterone is the principal endogenous androgen. Endogenous androgens are essential hormones that are responsible for the normal growth and development of the male sex organs and for maintenance of secondary sex characteristics, including the growth and maturation of the prostate, seminal vesicles, penis, and scrotum; development of male hair distribution, such as beard, pubic, chest, and axillary hair; laryngeal enlargement and thickening of the vocal cords; and alterations in body musculature and fat distribution.

Testosterone, like other androgenic anabolic hormones, also produces retention of nitrogen, potassium, sodium, and phosphorus; increases protein anabolism; and decreases amino acid catabolism and urinary calcium concentrations. Nitrogen balance is improved only when there is sufficient intake of calories and protein.

Androgens are responsible for the growth spurt that occurs during adolescence and for the eventual termination of linear growth that results from fusion of the epiphyseal growth centers. Although endogenous androgens accelerate linear growth rates in children, the drugs may cause a disproportionate advancement in bone maturation, and long-term administration of the drugs in prepubertal children may result in fusion of the epiphyseal growth centers and premature termination of the growth process.

Exogenous administration of androgens inhibits the release of endogenous testosterone via feedback inhibition of pituitary luteinizing hormone (LH). Following administration of large doses of exogenous androgens, spermatogenesis may also be suppressed as a result of feedback inhibition of pituitary follicle-stimulating hormone (FSH).

Androgens reportedly stimulate the production of erythrocytes, apparently by enhancing the production of erythropoietic-stimulating factor.

Endogenous serum testosterone concentrations vary from hour to hour, and periodic declines below the normal range can occur occasionally in otherwise healthy men. Serum concentrations of the hormone exhibit diurnal variation, with highest concentrations of circulating testosterone occurring in the early morning hours. For a reliable testosterone determination, use of 3 pooled morning serum testosterone samples can minimize errors attributable to variation in concentrations of the hormone. Testosterone circulates principally in bound form, mainly to sex hormone binding globulin (SHBG; testosterone-estradiol binding globulin, TEBG) and albumin. Testosterone is tightly bound to SHBG and is not biologically active, whereas the fraction associated with albumin is only weakly bound and can dissociate to unbound, active hormone. Only about 2% of endogenous testosterone circulates unbound while 30–40% circulates bound to SHBG and the rest is bound to albumin and other proteins.

PHARMACOKINETICS

For information on the pharmacokinetics of endogenous testosterone, see Pharmacology.

● *Absorption*

Following oral administration of testosterone, only small amounts of the drug reach systemic circulation unchanged. The low bioavailability of orally administered testosterone results from metabolism of the drug in the GI mucosa during absorption and on first pass through the liver. The synthetic androgens (i.e., fluoxymesterone, methyltestosterone) are less extensively metabolized following oral administration.

Esterification of testosterone generally results in less polar compounds. The enanthate ester of testosterone is absorbed slowly from the lipid tissue phase at the IM injection site, achieving peak serum concentrations about 72 hours after IM injection; thus, this preparation has a prolonged duration of action (i.e., up to 2–4 weeks) following IM administration. Because IM injection of testosterone esters causes local irritation, the rate of absorption may be erratic.

Testosterone is absorbed systemically through the skin following topical application as a gel, solution, or transdermal system. Following topical application of a hydroalcoholic gel formulation of testosterone (AndroGel®, Testim®, Vogelxo®) to the skin, the gel quickly dries on the skin surface, which serves as a reservoir for sustained release of the hormone into systemic circulation. Approximately 10% of a testosterone dose applied topically to the skin as a 1% gel is absorbed percutaneously into systemic circulation.

The manufacturer of AndroGel® states that increases in serum testosterone concentrations were apparent within 30 minutes of topical application of a 100-mg testosterone dose of the 1% gel, with physiologic concentrations being achieved in most patients within 4 hours (pretreatment concentrations were not described); percutaneous absorption continues for the entire 24-hour dosing interval. Serum testosterone concentrations approximate steady-state levels by the end of the initial 24 hours and are at steady state by the second or third day of dosing of the 1% gel. With daily topical application of the 1% gel (AndroGel®), serum testosterone concentrations 30, 90, and 180 days after initiating treatment generally are maintained in the eugonadal range. Administration of 10 or 5 g of the 1% gel (AndroGel®) daily results in average daily serum testosterone concentrations of 792 or 566 ng/dL, respectively, at day 30. Following discontinuance of such topical therapy, serum testosterone concentrations remain within the normal range for 24–48 hours but return to pretreatment levels by the fifth day after the last application. The manufacturer states that mean concentrations of the active metabolite dihydrotestosterone (DHT) were within or about 7% above the normal range 180 days after initiating daily topical application of 50 or 100 mg, respectively, of testosterone as the gel. Increases in DHT concentrations appeared to parallel those of testosterone, and the mean steady-state ratio of DHT to testosterone was maintained in the normal range during the 180-day treatment period.

Following administration of testosterone gel (Testim®), physiologic concentrations of testosterone are achieved within 24 hours; percutaneous absorption continues for the entire 24-hour dosing interval. Administration of 10 or 5 g of Testim® daily results in average daily serum testosterone concentrations of 612 or 365 ng/dL, respectively, at day 30. DHT concentrations increase in parallel with testosterone concentrations; DHT concentrations have remained within the normal range during a 90-day treatment period.

Following topical application of testosterone solution (Axiron®) to the skin, ethanol and isopropyl alcohol evaporate leaving testosterone on the skin surface, which serves as a reservoir for sustained release of the hormone into systemic circulation. Following topical application of testosterone solution daily, serum testosterone concentrations reach steady-state levels by approximately 14 days. Following discontinuance of such topical therapy, serum testosterone concentrations return to pretreatment levels by 7–10 days after the last application. DHT concentrations increase in parallel with testosterone concentrations; mean steady-state ratios of testosterone to DHT have remained within the normal range during a 120-day treatment period.

Following topical application of transdermal systems of testosterone, the hormone is absorbed percutaneously into systemic circulation. Although interindividual variation in percutaneous testosterone absorption occurs, serum testosterone concentrations achieved with recommended dosages of transdermal

systems of the drug generally reach the normal range during the first day of dosing and are maintained during continuous dosing without accumulation. Average daily serum testosterone concentrations in patients receiving Androderm® reportedly are 498 ng/dL at steady state. Mean ratios of testosterone to DHT are within the normal range.

With topical application of a transdermal preparation, the extent of percutaneous testosterone absorption varies according to the site of application, possibly secondary to regional differences in skin permeability, cutaneous blood flow, and/or degree of adhesion between the transdermal system and skin. In one study in which transdermal systems were applied to the abdomen, back, chest, shin, thigh, or upper arm, serum hormone profiles were qualitatively similar with each site, but steady-state serum concentrations showed significant differences, decreasing in order with the back, thigh, upper arm, abdomen, chest, and shin. Application of Androderm® transdermal systems to the abdomen, back, thighs, or upper arms results in achievement of similar serum testosterone concentration profiles, and these sites are recommended as optimal for rotation of application sites during chronic therapy. Daily nighttime (at approximately 10 p.m.) application of Androderm® transdermal system results in a serum testosterone concentration profile that mimics the endogenous diurnal pattern in healthy young men. In one study, showering 3 hours after application of Androderm® decreased peak plasma concentrations of testosterone by 0.4% compared with not showering 3 hours after application of the transdermal system. In addition, showering 3 hours after transdermal system application did not substantially alter the systemic exposure of testosterone.

Following intranasal administration of testosterone nasal gel (Natesto®), peak plasma concentrations occur approximately 40 minutes after administration. Average daily serum testosterone concentration in patients receiving 11 mg of the nasal gel 3 times daily is 421 ng/dL. DHT concentrations increase in parallel with testosterone concentrations; mean steady-state ratios of testosterone to DHT have remained within the normal range during a 90-day treatment period.

Following buccal (transmucosal) administration of testosterone (Striant®), the drug is absorbed transmucosally from the buccal mucosa; testosterone that is absorbed systemically via the oral mucosa bypasses first-pass metabolism. Following administration of testosterone buccal tablets every 12 hours, steady-state concentrations of testosterone are achieved after the second dose. Testosterone concentrations decrease to concentrations below the normal range about 2–4 hours after removal of the buccal tablet. Average daily serum testosterone concentrations in patients receiving the buccal tablet are 520–550 ng/dL at steady state. Increases in DHT concentrations appear to parallel those of testosterone, and mean steady-state ratios of testosterone to DHT are within the normal range.

Following IM administration of testosterone undecanoate (Aveed®), the drug is slowly absorbed from the lipid phase and hydrolyzed to testosterone. Following IM administration of testosterone undecanoate 750 mg, peak plasma concentrations of testosterone occur after a median of 7 days and steady-state concentrations are achieved after the third injection (14 weeks). Increases in DHT concentrations appear to parallel those of testosterone, and mean ratios of testosterone to DHT are within the normal range.

● *Distribution*

Circulating testosterone is chiefly bound in the serum to sex steroid binding globulin (sex hormone binding globulin, SHBG; testosterone-estradiol-binding globulin, TEBG) and albumin. Because testosterone easily dissociates from albumin, the albumin-bound drug is presumed to be pharmacologically active. The SHBG-bound portion is not considered to be pharmacologically active.

In serum, testosterone is bound with high affinity to SHBG and with low affinity to albumin. The amount of SHBG in serum and the total testosterone concentration determine the distribution of pharmacologically active and non-active forms of the androgen. SHBG-binding capacity is high in prepubertal children, declines during puberty and adulthood, and increases again during the later decades of life. Approximately 30–40% of testosterone in plasma is bound to SHBG, 2% remains unbound (free), and the rest is bound to albumin and other proteins.

● *Elimination*

The plasma half-life of testosterone reportedly ranges from 10–100 minutes. The plasma half-life of testosterone cypionate after IM injection is approximately 8 days. Following removal of an Androderm® transdermal system, plasma testosterone concentrations decline with an apparent half-life of approximately 70 minutes and hypogonadal concentrations are reached within 24 hours.

Testosterone is metabolized principally in the liver to various 17-ketosteroids via 2 different pathways. The major active metabolites of testosterone are estradiol and DHT. In many tissues, the activity of testosterone appears to depend on reduction to DHT, which binds to SHBG with greater affinity than does testosterone. Testosterone and its metabolites are excreted in urine and feces. Approximately 90% of an IM dose of testosterone is excreted in urine as glucuronic and sulfuric acid conjugates of the drug and its metabolites; approximately 6% of a dose is excreted in feces, principally as unconjugated drug.

CHEMISTRY AND STABILITY

● Chemistry

Testosterone is a naturally occurring androgenic anabolic steroid hormone. The drug may be obtained from animal testes but is usually prepared synthetically from cholesterol. Dehydroepiandrosterone is an intermediate in the synthesis of the drug that can be treated by chemical or microbiologic processes to form testosterone. Testosterone is commercially available as the base, and as the cypionate, enanthate, and propionate esters.

Testosterone occurs as white or slightly creamy white, odorless crystals or as a crystalline powder and is practically insoluble in water, freely soluble in dehydrated alcohol, and soluble in vegetable oils. Testosterone cypionate occurs as a white or creamy white, crystalline powder that is odorless or has a slight odor and is insoluble in water, freely soluble in alcohol, and soluble in vegetable oils. Testosterone enanthate occurs as a white or creamy white, crystalline powder that is odorless or has a faint odor characteristic of heptanoic acid and is insoluble in water and soluble in vegetable oils. Testosterone undecanoate occurs as a white to off-white, crystalline powder.

Parenteral Preparations

Testosterone cypionate injection is a sterile solution of the drug in a suitable vegetable oil (e.g., cottonseed oil), which may also contain benzyl alcohol as a preservative.

Testosterone enanthate injection is a sterile solution of the drug in a suitable vegetable oil (e.g., sesame oil), which may also contain chlorobutanol as a preservative.

Testosterone undecanoate injection is a sterile solution of the drug in a suitable vegetable oil (e.g., castor oil).

Transdermal Systems

Transdermal testosterone (Androderm®) is commercially available as a system that consists of an outer layer of metallized polyester, ethylene-methacrylic acid copolymer (Surlyn®), and ethylene vinyl acetate; a drug reservoir of testosterone, alcohol, glycerin, glycerol monooleate, methyl laurate, and purified water, gelled with an acrylic acid copolymer; a permeable polyethylene microporous membrane; and a peripheral layer of acrylic adhesive surrounding the central, active drug delivery area of the system. The central delivery surface of the system is sealed with a peelable laminate disk composed of a 5-layer laminate containing polyester, polyesterurethane adhesive, aluminum foil, polyesterurethane adhesive, and polyethylene; the disk is attached to and removed with the release liner, a silicone-coated polyester film that should be removed prior to application.

Topical Gel

Testosterone topical gel is a clear to translucent, colorless, hydroalcoholic gel containing testosterone. AndroGel® also contains alcohol, purified water, sodium hydroxide, carbomer 980, and isopropyl myristate; Testim® also contains alcohol 74%, purified water, pentadecactone, carbopol, acrylates, propylene glycol, glycerin, polyethylene glycol, and tromethamine; Fortesta® also contains alcohol, purified water, propylene glycol, 2-propanol, oleic acid, carbomer 1382, triethanolamine, and butylated hydroxytoluene; Vogelxo® also contains alcohol, oleyl alcohol, purified water, glycerin, carbomer copolymer Type B, carbomer homopolymer Type C, diisopropyl adipate, methyl laurate, polyethylene glycol, propylene glycol, and tromethamine. Each g of testosterone gel 1% contains 10 mg

of testosterone. Each g of testosterone gel 1.62% contains 16.2 mg of testosterone. Each g of testosterone gel 2% contains 20 mg of testosterone.

Topical Solution

Testosterone topical solution is a clear to colorless solution containing testosterone. Axiron® also contains alcohol, isopropyl alcohol, octisalate, and povidone. Each mL of testosterone solution contains 20 mg of testosterone.

Nasal Gel

Testosterone nasal gel is a slightly yellow gel containing testosterone. Natesto® also contains castor oil, oleoyl polyoxylglycerides, and colloidal silicon dioxide. Each g of testosterone nasal gel contains approximately 45 mg of testosterone.

Buccal Tablets

Testosterone buccal (transmucosal) preparations (Striant®) contain the drug in a system that provides controlled and extended release of testosterone as the buccal system gradually hydrates. In addition to testosterone, the system also contains lactose (anhydrous and monohydrate), carbomer 934P, hypromellose, magnesium stearate, polycarbophil, colloidal silicon dioxide, starch, and talc.

● Stability

Testosterone enanthate injection (Delatestryl®) should be stored at room temperature. A precipitate may form if the injection is stored at a low temperature; however, this will dissolve after warming and rolling the syringe or vial containing the drug between the palms of the hands. Testosterone undecanoate injection (Aveed®) should be stored at 25°C, but may be exposed to temperatures of 15–30°C. Testosterone cypionate injection (Depo®-testosterone) should be stored at 20–25°C.

Testosterone pellets (Testopel®) should be stored at 25°C, but may be exposed to temperatures of 15–30°C.

Testosterone topical gels (AndroGel®, Fortesta,® Testim®, Vogelxo®) should be stored at 20–25°C, but may be exposed to temperatures of 15–30°C. Testosterone topical solution (Axiron®) should be stored at 25°C, but may be exposed to temperatures of 15–30°C. Testosterone transdermal system (Androderm®) should be stored at 20–25°C and protected from excessive heat. Testosterone nasal gel (Natesto®) should be stored at 20–25°C, but may be exposed to temperatures of 15–30°C. Testosterone buccal (transmucosal) tablets (Striant®) should be stored at 20–25°C and should be protected from heat and moisture.

Testosterone transdermal systems, topical gels, topical solutions, nasal gels, and buccal tablets should be disposed of in household trash in a manner that prevents accidental application or ingestion by children or pets.

PREPARATIONS

Distribution of testosterone undecanoate injection (Aveed®) is restricted. (See REMS and also see Restricted Distribution Program under Administration: IM Injection, in Dosage and Administration.)

Most preparations containing testosterone or its salts, esters, or ethers are subject to control under the Federal Controlled Substances Act of 1970, as amended by the Anabolic Steroids Control Act of 1990 and 2004, as schedule III (C-III) drugs. (See Uses: Misuse and Abuse.) However, manufacturers of certain preparations containing androgenic anabolic steroid hormones (principally combinations that also include estrogens) have applied for and obtained for their products(s) an exemption from the record-keeping and other regulatory requirements of the Federal Controlled Substances Act. Under provisions of the Act, specific products can be exempted from such control by the Attorney General, in consultation with the Secretary of Health and Human Services, if the product is determined *not* to possess any significant potential for abuse because of concentration, preparation, combination, and/or delivery system. Because regulatory requirements for a given preparation containing an androgenic anabolic steroid may be subject to change based on these provisions, the manufacturer should be contacted when specific clarification about a preparation's status is required.

Excipients in commercially available drug preparations may have clinically important effects in some individuals; consult specific product labeling for details.

Testosterone

Buccal (Transmucosal)		
Tablets, extended-release	30 mg	**Striant®** (C-III), Columbia
Nasal		
Gel	5.5 mg	**Natesto®** (C-III), Aytu Bioscience
Parenteral		
Implant, pellets for subcutaneous use	75 mg	**Testopel®** (C-III), Endo
Topical		
Gel	1% (12.5 and 50 mg)*	**Testosterone Gel** (C-III)
		Vogelxo® (C-III), Upsher-Smith
	1% (25 and 50 mg)*	**AndroGel®** (C-III), AbbVie
		Testosterone Gel (C-III)
	1% (50 mg)*	**Testim®** (C-III), Endo
		Testosterone Gel (C-III)
	1.62% (20.25 and 40.5 mg)*	**AndroGel®** (C-III), AbbVie
	2% (10 mg)*	**Fortesta®** (C-III), Endo
Solution	30 mg/1.5 mL*	**Axiron®** (C-III), Lilly
		Testosterone Topical Solution (C-III)
Transdermal System	2 mg/24 hours (9.7 mg/32 cm²)	**Androderm®** (C-III), Allergan
	4 mg/24 hours (19.5 mg/39 cm²)	**Androderm®** (C-III), Allergan

* available from one or more manufacturer, distributor, and/or repackager by generic (nonproprietary) name

Testosterone Cypionate

Parenteral		
Injection (in oil)	200 mg/mL*	**Depo®-Testosterone** (C-III), Pfizer
		Testosterone Cypionate Injection (C-III)

* available from one or more manufacturer, distributor, and/or repackager by generic (nonproprietary) name

Testosterone Enanthate

Parenteral		
Injection (in oil)	200 mg/mL*	**Delatestryl®** (C-III), Endo
		Testosterone Enanthate Injection (C-III)

* available from one or more manufacturer, distributor, and/or repackager by generic (nonproprietary) name

Testosterone Undecanoate

Parenteral		
Injection (in oil)	250 mg/mL	**Aveed®** (C-III), Endo

† Use is not currently included in the labeling approved by the US Food and Drug Administration.

Selected Revisions November 27, 2017, © Copyright, January 1, 1959, American Society of Health-System Pharmacists, Inc.

Estrogen-Progestin Combinations

68:12 • CONTRACEPTIVES

■ Estrogen-progestin combinations are contraceptive combinations containing estrogenic and progestinic steroids.

USES

● Contraception

Oral, intravaginal, and transdermal estrogen-progestin combinations are used for prevention of conception in women who elect to use one of these preparations as a method of contraception. When taken according to the prescribed regimen, these contraceptives provide almost completely effective contraception.

The pregnancy rate in women using conventional-dosage oral contraceptives (containing 35 mcg or more of ethinyl estradiol or 50 mcg or more of mestranol) is generally reported as less than one pregnancy per 100 woman-years of use. Slightly higher rates (somewhat more than one pregnancy per 100 woman-years) reportedly occur with some oral preparations containing 35 mcg or less of ethinyl estradiol, and rates of about 3 pregnancies per 100 woman-years reportedly occur with oral contraceptives containing progestins only. The pregnancy rate in women using the vaginal contraceptive ring containing ethinyl estradiol and etonogestrel (NuvaRing®) is reported as 1–2 pregnancies per 100 women-years of use. The pregnancy rate in women using the transdermal contraceptive system containing ethinyl estradiol and norelgestromin (Ortho Evra®) is reported as approximately one pregnancy per 100 women-years of use. Five out of the 15 pregnancies reported in large clinical trials in women using the transdermal contraceptive system Ortho Evra® occurred in women with a baseline weight of 90 kg or more; these data suggest that Ortho Evra® may be less effective in such women than in those with a lower body weight. Pregnancy rates for other methods of contraception reportedly range from about less than 1–6 pregnancies per 100 woman-years for intrauterine devices (IUDs) to about 14–47 pregnancies per 100 woman-years for the calendar method of periodic abstinence (rhythm). The pregnancy rate when no method of contraception is used is about 60–80 pregnancies per 100 woman-years. Pregnancy rates are derived from various studies conducted by different investigators in different population groups and, therefore, cannot be compared precisely.

Because a positive association between the dose of estrogens in oral contraceptives and the risk of thromboembolism has been shown in at least 2 studies, it is prudent and therapeutically desirable to minimize exposure to estrogens; therefore, the oral contraceptive used in a given patient should be that preparation which contains the least amount of estrogen and is compatible with an acceptable pregnancy rate and patient acceptance. Following a recommendation by the US Food and Drug Administration's (FDA) Fertility and Maternal Health Drugs Advisory Committee, oral contraceptive preparations containing more than 50 mcg of estrogen were discontinued in 1988 since these formulations were considered no more effective than those containing lower dosages of estrogen.

Because the pharmacokinetic profile for the transdermal contraceptive system containing ethinyl estradiol and norelgestromin (Ortho Evra®) differs from the profile for oral contraceptive preparations (see Pharmacokinetics: Absorption), the clinician and patient must weigh the possible risks of higher estrogen exposure with Ortho Evra® against the possibility of pregnancy if the oral contraceptive is not taken according to the prescribed regimen. Increased exposure to estrogen may increase the risk of certain adverse effects (e.g., venous thromboembolism). (See Thromboembolic Disorders in Cautions: Cardiovascular Effects.)

The clinician and patient must weigh the possible risks of estrogen-progestin contraception against those of other methods of contraception or no contraception. In addition, potential noncontraceptive benefits associated with use of oral contraceptives can be considered. (See Pharmacology: Other Effects.)

For information on parenteral use of fixed combinations of medroxyprogesterone acetate and estradiol cypionate (e.g., Lunelle®), see Uses: Contraception in Females, in Medroxyprogesterone Acetate 68:32.

Postcoital Contraception

A short-course, high-dose regimen of an oral estrogen-progestin combination is used in women for the prevention of conception after unprotected intercourse (postcoital contraception, morning-after pills) as an emergency contraceptive (EC)†. If taken soon enough after intercourse (i.e., within 72–120 hours), the combination regimen can *prevent* not *terminate* pregnancy; therefore, the regimen is contraceptive not abortifacient.

Several regimens employing high-dose combinations of ethinyl estradiol and norgestrel or levonorgestrel have been used safely and effectively for postcoital contraception†. One widely studied and used regimen (the Yuzpe regimen) consists of administering 2 tablets containing 50 mcg of ethinyl estradiol and 0.5 mg of norgestrel each (i.e., a dose of 100 mcg and 1 mg, respectively) within 72 hours after unprotected intercourse, repeating this dose 12 hours later. Alternative combination regimens consisting of 100–120 mcg of ethinyl estradiol and 1.2 mg of norgestrel or 0.5–0.6 mg of levonorgestrel administered within 72 hours of intercourse and repeated 12 hours later also have been used. Raw pregnancy (failure) rates in trials employing such regimens have ranged from 0.2–7.4%. However, not all women given emergency postcoital contraception are at genuine risk for pregnancy, since unprotected intercourse that occurs in the early follicular or in the luteal phase is unlikely to result in conception. Therefore, a more accurate indication of efficacy would be based on the timing of unprotected intercourse and the probability that pregnancy would occur without treatment. When efficacy of postcoital contraception with such estrogen-progestin combination regimens is based on the likelihood of pregnancy (computed by matching the cycle day of unprotected intercourse with known conception rates for that cycle day), estimates from various studies of the proportionate reduction in pregnancy risk have ranged from about 55–94%, and pooled analysis of data from studies employing the Yuzpe regimen reveal that such therapy is approximately 74% (confidence interval: 68.2–79.3%) effective in preventing a single pregnancy. Because of study limitations of this pooled analysis, it is likely that true efficacy rates are higher than this estimate, perhaps exceeding 80%. However, postcoital (emergency) contraceptive regimens are not as effective as most other forms of long-term contraception. The efficacy of postcoital regimens employing lower estrogen/progestin doses currently is not known.

An emergency contraceptive regimen employing a progestin alone (levonorgestrel) appears to be more effective and better tolerated than the estrogen-progestin emergency contraceptive ("Yuzpe") regimen when the regimens are initiated within 72 hours of unprotected intercourse, and therefore, the progestin-alone regimen generally is preferred when readily available.

To prevent pregnancy, oral estrogen-progestin combination therapy ideally should begin within 72 hours following coitus. Studies show that emergency contraception is moderately effective when the first dose is administered up to 120 hours after unprotected intercourse. Postcoital contraceptive efficacy diminishes as the time period between intercourse and administration of the combination increases, with the regimen becoming completely ineffective by day 6 or 7, when implantation usually occurs.

Because of the short time frame for effective postcoital use, women should be informed of the availability of postcoital contraception before such use is warranted and offered advanced provision (e.g., provided a prescription for emergency contraception at the time of a routine gynecology visit), advised of the availability of an over-the-counter (OTC) emergency contraceptive preparation, or advised to contact a clinician immediately if the need arises. By informing women of this emergency option and advising them of steps to take to readily obtain the combinations before or when needed, effective postcoital contraception ultimately could reduce substantially the number of unintended pregnancies and induced abortions. Because of the high incidence of adverse effects (e.g., nausea and vomiting with estrogen-progestin combinations) decreased contraceptive efficacy compared with conventional long-term contraceptive methods, including cyclic use of estrogen-progestin combinations, postcoital contraception with the combinations generally should be limited to emergency situations following unprotected intercourse (e.g., rape, contraceptive failure, missed doses of oral or parenteral contraceptives, lack of planning). Postcoital contraceptive regimens should not be used as a routine method of contraception. Women should be informed that postcoital contraceptives do not protect against human immunodeficiency virus (HIV) infection or other sexually transmitted diseases. Women should be advised about various available routine methods of contraception when given emergency contraception and instructed as to when to begin an effective method of such contraception; the potential value of condoms as a supplement to other methods (e.g., to reduce the risk of sexually transmitted diseases) also should be discussed. Women who request emergency contraceptives repeatedly should be informed about other contraceptive options.

The American College of Obstetricians and Gynecologists (ACOG), other experts, and some states (e.g., Alaska, California, Hawaii, Maine, New Mexico, Washington) have advocated increased access to emergency postcoital contraception (e.g., nonprescription access via pharmacies, advance provision by clinicians) as a means of decreasing unintended pregnancy and abortion rates. There is some evidence that increased access to emergency postcoital contraception may not compromise conventional contraceptive use or sexual behavior, potentially allaying some concerns that have prompted others to advocate for restricted access. The US Food and Drug Administration (FDA) has approved one postcoital contraceptive (Plan B® One-Step; levonorgestrel) for nonprescription (OTC) status for women 17 years of age or older; the contraceptive will remain a prescription-only preparation for women younger than 17 years of age. For information on this preparation, see Progestins 68:12.

Use of high-dose oral estrogen-progestin combinations as emergency postcoital contraception may cause menstrual cycle disruption; if menstruation is delayed by a week or more, a sensitive pregnancy test should be performed. If pregnancy has already occurred, there is little, if any, evidence that postcoital regimens will adversely affect the fetus or pregnancy. (See Cautions: Pregnancy, Fertility, and Lactation.) Because postcoital regimens may not prevent ectopic (tubal or abdominal) pregnancies, women receiving such regimens should be informed that ectopic pregnancy is a medical emergency and to consult their clinician immediately if spotting or cramping occurs (usually beginning shortly after the first missed period with such pregnancy). Women should consult their clinician regarding when they can start or resume cyclic oral contraceptive regimens with a combination; they also should be instructed carefully regarding differences in administration schedule and any differences in formulation (e.g., potency, active versus inert tablets) of the preparations.

For the use of progestin-only therapy as a postcoital contraceptive, see Progestins 68:12.

● *Contraception and Folate Supplementation*

Certain estrogen-progestin combinations (Beyaz® [ethinyl estradiol 20 mcg in fixed combination with drospirenone 3 mg and levomefolate calcium 0.451 mg], Safyral®[ethinyl estradiol 30 mcg in fixed combination with drospirenone 3 mg and levomefolate calcium 0.451 mg]) are used in women choosing oral contraceptives as their method of contraception, for the additional purpose of increasing folate concentrations to reduce the risk of fetal neural tube defects when conception occurs while the woman is receiving the contraceptive or shortly after the contraceptive is discontinued. The US Preventive Services Task Force recommends that women of childbearing age receive supplemental folic acid at a dosage of at least 0.4 mg daily. Other folate supplementation that a woman may be taking should be considered before prescribing ethinyl estradiol in combination with drospirenone and levomefolate calcium (Beyaz®, Safyral®). Folate supplementation should be maintained if a woman discontinues this contraceptive because of pregnancy.

● *Acne Vulgaris*

Certain triphasic or estrophasic oral estrogen-progestin combinations (specifically, Ortho Tri-Cyclen® [ethinyl estradiol 35 mcg in fixed combination with norgestimate 0.18, 0.215, or 0.25 mg], or Estrostep® [ethinyl estradiol 20, 30, or 35 mcg in fixed combination with norethindrone acetate 1 mg]) can be used for the treatment of moderate acne vulgaris in females 15 years of age or older who have no known contraindications to oral contraceptive therapy, desire contraception, have achieved menarche, and are unresponsive to topical anti-acne medication. The manufacturer of Estrostep® states that the drug should be used for the treatment of acne vulgaris only in women who desire oral contraception and plan to take the drug for at least 6 months. Acne is a skin condition with a multifactorial etiology and the combination of ethinyl estradiol and norgestimate may increase sex hormone-binding globulin (SHBG) and decrease free testosterone serum concentrations. This may result in a decrease in the severity of facial acne in otherwise healthy women. In two double-blind, placebo-controlled, 6-month multicenter trials, therapy with the ethinyl estradiol/norgestimate combination resulted in clinically important decreases in inflammatory lesion count and total lesion count as compared with placebo (56.6% versus 36.6% and 49.6% versus 30.3%, respectively). In two 6-month, randomized, double-blind, placebo-controlled, multicenter studies in young women (mean age: 24 years) with acne vulgaris, therapy with the ethinyl estradiol/norethindrone combination or placebo resulted in a 52 or 41% reduction in inflammatory lesion count, respectively, and a 43 or 32% reduction in total lesion count, respectively.

The estrogen-progestin combinations (specifically, Yaz® [ethinyl estradiol 20 mcg in fixed combination with drospirenone 3 mg], Beyaz® [ethinyl estradiol 20 mcg in fixed combination with drospirenone 3 mg and levomefolate calcium 0.451 mg]) also are used for the treatment of moderate acne vulgaris in females at least 14 years of age who have no known contraindications to oral contraceptive therapy and who desire oral contraception and have achieved menarche.

● *Premenstrual Dysphoric Disorder*

The estrogen-progestin combinations (Yaz® [ethinyl estradiol 20 mcg in fixed combination with drospirenone 3 mg], Beyaz® [ethinyl estradiol 20 mcg in fixed combination with drospirenone 3 mg and levomefolate calcium 0.451 mg]) are used for the treatment of premenstrual dysphoric disorder (formerly known as late luteal phase dysphoric disorder) in women who desire oral contraception. Efficacy of ethinyl estradiol in combination with drospirenone (Yaz®) has been evaluated in 2 randomized, placebo-controlled, double-blind studies of 3 months' duration in adult women who met DSM-IV criteria for premenstrual dysphoric disorder. In these studies, ethinyl estradiol in combination with drospirenone was found to be superior to placebo in improving symptoms associated with this disorder. Efficacy of ethinyl estradiol 20 mcg in fixed combination with drospirenone 3 mg (Yaz®) or ethinyl estradiol 20 mcg in fixed combination with drospirenone 3 mg and levomefolate calcium 0.451 mg (Beyaz®) when used for more than 3 menstrual cycles has not been evaluated.

● *Other Uses*

Estrogen-progestin preparations have been used for the treatment of endometriosis† or dysfunctional uterine bleeding†.

DOSAGE AND ADMINISTRATION

● *Administration*

Estrogen-progestin combination contraceptives are administered orally, intravaginally, and percutaneously by topical application of a transdermal system to the skin.

Contraception
Oral Administration

To ensure maximum contraceptive efficacy, oral contraceptives should be taken as near as possible to the same time each day (i.e., at regular 24-hour intervals). Most oral contraceptives are commercially available in a mnemonic dispensing package that is designed to aid the user in complying with the prescribed dosage schedule; these containers should be used whenever possible.

To minimize nausea, oral contraceptives should be taken with or after the evening meal or at bedtime. As vomiting or diarrhea may decrease absorption of oral contraceptives and potentially result in treatment failures, a back-up method of contraception (e.g., condoms, foam, sponge) should be used until the next clinician contact.

Chewable tablets may be swallowed whole or chewed and consumed with 240 mL of liquid.

Intravaginal Administration

Patients receiving the vaginal contraceptive ring containing ethinyl estradiol and etonogestrel (NuvaRing®) should be carefully instructed in the use of the vaginal ring. To obtain optimum results, patients also should be given a copy of the patient information provided by the manufacturer. The ring should be inserted into the vagina by the patient; the manufacturer states that the exact position of the ring inside the vagina is not critical for its proper functioning. If the ring is accidentally expelled, it can be rinsed with cool or lukewarm water and reinserted or, if necessary, a new ring should be inserted as soon as possible; in either case, the administration schedule employed should be continued. If the contraceptive ring has been out of the vagina for longer than 3 hours, a back-up method of contraception (e.g., condoms, spermicides) must be used until the ring has been used continuously for 7 days.

Transdermal Administration

Women receiving the transdermal contraceptive containing ethinyl estradiol and norelgestromin (Ortho Evra®) should be instructed in the use of the transdermal system. To obtain optimum results, women also should be given a copy of the patient information provided by the manufacturer. The transdermal system is applied topically to a clean and dry area of intact skin on the buttock, abdomen, upper outer arm, or upper torso, by firmly pressing the system with the adhesive side touching the skin. The system should be pressed firmly in place with the palm of the hand for about 10 seconds, ensuring good contact, particularly around the edges. The application site should not be oily, damaged, or irritated. The transdermal system should *not* be applied to the breasts or to areas where tight clothing may cause the system to be rubbed off. If the system inadvertently gets detached during the period of use, and is off for less than one day, the system may be reapplied or, if necessary, a new system (if the system is no longer sticky) may be applied; in either case, the application schedule employed should be continued. If the system is off for longer than one day or for an unknown duration, a new system should be applied immediately and a new 4-week cycle should be started; a back-up method of contraception (e.g., condoms, spermicides, diaphragm) must be used for the first week of the new cycle. Patients should be instructed to handle the used transdermal system carefully (e.g., fold the system in half with the sticky sides together) and then discard the system.

Postcoital Contraception

Oral Administration

Postcoital contraceptive regimens usually consist of 2–5 tablets per dose† administered 12 hours apart. The first dose should be administered *as soon as possible but preferably within 72 hours* following unprotected intercourse; the second dose is administered 12 hours later. Women should be advised of the importance of taking the second dose 12 hours after the initial dose, and to schedule the first dose as conveniently as possible so that the likelihood of missing the second dose 12 hours later is minimized (e.g., if the first dose were taken at 3 p.m., the second dose would need to be taken at 3 a.m., which might present a problem of compliance for heavy sleepers). The first dose can be taken up to 120 hours after unprotected intercourse if necessary, but efficacy decreases as initiation of contraception becomes more remote from unprotected intercourse.

Because the high dosage in the combination regimens may cause severe nausea and vomiting in a substantial proportion of women, which could limit compliance with postcoital contraception, use of an antiemetic 1 hour prior to administration of the first dose of the combination should be considered. Administering the dose with food is not effective in reducing adverse GI effects (i.e., nausea). If vomiting does occur within 2 hours after administration of a dose of the estrogen-progestin combination, consideration should be given to repeating the dose.

Because of the short time frame of effective postcoital use (i.e., therapy must commence within 72–120 hours of unprotected intercourse), clinicians ideally should inform women of the availability of postcoital contraception before such use is warranted, advising them to contact a clinician immediately if the need for such contraception arises. Alternatively, women can be given an appropriate estrogen-progestin combination in advance, with careful instructions on how to safely and effectively use the combination for emergency postcoital contraception; if a supply of the drugs is given to a woman in advance, she also should be advised that postcoital contraceptives are for emergency situations (e.g., unprotected intercourse, missed doses of oral contraceptives, missed parenteral contraceptive dose, contraceptive failure) only and should not be employed as the primary method of contraception.

If the menstrual period is delayed by a week or more, or if persistent irregular bleeding or lower abdominal pain occurs, professional medical follow-up care should be obtained.

● Dosage

Contraception

Before initiating therapy, women receiving estrogen-progestin contraceptives should be given a copy of the patient labeling for the drugs.

Oral Dosage

Estrogen-progestin oral contraceptives are usually classified according to their formulation:

- those monophasic preparations containing 50 mcg of estrogen,
- those monophasic preparations containing less than 50 mcg of estrogen (usually 20–35 mcg),
- those containing less than 50 mcg of estrogen with 2 sequences of progestin doses (biphasic),
- those containing less than 50 mcg of estrogen with 3 sequences of progestin doses (triphasic), and
- those containing 3 sequences of estrogen (e.g., 20, 30, 35 mcg) with a fixed dose of progestin (estrophasic).

Although the progestin content of the formulations also varies, oral contraceptives usually are described in terms of their estrogen content. The estrogenic and progestinic dominance of oral contraceptives depends mainly on the amount of estrogen and the amount and specific progestin contained in the formulation. The estrogenic or progestinic dominance of an oral contraceptive may contribute

to hormone-related adverse effects and may be useful in selecting an alternate formulation when unacceptable adverse effects occur with a given formulation.

Whenever possible, the smallest dosage of estrogen and progestin should be used. The amount of both hormones should be considered in the choice of an oral contraceptive preparation. It is prudent and in keeping with good principles of therapeutics to minimize exposure to estrogen and progestin. The combination used should be one which contains the least amount of estrogen and progestin that is compatible with a low failure rate and with the individual needs of the woman. Common adverse effects are usually most pronounced during the first oral contraceptive cycle and generally disappear or diminish after 3 or 4 cycles; there does not appear to be any advantage in changing preparations during this period. If minor adverse effects persist after the fourth cycle, a different combination of drugs or a different dosage may be tried.

Most fixed combinations are available as 21- or 28-day dosage preparations (conventional-cycle oral contraceptives). Some 28-day preparations contain 21 hormonally active tablets and 7 inert or ferrous fumarate-containing tablets; other 28-day preparations contain 24 hormonally active tablets and 4 inert or ferrous fumarate-containing tablets. In establishing an oral contraceptive dosage cycle, the menstrual cycle is usually considered to be 28 days. The first day of bleeding is counted as the first day of the cycle.

One fixed-combination extended-cycle oral contraceptive (e.g., Seasonale®) is available as a 91-day dosage preparation containing 84 hormonally active tablets and 7 inert tablets. Other extended-cycle oral contraceptive preparations (e.g., LoSeasonique®, Seasonique®,) are available as 91-day preparations with 84 hormonally active tablets containing estrogen/progestin and 7 tablets containing low-dose estrogen.

One fixed-combination continuous-regimen (noncyclic) oral contraceptive (i.e., Lybrel®) is available as a 28-day dosage preparation containing 28 hormonally active tablets.

Conventional-cycle Oral Contraceptives

Administration of **monophasic** fixed-combination conventional-cycle oral contraceptives usually begins on the first day of the menstrual cycle or on the first Sunday after menstrual bleeding has started. A back-up method of contraception (e.g., condoms, foam, sponge) should be employed for 7 days following initiation of oral contraceptive therapy if the first dose of the oral contraceptive is begun on the first Sunday after menstrual bleeding starts. A back-up method of contraception is not needed if the first dosage cycle is initiated on the first day of the menstrual cycle. When the 21-day conventional-cycle preparations are used, tablets containing estrogen/progestin are administered once daily for 21 consecutive days, followed by up to 7 days without drugs. When the 28-day dosage preparations containing 21 hormonally active tablets are used, tablets containing estrogen/progestin are administered once daily for 21 consecutive days, followed by inert tablets or tablets containing ferrous fumarate for 7 days. When the 28-day dosage preparations containing 24 hormonally active tablets are used, tablets containing estrogen/progestin are administered once daily for 24 consecutive days, followed by inert tablets or tablets containing ferrous fumarate for 4 days. Withdrawal bleeding usually occurs within 2 or 3 days after the last hormonally active tablet has been taken. Repeat dosage cycles begin on the same day of the week as the initial cycle. Repeat cycles should generally begin regardless of whether menstruation has stopped; after several cycles of fixed-combination preparations, menstrual flow may be considerably reduced. If a repeat 21-day cycle is started later than the eighth day after taking the last hormonally active tablet (or later than the next day after taking the last inactive tablet with 28-day dosage preparations), a back-up method of contraception should be employed until the patient has taken a hormonally active tablet daily for 7 consecutive days.

When a **biphasic** oral contraceptive (e.g., Ortho-Novum® 10/11) is used, each dosage cycle consists of 2 sequentially administered fixed combinations; the first sequence consists of 10 tablets containing a fixed combination of low-dose estrogen and low-dose progestin and the second sequence consists of 11 tablets containing a fixed combination of low-dose estrogen and higher-dose progestin. Although biphasic oral contraceptives consist of 2 sequentially administered fixed combinations, they are *not* the same as previously available "sequential" oral contraceptives which consisted of an estrogen alone for the first sequence. Administration of a biphasic oral contraceptive usually begins on the first Sunday after or on which bleeding has started. Tablets from the first sequence are administered once daily for 10 consecutive days, followed by once-daily administration of tablets from the second sequence for 11 consecutive days and then a period of 7 days without drug; when a 28-day dosage preparation is used, inert tablets are administered during this latter 7-day period. A back-up method of contraception (e.g., condoms, foam, sponge) should be employed for 7 days following initiation of oral contraceptive therapy if the first dose of the oral contraceptive is begun on the first Sunday on or after menstrual bleeding starts; a back-up method of contraception is not necessary if the first dosage cycle is initiated on the first day of the menstrual cycle. Repeat dosage cycles begin on the eighth day after taking the last hormonally active tablet.

Triphasic oral contraceptives contain graduated sequences of progestin or estrogen. With most commercially available triphasic oral contraceptives (e.g., Ortho-Novum® 7/7/7, Ortho-Tri-Cyclen®, Ortho-Tri-Cyclen® Lo, Tri-Levlen®, Tri-Norinyl®, Triphasil®), each dosage cycle consists of 3 sequentially administered fixed combinations of the hormones in which the ratio of progestin to estrogen progressively increases with each sequence. The first sequence consists of tablets containing a fixed combination of low-dose estrogen and low-dose progestin, the second sequence consists of tablets containing a fixed combination of low-dose (i.e., Ortho-Novum 7/7/7, Ortho-Tri-Cyclen®, Ortho-Tri-Cyclen® Lo, Tri-Norinyl®) or low but slightly higher-dose estrogen (i.e., Tri-Levlen®, Triphasil®) and higher-dose progestin, and the third sequence consists of tablets containing low-dose estrogen and either an even higher-dose progestin (i.e., Ortho-Novum® 7/7/7, Ortho-Tri-Cyclen®, Ortho-Tri-Cyclen® Lo, Tri-Levlen®, Triphasil®) or low-dose progestin (i.e., Tri-Norinyl®).

Triphasic oral contraceptives in which the estrogen component progressively increases with each sequence also are available; such contraceptives have been referred to as "**estrophasic**". With the currently commercially available estrophasic oral contraceptive (e.g., Estrostep®), the first sequence consists of tablets containing a fixed combination of a progestin and low-dose estrogen, the second sequence consists of tablets containing a fixed combination of a progestin and a slightly higher dosage of an estrogen, and the third sequence consists of tablets containing a progestin and an even higher dosage of an estrogen.

Administration of a triphasic oral contraceptive usually begins on the first Sunday after or on which bleeding has started or on the first day of the menstrual cycle. Tablets from the first sequence of Ortho-Novum® 7/7/7, Ortho-Tri-Cyclen®, or Ortho-Tri-Cyclen® Lo are administered once daily for 7 consecutive days, followed by once-daily administration of tablets from the second sequence for 7 consecutive days and then once-daily administration of tablets from the third sequence for 7 consecutive days. Tablets from the first sequence of Tri-Norinyl® are administered once daily for 7 consecutive days, followed by once-daily administration of tablets from the second sequence for 9 consecutive days and then once-daily administration of tablets from the third sequence for 5 consecutive days. Tablets from the first sequence of Tri-Levlen® or Triphasil® are administered once daily for 6 consecutive days, followed by once-daily administration of tablets from the second sequence for 5 consecutive days and then once-daily administration of tablets from the third sequence for 10 consecutive days. Tablets from the first sequence of Estrostep® are administered once daily for 5 consecutive days, followed by once-daily administration of tablets from the second sequence for 7 consecutive days and then once-daily administration of tablets from the third sequence for 9 consecutive days. The 3 sequences are then followed by a period of 7 days without drug; when a 28-day dosage preparation is used, inert tablets are administered during this latter 7-day period. Repeat dosage cycles begin on the eighth day after taking the last hormonally active tablet. If a repeat 21-day cycle is started later than the eighth day after taking the last hormonally active tablet (or later than the next day after taking the last inactive tablet with 28-day dosage preparations), a back-up method of contraception should be employed until the patient has taken a hormonally active tablet daily for 7 consecutive days.

If oral contraceptives are first taken postpartum or later than the fifth day of the menstrual cycle, the contraceptive effect should not be relied on until after 7 consecutive days of drug administration, since there is a possibility that ovulation and conception may have occurred. In all patients, additional contraceptive measures may be advisable through the first week of the *initial* regimen. In determining whether to initiate oral contraceptive therapy in the postpartum period, the increased risk of thromboembolism during this period must be considered since use of oral contraceptives is also associated with an increased risk of thromboembolic and thrombotic disorders. (See Thromboembolic Disorders in Cautions: Cardiovascular Effects.)

If spotting or breakthrough bleeding occurs during oral contraceptive use, the dosage cycle should generally be continued. Spotting or breakthrough bleeding usually stops within one week. If bleeding persists or is prolonged, nonfunctional causes should be considered. (See Cautions: Genitourinary Effects.) For

information on the use of oral contraceptives when a menstrual period has been missed, see Cautions: Pregnancy, Fertility, and Lactation.

When a woman misses one estrogen/progestin tablet of a conventional cycle oral contraceptive, the missed dose should be taken as soon as it is remembered, followed by resumption of the regular schedule. Additional contraceptive methods are not necessary if only one tablet is missed. When 2 doses are missed during the first one or 2 weeks of the cycle, the 2 missed doses should both be taken as soon as they are remembered, then 2 tablets the next day, followed by resumption of the regular schedule. If 2 consecutive estrogen/progestin tablets are missed during the third or fourth week of a dosage cycle that was initiated on the first day of the menstrual cycle, the remainder of the tablets in the pack for that cycle should be discarded and a new dosage cycle started the same day. If 2 consecutive estrogen/progestin tablets are missed during the third or fourth week of a dosage cycle that was initiated on the first Sunday on or after menstruation started, the patient should continue to take one tablet daily until Sunday, then discard the remainder of the tablets for that cycle and start a new dosage cycle that same day. If 3 or more consecutive estrogen/progestin tablets are missed during a dosage cycle that was initiated on the first day of the menstrual cycle, the remainder of the tablets in that cycle should be discarded and a new dosage cycle started the same day. If 3 or more consecutive estrogen/progestin tablets are missed during a dosage cycle that was initiated on the first Sunday on or after menstruation started, the patient should continue to take one tablet daily until Sunday, then discard the remainder of the tablets for that cycle and start a new dosage cycle that same day. During the 28-day dosage cycle, any inactive tablets that are missed should be discarded and the patient should continue taking the remaining inactive tablets until the cycle is finished. A back-up contraceptive method is not required during the fourth week as a result of missed inactive tablets. With 28-day contraceptive cycles, a new cycle of tablets should be started the day after taking the last tablet of the previous 28-day dosage cycle (i.e., no days without tablets). If the patient is unsure of what drug regimen to take as a result of missed tablets, a back-up method of contraception should be used for each sexual encounter, and one active tablet should be taken each day until the next clinician contact.

Missed doses may cause light bleeding or spotting or amenorrhea, and ingestion of multiple tablets to make up for those missed (i.e., 2 doses at a time) may be associated with nausea. If breakthrough bleeding occurs following missed doses, it will usually be transient and of no consequence. If breakthrough bleeding resembling menstruation occurs during use of monophasic (conventional cycle) fixed-combination oral contraceptives, therapy should be discontinued, the remainder of the tablets in that cycle should be discarded, and the next cycle should be started on the next Sunday. There is little likelihood of ovulation when one dose is missed; however, the possibility of ovulation and spotting or breakthrough bleeding increases with each missed dose. Whenever 2 or more doses are missed, additional contraceptive methods should be used for the next 7 days.

In nonlactating postpartum women, oral contraceptives may be initiated no earlier than 28 days after delivery. In women who choose to breast-feed, oral contraceptives should not be given in the immediate postpartum period. Whenever possible, the use of oral contraceptives should be deferred until the infant has been weaned. (See Cautions: Pregnancy, Fertility, and Lactation.)

Extended-cycle Oral Contraceptives

When a fixed-combination extended-cycle oral contraceptive (e.g., LoSeasonique®, Seasonale®, Seasonique®) is used, the oral contraceptive is administered in a cyclic regimen using a 91-day cycle. Because extended-cycle oral contraceptives are administered using a 91-day cycle, women using these preparations should expect to have 4 menstrual periods per year. When an extended-cycle preparation is used, tablets containing estrogen/progestin are administered once daily for 84 days followed by administration of inert tablets or tablets containing 10 mcg of estrogen for 7 days. Administration of the extended-cycle preparation usually begins on the first Sunday after or on which bleeding begins. A back-up method of contraception (e.g., condom, spermicide) should be employed for 7 days following initiation of therapy. Withdrawal bleeding usually occurs during the 7 days after the last estrogen/progestin tablet. Repeat dosage cycles begin on the same day of the week (Sunday) as the initial cycle. If a repeat cycle is started later than the scheduled day, a back-up method of contraception should be employed until the patient has taken a hormonally active tablet daily for 7 consecutive days.

When a woman misses one estrogen/progestin tablet of an extended-cycle oral contraceptive (i.e., LoSeasonique®, Seasonale®, Seasonique®), the missed dose should be taken as soon as it is remembered, followed by resumption of the regular schedule. Additional contraceptive measures are not necessary if only one tablet is missed. When 2 estrogen/progestin tablets are missed, the 2 missed tablets should be taken as soon as they are remembered, then 2 tablets the next day, followed by resumption of the regular cycle. A back-up method of contraception (e.g., condom, spermicide) should be employed until the patient has taken an estrogen/progestin tablet daily for 7 consecutive days. When 3 or more consecutive estrogen/progestin tablets are missed, the patient should continue to take one tablet daily; the missed tablets should be discarded. A back-up method of contraception (e.g., condom, spermicide) should be employed when the patient misses a dose and until the patient has taken an estrogen/progestin tablet daily for 7 consecutive days. Inert tablets or estrogen-containing tablets that are missed should be discarded and the patient should continue taking the remaining tablets until the cycle is finished. A back-up contraceptive method is not required if the patient missed inert or estrogen-containing tablets. If the patient is unsure of what drug regimen to take as a result of missed tablets, a back-up method of contraception should be used for each sexual encounter, and one tablet taken each day until the next clinician contact. Missed doses may cause light bleeding or spotting, and ingestion of multiple tablets to make up for those missed doses may be associated with nausea.

In nonlactating postpartum women, fixed-combination extended-cycle oral contraceptives may be started no earlier than 28 days after delivery. Women may start taking fixed-combination extended-cycle oral contraceptives immediately following a complete first-trimester abortion; a back-up method of contraception is not needed.

Continuous-Regimen (Noncyclic) Oral Contraceptive

When a fixed-combination continuous-regimen oral contraceptive (i.e., Lybrel®) is used, the oral contraceptive is administered each day and continued daily without interruption (i.e., without a drug-free interval). Therefore, women using this preparation should expect no withdrawal menstruation-like bleeding; uterine bleeding and/or spotting does occur in some women. Administration of the continuous-regimen oral contraceptive usually begins on the first day of the menstrual cycle in women who did not use hormonal contraception in the preceding month. A back-up method of contraception is not needed if the oral contraceptive is started on the first day of the menstrual cycle. The manufacturer states that women switching from a cyclic estrogen-progestin oral contraceptive should start the continuous-regimen oral contraceptive on the first day of withdrawal bleeding, within 7 days of the last hormonally active tablet; a back-up method of contraception is not needed. Women switching from progestin-only oral contraceptives should start the continuous-regimen oral contraceptive on the day after the last dose of the progestin-only oral contraceptive. Women switching from a progestin-only implant should start the continuous-regimen oral contraceptive on the same day that the implant is removed. Women switching from a progestin-only contraceptive injection should start the continuous-regimen oral contraceptive on the day that the next contraceptive injection would have been due. A back-up method of contraception (e.g., condom, spermicide) is recommended in all women switching from progestin-only contraceptives until the fixed-combination continuous-regimen oral contraceptive has been used for 7 days.

When a woman misses one tablet of the fixed-combination continuous-regimen oral contraceptive (i.e., Lybrel®), the missed dose should be taken as soon as it is remembered, followed by resumption of the regular schedule (this may involve taking 2 tablets on one day). When 2 tablets are missed and the missed doses are remembered on the day of the second missed dose, the 2 missed tablets should be taken as soon as they are remembered, followed by resumption of the regular schedule. When 2 tablets are missed and the missed doses are remembered on the day after the second missed dose, the 2 missed tablets should be taken as soon as they are remembered, then 2 tablets the next day, followed by resumption of the regular schedule. When 3 or more tablets are missed, the patient should contact her clinician for advice and continue to take one tablet daily until the clinician is contacted. When one or more tablets are missed, a back-up method of contraception (e.g., condom, spermicide) should be used until the patient has taken the oral contraceptive for 7 days. If the patient is unsure of what drug regimen to take as a result of missed tablets, a back-up method of contraception should be used for each sexual encounter.

In nonlactating postpartum women, the fixed-combination continuous-regimen oral contraceptive may be started no earlier than 28 days after delivery. In addition, the continuous regimen oral contraceptive may be started no earlier than 28 days after a second-trimester abortion. A back-up method of contraception should be used until the patient has taken the oral contraceptive for 7 days. Women may start the continuous-regimen oral contraceptive immediately following a complete first-trimester abortion; a back-up method of contraception is not needed.

Intravaginal Dosage

Each vaginal contraceptive ring containing ethinyl estradiol and etonogestrel (NuvaRing®) is intended to be used for one cycle which consists of a 3-week period of continuous use of the ring followed by a 1-week ring-free period. When the vaginal ring is used for contraception, one ring (delivering ethinyl estradiol 0.015 mg/24 hours and etonogestrel 0.12 mg/24 hours) is inserted into the vagina at the beginning of the cycle. After 3 weeks, the vaginal ring is removed on the same day of the week as it was inserted and at about the same time of day. After a 1-week ring-free period, a new ring is inserted on the same day of the week as in the previous cycle. Withdrawal bleeding usually occurs within 2–3 days after removal of the ring. For contraceptive effectiveness, a new ring must be inserted 1 week after the previous ring was removed even if menstrual bleeding is not finished.

To initiate therapy, the vaginal ring (containing ethinyl estradiol and etonogestrel) usually is inserted on or before day 5 of the cycle (the first day of bleeding is counted as the first day of the menstrual cycle) in women who did not use hormonal contraception in the preceding month. During the first cycle, a back-up method of contraception (e.g., condom, spermicide) is recommended until the contraceptive ring has been used continuously for 7 days. The manufacturer states that women switching from estrogen-progestin oral contraceptives to the vaginal ring should insert the ring within 7 days of the last hormonally active tablet and no later than the day that a new oral contraceptive cycle would have been started; a back-up method of contraception is not needed. Women switching from progestin-only contraceptives to the vaginal ring should insert the ring on any day of the month if they are switching from a progestin-only oral contraceptive (without skipping any day between receiving the last progestin oral contraceptive and the initial administration of the vaginal ring). In addition, women switching from a progestin-only contraceptive injection should insert the vaginal ring on the same day as the next contraceptive injection would have been due. Women who are switching from a progestin-only implant or a progestin-containing intrauterine device should insert the vaginal ring on the same day as the implant or the intrauterine device is removed. A back-up method of contraception is recommended in all women switching from progestin-only contraceptives until the vaginal ring has been used continuously for 7 days.

When the woman forgets to insert a new vaginal ring at the start of any cycle, the ring should be inserted as soon as she remembers and back-up contraception must be employed until the ring has been used continuously for 7 days. If the vaginal ring is left in place for up to 1 extra week (up to 4 weeks total), the ring should be removed and a new ring can be inserted after a 1-week drug-free interval. If the ring is left in place for longer than 4 weeks, pregnancy should be ruled out and a back-up method of contraception must be used until a new ring has been used continuously for 7 days.

Women may start using the vaginal contraceptive ring in the first 5 days following a complete first-trimester abortion; a back-up method of contraception is not needed in these women. If the contraceptive preparation is not used within the mentioned 5 days, the woman should follow the general instructions for women who did not use hormonal contraception in the preceding month.

If a nonlactating woman chooses to initiate contraception postpartum with the contraceptive vaginal ring (NuvaRing®) before menstruation has started, the possibility that ovulation and conception may have occurred prior to initiation of contraceptive therapy should be considered, and back-up contraception must be employed for the first 7 days.

Transdermal Dosage

When the transdermal system containing ethinyl estradiol and norelgestromin (Ortho Evra®) is used for contraception, it is applied topically in a cyclic regimen using a 28-day cycle. One transdermal system (containing ethinyl estradiol 0.75 mg and norelgestromin 6 mg) is applied once weekly (same day each week) for 3 weeks, followed by a 1-week drug-free interval (drug-free interval should *not* exceed 7 days); then the regimen is repeated. Systemic exposure to estrogen is greater with the transdermal system (Ortho Evra®) than with oral contraceptive preparations because of differences in the pharmacokinetic profiles of the preparations. (See Pharmacokinetics: Absorption and see the introductory discussion under Cautions.)

Administration of the transdermal contraceptive system usually begins on the first day of the menstrual cycle or on the first Sunday after menstrual bleeding has started. A back-up method of contraception (condom, spermicide, diaphragm) should be employed for the first 7 days after application of the first system if therapy is started after day 1 of the menstrual cycle. A back-up method of contraception is not needed if the first system is applied on the first day of the menstrual cycle. The manufacturer states that women switching from estrogen-progestin oral contraceptives to the estrogen-progestin transdermal system should apply the transdermal system on the first day of withdrawal bleeding. If there is no withdrawal bleeding within 5 days of the last hormonally active tablet, pregnancy must be ruled out. If therapy with the transdermal system is initiated after the first day of bleeding, a back-up method of contraception should be used for 7 days. If more than 7 days elapse after receiving the last hormonally active tablet, the possibility of ovulation and conception should be considered.

When a woman has not adhered to the prescribed transdermal contraceptive regimen by not applying the estrogen and progestin-containing system at the initiation of any cycle (i.e., day 1/first week), the system should be applied as soon as it is remembered and a new dosage cycle started the same day; back-up contraception must be employed for the first 7 days of the new cycle. In addition, if the transdermal system has not been changed in the middle of the cycle (i.e., on day 8/week 2 or day 15/week 3) for 1–2 days (up to 48 hours), a new system should be applied as soon as it is remembered and the application schedule employed should be continued; back-up contraception is not needed. However, if the transdermal system has not been changed for more than 2 days (48 hours or more) in the middle of the cycle, a new dosage cycle should be started; back-up contraception must be employed for the first 7 days of the new cycle. When the transdermal system is not removed at the end of the application schedule (i.e., on day 22/week 4), the system should be removed as soon as it is remembered and the application schedule employed should be continued (i.e., system applied on day 28); back-up contraception is not needed.

Women may start using the transdermal contraceptive system immediately after a first-trimester abortion; a back-up method of contraception is not needed. If the contraceptive preparation is not used within 5 days of a first-trimester abortion, the woman should follow instructions as if initiating transdermal contraception for the first time.

Postcoital Contraception
Oral Dosage

Several regimens employing short-course, high-dose oral combinations of ethinyl estradiol and norgestrel or levonorgestrel have been used safely and effectively for postcoital contraception†. One widely studied and used regimen (the "Yuzpe" regimen) consists of an oral dose of 100 mcg of ethinyl estradiol and 1 mg of norgestrel (administered as 2 tablets each containing 50 mcg and 0.5 mg of the drugs, respectively) within 72 hours after unprotected intercourse, initiating the first dose at a time when it would make convenient administering the subsequent repeat dose 12 hours later. Alternative combination regimens that have been used consist of a dose of 120 mcg of ethinyl estradiol and 1.2 mg of norgestrel or 0.5–0.6 mg of levonorgestrel (e.g., administered as 4 tablets each containing 30 mcg of ethinyl estradiol and 0.3 mg of norgestrel or 0.125–0.15 mg of levonorgestrel) within 72 hours after intercourse, repeating the dose 12 hours later. Another combination regimen that has been used consists of a dose of 100 mcg of ethinyl estradiol and 0.5 mg of levonorgestrel (e.g., administered as 5 tablets each containing 20 mcg of ethinyl estradiol and 0.1 mg of levonorgestrel) within 72 hours after intercourse, repeating the dose 12 hours later. Because postcoital efficacy diminishes as the time between intercourse and initiation of estrogen-progestin combination therapy increases, such therapy should be initiated *as soon as possible but preferably within 72 hours* following unprotected intercourse. If necessary, the first dose can be given up to 120 hours after unprotected intercourse. Women should be advised that taking more than the prescribed dose probably will not further decrease the risk of pregnancy, but will increase the risk of severe adverse GI effects.

If women are given a conventional mnemonic package of an oral estrogen-progestin combination for use in taking a postcoital contraceptive regimen, they should be instructed carefully regarding the number and color of the tablets to be taken with each dose and that only a portion of the contents of the package actually will be used.

TABLE 1. Dosage of estrogen-progestin combinations for postcoital contraception

Estrogen-progestin combination formulation [brand name]	Number and color of tablets per dose [a]
Ethinyl estradiol (50 mcg) with norgestrel (0.5 mg) [Ovral®]	2 white tablets (any of 21 tablets)
Ethinyl estradiol (50 mcg) with norgestrel (0.5 mg) [Ovral®-28]	2 white tablets (any of *first* 21 tablets)
Ethinyl estradiol (30 mcg) with norgestrel (0.3 mg) [Lo-Ovral®]	4 white tablets (any of 21 tablets)
Ethinyl estradiol (30 mcg) with norgestrel (0.3 mg) [Lo-Ovral®-28]	4 white tablets (any of *first* 21 tablets)
Ethinyl estradiol (30 mcg) with levonorgestrel (0.15 mg) [Nordette®]	4 light-orange tablets (any of 21 tablets)
Ethinyl estradiol (30 mcg) with levonorgestrel (0.15 mg) [Nordette®-28]	4 light-orange tablets (any of *first* 21 tablets)
Ethinyl estradiol (30 mcg) with levonorgestrel (0.15 mg) [Levlen® 21]	4 light-orange tablets (any of 21 tablets)
Ethinyl estradiol (30 mcg) with levonorgestrel (0.15 mg) [Levlen® 28]	4 light-orange tablets (any of *first* 21 tablets)
Ethinyl estradiol (30 mcg) with levonorgestrel (0.125 mg) [Tri-Levlen® 21]	4 yellow tablets (any of *last* 10 tablets)
Ethinyl estradiol (30 mcg) with levonorgestrel (0.125 mg) [Tri-Levlen® 28]	4 yellow tablets (any of tablets 12–21)
Ethinyl estradiol (30 mcg) with levonorgestrel (0.125 mg) [Tri-Phasil® 21]	4 yellow tablets (any of *last* 10 tablets)
Ethinyl estradiol (30 mcg) with levonorgestrel (0.125 mg) [Tri-Levlen® 28]	4 yellow tablets (any of tablets 12–21)
Ethinyl estradiol (20 mcg) with levonorgestrel (0.1 mg) [Lessina® 28]	5 pink tablets (any of *first* 21 tablets)

[a] Dose is administered initially and then repeated 12 hours later

Contraception and Folate Supplementation
Oral Dosage

For increasing folate concentrations in women using oral contraceptives, the combination of ethinyl estradiol 20 mcg in fixed combination with drospirenone 3 mg and levomefolate calcium 0.451 mg (Beyaz®) or ethinyl estradiol 30 mcg in fixed combination with drospirenone 3 mg and levomefolate calcium 0.451 mg (Safyral®) is used in the same dosage and administration (i.e., timing of initiation of therapy) as used in contraception.

Acne Vulgaris
Oral Dosage

For the treatment of acne vulgaris, the triphasic oral estrogen-progestin combination of ethinyl estradiol 35 mcg in fixed combination with norgestimate 0.18, 0.215, or 0.25 mg (Ortho-Tri-Cyclen®) or norethindrone 1 mg in fixed combination with ethinyl estradiol 20, 30, or 35 mcg (Estrostep®) is used in the same dosage and administration (i.e., timing of initiation of therapy) as used in contraception.

For the treatment of acne vulgaris, the estrogen-progestin combination of ethinyl estradiol 20 mcg in fixed combination with drospirenone 3 mg (Yaz®) or ethinyl estradiol 20 mcg in fixed combination with drospirenone 3 mg and levomefolate calcium 0.451 mg (Beyaz®) is used in the same dosage and administration (i.e., timing of initiation of therapy) as used in contraception.

Premenstrual Dysphoric Disorder
Oral Dosage

For the treatment of premenstrual dysphoric disorder, the combination of ethinyl estradiol 20 mcg in fixed combination with drospirenone 3 mg (Yaz®) or ethinyl estradiol 20 mcg in fixed combination with drospirenone 3 mg and levomefolate calcium 0.451 mg (Beyaz®) is used in the same dosage and administration (i.e., timing of initiation of therapy) as used in contraception. (See Conventional-cycle Oral Contraceptives under Dosage: Contraception, in Dosage and Administration.)

CAUTIONS

The potential risks of estrogen-progestin contraceptive use have been established in women of reproductive age. The risks should be identical for postpubertal adolescents under 16 years of age and users 16 years of age or older. Estrogen-progestin combination contraceptives including short-term, high-dose postcoital contraceptives are not indicated before menarche.

Exposure to ethinyl estradiol and norelgestromin is higher in women receiving the Ortho-Evra® transdermal system than in women receiving an oral contraceptive preparation containing ethinyl estradiol 35 mcg and norgestimate 0.25 mg per tablet. Increased exposure to estrogen may increase the risk for adverse effects.

Exposure to ethinyl estradiol and levonorgestrel is higher in women receiving Lybrel® (a fixed-combination continuous-regimen oral contraceptive) than in women receiving a conventional-cycle oral contraceptive containing the same ethinyl estradiol dose and a similar dose of the progestin component; use of Lybrel® results in 13 additional weeks of hormone intake per year.

Epidemiologic data are not available to determine whether safety and efficacy associated with the vaginal route of administration of estrogen-progestin contraceptives differ from the oral route. Adverse effects similar to those with oral estrogen-progestin contraceptives generally are expected with vaginal estrogen-progestin contraceptives.

Information on the potential risks of estrogen-progestin contraceptive use (and associated cautions, precautions, and contraindications) is based principally on studies and experience with preparations that contained higher estrogen and/or progestin doses than those in currently available preparations. The relative risks associated with use of currently available lower-dose preparations remains to be determined. For example, while previous experience indicated that the risk of adverse cardiovascular effects associated with oral contraceptives was increased in *nonsmoking* women older than 40 years of age, this risk may have resulted in part from the high estrogen content of previously available preparations. It currently is not known whether such increased cardiovascular risk also is associated with use of currently available, low-dose preparations, but some experts consider the possible benefits of low-dose (containing no more than 35 mcg of estrogen) oral contraceptives to outweigh the potential risks of pregnancy in healthy *nonsmoking* women older than 40 years of age who have no other risk factors. The risk of serious morbidity or mortality is very small in healthy women without underlying risk factors. The risk of morbidity and mortality increases significantly in the presence of other risk factors (e.g., hypertension, hyperlipidemias, obesity, diabetes).

Common adverse effects of oral estrogen-progestin contraceptives appear to be mainly caused by the estrogen, are usually most pronounced during the first oral contraceptive cycle, and disappear or diminish after 3 or 4 cycles; there does not appear to be any advantage in changing preparations during this period of time. If minor adverse effects persist after the fourth cycle, a different combination of drugs or a different dosage may be tried. Although conventional-dosage preparations (containing 35 mcg or more of ethinyl estradiol or 50 mcg or more of mestranol) are generally associated with slightly lower pregnancy rates than reduced-dosage preparations, conventional-dosage preparations are generally more frequently associated with adverse effects (e.g., edema, nausea and vomiting, thromboembolic disorders) than reduced-dosage preparations; however, reduced-dosage preparations are more frequently associated with bleeding irregularities, including breakthrough bleeding, spotting, and menstrual irregularities, than conventional-dosage preparations. Because of the increased risk of thromboembolic disorders associated with conventional-dosage preparations, reduced-dosage preparations are recommended for initial use in patients who have not previously received oral contraceptives. Although numerous adverse effects have been reported in women receiving oral contraceptives, many of the reported effects are conditions that could occur spontaneously in women of childbearing age and a causal relationship has, in many instances, been difficult to establish.

It is not known if oral contraceptive combinations containing desogestrel or norgestimate cause fewer androgenic effects (e.g., acne, hirsutism, weight gain) than estrogen-progestin combinations containing conventional progestins (e.g., levonorgestrel, norethindrone). There is some evidence that oral contraceptives containing desogestrel may be associated with an increased risk of nonfatal venous thrombosis. (See Thromboembolic Disorders in Cautions: Cardiovascular Effects.)

Limited data are available concerning the risk of using short-course, high-dose estrogen-progestin combinations for emergency contraception. No serious or long-term complications have been associated with such postcoital regimens in Europe, where experience is extensive. In addition, some evidence indicates that emergency postcoital contraception may not compromise conventional

contraception use or sexual behavior (e.g., promiscuity, sexually transmitted disease [STD] risk).

● *GI Effects*

The most frequent adverse effect of oral contraceptives is nausea. In addition, nausea has been reported in women using vaginal or transdermal estrogen-progestin contraceptives.

The principal risk associated with currently recommended high-dose, postcoital estrogen-progestin combination regimens appears to be moderate to severe adverse GI effects including severe vomiting and nausea, which occur in 12–22 and 30–66%, respectively, of women receiving the short-course regimens and may limit compliance with, and effectiveness of, the regimens. In 2 prospective, randomized studies, nausea and vomiting were less common with a high-dose postcoital progestin-only regimen (0.75 mg levonorgestrel every 12 hours for 2 doses) than with a high-dose estrogen-progestin regimen (100 mcg ethinyl estradiol and 0.5 mg levonorgestrel every 12 hours for 2 doses).

Other adverse GI effects include vomiting, abdominal cramps, abdominal pain, bloating, diarrhea, constipation, and inflammatory bowel disease. Gingivitis and dry socket also have been reported. Changes in appetite and changes in weight also may occur.

● *Dermatologic Effects*

The most frequent dermatologic reaction to oral contraceptives is chloasma or melasma. Women who have had melasma during pregnancy appear to be most susceptible. Irregular brown macules may develop slowly on the face within 1 month to 2 years following initiation of oral contraceptive therapy. The macules fade more slowly than in melasma gravidarum and may be permanent.

Acne may improve during oral contraceptive therapy because of decreased sebum production and depression of sebaceous gland activity; however, it may increase in severity during initial therapy and may develop in some women who have not previously had acne.

Other dermatologic reactions include allergic rash, urticaria, erythema multiforme, erythema nodosum, hemorrhagic eruption, pruritus, and angioedema. Hirsutism and alopecia also have occurred. Herpes gestationis and porphyria cutanea have reportedly been adversely affected in women receiving oral contraceptives.

Application site reaction has occurred in women using the transdermal contraceptive system containing ethinyl estradiol and norelgestromin. The manufacturer states that if such skin irritation occurs, the transdermal system may be removed and a new patch applied to a different location until the next new application day.

● *Cardiovascular Effects*

A positive association between the amount of estrogen and progestin in oral contraceptives and the risk of adverse cardiovascular effects has been observed. Adverse effects similar to those with oral combination estrogen-progestin contraceptives generally are expected with vaginal or transdermal estrogen-progestin contraceptives.

Elevated Blood Pressure

Increases in blood pressure may occur in women receiving estrogen-progestin contraceptives. Blood pressure elevations are usually minor, but clinically important hypertension may occur in some women. Some women develop hypertension within 1–3 weeks after initiation of oral contraceptive therapy and become normotensive during the part of the oral contraceptive cycle when they do not receive the drugs. In others, blood pressure increases slowly and may not reach abnormal levels for several months. Elevated blood pressure may gradually decrease or persist after the oral contraceptive is discontinued.

The risk of hypertension increases with increasing duration of oral contraceptive use and is about 2.5–3 times greater in the fifth year of continual use than in the first year. Age also is positively correlated with the risk of hypertension in oral contraceptive users, becoming substantial in women about 35 years of age and older. Women with a history of hypertension, preexisting renal disease, a history of toxemia or elevated blood pressure during pregnancy, a familial tendency toward hypertension or its consequences, or a history of excessive weight gain or fluid retention during the menstrual cycle may be at increased risk of developing elevated blood pressure during estrogen-progestin contraceptive therapy and, therefore, should be monitored closely. Even though elevated blood pressure may remain within the normal range, the clinical implications of elevations should be considered in all patients. All women, but particularly those with other risk factors for cardiovascular disease or stroke, should have blood pressure measurements before an oral contraceptive is prescribed and at regular intervals during therapy.

Thromboembolic Disorders

Oral contraceptive use is associated with an increased risk of thromboembolic and thrombotic disorders. One study has shown an increased relative risk of fatal venous thromboembolism (VTE) and several other studies have shown an increased relative risk of nonfatal VTE in oral contraceptive users. Case-controlled studies estimated that the relative risk for developing fatal or nonfatal thromboembolism (ranging in severity from superficial thrombosis to pulmonary embolism) was 3–11 times greater in oral contraceptive users than in nonusers and 1.5–6 times greater in women predisposed to venous thromboembolic disorders. However, cohort studies suggest that the overall relative risk is somewhat lower, ranging from 3 times greater for new cases to 4.5 times greater for new cases requiring hospitalization in oral contraceptive users when compared with nonusers. A prospective review failed to show increased mortality rates from cardiovascular disorders in oral contraceptive users; however, when a selected subset of this study was analyzed in a retrospective, case-controlled fashion, an increased risk of VTE was associated with oral contraceptive use. Hereditary coagulation disorders, such as factor V Leiden mutation, increase the risk of thromboembolic disease. The risk of thromboembolic disease from oral contraceptive use is not related to the duration of use and disappears when oral contraceptive use is discontinued.

The pharmacokinetic profile for the transdermal contraceptive system containing ethinyl estradiol and norelgestromin (Ortho Evra®) differs from the profile for oral contraceptive preparations. Overall exposure to ethinyl estradiol and norelgestromin is higher in women receiving Ortho Evra® than in women receiving an oral contraceptive preparation containing ethinyl estradiol 35 mcg and norgestimate 0.25 mg per tablet. (See Pharmacokinetics: Absorption.) Increased exposure to estrogen may increase the risk of certain adverse effects (e.g., VTE). The risk of VTE in women using Ortho Evra® relative to the risk in women using an oral contraceptive containing norgestimate or levonorgestrel and ethinyl estradiol 30–35 mcg has been investigated in several epidemiologic, case-controlled studies. In one study that used data from health care claims, current use of Ortho Evra® was not associated with an increased risk of nonfatal VTE compared with use of an oral contraceptive (odds ratio [OR] 0.9; 95% confidence interval: 0.5–1.6). In a subsequent analysis that included an additional 17 months of data from this study, current use of Ortho Evra® was not associated with an increased risk of nonfatal VTE compared with use of an oral contraceptive (OR 1.1; 95% confidence interval: 0.6–2.1). In another study that used claims data and chart review, current use of Ortho Evra® was associated with an increased risk of VTE compared with use of an oral contraceptive (OR 2.4; 95% confidence interval: 1.1–5.5). Findings from another study that used claims data indicated current use of Ortho Evra® might be associated with an increased risk of idiopathic VTE compared with use of an oral contraceptive (OR 2; 95% confidence interval: 0.9–4.1).

Because the fixed-combination continuous-regimen oral contraceptive (Lybrel®) is administered daily (not cyclically), overall exposure to estrogen and progestin is higher in women receiving this preparation than in women receiving a conventional-cycle oral contraceptive containing the same dose of ethinyl estradiol and a similar dose of the progestin component.

A review conducted by the US Food and Drug Administration (FDA) indicates that the use of oral contraceptive combinations that contain the progestins desogestrel (Desogen®, Ortho-Cept®) or gestodene (not commercially available in the US) may be associated with an increased risk of nonfatal venous thrombosis compared with oral contraceptives containing conventional progestins (e.g., levonorgestrel, norethindrone). This conclusion was based on interim results of 3 unpublished comparative studies (i.e., by the World Health Organization [WHO], by the Boston Drug Surveillance Program, by the European Transnational study coordinated by McGill University of Canada). Interim results of these unpublished studies indicate that, while the overall risk of nonfatal venous thrombosis is lower than that reported in previous studies, estrogen-progestin combinations containing desogestrel or gestodene appear to be associated with a twofold increased risk of venous thrombosis compared with oral contraceptives containing conventional progestins. Some experts have recommended that estrogen-progestin combinations containing desogestrel or gestodene not be prescribed routinely for prevention of conception in women; however, other clinicians state that further analysis of data is needed for such a recommendation. Although the FDA does not recommend that women currently using oral contraceptives containing desogestrel discontinue such use or switch to another estrogen-progestin combination contraceptive, the FDA states that women using an oral contraceptive containing desogestrel should be advised

to discuss such use with their clinician, taking into consideration the relative risks and benefits associated with these oral contraceptives. It should be considered that the contraceptive vaginal ring (NuvaRing®) contains etonogestrel, the active metabolite of desogestrel; however, it is not known whether NuvaRing® is associated with an increased risk of venous thrombosis.

Another safety review conducted by the FDA indicates that use of combination oral contraceptives containing the progestin drospirenone may be associated with an increased risk of VTE compared with that of oral contraceptives containing levonorgestrel or other progestins. This conclusion was based on results of several epidemiologic studies (i.e., the US postapproval safety study by Ingenix, the European Active Surveillance Study [EURAS], the Long-Term Active Surveillance Study [LASS], 2 Danish cohort studies, the Dutch multiple environmental and genetic assessment of risk factors for venous thrombosis [MEGA] study, the UK General Practice Research Database [GPRD] study, the PharMetrics study, and the FDA-supported study) evaluating the risk of VTE in women using oral contraceptives containing drospirenone. These studies reported that the risk of VTE in such women ranged from no increase to a threefold increase in risk. The FDA's safety review was prompted by results of 2 recent case-control studies that showed a twofold to threefold increased risk of VTE (including deep-vein thrombosis and pulmonary embolism) in patients receiving oral contraceptives containing drospirenone compared with those receiving oral contraceptives containing the progestin levonorgestrel. These 2 studies evaluated cases of idiopathic VTE occurring in women 15–44 years of age who were current users of oral contraceptives containing 30 mcg of estrogen with either drospirenone or levonorgestrel; women with risk factors for VTE were excluded from the studies. The FDA has also reviewed data from a large US retrospective cohort study in more than 800,000 women evaluating thrombotic and thromboembolic risks (including VTE) associated with hormonal contraceptives. Final results from this study suggest an increased risk of VTE (hazard ratio greater than 1) in women using oral contraceptives containing drospirenone compared with women using other hormonal contraceptives. (See Cautions: Precautions and Contraindications.)

Given the conflicting results of the previous epidemiologic studies and the recent findings, the FDA held a joint meeting of the Reproductive Health Drugs Advisory Committee and the Drug Safety and Risk Management Advisory Committee on December 8, 2011, to review the risks and benefits of such therapy and specifically discuss the risk of VTE associated with drospirenone-containing hormonal contraceptives. The studies reviewed by the FDA did not provide consistent data for the comparative risk of thromboembolic events between oral contraceptives that contain drospirenone and those that do not. In addition, the studies did not account for important known and unknown patient characteristics that may influence prescribing patterns and may affect risk of VTE. For these reasons, the FDA states that it is unclear whether the increased risk of thromboembolic events observed in these epidemiologic studies actually resulted from use of drospirenone-containing oral contraceptives. At this time, the FDA has concluded that the risk of VTE may be higher for such oral contraceptives. The FDA will continue to communicate any new safety information as it becomes available.

An increased risk of cerebrovascular disorders, including thrombotic and hemorrhagic stroke, also is associated with oral contraceptive use, although the risk generally is greatest in older (i.e., older than 35 years of age), hypertensive women who also smoke. The use of estrogen-progestin contraceptives also is associated with an increased risk of stroke in women with other underlying risk factors. Hypertension is a risk factor in both users and nonusers of oral contraceptives for both thrombotic and hemorrhagic stroke, while smoking appears to increase the risk for hemorrhagic stroke. Although cigarette smoking alone has been associated with an increased risk of cerebrovascular disorders, concomitant cigarette smoking and oral contraceptive use is associated with a greater risk of these disorders than either alone. The relative risk of thrombotic stroke has been shown to range from 3 for normotensive users of oral contraceptives to 14 for users with hypertension. The relative risk of hemorrhagic stroke is reported to be 1.2 in nonsmoking women who use oral contraceptives, 2.6 in nonusers who do not smoke, 7.6 in users who smoke, 1.8 in normotensive users, and 25.7 in users with severe hypertension. The risk also appears to be greater in older women.

An increased relative risk of myocardial infarction has been associated with oral contraceptive use. In one study, oral contraceptive use was one of several risk factors for coronary artery disease which included cigarette smoking, hypertension, hypercholesterolemia, obesity, diabetes, and preeclamptic toxemia; the risk of myocardial infarction increased as the number of risk factors for coronary artery disease increased. The relative risk of developing fatal myocardial infarction has been estimated as twice as great in oral contraceptive users who do not smoke compared with nonusers who do not smoke, as 5 times greater in oral contraceptive users who smoke compared with users who do not smoke, and about 10–12 times greater in users who smoke compared with nonusers who do not smoke; women who smoke 15 or more cigarettes daily are especially at risk. However, other data suggest that the likelihood of myocardial infarction is not increased in young women who use oral contraceptives and do not smoke or have hypertension or diabetes.

A positive association between thromboembolic disorders and estrogen dosage of oral contraceptives also exists. The progestin content of oral contraceptives also appears to contribute to the risk of thromboembolic disorders. Use of oral contraceptive combinations that contain the progestins desogestrel or gestodene (not commercially available in the US) may be associated with an increased risk of nonfatal venous thrombosis compared with use of oral contraceptives containing conventional progestins (e.g., levonorgestrel, norethindrone). However, desogestrel has minimal androgenic activity and there is some evidence that the risk of myocardial infarction associated with oral contraceptives is lower when the progestin has minimal androgenic activity than when the activity is greater. A relationship between the estrogen and/or progestin dosage of oral contraceptives and the risk of myocardial infarction has not been established. However, a decrease in serum high-density lipoprotein (HDL) concentration has been reported with increasing progestational activity of oral contraceptives and decreased HDL has been associated with an increased risk of ischemic heart disease. (See Effects on Lipids and Lipoproteins, in Cautions: Endocrine and Metabolic Effects.)

The clinician and the woman using estrogen-progestin contraceptives should be alert to the earliest signs and symptoms of thromboembolic and thrombotic disorders (e.g., thrombophlebitis, pulmonary embolism, cerebrovascular insufficiency, coronary occlusion, retinal thrombosis, mesenteric thrombosis). Estrogen-progestin contraceptives should be discontinued immediately when any of these disorders occurs or is suspected. A two- to four-fold increased risk of postsurgery thromboembolic complications has been reported in oral contraceptive users; the risk in women predisposed to venous thromboembolic disorders is twice that in women who have no such predisposition. (See Cautions: Precautions and Contraindications.)

Other Cardiovascular Effects

Oral contraceptives may cause some degree of fluid retention and edema. Oral contraceptives should be used with caution in patients with conditions that might be aggravated by fluid retention. (See Cautions: Precautions and Contraindications.) Premature ventricular and supraventricular complexes and other ECG abnormalities have been reported in women receiving oral contraceptives; however, a causal relationship has not been established.

● *Endocrine and Metabolic Effects*

Endocrine function test results may be altered in patients receiving oral contraceptives. If results of endocrine function tests are abnormal, the tests should be repeated 2 months after the drug has been discontinued.

Effects on Glucose

Decreased glucose tolerance has been observed in a significant percentage of patients receiving oral contraceptives. Fasting blood glucose concentrations are not altered in most patients; however, increased plasma insulin and blood pyruvate concentrations may occur. Although decreased glucose tolerance appears to be directly related to the estrogen of oral contraceptives, estrogen alone does not appear to decrease glucose tolerance and therefore this effect appears to involve both estrogenic and progestinic components. Progestins increase insulin secretion and insulin resistance, and these effects vary among different progestin agents. Prediabetic and diabetic patients should be carefully monitored during estrogen-progestin contraceptive therapy.

Effects on Lipids and Lipoproteins

Increased concentrations of plasma triglyceride, low-density lipoproteins, and total phospholipids may occur during therapy with estrogen-progestin contraceptives. The clinical importance of these alterations in lipid and lipoprotein concentrations has not been established; however, it may be advisable to avoid use of oral contraceptives in women with elevated serum lipids. Generally, the progestin component of oral contraceptives has been shown to decrease high-density lipoprotein cholesterol (HDL-cholesterol), whereas the estrogen component has been shown to increase it; however, some newer progestins (e.g., desogestrel, norgestimate) also may increase HDL-cholesterol. Therefore, it has been suggested that the net effect of estrogen-progestin contraceptives on high-density lipoprotein cholesterol depends on the specific formulation.

Effects on Thyroid

The estrogenic component of estrogen-progestin contraceptives may produce elevations in thyroxine-binding globulin (TBG) resulting in elevated total circulating thyroid hormone, as measured by protein-bound iodine (PBI), thyroxine (T_4) (by column and radioimmunoassay), and butanol extractable iodine. Decreased triiodothyronine (T_3) resin uptake, reflecting elevated TBG, also occurs, while free T_4 concentrations are unaltered. Basal metabolic rate, cholesterol concentrations, iodine-131 uptake, and the free thyroxine index remain unchanged, suggesting that thyroid function is not affected. Abnormal thyroid function test results usually return to pretreatment levels within 2–4 months after estrogen therapy is discontinued.

Other Endocrine and Metabolic Effects

Estrogen-progestin contraceptives also affect other serum proteins. Serum albumin may be increased or decreased and variable effects on immunoglobulins have been reported. Serum cholinesterase, haptoglobulins, and orosomucoid decrease; transferrin, plasminogen, α_2-macroglobulin, and testosterone- and estradiol-binding globulins are increased. Estrogen-progestin contraceptive therapy causes decreased pregnanediol excretion. Ceruloplasmin elevations may give plasma a green color. Cryofibrinogenemia has also been reported. The renin substrate (angiotensinogen) concentration is increased and the aldosterone excretion rate is moderately elevated. Some patients may have hyporesponsive plasma renin activity with normal aldosterone excretion for a few weeks after oral contraceptives are discontinued. Estrogen-progestin contraceptives may cause increased serum magnesium, copper, zinc, and iron concentrations as well as total iron-binding capacity; however, the clinical importance of these increased mineral concentrations has not been determined.

Oral contraceptives may also decrease the response to the metyrapone test. (See Laboratory Test Interferences.)

Because drospirenone has antimineralocorticoid activity, the potential exists for hyperkalemia to occur in high-risk patients (e.g., those with renal or hepatic impairment, adrenal insufficiency) receiving oral contraceptives containing this progestin.

● *Hepatic Effects*

Liver function test results may be altered in patients receiving oral contraceptives and if results of these tests are abnormal, they should be repeated 2 months after the drugs have been discontinued. Increased sulfobromophthalein retention occurs frequently, as a result of interference with the transfer of dye conjugates from liver cells into bile; uptake, conjugation, and storage do not appear to be affected. Less frequently, increased serum aminotransferase and alkaline phosphatase concentrations may occur. Liver function test results usually return to normal within several weeks after oral contraceptives are discontinued; occasionally, however, abnormal test results may persist for longer periods.

Cholestatic jaundice has been reported during oral contraceptive use. Cholestasis is manifested by the development of malaise, anorexia, and pruritus about 2 weeks to 2 months after the start of therapy. Occasionally, arthralgia, fever, and rash may occur. Serum bilirubin concentration may range from 3–10 mg/dL and is mostly conjugated. Women with a history of jaundice during pregnancy have an increased risk of jaundice recurrence while receiving oral contraceptives. If jaundice occurs during oral contraceptive therapy, the drugs should be discontinued. Oral contraceptives may precipitate hepatic forms of porphyria and these drugs probably should not be used by women who have a familial history of hepatic porphyrias, since the occurrence of these conditions appears to be genetically determined. Budd-Chiari syndrome has also occurred in oral contraceptive users. Many patients who develop oral contraceptive- or pregnancy-associated Budd-Chiari syndrome also may have inherited or acquired thrombophilia. Steroid hormones (including oral contraceptives) may be poorly metabolized in patients with hepatic dysfunction; therefore, the drugs should be administered with caution to these individuals.

Liver tumors have been associated with oral contraceptive use. Liver tumors have been benign or malignant and have occurred during short-term and long-term use of oral contraceptives. Most commonly, liver tumors are benign hepatocellular adenomas. Long-term oral contraceptive users have an estimated annual incidence of hepatocellular adenoma of 3–4 per 100,000; risk appears to increase after 4 or more years of use. In several women who developed benign hepatocellular adenomas during oral contraceptive use, these tumors regressed following discontinuance of the drugs. Although benign hepatocellular adenomas are apparently uncommon findings in oral contraceptive users, they may result in death because of their vascularity which predisposes them to rupture and massive hemorrhage. Therefore, the presence of a liver tumor should be considered in women who develop sudden severe abdominal pain or shock. Patients with liver tumors have shown variable clinical features which may make preoperative diagnosis difficult; some of these patients have had right upper quadrant masses, while most have had signs and symptoms of acute intraperitoneal hemorrhage. Routine radiologic and laboratory test evaluations may not be helpful. Liver scans may show a focal defect, and hepatic arteriography may be useful in diagnosing primary liver neoplasm. Hepatocellular carcinoma has also been reported rarely in women receiving oral contraceptives, although a causal relationship to the drugs has not been clearly established. For women using oral contraceptives for 8 or more years, several epidemiologic studies have suggested a relative risk that is up to 7–20 times that of nonusers, although the occurrence of this tumor is rare. It also has not been clearly established whether hepatic adenoma induced by oral contraceptives can differentiate into hepatic carcinoma.

● Genitourinary Effects

Breakthrough bleeding and/or spotting (especially within the first 3 months of use), changes in menstrual flow, missed menses (during use), or amenorrhea (after use) may occur in women receiving hormonal contraceptives. Bleeding irregularities are more frequently associated with reduced-dosage preparations than with conventional-dosage preparations. Breakthrough bleeding that occurs early in the cycle generally is caused by a lack of adequate estrogenic stimulation, whereas bleeding after midcycle generally indicates progestin deficiency. Changes in the estrogen and/or progestin dose, ratio, and/or sequence may control or alleviate breakthrough bleeding. In women who develop breakthrough bleeding while receiving a biphasic oral contraceptive, switching to a triphasic oral contraceptive may control or alleviate bleeding since the progestin dose is increased after day 7 with the triphasic regimen. Once the possibility of pregnancy has been ruled out in women with missed menses (absence of withdrawal bleeding) (see Pregnancy, in Cautions: Pregnancy, Fertility, and Lactation), switching to a preparation with higher estrogenic activity or dose or to a triphasic preparation (since it allows endometrial proliferation during the initial 7-day, low-dose progestin period) may be beneficial. However, the risks (e.g., adverse cardiovascular effects) associated with increased estrogen and progestin doses must be considered, and increasing the dose to minimize bleeding irregularities should only be done if necessary.

While use of an extended-cycle oral contraceptive (e.g., LoSeasonique®, Seasonale®, Seasonique®) results in fewer planned menses (4 per year) than conventional-cycle oral contraceptives (13 per year), bleeding irregularities occur more frequently in women using the extended-cycle preparation than in women using the conventional-cycle preparation. Irregular bleeding occurs most often during the first few 91-day cycles. In one study in women who had used oral contraceptives, administration of Seasonale® resulted in 7 or more and 20 or more days of intramenstrual bleeding and/or spotting in 65 and 35% of women, respectively, during cycle 1 and in 42 and 15% of women, respectively, during cycle 4. In another study, administration of Seasonique® resulted in 7 or more and 20 or more days of intramenstrual bleeding and/or spotting in 64 and 29% of women, respectively, during cycle 1 and in 39 and 11% of women, respectively, during cycle 4. In women receiving a conventional-cycle oral contraceptive, intramenstrual bleeding and/or spotting for 7 or more and 20 or more days occurred in 38 and 6% of women, respectively, during cycles 1–4 and in 39 and 4% of women, respectively, during cycles 10–13.

Use of extended-cycle oral contraceptive preparations is associated with fewer menstrual symptoms than use of conventional-cycle oral contraceptive preparations. Whether adding 10 mcg of estradiol to the final 7 tablets in the cycle (LoSeasonique®, Seasonique®) will further reduce withdrawal symptoms (e.g., migraine headache) remains to be determined.

While use of a continuous-regimen (noncyclic) estrogen-progestin oral contraceptive (Lybrel®) eliminates withdrawal bleeding, irregular bleeding and/or spotting occurs in some women. In one study, administration of Lybrel® resulted in 4 or more and 7 or more days of bleeding and/or spotting in 67 and 54% of women, respectively, during the second 28-day dosing period and in 31 and 20% of women, respectively, during the thirteenth 28-day dosing period.

Adequate diagnostic procedures should be performed in patients with undiagnosed persistent or recurrent vaginal bleeding. When pathology has been excluded, time or change to another preparation may resolve the problem. Women with a history of oligomenorrhea or secondary amenorrhea or young women with irregular cycles may tend to remain anovulatory or to become amenorrheic after discontinuance of oral contraceptives; women with these preexisting problems should be advised of this possibility and encouraged to use other contraceptive methods.

Dysmenorrhea also may occur. Post-use anovulation, occasionally accompanied by galactorrhea, and a premenstrual-like syndrome has been reported. Post-use anovulation may be prolonged and may occur in women who had no previous irregularities. Galactorrhea and pituitary tumors (e.g., adenomas) have been associated with amenorrhea in former oral contraceptive users. One study showed a 16-fold increased prevalence of prolactin-secreting pituitary tumors (prolactinomas) among former users of oral contraceptives who had amenorrhea with galactorrhea compared with those without galactorrhea. In another study, the relative risk of prolactinoma was 1.3 when oral contraceptives were used for contraception and 7.7 when the drugs were used for menstrual regulation. In patients with breakthrough bleeding or irregular vaginal bleeding, nonfunctional causes should be considered.

Changes in cervical erosion and secretions and endocervical hyperplasia may occur during oral contraceptive therapy. In addition, preexisting uterine leiomyoma may increase in size in women receiving oral contraceptives. Vaginitis, impaired renal function, and backache and a cystitis-like syndrome have been reported but have not been definitely attributed to the drugs.

An increased incidence of *Candida* vaginitis has been associated with oral contraceptive therapy. Decreased motility and tonus of the upper urinary tract may occur in some patients leading to overdistention of the ureters, thus promoting bacteriuria and its complications and making treatment of the infection more difficult. Because oral contraceptives change the vaginal pH from acidic to alkaline, it has been suggested that there may be an increased risk of gonorrhea infection upon exposure; however, there is some evidence that progestins may inhibit growth of *Neisseria gonorrhoeae* in vitro and that oral contraceptives may have some protective effect against gonococcal pelvic inflammatory disease (PID). Although some clinicians have suggested that the risk of PID may be decreased in oral contraceptive users, there is some evidence that the frequency of cervical chlamydial infections may be increased several-fold in women receiving oral contraceptives compared with nonusers or women using barrier contraceptives, possibly secondary to cervical ectopy induced by the drugs; therefore, it should *not* be assumed that oral contraceptives provide protection against PID (i.e., that caused by *Chlamydia trachomatis*).

Although it has been suggested (based on very limited data) that use of multiphasic estrogen-progestin oral contraceptives may be associated with an increased risk of functional ovarian cysts, there currently is insufficient evidence to determine whether such increased risk exists. Epidemiologic evidence with monophasic estrogen-progestin oral contraceptives, principally high-dose estrogen preparations, indicates that monophasic contraceptives are associated with a reduced risk of developing functional ovarian risks when compared with nonusers of oral contraceptives. Epidemiologic studies and postmarketing surveillance currently are under way to determine the incidences of ovarian cysts in users of various types of oral contraceptives and in similar women not using the drugs.

Coital problems, device expulsion, and vaginal symptoms (discomfort, vaginitis, leukorrhea, foreign body sensation) have occurred in women using the contraceptive vaginal ring containing ethinyl estradiol and etonogestrel.

● Nervous System Effects

Mental depression may occur in women receiving oral contraceptives. In a few cases, mental depression has been severe and has led to suicidal behavior. Mental depression appears to occur most frequently in patients with a history of depression, including premenstrual depression; however, relief of premenstrual tension occurs in some women. Patients with a history of mental depression should be observed carefully and the estrogen-progestin contraceptive discontinued if severe depression recurs during use.

Fatigue, dizziness, nervousness, aggressiveness, anxiety, emotional lability, and irritability have been reported in women receiving estrogen-progestin contraceptives; changes in libido may also occur. Psychotic behavior, chorea, and cerebrovascular disease (with associated mitral valve prolapse) have also been reported; however, a causal relationship has not been established.

Headache, especially migraine headache, may occur during estrogen-progestin contraceptive therapy. Estrogen-progestin contraceptives should be discontinued and the cause evaluated when migraine occurs or is exacerbated, or when a new headache pattern develops which is recurrent, persistent, or severe.

● Ocular Effects

Oral contraceptives have been reported to produce harmful ocular effects in myopic women. In women who developed myopia at or near puberty and in whom myopia became stable in adulthood, the drugs have reportedly increased the refractive error 2- to 3-fold, usually after 6 months of use. In women who are myopic and have considerable astigmatism, oral contraceptives may produce marked changes in the astigmatic error, possibly leading to frank keratoconus. In addition, oral contraceptives may produce a rapid advancement of the ocular disorder in patients with a family history of marked myopic astigmatism or keratoconus. Contact lens wearers receiving estrogen-progestin contraceptives may have more difficulties with their contact lenses than do nonusers who wear contact lenses. Contact lens wearers who develop visual disturbances or changes in lens tolerance during estrogen-progestin contraceptive use should be assessed by an ophthalmologist; temporary or permanent cessation of contact lens wear should be considered.

Neuro-ocular lesions such as optic neuritis or retinal thrombosis have been associated with estrogen-progestin contraceptive use. If unexplained, sudden or gradual, partial or complete loss of vision; proptosis or diplopia; papilledema; or retinal vascular lesions occur during therapy with estrogen-progestin contraceptives, the drugs should be discontinued and evaluation for retinal vein thrombosis should be instituted immediately along with other appropriate diagnostic and therapeutic measures. Cataracts have also occurred during oral contraceptive use but have not been directly attributed to the drugs.

● *Hematologic Effects*

Changes in various blood factors and blood components have been observed in patients receiving oral contraceptives; however, further studies are required before the clinical importance of these changes can be established. Increases in fibrinogen and blood coagulation factors II, VII, VIII, IX, X, and XII levels and decreases in antithrombin III activity may occur in women receiving hormonal contraceptives. Blood coagulation factor levels may return to normal one to several weeks after the oral contraceptive is discontinued. Hematocrit may be slightly increased and an increased rate of blood coagulation may occur. The estrogen component of the contraceptive appears to enhance norepinephrine-induced platelet aggregation, whereas the progestin causes increased fibrinolytic activity. Anemia and sickle cell disease have also been reported during oral contraceptive use.

● *Other Adverse Effects*

Breast changes, including tenderness, enlargement, and secretion, may occur during estrogen-progestin contraceptive use.

Oral contraceptive use and estrogen use have appeared to be associated with an increased risk of gallbladder disease, especially in young women. In one study, an increased risk of gallbladder disease occurred after 2 years of use of the drugs and doubled after 4 or 5 years of use. In another study, an increased risk was apparent between 6–12 months of use. However, recent evidence suggests that the risk of gallbladder disease may be minimal in patients using formulations of oral contraceptives containing relatively low dosages of estrogens and/or progestins.

The relationship between oral contraceptive use and systemic lupus erythematosus (SLE) is not well-defined. Positive lupus erythematosus (LE) cell test results and antinuclear antibodies have been associated with oral contraceptive use in some women. Precipitation of SLE and exacerbation of preexisting disease have also been associated with oral contraceptive use in some women, and some clinicians recommend that other methods of contraception be used in women with a history of SLE. Rheumatic symptoms and synovitis have been associated with oral contraceptive use. Although several epidemiologic studies have suggested that oral contraceptive use appears to be associated with a decreased incidence of rheumatoid arthritis compared with nonuse, one epidemiologic study found no such association and the relationship, if any, between oral contraceptive use and rheumatoid arthritis remains to be determined.

Other reported adverse effects of estrogen-progestin contraceptives include Raynaud's phenomenon, auditory disturbances, hemolytic uremic syndrome, colitis, pancreatitis, upper respiratory tract infection, sinusitis, and rhinitis.

● *Precautions and Contraindications*

Use of estrogen-progestin oral contraceptives is associated with an increased risk of several serious conditions including thromboembolism, arterial thrombosis (e.g., stroke, myocardial infarction), liver tumor, gallbladder disease, visual disturbances, fetal abnormalities, and hypertension. The risk of thrombotic events is even higher in women with other risk factors for these events. Cigarette smoking increases the risk of serious adverse cardiovascular effects during oral contraceptive use. This risk increases with age and with heavy smoking (15 or more cigarettes daily) and is markedly greater in women older than 35 years of age. Women who are receiving estrogen-progestin contraceptives should be *strongly*

advised not to smoke. Women older than 35 years of age who smoke, and women with ischemic heart disease or a history of this disease, should not use estrogen-progestin contraceptives. Estrogen-progestin contraceptives should be used with caution in women with cardiovascular disease risk factors. Clinicians prescribing estrogen-progestin contraceptives should be aware of the risks associated with such use; the sections in Cautions and the manufacturers' labeling should be consulted for further discussion of these risks and associated precautions. In addition, potential noncontraceptive benefits associated with use of estrogen-progestin contraceptives can be considered. (See Pharmacology: Other Effects.)

Because of dose-related risks of vascular disease from oral contraceptives, the dosage regimen prescribed should contain the least amount of estrogen and progestin that is compatible with a low failure rate and the needs of the patient.

Adverse effects similar to those with oral combination estrogen-progestin contraceptives generally are expected with vaginal or transdermal estrogen-progestin contraceptives.

No data are available concerning the risk of using short-course, high-dose estrogen-progestin combinations for emergency contraception among women with contraindications to routine use of cyclic estrogen-progestin combinations for contraception. Since such postcoital contraceptive regimens do not appear to adversely affect clotting factors, vascular complications (e.g., abnormal blood clotting, stroke, myocardial infarction) are unlikely to occur. No serious or long-term complications have been associated with such postcoital contraceptive regimens in Europe, where experience is extensive. Most experts state that there currently is no real contraindication to postcoital (emergency) contraception with the recommended regimens and that the benefits generally outweigh any theoretical or proven risk.

Patients should be advised that emergency contraceptive regimens are not as effective as most other forms of long-term contraception and should not be used as a woman's routine form of contraception. Patients should be informed that as with all estrogen-progestin contraceptives and other nonbarrier contraceptive methods, emergency contraceptive regimens do not protect against human immunodeficiency virus (HIV) infection or other sexually transmitted diseases.

Women receiving estrogen-progestin contraceptives should be under supervision of a physician who should inform them of the possible risks involved. Women receiving these contraceptives also should be given a copy of the patient labeling for the drugs.

It is good medical practice that all women, including those receiving estrogen-progestin contraceptives, have a medical history and physical examination performed annually. The physical examination may be deferred until after initiation of these contraceptives if requested by the woman and judged appropriate by the clinician. Physical examination should include special attention to blood pressure, breasts, abdomen, and pelvic organs and should include a Papanicolaou test (Pap smear) and relevant laboratory tests.

Women receiving estrogen-progestin contraceptives (including drospirenone-containing oral contraceptives) should be advised to notify their clinician if signs or symptoms of thromboembolic or thrombotic disorders (e.g., thrombophlebitis, pulmonary embolism, cerebrovascular insufficiency, coronary occlusion, retinal thrombosis, mesenteric thrombosis) occur, including sudden severe headache or vomiting, disturbance of vision or speech, sudden partial or complete loss of vision, dizziness or faintness, weakness or numbness in an extremity, sharp or crushing chest pain, unexplained cough, hemoptysis, sudden shortness of breath, calf pain, or heaviness in the chest. Oral contraceptive combinations containing drospirenone should be discontinued if an arterial or venous thrombotic event occurs during therapy. Women currently receiving an oral contraceptive combination containing drospirenone should be informed of the potential risk of thromboembolic events. Patients also should be advised about the current information available regarding the risk of VTE with oral contraceptives containing drospirenone compared with those containing levonorgestrel. Known risk factors for development of VTE include smoking, obesity, family history, and other factors that contraindicate the use of oral contraceptive combinations. Patients should discuss their risk of VTE with their clinician before deciding which contraceptive method to use. The risk of thromboembolic disease associated with oral contraceptive use gradually disappears after such therapy is discontinued. However, the FDA states that patients should not discontinue oral contraceptives containing drospirenone without consulting a clinician.

Although the risk of VTE is higher in women using any oral contraceptives compared with nonusers, the risk remains lower than that associated with pregnancy and the postpartum period. The risk of VTE in women receiving estrogen-progestin oral contraceptives is estimated to be 3–9 per 10,000 woman-years.

In comparison, if 10,000 women who are not pregnant and not users of oral contraceptives are followed for one year, 1–5 of these women will develop a VTE. The risk of VTE is highest during the first year of oral contraceptive use. Results from a large, prospective cohort safety study of various estrogen-progestin oral contraceptives suggest that this increased risk is highest during the first 6 months of use compared with that in nonusers. Data from this safety study indicate that the highest risk of VTE occurs after initiation of estrogen-progestin oral contraceptive therapy or resumption of therapy (following a 4-week or longer drug-free interval) with the same or a different oral contraceptive combination. Before initiating use of an estrogen-progestin combination containing drospirenone in a new user or in a woman who is switching from an oral contraceptive not containing drospirenone, clinicians should consider the risks and benefits of drospirenone-containing oral contraceptives, including risk for developing VTE, specific to that woman.

Women receiving estrogen-progestin contraceptives should also be advised to inform their physician if severe abdominal pain or mass (indicating a possible liver tumor), jaundice, severe mental depression, edema, or unusual bleeding occurs. Because severe nausea and vomiting have occurred following postcoital use of high-dose estrogen-progestin combinations as emergency contraception, women taking such therapy should be instructed carefully regarding what to do if vomiting occurs after administering a dose, and concomitant use of an antiemetic should be considered. (See Dosage and Administration: Administration.) Women receiving estrogen-progestin contraceptives should be instructed in self-examination of their breasts and should report nodules or fibrocystic disease in the breast or abnormal breast radiographic or mammographic findings to their physician.

Estrogen-progestin contraceptives should be used with caution, and only with careful monitoring, in patients with conditions that might be aggravated by fluid retention (e.g., asthma, seizure disorders, migraine, or cardiac, renal, or hepatic insufficiency) and in patients being treated for hyperlipidemia, since control of the condition may become difficult. Women with a history of hypertension, hypertension-related diseases, or renal disease should be encouraged to use another method of contraception. Women with hypertension who elect to use estrogen-progestin contraceptives should be monitored closely, and if a clinically important elevation of blood pressure occurs, use of the drugs should be discontinued.

Because a twofold to fourfold increased risk of postsurgery thromboembolic complications has been reported in oral contraceptive users, estrogen-progestin contraceptives should be discontinued whenever feasible, at least 4 weeks before surgery that is associated with an increased risk of thromboembolism or prolonged immobilization; it is also recommended that patients wait 2 weeks after elective surgery associated with an increased risk of thromboembolism or after immobilization before resuming the use of these contraceptives.

Although the absolute rates for developing VTE are increased for users of hormonal contraceptives compared with nonusers, the rates for VTE development are even greater during pregnancy, especially during the postpartum period. Since the immediate postpartum period is associated with an increased risk of thromboembolism, estrogen-progestin contraceptive use should be started no earlier than 4 weeks after delivery in women who elect not to breastfeed their infants or in women who have had a midtrimester pregnancy termination. The risk of thromboembolism decreases while the risk of ovulation increases after the first 3 weeks postpartum.

Oral contraceptives containing the progestin drospirenone should not be used in patients who are predisposed to developing hyperkalemia (e.g., those with renal or hepatic impairment or adrenal insufficiency). If a drospirenone-containing oral contraceptive is used in women receiving daily, long-term therapy with agents that may increase serum potassium concentrations (e.g., angiotensin-converting enzyme (ACE) inhibitors, angiotensin II type 1 (AT_1) receptor antagonists, potassium-sparing diuretics, heparin, aldosterone antagonists [spironolactone], nonsteroidal anti-inflammatory agents [NSAIAs]), the serum potassium concentration should be determined during the first oral contraceptive cycle.

Five out of the 15 pregnancies reported in large clinical trials in women using the transdermal contraceptive system containing ethinyl estradiol and norelgestromin (Ortho Evra®) occurred in women with a baseline weight of 90 kg or more; these results suggest that the contraceptive preparation may be less effective in such women than in those with a lower body weight. The clinician and the woman with high body weight should discuss the individual needs of such a patient when choosing an appropriate contraceptive option.

The contraceptive vaginal ring containing ethinyl estradiol and etonogestrel (NuvaRing®) may not be suitable for women with conditions that make the vagina susceptible to vaginal irritation or ulceration.

Estrogen-progestin contraceptives are contraindicated in women who are hypersensitive to the drug or any ingredient in the formulation and in those with known or suspected pregnancy, undiagnosed abnormal genital bleeding, diplopia or any ocular lesion arising from ophthalmic vascular disease, classical migraine, active liver disease, or history of cholestatic jaundice with pregnancy or with prior use of oral contraceptives. The drugs also are contraindicated during breast-feeding and in women who have or have had thrombophlebitis or thromboembolic disorders, cerebrovascular or coronary artery disease (including myocardial infarction), severe hypertension, diabetes with vascular involvement, known or suspected carcinoma of the breast, known or suspected estrogen-dependent neoplasia (e.g., carcinoma of the endometrium), or benign or malignant liver tumor that developed during oral contraceptive or other estrogen use. Oral contraceptives containing the progestin drospirenone are contraindicated in women with renal impairment, hepatic tumors (benign or malignant) or hepatic disease, adrenal insufficiency, high risk of arterial or venous thrombotic diseases, undiagnosed abnormal uterine bleeding, history of breast cancer or other estrogen- or progestin-sensitive cancer, and in pregnancy.

● Pediatric Precautions

Safety and efficacy of estrogen-progestin contraceptives have been established in women of reproductive age. Safety and efficacy are expected to be identical for postpubertal adolescents under 16 years of age and users 16 years of age or older. The manufacturers of estrogen-progestin contraceptives containing drospirenone state that safety and efficacy are expected to be the same for postpubertal adolescents under 18 years of age and users 18 years of age or older. Estrogen-progestin contraceptives are not indicated before menarche.

● Geriatric Precautions

Oral contraceptives have not been evaluated in women 65 years of age and older and are not indicated in this population.

● Mutagenicity and Carcinogenicity

Chromosomal abnormalities determined in peripheral lymphocytes have been increased in women receiving oral contraceptives compared with nonusers.

Prolonged continuous administration of natural or synthetic estrogen in certain animal species increases the frequency of certain benign or malignant tumors including those of the breast, cervix, uterus, vagina, ovary, pituitary, and liver. Certain synthetic progestins (none currently contained in oral contraceptives) have increased the frequency of benign and malignant mammary nodules in dogs. Drospirenone has increased the frequency of benign and total (benign plus malignant) adrenal gland pheochromocytomas in rats and the frequency of carcinomas of the harderian gland in mice.

The manufacturers state that there is at present no consistent evidence from human studies of an increased risk of cancer associated with oral contraceptive use; whether this statement also applies to vaginal or transdermal estrogen-progestin contraceptives is not known. Close clinical surveillance of all women using estrogen-progestin contraceptives is, nevertheless, essential. Appropriate diagnostic measures should be undertaken to rule out malignancy in all women with undiagnosed persistent or recurrent abnormal vaginal bleeding. Women with a strong family history of breast cancer or who have breast nodules, fibrocystic disease, or abnormal mammographic findings should be closely monitored if they elect to use estrogen-progestin contraceptives.

Cervical Cancer

There is some evidence from epidemiologic studies that use of oral contraceptives may be associated with an increased risk of cervical carcinoma. In one study, the incidence of biopsy-proven cervical neoplasia (i.e., dysplasia, carcinoma *in situ*, or invasive carcinoma) was increased in long-term oral contraceptive users compared with women who used an intrauterine contraceptive device (IUD); it was recommended that particular attention to the importance of regular Papanicolaou tests be given in women who have used oral contraceptives for longer than 48 months. Although a causal relationship to the drugs could not be excluded, data from a population-based (Costa Rican women), case-control study suggest that the increased risk of carcinoma in situ associated with oral contraceptive use may have resulted from a detection bias secondary to more frequent use of Papanicolaou tests in oral contraceptive users. These data revealed no evidence of increased risk of invasive cervical cancer in users compared with nonusers. The FDA recommends that all estrogen-progestin contraceptive users be monitored carefully with physical examinations and Papanicolaou tests, at least yearly. (See Cautions: Precautions and Contraindications.)

Endometrial Cancer

Several retrospective case-controlled studies have shown an increased relative risk of endometrial carcinoma in postmenopausal women who received prolonged estrogen replacement therapy for relief of menopausal symptoms. Although an increased risk of adenocarcinoma of the endometrium has been associated with sequential oral contraceptive use (sequential oral contraceptives are no longer available in the US), no association between increased risk of endometrial cancer and use of currently available estrogen-progestin combination preparations or progestin-only preparations has been shown, although individual cases have been reported. The Cancer and Steroid Hormone Study of the US Centers for Disease Control and Prevention (CDC) and the National Institute of Child Health and Human Development (NICHD) showed that women who used estrogen-progestin oral contraceptives had *decreased* relative risk of epithelial endometrial cancer (i.e., adenocarcinoma, adenoacanthoma, and adenosquamous cancers) compared with nonusers; the protective effect occurred in women who had used combination oral contraceptives for at least 12 months, and it persisted for at least 15 years after discontinuance of oral contraceptives. This decreased risk of endometrial cancer was not evident in women who had used oral contraceptives for less than 12 months.

Ovarian Cancer

Several studies have shown a decreased risk of epithelial ovarian cancer in oral contraceptive users compared with nonusers. The Cancer and Steroid Hormone Study showed that women who used oral contraceptives had a *decreased* relative risk of epithelial ovarian cancer compared with nonusers; the protective effect occurred in women who had used oral contraceptives for as little as 3–6 months, and it persisted for at least 15 years after discontinuance of oral contraceptive use. The risk of ovarian cancer decreased with increasing duration of oral contraceptive use and did not appear to be affected by the age at the time of first use of oral contraceptives or the oral contraceptive type (i.e., combination or sequential) or specific formulation. Because of inadequate data, the association between use of oral contraceptives and nonepithelial (i.e., germ-cell, sex cord-stromal) ovarian cancers could not be fully assessed.

Breast Cancer

Many studies have shown *no* increased risk of breast cancer in women receiving oral contraceptives or estrogens. Some studies, however, have suggested an overall increased risk of breast cancer in women receiving oral contraceptives and some studies have suggested that certain subgroups of women who use oral contraceptives may be at increased risk (e.g., women younger than 45 years of age who have used oral contraceptives, women who begin oral contraceptive use early in their childbearing years, women who use oral contraceptives for extended periods of time, women who use oral contraceptives before a first full-term pregnancy); however, these findings have occurred in only some studies and other large studies have shown no such possible associations. Because of several studies suggesting an increased risk of breast cancer with oral contraceptive use, the FDA Fertility and Maternal Health Drugs Advisory Committee reviewed these data in early 1989. The Committee concluded at that time that existing data suggested no *overall* increased risk of breast cancer associated with oral contraceptive use and that a change in prescribing practices by clinicians or in the use of oral contraceptives by women was not justified.

The Cancer and Steroid Hormone (CASH) study showed no association between oral contraceptive use and the risk of breast cancer; the duration of oral contraceptive use, time since first use, or menopause status did not alter the user's risk of breast cancer. In addition, in the CASH study, oral contraceptive use before a woman's first full-term pregnancy did not increase her risk of breast cancer compared with other methods of delaying first pregnancy. In a population based, case-controlled (Women's CARE) study in women 35–64 years of age, current or former use of oral contraceptives was not associated with an increased risk of breast cancer. Findings from the Women's CARE study generally are in agreement with results from the Cancer and Steroid Hormone Study. In the Women's CARE study, the relative risk of breast cancer did not increase consistently with longer periods of use or higher dosages of estrogen, nor was the risk increased with initiation of oral contraceptives at young age or in those with history of breast cancer in a first-degree relative. There was no consistent difference in risk between white and black women. The age at last use, use in relation to the first term pregnancy, duration of use before the first term pregnancy, or type of progestin did not change the oral contraceptive user's risk of breast cancer. A case-control study by the University of Southern California Cancer Surveillance Program indicated that use of "high-progestin" combination oral contraceptives (relative progestin potency determined by delay in menses test) before 25 years of age was associated with an increased risk of breast cancer; however, the validity of this study has been questioned and the CASH study found *no* such association. In this latter study, neither the type of estrogen nor the type of progestin contained in oral contraceptives was associated with increased risk of breast cancer; the type of progestin also was not associated with an increased risk of breast cancer in the Women's CARE study. In these studies, the type of oral contraceptive used (i.e., combination, sequential, progestin only, or more than one type) did not increase the risk. Another

case-control study indicated that in women younger than 45 years of age use of oral contraceptives before their first full-term pregnancy was associated with an increased risk of breast cancer; the CASH study and the Women's CARE study found *no* such association. In a meta-analysis of numerous clinical trials, a small increase in the frequency of breast cancer localized to the breast was diagnosed in women within 10 years of current or past use of combined estrogen-progestin oral contraceptives. The Women's CARE study found no such association. No increase in the frequency of breast cancer was diagnosed in women who had not received estrogen-progestin combination oral contraception for at least 10 years.

While the relationship between breast cancer risk and use of oral contraceptives in women with a familial predisposition to breast cancer has not been precisely established, results from a multigenerational study suggest that women who used earlier formulations of oral contraceptives (i.e., high-dose formulations commercially available prior to 1975) and who also have a first-degree relative with breast cancer may be at increased risk of breast cancer. This multigenerational, historical cohort study included the relatives (i.e., daughters, sisters, granddaughters, nieces, women who married into the families) of over 400 women diagnosed with breast cancer between 1944 and 1952 (probands). In the entire cohort (i.e., daughters, sisters, granddaughters, nieces, women who married into the families), the relative risk (RR) of breast cancer was 1.4 in those who reported ever having used oral contraceptives. Risk was not influenced by duration of contraceptive use. After accounting for age and birth cohort, use of oral contraceptives was associated with an increased risk of breast cancer (RR of 3.3) among sisters and daughters of the probands but not among their nieces or granddaughters (RR of 1.2) or in women who married into the family (RR of 1.2). The risk to first-degree relatives increased with the number of relatives in the family with breast or ovarian cancer; the relative risk was 4.6 for families with at least 3 members who had breast or ovarian cancer and 11.4 for families with at least 5 members who had breast or ovarian cancer. The risk of breast cancer was not increased in first-degree relatives who reported use of oral contraceptives after 1975, although the small number of reported cases of cancer in this study (2 of 60 women who took oral contraceptives) limits the statistical reliability of this finding. While the increased risk of breast cancer among high-risk women in this study appeared to be limited to those who used earlier formulations containing higher dosages of estrogen and progestin than current oral contraceptives, the mean age for first-degree relatives who reported use of oral contraceptives after 1975 was 43 years, and breast cancer may not yet have occurred in many women in this group. The Women's CARE study found no association between use of oral combination contraceptives with high dose estrogen (50 mcg or more of ethinyl estradiol or 75 mcg or more of mestranol) and an increased risk of breast cancer in women with a family history of breast cancer. The relative risk of breast cancer in women with a family history of breast cancer who received high dose estrogen combinations for up to 15 years or longer was essentially the same as the relative risk in women with a family history of breast cancer who received lower-dose estrogen combinations for similar periods of time.

Other Cancers

Although an increased occurrence of malignant melanoma, urinary tract cancers, and thyroid cancers has been reportedly associated with oral contraceptive use, these findings have not been established. Although liver tumors (mainly hepatocellular adenomas) have been associated with oral contraceptive use, these liver tumors have usually been benign. (See Cautions: Hepatic Effects.)

● *Pregnancy, Fertility, and Lactation*
Pregnancy

Although preliminary evidence suggested that oral contraceptives could cause serious fetal toxicity when administered to pregnant women, current evidence does not suggest an association between inadvertent use of oral contraceptives in early pregnancy and teratogenic effects (including cardiovascular and limb defects, which have been reported following use of sex hormones). In addition, extensive epidemiologic studies have revealed no increased risk of birth defects in neonates born to women who used estrogen-progestin contraceptives prior to pregnancy. However, since the risks of estrogen-progestin contraceptive use clearly outweigh any possible benefit in women who are pregnant, these agents are contraindicated in such women. Although estrogens and/or progestins were previously used to treat threatened or habitual abortion, there is considerable evidence that estrogens are ineffective and no evidence from well-controlled studies that progestins are effective for these uses. Progestin-only or estrogen-progestin contraceptives should *not* be used to induce withdrawal bleeding as a test of pregnancy.

Data concerning pregnancy outcomes following unsuccessful emergency postcoital contraception with estrogen-progestin combinations are limited, in part because such women may choose abortion following failure of postcoital contraception. Pooled data from several controlled trials that followed pregnancies that occurred despite postcoital estrogen-progestin combinations indicate delivery of 45 healthy neonates, 1 neonate with absent left kidney, and 2 neonates with minor anomalies. In addition, numerous studies evaluating teratologic risk of conception during cyclic (routine) oral contraceptive regimens (for both currently available low-dose oral contraceptive regimens and older, high-dose preparations [e.g., 150 mcg of ethinyl estradiol daily] that are no longer available) indicate no increased fetal risks. Exposure to the amount of estrogen-progestin in postcoital contraceptive regimens is not large when compared with the total amount of the estrogen-progestin cyclic (routine) oral contraceptive regimens, and there currently is no evidence of substantial risk to the fetus with such short-term exposure. Estrogen-progestin postcoital contraceptive regimens are contraindicated in pregnancy because of lack of efficacy, not because of adverse effects on the fetus.

In women who have missed 2 consecutive menstrual periods during estrogen-progestin conventional-cycle contraceptive use, the drug should be withheld until pregnancy has been ruled out. In women using a fixed-combination extended-cycle oral contraceptive (e.g., LoSeasonique®, Seasonale®, Seasonique®), the possibility of pregnancy should be considered after one missed menstrual period. When the woman has not adhered to the prescribed oral contraceptive regimen, the possibility of pregnancy should be considered after one missed menstrual period and the drug should be withheld until pregnancy has been ruled out. A back-up method of contraception should be instituted until the possibility of pregnancy has been eliminated. If pregnancy is confirmed, the woman should be informed of the potential hazard to the fetus and the advisability of continuing the pregnancy should be weighed against the risks of exposure of the fetus to the drugs.

Fertility

Studies have found a slight delay in return to fertility but no absolute impairment of fertility following discontinuance of fixed-combination conventional-cycle oral contraceptives. A survey of pregnant women attending antenatal clinics in England reported that the time to conception following discontinuance of long-term (i.e., longer than 2 years) use of fixed-combination oral contraceptives (8.2 months) was twofold longer than time to conception following condom use (4.2 months).

Lactation

Estrogen-progestin contraceptives may decrease the quantity and quality of milk if given in the immediate postpartum period. Small amounts of the hormonal agents in estrogen-progestin contraceptives are distributed into milk and adverse effects such as jaundice and breast enlargement have been reported in nursing infants of women receiving cyclic regimens; therefore, because of the theoretical risk, some clinicians recommend that lactating women receiving high-dose postcoital contraceptive regimens use alternative milk sources for their infants for at least 24 hours after completion of the regimen. When possible, the use of cyclic estrogen-progestin contraceptives should be deferred until the infant has been weaned. Long-term follow-up after oral contraceptive use showed no apparent clinical effect on breast-feeding mothers or children whose mothers were breast-feeding and using oral contraceptives.

DRUG INTERACTIONS

● *Drugs Affecting Hepatic Microsomal Enzymes*

Clinically important drug interactions may occur when estrogen-progestin oral contraceptives are administered with other drugs metabolized by the hepatic microsomal cytochrome P-450 (CYP) enzyme system. Metabolism of estrogens is mediated by the CYP3A4 isoenzyme, and the possibility exists that drugs that induce this isoenzyme may reduce ethinyl estradiol concentrations.

Rifampin reportedly decreases contraceptive efficacy and increases breakthrough bleeding during concomitant use with oral contraceptives. These effects have been attributed to enhanced metabolism of both the estrogenic and progestinic components of oral contraceptives, presumably by induction of hepatic microsomal enzymes. It has been suggested that similar effects may occur during concomitant therapy with other known inducers of hepatic microsomal enzymes, including barbiturates, bosentan, carbamazepine, dexamethasone, griseofulvin, phenylbutazone (no longer commercially available in the US), phenytoin, felbamate, oxcarbazepine, rifabutin, modafinil, topiramate, and primidone. Because herbal supplements containing St. John's wort (*Hypericum perforatum*) may induce hepatic cytochrome P-450 isoenzymes and the *p*-glycoprotein transport

system, St. John's wort may decrease contraceptive efficacy of estrogen-progestin contraceptives, including that of high-dose estrogen-progestin postcoital contraceptive regimens, and increase breakthrough bleeding during concomitant use with estrogen-progestin contraceptives. Because of the risk of contraceptive failure during concomitant use of estrogen-progestin contraceptives with known inducers of hepatic microsomal enzymes, it has been suggested that alternate methods of contraception be considered in patients receiving these drugs or that oral contraceptive preparations with increased dosage be considered; however, the possibility that adverse effects may be increased with increased-dosage preparations should also be considered.

Data currently are not available concerning the effect of drugs that induce hepatic microsomal enzymes on the contraceptive efficacy of high-dose estrogen-progestin postcoital contraceptive regimens. However, because contraceptive failure has occurred during concomitant use of cyclic oral contraceptive regimens and known inducers of hepatic microsomal enzymes, some clinicians suggest that the dosage of postcoital estrogen-progestin contraceptive regimens may need to be increased, possibly doubled, in women receiving such inducers concomitantly.

Estrogens are inhibitors of the CYP enzyme and may alter the pharmacokinetics of drugs metabolized by this isoenzyme.

● *Anti-infective Agents*

Antiretroviral Agents

Concomitant use of oral contraceptives and some HIV-protease inhibitors or nonnucleoside reverse transcriptase inhibitors may result in substantial changes in the area under the plasma concentration-time curve (AUC) of the estrogen and/or progestin. Concomitant use of oral contraceptives and some HIV-protease inhibitors or nonnucleoside reverse transcriptase inhibitors may reduce the efficacy of the oral contraceptive; whether this precaution applies to vaginal or transdermal estrogen-progestin contraceptives is not known. For additional information, see the individual monographs in 8:18:08 Antiretroviral Agents.

Other Anti-infective Agents

It has been suggested that anti-infective agents which alter the GI bacterial flora may decrease the contraceptive efficacy of oral contraceptives and increase breakthrough bleeding. GI bacteria produce enzymes which hydrolyze conjugates of estrogens (e.g., ethinyl estradiol) that have been excreted into the GI tract via bile; hydrolysis of these conjugates allows enterohepatic circulation of the pharmacologically active drug. By disrupting the GI flora, anti-infective agents may decrease or eliminate enterohepatic circulation of oral contraceptives. The clinical importance of this potential interaction has not been determined; however, the manufacturers caution that concomitant use of anti-infective agents (e.g., ampicillin, chloramphenicol, neomycin, nitrofurantoin, penicillin V, sulfonamides, tetracyclines) with oral contraceptives may result in decreased efficacy of the contraceptive.

In one study in healthy women using the vaginal contraceptive ring containing ethinyl estradiol and etonogestrel (NuvaRing®), vaginal administration of a single oil-based suppository containing 1200 mg of miconazole nitrate on day 8 of the cycle increased the serum concentration of ethinyl estradiol or etonogestrel by 16 or 17%, respectively. While the clinical importance of these findings is unknown, the efficacy of the contraceptive vaginal ring is not expected to be affected. The effects of long-term administration of miconazole nitrate vaginal suppositories in women using the contraceptive vaginal ring are not known.

Fluconazole, itraconazole and ketoconazole also may increase plasma concentrations of contraceptive steroids.

Concurrent use of oral contraceptives and troleandomycin may increase the risk of cholestatic jaundice; therefore, the drugs should be used together cautiously.

● *Benzodiazepines*

Oral contraceptives appear to decrease oxidative metabolism by the liver of some benzodiazepines (e.g., diazepam, chlordiazepoxide), while they may increase metabolism of other benzodiazepines (e.g., lorazepam, oxazepam, temazepam) that undergo glucuronide conjugation in the liver. Although the clinical importance of these potential interactions between oral contraceptives and benzodiazepines has not been determined, alterations in benzodiazepine dosage may be necessary in some patients. Although interactions have not yet been documented, other benzodiazepines that undergo oxidative metabolism in the liver include alprazolam, clorazepate, flurazepam, halazepam (no longer commercially available in the US), and prazepam.

• *β-Adrenergic Blocking Agents*

Oral contraceptives have substantially increased the area under the plasma concentration-time curve (AUC) of orally administered metoprolol when the drugs were used concomitantly. It has been suggested that oral contraceptives decrease the first-pass metabolism of metoprolol. Although the clinical importance of this interaction has not been determined, women receiving oral contraceptives and metoprolol (and possibly other β-adrenergic blockers that undergo first-pass metabolism in the liver) concomitantly may require a decrease in the dosage of the β-adrenergic blocker.

• *Corticosteroids*

Estrogens have been reported to enhance the anti-inflammatory effect of hydrocortisone in patients with chronic inflammatory skin diseases. In addition, there is limited evidence that oral contraceptives decrease the metabolic clearance of prednisolone. Increased plasma concentrations of prednisolone and other corticosteroids have been observed when these drugs were used concomitantly with oral contraceptives. It has been suggested that estrogens and oral contraceptives may decrease the hepatic metabolism of corticosteroids and/or alter serum corticosteroid protein binding. Patients receiving concomitant oral contraceptive-corticosteroid therapy should be observed for signs of excessive corticosteroid effects, and alterations in corticosteroid dosage may be necessary when oral contraceptives are started or discontinued.

• *Other Drugs*

There is limited evidence that oral contraceptives may decrease the metabolism of tricyclic antidepressants; however, the clinical importance of this effect has not been determined. Although one report indicated that oral contraceptives may inhibit the metabolism of meperidine, a subsequent study was unable to confirm this finding.

The manufacturers caution that analgesics, isoniazid, antimigraine drugs, and tranquilizers may decrease the efficacy of oral contraceptives. Oral contraceptives may alter the effects of other drugs by impairing their metabolism, altering their protein binding, or by other mechanisms. Although the clinical importance of many of these interactions has not been determined, the manufacturers caution that concomitant use of oral contraceptives with oral anticoagulants, anticonvulsants, hypotensive agents (e.g., guanethidine), vitamins, or oral antidiabetic agents may result in decreased or increased effects of these drugs. Concomitant administration of atorvastatin with an oral contraceptive increased the area under the plasma concentration-time curve (AUC) of norethindrone and ethinyl estradiol by about 30 and 20%, respectively.

Increased plasma concentrations of cyclosporine and theophylline have been observed when these drugs were used concomitantly with oral contraceptives. Ascorbic acid or acetaminophen may increase plasma concentrations of some synthetic estrogens. Decreased plasma concentrations of acetaminophen and lamotrigine, and increased clearance of temazepam, salicylic acid, morphine, or clofibric acid have been observed when these drugs were administered concomitantly with oral contraceptives. The effects of oral contraceptives on plasma concentrations of lamotrigine may reduce seizure control in patients receiving concomitant therapy and dosage adjustment of lamotrigine may be necessary.

There is a potential for increased serum potassium concentrations in women receiving a drospirenone-containing oral contraceptive concomitantly with other drugs that increase serum potassium concentrations. In one study in mildly hypertensive postmenopausal women receiving enalapril maleate (10 mg twice daily) and drospirenone in fixed combination with ethinyl estradiol (Yasmin®) or placebo, mean serum potassium concentrations (evaluated every other day for 2 weeks) relative to baseline were 0.22 mEq/L higher in those receiving drospirenone in fixed combination with ethinyl estradiol than in those receiving placebo. If a drospirenone-containing oral contraceptive is used in women receiving daily, long-term therapy with agents that may increase serum potassium concentrations (e.g., angiotensin-converting enzyme (ACE) inhibitors, angiotensin II type 1 (AT$_1$) receptor antagonists, potassium-sparing diuretics, heparin, aldosterone antagonists [spironolactone], nonsteroidal anti-inflammatory agents [NSAIAs]), the serum potassium concentration should be determined during the first oral contraceptive cycle.

In one study in healthy women using the vaginal contraceptive ring containing ethinyl estradiol and etonogestrel (NuvaRing®), vaginal administration of a single dose of 100 mg of water-based nonoxynol 9 spermicide gel did not affect the serum concentrations of ethinyl estradiol or etonogestrel. The effects of long-term vaginal administration of nonoxynol 9 spermicide gel in women using the contraceptive vaginal ring are not known.

LABORATORY TEST INTERFERENCES

A decreased response to the metyrapone test may occur in women receiving oral contraceptives; however, the drugs do not interfere with the pituitary-adrenal reaction to stress. Because the adrenal responds to corticotropin, it appears that the estrogen acts on the adrenal gland to interfere with the metyrapone test. The estrogen component of oral contraceptives increases the level of circulating corticosteroid-binding globulin (transcortin) resulting in an increase in total plasma cortisol, a decrease in cortisol secretion rate, and a decrease in urinary excretion of 17-ketogenic steroids, 17-hydroxycorticosteroids, and 17-ketosteroids. Because plasma cortisol concentrations may be similar to those of patients with Cushing's syndrome and urinary steroids may suggest hypofunction, oral contraceptives should be discontinued for a few weeks before performing adrenal function tests. The dexamethasone suppression test, however, can exclude Cushing's syndrome and corticotropin tests can rule out primary adrenocortical insufficiency, even in patients receiving oral contraceptives.

Elevation in sex-hormone binding globulin (SHBG) concentration by combination estrogen-progestin contraceptives results in increased total circulating sex steroids and corticoids; however, free (unbound) concentrations of these steroids remain unchanged. Certain other endocrine and liver function tests may also be affected by oral contraceptives. (See Cautions: Endocrine and Metabolic Effects; Hepatic Effects.)

False-positive results in the nitro blue tetrazolium (NBT) test for the diagnosis of bacterial infection have occurred in women receiving oral contraceptives.

The manufacturers state that the pathologist should be advised of oral contraceptive use when relevant specimens from an oral contraceptive user are submitted.

ACUTE TOXICITY

Acute overdosage of large doses of oral contraceptives in children reportedly produces almost no toxicity except nausea and vomiting. Withdrawal bleeding may occur in females.

Because drospirenone has antimineralocorticoid properties, serum potassium and sodium concentrations and indicators of metabolic acidosis should be monitored in the event of overdosage with a drospirenone-containing oral contraceptive.

PHARMACOLOGY

The pharmacologic effects of estrogen-progestin contraceptives are complex and appear to depend on many variables including the specific drugs used, the amount and proportion of each drug, the age of the user, and the duration of administration. In general, estrogen-progestin combinations elicit, to varying degrees, many of the pharmacologic responses usually produced by endogenous estrogens and progesterone and produce numerous effects on many organs.

• *Contraceptive Effect*

Estrogen-progestin combinations produce a contraceptive effect mainly by suppressing the hypothalamic-pituitary system resulting in prevention of ovulation. The estrogen acts mainly by suppressing secretion of follicle-stimulating hormone (FSH), resulting in prevention of follicular development and the rise of plasma estradiol concentration which is thought to be the stimulus for release of luteinizing hormone (LH). In combination products, the progestin appears to act mainly by inhibiting the preovulatory rise of LH. Long-term administration of these combination products results in inhibition of both FSH and LH secretion. It has been suggested that oral contraceptives may also produce a direct effect on ovarian steroidogenesis or the response of the ovary to gonadotropins. In addition, changes in the cervical mucus may prevent sperm penetration; however, further studies are required to determine the precise effects of estrogen-progestin combinations on sperm activity.

Endometrial changes depend on the type of oral contraceptive administered. Conventional-cycle combination products are usually associated with a shortened period of endometrial proliferation followed by an early but brief and limited secretory activity in the epithelium of endometrial glands. After several oral contraceptive cycles, thinning or regression of the endometrium may occur, resulting in reduced menstrual flow or possible amenorrhea.

The precise mechanism of contraceptive activity of estrogen-progestin combinations administered *after* intercourse (postcoital) is not known. However, the effect is contraceptive, not abortifacient, in nature; therefore, timing is critical to efficacy. High-dosage estrogen-progestin combinations are only effective before pregnancy is established. Once implantation occurs (i.e., usually within 6–7 days after ovulation), the combinations would be ineffective in preventing pregnancy. Estrogen-progestin combinations in high dosage provide a short, potent burst of hormonal exposure that may effectively prevent conception by delaying or inhibiting ovulation, and/or producing changes in endometrial development that are hostile to uterine implantation of the fertilized ovum, depending on when the drugs are administered relative to the menstrual cycle and the time period since intercourse. Postcoital contraceptives taken before midcycle may inhibit ovulation by suppressing the midcycle surge in luteinizing hormone that is necessary for final follicular growth and ovulation. Endometrial biopsies in women receiving high-dose estrogen-progestin combination contraceptives at midcycle indicate that coordinated timing of the maturation of glandular epithelium and stroma of the endometrial lining is disrupted. Possible alterations in transport of the ovum through the fallopian tube, fertilization, and corpus luteum development and function have been reported with postcoital use of estrogen-progestin combinations, but these effects are inconsistent and are thought to be of secondary importance as mechanisms in preventing pregnancy.

Ovulation usually resumes within 3 menstrual cycles after oral contraceptives have been discontinued; however, anovulation and amenorrhea may persist for 6 months or longer in some women. After the drug is discontinued, pituitary function recovers first, followed by ovarian function; the endometrium may require up to 3 months to regain its normal histology and enzymatic activity.

● *Other Effects*

Oral contraceptives may produce a wide variety of metabolic changes, possibly as a result of a direct action on the liver. The drugs may produce alterations in carbohydrate and lipid metabolism, increased serum hormone concentrations, and alterations in serum metals and plasma proteins. The estrogen appears to cause most of these metabolic effects. In one study, oral contraceptives containing mestranol and ethynodiol diacetate were shown to produce an increase in cardiac index and stroke volume, a small rise in plasma volume, and an elevation in blood pressure. Urinary tract dilatation may also occur in women receiving oral contraceptives. In nursing women, oral contraceptives may decrease the quantity and quality of milk when given immediately postpartum.

Potential noncontraceptive benefits of oral contraceptives, as evidenced from epidemiologic studies, include effects on menses, effects related to inhibition of ovulation, and effects from long-term use. Use of the drugs has been associated with improved menstrual cycle regularity and decreased incidences of blood loss, iron deficiency anemia, and dysmenorrhea. A decreased incidence of functional ovarian cysts and of ectopic pregnancies also has been associated with use of the drugs. Long-term use of oral contraceptives has been associated with a decreased incidence of formation of fibroadenomas and fibrocystic disease of the breast, a decreased incidence of some (e.g., gonococcal) pelvic inflammatory disease (see Cautions: Genitourinary Effects), and a decreased incidence of some cancers (e.g., endometrial or ovarian cancer) (see Cautions: Mutagenicity and Carcinogenicity).

PHARMACOKINETICS

● *Absorption*
Oral Administration

Oral contraceptive steroids are generally well absorbed from the GI tract. Following oral administration, levonorgestrel is completely absorbed. Some oral contraceptive steroids are metabolized in the GI mucosa during absorption and on first pass through the liver. Desogestrel is metabolized in the intestinal mucosa and on first pass through the liver to 3-keto-desogestrel, a metabolite believed to be responsible for the pharmacologic activity of desogestrel. Following oral administration, the absolute bioavailability appears to be about 40% for ethinyl estradiol, 65% for norethindrone, and about 76% for desogestrel or drospirenone. Following oral administration, the relative bioavailability of desogestrel, as measured by serum concentrations of 3-keto-desogestrel (the active metabolite of desogestrel), reportedly is about 84%. Although the absolute bioavailabilities have not been determined, about 60% of norgestimate and 60% of ethynodiol diacetate are reportedly absorbed following oral administration.

Considerable interindividual variation in peak plasma concentrations attained and extent of absorption have been reported for oral contraceptive steroids. Peak plasma concentrations of 100–200 pg/mL are reached 1–2 hours after a 50-mcg dose of ethinyl estradiol; although higher plasma concentrations have been reported, these probably represent methodologic problems. Following single-dose oral administration of ethinyl estradiol 20 mcg (in a fixed combination with levonorgestrel 0.1 mg), mean peak serum concentration was reported to be 50–62 pg/mL at approximately 1.5 hours; at steady state, mean peak ethinyl estradiol concentration of 66–77 pg/mL was reported at approximately 1.3–1.4 hours after administration.

Peak plasma norethindrone concentrations of 1.7–5 ng/mL or 5–10 ng/mL have been reported following a 0.5- or a 1-mg oral dose, respectively. The time to peak plasma norethindrone concentrations varies between 0.5–4 hours, apparently being more delayed as the dose increases.

Following oral administration of a single 0.15-mg dose of desogestrel (given in fixed combination with 30 mcg of ethinyl estradiol), average peak plasma 3-keto-desogestrel concentrations of 2.8 ng/mL are reached within 1.4 hours; at steady state (attained after 19 days or more), average peak plasma 3-keto-desogestrel concentrations of 5.8 ng/mL are reached within 1.4 hours after a dose.

Peak plasma norgestimate and 17-deacetyl norgestimate (an active metabolite of norgestimate) concentrations of 0.1 and 3.6 ng/mL are reached within 1 and 1.5 hours, respectively, following oral administration of a single 0.36-mg dose of norgestimate (given in fixed combination with 70 mcg of ethinyl estradiol); at steady state, mean plasma 17-deacetyl norgestimate concentrations of 4.4 ng/mL are reached in about 1.4 hours after a dose. Following single-dose oral administration of levonorgestrel 0.1 mg (in a fixed combination with ethinyl estradiol 20 mcg), mean peak serum concentration was reported to be 2.4–2.8 ng/mL at approximately 1.3–1.6 hours; at steady state, mean peak levonorgestrel concentration of 4–6 ng/mL was reported at approximately 1–1.5 hours after administration.

Plasma concentrations of desogestrel, norethindrone, and levonorgestrel at steady state are higher than predicted from single-dose kinetics because of enhanced binding of these progestins following the induction of sex hormone binding globulin (SHBG) by ethinyl estradiol.

Following single-dose oral administration of drospirenone 3 mg (in fixed combination with ethinyl estradiol 30 mcg) in women, mean peak serum concentration was reported to be 36.9 ng/mL at about 1.7 hours; at steady state, mean peak drospirenone concentrations of 78.7–87.5 ng/mL are reached in about 1.6–1.8 hours after a dose. Although steady-state serum concentrations of drospirenone in women with mild renal impairment (creatinine clearance 50–80 mL/minute) generally are similar to those in women with normal renal function (creatinine clearance greater than or equal to 80 mL/minute), drug concentrations in women with moderate renal impairment (creatinine clearance 30–49 mL/minute) are about 37% higher than concentrations in women with normal renal function.

Vaginal Administration

Ethinyl estradiol and etonogestrel are absorbed systemically through the mucous membrane. Following administration of one vaginal ring delivering ethinyl estradiol 0.015 mg/24 hours and etonogestrel 0.12 mg/24 hours (NuvaRing®), peak serum concentrations of ethinyl estradiol are reached on day 2–3 and peak serum concentrations of etonogestrel are reached by day 7. Mean serum concentrations of ethinyl estradiol 1, 2, or 3 weeks after insertion of the ring are 19.1, 18.3, or 17.6 pg/mL, respectively and mean serum concentration of etonogestrel at these time points are 1578, 1476, or 1374 pg/mL, respectively. Following vaginal administration of the ring, bioavailability appears to be about 56% for ethinyl estradiol and 100% for etonogestrel.

Transdermal Administration

Ethinyl estradiol and norelgestromin are also absorbed systemically through the skin. Following topical application of one system containing ethinyl estradiol 0.75 mg and norelgestromin 6 mg (Ortho Evra®), peak serum concentrations of ethinyl estradiol and norelgestromin are reached within 48 hours and are maintained at approximately steady state throughout the application period (7 days). In clinical studies, steady state serum concentrations of ethinyl estradiol and norelgestromin were reached during the second week of patch wear; mean steady-state serum concentrations of ethinyl estradiol ranged from 11.2–137 pg/mL and steady-state concentrations of norelgestromin ranged from 0.305–1.53 pg/mL. Serum concentrations generally are consistent from all studies and application sites (i.e., abdomen, buttock, upper outer arm, upper torso). Results of multi-dose studies indicate that steady-state area under the plasma-concentration time curve (AUC) of ethinyl estradiol and norelgestromin may increase slightly over time compared with values from week 1 of cycle 1. Following 3 consecutive cycles of patch wear, mean steady-state serum concentrations of ethinyl estradiol were 49.6 pg/mL (coefficient of variation of 54.4%) and steady-state concentrations of norelgestromin were 0.7 ng/mL (coefficient of variation of 45.3%) at week 3. Health club activities (i.e., sauna, whirlpool, treadmill) or a cold water bath do not result in clinically important changes in the absorption of ethinyl estradiol or norelgestromin compared with normal wear.

The pharmacokinetic profile for the transdermal contraceptive system containing ethinyl estradiol and norelgestromin (Ortho Evra®) differs from the profile for oral contraceptive preparations. Overall exposure to ethinyl estradiol and norelgestromin is higher in women receiving Ortho Evra® than in women receiving an oral contraceptive preparation containing ethinyl estradiol 35 mcg and norgestimate 0.25 mg. The average plasma concentration and AUC (from 0–168 hours) of ethinyl estradiol at steady-state in women receiving Ortho Evra® are 55–60% higher and peak plasma concentrations are 25% lower than values in women receiving an oral contraceptive preparation containing ethinyl estradiol 35 mcg (average weekly exposure [AUC_{0-168}] to the oral contraceptive calculated as 7 times the AUC from 0–24 hours).

● Distribution

Contraceptive steroids are widely distributed into body tissues and fluids. The apparent volume of distribution for contraceptive steroids reportedly ranges from 1.5–4.3 L/kg.

Contraceptive steroids are extensively bound to plasma proteins. Ethinyl estradiol is about 98% protein bound, mainly to albumin. Norethindrone is highly (greater than 95%) protein bound to albumin and sex hormone binding globulin (SHBG). Levonorgestrel and 3-keto-desogestrel (the active metabolite of desogestrel) are 93–98 and 96% protein bound, respectively; levonorgestrel is about 34–50 or 48–65% bound to albumin or SHBG, respectively, while 3-keto-desogestrel is about 64 or 32% bound to albumin or SHBG, respectively. Drospirenone is about 97% protein bound, presumably to albumin. Etonogestrel is about 32% bound to SHBG and 66% bound to albumin. Norelgestromin is reportedly more than 97% bound to serum proteins (mainly albumin). Norgestimate, norelgestromin, drospirenone, and ethinyl estradiol do not appear to bind to SHBG. The binding capacity of SHBG for progestins is enhanced by ethinyl estradiol and by other enzyme-inducing drugs such as carbamazepine, phenobarbital, or rifampin. The binding of progestins to albumin and SHBG is low affinity, high capacity and high affinity, low capacity, respectively. Only the unbound fraction of contraceptive steroids is biologically active.

Contraceptive steroids may be distributed into bile. Small amounts of oral contraceptive steroids are also distributed into milk. The plasma-to-milk ratios of levonorgestrel and norethindrone concentrations are reportedly 100:15–100:25 and 100:10, respectively. It has been estimated that about 0.02% of a 50-mcg dose of ethinyl estradiol is distributed into milk.

● Elimination

The elimination half-life has been reported to be 11–45 hours for levonorgestrel, about 28 hours for norelgestromin, about 30 hours for drospirenone or etonogestrel, 5–14 hours for norethindrone, 6–45 hours for ethinyl estradiol, and 12–58 hours for 3-keto-desogestrel (the active metabolite of desogestrel). Serum concentrations of norethindrone return to near baseline levels 24 hours after a single 0.35-mg dose, making rigid adherence to once-daily administration necessary for efficacy. Plasma clearance of norethindrone and ethinyl estradiol each is about 0.4 L/hour per kg. Serum concentrations of norgestimate generally are below the lower detection limits of assay within 5 hours of single or multiple oral dosing, and determination of half-life of the drug may not be accurate. An elimination half-life of 12–30 hours has been reported for 17-acetyl norgestimate (an active metabolite of norgestimate). Following removal of the transdermal preparation containing ethinyl estradiol 0.75 mg and norelgestromin 6 mg (Ortho Evra®), serum concentrations of ethinyl estradiol and norelgestromin decline to low or undetectable concentrations within 3 days.

Oral contraceptive steroids are metabolized mainly in the liver and/or GI mucosa during absorption. Ethinyl estradiol and norethindrone appear to undergo extensive first-pass metabolism. Levonorgestrel does not appear to undergo first-pass metabolism.

Ethinyl estradiol is mainly metabolized via aromatic hydroxylation by hepatic microsomal isoenzyme cytochrome P-450 (CYP) 3A4. The major hydroxylated metabolite of ethinyl estradiol is 2-hydroxy-ethinylestradiol, which is thought to contribute to some of the adverse cardiovascular effects of the drug. The hydroxylated metabolite is further metabolized by methylation and glucuronidation prior to urinary and fecal excretion. Ethinyl estradiol and its metabolites undergo glucuronide and sulfate conjugation. The major first-pass metabolite of ethinyl estradiol is its sulfate conjugate. Ethinyl estradiol undergoes extensive enterohepatic circulation as glucuronide and sulfate conjugates. Bacteria in the GI tract hydrolyze these conjugates (excreted into the GI tract via bile), allowing reabsorption of ethinyl estradiol. Mestranol is rapidly metabolized mainly to ethinyl estradiol by demethylation; ethinyl estradiol is thought to be principally responsible for the estrogenic effects of mestranol. Following oral administration of a single 50- or 100-mcg dose of mestranol, the ratio of plasma mestranol to ethinyl estradiol concentrations is reportedly 0.24:1; in the usual oral dosages, mestranol and ethinyl estradiol are considered approximately equipotent.

Levonorgestrel and norethindrone are metabolized mainly by reduction, hydroxylation or oxidation, and glucuronide and sulfate conjugation. Unlike ethinyl estradiol, levonorgestrel and norethindrone do not undergo appreciable enterohepatic circulation; norethindrone is partially excreted, mainly as metabolites, in the feces via biliary elimination. Levonorgestrel and its metabolites are principally (40–68%) excreted in the urine. Desogestrel is rapidly and completely metabolized by hydroxylation in the intestinal mucosa and on first pass through the liver to 3-keto-desogestrel, a metabolite believed to be responsible for the pharmacologic actions of desogestrel; metabolites with no pharmacologic actions also have been identified and these metabolites may undergo glucuronide and sulfate conjugation. Norgestimate is metabolized extensively, mainly by hydrolysis, reduction, and hydroxylation to 17-deacetyl norgestimate, 3-keto-norgestimate, and levonorgestrel, metabolites that subsequently may undergo glucuronide and sulfate conjugation; however, it is believed that only 17-deactyl norgestimate contributes to the pharmacologic activity of norgestimate. Limited information is available on the pharmacokinetics of norethindrone acetate and ethynodiol diacetate; however, the drugs reportedly are rapidly metabolized to norethindrone. Drospirenone is metabolized to 2 major inactive metabolites, which according to one study are formed independently of the cytochrome P-450 enzyme system. The manufacturers state that drospirenone is metabolized only to a minor extent in vitro, mainly by CYP3A4. At least 20 metabolites have been detected in urine or feces.

Contraceptive steroids are excreted in urine and feces, principally as glucuronide and sulfate conjugates of the drugs and metabolites. Unchanged drug and unconjugated metabolites may also be excreted to some extent in urine and feces; although this may be particularly true for ethinyl estradiol, the metabolism and excretion of this and other oral contraceptive steroids is complex and variable, and specialized references should be consulted for more detailed information.

CHEMISTRY AND STABILITY

● Chemistry

Estrogen-progestin combination contraceptives contain estrogenic and progestinic steroids and are commercially available as oral tablets, an intravaginal ring, and a transdermal system.

The estrogenic component of commercially available oral contraceptive combinations is ethinyl estradiol or mestranol; the estrogenic component of vaginal and transdermal contraceptive combinations is ethinyl estradiol.

Ethinyl estradiol is a semisynthetic steroidal estrogen; the compound is the most orally active estrogenic drug currently available. The estrogenic potency of ethinyl estradiol is about 20 times that of diethylstilbestrol (no longer commercially available in the US). Mestranol, the 3-methyl ester of ethinyl estradiol, is slightly less active than ethinyl estradiol.

The progestinic component of commercially available oral contraceptive combinations is desogestrel, drospirenone, ethynodiol diacetate, levonorgestrel, norethindrone, norethindrone acetate, norgestimate, or norgestrel. These progestins are mainly derivatives of 19-nortestosterone; ethynodiol diacetate is a 17α-hydroxyprogesterone derivative, and drospirenone is structurally related to spironolactone. Norgestrel is a racemic mixture; levonorgestrel is the pharmacologically active isomer. In terms of oral progestational activity, desogestrel, levonorgestrel, and norgestrel are the most potent of these progestins and norethindrone is the least potent. Levonorgestrel and norgestrel have the greatest androgenic activity while norgestimate and norethindrone have the weakest androgenic activity. Desogestrel, etonogestrel, and norgestimate appear to have a substantially higher selectivity index (ratio of affinity for progesterone receptors versus affinity for androgen receptors) than conventional progestins (e.g., levonorgestrel, norethindrone). Drospirenone has progestational, antimineralocorticoid, and antiandrogenic activity.

The progestinic component of the commercially available transdermal system (Ortho Evra®) or contraceptive vaginal ring (NuvaRing®) is norelgestromin (the active metabolite of orally administered norgestimate) or etonogestrel (the active metabolite of desogestrel), respectively.

Intravaginal ethinyl estradiol in fixed combination with etonogestrel (NuvaRing®) is commercially available as a non-biodegradable, flexible ring that also contains magnesium stearate and ethylene vinyl acetate copolymers.

Transdermal ethinyl estradiol in fixed combination with norelgestromin (Ortho Evra®) is commercially available as a system that consists of an outer layer of polyethylene/polyester film and a drug reservoir consisting of ethinyl estradiol and norelgestromin in a polyisobutylene/polybutene adhesive matrix; a polyethylene terephthalate film is attached to the adhesive surface and should be removed prior to application.

● Stability

Estrogen-progestin combinations generally should be stored at room temperature in a well-closed container, unless otherwise specified by the manufacturer. Commercially available oral contraceptives are provided in mnemonic (memory-aid) dispensing packages which are exempted from the child-safety packaging requirements of the US Poison Prevention Packaging Act of 1970. Vaginal ethinyl estradiol in fixed combination with etonogestrel (Nuva Ring®) should be refrigerated at 2–8°C until dispensed. Once dispensed, the vaginal ring can be stored for up to 4 months at 25°C, but may be exposed to temperatures ranging from 15–30°C. Transdermal ethinyl estradiol in fixed combination with norelgestromin (Ortho Evra®) should be stored at 25°C, but may be exposed to temperatures ranging from 15–30°C. After removal from the protective pouch, the transdermal system should be applied immediately.

PREPARATIONS

Excipients in commercially available drug preparations may have clinically important effects in some individuals; consult specific product labeling for details.

Ethinyl Estradiol Combinations

Oral

Tablets, monophasic regimen	20 mcg with Drospirenone 3 mg*	Beyaz® (24 tablets with levomefolate calcium 0.451 mg plus 4 tablets containing only levomefolate calcium 0.451 mg), Bayer HealthCare
		Yaz® (24 tablets plus 4 inert tablets), Bayer HealthCare
	20 mcg with Levonorgestrel 0.09 mg	Lybrel® (28 tablets), Wyeth
	20 mcg with Levonorgestrel 0.1 mg	Alesse®-21 (21 tablets), Wyeth
		Alesse®-28 (21 tablets plus 7 inert tablets), Wyeth
		Aviane® 28 (21 tablets plus 7 inert tablets), Barr
		Lessina® 28 (21 tablets plus 7 inert tablets), Barr
		Levlite® 28 (21 tablets plus 7 inert tablets), Berlex
		LoSeasonique® (84 tablets plus 7 tablets containing ethinyl estradiol 10 mcg), Duramed
	20 mcg with Norethindrone Acetate 1 mg	Loestrin® 21 1/20 (21 tablets), Pfizer
		Loestrin® Fe 1/20 (21 tablets plus 7 tablets containing only ferrous fumarate 75 mg), Pfizer
		Loestrin® 24 Fe (24 tablets plus 4 tablets containing only ferrous fumarate 75 mg), Warner Chilcott
		Microgestin® Fe 1/20 (21 tablets plus 7 tablets containing only ferrous fumarate 75 mg), Watson
	30 mcg with Desogestrel 0.15 mg	Apri® 28 (21 tablets plus 7 inert tablets), Barr
		Desogen® (21 tablets plus 7 inert tablets), Organon
		Ortho-Cept® 28 (21 tablets plus 7 inert tablets), Janssen (formerly Ortho-McNeil)
	30 mcg with Drospirenone 3 mg*	Safyral® (21 tablets with levomefolate calcium 0.451 mg plus 7 tablets containing only levomefolate calcium 0.451 mg), Bayer HealthCare
		Yasmin® (21 tablets plus 7 inert tablets), Bayer HealthCare
	30 mcg with Levonorgestrel 0.15 mg	Levlen® 21 (21 tablets), Berlex
		Levlen® 28 (21 tablets plus 7 inert tablets), Berlex
		Levora® 0.15/30-28 (21 tablets plus 7 inert tablets), Watson
		Nordette®-28 (21 tablets plus 7 inert tablets), Monarch
		Portia® 28 (21 tablets plus 7 inert tablets), Barr
		Seasonale® (84 tablets plus 7 inert tablets), Duramed
		Seasonique® (84 tablets plus 7 tablets containing ethinyl estradiol 10 mcg), Duramed
	30 mcg with Norethindrone Acetate 1.5 mg	Loestrin® 21 1.5/30 (21 tablets), Pfizer
		Loestrin® Fe 1.5/30 (21 tablets plus 7 tablets containing only ferrous fumarate 75 mg), Pfizer
		Microgestin® Fe 1.5/30 (21 tablets plus 7 tablets containing only ferrous fumarate 75 mg), Watson
	30 mcg with Norgestrel 0.3 mg	Cryselle® (21 tablets plus 7 inert tablets), Barr
		Lo/Ovral® (21 tablets), Wyeth
		Lo/Ovral®-28 (21 tablets plus 7 inert tablets), Wyeth
		Low-Ogestrel® 28 (21 tablets plus 7 inert tablets), Watson
	35 mcg with Ethynodiol Diacetate 1 mg	Demulen 1/35®-21 (21 tablets), Pfizer
		Demulen 1/35®-28 (21 tablets plus 7 inert tablets), Pfizer
		Zovia® 1/35E-28 (21 tablets plus 7 inert tablets), Watson
	35 mcg with Norethindrone 0.4 mg	Ovcon®/35. 21-Day (21 tablets), Warner Chilcott
		Ovcon®/35 28-Day (21 tablets plus 7 inert tablets), Warner Chilcott
	35 mcg with Norethindrone 0.5 mg	Brevicon® 28-Day (21 tablets plus 7 inert tablets), Watson
		Modicon® 28 (21 tablets plus 7 inert tablets), Janssen (formerly Ortho-McNeil)
		Necon®-0.5/35-21 (21 tablets), Watson
		Necon®-0.5/35-28 (21 tablets plus 7 inert tablets), Watson
		Nelova® 0.5/35E 28 (21 tablets plus 7 inert tablets), Warner Chilcott
		Nortrel® 0.5/35 28 (21 tablets plus 7 inert tablets), Barr
	35 mcg with Norethindrone 1 mg	Necon®-1/35 28 (21 tablets plus 7 inert tablets), Watson
		Norinyl® 1+35 28-Day (21 tablets plus 7 inert tablets), Watson
		Nortrel® 1/35 21 (21 tablets), Barr
		Nortrel® 1/35 28 (21 tablets plus 7 inert tablets), Barr
		Ortho-Novum® 1/35 28 (21 tablets plus 7 inert tablets), Janssen (formerly Ortho-McNeil)
	35 mcg with Norgestimate 0.25 mg	MonoNessa® (21 tablets plus 7 inert tablets), Watson
		Ortho-Cyclen® 28 (21 tablets plus 7 inert tablets), Janssen (formerly Ortho-McNeil)
		Sprintec® (21 tablets plus 7 inert tablets), Barr

	50 mcg with Ethynodiol Diacetate 1 mg	**Demulen 1/50®-21** (21 tablets), Pfizer
		Demulen 1/50®-28 (21 tablets plus 7 inert tablets), Pfizer
		Zovia® 1/50E-28 (21 tablets plus 7 inert tablets), Watson
	50 mcg with Norethindrone 1 mg	**Ovcon®/50 28-Day** (21 tablets plus 7 inert tablets), Warner Chilcott
	50 mcg with Norgestrel 0.5 mg	**Ogestrel® 0.5/50-28** (21 tablets plus 7 inert tablets), Watson
		Ovral® (21 tablets), Wyeth
		Ovral®-28 (21 tablets plus 7 inert tablets), Wyeth
	20 mcg with Desogestrel 0.15 mg (21 tablets), and 10 mcg (5 tablets),	**Kariva®** (26 tablets plus 2 inert tablets), Barr
		Mircette® (26 tablets plus 2 inert tablets), Organon
Tablets, chewable	35 mcg with Norethindrone 0.4 mg	**Ovcon® 35 Fe** (21 tablets plus 7 tablets containing only ferrous fumarate 75 mg), Warner Chilcott
		Femcon® Fe (21 tablets plus 7 tablets containing only ferrous fumarate 75 mg), Warner Chilcott
Tablets, biphasic regimen	35 mcg with Norethindrone 0.5 mg (10 tablets) and 35 mcg with Norethindrone 1 mg (11 tablets)	**Necon® 10/11-21** (21 tablets), Watson
		Necon® 10/11-28 (21 tablets plus 7 inert tablets), Watson
Tablets, triphasic regimen	20 mcg with Norethindrone Acetate 1 mg (5 tablets), 30 mcg with Norethindrone Acetate 1 mg (7 tablets), and 35 mcg with Norethindrone Acetate 1 mg (9 tablets)	**Estrostep® 21** (21 tablets), Pfizer
		Estrostep® Fe (21 tablets plus 7 tablets containing only ferrous fumarate 75 mg), Pfizer
	25 mcg with Desogestrel 0.1 mg (7 tablets), 25 mcg with Desogestrel 0.125 mg (7 tablets), and 25 mcg with Desogestrel 0.150 mg (7 tablets)	**Cyclessa®** (21 tablets plus 7 inert tablets), Organon
	25 mcg with Norgestimate 0.18 mg (7 tablets), 25 mcg with Norgestimate 0.215 mg (7 tablets), and 25 mcg with Norgestimate 0.25 mg (7 tablets)	**Ortho Tri-Cyclen® Lo** (21 tablets plus 7 inert tablets), Janssen (formerly Ortho-McNeil)

	30 mcg with Levonorgestrel 0.05 mg (6 tablets), 40 mcg with Levonorgestrel 0.075 mg (5 tablets), and 30 mcg with Levonorgestrel 0.125 mg (10 tablets)	**Enpresse® 28** (21 tablets plus 7 inert tablets), Barr
		Tri-Levlen® 21 (21 tablets), Berlex
		Tri-Levlen® 28 (21 tablets plus 7 inert tablets), Berlex
		Triphasil®-21 (21 tablets), Wyeth
		Triphasil®-28 (21 tablets plus 7 inert tablets), Wyeth
		Trivora®-28 (21 tablets plus 7 inert tablets), Watson
	35 mcg with Norethindrone 0.5 mg (7 tablets), 35 mcg with Norethindrone 0.75 mg (7 tablets), and 35 mcg with Norethindrone 1 mg (7 tablets)	**Necon® 7/7/7** (21 tablets plus 7 inert tablets), Watson
		Ortho-Novum® 7/7/7 28 (21 tablets plus 7 inert tablets), Janssen (formerly Ortho-McNeil)
	35 mcg with Norethindrone 0.5 mg (7 tablets), 35 mcg with Norethindrone 1 mg (9 tablets), and 35 mcg with Norethindrone 0.5 mg (5 tablets)	**Tri-Norinyl®-28** (21 tablets plus 7 inert tablets), Watson
	35 mcg with Norgestimate 0.18 mg (7 tablets), 35 mcg with Norgestimate 0.215 mg (7 tablets), and 35 mcg with Norgestimate 0.25 mg (7 tablets)	**Ortho Tri-Cyclen® 28** (21 tablets plus 7 inert tablets), Janssen (formerly Ortho-McNeil)
		Tri-Sprintec® (21 tablets plus 7 inert tablets), Barr

| **Topical Transdermal System** | 0.75 mg with 6 mg Norelgestromin/20 cm² | **Ortho Evra®**, Janssen (formerly Ortho-McNeil) |
| **Vaginal Ring** | 0.015 mg with 0.12 mg Etonogestrel/24 hours (2.7 mg with 11.7 mg Etonogestrel/ring | **NuvaRing®**, Organon |

Mestranol Combinations

Oral Tablets, monophasic regimen	50 mcg with Norethindrone 1 mg	**Necon® 1/50-21** (21 tablets), Watson
		Necon® 1/50-28 (21 tablets plus 7 inert tablets), Watson
		Norinyl® 1+50 28-Day (21 tablets plus 7 inert tablets), Watson
		Ortho-Novum® 1/50 28 (21 tablets plus 7 inert tablets), Janssen (formerly Ortho-McNeil)

† Use is not currently included in the labeling approved by the US Food and Drug Administration.

Selected Revisions December 11, 2012, © Copyright, January 1, 1973, American Society of Health-System Pharmacists, Inc.

Progestins

68:12 · CONTRACEPTIVES

■ Etonogestrel, levonorgestrel, and norethindrone are synthetic progestin contraceptives.

USES

● **Contraception**

Oral Contraceptives

Norethindrone, in small doses (minipills), is used for the prevention of conception in women who elect to use oral contraceptives as a method of contraception. Progestin-only oral contraceptives are generally reserved for women who do not tolerate estrogens or in whom estrogens are contraindicated, since progestin-only oral contraceptives are less effective than estrogen-progestin combinations and require a high level of patient compliance. When taken according to the prescribed regimen, progestin-only oral contraceptives provide almost completely effective contraception. The efficacy of oral contraceptives mainly depends on compliance with the prescribed regimen. Progestin-only oral contraceptives must be taken daily, without interruption, to be effective.

Progestin-only oral contraceptives are reported to be somewhat less effective than estrogen-progestin combinations. The pregnancy rate in women using progestin-only oral contraceptives is generally reported to be about 3 pregnancies per 100 woman-years of use. For information on the pregnancy rates reported with other methods of contraception, including estrogen-progestin combinations, see Uses in Estrogen-Progestin Combinations 68:12. Pregnancy rates are derived from various studies conducted by different investigators in different population groups and, therefore, cannot be compared precisely.

In women receiving norethindrone, the pregnancy rate, especially during the first 6 months of use, is reportedly greater in women who had not previously received oral contraceptives than in those who had been immediately switched from an estrogen-progestin combination. The reported difference in pregnancy rates probably resulted from failure to comply with the prescribed regimen. Therefore, it is especially important that women who are prescribed progestin-only oral contraceptives as initial oral contraception be advised to strictly adhere to the prescribed regimen.

For the use of norethindrone or norethindrone acetate in combination with estrogens as an oral contraceptive, see Estrogen-Progestin Combinations 68:12. For the use of the drugs in the treatment of secondary amenorrhea, endometriosis, or abnormal uterine bleeding, see Norethindrone 68:32.

Intrauterine System

Levonorgestrel-releasing intrauterine system is used for prevention of conception in women who elect to use this method of contraception. The manufacturer states that the system is recommended for use in women who have had one or more children; are in a stable, mutually monogamous relationship; have no history of pelvic inflammatory disease (PID); and have no history of ectopic pregnancy or any condition that would predispose to ectopic pregnancy. Each system may be used for up to 5 years; thereafter, the system should be removed and may be replaced with a new system if continued contraception is desired. The pregnancy rate in women using the levonorgestrel-releasing intrauterine system is reported as up to 0.2 pregnancies per 100 women during the first year of use; the cumulative 5-year pregnancy rate is reported to be approximately 0.7 pregnancies per 100 women.

Subcutaneous Implants

Etonogestrel for subcutaneous implantation (Implanon®) is used for prevention of conception in women who elect to use this method of contraception. The system consists of a single rod containing etonogestrel that is implanted subcutaneously in the upper arm to provide contraception for up to 3 years.

Postcoital (Emergency) Contraception

Levonorgestrel is used as an emergency contraceptive (EC) to prevent pregnancy following unprotected intercourse or known or suspected contraceptive failure. To achieve optimal efficacy, the postcoital contraceptive regimen should be initiated as soon as possible within 72 hours of unprotected intercourse. Studies show

that emergency contraception is moderately effective when the regimen is administered up to 120 hours after unprotected intercourse. Postcoital contraceptive efficacy diminishes as the time period between intercourse and initiation of contraception increases.

An emergency contraceptive regimen employing a progestin alone (levonorgestrel) appears to be more effective and better tolerated than a common estrogen-progestin emergency contraceptive ("Yuzpe") regimen when the regimens are initiated within 72 hours of unprotected intercourse; therefore, the progestin-only regimen generally is preferred when readily available. In a double-blind, randomized multicenter study in women who reported unprotected intercourse within 72 hours of receiving emergency contraception, a single-dose of levonorgestrel 1.5 mg was as effective in preventing pregnancy as levonorgestrel 0.75 mg every 12 hours for 2 doses. In a double-blind, randomized, multicenter study in women who reported only one act of unprotected intercourse within 72 hours of receiving emergency contraception, the expected pregnancy (failure) rate of 8% (with no contraception) was reduced to approximately 1% with a progestin-only regimen (levonorgestrel 0.75 mg every 12 hours for 2 doses). In another prospective, randomized study in women who reported a single act of intercourse within 48 hours of receiving emergency contraception, failure rates with the 2-dose levonorgestrel regimen and Yuzpe regimens (levonorgestrel 0.5 mg and 0.1 mg ethinyl estradiol every 12 hours for 2 doses) were similar (2.6 versus 2.4%, respectively). The efficacy of treatment in both studies was greatest when the contraceptive was given during the first 24 hours after unprotected intercourse; efficacy declined during subsequent 24-hour periods. The 2-dose levonorgestrel regimen was better tolerated than the Yuzpe regimen. In these 2 studies, nausea occurred in 23.1 versus 50.5% and in 16.1 versus 46.5% of women receiving the 2-dose levonorgestrel regimen versus the Yuzpe regimen, respectively, while vomiting occurred in 5.6 versus 18.8% and in 2.7 versus 22.4% of women with the 2-dose levonorgestrel regimen or Yuzpe regimen, respectively.

Since unprotected intercourse that occurs outside the fertile period is unlikely to result in conception, not all women given emergency postcoital contraception are at genuine risk for pregnancy. Therefore, a more accurate indication of the efficacy of postcoital contraceptive regimens would be based on the timing of unprotected intercourse and the probability that pregnancy would occur without treatment. Analysis of data from the multicenter, progestin-only (levonorgestrel) study involving approximately 2000 women suggest that when efficacy of postcoital contraception is based on the observed versus expected number of pregnancies, the levonorgestrel-only regimen would prevent 85% of pregnancies; pooled analysis of observed-versus-expected pregnancy data from other studies employing the Yuzpe regimen suggest that such therapy is approximately 74% effective in preventing pregnancy. However, postcoital (emergency) contraceptive regimens are not as effective as most other forms of long-term contraception.

Since postcoital contraceptive efficacy diminishes as the time period between intercourse and administration of the regimen increases, available data suggest that as with combination estrogen-progestin regimens, progestin-only postcoital contraception should ideally begin within 72 hours of unprotected intercourse. Emergency contraception is moderately effective when the regimen is administered up to 120 hours after unprotected intercourse. The effectiveness of postcoital contraception administered after more than 120 hours has not been established.

The American College of Obstetricians and Gynecologists (ACOG), other experts, and some states (e.g., Alaska, California, Hawaii, Maine, New Mexico, Washington) have advocated increased access to emergency postcoital contraception (e.g., nonprescription access via pharmacies, advance provision by clinicians) as a means of decreasing unintended pregnancy and abortion rates. There is some evidence that increased access to emergency postcoital contraception may not compromise conventional contraceptive use or sexual behavior, potentially allaying some concerns that have prompted others to advocate for restricted access. The FDA has approved the single-dose levonorgestrel regimen (Plan B One-Step®) for nonprescription (over-the-counter [OTC]) status for women of childbearing potential regardless of age. Another FDA-approved product (Next Choice One Dose®) is commercially available as a single-dose levonorgestrel regimen for OTC status in women 17 years of age or older or as a prescription-only preparation in women younger than 17 years of age. A 2-dose levonorgestrel preparation is also commercially available as a prescription-only preparation for women younger than 17 years of age.

For information on the use of combination estrogen-progestin contraceptives for postcoital contraception, see Contraception: Postcoital Contraception under Uses, in Estrogen-Progestin Combinations 68:12.

DOSAGE AND ADMINISTRATION

● *Administration*

Norethindrone is administered orally once daily. The tablets should be taken at the same time each day and continued daily without interruption, including throughout all bleeding episodes. Women should be advised to inform a clinician if prolonged bleeding, amenorrhea, or severe abdominal pain occurs.

Levonorgestrel is administered orally or as a levonorgestrel-releasing intrauterine device.

If vomiting occurs within 2 hours following administration of levonorgestrel (e.g., Plan B One-Step®, Next Choice One Dose®) for postcoital contraception, a clinician should be contacted to discuss the need for repeating the dose. If vomiting occurs within 2 hours following administration of the first or second dose of the levonorgestrel 2-dose regimen for emergency contraception, a clinician should be contacted to discuss the need for taking another dose.

Levonorgestrel-releasing intrauterine system should be inserted into the uterine cavity under strict aseptic conditions following a complete review of the patient's medical and social histories, exclusion of pregnancy, and physical examination (including pelvic examination, Papanicolaou test [Pap smear], and appropriate laboratory tests for other genital diseases [e.g., gonorrhea, chlamydia] as indicated). Special attention should be given to determining whether the woman is at risk for ectopic pregnancy or pelvic inflammatory disease (PID). Patients should be reexamined shortly after the first menstrual period following insertion of the device to verify that the device is properly positioned. The manufacturer's labeling should be consulted for proper methods of inserting and removing the levonorgestrel-releasing intrauterine system and for associated precautions.

Etonogestrel is administered as a nonbiodegradable implant that is inserted subcutaneously in the inner aspect of the upper arm. The manufacturer's labeling should be consulted for the proper method of administration and associated precautions.

● *Dosage*

Contraception

Oral Dosage

The daily dose of progestin-only oral contraceptives is 0.35 mg of norethindrone. Therapy should begin on the first day of menstruation and should be continued each day of the year without interruption. If therapy begins on another day, the woman should be advised to use a back-up method of contraception (e.g., condom, spermicide) for each sexual encounter during the first 48 hours. Women who have had a miscarriage or an abortion may begin progestin-only oral contraceptives the next day. Women who are exclusively breast-feeding their infants may begin therapy 6 weeks after delivery; women whose infants are only partially breast-fed may begin therapy with the drug 3 weeks after delivery.

If a norethindrone dose is taken more than 3 hours late or if one or more consecutive doses are missed, the last missed dose should be taken as soon as it is remembered, followed by resumption of the regular schedule; a back-up method of contraception (e.g., condom, spermicide) should be used for each sexual encounter during the next 48 hours. If the woman is unsure of what drug regimen to take as a result of missed doses, a back-up method of contraception should be used for each sexual encounter, and one tablet should be taken each day until the clinician can be contacted.

If vomiting occurs soon after a dose, a back-up method of contraception (e.g., condom, spermicide) should be used for each sexual encounter during the next 48 hours.

If a menstrual period is delayed and norethindrone has not been taken exactly as directed, or if 45 days have elapsed since the beginning of the last menstrual period, the possibility of pregnancy should be excluded. If pregnancy is confirmed, the woman should be advised to discontinue the progestin-only oral contraceptive.

Intrauterine Dosage

Each levonorgestrel-releasing intrauterine system contains 52 mg of the drug and is intended to be used for periods of up to 5 years. When the levonorgestrel-releasing intrauterine system is used for contraception, the system is inserted into the uterine cavity within 7 days of the onset of menses. In postpartum women, the levonorgestrel-releasing intrauterine system should not be inserted until at least 6 weeks postpartum or until involution of the uterus is complete. The system may be inserted immediately after a first-trimester abortion, but insertion following a second-trimester abortion should be delayed until involution of the uterus is complete.

The levonorgestrel-releasing intrauterine system should be removed after 5 years of use, since contraceptive efficacy beyond 5 years has not been established. In women who wish to continue contraception with the levonorgestrel-releasing intrauterine system, a new system may be inserted immediately following removal of the existing system. The system can be removed and replaced with a new system at any time during the menstrual cycle. For women with regular menstrual cycles who wish to initiate an alternative contraceptive method, the intrauterine system should be removed during the first 7 days of a menstrual cycle and the new method started. For those with irregular cycles or amenorrhea or for those in whom the system is removed after the seventh day of the menstrual cycle, the new contraceptive method should be initiated at least 7 days before removal of the intrauterine system.

Subcutaneous Dosage

Etonogestrel implant contains 68 mg of the drug and is intended to be used for periods of up to 3 years.

When an etonogestrel implant is used for contraception, timing of insertion depends on the patient's history. To initiate therapy in women who did not use hormonal contraception in the preceding month, the etonogestrel implant usually is inserted on or before day 5 of the cycle (the first day of bleeding is counted as the first day of the menstrual cycle). When switching from other contraceptive methods, therapy with etonogestrel should be initiated in a manner that ensures continuous contraceptive coverage based on the mechanism of action of both methods (e.g., etonogestrel implant should be inserted within 7 days of the last hormonally active tablet, or removal of a transdermal patch or vaginal ring in women switching from combined estrogen-progestin contraceptives; etonogestrel implant may be inserted on any day of the month in women switching from a progestin-only oral contraceptive [without skipping any day between receiving the last progestin oral contraceptive and the initial administration of the implant]; etonogestrel implant should be inserted within the dosing period recommended for the parenteral contraceptive preparation in women switching from a progestin-only contraceptive injection; etonogestrel implant should be inserted on the same day as a progestin-containing intrauterine device is removed in women switching from this device). The implant may be inserted immediately after a first-trimester abortion or 21–28 days following a second-trimester abortion. Etonogestrel implant may be inserted 21–28 days postpartum in women who are only partially breast-feeding their infant or after the fourth postpartum week in women who are exclusively breast-feeding their infant. The manufacturer states that a back-up method of contraception is not needed when etonogestrel therapy is initiated according to one of these schedules. The implant is removed 3 years after insertion. In women who wish to continue contraception with etonogestrel implant, a new implant should be inserted on the same day as the existing implant is removed.

Postcoital (Emergency) Contraception

When levonorgestrel is used alone as a short-course, progestin-only emergency postcoital contraceptive, a single 1.5-mg dose of levonorgestrel is administered as soon as possible within 72 hours of unprotected intercourse. Alternatively, a levonorgestrel dose of 0.75 mg is administered as soon as possible within 72 hours of unprotected intercourse, followed by a repeat dose of 0.75 mg 12 hours after the first dose. Regardless of regimen, the first dose can be taken up to 120 hours after unprotected intercourse if necessary, but efficacy decreases as initiation of contraception becomes more remote from unprotected intercourse. Commercial preparations containing one levonorgestrel 1.5-mg tablet (e.g., Plan B® One-Step, Next Choice One Dose®) are available for this purpose. The FDA has approved Plan B® One-Step for nonprescription (over-the-counter [OTC]) status for women of childbearing potential regardless of age. A commercial preparation containing 2 levonorgestrel 0.75-mg tablets also is available for postcoital contraception. The levonorgestrel postcoital contraceptive regimens may be used at any time during the menstrual cycle. Since postcoital contraceptive efficacy diminishes as the time period between intercourse and administration of the regimen increases, postcoital contraception with levonorgestrel should begin as soon as possible but within 72–120 hours of unprotected intercourse. The effectiveness of postcoital contraception administered after more than 120 hours has not been established.

Repeated postcoital (emergency) contraception use indicates the need for counseling about other contraceptive options. Safety of recurrent use has not been established but the risk appears to be low, even within the same menstrual cycle. The possibility that risk of adverse effects (e.g., menstrual irregularities) may be increased with frequently repeated postcoital contraception should be considered.

CAUTIONS

● Adverse Effects

Although common adverse effects of estrogen-progestin oral contraceptives appear to be mainly caused by the estrogen, it has not been determined whether the adverse effects associated with low-dose oral progestin regimens differ from those resulting from administration of estrogen-progestin combinations. There is some evidence that the progestin component plays a major role in the development of some adverse effects of oral contraceptives when combined with estrogens. The potency and type of progestin in estrogen-progestin combinations appear to have important effects on lipoprotein lipids (high-density and low-density lipoproteins) and may contribute to the increased risk of arteriosclerotic disease in oral contraceptive users. Pending further accumulation of data on progestin-only oral contraceptives, the same precautions associated with estrogen-progestin combination therapy should be observed with progestin-only preparations. For a complete discussion of the cautions, precautions, and contraindications of oral contraceptives, see Cautions in Estrogen-Progestin Combinations 68:12.

The most frequent adverse effects of continuous oral low-dose progestin administration are menstrual irregularity, changes in menstrual flow, and/or amenorrhea, which may be difficult to differentiate from pregnancy. In clinical trials, these adverse effects caused a higher drop-out rate than that observed with estrogen-progestin oral contraceptives. Like the estrogen-progestin combination oral contraceptives, progestins can cause breakthrough bleeding, spotting, edema, weight gain, nausea, breast tenderness, headache, and mental depression; however, the incidence and severity of these adverse effects are much less with progestins than with estrogen-progestin combinations. Progestin-only oral contraceptives occasionally may alter lipid metabolism, resulting in decreased concentrations of high-density lipoprotein [HDL]-cholesterol, HDL$_2$, apolipoprotein A-I (apo A-I), and apolipoprotein A-II (apo A-II), and increased concentrations of hepatic lipase. There usually is no effect on concentrations of total cholesterol, HDL$_3$, low-density lipoprotein (LDL)-cholesterol, or very low-density lipoprotein (VLDL)-cholesterol.

Adverse effects reported in 5% or more of women using the levonorgestrel-releasing intrauterine system include abdominal pain, leukorrhea, headache, vaginitis, back pain, breast pain, acne, depression, hypertension, upper respiratory infection, nausea, nervousness, dysmenorrhea, weight increase, skin disorder, decreased libido, abnormal Papanicolaou test (Pap smear), and sinusitis.

Adverse effects reported in 5% or more of women using the etonogestrel implant include headache, vaginitis, weight increase, acne, breast pain, upper respiratory infection, abdominal pain, pharyngitis, leukorrhea, influenza-like symptoms, dizziness, dysmenorrhea, back pain, emotional lability, nausea, pain, nervousness, sinusitis, depression, and insertion site pain.

Limited data from 2 comparative studies in which women receiving emergency postcoital contraception with either an estrogen-progestin regimen (levonorgestrel 0.5 mg and 100 mcg ethinyl estradiol every 12 hours for 2 doses) or a progestin-only regimen (levonorgestrel 0.75 mg every 12 hours for 2 doses) indicate a lower incidence of nausea or vomiting with the progestin-only (levonorgestrel) regimen. In these 2 studies, nausea occurred in 23.1 versus 50.5% and in 16.1 versus 46.5% of women receiving the 2-dose levonorgestrel regimen versus the estrogen-progestin regimen, respectively, while vomiting occurred in 5.6 versus 18.8% and in 2.7 versus 22.4% of women with the levonorgestrel- or estrogen-progestin regimen, respectively. Other adverse effects occurring in one of these studies with the 2-dose levonorgestrel regimen included nausea (23% of patients), abdominal pain (17.6% of patients), fatigue (16.9% of patients), headache (16.8% of patients), heavier or lighter menstrual bleeding (13.8 or 12.5% of patients, respectively), dizziness (11.2% of patients), breast tenderness (10.7% of patients), vomiting (5.6% of patients), or diarrhea (5% of patients). Adverse effects reported with the single-dose levonorgestrel regimen include heavier menstrual bleeding (30.9% of patients), nausea (13.7% of patients), lower abdominal pain (13.3% of patients), fatigue (13.3% of patients), headache (10.3% of patients), dizziness (9.6% of patients), breast tenderness (8.2% of patients), or more than a 7-day delay in menses (4.5% of patients). In addition, some evidence indicates that emergency postcoital contraception may not compromise conventional contraception use or sexual behavior (e.g., promiscuity, sexually transmitted disease [STD] risk).

Other adverse reactions which have been reported in women receiving progestins are weight gain or loss, changes in cervical erosion and secretions, cholestatic jaundice, allergic rash with or without pruritus, melasma or chloasma, breast changes (tenderness, enlargement, and secretion), and hirsutism.

● Precautions and Contraindications

It is good medical practice that all women, including those receiving progestin-only oral contraceptives, have a complete medical history and physical examination performed periodically (e.g., annually); the physical examination may be deferred until after initiation of therapy if requested by the woman and judged appropriate by the clinician. Physical examination is not required prior to initiating therapy with oral levonorgestrel for postcoital (emergency) contraception. In women receiving the levonorgestrel-releasing intrauterine system, complete medical and social histories (including those of the partner) and physical examination (including pelvic examination, Papanicolaou test [Pap smear], and appropriate laboratory tests for other genital diseases [e.g., gonorrhea, chlamydia] as indicated) should be performed, and pregnancy should be excluded prior to insertion of the intrauterine system; special attention should be given to determining whether the woman is at risk for ectopic pregnancy or pelvic inflammatory disease (PID).

Safety and efficacy of progestin contraceptives have been established in women of reproductive age. Safety and efficacy of long-term progestin contraceptives are expected to be identical for postpubertal adolescents younger than 16 years of age and women 16 years of age or older. Safety and efficacy of progestin emergency contraceptives are expected to be identical for postpubertal adolescents younger than 17 years of age and women 17 years of age or older. Progestin contraceptives are not indicated before menarche.

Progestin contraceptives have not been evaluated in women older than 65 years of age and these drugs are not indicated for use in postmenopausal women.

Slight deterioration in glucose tolerance, coupled with increases in plasma insulin concentrations, may occur in some patients receiving progestin-only contraceptives. However, in women with diabetes mellitus receiving progestin-only contraceptives, insulin requirements generally are unchanged. Nevertheless, prediabetic or diabetic women should be carefully monitored while receiving these contraceptives.

Headache, including migraine headache, has been reported during progestin-only contraceptive therapy. Progestin-only oral contraceptives should be discontinued and the cause evaluated when migraine occurs or is exacerbated, or when severe, persistent, or recurrent headache develops.

Because the presence of organisms capable of causing PID cannot be determined by appearance, and because insertion of an intrauterine system may be associated with introduction of vaginal bacteria into the uterus, the levonorgestrel-releasing intrauterine system should be inserted under strict aseptic conditions. Administration of anti-infectives may be considered; however, the benefit of such prophylactic measure is unknown. Syncope, bradycardia, or other neurovascular episodes may occur during insertion or removal of the intrauterine system, particularly in women predisposed to these conditions or in those with cervical stenosis. If decreased pulse, perspiration, or pallor is observed, the woman should remain supine until these signs have disappeared. Women receiving the levonorgestrel-releasing intrauterine system who have certain types of valvular or congenital heart disease and surgically constructed systemic-pulmonary shunts are at increased risk of infective endocarditis and, possibly, septic embolism. Women with known congenital heart disease who may be at increased risk should receive appropriate anti-infectives at the time of insertion and removal of the intrauterine system. Women requiring chronic corticosteroid therapy or insulin for diabetes mellitus should be carefully monitored for development of infection. The levonorgestrel-releasing intrauterine system should be used with caution in women who have a coagulopathy or are receiving anticoagulants. Use of the intrauterine system in women with vaginitis or cervicitis should be postponed until appropriate treatment has eradicated the infection and until it has been determined that the cervicitis is not caused by *Neisseria gonorrhoeae* or *Chlamydia*.

Because the levonorgestrel-releasing intrauterine system may be displaced following insertion, women should be reexamined and evaluated shortly after the first postinsertion menses, but definitely within 3 months after insertion. During examination, the removal threads of the intrauterine system should be located; if the threads are not visible, location of the system should be verified (e.g., by radiograph or ultrasound, by gentle exploration of the uterine cavity with a probe). If the intrauterine system is in place with no evidence of perforation, no intervention is indicated. If the system is verified as displaced, it should be removed, and a new system may be inserted at that time or during the next menses if it is certain that conception has not occurred. If expulsion has occurred, the system may be replaced within 7 days of a menstrual period after pregnancy has been excluded. Partial or complete expulsion of any intrauterine system may result in bleeding or pain; however, expulsion may occur without the woman's knowledge.

Concomitant use of progestin-only contraceptives with drugs that induce hepatic microsomal enzymes (e.g., barbiturates, carbamazepine, phenytoin, HIV protease inhibitors, rifampin, St. John's wort [*Hypericum perforatum*]) reduces contraceptive efficacy, possibly resulting in unintended pregnancy or break-through bleeding. Effects of hepatic enzyme inducers on the contraceptive efficacy of the levonorgestrel-releasing intrauterine system have not been evaluated. No significant interaction has been found when progestin-only oral contraceptives are used concomitantly with broad-spectrum anti-infectives.

Women should be informed that progestin-only contraceptives do not protect against human immunodeficiency virus (HIV) infection or other sexually transmitted diseases.

Levonorgestrel 0.75 or 1.5 mg used for postcoital (emergency) contraception is not effective in terminating an existing pregnancy. Rapid return of fertility is likely following use of levonorgestrel for postcoital contraception. Routine methods of contraception should be continued or initiated as soon as possible following use of levonorgestrel to ensure ongoing pregnancy prevention.

Women receiving progestin-only oral contraceptives should be advised to take the tablets exactly as directed and at the same time every day, including throughout all bleeding episodes. (See Dosage and Administration.) Women should be advised to inform a clinician if prolonged bleeding, amenorrhea, or severe abdominal pain occurs. Although progestin-only oral contraceptives do not affect the quality or quantity of breast milk in lactating women, isolated cases of decreased milk production have been reported, and lactating women are advised to contact a clinician if they are not producing enough milk. The World Health Organization states that nursing women can continue to breast-feed without restriction during postcoital (emergency) contraceptive regimens.

Women considering use of the levonorgestrel-releasing intrauterine system should be encouraged to review the manufacturer's patient information and to discuss with a clinician the risks and benefits associated with the use of an intrauterine contraceptive system. Following insertion of the intrauterine system, women should be instructed on how to check after their menstrual period to ensure that the removal threads still protrude from the cervix and should be cautioned not to pull on the threads and displace the system.

Irregular menstrual patterns are common in women receiving progestin-only contraceptives. If genital bleeding patterns are suggestive of infection, malignancy, or other pathologic causes, such causes should be ruled out. If prolonged amenorrhea develops in women receiving progestin-only oral contraceptives, the possibility of pregnancy should be evaluated. In women using the levonorgestrel-releasing intrauterine system, the number of days of bleeding and spotting may be increased and bleeding patterns may be irregular during the first 3–6 months of use; thereafter, bleeding may remain irregular but the number of days with bleeding or spotting is decreased. If bleeding irregularities develop during prolonged use of the levonorgestrel-releasing intrauterine system, pathologic causes should be ruled out. Amenorrhea develops within 1 year in about 20% of women using the levonorgestrel-releasing intrauterine system. The possibility of pregnancy should be considered in women using this contraceptive method if menstruation does not occur within 6 weeks of the onset of the previous menstrual period. Once pregnancy has been excluded, repeated pregnancy tests are not required in women using the levonorgestrel-releasing intrauterine system in the absence of other evidence of pregnancy or unless pelvic pain is present.

Delayed atresia of ovarian follicles, with resulting follicular enlargement, may occur in patients receiving progestins. Follicular enlargement generally is asymptomatic or associated with mild abdominal pain and resolves spontaneously; in rare cases, surgery may be required.

The rate of ectopic pregnancy in women receiving progestin-only oral contraceptives has been reported as 5 ectopic pregnancies per 1000 woman-years of use. Up to 10% of pregnancies reported in clinical trials in women receiving progestin-only oral contraceptives have been ectopic. The possibility of ectopic pregnancy should be considered whenever a patient receiving a low-dose progestin oral contraceptive becomes pregnant or experiences severe lower abdominal pain. A follow-up physical or pelvic examination is recommended by the manufacturers if there is any question regarding the general health or pregnancy status of a woman following administration of levonorgestrel 0.75 or 1.5 mg for postcoital (emergency) contraception. The manufacturers state that a history of ectopic pregnancy does not need to be considered a contraindication to progestin-only oral contraceptives.

The rate of ectopic pregnancy in clinical trials in women using the levonorgestrel-releasing intrauterine system has been reported to be 1 ectopic pregnancy per 1000 woman-years of use, a rate not substantially different from that in sexually active women not using any contraceptive method. About one-half of the pregnancies reported during these clinical trials were ectopic. Patients with a history of ectopic pregnancy were excluded from clinical trials of the levonorgestrel-releasing

intrauterine system, and use of this contraceptive method is not recommended in women with a history of ectopic pregnancy or conditions that may predispose to ectopic pregnancy. Women using the levonorgestrel-releasing intrauterine system should be taught to recognize and report symptoms of ectopic pregnancy.

In women who have intrauterine pregnancies while using an intrauterine contraceptive device, septic abortion (resulting in septicemia, septic shock, and death) can occur. If pregnancy occurs in a woman using the levonorgestrel-releasing intrauterine system, the intrauterine system should be removed. Removal or manipulation of the system may result in pregnancy loss. If the system cannot be removed or if the woman chooses not to have the system removed, she should be advised that failure to remove the system increases the risk of miscarriage, sepsis, and premature labor and delivery, and she should be followed closely and advised to report immediately any flu-like symptoms, fever, chills, cramping, pain, bleeding, vaginal discharge, or leakage of fluid. The long-term effects on the fetus of leaving the levonorgestrel-releasing system in place as the pregnancy progresses are unknown. Clinical experience with pregnancy outcomes in such cases is limited, and the possibility of teratogenic effects cannot be completely excluded. Congenital anomalies have been reported infrequently when the levonorgestrel-releasing system was not removed; however, the role of the levonorgestrel-releasing system in the development of these anomalies has not been established.

Group A streptococcal sepsis has been reported rarely following insertion of the levonorgestrel-releasing intrauterine system. Severe pain has occurred within hours of insertion, followed by onset of sepsis within several days. Use of strict aseptic technique during insertion of the device is essential.

Use of intrauterine contraceptive devices is associated with an increased risk of PID, with the highest risk occurring shortly (generally within 20 days) after insertion of the device. The decision to use the levonorgestrel-releasing intrauterine system should include consideration of the risk of PID. If the woman or her partner has multiple sexual partners, risk of PID is increased and the levonorgestrel-releasing intrauterine system should not be used. Risk also is increased in women with a history of PID, and use of the device is contraindicated in such women unless there has been a subsequent intrauterine pregnancy. All women who are considering use of the levonorgestrel-releasing intrauterine system should be informed of the possibility of PID and long-term sequelae (tubal damage resulting in ectopic pregnancy or infertility or, less often, hysterectomy or death) and should be taught to recognize signs and symptoms of PID (e.g., prolonged or heavy bleeding, unusual vaginal discharge, abdominal or pelvic pain or tenderness, dyspareunia, chills, fever). PID may be asymptomatic but still result in tubal damage and long-term sequelae. If PID is suspected or confirmed, the patient should be promptly evaluated and appropriate treatment initiated.

Actinomycosis also has been reported in association with intrauterine contraceptive devices. If symptomatic actinomycosis occurs, the intrauterine system should be removed and appropriate anti-infective treatment initiated. Management of asymptomatic patients is controversial.

Partial penetration or embedment of the levonorgestrel-releasing intrauterine system in the myometrium may decrease contraceptive efficacy and make removal of the device difficult. If perforation of the uterus or cervix occurs, the device must be removed and surgery may be required. Potential complications include adhesions, peritonitis, intestinal perforation or obstruction, abscesses, and erosion of adjacent viscera. The risk of perforation is increased in lactating women. To decrease the risk of perforation in postpartum women and in women who have undergone a second-trimester abortion, insertion of the device should be delayed until uterine involution is complete.

The levonorgestrel-releasing intrauterine system should be removed if any of the following occur: menorrhagia and/or metrorrhagia producing anemia, HIV infection, sexually transmitted disease, pelvic infection, endometritis, symptomatic genital actinomycosis, intractable pelvic pain, severe dyspareunia, pregnancy, endometrial or cervical malignancy, or uterine or cervical perforation. Removal of the intrauterine system also should be considered if any of the following conditions arise for the first time: migraine, focal migraine with asymmetrical visual loss or other manifestations indicating transient cerebral ischemia, exceptionally severe headache, jaundice, marked increase of blood pressure, or severe arterial disease (e.g., stroke, myocardial infarction).

The manufacturers state that progestin-only oral contraceptives are contraindicated in women who are hypersensitive to the drug or any ingredient in the formulation and in those with known or suspected pregnancy, undiagnosed abnormal genital bleeding, active liver disease, benign or malignant liver tumor, or known or suspected carcinoma of the breast. In addition to the usual contraindications associated with oral progestin therapy, the levonorgestrel-releasing intrauterine system is contraindicated in patients with congenital or acquired uterine anomalies (including fibroids) if they distort the uterine cavity, acute PID or a history of

PID unless there has been a subsequent intrauterine pregnancy, postpartum endometritis or infected abortion in the previous 3 months, known or suspected uterine or cervical neoplasia or an unresolved abnormal Papanicolaou test (Pap smear) result, untreated acute cervicitis or vaginitis (including bacterial vaginosis or other lower genital tract infection until the infection is controlled), conditions associated with increased susceptibility to infection (e.g., leukemia, acquired immunodeficiency syndrome [AIDS], IV drug abuse), genital actinomycosis, or a history of ectopic pregnancy or any condition that would predispose to ectopic pregnancy. The levonorgestrel-releasing intrauterine system also is contraindicated if a previously inserted intrauterine contraceptive device has not been removed or if the woman or her partner has multiple sexual partners.

Most experts state that there currently is no real contraindication to postcoital (emergency) contraception with the recommended regimens and that the benefits generally outweigh any theoretical or proven risk. Levonorgestrel for emergency contraception should not be used as a woman's routine form of contraception. In addition, use of levonorgestrel for emergency contraception is not recommended in women who are hypersensitive to the drug or any ingredient in the formulation or in those with known or suspected pregnancy.

DRUG INTERACTIONS

For information on drug interactions associated with oral contraceptives, see Drug Interactions in Estrogen-Progestin Combinations 68:12.

LABORATORY TEST INTERFERENCES

For information on laboratory test interferences associated with oral contraceptives, see Laboratory Test Interferences in Estrogen-Progestin Combinations 68:12.

PHARMACOLOGY

Norethindrone shares the actions of progestins. Although the exact mechanism of action of progestin-only oral contraceptives is not known, norethindrone, when administered in usual contraceptive doses, appears to act principally by altering cervical mucus so that sperm migration into the uterus is inhibited. Progestational changes in the endometrium also occur which may inhibit implantation of the fertilized ovum in the uterus. In addition, continuous administration of low doses of norethindrone alters the rate of ovum transport by changing motility and secretion in fallopian tubes. Norethindrone prevents pregnancy even in the presence of ovulation. Norethindrone suppresses ovulation and causes ovarian and endometrial atrophy at high doses; the drug does not consistently suppress ovulation when administered in a continuous low-dose regimen. In low doses, norethindrone causes variable suppression of follicle-stimulating hormone (FSH) and luteinizing hormone (LH). Norethindrone has mild androgenic activity. At low doses, norethindrone also has some estrogenic activity.

The precise mechanism of contraceptive activity of levonorgestrel administered *after* intercourse (postcoital) is not known. Levonorgestrel has been shown to inhibit or delay ovulation or fertilization; other mechanisms of action for preventing pregnancy presumably are involved. Levonorgestrel is only effective before pregnancy is established. Once implantation occurs, levonorgestrel is ineffective in preventing pregnancy.

PHARMACOKINETICS

For a discussion on the absorption, distribution, and elimination of oral contraceptive steroids, including norethindrone, see Pharmacokinetics in Estrogen-Progestin Combinations 68:12.

Following insertion of an intrauterine system containing 52 mg of levonorgestrel (Mirena®), the drug is initially released into the uterine cavity at a rate of 20 mcg per day. The rate of drug release decreases progressively to about one-half of the initial rate after 5 years of use. Plasma levonorgestrel concentrations stabilize at 150–200 pg/mL a few weeks following insertion of the system; concentrations at 12, 24, and 60 months following insertion of the device reportedly average 180, 192, and 159 pg/mL, respectively.

Following subcutaneous insertion of etonogestrel implant, the drug is released at a rate of 60–70 mcg per day at week 5–6; the rate decreases to 35–45 mcg per day at the end of the first year, to 30–40 mcg per day at the end of the second year, and then to 25–30 mcg per day at the end of the third year. Plasma etonogestrel concentrations of 781–894 pg/mL are achieved within a few weeks following insertion

of the implant; concentrations at 12, 24, and 36 months following insertion of the device reportedly average 192–261, 154–194, and 156–177 pg/mL, respectively.

Following oral administration of a single 0.75- or 1.5-mg dose of levonorgestrel, the drug is rapidly and completely absorbed with peak plasma concentrations of 14 or 19 ng/mL achieved in 1.6 or 1.7 hours, respectively.

CHEMISTRY AND STABILITY

● Chemistry

Etonogestrel, levonorgestrel, and norethindrone are synthetic progestins which are used as contraceptives. Norethindrone occurs as a white to creamy white, crystalline powder and is practically insoluble in water and sparingly soluble in alcohol.

The commercially available levonorgestrel-releasing intrauterine system consists of a T-shaped polyethylene frame with a cylindrical drug reservoir around the vertical stem. The drug reservoir, a mixture of levonorgestrel and silicone, contains 52 mg of levonorgestrel and is covered by a silicone membrane. The polyethylene frame contains barium sulfate and is radiopaque. A monofilament polyethylene removal thread is attached to a loop at the end of the vertical stem of the frame.

Etonogestrel is commercially available as a nonbiodegradable implant. The implant is 4 cm long and has a diameter of 2 mm. The implant does not contain latex and is not radiopaque.

● Stability

Norethindrone tablets should be stored at a temperature of 25°C but may be exposed to temperatures ranging from 15–30°C. Commercially available oral contraceptives are provided in mnemonic dispensing packages which are exempted from the child safety packaging requirements of the US Poison Prevention Packaging Act. Levonorgestrel tablets should be stored at 20–25°C.

The levonorgestrel-releasing intrauterine system should be stored at a temperature of 25°C but may be exposed to temperatures ranging from 15–30°C. The system is supplied as a sterile device and should not be resterilized. The device should not be used if the inner package is damaged or has been opened.

Etonogestrel implant should be stored at a temperature of 25°C but may be exposed to temperatures ranging from 15–30°C.

PREPARATIONS

FDA has approved Next Choice One Dose® for nonprescription (over-the-counter [OTC]) status for women 17 years of age or older; the contraceptive will remain a prescription-only preparation for women younger than 17 years of age.

Excipients in commercially available drug preparations may have clinically important effects in some individuals; consult specific product labeling for details.

Etonogestrel

Parenteral		
Implant	68 mg	Implanon®, Organon

Levonorgestrel

Intrauterine		
Intrauterine System	52 mg	Mirena®, Berlex
Oral		
Tablets	0.75 mg*	Levonorgestrel Tablets (available in pack of 2 tablets), Perrigo
	1.5 mg*	Fallback Solo®, Lupin
		Levonorgestrel Tablets
		Next Choice One Dose®, Actavis
		Opcicon® One-Step, Sun
		Plan B One-Step®, Teva

* available from one or more manufacturer, distributor, and/or repackager by generic (nonproprietary) name

Norethindrone (Norethisterone)

Oral		
Tablets	0.35 mg	Micronor®, Ortho-McNeil
		Nor-Q.D.®, Watson

Estrogens General Statement

68:16.04 • ESTROGENS

■ Estrogens are naturally occurring hormones or synthetic steroidal and nonsteroidal compounds with estrogenic activity.

USES

● *Estrogen Replacement Therapy*

Estrogens are used for the treatment of moderate to severe vasomotor symptoms and other symptoms, including vulvar and vaginal atrophy, associated with menopause and for the prevention and treatment of osteoporosis. When estrogens are used alone, such therapy is referred to as estrogen replacement therapy (ERT); when estrogens are used in combination with progestins, such therapy usually is referred to as hormone replacement therapy (HRT) or postmenopausal hormone therapy. Another therapeutic option for postmenopausal women involves use of estrogens in combination with an estrogen agonist-antagonist (e.g., bazedoxifene); this combination is referred to as a tissue-selective estrogen complex (TSEC). Long-term therapy with estrogens is associated with an increased risk of endometrial hyperplasia and/or carcinoma in postmenopausal women; however, use of progestins in conjunction with estrogen therapy (HRT) substantially reduces the risk. Women with an intact uterus must receive progestin in addition to estrogen to avoid the increased risk of endometrial carcinoma; long-term use of estrogen alone in women with an intact uterus is not recommended. As an alternative to progestin therapy, the use of bazedoxifene (an estrogen agonist-antagonist) in fixed combination with conjugated estrogens reduces the risk of endometrial hyperplasia. HRT is associated with increased risks of myocardial infarction (MI), stroke, invasive breast cancer, pulmonary emboli, and deep-vein thrombosis. ERT is associated with increased risks of stroke and deep-vein thrombosis. Because of the potential risks associated with HRT and ERT, the benefit to risk should be assessed for each patient, considering alternative therapies as part of this assessment. If ERT or HRT is used, it should be prescribed at the lowest effective dosage and for the shortest duration consistent with treatment goals and risks for the individual woman.

In the past, estrogens were used for prevention of cardiovascular disease in postmenopausal women; however, recent data indicate that use of ERT or HRT does not decrease the incidence of cardiovascular disease, and estrogen replacement therapy alone (ERT) or combined with progestins (HRT) should *no longer* be used for the prevention of cardiovascular disease.

While estrogen or estrogen/progestin therapy is effective for the management of certain menopausal symptoms and for the prevention and treatment of osteoporosis, results of a recent controlled study (Women's Health Initiative [WHI] study of estrogen plus progestin) indicate that HRT, specifically conjugated estrogens 0.625 mg in conjunction with medroxyprogesterone acetate 2.5 mg daily, is associated with a small increase in the risk of breast cancer, cardiovascular disease, stroke, and venous thromboembolism. Results of the WHI study of estrogen alone indicate that ERT (specifically conjugated estrogens 0.625 mg daily) is associated with a small increase in the risk of stroke and deep-vein thrombosis. Results of the WHI also showed that HRT had no clinically important effect on measures of depression, insomnia, sexual function, or cognition (i.e., health-related quality-of-life measures) in women without menopausal symptoms. Based on the WHI findings, recommendations on the appropriate use of hormone therapy have been revised. Because the risks of hormone therapy exceed the benefits for the prevention of chronic diseases in postmenopausal women, experts state that ERT or HRT should not be used for the prevention of chronic conditions in postmenopausal women. The American Heart Association (AHA), the American College of Obstetricians and Gynecologists (ACOG), FDA, and manufacturers recommend that hormone therapy not be used to prevent heart disease in healthy women (primary prevention) or to protect women with preexisting heart disease (secondary prevention). ACOG, FDA, and the manufacturers also recommend that women receiving hormone therapy solely for the prevention of postmenopausal osteoporosis consider alternative therapy (e.g., alendronate, raloxifene, risedronate). Although these recommendations are based on results of the WHI study that evaluated one specific estrogen (conjugated estrogens 0.625 mg) and one estrogen/progestin preparation (conjugated estrogens 0.625 mg in conjunction with

medroxyprogesterone acetate 2.5 mg), the risks should be assumed to be similar with other hormonal regimens, including different dosages of these drugs as well as other estrogen/progestin combinations not studied in WHI, in the absence of comparable data to the contrary.

While the risks of HRT are likely to exceed the benefits in most women receiving these agents for prevention of chronic diseases (e.g., cardiovascular disease, osteoporosis), the long-term safety of short-term use of HRT for the management of menopausal symptoms remains to be precisely established. Estrogen or estrogen/progestin therapy is the most effective therapy for the relief of vasomotor symptoms such as hot flushes (flashes) and sleep disturbances. The fixed combination of conjugated estrogens with bazedoxifene acetate also is used for the management of moderate to severe vasomotor symptoms associated with menopause. (See Uses: Vasomotor Symptoms, in Bazedoxifene Acetate 68:16.12.) Estrogen or estrogen/progestin therapy also is effective in the treatment of genitourinary symptoms such as vaginal dryness; however, the use of topical vaginal preparations should be considered when only vulvar and vaginal symptoms are being treated. The decision to use estrogen or estrogen/progestin therapy for management of menopausal symptoms should be individualized taking into account the woman's preference, her risk for specific chronic diseases, and the presence and severity of menopausal symptoms. ACOG, FDA, and the manufacturers recommend that women who choose hormone therapy for the relief of menopausal symptoms receive such therapy for the shortest possible time and in the lowest effective dosage; women also should regularly consult their clinician and undergo regular breast cancer screenings. ACOG recommends against routine discontinuance of systemic estrogen therapy when a women reaches 65 years of age, since some women 65 years of age or older may continue to need systemic hormone therapy for management of vasomotor symptoms. Continuation of hormone therapy for management of vasomotor symptoms should be individualized taking into account the woman's symptoms and the risks and benefits of hormone therapy, regardless of age.

Regardless of a woman's age or duration of hormone therapy, discontinuance may be associated with recurrent vasomotor symptoms in approximately 50% of women. There is insufficient evidence to recommend one method of stopping hormone therapy (e.g., abrupt discontinuance, dosage tapering) over another to prevent recurrent symptoms.

Lifestyle modifications that may help reduce menopausal symptoms such as hot flushes include smoking cessation, dietary manipulation (avoid/limit spicy foods, caffeine, and alcohol), stress reduction, and loose or layered clothing. There is increasing evidence that drugs other than hormone preparations may alleviate certain menopausal symptoms. For women experiencing vasomotor symptoms, selective serotonin-reuptake inhibitors (SSRIs), selective serotonin- and norepinephrine-reuptake inhibitors (SNRIs), gabapentin, or clonidine has been used for treatment. SSRIs, SNRIs, and gabapentin have been shown to be effective for treatment of vasomotor symptoms in randomized, controlled trials, while evidence supporting the efficacy of clonidine is limited. For symptoms such as vaginal dryness, topical administration of estrogen alone usually is effective. Although only limited amounts of estrogen are systemically absorbed from vaginal tablets and rings, limited data are available regarding long-term safety of vaginally administered estrogen.

Estrogens also are used in the treatment of a variety of other conditions associated with a deficiency of estrogenic hormones, including female hypogonadism and castration and primary ovarian failure. In addition, estrogens also may be used in the treatment of abnormal uterine bleeding caused by hormonal imbalance not associated with organic pathology; however, progestins are usually preferred.

Osteoporosis

Prevention in Postmenopausal Women

Estrogen replacement therapy (ERT) is effective for the prevention of osteoporosis in women and has been shown to reduce bone resorption and retard or halt bone loss associated with estrogen deficiency in postmenopausal women. Oral estrogens (e.g., estradiol, estropipate, conjugated estrogens) and transdermal estrogens (e.g., estradiol) are used adjunctively with other therapeutic measures (e.g., diet, calcium, vitamin D, weight-bearing exercise, physical therapy) to retard further bone loss and the progression of osteoporosis in postmenopausal women. The fixed combination of conjugated estrogens with bazedoxifene acetate also is used for the prevention of osteoporosis. (See Prevention in Postmenopausal Women under Uses: Osteoporosis, in Bazedoxifene Acetate 68:16.12.)

In a placebo-controlled study in postmenopausal women, administration of estrogen replacement therapy (conjugated estrogens) with (HRT) or without (ERT) a progestin for 36 months was associated with a 1.7% increase in hip bone mineral density (BMD) and 3.5–5% increase in lumbar spine BMD compared with baseline, while placebo recipients lost an average of 1.7% in hip BMD and 1.8% in spinal BMD. Increases in BMD observed in women receiving estrogen replacement therapy without a progestin (ERT) generally have been essentially the same as those observed in women receiving combined estrogen/progestin therapy (HRT).

In case-controlled studies in Caucasian women, estrogen replacement therapy has been associated with a substantial (about 60%) reduction in the incidence of hip and wrist fractures in those in whom estrogen therapy was initiated within a few years of menopause; some studies suggest that estrogens may also reduce the incidence of vertebral fracture. In the WHI study, there was a 24% reduction in total fractures in postmenopausal women receiving HRT compared with those receiving placebo and a 30–39% reduction in total fractures in women receiving ERT compared with women receiving placebo. The number of cases of hip fracture per 10,000 patient-years of exposure was 10 or 15 in women receiving HRT or placebo, respectively. The number of cases of hip fracture per 10,000 patient-years of exposure was 11 or 17 in women receiving ERT or placebo, respectively. Estrogen replacement therapy reportedly prevents further estrogen deficiency-induced bone loss in postmenopausal women when started up to 6 years after menopause, but such therapy does not appear to restore bone mass to premenopausal levels. In addition, when estrogen therapy is discontinued, bone mass declines at a rate similar to that occurring in the immediate postmenopausal period. It has been suggested that optimum estrogen replacement therapy for the prevention of osteoporosis should be initiated within 5 years of menopause and be continued for long-term (exceeding 10 years); however, risks associated with such long-term use should be considered. (See Carcinogenicity.)

Caucasian or Asian women are at a higher risk for osteoporosis than black women. Other risk factors include premature ovarian failure; a family history of osteoporosis; a small, slim body frame; endocrine disorders such as thyrotoxicosis, hyperparathyroidism, Cushing's syndrome, hyperprolactinemia, insulin-dependent diabetes mellitus (type 1, IDDM); cigarette smoking; drinking excessive amounts of alcohol; a sedentary lifestyle and/or lack of physical exercise; low body weight; and low dietary calcium intake. Premature ovarian failure (surgical or nonsurgical) hastens the onset of osteoporosis, and estrogen deficiency in premenopausal women (e.g., secondary to anorexia nervosa- or exercise-induced amenorrhea or to hyperprolactinemia) induces bone loss and may reduce peak bone mass.

While estrogen or estrogen/progestin therapy is effective for the prevention of osteoporosis in postmenopausal women, results of a recent controlled study (WHI study) indicate that HRT, specifically conjugated estrogens 0.625 mg in conjunction with medroxyprogesterone acetate 2.5 mg daily, is associated with a small increase in the risk of breast cancer, cardiovascular disease, stroke, and venous thromboembolism. Results of the WHI estrogen-alone study indicate that ERT (specifically conjugated estrogens 0.625 mg daily) is associated with a small increase in the risk of stroke and deep-vein thrombosis. Because the risks of hormone therapy exceed the benefits for the prevention of chronic diseases in postmenopausal women, experts state that ERT or HRT should not be used for the prevention of chronic conditions (e.g., osteoporosis) in postmenopausal women. ACOG, FDA, and the manufacturers recommend that women receiving hormone therapy solely for the prevention of postmenopausal osteoporosis consider alternative therapy. Alternative agents that can be used for the prevention of osteoporosis include alendronate, raloxifene, or risedronate. However, experience with these agents is not as extensive as with HRT. (See Osteoporosis: Prevention in Postmenopausal Women, under Uses, in Alendronate 92:24, Raloxifene 68:16.12, and Risedronate 92:24.) In addition, alendronate and risedronate are associated with substantial adverse GI effects (e.g., esophagitis). (See Dosage and Administration: Administration, in Alendronate 92:24 and Risedronate 92:24.)

Women being considered for estrogen replacement therapy should have no contraindications to estrogen therapy and should fully understand the risks associated with estrogen use and agree to regular medical examinations. The choice of estrogen replacement therapy, alendronate, raloxifene, or risedronate for the prevention of postmenopausal osteoporosis should be individualized, taking into account differences in tolerability and safety and individual preference. For all women, lifestyle modifications for healthy bones include a diet high in calcium (postmenopausal women should receive 1.2–1.5 g of calcium daily), adequate intake of vitamin D (as supplied by a multivitamin), and regular weight-bearing exercise such as walking or jogging. Whether additional preventive therapy generally should be offered to all women or just recommended for selected women at highest risk of developing osteoporosis remains to be established.

Although there is no biologic reason to suspect that the effects of estrogens would differ in nonwhite women, the efficacy of estrogen replacement therapy in preventing osteoporosis in nonwhite women has not been established to date.

Treatment in Postmenopausal Women

Estrogen replacement therapy has been effective in the treatment of osteoporosis in postmenopausal women and has been recommended as first-line therapy for women with osteoporosis. However, results of a recent controlled study (WHI study) indicate that HRT, specifically conjugated estrogens 0.625 mg in conjunction with medroxyprogesterone acetate 2.5 mg daily, is associated with a small increase in the risk of breast cancer, cardiovascular disease, stroke, and venous thromboembolism. Results of the WHI estrogen-alone study indicate that ERT (specifically conjugated estrogens 0.625 mg daily) is associated with a small increase in the risk of stroke and deep-vein thrombosis. Based on these findings, recommendations on the appropriate use of hormone therapy are being revised. The risks and benefits of long-term use of hormone therapy in the management of osteoporosis should be evaluated taking into account the increased risk of breast cancer and cardiovascular disease, availability of other pharmacologic modalities (e.g., alendronate, calcitonin, calcium, raloxifene, risedronate, vitamin D), and life-style factors that can be modified.

Estrogen replacement therapy produces the most marked benefits when begun soon (e.g., within 5 years) following menopause; such therapy also appears to be effective even when initiated many years after menopause in older women. Some clinicians suggest that prolonged therapy (e.g., at least 5 years) with estrogens is necessary since the beneficial effects of estrogen replacement therapy do not appear to persist after discontinuance of treatment.

Various estrogen-containing therapies (e.g., conjugated estrogens, estrogen/progestin combinations) have been used concomitantly with bisphosphonates (e.g., alendronate, etidronate) and calcium in the treatment of osteoporosis in postmenopausal women. In several clinical trials in postmenopausal women with osteoporosis, the combination of estrogen-containing therapy and alendronate resulted in a greater degree of suppression of bone turnover than either therapy given alone. In a placebo-controlled, 2-year clinical trial comparing monotherapy with alendronate (10 mg daily) or conjugated estrogens (0.625 mg daily) with the combination of these drugs at the same monotherapy dosages in postmenopausal women with osteoporosis not currently receiving antiresorptive therapy, combination therapy increased bone mineral density (BMD) (as determined by dual-energy radiographic absorption measurements) in the lumbar spine and femoral neck compared with either agent given alone or placebo (calcium 500 mg daily). A bone histology study in these patients indicated that the bone formed during therapy was of normal quality. Compared with calcium supplementation alone, bone turnover after 18 months was suppressed by 98% with combined alendronate-estrogen replacement therapy, 94% with alendronate therapy alone, and 78% with estrogen replacement therapy alone. In another comparative study in postmenopausal women who had osteoporosis despite hormone replacement therapy with estrogen (conjugated estrogens) or estrogen plus progestin (medroxyprogesterone) for at least 1 year (mean duration about 10 years), the addition of alendronate (10 mg daily) increased BMD (as determined by dual-energy radiographic absorption measurements) in the lumbar spine and hip trochanter compared with hormone replacement therapy alone at 12 months; all patients also received calcium and vitamin D supplementation. In both trials, the incidence of new fractures was similar across treatment groups. In these trials, sample size and study duration may have been inadequate to detect differences in fracture incidence with combination therapy, monotherapy with alendronate or estrogen, or placebo, and further studies are needed. The safety of combination therapy was similar to that with each antiresorptive agent alone.

Prevention in Women with Anorexia Nervosa

Estrogens have been used in a limited number of anorexic women with chronic amenorrhea to reduce calcium loss† and, thereby, reduce the risks of osteoporosis. However, results of various controlled and uncontrolled studies indicate that estrogens appear to benefit only a subset of low-weight (initial body weight less than 70% of ideal body weight) women with anorexia nervosa. Because data supporting use of estrogen therapy for the treatment or prevention of osteoporosis in female children, adolescents, or adults with anorexia nervosa are limited or lacking, the American Psychiatric Association (APA) concludes that therapy with estrogens alone does not appear to reverse osteoporosis or osteopenia, and unless there is weight gain, such therapy does not prevent further bone loss. Furthermore, many clinicians state that the decision to initiate estrogen therapy in these patients should be deferred until weight gain and normal menses have been restored, since artificially inducing menses carries the risk of supporting or reinforcing a patient's denial that she does not need to gain weight. For a complete discussion of diagnosis and treatment of anorexia nervosa and other eating disorders, see Uses: Eating Disorders, in Fluoxetine 28:16.04.20.

Cardiovascular Risk Reduction

While results from earlier observational studies indicated that estrogen replacement therapy or combined estrogen/progestin therapy was associated with cardiovascular benefit in postmenopausal women, results of the Heart and Estrogen/Progestin Replacement Study (HERS) and the Women's Health Initiative (WHI) study indicate that use of estrogen replacement therapy (ERT) or combined estrogen/progestin replacement therapy (hormone replacement therapy, HRT) does *not* decrease the incidence of cardiovascular disease.

Substantial epidemiologic evidence has indicated that postmenopausal women receiving ERT may have a reduction of up to 50% in the risk of ischemic heart disease and a similar reduction in total mortality compared with women who have never received such therapy. In observational studies, the increase in life expectancy based on a reduced risk of coronary heart disease (CHD) in postmenopausal women receiving ERT has been estimated to be 2–3 years. While these studies generally enrolled healthy women, observational studies in women with preexisting coronary disease also suggest that ERT reduces the risk of reinfarction and CHD-related death. However, the conclusions of these studies have been criticized for methodological reasons.

Although some observational studies have shown a cardioprotective effect with estrogen alone or in combination with progestin, conflicting data have been reported in large prospective, randomized studies. In one of these studies (HERS), no overall cardiovascular benefit was reported with HRT in postmenopausal women with established coronary disease. In addition, results of the WHI study indicate that HRT, specifically conjugated estrogens 0.625 mg in conjunction with medroxyprogesterone acetate 2.5 mg daily, is associated with a small increase in the risk of cardiovascular disease and stroke in predominantly healthy postmenopausal women. Results from the WHI estrogen-alone study indicate that ERT (specifically conjugated estrogens 0.625 mg daily) does not affect the risk of CHD but is associated with a small increase in the risk of stroke in healthy postmenopausal women who have undergone a hysterectomy. In another randomized study, ERT (conjugated estrogens 0.625 mg daily) or HRT (conjugated estrogens 0.625 mg daily and medroxyprogesterone acetate 2.5 mg daily) was associated with reductions in LDL-cholesterol and increases in HDL-cholesterol concentrations but had no effect on progression of coronary atherosclerosis in women with established CHD.

In HERS, 2763 postmenopausal women with established CHD were randomized to receive HRT (conjugated estrogens 0.625 mg daily in conjunction with medroxyprogesterone acetate 2.5 mg daily) or placebo. After a follow-up averaging 6.8 years, HRT was not associated with an overall reduction in the rate of CHD events (e.g., nonfatal MI, CHD-related death). Based on year of randomization, women who received HRT experienced an increased incidence of CHD events during the first year and a lower incidence in the fourth year compared with women who received placebo. However, based on the entire 6.8 years of follow-up, a trend toward a lower or higher incidence of CHD over time was not evident. Analysis of data from 2 observational studies in postmenopausal women with cardiovascular disease (i.e., the Nurses' Health Study and a Group Health Cooperative study) indicate that the risk for a recurrent major coronary event in women with established coronary heart disease is increased early (up to 1 year) after initiation of HRT and decreases with long-term use. Women with CHD often have risk factors such as diabetes mellitus and obesity that influence the tendency to develop thrombosis, and any procoagulant effects of hormone therapy would be greatest in such women. Whether estrogen/progestin therapy (HRT) is associated in susceptible subgroups with immediate prothrombotic, proarrhythmic, or proischemic effects that are gradually outweighed by a beneficial effect on the underlying progression of atherosclerosis (perhaps as a result of favorable effects on lipoproteins) requires further study.

The WHI was a long-term study sponsored by the National Institutes of Health (NIH) that focused on strategies that can potentially reduce the incidence of heart disease, breast and colorectal cancer, and fractures in postmenopausal women. One part of this initiative followed 16,608 predominantly healthy women (with an intact uterus) who were 50–79 years of age who received HRT (i.e., conjugated estrogens 0.625 mg in conjunction with medroxyprogesterone acetate 2.5 mg daily) or placebo. The goal of this 8.5-year study was to evaluate the relationship between HRT and CHD, stroke, pulmonary embolism, breast cancer, endometrial carcinoma, colorectal cancer, hip fracture, and death from other causes. The study was stopped early because health risks exceeded benefits over an average follow-up of 5.2 years. At the time the study was stopped, the increased number of cases of invasive breast cancer, CHD, stroke, and pulmonary embolism in the estrogen/progestin group relative to the placebo group was not counterbalanced by reductions in the number of cases of hip fracture and colorectal cancer. Estrogen/progestin therapy did not affect all-cause mortality.

In the WHI estrogen plus progestin study, there was a 29% increase in the incidence of heart disease in postmenopausal women receiving HRT compared with those receiving placebo. The number of CHD events (e.g., MI) per 10,000 patient-years of exposure was 37 or 30 in women receiving HRT or placebo, respectively. In addition, there was a 41% increase in the incidence of stroke in postmenopausal women receiving HRT compared with those receiving placebo. The number of cases of stroke per 10,000 patient-years of exposure was 29 or 20 in women receiving HRT or placebo, respectively.

Another part of the WHI initiative followed 10,739 predominately healthy women who were 50–79 years of age and had undergone a prior hysterectomy, and received ERT (conjugated estrogens 0.625 mg daily) or placebo. The goal of this study was to evaluate the relationship between ERT and CHD, stroke, pulmonary embolism, breast cancer, colorectal cancer, hip fracture, and death from other causes. At the time the study was stopped (after nearly 7 years), results indicated that ERT did not affect the incidence of CHD or overall mortality but did increase the risk of stroke. There was a 39% increase in the incidence of stroke in women receiving ERT compared with those receiving placebo. Approximately 80% of all strokes were ischemic. The number of cases of stroke per 10,000 patient-years of exposure was 44 or 32 in women receiving ERT or placebo, respectively.

An ancillary substudy of the WHI examined the effect of ERT (conjugated estrogens 0.625 mg daily) or placebo on coronary-artery calcification in women 50–59 years of age at the time of randomization. Imaging of the coronary arteries 8.7 years after study start (7.4 years of treatment and 1.3 years after study completion) indicated that women who received estrogen had a lower prevalence and quantity of coronary-artery calcium than placebo-treated women. Intent-to-treat analysis showed that administration of estrogen reduced coronary calcification by 42%; in women with at least 80% adherence to study medication for 5 years, administration of estrogen reduced coronary calcification by 61%.

Based on the finding of no overall cardiovascular benefit observed in HERS and the WHI study and the lack of effect of ERT or HRT on angiographic progression of coronary artery disease, the AHA, ACOG, FDA, and manufacturers recommend that hormone therapy not be used to prevent heart disease in healthy women (primary prevention) or to protect women with preexisting heart disease (secondary prevention).

If a woman with cardiovascular disease receiving long-term HRT experiences an acute cardiovascular event (e.g., MI) or is immobilized, discontinuance of HRT or administration of venous thrombosis prophylaxis during hospitalization should be considered to reduce the risk of thromboembolism. Decisions to resume HRT should be based on established noncoronary risks and benefits and patient preference.

● Corticosteroid-induced Hypogonadism and Osteoporosis

Patients receiving long-term corticosteroid therapy may develop hypogonadism secondary to inhibition of secretion of luteinizing hormone (LH) and follicle-stimulating hormone (FSH) from the pituitary as well as secondary to direct effects on the ovaries and testes, and such hypogonadism may be associated with bone loss. Therefore, all patients receiving prolonged corticosteroid therapy should be assessed for possible hypogonadism, which should be corrected if present.

Hormone replacement therapy (HRT, combined estrogen and progestin therapy) has been effective in increasing lumbar spine but not femoral neck bone mass density (BMD) in postmenopausal women with asthma or rheumatoid arthritis who were receiving chronic corticosteroid therapy. HRT in a control group of women receiving long-term low-dose corticosteroid therapy in one study appeared to prevent BMD loss at the lumbar spine, hip, and distal radius over the course of 1 year. While there currently are no well-designed studies establishing the *preventive* efficacy of HRT on corticosteroid-induced bone loss and radiographic vertebral fractures, data from existing studies suggest that HRT is adequate to prevent bone loss in postmenopausal women receiving low-to-moderate-dose corticosteroid therapy†, and postmenopausal women receiving long-term corticosteroid therapy should be offered HRT if no contraindications exist. The protective efficacy of HRT in such women who are receiving moderate-to-high doses of corticosteroids remains to be established. Corticosteroid-treated women who develop fractures while receiving HRT or in whom HRT is not well tolerated should receive calcium and vitamin D supplementation along with bisphosphonate therapy (e.g., alendronate, risedronate) in an attempt to prevent bone loss and/or increase BMD as well as to prevent apoptosis of osteocytes and osteoblasts and reduce the risk of radiographic vertebral fractures.

There also currently are no controlled studies of HRT in premenopausal women receiving chronic corticosteroid therapy. However, observational studies in premenopausal female athletes with menstrual irregularities suggest that estrogen-progestin combination (e.g., oral contraceptive) use is associated with a higher adjusted bone mineral content and BMD relative to women who do not take estrogen-progestin combinations. Therefore, premenopausal women who develop menstrual irregularities (e.g., oligomenorrhea, amenorrhea) while receiving long-term corticosteroid therapy should be offered combined cyclic estrogen and progestin therapy (e.g., estrogen-progestin combination oral contraceptives) in an attempt to treat hypogonadism and possibly reduce the risk of corticosteroid-induced osteoporosis† when contraindications to estrogen-progestin therapy are not present. For additional information on the management of corticosteroid-induced osteoporosis, see Cautions: Musculoskeletal Effects in the Corticosteroids General Statement 68:04.

● Alzheimer's Disease

Some data from observational studies indicate that prior use of hormone replacement therapy (HRT), but not current HRT unless such use exceeds 10 years, is associated with reduced risk of Alzheimer's disease†. Estrogens have not been shown to prevent progression of Alzheimer's disease, and the American Academy of Neurology (AAN) recommends that estrogens not be used for the treatment of Alzheimer's disease.

Findings from the Women' Health Initiative Memory study (WHIMS; an ancillary study of the Women's Health Initiative [WHI] study in women 65 years of age or older without dementia at study entry) indicate that use of ERT (conjugated estrogens 0.625 mg daily) or HRT (conjugated estrogens 0.625 mg in conjunction with medroxyprogesterone acetate 2.5 mg daily) does not improve cognitive function relative to placebo in these women and may adversely affect cognition. In the WHIMS study, more women receiving ERT or HRT had substantial and clinically important declines in the Modified Mini-Mental State Examination total score compared with women receiving placebo, suggesting that some women receiving these hormonal therapies experience detrimental effects. In addition, the rate of probable dementia in women receiving ERT or HRT was higher than that in women receiving placebo. Women with relatively low baseline cognitive function were at particularly high risk for adverse cognitive effects. Use of hormone therapy to prevent dementia or cognitive decline in women 65 years of age or older is not recommended.

● Metastatic Breast Carcinoma

Estrogens are used in the palliative treatment of advanced, inoperable, metastatic carcinoma of the breast in postmenopausal women and in men. Estrogens are one of several second-line agents that can be used in certain postmenopausal women with metastatic breast cancer.

● Prostate Carcinoma

In males, estrogens are used for the palliative treatment of advanced carcinoma of the prostate; however, the risk of adverse cardiovascular effects of the drugs must be considered.

● Other Uses

Estrogens also are used in combination with progestins for ovulation control in the prevention of conception and for the treatment of moderate acne vulgaris; estrogen-progestin combinations also are used in short-course, high-dose regimens in women for the prevention of contraception after unprotected intercourse (postcoital contraception, "morning-after pills") as emergency contraceptives. (See Uses: Postcoital Contraception, in Estrogen-Progestin Combinations 68:12.)

Although in the past estrogens have been used for the prevention of postpartum breast engorgement†, FDA has withdrawn approval of estrogen-containing drugs for this indication since estrogens have not been shown to be safe for use in women with postpartum breast engorgement. Data from controlled studies indicate that the incidence of substantial painful engorgement is low in untreated women, and the condition usually responds to appropriate analgesic or other supportive therapy.

Estrogens have *not* been shown to be effective for any purpose during pregnancy.

For information on the uses of specific estrogens, see the individual monographs in 68:16.04.

DOSAGE AND ADMINISTRATION

● Administration

Estrogens may be administered orally, parenterally, intravaginally, or topically.

● Dosage

Dosage equivalencies for estrogens have not been clearly established, and reported comparative values vary greatly. The dosage range of estrogens is generally wide, and dosage should be individualized according to the condition being treated and the response and tolerance of the patient. To minimize the risk of adverse effects, the lowest possible effective dosage and the shortest duration of therapy consistent with treatment goals and risks for the individual woman should be used. When estrogen therapy is used in the management of vasomotor symptoms or vulvar and vaginal atrophy associated with menopause, the lowest dosage that will control such symptoms should be used. When short-term estrogen therapy is indicated (e.g., for the management of vasomotor symptoms associated with menopause vulvar and vaginal atrophy), therapy should be discontinued as soon as possible; attempts to reduce dosage or discontinue the drug should be made at 3- to 6-month intervals.

Estrogen therapy is administered in a continuous daily regimen or, alternatively, estrogens are administered cyclically. When estrogens are administered cyclically, the drugs are usually given once daily for 3 weeks, followed by 1 week without the drugs, and then this regimen is repeated as necessary. While estrogen therapy alone may be appropriate in women who have undergone a hysterectomy, a progestin generally is added to estrogen therapy in women with an intact uterus. Addition of a progestin for 10 or more days of a cycle of estrogen administration or daily with estrogen in a continuous regimen reduces the incidence of endometrial hyperplasia and the attendant risk of endometrial carcinoma in women with an intact uterus. Morphologic and biochemical studies of the endometrium suggest that 10–13 days of progestin are needed to provide maximum maturation of the endometrium and to eliminate any hyperplastic changes. When a progestin is used in conjunction with estrogen therapy, the usual precautions associated with progestin therapy should be observed. Clinicians prescribing progestins should be aware of the risks associated with these drugs and the manufacturers' labeling should be consulted. The choice and dosage of a progestin may be important factors in minimizing potential adverse effects.

As an alternative to progestins, the use of bazedoxifene (an estrogen agonist-antagonist) in fixed combination with conjugated estrogens reduces the risk of endometrial hyperplasia. When bazedoxifene is used in fixed combination with estrogen therapy, the usual precautions associated with bazedoxifene therapy should be observed.

CAUTIONS

Numerous adverse effects have been reported in patients receiving estrogens and these may be similar to the adverse effects associated with estrogen-progestin oral contraceptives. Most of the serious adverse effects of estrogen-progestin oral contraceptives (e.g., thromboembolic disorders, hepatocellular adenoma) generally have not been associated with postmenopausal estrogen therapy, which may reflect the comparatively low dosages of estrogens used in postmenopausal women. When larger dosages of estrogen are used (e.g., for the palliative treatment of carcinoma of the breast or prostate), an increased risk of the serious adverse effects may occur. For additional information on the adverse effects, precautions, and contraindications associated with estrogens, see Cautions in Estrogen-Progestin Combinations 68:12.

● GI Effects

Nausea has been frequently associated with estrogen therapy. Other adverse GI effects include vomiting, abdominal cramps, bloating, and diarrhea. Changes in appetite and changes in weight may also occur.

In patients with hypertriglyceridemia, estrogen therapy may be associated with further increases in plasma triglycerides resulting in pancreatitis and other complications. If acute pancreatitis occurs, estrogens should be discontinued. The risk of gallbladder disease appears to be increased 2- to 4-fold in postmenopausal women receiving estrogen replacement therapy. In one study, an increased risk of gallbladder disease occurred after 2 years of use of the drugs and doubled after 4 or 5 years of use. In another study, an increased risk of gallbladder disease was apparent between 6–12 months of use.

● Dermatologic Effects

The most frequent adverse dermatologic reaction associated with estrogen therapy is chloasma or melasma. Women who have had melasma during pregnancy appear to be most susceptible. Irregular brown macules may develop slowly on the face within 1 month to 2 years following initiation of estrogen therapy. The macules fade more slowly than in melasma gravidarum and may be permanent.

Other dermatologic reactions include erythema multiforme, erythema nodosum, and hemorrhagic eruption. Hirsutism and alopecia have also occurred. Porphyria cutanea has reportedly been adversely affected in some women receiving estrogen therapy.

● *Cardiovascular Effects*

In the absence of comparable data, the cardiovascular risks identified in the Women's Health Initiative (WHI) study with conjugated estrogens 0.625 mg daily alone or in conjunction with medroxyprogesterone acetate 2.5 mg daily should be assumed to be similar for other dosages of these drugs as well as for other combinations of estrogens and progestins.

Elevated Blood Pressure

There is no evidence that estrogen replacement therapy in postmenopausal women is associated with elevated blood pressure; in fact, unopposed estrogen therapy in postmenopausal women has been associated with blood pressure reductions in some studies. However, increases in blood pressure may occur in some women receiving estrogens, particularly if high dosages are used. Blood pressure elevations are usually minor, but clinically important hypertension may occur in some women. Elevated blood pressure may gradually decrease or persist after discontinuance of estrogen therapy. The precise cause of increased blood pressure is not known, but it may result from a stimulatory effect of estrogen on the renin-angiotensin system.

Women receiving high dosages of estrogens or those with a history of hypertension, preexisting renal disease, a history of toxemia or elevated blood pressure during pregnancy, a familial tendency toward hypertension or its consequences, or a history of excessive weight gain or fluid retention during the menstrual cycle may be at increased risk of developing elevated blood pressure during estrogen therapy and, therefore, should be monitored closely. Even though elevated blood pressure may remain within the normal range, the clinical implications of elevations should be considered in all patients. All women, but particularly those with other risk factors for cardiovascular disease or stroke and those receiving high dosages of estrogens, should have blood pressure measurements before an estrogen is prescribed and at regular intervals during therapy. Estrogens should be discontinued if the patient becomes hypertensive during therapy.

Results of a recent controlled study (WHI study) indicate that hormone replacement therapy, specifically conjugated estrogens 0.625 mg in conjunction with medroxyprogesterone acetate 2.5 mg daily, is associated with a small increase in the risk of cardiovascular disease. In the WHI estrogen plus progestin study, there was a 29% increase in the incidence of heart disease in postmenopausal women receiving hormone replacement therapy compared with those receiving placebo. The number of coronary heart disease (CHD) events (e.g., myocardial infarction [MI]) per 10,000 patient-years of exposure was 37 or 30 in women receiving hormone replacement therapy or placebo, respectively. In the WHI estrogen-alone study, ERT did not affect the incidence of CHD.

Thromboembolic Disorders

Oral contraceptive use is associated with an increased risk of thromboembolic and thrombotic disorders including thrombophlebitis, pulmonary embolism, stroke, subarachnoid hemorrhage, and MI. Retinal thrombosis and mesenteric thrombosis also have been reported in women receiving oral contraceptives. An increased risk of postsurgery thromboembolic complications has also been reported in patients receiving oral contraceptives.

Estrogen replacement therapy and hormone (estrogen/progestin) replacement therapy are associated with an increased risk of venous thromboembolic events. Results of some studies indicate that the risk of venous thromboembolic events with estrogen or hormone replacement therapy is about 2–3 times greater than that in women not receiving such therapy. In the WHI estrogen plus progestin study, the rate of venous thromboembolism, deep-vein thrombosis, or pulmonary embolism in women receiving hormone replacement therapy was twice the rate of these events in women receiving placebo. The number of cases of venous thromboembolism per 10,000 patient-years of exposure was 34 or 16 in women receiving hormone replacement therapy or placebo, respectively. In the WHI estrogen-alone study, the incidence of deep-vein thrombosis was increased in women receiving estrogen compared with women receiving placebo. Venous thrombosis is more likely to occur during the first year of therapy; patients with risk factors for thrombosis are at increased risk of venous thrombosis.

Data are conflicting on whether estrogen therapy alone or in combination with progestins is associated with an increased risk of stroke. While some studies suggest that estrogen replacement therapy may be associated with both an increased and a decreased risk of stroke in postmenopausal women, results from a large prospective study (the Nurses' Health Study) indicate no association between risk of stroke and use of estrogen replacement therapy either alone or in combination with progestins. In the WHI estrogen plus progestin study, there was a 41% increase in the incidence of stroke in postmenopausal women receiving hormone replacement therapy compared with those receiving placebo. The number of cases of stroke per 10,000 patient-years of exposure was 29 or 21 in women receiving hormone replacement therapy or placebo, respectively. In the WHI estrogen-alone study, there was a 39% increase in the incidence of stroke in women receiving estrogen compared with those receiving placebo. Approximately 80% of all strokes in the WHI estrogen-alone study were ischemic strokes. The number of cases of stroke per 10,000 patient-years of exposure was 44 or 32 in women receiving ERT or placebo, respectively; this represents an absolute excess risk of 12 additional strokes per 10,000 patient-years. The American Heart Association (AHA) states that hormone therapy should not be used to prevent stroke in postmenopausal women.

In a study in men, large dosages (i.e., 5 mg daily) of conjugated estrogens have been shown to increase the risk of nonfatal MI, pulmonary embolism, and thrombophlebitis.

The clinician and the patient using estrogens should be alert to the earliest signs and symptoms of thromboembolic and thrombotic disorders (e.g., thrombophlebitis, pulmonary embolism, cerebrovascular insufficiency, coronary occlusion, retinal thrombosis, mesenteric thrombosis). Estrogen therapy should be discontinued immediately when any of these disorders occurs or is suspected. (See Cautions: Precautions and Contraindications.)

Other Cardiovascular Effects

Estrogens may cause some degree of fluid retention. Estrogen therapy should therefore be used with caution in patients with conditions that might be aggravated by fluid retention. (See Cautions: Precautions and Contraindications.)

● *Endocrine and Metabolic Effects*

Endocrine function test results (e.g., glucose tolerance, thyroid function) may be altered in patients receiving large dosages of estrogens. (See Laboratory Test Interferences.)

Decreased glucose tolerance has occurred in women receiving estrogen-containing oral contraceptives and may occur in patients receiving large dosages of estrogens. Prediabetic and diabetic patients should be carefully monitored during estrogen therapy.

Increased serum triglyceride concentrations have occurred in some women receiving estrogen-containing oral contraceptives and may occur during therapy with estrogens. The clinical importance of these alterations in lipid and lipoprotein concentrations has not been established; however, women with elevated serum lipid concentrations who have decided to use estrogens in combination with progestins should be monitored closely.

Estrogens have reportedly caused severe hypercalcemia in patients with breast cancer and bone metastases. If severe hypercalcemia occurs, estrogen therapy should be discontinued and appropriate therapy to decrease serum calcium concentration should be instituted.

Estrogen therapy should be used with caution in women with hypoparathyroidism because estrogen-induced hypocalcemia may occur.

● *Hepatic Effects*

Liver function test results may be altered in patients receiving estrogen therapy; if results of these tests are abnormal, they should be repeated 2 months after discontinuance of the drug. Increased sulfobromophthalein retention has reportedly occurred in women receiving estrogen-containing oral contraceptives, as a result of interference with the transfer of dye conjugates from liver cells into bile; uptake, conjugation, and storage do not appear to be affected. Less frequently, increased serum aminotransferase and alkaline phosphatase concentrations have occurred. Liver function test results usually return to normal within several weeks after estrogen-containing oral contraceptives are discontinued; occasionally, however, abnormal test results may persist for longer periods. The possibility that these alterations in liver function test results may occur in patients receiving estrogens should be considered.

Cholestatic jaundice has been reported in women receiving estrogen-containing oral contraceptives, and the possibility that this effect may occur during estrogen therapy should be considered. Cholestasis is manifested by the development of malaise, anorexia, and pruritus about 2 weeks to 2 months after the start of therapy. Occasionally, arthralgia, fever, and rash may occur. Serum bilirubin may range from 3–10 mg/dL and is mostly conjugated. Women with a history of jaundice during pregnancy have an increased risk of jaundice recurrence while receiving estrogen-containing oral contraceptives. If jaundice occurs during estrogen therapy, the drug should be discontinued. Estrogens may precipitate hepatic forms of porphyria, and the drugs probably should not be used by women who have a familial history of hepatic porphyrias, since the occurrence of these conditions appears to be genetically determined. Steroid hormones (including estrogens) may be poorly metabolized in patients with hepatic dysfunction; therefore, estrogens should be administered with caution to these individuals.

Liver tumors have been associated with use of estrogen-containing oral contraceptives. Liver tumors have been benign or malignant and have occurred during short-term and long-term use of oral contraceptives. Most commonly, liver tumors are benign hepatocellular adenomas and occur only rarely in oral contraceptive users; however, they may result in death because their vascularity predisposes them to rupture and cause massive hemorrhage. Although benign hepatocellular adenomas have not been reported to date with estrogens, the possibility of a liver tumor should be considered in any patient receiving an estrogen who develops sudden severe abdominal pain or shock.

● Genitourinary Effects

Breakthrough bleeding, spotting, changes in menstrual flow, missed menses (during use), or amenorrhea (after use) may occur in women receiving estrogen therapy. Dysmenorrhea and a premenstrual-like syndrome also have been reported. In patients with breakthrough bleeding or irregular vaginal bleeding, nonfunctional causes should be considered. Appropriate diagnostic procedures should be performed in patients with undiagnosed persistent or recurrent vaginal bleeding.

Changes in cervical erosion and secretions may occur during estrogen therapy. In addition, preexisting uterine leiomyoma may increase in size in women receiving estrogens. A cystitis-like syndrome has been reported but has not been definitely attributed to estrogens. An increased incidence of *Candida* vaginitis has been associated with estrogen therapy.

The possibility that estrogen replacement therapy in postmenopausal women, particularly prolonged use, may be associated with an increased risk of endometrial or ovarian cancer should be considered. (See Cautions: Mutagenicity and Carcinogenicity.)

● Nervous System Effects

Mental depression may occur in patients receiving estrogens. In a few women receiving estrogen-containing oral contraceptives, mental depression was severe and led to suicidal behavior. Patients with a history of mental depression should be observed carefully and estrogens discontinued if severe depression recurs during use.

Dizziness, changes in libido, and chorea have been reported in patients receiving estrogens.

Headache, especially migraine headache, may occur during estrogen therapy. Estrogens should be discontinued and the cause evaluated when migraine occurs or is exacerbated, or when a new headache pattern develops that is recurrent, persistent, and/or severe.

● Ocular Effects

Estrogens have been reported to produce keratoconus (steepening or corneal curvature) and intolerance to contact lenses. Contact lens wearers who develop visual disturbances or changes in lens tolerance during estrogen therapy should be assessed by an ophthalmologist; temporary or permanent cessation of contact lens wear should be considered.

Retinal vascular thrombosis has been reported in patients receiving estrogens. If unexplained, sudden or gradual, partial or complete loss of vision; proptosis or diplopia; papilledema; or retinal vascular lesions occur during therapy with an estrogen, the drug should be discontinued and appropriate diagnostic and therapeutic measures instituted.

● Hematologic Effects

Changes in various blood factors and blood components have been observed in women receiving estrogen-containing oral contraceptives and may occur in patients receiving estrogens; however, further studies are required before the clinical importance of these changes can be established. Estrogen (ERT) and hormone replacement therapy (estrogen/progestin, HRT) are associated with an increased risk of venous thromboembolic events in postmenopausal women. Increases in prothrombin and blood coagulation factors VII, VIII, IX, and X levels may occur in patients receiving estrogens; decreases in antithrombin III activity and decreased fibrinolysis also have been reported. In a clinical study in patients receiving conjugated estrogens in conjunction with medroxyprogesterone acetate, factors VII and X concentrations and plasminogen activity were increased and antithrombin III activity usually was decreased following 1 year of therapy. Estrogens may also enhance norepinephrine-induced platelet aggregation.

● Other Adverse Effects

Breast changes, including tenderness, enlargement, and secretion, may occur during estrogen therapy. The incidence of breast pain may be increased in patients receiving estrogens in conjunction with progestins compared with those receiving estrogens alone; breast pain was reported in about 33% of women receiving conjugated estrogens concomitantly with medroxyprogesterone acetate compared to 12% of women receiving unopposed conjugated estrogen therapy.

● Precautions and Contraindications

Use of estrogens may be associated with an increased risk of several serious conditions including deep-vein thrombosis, stroke, MI, pulmonary embolism, liver tumor, gallbladder disease, visual disturbances, and malignancy. Clinicians prescribing estrogens should be aware of the risks associated with the use of estrogens; the manufacturers' labeling also should be consulted for further discussion of these risks and associated precautions. When estrogens are used in combination with other drugs (e.g., androgens, progestins, bazedoxifene), the usual precautions associated with the other drugs should also be observed. If a progestin is administered concomitantly with estrogen therapy, potential risks may include adverse effects on lipid metabolism, glucose tolerance, or possible enhancement of mitotic activity in breast epithelial tissue.

Because of the potential increased risk of cardiovascular events, breast cancer, and venous thromboembolic events, estrogen and estrogen/progestin therapy should be limited to the lowest effective doses and shortest duration of therapy consistent with treatment goals and risks for the individual woman. Therapy with estrogen, estrogen/progestin, or conjugated estrogens in fixed combination with bazedoxifene should be periodically reevaluated.

Patients receiving estrogens should be under the supervision of a physician who should inform them of the possible risks involved. Patients receiving estrogens should also be given a copy of the patient labeling for the drugs.

A complete medical and family history should be taken prior to initiation of estrogen therapy and periodically thereafter. Estrogens should generally not be prescribed for longer than 1 year without a repeat physical examination being performed. Physical examination should include special attention to blood pressure, breasts, abdomen, and pelvic organs and should include a Papanicolaou test (Pap smear) and relevant laboratory tests.

Patients receiving estrogens should be informed to notify their physician if signs or symptoms of thromboembolic or thrombotic disorders (e.g., thrombophlebitis, pulmonary embolism, cerebrovascular insufficiency, coronary occlusion, retinal thrombosis, mesenteric thrombosis) occur, including sudden severe headache or vomiting, disturbance of vision or speech, sudden partial or complete loss of vision, dizziness or faintness, weakness or numbness in an extremity, sharp or crushing chest pain, unexplained cough, hemoptysis, sudden shortness of breath, calf pain, or heaviness in the chest. If signs or symptoms consistent with a thromboembolic or thrombotic disorder occur, hormone replacement therapy (HRT) should be discontinued immediately. Use of ERT or HRT is not advised in women with a history of stroke or transient ischemic attacks. If hormone therapy is initiated or discontinued in a woman receiving oral anticoagulant therapy, effectiveness of the anticoagulant may be altered and dosage adjustment needed. Patients receiving estrogens should also be advised to inform their physician if abdominal pain, swelling, or tenderness (indicating possible gallbladder disease), or an abdominal mass (indicating a possible liver tumor), jaundice, severe mental depression, or unusual bleeding occurs. Since endometrial hyperplasia and endometrial carcinoma have been reported in women receiving estrogen therapy, adequate diagnostic tests should be performed in women with undiagnosed, persistent, or recurring abnormal vaginal bleeding. (See Carcinogenicity.) Women receiving estrogens should be instructed in self-examination of their breasts and should report lumps in the breast to their physician.

Estrogens should be used with caution, and only with careful monitoring, in patients with conditions that might be aggravated by fluid retention (e.g., cardiac or renal insufficiency); in patients with cerebrovascular or coronary artery disease (including MI); and in women with a strong family history of breast cancer or who have breast nodules, fibrocystic disease, or abnormal mammographic findings (see Cautions: Carcinogenicity).

Women undergoing surgery and those with fracture or who are immobilized have a relatively high risk of venous thromboembolic events. Therefore, estrogens should be discontinued, whenever feasible, at least 4–6 weeks prior to surgery that is associated with an increased risk of thromboembolism or prolonged immobilization. The decision as to when to resume estrogen therapy following major surgery or immobilization should be based on the risks of postsurgery thromboembolic complications and the need for such therapy. In addition, some clinicians recommend that women discontinue estrogen replacement therapy during immobilization due to fracture, stroke, or other severe illness; estrogen replacement therapy can be restarted when normal activity is resumed. Since acute pancreatitis, associated with increased triglyceride concentrations, has been reported in a few women receiving estrogens alone or in conjunction with a progestin, it is recommended that serum lipid concentrations be monitored prior to and during estrogen therapy. (See Cautions: GI Effects.)

Because estrogens influence the metabolism of calcium and phosphorus, the drugs should be used with caution in patients with renal insufficiency and in patients with metabolic bone diseases that are associated with hypercalcemia.

Metabolism of estrogens may be decreased in patients with impaired hepatic function. Caution is advised in patients with a history of cholestatic jaundice associated with estrogen use or pregnancy; if cholestatic jaundice recurs, estrogen therapy should be discontinued.

Estrogens may exacerbate asthma, diabetes mellitus, epilepsy, migraine, porphyria, systemic lupus erythematosus, and hepatic hemangiomas and should be used with caution in women with these conditions. Estrogens also may exacerbate symptoms of angioedema in women with hereditary angioedema.

Estrogens are contraindicated in patients with known or suspected pregnancy, undiagnosed abnormal genital bleeding, known or suspected breast cancer or a history of breast cancer (except when used for the palliative treatment of metastatic disease in appropriately selected individuals), or known or suspected estrogen-dependent neoplasia. Estrogens also are contraindicated in patients with active deep-vein thrombosis or pulmonary embolism; a history of deep-vein thrombosis or pulmonary embolism; active or recent (within the past year) arterial thromboembolic disease (e.g., stroke, MI); liver disease or impairment; known protein C, protein S, or antithrombin deficiency, or other known thrombophilic disorders; or known hypersensitivity to estrogen or any ingredient in the formulation.

● Pediatric Precautions

Estrogen therapy has been used for the induction of puberty in adolescents with some forms of pubertal delay. Safety and efficacy of estrogens in children have not otherwise been established. Estrogen therapy should be used with caution in young individuals in whom bone growth is not yet complete, since estrogens may cause premature closure of the epiphyses.

● Geriatric Precautions

When the total number of patients studied in the Women's Health Initiative (WHI) study is considered, 44–46% were 65 years of age or older, while 6.6–7.1% were 75 years of age or older. In the estrogen plus progestin WHI study, there was a higher relative risk of nonfatal stoke or breast cancer in women 75 years of age or older compared with women younger than 75 years of age.

● Mutagenicity and Carcinogenicity

Prolonged continuous administration of natural or synthetic estrogen in certain animal species increases the frequency of certain benign or malignant tumors including those of the breast, cervix, uterus, vagina, ovary, pituitary, and liver.

Endometrial Cancer

Several studies have shown an increased relative risk of endometrial carcinoma in postmenopausal women who received prolonged estrogen replacement therapy for relief of menopausal symptoms. This risk was independent of other known risk factors for endometrial carcinoma and appeared to depend on duration and dosage of estrogen therapy. While there appears to be no increased risk

of endometrial carcinoma in postmenopausal women receiving estrogen therapy for less than 1 year, prolonged estrogen therapy may be associated with an increased risk of such carcinoma. The risk of endometrial carcinoma reportedly is increased 2- to 12-fold in postmenopausal women receiving unopposed estrogen therapy compared with those not receiving estrogens; such increased risk may depend on dosage and duration of therapy and may be 15- to 24-fold higher in women receiving long-term (5 years or more) estrogen therapy. Limited data indicate that a substantial increased risk of endometrial carcinoma may persist for up to 15 years following discontinuance of estrogen therapy. Because of the increased risk of endometrial carcinoma associated with prolonged estrogen therapy, patients receiving prolonged treatment with the drugs should be evaluated at least twice yearly to reassess the need for continued therapy. Results of several studies indicate that when progestins are used concomitantly with estrogen replacement therapy, the incidence of endometrial hyperplasia and endometrial carcinoma is reduced substantially. In a randomized, controlled, multicenter study in postmenopausal women, endometrial hyperplasia occurred in 20 or 1% or less of women receiving estrogen therapy alone or in conjunction with progestins, respectively. In the WHI study, the incidence of endometrial carcinoma in women receiving hormone replacement therapy (conjugated estrogens 0.625 mg in conjunction with medroxyprogesterone acetate 2.5 mg daily) was similar to the incidence in women receiving placebo. As an alternative to progestins, the use of bazedoxifene (an estrogen agonist-antagonist) in fixed combination with conjugated estrogens reduces the risk of endometrial hyperplasia, which may be a precursor to endometrial carcinoma.

Although estrogen-associated risk of endometrial carcinoma is substantially reduced when estrogens are administered concomitantly with progestins or bazedoxifene, a risk still exists. Therefore, clinical surveillance and evaluation of all menopausal women receiving estrogen therapy is essential. Diagnostic tests, including endometrial sampling when indicated, should be performed to rule out malignancy in all women who have undiagnosed, persistent, or abnormal vaginal bleeding.

Currently, there is no evidence that estrogens derived from natural sources are more or less hazardous than synthetic estrogens at equiestrogenic dosages.

Breast Cancer

All women receiving estrogens should perform monthly self-examinations of their breasts and be monitored at least annually by a health-care provider for breast abnormalities and more frequently if there are any signs and symptoms. Periodic mammography should be scheduled based on patient age, risk factors, and prior mammogram results. Women with a strong family history of breast cancer or who have breast nodules, fibrocystic disease, or abnormal mammographic findings should be monitored particularly closely if they elect to use estrogens. Although the clinical importance remains to be established, therapy with estrogen/progestin increases mammographic breast density relative to therapy with estrogen alone or placebo.

Because breast tissue is sensitive to reproductive hormones, there has been long-standing concern about the risk of breast cancer in women receiving hormone replacement therapy (HRT). The estrogen/progestin arm of the WHI study recently was terminated prematurely because of an increased incidence of breast cancer in women receiving HRT. In the WHI study, the risk of invasive breast cancer was 26% higher in women receiving HRT (conjugated estrogens 0.625 mg in conjunction with medroxyprogesterone acetate 2.5 mg daily) compared with those receiving placebo; the estimated hazard ratio for breast cancer was 1.26. While there have been several observational studies evaluating the risk of breast cancer in women receiving HRT, conclusions are limited by healthy-user bias; variations in specific preparations, dosage, and duration of therapy; and differences in the methods used to determine breast cancer end points. In aggregate, breast cancer incidence is slightly increased among current (relative risk: 1.21–1.4) or long-term (longer than 5 years) recipients (relative risk: 1.23–1.35) compared with nonusers. Based on these findings, recommendations on the appropriate use of hormone therapy have been revised. Because the risks of hormone therapy exceed the benefits for the prevention of chronic diseases in postmenopausal women, experts state that ERT or HRT should not be used for the prevention of chronic conditions in postmenopausal women. The American Heart Association (AHA), the American College of Obstetricians and Gynecologists (ACOG), FDA, and manufacturers recommend that hormone therapy not be used to prevent heart disease in healthy women (primary prevention) or to protect women with preexisting heart disease (secondary prevention). ACOG, FDA, and the manufacturers also recommend that women receiving hormone therapy solely for the prevention of postmenopausal osteoporosis consider alternative therapy (e.g., alendronate, raloxifene, risedronate).

The decision to use estrogen or estrogen/progestin for management of menopausal symptoms should be individualized taking into account the women's preference, her risk for specific chronic diseases, and the presence and severity of menopausal symptoms.

Results of a large (involving more than 100,000 women) prospective cohort study (the Nurses' Health Study) in postmenopausal women who received conjugated estrogens indicated an increased risk of breast cancer in such women; in addition, an increased risk of breast cancer also was observed in individuals who received estrogen therapy in conjunction with progestins. The relative risk of breast cancer increased with age and duration of therapy, with the greatest risk being observed in women 60–64 years of age and in women who received estrogen replacement therapy for more than 10 years. In women receiving estrogens alone or in conjunction with progestins, the relative risk of developing breast cancer was 1.32 or 1.41, respectively. The relative risk of breast cancer was similar in women who had never received estrogen replacement therapy, women who received prior estrogen therapy, and women who received estrogen therapy for less than 5 years; however, the relative risk of developing breast cancer increased to 1.63 in women 60–64 years who received estrogens for at least 5 years. Results of this study also indicated that the relative risk of developing breast cancer was similar in women with and without a family history of the disease; consumption of alcohol did not affect results.

Data from the Nurses' Health Study, the Breast Cancer Detection Demonstration Project, and other studies indicate that estrogen/progestin regimens are associated with an increased risk of breast cancer beyond that associated with estrogen alone. In the Breast Cancer Detection Demonstration Project (a study that included 46,000 women), the relative risk of breast cancer in women who received estrogen or estrogen/progestin within the previous 4 years was 1.2 or 1.4, respectively. Similar to results from other studies, the increased risk was generally limited to current or recent recipients and was related to duration of use. The relative risk (adjusted for mammographic screening, age at menopause, body mass index [BMI], education, age) increased by 0.01 with each year of estrogen use and by 0.08 with each year of estrogen/progestin use in recent recipients. Among recent recipients of progestin for fewer than 15 days per month, the relative risk of breast cancer associated with therapy for less than 4 years was 1.1 while the relative risk associated with therapy for longer than 4 years was 1.5; estimates for risk were not available for recipients of progestins for 15 or more days per month due to insufficient data. The relative risk of breast cancer in recent recipients of estrogen or estrogen/progestin increased 0.03 or 0.12, respectively, each year in women with a BMI of 24.4 kg/m^2 or less; an increase in risk associated with duration of use was not observed in heavier women.

The WHI, a long-term study sponsored by the National Institutes of Health (NIH), followed 16,608 predominantly healthy women with an intact uterus who were 50–79 years of age and who received HRT (i.e., conjugated estrogens 0.625 mg in conjunction with medroxyprogesterone acetate 2.5 mg daily) or placebo with the goal of evaluating the relationship between HRT and coronary heart disease (CHD), stroke, pulmonary embolism, breast cancer, endometrial carcinoma, colorectal cancer, hip fracture, and death from other causes. The study was stopped early because health risks exceeded benefits over an average follow-up of 5.2 years. At the time the study was stopped, the increased number of cases of invasive breast cancer, CHD, stroke, and pulmonary embolism in the estrogen/progestin group relative to the placebo group was not counterbalanced by reductions in the number of cases of hip fracture and colorectal cancer. The WHI study is the first randomized, controlled study to confirm that estrogen/progestin therapy increases the risk of breast cancer in postmenopausal women and to quantify the risk. In the WHI estrogen plus progestin study, the risk of invasive breast cancer was 26% higher in women receiving HRT (conjugated estrogens 0.625 mg in conjunction with medroxyprogesterone acetate 2.5 mg daily) compared with those receiving placebo; the estimated hazard ratio for breast cancer was 1.26. The number of cases of breast cancer per 10,000 patient-years of exposure was 38 or 30 in women receiving HRT or placebo, respectively. The increase in breast cancer risk was apparent after 4 years of estrogen/progestin therapy, and the risk appeared to be cumulative. In addition, the risk associated with HRT appeared to increase at a higher rate than would be expected based on advancing age. The hazard ratio for HRT was not higher in women with a family history or other risk factors for breast cancer, except for prior postmenopausal hormone therapy. In the WHI estrogen-alone study, use of estrogen was not associated with an increased risk of breast cancer.

Whether the effect of hormone replacement therapy on breast cancer incidence varies among histologic types of invasive carcinomas remains to be established. Findings from the Breast Cancer Detection Demonstration Project and the WHI estrogen plus progestin study indicate that such therapy is associated with an increase in risk for the majority of invasive tumors classified as lobular and/or ductal carcinomas. Findings from other studies indicate that estrogen/progestin therapy is associated with an increased risk of invasive lobular carcinoma. While data from some studies (e.g., the Iowa Women's Health Study) suggest that estrogen/progestin therapy is associated with an increased risk of invasive breast cancer with a favorable prognosis, findings from the WHI indicate that such therapy is associated with cancers that are at least as invasive as those in women not receiving estrogen/progestin therapy. Analysis of breast cancer characteristics in women enrolled in the WHI indicate that the invasive breast cancers diagnosed in women receiving estrogen/progestin were similar in histology and grade but were larger (1.7 versus 1.5 cm, respectively) and were at a more advanced grade (regional/metastatic disease in 25.4 versus 16%, respectively) than those diagnosed in women receiving placebo.

The US Department of Health and Human Services 1985 DES Task Force concluded that the weight of evidence to date indicates that women who used diethylstilbestrol (DES) during pregnancy may subsequently experience an increased risk of breast cancer; however, because of limitations of current data and study methodologies, a causal relationship to the drug has not been established. Data from studies to date suggest an overall relative risk of breast cancer for DES-treated women ranging from 1.2–1.5 times that for untreated women, an excess risk that is similar to that associated with a number of other breast cancer risk factors; however, in epidemiologic analyses, these levels of excess risk are difficult to evaluate since various sources of bias that could be responsible for such excesses cannot be easily ruled out. It should be noted that conclusions regarding the likelihood of causality for this association between DES use and breast cancer could be substantially influenced by further follow-up of exposed women who have already been identified and studied and by initiation of studies of other exposed women which pay particular attention to matching DES-exposed and unexposed groups based on indications for DES use, to evaluating dose-latency relationships, and to the possibility of bias toward early diagnosis of breast cancer among exposed women. Initiation of studies that investigate interactions with other risk factors, considering possible additive and cumulative risks, and endocrinologic and immunologic considerations may also influence conclusions about the likelihood of causality.

Ovarian Cancer

While findings from epidemiologic (e.g., case-control) studies on the association between postmenopausal hormone replacement therapy and the risk of ovarian cancer have been inconsistent, results from 2 large, prospective cohort studies with average follow-up of 13–14 years indicate that postmenopausal estrogen use is associated with an increased risk of ovarian cancer.

In the American Cancer Society's Cancer Prevention Study II, which included over 200,000 postmenopausal women, women receiving oral estrogen replacement therapy at study entry (baseline) had higher death rates from ovarian cancer (adjusted rate ratio: 1.51) than women who had never received estrogen replacement therapy. Duration of estrogen use also was associated with increased risk; women who received estrogen replacement therapy for 10 or more years and who were receiving such therapy at baseline were more than twice as likely to have died from ovarian cancer as never users (adjusted rate ratio: 2.2). Estrogen use for less than 10 years was not associated with an increased risk of ovarian cancer mortality. Among women who discontinued estrogen after 10 or more years of use, the risk decreased with time; the adjusted rate ratio was 2.05 in those who received estrogen within the previous 15 years and 1.31 in those who had not received estrogen within the previous 15 years. Whether women receiving oral estrogen also received progestin was not evaluated in this study; however, most hormone replacement regimens for postmenopausal women contained only estrogenic compounds until the late 1970's and most women receiving hormone replacement therapy in 1982 (baseline) presumably were receiving unopposed estrogen therapy.

Data from the Breast Cancer Detection Demonstration Project also indicate that estrogen replacement therapy is associated with an increased risk of developing ovarian cancer and that the risk associated with estrogen-only hormone replacement therapy is greater than that associated with estrogen-progestin replacement therapy. In a study in over 40,000 postmenopausal women, those who received estrogen-only hormone replacement therapy were twice as likely to develop ovarian cancer as never users (adjusted relative risk: 2) with a lower risk (adjusted relative risk: 1.3) in women who received estrogen-progestin replacement therapy. Although the lifetime risk of ovarian cancer is low (1.7%), any increase in risk of ovarian cancer related to long-term estrogen therapy should be considered in the risk/benefit assessment of such therapy.

GI Cancers

Data from observational studies, the Heart and Estrogen/progestin Replacement Study (HERS), and the WHI estrogen plus progestin study indicate that hormone replacement therapy reduces the incidence of colorectal cancer. In the WHI estrogen plus progestin study, the risk of colorectal cancer was reduced by 37% in women receiving hormone replacement therapy (conjugated estrogens 0.625 mg in conjunction with medroxyprogesterone acetate 2.5 mg daily) compared with those receiving placebo. The number of cases of colorectal cancer per 10,000 patient-years of exposure was 10 or 16 in women receiving hormone replacement therapy or placebo, respectively. Results from the WHI estrogen-alone study indicate that ERT (conjugated estrogens 0.625 mg daily) does not affect the incidence of colorectal cancer.

● Pregnancy, Fertility, and Lactation

Pregnancy

Estrogens can cause fetal harm when administered to pregnant women. *In utero* exposure of females to diethylstilbestrol (DES [no longer commercially available in the US]), a nonsteroidal estrogen, is associated with an increased risk of developing a rare form of vaginal or cervical cancer (clear-cell adenocarcinoma) in later life. In addition, such exposure to DES causes epithelial changes in the vagina and cervix in 30–90% of these exposed female offspring.

In utero exposure of females to DES is also associated with an increased risk of developing a rare form of vaginal or cervical cancer (clear-cell adenocarcinoma) in later life. In addition, such exposure to DES causes epithelial changes (adenosis) in the vagina and cervix in 30–90% of these exposed female offspring. Experience from the National Collaborative Diethylstilbestrol Adenosis (DESAD) Project indicates that women exposed to DES *in utero* appear to have an increased risk of dysplasia and carcinoma *in situ* of the cervix and vagina; the rate of these changes was 15.7 versus 7.9 cases per 1000 person-years of follow-up for exposed and unexposed women, respectively, and was even higher in exposed women with squamous metaplasia extending to the outer half of the cervix or onto the vagina. The 1985 DES Task Force concluded that, based on the results of the DESAD Project, women exposed to DES *in utero* may be at increased risk of cervical and vaginal dysplasia, particularly if they have extensive metaplasia; however, further documentation and evaluation of this association are necessary, and the relationship between DES exposure *in utero* and subsequent risk of squamous cell carcinoma of the cervix remains unclear.

In utero exposure to DES in females has not been associated with an increased risk of developing cancer other than an increased risk of developing vaginal or cervical clear-cell adenocarcinoma. *In utero* exposure of males to DES has been associated with an increased incidence of genital tract abnormalities including epididymal cysts, maldescended testes, hypoplastic testes, varicoceles, low sperm counts, and spermatozoal defects (e.g., decreased motility, possibly abnormal forms). Similar data are not available for other estrogens, but it cannot be presumed that they would not induce similar changes.

Although estrogens were previously used to treat threatened or habitual abortion, there is no evidence that estrogens are effective for these uses; in addition, the potential for adverse effects of the drugs on the fetus exists. Estrogens should not be used during pregnancy.

Lactation

Administration of estrogens to nursing women has been associated with decreased amounts and lower quality of milk. In addition, detectable amounts of estrogens and progestins have been identified in milk of women receiving these drugs. Although estrogens were previously used for the prevention of postpartum breast engorgement, such use is no longer recommended. Caution is advised when estrogens are administered to nursing women. Conjugated estrogens in fixed combination with bazedoxifene should not be used in nursing women.

DRUG INTERACTIONS

● Drugs Affecting Hepatic Microsomal Enzymes

Metabolism of estrogen is mediated in part by cytochrome P-450 (CYP) isoenzyme 3A4, and the possibility exists that drugs that induce or inhibit this isoenzyme may affect plasma estrogen concentrations. Concomitant use of estrogens with drugs that induce CYP3A4 (e.g., carbamazepine, phenobarbital, rifampin, St. John's wort [*Hypericum perforatum*]) may result in decreased plasma concentrations of estrogen, resulting in decreased therapeutic effects and/or changes in uterine bleeding profile. Concomitant use of estrogen with drugs or foods that inhibit CYP3A4 (e.g., clarithromycin, erythromycin, grapefruit juice, itraconazole, ketoconazole) may result in increased plasma concentrations of estrogens and an increase in the incidence of adverse effects.

Rifampin reportedly decreases estrogenic activity during concomitant use with estrogens. This effect has been attributed to enhanced metabolism of estrogen, presumably by induction of hepatic microsomal enzymes.

● Corticosteroids

Estrogens have been reported to enhance the anti-inflammatory effect of hydrocortisone in patients with chronic inflammatory skin diseases. It has been suggested that estrogens may decrease the hepatic metabolism of corticosteroids and/or alter serum corticosteroid protein binding. Patients receiving concomitant estrogen and corticosteroid therapy should be observed for signs of excessive corticosteroid effects, and alterations in corticosteroid dosage may be necessary when estrogens are started or discontinued.

● Oral Anticoagulants

Estrogens may decrease the action of oral anticoagulants. When estrogen therapy is initiated in patients receiving anticoagulants, an increase in anticoagulant dosage may be required.

LABORATORY TEST INTERFERENCES

Estrogen-containing oral contraceptives have caused abnormal thyroid function test results. (See Effects on Thyroid in Cautions: Endocrine and Metabolic Effects, in Estrogen-Progestin Combinations 68:12.) Estrogen-containing oral contraceptives have altered response to the metyrapone test (see Laboratory Test Interferences in Estrogen-Progestin Combinations 68:12) and liver function test results (see Cautions: Hepatic Effects, in Estrogen-Progestin Combinations 68:12). Estrogen-containing oral contraceptives have also caused decreased pregnanediol excretion.

The manufacturers state that the pathologist should be advised of estrogen use when relevant specimens from a patient exposed to estrogens are submitted.

ACUTE TOXICITY

Acute overdosage of large doses of oral contraceptives in children reportedly produces almost no toxicity except nausea and vomiting. Acute overdosage of estrogens may cause nausea, and withdrawal bleeding may occur in females.

PHARMACOLOGY

Estrogens are hormones secreted principally by the ovarian follicles and also by the adrenals, corpus luteum, placenta, and testes, or are synthetic steroidal and nonsteroidal compounds. Estrogenic hormones are secreted at varying rates during the menstrual cycle throughout the period of activity of the ovaries. During pregnancy, the placenta becomes the main source of estrogens. At the menopause, ovarian secretion of estrogens declines at varying rates. The gonadotropins of the anterior pituitary regulate secretion of the ovarian hormones, estradiol and progesterone; hypothalamic control of pituitary gonadotropin production is in turn regulated by plasma concentrations of the estrogens and progesterone. This complex feedback system results in the cyclic phenomenon of ovulation and menstruation.

● Estrogen Receptors

Estrogens have an important role in the reproductive, skeletal, cardiovascular, and central nervous systems in women, and act principally by regulating gene expression. Biologic response is initiated when estrogen binds to a ligand-binding domain of the estrogen receptor resulting in a conformational change that leads to gene transcription through specific estrogen response elements (ERE) of target gene promoters; subsequent activation or repression of the target gene is mediated through 2 distinct transactivation domains (i.e., AF-1 and AF-2) of the receptor. The estrogen receptor also mediates gene transcription using different response elements (i.e., AP-1) and other signal pathways. Recent advances in the molecular pharmacology of estrogen and estrogen receptors have resulted in the development of selective estrogen receptor modulators (e.g., clomiphene, raloxifene, tamoxifen, toremifene), agents that bind and activate the estrogen receptor but that exhibit tissue-specific effects distinct from estrogen. Tissue-specific estrogen-agonist or -antagonist activity of these drugs appears to be related to structural differences in their estrogen receptor complex (e.g., specifically the surface topography of AF-2 for raloxifene) compared with the estrogen (estradiol)-estrogen receptor complex. A second estrogen receptor also has been identified, and existence of at least 2 estrogen receptors (ER$_\alpha$, ER$_\beta$) may contribute to the tissue-specific activity of selective modulators. While the role of the estrogen receptor in bone, cardiovascular tissue, and the CNS continues to be studied, emerging evidence indicates that the mechanism of action of estrogen receptors in these tissues differs from the manner in which estrogen receptors function in reproductive tissue.

Intracellular cytosol-binding proteins for estrogens have been identified in estrogen-responsive tissues including the female genital organs, breasts, pituitary, and hypothalamus. The estrogen-binding protein complex (i.e., cytosol-binding protein and estrogen) distributes into the cell nucleus where it stimulates DNA, RNA, and protein synthesis. The presence of these receptor proteins is responsible for the palliative response to estrogen therapy in women with metastatic carcinoma of the breast.

● Estrogenic Effects

Exogenous estrogens elicit, to varying degrees, all the pharmacologic responses usually produced by endogenous estrogens. Endogenous estrogens are essential hormones that are responsible for the normal growth and development of the female sex organs and for maintenance of secondary sex characteristics, including the growth and maturation of the vagina, uterus, and fallopian tubes; enlargement of the breasts; maintenance of tone and elasticity of urogenital structures; growth of axillary and pubic hair; and pigmentation of the nipples and genitals.

Although the mechanism(s) has not been elucidated, estrogens contribute to the shaping of body contours and the skeleton, to the growth spurt that occurs during adolescence, and to the eventual termination of linear growth that results from fusion of the epiphyseal centers. Estrogens cause an increase in cell height and secretions of the cervical mucosa, thickening and cornification of the vaginal mucosa, proliferation of the endometrium, and an increase in uterine tone. The estrogen-stimulated endometrium may bleed within 48–72 hours after discontinuance of estrogen therapy. Paradoxically, prolonged estrogen therapy may cause shrinkage of the endometrium and an increase in size of the myometrium.

Menstrual Effects

During the preovulatory or nonovulatory phase of the menstrual cycle, estrogen is the principal determinant in the onset of menstruation. A decline of estrogenic activity at the end of the menstrual cycle also may induce menstruation; however, the cessation of progesterone secretion is the most important factor during the mature ovulatory phase of the menstrual cycle.

Gonadotropic Effects

Although the precise actions of estrogens on secretory activity of the pituitary have not been fully characterized, estrogens affect the release of gonadotropins (e.g., follicle-stimulating hormone [FSH]) from the pituitary, apparently as a result of feedback inhibition; the effect of estrogens on luteinizing hormone (LH) is complex and biphasic. The effects of estrogens on pituitary secretion of gonadotropins result in inhibition of lactation, inhibition of ovulation, development of a proliferative endometrium and, by inhibiting androgen secretion, a reduction of sebaceous secretions.

● Anabolic and Metabolic Effects

Estrogens have a weak anabolic effect and may cause sodium retention with associated fluid retention and edema. Estrogens also affect bone by increasing calcium deposition and accelerating epiphyseal closure, following initial growth stimulation.

● Cardiovascular Effects

Estrogens have generally favorable effects on blood cholesterol and phospholipid concentrations. Estrogens reduce LDL-cholesterol and increase HDL-cholesterol concentrations in a dose-related manner. The decrease in LDL-cholesterol concentrations associated with estrogen therapy appears to result from increased

LDL catabolism, while the increase in triglyceride concentrations is caused by increased production of large, triglyceride-rich, very-low-density lipoproteins (VLDLs); changes in serum HDL-cholesterol concentrations appear to result principally from an increase in the cholesterol and apolipoprotein A-1 content of HDL$_2$- and a slight increase in HDL$_3$-cholesterol.

Results of several clinical studies in postmenopausal women indicate that replacement therapy with unopposed conjugated estrogens (estrogen replacement therapy, ERT) may reduce LDL-cholesterol and increase HDL-cholesterol by about 8–15%; however, use of progestins in conjunction with estrogen (hormone replacement therapy, HRT) may blunt these favorable effects on the lipid profile. In a 1-year prospective, randomized, double-blind study in healthy, postmenopausal, predominately white women at low risk for cardiovascular disease, HDL-cholesterol concentrations increased 14.1 or 4.4% in women receiving conjugated estrogens (0.625 mg daily) alone (ERT) or conjugated estrogens (0.625 mg daily) in conjunction with cyclic medroxyprogesterone acetate (5 mg daily on days 15–28 of the cycle) (HRT), respectively; decreases in LDL-cholesterol concentrations were similar in women receiving estrogens alone (ERT) or in conjunction with the progestin (HRT). In this study, serum triglyceride concentrations increased by 39.4 or 27.5% in women receiving estrogens alone (ERT) or in conjunction with the progestin (HRT), respectively. In addition, in a 3-year, placebo-controlled, multicenter study in postmenopausal women, HDL-cholesterol concentrations were higher in patients receiving conjugated estrogens alone (ERT) than in those receiving conjugated estrogens in conjunction with progestins (HRT); HDL-cholesterol concentrations were lower in patients receiving placebo than in those receiving estrogen replacement therapy. Concomitant progestin therapy blunts some of the favorable effects of estrogens on the lipid profile of postmenopausal women.

Although most experience to date on the lipid-lowering effect of estrogens included administration of conjugated estrogens, limited evidence indicates that postmenopausal women who received oral micronized estradiol (2 mg daily for 6 weeks) had changes in LDL- and HDL-cholesterol and triglyceride concentrations that were similar to those produced by low-dose conjugated estrogen therapy, but transdermal estradiol (0.1 mg twice weekly) did not substantially affect serum lipoprotein concentrations.

Other effects of estrogens that may contribute to effects on cardiovascular risk indicators include reduction of insulin and blood glucose concentrations and direct effects on blood vessels. Estrogen receptors have been identified in the heart and coronary arteries, suggesting that estrogens may have specific effects on these tissues.

The Women's Health Initiative (WHI) study provided evidence of increased cardiovascular risk associated with combined estrogen and progestin therapy (HRT). (See Cautions: Cardiovascular Effects.)

PHARMACOKINETICS

● Absorption

Following oral administration, the natural, unconjugated estrogens are inactivated in the GI tract and liver. Conjugated estrogens and some synthetic derivatives of the natural estrogens may be administered orally. Absorption and metabolism following oral administration of these drugs is rapid and daily doses are usually required. Chlorotrianisene (no longer commercially available in the US), however, has a prolonged duration of action which may result from the storage in and slow release of estrogenically active substance from adipose tissue. Similarly, quinestrol (no longer commercially available in the US) has a prolonged duration of action as a result of its extensive storage in and slow release from adipose tissue.

Following IM administration of estrogen oil solutions, absorption begins promptly and continues for several days. When estrogen is conjugated with aryl and alkyl groups, the rate of absorption of estrogen is slowed.

Estrogens are readily absorbed through the skin and mucous membranes. Depending on the amount of estrogen applied, systemic as well as local effects may occur following topical application.

● Distribution

Estrogens are distributed throughout most body tissues. Studies utilizing radioisotopes have indicated that the greatest concentrations of estrogens may occur in the fat deposits of the body; obese patients have demonstrated slower and more prolonged estrogen excretion. Estrogens are 50–80% bound to plasma proteins. Estriol is bound less to plasma proteins than is estrone or estradiol but all 3 estrogens are bound to approximately the same extent by erythrocytes. Studies using radioisotopes have demonstrated a rapid transfer of free estrone and estradiol between mother and fetus. Fetal estrogens appear to originate principally from the placenta and mother.

● **Elimination**

The steroidal estrogens are metabolized principally in the liver, although the kidneys, gonads, and muscle tissues may be involved to some extent. The steroids and their metabolites are conjugated at the hydroxyl group of the C 3 position with sulfuric or glucuronic acid; these conjugates may undergo further metabolic change. Conjugation increases water solubility and facilitates excretion in urine. Large amounts of free estrogens are also distributed into the bile, reabsorbed from the GI tract, and recirculated through the liver where further degradation occurs. Estrogens and their metabolites are excreted mainly in urine; however, small amounts are also present in feces.

The metabolic fate of the synthetic estrogens has not been fully elucidated. Diethylstilbestrol (no longer commercially available in the US) metabolism, however, appears to be similar to that of the natural estrogens with the drug being excreted mainly as the glucuronide in urine.

● **Chemistry**

Estrogens are naturally occurring hormones or synthetic steroidal and nonsteroidal compounds with estrogenic activity. The estrogens can be divided into 2 groups based on their chemical structures: steroidal and nonsteroidal compounds. All naturally occurring estrogens are steroids that contain a cyclopentanoperhydrophenanthrene ring structure with an unsaturated A ring, a methyl group at the C 13 position, a phenolic hydroxyl group at the C 3 position, and a ketone or hydroxyl group at the C 17 position. Only a limited number of changes can be made in this basic steroid structure without losing estrogenic activity. These changes are limited to an interconversion of the hydroxyl and ketone groups or the addition of various side chains at the C 3 and C 17 positions.

The natural steroidal estrogens (estradiol, estrone, estriol, equilin, and equilenin) and their conjugates are usually obtained from pregnant mares' urine or prepared synthetically. The natural steroidal estrogens, both those obtained exclusively from natural sources and those prepared synthetically, are insoluble in water but when conjugated as the sulfates or glucuronides, these hormones become water soluble. Synthetic derivatives of the natural steroidal estrogens were previously available. The nonsteroidal estrogens include diethylstilbestrol (DES) (no longer commercially available in the US) and dienestrol (no longer commercially available in the US).

For further information on chemistry and stability, pharmacology, pharmacokinetics, uses, cautions, and dosage and administration of estrogens, see the individual monographs in 68:16.04. See also Estrogen-Progestin Combinations 68:12.

---

† Use is not currently included in the labeling approved by the US Food and Drug Administration.

Selected Revisions November 27, 2017, © Copyright, May 1, 1969, American Society of Health-System Pharmacists, Inc.

Estradiol

68:16.04 • ESTROGENS

■ Estradiol (a principal endogenous estrogen) is a steroidal estrogen.

USES

● Estradiol

Oral, transdermal, or topical estradiol is used for the management of moderate to severe vasomotor symptoms associated with menopause and for the management of vulvar and vaginal atrophy (atrophic vaginitis, kraurosis vulvae). Oral or transdermal estradiol is used for the treatment of female hypoestrogenism due to hypogonadism, castration, or primary ovarian failure. If estrogens are used solely for the management of vulvar and vaginal atrophy, use of topical vaginal preparations should be considered. Estradiol also may be administered intravaginally as a cream or tablet for the management of vulvar and vaginal atrophy. Estradiol vaginal ring is used for the management of urogenital symptoms associated with postmenopausal atrophy of the vagina (i.e., dryness, burning, pruritus, dyspareunia) and/or lower urinary tract (i.e., urinary urgency, dysuria).

Oral or transdermal estradiol (Alora®, Climara®, Climara Pro®, Estraderm®, Menostar®, Vivelle®, Vivelle-Dot®) is used adjunctively with other therapeutic measures (e.g., diet, calcium, weight-bearing exercise [including walking, running], physical therapy) to retard further bone loss and the progression of osteoporosis associated with estrogen deficiency in postmenopausal women. While estrogen replacement therapy is effective for the prevention of osteoporosis in women and has been shown to reduce bone resorption and retard or halt bone loss in postmenopausal women, such therapy is associated with a number of adverse effects. (See Uses: Estrogen Replacement Therapy, in the Estrogens General Statement 68:16.04.) If prevention of postmenopausal osteoporosis is the sole indication for estrogen therapy, alternative therapy (e.g., alendronate, raloxifene, risedronate) also should be considered.

While results from earlier observational studies indicated that estrogen replacement therapy (ERT) or combined estrogen/progestin therapy (HRT) was associated with cardiovascular benefit in postmenopausal women, results from recent controlled studies indicate that hormone therapy does not decrease the incidence of cardiovascular disease. The American Heart Association (AHA), American College of Obstetricians and Gynecologists (ACOG), US Food and Drug Administration (FDA) and manufacturers recommend that hormone therapy not be used to prevent heart disease in healthy women (primary prevention) or to protect women with preexisting heart disease (secondary prevention). (See Cardiovascular Risk Reduction under Uses: Estrogen Replacement Therapy, in the Estrogens General Statement 68:16.04.)

Oral estradiol is used for the palliative treatment of advanced, inoperable, metastatic carcinoma of the breast in postmenopausal women and in men. Estrogens are one of several second-line agents that can be used in certain postmenopausal women with metastatic breast cancer.

Oral estradiol is used for the palliative treatment of advanced carcinoma of the prostate in men; however, the risk of adverse cardiovascular effects of estrogens must be considered.

● Estradiol Acetate

Oral estradiol acetate and estradiol acetate vaginal ring are used for management of moderate to severe vasomotor symptoms associated with menopause. Estradiol acetate vaginal ring also is used for the management of moderate to severe symptoms of vulvar and vaginal atrophy associated with menopause. If estradiol acetate vaginal ring is used solely for the management of vulvar and vaginal atrophy, use of an alternative topical vaginal preparation should be considered.

● Estradiol Cypionate

Estradiol cypionate is used for the management of moderate to severe vasomotor symptoms associated with menopause. Estradiol cypionate also is used for the management of female hypogonadism.

Estradiol cypionate in fixed combination with testosterone cypionate is used for the management of moderate to severe vasomotor symptoms associated with menopause. While estrogen/androgen combinations were found to be effective

for this indication under a determination made by the US Food and Drug Administration (FDA) in 1976, formal administrative proceedings were initiated by the FDA in April 2003 to examine the effectiveness of estrogen/androgen combinations for the management of vasomotor symptoms associated with menopause. FDA is undertaking this action because the agency does not believe there is substantial evidence available to establish the contribution of androgens to the effectiveness of estrogen/androgen combinations for the management of vasomotor symptoms in menopausal women who do not respond adequately to estrogen alone. The FDA will allow continued marketing of combination estrogen/androgen products while the matter is under study.

Estradiol cypionate in fixed combination with medroxyprogesterone acetate is used parenterally as a long-active contraceptive in women. For additional information on contraceptive use of estradiol cypionate in fixed combination with medroxyprogesterone acetate, see Uses: Contraception in Females in Medroxyprogesterone Acetate 68:32.

● Estradiol Valerate

In women, estradiol valerate is used for the management of moderate to severe vasomotor symptoms associated with menopause. Estradiol valerate also is used for the management of vulvar and vaginal atrophy, female hypogonadism and castration, and primary ovarian failure. If estrogens are used solely for the management of vulvar and vaginal atrophy, use of topical vaginal preparations should be considered.

Estradiol valerate is used for the palliative treatment of advanced carcinoma of the prostate in men; however, the risk of adverse cardiovascular effects of estrogens must be considered.

Although in the past estradiol valerate was used for the prevention of postpartum breast engorgement†, the FDA has withdrawn approval of estrogen-containing drugs for this indication since estrogens have not been shown to be safe for use in women with postpartum breast engorgement. Data from controlled studies indicate that the incidence of substantial painful engorgement is low in untreated women, and the condition usually responds to appropriate analgesic or other supportive therapy.

● Ethinyl Estradiol

Ethinyl estradiol in fixed combination with norethindrone acetate is used for the management of moderate to severe vasomotor symptoms associated with menopause. Ethinyl estradiol in fixed combination with norethindrone acetate also is used adjunctively with other therapeutic measures (e.g., diet, calcium, weight-bearing exercise [including walking, running], physical therapy) to retard further bone loss and the progression of osteoporosis associated with estrogen deficiency in postmenopausal women. While estrogen replacement therapy is effective for the prevention of osteoporosis in women and has been shown to reduce bone resorption and retard or halt bone loss in postmenopausal women, such therapy is associated with a number of adverse effects. (See Uses: Estrogen Replacement Therapy, in the Estrogens General Statement 68:16.04.) If prevention of postmenopausal osteoporosis is the sole indication for estrogen therapy, alternative therapy (e.g., alendronate, raloxifene, risedronate) also should be considered.

DOSAGE AND ADMINISTRATION

● Reconstitution and Administration

Estradiol is administered orally, intravaginally, percutaneously by topical application of a transdermal system, and by topical application of a gel, emulsion, or transdermal spray to the skin. Estradiol acetate is administered orally and intravaginally. Ethinyl estradiol is administered orally. Estradiol cypionate and estradiol valerate are administered IM.

Patients receiving a transdermal estradiol system should be carefully instructed in the use of the transdermal system. To obtain optimum results, patients should also be given a copy of the patient instructions provided by the manufacturer. To expose the adhesive surface of the system, the protective strip should be peeled and discarded prior to administration. The transdermal system is applied topically to a clean, dry, and not excessively hairy area of intact skin on the trunk of the body, preferably the abdomen or buttocks, by firmly pressing the system with the adhesive side touching the skin. The system should be applied immediately after removal from its protective pouch and removal of the protective liner. The system should be pressed firmly in place with the palm of the hand for about 10 seconds, ensuring good contact, particularly around the edges. The application site should not be oily, damaged, or irritated. The transdermal system should *not* be applied to the breasts, and application at the waistline should be avoided, since tight clothing may cause the system to be rubbed off. If the system should inadvertently come off during the period of use, it may be reapplied or, if necessary, a new system may be applied; in either case, the application schedule employed should be continued. To minimize and/or prevent potential skin irritation, each transdermal system should be applied at a different site, with an interval of at least 1 week allowed between applications to a particular site. Estradiol transdermal systems are applied once (Climara®, Climara Pro®, Estradiol Transdermal System [Mylan], Menostar®) or twice (Alora®, Combipatch®, Estraderm®, Vivelle®, Vivelle-Dot®) weekly; the system in use is removed and discarded and a new system is applied. The transdermal systems for application twice weekly are commercially available in a dispensing package that is designed to aid the user in complying with the prescribed dosage regimen (the same 2 days each week). If a system is not changed on a designated day, it should be replaced as soon as possible.

Patients receiving estradiol topical gel (Elestrin®, EstroGel®) should be instructed in use of the gel and given a copy of the patient instructions provided by the manufacturer. Estradiol topical gel should be applied topically once daily at the same time each day to clean, dry, intact skin. To apply a dose of Elestrin®, the pump should be held with the tip facing the arm and the pump should be firmly and fully depressed. Elestrin® gel is applied to the upper arm and shoulder using 2 fingers. To apply a dose of EstroGel®, the gel should be collected in the palm of the hand by pressing the pump firmly and fully. EstroGel® gel is applied to one arm from shoulder to wrist using the hand. The topical gel should not be applied to the breasts or in or around the vagina. The application site should be allowed to dry for up for 5 minutes before dressing. Hands should be washed with soap and water after application of the gel. It is not known how long bathing and swimming should be delayed after application of the gel. Therefore, estradiol topical gel should be applied after bathing; the time allowed between application of the gel and swimming should be as long as possible (at least 2 hours). Application of sunscreen 10 minutes prior to application of Elestrin® increases exposure to estradiol by 55%, and application of sunscreen 25 minutes after application of Elestrin® does not alter exposure to estradiol. Application of sunscreen for 7 days to the site of application of Elestrin® increased estradiol exposure twofold; this effect was noted when sunscreen was applied before and after application of Elestrin®. Concomitant application of EstroGel® and sunscreen preparations has not been evaluated.

Patients receiving estradiol topical emulsion (Estrasorb®) should be instructed in use of the emulsion and given a copy of the patient instructions provided by the manufacturer. Estradiol topical emulsion should be applied topically once daily every morning to clean, dry, intact skin. To apply a dose, the contents of one pouch should be placed on the left thigh. The emulsion should be rubbed into the entire left thigh and calf for 3 minutes using one or both hands. Any excess emulsion remaining on the hands can be rubbed onto the buttocks. The contents of another pouch should be placed on the right thigh. The emulsion should be rubbed into the entire right thigh and calf for 3 minutes using one or both hands. Any excess emulsion remaining on the hands can be rubbed onto the buttocks. The emulsion should be applied immediately after opening the pouch. The application site should be allowed to dry before dressing. Hands should be washed with soap and water after application of the emulsion. Estradiol topical emulsion should not be applied in close proximity to application of sunscreen. Application of sunscreen 10 minutes prior to application of estradiol topical emulsion increases exposure to estradiol by 35%, and application of sunscreen 25 minutes after application of estradiol topical emulsion increases exposure to estradiol by 15%.

Patients receiving estradiol transdermal spray (Evamist®) should be instructed in use of the spray and given a copy of the patient instructions provided by the manufacturer. Estradiol transdermal spray should be applied topically once daily at the same time each day to clean, dry, intact skin on the inside of the forearm between the elbow and the wrist. Prior to initial use, estradiol transdermal spray pump must be primed; it is not necessary to prime the pump before each daily dose. To prime the pump, the applicator is held upright with the cover on and the pump depressed three times. To apply a dose of estradiol transdermal spray, the cover should be removed, the applicator held upright and the cone section of the applicator placed flat against the skin; the pump should then be depressed. One, two, or three sprays may be applied to non-overlapping areas of the inner forearm, starting near the elbow. Estradiol transdermal spray should not be applied to any area other than the inner forearm; the spray should not be applied to the breasts or around the vagina. The application site should be allowed to dry for up for 2 minutes before dressing and 30 minutes before washing the area. The application site should not be massaged or rubbed. Other individuals should not be allowed to have direct contact with the skin at the site of spray application for at least 30

minutes following administration. Patients receiving estradiol transdermal spray should ensure that children and pets avoid contact with the skin at the application site to prevent inadvertent exposure to the drug. (See Cautions.) If a child comes in direct contact with the patient's forearm where Evamist® was applied, the general area of contact should be washed with soap and water as soon as possible. Patients who cannot avoid such contact with children should wear clothing with long sleeves to cover the application site. Application of sunscreen 1 hour after application of estradiol transdermal spray decreases exposure to estradiol by 11%; application of sunscreen 1 hour prior to application of estradiol transdermal spray does not alter exposure to estradiol.

● Dosage

Dosage of estradiol, estradiol acetate, estradiol cypionate, estradiol valerate, and ethinyl estradiol must be individualized according to the condition being treated and the tolerance and therapeutic response of the patient. To minimize the risk of adverse effects, the lowest possible effective dosage should be used. When short-term estrogen therapy is indicated (e.g., for the management of vasomotor symptoms associated with menopause; vulvar and vaginal atrophy), therapy should be discontinued as soon as possible; attempts to reduce dosage or discontinue the drug should be made at 3- to 6-month intervals. Because of the potential increased risk of cardiovascular events, breast cancer, and venous thromboembolic events, estrogen and estrogen/progestin therapy should be limited to the lowest effective doses and shortest duration of therapy consistent with treatment goals and risks for the individual woman. Estrogen and estrogen/progestin therapy should be periodically reevaluated.

Estrogen therapy is administered continuously or cyclically. While estrogen therapy alone may be appropriate in women who have undergone a hysterectomy, many clinicians currently recommend that a progestin be added to estrogen therapy in women with an intact uterus. Addition of progestin therapy for 10 or more days of a cycle of estrogen administration or daily with estrogen in a continuous regimen reduces the incidence of endometrial hyperplasia and the attendant risk of endometrial carcinoma in women with an intact uterus. Morphologic and biochemical studies of the endometrium suggest that 10–13 days of progestin are needed to provide maximum maturation of the endometrium and to eliminate any hyperplastic changes. The manufacturer of Menostar® recommends that women with an intact uterus receive a progestin for 14 days every 6–12 months. When a progestin is used in conjunction with an estrogen, the usual precautions associated with progestin therapy should be observed. Clinicians prescribing progestins should be aware of the risks associated with these drugs and the manufacturers' labeling should be consulted. The choice and dosage of a progestin may be important factors in minimizing adverse effects.

When long-acting parenteral preparations are used in the management of conditions associated with estrogen deficiency, the drugs are usually administered once every 3–4 weeks.

Estradiol
Oral Dosage

For the management of moderate to severe vasomotor symptoms associated with menopause or for the management of vulvar and vaginal atrophy, the usual initial oral dosage of estradiol is 1 or 2 mg daily in a cyclic regimen. For replacement therapy in female hypogonadism, female castration, or primary ovarian failure, the usual initial oral dosage of estradiol is 1 or 2 mg daily. Subsequent dosage should be adjusted according to the patient's therapeutic response, using the lowest possible effective maintenance dosage.

For the prevention of osteoporosis, an oral dosage of estradiol 0.5 mg daily in a cyclic regimen has been used. The lowest effective dosage of estradiol for this indication has not been determined.

When estradiol is used in fixed combination with norethindrone acetate (Activella®) for the management of moderate to severe vasomotor symptoms associated with menopause, the management of vulvar and vaginal atrophy associated with menopause, or prevention of postmenopausal osteoporosis, the usual dosage is 1 mg of estradiol combined with 0.5 mg of norethindrone acetate daily.

When estradiol is used in fixed combination with drospirenone (Angeliq®) for the management of moderate to severe vasomotor symptoms associated with menopause or for the management of vulvar and vaginal atrophy associated with menopause, the usual dosage is 1 mg of estradiol combined with 0.5 mg of drospirenone daily.

When estradiol is used with norgestimate (Prefest®) for the management of moderate to severe vasomotor symptoms associated with menopause, the management of vulvar and vaginal atrophy associated with menopause, or prevention of postmenopausal osteoporosis, the usual dosage is 1 mg of estradiol daily for 3 days followed by 1 mg of estradiol with 0.09 mg of norgestimate daily for 3 days; the regimen is continued without interruption.

For the palliative treatment of advanced, metastatic carcinoma of the breast in appropriately selected men and postmenopausal women, the usual oral dosage of estradiol is 10 mg 3 times daily. Estrogen therapy is usually continued in these patients for at least 3 months.

For the palliative treatment of advanced carcinoma of the prostate, the usual oral dosage of estradiol is 1–2 mg 3 times daily.

Transdermal System Dosage

Transdermal estradiol is commercially available as systems that are applied once or twice weekly. Estradiol transdermal systems that are applied twice weekly include Alora® (available as a system delivering 0.025 mg/24 hours, 0.05 mg/24 hours, 0.075 mg/24 hours, or 0.1 mg/24 hours), Estraderm® (available as a system delivering 0.05 mg/24 hours or 0.1 mg/24 hours), and Vivelle® and Vivelle-Dot® (available as a system delivering 0.025 mg/24 hours, 0.0375 mg/24 hours, 0.05 mg/24 hours, 0.075 mg/24 hours, or 0.1 mg/24 hours). Estradiol transdermal systems that are applied once weekly include Climara® (available as a system delivering 0.025 mg/24 hours, 0.0375 mg/24 hours, 0.05 mg/24 hours, 0.06 mg/24 hours, 0.075 mg/24 hours, or 0.1 mg/24 hours) and Menostar® (available as a system delivering 0.014 mg/24 hours). In addition, transdermal estradiol/norethindrone (CombiPatch®) is commercially available as a system delivering 0.05 mg/24 hours of estradiol and 0.14 mg/24 hours of norethindrone acetate and as a system delivering 0.05 mg/24 hours of estradiol and 0.25 mg/24 hours of norethindrone acetate. Transdermal estradiol/levonorgestrel (Climara Pro®) is commercially available as a system delivering 0.045 mg/24 hours of estradiol and 0.015 mg/24 hours of levonorgestrel.

When Alora® or Estraderm® is used for the management of moderate to severe vasomotor symptoms associated with menopause or for the management of vulvar and vaginal atrophy, the usual initial dosage of transdermal estradiol is one system delivering 0.05 mg/24 hours applied twice weekly in a continuous regimen in women who have undergone a hysterectomy or a cyclic regimen (3 weeks on drug followed by 1 week without the drug, and then the regimen is repeated as necessary) in women with an intact uterus.

When Climara® is used for the management of moderate to severe vasomotor symptoms associated with menopause, the usual initial dosage of transdermal estradiol is one system delivering 0.025 mg/24 hours applied once weekly in a continuous regimen. Subsequent dosage should be adjusted according to the severity of the symptoms and the patient's therapeutic response, using the lowest possible effective maintenance dosage.

When Vivelle® or Vivelle-Dot® is used for the management of moderate to severe vasomotor symptoms associated with menopause or for the management of vulvar and vaginal atrophy, the usual initial dosage of transdermal estradiol is one system delivering 0.0375 mg/24 hours applied twice weekly in a cyclic or continuous regimen. Subsequent dosage should be adjusted according to the patient's therapeutic response, using the lowest possible effective maintenance dosage. In women who have undergone hysterectomy, transdermal estradiol Vivelle-Dot® may be applied twice a week in a continuous regimen.

When estradiol/levonorgestrel (Climara Pro®) is used for the management of moderate to severe vasomotor symptoms associated with menopause in women with an intact uterus, one system delivering 0.045 mg/24 hours of estradiol and 0.015 mg/24 hours of levonorgestrel is applied once weekly in a continuous regimen.

When estradiol/norethindrone acetate (CombiPatch®) is used for the management of moderate to severe vasomotor systems associated with menopause, for the management of vulvar and vaginal atrophy, or for the treatment of hypoestrogenism secondary to hypogonadism, castration, or primary ovarian failure, CombiPatch® may be administered as a continuous combined regimen or as a continuous sequential regimen. In the continuous combined regimen, one CombiPatch® system delivering 0.05 mg/24 hours of estradiol and 0.14 mg/24 hours of norethindrone acetate is applied twice weekly in a continuous regimen. If necessary, the dosage of norethindrone acetate may be increased by using the dosage system that delivers 0.25 mg/24 hours of norethindrone acetate. In the continuous sequential regimen, one system of transdermal estradiol delivering 0.05 mg/24 hours (i.e., Vivelle®) is applied twice weekly for the first 14 days of a 28-day cycle then one estradiol/norethindrone acetate (CombiPatch®) system delivering 0.05 mg/24 hours of estradiol and 0.14 mg/24 hours of norethindrone acetate is applied twice weekly for the remaining 14 days of the cycle. If necessary, the dosage of norethindrone acetate may be increased by using the dosage system that delivers 0.25 mg/24 hours of norethindrone acetate.

When Alora® is used for the prevention of postmenopausal osteoporosis, the minimum dose that has been shown to be effective is one system delivering 0.025 mg/24 hours applied twice weekly in a continuous regimen.

When Climara® is used for the prevention of postmenopausal osteoporosis, the minimum dose that has been shown to be effective is one system delivering 0.025 mg/24 hours applied once weekly in a continuous regimen.

For the prevention of osteoporosis, the usual initial dosage of transdermal estradiol (Estraderm®) is one system delivering 0.05 mg/24 hours applied twice weekly in a cyclic regimen in women with an intact uterus. In women who have undergone hysterectomy, one Estraderm® system is applied twice weekly in a continuous regimen. Subsequent dosage can be adjusted according to the patient's response.

For the prevention of osteoporosis, the usual dosage of transdermal estradiol (Menostar®) is one system delivering 0.014 mg/24 hours applied once weekly in a continuous regimen.

When Vivelle® or Vivelle-Dot® is used for the prevention of postmenopausal osteoporosis, the usual dosage is one system delivering 0.025 mg/24 hours applied twice weekly.

When estradiol/levonorgestrel (Climara Pro®) is used for the prevention of postmenopausal osteoporosis in women with an intact uterus, one system delivering 0.045 mg/24 hours of estradiol and 0.015 mg/24 hours of levonorgestrel is applied once weekly in a continuous regimen.

In women who are currently not receiving an oral estrogen, transdermal estradiol therapy can be initiated immediately. In women who are currently receiving an oral estrogen, transdermal estradiol therapy can be initiated 1 week after discontinuance of oral therapy or sooner if symptoms reappear before the week has passed.

Topical Gel Dosage

Commercially available estradiol 0.06% topical gel (Elestrin®) is supplied in a non-aerosol metered-dose pump. Each depression of the pump delivers 0.87 g of gel containing 0.52 mg of estradiol. When estradiol gel (Elestrin®) is used for the management of moderate to severe vasomotor symptoms associated with menopause, the usual initial dosage is 0.87 g of gel (0.52 mg of estradiol) applied topically once daily. Prior to using the pump for the first time, the pump must be primed by fully depressing the pump 10 times; this gel should be discarded in a manner that avoids accidental exposure or ingestion by household members or pets.

Commercially available estradiol 0.06% topical gel (EstroGel®) is supplied in a non-aerosol metered-dose pump. Each depression of the pump delivers 1.25 g of gel containing 0.75 mg of estradiol. When estradiol gel (EstroGel®) is used for the management of moderate to severe vasomotor symptoms associated with menopause or the treatment of moderate to severe symptoms of vulvar and vaginal atrophy associated with menopause, 1.25 g of gel (0.75 mg of estradiol) is applied topically once daily. Prior to using the pump for the first time, the pump must be primed by fully depressing the 93-g pump twice or depressing the 25-g pump 3 times; this gel should be discarded in a manner that avoids accidental exposure or ingestion by household members or pets.

Topical Emulsion Dosage

Commercially available estradiol hemihydrate 0.25% topical emulsion (Estrasorb®) is supplied in foil-laminated pouches. Each pouch contains 1.74 g of emulsion. When estradiol topical emulsion (Estrasorb®) is used for the management of moderate to severe vasomotor symptoms associated with menopause, the contents of 2 pouches (delivering a total of 0.05 mg of estradiol/24 hours) are applied topically once daily.

Transdermal Spray Dosage

Commercially available estradiol transdermal spray (Evamist®) is supplied in a metered-dose pump. The metered pump delivers a metered 90-mcL spray that contains 1.53 mg of estradiol per actuation. When estradiol transdermal spray is used for the management of moderate to severe vasomotor symptoms associated with menopause, the recommended initial dose is one spray to the inner forearm once daily. Subsequent dosage is based on clinical response. One, two, or three sprays may be administered each morning to adjacent, non-overlapping areas of the inner forearm.

Vaginal Dosage

For the management of symptoms of vulvar and vaginal atrophy associated with menopause, 2–4 g of estradiol vaginal cream may be administered intravaginally once daily for 1–2 weeks, then gradually reduced to one-half the initial dosage for a similar period. Maintenance dosages of 1 g of estradiol vaginal cream administered intravaginally 1–3 times weekly may be used after restoration of the vaginal mucosa has occurred.

When estradiol vaginal ring (Estring®) is used for the management of post-menopausal urogenital symptoms, one ring (delivering estradiol 0.0075 mg/24 hours) is inserted into the upper third of the vaginal vault; the ring is to remain in place for 3 months. After 3 months, the ring should be removed and, if appropriate, replaced with a new ring. If the ring is expelled, the ring should be rinsed in lukewarm water and reinserted.

For the management of atrophic vaginitis, one vaginal tablet containing 25 mcg of estradiol (Vagifem®) is inserted intravaginally once daily (preferably at the same time each day) for 2 weeks (initial dosage). For maintenance therapy for this condition, one vaginal tablet containing 25 mcg of the drug is inserted intravaginally twice weekly.

Estradiol Acetate

Estradiol acetate (Femtrace®) is commercially available for oral administration as tablets containing 0.45, 0.9, or 1.8 mg of estradiol acetate; the tablets are administered once daily. When estradiol acetate tablets are used for the management of moderate to severe vasomotor symptoms associated with menopause, therapy should be initiated with the lowest dose.

Estradiol acetate vaginal ring (Femring®) is commercially available as a ring delivering estradiol 0.05 mg/24 hours or 0.1 mg/24 hours. When estradiol acetate vaginal ring (Femring®) is used for the management of moderate to severe vasomotor symptoms or symptoms of vulvar and vaginal atrophy associated with menopause, therapy should be initiated with the lowest dose. To initiate therapy, one ring delivering estradiol 0.05 mg/24 hours is inserted into the vaginal vault; the ring remains in place for 3 months. After 3 months, the ring should be removed and, if appropriate, replaced with a new ring.

Estradiol Cypionate

For the management of moderate to severe vasomotor symptoms associated with menopause, the usual dosage of estradiol cypionate is 1–5 mg administered IM once every 3–4 weeks.

For replacement therapy in female hypogonadism, the usual dosage of estradiol cypionate is 1.5–2 mg once every month.

When estradiol cypionate in fixed combination with testosterone cypionate is used for the management of moderate to severe vasomotor symptoms associated with menopause, the usual dosage of estradiol cypionate is 2 mg in combination with testosterone 50 mg administered IM every 4 weeks.

Estradiol Valerate

For the management of moderate to severe vasomotor symptoms or for the management of vulvar and vaginal atrophy associated with menopause, and for replacement therapy in female hypogonadism, female castration, or primary ovarian failure, the usual dosage of estradiol valerate is 10–20 mg once every 4 weeks as necessary.

For the palliative treatment of advanced carcinoma of the prostate, the usual dosage of estradiol valerate is 30 mg or more once every 1 or 2 weeks.

Ethinyl Estradiol
Estrogen-Progestin Combination Therapy

Ethinyl estradiol in fixed combination with norethindrone acetate (Femhrt®) is commercially available for oral administration as tablets containing 2.5 mcg of ethinyl estradiol with 0.5 mg of norethindrone acetate and as tablets containing 5 mcg of ethinyl estradiol with 1 mg of norethindrone acetate; the tablets are administered once daily. When ethinyl estradiol is used in combination with norethindrone acetate for the management of moderate to severe vasomotor symptoms associated with menopause or the prevention of postmenopausal osteoporosis, therapy should be initiated with the lowest dose.

CAUTIONS

Estradiol, estradiol acetate, estradiol cypionate, estradiol valerate, and ethinyl estradiol share the toxic potentials of other estrogens, and the usual cautions, precautions, and contraindications associated with estrogen therapy should be observed. (See Cautions in the Estrogens General Statement 68:16.04.) In addition, when estradiol or ethinyl estradiol is used in conjunction with progestins, the cautions, precautions, and contraindications associated with progestins must

be considered in addition to those associated with estrogens. For additional information, see Cautions in Estrogen-Progestin Combinations 68:12.

In clinical studies, the most common adverse effect reported with transdermal estradiol therapy was erythema and irritation at the application site. Dermatologic reactions have been reported in up to 97% of patients using transdermal systems. The irritation generally resolves completely within a day or so. Rash has been reported rarely in patients receiving transdermal estradiol therapy. Rotation of application sites minimizes and/or prevents potential skin irritation. If erythema persists or severe irritation or rash occurs, patients should contact their physician.

Estrace® 2-mg tablets contain the dye tartrazine (FD&C yellow No. 5), which may cause allergic reactions including bronchial asthma in susceptible individuals. Although the incidence of tartrazine sensitivity is low, it frequently occurs in patients who are sensitive to aspirin.

The US Food and Drug Administration (FDA) is reviewing reports of adverse effects associated with estradiol transdermal spray (Evamist®) in children and pets who may have been inadvertently exposed to the drug through skin contact with women receiving the drug. Children exposed to the drug may experience signs of premature puberty including nipple swelling and breast development in females and breast enlargement in males. If such a child shows signs of premature puberty (e.g., nipple or breast swelling, breast tenderness or enlargement), the parents should be advised to contact the child's clinician and to inform the clinician of the child's possible exposure to the drug.

Some estradiol topical preparations (e.g., gel, solution) contain alcohol. Preparations containing alcohol are flammable; exposure to open flame or lighted cigarettes should be avoided until the applied product has dried.

PHARMACOLOGY

Estradiol is the principal and most active endogenous estrogen. Ethinyl estradiol is one of the most potent synthetic estrogens, and unlike estradiol, ethinyl estradiol has similar activity following oral or parenteral administration. Following subcutaneous administration, ethinyl estradiol is equal in potency to estradiol, but following oral administration, ethinyl estradiol is 15–20 times more active than estradiol. The principal pharmacologic effects of estradiol, estradiol cypionate or valerate, and ethinyl estradiol are similar to those of other natural and synthetic estrogens. (See Pharmacology in the Estrogens General Statement 68:16.04.)

Estradiol valerate has a duration of action of 14–21 days, and estradiol cypionate has a duration of action of 14–28 days.

CHEMISTRY AND STABILITY

● Chemistry
Estradiol

Estradiol is a naturally occurring steroidal estrogen. The drug may be obtained from natural sources or prepared synthetically. Estradiol is structurally similar to estrone but differs from estrone in the substitution of a secondary alcohol group for the keto group at the 17 position on ring D of the steroid nucleus.

Estradiol occurs as white or creamy white, small crystals or as a crystalline powder, is odorless and hygroscopic, and is practically insoluble in water and has a solubility of approximately 35.7 mg/mL in alcohol at 25°C.

Transdermal estradiol (Alora®) is commercially available as a system that consists of an outer layer of polyethylene backing film and a drug reservoir consisting of estradiol and sorbitan monooleate dissolved in an acrylic adhesive matrix. A polyester overlapped release liner protects the adhesive matrix during storage and should be removed prior to application.

Transdermal estradiol (Climara®) is commercially available as a system that consists of an outer layer of translucent polyethylene film and an acrylate adhesive matrix that contains estradiol; a siliconized or fluoropolymer-coated polyester film is attached to the adhesive surface and should be removed prior to application.

Transdermal estradiol (Estraderm®) is commercially available as a system that consists of an outer layer of transparent polyester film; a drug reservoir of estradiol and alcohol gelled with hydroxypropyl cellulose; an ethylene-vinyl acetate copolymer membrane that controls the rate of diffusion of the drug; and a final adhesive layer consisting of light mineral oil and polyisobutylene. The adhesive layer is covered by a protective strip of siliconized polyester film which is removed prior to application.

Transdermal estradiol (Menostar®) is commercially available as a system that consists of an outer layer of translucent polyethylene film and an acrylate adhesive matrix that contains estradiol; a siliconized or fluoropolymer-coated polyester film is attached to the adhesive surface and should be removed prior to application.

Transdermal estradiol (Vivelle®, Vivelle-Dot®) is commercially available as a system that consists of an outer layer of translucent film and an adhesive formulation that contains estradiol; a polyester release liner is attached to the adhesive surface and should be removed prior to application.

Transdermal estradiol in fixed combination with levonorgestrel (Climara Pro®) is commercially available as a system that consists of an outer layer of translucent polyethylene film and an acrylate adhesive matrix that contains estradiol and levonorgestrel; a siliconized or fluoropolymer-coated polyester film is attached to the adhesive surface and should be removed prior to application.

Transdermal estradiol in fixed combination with norethindrone acetate (CombiPatch®) is commercially available as a system that consists of an outer layer of polyolefin film and a silicone and acrylic-based multipolymeric adhesive matrix that contains estradiol and norethindrone acetate; a protective liner is attached to the adhesive surface and should be removed prior to application.

Estradiol topical gel (Elestrin®) is commercially available as a hydroalcoholic gel containing estradiol 0.06%; the gel also contains purified water, alcohol, propylene glycol, diethylene glycol monoethyl ether, triethanolamine, carbomer 940, and edetate disodium. Elestrin® is supplied in a non-aerosol metered-dose pump. The pump contains 144 g of gel and delivers 100 metered doses of 0.87 g of gel.

Estradiol topical gel (EstroGel®) is commercially available as a clear, colorless, hydroalcoholic gel containing estradiol 0.06%; the gel also contains purified water, alcohol, triethanolamine, and carbomer 934P and is formulated to provide controlled release of estradiol. EstroGel® is supplied in a non-aerosol metered-dose pump. The pump containing 93 g of gel delivers 64 metered doses of 1.25 g of gel, and the pump containing 25 g of gel delivers 14 metered doses of 1.25 g of gel.

Estradiol topical emulsion (Estrasorb®) is commercially available as an emulsion containing estradiol hemihydrate 0.25%; estradiol is encapsulated using a micellar nanoparticle technology. The emulsion also contains soybean oil, water, polysorbate 80, and alcohol. Estradiol topical emulsion is supplied in foil-laminated pouches. Each pouch contains 1.74 g of emulsion and 4.35 mg of estradiol hemihydrate.

Estradiol transdermal spray (Evamist®) delivers a metered 90-mcL spray that contains 1.53 mg of estradiol per actuation. The commercially available pump contains 8.1 mL of solution and delivers 75 metered doses. The solution is packaged in a glass vial fitted with a metered-dose pump; this unit is encased in a plastic housing with a conical bell opening that controls the distance, angle, and area of application of the spray.

Estradiol also is commercially available as a vaginal tablet and as a vaginal ring that consists of estradiol, silicone polymers, and barium sulfate.

Estradiol Acetate

Estradiol acetate is commercially available as an oral tablet and as a vaginal ring that consists of estradiol acetate, silicone polymers, and barium sulfate.

Estradiol Cypionate

Estradiol cypionate is formed by esterification of estradiol with cyclopentanepropionic acid at C 17 on ring D of the steroid nucleus. Estradiol cypionate occurs as a white to practically white, crystalline powder, is odorless or may have a slight odor, and has solubilities of less than 0.1 mg/mL in water and approximately 25 mg/mL in alcohol at 25°C. The drug is also sparingly soluble in vegetable oils. Estradiol cypionate is commercially available alone and in fixed combination with testosterone cypionate for parenteral use. Commercially available estradiol cypionate injection is a sterile solution of the drug in a suitable oil (e.g., cottonseed oil); the injection may also contain chlorobutanol as a preservative.

Estradiol Valerate

Estradiol valerate is formed by esterification of estradiol with valeric acid at C 17 on ring D of the steroid nucleus. Estradiol valerate occurs as a white, crystalline powder and is usually odorless but may have a faint, fatty odor. The drug is practically insoluble in water and sparingly soluble in sesame oil and in peanut oil. Estradiol valerate injection is a sterile solution of the drug in a suitable vegetable oil (e.g., sesame oil, castor oil); commercially available injections may also contain chlorobutanol or benzyl benzoate and benzyl alcohol as preservatives.

Ethinyl Estradiol

Ethinyl estradiol is a semisynthetic estrogen. The presence of the ethinyl group at C 17 on ring D of the steroid nucleus prevents enzymatic degradation of the estradiol molecule and results in an orally active compound.

Ethinyl estradiol occurs as a white to creamy white, odorless, crystalline powder and is insoluble in water and soluble in alcohol and vegetable oils.

● *Stability*

Estradiol tablets should be stored in tight, light-resistant containers at a temperature of 20–25°C. The commercially available transdermal systems of estradiol should be stored at a temperature of 30°C or lower; after removal from the protective pouch, a transdermal system should be applied immediately and should not be stored. The commercially available transdermal systems of estradiol/norethindrone acetate should be refrigerated at 2–8°C until dispensed. Once dispensed, the transdermal systems may be stored at a temperature lower than 25°C for up to 6 months. The commercially available transdermal systems of estradiol/levonorgestrel should be stored at 20–25°C but may be exposed to temperatures ranging from 15–30°C. After removal from the protective pouch, the transdermal systems should be applied immediately and should not be stored. Estradiol vaginal ring should be stored at controlled room temperature (15–30°C). Estradiol topical gel, estradiol topical emulsion, estradiol transdermal spray, estradiol vaginal tablets, and estradiol acetate vaginal ring should be stored at a controlled room temperature of 25°C, but may be exposed to temperatures ranging from 15–30°C. Estradiol cypionate and estradiol valerate injections should be stored at room temperature. Estradiol acetate tablets should be stored at 25°C but may be exposed to temperatures ranging from 15–30°C.

For further information on chemistry, pharmacology, pharmacokinetics, cautions, acute toxicity, drug interactions, laboratory test interferences, and dosage and administration of estradiol and estradiol esters, see the Estrogens General Statement 68:16.04.

PREPARATIONS

Most preparations containing androgenic anabolic steroid hormones are subject to control under the Federal Controlled Substances Act of 1970, as amended by the Anabolic Steroids Control Act of 1990 and 2004, as schedule III (C-III) drugs. (See Uses: Misuse and Abuse, in Testosterone 68:08.) However, manufacturers of certain preparations containing androgenic anabolic steroids (principally combinations that also include estrogens) have applied for and obtained for their product(s) an exemption from the record-keeping and other regulatory requirements of the Federal Controlled Substances Act. (See the introductory paragraph under Preparations, in Testosterone 68:08.) Because regulatory requirements for a given preparation containing an androgenic anabolic steroid may be subject to change under the provisions of the Act, the manufacturer should be contacted when specific clarification about a preparation's status is required.

Excipients in commercially available drug preparations may have clinically important effects in some individuals; consult specific product labeling for details.

Estradiol

Topical		
Gel	0.06%	**Elestrin®**, Kenwood Therapeutics
		EstroGel®, Ascend Therapeutics
Solution	1.53 mg/meter spray	**Evamist®**, Ther-Rx
Transdermal System	0.014 mg/24 hours (1 mg/3.25 cm²)	**Menostar®**, Berlex
	0.025 mg/24 hours (0.77 mg/9 cm²)	**Alora®**, Watson
	0.025 mg/24 hours (2 mg/6.5 cm²)	**Climara®**, Berlex
	0.025 mg/24 hours (0.97 mg/7.75 cm²)*	**Estradiol Transdermal System** (once weekly)
	0.025 mg/24 hours (2.17 mg/7.25 cm²)	**Vivelle®**, Novartis
	0.025 mg/24 hours (0.39 mg/2.5 cm²)	**Vivelle-Dot®**, Novartis
	0.0375 mg/24 hours (2.85 mg/9.375 cm²)	**Climara®**, Berlex
	0.0375 mg/24 hours (1.46 mg/11.625 cm²)*	**Estradiol Transdermal System** (once weekly)

	0.0375 mg/24 hours (3.28 mg/11 cm²)	**Vivelle®**, Novartis
	0.0375 mg/24 hours (0.585 mg/3.75 cm²)	**Vivelle-Dot®**, Novartis
	0.05 mg/24 hours (1.5 mg/18 cm²)	**Alora®**, Watson
	0.05 mg/24 hours (3.8 mg/12.5 cm²)	**Climara®**, Berlex
	0.05 mg/24 hours (4 mg/10 cm²)	**Estraderm®**, Novartis
	0.05 mg/24 hours (1.94 mg/15.5 cm²)*	**Estradiol Transdermal System** (once weekly)
	0.05 mg/24 hours (4.33 mg/14.5 cm²)	**Vivelle®**, Novartis
	0.05 mg/24 hours (0.78 mg/5 cm²)	**Vivelle-Dot®**, Novartis
	0.06 mg/24 hours (4.55 mg/15 cm²)	**Climara®**, Berlex
	0.06 mg/24 hours (2.33 mg/18.6 cm²)*	**Estradiol Transdermal System** (once weekly)
	0.075 mg/24 hours (2.3 mg/27 cm²)	**Alora®**, Watson
	0.075 mg/24 hours (5.7 mg/18.75 cm²)	**Climara®**, Berlex
	0.075 mg/24 hours (2.91mg/23.25 cm²)*	**Estradiol Transdermal System** (once weekly)
	0.075 mg/24 hours (6.57 mg/22 cm²)	**Vivelle®**, Novartis
	0.075 mg/24 hours (1.17 mg/7.5 cm²)	**Vivelle-Dot®**, Novartis
	0.1 mg/24 hours (3 mg/36 cm²)	**Alora®**, Watson
	0.1 mg/24 hours (7.6 mg/25 cm²)	**Climara®**, Berlex
	0.1 mg/24 hours (8 mg/20 cm²)	**Estraderm®**, Novartis
	0.1 mg/24 hours (3.88 mg/31 cm²)*	**Estradiol Transdermal System** (once weekly)
	0.1 mg/24 hours (8.66 mg/29 cm²)	**Vivelle®**, Novartis
	0.1 mg/24 hours (1.56 mg/10 cm²)	**Vivelle-Dot®**, Novartis

Vaginal

Cream	0.01%	**Estrace®**, Warner Chilcott
Ring	2 mg/ring (0.0075 mg/24 hours)	**Estring®**, Pfizer

* available from one or more manufacturer, distributor, and/or repackager by generic (nonproprietary) name

Estradiol Combinations

Oral

Tablets, biphasic regimen	1 mg (15 tablets) and 1 mg with Norgestimate 0.09 mg (15 tablets)	**Prefest®**, Barr
Tablets, film-coated	1 mg with Norethindrone Acetate 0.5 mg	**Activella®** (28 tablets), Novo Nordisk
	1 mg with Drospirenone 0.5 mg	**Angeliq®** (28 tablets), Berlex

Topical

Transdermal System	0.045 mg and 0.015 mg Levonorgestrel/24 hours (4.4 mg and 1.39 mg Levonorgestrel/22 cm²)	**Climara Pro®**, Berlex

Topical

	0.05 mg and 0.14 mg Norethindrone Acetate/24 hours (0.62 mg and 2.7 mg Norethindrone Acetate/ 9 cm²)	**CombiPatch®**, Novartis
	0.05 mg and 0.25 mg Norethindrone Acetate/24 hours (0.51 mg and 4.8 mg Norethindrone Acetate/ 16 cm²)	**CombiPatch®**, Novartis

Estradiol (Hemihydrate)

Topical

Emulsion	0.25%	**Estrasorb®**, Espirit

Vaginal

Tablets, film-coated	25 mcg (of estradiol)	**Vagifem®** (available as disposable applicators), NovoNordisk

Estradiol (Micronized)

Oral

Tablets	0.5 mg*	**Estrace®** (scored), Warner Chilcott
	1 mg*	**Estrace®** (scored), Warner Chilcott
	2 mg*	**Estrace®** (scored), Warner Chilcott

* available from one or more manufacturer, distributor, and/or repackager by generic (nonproprietary) name

Estradiol Acetate

Oral

Tablets	0.45 mg	**Femtrace®**, Warner Chillcott
	0.9 mg	**Femtrace®**, Warner Chillcott
	1.8 mg	**Femtrace®**, Warner Chilcott

Vaginal

Ring	12.4 mg/ring (0.05 mg estradiol/24 hours)	**Femring®**, Warner Chilcott
	24.8 mg/ring (0.1 mg estradiol/24 hours)	**Femring®**, Warner Chilcott

Estradiol Cypionate

Parenteral

Injection (in oil)	5 mg/mL	**Depo®-Estradiol**, Pfizer

Estradiol Cypionate Combinations

Parenteral

Injection (in oil)	2 mg/mL with Testosterone Cypionate 50 mg/mL	**Depo-Testadiol®**, Pfizer

Estradiol Valerate

Parenteral

Injection (in oil)	10 mg/mL	**Delestrogen®**, Monarch
	20 mg/mL	**Delestrogen®**, Monarch
	40 mg/mL	**Delestrogen®**, Monarch

Ethinyl Estradiol Combinations

Oral

Tablets	2.5 mcg with Norethindrone Acetate 0.5 mg	**FemHRT®**, Warner Chillcott
	5 mcg with Norethindrone Acetate 1 mg	**FemHRT®**, Warner Chillcott

† Use is not currently included in the labeling approved by the US Food and Drug Administration.

Estrogens, Conjugated

68:16.04 • ESTROGENS

■ Conjugated estrogens is a mixture of estrogens that is available either as preparations that meet current official USP standards (i.e., conjugated estrogens USP) or as nonofficial preparations (i.e., synthetic conjugated estrogens A and synthetic conjugated estrogens B, which are prepared synthetically from plant sources).

USES

In women, oral conjugated estrogens USP and synthetic conjugated estrogens A are used for the management of moderate to severe vasomotor symptoms associated with menopause and for the management of vulvar and vaginal atrophy (atrophic vaginitis). If estrogens are used solely for the management of vulvar and vaginal atrophy, use of topical vaginal preparations should be considered. Synthetic conjugated estrogens B is used for the management of moderate to severe vasomotor symptoms and for the management of severe vaginal dryness, pain with sexual intercourse, and symptoms of vulvar and vaginal atrophy associated with menopause. Oral conjugated estrogens USP also is used for the management of female hypoestrogenism secondary to hypogonadism, castration, or primary ovarian failure.

Oral conjugated estrogens USP is used adjunctively with other therapeutic measures (e.g., diet, calcium, weight-bearing exercise [including walking, running], physical therapy) to retard further bone loss and the progression of osteoporosis associated with estrogen deficiency in postmenopausal women. While estrogen replacement therapy is effective for the prevention of osteoporosis in women and has been shown to reduce bone resorption and retard or halt bone loss in postmenopausal women, such therapy is associated with a number of adverse effects. (See Uses: Estrogen Replacement Therapy, in the Estrogens General Statement 68:16.04.) If prevention of postmenopausal osteoporosis is the sole indication for therapy with oral conjugated estrogens, alternative therapy (e.g., alendronate, raloxifene, risedronate) should be considered.

Another therapeutic option involves use of conjugated estrogens in combination with an estrogen agonist-antagonist (bazedoxifene) for the management of moderate to severe vasomotor symptoms associated with menopause and for prevention of osteoporosis. The combination of conjugated estrogens with bazedoxifene is referred to as a tissue-selective estrogen complex (TSEC).

While results from earlier observational studies indicated that estrogen replacement therapy (ERT) or combined estrogen/progestin therapy (hormone replacement therapy, HRT) was associated with cardiovascular benefit in postmenopausal women, results of the Heart and Estrogen/progestin Replacement Study (HERS) evaluating estrogen/progestin and the Women's Health Initiative (WHI) study evaluating estrogen alone and estrogen/progestin therapy indicate that hormone therapy does not decrease the incidence of cardiovascular disease. The American Heart Association (AHA), American College of Obstetricians and Gynecologists (ACOG), FDA, and manufacturers recommend that hormone therapy not be used to prevent heart disease in healthy women (primary prevention) or to protect women with preexisting heart disease (secondary prevention). (See Cardiovascular Risk Reduction under Uses: Estrogen Replacement Therapy, in the Estrogens General Statement 68:16.04.)

Oral conjugated estrogens USP is used for the palliative treatment of advanced, inoperable, metastatic carcinoma of the breast in postmenopausal women and in men. Estrogens are one of several second-line agents that can be used in certain postmenopausal women with metastatic breast cancer.

Oral conjugated estrogens USP is used for the palliative treatment of advanced carcinoma of the prostate in men; however, the risk of adverse cardiovascular effects of estrogens must be considered.

Conjugated estrogens USP may be administered IM or IV for the treatment of abnormal uterine bleeding caused by hormonal imbalance not associated with organic pathology.

Conjugated estrogens USP may be administered intravaginally for the management of atrophic vaginitis or kraurosis vulvae.

Although in the past oral conjugated estrogens has been used for the prevention of postpartum breast engorgement†, the FDA has withdrawn approval of estrogen-containing drugs for this indication since estrogens have not been shown to be safe for use in women with postpartum breast engorgement. Data from controlled studies indicate that the incidence of substantial painful engorgement is

low in untreated women, and the condition usually responds to appropriate analgesic or other supportive therapy.

DOSAGE AND ADMINISTRATION

● Reconstitution and Administration

Conjugated estrogens USP is usually administered orally, but may also be administered intravaginally or by deep IM or slow IV injection. Synthetic conjugated estrogens A and synthetic conjugated estrogens B are administered orally.

When parenteral administration of conjugated estrogens USP is required, IV injection is preferred because of the more rapid response obtained following this route of administration compared to IM injection. For direct IV injection, the drug should be administered slowly to avoid the occurrence of a flushing reaction.

For parenteral administration, conjugated estrogens USP powder for injection is reconstituted with 5 mL of sterile water for injection. Using aseptic technique, the diluent should then be slowly added, directing the flow against the inner wall of the vial (Secule®), while gently agitating the container to facilitate dissolution of the contents; vigorous shaking of the container should be avoided. Premarin® solutions should be used immediately after reconstitution.

Oral dosage preparations containing medroxyprogesterone acetate in combination with conjugated estrogens USP as monophasic or biphasic regimens are commercially available in a mnemonic dispensing package that is designed to aid the user in complying with the prescribed dosage schedule. The monophasic combination (Prempro®) is available in a 28-day dosage preparation that contains 28 tablets of conjugated estrogens USP (0.625 mg) in fixed combination with medroxyprogesterone acetate (2.5 or 5 mg). The monophasic combination (Prempro®) also is available in a 28-day dosage preparation that contains 28 tablets of conjugated estrogens USP (0.3 or 0.45 mg) in fixed combination with medroxyprogesterone acetate (1.5 mg). The biphasic combination (Premphase®) is available in a 28-day dosage preparation that contains 14 tablets of conjugated estrogens USP (0.625 mg) and 14 tablets of conjugated estrogens USP (0.625 mg) in fixed combination with medroxyprogesterone acetate (5 mg).

The oral dosage preparation containing conjugated estrogens in fixed combination with bazedoxifene acetate is commercially available in a 30-day package that includes 2 blister packs of 15 tablets each containing conjugated estrogens 0.45 mg in fixed combination with bazedoxifene acetate 22.6 mg (equivalent to 20 mg of bazedoxifene).

● Dosage

Dosage of conjugated estrogens USP, synthetic conjugated estrogens A, and synthetic conjugated estrogens B must be individualized according to the condition being treated and the tolerance and therapeutic response of the patient. To minimize the risk of adverse effects, the lowest possible effective dosage should be used. Because of the potential increased risk of cardiovascular events, breast cancer, and venous thromboembolic events, therapy with estrogen, estrogen/progestin, or conjugated estrogens in fixed combination with bazedoxifene should be limited to the lowest effective doses and shortest duration of therapy consistent with treatment goals and risks for the individual woman. Therapy with estrogen, estrogen/progestin, or conjugated estrogens in fixed combination with bazedoxifene should be periodically reevaluated.

Estrogen therapy is administered in a continuous daily dosage regimen or, alternatively, in a cyclic regimen. When estrogens are administered cyclically, the drugs usually are given once daily for 3 weeks followed by 1 week without the drugs or once daily for 25 days followed by 5 days off, and then the respective regimen is repeated as necessary.

While estrogen therapy alone (estrogen replacement therapy, ERT) may be appropriate in women who have undergone a hysterectomy, a progestin generally is added to estrogen therapy (hormone replacement therapy, HRT) in women with an intact uterus. Addition of a progestin for 10 or more days of a cycle of estrogen or daily with estrogen in a continuous regimen reduces the incidence of endometrial hyperplasia and the attendant risk of endometrial carcinoma in women with an intact uterus. Morphologic and biochemical studies of the endometrium suggest that 10–13 days of progestin are needed to provide maximum maturation of the endometrium and to eliminate any hyperplastic changes. As an alternative to progestins, the use of bazedoxifene (an estrogen agonist-antagonist) in fixed combination with conjugated estrogens reduces the risk of endometrial hyperplasia.

When estrogen therapy is used in conjunction with a progestin or in fixed combination with bazedoxifene, the usual precautions associated with progestins or bazedoxifene should be observed. Clinicians prescribing estrogens in conjunction with progestins or conjugated estrogens in fixed combination with bazedoxifene should be aware of the risks associated with these drugs and the manufacturers' labeling should be consulted. Clinical studies indicate that addition of a progestin to estrogen replacement therapy does not interfere with the efficacy of estrogen therapy in the management of vasomotor symptoms associated with menopause, treatment of vulvar and vaginal atrophy, or prevention of osteoporosis. The choice and dosage of a progestin may be important factors in minimizing potential adverse effects.

Exposure to conjugated estrogens USP vaginal cream has been reported to weaken latex condoms. The potential for conjugated estrogens USP vaginal cream to weaken and contribute to the protective failure of latex or rubber condoms, diaphragms, or cervical caps should be considered.

Menopausal Symptoms

Conjugated Estrogens USP

For the management of moderate to severe vasomotor symptoms and/or for the management of vulvar and vaginal atrophy associated with menopause, the usual initial oral dosage of conjugated estrogens USP is 0.3 mg daily. Subsequent dosage adjustment should be based on the patient's response. The drug may be administered in a continuous daily regimen or in a cyclic regimen (25 days on drug followed by 5 days off drug, then this regimen is repeated as necessary). Alternatively, for the management of vulvar and vaginal atrophy, 0.5–2 g of conjugated estrogens USP vaginal cream may be administered intravaginally once daily in the usual cyclic regimen.

When conjugated estrogens USP is used in conjunction with medroxyprogesterone for the management of moderate to severe vasomotor symptoms associated with menopause or for the management of vulvar and vaginal atrophy, conjugated estrogens USP is administered in a continuous daily dosage regimen while medroxyprogesterone may be administered in a continuous daily dosage regimen (Prempro®) or cyclically (Premphase®). When both drugs are administered in a continuous daily dosage regimen, conjugated estrogens is administered in a daily dosage of 0.3 mg in conjunction with oral medroxyprogesterone acetate in a daily dosage of 1.5 mg. Alternatively, conjugated estrogens is administered in a daily dosage of 0.45 mg in conjunction with medroxyprogesterone acetate in a daily dosage of 1.5 mg, or conjugated estrogens is administered in a daily dosage of 0.625 mg in conjunction with medroxyprogesterone acetate in a daily dosage of 2.5 or 5 mg. When conjugated estrogens USP is administered in a continuous daily dosage regimen and medroxyprogesterone is administered cyclically (Premphase®), conjugated estrogens USP is administered in a daily dosage of 0.625 mg, while oral medroxyprogesterone acetate is administered in a daily dosage of 5 mg on days 15–28 of the cycle. Therapy with conjugated estrogens in conjunction with medroxyprogesterone generally should be initiated with the lowest dosage (i.e., conjugated estrogens 0.3 mg in conjunction with medroxyprogesterone acetate 1.5 mg). Subsequent dosage should be adjusted based on the patient's therapeutic response and should be reevaluated periodically. If spotting or bleeding is problematic and has been appropriately evaluated, dosage can be adjusted.

When conjugated estrogens is used in conjunction with bazedoxifene for the treatment of moderate to severe vasomotor symptoms associated with menopause, conjugated estrogens is administered in a daily dosage of 0.45 mg in fixed combination with bazedoxifene 20 mg.

Synthetic Conjugated Estrogens A

For the management of moderate to severe vasomotor symptoms associated with menopause, the usual oral dosage of synthetic conjugated estrogens A is 0.45–1.25 mg daily. The usual initial oral dosage of synthetic conjugated estrogens A is 0.45 mg daily; subsequent dosage adjustment should be based on the patient's response. For the management of vulvar and vaginal atrophy, the usual oral dosage of synthetic conjugated estrogens A is 0.3 mg daily.

Synthetic Conjugated Estrogens B

For the management of moderate to severe vasomotor symptoms associated with menopause, the usual oral dosage of synthetic conjugated estrogens B is 0.3–1.25 mg daily. The usual initial oral dosage of synthetic conjugated estrogens B for this condition is 0.3 mg daily. Subsequent dosage adjustment should be based on the patient's response.

For the management of severe vaginal dryness, pain with sexual intercourse, and vulvar and vaginal atrophy associated with menopause, the usual oral dosage of synthetic conjugated estrogens B is 0.3 mg daily.

Osteoporosis

For the prevention of osteoporosis, the usual initial oral dosage of conjugated estrogens USP is 0.3 mg once daily. Subsequent dosage should be adjusted based on the patient's clinical and bone mineral density responses. The drug may be administered in a continuous daily regimen or in a cyclic regimen (25 days on drug followed by 5 days off drug, then this regimen is repeated as necessary).

When conjugated estrogens USP is used in conjunction with medroxyprogesterone, conjugated estrogens USP is administered in a continuous daily dosage regimen while medroxyprogesterone may be administered in a continuous daily dosage regimen (Prempro®) or cyclically (Premphase®). When both drugs are administered in a continuous daily dosage regimen, conjugated estrogens USP is administered in a daily dosage of 0.3 mg in conjunction with oral medroxyprogesterone acetate in a daily dosage of 1.5 mg. Alternatively, conjugated estrogens is administered in a daily dosage of 0.45 mg in conjunction with medroxyprogesterone acetate in a daily dosage of 1.5 mg, or conjugated estrogens is administered in a daily dosage of 0.625 mg in conjunction with medroxyprogesterone acetate in a daily dosage of 2.5 or 5 mg. When conjugated estrogens USP is administered in a continuous daily dosage regimen and medroxyprogesterone is administered cyclically, conjugated estrogens USP is administered in a daily dosage of 0.625 mg, while oral medroxyprogesterone acetate is administered in a daily dosage of 5 mg on days 15–28 of the cycle. Therapy with conjugated estrogens in conjunction with medroxyprogesterone generally should be initiated with the lowest dosage (i.e., conjugated estrogens 0.3 mg in conjunction with medroxyprogesterone acetate 1.5 mg). Subsequent dosage should be adjusted based on the patient's clinical and bone mineral density responses. If spotting or bleeding is problematic and has been appropriately evaluated, dosage can be adjusted.

When conjugated estrogens is used in conjunction with bazedoxifene for the prevention of osteoporosis, conjugated estrogens is administered once daily at a dosage of 0.45 mg in fixed combination with bazedoxifene 20 mg.

Female Hypoestrogenism

For replacement therapy in female hypoestrogenism, the usual oral dosage of conjugated estrogens USP is 0.3–0.625 mg daily in a cyclic regimen (3 weeks on drug, 1 week off). Dosage may be adjusted based on symptom severity and responsiveness of the endometrium.

For the management of female castration or primary ovarian failure, the usual initial oral dosage of conjugated estrogens USP is 1.25 mg daily in a cyclic regimen. Subsequent dosage should be adjusted according to the severity of the symptoms and the patient's therapeutic response, using the lowest possible effective maintenance dosage.

Inoperable Carcinoma of the Breast

For the palliative treatment of inoperable, advanced, metastatic carcinoma of the breast in appropriately selected men and postmenopausal women, the usual oral dosage of conjugated estrogens USP is 10 mg 3 times daily. Estrogen therapy is usually continued in these patients for at least 3 months.

Prostate Carcinoma

For the palliative treatment of advanced carcinoma of the prostate, the usual oral dosage of conjugated estrogens USP is 1.25–2.5 mg 3 times daily.

Abnormal Uterine Bleeding

For the emergency treatment of abnormal uterine bleeding caused by hormonal imbalance, the usual IV or IM dose of conjugated estrogens USP is 25 mg. If necessary, the dose may be repeated in 6–12 hours. The use of conjugated estrogens USP for this condition does not preclude the use of other appropriate measures.

CAUTIONS

Conjugated estrogens USP, synthetic conjugated estrogens A, and synthetic conjugated estrogens B share the toxic potentials of other estrogens, and the usual cautions, precautions, and contraindications associated with estrogen therapy should be observed. (See Cautions in the Estrogens General Statement 68:16.04.)

Conjugated estrogens is contraindicated in patients who are hypersensitive to the drug or any ingredient in the respective formulation.

PHARMACOLOGY

The principal pharmacologic effects of conjugated estrogens are similar to those of other natural and synthetic estrogens. (See Pharmacology in the Estrogens General Statement 68:16.04.)

CHEMISTRY AND STABILITY

● Chemistry

Conjugated estrogens is a mixture of estrogens that is available either as preparations that meet current official USP standards (i.e., conjugated estrogens USP) or as nonofficial preparations (i.e., synthetic conjugated estrogens A, synthetic conjugated estrogens B).

Conjugated estrogens obtained from natural sources occurs as a buff-colored, amorphous powder and is odorless or has a slight, characteristic odor. Conjugated estrogens that is prepared synthetically occurs as a white to light buff, crystalline or amorphous powder and is odorless or has a slight odor. Conjugated estrogens is soluble in water.

Conjugated Estrogens USP

Conjugated estrogens USP is a mixture containing the sodium salts of the water-soluble sulfate esters of estrone and equilin derived wholly or in part from equine urine or may be prepared synthetically from estrone and equilin. Conjugated estrogens USP also contains conjugated estrogenic substances of the type excreted by pregnant mares including 17α-dihydroequilin, 17α-estradiol, 17β-dihydroequilin, equilenin, 17α-dihydroequilenin, 17β-dihydroequilenin, δ^{8,9}-dehydroestrone, and 17β-estradiol. Conjugated estrogens USP contains 52.5–61.5% sodium estrone sulfate and 22.5–30.5% sodium equilin sulfate. Conjugated estrogens contains, as sodium sulfate conjugates, 13.5–19.5% 17α-dihydroequilin, 2.5–9.5% 17α-estradiol, and 0.5–4% 17β-dihydroequilin.

Conjugated estrogens USP currently is commercially available as preparations (Premarin®, Premphase®, Prempro®) containing mixtures of estrogens obtained exclusively from natural sources and which are present in the formulations as the sodium salts of water-soluble estrogen sulfates blended to represent the average composition of material derived from pregnant mare urine; according to USP standards, the formulations include a mixture of sodium estrone sulfate and sodium equilin sulfate as well as the concomitant components 17α-dihydroequilin, 17α-estradiol, and 17β-dihydroequilin as sodium sulfate conjugates.

Conjugated estrogens USP injection is commercially available as a sterile, lyophilized cake. The lyophilized cake also contains lactose, sodium citrate, and simethicone; in addition, sodium hydroxide and/or hydrochloric acid may be added during manufacture of the powder for injection to adjust the pH. A sterile diluent containing water for injection and benzyl alcohol as a preservative is provided for reconstitution.

Synthetic Conjugated Estrogens A

Synthetic conjugated estrogens A is a mixture of conjugated estrogens prepared synthetically from plant sources (i.e., soy and yams). Synthetic conjugated estrogens A is commercially available as preparations (Cenestin®) containing a mixture of 9 of the 10 known conjugated estrogenic substances present in currently available commercial preparations of conjugated estrogens USP. However, unlike currently available preparations of conjugated estrogens USP, the conjugated estrogenic substances present in synthetic conjugated estrogens A are prepared entirely synthetically.

Synthetic conjugated estrogens A is commercially available as preparations containing mixtures of estrogens prepared exclusively synthetically as the sodium salts of water-soluble estrogen sulfates blended into a 9-component mixture of estrone sulfate and sodium equilin sulfate as well as the concomitant components 17α-dihydroequilin, 17α-estradiol, 17β-dihydroequilin, 17α-dihydroequilenin, 17β-dihydroequilenin, equilenin, and 17β-estradiol as sodium sulfate conjugates.

Synthetic Conjugated Estrogens B

Synthetic conjugated estrogens B is a mixture of conjugated estrogens prepared synthetically from plant sources. Synthetic conjugated estrogens B is commercially available as preparations (Enjuvia®) containing a mixture of the 10 conjugated estrogenic substances present in currently available commercial preparations of conjugated estrogens USP. Unlike currently available preparations of conjugated estrogens USP, the conjugated estrogenic substances present in synthetic conjugated estrogens B are prepared entirely synthetically.

Synthetic conjugated estrogens B is commercially available as preparations containing mixtures of estrogens prepared exclusively synthetically as the sodium salts of water-soluble estrogen sulfates blended into a 10-component mixture of estrone sulfate and sodium equilin sulfate as well as the concomitant components 17α-dihydroequilin, 17α-estradiol, 17β-dihydroequilin, 17α-dihydroequilenin, 17β-dihydroequilenin, equilenin, 17β-estradiol, and δ^{8,9}-dehydroestrone as sodium sulfate conjugates.

● Stability

Commercially available conjugated estrogens USP tablets, synthetic conjugated estrogens A tablets, synthetic conjugated estrogens B tablets, and conjugated estrogens USP vaginal cream should be stored at controlled room temperature

(20–25°C). Conjugated estrogens USP powder for injection should be stored at a temperature of 2–8°C prior to reconstitution. Following reconstitution, solutions of the drug should be used immediately.

Conjugated estrogens USP injection is physically and chemically compatible with the following IV solutions: 5% dextrose, 0.9% sodium chloride, and invert sugar solutions; the injection is physically and/or chemically incompatible with protein hydrolysate, ascorbic acid, or any solution with an acid pH. Specialized references should be consulted for specific compatibility information.

For further information on chemistry, pharmacology, pharmacokinetics, cautions, acute toxicity, drug interactions, laboratory test interferences, and dosage and administration of conjugated estrogens, see the Estrogens General Statement 68:16.04.

PREPARATIONS

Excipients in commercially available drug preparations may have clinically important effects in some individuals; consult specific product labeling for details.

Conjugated Estrogens USP

Oral		
Tablets	0.3 mg	Premarin®, Pfizer
	0.45 mg	Premarin®, Pfizer
	0.625 mg	Premarin®, Pfizer
	0.9 mg	Premarin®, Pfizer
	1.25 mg	Premarin®, Pfizer
Parenteral		
For injection	25 mg	Premarin® Intravenous, Pfizer
Vaginal		
Cream	0.0625%	Premarin®, Pfizer

Conjugated Estrogens Combinations

Oral		
Tablets	0.45 mg with Bazedoxifene Acetate 20 mg (of bazedoxifene)	Duavee®, Pfizer
Tablets, monophasic regimen	0.3 mg with Medroxyprogesterone Acetate 1.5 mg (28 tablets)	Prempro®, Pfizer
	0.45 mg with Medroxyprogersterone Acetate 1.5 mg (28 tablets)	Prempro®, Pfizer
	0.625 mg with Medroxyprogesterone Acetate 2.5 mg (28 tablets)	Prempro®, Pfizer
	0.625 mg with Medroxyprogesterone Acetate 5 mg (28 tablets)	Prempro®, Pfizer
Tablets, biphasic regimen	0.625 mg (14 tablets Premarin®) and 0.625 mg with Medroxyprogesterone Acetate 5 mg (14 tablets)	Premphase®, Pfizer

Conjugated Estrogens A, Synthetic

Oral		
Tablets, film-coated	0.3 mg	Cenestin®, Teva
	0.45 mg	Cenestin®, Teva
	0.625 mg	Cenestin®, Teva
	0.9 mg	Cenestin®, Teva
	1.25 mg	Cenestin®, Teva

Conjugated Estrogens B, Synthetic

Oral		
Tablets, film-coated	0.3 mg	Enjuvia®, Teva
	0.45 mg	Enjuvia®, Teva
	0.625 mg	Enjuvia®, Teva
	0.9 mg	Enjuvia®, Teva
	1.25 mg	Enjuvia®, Teva

† Use is not currently included in the labeling approved by the US Food and Drug Administration.

Selected Revisions September 18, 2017, © Copyright, October 1, 1961, American Society of Health-System Pharmacists, Inc.

metFORMIN Hydrochloride

68:20.04 • BIGUANIDES

■ Metformin hydrochloride is a biguanide antidiabetic agent.

USES

● Type 2 Diabetes Mellitus

Metformin is used as monotherapy as an adjunct to diet and exercise to improve glycemic control in patients with type 2 diabetes mellitus. Metformin may also be used in combination with a glucagon-like peptide-1 (GLP-1) agonist, a sodium-glucose cotransporter-2 (SGLT2) inhibitor, a dipeptidyl peptidase-4 (DPP-4) inhibitor, a thiazolidinedione, a sulfonylurea, or a meglitinide (repaglinide, nateglinide) antidiabetic agent for the management of type 2 diabetes mellitus in patients who do not achieve adequate glycemic control on monotherapy with metformin or any of these drugs.

Metformin is commercially available in fixed combination with glyburide or glipizide for use as an adjunct to diet and exercise to improve glycemic control in adults with diabetes mellitus; such fixed-combination preparations may be used as initial therapy in patients whose hyperglycemia cannot be controlled by diet and exercise alone, or as second-line therapy in patients who do not achieve adequate control of hyperglycemia with metformin or sulfonylurea monotherapy. A thiazolidinedione may be added to metformin in fixed combination with glyburide in patients who have inadequate glycemic control with fixed-combination therapy.

Immediate-release metformin is commercially available in fixed combination with pioglitazone for use as an adjunct to diet and exercise in patients with type 2 diabetes mellitus when treatment with both pioglitazone and metformin is appropriate and also in those who are already receiving pioglitazone and metformin concurrently as separate components.

Metformin is commercially available in fixed combination with a DPP-4 inhibitor (e.g., alogliptin, linagliptin, saxagliptin, sitagliptin) for use when treatment with both drug components is appropriate.

Metformin is commercially available in fixed combination with the SGLT2 inhibitors canagliflozin, dapagliflozin, empagliflozin, or ertugliflozin for use when treatment with both drug components is appropriate.

Metformin also may be used as adjunctive therapy in patients with type 2 diabetes mellitus receiving insulin therapy to improve glycemic control and/or decrease the dosage of insulin needed to obtain optimal glycemic control.

The American Diabetes Association (ADA) currently classifies diabetes mellitus as type 1 (due to autoimmune β-cell destruction, usually leading to absolute insulin deficiency); type 2 (due to a progressive loss of β-cell insulin secretion, frequently on the background of insulin resistance); gestational diabetes mellitus (diabetes diagnosed in the second or third trimester of pregnancy that was not clearly overt diabetes prior to gestation); or specific types of diabetes due to other causes, such as monogenic diabetes syndromes (e.g., neonatal diabetes or maturity-onset diabetes of the young), diseases of the exocrine pancreas (e.g., cystic fibrosis, pancreatitis), or drug- or chemical-induced diabetes (e.g., diabetes associated with glucocorticoid use, the treatment of HIV/AIDS, or organ transplantation). According to ADA and other experts, a diagnosis of diabetes mellitus currently is established by a fasting plasma glucose of 126 mg/dL or greater, a 2-hour plasma glucose of 200 mg/dL or greater during an oral glucose tolerance test, or a glycosylated hemoglobin (hemoglobin A_{1c}; HbA_{1c}) concentration of 6.5% or greater; results should be confirmed by repeat testing in the absence of unequivocal hyperglycemia. Alternatively, a random plasma glucose of 200 mg/dL or greater in a patient with classic symptoms of hyperglycemia or hyperglycemic crisis is considered confirmation of the diagnosis of diabetes mellitus.

In both type 1 and type 2 diabetes mellitus, various genetic and environmental factors can result in the progressive loss of β-cell mass and/or function that manifests clinically as hyperglycemia. Epidemiologic data indicate that the incidence of type 2 diabetes mellitus is increasing in children and adolescents. Patients with type 2 diabetes mellitus have insulin resistance and usually have relative (rather than absolute) insulin deficiency. Most patients with type 2 diabetes mellitus (about 80–90%) are overweight or obese; obesity itself also contributes to the insulin resistance and glucose intolerance observed in these patients. Patients with type 2 diabetes mellitus who are not obese may have an increased percentage of abdominal fat, which is an indicator of increased cardiometabolic risk. While children with immune-mediated type 1 diabetes mellitus generally are not overweight, the incidence of obesity in children with this form of diabetes is increasing with the increasing incidence of obesity in the US population. Distinguishing between type 1 and type 2 diabetes mellitus in children may be difficult since obesity may occur with either type of diabetes mellitus, and autoantigens and ketosis may be present in a substantial number of children with features of type 2 diabetes mellitus (e.g., obesity, acanthosis nigricans).

Patients with type 2 diabetes mellitus are *not* dependent initially on insulin (although many patients eventually require insulin for glycemic control) nor are they prone to ketosis; however, insulin occasionally may be required for correction of symptomatic or persistent hyperglycemia that is not controlled by dietary regulation or oral antidiabetic agents (e.g., sulfonylureas), and ketosis occasionally may develop during periods of severe stress (e.g., acute infection, trauma, surgery, use of certain drugs [e.g., corticosteroids, atypical antipsychotics, SGLT2 inhibitors]). Type 2 diabetes mellitus is a heterogeneous subclass of the disease; hyperglycemia in these patients often is accompanied by other metabolic abnormalities such as obesity, hypertension, hyperlipidemia, and impaired fibrinolysis. Endogenous insulin is present in type 2 diabetic patients, although plasma insulin concentrations may be decreased, increased, or normal. In patients with type 2 diabetes mellitus, glucose-stimulated secretion of endogenous insulin is frequently, but not always, reduced and decreased peripheral sensitivity to insulin is almost always associated with glucose intolerance.

Glycemic Control and Microvascular Complications

Current evidence from epidemiologic and clinical studies supports an association between chronic hyperglycemia and the pathogenesis of microvascular complications in patients with diabetes mellitus, and results of randomized, controlled studies in patients with type 1 diabetes mellitus indicate that intensive management of hyperglycemia with near-normalization of blood glucose and glycosylated hemoglobin (hemoglobin A_{1c} [HbA_{1c}]) concentrations provides substantial benefits in terms of reducing chronic microvascular (e.g., neuropathy, retinopathy, nephropathy) complications associated with the disease. HbA_{1c} concentration reflects the glycosylation of other proteins throughout the body as a result of recent hyperglycemia and is used as a predictor of risk for the development of diabetic microvascular complications (e.g., neuropathy, retinopathy, nephropathy). Microvascular complications of diabetes are the principal causes of blindness and renal failure in developed countries and are more closely associated with hyperglycemia than are macrovascular complications.

In the Diabetes Control and Complications Trial (DCCT), a reduction of approximately 50–75% in the risk of development or progression of retinopathy, nephropathy, and neuropathy was demonstrated during an average 6.5 years of follow-up in patients with type 1 diabetes mellitus receiving intensive insulin treatment (3 or more insulin injections daily with dosage adjusted according to results of at least 4 daily blood glucose determinations, dietary intake, and anticipated exercise) compared with that in patients receiving conventional insulin treatment (1 or 2 insulin injections daily, self-monitoring of blood or urine glucose values, education about diet and exercise). However, the incidence of severe hypoglycemia, including multiple episodes in some patients, was 3 times higher in the intensive-treatment group than in the conventional-treatment group. The reduction in risk of microvascular complications in the DCCT study correlated continuously with the reduction in HbA_{1c} concentration (hemoglobin A_{1c}) produced by intensive insulin treatment (e.g., a 40% reduction in risk of microvascular disease for each 10% reduction in hemoglobin A_{1c}). These data imply that any decrease in HbA_{1c} levels is beneficial and that complete normalization of blood glucose concentrations may prevent diabetic microvascular complications.

The DCCT was terminated prematurely because of the pronounced benefits of intensive insulin regimens, and all treatment groups were encouraged to institute or continue such intensive insulin therapy. In the Epidemiology of Diabetes Interventions and Complications (EDIC) study, the long-term, open-label continuation phase of the DCCT, the reduction in the risk of microvascular complications (e.g., retinopathy, nephropathy, neuropathy) associated with intensive insulin therapy has been maintained throughout 7 years of follow-up. In addition, the prevalence of hypertension (an important consequence of diabetic nephropathy) in those receiving conventional therapy has exceeded that of those receiving intensive therapy. Patients receiving conventional insulin therapy in the DCCT were able to achieve a lower HbA_{1c} when switched to intensive therapy in the continuation study, although the average HbA_{1c} values achieved during the continuation study were higher (i.e., worse) than those achieved during the DCCT with intensive insulin therapy. Patients who remained on intensive insulin therapy during the EDIC continuation study were not able to maintain the degree of glycemic control achieved during the DCCT; by 5 years of follow-up in the EDIC study, HbA_{1c} values were similar in both intensive and conventional therapy groups. The EDIC study demonstrated that the greater the duration of chronically elevated plasma glucose concentrations (as determined by HbA_{1c} values), the greater the risk of microvascular complications. Conversely, the longer patients can maintain a target HbA_{1c} of 7% of less, the greater the delay in the onset of these complications.

In another randomized, controlled study (Stockholm Diabetes Intervention Study) in patients with type 1 diabetes mellitus who were evaluated for up to 7.5 years, blood glucose control (as determined by HbA_{1c} concentrations) was improved, and the incidence of microvascular complications (e.g., decreased visual acuity, retinopathy, nephropathy, decreased nerve conduction velocity) reduced, with intensive insulin treatment (e.g., at least 3 insulin injections daily accompanied by intensive educational efforts) compared with that in patients receiving standard treatment (e.g., generally 2 insulin injections daily without intensive educational efforts).

Data from the United Kingdom Prospective Diabetes Study (UKPDS) and the Action in Diabetes and VAscular disease: preterax and diamicroN modified release Controlled Evaluation (ADVANCE) study in patients with type 2 diabetes mellitus generally are consistent with the same benefits of oral hypoglycemic agents on microvascular complications as those observed in type 1 diabetics receiving insulin therapy in the DCCT.

The UKPDS evaluated middle-aged, newly diagnosed, overweight (exceeding 120% of ideal body weight) or non-overweight patients with type 2 diabetes mellitus who received conventional or intensive treatment regimens with an oral sulfonylurea agent and/or insulin; overweight patients also could be allocated to metformin therapy in the same proportions as those allocated to sulfonylureas and insulin. Initial therapy consisted of an oral antidiabetic agent (sulfonylurea or metformin) or insulin, with stepwise addition of metformin (or glyburide in those initially allocated to metformin) in those poorly controlled on initial therapy or conversion to insulin alone in patients not adequately controlled with 2 oral agents. Intensive treatment consisted of antidiabetic therapy targeted to a fasting plasma glucose concentration of less than 108 mg/dL or, in patients receiving insulin, preprandial glucose concentrations of 72–126 mg/dL. Conventional treatment consisted of antidiabetic therapy targeted to a fasting plasma glucose concentration of less than 270 mg/dL without symptoms of hyperglycemia. Results of UKPDS indicate greater beneficial effects on retinopathy, nephropathy, and possibly neuropathy with intensive glucose-lowering therapy (median achieved HbA_{1c} concentration: 7%) in type 2 diabetics compared with that in the conventional treatment group (median achieved HbA_{1c} concentration: 7.9%). The overall incidence of microvascular complications was reduced by 25% with intensive therapy. Epidemiologic analysis of UKPDS results indicates a continuous relationship between the risks of microvascular complications and glycemia, with a 35% reduction in risk for each 1% reduction in HbA_{1c}, and no evidence of a glycemic threshold.

The ADVANCE study also evaluated the relatively short-term effects (median follow-up: 5 years) of conventional or intensive therapy on the development of major vascular complications. The primary end point was the composite of major macrovascular (death from cardiovascular events, nonfatal myocardial infarction, or nonfatal stroke) and major microvascular (new or worsening nephropathy or retinopathy) events. While the incidence of the primary composite end point was reduced by approximately 10% in the ADVANCE study, the beneficial effect was due principally to a 21% reduction in microvascular events (nephropathy); there was no appreciable reduction in macrovascular outcomes. Intensive antidiabetic therapy (mean achieved HbA_{1c} concentration: 6.5%) was associated with a reduction in new or worsening nephropathy compared with conventional treatment (mean achieved HbA_{1c} concentration of 7.3%), but there was no effect on the development of new or worsening retinopathy. Results of the Veterans Affairs Diabetes Trial (VADT), another study similar in design to the ADVANCE study, also indicated that intensive therapy in patients with poorly controlled type 2 diabetes mellitus (median baseline HbA_{1c} concentration of 9.4%) did not lessen the rate of microvascular complications compared with standard antidiabetic therapy.

In UKPDS, fasting plasma glucose concentrations and HbA_{1c} values steadily increased over 10 years in the patients receiving conventional therapy, and more

than 80% of these patients eventually required antidiabetic therapy in addition to diet to maintain fasting plasma glucose concentrations within the desired goal of less than 270 mg/dL. In patients receiving intensive therapy initiated with chlorpropamide, glyburide, or insulin, fasting plasma glucose concentrations and HbA_{1c} values decreased during the first year of the study. Subsequent increases in these indices of glycemic control after the first year paralleled that in the conventional therapy group for the remainder of the study, indicating slow decline of pancreatic β-cell function and loss of glycemic control regardless of intensity of therapy. In contrast to UKPDS, no diminution in the effect on HbA_{1c} or fasting blood glucose concentrations with either intensive or conventional therapy was observed in ADVANCE or VADT over a median follow-up of 5 or 5.6 years, respectively.

Data from long-term follow-up (over 10 years) of middle-aged, newly diagnosed UKPDS patients with type 2 diabetes mellitus indicate that strict glycemic control (i.e., maintenance of fasting blood glucose concentrations below 108 mg/dL) was not achieved with initial intensive oral antidiabetic therapy (stepwise introduction of a sulfonylurea [i.e., chlorpropamide, glyburide], then insulin, or an oral sulfonylurea and insulin, or insulin alone to achieve fasting plasma glucose concentrations of 108 mg/dL) in most patients; at 3 and 9 years, 50 and 75%, respectively, of patients required combination therapy with sulfonylureas or initiation of insulin to maintain adequate glycemic control. While strict guidelines for insulin dosage adjustments were used in the DCCT study, adjustments of antidiabetic therapy dosage in UKPDS were not as frequent (dosage adjustments allowed every 3 months); in addition, the definition of secondary treatment failure with sulfonylureas and the time of institution of supplementary antidiabetic therapy changed as the study progressed. Because of the benefits of strict glycemic control, the goal of therapy for type 2 diabetes mellitus is to lower blood glucose to as close to normal as possible, which generally requires aggressive management efforts (e.g., mixing therapy with various antidiabetic agents including sulfonylureas, metformin, insulin, and/or possibly others) over time. For additional information on clinical studies demonstrating the benefits of strict glycemic control on microvascular complications in patients with type 1 or type 2 diabetes mellitus, see Glycemic Control and Microvascular Complications under Uses: Diabetes Mellitus, in the Insulins General Statement 68:20.08.

Macrovascular Outcomes and Cardiovascular Risk Reduction

Current evidence indicates that appropriate management of dyslipidemia, blood pressure, and vascular thrombosis provides substantial benefits in terms of reducing macrovascular complications associated with diabetes mellitus; intensive glycemic control generally has not been associated with appreciable reductions in macrovascular outcomes in controlled trials. Reduction in blood pressure to a mean of 144/82 mm Hg ("tight blood pressure control") in patients with diabetes mellitus and uncomplicated mild to moderate hypertension in UKPDS substantially reduced the incidence of virtually all macrovascular (e.g., stroke, heart failure) and microvascular (e.g., retinopathy, vitreous hemorrhage, renal failure) outcomes and diabetes-related mortality; blood pressure and glycemic control were additive in their beneficial effects on these end points. While intensive antidiabetic therapy titrated with the goal of reducing HbA_{1c} to near-normal concentrations (6–6.5% or less) has not been associated with appreciable reductions in cardiovascular events during the randomized portion of controlled trials examining such outcomes, results of long-term follow-up (10–11 years) from DCCT and UKPDS indicate a delayed cardiovascular benefit in patients treated with intensive antidiabetic therapy early in the course of type 1 or type 2 diabetes mellitus. Recent evidence suggests that therapy with certain SGLT2 inhibitors or GLP-1 agonists can reduce the risk of major cardiovascular events (e.g., MI, stroke, cardiovascular death) or the risk of hospitalization for heart failure in patients with type 2 diabetes mellitus and established cardiovascular disease. Patients with type 2 diabetes mellitus who have established (or are at a high risk for) ASCVD, established kidney disease, or heart failure should receive a GLP-1 receptor agonist or SGLT2 inhibitor with demonstrated cardiovascular disease benefit. (See Reduction in Risk of Major Adverse Cardiovascular Events under Uses: Type 2 Diabetes Mellitus, in Liraglutide 68:20.06 and also see Reduction in Risk of Heart Failure-Related Hospitalization under Uses: Type 2 Diabetes Mellitus, in Dapagliflozin 68:20.18.) Experts state that therapy with a GLP-1 receptor agonist or SGLT2 inhibitor should be considered for patients with the aforementioned comorbidities independently of the patients' baseline or target HbA_{1c}. For additional details regarding the effects of antidiabetic therapy on macrovascular outcomes, see Reduction in Risk of Major Adverse Cardiovascular Events under Uses: Type 2 Diabetes Mellitus, in Canagliflozin 68:20.18, and in Liraglutide 68:20.06.

Treatment Goals

ADA currently recommends target preprandial (fasting) and peak postprandial (1–2 hours after the *beginning* of a meal) *plasma* glucose concentrations of 80–130 and less than 180 mg/dL, respectively, and HbA$_{1c}$ concentrations of less than 7% (based on a nondiabetic range of 4–6%) *in general* in adults with type 1 or type 2 diabetes mellitus who are not pregnant. ADA states that these glycemic targets are appropriate for many patients but must be individualized based on key patient characteristics, such as potential risks of hypoglycemia and other adverse drug effects, disease duration, life expectancy, important comorbidities, established vascular complications, patient preference, and resources and support system. Patients with diabetes mellitus who have elevated HbA$_{1c}$ concentrations despite having adequate preprandial glucose concentrations should monitor glucose concentrations 1–2 hours after the start of a meal and receive treatments aimed at reducing postprandial glucose concentrations.

More stringent treatment goals (i.e., an HbA$_{1c}$ less than 6%) can be considered in selected patients (e.g., during the second and third trimester of pregnancy) if achievable without substantial hypoglycemia. An *individualized* HbA$_{1c}$ concentration goal that is closer to normal without risking substantial hypoglycemia is reasonable in patients with a short duration of diabetes mellitus, no appreciable cardiovascular disease, and a long life expectancy. Less stringent treatment goals may be appropriate in patients with long-standing diabetes mellitus in whom the general HbA$_{1c}$ concentration goal of less than 7% is difficult to obtain despite adequate education on self-management of the disease, appropriate glucose monitoring, and effective dosages of multiple antidiabetic agents, including insulin. For additional details on individualizing treatment in patients with diabetes mellitus, see Treatment Goals under Uses: Diabetes Mellitus, in the Insulins General Statement 68:20.08.

Considerations in Initiating and Maintaining Antidiabetic Therapy

Recognizing that lifestyle interventions often fail to achieve or maintain the target glycemic goal within the first year of initiation of such interventions, ADA currently suggests initiation of metformin concurrently with lifestyle interventions at the time of diagnosis of type 2 diabetes mellitus. ADA and other clinicians state that lifestyle interventions should remain a principal consideration in the management of diabetes even after pharmacologic therapy is initiated. The importance of regular physical activity also should be emphasized, and cardiovascular risk factors should be identified and corrective measures employed when feasible.

Metformin Monotherapy

Current guidelines for the treatment of type 2 diabetes mellitus generally recommend metformin as first-line therapy in addition to lifestyle modifications in patients with recent-onset type 2 diabetes mellitus or mild hyperglycemia because of its well-established safety and efficacy (i.e., beneficial effects on glycosylated hemoglobin [hemoglobin A$_{1c}$; HbA$_{1c}$], weight, and cardiovascular mortality). Potential advantages of metformin compared with sulfonylurea antidiabetic agents or insulin include a minimal risk of hypoglycemia, more favorable effects on serum lipids, reduction of hyperinsulinemia, and weight loss or lack of weight gain. Clinical studies indicate that metformin is as effective (approximately 1.5% decrease in HbA$_{1c}$ values) as a sulfonylurea antidiabetic agent (e.g., chlorpropamide [no longer commercially available in the US], glyburide, glipizide, tolbutamide) for the management of type 2 diabetes mellitus. Since metformin may stabilize or decrease body weight, the drug is particularly useful as initial monotherapy in obese individuals who might gain weight while receiving a sulfonylurea. Metformin is equally effective in lean or obese patients with type 2 diabetes mellitus. In patients receiving initial monotherapy with metformin, the incidence of primary and secondary failures appears to be less than or similar to that in patients receiving sulfonylurea monotherapy. Metformin may be effective as replacement monotherapy in some patients with primary or secondary failure to sulfonylureas. In patients with metformin contraindications or intolerance (e.g., risk of lactic acidosis, GI intolerance) or in selected other patients, some experts suggest that initial therapy with a drug from another class of antidiabetic agents (e.g., a GLP-1 receptor agonist, SGLT2 inhibitor, DPP-4 inhibitor, sulfonylurea, thiazolidinedione, basal insulin) may be acceptable based on patient factors. (See Type 2 Diabetes Mellitus: Combination Therapy, in Uses.)

The manufacturer states that metformin is *not* used for the treatment of type 1 diabetes mellitus or diabetic ketoacidosis. (See Cautions: Contraindications.)

In controlled studies of up to 8 months' duration in adults with type 2 diabetes mellitus, therapy with metformin hydrochloride (0.5–3 g daily) reduced fasting and postprandial glucose concentrations and HbA$_{1c}$ substantially more than did placebo. The antihyperglycemic effect of metformin does not appear to correlate with duration of diabetes, age, obesity, race, fasting insulin concentrations, or baseline plasma lipid concentrations. In a placebo-controlled study in pediatric (10–16 years of age) patients with type 2 diabetes mellitus, the mean net reduction at week 16 in fasting plasma glucose concentrations in patients receiving metformin hydrochloride (up to 2 g daily) or placebo for up to 16 weeks was 42.9 mg/dL, compared with an increase of 21.4 mg/dL in fasting plasma glucose concentrations in the placebo group. The mean reduction from baseline in body weight in patients receiving metformin (mean baseline body weight: 93 kg) or placebo (mean baseline body weight: 85.7 kg) in this study was approximately 1.5 or 0.9 kg, respectively. In a multicenter, randomized, controlled study in newly diagnosed, asymptomatic patients with type 2 diabetes mellitus, the efficacy of metformin therapy in reducing fasting plasma glucose (target value: less than 108 mg/dL) and HbA$_{1c}$ concentrations in a subgroup of obese patients was similar to that of therapy with a sulfonylurea (chlorpropamide, glyburide, or glipizide) or insulin in nonobese patients; all drug regimens improved glycemic control compared with conventional (diet only) therapy. However, unlike sulfonylurea or insulin therapy, metformin therapy generally decreased plasma insulin concentrations and was not associated with weight gain or an increased incidence of hypoglycemia. In this long-term study, gradual deterioration in glycemic control occurred with all therapies over the study period despite increases in drug dosage or combined drug therapy; HbA$_{1c}$ concentrations generally had increased to baseline levels after 4–5 years of therapy with any of the drug regimens. Such deterioration in glycemic control has been attributed to a progressive decline in pancreatic β-cell function rather than a reduction in insulin sensitivity.

Combination Therapy

Because of the progressive nature of type 2 diabetes mellitus, patients initially receiving an oral antidiabetic agent will eventually require multiple oral and/or injectable noninsulin antidiabetic agents of different therapeutic classes and/or insulin for adequate glycemic control. Metformin may be used concomitantly with one or more oral antidiabetic agents or insulin to improve glycemic control in patients with type 2 diabetes. Data suggest that the addition of each noninsulin agent to initial antidiabetic therapy lowers HbA$_{1c}$ by approximately 0.7–1%. Combined therapy with metformin and one or more other oral antidiabetic agents generally is used in patients with longstanding type 2 diabetes mellitus who have poor glycemic control with monotherapy. While usual practice generally has been to add additional antidiabetic agents in a sequential manner when metformin monotherapy no longer provides adequate glycemic control, initiating antidiabetic therapy with 2 agents (e.g., metformin plus another drug) may be appropriate in patients with an initial HbA$_{1c}$ exceeding 7.5% or at least 1.5% above the target level. In addition, early initiation of combination therapy may help more rapidly attain glycemic goals and extend the time to treatment failure. In metformin-intolerant patients with high initial HbA$_{1c}$ levels, some experts suggest initiation of therapy with 2 agents from other antidiabetic classes with complementary mechanisms of action. Experts state that the choice of which agent to add to metformin monotherapy is based on drug-specific effects and patient factors. Inclusion of a GLP-1 receptor agonist or SGLT2 inhibitor with demonstrated cardiovascular disease benefit may be preferred in patients with type 2 diabetes mellitus who have established (or are at a high risk for) ASCVD, established kidney disease, or heart failure. (See Reduction in Risk of Major Adverse Cardiovascular Events under Uses: Type 2 Diabetes Mellitus, in Liraglutide 68:20.06 and also see Reduction in Risk of Heart Failure-Related Hospitalization under Uses: Type 2 Diabetes Mellitus, in Dapagliflozin 68:20.18.) Experts state that therapy with a GLP-1 receptor agonist or SGLT2 inhibitor should be considered for patients with the aforementioned comorbidities independently of the patients' baseline or target HbA$_{1c}$. GLP-1 receptor agonists and SGLT2 inhibitors appear to have effects on the kidneys independent of their glycemic effects, and some experts suggest that an agent from one of these classes of drugs be considered in patients with type 2 diabetes mellitus and chronic kidney disease (CKD). (See Beneficial Effects on Renal Function and Cardiovascular Morbidity and Mortality in Diabetic Nephropathy under Uses: Type 2 Diabetes Mellitus, in Canagliflozin 68:20.18.) In patients *without* established ASCVD or indicators of high ASCVD risk, heart failure, or CKD, the decision regarding the addition of other antidiabetic agents (e.g., GLP-1 receptor agonist, SGLT2 inhibitor, DPP-4 inhibitor, thiazolidinedione, sulfonylurea, basal insulin) to metformin therapy should be based on avoidance of adverse effects, cost, and individual patient factors.

Combination Therapy with Oral and/or Injectable Noninsulin Antidiabetic Agents

Combined therapy with metformin and other noninsulin antidiabetic agents in patients not adequately controlled with monotherapy may reduce symptoms and serve as a means to delay or avoid institution of insulin. Factors to consider when selecting additional antidiabetic agents for combination therapy in patients with inadequate glycemic control on metformin monotherapy include patient comorbidities (e.g., atherosclerotic cardiovascular disease [ASCVD], established kidney disease, heart failure), hypoglycemia risk, impact on weight, cost, risk of adverse effects, and patient preference. When glycemic control is closer to the target HbA_{1c} goal with metformin monotherapy (e.g., HbA_{1c} less than 7.5%), some clinicians have suggested that an agent with a lesser potential to lower glycemia and/or slower onset of action may be considered (e.g., sulfonylurea, thiazolidinedione) as additional therapy to metformin. When the greater glucose-lowering effect of an injectable drug is needed in patients with type 2 diabetes mellitus, some experts currently state that an injectable GLP-1 receptor agonist is preferred over insulin in most patients because of beneficial effects on body weight and a lower risk of hypoglycemia, although adverse GI effects may diminish tolerability.

While addition of a GLP-1 receptor agonist may successfully control hyperglycemia, many patients will eventually require insulin therapy. Early introduction of insulin therapy should be considered when hyperglycemia is severe (e.g., blood glucose of at least 300 mg/dL or HbA_{1c} exceeding 9–10%), especially in the presence of catabolic manifestations (e.g., weight loss, hypertriglyceridemia, ketosis) or symptoms of hyperglycemia. (See Combination Therapy with Insulin under Type 2 Diabetes Mellitus: Combination Therapy, in Uses.) For additional information regarding the initiation of insulin therapy in patients with diabetes mellitus, see Uses: Diabetes Mellitus, in the Insulins General Statement 68:20.08.

Metformin is commercially available in fixed combination with glyburide or glipizide for use as initial therapy in the management of patients with type 2 diabetes mellitus whose hyperglycemia cannot be controlled by diet and exercise alone. In several comparative trials in such patients, therapy with metformin in fixed combination with glyburide or glipizide was more effective in improving glycemic control (as determined by HbA_{1c} values, fasting plasma glucose concentrations) than monotherapy with either component. A greater percentage of patients receiving metformin in fixed combination with glyburide or glipizide achieved strict glycemic control (e.g., HbA_{1c} values less than 7%) than patients receiving monotherapy with metformin, glyburide, or glipizide.

Metformin in fixed combination with glyburide or glipizide also is used to improve glycemic control in patients with type 2 diabetes mellitus who are inadequately controlled with either sulfonylurea or metformin monotherapy. In several comparative studies in such patients, greater glycemic control (as determined by HbA_{1c} values, fasting plasma glucose concentrations) was achieved with the fixed combination of metformin and glyburide or glipizide than with metformin, glyburide, or glipizide monotherapy. Strict glycemic control (e.g., HbA_{1c} values less than 7%) was achieved in a greater percentage of patients receiving fixed combinations of metformin with a sulfonylurea (glyburide or glipizide) than with sulfonylurea or metformin monotherapy. In a comparative clinical trial in pediatric patients (9–16 years of age) with type 2 diabetes mellitus, therapy with metformin in fixed combination with glyburide (titrated to a final mean daily dosage of 3.1 mg of glyburide and 623 mg of metformin hydrochloride) was no more effective in improving glycemic control (as determined by reductions in HbA_{1c} values) than monotherapy with either component (titrated to final mean daily dosages of 6.5 mg of glyburide or 1.5 g of metformin hydrochloride).

Immediate-release metformin is used in fixed combination with pioglitazone in patients with type 2 diabetes mellitus who have inadequate glycemic control with pioglitazone or metformin monotherapy or in those who are already receiving pioglitazone and metformin concurrently as separate components. No clinical trials have evaluated the fixed combination of immediate-release metformin and pioglitazone; efficacy and safety of the fixed combination has been established based on concurrent administration of the 2 agents given separately. Safety and efficacy of the fixed combination of immediate-release metformin and pioglitazone in patients with type 2 diabetes mellitus are extrapolated from clinical trials evaluating pioglitazone as add-on therapy to metformin.

Metformin also is used in combination with rosiglitazone in patients with type 2 diabetes mellitus when treatment with both metformin and rosiglitazone is appropriate. (See Combination Therapy under Uses: Type 2 Diabetes Mellitus, in Rosiglitazone 68:20.28.)

In a dose-ranging trial evaluating rosiglitazone 4 or 8 mg as add-on therapy to the maximum daily dosage of metformin hydrochloride, 28.1% of patients receiving the higher dosage of rosiglitazone concurrently with metformin achieved HbA_{1c} values of 7% or less.

A thiazolidinedione may be added to metformin in fixed combination with glyburide in patients with type 2 diabetes mellitus who have inadequate glycemic control with the fixed combination. In such patients, the addition of rosiglitazone to combined therapy with metformin and glyburide has reduced fasting glucose concentrations and HbA_{1c} values. Strict glycemic control (e.g., HbA_{1c} values less than 7%) was achieved in 42.4% of patients of receiving the triple combination of metformin, glyburide, and rosiglitazone compared with 13.5% of those receiving metformin and glyburide.

In a double-blind, controlled trial in patients with type 2 diabetes mellitus who had inadequate glycemic control with metformin monotherapy, add-on therapy with repaglinide resulted in greater glycemic control (as determined by HbA_{1c} values, fasting plasma glucose concentrations) than metformin or repaglinide monotherapy. Combined therapy with metformin and repaglinide resulted in a greater reduction in HbA_{1c} and fasting plasma glucose concentrations at a lower repaglinide dosage than with repaglinide monotherapy. However, the incidence of hypoglycemia with combined metformin and repaglinide therapy was higher than with repaglinide monotherapy. In addition, body weight increased in patients receiving repaglinide alone or combined with metformin but remained stable in those receiving metformin monotherapy.

In a clinical trial in patients who had inadequate glycemic control (HbA_{1c} exceeding 7.1%) with metformin monotherapy, addition of repaglinide to metformin therapy produced reductions in fasting plasma glucose concentrations and HbA_{1c} averaging 39.6 mg/dL and 1.4%, respectively, compared with reductions averaging 4.5 mg/dL and 0.33%, respectively, with metformin alone; patients receiving repaglinide therapy alone had an increase in fasting plasma glucose concentrations of 8.8 mg/dL and a reduction of 0.38% in HbA_{1c}. In a clinical trial in treatment-naive patients or patients who had previously received antidiabetic therapy (followed by a washout period of at least 2 months), combined therapy with metformin hydrochloride and nateglinide resulted in greater reductions in HbA_{1c} and fasting plasma glucose concentrations than metformin or nateglinide monotherapy.

In another clinical trial in patients with type 2 diabetes mellitus who had inadequate glycemic control with metformin, a sulfonylurea, or insulin, the combination of pioglitazone (30 mg daily) and metformin (and withdrawal of other antidiabetic therapy) reduced fasting plasma glucose concentrations and HbA_{1c} values compared with metformin therapy alone, regardless of whether patients were receiving lower (less than 2 g daily) or higher (2 g daily or more) dosages of metformin hydrochloride.

In a multicenter, controlled study in patients whose hyperglycemia was inadequately controlled by diet and metformin therapy, the addition of acarbose produced appreciable improvement in postprandial plasma glucose concentrations and modest improvement in HbA_{1c}. Fasting plasma glucose concentrations generally are not reduced by addition of acarbose to therapy with metformin since acarbose acts principally during a meal to delay carbohydrate absorption. Limited data suggest that combined therapy with metformin and a sulfonylurea is as effective or more effective in reducing fasting blood glucose and HbA_{1c} concentrations than combined therapy with acarbose and a sulfonylurea; however, acarbose may provide better control of postprandial blood glucose concentrations.

Metformin (immediate-release) is used in fixed combination with alogliptin in patients with type 2 diabetes mellitus when treatment with both drugs is appropriate. Efficacy and safety of this fixed combination have been established based on concurrent administration of the 2 agents given separately. (See Combination Therapy under Uses: Type 2 Diabetes Mellitus, in Alogliptin 68:20.05.)

Metformin (immediate- or extended-release) is used in fixed combination with linagliptin in patients with type 2 diabetes mellitus when treatment with both drugs is appropriate. Efficacy and safety of these fixed combinations have been established based on concurrent administration of the 2 agents given separately. (See Combination Therapy under Uses: Type 2 Diabetes Mellitus, in Linagliptin 68:20.05.)

Extended-release metformin is used in fixed combination with saxagliptin in patients with type 2 diabetes mellitus when treatment with both drugs is appropriate. Efficacy and safety of this fixed combination have been established based on concurrent administration of metformin and saxagliptin given as separate tablets.

(See Combination Therapy under Uses: Type 2 Diabetes Mellitus, in Saxagliptin 68:20.05.)

Metformin (immediate- or extended-release) is used in fixed combination with sitagliptin in patients with type 2 diabetes mellitus when treatment with both drugs is appropriate. Efficacy and safety of these fixed combinations have been established based on concurrent administration of the 2 agents given separately and extrapolations from clinical trials evaluating sitagliptin as add-on therapy to metformin. (See Combination Therapy under Uses: Type 2 Diabetes Mellitus, in Sitagliptin 68:20.05.)

Metformin is used in fixed combinations with the SGLT2 inhibitors canagliflozin, dapagliflozin, empagliflozin, or ertugliflozin. These fixed-combination preparations are used in patients with type 2 diabetes mellitus when treatment with both drugs is appropriate. Efficacy and safety of these fixed combinations have been established based on concurrent administration of the 2 drugs given separately. In clinical trials evaluating the efficacy of the combination of an SGLT2 inhibitor and metformin, patients who received both drugs had substantially greater improvements in HbA$_{1c}$ than when either drug component was administered alone. (See Combination Therapy under Uses: Type 2 Diabetes Mellitus, in the individual monographs on Canagliflozin 68:20.18, Dapagliflozin 68:20.18, Empagliflozin 68:20.18, and Ertugliflozin 68:20.18.)

Combination Therapy with Insulin

Combined therapy with insulin and metformin with or without other oral antidiabetic agents is one of several options for the management of hyperglycemia in patients with type 2 diabetes mellitus not responding adequately to oral monotherapy with metformin. Some experts state that patients with a HbA$_{1c}$ exceeding 9–10% who have symptoms secondary to hyperglycemia (polyuria, polydipsia, polyphagia) despite therapy with 2 antidiabetic agents would likely derive the greatest benefit from addition of insulin. When insulin therapy becomes necessary, some experts recommend that a single daily dose of basal insulin be added to the drug therapy regimen. Patients whose basal insulin-containing regimens (which may already include metformin) fail to provide adequate glycemic control may benefit from the addition of a GLP-1 receptor agonist, SGLT2 inhibitor, or DPP-4 inhibitor (if they not already taking one of these drugs). When glycemia is still not adequately controlled with the addition of other oral antidiabetic agents or a GLP-1 receptor agonist and basal insulin, therapy with additional short-acting or rapid-acting insulin injections at mealtimes may be required. Patients receiving combined therapy with metformin and insulin or insulin secretagogues (e.g., sulfonylureas) may require lower dosages of insulin or insulin secretagogues to minimize the risk of hypoglycemia. (See Cautions: Hypoglycemia.)

● Polycystic Ovary Syndrome

Metformin has been used in the management of metabolic and reproductive abnormalities associated with polycystic ovary syndrome†. However, adequate and well-controlled clinical trials evaluating metformin therapy for polycystic ovary syndrome remain limited, particularly regarding long-term efficacy, and available data are conflicting regarding the benefits of the drug in ameliorating various manifestations of the condition.

While metformin has beneficial effects on cardiovascular risk factors such as insulin resistance and obesity, evidence from pooled analyses of data suggest that the drug has limited overall benefits on reproductive outcomes (e.g., live birth rates) in women with polycystic ovary syndrome. As with diabetes mellitus, lifestyle changes (e.g., diet, exercise, weight loss in obese patients) are strongly recommended for the initial management of polycystic ovary syndrome; however, long-term success with such measures alone is difficult to achieve and drug therapy, including metformin, often is used for symptomatic management of this condition.

Polycystic ovary syndrome is characterized by chronic anovulation (generally manifested as oligomenorrhea or amenorrhea) and hyperandrogenism (excessive production of male hormones in women) with clinical manifestations of irregular menstrual cycles, infertility, hirsutism, acne, and dyslipidemia. While the principal etiology is unknown, insulin resistance with compensatory hyperinsulinemia is a prominent manifestation of polycystic ovary syndrome. Hyperinsulinemia stimulates ovarian and adrenal androgen secretion, leading to hyperandrogenism and its associated clinical manifestations. In addition, cardiovascular risk factors such as obesity and impaired glucose tolerance, including metabolic syndrome and type 2 diabetes mellitus, are present in a substantial proportion of women with polycystic ovary syndrome, making the use of insulin-sensitizing drugs such as metformin reasonable in the treatment of this condition.

Metformin and other insulin-sensitizing agents (e.g., thiazolidinedione antidiabetic agents) improve insulin resistance, which leads to a reduction in androgen production in ovarian theca cells and potential beneficial effects on metabolic and hormonal abnormalities associated with polycystic ovary syndrome. Although metformin therapy has not been shown specifically to reduce cardiovascular events in women with polycystic ovary syndrome, the drug's pharmacologic and clinical effects support its use as maintenance therapy to ameliorate insulin resistance and hyperinsulinemia in such women.

Estrogen-progestin oral contraceptives with or without an antiandrogen (e.g., spironolactone) traditionally have been used in the long-term management of polycystic ovary syndrome; however, such therapy may worsen preexisting insulin resistance and glucose tolerance and potentially increase cardiovascular risk. In a meta-analysis based on a small number of randomized, controlled trials in patients with polycystic ovary syndrome, oral contraceptive therapy (ethinyl estradiol with cyproterone acetate [not commercially available in the US] or norgestimate) for up to 12 months was associated with improvement in menstrual pattern and serum androgen concentrations compared with metformin, while metformin was more effective than oral contraceptives in reducing fasting insulin and triglyceride concentrations. However, a preference for either drug as maintenance therapy for polycystic ovary syndrome could not be determined because of a lack of adequate trial data. Another meta-analysis was unable to determine clinically important effects of metformin or thiazolidinedione therapy on metabolic or hyperandrogenism parameters such as fasting insulin or glucose concentrations, hirsutism, or hormone levels. Because of a lack of adequate long-term clinical trials, the effects of therapy with oral contraceptives or metformin on long-term outcomes such as diabetes, cardiovascular disease, or endometrial cancer in women with polycystic ovary syndrome have not been established.

Variable effects have been reported with metformin therapy used alone or in combination with fertility-enhancing drugs (e.g., clomiphene) for the treatment of infertility in women with polycystic ovary syndrome. Currently available evidence suggests that metformin hydrochloride dosages of 1.5–2.5 g daily in women with polycystic ovary syndrome increase the frequency of spontaneous ovulation, menstrual cyclicity, and ovulatory response after ovarian stimulation (e.g., with clomiphene, recombinant follicle-stimulating hormone). However, improvement in the rate of live births with metformin therapy generally has not been comparable to that associated with clomiphene therapy in such women. Results of a meta-analysis also indicated improvement in ovulation and clinical pregnancy rates with combined metformin and clomiphene treatment compared with clomiphene alone in women with polycystic ovary syndrome. However, another meta-analysis found only minimal improvement in ovulation rate and no improvement in pregnancy rate with metformin therapy. Some clinicians suggest that metformin therapy may be useful for inducing ovulation in women with polycystic ovary syndrome who desire pregnancy at a more distant time (e.g., more than 6 months away), and that clomiphene therapy may be preferable in those who desire to become pregnant much sooner. A potential advantage of metformin therapy over clomiphene for infertility is a reduced chance of twin or triplet pregnancy with metformin. Additional large, randomized, well-controlled studies are needed to establish the effectiveness of metformin alone or in combination with other therapies for treatment of infertility associated with polycystic ovary syndrome.

DOSAGE AND ADMINISTRATION

● Administration

Metformin hydrochloride is administered orally. In patients receiving metformin hydrochloride immediate-release tablets at a dosage of 2 g or less daily, the drug usually can be given as 2 divided doses daily; however, in patients who require more than 2 g daily, the drug may be better tolerated if administered in 3 divided doses daily. Immediate-release metformin hydrochloride in fixed combination with canagliflozin, dapagliflozin, empagliflozin, ertugliflozin, pioglitazone, alogliptin, linagliptin, or sitagliptin is administered in divided doses daily with meals to reduce the GI effects of the metformin hydrochloride component. Although food decreases the extent and slightly delays absorption of metformin immediate-release tablets, the manufacturer recommends that the drug be taken with meals to decrease adverse GI effects.

Metformin hydrochloride extended-release tablets usually are taken with the evening meal. The manufacturer of Fortamet® (metformin hydrochloride extended-release tablets) states that each dose of the drug should be taken with a full glass of water. The matrix core of some extended-release tablet preparations (e.g., Glumetza®) usually is broken up in the GI tract, but patients should be advised that occasionally the biologically inert components of the tablet may remain intact and be passed in the stool as a soft, hydrated mass. Occasionally, Glumetza® may be eliminated in the feces as a soft, hydrated mass or an insoluble shell. The membrane coating surrounding the core of another extended-release tablet (Fortamet®) remains intact through the GI tract and is excreted in feces as a soft mass that may resemble the original tablet. (See Chemistry and Stability: Stability.)

Extended-release metformin hydrochloride in fixed combination with canagliflozin, dapagliflozin, or empagliflozin is administered once daily with the morning meal.

The fixed combination of extended-release metformin hydrochloride and linagliptin should be administered once daily with a meal. The fixed combination of extended-release metformin hydrochloride and sitagliptin should be administered once daily with a meal, preferably with the evening meal. Extended-release metformin hydrochloride in fixed combination with saxagliptin should be administered once daily with the evening meal.

Extended-release metformin hydrochloride tablets and fixed-combination preparations containing the extended-release form of the drug must be swallowed whole and not chewed, cut, or crushed; inactive ingredients occasionally may be eliminated in feces as a soft mass that may resemble the original tablet.

● Dosage

Type 2 Diabetes Mellitus

Dosage of metformin hydrochloride must be individualized carefully based on patient response and tolerance. The goal of therapy should be to reduce both fasting glucose and glycosylated hemoglobin (hemoglobin A_{1c} [HbA_{1c}]) values to normal or near normal using the lowest effective dosage of metformin hydrochloride, either when used as monotherapy or combined with another antidiabetic agent. Patients should be monitored with regular laboratory evaluations, including fasting blood (or plasma) glucose determinations, to assess therapeutic response and the minimum effective dosage of metformin hydrochloride.

Following initiation of metformin therapy and dosage titration, determination of HbA_{1c} concentrations at intervals of approximately 3 months is useful for assessing the patient's continued response to therapy.

Since adverse GI effects with metformin appear to be dose related, it is recommended that dosage of the drug be increased gradually and that the drug be taken with meals. (See Cautions: GI Effects.)

Initial Dosage

For the management of type 2 diabetes mellitus in adults, the usual initial dosage of metformin hydrochloride as immediate-release tablets or immediate-release oral solution is 500 mg twice daily or 850 mg once daily with meals. Alternatively, an initial metformin hydrochloride dosage of 500 mg once daily has been suggested by some experts. Some manufacturers state that in general, clinically important responses are not observed at metformin hydrochloride dosages of less than 1.5 g daily.

When metformin hydrochloride is administered as an extended-release tablet preparation in adults, some manufacturers recommend an initial dosage of 500 mg once daily with the evening meal. The manufacturer of a certain extended-release tablet preparation (Fortamet®) recommends an initial dosage of 1 g once daily with the evening meal, although the manufacturer states that 500 mg once daily may be used when clinically appropriate. The recommended initial dosage of another extended-release preparation of metformin hydrochloride (Glumetza®) is 1 g once daily with the evening meal. Subsequent dosage of metformin hydrochloride should be adjusted according to the patient's therapeutic response, using the lowest possible effective dosage. (See Dosage: Dosage Titration, under Dosage and Administration.)

Although satisfactory control of blood glucose concentrations may be achieved within a few days after dosage adjustment, the full effects of the drug may not be observed for up to 2 weeks.

Initial dosages of metformin hydrochloride in geriatric patients should be conservative (initiated at the low end of the dosage range) and should be titrated carefully; limited data suggest reducing dosage by approximately 33% in geriatric patients.

For the management of type 2 diabetes mellitus in children or adolescents 10–16 years of age, the usual initial dosage of metformin hydrochloride as immediate-release tablets or the immediate-release oral solution is 500 mg twice daily given in the morning and evening with meals. Safety and efficacy of Fortamet® and certain other extended-release tablet preparations of metformin hydrochloride have not been established in patients younger than 17 years of age; refer to labeling of specific preparations for details. Safety and efficacy of Glumetza®, another extended-release tablet preparation, have not been established in patients younger than 18 years of age.

Transferring from Therapy with Other Antidiabetic Agents

When transferring from most sulfonylurea antidiabetic agents to metformin, a transition period generally is not required, and administration of the sulfonylurea antidiabetic agent may be abruptly discontinued. Because an exaggerated hypoglycemic response may occur in some patients during the transition from a sulfonylurea antidiabetic agent with a prolonged half-life (e.g., chlorpropamide [no longer commercially available in the US]) to metformin, patients being transferred from such agents should be monitored closely for the occurrence of hypoglycemia during the initial 2 weeks of the transition period.

Dosage Titration

In adults receiving an initial metformin hydrochloride dosage of 500 mg twice daily as immediate-release tablets or the immediate-release oral solution, daily dosage may be increased by 500 mg at weekly intervals until the desired fasting blood glucose concentration is achieved or a dosage of 2.55 g daily is reached. In adults receiving an initial dosage of 500 mg of metformin hydrochloride once or twice daily (with breakfast and/or dinner), some experts recommend increasing the dosage to 850 mg or 1 g twice daily after 5–7 days if additional glycemic control is needed and the drug is well tolerated (e.g., no adverse GI effects). If adverse GI effects appear during dosage titration of metformin hydrochloride, some experts suggest that dosage be decreased to the previous lower dosage, and further dosage increments attempted at a later time. In adults receiving an initial metformin hydrochloride dosage of 850 mg daily as immediate-release tablets or the immediate-release oral solution, daily dosage may be increased by 850 mg every other week (i.e., every 2 weeks) until the desired fasting blood glucose concentration is achieved or a total dosage of 2.55 g daily is reached. For patients requiring additional glycemic control with metformin hydrochloride, a maximum daily dosage of 2.55 g as immediate-release tablets or the immediate-release oral solution may be used.

In adults (17–18 years of age or older) receiving Glumetza® or certain other extended-release metformin hydrochloride preparations, daily dosage may be increased by 500 mg at weekly intervals until the desired glycemic response is achieved or a maximum of 2 g daily is reached. If glycemic control is not achieved with extended-release metformin hydrochloride tablets (e.g., Glumetza®) at a dosage of 2 g once daily, a dosage of 1 g twice daily should be considered. If a dosage exceeding 2 g daily is needed in patients receiving certain other extended-release metformin hydrochloride preparations, the manufacturers suggest that therapy be switched to immediate-release metformin hydrochloride tablets and dosage titrated up to a maximum dosage of 2.55 g daily in divided doses. Conversely, therapy with extended-release tablets may be substituted for immediate-release tablets at the same total daily dosage of immediate-release tablets, up to a dosage of 2 g once daily.

With another extended-release metformin hydrochloride preparation (Fortamet®), daily dosage may be increased by 500 mg at weekly intervals up to a maximum of 2.5 g once daily with the evening meal. In patients transferring from immediate-release tablets to an extended-release preparation, glycemic control should be closely monitored and dosage adjustments made accordingly.

Dosage in adults generally should not exceed 2.55 g daily when given as metformin hydrochloride immediate-release tablets or immediate-release oral solution, 2.5 g daily when given as certain extended-release tablets (e.g., Fortamet®), or 2 g daily when given as certain other extended-release tablet preparations. Metformin hydrochloride dosages of up to 3 g daily have been associated with modestly greater effectiveness than 1.7 g daily. However, adverse GI effects may limit the maximum dosage that can be tolerated. (Consult the manufacturer's labeling for product-specific details.) Dosages exceeding 2 g of metformin hydrochloride daily as immediate-release tablets or the immediate-release oral solution may be better tolerated if given in 3 divided doses daily with meals.

Metformin should be used with caution in geriatric patients since aging is associated with reduced renal function, and accumulation of the drug resulting in lactic acidosis may occur in patients with renal impairment. In addition, renal function should be monitored periodically in geriatric patients to determine the appropriate dosage of metformin hydrochloride. Any dosage adjustment in geriatric patients should be based on a careful assessment of renal function.

In children or adolescents 10–16 years of age receiving metformin hydrochloride 500 mg twice daily as immediate-release tablets or the immediate-release oral solution, daily dosage may be increased by 500 mg at weekly intervals until the desired glycemic response is achieved or a maximum dosage of 2 g daily given in 2 divided doses is reached.

Combination Therapy with Metformin and Sulfonylurea Antidiabetic Agents

While additional antidiabetic agents generally are added in a sequential manner to metformin monotherapy when such therapy no longer provides adequate glycemic control, initial antidiabetic therapy with 2 agents (e.g., metformin plus another drug) also may be appropriate in patients with high initial HbA$_{1c}$ values. (See Combination Therapy under Uses: Type 2 Diabetes Mellitus.)

The manufacturers of certain extended-release metformin hydrochloride tablets (Fortamet®, Glumetza®) suggest that gradual addition of an oral sulfonylurea agent be considered in patients not responding to 4 weeks of monotherapy with maximum dosages of metformin hydrochloride. Metformin hydrochloride should be continued at the maximum dosage in such patients even if prior primary or secondary failure to a sulfonylurea has occurred. Dosage of metformin hydrochloride (Fortamet®, Glumetza®) and the sulfonylurea should be adjusted to obtain the desired level of glycemic control with the minimum effective dosage. Concomitant metformin and sulfonylurea therapy may increase the risk of hypoglycemia; appropriate precautions should be taken. If the patient has not responded satisfactorily to 1–3 months of concomitant therapy with maximum dosages of metformin hydrochloride (Fortamet®, Glumetza®) and an oral sulfonylurea, therapeutic alternatives, including switching to insulin with or without metformin, should be considered.

If the fixed combination of metformin hydrochloride and glipizide is used as initial therapy in patients who have inadequate glycemic control with diet and exercise alone, the recommended initial dosage is 250 mg of metformin hydrochloride and 2.5 mg of glipizide once daily with a meal. In patients with more severe hyperglycemia (fasting plasma glucose concentrations of 280–320 mg/dL), an initial dosage of 500 mg of metformin hydrochloride and 2.5 mg of glipizide twice daily should be considered. The efficacy of metformin in fixed combination with glipizide has not been established in patients whose fasting plasma glucose concentrations exceed 320 mg/dL. Daily dosage may be increased in increments of one tablet (using the tablet strength at which therapy was initiated, either 2.5 mg of glipizide and 250 mg of metformin hydrochloride or 2.5 mg of glipizide and 500 mg of metformin hydrochloride) at 2-week intervals until the minimum effective dosage required to achieve adequate blood glucose control or a maximum dosage of 1 or 2 g of metformin hydrochloride and 10 mg of glipizide in divided doses is reached; there is no experience in clinical trials with the fixed combination using total daily dosages exceeding 2 g of metformin hydrochloride and 10 mg of glipizide as initial therapy.

In patients *not* already receiving therapy with either glyburide (or another sulfonylurea) or metformin hydrochloride, the fixed combination of metformin and glyburide should be initiated using a dosage of 250 mg of metformin hydrochloride and 1.25 mg of glyburide once or twice daily with a meal. For patients not adequately controlled on either glyburide (or another sulfonylurea) or metformin hydrochloride alone, the recommended initial dosage of the fixed combination is glyburide 2.5 mg and metformin hydrochloride 500 mg or glyburide 5 mg and metformin hydrochloride 500 mg orally twice daily with meals. For patients previously treated with the combination of glyburide (or another sulfonylurea) and metformin hydrochloride, the initial dosage of glyburide and metformin hydrochloride should not exceed the daily dosage of glyburide (or equivalent dose of another sulfonylurea) and metformin hydrochloride already being taken. Dosage of the fixed combination may be increased gradually based on glycemic control and tolerability up to a maximum daily dosage of 20 mg of glyburide and 2 g of metformin hydrochloride.

Therapy with metformin in fixed combination with glyburide should be used with caution in geriatric patients, since aging is associated with reduced renal function. The initial and maintenance dosages of metformin hydrochloride in fixed combination with glyburide should be conservative, starting at the low end of the dosage range, reflecting the greater frequency of decreased hepatic, renal, or cardiac function and of concomitant disease or other drug therapy and higher risk of hypoglycemia and lactic acidosis in the elderly.

Combination Therapy with Metformin and Pioglitazone

Dosage of the fixed combination of immediate-release metformin hydrochloride and pioglitazone should be based on the patient's current dosages of metformin hydrochloride and/or pioglitazone and on effectiveness and tolerability. For patients in whom combination therapy with metformin and pioglitazone is considered appropriate, the usual initial dosage of the fixed combination is metformin hydrochloride 500 mg and pioglitazone 15 mg twice daily or metformin hydrochloride 850 mg and pioglitazone 15 mg once daily. For patients inadequately controlled on metformin hydrochloride monotherapy, the usual initial dosage of the fixed combination is metformin hydrochloride 500 mg and pioglitazone 15 mg twice daily or metformin hydrochloride 850 mg and pioglitazone 15 mg once or twice daily (depending on the dosage of metformin hydrochloride already being taken). For patients inadequately controlled on pioglitazone monotherapy, the usual initial dosage of the fixed combination is metformin hydrochloride 500 mg and pioglitazone 15 mg twice daily or metformin hydrochloride 850 mg and pioglitazone 15 mg once daily. For patients switching from combination therapy with metformin hydrochloride and pioglitazone given as separate tablets, the dosage of the fixed combination should be as close as possible to the metformin hydrochloride and pioglitazone dosages already being taken.

For patients with New York Heart Association (NYHA) class I or II congestive heart failure, the recommended initial dosage of the fixed combination is metformin hydrochloride 500 mg and pioglitazone 15 mg or metformin hydrochloride 850 mg and pioglitazone 15 mg once daily. Initiation of the fixed combination of metformin and pioglitazone is contraindicated in patients with NYHA class III or IV congestive heart failure. (See Cautions: Precautions and Contraindications.)

Dosage of the fixed combination should be titrated gradually as needed based on adequacy of therapeutic response and tolerability up to a maximum daily dosage of 2.55 g of metformin hydrochloride and 45 mg of pioglitazone. Metformin hydrochloride dosages exceeding 2 g daily may be better tolerated if given in 3 divided doses daily.

Metformin Hydrochloride/Alogliptin Fixed-combination Therapy

Dosage of the fixed combination of metformin hydrochloride and alogliptin should be individualized based on the patient's current antidiabetic regimen, effectiveness, and tolerability. Dosage should be increased gradually to minimize the adverse GI effects of metformin. The maximum recommended dosage of the fixed combination of metformin hydrochloride and alogliptin is 2 g of metformin hydrochloride and 25 mg of alogliptin daily.

Metformin Hydrochloride/Linagliptin Fixed-combination Therapy

Dosage of the fixed combination of metformin hydrochloride and linagliptin should be individualized based on its effectiveness and patient tolerability. The dosage may be increased up to a maximum of 2 g of metformin hydrochloride and 5 mg of linagliptin daily.

In patients *not* currently receiving metformin hydrochloride, the recommended initial total daily dosage of the fixed combination is 1 g of metformin hydrochloride and 5 mg of linagliptin administered in 2 divided doses (when given as the fixed-combination preparation containing immediate-release metformin hydrochloride) or once daily (when given as the fixed-combination preparation containing extended-release metformin hydrochloride).

In patients currently receiving metformin hydrochloride, the recommended initial total daily dosage of the fixed combination is a total daily metformin hydrochloride dosage similar to what the patient is receiving and 5 mg of linagliptin, administered in 2 divided doses (when given as the fixed-combination preparation containing immediate-release metformin hydrochloride) or once daily (when given as the fixed-combination preparation containing extended-release metformin hydrochloride).

In patients currently receiving metformin hydrochloride and linagliptin, the recommended initial dosage of the fixed combination of immediate-release metformin hydrochloride and linagliptin is the same as the existing total daily dosage of each component administered in 2 divided doses daily. In patients already receiving linagliptin and metformin or the fixed combination of linagliptin and immediate-release metformin, the recommended initial dosage of the fixed combination of extended-release metformin hydrochloride and linagliptin is a total daily metformin hydrochloride dosage similar to the patient's existing dosage and 5 mg of linagliptin administered once daily.

Metformin Hydrochloride/Saxagliptin Fixed-combination Therapy

Dosage of extended-release metformin hydrochloride in fixed combination with saxagliptin hydrochloride should be individualized based on the patient's current antidiabetic regimen, clinical response, and tolerability. Any change in therapy should be undertaken with care and appropriate monitoring because changes in glycemic control can occur.

When the fixed-combination preparation containing extended-release metformin hydrochloride and saxagliptin is used in patients inadequately controlled on monotherapy with saxagliptin 5 mg daily, the recommended initial dosage of the fixed combination is 500 mg of extended-release metformin hydrochloride and 5 mg of saxagliptin once daily; dosage should be increased gradually to reduce adverse GI effects of metformin.

When the fixed-combination preparation containing extended-release metformin hydrochloride and saxagliptin is used in patients inadequately controlled on monotherapy with extended-release metformin hydrochloride, dosage of the fixed combination should provide metformin hydrochloride at the patient's current dosage or at the nearest therapeutically appropriate dosage. Following a switch from immediate-release to extended-release metformin, glycemic control should be closely monitored and dosage adjustments made accordingly.

In patients inadequately controlled on monotherapy with saxagliptin 2.5 mg daily, the recommended initial dosage of the fixed combination is 1 g of extended-release metformin hydrochloride and 2.5 mg of saxagliptin daily. Patients who require 2.5 mg of saxagliptin *and* who are either metformin naive or require a dose of metformin hydrochloride exceeding 1 g should use the individual components.

The maximum recommended dosages of extended-release metformin hydrochloride and saxagliptin in fixed combination are 2 g of extended-release metformin hydrochloride and 5 mg of saxagliptin daily.

When the fixed-combination preparation containing extended-release metformin hydrochloride and saxagliptin is used concomitantly with a potent cytochrome P-450 isoenzyme 3A4/5 (CYP3A4/5) inhibitor (e.g., atazanavir, clarithromycin, indinavir, itraconazole, ketoconazole, nefazodone, nelfinavir, ritonavir, saquinavir, telithromycin), dosage of saxagliptin should be limited to 2.5 mg once daily.

Metformin Hydrochloride/Sitagliptin Fixed-combination Therapy

Dosage of the fixed-combination preparation containing immediate- or extended-release metformin hydrochloride and sitagliptin (Janumet® or Janumet® XR) should be individualized based on the patient's current antidiabetic regimen, effectiveness, and tolerability. When the fixed combination containing immediate-release metformin hydrochloride and sitagliptin is used in patients *not* currently receiving metformin hydrochloride, the recommended initial dosage is 500 mg of immediate-release metformin hydrochloride and 50 mg of sitagliptin twice daily. When the fixed combination containing extended-release metformin hydrochloride and sitagliptin is used in patients *not* currently receiving metformin hydrochloride, the recommended initial dosage is 1 g of extended-release metformin hydrochloride and 100 mg of sitagliptin once daily. The dosage should be increased gradually to reduce adverse GI effects associated with the metformin hydrochloride component.

When the fixed combination of immediate-release metformin hydrochloride and sitagliptin is used in patients currently receiving metformin hydrochloride, the recommended initial dosage is 500 mg of metformin hydrochloride and 50 mg of sitagliptin or 1 g of metformin hydrochloride and 50 mg of sitagliptin twice daily, depending on the patient's existing dosage of metformin hydrochloride.

When the fixed combination of immediate-release metformin hydrochloride and sitagliptin is used in patients currently receiving immediate-release metformin hydrochloride 850 mg twice daily, the recommended initial dosage of the fixed combination is 1 g of immediate-release metformin hydrochloride and 50 mg of sitagliptin twice daily.

When the fixed combination of extended-release metformin hydrochloride and sitagliptin is used in patients currently receiving metformin hydrochloride, the recommended initial dosage of the fixed combination is 1 g of extended-release metformin hydrochloride and 100 mg of sitagliptin or 2 g of extended-release metformin hydrochloride and 100 mg of sitagliptin once daily, depending on the patient's existing dosage of metformin hydrochloride.

In patients currently receiving immediate-release metformin hydrochloride 850 or 1000 mg twice daily, the recommend initial dosage of the fixed combination containing extended-release metformin hydrochloride and sitagliptin is 2 g of extended-release metformin hydrochloride and 100 mg of sitagliptin once daily.

The same total daily dosage of sitagliptin and metformin hydrochloride should be maintained when transitioning between the fixed combination of immediate-release metformin hydrochloride and sitagliptin and the fixed combination of extended-release metformin hydrochloride and sitagliptin.

The safety and efficacy of transferring from therapy with other oral antidiabetic agents to the fixed combination of sitagliptin and immediate- or extended-release metformin hydrochloride have not been specifically established in clinical studies. Any change in the therapy of patients with type 2 diabetes mellitus should be undertaken with caution and appropriate monitoring, as changes in glycemic control can occur.

Concomitant administration of the fixed combination of immediate- or extended-release metformin hydrochloride and sitagliptin with a sulfonylurea or insulin may require reduced dosages of the sulfonylurea or insulin to reduce the risk of hypoglycemia.

Dosage of metformin hydrochloride in fixed combination with sitagliptin should be selected carefully in patients of advanced age, since aging is associated with reduced renal function. In geriatric patients, dosage adjustment should be based on careful and regular assessment of renal function.

Metformin Hydrochloride/Canagliflozin Fixed-combination Therapy

When the commercially available fixed combination of immediate-release metformin hydrochloride and canagliflozin (Invokamet®) is used in patients with type 2 diabetes mellitus in whom treatment with both drugs is appropriate, the initial dosage should be based on the patient's current regimen with canagliflozin and/or metformin hydrochloride. In patients with an estimated glomerular filtration rate (eGFR) of at least 60 mL/minute per 1.73 m², the dosage of the fixed-combination preparation may be gradually increased based on effectiveness and tolerability up to a maximum of 2 g of metformin hydrochloride and 300 mg of canagliflozin daily.

In patients *not* currently treated with either metformin hydrochloride or canagliflozin, the recommended initial total daily dosage of these drugs is 1 g of metformin hydrochloride and 100 mg of canagliflozin, administered in 2 divided doses (when given as the fixed-combination preparation containing immediate-release metformin hydrochloride) or once daily (when given as the fixed-combination preparation containing extended-release metformin hydrochloride).

In patients currently receiving metformin hydrochloride, the recommended initial total daily dosage of the fixed combination with canagliflozin is a metformin hydrochloride dosage similar to the patient's existing total daily dosage and 100 mg of canagliflozin, administered in 2 divided doses (when given as the fixed-combination preparation containing immediate-release metformin hydrochloride) or once daily (when given as the fixed-combination preparation containing extended-release metformin hydrochloride). Patients who are currently receiving an evening dose of extended-release metformin hydrochloride should skip their last dose prior to initiating therapy with the fixed combination of canagliflozin and metformin hydrochloride the following morning.

In patients currently receiving canagliflozin, the recommended initial total daily dosage of the fixed combination is 1 g of metformin hydrochloride and the same daily dosage of canagliflozin, administered in 2 divided doses (when given as the fixed-combination preparation containing immediate-release metformin hydrochloride) or once daily (when given as the fixed-combination preparation containing extended-release metformin hydrochloride).

In patients currently receiving metformin hydrochloride and canagliflozin as separate components, the recommended initial dosage of the fixed combination is a total daily metformin hydrochloride dosage similar to the patient's existing dosage and the same daily dosage of canagliflozin, administered in 2 divided doses (when given as the fixed-combination preparation containing immediate-release metformin hydrochloride) or once daily (when given as the fixed-combination preparation containing extended-release metformin hydrochloride).

Metformin Hydrochloride/Dapagliflozin Fixed-combination Therapy

When the commercially available fixed combination of extended-release metformin hydrochloride and dapagliflozin (Xigduo® XR) is used in patients with type 2 diabetes mellitus, the recommended initial dosage is based on the patient's current regimen of metformin hydrochloride and/or dapagliflozin. For patients *not* currently receiving dapagliflozin, the recommended initial dosage of the dapagliflozin component is 5 mg once daily. Dosage should be titrated gradually based on effectiveness and tolerability up to a maximum daily dosage of 2 g of extended-release metformin hydrochloride and 10 mg of dapagliflozin. Patients who are already receiving extended-release metformin hydrochloride in the evening who are switching to the fixed combination of dapagliflozin and metformin hydrochloride should skip their last dose of metformin hydrochloride before initiating therapy with the fixed combination the following morning.

Metformin Hydrochloride/Empagliflozin Fixed-combination Therapy

Dosage of metformin hydrochloride in fixed combination with empagliflozin should be individualized based on the patient's current antidiabetic regimen. The dosage of the fixed-combination preparation may be gradually increased based on effectiveness and tolerability up to a maximum of 2 g of metformin hydrochloride and 25 mg of empagliflozin daily.

In patients currently receiving metformin hydrochloride, the recommended initial total daily dosage of the fixed combination is a metformin hydrochloride dosage similar to the patient's existing total daily dosage and 10 mg of empagliflozin, administered in 2 divided doses (when given as the fixed-combination preparation containing immediate-release metformin hydrochloride) or once daily (when given as the fixed-combination preparation containing extended-release metformin hydrochloride).

In patients currently receiving empagliflozin, the recommended initial total daily dosage of the fixed combination is 1 g of metformin hydrochloride and the same daily dosage of empagliflozin administered in 2 divided doses (when given as the fixed-combination preparation containing immediate-release metformin hydrochloride) or once daily (when given as the fixed-combination preparation containing extended-release metformin hydrochloride).

In patients currently receiving metformin hydrochloride and empagliflozin as separate components, the recommended initial total daily dosage of the fixed combination is a metformin hydrochloride dosage similar to the patient's existing total daily dosage and the same daily dosage of empagliflozin, administered in 2 divided doses (when given as the fixed-combination preparation containing immediate-release metformin hydrochloride) or once daily (when given as the fixed-combination preparation containing extended-release metformin hydrochloride).

Metformin Hydrochloride/Ertugliflozin Fixed-combination Therapy

When the commercially available fixed-combination preparation containing immediate-release metformin hydrochloride and ertugliflozin (Segluromet®) is used in patients with type 2 diabetes mellitus, the recommended initial dosage is based on the patient's current regimen of metformin hydrochloride and/or ertugliflozin. The dosage of the fixed combination may be increased gradually based on effectiveness and tolerability up to a maximum of 2 g of metformin hydrochloride and 15 mg of ertugliflozin daily.

In patients currently receiving metformin hydrochloride, the recommended initial total daily dosage of the fixed combination is a metformin hydrochloride dosage similar to the patient's existing total daily dosage and 5 mg of ertugliflozin, administered in 2 divided doses.

In patients currently receiving ertugliflozin, the recommended initial total daily dosage of the fixed combination is 1 g of metformin hydrochloride and an ertugliflozin dosage similar to the patient's existing total daily dosage, administered in 2 divided doses.

For patients currently receiving metformin hydrochloride and ertugliflozin as separate components, the recommended initial total daily dosage of the fixed combination is a dosage of metformin hydrochloride similar to the patient's existing total daily dosage and the same daily dosage of ertugliflozin, administered in 2 divided doses.

Concomitant Therapy with Metformin and Insulin

In patients receiving insulin therapy in whom metformin is to be given concomitantly, the current insulin dosage should initially be continued. In such patients, some manufacturers recommend an initial metformin hydrochloride dosage of 500 mg once daily as extended-release tablets (Fortamet®, Glumetza®). For patients with inadequate glycemic response, the daily dosage of metformin hydrochloride may be increased by 500 mg at weekly intervals until glycemic control is

achieved or a maximum dosage of 2.5 or 2 g daily is reached with the extended-release tablet preparations Fortamet® or Glumetza®, respectively. When fasting plasma glucose concentrations decrease to less than 120 mg/dL in patients receiving combined metformin and insulin therapy, some manufacturers of metformin recommend that insulin dosage be decreased by 10–25%. Further dosage adjustments should be individualized based on glycemic response.

Polycystic Ovary Syndrome

In women with polycystic ovary syndrome†, metformin hydrochloride dosages of 1.5–2.25 g daily in divided doses generally have been used to ameliorate symptoms of insulin resistance and hyperinsulinemia and to increase the frequency of spontaneous ovulation, menstrual cyclicity, and ovulatory response after ovarian stimulation.

● Dosage in Renal and Hepatic Impairment

Because of the risk of lactic acidosis, which occurs rarely but may be fatal, metformin should not be used in patients with severe renal disease or dysfunction (eGFR less than 30 mL/minute per 1.73 m²) and should be avoided in those with clinical or laboratory evidence of hepatic disease. In patients with moderate renal disease, the benefits and risks of continuing metformin therapy should be assessed. (See Cautions: Lactic Acidosis.)

An FDA review of clinical studies evaluating the safety of metformin in patients with reduced kidney function suggests that metformin can be used safely in patients with mild impairment in kidney function and in some patients with moderate impairment in kidney function.

The manufacturers and FDA state that renal function (eGFR) should be assessed prior to initiation of metformin and at least annually; more frequent monitoring has been recommended in patients with an increased risk of developing renal impairment (e.g., geriatric patients). The manufacturers and FDA state that initiation of metformin therapy is not recommended in patients with an eGFR between 30–45 mL/minute per 1.73 m² and that the benefits and risks of continuing the drug should be assessed in those already receiving metformin whose eGFR falls below 45 mL/minute per 1.73 m². The manufacturers and FDA state that metformin is contraindicated in patients with an eGFR of less than 30 mL/minute per 1.73 m² and that the drug should be discontinued in patients whose eGFR falls below 30 mL/minute per 1.73 m² who are already receiving metformin.

CAUTIONS

Adverse effects, principally GI effects, reportedly occur in about 5–50% of patients receiving metformin therapy as immediate-release tablets in clinical trials and generally required discontinuance of the drug in 6% or less of patients.

● Lactic Acidosis

Accumulation of metformin may occur in patients with renal impairment, and such accumulation rarely can result in lactic acidosis, a serious, potentially fatal metabolic disease. The reported overall incidence of lactic acidosis in patients receiving metformin therapy is approximately 0.04 cases per 1000 patient-years of metformin therapy. (See Cautions: Precautions and Contraindications and also see Chemistry and Stability: Chemistry.) However, lactic acidosis constitutes a medical emergency requiring immediate hospitalization and treatment; in such cases, metformin should be discontinued and general supportive therapy (e.g., volume expansion, diuresis) initiated immediately. Prompt hemodialysis also is recommended. (See Acute Toxicity.)

Cases of metformin-associated lactic acidosis reported during postmarketing experience have resulted in death, hypothermia, hypotension, and resistant bradyarrhythmias. Metformin-associated lactic acidosis has been characterized by elevated blood lactate concentrations (exceeding 45 mg/dL), anion gap acidosis (without evidence of ketonuria or ketonemia), an increased lactate/pyruvate ratio. Lactic acidosis also may occur in association with a variety of pathophysiologic conditions, including diabetes mellitus, and generally whenever substantial tissue hypoperfusion and hypoxemia exist. Approximately 50% of cases of metformin-associated lactic acidosis have been reported to be fatal. However, it has been suggested that in such cases of lactic acidosis not accompanied by conditions predisposing to tissue anoxia (e.g., heart failure, renal or pulmonary disease), techniques for the elimination of metformin from the body may allow recovery rates exceeding 80%.

The manufacturer states that when metformin has been implicated as the cause of lactic acidosis, plasma metformin concentrations exceeding 5 mcg/mL generally have been observed. However, plasma metformin concentrations may not be an accurate indication of tissue accumulation of the drug in patients with metformin-induced lactic acidosis, and increased plasma concentrations of lactic acid or lactic acidosis have been demonstrated during metformin therapy despite normal plasma concentrations of the drug. Patients with lactic acidosis and normal plasma metformin concentrations also may have other conditions contributing to the development of lactic acidosis (e.g., hypoxia, dehydration). Some observational data suggest that neither plasma metformin concentrations nor plasma lactate concentrations are related to mortality in patients with lactic acidosis receiving metformin.

Lactic acidosis often has a subtle onset and may be accompanied only by nonspecific symptoms such as malaise, myalgias, respiratory distress, increasing somnolence, and nonspecific and unexplained abdominal distress with nausea and vomiting or diarrhea. Associated hypothermia (e.g., cold hands or feet), hypotension (e.g., dizziness or lightheadedness), and resistant bradyarrhythmias with more marked acidosis also may occur. Patients and clinicians should be aware of the possible importance of such symptoms, and patients should be instructed to notify their clinician immediately if these symptoms occur; metformin should be discontinued until the patient is hospitalized and a clinician has evaluated the patient's condition. Once a patient is stabilized at any dosage of metformin hydrochloride, GI symptoms, which are common during initiation of therapy, are unlikely to be drug related; later occurrence of GI symptoms could be manifestations of lactic acidosis or other serious disease.

Lactic acidosis associated with metformin therapy generally has occurred in diabetic patients with severe renal insufficiency; most cases of lactic acidosis have been reported in patients with concomitant medical and/or surgical problems who were receiving multiple drugs.

Some observational studies and meta-analyses suggest that the incidence of lactic acidosis in patients with type 2 diabetes mellitus who are receiving metformin therapy is similar to that in patients not receiving the drug. Analyses of pooled data that included all known prospective comparative trials and observational cohort studies of metformin therapy of at least 1 month's duration (up to 70,490 patient-years of metformin treatment) revealed no cases of fatal or nonfatal metformin-induced lactic acidosis; therefore, an incidence rate for metformin-associated lactic acidosis could not be calculated. While these analyses allowed for the inclusion of patients with at least one contraindication to metformin (e.g., renal insufficiency), information on the safety of metformin in the presence of such contraindications could not be evaluated because of the lack of information on the number of included patients with such conditions. In these analyses, all cases of lactic acidosis reportedly occurred in patients with comorbidities predisposing to lactic acidosis, suggesting that association of the condition with metformin use may be coincidental rather than causal.

The risk of lactic acidosis appears to increase with the degree of renal impairment and the patient's age; therefore, the risk of this condition can be minimized by periodic monitoring of renal function and cautious dosage selection (i.e., initiating drug therapy at the low end of the dosage range). Other risk factors for lactic acidosis include concomitant use of certain drugs (e.g., carbonic anhydrase inhibitors such as topiramate), age 65 years or older, undergoing radiological procedures with intravascular contrast agents, surgery and other procedures, hypoxic states, excessive alcohol consumption, and hepatic impairment. Metformin therapy should be withheld promptly in patients with any condition associated with hypoxemia, sepsis, or dehydration, or in any patient who becomes acutely unwell. Therapy with the drug alone or in fixed combinations also should be avoided in patients with clinical or laboratory evidence of hepatic impairment since elimination of lactate may be reduced substantially in such patients. Patients should be advised not to consume excessive amounts of alcohol, either acutely or chronically, since alcohol may potentiate the effects of metformin on lactate metabolism by decreasing hepatic gluconeogenesis.

The manufacturers, FDA, and other clinicians state that metformin-containing therapy should be discontinued before or at the time of an intravascular (e.g., IV, intra-arterial) iodinated contrast imaging procedure in patients with an estimated glomerular filtration rate (eGFR) of 30–60 mL/minute per 1.73 m^2 and in patients with a history of liver disease, alcoholism, or heart failure. Therapy with metformin-containing preparations also should be withheld temporarily in patients undergoing surgery. Renal function should be evaluated 48 hours after the imaging procedure and metformin therapy may be reinstituted if renal function is stable. (See Cautions: Precautions and Contraindications.)

● GI Effects

Adverse GI effects such as diarrhea, nausea, vomiting, flatulence, indigestion, and abdominal discomfort (e.g., bloating, abdominal cramping or pain) are the most common adverse effects associated with metformin-containing therapy as immediate-release tablets; diarrhea and nausea/vomiting are among the most common drug-related adverse effects reported in clinical trials with the extended-release tablets. Because substantial diarrhea and/or vomiting may cause dehydration and prerenal azotemia, metformin should be discontinued in patients who develop such potentially serious GI effects; persistent diarrhea resolves promptly upon discontinuance of the drug. Unpleasant or metallic taste (taste disorder/disturbance), which usually resolves spontaneously, has been reported in approximately 1–5% of patients receiving metformin immediate-release or extended-release tablets. Other adverse GI effects reported in 1–5% of patients receiving certain immediate-release or extended-release metformin tablet preparations include abnormal stools, abdominal pain, distended abdomen, constipation, dyspepsia/heartburn, and flatulence. Other adverse GI effects reported in 1–5% of patients receiving another metformin extended-release tablet (Fortamet®) include dyspepsia, flatulence, and abdominal pain. Anorexia also has been reported with metformin therapy.

Metformin-induced adverse GI effects appear to be dose related, generally occur at initiation of therapy, and usually subside spontaneously during continued metformin therapy; in some cases, a reduction in metformin hydrochloride dosage may be useful in hastening resolution of these effects. Diarrhea severe enough to require discontinuance of metformin occurred in about 6% of patients receiving the immediate-release tablets and in about 0.6% of those receiving the extended-release tablets in controlled clinical trials. Since adverse GI effects occurring during initiation of metformin therapy appear to be dose related, they may be reduced by gradual dosage escalation and administration of the drug with meals.

Diarrhea was reported in up to 7.5% of patients receiving combined therapy with metformin hydrochloride and sitagliptin in clinical trials.

● Hypoglycemia

Hypoglycemia is uncommon in patients receiving metformin as monotherapy; however, it may occur when metformin is used concomitantly with an insulin secretagogue (e.g., sulfonylurea antidiabetic agent), a thiazolidinedione, or insulin; when caloric intake is deficient; or when strenuous exercise is not accompanied by food intake. Symptoms of hypoglycemia (such as dizziness, shakiness, sweating, hunger) have occurred in 21.3, 11.4, or 37.7% of patients receiving glyburide (5.3 mg), glyburide in fixed combination with metformin hydrochloride (2.78 mg of glyburide, 557 mg of metformin hydrochloride), or glyburide in fixed combination with metformin hydrochloride at a final mean titrated dosage of 824 mg of metformin hydrochloride and 4.1 mg of glyburide in controlled clinical trials. In a controlled initial therapy trial of metformin hydrochloride in fixed combination with glipizide, symptomatic hypoglycemia and blood glucose concentrations 50 mg/dL or less occurred in 2.9, 0, 7.6, or 9.3% of patients receiving glipizide monotherapy (final mean dosage of 16.7 mg), metformin hydrochloride monotherapy (final mean dosage of 1.749 g of metformin hydrochloride), the fixed combination with glipizide (final mean dosage of 791 mg of metformin hydrochloride and 7.9 mg of glipizide), and the fixed combination with a higher dosage of the metformin hydrochloride component (final mean dosage of 1.477 g of metformin hydrochloride and 7.4 mg of glipizide). In a controlled trial in patients inadequately controlled by monotherapy with metformin hydrochloride or a sulfonylurea agent, documented hypoglycemia (as determined by blood glucose concentrations of 50 mg/dL or less) occurred in 0, 1.3, or 12.6% of patients receiving glipizide monotherapy (mean final dosage of 30 mg), metformin hydrochloride monotherapy (mean final dosage of 1.927 g), or metformin hydrochloride in fixed combination with glipizide at a final mean dosage of 1.747 g of metformin hydrochloride and 5 mg of glipizide. When rosiglitazone was added to fixed combination therapy of glyburide and metformin hydrochloride, documented hypoglycemia occurred in 22% of such patients compared to 3.3% of patients receiving glyburide in fixed combination with metformin hydrochloride. (See Cautions: Precautions and Contraindications.)

Hypoglycemia was reported in 16.4% of patients when sitagliptin was added to combined metformin hydrochloride and glimepiride therapy, compared with 0.9% of those receiving placebo in conjunction with metformin hydrochloride and glimepiride therapy.

● Hematologic Effects

Asymptomatic decreases in serum vitamin B_{12} concentration were reported in about 7–9% of patients receiving metformin alone, and in about 6% of those receiving metformin concomitantly with a sulfonylurea antidiabetic agent, during 29-week controlled clinical trials. Such decreases may be related to interference with absorption of vitamin B_{12} from B_{12}-intrinsic factor complex; however, they rarely are associated with anemia and are rapidly reversible following discontinuation of metformin or supplementation with vitamin B_{12}. Serum folic acid concentrations do not appear to decrease substantially in patients receiving metformin therapy. Megaloblastic anemia has been reported rarely in patients receiving metformin. No increased incidence of neuropathy has been observed in patients receiving the drug. Hematologic parameters (e.g., hemoglobin) should be monitored annually and serum vitamin B_{12} concentrations should be monitored every 2–3 years in patients receiving metformin; any apparent abnormalities should be appropriately investigated and managed (e.g., administration of supplemental vitamin B_{12} to those who develop neuropathy). Some individuals such as those who have inadequate vitamin B_{12} or calcium intake or absorption appear to be at an increased risk for developing subnormal vitamin B_{12} concentrations. Some clinicians have suggested that periodic supplementation with parenteral vitamin B_{12} be considered in such patients and in alcoholics. (See Cautions: Precautions and Contraindications.)

● Dermatologic Reactions

Rash has been reported in 1–5% of patients receiving immediate-release metformin in clinical trials.

● Nervous System Effects

Headache, agitation, dizziness, and tiredness were reported in a small comparative study in geriatric diabetic patients receiving metformin. Headache was reported in 4.7 or 5.1% of patients receiving metformin as an extended-release tablet preparation (Fortamet®) or as immediate-release tablets, respectively. Headache has been reported in 9.3 or 8.9% of patients receiving metformin or metformin in fixed combination with glyburide, respectively. Headache has been reported in 5.3 or 12.6% of patients receiving metformin or metformin in fixed combination with glipizide, respectively. Headache has been reported in 5.9% of patients receiving combined therapy with metformin and sitagliptin and 6.9% of patients receiving combined therapy with metformin, sitagliptin, and glimepiride in clinical trials. Dizziness has been reported in 3.8 or 5.5% of patients receiving metformin or metformin in fixed combination with glyburide, respectively. Dizziness has been reported in 3.8 or 5.5% of patients receiving metformin or metformin in fixed combination with glyburide, respectively.

● Respiratory Effects

Pneumonitis with vasculitis has been reported rarely with concomitant metformin and oral sulfonylurea (e.g., glyburide) therapy. Upper respiratory tract infection was reported in 16.3 or 17.3% of patients receiving metformin or metformin in fixed combination with glyburide, respectively. Upper respiratory tract infection was reported in 8.5 or 8.1–9.9% of patients receiving metformin or metformin in fixed combination with glipizide, respectively, as initial therapy for type 2 diabetes mellitus. Upper respiratory tract infection was reported in 10.7 or 10.3% of patients receiving metformin or metformin in fixed combination with glipizide, respectively, as second-line therapy for type 2 diabetes mellitus. Upper respiratory tract infection was reported in 5.2 or 6.2% of patients receiving metformin or metformin combined with sitagliptin, respectively, in clinical trials. Rhinitis was reported in 4.2 or 5.6% of patients receiving metformin as an extended-release tablet preparation (Fortamet®) or as immediate-release tablets, respectively. Infection was reported in 20.5 or 20.9% of patients receiving an extended-release tablet preparation (Fortamet®) or immediate-release tablets, respectively.

● Macrovascular Outcomes

The manufacturer states that there have been no clinical studies establishing conclusive evidence of macrovascular risk reduction with metformin.

● Other Adverse Effects

Urinary tract infection has been reported in 8 or 1.1% of patients receiving metformin alone or in fixed combination with glipizide, respectively. Hypertension has been reported in 5.6 or 2.9–3.5% of patients receiving metformin alone or in fixed combination with glipizide, respectively. Musculoskeletal pain has been reported in 6.7 or 8% of patients receiving metformin alone or in fixed combination with glipizide, respectively. Severe acute hepatitis associated with marked elevations in serum hepatic aminotransferase values and cholestasis has been reported following initiation of metformin therapy in a patient receiving glipizide and enalapril. Cholestatic, hepatocellular, and mixed hepatocellular liver injury have been reported during postmarketing experience with metformin therapy. Accidental injury was reported in 7.3 or 5.6% of patients receiving metformin as an extended-release tablet preparation (Fortamet®) or as immediate-release tablets, respectively.

● Precautions and Contraindications

When metformin hydrochloride is used in fixed combination with other drugs (e.g., sulfonylureas, thiazolidinediones, dipeptidyl peptidase-4 [DPP-4] inhibitors, meglitinides, sodium-glucose cotransporter 2 [SGLT2] inhibitors), the cautions, precautions, contraindications, and drug interactions associated with these concomitant agents must be considered in addition to those associated with metformin.

The diagnostic and therapeutic measures for managing diabetes mellitus that are necessary to ensure optimum control of the disease with insulin are generally necessary with metformin. Clinicians who prescribe metformin should be familiar with the indications, limitations, and patient-selection criteria for therapy with oral antidiabetic agents to ensure appropriate patient management. Patients receiving metformin should be monitored with regular laboratory evaluations, including blood glucose determinations, to determine the minimum effective dosage of metformin hydrochloride when used either as monotherapy or in combination with a sulfonylurea or thiazolidinedione antidiabetic agent. Glycosylated hemoglobin (hemoglobin A_{1c} [HbA_{1c}]) measurements also are useful, particularly for monitoring long-term control of blood glucose concentration.

Patients should be informed of the risks of lactic acidosis and conditions that predispose to its development. (See Cautions: Lactic Acidosis.) Since metformin is excreted substantially by the kidneys, accumulation of the drug resulting in lactic acidosis may occur in patients with renal impairment; the risk of lactic acidosis increases with degree of renal impairment. Hemodialysis has been used in patients with lactic acidosis to accelerate the clearance of metformin. (See Acute Toxicity.) The manufacturer states that eGFR (renal function) should be evaluated prior to initiation of therapy with metformin preparations and at least annually thereafter.

Extended-release metformin hydrochloride tablets or fixed-combination preparations containing the extended-release form of the drug should not be chewed, cut, or crushed; these dosage forms must be swallowed whole. Patients should be aware that the biologically inert components of the tablet may occasionally be eliminated in the feces as a soft, hydrated mass.

Some clinicians state that metformin should not be used in patients with heart failure requiring drug therapy (e.g., digoxin, furosemide), such as those with unstable or acute heart failure. These patients are at risk for hypoperfusion and hypoxemia, which may lead to lactic acidosis. It has been suggested that metformin may be reinstituted once acute heart failure has resolved and renal function is normal (as measured by creatinine clearance); the decision to continue metformin therapy in such patients should be individualized.

Iodinated contrast agents are a potential concern for furthering renal damage in patients with acute kidney injury, and in patients with severe chronic kidney disease (stage IV or stage V). Since administration of iodinated contrast media may lead to acute alteration of renal function and has been associated with lactic acidosis in patients receiving metformin, the manufacturers state that metformin-containing preparations should be discontinued before or at the time of the procedure in patients with an eGFR between 30–60 mL/minute per 1.73 m²; in patients with a history of liver disease, alcoholism, or heart failure; and in those receiving intra-arterial iodinated contrast agents. Renal function should be evaluated 48 hours after the imaging procedure and metformin therapy may be reinstituted if renal function is stable. However, the American College of Radiology states that in patients with no evidence of acute kidney injury and an eGFR of at least 30 mL/minute per 1.73 m², there is no need to discontinue metformin either prior to or following the administration of iodinated contrast media, nor is there a need to reassess the patient's renal function following the test or procedure.

Patients should be instructed to inform their clinicians that they are taking metformin or metformin-containing therapy prior to any surgical or radiological procedure since temporary discontinuation of the drug may be required. The manufacturers state that the drug should be reinitiated only when the patient's oral intake has resumed and renal function has been shown to be normal. In addition, any diabetic patient previously well controlled with metformin therapy who develops a clinical illness (especially one that is vague and poorly defined) or whose laboratory test results deviate from normal should be evaluated promptly for evidence of ketoacidosis or lactic acidosis. (See Cautions: Lactic Acidosis.) Such evaluation should include determinations of serum electrolytes and ketones, blood glucose, and if indicated, blood pH, lactate, pyruvate, and metformin concentrations. Since cardiovascular collapse (shock), heart failure, ischemic heart disease (e.g., acute myocardial infarction), peripheral vascular disease (e.g., claudication), obstructive airways disease, or other conditions that are likely to cause central hypoxemia or reduced peripheral perfusion have been associated with lactic acidosis and prerenal azotemia, metformin should be discontinued in patients developing such conditions.

Patients should be advised fully and completely about the nature of diabetes mellitus, what they must do to prevent and detect complications, and how to control their condition. Patients should be instructed about the importance of adherence to dietary instructions, of a regular exercise program, and of regular assessment of blood glucose, HbA_{1c}, renal function, and hematologic parameters.

Patients and responsible family members should be informed of the risks of hypoglycemia, symptoms and treatment of hypoglycemic reactions, and conditions that predispose to the development of such reactions, since these reactions occasionally may occur during therapy with metformin. Hypoglycemia occurs infrequently in patients receiving metformin therapy under usual conditions of use; the incidence of hypoglycemia with metformin is much lower than that in patients receiving sulfonylureas, meglitinides (e.g., repaglinide), or insulin. However, hypoglycemia may occur when the drug is used concomitantly with a sulfonylurea antidiabetic agent and/or insulin. In addition, certain other factors (e.g., deficient caloric intake, strenuous exercise not compensated by caloric supplementation, alcohol ingestion, adrenal or pituitary insufficiency) may predispose patients to the development of hypoglycemia. Debilitated, malnourished, or geriatric patients also may be particularly susceptible to hypoglycemia; this condition may be difficult to recognize in geriatric patients or in those receiving β-adrenergic blocking agents or other sympatholytic agents. (See Drug Interactions: β-Adrenergic Blocking Agents.)

To maintain control of diabetes during periods of stress (e.g., fever of any cause, trauma, infection, surgery), temporary discontinuance of metformin and administration of insulin may be required. Patients should contact a clinician promptly concerning changes in dosage requirements during periods of stress.

Since decreases in serum vitamin B_{12} concentrations have been reported in some patients receiving metformin, hematologic parameters (e.g., hemoglobin, hematocrit, erythrocyte indices) should be evaluated prior to initiation of metformin therapy and at least annually during treatment and any abnormality properly investigated. Vitamin B_{12} concentrations should be monitored every 2–3 years in patients receiving metformin therapy and any abnormalities managed. Some patients (i.e., those with an inadequate absorption or intake of vitamin B_{12} or calcium) appear to be predisposed to developing decreased vitamin B_{12} concentrations.

The potential for unplanned pregnancy should be discussed with premenopausal women since metformin-containing therapy may result in ovulation in some anovulatory women.

Metformin-containing therapy is contraindicated in patients with diabetes mellitus complicated by acute or chronic metabolic acidosis, including diabetic ketoacidosis with or without coma.

Metformin therapy is contraindicated in patients with an eGFR of less than 30 mL/minute per 1.73 m². In patients in whom development of impaired renal function is anticipated (e.g., those with blood glucose concentrations exceeding 300 mg/dL, who may develop renal dysfunction as a result of polyuria and volume depletion; geriatric patients), renal function should be monitored more frequently. In addition, drugs that may affect renal function, produce substantial hemodynamic changes, or interfere with metformin elimination (e.g., cimetidine) should be used with caution in patients receiving metformin. The National Kidney Foundation (NKF) Kidney Disease Outcomes Quality Initiative (KDOQI) recommends temporary discontinuance of potentially nephrotoxic and renally excreted drugs (e.g., angiotensin-converting enzyme [ACE] inhibitors, angiotensin II receptor antagonists, aldosterone inhibitors, direct renin inhibitors, diuretics, nonsteroidal anti-inflammatory agents [NSAIAs],

metformin, lithium, digoxin) in patients with a GFR less than 60 mL/minute per 1.73 m².

Metformin alone or in fixed combination with other drugs is contraindicated in patients with severe renal impairment (eGFR less than 30 mL/minute per 1.73 m²), which may result from conditions such as cardiovascular collapse (shock), acute myocardial infarction, or septicemia. Initiation of therapy with immediate-release metformin in fixed combination with pioglitazone is contraindicated in patients with New York Heart Association (NYHA) class III or IV heart failure. (See Heart Failure under Warnings/Precautions: Warnings, in Cautions in Pioglitazone 68:20.28.)

Metformin-containing therapy also is contraindicated in patients with known hypersensitivity to any ingredient in the respective formulations.

● *Pediatric Precautions*

Safety and efficacy of metformin immediate-release or certain extended-release tablets (e.g., Fortamet®) in pediatric patients younger than 10 or younger than 17 years of age, respectively, have not been established. Safety and efficacy of another extended-release preparation (Glumetza®) have not been established in pediatric patients younger than 18 years of age. Safety and efficacy of immediate-release metformin oral solution in children younger than 10 years of age have not been established. Data from a placebo-controlled clinical trial indicated a similar glycemic response and adverse effect profile for metformin in pediatric patients (10–16 years of age) as in adults. (See Type 2 Diabetes Mellitus: Metformin Monotherapy, in Uses.)

The safety and efficacy of metformin in fixed combination with glipizide, glyburide, pioglitazone, or sitagliptin in pediatric patients have not been established. Data from a comparative trial evaluating the safety and efficacy of metformin in fixed combination with glyburide compared with monotherapy with each agent in pediatric patients (9–16 years of age) with type 2 diabetes mellitus indicate no unexpected safety concerns with such combination therapy.

The American Diabetes Association (ADA) states that most pediatric diabetologists use oral antidiabetic agents in children with type 2 diabetes mellitus because of greater patient compliance and convenience for the patient's family and a lack of evidence demonstrating better efficacy of insulin as initial therapy for type 2 diabetes mellitus.

● *Geriatric Precautions*

Controlled clinical trials evaluating metformin hydrochloride immediate-release and extended-release tablets (Glumetza®) did not include sufficient numbers of geriatric patients to determine whether geriatric patients respond differently to metformin than younger patients, although other reported clinical experience has not identified any differences in response between geriatric and younger patients. Data from controlled clinical trials evaluating another metformin hydrochloride extended-release preparation (Fortamet®) indicate no overall differences in safety or efficacy in geriatric patients compared with younger adults. Data from controlled clinical trials with metformin in fixed combination with glyburide or glipizide have not revealed age-related differences in safety and efficacy of the combination, but greater sensitivity of geriatric patients to these fixed combinations cannot be ruled out. Since metformin is excreted principally by the kidneys and renal function declines with age, accumulation of the drug may occur in patients with renal impairment; the drug should be used with caution in geriatric patients. As geriatric patients are at risk for the development of lactic acidosis, metformin therapy should not be initiated in geriatric patients 80 years of age and older without confirmation of adequate renal function as measured by creatinine clearance. In addition, renal function should be monitored periodically and care should be taken in dosage selection for geriatric patients; such patients generally should not receive the maximum recommended dosage of metformin hydrochloride. (See Dosage: Dosage Titration in Dosage and Administration.)

● *Mutagenicity and Carcinogenicity*

No evidence of mutagenicity or chromosomal damage was observed in vivo in a micronucleus test in mice or in in vitro test systems, including microbial (Ames test) and mammalian (mouse lymphoma and human lymphocytes) assays.

No evidence of carcinogenic potential was seen in a 104-week study in male and female rats receiving metformin hydrochloride dosages up to and including 900 mg/kg daily or in a 91-week study in male and female mice receiving metformin hydrochloride at dosages up to and including 1500 mg/kg daily; these dosages are about 3 times the maximum recommended human daily dosage based on body surface area. However, an increased incidence of benign stromal uterine polyps was observed in female rats treated with 900 mg/kg of metformin hydrochloride daily.

● Pregnancy, Fertility, and Lactation

Pregnancy

Reproduction studies in rats and rabbits given metformin hydrochloride dosages of 600 mg/kg daily (about twice the maximum recommended human daily dosage based on body surface area or about 3 and 6 times the maximum recommended human daily dosage of extended-release tablets [2 g] based on body surface area comparisons with rats and rabbits, respectively) have not revealed evidence of harm (e.g., teratogenicity) to the fetus. Determination of fetal concentrations of metformin suggest that a partial placental barrier to the drug exists. Since abnormal maternal blood glucose concentrations during pregnancy may be associated with a higher incidence of congenital abnormalities, most experts recommend that insulin be used during pregnancy to maintain optimum control of blood glucose concentration.

The estimated background risk of major birth defects is 6–10% in women with pre-gestational diabetes mellitus who have an HbA_{1c} exceeding 7 and has been reported to be as high as 20–25% in women with a HbA_{1c} exceeding 10. The estimated background risk of miscarriage for the indicated population is unknown. In the US general population, the estimated background risk of major birth defects and miscarriage in clinically recognized pregnancies is 2–4% and 15–20%, respectively.

Available studies on the use of metformin in pregnant women have not reported a clear association with metformin and major birth defects, miscarriage, or adverse maternal or fetal outcomes. Limited data from uncontrolled or retrospective studies are conflicting with regard to the effects of long-term maternal therapy with metformin hydrochloride (1.5–3 g daily) on neonatal morbidity (e.g., congenital malformations) and mortality. Poorly controlled diabetes mellitus in pregnancy increases the maternal risk for diabetic ketoacidosis, pre-eclampsia, spontaneous abortions, preterm delivery, and delivery complications. Poorly controlled diabetes mellitus increases the fetal risk for major birth defects, stillbirth, and macrosomia-related morbidity. Metformin should be used during pregnancy only when clearly needed.

Lactation

Metformin is distributed into milk in lactating rats. Limited data indicate that small amounts of metformin also are distributed into breast milk in humans. In a study in 7 nursing women who received metformin hydrochloride (median dosage 1500 mg daily), the mean milk-to-plasma ratio for metformin was 0.35 and the overall average concentration in milk over the dosing interval was 0.27 mg/L. Metformin was present in low or undetectable amounts in the plasma of 4 breastfed infants, and no adverse effects were noted in 6 infants that were evaluated. In another study, mean peak and trough metformin concentrations in 4 nursing women receiving metformin hydrochloride 500 mg twice daily were 1.06 and 0.42 mcg/mL, respectively, in serum and 0.42 and 0.39 mcg/mL, respectively, in breast milk. The mean milk-to-serum ratio was 0.63 and the mean estimated infant dose as a percentage of the mother's weight-adjusted dose was 0.65%. Blood glucose concentrations obtained in 3 infants 4 hours after breastfeeding were within normal limits (47–77 mg/dL). The developmental and health benefits of breastfeeding should be considered along with mother's clinical need for the drug and potential adverse effects on the breastfed child (e.g., hypoglycemia). Breastfed infants should be monitored for signs of hypoglycemia (e.g., jitters, cyanosis, apnea, hypothermia, excessive sleepiness, poor feeding, seizures).

DRUG INTERACTIONS

● Antidiabetic Agents

Although hypoglycemia occurs infrequently in patients receiving metformin therapy alone, hypoglycemia may occur when the drug is used concomitantly with an insulin secretagogue such as a sulfonylurea antidiabetic agent (e.g., glyburide), a meglitinide (e.g., repaglinide), and/or insulin. (See Cautions: Precautions and Contraindications.)

In a single-dose study in patients with type 2 diabetes mellitus, concomitant administration of glyburide with metformin did not alter the pharmacokinetics or pharmacodynamics of metformin.

In a single-dose study, administration of metformin concomitantly with an α-glucosidase inhibitor (acarbose) resulted in an acute decrease in the bioavailability of metformin. Coadministration of guar gum (10 g) and metformin hydrochloride (1.7 g) with a standard meal in healthy individuals reduced and delayed the absorption of metformin from the GI tract.

● Diuretics

Thiazide diuretics can exacerbate diabetes mellitus, resulting in increased requirements of oral antidiabetic agents, temporary loss of diabetic control, or secondary failure to the antidiabetic agent. If control of diabetes is impaired by a thiazide diuretic, clinicians may consider substituting a less diabetogenic diuretic (e.g., potassium-sparing diuretic), reducing the dosage of or discontinuing the diuretic, or increasing the dosage of the oral antidiabetic agent.

In a single-dose study in healthy individuals, administration of furosemide concomitantly with metformin increased peak plasma and blood concentrations of metformin by approximately 22% and AUC of metformin by approximately 15%. Administration of metformin concomitantly with furosemide decreased peak plasma furosemide concentrations by approximately 31% and AUC by approximately 12%. The renal clearance of both drugs remained unchanged during such concomitant use, but the half-life of furosemide was decreased by 32%. The manufacturer states that no information is available on potential interactions between metformin and furosemide during long-term administration.

● Nifedipine

Concomitant administration of single doses of metformin and nifedipine in healthy individuals resulted in enhanced absorption of metformin, as indicated by increases of 20 and 9% in the peak plasma concentration and AUC, respectively, of metformin. Nifedipine also increased the urinary excretion of metformin; half-life and time to peak plasma concentration of metformin remained unchanged. Metformin appears to have minimal effects on the pharmacokinetics of nifedipine.

● Cationic Agents

Cimetidine may reduce the urinary excretion of metformin by competing for renal tubular organic cationic transport systems. In single- and multiple-dose studies in healthy individuals, concomitant administration of cimetidine and metformin increased the peak plasma and whole blood concentrations of metformin by approximately 60–81% and the area under the plasma or whole blood concentration-time curve (AUC) of metformin by approximately 40–50%. Metformin has negligible effects on cimetidine pharmacokinetics, possibly because cimetidine has a higher affinity for renal tubular transport sites. The manufacturer states that the possibility of other cationic drugs that undergo substantial tubular secretion (e.g., amiloride, digoxin, dolutegravir, morphine, procainamide, quinidine, quinine, ranolazine, ranitidine, triamterene, trimethoprim, vancomycin, vandetanib) decreasing the urinary excretion of metformin and increasing systemic exposure to the drug should be considered. Patients receiving metformin concomitantly with a cationic drug that is excreted by the proximal renal tubules should be monitored carefully and the need for possible dosage adjustment of either agent considered.

● β-Adrenergic Blocking Agents

In single-dose studies in healthy individuals, concomitant administration of metformin and propranolol did not alter the pharmacokinetics of either drug. However, several potential interactions between β-adrenergic blocking agents and oral antidiabetic agents (e.g., sulfonylureas, metformin) exist. β-Adrenergic blocking agents may impair glucose tolerance; increase the frequency or severity of hypoglycemia; block hypoglycemia-induced tachycardia but not hypoglycemic sweating, which may actually be increased; delay the rate of recovery of blood glucose concentration following drug-induced hypoglycemia; alter the hemodynamic response to hypoglycemia, possibly resulting in an exaggerated hypertensive response; and possibly impair peripheral circulation. Nonselective β- adrenergic blocking agents (e.g., propranolol, nadolol) without intrinsic sympathomimetic activity are more likely to affect glucose metabolism than more selective β-adrenergic blocking agents (e.g., metoprolol, atenolol) or those with intrinsic sympathomimetic activity (e.g., acebutolol, pindolol). Signs of hypoglycemia (e.g., achycardia, blood pressure changes, tremor, feelings of anxiety) mediated by catecholamines may be masked by either nonselective or selective β-adrenergic blocking agents. These drugs should be used with caution in patients with type 2 diabetes mellitus who are receiving antidiabetic agents, especially in those with labile disease or in those prone to hypoglycemia. Use of low-dose, selective $β_1$-adrenergic blockers (e.g., metoprolol) or β-adrenergic blocking agents with intrinsic sympathomimetic activity in patients receiving oral antidiabetic agents may theoretically decrease the risk of affecting glycemic control. When an oral antidiabetic agent and a β-adrenergic blocking agent are used concomitantly, the patient should be advised about and monitored closely for altered antidiabetic response.

Alcohol

Combined use of alcohol and metformin can increase the risk of hypoglycemia and lactic acidosis, since alcohol decreases lactate clearance and hepatic gluconeogenesis and may increase insulin secretion. (See Cautions: Lactic Acidosis.) Excessive alcohol intake, on an acute or chronic basis, should be avoided in patients receiving metformin therapy.

Angiotensin-Converting Enzyme Inhibitors

Angiotensin-converting enzyme (ACE) inhibitors (e.g., captopril, enalapril) may reduce fasting blood glucose concentrations in nondiabetic individuals and have been associated with unexplained hypoglycemia in patients whose diabetes had been controlled with insulin or oral antidiabetic agents, including combined therapy with glyburide and metformin. Testing in some of these patients indicated that the ACE inhibitor (e.g., captopril) apparently increased insulin sensitivity; the mechanism of this effect is not known. Other investigators have reported no alterations in glycemic control with concomitant use of an ACE inhibitor and oral antidiabetic agents or insulin in diabetic patients. The potential risk of precipitating hypoglycemia or hyperglycemia appears to be low but should be considered when therapy with an ACE inhibitor is initiated or withdrawn in diabetic patients; blood glucose concentrations should be monitored during dosage adjustments with either agent.

Clomiphene

In premenopausal patients with polycystic ovary syndrome, therapy with certain oral antidiabetic agents, including metformin, may result in the resumption of ovulation in a modest number of women. Ovulatory response is further increased in patients pretreated with metformin hydrochloride (500 mg 3 times daily for 35 days) receiving additional low-dose clomiphene (50 mg daily for 5 days); ovulation was associated with decreased insulin secretion and increased serum progesterone concentrations.

Carbonic Anhydrase Inhibitors

Topiramate and other carbonic anhydrase inhibitors (e.g., zonisamide, acetazolamide, dichlorphenamide) frequently cause a reduction in serum bicarbonate concentrations and induce non-anion gap, hyperchloremic metabolic acidosis. Concomitant use of these drugs with metformin hydrochloride tablets may increase the risk for lactic acidosis; consider more frequent monitoring in patients receiving these drugs in combination.

Drugs That May Antagonize Hypoglycemic Effects

Drugs that cause hyperglycemia and may lead to loss of glycemic control in patients with diabetes mellitus include thiazide and other diuretics, corticosteroids, phenothiazines, thyroid preparations, estrogens, oral contraceptives, phenytoin, niacin, sympathomimetics, calcium-channel blocking agents, and isoniazid. When such drugs are added to or withdrawn from therapy in patients receiving oral antidiabetic agents, patients should be observed closely for evidence of altered glycemic control.

ACUTE TOXICITY

Limited information is available on the acute toxicity of metformin. Hypoglycemia has been reported in approximately 10% of cases after acute oral ingestion of amounts exceeding 50 g of metformin hydrochloride; lactic acidosis has been reported in approximately 32% of metformin overdose cases. (See Cautions: Lactic Acidosis.) Since metformin is eliminated by dialysis (with a clearance of up to 170 mL per minute under good hemodynamic conditions), prompt hemodialysis

is recommended to correct acidosis and remove accumulated drug; such management often results in rapid reversal of symptoms and recovery.

PHARMACOLOGY

Antidiabetic Effects

Metformin hydrochloride, a biguanide antidiabetic agent, is chemically and pharmacologically unrelated to sulfonylurea antidiabetic agents. Unlike sulfonylureas, biguanides such as metformin lower blood glucose concentrations in patients with type 2 diabetes mellitus without increasing insulin secretion from pancreatic β cells; however, metformin is ineffective in the absence of some endogenous or exogenous insulin. Biguanides usually do not produce hypoglycemia in diabetic patients and do not affect normal blood glucose concentrations in nondiabetic individuals; metformin, even in excessive dosage, normally does not lower glucose concentrations below euglycemia, although hypoglycemia occasionally may occur with overdosage. (See Acute Toxicity.) Therefore, while biguanides as well as sulfonylureas historically have been referred to as oral hypoglycemic agents, biguanides such as metformin are more appropriately referred to as antihyperglycemic agents.

Type 2 diabetes mellitus is characterized by insulin resistance (impaired uptake and disposal of glucose by peripheral tissues and excessive glucose production by the liver), and abnormal insulin secretion, which may result in insulin deficiency (impaired secretion of insulin from pancreatic β cells) during the late stage of the disease. (See Uses.) Although the underlying pathophysiology of type 2 diabetes mellitus may be similar in obese and nonobese patients with the disease, severe peripheral and hepatic insulin resistance appears to predominate in obese patients, while nonobese patients tend to have milder degrees of insulin resistance but more marked insulin deficiency; however, both abnormalities eventually occur in the course of the disease. Obesity itself often is associated with insulin resistance and an elevated rate of fatty acid oxidation, which may contribute to the glucose intolerance observed in obese patients with type 2 diabetes mellitus.

Metformin lowers both basal (fasting) and postprandial glucose concentrations in patients with type 2 diabetes mellitus. Although the precise mechanism(s) by which metformin exerts its antihyperglycemic effect has not been fully established, current evidence suggests that the drug improves both peripheral and hepatic sensitivity to insulin. Improved insulin sensitivity occurs principally as a result of decreased hepatic glucose production and enhanced insulin-stimulated uptake and utilization of glucose by peripheral tissues (e.g., skeletal muscle, adipocytes); the relative contribution of these mechanisms to the antihyperglycemic effect of metformin has not been fully elucidated. Increases of 18–29% in the rate of insulin-stimulated glucose uptake (principally by skeletal muscle) have been reported in patients with type 2 diabetes mellitus with metformin hydrochloride and in normoglycemic insulin-resistant individuals in whom glucose utilization during therapy (0.5–3 g daily) generally was evaluated using a euglycemic, hyperinsulinemic clamp technique (a high-dose, continuous IV infusion of insulin administered concurrently with a glucose infusion titrated to maintain euglycemia). However, some studies in which insulin and/or glucose concentrations were not regulated during metformin therapy have reported no increases and/or even decreases in glucose uptake, possibly because of the nonphysiologic conditions inherent in the euglycemic, hyperinsulinemic clamp technique.

The apparent improvement in peripheral glucose disposal with metformin therapy has been attributed principally to improved metabolism of glucose via nonoxidative (anaerobic) pathways (e.g., glycogen formation in skeletal muscle, postprandial lactate production in splanchnic tissues, lipogenesis in adipose tissue). Studies in animals and humans indicate that metformin, unlike phenformin, enhances glucose oxidation and does not affect fasting lactate production in peripheral tissues. While increases in postprandial plasma lactate concentrations have been demonstrated in type 2 diabetic patients receiving metformin alone or in combination with a sulfonylurea (e.g., glyburide), plasma lactate concentrations generally remain within the normal range during metformin therapy. Postprandial increases in serum lactate concentration observed with metformin therapy may occur as a result of increased conversion of glucose to lactate and glycogen in the splanchnic bed by metformin. While most of the lactate from the portal circulation serves as a substrate for gluconeogenesis and is thus cleared, some may escape into the systemic circulation as increased amounts are presented to the liver after a meal. Metformin does not increase lactate production or alter lactate uptake or release from skeletal muscle; however, the drug reportedly decreases liver uptake of lactate, which may increase the risk of lactic acidosis especially in patients at risk for this condition. (See Cautions: Lactic Acidosis.)

Metformin reduces basal hepatic glucose production by decreasing gluconeogenesis and possibly glycogenolysis, thereby lowering fasting plasma glucose concentrations. Although some investigators have suggested that reduction of hepatic glucose production may be the drug's principal antihyperglycemic mechanism, this effect has not been demonstrated in all studies. In vitro studies in hepatocytes indicate that metformin, at concentrations similar to or higher than those observed with therapeutic dosages, enhances insulin-induced suppression of gluconeogenesis and decreases glucagon-stimulated gluconeogenesis. Insulin secretion usually remains unchanged during metformin therapy; fasting insulin concentrations and day-long plasma insulin response remain the same or may even decrease. The magnitude of the decrease in fasting blood glucose concentrations generally is proportional to the level of fasting baseline hyperglycemia. Metformin also may decrease plasma glucose concentrations by enhancing basal glucose disposal through insulin-independent mechanisms (e.g., a decrease in free fatty acid oxidation), but such effects appear to be modest.

Receptor binding of insulin is decreased in patients with type 2 diabetes mellitus, and some studies using radiolabeled insulin in rat and human cell cultures have demonstrated improved insulin binding with metformin. However, conflicting data also have been reported, and a direct correlation between increases in insulin binding and decreases in blood glucose concentration has not been observed. In in vitro studies in animal and human skeletal muscle cells or adipocytes, metformin has increased glucose uptake through enhancement of insulin-stimulated recruitment of specific glucose transporters (e.g., GLUT-1, GLUT-4) to the plasma membrane of insulin target cells (e.g., adipose tissue, skeletal muscle) and through increases in the activity of these glucose transporters. In in vitro studies using metformin concentrations within the therapeutic range, metformin has not consistently enhanced basal glucose uptake, which is noninsulin-mediated; however, in vitro data may not accurately reflect in vivo actions of the drug, and further study is needed to determine whether metformin acts through insulin-dependent or -independent pathways, or both, to affect basal glucose uptake.

Metformin accumulates in the walls of the intestine but does not appear to have clinically important effects on glucose absorption.

● Antilipemic Effects

Metformin has demonstrated modest favorable effects on serum lipids, which are often abnormal in patients with type 2 diabetes mellitus. In clinical studies, particularly in patients with elevated baseline serum lipid concentrations (e.g., patients with type II, type III, or type IV hyperlipoproteinemia), metformin alone or combined with a sulfonylurea antidiabetic agent lowered fasting serum triglyceride concentrations and total and LDL-cholesterol concentrations without adversely affecting other serum lipids. Modest reductions (e.g., 10–20%) in serum triglyceride concentrations noted with metformin therapy generally have been attributed to decreased hepatic synthesis of VLDL-cholesterol, particularly in patients with elevated baseline triglyceride concentrations. Characteristics of patients who are likely to exhibit a decrease in serum triglycerides with metformin therapy have not been determined, and correlation of potential antilipemic effect with the degree of glycemic control has been inconsistent. Small reductions (e.g., 5–10%) in serum total cholesterol also have been reported in some studies; these effects may be attributed to decreased LDL- or VLDL-cholesterol concentrations. Increases in HDL-cholesterol also have been reported with metformin therapy in nondiabetic patients and in those with type 2 diabetes mellitus. Consistent changes in plasma glycerol and free fatty acid concentrations have not been reported during metformin therapy in patients with type 2 diabetes mellitus or in nondiabetic individuals. A reduction in free fatty oxidation has been suggested as a possible mechanism for the decrease in plasma free fatty acids observed in some studies with metformin therapy.

● Hematologic Effects

Metformin may exert potentially beneficial effects on the fibrinolytic system by increasing the activity of tissue-type plasminogen activator (t-PA) and/or reducing concentrations of plasminogen activator inhibitor-1 (PAI-1) in nondiabetic, hypertensive patients and in patients with type 2 diabetes mellitus; serum fibrinogen concentrations do not appear to be affected by metformin therapy. Patients with type 2 diabetes mellitus, hypertension, and obesity often have hyperinsulinemia and a high incidence of vascular disease. PAI-1 concentrations, which are regulated by insulin, may be substantially increased in patients with type 2

diabetes mellitus and in obese individuals, and it has been suggested that the reduced fibrinolytic activity associated with elevated PAI-1 concentrations may be important in the pathogenesis of vascular disease in these individuals. Metformin has been shown to increase fibrinolytic activity (as measured by blood clot lysis time, euglobulin fibrinolytic activity, and by increases in t-PA activity) in patients with coronary artery disease, obese individuals, and in patients with mild hypertension; increases in fibrinolytic activity with metformin therapy generally occur in patients who have low fibrinolytic activity at baseline. Reduced platelet density, activation, and/or aggregation; decreased blood pressure; and decreased peripheral arterial resistance also have been reported in some normotensive patients with type 2 diabetes mellitus and in nondiabetic, mildly hypertensive patients receiving metformin; however, whether these effects are associated with the drug or are secondary to improvement in glycemic control or a reduction in body weight has not been determined.

● Other Effects

Therapy with metformin may be associated with weight stabilization or loss. Although the exact mechanism associated with such alterations in weight has not been established, suggested mechanisms include the absence of a hyperinsulinemic effect (which if present may increase appetite and/or lipogenesis) and decreased dietary intake associated with adverse GI effects of metformin. The antihyperglycemic effect of the drug does not appear to be related to weight loss in patients with type 2 diabetes mellitus receiving metformin, nor does weight loss appear to be dose related. Limited data from studies comparing metformin therapy with oral sulfonylurea (e.g., glyburide, chlorpropamide, tolbutamide) therapy indicate that patients with type 2 diabetes mellitus receiving oral sulfonylureas gained weight or lost less weight than patients receiving metformin.

Metformin has little or no effect on fasting plasma glucagon, somatostatin, serum growth hormone, or serum cortisol concentration in patients with normal renal function; glucagon, growth hormone, and cortisol concentrations are elevated in patients with lactic acidosis and renal failure who have been receiving metformin.

PHARMACOKINETICS

The pharmacokinetics of metformin in patients with normal renal function do not appear to be affected by sex, race, or the presence of diabetes mellitus. Following administration of a single 500-mg dose of metformin hydrochloride as immediate-release tablets with food in pediatric patients (12–16 years of age) with type 2 diabetes mellitus, mean peak plasma concentrations and area under the concentration-time curve (AUC) differed less than 5% compared with those values in healthy adults; all patients had normal renal function. In pediatric patients 11–16 years of age receiving a single dose of metformin in fixed combination with glyburide, mean dose-normalized glyburide peak plasma concentration and AUC differed less than 6% from historical values in healthy adults.

Bioequivalence has been demonstrated between the fixed combination of sitagliptin and metformin and each agent given concurrently. Bioequivalence also has been demonstrated between the fixed combination of pioglitazone and immediate-release metformin (ActoPlus Met®) and each agent (pioglitazone [Actos®] and immediate-release metformin [Glucophage®]) given concurrently. Results of a bioequivalence study indicate that the fixed-combination tablets of canagliflozin and immediate-release metformin hydrochloride are bioequivalent to the corresponding doses of canagliflozin and metformin hydrochloride given as individual tablets under fed conditions. Bioequivalence between the fixed combination of dapagliflozin and extended-release metformin hydrochloride (Xigduo® XR) and each agent (dapagliflozin and extended-release metformin hydrochloride) given concurrently as separate tablets has been demonstrated; however, the relative bioavailability of the fixed combination of dapagliflozin and extended-release metformin hydrochloride (Xigduo® XR) and concomitantly administered dapagliflozin and immediate-release metformin hydrochloride has not been established. Bioequivalence between the fixed-combination tablets of empagliflozin and immediate-release metformin hydrochloride and the corresponding doses of empagliflozin and metformin hydrochloride as individual tablets also has been established. In healthy individuals who received the extended-release metformin hydrochloride preparation (Glumetza®) in a single-dose crossover study, a 1-g tablet has been shown to be bioequivalent to two 500-mg tablets based on peak plasma concentrations and AUC.

Absorption

Metformin is slowly and incompletely absorbed from the GI tract, mainly from the small intestine; absorption is complete within 6 hours. The absolute oral bioavailability of the drug under fasting conditions is reported to be approximately 50–60% with metformin hydrochloride doses of 0.5–1.5 g; binding of the drug to the intestinal wall may explain the difference between the amount of drug absorbed (as determined by the urinary and fecal excretion of unchanged drug) and the amount bioavailable in some studies. In single-dose studies with metformin hydrochloride immediate-release tablets at doses of 0.5–1.5 g or 0.85–2.55 g, plasma metformin concentrations did not increase in proportion to increasing doses, suggesting an active saturable absorption process. Similarly, in single-dose studies with an extended-release tablet preparation (Glumetza®) at doses of 0.5–2.5 g, plasma metformin concentrations did not increase in proportion to increasing doses. At steady state after administration of a metformin hydrochloride extended-release tablet preparation, the AUC and peak plasma concentrations were not dose proportional within the range of 0.5–2 g. However, limited data from studies in animals and in human intestinal cell cultures suggest that transepithelial transfer of metformin in the intestine may occur through a passive, nonsaturable mechanism, possibly involving a paracellular route. In several studies with another metformin hydrochloride extended-release tablet preparation (Fortamet®) using doses of 1–2.5 g, metformin exposure was dose-related.

Food decreases and slightly delays the absorption of metformin immediate-release tablets; the clinical importance of these effects is unknown. (See Dosage and Administration: Administration.) Administration of metformin hydrochloride immediate-release tablets with food reportedly has decreased peak plasma concentrations of the drug by 35–40%, reduced area under the plasma concentration-time curve (AUC) by 20–25%, and delayed time to peak plasma drug concentration by 35–40 minutes compared with these parameters in fasting individuals receiving this metformin preparation. However, in one study, concomitant administration of the drug as immediate-release tablets with food had a less pronounced effect (average reduction in bioavailability of 10%) on absorption.

Following oral administration of metformin hydrochloride as an extended-release tablet preparation with food, the extent of absorption (as measured by AUC) increased by approximately 50%, but peak plasma concentrations and time to achieve peak plasma concentrations were not altered. Following administration of another metformin hydrochloride extended-release tablet formulation (Fortamet®) with food, the extent of absorption (as measured by AUC) increased by approximately 60%, peak plasma concentrations were increased by approximately 30%, and time to achieve peak plasma concentrations was prolonged (6.1 hours versus 4 hours) compared with those in the fasting state. The pharmacokinetics of a certain metformin extended-release tablet preparation were not affected by the fat content of meals. However, following administration of another metformin hydrochloride extended-release preparation (Glumetza®) with low-fat and high-fat meals, the AUCs increased by 38 and 73%, respectively, compared with those in the fasting state.

Following oral administration of metformin hydrochloride as an immediate-release oral solution with food, the extent of absorption (as measured by AUC) increased by approximately 17–21% compared with administration in the fasted state. Food delayed the time to achieve peak plasma concentrations by 1.4 hours compared with administration in the fasted state. The pharmacokinetics of immediate-release metformin oral solution were not appreciably affected by the fat content of meals.

Following oral administration of 0.5–1.5 g of metformin hydrochloride as immediate-release tablets in healthy individuals or in patients with type 2 diabetes mellitus, peak plasma drug concentrations of approximately 0.4–3 mcg/mL usually are attained within 2–4 hours. At usual clinical doses and dosing schedules of metformin hydrochloride, steady-state plasma concentrations of metformin are reached within 24 to 48 hours and are generally less than 1 mcg/mL. Following oral administration of a single dose of metformin hydrochloride as extended-release tablets, peak plasma drug concentrations usually are attained within a median of 7 hours. Following administration of a single dose (0.5–2.5 g) of another extended-release preparation (Glumetza®), peak plasma drug concentrations of 0.47–1.6 mcg/mL usually are attained within 7–8 hours. Peak plasma drug concentrations following administration of metformin extended-release tablets are approximately 20% lower than those following administration of the same dose as immediate-release tablets. The extent of absorption of metformin hydrochloride 2 g once daily as extended-release tablets is similar to that following administration of 1 g of the drug twice daily as immediate-release tablets.

Steady-state plasma concentrations with usual dosages of metformin hydrochloride as immediate-release tablets (e.g., 1.5–2.55 g daily in 1 to 3 divided doses) are attained within 24–48 hours and generally average about 1 mcg/mL or less.

A precise correlation between plasma metformin concentrations and the drug's antihyperglycemic effect has not been established. In addition, plasma metformin concentrations generally have shown no correlation with plasma lactate concentrations during metformin therapy in patients with type 2 diabetes mellitus. Although metformin-associated lactic acidosis generally has been associated with plasma metformin concentrations exceeding 5 mcg/mL (see Cautions: Lactic Acidosis), such high concentrations reportedly were not observed during controlled clinical trials with the drug, even at maximum dosage (2.5–2.55 g daily).

Satisfactory control of blood or plasma glucose concentration may occur within a few days to 1 week following initiation of metformin therapy in patients with type 2 diabetes mellitus, but the maximum antihyperglycemic effect may be delayed for up to 2 weeks. Following discontinuance of metformin therapy, blood glucose concentration increases within 2 weeks.

Distribution

Metformin is distributed rapidly in animals and humans into peripheral body tissues and fluids, particularly the GI tract; the drug also appears to distribute slowly into erythrocytes and into a deep tissue compartment (probably GI tissues). The highest tissue concentrations of metformin (at least 10 times the plasma concentration) occur in the GI tract (e.g., esophagus, stomach, duodenum, jejunum, ileum), with lower concentrations (twice the plasma concentration) occurring in kidney, liver, and salivary gland tissue. The drug distributes into salivary glands with a half-life of about 9 hours. Metformin concentrations in saliva are tenfold lower than those in plasma and may be responsible for the metallic taste reported in some patients receiving the drug. Any local effect of metformin on glucose absorption in the GI tract may be associated with the relatively high GI concentrations of the drug compared with those in other tissues. It is not known whether metformin crosses the blood-brain barrier or the placenta in humans or if the drug is distributed into human milk; however, in lactating rats, metformin is distributed into breast milk at levels comparable to those in plasma.

Following oral administration of single 850-mg doses of metformin hydrochloride as immediate-release tablets, the apparent volume of distribution has been reported to average 654 L. Volume of distribution reported after IV administration of the drug generally has been smaller (e.g., 63–276 L) than that with oral administration, perhaps because of less drug binding in the GI tract and/or different methods of determining volume of distribution in various studies. Unlike oral sulfonylurea antidiabetic agents, which are more than 90% bound to plasma proteins, metformin is negligibly bound to plasma proteins. Metformin equilibrates freely between erythrocytes and plasma, most likely as a function of time; drug bound to erythrocytes is approximately 5% of total blood concentration.

Elimination

Following oral administration of metformin hydrochloride (0.5–1.5 g) as immediate-release tablets in healthy individuals or in patients with type 2 diabetes mellitus, plasma concentrations decline in a triphasic manner. Following multiple-dose administration of metformin hydrochloride (500 mg twice daily for 7–14 days) as immediate-release tablets in a limited number of patients with type 2 diabetes mellitus, peak plasma concentrations remained unchanged, but trough drug concentrations were higher than with single-dose administration, suggesting some drug accumulation in a peripheral tissue compartment. (See Pharmacokinetics: Distribution.) No accumulation of metformin appears to occur following repeated oral doses of the drug as extended-release tablets. The principal plasma elimination half-life of metformin averages approximately 6.2 hours; 90% of the drug is cleared within 24 hours in patients with normal renal function. The decline in plasma metformin concentrations is slower after oral than after IV administration of the drug, indicating that elimination is absorption rate-limited. Urinary excretion data and data from whole blood indicate a slower terminal-elimination phase half-life of 8–20 hours (e.g., 17.6 hours) suggesting that the erythrocyte mass may be a compartment of distribution.

Metformin is not metabolized in the liver or GI tract and is not excreted in bile; no metabolites of the drug have been identified in humans. Renal elimination of metformin involves glomerular filtration and secretion by the proximal convoluted tubules as unchanged drug. Following single-dose oral administration of metformin hydrochloride (0.5–1.5 g) as immediate-release tablets, urinary recovery ranges from 35–52% of the total dose. Following administration of a single dose of metformin hydrochloride as an extended-release tablet (Fortamet®) in healthy individuals, urinary recovery was 40.9% over 24 hours. Approximately 20–33% of the total oral dose as immediate-release tablets is excreted in feces within 4–7 days. Total plasma clearance of metformin hydrochloride following single-dose oral administration (0.5–1.5 g) has ranged from 718–1552 mL/minute. Metformin is removed by hemodialysis with a clearance of up to 170 mL/minute under good hemodynamic conditions.

Renal clearance is approximately 3.5 times greater than creatinine clearance, indicating that tubular secretion is the principal route of metformin elimination. Following a single 850-mg oral dose of metformin hydrochloride, renal clearance averaged 552, 491, or 412 mL/minute in nondiabetic adults, diabetic adults, or healthy geriatric individuals, respectively. Renal impairment results in increased peak plasma concentrations of metformin, a prolonged time to peak plasma concentration, and a decreased volume of distribution. Renal clearance is decreased in patients with renal impairment (as measured by decreases in creatinine clearance) and, apparently because of reduced renal function with age, in geriatric individuals. In geriatric individuals, decreased renal and plasma clearance of metformin also results in increased plasma concentrations of the drug; volume of distribution remains unaffected. (See Cautions: Precautions and Contraindications.)

CHEMISTRY AND STABILITY

● Chemistry

Metformin hydrochloride, a dimethylbiguanide, is an orally active antidiabetic agent derived from guanidine. Guanidine occurs naturally in *Galega officinalis*, a medieval European remedy for diabetes mellitus.

Metformin is structurally and pharmacologically related to phenformin, a phenethylbiguanide (no longer commercially available in the US). However, the guanidinium group of metformin has 2 methyl substituents rather than a single hydrophobic phenethyl substituent as in phenformin, giving metformin improved water solubility and decreased binding affinity for biologic membranes (e.g., mitochondrial, plasma membranes) compared with phenformin. Consequently, metformin causes less disturbance to mitochondrial-mediated glucose oxidative pathways, resulting in a decrease in the formation of lactate from glucose via anaerobic metabolism and a reduced potential for the development of lactic acidosis compared with phenformin.

Metformin hydrochloride is commercially available as immediate- or extended-release tablets alone or in fixed combination with dipeptidyl peptidase-4 [DPP-4] inhibitors, sodium-glucose cotransporter 2 [SGLT2] inhibitors, sulfonylureas, or thiazolidinediones.

Certain extended-release tablet formulations (e.g., Glumetza®) contain hydrophilic polymer(s) that form a swellable gel matrix when in contact with gastric or intestinal fluids and release the drug by diffusion slowly over time. Another commercially available metformin hydrochloride extended-release tablet formulation (Fortamet®) contains the drug in an oral osmotic delivery system. This delivery system consists of an osmotically active core (comprised of a layer containing the drug and a coating that delays release of the drug from the core) surrounded by a semipermeable membrane with laser-drilled delivery orifices; the semipermeable membrane allows the passage of water but not higher molecular weight components of biological fluids. When exposed to water in the GI tract, the drug dissolves and is pushed out of the delivery orifices of the membrane into the GI tract at a constant rate. The rate of metformin hydrochloride delivery in the GI tract depends on the maintenance of a constant osmotic gradient across the membrane. The inert components of the drug delivery system (membrane coating) remain intact and are eliminated in feces.

Metformin is a weak base; the pH of a 1% aqueous solution of metformin hydrochloride is 6.68. The pK_a of metformin base is 12.4. Metformin hydrochloride is freely soluble in water and practically insoluble in acetone, ether, and chloroform.

● Stability

Commercially available metformin hydrochloride immediate-release (including fixed-combination preparations with glipizide) and extended-release tablets should be stored at a controlled room temperature of 20–25°C and protected from light but may be exposed to temperatures ranging from 15–30°C. Metformin hydrochloride immediate-release oral solution should be stored at

15–30°C. Fixed-combination preparations containing metformin hydrochloride and glyburide should be stored at a controlled room temperature up to 25°C and be protected from light. Immediate-release metformin hydrochloride in fixed combination with pioglitazone should be stored at 20–25°C and protected from moisture and humidity. Preparations containing metformin hydrochloride and canagliflozin, dapagliflozin, ertugliflozin, saxagliptin, or sitagliptin in fixed combination should be stored at 20–25°C but may be exposed to temperatures ranging from 15–30°C. The fixed combination of metformin hydrochloride and ertugliflozin should be protected from moisture and stored in a dry place. Preparations containing metformin hydrochloride and empagliflozin, alogliptin, or linagliptin in fixed combination should be stored at 25°C but may be exposed to temperatures ranging from 15–30°C. The fixed combination of metformin hydrochloride and linagliptin should be protected from exposure to high humidity.

PREPARATIONS

Excipients in commercially available drug preparations may have clinically important effects in some individuals; consult specific product labeling for details.

metFORMIN Hydrochloride

Oral

Solution	500 mg/5 mL*	metFORMIN Hydrochloride Solution
		Riomet®, Ranbaxy
Tablets, extended-release	500 mg*	Fortamet®, Shionogi Pharma
		Glumetza®, Depomed
		metFORMIN Hydrochloride Extended-Release Tablets
	750 mg*	metFORMIN Hydrochloride Extended-Release Tablets
	1 g*	Fortamet®, Shionogi Pharma
		Glumetza®, Depomed
		metFORMIN Hydrochloride Extended-Release Tablets
Tablets, film-coated	500 mg*	metFORMIN Hydrochloride Tablets
	625 mg*	metFORMIN Hydrochloride Tablets
	750 mg*	metFORMIN Hydrochloride Tablets
	850 mg*	metFORMIN Hydrochloride Tablets
	1 g*	metFORMIN Hydrochloride Tablets

* available from one or more manufacturer, distributor, and/or repackager by generic (nonproprietary) name

metFORMIN Hydrochloride Combinations

Oral

Tablets, extended-release	500 mg with Immediate-release Canagliflozin (anhydrous) 50 mg	Invokamet® XR, Janssen
	500 mg with Immediate-release Canagliflozin (anhydrous) 150 mg	Invokamet® XR, Janssen
	500 mg with Immediate-release Dapagliflozin Propanediol 5 mg (of dapagliflozin)	Xigduo® XR, AstraZeneca
	500 mg with Immediate-release Dapagliflozin Propanediol 10 mg (of dapagliflozin)	Xigduo® XR, AstraZeneca
	500 mg with Immediate-release Saxagliptin 5 mg	Kombiglyze® XR, AstraZeneca
	500 mg with Immediate-release Sitagliptin 50 mg	Janumet® XR, Merck

	1 g with Immediate-release Canagliflozin (anhydrous) 50 mg	**Invokamet® XR**, Janssen
	1 g with Immediate-release Canagliflozin (anhydrous) 150 mg	**Invokamet® XR**, Janssen
	1 g with Immediate-release Dapagliflozin Propanediol 2.5 mg (of dapagliflozin)	**Xigduo® XR**, AstraZeneca
	1 g with Immediate-release Dapagliflozin Propanediol 5 mg (of dapagliflozin)	**Xigduo® XR**, AstraZeneca
	1 g with Immediate-release Dapagliflozin Propanediol 10 mg (of dapagliflozin)	**Xigduo® XR**, AstraZeneca
	1 g with Immediate-release Empagliflozin 5 mg	**Synjardy® XR**, Boehringer Ingelheim
	1 g with Immediate-release Empagliflozin 10 mg	**Synjardy® XR**, Boehringer Ingelheim
	1 g with Immediate-release Empagliflozin 12.5 mg	**Synjardy® XR**, Boehringer Ingelheim
	1 g with Immediate-release Empagliflozin 25 mg	**Synjardy® XR**, Boehringer Ingelheim
	1 g with Immediate-release Linagliptin 2.5 mg	**Jentadueto® XR**, Boehringer Ingelheim
	1 g with Immediate-release Linagliptin 5 mg	**Jentadueto® XR**, Boehringer Ingelheim
	1 g with Immediate-release Saxagliptin 2.5 mg	**Kombiglyze® XR**, AstraZeneca
	1 g with Immediate-release Saxagliptin 5 mg	**Kombiglyze® XR**, AstraZeneca
	1 g with Immediate-release Sitagliptin 50 mg	**Janumet® XR**, Merck
	1 g with Immediate-release Sitagliptin 100 mg	**Janumet® XR**, Merck
Tablets, film-coated	250 mg with Glipizide 2.5 mg*	**metFORMIN Hydrochloride and Glipizide Tablets**
	250 mg with Glyburide 1.25 mg*	**metFORMIN Hydrochloride and Glyburide Tablets**
	500 mg with Alogliptin Benzoate 12.5 mg (of alogliptin)	**Kazano®**, Takeda
	500 mg with Canagliflozin (anhydrous) 50 mg	**Invokamet®**, Janssen
	500 mg with Canagliflozin (anhydrous) 150 mg	**Invokamet®**, Janssen
	500 mg with Empagliflozin 5 mg	**Synjardy®**, Boehringer Ingelheim
	500 mg with Empagliflozin 12.5 mg	**Synjardy®**, Boehringer Ingelheim
	500 mg with Ertugliflozin L-pyroglutamic Acid 2.5 mg (of ertugliflozin)	**Segluromet®**, Merck

	500 mg with Ertugliflozin L-pyroglutamic Acid 7.5 mg (of ertugliflozin)	**Segluromet®**, Merck
	500 mg with Glipizide 2.5 mg*	**metFORMIN Hydrochloride and Glipizide Tablets**
	500 mg with Glipizide 5 mg*	**metFORMIN Hydrochloride and Glipizide Tablets**
	500 mg with Glyburide 2.5 mg*	**metFORMIN Hydrochloride and Glyburide Tablets**
	500 mg with Glyburide 5 mg*	**MetFORMIN Hydrochloride and Glyburide Tablets**
	500 mg with Linagliptin 2.5 mg	**Jentadueto®**, Boehringer Ingelheim
	500 mg with Pioglitazone Hydrochloride 15 mg (of pioglitazone)	**Actoplus Met®**, Takeda
	500 mg with Sitagliptin Phosphate 50 mg (of sitagliptin)	**Janumet®**, Merck
	850 mg with Linagliptin 2.5 mg	**Jentadueto®**, Boehringer Ingelheim
	850 mg with Pioglitazone Hydrochloride 15 mg (of pioglitazone)	**Actoplus Met®**, Takeda
	1 g with Alogliptin Benzoate 12.5 mg (of alogliptin)	**Kazano®**, Takeda
	1 g with Canagliflozin (anhydrous) 50 mg	**Invokamet®**, Janssen
	1 g with Canagliflozin (anhydrous) 150 mg	**Invokamet®**, Janssen
	1 g with Empagliflozin 5 mg	**Synjardy®**, Boehringer Ingelheim
	1 g with Empagliflozin 12.5 mg	**Synjardy®**, Boehringer Ingelheim
	1 g with Ertugliflozin L-pyroglutamic Acid 2.5 mg (of ertugliflozin)	**Segluromet®**, Merck
	1 g with Ertugliflozin L-pyroglutamic Acid 7.5 mg (of ertugliflozin)	**Segluromet®**, Merck
	1 g with Linagliptin 2.5 mg	**Jentadueto®**, Boehringer Ingelheim
	1 g with Sitagliptin Phosphate 50 mg (of sitagliptin)	**Janumet®**, Merck

* available from one or more manufacturer, distributor, and/or repackager by generic (nonproprietary) name

† Use is not currently included in the labeling approved by the US Food and Drug Administration.

Selected Revisions June 21, 2021, © Copyright, June 1, 1996, American Society of Health-System Pharmacists, Inc.

Alogliptin Benzoate

68:20.05 · DIPEPTIDYL PEPTIDASE IV (DPP-4) INHIBITORS

■ Alogliptin benzoate, a dipeptidyl peptidase-4 (DPP-4) inhibitor, is an antidiabetic agent.

USES

● Type 2 Diabetes Mellitus

Alogliptin benzoate is used as monotherapy as an adjunct to diet and exercise to improve glycemic control in patients with type 2 diabetes mellitus. Alogliptin is used as initial therapy in combination with metformin hydrochloride or pioglitazone as an adjunct to diet and exercise to improve glycemic control in patients with type 2 diabetes mellitus when treatment with both alogliptin and metformin or pioglitazone is appropriate. Alogliptin also is used in combination with other oral antidiabetic agents (e.g., metformin, a sulfonylurea, a peroxisome proliferator-activated receptor$_\gamma$ [PPAR$_\gamma$] agonist [thiazolidinedione]) or insulin as an adjunct to diet and exercise in patients with type 2 diabetes mellitus who have not achieved adequate glycemic control.

Current guidelines for the treatment of type 2 diabetes mellitus generally recommend metformin as first-line therapy in addition to lifestyle modifications in patients with recent-onset type 2 diabetes mellitus or mild hyperglycemia because of its well-established safety and efficacy (i.e., beneficial effects on glycosylated hemoglobin [hemoglobin A$_{1c}$; HbA$_{1c}$], weight, and cardiovascular mortality). (See Uses: Type 2 Diabetes Mellitus, in Metformin 68:20.04.) In patients with contraindications or intolerance to metformin (e.g., risk of lactic acidosis, GI intolerance) or in selected other patients, some experts suggest that initial therapy with a drug from another class of antidiabetic agents (e.g., a glucagon-like peptide-1 [GLP-1] receptor agonist, sodium-glucose cotransporter 2 [SGLT2] inhibitor, DPP-4 inhibitor, sulfonylurea, thiazolidinedione, basal insulin) may be acceptable based on patient factors. Initiating antidiabetic therapy with 2 agents (e.g., metformin plus another agent) may be appropriate in patients with an initial HbA$_{1c}$ exceeding 7.5% or at least 1.5% above the target level. In metformin-intolerant patients with high initial HbA$_{1c}$ levels, some experts suggest initiation of therapy with 2 agents from other antidiabetic drug classes with complementary mechanisms of action.

Because of the progressive nature of type 2 diabetes mellitus, patients initially receiving an oral antidiabetic agent will eventually require multiple oral and/or injectable noninsulin antidiabetic agents of different therapeutic classes and/or insulin for adequate glycemic control. Patients who have inadequate glycemic control with initial (e.g., metformin) monotherapy should receive treatment with additional antidiabetic agents; data suggest that the addition of each noninsulin agent to initial therapy lowers HbA$_{1c}$ by approximately 0.7–1%. In addition, early initiation of combination therapy may help more rapidly attain glycemic goals and extend the time to treatment failure.

Factors to consider when selecting additional antidiabetic agents for combination therapy in patients with inadequate glycemic control on metformin monotherapy include patient comorbidities (e.g., atherosclerotic cardiovascular disease [ASCVD], established kidney disease, heart failure), hypoglycemia risk, impact on weight, cost, risk of adverse effects, and patient preference. Some experts recommend DPP-4 inhibitors as one of several classes of drugs for use in combination therapy, particularly in patients with both postprandial and fasting plasma glucose elevations. When the greater glucose-lowering effect of an injectable drug is needed in patients with type 2 diabetes mellitus, some experts currently state that an injectable GLP-1 receptor agonist is preferred over insulin in most patients because of beneficial effects on body weight and a lower risk of hypoglycemia, although adverse GI effects may diminish tolerability. While addition of a GLP-1 receptor agonist may successfully control hyperglycemia, many patients will eventually require insulin therapy. Early introduction of insulin therapy should be considered when hyperglycemia is severe (e.g., blood glucose of at least 300 mg/dL or HbA$_{1c}$ exceeding 9–10%), especially in the presence of catabolic manifestations (e.g., weight loss, hypertriglyceridemia, ketosis) or symptoms of hyperglycemia. For additional information regarding the initiation of insulin therapy in patients with diabetes mellitus, see Uses: Diabetes Mellitus, in the Insulins General Statement 68:20.08.

The manufacturer states that alogliptin is *not* indicated for the treatment of type 1 diabetes mellitus or diabetic ketoacidosis, as it would not be effective in these settings.

Alogliptin Monotherapy

Efficacy of alogliptin as monotherapy for the management of type 2 diabetes mellitus has been established in a double-blind, placebo-controlled study of 26 weeks' duration in a total of 329 patients. Alogliptin (12.5 or 25 mg once daily) improved glycemic control as evidenced by a reduction in glycosylated hemoglobin (HbA$_{1c}$) as well as in fasting plasma glucose concentrations compared with placebo. HbA$_{1c}$ was reduced by approximately 0.6% (from a mean baseline HbA$_{1c}$ concentration of about 8%) in patients receiving alogliptin 25 mg, compared with no change in HbA$_{1c}$ in those receiving placebo.

In a double-blind, active-controlled study of 52 weeks' duration in 441 patients 65–87 years of age, alogliptin (25 mg once daily) was noninferior to glipizide (5–10 mg daily) in reducing HbA$_{1c}$. Mean reductions in HbA$_{1c}$ from baseline (mean HbA$_{1c}$ of 7.5%) were 0.14% with alogliptin and 0.09% with glipizide. Patients receiving alogliptin also experienced lower risk of hypoglycemia and lost weight (loss of 0.62 kg) compared with patients receiving glipizide, who experienced weight gain (0.6 kg).

Combination Therapy

Efficacy of the combination of alogliptin and pioglitazone as *initial* therapy in patients with type 2 diabetes mellitus inadequately controlled with diet and exercise is supported by results of a 26-week randomized, active-controlled study. Patients receiving initial therapy with alogliptin (25 mg daily) in combination with pioglitazone (30 mg daily) had greater improvements in HbA$_{1c}$ and fasting plasma glucose than those receiving alogliptin monotherapy or pioglitazone monotherapy. Mean reductions in HbA$_{1c}$ from baseline (mean HbA$_{1c}$ of 8.8%) were 1% with alogliptin 25 mg once daily, 1.2% with pioglitazone 30 mg once daily, and 1.7% with alogliptin 25 mg once daily in combination with pioglitazone 30 mg once daily. The proportion of patients who achieved an HbA$_{1c}$ of 7% or less was greater with alogliptin and pioglitazone combination therapy (63%) than with alogliptin (24%) or pioglitazone (34%) monotherapy.

In another 26-week, randomized trial in patients who had inadequate glycemic control with diet and exercise, patients receiving *initial* therapy with the combination of alogliptin (12.5 mg twice daily) and metformin hydrochloride (500 mg or 1 g twice daily) had greater improvements in HbA$_{1c}$ and fasting plasma glucose than those receiving placebo, metformin monotherapy, or alogliptin monotherapy. Mean reductions in HbA$_{1c}$ from baseline (mean HbA$_{1c}$ of 8.4%) were 0.6% with alogliptin 12.5 mg twice daily, 0.7% with metformin hydrochloride 500 mg twice daily, 1.1% with metformin hydrochloride 1 g twice daily, 1.2% with alogliptin 12.5 mg and metformin hydrochloride 500 mg twice daily, and 1.6% with alogliptin 12.5 mg and metformin hydrochloride 1 g twice daily, while HbA$_{1c}$ increased by 0.1% with placebo. In this trial, 47% of patients receiving alogliptin 12.5 mg and metformin hydrochloride 500 mg twice daily and 59% of those receiving alogliptin 12.5 mg and metformin hydrochloride 1 g twice daily achieved a mean HbA$_{1c}$ of less than 7%, compared with 20% of those receiving alogliptin 12.5 mg twice daily as monotherapy and 27 or 34% of those receiving metformin hydrochloride 500 mg or 1 g twice daily as monotherapy.

Efficacy of alogliptin in combination with metformin, a sulfonylurea, or a thiazolidinedione in the management of type 2 diabetes mellitus (inadequately controlled with metformin monotherapy, metformin and a thiazolidinedione, or a sulfonylurea) has been established in several randomized, placebo- or active-controlled, double-blind studies. In these studies, addition of alogliptin (25 mg daily) to existing therapy improved glycemic control as evidenced by reductions in HbA$_{1c}$ as well as in fasting plasma glucose concentrations, compared with placebo or existing therapy. In a 26-week study in patients receiving metformin hydrochloride (dosage of at least 1.5 g daily or maximum tolerated dosage), the addition of alogliptin resulted in a reduction of 0.6% in HbA$_{1c}$ compared with a reduction of 0.1% in HbA$_{1c}$ with placebo. In a 26-week study in patients receiving metformin hydrochloride (at least 1.5 g daily), the addition of alogliptin and pioglitazone (15, 30, or 45 mg daily) resulted in reductions of 1.3–1.6% in HbA$_{1c}$; addition of pioglitazone alone, alogliptin alone, or placebo resulted in HbA$_{1c}$ reductions of 0.8–1, 0.9, or 0.1%, respectively.

In a 26-week study in patients receiving a thiazolidinedione alone or in combination with metformin or a sulfonylurea, addition of alogliptin (25 mg once daily) or placebo resulted in reductions of 0.8 or 0.2%, respectively, in HbA_{1c}. Patients receiving metformin or a sulfonylurea at baseline continued these agents at the same dosage throughout the study.

In a 52-week study in patients receiving metformin hydrochloride (at least 1.5 g daily or maximum tolerated dosage) and pioglitazone (30 mg daily), add-on therapy with alogliptin (25 mg daily) or increased dosage of pioglitazone (45 mg daily) resulted in a reduction of 0.7 or 0.3%, respectively, from a baseline HbA_{1c} of approximately 8.2%.

In a 26-week study in patients receiving glyburide, addition of alogliptin (25 mg daily) resulted in a reduction of 0.5% in HbA_{1c} compared with addition of placebo.

Efficacy of alogliptin in combination with insulin (with or without metformin) in the management of type 2 diabetes mellitus in patients who have inadequate glycemic control with insulin is supported by results of a 26-week, randomized, double-blind, placebo-controlled study. In this study, addition of alogliptin (25 mg once daily) to existing stable insulin (premixed insulin, or short-, intermediate- or long-acting [basal] insulin) therapy with or without metformin hydrochloride resulted in improvements in HbA_{1c} and fasting plasma glucose concentrations compared with the addition of placebo. Among patients also receiving metformin, addition of alogliptin reduced HbA_{1c} by 0.8% compared with 0.2% in those receiving add-on placebo; among patients receiving insulin monotherapy, addition of alogliptin reduced HbA_{1c} by 0.7% compared with 0.1% in those receiving add-on placebo.

DOSAGE AND ADMINISTRATION

● Administration

When administered as monotherapy, alogliptin may be administered orally once daily without regard to meals.

When alogliptin is administered in fixed combination with metformin hydrochloride, the combination should be administered twice daily with food; dosage should be titrated gradually to minimize adverse GI effects of the metformin component. Fixed-combination tablets should be swallowed whole and should not be split before swallowing.

When alogliptin is administered in fixed combination with pioglitazone, the combination should be administered once daily without regard to meals. Fixed-combination tablets should be swallowed whole and should not be split before swallowing.

If a dose of alogliptin alone or in combination with metformin or pioglitazone is missed, the missed dose should be taken as soon as it is remembered followed by resumption of the regular schedule. If the missed dose is not remembered until the time of the next dose, the missed dose should be skipped and the regular schedule resumed; the dose should not be doubled to replace a missed dose.

● Dosage

Type 2 Diabetes Mellitus

Dosage of alogliptin benzoate is expressed in terms of alogliptin.

Alogliptin Monotherapy

The recommended dosage of alogliptin for the management of type 2 diabetes mellitus is 25 mg once daily.

Combination Therapy with Metformin Hydrochloride

Dosage of alogliptin in fixed combination with metformin hydrochloride should be individualized based on the patient's current antidiabetic regimen, effectiveness, and tolerability. Dosage should be increased gradually to reduce adverse GI effects of metformin.

The maximum recommended dosage of alogliptin in fixed combination with metformin hydrochloride is 25 mg of alogliptin and 2 g of metformin hydrochloride daily.

Combination Therapy with Pioglitazone

When the fixed-combination preparation containing alogliptin and pioglitazone is used in patients who have inadequate glycemic control with diet and exercise,

the recommended initial dosage is 25 mg of alogliptin and 15 mg of pioglitazone once daily or 25 mg of alogliptin and 30 mg of pioglitazone once daily.

When the fixed-combination preparation containing alogliptin and pioglitazone is used in patients who have inadequate glycemic control on alogliptin monotherapy, the recommended initial dosage is 25 mg of alogliptin and 15 mg of pioglitazone once daily or 25 mg of alogliptin and 30 mg of pioglitazone once daily.

When the fixed-combination preparation containing alogliptin and pioglitazone is used in patients who have inadequate glycemic control on pioglitazone monotherapy, the recommended initial dosage is 25 mg of alogliptin and 15 mg of pioglitazone once daily, 25 mg of alogliptin and 30 mg of pioglitazone once daily, or 25 mg of alogliptin and 45 mg of pioglitazone once daily based on the patient's current antidiabetic therapy.

When the fixed-combination preparation containing alogliptin and pioglitazone is used in patients who have inadequate glycemic control on metformin monotherapy, the recommended initial dosage is 25 mg of alogliptin and 15 mg of pioglitazone once daily or 25 mg of alogliptin and 30 mg of pioglitazone once daily.

The maximum recommended daily dosage of alogliptin in fixed combination with pioglitazone is 25 mg of alogliptin and 45 mg of pioglitazone.

● Special Populations

No adjustment of alogliptin dosage is necessary in patients with mild renal impairment (creatinine clearance of 60 mL/minute or greater). In patients with moderate renal impairment (creatinine clearance of 30 to less than 60 mL/minute), the recommended dosage of alogliptin is 12.5 mg once daily. In patients with severe renal impairment (creatinine clearance of 15 to less than 30 mL/minute) or end-stage renal disease (creatinine clearance of 15 mL/minute or less or requiring hemodialysis), the recommended daily dosage is 6.25 mg once daily. Alogliptin may be administered without regard to the timing of hemodialysis.

The fixed combination of alogliptin and metformin hydrochloride is contraindicated in patients with renal impairment. Assessment of renal function is recommended prior to initiation of alogliptin therapy and periodically thereafter.

The fixed combination of alogliptin and pioglitazone is not recommended in patients with severe renal impairment or end-stage renal disease.

No adjustment of alogliptin dosage is recommended in patients with mild to moderate hepatic impairment; data are lacking in patients with severe hepatic impairment.

The fixed combination of alogliptin and metformin is not recommended in patients with hepatic impairment.

No dosage adjustment is necessary based on age, gender, or race.

The recommended initial dosage of the fixed combination of alogliptin and pioglitazone in patients with congestive heart failure (CHF) (New York Heart Association [NYHA] class I or II) is 25 mg of alogliptin and 15 mg of pioglitazone once daily.

CAUTIONS

● Contraindications

Known serious hypersensitivity (e.g., anaphylaxis, angioedema, severe adverse cutaneous reactions) to alogliptin.

● Warnings/Precautions

Pancreatitis and Pancreatic Precancerous Changes

Acute pancreatitis has been reported during postmarketing experience in patients receiving alogliptin. In clinical studies in patients with type 2 diabetes mellitus, acute pancreatitis was reported in 0.2% of patients receiving alogliptin 25 mg compared with less than 0.1% of patients receiving active comparators or placebo. In a randomized, double-blind study (EXAMINE) in 5380 patients with type 2 diabetes mellitus and recent acute coronary syndrome, acute pancreatitis was reported in 0.4 or 0.3% of patients receiving alogliptin or placebo, respectively. FDA has been evaluating unpublished findings suggesting an increased risk of pancreatitis and precancerous pancreatic cell changes (pancreatic duct metaplasia) in patients with type 2 diabetes mellitus receiving incretin mimetics (e.g., exenatide, liraglutide, sitagliptin, saxagliptin, alogliptin, linagliptin). These findings are based on examination of a small number of pancreatic tissue specimens taken from patients who died from unspecified causes while receiving an incretin mimetic. FDA will notify healthcare professionals of its conclusions and recommendations when the review is complete, or when the agency has additional information to report.

FDA has recommended that clinicians continue to follow the recommendations in the prescribing information for incretin mimetics. The manufacturer states that patients receiving alogliptin should be observed carefully for signs and symptoms of pancreatitis. If pancreatitis is suspected, alogliptin should be promptly discontinued and appropriate management instituted. It is not known whether patients with a history of pancreatitis are at increased risk for pancreatitis with alogliptin therapy.

Severe Arthralgia

Severe, disabling joint pain has been reported during postmarketing experience in patients receiving DPP-4 inhibitors (e.g., alogliptin, linagliptin, saxagliptin, sitagliptin). Onset of such symptoms has ranged from 1 day to years following initiation of therapy. Fever, chills, rash, and swelling accompanied joint pain in some patients, suggesting an immunologic reaction; some patients have required hospitalization. Symptoms resolved upon discontinuance of the DPP-4 inhibitor, usually in less than a month. In some patients, symptoms recurred when the same or another DPP-4 inhibitor was restarted. DPP-4 inhibitors should be considered as a possible cause of severe joint pain and should be discontinued if appropriate. (See Advice to Patients.)

Sensitivity Reactions

Hypersensitivity reactions (e.g., anaphylaxis, angioedema, severe adverse cutaneous reactions including Stevens-Johnson syndrome) have been reported in patients receiving alogliptin.

If a serious hypersensitivity reaction is suspected, alogliptin should be promptly discontinued, other potential causes of the event should be investigated, and alternative antidiabetic therapy should be instituted. (See Advice to Patients.) Alogliptin should be used with caution in patients with a history of angioedema to other dipeptidyl peptidase-4 inhibitors because it is unknown whether such patients will be predisposed to angioedema with alogliptin.

Hepatic Effects

Fatal and nonfatal hepatic failure have been reported during postmarketing experience in patients receiving alogliptin. In randomized controlled trials, serum alanine aminotransferase (ALT) elevations exceeding 3 times the upper limit of normal were observed in 1.3% of patients receiving alogliptin and 1.5% of all comparator-treated patients.

Patients with type 2 diabetes mellitus may have fatty liver disease, which may cause liver function test abnormalities; such patients may also have other forms of liver function disease, many of which can be treated or managed. Therefore, hepatic function should be assessed prior to initiation of alogliptin, and the drug should be initiated with caution in patients with abnormal liver function test results.

Liver function should be assessed promptly in patients who report signs or symptoms that may indicate liver injury (e.g., fatigue, anorexia, right upper abdominal discomfort, dark urine, jaundice). If the patient has clinically important liver enzyme elevations and if liver function test abnormalities persist or worsen, alogliptin therapy should be interrupted. Alogliptin should not be restarted in these patients without another explanation for the liver function test abnormalities.

Concomitant Therapy with Hypoglycemic Agents

When alogliptin is used in combination with an insulin secretagogue (e.g., a sulfonylurea) or insulin, the incidence of hypoglycemia is increased compared with sulfonylurea or insulin monotherapy. Therefore, patients receiving alogliptin may require a reduced dosage of the concomitant insulin secretagogue or insulin to reduce the risk of hypoglycemia.

Heart Failure Risk

Alogliptin may increase the risk of heart failure, particularly in patients who have a history of heart failure or renal impairment. In a randomized, double-blind study (EXAMINE) in which alogliptin or placebo was added to standard care in 5380 patients with type 2 diabetes mellitus and recent acute coronary syndrome,

3.9% of patients receiving alogliptin experienced at least one hospitalization for heart failure compared with 3.3% of patients receiving placebo. The average duration of follow-up in this study was 1.5 years.

The potential risks and benefits of alogliptin therapy should be considered prior to use in patients at higher risk for heart failure (e.g., history of heart failure or renal impairment). Patients receiving alogliptin-containing therapy should be monitored for manifestations of heart failure. (See Advice to Patients.) If heart failure develops, appropriate evaluation and management should be instituted according to current standards of care and consideration given to discontinuing alogliptin.

Macrovascular Outcomes

The manufacturer states that evidence of macrovascular risk reduction with alogliptin or any other antidiabetic agent has not been conclusively demonstrated in clinical trials.

Use of Fixed Combinations

When alogliptin is used in fixed combination with metformin hydrochloride or pioglitazone, the cautions, precautions, and contraindications associated with metformin hydrochloride or pioglitazone should be considered in addition to those associated with alogliptin.

Specific Populations

Pregnancy

Category B. (See Users Guide.)

Lactation

Alogliptin is distributed into milk in lactating rats at a milk-to-plasma ratio of 2:1; it is not known whether the drug is distributed into human milk. Caution is advised if alogliptin is administered in nursing women.

Pediatric Use

Safety and efficacy of alogliptin alone, in fixed combination with metformin, or in fixed combination with pioglitazone have not been established in pediatric patients younger than 18 years of age.

Geriatric Use

Of 8507 patients in clinical trials of alogliptin, 24.3% were 65 years of age and older; 4% were 75 years of age and older. No substantial differences in safety and efficacy relative to younger adults were observed, but increased sensitivity cannot be ruled out.

Hepatic Impairment

In patients with moderate hepatic impairment (Child-Pugh class B), alogliptin total exposure was approximately 10% lower than values in healthy individuals. Alogliptin has not been studied in patients with severe hepatic impairment (Child-Pugh class C). Caution should be exercised in patients with liver disease.

Renal Impairment

In patients with mild renal impairment (creatinine clearance of 60 to less than 90 mL/minute), area under the plasma concentration-time curve (AUC) of alogliptin increased approximately 1.2-fold; the manufacturer does not recommend dosage adjustment of alogliptin in patients with mild renal impairment.

However, dosage adjustment is recommended when the drug is used in patients with moderate or severe renal impairment or end-stage renal disease. (See Special Populations under Dosage and Administration: Dosage.) Plasma AUC of alogliptin was increased approximately twofold in patients with moderate renal impairment (creatinine clearance of 30 to less than 60 mL/minute), threefold in those with severe renal impairment (creatinine clearance of 15 to less than 30 mL/minute), and fourfold in those with end-stage renal disease (creatinine clearance of 15 mL/minute or less or requiring hemodialysis).

● Common Adverse Effects

Adverse effects reported in at least 4% of patients receiving alogliptin monotherapy and more commonly than with placebo include nasopharyngitis, headache, and upper respiratory tract infection.

Adverse effects reported in at least 4% of patients receiving alogliptin in combination with metformin and more commonly than with placebo include upper respiratory tract infection, nasopharyngitis, diarrhea, hypertension, headache, back pain, and urinary tract infection.

Adverse effects reported in at least 4% of patients receiving alogliptin in combination with pioglitazone and more commonly than with placebo include nasopharyngitis, back pain, and upper respiratory tract infection.

DRUG INTERACTIONS

Alogliptin is principally renally excreted; cytochrome P-450 (CYP)-related metabolism is negligible.

Drugs Affecting or Metabolized by Hepatic Microsomal Enzymes

Alogliptin does not induce CYP1A2, 2B6, 2C9, 2C19, or 3A4 and does not inhibit CYP1A2, 2C8, 2C9, 2C19, 3A4, or 2D6.

Concurrent administration of alogliptin (100 mg once daily for 7 days) with a single dose of a CYP1A2 substrate (caffeine 200 mg), a CYP2C9 substrate (tolbutamide 500 mg), a CYP2D6 substrate (dextromethorphan 30 mg), or a CYP3A4 substrate (midazolam 4 mg) did not meaningfully increase the peak plasma concentrations or area under the concentration-time curve (AUC) of caffeine, tolbutamide, dextromethorphan, or midazolam. The manufacturer states that no dosage adjustment is necessary with such concomitant therapy.

Drugs that are Substrates of P-glycoprotein Transport Systems

Concurrent administration of alogliptin (100 mg once daily for 7 days) with a single dose of a P-glycoprotein substrate (fexofenadine 80 mg) did not meaningfully increase the peak plasma concentration or AUC of fexofenadine. The manufacturer states that no dosage adjustment is necessary with such concomitant therapy.

Atorvastatin

Concurrent administration of alogliptin (25 mg once daily for 7 days) and atorvastatin (80 mg once daily for 7 days) did not meaningfully alter the peak plasma concentrations or AUC of alogliptin or atorvastatin. The manufacturer states that no dosage adjustment is necessary.

Cimetidine

Concurrent administration of alogliptin (100 mg once daily for 6 days) and cimetidine (400 mg once daily for 6 days) did not meaningfully alter the peak plasma concentrations or AUC of alogliptin or cimetidine. The manufacturer states that no dosage adjustment is necessary.

Contraceptives, Hormonal

Concurrent administration of alogliptin (25 mg once daily for 21 days) and an estrogen-progestin contraceptive (ethinyl estradiol 35 mcg and norethindrone 1 mg once daily for 21 days) did not meaningfully alter the peak plasma concentrations or AUC of ethinyl estradiol or norethindrone; no dosage adjustment is necessary.

Cyclosporine

Concurrent administration of a single dose of alogliptin (25 mg) and a single dose of cyclosporine (600 mg) did not meaningfully alter the peak plasma concentrations or AUC of alogliptin. The manufacturer states that no dosage adjustment is necessary.

Digoxin

Concurrent administration of alogliptin (25 mg once daily for 10 days) and digoxin (0.2 mg once daily for 10 days) did not meaningfully alter the peak plasma concentrations or AUC of alogliptin or digoxin. The manufacturer states that no dosage adjustment is necessary.

Fluconazole

Concurrent administration of a single dose of alogliptin (25 mg) and fluconazole (200 mg once daily for 7 days) did not meaningfully alter the peak plasma concentrations or AUC of alogliptin. The manufacturer states that no dosage adjustment is necessary.

Gemfibrozil

Concurrent administration of a single dose of alogliptin (25 mg) and gemfibrozil (600 mg twice daily for 7 days) did not meaningfully alter the peak plasma concentrations or AUC of alogliptin. The manufacturer states that no dosage adjustment is necessary.

Glyburide

Concurrent administration of alogliptin (25 mg once daily for 8 days) and a single dose of glyburide (5 mg) did not meaningfully alter the peak plasma concentrations or AUC of glyburide. No dosage adjustment is necessary.

Ketoconazole

Concurrent administration of a single dose of alogliptin (25 mg) and ketoconazole (400 mg once daily for 7 days) did not meaningfully alter the peak plasma concentrations or AUC of alogliptin. The manufacturer states that no dosage adjustment is necessary.

Metformin

Concurrent administration of alogliptin (100 mg once daily for 6 days) and metformin hydrochloride (1 g twice daily for 6 days) did not meaningfully alter the peak plasma concentrations or AUC of alogliptin or metformin. The manufacturer states that no dosage adjustment is necessary.

Pioglitazone

Concurrent administration of alogliptin (25 mg once daily for 12 days) and pioglitazone (45 mg once daily for 12 days) did not meaningfully alter the peak plasma concentrations or AUC of alogliptin or pioglitazone. No dosage adjustment is necessary.

Warfarin

Concurrent administration of alogliptin (25 mg once daily for 7 days) and warfarin sodium (stable dosage of 1–10 mg once daily for 7 days) did not alter the peak plasma concentrations or AUC of R- or S-warfarin; prothrombin time (PT) or international normalized ratio (INR) was not altered. The manufacturer states that no dosage adjustment is necessary.

DESCRIPTION

Alogliptin inhibits dipeptidyl peptidase-4 (DPP-4), an enzyme that inactivates the incretin hormones glucagon-like peptide-1 (GLP-1) and glucose-dependent insulinotropic polypeptide (GIP). Alogliptin selectively inhibits DPP-4 with no effect on DPP-8 or DPP-9 in vitro at concentrations approximating those from therapeutic exposures. Alogliptin increases circulating concentrations of GLP-1 and GIP in a glucose-dependent manner.

GLP-1 and GIP stimulate insulin secretion from pancreatic β-cells in a glucose-dependent manner (i.e., when glucose concentrations are elevated). GLP-1 also decreases glucagon secretion from pancreatic α-cells, leading to reduced hepatic glucose production.

Alogliptin did not increase the QT interval corrected for rate (QT$_c$) at daily dosages of 50 or 400 mg daily for 7 days in a randomized, placebo-controlled, active-comparator (moxifloxacin) study; the 400-mg dose produced plasma concentrations 19-fold higher than the maximum recommended clinical dose of 25 mg.

Following oral administration of a single dose of alogliptin (up to 800 mg) in healthy individuals, median time to peak plasma concentration was 1–2 hours; the drug has an absolute oral bioavailability of approximately 100%. Administration of alogliptin with food did not substantially alter total and peak exposure to the drug. Alogliptin does not undergo extensive metabolism; 60–80% of the dose is excreted unchanged. Following administration of a radiolabeled dose of alogliptin, approximately 89% of administered radioactivity was excreted in urine (76%) and feces (13%). Terminal elimination half-life of alogliptin is approximately 21 hours following a single dose of 25 mg.

ADVICE TO PATIENTS

Importance of patient reading medication guide before initiating therapy and each time the drug is dispensed.

Importance of informing patients of the potential risks and benefits of alogliptin. Importance of not using alogliptin in patients with type 1 diabetes mellitus or diabetic ketoacidosis.

Importance of informing patient about the possibility of acute pancreatitis, which may be severe or fatal, with alogliptin therapy. Importance of patient informing clinicians about a history of pancreatitis, gallstones, alcoholism, or kidney or liver problems. Importance of informing patients about signs and symptoms of pancreatitis, including persistent severe abdominal pain sometimes radiating to the back that may or may not be accompanied by vomiting; importance of patient discontinuing alogliptin and promptly notifying clinician if such signs or symptoms are present.

Importance of informing patients about possibility of heart failure with alogliptin therapy. Importance of clinicians asking patients about a history of heart failure or renal impairment prior to initiating alogliptin therapy. Importance of informing patients about signs and symptoms of heart failure (e.g., shortness of breath, weight gain, edema); importance of patients immediately contacting a clinician if manifestations of heart failure occur.

Importance of informing patients of the possibility of severe and disabling joint pain with DPP-4 inhibitors (e.g., alogliptin, linagliptin, saxagliptin, sitagliptin). Advise patients to contact a clinician promptly if severe and persistent joint pain occurs; patients should not discontinue the DPP-4 inhibitor without consulting their clinician.

Importance of informing patient of risk of hypoglycemia, particularly if concomitant therapy with a sulfonylurea antidiabetic agent (i.e., insulin secretagogue) or insulin is used.

Risk of serious allergic (hypersensitivity) reaction. If signs or symptoms of such reactions occur (e.g., rash, hives, swelling of the face, lips, tongue, and throat that may cause difficulty in breathing or swallowing), importance of discontinuing alogliptin therapy and informing clinician promptly.

Importance of informing patients about possibility of liver injury, sometimes fatal, with alogliptin. If signs or symptoms of liver injury (e.g., nausea, vomiting, abdominal pain, unusual/unexplained fatigue, anorexia, dark urine, jaundice) occur, importance of discontinuing alogliptin therapy and informing clinician promptly.

Importance of taking alogliptin exactly as directed by clinician. (See Dosage and Administration: Administration.)

Importance of women informing their clinicians if they are or plan to become pregnant or plan to breast-feed.

Importance of informing clinicians of existing or contemplated concomitant therapy, including prescription and OTC drugs and dietary or herbal supplements, as well as any concomitant illnesses.

Importance of informing patients of other important precautionary information. (See Cautions.)

PREPARATIONS

Excipients in commercially available drug preparations may have clinically important effects in some individuals; consult specific product labeling for details.

Alogliptin Benzoate

Oral

Tablets, film-coated	6.25 mg (of alogliptin)	Nesina®, Takeda
	12.5 mg (of alogliptin)	Nesina®, Takeda
	25 mg (of alogliptin)	Nesina®, Takeda

Alogliptin Benzoate Combinations

Oral

Tablets, film-coated	12.5 mg (of alogliptin) with Metformin Hydrochloride 500 mg	Kazano®, Takeda
	12.5 mg (of alogliptin) with Metformin Hydrochloride 1 g	Kazano®, Takeda
	12.5 mg (of alogliptin) with Pioglitazone Hydrochloride 15 mg (of pioglitazone)	Oseni®, Takeda
	12.5 mg (of alogliptin) with Pioglitazone Hydrochloride 30 mg (of pioglitazone)	Oseni®, Takeda
	12.5 mg (of alogliptin) with Pioglitazone Hydrochloride 45 mg (of pioglitazone)	Oseni®, Takeda
	25 mg (of alogliptin) with Pioglitazone Hydrochloride 15 mg (of pioglitazone)	Oseni®, Takeda
	25 mg (of alogliptin) with Pioglitazone Hydrochloride 30 mg (of pioglitazone)	Oseni®, Takeda
	25 mg (of alogliptin) with Pioglitazone Hydrochloride 45 mg (of pioglitazone)	Oseni®, Takeda

Selected Revisions June 21, 2021, © Copyright, November 26, 2013, American Society of Health-System Pharmacists, Inc.

Linagliptin

68:20.05 • DIPEPTIDYL PEPTIDASE IV (DPP-4) INHIBITORS

■ Linagliptin, a dipeptidyl peptidase-4 (DPP-4) inhibitor, is an antidiabetic agent.

USES

● Type 2 Diabetes Mellitus

Linagliptin is used as monotherapy as an adjunct to diet and exercise to improve glycemic control in patients with type 2 diabetes mellitus. Linagliptin also is used as initial therapy in combination with metformin hydrochloride as an adjunct to diet and exercise to improve glycemic control in patients with type 2 diabetes mellitus. Linagliptin also is used in combination with other oral antidiabetic agents (e.g., metformin, a sulfonylurea, a peroxisome proliferator-activated receptor$_\gamma$ [PPAR$_\gamma$] agonist [thiazolidinedione]) or insulin as an adjunct to diet and exercise in patients with type 2 diabetes mellitus who have not achieved adequate glycemic control with oral antidiabetic agent monotherapy. Linagliptin is commercially available in fixed combination with the sodium-glucose cotransporter 2 (SGLT2) inhibitor, empagliflozin (Glyxambi®) or immediate- or extended-release metformin hydrochloride (Jentadueto®, Jentadueto® XR, respectively); these fixed-combination preparations are used as adjuncts to diet and exercise to improve glycemic control in patients with type 2 diabetes mellitus when treatment with both drugs in the fixed combination is appropriate.

Current guidelines for the treatment of type 2 diabetes mellitus generally recommend metformin as first-line therapy in addition to lifestyle modifications in patients with recent-onset type 2 diabetes mellitus or mild hyperglycemia because of its well-established safety and efficacy (i.e., beneficial effects on glycosylated hemoglobin [hemoglobin A$_{1c}$; HbA$_{1c}$], weight, and cardiovascular mortality). (See Uses: Type 2 Diabetes Mellitus, in Metformin 68:20.04.) In patients with contraindications or intolerance to metformin (e.g., risk of lactic acidosis, GI intolerance) or in selected other patients, some experts suggest that initial therapy with a drug from another class of antidiabetic agents (e.g., a glucagon-like peptide-1 [GLP-1] receptor agonist, SGLT2 inhibitor, DPP-4 inhibitor, sulfonylurea, thiazolidinedione, basal insulin) may be acceptable based on patient factors. Initiating antidiabetic therapy with 2 agents (e.g., metformin plus another drug) may be appropriate in patients with an initial HbA$_{1c}$ exceeding 7.5% or at least 1.5% above the target level. In metformin-intolerant patients with high initial HbA$_{1c}$ levels, some experts suggest initiation of therapy with 2 agents from other antidiabetic drug classes with complementary mechanisms of action.

Because of the progressive nature of type 2 diabetes mellitus, patients initially receiving an oral antidiabetic agent will eventually require multiple oral and/or injectable noninsulin antidiabetic agents of different therapeutic classes and/or insulin for adequate glycemic control. Patients who have inadequate glycemic control with initial (e.g., metformin) monotherapy should receive treatment with additional antidiabetic agents; data suggest that the addition of each noninsulin agent to initial therapy lowers HbA$_{1c}$ by approximately 0.7–1%. In addition, early initiation of combination therapy may help to more rapidly attain glycemic goals and extend the time to treatment failure.

Factors to consider when selecting additional antidiabetic agents for combination therapy in patients with inadequate glycemic control on metformin monotherapy include patient comorbidities (e.g., atherosclerotic cardiovascular disease [ASCVD], established kidney disease, heart failure), hypoglycemia risk, impact on weight, cost, risk of adverse effects, and patient preference. Some experts recommend DPP-4 inhibitors as one of several classes of drugs for use in combination therapy, particularly in patients with both postprandial and fasting plasma glucose elevations. When the greater glucose-lowering effect of an injectable drug is needed in patients with type 2 diabetes mellitus, some experts currently state that an injectable GLP-1 receptor agonist is preferred over insulin in most patients because of beneficial effects on body weight and a lower risk of hypoglycemia, although adverse GI effects may diminish tolerability. While addition of a GLP-1 receptor agonist may successfully control hyperglycemia, many patients will eventually require insulin therapy. Early introduction of insulin therapy should be considered when hyperglycemia is severe (e.g., blood glucose of at least 300 mg/dL or HbA$_{1c}$ exceeding 9–10%), especially in the presence of catabolic manifestations

(e.g., weight loss, hypertriglyceridemia, ketosis) or symptoms of hyperglycemia. For additional information regarding the initiation of insulin therapy in patients with diabetes mellitus, see Uses: Diabetes Mellitus, in the Insulins General Statement 68:20.08.

The manufacturer states that linagliptin should *not* be used in patients with type 1 diabetes mellitus or for the treatment of diabetic ketoacidosis.

Linagliptin Monotherapy

Efficacy of linagliptin as monotherapy for the management of type 2 diabetes mellitus has been established in 2 double-blind, placebo-controlled studies of 18 or 24 weeks' duration. Linagliptin (5 mg once daily) improved glycemic control as evidenced by reductions in glycosylated hemoglobin (HbA$_{1c}$) as well as in fasting and 2-hour postprandial plasma glucose concentrations. HbA$_{1c}$ was reduced by a mean of 0.4% (from a mean baseline concentration of about 8%) in patients receiving linagliptin 5 mg daily, compared with an increase in HbA$_{1c}$ of 0.1–0.3% in those receiving placebo.

Combination Therapy

Efficacy of linagliptin in combination with metformin, an SGLT2 inhibitor, a sulfonylurea, or a thiazolidinedione in the management of type 2 diabetes mellitus has been established in several randomized, placebo- or active-controlled, double-blind studies. In these studies, the addition of linagliptin (5 mg once daily) to current therapy (metformin and/or a sulfonylurea; pioglitazone; metformin and empagliflozin) improved glycemic control as evidenced by reductions in HbA$_{1c}$ as well as in fasting and/or 2-hour postprandial plasma glucose concentrations.

Efficacy of the combination of linagliptin and metformin as *initial* therapy in patients with type 2 diabetes mellitus inadequately controlled with diet and exercise is supported by results of a 24-week, randomized, double-blind trial. In this trial, concurrent therapy with linagliptin and metformin hydrochloride improved glycemic control (as evidenced by reductions in HbA$_{1c}$ and fasting plasma glucose) compared with linagliptin or metformin hydrochloride monotherapy or placebo. Reductions in HbA$_{1c}$ were 1.2 or 1.6% with linagliptin 2.5 mg plus metformin hydrochloride 0.5 or 1 g twice daily, respectively; 0.5% with linagliptin 5 mg once daily; 0.6 or 1.1% with metformin hydrochloride 0.5 or 1 g twice daily, respectively; and 0.1% with placebo.

In a 24-week study in patients receiving metformin hydrochloride monotherapy (at least 1.5 g daily), add-on therapy with linagliptin resulted in a reduction of 0.5% in HbA$_{1c}$ compared with an increase of 0.15% in patients receiving metformin hydrochloride and add-on placebo. In a 104-week, active-controlled, noninferiority study in patients receiving metformin hydrochloride monotherapy (at least 1.5 g daily), add-on therapy with linagliptin was noninferior at 52 weeks and resulted in a reduction of 0.4% in HbA$_{1c}$ from baseline, compared with a reduction of 0.6% from baseline in patients receiving add-on therapy with glimepiride (initiated at 1 mg daily and titrated over 12 weeks to a maximum dosage of 4 mg daily [mean dosage: 3 mg daily]). At 104 weeks, add-on therapy with linagliptin resulted in a reduction of 0.2% in HbA$_{1c}$ from baseline, compared with a reduction of 0.4% from baseline in those receiving add-on glimepiride therapy. Patients receiving add-on linagliptin therapy had a mean decrease in body weight (loss of 1.1 kg), while those receiving add-on glimepiride had a mean increase in body weight (gain of 1.4 kg). In a 24-week study in treatment-naive patients with type 2 diabetes mellitus, initial therapy with linagliptin and metformin hydrochloride produced substantially greater reductions in HbA$_{1c}$ compared with linagliptin therapy alone (reduction of 2.9 versus 2%, respectively).

In a 24-week study in patients receiving pioglitazone monotherapy (30 mg daily), add-on linagliptin or placebo resulted in a reduction of 1.1 or 0.6%, respectively, in HbA$_{1c}$.

In an 18-week study in patients receiving a sulfonylurea antidiabetic agent (sulfonylurea not specified), add-on therapy with linagliptin resulted in a reduction of 0.5% in HbA$_{1c}$ compared with a reduction of 0.1% in patients receiving add-on placebo.

In a 24-week study in patients receiving metformin and a sulfonylurea (generally glimepiride, glyburide [glibenclamide], or gliclazide [not commercially available in the US]), add-on therapy with linagliptin or placebo resulted in a reduction of 0.7 or 0.1%, respectively, in HbA$_{1c}$.

In an international, phase 3, randomized, double-blind trial, add-on therapy with linagliptin and empagliflozin in fixed combination was more effective in reducing HbA$_{1c}$ and fasting plasma glucose concentrations than add-on linagliptin or empagliflozin monotherapy in 686 adults with type 2 diabetes mellitus inadequately controlled with metformin hydrochloride (dosage of at least 1.5 g daily, or maximum tolerated dosage, or maximum labeled dosage). At 24 weeks, reduction in mean HbA_{1c} from baseline was 1.19% with linagliptin 5 mg/empagliflozin 25 mg, 1.08% with linagliptin 5 mg/empagliflozin 10 mg, 0.62% with empagliflozin 25 mg, 0.66% with empagliflozin 10 mg, and 0.7% with linagliptin 5 mg. Glycemic efficacy (HbA_{1c} reductions) with the fixed combinations of linagliptin and empagliflozin was maintained at week 52. The fixed combinations of linagliptin and empagliflozin also were associated with reductions from baseline in systolic blood pressure compared with linagliptin monotherapy. Body weight was reduced in patients receiving the fixed combinations of empagliflozin/linagliptin compared with linagliptin but not empagliflozin monotherapy.

Efficacy of linagliptin in combination with insulin in patients with type 2 diabetes mellitus inadequately controlled with insulin (with or without oral antidiabetic agents) is supported by the results of a 24-week randomized, placebo-controlled trial. In this trial, addition of linagliptin (5 mg once daily) to existing stable therapy with insulin resulted in improvements in HbA_{1c} and fasting plasma glucose concentrations at week 24 compared with addition of placebo. Mean reductions in HbA_{1c} were 0.6% in patients receiving linagliptin and 0.1% in those receiving placebo.

DOSAGE AND ADMINISTRATION

• Administration

When administered as monotherapy, linagliptin is administered orally once daily without regard to meals.

The fixed combination of linagliptin and empagliflozin is administered orally once daily in the morning with or without food.

The fixed combination of linagliptin and *immediate-release* metformin hydrochloride is administered orally twice daily with meals.

The fixed combination of linagliptin and *extended-release* metformin hydrochloride is administered orally once daily with a meal.

If a dose of linagliptin alone or in fixed combination with empagliflozin or immediate- or extended-release metformin hydrochloride is missed, the missed dose should be taken as soon as it is remembered followed by resumption of the regular schedule. If the missed dose is not remembered until the time of the next dose, the missed dose should be skipped and the regular schedule resumed. The dose should not be doubled to replace a missed dose.

• Dosage
Type 2 Diabetes Mellitus
Linagliptin Monotherapy

When used as monotherapy for the management of type 2 diabetes mellitus, the recommended dosage of linagliptin is 5 mg once daily.

Combination Therapy with a Sulfonylurea

When used concomitantly with a sulfonylurea for the management of type 2 diabetes mellitus, the recommended dosage of linagliptin is 5 mg once daily; dosage of the sulfonylurea may need to be reduced to decrease risk of hypoglycemia.

Linagliptin/Empagliflozin Fixed-combination Therapy

The recommended initial dosage of the fixed combination of linagliptin and empagliflozin is 5 mg of linagliptin and 10 mg of empagliflozin once daily in the morning. If this dosage is well tolerated, the dosage may be increased to 5 mg of linagliptin and 25 mg of empagliflozin once daily.

Linagliptin/Immediate- or Extended-release Metformin Hydrochloride Fixed-combination Therapy

Dosage of the fixed combinations of linagliptin and immediate- or extended-release metformin hydrochloride should be individualized based on effectiveness and patient tolerability. Dosage of these fixed combinations may be increased up to a daily maximum of 5 mg of linagliptin and 2 g of metformin hydrochloride.

In patients *not* currently receiving metformin hydrochloride, the recommended initial total daily dosage of the fixed combination is 5 mg of linagliptin and 1 g of metformin hydrochloride administered *in 2 divided doses* (when given as the fixed combination containing *immediate-release* metformin hydrochloride)

or *once* daily (when given as the fixed combination containing *extended-release* metformin hydrochloride).

In patients currently receiving metformin hydrochloride, the recommended initial total daily dosage of the fixed combination is 5 mg of linagliptin and a total daily metformin hydrochloride dosage similar to the patient's existing dosage, administered *in 2 divided doses* (when given as the fixed combination containing *immediate-release* metformin hydrochloride) or *once* daily (when given as the fixed combination containing *extended-release* metformin hydrochloride).

In patients currently receiving linagliptin *and* metformin hydrochloride as individual components, the recommended initial dosage of the fixed combination of linagliptin and *immediate-release* metformin hydrochloride is the same total daily dosage of each component administered in 2 divided doses daily.

In patients currently receiving linagliptin *and* metformin hydrochloride as individual components *or* the fixed combination of linagliptin and *immediate-release* metformin, the recommended initial dosage of the fixed combination of linagliptin and *extended-release* metformin is 5 mg of linagliptin and a total daily dosage of metformin hydrochloride similar to the patient's existing dosage, administered once daily.

• Special Populations
Hepatic Impairment
Linagliptin Monotherapy

Dosage adjustment is not routinely required based on hepatic impairment.

Linagliptin/Empagliflozin Fixed-combination Therapy

The fixed combination of linagliptin and empagliflozin may be used in patients with hepatic impairment.

Linagliptin/Immediate- or Extended-release Metformin Hydrochloride Fixed-combination Therapy

The fixed combinations of linagliptin and immediate- or extended-release metformin hydrochloride are not recommended in patients with hepatic impairment.

Renal Impairment
Linagliptin Monotherapy

Dosage adjustment is not routinely required based on renal impairment.

Linagliptin/Empagliflozin Fixed-combination Therapy

Dosage adjustment of the fixed combination of linagliptin and empagliflozin is not necessary in patients with an estimated glomerular filtration rate (eGFR) of at least 45 mL/minute per 1.73 m^2.

The fixed combination of linagliptin and empagliflozin should not be initiated in patients with an eGFR less than 45 mL/minute per 1.73 m^2. The fixed combination should be discontinued if the eGFR is persistently less than 45 mL/minute per 1.73 m^2.

Linagliptin/Immediate- or Extended-release Metformin Hydrochloride Fixed-combination Therapy

Initiation of the fixed combinations of linagliptin and immediate- or extended-release metformin hydrochloride is not recommended in patients with an eGFR of 30–45 mL/minute per 1.73 m^2.

If the eGFR decreases to 30–45 mL/minute per 1.73 m^2 during therapy with a fixed combination of linagliptin and metformin hydrochloride, the risks and benefits of continuing therapy with the fixed combination should be assessed.

The fixed combinations of linagliptin and immediate- or extended-release metformin hydrochloride are contraindicated in patients with an eGFR less than 30 mL/minute per 1.73 m^2.

If a fixed combination of linagliptin and metformin is discontinued due to evidence of renal impairment, linagliptin may be continued as a single-entity tablet at the same total daily dosage of 5 mg.

Geriatric Patients
Linagliptin Monotherapy

Dosage adjustment of linagliptin is not recommended in geriatric patients based solely on age.

CAUTIONS

● Contraindications

Linagliptin is contraindicated in patients with a history of hypersensitivity reaction (e.g., anaphylaxis, urticaria, angioedema, bronchial hyperreactivity) to linagliptin.

● Warnings/Precautions

Pancreatitis and Pancreatic Precancerous Changes

Acute pancreatitis, including fatal pancreatitis, has been reported in patients receiving linagliptin therapy. In a multicenter, randomized, placebo-controlled trial evaluating linagliptin, acute pancreatitis was reported in 9 patients receiving linagliptin (0.3%) versus 5 patients receiving placebo (0.1%); 2 patients who developed acute pancreatitis while receiving linagliptin died.

FDA has been evaluating unpublished findings suggesting an increased risk of pancreatitis and precancerous pancreatic cell changes (pancreatic duct metaplasia) in patients with type 2 diabetes mellitus receiving incretin mimetics (alogliptin, exenatide, linagliptin, liraglutide, saxagliptin, and sitagliptin). These findings are based on examination of a small number of pancreatic tissue specimens taken from patients who died from unspecified causes while receiving an incretin mimetic. FDA will notify healthcare professionals of its conclusions and recommendations when the review is complete, or when the agency has additional information to report.

FDA has recommended that clinicians continue to follow the recommendations in the prescribing information for incretin mimetics. The manufacturer states that patients receiving linagliptin therapy should be monitored for signs and symptoms of pancreatitis. (See Advice to Patients.) If pancreatitis is suspected, linagliptin should be promptly discontinued and appropriate management instituted. Safety and efficacy of linagliptin have not been established in patients with a history of pancreatitis and it is not known whether such patients are at increased risk for pancreatitis with linagliptin therapy.

Severe Arthralgia

Severe, disabling joint pain has been reported during postmarketing experience in patients receiving dipeptidyl peptidase-4 (DPP-4) inhibitors (e.g., alogliptin, linagliptin, saxagliptin, sitagliptin). Onset of such symptoms has ranged from 1 day to years following initiation of therapy. Fever, chills, rash, and swelling accompanied joint pain in some patients, suggesting an immunologic reaction; some patients required hospitalization. Symptoms resolved upon discontinuance of the DPP-4 inhibitor, usually in less than a month. In some patients, symptoms recurred when the same or another DPP-4 inhibitor was restarted. DPP-4 inhibitors should be considered as a possible cause of severe joint pain and should be discontinued if appropriate. (See Advice to Patients.)

Heart Failure Risk

In cardiovascular outcomes studies conducted with 2 other DPP-4 inhibitors (alogliptin, saxagliptin) in patients with type 2 diabetes mellitus and ASCVD, an association between DPP-4 inhibitor treatment and heart failure was observed. The potential risks and benefits of linagliptin therapy should be considered prior to use in patients at risk for heart failure (e.g., history of heart failure or renal impairment). Patients receiving linagliptin-containing therapy should be monitored for manifestations of heart failure. (See Advice to Patients.) If heart failure develops, appropriate evaluation and management according to current standards of care should be instituted and consideration given to discontinuing linagliptin.

Concomitant Therapy with Hypoglycemic Agents

Use of linagliptin in combination with an insulin secretagogue (e.g., a sulfonylurea) was associated with a higher rate of hypoglycemia compared with placebo in a clinical trial. Use of linagliptin in combination with insulin in patients with severe renal impairment also was associated with a higher rate of hypoglycemia compared with placebo in another clinical trial. A reduced dosage of an insulin secretagogue or insulin may be required to decrease the risk of hypoglycemia when used in combination with linagliptin.

Dermatologic and Sensitivity Reactions

There have been postmarketing reports of serious allergic and hypersensitivity reactions (e.g., anaphylaxis, angioedema, exfoliative skin conditions) with linagliptin; rash also has been reported. The onset of such reactions usually was within the first 3 months following treatment initiation, but such reactions may occur after the first dose. (See Cautions: Contraindications.)

If a serious hypersensitivity reaction is suspected, promptly discontinue linagliptin, assess for other potential causes of the event, and initiate alternative antidiabetic therapy. (See Advice to Patients.) Linagliptin should be used with caution in patients with a history of angioedema with other DPP-4 inhibitors because it is unknown whether such patients will be predisposed to angioedema with linagliptin.

Cases of bullous pemphigoid requiring hospitalization have been reported with DPP-4 inhibitor use during postmarketing experience. These cases usually resolved after discontinuance of the DPP-4 inhibitor and treatment with topical or systemic immunosuppressive therapy. In a multicenter, randomized, placebo-controlled trial, bullous pemphigoid was reported in 7 patients (0.2%) receiving linagliptin versus none of the patients receiving placebo. Patients should be advised to report the development of blisters or erosions while receiving linagliptin. If bullous pemphigoid is suspected, the drug should be discontinued and referral to a dermatologist should be considered for diagnosis and appropriate treatment.

Macrovascular Outcomes

The manufacturer states that evidence of macrovascular risk reduction with linagliptin has not been conclusively demonstrated in clinical trials.

Use of Fixed Combinations

When linagliptin is used in fixed combination with empagliflozin, metformin hydrochloride, or other drugs, the cautions, precautions, contraindications, and interactions associated with the concomitant agent(s) should be considered in addition to those associated with linagliptin.

Specific Populations

Pregnancy

Data on use of linagliptin in pregnant women are insufficient to inform a drug-associated risk for major birth defects or miscarriage.

In animal reproduction studies, no adverse developmental effects were observed when linagliptin was administered to pregnant rats during the period of organogenesis.

Lactation

Linagliptin is distributed into milk in rats; it is not known whether the drug is distributed into human milk. The developmental and health benefits of breast-feeding and the importance of linagliptin to the woman should be considered along with any potential adverse effects on the breast-fed infant from the drug or from the underlying maternal condition.

Pediatric Use

Safety and efficacy of linagliptin alone or in fixed combination with empagliflozin or fixed combination with immediate- or extended-release metformin hydrochloride have not been established in patients younger than 18 years of age.

Geriatric Use

Of 4040 patients in clinical studies of linagliptin, 27% were 65 years of age and older and 3% were 75 years of age and older. No substantial differences in safety and efficacy relative to younger adults were observed, but increased sensitivity cannot be ruled out.

Hepatic Impairment

In patients with mild hepatic impairment (Child-Pugh class A), linagliptin area under the concentration-time curve (AUC) and peak plasma concentration were reduced by 25 and 36%, respectively, compared with values in healthy individuals. In patients with moderate hepatic impairment (Child-Pugh class B), linagliptin AUC and peak plasma concentration were reduced by 14 and 8%, respectively, compared with values in healthy individuals. In patients with severe hepatic impairment (Child-Pugh class C), linagliptin AUC was comparable to that in healthy individuals, and peak plasma concentration was reduced by 23% relative to that in healthy individuals.

The fixed combination of linagliptin and empagliflozin may be used in patients with hepatic impairment.

Use of the fixed combinations of linagliptin and immediate- or extended-release metformin hydrochloride is not recommended in patients with hepatic impairment.

Renal Impairment

In patients with mild renal impairment (creatinine clearance 50 to less than 80 mL/minute), linagliptin exposure was comparable to that in healthy individuals. In patients with moderate renal impairment (creatinine clearance 30 to less than 50 mL/minute), linagliptin AUC and peak plasma concentration were increased by 71 and 46%, respectively, compared with values in healthy individuals. In patients with severe renal impairment (creatinine clearance less than 30 mL/minute) and type 2 diabetes mellitus, linagliptin AUC and peak plasma concentration were increased by 42 and 35%, respectively, compared with those values in patients with type 2 diabetes mellitus and normal renal function.

The fixed combination of linagliptin and empagliflozin should not be initiated in patients with an estimated glomerular filtration rate (eGFR) less than 45 mL/minute per 1.73 m². (See Renal Impairment under Dosage and Administration: Special Populations.)

Initiation of the fixed combinations of linagliptin and immediate- or extended-release metformin hydrochloride is not recommended in patients with an eGFR between 30–45 mL/minute per 1.73 m² and is contraindicated in patients with an eGFR less than 30 mL/minute per 1.73 m². (See Renal Impairment under Dosage and Administration: Special Populations.)

• Common Adverse Effects

Adverse effects reported in at least 5% of patients receiving linagliptin monotherapy include nasopharyngitis.

Adverse effects reported in at least 2% of patients receiving linagliptin concomitantly with pioglitazone, a sulfonylurea, metformin, or basal insulin include nasopharyngitis, hyperlipidemia, cough, hypertriglyceridemia, weight gain, urinary tract infection, constipation, back pain, arthralgia, upper respiratory tract infection, headache, and pain in extremity.

Adverse effects reported in at least 5% of patients receiving linagliptin and empagliflozin in clinical trials include urinary tract infection, nasopharyngitis, and upper respiratory tract infection.

Adverse effects reported in at least 5% of patients receiving linagliptin and metformin hydrochloride in clinical trials include nasopharyngitis and diarrhea.

DRUG INTERACTIONS

• Drugs Affecting or Metabolized by Hepatic Microsomal Enzymes

Linagliptin is a weak to moderate inhibitor of cytochrome P-450 (CYP) isoenzyme 3A4; however, it does not inhibit or induce CYP isoenzymes 1A2, 2A6, 2B6, 2C8, 2C9, 2C19, 2D6, 2E1, or 4A11 in vitro.

In vivo studies indicate that drug interactions are unlikely with substrates of CYP isoenzymes 3A4, 2C9, or 2C8. No adjustment of linagliptin dosage is recommended based on results of pharmacokinetic studies.

Inducers of CYP3A4 (e.g., rifampin) decrease exposure to linagliptin, resulting in subtherapeutic and likely ineffective concentrations. The manufacturer states that alternatives to linagliptin are strongly recommended in patients who require therapy with potent CYP3A4 inducers.

• Drugs Affecting or Affected by P-glycoprotein Transport

Linagliptin is a P-glycoprotein substrate and inhibits P-glycoprotein-mediated transport of digoxin at high concentrations. At therapeutic concentrations, linagliptin is considered unlikely to cause interactions with other P-glycoprotein substrates; no adjustment of linagliptin dosage is recommended based on results of pharmacokinetic studies.

Inducers of P-glycoprotein (e.g., rifampin) decrease exposure to linagliptin, resulting in subtherapeutic and likely ineffective concentrations. The manufacturer states that alternatives to linagliptin are strongly recommended in patients who require therapy with potent P-glycoprotein inducers.

• Drugs Affected by Organic Cation Transporter

In vivo studies indicate that drug interactions are unlikely with substrates of organic cation transporter (OCT). No adjustment of linagliptin dosage is recommended based on results of pharmacokinetic studies.

• Digoxin

Concomitant use of linagliptin (5 mg once daily) and digoxin (0.25 mg once daily) in healthy individuals did not appreciably alter the pharmacokinetics of digoxin (e.g., a 2% increase in area under the concentration-time curve [AUC] and a 6% decrease in peak plasma concentration with concomitant use); no digoxin dosage adjustment is necessary.

• Estrogens or Progestins

Concomitant use of linagliptin (5 mg once daily) and an estrogen-progestin contraceptive (ethinyl estradiol 30 mcg with levonorgestrel 0.15 mg once daily) increased AUC and peak plasma concentration by 1 and 8%, respectively, for ethinyl estradiol and by 9 and 13%, respectively, for levonorgestrel. No dosage adjustments are necessary for ethinyl estradiol or levonorgestrel when given concomitantly with linagliptin.

• Metformin

Concomitant use of linagliptin (10 mg once daily) and metformin hydrochloride (850 mg 3 times daily) in healthy individuals increased linagliptin AUC and peak plasma concentration by 20 and 3%, respectively. Such concomitant use did not affect metformin AUC but reduced metformin peak plasma concentration by 11%. These alterations in pharmacokinetic parameters were not associated with clinically relevant effects (e.g., hypoglycemia), and no dosage adjustments are necessary for either drug.

• Pioglitazone

Concomitant use of linagliptin (10 mg once daily) and pioglitazone (45 mg once daily) in healthy individuals increased linagliptin AUC and peak plasma concentration by 13 and 7%, respectively. Pioglitazone AUC and peak plasma concentration were reduced by 6 and 14%, respectively, during concomitant linagliptin therapy; small changes (5% or less) in AUC and peak plasma concentrations of 2 pioglitazone active metabolites also occurred with such concomitant therapy. No dosage adjustments are necessary for either drug when given concomitantly.

• Rifampin

Concomitant use of linagliptin (5 mg once daily) and rifampin (600 mg once daily) reduced linagliptin AUC and peak plasma concentration by 40 and 44%, respectively; such concomitant therapy is not recommended. (See Drugs Affecting or Metabolized by Hepatic Microsomal Enzymes and see Drugs Affecting or Affected by P-glycoprotein Transport under Drug Interactions.)

• Ritonavir

Administration of a single dose of linagliptin (5 mg) to patients receiving ritonavir (200 mg twice daily) resulted in approximately a twofold increase in linagliptin AUC and approximately a threefold increase in linagliptin peak plasma concentration. The increase in exposure was not associated with an increase in linagliptin accumulation. No adjustment of linagliptin dosage is necessary when linagliptin is administered concurrently with ritonavir.

• Simvastatin

Concomitant use of linagliptin (10 mg once daily) and simvastatin (40 mg once daily) in healthy individuals increased simvastatin AUC and peak plasma concentration by 34 and 10%, respectively; these changes were not considered clinically important. No simvastatin dosage adjustment is necessary when given concomitantly with linagliptin.

• Sulfonylureas

When a sulfonylurea is administered concomitantly with linagliptin, reduction in the dosage of the sulfonylurea may be required to reduce the risk of hypoglycemia.

A single dose of glyburide (1.75 mg) given on day day 6 to healthy individuals receiving linagliptin therapy (5 mg once daily for 6 days) decreased glyburide exposure (AUC and peak plasma concentration) by about 14%; these changes were not considered clinically important. No dosage adjustments are necessary for either drug when given concomitantly.

• Warfarin

Administration of a single dose of warfarin sodium (10 mg) to healthy individuals receiving linagliptin (5 mg once daily) had no apparent effect (i.e., change of 3% or less) on R- or S-warfarin AUC and peak plasma concentration and no clinically relevant effect on international normalized ratio (INR) or prothrombin time (PT); no warfarin dosage adjustment is necessary.

DESCRIPTION

Linagliptin is a xanthine-derived inhibitor of dipeptidyl peptidase-4 (DPP-4), an enzyme that inactivates incretin hormones glucagon-like peptide-1 (GLP-1) and glucose-dependent insulinotropic polypeptide (GIP). The drug selectively inhibits DPP-4 with no effect on DPP-8 or DDP-9 in vitro at concentrations approximating those achieved with therapeutic dosages. Linagliptin increases the concentrations of active incretin hormones (e.g., GLP-1, GIP), stimulating the release of insulin in a glucose-dependent manner and decreasing circulating levels of glucagon. GLP-1 and GIP are secreted at low basal levels throughout the day, and levels increase immediately after a meal. Both incretin hormones increase insulin biosynthesis and secretion from pancreatic β-cells in the presence of normal and elevated blood glucose concentrations. GLP-1 also reduces glucagon secretion from pancreatic α-cells, resulting in a reduction in hepatic glucose output.

Linagliptin monotherapy usually is not associated with hypoglycemia or substantial changes in body weight.

Peak plasma linagliptin concentrations usually are attained within 1.5 hours after a 5-mg oral dose, and the drug has an absolute oral bioavailability of approximately 30%. Administration of linagliptin with a high-fat meal reduced peak plasma concentration by 15% and increased area under the concentration-time curve (AUC) by 4%; these changes are not considered clinically important. Metabolism represents a minor elimination pathway for linagliptin; approximately 90% of a dose is excreted unchanged. Following administration of a radiolabeled dose of linagliptin, approximately 85% of administered radioactivity was eliminated via the enterohepatic system (80%) or in urine (5%). Terminal half-life of linagliptin exceeds 100 hours; plasma concentrations decline in at least a biphasic manner. The effective half-life for accumulation of linagliptin based on 5-mg multiple oral dosing is approximately 12 hours.

Results of bioequivalence studies indicate that the fixed-combination tablets containing linagliptin and empagliflozin or linagliptin and immediate-release metformin hydrochloride are bioequivalent to single-entity tablets of linagliptin given concomitantly with single-entity tablets of empagliflozin or single-entity tablets of immediate-release metformin hydrochloride, respectively, in corresponding doses.

ADVICE TO PATIENTS

When linagliptin is used in fixed combination with other drugs, importance of informing patients of important cautionary information about the concomitant agent(s).

Importance of patient reading medication guide before initiating therapy and each time the drug is dispensed.

Importance of informing patients of the potential risks and benefits of linagliptin and of alternative therapies. Importance of not using linagliptin in patients with type 1 diabetes mellitus or diabetic ketoacidosis.

Importance of informing patient about possibility of acute pancreatitis, which may be severe or fatal, with linagliptin therapy. Importance of patient informing clinicians about a history of pancreatitis, gallstones, alcoholism, or high triglyceride levels. Importance of informing patients about signs and symptoms of pancreatitis, including persistent severe abdominal pain sometimes radiating to the back that may or may not be accompanied by vomiting; importance of patient discontinuing linagliptin and promptly notifying clinician if such signs or symptoms are present.

Importance of informing patients about possibility of heart failure with linagliptin therapy. Importance of clinicians asking patients about a history of heart failure or renal impairment prior to initiating linagliptin therapy. Importance of informing patients about signs and symptoms of heart failure (e.g., shortness of breath, weight gain, edema); importance of patients immediately contacting a clinician if manifestations of heart failure occur.

Importance of informing patients of the possibility of severe and disabling joint pain with dipeptidyl peptidase-4 (DPP-4) inhibitors (e.g., alogliptin, linagliptin,

saxagliptin, sitagliptin). Advise patients to contact a clinician promptly if severe and persistent joint pain occurs; patients should not discontinue the DPP-4 inhibitor without consulting their clinician.

Importance of informing patients that bullous pemphigoid may occur with the use of a DPP-4 inhibitor. Advise patients to contact a clinician if blisters or erosions occur.

Increased risk of hypoglycemia when linagliptin is used in combination with a sulfonylurea or insulin. Importance of informing patients that a lower dosage of the sulfonylurea or insulin may be required to reduce the risk of hypoglycemia if used concomitantly with linagliptin.

Risk of serious allergic (hypersensitivity) reactions, such as angioedema, anaphylaxis, and exfoliative skin conditions. If signs or symptoms of such reactions occur (e.g., rash, blisters, skin flaking or peeling/erosion, hives, swelling of the skin, swelling of the face, lips, tongue, and throat that may cause difficulty in breathing or swallowing), importance of discontinuing linagliptin-containing therapy and informing clinician promptly.

Importance of informing patients about the importance of adherence to dietary instructions, regular physical activity, periodic blood glucose monitoring and HbA$_{1C}$ testing, recognition and management of hypoglycemia and hyperglycemia, and assessment of complications of diabetes mellitus.

Importance of seeking medical advice promptly during periods of stress such as fever, trauma, infection, or surgery as medication requirements may change.

Importance of informing patients that response to all antidiabetic therapies should be monitored by periodic measurements of blood glucose and HbA$_{1C}$, with a goal of decreasing these levels toward the normal range.

Importance of informing clinicians if any unusual symptom develops or if any existing symptom persists or worsens.

Importance of women informing their clinicians if they are or plan to become pregnant or plan to breast-feed.

Importance of informing clinicians of existing or contemplated concomitant therapy, including prescription and OTC drugs and dietary or herbal supplements, as well as any concomitant illnesses.

Importance of informing patients of other important precautionary information. (See Cautions.)

PREPARATIONS

Excipients in commercially available drug preparations may have clinically important effects in some individuals; consult specific product labeling for details.

Linagliptin

Oral		
Tablet, film-coated	5 mg	Tradjenta®, Boehringer Ingelheim

Linagliptin Combinations

Oral		
Tablets, extended-release	2.5 mg with Extended-release Metformin Hydrochloride 1 g	Jentadueto® XR, Boehringer Ingelheim
	5 mg with Extended-release Metformin Hydrochloride 1 g	Jentadueto® XR, Boehringer Ingelheim
Tablets, film-coated	2.5 mg with Metformin Hydrochloride 500 mg	Jentadueto®, Boehringer Ingelheim
	2.5 mg with Metformin Hydrochloride 850 mg	Jentadueto®, Boehringer Ingelheim
	2.5 mg with Metformin Hydrochloride 1 g	Jentadueto®, Boehringer Ingelheim
	5 mg with Empagliflozin 10 mg	Glyxambi®, Boehringer Ingelheim
	5 mg with Empagliflozin 25 mg	Glyxambi®, Boehringer Ingelheim

Selected Revisions June 21, 2021, © Copyright, December 10, 2012, American Society of Health-System Pharmacists, Inc.

sAXagliptin Hydrochloride

68:20.05 · DIPEPTIDYL PEPTIDASE IV (DPP-4) INHIBITORS

■ Saxagliptin hydrochloride, a dipeptidyl peptidase-4 (DPP-4) inhibitor, is an antidiabetic agent.

USES

● Type 2 Diabetes Mellitus

Saxagliptin is used as monotherapy as an adjunct to diet and exercise to improve glycemic control in patients with type 2 diabetes mellitus. Saxagliptin also is used in fixed combination with dapagliflozin (Qtern®) or with dapagliflozin and extended-release metformin hydrochloride (Qternmet® XR) as an adjunct to diet and exercise to improve glycemic control in patients with type 2 diabetes mellitus. The manufacturer states that the fixed combination of dapagliflozin, saxagliptin, and extended-release metformin hydrochloride (Qternmet® XR) is intended for use only in patients currently receiving metformin hydrochloride.

Saxagliptin is used as initial therapy in combination with metformin (given separately or as the fixed combination of saxagliptin and extended-release metformin) as an adjunct to diet and exercise to improve glycemic control in patients with type 2 diabetes mellitus when treatment with both saxagliptin and metformin is appropriate. Saxagliptin also is used in combination with other oral antidiabetic agents (e.g., a sulfonylurea, a thiazolidinedione [peroxisome proliferator-activated receptor-γ agonist]) or insulin as an adjunct to diet and exercise in patients with type 2 diabetes mellitus who have not achieved adequate glycemic control with one or more oral antidiabetic agents and/or insulin.

In pivotal clinical trials, glycemic efficacy and safety of saxagliptin in patients with type 2 diabetes mellitus were evaluated at dosages of 2.5, 5, and 10 mg once daily as monotherapy or in combination with other antidiabetic agents. In these trials, the 10-mg daily dosage (currently not an FDA-labeled dosage) of saxagliptin did not demonstrate greater efficacy than the 5-mg daily dosage. (See Saxagliptin Monotherapy under Dosage: Type 2 Diabetes Mellitus, in Dosage and Administration.)

Current guidelines for the treatment of type 2 diabetes mellitus generally recommend metformin as first-line therapy in addition to lifestyle modifications in patients with recent-onset type 2 diabetes mellitus or mild hyperglycemia because of its well-established safety and efficacy (i.e., beneficial effects on glycosylated hemoglobin [hemoglobin A$_{1c}$; HbA$_{1c}$], weight, and cardiovascular mortality). (See Uses: Type 2 Diabetes Mellitus, in Metformin 68:20.04.) In patients with contraindications or intolerance to metformin (e.g., risk of lactic acidosis, GI intolerance) or in selected other patients, some experts suggest that initial therapy with a drug from another class of antidiabetic agents (e.g., a glucagon-like peptide-1 [GLP-1] receptor agonist, sodium-glucose cotransporter 2 [SGLT2] inhibitor, DPP-4 inhibitor, sulfonylurea, thiazolidinedione, basal insulin) may be acceptable based on patient factors. Initiating antidiabetic therapy with 2 agents (e.g., metformin plus another drug) may be appropriate in patients with an initial HbA$_{1c}$ exceeding 7.5% or at least 1.5% above the target level. In metformin-intolerant patients with high initial HbA$_{1c}$ levels, some experts suggest initiation of therapy with 2 agents from other antidiabetic drug classes with complementary mechanisms of action.

Because of the progressive nature of type 2 diabetes mellitus, patients initially receiving an oral antidiabetic agent will eventually require multiple oral and/or injectable noninsulin antidiabetic agents of different therapeutic classes and/or insulin for adequate glycemic control. Patients who have inadequate glycemic control with initial (e.g., metformin) monotherapy should receive treatment with additional antidiabetic agents; data suggest that the addition of each noninsulin agent to initial therapy lowers HbA$_{1c}$ by approximately 0.7–1%. In addition, early initiation of combination therapy may help to more rapidly attain glycemic goals and extend the time to treatment failure.

Factors to consider when selecting additional antidiabetic agents for combination therapy in patients with inadequate glycemic control on metformin monotherapy include patient comorbidities (e.g., atherosclerotic cardiovascular disease [ASCVD], established kidney disease, heart failure), hypoglycemia risk, impact on weight, cost, risk of adverse effects, and patient preference. Some experts recommend DPP-4 inhibitors as one of several classes of drugs for use in combination

therapy, particularly in patients with both postprandial and fasting plasma glucose elevations. When the greater glucose-lowering effect of an injectable drug is needed in patients with type 2 diabetes mellitus, some experts currently state that an injectable GLP-1 receptor agonist is preferred over insulin in most patients because of beneficial effects on body weight and a lower risk of hypoglycemia, although adverse GI effects may diminish tolerability. While addition of a GLP-1 receptor agonist may successfully control hyperglycemia, many patients will eventually require insulin therapy. Early introduction of insulin therapy should be considered when hyperglycemia is severe (e.g., blood glucose of at least 300 mg/dL or HbA$_{1c}$ exceeding 9–10%), especially in the presence of catabolic manifestations (e.g., weight loss, hypertriglyceridemia, ketosis) or symptoms of hyperglycemia. For additional information regarding the initiation of insulin therapy in patients with diabetes mellitus, see Uses: Diabetes Mellitus, in the Insulins General Statement 68:20.08.

The manufacturer states that saxagliptin is *not* indicated in patients with type 1 diabetes mellitus or for the treatment of diabetic ketoacidosis.

Saxagliptin Monotherapy

Efficacy of saxagliptin as monotherapy in treatment-naive patients with type 2 diabetes mellitus is supported by results of 2 double-blind, placebo-controlled trials of 24 weeks' duration. In these trials, saxagliptin (2.5 or 5 mg once daily) improved glycemic control as evidenced by mean reductions in glycosylated hemoglobin (hemoglobin A$_{1c}$; HbA$_{1c}$) of about 0.4–0.7% (from a mean baseline HbA$_{1c}$ of 7.9%) compared with a mean increase in HbA$_{1c}$ of about 0.2–0.3% with placebo.

Combination Therapy

Clinical trials evaluating the efficacy and safety of the *fixed combination* of saxagliptin and extended-release metformin hydrochloride (Kombiglyze® XR) in reducing HbA$_{1c}$ have not been conducted; unless otherwise specified, clinical trials of saxagliptin in combination with metformin discussed in this monograph were conducted using concomitantly administered saxagliptin and *immediate-release* metformin. Bioequivalence between the fixed combination of saxagliptin and extended-release metformin hydrochloride (Kombiglyze® XR) and each agent (saxagliptin and extended-release metformin hydrochloride) given concurrently as separate tablets has been demonstrated. (See Description.)

Efficacy of the combination of saxagliptin and metformin as *initial* therapy in patients with type 2 diabetes mellitus inadequately controlled with diet and exercise is supported by results of a 24-week randomized, active-controlled trial. In this trial, concurrent therapy with saxagliptin (5 or 10 mg once daily) and metformin hydrochloride (500 mg daily initially, titrated up to a maximum of 2 g daily given in 2 divided doses with meals) improved HbA$_{1c}$, fasting plasma glucose, and 2-hour postprandial glucose values compared with saxagliptin or metformin monotherapy. Mean reductions in HbA$_{1c}$ from baseline were 2.5% in patients receiving saxagliptin 5 mg daily plus metformin, 2.5% in patients receiving saxagliptin 10 mg daily plus metformin, 2% with metformin plus placebo, and 1.7% with saxagliptin 10 mg daily plus placebo. The proportion of patients achieving an HbA$_{1c}$ less than 7% at week 24 was approximately 60% in patients receiving saxagliptin 5 or 10 mg daily plus metformin, 32% in patients receiving saxagliptin 10 mg daily plus placebo, and 41% in patients receiving metformin plus placebo.

Efficacy of saxagliptin in combination with metformin, a sulfonylurea (glyburide), or a thiazolidinedione (pioglitazone or rosiglitazone) in patients with type 2 diabetes mellitus inadequately controlled on monotherapy with these drugs is supported by results of several long-term (24–52 weeks' duration), randomized, placebo- or active-controlled trials demonstrating improvements in HbA$_{1c}$ and fasting and/or 2-hour postprandial plasma glucose concentrations. In a trial in patients already receiving metformin hydrochloride (1.5–2.55 g daily), add-on therapy with saxagliptin (2.5 or 5 mg daily) resulted in a mean HbA$_{1c}$ decrease of about 0.6 or 0.7%, respectively, (from a mean baseline HbA$_{1c}$ of 8.1%) compared with a mean HbA$_{1c}$ increase of about 0.1% with add-on placebo. In patients receiving either pioglitazone (30–45 mg daily) or rosiglitazone (4–8 mg daily) therapy, addition of saxagliptin (2.5 or 5 mg daily) resulted in a mean HbA$_{1c}$ reduction of 0.7 or 0.9%, respectively, (from a mean baseline HbA$_{1c}$ of 8.3 or 8.4%, respectively) compared with a mean reduction of 0.3% (from a mean baseline HbA$_{1c}$ of 8.2%) with add-on placebo. In patients receiving a submaximal dosage of glyburide (7.5 mg daily as a fixed dosage), addition of saxagliptin (2.5 or 5 mg daily) resulted in a mean HbA$_{1c}$ reduction of 0.5 or 0.6%, respectively, (from a mean baseline HbA$_{1c}$ of 8.4 or 8.5%, respectively) compared with a mean increase of 0.1% with placebo added to glyburide 10 mg daily and titrated up to a maximum dosage of 15 mg daily (about 92% of patients had glyburide dosage titrated up to 15 mg daily within the initial 4 weeks of the trial).

In a 24-week trial in patients already receiving metformin and a sulfonylurea, addition of saxagliptin (5 mg once daily) resulted in a mean HbA₁c reduction of 0.7% (from a mean baseline HbA₁c of 8.4%) compared with a mean reduction of 0.1% with placebo (from a mean baseline HbA₁c of 8.2%).

In another 24-week, placebo-controlled trial in patients with inadequate glycemic control while receiving metformin hydrochloride (at least 1.5 g daily for at least 8 weeks) and dapagliflozin (10 mg daily), addition of saxagliptin (5 mg daily) resulted in greater reductions in HbA₁c from baseline compared with add-on placebo. A larger proportion of patients receiving saxagliptin add-on therapy (35.3%) achieved HbA₁c values below 7 compared with those receiving add-on placebo (23.1%).

In another trial comparing add-on therapy with saxagliptin versus add-on therapy with glipizide in patients already receiving metformin hydrochloride (1.5–3 g daily), addition of saxagliptin (5 mg daily) resulted in a mean HbA₁c reduction of 0.6% (from a mean baseline HbA₁c of 7.7%) versus a reduction of 0.7% (from a mean baseline HbA₁c of 7.6%) with add-on glipizide therapy (initial glipizide dosage of 5 mg daily, titrated up to a mean final dosage of 15 mg daily).

Efficacy of saxagliptin in combination with insulin in patients with type 2 diabetes mellitus inadequately controlled with insulin (with or without metformin) is supported by results of a 24-week, randomized, placebo-controlled trial. In this trial, addition of saxagliptin (5 mg once daily) to existing stable therapy with pre-mixed insulin or intermediate- or long-acting insulin (insulin given in combination with metformin in some patients) resulted in improvements in HbA₁c and 2-hour postprandial glucose concentrations at week 24 compared with addition of placebo. Mean reductions in HbA₁c were similar for patients receiving saxagliptin as add-on therapy with insulin alone or insulin with metformin (0.4% in both groups). The mean reduction from baseline in 2-hour postprandial glucose at week 24 was 27 mg/dL with add-on saxagliptin and 4 mg/dL with add-on placebo. The mean change from baseline in daily insulin dosage at the end of the study was 2 or 5 units with saxagliptin or placebo, respectively.

DOSAGE AND ADMINISTRATION

● Administration

When saxagliptin is administered as monotherapy or in fixed combination with dapagliflozin, the drug should be administered orally once daily without regard to meals. The fixed-combination tablets with dapagliflozin should be swallowed whole; they should not be cut, chewed, or crushed. If a dose of saxagliptin alone or in fixed combination with dapagliflozin is missed, the missed dose should be taken as soon as it is remembered followed by resumption of the regular schedule. If the missed dose is not remembered until the time of the next dose, the missed dose should be skipped and the regular schedule resumed; the dose should not be doubled to replace a missed dose.

When saxagliptin is administered in fixed combination with extended-release metformin, the combination should be administered orally once daily with the evening meal; dosage should be titrated gradually to minimize adverse GI effects of the metformin component. The fixed-combination tablets with extended-release metformin should be swallowed whole; they should not be cut, chewed, or crushed. If a dose is missed, the next dose should be taken as prescribed unless a healthcare provider instructs otherwise; an extra dose should not be taken the next day.

When saxagliptin is administered in fixed combination with extended-release metformin and dapagliflozin, the combination should be administered orally once daily in the morning with food; dosage should be individualized based on the patient's current drug regimen, effectiveness, and tolerability. The fixed-combination tablets with saxagliptin, extended-release metformin, and dapagliflozin should be swallowed whole; they should not be cut, chewed, or crushed. If a dose is missed and it is at least 12 hours before the next scheduled dose, the missed dose should be taken as soon as possible with food. If a dose is missed and it is less than 12 hours before the next scheduled dose, the missed dose should be skipped and the next dose taken at the usual time.

Patient receiving saxagliptin in fixed combination with extended-release metformin hydrochloride (Kombiglyze® XR) or with extended-release metformin hydrochloride and dapagliflozin (Qternmet® XR) should be advised that

occasionally, the inactive ingredients of the fixed-combination tablet will be eliminated in the feces as a soft, hydrated mass that may resemble the original tablet.

● Dosage

Dosage of saxagliptin hydrochloride (anhydrous) is expressed in terms of saxagliptin.

Type 2 Diabetes Mellitus

Saxagliptin Monotherapy

The recommended dosage of saxagliptin for the management of type 2 diabetes mellitus in adults is 2.5 or 5 mg once daily. In clinical trials, dosages higher than 5 mg daily (e.g., 10 mg once daily) did not provide additional benefit and are not recommended by the manufacturer.

When saxagliptin is used concomitantly with a potent inhibitor of cytochrome P-450 (CYP) isoenzymes 3A4/5 (e.g., atazanavir, clarithromycin, indinavir, itraconazole, ketoconazole, nefazodone, nelfinavir, ritonavir, saquinavir, telithromycin), dosage of saxagliptin should be limited to 2.5 mg once daily. (See Drug Interactions: Drugs Affecting or Metabolized by Hepatic Microsomal Enzymes.)

Combination Therapy with Dapagliflozin

When the fixed-combination preparation containing saxagliptin and dapagliflozin is used in patients not already receiving dapagliflozin, the recommended initial dosage is 5 mg of saxagliptin and 5 mg of dapagliflozin once daily.

If additional glycemic control is needed and the initial dosage is tolerated, the dosage may be increased to 5 mg of saxagliptin and 10 mg of dapagliflozin once daily.

The fixed combination of saxagliptin and dapagliflozin should not be used in patients receiving a potent CYP3A4/5 inhibitor. (See Drug Interactions: Drugs Affecting or Metabolized by Hepatic Microsomal Enzymes.)

Combination Therapy with Metformin Hydrochloride

Dosage of saxagliptin hydrochloride in fixed combination with extended-release metformin hydrochloride should be individualized based on the patient's current antidiabetic regimen, clinical response, and tolerability. Any change in therapy should be undertaken with caution and appropriate monitoring because changes in glycemic control can occur.

When the fixed-combination preparation containing saxagliptin and extended-release metformin hydrochloride is used in patients who have inadequate glycemic control on monotherapy with saxagliptin 5 mg daily, the recommended initial dosage of the fixed combination is 5 mg of saxagliptin and 500 mg of extended-release metformin hydrochloride once daily; dosage should be increased gradually to reduce adverse GI effects of metformin.

When the fixed-combination preparation containing saxagliptin and extended-release metformin hydrochloride is used in patients who have inadequate glycemic control on monotherapy with extended-release metformin hydrochloride, dosage of the fixed combination should provide metformin hydrochloride at the patient's current dosage, or the nearest therapeutically appropriate dosage. Following a switch from immediate-release to extended-release metformin, glycemic control should be closely monitored and dosage adjustments made accordingly.

In patients who have inadequate glycemic control on monotherapy with saxagliptin 2.5 mg daily, the recommended initial dosage of saxagliptin in fixed combination with extended-release metformin hydrochloride is 2.5 mg of saxagliptin and 1 g of extended-release metformin hydrochloride daily. Patients who require 2.5 mg of saxagliptin and who are either metformin naive or require a dose of metformin hydrochloride exceeding 1 g should use the individual components.

The maximum recommended dosage of saxagliptin in fixed combination with extended-release metformin hydrochloride is 5 mg of saxagliptin and 2 g of extended-release metformin hydrochloride daily. When this fixed-combination preparation is used concomitantly with a potent CYP3A4/5 inhibitor (e.g., atazanavir, clarithromycin, indinavir, itraconazole, ketoconazole, nefazodone, nelfinavir, ritonavir, saquinavir, telithromycin), dosage should be limited to 2.5 mg of saxagliptin and 1 g of extended-release metformin hydrochloride once daily. (See Drug Interactions: Drugs Affecting or Metabolized by Hepatic Microsomal Enzymes.)

Combination Therapy with Metformin Hydrochloride and Dapagliflozin

Dosage of saxagliptin hydrochloride in fixed combination with extended-release metformin hydrochloride and dapagliflozin should be individualized based on the patient's current antidiabetic regimen, clinical response, and tolerability.

When the fixed-combination preparation containing saxagliptin, extended-release metformin hydrochloride, and dapagliflozin is used in patients who are *not* currently receiving dapagliflozin, the recommended initial dosage is 5 mg of saxagliptin, either 1 or 2 g of extended-release metformin hydrochloride, and 5 mg of dapagliflozin once daily.

The maximum recommended dosage of saxagliptin in fixed combination with extended-release metformin hydrochloride and dapagliflozin is 5 mg of saxagliptin, 2 g of extended-release metformin hydrochloride, and 10 mg of dapagliflozin daily.

The fixed combination of saxagliptin, extended-release metformin hydrochloride, and dapagliflozin should *not* be used in patients receiving a potent CYP3A4/5 inhibitor. (See Drug Interactions: Drugs Affecting or Metabolized by Hepatic Microsomal Enzymes.)

● Special Populations

Assessment of renal function is recommended prior to initiation of saxagliptin and periodically thereafter. No dosage adjustment for saxagliptin is recommended in patients with creatinine clearance of 45 mL/minute per 1.73 m² or greater. In patients with creatinine clearance less than 45 mL/minute (including patients with moderate or severe renal impairment or with end-stage renal disease requiring hemodialysis), the recommended dosage of saxagliptin is 2.5 mg once daily regardless of meals. In patients undergoing hemodialysis, saxagliptin should be administered following the dialysis procedure. Data are lacking regarding the use of saxagliptin in patients undergoing peritoneal dialysis.

The manufacturer makes no recommendation regarding dosage adjustment of saxagliptin in patients with hepatic impairment.

No dosage adjustment is recommended for geriatric patients based solely on age; however, because of the greater frequency of decreased renal function in geriatric patients, dosage in geriatric patients should be selected with caution.

CAUTIONS

● Contraindications

Saxagliptin is contraindicated in patients with known serious hypersensitivity (e.g., anaphylaxis, angioedema, exfoliative skin reaction) to saxagliptin or any ingredient in the formulation.

● Warnings/Precautions

Pancreatitis and Pancreatic Precancerous Changes

Acute pancreatitis has been reported during postmarketing experience in patients receiving saxagliptin therapy. In a randomized, double-blind study (SAVOR) in 16,492 patients with type 2 diabetes mellitus and established atherosclerotic cardiovascular disease (ASCVD) or at high risk for the disease, acute pancreatitis was confirmed in 0.2 or 0.1% of patients receiving saxagliptin or placebo, respectively, in addition to standard care. Preexisting risk factors for pancreatitis were present in 88% of patients who developed pancreatitis while receiving saxagliptin and in 100% of those who developed pancreatitis while receiving placebo.

FDA has been evaluating unpublished findings suggesting an increased risk of pancreatitis and precancerous pancreatic cell changes (pancreatic duct metaplasia) in patients with type 2 diabetes mellitus receiving incretin mimetics (e.g., exenatide, liraglutide, sitagliptin, saxagliptin, alogliptin, linagliptin). These findings are based on examination of a small number of pancreatic tissue specimens taken from patients who died from unspecified causes while receiving an incretin mimetic. FDA will notify healthcare professionals of its conclusions and recommendations when the review is complete or when the agency has additional information to report.

FDA has recommended that clinicians continue to follow the recommendations in the prescribing information for incretin mimetics. The manufacturer states that patients receiving saxagliptin-containing therapy should be monitored for manifestations of pancreatitis. (See Advice to Patients.) If pancreatitis is suspected, saxagliptin should be promptly discontinued and appropriate management instituted. Safety and efficacy of saxagliptin have not been established in patients with a history of pancreatitis and it is not known whether such patients are at increased risk for pancreatitis with saxagliptin therapy.

Severe Arthralgia

Severe, disabling joint pain has been reported during postmarketing experience in patients receiving DPP-4 inhibitors (e.g., alogliptin, linagliptin, saxagliptin, sitagliptin). Onset of such symptoms has ranged from 1 day to years following initiation of therapy. Fever, chills, rash, and swelling accompanied joint pain in some patients, suggesting an immunologic reaction; some patients have required hospitalization. Symptoms resolved upon discontinuance of the DPP-4 inhibitor, usually in less than a month. In some patients, symptoms recurred when the same or another DPP-4 inhibitor was restarted. DPP-4 inhibitors should be considered as a possible cause of severe joint pain and should be discontinued if appropriate. (See Advice to Patients.)

Heart Failure Risk

Saxagliptin may increase the risk of heart failure, particularly in patients who have a history of heart failure or renal impairment. In a randomized, double-blind study (SAVOR) in which saxagliptin or placebo was added to standard care in 16,492 patients with type 2 diabetes mellitus and established ASCVD or at high risk for the disease, more patients receiving saxagliptin were hospitalized for heart failure than patients receiving placebo (3.5 or 2.8%, respectively). After a median of 2 years of follow-up, treatment with saxagliptin was associated with a 27% increased risk of hospitalization for heart failure; however, therapy with the drug was not associated with increased or decreased rates of cardiovascular death or other ischemic events. Patients with a history of heart failure or renal impairment had a higher risk of hospitalization for heart failure in this study regardless of treatment (saxagliptin or placebo).

The potential risks and benefits of saxagliptin therapy should be considered prior to use in patients at higher risk for heart failure (e.g., history of heart failure or renal impairment). Patients receiving saxagliptin-containing therapy should be monitored for manifestations of heart failure. (See Advice to Patients.) If heart failure develops, appropriate evaluation and management according to current standards of care should be instituted and consideration given to discontinuing saxagliptin.

Concomitant Therapy with Hypoglycemic Agents

When saxagliptin is added to therapy with an insulin secretagogue (e.g., a sulfonylurea) or insulin, the incidence of hypoglycemia is increased compared with sulfonylurea or insulin monotherapy. Therefore, patients receiving saxagliptin may require a reduced dosage of a concomitant insulin secretagogue (e.g., a sulfonylurea) or insulin to reduce the risk of hypoglycemia.

Reduction in Lymphocyte Count

Dose-related mean decreases in absolute lymphocyte count have been reported with saxagliptin dosages of 5 and 10 mg daily in clinical trials; clinical importance is not known. In most patients, recurrence of this effect was not observed with repeated exposure; however, some patients had reductions in lymphocyte count upon rechallenge that led to discontinuance of saxagliptin. Reductions in lymphocyte count were not associated with clinically relevant adverse effects. When clinically indicated (i.e., settings of unusual or prolonged infection), lymphocyte count should be measured.

Dermatologic and Sensitivity Reactions

Postmarketing cases of bullous pemphigoid requiring hospitalization have been reported with DPP-4 inhibitor use. The cases usually resolved after discontinuation of the DPP-4 inhibitor and treatment with topical or systemic immunosuppressive therapy. Patients should be advised to report the development of blisters or erosions while receiving saxagliptin. Saxagliptin should be discontinued if bullous pemphigoid is suspected, and referral of the patient to a dermatologist for diagnosis and appropriate treatment should be considered.

In a pooled analysis of data from 5 studies, hypersensitivity reactions (e.g., urticaria, facial edema) were reported in 1.5% of patients receiving saxagliptin 2.5 or 5 mg daily. In addition, there have been postmarketing reports of serious allergic and hypersensitivity reactions (e.g., anaphylaxis, angioedema, exfoliative skin conditions). The onset of such reactions usually was within the first 3 months following treatment initiation; some reactions occurred after the first dose. (See Cautions: Contraindications.)

If a serious hypersensitivity reaction is suspected, saxagliptin should be promptly discontinued, other potential causes of the event should be investigated, appropriate treatment for the reaction should be provided, and alternative antidiabetic therapy should be instituted. (See Advice to Patients.) Saxagliptin should be used with caution in patients with a history of angioedema to other dipeptidyl peptidase-4 inhibitors because it is unknown whether such patients will be predisposed to angioedema with saxagliptin.

Macrovascular Outcomes

In a pooled analysis of 8 randomized, phase 2 or 3 clinical trials (total of 4607 patients) designed to evaluate the relative risk of cardiovascular events (cardiovascular death, myocardial infarction, stroke) in patients receiving saxagliptin versus other antidiabetic agents (metformin, glyburide) or placebo, no increased cardiovascular risk was noted with saxagliptin therapy. The manufacturer states that evidence of macrovascular risk reduction with saxagliptin has not been conclusively demonstrated in clinical trials.

Use of Fixed Combinations

When saxagliptin is used in fixed combination with metformin, dapagliflozin, and/or other drugs, the cautions, precautions, contraindications, and drug interactions associated with the concomitant agent(s) should be considered in addition to those associated with saxagliptin.

Specific Populations
Pregnancy

Data on the use of saxagliptin in pregnant women are insufficient to determine a drug-associated risk for major birth defects or miscarriage. Poorly controlled diabetes mellitus in pregnancy increases the maternal risk for diabetic ketoacidosis, preeclampsia, spontaneous abortions, preterm delivery, stillbirth, and delivery complications. In addition, poorly controlled diabetes mellitus increases the fetal risk for major birth defects, stillbirth, and macrosomia-related morbidity.

No adverse developmental effects independent of maternal toxicity were observed when saxagliptin was administered to pregnant rats and rabbits during the period of organogenesis and in pregnant and lactating rats during the prenatal and postnatal period.

Lactation

Saxagliptin is distributed into milk in rats at a milk-to-plasma ratio of approximately 1:1. Data are lacking regarding the presence of saxagliptin in human milk and on the effects of the drug on the breastfed infant or on milk production. The developmental and health benefits of breastfeeding should be considered along with the mother's clinical need for saxagliptin and any potential adverse effects on the breastfed infant from saxagliptin or the underlying maternal condition.

Pediatric Use

Safety and efficacy of saxagliptin have not been established in patients younger than 18 years of age.

Geriatric Use

No substantial differences in safety and efficacy relative to younger adults have been observed, but increased sensitivity cannot be ruled out.

Saxagliptin and its active metabolite are eliminated in part by the kidneys; renal function should be assessed periodically since geriatric patients are more likely to have decreased renal function.

Hepatic Impairment

In patients with hepatic impairment (Child-Pugh class A, B, and C), mean peak concentrations and area under the plasma concentration-time curve (AUC) of saxagliptin were increased by up to 8 and 77%, respectively, compared with healthy individuals following a single 10-mg dose of the drug; peak concentrations and AUC of the active metabolite were increased by up to 59 and 33%, respectively. These differences were not considered clinically important.

Renal Impairment

Renal function should be assessed prior to initiation of saxagliptin therapy and periodically thereafter. Adjustment of saxagliptin dosage is recommended when the drug is used in patients with moderate (eGFR 30 to less than 45 mL/minute per 1.73 m^2) or severe renal impairment (eGFR 15 to less than 30 mL/minute per

1.73 m^2) or end-stage renal disease requiring hemodialysis. The fixed combination of saxagliptin and extended-release metformin is contraindicated in patients with severe renal impairment (eGFR less than 30 mL/minute per 1.73 m^2).

● Common Adverse Effects

In clinical trials, the incidence of hypoglycemic adverse reactions in patients receiving saxagliptin was based on all reports of hypoglycemia, although a concurrent glucose measurement was not required or was normal in some patients with reported hypoglycemic reactions; therefore, it is not possible to determine conclusively whether all these reports represent true hypoglycemic events. In the clinical trial in which saxagliptin or placebo was added to insulin therapy (with or without metformin), (see Uses: Type 2 Diabetes Mellitus) the incidence of adverse effects (except for confirmed hypoglycemia) was similar with add-on saxagliptin and add-on placebo. However, the incidence of confirmed hypoglycemia (as determined by fingerstick blood glucose of 50 mg/dL or less) in this trial was higher with saxagliptin 5 mg daily (5.3%) than with placebo (3.3%).

Adverse effects reported in at least 5% of patients in clinical trials receiving saxagliptin 5 mg daily as monotherapy or in combination with metformin, a thiazolidinedione (pioglitazone or rosiglitazone), or glyburide and more frequently than with placebo include upper respiratory tract infection, urinary tract infection, and headache.

Adverse effects reported in at least 5% of patients in clinical trials receiving saxagliptin in combination with immediate-release metformin and more frequently than with metformin alone include headache and nasopharyngitis.

DRUG INTERACTIONS

● Drugs Affecting or Metabolized by Hepatic Microsomal Enzymes

Saxagliptin and its active metabolite do not inhibit cytochrome P-450 (CYP) isoenzymes 1A2, 2A6, 2B6, 2C9, 2C19, 2D6, 2E1, or 3A4 and do not induce CYP1A2, 2B6, 2C9, or 3A4 in vitro. Pharmacokinetic interactions with drugs metabolized by these isoenzymes are unlikely.

Saxagliptin is metabolized principally via CYP3A4 and CYP3A5. Administration of a single dose of saxagliptin (100 mg) to healthy individuals receiving ketoconazole (200 mg every 12 hours for 9 days) decreased the peak steady-state plasma concentration and area under the plasma concentration-time curve (AUC) of ketoconazole by 16 and 13%, respectively, and increased the peak plasma concentration and AUC of saxagliptin by 62 and 145% (2.5-fold), respectively. Similar increases in saxagliptin plasma concentrations and AUC are anticipated with concomitant use of saxagliptin and other potent CYP3A4/5 inhibitors (e.g., atazanavir, clarithromycin, indinavir, itraconazole, nefazodone, nelfinavir, ritonavir, saquinavir, telithromycin). Saxagliptin dosage should be limited to 2.5 mg daily when the drug is used concomitantly with a potent CYP3A4/5 inhibitor.

● Inhibitors of P-glycoprotein Transport System

Saxagliptin is a substrate of the P-glycoprotein transport system but does not appreciably induce or inhibit P-glycoprotein.

● Antacids

Concurrent administration of a single dose of saxagliptin (10 mg) and a single dose of liquid antacid containing aluminum hydroxide (2.4 g), magnesium hydroxide (2.4 g), and simethicone (240 mg) decreased peak plasma concentrations of saxagliptin by 26% and AUC by 3%. The manufacturer states that no dosage adjustments are required with concurrent use.

● Dapagliflozin

Coadministration of saxagliptin (5-mg single dose) and dapagliflozin (10-mg single dose) decreased the AUC and peak plasma concentration of saxagliptin by 1 and 7%, respectively, and increased the AUC and peak plasma concentration of its active metabolite 5-hydroxy saxagliptin by 9 and 6%, respectively. The manufacturer states that no dosage adjustments are required with concomitant use.

● Digoxin

Concurrent administration of saxagliptin (10 mg once daily for 7 days) and digoxin (0.25 mg every 6 hours the first day, then 0.25 mg every 12 hours the second day, then 0.25 mg once daily for 5 days), a P-glycoprotein substrate, increased the AUC and peak plasma concentration of digoxin by 6 and 9%, respectively; the AUC of saxagliptin was increased by 5% and peak plasma saxagliptin concentrations decreased by 1%. The manufacturer states that no dosage adjustments are required with concurrent use.

● **Diltiazem**

Concurrent administration of saxagliptin (10-mg single dose) and a long-acting formulation of diltiazem (360 mg daily for 9 days) increased the peak steady-state plasma concentration of diltiazem by 16% and the AUC by 10%; in addition, peak plasma saxagliptin concentrations increased by 63% and saxagliptin AUC was increased by 2.1-fold. The manufacturer states that no dosage adjustments are required with concurrent use.

● **Famotidine**

Administration of a single dose of saxagliptin (10 mg) concurrently with a single dose of famotidine (40 mg) increased the peak plasma concentration of saxagliptin by 14% and AUC by 3%. The manufacturer states that no dosage adjustments are required with concurrent use.

● **Hormonal Contraceptives**

Concurrent administration of saxagliptin (5 mg once daily for 21 days) and an estrogen-progestin combination contraceptive (ethinyl estradiol 35 mcg in fixed combination with norgestimate 0.25 mg once daily for 21 days) did not appreciably alter the steady-state pharmacokinetics of ethinyl estradiol or the primary active progestin component, norelgestromin. The mean AUC and peak plasma concentration of norgestrel, an active metabolite of norelgestromin, were increased by 13 and 17%, respectively, which is not considered clinically important. The manufacturer states that no dosage adjustments are required with concurrent use.

● **Metformin**

Concomitant administration of a single dose of saxagliptin (100 mg) and metformin hydrochloride (1 g) decreased the peak plasma concentration of saxagliptin by 21% and the AUC by 2%; metformin AUC and peak plasma concentration were increased by 20 and 9%, respectively. The manufacturer states that no dosage adjustments are required with concurrent use.

● **Omeprazole**

Concurrent administration of saxagliptin (10 mg daily) and omeprazole (40 mg daily for 5 days) increased saxagliptin AUC by 13% and decreased peak plasma concentrations of the drug by 2%. The manufacturer states that no dosage adjustments are required with concurrent use.

● **Pioglitazone**

Concurrent administration of saxagliptin (10 mg once daily for 5 days) and pioglitazone (45 mg daily for 10 days) increased the peak plasma concentration of pioglitazone by 14% and the AUC by 8%. In addition, the AUC and peak plasma concentration of saxagliptin were each increased by 11%. The manufacturer states that no dosage adjustments are required with concurrent use.

● **Rifampin**

Concomitant administration of a single dose of saxagliptin (5 mg) with rifampin (600 mg daily for 6 days) decreased peak steady-state plasma concentrations and AUC of saxagliptin by 53 and 76%, respectively, while peak plasma concentration of the active metabolite was increased by 39%; there was no appreciable change in the AUC of the active metabolite of saxagliptin. The manufacturer states that no dosage adjustments are required with concurrent use.

● **Simvastatin**

Concomitant administration of saxagliptin (10 mg once daily for 4 days) and simvastatin (40 mg once daily for 8 days) increased the peak plasma concentration and AUC of saxagliptin by 21 and 12%, respectively, while simvastatin peak plasma concentrations were reduced by 12% and AUC was increased by 4%. The manufacturer states that no dosage adjustments are required with concurrent use.

● **Sulfonylureas**

Concomitant administration of single doses of saxagliptin (10 mg) and glyburide (5 mg) increased peak plasma concentrations of glyburide and saxagliptin by

16 and 8%, respectively; the AUC of glyburide was increased by 6% and that of saxagliptin was decreased by 2%. The manufacturer states that no dosage adjustments are required because of changes in systemic exposures when saxagliptin and glyburide are given concomitantly. However, in patients receiving saxagliptin concomitantly with a sulfonylurea antidiabetic agent, a reduced dosage of the sulfonylurea may be required to reduce the risk of hypoglycemia.

DESCRIPTION

Saxagliptin inhibits dipeptidyl peptidase-4 (DPP-4), an enzyme that inactivates incretin hormones glucagon-like peptide-1 (GLP-1) and glucose-dependent insulinotropic polypeptide (GIP). Both saxagliptin and its active metabolite (5-hydroxy saxagliptin) are more selective for inhibition of DPP-4 than for DPP-8 or DPP-9. Saxagliptin increases circulating levels of GLP-1 and GIP in a glucose-dependent manner.

GLP-1 and GIP stimulate insulin secretion from pancreatic β-cells in a glucose-dependent manner (i.e., when glucose concentrations are normal or elevated). GLP-1 also decreases glucagon secretion from pancreatic α-cells, leading to reduced hepatic glucose production.

Saxagliptin lowers fasting plasma glucose concentrations and reduces glucose excursions following a glucose load or meal in patients with type 2 diabetes mellitus.

Saxagliptin monotherapy usually is not associated with substantial changes in body weight.

Saxagliptin did not produce a clinically meaningful prolongation of the QT interval corrected for rate (QT$_c$) or heart rate at daily dosages up to 40 mg (8 times the maximum recommended human dose) in a randomized, double-blind, placebo-controlled, crossover active-comparator study using moxifloxacin in healthy individuals.

Following oral administration of a single dose of saxagliptin under fasted conditions, the median time to peak plasma concentration was 2 hours for saxagliptin and 4 hours for 5-hydroxy saxagliptin. Administration of saxagliptin with a high-fat meal increased the area under the plasma concentration-time curve (AUC) by 27% and delayed the time to peak plasma concentration by approximately 20 minutes. In vitro binding of saxagliptin and 5-hydroxy saxagliptin to serum proteins is negligible. Metabolism of saxagliptin is principally mediated by cytochrome P-450 (CYP) 3A4 and 3A5 isoenzymes. Mean plasma half-life of saxagliptin or 5-hydroxy saxagliptin is 2.5 or 3.1 hours, respectively. Saxagliptin is eliminated by both renal and hepatic pathways; following administration of a single radiolabeled dose, 75% of the dose was excreted in urine (including 24% as unchanged drug and 36% as 5-hydroxy saxagliptin). A total of 22% of administered radioactivity was recovered in feces, representing the fraction of the saxagliptin dose excreted in bile and/or unabsorbed drug from the GI tract.

Bioequivalence between the fixed combination of saxagliptin and extended-release metformin hydrochloride (Kombiglyze® XR) and each agent (saxagliptin and *extended-release* metformin hydrochloride) given concurrently as separate tablets has been demonstrated; however, the relative bioavailability of the fixed combination of saxagliptin and extended-release metformin hydrochloride (Kombiglyze® XR) and concomitantly administered saxagliptin and *immediate-release* metformin hydrochloride has not been established. Metformin immediate-release and extended-release tablets have a similar extent of absorption (AUC), but peak plasma concentrations of metformin following administration of the drug as extended-release tablets are approximately 20% lower than peak concentrations following administration of the same dose as immediate-release tablets.

ADVICE TO PATIENTS

Importance of patients reading medication guide before initiating therapy and each time the drug is dispensed.

Importance of informing patients of the potential risks and benefits of saxagliptin and of alternative therapies. Importance of not using saxagliptin in patients with type 1 diabetes mellitus or diabetic ketoacidosis.

Importance of informing patients about the possibility of acute pancreatitis, which may be severe or fatal, with saxagliptin therapy. Importance of patients advising clinicians about a history of pancreatitis, gallstones, alcoholism, or high triglyceride levels. Importance of informing patients about signs and symptoms of pancreatitis, including persistent severe abdominal pain sometimes radiating to the back that may or may not be accompanied by vomiting; importance of patient discontinuing saxagliptin and promptly notifying clinician if such signs or symptoms are present.

Importance of informing patients of the possibility of severe and disabling joint pain with DPP-4 inhibitors (e.g., alogliptin, linagliptin, saxagliptin, sitagliptin). Advise patients to contact a clinician promptly if severe and persistent joint pain occurs; patients should not discontinue the drug without consulting their clinician.

Importance of promptly informing clinician if skin blisters or erosion (breakdown of the outer layer of skin) occurs.

Importance of informing patients about possibility of heart failure with saxagliptin therapy. Importance of clinicians asking patients about a history of heart failure or renal impairment prior to initiating saxagliptin therapy. Importance of informing patients about signs and symptoms of heart failure (e.g., shortness of breath, unusual tiredness, rapid weight gain, edema especially in the feet, ankles, or legs); importance of patients immediately contacting a clinician if manifestations of heart failure occur.

Importance of informing clinician if hypoglycemia occurs, particularly if concomitant therapy with a sulfonylurea antidiabetic agent (i.e., insulin secretagogue) or insulin is used; a lower dosage of the sulfonylurea or insulin may be required in such cases.

Importance of informing patients about the importance of adherence to dietary instructions, regular physical activity, periodic blood glucose monitoring and glycosylated hemoglobin (hemoglobin A_{1c}; HbA_{1c}) testing, recognition and management of hypoglycemia and hyperglycemia, and assessment of diabetes complications.

Importance of seeking medical advice promptly during periods of stress such as fever, trauma, infection, or surgery as medication requirements may change.

Importance of informing patients that response to all diabetic therapies should be monitored by periodic measurements of blood glucose and HbA_{1c}, with a goal of decreasing these levels toward the normal range.

Importance of informing patients of the potential need to adjust their dosage based on changes in renal function over time.

Importance of informing their clinician if any unusual symptom develops or if any existing symptom persists or worsens.

Risk of serious allergic (hypersensitivity) reactions, such as angioedema, anaphylaxis, and exfoliative skin conditions. If signs or symptoms of such reactions occur (e.g., rash, skin flaking or peeling, hives, swelling of the skin, swelling of the face, lips, tongue, and throat that may cause difficulty in breathing or swallowing), importance of discontinuing saxagliptin-containing therapy and informing clinician promptly.

Importance of advising patient not to split or cut saxagliptin tablets. Importance of swallowing saxagliptin/metformin tablets whole and not cutting, crushing, or chewing them. Importance of advising patients receiving saxagliptin/ metformin that occasionally the inactive components of the tablet may remain intact and be passed in the stool as a soft, hydrated mass resembling the original tablet.

Importance of taking saxagliptin exactly as directed by clinician. Importance of informing patients that if they miss a dose, they should take the dose as soon as it is remembered unless it is almost time for the next dose. In that case, the missed dose should be skipped and the next dose taken at the regular time; patients should not take 2 doses at the same time unless instructed to do so by their clinician.

Importance of women informing their clinicians if they are or plan to become pregnant or plan to breast-feed.

Importance of informing clinicians of existing or contemplated concomitant therapy, including prescription (e.g., antibiotics, antifungals, antiretrovirals) and OTC drugs and dietary or herbal supplements, as well as any concomitant illnesses (e.g., allergies, kidney disease).

Importance of informing patients of other important precautionary information. (See Cautions.)

PREPARATIONS

Excipients in commercially available drug preparations may have clinically important effects in some individuals; consult specific product labeling for details.

sAXagliptin Hydrochloride

Oral

Tablets, film-coated	2.5 mg (of saxagliptin)	Onglyza®, Astra Zeneca
	5 mg (of saxagliptin)	Onglyza®, Astra Zeneca

sAXagliptin Hydrochloride Combinations

Oral

Tablets, extended-release	2.5 mg (of saxagliptin) with Metformin Hydrochloride extended-release 1 g	Kombiglyze® XR, AstraZeneca
	2.5 mg (of saxagliptin) with Metformin Hydrochloride extended-release 1 g and Dapagliflozin Propanediol 2.5 mg (of dapagliflozin)	Qternmet® XR, AstraZeneca
	2.5 mg (of saxagliptin) with Metformin Hydrochloride extended-release 1 g and Dapagliflozin Propanediol 5 mg (of dapagliflozin)	Qternmet® XR, AstraZeneca
	5 mg (of saxagliptin) with Metformin Hydrochloride extended-release 500 mg	Kombiglyze® XR, AstraZeneca
	5 mg (of saxagliptin) with Metformin Hydrochloride extended-release 1 g	Kombiglyze® XR, AstraZeneca
	5 mg (of saxagliptin) with Metformin Hydrochloride extended-release 1 g and Dapagliflozin Propanediol 5 mg (of dapagliflozin)	Qternmet® XR, AstraZeneca
	5 mg (of saxagliptin) with Metformin Hydrochloride extended-release 1 g and Dapagliflozin Propanediol 10 mg (of dapagliflozin)	Qternmet® XR, AstraZeneca
Tablets, film-coated	5 mg (of saxagliptin) with Dapagliflozin Propanediol 5 mg (of dapagliflozin)	Qtern®, AstraZeneca
	5 mg (of saxagliptin) with Dapagliflozin Propanediol 10 mg (of dapagliflozin)	Qtern®, AstraZeneca

Selected Revisions June 21, 2021, © Copyright, December 9, 2011, American Society of Health-System Pharmacists, Inc.

SITagliptin Phosphate

68:20.05 • DIPEPTIDYL PEPTIDASE IV (DPP-4) INHIBITORS

■ Sitagliptin phosphate, a dipeptidyl peptidase-4 (DPP-4) inhibitor, is an antidiabetic agent.

USES

● Type 2 Diabetes Mellitus

Sitagliptin is used as monotherapy as an adjunct to diet and exercise to improve glycemic control in patients with type 2 diabetes mellitus. Sitagliptin is used as initial therapy in combination with immediate- or extended-release metformin hydrochloride (given separately or as the fixed combination) as an adjunct to diet and exercise to improve glycemic control in patients with type 2 diabetes mellitus when treatment with both sitagliptin and metformin is appropriate. Sitagliptin also is used in fixed combination with ertugliflozin L-pyroglutamic acid (Steglujan®) as an adjunct to diet and exercise to improve glycemic control in patients with type 2 diabetes mellitus when treatment with both drugs is appropriate. Sitagliptin also may be used in combination with other oral antidiabetic agents (e.g., metformin, a sulfonylurea, a thiazolidinedione [peroxisome proliferator-activated receptor$_\gamma$ agonist]) or insulin as an adjunct to diet and exercise in patients with type 2 diabetes mellitus who have not achieved adequate glycemic control with one or more oral antidiabetic agents and/or insulin.

Current guidelines for the treatment of type 2 diabetes mellitus generally recommend metformin as first-line therapy in addition to lifestyle modifications in patients with recent-onset type 2 diabetes mellitus or mild hyperglycemia because of its well-established safety and efficacy (i.e., beneficial effects on glycosylated hemoglobin [hemoglobin A_{1c}; HbA_{1c}], weight, and cardiovascular mortality). (See Uses: Type 2 Diabetes Mellitus, in Metformin 68:20.04.) In patients with contraindications or intolerance to metformin (e.g., risk of lactic acidosis, GI intolerance) or in selected other patients, some experts suggest that initial therapy with a drug from another class of antidiabetic agents (e.g., a glucagon-like peptide-1 [GLP-1] receptor agonist, sodium-glucose cotransporter 2 [SGLT2] inhibitor, DPP-4 inhibitor, sulfonylurea, thiazolidinedione, basal insulin) may be acceptable based on patient factors. Initiating antidiabetic therapy with 2 agents (e.g., metformin plus another drug) may be appropriate in patients with an initial HbA_{1c} exceeding 7.5% or at least 1.5% above the target level. In metformin-intolerant patients with high initial HbA_{1c} levels, some experts suggest initiation of therapy with 2 agents from other antidiabetic drug classes with complementary mechanisms of action.

Because of the progressive nature of type 2 diabetes mellitus, patients initially receiving an oral antidiabetic agent will eventually require multiple oral and/or injectable noninsulin antidiabetic agents of different therapeutic classes and/or insulin for adequate glycemic control. Patients who have inadequate glycemic control with initial (e.g., metformin) monotherapy should receive treatment with additional antidiabetic agents; data suggest that the addition of each noninsulin agent to initial therapy lowers HbA_{1c} by approximately 0.7–1%. In addition, early initiation of combination therapy may help to more rapidly attain glycemic goals and extend the time to treatment failure.

Factors to consider when selecting additional antidiabetic agents for combination therapy in patients with inadequate glycemic control on metformin monotherapy include patient comorbidities (e.g., atherosclerotic cardiovascular disease [ASCVD], established kidney disease, heart failure), hypoglycemia risk, impact on weight, cost, risk of adverse effects, and patient preference. Some experts recommend DPP-4 inhibitors as one of several classes of drugs for use in combination therapy, particularly in patients with both postprandial and fasting plasma glucose elevations. When the greater glucose-lowering effect of an injectable drug is needed in patients with type 2 diabetes mellitus, some experts currently state that an injectable GLP-1 receptor agonist is preferred over insulin in most patients because of beneficial effects on body weight and a lower risk of hypoglycemia, although adverse GI effects may diminish tolerability. While addition of a GLP-1 receptor agonist may successfully control hyperglycemia, many patients will eventually require insulin therapy. Early introduction of insulin therapy should be considered when hyperglycemia is severe (e.g., blood glucose of at least 300 mg/dL or HbA_{1c} exceeding 9–10%), especially in the presence of catabolic manifestations (e.g., weight loss, hypertriglyceridemia, ketosis) or symptoms of hyperglycemia. For additional information regarding the initiation of insulin therapy in patients with diabetes mellitus, see Uses: Diabetes Mellitus, in the Insulins General Statement 68:20.08.

The manufacturer states that sitagliptin should *not* be used in patients with type 1 diabetes mellitus or for the treatment of diabetic ketoacidosis.

Sitagliptin Monotherapy

Efficacy of sitagliptin as monotherapy for the management of type 2 diabetes mellitus is supported by results of 2 controlled trials of 18 or 24 weeks' duration. Sitagliptin (100 or 200 mg once daily) improved glycemic control, as evidenced by reductions in glycosylated hemoglobin (hemoglobin A_{1c} [HbA_{1c}]) as well as fasting and 2-hour postprandial plasma glucose concentrations, compared with placebo. HbA_{1c} was reduced by 0.5–0.6% (from an average baseline value of about 8%) in patients receiving sitagliptin 100 mg daily, compared with an increase of 0.1–0.2% in those receiving placebo. Overall, use of a higher than recommended dosage of sitagliptin (200 mg daily) did not provide greater glycemic control than did the recommended dosage of 100 mg daily.

Combination Therapy

Efficacy of the combination of sitagliptin and metformin as *initial* therapy in patients with type 2 diabetes mellitus inadequately controlled with diet and exercise is supported by results of a 24-week randomized, placebo-controlled trial. In this trial, patients receiving initial therapy with sitagliptin (50 mg twice daily) in combination with metformin hydrochloride (500 mg or 1 g twice daily) had greater improvements in HbA_{1c}, fasting plasma glucose, and 2-hour postprandial glucose concentrations than those receiving placebo, metformin monotherapy, or sitagliptin monotherapy. Mean reductions in HbA_{1c} from baseline in patients not receiving an antihyperglycemic agent at trial entry were 1.1% with sitagliptin 100 mg once daily, 1.1% with metformin hydrochloride 500 mg twice daily, 1.2% with metformin hydrochloride 1 g twice daily, 1.6% with sitagliptin 50 mg twice daily in combination with metformin hydrochloride 500 mg twice daily, 1.9% with sitagliptin 50 mg twice daily in combination with metformin hydrochloride 1g twice daily, and 0.2% with placebo. In the same study, patients with more severe hyperglycemia (HbA_{1c} exceeding 11% or blood glucose exceeding 280 mg/dL) who received sitagliptin (50 mg twice daily) in combination with metformin hydrochloride (1 g twice daily) on an open-label basis achieved mean reductions from baseline of 2.9% in HbA_{1c}, 127 mg/dL in fasting plasma glucose, and 208 mg/dL in 2-hour postprandial glucose by the end of the trial (at 24 weeks).

In another 24-week, randomized trial in patients who had inadequate glycemic control with diet and exercise, *initial* therapy with the combination of sitagliptin (100 mg once daily) and pioglitazone (30 mg once daily) produced greater improvements in HbA_{1c}, fasting plasma glucose, and 2-hour postprandial glucose concentrations than pioglitazone monotherapy (30 mg once daily). In this trial, patients receiving the sitagliptin/pioglitazone combination achieved a 0.9% mean reduction in HbA_{1c} compared with those receiving pioglitazone monotherapy, and 60% of patients receiving sitagliptin/pioglitazone achieved a mean HbA_{1c} less than 7%, compared with 28% of those receiving pioglitazone monotherapy.

Efficacy and safety of the fixed combination of sitagliptin and metformin have been established based on concurrent administration of the 2 agents given separately and extrapolations from clinical trials evaluating sitagliptin as add-on therapy to metformin. Bioequivalence has been demonstrated between the fixed combination of sitagliptin and metformin hydrochloride and the drugs administered concurrently as separate tablets.

Efficacy of sitagliptin in combination with metformin, a sulfonylurea, and/or a thiazolidinedione in the management of type 2 diabetes mellitus (in patients inadequately controlled with metformin or thiazolidinedione monotherapy) is supported by results from several long-term (24 weeks' duration), randomized, placebo-controlled trials. In these trials, the addition of sitagliptin (100 mg once daily) to existing metformin and/or glimepiride therapy or to pioglitazone or rosiglitazone/metformin therapy improved glycemic control, as evidenced by reductions in HbA_{1c} as well as fasting and/or 2-hour postprandial plasma glucose concentrations, compared with placebo or existing therapy. In patients receiving metformin hydrochloride therapy (dosage of at least 1.5 g daily), the addition of sitagliptin resulted in a reduction of 0.7% in HbA_{1c}, while the addition of placebo resulted in no appreciable change in HbA_{1c}. In patients receiving glimepiride therapy (dosage of at least 4 mg daily), the addition of sitagliptin resulted in a reduction of 0.6% in HbA$_{1c}$ compared with addition of placebo. In patients receiving glimepiride (dosage of at least 4 mg daily) in combination with metformin hydrochloride (dosage of at least 1.5 g daily), the addition of sitagliptin resulted in a reduction of 0.9% in HbA$_{1c}$ compared with addition of placebo. In patients receiving pioglitazone therapy (30–45 mg daily), the addition of sitagliptin or placebo resulted in reductions of 0.9 or 0.2%, respectively, in HbA$_{1c}$. In patients receiving metformin and rosiglitazone therapy in a 54-week trial, addition of sitagliptin 100 mg once daily or placebo resulted in mean reductions in HbA$_{1c}$ of 1 or 0.3%, respectively; sulfonylurea (e.g., glipizide) rescue therapy was used in 18 or 40% of patients receiving sitagliptin or placebo, respectively. In a 52-week noninferiority trial in patients receiving metformin hydrochloride (dosage of at least 1.5 g daily), add-on therapy with sitagliptin (100 mg once daily) or glipizide (5–20 mg once daily; mean 10 mg once daily) was associated with similar mean reductions from baseline in HbA$_{1c}$ (intent-to-treat analysis); results may be applicable principally to patients with baseline HbA$_{1c}$ values less than 8–9%, comparable to those of this study population.

Efficacy and safety of the combination of sitagliptin and ertugliflozin (as initial or add-on therapy) for the management of type 2 diabetes mellitus have been established in several randomized, placebo-controlled and active comparator trials. In a 26-week, randomized, double-blind trial, concomitant therapy with sitagliptin (100 mg daily) and ertugliflozin (5 or 15 mg once daily) given as initial therapy in patients with type 2 diabetes mellitus inadequately controlled with diet and exercise substantially improved glycemic control (as evidenced by reductions in HbA$_{1c}$) compared with placebo. Reductions in HbA$_{1c}$ were 1.6 or 1.7% with ertugliflozin 5 or 15 mg once daily, respectively, plus sitagliptin and 0.4% with placebo. Additionally, a greater proportion of patients receiving sitagliptin and ertugliflozin combination therapy achieved an HbA$_{1c}$ of less than 7%, and greater reductions in fasting plasma glucose were observed with ertugliflozin and sitagliptin combination therapy compared with placebo.

In a trial evaluating the safety and efficacy of ertugliflozin in combination with sitagliptin in adults with type 2 diabetes mellitus inadequately controlled with metformin hydrochloride monotherapy (dosage of at least 1.5 g daily), the addition of ertugliflozin and sitagliptin combination therapy to existing metformin therapy substantially improved glycemic control compared with the addition of either ertugliflozin or sitagliptin alone. In this trial, patients received ertugliflozin 5 mg, ertugliflozin 15 mg, sitagliptin 100 mg, ertugliflozin 5 mg and sitagliptin 100 mg, or ertugliflozin 15 mg and sitagliptin 100 mg once daily. At week 26, patients who received concomitant therapy with ertugliflozin 5 or 15 mg and sitagliptin 100 mg had greater reductions in HbA$_{1c}$ (reduction of 1.4%) compared with those receiving ertugliflozin or sitagliptin alone (reduction of 1%). Additionally, a higher proportion of patients who received ertugliflozin 5 or 15 mg and sitagliptin 100 mg as an add-on to existing metformin therapy achieved an HbA$_{1c}$ of less than 7% (53 or 51%, respectively) compared with those who received ertugliflozin 5 or 15 mg or sitagliptin 100 mg alone (29, 34, or 39%, respectively).

Efficacy of sitagliptin in combination with insulin (with or without metformin) in the management of type 2 diabetes mellitus in patients who have inadequate glycemic control with insulin is supported by results of a 24-week, randomized, placebo-controlled trial. In this trial, addition of sitagliptin (100 mg once daily) to existing stable insulin (premixed insulin or intermediate- or long-acting insulin) therapy with or without metformin hydrochloride (dosage of at least 1.5 g daily) resulted in improvements in HbA$_{1c}$, fasting plasma glucose, and 2-hour postprandial glucose concentrations compared with addition of placebo. In patients who received sitagliptin as add-on therapy to metformin and insulin, 14% had HbA$_{1c}$ reductions to less than 7% compared with 5% of those receiving add-on placebo with metformin and insulin. Among patients also receiving metformin, the median daily dosage of insulin at baseline for patients treated with sitagliptin or placebo was 40 or 42 units, respectively; the median daily insulin dosage for both groups at the end of the study was unchanged. Patients in both treatment groups gained a mean of 0.1 kg of body weight over the study period; hypoglycemia was more common in patients receiving add-on sitagliptin therapy.

DOSAGE AND ADMINISTRATION

● General

The dosage of sitagliptin/metformin hydrochloride in fixed combination should be individualized according to clinician judgment based on the patient's current antidiabetic regimen, clinical response, and tolerability. Any change in therapy

should be undertaken with care and appropriate monitoring because changes in glycemic control can occur.

In patients receiving the fixed combination of sitagliptin and ertugliflozin, volume depletion should be corrected prior to initiating therapy.

● Administration

When sitagliptin is administered as monotherapy, the drug should be administered orally once daily with or without food. If a dose is missed, the missed dose should be taken as soon as it is remembered followed by resumption of the regular schedule. If the missed dose is remembered at the time of the next dose, the missed dose should be skipped and the regular schedule resumed. The dose should not be doubled to replace a missed dose.

When sitagliptin is administered in fixed combination with immediate-release metformin hydrochloride, the combination should be administered orally twice daily with meals, increasing dosage gradually to minimize the adverse GI effects of the metformin component. If a dose is missed, the missed dose should be taken with a meal as soon as it is remembered followed by resumption of the regular schedule. If a missed dose is not remembered until the time of the next dose, the missed dose should be skipped and the regular schedule resumed. The dose should not be doubled to replace a missed dose.

The manufacturer states that tablets of the fixed combination of sitagliptin and immediate- or extended-release metformin hydrochloride must not be split or divided before swallowing.

The fixed combination of sitagliptin and ertugliflozin should be administered orally once daily in the morning with or without food. If a dose of the fixed combination of sitagliptin and ertugliflozin is missed, the missed dose should be taken as soon as it is remembered followed by resumption of the regular schedule. If the missed dose is not remembered until the time of the next dose, the missed dose should be skipped and the regular schedule resumed; the dose should not be doubled to replace a missed dose.

● Dosage

Sitagliptin phosphate is commercially available as the monohydrate; dosage is expressed in terms of sitagliptin.

Type 2 Diabetes Mellitus

Sitagliptin Monotherapy

The recommended dosage of sitagliptin for the management of type 2 diabetes mellitus in adults is 100 mg once daily. In clinical trials, higher dosages of sitagliptin (200 mg daily) did not provide additional glycemic benefit, and the manufacturer states that 100 mg daily is the maximum recommended dosage.

Sitagliptin/Immediate-release Metformin Hydrochloride Fixed-combination Therapy

Dosage of sitagliptin in fixed combination with immediate-release metformin hydrochloride should be individualized based on the patient's current antidiabetic regimen, effectiveness, and tolerability. In patients not currently receiving metformin hydrochloride, the recommended initial dosage is 50 mg of sitagliptin and 500 mg of immediate-release metformin hydrochloride twice daily as the fixed combination, with gradual dosage escalation to reduce adverse GI effects associated with the metformin hydrochloride component.

When the fixed combination of sitagliptin and immediate-release metformin hydrochloride is used in patients currently receiving metformin hydrochloride, the recommended initial dosage is 50 mg of sitagliptin and 500 mg of metformin hydrochloride twice daily or 50 mg of sitagliptin and 1 g of metformin hydrochloride twice daily, depending on the patient's existing dosage of metformin hydrochloride. In patients currently receiving immediate-release metformin hydrochloride 850 mg twice daily, the recommended initial dosage is 50 mg of sitagliptin and 1 g of immediate-release metformin hydrochloride twice daily as the fixed combination.

The maximum recommended daily dosage of the fixed combination containing sitagliptin and immediate-release metformin hydrochloride is 100 mg of sitagliptin and 2 g of immediate-release metformin hydrochloride.

The same total daily dosage of sitagliptin and metformin hydrochloride should be maintained when transitioning between the fixed combination of sitagliptin and immediate-release metformin hydrochloride and the fixed combination of sitagliptin and extended-release metformin hydrochloride.

Sitagliptin/Extended-release Metformin Hydrochloride Fixed-combination Therapy

Dosage of sitagliptin in fixed combination with extended-release metformin hydrochloride should be individualized based on the patient's current antidiabetic regimen, effectiveness, and tolerability. In patients *not* currently receiving metformin hydrochloride, the recommended initial dosage of the fixed combination is 100 mg of sitagliptin and 1 g of extended-release metformin hydrochloride once daily, with gradual dosage escalation to reduce adverse GI effects associated with the metformin hydrochloride component.

When the fixed combination of sitagliptin and metformin hydrochloride is used in patients *currently receiving* metformin hydrochloride, the recommended initial dosage is 100 mg of sitagliptin and 1 g of extended-release metformin hydrochloride once daily or 100 mg of sitagliptin and 2 g of extended-release metformin hydrochloride once daily, depending on the patient's existing dosage of metformin hydrochloride. In patients currently receiving metformin hydrochloride 850 mg or 1 g twice daily, the recommended initial dosage of the fixed combination is 100 mg of sitagliptin and 2 g of metformin hydrochloride once daily.

The maximum recommended daily dosage of the fixed combination containing sitagliptin and extended-release metformin hydrochloride is 100 mg of sitagliptin and 2 g of extended-release metformin hydrochloride.

The same total daily dosage of sitagliptin and metformin hydrochloride should be maintained when transitioning between the fixed combination of sitagliptin and *immediate-release* metformin hydrochloride and the fixed combination of sitagliptin and *extended-release* metformin hydrochloride.

Sitagliptin/Ertugliflozin Fixed-combination Therapy

The recommended initial dosage of the fixed combination of sitagliptin and ertugliflozin is 100 mg of sitagliptin and 5 mg of ertugliflozin once daily in the morning with or without food. If tolerated, the dosage may be increased to a maximum of 100 mg of sitagliptin and 15 mg of ertugliflozin once daily in patients who require additional glycemic control.

In patients currently receiving ertugliflozin and switching to the fixed combination of sitagliptin and ertugliflozin, the current dosage of ertugliflozin can be maintained.

Combination Therapy with Sitagliptin and Other Oral Antidiabetic Agents or Insulin Given as Separate Components

When given in combination with metformin hydrochloride as separate tablets, a sitagliptin dosage of 100 mg once daily has been used.

When given as separate tablets in combination with a sulfonylurea with or without metformin hydrochloride, a sitagliptin dosage of 100 mg once daily has been used. Dosage of the concomitant sulfonylurea may need to be reduced to decrease risk of hypoglycemia. For additional details, see Uses: Type 2 Diabetes Mellitus.

When given as separate tablets in combination with a thiazolidinedione antidiabetic agent (e.g., pioglitazone, rosiglitazone) with or without metformin hydrochloride, a sitagliptin dosage of 100 mg once daily has been used. For additional details, see Uses: Type 2 Diabetes Mellitus.

When given in combination with insulin with or without metformin hydrochloride, a sitagliptin dosage of 100 mg once daily has been used. Dosage of concomitant insulin may need to be reduced to decrease risk of hypoglycemia.

• Special Populations

Hepatic Impairment

Dosage adjustments of sitagliptin alone or in fixed combination with ertugliflozin are not necessary in patients with mild to moderate hepatic impairment (Child-Pugh score of 9 or less). Data are lacking on use of sitagliptin or the fixed combination of sitagliptin and ertugliflozin in patients with severe hepatic impairment (Child-Pugh score greater than 9), and the manufacturer states that such use is *not* recommended.

The manufacturer states that the fixed combinations of sitagliptin and immediate- or extended-release metformin are *not* recommended in patients with hepatic impairment.

Renal Impairment
Sitagliptin Monotherapy

Dosage adjustment is recommended for patients with an estimated glomerular filtration rate (eGFR) less than 45 mL/minute per 1.73 m². Caution should be used to ensure that the correct dosage of sitagliptin is prescribed for patients with moderate or severe renal impairment or end-stage renal disease (ESRD) requiring hemodialysis or peritoneal dialysis. (See Worsening of Renal Function under Cautions: Warnings/Precautions.) In patients with moderate renal impairment (creatinine clearance of 30 to less than 45 mL/minute per 1.73 m²), the recommended dosage of sitagliptin is 50 mg once daily. In patients with severe renal impairment (creatinine clearance less than 30 mL/minute per 1.73 m², corresponding to serum creatinine concentrations greater than 3 mg/dL in men or greater than 2.5 mg/dL in women), the recommended sitagliptin dosage is 25 mg once daily. Patients with ESRD requiring hemodialysis or peritoneal dialysis should receive a dosage of 25 mg once daily. Sitagliptin may be administered without regard to the timing of dialysis.

Sitagliptin/Ertugliflozin Fixed-combination Therapy

No dosage adjustment or increased monitoring is needed in patients with mild renal impairment receiving the fixed combination of sitagliptin and ertugliflozin. The manufacturer states that *initiation* of therapy with the fixed combination of sitagliptin and ertugliflozin is not recommended in patients with an eGFR of 30 to less than 60 mL/minute per 1.73 m² and that *continued use* of the combination is not recommended when eGFR is persistently between 30 and less than 60 mL/minute per 1.73 m². Use of the fixed combination of sitagliptin and ertugliflozin is contraindicated in patients with eGFR less than 30 mL/minute per 1.73 m².

Sitagliptin/Immediate- or Extended-release Metformin Hydrochloride Fixed-combination Therapy

Renal function (eGFR) should be assessed prior to initiation of the fixed combination of sitagliptin and immediate- or extended-release metformin. (See Renal Impairment under Warnings/Precautions: Specific Populations, in Cautions.) The manufacturer states that the fixed combination of sitagliptin and *immediate-release* metformin hydrochloride is not recommended in patients with eGFR between 30 and less than 45 mL/minute per 1.73 m² because such patients require a lower dosage of sitagliptin than what is available in the fixed-combination preparation.

The manufacturer states that *initiation* of the fixed combination of sitagliptin and *extended-release* metformin hydrochloride is not recommended in patients with eGFR of 30–45 mL/minute per 1.73 m². In patients taking the fixed combination of sitagliptin and extended-release metformin hydrochloride whose eGFR later decreases to less than 45 mL/minute per 1.73 m², the dosage of the sitagliptin component should be limited to 50 mg daily and the benefit versus risk of continuing therapy with the fixed combination should be assessed. The fixed combination should be discontinued in patients whose eGFR decreases to less than 30 mL/minute per 1.73 m².

Use of the fixed combinations of sitagliptin and immediate- or extended-release metformin is contraindicated in patients with severe renal impairment (eGFR less than 30 mL/minute per 1.73 m²).

Geriatric Patients

Dosage should be selected with caution because of age-related decreases in renal function. (See Geriatric Use and also see Renal Impairment under Warnings/Precautions: Specific Populations, in Cautions.) Dosage should be titrated carefully to the minimum dosage necessary for adequate glycemic control. The fixed combination of sitagliptin and ertugliflozin is expected to have diminished efficacy in geriatric patients with renal impairment.

CAUTIONS

• Contraindications

Sitagliptin is contraindicated in patients with known serious hypersensitivity (e.g., anaphylaxis, angioedema) to sitagliptin or to any ingredient in the formulation.

● *Warnings/Precautions*

Pancreatitis and Pancreatic Precancerous Changes

Acute pancreatitis, including fatal and nonfatal hemorrhagic or necrotizing pancreatitis, has been reported during postmarketing experience in patients receiving sitagliptin with or without metformin. The most common manifestations associated with pancreatitis were abdominal pain, nausea, and vomiting. Hospitalization was required in 66% of 88 reported cases, including 2 cases of hemorrhagic or necrotizing pancreatitis that necessitated prolonged hospitalization and intensive-care unit (ICU) care. Pancreatitis occurred within 30 days of initiation of sitagliptin or sitagliptin/metformin therapy in 21% of cases; discontinuance of the drug led to resolution of pancreatitis in 53% of patients. At least one other risk factor (e.g., obesity, high cholesterol and/or triglyceride concentrations) was noted in 51% of cases.

FDA has been evaluating unpublished findings suggesting an increased risk of pancreatitis and precancerous pancreatic cell changes (pancreatic duct metaplasia) in patients with type 2 diabetes mellitus receiving incretin mimetics (e.g., exenatide, liraglutide, sitagliptin, saxagliptin, alogliptin, linagliptin). These findings are based on examination of a small number of pancreatic tissue specimens taken from patients who died from unspecified causes while receiving an incretin mimetic. FDA will notify healthcare professionals of its conclusions and recommendations when the review is complete or when the agency has additional information to report.

FDA has recommended that clinicians continue to follow the recommendations in the prescribing information for incretin mimetics. The manufacturer states that patients receiving sitagliptin-containing therapy should be monitored for manifestations of pancreatitis, such as nausea, vomiting, anorexia, and persistent severe abdominal pain, sometimes radiating to the back; persistent severe abdominal pain, sometimes radiating to the back, which may or may not be accompanied by vomiting, is the hallmark symptom of acute pancreatitis. If pancreatitis is suspected, sitagliptin should be promptly discontinued and appropriate management instituted. (e.g., including laboratory studies such as serum and urine amylase, amylase/creatinine clearance ratio, electrolytes, and serum calcium, glucose, and lipase). Safety and efficacy of sitagliptin have not been established in patients with a history of pancreatitis and it is not known whether such patients are at increased risk for pancreatitis with sitagliptin therapy.

Heart Failure Risk

In cardiovascular outcomes studies conducted with 2 other dipeptidyl peptidase-4 (DPP-4) inhibitors (alogliptin, saxagliptin) in patients with type 2 diabetes mellitus and atherosclerotic cardiovascular disease (ASCVD), an association between DPP-4 inhibitor treatment and heart failure was observed. The potential risks and benefits of sitagliptin therapy should be considered prior to use in patients at higher risk for heart failure (e.g., history of heart failure or renal impairment). Patients receiving sitagliptin-containing therapy should be monitored for manifestations of heart failure. (See Advice to Patients.) If heart failure develops, appropriate evaluation and management should be instituted according to current standards of care and consideration given to discontinuing sitagliptin.

Worsening of Renal Function

Renal function should be assessed prior to initiation of sitagliptin and periodically thereafter. Worsening of renal function, including acute renal failure that sometimes required dialysis, has been reported in some patients during postmarketing experience. A subset of these patients had renal insufficiency, some of whom were prescribed inappropriate dosages of sitagliptin. A return to baseline levels of renal insufficiency has been observed with supportive treatment and discontinuance of potentially causative agents. Cautious reinitiation of sitagliptin can be considered if another etiology is deemed likely to have precipitated the acute worsening of renal function. The manufacturer states that sitagliptin has not been found to be nephrotoxic in clinical trials or in preclinical studies at clinically relevant dosages.

Severe Arthralgia

Severe, disabling joint pain has been reported during postmarketing experience in patients receiving DPP-4 inhibitors (e.g., alogliptin, linagliptin, saxagliptin, sitagliptin). Onset of such symptoms has ranged from 1 day to years following initiation of therapy. Fever, chills, rash, and swelling accompanied joint pain in some

patients, suggesting an immunologic reaction; some patients have required hospitalization. Symptoms resolved upon discontinuance of the DPP-4 inhibitor, usually in less than a month. In some patients, symptoms recurred when the same or another DPP-4 inhibitor was restarted. DPP-4 inhibitors should be considered as a possible cause of severe joint pain and should be discontinued if appropriate. (See Advice to Patients.)

Concomitant Therapy with Hypoglycemic Agents

When sitagliptin was used in combination with a sulfonylurea or insulin, the incidence of hypoglycemia was greater than that in patients receiving placebo with a sulfonylurea or insulin. In a long-term (52-week) clinical noninferiority study, rates of hypoglycemia with sitagliptin/metformin combination therapy were lower than those observed with glipizide/metformin combination therapy. However, in a 24-week clinical study, rates of hypoglycemia in patients receiving sitagliptin and glimepiride with or without metformin were greater than those in patients receiving glimepiride and metformin. Patients receiving sitagliptin may require a lower dosage of a concomitant insulin secretagogue (e.g., sulfonylurea) or insulin to reduce the risk of hypoglycemia.

Dermatologic and Sensitivity Reactions

There have been postmarketing reports of serious allergic and hypersensitivity reactions (e.g., anaphylaxis, angioedema, exfoliative skin conditions such as Stevens-Johnson syndrome) in patients receiving sitagliptin; rash, urticaria, and cutaneous vasculitis also have been reported. The onset of such reactions usually has been within the first 3 months following treatment initiation, but such reactions may occur after the first dose. (See Cautions: Contraindications.)

If hypersensitivity reactions occur, promptly discontinue the drug, assess for other potential causes of the event, institute appropriate monitoring and treatment, and initiate alternative antidiabetic therapy. (See Advice to Patients.) Use caution in patients with a history of angioedema with other dipeptidyl peptidase-4 (DPP-4) inhibitors because it is unknown whether such patients will be predisposed to angioedema with sitagliptin.

Cases of bullous pemphigoid requiring hospitalization have been reported with DPP-4 inhibitor use during postmarketing experience. Patients in such cases usually recovered after discontinuation of the DPP-4 inhibitor and treatment with topical or systemic immunosuppressive therapy. Patients should be advised to report the development of blisters or erosions while receiving sitagliptin. If bullous pemphigoid is suspected, sitagliptin should be discontinued and consideration given to referring the patient to a dermatologist for diagnosis and appropriate treatment.

Loss of Glycemic Control

Loss of glycemic control may occur during periods of stress (e.g., fever, trauma, infection, surgery). (See Advice to Patients.)

Temporary discontinuance of sitagliptin and administration of insulin may be required. Sitagliptin therapy may be reinstituted after the acute episode of hyperglycemia has resolved.

Macrovascular Outcomes

The manufacturer states that evidence of macrovascular risk reduction with sitagliptin has not been conclusively demonstrated in controlled clinical trials.

Use of Fixed Combinations

When sitagliptin is used in fixed combination with metformin hydrochloride, ertugliflozin, or other drugs, the cautions, precautions, contraindications, and drug interactions associated with the concomitant agent(s) should be considered in addition to those associated with sitagliptin.

Specific Populations

Pregnancy

Data are lacking on the use of sitagliptin in pregnant women. In embryofetal developmental studies, no adverse developmental effects were observed during organogenesis when sitagliptin was administered to pregnant rats and rabbits during organogenesis at doses of 250 and 125 mg/kg, respectively (up to 30 and

20 times, respectively, the 100-mg clinical dosage based on AUC). Pregnancy registry may be contacted at 800-986-8999.

Lactation

Sitagliptin is distributed into milk in rats; data are lacking regarding the presence of the drug in human milk, the effects on the breastfed infant, or effects on milk production. The developmental and health benefits of breastfeeding should be considered along with the mother's clinical need for sitagliptin and any potential adverse effects on the breastfed infant from sitagliptin or the underlying maternal condition.

Pediatric Use

Safety and efficacy of sitagliptin alone or in fixed combination with metformin or ertugliflozin have not been established in children younger than 18 years of age.

Geriatric Use

No substantial differences in safety and efficacy of sitagliptin relative to younger adults, but increased sensitivity cannot be ruled out. Renal function should be assessed more frequently in geriatric patients. (See Renal Impairment under Warnings/Precautions: Specific Populations, in Cautions.)

Renal Impairment

Sitagliptin is substantially eliminated by the kidneys; renal function should be assessed prior to initiation of therapy and periodically thereafter. (See Worsening of Renal Function under Cautions: Warnings/Precautions.) Sitagliptin exposure is increased in patients with renal impairment; lower dosages of the drug are recommended in patients with eGFR less than 45 mL/minute per 1.73 m² and those with end-stage renal disease requiring dialysis. (See Renal Impairment under Dosage and Administration: Special Populations.)

● Common Adverse Effects

Adverse effects reported in at least 5% of patients receiving sitagliptin as monotherapy or add-on therapy with metformin and/or a thiazolidinedione or glimepiride and more commonly than with placebo include nasopharyngitis, upper respiratory tract infection, peripheral edema, and headache.

Adverse effects reported in at least 5% of patients receiving sitagliptin concomitantly with immediate-release metformin and more commonly than with placebo include diarrhea, upper respiratory infection, and headache.

Adverse effects reported in at least 5% of patients receiving sitagliptin given concomitantly with metformin and a sulfonylurea (glimepiride) and more commonly than with placebo include hypoglycemia and headache.

Adverse effects reported in clinical trials of sitagliptin given concomitantly with ertugliflozin were similar in type and incidence to those reported with ertugliflozin alone.

Adverse effects reported in at least 5% of patients receiving sitagliptin in combination with insulin and more commonly than with placebo include hypoglycemia.

DRUG INTERACTIONS

● Drugs Metabolized by Hepatic Microsomal Enzymes

Sitagliptin is metabolized to a limited extent by cytochrome P-450 (CYP) isoenzymes 3A4 and 2C8 to inactive metabolites. Sitagliptin does not inhibit CYP isoenzymes 1A2, 2B6, 2C8, 2C9, 2C19, 2D6, or 3A4 in vitro or induce CYP3A4. Pharmacokinetic interactions with drugs metabolized by these isoenzymes are unlikely.

● Drugs Secreted by Renal Tubular Cationic Transport

Sitagliptin is a substrate of the organic anion transport system; pharmacokinetic interactions are unlikely with substrates of the organic cationic transport system.

● Inhibitors of P-glycoprotein Transport System

Sitagliptin is a substrate of the P-glycoprotein transport system. There is a potential pharmacokinetic interaction (increased absorption and renal clearance of sitagliptin) with P-glycoprotein inhibitors.

Clinically important pharmacokinetic interactions with P-glycoprotein inhibitors appear to be unlikely. Sitagliptin does not appear to inhibit the P-glycoprotein transport system.

● Protein-bound Drugs

Pharmacokinetic interactions between sitagliptin and protein-bound drugs are unlikely.

● Cyclosporine

Concomitant administration of cyclosporine and sitagliptin may increase absorption and plasma concentrations of sitagliptin. However, this interaction is not considered clinically important and dosage adjustments are not required.

● Digoxin

Concomitant administration of sitagliptin (100 mg daily for 10 days) with digoxin (0.25 mg once daily for 10 days) resulted in a slight increase in plasma concentrations and area under the concentration-time curve (AUC) of digoxin (18 and 11%, respectively). While these increases are not considered clinically important, patients receiving digoxin should be monitored appropriately; however, no digoxin or sitagliptin dosage adjustment is needed.

● Hormonal Contraceptives, Oral

Sitagliptin has no clinically important effect on the pharmacokinetics of norethindrone or ethinyl estradiol.

● Metformin

Sitagliptin and metformin have a potential additive effect on active glucagon-like peptide (GLP-1) concentrations. Pharmacokinetic interactions are unlikely.

The relevance of these effects to glycemic control in patients with type 2 diabetes mellitus is unclear.

● Simvastatin

Pharmacokinetic interactions between sitagliptin and simvastatin are unlikely.

● Insulin Secretagogues or Insulin

The incidence of hypoglycemia was increased compared with placebo when sitagliptin was added to therapy with an insulin secretagogue (e.g., sulfonylurea) or insulin. (See Concomitant Therapy with Hypoglycemic Agents under Cautions: Warnings/Precautions.) Clinically important pharmacokinetic interactions between sitagliptin and sulfonylureas (e.g., glimepiride, glipizide, glyburide, tolbutamide) are unlikely.

● Thiazolidinediones

Pharmacokinetic interactions between sitagliptin and thiazolidinediones (e.g., rosiglitazone) are unlikely.

● Warfarin

Pharmacokinetic interactions between sitagliptin and warfarin are unlikely.

DESCRIPTION

Sitagliptin inhibits dipeptidyl peptidase-4 (DPP-4), an enzyme that inactivates glucagon-like peptide (GLP-1) and glucose-dependent insulinotropic polypeptide (GIP), which are incretin hormones. The drug inhibits DPP-4 selectively with no effect on DPP-8 or DDP-9 in vitro at concentrations approximating those from therapeutic dosage. Sitagliptin increases circulating concentrations of GIP and GLP-1 in a glucose-dependent manner. Coadministration of sitagliptin and metformin has an additive effect on active GLP-1 concentrations.

GIP and GLP-1 stimulate insulin synthesis and release from pancreatic β-cells in a glucose-dependent manner (i.e., when glucose concentrations are normal or elevated) by intracellular signaling pathways involving cyclic 3′,5′-adenosine monophosphate (cAMP). GLP-1 also decreases glucagon secretion from pancreatic α-cells in a glucose-dependent manner, leading to reduced hepatic glucose production.

Sitagliptin lowers fasting plasma glucose concentrations and reduces glucose excursions following glucose load or meal in patients with type 2 diabetes mellitus.

Sitagliptin monotherapy usually is not associated with hypoglycemia or substantial changes in body weight.

Peak plasma sitagliptin concentration is achieved within 3 hours following oral administration. Absolute bioavailability is approximately 87%. Administration of sitagliptin with a high-fat meal had no effect on the pharmacokinetics of the drug Sitagliptin is metabolized to a limited extent by CYP isoenzymes 3A4 and 2C8 to inactive metabolites. Terminal half-of sitagliptin is 12.4 hours following oral administration of a 100 mg oral dose. Following administration of a single radiolabeled dose, 87% of the dose was excreted in the urine (mainly as unchanged drug) and 13% was excreted in the feces.

ADVICE TO PATIENTS

Importance of patient reading medication guide before initiating therapy and each time the drug is dispensed.

Importance of informing patients of potential risks and benefits of sitagliptin-containing therapy and of alternative therapies. Importance of not using sitagliptin in patients with type 1 diabetes mellitus or diabetic ketoacidosis.

Importance of informing patient about the possibility of acute pancreatitis, which may be severe or fatal, with sitagliptin therapy. Importance of patients advising clinicians about a history of pancreatitis, gallstones, alcoholism, high triglyceride levels, or kidney problems. Importance of advising patients about signs and symptoms of pancreatitis, including persistent severe abdominal pain sometimes radiating to the back that may or may not be accompanied by vomiting; importance of patient discontinuing sitagliptin and promptly notifying clinician if such signs or symptoms are present.

Importance of informing patients of the possibility of severe and disabling joint pain with DPP-4 inhibitors (e.g., alogliptin, linagliptin, saxagliptin, sitagliptin). Advise patients to contact a clinician promptly if severe and persistent joint pain occurs; patients should not discontinue the DPP-4 inhibitor without consulting their clinician.

Importance of informing patients about possibility of heart failure with sitagliptin therapy. Importance of clinicians asking patients about a history of heart failure or renal impairment prior to initiating sitagliptin therapy. Importance of informing patients about signs and symptoms of heart failure (e.g., shortness of breath, unusual tiredness, rapid weight gain, edema especially in the feet, ankles, or legs); importance of patients immediately contacting a clinician if manifestations of heart failure occur.

Importance of informing patients that bullous pemphigoid may occur with the use of a DPP-4 inhibitor. Advise patients to promptly inform clinician if skin blisters or erosion (breakdown of the outer layer of skin) occurs.

Importance of patient informing clinician if hypoglycemia occurs, particularly if concomitant therapy with a sulfonylurea antidiabetic agent (i.e., insulin secretagogue) or insulin is used; a lower dosage of the sulfonylurea or insulin may be required in such cases.

Importance of instructing patients regarding self-monitoring of blood glucose, periodic HbA$_{1c}$ monitoring, adherence to meal planning, regular physical exercise, and management of hypoglycemia and hyperglycemia.

Discuss potential for alterations in dosage requirements in special situations (e.g., fever, trauma, infection, surgery, changes in renal function); importance of

informing clinician promptly if such situations occur. (See Loss of Glycemic Control under Cautions: Warnings/Precautions.)

Risk of allergic reactions (e.g., rash; hives; swelling of face, lips, tongue, throat that may cause difficulty in breathing or swallowing). If such reactions occur, importance of discontinuing sitagliptin and informing clinicians promptly. (See Dermatologic and Sensitivity Reactions under Cautions: Warnings/Precautions.)

Importance of women informing their clinicians if they are or plan to become pregnant or plan to breast-feed.

Importance of informing clinicians of existing or contemplated concomitant therapy, including prescription and OTC drugs and dietary or herbal supplements, as well as any concomitant illnesses (e.g., allergies, kidney problems, history of pancreatitis).

Importance of informing patients of other important precautionary information. (See Cautions.)

PREPARATIONS

Excipients in commercially available drug preparations may have clinically important effects in some individuals; consult specific product labeling for details.

SITagliptin Phosphate

Oral

Tablets, film-coated	25 mg (of sitagliptin)	Januvia®, Merck
	50 mg (of sitagliptin)	Januvia®, Merck
	100 mg (of sitagliptin)	Januvia®, Merck

SITagliptin Phosphate Combinations

Oral

Tablets, extended-release	50 mg (of sitagliptin) with Extended-release Metformin Hydrochloride 500 mg	Janumet® XR, Merck
	50 mg (of sitagliptin) with Extended-release Metformin Hydrochloride 1 g	Janumet® XR, Merck
	100 mg (of sitagliptin) with Extended-release Metformin Hydrochloride 1 g	Janumet® XR, Merck
Tablets, film-coated	50 mg (of sitagliptin) with Metformin Hydrochloride 500 mg	Janumet®, Merck
	50 mg (of sitagliptin) with Metformin Hydrochloride 1 g	Janumet®, Merck
	100 mg (of sitagliptin) with Ertugliflozin L-pyroglutamic Acid 5 mg (of ertugliflozin)	Steglujan®, Merck
	100 mg (of sitagliptin) with Ertugliflozin L-pyroglutamic Acid 15 mg (of ertugliflozin)	Steglujan®, Merck

Selected Revisions June 21, 2021, © Copyright, January 1, 2010, American Society of Health-System Pharmacists, Inc.

Dulaglutide

68:20.06 · INCRETIN MIMETICS

■ Dulaglutide, a long-acting glucagon-like peptide-1 (GLP-1) receptor agonist (incretin mimetic), is an antidiabetic agent.

USES

● Type 2 Diabetes Mellitus

Dulaglutide is used as an adjunct to diet and exercise to improve glycemic control in adults and pediatric patients ≥10 years of age with type 2 diabetes mellitus. Dulaglutide has been used alone or as add-on therapy with metformin, the combination of metformin and a sulfonylurea, the combination of metformin and a thiazolidinedione, a sodium-glucose cotransporter 2 (SGLT2) inhibitor with or without metformin, basal insulin with or without metformin, and prandial insulin with or without metformin.

Dulaglutide also is used to reduce the risk of major adverse cardiovascular events in adults with type 2 diabetes mellitus and established cardiovascular disease or multiple cardiovascular risk factors.

Glycemic Control

Current guidelines for the treatment of type 2 diabetes mellitus generally recommend metformin as first-line therapy in addition to lifestyle modifications in patients with recent-onset type 2 diabetes mellitus or mild hyperglycemia because of its well-established safety and efficacy (i.e., beneficial effects on glycosylated hemoglobin [hemoglobin A_{1c}; HbA_{1c}], weight, and cardiovascular mortality). In patients with contraindications or intolerance to metformin (e.g., risk of lactic acidosis, GI intolerance) or in selected other patients, some experts suggest that initial therapy with a drug from another class of antidiabetic agents (e.g., a GLP-1 receptor agonist, SGLT2 inhibitor, dipeptidyl peptidase-4 [DPP-4] inhibitor, sulfonylurea, thiazolidinedione, basal insulin) may be acceptable based on patient factors. Initiating antidiabetic therapy with 2 agents (e.g., metformin plus another drug) may be appropriate in patients with an initial HbA_{1c} exceeding 7.5% or at least 1.5% above the target level. In metformin-intolerant patients with high initial HbA_{1c} levels, some experts suggest initiation of therapy with 2 agents from other antidiabetic drug classes with complementary mechanisms of action.

Because of the progressive nature of type 2 diabetes mellitus, patients initially receiving an oral antidiabetic agent will eventually require multiple oral and/or injectable noninsulin antidiabetic agents of different therapeutic classes and/or insulin for adequate glycemic control. Patients who have inadequate glycemic control with initial (e.g., metformin) monotherapy should receive treatment with additional antidiabetic agents; data suggest that the addition of each noninsulin agent to initial therapy lowers HbA_{1c} by approximately 0.7–1%. In addition, early initiation of combination therapy may help to more rapidly attain glycemic goals and extend the time to treatment failure.

Factors to consider when selecting additional antidiabetic agents for combination therapy in patients with inadequate glycemic control on metformin monotherapy include patient comorbidities (e.g., atherosclerotic cardiovascular disease [ASCVD], established kidney disease, heart failure), hypoglycemia risk, impact on weight, cost, risk of adverse effects, and patient preference. When the greater glucose-lowering effect of an injectable drug is needed in patients with type 2 diabetes mellitus, some experts currently state that an injectable GLP-1 receptor agonist is preferred over insulin in most patients because of beneficial effects on body weight and a lower risk of hypoglycemia, although adverse GI effects may diminish tolerability. While addition of a GLP-1 receptor agonist may successfully control hyperglycemia, many patients will eventually require insulin therapy. Early introduction of insulin therapy should be considered when hyperglycemia is severe (e.g., blood glucose of at least 300 mg/dL or HbA_{1c} exceeding 9–10%), especially in the presence of catabolic manifestations (e.g., weight loss, hypertriglyceridemia, ketosis) or symptoms of hyperglycemia.

Patients with type 2 diabetes mellitus who have established (or are at a high risk for) ASCVD, established kidney disease, or heart failure should receive a GLP-1 receptor agonist or SGLT2 inhibitor with demonstrated cardiovascular disease benefit. Experts state that therapy with a GLP-1 receptor agonist or SGLT2

inhibitor should be considered for patients with the aforementioned comorbidities independently of the patients' HbA_{1c}. GLP-1 receptor agonists and SGLT2 inhibitors appear to have effects on the kidneys independent of their glycemic effects, and some experts suggest that an agent from one of these classes of drugs be considered in patients with type 2 diabetes mellitus and chronic kidney disease (CKD). In patients *without* established ASCVD or indicators of high ASCVD risk, heart failure, or CKD, the decision regarding the addition of other antidiabetic agents (e.g., GLP-1 receptor agonist, SGLT2 inhibitor, DPP-4 inhibitor, thiazolidinedione, sulfonylurea, basal insulin) to metformin therapy should be based on avoidance of adverse effects, cost, and individual patient factors.

Has not been studied in patients with a history of pancreatitis; consider other antidiabetic agents in such patients.

Data are lacking on the use of dulaglutide in patients with severe GI disease, including severe gastroparesis, and the drug is not recommended for use in patients with preexisting severe GI disease.

Dulaglutide is *not* indicated for the treatment of type 1 diabetes mellitus.

Dulaglutide Monotherapy in Adults

When given as monotherapy for the management of type 2 diabetes mellitus, dulaglutide improves glycemic control as evidenced by reductions from baseline in glycosylated hemoglobin (hemoglobin A_{1c}; HbA_{1c}). Efficacy and safety of dulaglutide as monotherapy have been established in a 52-week, randomized, double-blind, noninferiority study comparing dulaglutide (0.75 mg or 1.5 mg once weekly throughout the study) with metformin (median initial dosage of 1 g daily with upward titration to 1.5–2 g daily) in patients with type 2 diabetes mellitus. The primary study end point was the change in HbA_{1c} from baseline to week 26.

At week 26, HbA_{1c} was reduced in all treatment groups; both dosages of dulaglutide were noninferior to metformin at 26 and 52 weeks. Mean HbA_{1c} was reduced by 0.7 and 0.8% in patients receiving dulaglutide 0.75 and 1.5 mg, respectively, and by 0.6% in those receiving metformin. Patients in all 3 treatment groups also had decreased fasting plasma glucose and body weight at 26 and 52 weeks. Patients included in this trial had type 2 diabetes mellitus inadequately controlled by diet and exercise or one oral antidiabetic agent, and had a mean baseline HbA_{1c} of 7.6%. Approximately 75% of patients were taking an oral antidiabetic agent before the study; approximately 90% of these patients were receiving metformin and approximately 10% were receiving a sulfonylurea.

Combination Therapy in Adults

When given as add-on therapy in combination with one or more oral antidiabetic agents (e.g., metformin, a sulfonylurea, a thiazolidinedione), dulaglutide improved glycemic control more than sitagliptin or exenatide. Dulaglutide was noninferior to insulin glargine in reducing HbA_{1c} when added to prandial insulin with or without metformin or to other oral antidiabetic agents, and was noninferior to liraglutide when added to metformin. Safety and efficacy of dulaglutide as add-on therapy to other antidiabetic agents in the management of type 2 diabetes mellitus have been established in several randomized, active-controlled, double-blind or open-label studies lasting 24–104 weeks in over 4000 patients. In these studies, patients randomized to dulaglutide generally received either 0.75 or 1.5 mg once weekly with no dosage adjustments.

In a 24-week, double-blind study, add-on therapy with dulaglutide (1.5 mg once weekly) substantially reduced HbA_{1c} from baseline compared with placebo at 24 weeks (mean difference in HbA_{1c}: 1.1%) in patients receiving glimepiride. An HbA_{1c} less than 7% was achieved in 50 or 17% of patients receiving dulaglutide or placebo, respectively.

In a 104-week, randomized, double-blind study, patients who received dulaglutide in addition to existing metformin therapy (at least 1.5 g daily) experienced a substantially greater reduction in HbA_{1c} at the 52-week primary end point than those who received sitagliptin (100 mg once daily) as add-on therapy to metformin. Both 0.75- and 1.5-mg dosages of dulaglutide were superior to placebo and sitagliptin in reducing HbA_{1c}, with greater reduction in HbA_{1c} with the higher dulaglutide dosage. More patients achieved HbA_{1c} less than 7% in the dulaglutide groups than in the sitagliptin group; patients who received dulaglutide also had substantially lowered fasting plasma glucose and greater weight loss compared with those who received sitagliptin.

In a 52-week study in patients inadequately controlled on pioglitazone (30–45 mg daily) and metformin (at least 1.5 g daily) therapy, add-on therapy with dulaglutide (0.75 or 1.5 mg once weekly) was superior to placebo and add-on exenatide (5 mcg twice daily for 4 weeks, then 10 mcg twice daily) in reducing HbA$_{1c}$ at the 26-week primary end point. Superiority of dulaglutide over exenatide was maintained at 52 weeks. At 26 weeks, an HbA$_{1c}$ less than 7% was achieved in 66 or 78% of patients receiving dulaglutide 0.75 or 1.5 mg, respectively, compared with 52% of those receiving exenatide.

In another 24-week, double-blind study, add-on therapy with dulaglutide (0.75 or 1.5 mg once weekly) in patients receiving SGLT2 inhibitor therapy with or without metformin substantially reduced HbA$_{1c}$ from baseline compared with placebo at 24 weeks (mean difference in HbA$_{1c}$ of 0.7 or 0.8% in the 0.75- or 1.5-mg group, respectively). An HbA$_{1c}$ less than 7% was achieved in 59, 67, or 31% of patients receiving once-weekly dulaglutide 0.75 mg, dulaglutide 1.5 mg, or placebo, respectively. Mean reductions from baseline in fasting serum glucose at week 24 with dulaglutide 0.75 and 1.5 mg once weekly were 19 and 24 mg/dL, respectively, compared with placebo.

In a 78-week, randomized, open-label noninferiority study, dulaglutide (0.75 or 1.5 mg once weekly) was compared with insulin glargine (10 units daily initially, titrated to a fasting plasma glucose goal of less than 100 mg/dL) as add-on therapy to maximally tolerated dosages of metformin and glimepiride. At the 52-week primary end point, dulaglutide 1.5 mg was superior, and 0.75 mg noninferior to insulin glargine (mean daily dosage 29.4 units) as add-on therapy with regard to HbA$_{1c}$ reduction. Dulaglutide was associated with mean body weight losses of 1.3 and 1.9 kg for the 0.75- and 1.5-mg dosages, respectively, while insulin glargine treatment resulted in a mean body weight gain of 1.4 kg.

In a 52-week, randomized, open-label noninferiority trial in patients with moderate to severe chronic kidney disease, dulaglutide (0.75 or 1.5 mg once weekly) was compared with insulin glargine (initiated at 50% of the prerandomization total daily insulin dosage and titrated to a fasting plasma glucose of less than 100 mg/dL) as add-on therapy to prandial (3 times daily) insulin lispro with or without metformin. At the 26-week primary end point, HbA$_{1c}$ was reduced in all treatment groups; both dosages of dulaglutide were noninferior to insulin glargine. Overall estimated glomerular filtration rate (eGFR) in study patients at baseline was 38 mL/minute per 1.73 m^2; 30% of patients had an eGFR of less than 30 mL/minute per 1.73 m^2 and 45% had macroalbuminuria.

In a 26-week, open-label noninferiority study, dulaglutide (1.5 mg once weekly) was compared with liraglutide (titrated from 0.6 mg daily to 1.8 mg daily by week 3) as add-on therapy in patients with type 2 diabetes not adequately controlled with metformin (at least 1.5 g daily). At the 26-week primary end point, HbA$_{1c}$ was reduced in both groups; the dulaglutide 1.5-mg dosage was noninferior to liraglutide.

In a 28-week, double-blind study, dulaglutide (1.5 mg once weekly) added to therapy with basal insulin glargine with or without metformin was more effective than placebo in reducing HbA$_{1c}$ (1.4 versus 0.7% change from baseline). At week 28, HbA$_{1c}$ was less than 7% in 67 or 33% of patients receiving dulaglutide or placebo, respectively.

Use in Pediatric Patients

Efficacy and safety of dulaglutide in pediatric patients have been established in a 26-week randomized, double-blind, placebo-controlled trial with an open-label extension for an additional 26 weeks. In this study, 154 patients ≥10 years of age with type 2 diabetes mellitus who had inadequate glycemic control despite diet and exercise were randomized to receive dulaglutide (0.75 or 1.5 mg) or placebo once weekly by subcutaneous injection with or without concomitant metformin and/or basal insulin. Results at 26 weeks showed that dulaglutide was significantly more effective than placebo in reducing HbA$_{1c}$ from baseline (difference from placebo of -1.2% with dulaglutide 0.75 mg and -1.5% with dulaglutide 1.5 mg).

Reduction in Risk of Major Adverse Cardiovascular Events

Dulaglutide is used to reduce the risk of major adverse cardiovascular events in adults with type 2 diabetes mellitus and established cardiovascular disease or multiple cardiovascular risk factors. In addition to lowering blood glucose, GLP-1 receptor agonists appear to modify several nonglycemic cardiovascular risk factors such as blood pressure, body weight, and lipid profile. Additionally, GLP-1 receptor agonists may have beneficial endothelial effects.

In a double-blind, placebo-controlled study (REWIND) in 9901 adults with type 2 diabetes mellitus at risk for cardiovascular events or with a history of cardiovascular disease, add-on therapy with dulaglutide (1.5 mg subcutaneously once weekly for a median of 5.4 years) substantially reduced the primary composite

outcome (first occurrence of nonfatal myocardial infarction [MI], nonfatal stroke, or death from cardiovascular causes). The primary composite outcome occurred in 12 or 13.4% of patients receiving dulaglutide or placebo, respectively, representing a 12% risk reduction with dulaglutide therapy. All-cause mortality did not differ between treatment groups. Patients in the study were at least 50 years of age (mean age: 66 years) and approximately 32% of the patients had established cardiovascular disease. Approximately 95% of patients were receiving at least one antidiabetic drug (e.g., metformin, sulfonylurea, insulin); most patients were also receiving cardiovascular drugs at baseline (angiotensin-converting enzyme [ACE] inhibitor or angiotensin II receptor antagonist [81.5% of patients], β-adrenergic blocking agent [β-blocker; 45.6% of patients], calcium-channel blocker [34.4% of patients], diuretic [46.5% of patients], statin [66.1% of patients], antithrombotic agent [58.7% of patients], aspirin [51.7% of patients]).

Beneficial Effects on Renal Function

In several cardiovascular outcomes trials involving the use of GLP-1 receptor agonists (e.g., dulaglutide, liraglutide, semaglutide) in patients with type 2 diabetes mellitus at high risk for cardiovascular disease or with existing cardiovascular disease, beneficial effects on renal function have been observed as a secondary outcome. Some experts suggest that in patients with type 2 diabetes mellitus and CKD who are at increased risk for cardiovascular events, use of a GLP-1 receptor agonist may reduce risk of progression of albuminuria, cardiovascular events, or both†.

DOSAGE AND ADMINISTRATION

● General

Patient Monitoring

- Perform regular monitoring (e.g., blood glucose determinations, HbA$_{1c}$) to determine therapeutic response.

● Administration

Dulaglutide is administered by subcutaneous injection; the drug should *not* be administered IV or IM. Dulaglutide is administered once weekly, on the same day each week, at any time of day without regard to meals. The day of weekly administration may be changed if necessary; however, at least 3 days should elapse between doses.

If a dose is missed, the missed dose should be administered as soon as possible if there are at least 3 days (72 hours) remaining before the next scheduled dose; the regular weekly schedule should then be resumed. If less than 3 days remain before the next scheduled dose, the missed dose should be skipped and the next dose should be administered on the usual weekly day, followed by resumption of the regular weekly schedule.

Dulaglutide is administered by subcutaneous injection into the abdomen, thigh, or upper arm using a single-dose, prefilled injection pen. Rotate injection sites with each dose.

When using dulaglutide in combination with insulin, the drugs should be administered as separate injections; insulin and dulaglutide injections should never be mixed. Dulaglutide and insulin may be injected into the same body regions; however, the injections should not be adjacent to each other.

● Dosage

Type 2 Diabetes Mellitus in Adults

The recommended initial dosage of dulaglutide for the management of type 2 diabetes mellitus in adults is 0.75 mg subcutaneously once weekly. Increase the dosage to 1.5 mg once weekly for additional glycemic control. If further glycemic control is needed, dosage may be increased in 1.5-mg increments after at least 4 weeks on the current dosage. The maximum recommended dosage is 4.5 mg once weekly.

Type 2 Diabetes Mellitus in Pediatric Patients

The recommended initial dosage of dulaglutide for the management of type 2 diabetes mellitus in pediatric patients ≥10 years of age is 0.75 mg subcutaneously once weekly. If additional glycemic control is needed, the dosage may be increased to the maximum recommended dosage of 1.5 mg once weekly after at least 4 weeks on the 0.75 mg dosage.

● **Special Populations**

No dosage adjustment is necessary in patients with renal or hepatic impairment, including end-stage renal disease. However, clinicians should use caution in patients with end-stage renal disease.

CAUTIONS

● **Contraindications**

Dulaglutide is contraindicated in patients with a personal or family history of medullary thyroid carcinoma (MTC) and in patients with multiple endocrine neoplasia syndrome type 2 (MEN 2).

Dulaglutide is also contraindicated in patients with a prior serious hypersensitivity reaction to dulaglutide or to any of the product components.

● **Warnings/Precautions**

Warnings

Risk of Thyroid C-Cell Tumors

Glucagon-like peptide-1 (GLP-1) receptor agonists such as dulaglutide cause dose- and treatment duration-dependent thyroid C-cell tumors (adenomas and carcinomas) in rats and mice. It is unknown whether dulaglutide causes thyroid C-cell tumors, including MTC, in humans.

At least 1 case of MTC has been reported in a patient treated with dulaglutide. This patient had serum calcitonin concentrations approximately 8 times the upper limit of normal (ULN) prior to treatment. Very elevated serum calcitonin values may be indicative of MTC; patients with MTC usually have serum calcitonin values exceeding 50 ng/mL. Although routine monitoring of serum calcitonin is of uncertain value in patients treated with dulaglutide, patients should also be referred to an endocrinologist for further evaluation if serum calcitonin is found to be elevated.

Patients should be counseled about potential risk of MTC and informed about symptoms of thyroid tumors. Patients with thyroid nodules noted on physical examination or neck imaging also should be referred to an endocrinologist. The role of monitoring serum calcitonin concentrations or thyroid ultrasounds for the purpose of early detection of MTC in patients receiving dulaglutide is unknown.

Sensitivity Reactions

Serious hypersensitivity reactions (severe urticaria, systemic rash, facial edema, lip swelling), including anaphylactic reactions and angioedema, have been reported in patients receiving dulaglutide. If a hypersensitivity reaction occurs, the patient should discontinue dulaglutide, be treated promptly according to the standard of care, and be monitored until signs and symptoms have resolved. Caution should be exercised in patients with a history of anaphylaxis or angioedema to other GLP-1 receptor agonists, as it is unknown whether such patients will be predisposed to anaphylaxis with dulaglutide.

Other Warnings and Precautions

Risks During General Anesthesia and Deep Sedation

GLP-1 agonists are associated with adverse GI effects such as nausea, vomiting, and delayed gastric emptying; such effects are likely a result of rapid tachyphlaxis at the level of vagal nerve activation. Delayed gastric emptying from GLP-1 agonists can increase the risk of regurgitation and pulmonary aspiration of gastric contents during general anesthesia and deep sedation. Given these concerns, the American Society of Anesthesiologists (ASA) Task Force on Preoperative Fasting has issued a consensus-based guidance for the management of GLP-1 receptor agonists prior to elective surgery. The task force suggests that for patients on daily GLP-1 agonist dosing (irrespective of indication, dose, or type of surgery), consider holding the drug on the day of the procedure/surgery. For patients on weekly dosing (irrespective of indication, dose, or type of surgery), consider holding the GLP-1 agonist a week prior to the procedure/surgery.

If GLP-1 agonists prescribed for diabetes management are held for longer than the dosing schedule, consider consulting an endocrinologist for bridging the antidiabetic therapy to avoid hyperglycemia. These recommendations are based on limited evidence only (case reports). For patients requiring urgent or emergent procedures, the task force states to proceed and treat the patient as 'full stomach' and manage accordingly.

Pancreatitis and Pancreatic Precancerous Changes

Acute pancreatitis has been reported in association with dulaglutide.

In clinical trials, 5 cases of confirmed pancreatitis occurred among dulaglutide-treated patients compared with 1 case in patients treated with a non-incretin comparator drug (1.4 versus 0.88 cases per 1000 patient years, respectively).

Observe patients carefully for signs and symptoms of pancreatitis, including persistent severe abdominal pain, sometimes radiating to the back, which may or may not be accompanied by vomiting; if pancreatitis is suspected, dulaglutide should be discontinued promptly. If pancreatitis is confirmed, dulaglutide should not be restarted.

Efficacy and safety of dulaglutide have not been established in patients with a history of pancreatitis. Alternative antidiabetic therapy should be considered in such patients.

Use with Drugs Known to Cause Hypoglycemia

Patients receiving dulaglutide in combination with an insulin secretagogue (e.g., sulfonylurea) or insulin have an increased risk of hypoglycemia. A lower dosage of the concomitant insulin secretagogue or insulin may be required to reduce the risk of hypoglycemia.

Renal Effects

During postmarketing experience, acute renal failure and worsening of chronic renal failure (which sometimes required hemodialysis) have been reported with GLP-1 receptor agonists. Some of these events have occurred in patients without known underlying renal disease. Most of these events have occurred in patients experiencing nausea, vomiting, diarrhea, or dehydration. Because these GI effects may worsen renal function, clinicians should use caution when initiating dulaglutide or escalating dosage in patients with renal impairment.

GI Effects

Use of dulaglutide may be associated with adverse GI effects, sometimes severe. In clinical trials, more patients receiving dulaglutide (1.3–3.5%) discontinued treatment because of adverse GI effects than patients receiving placebo (0.2%). In a cardiovascular outcomes trial with a median follow-up of 5.4 years, cholelithiasis occurred at rates of 0.62 or 0.56 per 100 patient-years in patients receiving dulaglutide or placebo, respectively; serious acute cholecystitis occurred in 0.5 or 0.3%, respectively, of such patients. Data are lacking on the use of dulaglutide in patients with severe GI disease, including severe gastroparesis; the manufacturer states that the drug is not recommended in such patients.

Diabetic Retinopathy Complications

In a clinical study involving patients with type 2 diabetes mellitus and established cardiovascular disease or multiple cardiovascular risk factors (REWIND), a higher incidence of diabetic retinopathy complications was observed among patients who received dulaglutide compared with those who received placebo (1.9 versus 1.5%, respectively). Patients with a history of diabetic retinopathy at baseline had a greater absolute increase in risk for diabetic retinopathy complications compared with those without a known history of diabetic retinopathy. Rapid improvement in glucose control has been associated with a temporary worsening of diabetic retinopathy. Patients with a history of diabetic retinopathy should be monitored for progression of diabetic retinopathy while receiving dulaglutide.

Acute Gallbladder Disease

Acute events of gallbladder disease have been reported with GLP-1 receptor agonists, including dulaglutide, during clinical studies and postmarketing experience. If cholelithiasis is suspected, gallbladder studies and appropriate clinical follow-up are indicated.

Immunogenicity

In adult clinical trials of dulaglutide for the treatment of type 2 diabetes mellitus, anti-drug antibodies were detected in 1.6% of dulaglutide-treated patients; 0.9% of patients developed neutralizing antibodies and 0.9% of patients developed antibodies to native GLP-1. Such antibodies did not appear to have any clinically significant effects on the pharmacokinetics, pharmacodynamics, safety, or effectiveness of dulaglutide.

In the controlled clinical trial of dulaglutide for the treatment of type 2 diabetes mellitus in pediatric patients, 4% of dulaglutide-treated patients developed anti-drug antibodies; 1% of patients developed neutralizing antibodies and 3% developed antibodies against native GLP-1. Because of the low incidence, the effect of these antibodies on the pharmacokinetics, pharmacodynamics, safety, and/or effectiveness of dulaglutide is not known.

Specific Populations

Pregnancy

Data on the use of dulaglutide in pregnant women are not sufficient to determine a drug-associated risk for major birth defects and miscarriage. Poorly controlled diabetes mellitus during pregnancy increases maternal risks for diabetic ketoacidosis, preeclampsia, spontaneous abortion, preterm delivery, and delivery complications, and also increases the risk of major birth defects, stillbirth, and macrosomia-related morbidity in the fetus.

Based on studies in animals, there may be risks to the fetus from exposure to dulaglutide during pregnancy. Dulaglutide should be used during pregnancy only if the potential benefit justifies the potential risk to the fetus.

Lactation

Data are lacking regarding the distribution of dulaglutide into milk in humans, the effects on the breast-fed infant, or the effects on milk production. The developmental and health effects of breast-feeding should be considered along with the mother's clinical need for dulaglutide and any potential adverse effects on the breast-fed infant from the drug or the underlying maternal condition.

Pediatric Use

Use of dulaglutide in pediatric patients ≥10 years of age with type 2 diabetes mellitus is supported by a 26-week multicenter, randomized, double-blind, placebo-controlled trial. A higher incidence of injection site reactions have been reported in pediatric patients compared with adults receiving the drug. Efficacy and safety of dulaglutide have not been established in pediatric patients <10 years of age.

Geriatric Use

In adult clinical trials, 19% of dulaglutide-treated patients were 65 years of age and older and 2% were 75 years of age and older. No substantial differences in safety and efficacy relative to younger adults were observed in these patients.

Hepatic Impairment

Because of the limited clinical experience of dulaglutide in patients with hepatic impairment, the drug should be used with caution in such patients. In a single-dose pharmacokinetic study, systemic exposure of dulaglutide decreased by 23, 33, and 21% in patients with mild, moderate, and severe hepatic impairment, respectively, compared with that in patients with normal hepatic function. These findings were not considered clinically important, and no dosage adjustment is considered necessary in patients with hepatic impairment.

Renal Impairment

In clinical trials of dulaglutide, no overall differences in safety or efficacy were observed in patients with varying degrees of renal impairment.

In a single-dose pharmacokinetic study in individuals with renal impairment, systemic exposure to dulaglutide was increased by 20, 28, and 14% in patients with mild, moderate, and severe renal impairment, respectively, and by 12% in patients with end-stage renal disease compared with patients with normal renal function. Corresponding increases in peak plasma concentrations were 13, 23, and 20% in patients with mild, moderate, and severe renal impairment, respectively, and 11% in patients with end-stage renal disease. In addition, in a 52-week study in patients with type 2 diabetes mellitus and moderate to severe renal impairment, the pharmacokinetics of dulaglutide 0.75 and 1.5 mg once weekly were similar to those reported in prior clinical studies.

The manufacturer states that no dosage adjustment is necessary in patients with renal impairment including end-stage renal disease. However, caution is advised when the drug is used in patients with end-stage renal disease. Monitor renal function in patients with renal impairment reporting severe GI reactions.

Common Adverse Effects

Adverse effects reported in at least 5% of patients receiving dulaglutide include nausea, diarrhea, vomiting, abdominal pain, and decreased appetite.

DRUG INTERACTIONS

Effects on GI Absorption of Other Drugs

Dulaglutide delays gastric emptying and has the potential to reduce the rate of absorption of concomitantly administered oral drugs; the delay in gastric emptying is dose-dependent. Concentrations of orally administered drugs with a narrow therapeutic index (e.g., warfarin) should be monitored when such drugs are administered concomitantly with dulaglutide.

Acetaminophen

Concomitant administration of dulaglutide and acetaminophen did not meaningfully alter the peak plasma concentration or area under the concentration-time curve (AUC) of acetaminophen. The manufacturer states that no adjustment of concomitant acetaminophen dosage is necessary.

Atorvastatin

Concomitant administration of dulaglutide 1.5 mg and atorvastatin 40 mg decreased the AUC of atorvastatin by 21%, which is not considered clinically important. Peak plasma concentration of atorvastatin was reduced by 70%; the clinical importance of this is not known. The manufacturer states that no adjustment of concomitant atorvastatin dosage is necessary.

Digoxin

Concomitant administration of dulaglutide and digoxin did not meaningfully alter the peak plasma concentration or AUC of digoxin. The manufacturer states that no adjustment of concomitant digoxin dosage is necessary.

Insulin or Insulin Secretagogues

When initiating dulaglutide, consider reducing the dose of concomitantly administered insulin secretagogues (e.g., sulfonylureas) or insulin to reduce the risk of hypoglycemia.

Lisinopril

Concomitant administration of dulaglutide and lisinopril did not meaningfully alter the peak plasma concentration or AUC of lisinopril. The manufacturer states that no adjustment of concomitant lisinopril dosage is necessary.

Metformin

Concomitant administration of dulaglutide and metformin did not meaningfully alter the peak plasma concentration or AUC of metformin. The manufacturer states that no adjustment of concomitant metformin dosage is necessary.

Metoprolol

Concomitant administration of dulaglutide and metoprolol did not meaningfully alter the peak plasma concentration or AUC of metoprolol. The manufacturer states that no adjustment of concomitant metoprolol dosage is necessary.

Oral Contraceptives

Concomitant administration of dulaglutide and an oral contraceptive containing ethinyl estradiol and norgestimate did not substantially alter the AUC or peak plasma concentration of ethinyl estradiol or norelgestromin (a major metabolite of norgestimate); no adjustment of the concomitant oral contraceptive containing ethinyl estradiol and norgestimate dosage is necessary.

Sitagliptin

Administration of single doses of dulaglutide 1.5 mg with sitagliptin 100 mg at steady state resulted in increases of approximately 38 and 27% in dulaglutide AUC and peak plasma concentration, respectively, which was not considered clinically important; no dosage adjustment of either drug is necessary.

● *Warfarin*

Concomitant administration of dulaglutide 1.5 mg and single 10-mg doses of warfarin sodium did not meaningfully alter the AUC of *R*- or *S*-warfarin; the manufacturer states that no adjustment of concomitant warfarin dosage is necessary.

DESCRIPTION

Dulaglutide is a long-acting glucagon-like peptide-1 (GLP-1) receptor agonist prepared from mammalian cell culture. The drug is a recombinant fusion protein that consists of 2 identical disulfide-linked chains, each containing an N-terminal GLP-1 analog covalently linked to the Fc portion of a modified human immunoglobulin G_4 (IgG_4) heavy chain by a small peptide linker. Each GLP-1 analog is 90% homologous to human GLP-1 (7–37) with structural modifications conferring resistance to degradation by dipeptidyl peptidase-4 (DPP-4). Both resistance to DPP-4 degradation and large molecule size (approximately 63 kilodaltons) extend the half-life of dulaglutide, allowing for weekly dosing.

Activation of GLP-1 receptors by dulaglutide stimulates insulin release in the presence of elevated glucose concentrations, suppresses glucagon release, and slows gastric emptying, resulting in lower fasting and postprandial blood glucose concentrations in patients with type 2 diabetes mellitus. The delay in gastric emptying produced by dulaglutide is largest after the first dose and diminishes with subsequent dosing.

Peak plasma dulaglutide concentrations are achieved 24–72 hours following subcutaneous administration. Steady-state concentrations are achieved 2–4 weeks following weekly administration. Absolute bioavailability following subcutaneous administration of single doses of 0.75 and 1.5 mg are 65 and 47%, respectively. Dulaglutide is thought to be degraded into its component amino acids by general protein catabolism pathways. The elimination half-life of dulaglutide is approximately 5 days.

ADVICE TO PATIENTS

Importance of informing patients that dulaglutide causes benign and malignant thyroid C-cell tumors in rats and that relevance of this finding to humans is unknown. Patients should report symptoms of thyroid tumors (e.g., a lump in the neck, persistent hoarseness, dysphagia, dyspnea) to their clinician.

Importance of informing patients about the possibility of acute pancreatitis with dulaglutide therapy. Importance of patients informing clinicians if they have a history of pancreatitis. Importance of informing patients about signs and symptoms of pancreatitis, including persistent severe abdominal pain sometimes radiating to the back that may or may not be accompanied by vomiting; importance of patient discontinuing dulaglutide and promptly notifying clinician if such signs or symptoms occur.

Importance of informing patients of risk of hypoglycemia, particularly if concomitant therapy with an insulin secretagogue (e.g., sulfonylurea) or insulin is used. Importance of reviewing signs, symptoms, and management of hypoglycemia.

Importance of informing patients of possibility of hypersensitivity reactions. Patients should be instructed to discontinue dulaglutide and promptly seek medical advice if symptoms of hypersensitivity occur.

Inform patients of the potential risk for cholelithiasis or cholecystitis. Instruct patients to contact their physician if cholelithiasis or cholecystitis is suspected for appropriate clinical follow-up.

Importance of informing patients of potential risk of adverse GI effects and possibility of dehydration due to such adverse effects; patients should be advised to take precautions to avoid fluid depletion. Importance of informing patients of potential risk of worsening renal function, which may require dialysis in some cases.

Importance of informing patients to contact their clinician if they experience changes in vision during treatment with dulaglutide.

Importance of patients reading the manufacturer's instructions for use before starting dulaglutide therapy. Importance of instructing patients regarding proper use, storage, and disposal of injection pen. After dispensing, pens should be stored in the refrigerator or may be stored at room temperature for up to 14 days; injection pens should be protected from light and not frozen.

Importance of informing patients not to take an extra dose of dulaglutide to make up for a missed dose. If a dose is missed, patients should take the dose as soon as possible if there are at least 3 days (72 hours) until the next dose; the next dose can be taken on their usual weekly day. If there are less than 3 days until the next dose, the missed dose should be skipped and patient should take the next dose on their usual weekly day.

Importance of women informing clinicians if they are or plan to become pregnant or plan to breast-feed.

Importance of informing clinicians of existing or contemplated concomitant therapy, including prescription and OTC drugs, as well as any concomitant illnesses (e.g., pancreatitis, diabetic retinopathy, GI disease).

Importance of informing patients of other important precautionary information.

PREPARATIONS

Excipients in commercially available drug preparations may have clinically important effects in some individuals; consult specific product labeling for details.

Dulaglutide

Parenteral

Injection, for subcutaneous use only	0.75 mg/0.5 mL	Trulicity® (available as prefilled single-dose injection pen), Lilly
	1.5 mg/0.5 mL	Trulicity® (available as prefilled single-dose injection pen), Lilly
	3 mg/0.5 mL	Trulicity® (available as prefilled single-dose injection pen), Lilly
	4.5 mg/0.5 mL	Trulicity® (available as prefilled single-dose injection pen), Lilly

† Use is not currently included in the labeling approved by the US Food and Drug Administration.

Selected Revisions October 16, 2023, © Copyright, June 25, 2015, American Society of Health-System Pharmacists, Inc.

Exenatide

68:20.06 • INCRETIN MIMETICS

■ Exenatide, a synthetic, human glucagon-like peptide-1 (GLP-1) receptor agonist (incretin mimetic), is an antidiabetic agent.

USES

● Type 2 Diabetes Mellitus

Exenatide is used as an adjunct to diet and exercise to improve glycemic control in patients with type 2 diabetes mellitus. The drug is available as an injection for twice-daily administration (Byetta®) labeled for use in adults and as an extended-release for injectable suspension formulation for once-weekly administration labeled for use in adults and pediatric patients ≥10 years of age (Bydureon Bcise®).

Exenatide has been used as monotherapy or in combination with metformin, a sulfonylurea, or a thiazolidinedione; in combination with metformin and a sulfonylurea or a thiazolidinedione; or in combination with insulin glargine with or without metformin and/or a thiazolidinedione. The extended-release formulation of exenatide has been used as monotherapy or in combination with metformin, a sulfonylurea, or a thiazolidinedione; in combination with metformin and a sulfonylurea or a thiazolidinedione; in combination with an SGLT2 inhibitor and metformin; or in combination with basal insulin Because of the uncertain relevance to humans of thyroid C-cell tumors found in rodents given extended-release exenatide, this formulation of the drug is not recommended as *first-line* therapy for patients with inadequate glycemic control on diet and exercise alone.

Current guidelines for the treatment of type 2 diabetes mellitus generally recommend metformin as first-line therapy in addition to lifestyle modifications in patients with recent-onset type 2 diabetes mellitus or mild hyperglycemia because of its well-established safety and efficacy (i.e., beneficial effects on glycosylated hemoglobin [hemoglobin A_{1c}; HbA_{1c}], weight, and cardiovascular mortality). In patients with contraindications or intolerance to metformin (e.g., risk of lactic acidosis, GI intolerance) or in selected other patients, some experts suggest that initial therapy with a drug from another class of antidiabetic agents (e.g., GLP-1 receptor agonist, sodium-glucose cotransporter 2 [SGLT2] inhibitor, dipeptidyl peptidase-4 [DPP-4] inhibitor, sulfonylurea, thiazolidinedione, basal insulin) may be acceptable based on patient factors. Initiating antidiabetic therapy with 2 agents (e.g., metformin plus another agent) may be appropriate in patients with an initial HbA_{1c} exceeding 7.5% or at least 1.5% above the target level. In metformin-intolerant patients with high initial HbA_{1c} levels, some experts suggest initiation of therapy with 2 agents from other antidiabetic drug classes with complementary mechanisms of action.

Because of the progressive nature of type 2 diabetes mellitus, patients initially receiving an oral antidiabetic agent will eventually require multiple oral and/or injectable noninsulin antidiabetic agents of different therapeutic classes and/or insulin for adequate glycemic control. Patients who have inadequate glycemic control with initial (e.g., metformin) monotherapy should receive treatment with additional antidiabetic agents; data suggest that the addition of each noninsulin agent to initial therapy lowers HbA_{1c} by approximately 0.7–1%. In addition, early initiation of combination therapy may help to more rapidly attain glycemic goals and extend the time to treatment failure.

Factors to consider when selecting additional antidiabetic agents for combination therapy in patients with inadequate glycemic control on metformin monotherapy include patient comorbidities (e.g., atherosclerotic cardiovascular disease [ASCVD], established kidney disease, heart failure), hypoglycemia risk, impact on weight, cost, risk of adverse effects, and patient preference. When the greater glucose-lowering effect of an injectable drug is needed in patients with type 2 diabetes mellitus, some experts currently state that an injectable GLP-1 receptor agonist is preferred over insulin in most patients because of beneficial effects on body weight and a lower risk of hypoglycemia, although adverse GI effects may diminish tolerability. While addition of a GLP-1 receptor agonist may successfully control hyperglycemia, many patients will eventually require insulin therapy. Early introduction of insulin therapy should be considered when hyperglycemia is severe (e.g., blood glucose of at least 300 mg/dL or HbA_{1c} exceeding 9–10%), especially in the presence of catabolic manifestations (e.g., weight loss, hypertriglyceridemia, ketosis) or symptoms of hyperglycemia.

Experts recommend that patients with type 2 diabetes mellitus who have established (or are at a high risk for) ASCVD, established kidney disease, or heart failure should receive a GLP-1 receptor agonist or SGLT2 inhibitor with demonstrated cardiovascular disease benefit. Experts state that therapy with a GLP-1 receptor agonist or SGLT2 inhibitor should be considered for patients with the aforementioned comorbidities independently of the patients' HbA_{1c}. GLP-1 receptor agonists and SGLT2 inhibitors appear to have effects on the kidneys independent of their glycemic effects, and some experts suggest that an agent from one of these classes of drugs be considered in patients with type 2 diabetes mellitus and chronic kidney disease (CKD). In patients *without* established ASCVD or indicators of high ASCVD risk, heart failure, or CKD, the decision regarding the addition of other antidiabetic agents (e.g., GLP-1 receptor agonist, SGLT2 inhibitor, DPP-4 inhibitor, thiazolidinedione, sulfonylurea, basal insulin) to metformin therapy should be based on avoidance of adverse effects, cost, and individual patient factors.

Exenatide has not been studied in patients with a history of pancreatitis; other antidiabetic agents should be considered in such patients.

Exenatide is not indicated for the treatment of type 1 diabetes mellitus.

Exenatide (Byetta®) and extended-release exenatide (Bydureon Bcise®) should not be used concomitantly.

Exenatide

When given as monotherapy or add-on therapy, twice-daily exenatide improves glycemic control (e.g., as determined by changes in glycosylated hemoglobin [hemoglobin A_{1c}, HbA_{1c}]) more than placebo and similar to that of titrated insulin lispro or insulin aspart 70/30 therapy. In addition, therapy with GLP-1 receptor agonists such as exenatide generally is associated with weight loss compared with that observed with placebo and most other antidiabetic agents (e.g., sulfonylureas, thiazolidinediones, insulin).

Safety and efficacy of immediate-release exenatide as monotherapy in adults with type 2 diabetes mellitus have been established in a 24-week, randomized, double-blind, placebo-controlled study. In this study, patients with baseline HbA_{1c} concentrations of 6.5–10% (mean: 7.8–7.9%) received exenatide 5 or 10 mcg or placebo subcutaneously twice daily before the morning and evening meals. Patients assigned to receive exenatide 10 mcg twice daily received 5 mcg twice daily for 4 weeks, then 10 mcg twice daily. The primary study end point was the change in HbA_{1c} concentration from baseline to week 24 (or the last value at time of early discontinuance of therapy). At week 24, therapy with exenatide 5 or 10 mcg twice daily resulted in mean reductions of 0.7 or 0.9%, respectively, in HbA_{1c} compared with baseline. HbA_{1c} concentrations below 7% were achieved in 48, 53, or 38% of patients receiving exenatide 5 mcg, exenatide 10 mcg, or placebo, respectively. Patients receiving exenatide also experienced greater weight reduction than those receiving placebo (-2.8, -3.1, or -1.4 kg with twice-daily dosages of exenatide 5 mcg, 10 mcg, or placebo, respectively).

In several studies of 30 weeks' duration in which exenatide (5 or 10 mcg twice daily) was given in combination with maximally effective dosages of metformin hydrochloride, a sulfonylurea (e.g., glipizide, glyburide, glimepiride, tolazamide, chlorpropamide), or metformin hydrochloride in combination with a sulfonylurea, combined therapy with subcutaneous exenatide and these oral antidiabetic agents or regimens resulted in a reduction from baseline in HbA_{1c} and progressive weight loss compared with that achieved with existing oral antidiabetic therapy.

Safety and efficacy of exenatide as add-on therapy to other antidiabetic agents also have been established in other studies. In a 16-week, placebo-controlled study in patients who had not achieved adequate glycemic control with a thiazolidinedione with or without metformin, the addition of subcutaneous exenatide (5 or 10 mcg twice daily) to existing oral antidiabetic therapy resulted in a reduction from baseline in HbA_{1c} at week 16 compared with that achieved with existing oral antidiabetic therapy. In a 30-week, placebo-controlled study in patients with type 2 diabetes mellitus who had inadequate glycemic control on titrated insulin glargine with or without metformin and/or a thiazolidinedione (i.e., pioglitazone), addition of exenatide (5 or 10 mcg twice daily) to existing antidiabetic therapy reduced HbA_{1c} from baseline at week 30 compared with that achieved with existing antidiabetic therapy. In a 26-week randomized, open-label study in patients with type 2 diabetes mellitus receiving metformin therapy (baseline HbA_{1c} 6.5–10%), addition of exenatide (5 mcg twice daily for 4 weeks, then 10 mcg twice daily) was noninferior to addition of titrated, premixed insulin aspart (70% long-acting insulin aspart protamine, 30% rapid-acting insulin aspart) in improving HbA_{1c}

(least-squares mean HbA$_{1c}$ reduction of 1 or 1.14% with exenatide or insulin aspart 70/30, respectively). In addition, exenatide therapy was associated with less hypoglycemia than insulin aspart and resulted in weight reduction while insulin aspart 70/30 caused weight gain.

Extended-release Exenatide

Clinical studies indicate that the once-weekly extended-release formulation of exenatide generally is as effective as conventional regimens of metformin or pioglitazone and more effective than sitagliptin, titrated insulin glargine, insulin detemir, or twice-daily exenatide in improving glycemic control. Improvements in glycemic control have been maintained during long-term therapy (e.g., up to 6 years) with extended-release exenatide. In addition, compared with twice-daily exenatide, once-weekly extended-release exenatide generally has been associated with a similar degree of weight loss and GI adverse effects.

Safety and efficacy of once-weekly subcutaneous extended-release exenatide as monotherapy or in combination with other antidiabetic agents in adults have been established in several randomized, open-label or double-blind clinical studies generally of 24–30 weeks' duration (e.g., DURATION studies) in adults with type 2 diabetes mellitus; these studies were conducted with a previous formulation of extended-release exenatide. In the 6 DURATION studies, once-weekly therapy with subcutaneous extended-release exenatide was compared with subcutaneous insulin glargine, liraglutide, or twice-daily exenatide or with oral antidiabetic agents (metformin, sitagliptin, pioglitazone) in patients who had inadequate glycemic control (mean baseline HbA$_{1c}$ concentrations of 8.3–8.6%) with or without preexisting oral antidiabetic therapy. The primary efficacy end point in these studies was the mean change in HbA$_{1c}$ from baseline to the end of the study; extended-release exenatide reduced HbA$_{1c}$ by 1.3–1.9% compared with reductions of 0.9–1.5% for twice-daily exenatide, 1.2–1.6% for pioglitazone, 0.9–1.2% for sitagliptin, 1.5% for metformin, 1.3% for insulin glargine, and 1.5% for liraglutide. In general, extended-release exenatide was more effective than twice-daily exenatide overall in reducing HbA$_{1c}$ and fasting plasma glucose, while twice-daily exenatide had a greater effect on postprandial hyperglycemia. In addition, the proportion of patients achieving an HbA$_{1c}$ of less than 7% with extended-release exenatide in the DURATION studies generally was similar to that with pioglitazone and greater than that with sitagliptin or insulin glargine.

In the long-term therapy (up to 6 years) portions of the DURATION-1 study, improvements in glycemic control and weight generally were sustained in patients who continued once-weekly therapy with extended-release exenatide and sustained or enhanced in those whose therapy was switched from the twice-daily to the once-weekly formulation. Compared with insulin and most oral antidiabetic agents, therapy with subcutaneous extended-release exenatide resulted in slow but progressive weight loss, which was similar to that associated with twice-daily exenatide and sustained during long-term therapy. Extended-release exenatide therapy was well tolerated in these studies, with no major hypoglycemic episodes reported and a low risk of hypoglycemia compared with insulin and most other oral antidiabetic agent comparators; when hypoglycemic episodes occurred, patients generally were receiving concomitant sulfonylurea therapy.

Efficacy of extended-release exenatide in conjunction with basal insulin with or without metformin hydrochloride in the management of type 2 diabetes mellitus in adults with inadequate glycemic control despite treatment with titrated insulin glargine (dosage of at least 20 units daily) with or without metformin hydrochloride is supported by results of a 28-week, randomized, active-controlled study (DURATION-7). In this study, the addition of extended-release exenatide to existing therapy with insulin glargine with or without metformin hydrochloride resulted in substantially greater improvements in HbA$_{1c}$ compared with insulin glargine therapy with or without metformin (reduction of 0.88 versus 0.24%, respectively). Greater reductions in fasting plasma glucose concentrations and body weight also were observed among patients who received therapy with extended-release exenatide therapy.

Efficacy of extended-release exenatide in conjunction with dapagliflozin as add-on therapy to metformin hydrochloride in the management of type 2 diabetes mellitus in adults who have inadequate glycemic control (HbA$_{1c}$ concentration of 8 to less than 12%) with metformin hydrochloride is supported by results of a 28-week, randomized, active-controlled study (DURATION-8). In this study, the addition of dapagliflozin (10 mg daily) and extended-release exenatide (2 mg once weekly) to existing stable therapy with metformin hydrochloride (at least 1.5 g daily) resulted in substantially greater improvements in HbA$_{1c}$ and fasting plasma glucose compared with dapagliflozin or extended-release exenatide therapy

alone. In patients who received dapagliflozin 10 mg once daily and extended-release exenatide 2 mg once weekly as add-on therapy to metformin hydrochloride, addition of dapagliflozin and extended-release exenatide reduced HbA$_{1c}$ by 1.77%, versus a 1.3 or 1.42% reduction in those receiving add-on therapy with dapagliflozin or extended-release exenatide alone, respectively. More weight loss and greater reductions in systolic blood pressure also were observed among those who received add-on therapy with dapagliflozin and extended-release exenatide compared with add-on therapy with either drug alone.

A 28-week open-label (oral medication blinded) comparator- and placebo-controlled trial was conducted to evaluate the effects of the currently available extended-release formulation of exenatide to sitagliptan in adults with type 2 diabetes mellitus who had inadequate glycemic control despite metformin therapy. Patients were randomized to receive extended-release exenatide 2 mg once weekly, sitagliptan 100 mg daily, or placebo in addition to their existing metformin therapy. Treatment with extended-release exenatide resulted in a statistically significant mean reduction in HbA$_{1c}$ compared to placebo. The difference in HbA$_{1c}$ reduction from baseline with extended-release exenatide compared to sitagliptan was not statistically significant; sitagliptan did not show superiority over placebo in this study.

Efficacy and safety of extended-release exenatide in pediatric patients were evaluated in a 24-week, randomized, double-blind, placebo-controlled study with a previous formulation of extended-release exenatide and a 28-week open-label uncontrolled extension in 82 patients 10–17 years of age with type 2 diabetes mellitus treated with diet and exercise alone or in combination with a stable dosage of oral antidiabetic agents and/or insulin. At baseline mean HbA$_{1c}$ was 8.17%. After 24 weeks of treatment, exenatide was more effective than placebo in reducing HbA$_{1c}$ (difference of -0.71). Use of extended-release exenatide in the pediatric population is further supported by a pediatric pharmacokinetics study and studies in adults with type 2 diabetes mellitus.

A randomized, open-label study was conducted to compare the efficacy and safety of extended-release exenatide (Bydureon Bcise®) to immediate-release exenatide (Byetta®) in adults with type 2 diabetes and inadequate glycemic control with diet and exercise alone or with oral antidiabetic therapy including metformin, a sulfonylurea, a thiazolidinedione, or any combination of these therapies. Patients were randomized to extended-release exenatide 2 mg once weekly or immediate-release exenatide 10 mcg twice daily. Treatment with extended-release exenatide resulted in a statistically significantly greater reduction in HbA$_{1c}$ compared to immediate-release exenatide at 28 weeks. The mean reduction in HbA$_{1c}$ with extended-release exenatide was noninferior to the immediate-release formulation based on the prespecified noninferior margin.

Reduction in Risk of Major Adverse Cardiovascular Events

Some GLP-1 receptor agonists (e.g., liraglutide) have demonstrated the ability to reduce the risk of cardiovascular events in those patients with type 2 diabetes mellitus and established cardiovascular disease. While exenatide therapy has *not* been associated with reductions in major cardiovascular events in clinical trials, the extended-release formulation does not appear to *increase* the risk of such events in patients with type 2 diabetes mellitus with or without preexisting cardiovascular disease. In addition to lowering blood glucose, GLP-1 receptor agonists appear to modify several nonglycemic cardiovascular risk factors, such as blood pressure, body weight, and lipid profile. GLP-1 receptor agonists also may have beneficial endothelial effects. The Exenatide Study of Cardiovascular Event Lowering (EXSCEL) was designed to assess the cardiovascular safety and efficacy of extended-release exenatide in patients with type 2 diabetes mellitus with or without cardiovascular disease. This study included adults (mean age: 62 years) with type 2 diabetes mellitus; approximately 73% of patients had established cardiovascular disease (e.g., history of major clinical manifestation of coronary artery disease, ischemic cerebrovascular disease, atherosclerotic peripheral arterial disease). In this study, patients received 2 mg of extended-release exenatide or placebo subcutaneously once weekly. During the study, other antidiabetic agents also were used to achieve clinically appropriate HbA$_{1c}$ concentrations. Other oral antidiabetic drugs used in the study included metformin hydrochloride (76.6%), sulfonylurea (36.6%), DPP-4 inhibitors (14.9%), thiazolidinediones (3.9%), and SGLT2 inhibitors (0.9%). Approximately 46.3% of patients also received insulin therapy (13.8% with insulin alone and 32.6% with insulin and one or more oral antidiabetic agents). The use of concomitant cardiovascular medications (e.g., angiotensin-converting enzyme [ACE] inhibitors, angiotensin II receptor antagonists, diuretics, β-adrenergic blocking agents, calcium-channel blocking agents, antithrombotics and anticoagulants, and lipid-lowering agents) was similar between the extended-release exenatide treatment group and the placebo group. The primary outcome was the composite of time to first occurrence of cardiovascular death, nonfatal myocardial infarction (MI), and nonfatal stroke. In this study, treatment with extended-release exenatide did not increase the risk of a major cardiovascular adverse event; additionally, there was no substantial difference in the incidence of major cardiovascular adverse events between those who received extended-release exenatide and those who received placebo (event rate 11.4 versus 12.2%, respectively).

Beneficial Effects on Renal Function

In several cardiovascular outcomes trials involving the use of GLP-1 receptor agonists (e.g., dulaglutide, liraglutide, semaglutide) in patients with type 2 diabetes mellitus at high risk for cardiovascular disease or with existing cardiovascular disease, beneficial effects on renal function have been observed as a secondary outcome. Some experts state that in patients with type 2 diabetes mellitus and CKD who are at increased risk for cardiovascular events, use of a GLP-1 receptor agonist may reduce risk of progression of albuminuria, cardiovascular events, or both†.

DOSAGE AND ADMINISTRATION

● General
Patient Monitoring

Patients should be monitored regularly (e.g., blood glucose determinations, HbA$_{1c}$) to determine therapeutic response.

● Administration
Exenatide (Byetta®)

Exenatide is administered by subcutaneous injection into the abdomen, thigh, or upper arm; safety and efficacy of IV or IM administration have not been established.

Exenatide is administered within 60 minutes *before* the morning and evening meals (or before the 2 main meals of the day, approximately 6 hours or more apart); it should *not* be administered after a meal.

If a dose of exenatide is missed, that dose should be omitted and the next dose taken at the regularly scheduled time.

Exenatide should not be transferred from the injection pen to a syringe or vial. Exenatide should not be mixed with insulin in the same injection pen or vial even if they are taken at the same time. Exenatide should be used only if the solution is clear, colorless, and contains no particles.

Exenatide injection pens should be stored in the original carton and protected from light at 2–8°C before first use and at room temperature not exceeding 25°C after first use. Exenatide pens should not be frozen; the pen should be discarded if it has been frozen. Injection pens should be discarded 30 days after first use, even if some drug remains in the pen.

The manufacturer's instructions for use should be consulted for additional details about preparation and administration of exenatide.

Extended-release Exenatide (Bydureon Bcise®)

Extended-release exenatide is administered by subcutaneous injection into the abdomen, thigh, or back of upper arm region; the drug must not be administered IV or IM. Patients should use a different injection site each week when administering extended-release exenatide in the same region. Patients and caregivers must be trained on proper preparation and administration.

Extended-release exenatide may be administered at any time during the dosing day, with or without a meal. The day of weekly administration of extended-release exenatide may be changed if necessary, provided the last dose was administered at least 3 days previously.

Remove autoinjector from refrigerator 15 minutes prior to administration. Prepare the autoinjector by shaking vigorously for at least 15 seconds to mix the solution. Administer immediately

If a dose of extended-release exenatide is missed, the missed dose should be administered as soon as noticed provided there are at least 3 days until the next scheduled dose; the usual regimen of extended-release exenatide (once weekly) may then be resumed. If a dose is missed and the next regularly scheduled dose is

due in 1 or 2 days, the missed dose should *not* be administered; instead, the next dose should be taken on the regularly scheduled day.

Extended-release exenatide should be stored at 2–8°C up to the expiration date or until preparation for use. If needed, the drug can be stored for up to 4 weeks at room temperature *not* to exceed 25°C. Extended-release exenatide should be protected from light and should not be frozen; the drug should be discarded if it has been frozen.

The manufacturer's instructions for use should be consulted for additional details about preparation and administration of extended-release exenatide.

● Dosage
Type 2 Diabetes Mellitus
Exenatide

The recommended initial dosage of exenatide for the management of type 2 diabetes mellitus is 5 mcg subcutaneously twice daily. Based on clinical response, the dosage of exenatide may be increased to 10 mcg subcutaneously twice daily 1 month after treatment initiation.

Patients receiving exenatide in combination with a sulfonylurea may require a reduction in the dosage of the sulfonylurea to reduce the risk of hypoglycemia.

When exenatide is used in combination with insulin, the dosage of insulin should be evaluated. In patients at increased risk of hypoglycemia, a reduction in the dosage of insulin should be considered.

Extended-release Exenatide

The recommended dosage of extended-release exenatide for the management of type 2 diabetes mellitus in adults and pediatric patients ≥10 years of age is 2 mg subcutaneously once every 7 days (once weekly).

Patients receiving extended-release exenatide in combination with insulin or an insulin secretagogue (e.g., sulfonylurea) may require a reduction in the dosage of the sulfonylurea or insulin to reduce the risk of hypoglycemia.

If extended-release exenatide is initiated in an individual already receiving immediate-release exenatide, the immediate-release formulation should be discontinued. Patients changing from therapy with immediate-release exenatide to extended-release exenatide may experience transient elevations (lasting approximately 2–4 weeks) in blood glucose concentrations.

● Special Populations
Hepatic Impairment

The pharmacokinetics of exenatide have not been studied in patients with acute or chronic hepatic impairment. However, since exenatide is eliminated principally by the kidney, dosage adjustments are not expected to be necessary in patients with hepatic impairment.

Renal Impairment

No dosage adjustment of exenatide is required in patients with mild renal impairment (creatinine clearance 50–80 mL/minute). Caution should be used when initiating exenatide or increasing dosage from 5 mcg twice daily to 10 mcg twice daily in patients with moderate renal impairment (creatinine clearance 30–50 mL/minute). In a study of exenatide in patients with end-stage renal disease receiving dialysis, mean exenatide exposure increased by 3.4-fold compared with that in patients with normal renal function. Extended-release exenatide has not been studied in patients with severe renal impairment (creatinine clearance less than 30 mL/min) or in patients with end-stage renal disease receiving dialysis. However, population pharmacokinetic analysis of patients with renal impairment who received extended-release exenatide 2 mg indicates that exposure to the drug is increased by 62 or 33% in those with moderate or mild renal impairment, respectively. Exenatide and extended-release exenatide should not be used in patients with end-stage renal disease or severe renal impairment (creatinine clearance less than 30 mL/minute for exenatide or estimated glomerular filtration rate [eGFR] less than 45 mL/minute per 1.73 m² for extended-release exenatide) and should be used with caution in patients with moderate renal impairment or in those who have undergone renal transplantation.

Geriatric Patients

Careful dosage selection is recommended in geriatric patients due to possible age-related decrease in renal function and concomitant disease and drug therapy;

however, dosage requirements generally are similar in geriatric patients and younger adults. Caution should be used when initiating extended-release exenatide in geriatric patients.

Other Special Populations

Population pharmacokinetic analysis suggests that body mass index has no clinically important effect on the pharmacokinetics of exenatide, and sex and race do not affect steady-state concentrations of exenatide following administration of extended-release exenatide.

CAUTIONS

● Contraindications

Known hypersensitivity to exenatide or any ingredient in the formulation.

History of drug-induced immune-mediated thrombocytopenia from exenatide products.

Extended-release exenatide is contraindicated in patients with a personal or family history of medullary thyroid carcinoma (MTC) and in patients with multiple endocrine neoplasia syndrome type 2 (MEN 2).

● Warnings/Precautions

Warnings

Risk of Thyroid C-cell Tumors with Extended-release Exenatide

Extended-release exenatide causes a dose-dependent and treatment-duration-dependent increase in the incidence of thyroid C-cell tumors (adenomas and/or carcinomas) at clinically relevant exposures in male and female rats compared with controls. The manufacturer states the potential of extended-release exenatide to induce C-cell tumors in mice has not been established. Other glucagon-like peptide-1 (GLP-1) receptor agonists also have induced thyroid C-cell adenomas and carcinomas in male and female mice and rats at clinically relevant exposures. It is unknown whether extended-release exenatide causes thyroid C-cell tumors, including MTC, in humans. Serum calcitonin, a biologic marker of MTC, was not assessed in clinical trials evaluating the use of extended-release exenatide. Patients with MTC typically have serum calcitonin concentrations exceeding 50 ng/L. Patients receiving extended-release exenatide who have thyroid nodules noted on physical examination or neck imaging should be referred to an endocrinologist for further evaluation. Although routine monitoring of serum calcitonin or using thyroid ultrasound for early detection of MTC in patients receiving extended-release exenatide is of uncertain value, patients should also be referred to an endocrinologist for further evaluation if serum calcitonin is measured and found to be elevated.

Sensitivity Reactions

Generalized pruritus and/or urticaria and macular or papular rash have been reported during postmarketing experience with exenatide. Serious hypersensitivity reactions (e.g., angioedema, anaphylaxis) also have been reported. If a hypersensitivity reaction occurs, exenatide or extended-release exenatide and other suspect agents should be discontinued, and the patient should seek medical advice promptly. Patients with a history of anaphylaxis or angioedema with another GLP-1 receptor agonist should be monitored closely for allergic reactions; it is unknown whether such patients will be predisposed to anaphylaxis with extended-release exenatide.

Other Warnings and Precautions

Risks During General Anesthesia and Deep Sedation

GLP-1 agonists are associated with adverse GI effects such as nausea, vomiting, and delayed gastric emptying; such effects are likely a result of rapid tachyphlaxis at the level of vagal nerve activation. Delayed gastric emptying from GLP-1 agonists can increase the risk of regurgitation and pulmonary aspiration of gastric contents during general anesthesia and deep sedation. Given these concerns, the American Society of Anesthesiologists (ASA) Task Force on Preoperative Fasting has issued a consensus-based guidance for the management of GLP-1 receptor agonists prior to elective surgery. The task force suggests that for patients on daily GLP-1 agonist dosing (irrespective of indication, dose, or type of surgery), consider holding the

drug on the day of the procedure/surgery. For patients on weekly dosing (irrespective of indication, dose, or type of surgery), consider holding the GLP-1 agonist a week prior to the procedure/surgery. If GLP-1 agonists prescribed for diabetes management are held for longer than the dosing schedule, consider consulting an endocrinologist for bridging the antidiabetic therapy to avoid hyperglycemia. These recommendations are based on limited evidence only (case reports). For patients requiring urgent or emergent procedures, the task force states to proceed and treat the patient as 'full stomach' and manage accordingly.

Pancreatitis and Pancreatic Precancerous Changes

Acute pancreatitis, including fatal and nonfatal hemorrhagic or necrotizing pancreatitis requiring hospitalization, has been reported during postmarketing experience with exenatide. Persistent, severe abdominal pain, which may be accompanied by vomiting, is the hallmark symptom of acute pancreatitis. Most patients who have developed pancreatitis during exenatide therapy had at least one other risk factor for acute pancreatitis (e.g., gallstones, severe hypertriglyceridemia, alcohol use) and have required hospitalization. Some patients have developed serious complications including dehydration and renal failure, suspected ileus, phlegmon, and ascites. Acute or worsening pancreatitis has been associated temporally with an increase in exenatide dosage from 5 to 10 mcg twice daily, the maximum recommended dosage, in some patients. Symptoms of acute pancreatitis (e.g., nausea, vomiting, abdominal pain) recurred upon rechallenge with the drug in several patients; abdominal pain abated after permanent discontinuance of the drug in one patient. Most patients have improved upon discontinuance of exenatide.

If pancreatitis is suspected, therapy with exenatide should be promptly discontinued and appropriate therapy initiated. Exenatide should *not* be resumed if pancreatitis is confirmed.

Data are lacking on the use of exenatide in patients with a history of pancreatitis; other antidiabetic therapies should be considered in such patients.

Use with Drugs Known to Cause Hypoglycemia

The risk of hypoglycemia is increased when exenatide is used in combination with an insulin secretagogue (e.g., sulfonylurea) or insulin. The risk may be decreased with a reduction in dosage of sulfonylurea (or other concomitantly administered insulin secretagogue).

When exenatide is used in combination with insulin, the dosage of insulin should be evaluated. In a clinical trial in which exenatide was added to insulin glargine therapy, the dosage of insulin glargine was reduced by 20% in patients with HbA$_{1c}$ concentrations of 8% or less; however, some clinicians suggest that the relative safety and efficacy of this approach to dosage adjustment of basal insulin may not apply to patients with baseline HbA$_{1c}$ concentrations of less than 7%, those with a recent history of major hypoglycemia, or those receiving long-acting GLP-1 receptor agonists. In patients at increased risk of hypoglycemia, a reduction in the dosage of insulin should be considered.

Renal Effects

Deterioration of renal function (e.g., increased serum creatinine concentrations, renal impairment/insufficiency, worsened chronic renal failure, acute renal failure sometimes requiring hemodialysis or kidney transplantation) has been reported rarely with exenatide. Some of these events occurred in patients experiencing nausea, vomiting, and/or diarrhea with or without dehydration; these adverse effects may have contributed to development of altered renal function in these patients. Some of these events also occurred in patients receiving exenatide in combination with other agents known to affect renal function or hydration status (e.g., angiotensin-converting enzyme inhibitors, nonsteroidal anti-inflammatory agents, diuretics).

Exenatide has not been found to be directly nephrotoxic in preclinical or clinical studies. Renal effects usually have been reversible with supportive treatment and discontinuance of potentially causative agents, including exenatide. Altered renal function may be a consequence of diabetes mellitus, independent of any risk associated with exenatide therapy. Because exenatide or extended-release exenatide may induce nausea and vomiting with transient hypovolemia, treatment with this drug may worsen renal function.

Clinicians should closely monitor patients receiving exenatide for signs and symptoms of renal dysfunction and consider discontinuance of the drug if renal dysfunction is suspected and cannot be explained by other causes.

GI Effects

Data are lacking on the use of exenatide in patients with severe GI disease, including gastroparesis. Use of exenatide is commonly associated with adverse GI effects, including nausea, vomiting, and diarrhea. Nausea, vomiting, and/or diarrhea resulting in dehydration, abdominal distention, abdominal pain, eructation, constipation, flatulence, acute pancreatitis, and hemorrhagic and necrotizing pancreatitis sometimes resulting in death have been reported during postmarketing experience with exenatide. Use of exenatide or extended-release exenatide is not recommended in patients with severe GI disease.

Immunogenicity

Antibodies to exenatide have developed in patients receiving exenatide. Antibodies to exenatide were assessed in 90% of patients in the 30-, 16-, and 24-week clinical trials of exenatide with or without other antidiabetic therapy. Patients in these trials who had low-titer (e.g., less than 625) antibodies to exenatide (38, 31, or 28% of patients assessed for antibodies in the 3 clinical trials at 30, 16, or 24 weeks, respectively) generally had glycemic control (based on glycosylated hemoglobin [HbA$_{1c}$]) comparable to that of patients without antibodies. Of patients who had higher (e.g., 625 or higher) antibody titers (6, 9, or 2% of patients assessed for antibodies in the 3 clinical trials, respectively), 3, 4, or 1% of patients, respectively, appeared to have an attenuated glycemic response.

Anti-exenatide antibodies were measured in 2 controlled studies of extended-release exenatide in adults with type 2 diabetes mellitus. During the 28-week treatment period in these trials, 32% of exenatide-treated patients with evaluable anti-exenatide antibody measurements developed high titer antibodies and these patients had a lower glycemic response compared to exenatide-treated patients who did not have anti-drug antibodies during the treatment period. Injection-site reactions were more common in patients with high-titer antibodies compared with those with low-titer antibodies or no antibodies. There is insufficient data to determine the effects of antibody development on the severity of injection-site reactions or on the incidence and severity of hypersensitivity reactions. In a 52-week study of extended-release exenatide in pediatric patients with type 2 diabetes mellitus, 64% of exenatide-treated patients had high titer anti-exenatide antibodies at any time during the study and appeared to have a lower glycemic response compared with patients who did not develop anitbodies. There is insufficient data to assess whether the observed anti-exenatide antibodies in pediatric patients had an effect on the incidence or severity of hypersensitivity reactions or injection-site reactions.

Approximately 210 patients with anti-exenatide antibodies in clinical trials were evaluated for cross-reactive antibodies to GLP-1 and/or glucagon, and treatment-emergent cross-reactive antibodies were not observed across the range of titers.

If worsening glycemic control or failure to achieve targeted glycemic control occurs in patients receiving exenatide or extended-release exenatide therapy, alternative antidiabetic therapy should be considered.

Injection-site Reactions

Serious injection-site reactions (e.g., abscess, cellulitis, necrosis) with or without subcutaneous nodules have been reported during postmarketing experience in patients receiving extended-release exenatide; in isolated cases, surgical intervention was required. Injection-site reactions also have been reported with exenatide during postmarketing experience.

The incidence of injection-site reactions for patients treated with extended-release exenatide was similar for patients with antibodies to the drug and those without evidence of such antibody development (5.8 and 7%, respectively). In the 5 comparator-controlled clinical studies, injection-site reactions were observed more frequently in patients treated with extended-release exenatide (17.1%) than in patients treated with exenatide (12.7%), titrated insulin glargine (1.8%), or in those patients who received placebo injections (sitagliptin [10.6%], pioglitazone [6.4%], and metformin [13%] treatment arms). For patients treated with extended-release exenatide, injection-site reactions were more commonly observed in antibody-positive patients (14.2%) versus antibody-negative patients (3.1%), with a greater incidence in those with higher titer antibodies.

Risk Associated with Sharing of Injection Pens

Exenatide and extended-release exenatide injection pens must never be shared among patients, even if the needle has been changed. Sharing of injection pens poses a risk for transmission of blood-borne pathogens.

Acute Gallbladder Disease

Acute events of gallbladder disease have been reported with GLP-1 receptor agonist use, including exenatide, during clinical studies. In the EXSCEL study, 1.9% of patients who received extended-release exenatide and 1.4% of those who received placebo reported an acute event of gallbladder disease (e.g., cholelithiasis, cholecystitis). If cholelithiasis is suspected, the manufacturer states that gallbladder studies and appropriate clinical follow-up are indicated.

Drug-Induced Thrombocytopenia

Serious bleeding, which may be fatal, from drug-induced immune-mediated thrombocytopenia has been reported with exenatide use. Platelet destruction is caused by the presence of exenatide-dependent antiplatelet antibodies. If drug-induced thrombocytopenia is suspected, exenatide should be discontinued and the patient should not be re-exposed to the drug. Following discontinuance of extended-release exenatide, thrombocytopenia can persist due to the prolonged exenatide exposure (approximately 10 weeks).

Specific Populations

Pregnancy

Data are lacking on the use of exenatide or extended-release exenatide in pregnant women. In animal reproduction studies in rats, exenatide or extended-release exenatide use during pregnancy was associated with reduced fetal growth and skeletal ossification deficits. In animal reproduction studies in mice, exenatide use was associated with an increased number of neonatal deaths. Exenatide or extended-release exenatide should be used during pregnancy only if the potential benefit justifies the potential risk to the fetus.

Lactation

Exenatide is distributed into milk in mice. It is not known whether exenatide is distributed into human milk. The benefits of breast-feeding and the importance of exenatide or extended-release exenatide to the woman should be considered along with any potential adverse effects on the breast-fed infant from the drug or from the underlying maternal condition.

Pediatric Use

Safety and efficacy of immediate-release exenatide have not been established in patients. Safety and efficacy of extended-release exenatide have not been established in pediatric patients <10 years of age. Use of extended-release exenatide in pediatric patients ≥10 years of age is supported by a 24-week placebo-controlled trial with a previous formulation of extended-release exenatide and a 28-week open-label uncontrolled extension in 82 pediatric patients ≥10 years of age with type 2 diabetes, a pediatric pharmacokinetic study, and studies in adults with type 2 diabetes mellitus.

Geriatric Use

No substantial differences in safety and efficacy nor in pharmacokinetics have been observed in geriatric patients relative to younger adults. Because geriatric patients are more likely to have decreased renal function, caution should be used when initiating therapy with the drug in such patients.

Hepatic Impairment

Exenatide has not been studied in patients with a diagnosis of acute or chronic hepatic impairment. Because exenatide is cleared principally by the kidney, hepatic dysfunction is not expected to affect blood concentrations of the drug, and the manufacturer makes no specific dosage recommendations for patients with hepatic impairment.

Renal Impairment

Use of exenatide or extended-release exenatide is not recommended in patients with end-stage renal disease or severe renal impairment (creatinine clearance less than 30 mL/minute for exenatide or estimated glomerular filtration rate [eGFR] less than 45 mL/minute per 1.73 m^2 for extended-release exenatide); the drug should be used with caution in patients who have undergone renal transplantation. In patients with end-stage renal disease receiving dialysis, mean exenatide clearance was reduced to 0.9 L/hour compared with 9.1 L/hour in patients without renal disease, and single 5-mcg doses of exenatide were not well tolerated in patients with end-stage renal disease because of adverse GI effects. Because exenatide or extended-release exenatide may induce nausea and vomiting with transient hypovolemia, treatment with this drug may worsen renal function. Data are lacking on the use of extended-release exenatide in patients with end-stage renal disease or severe renal impairment.

In patients with mild renal impairment (creatinine clearance 50–80 mL/minute), no adjustment of exenatide dosage is required. Caution should be used when initiating exenatide or increasing exenatide dosage from 5 mcg twice daily to 10 mcg twice daily in patients with moderate renal impairment (creatinine clearance 30–50 mL/minute). Patients receiving extended-release exenatide who have mild renal impairment should be monitored for adverse effects (e.g., nausea and vomiting) that may lead to hypovolemia. In patients with mild to moderate renal impairment (creatinine clearance 30–80 mL/minute), systemic exposure to exenatide was similar to that in individuals with normal renal function.

Extended-release exenatide should be used with caution in patients with moderate renal impairment (creatinine clearance 30–50 mL/minute).

● Common Adverse Effects

The most common adverse effects (≥5%) in clinical trials of exenatide injection were nausea, hypoglycemia, vomiting, diarrhea, feeling jittery, dizziness, headache, dyspepsia, constipation, and asthenia. Nausea usually decreased over time.

The most common adverse effects (≥5%) in clinical trials of extended-release exanatide were injection-site nodule and nausea.

DRUG INTERACTIONS

● Effects on GI Absorption of Other Drugs

The effect of exenatide-induced slowing of gastric emptying may reduce the rate and extent of absorption of concomitantly administered oral drugs. Exenatide should be used with caution in patients receiving oral drugs that have a narrow therapeutic index or require rapid GI absorption. In patients receiving oral drugs for which efficacy depends on threshold concentrations, such as oral contraceptives and anti-infective agents, those drugs should be taken at least 1 hour before exenatide administration. If such drugs need to be administered with food, patients should take them with a meal or snack (e.g., lunch) at a time when exenatide is not administered.

Because of the potential for similar effects of extended-release exenatide on concomitant oral drug absorption, caution should be used with such concomitant use.

● Acetaminophen

When acetaminophen (1 g) was administered simultaneously with subcutaneous exenatide (10 mcg) or 1, 2, or 4 hours following exenatide injection, acetaminophen area under the concentration-time curve (AUC) decreased by 21, 23, 24, or 14%, respectively; peak plasma concentrations decreased by 37, 56, 54, or 41%, respectively; and time to peak plasma concentrations increased from 0.6 hours to 0.9, 4.2, 3.3, or 1.6 hours, respectively; however, acetaminophen AUC, peak plasma concentration, and time to peak plasma concentration were not appreciably changed when acetaminophen was given 1 hour prior to exenatide.

When acetaminophen (1 g) was administered either with or without a meal following 14 weeks of therapy with subcutaneous extended-release exenatide (2 mg once weekly), no substantial changes in acetaminophen AUC were observed compared with control. Acetaminophen peak plasma concentration was reduced by 16% (fasting) and 5% (fed), and time to peak plasma concentration was increased from approximately 1 hour in the control period to 1.4 and 1.3 hours in the fasting and fed states, respectively.

● Antidiabetic Agents

The risk of hypoglycemia is increased when exenatide is used in combination with an insulin secretagogue (e.g., sulfonylurea) or insulin; patients receiving these drugs concomitantly may require a reduction in the dosage of the sulfonylurea or insulin.

When exenatide is used in combination with insulin, the dosage of insulin should be evaluated; in patients at increased risk of hypoglycemia, a reduction in the dosage of insulin should be considered.

● Anti-infective Agents

The effect of exenatide-induced slowing of gastric emptying may reduce the rate and extent of absorption of concomitantly administered oral anti-infective agents. Oral anti-infective agents should be taken at least 1 hour before exenatide administration.

● Digoxin

Administration of exenatide (10 mcg subcutaneously twice daily) 30 minutes before digoxin (0.25 mg orally once daily) decreased the peak plasma concentration of digoxin by 17% and delayed the time to peak plasma concentration of digoxin by approximately 2.5 hours; however, there was no change in the overall steady-state AUC and renal clearance of digoxin.

● Lisinopril

In patients with mild to moderate hypertension receiving stable dosages of lisinopril (5–20 mg daily), exenatide (10 mcg subcutaneously twice daily) did not alter the steady-state AUC or peak plasma concentration of lisinopril or the 24-hour mean systolic and diastolic blood pressure. However, the steady-state time to peak plasma concentration of lisinopril was delayed by 2 hours.

● Lovastatin

Administration of exenatide (10 mcg subcutaneously twice daily) 30 minutes before lovastatin (single 40-mg oral dose) decreased the lovastatin AUC and peak plasma concentration by approximately 40 and 28%, respectively, and delayed the time to peak plasma concentration of lovastatin by 4 hours. In clinical trials, the use of exenatide in patients already receiving HMG-CoA reductase inhibitors (statins) was not associated with consistent changes in lipid profiles compared to baseline.

● Oral Contraceptives

In healthy women, repeated daily administration of a fixed-combination oral contraceptive (30 mcg of ethinyl estradiol and 150 mcg of levonorgestrel) 30 minutes after subcutaneous injection of exenatide (10 mcg twice daily) decreased the peak plasma concentrations of ethinyl estradiol and levonorgestrel by 45 and 27%, respectively, and delayed the time to peak plasma concentrations of ethinyl estradiol and levonorgestrel by 3 and 3.5 hours, respectively. Repeated daily administration of the fixed-combination oral contraceptive 1 hour prior to administration of exenatide decreased the mean peak plasma concentration of ethinyl estradiol by 15%; however, the mean peak plasma concentration of levonorgestrel was not substantially changed. Exenatide did not alter the mean trough concentrations of levonorgestrel following repeated daily administration of the fixed-combination oral contraceptive for both regimens; however, the mean trough concentration of ethinyl estradiol increased by 20% when the fixed-combination oral contraceptive was administered 30 minutes after exenatide injection. In this study, the effect of exenatide on the pharmacokinetics of oral contraceptives was confounded by the possible effect of food on oral contraceptives. Therefore, oral contraceptives should be administered at least 1 hour prior to exenatide administration.

● Warfarin

Increases in international normalized ratio [INR], sometimes associated with bleeding, have been reported during postmarketing experience with concomitant use of exenatide and warfarin. In a drug interaction study, no clinically important changes in warfarin (S- or R-enantiomer) AUC, peak plasma concentrations, or therapeutic response (as indicated by INR) were observed when warfarin sodium (single 25-mg dose) was administered 35 minutes after exenatide (5 mcg subcutaneously twice daily for 2 days, then 10 mcg twice daily for 7 days); however, the time to peak warfarin concentration was delayed by approximately 2 hours. In patients receiving warfarin, prothrombin time should be monitored more frequently after initiating or altering exenatide therapy; once a stable prothrombin time has been achieved, prothrombin times may be monitored at intervals usually recommended for patients receiving warfarin therapy.

Data are lacking on the effects of concomitant therapy with warfarin and extended-release exenatide. After initiation of extended-release exenatide in patients receiving warfarin concomitantly, the INR should be monitored more frequently. Once a stable INR has been documented, the INR can be monitored at intervals generally recommended for patients receiving warfarin therapy.

DESCRIPTION

Exenatide, a synthetic analog of a naturally occurring peptide isolated from the saliva of *Heloderma suspectum* (Gila monster), is a glucagon-like peptide-1 (GLP-1) mimetic (incretin mimetic). Exenatide has 53% amino acid similarity to human GLP-1 and is structurally and pharmacologically unrelated to insulin, sulfonylureas, meglitinides, biguanides, thiazolidinediones, and α-glucosidase inhibitors. Several antihyperglycemic actions of exenatide similar to the effects of human GLP-1 are involved in the lowering of fasting and postprandial glucose concentrations in patients with type 2 diabetes mellitus. The drug improves pancreatic β-cell function by increasing glucose-dependent insulin synthesis, secretion, and acute β-cell responsiveness (i.e., first phase insulin response). In contrast to sulfonylureas, stimulation of insulin secretion by exenatide subsides as blood glucose concentrations following a meal decrease and approach euglycemia. Exenatide inhibits inappropriately high glucagon secretion during episodes of hyperglycemia (e.g., after a meal) in patients with type 2 diabetes mellitus but does not impair the normal glucagon response to hypoglycemia. In addition, exenatide slows gastric emptying, which reduces the rate of glucose absorption from a meal, reduces food intake, and is associated with weight loss; the drug also may reduce appetite and promote early satiety. Exenatide does not appear to be associated with clinically important prolongation of the QT interval (corrected for rate using Bazett's formula [QT_c]).

Extended-release exenatide consists of exenatide incorporated in an extended-release microsphere formulation containing the 50:50 poly(D, L-lactide-co-glycolide) polymer along with sucrose. Each dose of extended-release exenatide contains 37.2 mg of the polymer and 0.8 mg of sucrose. Following a single dose of exenatide given as the extended-release formulation, the drug is released from the microspheres over approximately 10 weeks. Exenatide plasma concentration peaks around week 2 and week 6–7 after administration of the extended-release formulation, representing an initial surface-bound release and then a more gradual release of the drug from microspheres. Steady-state plasma concentrations of the drug are reached at approximately 6–7 weeks with once-weekly (every 7 days) administration. Plasma exenatide concentrations generally fall to undetectable levels approximately 10 weeks after discontinuance of dosing.

ADVICE TO PATIENTS

Importance of instructing patients on proper use and storage of the exenatide or extended-release exenatide injection pen or autoinjector, including proper injection technique to ensure delivery of a full dose, proper disposal of injection pens and autoinjectors using puncture-resistant containers, how and when to set up a new injection pen, and that only one setup step is necessary at initial use of exenatide. Importance of reading manufacturer's patient information (e.g., medication guide) and the injection pen user manual before starting therapy with exenatide or extended-release exenatide and of reviewing this information each time the prescription is refilled. Importance of patients not *self-administering* exenatide or extended-release exenatide if they are blind or unable to see well.

Importance of providing information regarding the potential risks and advantages of exenatide or extended-release exenatide therapy and of alternative modes of treatment. Importance of not using exenatide or extended-release exenatide in patients with type 1 diabetes mellitus or diabetic ketoacidosis.

Importance of providing instruction regarding diabetes self-management practices, such as regular physical activity, adhering to meal planning, periodic blood glucose monitoring, glycosylated hemoglobin (hemoglobin A_{1c} [HbA_{1c}]) testing, recognition and management of hypoglycemia and hyperglycemia, and assessment of other diabetic complications.

Importance of informing patients that extended-release exenatide causes benign and malignant thyroid C-cell tumors in rats and that the relevance of this finding in humans is unknown. Importance of not using extended-release exenatide in patients with a personal or family history of medullary thyroid cancer (MTC) or diagnosis of multiple endocrine neoplasia syndrome type 2 (MEN 2). Importance of advising patients receiving extended-release exenatide to report symptoms such as a lump or swelling in the neck, hoarseness, dysphagia, or dyspnea, which may be suggestive of thyroid cancer.

Importance of patients discontinuing exenatide or extended-release exenatide and other suspect drugs and seeking medical assistance immediately if signs and symptoms of a serious hypersensitivity reaction (e.g., anaphylaxis, angioedema) occur. Importance of patients informing their clinician if they have experienced a sensitivity reaction to exenatide or any ingredient in the formulations.

Importance of informing patients of the potential risk of acute pancreatitis, which may be severe and lead to death. Importance of patient informing clinicians about a history of pancreatitis, gallstones, alcoholism, or high triglyceride concentrations. Importance of patients discontinuing exenatide or extended-release exenatide and promptly informing clinician if unexplained, persistent, severe abdominal pain that may radiate to the back and may or may not be accompanied by nausea and vomiting occurs; these symptoms may be associated with acute pancreatitis. If pancreatitis is suspected, exenatide or extended-release exenatide should be promptly discontinued and not restarted if pancreatitis is confirmed.

Importance of informing patients of the potential risk for worsening renal function and about signs and symptoms of altered renal function (e.g., increased serum creatinine; changes in color, frequency, or amount of urination; unexplained swelling in extremities; increases in blood pressure; lethargy; changes in appetite or digestion; dull ache in the middle to lower back). Importance of patient informing clinician about development of nausea, vomiting, or diarrhea because of potential contribution of these effects to dehydration and consequent altered renal function. Importance of informing patients that chronic conditions such as hypertension or pancreatitis and concomitant therapy with nonsteroidal anti-inflammatory agents (NSAIAs), diuretics, or antihypertensive agents can increase the risk of developing altered renal function with exenatide therapy.

Importance of informing patients that drug-induced immune-mediated thrombocytopenia has been reported with exenatide use. Importance of informing patients to discontinue exenatide and promptly seek medical advice if symptoms of thrombocytopenia occur.

Importance of informing patients receiving exenatide that the dosage of concomitant insulin may need to be reduced in those at increased risk of hypoglycemia. Increased risk of hypoglycemia when exenatide or extended-release exenatide is used in combination with an agent that induces hypoglycemia, such as a sulfonylurea or other insulin secretagogue (e.g., meglitinide). Importance of informing patients that a lower dosage of sulfonylurea or other insulin secretagogue may be required to reduce the risk of hypoglycemia if used concomitantly with exenatide. Importance of reviewing with patients the symptoms, treatment, and conditions that predispose to development of hypoglycemia when initiating exenatide or extended-release exenatide treatment, especially when exenatide is administered concomitantly with a sulfonylurea or insulin; importance of clinician reinforcing instructions for management of hypoglycemia.

Importance of advising patients to seek medical advice if symptomatic subcutaneous injection-site nodules or any signs or symptoms of abscess, cellulitis, or necrosis occur.

Importance of informing patients of the potential risk for cholelithiasis or cholecystitis. Importance of instructing patients to contact a clinician for appropriate clinical follow-up if cholelithiasis or cholecystitis is suspected.

Importance of informing patients that reduced appetite, food intake, and/or body weight may occur with exenatide or extended-release exenatide therapy but do not require modification of dosage regimen. Importance of informing patient about occurrence of nausea, particularly upon initiation of exenatide or extended-release exenatide therapy, and that nausea decreases over time as the drug is continued.

Importance of informing patients that exenatide or extended-release exenatide injection pens should *not* be shared with another person, even if the needle has been changed. Sharing of the injection pen among patients may pose a risk of transmitting or acquiring infection.

Importance of informing patients regarding the timing of exenatide or extended-release exenatide administration with concomitant oral drugs, such as oral contraceptives and anti-infective agents, because of slowing of gastric emptying with these exenatide formulations.

Importance of not mixing exenatide with insulin.

Importance of advising patients what to do if a dose of exenatide or extended-release exenatide is missed.

Importance of informing patient that extended-release exenatide should be administered as a subcutaneous injection at any time on the dosing day, with or without meals. Importance of informing patients that the day of once-weekly administration (once every 7 days) can be changed if necessary, provided the last dose was administered 3 or more days previously.

Importance of informing patients to discontinue immediate-release exenatide once extended-release exenatide is initiated. Importance of informing patients that transient elevations in blood glucose concentrations may occur but generally improve within the first 2 weeks after initiation of extended-release exenatide therapy.

Importance of women informing clinicians if they are or plan to become pregnant or plan to breast-feed. Importance of informing women about enrolling in the pregnancy registry for exenatide or extended-release exenatide if they use the drugs at any time during pregnancy.

Importance of informing clinicians of existing or contemplated concomitant therapy, including prescription and OTC drugs, vitamins, and herbal supplements, as well as any concomitant illnesses (e.g., hypertension, history of liver disease, gastroparesis or serious digestive problems, severe kidney disease or kidney transplant).

Inform patients of other important precautionary information.

PREPARATIONS

Excipients in commercially available drug preparations may have clinically important effects in some individuals; consult specific product labeling for details.

Exenatide

Parenteral

Injection, for subcutaneous use	250 mcg/mL	**Byetta®** (available as 5 mcg per dose 1.2-mL prefilled pen or 10 mcg per dose 2.4-mL prefilled pen), AstraZeneca
Injection, extended-release, for subcutaneous use	2 mg/0.85 mL	**Bydureon Bcise®** (available as single-dose autoinjector), AstraZeneca

† Use is not currently included in the labeling approved by the US Food and Drug Administration.

Selected Revisions October 16, 2023, © Copyright, August 01, 2006, American Society of Health-System Pharmacists, Inc.

Liraglutide

68:20.06 • INCRETIN MIMETICS

■ Liraglutide, a synthetic, long-acting human glucagon-like peptide-1 (GLP-1) receptor agonist (incretin mimetic), is an antidiabetic agent and antiobesity drug.

USES

Liraglutide (Victoza®) is used as an adjunct to diet and exercise to improve glycemic control in patients with type 2 diabetes mellitus and also is used to reduce the risk of major adverse cardiovascular events (i.e., cardiovascular death, nonfatal myocardial infarction [MI], nonfatal stroke) in patients with type 2 diabetes mellitus and established cardiovascular disease. Liraglutide in fixed combination with insulin degludec (insulin degludec/liraglutide; Xultophy®) is used as an adjunct to diet and exercise to improve glycemic control in adults with type 2 diabetes mellitus.

Liraglutide (Saxenda®) is used for chronic weight management.

● Type 2 Diabetes Mellitus

Liraglutide is used as an adjunct to diet and exercise to improve glycemic control in adults and pediatric patients ≥10 years of age with type 2 diabetes mellitus. Liraglutide has been used alone or as add-on therapy with metformin, a sulfonylurea, insulin, or the combination of metformin and a sulfonylurea or thiazolidinedione. Various preparations of liraglutide are available; Victoza® injection and the fixed-combination injection of liraglutide and insulin degludec (Xultophy®) are specifically FDA-labeled for use in the management of diabetes mellitus.

Glycemic Control

Current guidelines for the treatment of type 2 diabetes mellitus generally recommend metformin as first-line therapy in addition to lifestyle modifications in patients with recent-onset type 2 diabetes mellitus or mild hyperglycemia because of its well-established safety and efficacy (i.e., beneficial effects on glycosylated hemoglobin [hemoglobin A_{1c}; HbA_{1c}], weight, and cardiovascular mortality). In patients with contraindications or intolerance to metformin (e.g., risk of lactic acidosis, GI intolerance) or in selected other patients, some experts suggest that initial therapy with a drug from another class of antidiabetic agents (e.g., a glucagon-like peptide-1 [GLP-1] receptor agonist, sodium-glucose cotransporter 2 [SGLT2] inhibitor, dipeptidyl peptidase-4 [DPP-4] inhibitor, sulfonylurea, thiazolidinedione, basal insulin) may be acceptable based on patient factors. Initiating antidiabetic therapy with 2 agents (e.g., metformin plus another agent) may be appropriate in patients with an initial HbA_{1c} exceeding 7.5% or at least 1.5% above the target level. In metformin-intolerant patients with high initial HbA_{1c} levels, some experts suggest initiation of therapy with 2 agents from other antidiabetic drug classes with complementary mechanisms of action.

Because of the progressive nature of type 2 diabetes mellitus, patients initially receiving an oral antidiabetic agent will eventually require multiple oral and/or injectable noninsulin antidiabetic agents of different therapeutic classes and/or insulin for adequate glycemic control. Patients who have inadequate glycemic control with initial (e.g., metformin) monotherapy should receive treatment with additional antidiabetic agents; data suggest that the addition of each noninsulin agent to initial therapy lowers HbA_{1c} by approximately 0.7–1%. In addition, early initiation of combination therapy may help more rapidly attain glycemic goals and extend the time to treatment failure.

Factors to consider when selecting additional antidiabetic agents for combination therapy in patients with inadequate glycemic control on metformin monotherapy include patient comorbidities (e.g., atherosclerotic cardiovascular disease [ASCVD], established kidney disease, heart failure), hypoglycemia risk, impact on weight, cost, risk of adverse effects, and patient preference. When the greater glucose-lowering effect of an injectable drug is needed in patients with type 2 diabetes mellitus, some experts currently state that an injectable GLP-1 receptor agonist is preferred over insulin in most patients because of beneficial effects on body weight and a lower risk of hypoglycemia, although adverse GI effects may diminish tolerability. While addition of a GLP-1 receptor agonist may successfully control hyperglycemia, many patients will eventually require insulin therapy. Early introduction of insulin therapy should be considered when hyperglycemia is severe (e.g., blood glucose of at least 300 mg/dL or HbA_{1c} exceeding 9–10%), especially in the presence of catabolic manifestations (e.g., weight loss, hypertriglyceridemia, ketosis) or symptoms of hyperglycemia.

Patients with type 2 diabetes mellitus who have established (or are at a high risk for) ASCVD, established kidney disease, or heart failure should receive a GLP-1 receptor agonist or SGLT2 inhibitor with demonstrated cardiovascular disease benefit. Experts state that therapy with a GLP-1 receptor agonist or SGLT2 inhibitor should be considered for patients with the aforementioned comorbidities independently of the patients' HbA_{1c}. GLP-1 receptor agonists and SGLT2 inhibitors appear to have effects on the kidneys independent of their glycemic effects, and some experts suggest that an agent from one of these classes of drugs be considered in patients with type 2 diabetes mellitus and chronic kidney disease (CKD). In patients *without* established ASCVD or indicators of high ASCVD risk, heart failure, or CKD, the decision regarding the addition of other antidiabetic agents (e.g., GLP-1 receptor agonist, SGLT2 inhibitor, DPP-4 inhibitor, thiazolidinedione, sulfonylurea, basal insulin) to metformin therapy should be based on avoidance of adverse effects, cost, and individual patient factors.

The manufacturer states that liraglutide or the fixed combination of insulin degludec and liraglutide (Xultophy®) is *not* indicated for the treatment of type 1 diabetes mellitus.

Liraglutide Monotherapy

When given as monotherapy for the management of type 2 diabetes mellitus, liraglutide improves glycemic control compared with glimepiride as evidenced by reductions from baseline in glycosylated hemoglobin (hemoglobin A_{1c}; HbA_{1c}) and fasting plasma glucose concentrations; liraglutide therapy also was associated with a reduction in body weight compared with an increase in body weight with glimepiride.

Efficacy and safety of liraglutide as monotherapy in adults with type 2 diabetes mellitus have been established in a 52-week randomized, double-blind, active-controlled, double-dummy trial. In this trial, 746 patients with a mean baseline HbA_{1c} concentration of 8.2% received liraglutide 1.2 or 1.8 mg subcutaneously once daily or glimepiride 8 mg orally once daily. All patients randomized to liraglutide received an initial dosage of 0.6 mg once daily for 1 week; dosage subsequently was titrated in increments of 0.6 mg weekly to a dosage of either 1.2 or 1.8 mg once daily. All patients randomized to glimepiride received an initial dosage of 2 mg once daily for 2 weeks, followed by 4 mg once daily for 2 weeks, and then 8 mg once daily. The primary study end point was the change in HbA_{1c} concentration from baseline to week 52 (or the last value at time of early discontinuance of therapy). At week 52, HbA_{1c} was reduced from baseline by about 0.8, 1.1, or 0.5% with once-daily liraglutide 1.2 mg, liraglutide 1.8 mg, or glimepiride 8 mg, respectively. HbA_{1c} concentrations below 7% were achieved in 43, 51, or 28% of patients receiving once-daily liraglutide 1.2 mg, liraglutide 1.8 mg, or glimepiride 8 mg, respectively. Body weight was reduced from baseline by 2.1 or 2.5 kg with liraglutide 1.2 or 1.8 mg once daily, respectively, but was increased by 1.1 kg in patients receiving glimepiride 8 mg once daily.

Combination Therapy

When given as add-on therapy to metformin and/or a sulfonylurea, metformin and a thiazolidinedione, or metformin and insulin detemir in clinical trials, liraglutide was more effective than placebo and at least as effective as add-on therapy with sitagliptin, glimepiride, or exenatide in improving glycemic control (as evidenced by reduction in HbA_{1c} concentrations).

Efficacy and safety of liraglutide (1.2 or 1.8 mg subcutaneously once daily) as add-on therapy with maximally effective dosages of metformin, a sulfonylurea (e.g., glimepiride), or metformin in combination with a sulfonylurea or a thiazolidinedione were established in several studies of 26 weeks' duration. Combined therapy with subcutaneous liraglutide and these oral antidiabetic agents or regimens resulted in improved glycemic control (as indicated by a reduction in HbA_{1c} from baseline values) compared with that achieved with existing oral antidiabetic therapy.

In a multicenter, randomized, open-label comparative study, adults with type 2 diabetes mellitus who received liraglutide 1.8 mg once daily in addition to their current therapy (metformin, a sulfonylurea, or both) experienced a greater reduction in HbA_{1c} than those who received exenatide 10 mcg twice daily in addition to current therapy (1.12 or 0.79% with liraglutide or exenatide, respectively). Mean reductions in weight were similar with liraglutide (3.24 kg) or exenatide (2.87 kg).

In a 26-week, randomized, open-label comparative study, adults with type 2 diabetes mellitus who received liraglutide 1.2 or 1.8 mg once daily in addition to their current therapy (metformin hydrochloride at least 1.5 g daily) experienced a greater reduction in HbA$_{1c}$ than those who received sitagliptin 100 mg once daily in addition to current therapy (HbA$_{1c}$ reduction of 1.2, 1.5, or 0.9% with liraglutide 1.2 mg, liraglutide 1.8 mg, or sitagliptin 100 mg once daily, respectively).

Safety and efficacy of liraglutide in combination with insulin (i.e., insulin detemir) were established in a study of 26 weeks' duration in adult patients receiving metformin hydrochloride (at least 1.5 g daily). Treatment with liraglutide 1.8 mg in addition to insulin detemir and metformin resulted in greater reduction in HbA$_{1c}$ than treatment with liraglutide 1.8 mg in addition to metformin (HbA$_{1c}$ reduction of 0.5% or 0, respectively).

In another study, pediatric patients at least 10 years of age (mean age: 14.6 years) with type 2 diabetes mellitus and a HbA$_{1c}$ of 7–11% (if previously treated with diet and exercise alone) or a HbA$_{1c}$ of 6.5–11% (if previously treated with metformin with or without insulin) were randomized to receive liraglutide or placebo once daily; all patients received metformin with or without basal insulin therapy. Liraglutide was initiated at a dosage of 0.6 mg subcutaneously once daily and increased by increments of 0.6 mg every week over the course of 2–3 weeks based on tolerability and fasting plasma glucose concentrations (goal fasting plasma glucose concentration: 110 mg/dL or less). Most patients did not receive the maximum dosage of liraglutide because fasting plasma glucose concentrations of 110 mg/dL or less were achieved with lower dosages. After 26 weeks of therapy, treatment with liraglutide was superior to placebo in reducing HbA$_{1c}$ from baseline (reduction of 0.64% or increase of 0.42%, respectively). Additionally, a larger proportion of patients who received liraglutide therapy obtained a HbA$_{1c}$ of less than 7% compared with those who received placebo (63.7 versus 36.5%, respectively).

In a 26-week, randomized, double-blind, placebo-controlled study, adults with type 2 diabetes mellitus and moderate renal impairment (eGFR 30–59 mL/minute per 1.73 m^2) who received liraglutide 1.8 mg once daily in addition to their current therapy (basal or premixed insulin and/or metformin, pioglitazone, or sulfonylurea) experienced a greater reduction in HbA$_{1c}$ than those who received placebo in addition to their current therapy (reduction of 0.9 versus 0.4%, respectively). There was no worsening of renal function in those who received liraglutide therapy.

If inadequate glycemic control or failure to achieve target glycemic control occurs with liraglutide, alternative antidiabetic therapy should be considered.

Fixed-combination Therapy with Insulin Degludec and Liraglutide

Current data indicate that the fixed combination of insulin degludec and liraglutide (insulin degludec/liraglutide) is more effective than either drug (as add-on therapy to one or more oral antidiabetic agents) in improving glycemic control (as determined by reductions in HbA$_{1c}$) in adults with type 2 diabetes mellitus. Safety and efficacy of insulin degludec/liraglutide for the treatment of type 2 diabetes mellitus have been established in 5 parallel, randomized, active- or placebo-controlled phase 3 clinical trials of 26 weeks' duration in adults with type 2 diabetes mellitus.

In 2 clinical studies, the use of insulin degludec/liraglutide substantially improved glycemic control in adults with type 2 diabetes mellitus who had inadequate glycemic control with oral antidiabetic agents and who were naive to basal insulin or GLP-1 receptor agonists. In the first study, all patients continued on prestudy treatment with metformin with or without pioglitazone. In addition to the prestudy treatment, patients also received insulin degludec/liraglutide (initial dosage: 10 units of insulin degludec and 0.36 mg liraglutide), liraglutide (initial dosage: 0.6 mg), or insulin degludec (initial dosage: 10 units) subcutaneously once daily. Patients in the fixed-combination group or the insulin degludec treatment group had their dosages titrated twice weekly towards a target fasting plasma glucose concentration of 72–90 mg/dL. Patients in the liraglutide treatment group followed a fixed-escalation scheme with weekly dosage increases of 0.6 mg until the liraglutide maintenance dosage of 1.8 mg was achieved. After 26 weeks, the reduction in HbA$_{1c}$ from baseline was 1.81, 1.35, or 1.21% in patients treated with the fixed combination of insulin degludec and liraglutide, insulin degludec, or liraglutide, respectively. In the second study, all patients continued on prestudy treatment with a sulfonylurea with or without metformin. In addition to the prestudy treatment, patients also received insulin degludec/liraglutide (initial dosage:

10 units of insulin degludec and 0.36 mg liraglutide) or placebo. Patients in the fixed-combination group had their dosage titrated twice weekly towards a target fasting plasma glucose concentration of 72–108 mg/dL. After 26 weeks, the reduction in HbA$_{1c}$ from baseline was 1.42 or 0.62% in patients treated with insulin degludec/liraglutide or placebo, respectively.

In another clinical trial, insulin-naive adults with type 2 diabetes mellitus who were inadequately controlled on metformin alone or in combination with pioglitazone and/or a sulfonylurea plus maximum-dose (or maximally tolerated) liraglutide (mean daily dose at baseline: 1.7 mg) continued to receive their pretrial therapy or had their therapy changed from liraglutide to insulin degludec/liraglutide. Oral antidiabetic agents were continued at pretrial dosages throughout the trial in both treatment groups. The starting dosage of the fixed combination was insulin degludec 16 units and liraglutide 0.58 mg once daily; dosage adjustments were performed twice weekly based on fasting blood glucose concentrations (end-of-trial dosage of the fixed combination: insulin degludec 44 units and liraglutide 1.58 mg daily). After 26 weeks, the reduction in HbA$_{1c}$ from baseline was 1.31 or 0.36% with insulin degludec/liraglutide versus liraglutide, respectively. A mean weight gain from baseline of 2 kg was observed in patients receiving insulin degludec/liraglutide compared with a weight loss of 0.8 kg in those receiving liraglutide. A higher rate of hypoglycemia was observed in the fixed-combination treatment group.

In another trial comparing insulin degludec/liraglutide with insulin degludec therapy in adults with type 2 diabetes mellitus who were inadequately controlled with basal insulin and metformin with or without a sulfonylurea or a meglitinide, patients who received the fixed combination at equivalent insulin dosages achieved superior glycemic control. In this trial, all basal insulins and oral antidiabetic drugs except for metformin hydrochloride (mean daily dose: 1984 mg) were discontinued at randomization; patients received a starting insulin degludec dosage of 16 units (given separately or in the fixed combination with liraglutide 0.58 mg) once daily, which was titrated biweekly based on fasting plasma glucose concentrations. After 26 weeks, the mean daily dosage of insulin degludec was 46 units (with liraglutide 1.66 mg in the fixed combination) in both treatment groups. The reductions in HbA$_{1c}$ from baseline were superior with insulin degludec/liraglutide compared with insulin degludec treatment (reduction of 1.94 versus 1.05 %, respectively). There was no substantial difference between the 2 treatment groups with regard to hypoglycemia.

In another trial comparing insulin degludec/liraglutide with insulin glargine therapy in adults with type 2 diabetes mellitus inadequately controlled on insulin glargine and metformin, patients who received the fixed combination of insulin degludec and liraglutide achieved substantially greater reductions in HbA$_{1c}$ compared with those who received insulin glargine therapy. Patients in this trial either continued treatment with insulin glargine or were switched to insulin degludec/liraglutide, both in conjunction with metformin. The starting insulin degludec dosage was 16 units daily (with liraglutide 0.58 mg in the fixed combination), irrespective of the patient's previous daily dosage of insulin glargine (mean insulin glargine pretrial dosage: 31 units daily). Patients whose therapy was switched from insulin glargine to insulin degludec/liraglutide showed no worsening of blood glucose control immediately following the switch, despite the initial reduction in insulin dosage for patients who received the fixed combination. Each treatment was titrated biweekly based on fasting blood glucose concentrations with no upper dosing limit in the insulin glargine group and a maximum daily dosage of 50 units of insulin degludec in the fixed-combination treatment group. The mean dosage of the fixed combination was insulin degludec 41 units and liraglutide 1.48 mg daily; mean dosage of insulin glargine was 66 units daily. The reductions in HbA$_{1c}$ from baseline were substantially greater with insulin degludec/liraglutide compared with insulin glargine (reduction of 1.67 versus 1.16%, respectively).

The manufacturer states that insulin degludec/liraglutide should not be used in combination with any other preparation containing liraglutide or another GLP-1 receptor agonist.

Reduction in Risk of Major Adverse Cardiovascular Events

Liraglutide is used to reduce the risk of major adverse cardiovascular events in adults with type 2 diabetes mellitus and established cardiovascular disease. In addition to lowering blood glucose, GLP-1 receptor agonists appear to modify several nonglycemic cardiovascular risk factors, such as blood pressure, body weight, and lipid profile. GLP-1 receptor agonists also may have beneficial endothelial effects. The Liraglutide Effect and Action in Diabetes: Evaluation of Cardiovascular Outcome Results (LEADER) study was designed to assess the cardiovascular safety and efficacy of liraglutide in patients with type 2 diabetes mellitus at high risk for or with cardiovascular disease. This study included adults with type 2 diabetes mellitus who were at least 50 years of age (mean age: 64 years) with at least one coexisting cardiovascular condition (e.g., coronary heart disease, cerebrovascular disease, peripheral vascular disease, CKD of stage 3 or greater, chronic heart failure New York Heart Association [NYHA] class II or III) or at least 60 years of age with at least one cardiovascular risk factor (e.g., microalbuminuria or proteinuria, hypertension and left ventricular hypertrophy, left ventricular systolic or diastolic dysfunction, an ankle-branchial index of less than 0.9). In this study, patients were randomized to receive liraglutide (1.8 mg [or maximally tolerated dose]) or placebo subcutaneously once daily for a median duration of 3.5 years. During the study, antidiabetic and cardiovascular therapies were modified to achieve standard of care treatment targets with respect to blood glucose, lipids, and blood pressure. Concomitant use of other standard of care treatments for diabetes mellitus (excluding DPP-4 inhibitors or other GLP-1 receptor agonists) and ASCVD (nondiuretic antihypertensives [92.4%], diuretics [41.8%], statins [72.1%], antiplatelet agents [66.8%]) was permitted. The primary outcome was the composite of time to first occurrence of cardiovascular death, nonfatal MI, and nonfatal stroke. In these studies, patients who received treatment with liraglutide had substantially lower rates of the primary cardiovascular outcome compared with those who received placebo (event rate 13 versus 14.9%). Deaths from cardiovascular causes were substantially reduced in the liraglutide group compared with placebo (event rate 4.7 versus 6%).

The manufacturer states that effects on cardiovascular morbidity and mortality have not been established in patients receiving liraglutide for management of obesity.

Beneficial Effects on Renal Function

In several cardiovascular outcomes trials involving the use of GLP-1 receptor agonists (e.g., dulaglutide, liraglutide, semaglutide) in patients with type 2 diabetes mellitus at high risk for cardiovascular disease or with existing cardiovascular disease, beneficial effects on renal function have been observed as a secondary outcome. Some experts state that in patients with type 2 diabetes mellitus and CKD who are at increased risk for cardiovascular events, use of a GLP-1 receptor agonist may reduce risk of progression of albuminuria, cardiovascular events, or both. In the LEADER study, liraglutide reduced the risk of new or worsening nephropathy (a composite of persistent macroalbuminuria, doubling of serum creatinine, end-stage renal disease, or death from end-stage renal disease)† by 22%.

● Chronic Weight Management

Liraglutide is used as an adjunct to a reduced-calorie diet and increased physical activity for the long-term management of body weight in adults who are obese (pretreatment body mass index [BMI] of 30 kg/m² or greater) or, in those who are overweight (pretreatment BMI of 27 kg/m² or greater) *and* have an underlying weight-related comorbid condition (e.g., hypertension, type 2 diabetes mellitus, dyslipidemia). Liraglutide also is used as an adjunct to a reduced-calorie diet and increased physical activity for chronic weight management in pediatric patients ≥12 years of age with body weight >60 kg and an initial BMI corresponding to 30 kg/m² for adults (obese) by international cut-offs.

Various preparations of liraglutide are available; Saxenda® injection is specifically FDA-labeled for use in chronic weight management.

The manufacturer states that the Saxenda® preparation of liraglutide is not intended for use in the treatment of type 2 diabetes mellitus. In addition, Saxenda® should not be used in combination with any other GLP-1 receptor agonist or with insulin.

Safety and efficacy of liraglutide in combination with other products used to promote weight loss, including prescription and nonprescription (OTC) drugs and dietary or herbal supplements, have not been established.

When used in conjunction with a reduced-calorie diet and increased exercise, liraglutide substantially decreases body weight compared with placebo in obese and overweight diabetic and nondiabetic patients. In clinical trials, weight loss with liraglutide therapy has been maintained over 56 weeks.

Efficacy and safety of liraglutide for the management of body weight in adults were evaluated in 3 randomized, double-blind, placebo-controlled studies of 56 weeks' duration (studies 1, 2, and 3) in a total of 4788 patients who were obese (defined as a BMI of 30 kg/m² or greater) or overweight (defined as a BMI of 27–29.9 kg/m²) with at least one weight-related comorbid condition such as

hypertension or dyslipidemia. All patients received instruction regarding a reduced-calorie diet (approximately 500 kcal/day deficit) and exercise counseling (recommended increased physical activity for at least 150 minutes per week) initially and throughout the study. In all 3 studies, liraglutide was initiated at 0.6 mg subcutaneously once daily and titrated over 4 weeks to a dosage of 3 mg once daily. Across all 3 studies, 27% of patients in the liraglutide group and 35% of patients in the placebo group discontinued treatment. Approximately 10 or 4% of patients treated with liraglutide or placebo, respectively, discontinued treatment due to an adverse reaction; most such discontinuances occurred during the first few months of treatment.

Study 1 compared liraglutide with placebo in addition to caloric restriction and increased physical activity in 3731 obese or overweight nondiabetic patients. The mean baseline body weight for both treatment groups was 106.2 kg and mean BMI was 38.3 kg/m². Other baseline characteristics were similar between groups; mean age was 45 years, 79% were female, 85% Caucasian, 10% African American, and 11% Hispanic or Latino. Principal measures of efficacy were mean percent change in body weight from baseline, the proportion of patients who lost at least 5% of their baseline body weight, and the proportion who lost at least 10% of their baseline body weight. At 56 weeks, liraglutide 3 mg daily reduced body weight by a greater percentage from baseline than placebo (a mean reduction of 7.4% versus 3%, respectively). A substantially greater proportion of patients receiving liraglutide lost 5% or more of their baseline body weight compared with patients receiving placebo (62.3 versus 34.4%, respectively). Similarly, more patients receiving liraglutide lost 10% or more of their baseline body weight compared with patients receiving placebo (33.9 versus 15.4%, respectively). In a subset of patients who had abnormal blood glucose concentrations at randomization (prediabetes), a substantially greater proportion of patients receiving liraglutide lost 5% or more of their baseline body weight at week 56, 160, or both 56 and 160 weeks compared with patients receiving placebo (56, 28, or 26 versus 25, 14, or 10%, respectively). More patients in the liraglutide treatment group regressed from prediabetes to normoglycemia by week 160 than those patients who received placebo. In addition, liraglutide was superior to placebo on several secondary measures of efficacy: deceased BMI, waist circumference, systolic and diastolic blood pressure, total cholesterol and triglyceride concentrations, and measures of glycemic control (glycosylated hemoglobin [HbA$_{1c}$], fasting glucose, fasting insulin).

Study 2 compared liraglutide with placebo in addition to caloric restriction and increased physical activity in 635 obese or overweight patients with type 2 diabetes mellitus. Patients had baseline HbA$_{1c}$ 7–10% and were treated with 1-3 oral antidiabetic agents (metformin, a sulfonylurea, a thiazolidinedione) or with diet and exercise alone. The mean baseline body weight was 105.9 kg and mean BMI was 37.1 kg/m²; mean age was 55 years, 50% were female, 83% Caucasian, 12% African American, and 10% Hispanic or Latino. Principal measures of efficacy were identical to those in study 1. At 56 weeks, liraglutide 3 mg daily reduced body weight by a greater percentage from baseline than placebo (a mean reduction of 5.4% versus 1.7%, respectively). More patients receiving liraglutide lost 5% or more (49%) or 10% or more (22.4%) of their baseline body weight compared with patients receiving placebo (16.4 or 5.5%, respectively). Liraglutide also improved several secondary measures of efficacy: waist circumference, systolic and diastolic blood pressure, total cholesterol and triglyceride concentrations, and measures of glycemic control (HbA$_{1c}$, fasting glucose).

Study 3 evaluated the effect of liraglutide or placebo in 422 obese or overweight nondiabetic patients who had lost at least 5% of their baseline body weight with diet and exercise. In this study, patients were initially treated with a low-calorie diet (total daily energy intake 1200–1400 kcal) and recommended physical activity of at least 150 minutes per week for up to 12 weeks. Patients who lost at least 5% of their baseline body weight received liraglutide 3 mg daily or placebo for 56 weeks in addition to a continued reduced-calorie diet (approximately 500 kcal/day deficit) and exercise counseling. The mean baseline body weight was 99.6 kg and mean BMI was 35.6 kg/m²; mean age was 46 years, 81% were female, 84% Caucasian, 13% African American, and 7% Hispanic or Latino. Principal measures of efficacy in this study were mean percent change in body weight from time of randomization, the proportion of patients that maintained their original weight loss (i.e., not gaining more than 0.5% body weight from time of randomization), and the proportion of patients who lost 5% or more of body weight after randomization. Liraglutide was superior to placebo on all primary efficacy end points at 56 weeks; liraglutide-treated patients experienced a weight loss of 4.9% of body weight at randomization compared with a weight gain of 0.3% in placebo recipients. A greater proportion of liraglutide-treated patients did not gain back more than 0.5% of their weight at randomization compared with placebo recipients, and more liraglutide-treated patients lost an additional 5% or more of their body weight at randomization compared with those who received placebo (44.2 versus 21.7%, respectively). Furthermore, a substantially greater proportion of patients receiving liraglutide lost 10% or more of their body weight at randomization compared with patients receiving placebo (25.4 versus 6.9%, respectively).

Efficacy and safety of liraglutide for weight management in pediatric patients 12 years of age or older with obesity were evaluated in a 56-week, double-blind, randomized, placebo-controlled trial in 251 pubertal patients with BMI corresponding to 30 kg/m² or greater for adults by international cut-off points and BMI of 95th percentile or greater for age and sex. The mean age of patients was 14.5 years; 40.6% were male, 87.6% were white. 0.8% were Asian, 8% were Black or African American, and 22.3% were of Hispanic or Latino ethnicity. The mean baseline body weight was 100.8 kg and mean BMI was 35.6 kg/m². The primary endpoint was change in BMI standard deviation score (SDS). Mean BMI SDS at baseline was 3.14 in the liraglutide group and 3.2 in the placebo group. The observed mean change in BMI SDS from baseline to week 56 was -0.23 in the liraglutide group and -0 in the placebo group (estimated treatment difference of -0.22 between liraglutide and placebo). Liraglutide treatment also resulted in beneficial effects on waist circumference and cardiometabolic parameters.

The STEP 8 trial was a 68-week, open-label, multicenter trial that compared once-weekly subcutaneous semaglutide 2.4 mg with once-daily subcutaneous liraglutide 3 mg in adults with BMI ≥30 kg/m² or BMI ≥ 27 kg/m² with 1 or more weight-related comorbidities (except diabetes). All patients received counseling to adhere to diet and physical activity recommendations. The study showed that weight loss with semaglutide was significantly greater than with liraglutide. The mean weight change from baseline at 68 weeks was -15.8% with semaglutide compared with -6.4% with liraglutide (difference of -9.4 percentage points).

Clinical Perspective

Clinical practice guidelines recommend treatment for obesity in patients with excess body weight and associated health risks. A comprehensive lifestyle intervention is an essential component of therapy and should be provided to all patients; pharmacologic therapy may be considered as an adjunct to behavioral modification in patients who fail to achieve or sustain clinically meaningful weight loss (generally defined as a loss of more than 4–5% of total body weight). Response to drug therapy should be evaluated after 3–4 months of treatment; if clinically meaningful weight loss is not achieved, it is generally recommended that a new treatment plan be considered because the patient is likely not responding to the drug.

DOSAGE AND ADMINISTRATION

● General

Patient Monitoring

- Patients receiving liraglutide for the management of type 2 diabetes mellitus should be monitored regularly (e.g., blood glucose determinations, HbA₁c) to determine therapeutic response.

- When used for chronic weight management, evaluate body weight after 16 weeks (in adults) and after 12 weeks (in pediatric patients). Discontinue treatment in adults who do not experience a meaningful weight loss (≥4% baseline weight); discontinue treatment in pediatric patients who do not experience a reduction in BMI of ≥1% from baseline.

- Observe patients carefully for signs and symptoms of pancreatitis (including persistent severe abdominal pain, sometimes radiating to the back and which may or may not be accompanied by vomiting).

● Administration

Liraglutide or the fixed combination of insulin degludec and liraglutide (insulin degludec/liraglutide) is administered by subcutaneous injection into the abdomen, thigh, or upper arm using a prefilled injection pen; the drug must *not* be administered IV or IM.

Liraglutide is administered once daily at any time of day, without regard to meals. The injection site and timing can be changed without dosage adjustment. Rotate injection sites within the same region to reduce the risk of cutaneous amyloidosis.

The fixed combination of insulin degludec/liraglutide is administered by subcutaneous injection once daily at the same time each day without regard to meals.

If a dose of liraglutide or insulin degludec/liraglutide is missed, the regular schedule should be resumed with the next scheduled dose; an extra dose or increase in dose should not be taken to replace a missed dose. If more than 3 days have elapsed since the last dose of liraglutide or insulin degludec/liraglutide, the initial dosage should be restarted and retitrated.

When using liraglutide in combination with insulin for the management of type 2 diabetes mellitus, the drugs should be administered as separate injections; insulin and liraglutide should never be mixed. Liraglutide and insulin may be injected in the same body regions; however, the injections should not be adjacent to each other. Liraglutide in fixed combination with insulin degludec is commercially available as Xultophy®. The fixed combination of insulin degludec and liraglutide should not be mixed with any other insulin preparations or solutions.

● Dosage

Type 2 Diabetes Mellitus

The recommended initial dosage of liraglutide for the management of type 2 diabetes mellitus in adults is 0.6 mg subcutaneously once daily. The 0.6-mg daily dosage of liraglutide is *not* effective for glycemic control and is intended only as a starting dosage to reduce GI intolerance. After one week, the dosage of liraglutide should be increased to 1.2 mg daily. If additional glycemic control is required, dosage may be increased to 1.8 mg daily after at least one week of treatment with the 1.2-mg daily dose.

The recommended initial dosage of liraglutide for the management of type 2 diabetes mellitus in children and adolescents ≥10 years of age is 0.6 mg subcutaneously once daily. After at least one week, the dosage may be increased by 0.6 mg increments. The maximum recommended dosage is 1.8 mg once daily.

If a dose is missed and more than 3 days have elapsed since the last dose of liraglutide, patients should be advised to reinitiate liraglutide at 0.6 mg subcutaneously once daily to minimize any adverse GI effects. Upon reinitiation, liraglutide should be titrated at the discretion of the clinician.

Fixed Combination of Insulin Degludec and Liraglutide (Xultophy®)

Dosage of the fixed combination of insulin degludec and liraglutide (insulin degludec/liraglutide) is expressed in terms of units of insulin degludec on the dose counter display of the Xultophy® injection pen; each dosage unit delivers 1 unit of insulin degludec and 0.036 mg of liraglutide.

The dosage of insulin degludec/liraglutide is based on the results of blood glucose determinations and should be carefully individualized to obtain optimum therapeutic effect. Dosage adjustments may be needed during acute illness or when used with other drugs or with changes in physical activity, meal patterns (i.e., macronutrient content or timing of food intake), or renal or hepatic function.

In adults with type 2 diabetes mellitus who are naive to basal insulin or a glucagon-like peptide-1 (GLP-1) receptor agonist, the recommended initial dosage of insulin degludec/liraglutide is 10 units (10 units of insulin degludec and 0.36 mg of liraglutide) once daily.

In adults with type 2 diabetes mellitus who are currently receiving basal insulin or a GLP-1 receptor agonist (e.g., liraglutide), such therapy must be discontinued prior to initiation of the fixed combination of insulin degludec/liraglutide. The recommended initial dosage of insulin degludec/liraglutide in these patients is 16 units (16 units of insulin degludec and 0.58 mg of liraglutide) once daily.

The dosage of insulin degludec in the fixed combination with liraglutide may be increased or decreased by 2 units (2 units of insulin degludec and 0.072 mg of liraglutide) every 3–4 days as needed. The fixed combination preparation should not be administered more than once daily. Adjustments in concomitant oral antidiabetic therapy may be needed. The maximum daily dosage of insulin degludec in the fixed combination with liraglutide is 50 units (50 units of insulin degludec and 1.8 mg of liraglutide).

Chronic Weight Management

The recommended maintenance dosage of liraglutide for the management of body weight in adults and pediatric patients ≥12 years of age is 3 mg subcutaneously once daily. To minimize adverse GI effects, dosage should be initiated at 0.6 mg daily for 1 week and then increased at weekly intervals until the maintenance dosage is reached. (See Table 1.)

TABLE 1. Dosage Escalation Schedule for Chronic Weight Management in Adults and Pediatric Patients ≥12 Years of Age

Week	Daily Dose
1	0.6 mg
2	1.2 mg
3	1.8 mg
4	2.4 mg
5 and onward	3 mg

If an increase in dosage is not tolerated (e.g., adverse GI effects) in adults, dosage escalation may be delayed for approximately 1 week. However, if a dosage of 3 mg daily is not tolerated, liraglutide should be discontinued, as efficacy has not been established at dosages lower than 3 mg daily. If pediatric patients do not tolerate an increased dose during dose escalation, the dose may be lowered to the previous level. Dose escalation for pediatric patients may take up to 8 weeks. In pediatric patients who do not tolerate a dosage of 3 mg daily, the maintenance dosage may be reduced to 2.4 mg daily; therapy should be discontinued if the patient cannot tolerate the 2.4 mg dose.

If a dose is missed and more than 3 days have elapsed since the last dose of liraglutide, the drug should be reinitiated at a dosage of 0.6 mg subcutaneously once daily to minimize any adverse GI effects; the dosage should then be retitrated to a maintenance dosage of 3 mg once daily.

Body weight should be evaluated 16 weeks after initiating liraglutide in adults. Treatment should be discontinued in patients who do not experience a meaningful reduction in weight (at least 4% of baseline body weight) after 16 weeks since such patients are unlikely to achieve and sustain meaningful weight loss with continued liraglutide therapy.

The change in BMI should be evaluated in pediatric patients after 12 weeks on the maintenance liraglutide dosage and treatment should be discontinued if the patient has not had a reduction in BMI of at least 1% from baseline, since it is unlikely that the patient will achieve and sustain clinically meaningful weight loss with continued treatment.

● Special Populations

No adjustment of liraglutide dosage is recommended in patients with renal or hepatic impairment or based solely on age or sex. However, clinicians should use caution when initiating liraglutide or escalating dosage in patients with renal impairment. Data are lacking on the use of the fixed combination of insulin degludec and liraglutide in patients with hepatic impairment. There is limited experience with the use of the fixed combination of insulin degludec and liraglutide in patients with mild or moderate renal impairment; glucose monitoring should be intensified and the dosage of the fixed combination individualized as required.

CAUTIONS

● Contraindications

Liraglutide alone or in fixed combination with insulin degludec (Xultophy®) is contraindicated in patients with a personal or family history of medullary thyroid carcinoma (MTC) and in patients with multiple endocrine neoplasia syndrome type 2 (MEN 2).

Liraglutide alone or in fixed combination with insulin degludec also is contraindicated in patients with a history of serious hypersensitivity to liraglutide or to any of the product components.

The fixed combination of insulin degludec and liraglutide is contraindicated during episodes of hypoglycemia.

Liraglutide is contraindicated for chronic weight management in women who are pregnant.

● Warnings/Precautions

Warnings

Risk of Thyroid C-Cell Tumors

Liraglutide causes dose-dependent and treatment duration-dependent thyroid C-cell tumors at clinically relevant exposures in both genders of rats and mice. Cases of MTC have been reported in patients receiving liraglutide during post-marketing experience; data from these reports are insufficient to establish or exclude a causal relationship between MTC and liraglutide use in humans. It is also unknown whether liraglutide causes thyroid C-cell tumors in humans, as relevance to humans of such tumors in rodents has not been determined. For this reason, liraglutide or the fixed combination of insulin degludec and liraglutide is contraindicated in patients with a history of MTC and in patients with MEN 2. In addition, liraglutide should not be used as first-line treatment for diabetes mellitus until additional studies are completed that support expanded use.

In clinical trials of diabetes mellitus treatment, adjusted mean serum calcitonin concentrations were higher in liraglutide-treated patients than in placebo-treated patients but not higher than in patients receiving an active comparator drug. Adjusted mean serum calcitonin concentrations were also higher in liraglutide-treated patients than in placebo-treated patients in clinical trials of obesity management. Very elevated serum calcitonin values may be indicative of MTC; patients with MTC usually have serum calcitonin values exceeding 50 ng/L. Although routine monitoring of serum calcitonin concentrations or thyroid ultrasounds for the purpose of early detection of MTC in patients receiving liraglutide is of uncertain value and may increase the risk of unnecessary procedures, patients should be further evaluated if serum calcitonin is measured and found to be elevated or thyroid nodules are noted on physical examination or neck imaging.

To specifically evaluate the risk of MTC, the FDA has required the manufacturer to establish a cancer registry to monitor the rate of this type of cancer in the US over a period of 15 years.

Sensitivity Reactions

Serious hypersensitivity reactions (anaphylaxis, angioedema) have been reported in patients receiving liraglutide. Asthma, bronchial hyperreactivity, bronchospasm, oropharyngeal swelling, facial swelling, pharyngeal edema, and type IV hypersensitivity reactions also have been reported with liraglutide therapy. Anaphylactic reactions with additional symptoms (e.g., hypotension, palpitations, dyspnea, edema) have been reported; anaphylactic reactions may be potentially life-threatening. If a hypersensitivity reaction occurs, patients should discontinue liraglutide-containing therapy and other suspect drugs and promptly seek medical advice.

Liraglutide should be used with caution in patients with a history of anaphylaxis or angioedema with another glucagon-like peptide-1 (GLP-1) receptor agonist, as it is unknown whether such patients will be predisposed to angioedema with liraglutide.

Other Warnings and Precautions

Use of Fixed Combinations

When liraglutide is used in fixed combination with other drugs (e.g., insulin degludec), cautions, precautions, contraindications, and interactions associated with the concomitant agent(s) should be considered in addition to those associated with insulin degludec.

Risks During General Anesthesia and Deep Sedation

GLP-1 agonists are associated with adverse GI effects such as nausea, vomiting, and delayed gastric emptying; such effects are likely a result of rapid tachyphlaxis at the level of vagal nerve activation. Delayed gastric emptying from GLP-1 agonists can increase the risk of regurgitation and pulmonary aspiration of gastric contents during general anesthesia and deep sedation. Given these concerns, the American Society of Anesthesiologists (ASA) Task Force on Preoperative Fasting has issued a consensus-based guidance for the management of GLP-1 receptor agonists prior to elective surgery. The task force suggests that for patients on daily GLP-1 agonist dosing (irrespective of indication, dose, or type of surgery), consider holding the drug on the day of the procedure/surgery. For patients on weekly dosing (irrespective of indication, dose, or type of surgery), consider holding the GLP-1 agonist a week prior to the procedure/surgery. If GLP-1 agonists prescribed for diabetes management are held for longer than the dosing schedule, consider consulting an endocrinologist for bridging the antidiabetic therapy to avoid hyperglycemia. These recommendations are based on limited evidence only (case reports). For patients requiring urgent or emergent procedures, the task force states to proceed and treat the patient as 'full stomach' and manage accordingly.

Pancreatitis and Pancreatic Precancerous Changes

Acute pancreatitis, including fatal and nonfatal hemorrhagic or necrotizing pancreatitis, has been reported during postmarketing experience with liraglutide.

In clinical trials with liraglutide in type 2 diabetes mellitus, there were 13 cases of pancreatitis (9 acute, 4 chronic) among liraglutide-treated patients compared with 1 case in a glimepiride-treated patient (2.7 versus 0.5 cases per 1000 patient-years, respectively). One case of pancreatitis with necrosis was fatal, though clinical causality could not be established. Some patients had other risk factors for pancreatitis, including a history of cholelithiasis or alcohol abuse. In clinical trials in adults with liraglutide for chronic weight management, acute pancreatitis was confirmed in 0.3% of liraglutide-treated patients (9 of 3291 patients) compared with 0.1% of patients who received placebo (1 of 1843 patients). In addition, there were 2 cases of acute pancreatitis in liraglutide-treated patients who withdrew prematurely from the clinical trials; these cases occurred 74 and 124 days after the last dose of liraglutide. Two additional cases of acute pancreatitis were reported during a follow-up period; one case occurred within 2 weeks of discontinuing liraglutide and the other occurred 106 days after completing treatment with liraglutide. In a clinical trial in pediatric patients receiving liraglutide for chronic weight management, pancreatitis was not independently adjudicated; pancreatitis was reported in 1 (0.8%) liraglutide-treated patient and resulted in treatment discontinuation.

Observe patients carefully for signs and symptoms of pancreatitis (including persistent severe abdominal pain, sometimes radiating to the back and which may or may not be accompanied by vomiting). If pancreatitis is suspected, liraglutide or the fixed combination of insulin degludec and liraglutide should be discontinued promptly and appropriate management initiated. If pancreatitis is confirmed, liraglutide or the fixed combination of insulin degludec and liraglutide should not be restarted.

Efficacy and safety of liraglutide or the fixed combination of insulin degludec and liraglutide have not been established in patients with a history of pancreatitis, and it is not known whether such patients would have an increased risk of pancreatitis while taking liraglutide. Liraglutide has been evaluated in a limited number of adults with a history of pancreatitis in clinical trials of the drug for chronic weight management; it is not known if patients with a history of pancreatitis are at increased risk for pancreatitis while receiving liraglutide.

Acute Gallbladder Disease

Liraglutide may increase the risk of acute gallbladder disease (e.g., cholelithiasis, cholecystitis). In clinical trials for obesity management, cholelithiasis was reported in 2.2% of patients receiving liraglutide and in 0.8% of placebo recipients, and cholecystitis occurred in 0.8% of liraglutide-treated patients compared with 0.4% of placebo recipients. Cholecystectomy was required in most liraglutide-treated patients experiencing cholelithiasis and cholecystitis. In the LEADER study, gallbladder disease (e.g., cholelithiasis or cholecystitis) occurred in 3.1% of liraglutide-treated patients compared with 1.9% of placebo recipients. Cholecystectomy or hospitalization was required in most liraglutide-treated patients experiencing gallbladder disease.

Although substantial or rapid weight loss can increase the risk of cholelithiasis, the incidence of acute gallbladder disease was greater in liraglutide-treated patients than in those who received placebo in clinical trials of obesity management, even after accounting for the degree of weight loss. If cholelithiasis is suspected, gallbladder studies and appropriate clinical follow-up are recommended.

Sharing of Injection Pens

Injection pens containing liraglutide (Victoza®, Saxenda®) or the fixed combination of insulin degludec and liraglutide (Xultophy®) must never be shared among patients, even if the needle has been changed. Sharing of injection pens poses a risk for transmission of blood-borne pathogens.

Hypoglycemia

Patients receiving liraglutide in combination with an insulin secretagogue (e.g., a sulfonylurea) or insulin may have an increased risk of hypoglycemia. In 5 clinical

trials of liraglutide for the treatment of diabetes mellitus, hypoglycemia requiring the assistance of another person for treatment occurred in 8 patients receiving liraglutide, and 7 of these patients were concomitantly receiving a sulfonylurea antidiabetic agent.

In pediatric patients 10 years of age or older with type 2 diabetes mellitus, the risk of hypoglycemia was higher with liraglutide regardless of concomitant antidiabetic therapies. In a clinical study in pediatric patients (mean age: 14.6 years) with type 2 diabetes mellitus, 21.2% of liraglutide-treated patients experienced hypoglycemia (blood glucose concentration less than 54 mg/dL) with or without symptoms. None of the patients experienced severe hypoglycemia (i.e., a hypoglycemic episode requiring assistance of another person).

In clinical trials of chronic weight management in adults *without* type 2 diabetes mellitus, spontaneously reported symptomatic episodes of unconfirmed hypoglycemia were reported by 1.6 or 1.1% of adults receiving liraglutide or placebo, respectively. The manufacturer states that in patients with type 2 diabetes mellitus receiving liraglutide for chronic weight management, blood glucose parameters should be monitored prior to starting and during treatment. If needed, dosage of coadministered antidiabetic drugs should be adjusted based on results of glucose monitoring and risk of hypoglycemia.

In a clinical trial of chronic weight management in pediatric patients without type 2 diabetes mellitus in which blood glucose meters were provided, 15.2% of liraglutide-treated patients had hypoglycemia with a blood glucose less than 70 mg/dL with symptoms compared to 4% of placebo-treated patients. No severe hypoglycemic episodes, defined as requiring assistance of another person to actively administer carbohydrate, glucagon, or other resuscitative actions, occurred in patients receiving liraglutide.

When initiating liraglutide in patients taking insulin secretagogues (e.g., a sulfonylurea) or insulin, the risk of hypoglycemia may be reduced by decreasing the dosage of the concomitant insulin secretagogue (e.g., by 50% in patients receiving the drug for obesity) or insulin. The manufacturer states that insulin should not be used concomitantly in patients receiving liraglutide for the management of obesity. Patients with type 2 diabetes mellitus should be monitored for an increase in blood glucose when liraglutide is discontinued.

Elevated Heart Rate

Liraglutide has been associated with increases in heart rate in patients receiving the drug for the management of type 2 diabetes mellitus or obesity. In clinical trials in such patients, liraglutide was associated with a mean increase in resting heart rate of 2–3 beats per minute compared with placebo. In a clinical pharmacology study in patients receiving liraglutide for management of obesity, liraglutide therapy was associated with an increase in heart rate of 4–9 beats per minute compared with placebo. Heart rate increases of more than 10 or 20 beats per minute at 2 consecutive study visits were reported in 34 or 5% of patients receiving liraglutide, respectively, compared with 19 or 2% of patients receiving placebo, respectively, in clinical studies of obesity management. At least one occurrence of resting heart rate exceeding 100 beats per minute was reported in 6% of liraglutide-treated patients compared with 4% of placebo recipients, and such heart rate increases occurred at 2 consecutive visits in 0.9 or 0.3% of liraglutide- or placebo-treated patients, respectively. Tachycardia was reported as an adverse effect in 0.6% of patients receiving liraglutide for management of obesity versus 0.1% of those receiving placebo. The clinical importance of elevated heart rate is unclear, especially in patients with cardiovascular or cerebrovascular disease who had limited exposure to the drug in clinical trials of obesity management. Heart rate should be monitored regularly in patients receiving liraglutide; the drug should be discontinued in patients who experience a sustained increase in resting heart rate.

Renal Effects

Acute renal failure and worsening of chronic renal failure, sometimes requiring hemodialysis, have been reported with GLP-1 receptor agonists, including liraglutide. Some of these events occurred in patients without known underlying renal disease. Most of these events occurred in patients experiencing nausea, vomiting, diarrhea, or dehydration. Some of these events occurred in patients receiving liraglutide in combination with one or more agents known to affect renal function or hydration status.

Liraglutide has not been found to be directly nephrotoxic in preclinical or clinical studies. Renal effects usually have been reversible with supportive treatment and discontinuance of potentially causative agents, including liraglutide.

Suicidality

Suicidal ideation was reported in 9 patients (0.3%) receiving liraglutide in clinical trials for chronic weight management and in 2 patients (0.1%) receiving placebo; suicide attempt was reported in one of these patients. Patients receiving liraglutide should be monitored for the emergence or worsening of depression, suicidal thoughts or behavior (suicidality), and/or any unusual changes in mood or behavior. If a patient experiences suicidal thoughts or behaviors while receiving liraglutide, the drug should be discontinued. Liraglutide should be avoided in patients with a history of suicidal attempts or active suicidal ideation.

Immunogenicity

As with all therapeutic proteins, there is a potential for immunogenicity with liraglutide or the fixed combination of insulin degludec and liraglutide. In 5 double-blind clinical studies in patients with type 2 diabetes mellitus, antibodies to liraglutide were assessed in 50–70% of liraglutide-treated patients at the end of treatment (week 26 or greater). Low titers of anti-liraglutide antibodies were detected in 8.6% of these liraglutide-treated patients. Anti-liraglutide antibodies were detected at a post-baseline assessment in 42 (2.8%) of 1505 patients receiving liraglutide for management of obesity. Antibodies that had a neutralizing effect on liraglutide in an in vitro assay occurred in 18 (1.2%) of 1505 liraglutide-treated patients. The presence of antibodies may be associated with a higher incidence of injection site reactions and reports of low blood glucose. In clinical trials, these events were usually classified as mild and resolved while patients continued on treatment. The development of cross-reacting anti-liraglutide antibodies to native GLP-1 peptide also has occurred; however, the potential for clinically important neutralization of native GLP-1 has not been assessed. Antibody formation has not been associated with reduced efficacy of liraglutide or an increase in adverse events potentially related to immunogenicity (e.g., urticaria, angioedema). In a clinical study in pediatric patients 10–17 years of age, anti-liraglutide antibodies were detected in 1.5% of liraglutide-treated patients after 26 weeks of treatment and 8.5% of liraglutide-treated patients after 53 weeks of treatment. None of these patients developed cross-reactive antibodies to native GLP-1 or had neutralizing antibodies.

Specific Populations

Pregnancy

Data are lacking on the use of liraglutide (Victoza®) in pregnant women. Reproduction studies in rats using liraglutide at dosages resulting in systemic exposures 0.8 times the exposure from the maximum recommended human dosage (1.8 mg daily) have shown teratogenic effects. Studies in rabbits have shown reduced growth and major abnormalities at systemic exposures below the maximum recommended human dosage. Liraglutide for the management of diabetes mellitus should be used during pregnancy only when the potential benefits justify the possible risks to the fetus.

The manufacturer states that liraglutide (Saxenda®) is contraindicated for the management of obesity in women who are pregnant because weight loss offers no potential benefit to pregnant women and may result in fetal harm. If a woman taking liraglutide for the management of obesity becomes pregnant or plans to become pregnant, the drug should be discontinued.

Lactation

Liraglutide is distributed into milk in rats. It is not known whether liraglutide is distributed into milk in humans; a decision should be made whether to discontinue nursing or the drug, taking into account the importance of the drug to the woman.

Pediatric Use

Safety and efficacy of liraglutide for the management of type 2 diabetes mellitus have not been established in children or adolescents younger than 10 years of age. Safety and efficacy of liraglutide for chronic weight management have not been established in children or adolescents younger than 18 years of age, and the manufacturer of Saxenda® states that the drug is not recommended for use in pediatric patients.

Safety and efficacy of the fixed combination of insulin degludec and liraglutide have not been established in pediatric patients.

Geriatric Use

No substantial differences in safety and efficacy relative to younger adults have been observed with liraglutide or the fixed combination of insulin degludec and liraglutide, but increased sensitivity of some older patients cannot be ruled out. Hypoglycemia may be difficult to recognize in geriatric patients.

Hepatic Impairment

Experience in patients with mild, moderate, or severe hepatic impairment is limited; liraglutide (as Victoza® or Saxenda®) or the fixed combination of insulin degludec and liraglutide should be used with caution in such patients.

Renal Impairment

In a clinical study of 26 weeks' duration, patients with moderate renal impairment (estimated glomerular filtration rate [eGFR] 30–59 mL/minute per 1.73m^2) who received liraglutide 1.8 mg once daily had no worsening of renal function. Data regarding the use of liraglutide in patients with severe renal impairment are lacking. Caution should be used when initiating or escalating doses of liraglutide in patients with renal impairment. Experience with the fixed combination of insulin degludec and liraglutide in patients with mild, moderate, or severe renal impairment is limited; the combination should be used with caution in such patients.

The manufacturer states that there is limited experience with liraglutide (as Saxenda®) in patients with mild, moderate, and severe renal impairment, including in patients with end-stage renal disease; Saxenda® should be used with caution in this patient population.

Patients with Gastroparesis

Liraglutide slows gastric emptying and potentially may affect absorption of concomitantly administered oral drugs. Liraglutide has not been studied in patients with preexisting gastroparesis.

● Common Adverse Effects

Adverse effects reported in at least 5% of patients receiving liraglutide monotherapy for the management of type 2 diabetes mellitus in clinical trials include nausea, diarrhea, vomiting, constipation, and headache.

Adverse effects reported in at least 2% of patients receiving liraglutide for the management of obesity and more frequently than with placebo include nausea, hypoglycemia (in patients with both obesity and type 2 diabetes mellitus), headache, diarrhea, constipation, dizziness, fatigue, vomiting, gastroenteritis, abdominal pain, urinary tract infection, abdominal distention, dyspepsia, upper abdominal pain, flatulence, decreased appetite, increased lipase, gastroesophageal reflux disease, insomnia, anxiety, viral gastroenteritis, dry mouth, asthenia, injection site reaction, eructation, and injection site erythema.

Adverse effects occurring in at least 5% of patients with type 2 diabetes mellitus who received the fixed combination of insulin degludec and liraglutide include nasopharyngitis, headache, nausea, diarrhea, increased lipase concentrations, and upper respiratory tract infection.

DRUG INTERACTIONS

● Effects on GI Absorption of Other Drugs

Potential pharmacokinetic interaction (altered absorption because of liraglutide-induced slowing of gastric emptying). In clinical trials, liraglutide did not affect the absorption of concomitantly administered oral drugs to any clinically relevant degree. However, caution should be exercised when liraglutide is administered concomitantly with oral drugs.

● Acetaminophen

Potential pharmacokinetic interaction (decreased acetaminophen peak plasma concentration and rate of absorption following a single dose of acetaminophen); no change in overall acetaminophen exposure (area under the serum concentration-time curve [AUC]).

● Antidiabetic Agents

The risk of serious hypoglycemia is increased when liraglutide is used in conjunction with an insulin secretagogue (e.g., sulfonylurea) or basal insulin; patients receiving liraglutide concomitantly with such agents may require a reduction in the dosage of the insulin secretagogue or insulin.

No pharmacokinetic interaction has been observed following administration of separate subcutaneous injections of insulin detemir (single dose of 0.5 units/kg) and liraglutide (1.8 mg at steady state) in patients with type 2 diabetes mellitus.

● **Atorvastatin**

Potential pharmacokinetic interaction (decreased atorvastatin peak plasma concentration and rate of absorption following a single dose of atorvastatin); no change in overall atorvastatin exposure (AUC).

● **Digoxin**

Potential pharmacokinetic interaction (decreased digoxin peak plasma concentration, AUC, and rate of absorption following a single dose of digoxin).

● **Griseofulvin**

Potential pharmacokinetic interaction (increased griseofulvin peak plasma concentration following a single dose of griseofulvin); no change in overall griseofulvin exposure (AUC).

● **Lisinopril**

Potential pharmacokinetic interaction (decreased lisinopril peak plasma concentration, AUC, and rate of absorption following a single dose of lisinopril).

● **Oral Contraceptives**

Potential pharmacokinetic interaction (decreased peak plasma concentrations and rates of absorption of ethinyl estradiol and levonorgestrel; increased AUC of levonorgestrel but no effect on AUC of ethinyl estradiol).

DESCRIPTION

Liraglutide is an acylated, long-acting, human glucagon-like peptide-1 (GLP-1) receptor agonist; the synthetic (recombinant DNA origin) peptide precursor of liraglutide has 97% amino acid sequence homology to endogenous human GLP-1-(7-37). Liraglutide is prepared by substituting arginine for lysine at position 34 and attaching palmitic acid with a glutamic acid spacer on the remaining lysine residue at position 26 of the peptide precursor. GLP-1-(7-37) represents less than 20% of total circulating endogenous GLP-1. Like GLP-1-(7-37), liraglutide binds to and activates the GLP-1 receptor in pancreatic β cells. Liraglutide also increases intracellular cyclic 3′,5′-adenosine monophosphate (cAMP) leading to insulin release in the presence of elevated glucose concentrations. This insulin secretion subsides as blood glucose concentrations decrease and approach euglycemia. In addition, liraglutide suppresses glucagon secretion in a glucose-dependent manner but does not impair normal glucagon response to hypoglycemia. Liraglutide delays gastric emptying, reducing the rate at which postprandial glucose appears in the circulation. As a result of these actions resulting in increased insulin secretion, suppression of glucagon secretion, and delays in gastric emptying, liraglutide effectively reduces fasting and postprandial plasma glucose concentrations in patients with type 2 diabetes mellitus.

GLP-1 is a physiological regulator of appetite and caloric intake. The GLP-1 receptor is located in several areas of the brain involved in appetite regulation. Weight loss effects of liraglutide are mediated by decreased calorie intake; the drug does not increase 24-hour energy expenditure.

Peak plasma liraglutide concentration is achieved an average of 11 hours (range: 8–12 hours) following subcutaneous administration. The average liraglutide steady-state concentration following administration of liraglutide in obese (body mass index [BMI] 30–40 kg/m²) individuals was approximately 116 ng/mL. Glucose-lowering activity is sustained for 24 hours after a dose of liraglutide at steady state. Liraglutide exposure increases proportionally in the dosage range of 0.6–3 mg; exposures were similar following subcutaneous injection into the upper arm, abdomen, or thigh. Absolute bioavailability following subcutaneous administration is approximately 55%. The mean apparent volume of distribution after subcutaneous administration of liraglutide 3 mg is 20-25 L (for an individual weighing approximately 100 kg). Liraglutide is extensively (greater than 98%) bound to plasma proteins. Liraglutide is endogenously metabolized in a similar manner to large proteins without a specific organ as a major route of elimination. The endogenous enzymes dipeptidyl peptidase-4 (DPP-4) and

neutral endopeptidase (NEP) are likely to be involved in degradation of the drug. The average terminal half-life of liraglutide is 13 hours following subcutaneous administration, making the drug suitable for once-daily administration. Following a dose of radiolabeled liraglutide, intact liraglutide was not detected in urine or feces, and only a minor amount of administered radioactivity was excreted as liraglutide-related metabolites in urine or feces (6 or 5%, respectively).

In a study of the effect of liraglutide on cardiac repolarization in healthy individuals, steady-state liraglutide concentrations attained with daily dosages of up to 1.8 mg did not produce QTc (QT interval corrected for rate, Bazett's formula) prolongation. The manufacturer states that maximum plasma liraglutide concentrations in overweight or obese individuals receiving liraglutide 3 mg daily are similar to those observed in the QTc study in healthy individuals.

ADVICE TO PATIENTS

When liraglutide is used in fixed combination with other drugs, importance of informing patients of important cautionary information about the concomitant agents.

Importance of reading manufacturer's medication guide and the injection pen's patient instructions for use before starting therapy with liraglutide or the fixed combination of insulin degludec and liraglutide and of reviewing this information each time the prescription is renewed. Importance of clinicians instructing patients in proper injection technique to reduce administration errors (e.g., needle sticks, incomplete dosing).

Importance of informing patients that liraglutide causes benign and malignant thyroid C-cell tumors in mice and rats and that relevance of this finding to humans is unknown. Importance of counseling patients to report symptoms of thyroid tumors (e.g., a lump in the neck, hoarseness, dysphagia, dyspnea) or a personal or family history of thyroid cancer, including medullary thyroid cancer (MTC) or multiple endocrine neoplasia type 2 (MEN 2), to their clinician.

Importance of informing patients of the potential risk of acute pancreatitis, which may be severe or fatal, with liraglutide therapy. Importance of patient informing clinicians about a history of pancreatitis. Importance of informing patients about signs and symptoms of pancreatitis, including persistent severe abdominal pain sometimes radiating to the back that may or may not be accompanied by vomiting. Importance of instructing patients to discontinue liraglutide or the fixed combination of insulin degludec and liraglutide promptly and contact their clinician if persistent, severe abdominal pain occurs.

Importance of informing patients of the risk of gallbladder disease, which can require cholecystectomy. Importance of informing patients that substantial or rapid weight loss increases the risk of cholelithiasis; however, cholelithiasis can occur in the absence of weight loss. Patients should be instructed to contact their clinician if they experience symptoms of gallbladder disease (e.g., abdominal pain, fever, jaundice, clay-colored stools).

Importance of informing patient of risk of hypoglycemia, particularly if concomitant therapy with an insulin secretagogue (e.g., a sulfonylurea) or insulin is used. Importance of reviewing signs, symptoms, and management of hypoglycemia.

Risk of increased resting heart rate; importance of advising patients that their heart rate should be measured periodically during therapy. Patients should be instructed to contact their clinician if they experience sustained palpitations or tachycardia at rest.

Importance of informing patients of possibility of risk of dehydration due to adverse GI reactions; patients should be advised to take precautions to avoid fluid depletion. Importance of informing patients of potential risk of worsening renal function, including renal failure that may require dialysis in some cases.

Importance of informing patients of possibility of serious hypersensitivity reactions. Patients should be instructed to discontinue liraglutide or the fixed combination of insulin degludec and liraglutide and promptly seek medical advice if symptoms of hypersensitivity occur.

Potential risk of suicidality; importance of patients being alert to and immediately reporting emergence or worsening of depression, suicidal thoughts or behavior, and/or unusual changes in mood or behavior. Importance of patient discontinuing liraglutide if suicidal thoughts or behaviors are experienced.

Importance of informing patients that they should never share an injection pen containing liraglutide or the fixed combination of insulin degludec and liraglutide with another person, even if the needle is changed; sharing of the pen may pose a risk of transmission of infection.

Importance of instructing patients with diabetes mellitus regarding self-monitoring of blood glucose, periodic glycosylated hemoglobin (hemoglobin A_{1c}, HbA_{1c}) monitoring, adherence to meal planning, and regular physical exercise.

Importance of informing patients of the most common adverse effects, including headache, nausea, and diarrhea. Nausea is most common when first starting liraglutide, but decreases over time in most patients and does not typically require discontinuance of the drug.

Importance of cautioning patients not to take an extra dose of liraglutide or the fixed combination of insulin degludec and liraglutide to make up for a missed dose. If a dose is missed, patients should resume the once-daily regimen with the next scheduled dose.

Importance of informing patients that if more than 3 days have passed since the last dose of liraglutide, the drug should be reinitiated at a dosage of 0.6 mg once daily to mitigate GI symptoms associated with reinitiation of treatment, then retitrated.

Importance of informing patients that if more than 3 days have passed since the last dose of the fixed combination of insulin degludec and liraglutide, the drug should be reinitiated at the starting dose to mitigate GI symptoms due to the liraglutide component.

Importance of instructing patients to discontinue use of liraglutide for the management of obesity if they have not achieved 4% weight loss after 16 weeks of therapy.

Response to all diabetic therapies should be monitored by periodic measurements of blood glucose and HbA_{1c} levels, with a goal of decreasing these levels towards the normal range.

Importance of women informing clinicians if they are or plan to become pregnant or plan to breast-feed.

Importance of informing clinicians of existing or contemplated concomitant therapy, including prescription and OTC drugs, as well as any concomitant illnesses (e.g., gallstones, hypertension, pancreatitis, history of alcoholism, high triglyceride concentrations, digestion problems, severe kidney disease, kidney transplant).

Inform patients of other important precautionary information.

PREPARATIONS

Excipients in commercially available drug preparations may have clinically important effects in some individuals; consult specific product labeling for details.

Liraglutide

Parenteral		
Injection, for subcutaneous use	6 mg/mL	Victoza® (available as prefilled single-patient-use 3 mL pen that delivers doses of 0.6 mg, 1.2 mg, or 1.8 mg), Novo Nordisk
	6 mg/mL	Saxenda® (available as prefilled single-patient-use 3 mL pen that delivers doses of 0.6 mg, 1.2 mg, 1.8 mg, 2.4 mg, or 3 mg), Novo Nordisk

Liraglutide Combinations

Parenteral		
Injection, for subcutaneous use	3.6 mg/mL with Insulin Degludec 100 units/mL	Xultophy® (available as prefilled single-patient-use 3 mL pen), Novo Nordisk

† Use is not currently included in the labeling approved by the US Food and Drug Administration.

Lixisenatide

68:20.06 • INCRETIN MIMETICS

■ Lixisenatide, a synthetic, short-acting glucagon-like peptide-1 (GLP-1) receptor agonist (incretin mimetic), is an antidiabetic agent.

USES

● Type 2 Diabetes Mellitus

Lixisenatide is used as an adjunct to diet and exercise to improve glycemic control in patients with type 2 diabetes mellitus. Lixisenatide also is commercially available in fixed combination with insulin glargine; the fixed combination is used as an adjunct to diet and exercise to improve glycemic control in patients with type 2 diabetes mellitus. Lixisenatide has been used alone or as add-on therapy in conjunction with other antidiabetic agents, including metformin with or without a sulfonylurea; a sulfonylurea or thiazolidinedione with or without metformin; basal insulin (insulin glargine, insulin detemir, or isophane [NPH] insulin) with or without metformin or a sulfonylurea; or insulin glargine with or without metformin with or without a thiazolidinedione.

Glycemic Control

Current guidelines for the treatment of type 2 diabetes mellitus generally recommend metformin as first-line therapy in addition to lifestyle modifications in patients with recent-onset type 2 diabetes mellitus or mild hyperglycemia because of its well-established safety and efficacy (i.e., beneficial effects on glycosylated hemoglobin [hemoglobin A_{1c}; HbA_{1c}], weight, and cardiovascular mortality). In patients with contraindications or intolerance to metformin (e.g., risk of lactic acidosis, GI intolerance) or in selected other patients, some experts suggest that initial therapy with a drug from another class of antidiabetic agents (e.g., a GLP-1 receptor agonist, sodium-glucose cotransporter 2 [SGLT2] inhibitor, dipeptidyl peptidase-4 [DPP-4] inhibitor, sulfonylurea, thiazolidinedione, basal insulin) may be acceptable based on patient factors. Initiating antidiabetic therapy with 2 agents (e.g., metformin plus another drug) may be appropriate in patients with an initial HbA_{1c} exceeding 7.5% or at least 1.5% above the target level. In metformin-intolerant patients with high initial HbA_{1c} levels, some experts suggest initiation of therapy with 2 agents from other antidiabetic drug classes with complementary mechanisms of action.

Because of the progressive nature of type 2 diabetes mellitus, patients initially receiving an oral antidiabetic agent will eventually require multiple oral and/or injectable noninsulin antidiabetic agents of different therapeutic classes and/or insulin for adequate glycemic control. Patients who have inadequate glycemic control with initial (e.g., metformin) monotherapy should receive treatment with additional antidiabetic agents; data suggest that the addition of each noninsulin agent to initial therapy lowers HbA_{1c} by approximately 0.7–1%. In addition, early initiation of combination therapy may help to more rapidly attain glycemic goals and extend the time to treatment failure.

Factors to consider when selecting additional antidiabetic agents for combination therapy in patients with inadequate glycemic control on metformin monotherapy include patient comorbidities (e.g., atherosclerotic cardiovascular disease [ASCVD], established kidney disease, heart failure), hypoglycemia risk, impact on weight, cost, risk of adverse effects, and patient preference. When the greater glucose-lowering effect of an injectable drug is needed in patients with type 2 diabetes mellitus, some experts currently state that an injectable GLP-1 receptor agonist is preferred over insulin in most patients because of beneficial effects on body weight and a lower risk of hypoglycemia, although adverse GI effects may diminish tolerability. While addition of a GLP-1 receptor agonist may successfully control hyperglycemia, many patients will eventually require insulin therapy. Early introduction of insulin therapy should be considered when hyperglycemia is severe (e.g., blood glucose of at least 300 mg/dL or HbA_{1c} exceeding 9–10%), especially in the presence of catabolic manifestations (e.g., weight loss, hypertriglyceridemia, ketosis) or symptoms of hyperglycemia.

Patients with type 2 diabetes mellitus who have established (or are at a high risk for) ASCVD, established kidney disease, or heart failure should receive a GLP-1 receptor agonist or SGLT2 inhibitor with demonstrated cardiovascular disease benefit. Experts state that therapy with a GLP-1 receptor agonist or SGLT2 inhibitor should be considered for patients with the aforementioned comorbidities independently of the patients' HbA_{1c}. GLP-1 receptor agonists and SGLT2 inhibitors appear to have effects on the kidneys independent of their glycemic effects, and some experts suggest that an agent from one of these classes of drugs be considered in patients with type 2 diabetes mellitus and chronic kidney disease (CKD). In patients *without* established ASCVD or indicators of high ASCVD risk, heart failure, or CKD, the decision regarding the addition of other antidiabetic agents (e.g., GLP-1 receptor agonist, SGLT2 inhibitor, DPP-4 inhibitor, thiazolidinedione, sulfonylurea, basal insulin) to metformin therapy should be based on avoidance of adverse effects, cost, and individual patient factors.

Data indicate that lixisenatide 20 mcg daily is capable of reducing glycosylated hemoglobin (hemoglobin A_{1c}; HbA_{1c}) by approximately 0.5–0.6% from a baseline of 8% after 6 months of therapy and is especially effective in reducing postprandial plasma glucose concentrations. Available data suggest that lixisenatide therapy may be useful for patients who need to lower their postprandial plasma glucose concentrations in order to achieve their goal HbA_{1c} despite having fasting plasma glucose concentrations that are within goal.

Safety and efficacy of lixisenatide alone or in combination with insulin glargine have *not* been established in patients with chronic pancreatitis or a history of unexplained pancreatitis. The manufacturer states that other antidiabetic therapies should be considered in patients with a history of pancreatitis.

The manufacturer states that lixisenatide alone or in combination with insulin glargine is *not* indicated for the treatment of type 1 diabetes mellitus.

Lixisenatide alone or in combination with insulin glargine is not recommended for use in patients with gastroparesis.

Lixisenatide Monotherapy

When given as monotherapy for the management of type 2 diabetes mellitus, lixisenatide improves glycemic control as evidenced by reductions from baseline in HbA_{1c}. Safety and efficacy of lixisenatide as monotherapy have been established in a 12-week, randomized, double-blind, placebo-controlled trial comparing lixisenatide (20 mcg once daily) with placebo in patients with a mean baseline HbA_{1c} concentration of 8.07%. At week 12, therapy with lixisenatide 20 mcg once daily was associated with a mean HbA_{1c} reduction of 0.83%. HbA_{1c} concentrations below 7% were achieved in 44 or 24% of patients receiving lixisenatide or placebo, respectively. There was no substantial difference in weight loss between lixisenatide and placebo treatment groups.

Combination Therapy

When given as add-on therapy in conjunction with one or more oral antidiabetic agents (e.g., metformin, a sulfonylurea, a thiazolidinedione) with or without basal insulin, lixisenatide improved glycemic control and had a beneficial effect on body weight (i.e., no weight gain or weight loss). In trials comparing add-on therapy with lixisenatide versus add-on exenatide or insulin glulisine, lixisenatide was noninferior to exenatide, and lixisenatide in conjunction with insulin glargine was noninferior to insulin glulisine (administered once or 3 times daily) in conjunction with insulin glargine with regard to HbA_{1c} reduction from baseline; however, lixisenatide add-on therapy was associated with smaller mean reductions in HbA_{1c} compared with exenatide or insulin glulisine (3 times daily) add-on therapy.

In several trials of 24 weeks' duration in which lixisenatide (20 mcg once daily) was added to therapy with metformin hydrochloride alone or with a sulfonylurea, combined therapy with lixisenatide and these oral antidiabetic agents resulted in greater reductions from baseline in HbA_{1c} compared with those achieved with existing oral antidiabetic therapy. In a trial comparing lixisenatide 20 mcg once daily and exenatide 10 mcg twice daily (both in conjunction with metformin), lixisenatide was noninferior to exenatide; however, lixisenatide therapy was associated with less HbA_{1c} reduction than exenatide therapy (reduction of 0.73 versus 0.9%, respectively). Additionally, weight loss was greater with exenatide compared with lixisenatide therapy.

Safety and efficacy of lixisenatide as add-on therapy also have been established in clinical trials with other antidiabetic agents. In a 24-week, placebo-controlled trial in patients who had not achieved adequate glycemic control with a sulfonylurea with or without metformin, the addition of lixisenatide (20 mcg once daily) resulted in a greater reduction from baseline in HbA_{1c} at week 24 than that achieved with existing oral antidiabetic therapy (HbA_{1c} reduction of 0.77 versus

0.18%, respectively). Lixisenatide therapy also was associated with a substantially greater reduction in mean body weight (reduction of 1.63 versus 0.83 kg, respectively). In a 24-week, placebo-controlled trial in patients with type 2 diabetes mellitus who had inadequate glycemic control on pioglitazone with or without metformin, addition of lixisenatide (20 mcg once daily) resulted in improved glycemic control (as indicated by a reduction in HbA$_{1c}$ from baseline) at week 24. There was no substantial difference in weight loss between the 2 treatment groups.

Safety and efficacy of lixisenatide in conjunction with basal insulin have been established in several trials of 24 or 26 weeks' duration in patients receiving insulin with or without oral antidiabetic agents (e.g., metformin, a sulfonylurea, a thiazolidinedione). In 2 trials of 24 weeks' duration, patients with type 2 diabetes mellitus who had inadequate glycemic control on basal insulin (e.g., insulin glargine, insulin detemir, NPH insulin) with or without metformin or a sulfonylurea demonstrated a reduction in HbA$_{1c}$ from baseline at week 24 with the addition of lixisenatide (20 mcg once daily) to existing antidiabetic therapy. In another trial of 24 weeks' duration, patients with type 2 diabetes mellitus who had inadequate glycemic control with insulin glargine and metformin with or without a thiazolidinedione had substantial reductions in HbA$_{1c}$ from baseline at week 24 with add-on lixisenatide (20 mcg once daily) compared with that achieved with existing antidiabetic therapy. In a 26-week, open-label trial, patients with type 2 diabetes mellitus who had inadequate glycemic control with insulin glargine with or without 1–3 oral antidiabetic agents (e.g., metformin, a dipeptidyl peptidase-4 [DPP-4] inhibitor, a sulfonylurea, a meglitinide) received lixisenatide 20 mcg once daily or insulin glulisine 1 or 3 times daily, all in conjunction with insulin glargine with or without metformin. Lixisenatide was noninferior to insulin glulisine (1 or 3 times daily) with regard to HbA$_{1c}$ reduction from baseline; however, the HbA$_{1c}$ reductions observed with lixisenatide were substantially less than those associated with insulin glulisine therapy administered 3 times daily (reduction of 0.6 versus 0.8%, respectively).

Fixed-combination Therapy with Insulin Glargine and Lixisenatide

Current data indicate that the fixed combination of insulin glargine and lixisenatide is more effective than monotherapy with either drug in improving glycemic control (as determined by reductions in HbA$_{1c}$) in patients with type 2 diabetes mellitus. Additionally, therapy with the fixed combination of insulin glargine and lixisenatide was associated with weight loss while weight gain was observed with insulin glargine monotherapy. Safety and efficacy of the fixed combination of insulin glargine and lixisenatide have been established in 2 clinical studies. In an open-label trial in approximately 740 patients with type 2 diabetes mellitus inadequately controlled on basal insulin (e.g., insulin detemir, insulin glargine, NPH insulin) alone or in conjunction with 1 or 2 oral antidiabetic agents (e.g., metformin, a sulfonylurea, a meglitinide, a sodium-glucose cotransporter 2 [SGLT2] inhibitor, a DPP-4 inhibitor). Patients underwent a 6-week run-in period in which all oral antidiabetic drugs (except metformin) were discontinued and therapy with insulin glargine was initiated and titrated prior to randomization. Patients then received treatment with the fixed combination of insulin glargine and lixisenatide or continued insulin glargine therapy. The dosages of insulin glargine or the fixed combination of insulin glargine and lixisenatide were titrated once weekly based on fasting plasma glucose concentrations (mean final dosages of insulin glargine alone or in combination with lixisenatide were equivalent at week 30 [46.7 units]). At week 30, there was a substantially greater reduction in HbA$_{1c}$ with the fixed combination of insulin glargine and lixisenatide than with insulin glargine alone (reduction of 1.1 versus 0.6%, respectively). Patients receiving therapy with the fixed combination of insulin glargine and lixisenatide had an average weight loss of 0.7 kg while those receiving insulin glargine monotherapy gained an average of 0.7 kg.

In another open-label trial of 30 weeks' duration, approximately 1170 patients with type 2 diabetes mellitus inadequately controlled on metformin with or without another antidiabetic agent (e.g., a sulfonylurea, a meglitinide, an SGLT2 inhibitor, a DPP-4 inhibitor) received therapy with the fixed combination of insulin glargine and lixisenatide, insulin glargine, or lixisenatide, all in conjunction with metformin. Greater reductions in HbA$_{1c}$ were observed with the fixed combination of insulin glargine and lixisenatide than with either component alone (reduction of 1.6, 1.3, or 0.9% for the fixed combination of insulin glargine and lixisenatide, insulin glargine, or lixisenatide therapy, respectively). Mean body weight was reduced by 0.3 or 2.3 kg in patients receiving the fixed combination of insulin glargine and lixisenatide or lixisenatide, respectively. Mean body weight was increased by 1.1 kg in patients receiving insulin glargine monotherapy.

The fixed combination of insulin glargine and lixisenatide is not recommended for use with any other drug preparation containing lixisenatide or another GLP-1 receptor agonist.

Macrovascular Outcomes and Cardiovascular Risk Reduction

Some GLP-1 receptor agonists (e.g., dulaglutide, liraglutide, semaglutide) have demonstrated the ability to reduce the risk of cardiovascular events in those patients with type 2 diabetes mellitus and established cardiovascular disease. In addition to lowering blood glucose, GLP-1 receptor agonists appear to modify several nonglycemic cardiovascular risk factors, such as blood pressure, body weight, and lipid profile. GLP-1 receptor agonists also may have beneficial endothelial effects. The manufacturer states that there have been no clinical studies establishing conclusive evidence of macrovascular risk reduction with lixisenatide.

Safety and efficacy of lixisenatide in patients with type 2 diabetes mellitus who had a recent acute coronary event (myocardial infarction [MI], hospitalization for unstable angina) were evaluated in a double-blind, placebo-controlled, multinational trial (The Evaluation of Lixisenatide in Acute Coronary Syndrome [ELIXA]). No substantial difference in the rate of cardiovascular events was demonstrated in patients receiving lixisenatide in addition to conventional antidiabetic therapy (e.g., oral antidiabetic agents, insulin) compared with conventional therapy without lixisenatide. In this trial, patients received lixisenatide 20 mcg or placebo subcutaneously once daily for a median of 22.4–23.3 months. Approximately 93.9% of patients were receiving one antidiabetic drug (e.g., metformin, a sulfonylurea, insulin) prior to starting the trial; additionally, most patients also were receiving cardiovascular drugs at baseline (platelet aggregation inhibitors [97.5%], statins [92.7%], angiotensin-converting enzyme [ACE] inhibitors and/or angiotensin II receptor antagonists [86.8%], β-adrenergic blocking agents [84.4%]). The primary end point was the composite of the first occurrence of death from cardiovascular causes, nonfatal MI, nonfatal stroke, or hospitalization for unstable angina, which occurred in 13.4 versus 13.2% of patients treated with or without lixisenatide, respectively.

DOSAGE AND ADMINISTRATION

• General

Patient Monitoring

- Periodically monitor blood glucose and glycosylated hemoglobin (hemoglobin HbA$_{1c}$) to determine therapeutic response in patients with type 2 diabetes mellitus.

- Monitor renal function when initiating or escalating dosage in patients with renal impairment or those reporting severe adverse GI effects.

- Closely monitor patients with a history of anaphylaxis or angioedema with another GLP-1 receptor agonist for allergic reactions during lixisenatide therapy.

- Observe patients carefully for signs and symptoms of pancreatitis.

• Administration

Lixisenatide or the fixed combination of insulin glargine and lixisenatide is administered by subcutaneous injection into the abdomen, thigh, or upper arm using a prefilled injection pen; the injection must *not* be administered IV, IM, or via an insulin pump. A planned rotation of injection sites within an area should be followed to reduce the risk of lipodystrophy and localized cutaneous amyloidosis.

Lixisenatide is administered once daily within 1 hour *before* the first meal of the day, preferably the same meal each day and the same time each day. If a dose of lixisenatide is missed, the dose should be administered within 1 hour before the next meal. The fixed combination of insulin glargine and lixisenatide is administered once daily within 1 hour *before* the first meal of the day. If a dose of the fixed combination of insulin glargine and lixisenatide is missed, the patient should resume the once-daily regimen with the next scheduled dose.

Lixisenatide or the fixed combination of insulin glargine and lixisenatide should be used only if the solution is clear, colorless (or almost colorless for the fixed combination of insulin glargine and lixisenatide), and contains no particles. The fixed combination of insulin glargine and lixisenatide should not be mixed with any other insulin or solution.

Injection pens containing lixisenatide or the fixed combination of insulin glargine and lixisenatide should be stored at 2–8°C in the original carton and protected from light before first use. After first use, injection pens containing lixisenatide or the fixed combination of insulin glargine and lixisenatide should be stored at room temperature not exceeding 30 or 25°C, respectively. The injection pens should not be frozen; the pen should be discarded if it has been frozen. Injection pens containing lixisenatide or the fixed combination of insulin glargine and lixisenatide should be discarded 14 or 28 days after first use, respectively, even if some drug remains in the pen.

The manufacturer's instructions for use should be consulted for additional details about the administration of lixisenatide or the fixed combination of insulin glargine and lixisenatide.

● **Dosage**

Lixisenatide Monotherapy

The recommended initial dosage of lixisenatide for the management of type 2 diabetes mellitus is 10 mcg subcutaneously once daily for 14 days. On day 15, the dosage should be increased to 20 mcg subcutaneously once daily.

Insulin Glargine/Lixisenatide Fixed-combination Therapy

The dosage of the fixed combination of insulin glargine and lixisenatide has been expressed in terms of the insulin glargine component; however, each mL of the fixed combination of insulin glargine and lixisenatide contains 100 units of insulin glargine *and* 33 mcg of lixisenatide.

Therapy with lixisenatide or basal insulin should be discontinued prior to initiating therapy with the fixed combination of insulin glargine and lixisenatide.

For patients who are naive to basal insulin or to a glucagon-like peptide-1 (GLP-1) receptor agonist who are currently on a GLP-1 receptor agonist, or who are inadequately controlled on less than 30 units of basal insulin daily, the recommended initial dosage of the fixed combination of insulin glargine and lixisenatide is 15 units (15 units insulin glargine and 5 mcg lixisenatide) subcutaneously once daily. For patients inadequately controlled on 30–60 units of basal insulin daily with or without a GLP-1 receptor agonist, the recommended initial dosage of the fixed combination of insulin glargine and lixisenatide is 30 units (30 units insulin glargine and 10 mcg lixisenatide) subcutaneously once daily. The dosage should be titrated by 2–4 units every week based on the patient's metabolic needs, blood glucose concentrations, and glycemic control goal. The recommended dosage of the fixed combination of insulin glargine and lixisenatide is 15–60 units (15–60 units insulin glargine and 5–20 mcg lixisenatide) once daily.

● **Special Populations**

Hepatic Impairment

Dosage adjustments of lixisenatide are not likely required in patients with hepatic impairment since hepatic impairment is not expected to affect the pharmacokinetics of the drug.

Frequent glucose monitoring and dosage adjustments may be required for patients with hepatic impairment receiving the fixed combination of insulin glargine and lixisenatide.

Renal Impairment

No adjustment of lixisenatide dosage is required in patients with mild or moderate renal impairment (estimated glomerular filtration rate [eGFR] 30–89 mL/minute per 1.73 m²). However, close monitoring for changes in renal function and for adverse effects (e.g., hypoglycemia, nausea, vomiting) is recommended in such patients when initiating lixisenatide or escalating dosage; such changes and adverse effects may lead to dehydration and acute renal failure or worsening of chronic renal failure in patients with moderate renal impairment. There is limited experience with the use of lixisenatide in patients with severe renal impairment (eGFR 15 to less than 30 mL/minute per 1.73 m²), and these patients should be closely monitored for the occurrence of adverse GI effects and changes in renal function with lixisenatide use. Data and experience are lacking on the use of lixisenatide in patients with end-stage renal disease (eGFR less than 15 mL/minute per 1.73 m²) and lixisenatide use is not recommended in such patients.

Frequent glucose monitoring and dosage adjustments may be required for patients with renal impairment receiving the fixed combination of insulin glargine

and lixisenatide. Data and experience are lacking on the use of the fixed combination of insulin glargine and lixisenatide in patients with end-stage renal disease; the fixed combination is not recommended in such patients.

CAUTIONS

● **Contraindications**

Lixisenatide and the fixed combination of insulin glargine and lixisenatide are contraindicated in patients with known severe hypersensitivity to lixisenatide or any ingredient in the formulation. The fixed combination of insulin glargine and lixisenatide also is contraindicated during episodes of hypoglycemia.

● **Warnings/Precautions**

Risks During General Anesthesia and Deep Sedation

GLP-1 agonists are associated with adverse GI effects such as nausea, vomiting, and delayed gastric emptying; such effects are likely a result of rapid tachyphlaxis at the level of vagal nerve activation. Delayed gastric emptying from GLP-1 agonists can increase the risk of regurgitation and pulmonary aspiration of gastric contents during general anesthesia and deep sedation. Given these concerns, the American Society of Anesthesiologists (ASA) Task Force on Preoperative Fasting has issued a consensus-based guidance for the management of GLP-1 receptor agonists prior to elective surgery. The task force suggests that for patients on daily GLP-1 agonist dosing (irrespective of indication, dose, or type of surgery), consider holding the drug on the day of the procedure/surgery. For patients on weekly dosing (irrespective of indication, dose, or type of surgery), consider holding the GLP-1 agonist a week prior to the procedure/surgery. If GLP-1 agonists prescribed for diabetes management are held for longer than the dosing schedule, consider consulting an endocrinologist for bridging the antidiabetic therapy to avoid hyperglycemia. These recommendations are based on limited evidence only (case reports). For patients requiring urgent or emergent procedures, the task force states to proceed and treat the patient as 'full stomach' and manage accordingly.

Pancreatitis

Acute pancreatitis, including fatal and nonfatal hemorrhagic or necrotizing pancreatitis, has been reported during postmarketing experience in patients treated with GLP-1 receptor agonists.

In clinical trials of lixisenatide, the incidence of pancreatitis in lixisenatide-treated patients versus patients who received other antidiabetic therapy was 21 versus 17 per 10,000 patient-years; some patients in these trials had risk factors for pancreatitis (e.g., history of cholelithiasis or alcohol abuse).

Observe patients carefully for signs and symptoms of pancreatitis (including persistent severe abdominal pain, sometimes radiating to the back and which may or may not be accompanied by vomiting). If pancreatitis is suspected, lixisenatide or the fixed combination of insulin glargine and lixisenatide should be discontinued promptly and appropriate management initiated. If pancreatitis is confirmed, therapy with lixisenatide or the fixed combination of insulin glargine and lixisenatide should not be restarted.

Data are lacking on use of lixisenatide in patients with chronic pancreatitis or a history of unexplained pancreatitis; other antidiabetic therapies should be considered in patients with a history of pancreatitis.

Sharing of Injection Pens

Injection pens containing lixisenatide or the fixed combination of insulin glargine and lixisenatide must never be shared among patients, even if the needle has been changed. Sharing of injection pens poses a risk for transmission of blood-borne pathogens.

Use with Drugs Known to Cause Hypoglycemia

The risk of hypoglycemia is increased when lixisenatide is used in conjunction with an insulin secretagogue (e.g., sulfonylurea) or basal insulin. Therefore, patients receiving lixisenatide in conjunction with a sulfonylurea (or other insulin secretagogue) or basal insulin may require a reduction in the dosage of the sulfonylurea or insulin to reduce the risk of hypoglycemia.

Medication Errors

Administration of the fixed combination of insulin glargine and lixisenatide in a dose exceeding 60 units (of the insulin glargine component) may result in an overdose of the lixisenatide component. The maximum dosage of lixisenatide (20 mcg daily) should not be exceeded, and the fixed combination of insulin glargine and lixisenatide should not be used in conjunction with another GLP-1 receptor agonist.

Renal Effects

Deterioration of renal function (e.g., acute kidney injury and worsened chronic renal failure, sometimes requiring hemodialysis) has been reported in patients receiving GLP-1 receptor agonists. Some of these events occurred in patients without known underlying renal disease. Most of these events occurred in patients experiencing nausea, vomiting, diarrhea, or dehydration.

Clinicians should monitor renal function when initiating or escalating dosage of lixisenatide or the fixed combination of insulin glargine and lixisenatide in patients with renal impairment and in those reporting severe adverse GI effects.

Immunogenicity

As with all therapeutic proteins, there is a potential for immunogenicity with lixisenatide or the fixed combination of insulin glargine and lixisenatide. Antibodies to lixisenatide have developed in patients receiving lixisenatide therapy. In a pooled analysis of 9 placebo-controlled studies, antibodies to lixisenatide were assessed in 70% of lixisenatide-treated patients at week 24. Patients in these studies who had higher antibody concentrations (exceeding 100 nmol/L) had an attenuated glycemic response. Additionally, a higher incidence of allergic reactions and injection-site reactions occurred in antibody-positive patients. After 30 weeks of treatment with the fixed combination of insulin glargine and lixisenatide in clinical trials, the incidence of anti-insulin glargine or anti-lixisenatide antibodies was 21–26.2 or 43%, respectively. Alternative antidiabetic therapy should be considered if there is worsening glycemic control, failure to achieve targeted glycemic control, or clinically important injection-site reactions or allergic reactions with the use of lixisenatide or the fixed combination of insulin glargine and lixisenatide.

Acute Gallbladder Disease

Acute events of gallbladder disease such as cholelithiasis or cholecystitis have been reported in clinical trials with GLP-1 receptor agonists and during post-marketing experience. In the ELIXA study, cholelithiasis occurred in 0.4% of lixisenatide-treated patients compared wtih 0.2% of placebo patients, and acute cholecystitis occurred in 0.3% of lixisenatide-treated patients compared wtih 0.2% of placebo patients. If cholelithiasis is suspected, gallbladder studies and appropriate clinical follow-up are indicated.

Sensitivity Reactions

Serious hypersensitivity reactions (e.g., anaphylaxis, angioedema) have been reported with lixisenatide. In clinical trials, 0.1% of patients experienced an anaphylactic reaction. Patients with a history of anaphylaxis or angioedema with another GLP-1 receptor agonist should be monitored closely for allergic reactions when receiving lixisenatide because it is unknown whether such patients will be predisposed to anaphylaxis with lixisenatide. If a hypersensitivity reaction occurs, lixisenatide or the fixed combination of insulin glargine and lixisenatide should be discontinued and the patient should seek medical attention promptly.

Specific Populations

Pregnancy

Data are lacking on the use of lixisenatide or the fixed combination of insulin glargine and lixisenatide in pregnant women. Lixisenatide has been associated with visceral closure and skeletal defects in rats and rabbits receiving the drug during organogenesis at dosages producing systemic exposures (based on plasma area under the concentration-time curve [AUC]) that were equal to or sixfold greater than, respectively, those achieved in humans at the highest recommended dosage (20 mcg daily). Lixisenatide or the fixed combination of insulin glargine and lixisenatide should be used during pregnancy only if the potential benefit justifies the potential risk to the fetus.

Lactation

Lixisenatide is distributed into milk in rats. It is not known whether lixisenatide is distributed into milk in humans. The benefits of breast-feeding and the importance of lixisenatide to the woman should be considered along with any potential adverse effects on the breast-fed infant from the drug or from the underlying maternal condition.

Pediatric Use

Safety and efficacy of lixisenatide or the fixed combination of insulin glargine and lixisenatide have not been established in patients younger than 18 years of age.

Geriatric Use

No substantial differences in safety and efficacy of lixisenatide or the fixed combination of insulin glargine and lixisenatide have been observed in geriatric patients relative to younger adults, but increased sensitivity cannot be ruled out. Caution should be used when the fixed combination of insulin glargine and lixisenatide is administered to geriatric patients; hypoglycemia may be difficult to recognize in such patients, and the initial dosing, dose increments, and maintenance dosage of the fixed combination of insulin glargine and lixisenatide should be conservative to prevent hypoglycemia.

Hepatic Impairment

Data are lacking on use of lixisenatide in patients with acute or chronic hepatic impairment. Because lixisenatide is presumed to be cleared principally by the kidney, hepatic dysfunction is not expected to affect the pharmacokinetics of the drug, and the manufacturer makes no specific dosage recommendations for patients with hepatic impairment.

The effect of hepatic impairment on the pharmacokinetics of the fixed combination of insulin glargine and lixisenatide have not been evaluated. Frequent glucose monitoring and dosage adjustments may be necessary in patients with hepatic impairment receiving the fixed combination of insulin glargine and lixisenatide.

Renal Impairment

Use of lixisenatide is not recommended in patients with end-stage renal disease (estimated glomerular filtration rate [eGFR] less than 15 mL/minute per 1.73 m²). In patients with mild, moderate, or severe renal impairment, lixisenatide plasma concentrations and systemic exposure were increased by 60, 42, or 83% and 34, 69, or 124%, respectively. The manufacturer recommends no dosage adjustments for patients with mild, moderate, or severe renal impairment receiving lixisenatide; however, the renal function of such patients should be closely monitored when initiating or escalating doses of lixisenatide and patients should be observed for adverse effects.

Frequent glucose monitoring and dosage adjustments may be necessary in patients with renal impairment receiving the fixed combination of insulin glargine and lixisenatide.

Patients with Gastroparesis

Lixisenatide slows gastric emptying and may affect absorption of concomitantly administered oral drugs. Safety and efficacy of lixisenatide or the fixed combination of insulin glargine and lixisenatide have not been established in patients with preexisting gastroparesis, and the manufacturer states that lixisenatide therapy is not recommended in patients with severe gastroparesis.

● Common Adverse Effects

Adverse effects reported in at least 5% of patients receiving lixisenatide include nausea, vomiting, headache, diarrhea, dizziness, and hypoglycemia.

Adverse effects reported in at least 5% of patients receiving insulin glargine in fixed combination with lixisenatide include hypoglycemia, nausea, nasopharyngitis, diarrhea, upper respiratory tract infection, and headache.

DRUG INTERACTIONS

In vitro, lixisenatide is neither an inducer nor an inhibitor of cytochrome P-450 (CYP) isoenzymes; lixisenatide is not metabolized by CYP isoenzymes.

● Effects on GI Absorption of Other Drugs

The effect of lixisenatide-induced slowing of gastric emptying may reduce the rate and extent of absorption of concomitantly administered oral drugs. Lixisenatide should be used with caution in patients receiving oral drugs that have a narrow therapeutic index or require careful clinical monitoring. In patients receiving oral drugs for which efficacy depends on threshold concentrations (e.g., anti-infective agents) or drugs for which a delay in effect would be undesirable (e.g., acetaminophen), those drugs should be taken at least 1 hour before the administration of lixisenatide or the fixed combination of insulin glargine and lixisenatide. If such drugs need to be administered with food, patients should take them with a meal or snack at a time when lixisenatide is not administered.

● Acetaminophen

Lixisenatide appears to reduce the rate but not the extent of acetaminophen absorption when the drugs are administered concurrently. With administration of a single 1-g oral dose of acetaminophen, acetaminophen area under the concentration-time curve (AUC) was not changed whether the dose of acetaminophen was administered before or after subcutaneous lixisenatide (10 mcg). In addition, peak plasma concentration and time to peak plasma concentration of acetaminophen were not affected when acetaminophen was administered 1 hour *before* lixisenatide. However, when acetaminophen was administered 1 or 4 hours *after* lixisenatide (10 mcg), the peak plasma concentration of acetaminophen was decreased by 29 or 31%, respectively, and the median time to acetaminophen peak plasma concentration was delayed by 2 or 1.75 hours, respectively. To facilitate a rapid onset of effect, acetaminophen should be administered at least 1 hour prior to injection of lixisenatide; no adjustment of acetaminophen dosage is necessary with concomitant lixisenatide.

● Antidiabetic Agents

The risk of hypoglycemia is increased when lixisenatide is used in conjunction with a sulfonylurea or basal insulin; patients receiving lixisenatide concomitantly with such agents may require a reduction in the dosage of the sulfonylurea or insulin.

● Anti-infective Agents

The effect of lixisenatide-induced slowing of gastric emptying may reduce the rate and extent of absorption of concomitantly administered oral anti-infective agents. Oral anti-infective agents should be taken at least 1 hour prior to subcutaneous injection of lixisenatide.

● Atorvastatin

Concurrent administration of subcutaneous lixisenatide (20 mcg) and oral atorvastatin (40 mg) once daily in the morning for 6 days did not alter atorvastatin AUC; however, the peak plasma concentration and the time to peak plasma concentration of atorvastatin were decreased by 31% and delayed by 3.25 hours, respectively. When atorvastatin was administered in the evening and lixisenatide was administered in the morning, no change in the time to peak plasma concentration of atorvastatin was observed; however, the AUC and peak plasma concentration of atorvastatin were increased by 27 and 66%, respectively. Atorvastatin should be administered at least 1 hour prior to lixisenatide.

● Digoxin

Subcutaneous injection of lixisenatide (20 mcg) 30 minutes before oral digoxin (0.25 mg) decreased the steady-state peak plasma digoxin concentration by 26% and delayed the time to peak plasma digoxin concentration by approximately 1.5 hours. However, there was no change in the overall steady-state AUC of digoxin. No change in digoxin dosage or timing of administration is necessary. Patients receiving such concomitant therapy should be monitored appropriately.

● Oral Contraceptives

Administration of a single dose of a fixed-combination oral contraceptive (30 mcg of ethinyl estradiol and 150 mcg of levonorgestrel) 1 hour *before* or 11 hours *after* subcutaneous injection of lixisenatide (10 mcg) did not affect the peak plasma concentrations, AUCs, or time to peak plasma concentrations of the oral contraceptive components. Administration of the same oral contraceptive 1 or 4 hours *after* subcutaneous injection of lixisenatide (10 mcg) did not affect AUCs or terminal half-lives of the oral contraceptive components; however, the peak plasma concentration of ethinyl estradiol was decreased by 52 or 39%, respectively, and the peak plasma concentration of levonorgestrel was decreased by 46 or 20%, respectively. Therefore, oral contraceptives should be administered at least 1 hour *before* or 11 hours *after* lixisenatide.

● Ramipril

Concomitant administration of subcutaneous lixisenatide (20 mcg) and oral ramipril (5 mg) for 6 days did not affect the AUC and peak plasma concentration of ramiprilat (the active metabolite of ramipril); however, such concomitant administration increased the ramipril AUC by 21% and decreased its peak plasma concentration by 63%. The time to peak plasma concentration of ramipril and ramiprilat was delayed by approximately 2.5 hours. No change in ramipril dosage or timing of administration is necessary.

● Warfarin

Concomitant administration of warfarin 25 mg during repeated dosing with lixisenatide 20 mcg had no affect on warfarin AUC or on international normalized ratio (INR); however, the peak plasma concentration of warfarin was decreased by 19% and the time to peak plasma concentration was delayed by 7 hours. No change in warfarin dosage or timing of administration is necessary. INR should be monitored frequently in patients receiving warfarin and lixisenatide concomitantly. (See Drug Interactions: Effects on GI Absorption of Other Drugs.)

DESCRIPTION

Lixisenatide, a synthetic analog of endogenous exendin-4 (a naturally occurring peptide isolated from the saliva of *Heloderma suspectum* [Gila monster]), is a short-acting, glucagon-like peptide-1 (GLP-1) receptor agonist. Lixisenatide is a 44-amino acid amidated peptide that is similar in structure to exendin-4 with the exception of the addition of 6 lysine residues at the C-terminal amino acid and the deletion of a proline at position 36. These structural changes increase lixisenatide's binding affinity to the GLP-1 receptor, prevent the degradation of the peptide by dipeptidyl peptidase-4 (DPP-4), and increase its circulating half-life. Lixisenatide has a fourfold higher affinity for the GLP-1 receptor than endogenous human GLP-1.

Activation of GLP-1 receptors stimulates insulin release in the presence of elevated glucose concentrations, suppresses glucose-dependent glucagon release, and slows gastric emptying, resulting in lower fasting and postprandial blood glucose concentrations and, potentially, weight loss in patients with type 2 diabetes mellitus. Long-acting GLP-1 agonists (e.g., albiglutide, dulaglutide, exenatide extended-release, liraglutide) induce marked reductions in fasting plasma glucose concentrations (by stimulating insulin secretion) and modest reductions in postprandial glucose concentrations, while short-acting GLP-1 agonists (e.g., exenatide, lixisenatide) have less of an effect on fasting plasma glucose concentrations and more of an effect on reducing postprandial glucose concentrations (by slowing gastric emptying and inhibiting glucagon secretion). Lixisenatide does not appear to be associated with clinically important prolongation of the corrected QT interval (QT$_c$, Bazett's formula) or increases in heart rate.

Peak plasma lixisenatide concentrations are achieved 1–3.5 hours following subcutaneous administration. Lixisenatide is thought to be eliminated through glomerular filtration and proteolytic degradation. The elimination half-life of lixisenatide is approximately 3 hours. The manufacturer states that the pharmacokinetics of lixisenatide are independent of age, body weight, sex, and race.

ADVICE TO PATIENTS

Importance of patients reading the medication guide and instructions for use prior to initiating therapy and each time drug is dispensed.

Importance of instructing patient and caregivers on preparation and use of the injection pen prior to first use; training should include a practice injection.

Importance of *not* mixing or diluting the fixed combination of insulin glargine and lixisenatide with any other insulin or solution.

Importance of informing patients of possibility of serious hypersensitivity reactions (e.g., anaphylaxis). Patients should be instructed to discontinue lixisenatide or the fixed combination of insulin glargine and lixisenatide and promptly seek medical advice if symptoms of hypersensitivity occur.

Importance of informing patients of the possibility of acute pancreatitis with lixisenatide therapy. Importance of patients informing clinicians about a history of pancreatitis, gallstones, or alcoholism. Importance of informing patients about signs and symptoms of pancreatitis, including persistent severe abdominal pain sometimes radiating to the back that may or may not be accompanied by vomiting; importance of patient discontinuing lixisenatide or the fixed combination of insulin glargine and lixisenatide and promptly notifying clinician if such signs or symptoms occur.

Importance of informing patients that they should never share injection pens containing lixisenatide or the fixed combination of insulin glargine and lixisenatide with another person, even if the needle is changed; sharing of the pen may pose a risk of transmitting or acquiring infection.

Importance of informing patients of the risk of hypoglycemia, particularly if concomitant therapy with an insulin secretagogue (e.g., sulfonylurea) or insulin is used.

Importance of informing patients of the potential risk of dehydration due to adverse GI effects; importance of advising patients to take precautions to avoid fluid depletion. Importance of informing patients of the potential risk for worsening renal function, which in some cases may require dialysis.

Importance of informing patients of the potential risk of cholelithiasis or cholecystitis. Instruct patients to contact their physician if cholelithiasis or cholecystitis is suspected for appropriate clinical follow-up.

Importance of women informing clinicians if they are or plan to become pregnant or plan to breast-feed.

Importance of informing clinicians of existing or contemplated concomitant therapy, including prescription and OTC drugs, as well as any concomitant illnesses.

Importance of informing patients of other important precautionary information. (See Cautions.)

PREPARATIONS

Excipients in commercially available drug preparations may have clinically important effects in some individuals; consult specific product labeling for details.

Lixisenatide

Parenteral

Kit, injection, for subcutaneous use	2 injection pens, 100 mcg/mL	Adlyxin® Pen Maintenance Pack (available as prefilled injection pens), Sanofi-Aventis
Kit, injection, for subcutaneous use	1 injection pen, 50 mcg/mL 1 injection pen, 100 mcg/mL	Adlyxin® Pen Starter Pack (available as prefilled injection pens), Sanofi-Aventis

Lixisenatide Combinations

Parenteral

Injection, for subcutaneous use	33 mcg/mL with Insulin Glargine 100 units/mL	Soliqua® 100/33 (available as prefilled injection pens), Sanofi-Aventis

Selected Revisions October 16, 2023, © Copyright, September 14, 2016, American Society of Health-System Pharmacists, Inc.

Semaglutide

68:20.06 • INCRETIN MIMETICS

On December 21, 2023, FDA issued a warning to consumers to not use counterfeit Ozempic® (semaglutide) injection 1 mg found in the US supply chain. The agency has seized thousands of units of counterfeit product. Additional investigation is ongoing, and FDA is working with the manufacturer to identify, investigate, and remove further suspected counterfeit semaglutide injectable products found in the U.S. For additional information, see https://www.fda.gov/drugs/drug-safety-and-availability/fda-warns-consumers-not-use-counterfeit-ozempic-semaglutide-found-us-drug-supply-chain

FDA has received adverse event reports related to the use of compounded semaglutide. Patients should not use a compounded drug if an approved drug is available. Patients and healthcare professionals should understand that the agency does not review compounded versions of these drugs for safety, effectiveness, or quality. Additionally, FDA has received reports that in some cases, compounders may be using salt forms of semaglutide, including semaglutide sodium and semaglutide acetate. The salt forms are different active ingredients than is used in the approved drugs, which contain the base form of semaglutide.

■ Semaglutide, a synthetic, long-acting glucagon-like peptide-1 (GLP-1) receptor agonist (incretin mimetic), is an antidiabetic agent.

USES

● Type 2 Diabetes Mellitus

Semaglutide is used as an adjunct to diet and exercise to improve glycemic control in adults with type 2 diabetes mellitus. Various preparations of semaglutide are available; Rybelsus® oral tablets and Ozempic® subcutaneous injection are specifically FDA-labeled for use in the management of diabetes mellitus. Semaglutide injection has been used alone or as add-on therapy in conjunction with other antidiabetic agents, including metformin, metformin and a sulfonylurea, metformin and/or a thiazolidinedione, and basal insulin. Semaglutide tablets have been used alone or in combination with metformin, sulfonylureas, sodium-glucose cotransporter 2 (SGLT2) inhibitors, insulins, and thiazolidinediones. Semaglutide injection also is indicated for the reduction of the risk of major adverse cardiovascular events in adults with type 2 diabetes mellitus and established cardiovascular disease.

Glycemic Control

Current guidelines for the treatment of type 2 diabetes mellitus generally recommend metformin as first-line therapy in addition to lifestyle modifications in patients with recent-onset type 2 diabetes mellitus or mild hyperglycemia because of its well-established safety and efficacy (i.e., beneficial effects on glycosylated hemoglobin [hemoglobin A_{1c}; HbA_{1c}], weight, and cardiovascular mortality). In patients with contraindications or intolerance to metformin (e.g., risk of lactic acidosis, GI intolerance) or in selected other patients, some experts suggest that initial therapy with a drug from another class of antidiabetic agents (e.g., a glucagon-like peptide-1 [GLP-1] receptor agonist, sodium-glucose cotransporter 2 [SGLT2] inhibitor, dipeptidyl peptidase-4 [DPP-4] inhibitor, sulfonylurea, thiazolidinedione, basal insulin) may be acceptable based on patient factors. Initiating antidiabetic therapy with 2 agents (e.g., metformin plus another drug) may be appropriate in patients with an initial HbA_{1c} exceeding 7.5% or at least 1.5% above the target level. In metformin-intolerant patients with high initial HbA_{1c} levels, some experts suggest initiation of therapy with 2 agents from other antidiabetic drug classes with complementary mechanisms of action.

Because of the progressive nature of type 2 diabetes mellitus, patients initially receiving an oral antidiabetic agent will eventually require multiple oral and/or injectable noninsulin antidiabetic agents of different therapeutic classes and/or insulin for adequate glycemic control. Patients who have inadequate glycemic control with initial (e.g., metformin) monotherapy should receive treatment with additional antidiabetic agents; data suggest that the addition of each noninsulin agent to initial therapy lowers HbA_{1c} by approximately 0.7–1%. In addition, early initiation of combination therapy may be considered to more rapidly attain glycemic goals and extend the time to treatment failure.

Factors to consider when selecting additional antidiabetic agents for patients with inadequate glycemic control on metformin monotherapy include patient comorbidities (e.g., atherosclerotic cardiovascular disease [ASCVD], established kidney disease, heart failure), hypoglycemia risk, impact on weight, cost, risk of adverse effects, and patient preference. When the greater glucose-lowering effect of an injectable drug is needed in patients with type 2 diabetes mellitus, some experts currently state that an injectable GLP-1 receptor agonist is preferred over insulin in most patients because of beneficial effects on body weight and a lower risk of hypoglycemia, although adverse GI effects may diminish tolerability. While addition of a GLP-1 receptor agonist may successfully control hyperglycemia, many patients will eventually require insulin therapy. Early introduction of insulin therapy should be considered when hyperglycemia is severe (e.g., blood glucose of at least 300 mg/dL or HbA_{1c} exceeding 9–10%), especially in the presence of catabolic manifestations (e.g., weight loss, hypertriglyceridemia, ketosis) or symptoms of hyperglycemia.

Patients with type 2 diabetes mellitus who have established (or are at a high risk for) ASCVD, established kidney disease, or heart failure should receive a GLP-1 receptor agonist or SGLT2 inhibitor with demonstrated cardiovascular disease benefit. Experts state that therapy with a GLP-1 receptor agonist or SGLT2 inhibitor should be considered for patients with the aforementioned comorbidities independently of the patients' HbA_{1c}.

GLP-1 receptor agonists and SGLT2 inhibitors appear to have effects on the kidneys independent of their glycemic effects, and some experts suggest that an agent from one of these classes of drugs be considered in patients with type 2 diabetes mellitus and chronic kidney disease (CKD).

In patients *without* established ASCVD or indicators of high ASCVD risk, heart failure, or CKD, the decision regarding the addition of other antidiabetic agents (e.g., GLP-1 receptor agonist, SGLT2 inhibitor, DPP-4 inhibitor, thiazolidinedione, sulfonylurea, basal insulin) to metformin therapy should be based on avoidance of adverse effects, cost, and individual patient factors.

Safety and efficacy of semaglutide have *not* been established in patients with a history of pancreatitis. The manufacturer states that other antidiabetic therapies should be considered in patients with a history of pancreatitis.

Semaglutide is not a substitute for insulin in insulin-requiring patients. The manufacturer states that semaglutide is not indicated in patients with type 1 diabetes mellitus.

Safety and efficacy of oral or subcutaneous semaglutide for glycemic control as monotherapy or in combination with other antidiabetic agents have been established in several randomized, open-label or double-blind, controlled clinical trials generally of 30 or 56 weeks' duration with subcutaneous semaglutide (e.g., SUSTAIN trials) or 52 weeks' duration (often with outcomes analysis at 26 weeks) with oral semaglutide (e.g., PIONEER trials) in adults with type 2 diabetes mellitus. These trials have demonstrated that semaglutide therapy (target dosage generally 7 or 14 mg orally once daily or 0.5 or 1 mg subcutaneously once weekly) improves glycemic control compared with placebo or comparator antidiabetic agents as evidenced by reductions in HbA_{1c} and also by the proportion of patients achieving HbA_{1c} reductions to less than 7%. Weight loss was also observed in those who received oral or subcutaneous semaglutide therapy, which may be an additional benefit in some patients with type 2 diabetes mellitus. Both oral and subcutaneous semaglutide appear to have a safety profile similar to that reported with other GLP-1 receptor agonists, with GI adverse effects (e.g., nausea) being most commonly reported.

Semaglutide Monotherapy

In a 30-week, randomized, double-blind, placebo-controlled trial (SUSTAIN-1) in adults with type 2 diabetes mellitus inadequately controlled with diet and exercise (mean baseline HbA_{1c} concentration of 8.05%), therapy with semaglutide 0.5 or 1 mg subcutaneously once weekly was associated with a mean HbA_{1c} reduction of 1.4 or 1.6%, respectively, at week 30 compared with a reduction of 0.1% among those who received placebo. HbA_{1c} concentrations less than 7% were achieved in a substantially higher proportion of patients receiving semaglutide (73–74 or 70–72% with 0.5 or 1 mg, respectively) than with placebo (25–28% of patients). At week 30, therapy with semaglutide 0.5 or 1 mg subcutaneously once weekly was associated with a reduction in body weight from baseline of 3.7–3.8 or 4.5–4.7 kg, respectively, compared with a reduction of 0.98–1.2 kg from baseline among those who received placebo. Adverse effects reported with semaglutide principally were GI in nature (e.g., nausea, which generally decreased over time with continued therapy), and were similar to those reported with other GLP-1 receptor agonists.

In a 26-week, randomized, double-blind, placebo-controlled trial (PIONEER 1) in adults with type 2 diabetes mellitus previously managed with only diet and exercise, therapy with oral semaglutide 7 or 14 mg or placebo once daily was associated with mean HbA_{1c} reductions of 1.2, 1.4, or 0.3%, respectively, at week 26 in the intent-to-treat population. HbA_{1c} concentrations of less than 7% were achieved in 69, 77, or 31% of patients receiving semaglutide 7 or 14 mg or placebo, respectively, once daily. At 26 weeks, reductions in body weight with oral semaglutide compared with placebo were dose dependent, averaging 0.9 or 2.3 kg with 7 or 14 mg of semaglutide once daily, respectively; substantially more patients achieved a loss in body weight of at least 5% with semaglutide therapy than with placebo. Safety and tolerability of oral semaglutide were similar to that of other GLP-1 receptor agonists.

Combination Therapy

When given as add-on therapy in adults with type 2 diabetes mellitus inadequately controlled with one or more oral antidiabetic agents (e.g., metformin, a sulfonylurea, a thiazolidinedione, an SGLT2 inhibitor) with or without basal insulin, oral or subcutaneous semaglutide improved glycemic control and reduced body weight compared with baseline therapy. In clinical trials comparing add-on therapy with oral or subcutaneous semaglutide (7 or 14 mg orally once daily, 0.5 or 1 mg subcutaneously once weekly) versus add-on therapy with sitagliptin, empagliflozin, extended-release exenatide, liraglutide, dulaglutide, or insulin glargine, semaglutide generally was superior to each of these comparator drugs in improving glycemic control and reducing body weight. While add-on therapy with subcutaneous semaglutide was associated with a greater reduction in HbA_{1c} and body weight than add-on insulin glargine in one of these trials (SUSTAIN-4), a limitation of this trial was that the dosage of insulin glargine was titrated to goal in only 26% of study patients by the primary end point at week 30, reaching a mean daily insulin dosage of 29 units. Effects of semaglutide on glycemic control and body weight do not appear to be altered in patients with renal or hepatic impairment. Adverse effects (e.g., usually GI effects) attributed to oral or subcutaneous semaglutide in clinical trials of combination therapy generally have been similar in frequency to those reported with other GLP-1 receptor agonist comparator drugs (e.g., dulaglutide, liraglutide).

Reduction in Risk of Major Adverse Cardiovascular Events in Patients with Type 2 Diabetes

Semaglutide is used by subcutaneous injection to reduce the risk of major adverse cardiovascular events in adults with type 2 diabetes mellitus and established cardiovascular disease. In addition to lowering blood glucose, GLP-1 receptor agonists such as semaglutide appear to modify several nonglycemic cardiovascular risk factors such as blood pressure, body weight, and lipid profile. Additionally, GLP-1 receptor agonists may have beneficial endothelial effects. Several GLP-1 receptor agonists, including semaglutide, have demonstrated either noninferiority or superiority to placebo with regard to reducing the risk of cardiovascular events in clinical trials in patients with type 2 diabetes mellitus and ASCVD and/or a high risk of cardiovascular events.

In a double-blind, placebo-controlled trial (SUSTAIN-6) in approximately 3300 adults with inadequately controlled type 2 diabetes mellitus and coexisting ASCVD on conventional antidiabetic therapy (e.g., oral antidiabetic agents, insulin), add-on therapy with semaglutide (0.5 or 1 mg subcutaneously once weekly for 104 weeks) was noninferior to add-on placebo with regard to the primary composite outcome (first occurrence of cardiovascular death, nonfatal myocardial infarction [MI], or nonfatal stroke). In addition, while analysis of results for superiority was not prespecified in the trial, the primary composite outcome occurred in 6.6 or 8.9% of patients receiving add-on semaglutide or add-on placebo, respectively, representing a 26% risk reduction (principally due to a reduction in nonfatal stroke) with semaglutide therapy. Patients in this trial had a high risk of cardiovascular events (i.e., at least 50 years of age with established, stable cardiovascular, cerebrovascular, peripheral artery, or chronic kidney disease or NYHA class II or III heart failure, or at least 60 years of age with other cardiovascular risk factors). Approximately 98.4% of patients were receiving at least one antidiabetic drug (e.g., metformin, a sulfonylurea, insulin) at baseline; most patients were also receiving cardiovascular drugs at baseline (antihypertensive drugs [93.5%], lipid-lowering drugs [76.5%], antithrombotic drugs [76.3%]).

In a double-blind, placebo-controlled trial of oral semaglutide (PIONEER 6) with a similar design and end points as the SUSTAIN-6 trial of subcutaneous semaglutide, oral semaglutide† (target dosage: 14 mg once daily) was noninferior to placebo in terms of major adverse cardiovascular event outcomes (i.e., first occurrence of cardiovascular death, nonfatal MI, or nonfatal stroke). The PIONEER 6 trial included approximately 3200 patients with inadequately controlled type 2 diabetes mellitus and ASCVD at high risk for cardiovascular events. Similarities in the hazard ratios for the primary outcomes in the PIONEER 6 trial (0.79, or a 21% risk reduction) and the SUSTAIN-6 trial (0.74, or a 26% risk reduction) and results of some analyses of pooled data suggest that the cardiovascular benefits of semaglutide may be independent of route of administration.

Beneficial Effects on Renal Function

Some experts suggest that a GLP-1 receptor agonist (e.g., dulaglutide, liraglutide, semaglutide†) or SGLT2 inhibitor (e.g., canagliflozin, dapagliflozin, empagliflozin) with demonstrated ability to reduce the risk of CKD progression†, cardiovascular events, or both† should be considered in patients with type 2 diabetes mellitus and CKD, in addition to metformin therapy or in those in whom metformin cannot be used. GLP-1 receptor agonists and SGLT2 inhibitors appear to have direct or indirect effects on the kidneys independent of their glycemic effects, and these classes of drugs have shown salutary effects on progression of CKD in clinical trials. In a number of cardiovascular outcomes trials involving the use of GLP-1 receptor agonists (e.g., liraglutide, semaglutide) in patients with type 2 diabetes mellitus at high risk for, or with existing, cardiovascular disease, beneficial effects on renal function have been observed as a secondary outcome. In the SUSTAIN-6 trial, semaglutide reduced the risk of new or worsening nephropathy† (a composite of persistent macroalbuminuria, doubling of serum creatinine, or end-stage renal disease) by 36%. Some GLP-1 receptor agonists may be used in patients with lower estimated glomerular filtration rate (eGFR) and may provide greater benefits for reduction of major adverse cardiovascular events than for CKD progression or heart failure.

● Overweight or Obesity

Weight Reduction

Semaglutide is used in combination with a reduced-calorie diet and increased physical activity to reduce excess body weight and maintain weight reduction long term in adults and pediatric patients 12 years of age and older with obesity or, in adults who are overweight *and* have at least one weight-related comorbid condition (e.g., hypertension, type 2 diabetes mellitus, dyslipidemia).

Various preparations of semaglutide are available; Wegovy® subcutaneous injection is specifically FDA-labeled for this use. The manufacturer states that the drug should not be used in combination with any other semaglutide-containing products or any other GLP-1 receptor agonist.

Efficacy and safety of semaglutide injection for weight reduction management in adults were evaluated in 5 randomized, double-blind, placebo-controlled studies of 68 weeks' duration (STEP studies). In 3 of the studies, patients were advised to begin a reduced-calorie diet (approximately 500 kcal/day deficit) and received exercise counseling initially and throughout the studies. When used in conjunction with a reduced-calorie diet and increased exercise, these studies showed that semaglutide substantially decreased body weight compared with placebo in patients who were obese or overweight (with or without diabetes mellitus). There are currently no cardiovascular outcomes data with semaglutide in patients without type 2 diabetes mellitus.

The STEP 1 study included 1961 adults without diabetes mellitus who were obese (BMI ≥30 kg/m²) or overweight (BMI 27–29.9 kg/m²) and had at least one weight-related comorbid condition such as hypertension or dyslipidemia. The mean baseline body weight was 105.3 kg and mean BMI was 37.9 kg/m². The mean age of patients was 46 years; 74% were female, 75% were White, 13% were Asian, 5.7% were Black or African American, and 12% were Hispanic or Latino. Semaglutide dosage was increased to a maintenance dosage of 2.4 mg subcutaneously once weekly over 16 weeks and then maintained on that dosage for another 52 weeks. The primary efficacy measures were the mean percent change in body weight from baseline and the proportion of patients who lost at least 5% of their baseline body weight. At 68 weeks, semaglutide reduced body weight by a greater percentage from baseline than placebo (mean reduction of 14.9% versus 2.4%, respectively). A substantially greater proportion of patients receiving semaglutide lost 5% or more of their baseline body weight compared with patients receiving placebo (83.5 versus 31.1%). Additionally, more patients receiving semaglutide lost 10% or more (66.1 versus 12%) or 15% or more (47.9 versus 4.8%) of their baseline body weight compared with those receiving placebo.

The STEP 2 study included 807 adults with type 2 diabetes mellitus and BMI ≥30 kg/m². Patients had baseline HbA$_{1c}$ 7–10% and were treated with 1-3 oral antidiabetic agents or with diet and exercise alone. The mean baseline body weight was 99.8 kg and mean BMI was 35.7 kg/m²; mean age was 55 years, 51% were female, 62% were White, 26% were Asian, 8% were Black or African American, and 13% were Hispanic or Latino. Semaglutide dosage was increased to a maintenance dosage of 2.4 mg subcutaneously once weekly over 16 weeks and then maintained on that dosage for another 52 weeks. The primary efficacy measures were mean percent change in body weight from baseline and the proportion of patients who lost at least 5% of their baseline body weight. At 68 weeks, semaglutide reduced body weight by a greater percentage from baseline than placebo (mean reduction of 9.6% versus 3.4%,). More patients receiving semaglutide lost 5% or more (67.4 versus 30.2%), 10% or more (44.5 versus 10.2%), or 15% or more (25.1 versus 4.3%) of their baseline body weight compared with patients receiving placebo.

The STEP 3 study included 611 adults without diabetes mellitus who were obese or overweight and had at least one weight-related comorbid condition such as hypertension or dyslipidemia. The mean baseline body weight was 105.8 kg and mean BMI was 38 kg/m²; mean age was 46 years, 81% were female, 76% were white, 19% were Black or African American, 1.8% were Asian, and 19.8% were Hispanic or Latino. Semaglutide dosage was increased to a maintenance dosage of 2.4 mg subcutaneously once weekly over 16 weeks and then maintained on that dosage for another 52 weeks. The primary efficacy measures were the mean percent change in body weight from baseline and the proportion of patients who lost at least 5% of their baseline body weight. At 68 weeks, semaglutide reduced body weight by a greater percentage from baseline than placebo (a mean reduction of 16% versus 5.7%). More patients receiving semaglutide lost 5% or more (84.8 versus 47.8%), 10% or more (73 versus 27.1%), or 15% or more (53.4 versus 13.2%) of their baseline body weight compared with patients receiving placebo.

The STEP 4 study included 902 adults without diabetes mellitus who were obese or overweight and had at least one weight-related comorbid condition such as hypertension or dyslipidemia. The mean baseline body weight was 106.8 kg and mean BMI was 38.3 kg/m²; mean age was 46 years, 79% were female, 83.7% were White, 13% were Black or African American, 2.4% were Asian, and 7.8% were Hispanic or Latino. In this study, semaglutide dosage was increased during a 20-week run-in period; patients who reached a dosage of 2.4 mg once weekly were randomized to continue treatment with the drug or placebo for 48 weeks. The primary efficacy measure was the mean percent change in body weight from randomization (week 20) to week 68. During this time period, treatment with semaglutide resulted in a statistically significant reduction in body weight compared with placebo (mean reduction of 7.9% with semaglutide compared with a mean increase of 6.9% with placebo). Because patients who discontinued semaglutide during titration and those who did not reach the 2.4 mg weekly dose were not eligible for the randomized treatment period, the manufacturer states that these results may not be reflective of the general population of patients who are first starting semaglutide.

The STEP 6 study included 401 East-Asian patients (Japan and South Korea) with BMI ≥35 kg/m² who had at least one weight-related comorbid condition or with BMI 27–34.9 kg/m²who had at least 2 weight-related comborbid conditions. At baseline, mean body weight was 87.5 kg and mean BMI was 31.9 kg/m²; 24.7% of patients had type 2 diabetes mellitus. Patients were randomized to receive semaglutide 2.4 mg, semaglutide 1.7 mg, or placebo once weekly. After 68 weeks, treatment with semaglutide 1.7 mg or 2.4 mg resulted in statistically significant reductions in body weight compared with placebo (mean reduction of 7.5% with the 1.7 mg dose and 11.1% with the 2.4 mg dose).

Patients who received semaglutide in these STEP studies also had greater improvement in cardiometabolic risk factors and physical functioning than those who received placebo. However, GI adverse effects were more frequent with semaglutide than placebo in all of the studies.

The STEP 8 trial was a 68-week open-label multicenter trial that compared once-weekly subcutaneous semaglutide 2.4 mg with once-daily subcutaneous liraglutide 3 mg in adults with BMI ≥30 or BMI ≥ 27 with 1 or more weight-related comorbidities (except diabetes). All patients received counseling to adhere to diet and physical activity recommendations. The study showed that weight loss with semaglutide was significantly greater than with liraglutide. The mean weight

change from baseline at 68 weeks was –15.8% with semaglutide compared with –6.4% with liraglutide (difference of –9.4 percentage points).

Safety and efficacy of semaglutide injection in pediatric patients were evaluated in a 68-week, double-blind, randomized, placebo-controlled multicenter study. The study included 201 pubertal pediatric patients (mean age of 15 years) with BMI corresponding to ≥95th percentile standardized for age and sex. After 68 weeks of treatment, patients who received semaglutide had a statistically significant reduction in percent BMI from baseline compared with placebo. Semaglutide also had beneficial effects on anthropometry and cardiometabolic parameters such as waist circumference, blood pressure, and lipid values.

Reduction in Risk of Major Adverse Cardiovascular Events in Overweight or Obese Patients

Semaglutide is used in combination with a reduced-calorie diet and increased physical activity to reduce the risk of major adverse cardiovascular events (MACE; cardiovascular death, non-fatal myocardial infarction [MI], or non-fatal stroke) in adults with established cardiovascular disease and either obesity or overweight.

Various preparations of semaglutide are available; Wegovy® subcutaneous injection is specifically FDA-labeled for this use. The manufacturer states that the drug should not be used in combination with any other semaglutide-containing products or any other GLP-1 receptor agonist.

Efficacy and safety of semaglutide for this indication are based on a multicenter, double-blind, randomized, placebo-controlled, event-driven trial in patients 45 years of age or older with an initial BMI of 27 kg/m² or greater and established cardiovascular disease (prior MI, prior stroke, or peripheral arterial disease), but no history of diabetes. The mean age of patients was 62 years; 72% were male, 84% were White, 4% were Black or African American, 8% were Asian, and 10% were Hispanic or Latino. At baseline, the mean body weight was 97 kg and mean BMI was 33 kg/m². A total of 17,604 patients were randomized to semaglutide (once weekly injections at a dose of 2.4 mg) or placebo; patients continued to receive the current standard of care for cardiovascular risk reduction including diet and physical activity. Results showed a significant reduction in the risk for first occurrence of MACE in patients receiving semaglutide compared with those receiving placebo (20% lower risk). At a mean follow-up of 39.8 months, the primary composite endpoint of cardiovascular death, nonfatal MI, or nonfatal stroke occurred in 6.5% of semaglutide-treated patients compared with 8% of placebo-recipients.

Clinical Perspective

Clinical practice guidelines recommend treatment for obesity in patients with excess body weight and associated health risks. A comprehensive lifestyle intervention is an essential component of therapy and should be provided to all patients; pharmacologic therapy may be considered as an adjunct to behavioral modification in patients who fail to achieve or sustain clinically meaningful weight loss (generally defined as a loss of more than 4–5% of total body weight). Response to drug therapy should be evaluated after 3–4 months of treatment; if clinically meaningful weight loss is not achieved, it is generally recommended that a new treatment plan be considered because the patient is likely not responding to the drug.

DOSAGE AND ADMINISTRATION

● *General*

Pretreatment Screening

- In patients with type 2 diabetes mellitus receiving semaglutide for chronic weight management, monitor blood glucose prior to initiating therapy.

Patient Monitoring

- Periodically monitor blood glucose and glycosylated hemoglobin (hemoglobin HbA$_{1c}$) to determine therapeutic response in patients with type 2 diabetes mellitus.

- In patients with type 2 diabetes mellitus receiving semaglutide for chronic weight management, monitor blood glucose during therapy.

- Monitor patients with a history of diabetic retinopathy for progression of diabetic retinopathy while receiving semaglutide.

- Monitor renal function when initiating semaglutide or escalating dosage in patients reporting severe adverse GI effects. Monitor renal function in patients with renal impairment reporting any adverse effect that could lead to volume depletion.
- Monitor heart rate regularly.
- Monitor for the emergence or worsening of depression, suicidal thoughts or behavior (suicidality), and/or any unusual changes in mood or behavior.

● *Administration*

Semaglutide is administered orally or by subcutaneous injection.

Oral Administration (Rybelsus®)

Patients should be instructed to take semaglutide tablets at least 30 minutes before the first food, beverage, or other oral drugs of the day, with no more than 120 mL of plain water. Taking semaglutide with, or less than 30 minutes before, food, beverages (other than plain water), or other oral drugs will decrease absorption of the drug and lessen the effect of the drug. Waiting more than 30 minutes to eat after taking the dose may increase semaglutide absorption. Semaglutide tablets should be swallowed whole; they should not be cut, crushed, or chewed.

If a dose of oral semaglutide is missed, the missed dose should be omitted and the next dose taken the following day.

Oral semaglutide tablets should be stored at 20–25°C in the original container, but may be exposed to temperatures ranging from 15–30°C; tablets should be protected from moisture.

Subcutaneous Administration

Ozempic® Preparation

Administer semaglutide injection once weekly into the abdomen, thigh, or upper arm using a prefilled, single patient-use, disposable injection pen; the injection should be administered in a different site each week when injecting in the same body region. If subcutaneous semaglutide is being administered at the same time as insulin, semaglutide and insulin should be administered as separate injections; the 2 drugs should not be mixed. Semaglutide and insulin may be administered subcutaneously in the same body region, but the injections should not be adjacent to each other.

Administer subcutaneous injections of semaglutide once weekly, on the same day each week, at any time of day without regard to meals. The day of weekly administration can be changed if necessary as long as the time between 2 doses is at least 2 days (more than 48 hours) apart. If a dose of subcutaneous semaglutide is missed, the dose should be administered as soon as possible within 5 days after the missed dose. If more than 5 days have passed, the missed dose should be skipped and the next dose should be administered on the regularly scheduled day. In each case, patients may then resume their regular once-weekly dosing schedule.

Inspect the solution visually prior to use; the injection should be used only if the solution is clear, colorless, and contains no particles.

Unopened injection pens containing semaglutide (Ozempic®) should be stored refrigerated at 2–8°C until the expiration date. When stored in a refrigerator, do not place semaglutide injection pens directly next to the cooling element. After first use, semaglutide injection pens may be stored at room temperature (15–30°C) or refrigerated (2–8°C) for up to 56 days. Injection pens containing semaglutide should not be subjected to freezing; if freezing has occurred, the pen should not be used.

Wegovy® Preparation

Administer semaglutide injections into the abdomen, thigh, or upper arm using a prefilled, single-use, disposable injection pen. If a dose is missed and the next scheduled dose is more than 2 days (48 hours) away, administer the missed dose as soon as possible; if the next scheduled dose is less than 2 days (48 hours) away, do not administer the missed dose. Resume dosing on the regularly scheduled day of the week. If 2 or more consecutive doses are missed, resume dosing as scheduled or, if needed, reinitiate therapy and follow the dose escalation schedule.

Administer injections once weekly, on the same day each week, at any time of day without regard to meals.

Inspect the solution visually prior to use; the injection should be used only if the solution is clear, colorless, and contains no particles.

Injection pens containing semaglutide (Wegovy®) should be stored refrigerated at 2–8°C; do not freeze and protect from light. If needed, the pen can be stored at 8–30°C for up to 28 days prior to cap removal. Store in the original carton until time of administration. Discard the single-use prefilled pen after use.

● *Oral Dosage*

Type 2 Diabetes Mellitus

Glycemic Control

The recommended initial oral dosage of semaglutide is 3 mg once daily for 30 days. The 3-mg dosage is for initiation of treatment *only* to reduce GI intolerance and is *not* effective for glycemic control. After 30 days, the dosage should be increased to 7 mg once daily. If the patient requires additional glycemic control after receiving 7 mg of semaglutide once daily for at least 30 days, the dosage may be increased to 14 mg once daily. The manufacturer states that taking two 7-mg tablets to achieve a 14-mg dose is not recommended.

Patients receiving semaglutide in conjunction with an insulin secretagogue (e.g., sulfonylurea) or insulin may require a reduction in the dosage of the insulin secretagogue or insulin to reduce the risk of hypoglycemia.

Patients receiving oral semaglutide 14 mg *once daily* may be switched to subcutaneous semaglutide 0.5 mg *once weekly*; the subcutaneous dosage should be started the day after the last dose of oral semaglutide is taken.

● *Subcutaneous Dosage*

Type 2 Diabetes Mellitus

Glycemic Control and Reduction in Risk of Major Adverse Cardiovascular Events

The recommended *initial* subcutaneous dosage of semaglutide for the management of type 2 diabetes mellitus and reduction in the risk of major adverse cardiovascular events in adults is 0.25 mg once weekly for 4 weeks. The 0.25 mg dose is intended for treatment initiation only; it is not effective for glycemic control and is intended only as a starting dosage to reduce GI intolerance. After 4 weeks, the dosage should be increased to 0.5 mg subcutaneously once weekly. Based on clinical response, the dosage of semaglutide may be further increased to 1 mg subcutaneously once weekly after the patient has received the 0.5 mg dose for at least 4 weeks. If additional glycemic control is needed after at least 4 weeks on the 1 mg dosage, the dosage may be increased to a maximum recommended dosage of 2 mg once weekly.

Patients receiving semaglutide in conjunction with an insulin secretagogue (e.g., sulfonylurea) or insulin may require a reduction in the dosage of the insulin secretagogue or insulin to reduce the risk of hypoglycemia.

Patients receiving 0.5 mg of semaglutide subcutaneously *once weekly* may be switched to 7 or 14 mg of oral semaglutide *once daily*. Patients may begin taking oral semaglutide up to 7 days after their last dose of subcutaneous semaglutide. The 1-mg subcutaneous dose of semaglutide has no equivalent oral dose.

Overweight or Obesity

Weight Reduction

The recommended *initial* dosage of semaglutide for weight reduction in adults and pediatric patients ≥12 years of age is 0.25 mg once weekly by subcutaneous injection; dosage should be escalated according to the schedule in Table 1 to minimize adverse GI effects. If the patient does not tolerate dose escalation, consider delaying the escalation for 4 weeks.

TABLE 1. Semaglutide (Wegovy®) Dosage Escalation Schedule

Weeks	Weekly Dosage
1–4	0.25 mg
5–8	0.5 mg
9–12	1 mg
13–16	1.7 mg
Week 17 and onward	2.4 mg

The recommended *maintenance* dosage of semaglutide for adults with overweight or obesity is 2.4 mg once weekly (preferred) or 1.7 mg once weekly. Consider treatment response and tolerability when selecting the maintenance dosage.

The recommended maintenance dosage in pediatric patients ≥12 years of age with obesity is 2.4 mg once weekly. If the patient does not tolerate the 2.4 mg once weekly dosage, the dosage may be reduced to 1.7 mg once weekly; discontinue therapy if the patient is unable to tolerate the once-weekly 1.7 mg dose.

Reduction in Risk of Major Adverse Cardiovascular Events

The recommended *initial* dosage of semaglutide for reduction in the risk of major adverse cardiovascular events (MACE) in adults with established cardiovascular disease and either obesity or overweight is 0.25 mg once weekly by subcutaneous injection; dosage should be escalated according to the schedule in Table 1 to minimize adverse GI effects. If the patient does not tolerate dose escalation, consider delaying the escalation for 4 weeks.

The recommended *maintenance* dosage of semaglutide for reduction in the risk of MACE in adults with established cardiovascular disease and either obesity or overweight is 2.4 mg once weekly (preferred) or 1.7 mg once weekly. Consider treatment response and tolerability when selecting the maintenance dosage.

● Special Populations

No dosage adjustment is necessary for patients with renal or hepatic impairment, including end-stage renal disease.

CAUTIONS

● Contraindications

- Patients with personal or family history of medullary thyroid carcinoma (MTC) or in patients with multiple endocrine neoplasia syndrome type 2 (MEN 2).
- Patients with prior serious hypersensitivity reaction to semaglutide or any ingredient in the formulation.

● Warnings/Precautions
Warnings
Risk of Thyroid C-Cell Tumors

Glucagon-like peptide-1 (GLP-1) receptor agonists such as semaglutide cause dose- and treatment duration-dependent thyroid C-cell tumors in rats and mice. Cases of MTC have been reported in patients receiving liraglutide, another GLP-1 receptor agonist, during postmarketing experience; data from these reports are insufficient to establish or exclude a causal relationship between MTC and liraglutide use in humans. It is unknown whether semaglutide causes thyroid C-cell tumors, including MTC, in humans. For these reasons, semaglutide is contraindicated in patients with a history of MTC and in patients with MEN 2. In addition, the manufacturer of oral semaglutide (Rybelsus®) states that the drug is not recommended as *first-line* treatment for diabetes mellitus inadequately controlled by diet and exercise.

In a 2-year carcinogenicity study in rats, a substantial increase in thyroid C-cell adenomas were observed at dosages resulting in systemic exposures lower than the maximum recommended human dosage and up to 6 times the maximum recommended human dosage. The human relevance of thyroid C-cell tumors in rats is unknown.

Very elevated serum calcitonin values may be indicative of MTC; patients with MTC usually have serum calcitonin values exceeding 50 ng/mL. Although routine monitoring of serum calcitonin is of uncertain value in patients treated with semaglutide, patients should be further evaluated if serum calcitonin is found to be elevated. Patients with thyroid nodules noted on physical examination or neck imaging also should be further evaluated. The role of monitoring serum calcitonin concentrations or thyroid ultrasounds for the purpose of early detection of MTC in patients receiving semaglutide is unknown.

Sensitivity Reactions

Serious hypersensitivity reactions (e.g., anaphylaxis, angioedema) have been reported in patients receiving semaglutide. If a hypersensitivity reaction occurs,

semaglutide should be discontinued and the patient should be treated according to the standard of care and monitored until manifestations resolve.

Anaphylaxis and angioedema have been reported with other GLP-1 receptor agonists. Semaglutide should be used with caution in patients with a history of angioedema or anaphylaxis with another GLP-1 receptor agonist; it is unknown whether such patients with be predisposed to anaphylaxis with semaglutide.

Other Warnings and Precautions
Risks During General Anesthesia and Deep Sedation

GLP-1 agonists are associated with adverse GI effects such as nausea, vomiting, and delayed gastric emptying; such effects are likely a result of rapid tachyphlaxis at the level of vagal nerve activation. Delayed gastric emptying from GLP-1 agonists can increase the risk of regurgitation and pulmonary aspiration of gastric contents during general anesthesia and deep sedation. Given these concerns, the American Society of Anesthesiologists (ASA) Task Force on Preoperative Fasting has issued a consensus-based guidance for the management of GLP-1 receptor agonists prior to elective surgery. The task force suggests that for patients on daily GLP-1 agonist dosing (irrespective of indication, dose, or type of surgery), consider holding the drug on the day of the elective procedure/surgery. For patients on weekly dosing (irrespective of indication, dose, or type of surgery), consider holding the GLP-1 agonist a week prior to the elective procedure/surgery. If GLP-1 agonists prescribed for diabetes management are held for longer than the dosing schedule, consider consulting an endocrinologist for bridging the antidiabetic therapy to avoid hyperglycemia. These recommendations are based on limited evidence only (case reports). For patients requiring urgent or emergent procedures, the task force states to proceed and treat the patient as 'full stomach' and manage accordingly.

Pancreatitis

Acute pancreatitis, including fatal and nonfatal hemorrhagic or necrotizing pancreatitis, has been reported in patients receiving GLP-1 receptor agonists including semaglutide. Cases of acute pancreatitis were reported in clinical studies; in addition, unpublished findings suggested an increased risk of pancreatitis and precancerous pancreatic cell changes (pancreatic duct metaplasia) in patients with type 2 diabetes mellitus receiving incretin mimetics (exenatide, liraglutide, sitagliptin, saxagliptin, alogliptin, or linagliptin). In one glycemic control trial, 7 cases of confirmed acute pancreatitis occurred among patients treated with subcutaneous semaglutide compared with 1 case in patients treated with a comparator drug (0.3 versus 0.2 cases per 100 patient years, respectively); 1 case of chronic pancreatitis was confirmed in another patient receiving semaglutide. In another clinical trial in patients with diabetes mellitus, 8 cases of confirmed pancreatitis occurred among patients treated with subcutaneous semaglutide compared with 10 cases in patients receiving placebo; all patients in this trial were receiving standard-of-care therapy in addition to semaglutide or placebo. In glycemic control clinical trials with oral semaglutide, pancreatitis was reported in 6 patients receiving semaglutide (0.1 events per 100 patient-years) versus 1 patient treated with a comparator drug (less than 0.1 events per 100 patient-years). Recent trials in which the risk of pancreatitis and pancreatic cancer has been assessed, as well as the results of meta-analyses of GLP-1 receptor agonist trials, have not confirmed safety concerns regarding these events with incretin mimetic therapy.

Carefully observe patients for manifestations of acute pancreatitis after initiation of the drug. Patients should contact their clinician promptly if they experience symptoms of pancreatitis, including persistent severe abdominal pain that sometimes radiates to the back and that may or may not be accompanied by vomiting. If pancreatitis is suspected, discontinue semaglutide promptly and initiate appropriate management. Do not restart therapy if pancreatitis is confirmed.

Efficacy and safety of semaglutide have not been established in patients with a history of pancreatitis. It is not known whether patients with a history of pancreatitis are at higher risk of developing this condition while receiving the drug. If used as an antidiabetic agent, the manufacturers state that alternative antidiabetic therapy should be considered in patients with a history of pancreatitis.

Diabetic Retinopathy Complications

In a 2-year clinical trial involving patients with type 2 diabetes mellitus and a high cardiovascular risk (SUSTAIN-6), a higher incidence of diabetic retinopathy complications was observed among patients who received subcutaneous semaglutide (Ozempic®) compared with those who received placebo (3 versus 1.8%, respectively). In a similar cardiovascular outcomes trial (PIONEER 6) in patients with type 2 diabetes mellitus receiving oral semaglutide, the rate of adverse events related to diabetic retinopathy was 7.1% of semaglutide-treated patients and 6.3% in those receiving placebo. In a pooled analysis of glycemic control trials with oral semaglutide, diabetic retinopathy-related adverse reactions were reported in 4.2% of patients receiving oral semaglutide and in 3.8% of those receiving a comparator drug. In a trial in patients with type 2 diabetes mellitus and BMI ≥27 kg/m², diabetic retinopathy occurred in 4% of patients receiving subcutaneous semaglutide (Wegovy®) compared with 2.7% of those receiving placebo. Patients with a history of diabetic retinopathy at baseline had a greater absolute risk increase for diabetic retinopathy complications compared with those without a known history of diabetic retinopathy in these studies.

Rapid improvement in glucose control has been associated with a temporary worsening of diabetic retinopathy. Data are lacking on the effect of long-term glycemic control with semaglutide on diabetic retinopathy. Monitor patients with a history of diabetic retinopathy for progression of diabetic retinopathy while receiving semaglutide.

Sharing of Injection Pens

Semaglutide injection pens must never be shared among patients, even if the needle has been changed. Sharing of injection pens poses a risk for transmission of blood-borne pathogens.

Hypoglycemia

Patients with diabetes mellitus receiving semaglutide in combination with an insulin secretagogue (e.g., sulfonylurea) or insulin have an increased risk of hypoglycemia, including severe hypoglycemia. Patients receiving such concomitant therapy should be cautioned about the risks and educated about the signs and symptoms of hypoglycemia. A lower dosage of the concomitant insulin secretagogue or insulin may be required to reduce the risk of hypoglycemia.

Renal Effects

During postmarketing experience, acute renal failure and worsening of chronic renal failure (which sometimes required hemodialysis) have been reported with GLP-1 receptor agonists. Patients with baseline renal impairment may be at greater risk; however, some patients did not have known underlying renal disease. Other factors (nausea, vomiting, diarrhea, or dehydration) were present in most patients. Because such adverse GI effects may worsen renal function, use caution and monitor renal function when initiating semaglutide or escalating dosage in patients reporting severe adverse GI effects. Monitor renal function in patients with renal impairment reporting any adverse effect that could lead to volume depletion.

In a pharmacokinetic study in patients with varying degrees of renal impairment, including end-stage renal disease (ESRD), adverse effects observed with oral semaglutide were consistent with those reported with other GLP-1 receptor agonists and no safety concerns were identified.

Elevated Heart Rate

Semaglutide has been associated with increases in heart rate in patients receiving the drug for diabetes mellitus or for weight management. Monitor heart rate regularly in patients receiving semaglutide. Advise patients to inform their clinician if palpitations or feelings of a racing heartbeat occur while at rest during semaglutide therapy; if a sustained increase in resting heart rate is experienced, discontinue therapy.

Suicidality

Suicidal behavior and ideation have been reported in clinical trials of other weight management agents. Monitor patients receiving semaglutide for the emergence or worsening of depression, suicidal thoughts or behavior (suicidality), and/or any unusual changes in mood or behavior. If a patient experiences suicidal thoughts or behaviors while receiving semaglutide, discontinue the drug. Avoid semaglutide in patients with a history of suicidal attempts or active suicidal ideation.

Acute Gallbladder Disease

Acute events of gallbladder disease such as cholelithiasis or cholecystitis have been reported in clinical trials with GLP-1 receptor agonists and during postmarketing experience. In placebo-controlled trials, cholelithiasis was reported in

1% of patients treated with semaglutide 7 mg (administered as the oral tablets for the treatment of type 2 diabetes mellitus). Cholelithiasis was not reported in semaglutide 14 mg or placebo-treated patients. In patients receiving semaglutide injection for weight loss management, the incidence of cholelithiasis and cholecystitis was higher in pediatric patients receiving the drug than in adults. If cholelithiasis issuspected, gallbladder studies and appropriate clinical follow-up are indicated.

Immunogenicity

As with all therapeutic proteins, there is a potential for immunogenicity with semaglutide. Antibodies to semaglutide have developed in patients receiving semaglutide therapy. During clinical trials with subcutaneous semaglutide for the treatment of type 2 diabetes mellitus, 32 patients (1%) developed anti-drug antibodies; of these 32 patients, 19 developed antibodies cross-reacting with native GLP-1. Among placebo- and active-control glycemic control trials in which antibodies to oral semaglutide were measured, 14 patients (0.5%) treated with oral semaglutide developed anti-drug antibodies to semaglutide. Of the 14 semaglutide-treated patients who developed such anti-drug antibodies, 7 patients (0.2% of the overall population) developed antibodies cross-reacting with native GLP-1. The presence of these antibodies has the potential to increase the risk of local skin reactions, hypersensitivity, or anaphylactic reactions and may also neutralize the therapeutic effects of GLP-1 receptor agonists; however, their clinical importance appears to be low in most patients. The in vitro neutralizing activity of the antibodies is unknown. In clinical studies of subcutaneous semaglutide for chronic weight management, 3% of patients who received the drug developed anti-drug antibodies, some of which cross-reacted with native GLP-1. No clinically significant effect of the antibodies on pharmacokinetics of semaglutide was observed.

Specific Populations

Pregnancy

Data are lacking on the use of semaglutide in pregnant women. However, reproduction studies in animals have shown teratogenic effects. Poorly controlled diabetes mellitus during pregnancy increases maternal risk for diabetic ketoacidosis, pre-eclampsia, spontaneous abortion, preterm delivery, and delivery complications. In addition, poorly controlled diabetes mellitus during pregnancy increases the risk of major fetal birth defects, stillbirth, and macrosomia-related morbidity.

Embryofetal mortality, structural abnormalities (e.g., visceral and skeletal abnormalities), and alterations to growth were observed in the offspring of rats who were administered semaglutide during organogenesis at dosages resulting in systemic exposures lower than the maximum recommended human dosage. In reproduction studies in rabbits and monkeys, early pregnancy loss and structural abnormalities (e.g., visceral and skeletal abnormalities) were observed at dosages below the maximum recommended human dosage and at dosages at least 5 times greater than the maximum recommended human dosage.

Salcaprozate sodium (SNAC), an absorption enhancer contained in semaglutide oral tablets, crosses the placenta and reaches fetal tissues in rats. In a prenatal and postnatal development study in pregnant Sprague Dawley rats, SNAC was administered orally at 1000 mg/kg per day (exposure levels were not measured) on gestation day 7 through lactation day 20. An increase in the length of gestation and number of stillbirths and a decrease in pup viability were observed.

The manufacturers of the semaglutide preparations used for diabetic management state the drug should be used during pregnancy only if the potential benefit justifies the potential risk to the fetus. Semaglutide should be discontinued in women for at least 2 months before a planned pregnancy due to the drug's long half-life. The manufacturer of the semaglutide preparation used for weight control management states that weight loss offers no benefit to a pregnant patient and may cause fetal harm; if a patient becomes pregnant while receiving the drug, treatment should be discontinued.

A pregnancy exposure registry has been established to monitor pregnancy outcomes in women exposed to Wegovy®; encourage pregnant women exposed to the drug to contact 1-800-727-6500.

Females and Males of Reproductive Potential

Discontinue semaglutide at least 2 months before a pregnancy is planned to account for the long half-life of the drug.

Lactation

Semaglutide is distributed into milk in rats at concentrations 3–12 fold lower than in maternal plasma. It is not known whether semaglutide is distributed into milk in humans or what the effects of the drug are on the breast-fed infant or on milk production. The benefits of breast-feeding and the importance of semaglutide to the woman should be considered along with any potential adverse effects on the breast-fed infant from the drug or from the underlying maternal condition.

SNAC, an absorption enhancer contained in semaglutide oral tablets, and/or its metabolites are concentrated in the milk of lactating rats. SNAC and/or its metabolites were detected in milk of lactating rats following a single maternal administration on lactation day 10. Mean levels of SNAC and/or its metabolites in milk were approximately 2–12 fold higher than in maternal plasma. There are no data on the presence of SNAC in human milk; however, substances present in animal milk are likely to be present in human milk. Since the activity of UGT2B7, an enzyme involved in SNAC clearance, is lower in infants than in adults, higher SNAC plasma concentrations may occur in neonates and infants. Because of the unknown potential for serious adverse reactions in the breast-fed infant due to the possible accumulation of SNAC from breast-feeding and because there are alternative formulations of semaglutide (e.g., injection) that can be used during lactation, patients should be advised that breast-feeding is not recommended during treatment with oral semaglutide.

Pediatric Use

Safety and efficacy of semaglutide for type 2 diabetes mellitus (Ozempic®, Rybelsus®) have not been established in children or adolescents <18 years of age.

The safety and efficacy of semaglutide (Wegovy®) as an adjunct to a reduced calorie diet and increased physical activity for chronic weight management have been established in pediatric patients ≥12 years of age with a BMI corresponding to ≥95th percentile standardized for age and sex. Use of semaglutide for this indication is supported by a 68-week, double-blind, placebo-controlled clinical trial in pediatric patients and from studies in adult patients with obesity. There are insufficient data in pediatric patients with type 2 diabetes treated with Wegovy® for obesity to determine if there is an increased risk of hypoglycemia with the drug similar to that reported in adults. Inform patients of the risk of hypoglycemia and educate them on the signs and symptoms of hypoglycemia. When initiating Wegovy® in pediatric patients ≥12 years of age with type 2 diabetes, consider reducing the dose of the concomitantly administered insulin secretagogue (such assulfonylureas) or insulin to reduce the risk of hypoglycemia.

Geriatric Use

In the pool of placebo- and active-controlled glycemic control clinical trials, 23.6% of patients receiving subcutaneous semaglutide and 29.9% of those receiving oral semaglutide were 65 years of age and older; 3.2% of those receiving subcutaneous semaglutide and 4.8% of those receiving oral semaglutide were 75 years of age and older. In a cardiovascular outcome trial (SUSTAIN-6) of subcutaneous semaglutide, 48% of patients were 65 years of age and older and 9.6% were 75 years of age and older; in a cardiovascular outcomes trial of oral semaglutide (PIONEER 6), 43.4 or 12.3% of patients were at least 65 or at least 75 years of age, respectively. In the trials of subcutaneous semaglutide (Wegovy), 8.8% of patients receiving the drug were 65–75 years of age and 0.9% were ≥75 years of age. No substantial differences in safety and efficacy relative to younger adults were observed in these patients, but increased sensitivity in some geriatric individuals cannot be ruled out.

Hepatic Impairment

No substantial differences in the pharmacokinetics of semaglutide administered orally or subcutaneously have been observed in patients with mild, moderate, or severe hepatic impairment.

Limited data indicate that exposure of SNAC, an absorption enhancer contained in oral semaglutide tablets, is increased with increasing hepatic impairment; however, this finding is not considered clinically relevant since SNAC has no anticipated systemic effects. Data on the long-term safety of SNAC in patients with hepatic impairment are lacking.

Renal Impairment

In a 26-week, placebo-controlled clinical trial (PIONEER 5) in patients with type 2 diabetes mellitus and moderate renal impairment (eGFR of 30–59 mL/minute

per 1.73 m²), oral semaglutide (dosage titrated to 14 mg once daily) added to the patient's pretrial antidiabetic regimen (metformin and/or sulfonylurea, or basal insulin with or without metformin) was more effective than placebo for glycemic control (mean HbA₁c reduction of 1% versus 0.2% with placebo at week 26) and reduction in body weight (mean decrease of 3.4 or 0.9 kg with semaglutide or placebo, respectively, at week 26); adverse effects, mainly GI effects, were similar to those reported with other GLP-1 receptor agonists.

No substantial differences in the pharmacokinetics of semaglutide administered orally or subcutaneously have been observed in patients with mild, moderate, or severe renal impairment, including patients with ESRD.

Limited data indicate that exposure of SNAC, an absorption enhancer contained in semaglutide oral tablets, generally increases with increasing renal impairment; however, this finding is not considered clinically relevant since SNAC has no anticipated systemic effects. Data on the long-term safety of SNAC in patients with renal impairment are lacking.

Hemodialysis does not appear to affect the pharmacokinetics of orally administered semaglutide or SNAC.

Disease of the Upper GI Tract

In a study in patients with type 2 diabetes mellitus, there were no clinically important differences in semaglutide pharmacokinetics between patients with or without upper GI disease (chronic gastritis and/or gastroesophageal reflux disease) who received oral semaglutide once daily for 10 consecutive days.

● Common Adverse Effects

Adverse effects reported in at least 5% of patients receiving subcutaneous semaglutide (Ozempic®) in placebo-controlled clinical trials include nausea, vomiting, diarrhea, abdominal pain, and constipation.

Adverse effects reported in at least 5% of patients receiving oral semaglutide in placebo-controlled clinical trials include nausea, abdominal pain/discomfort, diarrhea, decreased appetite, vomiting, and constipation.

Adverse effects reported in at least 5% of patients receiving sub-Q semaglutide (Wegovy®): nausea, diarrhea, vomiting, constipation, abdominal pain, headache, fatigue, dyspepsia, dizziness, abdominal distension, eructation, hypoglycemia in patients with type 2 diabetes, flatulence, gastroenteritis, gastroesophageal reflux disease, and nasopharyngitis.

DRUG INTERACTIONS

In vitro studies have demonstrated that semaglutide has a very low potential to inhibit or induce cytochrome P-450 (CYP) enzymes or to inhibit drug transporters.

● Orally Administered Drugs

The effect of semaglutide-induced slowing of gastric emptying may reduce the rate and extent of absorption of concomitantly administered oral drugs. In clinical pharmacology trials, subcutaneous semaglutide did not affect the absorption of orally administered drugs (e.g., atorvastatin, digoxin, metformin, ethinyl estradiol, levonorgestrel, warfarin) to any clinically important extent. Similarly, oral administration of semaglutide did not have clinically important effects on the absorption of other drugs (e.g., digoxin, ethinyl estradiol, levonorgestrel, furosemide, levothyroxine, lisinopril, metformin, omeprazole, rosuvastatin, warfarin) in drug interaction studies. Use caution and monitor the patient when oral medications are administered concomitantly with semaglutide.

Patients receiving oral semaglutide concomitantly with other oral drugs should be advised to closely follow administration instructions for oral semaglutide. Increased clinical or laboratory monitoring should be considered in patients receiving concomitant therapy with drugs that have a narrow therapeutic index or that require clinical monitoring.

● Antidiabetic Agents

The risk of hypoglycemia is increased when semaglutide is used in conjunction with a sulfonylurea or insulin; patients receiving semaglutide concomitantly with such agents may require a reduction in the dosage of the sulfonylurea or insulin. Concomitant administration of subcutaneous semaglutide (Ozempic®) at 1 mg steady-state exposure and metformin at 500 mg twice daily did not alter the absorption of metformin to any clinically important extent. In a pharmacokinetic study in healthy individuals receiving oral semaglutide (20 mg once daily), concomitant administration (at steady-state semaglutide exposure) of metformin hydrochloride (850 mg twice daily for 7 doses) resulted in a 32% increase in metformin exposure, which was not considered clinically relevant. Peak plasma concentration, time to peak concentration, and half-life of metformin were not affected by concomitant oral semaglutide administration. The addition of subcutaneous semaglutide (Wegovy®) in patients treated with insulin has not been evaluated.

No adjustment of metformin hydrochloride dosage is needed when administered concomitantly with oral or subcutaneous semaglutide.

● **Atorvastatin**

Concomitant administration of subcutaneous semaglutide (at 1 mg steady-state exposure) and atorvastatin (single dose of 40 mg) did not meaningfully alter the peak plasma concentration or area under the plasma concentration-time curve (AUC) of atorvastatin. No adjustment of atorvastatin dosage is needed when administered concomitantly with subcutaneous semaglutide.

● **Digoxin**

Concomitant administration of subcutaneous semaglutide (at 1 mg steady-state exposure) and oral digoxin (single dose of 0.5 mg) did not meaningfully alter the peak plasma concentration or AUC of digoxin. In a pharmacokinetic study in healthy individuals receiving oral semaglutide (20 mg once daily), concomitant administration (at steady-state semaglutide exposure) of a single dose of digoxin (0.5 mg) did not affect exposure of digoxin (as assessed by AUC or peak plasma concentration). In addition, neither time to peak concentration nor half-life of digoxin was affected by concomitant oral semaglutide administration. No adjustment of digoxin dosage is needed when administered concomitantly with subcutaneous semaglutide.

● **Levothyroxine**

Levothyroxine total exposure (AUC adjusted for endogenous levels) was increased 33% when a single dose of levothyroxine (0.6 mg) was administered concurrently with oral semaglutide in a drug interaction study; however, maximum exposure (peak plasma concentration) was unchanged.

● **Lisinopril**

In a pharmacokinetic study in healthy individuals receiving oral semaglutide (20 mg once daily), concomitant administration (at steady-state semaglutide exposure) of a single dose of lisinopril (20 mg) did not affect exposure of lisinopril (as assessed by AUC or peak plasma concentration). In addition, neither time to peak concentration nor half-life of lisinopril was affected by concomitant semaglutide administration. No adjustment of lisinopril dosage is needed when administered concomitantly with oral semaglutide.

● **Omeprazole**

In a randomized, parallel-group trial in healthy individuals receiving oral semaglutide (5 mg once daily for 5 days, then 10 mg once daily for 5 days) with or without omeprazole (40 mg once daily), there was no clinically important difference in semaglutide pharmacokinetics with concomitant omeprazole administration, although a slight increase in semaglutide exposure (peak plasma concentration and AUC) was observed. No adjustment of oral semaglutide dosage is likely to be needed with concomitant administration of omeprazole.

● **Oral Contraceptives**

Concomitant administration of subcutaneous semaglutide (at 1 mg steady-state exposure) and the fixed combination oral contraceptive ethinyl estradiol/levonorgestrel (0.03 mg/0.15 mg steady-state exposure) did not meaningfully alter the peak plasma concentration or AUC of the oral contraceptive. No adjustment of ethinyl estradiol/levonorgestrel dosage is needed when administered concomitantly with subcutaneous semaglutide.

● **Warfarin**

Concomitant administration of subcutaneous semaglutide (at 1 mg steady-state exposure) and warfarin (single dose of 25 mg) did not meaningfully alter the peak plasma concentration or AUC of warfarin. In a pharmacokinetic study in healthy individuals receiving oral semaglutide (20 mg once daily), concomitant administration (at steady-state semaglutide exposure) of a single dose of warfarin (25 mg) did not affect exposure of S- or R-warfarin (as assessed by AUC or peak plasma concentration). In addition, neither time to peak concentration nor half-life of warfarin was affected by concomitant oral semaglutide administration. No adjustment of warfarin dosage is needed when administered concomitantly with oral or subcutaneous semaglutide.

DESCRIPTION

Semaglutide is a long-acting, glucagon-like peptide-1 (GLP-1) receptor agonist modified from the active fragment of human GLP-1. Semaglutide is a peptide that is similar in structure (94% sequence homology) to endogenous GLP-1 with the exception of substituting arginine for lysine at position 34, the attachment of a long fatty acid derivative at position 26, and the substitution of amino-isobutyric acid for alanine at position 8 of the peptide backbone. These structural changes slow the degradation of the drug by dipeptidyl peptidase-4 (DPP-4) and increase its affinity for albumin, which prolongs the half-life of the drug and allows the drug to be administered once weekly.

Activation of GLP-1 receptors stimulates insulin release in the presence of elevated glucose concentrations, suppresses glucose-dependent glucagon release, and slows gastric emptying, resulting in lower fasting and postprandial blood glucose concentrations and weight loss in patients with type 2 diabetes mellitus. Long-acting GLP-1 receptor agonists (e.g., albiglutide [no longer commercially available in the US], dulaglutide, exenatide extended-release, liraglutide, semaglutide) induce marked reductions in fasting plasma glucose concentrations (by stimulating insulin secretion) and modest reductions in postprandial glucose concentrations, while short-acting GLP-1 receptor agonists (e.g., exenatide, lixisenatide) have less of an effect on fasting plasma glucose concentrations and more of an effect on reducing postprandial glucose concentrations (by slowing gastric emptying and inhibiting glucagon secretion). At an average exposure fourfold higher than that produced by the maximum recommended dosage in humans, semaglutide did not prolong the corrected QT interval (QT_c) to any clinically important extent.

Peak plasma semaglutide concentrations are achieved 1–3 days following subcutaneous administration. The absolute bioavailability of semaglutide following subcutaneous administration is 89–94%; similar exposure is achieved following subcutaneous administration in the abdomen, thigh, or upper arm. Semaglutide is more than 99% bound to plasma albumin. Steady-state concentrations are achieved 4–5 weeks following weekly subcutaneous administration.

Semaglutide oral tablets are formulated with salcaprozate sodium (SNAC) to facilitate the absorption of semaglutide following oral administration; semaglutide is absorbed predominantly in the stomach. Peak plasma semaglutide concentrations are achieved 1 hour after oral administration. The absolute bioavailability of semaglutide following oral administration is low, approximately 0.4–1%. Steady-state semaglutide concentrations are achieved after 4–5 weeks of oral dosing.

Semaglutide is mainly metabolized through proteolytic cleavage of the peptide backbone and sequential beta-oxidation of the fatty acid sidechain. The elimination half-life of semaglutide is approximately 1 week.

ADVICE TO PATIENTS

- Importance of patients reading the medication guide and instructions for use prior to initiating therapy and each time prescription is refilled.

- Importance of informing patients that semaglutide causes thyroid C-cell tumors in rats and that the relevance of this finding in humans is unknown. Importance of advising patients receiving semaglutide to report symptoms such as a lump in the neck, hoarseness, dysphagia, or dyspnea, which may be suggestive of thyroid cancer.

- Importance of informing patients of the possibility of pancreatitis with semaglutide therapy. Importance of informing patients about signs and symptoms of pancreatitis, including persistent severe abdominal pain sometimes radiating to the back that may or may not be accompanied by vomiting; importance of patient discontinuing semaglutide and promptly notifying clinician if such signs or symptoms occur.

- Importance of informing patients to contact a clinician if changes in vision are experienced during treatment with semaglutide.

- Importance of informing patients that they should never share injection pens containing semaglutide with another person, even if the needle is changed; sharing of the pen may pose a risk of transmitting or acquiring infection.

- Importance of informing patients of the potential risk of dehydration due to adverse GI effects; importance of advising patients to drink fluids to avoid dehydration. Importance of informing patients of the potential risk for worsening renal function, which in some cases may require dialysis.

- Importance of informing patients of possibility of serious allergic or hypersensitivity reactions (e.g., anaphylaxis). Patients should be instructed to discontinue semaglutide and promptly seek medical advice if symptoms of a serious hypersensitivity reaction (e.g., swelling of the face, lips, tongue, or throat; difficulty breathing or swallowing; severe rash or itching; fainting or feeling dizzy; very rapid heart rate) occur.

- Importance of providing information regarding the potential risks and advantages of semaglutide therapy and of alternative modes of treatment.

- If the drug is being used as an antidiabetic agent, instruct the patient regarding diabetes self-management practices, such as regular physical activity, adhering to meal planning, periodic blood glucose monitoring, HbA$_{1c}$ testing, recognition and management of hypoglycemia and hyperglycemia, and assessment of other diabetic complications. Advise patients to seek medical advice promptly during periods of stress (e.g., fever, trauma, infection, surgery) as medication requirements may change.

- Importance of advising patients that the most common adverse effects of oral semaglutide are nausea, abdominal pain, diarrhea, decreased appetite, vomiting, and constipation and that the most common adverse effects of sub-Q semaglutide therapy are nausea, vomiting, diarrhea, abdominal pain, and constipation. Advise patients that nausea, vomiting, and diarrhea are most common when first initiating oral or sub-Q semaglutide therapy but these effects decrease over time in most patients.

- Instruct patients to inform their healthcare providers of palpitations or feelings of a racing heartbeat while at rest during semaglutide treatment.

- Advise patients to report emergence or worsening of depression, suicidal thoughts or behavior, and/or any unusual changes in mood or behavior. Inform patients that if they experience suicidal thoughts or behaviors, they should stop taking the drug.

- Importance of women informing clinicians if they are or plan to become pregnant or plan to breast-feed. Breast-feeding is not recommended during treatment with oral semaglutide due to the unknown potential for serious adverse effects from accumulation of salcaprozate sodium (SNAC), an absorption enhancer in the oral formulation, in milk; alternative formulations of semaglutide (i.e., injection) are available for use during lactation.

Advise patients who are exposed to the Wegovy® preparation during pregnancy to contact the manufacturer at 1-800-727-6500.

- Importance of informing clinicians of existing or contemplated concomitant therapy, including prescription and OTC drugs, as well as any concomitant illnesses.

- Importance of informing patients of other important precautionary information.

PREPARATIONS

Excipients in commercially available drug preparations may have clinically important effects in some individuals; consult specific product labeling for details.

Semaglutide

Oral		
Tablets	3 mg	**Rybelsus®**, Novo Nordisk
	7 mg	**Rybelsus®**, Novo Nordisk
	14 mg	**Rybelsus®**, Novo Nordisk
Parenteral		
Injection, for subcutaneous use only	0.25 mg/0.5 mL	**Wegovy®** (available as single-dose prefilled injection pen), Novo Nordisk
	0.5 mg/0.5 mL	**Wegovy®** (available as single-dose prefilled injection pen), Novo Nordisk
	1 mg/0.5 mL	**Wegovy®** (available as single-dose prefilled injection pen), Novo Nordisk
	1.7 mg/0.75 mL	**Wegovy®** (available as single-dose prefilled injection pen), Novo Nordisk
	2.4 mg/0.75 mL	**Wegovy®** (available as single-dose prefilled injection pen), Novo Nordisk
	2 mg/3 mL (0.68 mg/mL)	**Ozempic®** (available as single patient-use prefilled injection pen that delivers 0.25 or 0.5 mg per injection), Novo Nordisk
	4 mg/3 mL (1.34 mg/mL)	**Ozempic®** (available as single patient-use prefilled injection pen that delivers 1 mg per injection), Novo Nordisk
	8 mg/3 mL (2.68 mg/mL)	**Ozempic®** (available as single patient-use prefilled injection pen that delivers 2 mg per injection), Novo Nordisk

† Use is not currently included in the labeling approved by the US Food and Drug Administration.

Selected Revisions June 10, 2024, © Copyright, December 18, 2017, American Society of Health-System Pharmacists, Inc.

Tirzepatide

68:20.06 • INCRETIN MIMETICS

■ Tirzepatide is a dual glucose-dependent insulinotropic polypeptide (GIP) receptor and glucagon-like peptide 1 (GLP-1) receptor agonist.

USES

● Type 2 Diabetes

Tirzepatide is used subcutaneously as an adjunct to diet and exercise to improve glycemic control in adults with type 2 diabetes. There are 2 preparations of tirzepatide that are commercially available; Mounjaro® subcutaneous injection is specifically FDA-labeled for use in the management of diabetes mellitus.

Tirzepatide has not been studied in patients with a history of pancreatitis, and is not indicated for use in patients with type 1 diabetes.

Clinical Experience

The efficacy of tirzepatide for the treatment of patients with type 2 diabetes was established in the SURPASS clinical trials, in which tirzepatide was studied as monotherapy, in combination with oral antihyperglycemic agents, or in combination with insulin with or without metformin. In the randomized, double-blind, phase 3 SURPASS-1 trial, adults with type 2 diabetes mellitus inadequately controlled with diet and exercise alone were randomized 1:1:1:1 to once weekly subcutaneous injections of tirzepatide 5 mg, tirzepatide 10 mg, tirzepatide 15 mg, or matching placebo. The primary outcome was change in hemoglobin A1c (HbA_{1c}) from baseline at 40 weeks. Among 478 participants in SURPASS-1, mean age was 54 years; 52% were male, 36% were white, 35% were Asian, and 25% were American Indians/Alaska Natives. Patients assigned to tirzepatide 5 mg, 10 mg, or 15 mg experienced substantially greater reductions in least-squares mean HbA_{1c} from baseline (1.8, 1.7, or 1.7%, respectively) than those assigned to placebo (0.1%). Patients assigned to tirzepatide also experienced substantially greater reductions in least-squares mean weight from baseline (ranging from 6.3–7.8 kg) than those assigned to placebo (1.0 kg).

In the randomized, open-label, phase 3 SURPASS-2 trial, adults with type 2 diabetes inadequately controlled with metformin alone were randomized 1:1:1:1 to add-on subcutaneous injections of tirzepatide 5 mg, tirzepatide 10 mg, or tirzepatide 15 mg (double-blinded to tirzepatide dose assignment), or semaglutide 1 mg, once weekly. The primary outcome was change in HbA_{1c} from baseline at 40 weeks. Among 1879 participants in SURPASS-2, mean age was 57 years; 47% were male, 83% were white, and 70% identified as Hispanic or Latino. Patients assigned to tirzepatide 10 mg or 15 mg experienced substantially greater reductions in least-squares mean HbA_{1c} from baseline (2.2 or 2.3%, respectively) than those assigned to semaglutide (1.9%). Patients assigned to tirzepatide also experienced substantially greater reductions in least-squares mean weight from baseline (ranging from 7.6–11.2 kg) than those assigned to semaglutide (5.7 kg).

In the randomized open-label, phase 3 SURPASS-3 trial, adults with type 2 diabetes inadequately controlled on metformin (with or without concomitant sodium-glucose cotransporter 2 [SGLT2] inhibitor therapy) were randomized 1:1:1:1 to add-on subcutaneous injections of tirzepatide 5 mg, tirzepatide 10 mg, or tirzepatide 15 mg once weekly, or insulin degludec 10 units (with subsequent adjustment to target blood glucose values) once daily. The primary outcome was change in HbA_{1c} from baseline at 52 weeks. Among 1444 participants in SURPASS-3, mean age was 57 years; 32% were receiving an SGLT2 inhibitor, 56% were male, 91% were white, and 29% identified as Hispanic or Latino. Patients assigned to tirzepatide 5 mg, 10 mg, or 15 mg experienced substantially greater reductions in least-squares mean HbA_{1c} from baseline (1.9, 2.0, or 2.1%, respectively) than those assigned to insulin degludec (1.3%). Patients assigned to tirzepatide also experienced substantially greater reductions in least-squares mean weight from baseline (ranging from 7.0–11.3 kg) than those assigned to insulin degludec (mean weight increase of 1.9 kg).

In the randomized, open-label, phase 3 SURPASS-4 trial, adults with type 2 diabetes mellitus with known or increased risk of cardiovascular events and inadequate glycemic control on monotherapy or any combination of metformin, a

sulfonylurea, and/or an SGLT2 inhibitor were randomized 1:1:1:3 to add-on subcutaneous injections of tirzepatide 5 mg, tirzepatide 10 mg, or tirzepatide 15 mg once weekly or insulin glargine 10 units (with subsequent adjustment to target blood glucose values) once daily. The primary outcome was change in HbA_{1c} from baseline to 52 weeks. Among 2002 participants in SURPASS-4, mean age was 64 years; 95% were receiving metformin, 54% were receiving a sulfonylurea, 25% were receiving an SGLT2 inhibitor, 63% were male, 82% were white, and 48% identified as Hispanic or Latino. Patients assigned to tirzepatide 5 mg, 10 mg, or 15 mg experienced substantially greater reductions in least-squares mean HbA_{1c} from baseline (2.1, 2.3, or 2.4%, respectively) than those assigned to insulin glargine (1.4%). Patients assigned to tirzepatide also experienced substantially greater reductions in least-squares mean weight from baseline (ranging from 6.4–10.6 kg) than those assigned to insulin glargine (mean weight increase of 1.7 kg).

In the randomized, double-blind, phase 3 SURPASS-5 trial, adults with type 2 diabetes inadequately controlled on insulin glargine (with or without metformin) were randomized 1:1:1:1 to add-on once weekly subcutaneous injections of tirzepatide 5 mg, tirzepatide 10 mg, or tirzepatide 15 mg, or matching placebo. The primary outcome was change in HbA_{1c} from baseline at 40 weeks. Among 475 participants in SURPASS-5, mean age was 61 years; 56% were male, 80% were white, 18% were Asian, and 5% identified as Hispanic or Latino. Patients assigned to tirzepatide 5 mg, 10 mg, or 15 mg experienced substantially greater reductions in least-squares mean HbA_{1c} from baseline (2.1, 2.4, or 2.3%, respectively) than those assigned to placebo (0.9%). Patients assigned to tirzepatide also experienced substantially greater reductions in least-squares mean weight from baseline (ranging from 5.4–8.8 kg) than those assigned to placebo (mean weight increase of 1.6 kg).

Clinical Perspective

The American Diabetes Association (ADA) publishes an annual guideline on diabetes management, which provides clinical practice recommendations for glucose-lowering therapies in patients with type 2 diabetes. The current guideline states that the pharmacologic approach that will provide adequate efficacy to achieve and maintain treatment goals should be considered, such as metformin or other agents, including combination therapy. Weight management and other healthy lifestyle behaviors should also be included in the treatment plan. When selecting an appropriate treatment regimen, clinicians should be guided by factors such as cardiovascular and renal comorbidities, drug efficacy, hypoglycemic risk, impact on weight, cost, access, and patient preferences. In adults with type 2 diabetes and established/high risk of atherosclerotic cardiovascular disease (ASCVD), heart failure, and/or chronic kidney disease, the treatment regimen should include agents that reduce cardiorenal risk. In general, higher-efficacy approaches have a greater likelihood of achieving glycemic goals. Tirzepatide is considered one of several agents with very high glucose-lowering efficacy and also very high efficacy for weight loss.

The American Association of Clinical Endocrinology (AACE) also publishes guidelines for the management of type 2 diabetes. The principles of diabetes management outlined in the guidelines are similar to those recommended by the ADA. The AACE guidelines state that in patients with type 2 diabetes whose primary treatment goal does not include managing risk factors for cardiorenal complications, metformin is considered front-line therapy; additional glucose-lowering therapy should be guided by glycemic and weight management goals, risk of hypoglycemia, and issues related to medication access and cost. Glucose-dependent insulinotropic polypeptide (GIP)/GLP-1 receptor agonists are one of several preferred agents for patients whose treatment goals include weight loss or who are considered to be at risk of hypoglycemia.

● Chronic Weight Management

Tirzepatide is used as an adjunct to a reduced-calorie diet and increased physical activity for chronic weight management in adults who are obese (pretreatment body mass index [BMI] ≥30 kg/m²) or, in adults who are overweight (pretreatment BMI ≥27 kg/m²) *and* who have at least one weight-related comorbid condition (e.g., hypertension, dyslipidemia, type 2 diabetes mellitus, obstructive sleep apnea, cardiovascular disease).

There are 2 preparations of tirzepatide that are commercially available; Zepbound® subcutaneous injection is specifically FDA-labeled for use in chronic weight management in adults. The manufacturer states that the drug should not be used in combination with any other tirzepatide-containing products or any other GLP-1 receptor agonist.

Safety and efficacy of tirzepatide in combination with other products used to promote weight loss have not been established. Tirzepatide also has not been studied in patients with a history of pancreatitis.

Clinical Experience

The SURMOUNT-1 trial was conducted In adults who were obese (BMI ≥30 kg/m^2) or overweight (BMI 27–29.9 kg/m^2) and had at least one weight-related comorbid condition (e.g., hypertension, dyslipidemia, obstructive sleep apnea, cardiovascular disease) except diabetes. Patients were randomized to receive once-weekly subcutaneous injections of tirzepatide (5 mg, 10 mg, or 15 mg) or placebo for 72 weeks in addition to lifestyle intervention. At baseline, the mean body weight was 104.8 kg; the mean BMI was 38 kg/m^2 and 94.5% of participants had a BMI of 30 or higher. The primary efficacy measures were the mean percent change in body weight from baseline and the proportion of patients who lost at least 5% of their baseline body weight. At 72 weeks, tirzepatide reduced body weight by a greater percentage from baseline than placebo (mean reductions of 15%, 19.5%, and 20.9% with tirzepatide 5 mg, tirzepatide 10 mg, and tirzepatide 15 mg, respectively, versus 3.1% with placebo). More participants treated with tirzepatide met body weight reduction thresholds of 5% or higher (85-91%) than those treated with placebo (35%). The most common adverse events in the study were GI effects (nausea, diarrhea, and constipation), which occurred more frequently in the tirzepatide groups than in the placebo group; however, these effects were transient and mild to moderate in severity, and were limited to primarily the dose-escalation period.

The SURMOUNT-2 trial was conducted in adults with obesity (BMI of 27 kg/m^2 or higher) and type 2 diabetes. Patients were randomized to receive once-weekly subcutaneous injections of tirzepatide (10 mg or 15 mg) or placebo for 72 weeks. The primary efficacy measures were the mean percent change in body weight from baseline and the proportion of patients who lost at least 5% of their baseline body weight. At baseline, the mean body weight was 100.7 kg and HbA$_{1c}$ was 8.02%. After 72 weeks of treatment, patients receiving tirzepatide experienced substantially greater reductions in least-squares mean weight from baseline (reduction of 12.8% with tirzepatide 10 mg and 14.7% with tirzepatide 15 mg) than those who received placebo (reduction of 3.2%). More participants treated with tirzepatide met body weight reduction thresholds of 5% or higher (79-83%) than those treated with placebo (32%). The most frequent adverse events with tirzepatide were GI-related (e.g., nausea, diarrhea, vomiting) and were mostly mild to moderate in severity, with few events resulting in treatment discontinuation.

Clinical Perspective

Clinical practice guidelines recommend treatment for obesity in patients with excess body weight and associated health risks. A comprehensive lifestyle intervention is an essential component of therapy and should be provided to all patients; pharmacologic therapy may be considered as an adjunct to behavioral modification in patients who fail to achieve or sustain clinically meaningful weight loss (generally defined as a loss of more than 4–5% of total body weight). Response to drug therapy should be evaluated after 3–4 months of treatment; if clinically meaningful weight loss is not achieved, it is generally recommended that a new treatment plan be considered because the patient is likely not responding to the drug.

DOSAGE AND ADMINISTRATION

● General

Pretreatment Screening

- If used for weight management, select patients for treatment based on baseline body mass index (BMI).
- In patients with type 2 diabetes mellitus receiving tirzepatide for chronic weight management, monitor blood glucose prior to initiating therapy.

Patient Monitoring

- Periodically monitor blood glucose and glycosylated hemoglobin (HbA$_{1c}$) to determine therapeutic response in patients with type 2 diabetes mellitus.
- Monitor for signs and symptoms of thyroid tumors, including a mass in the neck, dysphagia, dyspnea, and persistent hoarseness.

- Monitor for signs and symptoms of pancreatitis, such as persistent severe abdominal pain with or without vomiting.
- For patients with pre-existing renal impairment reporting severe GI adverse reactions, monitor renal function when initiating or escalating doses of tirzepatide.
- For patients with a history of diabetic retinopathy, monitor for progression of retinopathy.
- Monitor for signs and symptoms of hypoglycemia, particularly in patients receiving concomitant therapy with insulin or an insulin secretagogue.
- Monitor patients with a history of diabetic retinopathy for progression of diabetic retinopathy while receiving tirzepatide.
- Monitor for the emergence or worsening of depression, suicidal thoughts or behavior (suicidality), and/or any unusual changes in mood or behavior.

● Administration

Tirzepatide is administered via subcutaneous injection once weekly with or without meals. Tirzepatide for the treatment of type 2 diabetes (Mounjaro®) is available in pre-filled single-dose pens or single-dose vials in the following strengths per 0.5 mL: 2.5 mg, 5 mg, 7.5 mg, 10 mg, 12.5 mg, and 15 mg. Tirzepatide for weight management (Zepbound®) is available in pre-filled single-dose pens in the following strengths per 0.5 mL: 2.5 mg, 5 mg, 7.5 mg, 10 mg, 12.5 mg, and 15 mg. Tirzepatide is a clear, colorless to slightly yellow solution; do not use if particulate matter or discoloration is seen.

Train patients and/or caregivers on proper injection technique. Inject subcutaneously into the abdomen, thigh, or upper arm. Rotate injection sites with each dose.

Instruct patients using the single-dose vial to use an appropriate syringe for administration (e.g., a 1 mL syringe capable of measuring a 0.5 mL dose). When using tirzepatide with insulin, administer as separate injections and do not mix in the same syringe. Injections of tirzepatide and insulin can be given in the same body region but the injections should not be adjacent to one other.

If a dose is missed, administer as soon as possible within 4 days (96 hours) after the missed dose; then, resume the regular once weekly dosing schedule. If more than 4 days have passed, skip the missed dose and administer the next dose on the regularly scheduled day. The day of weekly administration can be changed, if necessary, as long as the time between the 2 doses is at least 3 days (72 hours).

Store tirzepatide vials and prefilled injection pens in a refrigerator at 2–8°C. If necessary, the drug can be stored out of the refrigerator at temperatures not to exceed 30°C for up to 21 days. Do not freeze or use if frozen. Store in the original carton to protect the drug from light.

● Dosage

Type 2 Diabetes

For the treatment of type 2 diabetes in adults, the recommended initial dosage of tirzepatide is 2.5 mg once weekly administered as a subcutaneous injection. The 2.5 mg dosage is for treatment initiation and is not intended for glycemic control. Increase the dosage to 5 mg once weekly after 4 weeks. For additional glycemic control, the dosage may be further increased in 2.5 mg increments after at least 4 weeks on the current dosage; the maximum recommended dosage is 15 mg once weekly.

Weight Management

When used for chronic weight management, the recommended adult dosage of tirzepatide is 2.5 mg once weekly administered as a subcutaneous injection. The 2.5 mg dosage is for treatment initiation and is not intended for chronic weight management. Increase the dosage to 5 mg once weekly after 4 weeks. The dosage may be further increased in 2.5 mg increments after at least 4 weeks on the current dosage. The recommended maintenance dosage in adults is 5 mg, 10 mg, or 15 mg once weekly; consider treatment response and tolerability when selecting an appropriate maintenance dosage. The maximum recommended dosage is 15 mg once weekly.

● Special Populations

Hepatic Impairment

No dosage adjustments are necessary in patients with hepatic impairment.

Renal Impairment

No dosage adjustments are necessary in patients with renal impairment, including those with end-stage renal disease.

Geriatric Use

The manufacturer makes no specific dosage recommendations for geriatric patients.

CAUTIONS

● Contraindications

● Personal or family history of medullary thyroid carcinoma (MTC) or in patients with multiple endocrine neoplasia syndrome type 2 (MEN 2).

● Known serious hypersensitivity to tirzepatide or any excipients.

● Warnings/Precautions

Risk of Thyroid C-Cell Tumors

Tirzepatide causes dose- and treatment duration-dependent thyroid C-cell tumors in rats; it is unknown whether the drug causes thyroid C-cell tumors, including medullary thyroid carcinoma (MTC), in humans. A boxed warning about this risk has been included in the prescribing information for tirzepatide.

Tirzepatide is contraindicated in patients with a personal or family history of MTC or in patients with multiple endocrine neoplasia syndrome type 2 (MEN 2). Counsel patients regarding the potential risk of MTC and inform them of symptoms of thyroid tumors (e.g., a mass in the neck, dysphagia, dyspnea, persistent hoarseness). Routine monitoring of serum calcitonin or thyroid ultrasound is of uncertain value for early MTC detection in patients treated with tirzepatide.

Risks During General Anesthesia and Deep Sedation

GLP-1 agonists are associated with adverse GI effects such as nausea, vomiting, and delayed gastric emptying; such effects are likely a result of rapid tachyphlaxis at the level of vagal nerve activation. Delayed gastric emptying from GLP-1 agonists can increase the risk of regurgitation and pulmonary aspiration of gastric contents during general anesthesia and deep sedation. Given these concerns, the American Society of Anesthesiologists (ASA) Task Force on Preoperative Fasting has issued a consensus-based guidance for the management of GLP-1 receptor agonists prior to elective surgery. The task force suggests that for patients on daily GLP-1 agonist dosing (irrespective of indication, dose, or type of surgery), consider holding the drug on the day of the elective procedure/surgery. For patients on weekly dosing (irrespective of indication, dose, or type of surgery), consider holding the GLP-1 agonist a week prior to the elective procedure/surgery. If GLP-1 agonists prescribed for diabetes management are held for longer than the dosing schedule, consider consulting an endocrinologist for bridging the antidiabetic therapy to avoid hyperglycemia. These recommendations are based on limited evidence only (case reports). For patients requiring urgent or emergent procedures, the task force states to proceed and treat the patient as 'full stomach' and manage accordingly.

Pancreatitis

Acute pancreatitis, including fatal and non-fatal hemorrhagic or necrotizing pancreatitis, has been observed in patients treated with glucagon-like peptide 1 (GLP-1) receptor agonists. In clinical studies, 14 events of acute pancreatitis were observed in 13 tirzepatide-treated patients (0.23 patients per 100 years of exposure) and 3 events were observed in 3 comparator-treated patients (0.11 patients per 100 years of exposure). Tirzepatide has not been studied in patients with a prior history of pancreatitis. It is unknown if patients with a history of pancreatitis are at higher risk for development of pancreatitis on tirzepatide.

After initiation of tirzepatide, observe patients carefully for signs and symptoms of pancreatitis (e.g., persistent severe abdominal pain that sometimes radiates to the back; may or may not be accompanied by vomiting). If pancreatitis is suspected, discontinue tirzepatide and initiate appropriate management.

Hypoglycemia

Tirzepatide lowers blood glucose and can cause hypglycemia.

Patients receiving tirzepatide in combination with an insulin secretagogue (e.g., sulfonylurea) or insulin may have an increased risk of hypoglycemia, including severe hypoglycemia. The risk of hypoglycemia may be lowered by reducing the dose of the insulin secretagogue or insulin. Inform patients using these concomitant medications of the risk of hypoglycemia and educate them on the signs and symptoms of hypoglycemia.

Hypersensitivity Reactions

Serious hypersensitivity reactions have been reported with tirzepatide (e.g., anaphylaxis, angioedema). If hypersensitivity reactions occur, discontinue tirzepatide; treat the reaction promptly per standard of care, and monitor until signs and symptoms resolve. Do not use tirzepatide in patients with a previous serious hypersensitivity reaction to tirzepatide or any of the excipients in the formulation.

Anaphylaxis and angioedema have been reported with other GLP-1 receptor agonists. Use tirzepatide with caution in patients with a history of angioedema or anaphylaxis with another GLP-1 receptor agonist, because it is unknown whether such patients will be predisposed to these reactions with tirzepatide.

Acute Kidney Injury

Tirzepatide has been associated with GI adverse reactions (e.g., nausea, vomiting, diarrhea); these events may lead to dehydration, which could cause acute kidney injury if severe. In patients treated with GLP-1 receptor agonists, there have been postmarketing reports of acute kidney injury and worsening of chronic renal failure, which may sometimes require hemodialysis. Some of these events have been reported in patients without known underlying renal disease. Most events occurred in patients who had experienced nausea, vomiting, diarrhea, or dehydration. Monitor renal function when initiating or escalating doses of tirzepatide in patients with renal impairment reporting severe GI adverse reactions.

Severe GI Disease

Use of tirzepatide has been associated with GI adverse reactions, sometimes severe. Tirzepatide has not been studied in patients with severe GI disease, including severe gastroparesis, and is therefore not recommended in these patients.

Diabetic Retinopathy Complications in Patients with a History of Diabetic Retinopathy

Rapid improvement in glucose control has been associated with a temporary worsening of diabetic retinopathy. Tirzepatide has not been studied in patients with non-proliferative diabetic retinopathy requiring acute therapy, proliferative diabetic retinopathy, or diabetic macular edema. Monitor patients with a history of diabetic retinopathy for progression of diabetic retinopathy.

Acute Gallbladder Disease

Acute events of gallbladder disease such as cholelithiasis or cholecystitis have been reported in GLP-1 receptor agonist trials and during postmarketing experience. In placebo-controlled trials of tirzepatide, acute gallbladder disease (cholelithiasis, biliary colic, and cholecystectomy) was reported by 0.6% of tirzepatide-treated patients and 0% of placebo-treated patients. If cholelithiasis is suspected, gallbladder diagnostic studies and appropriate clinical follow-up are indicated.

Suicidality

Suicidal behavior and ideation have been reported in clinical trials of other weight management agents. Monitor patients receiving tirzepatide for the emergence or worsening of depression, suicidal thoughts or behavior (suicidality), and/or any unusual changes in mood or behavior. If a patient experiences suicidal thoughts or behaviors while receiving semaglutide, discontinue the drug. Avoid tirzepatide in patients with a history of suicidal attempts or active suicidal ideation.

Immunogenicity

Anti-tirzepatide antibodies, including neutralizing antibodies, have been reported in patients receiving the drug. These antibodies did not impact the pharmacokinetics or effectiveness of tirzepatide; however, patients who developed anti-tirzepatide antibodies were more likely to experience hypersensitivity reactions or injection site reactions.

Specific Populations

Pregnancy

Available data with tirzepatide use in pregnant women are insufficient to inform a drug-associated risk of major birth defects, miscarriage, or other adverse maternal or fetal outcomes. Based on animal reproduction studies, there may be risks to the fetus from exposure to tirzepatide during pregnancy. In pregnant rats administered tirzepatide during organogenesis, fetal growth reductions and fetal abnormalities (including external, visceral, and skeletal malformations) occurred at clinically relevant exposures based on AUC. In rabbits administered tirzepatide during organogenesis, fetal growth reductions were observed at clinically relevant exposures based on AUC. Tirzepatide should be used during pregnancy only if the potential benefit justifies the potential risk to the fetus.

Lactation

There are no data on the presence of tirzepatide in animal or human milk, the effects on the breast-fed infant, or the effects on milk production. The developmental and health benefits of breastfeeding should be considered along with the mother's clinical need for tirzepatide and any potential adverse effects on the breast-fed infant from tirzepatide or from the underlying maternal condition.

Females and Males of Reproductive Potential

Tirzepatide may reduce the efficacy of oral hormonal contraceptives due to delayed gastric emptying; this delay is largest after the first dose and diminishes over time. Advise patients using oral hormonal contraceptives to switch to a non-oral contraceptive method or add a barrier method of contraception for 4 weeks after tirzepatide initiation and 4 weeks after each dose escalation.

Pediatric Use

Safety and effectiveness of tirzepatide have not been established in pediatric patients (<18 years of age).

Geriatric Use

In clinical trials of tirzepatide for diabetes mellitus, 30.1% of tirzepatide-treated patients were ≥65 years of age and 4.1% were ≥75 years of age. In clinical trials of tirzepatide for chronic weight management, 9% of tirzepatide-treated patients were ≥65 years of age and 0.5% were ≥75 years of age. No overall differences in safety or efficacy have been observed between geriatric patients and younger patients, but greater sensitivity of some older individuals cannot be ruled out.

Hepatic Impairment

Hepatic impairment (mild, moderate, or severe) does not impact the pharmacokinetics of tirzepatide.

Renal Impairment

Renal impairment, including end-stage renal disease, does not impact the pharmacokinetics of tirzepatide. Monitor renal function when initiating or escalating doses of tirzepatide in patients with renal impairment reporting severe adverse GI reactions.

● Common Adverse Effects

Adverse reactions reported in ≥5% of patients receiving tirzepatide for type 2 diabetes mellitus include nausea, diarrhea, decreased appetite, vomiting, constipation, dyspepsia, and abdominal pain.

Adverse reactions reported in ≥5% of patients receiving tirzepatide for chronic weight management include nausea, diarrhea, vomiting, constipation, abdominal pain, dyspepsia, injection site reactions, fatigue, hypersensitivity reactions, eructation, hair loss, and gastroesophageal reflux disease.

DRUG INTERACTIONS

In vitro studies have shown low potential for tirzepatide to inhibit or induce cytochrome P-450 (CYP) enzymes, and to inhibit drug transporters.

● Acetaminophen

Following a first dose of tirzepatide, acetaminophen maximum concentrations were reduced by 50%, and the median peak plasma concentration occurred 1 hour later. After coadministration at week 4, tirzepatide had no meaningful impact on acetaminophen maximum concentrations or time to maximum concentration. Overall acetaminophen exposure was not influenced.

● Insulin Secretagogues or Insulin

Patients receiving tirzepatide in combination with insulin or an insulin secretagogue (e.g., sulfonylureas) may have an increased risk for hypoglycemia. When initiating tirzepatide, consider reducing the dosage of concomitantly administered insulin secretagogues or insulin to reduce the risk of hypoglycemia.

● Orally Administered Drugs

Tirzepatide delays gastric emptying and has the potential to impact the absorption of concomitantly administered oral medications. The impact of tirzepatide on gastric emptying was greatest after a single 5-mg dose and diminished after subsequent doses.

Use caution when oral medications are administered concomitantly with tirzepatide. Monitor patients taking oral medications dependent on threshold concentrations for efficacy and those with a narrow therapeutic index (e.g., warfarin) when concomitantly administered with tirzepatide.

● Oral Hormonal Contraceptives

Following administration of a combined oral contraceptive (0.035 mg ethinyl estradiol and 0.25 mg norgestimate) in the presence of a single dose of tirzepatide 5 mg, the mean maximum concentration of ethinyl estradiol, norgestimate, and norelgestromin was reduced by 59, 66, and 55% respectively. The mean AUC was reduced by 20, 21, and 23% for ethinyl estradiol, norgestimate, and norelgestromin, respectively. Time to maximum concentration was delayed by 2.5–4.5 hours.

Advise patients taking oral hormonal contraceptives to switch to a non-oral contraceptive method or add a barrier method of contraception for 4 weeks after tirzepatide initiation and 4 weeks after each tirzepatide dose escalation. Hormonal contraceptives not administered orally should not be affected.

DESCRIPTION

Tirzepatide is a glucose-dependent insulinotropic polypeptide (GIP) receptor and glucagon-like peptide-1 (GLP-1) receptor agonist. The drug is a 39-amino-acid modified peptide based on the GIP sequence with a C20 fatty diacid moiety that enables albumin binding and prolongs the half-life.

In healthy individuals, plasma concentrations of endogenous GIP and GLP-1 rise 15–30 minutes following a meal; once produced, these peptides stimulate receptors on pancreatic cells to activate glucose-dependent insulin release. Tirzepatide selectively binds to and activates both GIP and GLP-1 receptors, the targets for native GIP and GLP-1. Tirzepatide enhances first- and second-phase insulin secretion and reduces glucagon levels, both in a glucose-dependent manner; it also increases insulin sensitivity and delays gastric emptying. The delay in gastric emptying is longest after the first dose, and diminishes over time.

Tirzepatide exposure increases in a dose-proportional manner. The time to maximum plasma concentration ranges from 8–72 hours. Steady-state plasma tirzepatide concentrations are achieved following 4 weeks of once weekly administration. The mean absolute bioavailability of tirzepatide following subcutaneous administration is 80%. Similar exposure was achieved with subcutaneous administration of tirzepatide in the abdomen, thigh, or upper arm.

Tirzepatide is 99% bound to plasma albumin. It is metabolized by proteolytic cleavage of the peptide backbone, beta oxidation of the C20 fatty diacid moiety, and amide hydrolysis. The primary excretion routes of tirzepatide metabolites are via urine and feces. Intact tirzepatide is not observed in urine or feces. The elimination half-life is approximately 5 days. Age, gender, race, ethnicity, and body weight do not have a clinically relevant impact on tirzepatide pharmacokinetics.

ADVICE TO PATIENTS

- Inform patients that tirzepatide causes thyroid C-cell tumors in rats and that the human relevance of this finding has not been determined. Counsel patients to report symptoms of thyroid tumors (e.g., a lump in the neck, persistent hoarseness, dysphagia, or dyspnea) to their healthcare provider.

- Inform patients of the potential risk for pancreatitis. Instruct patients to discontinue tirzepatide promptly and contact their healthcare provider if pancreatitis is suspected (severe abdominal pain that may radiate to the back; may or may not be accompanied by vomiting).

- Inform patients that the risk of hypoglycemia is increased when tirzepatide is used with an insulin secretagogue (such as a sulfonylurea) or insulin. Educate patients on the signs and symptoms of hypoglycemia.

- Inform patients that serious hypersensitivity reactions have been reported with use of tirzepatide. Advise patients on the symptoms of hypersensitivity reactions and instruct them to stop taking tirzepatide and seek medical advice promptly if such symptoms occur.

- Advise patients treated with tirzepatide of the potential risk of dehydration due to GI adverse reactions and take precautions to avoid fluid depletion. Inform patients of the potential risk for worsening renal function and explain the associated signs and symptoms of renal impairment, as well as the possibility of dialysis as a medical intervention if renal failure occurs.

- Inform patients of the potential risk of severe GI adverse reactions. Instruct patients to contact their healthcare provider if they have severe or persistent GI symptoms.

- Inform patients to contact their healthcare provider if changes in vision are experienced during treatment with tirzepatide.

- Inform patients of the risk of acute gallbladder disease. Instruct patients to contact their healthcare provider for appropriate clinical follow-up if gallbladder disease is suspected.

- Advise women to inform their clinician if they are or plan to become pregnant or plan to breast-feed. Advise a pregnant woman of the potential risk to a fetus.

- Use of tirzepatide may reduce the efficacy of oral hormonal contraceptives. Advise patients using oral hormonal contraceptives to switch to a non-oral contraceptive method or add a barrier method of contraception for 4 weeks after tirzepatide initiation and for 4 weeks after each dose escalation with tirzepatide.

- Instruct patients how to prepare and administer the correct dose of tirzepatide and assess their ability to inject subcutaneously to ensure the proper administration of tirzepatide. Instruct patients using the single-dose vial to use a syringe appropriate for dose administration (e.g., a 1 mL syringe capable of measuring a 0.5 mL dose).

- Advise patients to report emergence or worsening of depression, suicidal thoughts or behavior, and/or any unusual changes in mood or behavior. Inform patients that if they experience suicidal thoughts or behaviors, they should stop taking the drug.

- Inform patients that if a dose is missed, it should be administered as soon as possible within 4 days after the missed dose. If more than 4 days have passed, the missed dose should be skipped and the next dose should be administered on the regularly scheduled day. In each case, inform patients to resume their regular once weekly dosing schedule.

- Advise patient to inform their clinician of existing or contemplated concomitant therapy, including prescription and OTC drugs and dietary or herbal supplements, as well as any concomitant illnesses.

- Inform patients of other important precautionary information.

PREPARATIONS

Excipients in commercially available drug preparations may have clinically important effects in some individuals; consult specific product labeling for details.

Tirzepatide

Parenteral		
Injection, for subcutaneous use	2.5 mg/0.5 mL	Mounjaro® (available as single-dose prefilled injection pens and single-dose vials), Eli Lilly and Company
		Zepbound® (available as single-dose prefilled injection pens), Eli Lilly and Company
	5 mg/0.5 mL	Mounjaro® (available as single-dose prefilled injection pens and single-dose vials), Eli Lilly and Company
		Zepbound® (available as single-dose prefilled injection pens), Eli Lilly and Company
	7.5 mg/0.5 mL	Mounjaro® (available as single-dose prefilled injection pens and single-dose vials), Eli Lilly and Company
		Zepbound® (available as single-dose prefilled injection pens), Eli Lilly and Company
	10 mg/0.5 mL	Mounjaro® (available as single-dose prefilled injection pens and single-dose vials), Eli Lilly and Company
		Zepbound® (available as single-dose prefilled injection pens), Eli Lilly and Company
	12.5 mg/0.5 mL	Mounjaro® (available as single-dose prefilled injection pens and single-dose vials), Eli Lilly and Company
		Zepbound® (available as single-dose prefilled injection pens), Eli Lilly and Company
	15 mg/0.5 mL	Mounjaro® (available as single-dose prefilled injection pens and single-dose vials), Eli Lilly and Company
		Zepbound® (available as single-dose prefilled injection pens), Eli Lilly and Company

Selected Revisions November 20, 2023, © Copyright, December 22, 2021, American Society of Health-System Pharmacists, Inc.

Insulins General Statement

68:20.08 • INSULINS

■ Insulin is a hormone secreted by the beta cells of the pancreatic islets of Langerhans. Commercially available insulin preparations are classified as rapid-acting (insulin aspart, insulin glulisine, insulin lispro), short-acting (insulin human), intermediate-acting (insulin human isophane), or long-acting (insulin degludec, insulin detemir, insulin glargine).

USES

● Diabetes Mellitus

Overview

The American Diabetes Association (ADA) generally classifies diabetes mellitus as type 1 (due to autoimmune β-cell destruction, usually leading to absolute insulin deficiency); type 2 (due to a progressive loss of β-cell insulin secretion frequently on the background of insulin resistance); gestational diabetes mellitus (diabetes diagnosed in the second or third trimester of pregnancy that was not clearly overt diabetes prior to gestation); or specific types of diabetes due to other causes, such as monogenic diabetes syndromes (e.g., neonatal diabetes or maturity-onset diabetes of the young [MODY], diseases of the exocrine pancreas (e.g., cystic fibrosis, pancreatitis), or drug- or chemical-induced diabetes (e.g., that associated with glucocorticoid use, treatment of human immunodeficiency virus [HIV] /acquired immunodeficiency syndrome [AIDS], organ transplantation).

According to ADA and other experts, a diagnosis of diabetes mellitus currently is established by a fasting plasma glucose concentration of 126 mg/dL or greater, a 2-hour plasma glucose concentration of 200 mg/dL or greater during an oral glucose tolerance test, or a glycosylated hemoglobin (hemoglobin A_{1c}; HbA_{1c}) concentration of 6.5% or greater; results should be confirmed by repeat testing in the absence of unequivocal hyperglycemia. Alternatively, a random plasma glucose concentration of 200 mg/dL or greater in a patient with classic symptoms of hyperglycemia or hyperglycemic crisis is considered confirmation of the diagnosis of diabetes mellitus.

Type 1 diabetes mellitus was previously described as juvenile-onset diabetes mellitus, since it usually occurs during youth. Type 2 diabetes mellitus was previously described as adult-onset diabetes mellitus. However, type 1 or type 2 diabetes mellitus can occur at any age, and the current classification is based on pathogenesis (e.g., autoimmune destruction of pancreatic β cells, insulin resistance) and clinical presentation rather than on the age of onset. In both type 1 and type 2 diabetes mellitus, various genetic and environmental factors can result in the progressive loss of β-cell mass and/or function that manifests clinically as hyperglycemia. Many patients' diabetes mellitus does not easily fit into a single classification. Epidemiologic data indicate that the incidence of type 2 diabetes mellitus is increasing in children and adolescents.

Patients with type 2 diabetes mellitus (approximately 90–95% of all patients with diabetes mellitus) have insulin resistance and usually have relative (rather than absolute) insulin deficiency. Most patients with type 2 diabetes mellitus are overweight or obese; obesity itself also contributes to the insulin resistance and glucose intolerance observed in these patients. Patients with type 2 diabetes mellitus who are not obese may have an increased percentage of abdominal fat, which is an indicator of increased cardiometabolic risk. Distinguishing between type 1 and type 2 diabetes in children may be difficult since obesity may occur with either type of diabetes mellitus, and autoantigens and ketosis may be present in a substantial number of children with features of type 2 diabetes mellitus (e.g., obesity, acanthosis nigricans).

Considerations in Initiating Antidiabetic Therapy

Lifestyle modifications (e.g., self-management of diabetes mellitus, medical nutrition therapy [promoting healthy eating to achieve and maintain body weight goals], increased physical activity, smoking cessation, psychosocial care) are an important aspect of diabetes mellitus care in patients of all ages. Such lifestyle/behavioral modifications decrease cardiovascular risk and microvascular complications, improve glycemic control, and remain an indispensable part of the management of diabetes mellitus. Lipid management aimed at lowering low-density lipoprotein (LDL)-cholesterol, raising high-density lipoprotein (HDL)-cholesterol, and lowering triglycerides in patients with type 2 diabetes mellitus has been shown to reduce macrovascular disease and mortality. Although data on risk reduction are not as definitive in patients with type 1 diabetes mellitus, lipid-lowering therapy also should be considered in patients with type 1 diabetes. Efforts also should be aimed at blood pressure control in both adults and children, as reduction in blood pressure in uncomplicated mild to moderately hypertensive patients with diabetes mellitus has reduced the incidence of virtually all macrovascular (stroke, heart failure) and microvascular (retinopathy, vitreous hemorrhage, renal failure) outcomes and diabetes-related mortality. For information on the treatment of hypertension in patients with diabetes mellitus, see Uses: Hypertension, in Captopril 24:24.

Treatment with insulin is essential in all patients with type 1 diabetes mellitus. (See Insulin Monotherapy under Uses: Diabetes Mellitus.) Current guidelines for the treatment of type 2 diabetes mellitus generally recommend metformin as first-line therapy in addition to lifestyle modifications because of its well-established safety and efficacy (e.g., beneficial effects on HbA_{1c}, weight, and cardiovascular mortality) in patients with recent-onset or newly diagnosed type 2 diabetes mellitus or mild hyperglycemia. However, insulin therapy should be considered in patients with type 2 diabetes mellitus when hyperglycemia is severe (e.g., blood glucose concentration of 300 mg/dL or higher, HbA_{1c} of at least 10%), especially in the presence of catabolic manifestations (e.g., weight loss, hypertriglyceridemia, ketosis), or if symptoms of hyperglycemia are present. When the greater glucose-lowering effect of an injectable drug is needed, some experts currently suggest that glucagon-like peptide-1 (GLP-1) receptor agonists may be preferred over insulin because of a lower risk of hypoglycemia and beneficial effects on body weight, although they are associated with a greater risk of adverse GI effects. Because of the progressive nature of the disease, patients initially receiving an oral antidiabetic agent will eventually require multiple oral and/or injectable antidiabetic agents of different therapeutic classes and/or insulin for adequate glycemic control. (See Combination Therapy with Other Antidiabetic Agents under Uses: Diabetes Mellitus.)

Insulin Monotherapy

Insulin is used as replacement therapy in the management of diabetes mellitus. It supplements deficient concentrations of endogenous insulin and temporarily restores the ability of the body to properly utilize carbohydrates, fats, and proteins.

Insulin therapy is indicated in all cases of type 1 diabetes mellitus and is mandatory in the treatment of diabetic ketoacidosis and hyperosmolar hyperglycemic states. For additional information, see Diabetic Ketoacidosis and Hyperosmolar Hyperglycemic States under Dosage and Administration: Dosage, in Insulin Human 68:20.08.08. Insulin also is indicated in patients with type 2 diabetes mellitus when weight reduction, proper dietary regulation, and/or oral antidiabetic agents have failed to maintain satisfactory concentrations of blood glucose in both the fasting and postprandial state. In addition, insulin is indicated in otherwise stable, type 2 diabetic patients in the presence of major surgery, fever, severe trauma, infections, serious renal or hepatic dysfunction, hyperthyroidism or other endocrine dysfunction, gangrene, Raynaud's disease, or pregnancy.

In general, goals of insulin therapy in all patients should include maintenance of blood glucose as close as possible to euglycemia without an undue risk of hypoglycemia; avoidance of symptoms attributable to hyperglycemia, glycosuria, or ketonuria; and maintenance of ideal body weight and of normal growth and development in children.

Both conventional and intensive insulin treatment regimens have been used in patients with type 1 or severe type 2 diabetes mellitus. Conventional insulin therapy generally has consisted of 1 or 2 subcutaneous injections of insulin per day (e.g., before breakfast and/or dinner) using a mixture of an intermediate-acting insulin such as isophane (neutral protamine Hagedorn [NPH]) insulin and a short-acting (e.g., insulin human) or rapid-acting insulin (e.g., insulin lispro, insulin glulisine, insulin aspart). However, in most patients with type 1 diabetes mellitus who are able to understand and carry out the treatment regimen, who are not at increased risk for hypoglycemic episodes, and who do not have other characteristics that increase risk or decrease benefit, ADA and many clinicians currently recommend the use of physiologically based, intensive insulin regimens (i.e., 3 or more insulin injections daily of basal [intermediate- or long-acting] and prandial [short- or rapid-acting] insulin or continuous subcutaneous insulin infusion with dosage adjusted according to the results of multiple daily blood glucose determinations [e.g., 3 or 4 times daily], dietary intake, and anticipated exercise). (See Cautions: Precautions and Contraindications.)

The goal of intensive insulin therapy is to achieve near-normal glycemic control (some experts currently recommend a HbA$_{1c}$ target of less than 7% as a reasonable goal for nonpregnant adults); however, some clinicians recommend more stringent goals (i.e., HbA$_{1c}$ target of 6.5% or less), especially if this can be achieved without substantial hypoglycemia or other adverse effects. Because HbA$_{1c}$ is slightly lower in normal pregnancy than in normal nonpregnant women due to increased red blood cell turnover, ADA states that the ideal HbA$_{1c}$ in pregnant women is less than 6% but that target HbA$_{1c}$ may be relaxed to less than 7% to prevent hypoglycemia. ADA recommends a HbA$_{1c}$ target of less than 7.5% for older adults and even less stringent glycemic goals (i.e., HbA$_{1c}$ target of less than 8–8.5%) in older adults with multiple comorbidities, cognitive impairment, or functional dependence. In children and adolescents, ADA recommends an HbA$_{1c}$ target of less than 7.5% in those with type 1 diabetes mellitus (with individualization according to the needs of the patient and family), although a target less than 7% is reasonable if it can be achieved without excessive hypoglycemia. In children and adolescents with type 2 diabetes mellitus, ADA recommends an HbA$_{1c}$ target of less than 7% (or less than 6.5% if it can be achieved without substantial hypoglycemia or other adverse effects). (See Glycemic Control and Microvascular Complications under Uses: Diabetes Mellitus.)

Insulin regimens should be tailored to the specific clinical circumstances in individual patients. In patients without acute illness who are eating discrete meals, physiologic insulin requirements are composed of basal insulin (the amount of exogenous insulin per unit of time required to prevent unchecked gluconeogenesis and ketogenesis), meal-related (prandial or "bolus") insulin, and supplemental (correction-dose) insulin to cover premeal or between-meal hyperglycemia. Correction-dose insulin should not be confused with "sliding-scale" insulin regimens, which generally consist of set amounts of short-acting insulin given several times daily based on capillary blood glucose measurements without regard to timing of food, presence or absence of other insulin requirements, or consideration of individual patient sensitivity to insulin; such regimens have been ineffective in hospitalized diabetic patients and are not recommended. Use of such sliding-scale regimens treats existing hyperglycemia rather than preventing its occurrence and may lead to rapid changes in blood glucose concentrations, which exacerbates both hyperglycemia and hypoglycemia. In addition, studies have found that sliding-scale insulin regimens prescribed upon hospital admission are likely to be used throughout the hospital stay without modifications for risk factors for hypoglycemia or hyperglycemia, prehospital insulin treatment regimens, or patient's sensitivity to insulin.

In hospitalized patients, nutritional intake may not be provided principally as discrete meals, and insulin requirements should be considered to comprise basal and nutritional needs (e.g., IV dextrose, parenteral nutrition, enteral feedings, nutritional supplements, discrete meals). Determination of insulin requirements in hospitalized patients also must take into account counterregulatory responses to stress and/or illness and use of diabetogenic drugs (e.g., corticosteroids, vasopressors).

Subcutaneous insulin may be used to achieve glucose control in most noncritically ill hospitalized patients with diabetes mellitus, and various types of insulin may be used to achieve the daily insulin dose requirements. Subcutaneous insulin regimens in hospitalized patients generally consist of regularly scheduled injections of intermediate- or long-acting insulin to fulfill basal insulin requirements, with supplemental injections of rapid- or short-acting insulin as prandial and correction-dose insulin.

IV administration of regular insulin provides the greatest flexibility in dosing and is used in preference to subcutaneous administration in hospitalized patients with established diabetes mellitus or hyperglycemia (e.g., unrecognized diabetes mellitus, hospital-related hyperglycemia) for diabetic ketoacidosis, nonketotic hyperosmolar states, poorly controlled diabetes mellitus and widely fluctuating blood glucose concentrations, or severe insulin resistance. In critically ill patients, continuous IV insulin infusion has been demonstrated to be the most effective method for achieving glycemic control. Other situations that may require IV infusion of regular insulin include diabetic or hyperglycemic hospitalized patients who are not eating, have cardiogenic shock, or are experiencing exacerbated hyperglycemia during high-dose corticosteroid therapy. IV infusion of regular insulin also is used in general preoperative, intraoperative, and postoperative care, including heart or solid organ transplantation or surgery, or surgical patients requiring mechanical ventilation. IV regular insulin is also used as a dose-finding strategy in anticipation of initiation or reinitiation of subcutaneous insulin therapy in diabetic patients.

Combination Therapy with Other Antidiabetic Agents

Combined therapy with insulin and oral antidiabetic agents may be useful in some patients with type 2 diabetes mellitus whose blood glucose concentrations are not adequately controlled with maximal dosages of oral agent(s) and/or as a means of providing increased flexibility with respect to timing of meals and amount of food ingested. Some experts currently state that GLP-1 receptor agonists may be preferred over insulin in most patients who require the addition of a more potent glucose-lowering drug to achieve glycemic control. In clinical studies in patients receiving oral antidiabetic agents who required further blood glucose lowering, the efficacy of add-on therapy with a GLP-1 receptor agonist or insulin was similar. Additionally, use of GLP-1 receptor agonists was associated with beneficial effects on body weight and a lower risk of hypoglycemia compared with insulin, at the cost of a greater incidence of adverse GI effects.

Concomitant therapy with insulin (e.g., given as intermediate- or long-acting insulin at bedtime or rapid-acting insulin prior to meals) and one or more oral antidiabetic agents appears to improve glycemic control with lower dosages of insulin than would be required with insulin alone and may decrease the potential for body weight gain associated with insulin therapy. In addition, oral antidiabetic therapy combined with insulin therapy may delay progression to either more intensive insulin monotherapy or to a second daytime injection of insulin with oral antidiabetic agents. However, combined therapy may increase the risk of hypoglycemic reactions.

Patients who have inadequate glycemic control with basal insulin (with or without metformin) may benefit from the addition of a GLP-1 receptor agonist, a sodium glucose cotransporter-2 (SGLT2) inhibitor, or a dipeptidyl peptidase-4 (DPP-4) inhibitor (if not already receiving one of these agents). The combination of insulin and a DPP-4 inhibitor, GLP-1 receptor agonist, or SGLT2 inhibitor enhances blood glucose reductions and may minimize weight gain without increasing the risk of hypoglycemia. DPP-4 inhibitors and GLP-1 receptor agonists also increase endogenous insulin secretion in response to food, which may reduce postprandial hyperglycemia. Patients whose blood glucose concentrations remain uncontrolled despite treatment with basal insulin (e.g., given as intermediate-acting or long-acting insulin at bedtime or in the morning) in combination with oral antidiabetic agents or a GLP-1 receptor may require intensification of their insulin regimens through the addition of short-acting or rapid-acting insulin injections at mealtimes to control postprandial hyperglycemia.

Glycemic Control and Microvascular Complications

Current evidence from epidemiologic and clinical studies supports an association between chronic hyperglycemia and the pathogenesis of microvascular complications in patients with diabetes mellitus, and results of randomized, controlled studies in patients with type 1 diabetes mellitus indicate that intensive management of hyperglycemia with near-normalization of blood glucose and glycosylated hemoglobin (hemoglobin A$_{1c}$ [HbA$_{1c}$]) concentrations provides substantial benefits in terms of reducing chronic microvascular (e.g., neuropathy, retinopathy, nephropathy) complications associated with the disease. HbA$_{1c}$ concentration reflects the nonenzymatic glycosylation of other proteins throughout the body as a result of hyperglycemia over the previous 6–8 weeks and is used as a predictor of risk for the development of diabetic microvascular complications (e.g., neuropathy, retinopathy, nephropathy). Microvascular complications of diabetes are the principal causes of blindness and renal failure in developed countries and are more closely associated with hyperglycemia than are macrovascular complications.

In the Diabetes Control and Complications Trial (DCCT), a reduction of approximately 50–75% in the risk of development or progression of retinopathy, nephropathy, and neuropathy was demonstrated during an average 6.5 years of follow-up in patients with type 1 diabetes mellitus receiving intensive insulin treatment (3 or more insulin injections daily with dosage adjusted according to results of at least 4 daily blood glucose determinations, dietary intake, and anticipated exercise) compared with that in patients receiving conventional insulin treatment (1 or 2 insulin injections daily, self-monitoring of blood or urine glucose values, education about diet and exercise). However, the incidence of severe hypoglycemia, including multiple episodes in some patients, was 3 times higher in the intensive-treatment group than in the conventional-treatment group. The reduction in risk of microvascular complications in the DCCT correlated continuously with the reduction in HbA$_{1c}$ concentration produced by intensive insulin treatment (e.g., a 40% reduction in risk of microvascular disease for each 10% reduction in hemoglobin A$_{1c}$ concentration). These data imply that any reduction in HbA$_{1c}$ concentrations is beneficial and that complete normalization of blood glucose concentrations may prevent diabetic microvascular complications.

The DCCT was terminated prematurely because of the pronounced benefits of intensive insulin regimens, and all treatment groups were encouraged to institute or continue such intensive insulin therapy. In the Epidemiology of Diabetes Interventions and Complications (EDIC) study, the long-term, open-label continuation phase of the DCCT, the reduction in the risk of microvascular complications (e.g., retinopathy, nephropathy, neuropathy) associated with intensive insulin therapy has been maintained throughout 7 years of follow-up. In addition, the prevalence of hypertension (an important consequence of diabetic nephropathy) in those receiving conventional therapy has exceeded that of those receiving intensive therapy. Patients receiving conventional insulin therapy in the DCCT were able to achieve a lower HbA$_{1c}$ concentration when switched to intensive therapy in the continuation study, although the average HbA$_{1c}$ concentrations achieved during the continuation study were higher (i.e., worse) than those achieved during the DCCT with intensive insulin therapy. Patients who remained on intensive insulin therapy during the EDIC continuation study were not able to maintain the degree of glycemic control achieved during the DCCT; by 5 years of follow-up in the EDIC study, HbA$_{1c}$ concentrations were similar in both intensive and conventional therapy groups. The EDIC study demonstrated that the greater the duration of chronically elevated plasma glucose concentrations (as determined by HbA$_{1c}$ concentrations), the greater the risk of microvascular complications. Conversely, the longer patients can maintain a target HbA$_{1c}$ concentration of 7% or less, the greater the delay in the onset of these complications.

In another randomized, controlled study (Stockholm Diabetes Intervention Study) in patients with type 1 diabetes mellitus who were evaluated for up to 7.5 years, blood glucose control (as determined by HbA$_{1c}$ concentrations) was improved, and the incidence of microvascular complications (e.g., decreased visual acuity, retinopathy, nephropathy, decreased nerve conduction velocity) was reduced, with intensive insulin treatment (e.g., at least 3 insulin injections daily accompanied by intensive educational efforts) compared with that in patients receiving standard treatment (e.g., generally 2 insulin injections daily without intensive educational efforts).

Evidence from the United Kingdom Prospective Diabetes Study (UKPDS) and the Action in Diabetes and VAscular disease: preterax and diamicroN modified release Controlled Evaluation (ADVANCE) study in patients with type 2 diabetes mellitus generally is consistent with the same benefits of therapy with insulin and/or oral hypoglycemic agents on microvascular complications as those observed in type 1 diabetics receiving insulin therapy in the DCCT.

The UKPDS evaluated middle-aged, newly diagnosed, overweight (exceeding 120% of ideal body weight) or non-overweight patients with type 2 diabetes mellitus who received conventional or intensive treatment regimens with an oral antidiabetic agent and/or insulin. Intensive insulin (i.e., long-acting [UltraLente®, no longer commercially available in the US] or insulin human isophane [NPH] given once daily) therapy was initiated with a stepwise approach, in which the dosage of insulin is gradually increased, followed by addition of short-acting regular insulin at meals, and substitution of mixtures of short-acting and isophane (NPH) insulins given several times daily if preprandial or bedtime plasma glucose concentrations were above 126 mg/dL. Conventional treatment consisted of antidiabetic therapy targeted to a fasting plasma glucose concentration of less than 270 mg/dL without symptoms of hyperglycemia. Results of the UKPDS indicate greater beneficial effects on retinopathy, nephropathy, and possibly neuropathy with intensive glucose-lowering therapy (median achieved HbA$_{1c}$ concentration: 7%) in type 2 diabetics compared with that in the conventional treatment group (median achieved HbA$_{1c}$ concentration: 7.9%). The overall incidence of microvascular complications was reduced by 25% with intensive therapy. Epidemiologic analysis of the UKPDS results indicates a continuous relationship between the risks of microvascular complications and glycemia, with a 35% reduction in risk for each 1% reduction in HbA$_{1c}$ concentrations, and no evidence of a glycemic threshold.

The ADVANCE study also evaluated the relatively short-term effects (median follow-up: 5 years) of conventional or intensive therapy on the development of major vascular complications. The primary end point was the composite of major macrovascular (death from cardiovascular events, nonfatal myocardial infarction, or nonfatal stroke) and major microvascular (new or worsening nephropathy or retinopathy) events. While the incidence of the primary composite end point was reduced by approximately 10% in the ADVANCE study, the beneficial effect was due principally to a 21% reduction in microvascular events (nephropathy); there was no appreciable reduction in macrovascular outcomes. Intensive antidiabetic therapy (mean achieved HbA$_{1c}$ concentration: 6.5%) was associated with a reduction in new or worsening nephropathy compared with conventional treatment (mean achieved HbA$_{1c}$ concentration of 7.3%), but there was no effect on the development of new or worsening retinopathy. Results of the Veterans Affairs Diabetes Trial (VADT), another study similar in design to the ADVANCE study, also indicated that intensive therapy in patients with poorly controlled type 2 diabetes mellitus (median baseline HbA$_{1c}$ concentration of 9.4%) did not lessen the rate of microvascular complications compared with standard antidiabetic therapy.

In the UKPDS, fasting plasma glucose and HbA$_{1c}$ concentrations steadily increased over 10 years in the patients receiving conventional therapy, and more

than 80% of these patients eventually required antidiabetic therapy in addition to diet to maintain fasting plasma glucose concentrations within the desired goal of less than 270 mg/dL. In patients receiving intensive therapy initiated with insulin, chlorpropamide, or glyburide, fasting plasma glucose concentrations and HbA$_{1c}$ concentrations decreased during the first year of the study. Subsequent increases in these indices of glycemic control after the first year paralleled that in the conventional therapy group for the remainder of the study, indicating slow decline of pancreatic β-cell function and loss of glycemic control regardless of intensity of therapy. In contrast to UKPDS, no diminution in the effect on HbA$_{1c}$ or fasting blood glucose concentrations with either intensive or conventional therapy was observed in ADVANCE or VADT over a median follow-up of 5 or 5.6 years, respectively.

Macrovascular Outcomes and Cardiovascular Risk Reduction

Current evidence indicates that appropriate management of dyslipidemia, blood pressure, and vascular thrombosis provides substantial benefits in terms of reducing macrovascular complications associated with diabetes mellitus. In contrast to the demonstrated benefits of intensive glycemic control on microvascular complications, antidiabetic therapy titrated with the goal of reducing HbA$_{1c}$ to near-normal concentrations (6–6.5% or less) has not been associated with appreciable reductions in cardiovascular events during the randomized portion of controlled trials examining such outcomes. Data from recent, relatively short-term (median duration: 3.5–5.6 years) clinical trials (ADVANCE, VADT, Action to Control Cardiovascular Risk in Diabetes [ACCORD]) in patients with type 2 diabetes mellitus who were at high risk for cardiovascular disease (e.g., mean age 60–66 years, 8–12 years older than patients in UKPDS, disease duration of 8–11.5 years, known cardiovascular disease or multiple risk factors suggestive of atherosclerosis present in approximately one-third of patients) and were receiving intensive antidiabetic therapy (median achieved HbA$_{1c}$ concentrations of 6.3, 6.4, and 6.9% in ADVANCE, ACCORD, and VADT studies, respectively) have not demonstrated substantial reductions in the incidence of cardiovascular events beyond that associated with aggressive management of known cardiovascular risk factors (e.g., blood pressure control, dyslipidemia, smoking cessation).

However, results of long-term follow-up (10–11 years) from DCCT and UKPDS indicate a delayed cardiovascular benefit in patients treated with intensive antidiabetic therapy early in the course of type 1 or type 2 diabetes mellitus. Data from the DCCT-EDIC study, which reported the results of 11 years of follow-up from DCCT, have shown that patients with type 1 diabetes mellitus and without cardiovascular disease who were randomized to intensive insulin therapy at a relatively young age (13–40 years of age at time of randomization) had a 42% reduction in the risk of any cardiovascular event (i.e., myocardial infarction, stroke, angina, need for revascularization, cardiovascular death) and a 57% reduction in the risk of first nonfatal myocardial infarction, stroke, or cardiovascular death compared with those outcomes in patients randomized at baseline to conventional insulin therapy. Similarly, 10-year follow-up data from the UKPDS indicate that intensive therapy with sulfonylurea/insulin or metformin reduced the risk of myocardial infarction by 15 or 33%, respectively.

In middle-aged patients with well-established type 2 diabetes mellitus, some evidence of a cardiovascular benefit with intensive antidiabetic therapy also has been observed in certain subsets of patients with characteristics similar to those in the DCCT and UKPDS, such as those with a shorter duration of diabetes, lower baseline HbA$_{1c}$ concentrations, and/or absence of known cardiovascular disease. In the ACCORD study, prespecified subgroup analyses suggested that patients with no cardiovascular events at study entry and those with a baseline HbA$_{1c}$ concentration of 8% or less had a reduction in primary cardiovascular outcome (myocardial infarction, stroke, cardiovascular death). Posthoc subgroup analyses of the VADT suggested that patients with a duration of diabetes of less than 12 years appeared to have a cardiovascular benefit with intensive antidiabetic therapy while such therapy had a neutral or adverse effect on the development of cardiovascular disease in those with a longer duration of diabetes.

A relationship between glycemia (as determined by fasting glucose or HbA$_{1c}$ concentration) and vascular intima-media thickness, a surrogate marker for coronary and cerebrovascular disease, has been demonstrated in patients with and without diabetes mellitus. The delayed benefits of intensive antidiabetic therapy on risk of cardiovascular events in patients with diabetes mellitus in whom such therapy was initiated relatively early in the course of the disease may relate to reduction in the accumulation of advanced glycosylation end products that lead to the development of atherosclerosis over a period of years. Clinical data from long-term follow-up studies and subgroup analyses of relatively short-term studies suggest that intensive therapy may delay or prevent the progression of cardiovascular disease optimally in those without substantial atherosclerosis while providing minimal protection from cardiovascular events when the disease is well established. Subset analyses from EDIC and VADT examining carotid intima-media thickness and vascular calcification also suggest that intensive therapy reduces the progression of atherosclerosis in those with minimal or less advanced atherosclerosis. Data from the EDIC follow-up study to DCCT suggest that patients receiving intensive insulin therapy during DCCT had less progression of carotid intima-media thickness 6 years after completion of the DCCT than patients receiving conventional therapy. The lower HbA_{1c} concentration attained in the intensive therapy group during DCCT was associated with a decrease in the progression of carotid-intima media thickness at the end of the EDIC follow-up study. Limited data from VADT suggest that middle-aged patients with less coronary arterial calcification at baseline (coronary artery calcification Agatson scores of less than 100) had a reduction in cardiovascular events with intensive treatment. In contrast, patients in VADT with higher coronary arterial calcification at baseline (coronary artery calcification Agatson scores exceeding 100) did not have a reduction in cardiovascular events with intensive treatment.

Current strategies for intensive treatment of hyperglycemia and the associated increased risk of severe hypoglycemia in patients with advanced type 2 diabetes mellitus may have counterbalancing consequences for cardiovascular disease (e.g., myocardial ischemia/infarction, increased cardiovascular morbidity and mortality, weight gain, other metabolic changes). Potential risks of very intensive therapy may outweigh benefits in patients with a very long duration of diabetes; known history of severe hypoglycemia; advanced atherosclerosis or other cardiovascular disease; positive risk factors for cardiovascular disease; or advanced age or frailty. In the ACCORD study, patients with type 2 diabetes mellitus who were at high risk for cardiovascular disease and received intensive antidiabetic therapy had a 22 or 35% increase in the relative risk of all-cause or cardiovascular death, respectively, compared with that in patients receiving conventional antidiabetic therapy. Differences in mortality in patients receiving intensive therapy became apparent after 1 year and continued throughout follow-up until premature discontinuance of the intensive-therapy regimen after a mean of 3.5 years of follow-up. Exploratory analyses of episodes of severe hypoglycemia, differences in the use of ancillary drug therapy between those receiving conventional and intensive therapy, weight changes, achieved HbA_{1c} concentrations and rate of achievement of target HbA_{1c} concentrations, drug interactions, and other factors did not provide an explanation for the increased mortality observed in the ACCORD study. However, intensive therapy was not associated with an increase in mortality in the ADVANCE trial, another trial of similar design, despite achievement of a target HbA_{1c} concentration (median of 6.3%) that was similar to that achieved in the ACCORD trial (median of 6.4%). Differences in patient characteristics and study design between the ADVANCE and ACCORD trials may provide additional hypotheses regarding discrepancies between the effects of intensive therapy on mortality in these trials. Patients in the ADVANCE trial had less-advanced diabetes (disease duration 2–3 years shorter than in ACCORD) and had lower baseline HbA_{1c} despite use of insulin in only a small proportion of patients (1.5% of patients in the ADVANCE study were receiving insulin at baseline versus 35% of those in the ACCORD study). HbA_{1c} concentration was lowered more gradually to the target goal in the ADVANCE trial (several years versus 1 year to achieve maximum separation between HbA_{1c} in the ADVANCE or ACCORD trial, respectively); the target goal was achieved in the ADVANCE trial without appreciable weight gain and with fewer episodes of severe hypoglycemia than in ACCORD or VADT. Severe hypoglycemia occurred in less than 3%, approximately 16%, or 21% of patients receiving intensive therapy in ADVANCE, ACCORD, or VADT, respectively. Future combined analyses of the ADVANCE, ACCORD, and other trials should provide further insight into the effects of intensive antidiabetic therapy on the development of macrovascular events.

Data from clinical trials also support the use of certain oral antidiabetic agents (e.g., some SGLT2 inhibitors [canagliflozin, empagliflozin] or GLP-1 receptor agonists [liraglutide, semaglutide]) to reduce the risk of cardiovascular events in patients with type 2 diabetes mellitus and established cardiovascular disease. For further discussion on the use of certain SGLT2 inhibitors or GLP-1 receptor agonists for cardiovascular risk reduction, see the individual drug monographs in 68:20.

Treatment Goals

ADA generally recommends the same blood glucose and HbA_{1c} concentration goals for all nonpregnant adults with type 1 or type 2 diabetes mellitus but states that less stringent treatment goals may be appropriate for certain patients. ADA currently recommends target preprandial and peak postprandial (1–2 hours after

the *beginning* of a meal) *plasma* glucose concentrations of 80–130 and less than 180 mg/dL, respectively, and HbA_{1c} concentrations of less than 7% (based on a nondiabetic range of 4–6%) *in general* in adults with type 1 or 2 diabetes mellitus who are not pregnant. HbA_{1c} concentrations of 7% or greater should prompt clinicians to initiate or adjust antidiabetic therapy in nonpregnant patients with the goal of achieving HbA_{1c} concentrations of less than 7%. Patients with diabetes mellitus who have elevated HbA_{1c} concentrations despite having adequate preprandial glucose concentrations should monitor glucose concentrations 1–2 hours after the start of a meal.

More stringent treatment goals (i.e., HbA_{1c} concentrations even lower than the general goal of less than 7 or less than 6% in nonpregnant or pregnant patients, respectively, can be considered in selected patients. An *individualized* HbA_{1c} concentration goal that is closer to normal without risking severe hypoglycemia is reasonable in patients with a short duration of diabetes mellitus, no appreciable cardiovascular disease, and a long life expectancy. ADA recommends target preprandial and 2-hour postprandial blood glucose concentrations less than 95 and 120 mg/dL, respectively, in women with gestational diabetes mellitus. (See Cautions: Pregnancy and see Uses: Gestational Diabetes Mellitus.)

In hospitalized patients, ADA recommends a target blood glucose concentration of 140–180 mg/dL for the majority of critically ill and noncritically ill patients. Higher target glucose concentrations may be appropriate in terminally ill patients, those with severe comorbidities, and in patient care settings where frequent glucose monitoring is not feasible. An HbA_{1c} concentration should be obtained in all hospitalized diabetic patients if a current (previous 3 months) test is not available. Hospitalized patients who have hyperglycemia (random blood glucose concentration exceeding 140 mg/dL) should have a follow-up appointment with a clinician within 1 month of hospital discharge.

Treatment goals should be individualized, and specific target values for blood glucose and HbA_{1c} concentration appropriately adjusted, based on the patient's capacity to understand and adhere to the treatment regimen, the risk of severe hypoglycemia, and other patient factors that may increase risk or decrease benefit (e.g., young children [less than 6 years of age]; advanced age or frailty; cognitive or functional impairment; advanced microvascular or macrovascular complications or extensive comorbid conditions; other diseases that materially shorten life expectancy). Less stringent treatment goals may be appropriate in patients with long-standing diabetes mellitus in whom the general HbA_{1c} concentration goal of less than 7% is difficult to obtain despite adequate education on self-management of the disease, appropriate glucose monitoring, and effective dosages of multiple antidiabetic agents, including insulin. Achievement of HbA_{1c} concentrations less than 7% is not appropriate or practical for some patients, and clinical judgment should be used in designing a treatment regimen based on the potential benefits and risks (e.g., hypoglycemia) of more intensified therapy. Higher target blood glucose concentrations are advisable in patients with a history of recurrent, severe hypoglycemia and in patients with hypoglycemic unawareness, after they have been advised of the risks of intensive insulin therapy. Some clinicians consider it inappropriate to institute intensive therapy in these patients because they may have defective glucose counterregulatory responses. Severe or frequent hypoglycemia is an absolute indication for modification of treatment regimens, including setting higher glycemic goals. Clinicians should be vigilant in the prevention of severe hypoglycemia in patients with advanced diabetes mellitus and should not aggressively attempt to achieve near-normal HbA_{1c} concentrations in patients in whom such a target cannot be achieved with reasonable ease and safety.

Data from a decision model based on extrapolated benefits of intensive glycemic control in type 1 diabetic patients (i.e., as demonstrated in the Diabetes Control and Complications Trial [DCCT]) suggest substantial benefits (i.e., in terms of reduction in years of blindness or end-stage renal disease) of reducing HbA_{1c} to near-normal concentrations (e.g., from 9 to 7%) in patients with early-onset (i.e., at 40–50 years of age) type 2 diabetes mellitus. Geriatric patients with a life expectancy long enough to reap the benefits of long-term intensive diabetes management who are active, cognitively intact, and willing to self-manage diabetes mellitus should be treated using the same goals for younger adults with diabetes mellitus. For frail geriatric patients, patients with an intermediate remaining life expectancy, and those in whom the risks of intensive glycemic control appears to outweigh the benefits, a less stringent target HbA_{1c} concentration such as 8% is appropriate. An even less stringent target HbA_{1c} concentration (i.e., less than 8.5%) may be considered in geriatric patients in very poor health and with a limited life expectancy. Hyperglycemia leading to symptoms or risk of acute hyperglycemic complications should be avoided in all geriatric patients.

In children and adolescents with type 1 diabetes mellitus, ADA recommends target preprandial and bedtime/overnight plasma glucose concentrations of 90–130 and 90–150 mg/dL, respectively, and HbA$_{1c}$ concentrations of less than 7.5% (a lower goal of less than 7% may be reasonable if it can be achieved without excessive hypoglycemia). Special consideration should be given to the risk of hypoglycemia in young children (younger than 6 years of age) who may be unable to recognize, articulate, and/or manage hypoglycemia. However, some data indicate that young children can achieve target HbA$_{1c}$ concentrations without increased risk of severe hypoglycemia. In children and adolescents with type 2 diabetes mellitus, ADA recommends a target HbA$_{1c}$ concentration of less than 7% in those patients treated with oral antidiabetic agents alone; more stringent targets (i.e., less than 6.5%) may be appropriate for certain individuals who can achieve this concentration without substantial hypoglycemia or other adverse effects. Treatment goals should be individualized and the benefits of achieving a lower HbA$_{1c}$ concentration should be weighed against the risks of hypoglycemia and the developmental burdens of intensive antidiabetic regimens in children and adolescents.

Gestational Diabetes Mellitus

Gestational diabetes mellitus is a condition in which a woman without clearly overt diabetes mellitus prior to pregnancy develops glucose intolerance (i.e., elevated blood glucose concentrations) during pregnancy. (See Insulin Use during Pregnancy under Dosage and Administration: Dosage.) Gestational diabetes mellitus may be associated with macrosomia, birth complications, and an increased risk of maternal type 2 diabetes mellitus after pregnancy. (See Cautions: Pregnancy.) ADA states that insulin therapy is preferred in patients with gestational diabetes who, despite dietary management (medical nutrition therapy [MNT]), have fasting blood glucose concentrations of 95 mg/dL or higher, 1-hour postprandial blood glucose concentrations of 140 mg/dL or higher, or 2-hour postprandial blood glucose concentrations of 120 mg/dL or higher. Long-acting and intermediate-acting insulins used in gestational diabetes mellitus include NPH insulin, insulin glargine, and insulin detemir. When short-acting insulins are used, insulin lispro and insulin aspart are preferred over regular human insulin because of the former drugs' rapid onset of action. Oral antidiabetic agents (e.g., glyburide, metformin) are not recommended as first-line therapy because these drugs are able to cross the placenta and data on the safety of these drugs in offspring are lacking.

Women with gestational diabetes should be evaluated for prediabetes or persistent diabetes mellitus at least 4–12 weeks postpartum using a 75-g, 2-hour oral glucose tolerance test. Follow-up should be performed every 1–3 years thereafter if the results of the postpartum glucose tolerance test at 4–12 weeks are normal. Women with impaired glucose tolerance in the postpartum period should attempt lifestyle changes to prevent or delay the progression to diabetes mellitus; initiating therapy with metformin also may be considered. Subsequent pregnancies should be planned to ensure optimal glycemic control throughout pregnancy.

Critical Illness

Moderate glycemic control has been shown to reduce morbidity and mortality in hospitalized patients with critical illness† requiring intensive care. Randomized, clinical studies and meta-analyses of studies in surgical patients have indicated lower rates of mortality and stroke with a perioperative blood glucose target of less than 180 mg/dL compared with a target of less than 200 mg/dL; no substantial additional benefit was found with more stringent glycemic control (i.e., blood glucose concentration less than 140 mg/dL). Some experts recommend a blood glucose target of 140–180 mg/dL in most hospitalized patients; more stringent goals (i.e., 110–140 mg/dL) may be appropriate in selected patients if substantial hypoglycemia can be avoided. While some experts recommend initiating insulin therapy when blood glucose concentrations reach 180 mg/dL or higher, other clinicians recommend initiating therapy at lower blood glucose concentrations (e.g., 150 mg/dL or higher). When insulin is used in critically ill patients, most experts recommend that insulin be administered by continuous IV infusion.

Acute Myocardial Infarction

Data from several clinical trials in patients with ST-segment-elevation myocardial infarction (STEMI) suggest that blood glucose concentrations are positively correlated with mortality. Current data suggest that high-dose regular insulin in combination with IV potassium chloride and dextrose (D-glucose) (referred to as glucose-insulin-potassium or GIK therapy) is *not* beneficial in reducing mortality following ST-segment-elevation myocardial infarction (STEMI) and may even be harmful. The American College of Cardiology Foundation (ACCF) and American Heart Association (AHA) state that blood glucose levels should be maintained below 180 mg/dL if possible while avoiding hypoglycemia and that there is no established role for GIK infusions in patients with STEMI.

Hyperalimentation Adjunct

Regular insulin has been added to IV hyperalimentation solutions to assure proper utilization of glucose and reduce glycosuria in diabetic patients. Addition of insulin also may be beneficial in nondiabetic patients whose glycosuria cannot be controlled by adjustment of the infusion flow rate. Because not all nondiabetic patients receiving hyperalimentation therapy require insulin and because of variable adsorption of insulin to the IV infusion system, there is debate over the value of adding insulin to hyperalimentation solutions. If insulin is required in patients receiving hyperalimentation therapy, some clinicians prefer subcutaneous or direct IV injection. Since insulin requirements may vary abruptly in patients receiving hyperalimentation, insulin dosage must be carefully adjusted based on frequent determinations of blood and urine glucose concentrations.

Growth Hormone Reserve Test

IV injection of regular insulin is used as a provocative test for growth hormone secretion.

Hyperkalemia

Regular insulin has also been added to IV dextrose infusions to facilitate an intracellular shift of potassium in the treatment of severe hyperkalemia.

DOSAGE AND ADMINISTRATION

Administration

Insulin usually is administered by subcutaneous injection. The subcutaneous route is preferred to IM administration because it provides more prolonged absorption and is less painful. Regular insulin may be given IV or IM under medical supervision with close monitoring of blood glucose and potassium concentrations to avoid hypoglycemia and hypokalemia. Regular insulin also may be administered IV for general perioperative use and during the postoperative period following cardiac surgery or organ transplantation; in patients with diabetic ketoacidosis, nonketotic hyperosmolar state, cardiogenic shock, critical illness, or exacerbated hyperglycemia during high-dose corticosteroid therapy, or in those who are not eating; and to facilitate determination of optimal dosage prior to initiating or reinitiating subcutaneous insulin therapy in patients with type 1 or type 2 diabetes mellitus. Rapid-acting insulins (e.g., insulin lispro, insulin glulisine, insulin aspart) have been used IV, but such use offers no advantage over regular insulin (insulin human).

Subcutaneous administration of insulin has been made into the thighs, upper arms, buttocks, or abdomen using a 25- to 28-gauge needle 1.3–1.6 cm in length. With the availability of smaller 30- and 31-gauge needles, the needle tip may become bent to form a hook, which can lacerate tissue or break off to leave needle fragments within the skin. The medical consequences of these needle fragments are unknown but may increase the risk of lipodystrophy or other adverse effects. *It is essential to use only syringes calibrated for the particular concentration of insulin administered.* To avoid painful injections, patients should inject insulin that is at room temperature. To prevent air bubbles in an insulin pen, the injection pen should be primed with 2 units of insulin before injection; patients should avoid leaving a needle in the pen between injections. In most individuals, a fold of the skin is grasped lightly with the fingers at least 7.6 cm apart and the needle inserted at a 90° angle; thin individuals or children may need to pinch the skin and inject at a 45° angle to avoid IM injection of the dose, especially in the thigh area. Routine aspiration (to check for inadvertent intravascular injection as indicated by the presence of blood in the syringe) after subcutaneous injection of insulin generally is not necessary. The insulin should be injected over a period of at least 6 seconds; presence of air bubbles could interfere with accurate dosing. The push button of the insulin injection pen or other compatible insulin delivery device should continue to be depressed during drug delivery until the needle is withdrawn from the skin to ensure that the full dose has been delivered. Preparations of insulin suspensions that are injected slowly may clog the tip of the needle, preventing completion of the injection. The injection site should be pressed lightly for a few seconds after the needle is withdrawn but should not be rubbed. A planned rotation of sites within one area should be followed so that any one site is not injected more than once every 1–2 weeks. Rotating injection sites within one anatomic region (e.g., rotating injections systematically in the abdominal area) rather than selecting a different anatomic region is recommended to decrease day-to-day variability in insulin absorption. Variability in insulin absorption by injection site is reduced with insulin lispro compared with that with insulin human.

The American Diabetes Association (ADA) states that if an insulin injection seems particularly painful or if blood or clear fluid is observed after withdrawing the needle, patients should be instructed to apply pressure to the injection site for 5–8 seconds without rubbing and perform blood glucose monitoring more frequently that day. If the patient suspects that an appreciable portion of the insulin dose was not administered, blood glucose should be checked within a few hours after the injection and supplemental insulin administered if necessary. (See Dosage and Administration: Administration.)

Although most insulin syringes have been designed to eliminate dead-space volume, dosage errors attributable to the dead-space volume within some insulin syringes may result when 2 types of insulin are mixed in the syringes. Patients stabilized on a particular order of mixing and using a particular brand and design of syringe should not change these factors without first consulting their physician.

Alternatively, specialized delivery devices (e.g., subcutaneous controlled-infusion devices [pumps], insulin pens) have been used to administer insulins, and the manufacturers' instructions should be consulted for proper methods of assembly, administration (including dosage calibration), and care. For information on subcutaneous controlled-infusion devices, see Dosage and Administration: Administration, in Insulin Aspart 68:20.08/04 and also see Dosage and Administration: Administration, in Insulin Lispro 68:20.08.04.

● **Dosage**

Dosage of insulin injection is always expressed in USP units. The number of units in a given volume varies with the strength of the preparation employed. Commercially available insulin human (regular insulin) preparations contain 100 (U-100) or 500 (U-500) units per mL. All commercially available preparations have standardized label colors to facilitate identification. Concentrated (U-500) insulin human injection is indicated in diabetic patients with daily insulin requirements exceeding 200 units, so that a large dose may be administered subcutaneously in a relatively small volume.

Insulin Regimens

Both conventional and intensive insulin treatment regimens have been used in patients with type 1 or type 2 diabetes mellitus. (See Glycemic Control and Microvascular Complications under Uses: Diabetes Mellitus.) Conventional therapy generally consists of 1 or 2 subcutaneous doses of insulin per day (e.g., at breakfast and/or dinner), usually with a mixture of intermediate-acting and rapid- or short-acting insulin; blood glucose concentrations generally are monitored 1–4 times daily. Commercially available premixed insulin combinations may be used if the insulin ratio is appropriate to the patient's insulin requirements; these preparations may be especially useful in patients with type 2 diabetes mellitus who eat small lunches, geriatric patients, those unable to use more complex regimens, and those with visual impairment. Premixed insulins offer little flexibility for meal size and time, particularly in patients with severe insulin deficiency (i.e., most patients with type 1 diabetes mellitus), since such mixtures of insulins may not provide enough insulin for lunchtime needs.

The selection of a particular insulin treatment program is dependent on a number of factors including the age of the patient, the nature of the disease (ketoacidosis-prone or ketoacidosis-resistant), the presence or absence of symptoms of hyperglycemia, and the experience and judgment of the clinician. Initial total daily insulin dosages in adults and children with type 1 diabetes mellitus generally range from 0.4–1 units/kg; basal insulin requirements with an intermediate-acting or long-acting insulin usually comprise 40–60% of the total daily insulin dosage, with the remainder given preprandially as rapid- or short-acting insulin. Alternatively, some manufacturers recommend that basal insulin comprise approximately one-third to one-half of the total daily insulin dosage in insulin-naive patients with type 1 diabetes mellitus, with the remainder of the daily dosage given preprandially as rapid- or short-acting insulin.

To initiate therapy in patients with severe symptomatic diabetes, unstable type 1 diabetes, severe metabolic dysfunction, or diabetes with complications, hospitalization and the use of regular insulin may be advisable. Some clinicians suggest that in general, insulin therapy in adults of normal weight may be initiated with 15–20 units daily of an intermediate-acting (e.g., insulin human isophane [NPH]) or long-acting (e.g., insulin glargine, insulin detemir) insulin given subcutaneously before breakfast, dinner, or bedtime; obese patients, because of associated insulin resistance, may initially be given 25–30 units daily. Use of rapid- or short-acting insulin alone before meals may rarely be sufficient in newly diagnosed patients with diabetes mellitus who have some residual basal endogenous insulin secretion.

In patients with type 2 diabetes mellitus who have secondary failure to oral antidiabetic agent(s), an intermediate-acting or long-acting insulin may be added to the existing oral antidiabetic regimen; premixed insulin combinations containing insulin human isophane (NPH) may be given once daily with the evening meal in such patients. Initial dosage of a basal insulin (e.g., intermediate-acting insulin at bedtime, long-acting insulin at bedtime or morning) in patients with type 2 diabetes mellitus inadequately controlled on oral antidiabetic agent(s) generally is 0.1–0.2 units/kg daily or 10 units daily. Patients should be advised that initial insulin dosages are approximations and that frequent dosage adjustments will be required over the next few weeks. ADA recommends the use of an evidence-based insulin dosage titration algorithm (i.e., increase of 2 units every 3 days to achieve target fasting plasma glucose concentration).

Virtually all patients with type 1 diabetes mellitus and many with type 2 diabetes mellitus will require 2 or more insulin injections daily with intermediate-acting and/or rapid- or short-acting insulins to maintain adequate control of blood glucose throughout the night while avoiding daytime hypoglycemia. ADA currently recommends the same blood glucose and HbA$_{1c}$ concentration goals for all nonpregnant adults with type 1 or type 2 diabetes mellitus but states that less stringent treatment goals may be appropriate for certain patients. (See Treatment Goals under Uses: Diabetes Mellitus.) If a patient's HbA$_{1c}$ remains above target despite the use of adequately titrated basal insulin or daily basal insulin dosages exceeding 0.7–1 unit/kg, or despite achieving target fasting plasma glucose concentrations, prandial insulin should be initiated. Prandial insulin should be given with the largest meal of the day or the meal associated with the greatest postprandial plasma glucose concentration. More prandial insulin may be added in a stepwise manner (i.e., 2, then 3 additional injections) to a patient's regimen as needed. The recommended starting dose of prandial insulin in patients with type 2 diabetes mellitus is either 4 units or 10% of the basal dose at each meal.

Intensive insulin therapy generally refers to regimens consisting of 3 or more doses of insulin per day administered by subcutaneous injection or continuous subcutaneous infusion of insulin via an insulin pump, with dosage adjustments made according to the results of frequent (e.g., at least 3–4 times daily) self-monitored blood glucose determinations and anticipated dietary intake and exercise. Since patients receiving intensive insulin therapy generally will achieve greater postprandial glycemic control than those receiving conventional therapy because of increased use of rapid- or short-acting insulin, patients receiving conventional insulin regimens generally will require a smaller total daily insulin dosage when switched to an intensive insulin regimen.

In patients with type 1 diabetes mellitus who have been receiving conventional insulin therapy (e.g., twice-daily doses of intermediate-acting and rapid- or short-acting insulin given before breakfast and the evening meal), intensive insulin therapy may be initiated with a stepwise approach in which the number of insulin injections per day is gradually increased until near-normal postprandial and basal glycemic control is attained. Alternatively, a dose of long-acting insulin (e.g., insulin glargine) may be administered in the evening in conjunction with doses of a rapid-acting (e.g., insulin lispro, insulin aspart, insulin glulisine) or short-acting (e.g., regular) insulin before each meal. Because of insulin degludec's very long duration of action (e.g., 42 hours) and low variability in insulin concentrations over the dosing interval, it can be administered at any time of day in adults, which may provide greater dosing flexibility than other basal insulins such as insulin detemir or insulin glargine.

A subcutaneous insulin regimen in hospitalized patients is comprised of regularly scheduled subcutaneous injections (basal and prandial) and correctional (supplemental) injections as an adjunct to regularly scheduled insulin to meet nutritional needs. Premixed insulin regimens are not routinely recommended for in-hospital use. Daily insulin dose requirements can be met by various types of insulin, depending on the particular clinical situation. Since insulin human has a longer duration of action than more rapid-acting analogues, use of correctional insulin for premeal or between-meal hyperglycemia before previously administered regular insulin has reached a peak effect may lead to hypoglycemia.

IV insulin is considered the standard of care for management of hyperglycemia in critically ill patients. IV infusion of regular insulin may be used in hospitalized patients with diabetic ketoacidosis, nonketotic hyperosmolar states, cardiogenic shock, exacerbated hyperglycemia during high-dose corticosteroid therapy, poorly controlled diabetes mellitus and widely fluctuating blood glucose concentrations, severe insulin resistance, or as a dose-finding strategy prior to initiation or reinitiation of subcutaneous insulin therapy. IV administration of regular insulin also is recommended during general perioperative care and the postoperative period following cardiac surgery or organ transplantation or when a prolonged postoperative period with no oral intake is anticipated (e.g., cardiothoracic, major abdominal, CNS surgery). The initial perioperative maintenance insulin infusion rate in patients undergoing major surgery is 0.2 units/kg per hour. When regular insulin is administered by continuous IV infusion, bedside glucose testing should be performed every hour until blood glucose concentrations are stable for 6–8 hours; the frequency of testing can then be reduced to every 2–3 hours. Dosing algorithms should achieve correction of hyperglycemia in a timely manner, provide a method to adjust the insulin infusion rate required to maintain blood glucose concentrations within a defined target range, and allow for the adjustment of insulin infusion maintenance rate as patient's insulin sensitivity or carbohydrate intake changes.

When normoglycemia has been reached after IV insulin infusion in hospitalized patients, some patients will require subcutaneous insulin maintenance therapy and some patients with type 2 diabetes mellitus will have therapy transferred to oral antidiabetic agents. For those who require subcutaneous insulin, basal insulin should be administered 2–4 hours prior to discontinuance of the IV insulin infusion. Converting to basal insulin at 60–80% of the daily IV insulin infusion dose has been shown to be effective.

Data indicate that continuous subcutaneous insulin injection (i.e., insulin pump) may provide a slight advantage in reducing HbA_{1c} and the risk of severe hypoglycemia compared with multiple daily insulin injections. ADA recommends that most adults, children, and adolescents with type 1 diabetes mellitus should be treated with intensive insulin therapy with multiple daily insulin injections or an insulin pump. ADA also states that an insulin pump may be considered in all children and adolescents requiring insulin therapy, especially those younger than 7 years of age.

Any change of insulin preparation or dosage regimen should be made with caution and only under medical supervision. Should a brand of insulin become unavailable temporarily, the same insulin formulation from another manufacturer may be substituted. Although it is not possible to clearly identify which patients will require a change in dosage when therapy with a different preparation is started, it is known that a limited number of patients will require such a change. Adjustments may be needed with the first dose or may occur over a period of several weeks. In general, the usual initial dosage reduction in these patients is about 10–20%.

Considerations in Monitoring Insulin Therapy

Patients receiving intensive insulin regimens should self-monitor blood glucose concentrations prior to meals and snacks, at bedtime, occasionally postprandially, prior to exercise, when low blood glucose is suspected, after treating low blood glucose (until normoglycemic), and prior to critical tasks (e.g., driving); this may require patients to test up to 6–10 times daily. Patients not receiving intensive insulin regimens, such as those receiving basal insulin only, should at least assess fasting blood glucose concentrations in order to facilitate dosage adjustments; data regarding the exact number of times a patient should ideally check their blood glucose concentrations are lacking in this patient population. Blood glucose concentrations may be influenced by food consumption, exercise, stress, hormonal changes, illness, travel, insulin absorption rates, and insulin sensitivity.

If preprandial blood glucose concentrations consistently exceed 300 mg/dL, patients should be instructed to monitor for ketones in urine or blood (β-hydroxybutyric acid). The presence of ketones in urine or blood may indicate insulin deficiency or insulin resistance; in such cases, clinicians should consider possible causes of insulin deficiency, such as a missed insulin dose or illness, and supplement the dosage of insulin as appropriate. (See Diabetic Ketoacidosis and Hyperosmolar Hyperglycemic States under Dosage and Administration: Dosage, in Insulin Human 68:20.08.08.)

If blood glucose concentrations are unexpectedly high, additional doses of short- or rapid-acting insulin (e.g., up to 15% of the regular dose) may be necessary to reestablish glycemic control. Blood glucose concentrations should be reassessed approximately 4 hours after additional doses have been given. If blood glucose concentrations are still high, another dose of insulin (e.g., 5% of the regular dose) may be given to achieve glycemic control. Records of self-monitored blood glucose concentrations should be compared with clinician-obtained values for evidence of faulty injection technique or patient noncompliance. Patients should contact their clinician if extra insulin fails to reduce high blood glucose concentrations and/or ketonuria or ketonemia.

Insulin Use During Pregnancy

Insulin requirements generally increase, sometimes dramatically, in pregnant patients with diabetes. In addition, pregnancy may induce a temporary state of diabetes in patients not previously known to be diabetic (i.e., gestational diabetes mellitus). (See Uses: Gestational Diabetes Mellitus.) The increased need for insulin generally begins in the second trimester, and an insulin regimen should be established during preconception care visits. In high-risk pregnancies, hospitalization may be required to ensure an appropriate insulin regimen. Since the renal threshold for glucose may be decreased during pregnancy, blood glucose determinations are needed to ascertain the effectiveness of therapy.

In patients with gestational diabetes mellitus requiring insulin therapy, the usual initial total daily dosage is 0.7–1 units/kg, given in divided doses. In women with gestational diabetes, if fasting and postprandial hyperglycemia are present, an insulin regimen consisting of long-acting or intermediate-acting insulin in conjunction with short-acting insulin is recommended. In women with gestational diabetes mellitus who have only isolated high blood glucose concentrations at specific times of the day, an insulin regimen which focuses on the times when hyperglycemia occurs is preferred (e.g., administering short-acting insulin prior to certain meals of the day).

Maternal blood glucose monitoring in women with gestational diabetes mellitus should be instituted to assess glycemic control. Self-monitoring of fasting and postprandial blood glucose concentrations are recommended in women with gestational diabetes mellitus and pre-existing diabetes mellitus. Additionally, pregnant women who are using an insulin pump or basal-bolus insulin therapy should also test preprandial blood glucose concentrations in order to facilitate insulin dosage adjustments.

CAUTIONS

● Endocrine and Metabolic Effects

Hypoglycemia

Hypoglycemia is the most common adverse effect of insulins, and monitoring of blood glucose concentrations is recommended for all patients with diabetes. The timing of hypoglycemia depends on the time of peak action of insulin in relation to food intake (absorption) and/or exercise. The risk of hypoglycemia is increased in patients with unstable type 1 diabetes, autonomic neuropathy, or irregular eating patterns and in patients receiving intensive insulin therapy or who exercise without making appropriate insulin dosage adjustments or ingesting extra food. Hypoglycemia also may result from increased insulin absorption rates (e.g., increased skin temperature resulting from sunbathing or exposure to hot water). Hypoglycemic reactions also have been reported in patients who were transferred from beef to pork insulin or mixed beef-pork preparations or from pork insulin (no longer commercially available in the US) to insulin human; however, preparations containing beef insulin alone or in combination with pork insulin are no longer commercially available in the US. Hypoglycemia also may occur in association with increased insulin sensitivity that accompanies secondary adrenocortical insufficiency or Addison's disease.

Symptoms of hypoglycemia usually are manifested when the administered insulin reaches its peak action and may include hunger, pallor, fatigue, mild or profuse perspiration, headache, nausea, palpitation, numbness of the mouth, tingling in the fingers, tremors, muscle weakness, blurred or double vision, hypothermia, uncontrolled yawning, nervousness, irritability or agitation, difficulty in concentrating, mental confusion, aggressiveness, drowsiness, tachycardia, shallow breathing, seizures, and loss of consciousness. Insulin overdosage may result in psychic disturbances such as aphasia, personality changes, or maniacal behavior. Homeostatic responses to hypoglycemia include cessation of insulin release and mobilization of counterregulatory hormones such as glucagon, epinephrine, and less acutely, growth hormone and cortisol. These responses become defective, and early warning signs of hypoglycemia may be diminished or absent, in patients with long-standing type 1 diabetes mellitus diabetic neuropathy, and/or those receiving drugs such as β-adrenergic blocking agents that mask catecholamine-induced manifestations of hypoglycemia (e.g., tremors, palpitations) or intensive insulin therapy. If untreated, severe prolonged hypoglycemia can result in irreversible brain damage.

Hypoglycemic reactions in geriatric diabetic patients may mimic a cerebrovascular accident. In addition, because of an increased incidence of macrovascular disease in geriatric patients with type 2 diabetes mellitus, such patients may be more vulnerable to serious consequences of hypoglycemia, including fainting, seizures, falls, stroke, silent ischemia, myocardial infarction, or sudden death.

The more vigorous the attempt to achieve euglycemia, the greater the risk of hypoglycemia. In the Diabetes Control and Complications Trial (DCCT), the incidence of severe hypoglycemia, including multiple episodes in some patients, was 3 times higher in patients receiving intensive insulin treatment (3 or more insulin injections daily with dosage adjusted according to results of at least 4 daily blood glucose determinations, dietary intake, and anticipated exercise) than in those receiving conventional treatment (1 or 2 insulin injections daily, self-monitoring of blood or urine glucose values, education about diet and exercise). In the Action to Control Cardiovascular Risk in Diabetes (ACCORD) trial in patients with type 2 diabetes mellitus, the incidence of severe hypoglycemia (episodes requiring medical assistance) was 10.5 or 3.5% in patients receiving intensive (median achieved HbA_{1c} concentrations: 6.4%) or conventional (median achieved HbA_{1c} concentrations: 7.5%) treatment, respectively. Hypoglycemia is the major risk that must be considered against the benefits of intensive insulin therapy. An increased rate of mortality was noted among patients in the ACCORD trial receiving intensive treatment; preliminary exploratory analyses evaluating numerous variables, including hypoglycemia, were unable to identify an explanation for increased mortality in the intensive therapy group. However, in DCCT, there was no increase in mortality or permanent neuropsychologic morbidity associated with the increased rate of severe hypoglycemia in that study. Since symptoms of hypoglycemia may develop suddenly, diabetic patients should be instructed to carry a ready source of carbohydrate as well as some form of diabetic identification. Episodes of late postprandial hypoglycemia (i.e., 4–6 hours after a meal) observed with the use of short-acting insulin before meals occur as a consequence of hyperinsulinemia present when the meal has been almost totally absorbed. The potential for late postprandial hypoglycemia observed with short-acting insulin may be reduced by altering the timing, frequency, and content of meals, altering exercise patterns, frequently monitoring blood glucose concentrations, adjusting insulin dosage, and/or switching to a more rapid-acting insulin (e.g., insulin lispro, insulin glulisine).

Rebound Hyperglycemia

Hyperglycemia that occurs as a result of excessive counterregulatory hormone responses to hypoglycemia (Somogyi effect, posthypoglycemic hyperglycemia) appears to occur principally in patients with type 1 diabetes mellitus. While the exact mechanism of this effect is unknown and there is controversy regarding whether it even exists, it has been suggested that excessive doses of an intermediate-acting (e.g., isophane [NPH]) insulin in the evening lead to nocturnal hypoglycemia and a compensatory release of counterregulatory hormones (e.g., epinephrine, growth hormone, cortisol, glucagon), resulting in increased hepatic glucose production and rebound hyperglycemia the following morning. The existence of such "rebound" hyperglycemia and/or the frequency with which it occurs has been questioned since the effect often has not been reproducible in clinical studies (particularly in adults), and neuroendocrine counterregulatory responses to hypoglycemia are known to be reduced in patients with long-standing diabetes mellitus. Some clinicians suggest that morning hyperglycemia occurring after an episode of nocturnal hypoglycemia results principally from overzealous intake of carbohydrate in an attempt to correct the hypoglycemia; other proposed mechanisms for this effect include the waning action of the insulin that caused the hypoglycemia and hypoglycemia-induced insulin resistance.

Manifestations suggesting an excessive insulin dosage in patients with hyperglycemia include excessive appetite and weight gain, nocturnal hypoglycemia, extreme variations in glucose concentrations, and frequent ketosis (especially in the absence of glycosuria), with worsening of these manifestations when insulin dosage is increased. The Somogyi effect must be differentiated from the "dawn phenomenon," which is characterized by early morning hyperglycemia that appears related to nocturnal growth hormone release and the patient's inability to compensate for increased blood glucose concentrations with an increase in endogenous insulin secretion; differentiation of the Somogyi effect and the dawn phenomenon may be accomplished by monitoring blood glucose at 3 a.m. Recommended treatment for the Somogyi effect, if it is suspected, is gradual *reduction* of the evening intermediate-acting insulin dosage or addition of/increase in the size of the nighttime snack (with a slowly absorbable carbohydrate) in conjunction with continuous blood glucose monitoring. (See Dosage and Administration: Dosage.) The dawn phenomenon reflects a relative deficiency of insulin and is treated by *increasing* the evening intermediate-acting insulin dose and/or later administration of that dose (i.e., at bedtime rather than at dinner).

Potassium Effects

Hypokalemia may occur with insulin therapy since insulin promotes an intracellular shift of potassium as a result of stimulating cell membrane Na+- K+-ATPase. Untreated hypokalemia may result in respiratory paralysis, ventricular arrhythmia, and death.

● Dermatologic and Sensitivity Reactions

Localized allergic reactions such as pruritus, erythema, swelling, stinging or warmth at the site of injection may develop in patients receiving insulin. Localized allergic reactions may occur within 1–3 weeks after initiating insulin therapy, are relatively minor, and usually disappear within a few days to weeks. Poor injection technique may contribute to localized injection site reactions.

Manifestations of immediate hypersensitivity commonly occur within 30–120 minutes after the injection, may last for several hours or days, and usually subside spontaneously. True insulin allergy is rare and is characterized by generalized urticaria or bullae, dyspnea, wheezing, hypotension, tachycardia, diaphoresis, angioedema, and anaphylaxis. These reactions may represent a secondary anamnestic response and occur most frequently after intermittent insulin therapy or in patients with increased circulating insulin antibodies. Severe cases of generalized insulin allergy may be life-threatening. (See Cautions: Precautions and Contraindications.) There is some evidence that the incidence of allergic reactions has decreased with the availability of more purified insulin (e.g., insulin human, insulin lispro). In addition, several studies have shown insulin human and insulin lispro to be less immunogenic than animal-source insulin (i.e., purified pork insulin, beef insulin). Preparations containing beef or pork insulin are no longer commercially available in the US. (See Cautions: Immunogenicity, in Insulin Human 68:20.08.08 and Insulin Lispro 68:20.08.04.)

Atrophy or hypertrophy of subcutaneous fat tissue may occur at sites of frequent insulin injections. (See Cautions: Precautions and Contraindications.) Lipoatrophy is thought to be the result of an immune reaction to some contaminant of insulin.

● Insulin Resistance

Resistance to insulin in patients with type 1 diabetes mellitus occurs infrequently and may be caused by either immune or nonimmune factors. Patients with insulin resistance usually require more than 200 units of insulin daily; in comparison, data from a small number of patients who had undergone pancreatectomy indicate that 10–44 units of insulin daily were required to control secondary diabetes mellitus.

Insulin resistance in patients with type 2 diabetes mellitus is frequently associated with obesity. This type of resistance results from tissue insensitivity to insulin, which may be caused by a decrease in the number of insulin receptors or a decreased affinity of insulin for the receptors. The principal treatment for obesity-related insulin resistance is weight reduction.

Acute insulin resistance may develop in diabetic patients with infections, surgical or other trauma, emotional disturbances, or additional endocrine disorders (e.g., hyperthyroidism, acromegaly, Cushing's syndrome); therapy is aimed at relieving the intercurrent medical illness. Insulin requirements usually increase during pregnancy. (See Insulin Use during Pregnancy under Dosage and Administration: Dosage.)

Chronic insulin resistance resulting from immunity may occur when insulin therapy is reinstituted after a period of withdrawal. Most patients with chronic insulin resistance have been found to have markedly elevated concentrations of circulating insulin antibodies. Chronic insulin resistance resulting from immunity has been decreased by changing from beef (no longer commercially available in the US) to pork insulin (since some patients have selective resistance to beef insulin) or by changing to a purified insulin preparation (e.g., insulin human). Animal insulins are no longer commercially available in the US. Insulin lispro also has been effective in establishing glycemic control in patients with insulin resistance. (See Uses, in Insulin Lispro 68:20.08.04.) Patients with insulin immune resistance who are switched to another type of insulin should be started at a lower dosage because their dosage requirements may be greatly decreased. Although administration of corticosteroids has been associated with induction of diabetes mellitus and insulin resistance, these drugs have been used with limited success in the treatment of immune-mediated insulin resistance. Sulfated insulin (not commercially available in the US) has been used in patients with immune-mediated insulin resistance in whom other methods had failed.

● Ocular Effects

Transient presbyopia or blurred vision may occur in diabetic patients given insulin whose blood glucose concentrations have been uncontrolled for an extended period of time or in newly diagnosed diabetic patients in whom rapid glycemic control has been achieved. Patients with proliferative retinopathy who have hemoglobin A_{1c} (HbA_{1c}) concentrations exceeding 10% are at highest risk of worsening retinopathy. When blood glucose concentration is lowered in these patients, the osmotic equilibrium between the lens and ocular fluids occurs slowly but visual acuity will stabilize eventually. Some clinicians recommend that HbA$_{1c}$ concentrations be reduced slowly (2% per year) in such patients and that frequent ophthalmologic examinations (e.g., every 6 months or when symptoms appear) be performed to ensure aggressive treatment of progressive retinopathy. New eyeglasses should not be prescribed for these patients until vision has stabilized.

● Heart Failure

Peroxisome proliferator-activated receptor (PPAR)-γ agonists (e.g., thiazolidinediones) can cause dose-related fluid retention, particularly when used in combination with insulin. Fluid retention may lead to or exacerbate heart failure. Patients receiving insulin and a PPAR-γ agonist should be observed for manifestations of heart failure (e.g., excessive/rapid weight gain, shortness of breath, edema). If heart failure develops, it should be managed according to current standards of care, and discontinuance of the PPAR-γ agonist or reduction of the dosage must be considered. Concomitant use of rosiglitazone and insulin therapy is not recommended.

● Precautions and Contraindications

Formulation Considerations

Any change in insulin should be made cautiously and only under medical supervision. Patients should be informed of the reasons for any change in the insulin regimen and the potential need for additional glucose monitoring. Changes in insulin strength, manufacturer, type (e.g., regular, NPH), or method of manufacture may necessitate a change in dosage. Patients receiving insulin should be monitored with regular laboratory evaluations, including blood glucose determinations and glycosylated hemoglobin (hemoglobin A$_{1c}$ [HbA$_{1c}$]) concentrations, to determine the minimum effective dosage of insulin when used alone, with other insulins, or in combination with an oral antidiabetic agent.

Hypoglycemia and Hypokalemia

As hypoglycemia and hypokalemia may occur with insulin therapy, care should be taken in patients who are most at risk for the development of these effects, including patients who are fasting, those with defective counterregulatory responses (e.g., patients with autonomic neuropathy, adrenal or pituitary insufficiency, those receiving β-adrenergic blocking agents) or patients who are receiving potassium-lowering drugs. Insulin human is contraindicated during episodes of hypoglycemia. As IV insulin has a rapid onset of action, increased attention to hypoglycemia and hypokalemia is necessary. Blood glucose and potassium concentrations should be monitored closely when insulin is administered IV. Rapid changes in serum glucose concentrations may precipitate manifestations of hypoglycemia, regardless of glucose concentration. The potential for late postprandial hypoglycemia observed with short-acting insulin may be reduced by altering the timing, frequency, and content of meals, altering exercise patterns, frequently monitoring blood glucose concentrations, adjusting insulin dosage, and/or switching to a more rapid-acting insulin (e.g., insulin lispro, insulin glulisine). Patients with a history of hypoglycemic unawareness or recurrent, severe hypoglycemic episodes should be particularly vigilant in monitoring their blood glucose concentrations frequently, especially before activities such as driving; intensive insulin therapy should be used with caution in these patients. Maintenance of higher target blood glucose concentrations for at least several weeks is advisable in patients with a history of hypoglycemic unawareness or one or more episodes of severe hypoglycemia to avoid further hypoglycemia, partially reverse hypoglycemic unawareness, and reduce the risk of future episodes. Severe or frequent hypoglycemia is an absolute indication for the modification of treatment regimens, including setting higher glycemic goals. All adolescents with diabetes mellitus should monitor their blood glucose concentrations before driving and take corrective action to avoid hypoglycemia and cognitive-motor impairments. Such adolescents should carry a source of glucose in the car and should cease driving immediately should symptoms of hypoglycemia occur.

Management of Hypoglycemia

Oral administration of 15–20 g of dextrose is the preferred treatment for mild hypoglycemia, although any form of carbohydrate that contains glucose may be used, such as orange or other fruit juice, sugar, hard candy, regular nondiet soda, or dextrose gel or chewable tablets. The dose may be repeated in 15 minutes if blood glucose concentrations remain below 70 mg/dL (as determined by self-monitoring of blood glucose concentrations) or if symptoms of hypoglycemia are still present. Once blood glucose concentrations return to normal, ADA suggests that patients eat a meal or snack to prevent the recurrence of hypoglycemia.

In children and adolescents, administration of 15 g of an easily-absorbed carbohydrate followed by a protein-containing snack is sufficient for mild hypoglycemia; younger children may require about 10 g of carbohydrate to alleviate symptoms. Adjustments in the carbohydrate amounts should be based on blood glucose concentrations. Treatment of moderate hypoglycemia requires that someone other than the child or adolescent administer treatment, usually 20–30 g of glucose to restore blood glucose concentrations to greater than 80 mg/dL. Severe hypoglycemia (associated with altered states of consciousness, including coma and seizures) requires treatment with glucagon or IV dextrose solutions. (See Acute Toxicity: Treatment.)

Following a hypoglycemic reaction, patients should review the probable cause (e.g., excessive exercise, insufficient food intake, inappropriate insulin dosage) with their clinician and take action to prevent further such reactions. Alterations in snack patterns and adjustment in timing and/or dosage of insulin relative to activity levels should be discussed. (See Acute Toxicity.)

Sensitivity Reactions

Patients who have had severe allergic reactions to insulin (i.e., generalized rash, swelling, or breathing difficulty) should be skin-tested with *any new* insulin preparation before it is initiated. Desensitization may be required in patients with a potential for allergic reaction. Because patients may have selective allergic reactions to pork or beef insulin, or to protamine or proteins, further allergic reactions may be prevented by substitution of an insulin that contains less protein (i.e., purified insulins, including insulin human) or that does not contain protamine. Pure beef and mixed beef-pork insulins are no longer commercially available in the US.

Patient Instructions

It is important that the patient receive careful instruction in the importance of proper mixing and storage of insulin, timing of insulin dosing, adherence to meal planning, regular physical exercise, periodic HbA$_{1c}$ concentration testing, recognition and management of hypoglycemia and hyperglycemic reactions, and periodic assessment of diabetic complications.

Patients and their families should be informed of the potential risks and advantages of conventional and intensive insulin therapy. While an intensive insulin regimen consisting of multiple insulin injections daily may not be advisable clinically in certain patient populations, such a regimen also may be problematic in noncompliant patients (e.g., substance abusers, psychiatric patients) or patients who not capable of adjusting their insulin requirements based on frequent self-monitoring of blood glucose concentrations.

Patients should be aware of the need for possible changes in the dosage of insulin and the need for additional monitoring of blood glucose concentrations during an illness, emotional disturbances or stress, or travel. Adjustment of insulin dosage may be needed if patients change their physical activity or usual meal plan.

Patients should be aware of symptoms of diabetic ketoacidosis and should monitor blood ketones if preprandial blood glucose concentrations repeatedly exceed 250–300 mg/dL or if they have an acute illness. Patients should be advised about sick-day procedures to assist in managing their diabetes during acute illness. Patients should contact their physician if results of self-monitored blood glucose concentrations are consistently abnormal.

Administration Considerations

Careful instruction about insulin administration technique and periodic reevaluation can minimize the likelihood of local adverse effects associated with faulty technique (e.g., lipoatrophy, lipohypertrophy). (See Dosage and Administration: Administration.) Subcutaneous injection sites should be rotated to prevent tissue damage that can occur with repeated subcutaneous injections of insulin into the same site. Direct injection of insulin into the outside edge of the atrophied area may result in improvement or complete disappearance of the atrophy in some patients. Rotating injection sites within one anatomical region (e.g., rotating injections systematically in the abdominal area) rather than selecting a different anatomical region is recommended to decrease day-to-day variability in insulin absorption. Variability in insulin absorption by injection site is reduced with insulin lispro compared with that with insulin human. Patients should be instructed to contact their clinician if lipoatrophy, lipohypertrophy, or local adverse effects (e.g., burning, itching, swelling) occur at the site of injection. Direct injection of insulin into the outside edge of the atrophied area may result in improvement or complete disappearance of the atrophy in some patients.

● Pediatric Precautions

In young patients (i.e., those younger than 6 years of age) who may be unable to recognize, articulate, and/or manage hypoglycemia, the risk of hypoglycemia should be considered when setting glycemic targets. However, some data indicate that lower HbA$_{1c}$ targets can be achieved in young children without increased risk of severe hypoglycemia. The risks of hypoglycemia and the developmental burdens of intensive insulin regimens in children and adolescents should be weighed against the long-term health benefits associated with achieving a lower HbA$_{1c}$.

ADA generally recommends that all children and adolescents with type 1 diabetes mellitus be treated with intensive insulin regimens; all children and adolescents should self-monitor blood glucose concentrations multiple times daily (up to 6–10 times per day), including premeal and prebedtime determinations, as needed for safety (e.g., prior to exercise or driving), or during the presence of hypoglycemic symptoms. Continuous glucose monitoring should be considered in all children and adolescents with type 1 diabetes mellitus.

● Geriatric Precautions

Long-term studies conducted in geriatric patients with diabetes mellitus demonstrating the benefits of tight glycemic, blood pressure, and lipid control are lacking. Older adults are at an increased risk of developing hypoglycemia due to multiple factors such as renal insufficiency and cognitive deficits. It is important to prevent hypoglycemia in older adults to reduce the risk of cognitive decline and other adverse effects. Treatment goals for older patients should be individualized and should take into consideration multiple patient specific factors (e.g., comorbidities, cognitive function, functional status, life expectancy). Although control of hyperglycemia is important in geriatric patients with diabetes mellitus, greater reductions in morbidity and mortality may result from control of all cardiovascular risk factors. However, intensive management of diabetes mellitus and coexisting conditions may not be feasible in a proportion of geriatric patients, and clinicians may have to prioritize reduction of some of these risks. In frail geriatric patients with appreciable comorbid conditions, short life expectancy, cognitive or functional impairment, or noncompliance with treatment recommendations, clinicians may choose to enact treatment goals that enhance the quality of life and to treat symptoms or related conditions associated with diabetes mellitus.

● Pregnancy, Fertility, and Lactation

Pregnancy

Diabetic pregnancy is a high-risk state for both mother and fetus/infant. Women with diabetes mellitus who are pregnant or planning pregnancy require tight glycemic control. In women with preexisting diabetes mellitus or gestational diabetes mellitus, the ADA currently recommends a target fasting blood glucose concentrations of less than 95 mg/dL, a 1-hour postprandial blood glucose concentrations of less than 140 mg/dL, a 2-hour postprandial blood glucose concentration of less than 120 mg/dL, and a target HbA$_{1c}$ concentration of less than 6% in such women. If women cannot achieve these glycemic targets without substantial hypoglycemia, less stringent targets may be appropriate and should be individualized.

Patients with diabetes mellitus should inform their physician if they are pregnant or intend to become pregnant; preconception glycemic control is crucial in preventing congenital malformations and reducing the risk of other complications. Many experts recommend institution of strict glycemic control, including use of intensive insulin regimens as needed, before conception and throughout pregnancy in patients with diabetes. (See Insulin Use During Pregnancy under Dosage and Administration: Dosage.) Experts recommend the use of insulin for the management of both type 1 and type 2 diabetes mellitus in pregnant women. Newer rapid-acting insulin analogs have been used increasingly in pregnant women, and based on current evidence, insulin lispro and insulin aspart are not teratogenic. These rapid-acting insulin analogs have been shown to be safe and effective during pregnancy and may provide better postprandial glycemic control with less hypoglycemia than regular insulin. In an open-label clinical study of pregnant women with type 1 diabetes mellitus, insulin detemir therapy did not increase the risk of fetal abnormalities. Additionally, there was no difference in pregnancy outcomes or the health of the fetus and newborn with insulin detemir use. Experience with insulin degludec and insulin glargine in pregnant women is limited.

Maintenance of normal glycemia during pregnancy appears to reduce the risk of congenital malformations, fetal macrosomia and other neonatal morbidities (e.g., hypoglycemia, hypocalcemia, polycythemia, hyperbilirubinemia) as well as perinatal mortality (e.g., miscarriage, intrauterine death, stillbirth). Diabetic women of childbearing age should be informed about the risks of unplanned pregnancy and the appropriate use of contraception until glycemic control is achieved.

DRUG INTERACTIONS

● Drugs That May Have a Variable Effect on Glycemic Control

Anabolic steroids, lithium salts, pentamidine, clonidine, and β-adrenergic blocking agents have variable effects on glucose metabolism as such agents may impair glucose tolerance or increase the frequency or severity of hypoglycemia. In addition, β-adrenergic blocking agents may suppress hypoglycemia-induced tachycardia but not hypoglycemic sweating, which may actually be increased; delay the rate of recovery of blood glucose concentration following drug-induced hypoglycemia; alter the hemodynamic response to hypoglycemia, possibly resulting in an exaggerated hypertensive response; and possibly impair peripheral circulation.

Nonselective β-adrenergic blocking agents (e.g., propranolol, nadolol) without intrinsic sympathomimetic activity are more likely to affect glucose metabolism than more selective β-adrenergic blocking agents (e.g., metoprolol, atenolol) or those with intrinsic sympathomimetic activity (e.g., acebutolol, pindolol). Signs of hypoglycemia (e.g., tachycardia, blood pressure changes, tremor, feelings of anxiety) mediated by catecholamines may be masked by either nonselective or selective β-adrenergic blockade or by other sympatholytic agents such as centrally acting α-adrenergic blocking agents (e.g., clonidine) or reserpine. These drugs should be used with caution in patients with diabetes mellitus, especially in those with labile disease or in those prone to hypoglycemia. Use of low-dose, selective β$_1$-adrenergic blockers (e.g., metoprolol, atenolol) or β-adrenergic blocking agents with intrinsic sympathomimetic activity in patients receiving insulin may theoretically decrease the risk of affecting glycemic control. When insulin and a β-adrenergic blocking agent are used concomitantly, the patient should be advised about and monitored closely for altered glycemic control.

● Other Drugs Affecting Glycemic Control

The hypoglycemic activity of insulin may be potentiated by concomitant administration of alcohol, α-adrenergic blocking agents, certain antidepressants (e.g., monoamine oxidase inhibitors), glucagon-like peptide-1 (GLP-1) receptor agonists, guanethidine (no longer commercially available in the US), oral hypoglycemic agents, pramlintide, salicylates, sulfa antibiotics, certain angiotensin-converting enzyme inhibitors, angiotensin II receptor antagonists, and inhibitors of pancreatic function (e.g., octreotide). When such drugs are added to or withdrawn from therapy in patients receiving insulin, patients should be observed closely for evidence of altered glycemic control and possibly decreased insulin requirements.

Drugs with hyperglycemic activity that may antagonize the activity of insulin and exacerbate glycemic control in patients with diabetes mellitus include asparaginase, calcium-channel blocking agents, diazoxide, certain antilipemic agents (e.g., niacin), corticosteroids, danazol, estrogens, oral contraceptives, isoniazid, phenothiazines, sympathomimetics (e.g., epinephrine, albuterol, terbutaline), thiazide diuretics, furosemide, ethacrynic acid, and thyroid hormones. When such drugs are added to or withdrawn from therapy in patients receiving insulin, patients should be observed closely for evidence of altered glycemic control and possibly increased insulin requirements.

ACUTE TOXICITY

● Pathogenesis

Acute hypoglycemia may result from excessive insulin dosage relative to food intake and/or energy expenditure, and numerous conditions may predispose to the development of insulin-induced hypoglycemia (e.g., defective counterregulatory response, hypoglycemic unawareness, insulin dosage errors, excessive alcohol intake, diabetic nephropathy, adrenal insufficiency, gastroparesis). (See Cautions: Precautions and Contraindications.) Hypoglycemia may result from overinsulinization, irregular eating patterns, increased physical activity, and/or decreased carbohydrate content of meals.

● Manifestations

Hypoglycemia, which may be severe, is the principal manifestation of acute insulin overdosage. Symptoms of moderate hypoglycemia include aggressiveness, drowsiness, confusion, and autonomic symptoms. Severe hypoglycemia is associated with altered states of consciousness, including coma and seizures. Severe hypoglycemia may result in loss of consciousness and seizures, with resultant neurologic sequelae (e.g., cerebral damage, seizures); fatalities have been reported following severe, insulin-induced hypoglycemia Other complications reported with insulin overdosage include hypokalemia, respiratory insufficiency/failure, pulmonary edema, congestive heart failure, hypertension, and cerebral edema.

● Treatment

Mild hypoglycemia (symptoms of sweating, pallor, palpitations, tremors, headache, behavioral changes) may be relieved by oral administration of carbohydrate-containing food or drink (e.g., orange or other fruit juice, lump sugar, candy). (See Management of Hypoglycemia under Precautions and Contraindications: Hypoglycemia and Hypokalemia, in Cautions.)

Severe hypoglycemia (associated with altered states of consciousness, including coma and seizures) requires treatment with glucagon or IV dextrose solutions. Severe insulin-induced hypoglycemia occurs infrequently but constitutes a medical emergency requiring immediate treatment. Adults with severe hypoglycemia (e.g., symptoms of lethargy, headache, confusion, sweating, agitation, seizures) or who are comatose from insulin overdosage and have adequate liver glycogen stores should receive 1 unit (1 mg) of subcutaneous, IM, or IV glucagon; patients should have a vial of glucagon available for family members to administer in emergency situations. Family members should be instructed in the proper administration of glucagon and the indications for its use. Patients unresponsive to or unable to receive glucagon should be given approximately 10–25 g of glucose as 20–50 mL of 50% dextrose injection IV. Higher or repeated doses of IV dextrose may be required in severe cases (e.g., intentional overdosage), and subsequent continuous IV infusion of glucose at 5–10 g/hour may be necessary to maintain adequate blood glucose concentrations until the patient is conscious and able to eat. The patient should be monitored closely until complete recovery is assured as hypoglycemia may recur. To prevent late or recurrent hypoglycemic reactions, oral carbohydrate should be given as soon as the comatose patient awakens.

In children and adolescents with severe hypoglycemia, glucagon at a dose of 30 mcg/kg subcutaneously up to a maximum of 1 mg (1 unit) will increase blood glucose concentrations within 5–15 minutes but may be associated with nausea and vomiting. A lower glucagon dose of 10 mcg/kg results in a lower glycemic response but is associated with less nausea. Repeated episodes of hypoglycemia or longstanding diabetes mellitus may result in defective glucose counterregulation and hypoglycemia unawareness. In such patients, blood glucose should be monitored frequently to avoid recurrent episodes.

PHARMACOLOGY

Exogenous insulin elicits all the pharmacologic responses usually produced by endogenous insulin.

Insulin stimulates carbohydrate metabolism in skeletal and cardiac muscle and adipose tissue by facilitating transport of glucose into these cells. Nerve tissues, erythrocytes, and cells of the intestines, liver, and kidney tubules do not require insulin for transfer of glucose. In the liver, insulin facilitates phosphorylation of glucose to glucose-6-phosphate which is converted to glycogen or further metabolized.

Insulin also has a direct effect on fat and protein metabolism. The hormone stimulates lipogenesis and inhibits lipolysis and release of free fatty acids from adipose cells. Insulin also stimulates protein synthesis.

Administration of suitable doses of insulin to patients with type 1 (insulin-dependent) diabetes mellitus temporarily restores their ability to metabolize carbohydrates, fats, and proteins; to store glucose in the liver; and to convert glycogen to fat. When insulin is given in suitable doses at regular intervals to a patient with diabetes mellitus, blood glucose is maintained at a reasonable concentration, the urine remains relatively free of glucose and ketone bodies, and diabetic acidosis and coma are prevented. The action of insulin is antagonized by somatotropin (growth hormone), epinephrine, glucagon, adrenocortical hormones, thyroid hormones, and estrogens.

Insulin promotes an intracellular shift of potassium and magnesium and thereby appears to temporarily decrease elevated blood concentrations of these ions.

PHARMACOKINETICS

● Absorption

Because of its protein nature, insulin is destroyed in the GI tract and usually is administered parenterally; however, regular insulin also has been administered via oral inhalation. Regular insulin also has been administered intranasally† or transdermally† in a limited number of patients. Following subcutaneous or IM administration, insulin is absorbed directly into the blood. Rate of absorption depends on many factors including route of administration, site of injection, volume and concentration of the injection, and type of insulin. One study in lean, healthy, fasting adults indicates that regular insulin is absorbed more rapidly following IM administration than when it is given subcutaneously. Absorption may be delayed and/or decreased by the presence of insulin-binding antibodies, which develop in all patients after 2–3 months of insulin treatment. Absorption of regular insulin following intranasal or transdermal administration generally has been variable and incomplete, and absorption enhancers (e.g., bile salts) have been used to facilitate delivery of insulin given by these routes. Some data suggest that intrapulmonary absorption of insulin and other peptides may be enhanced in cigarette smokers.

Commercially available insulin preparations differ mainly in their onset, peak, and duration of action following *subcutaneous* administration. Currently available insulin preparations are classified as rapid-acting, short-acting, intermediate-acting, or long-acting. The values for onset, peak, and duration of action of insulin injections shown in Table 1 are only approximate; substantial interindividual and intraindividual variation in these values may occur based on site of injection, injection technique, tissue blood supply, temperature, presence of insulin antibodies, exercise, excipients in insulin formulations, and/or interindividual and intraindividual differences in response. In addition, human insulins may have a more rapid onset and shorter duration of action than porcine insulins (no longer commercially available in the US) in patients with diabetes. (See Pharmacokinetics, in Insulin Human 68:20.08.08.) Similarly, insulin aspart has a more rapid onset and shorter duration of effect than insulin human; differences in pharmacodynamics between the 2 types of insulins are not associated with differences in overall glycemic control.

TABLE 1.

	Onset (hours)	Peak (hours)	Duration (hours)
Rapid-Acting			
Insulin Aspart Injection	0.17–0.33	1–3	3–5
Insulin Glulisine Injection	0.41	0.75–0.8	4–5.3
Insulin Lispro Injection	0.25–0.5	0.5–2.5	3–6.5
Short-Acting			
Insulin Human Injection	0.5–1	1–5	6–10
Intermediate-Acting			
Insulin Human Isophane (NPH) Injection	1–2	6–14	16–24+
Long-Acting			
Insulin Degludec Injection (100 or 200 units/mL)	0.5–1.5	No pronounced peak	42+
Insulin Detemir Injection	1.1–2	No pronounced peak	5.7–24
Insulin Glargine Injection (100 units/mL)	1.1	No pronounced peak	24
Insulin Glargine Injection (300 units/mL)	6	No pronounced peak	36

The hypoglycemic effect of commercially available mixtures containing insulin human isophane (NPH) 70 units/mL and insulin human 30 units/mL (Novolin® 70/30, Humulin® 70/30) usually occurs within 30 minutes, peaks within 1.5–12 hours, and persists for up to 24 hours. The hypoglycemic effect of the commercially available mixture containing insulin human isophane (NPH) 50 units/mL and insulin human 50 units/mL usually occurs within 0.5–1 hour, peaks within 1.5–4.5 hours, and persists for 7.5–24 hours. The addition of insulin lispro protamine 75 units/mL to insulin lispro 25 units/mL in the commercially available mixture (Humalog® 75/25) or 50 units/mL of insulin lispro protamine to insulin lispro 50 units/mL in the commercially available mixture (Humalog® 50/50) does not affect the onset of hypoglycemic effect compared with that with insulin lispro alone, which usually occurs within 0.25–0.5 hours, peaks within 2 hours, and persists for more than 22 hours. The hypoglycemic effect of the commercially available mixture containing insulin aspart protamine 70 units/mL and insulin aspart 30 units/mL usually occurs within 10–20 minutes, peaks within 1–4 hours, and persists for up to 24 hours. When administered in fixed combination with insulin aspart protamine, rapid absorption of the insulin aspart component is preserved, and absorption of insulin aspart protamine component is prolonged.

● Distribution

Insulin is rapidly distributed throughout extracellular fluids. It is not known whether insulin aspart is distributed into milk. Insulin aspart is minimally bound to plasma proteins (0–9%).

● Elimination

Insulin has a plasma half-life of a few minutes in healthy individuals; however, the biologic half-life may be prolonged in diabetic patients, probably as a result of binding of the hormone to antibodies, and in patients with renal impairment as a result of altered degradation/decreased clearance. Following subcutaneous administration, the half-life of insulin aspart averages 81 minutes. The half-life of insulin aspart in fixed combination with insulin aspart protamine is about 8–9 hours. Data from a pharmacokinetic study in patients with a wide range of body mass index, indicate that clearance of insulin aspart is reduced by 28% in obese patients with type 1 diabetes mellitus compared with that in leaner patients.

Insulin is rapidly metabolized mainly in the liver by the enzyme glutathione insulin transhydrogenase and to a lesser extent in the kidneys and muscle tissue. In the kidneys, insulin is filtered at the glomerulus and almost completely (98%) reabsorbed in the proximal tubule. About 40% of this reabsorbed insulin is returned to venous blood and 60% is metabolized in the cells lining the proximal convoluted tubule. In normal patients, only a small amount (less than 2%) of a filtered insulin dose is excreted unchanged in the urine.

In a pharmacokinetic study in a limited number of patients receiving an IV infusion (1.5 milliunits/kg per minute for 120 minutes) of either insulin aspart or insulin human, the mean insulin clearance was similar for the 2 types of insulins (1.22–1.24 L/hour per kg).

CHEMISTRY AND STABILITY

● Chemistry

Insulin is a hormone secreted by the beta cells of the pancreatic islets of Langerhans. Insulin is a protein with a molecular weight of about 6000 and is composed of 2 chains (A and B chains) of amino acids connected by disulfide linkages.

The potency of insulin is standardized according to its ability to lower blood glucose concentrations of normal fasting rabbits as compared to the USP Insulin Reference Standard. Potency is expressed in USP units per mL.

Insulin Aspart

Insulin aspart is a rapid-acting, biosynthetic (recombinant DNA origin) insulin human analog that is structurally identical to insulin human except for the replacement of aspartic acid with proline at position 28 on the B chain of the molecule.

Insulin Degludec

Insulin degludec is a long-acting, biosynthetic (recombinant DNA origin) insulin human analog that is prepared using a process that includes expression of recombinant DNA in *Saccharomyces cerevisiae* followed by chemical modification. Insulin degludec differs structurally from insulin human by the deletion of threonine at position 30 on the B chain and by the acylation of lysine at position 29 on the B chain with hexadecandioic acid, a 16-carbon fatty acid, via a glutamic acid spacer.

Insulin Detemir

Insulin detemir is a long-acting, biosynthetic (recombinant DNA origin) insulin human analog that is prepared using a process that includes expression of

recombinant DNA in *Saccharomyces cerevisiae* followed by chemical modification. Insulin detemir differs structurally from insulin human by the deletion of threonine at position 30 on the B chain and by the acylation of lysine at position 29 on the B chain with myristic acid, a 14-carbon fatty acid.

Insulin Glargine

Insulin glargine is a long-acting, biosynthetic (recombinant DNA origin) insulin human analog that is prepared using special laboratory strains of nonpathogenic *E. coli*, insulin glargine that differs structurally from insulin human by the replacement of asparagine with glycine at position 21 of the A chain and the addition of 2 arginine groups to the C-terminus of the B chain.

Insulin Glulisine

Insulin glulisine is a rapid-acting, biosynthetic (recombinant DNA origin) insulin human analog that is structurally identical to insulin human except for the replacement of asparagine at position 3 on the B chain with lysine and by replacement of lysine at position 29 on the B chain with glutamic acid.

Insulin Human

Commercially available insulin human (regular insulin) is structurally identical to human insulin. Insulin human is *not* extracted from the human pancreas but rather is prepared biosynthetically using recombinant DNA technology and special laboratory strains of *Escherichia coli* or *Saccharomyces cerevisiae*. Biosynthetic insulin human isophane (NPH insulin) is an intermediate-acting, sterile suspension of zinc insulin crystals and protamine sulfate in buffered water for injection. (See Chemistry and Stability: Chemistry, in Insulin Human 68:20.08.08.)

Insulin Lispro

Insulin lispro is a rapid-acting, biosynthetic (recombinant DNA origin) insulin human analog that is structurally identical to insulin human except for transposition of the natural sequence of lysine and proline on the B chain of the molecule. (See Chemistry and Stability: Chemistry, in Insulin Lispro 68:20.08.04.)

● Stability

Insulin Human

Regular insulin (insulin human) injection may be mixed with other insulin preparations that have an approximately neutral pH (e.g., insulin human isophane [NPH]). Whenever regular insulin is mixed with other insulin preparations, regular insulin should be drawn into the syringe first in order to avoid transfer of the modified insulin preparation into the regular insulin vial.

When regular insulin is mixed with NPH insulin, binding of added regular insulin occurs in vitro because of excess protamine in the formulation of NPH. In vitro binding of regular insulin by NPH insulin is rapid and marked, occurring within about 5–15 minutes after mixing; however, these chemical changes appear to have no clinical importance since the onset and duration of action of mixtures containing regular and NPH insulins are similar to those observed when these insulins are administered separately.

Mixtures containing regular insulin and NPH insulin appear to be stable for at least 1 month when stored at room temperature or 3 months when stored at 2–8°C; however, the possibility of microbial contamination should be considered. Fixed combinations that contain 30 units/mL of insulin human injection and 70 units/mL of insulin human isophane (NPH) suspension (Humulin® 70/30, Novolin® 70/30), 25 units/mL of insulin lispro and 75 units/mL of insulin lispro protamine suspension (Humalog® mix 75/25), 30 units/mL of insulin aspart and 70 units/mL of insulin aspart protamine (Novolog® mix 70/30), 50 units/mL of insulin lispro and 50 units/mL of insulin lispro protamine (Humalog® mix 50/50), and those that contain 50 units/mL of insulin human injection and 50 units/mL of insulin human isophane (NPH) suspension (Humulin® 50/50) are commercially available. (See Insulin Human, Insulin Lispro, and Insulin Aspart 68:20.08.04.)

Regular insulin may be mixed in any proportion with water for injection or 0.9% sodium chloride injection for use in an insulin subcutaneous infusion pump. However, the mixtures should be used within 24 hours after preparation, since changes in pH and dilution of buffer may affect stability. Insulins are physically and chemically compatible with Lilly's insulin diluting fluids, and may be mixed in any proportion for use in an infusion pump. The mixtures using Lilly's insulin diluting fluids are stable for up to 4 weeks when stored at room temperature. Lilly's insulin diluting fluids are not commercially available; the preparations and specific information about their use should be obtained from the manufacturer. Regular insulin may form crystal deposits on the tubing of insulin infusion pumps.

Studies indicate that the addition of regular insulin to an IV infusion solution may result in adsorption of insulin to the container and tubing. The amount of an insulin dose lost by adsorption to an IV infusion system is highly variable and depends on the concentration of insulin, the type and surface area of the infusion system, the duration of contact time, and the flow rate of the infusion. The lesser the concentration of insulin in solution or the slower the rate of flow of solution, the greater the percentage of adsorption. Adding more insulin to the solution may saturate binding sites of the infusion system. Alternatively, insulin injection may be administered from a syringe directly into a vein or IV tubing with no significant loss due to adsorption. Insulin adsorption is decreased by the presence of negatively charged proteins, such as normal serum albumin. In one study, addition of 7 mL of 25% normal human serum albumin to 500 mL of 0.9% sodium chloride injection with 5, 10, 20, or 40 units of insulin prevented significant insulin adsorption.

Insulin Aspart, Insulin Glulisine, and Insulin Lispro

When a rapid-acting insulin is mixed with a longer-acting insulin (i.e., insulin human isophane [NPH]), the rapid onset of action of the rapid-acting insulin (i.e., insulin lispro, insulin aspart) is not affected; therefore, such insulins can be mixed. A slight decrease in absorption rate but not total bioavailability is seen when rapid-acting insulin and insulin human isophane (NPH) are mixed. In clinical trials, postprandial glycemic control was similar when a rapid-acting insulin was mixed with either insulin human isophane (NPH) or extended insulin human zinc (Ultralente®, no longer commercially available in the US). Insulin lispro has been administered with a longer-acting insulin (insulin human isophane [Humulin N®]) in the same syringe. Mixing of insulin lispro with other insulins may be associated with physicochemical changes (either immediately or over time) that could alter the physiologic response to the insulins. For additional information on the stability of insulin lispro or insulin mixtures containing insulin lispro, see Chemistry and Stability: Stability, in Insulin Lispro 68:20.08.04. Insulin aspart or insulin glulisine may be mixed with insulin human isophane (NPH). Although some attenuation of peak serum insulin aspart or insulin glulisine concentrations was observed when administered concomitantly with insulin human isophane (NPH) in the same syringe, the time to peak concentration and total bioavailability of insulin aspart were not substantially affected. If insulin aspart or insulin glulisine is mixed with insulin human isophane (NPH), insulin aspart should be drawn into the syringe first and the mixture administered immediately after mixing. The manufacturer states that the effect of mixing insulin aspart with insulins of animal origin (no longer commercially available in the US), insulins produced by other manufacturers, or crystalline insulin zinc formulations has not been studied. The manufacturer of insulin glulisine states that the effects of mixing insulin glulisine in the same syringe with insulins other than insulin human isophane (NPH), or mixing insulin glulisine with diluents or other insulins when used in external subcutaneous infusion pumps have not been studied.

Unopened insulin aspart alone or in fixed combination with insulin aspart protamine should be stored at 2–8°C until the expiration date and protected from light. Insulin aspart alone or in fixed combination with insulin aspart protamine should not be subjected to freezing; do not use insulin aspart if freezing has occurred or if exposed to temperatures exceeding 37°C. In-use vials, cartridges, or injection pens containing insulin aspart alone should be stored at temperatures below 30°C for up to 28 days. In-use vials containing insulin aspart in fixed combination with insulin aspart protamine vials may be stored at temperatures below 30°C for up to 28 days, provided such vials are kept as cool as possible and away from direct heat and light. Opened insulin aspart should not be exposed to excessive heat or sunlight; do not use the drug if exposure to temperatures exceeding 37°C has occurred. Opened vials of insulin aspart may be refrigerated. Cartridges of insulin aspart assembled into an injection pen or other compatible insulin delivery device should not be refrigerated. Punctured cartridges containing insulin aspart in fixed combination with insulin aspart protamine or Novolog® Mix 70/30 FlexPen® are stable for up to 14 days if stored

at temperatures below 30°C; do not refrigerate and keep away from direct heat and sunlight. Infusion bags containing insulin aspart or insulin human regular are stable at room temperature for 24 hours. A certain amount of insulin will be adsorbed initially to material of the infusion bag. The infusion set (tubing, reservoirs, catheters, needle) and the drug in the reservoir should be discarded at least every 48 hours or after exposure to temperatures exceeding 37°C.

When insulin aspart, insulin lispro, or insulin glulisine is used in an external subcutaneous insulin infusion pump, the drug should not be diluted or mixed with any other insulin. Malfunctioning of the external infusion pump or infusion set (e.g., infusion set occlusion, leakage, disconnection or kinking) or insulin degradation can lead to hyperglycemia or ketosis within a short time period because of the small subcutaneous depot of insulin with continuous infusion administration and the rapid onset and short duration of action of insulin aspart, insulin lispro, or insulin glulisine. Prompt identification and correction of the cause of hyperglycemia or ketosis is necessary. If these problems cannot be corrected promptly, patients should resume therapy with subcutaneous injections of insulin and contact their clinician. Patients who are switching from multiple-injection therapy or infusion with buffered regular insulin to subcutaneous infusion with insulin aspart may be particularly susceptible to hyperglycemia or ketosis, and interim therapy with subcutaneous injections with insulin aspart may be required.

In vitro studies have shown that pump malfunction, loss of cresol, and insulin degradation may occur with the use of insulin aspart or insulin glulisine for more than 2 days at 37°C. Insulin aspart, insulin glulisine, and insulin lispro should not be exposed to temperatures exceeding 37°C during administration. The temperature of insulin aspart or insulin glulisine may exceed ambient temperature when the pump housing, cover, tubing, or sport case is exposed to sunlight or radiant heat. Insulin aspart or insulin glulisine exposed to higher than recommended temperatures should be discarded. To avoid insulin degradation, infusion set occlusion, and loss of preservative (cresol), infusions sets (reservoir syringe, tubing, and catheter) and insulin aspart, insulin lispro, or insulin glulisine in the reservoir should be replaced and a new infusion site selected at least every 48 hours. The 3-mL insulin lispro cartridge used in the Disetronic®D-TRON® or Disetronic®D-TRON plus insulin infusion device should be discarded after 7 days, even if some drug still remains in the reservoir.

Insulin Degludec

The manufacturer states that insulin degludec must not be mixed with any other insulin or solution.

Insulin Detemir

The manufacturer states that insulin detemir must not be diluted or mixed with any other insulin or solution. Such dilution or mixing of insulin detemir may result in unpredictable alterations in the pharmacokinetic and/or pharmacodynamic characteristics (e.g., onset of action, time to peak effect) of insulin detemir and/or the mixed insulin.

Insulin Glargine

The manufacturer states that insulin glargine must not be diluted or mixed with any other insulin or solution. Such dilution or mixing of insulin glargine may result in clouding of the solution and unpredictable alterations in the pharmacokinetic and/or pharmacodynamic characteristics (e.g., onset of action, time to peak effect) of insulin glargine and/or the mixed insulin.

For the dosage of regular insulin in the treatment of severe diabetic ketoacidosis and coma, see Insulin Human 68:20.08.08. For further information on the chemistry and stability, uses, and dosage and administration of specific insulin preparations, see the individual monographs in 68:20.08.

† Use is not currently included in the labeling approved by the US Food and Drug Administration.

Insulin Aspart

68:20.08.04 • RAPID-ACTING INSULINS

■ Insulin aspart (rDNA origin) is a biosynthetic, rapid-acting insulin analog that is prepared using recombinant DNA technology and genetically modified *Saccharomyces cerevisiae*.

USES

● Diabetes Mellitus

Insulin aspart is used to control hyperglycemia in the management of diabetes mellitus. When administered subcutaneously, insulin aspart has a more rapid onset and shorter duration of action compared with insulin human (regular); therefore, insulin aspart is associated with greater relative reductions in postprandial blood glucose concentrations and may provide greater patient convenience in terms of the timing of insulin injections in relation to meals in patients with type 1 (insulin-dependent) and type 2 (noninsulin-dependent) diabetes mellitus. Because of its short onset and duration of action, insulin aspart usually is used in regimens that include an intermediate-acting (e.g., isophane [NPH] insulin) or long-acting insulin.

Safety and efficacy of insulin aspart administered immediately before meals has been demonstrated by comparison with insulin human (regular) administered 30 minutes before meals in open, clinical studies of 6 months' duration in adults with type 1 or type 2 diabetes mellitus; patients in these studies also received NPH insulin as the basal insulin supplement. Glycemic control (as determined by glycosylated hemoglobin [hemoglobin A_{1c}, HbA_{1c}]) was comparable or slightly improved in patients receiving insulin aspart compared with those receiving insulin human. Patients receiving insulin aspart required slightly higher total daily dosages of insulin (1–3 units daily), principally due to altered basal insulin requirements.

Insulin aspart also is administered by continuous subcutaneous infusion using an external controlled-infusion pump (e.g., Minimed® model 500 series, Disetronic H-TRON series or other equivalent pumps) in patients with type 1 or type 2 diabetes mellitus. Available data in patients with type 1 diabetes mellitus suggest that continuous subcutaneous administration of insulin aspart provides glycemic control (as measured by glycosylated hemoglobin) that is similar to that provided by continuous subcutaneous administration of buffered human insulin or insulin lispro† therapy. In an open-label, short-term trial (16 weeks) in patients with type 2 diabetes mellitus, glycemic control was similar during therapy with insulin aspart administered via an external subcutaneous continuous infusion pump or with preprandial injections of insulin aspart in conjunction with basal isophane insulin injections. These data indicate a similar incidence of hypoglycemia among patients receiving any type of study insulin via external infusion pumps versus a regimen of multiple daily injections.

Insulin aspart has been administered as an IV infusion in a limited number of patients with diabetes mellitus, but The American Diabetes Association (ADA) states that insulin aspart offers no advantage over regular crystalline insulin in patients who require IV insulin.

For additional information on the management of diabetes mellitus, see Uses in the Insulins General Statement 68:20.08.

DOSAGE AND ADMINISTRATION

● General

Dosage of insulin aspart alone (Novolog®) or in fixed combination with insulin aspart protamine (Novolog® Mix 70/30) must be individualized and should be regularly adjusted based on the results of blood glucose determinations. Whenever possible, patients should self-monitor blood glucose concentrations. Glucose monitoring is particularly important for patients receiving insulin via an external infusion pump. Patients previously receiving insulin may require a change in dosage if insulin therapy is changed to insulin aspart.

● Administration

Insulin aspart alone or in fixed combination with insulin aspart protamine is administered by subcutaneous injection using a conventional insulin syringe, an insulin injection pen (e.g., NovoPen® 3 PenMate, Novolog® FlexPen®), or a compatible insulin delivery device (Innovo®, InDuo®). The manufacturer states that NovoLog® or Novolog Mix 70/30 PenFill® cartridges are intended for use with NovoPen® 3 PenMate® or a compatible insulin delivery device (Innovo®, InDuo®).

Insulin aspart also is administered by continuous subcutaneous infusion using an external controlled-infusion device (e.g., Minimed® model 500 series, Disetronic H-TRON series or other equivalent pump). Insulin aspart is recommended for use in any reservoir and infusion sets that are compatible with insulin and the specific pump. Insulin aspart in fixed combination with insulin aspart protamine should not be used in insulin infusion pumps. For information on the stability of insulin aspart in external infusion pumps, see Insulin Aspart and Insulin Lispro under Chemistry and Stability: Stability, in the Insulins General Statement 68:20.08.

Because of its short duration of action, insulin aspart is used concomitantly with a longer-acting insulin (e.g., isophane [NPH] insulin human, insulin aspart protamine) to meet basal insulin needs in patients with diabetes mellitus and to provide more optimal glycemic control. Insulin aspart may be mixed with isophane insulin human. Although some attenuation of peak serum insulin aspart concentrations was observed when administered concomitantly with isophane insulin human in the same syringe, the time to peak concentration and total bioavailability of insulin aspart were not substantially affected. Whenever insulin aspart is mixed with isophane insulin human, insulin aspart should be drawn into the syringe first in order to avoid transfer of isophane insulin human into the insulin vial. The mixture should be administered immediately after mixing, and such mixtures should not be administered IV. The manufacturer states that the effect of mixing insulin aspart with insulins of animal origin, insulins produced by other manufacturers, or crystalline insulin zinc formulations has not been studied.

The manufacturer states that insulin aspart in fixed combination with insulin aspart protamine suspension (Novolog® Mix 70/30) is intended only for subcutaneous administration and should not be given IV. To resuspend the mixture in a vial immediately before use, the vial should be rolled gently between the hands 10 times until the suspension appears to be uniformly white and cloudy.

Before inserting the Novolog® PenFill® cartridge into a compatible delivery device, the cartridge should be rolled between the palms 10 times. The cartridge should then be turned upside down so that the glass ball inside the cartridge moves the length of the cartridge. This rolling and turning of the cartridge should be repeated at least 10 times or until the suspension appears to be uniformly white and cloudy. The dose should be injected immediately after resuspension, and the rolling and turning of the cartridge should be repeated before each subsequent injection.

Similarly, if using the Novolog® FlexPen®, the pen should be rolled between the palms 10 times. The injection pen should then be turned upside down so that the glass ball inside the pen moves from one end of the reservoir to the other. This rolling and turning procedure should be repeated at least 10 times or until the suspension appears uniformly white and cloudy. The dose should be injected immediately after resuspension, and the rolling and turning of the FlexPen® should be repeated before each subsequent injection.

Insulin aspart is administered immediately (within 5–10 minutes) before a meal. Insulin aspart in fixed combination with insulin aspart protamine (Novolog® Mix 70/30) generally is administered twice daily, 15 minutes before the morning and evening meals, with each dose intended to optimize glycemic control during 2 meals or a meal and a snack. Insulin aspart can be administered by subcutaneous injection into the abdominal wall, thigh, or upper arm. A planned rotation of injection sites within an area should be followed.

Insulin aspart may be administered by IV infusion under proper medical supervision in a clinical setting. For IV infusion in polypropylene infusion bags, insulin aspart is usually diluted to a concentration of 0.05–1 units/mL in 0.9% sodium chloride, 5% dextrose, or 10% dextrose injection with 40 mEq/L of potassium chloride.

Dispensing and Administration Precautions

Because of the similarity in names and product packaging between Novolog® (insulin aspart) and Novolog® Mix 70/30 (insulin aspart 30 units/mL with insulin aspart protamine 70 units/mL), the manufacturer has recently implemented color-branded labeling to help prevent dispensing errors. The current packaging for NovoLog® Mix 70/30 is very similar to the previous packaging and remains white with a blue band along the left side of the package. The previous packaging for NovoLog® was also white with a blue band. The current packaging for Novolog® is now white with an orange band along the left side of the package. Although color differentiation can help with product recognition, color should not be relied upon as the sole means of identification of the correct drug. Pharmacists should also use the drug name and NDC number and other measures to carefully distinguish between insulin formulations when dispensing. (See Dispensing and Administration Precautions under Warnings/Precautions: General Precautions, in Cautions.)

● Dosage

Because of its short duration of action, insulin aspart is used concomitantly with a longer-acting insulin (e.g., isophane [NPH] insulin human, insulin aspart protamine) to meet basal insulin needs in patients with diabetes mellitus and to provide more optimal glycemic control. Initial *total* daily insulin requirements may vary and generally range from 0.5–1 units/kg. When used in a meal-related subcutaneous injection regimen, 50–70% of the *total* daily insulin requirement may be provided by insulin aspart and the remainder by an intermediate-acting or long-acting insulin. Because of the comparatively rapid onset and short duration of activity of insulin aspart, some patients may require more basal insulin and more total daily insulin to prevent pre-meal hyperglycemia than when using insulin human (regular).

When insulin aspart is used in external infusion pumps, the initial dosage is based on the total daily insulin dosage of the previous regimen. Approximately 50% of the total dosage is given as meal-related injections and the remainder as a basal infusion. Adjustments in basal insulin injections or higher basal infusion rates may be necessary.

When insulin aspart in fixed combination with insulin aspart protamine is used as monotherapy in patients with type 1 or 2 diabetes mellitus, an initial total daily dosage of 0.4–0.6 units/kg given in 2 doses (before the morning and evening meal) has been recommended, with subsequent dosage titrated in increments of 2–4 units every 3–4 days to achieve the target fasting plasma glucose. When the fixed combination of insulin aspart and insulin aspart protamine is given in combination with oral antidiabetic agents, an initial total daily dosage of 0.2–0.3 units/kg has been recommended, with subsequent dosage titration to target glycemic goals. (See Treatment Goals under Uses: Diabetes Mellitus, in the Insulins General Statement 68:20.08.) Because of diurnal variation in insulin resistance and endogenous insulin secretion, variability in the time and content of meals, and variability in the time and extent of exercise, fixed-ratio insulin mixtures may not provide optimal glycemic control for all patients. The dose of the insulin mixture required to provide adequate glycemic control for one of the meals may result in hypoglycemia or hyperglycemia for the other meal. The pharmacodynamic profile of insulin aspart in fixed combination with insulin aspart protamine also may be inadequate for patients who require more frequent meals (e.g., pregnant women).

When the fixed combination of insulin aspart and insulin aspart protamine is used to replace isophane insulin alone or a biphasic insulin product (e.g., premixed isophane and regular insulin) in patients with adequate glycemic control, the initial dosage of insulin aspart in fixed combination with insulin aspart protamine should be identical to the previous insulin dosage, with subsequent adjustment of dosage as required. Patients inadequately controlled on isophane insulin may require increases of 10–20% in the dosage of the fixed combination of insulin aspart and insulin aspart protamine during the first week. In patients transferring from a multiple-daily-dose regimen consisting of an intermediate-acting (e.g., isophane) insulin and a rapid- or short-acting insulin at mealtimes, the initial dosage of the insulin aspart protamine component of the fixed combination should be same as the dosage of the previously used intermediate-acting insulin. Adjustments in the dosage or type of insulin may be needed during illness, emotional or physiologic stress, or changes in meals and exercise.

● Special Populations

In a pharmacokinetic study in a limited number of patients with or without renal impairment (creatinine clearance ranging from normal to less than 30 mL/minute but not requiring hemodialysis) who received a single subcutaneous dose of insulin aspart, peak serum drug concentrations and AUC were not affected; however, only 2 patients with severe renal impairment were studied. Similarly, coexisting hepatic impairment (Child-Pugh score 12 or less) did not affect the pharmacokinetics of insulin aspart. However, since increased circulating concentrations of insulin have been observed in patients with renal or hepatic failure who were receiving insulin human, careful monitoring of blood glucose and adjustment of insulin aspart dosage may be necessary in such patients. Dosage requirements for insulin aspart may be reduced in patients with hepatic or renal impairment.

Because of the greater frequency of decreased hepatic, renal, and/or cardiac function and of concomitant disease and drug therapy in geriatric patients, the

manufacturer suggests that patients in this age group receive initial dosages of insulin aspart at the lower end of the usual range.

CAUTIONS

● Contraindications

Known hypersensitivity to insulin aspart or any ingredient in the formulation. Contraindicated during episodes of hypoglycemia.

● Warnings/Precautions

Warnings

Formulation Considerations

Because insulin aspart has a more rapid onset and shorter duration of action than insulin human (regular), administration of insulin aspart should be *immediately* followed by a meal. In addition, a longer-acting insulin is required to maintain adequate glycemic control in patients with type 1 diabetes mellitus. Any change in insulin should be made cautiously and only under medical supervision. Insulin aspart in fixed combination with insulin aspart protamine should not be mixed with any other insulin. Patients previously receiving insulin may require a change in dosage if insulin therapy is changed to insulin aspart.

Hypoglycemia

Hypoglycemia is the most common adverse effect of insulins, including insulin aspart, and monitoring of blood glucose concentrations is recommended for all patients with diabetes mellitus.

Insulin Pumps

Pump or infusion set malfunction or insulin degradation may lead to hyperglycemia and ketosis in a short time period because of the small subcutaneous depot of insulin. Because of rapid absorption and short duration of action, such effects may occur when patients are switched from multiple injection therapy or infusion with buffered regular insulin. Prompt indentification and correction of hyperglycemia or ketosis is necessary; interim therapy with intermittent subcutaneous injections may be required.

Sensitivity Reactions

Dermatologic and Sensitivity Reactions

Localized allergic reactions (e.g., pruritus, erythema, swelling) at the injection site may develop in patients receiving insulins, including insulin aspart alone or in fixed combination with insulin aspart protamine. These reactions are relatively minor and usually resolve within a few days to a few weeks but occasionally may require discontinuance of insulin aspart. Poor injection technique or irritants in skin cleansing agents may contribute to localized injection site reactions. As with any insulin, atrophy or hypertrophy of subcutaneous fat tissue may occur at sites of frequent insulin injection. Injection site rotation within an area may reduce or prevent these effects.

Generalized hypersensitivity to insulin characterized by rash, pruritus, shortness of breath, wheezing, hypotension, tachycardia, and diaphoresis has occurred less frequently than localized reactions. Severe cases of generalized insulin allergy with anaphylaxis may be life-threatening. In several clinical studies in patients with type 1 and 2 diabetes mellitus receiving insulin human or insulin aspart alone or in fixed combination with insulin aspart protamine, formation of insulin aspart-specific or insulin human-specific antibodies was low in patients receiving either insulin, but among patients receiving insulin aspart-containing regimens, concentrations of cross-reactive antibodies increased after 3–6 months of therapy before returning to near-baseline levels at 12 months. It was not necessary to increase the dosage of insulin aspart in patients experiencing increased cross-reactive antibodies, and the manufacturer states that the clinical importance of these findings is unknown. No consistent relationship between antibody formation and glycemic control (as measured by HbA_{1c}) was observed, and dosage adjustments were not necessary to maintain glycemic control.

Localized reactions and generalized myalgias have been reported with the use of cresol, which is included in the NovoLog® (insulin aspart) and Novolog® Mix 70/30 formulations as an excipient.

General Precautions

Hypoglycemia and Hypokalemia

As hypoglycemia and hypokalemia may occur with insulin therapy, care should be taken in patients who are most at risk for the development of these effects, including patients who are fasting, patients with autonomic neuropathy, or patients who are receiving potassium-lowering drugs or drug therapy that may be affected by altered serum potassium concentrations. Untreated hypokalemia may cause respiratory paralysis, ventricular arrhythmia, and death. Since IV insulin aspart has a rapid onset of action, increased attention to hypoglycemia and hypokalemia is necessary. Serum glucose and potassium concentrations must be monitored closely when insulin aspart or any other insulin is administered IV.

Dispensing and Administration Precautions

Because of the similarity in names and product packaging between Humalog® and Humalog® 75/25, medication errors with these 2 drugs have been noted. The manufacturer of Novolog® Mix 70/30 and Novolog® has recently implemented color-branded labeling to help prevent dispensing errors. The current packaging for NovoLog® Mix 70/30 is very similar to the previous packaging and remains white with a blue band along the left side of the package. The packaging for Novo-Log® previously was also white with a blue band. The current packaging of Novo-log® is now white with an orange band along the left side of the package. Although color differentiation can help with product recognition, color should not be relied upon as the sole means of identification of the correct agent. Pharmacists should also use the drug name and NDC number and other measures (e.g., matching product name on the prescription to the pharmacy-issued label, separating agents with similar names on pharmacy shelves, counseling patients) to carefully distinguish between insulin formulations when dispensing. This recent packaging change will not help prevent name confusion errors involving these 2 agents (Novolog® and Novolog® Mix 70/30) or other insulin products (e.g., Novolog® Mix 70/30 and Novolin® 70/30, or Novolog® and Novolin®).

Dispensing errors involving Novolog® or Novolog® Mix 70/30 should be reported to the manufacturer (800-727-6500), the USP Medication Errors Reporting Program (800-233-7767), or the FDA MedWATCH program by phone (800-FDA-1088, 800-FDA-0178 [fax]) or online at http://www.fda.gov/Safety/MedWatch/default.htm.

Specific Populations

Pregnancy

Category C. (See Users' Guide.)

Lactation

It is unknown whether insulin aspart is distributed into milk; caution is advised if used in nursing women.

Pediatric Use

Safety and efficacy of insulin aspart in fixed combination with insulin aspart protamine not established in children. The comparative safety and efficacy of insulin aspart and insulin human (regular) have been demonstrated in a 24-week clinical study in children and adolescents 6–18 years of age with type 1 diabetes mellitus; children also received isophane insulin as the basal insulin supplement. Glycemic control (as determined by glycosylated hemoglobin [hemoglobin A_{1c}, HbA_{1c}]) was comparable in patients receiving insulin aspart or insulin human. In addition, safety and efficacy of insulin aspart were comparable with insulin human in another clinical study in adolescents 12–17 years of age with type 1 diabetes mellitus. In comparative study in a limited number of children 2–6 years of age, glycemic control (as measured by HbA_{1c}, fructosamine) was comparable in children receiving insulin aspart or insulin human. As observed in the 6- to 18-year age group, the rates of hypoglycemia in children 2-6 years of age were similar with insulin aspart or insulin human. In one pharmacokinetic study, insulin aspart had a more rapid onset and a shorter duration of action when compared with insulin human in a limited number of children and adolescents 6–17 years of age; such effects are similar to those observed in adults.

Geriatric Use

Experience in those 65 years of age and older insufficient to determine whether safety differs from younger adults. Efficacy of insulin aspart (as measured by HbA_{1c}) as compared to insulin human appears to be similar in geriatric and younger patients, particularly in patients with type 2 diabetes mellitus.

● Common Adverse Effects

Hypoglycemia, hypersensitivity reactions, lipodystrophy, pruritus, rash, and injection site reactions have been reported with insulin aspart monotherapy. In clinical studies, small but persistent elevations in alkaline phosphatase were observed in some patients with type 1 diabetes mellitus who received insulin aspart. However, the clinical importance, if any, of these findings has not been established. Injection site reactions have been reported in 7% of patients receiving insulin aspart in fixed combination with insulin aspart protamine. Data from comparative clinical trials evaluating insulin aspart in fixed combination with insulin aspart protamine (Novolog® Mix 70/30) and insulin human (regular) injection in fixed combination with isophane insulin human (Novolin® 70/30) did not reveal differences in the frequency of adverse effects between the 2 preparations.

DRUG INTERACTIONS

● Drugs Affecting Glycemic Control

Drugs that May Potentiate Hypoglycemic Effects

Angiotensin-converting enzyme (ACE) inhibitors, disopyramide, fibrate derivatives, fluoxetine, monoamine oxidase (MAO) inhibitors, oral antidiabetic agents, propoxyphene, salicylates, somatostatin derivatives (e.g., octreotide), sulfonamide anti-infectives.

Drugs that May Antagonize Hypoglycemic Effects

Corticosteroids, danazol, diuretics, estrogens and progestins (e.g., oral contraceptives), isoniazid, niacin, phenothiazines, somatropin, sympathomimetic agents (e.g., albuterol, epinephrine, terbutaline), thyroid hormones.

Drugs that May Have a Variable Effect of Glycemic Control

Alcohol, β-adrenergic blocking agents, clonidine, lithium salts, pentamidine.

Sympatholytic Agents

May decrease or eliminate the signs of hypoglycemia in patients receiving insulin aspart concomitantly with these drugs (e.g., β-adrenergic blocking agents, clonidine, guanethidine, reserpine).

DESCRIPTION

Insulin aspart (rDNA origin) is a biosynthetic, rapid-acting human insulin analog that is prepared using recombinant DNA technology and genetically modified *Saccharomyces cerevisiae*. Insulin aspart differs structurally from insulin human by the replacement of proline at position B28 with aspartic acid. This structural modification results in decreased tendency to form hexamers, more rapid absorption and onset of action, and a shorter duration of action compared with insulin human when given subcutaneously to patients with type 1 diabetes mellitus. Interindividual and intraindividual variation in rate of absorption and consequently, the onset of action of insulins, including insulin aspart alone or in fixed combination with insulin aspart protamine, may occur based on site of injection, tissue blood supply, temperature, and physical activity.

ADVICE TO PATIENTS

Provide information regarding the potential risks and advantages of insulin aspart-containing therapy.

Provide instructions to patient regarding use of subcutaneous insulin infusion devices (e.g., infusion pumps and accessories) and intensive insulin therapy with multiple injections.

Provide instructions regarding self-monitoring of blood glucose, insulin storage and injection technique, adherence to meal planning, regular physical exercise, periodic hemoglobin A_{1c} (HbA_{1c}) monitoring, and management of hypoglycemia or hyperglycemia.

Importance of *not* mixing insulin aspart with crystalline zinc insulin preparations, insulins of animal source, or preparations produced by other manufacturers. Importance of using insulin aspart only if solution is clear and colorless with no particles visible; resuspended insulin aspart in fixed combination with insulin aspart protamine must appear uniformly white and cloudy.

Importance of *not* mixing insulin aspart with other insulins or diluent when used in external subcutaneous infusion pumps.

Importance of administering insulin aspart or the fixed combination of insulin aspart and insulin aspart protamine within 5–10 minutes or within 15 minutes, respectively, of the start of a meal.

Discuss potential for alterations in insulin requirements in special situations (e.g., illness, emotional disturbances or other stresses).

Importance of informing clinicians of the development of skin reactions (erythema, pruritus, thickened skin) at infusion sites in patients using insulin infusion pumps. Importance of selection of a new infusion site, as continued infusion may increase skin reactions and/or alter the absorption of insulin aspart.

Importance of resumption of subcutaneous insulin injection therapy and of contacting a clinician if pump malfunctions occur and cannot be corrected promptly.

Importance of informing clinicians of existing or contemplated concomitant therapy, including prescription and OTC drugs. Importance of women informing clinicians if they are or plan to become pregnant or breast-feed.

Importance of informing patients of other important precautionary information. (See Cautions.)

PREPARATIONS

Excipients in commercially available drug preparations may have clinically important effects in some individuals; consult specific product labeling for details.

Insulin Aspart (Recombinant DNA Origin)

Parenteral

Injection for subcutaneous use	100 units/mL (U-100)	**NovoLOG®**, Novo Nordisk **NovoLOG® FlexPen®** (available as a 3 mL prefilled syringe preassembled into pen), Novo Nordisk
Injection, for use with NovoPen® 3 PenMate® or other compatible devices	100 units/mL (300 units)	**NovoLOG® Penfill®**, Novo Nordisk

Insulin Aspart Combinations (Recombinant DNA Origin)

Parenteral

Injectable Suspension	Insulin Aspart 30 units/mL with Insulin Aspart Protamine 70 units/mL	**NovoLOG® Mix 70/30**, Novo Nordisk **NovoLOG® Mix 70/30 FlexPen®** (available as a 3 mL prefilled syringe preassembled into pen), Novo Nordisk
Injectable Suspension, for use with NovoPen® 3 PenMate® or other compatible devices	100 units/mL (300 units)	**NovoLOG® Mix 70/30 Penfill®**, Novo Nordisk

† Use is not currently included in the labeling approved by the US Food and Drug Administration.

Selected Revisions January 1, 2009, © Copyright, January 1, 2001, American Society of Health-System Pharmacists, Inc.

Insulin Lispro

68:20.08.04 • RAPID-ACTING INSULINS

- Insulin lispro is a rapid-acting biosynthetic human insulin analog that is structurally identical to insulin human except for reversal of the sequence of lysine and proline on the B chain of the molecule; in insulin lispro, lysine and proline occur at positions 28 and 29, respectively, of the B chain.

USES

• Diabetes Mellitus

Insulin lispro is a rapid-acting insulin analog that is used to control hyperglycemia in the management of diabetes mellitus. In patients with type 1 diabetes mellitus, insulin lispro generally is used in conjunction with a longer-acting insulin (except when administered via an external insulin infusion device [pump]); in patients with type 2 diabetes mellitus, insulin lispro may be used without a longer-acting insulin when given with an oral sulfonylurea antidiabetic agent. (See Combination Therapy under Uses: Diabetes Mellitus, in the Insulins General Statement 68:20.08.) When administered subcutaneously, insulin lispro has a more rapid onset and shorter duration of action compared with insulin human (regular); therefore, insulin lispro is associated with greater relative reductions in postprandial blood glucose concentrations and may provide greater patient convenience in terms of the timing of insulin injections in relation to meals in patients with type 1 and type 2 diabetes mellitus. Because of its short onset and duration of action, insulin lispro usually is used in regimens that include a longer-acting insulin (i.e., isophane [NPH] insulin human, insulin lisproprotamine [as the fixed combination Humalog® Mix75/25®, Humalog® Mix50/50®], insulin glargine) in an attempt to provide more physiologic insulin levels throughout the day.

Insulin lispro also is administered by continuous subcutaneous infusion using selected external controlled-infusion devices (pumps) in patients with diabetes mellitus. Limited data in patients with type 1 diabetes mellitus suggest that continuous subcutaneous administration of insulin lispro provides greater glycemic control (as measured by glycosylated hemoglobin) than that provided by continuous subcutaneous administration of buffered human insulin or regular human insulin. These data indicate a similar incidence of hypoglycemia among patients receiving insulin lispro or regular or buffered human insulin via external infusion pumps. Available data suggest that continuous subcutaneous administration of insulin provides glycemic control similar to that provided by intensive, multiple-daily-dose insulin therapy. Insulin lispro administration via external controlled-infusion devices has not been studied in patients with type 2 diabetes mellitus.

The American Diabetes Association (ADA) currently classifies diabetes mellitus as type 1 (immune mediated or idiopathic), type 2 (predominantly insulin resistance with relative insulin deficiency to predominantly an insulin secretory defect with insulin resistance), gestational diabetes mellitus, or that associated with certain conditions or syndromes (e.g., drug- or chemical-induced, hormonal, that associated with pancreatic disease, infections, specific genetic defects or syndromes). Type 1 diabetes mellitus previously was described as juvenile-onset (JOD) diabetes mellitus, since it usually occurs during youth. Type 2 diabetes mellitus previously was described as adult-onset (AODM) diabetes mellitus. However, type 1 or type 2 diabetes mellitus can occur at any age, and the current classification is based on pathogenesis (e.g., autoimmune destruction of pancreatic β cells, insulin resistance) and clinical presentation rather than on age of onset. Many patients' diabetes mellitus does not easily fit into a single classification. Epidemiologic data indicate that the incidence of type 2 diabetes mellitus is increasing in children and adolescents such that 8–45% of children with newly diagnosed diabetes have nonimmune-mediated diabetes mellitus.

Comparative clinical studies in patients with type 1 or type 2 diabetes mellitus who received insulin lispro or insulin human (regular) indicate that insulin lispro is associated with improved control of postprandial blood glucose concentrations. However, while therapy with insulin lispro was associated with reduced postprandial (e.g., post-breakfast) blood glucose excursions in these patients, overall glycemic control (as measured by hemoglobin A_{1c} values) did not differ appreciably from that in patients receiving insulin human (regular). The clinical importance of increased glycemic control of postprandial glucose excursions in nonpregnant

diabetic patients with similar glycosylated hemoglobin (hemoglobin A_{1c} [HbA_{1c}]) values has not been established. Most comparative studies of insulin lispro and insulin human (regular) were of open, crossover design in which patients received either insulin lispro within approximately 15 minutes before a meal or insulin human (regular) 20–45 minutes before a meal in addition to an intermediate-acting (e.g., NPH insulin) or long-acting (Ultralente®) insulin as the basal insulin supplement. Main efficacy end points were 1–2 hour-postprandial blood glucose concentrations, glycosylated hemoglobin concentrations, frequency of hypoglycemia, and quality-of-life measures. However, in most of the larger studies conducted to date, patients were evaluated for only 3 months, which some clinicians state may not have been a sufficient period in which to assess changes in glycosylated hemoglobin. Since the duration of action of insulin lispro is brief, some clinicians have suggested that basal (e.g., intermediate-acting) insulin dosage be optimized to reflect the short duration of action of insulin lispro. The dosage or frequency of administration of the longer-acting insulin may be increased or the evening dose of longer-acting insulin may be delayed until bedtime; continuous subcutaneous infusion of insulin also may be used to manage increased preprandial and nighttime glucose concentrations (as compared with insulin human [regular]) observed with insulin lispro.

Some clinicians suggest that patient-related factors such as motivation and knowledge of the disease may be more important in determining glycemic control than the type of insulin or insulin regimen used, and that patients who are well-controlled on conventional short-acting insulin preparations without frequent hypoglycemia should not be routinely switched to insulin lispro. Patients likely to benefit from insulin lispro therapy include type 1 diabetics who would appreciate the more flexible injection schedule associated with insulin lispro's shorter onset and duration of activity, those with low glycosylated hemoglobin values who are at high risk for hypoglycemic episodes, and patients with recent-onset type 1 diabetes mellitus who have some residual β-cell function to provide basal insulin levels between meals.

Insulin lispro therapy generally has been associated with a reduced frequency of hypoglycemic episodes compared with insulin human (regular) in patients with type 1 diabetes mellitus and no change in hypoglycemic episodes in type 2 diabetics. In parallel-group clinical trials of insulin lispro and insulin human (regular) in patients with type 1 or type 2 diabetes mellitus, the overall incidence of hypoglycemia was not significantly different among patients receiving either of the 2 insulin preparations; however, patients with type 1 diabetes receiving insulin lispro had fewer late hypoglycemic episodes (i.e., between 12 midnight and 6 a.m.) than those receiving insulin human (regular), possibly because of higher nocturnal blood glucose concentrations (as reflected by a small increase in fasting blood glucose concentrations).

Limited evidence suggests that insulin lispro also may be effective in establishing glycemic control in patients with resistance to insulin human. Transfer from insulin human (regular) to insulin lispro resulted in a reduction in insulin requirements in a patient with excessive insulin antibodies whose response was refractory to insulin human (regular). Further study and experience are needed to determine whether insulin lispro has clinical advantages over regular insulin for the long-term management of diabetes mellitus.

For further information on indications for insulin therapy and considerations in selecting and monitoring such therapy in patients with diabetes mellitus, see the Insulins General Statement 68:20.08.

DOSAGE AND ADMINISTRATION

• Administration

Insulin lispro is administered by subcutaneous injection using a conventional insulin syringe or an injection pen (e.g., Humalog® Pen, Owen Mumford Auto pen®). Whenever possible, insulin should be self-administered by the patient. Patients should be instructed regarding proper administration and dosage of insulin lispro and given a copy of the patient information provided by the manufacturer. To improve accuracy of dosing in pediatric patients, insulin lispro may be diluted to a ratio of 1:10 or 1:2 with the sterile diluent supplied by the manufacturer. Use of injection pens may improve accuracy of insulin delivery and be more convenient in patients who are visually or neurologically impaired or who are receiving multiple daily injections of insulin. When a compatible delivery device is used for subcutaneous injection of insulin lispro, the labeling accompanying the delivery device should be consulted for proper methods of assembly, administration (including dose calibration), and care.

The manufacturer states that insulin lispro in fixed combination with insulin lispro protamine suspension (Humalog® Mix50/50®, Humalog Mix75/25®) is intended only for subcutaneous administration and should not be given IV. Before injecting the fixed combination of insulin lispro and insulin lispro protamine suspension using the injection pen, the pen should be rolled between the palms 10 times. The pen should then be turned upside down so that the glass ball inside the pen moves the length of the pen. This rolling and turning of the pen should be repeated at least 10 times or until the suspension appears to be uniformly white and cloudy.

Insulin lispro also is administered by continuous subcutaneous infusion using selected external controlled-infusion devices (pumps). The pumps deliver rapid- or short-acting insulin at a basal rate continuously throughout the day, with patient-initiated increased delivery of insulin prior to meals. The manufacturer states that insulin lispro is recommended for use in Disetronic H-TRON®plus V100 (with Disetronic 3.15-mL insulin reservoir), Disetronic D-TRON®, or Disetronic D-TRON®plus external infusion pumps with Disetronic Rapid® Infusion sets and in MiniMed model 506, 507, or 508 pumps with MiniMed Polyfin® infusion sets.

The safety and efficacy of insulin lispro following IV administration†, such as in the treatment of diabetic ketoacidosis, has not been adequately evaluated to date. Insulin lispro's favorable pharmacokinetic profile compared with insulin human (regular) is based on its more rapid subcutaneous absorption rather than on more rapid post-absorptive uptake to insulin receptor sites, and no clinical advantage of IV insulin lispro compared with IV insulin human (regular) has been identified. While insulin lispro and insulin human have similar hypoglycemic effects when given IV†, the manufacturer states that insulin lispro is intended for subcutaneous administration and that insulin human (regular) should be used when IV administration of insulin is required. Some clinicians suggest that insulin lispro should not be used IV, especially in patients with diabetic ketoacidosis, as data are limited concerning the IV use of insulin lispro.

The manufacturer states that the safety and efficacy of insulin lispro following IM† administration has not been evaluated in clinical trials.

For additional information concerning insulin administration, see Dosage and Administration: Administration, in the Insulins General Statement 68:20.08.

When used as a mealtime insulin alone or in fixed combination with isophane insulin human to control postprandial hyperglycemia, insulin lispro should be administered within 15 minutes prior to a meal. Because of its short duration of action, insulin lispro is used concomitantly with, but not necessarily administered at the same time as, a longer-acting insulin (e.g., isophane [NPH] insulin human) to meet basal insulin needs in patients with type 1 diabetes mellitus and to provide more optimal glycemic control. Insulin lispro alone or in fixed combination with isophane insulin human can be administered by subcutaneous injection into the abdominal wall, thigh, or upper arm. A planned rotation of injection sites within an area (injections should be spaced at least 0.5 inch from a previous injection site) should be followed.

Conflicting data have been reported regarding the effects of mixing insulin lispro and a longer-acting insulin on the pharmacodynamic effects of insulin lispro. Some data in healthy individuals indicate that mixing insulin lispro (Humalog®) and NPH insulin human (i.e., Humulin N®) in the same syringe results in a decreased rate of absorption, but no change in total bioavailability, of insulin lispro; this finding may be attributable to adsorption of insulin lispro to excess protamine in the NPH insulin formulation. Clinical studies in patients with type 1 diabetes mellitus indicate that mixtures of insulin lispro (Humalog®) and NPH insulin human (i.e., Humulin N®) either improve or produce similar effects on postprandial glycemic control compared with separate injection of these insulins. Concomitant administration of insulin lispro and Ultralente® (no longer commercially available in the US) insulin human in the same syringe reportedly did not affect the absorption of insulin lispro in healthy individuals who received these insulins immediately after mixing. The manufacturer states that the effect of mixing Humalog® (insulin lispro) with insulins of animal origin (no longer commercially available in the US) or human insulins produced by other manufacturers (i.e., other than Lilly) has not been studied. When insulin lispro is mixed with a longer-acting insulin preparation, insulin lispro should be drawn into the syringe first in order to prevent precipitation or turbidity of the insulin lispro solution by the longer-acting insulin. Insulin mixtures should not be administered IV.

● Dosage

Dosage of insulin lispro, which is always expressed in USP units, must be based on the results of blood glucose determinations and carefully individualized to attain optimum therapeutic effects. (*Glucose concentrations in plasma generally are 10–15% higher than those in whole blood; glucose concentrations also may vary*

according to the method and laboratory used for these determinations.) Patients should be monitored with regular laboratory evaluations, including fasting blood (or plasma) glucose determinations, to assess therapeutic response and obtain the minimum effective dosage of insulin lispro. Whenever possible, patients should self-monitor blood glucose concentrations. Urine glucose concentrations correlate poorly with blood glucose; therefore, urine glucose determinations should be used only when patients cannot or will not test blood glucose concentrations. Glucose monitoring is particularly important for patients receiving insulin lispro via an external infusion pump. Following initiation of insulin lispro therapy and dosage titration, determination of glycosylated hemoglobin (hemoglobin A_{1c} [HbA_{1c}]) concentrations at intervals of approximately 3 months is useful for assessing the patient's continued response to therapy.

For additional information on monitoring and management of insulin therapy, see Dosage: Considerations in Monitoring Insulin Therapy, in Dosage and Administration in the Insulins General Statement 68:20.08.

Both conventional and intensive insulin treatment regimens have been used in patients with type 1 or severe type 2 diabetes mellitus. (See Glycemic Control and Microvascular Complications of Diabetes Mellitus, in Uses in the Insulins General Statement 68:20.08.) Insulin lispro generally is administered in multiple daily doses in regimens that also include an intermediate- or long-acting insulin (e.g., NPH, Lente, Ultralente®) given in the morning and/or evening to provide basal insulin needs. Insulin lispro in fixed combination with insulin lispro protamine (Humalog® Mix75/25®) generally is administered twice daily with the morning and evening meal. Dosage of insulin lispro alone or in fixed combination with insulin lispro protamine must be based on the results of blood glucose determinations and carefully individualized to obtain optimum therapeutic effect. While absorption of insulin lispro is more rapid, and duration of action slightly shorter, when administered in abdominal compared with deltoid or thigh sites, variations in absorption related to site of administration are smaller with insulin lispro than with regular insulin when insulin lispro is not mixed with other insulins in the same syringe.

Transferring from Therapy with Other Insulins

Any change in insulin preparation or dosage regimen should be made with caution and only under medical supervision. When insulin lispro replaces insulin human (regular) in regimens consisting of multiple daily insulin doses, the initial dosage of insulin lispro can be identical to the previous insulin (regular) dosage with subsequent adjustment as required. However, patients in whom insulin lispro is initiated should be carefully advised regarding the difference in action profiles between insulin lispro and insulin human (regular); adjustments in the consumption and/or timing of snacks or exercise relative to that with the use of insulin (regular) may be necessary to avoid hypoglycemic episodes and/or prevent preprandial hyperglycemia. While pharmacokinetic and pharmacodynamic studies indicate that insulin lispro and insulin human are equipotent on a unit-for-unit basis with regard to glucose-lowering activity, changes in insulin purity, strength, brand, type, and/or species source or method of manufacture may necessitate a change in insulin dosage. Although it is not possible to clearly identify which patients will require a change in dosage when therapy with a different preparation is initiated, it is known that a limited number of patients will require such a change. Adjustments may be needed with the first dose or over a period of several weeks.

When insulin lispro is substituted for insulin human (regular) in patients receiving combination therapy with insulin human (regular) and a longer-acting insulin, adjustment of the dosage of the longer-acting insulin may be required because of the shorter duration of action of insulin lispro. Patients receiving intensive insulin therapy will achieve greater postprandial glycemic control than those receiving conventional therapy because of the increased use of rapid- or short-acting insulin; patients who previously were poorly controlled on conventional insulin therapy generally will require a smaller total daily insulin dosage when switched to an intensive insulin regimen.

● Dosage in Renal and Hepatic Impairment

Results from clinical trials in a limited number of patients with type 2 diabetes mellitus and renal or hepatic impairment who were receiving either insulin lispro or insulin human indicate that the pharmacokinetic differences between the 2 types of insulin generally were maintained. The presence of hepatic impairment does not affect the absorption or distribution of insulin lispro in patients with type 2 diabetes mellitus. However, increased circulating concentrations of insulin have been observed in patients with renal or hepatic impairment who were receiving insulin human; therefore, insulin lispro requirements may be reduced in these patients. Careful monitoring of blood glucose and adjustment of insulin lispro (alone or in fixed combination with isophane insulin human) dosage may be necessary in such patients.

For further information on the chemistry and stability, uses, and dosage and administration of specific insulin preparations, see the individual monographs in 68:20.08.

CAUTIONS

Insulin lispro shares the toxic potential of other insulins, and the usual precautions of insulin therapy should be observed with insulin lispro. (See Cautions in the Insulins General Statement 68:20.08.) The overall frequency and severity of adverse reactions to insulin lispro appear to be similar to those associated with insulin human (regular).

● *Hypoglycemia*

In comparative studies in patients with type 1 or type 2 diabetes mellitus, the overall rate of hypoglycemic reactions with insulin lispro was similar or somewhat less than that with insulin human; the frequency of nocturnal hypoglycemic reactions in patients with type 1 diabetes mellitus is less among those receiving insulin lispro. The lower rate of hypoglycemia observed with insulin lispro may be related to its shorter duration of action, resulting in a slightly greater degree of fasting hyperglycemia compared with insulin human.

● *Immunogenicity*

Several studies have shown that insulin lispro is no more immunogenic than insulin human. In one study in patients with type 1 or type 2 diabetes mellitus receiving insulin lispro or insulin human for 12 months, insulin specific antibody titers at endpoint were no different for each of the 2 insulin preparations. In large clinical trials, formation of insulin lispro-specific antibodies was low in patients receiving insulin lispro, but cross-reactive antibodies were observed in patients receiving insulin human or insulin lispro. The largest increase in antibody levels during year-long trials was observed in patients with type 1 diabetes mellitus who were receiving insulin therapy for the first time. In one study in rhesus monkeys, insulin antibody titers (IgG type) were found in 1 of 4 monkeys immunized with 6 weekly injections of insulin lispro (up to 100 mcg) prepared in Freund's adjuvant and in none of the monkeys receiving insulin human or purified pork insulin in Freund's adjuvant; none of the monkeys developed elevated insulin antibody titers of IgE type. As insulin allergies are mediated primarily by IgE insulin antibodies, use of insulin lispro is not expected to pose an increased risk for the development of insulin allergies.

● *Other Effects*

Localized reactions and generalized myalgias have been reported with the use of *m*-cresol, which is included in the Humalog®, Humalog® Mix75/25®, or Humalog® Mix50/50® (insulin lispro) formulations as an excipient.

● *Precautions and Contraindications*

Insulin lispro has a more rapid onset and shorter duration of action than insulin human (regular). Clinicians who prescribe rapid-acting insulins should be familiar with the indications, limitations, and patient-selection criteria for therapy with insulin to ensure appropriate patient management. Because insulin lispro has a short duration of action, patients with type 1 diabetes also require a longer-acting insulin to maintain adequate nighttime and preprandial blood glucose control.

Patients should read carefully and follow instructions regarding use of subcutaneous insulin infusion devices (e.g., infusion pumps and accessories) and intensive insulin therapy with multiple injections. Patients using insulin infusion devices should inform clinicians of the development of skin reactions (erythema, pruritus, thickened skin) at infusion sites. If such reactions occur, a new infusion site should be selected. Malfunctioning of the external-controlled infusion device or infusion set or insulin degradation can lead to hyperglycemia or ketosis within a short time period. If such symptoms occur, prompt identification and correction of the cause is necessary. Interim therapy with subcutaneous injections with insulin may be required if the cause of the symptoms cannot be promptly determined. (See Insulin Regimens under Dosage and Administration: Dosage, in the Insulins General Statement 68:20.08.) Complications such as undetected interruptions in insulin delivery may result in more frequent and more rapid ketotic episodes or unexplained hyperglycemia compared with multiple daily injections.

Any change in insulin should be made cautiously and only under medical supervision. Changes in insulin strength, manufacturer, type (e.g., regular,

NPH), species, (animal, human), or method of manufacture (rDNA versus animal-source insulin) may necessitate a change in dosage.

The manufacturer states that insulin lispro alone or in fixed combination with isophane insulin human (Humalog® Mix50/50®, Humalog® Mix75/25®) is contraindicated during episodes of hypoglycemia and in patients with hypersensitivity to the drug or any of its excipients. Patients with a history of hypersensitivity to *other* insulins should be given insulin lispro only if the clinician has determined that the possible benefits outweigh the potential adverse effects. (See Cautions: Dermatologic and Sensitivity Reactions, in the Insulins General Statement 68:20.08.) Patients should seek immediate medical assistance if they experience a generalized allergic reaction after injection of insulin lispro.

● *Pediatric Precautions*

The safety and efficacy of insulin lispro in fixed combination with insulin lispro protamine in children younger than 18 years of age have not been established. However, clinical trials with insulin lispro are ongoing in children aged 3–18 years of age with type 1 diabetes mellitus, and preliminary data suggest no unusual effects of insulin lispro therapy in adolescents receiving the drug. In several long-term (e.g., 8–9 months) comparative studies evaluating insulin lispro and insulin human in children and adolescents with diabetes mellitus, insulin lispro (given either immediately before or after meals) was as effective as insulin human (given 30–45 minutes before a meal) in improving glycemic control as determined by glycosylated hemoglobin (hemoglobin A_{1c} [HbA_{1c}]) concentrations. Adjustment of basal insulin dosage may be required in these children. (See Cautions: Pediatric Precautions, in the Insulins General Statement 68:20.08.)

● *Geriatric Precautions*

In clinical trials, the efficacy (as measured by HbA_{1c} values) of insulin lispro or incidence of hypoglycemia did not differ by age. Pharmacokinetic/pharmacodynamic studies to assess the effect of age on the onset of action of insulin lispro have not been performed. Subgroup analyses of large clinical trials have not revealed evidence of altered effectiveness of insulin lispro compared with insulin human based on age. However, some evidence suggests an increased risk of cardiovascular morbidity associated with hypoglycemia in geriatric patients receiving intensive insulin therapy. (See Cautions: Geriatric Precautions, in the Insulins General Statement 68:20.08.)

With insulin lispro in fixed combination with isophane insulin human, experience in those 65 years of age or older is insufficient to determine whether they respond differently from younger adults. However, dosage of insulin lispro in fixed combination with isophane insulin human should be selected carefully in geriatric patients, and the greater frequency of decreased hepatic, renal, and/or cardiac function and of concomitant disease and drug therapy observed in the elderly also should be considered.

● *Mutagenicity and Carcinogenicity*

No evidence of mutagenicity or chromosomal damage with insulin lispro was observed in vivo in a micronucleus test or chromosome aberration test or in in vitro test systems, including microbial (bacterial mutation tests) and mammalian (mouse lymphoma) assays. There was no increase in DNA repair when insulin lispro was tested in an unscheduled DNA synthesis test.. In addition, no evidence of carcinogenicity was observed in a study in rats receiving up to 200 units/kg daily of insulin lispro subcutaneously for 12 months.

● *Pregnancy, Fertility, and Lactation*
Pregnancy

Insulin lispro has been evaluated in a limited number of pregnant women with gestational diabetes. The American Diabetes Association (ADA) suggests that continuous subcutaneous insulin infusion with insulin lispro may improve glycemic control during pregnancy. Congenital abnormalities (including kidney dysplasia) have been reported in at least 2 infants of patients with type 1 diabetes mellitus who received insulin lispro and other insulins during pregnancy; a causal relationship to insulin lispro has not been established. Abnormal maternal blood glucose concentrations during pregnancy have been associated with a higher incidence of congenital abnormalities. Although glycemic control reportedly was well maintained during pregnancy in these women, optimization of glycemic control before conception and throughout pregnancy does not completely eliminate the risk of congenital anomalies. The manufacturer states that insulin lispro alone or in fixed combination with isophane insulin human should be used in pregnant women only when clearly needed.

Reproduction studies of insulin lispro in pregnant rats and rabbits using parenteral dosages of up to 4 or 0.3 times, respectively, the average human dosage (40 units daily) have not revealed evidence of fetal malformations. Modest decreases in food consumption and weight gain, and occasional instances of severe hypoglycemia and death, were noted when insulin lispro was administered subcutaneously at a dosage of 20 units/kg daily to male rats prior to cohabitation through two consecutive matings and to female rats prior to cohabitation and through gestational day 19; these effects were expected based on the pharmacologic effects of the drug. Transient decreases in fetal and newborn pup weights and an increased incidence of fetal runts per litter suggested a marginal effect on in utero growth at an insulin lispro dosage of 20 units/kg daily; however, no effects on pup growth were observed with dosages of 1–5 units/kg daily.

Fertility

Reproduction studies evaluating the effect of insulin lispro on fertility have not been conducted. Reproduction studies in male rats receiving subcutaneous injections of insulin lispro at doses up to 20 units/kg daily have not revealed evidence of impaired reproductive performance, testicular histopathology, or impaired fertility in the parental generation or in the untreated successive generation.

Lactation

Insulin lispro alone or in fixed combination with isophane insulin human should be used with caution in nursing women, since it is not known whether the drug is distributed into milk in humans. However, other insulins (e.g., insulin human) are distributed into milk. Patients with diabetes who are lactating may require adjustments in insulin lispro (alone or in fixed combination with isophane insulin human) dosage, meal plans, or both.

For additional information on the use of insulin in gestational diabetes mellitus and during the perinatal period, see Uses: Gestational Diabetes Mellitus and see Dosage: Insulin Use during Pregnancy, in the Insulins General Statement 68:20.20.

PHARMACOLOGY

Studies in animals, healthy adults, and patients with type 1 (insulin-dependent) diabetes mellitus indicate that insulin lispro has pharmacologic effects comparable to those of insulin human. The fixed combination of insulin lispro and insulin lispro protamine (Humalog® Mix75/25®) has glucose-lowering effects similar to those of the fixed combination of insulin human (regular) and isophane insulin human (Humulin® 70/30) on a unit-for-unit basis.

The potency of insulin lispro, with respect to its efficacy for replacement therapy in patients with type 1 diabetes mellitus, is similar to that of insulin human. Short-term, in vitro receptor-binding studies demonstrate that insulin lispro and insulin human have similar affinity for insulin receptor binding sites. However, the number and affinity of insulin receptors on circulating monocytes in a limited number of patients with type 1 diabetes mellitus increased to levels similar to those in healthy individuals following 3 months of therapy with insulin lispro, while patients receiving insulin human (regular) had a decrease in insulin receptor affinity and binding capacity. It has been suggested that the improvement in insulin receptor status during prolonged therapy with insulin lispro may be related to its more physiologic pharmacokinetic profile relative to that of regular insulin.

Insulin lispro and insulin human have similar short-term hypoglycemic effects when given IV. In patients with type 1 diabetes mellitus in whom hypoglycemia was induced experimentally, the counterregulatory hormone response to hypoglycemia was similar with insulin lispro and insulin human; similar counterregulatory hormone responses to ingestion of a meal have been reported in other studies. Limited data suggest that insulin lispro suppresses hepatic glucose production and promotes peripheral glucose utilization to a greater extent than does insulin human when the drugs are given subcutaneously. In patients with type 1 diabetes mellitus who received insulin lispro or insulin human (regular) by continuous subcutaneous infusion for 3 months, glycosylated hemoglobin (hemoglobin A_{1c} [HbA_{1c}]) values and postprandial blood glucose concentrations were lower with insulin lispro therapy; however, timing of insulin human administration was not optimized since both insulin human and insulin lispro were administered within 5 minutes before meals. (See Insulin Regimens, under Dosage and Administration: Dosage in the Insulins General Statement 68:20.08.) The incidence of hypoglycemic episodes was lower than baseline levels and similar for both drugs.

For further information on the pharmacology of insulin, see the Insulins General Statement 68:20.08.

PHARMACOKINETICS

● Absorption

Insulin lispro is more rapidly absorbed than soluble preparations of insulin human or insulins of animal origin following subcutaneous administration because of its ability to dissociate faster from the insulin hexamer in solution. Absorption of other insulins (e.g., insulin human) from subcutaneous sites is delayed by the time required for dissociation of insulin hexamers into dimers and monomers that can diffuse into the systemic circulation. Therefore, insulin lispro has a faster onset and shorter duration of action than other insulins and, when administered subcutaneously 15 minutes before a meal, more closely mimics the endogenous postprandial insulin response. After subcutaneous administration of 0.1–0.4 units/kg of insulin lispro or insulin human in healthy individuals or patients with type 1 diabetes mellitus, peak plasma insulin concentrations are higher and occur earlier with insulin lispro (at 30–90 minutes) than with insulin human (at 50–120 minutes). Addition of zinc to the commercially available formulation of insulin lispro reduces peak serum concentrations somewhat compared with an insulin lispro formulation without zinc (not commercially available in the US) but does not appreciably alter the time to peak concentration. Unlike with insulin human, the time to peak serum concentration following subcutaneous administration of insulin lispro does not increase with increasing doses. Serum concentrations of insulin lispro also exhibit less intraindividual and interindividual variability than those of insulin human, possibly because of differences in the intrinsic properties of these insulins.

The fixed combination of insulin lispro and insulin lispro protamine (Humalog® Mix75/25®, Humalog® Mix50/50®) exhibits 2 phases of absorption. The early phase represents insulin lispro and its rapid onset of action; the late phase represents the prolonged action of insulin lispro protamine suspension. In a limited number of nondiabetic individuals, peak serum insulin concentrations were observed 30–240 minutes (median: 60 minutes) following subcutaneous administration of the fixed combination (0.3 units/kg) of insulin lispro and insulin lispro protamine (Humalog® Mix75/25®); results were identical in diabetic patients. In patients with type 1 diabetes mellitus, peak serum (immunoreactive) insulin concentrations were observed at 45–120 minutes (median: 60 minutes) following administration of the Humalog® Mix50/50® fixed combination. The fixed combinations of insulin lispro and insulin lispro protamine (Humalog® Mix75/25®, Humalog® Mix50/50®) are absorbed more rapidly than the fixed combination of insulin human (regular) and isophane insulin human (Humulin® 70/30®, Humulin® 50/50), including in patients with type 1 diabetes mellitus. The duration of action of Humalog® Mix75/25® and Humalog® Mix50/50® also is similar to that of Humulin® 70/30® and Humulin® 50/50®.

The pharmacokinetics and pharmacodynamics of insulin human and insulin lispro are similar following IV administration in healthy individuals; however, the safety and efficacy of IV insulin lispro have not been evaluated in clinical trials in patients with diabetes mellitus. Following single IV doses of 0.1–0.2 units/kg, the absolute bioavailabilities of insulin lispro and insulin human were similar, ranging from 55–77%.

The onset of glycemic response following subcutaneous injection of insulin lispro in healthy individuals or in patients with type 1 or 2 diabetes mellitus generally ranges from 0.25–0.5 hours versus 0.5–1 hours for insulin human; peak glycemic response for insulin lispro or insulin human occurs at 0.5–2.5 or 1–5 hours, respectively. Following subcutaneous administration in these individuals or patients, the duration of hypoglycemic action of insulin lispro is 3–6.5 hours compared with 6–10 hours for insulin human. Many factors can affect the onset, degree, and duration of insulin activity, including injection technique, presence of insulin antibodies, site of injection, tissue blood supply, temperature, excipients in insulin formulations, and interindividual and intraindividual differences in response. After subcutaneous administration, onset of action of insulin lispro from abdominal, deltoid, and thigh sites is similar, and variations in absorption related to site of administration are smaller than those observed with regular insulin. However, the effects of age, obesity, gender, and type of diabetes mellitus on glycemic response do not appear to differ in patients receiving insulin lispro versus insulin human.

● Distribution

The volume of distribution of insulin lispro reportedly is identical to that of insulin human and ranges from 0.26–0.36 L/kg. Distribution of insulin lispro when given in the fixed-combination formulation containing protamine sulfate (Humalog® Mix75/25®) has not been determined. It is not known whether insulin lispro is distributed into human milk; however, other insulins (e.g., insulin human) are distributed into milk. In a study in a limited number of pregnant women with gestational diabetes, the drug did not appear to cross the placenta.

● **Elimination**

In healthy adults, the half-life of subcutaneously administered insulin lispro or insulin human is 1 or 1.5 hours, respectively, while systemic clearance of insulin lispro and insulin human is similar. Following IV administration, insulin lispro and insulin human reportedly exhibit identical dose-dependent elimination, with half-lives of 26 or 52 minutes at doses of 0.1 or 0.2 units/kg, respectively.

The metabolic fate of insulin lispro alone or in fixed combination with insulin lispro protamine has not been determined in humans; however, in animals, metabolism of insulin lispro is identical to that of insulin human.

Some studies with insulin human have shown increased circulating insulin concentrations in patients with renal or hepatic failure; information on the use of insulin lispro in such patients is limited. In a study in a limited number of patients with type 2 diabetes mellitus and various degrees of renal function, sensitivity to insulin lispro increased as renal function declined. (See Cautions: Precautions and Contraindications and see Dosage and Administration: Dosage in Renal and Hepatic Impairment.)

CHEMISTRY AND STABILITY

● **Chemistry**

Insulin lispro is a biosynthetic human insulin analog that is structurally identical to insulin human except for reversal of the sequence of lysine and proline on the B chain of the molecule; in insulin lispro, lysine and proline occur at positions 28 and 29, respectively, of the B chain. The inversion of lysine and proline in the amino acid sequence eliminates hydrophobic interactions and weakens some of the hydrogen bonds that contribute to the stability of dimer subunits composing the hexameric form of insulin lispro. Endogenous insulin is stored in the pancreas as a stable, zinc-containing hexamer; stabilization of insulin lispro in the commercial formulation is accomplished by addition of zinc and *m*-cresol. The hexamers formed with zinc and insulin lispro are weak compared with those of human insulin and dissociate rapidly into monomers of the insulin analog that are absorbed through vascular endothelial cells. Consequently, insulin lispro has a more rapid onset of action than insulin human when given subcutaneously while retaining the conformation of critical sites necessary for binding to and activating the insulin receptor.

Biosynthetic insulin lispro (Humalog®) is prepared using recombinant DNA technology and special laboratory strains of nonpathogenic *E. coli*. The *E. coli* bacteria have been genetically modified by the addition of plasmids that incorporate genes for the lispro form of human proinsulin.

Commercially available biosynthetic insulin lispro injection consists of zinc insulin lispro crystals that are prepared by precipitating insulin lispro in the presence of zinc oxide and dissolving the crystals in water for injection, resulting in a clear aqueous solution. Each mL contains 100 USP units of biosynthetic insulin lispro solution and 19.7 mcg of zinc. Each mL of insulin lispro also contains dibasic sodium phosphate 1.88 mg, glycerin 16 mg, *m*-cresol 3.15 mg, and trace amounts of phenol. Sodium hydroxide and/or hydrochloric acid may be added during manufacture of biosynthetic insulin lispro zinc injection to adjust pH to 7–7.8.

Insulin lispro also is commercially available in fixed combination with insulin lispro protamine (neutral protamine lispro [NPL]), an intermediate-acting insulin. Insulin lispro protamine is prepared by crystallizing insulin lispro with protamine sulfate to produce a suspension with similar pharmacokinetics as isophane (NPH) insulin human. Each mL of the fixed combination of insulin lispro and insulin lispro protamine suspension (Humalog® Mix75/25®) contains 100 USP units of insulin lispro, 25 mcg of zinc (as zinc oxide), and 0.28 mg of protamine sulfate. Each mL of Humalog® Mix75/25® also contains dibasic sodium phosphate 3.78 mg, glycerin 16 mg, cresol 1.76 mg, and phenol 0.715 mg. Sodium hydroxide and/or hydrochloric acid may be added during manufacture of Humalog® Mix75/25® or Humalog® Mix50/50® injection to adjust pH to 7–7.8. Each mL of Humalog® Mix50/50® contains 100 units of insulin lispro, 0.03 mg of zinc ion (as zinc oxide), and 0.19 mg of protamine sulfate. Each mL of Humalog® Mix50/50® also contains dibasic sodium phosphate 3.78 mg, glycerin 16 mg, m-cresol 2.2 mg, and phenol 0.89 mg.

● **Stability**

Insulin lispro injection should be dispensed in the original, unopened, multiple-dose vial, disposable injection pen, or injection cartridge supplied by the manufacturer. When stored as directed, the vials and cartridges have an expiration date of not later than 2 years after the date of manufacture. Unopened vials or disposable injection pens of insulin lispro alone or in fixed combination with insulin lispro protamine or cartridges of the drug that have not been placed in a delivery device should be stored at 2–8°C and should not be subjected to freezing; the drug vial or cartridge should be discarded if it is frozen. Vials or cartridges of insulin lispro that cannot be refrigerated or vials and disposable injection pens that are in use may be stored at room temperature not exceeding 30°C for up to 28 days; exposure to extremes in temperature or direct sunlight should be avoided. Disposable injection pens of insulin lispro in fixed combination with insulin lispro protamine (Humalog® Mix75/25® Pen, Humalog® Mix50/50® Pen) that are in use may be stored at room temperature (below 30°C) for up to 10 days; exposure to extremely hot temperatures or direct light should be avoided. The manufacturer states that, once assembled by placement in the injectable pen (Owen Mumford Autopen®), insulin lispro cartridges and the injection device should be stored at room temperature and should *not* be refrigerated *nor* exposed to extremely hot temperatures or direct sunlight. Any unused insulin lispro in unrefrigerated vials, disposable injection pens, or cartridges should be discarded after 28 days. With the fixed combination of insulin lispro and insulin lispro protamine in disposable injection pens (Humalog® Mix75/25® Pen, Humalog® Mix50/50® Pen) or in vials, any unused portion should be discarded after 10 or 28 days, respectively.

When insulin lispro is diluted with the sterile diluent supplied by the manufacturer for improved accuracy in preparing pediatric dosages (see Dosage and Administration: Administration), the diluted solution should be discarded after 28 days when stored at 5°C or after 14 days when stored at 30°C.

Insulin lispro injection should be inspected visually prior to administration whenever the solution and the container permit. If the solution exhibits discoloration, turbidity, or unusual viscosity, the vial or cartridge should be discarded, since these changes indicate deterioration or contamination. Insulin lispro in fixed combination with insulin lispro protamine should be not be used if resuspension cannot be achieved (suspension should appear uniformly cloudy). (See Dosage and Administration: Administration.) Patients observing unexplained increases in blood glucose concentrations during insulin therapy should be particularly vigilant for any indications of loss of insulin potency and should contact a clinician if insulin requirements change markedly.

The compatibility of insulin lispro injection with other drugs depends on several factors (e.g., pH of the injection, concentration of the drugs, specific diluents used, temperature, resulting pH); specialized references should be consulted for specific compatibility information. For convenience, insulin lispro has been administered with a longer-acting insulin (e.g., isophane [NPH] insulin human) in the same syringe. Mixing of insulin lispro with other insulins may be associated with physicochemical changes that could alter the physiologic response to the insulins. When insulin lispro (Humalog®) was mixed with isophane (NPH) insulin human (Humulin N®), binding of insulin lispro with stabilizers/excipients (e.g., zinc, protamine) in the NPH insulin decreased the absorption rate and the peak concentration, but not the total bioavailability, of insulin lispro. (See Dosage and Administration: Administration.) Mixtures of insulin lispro and a longer-acting insulin (e.g., NPH insulin human should be given within 5 minutes after mixing; insulin mixtures should not be given IV. The manufacturer states that the effect of mixing Humalog® with insulins of animal origin (no longer commercially available in the US) or human insulins produced by other manufacturers has not been studied. Whenever insulin lispro is mixed with a longer-acting insulin preparation, insulin lispro should be drawn into the syringe first in order to prevent precipitation or turbidity of the insulin lispro solution by the longer-acting insulin.

When insulin lispro is administered via an external subcutaneous controlled-infusion device (pump), the drug should not be diluted or mixed with any other insulin. Insulin lispro in the external infusion device should not be exposed to temperatures exceeding 37°C during administration. Infusions sets (reservoir syringe, tubing, and catheter), the Disetronic® D-TRON® or Disetronic® D-TRON®plus cartridge adapter, and insulin lispro in the pump reservoir should be replaced and a new infusion site selected at least every 48 hours. The 3-mL cartridges used in the Disetronic® D-TRON® or Disetronic® D-TRON®plus insulin pumps should be discarded after 7 days, even if some drug remains in the reservoir.

Simulated administration of insulin lispro by continuous subcutaneous infusion in several external infusion pump systems (i.e., Disetronic H-Tron, MiniMed Model 504 pumps) revealed no changes in the potency, purity, or physical stability of insulin lispro when stored within each of these devices for 48 hours. However, precipitation of insulin lispro on infusion catheters (i.e., Silhouette, Soft-Set catheters) has been noted in several patients who were receiving insulin lispro via one of several external pump systems (i.e., Disetronic H-Tron V-100, MiniMed 507C pumps).

PREPARATIONS

Excipients in commercially available drug preparations may have clinically important effects in some individuals; consult specific product labeling for details.

Insulin Lispro (Recombinant DNA Origin)

Parenteral

Injection	100 units/mL	**HumaLOG®** (available as 3-mL cartridge, 3-mL disposable delivery device, and 10-mL vial), Lilly

Insulin Lispro Combinations (Recombinant DNA Origin)

Parenteral

Injectable Suspension	Insulin Lispro 25 units/mL with Insulin Lispro Protamine 75 units/mL	**HumaLOG® Mix75/25** (available as 3-mL delivery device and 10-mL vial), Lilly
	Insulin Lispro 50 units/mL with Insulin Lispro Protamine 50 units/mL	**HumaLOG® Mix50/50** (available as 3-mL delivery device), Lilly

† Use is not currently included in the labeling approved by the US Food and Drug Administration.

Selected Revisions January 1, 2010, © Copyright, January 1, 1998, American Society of Health-System Pharmacists, Inc.

Insulin Human

68:20.08.08 · SHORT-ACTING INSULINS

■ Insulin human is a biosynthetic protein that is structurally identical to endogenous insulin secreted by the beta cells of the human pancreas; commercially available insulin human preparations are classified as short-acting or intermediate-acting.

USES

● Diabetes Mellitus

Insulin human is used as replacement therapy for the management of diabetes mellitus, including in the emergency treatment of diabetic ketoacidosis or hyperosmolar hyperglycemic states when rapid control of hyperglycemia is required. Insulin human may be used in all patients with type 1 (insulin-dependent) diabetes mellitus, including all newly diagnosed patients requiring insulin therapy. In patients with type 1 diabetes mellitus, insulin human generally should be used in conjunction with a longer-acting insulin. In patients with type 2 diabetes mellitus, insulin human may be used in combination with oral antidiabetic agents and/or longer-acting insulins. Human insulin manufactured using recombinant DNA technology has replaced animal-source insulin (no longer commercially available in the US).

Safety and efficacy of insulin human injection have been established during short-term and long-term use.

Concentrated (U-500) insulin human (regular) is used in patients with marked insulin resistance (daily insulin requirements exceeding 200 units) so that a large dose may be administered subcutaneously in a reasonable volume.

The American Diabetes Association (ADA) states that human insulin is preferred for use in pregnant women, women considering pregnancy, individuals with allergies or immune resistance to animal-derived insulins, those initiating insulin therapy, and those expected to use insulin only intermittently. Use of insulin human has been associated with a reduction in insulin requirements in some diabetic patients with excessive insulin antibodies whose response was refractory to purified pork insulin (no longer commercially available in US).

Gestational Diabetes Mellitus

ADA recommends that insulin therapy (using insulin human) be considered in patients with gestational diabetes who, despite dietary management, have fasting plasma glucose concentrations exceeding 105 mg/dL or 2-hour postprandial plasma glucose concentrations exceeding 130 mg/dL.

● Hospitalized Patients

IV administration of regular crystalline insulin provides the greatest flexibility in dosing and is used in preference to subcutaneous administration in hospitalized patients with hyperglycemia (e.g., unrecognized diabetes mellitus, hospital-related hyperglycemia), diabetic ketoacidosis, nonketotic hyperosmolar states, poorly controlled diabetes mellitus and widely fluctuating blood glucose concentrations, or severe insulin resistance. Other situations that may require IV infusion of insulin include use in diabetic or hyperglycemic hospitalized patients who are not eating and those with hyperkalemia or critical illness requiring intensive care. IV insulin infusion also is used in general preoperative, intraoperative, and postoperative care, including heart or solid organ transplantation or surgery, or surgical patients requiring mechanical ventilation.

● Cardiovascular Disease

While insulin human (regular) has been used in combination with IV potassium chloride and dextrose (D-glucose) (referred to as glucose-insulin-potassium or GIK therapy) early in the course of suspected acute ST-segment-elevation myocardial infarction† (STEMI) for metabolic modulation and potential beneficial effects on morbidity and mortality, current data from a large randomized trial suggest that high-dose GIK therapy is not beneficial in reducing mortality following acute STEMI.

IV infusion of insulin also may be required in diabetic hospitalized patients with cardiogenic shock or hemodynamic instability.

DOSAGE AND ADMINISTRATION

● Administration

Insulin Human (Regular)

Insulin human (regular) injection is usually administered by subcutaneous injection. Insulin human (regular) also may be administered IV or IM† under medical supervision with close monitoring of blood glucose and potassium concentrations to avoid hypoglycemia or hypokalemia.

Parenteral Administration

Excessive agitation of the vial prior to withdrawing the insulin dose should be avoided since loss of potency, clumping, frosting, or precipitation may occur. Warming refrigerated insulin to room temperature prior to use will limit local irritation at the injection site.

For IV infusion, insulin human (regular) injection is usually diluted to a concentration of 0.05–1 unit/mL in 0.9% sodium chloride or 5 or 10% dextrose injection with 40 mEq/L of potassium chloride in polypropylene infusion bags.

The manufacturer of Novolin® R states that the injection should not be used in continuous infusion pumps, as such use may result in adsorption onto pump catheters.

When concentrated (U-500) insulin human (regular) injection is used in patients with marked insulin resistance (i.e., daily insulin requirements exceeding 200 units), extreme caution must be exercised in dosage measurement because inadvertent overdosage may result in irreversible insulin shock. The manufacturer further warns that serious consequences may result if this concentrated injection were used other than under constant medical supervision.

Standardize 4 Safety

Standardized concentrations for insulin (regular) have been established through Standardize 4 Safety (S4S), a national patient safety initiative to reduce medication errors, especially during transitions of care. Multidisciplinary expert panels were convened to determine recommended standard concentrations. Because recommendations from the S4S panels may differ from the manufacturer's prescribing information, caution is advised when using concentrations that differ from labeling, particularly when using rate information from the label. For additional information on S4S (including updates that may be available), see https://www.ashp.org/pharmacy-practice/standardize-4-safety-initiative.

TABLE 1. Standardize 4 Safety Continuous IV Infusion Standard Concentrations for Insulin (Regular)

Patient Population	Concentration Standards	Dosing Units
Adults	1 unit /mL	units/hour[a]
Pediatric patients (<50 kg)	0.2 units/mL	units/kg/hour
	1 unit/mL	

[a] DKA protocols may require units/kg/hour

Isophane Insulin Human

Parenteral Administration

Isophane insulin human suspension is usually administered subcutaneously; this form of insulin must *not* be administered IV. Since the active ingredient in isophane insulin suspensions is in the precipitate and not in the clear supernatant liquid, the vial should be gently agitated to assure a homogeneous mixture for accurate measurement of each dose. This may be done by slowly rotating and inverting or *carefully* shaking the vial several times before withdrawal of each dose. Vigorous shaking should be avoided since this causes frothing, which interferes with correct measurement of a dose.

Preparations of isophane insulin suspensions that are slowly injected subcutaneously may clog the tip of the needle, resulting in an inability to complete the injection. Since this is less likely to occur when the insulin is injected subcutaneously more rapidly, the dose should be injected over a period of less than 5 seconds.

When a compatible delivery device is used for subcutaneous injection of isophane insulin human suspension (e.g., Humulin® N pen) or the fixed combination containing insulin human (regular) injection and isophane insulin human suspension (Humulin® 70/30 Pen®), the accompanying labeling should be consulted for proper methods of assembly, administration, and care.

● **Dosage**

Diabetes Mellitus

Any change in insulin preparation or dosage regimen should be made with caution and only under medical supervision. Changes in strength, brand, type, and/or method of manufacture may necessitate a change in dosage. Illness, particularly nausea and vomiting, and changes in eating patterns may alter insulin requirements. Although it is not possible to clearly identify which patients will require a change in dosage when therapy with a different preparation is initiated, it is known that a limited number of patients will require such a change. Adjustments may be needed with the first dose or may occur over a period of several weeks.

Parenteral Dosage

Dosage of insulin human as the injection is always expressed in USP units. Dosage of insulin should be individualized to attain optimum therapeutic effect.

Initial total daily insulin dosages in adults and children with type 1 diabetes mellitus range from 0.2–1 units/kg. Children with newly diagnosed type 1 diabetes usually require an initial total daily dosage of approximately 0.5–1 units/kg; the dosage requirement can be much lower during the period of partial remission. In severe insulin resistance (e.g., puberty, obesity), the daily insulin dosage may be substantially higher. In patients with type 2 diabetes mellitus, the initial total daily insulin dosage ranges from 0.2–0.4 units/kg.

Diabetic Ketoacidosis and Hyperosmolar Hyperglycemic States

Because it has a relatively rapid onset of action and can be administered IV, regular insulin (e.g., insulin human [regular]) is the insulin of choice in the treatment of diabetic emergencies such as diabetic ketoacidosis or hyperosmolar hyperglycemic coma. Prompt correction of hyperglycemia with adequate doses of insulin, correction of dehydration and electrolyte imbalances with IV fluid and electrolyte therapy, and frequent monitoring of clinical and laboratory data are essential to successful treatment of these hyperglycemic crises. Hydration status should be carefully monitored in patients with diabetic ketoacidosis or hyperosmolar hyperglycemia, and 0.9% sodium chloride injection generally should be infused IV (in the absence of cardiac compromise) if serum sodium concentrations (corrected for the effect of hyperglycemia) are low; 0.45% sodium chloride injection may be used if serum sodium concentrations are normal or elevated. Since diabetic ketoacidosis often is associated with hypokalemia, the possibility of potassium imbalance should be evaluated and, if present, corrected before administration of insulin as long as adequate renal function is assured. Blood pH should be determined, and if acidosis is severe (blood pH less than 7), patients should receive IV sodium bicarbonate until blood pH exceeds 7.

Adults

For the treatment of *moderate to severe* diabetic ketoacidosis (plasma glucose exceeding 250 mg/dL with arterial pH of 7–7.24 or less and serum bicarbonate of 10–15 mEq/L or less) or hyperosmolar hyperglycemia in adults, the American Diabetes Association (ADA) recommends a loading dose of 0.15 units/kg of regular insulin by direct IV injection, followed by continuous IV infusion of 0.1 units/kg per hour. Plasma glucose should decrease at a rate of 50–75 mg/dL per hour. If plasma glucose concentrations do not fall by 50 mg/dL within the first hour of insulin therapy, the insulin infusion rate may be doubled every hour, provided the patient is adequately hydrated, until plasma glucose decreases steadily by 50–75 mg/dL per hour. When a plasma glucose concentration of 250 or 300 mg/dL is achieved in patients with diabetic ketoacidosis or hyperosmolar hyperglycemia, respectively, the insulin infusion rate may be decreased to 0.05–0.1 units/kg per hour. Once these target glucose concentrations have been achieved, infusion with 0.9% sodium chloride injection may be changed to dextrose 5% with

0.45% sodium chloride solution and administered with insulin to maintain serum glucose concentrations between 150–200 mg/dL in patients with diabetic ketoacidosis or 250–300 mg/dL in those with hyperosmolar hyperglycemia. Serum determinations of electrolytes, BUN, creatinine, osmolality, and glucose should be made every 2–4 hours until the patient is stable; monitoring of serum osmolality and cardiac, renal, and mental status is particularly important in patients with renal or cardiac compromise to avoid iatrogenic fluid overload. The rate of insulin administration or the concentration of dextrose may need to be adjusted to maintain glucose concentration until resolution of diabetic ketoacidosis (i.e., serum glucose less than 200 mg/dL, venous pH exceeding 7.3, serum bicarbonate of at least 18 mEq/L or hyperosmolar hyperglycemia (i.e., patient mentally alert, serum osmolality of 315 mOsm/kg or less).

For the treatment of *mild* diabetic ketoacidosis (plasma glucose exceeding 250 mg/dL with an arterial pH of 7.25–7.3 and serum bicarbonate of 15–18 mEq/L), ADA states that regular insulin given subcutaneously or IM† every hour is as effective as IV insulin administration in reducing hyperglycemia and ketonemia. A loading dose of regular insulin 0.4–0.6 units/kg may be administered in 2 doses, with 50% given by direct IV injection and 50% by subcutaneous or IM† injection. After the loading dose, 0.1 units/kg per hour of regular insulin may be given subcutaneously or IM†.

After resolution of diabetic ketoacidosis (i.e., plasma glucose less than 200 mg/dL, venous pH exceeding 7.3, serum bicarbonate of 18 mEq/L or greater) or hyperosmolar hyperglycemia in patients who are unable to eat, IV insulin and fluid replacement is continued, and subcutaneous regular insulin may be given as needed every 4 hours. Regular insulin may be given subcutaneously in 5-unit increments for every 50 mg/dL increase in blood glucose concentrations above 150 mg/dL, to a dose of up to 20 units of insulin for a blood glucose of 300 mg/dL or higher. When the patient is able to eat, a multiple-dose, subcutaneous insulin regimen consisting of a short- or rapid-acting insulin and an intermediate- or long-acting insulin is initiated. Regular insulin is continued IV for 1–2 hours after initiation of the subcutaneous insulin regimen to ensure adequate plasma insulin concentrations during the transition from IV to subcutaneous insulin; otherwise, abrupt discontinuance of IV insulin with the institution of delayed-onset subcutaneous insulin may lead to worsened glycemic control. Patients with known diabetes mellitus may reinstitute the insulin regimen they were receiving before the onset of diabetic ketoacidosis or hyperosmolar hyperglycemia, and the regimen may then be adjusted further as needed for adequate glycemic control.

Patients with newly diagnosed diabetes mellitus should receive a total insulin dosage of 0.5–1 units/kg daily as part of a multiple-dose regimen of short- and long-acting insulin until an optimal dosage is established. Some patients with newly diagnosed type 2 diabetes mellitus may be managed with diet therapy and oral antidiabetic agents following resolution of hyperglycemic crises.

Pediatric Patients

In pediatric patients (younger than 20 years of age) with diabetic ketoacidosis or hyperosmolar hyperglycemia, ADA recommends initiation of insulin therapy with an IV infusion of regular insulin at a rate of 0.1 units/kg per hour; an initial direct IV injection of insulin is *not* recommended in pediatric patients. If IV access is unavailable, insulin may be given IM in an initial dose of 0.1 units/kg, followed by 0.1 units/kg per hour subcutaneously or IM until acidosis is resolved (i.e., venous pH exceeds 7.3, serum bicarbonate concentration exceeds 15 mEq/L). Upon resolution, the insulin infusion rate should be decreased to 0.05 units/kg per hour until subcutaneous replacement insulin therapy (using a multiple-dose regimen of short- and intermediate-acting insulins) is initiated. When a serum glucose concentration of 250 mg/dL is achieved in pediatric patients with diabetic ketoacidosis or hyperosmolar hyperglycemia, dextrose 5–10% with 0.45–0.75% sodium chloride injection is administered to complete rehydration in 48 hours and maintain serum glucose concentrations between 150–250 mg/dL. Serum electrolyte and glucose concentrations should be determined every 2–4 hours until the patient is stable. After diabetic ketoacidosis in pediatric patients has resolved, subcutaneous insulin may be initiated at a dosage of 0.5–1 units/kg daily in divided doses ((2/3) of the daily dosage in the morning [(1/3) as short-acting insulin, (2/3) as intermediate-acting insulin] and (1/3) in the evening [½ as short-acting insulin, ½ as intermediate-acting insulin]). In pediatric patients with newly diagnosed diabetes mellitus, regular insulin 0.1–0.25 units/kg may be given every 6–8 hours during the first 24 hours to determine insulin requirements.

CAUTIONS

Insulin human shares the toxic potentials of other insulins, and the usual precautions of insulin therapy should be observed with insulin human.

Frequency and severity of adverse reactions to insulin human appear to be similar to those associated with purified pork insulin (no longer commercially available in the US).

● *Immunogenicity*

Several studies have shown parenteral insulin human to be less immunogenic than purified pork insulin (no longer commercially available in the US). Data from several studies in patients with diabetes mellitus have shown that insulin antibodies (IgE type) develop less frequently following administration of insulin human than following purified animal insulins (no longer commercially available in the US). Although a few patients in these studies developed elevated insulin antibody titers (IgE type) following administration of insulin human, they did not develop any signs or symptoms of insulin allergy or adverse reactions to insulin human. In one study in patients with diabetes mellitus who had not previously received insulin therapy, insulin human was associated with relatively weaker immunogenicity than purified pork insulin as determined by fasting insulin antibody levels.

Insulin human is contraindicated in patients who are hypersensitive to insulin human or to any ingredient in the formulation.

PHARMACOLOGY

Studies in animals, healthy adults, and patients with type 1 (insulin-dependent) diabetes mellitus have shown insulin human to have essentially identical pharmacologic effects compared with purified pork insulin (no longer commercially available in the US). Potency of insulin human, with respect to its efficacy for replacement therapy in patients with type 1 diabetes mellitus, is similar to that of purified pork insulin.

PHARMACOKINETICS

The pharmacokinetic profile of insulin human has been shown to be essentially identical to that of purified pork insulin (no longer commercially available in the US). No clinically important differences in total body clearance rates, plasma half-lives, apparent volume of distribution, or effect on blood glucose concentration have been observed following administration of insulin human or purified pork insulin. In vitro studies have shown that the binding affinities for human erythrocyte receptors and for receptors on porcine hepatocytes are similar for insulin human and purified pork insulin.

CHEMISTRY AND STABILITY

● *Chemistry*

Insulin human is a biosynthetic protein that is structurally identical to endogenous insulin secreted by the beta cells of the human pancreas. Although structurally identical to endogenous human insulin, commercially available insulin human is *not* extracted from the human pancreas, but is prepared biosynthetically from cultures of genetically modified *Escherichia coli* or *Saccharomyces cerevisiae*.

Biosynthetic insulin human (Humulin®) is prepared using recombinant DNA technology and special laboratory strains of nonpathogenic *E. coli*; the A and B chains of human insulin are synthesized by different strains of *E. coli*. The bacteria have been genetically modified by the addition of plasmids that incorporate genes for human insulin synthesis. Biosynthetic insulin human (Novolin® [formerly available as semisynthetic insulin]) is prepared using recombinant DNA technology and strains of *Saccharomyces cerevisiae*. The bacteria have been genetically modified by the addition of plasmids that incorporate genes for human insulin synthesis. Unlike the process used for the production of animal insulins (no longer commercially available in the US), the commercial process using recombinant DNA technology to produce insulin human avoids contamination with

glucagon, somatostatin, and proinsulin. Although a possible theoretical source of protein contamination (i.e., *E. coli* polypeptides [ECPs]) of certain biosynthetic insulin human (i.e., Humulin®) could be derived from the *E. coli* organism used in its manufacture, this commercially available biosynthetic insulin human contains less than 4 ppm of immunoreactive ECPs.

Each mg of insulin human has a biologic potency of not less than 27.5 USP insulin human units calculated on a dried basis.

● *Insulin (Regular)*

Biosynthetic

Biosynthetic insulin human (regular) injection consists of zinc insulin crystals that are prepared by precipitating insulin in the presence of zinc chloride. Commercially available insulin human (regular) injections containing 100 units/mL are clear and colorless. Each 100 USP units of biosynthetic insulin human (regular) contains 10–40 mcg of zinc. However, Novolin® R contains approximately 7 mcg/mL of zinc chloride. Humulin® R also contains 1.4–1.8% glycerin and 0.225–0.275% cresol and has a pH of 7–7.8. Novolin® R also contains 16 mg/mL of glycerin and 3 mg/mL of metacresol and has a pH of 7.4.

● *Insulin, Isophane*

Biosynthetic

Biosynthetic isophane insulin human is an intermediate-acting, sterile suspension of zinc insulin crystals and protamine sulfate in buffered water for injection, combined in a manner such that the solid phase of the suspension consists of crystals composed of insulin, protamine, and zinc. Biosynthetic isophane insulin human suspension is a cloudy or milky suspension of rod-shaped crystals free from large aggregates of crystals following moderate agitation. When examined microscopically, the insoluble material in biosynthetic isophane insulin human suspension (Humulin® N) is crystalline and contains not more than trace amounts of amorphous material. Each 100 USP units of biosynthetic isophane insulin human (Humulin® N) contains 10–40 mcg of zinc and 0.15–0.25% dibasic sodium phosphate. In addition, it contains 1.4–1.8% glycerin, 0.15–0.175% cresol, and 0.05–0.07% phenol. Biosynthetic isophane insulin human (Humulin® N) suspension has a pH of 7.1–7.4. Biosynthetic isophane insulin human (Novolin® N) has a pH of 7–7.8 and contains unspecified amounts of zinc, dibasic sodium phosphate, glycerin, cresol, and phenol.

● *Stability*

Insulin human injections and suspensions should be dispensed in the original, unopened, multiple-dose containers supplied by the manufacturers and have an expiration date of not later than 24–36 months, depending on the specific preparation, after the vial was filled. Unopened vials of insulin human injections, pre-filled syringes, and suspensions should be stored at 2–8°C and should not be subjected to freezing or exposed to heat and sunlight; freezing will cause isophane insulin human to resuspend improperly, preventing accurate measurement of a dose. Unopened solutions and suspensions that have been frozen should be discarded. In addition, agglomeration of particles may occur, altering absorption from the injection site. The insulin vial in use may be kept at room temperature for up to 1 month; exposure to extremes in temperature (less than 2 °C or greater than 30 °C) or direct sunlight should be avoided. Insulin vials in use and stored in the refrigerator may be used beyond 30 days. Length of storage of refrigerated insulin vials is dependent on light, agitation, and technique used for dose preparation. Warming refrigerated insulin to room temperature prior to use will limit local irritation at the injection site. Because of possible microbial contamination, a partially empty vial should be discarded if it has not been used for several weeks. Insulin human (regular) injection exhibiting discoloration, turbidity, or unusual viscosity should be discarded, since these changes indicate deterioration or contamination. Isophane insulin human suspension alone or in combination with insulin human should be discarded if the suspension is clear and remains clear after the vial is rotated or if the precipitate has become clumped or granular in appearance or has formed a deposit of solid particles on the wall of the vial.

The individual manufacturer's labeling should be consulted for instructions regarding storage of specific disposable insulin pens or other insulin delivery systems preassembled with cartridges (e.g., Humulin® N Pen, Humulin® 70/30 Pen).

Infusion bags containing insulin human (regular) are stable at room temperature for 24 hours. A certain amount of insulin will initially be adsorbed onto the walls of the infusion bag.

The compatibility of insulin human (regular) injection with other drugs depends on several factors (e.g., pH of the insulin injection used, concentration of the drugs, specific diluents used, temperature, resulting pH); specialized references should be consulted for specific compatibility information.

PREPARATIONS

Excipients in commercially available drug preparations may have clinically important effects in some individuals; consult specific product labeling for details.

Insulin Human (Regular) (Recombinant DNA Origin)

Parenteral		
Injection	100 units/mL	**HumuLIN® R**, Lilly
		NovoLIN® R, Novo Nordisk
	500 units/mL	**HumuLIN® R** (concentrated U-500), Lilly

Isophane Insulin Human (Recombinant DNA Origin)

Parenteral		
Injectable Suspension	100 units/mL	**HumuLIN® N**, Lilly
		HumuLIN® N Pen (available as prefilled cartridge preassembled into pen), Lilly
		NovoLIN® N, Novo Nordisk

Insulin Human Combinations (Recombinant DNA Origin)

Parenteral		
Injectable Suspension	Insulin Human (Regular) 30 units/mL with Isophane Insulin Human 70 units/mL	**HumuLIN® 70/30**, Lilly
		HumuLIN® 70/30 Pen (available as cartridge preassembled into pen), Lilly
		NovoLIN® 70/30, Novo Nordisk

† Use is not currently included in the labeling approved by the US Food and Drug Administration.

Selected Revisions October 10, 2024, © Copyright, April 1, 1984, American Society of Health-System Pharmacists, Inc.

Insulin Degludec

68:20.08.16 • LONG-ACTING INSULINS

■ Insulin degludec is a biosynthetic (rDNA origin), long-acting human insulin analog.

USES

● *Diabetes Mellitus*

Insulin degludec is used to improve glycemic control in the management of type 1 or type 2 diabetes mellitus in patients who require a long-acting insulin. Insulin degludec also is commercially available in fixed combination with liraglutide (Xultophy®); the fixed combination is used as an adjunct to diet and exercise to improve glycemic control in adults with type 2 diabetes mellitus.

Insulin degludec is *not* indicated for the treatment of diabetic ketoacidosis; a short-acting insulin (e.g., insulin human) is the preferred agent. Insulin degludec also is not recommended for use in pediatric patients who require less than 5 units of insulin degludec daily.

Insulin Degludec

Insulin degludec appears to be at least as effective for glycemic control as insulin glargine or insulin detemir (as determined by glycosylated hemoglobin [hemoglobin A_{1c}, HbA_{1c}]) in adult and pediatric (1 year and older) patients with type 1 or type 2 diabetes mellitus and is more effective in adults with type 2 diabetes mellitus than the oral antidiabetic agent, sitagliptin. Current evidence suggests that the prolonged duration of action and low variability in insulin degludec concentrations over the dosing interval may contribute to potentially lower rates of hypoglycemia (particularly nocturnal hypoglycemia) compared with other basal insulins. The peakless pharmacokinetic profile of insulin degludec allows for the timing of a once-daily injection to be varied from day to day in adults (when required) without increasing the risk of hypoglycemia (see Description); this flexibility in dosing may make insulin therapy less demanding and more acceptable to some patients, potentially improving patient compliance and glycemic control. Some clinicians suggest that insulin degludec may be a more suitable option than other basal insulins (i.e., insulin detemir, insulin glargine) in individuals who are prone to hypoglycemia and in those who require twice-daily administration of a basal insulin for adequate glycemic control, as well as in patients who experience variability in glycemic control with other basal insulins.

Type 1 Diabetes Mellitus

Safety and efficacy of insulin degludec for the treatment of type 1 diabetes mellitus has been demonstrated in comparisons with insulin detemir or insulin glargine in 3 randomized, open-label, noninferiority phase 3 trials of 26 or 52 weeks' duration in adults and a study in pediatric patients 1–17 years of age; patients also received mealtime insulin aspart during these trials. In a phase 3 trial in adults with type 1 diabetes mellitus who had been treated with basal and rapid-acting ("bolus") insulins for at least 1 year, patients received insulin degludec once daily with the evening meal or insulin glargine once daily at the same time each day, both in conjunction with mealtime insulin aspart. Basal insulin dosages were titrated based upon fasting plasma glucose concentrations. After 52 weeks of therapy, the decrease in HbA_{1c} from baseline was similar between treatment groups (average reduction in HbA_{1c} of 0.36 and 0.34% for insulin degludec and insulin glargine, respectively). The rate of nocturnal hypoglycemia (per patient-year of exposure) with insulin degludec in this trial was 25% lower than that with insulin glargine; however, the rate of severe hypoglycemic episodes did not differ substantially between the treatment groups. In another similar phase 3 trial, adults with type 1 diabetes mellitus received insulin degludec or insulin detemir once daily between the evening meal and bedtime, both in conjunction with mealtime insulin aspart. Patients who received insulin detemir were eligible to receive a second dose daily if there was inadequate glycemic control after at least 8 weeks of therapy. Basal insulin dosages were titrated based upon fasting blood glucose concentrations. After 26 weeks of therapy, the decrease in HbA_{1c} from baseline was similar between treatment groups (average reduction in HbA_{1c} of 0.71 and 0.61% for insulin degludec and insulin detemir treatment groups, respectively). Treatment with insulin degludec was associated with a substantially lower rate of nocturnal hypoglycemia than insulin detemir. In a third phase 3 trial, adults with type 1 diabetes mellitus received insulin degludec once daily (at the same time each day

or at alternating times daily [minimum of 8 and maximum of 40 hours between doses]) or insulin glargine once daily, all in conjunction with mealtime insulin aspart. Basal insulin dosages were titrated based upon fasting plasma glucose concentrations. After 26 weeks of therapy, the treatment group that received insulin degludec at varying times of the day had similar reductions in HbA_{1c} as those patients who received insulin degludec or insulin glargine injections at the same time every day (average reduction in HbA_{1c} of 0.41, 0.4, and 0.57% for insulin degludec administered at the same time each day, insulin degludec administered at varying times, and insulin glargine treatment groups, respectively). The treatment group receiving insulin degludec at varying times of the day had lower rates of nocturnal hypoglycemia than the insulin glargine treatment group.

In another study, pediatric patients 1–17 years of age (mean age: 10 years) with type 1 diabetes mellitus received insulin degludec once daily or insulin detemir once or twice daily, all in conjunction with mealtime insulin aspart. After 26 weeks of therapy, the mean decrease in HbA_{1c} from baseline did not differ substantially between treatment groups (reduction in HbA_{1c} of 0.19 and 0.34% for insulin degludec and insulin detemir treatment groups, respectively). At the conclusion of the additional 26-week extension period of this study, the observed mean decrease in HbA_{1c} remained similar between the 2 treatment groups; no substantial difference in the rates of hypoglycemia between groups was observed.

Type 2 Diabetes Mellitus

Safety and efficacy of insulin degludec administered once daily in adults with type 2 diabetes mellitus have been established in 6 open-label, randomized clinical trials of 26 or 52 weeks' duration that compared insulin degludec with sitagliptin or with other basal insulins (i.e., insulin detemir or insulin glargine) in conjunction with oral antidiabetic agents or mealtime insulin. In a noninferiority trial in insulin-naive patients with type 2 diabetes mellitus who were inadequately controlled with oral antidiabetic therapy, once-daily therapy with insulin degludec or insulin glargine was added to existing therapy with metformin with or without a dipeptidyl peptidase-4 (DPP-4) inhibitor. Insulin degludec and insulin glargine provided similar improvements in glycemic control (as measured by HbA_{1c}, the primary clinical end point) in this trial. The proportion of patients attaining target HbA_{1c} values of less than 7% at trial end point was similar across treatment groups. The risk of nocturnal hypoglycemia was lower with insulin degludec compared with that observed with insulin glargine.

In another noninferiority trial in insulin-naive Asian patients with type 2 diabetes mellitus who were inadequately controlled with oral antidiabetic therapy, once-daily therapy with insulin degludec or insulin glargine was added to existing therapy with 1 or more oral antidiabetic agents (metformin, a sulfonylurea, a meglitinide, or an alpha-glucosidase inhibitor). Patients receiving a glucagon-like peptide-1 (GLP-1) receptor agonist (exenatide or liraglutide) or a thiazolidinedione within 3 months of trial screening were excluded from the trial. All patients received an initial insulin degludec or insulin glargine dosage of 10 units subcutaneously once daily. Insulin dosages were titrated once weekly based on fasting plasma glucose concentrations. After 26 weeks of treatment, the observed mean HbA_{1c} and fasting plasma glucose concentrations were similar for insulin degludec and insulin glargine. Additionally, there was no substantial difference in the proportion of patients achieving an HbA_{1c} less than 7%.

In a trial evaluating the safety and efficacy of varying the daily injection time of insulin degludec, adults with type 2 diabetes mellitus inadequately controlled on basal insulin, oral antidiabetic agents, or a combination of these agents received insulin degludec once daily with the evening meal, insulin degludec once daily at varying times, or insulin glargine once daily. Patients who received insulin degludec at varying times were given alternating morning and evening injections (minimum of 8 hours and maximum of 40 hours maintained between injections). Patients receiving once-daily basal insulin prior to the study were transitioned to insulin degludec or insulin glargine on a unit-for-unit basis. Insulin dosages were titrated individually once a week throughout the trial based upon fasting plasma glucose concentrations. Patients receiving oral antidiabetic agents were allowed to continue treatment with up to 3 oral antidiabetic agents (metformin, a sulfonylurea, a meglitinide, or a thiazolidinedione) during the trial. Overall, insulin degludec given at variable dosing intervals resulted in similar glycemic control, hypoglycemic risk, and weight gain compared with either insulin glargine or insulin degludec given at fixed dosing intervals. There was no substantial difference in HbA_{1c} between patients who received insulin degludec once daily, insulin degludec once daily at varying administration times, or insulin glargine once daily.

In a noninferiority trial in adults with type 2 diabetes mellitus inadequately controlled on insulin and/or oral antidiabetic agents, no difference in overall glycemic control (as assessed by HbA_{1c}) was observed in patients receiving therapy with insulin degludec or insulin glargine; however, insulin degludec therapy was associated with a lower risk of hypoglycemia than insulin glargine. In this trial, patients received once-daily insulin degludec or once-daily insulin glargine, both in combination with mealtime insulin aspart, with or without oral antidiabetic agents (metformin, pioglitazone, or both). After 52 weeks of treatment, HbA_{1c} decreased by 1.1 and 1.2% in the insulin degludec and insulin glargine treatment groups, respectively. Rates of overall, nocturnal, and diurnal hypoglycemia were substantially lower in patients treated with insulin degludec versus insulin glargine.

In a trial comparing the efficacy of insulin degludec with sitagliptin in insulin-naive adults with type 2 diabetes mellitus, insulin degludec improved glycemic control and was superior to sitagliptin in terms of lowering HbA_{1c}. Patients in this trial received add-on treatment with subcutaneous insulin degludec once daily at any time of the day (minimum of 8 hours and maximum of 40 hours between injections) or sitagliptin 100 mg orally once daily; all patients were receiving stable therapy with 1–2 oral antidiabetic agents (metformin, a meglitinide, a sulfonylurea, or pioglitazone) at baseline. The starting dosage of insulin degludec was 10 units once daily, which was titrated weekly based upon fasting plasma glucose concentrations. Sitagliptin was administered at a dosage of 100 mg orally once daily. After 26 weeks of treatment, HbA_{1c} was reduced by 1.52 and 1.09% in patients receiving insulin degludec and sitagliptin therapy, respectively. Patients receiving insulin degludec therapy also had a lower fasting blood glucose after 26 weeks of treatment compared with those receiving sitagliptin therapy (mean fasting glucose 112 versus 154 mg/dL, respectively).

Insulin Degludec/Liraglutide Fixed-combination Therapy

Current data indicate that the fixed combination of insulin degludec and liraglutide is more effective than either drug (as add-on therapy to one or more oral antidiabetic agents) in improving glycemic control (as determined by reductions in HbA_{1c}) in patients with type 2 diabetes mellitus. Safety and efficacy of insulin degludec and liraglutide in fixed combination for the treatment of type 2 diabetes mellitus have been established in 5 parallel, randomized, active- or placebo-controlled phase 3 clinical trials of 26 weeks' duration in adults with type 2 diabetes mellitus.

In 2 clinical studies, the use of the fixed combination of insulin degludec and liraglutide substantially improved glycemic control in adults with type 2 diabetes mellitus who had inadequate glycemic control with oral antidiabetic agents and who were naive to therapy with a basal insulin or GLP-1 receptor agonist. In the first study, all patients continued on prestudy treatment with metformin with or without pioglitazone. In addition to the prestudy treatment, patients also received insulin degludec and liraglutide in fixed combination (initially 10 units of insulin degludec and 0.36 mg liraglutide), liraglutide (initially 0.6 mg), or insulin degludec (initially 10 units) subcutaneously once daily. Patients in the fixed-combination group or the insulin degludec treatment group had their dosages titrated twice weekly towards a target fasting plasma glucose concentration of 72–90 mg/dL. Patients in the liraglutide treatment group followed a fixed-escalation scheme with weekly dosage increases of 0.6 mg until the maintenance dosage of 1.8 mg once daily was achieved. After 26 weeks, the reduction in HbA_{1c} from baseline was 1.81, 1.35, or 1.21% in patients treated with the fixed combination of insulin degludec and liraglutide, insulin degludec, or liraglutide, respectively. In the second study, all patients continued on prestudy treatment with a sulfonylurea with or without metformin. In addition to the prestudy treatment, patients also received insulin degludec and liraglutide in fixed combination (initially 10 units of insulin degludec and 0.36 mg liraglutide) or placebo once daily. Patients in the fixed-combination group had their dosage titrated twice weekly towards a target fasting plasma glucose concentration of 72–108 mg/dL. After 26 weeks, the reduction in HbA_{1c} from baseline was 1.42 or 0.62% in patients treated with the fixed combination of insulin degludec and liraglutide or placebo, respectively.

In another trial, insulin-naive adults with type 2 diabetes mellitus who were inadequately controlled on metformin alone or in combination with pioglitazone and/or a sulfonylurea plus maximum-dose (or maximally tolerated) liraglutide (mean daily dosage at baseline: 1.7 mg) continued to receive their pretrial therapy or had their therapy converted from liraglutide to the fixed combination of insulin degludec and liraglutide. Oral antidiabetic agents were continued at pretrial dosages throughout the trial in both treatment groups. The starting dosage of the fixed combination was insulin degludec 16 units and liraglutide 0.58 mg once daily; dosage adjustments were performed twice weekly based on fasting blood glucose concentrations (end-of-trial dosage of the fixed combination: insulin degludec 44 units and liraglutide 1.58 mg daily). After 26 weeks, the reduction in HbA_{1c} from baseline was 1.31 or 0.36% with the fixed combination of insulin degludec and liraglutide versus liraglutide, respectively. A mean weight gain from baseline of 2 kg was observed in patients receiving the fixed combination

of insulin degludec and liraglutide compared with a weight loss of 0.8 kg in those receiving liraglutide. A higher rate of hypoglycemia was observed in the fixed-combination treatment group.

In another trial comparing the fixed combination of insulin degludec and liraglutide with insulin degludec therapy in adults with type 2 diabetes mellitus who were inadequately controlled with basal insulin and metformin with or without a sulfonylurea or a meglitinide, patients who received the fixed combination at equivalent insulin dosages achieved superior glycemic control. In this trial, all basal insulins and oral antidiabetic drugs except for metformin hydrochloride (mean daily dosage: 1984 mg) were discontinued at randomization; patients received a starting insulin degludec dosage of 16 units (given separately or in fixed combination with liraglutide 0.58 mg) once daily, which was titrated biweekly based on fasting plasma glucose concentrations. After 26 weeks, the mean daily dosage of insulin degludec was 46 units (with liraglutide 1.66 mg in the fixed combination) in both treatment groups. The reductions in HbA_{1c} from baseline were superior with the fixed combination of insulin degludec and liraglutide compared with insulin degludec treatment (reduction of 1.94 versus 1.05%, respectively). There was no substantial difference between the 2 treatment groups with regard to hypoglycemia.

In another trial comparing the fixed combination of insulin degludec and liraglutide with insulin glargine therapy in adults with type 2 diabetes mellitus inadequately controlled on insulin glargine and metformin, patients who received the fixed combination of insulin degludec and liraglutide achieved substantially greater reductions in HbA_{1c} compared with those who received insulin glargine. Patients in this trial either continued treatment with insulin glargine or were switched to the fixed combination of insulin degludec and liraglutide, both in conjunction with metformin. The starting insulin degludec dosage was 16 units daily (with liraglutide 0.58 mg in the fixed combination), irrespective of the patient's previous daily dosage of insulin glargine (mean insulin glargine pretrial dosage: 31 units daily). Patients whose therapy was switched from insulin glargine to the fixed combination of insulin degludec and liraglutide showed no worsening of blood glucose control immediately following the switch, despite the initial reduction in insulin dosage for patients who received the fixed combination. Each treatment was titrated biweekly based on fasting blood glucose concentrations with no upper dosing limit in the insulin glargine group and a maximum daily dosage of 50 units of insulin degludec in the fixed-combination treatment group. The mean dosage of the fixed combination of insulin degludec and liraglutide or insulin glargine was 41 units insulin degludec and 1.48 mg liraglutide or 66 units of insulin glargine daily, respectively. The reductions in HbA_{1c} from baseline were substantially greater with the fixed combination of insulin degludec and liraglutide compared with insulin glargine (reduction of 1.67 versus 1.16 %, respectively).

Insulin degludec and liraglutide in fixed combination should not be used for the treatment of diabetic ketoacidosis or for the treatment of type 1 diabetes mellitus. The fixed combination also should not be used with any other preparation containing liraglutide or another GLP-1 receptor agonist. Data are lacking on the use of the fixed combination of insulin degludec and liraglutide with prandial insulin.

DOSAGE AND ADMINISTRATION

● *General*

The dosage of insulin degludec is expressed in units. Each mL of insulin degludec injection contains 100 or 200 units of insulin degludec. Each mL of the fixed combination of insulin degludec and liraglutide contains 100 units of insulin degludec and 3.6 mg of liraglutide.

Dosage of insulin degludec should be carefully individualized to obtain optimum therapeutic effect based on the patient's metabolic needs, blood glucose determinations, and glycemic control goals. Glucose monitoring is recommended for all patients with diabetes mellitus.

Dosage adjustments of insulin degludec or the fixed combination of insulin degludec and liraglutide may be needed when used with other drugs or with intercurrent conditions (e.g., illness, stress, emotional disturbances), changes in physical activity, changes in meal patterns (i.e., macronutrient content or timing of food intake), or changes in weight or renal or hepatic function.

The 100-units/mL and 200-units/mL formulations of insulin degludec are pharmacodynamically and pharmacokinetically bioequivalent and have shown similar effects on glycemic control at equivalent dosages in clinical trials. Dose conversions between the insulin degludec 100- and 200-units/mL FlexTouch® injection pens based on differences in insulin concentration are not necessary and should *not* be performed. The dose window for the insulin degludec 100- and 200-units/mL FlexTouch® injection pens displays the number of insulin degludec units to be delivered independent of insulin concentration, and no conversion is needed to calculate the dose using either injection pen.

● Administration

Insulin degludec is administered by subcutaneous injection once daily using a FlexTouch® injection pen. Because of its delayed absorption and long duration of action, insulin degludec may be administered at any time of the day in adults. However, in pediatric patients, the drug should be administered once daily at the same time every day.

The fixed combination of insulin degludec and liraglutide is administered by subcutaneous injection once daily at the same time each day without regard to meals in adults; the injection is administered using the Xultophy® injection pen.

Insulin degludec or the fixed combination of insulin degludec and liraglutide should *not* be given IV or IM, nor should it be given via an insulin infusion pump. (See Description.) Insulin degludec or the fixed combination with liraglutide should not be mixed with any other insulin preparations or solutions.

Insulin degludec or the fixed combination of insulin degludec and liraglutide is administered subcutaneously into the thigh, abdomen, or upper arm. A planned rotation of sites within an area should be followed to reduce the risk of lipodystrophy.

The accompanying labeling should be consulted for proper methods of administration and care of the FlexTouch® or Xultophy® injection pen. These injection pens are used with NovoFine® or NovoTwist® needles. Insulin degludec should *not* be transferred from the FlexTouch® injection pen into a syringe for administration. (See Hypoglycemia: Hypoglycemia Due to Medication Errors under Warnings/Precautions, in Cautions.)

For adults who miss a dose of insulin degludec, the missed dose should be injected as soon as remembered during waking hours if at least 8 hours have elapsed between consecutive doses. If a pediatric patient misses a dose of insulin degludec, the patient or a parent or caregiver should be instructed to contact the child's clinician for guidance about dosing and monitoring blood glucose concentrations more frequently until the next scheduled insulin degludec dose. Patients who miss a dose of the fixed combination of insulin degludec and liraglutide should be instructed to resume the once-daily regimen as prescribed with the next scheduled dose; however, if more than 3 days have elapsed since the last dose, the fixed combination of insulin degludec and liraglutide should be reinitiated at the starting dose to mitigate GI symptoms related to the liraglutide component.

Unopened injection pens containing insulin degludec or the fixed combination of insulin degludec and liraglutide should be stored at 2–8°C until the expiration date. Alternatively, unopened insulin degludec injection pens may be stored at room temperature (up to 30°C) for up to 56 days. Injection pens containing insulin degludec or the fixed combination of insulin degludec and liraglutide should not be subjected to freezing; if freezing has occurred, the pen should not be used. In-use insulin degludec pens may be stored at room temperature (up to 30°C) or under refrigeration (2–8°C) away from direct heat and light for up to 56 days. In-use pens containing the fixed combination of insulin degludec and liraglutide may be stored at room temperature (15–30°C) or under refrigeration (2–8°C) away from heat or light for up to 21 days.

● Dosage

Insulin Degludec Therapy

Dosage of insulin degludec may be increased every 3–4 days as needed.

Insulin-Naive Patients

In patients with type 1 diabetes mellitus, insulin degludec should be administered once daily concomitantly with a prandial, shorter-acting ("bolus") insulin to provide more optimal postprandial glycemic control. In patients with type 2 diabetes mellitus, insulin degludec can be administered alone or concomitantly with oral antidiabetic agents or with a shorter-acting insulin. When used in a meal-related subcutaneous insulin regimen in patients with type 1 diabetes mellitus, an initial insulin degludec dosage usually comprises one-third to one-half of the total daily insulin dosage, with the remainder given preprandially in divided doses as a rapid- or short-acting insulin. An initial *total* daily dosage of insulin (total combined dosages of basal and rapid- or short-acting insulins) of 0.2–0.4 units/kg generally is recommended for insulin-naive patients with type 1 diabetes mellitus. The dosage of insulin degludec should be titrated based upon the patient's metabolic needs, blood glucose monitoring results, and glycemic control goal.

In insulin-naive adult and pediatric patients with type 2 diabetes mellitus, the recommended initial dosage of insulin degludec is 10 units once daily, with subsequent dosage adjustments to achieve glycemic goals.

Transferring from Therapy with Other Insulins

When insulin degludec is substituted for another intermediate- or long-acting insulin in adults with type 1 or type 2 diabetes mellitus, the manufacturer states that the initial dosage of insulin degludec for adults can be identical (on a unit-for-unit basis) to the total daily dosage of the previous longer-acting insulin. The dosage and timing of concurrent short- or rapid-acting insulins or other concomitant antidiabetic agents may need to be adjusted with the initiation of insulin degludec therapy.

For pediatric patients 1 year of age and older with type 1 or type 2 diabetes mellitus, the manufacturer recommends initiating insulin degludec at 80% of the previous total daily intermediate- or long-acting insulin dose to reduce the risk of hypoglycemia. The dosage of insulin degludec should then be adjusted according to blood glucose determinations to achieve glycemic goals. Close monitoring of blood glucose concentrations is recommended during the transition to insulin degludec from other insulin therapies. Additionally, adjustments to the dose and timing of concurrent short- or rapid-acting insulin or other glucose-lowering treatments (e.g., oral antidiabetic agents) may also be required.

For additional information on monitoring and management of insulin therapy, see Dosage: Considerations in Monitoring Insulin Therapy, in Dosage and Administration in the Insulins General Statement 68:20.08.

Insulin Degludec/Liraglutide Fixed-combination Therapy

In adults with type 2 diabetes mellitus who are naive to basal insulin or a glucagon-like peptide-1 (GLP-1) receptor agonist, the recommended initial dosage of the fixed combination of insulin degludec and liraglutide (Xultophy®) is 10 units (10 units of insulin degludec and 0.36 mg of liraglutide) once daily.

In adults with type 2 diabetes mellitus who are currently receiving basal insulin or a GLP-1 receptor agonist (e.g., liraglutide), such therapy must be discontinued prior to initiation of the fixed combination of insulin degludec and liraglutide. The recommended initial dosage of the fixed combination in these patients is 16 units (16 units of insulin degludec and 0.58 mg of liraglutide) once daily.

Dosage of insulin degludec in the fixed combination with liraglutide may be increased or decreased by 2 units (2 units of insulin degludec and 0.072 mg of liraglutide) every 3–4 days as needed. The fixed combination of insulin degludec and liraglutide should not be administered more than once daily. Adjustments in concomitant oral antidiabetic therapy may be needed.

The maximum daily dosage of insulin degludec in fixed combination with liraglutide is 50 units (50 units of insulin degludec and 1.8 mg of liraglutide).

● Special Populations

Hepatic Impairment

As with all insulin preparations, glucose monitoring should be intensified and the dosage of insulin degludec adjusted on an individual basis in patients with hepatic impairment. Safety and efficacy of the fixed combination of insulin degludec and liraglutide have not been established in patients with hepatic impairment.

Renal Impairment

As with all insulin preparations (including combination preparations), glucose monitoring should be intensified and the dosage of insulin degludec adjusted on an individual basis in patients with renal impairment. Safety and efficacy of the fixed combination of insulin degludec and liraglutide have not been established in patients with renal impairment.

Geriatric Patients

In geriatric patients, the initial dosage, dose increments, and maintenance dosage of insulin degludec or the fixed combination of insulin degludec and liraglutide should be conservative in order to avoid hypoglycemia.

CAUTIONS

● Contraindications

Insulin degludec alone or in fixed combination with liraglutide is contraindicated in patients with known hypersensitivity to insulin degludec or to any ingredient in the formulation. Insulin degludec alone or in fixed combination with liraglutide also is contraindicated during episodes of hypoglycemia.

The fixed combination of insulin degludec and liraglutide is contraindicated in patients with a personal or family history of medullary thyroid carcinoma (MTC) or in patients with multiple endocrine neoplasia type 2 (MEN 2).

● *Warnings/Precautions*

Use of Fixed Combinations

When insulin degludec is used in fixed combination with liraglutide or other drugs, the cautions, precautions, contraindications, and interactions associated with the concomitant agent(s) should be considered in addition to those associated with insulin degludec.

Hypoglycemia

Hypoglycemia is the most common adverse effect of insulins, including insulin degludec, and monitoring of blood glucose concentrations is recommended for all patients with diabetes mellitus. Severe hypoglycemia can cause seizures, may be life-threatening, or cause death. The onset of hypoglycemia depends on the action profile of the insulin used and may change when the treatment regimen or timing of dosing of the insulin is changed. (See Transferring from Therapy with Other Insulins under Dosage: Insulin Degludec Therapy, in Dosage and Administration.) As with all insulin preparations, the time course of the glucose-lowering effect of insulin degludec or the fixed combination of insulin degludec and liraglutide may vary among different individuals or at different times in the same individual and depends on many conditions (e.g., the area of injection, the injection site blood supply and temperature). The risk of hypoglycemia generally increases with the intensity of glycemic control. Other factors that may increase a patient's risk of hypoglycemia include changes in meal patterns, changes in level of physical activity, or changes to concomitant drug therapy. Patients with renal or hepatic impairment may be at higher risk of hypoglycemia. (See Renal Impairment and also see Hepatic Impairment under Dosage and Administration: Special Populations.) Some evidence suggests that insulin degludec may be associated with a lower risk of hypoglycemia, particularly nocturnal hypoglycemia, than insulin glargine and insulin detemir. (For more information on the symptoms associated with hypoglycemia, see Hypoglycemia under Cautions: Endocrine and Metabolic Effects, in the Insulins General Statement 68:20.08.)

Hypoglycemia Due to Medication Errors

Confusion between basal insulin preparations and other insulins, particularly rapid-acting insulins, has caused medication errors. To avoid such errors, patients should be advised to check the label on all insulin preparations to confirm the correct formulation and strength prior to administration. Insulin degludec should *not* be transferred from the FlexTouch® injection pen into an insulin syringe; the insulin syringe will not measure the dose correctly, and may cause an overdose and severe hypoglycemia.

Formulation Considerations

Any change in insulin should be made cautiously and only under medical supervision. Insulin degludec should not be diluted or mixed with any other insulins or solutions. Changes in insulin type, manufacturer, and/or method of administration may predispose patients to hypoglycemia or hyperglycemia. The frequency of blood glucose monitoring should be increased when changing a patient's insulin regimen. Adjustments to the dosage and timing of concurrent short- or rapid-acting insulin or other glucose-lowering treatments (e.g., oral antidiabetic agents) may be required. (See Transferring from Therapy with Other Insulins under Dosage: Insulin Degludec Therapy, in Dosage and Administration.)

Sharing of Injection Pens

Injection pens containing insulin degludec or the fixed combination of insulin degludec and liraglutide must never be shared among patients, even if the needle has been changed. Sharing of injection pens poses a risk for transmission of blood-borne pathogens.

Hypokalemia

All insulin preparations, including insulin degludec, cause a shift in potassium from the extracellular to intracellular space, possibly leading to hypokalemia. Untreated hypokalemia may cause respiratory paralysis, ventricular arrhythmia, and death. Serum potassium concentrations should be monitored in patients at risk for hypokalemia (e.g., patients receiving potassium-lowering drugs, patients taking drugs with effects sensitive to serum potassium concentrations).

Metabolic Effects

Insulin therapy may cause sodium retention and edema. Insulin therapy, including insulin degludec, also may cause weight gain attributable to the anabolic effects of insulin.

Heart Failure

Peroxisome proliferator-activated receptor (PPAR)-γ agonists (e.g., thiazolidinediones) can cause dose-related fluid retention, particularly when used in combination with insulin. Fluid retention may lead to or exacerbate heart failure. Patients treated with insulins, including insulin degludec, and a PPAR-γ agonist should be observed for manifestations of heart failure (e.g., excessive/rapid weight gain, shortness of breath, edema). If heart failure develops, it should be managed according to current standards of care and discontinuance or reduction of the dosage of the PPAR-γ agonist must be considered. Concomitant use of rosiglitazone and insulin therapy is not recommended.

Immunogenicity

As with all therapeutic proteins, there is a potential for immunogenicity with insulin degludec or the fixed combination of insulin degludec and liraglutide. In studies in patients with type 1 and type 2 diabetes mellitus, anti-insulin antibodies were detected in patients receiving insulin degludec therapy, including some patients who had anti-insulin antibodies at baseline. The presence of antibodies that affect clinical efficacy may require dosage adjustments to correct for tendencies toward hyperglycemia or hypoglycemia. The incidence of anti-insulin degludec antibodies has not been established.

Antiliraglutide antibodies have been found in patients who received the fixed combination of insulin degludec and liraglutide; however, this antibody formation has not been associated with reduced efficacy of the fixed combination.

Sensitivity Reactions

Dermatologic and Hypersensitivity Reactions

As with any insulin therapy, lipodystrophy may occur at sites of insulin injections and may affect insulin absorption. Injection site rotation may reduce the risk of lipodystrophy. Localized allergic reactions (e.g., pruritus, erythema, swelling) at the injection site may develop in patients receiving insulin, including insulin degludec. Pain, hematoma, hemorrhage, discoloration, warmth, injection site mass, and nodules at the injection site of insulin degludec or the fixed combination of insulin degludec and liraglutide also have been reported.

Severe, life-threatening, generalized allergic reactions, including anaphylaxis, angioedema, bronchospasm, hypotension, and shock, may occur with insulin preparations, including insulin degludec. If hypersensitivity reactions occur, insulin degludec therapy or the fixed combination of insulin degludec and liraglutide should be discontinued and appropriate treatment initiated; patients should be monitored until the hypersensitivity reaction resolves.

Specific Populations

Pregnancy

Data are lacking on the use of insulin degludec in pregnant women. In reproduction studies in animals, insulin degludec caused pre- and post-implantation loss and visceral/skeletal abnormalities in the offspring of pregnant rats and rabbits at maternal plasma concentrations 5–10 times higher than those achieved with a subcutaneous human dosage of 0.75 units/kg per day. The manufacturer states that these effects are probably secondary to maternal hypoglycemia. Insulin degludec should be used during pregnancy only if the potential benefit justifies the potential risk to the fetus.

Data are lacking on the use of the fixed combination of insulin degludec and liraglutide in pregnant women. Animal studies suggest that there may be risks to the fetus from exposure to liraglutide during pregnancy. The fixed combination of insulin degludec and liraglutide should be used during pregnancy only if the potential benefit justifies the potential risk to the fetus.

Lactation

Insulin degludec is distributed into milk in rats; it is not known whether the drug is distributed into human milk. The benefits of breast-feeding and the importance of insulin degludec to the woman should be considered along with any potential adverse effects on the breast-fed infant from the drug or from the underlying maternal condition.

Pediatric Use

Safety and efficacy of insulin degludec have not been established in pediatric patients younger than 1 year of age. Insulin degludec is not recommended for pediatric patients who require less than 5 units of insulin degludec daily; in clinical trials, pediatric patients receiving less than 5 units daily had their dosages titrated in 0.5-unit increments, which cannot be measured accurately with the commercially available FlexTouch® injection pen. In pediatric patients whose therapy is being transferred from another long- or intermediate-acting insulin to insulin degludec, the drug should be initiated at a reduced dosage to minimize the risk of hypoglycemia. (See Transferring from Therapy with Other Insulins under Dosage: Insulin Degludec Therapy, in Dosage and Administration.)

Safety and efficacy of insulin degludec in pediatric patients 1 year of age and older are based on a noninferiority clinical study of 12 months' duration in patients 1–17 years of age with type 1 diabetes mellitus, a pharmacokinetic study that included approximately 200 patients 1–17 years of age with type 1 diabetes mellitus, and data from clinical trials conducted in adults with type 2 diabetes mellitus. In the noninferiority study, insulin degludec and insulin detemir provided similar glycemic control (as determined by glycosylated hemoglobin [hemoglobin A_{1c}, HbA_{1c}]). Adverse effects reported in pediatric patients with type 1 diabetes mellitus who were receiving insulin degludec therapy were similar to those reported in adults.

Safety and efficacy of the fixed combination of insulin degludec and liraglutide have not been established in pediatric patients.

Geriatric Use

No substantial differences in safety and efficacy of insulin degludec or the fixed combination of insulin degludec and liraglutide have been observed in geriatric patients relative to younger patients; however, increased sensitivity of some older patients cannot be ruled out. Data indicate that the pharmacokinetic and pharmacodynamic properties of insulin degludec at steady sate are similar in younger adults and geriatric patients; however, greater variability has been observed among geriatric patients. Initial dosage, dose increments, and maintenance dosage should be conservative to avoid hypoglycemia. Hypoglycemia may be difficult to recognize in geriatric patients.

Renal Impairment

In a pharmacokinetic study in patients with or without renal impairment (including some patients with end-stage renal disease) who received a single subcutaneous dose of insulin degludec, there was no clinically relevant difference in the pharmacokinetic parameters in the renally impaired patients compared with healthy individuals. Blood glucose concentrations should be monitored closely; adjustment of insulin degludec dosage may be necessary.

Experience with the fixed combination of insulin degludec and liraglutide in patients with mild, moderate, or severe renal impairment is limited; the drug should be used with caution in such patients. (See Dosage and Administration: Special Populations.)

Hepatic Impairment

In a pharmacokinetic study in patients with or without hepatic impairment (mild to severe hepatic impairment) who received a single subcutaneous dose of insulin degludec, there was no clinically relevant difference in the pharmacokinetic parameters in the hepatically impaired patients compared with healthy individuals. Blood glucose concentrations should be monitored closely; adjustment of insulin degludec dosage may be necessary.

Experience with the fixed combination of insulin degludec and liraglutide in patients with mild, moderate, or severe hepatic impairment is lacking. (See Dosage and Administration: Special Populations.)

● Common Adverse Effects

Common adverse effects associated with insulin degludec during clinical trials include hypoglycemia, allergic reactions, injection site reactions, lipodystrophy, pruritus, rash, edema, and weight gain. Adverse effects occurring in at least 5% of patients with type 1 or type 2 diabetes mellitus who received insulin degludec during clinical trials include nasopharyngitis, headache, and upper respiratory tract infection. Sinusitis and gastroenteritis also were reported in at least 5% of patients with type 1 diabetes mellitus who received insulin degludec during clinical trials. Diarrhea was reported in at least 5% of patients with type 2 diabetes mellitus who received insulin degludec during clinical trials.

Adverse effects occurring in at least 5% of patients with type 2 diabetes mellitus who received the fixed combination of insulin degludec and liraglutide include nasopharyngitis, headache, nausea, diarrhea, increased lipase concentrations, and upper respiratory tract infection.

DRUG INTERACTIONS

● Drugs Affecting Glycemic Control

Drugs that May Potentiate Hypoglycemic Effects

Angiotensin-converting enzyme (ACE) inhibitors, angiotensin II receptor antagonists, antidiabetic agents, dipeptidyl peptidase-4 (DPP-4) inhibitors, disopyramide, fibrate derivatives, fluoxetine, glucagon-like peptide-1 (GLP-1) receptor agonists, monoamine oxidase (MAO) inhibitors, pentoxifylline, pramlintide, propoxyphene (no longer commercially available in US), salicylates, sodium-glucose cotransporter 2 (SGLT2) inhibitors, somatostatin analogs (e.g., octreotide), sulfonamide anti-infectives. Dosage reductions and increased frequency of glucose monitoring may be required if insulin degludec or the fixed combination of insulin degludec and liraglutide is used concomitantly with these drugs.

Drugs that May Antagonize Hypoglycemic Effects

Atypical antipsychotics (e.g., olanzapine, clozapine), corticosteroids, danazol, diuretics (e.g., thiazides), estrogens or progestins (e.g., oral contraceptives), glucagon, niacin, phenothiazines, protease inhibitors, somatropin, sympathomimetic agents (e.g., albuterol, epinephrine, terbutaline), thyroid hormones. Insulin degludec dosage increases and increased frequency of glucose monitoring may be required if insulin degludec is used concomitantly with these drugs.

Drugs With a Variable Effect on Glycemic Control

Alcohol, β-adrenergic blocking agents (β-blockers), clonidine, lithium salts, pentamidine. Adjustments of insulin degludec dosage and increased frequency of glucose monitoring may be required if insulin degludec is used concomitantly with these drugs.

Sympatholytic Agents

May decrease or eliminate the signs and symptoms of hypoglycemia in patients receiving insulin degludec concomitantly with these drugs (e.g., β-blockers, clonidine, guanethidine, reserpine). Increased frequency of glucose monitoring may be required if insulin degludec is used concomitantly with these drugs.

● Peroxisome Proliferator-activated Receptor-γ Agonists

Peroxisome proliferator-activated receptor (PPAR)-γ agonists (e.g., thiazolidinediones) can cause dose related fluid retention, particularly when used in combination with insulin. Fluid retention may lead to or exacerbate heart failure. Patients treated with insulin, including insulin degludec, and a PPAR-γ agonist should be observed for manifestations of heart failure (e.g., excessive/rapid weight gain, shortness of breath, edema). (See Heart Failure under Cautions: Warnings/Precautions.) Concomitant use of rosiglitazone and insulin therapy is not recommended.

● Protein-bound Drugs

No clinically relevant interaction suggested by in vitro binding studies with other protein-bound drugs.

DESCRIPTION

Insulin degludec is a biosynthetic (rDNA origin), long-acting insulin human analog that is prepared using a process that includes expression of recombinant DNA in *Saccharomyces cerevisiae* followed by chemical modification. Insulin degludec differs structurally from insulin human by the deletion of threonine at position 30 on the B chain and by the acylation of lysine at position 29 on the B chain with hexadecandioic acid, a 16-carbon fatty acid, via a glutamic acid spacer.

Insulin degludec has pharmacologic effects comparable to those of insulin human. (See the Insulins General Statement 68:20.08.) The prolonged duration of action of insulin degludec is dependent in part on slow systemic absorption, predominantly due to the formation of a depot of soluble multihexamer chains after subcutaneous injection and to a lesser extent due to binding of insulin degludec to circulating albumin. The fatty acid side chain modification of insulin degludec favors the formation of stable dihexamers while in solution at a neutral pH in the presence of phenol and zinc. After subcutaneous injection, these dihexamers assemble into long multihexamers; the large molecular weight of these multihexamers slows absorption, which creates a subcutaneous depot of insulin degludec from which monomers slowly dissociate in circulation. Insulin degludec has a long, flat, stable glucose lowering-profile, with a duration of action exceeding 42 hours and a terminal elimination half-life of approximately 25 hours. Due to the prolonged pharmacodynamics of insulin degludec, under steady state conditions the overlapping effect of daily injections results in less variability in glucose-lowering effect. Total exposure (in terms of area under the concentration-time curve [AUC]) and glucose-lowering effect of insulin degludec have been shown to be more evenly distributed than other basal insulins across a 24-hour dosing interval (i.e., peakless) in patients with type 1 or type 2 diabetes mellitus. Insulin degludec has a longer duration of action than insulin detemir and insulin glargine, and insulin degludec therapy is associated with less pharmacodynamic variability than other basal insulins. Insulin degludec has been associated with a fourfold lower within-patient day-to-day variability with regard to total glucose lowering effect compared to insulin glargine.

ADVICE TO PATIENTS

When insulin degludec is used in fixed combination with other drugs, importance of informing patients of important cautionary information about the concomitant agents.

Importance of providing patient a copy of manufacturer's patient information. Importance of advising patient to read the manufacturer's medication guide before beginning treatment with insulin degludec in fixed combination with liraglutide and of reviewing this information each time the prescription is refilled.

Importance of instructing patients not to administer the fixed combination of insulin degludec and liraglutide concurrently with other glucagon-like peptide-1 (GLP-1) receptor agonists. Importance of advising patients that dosages of insulin degludec exceeding 50 units daily given as the fixed combination with liraglutide can result in an overdose of the liraglutide component.

Importance of informing patients that serious hypersensitivity reactions have been reported with insulin degludec or the fixed combination of insulin degludec and liraglutide; importance of instructing patients to stop taking insulin degludec or the fixed combination and seek prompt medical attention if such adverse reactions occur.

Importance of advising patients to refer to patient information for additional information about the potential side effects of insulin therapy, including lipodystrophy (and the need to rotate injection sites within the same body region), weight gain, allergic reactions, and hypoglycemia.

Importance of informing patients that they should never share an injection pen containing insulin degludec or the fixed combination of insulin degludec and liraglutide with another person, even if the needle is changed; sharing of the pen may pose a risk of transmission of infection.

Importance of informing patients that hypoglycemia is the most common adverse effect of insulin. Importance of informing patients of the symptoms of hypoglycemia; the ability to concentrate and react may be impaired as a result of hypoglycemia, which may pose a risk in situations where these abilities are especially important (e.g., driving, operating machinery). Importance of advising patients who experience frequent hypoglycemia or reduced or absent warning signs of hypoglycemia to use caution when driving or operating machinery.

Importance of advising patients that changes in insulin regimen can predispose to hyperglycemia or hypoglycemia. Importance of changing insulin dosage with caution and only under medical supervision.

Discuss potential for alterations in insulin requirements in special situations (e.g., illness, emotional disturbances, other stresses). Discuss potential for alterations in insulin requirements as a result of inadequate or skipped doses, or inadvertent administration of an incorrect dose.

Importance of advising patients regarding what to do in the event of missed or delayed doses. (See Dosage and Administration: Administration.)

Importance of *not* mixing insulin degludec or the fixed combination of insulin degludec and liraglutide with other insulins or solutions. Importance of using insulin degludec or the fixed combination of insulin degludec and liraglutide only if the solution is clear and colorless with no visible particles.

Importance of informing patients to always check the insulin label prior to each injection; insulin degludec is available in concentrations of 100 and 200 units/mL. Importance of informing patients that the dose window of the insulin degludec FlexTouch® injection pen displays the number of units to be injected independent of insulin concentration; no recalculation of the dose is required to convert between different concentrations of insulin degludec. Importance of informing patients that the dose window of the injection pen containing the fixed combination of insulin degludec and liraglutide shows the number of units of insulin degludec to be injected; with each unit of insulin degludec, the pen also delivers 0.036 mg of liraglutide.

Provide instructions regarding self-management procedures including glucose monitoring, proper injection technique, and management of hypoglycemia and hyperglycemia.

Provide instructions to patient regarding use of the subcutaneous injection devices containing insulin degludec or the fixed combination of insulin degludec and liraglutide. Patients should be cautioned against reuse of needles. Importance of advising patients to never use a syringe to remove insulin degludec from the FlexTouch® injection pen.

Importance of informing clinicians of existing or contemplated concomitant therapy, including prescription and OTC drugs.

Importance of women informing clinicians if they are or plan to become pregnant or plan to breast-feed.

Importance of informing patients of other important precautionary information. (See Cautions.)

PREPARATIONS

Excipients in commercially available drug preparations may have clinically important effects in some individuals; consult specific product labeling for details.

Insulin Degludec (Recombinant DNA Origin)

Parenteral		
Injection, for subcutaneous use	100 units/mL	Tresiba® (available as FlexTouch® prefilled pens), Novo Nordisk
	200 units/mL	Tresiba® (available as FlexTouch® prefilled pens), Novo Nordisk

Insulin Degludec (Recombinant DNA Origin) Combinations

Parenteral		
Injection, for subcutaneous use	100 units/mL with Liraglutide 3.6 mg/mL	Xultophy® (available as prefilled injection pens), Novo Nordisk

Selected Revisions November 18, 2019, © Copyright, September 14, 2016, American Society of Health-System Pharmacists, Inc.

Insulin Glargine

68:20.08.16 • LONG-ACTING INSULINS

■ Insulin glargine is a biosynthetic (rDNA origin), long-acting human insulin analog.

USES

Insulin glargine is commercially available as Lantus® (100 units/mL), a "follow-on" preparation (Basaglar®; 100 units/mL), and a concentrated preparation (Toujeo®; 300 units/mL).

Lantus® and Basaglar® are structurally and pharmacologically similar drugs that contain a related drug substance. Basaglar® was licensed by the US Food and Drug Administration (FDA) through an abbreviated approval pathway [505(b) (2)] that relies in part on FDA's finding of safety and effectiveness for Lantus®. Comparative studies have found no substantial differences between the pharmacokinetics, immunogenicity, or toxicity of Lantus® and Basaglar®. Although Basaglar® is highly similar to Lantus® in terms of composition, strength, presentation, structure, and physicochemical and biological properties, it was *not* approved as a biosimilar or an interchangeable biologic product. Insulin is classified by FDA as a chemical, not a biologic product, so there is no biologic reference product for insulin glargine; thus, biosimilarity to insulin glargine cannot be established. Instead, Basaglar® is referred to as a "follow-on" insulin glargine preparation; FDA determined that there was no need to use a different nonproprietary name (insulin glargine) for Basaglar® at this time.

● *Diabetes Mellitus*

Insulin glargine 100-unit/mL preparations (Basaglar® and Lantus®) are used for the treatment of type 1 diabetes mellitus in adults and pediatric patients or type 2 diabetes mellitus in adults who require long-acting insulin for control of hyperglycemia. The 300-unit/mL preparation of insulin glargine (Toujeo®) is used for the treatment of type 1 or type 2 diabetes mellitus in adults who require long-acting insulin for control of hyperglycemia.

Insulin glargine in fixed combination with lixisenatide (Soliqua® 100/33) is used as an adjunct to diet and exercise to improve glycemic control in adults with type 2 diabetes mellitus inadequately controlled on lixisenatide or on less than 60 units daily of basal insulin.

For additional information on the management of diabetes mellitus, see Uses in the Insulins General Statement 68:20.08.

Insulin Glargine

Efficacy of insulin glargine administered once daily at bedtime (as Lantus®) in patients with type 1 diabetes mellitus has been demonstrated in comparisons with isophane (NPH) insulin human administered once or twice daily in 3 open-label, randomized studies of up to 28 weeks' duration in adults and one study in pediatric patients 6–15 years of age; patients also received regular insulin or insulin lispro before meals during these studies. Glycemic control (as determined by glycosylated hemoglobin [hemoglobin A$_{1c}$, HbA$_{1c}$]) was similar in patients receiving insulin glargine or isophane insulin human.

Efficacy of insulin glargine administered once daily at bedtime (as Lantus®) in adults with type 2 diabetes mellitus has been established in 2 open-label, randomized clinical studies comparing insulin glargine with isophane insulin human administered once or twice daily; patients continued to receive regular insulin or oral antidiabetic agents during these studies. Insulin glargine achieved a level of glycemic control similar to that of isophane insulin human as measured by HbA$_{1c}$.

Glycemic control with insulin glargine appears to be similar regardless of which meal it is administered before during the day. In a 24-week, open-label, randomized clinical study in adults with type 1 diabetes mellitus, insulin glargine (as Lantus®) was administered prior to breakfast, dinner, or bedtime; patients received supplemental insulin lispro at mealtimes. Glycemic control (as determined by HbA$_{1c}$ values at the end of the study, the primary end point) was not significantly different among the 3 treatment groups; only minor reductions in HbA$_{1c}$ occurred. Symptomatic and documented nocturnal hypoglycemia occurred in fewer patients receiving insulin glargine before breakfast than in the other 2 groups. However, 5% of patients in the before-breakfast group discontinued treatment because of lack of efficacy.

In another open-label, randomized, 24-week clinical study in patients with type 2 diabetes mellitus poorly controlled on oral antidiabetic agents, insulin glargine (as Lantus®) given prior to breakfast was more effective in reducing HbA$_{1c}$ than insulin glargine or isophane (NPH) insulin human given at bedtime. All patients were switched to or continued to receive glimepiride (3 mg daily in the morning) for 4 weeks prior to the addition of insulin therapy, and glimepiride therapy was continued throughout the remainder of the study. The incidence of hypoglycemia (primary safety end point) was similar across all treatment groups.

In an open-label study of 5 years' duration comparing therapy with once-daily insulin glargine (as Lantus®) to twice-daily NPH insulin in patients with type 2 diabetes mellitus, the progression of diabetic retinopathy was similar between the 2 treatment groups.

In a study evaluating the cardiovascular safety of insulin glargine (Outcome Reduction with Initial Glargine Intervention [ORIGIN]), the early use of insulin glargine to achieve normal plasma glucose concentrations in patients with dysglycemia neither reduced nor increased adverse cardiovascular outcomes as compared with guideline-suggested glycemic control. In this study, approximately 12,500 adults with cardiovascular risk factors in addition to impaired fasting glucose, impaired glucose tolerance, or type 2 diabetes mellitus received treatment with insulin glargine (as Lantus®, median dosage: 0.45 units/kg daily) or standard care (antidiabetic drugs other than insulin glargine in patients with a diagnosis of type 2 diabetes mellitus) for a median duration of 6 years. Patients who received standard care were not able to receive insulin therapy until maximal dosages of 2 different oral antidiabetic drugs had been used. There were 2 coprimary composite end points in this study: the composite of death from cardiovascular causes, nonfatal myocardial infarction [MI], and nonfatal stroke, and a composite of any of the previously mentioned cardiovascular adverse events, a revascularization procedure, or hospitalization due to heart failure. At a median follow-up of 6.2 years, there was no substantial difference between the 2 treatment groups in terms of major adverse cardiovascular outcomes or all-cause mortality. Additionally, the incidence of cancer or death from cancer was similar between treatment groups. Therapy with insulin glargine reduced the incidence of diabetes mellitus; however, the long-term clinical benefits of this reduction is unknown.

Safety and efficacy of the "follow-on" 100-unit/mL preparation of insulin glargine (Basaglar®) have been established by studies demonstrating its similarity to Lantus® and by the clinical trials that established the safety and efficacy of Lantus®, as well as by 2 clinical trials conducted using Basaglar® in patients with type 1 or type 2 diabetes mellitus. In these studies, Basaglar® was deemed sufficiently similar to Lantus® in terms of pharmacokinetics, toxicity, and immunogenicity and provided comparable glycemic control.

Safety and efficacy of the 300-unit/mL preparation of insulin glargine (Toujeo®) administered once daily in adults with type 1 or type 2 diabetes mellitus have been established in 4 open-label, controlled trials comparing a 100-unit/mL insulin glargine preparation (Lantus®) to Toujeo®. In these trials, the 300-unit/mL preparation of insulin glargine provided similar glycemic control as the 100-unit/mL preparation (as assessed by reductions in HbA$_{1c}$). Patients treated with insulin glargine 300 unit/mL required approximately 11–17.5% higher insulin dosages after 6 months of therapy compared with those receiving the 100-unit/mL preparation. Additionally, there were no clinically important differences in weight gain between the 2 insulin groups.

Insulin glargine is *not* the insulin of choice for treatment of diabetic ketoacidosis; a short-acting insulin (e.g., insulin regular) is the preferred agent.

Insulin Glargine/Lixisenatide Fixed-combination Therapy

Current data indicate that treatment with the fixed combination of insulin glargine and lixisenatide (insulin glargine/lixisenatide) is more effective than monotherapy with either drug in improving glycemic control (as determined by reductions in HbA$_{1c}$) in patients with type 2 diabetes mellitus. Additionally, therapy with insulin glargine/lixisenatide was associated with weight loss while weight gain was observed with insulin glargine monotherapy. Safety and efficacy of insulin glargine/lixisenatide have been established in an open-label trial in approximately 740 patients with type 2 diabetes mellitus inadequately controlled on basal insulin (e.g., insulin glargine, NPH insulin, insulin detemir) alone or in conjunction with 1 or 2 oral antidiabetic agents (e.g., metformin, a sulfonylurea, a meglitinide, a sodium-glucose cotransporter 2 [SGLT2] inhibitor, a dipeptidyl peptidase-4 [DPP-4] inhibitor). Patients underwent a 6-week run-in period in which all oral antidiabetic drugs (except metformin) were discontinued and therapy with insulin glargine was initiated and titrated prior to randomization. Patients then received treatment with insulin glargine/lixisenatide or continued insulin glargine therapy. The dosages of insulin glargine or insulin glargine/lixisenatide were titrated once weekly based upon fasting plasma glucose concentrations (mean final dosages of insulin glargine/lixisenatide or insulin glargine were equivalent at week 30 [46.7 units]). At week 30, there was a substantially greater reduction in HbA$_{1c}$ with insulin glargine/lixisenatide than with insulin glargine alone (reduction of 1.1 versus 0.6%, respectively). Patients receiving insulin glargine/lixisenatide had an average weight loss of 0.7 kg while those receiving insulin glargine monotherapy gained an average of 0.7 kg.

In another open-label trial of 30 weeks' duration, approximately 1170 patients with type 2 diabetes mellitus inadequately controlled on metformin with or without another antidiabetic agent (e.g., a sulfonylurea, a meglitinide, an SGLT2 inhibitor, a DPP-4 inhibitor) received therapy with insulin glargine/lixisenatide, insulin glargine, or lixisenatide, all in conjunction with metformin. Greater reductions in HbA$_{1c}$ were observed with insulin glargine/lixisenatide than with either component alone (reduction of 1.6, 1.3, or 0.9% with insulin glargine/lixisenatide, insulin glargine, or lixisenatide therapy, respectively). Mean body weight was reduced by 0.3 or 2.3 kg in patients receiving insulin glargine/lixisenatide or lixisenatide, respectively. Mean body weight was increased by 1.1 kg in patients receiving insulin glargine monotherapy.

The manufacturer states that insulin glargine/lixisenatide should not be used in patients with type 1 diabetes mellitus or for the treatment of diabetic ketoacidosis. The safety and efficacy of insulin glargine/lixisenatide in conjunction with short-acting (e.g., prandial) insulin have not been established, and such concomitant use is not recommended. Insulin glargine/lixisenatide is not recommended for use with any other drug preparations containing lixisenatide or another glucagon-like peptide-1 (GLP-1) receptor agonist.

DOSAGE AND ADMINISTRATION

● General

The dosage of insulin glargine is expressed in units. Each unit of insulin glargine is approximately equal to 0.036 mg of the drug. The dosage of the fixed combination of insulin glargine and lixisenatide (insulin glargine/lixisenatide) has been expressed in terms of the insulin glargine component; however, each mL of insulin glargine/lixisenatide contains 100 units of insulin glargine *and* 33 mcg of lixisenatide.

Therapy with lixisenatide or basal insulin should be discontinued prior to initiating therapy with insulin glargine/lixisenatide.

● Administration

Insulin glargine is administered by subcutaneous injection once daily into the abdomen, thigh, or upper arm at the same time each day using a conventional insulin syringe or the appropriate injection pen (e.g., SoloStar®, KwikPen®).

Insulin glargine/lixisenatide is administered by subcutaneous injection once daily using a prefilled injection pen. Insulin glargine/lixisenatide should be administered within 1 hour *before* the first meal of the day. If a dose of insulin glargine/lixisenatide is missed, the patient should resume the once-daily regimen with the next scheduled dose.

Insulin glargine or insulin glargine/lixisenatide should *not* be administered IV, IM, or via an infusion pump. A planned rotation of sites within an area should be followed so that any one site is not injected more than once every 1–2 weeks to reduce the risk of lipodystrophy. Clinical studies have not indicated important differences in absorption of insulin glargine from the various injection areas (e.g., abdomen, thigh, upper arm). It is *not* necessary to shake the vial of insulin glargine prior to measuring the dosage. Insulin glargine or insulin glargine/lixisenatide should not be mixed with other insulins, other drugs, or diluted with other solutions.

Insulin glargine injection should be inspected visually for particulate matter and discoloration before administration whenever solution and container permit. Insulin glargine or insulin glargine/lixisenatide should be administered only if the solution is clear, colorless, and without particulates.

Unopened injection pens and vials containing insulin glargine 100 units/mL should be stored at 2–8°C and protected from direct heat and light until the expiration date; the drug should *not* be frozen. Alternatively, unopened injection pens and vials containing insulin glargine 100 units/mL may be stored at room temperature (below 30°C) and away from direct heat and light for up to 28 days. Opened (in-use) *vials* containing insulin glargine 100 units/mL should be stored at 2–8°C for up to 28 days. Alternatively, such in-use *vials* may be stored at room temperature away from direct heat and light for up to 28 days. In-use *injection*

pens of insulin glargine 100 units/mL (Kwikpen®, SoloStar®) should be stored at room temperature away from heat and direct light for up to 28 days; in-use *injection pens* should *not* be refrigerated.

Unopened injection pens of insulin glargine 300 units/mL (Toujeo®) should be stored at 2–8°C and protected from light until the expiration date; the drug should *not* be frozen. In-use injection pens of insulin glargine 300 units/mL should be stored at room temperature away from heat and direct light for up to 42 days; such in-use injection pens should *not* be refrigerated.

Injection pens containing insulin glargine/lixisenatide should be stored at 2–8°C in the original carton and protected from light before first use; after first use, the injection pens should be stored at room temperature below 25°C. The injection pens should not be frozen; they should not be used if freezing has occurred. Injection pens of insulin glargine/lixisenatide should be discarded 28 days after first use, even if some drug remains in the pen.

The accompanying labeling should be consulted for additional details about the administration of insulin glargine or insulin glargine/lixisenatide.

● Dosage

Insulin Glargine Therapy

In patients with type 1 diabetes mellitus, insulin glargine must be used concomitantly with short-acting (e.g., prandial) insulin. In general, an initial total daily insulin dosage of 0.2–0.4 units/kg may be used in insulin-naive patients with type 1 diabetes mellitus. When used in conjunction with short-acting insulin, the manufacturers state that an initial insulin glargine dosage should be approximately one-third or one-third to one-half of the total daily insulin dosage for the 100- or 300-unit/mL preparations, respectively. The remainder of the daily insulin dosage should be given preprandially as rapid- or short-acting insulin.

In insulin-naive patients with type 2 diabetes mellitus, the recommended initial dosage of the 100-unit/mL preparation of insulin glargine is 0.2 unit/kg or up to 10 units given once daily. The recommended initial dosage of the 300-unit/mL preparation of insulin glargine in insulin-naive patients with type 2 diabetes mellitus is 0.2 units/kg once daily. The dosage of insulin glargine should be titrated based upon a patient's metabolic needs, blood glucose concentrations, and glycemic control goal.

The dosage of the 300-unit/mL preparation of insulin glargine should be increased no more frequently than every 3–4 days to minimize the risk of hypoglycemia. The maximum glucose-lowering effect of a dose of insulin glargine 300 units/mL may take 5 days to fully manifest, and the first dose of the 300-unit/mL preparation may not be able to fulfill the metabolic needs of the patient in the first 24 hours of use. Therefore, blood glucose concentrations should be monitored and dosages of coadministered antidiabetic drugs should be adjusted per the standard of care.

The dosage and timing of concurrent short- or rapid-acting insulins or other concomitant antidiabetic agents may need to be adjusted in patients receiving insulin glargine. Insulin requirements may be altered with changes in physical activity, changes in meal patterns (i.e., macronutrient content or timing of food intake), or during illness, emotional disturbances, or other stresses.

Transferring from Therapy with Other Insulins

When insulin glargine is substituted for another intermediate- or long-acting insulin in patients with diabetes mellitus, a change in the dosage of the basal insulin may be required. The dosage and timing of concurrent short- or rapid-acting insulin or other concomitant antidiabetic agents may also need to be adjusted.

In patients transferring from another 100-unit/mL preparation of insulin glargine (e.g., Lantus®) to Basaglar®, the dosage of Basaglar® should be the same as the other preparation, and the administration time should be determined by the clinician. In patients currently receiving once-daily isophane (NPH) insulin, the 100-unit/mL preparation of insulin glargine administered once daily may be substituted on a unit-for-unit basis for NPH insulin. In patients currently receiving twice-daily NPH insulin, the recommended initial dosage of the 100-unit/mL preparation of insulin glargine once daily is 80% of the total daily NPH insulin dosage that is being discontinued. For patients transferring from the 300-unit/mL preparation of insulin glargine to the 100-unit/mL preparation of insulin glargine, the recommended initial dosage of the 100-unit/mL insulin glargine preparation is 80% of the insulin glargine 300-unit/mL preparation dosage.

On a unit-for-unit basis, the 300-unit/mL preparation of insulin glargine has less of a glucose-lowering effect than the 100-unit/mL preparation. In patients currently receiving once-daily insulin glargine (100 units/mL) or an intermediate-acting insulin preparation, the recommended initial dosage of the 300-unit/mL preparation of insulin glargine is the same as the current long-acting insulin dosage. For patients controlled on the 100-unit/mL preparation of insulin glargine, a higher daily dose of the 300-unit/mL preparation of insulin glargine will be needed to maintain the current level of glycemic control. Patients transferring from other basal insulins to the 300-unit/mL preparation of insulin glargine may experience higher average fasting plasma glucose concentrations during the first weeks of therapy. In patients currently receiving twice-daily NPH insulin, the recommended initial dosage of the 300-unit/mL preparation of insulin glargine once daily is 80% of the total daily NPH insulin dosage that is being discontinued. Close monitoring of blood glucose concentrations is recommended during the transition to insulin glargine and in the initial weeks thereafter.

For patients with type 1 diabetes mellitus transitioning from IV insulin to the 300-unit/mL preparation of insulin glargine, the longer onset of action of the 300-unit/mL preparation of insulin glargine (onset of action develops over 6 hours) should be considered before stopping IV insulin. The full glucose-lowering effect of the 300-unit/mL preparation of insulin glargine may not be apparent for at least 5 days.

Insulin Glargine/Lixisenatide Fixed-combination Therapy

The recommended initial dosage of insulin glargine/lixisenatide for patients with type 2 diabetes mellitus inadequately controlled on less than 30 units of basal insulin or on lixisenatide is 15 units (15 units insulin glargine/5 mcg lixisenatide) subcutaneously once daily. For patients inadequately controlled on 30–60 units of basal insulin, the recommended initial dosage of insulin glargine/lixisenatide is 30 units (30 units insulin glargine/10 mcg lixisenatide) subcutaneously once daily. The dosage should be titrated by 2–4 units every week based on the patient's metabolic needs, blood glucose concentrations, and glycemic control goal. The recommended daily dosage of insulin glargine/lixisenatide is 15–60 units (15–60 units insulin glargine/5–20 mcg lixisenatide) once daily. Alternative antidiabetic therapy should be used if the patient requires a daily dosage of insulin glargine/lixisenatide of less than 15 units (15 units insulin glargine/5 mcg lixisenatide) or exceeding 60 units (60 units insulin glargine/20 mcg lixisenatide) daily.

● Special Populations

Hepatic Impairment

Data regarding the effects of hepatic impairment on the pharmacokinetics of insulin glargine in patients with diabetes mellitus are lacking. Careful monitoring of blood glucose and adjustment of insulin glargine or insulin glargine/lixisenatide dosage may be necessary in such patients.

Renal Impairment

Data regarding the effects of renal impairment on the pharmacokinetics of insulin glargine in patients with diabetes mellitus are lacking. However, increased circulating concentrations of insulin have been observed in patients with renal impairment who were receiving insulin human; therefore, insulin glargine requirements may be reduced in these patients. Careful monitoring of blood glucose and adjustment of insulin glargine or insulin glargine/lixisenatide dosage may be necessary in such patients. Safety and efficacy of insulin glargine/lixisenatide have not been established in patients with end-stage renal disease (estimated glomerular filtration rate [eGFR] less than 15 mL/minute per 1.73 m²); the fixed combination is not recommended for use in such patients.

Geriatric Patients

In geriatric patients, the initial dosage, dose increments, and maintenance dosage of insulin glargine or insulin glargine/lixisenatide should be conservative in order to avoid hypoglycemia.

CAUTIONS

● Contraindications

Known hypersensitivity to insulin glargine or any ingredient in the preparation. Contraindicated during episodes of hypoglycemia.

● Warnings/Precautions

Hypoglycemia

Hypoglycemia is the most common adverse effect of insulins, including insulin glargine, and monitoring of blood glucose concentrations is recommended for all patients with diabetes mellitus. The prolonged effect of subcutaneous insulin glargine may delay recovery from hypoglycemia. Severe hypoglycemia requiring the assistance of another person, IV glucose infusions, or glucagon administration has occurred with insulin therapy, including insulin glargine. As with all insulin preparations, the time course of the glucose-lowering effect of insulin

glargine or insulin glargine/lixisenatide may vary among different individuals or at different times in the same individual and depends on many factors (e.g., area of injection, injection site blood supply, temperature). The risk of hypoglycemia generally increases with the intensity of glycemic control. Other factors that may increase a patient's risk of hypoglycemia include changes in meal patterns (e.g., macronutrient content, timing of meals), level of physical activity, and concomitant drug therapy. Patients with renal or hepatic impairment may be at a higher risk of hypoglycemia. In comparative studies, the overall rate of hypoglycemic reactions with insulin glargine was similar to that with isophane insulin human. For more information on the symptoms associated with hypoglycemia, See Hypoglycemia under Cautions: Endocrine and Metabolic Effects, in the Insulins General Statement 68:20.08.

Hypoglycemia Due to Medication Errors

Confusion between basal insulin preparations and other insulins, particularly rapid-acting insulins, has caused medication errors. To avoid such errors, patients should be advised to check the label on all insulin preparations to confirm the correct preparation and strength prior to administration.

Formulation Considerations

Any change in insulin should be made cautiously and only under medical supervision. Insulin glargine should not be diluted or mixed with any other insulin. Patients previously receiving insulin may require a change in dosage if insulin therapy is changed to insulin glargine. Likewise, adjustment of oral antidiabetic dosage may be necessary in patients receiving concomitant therapy with insulin glargine. Changes in insulin strength, manufacturer, type, and/or method of administration may necessitate a change in insulin dosage.

On a unit-for-unit basis, the 300-unit/mL preparation of insulin glargine has less of a glucose lowering effect than the 100-unit/mL preparation. To minimize the risk of hyperglycemia when initiating insulin glargine 300 unit/mL, blood glucose concentrations should be monitored daily, the dosage of the 300-unit/mL insulin glargine preparation should be titrated appropriately, and dosage of coadministered antidiabetic drugs should be adjusted per the standard of care. (See Transferring from Therapy with Other Insulins under Dosage: Insulin Glargine Therapy, in Dosage and Administration.)

Sharing of Injection Pens

Injection pens containing insulin glargine or insulin glargine/lixisenatide must never be shared among patients, even if the needle has been changed. Sharing of injection pens poses a risk for transmission of blood-borne pathogens.

Hypokalemia

All insulin preparations, including insulin glargine, cause a shift in potassium from the extracellular to the intracellular space, possibly leading to hypokalemia. Untreated hypokalemia can lead to respiratory paralysis, ventricular arrhythmias, and death. Serum potassium concentrations should be monitored in patients at risk for hypokalemia (e.g., patients receiving potassium-lowering drugs, patients taking drugs with effects sensitive to serum potassium concentrations).

Metabolic Effects

Insulin may cause sodium retention and edema, particularly if metabolic control is improved by intensive insulin therapy. Insulin therapy, including insulin glargine, also may cause weight gain attributable to the anabolic effects of insulin and the decrease in glucosuria.

Heart Failure

Peroxisome proliferator-activated receptor (PPAR)-γ agonists (e.g., thiazolidinediones) can cause dose-related fluid retention, particularly when used in conjunction with insulin. Fluid retention may lead to or exacerbate heart failure. Patients treated with insulin, including insulin glargine, and a PPAR-γ agonist should be observed for manifestations of heart failure (e.g., excessive/rapid weight gain, shortness of breath, edema). If heart failure develops, it should be managed according to current standards of care, and discontinuance or reduction of the dosage of the PPAR-γ agonist must be considered. Concomitant use of rosiglitazone and insulin therapy is not recommended.

Immunogenicity

As with all therapeutic proteins, there is a potential for immunogenicity with insulin glargine or insulin glargine/lixisenatide. Insulin antibodies may increase or decrease the efficacy of insulin, and insulin dosage adjustments may be required.

During phase 3 clinical trials of insulin glargine (as Lantus®), the incidence of insulin antibody development with insulin glargine therapy was similar to the incidence observed with isophane (NPH) insulin. Insulin antibodies have also been detected in patients receiving other insulin glargine preparations (Basaglar® or Toujeo®).

Potential Carcinogenicity

FDA has notified healthcare professionals and patients about the results of several observational studies suggesting an increased risk of cancer in patients with diabetes receiving insulin glargine; however, upon further analysis, FDA states that the results of these studies are inconclusive due to limitations in how the studies were designed and carried out and in the data available for analysis. At this time, FDA states that it has *not* concluded that insulin glargine increases the risk of cancer.

In a health insurance database cohort of over 127,000 diabetic patients in Germany, a positive, dose-related association was found between diagnosis of a malignant neoplasm and use of insulin human or an insulin analog (insulin glargine, insulin aspart, insulin lispro) over a mean follow-up period of 1.63 years. After adjusting for insulin dosage, patients who had received insulin glargine dosages of 10, 30, or 50 units daily had a 9, 19, or 31% increase, respectively, in cancer risk compared with that for insulin human; no such increased risk was found for insulin aspart or insulin lispro. The results of this study prompted similar reviews of patient databases in Sweden and Scotland, both of which also suggested a positive association between cancer (e.g., of the breast) and use of insulin glargine. Review of a third database of patients in the United Kingdom and post hoc analysis of data from a controlled trial in patients with type 2 diabetes mellitus receiving insulin glargine or isophane (NPH) insulin human for a mean cumulative period exceeding 4 years did not reveal such an association. Potentially confounding factors (e.g., patient age, blood pressure, weight, concomitant antidiabetic therapy) and other limitations of retrospective analyses prevent firm conclusions based on these data. However, in vitro studies indicating that insulin promotes the growth of cancer cells and that insulin glargine is more mitogenic than insulin human support the concerns raised by these observations. and additional epidemiologic analyses worldwide have been called for to further examine any association between insulin analogs such as insulin glargine and cancer. In a study evaluating the cardiovascular safety of insulin glargine (Outcomes Reduction with Initial Glargine Intervention [ORIGIN]), the overall incidence of cancer or death from cancer was similar among patients who received insulin glargine and those who received other antidiabetic drugs (e.g., oral antidiabetic agents, insulin other than insulin glargine).

Based on currently available data, FDA recommends that patients *not* stop taking their insulin therapy without consulting a clinician, since uncontrolled hyperglycemia can have both immediate and long-term serious adverse effects. Some clinicians suggest that use of a long-acting human insulin (e.g., isophane [NPH] insulin human) or a combination of a long- and short-acting insulin twice daily may be considered as an alternative to insulin glargine therapy. FDA is continuing to evaluate the long-term risk, if any, for cancer associated with the use of insulin glargine. FDA encourages both healthcare professionals and patients to report adverse effects with the use of insulin glargine to the FDA's MedWatch Adverse Event Reporting Program (http://www.fda.gov/Safety/MedWatch/default.htm).

Use of Fixed Combinations

When insulin glargine is used in fixed combination with lixisenatide or other drugs, the cautions, precautions, contraindications, and interactions associated with the concomitant agent(s) should be considered in addition to those associated with insulin glargine.

Sensitivity Reactions

Dermatologic and Sensitivity Reactions

As with any insulin therapy, lipodystrophy may occur at sites of insulin injections and may affect insulin absorption. Injection site rotation within an area may reduce or prevent these effects. Pain at the injection site was reported among 2.7% of patients receiving insulin glargine (as Lantus®) compared with 0.7% of those receiving isophane insulin human in clinical studies. Other adverse local reactions reported with insulin glargine include redness, itching, urticaria, edema, and inflammation.

Hypersensitivity characterized by generalized skin reactions, angioedema, anaphylaxis, bronchospasm, hypotension, or shock may occur with insulin glargine therapy and may be life-threatening. If hypersensitivity reactions occur, insulin glargine or insulin glargine/lixisenatide should be discontinued and the patient should be treated per standard of care until hypersensitivity manifestations resolve.

Specific Populations

Pregnancy

Data are lacking on the use of insulin glargine or insulin glargine/lixisenatide in pregnant women. In animal reproduction studies in rats and rabbits, insulin glargine (100 units/mL) administered during pregnancy at dosages 2–7 times the human dose of 10 units daily did not cause any effects different than those seen with insulin human (regular). However, dilation of the cerebral ventricles was observed in some rabbit fetuses. Insulin glargine or insulin glargine/lixisenatide should be used during pregnancy only if the potential benefit justifies the potential risk to the fetus.

Lactation

It is unknown whether insulin glargine is distributed into milk; caution is advised if used in nursing women. Use of insulin glargine is compatible with breast-feeding; however, women who are lactating may require adjustments of their insulin dose.

Pediatric Use

Safety and efficacy of the 100-unit/mL preparations of insulin glargine (Lantus®, Basaglar®) have not been established in children younger than 6 years of age with type 1 diabetes mellitus or in pediatric patients with type 2 diabetes mellitus. Safety and efficacy of the 300-unit/mL preparation of insulin glargine (Toujeo®) or of insulin glargine/lixisenatide have not been established in pediatric patients.

Geriatric Use

Initial dosage, dose increments, and maintenance dosage of insulin glargine or insulin glargine/lixisenatide should be conservative to avoid hypoglycemia.

● Common Adverse Effects

Common adverse effects associated with insulin glargine therapy during clinical trials include hypoglycemia, allergic reactions, injection site reactions, lipodystrophy, pruritus, rash, edema, and weight gain.

Adverse effects occurring in at least 5% patients receiving insulin glargine/lixisenatide in clinical trials include hypoglycemia, nausea, nasopharyngitis, diarrhea, upper respiratory tract infection, and headache.

DRUG INTERACTIONS

● Drugs Affecting Glycemic Control

Drugs That May Potentiate Hypoglycemic Effects

Drug interactions are possible with drugs that may potentiate hypoglycemic effects of insulin glargine (e.g., angiotensin-converting enzyme [ACE] inhibitors, angiotensin II receptor antagonists, disopyramide, fibrate derivatives, fluoxetine, monoamine oxidase [MAO] inhibitors, oral antidiabetic agents, pentoxifylline, pramlintide, propoxyphene [no longer commercially available in the US], salicylates, somatostatin derivatives [e.g., octreotide], sulfonamide anti-infectives). Dosage reductions and increased frequency of glucose monitoring may be required if insulin glargine is used concomitantly with these drugs.

Drugs That May Antagonize Hypoglycemic Effects

Drug interactions are possible with drugs that may antagonize hypoglycemic effects such as atypical antipsychotics (e.g., olanzapine, clozapine), corticosteroids, danazol, diuretics, estrogens and progestins (e.g., oral contraceptives), glucagon, isoniazid, niacin, phenothiazines, protease inhibitors, somatropin, sympathomimetic agents (e.g., albuterol, epinephrine, terbutaline), and thyroid hormones. Dosage increases and increased frequency of glucose monitoring may be required if insulin glargine is used concomitantly with these drugs.

Drugs That May Have a Variable Effect on Glycemic Control

Drug interactions are possible with drugs that may have a variable effect on glycemic control (e.g., alcohol, β-adrenergic blocking agents, clonidine, lithium salts, pentamidine). Dosage adjustments and increased frequency of glucose monitoring may be required if insulin glargine is used concomitantly with these drugs.

Sympatholytic Agents

Sympatholytic agents (e.g., β-adrenergic blocking agents, clonidine, guanethidine, reserpine) may decrease or eliminate the signs of hypoglycemia. Increased frequency of glucose monitoring may be required when insulin glargine is used concomitantly with these drugs.

PHARMACOKINETICS

● *Absorption*

Bioavailability

Following injection into subcutaneous tissue, neutralization of insulin glargine solution results in formation of microprecipitates from which the drug is slowly released.

Following subcutaneous injection, absorption of insulin glargine is slower and more prolonged compared with that of isophane (NPH) insulin human; the serum concentration-time profile for the 100- or 300-unit/mL preparation of insulin glargine is relatively constant over 24 or 36 hours, respectively.

The absorption of the 300-unit/mL preparation of insulin glargine is more prolonged than that of the 100-unit/mL preparation.

Onset

Following subcutaneous injection of the 100-unit/mL preparation of insulin glargine, onset of hypoglycemic action is 1.1 hours. Following subcutaneous injection of the 300-unit/mL preparation of insulin glargine, the onset of glucose-lowering action develops over 6 hours. Substantial interindividual and intraindividual variation may occur based on tissue blood supply, temperature, exercise, and/or interindividual and intraindividual differences in response.

Duration

Following subcutaneous injection of the 100- or 300-unit/mL preparation of insulin glargine, duration of hypoglycemic action is approximately 24 or 36 hours, respectively. Duration of action is similar following subcutaneous injection at abdominal, deltoid, or thigh sites. Substantial interindividual and intraindividual variation in duration may occur based on tissue blood supply, temperature, exercise, and/or interindividual and intraindividual differences in response.

● *Elimination*

Metabolism

In the subcutaneous tissue depot, insulin glargine is partially metabolized to form 2 metabolites with activity similar to that of insulin. There are no differences in metabolism of insulin glargine when administered as the 100- or 300-unit/mL preparation.

DESCRIPTION

Insulin glargine is a biosynthetic (rDNA origin), long-acting human insulin analog that is prepared using recombinant DNA technology and a special laboratory strain of nonpathogenic *Escherichia coli* (K12). Insulin glargine differs structurally from insulin human by the replacement of asparagine at position A21 with glycine and the addition of 2 arginines to the C-terminus of the B-chain. Insulin glargine has pharmacologic effects comparable to those of insulin human. (See the Insulins General Statement 68:20.08.) In clinical studies, the glucose-lowering effect of the 100-unit/mL preparation of insulin glargine was approximately the same as insulin human on a molar basis.

Insulin glargine is commercially available as an acidic solution with a pH of approximately 4. Neutralization of the acidic insulin glargine solution following injection into subcutaneous tissue results in the formation of microprecipitates of the drug from which small amounts of insulin glargine are slowly released. This results in a relatively constant concentration-time profile over 24–36 hours (dependent upon insulin concentration) with no pronounced peak. Compared with the 100-unit/mL preparation of insulin glargine, the pharmacokinetic and pharmacodynamic profiles of the 300-unit/mL preparation of insulin glargine demonstrate a less variable response and a longer duration of action (36 versus 24 hours).

ADVICE TO PATIENTS

Provide copy of manufacturer's patient information.

Importance of *not* mixing or diluting insulin glargine or the fixed combination of insulin glargine and lixisenatide (insulin glargine/lixisenatide) with any other insulin or solution. Importance of using insulin glargine or insulin glargine/lixisenatide only if solution is clear and colorless with no particles visible.

Provide instructions regarding proper glucose monitoring, injection technique, and management of hyperglycemia or hypoglycemia. Discuss insulin requirements in special situations such as intercurrent conditions (illness, stress,

emotional disturbances), missed doses, or inadvertent administration of incorrect doses. Risk of inadequate, or variable timing of, food intake.

Importance of advising patients to refer to patient information for additional information about the potential adverse effects of insulin therapy, including lipodystrophy (and the need to rotate injection sites within the same body region), weight gain, allergic reactions, and hypoglycemia.

Provide instructions to patient regarding use of the subcutaneous insulin glargine devices. Patients should be cautioned against reuse of needles. Importance of advising patients to never use a syringe to remove insulin glargine from the SoloStar® injection pen.

Importance of informing patients that they should never share injection pens containing insulin glargine or insulin glargine/lixisenatide with another person, even if the needle has been changed; sharing of the pen may pose a risk of transmission of infection.

Importance of informing patients that changes to insulin regimens should be made cautiously and only under medical supervision. Importance of advising patients that changes in insulin regimen can predispose to hyperglycemia or hypoglycemia.

Importance of informing patients that their ability to concentrate and react may be impaired as a result of hypoglycemia, which may pose a risk in situations where these abilities are especially important (e.g., driving, operating machinery). Importance of advising patients who experience frequent hypoglycemia or reduced or absent warning signs of hypoglycemia to use caution when driving or operating machinery.

Importance of advising patients to always check the insulin label prior to each injection; medication errors involving confusion between insulins, particularly long- and short-acting insulins, have occurred.

Importance of informing patients that the 300-unit/mL preparation of insulin glargine (Toujeo®) contains 3 times as much insulin in 1 mL as standard insulin preparations (100 units/mL).

Importance of informing patients that the dose counter of the Toujeo® SoloStar® injection pen displays the number of units to be injected; no recalculation of the dose is required to convert between different concentrations of insulin glargine.

Importance of informing patients that if they are transitioned to the 300-unit/mL preparation of insulin glargine (Toujeo®) from other basal insulins, they may experience higher average fasting plasma glucose concentrations during the first weeks of therapy. Importance of advising patients to monitor glucose concentrations daily when initiating insulin glargine.

Importance of informing clinicians of existing or contemplated concomitant therapy, including prescription and OTC drugs.

Importance of women informing clinicians if they are or plan to become pregnant or breast-feed.

Importance of informing patients of other important precautionary information. (See Cautions.)

PREPARATIONS

Excipients in commercially available drug preparations may have clinically important effects in some individuals; consult specific product labeling for details.

Insulin Glargine (Recombinant DNA Origin)

Parenteral		
Injection, for subcutaneous use only	100 units/mL (U-100)	**Basaglar®** (in prefilled KwikPen® pens), Lilly
		Lantus® (in vials and prefilled SoloStar® pens), Sanofi-Aventis
	300 units/mL (U-300)	**Toujeo®** (in prefilled SoloStar® pens), Sanofi-Aventis

Insulin Glargine (Recombinant DNA Origin) Combinations

Parenteral		
Injection, for subcutaneous use	100 units/mL with Lixisenatide 33 mcg/mL	**Soliqua® 100/33** (available as prefilled injection pens), Sanofi-Aventis

Selected Revisions July 30, 2018, © Copyright, August 1, 2000, American Society of Health-System Pharmacists, Inc.

Canagliflozin

68:20.18 • SODIUM-GLUCOSE COTRANSPORTER 2 (SGLT2) INHIBITORS

■ Canagliflozin, a sodium-glucose cotransporter 2 (SGLT2) inhibitor, is an antidiabetic agent.

USES

● Type 2 Diabetes Mellitus

Canagliflozin is used as monotherapy as an adjunct to diet and exercise to improve glycemic control in patients with type 2 diabetes mellitus. In addition, canagliflozin is used to reduce the risk of major cardiovascular events (e.g., cardiovascular death, nonfatal myocardial infarction [MI], nonfatal stroke) in patients with type 2 diabetes mellitus and established cardiovascular disease. In addition, canagliflozin is used to reduce the risk of end-stage renal disease (ESRD), doubling of serum creatinine, cardiovascular death, and hospitalization for heart failure in adults with type 2 diabetes mellitus and diabetic nephropathy with albuminuria (exceeding 300 mg/day).

Canagliflozin is commercially available in fixed combination with immediate- or extended-release metformin hydrochloride (Invokamet® or Invokamet® XR); the fixed combination is used when treatment with both drugs is appropriate. Canagliflozin also is used in combination with other antidiabetic agents (e.g., metformin, a sulfonylurea, a peroxisome proliferator-activated receptor$_\gamma$ [PPAR$_\gamma$] agonist [thiazolidinedione]) or insulin as an adjunct to diet and exercise in patients with type 2 diabetes mellitus who have not achieved adequate glycemic control.

Glycemic Control

Current guidelines for the treatment of type 2 diabetes mellitus generally recommend metformin as first-line therapy in addition to lifestyle modifications in patients with recent-onset type 2 diabetes mellitus or mild hyperglycemia because of its well-established safety and efficacy (i.e., beneficial effects on glycosylated hemoglobin [hemoglobin A$_{1c}$; HbA$_{1c}$], weight, and cardiovascular mortality). (See Uses: Type 2 Diabetes Mellitus, in Metformin 68:20.04.) In patients with contraindications or intolerance to metformin (e.g., risk of lactic acidosis, GI intolerance) or in selected other patients, some experts suggest that initial therapy with a drug from another class of antidiabetic agents (e.g., a glucagon-like peptide-1 [GLP-1] receptor agonist, SGLT2 inhibitor, dipeptidyl peptidase-4 [DPP-4] inhibitor, sulfonylurea, thiazolidinedione, basal insulin) may be acceptable based on patient factors. Initiating antidiabetic therapy with 2 agents (e.g., metformin plus another agent) may be appropriate in patients with an initial HbA$_{1c}$ exceeding 7.5% or at least 1.5% above the target level. In metformin-intolerant patients with high initial HbA$_{1c}$ levels, some experts suggest initiation of therapy with 2 agents from other antidiabetic classes with complementary mechanisms of action.

Because of the progressive nature of type 2 diabetes mellitus, patients initially receiving an oral antidiabetic agent will eventually require multiple oral and/or injectable noninsulin antidiabetic agents of different therapeutic classes and/or insulin for adequate glycemic control. Patients who have inadequate glycemic control with initial (e.g., metformin) monotherapy should receive treatment with additional antidiabetic agents; data suggest that the addition of each noninsulin agent to initial therapy lowers HbA$_{1c}$ by approximately 0.7–1%. In addition, early initiation of combination therapy may help to more rapidly attain glycemic goals and extend the time to treatment failure.

Factors to consider when selecting additional antidiabetic agents for combination therapy in patients with inadequate glycemic control on metformin monotherapy include patient comorbidities (e.g., atherosclerotic cardiovascular disease [ASCVD], established kidney disease, heart failure), hypoglycemia risk, impact on weight, cost, risk of adverse effects, and patient preference. When the greater glucose-lowering effect of an injectable drug is needed in patients with type 2 diabetes mellitus, some experts currently state that an injectable GLP-1 receptor agonist is preferred over insulin in most patients because of beneficial effects on body weight and a lower risk of hypoglycemia, although adverse GI effects may diminish tolerability. While addition of a GLP-1 receptor agonist may successfully control hyperglycemia, many patients will eventually require insulin therapy. Early introduction of insulin therapy should be considered when hyperglycemia is severe (e.g., blood glucose of at least 300 mg/dL or HbA$_{1c}$ exceeding 9–10%), especially in the presence of catabolic manifestations (e.g., weight loss, hypertriglyceridemia, ketosis) or symptoms of hyperglycemia. For additional information regarding the initiation of insulin therapy in patients with diabetes mellitus, see Uses: Diabetes Mellitus, in the Insulins General Statement 68:20.08.

Patients with type 2 diabetes mellitus who have established (or are at a high risk for) ASCVD, established kidney disease, or heart failure should receive a GLP-1 receptor agonist or SGLT2 inhibitor with demonstrated cardiovascular disease benefit. (See Reduction in Risk of Major Adverse Cardiovascular Events under Uses: Type 2 Diabetes Mellitus, in Liraglutide 68:20.06 and also see Reduction in Risk of Heart Failure-Related Hospitalization under Uses: Type 2 Diabetes Mellitus, in Dapagliflozin 68:20.18.) Experts state that therapy with a GLP-1 receptor agonist or SGLT2 inhibitor should be considered for patients with the aforementioned comorbidities independently of the patients' HbA$_{1c}$. GLP-1 receptor agonists and SGLT2 inhibitors appear to have effects on the kidneys independent of their glycemic effects, and some experts suggest that an agent from one of these classes of drugs be considered in patients with type 2 diabetes mellitus and chronic kidney disease (CKD). (See Beneficial Effects on Renal Function and Cardiovascular Morbidity and Mortality in Diabetic Nephropathy under Uses: Type 2 Diabetes Mellitus.) In patients *without* established ASCVD or indicators of high ASCVD risk, heart failure, or CKD, the decision regarding the addition of other antidiabetic agents (e.g., GLP-1 receptor agonist, SGLT2 inhibitor, DPP-4 inhibitor, thiazolidinedione, sulfonylurea, basal insulin) to metformin therapy should be based on avoidance of adverse effects, cost, and individual patient factors.

The manufacturer states that canagliflozin should *not* be used for the treatment of type 1 diabetes mellitus or diabetic ketoacidosis.

Canagliflozin Monotherapy

When given as monotherapy for the management of type 2 diabetes mellitus, canagliflozin improves glycemic control compared with placebo as evidenced by reductions in glycosylated hemoglobin HbA$_{1c}$ and in fasting and 2-hour postprandial plasma glucose concentrations. Efficacy of canagliflozin as monotherapy for the management of type 2 diabetes mellitus has been established in a double-blind, placebo-controlled study of 26 weeks' duration. Canagliflozin (100 or 300 mg once daily) improved glycemic control as evidenced by reductions in HbA$_{1c}$ and fasting and 2-hour postprandial plasma glucose concentrations. HbA$_{1c}$ was reduced by 0.77 or 1% in patients receiving canagliflozin 100 or 300 mg once daily, respectively, compared with an increase of 0.1% in those receiving placebo. Patients receiving canagliflozin 100 or 300 mg once daily also lost substantially more body weight (2.8 or 3.9%, respectively) than those receiving placebo (0.6%).

Combination Therapy

When given in combination with one or more oral antidiabetic agents or insulin, canagliflozin improves glycemic control compared with monotherapy with these drugs and generally is associated with reductions in body weight. Canagliflozin generally is well tolerated, although genital mycotic infections appear to be more common with canagliflozin than with other antidiabetic agents. (See Genital Mycotic Infections under Cautions: Warnings/Precautions.)

Efficacy of canagliflozin in combination with metformin, a sulfonylurea, and/or a thiazolidinedione for the management of type 2 diabetes mellitus (in patients inadequately controlled with metformin, a sulfonylurea, and/or a thiazolidinedione monotherapy) is supported by results from several long-term, randomized, active- or placebo-controlled trials. In these trials, the addition of canagliflozin (100 or 300 mg once daily) to existing therapy improved glycemic control as evidenced by reductions in HbA$_{1c}$, fasting plasma glucose, 2-hour postprandial plasma glucose concentrations, and/or body weight compared with placebo. In a 26-week study in patients receiving metformin hydrochloride therapy (dosage of at least 1.5 g daily), the addition of canagliflozin resulted in a reduction of 0.8–0.9% in HbA$_{1c}$, while HbA$_{1c}$ was increased by 0.1% with add-on placebo. In a 52-week study in patients receiving metformin hydrochloride therapy (dosage of at least 1.5 g daily), canagliflozin 100 mg once daily was noninferior to glimepiride (titrated to 6 or 8 mg once daily), and canagliflozin 300 mg once daily was superior to glimepiride, in reducing HbA$_{1c}$; patients achieved reductions of 0.8, 0.9, or 0.8% in HbA$_{1c}$ with canagliflozin 100 mg, canagliflozin 300 mg, or glimepiride, respectively. In an 18-week trial in patients receiving a sulfonylurea (generally glimepiride, glyburide [glibenclamide], or gliclazide [not commercially available in the US]), add-on therapy with canagliflozin 100 or 300 mg once daily resulted in a reduction in HbA$_{1c}$ of 0.74 or 0.83%, respectively, compared with placebo.

Efficacy and safety of the combination of canagliflozin and metformin as initial therapy in patients with type 2 diabetes mellitus inadequately controlled with diet and exercise is supported by results of a 26-week, randomized, double-blind trial. In this trial, concurrent therapy with canagliflozin (100 or 300 mg once daily) and metformin hydrochloride extended-release (dosage of at least 1.5 g daily; 90% of patients achieved a dosage of 2 g daily) substantially improved glycemic control (as evidenced by reductions in HbA$_{1c}$) compared with canagliflozin or metformin hydrochloride monotherapy. Reductions in HbA$_{1c}$ were 1.77 or 1.78% with canagliflozin 100 or 300 mg once daily, respectively, plus metformin hydrochloride; 1.37 or 1.42% with canagliflozin 100 or 300 mg once daily, respectively; and 1.3% with metformin hydrochloride monotherapy. Additionally, a greater percentage of patients achieved an HbA$_{1c}$ of less than 7% with canagliflozin and metformin combination therapy compared with canagliflozin or metformin hydrochloride monotherapy.

In a 26-week trial in patients receiving metformin hydrochloride (dosage of at least 1.5 g daily) and a sulfonylurea (sulfonylurea not specified), addition of canagliflozin 100 or 300 mg once daily resulted in a reduction in HbA$_{1c}$ of 0.85 or 1.06%, respectively, compared with a 0.13% reduction in HbA$_{1c}$ with placebo. In a 52-week study in patients receiving metformin hydrochloride (dosage of at least 1.5 g daily) and a sulfonylurea (generally glipizide, glyburide [glibenclamide], or gliclazide [not commercially available in the US]), addition of canagliflozin 300 mg or sitagliptin 100 mg resulted in a reduction in HbA$_{1c}$ of 1 or 0.6%, respectively. Canagliflozin was noninferior to sitagliptin and demonstrated superiority to sitagliptin in reducing HbA$_{1c}$ in subsequent analyses. In a 26-week trial in patients inadequately controlled on metformin hydrochloride (dosage of at least 1.5 g daily) and sitagliptin (100 mg daily), the addition of canagliflozin (100 mg daily titrated to 300 mg daily) resulted in a substantial reduction in HbA$_{1c}$ from baseline at 26 weeks compared with the addition of placebo (reduction of 0.83 versus 0.03%, respectively).

In a 26-week trial in patients receiving metformin hydrochloride (dosage of at least 1.5 g daily) and pioglitazone (30 or 45 mg daily), addition of canagliflozin 100 or 300 mg once daily or placebo resulted in a reduction in HbA$_{1c}$ of approximately 0.9, 1, or 0.3%, respectively.

Efficacy of canagliflozin in combination with insulin in the management of type 2 diabetes mellitus in patients who have inadequate glycemic control with insulin is supported by results of an 18-week, randomized, placebo-controlled trial. In this trial, addition of canagliflozin (100 or 300 mg daily) to existing insulin therapy resulted in improvements in HbA$_{1c}$, fasting plasma glucose, and body weight. In patients who received canagliflozin 100 or 300 mg as add-on therapy to insulin, 20 or 25%, respectively, had HbA$_{1c}$ reductions to less than 7%, compared with 8% of patients receiving add-on placebo.

Reduction in Risk of Major Adverse Cardiovascular Events

Canagliflozin is used to reduce the risk of major cardiovascular events (e.g., cardiovascular death, nonfatal myocardial infarction [MI], nonfatal stroke) in patients with type 2 diabetes mellitus and established cardiovascular disease. In addition to lowering blood glucose, SGLT2 inhibitors appear to modify several nonglycemic cardiovascular risk factors such as blood pressure, body weight, adiposity, and arterial stiffness. While canagliflozin reduces the risk of adverse cardiovascular and renal outcomes in patients with type 2 diabetes mellitus and increased cardiovascular risk, such therapy is associated with an increased risk of lower extremity amputations. The Canagliflozin Cardiovascular Assessment Studies (CANVAS and CANVAS-R) were designed to assess the cardiovascular safety and efficacy of canagliflozin in patients with type 2 diabetes mellitus. In CANVAS and CANVAS-R, adults (mean age: 63.3 years) with type 2 diabetes mellitus and established cardiovascular disease (i.e., secondary prevention treatment group) or at high risk for cardiovascular disease (i.e., primary prevention treatment group [at least 50 years of age with at least 2 risk factors for cardiovascular disease]) received canagliflozin (100 or 300 mg) once daily or placebo for a mean of 149 weeks. During the studies, antidiabetic and cardiovascular therapies were modified to achieve standard-of-care treatment targets with respect to blood glucose, lipids, and blood pressure. Concomitant use of other standard-of-care treatments for diabetes mellitus and atherosclerotic cardiovascular disease (renin-angiotensin system inhibitors [80%], β-blockers [53%], loop diuretics [36%], statins [75%], antiplatelet agents [74%]) was permitted. The primary

outcome was the composite of death from cardiovascular causes, nonfatal MI, or nonfatal stroke. In these studies, patients who received treatment with canagliflozin had substantially lower rates of the primary cardiovascular outcome compared with those who received placebo (event rate 9.2 versus 10.4%). However, canagliflozin therapy was associated with a twofold increase in the risk of lower limb amputations in these studies.

Beneficial Effects on Renal Function and Cardiovascular Morbidity and Mortality in Diabetic Nephropathy

Canagliflozin is used to reduce the risk of ESRD, doubling of serum creatinine, cardiovascular death, and hospitalization for heart failure in patients with type 2 diabetes mellitus and diabetic nephropathy with albuminuria exceeding 300 mg/day. SGLT2 inhibitors such as canagliflozin reduce renal tubular glucose reabsorption, weight, systemic blood pressure, intraglomerular pressure, and albuminuria and slow glomerular filtration rate (GFR) loss through mechanisms that appear to be independent of glucose-lowering effects. Some experts state that use of an SGLT2 inhibitor should be considered to reduce the risk of CKD progression, cardiovascular events, or both in patients with type 2 diabetes mellitus and diabetic kidney disease with albuminuria (an eGFR of at least 30 mL/minute per 1.73 m² and urinary albumin exceeding 30 mg/g creatinine, particularly urinary albumin exceeding 300 mg/g creatinine).

The effects of canagliflozin on renal outcomes have been evaluated in a randomized, double-blind, placebo-controlled study (CREDENCE) in approximately 4400 patients with type 2 diabetes mellitus, CKD (eGFR 30–89 mL/minute per 1.73 m²; mean: 56.2 mL/minute per 1.73 m²), and albuminuria (urine albumin:creatinine ratio exceeding 300 but less than 5000 mg/g). In this study, patients received canagliflozin 100 mg orally or placebo once daily in conjunction with the standard of care for glycemic control. Patients also had to have been receiving a stable dosage of an angiotensin-converting enzyme (ACE) inhibitor or an angiotensin II receptor antagonist for at least 4 weeks prior to randomization. The primary outcome was the composite of ESRD, doubling of serum creatinine concentrations from baseline, or death from renal or cardiovascular disease. The study was stopped early after a planned interim analysis (median follow-up: 2.6 years) at which the relative risk of the primary outcomes was found to be 30% lower in the canagliflozin group than in the placebo group. Additionally, treatment with canagliflozin reduced the relative risk of hospitalization for heart failure by 39%. These outcomes were observed despite very small differences in blood glucose control, weight, and blood pressure between the canagliflozin and placebo groups. These findings suggest that the beneficial renal effects of SGLT2 inhibitors may be independent of glucose homeostasis and may be related to other mechanisms, such as a reduction in intraglomerular pressure.

In several cardiovascular outcomes trials involving the use of SGLT2 inhibitors (e.g., canagliflozin, dapagliflozin, empagliflozin) in patients with type 2 diabetes mellitus at high risk for cardiovascular disease or with existing cardiovascular disease, beneficial effects on renal function have been observed as a secondary outcome. In the CANVAS trials (see Reduction in Risk of Major Adverse Cardiovascular Events under Uses: Type 2 Diabetes Mellitus), canagliflozin therapy was associated with a 27% reduction in the risk of progression of albuminuria; in addition, regression of albuminuria occurred more frequently among those receiving canagliflozin versus placebo. The composite outcome of a sustained 40% reduction in eGFR, the need for renal replacement therapy, or death from renal causes also occurred less frequently among those receiving canagliflozin compared with placebo.

DOSAGE AND ADMINISTRATION

● Administration

Canagliflozin should be administered orally once daily, before the first meal of the day. The fixed combination of canagliflozin and immediate-release metformin hydrochloride should be administered twice daily with meals. The fixed combination of canagliflozin and extended-release metformin hydrochloride should be administered once daily with the morning meal; the tablet should be swallowed whole and should not be crushed, chewed, or cut.

If a dose is missed, the missed dose should be taken as soon as it is remembered followed by resumption of the regular schedule. If the missed dose is not remembered until the time of the next dose, the missed dose should be skipped and the regular schedule resumed; the dose should not be doubled to replace a missed dose.

● *Dosage*

Dosage of canagliflozin is expressed in terms of anhydrous canagliflozin.

Type 2 Diabetes Mellitus

Patients with volume depletion should have this condition corrected before initiation of canagliflozin therapy.

Canagliflozin Monotherapy

The recommended initial dosage of canagliflozin in patients with type 2 diabetes mellitus and an estimated glomerular filtration rate (eGFR) of at least 60 mL/minute per 1.73 m^2 is 100 mg once daily, taken before the first meal of the day. If this initial dosage is well tolerated and additional glycemic control is needed in such patients, the dosage may be increased to 300 mg once daily.

In patients with an eGFR of at least 60 mL/minute per 1.73 m^2 who are receiving concurrent therapy with a uridine diphosphate-glucuronosyltransferase (UGT) enzyme inducer (e.g., phenobarbital, phenytoin, rifampin, ritonavir), the dosage of canagliflozin should be increased to 200 mg once daily in patients who are tolerating a dosage of 100 mg once daily. The dosage of canagliflozin may be increased to 300 mg once daily in patients who require additional glycemic control and who are tolerating a dosage of 200 mg once daily. (See Drug Interactions: Uridine Diphosphate-glucuronosyltransferase Enzyme Inducers.)

Canagliflozin/Metformin Hydrochloride Fixed-combination Therapy

Dosage of canagliflozin in fixed combination with metformin hydrochloride should be individualized based on the patient's current antidiabetic regimen. In patients with an eGFR of at least 60 mL/minute per 1.73 m^2, the dosage of the fixed-combination preparation may be increased gradually based on effectiveness and tolerability up to a maximum of 300 mg of canagliflozin and 2 g of metformin hydrochloride daily.

In patients *not* currently receiving treatment with either canagliflozin or metformin hydrochloride, the recommended initial dosage of the fixed combination of canagliflozin and *immediate-release* metformin hydrochloride (Invokamet®) is 50 mg of canagliflozin and 500 mg of metformin hydrochloride twice daily; the recommended initial dosage of the fixed combination of canagliflozin and *extended-release* metformin hydrochloride (Invokamet® XR) is 100 mg of canagliflozin and 1 g of metformin hydrochloride once daily.

In patients currently receiving metformin hydrochloride, the recommended initial total daily dosage of the fixed combination is 100 mg of canagliflozin and a metformin hydrochloride dosage similar to the patient's existing total daily dosage, administered in 2 divided doses (when given as the fixed combination containing *immediate-release* metformin hydrochloride) or once daily (when given as the fixed combination containing *extended-release* metformin hydrochloride). Patients who are currently receiving an evening dose of extended-release metformin hydrochloride should skip their last dose prior to initiating therapy with the fixed combination of canagliflozin and metformin hydrochloride the following morning.

In patients currently receiving canagliflozin, the recommended initial total daily dosage of the fixed combination is the same daily dosage of canagliflozin and 1 g of metformin hydrochloride, administered in 2 divided doses (when given as the fixed combination containing *immediate-release* metformin hydrochloride) or once daily (when given as the fixed combination containing *extended-release* metformin hydrochloride).

In patients currently receiving both canagliflozin and metformin hydrochloride as separate components, the recommended initial total daily dosage of the fixed combination is the same daily dosage of canagliflozin and a metformin hydrochloride dosage similar to the patient's existing total daily dosage, administered in 2 divided doses (when given as the fixed combination containing *immediate-release* metformin hydrochloride) or once daily (when given as the fixed combination containing *extended-release* metformin hydrochloride).

In patients currently receiving both canagliflozin and metformin hydrochloride who have an eGFR of at least 60 mL/minute per 1.73 m^2 and who are receiving concurrent therapy with a UGT enzyme inducer (e.g., phenobarbital, phenytoin, rifampin, ritonavir), the total daily dosage of canagliflozin should be increased to 200 mg in patients who are tolerating a canagliflozin dosage of 100 mg daily. The total daily dosage of canagliflozin may be increased to a maximum of 300 mg in patients who are tolerating a daily canagliflozin dosage of 200 mg and require additional glycemic control. (See Drug Interactions: Uridine Diphosphate-glucuronosyltransferase Enzyme Inducers.)

● *Special Populations*

Hepatic Impairment

Canagliflozin Monotherapy

No dosage adjustment is necessary in patients with mild or moderate hepatic impairment. Data are lacking on use of canagliflozin in patients with severe hepatic impairment, and the manufacturer states that use in such patients is not recommended.

Canagliflozin/Metformin Hydrochloride Fixed-combination Therapy

Use of the fixed-combination preparations of canagliflozin and metformin hydrochloride is not recommended in patients with hepatic impairment.

Renal Impairment

Canagliflozin Monotherapy

No dosage adjustment is necessary in patients with mild renal impairment (eGFR of at least 60 mL/minute per 1.73 m^2). In patients with moderate renal impairment (eGFR of 45 to less than 60 mL/minute per 1.73 m^2), the dosage of canagliflozin should not exceed 100 mg daily. The manufacturer states there are insufficient data to support dosage recommendations for the *initiation* of canagliflozin therapy in patients who have (1) an eGFR of less than 30 mL/minute per 1.73 m^2 with albuminuria exceeding 300 mg/day or (2) an eGFR of 30 to less than 45 mL/minute per 1.73 m^2 with albuminuria of 300 mg/day or less. In patients already receiving canagliflozin therapy who have a reduction in eGFR to less than 30 mL/minute per 1.73 m^2 and who have albuminuria exceeding 300 mg/day, canagliflozin therapy can be continued at a dosage of 100 mg once daily. Canagliflozin use is contraindicated in patients with severe renal impairment (an eGFR less than 30 mL/minute per 1.73 m^2) when used for glycemic control. Canagliflozin also is contraindicated in patients with end-stage renal disease (ESRD) on dialysis.

In patients with an eGFR of less than 60 mL/minute per 1.73 m^2 who are receiving concomitant therapy with a UGT enzyme inducer (e.g., phenobarbital, phenytoin, rifampin, ritonavir), the total daily dosage of canagliflozin may be increased to 200 mg in patients who are tolerating a dosage of 100 mg daily. In patients who require additional glycemic control, addition of another antihyperglycemic agent should be considered. (See Drug Interactions: Uridine Diphosphate-glucuronosyltransferase Enzyme Inducers.)

Canagliflozin/Metformin Hydrochloride Fixed-combination Therapy

In patients with moderate renal impairment (eGFR 45 to less than 60 mL/minute per 1.73 m^2), the dosage of the canagliflozin component should not exceed 100 mg daily. In patients with an eGFR of 30 to less than 45 mL/minute per 1.73 m^2 and albuminuria exceeding 300 mg/day, the benefits and risks of continuing canagliflozin and metformin hydrochloride should be considered;, additionally, the dosage of canagliflozin in these patients should be limited to 100 mg daily. Use of the fixed-combination preparation of canagliflozin and metformin hydrochloride is contraindicated in patients with an eGFR of less than 30 mL/minute per 1.73 m^2 and in patients on dialysis.

In patients with an eGFR of less than 60 mL/minute per 1.73 m^2 who are receiving concurrent therapy with a UGT enzyme inducer (e.g., phenobarbital, phenytoin, rifampin, ritonavir), the total daily dosage of canagliflozin should be increased to a maximum of 200 mg in patients who are tolerating a dosage of 100 mg daily. (See Drug Interactions: Uridine Diphosphate-glucuronosyltransferase Enzyme Inducers.)

Geriatric Patients

Canagliflozin Monotherapy

The manufacturer makes no specific dosage recommendations for geriatric patients.

Canagliflozin/Metformin Hydrochloride Fixed-combination Therapy

Renal function should be monitored frequently after initiating the fixed-combination preparation; the dosage should be adjusted according to the patient's renal function. (See Renal Impairment under Dosage and Administration: Special Populations.)

CAUTIONS

● Contraindications

History of serious hypersensitivity reactions (e.g., anaphylaxis, angioedema) to canagliflozin.

Severe renal impairment (estimated glomerular filtration rate [eGFR] less than 30 mL/minute per 1.73 m^2) in patients who are being treated for glycemic control or on dialysis.

● Warnings/Precautions

Warnings

Lower Limb Amputation

In 2 randomized, placebo-controlled studies (Canagliflozin Cardiovascular Assessment Study [CANVAS] and CANVAS-R) evaluating the effects of canagliflozin on the risk of cardiovascular disease and the overall safety and tolerability of the drug, canagliflozin-treated patients had a twofold increased risk of lower limb (leg and foot) amputations (mostly affecting the toes and midfoot) compared with placebo. In the CANVAS study, canagliflozin- or placebo-treated patients had 5.9 or 2.8 amputations per 1000 patients per year, respectively; the amputation rate in the CANVAS-R trial was 7.5 or 4.2 per 1000 patients per year with canagliflozin or placebo, respectively. Amputations below and above the knee also occurred, and some patients had more than one amputation (some involving both lower limbs). The increased risk of lower limb amputation was observed with both the 100- and 300-mg daily dosage regimens. Patients with a baseline history of prior amputation, peripheral vascular disease, or neuropathy were at greatest risk for amputation. The most common precipitating medical events leading to an amputation were lower limb infections, gangrene, diabetic foot ulcers, and ischemia.

Prior to initiating therapy with canagliflozin, clinicians should consider patient factors that may predispose them to the need for amputation, such as a history of amputation, peripheral vascular disease, neuropathy, or diabetic foot ulcers. Clinicians should monitor patients receiving canagliflozin for the presence of infection (including osteomyelitis), new pain or tenderness, and sores or ulcers involving the lower limbs; canagliflozin should be discontinued if such complications occur. Patients should also be counseled on the importance of routine preventative foot care.

Sensitivity Reactions

Hypersensitivity reactions (e.g., generalized urticaria), some serious, have been reported with canagliflozin treatment. These reactions generally occurred within hours to days of canagliflozin initiation. If a hypersensitivity reaction occurs, the drug should be discontinued, appropriate treatment instituted, and the patient monitored until signs and symptoms resolve.

Other Warnings/Precautions

Use of Fixed Combinations

When canagliflozin is used in fixed combination with other drugs (e.g., metformin), the cautions, precautions, contraindications, and interactions associated with the concomitant agent(s) must be considered in addition to those associated with canagliflozin.

Ketoacidosis

Use of sodium glucose cotransporter 2 (SGLT2) inhibitors (canagliflozin, dapagliflozin, empagliflozin) in patients with type 2 diabetes mellitus may lead to ketoacidosis requiring hospitalization. Ketoacidosis associated with use of SGLT2 inhibitors may be present without markedly elevated blood glucose concentrations (e.g., less than 250 mg/dL).

FDA identified 73 cases of acidosis (reported as diabetic ketoacidosis [DKA], ketoacidosis, or ketosis) associated with SGLT2 inhibitor use in the FDA Adverse Event Reporting System (FAERS) between March 2013 and May 2015. DKA had an atypical presentation in most of the reported cases in that type 2 diabetes mellitus was noted as the indication for the drug, and glucose concentrations were only slightly elevated (median: 211 mg/dL); type 1 diabetes mellitus was named as the indication in a few cases, and in some reports the indication was not specified. The median time to onset of symptoms of acidosis following initiation or increase in dosage of the SGLT2 inhibitor was 43 days (range: 1–365 days). No trend

demonstrating a relationship between the dosage of an SGLT2 inhibitor and the risk of ketoacidosis was identified. In all reported episodes, a diagnosis of DKA or ketoacidosis was made by the clinician and hospitalization or treatment in an emergency department was warranted. In most cases, at least 1 diagnostic laboratory criterion suggestive of ketoacidosis (e.g., high anion gap metabolic acidosis, ketonemia, reduced serum bicarbonate) was reported. Most cases of ketoacidosis were associated with a concurrent event, most commonly dehydration, infection, or change in insulin dosage. Potential factors for development of ketoacidosis with SGLT2 inhibitor therapy identified in the 73 cases included infection, low carbohydrate diet or reduced caloric intake, surgery, pancreatic disorders suggesting insulin deficiency (e.g., type 1 diabetes mellitus, history of pancreatitis, pancreatic surgery), reduced dosage or discontinuance of insulin, discontinuance of an oral insulin secretagogue, and alcohol use.

Prior to initiating therapy with an SGLT2 inhibitor, clinicians should consider patient factors that may predispose the patient to ketoacidosis, such as pancreatic insulin deficiency from any cause, reduced caloric intake, and alcohol abuse.

Clinicians should evaluate for the presence of acidosis, including ketoacidosis, in patients experiencing signs or symptoms of acidosis while receiving SGLT2 inhibitors, regardless of the patient's blood glucose concentration. For patients who are to undergo scheduled surgery, discontinuation of canagliflozin at least 3 days prior to surgery should be considered. Clinicians should consider monitoring for ketoacidosis and temporarily discontinuing therapy with an SGLT2 inhibitor in other clinical situations known to predispose individuals to ketoacidosis (e.g., prolonged fasting due to acute illness or post-surgery). If acidosis is confirmed, the SGLT2 inhibitor should be discontinued and appropriate treatment initiated to correct the acidosis; glucose concentrations should be monitored appropriately. In addition, supportive medical treatment should be instituted to treat and correct factors that may have precipitated or contributed to the metabolic acidosis. Risk factors for ketoacidosis should be resolved prior to restarting canagliflozin.

Euglycemic DKA associated with SGLT2 inhibitors may be detected and potentially prevented by having patients monitor urine and/or plasma ketone levels if they feel unwell, regardless of ambient glucose concentrations. Clinicians should inform patients and caregivers of the signs and symptoms of ketoacidosis (e.g., tachypnea or hyperventilation, anorexia, abdominal pain, nausea, vomiting, lethargy, mental status changes) and instruct patients to discontinue the SGLT2 inhibitor and immediately seek medical attention should they experience such signs or symptoms.

Hypotension

Canagliflozin may cause intravascular volume contraction. Following initiation of canagliflozin, symptomatic hypotension can occur, particularly in patients with impaired renal function (eGFR less than 60 mL/minute per 1.73 m^2), geriatric patients, patients receiving diuretics or drugs that interfere with the renin-angiotensin-aldosterone system (e.g., angiotensin-converting enzyme [ACE] inhibitors, angiotensin II receptor antagonists), or patients with low systolic blood pressure. (See Drug Interactions: Drugs Affecting the Renin-Angiotensin System, and also see Drug Interactions: Diuretics.) Prior to initiating canagliflozin in such patients, intravascular volume should be assessed and corrected. Patients should be monitored for signs and symptoms of hypotension after initiating canagliflozin therapy.

Renal Effects

Canagliflozin causes intravascular volume contraction and can cause acute kidney injury. Initiation of canagliflozin may cause an increase in serum creatinine and decrease in eGFR. In patients with moderate renal impairment, the increase in serum creatinine generally does not exceed 0.2 mg/dL, occurs within the first 6 weeks of starting therapy, and then stabilizes. Increases in serum creatinine that do not fit this pattern should be evaluated to exclude the possibility of acute kidney injury. Renal function should be evaluated prior to initiation of canagliflozin and monitored periodically thereafter. If acute kidney injury occurs during canagliflozin therapy, the drug should be discontinued and appropriate treatment initiated.

FDA identified 101 cases of acute kidney injury associated with canagliflozin or dapagliflozin therapy in FAERS between March 2013 and October 2015. Hospitalization for evaluation and management of kidney injury was warranted in most cases, and some cases required admission to an intensive care unit and initiation of dialysis. In approximately half of the cases, onset of acute kidney injury occurred within 1 month or less of initiating canagliflozin or dapagliflozin therapy, and most patients' kidney function improved after stopping the drug. However, kidney injury may not be fully reversible in some situations and has led to death in some patients.

Prior to initiating canagliflozin therapy, clinicians should consider patient factors that may predispose the patient to acute kidney injury, including hypovolemia, chronic renal insufficiency, heart failure, and concomitant drug therapy (e.g., diuretics, angiotensin converting enzyme [ACE] inhibitors, angiotensin II receptor antagonists, nonsteroidal anti-inflammatory agents [NSAIAs]). Clinicians should consider temporarily discontinuing canagliflozin in any setting of reduced oral intake (e.g., acute illness, fasting) or fluid losses (e.g., GI illness, excessive heat exposure).

Concomitant Therapy with Hypoglycemic Agents

When canagliflozin is added to therapy with an insulin secretagogue (e.g., a sulfonylurea) or insulin, the risk of hypoglycemia is increased compared with sulfonylurea or insulin monotherapy. Therefore, patients receiving canagliflozin may require a reduced dosage of the concomitant insulin secretagogue or insulin to reduce the risk of hypoglycemia. (See Drug Interactions: Antidiabetic Agents.)

Fournier Gangrene

Fournier gangrene (necrotizing fasciitis of the perineum), a rare but serious or life-threatening bacterial infection requiring urgent surgical intervention, has been reported during postmarketing surveillance in men and women with type 2 diabetes mellitus receiving an SGLT2 inhibitor, including canagliflozin. Permanent disfigurement, prolonged hospitalization, disability, and complications from sepsis all may be associated with Fournier gangrene. Although diabetes mellitus is a risk factor for developing Fournier gangrene, this condition is still rare among patients with diabetes mellitus.

FDA identified 12 cases of Fournier gangrene in patients taking an SGLT2 inhibitor reported in FAERS and the medical literature between March 2013 and May 2018. Since FDA's review, additional cases of Fournier gangrene have been reported. In the initial cases reviewed by FDA, the average time to onset of infection was 9.2 months (range 7 days to 25 months) after initiation of therapy with an SGLT2 inhibitor. Some experts speculate that the variation in time to diagnosis of Fournier gangrene might be due to fluctuating glycemic control, microvascular complications, or an inciting event associated with SGLT2 inhibitors (e.g., urinary tract infection, mycotic infection, skin or mucosal breakdown due to pruritus). In all reported cases, hospitalization and surgery were required. Among these cases, some patients required multiple disfiguring surgeries, some developed complications (e.g., diabetic ketoacidosis, acute kidney injury, septic shock), and 1 patient died. In a review of other antidiabetic drugs (e.g., insulin, biguanides, sulfonylureas, dipeptidyl peptidase-4 inhibitors) over a period of more than 30 years, only 6 cases of Fournier gangrene were identified; all of theses cases occurred in men.

Patients receiving canagliflozin who develop pain or tenderness, erythema, or swelling in the genital or perineal area, in addition to fever or malaise, should be assessed for necrotizing fasciitis. If Fournier gangrene is suspected, canagliflozin should be discontinued and treatment should be initiated with broad-spectrum antibiotics; surgical debridement should be performed if necessary. Blood glucose concentrations should be closely monitored; alternative antidiabetic agents should be initiated to maintain glycemic control.

Genital Mycotic Infections

Canagliflozin may increase the risk of genital mycotic infections in males (e.g., balanoposthitis, candidal balanitis) and females (e.g., vulvovaginal candidiasis, vulvovaginal mycotic infection, vulvovaginitis). In clinical trials, patients with a history of genital mycotic infections and uncircumcised males were more likely to develop such infections. Patients should be monitored for genital mycotic infections and appropriate treatment should be instituted if these infections occur.

Urosepsis and Pyelonephritis

Treatment with an SGLT2 inhibitor (e.g., canagliflozin) increases the risk for serious urinary tract infections.

Cases of serious urinary tract infections, including urosepsis and pyelonephritis, have been reported in patients receiving an SGLT2 inhibitor. FDA identified 19 cases of urosepsis and pyelonephritis, which began as urinary tract infections

associated with SGLT2 inhibitor use, in FAERS between March 2013 and October 2014. In all cases reported, hospitalization was warranted and some patients required admission to an intensive care unit or dialysis for treatment. The median time to onset of infection following initiation of the SGLT2 inhibitor was 45 days (range: 2–270 days).

Prior to initiating therapy with an SGLT2 inhibitor, clinicians should consider patient factors that may predispose them to serious urinary tract infections, such as a history of difficulty urinating or infections of the bladder, kidneys, or urinary tract. Patients should be monitored for urinary tract infections and treatment instituted if indicated.

Risk of Bone Fracture

In the CANVAS study, an increased risk of bone fracture was observed in patients receiving canagliflozin 100 or 300 mg once daily. Fractures were observed as early as 12 weeks after initiation of treatment and were more likely to affect the distal portion of upper and lower extremities and be associated with minor trauma (e.g., falls from no greater than standing height). Dose-related decreases in bone mineral density (e.g., hip and lumbar spine) also have been observed in older adults (mean age: 64 years) receiving canagliflozin therapy over a period of 2 years. Clinicians should consider factors that contribute to fracture risk and counsel patients about such factors prior to initiating canagliflozin therapy. (See Advice to Patients.)

Laboratory Test Interferences

SGLT2 inhibitors such as canagliflozin increase urinary glucose excretion and will result in false-positive urine glucose tests. Data from healthy individuals receiving a single 300-mg dose of canagliflozin indicate that the elevation in urinary glucose excretion approaches baseline after approximately 3 days. In addition, the manufacturer states that the 1,5-anhydroglucitol assay is unreliable for monitoring glycemic control in patients taking SGLT2 inhibitors. Alternative methods of monitoring glycemic control should be used in patients receiving SGLT2 inhibitors.

Specific Populations

Pregnancy

Based on the results of reproductive and developmental toxicity studies in animals, canagliflozin use during pregnancy may affect renal development and maturation, especially during the second and third trimesters of pregnancy. Limited data with canagliflozin in pregnant women are not sufficient to determine a drug-associated risk for major birth defects or miscarriage, and poorly controlled diabetes mellitus during pregnancy carries risks to the mother and fetus; however, canagliflozin therapy is not recommended in pregnant women during the second and third trimesters of pregnancy.

Lactation

Canagliflozin is distributed into milk in rats; it is not known whether the drug is distributed into human milk. Because many drugs are distributed into human milk and because of the potential for serious adverse reactions in nursing infants from canagliflozin, use of the drug is not recommended while breastfeeding.

Pediatric Use

Safety and efficacy of canagliflozin have not been established in pediatric patients younger than 18 years of age.

Geriatric Use

Among patients in 13 clinical trials, 2294 were 65 years of age or older and 351 were 75 years of age or older, including one trial in patients 55 to 80 years of age. Geriatric patients experienced reduced efficacy of canagliflozin compared with younger patients, which may be related to decreased renal function in geriatric patients. Geriatric patients also were more likely to experience certain adverse effects related to reduced intravascular volume (e.g., hypotension, postural dizziness, orthostatic hypotension, syncope, dehydration) with canagliflozin, particularly those receiving 300 mg daily.

Hepatic Impairment

Compared with values in individuals with normal hepatic function, canagliflozin area under the concentration-time curve (AUC) and peak plasma concentrations were increased by 10 and 7%, respectively (based on geometric mean ratios), in patients with mild hepatic impairment (Child-Pugh class A) following a single 300-mg dose of the drug; canagliflozin AUC was increased by 11% and peak plasma concentration was decreased by 4% in patients with moderate hepatic impairment (Child-Pugh class B). These differences were not considered clinically important.

Data are lacking on the use of canagliflozin in patients with severe hepatic impairment (Child-Pugh class C), and such use is not recommended.

Renal Impairment

Safety and efficacy of canagliflozin for glycemic control were evaluated in a study that included 269 patients with moderate renal impairment (eGFR 30 to less than 50 mL/minute per 1.73 m^2) and type 2 diabetes mellitus. These patients experienced less overall improvement in glycemic control and had higher rates of adverse effects related to reduced intravascular volume, renal-related adverse effects, and decreases in eGFR compared with those who had mild renal impairment or normal renal function. Patients receiving canagliflozin 300 mg were more likely to experience increases in serum potassium concentrations.

Renal impairment did not affect peak plasma concentrations of canagliflozin. In patients with mild (eGFR 60 to less than 90 mL/minute per 1.73 m^2), moderate (eGFR 30 to less than 60 mL/minute per 1.73 m^2), or severe renal impairment (eGFR less than 30 mL/minute per 1.73 m^2), canagliflozin AUC was increased by 15, 29, or 53%, respectively, compared with that in healthy individuals following a single 200-mg dose of the drug.

Renal function should be assessed prior to initiation of therapy and periodically thereafter. Reduction of canagliflozin dosage is required for patients with an eGFR less than 60 mL/minute per 1.73 m^2. (See Renal Impairment under Dosage and Administration: Special Populations.)

The fixed combination of canagliflozin and metformin is contraindicated in patients with eGFR less than 30 mL/minute per 1.73 m^2.

● Common Adverse Effects

Adverse effects reported in at least 2% of patients receiving canagliflozin in clinical trials and more frequently than with placebo include female genital mycotic infections, urinary tract infection, increased urination, male genital mycotic infections, vulvovaginal pruritus, thirst, constipation, and nausea.

DRUG INTERACTIONS

The major metabolic elimination pathway for canagliflozin is O-glucuronidation; the drug is mainly glucuronidated by uridine diphosphate-glucuronosyltransferase (UGT) isoenzymes UGT1A9 and UGT2B4.

Canagliflozin is a P-glycoprotein substrate and weakly inhibits P-glycoprotein. Canagliflozin also is a substrate of MRP2.

● Drugs Affecting or Metabolized by Hepatic Microsomal Enzymes

Canagliflozin did not induce cytochrome P-450 (CYP) isoenzymes 3A4, 2C9, 2C19, 2B6, or 1A2 in cultured human hepatocytes. Canagliflozin also does not inhibit CYP isoenzymes 1A2, 2A6, 2C19, 2D6, or 2E1 but weakly inhibits CYP2B6, 2C8, 2C9, and 3A4 in human hepatic microsomes.

● Drugs Affecting the Renin-Angiotensin System

Concomitant use of canagliflozin with drugs that interfere with the renin-angiotensin-aldosterone system, including angiotensin-converting enzyme (ACE) inhibitors or angiotensin II receptor antagonists, may increase the incidence of symptomatic hypotension. Prior to initiating canagliflozin in such patients, intravascular volume should be assessed and corrected; patients should be monitored for signs and symptoms of hypotension after initiating therapy. (See Hypotension under Cautions: Warnings/Precautions.) These drugs also may cause hyperkalemia in patients with moderate renal impairment. Serum potassium concentrations should be monitored periodically following initiation of canagliflozin in patients predisposed to hyperkalemia due to drug therapy. (See Hyperkalemia under Cautions: Warnings/Precautions.)

● Uridine Diphosphate-glucuronosyltransferase Enzyme Inducers

Concomitant use of canagliflozin with an inducer of UGT enzymes may decrease the efficacy of canagliflozin. When a single dose of canagliflozin (300 mg) was administered to patients receiving rifampin (600 mg once daily for 8 days), a nonselective inducer of UGT isoenzymes 1A9 and 2B4, canagliflozin area under the concentration-time curve (AUC) was decreased by 51% and peak plasma concentration was reduced by 28% (based on geometric mean ratios). If a UGT enzyme inducer (e.g., phenobarbital, phenytoin, rifampin, ritonavir) is used concomitantly with canagliflozin in patients who are currently tolerating canagliflozin 100 mg once daily, the dosage of canagliflozin should be increased to 200 mg once daily in patients with an estimated glomerular filtration rate (eGFR) of at least 60 mL/minute per 1.73 m^2. The dosage may be increased to 300 mg once daily in patients currently tolerating canagliflozin 200 mg daily who require additional glycemic control. In patients with an eGFR less than 60 mL/minute per 1.73 m^2 who are receiving concomitant therapy with a UGT enzyme inducer and currently tolerating canagliflozin 100 mg once daily, the dosage of canagliflozin should be increased to 200 mg once daily. The addition of another antidiabetic agent should be considered in such patients who require additional glycemic control.

● Acetaminophen

Administration of a single dose of acetaminophen (1 g) to individuals receiving canagliflozin (300 mg twice daily for 25 days) had no effect on peak plasma acetaminophen concentration; acetaminophen AUC increased by 6% (based on geometric mean ratios). No adjustment of concomitant acetaminophen dosage is necessary.

● Antidiabetic Agents

When canagliflozin is added to therapy with an insulin secretagogue (e.g., a sulfonylurea) or insulin, the incidence of hypoglycemia is increased compared with sulfonylurea or insulin monotherapy. Patients receiving canagliflozin may require a reduced dosage of the concomitant insulin secretagogue or insulin to reduce the risk of hypoglycemia.

Administration of a single dose of glyburide (1.25 mg) to individuals receiving canagliflozin (200 mg once daily for 6 days) increased glyburide AUC by 2% (based on geometric mean ratios) and decreased peak plasma concentrations by 7% (based on geometric mean ratios). No adjustment of glyburide dosage is necessary with concomitant canagliflozin.

● Cyclosporine

Administration of a single dose of cyclosporine (400 mg) to individuals receiving canagliflozin (300 mg once daily for 8 days) increased canagliflozin AUC and peak plasma concentrations by 23 and 1%, respectively (based on geometric mean ratios). No adjustment of canagliflozin dosage is necessary with concomitant cyclosporine.

● Digoxin

Concomitant use of canagliflozin (300 mg once daily for 7 days) and digoxin (0.5 mg once daily for one day, then 0.25 mg once daily for 6 days) increased AUC and mean peak plasma concentration of digoxin by 20 and 36%, respectively (based on geometric mean ratios). Patients should be monitored appropriately when receiving canagliflozin and digoxin concomitantly.

● Diuretics

Concomitant use of canagliflozin with diuretics may increase the incidence of symptomatic hypotension. Prior to initiation of canagliflozin, volume status should be assessed and corrected in patients receiving diuretics. Patients should be monitored for signs and symptoms of symptomatic hypotension following initiation of canagliflozin therapy.

Patients with moderate renal impairment receiving potassium-sparing diuretics are more likely to develop hyperkalemia. Serum potassium concentrations should be monitored periodically following initiation of canagliflozin in patients predisposed to hyperkalemia due to drug therapy.

● Hormonal Contraceptives

Administration of a single dose of ethinyl estradiol (0.03 mg) and levonorgestrel (0.15 mg) to individuals receiving canagliflozin (200 mg once daily for 6 days) increased ethinyl estradiol and levonorgestrel AUC (7 and 6%, respectively, based on geometric mean ratios) and peak plasma concentration (22% for both drugs, based on geometric mean ratios) and decreased canagliflozin AUC and peak plasma concentration (9 and 8%, respectively, based on geometric mean ratios). No dosage adjustment is necessary for any of the drugs.

● *Hydrochlorothiazide*

Concurrent use of hydrochlorothiazide (25 mg once daily for 35 days) and canagliflozin (300 mg once daily for 7 days) increased canagliflozin AUC and peak plasma concentrations (12 and 15%, respectively, based on geometric mean ratios) and decreased hydrochlorothiazide AUC and peak plasma concentrations (1 and 6%, respectively, based on geometric mean ratios). No dosage adjustment is necessary for either drug. (See also Drug Interactions: Diuretics.)

● *Metformin*

In individuals receiving canagliflozin (300 mg once daily for 8 days), a single dose of metformin hydrochloride (2 g) increased canagliflozin and metformin AUCs (10 and 20%, respectively, based on geometric mean ratios) and peak plasma concentrations (5 and 6%, respectively, based on geometric mean ratios). No dosage adjustment is necessary for either drug.

● *Probenecid*

Concomitant use of probenecid (500 mg twice daily for 3 days) and canagliflozin (300 mg once daily for 17 days) increased canagliflozin AUC and peak plasma concentration by 21 and 13%, respectively (based on geometric mean ratios). No adjustment of canagliflozin dosage is necessary.

● *Simvastatin*

Administration of a single dose of simvastatin (40 mg) in individuals receiving canagliflozin (300 mg once daily for 7 days) increased simvastatin AUC and peak plasma concentration by 12 and 9%, respectively (based on geometric mean ratios). No simvastatin dosage adjustment is necessary.

● *Warfarin*

Administration of a single dose of warfarin (30 mg) in individuals receiving canagliflozin (300 mg once daily for 12 days) slightly increased *R*- and *S*-warfarin AUC (1 and 6%, respectively, based on geometric mean ratios) and peak plasma concentrations (3 and 1%, respectively, based on geometric mean ratios). No warfarin dosage adjustment is necessary.

DESCRIPTION

Canagliflozin inhibits sodium-glucose cotransporter 2 (SGLT2), a transporter that is expressed in the proximal renal tubules and is responsible for most of the reabsorption of filtered glucose from the tubular lumen. Through inhibition of SGLT2, canagliflozin reduces reabsorption of filtered glucose and lowers the renal threshold for glucose in a dose-dependent manner, leading to increased urinary glucose excretion; increased glucose excretion is independent of insulin secretion. Canagliflozin also may delay oral glucose absorption through transient inhibition of SGLT1 in the intestinal lumen.

Canagliflozin also increases the delivery of sodium to the distal tubule by blocking SGLT2-dependent glucose and sodium reabsorption. This effect may increase tubuloglomerular feedback and reduce intraglomerular pressure.

Following oral administration of a single dose of canagliflozin, the median time to peak plasma concentration was 1–2 hours; mean absolute oral bioavailability of the drug is 65%. Administration of canagliflozin with a high-fat meal had no effect on the pharmacokinetics of the drug; canagliflozin may be administered with or without food. However, based on the potential of the drug to reduce postprandial plasma glucose excursions due to delayed intestinal glucose absorption, the manufacturer recommends that canagliflozin be taken with the first meal of the day. Following administration of a radiolabeled dose of canagliflozin, the dose was recovered in feces as unchanged drug (41.5%), a hydroxylated metabolite (7%), and an *O*-glucuronide metabolite (3.2%) and in urine as the *O*-glucuronide metabolites (30.5%) and unchanged drug (less than 1%). Terminal elimination half-life of canagliflozin was 10.6 and 13.1 hours for single doses of 100 and 300 mg, respectively.

The fixed combination of canagliflozin and extended-release metformin hydrochloride (Invokamet® XR) contains immediate-release canagliflozin and extended-release metformin hydrochloride. Results of a bioequivalence study indicate that the fixed-combination tablets containing canagliflozin and immediate-release metformin hydrochloride (Invokamet®) are bioequivalent to individual tablets of canagliflozin and metformin hydrochloride administered concomitantly in equivalent doses under fed conditions.

ADVICE TO PATIENTS

When canagliflozin is used in fixed combination with other drugs, importance of informing patients of important cautionary information about the concomitant agent(s).

Importance of patient reading medication guide before initiating therapy and each time the drug is dispensed.

Importance of informing patients of the potential risks and benefits of canagliflozin and of alternative therapies. Importance of *not* using canagliflozin in patients with type 1 diabetes mellitus or diabetic ketoacidosis.

Importance of informing patients that if a dose of canagliflozin or the fixed combination of canagliflozin and metformin hydrochloride is missed, it should be taken as soon as it is remembered; if it is almost time for the next dose, the patient should skip the missed dose and take the drug at the next regularly scheduled time. Advise patients not to take 2 doses of the drug at the same time.

Importance of informing patients that ketoacidosis, which can be a life-threatening condition and is sometimes associated with illness or surgery among other risk factors, has been reported with canagliflozin therapy. Importance of informing patients receiving canagliflozin and their caregivers about the signs and symptoms of ketoacidosis (e.g., tachypnea or hyperventilation, anorexia, abdominal pain, nausea, vomiting, lethargy, mental status changes) and of instructing patients to discontinue canagliflozin and seek medical attention immediately should they experience any such signs or symptoms. Advise patients to use a ketone dipstick to check for ketones in their urine (when possible) if symptoms of ketoacidosis occur, even if blood glucose is not elevated (i.e., less than 250 mg/dL).

Importance of informing patients that canagliflozin therapy is associated with an increased risk of requiring lower limb amputations; risk may be higher in some patients, including those with peripheral vascular disease, neuropathy, diabetic foot ulcers, or a history of amputation. Importance of counseling patients on the importance of routine preventative foot care. Advise patients to monitor for new pain or tenderness, sores or ulcers, or infections involving the leg or foot and to seek medical attention immediately should they experience such signs or symptoms.

Importance of informing patients that symptomatic hypotension may occur with canagliflozin and to report such symptoms to their clinicians. Inform patients that canagliflozin-induced dehydration may increase the risk of hypotension and that patients should maintain adequate fluid intake.

Importance of informing patients that acute kidney injury has been reported with canagliflozin therapy. Advise patients to seek medical attention immediately if they experience decreased urine output, or swelling of the legs or feet. Advise patients to seek medical advice immediately if they have reduced oral intake (such as due to acute illness or fasting) or increased fluid losses (such as due to vomiting, diarrhea, or excessive heat exposure), as it may be appropriate to temporarily discontinue canagliflozin in those settings.

Importance of informing patients that yeast infection may occur (e.g., vulvovaginitis, balanitis, balanoposthitis). Importance of informing female patients of the signs and symptoms of vaginal yeast infections (e.g., vaginal discharge, odor, itching) and male patients of the signs and symptoms of balanitis or balanoposthitis (e.g., rash or redness of the glans or foreskin of the penis). Advise patients of treatment options and when to seek medical advice.

Importance of informing patients of the potential for urinary tract infections, which may be serious, with canagliflozin therapy. Advise patients of the signs and symptoms of urinary tract infection and the need to contact a clinician promptly if such signs and symptoms occur.

Importance of informing patients that necrotizing infections of the perineum (Fournier gangrene) have occurred with canagliflozin therapy. Advise patients to seek prompt medical attention if they experience any symptoms of tenderness, redness, or swelling of the genitals or the area from the genitals back to the rectum, occurring with a fever above 38°C or malaise.

Importance of informing patients that due to the mechanism of action of canagliflozin, patients taking the drug will test positive for glucose in urine. Importance of not using urine glucose tests to monitor glycemic status while taking canagliflozin. (See Laboratory Test Interferences under Cautions: Warnings/Precautions.)

Risk of serious hypersensitivity reactions, such as rash, urticaria, and swelling of the face, lips, tongue, and throat that may result in difficulty breathing or swallowing. If signs or symptoms of such a reaction or anaphylaxis or angioedema occur, importance of discontinuing canagliflozin and informing clinician promptly.

Importance of informing patients about the potential for bone fractures (e.g., hip, lumbar spine) with canagliflozin therapy and of providing them with information about factors contributing to fracture risk.

Importance of informing patients about the importance of adherence to dietary instructions, regular physical activity, periodic blood glucose monitoring and glycosylated hemoglobin (hemoglobin A_{1c}; HbA_{1c}) testing, recognition and management of hypoglycemia and hyperglycemia, and assessment of diabetes complications.

Importance of seeking medical advice promptly during periods of stress such as fever, trauma, infection, or surgery as drug dosage requirements may change.

Importance of taking canagliflozin exactly as directed by clinician. Importance of advising patients not to discontinue canagliflozin without first discussing it with the prescribing clinician.

Importance of women informing their clinicians if they are or plan to become pregnant or plan to breast-feed. Advise pregnant women and women of childbearing potential of the possible risk to the fetus with canagliflozin therapy. Advise women that breastfeeding is not recommended during canagliflozin therapy.

Importance of informing clinicians of existing or contemplated concomitant therapy, including prescription (e.g., diuretics, rifampin, phenytoin, phenobarbital, ritonavir, digoxin) and OTC drugs and dietary or herbal supplements, as well as any concomitant illnesses.

Importance of informing patients of other important precautionary information. (See Cautions.)

PREPARATIONS

Excipients in commercially available drug preparations may have clinically important effects in some individuals; consult specific product labeling for details.

Canagliflozin

Oral		
Tablet, film-coated	100 mg (of anhydrous canagliflozin)	Invokana®, Janssen
	300 mg (of anhydrous canagliflozin)	Invokana®, Janssen

Canagliflozin Combinations

Oral		
Tablets, extended-release	50 mg (of anhydrous canagliflozin) with Extended-release Metformin Hydrochloride 500 mg	Invokamet® XR, Janssen
	50 mg (of anhydrous canagliflozin) with Extended-release Metformin Hydrochloride 1 g	Invokamet® XR, Janssen
	150 mg (of anhydrous canagliflozin) with Extended-release Metformin Hydrochloride 500 mg	Invokamet® XR, Janssen
	150 mg (of anhydrous canagliflozin) with Extended-release Metformin Hydrochloride 1 g	Invokamet® XR, Janssen
Tablets, film-coated	50 mg (of anhydrous canagliflozin) with Metformin Hydrochloride 500 mg	Invokamet®, Janssen
	50 mg (of anhydrous canagliflozin) with Metformin Hydrochloride 1 g	Invokamet®, Janssen
	150 mg (of anhydrous canagliflozin) with Metformin Hydrochloride 500 mg	Invokamet®, Janssen
	150 mg (of anhydrous canagliflozin) with Metformin Hydrochloride 1 g	Invokamet®, Janssen

Dapagliflozin Propanediol

68:20.18 • SODIUM-GLUCOSE COTRANSPORTER 2 (SGLT2) INHIBITORS

■ Dapagliflozin propanediol, a sodium-glucose cotransporter 2 (SGLT2) inhibitor, is an antidiabetic agent.

USES

● Type 2 Diabetes Mellitus

Dapagliflozin propanediol is used as monotherapy as an adjunct to diet and exercise to improve glycemic control in patients with type 2 diabetes mellitus. Dapagliflozin also is used in combination with other antidiabetic agents (e.g., metformin and/or a sulfonylurea, a peroxisome proliferator-activated receptor$_\gamma$ [PPAR$_\gamma$] agonist [thiazolidinedione], a dipeptidyl peptidase-4 [DPP-4] inhibitor, a glucagon-like peptide [GLP-1] receptor agonist, insulin) as an adjunct to diet and exercise in patients with type 2 diabetes mellitus who have not achieved adequate glycemic control with dapagliflozin monotherapy. Dapagliflozin is commercially available in fixed combination with extended-release metformin hydrochloride, saxagliptin, or both extended-release metformin hydrochloride and saxagliptin. The fixed combination of dapagliflozin and extended-release metformin hydrochloride, dapagliflozin and saxagliptin, or dapagliflozin, saxagliptin, and extended-release metformin hydrochloride is used as an adjunct to diet and exercise to improve glycemic control in patients with type 2 diabetes mellitus. The manufacturer states that the fixed-combination preparation containing dapagliflozin, saxagliptin, and extended-release metformin hydrochloride is intended only for patients currently taking metformin hydrochloride.

Dapagliflozin also is used as monotherapy or in fixed combination with extended-release metformin hydrochloride to reduce the risk of hospitalization for heart failure in patients with type 2 diabetes mellitus and established cardiovascular disease or multiple cardiovascular risk factors. In addition, dapagliflozin is used to reduce the risk of cardiovascular death and hospitalization for heart failure in patients with heart failure (New York Heart Association [NYHA] class II–IV) and reduced ejection fraction.

Glycemic Control

Current guidelines for the treatment of type 2 diabetes mellitus generally recommend metformin as first-line therapy in addition to lifestyle modifications in patients with recent-onset type 2 diabetes mellitus or mild hyperglycemia because of its well-established safety and efficacy (i.e., beneficial effects on glycosylated hemoglobin [hemoglobin A$_{1c}$; HbA$_{1c}$], weight, and cardiovascular mortality). (See Uses: Type 2 Diabetes Mellitus, in Metformin 68:20.04.) In patients with contraindications or intolerance to metformin (e.g., risk of lactic acidosis, GI intolerance) or in selected other patients, some experts suggest that initial therapy with a drug from another class of antidiabetic agents (e.g., a glucagon-like peptide-1 (GLP-1) receptor agonist, SGLT2 inhibitor, dipeptidyl peptidase-4 (DPP-4) inhibitor, sulfonylurea, thiazolidinedione, basal insulin) may be acceptable based on patient factors. Initiating antidiabetic therapy with 2 agents (e.g., metformin plus another agent) may be appropriate in patients with an initial HbA$_{1c}$ exceeding 7.5% or at least 1.5% above the target level. In metformin-intolerant patients with high initial HbA$_{1c}$ levels, some experts suggest initiation of therapy with 2 agents from other antidiabetic classes with complementary mechanisms of action.

Because of the progressive nature of type 2 diabetes mellitus, patients initially receiving an oral antidiabetic agent will eventually require multiple oral and/or injectable noninsulin antidiabetic agents of different therapeutic classes and/or insulin for adequate glycemic control. Patients who have inadequate glycemic control with initial (e.g., metformin) monotherapy should receive treatment with additional antidiabetic agents; data suggest that the addition of each noninsulin agent to initial therapy lowers HbA$_{1c}$ by approximately 0.7–1%. In addition, early initiation of combination therapy may help to more rapidly attain glycemic goals and extend the time to treatment failure.

Factors to consider when selecting additional antidiabetic agents for combination therapy in patients with inadequate glycemic control on metformin monotherapy include patient comorbidities (e.g., atherosclerotic cardiovascular disease [ASCVD], established kidney disease, heart failure), hypoglycemia risk, impact on weight, cost, risk of adverse effects, and patient preference. When the greater glucose-lowering effect of an injectable drug is needed in patients with type 2 diabetes mellitus, some experts currently state that an injectable GLP-1 receptor agonist is preferred over insulin in most patients because of beneficial effects on body weight and a lower risk of hypoglycemia, although adverse GI effects may diminish tolerability. While addition of a GLP-1 receptor agonist may successfully control hyperglycemia, many patients will eventually require insulin therapy. Early introduction of insulin therapy should be considered when hyperglycemia is severe (e.g., blood glucose of at least 300 mg/dL or HbA$_{1c}$ exceeding 9–10%), especially in the presence of catabolic manifestations (e.g., weight loss, hypertriglyceridemia, ketosis) or symptoms of hyperglycemia. For additional information regarding the initiation of insulin therapy in patients with diabetes mellitus, see Uses: Diabetes Mellitus, in the Insulins General Statement 68:20.08.

Patients with type 2 diabetes mellitus who have established (or are at a high risk for) ASCVD, established kidney disease, or heart failure should receive a GLP-1 receptor agonist or SGLT2 inhibitor with demonstrated cardiovascular disease benefit. (See Reduction in Risk of Major Adverse Cardiovascular Events under Uses: Type 2 Diabetes Mellitus, in Liraglutide 68:20.06 and also see Reduction in Risk of Heart Failure-Related Hospitalization under Uses.) Experts state that therapy with a GLP-1 receptor agonist or SGLT2 inhibitor should be considered for patients with the aforementioned comorbidities independently of the patients' HbA$_{1c}$. GLP-1 receptor agonists and SGLT2 inhibitors appear to have effects on the kidneys independent of their glycemic effects, and some experts suggest that an agent from one of these classes of drugs be considered in patients with type 2 diabetes mellitus and chronic kidney disease (CKD). (See Beneficial Effects on Renal Function under Uses: Type 2 Diabetes Mellitus.) In patients *without* established ASCVD or indicators of high ASCVD risk, heart failure, or CKD, the decision regarding the addition of other antidiabetic agents (e.g., GLP-1 receptor agonist, SGLT2 inhibitor, DPP-4 inhibitor, thiazolidinedione, sulfonylurea, basal insulin) to metformin therapy should be based on avoidance of adverse effects, cost, and individual patient factors.

The manufacturer states that dapagliflozin or the fixed combinations of dapagliflozin with extended-release metformin hydrochloride, saxagliptin, or both extended-release metformin hydrochloride and saxagliptin are *not* indicated for the treatment of type 1 diabetes mellitus or diabetic ketoacidosis.

Dapagliflozin Monotherapy

When given as monotherapy for the management of type 2 diabetes mellitus, dapagliflozin improves glycemic control compared with placebo as evidenced by reductions in glycosylated hemoglobin (hemoglobin A$_{1c}$; HbA$_{1c}$) and in fasting and 2-hour postprandial plasma glucose concentrations. Efficacy of dapagliflozin as monotherapy has been established in 2 double-blind, placebo-controlled studies of 24-weeks' duration in 840 treatment-naive patients with type 2 diabetes mellitus and baseline HbA$_{1c}$ concentrations of 7–10%. In the first study, HbA$_{1c}$ was reduced by 0.8 or 0.9% in patients receiving dapagliflozin 5 or 10 mg once daily, respectively, compared with a decrease of 0.2% in those receiving placebo. In patients who received dapagliflozin 5 or 10 mg, approximately 44 or 51%, respectively, had HbA$_{1c}$ reductions to less than 7%, compared with approximately 32% of patients receiving placebo. In the second study, mean HbA$_{1c}$ reduction at week 24 was 0.68, 0.72, or 0.82% in patients receiving 1, 2.5, or 5 mg of dapagliflozin, respectively, compared with an increase of 0.02% in those receiving placebo.

Combination Therapy

Clinical trials evaluating the safety and efficacy of the fixed combination of dapagliflozin and extended-release metformin hydrochloride (Xigduo® XR) in reducing HbA$_{1c}$ have not been conducted; unless otherwise specified, clinical trials of dapagliflozin in combination with metformin discussed in this monograph were conducted using concomitantly administered dapagliflozin and immediate- or extended-release metformin hydrochloride. Bioequivalence between the fixed combination of dapagliflozin and extended-release metformin hydrochloride and each agent (dapagliflozin and extended-release metformin hydrochloride) given concurrently as separate tablets has been demonstrated. (See Description.) Safety and efficacy of the fixed combination of dapagliflozin and saxagliptin (Qtern®) have been established by clinical studies evaluating treatment with saxagliptin as add-on therapy to treatment with dapagliflozin and metformin hydrochloride or with dapagliflozin and saxagliptin as add-on therapy to treatment with metformin.

When given in combination with one or more oral antidiabetic agents (e.g., metformin, a sulfonylurea, a thiazolidinedione, a DPP-4 inhibitor) and/or insulin or a GLP-1 receptor agonist (e.g., exenatide), dapagliflozin improves glycemic control compared with monotherapy with these drugs and generally is associated with reductions in body weight and systolic blood pressure. Dapagliflozin generally is well tolerated, although genital mycotic infections appear to be more common with dapagliflozin than with other antidiabetic therapy.

Efficacy of dapagliflozin in combination with other antidiabetic agents for the management of type 2 diabetes mellitus is supported by results from several randomized, active- or placebo-controlled studies in patients receiving dapagliflozin with metformin, a sulfonylurea, metformin and a sulfonylurea, a thiazolidinedione, a DPP-4 inhibitor, a GLP-1 receptor agonist, or insulin. In these studies, initial combined therapy with dapagliflozin (5 or 10 mg once daily) and one or more antidiabetic drugs or addition of dapagliflozin to existing therapy improved glycemic control as evidenced by reductions in HbA_{1c}, fasting plasma glucose, and 2-hour postprandial plasma glucose concentrations; combined therapy also had beneficial effects on weight reduction and blood pressure compared with placebo and/or monotherapy.

In two 24-week studies in treatment-naive patients with baseline mean HbA_{1c} concentrations of 9–9.2%, the combination of extended-release metformin hydrochloride (up to 2 g daily) and dapagliflozin 5 or 10 mg once daily resulted in a reduction of 2.1 or 2%, respectively, in HbA_{1c} compared with a reduction of 1.5, 1.2 or 1.4% in HbA_{1c} with dapagliflozin 10 mg, dapagliflozin 5 mg, or extended-release metformin hydrochloride alone, respectively. Dapagliflozin 10 mg once daily was noninferior to metformin in reducing HbA_{1c}, and superior in reducing fasting plasma glucose; dapagliflozin in this dosage also was associated with substantially greater weight loss than metformin monotherapy.

In a 24-week study in patients with HbA_{1c} concentrations of 7–10% while receiving metformin hydrochloride (dosage of at least 1.5 g daily), the addition of dapagliflozin 5 or 10 mg resulted in a reduction of 0.7 or 0.8%, respectively, in HbA_{1c} compared with a 0.3% HbA_{1c} reduction with placebo. In these patients, add-on therapy with dapagliflozin 5 or 10 mg resulted in HbA_{1c} reductions to less than 7% in 37.5 or 40.6% of patients, respectively, compared with 25.9% of patients receiving add-on placebo. In a 78-week extension of this study, add-on dapagliflozin was associated with sustained reductions in HbA_{1c}, fasting plasma glucose, and body weight.

In a study in patients with HbA_{1c} concentrations of approximately 6.5–10% while receiving metformin hydrochloride (dosage of at least 1.5 g daily), add-on therapy with dapagliflozin (titrated to 10 mg once daily) was noninferior to add-on glipizide (titrated to 20 mg once daily) in reducing HbA_{1c} after 52 weeks of therapy. In addition, weight loss with add-on dapagliflozin therapy (3.2 kg) was superior to that with add-on glipizide therapy (1.4 kg).

In a 24-week study in patients who had inadequate glycemic control (HbA_{1c} concentration of 7–10%) while receiving a sulfonylurea antidiabetic agent (glimepiride), add-on therapy with dapagliflozin 2.5, 5, or 10 mg once daily resulted in a reduction of approximately 0.6, 0.6, or 0.8%, respectively, in HbA_{1c} compared with a reduction of approximately 0.1% with add-on placebo. In a 24-week study in patients who had inadequate glycemic control (HbA_{1c} concentration of 7–10.5%) on pioglitazone (30 or 45 mg daily), the addition of dapagliflozin 5 or 10 mg resulted in a reduction of 0.8 or 1%, respectively, in HbA_{1c} compared with a reduction of 0.4% with add-on placebo. Dapagliflozin also improved postprandial and fasting plasma glucose concentrations as well as reducing body weight and systolic blood pressure. In a 24-week study in patients who were treatment naive or who had inadequate glycemic control (HbA_{1c} concentration of 7–10%) while receiving sitagliptin (100 mg once daily) with or without metformin hydrochloride (dosage of at least 1.5 g daily), addition of dapagliflozin 10 mg once daily reduced HbA_{1c} by 0.45%, while patients receiving add-on placebo experienced no appreciable change. Patients receiving dapagliflozin add-on therapy also showed improved fasting plasma glucose and reduced body weight.

In a 24-week study in patients who had inadequate glycemic control (HbA_{1c} concentration 7–10.5%) while receiving immediate- or extended-release metformin hydrochloride (at least 1.5 g daily) plus a sulfonylurea antidiabetic agent at the maximum tolerated dosage (and at least 50% of the maximum dosage), add-on therapy with dapagliflozin 10 mg once daily was associated with a 0.7% reduction in HbA_{1c} compared with add-on placebo at 24 weeks. Add-on dapagliflozin therapy also was associated with reductions in fasting plasma glucose and body weight at week 24, and systolic blood pressure at week 8 compared with placebo.

In a 24-week study examining the effects of dapagliflozin on total body weight in patients with inadequate glycemic control on metformin hydrochloride,

addition of dapagliflozin 10 mg once daily reduced total body weight by 2.96 kg compared with a reduction of 0.88 kg in those receiving add-on placebo.

Efficacy of dapagliflozin as add-on therapy to insulin in the management of type 2 diabetes mellitus in patients who have inadequate glycemic control (HbA_{1c} concentration of 7.5–10.5%) with insulin is supported by results of a 24-week, randomized, placebo-controlled study. In this study, addition of dapagliflozin (5 or 10 mg daily) to existing stable therapy with insulin (mean daily dosage of at least 30 units) with or without up to 2 additional oral antidiabetic agents resulted in improvements in HbA_{1c}, fasting plasma glucose, 2-hour postprandial plasma glucose concentrations, and body weight. In patients who received dapagliflozin 5 or 10 mg as add-on to insulin therapy with or without 1 or 2 additional antidiabetic agents, addition of dapagliflozin 5 or 10 mg reduced HbA_{1c} by 0.8 or 0.9%, respectively, compared with a 0.3% reduction in those receiving add-on placebo. During extended treatment and follow-up in this study, reductions in HbA_{1c}, body weight, and insulin dosage were maintained for 104 weeks with dapagliflozin therapy.

In a 12-week randomized, double-blind study in patients receiving insulin with or without up to 2 oral antidiabetic agents, HbA_{1c} was reduced by 0.7 or 0.78% with addition of dapagliflozin 10 or 20 mg once daily, respectively, to existing therapy compared with addition of placebo. The mean change from baseline in body weight at the end of the study was 4.5, 4.3, or 1.9 kg with dapagliflozin 10 mg, 20 mg, or placebo, respectively. Patients receiving add-on dapagliflozin 10 or 20 mg had mean *reductions* in insulin dosage from baseline of 1.4 and 0.8 units, respectively, at the end of the study compared with a mean *increase* from baseline of 1.7 units in those receiving add-on placebo.

Efficacy of the combination of dapagliflozin and saxagliptin with metformin hydrochloride for the management of type 2 diabetes mellitus is supported by several randomized, controlled clinical studies. In a 24-week study in patients with inadequate glycemic control (HbA_{1c} concentration of 7.5–10%) despite treatment with metformin hydrochloride, the addition of dapagliflozin and saxagliptin to existing therapy with metformin hydrochloride substantially improved glycemic control. Patients who received triple therapy with dapagliflozin, saxagliptin, and metformin hydrochloride had an HbA_{1c} reduction of 1.02% compared with a reduction of 0.62 or 0.69% in those who received dual therapy with dapagliflozin and metformin hydrochloride or saxagliptin and metformin hydrochloride, respectively. Additionally, a larger proportion of patients who received triple therapy achieved HbA_{1c} below 7% compared with those who received dual therapy.

In another clinical study of 24 weeks' duration, adults with type 2 diabetes mellitus who had inadequate glycemic control on metformin alone (HbA_{1c} 8–12%) received add-on therapy with 10 mg of dapagliflozin and 5 mg of saxagliptin, 10 mg of dapagliflozin, or 5 mg of saxagliptin. After 24 weeks, concomitant therapy with dapagliflozin and saxagliptin resulted in substantial decreases in HbA_{1c}, and a greater proportion of patients receiving this therapy achieved an HbA_{1c} below 7% compared with those receiving add-on therapy with dapagliflozin or saxagliptin.

In a clinical study evaluating the efficacy of add-on therapy with saxagliptin in adults (mean age: 54.6 years, 52.7% female, 87.9% Caucasian) with type 2 diabetes mellitus (mean HbA_{1c}: 7.9%) already receiving concomitant dapagliflozin and metformin therapy, the addition of saxagliptin resulted in substantial reductions in HbA_{1c}. The combination of the 3 agents was well tolerated, and patients receiving therapy with all 3 agents had a reduction in HbA_{1c} of 0.5% compared with a reduction of 0.2% in patients receiving dapagliflozin and metformin therapy.

Efficacy of dapagliflozin in conjunction with extended-release exenatide as add-on therapy to metformin hydrochloride in the management of type 2 diabetes mellitus in patients who have inadequate glycemic control (HbA_{1c} concentration of 8 to less than 12%) with metformin hydrochloride is supported by results of a 28-week, randomized, active-controlled study. In this study, addition of dapagliflozin (10 mg daily) and extended-release exenatide (2 mg subcutaneously every week) to existing stable therapy with metformin hydrochloride (at least 1.5 g daily) resulted in substantially greater improvements in HbA_{1c} and fasting plasma glucose compared with dapagliflozin or extended-release exenatide alone. In patients who received dapagliflozin 10 mg once daily and extended-release exenatide 2 mg once weekly as add-on to metformin hydrochloride therapy, addition of dapagliflozin and extended-release exenatide reduced HbA_{1c} by 1.8% compared with a 1.3 or 1.4% reduction in those receiving add-on therapy with dapagliflozin or extended-release exenatide alone, respectively. More weight loss and greater reductions in systolic blood pressure also were observed among those who received add-on therapy with dapagliflozin and extended-release exenatide compared with add-on therapy with either drug alone.

Reduction in Risk of Heart Failure-Related Hospitalization

Dapagliflozin is used to reduce the risk of hospitalization for heart failure in patients with type 2 diabetes mellitus and established cardiovascular disease or multiple cardiovascular risk factors. In addition to lowering blood glucose, SGLT2 inhibitors such as dapagliflozin appear to modify several nonglycemic cardiovascular risk factors such as blood pressure, body weight, adiposity, and arterial stiffness.

In a randomized, placebo-controlled trial in adults with type 2 diabetes mellitus and established ASCVD or multiple (2 or more) ASCVD risk factors (DECLARE-TIMI 58), dapagliflozin demonstrated a beneficial effect specifically related to the risk of heart failure; a lower risk of major adverse cardiovascular events compared with placebo was *not* observed. In this study, patients 40 years of age or older with type 2 diabetes mellitus who had or were at risk for ASCVD received dapagliflozin 10 mg once daily or placebo for a median of 4.2 years. The use of other antidiabetic agents was at the discretion of the treating clinician. Approximately 59% of patients had multiple risk factors for ASCVD (but not *established* ASCVD); 10% of patients had a history of heart failure. The primary efficacy outcomes were major adverse cardiovascular events (e.g., cardiovascular death, myocardial infarction [MI], ischemic stroke) and the composite of cardiovascular death or hospitalization for heart failure. Dapagliflozin was noninferior to placebo with regard to the risk of major adverse cardiovascular effects but did not significantly reduce or increase the risk of such events compared with placebo (event rate: 8.8 versus 9.4%, respectively). However, dapagliflozin therapy was associated with a reduction in the risk of the composite outcome of cardiovascular death or hospitalization for heart failure, which was attributable to a 27% relative risk reduction in hospitalization for heart failure; there was no difference between placebo and dapagliflozin with regard to the risk of cardiovascular death.

Beneficial Effects on Renal Function

SGLT2 inhibitors reduce renal tubular glucose reabsorption, weight, systemic blood pressure, intraglomerular pressure, and albuminuria and slow glomerular filtration rate (GFR) loss through mechanisms that appear to be independent of glucose lowering effects. In several cardiovascular outcomes trials involving the use of SGLT2 inhibitors (e.g., canagliflozin, dapagliflozin, empagliflozin) in patients with type 2 diabetes mellitus at high risk for cardiovascular disease or with existing cardiovascular disease, beneficial effects on renal function have been observed as a secondary outcome. Some experts state that the use of an SGLT2 inhibitor should be considered to reduce the risk of CKD progression, cardiovascular events, or both in patients with type 2 diabetes mellitus and diabetic kidney disease with albuminuria† (an eGFR of at least 30 mL/minute per 1.73 m² and urinary albumin exceeding 30 mg/g creatinine, particularly urinary albumin exceeding 300 mg/g creatinine).

In the DECLARE-TIMI 58 study, dapagliflozin therapy was associated with a lower incidence of a secondary composite renal outcome (at least a 40% decrease in eGFR to less than 60 mL/minute per 1.73 m², end-stage renal disease (ESRD), or death from renal or cardiovascular causes), which occurred in 4.3% of dapagliflozin-treated patients versus 5.6% of those receiving placebo. In a clinical study evaluating the use of another SGLT2 inhibitor, canagliflozin, in patients with type 2 diabetes mellitus, CKD (eGFR 30–89 mL/minute per 1.73 m²; mean 56.2 mL/minute per 1.73 m²), and albuminuria (urine albumin:creatinine ratio exceeding 300 but less than 5000 mg/g), canagliflozin therapy reduced the risk of end-stage kidney disease, doubling of serum creatinine, cardiovascular death, and hospitalization for heart failure.

● Reduction in Risk of Cardiovascular Death and Heart Failure-Related Hospitalization

Dapagliflozin is used to reduce the risk of cardiovascular death and hospitalization for heart failure in patients with heart failure (NYHA class II–IV) and reduced ejection fraction.

In a double-blind, placebo-controlled study (Dapagliflozin And Prevention of Adverse outcomes in Heart Failure [DAPA-HF]) in patients with chronic heart failure (NYHA class II–IV) and reduced ejection fraction (left ventricular ejection fraction [LVEF] of 40% or less), dapagliflozin therapy reduced the risk of worsening heart failure or death from cardiovascular causes in patients with or without type 2 diabetes mellitus. In this study, approximately 4700 patients with chronic heart failure (68% NYHA class II, 32% class III, and 1% class IV) and reduced ejection fraction (median baseline LVEF: 32%) received dapagliflozin 10 mg orally once daily or placebo in conjunction with standard medical and medical device therapy for heart failure for a median duration of 18.2 months. Initially, 42% of enrolled patients had a history of type 2 diabetes mellitus and an additional 3% of patients in each group received a diagnosis of type 2 diabetes mellitus

(based on a HbA₁c of at least 6.5%) during the enrollment process. At baseline, most patients were receiving an angiotensin-converting enzyme (ACE) inhibitor, angiotensin II receptor antagonist, or angiotensin receptor-neprilysin inhibitor (ARNI); a β-adrenergic blocking agent (β-blocker); a mineralocorticoid receptor antagonist; and a diuretic; 26% had an implantable cardiac device. The primary outcome was a composite of cardiovascular death, hospitalization for heart failure, or urgent heart failure visit (i.e., urgent, unplanned clinician assessment requiring treatment for worsening heart failure). Among patients who received dapagliflozin therapy, the incidence of the primary end point was reduced by 26%. All three components of the primary composite end point contributed individually to the treatment effect, and the results were applicable to all subgroups analyzed, including patients with or without type 2 diabetes mellitus.

DOSAGE AND ADMINISTRATION

● General

Volume depletion should be corrected before initiating dapagliflozin. In addition, renal function should be assessed prior to treatment and then as clinically indicated. (See Dosage and Administration: Special Populations.)

● Administration

Dapagliflozin or the fixed combination of dapagliflozin and saxagliptin is administered orally once daily in the morning, with or without food. The fixed combination of dapagliflozin and extended-release metformin hydrochloride or dapagliflozin, saxagliptin, and extended-release metformin hydrochloride is administered once daily in the morning with food to reduce the adverse GI effects of the metformin hydrochloride component.

The fixed-combination tablets of dapagliflozin and extended-release metformin hydrochloride, dapagliflozin and saxagliptin, or dapagliflozin, extended-release metformin hydrochloride, and saxagliptin should be swallowed whole; tablets should not be crushed, cut, or chewed. Occasionally, inactive ingredients in the fixed-combination tablets containing extended-release metformin hydrochloride may be eliminated in feces as a soft mass that may resemble the original tablet.

If a dose of dapagliflozin, the fixed combination of dapagliflozin and extended-release metformin hydrochloride, or the fixed-combination of dapagliflozin and saxagliptin is missed, the missed dose should be taken as soon as it is remembered followed by resumption of the regular schedule. If the missed dose is not remembered until it is almost time for the next dose, the missed dose should be skipped and the regular schedule resumed; the dose should not be doubled to replace a missed dose. If a dose of the fixed combination of dapagliflozin, extended-release metformin hydrochloride, and saxagliptin is missed and it is 12 hours or more until the next dose, the dose should be taken. If a dose if missed and it is less than 12 hours until the next dose, the missed dose should be skipped and the next dose taken at the usual time; patients should be advised not to take 2 doses at the same time.

● Dosage

Dosage of dapagliflozin propanediol is expressed in terms of dapagliflozin.

Type 2 Diabetes Mellitus

Glycemic Control

The recommended initial dosage of dapagliflozin as monotherapy for the management of type 2 diabetes mellitus in adults is 5 mg once daily in the morning. If well tolerated, the dosage may be increased to 10 mg once daily in the morning in patients who require additional glycemic control.

When the commercially available fixed-combination preparation containing dapagliflozin and extended-release metformin hydrochloride (Xigduo® XR) is used for glycemic control in patients with type 2 diabetes mellitus, the recommended initial dosage is based on the patient's current regimen of dapagliflozin and/or metformin hydrochloride. For patients *not* currently receiving dapagliflozin, the recommended initial dosage of the dapagliflozin component is 5 mg once daily in the morning. Dosage should be titrated gradually based on effectiveness and tolerability, up to a maximum daily dosage of 10 mg of dapagliflozin and 2 g of extended-release metformin hydrochloride. Patients who are already receiving extended-release metformin hydrochloride in the evening and are switching to the fixed combination of dapagliflozin and metformin hydrochloride should skip their last dose of metformin hydrochloride before initiating therapy with the fixed combination the following morning.

In patients *not* already receiving dapagliflozin therapy, the recommended initial dosage of the fixed combination of dapagliflozin and saxagliptin (Qtern®) is 5 mg of dapagliflozin and 5 mg of saxagliptin once daily in the morning. In patients who tolerate the initial dosage and require additional glycemic control, the dosage of the fixed combination may be increased to 10 mg of dapagliflozin and 5 mg of saxagliptin once daily in the morning.

The fixed combination of dapagliflozin and saxagliptin should *not* be used in patients receiving concomitant therapy with a potent cytochrome P-450 (CYP) 3A4/5 inhibitor (e.g., atazanavir, clarithromycin, indinavir, itraconazole, ketoconazole, nefazodone, nelfinavir, ritonavir, saquinavir, telithromycin). (See Drug Interactions: Drugs Affecting or Metabolized by Hepatic Microsomal Enzymes, in Saxagliptin 68:20.05.)

When the fixed-combination preparation containing dapagliflozin, saxagliptin, and extended-release metformin hydrochloride (Qternmet® XR) is used in patients with type 2 diabetes mellitus, the recommended initial dosage is based on the patient's current antidiabetic drug regimen. For patients *not* currently receiving dapagliflozin, the recommended initial total daily dosage of the fixed combination is dapagliflozin 5 mg, saxagliptin 5 mg, and extended-release metformin hydrochloride 1 or 2 g once daily in the morning. Dosage should be titrated gradually based on effectiveness and tolerability, up to a maximum daily dosage of 10 mg of dapagliflozin, 5 mg of saxagliptin, and 2 g of extended-release metformin hydrochloride. The manufacturer states that the fixed-combination preparation containing dapagliflozin, saxagliptin, and extended-release metformin is intended only for patients currently taking metformin.

The fixed combination of dapagliflozin, saxagliptin, and extended-release metformin should *not* be used in patients receiving concomitant therapy with a potent cytochrome P-450 (CYP) 3A4/5 inhibitor (e.g., atazanavir, clarithromycin, indinavir, itraconazole, ketoconazole, nefazodone, nelfinavir, ritonavir, saquinavir, telithromycin). (See Drug Interactions: Drugs Affecting or Metabolized by Hepatic Microsomal Enzymes, in Saxagliptin 68:20.05.)

Reduction in Heart Failure-Related Hospitalization in Type 2 Diabetes Mellitus

The recommended dosage of dapagliflozin for the reduction of heart failure-related hospitalization in adults with type 2 diabetes mellitus and established cardiovascular disease or multiple cardiovascular risk factors is 10 mg once daily.

Reduction in Cardiovascular Death and Heart Failure-Related Hospitalization

The recommended dosage of dapagliflozin for reduction in cardiovascular death and hospitalization for heart failure in adults with heart failure (NYHA class II–IV) and reduced ejection fraction is 10 mg once daily.

● Special Populations

Dosage adjustments for dapagliflozin or the fixed combination of dapagliflozin and saxagliptin are not necessary in patients with mild, moderate, or severe hepatic impairment. Use of the fixed-combination preparations containing dapagliflozin and extended-release metformin hydrochloride or dapagliflozin, saxagliptin, and extended-release metformin hydrochloride should be avoided in patients with hepatic impairment.

When dapagliflozin is used for glycemic control in patients *without* established cardiovascular disease or cardiovascular risk factors, dosage adjustments are not needed if patients have an estimated glomerular filtration rate (eGFR) of at least 45 mL/minute per 1.73 m². Dapagliflozin is not recommended in such patients who have an eGFR of 30 to less than 45 mL/minute per 1.73 m², and the drug is contraindicated in patients with severe renal impairment (eGFR less than 30 mL/minute per 1.73 m²) and in those with end-stage renal disease (ESRD) or undergoing dialysis.

When dapagliflozin is used to reduce the risk of heart failure-related hospitalization in patients with type 2 diabetes mellitus and cardiovascular disease or multiple cardiovascular risk factors, dosage adjustments are not needed in patients with an eGFR of at least 45 mL/minute per 1.73 m². There are insufficient data to support a dapagliflozin dosage recommendation in patients with an eGFR less than 45 mL/minute per 1.73 m²; dapagliflozin is contraindicated in patients with ESRD or undergoing dialysis.

When dapagliflozin is used to reduce the risk of cardiovascular death or heart failure-related hospitalization in patients with or without type 2 diabetes mellitus who have heart failure and a reduced ejection fraction, no dosage adjustment

is needed in patients with an eGFR of at least 30 mL/minute per 1.73 m². There are insufficient data to support a dosage recommendation in patients with an eGFR less than 30 mL/minute per 1.73 m², and dapagliflozin is contraindicated in patients with ESRD or undergoing dialysis.

Dosage adjustments for the fixed combination of dapagliflozin and extended-release metformin hydrochloride or the fixed combination of dapagliflozin and saxagliptin are not necessary in patients with an eGFR of at least 45 mL/minute per 1.73 m². The fixed combination of dapagliflozin and metformin hydrochloride should not be used in patients with an eGFR of less than 45 mL/minute per 1.73 m². Use of the fixed combination of dapagliflozin and metformin hydrochloride is contraindicated in patients with an eGFR of less than 30 mL/minute per 1.73 m². The fixed combination of dapagliflozin and saxagliptin is contraindicated in patients with an eGFR of less than 45 mL/minute per 1.73 m².

No adjustment of dapagliflozin dosage is necessary based solely on age. In addition, dosage adjustment is not recommended based solely on sex, race, or body weight.

CAUTIONS

● Contraindications

History of serious hypersensitivity reaction to dapagliflozin or any ingredient in the formulation.

Dapagliflozin is contraindicated in patients receiving the drug for glycemic control who have severe renal impairment (estimated glomerular filtration rate [eGFR] less than 30 mL/minute per 1.73 m²) without established cardiovascular disease or multiple cardiovascular risk factors.

Dapagliflozin is contraindicated in patients with end-stage renal disease (ESRD) or undergoing dialysis.

● Warnings/Precautions

Volume Depletion and Renal Effects

Dapagliflozin can cause intravascular volume depletion, which may manifest as symptomatic hypotension or acute transient changes in serum creatinine concentration. Patients with impaired renal function (eGFR less than 60 mL/minute per 1.73 m²), geriatric patients, and patients receiving loop diuretics may be at an increased risk for volume depletion or hypotension. (See Drug Interactions: Diuretics.) Intravascular volume status should be assessed and corrected prior to initiating dapagliflozin.

Acute kidney injury, sometimes requiring hospitalization and dialysis, has been reported in patients with type 2 diabetes mellitus receiving canagliflozin or dapagliflozin. FDA identified 101 cases of acute kidney injury associated with canagliflozin or dapagliflozin therapy in FAERS between March 2013 and October 2015. Hospitalization for evaluation and management of kidney injury was warranted in most cases, and some cases required admission to an intensive care unit and dialysis. In approximately half of the cases, onset of acute kidney injury occurred within 1 month or less of initiating dapagliflozin therapy, and most patients' kidney function improved after stopping the drug. However, kidney injury may not be fully reversible in some situations and has led to death in some patients.

Prior to initiating dapagliflozin therapy, clinicians should consider patient factors that may predispose the patient to acute kidney injury, including hypovolemia, chronic renal insufficiency, heart failure, and concomitant medications (e.g., diuretics, angiotensin converting enzyme [ACE] inhibitors, angiotensin II receptor antagonists, nonsteroidal anti-inflammatory agents [NSAIAs]). Clinicians should consider temporarily discontinuing dapagliflozin in any setting of reduced oral intake (e.g., acute illness, fasting) or fluid losses (e.g., GI illness, excessive heat exposure). Patients should be monitored for signs and symptoms of hypotension and effects on renal function as clinically indicated after initiating therapy with dapagliflozin. If patients develop acute kidney injury, dapagliflozin should be discontinued and appropriate treatment initiated for such injury.

Ketoacidosis in Patients with Diabetes Mellitus

Use of sodium glucose cotransporter 2 (SGLT2) inhibitors in patients with type 2 diabetes mellitus may lead to ketoacidosis requiring hospitalization. Fatal cases of ketoacidosis have been reported in patients receiving dapagliflozin. Ketoacidosis associated with use of SGLT2 inhibitors may be present without markedly elevated blood glucose concentrations (e.g., less than 250 mg/dL).

FDA identified 73 cases of acidosis (reported as diabetic ketoacidosis [DKA], ketoacidosis, or ketosis) associated with SGLT2 inhibitor use in the FDA Adverse Event Reporting System (FAERS) between March 2013 and May 2015. DKA had an atypical presentation in most of the reported cases in that type 2 diabetes mellitus was noted as the indication for the drug, and glucose concentrations were only slightly elevated (median: 211 mg/dL); type 1 diabetes mellitus was named as the indication in a few cases, and in some reports the indication for use was not specified. The median time to onset of symptoms of acidosis following initiation or increase in dosage of the SGLT2 inhibitor was 43 days (range: 1–365 days). No trend demonstrating a relationship between the dosage of an SGLT2 inhibitor and the risk of ketoacidosis was identified. In all reported episodes, a diagnosis of DKA or ketoacidosis was made by the clinician and hospitalization or treatment in an emergency department was warranted. In most cases, at least 1 diagnostic laboratory criterion suggestive of ketoacidosis (e.g., high anion gap metabolic acidosis, ketonemia, reduced serum bicarbonate) was reported. Potential factors for the development of ketoacidosis with SGLT2 inhibitor therapy identified in the 73 cases included infection, low carbohydrate diet or reduced caloric intake (due to illness or surgery), pancreatic disorders suggesting insulin deficiency (e.g., type 1 diabetes mellitus, history of pancreatitis, pancreatic surgery), reduced dosage or discontinuance of insulin, discontinuance of an oral insulin secretagogue, and alcohol use.

Prior to initiating therapy with an SGLT2 inhibitor, clinicians should consider patient factors that may predispose the patient to ketoacidosis such as pancreatic insulin deficiency from any cause, reduced caloric intake, and alcohol abuse.

Clinicians should evaluate for the presence of acidosis, including ketoacidosis, in patients experiencing signs or symptoms of acidosis while receiving SGLT2 inhibitors, regardless of the patient's blood glucose concentration. For patients who undergo scheduled surgery, temporary discontinuation of dapagliflozin for at least 3 days prior to surgery should be considered. Clinicians should consider monitoring for ketoacidosis and temporarily discontinuing therapy with an SGLT2 inhibitor in other clinical situations known to predispose individuals to ketoacidosis (e.g., prolonged fasting due to acute illness or post-surgery). If acidosis is confirmed, the SGLT2 inhibitor should be discontinued and appropriate treatment initiated to correct the acidosis; glucose concentrations should be monitored appropriately. In addition, supportive medical treatment should be instituted to treat and correct factors that may have precipitated or contributed to the metabolic acidosis. Risk factors for the development of ketoacidosis should be resolved prior to restarting dapagliflozin therapy.

Euglycemic DKA associated with SGLT2 inhibitors may be detected and potentially prevented by having patients monitor urine and/or plasma ketone levels if they feel unwell, regardless of ambient glucose concentrations. Clinicians should inform patients and caregivers of the signs and symptoms of ketoacidosis (e.g., tachypnea or hyperventilation, anorexia, abdominal pain, nausea, vomiting, lethargy, mental status changes) and instruct patients to discontinue the SGLT2 inhibitor and immediately seek medical attention should they experience such signs or symptoms.

Urosepsis and Pyelonephritis

Dapagliflozin may increase the risk of serious urinary tract infections; urosepsis and pyelonephritis have been reported with SGLT2 inhibitors, including dapagliflozin.

FDA identified 19 cases of urosepsis and pyelonephritis, which began as urinary tract infections associated with SGLT2 inhibitor use, in FAERS between March 2013 and October 2014. In all cases reported, hospitalization was warranted and some patients required admission to an intensive care unit or dialysis for treatment. The median time to onset of infection following initiation of the SGLT2 inhibitor was 45 days (range: 2–270 days).

Prior to initiating therapy with an SGLT2 inhibitor, clinicians should consider patient factors that may predispose the patient to serious urinary tract infections such as a history of difficulty urinating or infections of the bladder, kidneys, or urinary tract. Patients should be monitored for urinary tract infections and treatment instituted if indicated.

Concomitant Therapy with Insulin or Insulin Secretagogues

When dapagliflozin is added to therapy with an insulin secretagogue (e.g., a sulfonylurea) or insulin, the incidence of hypoglycemia is increased compared with sulfonylurea or insulin monotherapy. Therefore, patients receiving dapagliflozin may require a reduced dosage of the concomitant insulin secretagogue or insulin to reduce the risk of hypoglycemia. (See Drug Interactions: Antidiabetic Agents.)

Necrotizing Fasciitis of the Perineum

Necrotizing fasciitis of the perineum (Fournier gangrene), a rare but serious or life-threatening bacterial infection requiring urgent surgical intervention, has been reported during postmarketing surveillance in men and women with type 2 diabetes mellitus receiving an SGLT2 inhibitor, including dapagliflozin. Permanent disfigurement, prolonged hospitalization, disability, and complications from sepsis all may be associated with Fournier gangrene. Although diabetes mellitus is a risk factor for developing Fournier gangrene, this condition is still rare among patients with diabetes mellitus.

FDA identified 12 cases of Fournier gangrene in patients taking an SGLT2 inhibitor reported in FAERS and the medical literature between March 2013 and May 2018. Since FDA's review, additional cases of Fournier gangrene have been reported. In the initial cases reviewed by FDA, the average time to onset of infection was 9.2 months (range 7 days to 25 months) after initiation of therapy with an SGLT2 inhibitor. Some experts speculate that the variation in time to diagnosis of Fournier gangrene might be due to fluctuating glycemic control, microvascular complications, or an inciting event associated with SGLT2 inhibitors (e.g., urinary tract infection, mycotic infection, skin or mucosal breakdown due to pruritus). In all reported cases, hospitalization and surgery were required. Among these cases, some patients required multiple disfiguring surgeries, some developed complications (e.g., diabetic ketoacidosis, acute kidney injury, septic shock), and 1 patient died. In a review of other antidiabetic drugs (e.g., insulin, biguanides, sulfonylureas, dipeptidyl peptidase-4 inhibitors) over a period of more than 30 years, only 6 cases of Fournier gangrene were identified; all of theses cases occurred in men.

Patients receiving dapagliflozin who develop pain or tenderness, erythema, or swelling in the genital or perineal area, in addition to fever or malaise, should be assessed for necrotizing fasciitis. If Fournier gangrene is suspected, dapagliflozin should be discontinued and immediate treatment with broad-spectrum antibiotics should be initiated; surgical debridement should be performed if necessary. Blood glucose concentrations should be closely monitored; alternative antidiabetic agents should be initiated to maintain glycemic control.

Genital Mycotic Infections

Dapagliflozin may increase the risk of genital mycotic infections in males (e.g., balanitis) and females (e.g., vulvovaginal mycotic infection). In glycemic control clinical trials, patients with a history of genital mycotic infections were more likely to develop such infections. Patients should be monitored for genital mycotic infections and appropriate treatment should be instituted if these infections occur.

Risk of Bone Fracture

An increased risk of bone fracture, along with dose-related decreases in bone mineral density in older adults, has been observed in patients receiving another drug in the SGLT2 inhibitor class (canagliflozin). (See Risk of Bone Fracture under Cautions: Warnings/Precautions, in Canagliflozin 68:20.18.) In a clinical trial in patients with renal impairment (eGFR of 30 to less than 60 mL/minute per 1.73 m^2), a greater incidence of bone fractures was observed in patients receiving dapagliflozin compared with those receiving placebo. FDA is continuing to evaluate the risk of bone fracture with SGLT2 inhibitors.

Laboratory Test Interferences

SGLT2 inhibitors, including dapagliflozin, increase urinary glucose excretion and will result in false-positive urine glucose tests. In addition, the manufacturer states that the 1,5-anhydroglucitol assay is unreliable for monitoring glycemic control in patients taking SGLT2 inhibitors. Alternative methods of monitoring glycemic control should be used in patients receiving SGLT2 inhibitors.

Initiation of therapy with an SGLT2 inhibitor, including dapagliflozin, may cause small increases in serum creatinine concentration and decreases in eGFR. In patients with normal or mildly impaired renal function, these changes in serum creatinine and eGFR generally occur within weeks of starting dapagliflozin therapy and then stabilize. Increases that do not fit this pattern should prompt further evaluation to exclude the possibility of acute kidney injury. (See Warnings/Precautions: Volume Depletion and Renal Effects, under Cautions.) The acute effect on eGFR reverses after dapagliflozin discontinuation, suggesting that acute hemodynamic changes may play a role in the renal function changes observed with dapagliflozin.

Use of Fixed Combinations

When dapagliflozin is used in fixed combination with metformin hydrochloride, saxagliptin, or other drugs, the cautions, precautions, contraindications, and interactions associated with the concomitant agent(s) must be considered in addition to those associated with dapagliflozin.

Sensitivity Reactions

Hypersensitivity reactions (e.g., angioedema, urticaria, hypersensitivity), some serious, have been reported with dapagliflozin treatment. If a hypersensitivity reaction occurs, the drug should be discontinued, appropriate treatment instituted, and the patient monitored until signs and symptoms resolve.

Specific Populations

Pregnancy

Data are lacking on the use of dapagliflozin in pregnant women. Based on the results of reproductive and developmental toxicity studies in animals, dapagliflozin use during pregnancy may affect renal development and maturation, especially during the second and third trimesters of pregnancy. Poorly controlled diabetes mellitus and untreated heart failure also are associated with risks to the mother and fetus. The manufacturer states that dapagliflozin therapy is not recommended in pregnant women during the second and third trimesters of pregnancy.

Lactation

Dapagliflozin is distributed into milk in rats; it is not known whether the drug is distributed into human milk. Since human kidney maturation occurs in utero and during the first 2 years of life when lactational exposure may occur, there may be risk to the developing human kidney. Use of dapagliflozin in women who are breast-feeding is not recommended.

Pediatric Use

Safety and efficacy of dapagliflozin have not been established in pediatric patients younger than 18 years of age.

Geriatric Use

Among patients with type 2 diabetes mellitus in 21 clinical trials, 1424 (24%) were 65 years of age or older and 207 (3.5%) were 75 years of age or older. Efficacy of dapagliflozin was similar for patients younger than 65 years of age and those 65 years of age or older after controlling for renal function (eGFR). Geriatric patients receiving dapagliflozin for glycemic control were more likely to experience hypotension compared with patients treated with placebo. In the DAPA-HF study, 57% of patients were older than 65 years of age; safety and efficacy in these patients were similar to those in patients younger than 65 years of age.

Hepatic Impairment

The benefits versus risks of using dapagliflozin or the fixed combination of dapagliflozin and saxagliptin in patients with severe hepatic impairment should be individually assessed since the safety and efficacy of these preparations have not been established in this population.

Compared with values in healthy individuals, values for peak plasma dapagliflozin concentration were increased by 40% in patients with severe hepatic impairment (Child-Pugh class C) following a single 10-mg dose of the drug. The area under the concentration-time curve (AUC) of dapagliflozin was increased by 67% in patients with severe hepatic impairment compared with that in healthy individuals. Differences in peak plasma concentration and AUC of the drug in patients with mild or moderate hepatic impairment were not considered clinically important.

Use of the fixed-combination preparations containing dapagliflozin and extended-release metformin or dapagliflozin, saxagliptin, and extended-release metformin should be avoided in patients with clinical or laboratory evidence of hepatic impairment.

Renal Impairment

Safety and efficacy of dapagliflozin were evaluated in 2 randomized, placebo-controlled studies that included patients with type 2 diabetes mellitus and moderate renal impairment (eGFR of 45 to less than 60 mL/minute per 1.73 m^2 or eGFR of 30 to less than 60 mL/minute per 1.73 m^2). Patients with an eGFR of 45 to less than 60 mL/minute per 1.73 m^2 experienced adverse effects similar to those observed in patients without renal impairment. Additionally, these patients also experienced a substantial reduction in glycosylated hemoglobin (hemoglobin A_{1c}; HbA_{1c}) compared with placebo. Patients in this study who received dapagliflozin

therapy had a greater reduction in eGFR compared with those who received placebo; however, renal function generally increased back to baseline values after discontinuing treatment with dapagliflozin. Patients with renal impairment receiving dapagliflozin may be more likely to experience hypotension and may be at an increased risk for acute kidney injury.

In patients with type 2 diabetes mellitus with mild, moderate, or severe renal impairment, geometric mean systemic exposures of dapagliflozin at steady state (20 mg once daily for 7 days) were 45%, 2.04-fold, or 3.03-fold higher, respectively, compared with patients with type 2 diabetes mellitus and normal renal function. Higher systemic exposure of dapagliflozin did not result in a correspondingly higher 24-hour urinary glucose excretion.

The impact of hemodialysis on dapagliflozin exposure is not known. (See Cautions: Contraindications.)

Renal function should be assessed prior to initiation of therapy and then as clinically indicated. The manufacturer states that dapagliflozin therapy is not recommended for glycemic control in patients without established cardiovascular disease or cardiovascular risk factors who have an eGFR of less than 45 mL/minute per 1.73 m^2; the drug is contraindicated in patients with severe renal impairment (eGFR less than 30 mL/minute per 1.73 m^2).

The fixed combination of dapagliflozin and metformin hydrochloride is not recommended in patients with an eGFR of less than 45 mL/minute per 1.73 m^2 and is contraindicated in patients with severe renal impairment (eGFR of less than 30 mL/minute per 1.73 m^2). The fixed combination of dapagliflozin and saxagliptin is contraindicated in patients with moderate to severe renal impairment (eGFR of less than 45 mL/minute per 1.73 m^2).

● Common Adverse Effects

Adverse effects reported in at least 2% of patients receiving dapagliflozin in clinical trials and more commonly than with placebo include female genital mycotic infection, nasopharyngitis, urinary tract infection, back pain, increased urination, male genital mycotic infection, nausea, dyslipidemia, constipation, discomfort with urination, and pain in extremity.

Adverse effects reported in at least 2% of patients receiving dapagliflozin in combination with metformin hydrochloride and more commonly than with placebo in combination with metformin hydrochloride include female genital mycotic infection, nasopharyngitis, urinary tract infection, diarrhea, headache, male genital mycotic infection, influenza, nausea, back pain, dizziness, cough, constipation, dyslipidemia, pharyngitis, increased urination, and discomfort with urination.

Adverse effects reported in at least 2% of patients receiving dapagliflozin in combination with saxagliptin and metformin hydrochloride include upper respiratory tract infection, urinary tract infection, dyslipidemia, headache, diarrhea, back pain, genital infection, and arthralgia.

DRUG INTERACTIONS

The metabolism of dapagliflozin is primarily mediated by uridine diphosphate-glucuronosyltransferase (UGT) isoenzyme 1A9.

● Drugs Affecting or Metabolized by Hepatic Microsomal Enzymes

Dapagliflozin and dapagliflozin 3-O-glucuronide, an inactive metabolite of dapagliflozin, did not inhibit cytochrome P-450 (CYP) isoenzymes 1A2, 2A6, 2B6, 2C8, 2C9, 2C19, 2D6 or 3A4 in in vitro studies. Dapagliflozin also does not induce CYP isoenzymes 1A2, 2B6, or 3A4 in vitro.

● Drugs Affected by Organic Anion Transporter

Dapagliflozin 3-O-glucuronide is a substrate of organic anion transport (OAT) 3. Dapagliflozin and dapagliflozin 3-O-glucuronide did not meaningfully inhibit OAT1 or OAT3 active transporters; pharmacokinetic interactions are unlikely with substrates of OAT1 or OAT3.

● Drugs Affected by Organic Cation Transporter

Dapagliflozin and dapagliflozin 3-O-glucuronide did not meaningfully inhibit organic cation transporter (OCT) 2; pharmacokinetic interactions are unlikely with substrates of OCT2.

● Drugs Affected by P-glycoprotein Transport

Dapagliflozin is a weak P-glycoprotein substrate, but does not meaningfully inhibit P-glycoprotein. The manufacturer states that dapagliflozin is unlikely to affect the pharmacokinetics of concurrently administered P-glycoprotein substrates.

● Antidiabetic Agents

When dapagliflozin is added to therapy with an insulin secretagogue (e.g., a sulfonylurea) or insulin, the incidence of hypoglycemia is increased compared with sulfonylurea or insulin monotherapy. Patients receiving dapagliflozin may require a reduced dosage of the concomitant insulin secretagogue or insulin to reduce the risk of hypoglycemia.

● Diuretics

Concomitant use of dapagliflozin with loop diuretics may increase the incidence of symptomatic hypotension. Prior to initiation of dapagliflozin, volume status should be assessed and corrected in patients receiving diuretics. Patients should be monitored for signs and symptoms of symptomatic hypotension following initiation of dapagliflozin therapy.

● Bumetanide

Administration of a single dose of bumetanide (1 mg) to individuals receiving dapagliflozin (10 mg once daily for 7 days) increased bumetanide area under the concentration-time curve (AUC) and peak plasma concentrations by 13%. The manufacturer states that no adjustment of dapagliflozin or bumetanide dosage is necessary. (See also Drug Interactions: Diuretics.)

● Digoxin

Administration of a single dose of digoxin (0.25 mg) with dapagliflozin (20 mg loading dose, then 10 mg once daily for 7 days) did not have a clinically meaningful effect on the AUC or peak plasma concentration of digoxin. The manufacturer states that no adjustment of digoxin dosage is necessary.

● Glimepiride

Administration of a single dose of glimepiride (4 mg) with a single dose of dapagliflozin (20 mg) increased glimepiride AUC by 13%; no dosage adjustment for either drug is necessary.

● Hydrochlorothiazide

Administration of a single dose of hydrochlorothiazide (25 mg) with a single dose of dapagliflozin (50 mg) did not have a clinically important effect on the pharmacokinetics of hydrochlorothiazide or dapagliflozin. The manufacturer states that no adjustment of dapagliflozin or hydrochlorothiazide dosage is necessary. (See also Drug Interactions: Diuretics.)

● Mefenamic Acid

Concurrent use of mefenamic acid (loading dose of 500 mg, then 250 mg every 6 hours for 14 doses) and a single dose of dapagliflozin (10 mg) increased dapagliflozin peak plasma concentration and AUC by 13 and 51%, respectively. No adjustment of dapagliflozin dosage is necessary.

● Metformin

Administration of a single dose of metformin (1 g) with a single dose of dapagliflozin (20 mg) did not have a clinically meaningful effect on the pharmacokinetics of dapagliflozin or metformin. No dosage adjustment for either drug is necessary.

● Pioglitazone

Administration of a single dose of pioglitazone (45 mg) with a single dose of dapagliflozin (50 mg) decreased pioglitazone peak plasma concentration by 7%. No dosage adjustment for either drug is necessary.

● Rifampin

Administration of rifampin (600 mg once daily for 6 days) with a single dose of dapagliflozin (10 mg) decreased dapagliflozin peak plasma concentration and AUC by 7 and 22%, respectively. No adjustment of dapagliflozin dosage is necessary.

● Simvastatin

Administration of a single dose of simvastatin (40 mg) with a single dose of dapagliflozin (20 mg) increased simvastatin AUC by 19%. The manufacturer states that no adjustment of dapagliflozin or simvastatin dosage is necessary.

● Sitagliptin

Administration of a single dose of sitagliptin (100 mg) with a single dose of dapagliflozin (20 mg) did not have a clinically meaningful effect on the pharmacokinetics of dapagliflozin or sitagliptin. No dosage adjustment for either drug is necessary.

● Valsartan

Administration of a single dose of valsartan (320 mg) with a single dose of dapagliflozin (20 mg) decreased peak plasma concentrations of valsartan and dapagliflozin by 6 and 12%, respectively, and increased valsartan AUC by 5%. The manufacturer states that no adjustment of dapagliflozin or valsartan dosage is necessary.

● Voglibose

Concomitant administration of voglibose (0.2 mg three times daily; not commercially available in the US) with a single dose of dapagliflozin (10 mg) did not have a clinically meaningful effect on the pharmacokinetics of dapagliflozin.

● Warfarin

Administration of a single dose of warfarin (25 mg) in individuals receiving dapagliflozin (20 mg loading dose, then 10 mg once daily for 7 days) did not have a clinically meaningful effect on the pharmacokinetics or pharmacodynamics of warfarin. No warfarin dosage adjustment is necessary.

DESCRIPTION

Dapagliflozin propanediol is a potent, competitive, reversible and highly selective inhibitor of sodium-glucose cotransporter 2 (SGLT2), a transporter that is expressed in the proximal renal tubules and is responsible for most of the reabsorption of filtered glucose from the tubular lumen. Through inhibition of SGLT2, dapagliflozin reduces reabsorption of filtered glucose and lowers the renal threshold for glucose in a dose-dependent manner, leading to increased urinary glucose excretion; increased glucose excretion is independent of insulin secretion. After discontinuation of a 10-mg dose of dapagliflozin, the elevation in urinary glucose excretion approaches baseline in an average of about 3 days for the 10-mg dose. Reduction of plasma glucose with dapagliflozin to induce glucosuria improves sensitivity of muscle to insulin; however, glucosuria induction appears to be associated with a paradoxical increase in endogenous glucose production. Following dapagliflozin treatment, endogenous glucose production increased, accompanied by an increase in fasting plasma glucagon concentration.

Following oral administration of dapagliflozin in the fasting state, peak plasma concentration is usually attained within 2 hours. Following administration of a 10-mg dose, the absolute oral bioavailability of the drug is 78%. Administration of dapagliflozin with a high-fat meal decreased peak plasma concentration by up to 50% and prolonged time to peak plasma concentration by approximately 1 hour, but did not alter the area under the concentration-time curve (AUC). These changes are not considered clinically meaningful and dapagliflozin can be administered with or without food. Dapagliflozin is approximately 91% protein bound. Following administration of a single 50-mg radiolabeled dose of dapagliflozin, 75% and 21% total radioactivity is excreted in urine and feces, respectively, with less than 2% in urine as parent drug and approximately 15% in feces as parent drug. The mean terminal elimination half-life of dapagliflozin was approximately 12.9 hours following a single oral 10-mg dose.

Bioequivalence between the fixed combination of dapagliflozin and extended-release metformin hydrochloride (Xigduo® XR) and each agent (dapagliflozin and extended-release metformin hydrochloride) given concurrently as separate tablets has been demonstrated; however, the relative bioavailability of the fixed combination of dapagliflozin and extended-release metformin hydrochloride (Xigduo® XR) and concomitantly administered dapagliflozin and immediate-release metformin hydrochloride has not been established. Metformin hydrochloride immediate-release and extended-release tablets have a similar extent of absorption (AUC), but peak plasma concentrations of metformin following administration of the drug as extended-release tablets are approximately 20% lower than peak concentrations following administration of the same dose as immediate-release tablets. The overall pharmacokinetics of dapagliflozin, saxagliptin, and metformin were not affected in a clinically relevant manner when administered in fixed combination (as Qternmet® XR).

ADVICE TO PATIENTS

Importance of patient reading medication guide before initiating therapy and each time the drug is dispensed.

When dapagliflozin is used in fixed combination with other drugs, importance of informing patients of important cautionary information about the concomitant agent(s).

Importance of informing patients of the potential risks and benefits of dapagliflozin and of alternative therapies. Importance of *not* using dapagliflozin in patients with type 1 diabetes mellitus or diabetic ketoacidosis.

Importance of informing patients that ketoacidosis, which can be a life-threatening condition, has been reported with dapagliflozin therapy in patients with diabetes mellitus (sometimes associated with illness or surgery among other risk factors). Importance of informing patients receiving dapagliflozin and their caregivers of the signs and symptoms of ketoacidosis (e.g., tachypnea or hyperventilation, anorexia, abdominal pain, nausea, vomiting, lethargy, mental status changes) and of instructing patients to discontinue dapagliflozin and seek medical advice immediately should they experience any such signs or symptoms. Advise patients to use a ketone dipstick to check for ketones in their urine (when possible) if symptoms of ketoacidosis occur, even if blood glucose is not elevated (e.g., less than 250 mg/dL).

Importance of informing patients that symptomatic hypotension may occur with dapagliflozin and advising patients to report such symptoms to their clinician. Inform patients that dapagliflozin-induced dehydration may increase the risk of hypotension and changes in kidney function and that they should maintain adequate fluid intake.

Importance of informing patients that acute kidney injury has been reported with dapagliflozin therapy. Advise patients to seek medical attention immediately if they experience decreased urine output, or swelling of the legs or feet. Advise patients to seek medical advice immediately if they have reduced oral intake (such as due to acute illness or fasting) or increased fluid losses (such as due to vomiting, diarrhea, or excessive heat exposure), as it may be appropriate to temporarily discontinue dapagliflozin in those settings.

Importance of informing patients that necrotizing infections of the perineum (Fournier gangrene) have occurred with sodium-glucose cotransporter 2 (SGLT2) inhibitor therapy in patients with diabetes mellitus. Advise patients to promptly seek medical attention if they develop pain or tenderness, redness, or swelling of the genitals or the area from the genitals back to the rectum, in addition to fever (above 38°C) or malaise.

Importance of informing patients that yeast infection may occur (e.g., vulvovaginitis, balanitis, balanoposthitis). Importance of informing female patients of the signs and symptoms of vaginal yeast infections (e.g., vaginal discharge, odor, itching) and male patients of the signs and symptoms of balanitis or balanoposthitis (e.g., rash or redness of the glans or foreskin of the penis). Advise patients of treatment options and when to seek medical advice.

Importance of informing patients of the potential for urinary tract infections, which may be serious, with dapagliflozin therapy. Advise patients of the signs and symptoms of urinary tract infection and the need to contact a clinician if such signs and symptoms occur.

Importance of informing patients that due to the mechanism of action of dapagliflozin, patients taking the drug will test positive for glucose in their urine. Importance of not using urine glucose tests to monitor glycemic status while taking dapagliflozin. (See Laboratory Test Interferences under Cautions: Warnings/Precautions.)

Risk of serious hypersensitivity reactions, such as urticaria and angioedema. If signs or symptoms of such a reaction or angioedema occur, importance of discontinuing dapagliflozin and promptly informing clinician.

Importance of informing patients about the importance of adherence to dietary instructions, regular physical activity, periodic blood glucose monitoring

and glycosylated hemoglobin (hemoglobin A_{1c}; HbA_{1c}) testing, recognition and management of hypoglycemia and hyperglycemia, and assessment of diabetes complications.

Importance of promptly seeking medical advice during periods of stress such as fever, trauma, infection, or surgery as medication requirements may change.

Importance of taking dapagliflozin exactly as directed by clinician. (See Dosage and Administration: Administration.)

Importance of women informing their clinicians immediately if they are or plan to become pregnant or plan to breast-feed.

Importance of informing clinicians of existing or contemplated concomitant therapy, including prescription and OTC drugs and dietary or herbal supplements, as well as any concomitant illnesses (e.g., severe kidney disease).

Importance of informing patients of other important precautionary information. (See Cautions.)

PREPARATIONS

Excipients in commercially available drug preparations may have clinically important effects in some individuals; consult specific product labeling for details.

Dapagliflozin Propanediol

Oral			
Tablets, film-coated	5 mg (of dapagliflozin)		Farxiga®, AstraZeneca
	10 mg (of dapagliflozin)		Farxiga®, AstraZeneca

Dapagliflozin Propanediol Combinations

Oral		
Tablets, extended-release	2.5 mg (of dapagliflozin) with Extended-release Metformin Hydrochloride 1 g	Xigduo® XR, AstraZeneca
	2.5 mg (of dapagliflozin) with Extended-release Metformin Hydrochloride 1 g and Saxagliptin 2.5 mg	Qternmet® XR, AstraZeneca
	5 mg (of dapagliflozin) with Extended-release Metformin Hydrochloride 500 mg	Xigduo® XR, AstraZeneca
	5 mg (of dapagliflozin) with Extended-release Metformin Hydrochloride 1 g	Xigduo® XR, AstraZeneca
	5 mg (of dapagliflozin) with Extended-release Metformin Hydrochloride 1 g and Saxagliptin 2.5 mg	Qternmet® XR, AstraZeneca
	5 mg (of dapagliflozin) with Extended-release Metformin Hydrochloride 1 g and Saxagliptin 5 mg	Qternmet® XR, AstraZeneca
	10 mg (of dapagliflozin) with Extended-release Metformin Hydrochloride 500 mg	Xigduo® XR, AstraZeneca
	10 mg (of dapagliflozin) with Extended-release Metformin Hydrochloride 1 g	Xigduo® XR, AstraZeneca
	10 mg (of dapagliflozin) with Extended-release Metformin Hydrochloride 1 g and Saxagliptin 5 mg	Qternmet® XR, AstraZeneca
Tablets, film-coated	5 mg (of dapagliflozin) with Saxagliptin 5 mg	Qtern®, AstraZeneca
	10 mg (of dapagliflozin) with Saxagliptin 5 mg	Qtern®, AstraZeneca

† Use is not currently included in the labeling approved by the US Food and Drug Administration.

Selected Revisions June 21, 2021, © Copyright, December 11, 2014, American Society of Health-System Pharmacists, Inc.

Empagliflozin

68:20.18 • SODIUM-GLUCOSE COTRANSPORTER 2 (SGLT2) INHIBITORS

■ Empagliflozin, a sodium-glucose cotransporter 2 (SGLT2) inhibitor, is an antidiabetic agent.

USES

● Type 2 Diabetes Mellitus

Empagliflozin is used as monotherapy as an adjunct to diet and exercise to improve glycemic control in patients with type 2 diabetes mellitus. Empagliflozin also is used to reduce the risk of cardiovascular death in patients with type 2 diabetes mellitus and established cardiovascular disease. Empagliflozin is commercially available in fixed combination with immediate- or extended-release metformin hydrochloride (Synjardy® or Synjardy® XR, respectively) or linagliptin (Glyxambi®); the fixed-combination preparations are used as an adjunct to diet and exercise to improve glycemic control in patients with type 2 diabetes mellitus when treatment with both drugs is appropriate. The manufacturer states that the effectiveness of the fixed combination of empagliflozin and immediate- or extended-release metformin hydrochloride or linagliptin in reducing the risk of cardiovascular death in patients with type 2 diabetes mellitus and cardiovascular disease has not been established. Empagliflozin also is used in combination with other antidiabetic agents (e.g., metformin, a sulfonylurea, a peroxisome proliferator-activated receptor$_\gamma$ [PPAR$_\gamma$] agonist [thiazolidinedione], a dipeptidylpeptidase-4 [DPP-4] inhibitor) or insulin as an adjunct to diet and exercise in patients with type 2 diabetes mellitus who have not achieved adequate glycemic control.

Glycemic Control

Current guidelines for the treatment of type 2 diabetes mellitus generally recommend metformin as first-line therapy in addition to lifestyle modifications in patients with recent-onset type 2 diabetes mellitus or mild hyperglycemia because of its well-established safety and efficacy (i.e., beneficial effects on glycosylated hemoglobin [hemoglobin A$_{1c}$; HbA$_{1c}$], weight, and cardiovascular mortality). (See Uses: Type 2 Diabetes Mellitus, in Metformin 68:20.04.) In patients with contraindications or intolerance to metformin (e.g., risk of lactic acidosis, GI intolerance) or in selected other patients, some experts suggest that initial therapy with a drug from another class of antidiabetic agents (e.g., a glucagon-like peptide-1 (GLP-1) receptor agonist, SGLT2 inhibitor, dipeptidyl peptidase-4 (DPP-4) inhibitor, sulfonylurea, thiazolidinedione, basal insulin) may be acceptable based on patient factors. Initiating antidiabetic therapy with 2 agents (e.g., metformin plus another agent) may be appropriate in patients with an initial HbA$_{1c}$ exceeding 7.5% or at least 1.5% above the target level. In metformin-intolerant patients with high initial HbA$_{1c}$ levels, some experts suggest initiation of therapy with 2 agents from other antidiabetic classes with complementary mechanisms of action.

Because of the progressive nature of type 2 diabetes mellitus, patients initially receiving an oral antidiabetic agent will eventually require multiple oral and/or injectable noninsulin antidiabetic agents of different therapeutic classes and/or insulin for adequate glycemic control. Patients who have inadequate glycemic control with initial (e.g., metformin) monotherapy should receive treatment with additional antidiabetic agents; data suggest that the addition of each noninsulin agent to initial therapy lowers HbA$_{1c}$ by approximately 0.7–1%. In addition, early initiation of combination therapy may help to more rapidly attain glycemic goals and extend the time to treatment failure.

Factors to consider when selecting additional antidiabetic agents for combination therapy in patients with inadequate glycemic control on metformin monotherapy include patient comorbidities (e.g., atherosclerotic cardiovascular disease [ASCVD], established kidney disease, heart failure), hypoglycemia risk, impact on weight, cost, risk of adverse effects, and patient preference. When the greater glucose-lowering effect of an injectable drug is needed in patients with type 2 diabetes mellitus, some experts currently state that an injectable GLP-1 receptor agonist is preferred over insulin in most patients because of beneficial effects on body weight and a lower risk of hypoglycemia, although adverse GI effects may diminish tolerability. While addition of a GLP-1 receptor agonist may successfully control hyperglycemia, many patients will eventually require insulin therapy.

Early introduction of insulin therapy should be considered when hyperglycemia is severe (e.g., blood glucose of at least 300 mg/dL or HbA$_{1c}$ exceeding 9–10%), especially in the presence of catabolic manifestations (e.g., weight loss, hypertriglyceridemia, ketosis) or symptoms of hyperglycemia. For additional information regarding the initiation of insulin therapy in patients with diabetes mellitus, see Uses: Diabetes Mellitus, in the Insulins General Statement 68:20.08.

Patients with type 2 diabetes mellitus who have established (or are at a high risk for) ASCVD, established kidney disease, or heart failure should receive a GLP-1 receptor agonist or SGLT2 inhibitor with demonstrated cardiovascular disease benefit. (See Reduction in Risk of Major Adverse Cardiovascular Events under Uses: Type 2 Diabetes Mellitus, in Liraglutide 68:20.06 and also see Reduction in Risk of Heart Failure-Related Hospitalization under Uses: Type 2 Diabetes Mellitus, in Dapagliflozin 68:20.18.) Experts state that therapy with a GLP-1 receptor agonist or SGLT2 inhibitor should be considered for patients with the aforementioned comorbidities independently of the patients' HbA$_{1c}$. GLP-1 receptor agonists and SGLT2 inhibitors appear to have effects on the kidneys independent of their glycemic effects, and some experts suggest that an agent from one of these classes of drugs be considered in patients with type 2 diabetes mellitus and chronic kidney disease (CKD). (See Beneficial Effects on Renal Function and Cardiovascular Morbidity and Mortality in Diabetic Nephropathy under Uses: Type 2 Diabetes Mellitus, in Canagliflozin 68:20.18.) In patients *without* established ASCVD or indicators of high ASCVD risk, heart failure, or CKD, the decision regarding the addition of other antidiabetic agents (e.g., GLP-1 receptor agonist, SGLT2 inhibitor, DPP-4 inhibitor, thiazolidinedione, sulfonylurea, basal insulin) to metformin therapy should be based on avoidance of adverse effects, cost, and individual patient factors.

The manufacturer states that empagliflozin is *not* indicated for the treatment of type 1 diabetes mellitus or diabetic ketoacidosis.

Empagliflozin Monotherapy

When given as monotherapy for the management of type 2 diabetes mellitus, empagliflozin improves glycemic control compared with placebo as evidenced by reductions in glycosylated hemoglobin (hemoglobin A$_{1c}$ [HbA$_{1c}$]) and fasting plasma glucose concentrations, and also reduces body weight. Efficacy of empagliflozin as monotherapy for the management of type 2 diabetes mellitus has been established in a phase 3, double-blind, placebo-controlled study of 24 weeks' duration in 986 adults with previously untreated type 2 diabetes mellitus (defined as receiving no oral or injected antidiabetic agents for 12 weeks prior to randomization or initiation of open-label treatment). Empagliflozin (10 mg or 25 mg once daily) improved glycemic control as evidenced by reductions in HbA$_{1c}$, fasting plasma glucose concentrations, and body weight. Patients with HbA$_{1c}$ concentrations exceeding 10% were assigned open-label treatment with empagliflozin 25 mg once daily with no placebo run-in phase. Patients with HbA$_{1c}$ concentrations of 7–10% entered a placebo run-in period for 2 weeks, and those who remained inadequately controlled received empagliflozin 10 mg once daily, empagliflozin 25 mg once daily, sitagliptin 100 mg once daily, or placebo. The primary end point of the study was change from baseline in HbA$_{1c}$ at week 24. At 24 weeks, reductions (adjusted mean) in HbA$_{1c}$ were 0.7, 0.8, or 0.7% in patients who received empagliflozin 10 mg, empagliflozin 25 mg, or sitagliptin 100 mg once daily, respectively; an increase (adjusted mean) in HbA$_{1c}$ of 0.1% was observed in patients who received placebo. Also, at 24 weeks, the reduction (adjusted mean) in fasting plasma glucose concentrations was 19 or 25 mg/dL in patients who received empagliflozin 10 or 25 mg once daily, respectively, compared with an increase of 12 mg/dL in those receiving placebo. Patients who received empagliflozin 10 mg, empagliflozin 25 mg, or placebo once daily had reductions (adjusted mean) in body weight of 2.8, 3.2, or 0.4%, respectively, at week 24; systolic blood pressure was reduced by 2.6 mm Hg in patients who received empagliflozin 10 mg once daily and by 3.4 mm Hg in those who received empagliflozin 25 mg once daily compared with that in placebo recipients.

Combination Therapy

When given in combination with one or more oral antidiabetic agents (e.g., metformin, a sulfonylurea, a thiazolidinedione, a DPP-4 inhibitor) or insulin, empagliflozin improves glycemic control compared with monotherapy with these drugs and generally is associated with reductions in body weight and systolic blood pressure. In a 24-week phase 3, randomized, double-blind, placebo-controlled study in 637 adults with inadequately controlled type 2 diabetes mellitus who were receiving metformin hydrochloride (at least 1.5 g daily, or maximum tolerated dosage, or maximum labeled dosage), addition of empagliflozin 10 or 25 mg once daily resulted in reductions of HbA$_{1c}$ compared with placebo. Patients with HbA$_{1c}$ concentrations exceeding 10% were assigned open-label treatment with empagliflozin 25 mg once daily without a placebo run-in phase. Patients with HbA$_{1c}$ concentrations of 7–10%

entered a placebo run-in period for 2 weeks, and those who remained inadequately controlled following the run-in phase received empagliflozin 10 mg, empagliflozin 25 mg, or placebo once daily for 24 weeks. The primary end point of the study was change from baseline in HbA$_{1c}$ at week 24. Following 24 weeks of therapy, the addition of empagliflozin to current metformin treatment resulted in reductions (adjusted mean) in HbA$_{1c}$ of 0.7, 0.8, and 0.1% in patients who received empagliflozin 10 mg once daily, empagliflozin 25 mg once daily, and placebo, respectively. In addition, at 24 weeks, the reduction (adjusted mean) in fasting plasma glucose concentration was 20 or 22 mg/dL in patients who received empagliflozin 10 or 25 mg once daily, respectively, compared with an increase of 6 mg/dL in those receiving placebo. Patients who received empagliflozin 10 mg, empagliflozin 25 mg, or placebo experienced reductions (adjusted mean) in body weight of 2.5, 2.9, or 0.5%, respectively, at week 24; systolic blood pressure was reduced compared with placebo by 4.1 mm Hg in patients who received empagliflozin 10 mg and by 4.8 mm Hg in those who received empagliflozin 25 mg.

Efficacy and safety of the combination of empagliflozin and metformin hydrochloride as initial therapy in treatment-naive patients with type 2 diabetes mellitus are supported by results of a 24-week, randomized, double-blind trial. In this trial, concurrent therapy with empagliflozin (10 or 25 mg once daily) and metformin hydrochloride (1 or 2 g daily) substantially improved glycemic control (as evidenced by reductions in HbA$_{1c}$), compared with empagliflozin or metformin hydrochloride monotherapy. Reductions in HbA$_{1c}$ were 2 or 2.1% with 1 or 2 g daily, respectively, of metformin hydrochloride plus empagliflozin 10 mg once daily; 1.9 or 2.1% with 1 or 2 g daily, respectively, of metformin hydrochloride plus empagliflozin 25 mg once daily; 1.2 or 1.8% with 1 or 2 g daily, respectively, of metformin hydrochloride; and 1.4% with empagliflozin 10 or 25 mg once daily.

Efficacy of empagliflozin 10 or 25 mg once daily in combination with metformin hydrochloride (dosage of at least 1.5 g daily, or maximum tolerated dosage, or maximum labeled dosage) plus a sulfonylurea was established in 666 adults with type 2 diabetes mellitus in an international 24-week, phase 3, randomized, double-blind, placebo-controlled study. Patients with HbA$_{1c}$ concentrations exceeding 10% were assigned open-label treatment with empagliflozin 25 mg. Patients with HbA$_{1c}$ concentrations of 7–10% entered a placebo run-in period for 2 weeks, and those who remained inadequately controlled received empagliflozin 10 mg, empagliflozin 25 mg, or placebo once daily. The primary end point of the study was change from baseline in HbA$_{1c}$ at week 24. Following 24 weeks of therapy, add-on therapy with empagliflozin reduced HbA$_{1c}$ by 0.8, 0.8, or 0.2% (adjusted mean values) in patients who received empagliflozin 10 mg, empagliflozin 25 mg, or placebo once daily, respectively. Also, at 24 weeks, the reduction (adjusted mean) in fasting plasma glucose concentrations was 23 mg/dL in patients who received empagliflozin 10 or 25 mg once daily, compared with an increase of 6 mg/dL in those receiving placebo. Patients who received empagliflozin 10 mg, empagliflozin 25 mg, or placebo once daily had reductions (adjusted mean) in body weight of 2.9, 3.2, or 0.5%, respectively, at week 24.

Efficacy of empagliflozin 25 mg in combination with metformin hydrochloride (dosage of at least 1.5 g daily, or maximum tolerated dosage, or maximum labeled dosage) in an international phase 3, randomized, double-blind study was established in 1545 adults with type 2 diabetes mellitus. Patients with inadequately controlled type 2 diabetes mellitus (HbA$_{1c}$ concentration of 7–10%) received empagliflozin 25 mg once daily or glimepiride 1–4 mg once daily (mean daily dosage of 2.7 mg) following a 2-week run-in period. The primary end point was change from baseline in HbA$_{1c}$ concentrations at weeks 52 and 104. At week 52, add-on therapy with empagliflozin 25 mg or glimepiride 1–4 mg in patients receiving metformin resulted in a reduction in HbA$_{1c}$ concentration of 0.7% for both drugs. At week 52, add-on therapy with empagliflozin 25 mg or glimepiride 1–4 mg reduced fasting plasma glucose concentrations by 19 or 9 mg/dL, respectively. Body weight was reduced by 3.9 or increased by 2% in those who received empagliflozin 25 mg or glimepiride 1–4 mg, respectively, plus metformin at week 52. At week 52, the reduction in systolic blood pressure in patients who received empagliflozin (3.6 mm Hg) was not appreciably different from that in patients who received glimepiride (2.2 mm Hg). Empagliflozin demonstrated noninferiority to glimepiride in glycemic control at weeks 52 and 104; the reduction (adjusted mean) in HbA$_{1c}$ with empagliflozin was 0.11% greater than that with glimepiride at week 104.

In a 24-week, double-blind, placebo-controlled study in 498 adults with type 2 diabetes mellitus receiving pioglitazone (dosage of at least 30 mg daily, or maximum tolerated dosage, or maximum labeled dosage) with or without metformin hydrochloride (dosage of at least 1.5 g daily, or maximum tolerated dosage, or maximum labeled dosage), addition of empagliflozin 10 or 25 mg once daily reduced HbA$_{1c}$, fasting plasma glucose concentrations, and body weight. Following an open-label placebo run-in period of 2 weeks, patients with inadequate

glycemic control (HbA$_{1c}$ concentrations of 7–10%) received empagliflozin 10 mg, empagliflozin 25 mg, or placebo once daily, in addition to existing antidiabetic therapy with pioglitazone with or without metformin. The primary end point was change from baseline in HbA$_{1c}$ concentrations at week 24. Addition of empagliflozin 10 or 25 mg to existing antidiabetic therapy resulted in reductions (adjusted mean) in HbA$_{1c}$ of 0.6 or 0.7%, respectively, at week 24 compared with a reduction of 0.1% in patients receiving placebo. Patients receiving empagliflozin 10 or 25 mg had reductions (adjusted mean) in fasting plasma glucose concentrations of 17 or 22 mg/dL, respectively, at week 24 compared with an increase of 7 mg/dL with placebo. Reductions in body weight were 2.0, 1.8, or 0.6% in patients who received empagliflozin 10 mg, empagliflozin 25 mg, or placebo once daily, respectively.

In an international, phase 3, randomized, double-blind trial, add-on therapy with empagliflozin and linagliptin in fixed combination was more effective in reducing HbA$_{1c}$ and fasting plasma glucose concentrations than add-on empagliflozin or linagliptin monotherapy in 686 adults with type 2 diabetes mellitus inadequately controlled with metformin hydrochloride (dosage of at least 1.5 g daily, or maximum tolerated dosage, or maximum labeled dosage). At 24 weeks, reduction in mean HbA$_{1c}$ from baseline was 1.19% with empagliflozin 25 mg/linagliptin 5 mg, 1.08% with empagliflozin 10 mg/linagliptin 5 mg, 0.62% with empagliflozin 25 mg, 0.66% with empagliflozin 10 mg, and 0.7% with linagliptin 5 mg. Glycemic efficacy (HbA$_{1c}$ reductions) with the fixed combinations of empagliflozin/linagliptin was maintained at week 52. The fixed combinations of empagliflozin and linagliptin also were associated with reductions from baseline in systolic blood pressure compared with linagliptin monotherapy. Body weight was reduced in patients receiving the fixed combinations of empagliflozin/linagliptin compared with linagliptin but not empagliflozin monotherapy.

In a double-blind, placebo-controlled study in 494 adults with inadequately controlled type 2 diabetes mellitus while receiving insulin with or without metformin and/or a sulfonylurea, add-on therapy with empagliflozin 10 or 25 mg once daily reduced HbA$_{1c}$, fasting plasma glucose concentrations, and body weight after 18 and 78 weeks of treatment. Following a 2-week placebo run-in period on basal insulin (e.g., insulin glargine, insulin detemir, or NPH insulin) with or without metformin and/or sulfonylurea therapy, patients received empagliflozin 10 or 25 mg or placebo once daily in addition to existing antidiabetic therapy. Patients were maintained on a stable dose of insulin prior to enrollment, during the run-in period, and during the first 18 weeks of treatment; for the remaining 60 weeks, adjustment of insulin dosage was permitted. Mean total daily insulin dosages at baseline for patients receiving empagliflozin 10 mg, empagliflozin 25 mg, or placebo were 45, 48, or 48 units, respectively. At 18 weeks, add-on therapy with empagliflozin 10 or 25 mg reduced HbA$_{1c}$ concentration by 0.6 or 0.7% (adjusted mean values), respectively, compared with no change in HbA$_{1c}$ concentration in patients who received placebo. Also, at 78 weeks, addition of empagliflozin 10 or 25 mg reduced HbA$_{1c}$ concentration by 0.4 or 0.6% (adjusted mean values), respectively, compared with an increase of 0.1% in patients who received placebo. Following 18 weeks of treatment, the reduction in fasting plasma glucose concentrations in patients who received empagliflozin 10 or 25 mg plus existing antidiabetic therapy was 17.9 or 19.1 mg/dL, compared with an increase of 10.4 mg/dL in those who received placebo; at 78 weeks, the reduction in fasting plasma glucose concentrations in patients who received empagliflozin 10 or 25 mg was 10.1 or 15.2 mg/dL, compared with an increase of 2.8 mg/dL in those receiving placebo. Furthermore, reductions in body weight at 18 weeks in patients who received empagliflozin 10 mg, empagliflozin 25 mg, or placebo were 1.8, 1.4, or 0.1%, respectively; at 78 weeks, patients who received empagliflozin 10 or 25 mg had reductions of 2.4% in body weight, while those receiving placebo had an increase of 0.7% in body weight.

In a randomized, double-blind, placebo-controlled, international study in 563 obese patients (body mass index [BMI] of 30–45 kg/m^2) with inadequately controlled type 2 diabetes mellitus (HbA$_{1c}$ concentrations 7.5–10%) despite multiple daily injections of insulin with or without metformin, add-on therapy with empagliflozin reduced HbA$_{1c}$ and body weight. Following a 2-week, open-label, placebo run-in period, patients received empagliflozin 10 or 25 mg or placebo once daily as add-on therapy to insulin, with or without metformin hydrochloride (dosage of at least 1.5 g daily, maximum tolerated dosage, or maximum labeled dosage), for 52 weeks. The total daily dosage of insulin was adjusted to achieve a preprandial glucose target of less than 100 mg/dL and a postprandial glucose target of less than 140 mg/dL, except during the first 18 weeks (adjusted to be within 10% of prescribed dosage at randomization) and during weeks 41–52 (adjusted to be within 10% of the prescribed dosage at week 40 except for safety reasons). Metformin hydrochloride dosage was not adjusted during the study, although rescue therapy (e.g., metformin, insulin) could be initiated at any time during treatment if patients experienced clinically important hyperglycemia. The primary end point of the study was change from baseline in HbA$_{1c}$ at week 18. At week 18, the reduction in HbA$_{1c}$ was 0.94 or 1.02% in patients who received empagliflozin 10 or 25 mg once daily, respectively, as add-on therapy, compared with a reduction of 0.5% in patients who received placebo. At week 52, insulin titration resulted in additional reductions in HbA$_{1c}$ of 1.18, 1.27, or 0.81% in those who received empagliflozin 10 mg, empagliflozin 25 mg, or placebo once daily, respectively. Also, at week 52, patients who received empagliflozin 10 or 25 mg once daily experienced reductions in body weight of 1.95 or 2.04 kg, respectively, compared with an increase in body weight of 0.44 kg in patients receiving placebo.

Efficacy and safety of empagliflozin in 738 adults with inadequately controlled type 2 diabetes mellitus (HbA$_{1c}$ concentrations of 7–10%) and renal impairment were established in a phase 3, randomized, double-blind, placebo-controlled study. Patients with an estimated glomerular filtration rate (eGFR) of 60–89 mL/minute per 1.73 m^2 (mild renal impairment) received empagliflozin 10 or 25 mg or placebo once daily in addition to existing antidiabetic therapy. Patients with an eGFR of 30–59 mL/minute per 1.73 m^2 (moderate renal impairment) or 15–29 mL/minute per 1.73 m^2 (severe renal impairment) received empagliflozin 25 mg once daily or placebo. The primary end point was change from baseline in HbA$_{1c}$ at week 24. At 24 weeks, empagliflozin 25 mg reduced HbA$_{1c}$ concentration by 0.5% in the combined group of patients with mild or moderate renal impairment. Empagliflozin 25 mg also reduced HbA$_{1c}$ concentration in patients with either mild (0.7% reduction) or moderate (0.4% reduction) renal impairment, and empagliflozin 10 mg reduced HbA$_{1c}$ concentration by 0.5% in patients with mild renal impairment. Antihyperglycemic efficacy of empagliflozin 25 mg was reduced with decreasing level of renal function in the mild to moderate range. Mean reductions in HbA$_{1c}$ at 24 weeks were 0.6, 0.5, and 0.2% for those with a baseline eGFR of 60–89 mL/minute per 1.73 m^2, 45–59 mL/minute per 1.73 m^2, and 30–44 mL/minute per 1.73 m^2, respectively, for patients receiving empagliflozin 25 mg. In contrast, mean HbA$_{1c}$ at 24 weeks increased by 0.1 or 0.2% in patients with a baseline eGFR of 60–89 mL/minute per 1.73 m^2 or 30–44 mL/minute per 1.73 m^2, respectively, and decreased by 0.1% in patients with a baseline eGFR of 45–59 mL/minute per 1.73 m^2 for patients receiving placebo. For patients with severe renal impairment, the analyses of changes in HbA$_{1c}$ and fasting plasma glucose concentrations showed no discernible treatment effect of empagliflozin 25 mg compared with placebo.

Reduction in Risk of Cardiovascular Death

Empagliflozin is used to reduce the risk of cardiovascular death in patients with type 2 diabetes mellitus and established cardiovascular disease.

Empagliflozin and some other SGLT2 inhibitors have demonstrated the ability to reduce the risk of cardiovascular events in patients with type 2 diabetes mellitus and established cardiovascular disease. In addition to lowering blood glucose, SGLT2 inhibitors appear to modify several nonglycemic cardiovascular risk factors such as blood pressure, body weight, adiposity, and arterial stiffness. In the EMPA-REG OUTCOME study, adults (mean age: 63 years; 72% Caucasian) with type 2 diabetes mellitus and established, stable ASCVD (documented history of coronary artery disease [76%], stroke [23%], or peripheral artery disease [21%]) received empagliflozin (10 or 25 mg) once daily or placebo for a median duration of 2.6 years. During the study, additional antidiabetic agents and cardiovascular therapies were modified to achieve standard-of-care treatment targets with respect to blood glucose, lipids, and blood pressure. Concomitant use of other standard-of-care treatments for diabetes mellitus and ASCVD (renin-angiotensin system inhibitors [81%], β-blockers [65%], diuretics [43%], statins or ezetimibe [77%], antiplatelet agents [86%]) was permitted. A greater proportion of patients in the placebo group received additional antidiabetic agents (e.g., sulfonylurea, insulin), antihypertensive agents (e.g., diuretics), and anticoagulants during the study than those in the empagliflozin group. The primary outcome was the composite of death from cardiovascular causes, nonfatal myocardial infarction, or nonfatal stroke. In this study, patients who received empagliflozin had substantially lower rates of the primary cardiovascular outcome compared with those who received placebo (event rate 10.5 versus 12.1%, respectively). The lower rate of the composite outcome was driven by the substantial reduction in death from cardiovascular causes; there was no substantial difference between groups with regard to myocardial infarction or stroke. Patients receiving empagliflozin had an increased rate of genital infections but not in other adverse events.

Beneficial Effects on Renal Function

SGLT2 inhibitors reduce renal tubular glucose reabsorption, weight, systemic blood pressure, intraglomerular pressure, and albuminuria and slow glomerular filtration rate (GFR) loss through mechanisms that appear to be independent of glucose-lowering effects. In several cardiovascular outcomes trials involving the use of SGLT2 inhibitors (e.g., canagliflozin, dapagliflozin, empagliflozin) in patients with type 2 diabetes mellitus at high risk for cardiovascular disease or with existing cardiovascular disease, beneficial effects on renal function have been observed as a secondary outcome. Some experts state that the use of an SGLT2 inhibitor should be considered to reduce the risk of CKD progression, cardiovascular events, or both in patients with type 2 diabetes mellitus and diabetic kidney disease with albuminuria† (an eGFR of at least 30 mL/minute per 1.73 m^2 and urinary albumin exceeding 30 mg/g creatinine, particularly in those with urinary albumin exceeding 300 mg/g creatinine.

A clinical study evaluating the use of canagliflozin in patients with type 2 diabetes mellitus, CKD (eGFR 30–89 mL/minute per 1.73 m^2; mean: 56.2 mL/minute per 1.73 m^2), and albuminuria (urine albumin:creatinine ratio exceeding 300 but less than 5000 mg/g) found that canagliflozin therapy reduced the risk of end-stage kidney disease, doubling of serum creatinine, cardiovascular death, and hospitalization for heart failure. In another study (EMPA-REG OUTCOME) (see Reduction in Risk of Cardiovascular Death under Uses: Type 2 Diabetes Mellitus), empagliflozin therapy was associated with slower progression of kidney disease and lower rates of renal events. Compared with placebo, empagliflozin reduced the risk of incident or worsening nephropathy (composite of urine:creatinine ratio exceeding 300 mg/g creatinine, doubling of serum creatinine, end-stage renal disease, or death from end-stage renal disease) by 39%.

DOSAGE AND ADMINISTRATION

● General

Volume depletion should be corrected before initiating empagliflozin. In addition, renal function should be assessed prior to treatment and periodically thereafter. (See Special Populations under Dosage and Administration: Dosage.)

● Administration

Empagliflozin or the fixed combination of empagliflozin and linagliptin is administered orally once daily in the morning, with or without food. The fixed combination of empagliflozin and immediate-release metformin hydrochloride should be administered twice daily with meals. The fixed combination of empagliflozin and extended-release metformin hydrochloride should be administered once daily with the morning meal; the tablet should be swallowed whole and should not be crushed, chewed, or cut.

If a dose is missed, the missed dose should be taken as soon as it is remembered followed by resumption of the regular schedule. If the missed dose is not remembered until it is almost time for the next dose, the missed dose should be skipped and the regular schedule resumed; the dose should not be doubled to replace a missed dose.

● Dosage

Type 2 Diabetes Mellitus
Empagliflozin Monotherapy

The recommended dosage of empagliflozin for the management of type 2 diabetes mellitus in adults is 10 mg once daily in the morning. If this dosage is well tolerated, the dosage may be increased to 25 mg once daily in patients who require additional glycemic control.

Empagliflozin/Linagliptin Fixed-combination Therapy

The recommended dosage of the fixed-combination preparation is 10 mg of empagliflozin and 5 mg of linagliptin once daily in the morning. If this dosage is well tolerated, the dosage may be increased to 25 mg of empagliflozin and 5 mg of linagliptin once daily.

Empagliflozin/Metformin Hydrochloride Fixed-combination Therapy

The dosage of empagliflozin in fixed combination with metformin hydrochloride should be individualized based on the patient's current antidiabetic regimen. The dosage of the fixed-combination preparation may be increased gradually based on effectiveness and tolerability up to a maximum of 25 mg of empagliflozin and 2 g of metformin hydrochloride daily.

In patients currently receiving metformin hydrochloride, the recommended initial total daily dosage of the fixed combination is 10 mg of empagliflozin and a metformin hydrochloride dosage similar to the patient's existing total daily dosage, administered in 2 divided doses (when given as the fixed combination containing *immediate-release* metformin hydrochloride) or once daily (when given as the fixed combination containing *extended-release* metformin hydrochloride).

In patients currently receiving empagliflozin, the recommended initial total daily dosage of the fixed combination is the same daily dosage of empagliflozin and 1 g metformin hydrochloride, administered in 2 divided doses (when given as the fixed combination containing *immediate-release* metformin hydrochloride) or once daily (when given as the fixed combination containing *extended-release* metformin hydrochloride).

In patients currently receiving both empagliflozin and metformin hydrochloride, the recommended initial total daily dosage of the fixed combination is the same daily dosage of empagliflozin and a metformin hydrochloride dosage similar to the patient's total daily existing dosage, administered in 2 divided doses (when given as the fixed combination containing *immediate-release* metformin hydrochloride) or once daily (when given as the fixed combination containing *extended-release* metformin hydrochloride).

● **Special Populations**

Body mass index, gender, and race do not have a clinically meaningful effect on the pharmacokinetics of empagliflozin.

Hepatic Impairment

Empagliflozin Monotherapy

Empagliflozin may be used in patients with hepatic impairment. No dosage adjustment is necessary in patients with mild, moderate, or severe hepatic impairment.

Empagliflozin/Linagliptin Fixed-combination Therapy

The fixed combination of empagliflozin and linagliptin may be used in patients with hepatic impairment.

Empagliflozin/Metformin Hydrochloride Fixed-combination Therapy

Use of the fixed-combination preparation of empagliflozin and immediate- or extended-release metformin hydrochloride is not recommended in patients with hepatic impairment.

Renal Impairment

Empagliflozin Monotherapy

No dosage adjustment is necessary in patients with an estimated glomerular filtration rate (eGFR) of at least 45 mL/minute per 1.73 m². Empagliflozin should not be initiated in patients with an eGFR of less than 45 mL/minute per 1.73 m². (See Renal Impairment under Warnings/Precautions: Specific Populations, in Cautions.) The drug should be discontinued if the eGFR is persistently less than 45 mL/minute per 1.73 m². Renal function should be assessed before initiating empagliflozin and during therapy. More frequent monitoring is recommended in patients with eGFR less than 60 mL/minute per 1.73 m².

Empagliflozin/Linagliptin Fixed-combination Therapy

No dosage adjustment is necessary in patients with an eGFR of at least 45 mL/minute per 1.73 m². The fixed combination should not be initiated in patients with an eGFR less than 45 mL/minute per 1.73 m². The fixed-combination preparation should be discontinued if the eGFR is persistently less than 45 mL/minute per 1.73 m².

Empagliflozin/Metformin Hydrochloride Fixed-combination Therapy

No dosage adjustment is necessary in patients with an eGFR of at least 45 mL/minute per 1.73 m². Use of the fixed-combination preparation of empagliflozin and immediate- or extended-release metformin hydrochloride is contraindicated in patients with an eGFR less than 45 mL/minute per 1.73 m².

Geriatric Patients

Empagliflozin Monotherapy

No dosage adjustment is necessary based solely on age.

Empagliflozin/Metformin Hydrochloride Fixed-combination Therapy

Renal function should be monitored frequently after initiating the fixed-combination preparation of empagliflozin and immediate- or extended-release metformin hydrochloride.

CAUTIONS

● **Contraindications**

History of serious hypersensitivity reaction to empagliflozin or any ingredient in the formulation.

Severe renal impairment (estimated glomerular filtration rate [eGFR] less than 30 mL/minute per 1.73 m²), end-stage renal disease, or dialysis.

● **Warnings/Precautions**

Ketoacidosis

Use of sodium glucose cotransporter 2 (SGLT2) inhibitors (canagliflozin, dapagliflozin, empagliflozin) in patients with type 2 diabetes mellitus may lead to ketoacidosis requiring hospitalization. Ketoacidosis associated with use of SGLT2 inhibitors may be present without markedly elevated blood glucose concentrations (e.g., less than 250 mg/dL).

FDA identified 73 cases of acidosis (reported as diabetic ketoacidosis [DKA], ketoacidosis, or ketosis) associated with SGLT2 inhibitor use in the FDA Adverse Event Reporting System (FAERS) between March 2013 and May 2015. DKA had an atypical presentation in most of the reported cases in that type 2 diabetes mellitus was noted as the indication for the drug, and glucose concentrations were only slightly elevated (median: 211 mg/dL); type 1 diabetes mellitus was named as the indication in a few cases, and in some reports the indication was not specified. The median time to onset of symptoms of acidosis following initiation or increase in dosage of the SGLT2 inhibitor was 43 days (range: 1–365 days). No trend demonstrating a relationship between the dosage of an SGLT2 inhibitor and the risk of ketoacidosis was identified. In all reported episodes, a diagnosis of DKA or ketoacidosis was made by the clinician and hospitalization or treatment in an emergency department was warranted. In most cases, at least 1 diagnostic laboratory criterion suggestive of ketoacidosis (e.g., high anion gap metabolic acidosis, ketonemia, reduced serum bicarbonate) was reported. Most cases of ketoacidosis were associated with a concurrent event, most commonly dehydration, infection, or change in insulin dosage. Potential factors for the development of ketoacidosis with SGLT2 inhibitor therapy identified in the 73 cases included infection, low carbohydrate diet or reduced caloric intake, surgery, pancreatic disorders suggesting insulin deficiency (e.g., type 1 diabetes mellitus, history of pancreatitis, pancreatic surgery), reduced dosage or discontinuance of insulin, discontinuance of an oral insulin secretagogue, and alcohol use.

Prior to initiating therapy with an SGLT2 inhibitor, clinicians should consider patient factors that may predispose the patient to ketoacidosis such as pancreatic insulin deficiency from any cause, reduced caloric intake, and alcohol abuse.

Clinicians should evaluate for the presence of acidosis, including ketoacidosis, in patients experiencing signs or symptoms of acidosis while receiving SGLT2 inhibitors, regardless of the patient's blood glucose concentration. For patients who undergo scheduled surgery, temporary discontinuation of empagliflozin for at least 3 days prior to surgery should be considered. Clinicians should consider monitoring for ketoacidosis and temporarily discontinuing therapy with an SGLT2 inhibitor in other clinical situations known to predispose individuals to ketoacidosis (e.g., prolonged fasting due to acute illness or post-surgery). If acidosis is confirmed, the SGLT2 inhibitor should be discontinued and appropriate treatment initiated to correct the acidosis; glucose concentrations should be monitored appropriately. In addition, supportive medical treatment should be instituted to treat and correct factors that may have precipitated or contributed to the metabolic acidosis. Risk factors for the development of ketoacidosis should be resolved prior to restarting empagliflozin therapy.

Euglycemic DKA associated with SGLT2 inhibitors may be detected and potentially prevented by having patients monitor urine and/or plasma ketone levels if they feel unwell, regardless of ambient glucose concentrations. Clinicians should inform patients and caregivers of the signs and symptoms of ketoacidosis (e.g., tachypnea or hyperventilation, anorexia, abdominal pain, nausea, vomiting, lethargy, mental status changes) and instruct patients to discontinue the SGLT2 inhibitor and immediately seek medical attention should they experience such signs or symptoms.

Hypotension

Empagliflozin causes intravascular volume contraction. Following initiation of empagliflozin, symptomatic hypotension may occur, particularly in patients with impaired renal function, geriatric patients, patients with low systolic blood pressure, or patients receiving diuretics. (See Drug Interactions: Diuretics.) Prior to initiating empagliflozin, intravascular volume should be assessed and corrected if necessary. Patients should be monitored for signs and symptoms of hypotension after initiating therapy; monitoring should be increased in clinical situations in which volume contraction is expected.

Renal Effects

Empagliflozin causes intravascular volume contraction and can cause renal impairment. Empagliflozin may increase serum creatinine concentration and decrease eGFR; patients with hypovolemia may be more susceptible to these changes. Abnormalities in renal function can occur following initiation of the drug. Patients should be monitored for acute kidney injury, and more frequent monitoring is recommended for patients with an eGFR less than 60 mL/minute per 1.73 m². If acute kidney injury occurs during empagliflozin therapy, the drug should be discontinued and appropriate therapy initiated.

There have been postmarketing reports of acute kidney injury in patients receiving SGLT2 inhibitors, including empagliflozin. FDA identified 101 cases of acute kidney injury associated with canagliflozin or dapagliflozin therapy in FAERS between March 2013 and October 2015. Hospitalization for evaluation and management of kidney injury was warranted in most cases, and in some cases required admission to an intensive care unit and initiation of dialysis. In approximately half of the cases, onset of acute kidney injury occurred within 1 month or less of initiating canagliflozin or dapagliflozin therapy, and most patients' kidney function improved after stopping the drug.

Prior to initiating empagliflozin therapy, clinicians should consider patient factors that may predispose the patient to acute kidney injury, including hypovolemia, chronic renal insufficiency, heart failure, and concomitant drug therapy (e.g., diuretics, angiotensin-converting enzyme [ACE] inhibitors, angiotensin II receptor antagonists, nonsteroidal anti-inflammatory agents [NSAIAs]). Clinicians should consider temporarily discontinuing empagliflozin in any setting of reduced oral intake (e.g., acute illness, fasting) or fluid losses (e.g., GI illness, excessive heat exposure).

Concomitant Therapy with Hypoglycemic Agents

When empagliflozin is added to therapy with an insulin secretagogue (e.g., a sulfonylurea) or insulin, the risk of hypoglycemia is increased compared with sulfonylurea or insulin monotherapy. Therefore, patients receiving empagliflozin may require a reduced dosage of the concomitant insulin secretagogue or insulin to reduce the risk of hypoglycemia.

Fournier Gangrene

Fournier gangrene (necrotizing fasciitis of the perineum), a rare but serious or life-threatening bacterial infection requiring urgent surgical intervention, has been reported during postmarketing surveillance in men and women with type 2 diabetes mellitus receiving an SGLT2 inhibitor, including empagliflozin. Permanent disfigurement, prolonged hospitalization, disability, and complications from sepsis all may be associated with Fournier gangrene. Although diabetes mellitus is a risk factor for developing Fournier gangrene, this condition is still rare among patients with diabetes mellitus.

FDA identified 12 cases of Fournier gangrene in patients taking an SGLT2 inhibitor reported in FAERS and the medical literature between March 2013 and May 2018. Since FDA's review, additional cases of Fournier gangrene have been reported. In the initial cases reviewed by FDA, the average time to onset of infection was 9.2 months (range 7 days to 25 months) after initiation of therapy with an SGLT2 inhibitor. Some experts speculate that the variation in time to diagnosis of Fournier gangrene might be due to fluctuating glycemic control, microvascular complications, or an inciting event associated with SGLT2 inhibitors (e.g., urinary tract infection, mycotic infection, skin or mucosal breakdown due to pruritus). In all reported cases, hospitalization and surgery were required. Among these cases, some patients required multiple disfiguring surgeries, some developed complications (e.g., diabetic ketoacidosis, acute kidney injury, septic shock), and 1 patient died. In a review of other antidiabetic drugs (e.g., insulin, biguanides, sulfonylureas, dipeptidyl peptidase-4 inhibitors) over a period of more than 30 years, only 6 cases of Fournier gangrene were identified; all of theses cases occurred in men.

Patients receiving empagliflozin who develop pain or tenderness, erythema, or swelling in the genital or perineal area, in addition to fever or malaise, should be assessed for necrotizing fasciitis. If Fournier gangrene is suspected, empagliflozin should be discontinued and treatment should be initiated with broad-spectrum antibiotics; surgical debridement should be performed if necessary. Blood glucose concentrations should be closely monitored; alternative antidiabetic agents should be initiated to maintain glycemic control.

Genital Mycotic Infections

Empagliflozin may increase the risk of genital mycotic infections (e.g., vaginal mycotic infection, vaginal infection, genital fungal infection, vulvovaginal candidiasis, fungal vulvitis). In clinical trials, patients with a history of chronic or recurrent genital mycotic infections were more likely to develop such infections. Genital mycotic infections also occurred more frequently in female than male patients. Patients should be monitored for genital mycotic infections and appropriate treatment should be instituted if these infections occur.

Urosepsis and Pyelonephritis

Empagliflozin may increase the risk of serious urinary tract infections.

FDA identified 19 cases of urosepsis and pyelonephritis, which began as urinary tract infections associated with SGLT2 inhibitor use, in FAERS between March 2013 and October 2014. In all cases reported, hospitalization was warranted and some patients required admission to an intensive care unit or dialysis for treatment. The median time to onset of infection following initiation of the SGLT2 inhibitor was 45 days (range: 2–270 days). In clinical studies of empagliflozin, urinary tract infections occurred more frequently in female patients compared with male patients, and risk of urinary tract infections increased in patients 75 years of age or older. Patients with a history of chronic or recurrent urinary tract infections were also more likely to develop such infections.

Prior to initiating therapy with an SGLT2 inhibitor, clinicians should consider patient factors that may predispose the patient to serious urinary tract infections such as a history of difficulty urinating; or infections of the bladder, kidneys, or urinary tract. Patients should be monitored for urinary tract infections and treatment instituted if indicated.

Effects on Lipoproteins

Dose-related increases in low-density lipoprotein (LDL)-cholesterol concentration have been observed during empagliflozin therapy. Serum LDL-cholesterol concentrations should be monitored during treatment with empagliflozin and such lipid elevations should be treated according to the standard of care.

Potential Risk of Bone Fracture

An increased risk of bone fracture, along with dose-related decreases in bone mineral density in older adults, has been observed in patients receiving another drug in the SGLT2 inhibitor class (canagliflozin). (See Risk of Bone Fracture under Cautions: Warnings/Precautions, in Canagliflozin.) FDA is continuing to evaluate the risk of bone fracture with SGLT2 inhibitors.

Laboratory Test Interferences

SGLT2 inhibitors such as empagliflozin increase urinary glucose excretion and will result in false-positive urine glucose tests. Data from healthy volunteers receiving a single 10- or 25-mg dose of empagliflozin indicate the elevation in urinary glucose excretion approaches baseline in approximately 3 days. In addition, the manufacturer states that the 1,5-anhydroglucitol assay is unreliable for monitoring glycemic control in patients taking SGLT2 inhibitors. Alternative methods of monitoring glycemic control should be used in patients receiving SGLT2 inhibitors.

Use of Fixed Combinations

When empagliflozin is used in fixed combination with metformin hydrochloride, linagliptin, or other drugs, the cautions, precautions, contraindications, and interactions associated with the concomitant agent(s) must be considered in addition to those associated with empagliflozin.

Sensitivity Reactions

Serious hypersensitivity reactions (e.g., angioedema, urticaria) have been reported with empagliflozin treatment. If a hypersensitivity reaction occurs, the drug should be discontinued, appropriate treatment instituted, and the patient monitored until signs and symptoms resolve. Empagliflozin is contraindicated in patients with a previous serious hypersensitivity reaction to empagliflozin or any excipient in the drug formulation.

Specific Populations
Pregnancy

Data on the use of empagliflozin in pregnant women are lacking. Based on the results of reproductive and developmental toxicity studies in animals, empagliflozin use during pregnancy may affect renal development and maturation, especially during the second and third trimesters of pregnancy. Limited data with empagliflozin in pregnant women are not sufficient to determine a drug-associated risk for major birth defects or miscarriage, and poorly controlled diabetes mellitus during pregnancy carries risks to the mother and fetus; however, empagliflozin therapy is not recommended in pregnant women during the second and third trimesters of pregnancy.

Lactation

Empagliflozin is distributed into milk in rats; it is not known whether the drug is distributed into human milk. Because many drugs are distributed into human milk and because of the potential for serious adverse reactions in nursing infants from empagliflozin, a decision should be made whether to discontinue nursing or the drug, taking into account the importance of the drug to the woman.

Pediatric Use

Safety and efficacy of empagliflozin have not been established in pediatric patients younger than 18 years of age.

Geriatric Use

In clinical studies, 2721 (32%) patients treated with empagliflozin were 65 years of age or older and 491 (6%) were 75 years of age or older. Geriatric patients with renal impairment are expected to experience reduced efficacy when treated with empagliflozin. The risk of volume depletion-related adverse effects and urinary tract infections is increased in patients 75 years of age or older.

Hepatic Impairment

Empagliflozin may be used in patients with hepatic impairment. Compared with values in individuals with normal hepatic function, empagliflozin area under the concentration-time curve (AUC) was increased by approximately 23, 47, or 75% in patients with mild, moderate, or severe (Child-Pugh class A, B, or C) hepatic impairment, respectively; peak plasma concentrations of the drug in patients with mild, moderate, or severe hepatic function were increased by approximately 4, 23, or 48%, respectively.

Renal Impairment

Safety and efficacy of empagliflozin were evaluated in a study that included patients with mild or moderate renal impairment. Of those who received empagliflozin, 195 patients had an eGFR of 60–90 mL/minute per 1.73 m², 91 patients had an eGFR of 45–60 mL/minute per 1.73 m², and 97 patients had an eGFR of 30–45 mL/minute per 1.73 m². The glucose-lowering effect of empagliflozin 25 mg was reduced in patients with worsening renal function. In addition, the risk of renal impairment and of adverse effects related to volume depletion, and urinary tract infection increased with worsening renal function.

In patients with mild (eGFR 60 to less than 90 mL/minute per 1.73 m²), moderate (eGFR 30 to less than 60 mL/minute per 1.73 m²), or severe (eGFR less than 30 mL/minute per 1.73 m²) renal impairment, and in patients with renal failure/end-stage renal disease, AUC of empagliflozin increased by approximately 18, 20, 66, and 48%, respectively, compared with those with normal renal function. Peak plasma concentrations of empagliflozin were similar in patients with moderate renal impairment or renal failure/end-stage renal disease compared with those with normal renal function; however, peak plasma concentrations of empagliflozin were approximately 20% higher in patients with mild or severe renal impairment compared with such concentrations in individuals with normal renal function.

Population pharmacokinetic studies demonstrated that the apparent oral clearance of empagliflozin was reduced, with a reduction in eGFR resulting in an increase in drug exposure. However, the fraction of empagliflozin excreted unchanged in urine and urinary glucose excretion declined with decrease in eGFR.

Efficacy and safety of empagliflozin have not been established in patients with severe renal impairment or end-stage renal disease, or in those receiving dialysis; empagliflozin is not expected to be effective in these patients.

● Common Adverse Effects

Adverse effects reported in at least 2% of patients receiving empagliflozin in clinical trials and more commonly than with placebo include urinary tract infection, female genital mycotic infections, upper respiratory tract infection, increased urination, dyslipidemia, arthralgia, male genital mycotic infections, and nausea.

Adverse effects reported in at least 5% of patients receiving empagliflozin and linagliptin in clinical trials include urinary tract infection, nasopharyngitis, and upper respiratory tract infection.

Adverse effects reported in at least 5% of patients receiving empagliflozin concomitantly with metformin and a sulfonylurea include hypoglycemia, urinary tract infection, and nasopharyngitis.

DRUG INTERACTIONS

The major metabolic pathway for empagliflozin is glucuronidation; the drug is principally glucuronidated by uridine diphosphate-glucuronosyltransferase (UGT) isoenzymes 2B7, 1A3, 1A8, and 1A9.

● Drugs Affecting or Metabolized by Hepatic Microsomal Enzymes

Empagliflozin did not inhibit, inactivate, or induce cytochrome P-450 (CYP) isoforms in vitro; no effect of empagliflozin is expected on concomitantly administered drugs that are substrates of the major CYP isoforms.

● Drugs Affecting or Affected by Organic Anion Transporters

Empagliflozin is a substrate of organic anion transporter (OAT) 3 and organic anion transport proteins (OATP) 1B1 and 1B3. Empagliflozin is not a substrate of OAT1. Empagliflozin does not inhibit any of these transporters at clinically relevant plasma concentrations, and no effect of empagliflozin is expected on concomitantly administered drugs that are substrates of these uptake transporters.

● Drugs Affecting or Affected by Organic Cation Transporters

Empagliflozin is not a substrate of organic cation transporter (OCT) 2, nor does it inhibit OCT2 at clinically relevant plasma concentrations; no effect of empagliflozin is expected on concomitantly administered drugs that are substrates of this uptake transporter.

● Drugs Affecting or Metabolized by Uridine Diphosphate-glucuronosyltransferase

Empagliflozin does not inhibit UGT isoenzymes 1A1, 1A3, 1A8, 1A9, or 2B7, and no effect of empagliflozin is expected on concomitantly administered drugs that are substrates of these UGT isoenzymes. The manufacturer states the effect of UGT induction on empagliflozin exposure has not been established.

● Drugs Affecting or Affected by P-glycoprotein Transport

Empagliflozin is a substrate of P-glycoprotein (P-gp), but it does not inhibit P-gp at therapeutic doses. Empagliflozin is considered unlikely to cause interactions with drugs that are P-gp substrates based on in vitro studies.

● Drugs Affecting or Affected by Breast Cancer Resistance Protein

Empagliflozin is a substrate of breast cancer resistance protein (BCRP), but it does not inhibit BCRP at therapeutic doses.

● Antidiabetic Agents

Concomitant use of empagliflozin with insulin or insulin secretagogues increases the risk for hypoglycemia. Patients receiving empagliflozin may require a reduced dosage of the concomitant insulin secretagogue or insulin to reduce the risk of hypoglycemia.

● Digoxin

Administration of a single dose of digoxin (0.5 mg) in healthy individuals receiving empagliflozin 25 mg once daily did not have a clinically relevant effect on the pharmacokinetics of digoxin. No adjustment of digoxin dosage is necessary.

● Diuretics

Concomitant use of empagliflozin with diuretics may increase urine volume and frequency of urination, which may increase the risk of volume depletion. Patients should be assessed for volume contraction, and volume status should be corrected if indicated before initiating empagliflozin. Patients should be monitored for signs and symptoms of hypotension after initiating therapy, and monitoring should be increased in clinical situations where volume contraction is expected.

● Gemfibrozil

Concomitant administration of gemfibrozil 600 mg twice daily and a single dose of empagliflozin 25 mg resulted in an increase in area under the concentration-time curve (AUC) of empagliflozin, although this effect was not considered clinically relevant. No adjustment of empagliflozin dosage is necessary when administered with gemfibrozil.

● Glimepiride

Administration of a single dose of glimepiride (1 mg) in healthy individuals receiving empagliflozin 50 mg once daily did not have a clinically relevant effect on the pharmacokinetics of glimepiride or empagliflozin. No adjustment in either drug's dosage is necessary.

● Hormonal Contraceptives

Administration of 30 mcg of ethinyl estradiol once daily in healthy individuals receiving empagliflozin 25 mg once daily did not have a clinically relevant effect on the pharmacokinetics of ethinyl estradiol. Also, concomitant administration of levonorgestrel 150 mcg once daily and empagliflozin 25 mg once daily had no clinically relevant effect on the pharmacokinetics of levonorgestrel. No adjustment of ethinyl estradiol or levonorgestrel dosage is necessary when administered concomitantly with empagliflozin.

● Hydrochlorothiazide

Administration of hydrochlorothiazide 25 mg once daily in healthy individuals receiving empagliflozin 25 mg once daily did not have a clinically relevant effect on the pharmacokinetics of hydrochlorothiazide or empagliflozin. No adjustment in either drug's dosage is necessary. (See also Drug Interactions: Diuretics.)

● Linagliptin

Administration of linagliptin 5 mg once daily in healthy individuals receiving empagliflozin 50 mg once daily did not have a clinically relevant effect on the pharmacokinetics of linagliptin or empagliflozin. No adjustment in either drug's dosage is necessary.

● Metformin

Administration of metformin hydrochloride 1 g twice daily in healthy individuals receiving empagliflozin 50 mg once daily did not have a clinically relevant effect on the pharmacokinetics of metformin or empagliflozin. No adjustment in either drug's dosage is necessary.

● Pioglitazone

Concomitant use of pioglitazone 45 mg once daily in healthy individuals receiving empagliflozin 50 mg once daily did not have a clinically relevant effect on the pharmacokinetics of empagliflozin. Similarly, administration of pioglitazone 45 mg once daily in patients receiving empagliflozin 25 mg once daily did not have a clinically relevant effect on the pharmacokinetics of pioglitazone. No adjustment of empagliflozin dosage is necessary.

● Probenecid

Concomitant use of probenecid 500 mg twice daily in healthy individuals receiving a single dose of empagliflozin 10 mg resulted in an increase in AUC of empagliflozin. However, this effect was not clinically relevant. No adjustment of empagliflozin dosage is necessary when administered with probenecid. In patients with normal renal function, concomitant use of empagliflozin with probenecid resulted in a 30% decrease in the fraction of empagliflozin excreted in urine without any effect on 24-hour urinary glucose excretion. The manufacturer states that the relevance of this observation to patients with renal impairment is not known.

● Ramipril

Concomitant use of ramipril 5 mg once daily in healthy individuals receiving empagliflozin 25 mg once daily did not have a clinically relevant effect on the pharmacokinetics of ramipril or its active metabolite ramiprilat, or on

empagliflozin pharmacokinetics. No adjustment of ramipril or empagliflozin dosage is necessary.

● Rifampin

Administration of a single dose of rifampin 600 mg in healthy individuals also receiving a single dose of empagliflozin 10 mg resulted in an increase in AUC of empagliflozin. However, this effect was not clinically relevant. No adjustment of empagliflozin dosage is necessary when administered with rifampin.

● Simvastatin

Administration of a single dose of simvastatin 40 mg in healthy individuals also receiving a single dose of empagliflozin 25 mg did not have a clinically relevant effect on the pharmacokinetics of simvastatin or its active metabolite simvastatin acid, or on empagliflozin pharmacokinetics. No adjustment of simvastatin or empagliflozin dosage is necessary.

● Sitagliptin

Concomitant administration of sitagliptin 100 mg once daily in healthy individuals receiving empagliflozin 50 mg once daily did not have a clinically relevant effect on the pharmacokinetics of sitagliptin or empagliflozin. No adjustment in either drug's dosage is necessary.

● Torsemide

Concomitant use of torsemide 5 mg once daily in healthy individuals receiving empagliflozin 25 mg once daily did not have a clinically relevant effect on the pharmacokinetics of torsemide or empagliflozin. No adjustment in either drug's dosage is necessary.

● Verapamil

Administration of a single dose of verapamil 120 mg in healthy individuals also receiving a single dose of empagliflozin 25 mg did not have a clinically relevant effect on the pharmacokinetics of empagliflozin. No adjustment of verapamil dosage is necessary.

● Warfarin

Administration of a single dose (25 mg) of warfarin sodium in healthy individuals also receiving empagliflozin 25 mg once daily did not have a clinically relevant effect on the pharmacokinetics of R- or S-warfarin or on the pharmacokinetics of empagliflozin. No adjustment in either drug's dosage is necessary.

DESCRIPTION

Empagliflozin is an orally active inhibitor of sodium-glucose cotransporter 2 (SGLT2), the transporter principally responsible for the reabsorption of glucose from the glomerular filtrate back into the circulation. Through inhibition of SGLT2, empagliflozin reduces renal reabsorption of filtered glucose and lowers the renal threshold for glucose, thereby increasing urinary glucose excretion and reducing blood glucose concentrations, independent of insulin secretion.

Following oral administration of empagliflozin 10 or 25 mg under fasting conditions, empagliflozin is rapidly absorbed; median time to peak plasma concentration of the drug was 1 hour for both doses. Empagliflozin exposure increased in proportion to the dose. Administration of empagliflozin 25 mg following intake of a high-fat and high-calorie meal resulted in slightly lower exposure. Peak concentration and area under the concentration-time curve decreased by approximately 37 and 16%, respectively, compared with fasting conditions. Effect of food on empagliflozin pharmacokinetics was not considered clinically relevant, and empagliflozin can be administered with or without food. Empagliflozin is 86.2% bound to plasma proteins. The apparent terminal elimination half-life of empagliflozin is approximately 12.4 hours. Following administration of a radiolabeled dose of empagliflozin, 41.2% of the administered dose was eliminated in feces and 54.4% was eliminated in urine.

Results of bioequivalence studies indicate that the fixed-combination tablets containing empagliflozin and immediate-release metformin hydrochloride or empagliflozin and linagliptin are bioequivalent to corresponding doses of empagliflozin, metformin hydrochloride, or linagliptin given concurrently as individual tablets.

ADVICE TO PATIENTS

When empagliflozin is used in fixed combination with other drugs, importance of informing patients of important cautionary information about the concomitant agent(s).

Importance of patient reading medication guide before initiating therapy and each time the drug is dispensed.

Importance of informing patients of the potential risks and benefits of empagliflozin and of alternative therapies. Importance of informing patients that use of empagliflozin with other antidiabetic agents may increase risk of hypoglycemia. Importance of *not* using empagliflozin in patients with type 1 diabetes mellitus or diabetic ketoacidosis.

Importance of informing patients that ketoacidosis, which can be a life-threatening condition, has been reported with empagliflozin therapy (sometimes associated with illness or surgery among other risk factors). Importance of informing patients receiving empagliflozin and their caregivers of the signs and symptoms of ketoacidosis (e.g., tachypnea or hyperventilation, anorexia, abdominal pain, nausea, vomiting, lethargy, mental status changes). If signs or symptoms of acidosis occur, importance of discontinuing empagliflozin and seeking medical attention immediately. Advise patients to use a ketone dipstick to check for ketones in their urine (when possible) if symptoms of ketoacidosis occur, even if blood glucose is not elevated (e.g., less than 250 mg/dL).

Importance of informing patients that hypotension may occur with empagliflozin and to report such symptoms to their clinicians. Inform patients that empagliflozin-induced dehydration may increase the risk of hypotension and that patients should maintain adequate fluid intake.

Importance of informing patients that acute kidney injury has been reported with empagliflozin therapy. Advise patients to seek medical advice immediately if they have reduced oral intake (such as due to acute illness or fasting) or increased fluid losses (such as due to vomiting, diarrhea, or excessive heat exposure), as it may be appropriate to temporarily discontinue empagliflozin in those situations.

Importance of informing female patients that vaginal yeast infections (e.g., vulvovaginitis) may occur. Importance of informing male patients that yeast infections may occur (e.g., balanitis, balanoposthitis), especially in uncircumcised males. Importance of informing patients that yeast infections occur more frequently in females and in patients with chronic and recurrent infections. Importance of informing female patients of the signs and symptoms of vaginal yeast infections (e.g., vaginal discharge, odor, itching) and male patients of the signs and symptoms of balanitis or balanoposthitis (e.g. rash or redness of the glans or foreskin of the penis, foul-smelling discharge from the penis, pain in skin around penis). Advise patients of treatment options and when to seek medical advice.

Importance of informing patients of the potential for urinary tract infections, which may be serious, with empagliflozin therapy. Advise patients of the signs and symptoms of urinary tract infection (e.g., dysuria, cloudy urine, pelvic or back pain) and the need to contact a clinician if such signs and symptoms occur.

Importance of informing patients that necrotizing infections of the perineum (Fournier gangrene) have occurred with empagliflozin therapy. Advise patients to seek prompt medical attention if they experience any symptoms of tenderness, redness, or swelling of the genitals or the area from the genitals back to the rectum, occurring with a fever above 38°C or malaise.

Risk of serious hypersensitivity reactions, such as urticaria and angioedema. If signs or symptoms of such reactions occur, importance of discontinuing empagliflozin and informing clinician promptly.

Importance of informing patients that due to the mechanism of action of empagliflozin, patients taking the drug will test positive for glucose in urine. Importance of not using urine glucose tests to monitor glycemic status while taking empagliflozin. (See Laboratory Test Interferences under Cautions: Warnings/Precautions.)

Importance of informing patients about the importance of adherence to dietary instructions, regular physical activity, periodic blood glucose monitoring and glycosylated hemoglobin (hemoglobin A_{1c} [HbA_{1c}]) testing, recognition and management of hypoglycemia and hyperglycemia, and assessment of diabetes complications.

Importance of seeking medical advice promptly during periods of stress such as fever, trauma, infection, or surgery as drug dosage requirements may change.

Importance of informing patient *not* to take empagliflozin if allergic to the drug or any ingredients in the formulation.

Importance of taking empagliflozin exactly as directed by clinician. Importance of informing patients that if a dose is missed, it should be taken as soon as remembered; the dose should not be doubled to make up for the missed dose. (See Dosage and Administration: Administration.)

Importance of informing patients that renal function should be assessed prior to initiation of empagliflozin and monitored periodically thereafter.

Importance of women informing their clinicians if they are or plan to become pregnant or plan to breast-feed.

Importance of informing clinicians of existing or contemplated concomitant therapy, including prescription and OTC drugs and dietary or herbal supplements, as well as any concomitant illnesses.

Importance of informing patients of other important precautionary information. (See Cautions.)

PREPARATIONS

Excipients in commercially available drug preparations may have clinically important effects in some individuals; consult specific product labeling for details.

Empagliflozin

Oral

Tablets, film-coated	10 mg	Jardiance®, Boehringer Ingelheim
	25 mg	Jardiance®, Boehringer Ingelheim

Empagliflozin Combinations

Oral

Tablets, extended-release	5 mg with Extended-release Metformin Hydrochloride 1 g	Synjardy® XR, Boehringer Ingelheim
	10 mg with Extended-release Metformin Hydrochloride 1 g	Synjardy® XR, Boehringer Ingelheim
	12.5 mg with Extended-release Metformin Hydrochloride 1 g	Synjardy® XR, Boehringer Ingelheim
	25 mg with Extended-release Metformin Hydrochloride 1 g	Synjardy® XR, Boehringer Ingelheim
Tablets, film-coated	5 mg with Metformin Hydrochloride 500 mg	Synjardy®, Boehringer Ingelheim
	5 mg with Metformin Hydrochloride 1 g	Synjardy®, Boehringer Ingelheim
	10 mg with Linagliptin 5 mg	Glyxambi®, Boehringer Ingelheim
	12.5 mg with Metformin Hydrochloride 500 mg	Synjardy®, Boehringer Ingelheim
	12.5 mg with Metformin Hydrochloride 1 g	Synjardy®, Boehringer Ingelheim
	25 mg with Linagliptin 5 mg	Glyxambi®, Boehringer Ingelheim

† Use is not currently included in the labeling approved by the US Food and Drug Administration.

Selected Revisions December 01, 2022, © Copyright, December 07, 2015, American Society of Health-System Pharmacists, Inc.

Ertugliflozin L-pyroglutamic Acid

68:20.18 • SODIUM-GLUCOSE COTRANSPORTER 2 (SGLT2) INHIBITORS

■ Ertugliflozin L-pyroglutamic acid, a sodium-glucose cotransporter 2 (SGLT2) inhibitor, is an antidiabetic agent.

USES

● Type 2 Diabetes Mellitus

Ertugliflozin is used as monotherapy as an adjunct to diet and exercise to improve glycemic control in patients with type 2 diabetes mellitus. Ertugliflozin also is used in combination with other antidiabetic agents (e.g., metformin, sitagliptin) as an adjunct to diet and exercise in patients with type 2 diabetes mellitus who have not achieved adequate glycemic control. Ertugliflozin is commercially available in fixed combination with metformin hydrochloride (Segluromet®) or sitagliptin (Steglujan®). The fixed combination of ertugliflozin and metformin hydrochloride is used as an adjunct to diet and exercise to improve glycemic control in patients with type 2 diabetes mellitus who are not adequately controlled with ertugliflozin or metformin monotherapy, or in patients who are already receiving therapy with both drugs. The fixed combination of ertugliflozin and sitagliptin is used as an adjunct to diet and exercise to improve glycemic control in patients with type 2 diabetes mellitus when treatment with both drugs is appropriate.

Glycemic Control

Current guidelines for the treatment of type 2 diabetes mellitus generally recommend metformin as first-line therapy in addition to lifestyle modifications in patients with recent-onset type 2 diabetes mellitus or mild hyperglycemia because of its well-established safety and efficacy (i.e., beneficial effects on glycosylated hemoglobin [hemoglobin A_{1c}; HbA_{1c}], weight, and cardiovascular mortality). (See Uses: Type 2 Diabetes Mellitus, in Metformin 68:20.04.) In patients with contraindications or intolerance to metformin (e.g., risk of lactic acidosis, GI intolerance) or in selected other patients, some experts suggest that initial therapy with a drug from another class of antidiabetic agents (e.g., a glucagon-like peptide-1 [GLP-1] receptor agonist, SGLT2 inhibitor, dipeptidyl peptidase-4 [DPP-4] inhibitor, sulfonylurea, thiazolidinedione, basal insulin) may be acceptable based on patient factors. Initiating antidiabetic therapy with 2 agents (e.g., metformin plus another drug) may be appropriate in patients with an initial HbA_{1c} exceeding 7.5% or at least 1.5% above the target level. In metformin-intolerant patients with high initial HbA_{1c} levels, some experts suggest initiation of therapy with 2 agents from other antidiabetic classes with complementary mechanisms of action.

Because of the progressive nature of type 2 diabetes mellitus, patients initially receiving an oral antidiabetic agent will eventually require multiple oral and/or injectable noninsulin antidiabetic agents of different therapeutic classes and/or insulin for adequate glycemic control. Patients who have inadequate glycemic control with initial (e.g., metformin) monotherapy should receive treatment with additional antidiabetic agents; data suggest that the addition of each noninsulin agent to initial therapy lowers HbA_{1c} by approximately 0.7–1%. In addition, early initiation of combination therapy may help to more rapidly attain glycemic goals and extend the time to treatment failure.

Factors to consider when selecting additional antidiabetic agents for combination therapy in patients with inadequate glycemic control on metformin monotherapy include patient comorbidities (e.g., atherosclerotic cardiovascular disease [ASCVD], established kidney disease, heart failure), hypoglycemia risk, impact on weight, cost, risk of adverse effects, and patient preference. When the greater glucose-lowering effect of an injectable drug is needed in patients with type 2 diabetes mellitus, some experts currently state that an injectable GLP-1 receptor agonist is preferred over insulin in most patients because of beneficial effects on body weight and a lower risk of hypoglycemia, although adverse GI effects may diminish tolerability. While addition of a GLP-1 receptor agonist may successfully control hyperglycemia, many patients will eventually require insulin therapy. Early introduction of insulin therapy should be considered when hyperglycemia

is severe (e.g., blood glucose of at least 300 mg/dL or HbA_{1c} exceeding 9–10%), especially in the presence of catabolic manifestations (e.g., weight loss, hypertriglyceridemia, ketosis) or symptoms of hyperglycemia. For additional information regarding the initiation of insulin therapy in patients with diabetes mellitus, see Uses: Diabetes Mellitus, in the Insulins General Statement 68:20.08.

Patients with type 2 diabetes mellitus who have established (or are at a high risk for) ASCVD, established kidney disease, or heart failure should receive a GLP-1 receptor agonist or SGLT2 inhibitor with demonstrated cardiovascular disease benefit. (See Reduction in Risk of Major Adverse Cardiovascular Events under Uses: Type 2 Diabetes Mellitus, in Liraglutide 68:20.06 and also see Reduction in Risk of Heart Failure-Related Hospitalization under Uses: Type 2 Diabetes Mellitus, in Dapagliflozin 68:20.18.) Experts state that therapy with a GLP-1 receptor agonist or SGLT2 inhibitor should be considered for patients with the aforementioned comorbidities independently of the patients' HbA_{1c}. GLP-1 receptor agonists and SGLT2 inhibitors appear to have effects on the kidneys independent of their glycemic effects, and some experts suggest that an agent from one of these classes of drugs be considered in patients with type 2 diabetes mellitus and chronic kidney disease (CKD). (See Beneficial Effects on Renal Function and Cardiovascular Morbidity and Mortality in Diabetic Nephropathy under Uses: Type 2 Diabetes Mellitus, in Canagliflozin 68:20.18.) In patients *without* established ASCVD or indicators of high ASCVD risk, heart failure, or CKD, the decision regarding the addition of other antidiabetic agents (e.g., GLP-1 receptor agonist, SGLT2 inhibitor, DPP-4 inhibitor, thiazolidinedione, sulfonylurea, basal insulin) to metformin therapy should be based on avoidance of adverse effects, cost, and individual patient factors.

The manufacturer states that ertugliflozin is *not* indicated for treatment of type 1 diabetes mellitus or diabetic ketoacidosis.

Ertugliflozin Monotherapy

When given as monotherapy for the management of type 2 diabetes mellitus, ertugliflozin improves glycemic control compared with placebo as evidenced by reductions in HbA_{1c} and in fasting and 2-hour postprandial plasma glucose concentrations. Efficacy of ertugliflozin as monotherapy has been established in a double-blind, placebo-controlled trial of 26-weeks' duration in approximately 460 patients with type 2 diabetes mellitus and a mean baseline HbA_{1c} of 8.21%. Patients were either treatment naive or were not receiving any antidiabetic agents for at least 8 weeks prior to trial screening. Ertugliflozin (5 or 15 mg once daily) improved glycemic control as evidenced by reductions in HbA_{1c} and fasting and 2-hour postprandial plasma glucose concentrations. HbA_{1c} was reduced by 0.7 or 0.8% in patients receiving ertugliflozin 5 or 15 mg once daily, respectively, compared with a reduction of 0.2% in those receiving placebo. In patients who received ertugliflozin 5 or 15 mg, approximately 30 or 39%, respectively, had HbA_{1c} reductions to less than 7% compared with approximately 17% of patients receiving placebo. Patients receiving ertugliflozin 5 or 15 mg once daily also lost substantially more body weight (reduction of 3 or 3.1 kg, respectively) than those receiving placebo (reduction of 1 kg).

Combination Therapy

When given in combination with one or more oral antidiabetic agents, ertugliflozin improves glycemic control compared with monotherapy with these drugs and generally is associated with reductions in body weight and systolic blood pressure. Ertugliflozin generally is well tolerated, although genital mycotic infections appear to be more common with SGLT2 inhibitors such as ertugliflozin than with other classes of antidiabetic drugs.

Efficacy of ertugliflozin in combination with other antidiabetic agents for the management of type 2 diabetes mellitus is supported by results from several randomized, active- or placebo-controlled trials in patients receiving ertugliflozin with metformin, sitagliptin, or metformin and sitagliptin. In these trials, initial combined therapy with ertugliflozin (5 or 15 mg once daily) and one or more antidiabetic drugs or addition of ertugliflozin to existing therapy improved glycemic control as evidenced by reductions in HbA_{1c}, fasting plasma glucose, and 2-hour postprandial plasma glucose concentrations; combined therapy also had beneficial effects on weight reduction and blood pressure compared with placebo and/or monotherapy.

In a 26-week, randomized, double-blind trial in patients with type 2 diabetes mellitus inadequately controlled with metformin monotherapy, concomitant therapy with ertugliflozin (5 or 15 mg once daily) and existing metformin hydrochloride therapy (dosage of at least 1.5 g daily) substantially improved glycemic control (as evidenced by reductions in HbA_{1c}) compared with metformin monotherapy. Reductions in HbA_{1c} were 0.7 or 0.9% with ertugliflozin 5 or 15 mg once daily, respectively, plus metformin and 0.2% with existing metformin hydrochloride monotherapy. In patients who received metformin in conjunction with ertugliflozin 5 or 15 mg, approximately 36 or 43%, respectively, had HbA_{1c} reductions to less than 7%, compared with approximately 18% of patients receiving metformin monotherapy. The addition of ertugliflozin to existing metformin therapy also was associated with greater reductions in fasting plasma glucose, body weight, and blood pressure.

In a noninferiority trial of 52 weeks' duration in patients with type 2 diabetes mellitus who were inadequately controlled with metformin hydrochloride monotherapy (dosage of at least 1.5 g daily), once-daily therapy with ertugliflozin (5 or 15 mg) or glimepiride (mean daily dose 3 mg) was added to existing therapy with metformin. Ertugliflozin and glimepiride provided similar improvements in glycemic control (as measured by HbA_{1c}) and ertugliflozin 15 mg once daily was noninferior to glimepiride therapy. At week 52, approximately 48, 40, and 42% of patients in the glimepiride, ertugliflozin 5 mg, and ertugliflozin 15 mg treatment groups, respectively, had an HbA_{1c} of less than 7%. Greater reductions in body weight and systolic blood pressure from baseline also were observed in those patients who received ertugliflozin.

In a trial evaluating the safety and efficacy of ertugliflozin in combination with sitagliptin in adults with type 2 diabetes mellitus inadequately controlled with metformin hydrochloride monotherapy (dosage of at least 1.5 g daily), the addition of ertugliflozin and sitagliptin combination therapy to existing metformin therapy substantially improved glycemic control compared with the addition of either ertugliflozin or sitagliptin alone. In this trial, patients received ertugliflozin 5 mg, ertugliflozin 15 mg, sitagliptin 100 mg, ertugliflozin 5 mg and sitagliptin 100 mg, or ertugliflozin 15 mg and sitagliptin 100 mg once daily. At week 26, patients who received concomitant therapy with ertugliflozin 5 or 15 mg and sitagliptin 100 mg had greater reductions in HbA_{1c} (reduction of 1.4%) compared with those receiving ertugliflozin or sitagliptin alone (reduction of 1%). Additionally, a higher proportion of patients who received ertugliflozin 5 or 15 mg and sitagliptin 100 mg as an add-on to existing metformin therapy achieved an HbA_{1c} of less than 7% (53 or 51%, respectively) compared with those who received ertugliflozin 5 or 15 mg or sitagliptin 100 mg alone (29, 34, or 39%, respectively).

In a 26-week trial in patients receiving metformin hydrochloride (dosage of at least 1.5 g daily) and sitagliptin (100 mg once daily), the addition of ertugliflozin 5 or 15 mg once daily resulted in a reduction in HbA_{1c} of 0.7 or 0.8%, respectively, compared with a 0.2% reduction in HbA_{1c} with placebo. Approximately 35 or 42% of patients who received ertugliflozin 5 or 15 mg, respectively, had HbA_{1c} reductions to less than 7%, compared with approximately 20% of patients receiving placebo. Patients receiving ertugliflozin 5 or 15 mg once daily also had greater reductions in fasting plasma glucose, body weight, and systolic blood pressure than those receiving placebo.

Efficacy and safety of the combination of ertugliflozin and sitagliptin as initial therapy in patients with type 2 diabetes mellitus inadequately controlled with diet and exercise are supported by results of a 26-week, randomized, double-blind, placebo-controlled trial. In this trial, concomitant therapy with ertugliflozin (5 or 15 mg once daily) and sitagliptin (100 mg daily) substantially improved glycemic control (as evidenced by reductions in HbA_{1c}) compared with placebo. Reductions in HbA_{1c} were 1.6 or 1.7% with ertugliflozin 5 or 15 mg once daily, respectively, plus sitagliptin and 0.4% with placebo. Additionally, a greater proportion of patients receiving ertugliflozin and sitagliptin combination therapy achieved an HbA_{1c} of less than 7%, and greater reductions in fasting plasma glucose were observed with ertugliflozin and sitagliptin combination therapy compared with placebo.

Reduction in Risk of Cardiovascular Events

Some SGLT2 inhibitors (e.g., canagliflozin, empagliflozin) have demonstrated the ability to reduce the risk of cardiovascular events† in patients with type 2 diabetes mellitus and established cardiovascular disease. In addition to lowering blood glucose, SGLT2 inhibitors appear to modify several nonglycemic cardiovascular risk factors such as blood pressure, body weight, adiposity, and arterial stiffness.

The manufacturer states that data on the use of ertugliflozin for macrovascular risk reduction are lacking. For further discussion on the use of SGLT2 inhibitors for cardiovascular risk reduction, see Reduction in Risk of Major Adverse Cardiovascular Events under Uses: Type 2 Diabetes Mellitus, in Canagliflozin 68:20.18.

Beneficial Effects on Renal Function

SGLT2 inhibitors reduce renal tubular glucose reabsorption, body weight, systemic blood pressure, intraglomerular pressure, and albuminuria and slow glomerular filtration rate (GFR) loss through mechanisms that appear to be independent of glucose-lowering effects. In several cardiovascular outcomes trials involving the use of SGLT2 inhibitors (e.g., canagliflozin, dapagliflozin, empagliflozin) in patients with type 2 diabetes mellitus at high risk for cardiovascular disease or with existing cardiovascular disease, beneficial effects on renal function were observed as a secondary outcome. Some experts state that the use of an SGLT2 inhibitor should be considered to reduce the risk of CKD progression, cardiovascular events, or both in patients with type 2 diabetes mellitus and diabetic kidney disease with albuminuria† (an eGFR of at least 30 mL/minute per 1.73 m² and urinary albumin exceeding 30 mg/g creatinine, particularly urinary albumin exceeding 300 mg/g creatinine).

A clinical study evaluating the use of canagliflozin in patients with type 2 diabetes mellitus, CKD (eGFR 30–89 mL/minute per 1.73 m²; mean: 56.2 mL/minute per 1.73 m²), and albuminuria (urine albumin:creatinine ratio exceeding 300 but less than 5000 mg/g) found that canagliflozin therapy reduced the risk of end-stage kidney disease, doubling of serum creatinine, cardiovascular death, and hospitalization for heart failure. For further discussion of the beneficial effects on renal function of SGLT2 inhibitors, see Beneficial Effects on Renal Function and Cardiovascular Morbidity and Mortality in Diabetic Nephropathy under Uses: Type 2 Diabetes Mellitus, in Canagliflozin 68:20.18 and in Empagliflozin 68:20.18.

DOSAGE AND ADMINISTRATION

● General

Volume depletion should be corrected before initiating ertugliflozin. In addition, renal function should be assessed prior to treatment and periodically thereafter. (See Renal Impairment under Dosage and Administration: Special Populations.)

● Administration

Ertugliflozin or the fixed combination of ertugliflozin and sitagliptin is administered orally once daily in the morning, with or without food.

The fixed combination of ertugliflozin and metformin hydrochloride is administered orally twice daily with meals to reduce the adverse GI effects of the metformin hydrochloride component.

If a dose of ertugliflozin, the fixed combination of ertugliflozin and metformin hydrochloride, or the fixed combination of ertugliflozin and sitagliptin is missed, the missed dose should be taken as soon as it is remembered followed by resumption of the regular schedule. If the missed dose is not remembered until it is almost time for the next dose, the missed dose should be skipped and the regular schedule resumed; the dose should not be doubled to replace a missed dose.

● Dosage

Type 2 Diabetes Mellitus

Dosage of ertugliflozin L-pyroglutamic acid is expressed in terms of ertugliflozin.

Ertugliflozin Monotherapy

The recommended initial dosage of ertugliflozin for the management of type 2 diabetes mellitus in adults is 5 mg once daily. If well tolerated, the dosage may be increased to 15 mg once daily in patients who require additional glycemic control.

Ertugliflozin/Metformin Hydrochloride Fixed-combination Therapy

When the commercially available fixed-combination preparation containing ertugliflozin and immediate-release metformin hydrochloride (Segluromet®) is used in patients with type 2 diabetes mellitus, the recommended initial dosage is based on the patient's current regimen of ertugliflozin and/or metformin hydrochloride. The dosage of the fixed combination may be increased gradually based on effectiveness and tolerability. The total dosage of the drugs in the fixed combination should not exceed 15 mg of ertugliflozin and 2 g of metformin hydrochloride daily.

For patients currently receiving metformin hydrochloride, the recommended initial total daily dosage of the fixed combination is 5 mg of ertugliflozin (using the fixed-combination tablets containing 2.5 mg of ertugliflozin) and a metformin hydrochloride dosage similar to the patient's existing total daily dosage, administered in 2 divided doses.

For patients currently receiving ertugliflozin, the recommended initial total daily dosage of the fixed combination is 1 g of metformin hydrochloride and an ertugliflozin dosage similar to the patient's existing total daily dosage, administered in 2 divided doses.

For patients currently receiving both ertugliflozin and metformin hydrochloride as separate components, the initial total daily dosage of the fixed combination is the same daily dosage of ertugliflozin and a metformin hydrochloride dosage similar to the patient's existing total daily dosage, administered in 2 divided doses.

Ertugliflozin/Sitagliptin Fixed-combination Therapy

The recommended initial dosage of the fixed combination of ertugliflozin and sitagliptin is 5 mg of ertugliflozin and 100 mg of sitagliptin once daily in the morning without regard to meals. If tolerated, the dosage may be increased to a dosage of 15 mg of ertugliflozin and 100 mg of sitagliptin in patients who require additional glycemic control. In patients currently receiving ertugliflozin and switching to the fixed combination of ertugliflozin and sitagliptin therapy, the current dosage of ertugliflozin can be maintained.

● Special Populations

Hepatic Impairment

Dosage adjustments of ertugliflozin or the fixed combination of ertugliflozin and sitagliptin are not necessary in patients with mild or moderate hepatic impairment. Data are lacking on use of ertugliflozin or the fixed combination of ertugliflozin and sitagliptin in patients with severe hepatic impairment, and the manufacturer states that such use is not recommended. The manufacturer states that the use of the fixed combination of ertugliflozin and metformin hydrochloride is not recommended in patients with hepatic impairment.

Renal Impairment

Dosage adjustments of ertugliflozin or the fixed combinations of ertugliflozin and metformin hydrochloride or ertugliflozin and sitagliptin are not necessary in patients with mild renal impairment (estimated glomerular filtration rate [eGFR] 60–89 mL/minute per 1.73 m²). Initiation of ertugliflozin or the fixed combinations of ertugliflozin and metformin hydrochloride or ertugliflozin and sitagliptin is not recommended in patients with an eGFR of 30 to less than 60 mL/minute per 1.73 m². Continued use of ertugliflozin or the fixed combinations of ertugliflozin and metformin hydrochloride or ertugliflozin and sitagliptin is not recommended in patients with an eGFR persistently between 30 and less than 60 mL/minute per 1.73 m². The use of ertugliflozin or the fixed combinations of ertugliflozin and metformin hydrochloride or ertugliflozin and sitagliptin is contraindicated in patients with an eGFR less than 30 mL/minute per 1.73 m². (See Renal Impairment under Warnings/Precautions: Specific Populations, in Cautions.)

CAUTIONS

● Contraindications

History of serious hypersensitivity reaction to ertugliflozin or any ingredient in the formulation.

Severe renal impairment (estimated glomerular filtration rate [eGFR] less than 30 mL/minute per 1.73 m²), end-stage renal disease (ESRD), or on dialysis.

● Warnings/Precautions

Hypotension

Ertugliflozin may cause intravascular volume contraction. Following initiation of ertugliflozin, symptomatic hypotension can occur, particularly in patients with impaired renal function (eGFR less than 60 mL/minute per 1.73 m²), geriatric patients, patients with low systolic blood pressure, or patients receiving diuretics. (See Drug Interactions: Diuretics.) Prior to initiating ertugliflozin in such patients, intravascular volume status should be assessed and corrected. Patients should be monitored for signs and symptoms of hypotension after initiating ertugliflozin therapy.

Ketoacidosis

Use of sodium glucose cotransporter 2 (SGLT2) inhibitors in patients with type 1 or 2 diabetes mellitus may lead to ketoacidosis requiring hospitalization. In clinical studies, ketoacidosis was reported in 0.1% of patients who received ertugliflozin; ketoacidosis was not reported in any of the comparator-treated patients. Ketoacidosis associated with use of SGLT2 inhibitors may be present without markedly elevated blood glucose concentrations (e.g., less than 250 mg/dL).

FDA identified 73 cases of acidosis (reported as diabetic ketoacidosis [DKA], ketoacidosis, or ketosis) associated with SGLT2 inhibitor use in the FDA Adverse Event Reporting System (FAERS) between March 2013 and May 2015. DKA had an atypical presentation in most of the reported cases in that type 2 diabetes mellitus was noted as the indication for the drug, and glucose concentrations were only slightly elevated (median: 211 mg/dL); type 1 diabetes mellitus was named as the indication in a few cases, and in some reports the indication was not specified. The median time to onset of symptoms of acidosis following initiation or increase in dosage of the SGLT2 inhibitor was 43 days (range: 1–365 days). No trend demonstrating a relationship between the dosage of an SGLT2 inhibitor and the risk of ketoacidosis was identified. In all reported episodes, a diagnosis of DKA or ketoacidosis was made by the clinician and hospitalization or treatment in an emergency department was warranted. In most cases, at least 1 diagnostic laboratory criterion suggestive of ketoacidosis (e.g., high anion gap metabolic acidosis, ketonemia, reduced serum bicarbonate) was reported. Potential factors for the development of ketoacidosis with SGLT2 inhibitor therapy identified in the 73 cases included infection, low carbohydrate diet or reduced caloric intake (due to illness or surgery), pancreatic disorders suggesting insulin deficiency (e.g., type 1 diabetes mellitus, history of pancreatitis, pancreatic surgery), reduced dosage or discontinuance of insulin, discontinuance of an oral insulin secretagogue, and alcohol use.

Prior to initiating therapy with an SGLT2 inhibitor, clinicians should consider patient factors that may predispose the patient to ketoacidosis such as pancreatic insulin deficiency from any cause, reduced caloric intake, and alcohol abuse.

Clinicians should evaluate for the presence of acidosis, including ketoacidosis, in patients experiencing signs or symptoms of acidosis while receiving SGLT2 inhibitors, regardless of the patient's blood glucose concentration. For patients who undergo scheduled surgery, temporary discontinuation of ertugliflozin for at least 4 days prior to surgery should be considered. Clinicians should consider monitoring for ketoacidosis and temporarily discontinuing therapy with an SGLT2 inhibitor in other clinical situations known to predispose individuals to ketoacidosis (e.g., prolonged fasting due to acute illness or post-surgery). If acidosis is confirmed, the SGLT2 inhibitor should be discontinued and appropriate treatment initiated to correct the acidosis; glucose concentrations should be monitored appropriately. In addition, supportive medical treatment should be instituted to treat and correct factors that may have precipitated or contributed to the metabolic acidosis. Risk factors for the development of ketoacidosis should be resolved prior to restarting ertugliflozin therapy.

Euglycemic DKA associated with SGLT2 inhibitors may be detected and potentially prevented by having patients monitor urine and/or plasma ketone levels if they feel unwell, regardless of ambient glucose concentrations. Clinicians should inform patients and caregivers of the signs and symptoms of ketoacidosis (e.g., tachypnea or hyperventilation, anorexia, abdominal pain, nausea, vomiting, lethargy, mental status changes) and instruct patients to discontinue the SGLT2 inhibitor and immediately seek medical attention should they experience such signs or symptoms.

Renal Effects

Ertugliflozin causes intravascular volume contraction and can cause renal impairment. Ertugliflozin increases serum creatinine concentrations and decreases eGFR; patients with impaired renal function may be more susceptible to these changes. Adverse effects related to renal function can occur following initiation of the drug. Renal function should be evaluated prior to initiation of ertugliflozin and periodically thereafter.

FDA identified 101 cases of acute kidney injury associated with canagliflozin or dapagliflozin therapy in FAERS between March 2013 and October 2015. Hospitalization for evaluation and management of kidney injury was warranted in most cases, and some cases required admission to an intensive care unit and dialysis. In approximately half of the cases, onset of acute kidney injury occurred within 1 month or less of initiating canagliflozin or dapagliflozin therapy, and most patients' kidney function improved after stopping the drug. However, kidney injury may not be fully reversible in some situations and has led to death in some patients.

Prior to initiating ertugliflozin therapy, clinicians should consider patient factors that may predispose the patient to acute kidney injury, including hypovolemia, chronic renal insufficiency, heart failure, and concomitant medications (e.g., diuretics, angiotensin-converting enzyme [ACE] inhibitors, angiotensin II receptor antagonists, nonsteroidal anti-inflammatory agents [NSAIAs]). Clinicians should consider temporarily discontinuing ertugliflozin in any setting of reduced oral intake (e.g., acute illness, fasting) or fluid losses (e.g., GI illness, excessive heat exposure). Patients should be monitored for acute kidney injury and the drug should be discontinued and appropriate treatment should be initiated if such injury occurs.

Urosepsis and Pyelonephritis

Treatment with an SGLT2 inhibitor increases the risk for urinary tract infections.

Cases of serious urinary tract infections, including urosepsis and pyelonephritis, have been reported in patients receiving an SGLT2 inhibitor. FDA identified 19 cases of urosepsis and pyelonephritis, which began as urinary tract infections associated with SGLT2 inhibitor use, in FAERS between March 2013 and October 2014. In all cases reported, hospitalization was warranted and some patients required admission to an intensive care unit or dialysis for treatment. The median time to onset of infection following initiation of the SGLT2 inhibitor was 45 days (range: 2–270 days).

Prior to initiating therapy with an SGLT2 inhibitor, clinicians should consider patient factors that may predispose the patient to serious urinary tract infections such as a history of difficulty urinating or infections of the bladder, kidneys, or urinary tract. Patients should be monitored for urinary tract infections and treatment instituted if indicated.

Lower Limb Amputation

In 2 randomized, placebo-controlled studies evaluating the effects of another drug in the SGLT2 inhibitor class (canagliflozin) on the risk of cardiovascular disease and the overall safety and tolerability of the drug, canagliflozin-treated patients had a twofold increased risk of lower limb (leg and foot) amputations (mostly affecting the toes and midfoot) compared with placebo recipients. (See Lower Limb Amputation under Warnings/Precautions: Warnings, in Cautions, in Canagliflozin 68:20.18.) In clinical trials conducted with ertugliflozin, nontraumatic lower limb amputations were reported in 0.2 or 0.5% of patients receiving ertugliflozin 5 or 15 mg daily, respectively, compared with 0.1% of patients receiving a comparator drug. A causal association between ertugliflozin and lower limb amputation has not been established. Prior to initiating therapy with ertugliflozin, clinicians should consider patient factors that may predispose them to the need for amputation, such as a history of amputation, peripheral vascular disease, neuropathy, or diabetic foot ulcers. Clinicians should monitor patients receiving ertugliflozin for the presence of infection (including osteomyelitis), new pain or tenderness, and sores or ulcers involving the lower limbs; ertugliflozin should be discontinued if such complications occur. Patients should also be counseled on the importance of routine preventative foot care.

Concomitant Therapy with Hypoglycemic Agents

When ertugliflozin is added to therapy with an insulin secretagogue (e.g., a sulfonylurea) or insulin, the incidence of hypoglycemia is increased compared with sulfonylurea or insulin monotherapy. Therefore, patients receiving ertugliflozin may require a reduced dosage of the concomitant insulin secretagogue or insulin to reduce the risk of hypoglycemia.

Fournier Gangrene

Fournier gangrene (necrotizing fasciitis of the perineum), a rare but serious or life-threatening bacterial infection requiring urgent surgical intervention, has been reported during postmarketing surveillance in men and women with type 2 diabetes mellitus receiving an SGLT2 inhibitor. Permanent disfigurement, prolonged hospitalization, disability, and complications from sepsis all may be caused by Fournier gangrene. Although diabetes mellitus is a risk factor for developing Fournier gangrene, this condition is still rare among patients with diabetes mellitus.

FDA identified 12 cases of Fournier gangrene in patients taking an SGLT2 inhibitor reported in FAERS and medical literature between March 2013 and May 2018. Since FDA's review, additional cases of Fournier gangrene have been reported. In the initial cases reviewed by FDA, the average time to onset of infection was 9.2 months (range 7 days to 25 months) after initiating therapy with an SGLT2 inhibitor. Some experts speculate that the variation in time to diagnosis of Fournier gangrene might be due to fluctuating glycemic control, microvascular complications, or an inciting event associated with SGLT2 inhibitors (e.g., urinary tract infection, mycotic infection, skin or mucosal breakdown due to pruritus). In all cases reported, hospitalization and surgery were required. Among these cases, some patients required multiple disfiguring surgeries, some developed complications (e.g., diabetic ketoacidosis, acute kidney injury, septic shock), and 1 patient died. In a review of other antidiabetic drugs (e.g., insulin, biguanides, sulfonylureas, dipeptidyl peptidase-4 inhibitors) over a period of more than 30 years, only 6 cases of Fournier gangrene were identified; all of theses cases occurred in men.

Patients receiving ertugliflozin who develop pain or tenderness, erythema, or swelling in the genital or perineal area, in addition to fever or malaise, should be assessed for necrotizing fasciitis. If Fournier gangrene is suspected, ertugliflozin should be discontinued and treatment should be initiated with broad-spectrum antibiotics; surgical debridement should be performed if necessary. Blood glucose concentrations should be closely monitored; alternative antidiabetic agents should be initiated to maintain glycemic control.

Genital Mycotic Infections

Ertugliflozin increases the risk of genital mycotic infections in males (e.g., balanitis) and females (e.g., vulvovaginal mycotic infection). Patients with a history of genital mycotic infections and uncircumcised males are at an increased risk for developing genital mycotic infections. Patients should be monitored for genital mycotic infections and appropriate treatment should be instituted if these infections occur.

Risk of Bone Fracture

An increased risk of bone fracture, along with dose-related decreases in bone mineral density in older adults, has been observed in patients receiving another drug in the SGLT2 inhibitor class (canagliflozin). (See Risk of Bone Fracture under Warnings/Precautions: Other Warnings/Precautions, in Cautions, in Canagliflozin 68:20.18.) FDA is continuing to evaluate the risk of bone fracture with SGLT2 inhibitors.

Effects on Lipoproteins

Increases in low-density lipoprotein (LDL)-cholesterol can occur during ertugliflozin therapy. Serum LDL-cholesterol concentrations should be monitored during treatment with ertugliflozin and such lipid elevations treated according to the standard of care.

Laboratory Test Interferences

SGLT2 inhibitors such as ertugliflozin increase urinary glucose excretion and will result in false-positive urine glucose tests. In addition, the manufacturer states that the 1,5-anhydroglucitol assay is unreliable for monitoring glycemic control in patients taking SGLT2 inhibitors. Alternative methods of monitoring glycemic control should be used in patients receiving SGLT2 inhibitors.

Use of Fixed Combinations

When ertugliflozin is used in fixed combination with metformin, sitagliptin, or other drugs, the cautions, precautions, contraindications, and interactions associated with the concomitant agent(s) should be considered in addition to those associated with ertugliflozin.

Specific Populations

Pregnancy

Based on the results of reproductive and developmental toxicity studies in animals, ertugliflozin use during pregnancy may affect renal development and maturation, especially during the second and third trimesters of pregnancy. Limited data with ertugliflozin in pregnant women are not sufficient to determine a drug-associated risk for major birth defects or miscarriage, and poorly controlled diabetes mellitus during pregnancy carries risks to the mother and fetus; however, ertugliflozin therapy is not recommended in pregnant women during the second and third trimesters of pregnancy.

Lactation

Ertugliflozin is distributed into milk in rats; it is not known whether the drug is distributed into human milk. Because many drugs are distributed into human milk and because of the potential for serious adverse reactions in nursing infants from ertugliflozin, a decision should be made whether to discontinue nursing or the drug, taking into account the importance of the drug to the woman.

Pediatric Use

Safety and efficacy of ertugliflozin have not been established in pediatric patients younger than 18 years of age.

Geriatric Use

In clinical trials, 25.7% of patients were 65 years of age or older and 4.5% were 75 years of age or older. Geriatric patients receiving ertugliflozin were more likely to experience certain adverse reactions related to volume depletion compared with younger patients. Ertugliflozin is expected to have diminished efficacy in geriatric patients with renal impairment.

Hepatic Impairment

Compared with values in individuals with normal hepatic function, ertugliflozin area under the concentration-time curve (AUC) and peak plasma concentrations were decreased by 13 and 21%, respectively, in patients with moderate hepatic impairment (Child-Pugh class B); however, these decreases are not considered clinically meaningful. The plasma protein binding of ertugliflozin is unaffected in patients with moderate hepatic impairment. Data are lacking on the use of ertugliflozin in patients with severe hepatic impairment (Child-Pugh class C), and such use is not recommended.

Renal Impairment

Renal function should be assessed prior to initiation of ertugliflozin therapy and periodically thereafter.

Safety and efficacy of ertugliflozin have not been established in patients with moderate renal impairment (estimated glomerular filtration rate [eGFR] 30–59 mL/minute per 1.73 m²). The safety and efficacy of ertugliflozin were evaluated in adults with moderate renal impairment (mean eGFR: 47 mL/minute per 1.73 m²) and type 2 diabetes mellitus inadequately controlled on diet and exercise with or without other antidiabetic agents (a biguanide [24.6%], a dipeptidyl peptidase-4 [DPP-4] inhibitor [13.5%], a glucagon-like peptide-1 [GLP-1] receptor agonist [2.8%], insulin [55.9%], a sulfonylurea [40.3%], other [5.4%]). The addition of ertugliflozin 5 or 15 mg administered once daily to background antidiabetic agents did not improve glycemic control compared with placebo. Additionally, patients who received ertugliflozin had an increased risk of renal impairment, renal-related adverse effects, and adverse effects related to volume depletion compared with placebo-treated patients.

Ertugliflozin is not expected to be effective in patients with severe renal impairment (including those with end-stage renal disease [ESRD]) or those undergoing dialysis; the drug is contraindicated in such patients. (See Contraindications.)

In patients with mild (eGFR 60–89 mL/minute per 1.73 m²), moderate (eGFR 30–59 mL/minute per 1.73 m²), or severe (eGFR less than 30 mL/minute per 1.73 m²) renal impairment, AUC of ertugliflozin was increased by 1.6-, 1.7-, or 1.6-fold, respectively, compared with those with normal renal function. However, these increases are not considered clinically important. In patients receiving ertugliflozin, 24-hour urinary glucose excretion declined with increasing severity of renal impairment. Plasma protein binding of ertugliflozin was unaffected in patients with renal impairment.

● Common Adverse Effects

Adverse effects reported in at least 2% of patients receiving ertugliflozin in clinical trials and more commonly than with placebo include female genital mycotic infection, male genital mycotic infection, urinary tract infection, headache, vaginal pruritus, increased urination, nasopharyngitis, back pain, decreased weight, and thirst.

DRUG INTERACTIONS

The major metabolic pathway for ertugliflozin is glucuronidation; the drug is principally glucuronidated by uridine diphosphate-glucuronosyltransferase (UGT) isoenzymes 1A9 and 2B7.

● Drugs Affecting or Metabolized by Hepatic Microsomal Enzymes

Ertugliflozin in minimally metabolized by cytochrome P-450 (CYP) isoenzymes. Ertugliflozin and ertugliflozin glucuronides (clinically inactive metabolites) did not inhibit CYP isoenzymes 1A2, 2B6, 2C9, 2C19, 2C8, 2D6, or 3A4 and did not induce CYP isoenzymes 1A2, or 3A4 in vitro. Additionally, the drug is not a time-dependent inhibitor of CYP3A in vitro. Pharmacokinetic interactions are unlikely with drugs that are metabolized by these CYP isoenzymes.

● Drugs Affecting or Affected by Organic Anion Transporters

Ertugliflozin is not a substrate of organic anion transporter (OAT) 1 or OAT3. Ertugliflozin and ertugliflozin glucuronides did not meaningfully inhibit OAT1 or OAT3; pharmacokinetic interactions are unlikely with substrates of OAT1 or OAT3.

● Drugs Affecting or Affected by Organic Cation Transporters

Ertugliflozin is not a substrate of organic cation transporter (OCT) 1 or OCT2. Ertugliflozin and ertugliflozin glucuronides did not meaningfully inhibit OCT2; pharmacokinetic interactions are unlikely with substrates of OCT2.

● Drugs Affecting or Affected by P-glycoprotein Transport

Ertugliflozin is a P-glycoprotein (P-gp) substrate. Ertugliflozin and ertugliflozin glucuronides did not meaningfully inhibit P-gp. Ertugliflozin is unlikely to affect the pharmacokinetics of concomitantly administered P-gp substrates.

● Drugs Affected by Uridine Diphosphate-glucuronosyltransferase

Ertugliflozin did not inhibit UGT isoenzymes 1A6, 1A9, or 2B7 in vitro and was a weak inhibitor of UGT1A1 and 1A4. Ertugliflozin glucuronides did not inhibit UGT1A1, 1A4, 1A6, 1A9, or 2B7 in vitro. Pharmacokinetic interactions are unlikely with drugs that are metabolized by these enzymes.

● Drugs Affecting Breast Cancer Resistance Protein

Ertugliflozin is a substrate of breast cancer resistance protein (BCRP).

● Drugs Affecting or Affected by Organic Anion Transport Polypeptides

Ertugliflozin is not a substrate of organic anion transport polypeptides (OATP) 1B1 or 1B3. Ertugliflozin and ertugliflozin glucuronides did not meaningfully inhibit OATP1B1 or OATP1B3; pharmacokinetic interactions are unlikely with substrates of OATP1B1 or OATP1B3.

● Diuretics

Concomitant use of ertugliflozin with diuretics may increase the incidence of symptomatic hypotension. Prior to initiation of ertugliflozin, volume status should be assessed and corrected in patients receiving diuretics. Patients should be monitored for signs and symptoms of symptomatic hypotension following initiation of ertugliflozin therapy.

● Mefenamic Acid

Concomitant use of mefenamic acid, a UGT inhibitor, and ertugliflozin increased ertugliflozin peak plasma concentration and area under the concentration-time curve (AUC) by 1.51- and 1.19-fold, respectively. These increases are not considered to be clinically relevant.

● *Metformin*

Administration of a single dose of metformin hydrochloride (1 g) with a single dose of ertugliflozin (15 mg) did not have a clinically meaningful effect on the pharmacokinetics of ertugliflozin or metformin. No adjustment of ertugliflozin dosage is necessary when used concomitantly with metformin.

● *Rifampin*

Administration of rifampin (600 mg once daily) with a single dose of ertugliflozin (15 mg) decreased ertugliflozin peak plasma concentration and AUC by 15 and 39%, respectively. No adjustment of ertugliflozin dosage is necessary when used concomitantly with rifampin.

● *Simvastatin*

Administration of a single dose of simvastatin (40 mg) with a single dose of ertugliflozin (15 mg) did not have a clinically meaningful effect on the pharmacokinetics of ertugliflozin or simvastatin. No adjustment of ertugliflozin dosage is necessary when used concomitantly with simvastatin.

● *Sitagliptin*

Administration of a single dose of sitagliptin (100 mg) with a single dose of ertugliflozin (15 mg) did not have a clinically meaningful effect on the pharmacokinetics of ertugliflozin or sitagliptin. No adjustment of ertugliflozin dosage is necessary when used concomitantly with sitagliptin.

● *Sulfonylureas or Insulin*

When ertugliflozin is added to therapy with an insulin secretagogue (e.g., a sulfonylurea) or insulin, the incidence of hypoglycemia is increased compared with sulfonylurea or insulin monotherapy. Patients receiving ertugliflozin may require a reduced dosage of the concomitant insulin secretagogue or insulin to reduce the risk of hypoglycemia.

Glimepiride

Administration of a single dose of glimepiride (1 mg) with a single dose of ertugliflozin (15 mg) did not have a clinically important effect on the pharmacokinetics of glimepiride or ertugliflozin.

DESCRIPTION

Ertugliflozin is a reversible and highly selective inhibitor of sodium-glucose cotransporter 2 (SGLT2), a transporter that is expressed in the proximal renal tubules and is responsible for most of the reabsorption of filtered glucose from the tubular lumen. Through inhibition of SGLT2, ertugliflozin reduces reabsorption of filtered glucose and lowers the renal threshold for glucose in a dose-dependent manner, leading to increased urinary glucose excretion; increased glucose excretion is independent of insulin secretion.

Following oral administration of ertugliflozin in the fasting state, peak plasma concentration is attained in 1 hour. Following oral administration of a 15-mg dose of ertugliflozin, the absolute oral bioavailability of the drug is 100%. Administration of ertugliflozin with a high-fat, high-calorie meal decreased peak plasma ertugliflozin concentration by 29% and prolonged time to peak plasma concentration by 1 hour, but did not alter the area under the concentration-time curve (AUC). These changes are not considered clinically meaningful and ertugliflozin can be administered with or without food. Ertugliflozin is 93.6% protein bound. Renal or hepatic impairment does not meaningfully alter plasma protein binding. Ertugliflozin is principally metabolized by uridine diphosphate-glucuronosyltransferase (UGT) 1A9 and UGT2B7 to inactive metabolites. Following oral administration of a radiolabeled 25-mg dose of ertugliflozin, 41% of the total radioactivity was excreted in urine and 50% was excreted in feces, with 1.5 or approximately 33.8% of the administered dose recovered as parent drug in urine or feces, respectively. The mean elimination half-life of ertugliflozin is approximately 16.6 hours.

ADVICE TO PATIENTS

When ertugliflozin is used in fixed combination with other drugs, importance of informing patients of important cautionary information about the concomitant agent(s).

Importance of patient reading medication guide before initiating therapy and each time the drug is dispensed.

Importance of informing patients of the potential risks and benefits of ertugliflozin-containing therapy and of alternative therapies.

Importance of informing patients about the importance of adherence to dietary instructions, regular physical activity, periodic blood glucose monitoring and glycosylated hemoglobin (hemoglobin A_{1c}; HbA_{1c}) testing, recognition and management of hypoglycemia and hyperglycemia, and assessment of diabetes mellitus complications.

Importance of promptly seeking medical advice during periods of stress such as fever, trauma, infection, or surgery as medication requirements may change.

Importance of taking ertugliflozin exactly as directed by the clinician. Importance of advising patients about what to do if a dose of ertugliflozin is missed. (See Dosage and Administration: Administration.)

Importance of informing patients that the incidence of hypoglycemia may be increased if ertugliflozin is used concomitantly with insulin and/or an insulin secretagogue. Importance of informing patients that a lower dosage of insulin or insulin secretagogue may be required to reduce the risk of hypoglycemia if used concomitantly with ertugliflozin.

Importance of informing patients that symptomatic hypotension may occur with ertugliflozin and advising patients to report such symptoms to their clinician. Inform patients that ertugliflozin-induced dehydration may increase the risk of hypotension and that patients should maintain adequate fluid intake.

Importance of informing patients that ketoacidosis, which can be a life-threatening condition, has been reported with ertugliflozin therapy (sometimes associated with illness or surgery, among other risk factors). Importance of informing patients receiving ertugliflozin and their caregivers of the signs and symptoms of ketoacidosis (e.g., tachypnea or hyperventilation, anorexia, abdominal pain, nausea, vomiting, lethargy, mental status changes) and importance of instructing patients to discontinue ertugliflozin and seek medical attention immediately should they experience any such signs or symptoms. Advise patients to use a ketone dipstick to check for ketones in their urine (when possible) if symptoms of ketoacidosis occur, even if blood glucose is not elevated (e.g., less than 250 mg/dL).

Importance of informing patients that acute kidney injury has been reported with ertugliflozin therapy. Advise patients to seek medical advice immediately if they have reduced oral intake (such as due to acute illness or fasting) or increased fluid losses (such as due to vomiting, diarrhea, or excessive heat exposure), as it may be appropriate to temporarily discontinue ertugliflozin in those settings. Importance of regular renal function testing during ertugliflozin therapy.

Importance of informing patients receiving ertugliflozin of the potential for urinary tract infections, which may be serious. Advise patients of the signs and symptoms of urinary tract infection and the need to contact a clinician if such signs and symptoms occur.

Importance of informing patients of the potentially increased risk of amputation with ertugliflozin therapy. Advise patients of the importance of routine preventative foot care. Advise patients to monitor for new pain, tenderness, sores or ulcers, or infections involving the leg or foot, and to seek prompt medical advice if such signs or symptoms develop.

Importance of informing patients that necrotizing infections of the perineum (Fournier gangrene) have occurred with sodium-glucose cotransporter 2 (SGLT2) inhibitor therapy. Advise patients to promptly seek medical attention if they develop pain or tenderness, redness, or swelling of the genitals or the area from the genitals back to the rectum, in addition to fever (above 38°C) or malaise.

Importance of informing patients that yeast infection may occur (e.g., vulvovaginitis, balanitis, balanoposthitis). Importance of informing female patients of the signs and symptoms of vaginal yeast infections (e.g., vaginal discharge, odor, itching) and male patients of the signs and symptoms of balanitis or balanoposthitis (e.g., rash or redness of the glans or foreskin of the penis). Advise patients of treatment options and when to seek medical advice.

Importance of informing patients that due to the mechanism of action of ertugliflozin, patients taking the drug will test positive for glucose in their urine. Importance of not using urine glucose tests to monitor glycemic status while taking ertugliflozin. (See Laboratory Test Interferences under Cautions: Warnings/Precautions.)

Importance of women informing their clinicians immediately if they are or plan to become pregnant or plan to breast-feed. Advise patients that ertugliflozin use is not recommended while breast-feeding. Importance of advising pregnant women about the potential risks to the fetus if ertugliflozin is used during pregnancy. All women of childbearing potential should be advised to report pregnancy to their clinician as soon as possible. (See Specific Populations under Cautions: Warnings/Precautions.)

Importance of informing clinicians of existing or contemplated concomitant therapy, including prescription and OTC drugs and dietary or herbal supplements, as well as any concomitant illnesses.

Importance of informing patients of other important precautionary information. (See Cautions.)

PREPARATIONS

Excipients in commercially available drug preparations may have clinically important effects in some individuals; consult specific product labeling for details.

Ertugliflozin L-pyroglutamic Acid

Oral		
Tablets, film-coated	5 mg (of ertugliflozin)	**Steglatro®**, Merck
	15 mg (of ertugliflozin)	**Steglatro®**, Merck

Ertugliflozin L-pyroglutamic Acid Combinations

Oral		
Tablets, film-coated	2.5 mg (of ertugliflozin) with Metformin Hydrochloride 500 mg	**Segluromet®**, Merck
	2.5 mg (of ertugliflozin) with Metformin Hydrochloride 1 g	**Segluromet®**, Merck
	5 mg (of ertugliflozin) with Sitagliptin Phosphate 100 mg (of sitagliptin)	**Steglujan®**, Merck
	7.5 mg (of ertugliflozin) with Metformin Hydrochloride 500 mg	**Segluromet®**, Merck
	7.5 mg (of ertugliflozin) with Metformin Hydrochloride 1 g	**Segluromet®**, Merck
	15 mg (of ertugliflozin) with Sitagliptin Phosphate 100 mg (of sitagliptin)	**Steglujan®**, Merck

† Use is not currently included in the labeling approved by the US Food and Drug Administration.

Selected Revisions June 21, 2021, © Copyright, January 8, 2018, American Society of Health-System Pharmacists, Inc.

glipiZIDE

68:20.20 · SULFONYLUREAS

■ Glipizide is a sulfonylurea antidiabetic agent.

USES

● Type 2 Diabetes Mellitus

Glipizide is used as an adjunct to diet for the management of type 2 diabetes mellitus in patients whose hyperglycemia cannot be controlled by diet and exercise alone. Sulfonylureas, including glipizide, may be used in combination with one or more other oral antidiabetic agents (e.g., metformin, thiazolidinedione derivatives, α-glucosidase inhibitors) or insulin as an adjunct to diet and exercise for the management of type 2 diabetes mellitus in patients who do not achieve adequate glycemic control with diet, exercise, and oral antidiabetic agent monotherapy. Glipizide is commercially available in fixed combination with metformin for use as initial therapy in patients with type 2 diabetes mellitus whose hyperglycemia cannot be controlled by diet and exercise alone and as second-line therapy in patients with type 2 diabetes who are inadequately controlled with either sulfonylurea or metformin monotherapy.

The American Diabetes Association (ADA) currently classifies diabetes mellitus as type 1 immune mediated or idiopathic), type 2 (predominantly insulin resistance with relative insulin deficiency to predominantly an insulin secretory defect with insulin resistance), gestational diabetes mellitus, or that associated with certain conditions or syndromes (e.g., drug- or chemical-induced, hormonal, that associated with pancreatic disease, infections, specific genetic defects or syndromes). Type 1 diabetes mellitus was previously described as juvenile-onset (JOD) diabetes mellitus, since it usually occurs during youth. Type 2 diabetes mellitus was previously described as adult-onset (AODM) diabetes mellitus. However, type 1 or type 2 diabetes mellitus can occur at any age, and the current classification is based on pathogenesis (e.g., autoimmune destruction of pancreatic β cells, insulin resistance) and clinical presentation rather than on age of onset. Epidemiologic data indicate that the incidence of type 2 diabetes mellitus is increasing in children and adolescents such that 8–45% of children with newly diagnosed diabetes have nonimmune-mediated diabetes mellitus; most of these individuals have type 2 diabetes mellitus, although other types, including idiopathic or nonimmune-mediated type 1 diabetes mellitus, also have been reported.

Patients with type 2 diabetes mellitus have insulin resistance and usually have relative (rather than absolute) insulin deficiency. Most patients with type 2 diabetes mellitus (about 80–90%) are overweight or obese; obesity itself also contributes to the insulin resistance and glucose intolerance observed in these patients. Patients with type 2 diabetes mellitus who are not obese may have an increased percentage of abdominal fat, which is an indicator of increased cardiometabolic risk. While children with immune-mediated type 1 diabetes generally are not overweight, the incidence of obesity in children with this form of diabetes is increasing with the increasing incidence of obesity in the US population. Distinguishing between type 1 and type 2 diabetes in children may be difficult since obesity may occur with either type of diabetes mellitus, and autoantigens and ketosis may be present in a substantial number of children with features of type 2 diabetes mellitus (e.g., obesity, acanthosis nigricans).

Oral antidiabetic agents are *not* effective as sole therapy in patients with type 1 diabetes mellitus; insulin is necessary in these patients. Sulfonylurea antidiabetic agents are not routinely recommended in hospitalized patients with diabetes mellitus. Because of their long duration of action (24 hours with glipizide), sulfonylureas do not allow rapid dosage adjustments to meet changing needs of hospitalized patients. In addition, the risk of hypoglycemia during sulfonylurea therapy is increased in such patients with irregular eating patterns.

Patients with type 2 diabetes mellitus are *not* dependent initially on insulin (although many patients eventually require insulin for glycemic control) nor are they prone to ketosis; however, insulin may occasionally be required for correction of symptomatic or persistent hyperglycemia that is not controlled by dietary regulation or oral antidiabetic agents (e.g., sulfonylureas), and ketosis occasionally may develop during periods of severe stress (e.g., acute infections, trauma, surgery). Type 2 diabetes mellitus is a heterogeneous subclass of the disease, and subclassification criteria (e.g., basal and stimulated plasma insulin concentrations, insulin resistance)

remain to be clearly established. Endogenous insulin is present in type 2 diabetic patients, although plasma insulin concentrations may be decreased, increased, or normal. In type 2 diabetic patients, glucose-stimulated secretion of endogenous insulin is frequently, but not always, reduced and decreased peripheral sensitivity to insulin is almost always associated with glucose intolerance.

Glycemic Control and Microvascular Complications

Current evidence from epidemiologic and clinical studies supports an association between chronic hyperglycemia and the pathogenesis of microvascular complications in patients with diabetes mellitus, and results of randomized, controlled studies in patients with type 1 or type 2 diabetes mellitus indicate that intensive management of hyperglycemia with near-normalization of blood glucose and glycosylated hemoglobin (hemoglobin A_{1c} [HbA_{1c}]) concentrations provides substantial benefits in terms of reducing chronic microvascular (e.g., retinopathy, nephropathy, neuropathy) complications associated with the disease. HbA_{1c} concentration reflects the glycosylation of other proteins throughout the body as a result of recent hyperglycemia and is used as a predictor of risk for development of diabetic microvascular complications. Microvascular complications of diabetes are the principal causes of blindness and renal failure in developed countries and are more closely associated with hyperglycemia than are macrovascular complications.

In the Diabetes Control and Complications Trial (DCCT), the reduction in risk of microvascular complications in patients with type 1 diabetes mellitus correlated continuously with the reduction in HbA_{1c} concentration produced by intensive insulin treatment (e.g., a 40% reduction in risk of microvascular disease for each 10% reduction in HbA_{1c}). These data imply that any decrease in HbA_{1c} levels is beneficial and that complete normalization of blood glucose concentrations may prevent diabetic complications. Data from the largest United Kingdom Prospective Diabetes Study (UKPDS) and other smaller studies in patients with type 2 diabetes mellitus generally are consistent with the same benefits on microvascular complications as those observed with type 1 diabetes mellitus in the DCCT study.

Data from long-term follow-up (over 10 years) of UKPDS patients with type 2 diabetes mellitus who received initial therapy with conventional (diet and oral antidiabetic agents or insulin to achieve fasting plasma glucose concentrations below 270 mg/dL without symptoms of hyperglycemia) antidiabetic treatment or intensive (stepwise introduction of a sulfonylurea [i.e., chlorpropamide, glyburide], then insulin, or an oral sulfonylurea and insulin, or insulin alone to achieve fasting plasma glucose concentrations of 108 mg/dL) antidiabetic regimens indicate that intensive treatment with monotherapy generally is not capable of maintaining strict glycemic control (i.e., maintenance of blood glucose concentrations of 108 mg/dL or normal values) over time and that combination therapy eventually becomes necessary in most patients to attain target glycemic levels in the long term; in UKPDS, intensive treatment that eventually required combination therapy in most patients resulted in median HbA_{1c} concentrations of 7%. Because of the benefits of strict glycemic control, the goal of therapy for type 2 diabetes mellitus is to lower blood glucose to as close to normal as possible, which generally requires aggressive management efforts (e.g., mixing therapy with various antidiabetic agents including sulfonylureas, metformin, insulin, and/or possibly others) over time. For additional information on clinical studies demonstrating the benefits of strict glycemic control on microvascular complications in patients with type 1 or 2 diabetes mellitus, see Glycemic Control and Microvascular Complications under Uses: Diabetes Mellitus, in Metformin 68:20.04.

Glycemic Control and Macrovascular Complications

Current evidence indicates that appropriate management of dyslipidemia, blood pressure, and vascular thrombosis provides substantial benefits in terms of reducing macrovascular complications associated with diabetes mellitus; intensive glycemic control generally has not been associated with appreciable reductions in macrovascular outcomes in controlled trials. Reduction in blood pressure to a mean of 144/82 mm Hg ("tight blood pressure control") in patients with diabetes mellitus and uncomplicated mild to moderate hypertension in UKPDS substantially reduced the incidence of virtually all macrovascular (e.g., stroke, heart failure) and microvascular (e.g., retinopathy, vitreous hemorrhage, renal failure) outcomes and diabetes-related mortality; blood pressure and glycemic control were additive in their beneficial effects on these end points. While intensive antidiabetic therapy titrated with the goal of reducing HbA_{1c} to near-normal concentrations (6–6.5% or less) has not been associated with appreciable reductions in cardiovascular events during the randomized portion of controlled trials examining such outcomes, results of long-term follow-up (10–11 years) from DCCT and UKPDS indicate a delayed cardiovascular benefit in patients treated with intensive antidiabetic therapy early in the course of type 1 or type 2 diabetes mellitus. For additional details regarding the effects of intensive antidiabetic therapy on macrovascular outcomes, see Glycemic Control and Macrovascular Complications, under Uses: Diabetes Mellitus, in Metformin 68:20.04.

Treatment Goals

The ADA currently states that it is reasonable to attempt to achieve in patients with type 2 diabetes mellitus the same blood glucose and HbA$_{1c}$ goals recommended for patients with type 1 diabetes mellitus. Based on target values for blood glucose and HbA$_{1c}$ used in clinical trials (e.g., DCCT) for type 1 diabetic patients, modified somewhat to reduce the risk of severe hypoglycemia, ADA currently recommends target preprandial (fasting) and peak postprandial (1–2 hours after the *beginning* of a meal) *plasma* glucose concentrations of 70–130 and less than 180 mg/dL, respectively, and HbA$_{1c}$ concentrations of less than 7% (based on a nondiabetic range of 4–6%) *in general* in patients with type 1 or type 2 diabetes mellitus who are not pregnant. HbA$_{1c}$ concentrations of 7% or greater should prompt clinicians to initiate or adjust antidiabetic therapy in nonpregnant patients with the goal of achieving HbA$_{1c}$ concentrations of less than 7%. Patients with diabetes mellitus who have elevated HbA$_{1c}$ concentrations despite having adequate preprandial glucose concentrations should monitor glucose concentrations 1–2 hours after the start of a meal. Treatment with agents (e.g., α-glucosidase inhibitors, exenatide, pramlintide) that principally lower postprandial glucose concentrations to within target ranges also should reduce HbA$_{1c}$.

More stringent treatment goals (i.e., an HbA$_{1c}$ less than 6%) may be considered in selected patients. An *individualized* HbA$_{1c}$ concentration goal that is closer to normal without risking substantial hypoglycemia is reasonable in patients with a short duration of diabetes mellitus, no appreciable cardiovascular disease, and a long life expectancy. Less stringent treatment goals may be appropriate in patients with long-standing diabetes mellitus in whom the general HbA$_{1c}$ concentration goal of less than 7% is difficult to obtain despite adequate education on self-management of the disease, appropriate glucose monitoring, and effective dosages of multiple antidiabetic agents, including insulin. Achievement of HbA$_{1c}$ values of less than 7% is not appropriate or practical for some patients, and clinical judgment should be used in designing a treatment regimen based on the potential benefits and risks (e.g., hypoglycemia) of more intensified therapy. For additional details on individualizing treatment in patients with diabetes mellitus, see Treatment Goals under Uses: Diabetes Mellitus, in Metformin 68:20.04.

Considerations in Initiating and Maintaining Antidiabetic Therapy

When initiating therapy for patients with type 2 diabetes mellitus who do not have severe symptoms, most clinicians recommend that diet be emphasized as the primary form of treatment; caloric restriction and weight reduction are essential in obese patients. Although appropriate dietary management and weight reduction alone may be effective in controlling blood glucose concentration and symptoms of hyperglycemia, many patients receiving dietary advice fail to achieve and maintain adequate glycemic control with dietary modification alone.

Recognizing that lifestyle interventions often fail to achieve or maintain the target glycemic goal within the first year of initiation of such interventions, ADA currently suggests initiation of metformin concurrently with lifestyle interventions at the time of diagnosis of type 2 diabetes mellitus. Other experts suggest concurrent initiation of lifestyle interventions and antidiabetic agents only when HbA$_{1c}$ levels of 9% or greater are present at the time of diagnosis of type 2 diabetes mellitus. ADA and other clinicians state that lifestyle interventions should remain a principal consideration in the management of diabetes even after pharmacologic therapy is initiated. The manufacturer states that patients and clinicians should recognize that dietary management is the principal consideration in the management of diabetes mellitus and that antidiabetic therapy is used only as an adjunct to, and not as a substitute for or a convenient means to avoid, proper dietary management. In addition, loss of blood glucose control on diet alone may be temporary in some patients, requiring only short-term management with drug therapy. The importance of regular physical activity should be emphasized, and cardiovascular risk factors should be identified and corrective measures employed when feasible.

If lifestyle interventions alone are initiated and these interventions fail to reduce symptoms and/or blood glucose concentration, initiation of monotherapy with an oral antidiabetic agent (e.g., sulfonylurea, metformin, acarbose) or insulin should be considered. For more information on the stepwise approach to the management of type 2 diabetes mellitus, See Uses: Diabetes Mellitus, in Metformin 68:20.04.

Several large, long-term studies have evaluated the cardiovascular risks associated with the use of oral sulfonylurea antidiabetic agents. For information on these studies and associated recommendations, see Cautions: Precautions and Contraindications, in Glyburide 68:20.20. The ADA currently considers the beneficial effects of intensive glycemic control with insulin or sulfonylureas and blood pressure control in diabetic patients to outweigh the risks overall.

Glipizide Monotherapy

Clinical studies indicate that glipizide is as effective as chlorpropamide, glyburide, tolazamide, or tolbutamide for the management of type 2 diabetes mellitus. A relative advantage of glipizide compared with other sulfonylurea antidiabetic agents has not been clearly established. Although the glipizide-induced increase in glucose- or meal-stimulated secretion of endogenous insulin appears to be sustained during long-term therapy, the clinical importance of this effect in the long-term efficacy of the drug and any resultant therapeutic difference compared with other sulfonylureas remain to be determined. Reversal of basement-membrane thickening of muscle capillaries in asymptomatic individuals with impaired glucose tolerance (chemical diabetes) treated with glipizide has been reported, suggesting that early drug therapy to improve control of blood glucose concentration might reverse or delay microangiopathy, but this finding requires further evaluation.

Clinical trial data indicate that sulfonylureas are as effective as metformin in managing hyperglycemia (approximately 1.5% average reduction in HbA$_{1c}$ values), but sulfonylurea use is associated with hypoglycemia and weight gain. ADA generally recommends metformin as initial oral antidiabetic therapy because of the absence of weight gain or hypoglycemia, relatively low expense, and generally low adverse effect profile compared with other oral antidiabetic agents. (See Uses: Diabetes Mellitus, in Metformin 68:20.04)

Glipizide may be useful in some patients with type 2 diabetes mellitus who have primary or secondary failure to other sulfonylurea antidiabetic agents; however, primary or secondary failure to glipizide also may occur. Adequate adjustment of dosage and adherence to diet should be assessed before determining if secondary failure to glipizide has occurred. If primary or secondary failure to glipizide extended-release tablets has occurred, another oral antidiabetic agent may be added to glipizide therapy. Patients with secondary failure to one oral antidiabetic agent occasionally may respond to another agent.

Secondary failure to sulfonylurea antidiabetic agents is characterized by progressively decreasing diabetic control following 1 month to several years of good control. Interim data from a substudy (UKPD 26) of the UKPD study in newly diagnosed type 2 diabetic patients receiving intensive therapy (maintenance of fasting plasma glucose below 108 mg/dL by increasing doses of either a sulfonylurea [i.e., glyburide or chlorpropamide] to maximum recommended dosage) showed that secondary failure (defined as fasting plasma glucose exceeding 270 mg/dL or symptoms of hyperglycemia despite maximum recommended daily dosage of 20 mg of glyburide or 500 mg of chlorpropamide) occurred overall at about 7% per year. The failure rate at 6 years was 48% among patients receiving glyburide and about 40% among patients receiving chlorpropamide. In the UKPD studies, stepwise addition of insulin or metformin to therapy with maximal dosage of a sulfonylurea was required periodically over time to improve glycemic control. In another substudy (UKPD 49), progressive deterioration in diabetes control was such that monotherapy was effective in only about 50% of patients after 3 years and in only about 25% of patients after 9 years; thus, most patients require multiple-drug antidiabetic therapy over time to maintain such target levels of disease control. At diagnosis, risk factors predisposing toward sulfonylurea failure included higher fasting plasma glucose concentrations, younger age, and lower pancreatic β-cell reserve.

In some type 2 diabetic patients who are being treated with insulin, glipizide alone may be effective alternative therapy. However, glipizide is *not* effective as sole therapy in patients with diabetes mellitus complicated by acidosis, ketosis, or coma; management of these conditions requires the use of insulin.

Combination Therapy with Metformin or Other Oral Antidiabetic Agents

Sulfonylureas may be used in combination with one or more other oral antidiabetic agents (e.g., metformin, thiazolidinedione derivatives, α-glucosidase inhibitors) as an adjunct to diet and exercise for the management of type 2 diabetes mellitus in patients who do not achieve adequate glycemic control with diet, exercise, and oral antidiabetic agent monotherapy. Combined therapy with metformin or other oral antidiabetic agents generally is used in patients with longstanding type 2 diabetes mellitus who have poor glycemic control with monotherapy.

The sequence in which metformin or a sulfonylurea is used at initiation of therapy does not appear to alter the effectiveness of combined therapy with the drugs. However, ADA and other clinicians currently recommend initiating therapy with metformin and adding another antidiabetic agent, such as a sulfonylurea, insulin, or a thiazolidinedione, if patients fail to achieve or maintain target HbA$_{1c}$ goals. Optimal benefit generally is obtained by addition of a second antidiabetic agent as soon as monotherapy with metformin at the maximum tolerated dosage no longer provides adequate glycemic control (i.e., when the target glycemic goal is not achieved within 2–3 months of initiation of therapy with metformin or at any other time when the HbA$_{1c}$ goal is not achieved).

A major factor in choosing additional therapy is the degree of glycemic control obtained during metformin monotherapy. In patients with a HbA$_{1c}$ exceeding 8.5% or symptoms secondary to hyperglycemia despite metformin monotherapy, ADA states that consideration should be given to adding insulin. When glycemic control is closer to the target HbA$_{1c}$ goal with metformin monotherapy (e.g., HbA$_{1c}$ less than 7.5%), agents with a lesser potential to lower hyperglycemia and/or slower onset of action may be considered (e.g., sulfonylurea, thiazolidinedione) as additional therapy to metformin. ADA states that other antidiabetic agents such as α-glucosidase inhibitors, meglitinides, exenatide, and pramlintide generally are less effective, less well studied, and/or more expensive than recommended therapies (i.e., metformin, sulfonylurea, thiazolidinedione, insulin). However, these agents may be appropriate for treatment of type 2 diabetes mellitus in selected patients.

Glipizide is used in fixed combination with metformin as initial therapy in the management of patients with type 2 diabetes mellitus whose hyperglycemia cannot be controlled by diet and exercise alone. In a comparative study in such patients, therapy with the fixed combination of glipizide and metformin was more effective in improving glycemic control (as determined by HbA$_{1c}$ values, fasting plasma glucose concentrations) than monotherapy with either component. A greater percentage of patients receiving the fixed combination achieved strict glycemic control (HbA$_{1c}$ values below 7%) than did those receiving metformin or glipizide monotherapy.

Glipizide also is used in fixed combination with metformin as second-line therapy in patients with type 2 diabetes whose hyperglycemia is inadequately controlled with either sulfonylurea or metformin monotherapy. In a comparative study, greater glycemic control (as determined by HbA$_{1c}$ values and fasting plasma glucose concentrations) was achieved with the fixed combination of glipizide and metformin than with either drug as monotherapy. Strict glycemic control (e.g., HbA$_{1c}$ values less than 7%) also was achieved in a greater percentage of patients receiving the fixed combination of glipizide and metformin.

When lifestyle interventions, metformin, and a second oral antidiabetic agent are not effective in maintaining the target glycemic goal in patients with type 2 diabetes mellitus, ADA and other clinicians generally recommend the addition of insulin therapy. In patients whose HbA$_{1c}$ is close to the target level (less than 8%) on metformin and a second oral antidiabetic agent, addition of a third oral antidiabetic agent instead of insulin may be considered. However, ADA states that triple combination oral antidiabetic therapy is more costly and potentially not as effective as adding insulin therapy to dual combination oral antidiabetic therapy.

Combination Therapy with Insulin

Combined therapy with insulin and oral antidiabetic agents may be useful in some patients with type 2 diabetes mellitus whose blood glucose concentrations are not adequately controlled with maximal dosages of the oral agent and/or as a means of providing increased flexibility with respect to timing of meals and amount of food ingested. Concomitant therapy with insulin (e.g., given as intermediate- or long-acting insulin at bedtime or rapid-acting insulin at meal times) and one or more oral antidiabetic agents appears to improve glycemic control with lower dosages of insulin than would be required with insulin alone and may decrease the potential for body weight gain associated with insulin therapy. Oral antidiabetic therapy combined with insulin therapy may delay progression to either intensive insulin monotherapy or to a second daytime injection of insulin combined with oral antidiabetic agents. Preliminary data indicate that combination therapy with glipizide and insulin may be useful in some type 2 diabetic patients. However, combined therapy may increase the risk of hypoglycemic reactions.

ADA and other clinicians state that combined therapy with insulin and metformin with or without other oral antidiabetic agents is one of several options for the management of hyperglycemia in patients not responding adequately to oral monotherapy with metformin, the preferred initial oral antidiabetic agent. In patients with a HbA$_{1c}$ exceeding 8.5% or symptoms secondary to hyperglycemia despite metformin monotherapy, ADA states that consideration should be given to adding insulin. When patients are not controlled with metformin with or without other oral antidiabetic agents (i.e., sulfonylurea, thiazolidinedione) and basal insulin (e.g., given as intermediate- or long-acting insulin at bedtime or in the morning), therapy with insulin should be intensified by adding additional short-acting or rapid-acting insulin injections at mealtimes. Therapy with insulin secretagogues (i.e., sulfonylureas, meglitinides) should be tapered and discontinued when intensive insulin therapy is initiated, as insulin secretagogues do not appear to be synergistic with such insulin therapy.

For additional information on combination therapy with sulfonylureas and other oral antidiabetic agents, see the sections on combination therapy in Uses in the individual monographs in 68:20.

DOSAGE AND ADMINISTRATION

● Administration

Glipizide is administered orally. The extended-release tablets should be swallowed whole and should *not* be divided, chewed, or crushed. Patients receiving the extended-release tablets become alarmed if they notice a tablet-like substance in their stools; this is normal since the tablet containing the drug is designed to remain intact and slowly release the drug from a nonabsorbable shell during passage through the GI tract.

Extended-release tablets of glipizide are administered once daily, generally with breakfast. Conventional tablets of the drug usually are administered as a single daily dose given each morning before breakfast. It is generally recommended that glipizide be administered approximately 30 minutes before a meal(s) to achieve the maximum reduction in postprandial blood glucose concentration. Once-daily dosing of glipizide at dosages up to 15–20 mg daily provides adequate control of blood glucose concentration throughout the day in most patients with usual meal patterns; however, some patients may have a more satisfactory response when the drug is administered in 2 or 3 divided doses daily as conventional tablets. When glipizide dosage exceeds 15–20 mg daily as conventional tablets, the drug should usually be administered in divided doses before meals of sufficient caloric content. The maximum once-daily dose as conventional tablets recommended by the manufacturer is 15 mg. When a divided-dosing regimen as conventional tablets is employed in patients receiving more than 15 mg of glipizide daily, the doses and schedule of administration should be individualized according to the patient's meal pattern and response. Dosages greater than 30 mg daily have been given safely in twice-daily dosing regimens for prolonged periods.

● Dosage

Dosage of glipizide must be based on blood and urine glucose determinations and must be carefully individualized to obtain optimum therapeutic effect. Patients must be closely monitored (i.e., glycosylated hemoglobin [hemoglobin A$_{1c}$, HbA$_{1c}$], fasting blood glucose concentrations) to determine the minimum effective glipizide dosage and to detect primary or secondary failure to the drug. Self-monitoring of blood glucose concentrations may provide useful information to the patient and their clinician. *If appropriate glipizide dosage regimens are not followed, hypoglycemia may be precipitated.*

Patients receiving glipizide should be monitored carefully to determine the need for continued therapy and to ensure that the drug continues to be effective; if adequate lowering of blood glucose concentration is no longer achieved during maintenance therapy, the drug should be discontinued. Following initiation of glipizide therapy and dosage titration, determination of HbA$_{1c}$ concentrations at intervals of approximately 3 months is the preferred method for assessing the patient's continued response to therapy. While fasting blood glucose concentrations generally reach steady-state following initiation or change in glipizide dosage, a single fasting blood glucose determination may not accurately assess glycemic response. If fasting blood glucose concentrations are used to assess the need for dosage adjustments, 2 consecutive determinations of similar value should be obtained 7 or more days after the previous dosage adjustment. Patients who do not adhere to their prescribed dietary and drug regimens are more likely to have an unsatisfactory response to therapy. In patients usually well controlled by dietary management alone, short-term therapy with glipizide may be sufficient during periods of transient loss of diabetic control.

Initial Dosage in Previously Untreated Patients

For the management of type 2 diabetes mellitus in patients not previously receiving insulin or sulfonylurea antidiabetic agents, the recommended initial adult dosage of glipizide is 5 mg daily as conventional or extended-release tablets; in geriatric patients or those with hepatic disease, an initial dosage of 2.5 or 5 mg daily as conventional or extended-release tablets, respectively, may be used. Initial glipizide dosage should be conservative in debilitated, malnourished, or geriatric patients, patients with impaired renal or hepatic function, or those who may otherwise be more sensitive to oral hypoglycemic agents because of an increased risk of hypoglycemia in these patients. (See Cautions: Precautions and Contraindications.) Subsequent dosage should be adjusted according to the patient's tolerance and therapeutic response; dosage adjustments in increments of 2.5–5 mg daily at intervals of at least several days (usually 3–7 days) are recommended when conventional tablets are used. The manufacturer of extended-release glipizide tablets states that if fasting plasma glucose determinations are used to monitor response, dosage adjustment should be based on at least 2 similar consecutive values obtained at least 7 days after the previous dose adjustment.

Initial Dosage in Patients Transferred from Conventional to Extended-release Tablets

Based on results of a randomized crossover study, patients receiving conventional glipizide tablets may be switched safely to extended-release glipizide tablets by giving the nearest equivalent total daily dose once daily. Alternatively, dosage can be titrated beginning with an initial dosage of 5 mg once daily as extended-release tablets. The decision to switch to the nearest equivalent dosage versus re-titration should be individualized using clinical judgment.

Initial Dosage in Patients Transferred from Other Antidiabetic Agents

A transition period generally is not required when transferring from other sulfonylurea antidiabetic agents to glipizide, and administration of the other agent may be abruptly discontinued. Because of the prolonged elimination half-life of chlorpropamide, an exaggerated hypoglycemic response may occur in some patients during the transition from chlorpropamide to glipizide, and patients being transferred from chlorpropamide should be closely monitored for the occurrence of hypoglycemia during the initial 2 weeks of the transition period with conventional glipizide tablets or 1–2 weeks with extended-release glipizide tablets. A drug-free interval of 2–3 days may be advisable before glipizide therapy is initiated as conventional tablets in patients being transferred from chlorpropamide, particularly if blood glucose concentration was adequately controlled with chlorpropamide. An initial or loading dose of glipizide is *not* necessary when transferring from other sulfonylurea antidiabetic agents to glipizide. The transfer should be performed conservatively.

For the management of type 2 diabetes mellitus in patients previously receiving other sulfonylurea antidiabetic agents, the usual initial dosage of glipizide is 5–10 mg daily, but the initial dosage is variable and must be carefully individualized. Subsequent dosage is adjusted according to the patient's tolerance and therapeutic response. Although an exact dosage relationship between glipizide and other sulfonylurea antidiabetic agents does not exist, approximate dosage equivalencies have been estimated. (See Pharmacology: Antidiabetic Effect.)

In general, patients who were previously maintained on insulin dosages up to 20 units daily may be transferred directly to the usual recommended initial dosage of glipizide, and administration of insulin may be abruptly discontinued. In patients requiring insulin dosages greater than 20 units daily, the usual recommended initial dosage of glipizide should be started and insulin dosage reduced by 50%. Subsequently, insulin is withdrawn gradually and dosage of glipizide is adjusted in increments of 2.5–5 mg daily at intervals of at least several days, according to the patient's tolerance and therapeutic response. During the period of insulin withdrawal, patients should test their urine at least 3 times daily for glucose and ketones, and should be instructed to report the results to their physician so that appropriate adjustments in therapy may be made, if necessary; when feasible, patient or laboratory monitoring of blood glucose concentration is preferable. The presence of persistent ketonuria with glycosuria, ketosis, and/or inadequate lowering or persistent elevation of blood glucose concentration indicates that the patient requires insulin therapy. In some patients, especially those requiring greater than 40 units of insulin daily, the manufacturer suggests that it may be advisable to consider hospitalization during the transition from insulin to glipizide; however, some clinicians believe that hospitalization should rarely be necessary.

Maintenance Dosage

The adult maintenance dosage of glipizide for the management of type 2 diabetes mellitus varies considerably, ranging from 2.5–40 mg daily. Most patients appear to require 5–25 mg daily as conventional tablets or 5–10 mg daily as extended-release tablets, but some clinicians report that higher dosages may be necessary in many patients. Dosage adjustments in patients receiving glipizide extended-release tablets may be made at approximately 3-month intervals, based on HbA$_{1c}$ measurements. In patients receiving an initial dosage of 5 mg daily of extended-release glipizide tablets, dosage may be increased to 10 mg daily after 3 months if glycemic response is inadequate, based on a HbA$_{1c}$ measurement. Subsequent dosage should be adjusted according to patient's therapeutic response, using the lowest possible effective dosage. If an enhanced glycemic response is not observed after 3 months at a higher dosage, the dosage should be decreased to the previous equally effective dosage.

Maintenance dosage of glipizide should be conservative in debilitated, malnourished, or geriatric patients or patients with impaired renal or hepatic function because of an increased risk of hypoglycemia in these patients. (See Cautions: Precautions and Contraindications.) The maximum recommended dosage is 40 mg daily as conventional tablets or 20 mg daily as extended-release tablets. While glycemic control may improve with glipizide extended-release tablets in certain patients receiving dosages exceeding 10 mg daily, clinical studies to date have not demonstrated an additional group average reduction in HbA$_{1c}$ beyond what was achieved with the 10-mg daily dosage. Dosages up to 50 mg daily have been employed in some patients. Although the mechanism(s) has not been elucidated and further documentation is needed, some clinicians have reported that an increase in glipizide maintenance dosage actually resulted in a worsening of diabetic control in a few patients.

Combination Therapy with Other Oral Antidiabetic Agents

Glipizide may be used in combination with other oral antidiabetic agents if glycemic control is inadequate with glipizide, either upon initiation of therapy or after a period of effectiveness. The second oral antidiabetic agent should be added to glipizide at the lowest recommended dosage, and patients should be observed carefully. Titration of the additional oral antidiabetic agent should be based on clinical judgment.

When glipizide is added to therapy with other antidiabetic agents, glipizide extended-release tablets may be initiated at a dosage of 5 mg daily. Initiation of therapy with glipizide extended-release tablets at a lower dosage may be appropriate in patients who may be more sensitive to oral hypoglycemic agents. Titration of glipizide as add-on therapy to another oral antidiabetic agent should be based on clinical judgment.

If the fixed combination of glipizide and metformin is used as initial therapy, the recommended initial dosage is 2.5 mg of glipizide and 250 mg of metformin hydrochloride once daily with a meal. In patients with more severe hyperglycemia (i.e., fasting plasma glucose concentrations of 280–320 mg/dL), an initial dosage of 2.5 mg of glipizide and 500 mg of metformin hydrochloride twice daily may be considered. Dosage may be increased in increments of one tablet (using the tablet strength at which therapy was initiated, either 2.5 mg glipizide/250 mg metformin hydrochloride or 2.5 mg glipizide/500 mg metformin hydrochloride) daily every 2 weeks until the minimum effective dosage required to achieve adequate glycemic control or a maximum daily dosage of 10 mg of glipizide and 2 g of metformin hydrochloride given in divided doses is reached. A total daily dosage exceeding 10 mg of glipizide and 2 g of metformin hydrochloride has not been evaluated in clinical trials in patients receiving the fixed-combination preparation as initial therapy. The efficacy of glipizide in fixed combination with metformin hydrochloride has not been established in patients with fasting plasma glucose concentrations exceeding 320 mg/dL.

When the commercially available fixed-combination preparation is used as second-line therapy in patients with type 2 diabetes mellitus whose blood glucose is not adequately controlled by therapy with a sulfonylurea antidiabetic agent or metformin alone, the recommended initial dosage in previously treated patients is 2.5 or 5 mg of glipizide and 500 mg of metformin hydrochloride twice daily with the morning and evening meals. In order to minimize the risk of hypoglycemia, the initial dosage of glipizide and metformin hydrochloride in fixed combination should not exceed the daily dosage of glipizide or metformin hydrochloride previously received. The dosage of glipizide and metformin hydrochloride in fixed combination should be titrated upward in increments not exceeding 5 mg of glipizide and 500 mg of metformin hydrochloride until adequate glycemic control or a maximum daily dosage of 20 mg of glipizide and 2 g of metformin hydrochloride is reached.

For patients being switched from combination therapy using separate preparations of glipizide (or another sulfonylurea antidiabetic agent) and metformin, the initial dosage of the fixed-combination preparation should not exceed the daily dosages of glipizide (or equivalent dosage of another sulfonylurea) and metformin hydrochloride currently being taken. Such patients should be monitored for signs and symptoms of hypoglycemia following the switch. In the transfer from previous antidiabetic therapy to the fixed combination of glipizide and metformin hydrochloride, the decision to switch to the nearest equivalent dosage or to titrate dosage is based on clinical judgment. Hypoglycemia or hyperglycemia are possible in such patients, and any change in the therapy of type 2 diabetic patients should be undertaken with appropriate monitoring. The safety and efficacy of switching from combined therapy with separate preparations of glipizide (or another sulfonylurea antidiabetic agent) and metformin hydrochloride to the fixed-combination preparation containing these drugs have not been established in clinical studies.

CAUTIONS

When glipizide is used in fixed combination with metformin, the cautions, precautions, and contraindications associated with metformin must be considered in addition to those associated with glipizide.

● Hypoglycemia

Hypoglycemia may occur in patients receiving glipizide alone or in fixed combination with metformin. Hypoglycemia (defined as blood glucose of less than 60 mg/dL or symptoms associated with hypoglycemia) occurred in 3.4% of patients receiving glipizide extended-release tablets in clinical trials. *Appropriate patient selection and careful attention to dosage are important to avoid glipizide-induced hypoglycemia.* (See Cautions: Precautions and Contraindications.) Hypoglycemia may occur as a result of excessive glipizide dosage; however, since the development of hypoglycemia is a function of many factors, including diet, or exercise without adequate caloric supplementation, this effect may occur in some patients receiving usual dosages of the drug. Although glipizide-induced hypoglycemia has been reported infrequently and has usually been mild, severe hypoglycemia has occurred, principally in patients with predisposing conditions (e.g., impaired renal and/or hepatic function).

Management of glipizide-induced hypoglycemia depends on the severity of the reaction; patients with severe reactions require immediate hospitalization and treatment and observation until complete recovery is assured. Because of glipizide's elimination characteristics, the risk of prolonged hypoglycemia is likely to be low. Hypoglycemia is usually, but not always, readily controlled by administration of glucose. If hypoglycemia occurs during therapy with the drug, immediate reevaluation and adjustment of glipizide dosage and/or the patient's meal pattern are necessary.

For further discussion of the pathogenesis, manifestations, and treatment of glipizide-induced hypoglycemia, see Acute Toxicity.

● Other Endocrine and Metabolic Effects

Therapy with sulfonylureas, including glipizide, may be associated with weight gain. Although the exact mechanisms associated with such alterations in weight have not been established, suggested mechanisms include an increase in insulin secretion (which may increase appetite), stimulation of lipogenesis in fat tissue, or an increase in blood leptin concentrations. Data from the United Kingdom Prospective Diabetes (UKPD) study in patients receiving long-term therapy (over 10 years) with glyburide and other antidiabetic agents indicate that weight gain was greatest in those receiving intensive therapy (stepwise introduction of a sulfonylurea then insulin or an oral sulfonylurea and insulin, or insulin alone to achieve fasting glucose concentrations of 108 mg/dL) than conventional therapy (diet and oral antidiabetic agents or insulin to achieve fasting plasma glucose concentrations less than 270 mg/dL without symptoms of hyperglycemia), and weight gain was greatest in those initially receiving insulin or chlorpropamide compared with those receiving glyburide.

● GI Effects

Adverse GI effects such as nausea, anorexia, vomiting, pyrosis, gastralgia, diarrhea, and constipation are the most common adverse reactions to glipizide conventional tablets, occurring in about 1–2% of patients. Diarrhea or flatulence occurred in 5 or 3%, respectively, of patients receiving extended-release glipizide tablets in controlled clinical trials. Diarrhea was reported in 2.3–5.2 or 8.5% of patients receiving the fixed combination of glipizide and metformin or metformin monotherapy, respectively, as initial therapy for type 2 diabetes mellitus, and in 18.4 or 17.3% of patients receiving the fixed combination of glipizide and metformin or metformin monotherapy, respectively, as second-line therapy. Abdominal pain occurred in 5.7 or 6.7% of patients receiving the fixed combination of

glipizide and metformin or metformin monotherapy, respectively, in clinical trials as second-line therapy for type 2 diabetes mellitus. Nausea, dyspepsia, constipation, or vomiting occurred in less than 3% of patients receiving extended-release glipizide tablets in clinical trials. Anorexia, thirst, or trace blood in the stool has been reported in less than 1% of patients receiving extended-release glipizide in clinical trials. Nausea or vomiting was reported in 0.6–1.7 or 5.1% of patients receiving the fixed combination of glipizide and metformin or metformin monotherapy, respectively, as initial therapy for type 2 diabetes mellitus, and in 8% of patients receiving either the fixed combination of glipizide and metformin or metformin monotherapy as second-line therapy. Glipizide-induced adverse GI effects appear to be dose related and may subside following a reduction in dosage or administration of the drug in divided doses.

● Dermatologic Effects

Allergic skin reactions including pruritus, erythema, eczema, urticaria, and morbilliform or maculopapular eruptions occur in about 1.5% of patients receiving glipizide conventional tablets. Rash or urticaria has been reported in less than 1% of patients receiving extended-release glipizide tablets in clinical trials. Glipizide-induced adverse dermatologic effects may be transient and disappear despite continued therapy; however, if adverse dermatologic effects persist with continued glipizide therapy, the drug should be discontinued. Photosensitivity reactions and porphyria cutanea tarda have been reported with other sulfonylurea antidiabetic agents.

● Hepatic Effects

One case of glipizide-associated jaundice has been reported. Cholestatic jaundice has occurred with other sulfonylureas and is an indication for discontinuing glipizide. Although a causal relationship has not been established, mild to moderate increases in serum LDH, AST (SGOT), and alkaline phosphatase concentration have occurred occasionally in patients receiving glipizide. Exacerbation of hepatic porphyria has been reported with other sulfonylurea antidiabetic agents, but has not been reported to date with glipizide.

● Hematologic Effects

Like other sulfonylurea antidiabetic agents, glipizide may rarely cause leukopenia, thrombocytopenia, pancytopenia, agranulocytosis, aplastic anemia, and hemolytic anemia.

● Nervous System Effects

Dizziness, drowsiness, and headache have been reported in about 2% of patients receiving glipizide conventional tablets, usually as manifestations of mild hypoglycemia. Asthenia, headache, dizziness, nervousness, pain, or tremor has been reported in 10, 9, 7, or 4% of patients receiving glipizide extended-release tablets in controlled clinical trials. Headache has been reported in 12.6 or 5.3% of patients receiving the fixed combination of glipizide and metformin or metformin monotherapy, respectively, as second-line therapy for type 2 diabetes mellitus. Dizziness has been reported in 1.7–5.2 or 1.1% of patients receiving the fixed combination of glipizide and metformin or metformin monotherapy, respectively, in clinical trials as initial therapy for type 2 diabetes mellitus. Insomnia, paresthesia, anxiety, depression, and hypesthesia have been reported in less than 3% of patients receiving glipizide extended-release tablets in clinical trials. Chills, hypertonia, confusion, vertigo, somnolence, or gait abnormality has been reported in less than 1% of patients receiving extended-release glipizide in clinical trials.

● Other Adverse Effects

Arthralgia, leg cramps, or myalgia has been reported in less than 3% of patients receiving extended-release glipizide in clinical trials. Musculoskeletal pain has been reported in 8 or 6.7% of patients receiving the fixed combination of glipizide and metformin or metformin monotherapy, respectively, as second-line therapy for type 2 diabetes mellitus. Syncope has been reported in less than 3%, and arrhythmia, migraine, flushing, hypertension, or edema has been reported less than 1% of patients receiving extended-release glipizide tablets in clinical trials. Hypertension has been reported in 2.9–3.5 or 5.6 % of patients receiving glipizide in fixed combination with metformin or metformin alone, respectively, as initial therapy for type 2 diabetes mellitus. Rhinitis has been reported in less than 3%, and pharyngitis or dyspnea has been reported in than 1% of patients receiving extended-release glipizide tablets in clinical trials. Upper respiratory tract infection was reported in 8.1–9.9 or 8.5% of patients receiving the fixed combination of glipizide and metformin or metformin monotherapy, respectively, as initial therapy for type 2 diabetes mellitus, and in 10.3 or 10.7% of patients receiving the fixed combination of glipizide and metformin or metformin monotherapy, respectively, as second-line therapy. Blurred vision has been reported in less than 3%, and ocular pain, conjunctivitis, or retinal hemorrhage has been reported in less than 1% of patients receiving extended-release glipizide tablets in clinical trials. Although a causal relationship has not been established, mild to moderate increases in BUN and serum creatinine concentration have occurred occasionally in patients receiving glipizide. Urinary tract infection has been reported in 1.1 or 8% of patients receiving the fixed combination of glipizide and metformin or metformin monotherapy, respectively, as second-line therapy for type 2 diabetes mellitus. Decreased libido or polyuria has been reported in less than 3%, and dysuria has been reported in less than 1% of patients receiving extended-release glipizide tablets in clinical trials.

Like other sulfonylureas, hyponatremia and the syndrome of inappropriate secretion of antidiuretic hormone (SIADH) have occurred in patients receiving glipizide.

● Precautions and Contraindications

Glipizide shares the toxic potentials of other sulfonylurea antidiabetic agents, and the usual precautions associated with their use should be observed. The diagnostic and therapeutic measures for managing diabetes mellitus that are necessary to ensure optimum control of the disease with insulin generally are necessary with glipizide. Glipizide should only be prescribed for carefully selected patients by clinicians who are familiar with the indications, limitations, and patient-selection criteria for therapy with oral sulfonylurea antidiabetic agents.

Patients receiving glipizide should be monitored with regular clinical and laboratory evaluations, including blood and urine glucose determinations, to determine the minimum effective dosage and to detect primary failure (inadequate lowering of blood glucose concentration at the maximum recommended dosage) or secondary failure (loss of control of blood glucose concentration following an initial period of effectiveness) to the drug. Glycosylated hemoglobin (hemoglobin A_{1c} [HbA_{1c}]) measurements may also be useful for monitoring the patient's response to glipizide therapy. During the withdrawal period in patients in whom glipizide is replacing insulin, patients should be instructed to test their urine for glucose and ketones at least 3 times daily, and to report the results to their physician; when feasible, patient or laboratory monitoring of blood glucose concentration is preferable. Care should be taken to avoid ketosis, acidosis, and coma during the withdrawal period in patients being switched from insulin to glipizide. If adequate lowering of blood glucose concentration is no longer achieved during maintenance therapy with glipizide, the drug should be discontinued. When use of glipizide in asymptomatic type 2 diabetic patients is being considered, it should be recognized that control of blood glucose concentration in these patients has not been definitely established as effective for prevention of long-term cardiovascular or nervous system complications of the disease. There is limited evidence that sulfonylureas may reverse basement-membrane thickening of muscle capillaries in asymptomatic individuals with impaired glucose tolerance (chemical diabetes) and possibly reverse or retard the progression of microangiopathy in type 2 diabetic patients, but these findings require further evaluation.

Several large, long-term studies have evaluated the cardiovascular risks associated with the use of oral sulfonylurea antidiabetic agents. In 1970, the University Group Diabetes Program (UGDP) reported that administration of oral antidiabetic agents (i.e., tolbutamide or phenformin) was associated with increased cardiovascular mortality as compared to treatment with dietary regulation alone or with dietary regulation and insulin. The UGDP reported that type 2 diabetic patients who were treated for 5–8 years with dietary regulation and a fixed dose of tolbutamide (1.5 g daily) had a cardiovascular mortality rate approximately 2.5 times that of patients treated with dietary regulation alone; although a substantial increase in total mortality was not observed, the use of tolbutamide was discontinued because of the increase in cardiovascular mortality, thereby limiting the ability of the study to show an increase in total mortality. The results of the UGDP study have been exhaustively analyzed, and there has been general disagreement in the scientific and medical communities regarding the study's validity and clinical importance. However, recent results from the United Kingdom Prospective Diabetes (UKPD) study, a large, long-term (over 10 years) study in newly diagnosed type 2 diabetic patients, did not confirm an increase in cardiovascular events or mortality in the group treated intensively with sulfonylureas, insulin, or combination therapy compared with less intensive conventional antidiabetic therapy.

In the UKPD study, the overall aggregate rates of death from macrovascular diseases such as myocardial infarction, sudden death, stroke, or peripheral

vascular disease were not appreciably different among either intensive therapies (stepwise introduction of a sulfonylurea [i.e., chlorpropamide, glyburide] then insulin, or an oral sulfonylurea and insulin, or insulin alone to achieve fasting plasma glucose concentrations of 108 mg/dL) or less intensive conventional therapy (diet and oral antidiabetic agents or insulin to achieve fasting plasma glucose concentrations below 270 mg/dL without symptoms of hyperglycemia). However, a trend in reduction in fatal and nonfatal myocardial infarction with intensive therapy was noted with sulfonylurea or insulin, and epidemiologic analysis of the data indicate that each 1% decrease in HbA_{1c} was associated with an 18% reduction of fatal and nonfatal myocardial infarction. Among the single end points, the incidence of angina increased among patients receiving chlorpropamide, and blood pressure also was higher with chlorpropamide compared with glyburide or insulin intensive therapies. As a result of these and other findings (e.g., beneficial effects on microvascular [retinopathy, nephropathy, and possibly neuropathy] complications, confirmation of the beneficial effects of concomitant antihypertensive therapy and blood pressure lowering) of the UKDP study, the American Diabetes Association (ADA) currently considers the beneficial effects of intensive glycemic control with insulin or sulfonylureas and blood pressure control in diabetic patients to outweigh the risks overall.

Patients should be fully and completely advised about the nature of diabetes mellitus, what they must do to prevent and detect complications, and how to control their condition. *Patients should be informed of the potential risks and advantages of glipizide therapy and alternative forms of treatment.* Patients should be instructed that dietary regulation is the principal consideration in the management of diabetes, and that glipizide therapy is only used as an adjunct to, and not a substitute for or a convenient means to avoid, proper dietary regulation. Patients should also be advised that they should not neglect dietary restrictions, develop a careless attitude about their condition, or disregard instructions about body-weight control, exercise, hygiene, and avoidance of infection. Primary and secondary failure to oral sulfonylurea antidiabetic agents should also be explained to patients.

Patients and responsible family members should be informed of the risks of hypoglycemia, the symptoms and treatment of hypoglycemic reactions, and conditions that predispose to the development of hypoglycemic reactions, since these reactions may occasionally occur during therapy with glipizide. *Appropriate patient selection and careful attention to dosage are important to avoid glipizide-induced hypoglycemia.* Debilitated, malnourished, or geriatric patients and patients with impaired hepatic or renal function should be carefully monitored and dosage of glipizide should be carefully adjusted in these patients, since they may be predisposed to developing hypoglycemia (sometimes severe). Renal or hepatic insufficiency may cause increased serum concentrations of glipizide and hepatic insufficiency may also diminish gluconeogenic capacity, both of which increase the risk of severe hypoglycemic reactions. Alcohol ingestion, severe or prolonged exercise, deficient caloric intake, use of more than one antidiabetic agent, and adrenal or pituitary insufficiency may also predispose patients to the development of hypoglycemia. Hypoglycemia may be difficult to recognize in geriatric patients or in patients receiving β-adrenergic blocking agents. Intensive treatment (e.g., IV dextrose) and close medical supervision may be required in some patients who develop severe hypoglycemia during glipizide therapy. (See Acute Toxicity: Treatment.)

To maintain control of diabetes during periods of stress (e.g., fever of any cause, trauma, infection, surgery), temporary discontinuance of glipizide and administration of insulin may be required.

As with other nondeformable material, extended-release glipizide tablets should be used with caution in patients with severe preexisting GI narrowing, since obstruction may occur. The inert portion of glipizide extended-release tablets is not absorbed and is excreted in feces where it may be noticeable. If cholestatic jaundice occurs or if adverse dermatologic effects occur and persist during glipizide therapy, the drug should be discontinued. Glipizide is contraindicated as sole therapy in patients with type 1 diabetes mellitus or in those with diabetes complicated by ketosis, acidosis, or diabetic coma. Like other sulfonylureas, glipizide is generally contraindicated in patients with severe renal or hepatic impairment. Glipizide is also contraindicated in patients with known hypersensitivity or allergy to the drug.

● Pediatric Precautions

The manufacturer states that safety and efficacy of glipizide alone or in fixed combination with metformin in children have not been established. However, the American Diabetes Association (ADA) states that most pediatric diabetologists use oral antidiabetic agents in children with type 2 diabetes mellitus because of greater patient compliance and convenience for the patient's family and a lack of evidence demonstrating better efficacy of insulin as initial therapy for type 2 diabetes mellitus.

● Geriatric Precautions

Safety and efficacy of glipizide extended-release tablets in geriatric patients have not been specifically studied to date; however, in clinical studies of the drug, approximately 33% of patients were 65 years of age or older. It has not been determined whether clinical trials of glipizide conventional tablets did not include sufficient numbers of patients 65 years and older to determine whether they respond differently than younger adults. Although no overall differences in safety or efficacy were observed between geriatric and younger patients in clinical studies of glipizide extended-release tablets, the possibility that some older patients may exhibit increased sensitivity cannot be ruled out. Because of the greater frequency of decreased hepatic, renal, and/or cardiac function and of concomitant disease and drug therapy in geriatric patients, the manufacturer suggests that patients in this age group receive initial dosages of the drug in the lower end of the usual range. Geriatric patients should be carefully monitored and dosage of glipizide should be carefully adjusted in these patients, since they may be predisposed to developing hypoglycemia (sometimes severe).

● Mutagenicity and Carcinogenicity

It is not known if glipizide is mutagenic or carcinogenic in humans. The drug did not exhibit mutagenic activity in the Ames microbial mutagen test or in vivo in animal tests. Evidence of carcinogenicity was not observed in rats or mice receiving up to 75 times the maximum human dosage of glipizide daily for 20 or 18 months, respectively.

● Pregnancy, Fertility, and Lactation

Although there are no adequate and controlled studies to date in humans, glipizide has been shown to be mildly fetotoxic in rats when given at doses of 5–50 mg/kg; the fetotoxic effect is perinatal and similar to that of some other sulfonylureas, and is believed to be directly related to the hypoglycemic effect of the drug. No teratogenic effects were observed in reproduction studies in rats or rabbits. Since abnormal maternal blood glucose concentrations during pregnancy may be associated with a higher incidence of congenital abnormalities, many experts recommend that insulin be used during pregnancy to maintain optimum control of blood glucose concentration. Use of glipizide in pregnant women is generally *not* recommended, and the drug should be used during pregnancy only when clearly necessary (e.g., when insulin therapy is infeasible). Prolonged, severe hypoglycemia lasting 4–10 days has been reported in some neonates born to women who were receiving other sulfonylurea antidiabetic agents up to the time of delivery; this effect has been reported more frequently with the use of those agents having prolonged elimination half-lives. To minimize the risk of neonatal hypoglycemia if glipizide is used during pregnancy, the manufacturer recommends that the drug be discontinued at least 1 month before the expected delivery date.

Reproduction studies in rats using glipizide doses up to 75 times the usual human dose have not revealed evidence of impaired fertility.

Although it is not known whether glipizide is distributed into milk in humans, some sulfonylurea antidiabetic agents are distributed into milk. Because of the potential for hypoglycemia in nursing infants, a decision should be made whether to discontinue nursing or the drug, taking into account the importance of the drug to the woman. If glipizide is discontinued, and if dietary management alone is inadequate for controlling blood glucose concentration, administration of insulin should be considered.

DRUG INTERACTIONS

● Protein-bound Drugs

Because glipizide is highly protein bound, it theoretically could be displaced from binding sites by, or could displace from binding sites, other protein-bound drugs such as oral anticoagulants, hydantoins, salicylate and other nonsteroidal anti-inflammatory agents, and sulfonamides. However, unlike the protein binding of some other sulfonylurea antidiabetic agents (e.g., acetohexamide, chlorpropamide, tolazamide, tolbutamide) and like that of glyburide, the protein binding of glipizide is principally nonionic; in addition, glipizide appears to bind to different but closely related sites on serum albumin than does tolbutamide. Consequently, glipizide may be less likely to be displaced from binding sites by, or displace from binding sites,

other highly protein-bound drugs whose protein binding is ionic in nature. In vitro studies indicate that glipizide does not displace dicumarol or salicylate from plasma proteins. Whether any differences in protein binding demonstrated in vitro will result in fewer clinically important drug interactions in vivo has not been established. There appears to be no clinically important interaction between indoprofen and glipizide. Patients receiving highly protein-bound drugs should be observed for adverse effects when glipizide therapy is initiated or discontinued and vice versa.

● Cimetidine

Preliminary data indicate that cimetidine may potentiate the hypoglycemic effects of glipizide. The exact mechanism(s) of this interaction is not known, but cimetidine may inhibit hepatic metabolism of the sulfonylurea. Oral cimetidine has been shown to substantially increase the area under the plasma glipizide concentration-time curve and was associated with a substantial reduction in the postprandial increase in blood glucose concentration in diabetic patients receiving the drugs concomitantly. If cimetidine is administered concomitantly with glipizide, the patient should be closely monitored for signs and symptoms of hypoglycemia; dosage adjustment of glipizide may be necessary when cimetidine therapy is initiated or discontinued.

● Thiazide Diuretics

Thiazide diuretics may exacerbate diabetes mellitus, resulting in increased requirements of sulfonylurea antidiabetic agents, temporary loss of diabetic control, or secondary failure to the antidiabetic agent. When thiazide diuretics are administered concomitantly with sulfonylurea antidiabetic agents, caution should be used.

● Alcohol

Disulfiram-like reactions have occurred very rarely following the concomitant use of alcohol and glipizide.

● β-Adrenergic Blocking Agents

Several potential interactions between β-adrenergic blocking agents and sulfonylurea antidiabetic agents exist. β-Adrenergic blocking agents may impair glucose tolerance; increase the frequency or severity of hypoglycemia; block hypoglycemia-induced tachycardia, but not hypoglycemic sweating which may actually be increased; delay the rate of recovery of blood glucose concentration following drug-induced hypoglycemia;alter the hemodynamic response to hypoglycemia, possibly resulting in an exaggerated hypertensive response; and possibly impair peripheral circulation. There is some evidence that many of these effects may be minimized by use of a β_1-selective adrenergic blocking agent rather than a nonselective β-adrenergic blocking agent. In one study in type 2 diabetic patients, tolbutamide-induced insulin secretion was not affected by short-term propranolol therapy, but the hypoglycemic action of a single dose of glipizide in conjunction with an oral glucose load appeared to be slightly reduced. It generally is recommended that concomitant use of β-adrenergic blocking agents and sulfonylurea antidiabetic agents be avoided when possible; if concomitant therapy is necessary, use of a β_1-selective adrenergic blocking agent may be preferred. When glipizide and a β-adrenergic blocking agent are used concomitantly, the patient should be monitored closely for altered antidiabetic response.

● Antifungal Antibiotics

Concomitant use of certain antifungal antibiotics (i.e., miconazole, fluconazole) and oral antidiabetic agents has resulted in increased plasma concentrations of glipizide and/or hypoglycemia. In a study in healthy individuals, the area under the plasma concentration-time curve (AUC) of glipizide increased by 57% following concomitant administration with fluconazole (100 mg daily for 7 days). Clinically important hypoglycemia may be precipitated by concomitant use of oral hypoglycemic agents and fluconazole, and at least one fatality has been reported from hypoglycemia in a patient receiving glyburide and fluconazole concomitantly. (See Drug Interactions: Sulfonylurea Antidiabetic Agents in Fluconazole in 8:14.08).

● Other Drugs

Drugs that may enhance the hypoglycemic effect of sulfonylurea antidiabetic agents, including glipizide, include chloramphenicol, monoamine oxidase inhibitors, and probenecid. When these drugs are administered or discontinued in patients receiving glipizide, the patient should be observed closely for hypoglycemia or loss of diabetic control, respectively. When glipizide was administered to counter the hyperglycemic effect of diazoxide in several severely hypertensive nondiabetic patients with impaired renal function, hypoglycemic reactions resulted, prompting some clinicians to recommend that the drugs not be used concomitantly in such circumstances.

Drugs that may decrease the hypoglycemic effect of sulfonylurea antidiabetic agents, including glipizide, include nonthiazide diuretics (e.g., furosemide), corticosteroids, phenothiazines, thyroid agents, estrogens, oral contraceptives, phenytoin, nicotinic acid, sympathomimetic agents, calcium-channel blocking agents, rifampin, and isoniazid. When these drugs are administered or discontinued in patients receiving glipizide, the patient should be observed closely for loss of diabetic control or hypoglycemia, respectively.

Preliminary data suggest that glipizide may reduce the rate and/or extent of absorption of concomitantly administered oral xylose in type 2 diabetic patients.

ACUTE TOXICITY

● Pathogenesis

There is no well documented experience to date with glipizide overdosage. The oral LD$_{50}$ of the drug was greater than 4 g/kg in all animal species tested. Acute glipizide toxicity may result from excessive dosage, and numerous conditions may predispose patients to the development of glipizide-induced hypoglycemia. (See Cautions: Precautions and Contraindications.) Severe glipizide-induced hypoglycemia has reportedly occurred almost exclusively in patients with predisposing conditions (e.g., impaired renal and/or hepatic function).

● Manifestations

Acute glipizide overdosage is manifested principally as hypoglycemia, which is usually mild but occasionally may be severe. Severe sulfonylurea-induced hypoglycemia may result in loss of consciousness and seizures, with resultant neurologic sequelae. Because of glipizide's elimination characteristics, the risk of prolonged hypoglycemia is likely to be low. In some cases, hypoglycemia may persist despite continuous IV administration of dextrose.

● Treatment

Treatment of acute glipizide overdosage consists principally of administration of glucose and supportive therapy. *The patient should be monitored closely until complete recovery is assured.*

Patients with mild hypoglycemic symptoms without loss of consciousness or adverse neurologic effects should be treated aggressively with orally administered glucose, and glipizide dosage and/or the patient's meal pattern should be appropriately adjusted. Severe glipizide-induced hypoglycemia with coma, seizures, or other neurologic impairment occurs infrequently, but constitutes a medical emergency requiring immediate hospitalization and treatment. If hypoglycemic coma is diagnosed or suspected, 50% dextrose injection (e.g., 50 mL) should be administered IV rapidly, followed immediately by a continuous IV infusion of 10% dextrose injection at a rate sufficient to maintain a blood glucose concentration greater than 100 mg/dL. In some patients, subsequent administration of IV glucagon and/or corticosteroids may also be necessary. Blood glucose concentrations should be monitored at least every 3 hours during the first 24 hours and as often as necessary thereafter. Care should be taken to avoid inducing excessive hyperglycemia. Other symptomatic therapy (e.g., anticonvulsants) should be administered as necessary. Glipizide is effectively adsorbed by activated charcoal in vitro. Experimental studies using chlorpropamide suggest that if sulfonylurea overdosage is the result of an acute ingestion, administration of activated charcoal within several hours of the ingestion may be effective in reducing sulfonylurea absorption. Because glipizide is highly protein bound, dialysis is not likely to enhance elimination of the drug. Since hypoglycemia may occur after apparent clinical recovery, patients must be closely monitored for *at least* 24–48 hours; in patients with substantial renal or hepatic dysfunction, longer periods of monitoring may be necessary.

PHARMACOLOGY

● Antidiabetic Effect

Like other sulfonylurea antidiabetic agents, glipizide lowers blood glucose concentration in diabetic and nondiabetic individuals. Although the hypoglycemic action of the various sulfonylureas is generally similar, the drugs may differ quantitatively and/or possibly qualitatively in the extent to which they produce specific effects, and the effects may vary as a function of duration of treatment. On a weight basis, glipizide is one of the most potent of the sulfonylurea antidiabetic agents; although an exact dosage relationship does not exist, a daily glipizide dose of 5 mg controls blood glucose concentration to approximately the same degree as

daily doses of acetohexamide 500 mg, chlorpropamide or tolazamide 250 mg, glyburide 2.5–5 mg, or tolbutamide 0.5–1 g.

The precise mechanism(s) of hypoglycemic action of sulfonylurea antidiabetic agents has not been clearly established, but the drugs, including glipizide, initially appear to lower blood glucose concentration principally by stimulating secretion of endogenous insulin from the beta cells of the pancreas. Glipizide also appears to enhance peripheral insulin action at postreceptor (probably intracellular) site(s) during short-term therapy. Like other sulfonylureas, glipizide alone is ineffective in the absence of functioning beta cells.

The mechanism(s) of action of glipizide during prolonged administration has not been fully established. The glipizide-induced increase in glucose- or meal-stimulated secretion of endogenous insulin appears to be sustained during prolonged administration and has persisted in most diabetic patients for up to at least 2 years. The prolonged effect of glipizide on secretion of endogenous insulin is unlike that of most other sulfonylureas, but its clinical importance in the long-term efficacy of the drug remains to be clearly determined; while this effect likely contributes to the improvement in glucose tolerance in many patients during prolonged glipizide therapy, it alone does not appear to be sufficient for a long-term, effective response to the drug and glucose tolerance can improve in some patients without an increase in insulin secretion. Fasting plasma insulin concentrations are usually not increased during prolonged glipizide therapy but have been reported to be slightly increased in some patients. The drug generally does not appear to alter glucagon secretion. During prolonged administration of sulfonylureas, including glipizide, extrapancreatic effects appear to substantially contribute to the hypoglycemic action of the drugs. Many extrapancreatic effects of the drugs have been proposed and/or studied, but the principal effects appear to include enhanced peripheral sensitivity to insulin and reduction of basal hepatic glucose production; however, the nature of the long-term hypoglycemic effect and the mechanism(s) involved remain to be fully elucidated. There is evidence that glipizide enhances the peripheral action of insulin at postreceptor (probably intracellular) site(s) during long-term administration, and this appears to be a principal mechanism of action during prolonged therapy. An increase in insulin binding in erythrocytes obtained from diabetic patients receiving long-term therapy with the drug has also been reported.

● Other Effects

In patients with type 2 diabetes mellitus, glipizide-induced improvement in plasma glucose concentration is associated with a reduction in plasma total and very low-density lipoprotein (VLDL) triglyceride concentrations and plasma low-density lipoprotein (LDL) cholesterol concentration; mean serum or plasma total, LDL, and high-density lipoprotein (HDL) cholesterol concentrations generally do not appear to be changed during therapy with the drug, but the ratio of plasma HDL cholesterol to total cholesterol may be slightly increased. The effects of glipizide on plasma lipids are apparently secondary to improved control of plasma glucose concentration.

Glipizide has been reported to slightly enhance renal free water clearance in healthy individuals, possibly by increasing electrolyte reabsorption in the loop of Henle.

In vitro, glipizide reportedly inhibits platelet aggregation induced by collagen or adenosine diphosphate (ADP). The effect, if any, of the drug on platelet aggregation in vivo has not been determined to date.

PHARMACOKINETICS

● Absorption

Glipizide is rapidly and essentially completely absorbed from the GI tract. First-pass metabolism of glipizide appears to be minimal, and the absolute oral bioavailability of the drug is reported to be 80–100%. Food delays the absorption of glipizide but does not affect peak serum concentrations achieved or the extent of absorption of the drug.

Following oral administration of a single 5-mg dose of glipizide as conventional tablets in fasting and nonfasting individuals, the drug appears in plasma or serum within 15–30 minutes and average peak plasma or serum concentrations of approximately 310–450 ng/mL usually are attained within 1–3 hours (range: 1–6 hours). Peak serum concentrations generally are delayed 20–40 minutes in the nonfasting state compared with the fasting state. A few reports indicate that biphasic peak serum concentrations may occur in some patients, suggesting that the drug may undergo enterohepatic circulation. The area under the serum concentration-time curve (AUC) for glipizide increases in proportion to increasing doses. Time to reach steady-state plasma glipizide concentrations following administration of glipizide extended-release tablets was delayed by 1–2 days in geriatric patients compared with younger patients.

Following administration of glipizide extended-release tablets in men with type 2 diabetes mellitus and patients younger than 65 years of age, steady-state plasma glipizide concentrations were achieved by at least the fifth day of dosing.

Following single oral doses of glipizide as conventional tablets in nonfasting diabetic or healthy individuals, plasma insulin concentration generally begins to increase within 10–30 minutes and is maximal within 0.5–2 hours; increased plasma insulin concentrations generally do not persist beyond the time of the meal challenge. Following single oral doses in fasting healthy individuals, the hypoglycemic action of glipizide generally begins within 15–30 minutes and is maximal within 1–2 hours. In nonfasting diabetic patients, the hypoglycemic action of a single morning dose of the drug may persist for up to 24 hours. Although a correlation between the plasma concentration of glipizide and its hypoglycemic effect has not been established, plasma insulin concentration was increased only when the plasma glipizide concentration was 200 ng/mL or higher in one study.

● Distribution

Distribution of glipizide into human body tissues and fluids has not been fully characterized. Following IV administration of glipizide in mice, highest concentrations of the drug were attained in the liver and blood, with lower concentrations in the lungs, kidneys, adrenals, myocardium, salivary glands, and retroscapular fat; the drug was not detected in the brain or spinal cord. In humans, small amounts of glipizide are apparently distributed into bile and very small amounts are distributed into erythrocytes and saliva. Although glipizide apparently did not cross the placenta in mice in one study, the drug was detected in the fetuses of pregnant rats given the drug. It is not known if glipizide is distributed into milk in humans.

Following IV administration in humans, glipizide undergoes rapid distribution. Following IV administration of the drug, the volumes of distribution in the central compartment and at steady-state average 4.2–4.6 L (range: 3.5–13.2 L) and 10.2–11.7 L (range: 4.6–15.1 L), respectively, suggesting that the drug is distributed principally within extracellular fluid. Although pharmacokinetic data from one single-dose study suggest that glipizide might accumulate in a deep tissue compartment, data from other single-dose studies suggest that the drug does not accumulate in tissue depots.

At a concentration of 9–612 ng/mL, glipizide is approximately 92–99% bound to plasma proteins. Glipizide has a lower affinity for binding to serum albumin than does glyburide. Unlike the protein binding of some other sulfonylurea antidiabetic agents (e.g., acetohexamide, chlorpropamide, tolazamide, tolbutamide) and like that of glyburide, the protein binding of glipizide appears to be principally nonionic; consequently, glipizide may be less likely to be displaced from binding sites by, or displace from binding sites, other highly protein-bound drugs whose protein binding is ionic in nature. (See Drug Interactions: Protein-Bound Drugs.)

● Elimination

Following IV administration, serum concentrations of glipizide decline in a biphasic manner. Following IV administration of glipizide in healthy individuals or diabetic patients with normal renal and hepatic function, the half-life of the drug averages 8.4–36 minutes (range: 4–36 minutes) in the initial phase and 2.1–3.6 hours (range: 1.1–3.7 hours) in the terminal phase. Following oral administration in healthy individuals or diabetic patients with normal renal and hepatic function, the terminal elimination half-life of glipizide averages 3–4.7 hours (range: 2–7.3 hours). The terminal elimination half-life of total glipizide metabolites reportedly ranges from 2–6 hours in patients with normal renal and hepatic function. Serum glipizide concentrations may be increased in patients with renal or hepatic insufficiency. Data are limited, but the terminal elimination half-life of unchanged glipizide does not appear to be substantially increased in patients with impaired renal function. The terminal elimination half-life of total glipizide metabolites may be prolonged to greater than 20 hours in patients with impaired renal function; however, since glipizide metabolites are considered essentially inactive, this is probably of little clinical importance, at least in patients with moderate renal impairment.

Glipizide is almost completely metabolized, mainly in the liver. The drug is metabolized principally at the cyclohexyl ring to 4-trans-hydroxyglipizide; the drug is also metabolized to the 3-cis-hydroxy derivative, N-(2-acetylaminoethylphenyl-sulfonyl)-N'-cyclohexyl urea (DCDA), and at least 2 unidentified metabolites.

Glipizide and its metabolites are excreted principally in urine. The drug and its metabolites are also excreted in feces, apparently almost completely via biliary elimination; only small amounts may be excreted in feces as unabsorbed drug following oral administration. Most urinary excretion occurs within the first 6–24 hours after oral administration of the drug. Following oral administration of a single 5-mg dose of glipizide in individuals with normal renal and hepatic function, approximately 60–90% of the dose is excreted in urine as unchanged drug and metabolites within 24–72 hours and about 5–20% is excreted in feces within 24–96 hours; less than 10% of a dose is excreted in urine as unchanged drug within 24 hours, about 20–60% as the 4-trans-hydroxy metabolite, 10–15% as the 3-cis-hydroxy metabolite, 1–2% as DCDA, and the remainder as unidentified metabolites.

Total plasma or serum clearance of glipizide reportedly averages 21–38 mL/hour per kg in individuals with normal renal and hepatic function. Renal clearance of unchanged glipizide increases substantially with increasing urinary pH, but is only about 5% of total plasma clearance at urinary pH of 5–6; the low renal clearance indicates that the drug undergoes renal tubular reabsorption. The effects have not been fully evaluated, but elimination of glipizide may be reduced in patients with impaired renal and/or hepatic function. Limited data indicate that renal excretion and terminal elimination half-life of glipizide metabolites are substantially decreased and increased, respectively, in patients with severe renal impairment.

CHEMISTRY AND STABILITY

● Chemistry

Glipizide is a sulfonylurea antidiabetic agent. The drug is structurally similar to acetohexamide and glyburide. Glipizide occurs as a whitish powder and is practically insoluble in water and in alcohol. The drug has a pK_a of 5.9.

● Stability

Glipizide tablets should be stored in tight, light-resistant containers at a temperature less than 30°C. Glipizide extended-release tablets should be stored at controlled room temperatures of 15–30°C and protected from moisture and humidity.

PREPARATIONS

Excipients in commercially available drug preparations may have clinically important effects in some individuals; consult specific product labeling for details.

glipiZIDE

Oral		
Tablets	5 mg*	glipiZIDE Tablets
		Glucotrol® (scored), Pfizer
	10 mg*	glipiZIDE Tablets
		Glucotrol® (scored), Pfizer
Tablets, extended-release	2.5 mg*	glipiZIDE Tablets ER
		Glucotrol XL®, Pfizer
	5 mg*	glipiZIDE Tablets ER
		Glucotrol XL®, Pfizer
	10 mg*	glipiZIDE Tablets ER
		Glucotrol XL®, Pfizer

* available from one or more manufacturer, distributor, and/or repackager by generic (nonproprietary) name

glipiZIDE Combinations

Oral		
Tablets, film-coated	2.5 mg with 250 mg Metformin Hydrochloride*	glipiZIDE with Metformin Hydrochloride Tablets
		Metaglip®, Bristol-Myers Squibb
	2.5 mg with 500 mg Metformin Hydrochloride*	glipiZIDE with Metformin Hydrochloride Tablets
		Metaglip®, Bristol-Myers Squibb
	5 mg with 500 mg Metformin Hydrochloride*	glipiZIDE with Metformin Hydrochloride Tablets
		Metaglip®, Bristol-Myers Squibb

* available from one or more manufacturer, distributor, and/or repackager by generic (nonproprietary) name

Selected Revisions January 1, 2010, © Copyright, November 1, 1984, American Society of Health-System Pharmacists, Inc.

Pioglitazone Hydrochloride

68:20.28 • THIAZOLIDINEDIONES

■ Pioglitazone is a thiazolidinedione (glitazone) antidiabetic agent that is structurally and pharmacologically related to troglitazone and rosiglitazone.

USES

● Type 2 Diabetes Mellitus

Pioglitazone is used alone (monotherapy) or in combination with a sulfonylurea antidiabetic agent, metformin (either as a fixed-combination preparation or as individual drugs given concurrently), or insulin as an adjunct to diet and exercise to improve glycemic control in patients with type 2 diabetes mellitus. Pioglitazone also is used in fixed combination with glimepiride in patients with type 2 diabetes mellitus who are already receiving a thiazolidinedione and a sulfonylurea separately or who are inadequately controlled on a sulfonylurea or a thiazolidinedione alone. In patients whose hyperglycemia cannot be controlled with these other antidiabetic agents, pioglitazone should be added to, not substituted for, such antidiabetic therapy.

Current guidelines for the treatment of type 2 diabetes mellitus generally recommend metformin as first-line therapy in addition to lifestyle modifications in patients with recent-onset type 2 diabetes mellitus or mild hyperglycemia because of its well-established safety and efficacy (i.e., beneficial effects on glycosylated hemoglobin [hemoglobin A_{1c}; HbA_{1c}], weight, and cardiovascular mortality). (See Uses: Type 2 Diabetes Mellitus, in Metformin 68:20.04.) In patients with contraindications or intolerance to metformin (e.g., risk of lactic acidosis, GI intolerance) or in selected other patients, some experts suggest that initial therapy with a drug from another class of antidiabetic agents (e.g., a glucagon-like peptide-1 [GLP-1] receptor agonist, sodium-glucose cotransporter 2 [SGLT2] inhibitor, dipeptidyl peptidase-4 [DPP-4] inhibitor, sulfonylurea, thiazolidinedione, basal insulin) may be acceptable based on patient factors. Initiating antidiabetic therapy with 2 agents (e.g., metformin plus another drug) may be appropriate in patients with an initial HbA_{1c} exceeding 7.5% or at least 1.5% above the target level. In metformin-intolerant patients with high initial HbA_{1c} levels, some experts suggest initiation of therapy with 2 agents from other antidiabetic drug classes with complementary mechanisms of action.

Because of the progressive nature of type 2 diabetes mellitus, patients initially receiving an oral antidiabetic agent will eventually require multiple oral and/or injectable noninsulin antidiabetic agents of different therapeutic classes and/or insulin for adequate glycemic control. Patients who have inadequate glycemic control with initial (e.g., metformin) monotherapy should receive treatment with additional antidiabetic agents; data suggest that the addition of each noninsulin agent to initial therapy lowers HbA_{1c} by approximately 0.7–1%. In addition, early initiation of combination therapy may help to more rapidly attain glycemic goals and extend the time to treatment failure.

Factors to consider when selecting additional antidiabetic agents for combination therapy in patients with inadequate glycemic control on metformin monotherapy include patient comorbidities (e.g., atherosclerotic cardiovascular disease [ASCVD], established kidney disease, heart failure), hypoglycemia risk, impact on weight, cost, risk of adverse effects, and patient preference. When the greater glucose-lowering effect of an injectable drug is needed in patients with type 2 diabetes mellitus, some experts currently state that an injectable GLP-1 receptor agonist is preferred over insulin in most patients because of beneficial effects on body weight and a lower risk of hypoglycemia, although adverse GI effects may diminish tolerability. While addition of a GLP-1 receptor agonist may successfully control hyperglycemia, many patients will eventually require insulin therapy. Early introduction of insulin therapy should be considered when hyperglycemia is severe (e.g., blood glucose of at least 300 mg/dL or HbA_{1c} exceeding 9–10%), especially in the presence of catabolic manifestations (e.g., weight loss, hypertriglyceridemia, ketosis) or symptoms of hyperglycemia. For additional information regarding the initiation of insulin therapy in patients with diabetes mellitus, see Uses: Diabetes Mellitus, in the Insulins General Statement 68:20.08.

Some data suggest a possible protective effect of pioglitazone with regard to certain cardiovascular outcomes (e.g., death, myocardial infarction, stroke) in patients with type 2 diabetes mellitus. In a randomized, controlled study in over 5000 patients with type 2 diabetes mellitus who were at high risk for macrovascular complications, addition of pioglitazone to existing antidiabetic therapy was associated with a reduction in the secondary composite end point of all-cause mortality, nonfatal myocardial infarction, and stroke compared with placebo; no difference between the study groups was observed with respect to the primary composite study end point (all-cause mortality, nonfatal myocardial infarction, stroke, acute coronary syndrome, endovascular or surgical intervention on the coronary or leg arteries, or above-the-ankle amputation). Results of a meta-analysis of data from randomized, placebo- or active-controlled trials in over 16,000 patients indicated an 18% lower risk of the primary composite end point of death, myocardial infarction, or stroke with pioglitazone therapy. The incidence of serious heart failure was increased with pioglitazone therapy but without an associated increase in mortality. While an increased risk of myocardial ischemic events has not been documented to date with pioglitazone therapy in patients with type 2 diabetes mellitus, both pioglitazone and rosiglitazone, alone or in combination with other antidiabetic agents, can cause fluid retention and other cardiovascular effects that may lead to or exacerbate heart failure. Therefore, the potential risks and benefits of thiazolidinediones versus other second-line antidiabetic agents (sulfonylureas, insulin) should be carefully considered. (See Heart Failure under Warnings/Precautions: Warnings, in Cautions.)

The manufacturer states that pioglitazone should *not* be used for the treatment of type 1 diabetes mellitus or diabetic ketoacidosis because it will not be effective in treating these conditions.

Pioglitazone Monotherapy

Efficacy as monotherapy for the management of type 2 diabetes mellitus was established in 3 controlled studies of 16–26 weeks' duration. Pioglitazone improved glycemic control as measured by fasting glucose and glycosylated hemoglobin (HbA_{1c}) concentrations.

Combination Therapy

Efficacy of pioglitazone in combination with a sulfonylurea antidiabetic agent, metformin, or insulin in patients whose type 2 diabetes mellitus was inadequately controlled by therapy with one or more of these agents was established in several controlled studies in which combined therapy improved glycemic control regardless of the dosage of the other antidiabetic agent(s). A thiazolidinedione such as pioglitazone also may be added to therapy with the fixed combination of glyburide and metformin in patients whose hyperglycemia is not adequately controlled with the fixed combination. A thiazolidinedione antidiabetic agent also may be used concomitantly with repaglinide in patients whose hyperglycemia is inadequately controlled with diet, exercise, and monotherapy with metformin, a sulfonylurea, repaglinide, or a thiazolidinedione antidiabetic agent. In a clinical trial in patients with type 2 diabetes mellitus poorly controlled (as determined by HbA_{1c} concentrations exceeding 7%) by metformin or sulfonylurea monotherapy, the combination of repaglinide and pioglitazone reduced fasting plasma glucose and HbA_{1c} concentrations compared with pioglitazone or repaglinide monotherapy. Greater glycemic control was achieved with the combination of pioglitazone (fixed dosage: 30 mg daily) and repaglinide at a lower daily dosage of repaglinide (final median dosage: 6 mg daily) than with repaglinide monotherapy (final median dosage: 10 mg daily).

Pioglitazone also is used in fixed combination with metformin in patients with type 2 diabetes mellitus who have inadequate glycemic control with pioglitazone or metformin monotherapy or in those who are already receiving pioglitazone and metformin concurrently as separate components. Efficacy and safety of pioglitazone in fixed combination with metformin were established in a 24-week, randomized clinical study in 600 patients with type 2 diabetes mellitus (mean baseline HbA_{1c} 8.7%) inadequately controlled with diet and exercise. Substantial improvements in fasting plasma glucose and HbA_{1c} were observed in patients receiving the fixed combination of pioglitazone and metformin compared with each individual component alone. Efficacy and safety of the fixed combination also have been established based on concurrent administration of the 2 agents given separately and extrapolations from clinical trials evaluating pioglitazone as add-on therapy to metformin. Bioequivalence has been demonstrated between the fixed combination of pioglitazone and metformin and each agent given concurrently.

Pioglitazone also is used in fixed combination with glimepiride in patients with type 2 diabetes mellitus who are already receiving a thiazolidinedione and a sulfonylurea separately or who are inadequately controlled on a sulfonylurea or a thiazolidinedione alone. No clinical trials have been conducted evaluating the fixed combination of pioglitazone and glimepiride as second-line therapy in patients who are inadequately controlled on monotherapy with a sulfonylurea. Safety and efficacy of the fixed combination of pioglitazone and glimepiride in patients with type 2 diabetes mellitus who are inadequately controlled on a sulfonylurea alone have been extrapolated from clinical trials evaluating pioglitazone as add-on therapy to a sulfonylurea.

DOSAGE AND ADMINISTRATION

● *General*

Dosage should be carefully individualized based on patient response and tolerance. Hepatic function should be assessed before initiating pioglitazone therapy. (See Hepatic Effects under Warnings/Precautions: Other Warnings/Precautions, in Cautions.) Following initiation of pioglitazone therapy or dosage increases, patients should be carefully monitored for adverse effects related to fluid retention. (See Heart Failure under Warnings/Precautions: Warnings, in Cautions.)

Fasting plasma glucose (FPG) concentrations should be monitored periodically to determine the patient's response. Periodic glycosylated hemoglobin (hemoglobin A_{1c} [HbA_{1c}]) determinations also should be performed; HbA_{1c} is a better indicator of long-term glycemic control than fasting plasma glucose concentrations alone.

● *Administration*

Pioglitazone hydrochloride is administered orally once daily and can be taken without regard to meals. Pioglitazone in fixed combination with immediate-release metformin hydrochloride is administered once or twice daily with meals to reduce the GI effects of the metformin hydrochloride component. Pioglitazone in fixed combination with glimepiride is administered once daily with the first main meal.

● *Dosage*

Type 2 Diabetes Mellitus

Dosage of pioglitazone hydrochloride is expressed in terms of pioglitazone. Bioequivalence has been demonstrated between the fixed combination of pioglitazone and immediate-release metformin hydrochloride and each agent given concurrently as separate tablets at the currently approved dosage strengths (500 or 850 mg of metformin hydrochloride and 15 mg of pioglitazone). Bioequivalence also has been demonstrated between the fixed combination of pioglitazone and glimepiride and each agent given concurrently as separate tablets at the currently approved dosage strengths (2 or 4 mg of glimepiride and 30 mg of pioglitazone).

Pioglitazone Monotherapy

The recommended initial dosage of pioglitazone as monotherapy in patients *without* congestive heart failure is 15 or 30 mg once daily; lower initial dosages should be used in patients with NYHA class I or II heart failure. (See Dosage: Special Populations.) If the response is inadequate, dosage may be increased in increments of 15 mg based on glycemic response as determined by HbA_{1c} up to the maximum recommended dosage of 45 mg daily.

Combination Therapy with Other Oral Antidiabetic Agents or Insulin

The usual initial dosage of pioglitazone in combination with a sulfonylurea antidiabetic agent, metformin hydrochloride, or insulin (as separate components) is 15 or 30 mg once daily. Pioglitazone dosage should not exceed 45 mg daily.

Should hypoglycemia occur during combination therapy with an insulin secretagogue (e.g., sulfonylurea), the dosage of the insulin secretagogue should be decreased. If hypoglycemia occurs in patients receiving pioglitazone alone or concomitantly with metformin hydrochloride or glimepiride and insulin therapy, the dosage of insulin should be reduced by 10–25%; further adjustments to insulin dosage should be individualized according to glycemic response. (See Hypoglycemia under Warnings/Precautions: Other Warnings/Precautions, in Cautions.)

When the commercially available fixed-combination preparation containing pioglitazone and immediate-release metformin hydrochloride is used, dosage of the fixed combination is based on the patient's existing dosages of pioglitazone and/or metformin hydrochloride and on usual initial dosages of these drugs,

effectiveness, and tolerability. Metformin hydrochloride doses exceeding 2 g may be better tolerated when administered three times daily.

The usual initial dosage of the fixed combination containing pioglitazone and immediate-release metformin hydrochloride is pioglitazone 15 mg/metformin hydrochloride 500 mg twice daily or pioglitazone 15 mg/metformin hydrochloride 850 mg once daily.

When the commercially available preparation containing pioglitazone in fixed combination with immediate-release metformin hydrochloride is used to replace metformin monotherapy, the usual initial dosage is pioglitazone 15 mg/metformin hydrochloride 500 mg twice daily or pioglitazone 15 mg/metformin hydrochloride 850 mg once or twice daily depending on the patient's existing metformin hydrochloride dosage. The usual initial dosage of the fixed combination in patients currently receiving pioglitazone monotherapy is pioglitazone 15 mg/metformin hydrochloride 500 mg twice daily or pioglitazone 15 mg/metformin hydrochloride 850 mg once daily. When the fixed combination is used to replace therapy with separate tablets given concurrently, the dosage of the fixed combination is based on the patient's existing dosage of metformin and pioglitazone. Dosage should be titrated gradually after assessing adequacy of therapeutic response and tolerability, up to a maximum daily dosage of 45 mg of pioglitazone and 2.55 g of immediate-release metformin hydrochloride.

The safety and efficacy of transferring from therapy with other oral antidiabetic agents to the fixed combination of pioglitazone and metformin hydrochloride have not been established in clinical studies. Any change in the therapy of type 2 diabetic patients should be undertaken with caution and appropriate monitoring, as changes in glycemic control can occur.

The initial dosage of pioglitazone in fixed combination with glimepiride should be based on the patient's existing regimen with pioglitazone and/or a sulfonylurea. (See also Dosage: Special Populations.) When the commercially available preparation containing pioglitazone in fixed combination with glimepiride is used in patients inadequately controlled on glimepiride monotherapy, the usual initial dosage of the fixed combination is 30 mg of pioglitazone and 2 or 4 mg of glimepiride once daily with the first main meal. The usual initial dosage of the fixed combination in patients inadequately controlled on pioglitazone monotherapy is 30 mg of pioglitazone and 2 mg of glimepiride once daily. When the fixed combination is used to replace concurrent therapy as separate tablets, the dosage of the fixed combination should be as close as possible to the patient's existing dosage of glimepiride and pioglitazone. Therapy may be initiated with 2 or 4 mg of glimepiride and 30 mg of pioglitazone once daily. Following initiation of therapy with the fixed combination in patients previously receiving monotherapy with pioglitazone or a sulfonylurea or combination therapy with each component given separately, subsequent dosage should be adjusted according to the patient's therapeutic response and tolerability. For patients transferring from monotherapy with a sulfonylurea other than glimepiride or from combination therapy with pioglitazone and a sulfonylurea other than glimepiride, the usual initial dosage of the fixed combination is 30 mg of pioglitazone and 2 mg of glimepiride once daily. Because an exaggerated hypoglycemic response may occur in some patients during the transition from a sulfonylurea antidiabetic agent with a prolonged half-life (e.g., chlorpropamide, no longer commercially available in the US) to glimepiride in fixed combination with pioglitazone, it has been recommended that patients being transferred from such agents be monitored closely for the occurrence of hypoglycemia during the initial 1–2 weeks of the transition period.

If additional glycemic control is needed, dosage may be increased to a maximum total daily dosage of 8 mg of glimepiride and 45 mg of pioglitazone.

Concomitant Therapy with Potent CYP2C8 Inhibitors or Inducers

Because concomitant use of pioglitazone and potent inhibitors of cytochrome P-450 (CYP) isoenzyme 2C8 (e.g., gemfibrozil) increases exposure to pioglitazone, the maximum recommended dosage of pioglitazone in patients taking potent CYP2C8 inhibitors is 15 mg once daily. Patients receiving pioglitazone in fixed combination with glimepiride and a potent CYP2C8 inhibitor should be switched to therapy with the individual drug components administered separately because the minimum dose of pioglitazone in the fixed-combination preparation exceeds 15 mg. The maximum recommended dosage of pioglitazone in fixed combination with immediate-release metformin hydrochloride is pioglitazone 15 mg/metformin hydrochloride 850 mg once daily when used in combination with a potent CYP2C8 inhibitor.

If treatment with a CYP2C8 inducer (e.g., rifampin) is initiated or discontinued during pioglitazone therapy, changes in antidiabetic therapy may be required based on clinical response; however, the dosage of pioglitazone should not exceed the maximum recommended dosage of 45 mg daily. (See Drug Interactions: Drugs Affecting Hepatic Microsomal Enzymes.)

● Special Populations

Hepatic Impairment

Pioglitazone dosage adjustment is not necessary in patients with hepatic impairment when the drug is given as monotherapy. Pioglitazone should be initiated with caution in patients with hepatic impairment. (See Hepatic Effects under Warnings/Precautions: Other Warnings/Precautions, in Cautions.) If the fixed combination of glimepiride and pioglitazone is considered for use in patients with hepatic impairment, the drug should be initiated and dosage increased with caution. Patients with hepatic impairment should be closely monitored for hypoglycemia during initiation and subsequent dosage adjustment of such combination therapy. The use of the fixed combination of metformin hydrochloride and pioglitazone is not recommended in patients with hepatic impairment.

Renal Impairment

Pioglitazone dosage adjustment is not necessary in patients with renal impairment. Due to the risk of lactic acidosis with metformin hydrochloride therapy, the manufacturers state that the initiation of pioglitazone in fixed combination with metformin hydrochloride is not recommended in patients with an estimated glomerular filtration rate (eGFR) of 30–45 mL/minute per 1.73 m²; the benefits and risks of continuing the drug should be assessed in those with an eGFR in this range who are already receiving the drug. The manufacturers state that pioglitazone in fixed combination with metformin hydrochloride should not be used in patients with an eGFR of less than 30 mL/minute per 1.73 m². If the fixed combination of glimepiride and pioglitazone is considered for use in patients with renal impairment, the initial dosage, dose increments, and maintenance dosage of the drug should be conservative. Patients with renal impairment should be closely monitored for hypoglycemia during initiation and subsequent dosage adjustment of such combination therapy.

Geriatric Patients

Pioglitazone dosage adjustment is not necessary for geriatric patients solely because of age. Pioglitazone in fixed combination with metformin hydrochloride should be used with caution in geriatric patients since aging is associated with reduced renal function. Initial and maintenance dosages of the fixed combination should be conservative and should be titrated carefully.

As geriatric patients are particularly susceptible to hypoglycemia, the initial and maintenance dosages of pioglitazone in fixed combination with glimepiride should be conservative. Blood glucose concentrations of such patients should be closely monitored prior to and after initiation of therapy to avoid hypoglycemia.

Debilitated or Malnourished Patients

Caution should be used when initiating and increasing the dosage of pioglitazone in fixed combination with glimepiride in patients who are debilitated or malnourished and in those with adrenal, pituitary, or hepatic impairment. Such patients are particularly susceptible to the hypoglycemic effect of glucose-lowering drugs.

Patients with Heart Failure

The recommended initial dosage of pioglitazone in patients with New York Heart Association (NYHA) class I or II heart failure is 15 mg once daily. If subsequent dosage escalation is necessary, the dosage should be increased in increments of 15 mg up to a maximum dosage of 45 mg daily according to glycemic response based on HbA$_{1c}$. For patients with NYHA class I or II heart failure, the recommended initial dosage of the fixed combination containing pioglitazone and immediate-release metformin hydrochloride is pioglitazone 15 mg/metformin hydrochloride 500 mg or pioglitazone 15 mg/metformin hydrochloride 850 mg once daily. Following initiation of pioglitazone and any increase in dosage, patients should be monitored carefully for weight gain, edema, and other manifestations of congestive heart failure (CHF). Initiation of pioglitazone therapy in patients with more severe heart failure (NYHA class III or IV) is contraindicated. (See Heart Failure under Warnings/Precautions: Warnings, in Cautions and see Cautions: Contraindications.)

Before receiving therapy with the fixed-combination preparation containing glimepiride 2 mg and pioglitazone 30 mg, patients with diabetes mellitus and systolic dysfunction should receive pioglitazone 15 mg once daily as monotherapy and should safely tolerate dosage titration to 30 mg once daily as monotherapy. If subsequent dosage adjustment is necessary with the fixed-combination preparation, patients should be closely monitored for weight gain, edema, or other signs or symptoms of exacerbation of CHF.

CAUTIONS

● Contraindications

Known serious hypersensitivity reaction to pioglitazone or any ingredient in the formulation.

Initiation of therapy with pioglitazone is contraindicated in patients with New York Heart Association (NYHA) class III or IV heart failure. (See Heart Failure under Warnings/Precautions: Warnings, in Cautions.)

● Warnings/Precautions

Warnings

Heart Failure

Thiazolidinediones, including pioglitazone, alone or in combination with other antidiabetic agents, can cause dose-related fluid retention, which may lead to or exacerbate heart failure. Use of thiazolidinediones is associated with an approximately twofold increased risk of heart failure. (See Edema under Warnings/Precautions: Warnings, in Cautions.) Fluid retention is most common when pioglitazone is used in combination with insulin. Patients should be observed for signs and symptoms of heart failure (e.g., dyspnea, rapid weight gain, edema, unexplained cough or fatigue), especially during initiation of therapy and dosage titration. If signs and symptoms of heart failure develop, the disorder should be managed according to current standards of care. In addition, a decrease in the dosage or discontinuance of pioglitazone must be considered in such patients.

Patients with NYHA class III or IV cardiac status with or without congestive heart failure (CHF) or with an acute coronary event were not studied in clinical trials of pioglitazone; initiation of therapy with the drug is contraindicated in patients with NYHA class III or IV heart failure. Use of pioglitazone is *not* recommended in patients with symptomatic heart failure. Caution should be exercised in patients with edema and in those who are at risk for heart failure. Thiazolidinedione therapy should not be initiated in hospitalized patients with diabetes mellitus because of the delayed onset of action and because possible drug-related increases in vascular volume and CHF may complicate care of patients with hemodynamic changes induced by coexisting conditions or in-hospital interventions.

Findings from a meta-analysis of randomized controlled studies that assessed the risk of development of CHF and death from cardiovascular causes in patients receiving thiazolidinediones indicate that the risk of CHF is higher in patients receiving thiazolidinediones (relative risk of 1.72; 95% confidence interval: 1.21–2.42) than in controls (individuals receiving other antidiabetic agents or placebo). The relative risk for CHF was increased across a wide background of cardiovascular risk (i.e., patients with prediabetes, with type 2 diabetes mellitus without cardiovascular disease, with type 2 diabetes mellitus and cardiovascular disease other than CHF, or with type 2 diabetes mellitus and CHF [NYHA class I and II] and ejection fraction less than 40%). In contrast to the increased risk for CHF observed in thiazolidinedione-treated patients, the risk of cardiovascular death was not increased in patients receiving these agents.

In a 16-week, controlled study in patients with type 2 diabetes mellitus, CHF was reported in 1.1% of patients receiving combined therapy with pioglitazone and insulin and in none of the patients receiving insulin therapy alone; all patients who experienced CHF had a history of cardiac disease (e.g., coronary artery disease, previous coronary artery bypass graft procedures, myocardial infarction).

CHF has been reported during postmarketing experience in pioglitazone-treated patients who did or did not have previously known heart disease and who did or did not receive concomitant insulin therapy. In a 24-week postmarketing safety study in patients with NYHA class II and III heart failure and poorly controlled diabetes despite use of pioglitazone or glyburide, a higher incidence of CHF requiring hospitalization was observed in those receiving pioglitazone (9.9% of patients) than in those receiving glyburide (4.7% of patients). Patients who were older than 64 years of age or receiving insulin at study entry were particularly susceptible to this adverse event. No differences in cardiovascular mortality were noted between pioglitazone and glyburide therapy.

Data from a long-term (34.5 months) cardiovascular outcomes study (PROspective pioglitAzone Clinical Trial In macroVascular Events [PROACTIVE]) in patients with a history of macrovascular disease (those with NYHA class II–IV heart failure were excluded) receiving pioglitazone or placebo in addition to existing antidiabetic therapy (e.g., insulin, metformin, sulfonylureas) and cardiovascular agents indicated a higher incidence of serious heart failure (e.g., requiring hospitalization or prolonging hospital stay, fatal or life-threatening, resulting in substantial disability) in patients receiving pioglitazone than in those receiving placebo. Serious heart failure occurred in 5.7 or 4.1% of patients receiving pioglitazone or placebo, respectively; mortality rates from heart failure did not differ between pioglitazone or placebo recipients.

Edema

Fluid retention can occur and may lead to or exacerbate CHF in patients receiving a thiazolidinedione, including pioglitazone, alone or in combination with other antidiabetic agents, including insulin. Diuretic therapy may be necessary for management of fluid retention. Caution should be exercised in patients with edema and those at risk for CHF. (See Heart Failure under Warnings/Precautions: Warnings, in Cautions.)

All patients receiving thiazolidinedione therapy (e.g., rosiglitazone, pioglitazone) should be advised to monitor for weight gain and edema. Other potential causes of edema should be excluded. Pioglitazone-induced edema is reversible when the drug is discontinued. Hospitalization for edema usually is not required unless there is coexisting CHF.

Weight Gain

Dose-related weight gain, probably involving a combination of fluid retention and fat accumulation, has been observed during therapy with pioglitazone alone or in combination with other antidiabetic agents (e.g., metformin, sulfonylureas, insulin). Unusually rapid increases in weight and increases in excess of that usually observed in clinical trials have been reported during postmarketing experience. Patients who experience rapid or excessive weight gain should be assessed for fluid accumulation and volume-related events such as excessive edema and CHF.

Other Warnings/Precautions

Hepatic Effects

No evidence of drug-induced hepatotoxicity has been noted with pioglitazone in the controlled clinical trial database to date. However, hepatic failure with or without fatalities has been reported during postmarketing experience with the drug, although insufficient information is available to establish a cause. Patients with type 2 diabetes mellitus may have fatty liver disease or cardiac disease with episodic CHF, both of which may cause liver test abnormalities; such patients also may have other forms of liver disease, many of which can be treated or managed. Liver function tests (serum ALT and AST, alkaline phosphatase, total bilirubin) should be obtained prior to initiation of pioglitazone therapy. If results of such tests are abnormal, pioglitazone therapy should be initiated with caution.

Development of manifestations suggestive of hepatic dysfunction (e.g., right upper abdominal discomfort, fatigue, anorexia, dark urine, jaundice) should lead to prompt rechecking of liver function. If such symptoms are accompanied by serum ALT increases exceeding 3 times the upper limit of normal, pioglitazone therapy should be interrupted and investigation done to establish the probable cause of the abnormal test results; the drug should not be restarted in such patients without another explanation for the liver test abnormalities. Patients receiving pioglitazone who have serum ALT concentrations exceeding 3 times the reference range and serum total bilirubin concentrations exceeding twice the reference range without alternative explanations are at risk for severe drug-induced liver injury; the drug should not be restarted in such patients. The manufacturer states that pioglitazone may be used with caution in patients with lesser elevations of serum ALT or bilirubin who have an alternative probable cause for such elevations.

Musculoskeletal Effects

Thiazolidinedione use is associated with bone loss and fractures in women and possibly in men with type 2 diabetes mellitus. In a long-term (34.5 months of follow-up) cardiovascular outcomes study (PROACTIVE) in patients with type 2 diabetes mellitus (mean duration of diabetes: 9.5 years), 5.1 or 2.5% of women receiving pioglitazone or placebo, respectively, experienced a fracture. Such effects were noted after the first year of treatment and persisted throughout the study. The majority of fractures observed in female patients receiving pioglitazone were

nonvertebral, occurring in a distal upper limb (i.e., forearm, hand, wrist) or distal lower limb (i.e., foot, ankle, fibula, tibia). In an observational study in the United Kingdom in men and women (mean age: 60.7 years) with diabetes mellitus, use of pioglitazone or rosiglitazone for approximately 12–18 months (as estimated from prescription records) was associated with a twofold to threefold increase in fractures, particularly of the hip and wrist. The overall risk of fracture was similar among men and women and was independent of body mass index, comorbid conditions, diabetic complications, duration of diabetes mellitus, and use of other oral antidiabetic drugs.

Risk of fracture should be considered when initiating or continuing thiazolidinedione therapy, particularly in female patients. Bone health should be assessed and maintained according to current standards of care.

Risk of Bladder Cancer

Although the results of various clinical studies evaluating the association of pioglitazone use and bladder cancer have varied, overall findings from studies in animals and humans suggest that pioglitazone therapy may be associated with an increased risk of bladder cancer. There are insufficient data to determine whether pioglitazone is a tumor promoter for urinary bladder tumors.

In preclinical carcinogenicity studies of pioglitazone, bladder tumors were observed in male rats receiving doses of pioglitazone that produced blood concentrations of pioglitazone approximately equivalent to those resulting from the maximum recommended clinical dose in humans. In addition, results from two 3-year controlled clinical studies of pioglitazone (the PROACTIVE study and a liver safety study) demonstrated a higher percentage of bladder cancer cases in patients receiving pioglitazone versus comparator drugs. However, an increased risk of bladder cancer was not observed when patients who completed the PROACTIVE study were observed for an additional 10 years, with minimal exposure to pioglitazone.

A 10-year epidemiologic study conducted by the manufacturer concluded that there was no statistically significant association overall between pioglitazone exposure and bladder cancer. However, there was a slight trend towards higher risk of bladder cancer with increasing duration of pioglitazone use. The median duration of therapy among pioglitazone-treated patients in this study was 2.8 years (range 0.2–13.2 years). In addition, results of a retrospective cohort (nested case-control design) study involving more than 115,000 patients in a United Kingdom general practice database found a statistically significant 83% increase in the rate of bladder cancer with ever use of pioglitazone, but no increased risk with rosiglitazone therapy. This cohort study found a dose-response relationship for cumulative duration of pioglitazone use, with the highest risk observed in patients who received the drug for more than 24 months. Similarly, another retrospective cohort study involving more than 145,000 patients found a 63% increase in the rate of bladder cancer with pioglitazone therapy and no increased risk with rosiglitazone therapy. A duration-response and dose-response relationship also was evident in this study; substantial increases in the risk of bladder cancer were observed with increasing cumulative duration of use and cumulative dose of pioglitazone.

The manufacturer and FDA state that pioglitazone should not be used in patients with active bladder cancer; in addition, the drug should be used with caution in patients who have a history of bladder cancer, weighing the benefits of glycemic control against the unknown risks of cancer recurrence with pioglitazone therapy. Patients who are concerned about the possible risks associated with using pioglitazone should be advised to consult their healthcare professional.

Hypoglycemia

Concomitant therapy with pioglitazone and insulin or other antidiabetic drugs (particularly insulin secretagogues such as sulfonylureas) increases the risk for hypoglycemia. A reduced dosage of the concomitant antidiabetic agent may be needed to decrease the risk of hypoglycemia. (See Combination Therapy with Other Oral Antidiabetic Agents or Insulin under Dosage and Administration: Dosage.) Hypoglycemia can also occur when caloric intake is deficient or when strenuous exercise is not compensated by caloric supplement. Hypoglycemia may be difficult to recognize in geriatric patients and in individuals taking β-adrenergic blocking drugs.

Ocular Effects

During postmarketing experience, rare cases of new-onset or worsening (diabetic) macular edema with decreased visual acuity have been reported with pioglitazone or another thiazolidinedione; most patients had concurrent peripheral edema. Some patients with macular edema presented with symptoms of blurred vision or decreased visual acuity, but other cases were detected by routine ophthalmologic examination. Symptoms improved in some patients following discontinuance of pioglitazone. Patients with diabetes mellitus should have regular eye examinations by an ophthalmologist according to current standards of care. Patients receiving pioglitazone who report any visual symptoms should be referred promptly to an ophthalmologist, regardless of the presence of other concurrent therapy or physical findings.

Ovulatory Effects

Like other thiazolidinediones, pioglitazone may promote ovulation in some premenopausal anovulatory women. Premenopausal women receiving pioglitazone should be advised of the potential for an unintended pregnancy.

Macrovascular Outcomes

Evidence of macrovascular risk reduction with pioglitazone has not been conclusively demonstrated in controlled clinical trials.

Laboratory Abnormalities

Dose-related decreases in hemoglobin and hematocrit usually becomes evident 4–12 weeks after initiation of therapy and values remain stable thereafter. These effects may be related to plasma volume expansion and have rarely been associated with clinically important hematologic manifestations.

Isolated elevations in serum creatine kinase (CK, creatine phosphokinase, CPK) exceeding 10 times the upper limit of normal were noted rarely during protocol-specified measurements in clinical trials. Such elevations resolved in most patients without apparent sequelae despite continued therapy; any relationship to pioglitazone therapy is unknown.

Use of Fixed Combinations

When pioglitazone is used in fixed combination with other drugs (e.g., metformin, glimepiride), the cautions, precautions, and contraindications associated with those drugs must be considered in addition to those associated with pioglitazone.

Specific Populations

Pregnancy

Data are lacking on the use of pioglitazone in pregnant women. Blood glucose abnormalities during pregnancy are associated with an increased incidence of congenital anomalies and neonatal morbidity and mortality. In reproduction studies in rats and rabbits, pioglitazone administered during organogenesis at exposures up to 5 and 35 times the maximum recommended human dose, respectively, was not associated with adverse developmental effects. However, delayed parturition and reduced embryofetal viability were observed with pioglitazone dosages at least 9 times the maximum recommended human dose. Offspring of pregnant rats who were administered pioglitazone at dosages at least 2 times the maximum recommended human dose during late gestation and lactation had delayed postnatal development attributed to decreased body weight.

Lactation

Pioglitazone is distributed into milk in rats; it is unknown whether pioglitazone is distributed into human milk. The benefits of breast-feeding should be weighed against the potential risk of adverse effects on the breast-fed infant from pioglitazone.

Pediatric Use

Safety and efficacy of pioglitazone have not been established in children or adolescents younger than 18 years of age; use in this age group currently is not recommended by the manufacturer because of adverse effects observed in adults (e.g., fluid retention and heart failure, fractures, urinary bladder tumors). However, the American Diabetes Association (ADA) states that most pediatric diabetologists use oral antidiabetic agents in children with type 2 diabetes mellitus because of greater patient compliance with therapy and convenience for the patient's family and a lack of evidence demonstrating better efficacy of insulin as initial therapy for type 2 diabetes mellitus.

Geriatric Use

Pharmacokinetic, efficacy, and adverse effect profiles in geriatric patients are similar to those in younger adults, although small sample sizes in studies of patients 75 years or older limit conclusions. While pioglitazone area under the concentration-time

curve (AUC) is about 21% higher in healthy geriatric individuals than in younger individuals and mean terminal half-life is also prolonged (10 hours versus 7 hours, respectively), these changes are not considered clinically relevant.

Hepatic Impairment

Pioglitazone therapy should be initiated with caution in patients with abnormal liver function test results. Pioglitazone therapy should be interrupted if ALT exceeds 3 times the upper limit of normal and the cause of liver test abnormalities should be investigated. (See Hepatic Effects under Warnings/Precautions: Other Warnings/Precautions, in Cautions.)

● Common Adverse Effects

Adverse effects (not dose related) occurring in at least 5% of patients receiving pioglitazone and more frequently than with placebo include upper respiratory tract infection, headache, sinusitis, myalgia, pharyngitis, and edema. Adverse effects generally were similar with pioglitazone monotherapy versus combined therapy with sulfonylureas, metformin, or insulin; however, edema was more common during pioglitazone monotherapy and during all combined therapies than with placebo. Pioglitazone-induced reductions in hyperglycemia are associated with mild weight gain.

DRUG INTERACTIONS

● Drugs Affecting Hepatic Microsomal Enzymes

Inhibitors or Inducers of CYP3A4

Potential pharmacokinetic interaction with inhibitors or inducers of cytochrome P-450 (CYP) isoenzyme 3A4.

Concomitant use of pioglitazone (45 mg daily for 7 days) and ketoconazole (200 mg twice daily for 7 days), an inhibitor of CYP3A4, increased peak plasma concentration and area under the concentration-time curve (AUC) of pioglitazone by 14 and 34%, respectively.

Concomitant use of ranitidine (150 mg twice daily for 4 days), a relatively weak CYP3A4 inhibitor, and pioglitazone (45 mg daily for 7 days) reduced pioglitazone AUC and peak plasma concentration by 13 and 16%, respectively; pioglitazone had a negligible effect on ranitidine pharmacokinetics.

CYP3A4 Substrates

Pioglitazone is a weak inducer of CYP3A4. Potential pharmacokinetic interaction (reduction in peak plasma concentration and AUC) with CYP3A4 substrates (e.g., atorvastatin, midazolam, ethinyl estradiol, nifedipine).

Concomitant use of pioglitazone (45 mg daily for 7 days) and atorvastatin (80 mg daily for 7 days) resulted in reductions of 14 and 23% in atorvastatin AUC and peak plasma concentration, respectively; pioglitazone AUC and peak plasma concentration were reduced by 24 and 31%, respectively.

Administration of pioglitazone (45 mg daily for 7 days) and midazolam (single dose of 7.5 mg on day 15) reduced midazolam AUC and peak plasma concentration each by 26%.

Administration of pioglitazone (45 mg daily for 4 days) with extended-release nifedipine (30 mg daily for 4 days) reduced nifedipine AUC and peak plasma concentration by 13 and 17%, respectively; pioglitazone AUC and peak plasma concentration were increased by 5 and 4%, respectively, with concomitant use of pioglitazone (45 mg daily for 7 days) and extended-release nifedipine (30 mg daily for 7 days).

Concomitant use of an estrogen-progestin contraceptive (ethinyl estradiol 0.035 mg with norethindrone 1 mg daily for 21 days) and pioglitazone (45 mg daily for 21 days) resulted in small decreases in peak plasma concentration (13%) and AUC (11%) of ethinyl estradiol. The clinical importance of these changes is unknown.

Inhibitors or Inducers of CYP2C8

Pioglitazone is a CYP2C8 substrate; potential pharmacokinetic interaction with inhibitors (e.g., gemfibrozil) or inducers (e.g., rifampin) of CYP2C8. Adjustments in pioglitazone dosage may be needed during initiation or discontinuance of an inhibitor or inducer of CYP2C8. (See Concomitant Therapy with Potent CYP2C8 Inhibitors or Inducers under Dosage and Administration: Dosage.)

Concomitant use of pioglitazone (single 15-mg dose) and gemfibrozil (600 mg twice daily for 2 days) resulted in a 3.2-fold increase in AUC of pioglitazone and a 6% increase in pioglitazone peak plasma concentration; half-life of pioglitazone also increased from 8.3 to 22.7 hours.

Concomitant use of pioglitazone (single 30-mg dose) and rifampin (600 mg daily for 5 days) resulted in a 54% decrease in AUC and a 5% decrease in peak plasma concentration of pioglitazone.

CYP2C9 or CYP1A2 Substrates

Pharmacokinetic interaction is unlikely with CYP2C9 substrates (e.g., warfarin). Concomitant therapy with warfarin sodium (dosage adjusted to achieve therapeutic anticoagulation [Quick's prothrombin value of 35 ± 5%]) and pioglitazone (45 mg daily for 7 days) resulted in changes of 3% or less in AUC and peak plasma concentration of R- or S-warfarin.

Pharmacokinetic interaction is unlikely with theophylline, a CYP1A2 substrate. Concomitant use of pioglitazone (45 mg daily for 7 days) and theophylline (400 mg twice daily for 7 days) did not appreciably alter (i.e., 5% or less change) AUC and peak plasma concentration of pioglitazone or theophylline.

● *Antidiabetic Agents*

Potential pharmacodynamic interaction (risk of hypoglycemia) with insulin or oral hypoglycemic agents; reduction in the dose of the concomitant agent may be necessary.

Pharmacokinetic interaction with metformin or glipizide is unlikely. With concomitant use of pioglitazone (45 mg daily for 7 days) and glipizide (5 mg daily for 7 days), glipizide AUC and peak plasma concentration were reduced by 3 and 8%, respectively. Concomitant administration of pioglitazone (45 mg daily for 8 days) and metformin hydrochloride (single 1-g dose on day 8) resulted in reductions of 3 and 5% in metformin AUC and peak plasma concentration, respectively.

● *Digoxin*

Concomitant therapy with digoxin (0.2 mg for 2 doses as a loading dose, then 0.25 mg daily for 7 days) and pioglitazone (45 mg daily for 7 days) resulted in increases of 15 and 17% in digoxin AUC and peak plasma concentration, respectively.

● *Fexofenadine*

Concomitant administration of pioglitazone (45 mg daily for 7 days) and fexofenadine hydrochloride (60 mg twice daily for 7 days) resulted in an increase of 30 and 37% in fexofenadine AUC and peak plasma concentration, respectively; fexofenadine had no appreciable effect on pioglitazone pharmacokinetics.

● *Topiramate*

Concomitant administration of pioglitazone (30 mg daily for 7 days) and topiramate (96 mg twice daily for 7 days) resulted in a 15% decrease in the AUC of pioglitazone; in addition, AUC of its M-III (keto derivative) and M-IV (hydroxyl derivative) active metabolites was decreased by 60 and 16%, respectively. Although the clinical relevance of this decrease is unknown, patients receiving pioglitazone and topiramate concomitantly should be monitored for adequate glycemic control.

DESCRIPTION

Pioglitazone is a thiazolidinedione (glitazone) antidiabetic agent that is structurally and pharmacologically related to troglitazone and rosiglitazone but unrelated to other antidiabetic agents, including sulfonylureas, biguanides, and α-glucosidase inhibitors.

Pioglitazone acts principally by increasing insulin sensitivity in target tissues, as well as decreasing hepatic gluconeogenesis. Pioglitazone is a peroxisome proliferator-activated receptor$_\gamma$ (PPAR$_\gamma$) agonist that increases transcription of insulin-responsive genes and increases insulin sensitivity. Pioglitazone, like other thiazolidinediones, ameliorates insulin resistance associated with type 2 diabetes mellitus without stimulating insulin release from pancreatic β cells, thus avoiding

the risk of hypoglycemia. Because pioglitazone does not lower glucose concentrations below euglycemia, the drug is appropriately referred to as an antidiabetic agent rather than a hypoglycemic agent. Some evidence suggests that the glucoregulatory effects of thiazolidinediones are mediated in part via enhanced hepatic and peripheral glucose uptake and reduced systemic and tissue lipid availability.

Following oral administration of pioglitazone, peak plasma concentrations are achieved within 2 hours. Food delays time to peak concentrations to 3–4 hours but does not alter AUC. Pioglitazone is extensively metabolized via hydroxylation and oxidation, principally via the cytochrome P-450 (CYP) 2C8 and CYP3A4 isoenzymes, with involvement of several other isoforms, including CYP1A1 (mainly an extrahepatic isoenzyme). The major circulating active metabolites of pioglitazone are M-III (keto derivative) and M-IV (hydroxyl derivative).

ADVICE TO PATIENTS

When pioglitazone is used in fixed combination with other drugs, importance of informing patients of important cautionary information about the concomitant agent(s).

Importance of reading medication guide provided by the manufacturer before starting pioglitazone and each time prescription is refilled.

Importance of informing patients of potential risks and advantages of therapy and of alternative therapies.

Discuss potential for alterations in dosage requirements during periods of stress (e.g., fever, trauma, infection, surgery); importance of contacting a clinician promptly.

Importance of informing patients that pioglitazone must not be used in patients with severe heart failure (NYHA class III or IV). Importance of identifying and reporting to clinicians potential symptoms of heart failure, such as unusually rapid increase in weight, edema (especially in ankles or legs), unusual fatigue, trouble breathing, or shortness of breath (especially when lying down).

Importance of immediate reporting of potential manifestations of hepatotoxicity (e.g., unexplained nausea or vomiting, abdominal pain, fatigue, loss of appetite, or dark urine, yellowing of skin or whites of eyes).

Increased risk of bladder cancer with pioglitazone therapy. Importance of patient not taking pioglitazone if receiving treatment for bladder cancer. Importance of patient reporting any sign of macroscopic hematuria or symptoms such as dysuria or urinary urgency that develop or increase during pioglitazone treatment.

Importance of taking exactly as prescribed. If a dose is missed on one day, take the next dose as prescribed unless otherwise instructed by your clinician; do not double the dose to make up for the missed dose. Importance of changing dosage only under medical supervision. Importance of immediately contacting a clinician if accidental overdosage occurs.

Risk of hypoglycemia in patients receiving concomitant insulin or other antidiabetic therapy. Provide instructions to patients and responsible family members regarding management of hypoglycemia, including recognition of symptoms, predisposing conditions, and treatment.

Risk of pregnancy in premenopausal anovulatory women.

Importance of diet and exercise regimen adherence. Importance of regular monitoring (preferably self-monitoring) of blood glucose and of glycosylated hemoglobin (HbA$_{1c}$) concentrations.

Risk of fractures (e.g., hand, upper arm, foot) in women.

Importance of regular eye examinations. Importance of reporting changes in vision.

Importance of informing clinicians of existing or contemplated concomitant therapy, including prescription and OTC drugs, as well as any concomitant illnesses.

Importance of women informing their clinician if they are or plan to become pregnant or plan to breast-feed.

Importance of informing patients of other important precautionary information. (See Cautions.)

PREPARATIONS

Excipients in commercially available drug preparations may have clinically important effects in some individuals; consult specific product labeling for details.

Pioglitazone Hydrochloride

Oral		
Tablets, film-coated	15 mg (of pioglitazone)*	Actos®, Takeda
		Pioglitazone Hydrochloride
	30 mg (of pioglitazone)*	Actos®, Takeda
		Pioglitazone Hydrochloride
	45 mg (of pioglitazone)*	Actos®, Takeda
		Pioglitazone Hydrochloride

* available from one or more manufacturer, distributor, and/or repackager by generic (nonproprietary) name

Pioglitazone Hydrochloride Combinations

Oral		
Tablets	15 mg (of pioglitazone) with Metformin Hydrochloride 500 mg*	Actoplus Met®, Takeda
		Pioglitazone Hydrochloride with Metformin Hydrochloride
	15 mg (of pioglitazone) with Metformin Hydrochloride 850 mg*	Actoplus Met®, Takeda
		Pioglitazone Hydrochloride with Metformin Hydrochloride
	30 mg (of pioglitazone) with Glimepiride 2 mg*	Duetact®, Takeda
		Pioglitazone Hydrochloride with Glimepiride
	30 mg (of pioglitazone) with Glimepiride 4 mg*	Duetact®, Takeda
		Pioglitazone Hydrochloride with Glimepiride

* available from one or more manufacturer, distributor, and/or repackager by generic (nonproprietary) name

Selected Revisions June 21, 2021, © Copyright, September 1, 1999, American Society of Health-System Pharmacists, Inc.

Rosiglitazone Maleate

68:20.28 • THIAZOLIDINEDIONES

■ Rosiglitazone is a thiazolidinedione (glitazone) antidiabetic agent that is structurally and pharmacologically related to pioglitazone and troglitazone.

USES

● Type 2 Diabetes Mellitus

Rosiglitazone is used as monotherapy or in combination with a sulfonylurea, metformin hydrochloride, or a sulfonylurea and metformin as an adjunct to diet and exercise to improve glycemic control in patients with type 2 diabetes mellitus.

Rosiglitazone may be added to therapy with the fixed combination of glyburide and metformin hydrochloride in patients whose hyperglycemia is not adequately controlled on therapy with the fixed combination. (See Concomitant Glyburide and Metformin Therapy under Dosage and Administration: Dosage, in Glyburide 68:20.20.)

Current guidelines for the treatment of type 2 diabetes mellitus generally recommend metformin as first-line therapy in addition to lifestyle modifications in patients with recent-onset type 2 diabetes mellitus or mild hyperglycemia because of its well-established safety and efficacy (i.e., beneficial effects on glycosylated hemoglobin [hemoglobin A_{1c}; HbA_{1c}], weight, and cardiovascular mortality). (See Uses: Type 2 Diabetes Mellitus, in Metformin 68:20.04.) In patients with contraindications or intolerance to metformin (e.g., risk of lactic acidosis, GI intolerance) or in selected other patients, some experts suggest that initial therapy with a drug from another class of antidiabetic agents (e.g., a glucagon-like peptide-1 [GLP-1] receptor agonist, sodium-glucose cotransporter 2 [SGLT2] inhibitor, dipeptidyl peptidase-4 [DPP-4] inhibitor, sulfonylurea, thiazolidinedione, basal insulin) may be acceptable based on patient factors. Initiating antidiabetic therapy with 2 agents (e.g., metformin plus another drug) may be appropriate in patients with an initial HbA_{1c} exceeding 7.5% or at least 1.5% above the target level. In metformin-intolerant patients with high initial HbA_{1c} levels, some experts suggest initiation of therapy with 2 agents from other antidiabetic drug classes with complementary mechanisms of action.

Because of the progressive nature of type 2 diabetes mellitus, patients initially receiving an oral antidiabetic agent will eventually require multiple oral and/or injectable noninsulin antidiabetic agents of different therapeutic classes and/or insulin for adequate glycemic control. Patients who have inadequate glycemic control with initial (e.g., metformin) monotherapy should receive treatment with additional antidiabetic agents; data suggest that the addition of each noninsulin agent to initial therapy lowers HbA_{1c} by approximately 0.7–1%. In addition, early initiation of combination therapy may help more rapidly attain glycemic goals and extend the time to treatment failure.

Factors to consider when selecting additional antidiabetic agents for combination therapy in patients with inadequate glycemic control on metformin monotherapy include patient comorbidities (e.g., atherosclerotic cardiovascular disease [ASCVD], established kidney disease, heart failure), hypoglycemia risk, impact on weight, cost, risk of adverse effects, and patient preference. When the greater glucose-lowering effect of an injectable drug is needed in patients with type 2 diabetes mellitus, some experts currently state that an injectable GLP-1 receptor agonist is preferred over insulin in most patients because of beneficial effects on body weight and a lower risk of hypoglycemia, although adverse GI effects may diminish tolerability. While addition of a GLP-1 receptor agonist may successfully control hyperglycemia, many patients will eventually require insulin therapy. Early introduction of insulin therapy should be considered when hyperglycemia is severe (e.g., blood glucose of at least 300 mg/dL or HbA_{1c} exceeding 9–10%), especially in the presence of catabolic manifestations (e.g., weight loss, hypertriglyceridemia, ketosis) or symptoms of hyperglycemia. For additional information regarding the initiation of insulin therapy in patients with diabetes mellitus, see Uses: Diabetes Mellitus, in the Insulins General Statement 68:20.08.

Rosiglitazone Monotherapy

Efficacy of rosiglitazone as monotherapy for the management of type 2 diabetes mellitus was established in 6 controlled studies of 8–52 weeks' duration.

Rosiglitazone improved glycemic control as measured by fasting glucose and HbA_{1c} concentrations. Some evidence suggests that rosiglitazone has a more durable glycemic effect than sulfonylureas or metformin. In a long-term (4–6 years' duration) randomized, controlled clinical trial (A Diabetes Outcome Progression Trial [ADOPT]) evaluating the duration of glycemic control after initiation of monotherapy with rosiglitazone, metformin, or glyburide, the cumulative incidence of treatment failure (i.e., defined as confirmed fasting plasma glucose concentrations exceeding 180 mg/dL on consecutive testing after at least 6 weeks of treatment at the maximum dictated or tolerated dosage of the study drug) at 5 years was 15, 21, and 34%, respectively; this represents a risk reduction with rosiglitazone monotherapy of 32% or 63% compared with metformin or glyburide monotherapy, respectively. However, the use of fasting glucose concentrations as a measure of treatment failure rather than HbA_{1c} concentration, which correlates more closely with diabetic complications, has been criticized; also, differences among the treatment groups in mean HbA_{1c} concentration at 4 years were less pronounced, particularly between rosiglitazone and metformin.

The manufacturer states that rosiglitazone should *not* be used in patients with type 1 diabetes mellitus or for the treatment of diabetic ketoacidosis.

Combination Therapy

Data from a number of comparative trials evaluating combination therapy with rosiglitazone and metformin or a sulfonylurea agent indicate that such combination therapy may result in an additive effect on glycemic control. Efficacy of the combination of rosiglitazone and metformin in patients whose type 2 diabetes mellitus was inadequately controlled with metformin alone was established in several controlled studies of 26 weeks' duration in which combined therapy improved glycemic control without affecting serum insulin concentrations. In patients inadequately controlled with sulfonylurea (e.g., glyburide, glipizide, glimepiride) monotherapy, the combination of rosiglitazone and a sulfonylurea reduced fasting glucose and HbA_{1c} concentrations compared with monotherapy with a sulfonylurea alone.

Substantial improvements in fasting plasma glucose and HbA_{1c} concentrations have been observed in patients receiving concurrent rosiglitazone and metformin therapy compared with those receiving metformin alone. In a dose-ranging trial evaluating rosiglitazone 4 or 8 mg as add-on therapy to the maximum daily dosage of metformin hydrochloride, 28.1% of patients receiving the higher dosage of rosiglitazone concurrently with metformin achieved HbA_{1c} values not exceeding 7%.

In patients inadequately controlled with sulfonylurea (e.g., glyburide, glipizide, glimepiride) monotherapy, the combination of rosiglitazone and a sulfonylurea reduced fasting glucose and HbA_{1c} concentrations compared with monotherapy with a sulfonylurea alone. In a 2-year study in geriatric patients (59–89 years of age) who were inadequately controlled on glipizide at half the maximum recommended dosage (10 mg twice daily), the addition of rosiglitazone (4–8 mg daily) was more effective in preventing loss of glycemic control (defined as fasting plasma glucose concentrations of at least 180 mg/dL, the primary clinical end point) than continued upward titration of glipizide (maximum of 20 mg twice daily).

DOSAGE AND ADMINISTRATION

● General

Following initiation of rosiglitazone therapy or dosage increases, patients should be monitored for adverse effects related to fluid retention. (See Congestive Heart Failure under Warnings/Precautions: Warnings, in Cautions.) Fasting blood glucose (FPG) and glycosylated hemoglobin (hemoglobin A_{1c} [HbA_{1c}]) concentrations should be monitored periodically to determine the patient's response to therapy.

Following initiation of rosiglitazone therapy or dosage increases, sufficient time should be allowed to assess therapeutic response to rosiglitazone (8–12 weeks using FPG concentrations).

● Administration

Rosiglitazone maleate is administered orally once daily or in divided doses twice daily, without regard to meals. If the patient misses a dose of rosiglitazone, the missed dose should be taken as soon as it is remembered. If the missed dose is remembered at the time of the next dose, the regularly scheduled dose should be taken; a double dose should *not* be taken to make up for the missed dose.

● Dosage

Type 2 Diabetes Mellitus

Dosage of rosiglitazone maleate is expressed in terms of the base.

Rosiglitazone Monotherapy

The recommended initial dosage of rosiglitazone is 4 mg once daily or 2 mg twice daily. If the response is inadequate after 8–12 weeks, dosage may be increased to 8 mg daily as a single dose or 2 divided doses daily. The maximum recommended dosage is 8 mg daily; studies suggest no additional benefit from 12-mg daily dosages.

Combination Therapy

A thiazolidinedione such as rosiglitazone may be added to the antidiabetic regimen in patients who have inadequate glycemic control with repaglinide monotherapy. Conversely, if glycemic control with thiazolidinedione monotherapy is inadequate, repaglinide may be added to the antidiabetic regimen. (See Type 2 Diabetes Mellitus under Dosage and Administration: Dosage, in Repaglinide 68:20.16.) To minimize the risk of hypoglycemia, the dosage of each agent should be carefully adjusted to determine the minimal dosage required to achieve glycemic control.

For patients who have inadequate glycemic control on the fixed combination of glyburide and metformin hydrochloride, a thiazolidinedione such as rosiglitazone may be added at its recommended initial dosage and the dosage of the fixed combination may be continued unchanged. In patients requiring further glycemic control, the dosage of rosiglitazone may be titrated upward according to the manufacturer's recommendations. Triple therapy with glyburide, metformin hydrochloride, and a thiazolidinedione may increase the potential for hypoglycemia at any time of day. If hypoglycemia develops with such triple therapy, consideration should be given to reducing the dosage of the glyburide component; adjustment of the dosage of the other components of the antidiabetic regimen also should be considered as clinically indicated.

● Special Populations

Rosiglitazone maleate should be initiated (or continued) with caution in patients with mild hepatic enzyme elevations (ALT not exceeding 2.5 times the upper limit of normal) but no evidence of active liver disease. Therapy with rosiglitazone should not be initiated in patients with baseline ALT concentrations exceeding 3 times the upper limit of normal. (See Hepatic Effects under Warnings/Precautions: General Precautions, in Cautions.)

Adjustment of rosiglitazone dosage is *not* necessary for patients with renal impairment *nor* for geriatric patients.

CAUTIONS

● Contraindications

Initiation of therapy with rosiglitazone is contraindicated in patients with New York Heart Association (NYHA) class III or IV heart failure. (See Congestive Heart Failure under Warnings/Precautions: Warnings, in Cautions.)

Rosiglitazone is contraindicated in patients with a history of hypersensitivity to the drug or to any ingredient in the formulation.

● Warnings/Precautions

Warnings

Congestive Heart Failure

Thiazolidinediones, including rosiglitazone, alone or in combination with other antidiabetic agents, can cause fluid retention and may lead to or exacerbate congestive heart failure (CHF). Use of thiazolidinediones is associated with an approximately twofold increased risk of CHF. (See Edema under Warnings/Precautions: General Precautions, in Cautions.) Patients should be observed for signs and symptoms of CHF (e.g., dyspnea, rapid weight gain, edema, unexplained cough or fatigue), especially during initiation of therapy and dosage titration. If

signs and symptoms of CHF develop, the disorder should be managed according to current standards of care. In addition, a decrease in the dosage of rosiglitazone or discontinuance of the drug should be considered.

Initiation of therapy with rosiglitazone is contraindicated in patients with NYHA class III or IV heart failure. Patients with NYHA class III or IV cardiac status with or without CHF or with acute coronary syndromes were not studied in clinical trials of rosiglitazone; use of rosiglitazone is *not* recommended in these patients. If an acute coronary event occurs, the manufacturer states that discontinuance of rosiglitazone should be considered during the acute phase of a coronary event, as such patients are at risk for development of CHF. In addition, use of rosiglitazone is *not* recommended in patients with symptomatic heart failure. Caution should be exercised in patients with edema and in those who are at risk for CHF. Thiazolidinedione therapy should not be initiated in hospitalized patients with diabetes mellitus because of the delayed onset of action and because possible drug-related increases in vascular volume and CHF may complicate care of patients with hemodynamic changes induced by coexisting conditions or in-hospital interventions.

Findings from a meta-analysis of randomized controlled studies that assessed the risk of development of CHF and death from cardiovascular causes in patients receiving thiazolidinediones indicate that the risk of CHF is higher in patients receiving thiazolidinediones (relative risk of 1.72; 95% confidence interval: 1.21–2.42) than in controls (individuals receiving other antidiabetic agents or placebo). The relative risk for CHF was increased across a wide background of cardiovascular risk (i.e., patients with prediabetes, with type 2 diabetes mellitus without cardiovascular disease, with type 2 diabetes mellitus and cardiovascular disease other than CHF, or with type 2 diabetes mellitus and CHF [NYHA class I or II] and ejection fraction less than 40%). In contrast to the increased risk for CHF observed in thiazolidinedione-treated patients, the risk of cardiovascular death was not increased in patients receiving these agents.

In a placebo-controlled echocardiographic study in patients with type 2 diabetes mellitus and NYHA class I or II heart failure receiving rosiglitazone in addition to other antidiabetic and CHF therapy, an increased incidence of adverse cardiovascular events (e.g., edema, need for additional CHF therapy) was reported in patients receiving rosiglitazone compared with patients receiving placebo. Changes in the left ventricular ejection fraction from baseline did not differ among rosiglitazone- or placebo-treated patients. In a long-term, cardiovascular outcomes trial in patients with type 2 diabetes mellitus, heart failure was reported in 2.7% of patients receiving rosiglitazone compared with 1.3% of those receiving active control (metformin plus a sulfonylurea).

An increased incidence of CHF has been observed in a number of clinical trials (duration of 16–26 weeks) in patients receiving rosiglitazone as add-on therapy to insulin compared with that in patients receiving insulin monotherapy. These trials included patients with long-standing diabetes mellitus (median duration: 12 years) and a high prevalence of preexisting medical conditions, including peripheral neuropathy, retinopathy, ischemic heart disease, vascular disease, and CHF. The incidence of emergent symptomatic heart failure was at least twofold higher with concurrent rosiglitazone and insulin therapy compared with that observed with insulin therapy alone. The manufacturer states that concurrent administration of rosiglitazone and insulin therapy is *not* recommended.

Some observational studies have indicated a substantially increased risk of heart failure requiring hospitalization in geriatric patients 65 years of age or older receiving rosiglitazone compared with another thiazolidinedione antidiabetic agent (pioglitazone).

General Precautions

Major Adverse Cardiovascular Events

The cardiovascular safety of rosiglitazone has been an area of ongoing concern and study. Findings from several meta-analyses of principally short-term trials and observational studies suggested that rosiglitazone may be associated with an increased risk of myocardial infarction (MI) and other adverse cardiovascular events. However, although some uncertainty remains regarding the cardiovascular risk of rosiglitazone, FDA states that concerns have been substantially reduced in light of the readjudicated findings of a dedicated cardiovascular outcomes trial (the Rosiglitazone Evaluated for Cardiac Outcomes and Regulation of Glycemia in Diabetes [RECORD]). FDA has therefore removed previous prescribing and dispensing restrictions for the drug. Despite some limitations, the RECORD trial is considered to represent a higher level of evidence regarding cardiovascular risk than meta-analyses and observational studies, and therefore provides some reassurance that rosiglitazone does not increase the risk of MI or other adverse cardiovascular effects compared with other antidiabetic agents.

In a meta-analysis of 52 randomized, double-blind trials (mean duration: 6 months), a substantially increased risk of MI was observed with rosiglitazone versus placebo; in addition, major adverse cardiovascular events (MACE) occurred more frequently in patients receiving rosiglitazone than in those receiving comparator agents, although the difference was not statistically significant. As a result of these findings, the US Food and Drug Administration (FDA) restricted use of rosiglitazone in 2010 to patients who were unable to achieve glycemic control with other antidiabetic agents. However, evidence regarding the cardiovascular risk of rosiglitazone has been conflicting, and the findings observed in previous meta-analyses have not been confirmed in long-term (greater than 3 years' duration), prospective randomized studies. These studies, which include the RECORD study, generally have found no evidence of an increased risk of mortality or MACE with rosiglitazone compared with metformin and/or a sulfonylurea. In the RECORD study, rosiglitazone was noninferior to the combination of metformin and a sulfonylurea with respect to the primary composite end point of cardiovascular hospitalization or cardiovascular death. During the course of FDA's original review of the RECORD study, important questions arose about potential bias in the identification of cardiovascular events, prompting FDA to commission outside experts to perform an independent readjudication of the data. Results of this comprehensive reanalysis confirmed the original findings that failed to show an increased risk of MI with rosiglitazone versus metformin and a sulfonylurea. While some component end points appeared to favor rosiglitazone (i.e., cardiovascular deaths, nonfatal strokes, all-cause mortality) or metformin/sulfonylurea (i.e., nonfatal MI), these findings were not statistically significant. Results of 2 other long-term, prospective randomized studies also showed no statistically significant differences in MACE or its individual components between rosiglitazone and placebo (the Diabetes Reduction Assessment with Ramipril and Rosiglitazone Medication [DREAM] trial in patients with impaired glucose tolerance) or between rosiglitazone and metformin or a sulfonylurea (the Diabetes Outcome Progression Trial [ADOPT] in patients with type 2 diabetes mellitus who were initiating oral antidiabetic monotherapy).

Edema

Fluid retention can occur and may lead to or exacerbate heart failure in patients receiving a thiazolidinedione, including rosiglitazone, alone or in combination with other antidiabetic agents, including insulin. Patients with ongoing edema are more likely to have adverse events associated with edema if therapy with rosiglitazone in combination with insulin is initiated. Diuretic therapy may be necessary for management of fluid retention. Weight gain possibly associated with fluid retention and fat accumulation has been observed during therapy with rosiglitazone alone or in combination with other antidiabetic agents (e.g., metformin, sulfonylureas, insulin). Caution should be exercised in patients with edema and those at risk for CHF. (See Congestive Heart Failure under Warnings/Precautions: Warnings, in Cautions.)

All patients receiving thiazolidinedione therapy (e.g., rosiglitazone, pioglitazone) should be advised to monitor for weight gain and edema. Any patient developing edema within the first few months of therapy should be evaluated for possible CHF. Other potential causes of edema should be excluded.

Musculoskeletal Effects

Thiazolidinedione use is associated with bone loss and fractures in women and possibly in men with type 2 diabetes mellitus. In long-term comparative clinical trials in patients with type 2 diabetes mellitus, the incidence of bone fracture was increased in patients (particularly women) receiving rosiglitazone versus comparator agents (glyburide and/or metformin). Such effects were noted after the first year of treatment and persisted throughout the study. The majority of fractures observed in patients taking thiazolidinediones were in a distal upper limb (i.e., forearm, hand, wrist) or distal lower limb (i.e., foot, ankle, fibula, tibia). In an observational study in the United Kingdom in men and women (mean age: 60.7 years) with diabetes mellitus, use of pioglitazone or rosiglitazone for approximately 12–18 months (as estimated from prescription records) was associated with a twofold to threefold increase in fractures, particularly of the hip and wrist. The overall risk of fracture was similar among men and women and was independent of body mass index, comorbid conditions, diabetic complications, duration of diabetes mellitus, and use of other oral antidiabetic drugs.

Risk of fractures should be considered when initiating or continuing thiazolidinedione therapy in female patients with type 2 diabetes mellitus. Bone health should be assessed and maintained according to current standards of care. Although increased risk of fracture may also apply to men, the risk appears to be higher among women than men.

Ovulatory Effects

Risk for pregnancy unless contraceptive measures initiated; anovulatory premenopausal women with insulin resistance may resume ovulation during therapy. The frequency of resumption of ovulation with rosiglitazone therapy has not been evaluated in clinical studies, and, therefore, is unknown. If menstrual dysfunction occurs, weigh risks versus benefits of continued rosiglitazone.

Hepatic Effects

No evidence of hepatotoxicity has been noted with rosiglitazone in clinical studies to date, including a long-term (4–6 years) study (ADOPT) in patients with recently diagnosed type 2 diabetes mellitus. In the ADOPT study, the incidence of ALT elevation exceeding 3 times the upper limit of normal was similar in patients receiving rosiglitazone or active comparators (i.e., glyburide or metformin). However, hepatitis, elevations in hepatic enzymes to at least 3 times the upper limit of normal, and liver failure with or without fatalities have been reported during postmarketing experience with rosiglitazone.

Liver function tests are recommended in patients receiving rosiglitazone (prior to therapy, then periodically according to clinician judgment). Therapy with rosiglitazone should not be initiated if baseline ALT concentrations exceed 2.5 times the upper limit of normal. Patients with mildly elevated liver enzymes (e.g., ALT not exceeding 2.5 times the upper limit of normal) prior to or during therapy should be evaluated to determine the cause of the elevation; rosiglitazone should be initiated or continued in such patients with caution and close clinical monitoring.

If ALT increases to more than 3 times the upper limit of normal at any time during therapy, liver function tests should be rechecked as soon as possible. Development of manifestations suggestive of hepatic dysfunction (e.g., unexplained nausea, vomiting, abdominal pain, fatigue, anorexia, dark urine) also should prompt rechecking of liver function. The decision whether to continue therapy should be guided by clinical judgment pending laboratory evaluation. If ALT increases to 3 times the upper limit of normal during therapy and remains elevated, or if jaundice develops, rosiglitazone should be discontinued.

Hematologic Effects

Dose-related decreases in hemoglobin (not exceeding 1 g/dL) and hematocrit (not exceeding 3.3%) usually become evident within the first 3 months after initiation of therapy with rosiglitazone alone and in combination with other antidiabetic agents. Slight decreases in leukocyte counts have been observed in patients receiving rosiglitazone. These effects may be related to plasma volume expansion.

Ocular Effects

During postmarketing experience, rare cases of new-onset or worsening (diabetic) macular edema with decreased visual acuity have been reported with rosiglitazone or another thiazolidinedione; such patients frequently reported concurrent peripheral edema. Some patients with macular edema presented with symptoms of blurred vision or decreased visual acuity, but other cases were detected by routine ophthalmologic examination. Symptoms improved in some patients following discontinuance of rosiglitazone or, rarely, after dosage reduction. Patients with diabetes mellitus should have regular eye examinations by an ophthalmologist. Patients receiving rosiglitazone who report any visual symptoms should be referred promptly to an ophthalmologist, regardless of the presence of other concurrent therapy or physical findings.

Specific Populations

Pregnancy

Category C. The background risk of birth defects, pregnancy loss, or other adverse outcomes is increased in pregnancies complicated by hyperglycemia and may be decreased with good glycemic control. Most clinicians recommend use of insulin monotherapy for maintenance of optimum blood glucose concentrations during pregnancy. Women with diabetes mellitus or a history of gestational diabetes who are pregnant or planning pregnancy require excellent blood glucose control before conception and throughout pregnancy. Careful monitoring of blood glucose concentration is essential in such patients. Rosiglitazone should be used during pregnancy only when the potential benefits justify the possible risk to the fetus.

Lactation

Rosiglitazone-related material is distributed into milk in rats; it is not known whether the drug is distributed into human milk. Because many drugs are distributed into human milk, a decision should be made whether to discontinue nursing or the drug, taking into account the importance of the drug to the woman.

Pediatric Use

Rosiglitazone has been studied in children and adolescents 10–17 years of age; data are insufficient to recommend use in pediatric patients younger than 18 years of age. The manufacturer states that safety and efficacy of rosiglitazone have not been established in pediatric patients. However, the American Diabetes Association (ADA) states that most pediatric diabetologists use oral antidiabetic agents in children with type 2 diabetes mellitus because of greater patient compliance with therapy and convenience for the patient's family and a lack of evidence demonstrating better efficacy of insulin as initial therapy for type 2 diabetes mellitus.

Geriatric Use

Pharmacokinetic and adverse effect profiles of rosiglitazone similar to those in younger adults. Dosage adjustment based solely on age is not necessary in geriatric patients receiving rosiglitazone alone.

Data from several observational studies suggest that the risk of all-cause mortality may be increased in geriatric diabetic patients 65 years of age or older receiving rosiglitazone versus another thiazolidinedione antidiabetic agent (pioglitazone).

Hepatic Impairment

Rosiglitazone should be used with caution in patients with mild hepatic impairment; use is not recommended in moderate to severe hepatic impairment (ALT exceeding 2.5 times upper limit of normal, or active liver disease). (See Hepatic Effects under Warnings/Precautions: General Precautions, in Cautions.)

● Common Adverse Effects

Adverse effects of rosiglitazone occurring in at least 2% of patients include upper respiratory tract infection, injury, headache, edema, back pain, hyperglycemia, fatigue, sinusitis, and diarrhea. Anemia and edema generally were mild to moderate and usually did not require discontinuance. Rosiglitazone-induced reductions in hyperglycemia are associated with mild weight gain. Increased total, low-density lipoprotein (LDL)-, and high-density lipoprotein (HDL)-cholesterol; LDL/HDL-cholesterol ratio generally decreases after initial increase.

Adverse effects generally were similar with rosiglitazone monotherapy versus combined therapy with metformin; however, anemia was more common during combined therapy (7.1 versus 1.9%) with metformin compared with that in patients receiving rosiglitazone monotherapy or combination therapy with a sulfonylurea. Hypoglycemia occurs infrequently with rosiglitazone therapy. However, hypoglycemia was more common during combined therapy with rosiglitazone and metformin, a sulfonylurea, or insulin. In addition, self-monitored blood glucose measurements of 50 mg/dL or less were reported by 22% of patients receiving the fixed combination of glyburide and metformin hydrochloride plus rosiglitazone compared with 3.3% of patients receiving the fixed combination of glyburide and metformin hydrochloride. Hypoglycemia, confirmed by capillary blood glucose concentrations of 50 mg/dL or less, was reported by 12 or 14% of patients receiving combination therapy with insulin and rosiglitazone at dosages of 4 or 8 mg, respectively, compared with 6% of patients receiving insulin alone.

DRUG INTERACTIONS

● Drugs Affecting Hepatic Microsomal Enzymes

Inhibitors (e.g., gemfibrozil) or inducers (e.g., rifampin) of cytochrome P-450 (CYP) isoenzyme 2C8; potential pharmacokinetic interaction. With concurrent

gemfibrozil, potential pharmacokinetic interaction (increased area under the concentration-time curve [AUC] for rosiglitazone). With concurrent rifampin, potential pharmacokinetic interaction (decreased AUC for rosiglitazone). Adjustments in rosiglitazone dosage may be needed during initiation or discontinuance of an inhibitor or inducer of CYP2C8.

Because rosiglitazone does *not* affect CYP3A4, pharmacokinetic interactions unlikely with drugs metabolized mainly via this isoenzyme (e.g., nifedipine, estrogen-progestin combination contraceptives).

● Antidiabetic Agents

Additive glycemic control with metformin; no pharmacokinetic interaction.

Additive glycemic control with glimepiride; no pharmacokinetic interaction.

Acarbose reduced extent of absorption and prolonged half-life, but not considered clinically important; effect of combined rosiglitazone and acarbose on glycemic control remains to be established.

Although the manufacturer states that glyburide-induced reductions in blood glucose are unaltered by short-term (7 days) rosiglitazone in patients stabilized on the sulfonylurea, rosiglitazone can improve glycemic control during long-term combined therapy. With concurrent glyburide in Caucasian individuals, potential pharmacokinetic interaction (decreased glyburide concentrations). With concurrent glyburide in Japanese individuals, potential pharmacokinetic interaction (slightly increased glyburide concentrations).

Increased risk of congestive heart failure (CHF) with concomitant insulin therapy. Concomitant use of rosiglitazone and insulin therapy is not recommended. (See Congestive Heart Failure under Warnings/Precautions: Warnings, in Cautions.)

● Alcohol

Rosiglitazone-exacerbated hypoglycemia unlikely.

● Digoxin

Pharmacokinetic interaction unlikely.

● Ranitidine

Pharmacokinetic interaction unlikely.

● Warfarin

Pharmacokinetic interaction unlikely.

DESCRIPTION

Rosiglitazone is a thiazolidinedione (glitazone) antidiabetic agent that is structurally and pharmacologically related to pioglitazone and troglitazone but unrelated to other antidiabetic agents, including sulfonylureas, biguanides, and α-glucosidase inhibitors.

Rosiglitazone acts principally by increasing insulin sensitivity in target tissues, as well as decreasing hepatic gluconeogenesis. Rosiglitazone is a peroxisome proliferator-activated receptor$_\gamma$ (PPAR$_\gamma$) agonist that increases transcription of insulin-responsive genes and increases insulin sensitivity. Rosiglitazone, like other thiazolidinediones, ameliorates insulin resistance associated with type 2 diabetes mellitus without stimulating insulin release from pancreatic β cells, thus avoiding the risk of hypoglycemia. Because rosiglitazone does not lower glucose concentrations below euglycemia, the drug is appropriately referred to as an antidiabetic agent rather than a hypoglycemic agent. Some evidence suggests that the glucoregulatory effects of thiazolidinediones are mediated in part via reduced systemic and tissue lipid availability. Circulating concentrations of insulin and C-peptide are reduced during rosiglitazone therapy. Rosiglitazone is extensively metabolized, principally via the cytochrome P-450 (CYP) 2C8 isoenzyme; unlike troglitazone, rosiglitazone does not induce CYP3A4-mediated metabolism. Because of the delayed onset of action of rosiglitazone (2 weeks) and other thiazolidinediones and potential adverse effects, therapy with the drugs should not be initiated in hospitalized patients with diabetes mellitus. (See Congestive Heart Failure under Warnings/Precautions: Warnings, in Cautions.)

ADVICE TO PATIENTS

Importance of patient reading medication guide before starting rosiglitazone and each time the prescription is refilled.

Importance of informing patients of the current state of knowledge regarding the cardiovascular risks of rosiglitazone, and that although there is some evidence suggesting an increased risk of myocardial infarction compared with placebo, data from long-term clinical trials, including a cardiovascular outcomes trial, generally have not confirmed these findings. (See General Precautions: Major Adverse Cardiovascular Events, under Warnings/Precautions in Cautions.)

Importance of informing patients that rosiglitazone is not recommended for patients with symptomatic heart failure. Importance of identifying and reporting to clinicians potential symptoms of congestive heart failure (CHF), such as unusually rapid increase in weight, edema, unusual fatigue, or shortness of breath.

Importance of patients not taking rosiglitazone if they are allergic to the drug or any ingredients in the tablet. Signs and symptoms of a severe allergic reaction to rosiglitazone include swelling of the face, lips, tongue, or throat; problems breathing or swallowing; rash, itching, or hives; blisters on the skin or in the mouth, nose, or eyes; skin peeling; faintness or dizziness; rapid heartbeat.

Importance of taking exactly as prescribed. Importance of taking a missed dose as soon as possible, unless it is almost time for next dose. Do not double dose to make up for the missed dose. Importance of immediately contacting a clinician or a poison control center if accidental overdosage occurs.

Importance of continuing rosiglitazone therapy even if response is not evident within 2 weeks; full therapeutic response may not be evident for 2–3 months after initiation of therapy.

Risk of pregnancy in premenopausal anovulatory women with insulin resistance. Advise patients regarding use of effective contraception during therapy.

Importance of diet and exercise regimen adherence. Importance of regular monitoring (preferably self-monitoring) of blood glucose and glycosylated hemoglobin (HbA$_{1c}$) concentrations.

Importance of informing patients that rosiglitazone is not recommended in patients taking insulin due to potentially increased risk of CHF.

Risk of hypoglycemia in patients receiving concomitant antidiabetic agent therapy. Provide instructions regarding management of hypoglycemia, including recognition of symptoms, predisposing conditions, and treatment.

Importance of liver function test monitoring and immediate reporting of potential manifestations of hepatotoxicity (e.g., nausea or vomiting, abdominal pain, unusual fatigue, loss of appetite, dark urine, yellowing of skin or whites of eyes).

Risk of fractures (e.g., hand, upper arm, foot) in women.

Importance of regular eye examinations. Importance of reporting changes in vision to clinician.

Importance of informing clinicians of existing or contemplated concomitant therapy, including prescription (e.g., drugs that affect blood glucose concentrations; nitrates; antihypertensive agents; antilipemic agents; agents for CHF or prevention of coronary heart disease or stroke) and dietary or herbal supplements, as well as any concomitant illnesses (e.g., CHF or other cardiac disease, type 1 diabetes mellitus, history of diabetic ketoacidosis, macular edema, liver disease, history of liver disease associated with troglitazone, irregular menstrual periods).

Importance of women informing their clinician if they are or plan to become pregnant or plan to breast-feed.

Importance of informing patients of other important precautionary information. (See Cautions.)

PREPARATIONS

Excipients in commercially available drug preparations may have clinically important effects in some individuals; consult specific product labeling for details.

Rosiglitazone Maleate

Oral

Tablets, film-coated	2 mg (of rosiglitazone)	**Avandia®**, GlaxoSmithKline
	4 mg (of rosiglitazone)	**Avandia®**, GlaxoSmithKline
	8 mg (of rosiglitazone)	**Avandia®**, GlaxoSmithKline

Selected Revisions June 21, 2021, © Copyright, July 1, 1999, American Society of Health-System Pharmacists, Inc.

Glucagon

68:22.12 • GLYCOGENOLYTIC AGENTS

■ Glucagon, an antihypoglycemic agent, is a hormone synthesized and secreted by the α_2 cells of the pancreatic islets of Langerhans that increases blood glucose concentration by stimulating hepatic glycogenolysis.

USES

● Hypoglycemia

Glucagon is used for the emergency treatment of severe hypoglycemia in patients with diabetes mellitus. Glucagon is only effective in patients with hypoglycemia if liver glycogen is available; the drug is of little or no value in patients with chronic hypoglycemia or in those with hypoglycemia associated with starvation or adrenal insufficiency. Following glucagon administration, supplemental carbohydrate should be administered as soon as possible, especially to pediatric patients. The hyperglycemic response produced by glucagon may be reduced in emaciated or undernourished patients or in those with uremia or hepatic disease. Unlike IV dextrose, parenteral administration of glucagon results in a smooth, gradual termination of insulin coma. Glucagon is convenient for use in emergency situations when dextrose cannot be administered IV. The availability of more stable parenteral and intranasal formulations of glucagon that do not require reconstitution prior to use provide opportunities to expand the use of this hormone in managing insulin-induced hypoglycemia in nonhospital settings. The American Diabetes Association states that glucagon should be prescribed for all patients with diabetes mellitus who are at increased risk of level 2 (glucose concentration less than 54 mg/dL) or level 3 hypoglycemia (severe events characterized by altered mental and/or physical status requiring assistance for treatment of hypoglycemia) so that the drug is available if needed.

Depending on the stage of coma and the route of administration, patients usually become conscious within 5–20 minutes following parenteral administration of glucagon. After the patient responds, supplemental carbohydrate should be administered to restore liver glycogen and prevent secondary hypoglycemia. In patients in very deep coma, IV dextrose should be administered in addition to glucagon. If an unconscious diabetic patient suspected of being in insulin coma does not awaken following administration of glucagon, an additional dose of glucagon can be administered; emergency assistance should be sought. Other causes of coma should be considered. Failure of glucagon to relieve the coma may be caused by marked depletion of hepatic glycogen stores or irreversible brain damage resulting from prolonged hypoglycemia. In emergency situations in which hypoglycemia is suspected but not established, glucagon should *not* be substituted for IV dextrose.

Safety and efficacy of parenterally administered glucagon have been established in patients with diabetes mellitus. In several studies, almost all patients who received glucagon had a successful increase in plasma glucose concentrations within 30 minutes of administration. In 2 crossover studies in adults with type 1 diabetes mellitus, a single subcutaneous dose of glucagon (1 mg) administered following induction of hypoglycemia with insulin (target blood glucose concentration of less than 50 mg/dL; mean baseline concentration of 45–49 mg/dL) increased blood glucose to a concentration exceeding 70 mg/dL or by at least 20 mg/dL within 30 minutes in approximately 97–100% of patients. The mean time to reversal of hypoglycemia was 10–14 minutes. In another study, pediatric patients 2–17 years of age with type 1 diabetes mellitus received a single subcutaneous dose of glucagon (0.5 or 1 mg in those 12 years of age or older; 0.5 mg in those younger than 12 years of age) following insulin-induced reduction of blood glucose concentration to less than 80 mg/dL. In all patients, blood glucose concentration increased by at least 25 mg/dL following glucagon administration. Glucose response was similar across age groups.

Safety and efficacy of intranasal glucagon have been established in multiple clinical studies in patients with type 1 or type 2 diabetes mellitus. In 2 open-label, crossover studies in adults with type 1 or type 2 diabetes mellitus, a single 3-mg intranasal dose of glucagon was noninferior to a single 1-mg IM dose of the drug in reversing insulin-induced hypoglycemia. Following induction of hypoglycemia (target baseline blood glucose concentration of less than 50 or 60 mg/dL; mean baseline concentration of 44–47 or 54–56 mg/dL, respectively), intranasal or IM administration of glucagon increased blood glucose concentration to at least 70 mg/dL or by at least 20 mg/dL within 30 minutes in 99–100 or 100% of patients, respectively. The mean time to reversal of hypoglycemia was 12–16 minutes following intranasal administration compared with 10–12 minutes following IM administration. In another study, pediatric patients 4 years of age or older with type 1 diabetes mellitus were randomized to receive intranasal glucagon (3 mg) or IM glucagon (0.5 or 1 mg depending on body weight) following insulin-induced reduction of blood glucose concentration to less than 80 mg/dL; both formulations of glucagon increased blood glucose concentration in all patients in all age groups by at least 20 mg/dL within 20 minutes following administration (mean time of 11–14 or 11–12 minutes with intranasal or IM administration, respectively).

● Radiographic Examination of the GI Tract

Glucagon is used as a diagnostic aid in the radiographic examination of the stomach, duodenum, small intestine, and colon when a hypotonic state would be advantageous. Concomitant administration of glucagon used as a diagnostic aid and anticholinergic agents is not recommended because of the possibility of increased adverse GI effects.

● β-Adrenergic or Calcium-channel Blocking Agent Overdosage

Glucagon has been used with some success as a cardiac stimulant for the management of cardiac manifestations (e.g., bradycardia, hypotension, myocardial depression) associated with β-adrenergic blocking agent overdosage† or calcium-channel blocking agent overdosage†. Resuscitation following cardiac arrest from β-blocker or calcium-channel blocker overdosage should follow standard basic life support (BLS) and advanced cardiac life support (ACLS) algorithms. Some data indicate that administration of glucagon may be useful in treating severe cardiovascular instability associated with β-blocker overdosage that is refractory to standard measures, including vasopressors, and some experts state that such use is reasonable. Evidence of efficacy in calcium-channel blocker overdosage is more limited; however, some experts state that treatment with glucagon also may be considered in patients with severe, refractory cardiovascular instability associated with calcium-channel blocker overdosage.

● Sensitivity Reactions

Glucagon has been used in the treatment of anaphylaxis that is unresponsive to epinephrine in patients receiving β-adrenergic blocking agents†. Although evidence of efficacy is limited, glucagon is thought to exert a beneficial effect by directly activating adenylate cyclase and therefore bypassing the β-adrenergic receptor blockade.

DOSAGE AND ADMINISTRATION

● Reconstitution and Administration

Glucagon and glucagon hydrochloride may be administered by subcutaneous, IM, or IV injection. Glucagon also is administered intranasally. The drug also has been administered by continuous IV infusion for the treatment of β-adrenergic or calcium-channel blocking agent overdosage†.

Patients with diabetes mellitus and their caregivers should be informed of the signs and symptoms of severe hypoglycemia. Because effective treatment of severe hypoglycemia requires assistance from other individuals, patients should be advised to inform family members and friends about the availability of glucagon and provide them with instructions for use of the drug. Glucagon should be administered as soon as possible after severe hypoglycemia is recognized. Immediately following administration, emergency assistance should be summoned. If the patient has not responded within 15 minutes after the initial dose, an additional dose may be administered while awaiting emergency assistance. Once the patient has responded to treatment, oral carbohydrates should be administered to restore liver glycogen stores and to prevent recurrence of hypoglycemia.

Following radiographic examinations requiring use of glucagon as a diagnostic aid, patients who have been fasting should be given oral carbohydrate if compatible with the procedure.

Parenteral Administration

Glucagon or Glucagon Hydrochloride for Injection

Glucagon for injection is reconstituted by adding 1 mL of the sterile diluent provided by the manufacturer to a vial labeled as containing 1 mg of the drug to provide a solution containing 1 mg of glucagon per mL. The vial should be swirled gently until the powder is completely dissolved. The reconstituted solution should be inspected visually for particulate matter and discoloration; the solution should appear clear with a water-like consistency, and should not be used if it is cloudy or contains particulate matter.

Glucagon hydrochloride for injection (e.g., GlucaGen®) is reconstituted by adding 1 mL of sterile water for injection to a vial labeled as containing 1 mg of glucagon to provide a solution containing 1 mg of glucagon per mL. The vial should be shaken gently until the powder is completely dissolved. The reconstituted solution should be inspected visually for particulate matter and discoloration; the solution should appear clear and colorless, and should not be used if it is cloudy or contains particulate matter.

Reconstituted solutions of glucagon or glucagon hydrochloride may be administered IV (under medical supervision only) or by IM or subcutaneous injection into the upper arms, thighs, or buttocks. The solutions should be used immediately after reconstitution, and any unused portion should be discarded.

To prepare a continuous IV infusion solution for treatment of β-adrenergic blocking agent overdosage, reconstituted glucagon should be diluted in 5% dextrose injection.

Glucagon Injection

Glucagon injection in prefilled syringes and auto-injectors (Gvoke®) is for subcutaneous use only. Each syringe or auto-injector contains one 0.5- or 1-mg dose of glucagon and cannot be reused. The prefilled syringes and auto-injectors should be kept in the foil pouch until time of administration. Glucagon injection should be inspected visually prior to administration. The solution should appear clear and colorless to pale yellow and be free of particles; the solution should be discarded if it is discolored or contains particulate matter. The appropriate dose should be injected subcutaneously into the lower abdomen, outer thigh, or outer upper arm.

Intranasal Administration

Each glucagon intranasal device (Baqsimi®) contains one 3-mg dose of glucagon and cannot be reused. The intranasal device should be kept in the shrink-wrapped tube until time of administration and should not be tested prior to administration. If the tube has been opened and the device exposed to moisture, the drug may not work as expected. The drug should be administered by inserting the tip of the intranasal device into one nostril and pressing the device plunger all the way down until the green line is no longer showing. The patient does not need to inhale the dose. The manufacturer's prescribing information should be consulted for additional instructions on use of the intranasal device.

● Dosage

Dosage of glucagon or glucagon hydrochloride is expressed in terms of glucagon.

Hypoglycemia

Parenteral Dosage

For the treatment of severe hypoglycemia, the recommended subcutaneous, IM, or IV dose of glucagon administered as reconstituted glucagon for injection is 1 mg in adults and children weighing at least 20 kg and 0.5 mg in children weighing less than 20 kg; alternatively, a dose of 20–30 mcg/kg can be administered in children weighing less than 20 kg.

For the treatment of severe hypoglycemia, the recommended subcutaneous, IM, or IV dose of glucagon administered as reconstituted glucagon hydrochloride for injection (e.g., GlucaGen®) is 1 mg in adults and children weighing 25 kg or more and 0.5 mg in children weighing less than 25 kg. If the weight of the child is unknown, children younger than 6 years of age should receive a dose of 0.5 mg and those 6 years of age or older should receive 1 mg.

When glucagon prefilled syringes or auto-injectors (Gvoke®) are used for the treatment of severe hypoglycemia, the recommended subcutaneous dose of

glucagon in adults and adolescents at least 12 years of age is 1 mg; in children 2 to less than 12 years of age, the recommended subcutaneous dose is 1 mg in those weighing at least 45 kg and 0.5 mg in those weighing less than 45 kg.

If the patient has not responded to the initial dose of glucagon after 15 minutes, an additional dose of the drug (equivalent to the initial dose) may be administered.

Intranasal Dosage

For the treatment of severe hypoglycemia in adults and children 4 years of age and older, the recommended intranasal dosage of glucagon is 3 mg (one actuation of the Baqsimi® intranasal device) administered into one nostril. If the patient has not responded to the initial dose after 15 minutes, a second 3-mg dose may be administered.

Radiographic Examination of the GI Tract

When glucagon is used as a diagnostic aid in the radiographic examination of the stomach, duodenum, and small intestine in adults, the dose depends on the onset of action and duration of effect required for the specific examination. The onset of action after the injection depends on the organ under examination and the route of administration. The usual dose is 0.2–0.5 mg IV or 1 mg IM, although IV or IM doses up to 2 mg may be used if required. (See Pharmacokinetics: Absorption.)

For relaxation of the stomach, one manufacturer recommends a dose of 0.5 mg IV or 2 mg IM since the stomach is less sensitive to the effects of the drug. To facilitate a more satisfactory radiographic examination of the colon, a dose of 2 mg may be given as a single IM injection approximately 10 minutes prior to initiation of the procedure. Alternatively, other manufacturers state the usual dose to relax the colon is 0.5–0.75 mg IV or 1–2 mg IM. Glucagon doses of 2 mg are associated with a higher incidence of nausea and vomiting than lower doses of the drug.

β-Adrenergic or Calcium-channel Blocking Agent Overdosage

For the management of cardiac manifestations of β-blocker overdosage† in adults, glucagon has been administered as a direct IV injection at a dose of 3–10 mg administered slowly over 3–5 minutes, followed by an IV infusion of 2–5 mg/hour. Because of the amount of glucagon required to sustain this therapy, the availability of an adequate supply of glucagon must be considered.

For the management of cardiac manifestations of calcium-channel blocker overdosage† in adults, glucagon has been administered as a direct IV injection at a dose of 3–10 mg over 3–5 minutes, followed by an IV infusion of 3–5 mg/hour.

CAUTIONS

● Adverse Effects

Injection site reactions (e.g., edema, erythema, pain, discomfort), hypoglycemia or hypoglycemic coma, adverse GI effects (nausea, vomiting, abdominal pain, diarrhea), adverse cardiovascular effects (hypotension, hypertension, tachycardia), pallor, headache, dizziness, asthenia, and somnolence have been reported in patients receiving parenteral glucagon, although causality and frequency of such effects have not been fully established. Nausea and vomiting may be more common in patients receiving higher (2 mg) doses of the drug. Hypotension has been reported up to 2 hours following parenteral administration of glucagon as a diagnostic aid for upper GI endoscopic procedures. The risk of hypoglycemia may be increased in patients receiving indomethacin. (See Indomethacin under Drug Interactions.)

Hypersensitivity reactions, including generalized rash, urticaria, and anaphylaxis with respiratory distress and hypotension, have been reported in patients receiving glucagon.

In pediatric patients and adults receiving intranasal glucagon, nausea, headache, or vomiting has occurred in 15–31% of patients and upper respiratory tract irritation (rhinorrhea, nasal discomfort, nasal congestion, cough, epistaxis, sneezing) has occurred in 12–17% of patients. When symptoms were solicited by questionnaire, watery eyes or nasal congestion was reported in 42–59% of patients; runny nose, ocular redness, ocular or nasal pruritus, or sneezing was reported in 14–39% of patients; and aural or throat pruritus was reported in 3–12% of patients. Dysgeusia, pruritus, tachycardia, hypertension, throat irritation, and parosmia also have been reported.

Necrolytic migratory erythema (NME), a rash commonly associated with glucagonomas and characterized by scaly, pruritic, erythematous plaques, bullae, and erosions, has been reported in patients receiving continuous IV infusions of glucagon. NME lesions may affect the face, groin, perineum, and legs or may be more widespread. Reported cases of NME have resolved following discontinuance of glucagon therapy; treatment with corticosteroids has not been shown to be effective. If NME occurs, the risks and benefits of continued treatment with continuous IV infusions of glucagon should be considered.

● Precautions and Contraindications

Glucagon is contraindicated in patients with insulinoma. Although administration of glucagon may produce an initial increase in blood glucose concentration in patients with insulinoma, the drug may cause hypoglycemia by directly or indirectly (through an initial increase in blood glucose concentration) stimulating exaggerated insulin release from an insulinoma. If a patient develops symptoms of hypoglycemia after receiving glucagon, oral or IV glucose should be administered.

Because administration of glucagon may stimulate tumor release of catecholamines in patients with pheochromocytoma, which may cause a marked increase in blood pressure, glucagon is contraindicated in patients with pheochromocytoma. If a patient experiences a substantial increase in blood pressure after receiving glucagon and a previously undiagnosed pheochromocytoma is suspected, IV administration of 5–10 mg of phentolamine mesylate has been used effectively to lower blood pressure for the short time that control would be needed.

Because of the potential for hypoglycemia, use of glucagon as a diagnostic aid is contraindicated in patients with glucagonoma. In patients suspected of having glucagonoma, blood concentrations of glucagon should be determined prior to administration of glucagon and blood glucose concentrations should be monitored during glucagon treatment. If symptoms of hypoglycemia develop, oral or IV glucose should be administered.

In patients with cardiac disease, glucagon may increase myocardial oxygen demand, blood pressure, and heart rate, which may be life-threatening and may require treatment. When glucagon is used as a diagnostic aid in patients with cardiac disease, cardiac monitoring is recommended.

Use of glucagon as a diagnostic aid in patients with diabetes mellitus may result in hyperglycemia; blood glucose concentrations should be monitored and treated if indicated.

When glucagon is used for the treatment of hypoglycemia, liver glycogen must be available. Patients in states of starvation, with adrenal insufficiency, or with chronic hypoglycemia may not have adequate stores of hepatic glycogen for glucagon administration to be effective. Patients with these conditions should be treated with glucose.

Patients with diabetes mellitus should be fully and completely advised about the nature of the disease, what they must do to prevent and detect complications, and how to control their condition. Patients should be properly instructed in the early detection and treatment of hypoglycemia, and should be advised to routinely carry sugar, candy, or other readily absorbable carbohydrate so that it may be taken at the first sign of a developing hypoglycemic reaction. Patients (and their families or caregivers and other close contacts) should be properly instructed in the technique of preparing and administering glucagon before an emergency situation occurs. Patients should be instructed to notify their clinician when hypoglycemic reactions occur so that appropriate adjustment of insulin dosage can be made.

Since glucagon is a protein, the possibility of immunogenicity should be considered. Antibodies to glucagon have been detected in some patients receiving intranasal glucagon; however, no neutralizing antibodies have been detected.

Glucagon is contraindicated in patients with known hypersensitivity to the drug or any ingredient in the formulation.

● Pediatric Precautions

Glucagon has been used safely and effectively for the treatment of hypoglycemia in children. Prefilled syringes and auto-injectors of glucagon have been used safely in children 2 years of age and older. Safety and efficacy of intranasal glucagon have been established in children 4 years of age and older. Safety and efficacy of glucagon in diagnostic procedures in children have not been established.

● Geriatric Precautions

There is insufficient experience from clinical trials in patients 65 years of age or older to determine whether geriatric patients respond differently than younger patients. However, other clinical experience has not identified differences in response between geriatric patients and younger patients.

When glucagon is used as a diagnostic aid in geriatric patients, dosage of the drug should be selected with caution because of the greater frequency of decreased hepatic, renal, and/or cardiac function and of concomitant disease and drug therapy in geriatric patients.

● Pregnancy, Fertility, and Lactation

Available data from case reports and a limited number of observational studies involving administration of glucagon in pregnant women over decades of use have not identified a drug-associated risk of major birth defects, spontaneous abortion, or adverse maternal or fetal outcomes. Multiple small studies have demonstrated that endogenous glucagon is not transferred across the human placenta during early gestation. No embryofetal toxicity was observed in reproduction studies in rats and rabbits at glucagon doses up to 100 and 200 times, respectively, the human dose (based on body surface area).

It is not known whether glucagon is distributed into human milk. Effects of the drug on breast-fed infants and on milk production also are unknown. However, because glucagon is a peptide and would be expected to be broken down to its constituent amino acids in the infant's digestive tract, the drug is unlikely to harm an exposed infant.

DRUG INTERACTIONS

● Anticholinergic Agents

The inhibitory effects of anticholinergic agents and glucagon on GI motility may be additive, potentially increasing the risk of adverse GI effects; concomitant use of the drugs during radiographic examinations is not recommended.

● β-Adrenergic Blocking Agents

Patients receiving β-adrenergic blocking agents may experience a transient increase in pulse and blood pressure after receiving glucagon. Treatment of these increases in blood pressure and heart rate may be required in patients with coronary artery disease.

● Decongestants

In patients with the common cold, use of nasal decongestants did not alter the pharmacokinetics or pharmacodynamics of intranasally administered glucagon.

● Indomethacin

Glucagon may be ineffective for increasing blood glucose concentration or may even produce hypoglycemia in patients receiving indomethacin. Blood glucose concentrations should be monitored when glucagon is administered to patients receiving indomethacin.

● Insulin

Because insulin and glucagon have antagonistic effects, blood glucose concentration should be monitored when glucagon is used as a diagnostic aid during radiographic examinations in patients receiving insulin.

● Warfarin

Glucagon may increase the anticoagulant effect of warfarin. Patients should be monitored for unusual bruising or bleeding; adjustment of warfarin dosage may be required.

PHARMACOLOGY

Exogenous glucagon elicits all the pharmacologic responses usually produced by endogenous glucagon.

Glucagon is an antihypoglycemic agent that increases blood glucose concentration by stimulating hepatic glycogenolysis. Some of the metabolic effects produced by glucagon in various tissues (e.g., liver, adipose tissue) are similar to those of epinephrine. Glucagon stimulates the formation of adenylate cyclase, which catalyzes the conversion of ATP to cAMP, particularly in the liver and in adipose tissue. Formation of cAMP initiates a series of intracellular reactions including activation of phosphorylase, which promote the degradation of glycogen to glucose. The increase in blood glucose concentration occurs within minutes. Endogenous secretion of glucagon is stimulated when blood glucose concentration is low or when serum insulin concentration is increased. In general, the actions of glucagon are antagonistic to those of insulin; however, glucagon has been reported to stimulate insulin secretion in healthy individuals and in patients with type 2 diabetes mellitus. Glucagon also has been reported to enhance peripheral utilization of glucose. The intensity of the hyperglycemic effect of glucagon depends on hepatic glycogen reserve and the presence of phosphorylases. The action of glucagon is not blocked by sympatholytic agents such as dihydroergotamine. The hyperglycemic effect of glucagon is increased and prolonged by concomitant administration of epinephrine.

Glucagon produces extrahepatic effects that are independent of its hyperglycemic action. Although the exact mechanism(s) of action has not been conclusively determined, glucagon produces relaxation of smooth muscle of the stomach, duodenum, small intestine, and colon. The drug has also been shown to inhibit gastric and pancreatic secretions.

Glucagon has a positive inotropic and chronotropic effect. Following rapid IV administration in anesthetized animals, glucagon causes a decrease in blood pressure. Glucagon has also been shown to decrease plasma amino nitrogen concentration; enhance renal excretion of electrolytes; decrease synthesis of protein and fat; increase the metabolic rate; and, following prolonged administration, to produce a diabetic effect, which may persist for several days.

PHARMACOKINETICS

● Absorption

Because of its polypeptide nature, glucagon is destroyed in the GI tract, and therefore must be administered parenterally or intranasally.

Following parenteral administration of glucagon, blood glucose concentration increases within 10 minutes and peak blood glucose concentrations occur within 30 minutes; hyperglycemic activity persists for 60–90 minutes following IV or IM injection. Following intranasal administration of glucagon, glucose concentration increases within 10 minutes and peak glucose concentrations are attained within approximately 60 minutes.

Following IV administration of a single 0.25- to 0.5-mg or 2-mg dose of the drug, relaxation of GI smooth muscle occurs within 1 minute and persists for 9–17 or 22–25 minutes, respectively. Following IM administration of a single 1-mg dose of the drug, relaxation of GI smooth muscle occurs within 8–10 minutes and persists for 12–27 minutes; after a single 2-mg IM dose, relaxation of GI smooth muscle occurs within 4–7 minutes and persists for 21–32 minutes.

Peak plasma glucagon concentrations are obtained in about 10–13, 15–20, or 10–50 minutes following IM, intranasal, or subcutaneous administration.

Nasal congestion associated with the common cold does not alter the pharmacokinetics or pharmacodynamics of intranasally administered glucagon.

● Elimination

Glucagon has a plasma half-life of about 8–18, 26–45, or 32–42 minutes following IV, IM, or subcutaneous administration, respectively. Following intranasal administration, the median half-life is approximately 35 minutes in adults and 21–31 minutes in pediatric patients. Glucagon is extensively degraded in the liver, kidney, and plasma.

CHEMISTRY AND STABILITY

● Chemistry

Glucagon is a hormone synthesized and secreted by the a_2 cells of the pancreatic islets of Langerhans. Glucagon is a straight-chain polypeptide with a molecular weight of 3483 and contains 29 amino acids; histidine is the N-terminal acid and threonine is the C-terminal residue of the molecule. Glucagon is *not* chemically or structurally related to insulin; unlike insulin, glucagon does not contain cysteine and has no disulfide linkages. Although structurally identical to endogenous human glucagon, commercially available glucagon is prepared synthetically (e.g., via solid-phase peptide synthesis) or using recombinant DNA technology and special laboratory strains of nonpathogenic *Escherichia coli* or *Saccharomyces cerevisiae*. One mg of glucagon is equivalent to 1 International Unit (IU, unit).

Glucagon occurs as a fine, white or off-white, crystalline powder; is practically odorless and tasteless; and is practically insoluble in water and soluble in dilute alkali and acid solutions. Commercially available glucagon for injection is a sterile, white to off-white, lyophilized powder for reconstitution for IV, IM, or subcutaneous administration; a sterile diluent containing glycerin, hydrochloric acid, and sterile water for injection is provided by the manufacturer for reconstitution. Commercially available glucagon hydrochloride for injection is commercially available as a sterile, white, lyophilized powder for reconstitution for IV, IM, or subcutaneous administration; glucagon hydrochloride for injection is supplied in single-dose vials either alone or in kits that also include sterile water for injection for reconstitution. Glucagon injection is commercially available as a clear, colorless to pale yellow solution in prefilled syringes and auto-injectors for subcutaneous injection. Glucagon also is commercially available as a preservative-free white powder in a single-use intranasal device.

● Stability

Glucagon lyophilized powder for injection should be stored at 20–25°C and should not be used past the expiration date. Glucagon hydrochloride lyophilized powder for injection is stable for at least 24 months following the date of manufacture when stored at 20–25°C. The lyophilized powders should not be frozen and should be kept in the original packages for protection from light. Following reconstitution, solutions of glucagon or glucagon hydrochloride should be used immediately.

Glucagon injection in prefilled syringes or auto-injectors should be stored at 20–25°C but may be exposed to temperatures ranging from 15–30°C. Glucagon injection should not be refrigerated or frozen, and should not be exposed to extreme temperatures. The prefilled syringes and auto-injectors should be stored in the original sealed foil pouch until time of use.

Glucagon nasal powder should be stored at temperatures up to 30°C; the intranasal device should be stored in the shrink-wrapped tube provided by the manufacturer for protection from moisture until time of use.

PREPARATIONS

Excipients in commercially available drug preparations may have clinically important effects in some individuals; consult specific product labeling for details.

Glucagon (rDNA)

Parenteral		
For injection	1 mg (1 unit)*	Glucagon for Injection Emergency Kit (with 1 mL diluent)

Glucagon (synthetic)

Nasal		
Powder, for intranasal use	3 mg	Baqsimi®, Lilly

Parenteral		
Injection	0.5 mg/0.1 mL (0.5 and 1 mg)	Gvoke®, Xeris (available as prefilled syringes and auto-injectors)

Glucagon Hydrochloride (rDNA)

Parenteral

For injection	1 mg (of glucagon)	**GlucaGen®**, Boehringer Ingelheim
		GlucaGen® Diagnostic Kit (with 1 mL sterile water for injection diluent), Boehringer Ingelheim
		GlucaGen® HypoKit® (with 1 mL sterile water for injection diluent), Novo Nordisk

Glucagon Hydrochloride (synthetic)

Parenteral

For injection	1 mg (of glucagon)*	**Glucagon Hydrochloride for Injection**
		Glucagon Hydrochloride for Injection Diagnostic Kit (with 1 mL sterile water for injection diluent)
		Glucagon Hydrochloride for Injection Emergency Kit (with 1 mL sterile water for injection diluent)

† Use is not currently included in the labeling approved by the US Food and Drug Administration.

* available from one or more manufacturer, distributor, and/or repackager by generic (nonproprietary) name

Selected Revisions August 19, 2022, © Copyright, March 1, 1969, American Society of Health-System Pharmacists, Inc.

Desmopressin Acetate

68:28 • PITUITARY

■ Desmopressin, a synthetic polypeptide structurally related to arginine vasopressin (antidiuretic hormone), the natural human posterior pituitary hormone, elicits a greater antidiuretic response, on a weight basis, than does arginine vasopressin, and, among other pharmacologic effects, causes a dose-dependent increase in plasma factor VIII (antihemophilic factor) activity.

USES

● Polyuria and Polydipsia

Desmopressin is used intranasally, orally, or parenterally to prevent or control polydipsia, polyuria, and dehydration in patients with diabetes insipidus caused by a deficiency of endogenous posterior pituitary vasopressin (antidiuretic hormone) (neurohypophyseal diabetes insipidus) and to manage temporary polyuria and polydipsia associated with trauma or surgery in the pituitary region. Because of its relatively long duration of action and relative lack of adverse effects, many experts consider intranasal desmopressin the drug of choice for chronic treatment in patients with mild to severe neurohypophyseal diabetes insipidus. In children, intranasal desmopressin is preferred to vasopressin injection and to oral antidiuretic agents such as chlorpropamide because of the frequency of adverse effects of these agents in pediatric patients. Although intranasal administration of the drug is preferred for chronic therapy, parenteral administration of the drug may be useful when factors that can make nasal insufflation ineffective or inappropriate are present; these include poor intranasal absorption, nasal congestion and blockage, nasal discharge, atrophy of nasal mucosa, and severe atrophic rhinitis. In addition, parenteral administration of the drug may be preferred when the patient has an impaired level of consciousness. Parenteral administration of the drug also may be necessary during recovery from surgery or when nasal packing is present in patients who have undergone cranial surgical procedures such as transsphenoidal hypophysectomy.

Desmopressin is not effective in controlling polyuria caused by renal disease, nephrogenic diabetes insipidus, hypokalemia, or hypercalcemia. In uncontrolled studies, desmopressin had variable effectiveness in controlling polyuria secondary to administration of lithium.

● Primary Nocturnal Enuresis

Desmopressin is used orally for the management of primary nocturnal enuresis. It may be used alone or as an adjunct to behavioral therapy and/or other nondrug measures, and has been shown to be effective in some cases refractory to standard therapies (e.g., imipramine, enuresis alarms).

Some desmopressin intranasal preparations (i.e., nasal solutions containing 0.1 mg of desmopressin acetate per mL) initially received approval from the US Food and Drug Administration (FDA) for the treatment of primary nocturnal enuresis. However in late 2007, FDA withdrew its prior approval for the treatment of primary nocturnal enuresis due to the risk of serious hyponatremia that may result in seizures and death, particularly in children, following a review of 61 postmarketing cases of hyponatremia-related seizures associated with the use of desmopressin. FDA requested that prescribing information for desmopressin be revised to include information about the risk of severe hyponatremia and seizures and the safe use of desmopressin, and to state that these desmopressin intranasal preparations are no longer indicated for the treatment of primary nocturnal enuresis. FDA states that the status of all other approved indications for the individual desmopressin intranasal preparations has not changed. (See Cautions: Adverse Effects and Precautions and Contraindications.)

The etiology of nocturnal enuresis is not precisely known, but appears to be related to delayed maturation of the cortical mechanisms that allow voluntary control of the micturition reflex. The condition is characterized by nocturnal incontinence without overt daytime voiding symptoms and is usually 3 times more common in boys than in girls. Primary nocturnal enuresis is diagnosed when a child never has experienced a period of consistent nighttime continence; the condition is considered secondary when nocturnal enuresis occurs in a formerly "dry" child, and usually is associated with an emotionally disruptive event.

Treatment is not usually indicated until a child reaches the age of 6; the condition will then spontaneously remit in 15% of patients every year thereafter. The frequency of this condition in adults is less than 1%. Other possible etiologies for nocturnal enuresis (e.g., neurologic and/or spinal abnormalities, diabetes insipidus or diabetes mellitus, chronic renal failure, bacteriuria [especially in girls]) should be ruled out before initiation of drug therapy.

Controlled studies of oral desmopressin in doses of 0.2–0.6 mg daily for 2 weeks in patients 5–17 years of age with primary nocturnal enuresis indicated that patients experienced about 27–40% fewer nights of incontinence while receiving the drug versus placebo; a greater response was observed with increasing dosages up to 0.6 mg daily. In an open-label extension study of 6 months' duration in patients completing the placebo-controlled studies, 11% of patients receiving desmopressin achieved a complete or near complete response (no more than 2 nights of incontinence/2 weeks) and did not require titration to the 0. 6-mg daily dose. The majority of patients (86%) were titrated to the 0. 6-mg daily dose. When all dosage arms were combined (0.2–0.6 mg daily), 56% of patients receiving desmopressin experienced at least a 50% reduction in the number of nights of incontinence/2 weeks, while 38% of patients achieved a complete or near complete response. Although limited data demonstrate that desmopressin is effective for the control of primary nocturnal enuresis, the relapse rate after cessation of desmopressin therapy is high (with rates of nocturnal incontinence sometimes approaching incontinence rates before treatment); enuresis alarms have been observed to be the most effective treatment for nocturnal enuresis.

● Hemophilia A

Desmopressin acetate is used intranasally or parenterally for the management of spontaneous or trauma-induced bleeding episodes such as hemarthrosis, intramuscular hematoma, or mucosal bleeding in patients with mild hemophilia A. The drug is designated an orphan drug by the US Food and Drug Administration (FDA) for use in this condition. Desmopressin acetate also is used parenterally or intranasally to maintain hemostasis during surgical procedures and postoperatively in patients with hemophilia A. The drug is not indicated for patients with hemophilia B or those with factor VIII antibodies. Desmopressin acetate generally is indicated in patients with hemophilia A whose plasma factor VIII activity is greater than 5%. Although use of desmopressin may be justified in certain clinical situations in patients with hemophilia A whose factor VIII activity is between 2–5%, these patients should be carefully monitored if the drug is used. Desmopressin is ineffective in patients with severe hemophilia A.

The National Hemophilia Foundation's Medical and Scientific Advisory Council (MASAC) currently recommends that parenteral or intranasal desmopressin be used whenever possible for the treatment of mild hemophilia A. When desmopressin does not provide adequate treatment, patients should be treated with antihemophilic factor (recombinant) or antihemophilic factor (human). MASAC states that cryoprecipitate is not recommended as a treatment alternative for the management of hemophilia A. Despite the fact the donor units used to prepare cryoprecipitate are screened for antibody to HIV-1, HIV-2, hepatitis C virus, and hepatitis B surface antigen (HBsAg), cryoprecipitate may still be infectious for several reasons, including the several months' delay in seroconversion after HIV or hepatitis C infection.

● von Willebrand Disease

Desmopressin acetate is used intranasally or parenterally for the management of spontaneous or trauma-induced bleeding episodes in patients with mild to moderate type 1 von Willebrand disease. The drug is designated an orphan drug by the FDA for use in this condition. The drug also is used parenterally to maintain hemostasis during surgical procedures and postoperatively in these patients. MASAC and other experts state that desmopressin acetate is the treatment of choice for the management of mild to moderate type 1 von Willebrand disease, especially those whose plasma factor VIII activity is greater than 5%. Patients least likely to respond to the drug are those with severe homozygous von Willebrand disease whose factor VIII and factor VIII/von Willebrand factor activities are less than 1%; the response of other patients may be variable depending on the type of molecular defect associated with their disease. Desmopressin acetate is not indicated for patients with severe type 1 von Willebrand disease or when there is evidence of an abnormal molecular form of factor VIII antigen. Bleeding time, factor VIII and ristocetin cofactor activities, and von Willebrand factor antigen should be monitored during desmopressin therapy to ensure that an adequate response is being achieved. If individuals with type 1 disease become transiently unresponsive to desmopressin acetate, many experts recommend use of antihemophilic factor (human) preparations rich in von Willebrand factor (i.e., Alphanate®, Humate-P®, Koate®-DVI).

Desmopressin acetate may be effective for the management of bleeding in some, but not all, individuals with type 2A, 2M, or 2N von Willebrand disease†. Although desmopressin acetate reportedly has been used effectively in some patients with type 2B von Willebrand disease, the drug usually is not used in these individuals because of an increased risk of thromboembolic events. Desmopressin acetate is ineffective for the management of bleeding in individuals with type 3 von Willebrand disease. Experts generally recommend use of antihemophilic factor (human) preparations rich in von Willebrand factor if prevention or control of bleeding is necessary in individuals with type 2A, 2M, or 2N von Willebrand disease who do not respond to desmopressin acetate or when prevention or control of bleeding is considered necessary in those with type 2B or type 3 von Willebrand disease (e.g., in surgical situations). These antihemophilic factor (human) preparations are particularly useful for the management of von Willebrand disease in pediatric patients who are too young to receive desmopressin acetate. (See Cautions: Pediatric Precautions.) Cryoprecipitate should not be used in the management of von Willebrand disease except in emergency, life- or limb-threatening situations when desmopressin acetate or appropriate preparations of antihemophilic factor (human) are not available.

● **Other Uses**

Intranasal desmopressin has been used in adults and children to evaluate the ability of the kidneys to concentrate urine†. Use of the drug for this purpose is easier and more rapid but may be less accurate than the Mosenthal concentrating test.

Intranasal desmopressin has been used in a small number of patients with sickle cell anemia to induce hyponatremia for the prevention and treatment of sickle cell crisis†; however, further studies are needed to establish the safety and efficacy of the drug for this condition. In a few patients, chronic hyponatremia induced by desmopressin reduced the frequency of painful crises, and acutely induced hyponatremia shortened the duration of crises; however, successful therapy requires strict dietary regulation and patient supervision. Because of the need for further studies and the potential complications of hyponatremia (e.g., seizures), use of intranasal desmopressin for the management of patients with sickle cell disease should be limited to severely afflicted patients who can be treated and evaluated in a strictly supervised setting.

In one randomized, placebo-controlled study in uremic patients† with prolonged bleeding times and hemorrhagic tendencies, IV desmopressin increased factor VIII activity and reduced bleeding time; in some additional uremic patients who received IV desmopressin before surgery or renal biopsy, bleeding time was reduced and associated with normal hemostasis.

DOSAGE AND ADMINISTRATION

● **Administration**

Desmopressin acetate is administered intranasally, orally, by subcutaneous injection, direct IV injection, or slow IV infusion.

Intranasal Administration

Desmopressin acetate intranasal preparations should be administered in children under adult supervision in order to monitor the dose and fluid intake.

Desmopressin acetate nasal solutions containing 0.1 mg of the drug per mL are used for the treatment of diabetes insipidus; desmopressin acetate nasal solution containing 1.5 mg of the drug per mL is used for the treatment of hemophilia A or von Willebrand disease. Desmopressin acetate nasal solutions containing 0.1 or 1.5 mg/mL are administered using the spray pump supplied by the manufacturers; alternatively, desmopressin acetate nasal solutions containing 0.1 mg/mL can be administered using a calibrated nasal tube supplied by the manufacturers.

The intranasal spray pump provided by the manufacturers delivers 0.1 mL of solution per actuation. When the nasal solution containing 0.1 mg/mL is administered using the spray pump, each 0.1-mL spray delivers a dose of 10 mcg of desmopressin acetate; if a dose other than a multiple of 10 mcg is required, the solution should be administered using a nasal tube. The nasal tube has 4 graduation markings that measure 0.05, 0.1, 0.15, or 0.2 mL and can be used to administer 5, 10, 15, or 20 mcg, respectively. When the nasal solution containing 1.5 mg/mL is administered using the spray pump, each 0.1-mL spray delivers a dose of 150 mcg of desmopressin acetate; if a dose other than a multiple of 150 mcg is required, parenteral desmopressin acetate therapy should be used.

Desmopressin acetate nasal solution should be administered intranasally according to the manufacturer's instructions to ensure that the drug is deposited high in the nasal cavity and does not pass down the throat. The patient must be carefully instructed in the proper use of the nasal tube or spray pump in order to obtain optimum results. Desmopressin generally should not be administered intranasally when changes in the nasal mucosa such as scarring, edema, or other condition may cause erratic, unreliable absorption of the drug. The drug should not be administered intranasally when nasal congestion and blockage, nasal discharge, atrophy of nasal mucosa, or severe atrophic rhinitis is present. Intranasal therapy also may be inappropriate when the patient has impaired consciousness. In addition, cranial surgical procedures, such as transphenoidal hypophysectomy, create situations in which an alternative route of administration is needed as in cases of nasal packing or recovery from surgery.

Parenteral Administration

For IV infusion, the appropriate dose of desmopressin acetate should be diluted in 10 or 50 mL of 0.9% sodium chloride injection for administration in children weighing 10 kg or less or in adults and children weighing more than 10 kg, respectively; the solution is then infused IV slowly over 15–30 minutes. Blood pressure and pulse should be monitored during infusion of the drug.

● **Dosage**

Polyuria and Polydipsia

The intranasal, oral, or parenteral dose of desmopressin acetate required for antidiuresis is variable and must be adjusted according to the patient's requirements and response. Morning and evening doses must be adjusted separately for an adequate diurnal rhythm of water turnover. Response is generally estimated by duration of sleep and adequate, not excessive, turnover of water.

Intranasal Dosage

For the management of neurohypophyseal diabetes insipidus, the usual adult maintenance dosage of desmopressin acetate recommended by the manufacturer is 10–40 mcg (0.1–0.4 mL or 1–4 sprays from the spray pump of a solution containing 0.1 mg/mL) given intranasally in 1–3 divided doses daily. Some clinicians have recommended an adult desmopressin acetate maintenance dosage of 5–40 mcg (0.05–0.4 mL of a solution containing 0.1 mg/mL). Most adults require 20 mcg daily administered in 2 divided doses in the morning and the evening. In children 3 months to 12 years of age, the initial dose of desmopressin acetate is 5 mcg or less (0.05 mL of a solution containing 0.1 mg/mL) administered intranasally in the evening. In children 3 months to 12 years of age, the usual intranasal dosage is 5–30 mcg (0.05–0.3 mL of a solution containing 0.1 mg/mL) daily in a single evening dose or divided in 2 doses. About 25–33% of adults and children can be controlled with a single daily dose. The lowest effective dosage should be used. Fluid intake should be restricted. (See Cautions: Precautions and Contraindications.)

Parenteral Dosage

If the drug is administered by subcutaneous or direct IV injection in adults or children 12 years of age or older for the management of diabetes insipidus, the usual maintenance dosage is 2–4 mcg daily given in 2 divided doses. The parenteral dosage for the management of diabetes insipidus in children younger than 12 years of age has not been established. (See Cautions: Pediatric Precautions.) Patients with diabetes insipidus being switched from intranasal to subcutaneous or IV administration of the drug should generally receive one-tenth their maintenance intranasal dosage parenterally. The lowest effective parenteral dosage should be given. During long-term use, patients rarely may develop tolerance to the drug and require cautious increase in dosage to achieve an adequate therapeutic response. Fluid intake should be restricted. (See Cautions: Precautions and Contraindications.)

Oral Dosage

If oral desmopressin acetate is used for the management of diabetes insipidus in patients who previously received the drug intranasally, oral therapy should be initiated 12 hours after the last intranasal dose. The usual initial oral dosage of desmopressin acetate for adults and pediatric patients is 0.05 mg twice daily, and subsequent dosage should be adjusted according to response. In clinical studies, the optimal dosage range for most patients was 0.1–0.8 mg daily given in divided doses. Each dose should be adjusted separately for an adequate diurnal rhythm of water turnover. Total oral daily dosage should be increased or decreased in the range of 0.1–1.2 mg divided into 2 or 3 daily doses as needed to obtain adequate antidiuresis. Fluid intake should be restricted. (See Cautions: Precautions and Contraindications.)

Primary Nocturnal Enuresis

If oral desmopressin acetate is used for the treatment of primary nocturnal enuresis in patients who previously received the drug intranasally, oral therapy should be initiated the night following (24 hours after) the last intranasal dose. The usual initial oral dose of desmopressin acetate for adults and pediatric patients 6 years of age or older is 0.2 mg at bedtime. The dose may be titrated up to 0.6 mg to achieve the desired response. Duration of desmopressin therapy has not been established in pediatric patients responding to therapy; some experts have suggested that it is reasonable to continue therapy for 3–6 months; after 3–6 months, therapy can be withdrawn and the patient reevaluated.

Fluid restriction should be in effect for a minimum of 1 hour before desmopressin administration and continued until the next morning or at least 8 hours after desmopressin administration. Some experts recommend that not more than 240 mL of fluid should be consumed on any night when desmopressin is used. Desmopressin therapy should be interrupted during episodes of fluid and/or electrolyte imbalance (e.g., systemic infections, fever, recurrent vomiting or diarrhea) and under conditions associated with increased water intake (e.g., extremely hot weather, vigorous exercise). (See Cautions: Precautions and Contraindications.)

Hemophilia A and von Willebrand Disease

For the management of bleeding in patients with hemophilia A or mild to moderate type 1 von Willebrand disease, dosage of desmopressin acetate should be adjusted according to response. Factor VIII and factor VIII/ristocetin cofactor activities, factor VIII antigen levels, and activated partial thromboplastin activity should be monitored in patients with hemophilia A, and factor VIII and factor VIII/ristocetin cofactor activities and factor VIII/von Willebrand factor antigen levels should be monitored in patients with von Willebrand disease. Determination of bleeding time may also be useful in monitoring therapy in patients with von Willebrand disease.

The usual parenteral dose for adults and children 3 months of age and older with hemophilia A or type 1 von Willebrand disease is 0.3 mcg/kg given by slow IV infusion; if the dose is administered preoperatively, the drug should be injected 30 minutes prior to the scheduled procedure. Fluid intake should be restricted. (See Cautions: Precautions and Contraindications.)

The usual intranasal dosage of desmopressin acetate for the management of hemophilia A or type 1 von Willebrand disease is 300 mcg (0.1 mL or 1 spray from the spray pump into each nostril of a solution containing 1.5 mg/mL). A dosage of 150 mcg (0.1 mL or 1 spray from the spray pump into a single nostril of a solution containing 1.5 mg/mL) may be sufficient in patients who weigh less than 50 kg. If intranasal desmopressin acetate is used preoperatively, the drug should be administered 2 hours prior to surgery.

The need for additional doses of the desmopressin acetate or use of blood products for hemostasis should be determined by the clinical response of the patient and the response as determined by appropriate laboratory tests. The tendency toward tachyphylaxis (decreasing responsiveness) when doses of desmopressin are repeated more frequently than every 48 hours should be considered. When desmopressin acetate is used for the management of von Willebrand disease, the National Hemophilia Foundation' Medical and Scientific Advisory Council (MASAC) recommends that the drug be administered no more frequently than once every 24 hours and used for no more than 3 consecutive days unless such therapy is recommended by a clinician with expertise in the treatment of the disease.

Other Uses

To evaluate the urine concentrating ability of the kidneys†, fasting or nonfasting adults have been given 10–40 mcg (0.1–0.4 mL of 0.01% solution or 1–4 sprays from the spray pump) intranasally; nonfasting children 2–15 years of age have been given 20 mcg (0.2 mL of 0.01% solution); and nonfasting infants 1–12 weeks of age have been given 10 mcg (0.1 mL of 0.01% solution or 1 spray from the spray pump) intranasally. Then, a urine sample is collected in 1–5 hours and specific gravity of the urine is determined. Under test conditions, the average individual should concentrate the urine to a specific gravity of at least 1.020.

CAUTIONS

● Adverse Effects

In late 2007, the US Food and Drug Administration (FDA) reported the results of a review of 61 postmarketing cases of hyponatremia-related seizures associated with the use of desmopressin. In 55 cases, sodium concentrations ranged from 104–130 mEq/L during the seizure event. Two of these 55 cases were fatal; although both patients experienced hyponatremia and seizures, the direct contribution of desmopressin to the fatalities is not clear. Intranasal formulations were used in 36 cases; 25 of these cases involved pediatric patients (i.e., patients younger than 17 years of age). The most commonly reported indication for use of desmopressin in the 25 pediatric patients was nocturnal enuresis. In 39 of the 61 cases, the patient received at least one concomitant drug or had diseases associated with hyponatremia and/or seizures. As a result, FDA withdrew its prior approval for the treatment of primary nocturnal enuresis from desmopressin *intranasal* preparations; there is no change in the other approved indications for the individual intranasal preparations. (See Cautions: Precautions and Contraindications.)

Intranasal Administration

Adverse effects reported with intranasal desmopressin have been infrequent and mild. Rarely, conjunctivitis, ocular edema, lacrimation disorder, transient headache, dizziness, asthenia, chills, nasal congestion, nostril pain, rhinitis, epistaxis, sore throat, cough, upper respiratory infection, flushing, nausea, vomiting, mild abdominal cramps or pain, GI disorder, somnolence, insomnia, pain, chest pain, palpitations, tachycardia, agitation, balanitis, and vulval pain have occurred with usual intranasal doses. Unlike vasopressin and lypressin, usual doses of desmopressin do not cause skin pallor or severe smooth muscle or abdominal cramps. With large intranasal doses, blood pressure may increase. Severe hyponatremia was reported in one patient with neurohypophyseal diabetes insipidus who abused intranasal desmopressin and in one pediatric patient receiving the drug for primary nocturnal enuresis; the pediatric patient also experienced a single tonic-clonic seizure. Hyponatremia, convulsion, and coma were reported in a 13-year-old patient with cystic fibrosis also receiving the drug for primary nocturnal enuresis. Adverse effects with intranasal desmopressin usually disappear when the dose or the frequency of administration is decreased but, rarely, necessitate discontinuance of the drug.

Oral Administration

Desmopressin acetate generally is well tolerated when administered orally. In patients with diabetes insipidus who received desmopressin acetate tablets for up to 44 months, transient increases in AST (SGOT) (up to 1.5 times the normal upper limit) occurred occasionally but returned to the normal range despite continued administration of the drug. In clinical studies evaluating use of oral desmopressin for the treatment of primary nocturnal enuresis, the only adverse effect reported in 3% or more of patients that was probably, possibly, or remotely related to the drug was headache (4% in those receiving desmopressin acetate and 3% in those receiving placebo). Abnormal thinking, diarrhea, and edema-weight gain have been reported in patients receiving oral desmopressin acetate but a causal relationship has not been established.

Parenteral Administration

Adverse effects following parenteral administration of desmopressin have generally been infrequent and mild; however, there have been rare reports of thrombotic events (e.g., acute cerebrovascular thrombosis, acute myocardial infarction) following injection of the drug in patients predisposed to such events. Other reported adverse effects include transient headache, nausea, mild abdominal cramps, and vulval pain; these symptoms usually disappear with a reduction in dosage. Local erythema, swelling, and burning pain have been reported occasionally at the site of injection. Severe pain along the injected vein has been reported with large IV doses. Facial flushing has been reported occasionally following parenteral administration of the drug and slight increases in blood pressure, which disappeared with a reduction in dosage or slight decreases in blood pressure (with compensatory increases in heart rate), have been reported infrequently. With large IV doses of desmopressin, tachycardia, hypotension, and facial flushing have been reported. Water intoxication and hyponatremia are possible in patients who do not require vasopressin for its antidiuretic effect. (See Cautions: Precautions and Contraindications.) Excessive water retention occurred in a hemophiliac patient who received an IV dose of desmopressin acetate of 0.5 mcg/kg for bleeding.

Severe allergic reactions, including anaphylaxis, have been reported rarely with parenteral and intranasal desmopressin acetate. In addition, fatal anaphylaxis has been reported in patients receiving parenteral desmopressin.

● Precautions and Contraindications

Desmopressin acetate intranasal preparations should be reserved for situations in which oral therapy is not feasible.

All desmopressin preparations should be used cautiously in patients at risk for water intoxication with hyponatremia. Hyponatremia has been reported very rarely during international postmarketing surveillance in patients receiving desmopressin acetate. (See Cautions: Adverse Effects.) Desmopressin is a potent antidiuretic; use of desmopressin may result in water intoxication and/or hyponatremia, and hyponatremia may be fatal unless properly diagnosed and treated. Therefore, fluid restriction is recommended and should be discussed with the patient and/or guardian; careful medical supervision is required. The patient should promptly contact the clinician if water intake changes.

Fluid intake should be carefully restricted, particularly in pediatric and geriatric patients, to reduce the risk of potential water intoxication and hyponatremia. All patients receiving desmopressin therapy should be observed for signs and symptoms associated with hyponatremia (i.e., headache, nausea/vomiting, decreased serum sodium, weight gain, restlessness, fatigue, lethargy, disorientation, depressed reflexes, appetite loss, irritability, muscle weakness, spasms or cramps, abnormal mental status [e.g., hallucinations, decreased consciousness, confusion]); severe symptoms may include seizure, coma, and/or respiratory arrest. An extreme decrease in plasma osmolality that may result in seizures, which may lead to coma, has occurred rarely, and this possibility should be considered.

Desmopressin should be used with caution in patients with habitual or psychogenic polydipsia and in patients who are receiving certain drugs (e.g., tricyclic antidepressants, selective serotonin-reuptake inhibitors [SSRIs]) as these patients may be more likely to drink excessive amounts of water resulting in an increased risk for hyponatremia. (See Drug Interactions.)

Desmopressin should be used with caution in patients with conditions associated with fluid and electrolyte imbalances (e.g., cystic fibrosis, heart failure, renal disorders); these patients are prone to hyponatremia.

When fluid intake is not excessive, there is little danger of water intoxication and hyponatremia with usual intranasal or parenteral doses of desmopressin used to control diabetes insipidus. When the drug is used for its hemostatic effect in patients who do not require exogenous vasopressin for its antidiuretic effect, the risk of potential water intoxication and hyponatremia may be increased and these patients should be cautioned to ingest only enough fluid to satisfy their thirst. Water retention can usually be controlled by decreasing the dosage of desmopressin; severe water retention caused by overdosage may be treated with a diuretic such as furosemide.

Although vasoactive effects are minimal or absent with usual intranasal antidiuretic doses of desmopressin and also are minimal and infrequent and usually respond to dosage reduction when usual parenteral hemostatic doses of the drug are used, caution should be exercised in patients with coronary artery insufficiency and/or hypertensive cardiovascular disease. Desmopressin also should be used with caution in these patients and in patients predisposed to thrombotic events because of the drug's potential prothrombotic effect; although a causal relationship to the drug has not been determined, thrombotic events have been reported rarely in patients predisposed to thrombus formation.

In patients with diabetes insipidus or polyuria and polydipsia associated with head surgery or trauma, urine volume and osmolality and, in some cases, plasma osmolality should be monitored periodically during desmopressin therapy. In otherwise healthy patients with primary nocturnal enuresis, serum electrolytes should be checked at least once if therapy is continued beyond 7 days.

In patients with hemophilia A, factor VIII and factor VIII/ristocetin cofactor (von Willebrand factor) activities, factor VIII antigen levels, and activated partial thromboplastin time should be monitored during desmopressin therapy. Factor VIII activity should be determined prior to initiating desmopressin therapy for hemostasis; desmopressin therapy should not be relied on in patients with a factor VIII activity less than 5% of normal.

In patients with von Willebrand disease, factor VIII and factor VIII/ristocetin cofactor activities and factor VIII/von Willebrand factor antigen levels should be monitored during desmopressin therapy. Determination of bleeding time may also be useful in monitoring therapy in these patients.

Desmopressin is contraindicated in patients with hypersensitivity to the drug or any ingredient in the formulation. Desmopressin also is contraindicated in patients with moderate to severe renal impairment (creatinine clearance less than 50 mL/minute) and in patients with hyponatremia or a history of hyponatremia. Because of the risk of platelet aggregation and thrombocytopenia, the drug also should not be used in patients with type 2B or platelet-type (pseudo) von Willebrand disease. (See Pharmacology.)

● Pediatric Precautions

Fluid intake should be carefully restricted in pediatric patients to prevent possible hyponatremia and water intoxication; fluid restriction should be discussed with the patient and/or guardian. (See Cautions: Precautions and Contraindications.)

Desmopressin acetate nasal solutions containing 0.1 mg of desmopressin acetate per mL have been used in children with diabetes insipidus. However, pediatric dosage must be carefully adjusted according to individual patient needs and tolerance, with particular attention to the risk of an extreme decrease in plasma osmolality and resulting seizures in young children. There have been occasional reports of a change in response to desmopressin therapy over time, usually after periods exceeding 6 months. Some patients show a decreased responsiveness to the drug, while others show a shortened duration of effect. There is no evidence that this change in responsiveness results from the development of binding antibodies, but it may result from a local inactivation of the peptide.

Desmopressin acetate nasal solution containing 1.5 mg of desmopressin acetate per mL can be used for the treatment of hemophilia A or von Willebrand disease in children 11 months of age or older; however, safety and efficacy of the nasal solution have not been established in children younger than 11 months of age.

Desmopressin acetate tablets have been used safely for up to 44 months in pediatric patients 4 years of age or older with diabetes insipidus. In younger patients, dosage adjustment of oral desmopressin should be individualized to prevent an excessive decrease in plasma osmolality leading to hyponatremia and possible seizures.

Desmopressin acetate tablets have been used safely for up to 6 months in pediatric patients 6 years of age and older with primary nocturnal enuresis. In patients with primary nocturnal enuresis, desmopressin therapy should be interrupted during acute intercurrent illness characterized by fluid and/or electrolyte imbalance (e.g., systemic infections, fever, recurrent vomiting or diarrhea) and under conditions associated with increased water intake (e.g., extremely hot weather, vigorous exercise). (See Cautions: Precautions and Contraindications.)

Safety and efficacy of *parenteral* desmopressin for the management of *diabetes insipidus* in children younger than 12 years of age have not been established.

The manufacturers state that desmopressin acetate injection should not be used in the management of hemophilia A or von Willebrand disease in children younger than 3 months of age.

● Geriatric Precautions

Fluid intake should be carefully restricted in geriatric patients to prevent possible hyponatremia and water intoxication; fluid restriction should be discussed with the patient. (See Cautions: Precautions and Contraindications.)

Clinical studies of desmopressin did not include sufficient numbers of patients 65 years of age and older to determine whether geriatric patients respond differently than younger patients. While other clinical experience has not revealed age-related differences in response, drug dosage generally should be titrated carefully in geriatric patients, usually initiating therapy at the low end of the dosage range. The greater frequency of decreased hepatic, renal, and/or cardiac function and of concomitant disease and drug therapy observed in the elderly also should be considered. Desmopressin is known to be substantially excreted by the kidney and the risk of severe adverse reactions to the drug may be increased in patients with impaired renal function. Because geriatric patients may have decreased renal function, renal function should be monitored and dosage adjusted accordingly.

● Pregnancy, Fertility, and Lactation

Safe use of desmopressin during pregnancy or lactation has not been established. Reproduction studies in rats and rabbits using desmopressin dosages up to 12.5 times the usual human hemostatic dosage or 125 times the usual human antidiuretic dosage have not revealed evidence of harm to the fetus. There are no adequate and controlled studies to date using desmopressin in pregnant women; however, the drug has been used throughout pregnancy without adverse effect to mother or fetus and has been used during lactation without adverse effect to the lactating woman or nursing infant. Although published reports state that desmopressin, unlike preparations containing the natural hormones, has no uterotonic effect at usual antidiuretic doses, the physician must weigh the potential therapeutic benefits against the possible risks. Because it is not known whether desmopressin is distributed into milk, the drug should be used with caution in nursing women.

DRUG INTERACTIONS

Although drug interactions have been reported with vasopressin, few specific interactions have been reported with desmopressin. Desmopressin should be used cautiously in patients who are receiving lithium, large doses of epinephrine, demeclocycline, heparin, or alcohol, because the antidiuretic response to desmopressin may be decreased; drugs such as chlorpropamide, urea, or fludrocortisone may potentiate the antidiuretic response. Concurrent administration of clofibrate with desmopressin reportedly potentiates and prolongs the antidiuretic effect of desmopressin. In one patient, prior administration of carbamazepine decreased the duration of action of desmopressin. Patients receiving large doses of desmopressin (e.g., 0.3 mcg/kg) should be carefully monitored if the drug is administered concurrently with other vasopressor agents. Desmopressin has been used with aminocaproic acid without adverse effects.

Concomitant use of drugs that may increase the risk of water intoxication with hyponatremia (e.g., tricyclic antidepressants, selective serotonin-reuptake inhibitors [SSRIs], chlorpromazine, opiates, nonsteroidal anti-inflammatory agents [NSAIAs], lamotrigine, carbamazepine) with desmopressin should be undertaken with caution. Hyponatremic seizures have been reported rarely in patients receiving desmopressin and imipramine or oxybutynin during postmarketing surveillance.

PHARMACOLOGY

Desmopressin elicits a greater antidiuretic response, on a weight basis, than does arginine vasopressin. One important physiologic role of vasopressin is to maintain serum osmolality within a normal range. The antidiuretic potency of IV desmopressin is about 10 times that following intranasal administration of the drug. Vasopressin increases reabsorption of water by the collecting ducts in the kidneys resulting in increased urine osmolality and decreased urinary flow rate. In patients with neurohypophyseal diabetes insipidus, desmopressin has the same effects on water reabsorption as does vasopressin. Therapeutic doses of desmopressin do not directly affect urinary sodium or potassium excretion, or serum sodium, potassium, or creatinine concentrations.

Structural modifications of vasopressin present in desmopressin result in reduced smooth muscle contracting and vasopressor properties compared with vasopressin and lypressin. Intranasal doses of 20 mcg of desmopressin acetate have no effect on blood pressure or pulse rate, but mean arterial pressure may increase as much as 15 mm Hg with doses of 40 mcg or more. Desmopressin has not been reported to stimulate uterine contractions.

Desmopressin, unlike vasopressin, does not stimulate adrenocorticotropic hormone release or increase plasma cortisol concentrations. In children, intranasal administration of desmopressin has no effect on growth hormone, prolactin, or luteinizing hormone concentrations.

Desmopressin causes a dose-dependent increase in plasma factor VIII (antihemophilic factor), plasminogen activator, and, to a smaller degree, factor VIII-related antigen and ristocetin cofactor activities. Large IV doses of desmopressin acetate (0.2–0.5 mcg/kg) increase factor VIII activity in healthy individuals, in patients with mild to moderate hemophilia A and B, in patients with certain types of von Willebrand disease, and in patients with uremia. Desmopressin elicits a greater increase in plasma factor VIII activity, on a weight basis, than does arginine vasopressin in patients with hemophilia or type I von Willebrand's disease. The percentage increase in plasma factor VIII activity in patients with mild hemophilia A or type 1 von Willebrand disease is reportedly similar to that in healthy individuals following IV infusion of a 0.3-mcg/kg dose of the drug over 10 minutes. A gradual diminution in the magnitude of the desmopressin-induced increase in plasma factor VIII activity generally occurs when administration of the drug is repeated every 12–24 hours, but the magnitude is usually the same as the initial response when a period of 2–3 days elapses between administration. Patients with moderate, rather than mild, hemophilia A may or may not respond with an adequate increase in factor VIII to ensure clotting, and patients with type 1 von Willebrand disease may respond better than those with type 2 disease. Patients with severe hemophilia or severe von Willebrand disease are unresponsive to desmopressin. Following intranasal (2–4 mcg/kg) or IV (0.2 mcg/kg) administration of single doses of desmopressin in one study, 3/3 healthy individuals, 27/31 patients with mild or moderate von Willebrand disease, and 6/7 patients with mild to moderate hemophilia A had a greater than 200% increase in plasma factor VIII activity; a lesser but substantial increase in factor VIII-related antigen and ristocetin cofactor also occurred. In this study, 2 patients with severe von

Willebrand disease were unresponsive to desmopressin. Although plasminogen activator activity increases rapidly after desmopressin administration, clinically important fibrinolysis has not been reported to date in patients being treated with the drug.

In patients with type 2B von Willebrand disease, desmopressin has been reported to induce platelet aggregation and thrombocytopenia; it was suggested that platelet aggregation resulted from desmopression-induced release of the larger multimers of factor VIII/von Willebrand factor which subsequently were adsorbed to platelets. The drug has also been reported to induce platelet aggregation and thrombocytopenia in patients with platelet-type (pseudo) von Willebrand disease; however, the specific mechanism of this effect may be different in these patients.

Desmopressin has also reportedly increased factor VIII activity and, to a lesser extent, factor VIII-related antigen and ristocetin cofactor in patients with uremia; these changes were accompanied by a shortening of bleeding time. In addition, the drug induced the release into plasma of the larger multimers of factor VIII/von Willebrand factor in these patients.

In a few patients with sickle cell anemia, hyponatremia induced by intranasal desmopressin has resulted in decreased mean corpuscular hemoglobin concentration and a decreased degree of sickling.

PHARMACOKINETICS

● Absorption

Following intranasal administration of desmopressin acetate as directed by the manufacturer, approximately 10–20% of a dose is absorbed through the nasal mucosa. The manufacturer states that nasal congestion does not interfere with the effectiveness of the drug; however, investigators have reported that patients with nasal congestion may require an increased dosage. Following intranasal administration of usual doses of desmopressin acetate in patients with neurohypophyseal diabetes insipidus, antidiuretic effects occur within 15–60 minutes, peak in 1–5 hours, persist 5–21 hours, and then abruptly end over a period of 60–90 minutes. Duration of action varies among individuals with a specific dose. The relatively prolonged duration of action of desmopressin may result from slower enzymatic inactivation of desmopressin than vasopressin or from sequestration of desmopressin in a membrane compartment. Studies using the nasal solution containing 1.5 mg of desmopressin acetate per mL indicate that bioavailability of the drug is 3.3–4.1% and peak plasma concentrations are attained 40–45 minutes after a dose. Following intranasal administration of 150–450 mcg of desmopressin acetate (1–3 sprays of a solution containing 1.5 mg/mL), increases in plasma concentrations of factor VIII and von Willebrand factor are evident within 30 minutes and peak at about 1.5 hours.

Following oral administration of desmopressin acetate tablets, the drug is only minimally absorbed from the GI tract, and bioavailability is about 5% compared with intranasal administration and about 0.16% compared with IV administration of the drug. Peak plasma concentrations of desmopressin acetate are attained 0.9 or 1.5 hours following oral or intranasal administration, respectively. Antidiuretic effects occur at about 1 hour and peak at about 4–7 hours after an oral dose of the drug.

Following IV infusion of desmopressin, the increase in plasma factor VIII activity occurs within 15–30 minutes and peaks between 90 minutes and 2 hours after administration; the increase in factor VIII activity is dose dependent, with a 300–400% maximum increase reportedly occurring after IV infusion of a 0.4-mcg/kg dose.

● Distribution

Distribution of desmopressin has not been fully characterized. It is not known if desmopressin crosses the placenta. The drug is distributed into milk.

● Elimination

Desmopressin is excreted principally in the urine.

Following intranasal administration of 150–450 mcg of desmopressin acetate (1–3 sprays of a solution containing 1.5 mg/mL), half-life of the drug is 3.3–3.5 hours.

Following oral administration, half-life of desmopressin acetate is independent of dosage and averages 1.5–2.5 hours.

After IV administration of 2–3 mcg of desmopressin acetate in patients with neurohypophyseal diabetes insipidus, plasma concentrations decline in a biphasic manner with a mean initial plasma half-life of 7.8 minutes and a mean terminal plasma half-life of 75.5 minutes (range: 0.4–4 hours).

The metabolic fate of desmopressin is unknown. Unlike vasopressin, desmopressin apparently is not degraded by aminopeptidases or other peptidases that cleave oxytocin and endogenous vasopressin in the plasma during late pregnancy.

Renal clearance of desmopressin decreases with decreasing renal function. Following administration of a single IV dose of 2 mcg of desmopressin acetate in individuals with normal renal function (average creatinine clearance of 103 mL/minute), mild renal impairment (average creatinine clearance of 72 mL/minute), moderate renal impairment (average creatinine clearance of 37 mL/minute), or severe renal impairment (average creatinine clearance of 16 mL/minute; not on dialysis), terminal half-lives of desmopressin averaged 3.7, 4.8, 7.2, or 10 hours, respectively.

CHEMISTRY AND STABILITY

● Chemistry

Desmopressin is a synthetic polypeptide structurally related to arginine vasopressin (antidiuretic hormone), the natural human posterior pituitary hormone. Desmopressin acetate is commercially available as nasal solutions for intranasal administration, tablets for oral administration, and injections for parenteral administration.

Desmopressin acetate nasal solutions are aqueous solutions of the drug. For the treatment of central cranial diabetes insipidus, desmopressin acetate is commercially available as nasal solutions containing 0.1 mg of the drug per mL with 0.75 or 0.9% sodium chloride for administration via a spray pump or nasal tube; for the treatment of hemophilia A or von Willebrand disease, desmopressin acetate is commercially available as a nasal solution containing 1.5 mg of the drug per mL with 0.75% sodium chloride for administration via a spray pump. These nasal solutions contain either benzalkonium chloride or chlorobutanol as preservatives.

Desmopressin acetate injection is a sterile, aqueous solution containing 4 mcg of the drug per mL with 0.9% sodium chloride. Hydrochloric acid is added during the manufacture of the injection to adjust the pH to approximately 4; the injection also may contain chlorobutanol as a preservative.

● Stability

Commercially available nasal solutions of desmopressin acetate preserved with benzalkonium chloride should be stored at controlled room temperature (20–25°C, not to exceed 25°C). Commercially available nasal solutions containing 1.5 mg of the drug per mL should be discarded 6 months after opening. Commercially available nasal solutions of desmopressin acetate preserved with chlorobutanol should be refrigerated at 2–8°C; when

traveling, closed bottles are stable for 3 weeks at controlled room temperature (20–25°C).

Desmopressin acetate tablets should be stored at 20–25°C; exposure to excessive heat or light should be avoided.

Commercially available desmopressin acetate injection should be refrigerated at 2–8°C; freezing should be avoided.

PREPARATIONS

Excipients in commercially available drug preparations may have clinically important effects in some individuals; consult specific product labeling for details.

Desmopressin Acetate

Nasal		
Solution	0.1 mg/mL*	**DDAVP® Nasal Spray** (with spray pump), Sanofi-Aventis
		DDAVP® Rhinal Tube (with 2 calibrated nasal tubes; refrigerate), Sanofi-Aventis
		Desmopressin Acetate Nasal Spray, Apotex, Bausch & Lomb
		Desmopressin Acetate Rhinal Tube (with 2 calibrated nasal tubes; refrigerate), Ferring
		Minirin®, Ferring
	1.5 mg/mL*	**Desmopressin Acetate Nasal Spray**
		Stimate® Nasal Spray (with spray pump), CSL Behring
Oral		
Tablets	0.1 mg*	**DDAVP®,** Sanofi-Aventis
		Desmopressin Acetate Tablets
	0.2 mg*	**DDAVP®,** Sanofi-Aventis
		Desmopressin Acetate Tablets
Parenteral		
Injection	4 mcg/mL*	**DDAVP®,** Sanofi-Aventis
		Desmopressin Acetate Injection

* available from one or more manufacturer, distributor, and/or repackager by generic (nonproprietary) name

† Use is not currently included in the labeling approved by the US Food and Drug Administration.

Selected Revisions January 1, 2009, © Copyright, March 1, 1979, American Society of Health-System Pharmacists, Inc.

Somatropin

68:28 • PITUITARY

■ Somatropin is a recombinant human growth hormone (hGH) with an amino acid sequence identical to that of hGH of pituitary origin.

USES

Somatropin is used in the treatment of short stature or growth failure due to growth hormone deficiency or other conditions. Other indications for the drug include the treatment of HIV patients with wasting or cachexia or for the treatment of short bowel syndrome in adults. There are multiple recombinant growth hormone preparations commercially available in the US. Although clinically similar, differences exist among the products in FDA-approved indications, administration, and dosing schedules. Disease-specific treatment risks also vary among the various growth failure indications; consult guidelines and preparation-specific labeling for additional guidance.

● *Short Stature or Growth Failure in Pediatric Patients*

Somatropin is FDA-labeled for use in various conditions associated with growth failure or short stature in pediatric patients.

Growth Hormone Deficiency

Somatropin is used to treat growth failure in children due to inadequate secretion of endogenous growth hormone. Somatropin is designated an orphan drug by FDA for this use.

Growth hormone deficiency (GHD) in children is most often recognized through short stature and/or growth failure, and may be the result of genetics, pituitary malfunction, pituitary gland insult (e.g., brain surgery, irradiation, tumors), or unknown causes. The Pediatric Endocrine Society guideline recommends the use of growth hormone treatment (somatropin) to normalize adult height and avoid extreme shortness in children and adolescents with GHD because the benefits, impact on physical and psychosocial disability, outweigh potential harms. The primary objectives of growth hormone treatment in children diagnosed with GHD are growth velocity acceleration to promote normalization of growth and stature during childhood and attainment of normal adult height appropriate for the child's genetic potential.

Efficacy and safety of somatropin in pediatric patients with growth failure due to inadequate secretion of endogenous growth hormone are supported by multiple open-label studies that were conducted in children who were treatment-naïve or had previously received growth hormone treatment. Clinical trials conducted for FDA approval for this indication varied in patient population characteristics (e.g., age at enrollment, pubertal status, growth hormone naïve or non-naïve) and dosage of somatropin, which ranged from 0.175 to 0.7 mg/kg per week, divided and administered daily or 3 times a week; the highest dosage was studied in pubertal patients. Following treatment with somatropin, measures of response such as height velocity, height velocity standard deviation score (SDS), and height SDS increased from baseline, with the greatest responses generally observed during the first year of treatment.

Data on the effect of growth hormone treatment on adult height are available from postmarketing surveillance registries, a population-based registry, a cancer survivor registry, and clinic/hospital-based case series. When these studies were analyzed collectively, more than 4520 patients were treated to adult height (mean height SDS approximately -1) for a mean duration of 7 years (range 2–15.4 years) using a mean growth hormone dosage of 0.25 mg/kg per week (range 0.14–0.7 mg/kg per week).

Turner Syndrome

Somatropin is used to treat pediatric patients with short stature associated with Turner syndrome. Somatropin is designated an orphan drug by FDA for this use. Turner syndrome is characterized by a partial or complete absence of one X chromosome in females resulting in a constellation of issues such as lack of spontaneous pubertal development and short stature.

Clinical studies establishing the efficacy of somatropin for this indication include one randomized controlled trial with an untreated control group, one randomized, blinded, dose-response study, and two long-term studies with a matched historical control (untreated); all studies were open-label and pubertal induction varied amongst the studies. Somatropin dosages administered were 0.3 mg/kg per week given in divided doses 6 times a week; 0.375 mg/kg per week given in divided doses either 3 times a week or daily or 0.27 mg/kg or 0.36 mg/kg administered in divided doses 3 or 6 times weekly depending on the study. Average height gains in the 4 studies combined (which included a total of 249 patients treated to adult height) ranged from 5 to 8.3 cm. Additional randomized open-label studies were conducted with other somatropin products; results of these studies demonstrated statistically significant increases from baseline in growth variables evaluated (e.g., height velocity, height velocity SDS, height SDS).

Idiopathic Short Stature

Somatropin is used to treat pediatric patients with idiopathic short stature (ISS) when height SDS is less than -2.25 and is associated with growth rates unlikely to permit attainment of adult height in the normal range; the drug should be used in patients whose epiphyses are not closed and for whom other causes of short stature are excluded. The height cut-off of -2.25 SDS (1.2nd percentile) translates to an adult height of 63 inches in men and 59 inches in women.

The Pediatric Endocrine Society guideline suggests a shared decision-making approach instead of routine use of somatropin for children with ISS. The guideline discourages use of the drug for increasing height in children not meeting the criteria for ISS due to the lack of data showing that additional height significantly improves quality of life or provides any other benefit that must be weighed against the risk of harm, psychological and physical burdens, and costs of therapy.

Clinical studies establishing the efficacy of somatropin for this indication include a double-blind, randomized, placebo-controlled study and a randomized, dose-response study; all patients were diagnosed with ISS after excluding other known causes (e.g., GHD). Patients enrolled in the placebo-controlled trial had a mean age of 12.4 years and were predominantly prepubertal (Tanner I, 45%) or in early puberty (Tanner II, 47%) at baseline. Patients received somatropin 0.22 mg/kg per week or placebo in divided doses 3 times per week until height velocity decreased to ≤1.5 cm/year (also known as final height); mean treatment duration in those achieving final height was 4.4 (range 0.1–9.1) years. Final height measurements were only available for 33 patients (22 treated with somatropin, 11 treated with placebo). The number of patients who gained at least 1 SDS unit in height across the duration of the study (50% versus 0%) and those whose final height was above the 5th percentile of the general population height standard for age and sex (41% versus 0%) was significantly greater in the somatropin group compared to placebo, respectively.

Patients enrolled in the dose-response study had a mean age of 9.8 years, height SDS of -3.21, predicted adult height SDS of -2.63, and height velocity SDS of -1.09 at baseline; all but 3 of the 239 patients were prepubertal and no patients had a baseline height above the 5th percentile.

Somatropin dosages were 0.24 mg/kg per week, 0.24 mg/kg per week for 1 year followed by 0.37 mg/kg per week, and 0.37 mg/kg per week given in divided doses 6 times per week. Height velocity was assessed during the first 2 years, then 50 patients were followed to final height. Of the evaluable patients, mean height velocity and the mean difference between final height and baseline predicted height at 2 years was significantly greater in the 0.37 mg/kg per week group compared with the 0.24 mg/kg per week group (4.04 versus 3.27 cm/year and 7.2 versus 5.4 cm, respectively). Final height above the 5th percentile of the general population height standards was achieved in 82% and 47% of patients in the 0.37 mg/kg per week group compared with the 0.24 mg/kg per week group, respectively.

Short Stature Homeobox-Containing Gene Deficiency

Somatropin (e.g., Humatrope®, Zomacton®) is used to treat pediatric patients with short stature or growth failure in short stature homeobox-containing gene deficiency (SHOX-D). Somatropin is designated an orphan drug by FDA for this use. SHOX-D is responsible for an average 20-cm height deficit in untreated females with Turner Syndrome and is also the primary cause of short stature in most patients with Léri-Weill syndrome (LWS).

Efficacy and safety of somatropin in pediatric patients with SHOX deficiency who are not growth hormone-deficient were evaluated in a single randomized, controlled, open-label study. Pre-pubertal patients >3 years of age without chronic disease, no GHD, no known growth-influencing medications, and short stature (with low height or height velocity percentile) with confirmed SHOX-D were stratified and randomized based on LWS diagnosis. Three groups of patients were compared: a somatropin-treatment group (SHOX-D group), a no treatment group, and a group of patients wtih Turner syndrome who received somatropin treatment. Among enrolled patients, there was no difference in male to female ratio (with the exception of all Turner Syndrome patients who were females), bone age, baseline height, or proportion of patients with LWS; mean patient ages were 7.3 years in the somatropin-SHOX-D group, 7.5 years in the no treatment group, and 7.5 years in the somatropin-Turner syndrome group. SHOX-D and Turner syndrome patients were treated with subcutaneous somatropin 0.05 mg/kg per day; patients in the no treatment group did not receive placebo injections. The mean first-year height velocity of treated patients with SHOX-D was significantly greater than that of the untreated patients and similar to that of Turner syndrome patients receiving somatropin therapy. Second-year mean height velocity also was significantly greater with somatropin versus no treatment in patients with SHOX-D, and similar when compared with Turner syndrome patients receiving the drug.

This 2-year study was followed by an extension where all patients (untreated and treated) were offered somatropin 0.05 mg/kg per day until achieving final height or study closure; 49 SHOX-D and 24 Turner syndrome patients continued in the extension period. Due to delayed somatropin initiation in the untreated SHOX-D population, mean bone age and mean chronologic age differed at baseline. When all SHOX-D patients were combined and compared to Turner syndrome patients, bone age and chronologic age at baseline were similar. Final height was achieved in 64% of all extension patients and 14% of those who completed the extension study without achieving final height; the remaining patients discontinued the study before attaining final height or study closure.

Small for Gestational Age

Somatropin is used to treat pediatric patients with short stature born small for gestational age (SGA) with no catch-up growth by 2 to 4 years of age. Somatropin is designated an orphan drug by FDA for this use. Small for gestational age is defined as weight and/or length (height) less than or equal to -2 SDS below the mean for gestational age. Infants born SGA may achieve normal height following a catch-up growth period; those who fail to achieve catch-up growth within their first 2 years have a high risk of short stature later in life.

Efficacy and safety of somatropin for the treatment of SGA have been evaluated in multiple (mostly open-label or dose-response) studies, which were performed in children of various ages selected following exclusion of other growth-restricting conditions (e.g., Turner syndrome, malnutrition, diabetes mellitus, renal disease, GHD). Important factors for somatropin success in SGA patients with no catch-up growth, in order of importance, are higher dosage, early treatment, and treatment duration.

In 4 randomized, open-label, controlled clinical trials, patients 2–8 years of age were observed for 12 months and then randomized to somatropin 0.24 or 0.48 mg/kg per week in divided daily doses or no treatment for 24 months. Somatropin treatment resulted in significant increases in growth during the first 24 months of study compared with no treatment. Patients who received somatropin 0.48 mg/kg/week demonstrated a significant improvement in height SDS compared with those treated with 0.24 mg/kg/week.

Noonan Syndrome

Somatropin (e.g., Norditropin®) is used to treat pediatric patients with short stature associated with Noonan syndrome. Somatropin is designated an orphan drug by FDA for this use.

Noonan syndrome is a genetic multisystem condition with clinical features including short stature, a characteristic facial appearance, congenital heart disease, and skeletal anomalies. Although birth weight and length are usually normal, short stature, impacted by delayed or attenuated growth spurt, becomes more noticeable during the age of normal puberty.

Efficacy of somatropin in the treatment of Noonan syndrome was established in a small prospective, open-label, randomized study. Pre-pubertal patients were included in the study if there was no significant bone age acceleration, height SDS was less than -2, and height velocity SDS was <1 during the 12 months prior to treatment. Patients received a somatropin dosage of 0.033 or 0.066 mg/kg per day,

which could be adjusted for growth response after the initial 2 years. There were 24 enrolled patients, 3 to 14 years of age; 50% were male. Year 1 height velocity for the 0.033 mg/kg per day treatment group compared with the 0.066 mg/kg/day treatment group was 8.55 versus 10.1 cm/year, and year 2 height velocity for these treatment groups was 6.7 versus 7.6 cm/year.

Data from 2 similarly-designed, observational studies were combined to assess the long-term (more than 4 years) efficacy and safety of daily growth hormone treatment in Noonan syndrome patients. Patients enrolled in the study had a mean age of 8.38 years, height SDS of -2.76, and bone age of 7 years; 80% were male, 75% of patients had a treatment duration of <7 years, and the mean growth hormone treatment dose was 0.042 mg/kg per day. Mean height SDS increased from baseline to -1.66 by year 3, placing patients within the normal range; however, height SDS plateaued or decreased from years 5–6 and beyond.

Prader-Willi Syndrome

Somatropin is used to treat pediatric patients with growth failure due to Prader-Willi syndrome. The diagnosis of Prader-Willi syndrome should be confirmed by appropriate genetic testing. Somatropin is designated an orphan drug by FDA for this use. Prader-Willi syndrome is a multi-system genetic disorder with clinical features that include developmental delays, behavioral problems, hyperphagia, and GHD resulting in short stature; if left untreated, hyperphagia with childhood onset obesity may result in life-threatening obesity.

The efficacy of somatropin in the treatment of Prader-Willi syndrome was established in 2 randomized, open-label, controlled trials. The control groups received no treatment for year 1 and daily somatropin during year 2, and the treatment groups received daily somatropin injections for 2 years.

The first study evaluated a somatropin dosage of 0.24 mg/kg per week divided into daily injections. At the end of 12 months, mean linear growth increased by 11.6 cm and height SDS improved from -1.6 to -0.5 compared to 5 cm linear growth and no change in height SDS in the untreated control group. In addition, somatropin-treated patients achieved statistically significant improved changes from baseline in fat mass, lean body mass, and ratio of lean body mass/fat mass; body weight change from baseline was significant. The second study evaluated a somatropin dosage of 0.36 mg/kg per week divided into daily injections. At the end of 12 months, mean linear growth increased by 10.7 cm and height SDS improved from -2.6 to -1.4 compared to 4.3 cm linear growth and no change in height SDS in the untreated control group. In both studies, when untreated patients converted to somatropin treatment, linear growth continued to increase regardless of 1st year treatment status; somatropin treatment, compared to no treatment, did not accelerate bone age. In a larger 4-year multicenter prospective trial, somatropin 1 mg/m^2 per day administered to 55 prepubertal Prader-Willi syndrome patients (mean age 5.9 years) resulted in significantly improved body fat percentage, body mass index, and normalized mean height SDS from -2.27 to -0.24; although lean body mass increased during year 1, it returned to baseline during year 2 and remained unchanged thereafter.

Growth Failure Secondary to Chronic Kidney Disease

Somatropin (e.g., Nutropin® AQ) is used to treat pediatric patients with growth failure associated with chronic kidney disease (CKD), in conjunction with optimal CKD management, up to the time of renal transplantation. Somatropin is designated an orphan drug by FDA for this use.

Growth failure is a common complication of CKD in children. There are many factors (e.g., protein-calorie malnutrition, bone and mineral disorders, hormone axes disturbances) that can contribute to impairment of growth in such children. Children with advanced CKD experience insulin-like growth factor-1 (IGF-1) deficiency resulting in a state of growth hormone insensitivity that may be overcome by supraphysiologic exogenous growth hormone administration.

The efficacy of somatropin in the treatment of children with CKD prior to renal transplantation was established in 2 multi-center, randomized trials (a double-blind trial and an open-label, randomized trial). Somatropin 0.05 mg/kg per day was compared to placebo in the double-blind trial, and compared to untreated patients in the open-label trial. At the end of 2 years, patient data from both trials were combined. First year and second year growth rates were significantly improved in patients who received somatropin (10.8 and 7.8 cm/year) compared with the control groups (6.5 and 5.5 cm/year). From baseline to 2 years, mean height SDS improved significantly from -2.9 to -1.5 in the somatropin groups, but not in the the control groups (-2.8 to -2.9).

A systematic review was conducted in 2011 to evaluate the benefits and harms of recombinant growth hormone therapy in children diagnosed with CKD. The review included 16 randomized controlled trials that compared somatropin treatment with placebo or no treatment, or compared 2 different doses of somatropin in 809 children with CKD (pre-dialysis, on dialysis, and post-transplantation). In 8 studies (391 patients) that reported height SDS improvement from baseline at 1 year, this measure increased by a mean difference of 0.82 with somatropin compared to no treatment/placebo; this approximates a single-year growth of 5 cm in a 10 year old patient. In 7 studies (287 patients) that reported increases in height velocity over 1 year, this measure increased by a mean difference of 3.88 cm/year.

Growth Hormone Deficiency in Adults

Somatropin is used for the replacement of endogenous growth hormone in adults with GHD. Somatropin is designated an orphan drug by FDA for treatment of adults with GHD, including those with childhood onset GHD following epiphyseal closure.

GHD in adults is the result of decreased growth hormone secretion from the anterior pituitary gland in excess of the expected physiologic decline associated with aging. Adults can be diagnosed with GHD in childhood (childhood-onset GHD) or adulthood (adult-onset GHD). Adults with childhood onset GHD caused by structural pituitary issues or brain tumors should be followed closely during the transition to adult care, following achievement of final height.

Benefits of growth hormone treatment in adults with childhood-onset or adult-onset GHD include improved body composition (e.g., decreased body fat, increased lean body mass), bone health, exercise capacity, and quality of life. The diagnosis of adult onset GHD, including continued treatment for childhood-onset GHD beyond epiphyses closure, involves an appropriate growth hormone provocative test unless the patient has multiple pituitary hormone deficiencies or has congenital/genetic GHD. Patients with childhood-onset GHD who have closed epiphyses require re-evaluation before proceeding with somatropin treatment.

The American Association of Clinical Endocrinologists (AACE)/American College of Endocrinology (ACE) and Endocrine Society (ES) issued guidelines for the evaluation and management of GHD in adults, which includes recommendations for patients transitioning from pediatric to adult care. The guidelines recommend individualized, non-weight-based somatropin dosing, starting with a dose appropriate for age and comorbid condition (e.g., obesity, diabetes mellitus), and then titrating according to clinical response, adverse effects, and age- and gender-adjusted serum IGF-1 levels. The guidelines state no preference for use of any particular growth hormone preparation over another.

Multiple studies of somatropin in adults with GHD (childhood- or adult-onset) support the use of growth hormone to improve body composition, exercise capacity, bone health, and cardiovascular risk factors. Clinical trials conducted for FDA approval for this indication varied in patient population characteristics (e.g., cause of GHD, age at enrollment, age of GHD onset, history of prior growth hormone treatment) and somatropin dosage. Dosage of the drug ranged from 0.056 to 0.175 mg/kg per week divided and administered daily; during the first month of treatment, the initial weekly dosage was 33–50% lower.

In 4 randomized, blinded, placebo-controlled studies, patients with adult-onset GHD (2 studies) and childhood-onset GHD (2 studies) were treated with placebo or somatropin (0.00625 mg/kg per day during the first month followed by 0.0125 mg/kg per day for the next 5 months). At 6 months, all patients received open-label somatropin for 12 months. Adult-onset and childhood-onset patients differed by diagnosis (organic versus idiopathic pituitary disease), body size, weight, and age. The primary outcomes were lean body mass, fat mass, and lipid panel parameters (e.g., total cholesterol [TC], high-density lipoprotein [HDL], and low-density lipoprotein [LDL]). In patients with adult-onset GHD, mean lean body mass increased and body fat decreased from baseline with somatropin compared with placebo (2.59 versus -0.22 kg and -3.27 versus 0.56 kg, respectively). Similar improvements were observed in the childhood-onset population. In both populations, low baseline serum HDL concentrations improved significantly, but TC and LDL did not.

In early studies of growth hormone replacement therapy in adults, weight-based somatropin dosages were administered and subsequently reduced because of adverse events such as peripheral edema and carpal tunnel syndrome; single-center studies have suggested that starting with low daily non-weight-based dosages (0.17–0.33 mg/day), titrating the dosage based on IGF-1 levels and clinical response, may result in similar efficacy with fewer adverse reactions. In a large multinational, parallel, open-label study, patients with adult- and childhood-onset GHD were randomized to weight-based or non-weight-based somatropin; titration over 8- or 16-week intervals occurred in 0.004 mg/kg/day or 0.2 mg/day increments, respectively. Dosage adjustments for adverse reactions or serum IGF-1 levels exceeding the upper limit of normal of the age- and sex-adjusted reference range in the weight-based group were performed in 25% or 50% increments; in the non-weight based group, adjustments in 0.1 or 0.2 mg/day increments also occurred upon the presence or absence of perceived clinical benefit. At the end of the study, mean somatropin doses were significantly lower in the non-weight-based group compared with the weight-based group (0.54 and 0.70 mg/day, respectively). The primary outcome of fat mass was significantly decreased from baseline in both groups; when broken down by sex, fat mass decreased significantly more in males in the weight-based group, but there was no difference between groups in females. Waist circumference was significantly decreased from baseline in both groups; when broken down by sex, waist circumference decreased significantly more in females in the weight-based group, but there was no difference between groups in males. Adverse reactions were similar with the exception of a significantly reduced occurrence of peripheral edema and rash in the non-weight-based group compared with the weight-based group.

HIV-associated Wasting or Cachexia

Somatropin (e.g., Serostim®) is used for the treatment of HIV patients with wasting or cachexia to increase lean body mass and body weight, and improve physical endurance; concomitant antiretroviral therapy is necessary. Somatropin is designated an orphan drug by FDA for treatment of HIV-associated catabolism/weight loss. HIV-related wasting, defined as ≥10% involuntary weight loss, includes loss of both lean and fat mass and is associated with morbidity and mortality.

Efficacy of somatropin in patients with HIV-related wasting or cachexia was evaluated in two 12-week, randomized, double-blind, placebo-controlled clinical studies. One study (Trial 1) was conducted in the era preceding highly active antiretroviral therapy (HAART) and the other study (Trial 2) was conducted in patients receiving HAART.

Trial 1 compared somatropin 0.1 mg/kg daily to placebo in patients with severe HIV wasting (defined as unintentional weight loss of ≥10% or weight <90% of the lower limit of ideal body weight) taking nucleoside analogue therapy. The average baseline CD4 T-cell count was 85 cells/mm³; 96% of patients were male. The primary endpoint was body weight and secondary endpoints included body composition assessed by dual energy X-ray absorptiometry (DXA) and physical function assessed by treadmill exercise testing. Mean increase in weight and lean body mass, and mean decrease in body fat, were significantly greater in the somatropin-treated group than in the placebo group. The mean difference between somatropin and placebo was a 1.6 kg increase in body weight, 3.1 kg increase in lean body mass, and 1.7 kg decrease in body fat. No significant body composition changes were observed in those enrolled in the 12-week, open-label, extension study. The median treadmill work output did not increase in the placebo group, but increased by 13% in somatropin-treated patients.

Trial 2 compared somatropin 0.1 mg/kg daily (daily dose), somatropin 0.1 mg/kg every other day (alternate day dose), and placebo in patients with 10% unintentional body weight loss, body mass index (BMI) <20 kg/m² or body weight <90% of ideal body weight. The maximum daily somatropin dose was 6 mg. The average baseline CD4 T-cell count was 446 cells/mm³, 91% of patients were male, and 88% were on HAART. The primary endpoint was physical function as measured by cycle ergometry work output, and secondary endpoints included body composition assessed by bioelectrical impedance spectroscopy (BIS) or dual energy X-ray absorptiometry (DXA). Cycle work output increased from baseline by 9.1%, 8.9%, and 0.2% in the daily dose, alternate day dose, and placebo groups, respectively. Mean lean body mass significantly increased by 3.89 kg and 5.84 kg in the alternate day dose and daily dose somatropin groups, respectively, compared to an increase of 0.97 kg in the placebo group; this was accompanied by an increase in body weight and decrease in fat mass compared to placebo. Body composition changes were dose-related. Both treatment groups also experienced improved quality of life compared to placebo. In an open-label, extension phase (12–48 weeks), patients who were originally randomized to placebo were re-randomized to alternate day or daily somatropin. Cycle work output, lean body mass, body weight, and fat mass were further improved or maintained throughout the extension phase.

● Short Bowel Syndrome in Adults

Somatropin (e.g., Zorbtive®) is used for the treatment of short bowel syndrome (SBS) in adults receiving specialized nutritional support. Somatropin is designated an orphan drug by FDA for use alone or in combination with glutamine in the treatment of SBS. SBS is defined as a loss of two-thirds or more of the small bowel resulting in malabsorption of fluid, electrolytes, and other essential nutrients, severe diarrhea, dehydration, and progressive malnutrition; patients may require parenteral nutrition, the duration of which will be based on several factors (e.g., length of remaining bowel, malabsorption, diet). Growth hormone enhances transmucosal transport of water electrolytes, and nutrients; when combined with glutamine and an optimal oral diet, growth hormone may improve macronutrient and fluid absorption in patients with SBS.

Efficacy and safety of somatropin in patients with SBS have been evaluated in a single, randomized, double-blind, placebo-controlled, phase 3 clinical study. Adult patients with BMI 17–28 kg/m², small intestine length ≤200 cm, and the ability to ingest solid food while requiring ≥3000 parenteral nutrition calories/week who were at least ≥6 months from bowel resection surgery were eligible for randomization. After a 2-week baseline stabilization period, patients were randomized to 4 weeks of subcutaneous growth hormone placebo plus oral glutamine 30 g/day, subcutaneous somatropin 0.1 mg/kg per day plus oral glutamine placebo, or subcutaneous somatropin 0.1 mg/kg per day plus oral glutamine 30 g/day; the maximum daily somatropin dose was 8 mg/day. The study was conducted in a treatment facility over a 6-week period, including the 2-week baseline period, with controlled optimal diet and standardized monitoring. After 6 weeks, patients were discharged on the same parenteral nutrition prescription received during the last study week and optimized diet and oral glutamine or glutamine placebo, and monitored for 3 months; parenteral nutrition adjustments were made based on nutritional and hydration status. The primary endpoint was change in parenteral nutrition volume measured in week 2 (last week of baseline period) versus week 6 (last week of treatment); secondary endpoints were changes in parenteral nutrition calories and frequency of administration. All 3 of the following were required before parenteral nutrition adjustment: 1) maintenance of normal hydration, 2) stabilization of serum electrolyte and blood urea nitrogen (BUN), and 3) maintenance of a stable body weight. After 4 weeks, patients receiving placebo plus glutamine, somatropin plus placebo, and somatropin plus glutamine experienced a mean change in parenteral nutrition volume of -3.8, -5.9, and -7.7 L/week, respectively, and parenteral nutrition infusion days/week were decreased by 2, 3, and 4 days, respectively. Calories per week (parenteral nutrition) decreased by 2633, 4338, and 5751 in those receiving placebo plus glutamine, somatropin plus placebo, and somatropin plus glutamine, respectively. At the end of the 3-month follow-up period where no somatropin was administered, parenteral nutrition volume, calories, and frequency increased slightly, but remained reduced relative to pretreatment values.

● Other Uses

The American Association of Clinical Endocrinologists (AACE)/American College of Endocrinology (ACE) strongly recommends against marketing, distributing, or administering human growth hormone for athletic performance enhancement†, or to treat aging (or aging related conditions)† in patients without a recognized medical condition. The World Anti-Doping Agency and the International Olympic Committee have barred athletes from using human growth hormone in the US.

DOSAGE AND ADMINISTRATION

● General

Pretreatment Screening

- Perform fundoscopic examination to exclude preexisting papilledema.

- Obtain a baseline serum insulin-like growth factor-1 (IGF-1) concentration.

- Obtain hip X-rays prior to initiating somatropin therapy in pediatric patients with short stature due to chronic kidney disease.

- Evaluate for signs of upper airway obstruction and sleep apnea in patients with Prader-Willi syndrome.

Patient Monitoring

- Perform periodic fundoscopic examination.

- Monitor for signs and symptoms of intracranial hypertension (e.g., visual changes, headache, nausea and/or vomiting).

- Monitor glucose levels periodically in all patients, especially in those with risk factors for type 2 diabetes mellitus (e.g., obesity, family history, Turner syndrome).

- Monitor patients with preexisting diabetes mellitus or impaired glucose tolerance, and adjust antihyperglycemic drug doses as needed.

- Perform standard cancer screening and monitor for malignancy development. Monitor patients with preexisting tumors for progression or recurrence.

- Monitor patients for reduced cortisol levels.

- Perform periodic thyroid function tests.

- Monitor for cardiovascular disorders and otitis media in patients with Turner syndrome.

- Monitor serum inorganic phosphorous, alkaline phosphatase, and parathyroid hormone as appropriate.

- In pediatric patients, assess compliance and evaluate other causes of poor growth such as hypothyroidism, under-nutrition, advanced bone age, and antibodies to recombinant human growth hormone if patients experience failure to increase height velocity, particularly during the first year of treatment.

- In adults with growth hormone deficiency (GHD), monitor serum IGF-1 concentrations periodically every 1-2 months during dosage titration, then every 6 to 12 months once maintenance dose is achieved.

Other General Considerations

- Somatropin treatment should be supervised by a physician experienced in the diagnosis and management of the specific indication for which the drug is being used.

- Somatropin products are not considered biosimilar to one another and are not interchangeable.

● Administration

Somatropin is administered by subcutaneous injection. Subcutaneous injections should be made into the back of the upper arm, abdomen, buttock, or thigh with regular rotation of injection sites to avoid lipoatrophy.

The manufacturer of Zorbtive® states to administer the drug by subcutaneous injection at a 90° angle into the top side of the thigh, the areas around the belly button, the back of the upper arms, or the buttocks or hips. Rotate injection sites; do not administer injections into areas where the skin is tender, bruised, red, or hard.

Somatropin is commercially available in various dosage forms for subcutaneous administration including single-dose or multi-dose vial kits containing lyophilized powder and diluent vials, two-chamber cartridges containing lyophilized powder and diluent, and cartridge kits containing lyophilized powder and diluent in prefilled syringes; all powder formulations require reconstitution prior to administration, and some require product specific delivery devices.

Somatropin is also available as a solution for subcutaneous administration in ready-to-use prefilled pens, injection devices, or cartridges.

Prior to the first injection of somatropin, store preparations and diluent (if supplied) at 2–8°C in the original carton for protection from light and physical damage; exceptions include storing Serostim®, Saizen®, and Zorbtive® at 15–30°C until the expiration date on the manufacturer's label and Genotropin Miniquick®, which may be stored at or below 25°C for up to 3 months after dispensing. Avoid storage under conditions of extreme heat or cold, and do not shake or freeze the drug; protect from light.

Patients and/or their caregivers should be cautioned against sharing or reusing syringes, needles, and/or devices. Carefully instruct patients on the proper, safe disposal of needles, syringes, and unused drug. Patients should be supplied with a puncture-resistant container for the proper, safe disposal of such equipment after use.

● Dosage

Pediatric Patients

Growth Hormone Deficiency Due to Inadequate Endogenous Growth Hormone

Somatropin dosage is weight-based and expressed in weekly dosages that should be divided and administered in equal doses. The weekly dosage should be divided and administered daily 3 to 7 times a week;

The Pediatric Endocrine Society guideline recommends an initial somatropin dosage of 0.16–0.24 mg/kg per week for the management of GHD due to inadequate endogenous growth hormone in children; subsequent dosing should be individualized. Dosages as high as 0.3 mg/kg per week or up to 0.7 mg/kg per week in pubertal patients may be found in the FDA-approved labeling of some preparations.

The Pediatric Endocrine Society guideline recommends using the lowest effective dosage of somatropin based on growth response, but makes no recommendation for insulin-like growth factor-1 (IGF-1)-based dosing, other than suggesting dosage reduction if age- and gender-based levels are exceeded, due to insufficient data in pediatric patients.

Once epiphyseal fusion has occurred, discontinue somatropin for stimulation of linear growth.

Turner Syndrome

For the management of pediatric patients with short stature associated with Turner syndrome, a weekly somatropin dosage up to 0.375 mg/kg per week is commonly recommended; lower (0.33 mg/kg per week) and higher (0.47 mg/kg per week) weekly dosages are also found in the FDA approved labeling of some preparations. The weekly dosage should be divided and administered as daily subcutaneous injections 3–7 times a week.

Idiopathic Short Stature

For the management of idiopathic short stature (ISS) in pediatric patients, the Pediatric Endocrine Society guideline recommends an initial somatropin dosage of 0.24 mg/kg per week divided and administered daily; some patients may require up to 0.47 mg/kg per week, however, there are no data to support doses greater than 0.47 mg/kg per week.

Weekly dosages up to 0.3 mg/kg, 0.37 mg/kg, or 0.47 mg/kg are recommended in the FDA approved labeling of somatropin preparations indicated for use in patients with ISS; most manufacturers recommended dividing the weekly dosage into 6 or 7 daily subcutaneous injections; the manufacturer of Zomacton® states to divide the weekly dosage into equal doses given either 3, 6, or 7 days per week.

Once epiphyseal fusion has occurred, discontinue somatropin for stimulation of linear growth.

Short Stature Homeobox-containing Gene (SHOX) Deficiency

For the management of short stature or growth failure in short stature homeobox-containing gene (SHOX) deficiency in pediatric patients, the usual somatropin dosage is 0.35 mg/kg per week divided and administered in equal doses given over 3, 6 or 7 daily subcutaneous doses per week.

Once epiphyseal fusion has occurred, discontinue somatropin for stimulation of linear growth.

Small for Gestational Age

For the management of short stature born small for gestational age (SGA), the recommended somatropin dosage is up to 0.47 or 0.48 mg/kg per week divided and administered in equal doses given 3, 6, or 7 days a week.

In patients <4 years of age with baseline height standard deviation score (SDS) values between -2 and -3, consider initiating therapy with a lower initial dosage; titrate dosage as needed.

Consider a gradual reduction in dosage if substantial catch-up growth is observed during the first few years of therapy.

Once epiphyseal fusion has occurred, discontinue somatropin for stimulation of linear growth.

Noonan Syndrome

For the management of short stature associated with Noonan syndrome, the recommended somatropin dosage is up to 0.46 mg/kg per week divided and administered in equal doses given 6 or 7 days a week.

Once epiphyseal fusion has occurred, discontinue somatropin for stimulation of linear growth.

Prader-Willi Syndrome

For the management of growth failure due to Prader-Willi syndrome, the recommended somatropin dosage is 0.24 mg/kg per week divided and administered in equal doses given 6 or 7 days a week.

Once epiphyseal fusion has occurred, discontinue somatropin for stimulation of linear growth.

Growth Failure Secondary to Chronic Kidney Disease

For the management of growth failure secondary to chronic kidney disease (CKD), a weekly somatropin dosage up to 0.35 mg/kg is recommended; the weekly dosage should be divided and administered in equal daily doses.

In order to optimize therapy for patients who require dialysis, the following guidelines for injection schedule are recommended:

Hemodialysis Patients: Administer injection at night just prior to going to sleep or at least 3–4 hours after hemodialysis to prevent hematoma formation due to heparin.

Chronic Cycling Peritoneal Dialysis (CCPD) Patients: Administer injection in the morning after dialysis completion.

Chronic Ambulatory Peritoneal Dialysis (CAPD) Patients: Administer injection in the evening at the time of the overnight exchange.

Adults

Growth Hormone Deficiency

Somatropin dosing for the management of GHD in adults (childhood- or adult-onset) may be non-weight-based or weight-based. Individualize dosage of growth hormone treatment based on age, gender, body mass index (BMI), and various other characteristics to improve effectiveness and reduce adverse effects of therapy.

Non-weight-based dosing: the American Association of Clinical Endocrinologists (AACE)/American College of Endocrinology (ACE) and Endocrine Society guidelines recommend individualized, non-weight-based dosing, starting with a dose that is appropriate for age and comorbid condition (e.g., obesity, diabetes mellitus), and then titrating according to clinical response, adverse effects, and age- and gender-adjusted serum IGF-1 levels. The initial recommended non-weight-based somatropin dosage is 0.2 mg/day (range 0.15 mg/day to 0.3 mg/day). The AACE/ACE and Endocrine Society guidelines recommend an initial dosage of 0.4–0.5 mg/day for patients <30 years of age, 0.2–0.3 mg/day for patients between 30 and 60 years of age, and 0.1–0.2 mg/day for those >60 years of age, or with concurrent diabetes mellitus, previous gestational diabetes, or obesity; younger patients and females taking oral estrogen replacement therapy may require higher doses. Increase the dosage by increments of approximately 0.1–0.2 mg/day every 1–2 months based on clinical response, adverse effects, and IGF-1 levels; consider smaller dose increment increases, and/or longer time intervals, for geriatric patients.

Weight-based dosing: Initial recommended weight-based somatropin dosage range is 0.004–0.006 mg/kg per day; weight-based dosing is not recommended in obese patients because they are more likely to experience adverse reactions. Titrate the dose according to individual patient requirements at 4–8 week intervals to a maximum dosage range of 0.01–0.016 mg/kg per day; in patients receiving Nutropin AQ®, the manufacturer states that the maximum dosage is 0.025 mg/kg per day in patients ≤35 years of age and 0.0125 mg/kg per day in patients >35 years of age.

In patients transitioning from pediatric to adult treatment, after epiphyseal closure and re-evaluation of need for treatment continuation, the AACE/ACE guideline recommends somatropin resumption at 50% of the dosage used in childhood.

Maintenance dosages are expected to vary among patients, and between male and female patients.

Titration should be based on clinical response, adverse effects, and IGF-1 levels.

HIV-associated Wasting or Cachexia

For the management of HIV-associated wasting or cachexia in adults, the recommended starting dosage of somatropin (Serostim®) is 0.1 mg/kg once daily (up to a total dose of 6 mg) at bedtime as described in Table 1.

TABLE 1. Weight-based Somatropin (Serostim®) Dosage for HIV-associated Wasting or Cachexia

Weight (kg)	Subcutaneous Dosage
>55	6 mg daily
45–55	5 mg daily
35–45	4 mg daily
<35	0.1 mg/kg daily

In patients at increased risk for growth hormone-induced adverse effects (e.g., glucose intolerance), consider initiating treatment with 0.1 mg/kg every other day. For those experiencing adverse effects potentially related to growth hormone, consider reducing the total daily somatropin dose or the number of somatropin doses administered per week.

In clinical studies, most of the effect of somatropin on work output and lean body mass was apparent after 12 weeks of treatment, and the effect was maintained during an additional 12 weeks of therapy. There are no safety or efficacy data available from controlled studies in which patients were treated with somatropin continuously for more than 48 weeks. There are also no data on patients with HIV wasting or cachexia receiving intermittent treatment with somatropin.

Short Bowel Syndrome

For the management of short bowel syndrome in adults receiving specialized nutritional support, the recommended somatropin (Zorbtive®) dosage is 0.1 mg/kg once daily to a maximum dosage of 8 mg once daily for 4 weeks.

Dosage adjustment for fluid retention and arthralgia/carpal tunnel syndrome (moderate toxicity): Treat symptomatically with analgesics or reduce the somatropin dosage to 0.05 mg/kg (maximum total dose of 4 mg) once daily. For patients experiencing severe toxicity, discontinue somatropin for up to 5 days; upon symptom resolution, resume at a dosage of 0.05 mg/kg (maximum total dose of 4 mg) once daily. Permanently discontinue therapy if severe toxicity recurs or does not disappear within 5 days.

● Special Populations

Hepatic Impairment

The manufacturer makes no specific dosage recommendations for patients with hepatic impairment.

Renal Impairment

The manufacturer makes no specific dosage recommendations for patients with renal impairment.

Geriatric Patients

Elderly patients may be more sensitive to somatropin and may be more prone to develop adverse reactions; lower initial doses and smaller dose adjustment increments are recommended.

CAUTIONS

● Contraindications

- Acute critical illness after open heart surgery, abdominal surgery, or multiple accidental trauma, or acute respiratory failure.

- Hypersensitivity to somatropin or any of the excipients.
- Active malignancy.
- Active proliferative or severe non-proliferative diabetic retinopathy.
- Pediatric patients with closed epiphyses.
- Pediatric patients with Prader-Willi syndrome who are severely obese, have a history of upper airway obstruction or sleep apnea or have severe respiratory impairment, due to the risk of sudden death.

● Warnings/Precautions

Increased Mortality in Patients with Acute Critical Illness

Increased mortality has been reported in patients continuing pharmacologic somatropin doses while experiencing acute critical illness following open heart surgery, abdominal surgery, or multiple accidental trauma, or those with acute respiratory failure. In non-growth hormone deficient adults requiring intensive care in one study, mortality rate was 42% in the somatropin group (doses of 5.3–8.0 mg/day) versus 19% in the placebo group. The safety of continuing growth hormone replacement dosages of somatropin in growth hormone deficient patients experiencing concurrent acute critical illness has not been established. In non-growth hormone deficient adults, weigh potential risks against the potential benefit of somatropin continuation in patients experiencing concurrent acute critical illnesses.

The manufacturer of some somatropin preparations (e.g., Zorbtive®) recommends discontinuing the drug in patients with acute critical illness.

Sudden Death in Pediatric Patients with Prader-Willi Syndrome

Sudden death after somatropin initiation has been reported in pediatric patients with Prader-Willi syndrome who had at least one of the following risk factors: severe obesity, history of upper airway obstruction or sleep apnea, or unidentified respiratory infection. Male patients with one or more of these factors may be at greater risk.

Before initiating somatropin therapy, evaluate patients with Prader-Willi syndrome for signs of upper airway obstruction and sleep apnea. If the patient shows signs of upper airway obstruction (including onset of, or increased, snoring) and/or new onset sleep apnea during treatment, somatropin treatment should be interrupted. Monitor all patients with Prader-Willi syndrome for signs of respiratory infection, which should be diagnosed as early as possible and treated aggressively.

Patients with Prader-Willi syndrome who are treated with somatropin should have effective weight control.

Increased Risk of Neoplasms – Active Malignancy

Due to the increased risk of malignancy progression with somatropin in patients with active malignancy, treatment of any malignancies should be completed and any preexisting malignancy should be inactive before initiating the drug. If malignancy recurs during somatropin therapy, the drug should be discontinued.

The American Association of Clinical Endocrinologists (AACE)/American College of Endocrinology (ACE) and Growth Hormone Research Society guidelines suggest that low-dose growth hormone therapy should be considered only after achieving 5 years of cancer remission; however, treatment should be individualized based on clinical status and tumor type.

For children and adolescents with acquired growth hormone deficiency (GHD) due to effects of a primary malignancy, the Pediatric Endocrine Society guidelines recommend a 12-month waiting period before initiating growth hormone treatment following completion of tumor therapy with no evidence of ongoing tumor.

Discontinue somatropin if malignancy recurs.

Increased Risk of Neoplasms – Risk of Second Neoplasm in Pediatric Patients

An increased risk of a second neoplasm has been reported in pediatric cancer survivors with acquired GHD who were treated with somatropin following radiation to the brain/head for their first neoplasm; intracranial tumors, in particular meningiomas, were the most common of these second neoplasms.

In adults, it is unknown whether there is any relationship between somatropin replacement therapy and CNS tumor recurrence.

Monitor all patients with a history of GHD secondary to intracranial neoplasm for progression or recurrence of the tumor.

Increased Risk of Neoplasms – New Malignancy during Treatment

Consider the risks and benefits of starting somatropin in children with certain rare genetic causes of short stature that are associated with an intrinsically increased risk of developing malignancies (e.g., Noonan syndrome) and monitor these patients carefully for neoplasm development; some experts recommend counseling patients and/or caregivers regarding the lack of evidence in this population for a growth hormone effect on malignancy risk.

The manufacturer of Serostim® states to consider the risks and benefits of starting somatropin because malignancies are more common in HIV-positive patients.

In the observational KIMS (Pfizer International Metabolic Database) cohort of adult and adolescent GHD patients treated with growth hormone, of the 14,533 patients (mean follow-up 5.3 years) who did not have a prior history of cancer, 471 (3.2%) were diagnosed with cancer during the study; nonmelanoma and melanoma skin cancers were diagnosed in 57 (0.39%) and 25 (0.17%) patients, respectively.

An increase in size or number of cutaneous nevi has been reported in patients receiving somatropin; monitor patients carefully for increased growth, or potential malignant changes, of preexisting nevi. Advise all patients to report marked changes in behavior, onset of headaches, vision disturbances and/or changes in skin pigmentation.

Some experts recommend that standard cancer screening and long-term monitoring be performed in adults receiving growth hormone replacement therapy.

Glucose Intolerance and Diabetes Mellitus

Somatropin may decrease insulin sensitivity, particularly at higher doses, and/or unmask previously undiagnosed pre-diabetes, impaired glucose tolerance, or overt type 2 diabetes mellitus (DM).

New onset type 2 DM, new onset impaired glucose intolerance, and exacerbation of preexisting DM have been reported in patients taking somatropin. Some patients developed diabetic ketoacidosis and diabetic coma; clinical improvement occurred in some cases following drug discontinuance.

Monitor glucose levels periodically in all patients, especially in those with risk factors for type 2 DM (e.g., obesity, family history, Turner syndrome). Monitor patients with preexisting type 1 DM, type 2 DM, pre-diabetes, or impaired glucose tolerance closely and adjust antihyperglycemic drugs and/or doses as needed following somatropin initiation. The Pediatric Endocrine Society guideline suggests that monitoring for potential development of DM with blood glucose testing and/or hemoglobin A1c levels should be focused on growth hormone recipients at high risk. To avoid impairment of glucose metabolism, the AACE/ACE guideline suggests initiating daily growth hormone at lower starting dosages in adult patients with concurrent DM, obesity, older age, and previous gestational DM.

In patients with wasting or cachexia due to HIV infection, mean fasting blood glucose concentrations increased approximately 10 mg/dL and 6 mg/dL in those treated with somatropin (Serostim®) 0.1 mg/kg daily and every other day, respectively; increases occurred early in treatment. Antihyperglycemic drug initiation or dosage adjustment may be required. Closely monitor patients with risk factors for glucose intolerance, other than wasting/cachexia. Dose-dependent glucose intolerance and related adverse reactions were observed in an unapproved population of patients with HIV-associated lipodystrophy receiving Serostim® dosages of 4 mg daily or every other day.

Intracranial Hypertension

Intracranial hypertension with papilledema, visual changes, headache, nausea, and/or vomiting have been reported in patients treated with somatropin. A higher rate is observed in patients with chronic renal insufficiency, Turner syndrome, Prader-Willi syndrome, and organic GHD. Symptoms usually occur within 8 weeks after somatropin initiation, or dosage increases, and resolve rapidly after cessation of therapy or a dosage reduction.

To exclude preexisting papilledema, perform fundoscopic examination before initiating somatropin; reassess periodically thereafter.

If symptoms of intracranial hypertension (e.g., visual changes, headache, nausea and/or vomiting) occur, perform fundoscopic examination and stop treatment if papilledema is observed. If growth hormone-induced intracranial hypertension is confirmed, treatment may be resumed at a lower dosage after associated signs and symptoms have resolved.

Although no cases of intracranial hypertension have been observed among patients with short bowel syndrome treated with somatropin (Zorbtive®) to date, if papilledema is observed by fundoscopy, the manufacturer states to discontinue treatment.

Hypersensitivity Reactions

Post-marketing cases of serious hypersensitivity reactions, including anaphylactic reactions and angioedema, have been reported with the use of somatropin preparations.

Advise patients and caregivers of the potential for these reactions and to seek prompt medical attention if they occur.

Do not use somatropin in patients with known hypersensitivity to the drug or any of the excipients, including those with hypersensitivity to diluent excipients (e.g., metacresol, glycerin).

Fluid Retention/Carpal Tunnel Syndrome/Arthralgia

Fluid retention during somatropin therapy may occur frequently. Clinical manifestations (e.g., edema, arthralgia, myalgia, nerve compression syndromes including carpal tunnel syndrome/paresthesia) are usually transient, dose-dependent, and may occur more frequently with weight-based somatropin dosing regimens in obese or older adult patients with GHD.

In an observational cohort of adult and adolescent patients with GHD who were treated with growth hormone, all-cause edema and treatment-related peripheral edema were reported in 3.9% and 3.1% of patients, respectively.

Such effects may resolve spontaneously or resolve following treatment with analgesics, or after reducing the frequency of dosing.

Carpal tunnel syndrome may occur because of increased tissue turgor in the hands. In the trial comparing somatropin with placebo in patients with HIV-associated wasting, carpal tunnel syndrome occurred in 1.9–4.7% of patients who received the drug compared with none of the patients who received placebo. In patients treated with somatropin for short bowel syndrome, peripheral edema and arthralgia were common, but few patients developed carpal tunnel syndrome.

If symptoms of carpal tunnel syndrome do not resolve by decreasing the dosage of somatropin, treatment discontinuance is recommended by some manufacturers.

Hypoadrenalism

Patients receiving somatropin therapy with or at risk for pituitary hormone deficiency may have an increased risk of reduced serum cortisol levels and/or unmasking of central (secondary) hypoadrenalism.

Patients treated with glucocorticoid replacement for previously diagnosed hypoadrenalism may require an increase in their maintenance or stress doses following somatropin initiation.

Monitor patients for reduced serum cortisol levels and/or need for glucocorticoid dose increases in patients with known hypoadrenalism.

The Pediatric Endocrine Society guideline strongly recommends re-assessment of the adrenal axis after initiation of growth hormone therapy in pediatric patients whose cause of GHD is associated with possible multiple pituitary hormone deficiencies.

Hypothyroidism

Undiagnosed or untreated hypothyroidism may prevent optimal response to somatropin (e.g., growth response in children); patients with Turner syndrome have an increased risk of autoimmune thyroid disease and primary hypothyroidism.

Growth hormone increases extrathyroidal conversion of T4 to T3, decreasing T4 levels resulting in the potential to unmask central hypothyroidism in hypopituitary patients. In patients with GHD, central (secondary) hypothyroidism may first become evident or worsen during somatropin treatment; perform periodic thyroid function tests and initiate or appropriately adjust thyroid hormone replacement therapy when indicated. The Pediatric Endocrine Society guideline strongly recommends re-assessment of the thyroid axis after initiation of growth hormone therapy in pediatric patients whose cause of GHD is associated with possible multiple pituitary hormone deficiencies.

The manufacturer of Zorbtive® states that in patients with suspected and/or diagnosed hypopituitarism, evaluate thyroid function before initiation and following 4 weeks of somatropin treatment for short bowel syndrome; correct thyroid function when indicated.

Slipped Capital Femoral Epiphysis in Pediatric Patients

Slipped capital femoral epiphysis may occur more frequently in pediatric patients undergoing rapid growth or in those with endocrine disorders (e.g., GHD, Turner syndrome). Evaluate pediatric patients at the onset of a limp or complaints of persistent hip or knee pain.

The Pediatric Endocrine Society strongly recommends performing a physical examination at each follow-up visit to monitor for slipped capital femoral epiphysis in patients with GHD receiving somatropin.

Progression of Preexisting Scoliosis in Pediatric Patients

Progression of existing scoliosis can occur in patients who experience rapid growth. Scoliosis with or without other skeletal abnormalities are commonly seen in patients with untreated Turner syndrome or Prader-Willi syndrome. Somatropin has not been shown to increase the occurrence of scoliosis.

Monitor pediatric patients with a history of scoliosis for disease progression; the Pediatric Endocrine Society strongly recommends performing a physical examination at each follow-up visit to monitor for scoliosis progression in patients with GHD receiving somatropin.

Pancreatitis

Pancreatitis has been reported in pediatric patients and adults receiving somatropin; the risk is potentially greater in pediatric patients. Girls who have Turner syndrome may be at greater risk than other somatropin-treated patients.

Consider the possibility of pancreatitis in patients who develop persistent severe abdominal pain.

Lipoatrophy

When somatropin is administered subcutaneously at the same site over a prolonged time period, lipoatrophy may result; rotate injection sites to reduce this risk.

Cardiovascular Disorders in Patients with Turner Syndrome

Patients with Turner syndrome should be monitored closely for the occurrence of cardiovascular disorders (e.g., hypertension, aortic aneurysm or dissection, stroke) as these patients are at increased risk.

Otitis Media in Patients with Turner Syndrome

Patients with Turner syndrome should be evaluated carefully for otitis media and other ear disorders, as these patients have an increased risk of ear and hearing disorders; somatropin treatment may increase the occurrence of otitis media in patients with Turner syndrome.

Osteodystrophy in Pediatric Patients with Chronic Kidney Disease

Children with growth failure secondary to chronic kidney disease (CKD) should be examined periodically for evidence of progression of renal osteodystrophy.

Slipped capital femoral epiphysis or avascular necrosis of the femoral head may be seen in children with advanced renal osteodystrophy; it is uncertain whether these conditions are affected by somatropin therapy.

Obtain hip X-rays prior to initiating somatropin in patients with CKD; physicians and parents should monitor patients for the development of a limp or complaints of hip or knee pain.

Benzyl Alcohol

Benzyl alcohol may be a component of some somatropin preparations or the diluent used for reconstitution.

Benzyl alcohol has been associated with serious adverse events and death; "gasping syndrome," (characterized by CNS depression, metabolic acidosis, gasping respirations, and high levels of benzyl alcohol and its metabolites found in the blood and urine) has been associated with dosages >99 mg/kg per day in neonates and low-birth weight neonates. Additional symptoms may include gradual neurological deterioration, seizures, intracranial hemorrhage, hematologic abnormalities, skin breakdown, hepatic and renal failure, hypotension, bradycardia, and cardiovascular collapse. The combined daily metabolic load of benzyl alcohol from all sources should be considered.

To decrease benzyl alcohol exposure in high-risk patients, consult somatropin preparation-specific labeling to find a benzyl alcohol-free product or alternative diluents for reconstitution.

Confirmation of Childhood-Onset Adult Growth Hormone Deficiency

Patients with epiphyseal closure who were treated with somatropin in childhood should be re-evaluated.

Except for adults with multiple other pituitary hormone deficiencies due to organic disease or patients with congenital/genetic GHD, appropriate growth hormone provocative testing is required to confirm the diagnosis of adult GHD.

Laboratory Tests

Serum levels of inorganic phosphorus, alkaline phosphatase, parathyroid hormone, and IGF-1 may increase after somatropin treatment; monitor patients as appropriate if any abnormalities occur.

Concomitant Antiretroviral Therapy in Patients Receiving Serostim® for HIV-associated Wasting or Cachexia

Somatropin has been shown to potentiate HIV replication in vitro at concentrations ranging from 50–250 ng/mL. When antiretroviral agents (zidovudine, didanosine, or lamivudine) were added to the culture medium, there was no increase in virus production.

No significant somatropin-associated increase in viral burden was observed in controlled clinical trials of patients on concomitant antiretroviral therapy. Patients with HIV should be maintained on antiretroviral therapy for the duration of somatropin (Serostim®) treatment.

Immunogenicity

There is a potential for the development of immunogenicity to somatropin. Antibodies with binding capacities <2 mg/L have not been associated with growth attenuation; in small numbers of patients treated with somatropin, interference with growth response was observed when binding capacity was >2 mg/L.

The number of somatropin-treated patients who develop specific antibodies has been reported by a variety of trials. These trials have been conducted on naïve and treatment-experienced patients with a range of short stature conditions (e.g., GHD, CKD, Turner syndrome, idiopathic short stature, small for gestational age [SGA]). In one trial, 1.6% of treatment-naïve patients developed specific antibodies to somatropin after 6 months of treatment with the drug; another trial reported an antibody development rate of 24% in patients with SGA-associated short stature.

The effects of antibodies on adverse effects of somatropin (Nutropin AQ®) were evaluated in a population of pediatric patients with CKD. No adverse effects were noted in this study.

After 12 weeks of treatment with somatropin (Serostim®), none of the 651 treatment-naïve patients with HIV-associated wasting developed detectable antibodies to growth hormone (>4 pg binding). Patients were not rechallenged, and data beyond 3 months are not available.

Specific Populations

Pregnancy

Available data with somatropin use in pregnant women are insufficient to determine a drug-associated risk of adverse developmental outcomes or any impact on reproductive capacity.

The American Association of Clinical Endocrinologists (AACE)/American College of Endocrinology (ACE) and Endocrine Society guidelines state that due to insufficient evidence of safety or efficacy, routine use of somatropin for conception or continued use during pregnancy in women with GHD is not recommended.

Benzyl alcohol is rapidly metabolized in pregnancy; therefore, exposure to the fetus is unlikely. Intravenously administered drugs containing benzyl alcohol have caused adverse reactions in premature neonates and low birth weight infants. To avoid fetal exposure to benzyl alcohol in women continuing somatropin during pregnancy, consult the preparation-specific labeling to find a benzyl alcohol-free product or alternative diluents.

Animal reproduction studies were conducted with various somatropin preparations at doses in excess of normal human doses (e.g., 1 mg/kg per day, 3.3 mg/kg per day), resulting in growth hormone blood levels in excess of human therapeutic levels (e.g., 19 and 24 times higher, respectively), and administered at different time frames corresponding to the periods of organogenesis or gametogenesis. No adverse effects were observed on gestation, morphogenesis, parturition, lactation, postnatal development, or reproductive capacity of the offspring.

Lactation

There is no information regarding the presence of somatropin in human milk; limited data indicate that exogenous somatropin does not increase normal breast-milk concentrations of growth hormone, and no adverse effects on the breastfed infant have been reported with somatropin.

Consider the benefits of breast-feeding and the importance of somatropin to the woman along with the potential adverse effects on the breast-fed infant from the drug or underlying maternal condition.

Benzyl alcohol is rapidly metabolized in lactating women; therefore, exposure in the breast-fed infant is unlikely. Intravenously administered drugs containing benzyl alcohol have caused adverse reactions in premature neonates and low birth weight infants.

To avoid infant exposure to benzyl alcohol from women continuing somatropin while breast-feeding, consult the preparation-specific labeling to find a benzyl alcohol-free product or alternative diluents.

Pediatric Use

Safety and efficacy of somatropin for the management of children with growth failure due to inadequate secretion of endogenous growth hormone are supported by 3 open-label, multicenter trials conducted over a duration of 2 years (2 trials) and 8 years (1 trial).

Safety and efficacy of somatropin for the management of children with short stature associated with Turner syndrome are supported by one long-term, randomized, dose-response study and 3 long-term, open-label, multicenter studies with concurrent or historical controls.

Safety and efficacy of somatropin for the management of children with idiopathic short stature are supported by one dose-response study, one placebo-controlled study, and 3 randomized studies.

Safety and efficacy of somatropin for the management of children with short stature or growth failure in SHOX deficiency are supported by a single randomized, controlled, 2-year, 3-arm, open-label study in 52 patients.

Safety and efficacy of somatropin for the management of short stature in children born small for gestational age with no catch-up growth by 2 to 4 years of age are supported by 4 clinical studies. One study was a randomized, double-blind, 2-arm study and another was a randomized study of prepubertal, non-GHD, Japanese pediatric patients.

Safety and efficacy of somatropin for the management of short stature associated with Noonan syndrome are supported by a prospective, open-label, randomized, parallel group, 2-year study in 21 pediatric patients.

Safety and efficacy of somatropin for the management of growth failure due to Prader-Willi syndrome are supported by 2 randomized, open label, controlled clinical trials. Sudden death after somatropin initiation has been reported in pediatric patients with Prader-Willi syndrome who had at least one of the following risk factors: severe obesity, history of upper airway obstruction or sleep apnea, or unidentified respiratory infection.

Safety and efficacy of somatropin in pediatric patients with HIV have not been established. Treatment appeared to be well tolerated and consistent with safety observations of adults treated with somatropin for HIV-associated wasting in 2 small studies of 11 children with HIV-associated failure to thrive who received somatropin 0.04 mg/kg per day for 26 weeks or somatropin 0.07 mg/kg per day for 4 weeks.

Safety and efficacy of somatropin in pediatric patients with short bowel syndrome have not been established.

Risks of growth hormone therapy specific to pediatric patients include risk of sudden death in pediatric patients with Prader-Willi syndrome, increased risk of second neoplasm in pediatric cancer survivors treated with radiation to the brain and/or head, intracranial hypertension, slipped capital femoral epiphysis, progression of preexisting scoliosis, and pancreatitis.

Benzyl alcohol may be a component of somatropin products or the diluent used for reconstitution. Benzyl alcohol has been associated with serious adverse events and death; "gasping syndrome," (characterized by CNS depression, metabolic acidosis, gasping respirations, and high levels of benzyl alcohol and its metabolites found in the blood and urine) has been associated with dosages >99 mg/kg per day in neonates and low-birth weight neonates. Additional symptoms may include gradual neurological deterioration, seizures, intracranial hemorrhage, hematologic abnormalities, skin breakdown, hepatic and renal failure, hypotension, bradycardia, and cardiovascular collapse. The combined daily metabolic load of benzyl alcohol from all sources should be considered. To decrease benzyl alcohol exposure in high-risk patients, consult the preparation-specific labeling to find a benzyl alcohol-free product or alternative diluents.

Geriatric Use

Experience in patients ≥65 years of age is insufficient to determine whether they respond differently to somatropin than younger patients.

Elderly patients may be more sensitive to somatropin, may be more prone to develop adverse reactions, and lower initial doses with smaller dosage adjustment increments are recommended.

Hepatic Impairment

Patients with hepatic dysfunction exhibit decreased somatropin clearance compared to those with normal hepatic function; the clinical significance of this is unknown.

Renal Impairment

Chronic kidney disease or end-stage renal disease in pediatric and adult patients is associated with decreased somatropin clearance compared to those with normal renal function; the clinical significance of this is unknown.

● Common Adverse Effects

Common adverse reactions reported in adult and pediatric patients receiving somatropin include upper respiratory infection, fever, pharyngitis, headache, injection site reactions (such as pain, numbness, redness, and swelling), rashes, lipoatrophy, otitis media, edema, flatulence, abdominal pain, arthralgia, carpal tunnel syndrome, paresthesia, myalgia, peripheral edema, flu syndrome, and impaired glucose tolerance.

DRUG INTERACTIONS

Somatropin is not known to be metabolized by cytochrome P-450 (CYP) isoenzymes or other drug metabolizing enzymes, however growth hormone can induce changes in CYP activity.

● Drugs Affecting or Affected by Hepatic Microsomal Enzymes

Growth hormone has been shown to increase CYP-mediated antipyrine clearance and, therefore, may alter the clearance of drugs (e.g., anticonvulsants, corticosteroids, cyclosporine, sex hormones) known to be metabolized by CYP isoenzymes.

Careful monitoring is recommended if somatropin is used concomitantly with drugs metabolized by CYP isoenzymes.

Due to the lack of formal drug interaction studies, no data are available on drug interactions between somatropin and HIV protease inhibitors or the non-nucleoside reverse transcriptase inhibitors.

● Glucocorticoid Replacement Therapy

Growth hormone is a known inhibitor of 11β-hydroxysteroid dehydrogenase type 1, the microsomal enzyme required for conversion of cortisone to its active metabolite, cortisol.

Following initiation of somatropin, patients treated with glucocorticoid replacement therapy (particularly with cortisone acetate or prednisone) for established hypoadrenalism may require an increase in maintenance glucocorticoid dosage or supplemental stress-related glucocorticoid doses.

● Pharmacologic Glucocorticoid Therapy and Supraphysiologic Glucocorticoid Treatment in Pediatric Patients

Pharmacologic glucocorticoid therapy and supraphysiologic glucocorticoid treatment may attenuate the growth-promoting effects of somatropin in pediatric patients.

Carefully adjust glucocorticoid dosing in pediatric patients, including those with chronic kidney disease, to avoid both hypoadrenalism and an inhibitory effect on growth.

● Oral Estrogen

Oral estrogen may reduce the serum insulin-like growth factor-1 (IGF-1) response to somatropin and higher somatropin dosages may be required in those receiving oral estrogen replacement.

● Insulin and/or Other Antihyperglycemic Agents

Treatment with somatropin may decrease insulin sensitivity, particularly at higher doses; insulin and/or other antihyperglycemic agent dosage adjustments may be required for patients with diabetes mellitus.

DESCRIPTION

Somatropin (recombinant) is a human growth hormone (hGH) prepared using recombinant DNA technology, with an amino acid sequence identical to that of human growth hormone of pituitary origin.

Somatropin binds to the hGH receptor in the cell membrane of target cells resulting in a cascade of direct and indirect pharmacodynamic effects including normalization of insulin-like growth factor-1 (IGF-1) concentrations, stimulation of chondrocyte differentiation and proliferation, stimulation of hepatic glucose output, protein synthesis, and lipolysis.

Growth hormone and IGF-1 receptors are found in intestinal mucosa; the transmucosal transport of water, electrolytes, and nutrients is enhanced by growth hormone administration.

The stimulation of skeletal growth increases linear growth rate (height velocity) in most somatropin-treated pediatric patients (e.g., growth hormone deficiency [GHD], Turner syndrome, small for gestational age, idiopathic short stature, chronic kidney disease [CKD], Prader-Willi syndrome). In adults with GHD, somatropin treatment results in reduced fat mass, increased lean body mass, metabolic alterations that include beneficial changes in lipid metabolism, reduction in body fat stores, and normalization of IGF-1 concentrations. In adults with HIV-associated wasting or cachexia, somatropin treatment results in improved nitrogen balance and increased protein-sparing lipid oxidation; decreased trunk fat, decreased total body fat, and increased lean body mass were observed in these patients.

The absolute bioavailability of somatropin after subcutaneous injection ranges between 70-90%. Somatropin undergoes protein catabolism in both the liver and kidneys; extensive metabolism studies have not been conducted. In pharmacokinetic studies of various somatropin preparations in various patient populations (e.g., adult GHD, HIV-associated wasting) or healthy volunteers, the half-life of subcutaneously administered somatropin ranged from 2 to 10 hours; the median reported half-life was 3 hours. Limited published pharmacokinetic data do not suggest differences in somatropin plasma clearance and average steady-state plasma concentrations between young and elderly patients. Available published literature suggests that somatropin clearance is similar in adults and pediatric patients; no pharmacokinetic studies have been conducted in pediatric patients with short bowel syndrome or those with HIV. Available literature suggests somatropin clearance may be similar or higher in males, however sex-based analysis is not available in normal volunteers, patients infected with HIV, or patients with short bowel syndrome. Decreased somatropin clearance has been observed in children and adults with CKD and end-stage renal disease (ESRD); in a study of 6 pediatric patients (7–11 years of age) somatropin clearance was reduced 22.6% after subcutaneous injection compared to normal healthy adults. Somatropin accumulation has not been reported at this time in children with CKD or ESRD dosed with current regimens. Reduced somatropin clearance has been noted in patients with severe liver dysfunction; the clinical significance of this is unknown. Somatropin clearance and mean terminal half-life in healthy adults and children are similar to patients with GHD.

ADVICE TO PATIENTS

● Advise patients and caregivers to refer to the instructions for use that accompanies the somatropin preparation, including device specific instructions. Consult the manufacturer or specialty pharmacy customer support services for assistance or additional training, if needed.

● Advise patients and caregivers of proper needle disposal, caution against any reuse of needles, sharing of devices and/or needles, and disposal of used cartridges and needles in an appropriate container.

● Advise childhood cancer survivors and caregivers of the increased risk of secondary neoplasms and to immediately report marked changes in behavior, onset of headaches, vision disturbances, and/or changes in skin pigmentation or changes in the appearance of preexisting nevi.

● Advise patients and caregivers that impaired glucose intolerance, type 2 diabetes mellitus, or exacerbation of preexisting diabetes mellitus can occur and to monitor blood glucose.

● Advise patients and caregivers that somatropin can cause intracranial hypertension and to immediately report any visual changes, headache, and nausea and/or vomiting to their healthcare provider.

● Advise patients and caregivers that fluid retention may occur and to contact their healthcare provider if symptoms (e.g., edema, arthralgia, myalgia, nerve compression syndromes including carpal tunnel syndrome/paresthesia) occur.

● Advise patients and caregivers that hypoadrenalism may develop in those at risk and to report hyperpigmentation, extreme fatigue, dizziness, weakness, or weight loss to their healthcare provider.

● Advise patients and caregivers that periodic thyroid function tests may be required in those at risk.

● Advise patients and caregivers that pancreatitis may develop and to report any new onset abdominal pain to their healthcare provider.

● Advise patients and caregivers that hypersensitivity reactions (anaphylaxis and angioedema) are possible, and to seek prompt medical attention if an allergic reaction occurs.

● Advise caregivers to report the development of a limp or complaints of hip or knee pain in somatropin-treated children with chronic kidney disease.

● Advise patients and caregivers to rotate injection sites to decrease the risk of lipoatrophy; do not inject into skin that is tender, bruised, red, or hard.

● Advise patients to inform their clinicians of existing or contemplated concomitant therapy, including prescription and OTC drugs and dietary or herbal supplements, as well as any concomitant illnesses.

● Advise women to inform their clinicians if they are or plan to become pregnant or plan to breast-feed.

● Inform patients of other important precautionary information.

PREPARATIONS

Human growth hormone is not subject to control under the Federal Controlled Substances Act of 1970; however, distribution and possession for use other than recognized indications is criminalized.

Excipients in commercially available drug preparations may have clinically important effects in some individuals; consult specific product labeling for details.

Somatropin

Parenteral

For injection, for subcutaneous use	0.2 mg, 0.4 mg, 0.6 mg, 0.8 mg, 1 mg, 1.2 mg, 1.4 mg, 1.6 mg, 1.8 mg, and 2 mg	**Genotropin Miniquick®** (supplied as a single-use syringe device with cartridge and diluent), Pfizer
	4 mg, 5 mg, and 6 mg	**Serostim®** (supplied as single-dose or multi-dose vials), EMD Serono
	5 mg and 12 mg	**Genotropin®** (supplied in a cartridge with diluent, for use with Genotropin Pen®), Pfizer
	5 mg, 6 mg, 12 mg, and 24 mg	**Humatrope®** (5-mg strength is available in a vial with separate diluent vial; 6, 12, and 24 mg strengths are available as a cartridge with prefilled diluent syringe), Eli Lilly
	5 mg and 8.8 mg	**Saizen®** (8.8 mg strength also available with the Saizenprep® reconstitution device), EMD Serono
	5 mg and 10 mg	**Zomacton®** (supplied with diluent), Ferring
	5.8 mg	**Omnitrope®** (supplied with diluent), Sandoz
	8.8 mg	**Zorbtive®** (supplied in single-patient-use vials with diluent), EMD Serono
Injection, for subcutaneous use	5 mg/1.5 mL, 10 mg/1.5 mL, 15 mg/1.5 mL, and 30 mg/3 mL	**Norditropin®** (supplied in single-patient-use FlexPro pen), Novo Nordisk
	5 mg/1.5 mL and 10 mg/1.5 mL	**Omnitrope®** (supplied as prefilled cartridge), Sandoz
	5 mg/2 mL, 10 mg/2 mL, and 20 mg/2 mL	**Nutropin AQ® NuSpin®** (supplied as NuSpin prefilled injection device), Genentech
	10 mg/2 mL and 20 mg/2 mL	**Nutropin AQ®** (supplied as pen cartridge), Genentech

† Use is not currently included in the labeling approved by the US Food and Drug Administration.

Selected Revisions May 10, 2024, © Copyright, May 1, 2023, American Society of Health-System Pharmacists, Inc.

Vasopressin

68:28 • PITUITARY

■ Vasopressin (antidiuretic hormone) is a polypeptide hormone secreted by the neurons of the supraoptic and paraventricular nuclei of the hypothalamus and stored in the posterior pituitary (neurohypophysis) in mammals; the primary physiologic role of vasopressin is to maintain serum osmolality within a normal range, but the hormone also causes vasoconstriction.

USES

• Vasodilatory Shock

Vasopressin is used for its vasoconstrictive effects to increase blood pressure in patients with vasodilatory shock (e.g., postcardiotomy shock, septic shock); the drug is considered a second-line therapy in patients who remain hypotensive despite adequate fluid resuscitation and treatment with catecholamines (e.g., norepinephrine).

Evidence supporting the use of vasopressin in the management of vasodilatory shock is based principally on studies from the published literature, including 7 studies in adults with septic shock and 8 studies in adults with vasodilatory shock after cardiac surgery (i.e., postcardiotomy shock). While these studies had some limitations, vasopressin (administered in doses of 0.01 to 0.1 units/minute by continuous IV infusion) was shown to consistently increase mean arterial pressure (MAP) in patients with these hypotensive states. Although vasopressin appears to have a catecholamine-sparing effect, the effect of the drug on mortality remains unclear. In a randomized double-blind study comparing the effects of vasopressin (0.01–0.03 units/minute) and norepinephrine (5–10 mcg/minute) in patients with septic shock, no substantial difference in 28-day mortality was observed between the vasopressors. Large studies comparing vasopressin to other vasopressors for the treatment of septic shock generally are lacking.

The Surviving Sepsis Campaign International Guidelines for Management of Sepsis and Septic Shock recommend norepinephrine as the first-line vasopressor of choice in adults with septic shock. Vasopressin may be added if further increase in MAP is required or to reduce dosage requirements of norepinephrine. The guidelines recommend that vasopressin be used with caution in patients who are not euvolemic. Because of the risk of ischemic complications, use of vasopressin dosages greater than 0.03 units/minute should be reserved for situations in which alternative vasopressors have failed.

• Advanced Cardiovascular Life Support

Vasopressin has been used for its vasopressor effects as a nonadrenergic peripheral vasoconstrictor in patients with cardiac arrest†.

High-quality cardiopulmonary resuscitation (CPR) and defibrillation are integral components of advanced cardiovascular life support (ACLS) and the only proven interventions to increase survival to hospital discharge. Other resuscitative efforts, including drug therapy, are considered secondary and should be performed without compromising the quality and timely delivery of chest compressions and defibrillation. The principal goal of pharmacologic therapy during cardiac arrest is to facilitate return of spontaneous circulation (ROSC), and epinephrine is considered the drug of choice for this use. In previous ACLS guidelines, vasopressin was recommended as a substitute for epinephrine, with one dose of vasopressin (40 units by IV or intraosseous [IO] injection) replacing either the first or second dose of epinephrine, in the treatment of adult cardiac arrest. While some clinicians have suggested that vasopressin may be more effective than epinephrine in asystolic arrest because of underlying differences in the mechanism of action and cardiovascular effects of the drugs (e.g., epinephrine consumes oxygen whereas vasopressin increases coronary blood flow), current evidence indicates that vasopressin offers no advantage compared with epinephrine in patients with cardiac arrest. Results of several randomized controlled studies demonstrated no difference in outcomes (ROSC, survival to discharge or neurologic outcome) when vasopressin (used alone or in combination with epinephrine) was compared with epinephrine alone. In one of these studies in patients with out-of-hospital ventricular fibrillation, a larger proportion of patients initially treated with vasopressin

(40 units IV) were successfully resuscitated and survived 24 hours compared with those treated with epinephrine (1 mg IV); however, there was no difference in survival to hospital discharge. In another large (1186 patients), multinational, European study in adults with out-of-hospital cardiac arrest, vasopressin (up to 2 initial 40-unit IV doses) and epinephrine (up to 2 initial 1-mg IV doses) were comparably effective in the primary end point of survival to hospital admission as well as the secondary end point of survival to hospital discharge in patients with ventricular fibrillation (patients who responded successfully to electrical defibrillation were excluded) or pulseless electrical activity. Although a post-hoc analysis found that vasopressin was more effective than epinephrine for survival to hospital admission as well as hospital discharge in patients with asystolic cardiac arrest, vasopressin did not improve neurologically intact survival. Because of the equivalence of effect of vasopressin and epinephrine and efforts to simplify the management approach when therapies are found to be equivalent, vasopressin has been removed from the current ACLS treatment algorithm for adult cardiac arrest. There is insufficient evidence to recommend for or against routine use of vasopressin during cardiac arrest in pediatric patients.

Vasopressin has been used in the treatment of drug-induced distributive shock† associated with drug-induced cardiovascular emergencies or altered vital signs.

Vasopressin also has been used in severely hypotensive patients with anaphylaxis† as a potential therapy to prevent cardiopulmonary arrest.

• Diabetes Insipidus

Vasopressin has been used in the management of central diabetes insipidus†, a disorder caused by a deficiency of endogenous vasopressin, to control symptoms of polydypsia, polyuria, and dehydration. However, desmopressin, a synthetic analog of vasopressin that has a longer duration of action and lower incidence of adverse effects, is considered the drug of choice for this use. Although vasopressin injection may be used in the initial or emergency treatment of the disease, chronic therapy with the drug is impractical because of its short duration of action. Vasopressin is not effective in controlling polyuria caused by renal disease, nephrogenic diabetes insipidus, hypokalemia or hypercalcemia, or polyuria secondary to the administration of demeclocycline or lithium carbonate.

• Abdominal Distention and Abdominal Radiographic Procedures

Vasopressin injection has been used to stimulate peristalsis in the prevention or treatment of intestinal paresis†, postoperative abdominal distention†, and distention complicating pneumonias or toxemias†. In addition, the drug has been used prior to abdominal radiographic procedures† including IV urography, cholecystography, and kidney biopsy to dispel interfering gas shadows and/or to concentrate the contrast media.

• Diagnostic Uses

Vasopressin injection has been used in the past as a provocative test for pituitary release of growth hormone and corticotropin†; however, other diagnostic tests (e.g., insulin tolerance test) are considered more reliable diagnostic indicators of growth hormone reserve.

• GI Hemorrhage

Vasopressin has been administered IV or intra-arterially† into the superior mesenteric artery as an adjunct in the treatment of acute, massive GI hemorrhage† caused by various conditions including esophageal varices, inflammatory bowel disease, peptic ulcer disease, esophagogastritis, esophageal laceration, acute gastritis, colitis associated with Behcet's disease, colonic diverticulosis, Mallory-Weiss syndrome, and intestinal perforation. The drug also has been infused into the mesenteric artery prior to and during portosystemic shunt surgery for esophageal varices. Use of vasopressin in such situations is a temporary measure, intended to decrease portal venous pressure and increase clotting and hemostasis. There is no evidence that the drug substantially improves overall survival. Although vasopressin is a potent splanchnic vasoconstrictor that may provide effective control of bleeding, the clinical usefulness of the drug is limited because of its adverse effects. In addition, there is a high recurrence of bleeding when the drug is discontinued. Current management of acute GI hemorrhage usually includes endoscopic therapy or a combination of endoscopy and pharmacologic therapy with a splanchnic vasoconstrictor (e.g., most commonly octreotide because of its longer duration of action and favorable adverse effect profile).

DOSAGE AND ADMINISTRATION

• Administration

Vasopressin is administered by IV infusion for the management of vasodilatory shock. The drug also has been administered by IM† or subcutaneous† injection for other uses (e.g., postoperative abdominal distention, diabetes insipidus).

Vasopressin also has been applied topically† to the nasal mucosa (e.g., with a cotton pledget, nasal spray, or dropper) in the treatment of diabetes insipidus.

Vasopressin has been administered by intraosseous (IO)† injection for advanced cardiovascular life support (ACLS)†, generally when IV access is not readily available; onset of action and systemic concentrations of the drug are comparable to those achieved with venous administration. Vasopressin also has been administered endotracheally† when vascular (IV or IO) access cannot be established during cardiac arrest; however, IV or IO administration is preferred whenever possible because of more predictable drug delivery and pharmacologic effect.

In addition, the drug has been administered by intra-arterial infusion† in the management of GI hemorrhage†. Intra-arterial infusion of the drug requires specialized techniques, including angiographic placement of the catheter, and should only be performed by clinicians familiar with this method of administration and the management of potential complications.

IV Administration

For IV administration, vasopressin is commercially available as a 20-units/mL injection that should be further diluted with 0.9% sodium chloride or 5% dextrose injection prior to administration. The manufacturer recommends dilution to a final concentration of 0.1 or 1 unit/mL depending on the patient's fluid status. In patients who are not fluid restricted, a concentration of 0.1 units/mL may be prepared by mixing 50 units (2.5 mL) of vasopressin injection with 500 mL of diluent. In patients who are fluid restricted, a more concentrated solution of 1 unit/mL may be prepared by mixing 100 units (5 mL) of vasopressin injection with 100 mL of diluent.

Unused portions of the diluted solution should be discarded after 18 hours at room temperature or 24 hours under refrigeration. Vasopressin solutions should be inspected visually for particulate matter and discoloration prior to administration.

Standardize 4 Safety

Standardized concentrations for vasopressin have been established through Standardize 4 Safety (S4S), a national patient safety initiative to reduce medication errors, especially during transitions of care. Multidisciplinary expert panels were convened to determine recommended standard concentrations. Because recommendations from the S4S panels may differ from the manufacturer's prescribing information, caution is advised when using concentrations that differ from labeling, particularly when using rate information from the label. For additional information on S4S (including updates that may be available), see

https://www.ashp.org/pharmacy-practice/standardize-4-safety-initiative.

TABLE 1. Standardize 4 Safety Continuous IV Infusion Standard Concentrations for Vasopressin

Patient Population	Concentration Standards	Dosing Units
Adults	0.2 units/mL	units/min or units/kg/min [a]
	0.4 units/mL	
	1 unit/mL	
Pediatric patients (<50 kg)	0.05 units/mL	milliunits/kg/min for vasoconstriction/GI bleed or milliunits/kg/hr for diabetes insipidus [b]
	0.2 units/mL	
	1 unit/mL	

[a] The S4S panel recommends trying to standardize dosing units but understands that some protocols may use "flat" dosing while others may require weight-based dosing.

[b] dosing units differ from concentration units

• Dosage

Vasopressin dosage requirements are variable and must be adjusted according to patient response. In order to avoid adverse effects, it is desirable to give doses that are just sufficient to elicit the desired response.

Vasodilatory Shock

The manufacturer states that dosage of vasopressin is empiric for the management of vasodilatory shock; in general, dosage should be titrated to the lowest dose compatible with a clinically acceptable response. The goal of therapy is to optimize and maintain perfusion to critical organs without causing ischemic complications.

The manufacturer recommends an initial vasopressin dosage of 0.03 units/minute in adults with postcardiotomy shock and 0.01 units/minute in adults with septic shock. If target blood pressure response is not achieved, the infusion rate may be increased by 0.005 units/minute at intervals of 10–15 minutes to a maximum dosage of 0.1 units/minute for postcardiotomy shock or 0.07 units/minute for septic shock. Some experts recommend that infusion rates higher than 0.03 units/minute be used with caution because of the risk of cardiac and peripheral ischemia. After target blood pressure has been maintained for 8 hours without the use of catecholamines, the vasopressin infusion rate should be tapered by 0.005 units/minute every hour as tolerated to maintain target blood pressure.

Advanced Cardiovascular Life Support

For advanced cardiovascular life support (ACLS) in patients with cardiac arrest†, vasopressin has been given in a single dose of 40 units by IV or IO† injection as a replacement for the first or second dose of epinephrine.

Diabetes Insipidus

For the treatment of central diabetes insipidus†, vasopressin has been given in an adult dosage of 5–10 units 2–3 times daily as needed by IM or subcutaneous injection. Dosage has ranged from 5–60 units daily. In children, vasopressin has been given in proportionately reduced doses of 2.5–10 units by IM or subcutaneous injection 2–4 times daily. For the treatment of diabetes insipidus, vasopressin also has been administered intranasally at individualized dosages.

Abdominal Distention and Abdominal Radiographic Procedures

For the management of postoperative abdominal distention† in adults, vasopressin has been administered at an initial dose of 5 units by IM injection

. Subsequent injections have been given every 3–4 hours with doses increased to 10 units if necessary. In children, proportionately reduced doses have been used.

For use in abdominal roentgenography†, it has been suggested that two 10-unit IM or subcutaneous injections of vasopressin be administered, the first injection at 2 hours and the second injection at 30 minutes, prior to exposure of the radiograph; many clinicians recommend giving an enema prior to the first dose of vasopressin.

Diagnostic Uses

When used as a provocative test for growth hormone and corticotropin release†, vasopressin injection has been given IM in a dose of 10 units for adults and 0.3 units/kg for children.

GI Hemorrhage

For the management of GI hemorrhage†, vasopressin has been administered by continuous IV or intra-arterial infusion after dilution with 0.9% sodium chloride or 5% dextrose injection to a concentration of 0.1–1 unit/mL. Continuous IV rather than intra-arterial infusion of the drug is preferred.

For IV infusion in patients with GI hemorrhage, vasopressin has been infused into a peripheral vein via a controlled infusion device. For continuous intra-arterial infusion in patients with esophageal varices or upper GI bleeding, the drug has been infused into the superior or inferior mesenteric artery via a controlled infusion device.

For the management of GI bleeding†, dosage of vasopressin is empiric and must be individualized according to the response and tolerance of the patient. Because many of the adverse effects of vasopressin are dose related, the lowest possible effective dosage should be used. Some experts recommend continuous use of vasopressin for no longer than 24 hours. IV dosage generally has been initiated at 0.2–0.4 units/minute and progressively increased to a maximum of 0.6–0.9 units/minute if necessary based on individual patient response. To minimize adverse effects, some experts recommend concomitant use of IV nitroglycerin (initiated at 40 mcg/minute, increased to a maximum of 400 mcg/minute). When vasopressin is administered by intra-arterial infusion, a dosage of 0.1–0.5 units/minute has been used.

● Dosage in Hepatic and Renal Impairment

There is limited information regarding exposure of vasopressin in patients with hepatic impairment and no specific dosage recommendations are available for such patients; dosage should be titrated to effect.

There is limited information regarding exposure of vasopressin in patients with renal impairment and no specific dosage recommendations are available for such patients; dosage should be titrated to effect.

CAUTIONS

● Adverse Effects

Adverse effects associated with low doses of vasopressin are infrequent and mild, but increase in frequency and severity with high doses. Reported adverse effects include circumoral pallor, sweating, tremor, pounding in the head, abdominal cramps, passage of gas, vertigo, nausea, vomiting, and eructation. In addition, diarrhea, intestinal hyperactivity, and uterine cramps may occur. Some manufacturers state that blanching of the skin, abdominal cramps, and nausea that may occur following subcutaneous or IM injection of the drug can be minimized by drinking 1 or 2 glasses of water at the time of vasopressin administration. Vasopressin may also increase plasma cortisol concentrations and serum concentrations of growth hormone.

In large doses, vasopressin may produce increased blood pressure, bradycardia, minor arrhythmias, premature atrial contraction, heart block, peripheral vascular constriction or collapse, coronary insufficiency, decreased cardiac output, myocardial ischemia, or myocardial infarction. In patients with vascular disease (especially of the coronary arteries), even small doses of the drug can precipitate angina. Coronary vasodilators (e.g., nitroglycerin) may be used to treat angina if it occurs. An ECG should be used to monitor the hormone's cardiac effects during IV or intra-arterial therapy.

Adverse effects reported in the published literature with IV vasopressin in patients with vasodilatory shock include hemorrhagic shock, decreased platelets, intractable bleeding, right heart failure, atrial fibrillation, bradycardia, myocardial ischemia, mesenteric ischemia, increased bilirubin levels, acute renal insufficiency, distal limb ischemia, hyponatremia, and ischemic lesions.

When fluid intake is not excessive, there is little danger involved in the use of small antidiuretic doses of vasopressin to control diabetes insipidus. Overhydration was more likely to occur with the long-acting suspension of vasopressin tannate (no longer commercially available in the US) than with vasopressin injection; infants and children are often much more susceptible to such volume disturbances than are adults. If water intoxication occurs, some experts have recommended that vasopressin be discontinued and fluid intake restricted until the specific gravity of the urine decreases to less than 1.015 and polyuria occurs. In severe overhydration, osmotic diuresis with mannitol, hypertonic dextrose, or urea, alone or in conjunction with furosemide, is often effective in rapidly decreasing fluid overload. Hypertonic saline solutions are not indicated unless immediate correction of hyponatremia is required.

Hypersensitivity reactions characterized by urticaria, angioedema, bronchoconstriction, fever, rash, wheezing, dyspnea, circulatory collapse, cardiac arrest, and anaphylaxis have been reported with vasopressin administration. Appropriate agents for the treatment of hypersensitivity reactions should be readily available.

Coronary thrombosis, mesenteric infarction, venous thrombosis, infarction and necrosis of the small bowel, and peripheral emboli resulting from intra-arterial catheterization have been reported following infusion of vasopressin injection into the superior mesenteric artery. In one patient, intra-arterial injection of vasopressin produced mottling and cyanosis of the left foot. Several patients reportedly developed signs of cutaneous gangrene proximal to the site of IV infusion of the drug. Bilateral nipple necrosis, which gradually resolved over 10–14 days after discontinuance of the drug, has occurred in at least 2 patients during IV infusion of the drug. Reversible ischemic colitis has been reported in a patient receiving IV infusion of the drug for the management of variceal hemorrhage.

● Precautions and Contraindications

Vasopressin should be used cautiously in preoperative and postoperative polyuric patients, since hormone requirements in these patients may be considerably less than normal. Fluid intake and output should be monitored closely, especially in comatose or semicomatose patients. Electrolyte balance also should be monitored periodically. Patients receiving vasopressin should be observed for early signs of water intoxication such as drowsiness, listlessness, headache, confusion, anuria, and weight gain in order to prevent ensuing seizures, coma, and death.

Vasopressin should be used cautiously in patients with seizure disorders, migraine, asthma, heart failure, vascular disease (especially of the coronary arteries), angina pectoris, coronary thrombosis, renal disease, goiter with cardiac complications, arteriosclerosis, or any other disease in which rapid addition to extracellular fluids may be hazardous. ECG monitoring should be performed periodically during therapy with the drug. Patients with impaired cardiac response may experience worsening cardiac output.

Aggressive treatment with vasopressin in patients with vasodilatory shock can compromise perfusion of organs, including those of the GI tract, whose function is difficult to monitor. Dosage should be titrated to the lowest dose compatible with a clinically acceptable response.

Geriatric patients and children are particularly sensitive to the effects of vasopressin; therefore, the drug should be used cautiously in these patients.

Vasopressin is contraindicated in patients with known allergy or hypersensitivity (e.g., anaphylaxis) to synthetic vasopressin (8-L-arginine vasopressin) or chlorobutanol (a preservative in the formulation). Some manufacturers have stated that the drug is also contraindicated in patients with chronic nephritis accompanied by nitrogen retention and should not be used until reasonable nitrogen concentrations are attained.

● Pediatric Precautions

The manufacturer states that safety and efficacy of vasopressin in pediatric patients with vasodilatory shock have not been established. Although the drug has been evaluated in several studies for the treatment of pediatric vasodilatory shock, inconclusive results were reported and a wide range of doses were employed.

● Geriatric Precautions

Clinical studies of vasopressin did not include sufficient numbers of patients 65 years of age and older to determine whether geriatric patients respond differently than younger patients. Clinical experience to date has not identified any differences in response between geriatric and younger patients. In general, dosage selection in geriatric patients should be cautious, usually starting at the low end of the dosage range, since renal, hepatic, and cardiovascular dysfunction and concomitant disease or other drug therapy are more common in this age group.

● Pregnancy, Fertility, and Lactation

Pregnancy

There are no adequate or well-controlled studies of vasopressin in pregnant women, and animal reproduction studies with the drug have not been conducted. It is not known whether vasopressin can cause fetal harm when administered to pregnant women or can affect reproduction capacity; the drug should be used during pregnancy only if the potential benefits justify the potential risks to a fetus.

Vasopressin may produce tonic uterine contractions that could threaten the continuation of pregnancy.

Clearance of vasopressin is increased in the second and third trimester of pregnancy; dosages exceeding 0.1 units/minute may be required in patients with postcardiotomy shock and dosages exceeding 0.07 units/minute may be required in patients with septic shock.

Lactation

It is not known whether vasopressin is distributed into human milk. Some manufacturers recommend that the drug be used with caution in nursing women.

Oral absorption of vasopressin in a nursing infant is considered unlikely since the drug is rapidly destroyed in the GI tract. Consideration may be given to advising a lactating woman to pump and discard her breast milk for 1.5 hours after receiving vasopressin to minimize potential exposure to the infant.

DRUG INTERACTIONS

● Alcohol

Alcohol may decrease the antidiuretic effects of vasopressin.

● Catecholamines

Concomitant use of catecholamines and vasopressin is expected to result in additive effects on mean arterial blood pressure and other hemodynamic parameters.

● Drugs Causing Diabetes Insipidus

Drugs suspected of causing diabetes insipidus (e.g., demeclocycline, lithium, foscarnet, clozapine) may decrease the pressor effect and antidiuretic activity of vasopressin.

● Drugs Causing Syndrome of Inappropriate Secretion of Antidiuretic Hormone

Drugs suspected of causing syndrome of inappropriate secretion of antidiuretic hormone (SIADH) (e.g., selective serotonin-reuptake inhibitors [SSRIs], tricyclic antidepressants, haloperidol, chlorpropamide, enalapril, methyldopa, pentamidine, vincristine, cyclophosphamide, ifosfamide, felbamate) may increase the pressor effect and antidiuretic activity of vasopressin.

● Furosemide

Furosemide increases the effect of vasopressin on osmolar clearance and urine flow. Furosemide increased osmolar clearance and urine flow by 4 and 9 times, respectively, in healthy subjects receiving vasopressin.

● Ganglionic Blocking Agents

Ganglionic blocking agents may markedly increase sensitivity to the pressor effects of vasopressin. In healthy individuals, administration of tetra-ethylammonium (a ganglionic blocking agent) increased the pressor effect of vasopressin by 20%.

● Heparin

Heparin may decrease the antidiuretic effects of vasopressin.

● Indomethacin

Indomethacin may prolong the effects of vasopressin on peripheral vascular resistance and cardiac output.

● Norepinephrine

Norepinephrine may decrease the antidiuretic effects of vasopressin.

PHARMACOLOGY

Exogenous vasopressin elicits all the pharmacologic responses usually produced by endogenous vasopressin (antidiuretic hormone). The primary physiologic role of vasopressin is to maintain serum osmolality within a normal range. The hormone produces relatively concentrated urine by increasing reabsorption of water by the renal tubules. Its action in regulating body fluid balance is mediated by renal vasopressin V_2 receptors, which are coupled to adenyl cyclase and the generation of cyclic AMP. At the tubular level, vasopressin stimulates adenyl cyclase activity, leading to increases in cyclic adenosine monophosphate (AMP). Cyclic AMP increases water permeability at the luminal surface of the distal convoluted tubule and collecting duct, resulting in increased urine osmolality and decreased urinary flow rate. The antidiuretic activity of vasopressin conserves up to 90% of the water that might otherwise be excreted in the urine. Vasopressin also increases reabsorption of urea by the collecting ducts. Although solute diuresis does not generally occur, increased sodium and decreased potassium reabsorption have been induced by vasopressin. Vasopressin, however, plays no etiologic role in edema formation.

In doses greater than those required for antidiuretic effects, vasopressin directly stimulates contraction of smooth muscle V_1 receptors. The vasoconstrictive action of vasopressin is mediated by vascular V_1 receptors; the vascular receptors are coupled to phospholipase C, resulting in release of calcium from sarcoplasmic reticulum in smooth muscle cells, leading to vasoconstriction. The hormone exhibits relatively little vasoconstrictor effect in hemodynamically normal individuals, but is an important endogenous vasopressor when arterial pressure is threatened. Vasopressin causes vasoconstriction, particularly of capillaries and of small arterioles, resulting in decreased blood flow to the splanchnic, coronary, GI, pancreatic, skin, and muscular systems. At therapeutic doses, vasopressin elicits a vasoconstrictive effect in most vascular beds, including the splanchnic, renal, and cutaneous circulation. When administered into the celiac or superior mesenteric arteries, vasopressin constricts gastroduodenal, left gastric, superior mesenteric, and splenic arteries; however, hepatic arteries are not constricted and, instead, hepatic blood flow often increases. When used to produce antidiuresis, vasopressin has little effect on blood pressure. The drug indirectly decreases coronary blood flow and may precipitate myocardial infarction. In addition, the hormone can decrease heart rate and cardiac output and increase pulmonary arterial pressure and blood pressure.

Patients with septic shock or postcardiotomy shock appear to have a relative deficiency of endogenous vasopressin, which can contribute to the vasodilatory hypotension observed in these shock states. When administered in therapeutic doses to patients with vasodilatory shock, vasopressin increases systemic vascular resistance and mean arterial blood pressure. In addition, the drug tends to decrease heart rate and cardiac output. The pressor effect of vasopressin is proportional to the infusion rate of the drug. No evidence of tachyphylaxis or tolerance to the pressor effect of vasopressin has been observed.

Endogenous vasopressin concentrations in patients undergoing cardiopulmonary resuscitation (CPR) are higher in those who survive than in those who do not have return to spontaneous circulation (ROSC). This finding suggested that exogenous vasopressin might be beneficial during cardiac arrest. After ventricular fibrillation of short duration, administration of vasopressin during CPR has increased coronary perfusion pressure, vital organ blood flow, ventricular fibrillation median frequency, and cerebral oxygen delivery. Similar findings have been reported with prolonged cardiac arrest and pulseless electrical activity. The hormone did not result in bradycardia after ROSC. Interaction of vasopressin with V_1 receptors during CPR causes intense peripheral vasoconstriction of skin, skeletal muscle, intestine, and fat with relatively less vasoconstriction of coronary and renal vascular beds and vasodilatation of cerebral vasculature. Vasopressin does not exhibit β-adrenergic activity and therefore does not produce skeletal muscle vasodilatation or increased myocardial oxygen consumption during CPR.

At pressor doses, vasopressin triggers contraction of smooth muscles in the GI tract mediated by muscular V_1 receptors and release of prolactin and ACTH via V_3 receptors. In the intestinal tract, vasopressin increases peristaltic activity, particularly of the large bowel. Vasopressin also causes an increase in GI sphincter pressure and a decrease in gastric secretion but has no effect on gastric acid concentration.

The oxytocic properties of vasopressin are minimal, but in large doses the drug may stimulate uterine contraction. The hormone also possesses slight milk ejecting properties but its role during lactation is negligible.

In addition to its peripheral effects, vasopressin causes release of corticotropin, growth hormone, and follicle-stimulating hormone.

PHARMACOKINETICS

● Absorption

Vasopressin is destroyed by trypsin, which is found in the GI tract, and, therefore, must be administered parenterally or intranasally. Absorption of vasopressin through the nasal mucosa is relatively poor. Following subcutaneous or IM administration of vasopressin injection, the duration of antidiuretic activity is variable but effects are usually maintained for 2–8 hours. Urine isotonicity is maintained when plasma concentrations of vasopressin are approximately 1 microunit/mL, while plasma concentrations of 4.5–6 microunits/mL produce maximum concentration of urine. Following IV infusion of vasopressin in patients with vasodilatory shock, onset of the pressor effect is rapid, with peak effects occurring within 15 minutes. Pressor effects fade within 20 minutes following discontinuance of infusion.

● Distribution

Vasopressin is distributed throughout the extracellular fluid; there is no evidence of plasma protein binding.

It is not known whether vasopressin is distributed into human milk.

● Elimination

Vasopressin is predominantly metabolized by the liver and kidneys. The drug is cleaved by serine protease, carboxipeptidase, and disulfide oxidoreductase at relevant sites for its pharmacologic activity; resulting metabolites are not expected to be pharmacologically active. Vasopressin has a plasma half-life of about 10–20 minutes. When administered by IV infusion at usual rates for vasodilatory shock (e.g., 0.1–1 units/minute), the apparent half-life is 10 minutes or less. Oxytocinase, a circulating enzyme produced early in pregnancy, is capable of cleaving the polypeptide; otherwise, plasma inactivation of vasopressin is negligible. Approximately 5% of a subcutaneous dose of vasopressin is excreted in urine unchanged after 4 hours, and following IV administration, 5–15% of the total vasopressin dosage appears in urine.

CHEMISTRY AND STABILITY

● Chemistry

Vasopressin is a polypeptide hormone secreted by the neurons of the supraoptic and paraventricular nuclei of the hypothalamus and stored in the posterior pituitary (neurohypophysis) in mammals. In humans and most other mammals, the natural hormone is arginine vasopressin. Commercially available vasopressin injection is an aqueous solution of synthetic arginine vasopressin. The potency of vasopressin (arginine) is standardized according to its pressor activity in rats and is expressed in USP Posterior Pituitary (pressor) Units. Antidiuretic activity of the commercially available preparations may be variable.

Vasopressin is soluble in water. Vasopressin injection for IV infusion contains a sodium acetate buffer to adjust the pH to 3.8. Vasopressin injection solution contains chlorobutanol (anhydrous) as a preservative; glacial acetic acid and/or sodium hydroxide may be added during manufacture to adjust the pH to 2.5–4.5.

● Stability

Vasopressin injection for IV infusion should be stored at 2–8°C and should not be frozen. Unopened vials may be stored at room temperature (20–25°C) for up to 12 months or up to the manufacturer's labeled expiration date (whichever comes first); once removed from the refrigerator, the vials should be marked to indicate the revised 12-month expiration date (if it occurs before the manufacturer's labeled expiration date). Unused diluted solutions should be discarded after 18 hours at room temperature or after 24 hours under refrigeration.

PREPARATIONS

Excipients in commercially available drug preparations may have clinically important effects in some individuals; consult specific product labeling for details.

Vasopressin

Parenteral

Injection, for IV infusion	20 units/mL	Vasostrict®, Par

† Use is not currently included in the labeling approved by the US Food and Drug Administration.

Selected Revisions November 10, 2024, © Copyright, May 1, 1977, American Society of Health-System Pharmacists, Inc.

Progestins General Statement

68:32 • PROGESTINS

■ Progestins elicit, to varying degrees, all the pharmacologic responses usually produced by progesterone.

USES

Progesterone is used to support embryo implantation and early pregnancy by supplementing corpus luteal function as part of assisted reproductive technology (ART) treatment of infertile women.

Progestins are used in the treatment of functional uterine bleeding caused by hormonal imbalance and involving a hyperplastic nonsecretory endometrium and the absence of underlying organic pathology such as fibroids or uterine cancer, and for the treatment of primary and secondary amenorrhea in the presence of estrogen. Medroxyprogesterone also is used in the adjunctive and palliative treatment of some cancers. (See the individual monographs in 68:32.) Some progestins are used alone or in combination with estrogens for the prevention of conception. (See Progestins 68:12 and Estrogen-Progestin Combinations 68:12.) Medroxyprogesterone prevents follicular maturation and ovulation following IM administration, and the drug has been used parenterally for contraception. (See Uses: Contraception in Females in Medroxyprogesterone Acetate 68:32.)

Progestins (e.g., drospirenone, medroxyprogesterone, norethindrone acetate, norgestimate, progesterone) are used to reduce the incidence of endometrial hyperplasia and the attendant risk of endometrial carcinoma in postmenopausal women receiving estrogen replacement therapy. (See Uses: Prevention of Endometrial Changes Associated with Estrogens in Medroxyprogesterone Acetate 68:32.) Morphologic and biochemical studies of the endometrium suggest that 10–13 days of progestin are needed to provide maximum maturation of the endometrium and to eliminate any hyperplastic changes.

For other uses of progestins, see Uses in Medroxyprogesterone Acetate 68:32.

Although progestins have been used beginning in the first trimester of pregnancy to prevent habitual abortion or to treat threatened abortion, there is no adequate evidence from well-controlled studies to substantiate the efficacy of progestins for these uses; however, there is evidence of potential adverse effects on the fetus when these drugs are administered during the first 4 months of pregnancy. (See Cautions: Pregnancy and Lactation.) Although some progestins were previously used to induce withdrawal bleeding as a test for pregnancy when laboratory tests were not readily available, progestins are currently *contraindicated* for this use.

CAUTIONS

● Adverse Effects

Progestins may cause breakthrough bleeding, spotting, changes in menstrual flow, amenorrhea, changes in cervical erosion and secretions, edema, weight gain or loss, nausea, cholestatic jaundice, allergic rash with or without pruritus, anaphylactoid reactions and anaphylaxis, melasma or chloasma, pyrexia, somnolence or insomnia, and mental depression.

An association between pulmonary embolism and cerebral thrombosis and embolism and use of estrogen-progestin combination preparations has been shown. (See Thromboembolic Disorders in Cautions: Cardiovascular Effects, in Estrogen-Progestin Combinations 68:12.) The possibility that thromboembolic disorders may occur in patients receiving progestins should be considered and patients should be carefully observed for these effects during therapy with the drugs. (See Cautions: Precautions and Contraindications.)

Although available evidence suggests that an association exists between neuro-ocular lesions such as optic neuritis or retinal thrombosis and use of estrogen-progestin combination preparations, such a relationship has been neither confirmed nor refuted. Increased blood pressure in susceptible individuals, premenstrual-like syndrome, changes in libido or appetite, cystitis-like syndrome, headache, nervousness, dizziness, fatigue, backache, hirsutism, loss of scalp hair,

erythema multiforme or nodosum, hemorrhagic skin eruption, and itching have occurred in patients receiving estrogen-progestin combination preparations. Use of estrogen-progestin combinations has also been associated with increased levels of coagulation factors VII, VIII, IX, and X. The possibility that these effects may occur in patients receiving progestins should be considered and patients should be carefully observed for these effects during therapy with the drugs.

Because drospirenone has antimineralocorticoid activity, the potential exists for hyperkalemia to occur in high-risk patients (e.g., those with renal or hepatic impairment, adrenal insufficiency) receiving this progestin.

● Precautions and Contraindications

Because oral contraceptive combinations contain progestins, the precautions associated with oral contraceptives should generally be considered in patients receiving progestins. (See Cautions in Estrogen-Progestin Combinations 68:12.) Prior to initiation of therapy with progestins in women, a physical examination should be performed, including special attention to the breasts and pelvic organs and a Papanicolaou test (Pap smear). Women receiving progestins should be given a copy of the patient labeling for the drugs.

Progestins should be used with caution, and only with careful monitoring, in patients with conditions that might be aggravated by fluid retention (e.g., asthma, seizure disorders, migraine, or cardiac or renal dysfunction). Progestins should also be used with caution in patients with a history of mental depression; the drugs should be discontinued if depression recurs to a serious degree during progestin therapy.

When breakthrough bleeding or irregular vaginal bleeding occurs during progestin therapy, nonfunctional causes should be considered. Adequate diagnostic procedures should be performed in patients with undiagnosed vaginal bleeding.

The effect of long-term progestin therapy on pituitary, ovarian, adrenal, hepatic, or uterine function has not been determined. Diabetic patients should be carefully monitored during progestin therapy, since decreased glucose tolerance has been observed in women receiving estrogen-progestin combinations. Progestins may mask the onset of climacteric in women.

The clinician and the patient using progestins should be alert to the earliest signs and symptoms of thromboembolic and thrombotic disorders (e.g., thrombophlebitis, pulmonary embolism, cerebrovascular insufficiency, coronary occlusion, retinal thrombosis, mesenteric thrombosis). Progestins should be discontinued immediately when any of these disorders occurs or is suspected.

A safety review conducted by the US Food and Drug Administration (FDA) indicates that use of combination oral contraceptives containing the progestin drospirenone may be associated with an increased risk of venous thromboembolism (VTE) compared with that of oral contraceptives containing levonorgestrel or other progestins. This conclusion was based on results of several epidemiologic studies evaluating the risk of VTE in women using oral contraceptives containing drospirenone. These studies reported that the risk of VTE in such women ranged from no increase to a threefold increase in risk. The FDA's safety review was prompted by results of 2 recent case-control studies that showed a twofold to threefold increased risk of VTE (including deep-vein thrombosis and pulmonary embolism) in patients receiving oral contraceptives containing drospirenone compared with those receiving oral contraceptives containing the progestin levonorgestrel. These studies evaluated cases of idiopathic VTE occurring in women 15–44 years of age who were current users of oral contraceptives containing 30 mcg of estrogen with either drospirenone or levonorgestrel; women with risk factors for VTE were excluded from the studies. The FDA has also reviewed data from a large US retrospective cohort study in more than 800,000 women evaluating thrombotic and thromboembolic risks (including VTE) associated with hormonal contraceptives. Final results from this study suggest an increased risk of VTE (hazard ratio greater than 1) in women using oral contraceptives containing drospirenone compared with women using other hormonal contraceptives.

Given the conflicting results of the previous epidemiologic studies and the recent findings, the FDA held a joint meeting of the Reproductive Health Drugs Advisory Committee and the Drug Safety and Risk Management Advisory Committee on December 8, 2011, to review the risks and benefits of such therapy and specifically to discuss the risk of VTE associated with drospirenone-containing hormonal contraceptives. The studies reviewed by the FDA did not provide consistent data for the comparative risk of thromboembolic events between oral contraceptives that contain drospirenone and those that do not. In addition, the studies did not account for important known and unknown patient characteristics that may influence prescribing patterns and may affect risk of VTE. For these reasons, the FDA states that it is unclear whether the increased risk of thromboembolic events observed in these epidemiologic studies actually resulted from use of drospirenone-containing oral contraceptives. At this time, the FDA has concluded that the risk of VTE may be higher for such oral contraceptives and will continue to communicate any new safety information as it becomes available.

Oral contraceptive combinations containing drospirenone should be discontinued if an arterial or venous thrombotic event occurs during therapy. The risk of VTE is highest during the first year of oral contraceptive use. Results from a large, prospective cohort safety study of various estrogen-progestin oral contraceptives suggest that this increased risk is highest during the first 6 months of use compared with that in nonusers. Data from this safety study indicate that the highest risk of VTE occurs after initiation of estrogen-progestin oral contraceptive therapy or resumption of therapy (following a 4-week or longer drug-free interval) with the same or a different oral contraceptive combination. Before initiating use of an estrogen-progestin combination containing drospirenone in a new user or in a woman who is switching from an oral contraceptive not containing drospirenone, clinicians should consider the risks and benefits of drospirenone-containing oral contraceptives, including risk for developing VTE, specific to that woman.

Women currently receiving an oral contraceptive combination containing drospirenone should be informed of the potential risk of thromboembolic events. Patients also should be advised about the current information available regarding the risk of VTE with oral contraceptives containing drospirenone compared with those containing levonorgestrel. Patients should contact a clinician if they experience any signs or symptoms of VTE (e.g., persistent leg pain, severe chest pain, sudden shortness of breath). Known risk factors for development of VTE include smoking, obesity, family history, and other factors that contraindicate the use of oral contraceptive combinations. Patients should discuss their risk of VTE with their clinician before deciding which contraceptive method or hormonal contraceptive to use. The risk of thromboembolic disease associated with oral contraceptive use gradually disappears after such therapy is discontinued. However, the FDA states that patients should not discontinue oral contraceptives containing drospirenone without consulting a clinician.

If unexplained, sudden or gradual, partial or complete loss of vision; proptosis or diplopia; papilledema; retinal vascular lesions; or migraine occur during therapy with progestins, the drugs should be discontinued and appropriate diagnostic and therapeutic measures instituted. Because steroidal hormones are metabolized in the liver, progestins should be used with caution in patients with impaired liver function.

Drospirenone should not be used in patients who are predisposed to developing hyperkalemia (e.g., those with renal or hepatic impairment or adrenal insufficiency). If drospirenone is used in women receiving daily, long-term therapy with agents that may increase serum potassium concentrations (e.g., angiotensin-converting enzyme (ACE) inhibitors, angiotensin II type 1 (AT₁) receptor antagonists, potassium-sparing diuretics, potassium supplements, heparin, aldosterone antagonists [spironolactone], nonsteroidal anti-inflammatory agents [NSAIAs]), the serum potassium concentration should be determined during the first treatment cycle.

Progestins are contraindicated in patients with thrombophlebitis, thromboembolic disorders, cerebral apoplexy, or a history of these conditions. The drugs are also contraindicated in patients with undiagnosed vaginal bleeding, missed abortion, known sensitivity to the drug or any ingredient in the formulation, markedly impaired liver function or liver disease, or carcinoma of the breast or for use as a pregnancy test.

● Mutagenicity and Carcinogenicity

The carcinogenic and mutagenic potentials of progestins have not been fully determined.

Administration of medroxyprogesterone to beagles has been associated with the development of mammary nodules, some of which were malignant. Although nodules occasionally occurred in control beagles, they were intermittent in nature; nodules in drug-treated beagles were larger, more numerous, persistent, and occasionally malignant with metastases. The clinical relevance of these findings to humans has not been established. For additional information on the carcinogenic potential of progestins, see Cautions: Mutagenicity and Carcinogenicity, in Medroxyprogesterone Acetate 68:32.

● Pregnancy, Fertility, and Lactation
Pregnancy

Progesterone is used to support embryo implantation and maintain pregnancy as a component of assisted reproductive technology (ART) treatment in infertile women. Such use is associated with increased ongoing pregnancy rates.

Although progestins have been used beginning in the first trimester of pregnancy to prevent habitual abortion or to treat threatened abortion, there is no

adequate evidence from well-controlled studies to substantiate the efficacy of progestins for these uses; however, there is evidence of potential adverse effects on the fetus when these drugs are administered during the first 4 months of pregnancy. In addition, in most women, the cause of abortion is a defective ovum, which progestins could not be expected to influence. Because of their uterine-relaxant effects, progestins may delay spontaneous abortion of fertilized defective ova. Masculinization of the female fetus has reportedly occurred when progestins were used during pregnancy. Clitoral hypertrophy and fusion of the labia have been reported in a few female neonates born to women who had received medroxyprogesterone during pregnancy; hypospadias in male neonates born to women receiving progestational agents occurs at approximately twice the rate of occurrence in male neonates born to women not receiving the drugs. An association between intrauterine exposure to female sex hormones and congenital anomalies, including cardiovascular and limb defects, has been suggested. (See Cautions: Pregnancy, Fertility, and Lactation, in Estrogen-Progestin Combinations 68:12.) Use of progestins generally is not recommended during the first 4 months of pregnancy. If a woman becomes pregnant while receiving progestins or is inadvertently exposed to the drugs during the first 4 months of pregnancy, she should be advised of the potential risks to the fetus.

Progestins should *not* be used to induce withdrawal bleeding as a test for pregnancy.

Lactation

Progestins are reportedly distributed into milk. The possible effects of progestins in milk on nursing infants have not been determined.

LABORATORY TEST INTERFERENCES

Estrogen-progestin combinations have caused abnormal thyroid function test results. (See Effects on Thyroid in Cautions: Endocrine and Metabolic Effects, in Estrogen-Progestin Combinations 68:12.) Estrogen-progestin combinations have altered the metyrapone test (see Laboratory Test Interferences in Estrogen-Progestin Combinations 68:12) and liver function test results (see Cautions: Hepatic Effects, in Estrogen-Progestin Combinations 68:12). These combinations have also caused decreased pregnanediol excretion.

The pathologist should be advised of progestin use when relevant specimens from a patient exposed to the drug are submitted.

PHARMACOLOGY

Progestins elicit, to varying degrees, all the pharmacologic responses usually produced by progesterone: induction of secretory changes in the endometrium, increase in basal body temperature (thermogenic action), production of histologic changes in vaginal epithelium, relaxation of uterine smooth muscle, stimulation of mammary alveolar tissue growth, pituitary inhibition, and production of withdrawal bleeding in the presence of estrogen. For further discussion on the pharmacologic effects of progestins, see Progesterone and the other individual monographs in 68:32.

● Chemistry

The use of progesterone, a hormone secreted by the corpus luteum, is well established in medicine. Its relative inactivity following oral administration and the local reactions and pain sometimes produced upon injection have led to the synthesis of chemical derivatives that are effective orally, are more potent, more specific in action, or have a longer duration of action.

Ethisterone was the first synthetic progestin developed; the drug is not currently available. 19-Nor,17-acetoxy, and 6-methyl derivatives, which exhibit interesting structural-pharmacologic relationships, have been synthesized. Some estrogenic or androgenic activity, anabolic effects, nitrogen retention, and weight gain are exhibited by the 19-nor derivatives. The 17-hydroxy or acetoxy compounds, on the other hand, elicit responses more nearly resembling those of progesterone. They have little or no estrogenic or androgenic activity and may produce catabolic and slight diuretic effects. The 19-nor derivatives are more effective in postponing the normal menstrual period.

For further information on chemistry and stability, pharmacology, uses, cautions, and dosage and administration of progestins, see the individual monographs in 68:32 and the monographs on Estrogen-Progestin Combinations and Progestins in 68:12.

medroxyPROGESTERone Acetate

68:32 • PROGESTINS

■ Medroxyprogesterone acetate is a synthetic progestin.

USES

• Prevention of Endometrial Changes Associated with Estrogens

Medroxyprogesterone acetate is used orally to reduce the incidence of endometrial hyperplasia and the attendant risk of endometrial carcinoma in postmenopausal women receiving estrogen replacement therapy. When estrogens are used in combination with progestins, such therapy usually is referred to as hormone replacement therapy (HRT) or postmenopausal replacement therapy. Evidence from the Women's Health Initiative (WHI) study indicates that combined estrogen (conjugated estrogens 0.625 mg daily) and medroxyprogesterone acetate (2.5 mg daily) therapy in postmenopausal women is associated with increased risks of myocardial infarction, stroke, invasive breast cancer, pulmonary emboli, and deep-vein thrombosis. The risks identified in this study should be assumed to be similar with other hormonal regimens, including different dosages of these drugs as well as other estrogen/progestin combinations not studied in WHI, in the absence of comparable data to the contrary. If HRT is used, it should be prescribed in the lowest effective dosage and for the shortest duration consistent with treatment goals and risks for the individual women. (See Uses: Estrogen Replacement Therapy in the Estrogens General Statement 68:16.04.)

While there appears to be no increased risk of endometrial carcinoma in postmenopausal women receiving estrogen therapy for less than 1 year, prolonged estrogen therapy may be associated with an increased risk of such carcinoma. The risk of endometrial cancer reportedly is increased 2- to 12-fold in postmenopausal women receiving unopposed estrogen compared with those not receiving estrogens; such increased risk may depend on dosage and duration of estrogen therapy and may be increased 15- to 24-fold in women receiving long-term (5 years or more) estrogen therapy. Limited data indicate that a substantial increased risk of endometrial carcinoma may persist for up to 15 years following discontinuance of estrogen therapy. Results of several studies indicate that addition of a progestin (e.g., medroxyprogesterone acetate) to estrogen replacement therapy reduces the incidence of endometrial hyperplasia and risk of endometrial carcinoma in women with an intact uterus. In a randomized, double-blind, controlled, multicenter study in postmenopausal women, endometrial hyperplasia occurred in 20 or 1% or less of women receiving conjugated estrogens alone or in conjunction with medroxyprogesterone acetate, respectively. Although estrogen-associated risk of endometrial carcinoma is substantially reduced when estrogens are administered concomitantly with progestins, a risk still exists. Therefore, clinical evaluation of all menopausal women receiving estrogen therapy in conjunction with a progestin is essential. Existing data do not support addition of a progestin in women who have undergone hysterectomy and are receiving estrogen replacement therapy.

Clinical studies indicate that use of a progestin in conjunction with estrogen replacement therapy does not interfere with the efficacy of the estrogen in the management of vasomotor symptoms associated with menopause, treatment of vulvar and vaginal atrophy, or prevention of osteoporosis. However, addition of a progestin to estrogen therapy may adversely affect some metabolic effects associated with long-term estrogen therapy and potential risks of concomitant therapy may include adverse effects on lipid metabolism and glucose tolerance. Results of several clinical studies in postmenopausal women indicate that replacement therapy with unopposed conjugated estrogens may reduce LDL-cholesterol and increase HDL-cholesterol by about 8–15%; concomitant progestin therapy may blunt some of the favorable effects of estrogens on the lipid profile of menopausal women. (See Pharmacology in the Estrogens General Statement 68:16.04.) Data from several studies suggest that administration of a progestin concomitantly with estrogen therapy is associated with an increased risk of breast cancer beyond that associated with estrogen alone. (See Carcinogenicity in the Estrogens General Statement 68:16.04.)

• Contraception in Females

Medroxyprogesterone acetate (alone or in fixed combination with estradiol cypionate) is used parenterally as a long-acting contraceptive in women.

Medroxyprogesterone acetate (e.g., Depo-Provera® Contraceptive, depo-subQ provera 104®) is used parenterally for the prevention of conception. However, long-term use of parenteral medroxyprogesterone is associated with loss in bone mineral density (BMD). The loss of BMD in women of all ages and the possible impact on peak bone mass in adolescents should be considered when assessing the risks versus benefits of this contraceptive method. Parenteral medroxyprogesterone should be used as a long-term contraceptive method (e.g., longer than 2 years) *only* if other contraceptive methods are inadequate and the benefits are expected to outweigh the risks. (See Cautions: Precautions and Contraindications). Contraceptive measures other than parenteral medroxyprogesterone should be considered in women at risk for osteoporosis. When used according to the prescribed regimen (once every 3 months), parenteral medroxyprogesterone used alone provides almost completely effective contraception. The pregnancy rate in women using the drug alone generally is reported as less than 1 pregnancy per 100 women-years of use (as calculated via the Pearl index method) or as ranging from 0–0.7% during the first year of use (as calculated via life-table analysis). Compared with common contraceptive methods (e.g., estrogen-progestin combinations, condoms) other than intrauterine devices, implants, and sterilization, for which efficacy depends in large part on the reliability of appropriate use (patient compliance), contraceptive efficacy of parenteral medroxyprogesterone monotherapy depends on substantially less frequent patient-initiated actions (i.e., compliance with receipt of the injection only once every 3 months).

Medroxyprogesterone has been used extensively and effectively worldwide for many years as a contraceptive and has been recommended for this use by the World Health Organization (WHO) and the International Planned Parenthood Federation (IPPF); contraceptive use of medroxyprogesterone was added to the labeling approved by the US Food and Drug Administration (FDA) in the early 1990s. FDA's delay of approval of medroxyprogesterone for use as a contraceptive was based on questions of safety raised by studies in beagles in which the drug was associated with an increased incidence of mammary tumors; the availability of safer alternate methods for contraception and the lack of clear evidence that a substantial patient population in need of the drug exists in the US; the possibility that increased drug-induced bleeding disturbances may necessitate concomitant administration of an estrogen, imposing an additional risk and decreasing the benefits of progestin-only contraception; the possibility that exposure (possibly prolonged) of the fetus to the drug, if contraception fails, poses a risk of congenital malformation; and concerns that postmarketing surveillance for breast and cervical carcinoma might not provide meaningful data. Subsequently, the WHO Toxicology Review Panel, the IPPF, and several scientific advisory panels concluded that available evidence does not indicate a risk of adverse effects associated with parenteral medroxyprogesterone that would preclude its use as a contraceptive. These conclusions generally have been confirmed by various epidemiologic studies, including those conducted by WHO regarding the risk of various neoplasms and contraceptive steroid use. (See Cautions: Mutagenicity and Carcinogenicity and also see Pregnancy, Fertility, and Lactation.)

Medroxyprogesterone in a fixed combination with estradiol is used parenterally for the prevention of conception. In clinical trials with the fixed combination containing medroxyprogesterone acetate and estradiol cypionate (Lunelle®), the 12-month pregnancy rate reportedly was less than 0.2%. Because of limitations of the available data (e.g., loss to follow-up, lack of pregnancy testing, use of barrier contraceptives, concomitant drug therapy), it is not possible to estimate precisely the contraceptive failure rate, but the failure rate is likely to range from 0.1–1%. As with other estrogen-progestin contraceptives, the efficacy of medroxyprogesterone acetate in fixed combination with estradiol cypionate depends largely on adherence to the recommended dosage schedule. To ensure that the fixed combination of medroxyprogesterone acetate and estradiol cypionate is not inadvertently administered to a pregnant woman, the first injection should be given during the first 5 days of a normal menstrual period. (See Pregnancy, Fertility, and Lactation: Pregnancy, in Cautions.)

• Endometriosis

Medroxyprogesterone acetate (depo-subQ provera 104®) is used parenterally in the management of pain associated with endometriosis. In controlled clinical studies, medroxyprogesterone acetate (104 mg administered subcutaneously every 3 months for 6 months) was effective in relieving clinical symptoms (e.g., dysmenorrhea, dyspareunia, pelvic pain) and signs (e.g., pelvic tenderness, pelvic induration) of endometriosis. Long-term use of parenteral medroxyprogesterone is associated with loss in bone mineral density (BMD). The loss of BMD in women of all ages and the possible impact on peak bone mass in adolescents should be considered when assessing the risks versus benefits of therapy with medroxyprogesterone. (See Cautions: Precautions and Contraindications).

● *Amenorrhea and Uterine Bleeding*

Medroxyprogesterone acetate is used orally for the treatment of secondary amenorrhea and for the treatment of abnormal uterine bleeding caused by hormonal imbalance in patients without underlying organic pathology such as fibroids or uterine cancer.

● *Endometrial or Renal Carcinoma*

Medroxyprogesterone acetate is used parenterally as adjunctive and palliative therapy for the treatment of inoperable, recurrent, and metastatic endometrial carcinoma. The initial treatment of the early stages (I and II) of endometrial carcinoma is surgery, sometimes combined with radiation therapy. In advanced endometrial carcinoma that is no longer amenable to surgery or radiation, hormonal therapy with progestins or chemotherapy should be considered.

Although medroxyprogesterone has been used in the treatment of metastatic renal cell carcinoma, other agents are considered more effective for the systemic treatment of this cancer. (See Interferon Alfa 10:00 and Aldesleukin 10:00.)

● *Paraphilia in Males*

Medroxyprogesterone acetate has been used parenterally (e.g., 100–500 mg IM weekly) for the management of paraphilia (e.g., homosexual, heterosexual, or bisexual pedophilia; heterosexual voyeurism, sexual sadism, or exhibitionism; transvestism) in males†. The drug has been shown to decrease the frequency of erotic imagery and the intensity of erotic cravings in most of these males. Sexual deviance generally returns following discontinuance of the drug.

● *Other Uses*

Medroxyprogesterone acetate has been used for the management of both GnRH-dependent (central) and -independent (peripheral) forms of precocious puberty† and was the most widely used drug for the management of various forms of precocity. However, use of medroxyprogesterone in the management of central (true) precocious puberty† generally has been supplanted by GnRH analogs (e.g., leuprolide) because of the improved pharmacologic specificity and adverse effect profile of these latter drugs; occasionally, medroxyprogesterone continues to be used for central precocity in patients who do not tolerate GnRH analog therapy. The optimum therapeutic regimen for the management of familial male precocious puberty† (testotoxicosis) or for McCune-Albright syndrome†, both GnRH-independent forms of precocity, remains to be established, and medroxyprogesterone is one of several therapeutic regimens (e.g., medroxyprogesterone, testolactone/spironolactone, testolactone/flutamide, or ketoconazole for familial male precocity; medroxyprogesterone or testolactone for McCune-Albright syndrome) currently being employed. While comparative safety and efficacy have not been established by controlled studies, medroxyprogesterone may be less likely than other regimens to favorably affect growth rate and skeletal maturation and more likely to adversely affect adrenocortical function.

Medroxyprogesterone acetate also has been used in the management of postmenopausal symptoms in females†, obesity-hypoventilation syndrome† (Pickwickian syndrome), obstructive sleep apnea syndrome and hypersomnolence in adults†, hirsutism† and homozygous sickle-cell disease†.

DOSAGE AND ADMINISTRATION

● *Administration*

Medroxyprogesterone acetate (alone or in fixed combination with estrogens [i.e., conjugated estrogens, estradiol cypionate]) is administered orally, subcutaneously, or IM. When used as a contraceptive in females, medroxyprogesterone acetate is administered subcutaneously or IM; the drug is administered subcutaneously for the management of pain associated with endometriosis. Medroxyprogesterone acetate is administered IM in the treatment of cancer or male sexual deviance† (paraphilia). Because of the prolonged action, parenteral administration of the drug is not recommended for the treatment of secondary amenorrhea or abnormal uterine bleeding.

Medroxyprogesterone acetate injectable suspension (containing medroxyprogesterone acetate alone or in fixed combination with estradiol cypionate) must be vigorously shaken immediately before each use to ensure complete suspension of the drug(s). IM injection of medroxyprogesterone acetate alone (Depo-Provera® Contraceptive, Depo-Provera®, Medroxyprogesterone Acetate Contraceptive) or in combination with estradiol cypionate (Lunelle® Monthly Contraceptive) should be made deep into the gluteal, deltoid, or anterior thigh muscle. Subcutaneous injection of medroxyprogesterone acetate (depo-subQ provera 104®) is made into the anterior thigh or abdomen; the preparation for subcutaneous administration should not be administered IM.

Oral dosage preparations containing medroxyprogesterone acetate in combination with conjugated estrogens as monophasic or biphasic regimens are commercially available in a mnemonic dispensing package that is designed to aid the user in complying with the prescribed dosage schedule. The monophasic combination (Prempro®) is available in a 28-day dosage preparation that contains 28 tablets of conjugated estrogens (0.625 mg) in fixed combination with medroxyprogesterone acetate (2.5 or 5 mg). The monophasic combination (Prempro®) also is available in a 28-day dosage preparation that contains 28 tablets of conjugated estrogens USP (0.3 or 0.45 mg) in fixed combination with medroxyprogesterone acetate (1.5 mg). The biphasic combination (Premphase®) also is available in a 28-day dosage preparation that contains 14 tablets of conjugated estrogens (0.625 mg) and 14 tablets of conjugated estrogens (0.625 mg) in fixed combination with medroxyprogesterone acetate (5 mg).

● *Dosage*

Prevention of Endometrial Changes Associated with Estrogens

When medroxyprogesterone acetate is used in conjunction with estrogen replacement therapy, medroxyprogesterone may be administered in a monophasic (Prempro®) or biphasic (Premphase®) manner. In the monophasic regimen, oral conjugated estrogens is administered in a daily dosage of 0.3 mg in conjunction with oral medroxyprogesterone acetate in a daily dosage of 1.5 mg. Alternatively, conjugated estrogens is administered in a daily dosage of 0.45 mg in conjunction with medroxyprogesterone acetate in a daily dosage of 1.5 mg, or conjugated estrogens is administered in a daily dosage of 0.625 mg in conjunction with medroxyprogesterone acetate in a daily dosage of 2.5 or 5 mg. In the biphasic regimen (Premphase®) oral conjugated estrogens is administered in a daily dosage of 0.625 mg, while oral medroxyprogesterone acetate is administered in a dosage of 5 mg daily on days 15–28 of the cycle.

Contraception in Females

When medroxyprogesterone acetate injectable suspension (Depo-Provera® Contraceptive, Medroxyprogesterone Acetate Contraceptive) is used for the prevention of conception in women, the recommended dosage of medroxyprogesterone acetate is 150 mg IM every 3 months. The possibility of pregnancy should be excluded prior to administering the first dose of medroxyprogesterone and whenever more than 13 weeks has elapsed since the previous dose. To avoid inadvertent administration of the contraceptive to a pregnant woman, the initial injection should be given during the first 5 days of a normal menstrual cycle, within 5 days postpartum in those who do not breast-feed, or during the sixth postpartum week in women who breast-feed. (See Pregnancy, Fertility, and Lactation: Pregnancy, in Cautions.) Parenteral medroxyprogesterone should be used as a long-term contraceptive method (e.g., longer than 2 years) *only* if other contraceptive methods are inadequate and the benefits are expected to outweigh the risks. (See Cautions: Precautions and Contraindications.)

When medroxyprogesterone acetate injectable suspension (depo-subQ provera 104®) is used for the prevention of conception in women, the recommended dosage of medroxyprogesterone acetate is 104 mg administered subcutaneously every 3 months (12–14 weeks). The possibility of pregnancy should be excluded prior to administering the first dose of medroxyprogesterone and whenever more than 14 weeks has elapsed since the previous dose. To avoid inadvertent administration of the contraceptive to a pregnant woman, the initial injection should be given during the first 5 days of a normal menstrual cycle. In addition, the initial injection should be given no earlier than 6 weeks postpartum in women who breast-feed. (See Pregnancy, Fertility, and Lactation: Pregnancy, in Cautions.) When switching from other contraceptive methods, the manufacturer recommends that therapy with medroxyprogesterone acetate (depo-subQ provera 104®) be initiated in a manner that ensures continuous contraceptive coverage based on the mechanism of action of both methods (e.g., patients switching from combined estrogen-progestin contraceptives should be given an initial injection within 7 days after taking the last hormonally active tablet or removal of a transdermal patch or vaginal ring; patients switching from IM injections of medroxyprogesterone acetate [Depo-Provera® Contraceptive] to depo-subQ provera 104® should be given an initial injection of depo-subQ provera 104® within the dosing period recommended for the IM contraceptive preparation). Parenteral medroxyprogesterone should be used as a long-term contraceptive method (e.g., longer than 2 years) *only* if other contraceptive methods are inadequate and the benefits are expected to outweigh the risks. (See Cautions: Precautions and Contraindications.)

When Lunelle® is used for the prevention of conception in women, the usual dosage of medroxyprogesterone acetate is 25 mg (in fixed combination with 5 mg of estradiol cypionate per 0.5 mL) IM monthly. To avoid inadvertent administration of the contraceptive to a pregnant woman, the initial injection should be given during the first 5 days of a normal menstrual cycle or within 5 days of a complete first-trimester abortion. In addition, the initial injection should be given no earlier than 6 weeks postpartum in women who breast-feed and no earlier than 4 weeks postpartum in those who do not breast-feed. Subsequent injections should be given monthly (every 28–30 days, but no more than 33 days after the previous injection); the dosage schedule should be determined by the number of days between injections and not by bleeding episodes. If the patient has not adhered to the prescribed administration schedule (i.e., if more than 33 days have elapsed since the previous injection), an alternative (i.e., barrier) method of contraception should be instituted, and pregnancy ruled out, prior to continuation of Lunelle® (medroxyprogesterone acetate-estradiol cypionate) therapy. It should be noted that shortening of the injection interval may result in a change in menstrual pattern. When switching from other contraceptive methods, the manufacturer recommends that therapy with the fixed combination of medroxyprogesterone acetate and estradiol cypionate be initiated in a manner that ensures continuous contraceptive coverage based on the mechanism of action of both methods (e.g., patients switching from oral contraceptives should be given an initial injection within 7 days after taking the last hormonally active tablet).

Endometriosis

When medroxyprogesterone acetate injectable suspension (depo-subQ provera 104®) is used for the management of pain associated with endometriosis, the recommended dosage of medroxyprogesterone acetate is 104 mg administered subcutaneously every 3 months (12–14 weeks). The possibility of pregnancy should be excluded prior to administering the first dose of medroxyprogesterone and whenever more than 14 weeks has elapsed since the previous dose. To avoid inadvertent administration of the drug to a pregnant woman, the initial injection should be given during the first 5 days of a normal menstrual cycle. In addition, the initial injection should be given no earlier than 6 weeks postpartum in women who breast-feed. Efficacy of medroxyprogesterone acetate (depo-subQ provera 104®) for the management of pain associated with endometriosis was established in studies of 6 months' duration; data establishing continued efficacy with use beyond 6 months are lacking. Therapy with the drug for longer than 2 years is not recommended because of concerns about the potential long-term effects on bone density. If retreatment is considered following recurrence of endometriosis, bone density should be assessed. (See Effects on Bone under Cautions: Adverse Effects in Women.)

Amenorrhea and Uterine Bleeding

For the treatment of secondary amenorrhea, the usual oral dosage of medroxyprogesterone acetate is 5–10 mg daily for 5–10 days; although one manufacturer states that therapy may be initiated at any time, the drug is usually started during the assumed latter half (e.g., 16th to 21st day) of the menstrual cycle. In patients with a poorly developed endometrium, conventional estrogen therapy may be used in conjunction with medroxyprogesterone acetate. To induce optimum secretory transformation of an endometrium that has been adequately primed with endogenous or exogenous estrogen, one manufacturer recommends an oral dosage of 10 mg daily for 10 days. Progestin-induced withdrawal bleeding usually occurs within 3–7 days after discontinuing therapy with the drug.

For the treatment of abnormal uterine bleeding, 5–10 mg of medroxyprogesterone acetate may be given orally for 5–10 days beginning on the assumed or calculated 16th or 21st day of the menstrual cycle. When bleeding is caused by a deficiency of estrogen and progestin, as indicated by a poorly proliferative endometrium, estrogens should be used in conjunction with medroxyprogesterone acetate; if bleeding is controlled satisfactorily, 2 subsequent cycles of combined therapy should be given. To induce optimum secretory transformation of an endometrium that has been adequately primed with endogenous or exogenous

estrogen, one manufacturer recommends that 10 mg of the drug may be given orally for 10 days beginning on the calculated 16th day of the cycle. Progestin-induced withdrawal bleeding usually occurs within 3–7 days after discontinuing therapy with the drug. Patients with a history of recurrent episodes of abnormal uterine bleeding may benefit from planned menstrual cycling with medroxyprogesterone acetate.

Endometrial or Renal Carcinoma

For the adjunctive and palliative treatment of advanced, inoperable endometrial or renal carcinoma, an initial IM medroxyprogesterone acetate dosage of 400–1000 mg/week has been recommended. If improvement is noted within a few weeks or months and the disease appears to have stabilized, it may be possible to maintain response with as little as 400 mg/month. Medroxyprogesterone acetate is not recommended as primary therapy, but as adjunctive and palliative therapy in advanced inoperable cases including those with recurrent or metastatic disease.

Paraphilia in Males

For the management of paraphilia in males†, initial IM dosages of 200 mg 2 or 3 times daily or 500 mg weekly have been used. Dosage is generally adjusted according to patient response and tolerance and/or plasma testosterone concentration. Generally, the dose and/or frequency of administration is decreased to an effective maintenance level. In one study, maintenance dosages ranged from 100 mg once weekly to once monthly. Published protocols should be consulted for more specific dosage information in these males.

CAUTIONS

● Adverse Effects in Women

Genitourinary Effects

In women receiving parenteral medroxyprogesterone for contraception (alone or in fixed combination with estradiol cypionate) or the management of pain associated with endometriosis, the most common adverse effects are menstrual abnormalities. Irregular and unpredictable menstrual bleeding pattern, including spotting, occurs frequently during the first months of therapy with the drug. In women receiving IM medroxyprogesterone acetate in fixed combination with estradiol cypionate, about 59% experienced alterations in menstrual bleeding pattern (e.g., amenorrhea; frequent, irregular, prolonged, or infrequent bleeding) after 1 year of use; the incidence of irregular bleeding remained relatively constant at approximately 30% throughout the first year of use. If abnormal bleeding persists or is severe, appropriate steps to investigate the possibility of organic pathology should be undertaken, and appropriate therapy instituted as necessary.

Amenorrhea also occurs frequently in women receiving the drug for contraception or the management of pain associated with endometriosis, and as the duration of therapy increases the likelihood of intermenstrual bleeding decreases and that of amenorrhea increases; up to about 60 and 70% of women reportedly have amenorrhea after 1 and 2 years, respectively, of contraceptive therapy with medroxyprogesterone.

Although concomitant use of low doses of estrogens has been suggested to treat medroxyprogesterone-induced menstrual disturbances, the evidence for efficacy of this therapy is equivocal. Contraceptive use of the drug should be discontinued in women who do not tolerate irregular and unpredictable bleeding or amenorrhea.

Heavy or continuous vaginal bleeding may occur in some women receiving medroxyprogesterone, but rarely requires estrogen therapy. Impaired fertility persists long after discontinuance of the drug. (See Cautions: Pregnancy, Fertility, and Lactation.)

Effects on Bone

Use of parenteral medroxyprogesterone acetate (e.g., Depo-Provera® Contraceptive, depo-subQ provera 104®) reduces serum estrogen concentrations and is associated with loss of bone mineral density (BMD) as bone metabolism adjusts to lower serum estrogen concentrations. Bone loss is greater with increasing duration of medroxyprogesterone therapy and may not be completely reversible following discontinuance. In one clinical study, adult women receiving parenteral medroxyprogesterone (Depo-Provera® Contraceptive) for up to 5 years experienced a 5–6% loss in BMD of lumbar spine, total hip, and femoral neck; clinically important changes in BMD were not observed in a control group of women not receiving a hormonal contraceptive. The decline in BMD was more pronounced during the first 2 years of use of medroxyprogesterone; smaller declines were observed in subsequent years. Bone loss during the first 2 years of therapy with depo-subQ provera 104® is similar to that observed during the first 2 years of therapy with Depo-Provera® Contraceptive. In one comparative study, women receiving depo-subQ provera 104® for the management of endometriosis experienced a loss in BMD of lumbar spine and total hip of 0.03–1.2% over 6 months of therapy compared with a loss in BMD of 1.8–4.1% in women receiving leuprolide for the same period of time.

Evaluation of BMD 2 years after discontinuance of medroxyprogesterone indicates that BMD increases toward baseline values over this time period. However, longer duration of medroxyprogesterone therapy is associated with less complete recovery of BMD over the 2-year period after discontinuance of the drug. In an ongoing, open-label, self-selected, non-randomized study in adolescent females 12–18 years of age, use of parenteral medroxyprogesterone (Depo-Provera® Contraceptive) was associated with decreased bone density at the lumbar spine, total hip, and femoral neck; adolescents usually increase BMD during growth following menarche. Limited data indicate that BMD increases following discontinuance of medroxyprogesterone in these females. However, loss of BMD is of particular concern during adolescence and early adulthood.

It remains to be determined whether use of parenteral medroxyprogesterone in younger women will reduce peak bone mass and increase the risk of fractures secondary to osteoporosis later in life. Osteoporosis, including osteoporotic fractures, rarely has been reported during postmarketing surveillance of patients receiving IM medroxyprogesterone for contraception. (For information on women at risk for osteoporosis, see Cautions: Precautions and Contraindications.) The effect of BMD changes in women receiving medroxyprogesterone acetate in fixed combination with estradiol cypionate remains to be determined.

Effects on Body Weight

Weight changes (e.g., gain) also occur commonly during use of parenteral medroxyprogesterone (Depo Provera® Contraceptive, depo-subQ provera 104®). From an initial body weight averaging 61.8 kg, average weight gains of 2.45, 3.68, 6.27, and 7.5 kg occur after completion of 1, 2, 4, and 6 years of contraceptive use, respectively. In several large studies, 2–6% of women discontinued therapy with medroxyprogesterone alone or in fixed combination with estradiol cypionate because of excessive weight gain.

Other Adverse Effects

Medroxyprogesterone, like other progestins, may cause cholestatic jaundice, melasma or chloasma, and mental depression. Breast tenderness or galactorrhea has occasionally occurred. Alopecia, acne, and hirsutism have been reported rarely. Adverse CNS effects including nervousness, insomnia, somnolence, fatigue, and dizziness have occasionally occurred. Rarely, headache, hyperpyrexia, nausea, or jaundice, including neonatal jaundice, has been reported. Hypersensitivity reactions including urticaria, pruritus, angioedema, generalized rash (with or without pruritus), and anaphylactoid reactions and anaphylaxis have occasionally occurred in patients receiving the drug. Adverse local effects at the site of injection include residual lump, skin discoloration, and sterile abscess.

Other adverse effects reported during contraceptive use of medroxyprogesterone alone or in fixed combination with estradiol cypionate include abdominal pain or discomfort (e.g., bloating, enlarged abdomen), changes in mood or libido, emotional lability, anorgasmia, asthenia (weakness or fatigue), hot flushes (flashes), edema, absent hair growth, leukorrhea, vaginitis (e.g., candidiasis), vulvovaginal disorder, pelvic pain, breast pain, leg cramps, and backache. Infrequent (in less than 1% of patients) adverse effects associated with contraceptive use of medroxyprogesterone include seizures, appetite changes, GI disturbances, genitourinary infections, vaginal cysts, dyspareunia, paresthesia, chest pain, pulmonary embolus, anemia, and drowsiness. Other infrequent adverse effects associated with such use include syncope, dyspnea and asthma, tachycardia, fever, excessive sweating or body odor, dry skin, chills, increased or decreased libido, excessive thirst, hoarseness, pain at the injection site, blood dyscrasia, rectal bleeding, changes in breast size, breast lumps or nipple bleeding, axillary swelling, breast cancer, prevention of lactation, sensation of pregnancy, lack of return to fertility, accidental pregnancy, uterine hyperplasia, cervical cancer, thrombophlebitis, deep vein thrombosis, varicose veins, dysmenorrhea, paralysis, scleroderma, and osteoporosis.

Other adverse effects reported with noncontraceptive use of estrogen-progestin combination preparations include increased blood pressure in susceptible individuals, premenstrual-like syndrome, changes in libido or appetite, cystitis-like syndrome, backache, loss of scalp hair, erythema multiforme or nodosum, hemorrhagic skin eruption, and itching.

Allergic reactions reported with the injectable fixed combination of medroxyprogesterone acetate and estradiol cypionate (Lunelle®) have been principally dermatologic rather than respiratory in nature. If an anaphylactic reaction occurs, appropriate measures should be instituted; serious anaphylactic reactions require emergency medical treatment.

Cholecystitis and cholelithiasis have been reported in women receiving the fixed combination of medroxyprogesterone acetate and estradiol cypionate for up to 15 months. Other adverse effects reported with IM medroxyprogesterone acetate in fixed combination with estradiol cypionate generally are similar to those reported with estrogen-progestin oral contraceptives. For additional information on adverse effects associated with such combinations, see Cautions in Estrogen-Progestin Combinations 68:12.

Thromboembolic disorders including thrombophlebitis and pulmonary embolism have occurred in patients receiving medroxyprogesterone. An association between thrombophlebitis, pulmonary embolism, and cerebral thrombosis and embolism and use of estrogen-progestin combination preparations has been shown. (See Thromboembolic Disorders in Cautions: Cardiovascular Effects, in the Estrogen-Progestin Combinations 68:12.) The possibility that thromboembolic disorders may occur in patients receiving medroxyprogesterone should be considered and patients should be carefully observed for these effects during therapy with the drug.

Although available evidence suggests that an association exists between neuro-ocular lesions such as optic neuritis or retinal thrombosis and use of estrogen-progestin combination preparations, such a relationship has been neither confirmed nor refuted.

Use of estrogen-progestin combinations has also been associated with increased levels of coagulation factors VII, VIII, IX, and X. The possibility that these effects may occur in patients receiving medroxyprogesterone should be considered and patients should be carefully observed for these effects during therapy with the drug.

● Adverse Effects in Males

In males receiving parenteral medroxyprogesterone for the management of paraphilia, fatigue and weight gain occur commonly. Plasma testosterone concentrations decrease in most patients receiving the drug, and the decrease is generally associated with a diminution in the frequency and quality of erection and ejaculation; in one study, impotence generally occurred when plasma testosterone concentration decreased to one-fourth the pretreatment concentration. The drug is reportedly nonfeminizing in these males. Other adverse effects reported in these males include hot and cold flashes, headache, insomnia, nausea, and phlebitis.

● Precautions and Contraindications

Medroxyprogesterone acetate shares the toxic potentials of progestins, and the usual precautions of progestin therapy should be observed. Because oral contraceptive combinations contain progestins, the precautions associated with oral contraceptives should generally be considered in patients receiving progestins. (See Cautions in Estrogen-Progestin Combinations 68:12.) In addition, when medroxyprogesterone is used in conjunction with estrogens (i.e., conjugated estrogens, estradiol cypionate), the cautions, precautions, and contraindications associated with estrogens must be considered in addition to those associated with medroxyprogesterone.

Prior to initiation of therapy with medroxyprogesterone-containing preparations in women and annually thereafter during continued use (e.g., as a contraceptive, for the management of endometriosis, in conjunction with estrogen replacement therapy), a history should be obtained and physical examination performed, including special attention to the breasts and pelvic organs and a Papanicolaou test (Pap smear). Women receiving medroxyprogesterone-containing preparations should be given a copy of the patient labeling for the drug. In addition, women receiving the drug alone or in fixed combination with estradiol cypionate for contraceptive purposes or for management of endometriosis should be advised of anticipated effects on menstruation (e.g., initial irregular and unpredictable bleeding pattern), with the eventual development of amenorrhea in a large proportion of such women as use of the drug continues, and of the likelihood of weight gain during such use. (See Cautions: Adverse Effects Associated with Contraceptive Use in Women.) Women receiving parenteral medroxyprogesterone acetate alone or in fixed combination with estradiol cypionate for contraceptive purposes also should be advised that the contraceptive efficacy of such therapy depends on adherence to the recommended dosage schedule. Women with a family history of breast cancer or who have breast nodules should be monitored with particular care, and appropriate diagnostic measures should be employed if abnormal vaginal bleeding persists or recurs during therapy with the drug. In addition, women also should be advised that the contraceptive effect of parenteral medroxyprogesterone is prolonged, persisting long after the last dose of the drug. (See Pregnancy, Fertility, and Lactation: Fertility, in Cautions.) When medroxyprogesterone is to be used in conjunction with estrogen replacement therapy, potential risks may include adverse effects on lipid metabolism and glucose tolerance; addition of a progestin may adversely affect some beneficial metabolic effects associated with long-term estrogen therapy. Addition of medroxyprogesterone to estrogen replacement therapy appears to increase the risk of breast cancer beyond that associated with estrogen alone. (See Carcinogenicity in the Estrogens General Statement 68:16.04.) In addition, it should be considered that although estrogen-associated risk of endometrial carcinoma is substantially reduced when estrogens are administered concomitantly with progestins, such risk still exists, therefore, clinical evaluation of all menopausal women receiving estrogen therapy in conjunction with a progestin is essential. Diagnostic tests, including endometrial sampling when indicated, should be performed in all women who have undiagnosed, persistent, or abnormal vaginal bleeding.

Long-term use of parenteral medroxyprogesterone is associated with loss of bone mineral density (BMD). Parenteral medroxyprogesterone should be used as a long-term contraceptive method (e.g., longer than 2 years) *only* if other contraceptive methods are inadequate and the benefits are expected to outweigh the risks. Use of medroxyprogesterone (depo-subQ provera 104®) for the management of endometriosis for longer than 2 years is not recommended. BMD should be evaluated periodically when medroxyprogesterone is used long term; the patient's age (adult or adolescent) and skeletal maturity should be considered when evaluating BMD results. If retreatment with medroxyprogesterone is considered following recurrence of endometriosis, bone density should be assessed. Therapies other than parenteral medroxyprogesterone should be considered in women with pre-existing risk factors for osteoporosis; use of medroxyprogesterone may be an additional risk in women at risk for osteoporosis. Risk factors for osteoporosis include metabolic bone disease, drinking excessive amounts of alcohol, cigarette smoking, anorexia nervosa, a family history of osteoporosis, and long-term use of drugs that can reduce BMD (e.g., anticonvulsants, corticosteroids). Whether supplemental calcium and vitamin D can reduce BMD loss that occurs in women using long-term medroxyprogesterone remains to be determined; all women should have adequate intake of calcium and vitamin D.

If medroxyprogesterone is to be used for the treatment of cancer, patients should be referred to physicians who are actively engaged in investigation of the disease and are therefore familiar with the latest and most advantageous forms of therapy.

Medroxyprogesterone should be used with caution, and only with careful monitoring, in patients with conditions that might be aggravated by fluid retention (e.g., asthma, seizure disorders, migraine, or cardiac or renal dysfunction). The drug should also be used with caution in patients with a history of mental depression; medroxyprogesterone should be discontinued if depression recurs to a serious degree during therapy with the drug. While a causal relationship to the drug and the possible contribution of a preexisting condition remain unclear, the possibility of seizures during medroxyprogesterone use should be considered.

When breakthrough bleeding or irregular vaginal bleeding occurs during medroxyprogesterone therapy, nonfunctional causes should be considered. Adequate diagnostic procedures should be performed in patients with undiagnosed vaginal bleeding.

The manufacturers caution that the effect of long-term medroxyprogesterone therapy on pituitary, ovarian, adrenal, hepatic, or uterine function has not been determined. Diabetic patients should be carefully monitored during medroxyprogesterone therapy, since decreased glucose tolerance has been observed in women receiving estrogen-progestin combinations. Medroxyprogesterone may mask the onset of climacteric in women.

The clinician and the patient using medroxyprogesterone should be alert to the earliest signs and symptoms of thromboembolic and thrombotic disorders (e.g., thrombophlebitis, pulmonary embolism, cerebrovascular insufficiency, coronary occlusion, retinal thrombosis, mesenteric thrombosis). The drug should be discontinued immediately when any of these disorders occurs or is suspected. The clinician and patient also should be alert to the earliest manifestations of hepatic dysfunction (e.g., jaundice) during use of the drug. The drug should be discontinued and the patient's status reevaluated if such manifestations occur or are suspected. The manufacturer states that medroxyprogesterone acetate in fixed combination with estradiol cypionate (Lunelle®) should not be readministered to women in whom thromboembolic or thrombotic disorders have occurred or are suspected.

If unexplained, sudden or gradual, partial or complete loss of vision; proptosis or diplopia; papilledema; retinal vascular lesions; or migraine occur during

therapy with medroxyprogesterone, the drug should be discontinued and appropriate diagnostic and therapeutic measures instituted. If ocular examination reveals evidence of papilledema or retinal vascular lesions, medroxyprogesterone therapy should *not* be reinitiated.

The onset or exacerbation of migraine or development of headache with a new pattern that is recurrent, persistent, or severe requires evaluation of the cause before further administration of medroxyprogesterone acetate in fixed combination with estradiol cypionate for contraceptive purposes.

Medroxyprogesterone is contraindicated in patients with active thrombophlebitis or a current or past history of thromboembolic disorders or of cerebral vascular disease or apoplexy. The drug is also contraindicated in patients with undiagnosed vaginal bleeding, missed abortion, liver dysfunction or disease or with known or suspected malignancy of the genital organs, known sensitivity to the drug or any ingredient in the formulation, or known or suspected pregnancy or carcinoma of the breast, or for use as a pregnancy test. The manufacturer states that use of medroxyprogesterone acetate in combination with estradiol cypionate for contraceptive purposes also is contraindicated in patients with carcinoma of the endometrium, severe hypertension, diabetes mellitus with vascular involvement, headaches with focal neurologic symptoms, valvular heart disease with complications, and those 35 years of age or older who smoke 15 cigarettes or more daily. Women receiving medroxyprogesterone acetate in fixed combination with estradiol cypionate should be strongly advised not to smoke.

● *Mutagenicity and Carcinogenicity*

Administration of medroxyprogesterone to beagles has been associated with the development of mammary nodules, some of which were malignant. Although nodules occasionally occurred in control beagles, they were intermittent in nature; nodules in drug-treated beagles were larger, more numerous, persistent, and occasionally malignant with metastases. The clinical relevance of these findings to humans has not been established. In addition, there is evidence of species differences in the response of beagles and humans to medroxyprogesterone; because of these species differences, some experts state that it is not possible to draw conclusions from the observations in beagles. In long-term (10 years) toxicology studies in monkeys, 2 of the animals developed undifferentiated carcinoma of the uterus following administration of 150 mg/kg every 90 days. The relevance of this finding has been questioned since progestins are thought to protect against the development of endometrial cancer and because of the unusual nature of the cancer in these monkeys; additional study is needed to determine the relevance to humans. Transient mammary nodules occurred in control monkeys and those receiving 3 or 30 mg/kg every 90 days, but not in those receiving 150 mg/kg. At sacrifice, nodules still existed in 3 monkeys; histopathologic examination showed the nodules to be hyperplastic. No evidence of uterine or breast abnormalities was revealed in rats.

Analysis of worldwide epidemiologic evidence on the relationship between the risk of breast cancer and postmenopausal hormone replacement therapy and results of most, but not all, studies indicate that prolonged use of postmenopausal hormone replacement therapy is associated with an increased risk of breast cancer in current or recent recipients. In the Women's Health Initiative (WHI) study evaluating estrogen/progestin therapy, there was a small increase in the risk of breast cancer in postmenopausal women receiving hormone replacement therapy (i.e., conjugated estrogens 0.625 mg in conjunction with medroxyprogesterone acetate 2.5 mg daily) compared with those receiving placebo. (See Cautions: Mutagenicity and Carcinogenicity, in the Estrogens General Statement 68:16.04.) The increase in breast cancer risk was apparent after 4 years of estrogen/progestin therapy, and the risk appeared to be cumulative. Results of a large (involving more than 100,000 women) prospective cohort study (the Nurses' Health Study) in postmenopausal women who received conjugated estrogens indicated that while there appears to be no increased risk of breast cancer in postmenopausal women with prior or relatively short-term use of estrogens, long-term (exceeding 5 years) estrogen therapy may be associated with an increased risk of such carcinoma, especially in women 55 years and older. Addition of progestins to estrogen replacement therapy appears to increase the risk of breast cancer beyond that associated with estrogen alone. (See: Carcinogenicity in the Estrogens General Statement 68:16.04.)

In one retrospective study in black women who received sterile medroxyprogesterone acetate suspension for contraception, there was no evidence of an increased risk of developing cancer of the breast, uterine corpus, or ovary. Although the study indicated that there was no strong association between medroxyprogesterone and these cancers, limitations of the study included inability to detect a weak carcinogenic effect of the drug or a carcinogenic effect that would become evident only after a long latent period.

Long-term case-controlled studies conducted by the World Health Organization (WHO) in other users of medroxyprogesterone contraception have revealed slight or no evidence of increased overall risk of breast cancer and no evidence of increased overall risk of ovarian or cervical cancer. While there also was no evidence of an increased overall risk of liver cancer among users in populations in which hepatitis B infection was endemic, the relevance of these findings to populations in which this infection is not endemic currently is not known since relative risks of live cancer associated with use of oral estrogen-progestin combinations have been estimated to be lower among populations in which this infection is endemic compared with nonendemic populations. In the case-control study assessing the risk of breast cancer, there was evidence of an increased risk of breast cancer within the first 4 years of initial exposure to medroxyprogesterone, principally among those younger than 35 years of age. The relative risk estimated for users whose first exposure to the drug was within the previous 4 years was 2.19 times that in nonusers; this would represent an increase in the annual risk of breast cancer from 26.7 cases per 100,000 women among nonusers to 58.5 cases per 100,000 women among medroxyprogesterone users. Thus, the attributable annual risk for breast cancer among users in the US is 3.18 per 10,000 women. In the case-control study assessing the risk of cervical cancer, while there was no evidence of an increased overall risk of this cancer among medroxyprogesterone users (even after more than 12 years since initial use), there was a statistically insignificant increase in the relative risk (to 1.22–1.28) of invasive squamous cell carcinoma among users who were first exposed to the drug before age 35; however, no trends in risk with duration of use or times since initial or most recent use were observed.

There also is evidence from a long-term case-control study conducted by WHO in users of medroxyprogesterone contraception of a prolonged (e.g., for at least 8 years after discontinuance of the drug) protective effect manifested as a reduced risk of endometrial cancer among users; however, this possible protective effect of medroxyprogesterone may be reduced by concomitant estrogen use.

● Pregnancy, Fertility, and Lactation

Pregnancy

Although progestins have been used beginning in the first trimester of pregnancy to prevent habitual abortion or to treat threatened abortion, there is no adequate evidence from well-controlled studies to substantiate the efficacy of progestins for these uses; however, there is evidence of potential adverse effects on the fetus when these drugs are administered within the first 4 months of pregnancy. In addition, in most women, the cause of abortion is a defective ovum, which progestins could not be expected to influence. Because of their uterine-relaxant effects, progestins may delay spontaneous abortion of fertilized defective ova. Masculinization of the female fetus has reportedly occurred when progestins were used during pregnancy. Clitoral hypertrophy and fusion of the labia have been reported in a few female neonates born to women who had received medroxyprogesterone during pregnancy; hypospadias in male neonates born to women receiving progestational agents occurs at approximately twice the rate of occurrence in male neonates born to women not receiving the drugs. Postpartum bleeding, postabortal bleeding, and missed abortion have been reported in women who received the drug during pregnancy. An association between intrauterine exposure to female sex hormones and congenital anomalies, including cardiovascular and limb defects, has been suggested. (See Cautions: Pregnancy, Fertility, and Lactation, in Estrogen-Progestin Combinations 68:12.) Use of progestins, including medroxyprogesterone, is not recommended during the first 4 months of pregnancy. If a woman becomes pregnant while receiving medroxyprogesterone or is inadvertently exposed to the drug during the first 4 months of pregnancy, she should be advised of the potential risks to the fetus. To increase ensurance that the drug is not administered inadvertently to a pregnant woman, it is important that use of the drug be initiated only during the first 5 days after onset of normal menses, within 5 days postpartum if the woman is not lactating, or at the sixth postpartum week if she is. If more than 13–14 weeks has elapsed since the last dose of medroxyprogesterone, appropriate assessment should be performed to ensure that the woman is not pregnant prior to administering a dose.

When medroxyprogesterone is used as a contraceptive, unintended pregnancies that occur within 1–2 months after IM injection of the drug may be characterized by impaired fetal growth as evidenced by low birthweights, which theoretically could result in an increased risk of neonatal death. However, the attributable risk of this adverse effect is low because such pregnancies are unlikely. The risk of low birthweight was particularly evident when conception was estimated to occur within 4 weeks of medroxyprogesterone injection. While an increase in polysyndactyly, particularly among offspring of women younger than 30 years of age, and chromosomal anomalies also have been observed in neonates born to women who received IM medroxyprogesterone contraception, the unrelated nature of these effects, the lack of confirmation from other studies, the prolonged period of time between use of the drug and conception in many cases, and chance effects resulting from the multiple statistical comparisons applied make an association between these effects and the drug unlikely.

The possibility of ectopic pregnancy should be considered in any women using medroxyprogesterone contraception if pregnancy occurs or the woman develops complaints of severe abdominal pain.

Medroxyprogesterone should *not* be used to induce withdrawal bleeding as a test for pregnancy.

Fertility

Impairment of fertility persists for prolonged periods after the last dose of parenteral medroxyprogesterone in women receiving the drug for contraception or the management of endometriosis. Life-table analysis of data from one study in which follow-up was available in 61% of participants who received IM medroxyprogesterone indicated that, in women who intend to become pregnant following discontinuance of the drug, 68, 83, and 93% of women who successfully conceive are likely to do so within 12, 15, and 18 months, respectively, after the last dose. The median time to conception for those who do conceive is 10 months (range: 4–31 months) after the last dose and is unrelated to the duration of contraceptive medroxyprogesterone use. However, pregnancy (e.g., unintended) can occur rarely within 4 weeks after a dose of the drug. The median time to ovulation in women who received several doses of depo-subQ provera 104® was 10 months after the last injection; 80% of women ovulated within 1 year after the last injection. Ovulation may occur as early as 14 weeks after a single dose of depo-subQ provera 104®.

Lactation

Progestins reportedly are distributed into milk, and detectable amounts of medroxyprogesterone have been identified in milk of lactating women receiving the drug IM. Milk composition, quality, and volume are not affected adversely by medroxyprogesterone use. While the manufacturers warn that the possible effects of progestins in milk on nursing infants have not been determined, study of infants exposed to the drug via breast milk has revealed no evidence of adverse developmental or behavioral effects through puberty.

The effects of combined medroxyprogesterone acetate and estradiol cypionate therapy on lactation and nursing infants have not been established. However, because adverse effects such as jaundice and breast enlargement have been reported in nursing infants of women receiving estrogen-progestin combination oral contraceptives, the usual cautions and precautions associated with estrogens must be considered in lactating women receiving IM medroxyprogesterone acetate in fixed combination with estradiol cypionate. The manufacturer states that use of estrogen-progestin combination contraceptives should be deferred until 6 weeks postpartum. For additional information, see Cautions: Pregnancy, Fertility, and Lactation, in Estrogen-Progestin Combinations 68:12.

LABORATORY TEST INTERFERENCES

The manufacturers caution that estrogen-progestin combinations have caused abnormal thyroid function test results. (See Effects on Thyroid in Cautions: Endocrine and Metabolic Effects, in Estrogen-Progestin Combinations 68:12.) The manufacturers also caution that estrogen-progestin combinations have altered the metyrapone test (see Laboratory Test Interferences in Estrogen-Progestin Combinations 68:12), and that these combinations have altered liver function test results (see Cautions: Hepatic Effects, in Estrogen-Progestin Combinations 68:12). These combinations have also caused decreased pregnanediol excretion.

The manufacturers state that the pathologist should be advised of medroxyprogesterone use when relevant specimens from a patient exposed to the drug are submitted.

PHARMACOLOGY

Medroxyprogesterone shares the pharmacologic actions of the progestins. In women with adequate endogenous estrogen, medroxyprogesterone transforms a proliferative endometrium into a secretory one. Medroxyprogesterone has been shown to have slight androgenic activity in animals. Anabolic effects have also been reported, but the drug apparently lacks appreciable estrogenic activity in humans. In animals, the drug exhibits pronounced adrenocorticoid activity, but a clinically important effect has not been observed in humans. Medroxyprogesterone inhibits the secretion of pituitary gonadotropins following usual IM or subcutaneous dosages (e.g., 150 or 104 mg every 3 months), thus preventing follicular maturation and ovulation and resulting in endometrial thinning; these effects result in contraceptive activity. Available evidence indicates that these effects do not occur following oral administration of usual dosages (i.e., 5–10 mg daily as single daily doses) of the drug. High doses of medroxyprogesterone inhibit pituitary secretion of luteinizing hormone (LH) and follicle-stimulating hormone (FSH), and will prevent cyclic gonadotropin surges that occur during the normal menstrual cycle. It has been suggested that the drug acts at the hypothalamus since it does not suppress the release of LH and FSH following administration of gonadotropin-releasing hormone and since basal concentrations of LH and FSH remain within the low normal range when the drug is used as a contraceptive. Although the mechanism of action has not been determined, medroxyprogesterone has antineoplastic activity against some cancers (e.g., endometrial carcinoma, renal carcinoma).

CHEMISTRY AND STABILITY

● Chemistry

Medroxyprogesterone acetate is a synthetic progestin. Medroxyprogesterone acetate is a derivative of 17 α-hydroxyprogesterone that differs structurally by the addition of a 6 α-methyl group and a 17 α-acetate group.

Medroxyprogesterone acetate occurs as a white to off-white, odorless, crystalline powder and is insoluble in water and sparingly soluble in alcohol. Medroxyprogesterone acetate is commercially available alone and in fixed combination with estrogens (i.e., conjugated estrogens, estradiol cypionate). Medroxyprogesterone acetate suspension is a sterile suspension of the drug in a suitable aqueous medium. The commercially available medroxyprogesterone acetate injectable suspension containing 150 mg/mL also contains polyethylene glycol 3350, polysorbate 80, sodium chloride, and parabens as a preservative; the sterile suspension containing 400 mg/mL also contains polyethylene glycol 3350, sodium sulfate, and myristyl-gamma-picolinium chloride as a preservative. The commercially available medroxyprogesterone acetate injectable suspension containing 104 mg/0.65 mL contains polyethylene glycol, sodium chloride, povidone, polysorbate 80, parabens as a preservative, methionine, and phosphate buffers. The commercially available injection containing medroxyprogesterone acetate in fixed combination with estradiol cypionate is available as a sterile aqueous suspension; the injection also contains polyethylene glycol, polysorbate (Tween®) 80, sodium chloride, and parabens as preservatives. Sodium hydroxide and/or hydrochloric acid may be added during the manufacture of the sterile suspensions to adjust the pH to 3–7.

● Stability

Sterile medroxyprogesterone acetate suspensions should be stored at 20–25°C. The sterile injectable suspension containing medroxyprogesterone acetate in fixed combination with estradiol cypionate should be stored at 25°C, but may be exposed to temperatures ranging from 15–30°C. Medroxyprogesterone acetate tablets should be stored in well-closed containers at 20–25°C.

PREPARATIONS

Excipients in commercially available drug preparations may have clinically important effects in some individuals; consult specific product labeling for details.

medroxyPROGESTERone Acetate

Oral

Tablets	2.5 mg*	Medroxyprogesterone Acetate Tablets
		Provera® (scored), Pfizer
	5 mg*	Medroxyprogesterone Acetate Tablets
		Provera® (scored), Pfizer
	10 mg*	Medroxyprogesterone Acetate Tablets
		Provera® (scored), Pfizer

Parenteral

Injectable suspension	104 mg/0.65 mL	depo-subQ provera 104® (available in prefilled syringes with UltraSafe Passive® needle guard), Pfizer
	150 mg/mL*	Depo-Provera® Contraceptive, Pfizer
		Medroxyprogesterone Acetate Contraceptive
	400 mg/mL	Depo-Provera®, Pfizer

* available from one or more manufacturer, distributor, and/or repackager by generic (nonproprietary) name

medroxyPROGESTERone Acetate Combinations

Oral

Tablets, monophasic regimen	1.5 mg with Conjugated Estrogens 0.3 mg (28 tablets)	Prempro®, Wyeth
	1.5 mg with Conjugated Estrogens 0.45 mg (28 tablets)	Prempro®, Wyeth
	2.5 mg with Conjugated Estrogens 0.625 mg (28 tablets)	Prempro®, Wyeth
	5 mg with Conjugated Estrogens 0.625 mg (28 tablets)	Prempro®, Wyeth
Tablets, biphasic regimen	5 mg with Conjugated Estrogens 0.625 mg (14 tablets) and Conjugated Estrogens 0.625 mg (14 tablets)	Premphase®, Wyeth

Parenteral

| Injectable suspension | 25 mg/0.5 mL with Estradiol Cypionate 5 mg/0.5 mL | Lunelle® Monthly Contraceptive Injection, Pfizer |

† Use is not currently included in the labeling approved by the US Food and Drug Administration.

Selected Revisions January 1, 2009, © Copyright, April 1, 1965, American Society of Health-System Pharmacists, Inc.

Norethindrone Acetate

68:32 · PROGESTINS

■ Norethindrone acetate is a synthetic progestin.

USES

Norethindrone acetate is used for the treatment of secondary amenorrhea and for the treatment of abnormal uterine bleeding caused by hormonal imbalance in patients without underlying organic pathology such as fibroids or uterine cancer. The drug also is used for the treatment of endometriosis.

For the use of low-dose norethindrone as a progestin-only oral contraceptive, see Progestins 68:12. For the use of norethindrone or norethindrone acetate in combination with estrogens as an oral contraceptive, see Estrogen-Progestin Combinations 68:12.

DOSAGE AND ADMINISTRATION

● Administration

Norethindrone acetate is administered orally.

● Dosage

Amenorrhea and Uterine Bleeding

In establishing the dosage cycle for the treatment of secondary amenorrhea or abnormal uterine bleeding, the menstrual cycle is considered to be 28 days. The first day of bleeding is counted as the first day of the cycle. For the treatment of secondary amenorrhea or abnormal uterine bleeding, the usual oral dosage of norethindrone acetate is 2.5–10 mg daily for 5–10 days, beginning during the assumed latter half of the menstrual cycle to produce an optimum secretory transformation of an endometrium that has been adequately primed with endogenous or exogenous estrogen. Progestin-induced withdrawal bleeding usually occurs within 3–7 days after discontinuing therapy with the drug. Patients with a history of recurrent episodes of uterine bleeding may benefit from planned cycling with the drug.

Endometriosis

For the treatment of endometriosis, the usual initial oral dosage of norethindrone acetate is 5 mg daily for 14 consecutive days. Norethindrone acetate therapy may be increased by 2.5 mg daily at 14-day intervals until a maximum dosage of 15 mg daily is reached. Daily therapy may then be continued consecutively (no cyclic drug-free periods) for 6–9 months; if annoying breakthrough bleeding occurs, therapy should be temporarily discontinued.

CAUTIONS

● Adverse Effects

Norethindrone, like other progestins, may cause breakthrough bleeding, spotting, changes in menstrual flow, amenorrhea, changes in cervical erosion and secretions, edema, weight gain or loss, cholestatic jaundice, allergic rash with or without pruritus, melasma or chloasma, and mental depression.

An association between thrombophlebitis, pulmonary embolism, and cerebral thrombosis and embolism and use of estrogen-progestin combination preparations has been shown. (See Thromboembolic Disorders in Cautions: Cardiovascular Effects, in Estrogen-Progestin Combinations 68:12.) The possibility that thromboembolic disorders may occur in patients receiving norethindrone should be considered and patients should be carefully observed for these effects during therapy with the drug. Although available evidence suggests that an association exists between neuro-ocular lesions such as optic neuritis or retinal thrombosis and use of estrogen-progestin combination preparations, such a relationship has been neither confirmed nor refuted. Increased blood pressure in susceptible individuals, premenstrual-like syndrome, changes in libido or appetite, cystitis-like syndrome, headache, nervousness, dizziness, fatigue, backache, hirsutism, loss of scalp hair, erythema multiforme or nodosum, hemorrhagic skin eruption, and itching have occurred in patients receiving estrogen-progestin combination preparations. Use of estrogen-progestin combinations has also been associated with increased levels of coagulation factors VII, VIII, IX, and X. The possibility that these effects may occur in patients receiving norethindrone should be considered and patients should be carefully observed for these effects during therapy with the drug.

● Precautions and Contraindications

Norethindrone shares the toxic potentials of progestins, and the usual precautions of progestin therapy should be observed. Because oral contraceptive combinations contain progestins, the precautions associated with oral contraceptives should generally be considered in patients receiving progestins. (See Cautions in Estrogen-Progestin Combinations 68:12.) Prior to initiation of therapy with norethindrone in women, a physical examination should be performed, including special attention to the breasts and pelvic organs and a Papanicolaou test (Pap smear). Women receiving norethindrone should be given a copy of the patient labeling for the drug.

Norethindrone should be used with caution, and only with careful monitoring, in patients with conditions that might be aggravated by fluid retention (e.g., asthma, seizure disorders, migraine, or cardiac or renal dysfunction). The drug should also be used with caution in patients with a history of mental depression; norethindrone should be discontinued if depression recurs to a serious degree during therapy with the drug.

When breakthrough bleeding or irregular vaginal bleeding occurs during norethindrone therapy, nonfunctional causes should be considered. Adequate diagnostic procedures should be performed in patients with undiagnosed vaginal bleeding.

The manufacturers caution that the effect of long-term norethindrone therapy on pituitary, ovarian, adrenal, hepatic, or uterine function has not been determined. Diabetic patients should be carefully monitored during norethindrone therapy, since decreased glucose tolerance has been observed in women receiving estrogen-progestin combinations. Norethindrone may mask the onset of climacteric in women.

The clinician and the patient using norethindrone should be alert to the earliest signs and symptoms of thromboembolic and thrombotic disorders (e.g., thrombophlebitis, pulmonary embolism, cerebrovascular insufficiency, coronary occlusion, retinal thrombosis, mesenteric thrombosis). The drug should be discontinued immediately when any of these disorders occurs or is suspected.

If unexplained, sudden or gradual, partial or complete loss of vision; proptosis or diplopia; papilledema; retinal vascular lesions; or migraine occur during therapy with norethindrone, the drug should be discontinued and appropriate diagnostic and therapeutic measures instituted. Because steroidal hormones are metabolized in the liver, norethindrone should be used with caution in patients with impaired liver function.

Norethindrone is contraindicated in patients with thrombophlebitis, thromboembolic disorders, cerebral apoplexy, or a history of these conditions. The drug is also contraindicated in patients with undiagnosed vaginal bleeding, missed abortion, known sensitivity to the drug or any ingredient in the formulation, markedly impaired liver function or liver disease, or carcinoma of the breast or for use as a pregnancy test.

● Mutagenicity and Carcinogenicity

The carcinogenic and mutagenic potentials of norethindrone have not been specifically determined.

Administration of medroxyprogesterone to beagles has been associated with the development of mammary nodules, some of which were malignant. Although nodules occasionally occurred in control beagles, they were intermittent in nature; nodules in drug-treated beagles were larger, more numerous, persistent, and occasionally malignant with metastases. The clinical relevance of these findings to humans has not been established. For additional information on the carcinogenic potential of progestins, see Cautions: Mutagenicity and Carcinogenicity, in Medroxyprogesterone Acetate 68:32.

● Pregnancy, Fertility, and Lactation
Pregnancy

Although progestins have been used beginning in the first trimester of pregnancy to prevent habitual abortion or to treat threatened abortion, there is no adequate evidence from well-controlled studies to substantiate the efficacy of progestins for these uses; however, there is evidence of potential adverse effects on the fetus when these drugs are administered during the first 4 months of pregnancy. In addition, in most women, the cause of abortion is a defective ovum, which progestins could not be expected to influence. Because of their uterine-relaxant effects, progestins may delay spontaneous abortion of fertilized defective ova. Masculinization of the female fetus has reportedly occurred when progestins were used during pregnancy. Clitoral hypertrophy and fusion of the labia have been reported in a few female neonates born to women who had received medroxyprogesterone during pregnancy; hypospadias in male neonates born to women receiving progestational agents occurs at approximately twice the rate of occurrence in male neonates born to women not receiving the drugs. An association between intrauterine exposure to female sex hormones and congenital anomalies, including cardiovascular and limb defects, has been suggested. (See Cautions: Pregnancy, Fertility, and Lactation, in Estrogen-Progestin Combinations 68:12.) Use of progestins, including norethindrone, is not recommended during the first 4 months of pregnancy. If a woman becomes pregnant while receiving norethindrone or is inadvertently exposed to the drug during the first 4 months of pregnancy, she should be advised of the potential risks to the fetus.

Norethindrone should *not* be used to induce withdrawal bleeding as a test for pregnancy.

Lactation

Progestins are reportedly distributed into milk. The manufacturers warn that the possible effects of progestins in milk on nursing infants have not been determined.

PHARMACOLOGY

Norethindrone shares the pharmacologic actions of the progestins. In women with adequate endogenous estrogen, norethindrone transforms a proliferative endometrium into a secretory one. Norethindrone has been shown to have some estrogenic, androgenic, and anabolic activity. The drug inhibits the secretion of pituitary gonadotropins at usual dosages and thus prevents follicular maturation and ovulation.

CHEMISTRY AND STABILITY

● Chemistry

Norethindrone is a synthetic progestin. The drug is the 17α-ethinyl derivative of 19-nortestosterone which differs structurally from norethynodrel only in the position of the double bond in the A ring of the steroid. Norethindrone acetate is the acetic acid ester of norethindrone.

Norethindrone acetate occurs as a white to creamy white, odorless, crystalline powder and is practically insoluble in water and soluble in alcohol. Norethindrone acetate is about twice as potent as norethindrone.

● Stability

Norethindrone acetate tablets should be stored in well-closed containers at room temperature (approximately 25°C).

PREPARATIONS

Excipients in commercially available drug preparations may have clinically important effects in some individuals; consult specific product labeling for details.

Norethindrone Acetate

Oral		
Tablets	5 mg*	Aygestin® (scored), Duramed
		Norethindrone Acetate Tablets (scored)

* available from one or more manufacturer, distributor, and/or repackager by generic (nonproprietary) name

Selected Revisions January 1, 2009, © Copyright, April 1, 1965, American Society of Health-System Pharmacists, Inc.

Progesterone

68:32 · PROGESTINS

■ Progesterone is a naturally occurring progestin secreted by the corpus luteum and is the prototype of the progestins.

USES

Progesterone is used orally to reduce the incidence of endometrial hyperplasia in postmenopausal women receiving estrogen replacement therapy.

Progesterone is used orally or intravaginally for the management of secondary amenorrhea.

Progesterone is used intravaginally to support embryo implantation and early pregnancy by supplementing corpus luteal function as part of assisted reproductive technology (ART) treatment of infertile women. Efficacy of progesterone vaginal insert for this indication has not been established in women 35 years of age or older.

Progesterone is used parenterally for the treatment of amenorrhea and for the treatment of abnormal uterine bleeding caused by hormonal imbalance in patients without underlying organic pathology such as fibroids or uterine cancer. Progesterone also is used parenterally to support embryo implantation and early pregnancy by supplementing corpus luteal function as part of ART treatment† of infertile women.

DOSAGE AND ADMINISTRATION

● Administration

Progesterone is administered by orally, intravaginally, and by IM injection.

Progesterone capsules are administered orally once daily at bedtime. Women who have difficulty swallowing the capsules should be advised to swallow progesterone capsules while in an upright position and with adequate amounts of fluid (e.g., a glass of water). Administration at bedtime may alleviate some of the adverse effects (e.g., dizziness, blurred vision) associated with the drug.

Progesterone vaginal gel should *not* be administered concurrently with other intravaginal preparations. If therapy with another agent administered intravaginally is needed, such therapy should be administered 6 hours before or 6 hours after progesterone vaginal gel.

Concomitant use of progesterone vaginal inserts with other preparations that are administered intravaginally is *not* recommended. Although specific studies have not been undertaken, the possibility exists that concomitant administration of a progesterone vaginal insert with another preparation administered intravaginally may alter the release and absorption of progesterone from the vaginal insert.

● Dosage
Amenorrhea

When progesterone capsules are used in the management of secondary amenorrhea, the recommended dosage of progesterone is 400 mg once daily at bedtime for 10 days.

When progesterone vaginal gel is used for the management of secondary amenorrhea, the contents of one prefilled applicator of progesterone 4% vaginal gel (approximately 1.125 g of gel containing 45 mg of progesterone) should be inserted intravaginally every other day for a total of 6 doses. Women who do not respond to the 4% gel may be given progesterone 8% vaginal gel. For these women, the contents of one prefilled applicator of the 8% vaginal gel (approximately 1.125 g of gel containing 90 mg of progesterone) should be inserted intravaginally every other day for a total of 6 doses. Women who require the higher dose should receive the 8% vaginal gel; increasing the volume of the 4% gel will not achieve the same progesterone concentrations as administration of the 8% gel.

When parenteral progesterone is used for the treatment of amenorrhea, the usual dosage of progesterone is 5–10 mg administered IM daily for 6–8 days. When sufficient ovarian activity is present to produce a proliferative endometrium, withdrawal bleeding will usually occur within 48–72 hours after discontinuing therapy with the drug. Spontaneous normal cycles may occur in some patients after a single course of therapy.

Assisted Reproductive Technology Treatment

When progesterone vaginal gel is used as part of an assisted reproductive technology (ART) treatment regimen in women who require progesterone supplementation, the contents of one prefilled applicator of progesterone 8% vaginal gel (approximately 1.125 g of gel containing 90 mg of progesterone) should be inserted intravaginally once daily. When progesterone vaginal gel is used in women with partial or complete ovarian failure who require progesterone replacement, the contents of one prefilled applicator of progesterone 8% vaginal gel (approximately 1.125 g of gel containing 90 mg of progesterone) should be inserted intravaginally twice daily. If pregnancy occurs, treatment with progesterone gel may be continued until placental autonomy is achieved, up to 10–12 weeks.

When progesterone vaginal inserts are used as part of an ART treatment regimen in women younger than 35 years of age, one vaginal insert containing 100 mg of progesterone is inserted intravaginally 2 or 3 times daily, starting at oocyte retrieval. Therapy may be continued for up to 10 weeks. The appropriate dosage for women 35 years of age or older has not been established.

Prevention of Endometrial Changes Associated with Estrogens

When progesterone capsules are used in conjunction with estrogen replacement therapy, progesterone is administered in a dosage of 200 mg once daily at bedtime for 12 consecutive days (e.g., days 17–28) of the 28-day cycle.

Uterine Bleeding

When parenteral progesterone is used for the treatment of abnormal uterine bleeding, the usual dosage of progesterone is 5–10 mg administered IM daily for 6 days. When estrogen therapy is used concomitantly with progesterone, progesterone therapy is usually initiated after 2 weeks of estrogen therapy. Therapy with progesterone is usually discontinued if menses occurs during the series of injections.

CAUTIONS

● Adverse Effects

Adverse effects reported in patients receiving oral progesterone include dizziness, breast pain, headache, abdominal pain, fatigue, viral infection, abdominal distention, musculoskeletal pain, emotional lability, irritability, and upper respiratory tract infection. Extreme dizziness and/or drowsiness, blurred vision, slurred speech, difficulty walking, loss of consciousness, vertigo, confusion, disorientation, and shortness of breath have been reported in a few women receiving the drug. Hypotension and syncope have occurred rarely in women receiving progesterone capsules.

Adverse effects reported in patients receiving progesterone vaginal gel include breast pain/enlargement, somnolence, constipation, nausea, headache, and perineal pain.

Adverse effects reported in patients receiving progesterone vaginal insert include abdominal pain, nausea, and ovarian hyperstimulation syndrome.

Adverse effects reported in patients receiving IM progesterone include breakthrough bleeding, spotting, changes in menstrual flow, amenorrhea, changes in cervical erosion and secretions, edema, weight gain or loss, cholestatic jaundice, allergic rash with or without pruritus, breast tenderness, galactorrhea, alopecia, hirsutism, pyrexia, sleep disturbances, nausea, and mental depression. Pain and swelling at the site of injection may occur following IM administration of progesterone. Large doses (50–100 mg daily) of progesterone may cause a moderate catabolic effect and a transient increase in sodium and chloride excretion.

An association between pulmonary embolism and cerebral thrombosis and embolism and use of estrogen-progestin combination preparations has been shown. (See Thromboembolic Disorders in Cautions: Cardiovascular Effects, in Estrogen-Progestin Combinations 68:12.) The possibility that thromboembolic disorders may occur in patients receiving progesterone should be considered and patients should be carefully observed for these effects during therapy with the drug. Although available evidence suggests that an association exists between neuro-ocular lesions such as optic neuritis or retinal thrombosis and use of estrogen-progestin combination preparations, such a relationship has been neither confirmed nor refuted.

● Precautions and Contraindications

Progesterone shares the toxic potentials of progestins, and the usual precautions of progestin therapy should be observed. Prior to initiation of therapy with progesterone in women, a physical examination should be performed, including special attention to the breasts and pelvic organs and a Papanicolaou test (Pap smear). Women receiving progesterone should be given a copy of the patient labeling for the drug.

Progesterone should be used with caution, and only with careful monitoring, in patients with conditions that might be aggravated by fluid retention (e.g., asthma, seizure disorders, migraine, or cardiac or renal dysfunction). The drug should also be used with caution in patients with a history of mental depression; progesterone should be discontinued if depression recurs to a serious degree during therapy with the drug.

When breakthrough bleeding or irregular vaginal bleeding occurs during progesterone therapy, nonfunctional causes should be considered. Adequate diagnostic procedures should be performed in patients with undiagnosed vaginal bleeding.

Diabetic patients should be carefully monitored during progesterone therapy, since decreased glucose tolerance has been observed in women receiving estrogen-progestin combinations. Progesterone may mask the onset of climacteric in women.

The clinician and the patient using progesterone should be alert to the earliest signs and symptoms of myocardial infarction, cerebrovascular disorders, thromboembolism (e.g., venous thromboembolism, pulmonary embolism), thrombophlebitis, or retinal thrombosis. The drug should be discontinued immediately when any of these disorders occurs or is suspected.

If unexplained, sudden or gradual, partial or complete loss of vision; proptosis or diplopia; papilledema; retinal vascular lesions; or migraine occur during therapy with progesterone, the drug should be discontinued and appropriate diagnostic and therapeutic measures instituted.

Because dizziness has been reported during therapy with oral progesterone, patients receiving such therapy should be advised to use caution while driving or operating machinery.

Progesterone is contraindicated in patients with thrombophlebitis, thromboembolic disorders, cerebral apoplexy, or a history of these conditions. The drug is also contraindicated in patients with undiagnosed vaginal bleeding, missed abortion, known sensitivity to the drug or any ingredient in the formulation, markedly impaired liver function or liver disease, or carcinoma of the breast or for use as a pregnancy test.

Progesterone capsules are contraindicated in individuals with known hypersensitivity to peanuts because the capsules contain peanut oil.

● *Mutagenicity and Carcinogenicity*

The carcinogenic and mutagenic potentials of progesterone have not been specifically determined.

Administration of medroxyprogesterone to beagles has been associated with the development of mammary nodules, some of which were malignant. Although nodules occasionally occurred in control beagles, they were intermittent in nature; nodules in drug-treated beagles were larger, more numerous, persistent, and occasionally malignant with metastases. The clinical relevance of these findings to humans has not been established. For additional information on the carcinogenic potential of progestins, see Cautions: Mutagenicity and Carcinogenicity, in Medroxyprogesterone Acetate 68:32.

● *Pregnancy, Fertility, and Lactation*

Pregnancy

Progesterone is used to support embryo implantation and maintain pregnancy as a component of assisted reproductive technology (ART) treatment in infertile women. Such use is associated with increased ongoing pregnancy rates.

Although progestins have been used beginning in the first trimester of pregnancy to prevent habitual abortion or to treat threatened abortion, there is no adequate evidence from well-controlled studies to substantiate the efficacy of progestins for these uses; however, there is evidence of potential adverse effects on the fetus when these drugs are administered during the first 4 months of pregnancy. In addition, in most women, the cause of abortion is a defective ovum, which progestins could not be expected to influence. Because of their uterine-relaxant effects, progestins may delay spontaneous abortion of fertilized defective ova. Masculinization of the female fetus has reportedly occurred when progestins were

used during pregnancy. Clitoral hypertrophy has been reported in a few female neonates born to women who had received medroxyprogesterone during pregnancy. An association between intrauterine exposure to female sex hormones and congenital anomalies, including cardiovascular and limb defects, has been suggested. (See Cautions: Pregnancy, Fertility, and Lactation, in Estrogen-Progestin Combinations 68:12.) Use of progestins generally is not recommended during the first 4 months of pregnancy.

Progesterone should *not* be used to induce withdrawal bleeding as a test for pregnancy.

Lactation

Progestins are reportedly distributed into milk. The manufacturers warn that the possible effects of progestins in milk on nursing infants have not been determined.

LABORATORY TEST INTERFERENCES

The manufacturers caution that estrogen-progestin combinations have caused abnormal thyroid function test results. (See Effects on Thyroid in Cautions: Endocrine and Metabolic Effects, in Estrogen-Progestin Combinations 68:12.) The manufacturers also caution that estrogen-progestin combinations have altered the metyrapone test (see Laboratory Test Interferences in Estrogen-Progestin Combinations 68:12), and that these combinations have altered liver function test results (see Cautions: Hepatic Effects, in Estrogen-Progestin Combinations 68:12). These combinations have also caused decreased pregnanediol excretion.

The manufacturers state that the pathologist should be advised of progesterone use when relevant specimens from a patient exposed to the drug are submitted.

PHARMACOLOGY

Progesterone is a progestinic hormone secreted mainly from the corpus luteum of the ovary during the latter half of the menstrual cycle. Progesterone is formed from steroid precursors in the ovary, testis, adrenal cortex, and placenta. Luteinizing hormone (LH) stimulates the synthesis and secretion of progesterone from the corpus luteum. Progesterone is necessary for nidation (implantation) of the ovum and for maintenance of pregnancy. Although the hormone is secreted mainly during the luteal phase of the menstrual cycle, small amounts of progesterone are also secreted during the follicular phase. High concentrations of the hormone are secreted during the latter part of pregnancy. Amounts comparable to those secreted in women during the follicular phase have been shown to be secreted in males.

Progesterone shares the pharmacologic actions of the progestins. In women with adequate endogenous estrogen, progesterone transforms a proliferative endometrium into a secretory one. The abrupt decline in the secretion of progesterone at the end of the menstrual cycle is principally responsible for the onset of menstruation. Progesterone also stimulates the growth of mammary alveolar tissue and relaxes uterine smooth muscle. Progesterone has minimal estrogenic and androgenic activity.

Progesterone has a short plasma half-life of several minutes. The hormone is reduced to pregnanediol in the liver and conjugated with glucuronic acid, and then excreted mainly in urine.

CHEMISTRY AND STABILITY

● *Chemistry*

Progesterone is a naturally occurring progestin secreted by the corpus luteum. Progesterone is the prototype of the progestins. The drug may be obtained from animal ovaries but is usually prepared synthetically from stigmasterol or from diosgenin (extracted from *Dioscorea mexicana*, a Mexican yam).

Progesterone occurs as a white or creamy white, crystalline powder and is practically insoluble in water, soluble in alcohol, and sparingly soluble in vegetable oils. Progesterone injection is a sterile solution of the drug in a suitable solvent.

● Stability

Progesterone is stable when exposed to air. The drug should be stored in tight, light-resistant containers. Parenteral progesterone preparations, progesterone capsules, progesterone vaginal inserts, and progesterone vaginal gel should be stored at 15–30°C.

PREPARATIONS

Excipients in commercially available drug preparations may have clinically important effects in some individuals; consult specific product labeling for details.

Progesterone

Powder		
		Progesterone Powder Micronized or Microcrystalline for Prescription Compounding
Oral		
Capsules	100 mg	Prometrium®, Abbott
	200 mg	Prometrium®, Abbott

Parenteral		
Injection	50 mg/mL*	Progesterone Injection
Vaginal		
Gel	4%	Crinone® (available in prefilled, disposable applicators), Watson
	8%	Crinone® (available in prefilled, disposable applicators), Watson
Insert	100 mg	Endometrin® (with disposable applicators), Ferring Pharmaceuticals

* available from one or more manufacturer, distributor, and/or repackager by generic (nonproprietary) name

† Use is not currently included in the labeling approved by the US Food and Drug Administration.

Selected Revisions November 2, 2012, © Copyright, October 1, 1961, American Society of Health-System Pharmacists, Inc.

Thyroid Agents General Statement

68:36.04 • THYROID AGENTS

■ Thyroid agents are natural or synthetic preparations containing tetraiodothyronine (thyroxine, T_4) and/or triiodothyronine (T_3).

USES

● Hypothyroidism

Thyroid agents are used for supplementation or replacement of diminished or absent thyroid function resulting from primary causes including functional deficiency, primary atrophy, or partial or complete absence of the gland, or from the effects of surgery, radiation, or antithyroid agents; the drugs are not used for the management of transient hypothyroidism during the recovery phase of subacute thyroiditis. Thyroid agents also are used for replacement or supplemental therapy in patients with secondary (pituitary) or tertiary (hypothalamic) hypothyroidism and subclinical hypothyroidism. Therapy must be maintained continuously to control the symptoms of hypothyroidism. Levothyroxine sodium generally is the preferred thyroid agent for replacement therapy because its hormonal content is standardized and its effect is therefore predictable. Levothyroxine sodium also is considered the thyroid agent of choice for the treatment of congenital hypothyroidism (cretinism); however, other thyroid agents have been used. The earlier replacement therapy is initiated in congenital hypothyroidism, the greater is the potential for normal growth and development. (See Cautions: Pediatric Precautions.)

Levothyroxine sodium IV injection is used in the treatment of myxedema coma. Levothyroxine sodium injection has been used in other conditions when rapid thyroid replacement is required†; however, this is not an FDA-labeled use for the currently available injection.

● Pituitary TSH Suppression

Thyroid agents may be beneficial in the management or prevention of various types of euthyroid goiters, including thyroid nodules, subacute or chronic lymphocytic thyroiditis (Hashimoto's thyroiditis), and multinodular goiter. In these conditions, thyroid agents act as replacement therapy and may cause a reduction in goiter size by suppressing the secretion of thyrotropin.

Thyroid agents also may be used in conjunction with surgery and radioactive iodine therapy in the management of thyrotropin-dependent well-differentiated, papillary or follicular carcinoma of the thyroid.

● Other Uses

Thyroid agents may be used in combination with antithyroid agents in the treatment of thyrotoxicosis to prevent goitrogenesis and hypothyroidism. While administration of thyroid agents may occasionally be useful to prevent antithyroid agent-induced hypothyroidism in the management of thyrotoxicosis during pregnancy, combination therapy generally is considered unnecessary since it may increase the requirement for antithyroid agents and therefore the risk of fetal hypothyroidism, which is not amenable to exogenous thyroid agent therapy.

Thyroid agents may be used diagnostically in suppression tests to differentiate suspected hyperthyroidism from euthyroidism in patients with clinical signs and symptoms compatible with mild hyperthyroidism in whom baseline laboratory tests do not confirm the diagnosis, or to determine thyroid gland autonomy in patients with eye changes compatible with Graves' ophthalmology who are clinically and biochemically euthyroid and in whom demonstration of thyroid gland autonomy would support the diagnosis.

The use of thyroid agents, alone or in combination with other drugs, in the treatment of obesity and for weight loss is unjustified and has been shown to be ineffective. (See Cautions: Precautions and Contraindications.) The use of thyroid agents for the treatment of male or female infertility also is not justified unless the condition is accompanied by hypothyroidism.

DOSAGE AND ADMINISTRATION

● Administration

Thyroid agents usually are administered orally. Levothyroxine sodium (and occasionally liothyronine sodium) may be given by IV injection. Levothyroxine sodium also has been administered by IM injection†, however, the IV route is preferred since absorption may be variable following IM administration. IM administration is not an FDA-labeled route of administration for the currently available levothyroxine sodium injection. Oral therapy should replace parenteral therapy as soon as possible.

● Dosage

Dosage of thyroid agents must be carefully adjusted according to individual requirements and response. (See Cautions: Precautions and Contraindications.) The age and general physical condition of the patient and the severity and duration of hypothyroid symptoms determine the initial dosage and the rate at which dosage may be increased to the eventual maintenance dosage. Dosage should be initiated at a lower level in geriatric patients; in patients with long-standing disease, other endocrinopathies, or functional or ECG evidence of cardiovascular disease; and in patients with severe hypothyroidism. Adjustment of thyroid replacement therapy should be determined mainly by the patient's clinical response and confirmed by appropriate laboratory tests.

In infants and children, it is essential to achieve rapid and complete thyroid replacement because of the critical importance of thyroid hormone in sustaining growth and maturation. In general, despite the smaller body size of children, the dosage (on a weight basis) required to sustain a full rate of growth, development, and general thriving is higher in children than in adults.

● Laboratory Monitoring

Thyroid function status must be assessed periodically in patients receiving thyroid agents as a guide to therapy. Various laboratory tests are available to monitor thyroid function, and clinicians should consult specialized references for information on specific tests and their use and interpretation. Selection of appropriate tests for the diagnosis and management of hypothyroidism or hyperthyroidism depends on patient-specific variables (e.g., signs and symptoms of thyroid disease, pregnancy, concomitant administration of drugs). A combination of sensitive thyrotropin (thyroid-stimulating hormone, TSH) assay *plus* free thyroxine (T_4) and/or total or free triiodothyronine (T_3) assay usually is recommended to confirm a diagnosis of thyroid disease. TSH assay alone may be used initially to screen for thyroid disease and to monitor during drug therapy. Other thyroid function tests that may be used include total serum concentrations of T_4 triiodothyronine resin uptake, free T_4 index (the product of total serum T_4 multiplied by the percentage of serum T_3 resin uptake), and thyrotropin-releasing hormone (TRH) stimulation test.

CAUTIONS

Adverse reactions to thyroid agents result principally from overdosage. (See Toxicity.)

● Toxicity

Manifestations

Adverse reactions to thyroid agents result from overdosage and are manifested principally as signs and symptoms of hyperthyroidism including fatigue, weight loss, increased appetite, palpitations, nervousness, hyperactivity, anxiety, irritability, emotional lability, diarrhea, abdominal cramps, vomiting, elevated liver transaminase concentrations, sweating, tachycardia, increased pulse and blood pressures, angina pectoris, cardiac arrhythmias, tremors, muscle weakness, headache, insomnia, intolerance to heat, fever, hair loss, flushing, decreased bone mineral density, impaired fertility, and menstrual irregularities. Complications of severe overdosage may include cardiac decompensation, cardiac failure, myocardial infarction, cardiac arrest, and possibly death secondary to cardiac arrhythmia or failure. Seizures have been reported rarely with levothyroxine therapy. The effects of levothyroxine sodium, thyroid, or thyroglobulin may not appear for 1–3 weeks following initiation of therapy or an increase in dosage, but may appear within 24–72 hours after initiation of therapy or an increase in dosage with liothyronine sodium.

Treatment

Manifestations of overdosage are usually readily reversible following temporary discontinuance of therapy and are obviated by a reduction in dosage. If manifestations of overdosage appear with levothyroxine sodium, thyroid, or thyroglobulin, the drug should be discontinued for 2–7 days, and for 2–3 days in the case of liothyronine sodium, and then resumed at a lower dosage. For information on the treatment of acute overdosage of thyroid agents, see Acute Toxicity: Treatment.

● Other Adverse Effects

Hypersensitivity reactions to excipients in formulations of thyroid agents have been reported rarely. Manifestations include urticaria, pruritus, skin rash, flushing, angioedema, various GI symptoms (e.g., abdominal pain, nausea, vomiting, diarrhea), fever, arthralgia, serum sickness, and wheezing. Thyroid also may rarely cause GI intolerance in patients highly sensitive to pork. One manufacturer states that GI intolerance may also rarely occur in patients highly sensitive to corn.

● Precautions and Contraindications

Because thyroid agents have a narrow therapeutic index, dosage must be carefully adjusted to avoid the consequences of under or over treatment, including adverse effects on growth and development in pediatric patients, cardiovascular function, bone metabolism, reproductive function, cognitive function, emotional state, GI function, and glucose and lipid metabolism.

Patients receiving thyroid agents must be closely monitored and thyroid function status must be periodically assessed by appropriate laboratory studies. (See Dosage and Administration: Laboratory Monitoring.) Since hypothyroid patients, especially those with myxedema, are particularly sensitive to thyroid agents, replacement therapy should be initiated with low doses and subsequent dosage should be gradually increased in such patients.

Thyroid agents should be used with extreme caution and in reduced dosage in patients with angina pectoris or other cardiovascular disease, including hypertension. If chest pain or other aggravation of cardiovascular disease occurs in patients receiving thyroid agents, dosage should be reduced or temporarily withheld and reinstituted at a lower dosage. Overtreatment with thyroid agents may result in adverse cardiovascular effects (e.g., increased heart rate, cardiac wall thickness, cardiac contractility) and may precipitate angina pectoris or arrhythmias. Because the possibility of precipitating cardiac arrhythmias may be greater in patients receiving thyroid agents, patients with coronary artery disease should be closely monitored during surgery. Thyroid agents should be used with caution in geriatric patients since occult cardiac disease may be present.

Morphologic hypogonadism and nephroses should be ruled out before thyroid agents are administered. In patients whose hypothyroidism is secondary to hypopituitarism, adrenal insufficiency is likely to be present. When adrenal insufficiency and hypothyroidism exist concomitantly, adrenal insufficiency must be corrected by administration of corticosteroids before therapy with thyroid agents is initiated. Initiation of thyroid hormone therapy without prior treatment with corticosteroids may result in increased metabolic clearance of corticosteroids and, thus, may precipitate an acute adrenal crisis. Hypopituitarism, adrenal insufficiency, and other endocrine disorders such as diabetes mellitus and diabetes insipidus are characterized by signs and symptoms which may be diminished in severity or obscured by hypothyroidism. Thyroid agents may aggravate the intensity of previously obscured symptoms in patients with endocrine disorders, and appropriate adjustment of therapy for these concomitant disorders may be required.

Except in patients with transient hypothyroidism or in those receiving a therapeutic trial with an agent, patients should be advised that replacement therapy with a thyroid agent must be maintained continuously to control the symptoms of hypothyroidism and that clinical improvement may not occur until after several weeks of therapy. Patients should be instructed to immediately report any signs or symptoms of thyroid toxicity (hyperthyroidism) (e.g., chest pain, increased pulse rate, palpitations, excessive sweating, heat intolerance, nervousness) or any unusual event which occurs during therapy with a thyroid agent. (See Cautions: Toxicity and Other Adverse Effects.) Because dosage of antidiabetic agents (i.e., insulin, sulfonylureas) may require adjustment during thyroid agent replacement therapy, patients with diabetes mellitus receiving an antidiabetic agent concomitantly should be advised to closely monitor urinary and/or blood glucose concentrations during concomitant therapy. Hypoglycemia may occur in these patients if therapy with a thyroid agent is stopped. Patients should be advised that partial loss of hair may occur during the first few months of therapy, but this effect is usually transient and subsequent regrowth usually occurs. When surgery is required,

patients should be advised to inform the attending clinician (e.g., physician, dentist) that they are receiving thyroid hormone therapy.

Although thyroid agents have been used alone and in combination with other drugs for the treatment of obesity, dosages of thyroid agents within the usual range of daily requirements are *ineffective* for weight reduction in euthyroid individuals. Higher dosages may produce serious and even life-threatening manifestations of toxicity, especially when given in conjunction with sympathomimetic agents (e.g., amphetamines) used for their anorectic effect. The use of thyroid agents for the treatment of obesity or for weight loss is unjustified and contraindicated.

Thyroid agents are generally contraindicated in the presence of thyrotoxicosis and in acute myocardial infarction uncomplicated by hypothyroidism. When hypothyroidism is a complicating or causative factor in myocardial infarction, judicious use of small doses of thyroid agents may be considered. Thyroid agents are contraindicated in patients with uncorrected adrenal insufficiency because the drugs increase tissue demands for adrenal hormones and may precipitate an acute adrenal crisis in these patients. Although there is no well-documented evidence of true allergic or idiosyncratic reactions to thyroid agents, a particular agent should not be used in patients with apparent hypersensitivity to that agent or any ingredient in the formulation.

● Pediatric Precautions

Little, if any, maternal thyroid hormone is distributed to the fetus. The incidence of congenital hypothyroidism is relatively high (1:4000) and the hypothyroid fetus probably does not derive any benefit from the small amounts of thyroid hormones that may cross the placental barrier. Routine determination of serum thyroxine and/or thyrotropin (thyroid-stimulating hormone, TSH) concentrations is strongly advised in neonates because of the deleterious effects of thyroid deficiency on growth and development. Normal adult ranges for serum thyroxine concentrations must *not* be used to evaluate neonatal thyroid function, since failure to diagnose the condition may occur and result in disastrous effects on the prognosis. The Committee on Drugs of the American Academy of Pediatrics (AAP) recommends that physicians caring for children participate in state or regional screening programs for hypothyroidism and maintain a high level of clinical suspicion to assure the earliest possible diagnosis of congenital hypothyroidism. Signs and symptoms of congenital hypothyroidism include lethargy, hypothermia, feeding problems, failure to gain weight, dry skin, skin mottling, thick tongue, hoarse cry, umbilical hernia, persistence of mild jaundice, respiratory problems, and a large anterior and posterior fontanel.

Treatment, preferably with levothyroxine sodium, should be initiated immediately upon diagnosis, and maintained for life, unless transient hypothyroidism is suspected. If receipt of laboratory results will be delayed for several days or weeks, thyroid agent therapy may be initiated in neonates with suspected hypothyroidism pending the results of confirmative tests. The earlier replacement therapy is initiated in congenital hypothyroidism, the greater the potential for normal growth and development. If a positive diagnosis cannot be made on the basis of laboratory findings but there is a strong clinical suspicion of congenital hypothyroidism, a conservative approach would be to ensure euthyroidism with replacement therapy until the child is 1–2 years of age. Thyroid agent therapy can then be discontinued while diagnostic tests are carried out, and reinstituted if indicated; this treatment approach avoids the potential risk of the infant incurring serious, permanent brain damage. When transient hypothyroidism is suspected, therapy may be interrupted (or dosage of the thyroid agent reduced by half in suspected severe hypothyroidism) for 4–8 weeks to reassess the condition when the child is older than 3 years of age. If the diagnosis of permanent hypothyroidism is confirmed, full replacement therapy should be reinstituted. However, if serum concentrations of T₄ and TSH are normal, thyroid agent therapy may be discontinued, and the patient should be carefully monitored; thyroid function tests should be repeated if manifestations of hypothyroidism develop.

During the first 2 weeks of thyroid agent therapy, infants should be closely monitored for cardiac overload, arrhythmias, and aspiration resulting from avid suckling. Evaluation of the infant's clinical response to thyroid agent therapy should be performed about 6 weeks after initiation of therapy; additional examinations should be performed at least at 6 and 12 months of age and yearly thereafter. Achievement of normal serum thyrotropin concentration must *not* be used as the sole criterion of the adequacy of the dose in children with congenital hypothyroidism, since thyrotropin concentrations may remain elevated for several months during replacement therapy using proper or even excessive dosages of the thyroid agent. The goal of replacement therapy in these children is to maintain the serum thyroxine concentration at levels appropriate for age throughout infancy and childhood and to achieve and maintain normal intellectual and physical growth and development. Patients should be monitored closely to avoid undertreatment or overtreatment. Undertreatment may result in poor school performance (due to impaired concentration and slowed mentation) and reduced adult height. Overtreatment may result in craniosynostosis in infants and accelerate the aging of bones, resulting in premature epiphyseal closure and compromised adult stature.

Treated children may manifest a period of catch-up growth, which may be adequate in some cases to achieve normal adult height. In children with severe or long-standing hypothyroidism, catch-up growth may not be adequate to achieve normal adult height.

Pseudotumor cerebri and slipped capital femoral epiphysis have been reported in children receiving thyroid agent therapy.

● Mutagenicity and Carcinogenicity

Animal studies to determine the mutagenic or carcinogenic potential of thyroid agents have not been performed. Although an apparent association between prolonged thyroid therapy and breast cancer has been reported, the validity of the report has been seriously questioned. Patients receiving thyroid agents for established indications should not discontinue therapy.

● Pregnancy, Fertility, and Lactation

Pregnancy

Thyroid agents do not readily cross the placenta, and clinical experience does not indicate any adverse effect on the fetus when thyroid agents are administered during pregnancy. Thyroid agent replacement therapy for hypothyroidism should be continued throughout pregnancy, and if hypothyroidism is diagnosed during pregnancy, treatment should be initiated. Serum thyroxine concentrations are lower than normal during pregnancy, and the diagnosis should be confirmed by determination of serum thyrotropin concentration. In pregnant women dependent on thyroid replacement therapy, increased dosage may be required.

If myxedema coma develops during pregnancy, patients should be treated with IV levothyroxine sodium. Although the manufacturer states that there are no reports of levothyroxine sodium injection use in pregnant women with myxedema, nontreatment is associated with a high probability of maternal or fetal morbidity or mortality.

Lactation

Although only minimal amounts of thyroid hormones are distributed into milk, thyroid agents should be used with caution in nursing women.

Lactating women who develop myxedema coma should be treated with IV levothyroxine sodium. Although the manufacturer states that there are no reports of levothyroxine sodium injection use in lactating women with myxedema coma, nontreatment is associated with a high probability of maternal morbidity or mortality.

ACUTE TOXICITY

● Manifestations

In general, acute overdosage of thyroid agents may be expected to produce signs and symptoms of hyperthyroidism. (See Toxicity.) Cerebral embolism, shock, coma, and death have been reported. In addition, confusion and disorientation may occur. Seizures have occurred in a child who ingested approximately 18 mg of levothyroxine; manifestations of toxicity may not necessarily be evident or may not appear until several days after ingestion of levothyroxine sodium.

● Treatment

In the treatment of acute thyroid agent overdosage, symptomatic and supportive therapy should be instituted immediately. Treatment consists principally of reducing GI absorption of the drugs and counteracting central and peripheral effects, mainly those of increased sympathetic activity. Initially, the stomach should be emptied immediately by inducing emesis or by gastric lavage; activated charcoal or cholestyramine resin also may be used to decrease absorption. If the patient is comatose, having seizures, or lacks the gag reflex, gastric lavage may be performed if an endotracheal tube with cuff inflated is in place to prevent aspiration of gastric contents. Oxygen may be administered and ventilation maintained. If congestive heart failure develops, cardiac glycosides may be administered. Measures to control arrhythmia,

fever, hypoglycemia, or fluid loss should be initiated as necessary. β-Adrenergic blocking agents (e.g., propranolol) are useful to counteract many of the effects of increased sympathetic activity. Large doses of antithyroid drugs (e.g., methimazole, propylthiouracil) followed in 1–2 hours by large doses of iodine may be administered to inhibit synthesis and release of thyroid hormones. Corticosteroids may be given to inhibit the conversion of T_4 to triiodothyronine (T_3). Plasmapheresis, charcoal hemoperfusion, and exchange transfusion have been reserved for cases in which continued clinical deterioration occurs despite conventional therapy. Because T_4 is highly protein bound, very little drug will be removed by dialysis.

DRUG INTERACTIONS

In addition to the drug interactions described in this section, some drugs can interfere with thyroid function test results and their interpretation. (See Laboratory Test Interferences.)

● Oral Anticoagulants

Thyroid agents may potentiate the hypoprothrombinemic effect of warfarin and other oral anticoagulants, apparently by increasing catabolism of vitamin K-dependent clotting factors. When thyroid agents are administered to patients receiving oral anticoagulants, the prothrombin time should be determined frequently and anticoagulant dosage adjusted accordingly, and patients should be observed closely for adverse effects. It has been suggested that the dosage of the oral anticoagulant be reduced by one-third when thyroid therapy is started. No special precautions appear to be necessary when oral anticoagulant therapy is initiated in patients already stabilized on maintenance thyroid replacement therapy.

● Antidepressants

Concomitant use of tricyclic (e.g., amitriptyline) or tetracyclic (e.g., maprotiline) antidepressants and levothyroxine may increase the therapeutic and toxic effects (e.g., increased risk of cardiac arrhythmias and CNS stimulation) of both classes of drugs, possibly secondary to increased receptor sensitivity to catecholamines; onset of action of tricyclic antidepressants may be accelerated. Concomitant use of selective serotonin-reuptake inhibitors (SSRIs, e.g., sertraline) in patients stabilized on levothyroxine may result in increased levothyroxine requirements.

● Antidiabetic Agents

Hypothyroidism may reduce the severity of diabetes mellitus, resulting in decreased requirements of insulin or oral antidiabetic agents (e.g., sulfonylureas). Administration of thyroid agents to patients with diabetes mellitus may cause an increase in the required dosage of insulin or oral antidiabetic agents. When therapy with thyroid agents is initiated or discontinued or when dosage of a thyroid agent is adjusted in diabetic patients receiving insulin or an oral antidiabetic agent, patients should be closely monitored and appropriate adjustments in dosage of insulin or the oral antidiabetic agent made accordingly if necessary.

● Sympathomimetic Agents

Parenteral administration of sympathomimetic agents (e.g., epinephrine) to patients with coronary artery disease may precipitate an episode of coronary insufficiency. Because this reaction may be enhanced in patients receiving thyroid agents, patients with coronary artery disease who are receiving thyroid agents should be carefully observed when catecholamines are administered.

● Bile Acid Sequestrants

Bile acid sequestrants (e.g., cholestyramine resin, colestipol) bind thyroid agents in the GI tract and substantially impair their absorption. In vitro studies indicate that the binding is not readily reversible. To minimize or prevent this interaction, these agents should be administered at least 4 hours apart when the drugs must be used concurrently.

● GI Drugs

Antacids (e.g., aluminum hydroxide, magnesium hydroxide, calcium carbonate), simethicone, and sucralfate bind thyroid agents in the GI tract and delay or prevent their absorption. Calcium carbonate may form an insoluble chelate with levothyroxine, resulting in decreased levothyroxine absorption and increased serum thyrotropin concentrations; in vitro studies indicate that levothyroxine binds to calcium carbonate at acidic pH levels. To minimize or prevent this interaction, some clinicians recommend that these agents be administered approximately 4 hours apart when the drugs must be used concurrently with thyroid agents.

● Drugs Affecting Hepatic Microsomal Enzymes

Drugs that induce hepatic microsomal enzymes (e.g., carbamazepine, phenytoin, phenobarbital, rifampin) may accelerate metabolism of thyroid agents, resulting in increased thyroid agent dosage requirements. Phenytoin and carbamazepine also reduce serum protein binding of levothyroxine, and total- and free-T_4 may be reduced by 20–40%, but most patients have normal serum concentrations of thyrotropin (thyroid-stimulating hormone, TSH) and are clinically euthyroid.

● Cardiac Glycosides

Serum concentrations of digitalis glycosides may be decreased in patients with hyperthyroidism or in patients with hypothyroidism in whom a euthyroid state has been achieved. Thus, therapeutic effects of digitalis glycosides may be reduced in these patients.

● Growth Hormones

Excessive use of thyroid agents with growth hormones (e.g., somatropin) may accelerate epiphyseal closure. However, untreated hypothyroidism may interfere with growth response to growth hormone.

● Xanthine Derivatives

Decreased clearance of xanthine derivatives (e.g., theophylline) may occur in hypothyroid patients; clearance returns to normal when the euthyroid state is achieved.

● Other Drugs

Cation-exchange resins (e.g., sodium polystyrene sulfonate) and ferrous sulfate bind thyroid agents in the GI tract and delay or prevent their absorption. To minimize or prevent this interaction, thyroid agents should be administered at least 4 hours apart from these drugs.

Concomitant use of ketamine with thyroid agents may produce marked hypertension and tachycardia; caution is advised when the drug is administered in patients receiving thyroid hormone therapy.

LABORATORY TEST INTERFERENCES

● Drugs Affecting Thyroid Function or Thyroid Function Tests

Certain drugs and various pathologic and physiologic conditions can interfere with thyroid function tests and their interpretation, and the resultant effects must be considered.

Use of dopamine hydrochloride (at dosages of 1 mcg/kg per minute or greater), corticosteroids (at hydrocortisone-equivalent dosages of 100 mg daily or greater), or octreotide (at dosages exceeding 100 mcg daily) may result in a transient reduction in thyrotropin (thyroid-stimulating hormone, TSH) secretion. However, because these effects are transient, hypothyroidism is not expected to occur.

Drugs that may decrease thyroid hormone secretion (e.g., aminoglutethimide, amiodarone, iodide [including iodine-containing radiographic contrast agents], lithium, sulfonamides, tolbutamide) may be associated with hypothyroidism. Long-term lithium therapy can result in goiter in up to 50% of patients, and in subclinical or overt hypothyroidism, each in up to 20% of patients. The fetus, neonates, geriatric patients, and euthyroid patients with underlying thyroid disease (e.g., Hashimoto's thyroiditis, Grave's disease previously treated with radioiodine or surgery) are particularly susceptible to iodine-induced hypothyroidism. Oral cholecystographic agents and amiodarone are excreted slowly, producing more prolonged hypothyroidism than parenterally administered iodinated contrast agents. Long-term aminoglutethimide therapy may minimally decrease concentrations of T_4 and triiodothyronine (T_3) and increase concentrations of thyrotropin, although all values remain within normal limits in most patients.

Iodide (including iodine-containing radiographic contrast agents) and drugs that contain pharmacologic amounts of iodide may cause hyperthyroidism in euthyroid patients with Grave's disease previously treated with antithyroid drugs or in euthyroid patients with thyroid autonomy (e.g., multinodular goiter or hyperfunctioning thyroid adenoma). Hyperthyroidism may develop over several weeks and may persist for several months following discontinuance of therapy. Amiodarone may induce hyperthyroidism by causing thyroiditis.

Pregnancy, estrogens, estrogen-containing oral contraceptives, methadone, fluorouracil, mitotane, and tamoxifen increase serum concentrations of thyroxine-binding globulin; in patients with normal thyroid function only a transient decrease in free serum thyroxine concentration results, but in patients receiving thyroid replacement therapy, an increase in thyroid agent dosage may be necessary. Chronic active hepatitis, neonatal state, acute intermittent porphyria, and genetic factors also may increase thyroxine-binding globulin concentrations. Androgens, usual doses of corticosteroids, asparaginase, and sustained release niacin decrease serum concentrations of thyroxine-binding globulin; decreases in serum concentrations of thyroxine-binding globulin also occur in nephrosis, cirrhosis, and acromegaly. Some drugs (e.g., phenylbutazone [no longer commercially available in the US], salicylates) competitively bind to thyroxine-binding globulin and/or thyroxine-binding prealbumin. Familial hyper- or hypo-thyroxine-binding-globulinemias also have been reported.

Concomitant use of levothyroxine sodium with furosemide (at IV dosages exceeding 80 mg), heparin, hydantoins, nonsteroidal anti-inflammatory agents (NSAIAs, e.g., fenamates, phenylbutazone), or salicylates (at dosages exceeding 2 g daily) results in an initial transient increase in concentrations of free T_4. Continued administration results in a decrease in serum T_4 and normal free T_4 and TSH concentrations; therefore, patients are clinically euthyroid. Salicylates inhibit binding of T_4 and T_3 to thyroxine-binding globulin (TBG) and transthyretin. An initial increase in serum free T_4 is followed by return of free T_4 to normal levels with sustained therapeutic serum salicylate concentrations, although total T_4 concentrations may decrease by as much as 30%.

Concomitant use of thyroid agents with amiodarone, β-adrenergic blocking agents (e.g., propranolol hydrochloride at dosages exceeding 160 mg daily), or corticosteroids (e.g., dexamethasone at dosages of 4 mg daily or greater) decreases peripheral conversion of T_4 to T_3, resulting in decreased T_3 concentrations. However, serum T_4 concentrations usually remain within normal range but may occasionally be slightly increased. In patients treated with large doses of propranolol hydrochloride (i.e., exceeding 160 mg/day), T_3 and T_4 concentrations change slightly, TSH levels remain normal, and patients are clinically euthyroid. It should be noted that actions of particular β-adrenergic blocking agents may be impaired when the hypothyroid patient is converted to the euthyroid state. Short-term administration of large doses of corticosteroids may decrease serum T_3 concentrations by 30% with minimal change in serum T_4 levels. However, long-term corticosteroid therapy may result in slightly decreased T_3 and T_4 concentrations because of decreased TBG production.

Therapy with interferon alfa has been associated with the development of antithyroid microsomal antibodies in 20% of patients, and some experience transient hypothyroidism, hyperthyroidism, or both. Patients who have antithyroid antibodies prior to treatment with thyroid agents are at higher risk for thyroid dysfunction during treatment. Interleukin 2 (e.g., aldesleukin) has been associated with transient painless thyroiditis in 20% of patients. Interferon beta and gamma have not been reported to cause thyroid dysfunction.

Other agents that have been associated with alterations in thyroid hormone and/or TSH concentrations include chloral hydrate, diazepam, ethionamide, lovastatin, metoclopramide, mercaptopurine, nitroprusside, aminosalicylate sodium, perphenazine, resorcinol (excessive topical use), and thiazide diuretics.

● Other Laboratory Test Interferences

Radioactive iodine uptake tests used in evaluating thyroid function can be interfered with by dietary sources of iodine or iodine- or iodide-containing medications (e.g., potassium iodide).

Thyroid hormones may reduce the uptake of ^{123}I, ^{131}I, and ^{99m}Tc.

PHARMACOLOGY

● Thyroid Hormone Synthesis and Regulation

The extracts of the thyroid gland and hormones secreted by the gland or prepared synthetically are essential hormones that affect the rate of many physiologic processes. The amounts of thyroxine and triiodothyronine released into the circulation from the normally functioning thyroid gland are regulated by thyrotropin (thyroid-stimulating hormone, TSH), which is secreted by the anterior pituitary. Secretion of thyrotropin is in turn controlled by a feedback mechanism effected by concentrations of circulating thyroid hormones and by secretion of thyrotropin-releasing hormone (TRH) from the hypothalamus. Endogenous thyroid hormone secretion is suppressed when exogenous thyroid hormones are administered to euthyroid individuals in excess of the gland's normal secretion.

Tetraiodothyronine (thyroxine, T_4) and triiodothyronine (T_3) are produced in the thyroid gland by the iodination and coupling of the amino acid tyrosine. Iodine is an essential component of thyroid hormones, thyroxine and triiodothyronine, comprising 65 and 59% of the weights, respectively. Thyroid hormones and thus iodine are essential for human life. The hormones regulate many key biochemical reactions, especially protein synthesis and enzymatic activity, and target the developing brain, muscle, heart, pituitary, and kidneys.

The thyroid gland selectively concentrates iodide in amounts required for adequate thyroid hormone synthesis, with most of the remaining iodide being excreted renally. A sodium/iodide transporter in the thyroidal basal membrane is responsible for iodine concentration in the gland, transferring iodide from systemic circulation into the thyroid gland at a concentration gradient of 20–50 times that of plasma to ensure that the gland receives adequate amounts of iodine for hormone synthesis. During iodine deficiency, the thyroid gland concentrates most of the iodine available from plasma. Iodide participates in a complex series of reactions in the thyroid gland to produce thyroid hormones. Thyroglobulin is synthesized in thyroid cells and serves as an iodination vehicle. Thyroperoxidase and hydrogen peroxide promote the oxidation of iodide and its attachment to tyrosyl residues within the thyroglobulin molecule to produce the hormone precursors diiodotyrosine and monoiodotyrosine. Thyroperoxidase further catalyzes intramolecular coupling of 2 molecules of diiodotyrosine to produce thyroxine (T_4) and coupling of a molecule of diiodotyrosine and a molecule of monoiodotyrosine to produce triiodothyronine (T_3). The average adult thyroid gland in individuals residing in an iodine-sufficient geographic region contains about 15 mg of iodine. Iodine is not released into systemic circulation but instead is stored principally in diiodo and monoiodo tyrosine precursors, removed from the tyrosine moiety by a specific deiodinase, and then recycled within the thyroid gland as a mechanism of iodine conservation.

Once in systemic circulation, thyroxine and triiodothyronine attach to several binding proteins (e.g., thyronine-binding globulin, transthyretin, albumin), which then migrate to target tissues where thyroxine is deiodinated to triiodothyronine, the metabolically active form of thyroid hormone. The iodine that is removed from thyroxine returns to the serum iodine pool and follows the usual iodine cycle or is excreted renally. Thyrotropin is the major thyroid function regulator. Thyrotropin affects several sites within thyrocytes, the principal actions of which are to increase thyroidal uptake of iodine and to break down thyroglobulin to release thyroid hormone into systemic circulation. An elevated serum thyrotropin concentration indicates primary hypothyroidism and a decreased serum concentration indicates hyperthyroidism. The normal thyroid gland takes up the amount of systemically circulating iodine necessary to make the amount of thyroid hormone for the body's needs. In iodine deficiency, the thyroid gland will concentrate more iodine, and the gland will concentrate less in iodine excess. When iodine equilibrium is present, the mean daily thyroid iodine accumulation and release are similar.

● Pharmacologic Effects of Exogenous Thyroid Hormones

The principal pharmacologic effect of exogenous thyroid hormones is to increase the metabolic rate of body tissues. Thyroid hormones affect protein and carbohydrate metabolism, promoting gluconeogenesis, increasing the utilization and mobilization of glycogen stores, and stimulating protein synthesis. Thyroid hormones affect lipid metabolism by decreasing hepatic and serum cholesterol concentrations. Thyroid hormones are also involved in the regulation of cell growth and differentiation. The hormones aid in the development of the brain and CNS (particularly axonal and dendritic networks and myelination), and are involved with somatotropin in the development of bones and teeth and in the broad aspect of growth.

Although the exact mechanism of action by which thyroid hormones affect metabolism and cellular growth and differentiation is not clearly established, it is known that these physiologic effects are mediated at the cellular level, principally via triiodothyronine. A major portion of triiodothyronine (approximately 70–90%) is derived from thyroxine by deiodination in peripheral tissues; approximately 35% of secreted thyroxine is monodeiodinated peripherally to triiodothyronine. Thyroxine is the major component of normal secretions of the thyroid gland and is therefore the principal determinant of normal thyroid function. In normal human thyroid tissue, the thyroxine:triiodothyronine ratio is 10:1 to 15:1; in hyperthyroid patients with Graves' disease, the ratio is decreased to about 5:1.

Thyroid hormones also exhibit a cardiostimulatory effect which may be the result of a direct action on the heart. Thyroid hormones also may increase the sensitivity of the heart to catecholamines and/or increase the number of myocardial β-adrenergic receptors. Thyroid hormones increase cardiac output, in part, secondary to increased peripheral oxygen consumption. Thyroid hormones may increase renal blood flow and glomerular filtration rate in hypothyroid patients, resulting in a diuresis within 24 hours following administration.

Thyroid hormones will reverse the signs and symptoms of hypothyroidism and myxedema; in hypothyroid children, the hormones increase epiphyseal growth and bone ossification. For thyroid hormones to prevent the developmental abnormalities associated with congenital hypothyroidism (e.g., mental and growth retardation), the condition must be diagnosed and therapy initiated early.

PHARMACOKINETICS

● Absorption

Levothyroxine sodium is variably absorbed from the GI tract (range 40–80%) following oral administration. The extent of absorption is increased in the fasting state and decreased in malabsorption states. Liothyronine sodium is almost completely absorbed from the GI tract (about 95%) following oral administration. The absorption of hormones contained in the natural thyroid agent preparations is similar to that of the synthetic hormones. Absorption of levothyroxine sodium or liothyronine sodium following IM administration may be variable and poor. Thyroxine apparently undergoes enterohepatic circulation.

In healthy individuals, total serum thyroxine (endogenous) concentrations range from about 5–12 mcg/dL, and free (unbound) serum thyroxine concentrations range from about 1–3 ng/dL (about 0.02% of total). Total serum triiodothyronine (endogenous) concentrations range from 70–200 ng/dL (considerable interlaboratory variation) in healthy individuals, and free serum triiodothyronine concentrations range from 0.2–0.4 ng/dL (about 0.2% of total). Total serum reverse triiodothyronine (See Pharmacokinetics: Elimination) concentrations range from 10–60 ng/dL, and free serum reverse triiodothyronine concentrations range from about 0.05–0.15 ng/dL (about 0.5% of total). Serum triiodothyronine concentrations appear to decline slightly with age, are slightly increased in obese individuals, and are decreased in the fetus and neonates. Serum reverse triiodothyronine concentrations appear to be increased in healthy individuals older than 70 years of age and markedly increased in the fetus and neonates. Age-adjusted normal range values for serum thyroid hormone concentrations may be required for proper interpretation of such measurements. Although the normal range for endogenous thyroid hormones is the therapeutic range for exogenously administered hormones in hypothyroid patients, free hormone concentrations are often not easily measured and other measures of thyroid function (e.g., resin triiodothyronine uptake, free thyroxine index) are generally used to monitor thyroid hormone replacement therapy.

The maximum effects of liothyronine sodium are apparent within 24–72 hours following initiation of oral therapy and persist for up to 72 hours following discontinuance of the drug. Levothyroxine sodium, thyroid, and thyroglobulin have a much slower onset and longer duration of action than liothyronine sodium. The full effects of levothyroxine sodium, thyroid, and thyroglobulin do not occur for 1–3 weeks following initiation of oral therapy, and effects are maintained for a similar period of time following discontinuance of the drugs.

● Distribution

Distribution of thyroid hormones into human body tissues and fluids has not been fully characterized. Thyroxine is distributed into most body tissues and fluids with highest concentrations in the liver and kidneys. Thyroid hormones do not readily cross the placenta. Placental transfer of thyroid hormones is slow and the importance has not been precisely determined; the mother provides little, if any, thyroid hormone to the developing fetus. Minimal amounts of thyroid hormones are distributed into milk.

Thyroxine and triiodothyronine are more than 99% bound to serum proteins, principally thyronine-binding globulin (thyroxine-binding globulin, TBG) and transthyretin (thyroxine-binding prealbumin, TBPA) (and to a small extent albumin), whose capacities and affinities for the hormones vary. Thyroxine is more extensively and firmly bound than is triiodothyronine. The high affinity of thyroxine for TBG and TBPA is responsible for thyroxine's high serum concentration and slow metabolic clearance. Certain drugs and various pathologic and physiologic conditions can alter the binding of thyroid hormones to serum proteins and/or the concentrations of the serum proteins that bind the hormones; these effects must be considered when interpreting the results of thyroid function tests. (See Laboratory Test Interferences.)

● *Elimination*

The usual plasma half-lives of thyroxine and triiodothyronine are approximately 6–8 and 1–2 days, respectively. The plasma half-lives of thyroxine and triiodothyronine are decreased in patients with hyperthyroidism and increased in those with hypothyroidism.

In humans, endogenous thyroglobulin within the thyroid gland is proteolytically hydrolyzed, resulting in the release of thyroxine and triiodothyronine into the circulation. Thyroxine is conjugated with glucuronic and sulfuric acids in the liver and distributed into bile; a portion is then hydrolyzed in the intestine and reabsorbed, and a portion reaches the colon unchanged, where it is then hydrolyzed and eliminated unchanged in the feces. About 20–40% of thyroxine is eliminated in feces. About 35% of secreted thyroxine is monodeiodinated at the 5' position of the phenolic (outer) ring in peripheral tissues, principally liver and kidney, to form triiodothyronine; this accounts for about 80% of the total daily production of triiodothyronine. Thyroxine also undergoes peripheral monodeiodination at the 5 position of the tyrosyl (inner) ring to form reverse triiodothyronine (reverse T_3, rT_3), which is calorigenically inactive. About 85% of thyroxine metabolized daily is deiodinated. Deiodination is apparently an enzymatic process, and probably involves separate iodothyronine 5'- and 5-deiodinases which have a high capacity and are probably subject to some form(s) of regulation. The metabolic fate of triiodothyronine is not clearly established. Triiodothyronine and reverse triiodothyronine undergo peripheral monodeiodination to form 3,3'-diiodothyronine. Additional thyroid hormone metabolites in which the diphenyl ether linkage is either intact or broken have also been detected. Iodine liberated by deiodination reactions is utilized by the thyroid gland for hormone synthesis or is excreted in feces via bile or in urine.

● *Chemistry*

Thyroid agents are natural or synthetic preparations containing tetraiodothyronine (thyroxine, T_4) and/or triiodothyronine (T_3). Thyroxine and triiodothyronine are produced in the human thyroid gland; the commercially available synthetic preparations of these hormones, levothyroxine sodium and liothyronine sodium, respectively, are the sodium salts of the L-isomers of the hormones. Thyroxine and triiodothyronine are produced in the thyroid gland by the iodination and coupling of the amino acid tyrosine. Thyroxine contains 4 iodine atoms and is formed by the coupling of 2 molecules of diiodotyrosine. Triiodothyronine contains 3 iodine atoms and is formed by the coupling of one molecule of diiodotyrosine with one molecule of monoiodotyrosine. Thyroxine and triiodothyronine are stored in the thyroid colloid as thyroglobulin.

Natural thyroid agent preparations, which are derived from animal thyroid, include thyroid and thyroglobulin. USP previously required that thyroid and thyroglobulin be standardized only by their iodine content which is only an indirect indicator of true hormonal biologic activity. Some manufacturers of thyroid perform bioassays of their preparations to assure batch-to-batch reproducibility of metabolic potency, and the manufacturer of thyroglobulin standardizes the levothyroxine and liothyronine contents of

the preparation by chromatographic analysis; however, the concentrations of levothyroxine and liothyronine and the ratio of these hormones in these commercially available preparations may vary considerably. Even preparations that are standardized for metabolic potency via a bioassay may differ from other bioassay preparations in the ratio of levothyroxine:liothyronine concentration. Current USP standards specify the measurable amounts of levothyroxine and liothyronine in each 65 mg of thyroid or thyroglobulin; however, because of difficulty in measuring the actual hormonal content of thyroid USP or thyroglobulin USP, these measurable amounts may be less than the clinical equivalent. In guiding dosage adjustment, the clinical equivalent and not the measurable amount should be used.

Synthetic thyroid agent preparations include levothyroxine sodium, liothyronine sodium, and liotrix, a combination preparation containing a ratio of levothyroxine sodium to liothyronine sodium of 4:1 by weight; however, current USP standards do not specify the ratio of levothyroxine sodium and liothyronine sodium in liotrix.

Because some thyroid agent preparations currently may not be standardized by their levothyroxine and/or liothyronine contents and because the measurable amounts of these drugs in thyroid and thyroglobulin may be less than the clinical equivalent, thyroid agent preparations are not necessarily directly comparable; however, the following equivalencies have been suggested based on clinical response:

Thyroid Agent	Approximate Equivalent Dosage
Levothyroxine Sodium	100 mcg or less
Liothyronine Sodium	25 mcg
Liotrix (Levothyroxine Sodium/ Liothyronine Sodium)	50 mcg/12.5 mcg (Thyrolar®)
Thyroglobulin	65 mg
Thyroid	60–65 mg (1 grain)

These approximate clinical equivalents should be used in guiding dosage adjustment; following a change from one type of thyroid hormone preparation to another, patients still may require fine adjustment of dosage since the equivalents are only estimates.

For further information on chemistry and stability, pharmacology, pharmacokinetics, uses, cautions, and dosage and administration of thyroid agents, see the individual monographs in 68:36.04.

† Use is not currently included in the labeling approved by the US Food and Drug Administration.

Selected Revisions December 8, 2015, © Copyright, July 1, 1970, American Society of Health-System Pharmacists, Inc.

Levothyroxine Sodium

68:36.04 • THYROID AGENTS

■ Levothyroxine sodium, the sodium salt of the L-isomer of thyroxine, is a thyroid agent.

USES

● Hypothyroidism

Levothyroxine sodium is used as replacement or supplemental therapy in congenital or acquired hypothyroidism of any etiology, except transient hypothyroidism during the recovery phase of subacute thyroiditis. Levothyroxine sodium is specifically indicated for use in the management of subclinical hypothyroidism and primary (thyroidal), secondary (pituitary), and tertiary (hypothalamic) hypothyroidism. Primary hypothyroidism may result from functional deficiency, primary atrophy, partial or complete absence of the thyroid gland, or from the effects of surgery, radiation, or antithyroid agents, with or without the presence of goiter.

Replacement therapy with levothyroxine sodium must be maintained continuously to control the symptoms of hypothyroidism. Levothyroxine sodium generally is the preferred thyroid agent for replacement therapy because its hormonal content is standardized and its effect is therefore predictable.

Levothyroxine sodium also is considered the drug of choice for the treatment of congenital hypothyroidism (cretinism). For a discussion on the use of levothyroxine in the treatment of congenital hypothyroidism, see Cautions: Pediatric Precautions, in the Thyroid Agents General Statement 68:36.04.

Levothyroxine sodium IV injection is used in the treatment of myxedema coma. Levothyroxine sodium injection has been used in other conditions when rapid thyroid replacement is required†; however, this is not an FDA-labeled use for the currently available injection.

Levothyroxine sodium may be used with antithyroid agents in the treatment of thyrotoxicosis to prevent goitrogenesis and hypothyroidism. While administration of levothyroxine occasionally may be useful to prevent antithyroid agent-induced hypothyroidism in the management of thyrotoxicosis during pregnancy, combination therapy generally is considered unnecessary since it may increase the requirement for antithyroid agents and therefore the risk of fetal hypothyroidism, which is not amenable to exogenous thyroid agent therapy.

● Pituitary TSH Suppression

Levothyroxine sodium may be used to suppress the secretion of thyrotropin (thyroid-stimulating hormone, TSH) in the treatment or prevention of various types of euthyroid goiters, including thyroid nodules, subacute or chronic lymphocytic thyroiditis (Hashimoto's thyroiditis), and multinodular goiter. Levothyroxine sodium also is used as an adjunct to surgery and radioiodine therapy in the management of thyrotropin-dependent well-differentiated (papillary and follicular) thyroid cancer.

DOSAGE AND ADMINISTRATION

● Reconstitution and Administration

Levothyroxine sodium is administered orally or by IV injection. The drug also has been administered by IM injection†; however, the IV route is preferred since absorption may be variable following IM administration. IM administration is not an FDA-labeled route of administration for the currently available levothyroxine sodium injection.

Oral Administration

Levothyroxine sodium usually is administered orally on an empty stomach, preferably one-half to one hour before breakfast or the first food of the day. Because Levoxyl® tablets may rapidly swell and disintegrate following oral administration (resulting in choking, gagging, or difficulty in swallowing), the manufacturer states that Levoxyl® tablets should be taken with a full glass of water.

In individuals who are unable to swallow the intact tablets (e.g., pediatric patients), the appropriate dose of levothyroxine tablets may be crushed and placed in a small amount (5–10 mL) of water; the resultant suspension should be administered by spoon or dropper immediately and should not be stored.

Foods that decrease absorption of levothyroxine (e.g., soybean infant formula, soybean flour, cotton seed meal) should not be used for administering levothyroxine. (See Pharmacokinetics: Absorption.) Oral levothyroxine sodium should be administered at least 4 hours apart from drugs that are known to interfere with its absorption (e.g., antacids, bile acid sequestrants, cation-exchange resins, ferrous sulfate, sucralfate, simethicone, calcium carbonate). See Drug Interactions in the Thyroid Agents General Statement 68:36.04.

IV Administration

Levothyroxine sodium also is administered by IV injection.

Levothyroxine sodium powder for injection should be reconstituted by adding 5 mL of 0.9% sodium chloride injection to a vial labeled as containing 100, 200, or 500 mcg of the drug, and shaking the vial to mix completely. The resultant solutions contain approximately 20, 40, or 100 mcg/mL, respectively, of levothyroxine sodium. Prior to administration, the reconstituted solution should be inspected visually for particulate matter and discoloration whenever solution and container permit. Reconstituted solutions of levothyroxine sodium should be used immediately and any unused portions discarded; the solutions should *not* be admixed with IV infusion solutions. (See Chemistry and Stability: Stability.)

● Dosage

The FDA states that all approved levothyroxine sodium preparations should be considered therapeutically *in*equivalent unless equivalence has been established and noted in FDA's *Approved Drug Products with Therapeutic Equivalence Evaluations* (Orange Book). Theoretically, such preparations can be used interchangeably, and in some cases, pharmacists may be able to substitute generic for proprietary (brand) preparations without notifying the prescriber. However, because of the narrow therapeutic index of the drug, the American Thyroid Association (ATA) and the American Association of Clinical Endocrinologists (AACE) state that levothyroxine sodium preparations generally should *not* be used interchangeably. If a patient switches levothyroxine sodium preparations (e.g., from brand to generic), pharmacists are encouraged to notify the patient and prescriber of the switch. In addition, serum thyrotropin (thyroid-stimulating hormone, TSH) concentration should be measured about 4–8 weeks after starting the new preparation and the levothyroxine dosage adjusted if needed.

Dosage of levothyroxine sodium must be carefully adjusted according to individual requirements and response. The age, body weight, and general physical condition of the patient and the severity and duration of hypothyroid symptoms determine the initial dosage and rate at which dosage may be increased to the eventual maintenance dosage. Under- or over-treatment, which may result in adverse effects on growth and development in pediatric patients, cardiovascular function, bone metabolism, reproductive function, cognitive function, emotional state, GI function, and glucose and lipid metabolism, should be avoided.

Dosage should be initiated at a lower level in geriatric patients, in patients with functional or ECG evidence of cardiovascular disease, and in patients with severe, long-standing hypothyroidism, since an abrupt increase in metabolic rate and demand for increased cardiac output associated with levothyroxine therapy may precipitate angina pectoris, myocardial infarction, congestive heart failure, arrhythmias, or sudden cardiac death in such patients. In patients with severe, long-standing hypothyroidism in whom pituitary and adrenal function may be secondarily decreased, rapid replacement therapy with levothyroxine sodium also may precipitate adrenal insufficiency; in addition, psychosis or agitation occasionally may develop during initiation of levothyroxine therapy, necessitating a lower initial dosage in these patients. Adjustment of thyroid replacement therapy should be determined mainly by the patient's clinical response and confirmed by appropriate laboratory tests.

The manufacturer of levothyroxine sodium for injection states that caution should be used when switching patients from oral to IV levothyroxine sodium since the relative bioavailability and an accurate dosing conversion between the oral and IV preparations have not been established. Relative bioavailability between oral and IV administration has been estimated to range from 48–74%.

Hypothyroidism

Adult Dosage

For the management of hypothyroidism in otherwise healthy individuals younger than 50 years of age and in those older than 50 years of age who have been recently treated for hyperthyroidism or who have been hypothyroid for only a short time (i.e., several months), the usual initial oral dosage (full replacement dosage) of levothyroxine sodium is 1.7 mcg/kg daily (e.g., 100–125 mcg daily for a 70-kg adult) given as a single dose. Older patients may require less than 1 mcg/kg daily.

In one study, the usual maintenance dosage for geriatric patients was about 25% less than that for younger and heavier adults. Some manufacturers state that levothyroxine sodium dosages greater than 200 mcg daily are seldom required, and that failure to respond adequately to oral dosages of 300 mcg daily or greater is rare and should prompt reevaluation of the diagnosis, or suggest the presence of malabsorption, patient noncompliance, and/or drug interactions.

Patients should be evaluated initially about every 6–8 weeks to monitor the response to therapy. Once normalization of thyroid function and serum thyrotropin (thyroid-stimulating hormone, TSH) concentrations has been achieved, patients may be evaluated less frequently (i.e., every 6–12 months). However, if the dosage of levothyroxine sodium tablets is changed, serum TSH concentrations should be measured after 8–12 weeks or 4–8 weeks after switching from one levothyroxine sodium preparation to another.

For most patients older than 50 years of age or in patients younger than 50 years of age with underlying cardiovascular disease, the usual initial oral dosage of levothyroxine sodium is 25–50 mcg daily given as a single dose; dosage may be increased at intervals of 6–8 weeks. The usual initial dosage in geriatric patients with underlying cardiovascular disease is 12.5–25 mcg daily, with gradual dosage increments at intervals of 4–6 weeks. Dosage may be increased by increments of 12.5–25 mcg at recommended intervals until the patient becomes euthyroid and serum TSH concentrations return to normal.

For the management of severe, long-standing hypothyroidism in adults, the usual initial oral dosage of levothyroxine sodium is 12.5–25 mcg daily given as a single dose. Although the manufacturers state that dosage may be increased by increments of 25 mcg at intervals of 2–4 weeks until serum TSH concentrations return to normal, some clinicians suggest that dosage may be adjusted at intervals of 4–8 weeks.

If treatment is considered necessary in patients with subclinical hypothyroidism, the manufacturers state that lower initial levothyroxine dosages (e.g., 1 mcg/kg daily) may be adequate to normalize TSH concentrations. If levothyroxine replacement therapy is not initiated, patients still should be monitored annually for changes in clinical status and thyroid laboratory parameters.

Although the average full replacement dosage of levothyroxine sodium is about 1.6–1.7 mcg/kg daily, some patients (e.g., younger pediatric patients, pregnant women) may require higher dosages.

Pediatric Dosage

Despite the smaller body size of pediatric patients, the dosage of levothyroxine sodium (on a weight basis) required to sustain a full rate of growth, development, and general thriving is higher in these patients than in adults. In general, levothyroxine sodium therapy should be initiated at full replacement dosages in pediatric patients as soon as possible after diagnosis of hypothyroidism to prevent deleterious effects on intellectual and physical growth and development; however, dosage should be initiated at a lower level in children with long-standing or severe hypothyroidism.

For the treatment of congenital hypothyroidism (cretinism) or acquired hypothyroidism in pediatric patients, levothyroxine sodium therapy usually is initiated at full replacement dosages; daily dose per body weight decreases with age. The following dosages have been recommended:

Age	Daily Dose
0–3 months	10–15 mcg/kg
3–6 months	25–50 mcg or 8–10 mcg/kg
6–12 months	50–75 mcg or 6–8 mcg/kg
1–5 years	75–100 mcg or 5–6 mcg/kg
6–12 years	100–150 mcg or 4–5 mcg/kg
Older than 12 years	> 150 mcg or 2–3 mcg/kg
Growth and puberty complete	1.6–1.7 mcg/kg

The usual initial oral dosage of levothyroxine sodium in otherwise healthy, full-term neonates is 10–15 mcg/kg daily given as a single dose. A lower initial dosage (e.g., 25 mcg daily) should be considered in neonates at risk of cardiac failure; dosage may be increased at intervals of 4–6 weeks as needed based on clinical and laboratory response to treatment. In neonates with very low (less than 5

mcg/dL) or undetectable serum thyroxine (T_4) concentrations, the usual initial dosage is 50 mcg daily.

The manufacturers state that hyperactivity in an older child may be minimized by initiating therapy at a dosage approximately one-fourth of the recommended full replacement dosage; the dosage may then be increased by an amount equal to one-fourth the full recommended replacement dosage at weekly intervals until the full recommended replacement dosage is reached.

For the treatment of severe, long-standing hypothyroidism in pediatric patients, the usual initial oral dosage of levothyroxine sodium is 25 mcg daily. Dosage may be increased in increments of 25 mcg at intervals of 2–4 weeks until the desired response is obtained.

Myxedema Coma

For the treatment of myxedema coma, levothyroxine sodium is given by IV injection; oral administration is not recommended because absorption of the drug from the GI tract is unpredictable in such patients.

Initial and maintenance dosages of IV levothyroxine sodium should be selected after taking into account the age, general physical condition, and cardiac risk factors of the patient, as well as the clinical severity and duration of myxedema symptoms. The manufacturer states that the initial adult IV loading dose for the treatment of myxedema coma is 300–500 mcg; however, some clinicians recommend an initial dose of 100–500 mcg. Lower IV maintenance dosages of 50–100 mcg once daily should be administered thereafter as clinically indicated until the patient's condition is stabilized and the drug can be given orally.

In the geriatric population and in patients with underlying cardiovascular disease, administration of IV levothyroxine sodium, especially loading doses exceeding 500 mcg, may precipitate severe adverse cardiovascular effects (e.g., arrhythmias, tachycardia, myocardial ischemia or infarction, worsening of heart failure, death). The manufacturer states that cautious use (e.g., dosages in the lower end of the recommended range) of IV levothyroxine sodium may be warranted in geriatric patients and in those with known cardiac risk factors.

Pituitary TSH Suppression

Some manufacturers caution that the target level for TSH suppression in the management of well-differentiated thyroid cancer and thyroid nodules has not been established. In addition, the efficacy of TSH suppression for benign nodular disease remains controversial. Therefore, dosage of levothyroxine sodium used for TSH suppression should be individualized based on patient characteristics and the nature of the disease.

For the management of thyrotropin-dependent well-differentiated (papillary and follicular) thyroid cancer, an oral levothyroxine sodium replacement dosage of greater than 2 mcg/kg daily given as a single dose has been recommended to suppress TSH concentrations to less than 0.1 mU/L. In patients with high-risk tumors, the target level for TSH suppression may be less than 0.01 mU/L.

For the management of benign nodules and nontoxic multinodular goiter, TSH concentrations generally are suppressed to a higher target (e.g., 0.1–0.5 mU/L for nodules and 0.5–1 mU/L for multinodular goiter) than that used for the treatment of thyroid cancer.

CAUTIONS

Levothyroxine sodium shares the toxic potentials of other thyroid agents and the usual precautions of thyroid agent therapy should be observed. (See Cautions in the Thyroid Agents General Statement 68:36.04.) Adverse reactions to levothyroxine sodium result from overdosage and are manifested principally as signs and symptoms of hyperthyroidism (e.g., chest pain, palpitations, cardiac arrhythmias, difficulty in sleeping). Hyperthyroidism is a risk factor for osteoporosis. Evidence from several studies in premenopausal women receiving levothyroxine sodium for replacement or suppressive therapy suggests that subclinical hyperthyroidism is associated with bone loss. Therefore, to minimize the risk of osteoporosis, dosage of levothyroxine sodium should be titrated to the lowest possible effective level. (See Dosage and Administration: Dosage.) In addition, hypothyroidism manifested by severe depression, fatigue, weight gain, constipation, cold intolerance, edema, and difficulty in concentration may occur in patients receiving levothyroxine sodium preparations with inadequate potency.

Choking, gagging, dysphagia, or lodging of a tablet in the throat has been reported with Levoxyl®, particularly when the tablets were not administered with water. Therefore, the manufacturer states that Levoxyl® tablets should be taken with a full glass of water.

Patients with a history of lactose intolerance may be sensitive to Levothroid®, Synthroid®, and Unithroid® tablets, since lactose is used in the manufacture of the tablets.

PHARMACOLOGY

The principal pharmacologic effect of exogenous thyroid hormones is to increase the metabolic rate of body tissues. Thyroid hormones are also involved in the regulation of cell growth and differentiation. Although the precise mechanism of action by which thyroid hormones affect metabolism and cellular growth and differentiation is not clearly established, it is known that these physiologic effects are mediated at the cellular level, principally via triiodothyronine; a major portion of triiodothyronine is derived from thyroxine by deiodination in peripheral tissues. Thyroxine is the major component of normal secretions of the thyroid gland and is therefore the principal determinant of normal thyroid function. For further information, see Pharmacology in the Thyroid Agents General Statement 68:36.04.

PHARMACOKINETICS

● Absorption

Levothyroxine is variably absorbed from the GI tract (range: 40–80%). In animals, levothyroxine is absorbed in the proximal and middle jejunum; the drug is not absorbed from the stomach or distal colon and little, if any, absorption occurs in the duodenum. Studies in humans indicate that levothyroxine is absorbed from the jejunum and ileum and some absorption also occurs in the duodenum. The degree of absorption of levothyroxine from the GI tract depends on the product formulation and type of intestinal contents, including plasma protein and soluble dietary factors that may bind thyroid hormone and make it unavailable for diffusion. In addition, concurrent oral administration of infant soybean formula, soybean flour, cotton seed meal, walnuts, foods containing large amounts of fiber, ferrous sulfate, antacids, sucralfate, calcium carbonate, cation-exchange resins (e.g., sodium polystyrene sulfonate), simethicone, or bile acid sequestrants may decrease absorption of levothyroxine. The extent of levothyroxine absorption is increased in the fasting state and decreased in malabsorption states (e.g., sprue); absorption also may decrease with age.

The absorption of levothyroxine is variable following IM administration (not an FDA-labeled route of administration for the currently available levothyroxine sodium injection).

In the past, results of studies evaluating the bioequivalence and interchangeability of various commercially available oral preparations of levothyroxine have been conflicting. Results of several early studies indicated that various commercially available levothyroxine sodium tablets (i.e., Levothroid®, Synthroid® [formulation available prior to 1982], several nonproprietary [generic] preparations) were not bioequivalent based on measurements of thyroxine content in the tablets and of thyroid function in patients receiving the preparations. Potency of oral levothyroxine sodium preparations manufactured in the US after 1985 reportedly was more uniform since USP required all manufacturers of the drug to monitor levothyroxine content and ensure tablet potency. Several reports published after 1984 indicated that the drug content of various levothyroxine preparations (Synthroid®, Levothroid®, Levoxine®, and certain nonproprietary preparations) was within FDA specifications (i.e., no less than 90% and no more than 110% of labeled potency). However, the FDA concluded in 1997 that stability problems with oral levothyroxine sodium preparations commercially available at that time continued to result in unpredictable drug potency and announced that orally administered levothyroxine sodium products are considered new drugs; manufacturers wishing to market levothyroxine preparations were required to submit a new drug application (NDA) to the FDA. (See Chemistry and Stability: Stability.) Results of one single-blind, randomized, 4-way cross-over study in women with hypothyroidism who were clinically and chemically euthyroid and who received levothyroxine sodium 100 or 150 mcg daily for a minimum of 3 months prior to study entry suggested that the commercially available levothyroxine sodium tablets tested in this study (i.e., Levoxyl® [formerly Levoxine®], Synthroid®, 2 nonproprietary preparations) were bioequivalent and interchangeable in the majority of patients receiving such preparations, based on measurements of levothyroxine sodium content in the tablets and of patient thyroid function. However, the FDA states that all approved levothyroxine sodium preparations should be considered therapeutically *in*equivalent unless equivalence has been established and noted in

FDA's *Approved Drug Products with Therapeutic Equivalence Evaluations* (Orange Book). (See Dosage and Administration: Dosage.)

● Distribution

Because thyroxine is more highly and firmly protein bound than triiodothyronine, levothyroxine has a much slower onset of pharmacologic action and a longer duration of action than liothyronine.

● Elimination

The usual plasma half-lives of thyroxine and triiodothyronine are 6–7 days and approximately 1–2 days, respectively. The plasma half-lives of thyroxine and triiodothyronine are decreased in patients with hyperthyroidism and increased in those with hypothyroidism.

CHEMISTRY AND STABILITY

● Chemistry

Levothyroxine sodium is commercially available as tablets for oral administration and as a lyophilized powder for injection for IV administration.

Levothyroxine sodium is the monosodium salt of the *levo* isomer of thyroxine, the principal secretion of the thyroid gland. The commercially available drug is prepared synthetically. Structurally, levothyroxine sodium differs from liothyronine sodium only in the presence of an iodine atom in the 5′ position.

Levothyroxine sodium occurs as a light yellow to buff-colored, odorless, tasteless, hygroscopic powder and is very slightly soluble in water and slightly soluble in alcohol.

● Stability

Levothyroxine sodium is stable in dry air but may acquire a slight pink color upon exposure to light. Commercially available preparations of levothyroxine sodium should be stored in tight, light-resistant containers. Levothyroxine sodium is unstable in the presence of light, heat, air, and humidity. The manufacturers' labeling should be consulted for recommended storage temperatures, which can vary depending on the specific manufacturer and preparation. In some cases, tablets of the drug have been unstable even at room temperature, and storage at temperatures of 8–15°C were required to maintain potency.

In 1997, the FDA determined that important stability and potency problems existed for oral levothyroxine sodium preparations, and such problems potentially could result in serious health consequences because of inconsistent drug potency. It appeared that many oral levothyroxine sodium preparations that were commercially available at that time failed to maintain potency throughout their customary 2-year shelf-life even when stored as directed, and it was suggested that this shelf-life might not be appropriate for these preparations because of accelerated degradation secondary to a variety of factors (e.g., light, temperature, air, humidity). In addition, some excipients contained in oral levothyroxine sodium preparations might hasten such degradation. Results of some stability studies indicate that levothyroxine sodium exhibits biphasic, first-order degradation with an initial fast degradation rate (which is temperature dependent), followed by a slower terminal phase. To compensate for the initial fast degradation rate, some manufacturers used excessive amounts of active ingredient, which could result in superpotency. It appeared that oral levothyroxine sodium preparations failed to maintain potency throughout their shelf-life, and the amount of active ingredient varied from lot to lot in identical-strength tablets supplied by the same manufacturer. As a result of stability problems and manufacturing practices used to compensate for instability of the drug, potency of a given preparation could not be ensured, even when the same brand of oral levothyroxine sodium preparation was used.

Levothyroxine sodium was introduced into the US market before 1962 without an approved new drug application (NDA), apparently with the belief that it was not a new drug. In patients with diminished or absent thyroid function, uniform potency and bioavailability of levothyroxine sodium tablets are very important since hypothyroidism or hyperthyroidism may result from administration of preparations with less or more than the specified potency and bioavailability, respectively. (See Cautions.) Between 1987 and 1994, the FDA received 58 reports of adverse drug reactions (e.g., manifestations of hypothyroidism or hyperthyroidism) apparently associated with irregular potency, mainly subpotency but also superpotency, of levothyroxine sodium preparations. Some of these adverse effects occurred following a switch in the brand of levothyroxine sodium, while others may have occurred secondary to inconsistent stability, potency, and bioavailability of a given preparation supplied by the same manufacturer. Since levothyroxine sodium preparations were marketed without an approved NDA, manufacturers were required to report only unexpected and severe adverse drug reactions to FDA; therefore, it is believed that this reported incidence of adverse effects secondary to potency problems may be conservative because of underreporting of such effects. In addition, since manufacturers were not required to obtain FDA approval to reformulate preparations containing levothyroxine sodium, preparations with substantially increased potency and associated severe adverse effects occasionally were marketed.

Because of reported potency and stability problems, the FDA announced in 1997 that oral preparations containing levothyroxine sodium were considered new drugs. Manufacturers who wished to continue marketing oral preparations containing levothyroxine sodium were required to submit an NDA to the FDA by August 14, 2000. Oral levothyroxine sodium preparations commercially available in the US after August 14, 2003 have been approved by the FDA and are considered to be safe and effective for their intended uses. The current edition of FDA's *Approved Drug Products with Therapeutic Equivalence Evaluations* (Orange Book; http://www.accessdata.fda.gov/scripts/cder/ob/default.cfm) should be consulted to determine which levothyroxine sodium preparations the FDA has evaluated and deemed as being therapeutically equivalent (i.e., as bioequivalent and expected to have the same clinical effect and safety profile when administered appropriately). (See Dosage and Administration: Dosage.)

Levothyroxine sodium powder for injection should be stored at 20–25°C and protected from light. Following reconstitution, the drug is stable for 4 hours; however, the manufacturer states that reconstituted solutions of levothyroxine sodium should be used immediately and should not be added to other IV fluids. Any unused portion should be discarded.

For further information on chemistry, pharmacology, pharmacokinetics, uses, toxicity, cautions, acute toxicity, drug interactions, laboratory test interferences, and dosage and administration of levothyroxine sodium, see the Thyroid Agents General Statement 68:36.04.

PREPARATIONS

Excipients in commercially available drug preparations may have clinically important effects in some individuals; consult specific product labeling for details.

Levothyroxine Sodium

Oral		
Tablets	25 mcg*	Levothroid®, Forest
		Levothyroxine Sodium Tablets
		Levoxyl® (scored), Jones
		Synthroid® (scored), Abbott
		Unithroid®, Watson
	50 mcg*	Levothroid®, Forest
		Levothyroxine Sodium Tablets
		Levoxyl® (scored), Jones
		Synthroid® (scored), Abbott
		Unithroid®, Watson
	75 mcg*	Levothroid®, Forest
		Levothyroxine Sodium Tablets
		Levoxyl® (scored), Jones
		Synthroid® (scored), Abbott
		Unithroid®, Watson
	88 mcg*	Levothroid®, Forest
		Levothyroxine Sodium Tablets
		Levoxyl® (scored), Jones
		Synthroid® (scored), Abbott
		Unithroid®, Watson
	100 mcg*	Levothroid®, Forest
		Levothyroxine Sodium Tablets
		Levoxyl® (scored), Jones
		Synthroid® (scored), Abbott
		Unithroid®, Watson
	112 mcg*	Levothroid®, Forest
		Levothyroxine Sodium Tablets
		Levoxyl® (scored), Jones
		Synthroid® (scored), Abbott
		Unithroid®, Watson
	125 mcg*	Levothroid®, Forest
		Levothyroxine Sodium Tablets
		Levoxyl® (scored), Jones
		Synthroid® (scored), Abbott
		Unithroid®, Watson
	137 mcg*	Levothroid®, Forest
		Levothyroxine Sodium Tablets
		Levoxyl® (scored), Jones
		Synthroid® (scored), Abbott
	150 mcg*	Levothroid®, Forest
		Levothyroxine Sodium Tablets
		Levoxyl® (scored), Jones
		Synthroid® (scored), Abbott
		Unithroid®, Watson
	175 mcg*	Levothroid®, Forest
		Levothyroxine Sodium Tablets
		Levoxyl® (scored), Jones
		Synthroid® (scored), Abbott
		Unithroid®, Watson
	200 mcg*	Levothroid®, Forest
		Levothyroxine Sodium Tablets
		Levoxyl® (scored), Jones
		Synthroid® (scored), Abbott
		Unithroid®, Watson
	300 mcg*	Levothroid®, Forest
		Levothyroxine Sodium Tablets
		Levoxyl® (scored), Jones
		Synthroid® (scored), Abbott
		Unithroid®, Watson

Parenteral		
For injection	100 mcg*	Levothyroxine Sodium for Injection
	200 mcg*	Levothyroxine Sodium for Injection
	500 mcg*	Levothyroxine Sodium for Injection

* available from one or more manufacturer, distributor, and/or repackager by generic (nonproprietary) name

† Use is not currently included in the labeling approved by the US Food and Drug Administration.

Selected Revisions December 7, 2015, © Copyright, April 1, 1968, American Society of Health-System Pharmacists, Inc.

Potassium Iodide

68:36.08 · ANTITHYROID AGENTS

■ Potassium iodide is an antithyroid agent, antisporotrichotic agent, and expectorant.

USES

● Hyperthyroidism

Oral potassium iodide is used in the preoperative management of hyperthyroidism in patients with Graves' disease undergoing thyroidectomy†, usually as an adjunct to other antithyroid agents (e.g., methimazole, propylthiouracil) and/or β-adrenergic blocking agents (e.g., propranolol). The American Thyroid Association (ATA), American Association of Clinical Endocrinologists (AACE), and others recommend that patients with Graves' disease scheduled for thyroidectomy be rendered euthyroid using other antithyroid agents (preferably methimazole) and then receive oral potassium iodide for 7–14 days (usually 10 days) in the immediate preoperative period. In exceptional circumstances when the euthyroid state cannot be achieved prior to thyroidectomy (e.g., urgent need for surgery, allergy to antithyroid drugs), these experts recommend that oral potassium iodide and a β-adrenergic blocking agent (e.g., propranolol) be administered in the immediate preoperative period. Preoperative potassium iodide has traditionally been used in Graves' disease patients undergoing surgery in an attempt to decrease thyroid blood flow, vascularity, and intraoperative blood loss; however, the necessity and benefits of this strategy have been questioned. Because of the risk of exacerbating hyperthyroidism, preoperative potassium iodide is not indicated in patients with toxic multinodular goiter or toxic adenoma undergoing thyroidectomy.

Oral potassium iodide also is used in the management of severe, life-threatening thyrotoxicosis† (thyroid storm, thyrotoxicosis crisis) in conjunction with other antithyroid agents (e.g., methimazole, propylthiouracil), β-adrenergic blocking agents (e.g., propranolol), corticosteroids (hydrocortisone, dexamethasone), treatment of hyperpyrexia, and appropriate fluid, electrolyte, and respiratory support. Other antithyroid agents (e.g., methimazole, propylthiouracil) are initiated first to block thyroid hormone synthesis and conversion of tetraiodothyronine (thyroxine, T_4) to triiodothyronine (T_3); potassium iodide is initiated 1 hour after the other antithyroid agents and is used to block new hormone synthesis and thyroid hormone release.

● Radiation Emergency

Oral potassium iodide is used during a radiation emergency to block thyroidal uptake of radioactive isotopes of iodine (e.g., I 131) that may be released into the environment (e.g., from a nuclear power plant) and thus minimize the risk of radiation-induced thyroid neoplasms related to *internal* exposures to radioiodines (inhaled or ingested). *Although potassium iodide provides protection for the thyroid from radioiodines, the drug has no impact on body uptake of other radioactive materials and does not provide protection against external irradiation of any kind.*

The extent of protection that oral potassium iodide can provide against inhaled or ingested radioiodines depends on several factors, including how quickly the drug is initiated and the total dose of radioactivity involved in the exposure. Thyroidal uptake of radioiodine can be reduced by more than 90–99% by oral intake of 130 mg of potassium iodide daily initiated shortly before or within 1–2 hours after acute exposure. Potassium iodide may still provide substantial protection if taken 3–4 hours after exposure; however, although some data indicate that the drug may be about 40% effective if taken 8 hours after exposure, it may offer little protection if taken 12 hours or more after exposure. The thyroid-blocking effect of a single 130-mg dose of potassium iodide persists for about 24 hours. If the exposure lasts longer than 24 hours and involves continuing or ongoing contamination, additional doses may be necessary until the risk of significant exposure to radioiodines no longer exists.

The US Food and Drug Administration (FDA) issued updated recommendations in December 2001 on the use of potassium iodide in the event of a radiation emergency involving the release of radioactive iodine. These recommendations provide guidance to other federal agencies, including the Environmental Protection Agency (EPA) and Nuclear Regulatory Commission (NRC), and to state and local governments on safe and effective dosages of potassium iodide as an adjunct to other protective measures (e.g., evacuation, sheltering, assurance of

uncontaminated milk and food). FDA recommendations issued in 1978 and 1982 were based on studies that estimated *external* thyroid exposure to radiation resulting from nuclear detonations in Hiroshima and Nagasaki and analogous studies in children who received therapeutic radiation to the head and neck. The 2001 recommendations were derived from much more comprehensive and reliable data relating *internal* radioiodine exposure (e.g., through inhalation or ingestion) to thyroid cancer risk following the 1986 Chernobyl nuclear reactor accident. Data from the Chernobyl incident indicated that the risk of thyroid cancer following a radiation emergency (e.g., nuclear reactor accident) is inversely related to age and that exposure to relatively small doses of radioiodine may lead to dramatic increases in thyroid cancer among exposed children. The revised FDA guidelines therefore recommend potassium iodide prophylaxis at predicted radiation exposures that are lower than previously recommended (particularly for children) and, to reduce the risk of hypothyroidism, lower dosage of potassium iodide for neonates, infants, and children compared with previous FDA recommendations. In addition, FDA no longer recommends emergency use of potassium iodide in adults over 40 years of age, unless a large internal radiation dose (e.g., at least 500 centigrays [cGy]) is anticipated. Potassium iodide is used as an adjunct to other protective measures (e.g., evacuation, sheltering, assurance of uncontaminated milk and food). The FDA recommends that individuals who are intolerant of potassium iodide and those for whom repeat doses of the drug are a concern (e.g., neonates 1 month of age or younger, pregnant or lactating women) be given priority with regard to these other protective measures.

If a radiation emergency related to a US nuclear power plant occurs, decisions to recommend use of protective measures for public health and safety (including use of potassium iodide for thyroidal blockade) reside with state and/or local government authorities responsible for radiological emergency planning and response. These authorities should inform the public of the nature of the radiation hazard and potential benefits and adverse effects of potassium iodide. For use in radiation emergencies, potassium iodide is commercially available in appropriate dosage forms (see Radiation Emergency under Dosage and Administration: Dosage) and may also be retained in state or local stockpiles.

● Exposure to Radiopharmaceuticals

Oral potassium iodide is used for protection of the thyroid during diagnostic or therapeutic use of radiopharmaceuticals or drugs that have radioactive components† (e.g., iodine I 131 tositumomab; no longer commercially available in the US). Potassium iodide treatment is initiated prior to use of the radiolabeled diagnostic or therapeutic agent to saturate the thyroid and protect it from uptake of radioiodide and is continued until the estimated activity of the radiolabeled agent has decreased to acceptable levels after the procedure or treatment has been completed. In some cases, oral potassium iodide has been used in conjunction with other thyroid protective agents (e.g., methimazole, thyroxine).

● Sporotrichosis

Oral potassium iodide is used for the treatment of cutaneous sporotrichosis† (localized to skin; also known as fixed cutaneous sporotrichosis) and lymphocutaneous sporotrichosis† (involves skin, subcutaneous tissues, regional lymphatics) caused by *Sporothrix schenckii*. Since it is inexpensive and generally has been effective, potassium iodide (oral solution containing 1 g/mL; also known as saturated solution of potassium iodide [SSKI®]) has historically been considered a standard of care for the treatment of cutaneous and lymphocutaneous sporotrichosis and continues to be a drug of first choice for these infections in some resource-limited settings and countries where the disease is endemic. However, compliance with the long-term treatment regimen can be a problem since the drug is associated with a substantial number of adverse effects (e.g., nausea, rash, fever, bitter or metallic taste, salivary gland enlargement, risk of iodism or potassium toxicity with prolonged use). In addition, safety and efficacy of oral potassium iodide for the treatment of cutaneous or lymphocutaneous sporotrichosis have not been established in randomized, controlled clinical studies and efficacy of the drug compared with that of other antifungals used for the treatment of these infections (e.g., itraconazole, terbinafine, fluconazole) has not been established.

The Infectious Diseases Society of America (IDSA) and other experts state that oral itraconazole is the drug of choice for the treatment of cutaneous and lymphocutaneous sporotrichosis and oral terbinafine and potassium iodide (oral solution containing 1 g/mL; also known as saturated solution of potassium iodide [SSKI®]) are the preferred alternatives. For the treatment of cutaneous sporotrichosis, local hyperthermia (i.e., direct application of heat using a pocket warmer, infrared or far-infrared heater, or similar device that warms tissue to 42–43°C) is another alternative that can be used when antifungal agents or potassium iodide cannot be used (e.g., pregnant or nursing women).

Oral potassium iodide is not effective for and should not be used for the treatment of extracutaneous sporotrichosis† (osteoarticular, pulmonary, meningeal) or disseminated sporotrichosis†. IV amphotericin B and oral itraconazole are the drugs of choice for these forms of sporotrichosis.

● Cough

Oral potassium iodide (oral solution containing 1 g/mL; also known as saturated solution of potassium iodide [SSKI®]) has been used as an expectorant in the symptomatic management of chronic pulmonary diseases where tenacious mucus complicates the condition (e.g., bronchial asthma, bronchitis, pulmonary emphysema); however, the drug has generally been replaced by more effective and safer expectorants. Although there is limited evidence that saline expectorants like potassium iodide can increase respiratory tract secretions, possibly as a reflex response to drug-induced gastric irritation, such evidence is sparse and inconclusive. In addition, there currently is insufficient evidence from well-designed studies to support the efficacy of potassium iodide as an expectorant.

DOSAGE AND ADMINISTRATION

● Administration

Potassium iodide is administered orally.

For use during a radiation emergency, potassium iodide is commercially available as tablets containing 65 or 130 mg of the drug and as an oral solution containing 65 mg/mL. If the oral solution containing 65 mg/mL is used, the dose should be administered undiluted using the calibrated dropper provided by the manufacturer.

For other indications, an oral solution of potassium iodide containing 1 g/mL (also known as saturated solution of potassium iodide [SSKI®]) also is available. If this oral solution is used, the dose should be administered in a glassful of water, fruit juice, or milk. To minimize GI irritation, the dose should be taken with food or milk. A calibrated dropper marked to deliver 300 mg (0.3 mL) or 600 mg (0.6 mL) of the drug is provided by the manufacturer. If a dose of the oral solution containing 1 g/mL is administered using a standard medicinal dropper, each drop (0.05 mL) contains 50 mg of potassium iodide.

Potassium iodide may be available as strong iodine solution (also known as Lugol's solution), an oral solution containing 50 mg of iodine and 100 mg of potassium iodide per mL; this preparation may be commercially available but is not approved by the US Food and Drug Administration (FDA). Doses of strong iodine solution should be diluted in water or juice. If a dose of strong iodine solution is administered using a standard medicinal dropper, each drop contains 8 mg of iodide.

Extemporaneous Oral Solutions

For use during a radiation emergency in infants, small children, and others who cannot swallow tablets, oral solutions (liquid mixtures) of potassium iodide can be prepared extemporaneously using 65- or 130-mg tablets of the drug.

To prepare an oral solution containing 8.125 mg/5 mL (8.125 mg/teaspoon), the manufacturers state that a single 65-mg tablet of potassium iodide should be pulverized in a small bowl using the back of a teaspoon; 4 teaspoons (20 mL) of water should then be added to the bowl and mixed until the tablet dissolves. This potassium iodide mixture should then be added to 4 teaspoons (20 mL) of milk (low-fat white or chocolate), orange juice, flat soda, raspberry syrup, or infant formula.

To prepare an oral solution containing 16.25 mg/5 mL (16.25 mg/teaspoon), the manufacturers state that a single 130-mg tablet of potassium iodide should be pulverized in a small bowl using the back of a teaspoon; 4 teaspoons (20 mL) of water should then be added to the bowl and mixed until the tablet dissolves. This potassium iodide mixture should then be added to 4 teaspoons (20 mL) of milk (low-fat white or chocolate), orange juice, flat soda, raspberry syrup, or infant formula.

Alternatively, the FDA states that an oral solution containing 16.25 mg/5 mL (16.25 mg/teaspoon) can be prepared by putting two 65-mg tablets or one 130-mg tablet in a small bowl and adding 4 teaspoons (20 mL) of water to the bowl. After soaking in the water for 1 minute, the tablet(s) should be crushed using the back of the teaspoon until no large pieces remain. This potassium iodide mixture should then be added to 4 teaspoons (20 mL) of milk (white or chocolate), orange juice, soda (e.g., cola), infant formula, raspberry syrup, or water.

These extemporaneous oral solutions of potassium iodide should be stored in a refrigerator and used within 7 days.

● Dosage

Hyperthyroidism

When oral potassium iodide is used in the preoperative management of hyperthyroidism in patients with Graves' disease undergoing thyroidectomy†, the drug is administered for 7–14 days (usually 10 days) in the immediate preoperative period (see Uses: Hyperthyroidism). If the potassium iodide oral solution containing 1 g/mL (also known as saturated solution of potassium iodide [SSKI®]) is used, the recommended dosage is 50–100 mg (1–2 drops or 0.05–0.1 mL) 3 times daily in adults or 150–350 mg (3–7 drops or 0.15–0.35 mL) 3 times daily in children. Alternatively, if strong iodine solution (also known as Lugol's solution; commercially available but not FDA approved) is used, the recommended dosage in adults is 5–7 drops (0.25–0.35 mL) 3 times daily.

When oral potassium iodide is used in the management of severe, life-threatening thyrotoxicosis† (thyroid storm, thyrotoxicosis crisis), the drug is initiated 1 hour after the initial dose of other antithyroid agents (see Uses: Hyperthyroidism). If the potassium iodide oral solution containing 1 g/mL (also known as saturated solution of potassium iodide [SSKI®]) is used, the recommended adult dosage is 250 mg (5 drops or 0.25 mL) every 6 hours. For the treatment of thyrotoxicosis in children, some experts recommend that the oral solution containing 1 g/mL (also known as saturated solution of potassium iodide [SSKI®]) be administered in a dosage of 50–250 mg (1–5 drops or 0.05–0.25 mL) 3 times daily.

Radiation Emergency

The dosage and duration of potassium iodide recommended during a radiation emergency and potential *internal* (inhalation or ingestion) exposure to radioiodines is based on predicted thyroid exposure, age and/or weight, and pregnancy and lactation status.

For use during a radiation emergency, potassium iodide is available as 65- or 130-mg tablets or as a solution containing 65 mg/mL. If necessary in an emergency situation for an infant, small child, or other individual who cannot swallow tablets, the manufacturers and FDA have provided instructions on how to prepare extemporaneous oral solutions (liquid mixtures) using potassium iodide tablets. (See Extemporaneous Oral Solutions under Dosage and Administration: Administration.)

For optimal protection against inhaled radioiodines, oral potassium iodide should be administered before or immediately coincident with passage of a radioactive cloud; potassium iodide may still have a substantial protective effect if administered 3–4 hours after exposure. The protective effect of potassium iodide persists for about 24 hours.

Potassium iodide should be administered once daily until a risk of substantial exposure to inhaled or ingested radioiodines no longer exists. However, to minimize the risk of hypothyroidism during a period of critical brain development, repeat administration of potassium iodide should be avoided in neonates 1 month of age or younger, unless other protective measures are not available. (See Cautions: Pediatric Precautions.) In addition, repeat administration of the drug should be avoided in pregnant and lactating women, unless other protective measures are not available. (See Cautions: Pregnancy and Lactation.)

Adult Dosage

The recommended adult dosage of oral potassium iodide for a radiation emergency is 130 mg once daily (one 130-mg tablet or two 65-mg tablets once daily). If the commercially available oral solution containing 65 mg/mL is used, adults should receive 130 mg once daily (2 mL once daily). Alternatively, if an extemporaneous oral solution containing 16.25 mg/5 mL (16.25 mg/teaspoon) is used, adults should receive a dosage of 130 mg once daily (40 mL or 8 teaspoons once daily).

During a radiation emergency, the FDA recommends use of potassium iodide in adults 19 through 40 years of age if predicted thyroid exposure is 10 centigrays (cGy) or more and in pregnant or lactating women if predicted thyroid exposure is 5 cGy or more. Because of the risk of hypothyroidism, the FDA recommends potassium iodide in adults older than 40 years of age only if predicted thyroid exposure is 500 cGy or more.

Pediatric Dosage

For a radiation emergency, adolescents older than 12 through 18 years of age should receive oral potassium iodide in a dosage of 130 mg once daily if they weigh 70 kg (150 lbs) or more or a dosage of 65 mg once daily if they weigh less than 70 kg (150 lbs). (See Table 1 and Table 2.) The FDA recommends use of potassium iodide in adolescents if predicted thyroid exposure is 5 cGy or more.

For a radiation emergency, neonates and children through 12 years of age should receive potassium iodide in a dosage based on age. (See Table 1 and Table 2.) The FDA recommends use of potassium iodide in neonates and children 12 years of age or younger if predicted thyroid exposure is 5 cGy or more.

TABLE 1. Recommended Pediatric Dosage of Potassium Iodide for Radiation Emergency (65- or 130-mg Tablets or Oral Solution Containing 65 mg/mL)

Age and Weight	Potassium Iodide Tablets (Iosat®, ThyroSafe®)	Potassium Iodide Oral Solution Containing 65 mg/mL (Thyroshield®)
Birth to 1 month	(See Table 2)	16.25 mg once daily (0.25 mL)
>1 month to 3 years	(See Table 2)	32.5 mg once daily (0.5 mL)
>3 through 12 years	65 mg once daily (one 65-mg tablet or ½ of 130-mg tablet)	65 mg once daily (1 mL)
>12 through 18 years weighing <70 kg (150 lbs)	65 mg once daily (one 65-mg tablet or ½ of 130-mg tablet)	65 mg once daily (1 mL)
>12 through 18 years weighing ≥70 kg (150 lbs)	130 mg once daily (two 65-mg tablets or one 130-mg tablet)	130 mg once daily (2 mL)

TABLE 2. Recommended Pediatric Dosage of Potassium Iodide for Radiation Emergency (Extemporaneous Oral Solutions)

Age and Weight	Extemporaneous Oral Solution Containing 8.125 mg/5 mL (8.125 mg/teaspoon)	Extemporaneous Oral Solution Containing 16.25 mg/5 mL (16.25 mg/teaspoon)
Birth to 1 month	16.25 mg once daily (10 mL or 2 teaspoons)	16.25 mg once daily (5 mL or 1 teaspoon)
>1 month to 3 years	32.5 mg once daily (20 mL or 4 teaspoons)	32.5 mg once daily (10 mL or 2 teaspoons)
>3 through 12 years	65 mg once daily (40 mL or 8 teaspoons)	65 mg once daily (20 mL or 4 teaspoons)
>12 through 18 years weighing <70 kg (150 lbs)	65 mg once daily (40 mL or 8 teaspoons)	65 mg once daily (20 mL or 4 teaspoons)
>12 through 18 years weighing ≥70 kg (150 lbs)	Use alternative preparation	130 mg once daily (40 mL or 8 teaspoons)

Sporotrichosis

For the treatment of cutaneous or lymphocutaneous sporotrichosis† caused by *Sporothrix schenckii*, the Infectious Diseases Society of America (IDSA) and other clinicians state that the usual initial dosage of potassium iodide oral solution containing 1 g/mL (also known as saturated solution of potassium iodide [SSKI®]) in adults is 250 mg (5 drops or 0.25 mL) 3 times daily; dosage may then be increased gradually as tolerated to a maximum of 2–2.5 g (40–50 drops or 2–2.5 mL) 3 times daily. For the treatment of cutaneous or lymphocutaneous sporotrichosis in children, some experts recommend that the oral solution containing 1 g/mL (also known as saturated solution of potassium iodide

[SSKI®]) be given in an initial dosage of 50 mg (1 drop or 0.05 mL) 3 times daily; dosage may then be increased gradually as tolerated. The IDSA states that the maximum pediatric dosage of the oral solution containing 1 g/mL is 1 drop/kg 3 times daily or 2–2.5 g (40–50 drops or 2–2.5 mL) 3 times daily, whichever is lowest.

The usual duration of oral potassium iodide therapy for the treatment of cutaneous or lymphocutaneous sporotrichosis† is 3–6 months. The IDSA recommends that potassium iodide be continued for 2–4 weeks after cutaneous lesions resolve; other experts recommend that the drug be continued for 4–6 weeks after cutaneous lesions resolve.

Cough

If the potassium iodide oral solution containing 1 g/mL (also known as saturated solution of potassium iodide [SSKI®]) is used as an expectorant, the usual adult dosage is 300 or 600 mg (0.3 or 0.6 mL) 3 or 4 times daily.

CAUTIONS

● Adverse Effects

Hypersensitivity reactions to iodides may occur and may be manifested by angioedema, cutaneous and mucosal hemorrhage, and signs and symptoms resembling serum sickness, such as fever, arthralgia, lymph node enlargement, and eosinophilia. Urticaria, thrombotic thrombocytopenic purpura, and fatal periarteritis have also been attributed to iodide hypersensitivity. Hypocomplementemic vasculitis in some patients with chronic urticaria or systemic lupus erythematosus has been associated with iodide sensitivity, and some clinicians caution that potassium iodide may precipitate severe systemic illness in such patients. Jodbasedow or iodine-induced thyrotoxicosis may occur with low doses of iodides (i.e., less than 25 mg of iodine daily); this effect is uncommon in the US but more frequent in areas with endemic iodine deficiency.

Manifestations of iodism (chronic iodine poisoning) may occur when potassium iodide is given in large doses or over extended periods of time. Iodism is usually manifested as a metallic taste, burning in the mouth and throat, soreness of the teeth and gums, increased salivation, coryza, sneezing, and irritation of the eyes with swelling of the eyelids. Severe headache, productive cough, pulmonary edema, dyspnea, bronchospasm, and swelling and tenderness of the parotid and submaxillary glands may occur. The throat, pharynx, larynx, and tonsils may become inflamed. Mild acneiform eruptions may occur, usually in seborrheic areas; rarely, severe and sometimes fatal eruptions (ioderma) may occur. Gastric irritation is common and diarrhea, sometimes bloody, may also occur. Signs and symptoms of iodism generally subside spontaneously within a few days of discontinuing the drug; symptomatic and supportive therapy, including abundant fluid and salt intake to help eliminate iodide, may be necessary.

Prolonged use of iodides or excessive doses may result in thyroid gland hyperplasia, thyroid adenoma, goiter, and severe hypothyroidism. Prolonged use of iodides may also induce hyperthyroidism, particularly in older individuals, patients with preexisting nontoxic nodular goiter, and patients residing in areas with endemic iodine deficiency.

● Precautions and Contraindications

Potassium iodide is contraindicated in individuals with known sensitivity to iodides or any ingredient in the formulation.

Potassium iodide also is contraindicated in patients with dermatitis herpetiformis, hypocomplementemic vasculitis, or nodular thyroid disease (e.g., multinodular goiter) *with* heart disease.

Since some individuals are markedly sensitive to iodides, initial potassium iodide doses should be administered with caution. Patients at risk for iodine-induced adverse effects (e.g., hyperthyroidism, thyrotoxicosis) include older patients and those with goiter or autoimmune thyroid disease. Potassium iodide, especially when indicated for more than a few days, should be used with caution in patients with multinodular goiter, Graves' disease, or autoimmune thyroiditis.

In the event of a radiation emergency, potassium iodide should be used with caution and as directed by public authorities. For radiation emergencies, potassium iodide may be used in patients with preexisting thyroid diseases if they do not have nodular thyroid conditions *with* heart disease; however, careful supervision by clinicians is recommended if therapy must be administered for more than a few days.

Vesication and desquamation may occur if strong iodine solution (also known as Lugol's solution; commercially available but not approved by the US Food and Drug Administration [FDA]) is allowed to pool in contact with skin. If accidental contact of strong iodine solution with skin or eyes occurs, the skin or eyes should be flushed with copious amounts of water for 15 minutes.

● Pediatric Precautions

Safety and efficacy of potassium iodide oral solution containing 1 g/mL (also known as saturated solution of potassium iodide [SSKI®]) have not been established in children. Potassium iodide oral solution containing 1 g/mL has been used for the treatment of cutaneous and lymphocutaneous sporotrichosis in children† and is recommended by the Infectious Disease Society of America (IDSA) as an alternative for the treatment of these infections in children. (See Uses: Sporotrichosis.)

Children are more susceptible to the dangerous effects of radioactive iodide than adults and the benefits of potassium iodide during a radiation emergency exceed the risks. However, to minimize the risk of hypothyroidism during a period of critical brain development, repeat administration of potassium iodide should be avoided in neonates 1 month of age or younger, unless other protective measures are not available. If potassium iodide is used in a neonate 1 month of age or younger, the neonate should be monitored for the potential development of hypothyroidism by measuring thyrotropin (thyroid-stimulating hormone, TSH) and, if indicated, free thyroxine (free T_4) and thyroid replacement therapy should be instituted if hypothyroidism occurs.

In a radiation emergency, children and neonates unable to tolerate potassium iodide and neonates in whom repeat administration of the drug is a concern should be given priority with regard to other protective measures (e.g., evacuation, sheltering, assurance of uncontaminated milk and food).

● Pregnancy, Fertility, and Lactation

Pregnancy

Iodides readily cross the placenta and may result in abnormal thyroid function and/or goiter in the neonate. Fetal thyroid may be most susceptible to the effects of excess iodine at the end of gestation.

Some experts state that potassium iodide is contraindicated in pregnant women. The American Academy of Pediatrics (AAP) states that use of potassium iodide as an expectorant is contraindicated during pregnancy.

There is no evidence that short-term use (e.g., 10 days) of potassium iodide for preoperative management of hyperthyroidism in pregnant women with Graves' disease undergoing thyroidectomy† is harmful to the fetus. If thyroidectomy is necessary for the treatment of hyperthyroidism during pregnancy, the American Thyroid Association (ATA) and American Association of Clinical Endocrinologists (AACE) recommend that the surgery be performed during the second trimester.

The FDA recommends that pregnant women receive potassium iodide during a radiation emergency for their own protection and that of the fetus; however, repeat administration should be avoided during pregnancy, unless other protective measures are not available. When repeat administration is indicated in a pregnant woman, consultation with a clinician is recommended and thyroid function monitoring may be indicated in the neonate.

If potassium iodide is used during pregnancy or if the patient becomes pregnant while receiving the drug, the patient should be informed of the potential risks to the fetus.

Lactation

Potassium iodide is distributed into milk and may cause rash and thyroid suppression in nursing infants.

The AAP considers potassium iodide to be compatible with breast-feeding.

In a radiation emergency, the FDA recommends that lactating women receive potassium iodide for their own protection. However, repeat administration should be avoided in lactating women unless other protective measures are not available. If repeat administration is indicated in a nursing woman, consultation with a clinician is recommended; thyroid function monitoring may be indicated in a breast-fed neonate.

Because radioactive iodine is distributed into milk, some experts (including the AAP) recommend that lactating women temporarily *not* breast-feed after a radiation emergency, unless no alternative is available. Breast-feeding can then be resumed when public authorities declare it safe to do so. The fact that administration of potassium iodide to lactating women potentially can reduce the radioiodine content of milk should be considered.

DRUG INTERACTIONS

Concomitant use of lithium salts and iodides may result in additive or synergistic hypothyroid effects. Hypothyroidism has been reported in several patients who received the drugs concomitantly. A lithium salt and potassium iodide generally should not be used concomitantly; if the drugs are used together, the patient should be monitored closely for signs and symptoms of hypothyroidism.

Concomitant use of antithyroid agents (e.g., methimazole) and potassium iodide may result in additive hypothyroid and goitrogenic effects.

Concomitant use of potassium iodide and potassium-containing drugs, potassium-sparing diuretics, or angiotensin-converting enzyme (ACE) inhibitors may be associated with hyperkalemia, which may result in cardiac arrhythmias or cardiac arrest.

PHARMACOLOGY

● Thyroid Hormone Synthesis and Regulation

Iodine is an essential component of thyroid hormones, tetraiodothyronine (thyroxine, T_4) and triiodothyronine (T_3), comprising 65 and 59% of the weights, respectively. Thyroxine and triiodothyronine are produced in the thyroid gland by the iodination and coupling of the amino acid tyrosine. (See Chemistry in the Thyroid Agents General Statement.) Thyroid hormones and thus iodine are essential for human life. The hormones regulate many key biochemical reactions, especially protein synthesis and enzymatic activity, and target the developing brain, muscle, heart, pituitary, and kidneys.

Iodine is ingested in a variety of chemical forms, but because its content in most food sources is low, iodine present in iodized salt or in processed foods from the addition of iodized salt or other additives (potassium iodate, calcium iodate, cuprous iodide) is its principal source in humans in developed countries. Iodine also is available in dietary supplements and from other sources (e.g., drugs such as thyroid agents [hormones] and amiodarone). Most ingested iodine is reduced in the GI tract and absorbed almost completely. Under normal conditions, the absorption of dietary iodine exceeds 90%. Once absorbed systemically, iodide is removed principally by the thyroid gland and kidneys. The thyroid gland selectively concentrates iodide in amounts required for adequate thyroid hormone synthesis, with most of the remaining iodide being excreted renally. Salivary glands, breast, choroid plexus, and gastric mucosa also can concentrate iodide; however, other than the lactating breast, these tissues are minor pathways of uncertain importance.

A sodium/iodide transporter in the thyroidal basal membrane is responsible for iodine concentration in the gland, transferring iodide from systemic circulation into the thyroid gland at a concentration gradient of 20–50 times that of plasma to ensure that the gland receives adequate amounts of iodine for hormone synthesis. During iodine deficiency, the thyroid gland concentrates most of the iodine available from plasma. Iodide participates in a complex series of reactions in the thyroid gland to produce thyroid hormones. Thyroglobulin is synthesized in thyroid cells and serves as an iodination vehicle. Thyroperoxidase and hydrogen peroxide promote the oxidation of iodide and its attachment to tyrosyl residues within the thyroglobulin molecule to produce the hormone precursors diiodotyrosine and monoiodotyrosine. Thyroperoxidase further catalyzes intramolecular coupling of 2 molecules of diiodotyrosine to produce T_4 and coupling of a molecule of diiodotyrosine and a molecule of monoiodotyrosine to produce T_3. The average adult thyroid gland in individuals residing in an iodine-sufficient geographic region contains about 15 mg of iodine. Iodine is not released into systemic circulation but instead is stored principally in diiodo and monoiodo tyrosine precursors, removed from the tyrosine moiety by a specific deiodinase, and then recycled within the thyroid gland as a mechanism of iodine conservation.

Once in systemic circulation, thyroxine and triiodothyronine attach to several binding proteins (e.g., thyronine-binding globulin, transthyretin, albumin), which then migrate to target tissues where thyroxine is deiodinated to triiodothyronine, the metabolically active form of thyroid hormone. The iodine that is removed from thyroxine returns to the serum iodine pool and follows the usual iodine cycle or is excreted renally. Thyrotropin (TSH) is the major thyroid function regulator. Thyrotropin affects several sites within thyrocytes, the principal actions of which are to increase thyroidal uptake of iodine and to break down thyroglobulin to release thyroid hormone into systemic circulation. An elevated serum thyrotropin concentration indicates primary hypothyroidism and a decreased serum concentration indicates hyperthyroidism.

The normal thyroid gland takes up the amount of systemically circulating iodine necessary to make the necessary amount of thyroid hormone for the body's needs. In iodine deficiency, the thyroid gland will concentrate more radioactive iodine, and the gland will concentrate less in iodine excess. However, other factors can influence radioactive iodine uptake, including thyroidal overproduction of hormone (hyperthyroidism), hypothyroidism, subacute thyroiditis, and many chemical and medicinal products. When iodine equilibrium is present, the mean daily thyroid iodine accumulation and release are similar.

● Effects in Hyperthyroidism

In patients with hyperthyroidism, iodide rapidly inhibits the release of thyroid hormones via a direct effect on the thyroid gland and inhibits the synthesis of thyroid hormones. Iodide apparently attenuates the effects of thyrotropin that are mediated via cAMP. The vascularity of the thyroid gland is reduced, the gland becomes much firmer, the cells become smaller, colloid reaccumulates in the follicles, and the quantity of bound iodine increases. The effects of potassium iodide on thyroid function are usually observed within 24 hours and are maximal after 10–15 days of continuous therapy; however, the drug does not completely control the manifestations of hyperthyroidism, and after a variable period of time the salutary effects subside.

● Effects in Radiation Emergencies

In the event of a radiation emergency, isotopes of iodine may be released into the environment. Radioactive iodine is taken up and stored in the thyroid gland in the same manner as stable iodine. (See Pharmacology: Thyroid Hormone Synthesis and Regulation.) The selective and rapid concentration and storage of radioactive iodine in the thyroid gland results in internal radiation exposure to the thyroid and increased risk of thyroid cancer and benign nodules and, at high doses, hypothyroidism. Administration of stable iodine (potassium iodide) before or promptly after intake of radioactive iodine blocks or reduces accumulation of radioactive iodine in the thyroid gland.

● Antifungal Effects

The mechanism of action of potassium iodide in the treatment of cutaneous or lymphocutaneous sporotrichosis† caused by *Sporothrix schenckii* has not been determined. In vitro, potassium iodide does not appear to increase monocyte or neutrophil killing of *S. schenckii*. However, exposure of the yeast form of *S. schenckii* to various concentrations of iodine (iodine and potassium iodide solution) in vitro has resulted in rapid cell destruction.

● Effects on Respiratory Tract Secretions

Potassium iodide is thought to act as an expectorant by increasing respiratory tract secretions and thereby decreasing the viscosity of mucus; however, this remains to be clearly established.

CHEMISTRY AND STABILITY

● Chemistry

Potassium iodide occurs as hexahedral crystals, either transparent and colorless or somewhat opaque and white, or as a white, granular powder. The drug is slightly hygroscopic. Potassium iodide is very soluble in water and soluble in alcohol. Each gram of potassium iodide contains about 6 mEq of potassium.

Potassium iodide is commercially available as tablets containing 65 or 130 mg of the drug and as an oral solution containing 65 mg/mL in a black raspberry-flavored solution. An aqueous oral solution of potassium iodide containing 1 g/mL also is commercially available; this preparation is known as saturated solution of potassium iodide (SSKI®).

Potassium iodide may be available as strong iodine solution (also known as Lugol's solution), a solution containing 50 mg of iodine and 100 mg of potassium iodide per mL. Strong iodine solutions may be commercially available for oral or topical administration, but these preparations are not approved by the US Food and Drug Administration (FDA).

● Stability

Potassium iodide tablets should be stored at 20–25°C in their original foil pack and protected from moisture.

Potassium iodide oral solution containing 65 mg/mL should be stored at 25°C, but may be exposed to 15–30°C; the solution should be stored in a tight container and protected from light.

Potassium iodide oral solution containing 1 g/mL (also known as saturated solution of potassium iodide [SSKI®]) should be stored at 15–30°C in a tight container and protected from light. The oral solution may crystallize if exposed to cold temperatures; however, crystals will dissolve if the solution is warmed and shaken. The solution should be discarded if it turns brownish-yellow in color.

Oral solutions of potassium iodide prepared extemporaneously using 65- or 130-mg tablets (see Extemporaneous Oral Solutions under Dosage and Administration: Administration) should be stored in the refrigerator and any unused solution discarded after 7 days.

PREPARATIONS

Excipients in commercially available drug preparations may have clinically important effects in some individuals; consult specific product labeling for details.

Potassium Iodide

Oral		
Solution	65 mg/mL	ThyroShield®, Fleming
	1 g/mL	SSKI®, Upsher-Smith
Tablets	65 mg	Iosat® (scored), Anbex
		ThyroSafe® (scored), Recipharm
	130 mg	Iosat® (scored), Anbex

Strong Iodine Solution

Oral		
Solution	Iodine 50 mg/mL and Potassium Iodide 100 mg/mL	Strong Iodine Solution Lugol's Solution

† Use is not currently included in the labeling approved by the US Food and Drug Administration.

Selected Revisions May 29, 2014, © Copyright, January 1, 1959, American Society of Health-System Pharmacists, Inc.

Propylthiouracil

68:36.08 • ANTITHYROID AGENTS

■ Propylthiouracil is a thiourea-derivative antithyroid agent.

USES

● Hyperthyroidism

Propylthiouracil is used in patients with Graves' disease with hyperthyroidism or toxic multinodular goiter who are intolerant of methimazole and for whom surgery or radioactive iodine therapy is not an appropriate treatment option. The drug also is used to ameliorate symptoms of hyperthyroidism in preparation for thyroidectomy or radioactive iodine therapy in patients who are intolerant of methimazole.

Because use of propylthiouracil is associated with a higher risk of clinically serious or fatal liver injury in adult and pediatric patients compared with methimazole, propylthiouracil should be reserved for patients who cannot tolerate methimazole and for whom radioactive iodine therapy or surgery are not appropriate for the management of hyperthyroidism. (See Cautions: Hepatic Effects and also see Cautions: Precautions and Contraindications.) Propylthiouracil is not recommended for use in pediatric patients except in rare instances in which methimazole is not well tolerated and surgery or radioactive iodine therapy are not appropriate therapies. (See Cautions: Hepatic Effects and also see Cautions: Pediatric Precautions.)

Because of the risk of fetal abnormalities associated with methimazole, propylthiouracil is the preferred agent when an antithyroid drug is indicated during or just prior to the first trimester of pregnancy (during organogenesis). However, it may be preferable to switch from propylthiouracil to methimazole for the second and third trimesters (i.e., after the first trimester) because of the risk of maternal adverse effects associated with propylthiouracil (e.g., hepatotoxicity). (See Pregnancy under Cautions: Pregnancy and Lactation.)

Thioamide antithyroid agents (e.g., propylthiouracil, methimazole) are used to control the symptoms of hyperthyroidism associated with Graves' disease and maintain the patient in a euthyroid state for a period of several years (generally 1–2 years) until a spontaneous remission occurs. Thioamide antithyroid agents do not affect the underlying cause of hyperthyroidism. Spontaneous remission does not occur in all patients receiving therapy with thioamide antithyroid agents, and most patients eventually require ablative therapy (i.e., surgery, radioactive iodine). The minimum duration of thioamide therapy necessary before assessing whether spontaneous remission has occurred is not clearly established. However, some clinicians suggest that the optimum duration of antithyroid drug therapy in patients with Graves' disease generally is 12–18 months.

Propylthiouracil returns the hyperthyroid patient to a normal metabolic state prior to thyroidectomy and controls the thyrotoxic crisis that may accompany thyroidectomy. (See Thyrotoxic Crisis under Uses: Hyperthyroidism.)

Propylthiouracil also controls symptoms of hyperthyroidism prior to and after administration of radioactive iodine until the ablative effects of the iodine occur. However, the beneficial and detrimental effects and optimal sequencing of antithyroid drugs before or after radioactive iodine therapy have not been clearly established. In addition, pretreatment with propylthiouracil may increase the radioresistance of the thyroid and the risk of radioactive iodine treatment failure.

Antithyroid agents do not induce remission in patients with nodular thyroid disease (i.e., toxic adenoma†, toxic multinodular goiter), and discontinuance of therapy results in relapse. Therefore, some clinicians suggest that adults with overt toxic adenoma or toxic multinodular goiter be treated with either radioactive iodine therapy or thyroidectomy.

Thyrotoxic Crisis

In the management of thyrotoxic crisis, thioamide antithyroid agents are used to inhibit thyroid hormone synthesis. Because propylthiouracil also blocks the peripheral conversion of thyroxine to triiodothyronine, it theoretically may be more useful than methimazole or carbimazole (not commercially available in the US) in the management of thyrotoxic crisis. Iodides (e.g., potassium iodide, strong iodine solution) are given to inhibit the release of thyroid hormone from the gland but may subsequently be used as a substrate for thyroid hormone synthesis; therefore, treatment with a thioamide antithyroid agent is usually initiated

before iodide therapy. A β-adrenergic blocking agent (e.g., propranolol) is also usually given concomitantly to manage peripheral signs and symptoms of hyperthyroidism, particularly cardiovascular effects (e.g., tachycardia).

● Alcoholic Liver Disease

Propylthiouracil has been studied in patients with alcoholic liver disease†. However, analysis of data from 6 randomized clinical trials with propylthiouracil found that no substantial benefit has been demonstrated on any clinically important outcomes of alcoholic liver disease (e.g., all-cause mortality, liver-related mortality, complications associated with the liver disease, liver histology) and that the currently available evidence does not support its use outside of randomized clinical studies. Additional research (e.g., large clinical trials with adequate methodology, several years of treatment, independent and close monitoring of efficacy and safety) is needed to determine the safety and efficacy of propylthiouracil in patients with alcoholic liver disease.

DOSAGE AND ADMINISTRATION

● Administration

Propylthiouracil is administered orally; daily dosage is usually given in 3 equally divided doses at approximately 8-hour intervals. In some cases, more frequent administration (e.g., at 4- or 6-hour intervals) may be necessary.

● Dosage

Adult Dosage

For the treatment of hyperthyroidism, the manufacturer states that the usual initial adult dosage of propylthiouracil is 300 mg daily, usually given in 3 equally divided doses at approximately 8-hour intervals. The manufacturer also states that in patients with severe hyperthyroidism and/or very large goiters, the initial dosage may be increased to 400 mg daily; however, initial dosages of 600–900 mg daily occasionally may be required. Alternatively, for the treatment of Graves' disease, some clinicians recommend an initial adult dosage of 50–150 mg 3 times daily, depending on the severity of the hyperthyroidism. In general, most patients improve considerably or achieve normal thyroid function following 4–12 weeks of therapy, after which dosage may be decreased while maintaining normal thyroid function. Subsequent dosage should be carefully adjusted according to the patient's tolerance and therapeutic response. The manufacturer states that the usual adult maintenance dosage is 100–150 mg daily, given in 3 equally divided doses at approximately 8-hour intervals. Alternatively, as the clinical findings and thyroid function tests return to normal, some clinicians state that reducing the maintenance dosage to 50 mg 2 or 3 times daily is usually possible for treatment of Graves' disease. (See Cautions: Precautions and Contraindications and also see Cautions: Adverse Effects.) The optimum duration of antithyroid therapy remains to be clearly established. However, some clinicians suggest that the optimum duration of antithyroid drug therapy in patients with Graves' disease generally is 12–18 months.

If propylthiouracil is used during pregnancy for the management of hyperthyroidism, the manufacturer states that a sufficient, but not excessive, dosage of propylthiouracil is necessary. The manufacturer states that because thyroid dysfunction diminishes in many women as pregnancy proceeds, a reduction in dosage may be possible, and, in some patients, propylthiouracil can be discontinued several weeks or months before delivery. (See Pregnancy under Cautions: Pregnancy and Lactation.)

Dosage of propylthiouracil should be selected with caution in geriatric patients because of the greater frequency of decreased hepatic, renal, and/or cardiac function and of concomitant disease and drug therapy. (See Cautions: Geriatric Precautions.)

For the treatment of thyrotoxic crisis (i.e., thyroid storm) in adults, some clinicians recommend a propylthiouracil loading dose of 500 mg to 1 g, followed by 250 mg every 4 hours.

If propylthiouracil is used prior to thyroidectomy to render adults euthyroid, propylthiouracil should be discontinued at the time of the procedure.

If propylthiouracil is used as pretreatment prior to radioactive iodine therapy in adults, some clinicians recommend that propylthiouracil be discontinued 2–7 days before administration of radioactive iodine, restarted 3–7 days after radioactive iodine, and discontinued once thyroid function has normalized.

Pediatric Dosage

Propylthiouracil generally is not recommended for use in pediatric patients except in rare instances in which alternative therapies are not appropriate options. The manufacturer states that studies evaluating appropriate dosage regimens have not been conducted in the pediatric population, although general practice would suggest initiation of therapy in children 6 years of age or older at a dosage of 50 mg daily with careful upward titration based on clinical response and evaluation of thyrotropin (thyroid stimulating hormone, TSH) and free thyroxine (T_4) concentrations. Although cases of severe liver injury have been reported with dosages as low as 50 mg daily, most cases were associated with dosages of 300 mg daily and higher. (See Cautions: Pediatric Precautions and also see Cautions: Hepatic Effects.)

CAUTIONS

Adverse Effects

Minor adverse effects of propylthiouracil include rash, urticaria, pruritus, abnormal hair loss, skin pigmentation, edema, nausea, vomiting, epigastric distress, loss of taste, taste perversion, arthralgia, myalgia, paresthesia, and headache. Drowsiness, neuritis, vertigo, sialadenopathy, lymphadenopathy, and jaundice also have occurred in patients receiving the drug. (See Cautions: Hepatic Effects.)

Although reported much less frequently, severe adverse effects of propylthiouracil include liver injury (resulting in hepatitis, liver failure, a need for liver transplantation, or death [see Cautions: Hepatic Effects]); inhibition of myelopoiesis with resultant agranulocytosis (see Cautions: Agranulocytosis), granulocytopenia, and thrombocytopenia; aplastic anemia; drug fever; lupus-like syndrome (including splenomegaly and vasculitis); hepatitis; periarteritis; and hypoprothrombinemia and bleeding. Nephritis, glomerulonephritis, interstitial pneumonitis, exfoliative dermatitis, and erythema nodosum also have been reported.

A vasculitic syndrome associated with the presence of antineutrophil cytoplasmic antibodies (ANCA) has been reported. Manifestations of ANCA-positive vasculitis may include rapidly progressive glomerulonephritis (crescentic and pauci-immune necrotizing glomerulonephritis), sometimes resulting in acute renal failure; pulmonary infiltrates or alveolar hemorrhage; skin ulcers; and leukocytoclastic vasculitis. Cutaneous vasculitis, which may manifest as purpuric and/or bullous hemorrhagic lesions or erythema nodosum, and possibly may progress to necrotic ulcerations, and polymyositis also have occurred.

Hepatic Effects

Liver injury (including severe liver injury) resulting in hepatitis, liver failure (including acute liver failure), liver transplantation, or death has been reported with propylthiouracil therapy in adult and pediatric patients. An analysis of adverse event reports received by the US Food and Drug Administration (FDA) found that, while severe propylthiouracil-associated hepatotoxicity has been reported among patients in all age groups, the reports and signals of hepatotoxicity were highest among those younger than 17 years of age. No cases of liver failure have been reported with the use of methimazole, another antithyroid drug, in pediatric patients. For this reason, propylthiouracil is not recommended for use in pediatric patients except in rare instances in which methimazole is not well tolerated and surgery or radioactive iodine therapy are not appropriate therapies. (See Cautions: Pediatric Precautions.)

Cases of liver injury, including liver failure and death, have been reported in women receiving propylthiouracil during pregnancy. Two cases of in utero exposure to the drug with liver failure and death of a newborn have been reported. The use of an alternative antithyroid drug (e.g., methimazole) may be advisable after the first trimester of pregnancy. (See Pregnancy under Cautions: Pregnancy and Lactation.)

The extent of propylthiouracil-induced hepatitis and the true incidence of severe liver injury in patients receiving propylthiouracil is not known. The total annual number of cases of propylthiouracil-induced hepatitis in the United States has been estimated to be approximately 40–50 (31 adults, 4–8 pregnant women, 4 children) based on a 0.1% incidence of severe hepatitis; the total number of annual cases could range from 20–100 depending on the frequency of propylthiouracil-induced hepatitis and the prevalence of propylthiouracil use. In addition, propylthiouracil-induced acute liver failure has been estimated to occur in approximately 0.01% of adults and 0.025–0.05% of children receiving the drug. Between 1969 and June 2009, a total of 34 cases (23 adult and 11 pediatric) of serious liver injury associated with propylthiouracil use was reported to the FDA Adverse Event Reporting System (AERS). Among the 23 adult cases, 13 resulted in death and 5 resulted in liver transplantation; among the 11 pediatric cases, 2 resulted in death and 7 resulted in liver transplantation (one patient died while awaiting transplantation). In contrast, 5 AERS cases of serious liver injury were identified for methimazole; all cases were in adults and 3 resulted in death. Based on these results and a review of the medical literature, FDA has concluded that

use of propylthiouracil is associated with a higher risk for clinically serious or fatal liver injury compared with methimazole in both adult and pediatric patients. According to the United Network for Organ Sharing (UNOS) and the Organ Procurement and Transplantation Network (OPTN), liver transplantation was performed in 16 adults and 7 children between 1990 and 2007 as a result of propylthiouracil-induced liver failure; no liver transplantation attributed to methimazole toxicity occurred during this same time period.

Propylthiouracil-induced liver failure may occur at any time during therapy with a sudden onset, rapid progression, and a low chance of reversibility. According to data from the AERS database, liver failure occurred after 6–450 days of propylthiouracil therapy (median: 120 days). Although the effect of dosage on the risk of hepatotoxicity has not been clearly elucidated, the reported average daily dosage of propylthiouracil associated with liver failure in the AERS database was approximately 300 mg in both children and adults. Biochemical monitoring of liver function (bilirubin, alkaline phosphatase) and hepatocellular integrity (ALT, AST) is not expected to attenuate the risk of severe liver injury due to its rapid and unpredictable onset. (See Cautions: Precautions and Contraindications.)

Agranulocytosis

Agranulocytosis occurs in approximately 0.2–0.5% of patients receiving propylthiouracil and is a potentially life-threatening adverse effect of the drug. Agranulocytosis typically occurs within the first 3 months of therapy, but rarely may occur after 4 months of therapy. Agranulocytosis may occur irrespective of dosage, length of treatment, or previous exposure to the antithyroid drug, and may occur more frequently in geriatric patients. Although the mechanism(s) of propylthiouracil-induced agranulocytosis has not been determined, antigranulocyte antibodies have been reported in some patients with thioamide-induced agranulocytosis; a direct toxic effect of these drugs on bone marrow has not been excluded as an additional possible cause.

Hypothyroidism

Propylthiouracil may cause hypothyroidism necessitating routine monitoring of thyrotropin (thyroid stimulating hormone, TSH) and free thyroxine (T_4) concentrations; dosage should be adjusted to maintain a euthyroid state. (See Cautions: Precautions and Contraindications.) Because propylthiouracil readily crosses the placenta, the drug can cause fetal goiter and cretinism when administered to a pregnant woman. (See Pregnancy under Cautions: Pregnancy and Lactation.)

Precautions and Contraindications

Some clinicians suggest that liver function tests, including alkaline phosphatase, aminotransferase, and bilirubin, be performed prior to initiating antithyroid drug therapy in patients with Graves' disease. Patients receiving propylthiouracil should be closely monitored for signs and symptoms of liver injury, particularly during the first 6 months following initiation of therapy. (See Cautions: Hepatic Effects.) Routine biochemical monitoring of liver function (bilirubin, alkaline phosphatase) and hepatocellular integrity (ALT, AST) may not be effective in identifying patients at risk of developing propylthiouracil-induced liver failure and is not expected to attenuate the risk of severe liver injury because of its rapid and unpredictable onset; however, such tests should be performed in symptomatic patients. Patients should be informed of the risk of liver failure associated with propylthiouracil and advised to immediately discontinue the drug and promptly contact their clinician if signs and symptoms of liver injury or hepatic dysfunction (e.g., fatigue, weakness, vague abdominal pain, right upper quadrant pain, anorexia, pruritus, easy bruising, jaundice, pruritic rash, light-colored stool, dark urine, joint pain, bloating, nausea) occur, particularly in the first 6 months of therapy. Propylthiouracil should be discontinued immediately if a patient develops these symptoms, and the patient should be promptly evaluated for evidence of liver injury, including evaluation of liver function (bilirubin, alkaline phosphatase) and hepatocellular integrity (ALT, AST), and should be provided supportive care. Some clinicians state that propylthiouracil should be discontinued if aminotransferase concentrations (whether elevated at initiation of therapy, found incidentally, or measured as clinically indicated) increase to 2–3 times the upper limit of normal and fail to improve within 1 week with repeat testing. Following discontinuance of the drug, liver function (i.e., alkaline phosphatase, bilirubin, transaminases) should be monitored weekly until there is evidence of resolution. If resolution is not evident, prompt referral to a gastroenterologist or hepatologist is warranted.

Some clinicians suggest that a baseline complete blood count, including white count with differential, should be performed prior to initiating antithyroid drug therapy in patients with Graves' disease. Patients receiving propylthiouracil should be closely monitored and should be instructed to contact their clinician immediately if signs or symptoms of illness, particularly sore throat, skin eruptions, fever, chills, headache, or general malaise, occur; it is particularly important to carefully monitor for these signs and symptoms during the early stages of propylthiouracil therapy since propylthiouracil-induced agranulocytosis usually occurs during the first several months of therapy. Leukopenia, thrombocytopenia, and/or aplastic anemia (pancytopenia) also may occur. Leukocyte and differential counts should be performed in patients who develop fever or sore throat or other signs or symptoms of illness while receiving the drug. Leukopenia (i.e., leukocyte count less than 4000/mm³) occurs in 10% of untreated hyperthyroid patients and often is associated with relative granulocytopenia; this should be considered when evaluating the patient's myelopoietic response to the drug. Propylthiouracil should be used with extreme caution in patients receiving concomitant drugs known to be associated with agranulocytosis. The manufacturer states that propylthiouracil should be discontinued if agranulocytosis, aplastic anemia (pancytopenia), ANCA-positive vasculitis, hepatitis, interstitial pneumonitis, fever, or exfoliative dermatitis is suspected, and the patient's bone marrow indices should be obtained. Some clinicians state that patients should be informed of the adverse effects associated with propylthiouracil (e.g., agranulocytosis) and advised to immediately discontinue the drug and promptly contact their clinician if fever or pharyngitis occurs. In a patient who develops agranulocytosis or other serious adverse effects while receiving either methimazole or propylthiouracil, some clinicians state that use of the other drug also is contraindicated because of the risk of cross-sensitivity between the two drugs.

Because propylthiouracil may cause hypoprothrombinemia and bleeding, monitoring of prothrombin time should be considered during therapy with the drug, particularly prior to surgery (see Drug Interactions: Anticoagulants).

Thyroid function should be monitored periodically in patients receiving propylthiouracil. In patients with Graves' disease, some clinicians state that thyroid function (e.g., serum free T_4, serum free or total triiodothyronine [T_3], TSH) should be monitored before initiating therapy and then every 4–8 weeks thereafter (with subsequent dosage adjustments as needed) until thyroid function is stable or the patient is euthyroid; once the patient is euthyroid, thyroid function may be monitored every 2–3 months. Early in the course of antithyroid therapy, serum TSH concentration is not a reliable parameter to monitor because it may remain suppressed for several months after initiation of therapy despite normalization of free T_4 concentrations. The finding of a suppressed TSH concentration during this period, therefore, does not indicate a need for a dosage increase. However, once clinical evidence of resolution of hyperthyroidism occurs, the finding of an elevated serum TSH concentration indicates that a lower maintenance dosage of propylthiouracil should be employed. Monitoring serum T_3 concentrations may sometimes be useful for dosage adjustment; in patients in whom total or free T_3 concentrations remain elevated despite low, normal, or reduced free T_4 concentrations, an increase in antithyroid dosage may be necessary.

Patients should inform clinicians of existing or contemplated concomitant therapy, including prescription and OTC drugs, as well as any concomitant illnesses. Patients also should be advised not to discontinue propylthiouracil therapy unless instructed to do so by their clinician.

Propylthiouracil is contraindicated in patients who are hypersensitive to the drug or any ingredient in the formulation. Cross-sensitivity between thioamides may occur (i.e., in approximately 50% of patients switched from one thioamide agent to the other). In patients who develop agranulocytosis or other serious adverse effects while receiving either propylthiouracil or methimazole, some clinicians state that use of the other drug also is contraindicated because of the risk of cross-sensitivity between the two drugs. In patients experiencing serious allergic reactions to propylthiouracil, some clinicians state that using the alternative antithyroid drug (i.e., methimazole) is not recommended.

● Pediatric Precautions

During postmarketing experience, cases of severe liver injury, including hepatic failure requiring liver transplantation or resulting in death, have been reported in pediatric patients receiving propylthiouracil; however, no such cases have been reported in pediatric patients treated with methimazole. Therefore, propylthiouracil is not recommended for use in pediatric patients except in rare instances in which methimazole is not well tolerated and surgery or radioactive iodine therapy are not appropriate therapies. In addition, some experts state that alternative therapy should be considered for children who are currently receiving propylthiouracil and that it is reasonable and prudent to discontinue propylthiouracil use in children receiving this drug for the treatment of Graves' disease. When propylthiouracil is used in children, parents and patients should be informed of the risk of liver failure. If patients receiving propylthiouracil develop tiredness, nausea, anorexia, fever, pharyngitis, or malaise, propylthiouracil should be discontinued

immediately, a clinician should be contacted, and a leukocyte count, liver function tests, and transaminase concentrations obtained. (See Cautions: Hepatic Effects and also see Cautions: Precautions and Contraindications.)

● Geriatric Precautions

Clinical studies of propylthiouracil did not include sufficient numbers of patients 65 years of age and older to determine whether geriatric patients respond differently than younger patients. Other reported clinical experience has not identified differences in responses between geriatric and younger patients. Dosage of propylthiouracil generally should be selected with caution in geriatric patients because of the greater frequency of decreased hepatic, renal, and/or cardiac function and of concomitant disease and drug therapy.

● Pregnancy, Fertility, and Lactation
Pregnancy

Propylthiouracil crosses the placenta and may cause fetal harm when administered to pregnant women; the drug can induce goiter and hypothyroidism (cretinism) in the developing fetus. In April 2010, FDA reported a review of postmarketing data analyzing the potential for birth defects associated with use of propylthiouracil or methimazole during pregnancy. FDA found that congenital malformations were reported approximately 3 times more often with prenatal exposure to methimazole compared with propylthiouracil (29 cases with methimazole; 9 cases with propylthiouracil). In addition, there was a distinct and consistent pattern of congenital malformations associated with the use of methimazole that was not found with propylthiouracil. Approximately 90% of the congenital malformations with methimazole were craniofacial malformations (e.g., scalp epidermal aplasia [aplasia cutis], facial dysmorphism, choanal atresia). In most of the cases, there were multiple malformations that frequently included a combination of craniofacial defects and GI atresia or aplasia. These specific birth defects were associated with the use of methimazole during the first trimester of pregnancy but were not found when the drug was administered later in pregnancy. In contrast, FDA did not find a consistent pattern of birth defects associated with the use of propylthiouracil and concluded that there is no convincing evidence of an association between propylthiouracil use and congenital malformations, even with use during the first trimester.

Despite the potential fetal hazard, antithyroid agents are still considered the therapy of choice for the management of hyperthyroidism during pregnancy. Since methimazole may be associated with the rare development of fetal abnormalities, such as aplasia cutis and choanal atresia, propylthiouracil is the preferred agent when an antithyroid drug is indicated during organogenesis in the first trimester of pregnancy or just prior to the first trimester of pregnancy. Patients receiving methimazole should be switched to propylthiouracil if pregnancy is confirmed in the first trimester. Because of the potential adverse maternal effects of propylthiouracil (e.g., hepatotoxicity), however, it may be preferable to switch from propylthiouracil to methimazole for the second and third trimesters (i.e., after the first trimester). If the patient is switching from propylthiouracil to methimazole, thyroid function should be assessed after 2 weeks and then every 2–4 weeks thereafter. It is not known if the risk of methimazole-induced aplasia cutis or embryopathy outweighs the risk of propylthiouracil-induced hepatotoxicity.

If propylthiouracil is used during pregnancy for the management of hyperthyroidism, the manufacturer states that a sufficient, but not excessive, dosage of propylthiouracil is necessary. Some clinicians state that antithyroid drug therapy should be initiated or adjusted to maintain maternal free thyroxine (T_4) concentrations at or just above the upper limit of normal (ULN) of the nonpregnant reference range, or to maintain total T_4 concentrations at 1.5 times the ULN or the free T_4 index in the ULN, while using the lowest possible dosage of antithyroid drugs. In women receiving antithyroid drugs during pregnancy, free T_4 and TSH concentrations should be monitored approximately every 2–6 weeks. The manufacturer states that because thyroid dysfunction diminishes in many women as pregnancy proceeds, a reduction in dosage may be possible, and, in some patients, propylthiouracil can be discontinued several weeks or months before delivery.

Patients should be advised to contact their clinician immediately about their therapy if they are or plan to become pregnant while receiving an antithyroid drug. If propylthiouracil is used during pregnancy or if the patient becomes pregnant while receiving the drug, the patient should be advised of the rare potential hazard of liver damage in the mother and fetus; in addition, when considering antithyroid drug use during pregnancy, the patient should be informed of this potential risk, as well as the risks of methimazole-associated fetal malformations. Although liver toxicity may appear abruptly, some clinicians state that it is reasonable to monitor liver function every 3–4 weeks in pregnant women receiving propylthiouracil and to encourage patients to promptly report any new symptoms. (See Cautions: Hepatic Effects and also see Cautions: Precautions and Contraindications.)

Lactation

The manufacturer and some clinicians state that propylthiouracil is distributed into milk to a small extent and, therefore, is unlikely to result in clinically important doses in the nursing infant. In one study in 9 lactating women who received a single 400-mg dose of propylthiouracil orally, the mean amount of propylthiouracil distributed into milk during 4 hours following drug administration was 0.025% (range: 0.007–0.077%) of the administered dose.

Propylthiouracil generally is compatible with breast-feeding, and moderate dosages of the drug (i.e., less than 300 mg daily) appear to be safe during breast-feeding. However, some clinicians consider propylthiouracil to be a second-line agent in nursing women because of concerns regarding severe hepatotoxicity (i.e., hepatic necrosis in either woman or child) following maternal use of the drug; these clinicians state that methimazole is the preferred antithyroid drug in nursing women. If an antithyroid drug is used in nursing women, some clinicians recommend that the drug be administered *after* a feeding and in divided doses, and that thyroid function be monitored in nursing infants.

DRUG INTERACTIONS

● Drugs Known to be Associated with Agranulocytosis

Propylthiouracil should be used with extreme caution in patients receiving concomitant treatment with drugs known to be associated with agranulocytosis. (See Cautions: Agranulocytosis and also see Cautions: Precautions and Contraindications.)

● Anticoagulants

Because of the potential inhibition of vitamin K activity by propylthiouracil, the activity of oral anticoagulants (e.g., warfarin) may be increased. However, propylthiouracil also may decrease the anticoagulant effect of warfarin. Additional monitoring of prothrombin time (PT)/international normalized ratio (INR) should be considered, particularly prior to surgery. Adjustment of warfarin dosage may be necessary.

● β-Adrenergic Blocking Agents

Hyperthyroidism may cause an increased clearance of β-adrenergic blocking agents with a high extraction ratio. Dosage reduction of the β-adrenergic blocking agent may be needed when a hyperthyroid patient becomes euthyroid.

● Digitalis Glycosides

Serum digitalis concentrations may be increased when hyperthyroid patients receiving a stable digitalis glycoside regimen become euthyroid; dosage reduction of the digitalis glycoside may be needed.

● Theophylline

Theophylline clearance may decrease when hyperthyroid patients receiving a stable theophylline regimen become euthyroid; dosage reduction of theophylline may be needed.

ACUTE TOXICITY

● Manifestations

In general, overdosage of propylthiouracil may be expected to produce effects that are extensions of common adverse reactions. Nausea, vomiting, epigastric distress, headache, fever, arthralgia, pruritus, edema, and pancytopenia have been reported. Agranulocytosis is the most serious adverse effect associated with propylthiouracil overdosage. Exfoliative dermatitis, hepatitis, neuropathies, or CNS stimulation or depression may occur rarely.

● Treatment

Treatment of propylthiouracil overdosage generally involves appropriate supportive care as dictated by the patient's medical status. Clinicians should consider consulting a poison control center for the most current information on the management of propylthiouracil overdosage.

PHARMACOLOGY

Propylthiouracil inhibits the synthesis of thyroid hormones by interfering with the incorporation of iodine into tyrosyl residues of thyroglobulin; the drug also inhibits the coupling of these iodotyrosyl residues to form iodothyronine. Although the exact mechanism(s) has not been fully elucidated, propylthiouracil

may interfere with the oxidation of iodide ion and iodotyrosyl groups. Based on limited evidence it appears that the coupling reaction is more sensitive to antithyroid agents than the iodination reaction. Propylthiouracil does not inhibit the action of thyroid hormones already formed and present in the thyroid gland or circulation nor does the drug interfere with the effectiveness of exogenously administered thyroid hormones. Patients whose thyroid gland contains relatively high concentration of iodine (e.g., from prior ingestion or from administration during diagnostic radiologic procedures) may respond relatively slowly to antithyroid agents. Unlike methimazole, propylthiouracil inhibits the peripheral deiodination of thyroxine to triiodothyronine. Although the importance of this inhibition has not been established, propylthiouracil has a theoretical advantage compared with methimazole or carbimazole in patients with thyrotoxic crisis, since a decreased rate of conversion of circulating thyroxine to triiodothyronine may be clinically beneficial in these patients.

PHARMACOKINETICS

● Absorption

Propylthiouracil is rapidly and readily absorbed from the GI tract following oral administration with peak plasma concentrations of about 6–9 mcg/mL occurring within 1–1.5 hours after a single dose of 200–400 mg. In one study in which the drug was administered orally and IV, about 75% of the oral dose was absorbed. Plasma concentrations of the drug do not appear to correlate with the therapeutic effects.

● Distribution

Although distribution of propylthiouracil into human body tissues and fluids has not been fully characterized, the drug appears to be concentrated in the thyroid gland. Propylthiouracil readily crosses the placenta. The manufacturer states that propylthiouracil is distributed into milk to a small extent; one study indicated that the extent of distribution is about 0.007–0.077% of a single dose. (See Cautions: Pregnancy and Lactation.)

● Elimination

The elimination half-life of propylthiouracil has generally been reported to be about 1–2 hours.

Although the exact metabolic fate of propylthiouracil has not been fully established, the drug is extensively metabolized to its glucuronide conjugate and other minor metabolites. The drug and its metabolites are excreted in urine, with about 35% of a dose excreted within 24 hours.

CHEMISTRY AND STABILITY

● Chemistry

Propylthiouracil is a thiourea-derivative antithyroid agent. The drug differs chemically and structurally from methimazole in that propylthiouracil has a 6-membered ring instead of a 5-membered ring. Although presence of a thioamide group appears to be sufficient for antithyroid activity, propylthiouracil, like methimazole and carbimazole, contains the thioureylene moiety.

Propylthiouracil is a white, crystalline substance with a bitter taste. The drug is very slightly soluble in water.

● Stability

Commercially available propylthiouracil tablets should be stored in well-closed containers at 25°C but may be exposed to temperatures ranging from 15–30°C.

PREPARATIONS

Excipients in commercially available drug preparations may have clinically important effects in some individuals; consult specific product labeling for details.

Propylthiouracil

Oral		
Tablets	50 mg*	Propylthiouracil Tablets

* available from one or more manufacturer, distributor, and/or repackager by generic (nonproprietary) name

† Use is not currently included in the labeling approved by the US Food and Drug Administration.

Selected Revisions November 27, 2013, © Copyright, July 1, 1963, American Society of Health-System Pharmacists, Inc.

Angiotensin II Acetate

68:44 • RENIN-ANGIOTENSIN-ALDOSTERONE SYSTEM

■ Angiotensin II acetate is a synthetic form of endogenous angiotensin II, a peptide hormone of the renin-angiotensin-aldosterone system (RAAS) that causes vasoconstriction and increased blood pressure.

USES

● Shock

Angiotensin II acetate is used for its vasoconstrictive effects to increase blood pressure in patients with septic or other forms of distributive shock.

Vasopressors are used as standard therapy in the management of septic shock when fluid resuscitation alone fails to restore blood pressure. Current treatment guidelines recommend norepinephrine as the first-line vasopressor of choice in adults with septic shock. Angiotensin II may provide an additional treatment option for patients who do not respond adequately to traditional vasopressors.

In a randomized, double-blind, placebo-controlled study (Angiotensin II for the Treatment of High-Output Shock [ATHOS-3]), angiotensin II substantially increased mean arterial pressure (MAP) in patients with distributive shock (91% of cases caused by sepsis) who remained hypotensive (MAP of 55–70 mm Hg) despite fluid and vasopressor therapy. A total of 321 adults who were receiving more than 0.2 mcg/kg per minute of norepinephrine or an equivalent dosage of another vasopressor for at least 6 hours but no longer than 48 hours were enrolled in the study and received an IV infusion of angiotensin II (initial dosage of 20 ng/kg per minute) or placebo. During the first 3 hours of treatment, dosage of angiotensin II was titrated to achieve a target MAP of at least 75 mm Hg, while dosages of other vasopressors were maintained; in the subsequent 3 to 48 hours, dosage of angiotensin II was titrated to maintain MAP of 65–70 mm Hg, while dosages of other vasopressors were reduced or discontinued. The primary end point was MAP response (defined as a MAP of at least 75 mm Hg or an increase in MAP from baseline of at least 10 mm Hg, without an increase in baseline vasopressor therapy) at 3 hours. The primary end point was achieved in 70% of patients receiving angiotensin II compared with 23% of patients receiving placebo. The median time to reach target MAP with angiotensin II was approximately 5 minutes. The rapid treatment effect permitted reductions in both the dosage of angiotensin II and dosages of concomitant vasopressors. At 30 minutes, the median dosage of angiotensin II was 10 ng/kg per minute. Patients who received angiotensin II had lower catecholamine requirements compared with those who received placebo. In addition, there was a trend toward a 28-day mortality benefit with angiotensin II compared with placebo (mortality rate of 46 versus 54%, respectively); however, the difference was not statistically significant.

Additional studies are needed to further elucidate the role of angiotensin II in the management of shock, particularly in regard to the patient populations that are most likely to benefit, the optimal timing of administration, long-term benefits and harm, and comparative efficacy with other vasopressors.

DOSAGE AND ADMINISTRATION

● Administration

Angiotensin II acetate is administered by continuous IV infusion. It is recommended that the drug be infused through a central venous line.

Prior to administration, the commercially available injection concentrate must be diluted in 0.9% sodium chloride injection to a final concentration of 5000 or 10,000 ng/mL depending on the patient's fluid status. In patients who are not fluid restricted, a concentration of 5000 ng/mL may be prepared by adding 1 mL (2.5 mg) of the injection concentrate to an infusion bag containing 500 mL of 0.9% sodium chloride injection. In patients who are fluid restricted, a concentration of 10,000 ng/mL may be prepared by adding 1 mL (2.5 mg) of the injection concentrate to an infusion bag containing 250 mL of 0.9% sodium chloride injection. Diluted solutions may be stored at room temperature or under refrigeration for up to 24 hours.

Solutions of angiotensin II should be inspected visually for particulate matter and discoloration prior to administration.

● Dosage

Dosage of angiotensin II acetate is expressed in terms of angiotensin II.

Shock

The recommended initial dosage of angiotensin II in adults with septic or other distributive shock is 20 ng/kg per minute by continuous IV infusion. Dosage should be titrated based on blood pressure response. The infusion rate may be increased by increments of up to 15 ng/kg per minute as frequently as every 5 minutes as needed to achieve or maintain the target blood pressure. During the first 3 hours of treatment, dosage should not exceed 80 ng/kg per minute. Once the underlying shock has sufficiently improved, the infusion rate should be titrated downward by decrements of up to 15 ng/kg per minute every 5 to 15 minutes as tolerated to maintain target blood pressure. During maintenance therapy, dosage should not exceed 40 ng/kg per minute. Dosages as low as 1.25 ng/kg per minute may be used.

In the ATHOS-3 study, mean arterial pressure (MAP) increased rapidly following administration of angiotensin II, allowing for rapid down-titration of the initial dosage of 20 ng/kg per minute in 67% of the patients within 30 minutes; the median dosage at 30 minutes was 10 ng/kg per minute.

● Special Populations

The manufacturer makes no special population dosage recommendations at this time.

CAUTIONS

● Contraindications

The manufacturer states that there are no known contraindications to the use of angiotensin II acetate.

● Warnings/Precautions

Thromboembolic Risk

An increased incidence of arterial and venous thromboembolic events, particularly deep venous thrombosis (DVT), was reported in patients receiving angiotensin II compared with those receiving placebo in the ATHOS-3 study (13 versus 5%, respectively). DVT occurred in 7 (4.3%) patients who received angiotensin II compared with none of the patients who received placebo. Preclinical studies and studies in healthy individuals also have demonstrated prothrombotic effects of the drug.

Concurrent use of venous thromboembolism (VTE) prophylaxis is recommended during angiotensin II therapy.

Specific Populations

Pregnancy

There are insufficient data in pregnant women to determine whether angiotensin II is associated with a risk of adverse developmental effects. Animal reproduction studies have not been conducted with the drug.

Septic or other distributive shock is a medical emergency that can be fatal if untreated; a delay in treatment in pregnant women with hypotension associated with shock is likely to increase the risk of maternal and fetal morbidity and mortality.

Lactation

It is not known whether angiotensin II is distributed into human milk of if the drug has any effects on the nursing infant or on milk production.

Pediatric Use

Safety and efficacy of angiotensin II have not been established in pediatric patients.

Geriatric Use

In the ATHOS-3 study, 48% of the total patient population was 65 years of age or older. No substantial differences in safety or efficacy of angiotensin II have been observed between geriatric patients (65 years of age or older) and younger adults.

Hepatic Impairment

The pharmacokinetics of angiotensin II are not expected to be altered by hepatic impairment.

Renal Impairment

The pharmacokinetics of angiotensin II are not expected to be altered by renal impairment.

● *Common Adverse Effects*

Adverse reactions reported in 4% or more of patients receiving angiotensin II in clinical studies include thromboembolic events (e.g., DVT), thrombocytopenia, tachycardia, fungal infection, delirium, acidosis, hyperglycemia, and peripheral ischemia.

DRUG INTERACTIONS

No drug interaction studies have been performed to date with angiotensin II acetate. Concomitant use of angiotensin-converting enzyme (ACE) inhibitors may increase the response to angiotensin II and concomitant use of angiotensin II receptor antagonists (ARBs) may decrease the response to angiotensin II.

DESCRIPTION

Angiotensin II acetate is a synthetic preparation of endogenous human angiotensin II, a peptide hormone of the renin-angiotensin-aldosterone system (RAAS) that plays an essential role in blood pressure regulation. The drug is a potent vasoconstrictor that is used to increase blood pressure in patients with septic or other forms of distributive shock.

In patients with septic shock, a variety of physiologic responses are activated to restore effective circulating volume, vascular resistance, and arterial pressure, including activation of RAAS and production of angiotensin II. There is some evidence suggesting that patients with septic shock may have a relative deficiency of angiotensin II that may be reversed with exogenous administration of angiotensin II. Angiotensin II increases blood pressure through direct vasoconstriction of the peripheral vasculature in addition to other mechanisms (e.g., aldosterone secretion, vasopressin release, activation of the sympathetic nervous system). The physiologic effects of angiotensin II are mediated by specific G protein-coupled receptors located in the kidneys, vascular smooth muscle, lung, heart, brain, adrenal gland, pituitary gland, and liver. The angiotensin II receptor type 1 (AT1 receptor) is responsible for the vasoconstrictive effects of angiotensin II; activation of the receptor stimulates calcium/calmodulin-dependent phosphorylation of myosin and causes smooth muscle contraction. Angiotensin II also has been shown to have cardiac remodeling properties and preferential vasoconstrictive effects on renal efferent arterioles.

Following IV infusion, angiotensin II is rapidly metabolized by aminopeptidase A to angiotensin 2-8 (angiotensin III) and by angiotensin-converting enzyme 2 to angiotensin 1-7 in plasma, erythrocytes, and many other major organs (e.g., intestine, kidney, liver, lungs). Angiotensin III retains approximately 40% of the activity of angiotensin II, while angiotensin 1-7 exhibits opposing actions to angiotensin II and causes vasodilation, natriuresis, and reduced blood pressure. The plasma half-life of angiotensin II is less than 1 minute. Elimination of the drug is not dependent on renal or hepatic routes.

ADVICE TO PATIENTS

Importance of informing clinicians of existing or contemplated concomitant therapy, including prescription and OTC drugs as well as any concomitant illnesses.

Importance of women informing clinicians if they are or plan to become pregnant or plan to breast-feed.

Importance of informing patients of other important precautionary information. (See Cautions.)

PREPARATIONS

Excipients in commercially available drug preparations may have clinically important effects in some individuals; consult specific product labeling for details.

Angiotensin II Acetate

Parenteral

Concentrate for injection, for IV infusion	2.5 mg/mL (of angiotensin II)	Giapreza®, La Jolla

Selected Revisions November 4, 2019, © Copyright, February 12, 2018, American Society of Health-System Pharmacists, Inc.

Table of Contents

§ Omitted from the print version of *AHFS Drug Information®* because of space limitations. This monograph is available on the *AHFS Drug Information®* website, http://ahfsdruginformation.com.

Mifepristone

76:00 · OXYTOCICS

■ Mifepristone, a synthetic derivative of the progestin norethindrone, is a progesterone- and glucocorticoid-receptor antagonist.

REMS

FDA approved a REMS for mifepristone (Mifeprex® and approved generic tablets) to ensure that the benefits outweigh the risks. The REMS may apply to one or more preparations of mifepristone and consists of the following: elements to assure safe use and implementation system. See the FDA REMS page (https://www.accessdata.fda.gov/scripts/cder/rems/index.cfm).

USES

● Termination of Pregnancy

Mifepristone (Mifeprex® and generics) is FDA-labeled for use in conjunction with misoprostol for the medical termination of intrauterine pregnancy (i.e., medical abortion) through 70 days of gestation as dated from the first day of the last menstrual period; duration of pregnancy may be determined by menstrual history or clinical examination, or with an ultrasonographic scan if duration of pregnancy is uncertain or ectopic pregnancy is suspected. For termination of pregnancy, a single dose of mifepristone is administered, followed by misoprostol administered 24–48 hours after the mifepristone dose. Misoprostol must be administered 24–48 hours following mifepristone administration. Misoprostol, a prostaglandin E_1 analog, induces uterine contractions and expulsion of the products of conception.

In clinical studies in women with pregnancies of up to 70 days of gestation, oral mifepristone followed by oral misoprostol was effective for medical termination of pregnancy (i.e., complete expulsion of pregnancy without the need for surgical intervention) in approximately 96–97% of the women. The remaining patients later had surgical intervention due to incomplete abortion, excessive bleeding, ongoing pregnancy, medical necessity, or at the patient's request. As gestational age increased, efficacy of the mifepristone and misoprostol regimen decreased; complete medical abortion was reported in 98.1% of pregnancies at less than 49 days of gestation compared with 96.8, 94.7, and 92.7% of pregnancies at 50–56, 57–63, and 64–70 days of gestation, respectively. Surgical intervention for ongoing pregnancy was reported for 0.3, 0.8, 2, and 3.1% of pregnancies at less than 49, 50–56, 57–63, and 64–70 days of gestation, respectively. In one study that included pregnancies through 70 days of gestation, 23–38% of patients reported expulsion of the products of conception within 3 hours, and over 90% of patients reported expulsion within 24 hours of misoprostol administration.

Although the manufacturer of *misoprostol* states that it has not conducted and does not intend to conduct research to support use in pregnancy (e.g., termination of pregnancy), mifepristone is labeled by FDA for use with misoprostol for termination of pregnancy, and the American College of Obstetricians and Gynecologists (ACOG) states that the medication abortion regimen supported by major medical organizations nationally and internationally includes mifepristone and misoprostol; if mifepristone is unavailable, then a misoprostol-only regimen is an acceptable alternative.

Mifepristone also has been used for termination of pregnancy during the second or third trimester†, induction of labor†, postcoital contraception†, endometriosis†, leiomyoma†, and meningioma†. Mifepristone also has been used with intravaginal misoprostol (using tablets formulated for oral administration) for termination of pregnancy; however, such use very rarely has resulted in *fatal* bacterial infection and sepsis.

● Hyperglycemia Secondary to Cushing's Syndrome

Mifepristone (Korlym®) is used for the management of hyperglycemia secondary to hypercortisolism in adults with endogenous Cushing's syndrome who have type 2 diabetes mellitus or glucose intolerance and have failed surgery or are not surgical candidates. Mifepristone is designated an orphan drug by FDA for the treatment of clinical manifestations of endogenous Cushing's syndrome.

Mifepristone is *not* indicated for treatment of type 2 diabetes mellitus that is not secondary to Cushing's syndrome.

Efficacy and safety of mifepristone for the management of hyperglycemia secondary to Cushing's syndrome were evaluated in an uncontrolled, open-label, multicenter study of 24 weeks' duration in adults with endogenous Cushing's syndrome and associated type 2 diabetes mellitus, impaired glucose tolerance (defined as blood glucose concentration of 140–199 mg/dL following a 2-hour oral glucose tolerance test [oGTT]), or hypertension. Patients in this study had failed surgery, experienced disease recurrence, or were not considered surgical candidates. Of the 50 patients enrolled in the study, 29 had type 2 diabetes mellitus or impaired glucose tolerance (diabetes cohort), and 21 had hypertension (hypertension cohort). All patients received an initial mifepristone dosage of 300 mg once daily; dosage could be increased to 600 mg once daily after 2 weeks and then increased, based on tolerability and clinical response, in 300-mg increments every 4 weeks to a maximum of 900 or 1200 mg once daily in patients weighing less than or greater than 60 kg, respectively. Existing antidiabetic therapy was continued throughout the study, without dosage increases or additions to therapy.

The primary end point for the diabetes cohort was the proportion of patients who experienced at least a 25% reduction in glucose area under the plasma concentration-time curve (AUC) following oGTT from baseline to week 24. For the hypertension cohort, the primary end point was change in diastolic blood pressure from baseline to week 24; a response was defined as a decrease of at least 5 mm Hg. At week 24, 60% of patients in the diabetes cohort achieved at least 25% reduction in glucose AUC. Mifepristone treatment also substantially decreased glycosylated hemoglobin (hemoglobin A_{1c}; HbA_{1c}); of the 24 patients with HbA_{1c} measurements, the mean reduction in HbA_{1c} was 1.1%. In the 15 patients receiving antidiabetic agents at baseline, either dosage of the antidiabetic agent was reduced or antidiabetic therapy remained stable. There were no substantial changes in mean systolic and diastolic blood pressures in the hypertension cohort.

DOSAGE AND ADMINISTRATION

● General

Mifepristone (Mifeprex® and generics) is used for the medical termination of pregnancy and is intended for use by clinicians who are able to assess the gestational age of an embryo and to diagnose ectopic pregnancy. If necessary, clinicians also must be able to provide surgical intervention in cases of incomplete abortion or severe bleeding or ensure that such services are available from others, and patients must have access to medical facilities equipped to provide blood transfusions and resuscitation. Any intrauterine contraceptive device (IUD) should be removed prior to administration of mifepristone for termination of pregnancy.

Mifepristone (Korlym®) is used for the management of hyperglycemia secondary to Cushing's syndrome. Women of childbearing potential should be evaluated for pregnancy prior to initiation of the drug.

Because mifepristone may cause hypokalemia in patients with Cushing's syndrome, serum potassium concentrations should be monitored and corrected prior to initiation of mifepristone (Korlym®), 1–2 weeks after initiation of the drug or dosage increases, and periodically during therapy.

Because of the long half-life of mifepristone at steady state, the manufacturer of mifepristone (Korlym®) states at least 2 weeks must elapse between discontinuance of mifepristone and initiation or dosage increases of any interacting concomitant drugs.

Mifepristone REMS Program

For termination of pregnancy, mifepristone (Mifeprex® and generics) is only available through the Mifepristone Risk Evaluation and Mitigation Strategy (REMS) Program. The goal of the Mifepristone REMS Program is to mitigate the risk of serious complications associated with mifepristone when used for medical termination of pregnancy through 10 weeks gestation by requiring that prescribers have the necessary qualifications to assess whether patients are appropriate candidates for the drug and to provide necessary intervention in case of complications, ensuring that mifepristone is only dispensed by certified pharmacies or by or under the supervision of certified prescribers, and requiring that patients be informed of the risks of the treatment regimen. Although a causal association has not been determined, serious adverse events have been reported in patients receiving mifepristone, including 2 cases of ectopic pregnancy resulting in death and several fatal cases of severe systemic infection.

Under the Mifepristone REMS, clinicians must be certified to prescribe the drug; pharmacists must be certified to dispense the drug; and patients must review the patient agreement form and manufacturer's medication guide before they can receive the drug. The previous requirement for mifepristone to be dispensed only in certain health care settings (e.g., clinics, medical offices, hospitals) has been removed from the current REMS, and certified pharmacies may now dispense mifepristone directly to patients upon receipt of a prescription from a certified prescriber. Additional information about the Mifepristone REMS Program is available at 877-432-7596 or https://www.earlyoptionpill.com/.

● Administration

Termination of Pregnancy

Mifepristone (Mifeprex® and generics) is administered orally as a single dose, followed by intrabuccal administration of misoprostol 24–48 hours later. The effectiveness of the regimen may be reduced if misoprostol is administered less than 24 hours or more than 48 hours after the mifepristone dose.

For intrabuccal administration of misoprostol, patients should be instructed to place 2 misoprostol tablets in each side of the mouth between the cheek and gums for 30 minutes, then swallow any remnants with water or another liquid.

Misoprostol should be administered in an appropriate setting for the patient, taking into account that expulsion of uterine contents could begin within 2 hours of misoprostol administration. Medications for treatment of adverse effects (e.g., cramping, GI symptoms) may be needed in the period immediately following misoprostol administration.

Patients should be advised regarding appropriate actions to take if severe discomfort, excessive vaginal bleeding, or other adverse reactions occur. The name and telephone number of the clinician who will be handling emergencies and a telephone number to call with any questions following administration of misoprostol also should be provided to the patient.

The manufacturers state that patients must return for a follow-up clinical examination approximately 7–14 days after receiving mifepristone and misoprostol to confirm complete termination of pregnancy and to assess severity of any continued bleeding. However, some experts state that the type of follow-up visit after medical abortion has evolved over time, and routine in-person follow-up is not necessary after an uncomplicated medication abortion. Termination of pregnancy may be confirmed by medical history, clinical examination, human chorionic gonadotropin (hCG) testing, or ultrasonographic scan. Persistence of moderate to heavy vaginal bleeding at this follow-up visit could indicate an incomplete abortion. Lack of bleeding following the mifepristone and misoprostol regimen usually indicates treatment failure; however, prolonged or heavy bleeding is not proof of a complete abortion. Surgical termination is recommended to manage failure of medical abortion after the mifepristone and misoprostol regimen. Debris seen in the uterus on ultrasonography following the regimen will not necessarily require surgery for removal.

Hyperglycemia Secondary to Cushing's Syndrome

Mifepristone (Korlym®) is administered orally once daily with a meal. Tablets should be swallowed whole and should *not* be split, crushed, or chewed.

● Dosage

Termination of Pregnancy

The recommended dosage of mifepristone (Mifeprex® and generics) for the medical termination of pregnancy is 200 mg orally as a single dose followed by intrabuccal administration of misoprostol (800 mcg as a single dose given 24–48 hours after the mifepristone dose).

If complete expulsion of the products of conception has not occurred at the follow-up examination, and the pregnancy is not ongoing, another intrabuccal dose of misoprostol (800 mcg) may be administered. Uterine rupture has been reported rarely in women receiving mifepristone and misoprostol for termination of pregnancy, including women with prior uterine rupture or scarring and those receiving multiple doses of misoprostol within 24 hours. Patients should return for a follow-up examination approximately 7 days after administration of the repeated misoprostol dose to assess for complete pregnancy termination.

Hyperglycemia Secondary to Cushing's Syndrome

The recommended initial dosage of mifepristone (Korlym®) for the management of hyperglycemia secondary to hypercortisolism in adults with endogenous Cushing's syndrome is 300 mg once daily. Dosage may be increased in increments of 300 mg at intervals of no less than 2–4 weeks based on clinical response and tolerability up to a maximum dosage of 20 mg/kg daily. The maximum recommended dosage of mifepristone is 1200 mg once daily.

Careful and gradual dosage titration and monitoring for adverse reactions may reduce the risk of severe adverse effects. Interruption of therapy and/or dosage reduction may be necessary in some clinical situations. If treatment is interrupted, mifepristone should be reinitiated at the lowest dosage (i.e., 300 mg once daily). If treatment is interrupted as a result of adverse effects, the drug should be titrated to a lower dosage.

Changes in glucose control, antidiabetic medication requirements, serum insulin concentration, and psychiatric symptoms may provide an early assessment of response (i.e., within 6 weeks) and may help guide early dosage titration. Improvements in cushingoid appearance, acne, hirsutism, striae, and body weight occur over a longer period of time and, along with measures of glucose control, may be used to determine dosage adjustments beyond the first 2 months of therapy.

Dosage Modification for Concomitant Use with Cytochrome P-450 (CYP) 3A Inhibitors

Mifepristone (Korlym®) should be used concomitantly with drugs that are potent inhibitors of cytochrome P-450 (CYP) isoenzyme 3A only when necessary. If concomitant use is clinically warranted, the manufacturer of mifepristone (Korlym®) recommends that mifepristone dosage should not exceed 600 mg once daily.

If mifepristone therapy is initiated for management of hyperglycemia secondary to Cushing's syndrome in a patient who is already receiving a potent CYP3A inhibitor, the recommended starting dosage of mifepristone is 300 mg once daily. If clinically indicated, the dosage of mifepristone may be titrated to a maximum of 600 mg once daily in such patients.

If a potent CYP3A inhibitor is initiated in a patient who is already receiving mifepristone therapy for management of hyperglycemia secondary to Cushing's syndrome, dosage adjustment of mifepristone may be necessary. In patients already receiving mifepristone 300 mg once daily, no dosage adjustment is required. In those already receiving mifepristone 600 mg once daily, dosage should be reduced to 300 mg once daily; dosage may be titrated to a maximum of 600 mg once daily if clinically indicated. For patients already receiving mifepristone 900 or 1200 mg once daily, dosage should be reduced to 600 mg once daily.

● Special Populations

The manufacturer of mifepristone (Mifeprex®) makes no special population dosage recommendations for use of mifepristone for the medical termination of pregnancy.

If mifepristone (Korlym®) is used for the management of hyperglycemia secondary to Cushing's syndrome in patients with renal impairment or mild to moderate hepatic impairment, the maximum recommended mifepristone dosage is 600 mg once daily; initial dosage adjustment is not necessary. Mifepristone for the management of hyperglycemia secondary to Cushing's syndrome in patients with severe hepatic impairment is not recommended; the drug has not been studied in this patient population.

CAUTIONS

● Contraindications

● Mifepristone (Mifeprex® and generics) for medical termination of intrauterine pregnancy is contraindicated in patients with known hypersensitivity to mifepristone, misoprostol, or other prostaglandins. The drug also is contraindicated in patients with confirmed or suspected ectopic pregnancy, undiagnosed adnexal mass, or intrauterine contraceptive device (IUD) currently in place; chronic adrenal failure or concurrent long-term corticosteroid therapy; and hemorrhagic disorders, inherited porphyrias, or concurrent anticoagulant therapy.

- Mifepristone (Korlym®) for management of hyperglycemia secondary to Cushing's syndrome is contraindicated in patients with known hypersensitivity to mifepristone or any ingredient in the preparation. The drug also is contraindicated in women who are pregnant and women with a history of unexplained vaginal bleeding or endometrial hyperplasia with atypia or endometrial carcinoma. In addition, mifepristone is contraindicated in patients who require concomitant therapy with systemic corticosteroids for serious medical conditions (e.g., immunosuppression after organ transplantation) and in those receiving simvastatin, lovastatin, or other cytochrome P-450 (CYP) isoenzyme 3A substrates with a narrow therapeutic index (see Drug Interactions).

● *Warnings/Precautions*

Warnings

Fetal/Neonatal Morbidity and Mortality

Mifepristone causes termination of pregnancy and, when used for management of hyperglycemia secondary to Cushing's syndrome, is contraindicated during pregnancy. A boxed warning about this risk has been included in the prescribing information for the mifepristone preparation used in the treatment of Cushing's syndrome (Korlym®).

Pregnancy must be excluded prior to initiation of mifepristone (Korlym®), and women of childbearing potential should use effective, nonhormonal contraception during therapy and for 1 month after discontinuance of the drug, unless the woman has undergone surgical sterilization. In addition, such patients should be reevaluated for pregnancy if therapy is interrupted for more than 14 days.

If mifepristone (Korlym®) is used during pregnancy or if the patient becomes pregnant while receiving the drug, the patient should be apprised of the potential fetal hazard.

Hemorrhage

Serious and sometimes fatal bleeding can occur rarely following spontaneous, surgical, and medical abortions, including use of mifepristone. A causal relationship to mifepristone and misoprostol has not been established. A boxed warning about this risk has been included in the prescribing information for the mifepristone preparation used for the medical termination of intrauterine pregnancy (Mifeprex® and generics).

Uterine bleeding occurs in almost all women receiving mifepristone in conjunction with misoprostol for termination of pregnancy. Based on clinical studies, bleeding or spotting should be expected for an average of 9–16 days; heavy bleeding has been reported for a median duration of 2 days. Although more bleeding occurs after pregnancy termination with the mifepristone and misoprostol regimen than after a surgical abortion, in most patients the total blood loss is not clinically important and is indistinguishable from that associated with a spontaneous miscarriage. However, in about 8% of patients, bleeding continued 30 days or longer, and the duration of bleeding and spotting generally increased as the duration of pregnancy increased. Severity of uterine bleeding should be assessed when the patient returns for follow-up examination approximately 7–14 days after the mifepristone and misoprostol regimen.

Severe uterine bleeding may occur following spontaneous, surgical, or medical abortion (including following mifepristone administration). Prolonged heavy vaginal bleeding (i.e., soaking through 2 thick full-size sanitary pads per hour for 2 consecutive hours) may be a sign of incomplete abortion or other complications, and prompt medical or surgical intervention may be required to prevent the development of hypovolemic shock. Patients should be advised to seek immediate medical attention if prolonged heavy vaginal bleeding or syncope occurs following mifepristone administration. Decreases in hemoglobin concentration, hematocrit, and red blood cell count may occur in women who experience heavy bleeding.

Excessive uterine bleeding usually requires treatment with uterotonics, vasoconstrictors, saline infusions, and/or blood transfusions or surgical uterine evacuation. In approximately 1% of patients, heavy bleeding requiring surgical uterine evacuation occurs, and caution should be exercised in patients with hemostatic disorders, hypocoagulability, or severe anemia.

Infection and Sepsis

Serious and sometimes fatal bacterial (e.g., *Clostridium sordellii*) infections and sepsis, which can present without fever, bacteremia, or significant findings on pelvic examination, can occur rarely following spontaneous, surgical, and medical abortions, including use of mifepristone; a causal relationship to mifepristone and misoprostol has not been established. A boxed warning about this risk has been included in the prescribing information for the mifepristone preparation used for the medical termination of intrauterine pregnancy (Mifeprex® and generics).

Serious bacterial (e.g., *Clostridium sordellii*) infection and sepsis can present without fever, bacteremia, or substantial findings on pelvic examination. Deaths have been reported very rarely in patients who presented without fever, with or without abdominal pain, but with leukocytosis with a marked left shift, tachycardia, hemoconcentration, and general malaise. These deaths occurred in women who received intravaginal misoprostol; however, a causal relationship between use of mifepristone and misoprostol and risk of infection or death has not been established. Furthermore, *C. sordellii* infections also have been reported very rarely following childbirth (vaginal delivery and cesarean section) and in other gynecologic and nongynecologic conditions.

Clinicians should maintain a high index of suspicion to rule out serious infection and sepsis if sustained fever (temperature of 38°C or higher persisting for more than 4 hours), severe abdominal pain, or pelvic tenderness occurs within several days of medical abortion, *or* if abdominal pain/discomfort or general malaise (including weakness, nausea, vomiting, or diarrhea), with or without fever, occurs more than 24 hours after administration of misoprostol.

The American College of Obstetricians and Gynecologists (ACOG) states that the routine use of prophylactic antibiotics is not recommended in patients undergoing medical abortion. Following concerns about serious, rare, and deadly infection with clostridial bacteria in patients undergoing medical abortion, ACOG states that there is no evidence of a specific connection between clostridial organisms and medical abortion.

Other Warnings and Precautions

Ectopic Pregnancy

Mifepristone is *not* effective for the termination of ectopic pregnancy and is contraindicated for use in patients with confirmed or suspected ectopic pregnancy. The manufacturer states that, despite the clinician's best effort to rule out ectopic pregnancy, the possibility that such a condition may be present during the treatment period should be considered; some of the expected symptoms experienced with a medical abortion (e.g., abdominal pain, uterine bleeding) may be similar to those of a ruptured ectopic pregnancy.

Patients who became pregnant with an IUD in place should be evaluated for ectopic pregnancy.

Adrenal Insufficiency

Adrenal insufficiency may occur in patients receiving mifepristone for management of hyperglycemia secondary to Cushing's syndrome. In patients with Cushing's syndrome, serum cortisol concentrations remain elevated and may increase during treatment with mifepristone resulting from blockade of glucocorticoid receptors; therefore, serum cortisol concentrations are not a reliable parameter for assessment of adrenal insufficiency. Patients should be closely monitored for manifestations of adrenal insufficiency, including weakness, nausea, increased fatigue, hypotension, and hypoglycemia.

If adrenal insufficiency is suspected, mifepristone should be immediately discontinued and glucocorticoid therapy initiated; patients should be evaluated for precipitating causes of adrenal insufficiency (e.g., infection, trauma). High dosages of glucocorticoid may be necessary to overcome glucocorticoid-receptor blockade produced by mifepristone. Duration of glucocorticoid therapy should take into account the long half-life of mifepristone (85 hours). Upon resolution of adrenal insufficiency, mifepristone therapy may be resumed at a lower dosage.

Hypokalemia

Hypokalemia has been reported in 44% of patients with Cushing's syndrome receiving mifepristone and can occur at any time during mifepristone therapy.

Serum potassium concentrations should be monitored and corrected prior to initiating mifepristone in patients with Cushing's syndrome, 1–2 weeks after initiation of therapy or dosage increases, and periodically during therapy. Hypokalemia may be treated with IV or oral potassium supplementation, based on clinical severity. If hypokalemia persists despite potassium supplementation, addition of mineralocorticoid (aldosterone) antagonist therapy should be considered.

Vaginal Bleeding and Endometrial Changes

Progesterone-receptor blockade by mifepristone promotes unopposed endometrial proliferation and may result in endometrial thickening, cystic dilatation of endometrial glands, and uterine bleeding in women not undergoing medical abortion. Women receiving mifepristone for management of clinical manifestations of Cushing's syndrome who experience unexplained vaginal bleeding during therapy with the drug should be referred to a gynecologist for further evaluation.

Uterine rupture has been reported rarely in women receiving mifepristone and misoprostol for termination of pregnancy, including women with prior uterine rupture or scarring and those receiving multiple doses of misoprostol within 24 hours. Women who choose to use a repeat dose of misoprostol should have a follow-up visit with their healthcare provider in approximately 7 days to assess for complete termination.

Prolongation of QT Interval

Mifepristone and its metabolites block the rapidly activating delayed rectifier potassium current I_{kr} and produce dose-related prolongation of the QT interval. Data on the effects of high mifepristone dosages, concomitant use of other drugs that prolong the QT interval, or use in patients with long QT interval are limited.

The manufacturer of mifepristone (Korlym®) states that the lowest possible effective dosage of mifepristone should be used to minimize risk of QT-interval prolongation, and the drug should be avoided in patients with potassium channel variants resulting in a long QT interval. In addition, concomitant use of mifepristone and drugs that prolong the QT interval should be avoided.

Exacerbation/Deterioration of Conditions Treated with Corticosteroids

Mifepristone antagonizes the effects of glucocorticoids; therefore, use of mifepristone for management of hyperglycemia secondary to Cushing's syndrome in patients receiving corticosteroid therapy for other conditions (e.g., autoimmune disorders) may lead to exacerbation or deterioration of such conditions. Use of mifepristone in patients with Cushing's syndrome is contraindicated in patients with conditions where corticosteroid therapy is considered lifesaving (e.g., immunosuppression in organ transplantation).

Concomitant Use with Potent CYP3A Inhibitors

Mifepristone (Korlym®) should be used with caution in patients receiving ketoconazole or other potent inhibitors of CYP3A, since concomitant use may increase mifepristone systemic exposure. The benefits of such concomitant use should be carefully weighed against the potential risks. Mifepristone (Korlym®) should be used concomitantly with potent CYP3A inhibitors only when necessary; if concomitant use is clinically warranted, the dosage of mifepristone should not exceed 600 mg once daily.

Suppression of Rh Isoimmunization

As with a surgical abortion, preventive measures to suppress formation of anti-$Rh_o(D)$ antibodies (e.g., administration of $Rh_o[D]$ immune globulin) should be considered in $Rh_o(D)$-negative women who receive the mifepristone and misoprostol regimen for medical abortion.

Death

As of December 31, 2018, 24 deaths have been reported in women receiving mifepristone for the medical termination of pregnancy, including 2 cases of ectopic pregnancy. In addition, there were several reported cases of sepsis that also resulted in some fatalities. A causal relationship to mifepristone has not been established because of concomitant use of other drugs, other medical or surgical treatments, concurrent medical conditions, and lack of information about the patient's health status and clinical management.

Pending further investigation, clinicians and patients should be aware of the specific circumstances and directions for use as well as risks (e.g., sepsis) associated with mifepristone therapy. In addition, clinicians should inform patients of early potential manifestations that may warrant immediate medical evaluation.

Pneumocystis jirovecii Pneumonia

Patients with endogenous Cushing's syndrome receiving mifepristone have an increased risk of opportunistic infections such as *Pneumocystis jirovecii* (formerly known as *Pneumocystis carinii*) pneumonia (PCP). Patients should be monitored closely for possible PCP, including respiratory distress early in treatment; if PCP is diagnosed, appropriate therapy should be provided.

Effects of Hypercortisolism

In patients with Cushing's syndrome, serum cortisol concentrations remain elevated and may increase during mifepristone therapy. Elevated serum cortisol concentrations may activate mineralocorticoid (aldosterone) receptors that are expressed in cardiac tissues. Caution should be used in patients with underlying cardiac conditions, including heart failure and coronary vascular disease.

Specific Populations

Pregnancy

Mifepristone (Mifeprex® and generics) is used in conjunction with misoprostol for the medical termination of pregnancy (through 70 days of gestation) and is not labeled by FDA for any other indication during pregnancy. The drug is contraindicated in women with a confirmed or suspected ectopic pregnancy.

Mifepristone (Korlym®) is contraindicated in pregnancy. Pregnancy must be excluded prior to initiation of the drug for the management of hyperglycemia secondary to Cushing's syndrome in women of childbearing potential and such women should use nonhormonal contraceptives during and for 1 month after the drug is discontinued.

Lactation

Mifepristone is distributed into milk at low to undetectable concentrations. Limited data indicate the weight-adjusted infant dose in milk may be no more than 0.5% of the maternal dose.

Data are not available on the effects of mifepristone (Mifeprex®) used in conjunction with misoprostol for termination of pregnancy on a breast-fed infant or on milk production. The developmental and health benefits of breast-feeding should be considered along with any potential adverse effects on the breast-fed child from mifepristone used in conjunction with misoprostol.

Because of the potential for serious adverse reactions to mifepristone in nursing infants, the manufacturer of mifepristone (Korlym®) states that a decision should be made whether to discontinue nursing or the drug in women with hyperglycemia secondary to Cushing's syndrome.

Pediatric Use

Safety and efficacy of mifepristone (Mifeprex®) for termination of pregnancy have been established in pregnant females, including those younger than 17 years of age.

Safety and efficacy of mifepristone (Korlym®) for management of hyperglycemia secondary to Cushing's syndrome have not been established in pediatric patients.

Geriatric Use

Clinical studies of mifepristone (Korlym®) did not include sufficient numbers of patients ≥65 years of age to determine whether geriatric patients respond differently than younger patients.

Hepatic Impairment

Moderate hepatic impairment (Child-Pugh class B) did not appear to substantially affect the pharmacokinetics of mifepristone in single- and multiple-dose pharmacokinetic studies; however, there was high interpatient variability in the exposure of mifepristone and its metabolites. Because of limited information on safety in patients with hepatic impairment, dosage of mifepristone for the management of hyperglycemia secondary to Cushing's syndrome should not exceed 600 mg once daily in patients with mild or moderate hepatic impairment. Mifepristone has not been evaluated in patients with severe hepatic impairment.

Renal Impairment

Systemic exposure of mifepristone is increased 31% in patients with severe renal impairment (creatinine clearance less than 30 mL/minute not requiring dialysis) compared with individuals with normal renal function. Dosage of mifepristone in patients with hyperglycemia secondary to Cushing's syndrome in patients with renal impairment should not exceed 600 mg once daily.

● *Common Adverse Effects*

Mifepristone (Mifeprex®): Vaginal bleeding and abdominal pain/cramping are expected effects when mifepristone is used for termination of pregnancy. Adverse effects occurring in over 15% of patients receiving mifepristone in conjunction with misoprostol for termination of pregnancy in clinical studies include nausea, weakness, fever/chills, vomiting, headache, diarrhea, and dizziness.

Mifepristone (Korlym®): Adverse effects occurring in 20% or more of patients with Cushing's syndrome receiving mifepristone in the open-label study include nausea, fatigue, headache, hypokalemia, arthralgia, vomiting, peripheral edema, hypertension, dizziness, decreased appetite, and endometrial hypertrophy.

DRUG INTERACTIONS

Mifepristone is metabolized primarily by cytochrome P-450 (CYP) isoenzyme 3A4. In vitro studies demonstrate that mifepristone inhibits and induces CYP3A. The drug also inhibits CYP isoenzymes 2C8, 2C9, and 2B6 in vitro. In vitro studies indicate potential drug interactions with substrates of CYP isoenzymes 1A2, 2A6, 2B6, 2C8, 2C9, 2C19, 2D6, 2E1, and 3A4.

In vitro studies indicate potential interactions between mifepristone and drugs transported by P-glycoprotein (P-gp) and breast cancer resistance protein (BCRP).

Because of the long half-life of mifepristone at steady state, the manufacturer states at least 2 weeks should elapse between discontinuance of mifepristone for management of hyperglycemia secondary to Cushing's syndrome and initiation or dosage increases of any interacting concomitant drugs.

● *Drugs Affecting or Metabolized by Hepatic Microsomal Enzymes*

CYP3A Inhibitors

Concomitant use of mifepristone and potent inhibitors of CYP3A4 may increase plasma concentrations of mifepristone and dosage reduction of mifepristone may be required.

Mifepristone should be used with caution and only when necessary in patients currently or recently receiving therapy with potent CYP3A4 inhibitors. If concomitant use of a *potent* CYP3A inhibitor (e.g., atazanavir, clarithromycin, conivaptan, fosamprenavir, indinavir, itraconazole, ketoconazole, the fixed combination of lopinavir and ritonavir [lopinavir/ritonavir], nefazodone, nelfinavir, posaconazole, ritonavir, saquinavir, voriconazole) is clinically warranted, the manufacturer of mifepristone (Korlym®) states that the maximum recommended dosage of the drug for the management of hyperglycemia in patients with Cushing's syndrome is 600 mg once daily.

Grapefruit juice should be avoided in patients receiving mifepristone.

Cimetidine

Concomitant use of mifepristone (300 mg daily for 14 days) and cimetidine (800 mg daily; a weak CYP3A inhibitor) slightly decreased peak plasma concentrations and systemic exposure of mifepristone; the manufacturer of mifepristone (Korlym®) states dosage adjustment is not required during concomitant use.

CYP3A Inducers

Concomitant use of mifepristone and inducers of CYP3A4 (e.g., carbamazepine, dexamethasone, phenobarbital, phenytoin, rifampin, St. John's wort [*Hypericum perforatum*]) may result in increased mifepristone metabolism and decreased serum mifepristone concentrations.

Clinical effects of such an interaction on termination of pregnancy are unknown.

Concomitant use of *daily* mifepristone for management of hyperglycemia secondary to Cushing's syndrome and CYP3A4 inducers should be avoided.

CYP3A Substrates

Concomitant use of mifepristone with drugs that are metabolized by CYP3A4 may result in increased systemic exposure of the substrate drug. Concomitant use of *daily* mifepristone for management of hyperglycemia secondary to Cushing's syndrome and substrates of CYP3A4 that have a narrow therapeutic index

(e.g., cyclosporine, dihydroergotamine, ergotamine, fentanyl, pimozide, quinidine, sirolimus, tacrolimus) is contraindicated. Because of the increased risk of rhabdomyolysis, concomitant use of *daily* mifepristone and simvastatin or lovastatin in patients with Cushing's syndrome also is contraindicated. Caution should be exercised if single-dose mifepristone for the termination of pregnancy is used concomitantly with substrates of CYP3A4 that have a narrow therapeutic index.

Drugs that undergo extensive first-pass metabolism that are metabolized by CYP3A (e.g., midazolam, sildenafil, triazolam) should be used with extreme caution in patients with Cushing's syndrome receiving *daily* mifepristone. If concomitant use cannot be avoided, the manufacturer of mifepristone (Korlym®) recommends using the lowest effective dosage of the CYP3A substrate; therapeutic drug monitoring of the CYP3A substrate is recommended when possible. An alternative to such CYP3A substrates also is advised for concomitant use with *daily* mifepristone when possible.

If *daily* mifepristone for management of hyperglycemia secondary to Cushing's syndrome is used concomitantly with drugs that undergo minimal first-pass metabolism via CYP3A or are metabolized by CYP3A to a lesser extent, the manufacturer recommends using the lowest effective dose of the concomitant drug and/or decreased dosing frequency of the CYP3A substrate and monitoring for adverse effects; therapeutic drug monitoring of the CYP3A substrate is recommended when possible.

Alprazolam

Concomitant use of mifepristone (1200 mg daily for 10 days) and alprazolam (single 1-mg dose; a CYP3A substrate with minimal first-pass effect) increased systemic exposure of alprazolam by 80% and decreased 4-hydroxy-alprazolam exposure by 24%.

Simvastatin

In healthy individuals, concomitant use of mifepristone (1200 mg daily for 10 days) and simvastatin (single 80-mg dose; a CYP3A substrate with extensive first-pass effect) increased systemic exposure to simvastatin and simvastatin acid by approximately 10.4- and 15.7-fold, respectively. Concomitant use of mifepristone and simvastatin is contraindicated.

CYP2B6 Substrates

Concomitant use of mifepristone with drugs that are metabolized by CYP2B6 (e.g., bupropion, efavirenz) may result in increased systemic exposure of such drugs. Caution is advised if mifepristone is used concomitantly with substrates of CYP2B6.

CYP2C8 and/or 2C9 Substrates

Concomitant use of mifepristone with drugs that are metabolized principally by CYP2C8 and/or 2C9 (e.g., nonsteroidal anti-inflammatory agents [NSAIAs], repaglinide, warfarin) may result in increased systemic exposure of such drugs. If *daily* mifepristone for management of hyperglycemia secondary to Cushing's syndrome is used concomitantly with drugs that are substrates of CYP2C8 and/or 2C9, the manufacturer recommends the CYP2C8 and/or 2C9 substrates be given at the lowest effective dosage and the patient closely monitored for adverse effects.

Fluvastatin

In healthy individuals, concomitant use of mifepristone (1200 mg daily for 7 days) and fluvastatin (single 40-mg dose; a CYP2C8 and 2C9 substrate) increased systemic exposure of fluvastatin by approximately 3.6-fold.

● *Drugs that Prolong the QT Interval*

Effects of concomitant use of mifepristone and drugs that prolong the QT interval are not known; concomitant use should be avoided.

● *Digoxin*

Concomitant use of mifepristone (1200 mg daily for 10 days) and digoxin (0.125 mg daily) increased systemic exposure and peak plasma concentration of digoxin 1.4- and 1.6-fold, respectively. The manufacturer of mifepristone (Korlym®) recommends that plasma digoxin concentrations should be assessed after 1–2 weeks of concomitant use and periodically as clinically appropriate.

• *Hormonal Contraceptives*

Mifepristone is a progesterone-receptor antagonist and may reduce the efficacy of hormonal contraceptives. Nonhormonal methods of contraception should be used in women of childbearing potential with Cushing's syndrome who are receiving *daily* mifepristone.

DESCRIPTION

Mifepristone, a synthetic derivative of the progestin norethindrone, is a progesterone- and glucocorticoid-receptor antagonist. Mifepristone is a selective antagonist of the progesterone receptor at lower dosages and exhibits antiglucocorticoid activity at higher dosages. At higher dosages, mifepristone acts as a glucocorticoid-receptor antagonist but exhibits little affinity for the mineralocorticoid (aldosterone) receptor. At dosages of 1 mg/kg or higher, mifepristone antagonizes the endometrial and myometrial effects of progesterone in women; dosages of 4.5 mg/kg or higher cause compensatory elevation of corticotropin (ACTH) and cortisol in humans. The drug also has been shown to have weak antiandrogenic activity. Mifepristone exhibits little to no affinity for estrogen, muscarinic, histamine, or monoamine receptors.

Mifepristone binds to the progesterone receptor with greater affinity than progesterone, competitively antagonizing the endometrial and myometrial effects of progesterone and resulting in down-regulation of progesterone-dependent genes. Since the continuance of a viable pregnancy depends on progesterone, detachment of the products of conception and termination of pregnancy result. In addition, mifepristone promotes uterine contractions and softening of the cervix and sensitizes the myometrium to effects of prostaglandins (e.g., misoprostol) that stimulate uterine contractions and expulsion of the products of conception. In the absence of progesterone, mifepristone acts as a partial progestin agonist.

Mifepristone (Mifeprex®) is rapidly absorbed following oral administration and reaches peak plasma concentrations approximately 45 and 90 minutes following single 200- and 600-mg doses, respectively. Time to peak plasma concentration occurs 1–2 and 1–4 hours following single and multiple 600-mg oral doses of mifepristone (Korlym®), respectively; peak plasma concentrations of the active metabolites occur 2–8 hours following multiple 600-mg oral doses. Administration with food substantially increases plasma concentrations of mifepristone. The absolute oral bioavailability of a single 20-mg dose of mifepristone in women of childbearing age is 69%. Mifepristone is 98–99% bound to plasma proteins (mainly albumin and α₁-acid glycoprotein); binding of the drug and its active metabolites is concentration dependent. Mifepristone and its metabolites are distributed into milk and other tissues, including the CNS. Mifepristone is extensively metabolized, principally via the cytochrome P-450 (CYP) 3A4 isoenzyme into 3 known active metabolites. The drug and its metabolites are excreted mainly in feces (83–90%) with smaller amounts excreted in urine (9%). The initial half-life of the drug is 12–72 hours; the terminal elimination half-life is 18 hours. The half-life following multiple doses of 600 mg daily is 85 hours.

ADVICE TO PATIENTS

- Importance of advising patients receiving mifepristone (Mifeprex® and generics) in conjunction with misoprostol for termination of pregnancy to read the medication guide and to read and sign the patient agreement form before receiving the drug If visiting an emergency room or clinician other than the original prescriber, present medication guide to alert clinician of recent medical abortion.

- For termination of pregnancy, importance of taking misoprostol 24–48 hours after receiving mifepristone (Mifeprex®), and following up with a clinician approximately 7–14 days following the mifepristone and misoprostol regimen.

- Importance of understanding procedures for emergency situations and of obtaining a telephone number for emergency contact with clinicians.

- Vaginal bleeding is not proof of complete abortion. Possible need for surgical intervention if complete abortion does not occur following mifepristone and misoprostol regimen. Unknown risk of fetal malformation if pregnancy continues.

- Risk of severe infection and bleeding following termination of pregnancy. Contact clinician (or visit emergency room if clinician is unavailable) if sustained fever (temperature ≥38°C persisting for >4 hours), severe abdominal pain, or prolonged heavy bleeding (soaking through 2 thick full-size sanitary pads per hour for 2 consecutive hours) occurs *or* if abdominal pain/discomfort or general malaise (including weakness, nausea, vomiting, or diarrhea), with or without fever, occurs >24 hours after administration of misoprostol.

- Importance of initiating contraception immediately after confirmation of abortion or before resuming sexual intercourse; risk of pregnancy exists *immediately* after termination of existing pregnancy and before normal menses begin.

- Importance of advising patients receiving mifepristone for management of Cushing's syndrome (Korlym®) to read the medication guide.

- Importance of informing patients that mifepristone causes termination of pregnancy. Necessity of women of childbearing potential receiving mifepristone (Korlym®) for management of hyperglycemia secondary to Cushing's syndrome to avoid pregnancy and to use effective nonhormonal methods of contraception while receiving mifepristone and for at least 1 month following discontinuance of the drug. Importance of patients informing their clinicians if they are or suspect they may be pregnant.

- Potential risk of adrenal insufficiency when used in patients with Cushing's syndrome. Contact clinician if manifestations of adrenal insufficiency (e.g., nausea, fatigue, weakness, hypotension, hypoglycemia) develop.

- Potential risk of hypokalemia when used in patients with Cushing's syndrome. Contact clinician if manifestations of hypokalemia (e.g., muscle weakness, aches, cramps, palpitations) occur.

- Importance of women with Cushing's syndrome who are receiving mifepristone to contact a clinician if unusual vaginal bleeding occurs.

- Importance of informing clinicians of existing or contemplated concomitant therapy, including prescription and OTC drugs (e.g., corticosteroids, cyclosporine, fentanyl, lovastatin, simvastatin) and dietary or herbal supplements (e.g., St. John's wort), as well as any concomitant illnesses (e.g., hepatic or renal impairment, cardiovascular disease).

- Importance of women informing their clinician if they are breast-feeding.

- Importance of informing patients of other important precautionary information. (See Cautions.)

PREPARATIONS

Distribution of mifepristone (Mifeprex® and generics) is restricted. The drug can be obtained only through the Mifepristone REMS program.

Mifepristone (Korlym®) is available through a designated specialty pharmacy. Information regarding distribution of the drug is available from the manufacturer at 855-456-7596 or https://www.korlym.com/access-financial-support/support-program-for-access-and-reimbursement-for-korlym-spark/.

Excipients in commercially available drug preparations may have clinically important effects in some individuals; consult specific product labeling for details.

Mifepristone

Oral		
Tablets	200 mg*	**Mifeprex®**, Danco **Mifepristone Tablets**
	300 mg	**Korlym®**, Corcept Therapeutics

* available from one or more manufacturer, distributor, and/or repackager by generic (nonproprietary) name

† Use is not currently included in the labeling approved by the US Food and Drug Administration.

Selected Revisions January 18, 2023, © Copyright, December 01, 2000, American Society of Health-System Pharmacists, Inc.

Oxytocin

76:00 · OXYTOCICS

■ Oxytocin, a nonapeptide hormone secreted by the neurons of the supra-optic and paraventricular nuclei of the hypothalamus and stored in the posterior pituitary (neurohypophysis) in mammals, indirectly stimulates contraction of uterine smooth muscle.

USES

● Antepartum Uses

IV infusion of dilute solutions of oxytocin is the method of choice for inducing labor at term and stimulating uterine contractions during the first and second stages of labor.

Induction of Labor

Induction of labor with oxytocin infusion is indicated in term or near-term pregnancies associated with hypertension (e.g., preeclampsia, eclampsia, cardiovascular-renal disease), erythroblastosis fetalis, maternal or gestational diabetes mellitus, antepartum bleeding, or preterm, premature rupture of the membranes in which spontaneous labor does not ensue. Routine induction of labor with oxytocin may be indicated in prolonged pregnancies (greater than 42 weeks' gestation). *Elective induction of labor merely for physician or patient convenience is not a valid indication for oxytocin use.* In patients with eclampsia, if delivery is not imminent within 12 hours following an initial oxytocin infusion, some clinicians recommend cesarean section be done rather than continue administration of oxytocin.

Induction of labor also may be indicated in cases of uterine fetal death, fetal growth retardation, or static or decreasing maternal weight. However, in cases of missed abortion, intrauterine fetal death in late pregnancy, benign hydatidiform mole, or fetuses with anencephaly or erythroblastosis fetalis with hydrops or other congenital abnormalities incompatible with life, some clinicians recommend intravaginal dinoprostone because oxytocin may be relatively ineffective.

Pelvic adequacy and other maternal and fetal conditions (including fetal lung maturity) must be evaluated carefully whenever induction of labor is considered. Oxytocin should not be used to induce labor when the benefit-to-risk ratio for the mother or child favors surgical intervention. Induction of labor is contraindicated in cases of cephalopelvic disproportion, unfavorable fetal position or presentation (e.g., transverse lies), uterine or cervical scarring from previous cesarean section or major cervical or uterine surgery, fetal distress when delivery is not imminent, unengaged fetal head, when vaginal delivery is contraindicated (e.g., total placenta previa, vasa previa, cord presentation or prolapse, active genital herpes infection), or when uterine activity fails to progress adequately. Except in unusual circumstances requiring the clinician's judgment, the manufacturers warn that labor generally should not be induced with oxytocin when pregnancy is complicated by fetal distress, hydramnios, partial placenta previa, prematurity, borderline cephalopelvic disproportion, previous major surgery of the cervix or uterus (including cesarean section), overdistension of the uterus, grand multiparity, invasive cervical carcinoma, or history of uterine sepsis or traumatic delivery. Oxytocin should not be administered for prolonged periods in cases of severe toxemia.

Augmentation of Labor

During the first and second stages of labor, IV oxytocin infusion may be used to augment contractions if labor is prolonged or if dysfunctional uterine inertia occurs. Use of oxytocin is not recommended when labor is progressing normally during the first and second stages or when hypertonic patterns of labor occur, especially since response to the drug may be accentuated during the second stage of labor. In cases of uterine inertia, the drug should not be administered for prolonged periods (usually not more than 6–8 hours). Oxytocin should not be used to augment labor when vaginal delivery is contraindicated (e.g., total placenta previa).

● Postpartum Uses

Oxytocin infusions have been used to shorten the third stage of labor immediately following delivery of the infant (when the absence of additional fetuses is established), but some clinicians warn that oxytocics may inhibit, rather than assist in, expulsion of the placenta and increase the risk of hemorrhage and infection. If an oxytocic is used for this purpose, however, most clinicians recommend oxytocin.

Infusion of oxytocin is routinely used postpartum or following cesarean section to stimulate immediate contractions of the uterus and to control uterine bleeding. However, for the management of postpartum hemorrhage and uterine atony, most clinicians prefer ergonovine or methylergonovine to oxytocin unless an immediate contractile response is desired, because the amine ergot alkaloids produce more sustained contractions and higher uterine tonus than does oxytocin. Some clinicians prefer to manage postpartum bleeding with dilute IV oxytocin followed by an amine ergot alkaloid administered IM.

● Other Uses of Parenteral Oxytocin

Oxytocin infusion has been used following prostaglandin or hypertonic abortifacients to shorten the induction-to-abortion time when these abortifacients are being used to induce second trimester abortions, to induce abortion when a patient has failed to respond to the abortifacient, or to induce abortion after membranes have ruptured. Oxytocin also has been used as an adjunct in cases of incomplete abortion when the placenta fails to abort spontaneously within 1 hour after abortion of the fetus; however, some clinicians maintain that oxytocin may hinder rather than assist in expulsion of the placenta. Because concurrent use of oxytocin with abortifacients may produce uterine contractions of such intensity that uterine rupture or cervical laceration may be more likely to occur, oxytocin usually should not be administered until the oxytocic effect of the abortifacient has subsided, and patients should be carefully monitored. Oxytocin, however, is routinely used in conjunction with hypertonic urea- and dinoprostone-induced abortions.

Oxytocin infusion has been used with success to evaluate the adequacy of fetal respiratory capabilities in high-risk pregnancies of greater than 31 weeks gestation†. By inducing uterine contractions, oxytocin transiently impedes uterine blood flow. If placental reserve is low, a late deceleration in fetal heart rate may occur following oxytocin administration, indicating chronic hypoxia (positive response). If fetal heart rate is unchanged (negative response) by the oxytocin challenge, adequate placental support is probably available. The test should be repeated in 1 week to reassess fetal response. A positive response indicates that there may be fetal distress and may be an indication for termination of pregnancy, especially if a lecithin-sphingomyelin ratio of greater than 1.5 can be demonstrated.

DOSAGE AND ADMINISTRATION

● Administration

As an oxytocic, oxytocin should be given by IV infusion using a controlled-infusion device. Although oxytocin has been given IM, most clinicians believe this route of administration should *not* be used for augmentation or induction of labor because the effects it produces are unpredictable and difficult to control.

IV Administration

Prior to IV administration, the commercially available injection *must* be diluted. Generally, oxytocin infusions containing 10 milliunits/mL are used for induction or augmentation of labor. This solution may be prepared by adding 10 units (1 mL of the commercially available injection) to 1 L of 0.9% sodium chloride, lactated Ringer's, or 5% dextrose injection. Except under unusual circumstances, a physiologic electrolyte solution preferably should be used for preparing IV infusions of the drug intended for use in the induction or augmentation of labor. Infusions containing 20 milliunits/mL are used to produce intense uterine contractions and reduce postpartum bleeding, and as adjuncts to prostaglandin or hypertonic abortifacients. This solution may be prepared by adding 10 units (1 mL of the commercially available injection) to 500 mL of one of the above IV infusion solutions.

Standardize 4 Safety

Standardized concentrations for oxytocin have been established through Standardize 4 Safety (S4S), a national patient safety initiative to reduce medication errors, especially during transitions of care. Multidisciplinary expert panels were convened to determine recommended standard concentrations. Because recommendations from the S4S panels may differ from the manufacturer's prescribing information, caution is advised when using concentrations that differ from labeling, particularly when using rate information from the label. For additional information on S4S (including updates that may be available), see https://www.ashp.org/pharmacy-practice/standardize-4-safety-initiative.

TABLE 1. Standardize 4 Safety Continuous IV Infusion Standard Concentrations for Oxytocin

Patient Population	Concentration Standards	Dosing Units
Adults[a]	0.06 units/mL	milliunits/min[b]

[a] See ISMP for best practices. https://www.ismp.org/resources/taking-closer-look-medication-errors-involve-oxytocin; https://www.ncbi.nlm.nih.gov/pmc/articles/PMC3956395/

[b] dosing units differ from concentration units

● Dosage

Antepartum Uses

Oxytocin dosage and rate of infusion are determined by uterine response. The drug should be discontinued if prolonged uterine contractions (greater than 90 seconds in duration) or rising intrauterine pressure occur or if uterine motility interferes with fetal heart rate; in addition, oxygen should be administered to the mother, who preferably should be in the lateral position, and other appropriate measures taken as necessary. For induction of labor, oxytocin usually is infused at an initial rate of 0.5–1 milliunit/minute. The infusion rate generally is increased in 1- to 2-milliunit/minute increments at 30- to 60-minute intervals until a response is observed. When the desired frequency of contractions is established (a uterine pattern comparable to spontaneous labor), without evidence of fetal distress, and labor has progressed to 5–6 cm dilation, the rate of oxytocin infusion may be reduced by similar increments. IV infusion rates up to 6 milliunits/minute have been shown to produce oxytocin concentrations in maternal plasma comparable to those associated with spontaneous labor. At term, higher rates of infusion should be employed with caution, and rates exceeding 9–10 milliunits/minute rarely are required. Before term, when uterine sensitivity to oxytocin is reduced secondary to decreased oxytocin receptors, higher infusion rates may be necessary.

Postpartum Uses

To produce intense uterine contractions and reduce postpartum bleeding after expulsion of the placenta, a total of 10 units of oxytocin may be infused at a rate of 20–40 milliunits/minute after delivery of the infant(s) (when the absence of additional fetuses is established); rate is adjusted to maintain uterine contraction and control uterine atony. Most clinicians recommend that oxytocin not be given until after delivery of the placenta.

Other Uses of Parenteral Oxytocin

When used to shorten the induction-to-abortion time, to induce abortion in patients who have failed to abort following administration of second trimester abortifacients, or to induce abortion after membranes have ruptured, IV oxytocin infusions of 10–100 milliunits/minute have been used. However, it is recommended that cumulative dose in a 12-hour period not exceed 30 units because of the risk of water intoxication.

To evaluate fetal distress† using the oxytocin challenge test, 5–10 units of oxytocin (0.5–1.0 mL of the commercially available injection) is diluted with 1 L of 5% dextrose injection; the resultant solution contains 5–10 milliunits/mL. Initially the drug is infused IV in the mother at a rate of 0.5 milliunit/minute. The infusion rate may be gradually increased at 15- to 30-minute intervals to a maximum of 20 milliunits/minute. Fetal heart rate and uterine contractions should be monitored immediately before and during the oxytocin infusion. When 3 moderate uterine contractions occur within one 10-minute interval, the infusion should be

discontinued and baseline and oxytocin-induced fetal heart rates should be compared. If no change in fetal heart rate occurs, the test should be repeated in 1 week. If a late deceleration in fetal heart rate occurs, termination of the pregnancy may be indicated.

CAUTIONS

● Adverse Effects

When oxytocin is administered in excessive dosage, with abortifacients or to sensitive patients, hyperstimulation of the uterus, with strong (hypertonic) and/or prolonged (tetanic) contractions, or a resting uterine tone of 15–20 mm H_2O between contractions may occur, possibly resulting in uterine rupture, cervical and vaginal lacerations, postpartum hemorrhage, abruptio placentae, impaired uterine blood flow, amniotic fluid embolism, and fetal trauma including intracranial hemorrhage. Increased uterine motility also may cause adverse fetal effects, including sinus bradycardia, tachycardia, premature ventricular complexes and other arrhythmias, permanent CNS or brain damage, and death secondary to asphyxia. Excessive maternal dosage or administration of the drug to sensitive women also can cause uteroplacental hypoperfusion and variable deceleration of fetal heart rate, fetal hypoxia, perinatal hepatic necrosis, and fetal hypercapnia. Rare incidents of pelvic hematoma have been reported, but these were probably also related to the high incidence of operative vaginal deliveries in primiparas, the fragility of engorged pelvic veins (especially if varicosed), and faulty episiotomy repair.

When large amounts of oxytocin are administered, severe decreases in maternal systolic and diastolic blood pressure, increases in heart rate, systemic venous return and cardiac output, and arrhythmia may occur; these effects may be particularly hazardous to patients with valvular heart disease and those receiving spinal and epidural anesthesia.

Postpartum bleeding may be increased by administration of oxytocin; this effect may be related to reports of oxytocin-induced thrombocytopenia, afibrinogenemia, and hypoprothrombinemia. By carefully controlling delivery, the incidence of postpartum bleeding may be minimized.

Nausea, vomiting, maternal sinus bradycardia, and premature ventricular complexes reported in patients receiving oxytocin are probably related to labor and not the drug. The risk of neonatal hyperbilirubinemia appears to be about 1.6 times greater following oxytocin-induced labor than that following spontaneous labor, and neonatal jaundice has occurred. Other adverse neonatal effects from oxytocin-induced labor include retinal hemorrhage and low Apgar scores at 5 minutes.

Severe water intoxication with seizures, coma, and death has been reported following prolonged IV infusion of oxytocin with an excessive volume of fluid. Neonatal seizures also have been reported. Injudicious use of oxytocin has also resulted in maternal deaths secondary to hypertensive episodes and subarachnoid hemorrhage.

Anaphylactic and other allergic reactions have occurred in patients receiving oxytocin and may rarely be fatal.

● Precautions and Contraindications

Parenteral oxytocin should be used only by qualified professional personnel in a hospital where intensive care and surgical facilities are immediately available. During administration of oxytocin, uterine contractions, fetal and maternal heart rate, maternal blood pressure, and, if possible, intrauterine pressure should be continuously monitored to avoid complications. If uterine hyperactivity occurs, oxytocin administration should be immediately discontinued; oxytocin-induced stimulation of uterine contractions usually decreases soon after discontinuance of the drug. Electronic monitoring of the fetus is the best method for early detection of oxytocin overdosage. However, accurate measurement of intrauterine pressure during contractions requires intrauterine pressure recording. Determination of fetal heart rate via a fetal scalp electrode is more dependable than via external monitoring.

Since oxytocin may produce some antidiuretic effects, some clinicians recommend restricting fluid intake, avoiding administration of low-sodium infusion fluids and high oxytocin doses for prolonged periods, and monitoring fluid intake and output during administration of the drug.

Oxytocin should not be given simultaneously by more than one route of administration. Oxytocin is contraindicated in patients with a history of hypersensitivity to the drug. *For additional discussion on the precautions and contraindications associated with oxytocin, see Uses.*

● Mutagenicity and Carcinogenicity

The mutagenic and carcinogenic potentials of oxytocin have not been determined.

● Pregnancy, Fertility, and Lactation

Pregnancy

Animal reproduction studies have not been performed with oxytocin; however, the manufacturers state that the drug is not indicated for use during the first or second trimester of pregnancy other than in relation to spontaneous or induced abortion. Based on wide experience with oxytocin and on its chemical and pharmacologic properties, the drug would not be expected to cause fetal abnormalities when used as indicated. Oxytocin can, however, cause nonteratogenic adverse effects. (See Cautions: Adverse Effects.)

Fertility

It is not known whether oxytocin affects fertility.

Lactation

Oxytocin may be distributed in small quantities into milk. If oxytocin therapy is required postpartum (e.g., to control severe bleeding), commencement of nursing should be delayed for at least 1 day after the drug has been discontinued.

DRUG INTERACTIONS

Severe hypertension has been reported when oxytocin was given 3–4 hours following prophylactic administration of a vasoconstrictor in conjunction with caudal block anesthesia. Cyclopropane anesthesia may modify oxytocin's cardiovascular effects, producing less pronounced tachycardia but more severe hypotension than occurs with oxytocin alone; maternal sinus bradycardia with abnormal atrioventricular rhythms has been noted when oxytocin was used concomitantly with cyclopropane anesthesia. Oxytocin reportedly has delayed induction of thiopental (no longer commercially available in the US) anesthesia by producing venous spasm that caused peripheral pooling of thiopental; however, this interaction has not been conclusively established.

PHARMACOLOGY

Exogenous oxytocin elicits all the pharmacologic responses usually produced by endogenous oxytocin.

Oxytocin indirectly stimulates contraction of uterine smooth muscle by increasing the sodium permeability of uterine myofibrils. High estrogen concentrations lower the threshold for uterine response to oxytocin. Uterine response to oxytocin increases with the duration of pregnancy and is greater in patients who are in labor than those not in labor; only very large doses elicit contractions in early pregnancy. Contractions produced in the term uterus by oxytocin are similar to those occurring during spontaneous labor. In the term uterus, oxytocin increases the amplitude and frequency of uterine contractions which in turn tend to decrease cervical activity producing dilation and effacement of the cervix and to transiently impede uterine blood flow.

Oxytocin contracts myoepithelial cells surrounding the alveoli of the breasts, forcing milk from the alveoli into the larger ducts and thus facilitating milk ejection. The drug possesses no galactopoietic properties.

Oxytocin produces vasodilation of vascular smooth muscle, increasing renal, coronary, and cerebral blood flow. Blood pressure is usually unchanged, but following IV administration of very large doses or undiluted solutions, blood pressure may decrease transiently, and tachycardia and an increase in cardiac output may be reflexly induced. Any initial fall in blood pressure is usually followed by a small but sustained increase in blood pressure.

In contrast to vasopressin, oxytocin has minimal antidiuretic effects; however, water intoxication may occur when oxytocin is administered with an excessive volume of electrolyte-free IV fluids and/or at too rapid a rate.

PHARMACOKINETICS

● Absorption

Oxytocin is destroyed by chymotrypsin in the GI tract. Uterine response occurs almost immediately and subsides within 1 hour following IV administration of oxytocin. Following IM injection of the drug, uterine response occurs within 3–5 minutes and persists for 2–3 hours. Following intranasal application of 10–20 units of oxytocin (nasal preparations are no longer commercially available in the US), contractions of myoepithelial tissue surrounding the alveoli of the breasts begin within a few minutes and continue for 20 minutes; IV oxytocin produces the same effect with a dose of 100–200 milliunits.

● Distribution

Like vasopressin, oxytocin is distributed throughout the extracellular fluid. Small amounts of oxytocin probably reach the fetal circulation.

● Elimination

Oxytocin has a plasma half-life of about 3–5 minutes. Most of the drug is rapidly destroyed in the liver and kidneys. Oxytocinase, a circulating enzyme produced early in pregnancy, is also capable of inactivating the polypeptide. Only small amounts of oxytocin are excreted in urine unchanged.

CHEMISTRY AND STABILITY

● Chemistry

Oxytocin is a nonapeptide hormone secreted by the neurons of the supraoptic and paraventricular nuclei of the hypothalamus and stored in the posterior pituitary (neurohypophysis) in mammals. Commercially available oxytocin preparations are prepared synthetically. Although the highly purified synthetic preparations are substantially free from the pressor and antidiuretic principles of the posterior pituitary, even these preparations may contain some impurities with inherent pressor and antidiuretic properties which may be manifested following administration of large doses. The potency of oxytocin is standardized according to its vasodepressor activity in chickens (which closely parallels oxytocic activity) and is expressed in USP Posterior Pituitary units. Each unit is equivalent to about 2–2.2 mcg of the pure hormone.

Oxytocin occurs as a white powder and is soluble in water. During manufacture, the pH of commercially available oxytocin injection is adjusted to 2.5–4.5 with acetic acid.

● Stability

Oxytocin injection should be stored at temperatures less than 15–25°C but should not be frozen. Pitocin® should be refrigerated at 2–8°C but may be exposed to temperatures ranging from 15–25°C for up to 30 days; Pitocin® exposed to this latter temperature range for longer periods should be discarded.

Oxytocin injection appears to be compatible with most IV infusion fluids but is reported to be physically incompatible with fibrinolysin, norepinephrine bitartrate, prochlorperazine edisylate, and warfarin sodium. Oxytocin injection has also been reported to be incompatible with various other drugs, but the compatibility depends on several factors (e.g., the concentration of the drugs, resulting pH, temperature). Specialized references should be consulted for more specific compatibility information.

PREPARATIONS

Excipients in commercially available drug preparations may have clinically important effects in some individuals; consult specific product labeling for details.

Oxytocin

Parenteral		
Injection	10 units/mL*	Oxytocin Injection Pitocin®, Monarch

* available from one or more manufacturer, distributor, and/or repackager by generic (nonproprietary) name

† Use is not currently included in the labeling approved by the US Food and Drug Administration.

Selected Revisions June 10, 2024, © Copyright, July 1, 1978, American Society of Health-System Pharmacists, Inc.

Table of Contents

80:00 ANTITOXINS, IMMUNE GLOBULINS, TOXOIDS, AND VACCINES

§ Omitted from the print version of *AHFS Drug Information*® because of space limitations. This monograph is available on the *AHFS Drug Information*® website, http://ahfsdruginformation.com.

Table of Contents

84:00 SKIN AND MUCOUS MEMBRANE AGENTS

§ Omitted from the print version of *AHFS Drug Information*® because of space limitations. This monograph is available on the *AHFS Drug Information*® website, http://ahfsdruginformation.com.

Table of Contents

Table of Contents

90:00 IMMUNOMODULATORY AGENTS

§ Omitted from the print version of *AHFS Drug Information*® because of space limitations. This monograph is available on the *AHFS Drug Information*® website, http://ahfsdruginformation.com.

Natalizumab

90:04.04 • MONOCLONAL ANTIBODIES

REMS

FDA approved a REMS for natalizumab and natalizumab-sztn to ensure that the benefits outweigh the risks. The REMS may apply to one or more preparations of natalizumab and consists of the following: medication guide, elements to assure safe use, and implementation system. See the FDA REMS page (https://www.accessdata.fda.gov/scripts/cder/rems/index.cfm).

- Natalizumab and natalizumab-sztn, recombinant humanized anti-α4-integrin monoclonal antibodies, are biologic response modifiers.

- Natalizumab-sztn (Tyruko®) is biosimilar to natalizumab (Tysabri®). FDA defines a biosimilar as a biological product that is highly similar to an FDA-licensed reference biological with the exception of minor differences in clinically inactive components and for which there are no clinically meaningful differences in safety, purity, or potency. The claim of biosimilarity is based on a totality-of-evidence approach, which includes consideration of data from analytical, animal, and clinical studies (e.g., human pharmacokinetic and pharmacodynamic studies, clinical immunogenicity assessment, additional comparative clinical studies). Therefore, biosimilarity may be established even when there are formulation or minor structural differences as long as these differences are not clinically meaningful. Biosimilars are approved through an abbreviated licensure pathway that establishes biosimilarity between the proposed biological and the reference biological but does not independently establish safety and effectiveness of the proposed biological. In order to be considered an interchangeable biosimilar, a biological product must meet additional requirements beyond demonstrating biosimilarity to its reference product; these requirements include demonstrating that the biological product can be expected to produce the same clinical results as the reference product in any given patient and, for a biological product that is administered more than once to an individual, the risk in terms of safety or diminished efficacy of alternating or switching between use of the biological product and the reference product is no greater than the risk of using the reference product without such alternation or switch. Biosimilar products that are interchangeable can be substituted for the reference product without the intervention of the healthcare provider who prescribed the reference product. The currently available natalizumab biosimilar does not have interchangeable data at this time.

- In this monograph, unless otherwise stated, the term "natalizumab products" refers to natalizumab (the reference drug) and its biosimilar (natalizumab-sztn).

USES

A single natalizumab biosimilar is available. Biosimilarity of this product has been demonstrated for both approved indications of originator natalizumab (multiple sclerosis [MS] and Crohn disease). Biosimilarity to originator natalizumab is additionally supported by a comparative clinical study in patients with relapsing-remitting MS.

● Multiple Sclerosis

Natalizumab products are used as monotherapy in the management of relapsing forms of multiple sclerosis (MS), to include clinically isolated syndrome, relapsing-remitting disease, and active secondary progressive disease, in adults; the drug has been shown in clinical studies to delay the accumulation of physical disability and reduce the frequency of clinical exacerbations in patients with relapsing forms of MS. Because natalizumab increases the risk of progressive multifocal leukoencephalopathy (PML), an opportunistic viral infection of the brain that usually leads to death or severe disability, clinicians should consider whether the expected benefits of the drug are sufficient to outweigh this risk when initiating or continuing therapy.

Natalizumab (Tysabri®) was initially approved by the FDA in November 2004 for the treatment of relapsing-remitting MS; however, the manufacturer voluntarily withdrew the drug from the US market in February 2005 after 2 cases of PML were reported in patients who were receiving natalizumab in conjunction with interferon beta-1a (Avonex®). Following subsequent review of the efficacy and safety data, FDA allowed the drug to be reintroduced into the US market under restricted conditions of use. Given that the 2 cases of PML occurred in patients receiving natalizumab concomitantly with interferon beta-1a, the current indication for use is restricted to monotherapy as a prudent measure, although it is not certain whether the risk of PML in the monotherapy setting is less than when natalizumab is used concomitantly with other MS treatments.

Clinical Experience

Safety and efficacy of natalizumab were evaluated in 2 randomized, double-blind, placebo-controlled studies (MS1 and MS2) in adults with clinically active relapsing-remitting MS (i.e., at least 1 clinical relapse during the prior year) and Expanded Disability Status Scale (EDSS) scores of 0–5. Median duration of natalizumab therapy in both studies was 120 weeks. Neurologic evaluations were performed every 12 weeks and at the time of suspected clinical relapse. Annual MRI evaluations for T1-weighted gadolinium-enhancing lesions and T2-hyperintense lesions also were performed. The primary efficacy end point at 2 years was time to onset of sustained increase in disability (defined as an increase of at least 1 point on the EDSS from a baseline of 1 or greater or an increase of at least 1.5 points from a baseline of 0, sustained for 12 weeks).

The MS1 study included patients who had not received any interferon beta or glatiramer acetate for at least the previous 6 months (approximately 94% had never received these agents). The median age of patients in this study was 37 years and the median disease duration was 5 years. Patients were randomized in a 2:1 ratio to receive natalizumab (300 mg IV once every 4 weeks) or placebo for up to 28 months (30 infusions). At 2 years, the annualized relapse rate was 67% lower in those receiving natalizumab (0.22 relapse per year) compared with those receiving placebo (0.67 relapse per year). Patients receiving natalizumab had a 42% decrease in the risk of sustained progression of disability. The cumulative probability of progression at 2 years (based on Kaplan-Meier analysis) was 17% in those receiving natalizumab compared with 29% in those receiving placebo. Approximately 67% of those receiving natalizumab were free of relapses at 2 years compared with 41% of those receiving placebo. Study results also indicated that natalizumab therapy had beneficial effects on several MRI measures of disease activity. No new or enlarging T2-hyperintense lesions developed in 57% of patients receiving natalizumab compared with 15% of those receiving placebo. No gadolinium-enhancing lesions developed in 97% of patients receiving natalizumab compared with 72% of those receiving placebo.

In the MS2 study, adults with relapsing-remitting MS who had been receiving interferon beta-1a for at least 12 months and had at least 1 relapse during the 12-month period immediately prior to the study were randomly assigned to receive natalizumab (300 mg IV once every 4 weeks) or placebo in addition to their interferon beta-1a regimen (30 mcg IM once weekly) for up to 28 months (30 infusions). The median age of patients was 39 years and the median disease duration was 7 years. At 2 years, the annualized relapse rate was 56% lower in those receiving the combined regimen of natalizumab and interferon beta-1a (0.33 relapse per year) compared with those receiving interferon beta-1a and placebo (0.75 relapse per year). At 2 years, 54% of those receiving the combined regimen remained free of relapses compared with 32% of those receiving interferon beta-1a with placebo. Patients receiving the combined regimen had a 24% decrease in the risk of sustained disability progression over 2 years compared with those receiving interferon beta-1a and placebo. Kaplan-Meier estimates of the cumulative probability of sustained disability progression at 2 years were 23% in those receiving the combined regimen and 29% in those receiving interferon beta-1a with placebo. MRI studies indicated that 67% of those receiving natalizumab in conjunction with interferon beta-1a had no new or enlarging T2-hyperintense lesions at 2 years compared with 30% of those receiving interferon beta-1a and placebo. In addition, 96% of those receiving the combined regimen had no gadolinium-enhancing lesions at 2 years compared with 75% of those receiving interferon beta-1a and placebo.

Clinical Perspective

Natalizumab is one of several disease-modifying therapies used in the management of relapsing forms of MS. Although not curative, these therapies have all been shown to modify several measures of disease activity, including relapse rates, new or enhancing magnetic resonance imaging (MRI) lesions, and disability progression. The American Academy of Neurology (AAN) recommends that disease-modifying therapy be offered to patients with relapsing forms of MS who have had recent relapses and/or MRI activity; these experts state that the benefits versus risks (e.g., adverse effects or burden of taking a long-term medication) of treatment in patients who have not relapsed in 2 or more years and do not have active MRI lesions are not known. Because CNS damage occurs early and continues throughout the course of MS, other clinicians recommend that disease-modifying therapy be initiated as soon as possible following diagnosis and continued indefinitely unless there is a clear lack of benefit, adverse effects are intolerable, the patient is unable to adhere to the recommended treatment regimen, or a more appropriate treatment becomes available. Clinicians should consider the adverse effects, tolerability, method of administration, safety, efficacy, and cost of the drugs in addition to patient preferences when selecting an appropriate disease-modifying therapy.

Natalizumab has been used concomitantly with other disease-modifying therapies (e.g., glatiramer acetate)† in a limited number of adults with relapsing-remitting MS. .

● *Crohn Disease*

Natalizumab products are used to induce and maintain clinical response and remission in adults with moderately to severely active Crohn disease with evidence of inflammation who have had an inadequate response to or who do not tolerate conventional therapies and inhibitors of tumor necrosis factor (TNF; TNF-α).

Natalizumab should not be used in combination with immunosuppressants (e.g., mercaptopurine, azathioprine, cyclosporine, methotrexate) or TNF-α inhibitors in patients with Crohn disease, because of the potential for increased risk of PML and other infections. Aminosalicylates may be used in patients receiving natalizumab.

Clinical Experience

Safety and efficacy of natalizumab were evaluated in 3 randomized, double-blind, placebo-controlled studies (CD1, CD2, CD3) in adults with moderately to severely active Crohn disease (Crohn Disease Activity Index [CDAI] 220–450 in studies CD1 and CD2). The CDAI score is based on subjective observations by the patient (e.g., the daily number of liquid or very soft stools, severity of abdominal pain, general well-being) and objective evidence (e.g., number of extraintestinal manifestations, presence of an abdominal mass, use or nonuse of antidiarrheal drugs, hematocrit, body weight). Induction of clinical response was evaluated in studies CD1 and CD2 and maintenance of response was evaluated in study CD3. Concomitant use of inhibitors of TNF-α were not permitted. However, concomitant stable doses of aminosalicylates, corticosteroids, and/or immunosuppressants (e.g., mercaptopurine, azathioprine, methotrexate) were permitted and 89% of patients received at least one of these drugs in the studies. Although permitted in the clinical trials, concomitant use of natalizumab with immunosuppressants is not recommended by the manufacturer.

In study CD1, 905 patients were randomized in a 4:1 ratio to receive monthly 300-mg IV infusions of natalizumab or placebo on weeks 0, 4, and 8 and were followed until week 12. At week 10, 56% of patients receiving natalizumab achieved clinical response (defined as a reduction from baseline CDAI of at least 70 points) compared with 49% of those receiving placebo. In a post hoc analysis of a subset of 653 patients with elevated baseline C-reactive protein (CRP), indicative of active inflammation, 57% of patients receiving natalizumab achieved response compared with 45% of those receiving placebo.

In study CD2, 509 patients with elevated CRP were randomized in a 1:1 ratio to receive monthly 300-mg IV infusions of natalizumab or placebo (on weeks 0, 4, and 8). Clinical response (defined as a reduction from baseline CDAI of at least 70 points) and clinical remission (defined as a CDAI score less than 150) were required to be met at both weeks 8 and 12. Clinical response at both weeks 8 and 12 was achieved in 48% of patients receiving natalizumab compared with 32% of those receiving placebo, while clinical remission at both weeks 8 and 12 was achieved in 26% of patients receiving natalizumab compared with 16% of those receiving placebo.

Maintenance therapy was evaluated in study CD3. In this study, 331 patients from study CD1 who had a CDAI score of 0–220 at week 12 and a clinical response to natalizumab at both weeks 10 and 12 (without need for intervention) were re-randomized in a 1:1 ratio to receive 300-mg IV infusions of natalizumab

or placebo every 4 weeks from weeks 12 through 56 and were followed until week 60. Dosages of all concurrent drugs (except corticosteroids) remained constant. Patients receiving concomitant corticosteroids were required to attempt discontinuance according to a fixed tapering regimen.

Maintenance of response was assessed by the proportion of patients who did not lose clinical response at any study visit for an additional 6 and 12 months of treatment (i.e., month 9 [week 36] and 15 [week 60] after initial natalizumab treatment). The study also assessed the proportion of patients, within the subset of those who were in remission at study entry, who did not lose clinical remission at any study visit. Clinical response through months 9 and 15 was achieved in 61 and 54%, respectively, of patients receiving natalizumab compared with 29 and 20%, respectively, of those receiving placebo. Clinical remission through months 9 and 15 was achieved in 45 and 40%, respectively, of patients receiving natalizumab compared with 26 and 15%, respectively, of those receiving placebo.

For subgroups in study CD3 defined either by prior use or inadequate response to prior therapies (i.e., corticosteroids, immunosuppressants, inhibitors of TNF-α), treatment response generally was similar to that seen in the entire study population. In addition, in the subgroup of patients who were not receiving concomitant immunosuppressants or corticosteroids, treatment response was generally similar to that observed in the entire study population. In both the treatment and placebo groups, patients who had an inadequate response to prior therapy with inhibitors of TNF-α appeared to be less likely to maintain clinical response and clinical remission. For patients in study CD3 who had an inadequate response to prior treatment with inhibitors of TNF-α, maintenance of clinical response and clinical remission through month 9 was observed in 52 and 30%, respectively, of those randomized to natalizumab.

Clinical Perspective

The American College of Gastroenterology (ACG) and the American Gastroenterological Association (AGA) have issued guidelines for the medical treatment of Crohn disease. Treatment of Crohn disease is typically divided into 2 phases: induction therapy (where control of inflammation is rapidly achieved) and maintenance therapy (where control of inflammation is sustained for a prolonged period of time). Specific treatments for Crohn disease are selected according to the patient's risk profile and disease severity. Drug classes used to treat Crohn disease include 5-aminosalicylates, antibiotics, corticosteroids, immunomodulators (e.g., thiopurines, immunomodulators), and biologic agents, including tumor necrosis factor (TNF; TNF-α) blocking agents, ustekinumab, vedolizumab, and natalizumab.

The ACG guideline states that for moderate to severe disease/moderate to high risk disease, natalizumab is more effective than placebo and should be considered for induction of symptomatic response and remission in patients with active Crohn disease. Natalizumab should also be used for maintenance of natalizumab-induced remission of Crohn disease only if the antibody to JC virus is negative. Clinicians should repeat testing for anti-JC virus antibody every 6 months and discontinue therapy for a positive result. The guideline also recommends consideration of natalizumab for maintenance of natalizumab-induced remission of Crohn disease in severe/fulminant disease only if the JC virus test is negative.

The AGA guideline suggests against the use of natalizumab over no treatment for the induction and maintenance of remission in adult outpatients with moderate to severe Crohn disease. This suggestion is mainly due to the evidence of harm from PML and the availability of other drugs without this concern. The guideline also states that natalizumab may be considered for patients who are JC virus antibody negative who put a high value on the potential benefits of natalizumab therapy and lower value on PML risk and who will adhere to ongoing monitoring for JC virus positivity.

DOSAGE AND ADMINISTRATION

● *General*

Patient Monitoring

- Monitor patients for signs and symptoms of infection during therapy.

- Assess patients for bleeding abnormalities.

- Monitor for any new signs or symptoms that may be suggestive of progressive multifocal leukoencephalopathy (PML).

- Monitor for the development of immune reconstitution inflammatory syndrome (IRIS).
- Monitor patients during infusion.. Observe patients for 1 hour after the infusion is complete for the first 12 infusions. For patients who have received 12 infusions without evidence of hypersensitivity, the need for subsequent monitoring should be guided by clinical judgment.

REMS

- Because of risk of progressive multifocal leukoencephalopathy (PML), natalizumab products are available only through a restricted distribution program (TOUCH® Prescribing Program for Tysabri® and the TYRUKO REMS program for Tyruko®).
- Clinicians, pharmacies, infusion centers, and patients must enroll in and meet all conditions of the TOUCH® or TYRUKO REMS program before they can prescribe, dispense, infuse, or receive natalizumab.
- Information about the TOUCH® program (MS TOUCH® and CD TOUCH®) is available at 800-456-2255 or http://www.tysabri.com. Information about the TYRUKO REMS program is available at 800-489-7856 or https://tyruko-rems.com.

● Administration

Natalizumab is administered by IV infusion. The drug should *not* be administered by rapid IV injection.

Natalizumab solutions should be inspected visually prior to dilution and administration and should be discarded if there are visible particles and/or discoloration. Use of filtration devices during IV infusion of natalizumab has not been evaluated.

Natalizumab should not be infused or admixed with any other drug.

Following completion of the infusion, the infusion set should be flushed with 0.9% sodium chloride injection.

Store single-dose vials at 2-8°C and protect from light.

Dilution

Commercially available natalizumab concentrate products containing 300 mg/15 mL must be diluted in 0.9% sodium chloride injection prior to IV infusion; no other IV diluents should be used to prepare IV infusions of the drug.

Solutions for IV infusion are prepared by withdrawing 15 mL of the concentrate from a single-use vial containing 300 mg/15 mL and adding the concentrate to 100 mL of 0.9% sodium chloride injection (final concentration: 2.6 mg/mL). The diluted solution should be inverted gently to mix and should not be shaken. Because the drug contains no preservative, strict aseptic technique must be observed when preparing these solutions.

Diluted natalizumab solutions should be infused immediately or may be refrigerated at 2–8°C and used within 48 hours for Tysabri® and 4 hours for Tyruko®; these solutions should *not* be frozen. If refrigerated, solutions should be allowed to warm to room temperature prior to administration.

Rate of Administration

IV infusions of natalizumab should be given over approximately 1 hour (infusion rate approximately 5 mg/minute).

● Dosage

Multiple Sclerosis

The recommended dosage of natalizumab products for the treatment of relapsing forms of multiple sclerosis (MS) in adults is 300 mg once every 4 weeks by IV infusion.

Crohn Disease

The recommended adult dosage of natalizumab products for the treatment of moderately to severely active Crohn disease with evidence of inflammation is 300 mg once every 4 weeks by IV infusion.

Natalizumab should *not* be used in combination with immunosuppressants (e.g., azathioprine, cyclosporine, mercaptopurine, methotrexate), or tumor necrosis factor (TNF) inhibitors; however, aminosalicylates may be continued during treatment. Patients with Crohn disease who initiate natalizumab while receiving chronic oral corticosteroid therapy should start tapering corticosteroid dosage as soon as a therapeutic benefit of natalizumab occurs. Natalizumab should be discontinued if the patient cannot be tapered off oral corticosteroids within 6 months of initiating natalizumab. Consideration should be given to discontinuance of natalizumab in patients who require additional corticosteroid use that exceeds 3 months in a calendar year to control Crohn disease (other than the 6-month corticosteroid taper). Natalizumab should be discontinued if the patient with Crohn disease has not experienced therapeutic benefit by 12 weeks of induction therapy.

● Special Populations

Hepatic Impairment

No dosage adjustments recommended in patients with hepatic impairment.

Renal Impairment

No dosage adjustments recommended in patients with renal impairment.

Geriatric Patients

No dosage adjustments recommended in geriatric patients.

CAUTIONS

● Contraindications

- Known hypersensitivity to natalizumab products.
- Current or previous history of progressive multifocal leukoencephalopathy (PML).

● Warnings/Precautions

Warnings

Progressive Multifocal Leukoencephalopathy

Progressive multifocal leukoencephalopathy (PML), an opportunistic infection of the brain caused by the JC virus, has been reported in patients receiving natalizumab. PML typically occurs in immunocompromised patients (e.g., patients with HIV infection), and usually leads to death or severe disability. The prescribing information for natalizumab products contains a boxed warning regarding the risk of PML.

As of January 2012, 201 cases of PML had been reported among 96,582 patients treated with natalizumab worldwide. During initial clinical trials in patients with relapsing-remitting multiple sclerosis (MS), 2 cases of PML (1 fatal) occurred among 1869 study patients who received natalizumab for a median of 120 weeks. An additional fatal case of PML occurred in an initial study evaluating natalizumab in 1043 patients with Crohn disease. One of the MS patients had a possible PML lesion identified on MRI after 28 doses of natalizumab therapy; this patient survived but developed substantial deficits (disabling ataxia, cognitive impairment, mild neglect, mild left hemiparesis). The second MS patient was receiving natalizumab in conjunction with interferon beta-1a and had received 37 doses of natalizumab before the drug was discontinued; the neurologic status of this patient declined and the patient died. The patient with Crohn disease had received 8 doses of natalizumab and had previously received immunosuppressive therapy; this patient deteriorated rapidly and died. In the postmarketing setting, additional cases of PML have been identified in MS and Crohn disease patients who were not receiving concomitant immunomodulatory therapy. JC virus granule cell neuronopathy with or without concomitant PML also has been reported.

The 3 factors known to increase the risk of PML in natalizumab-treated patients are longer treatment duration (especially beyond 2 years), prior treatment with immunosuppressants (e.g., mitoxantrone, azathioprine, methotrexate, cyclophosphamide, mycophenolate mofetil), and presence of anti-JC virus antibodies. The risks and benefits of initiating or continuing natalizumab therapy in patients with these risk factors should be considered. Based on postmarketing data from approximately 100,000 patients exposed to natalizumab, the estimated incidence of PML in patients positive for anti-JC virus antibody who have received 1–24, 25–48, 49–72, or 73-96 months of natalizumab treatment is less than 1, 2, 4, or 2 cases per 1000 patients, respectively, in those with no history of immunosuppressant treatment, and 1, 6, 7, or 6 cases per 1000 patients, respectively, in those who previously received immunosuppressant therapy. The estimated incidence of PML in patients negative for anti-JC virus antibody is 1 case per 10,000 patients.

Because presence of anti-JC virus antibodies has been identified as a risk factor for PML, consideration should be given to testing patients for anti-JC virus antibody status prior to initiating natalizumab or during natalizumab treatment if the antibody status of the patient is unknown. A positive anti-JC virus antibody test indicates that the individual has been exposed to JC virus in the past. For the purposes of risk assessment, a patient with a positive anti-JC virus antibody test at any time should be considered to be anti-JC virus antibody positive, regardless of results of any prior or subsequent anti-JC virus antibody test. Patients with negative anti-JC virus antibody tests should be retested periodically. Although a negative anti-JC virus antibody test indicates that exposure to JC virus has not been detected, such patients are still at risk for PML because of the potential for subsequent JC virus infection or possibility of a false-negative test result for anti-JC virus antibody.

When anti-JC virus antibody testing is performed, an analytically and clinically validated immunoassay should be used. An anti-JC virus antibody test (Stratify JCV antibody ELISA test) received FDA approval in January 2012. In patients undergoing plasma exchange, anti-JC virus antibody testing should not be performed during or for at least 2 weeks after the procedure since serum antibodies may have been removed during the procedure, which may cause false-negative results. In patients receiving IV immunoglobulin, at least 6 months should elapse before anti-JC virus antibody testing is performed to allow the immunoglobulin to clear and avoid false-positive results.

Natalizumab ordinarily should *not* be used in patients receiving chronic immunosuppressant or immunomodulatory therapy or in those with systemic medical conditions that result in a clinically important compromised immune system. Although the risk of PML is increased in patients who received immunosuppressant therapy (e.g., azathioprine, cyclophosphamide, methotrexate, mitoxantrone, mycophenolate) prior to receiving natalizumab, the effect of prior immunomodulatory therapy (e.g., glatiramer acetate, interferon beta) or prior treatment with short courses of corticosteroids (e.g., to treat MS flares) on the risk of PML is unknown.

There are no known interventions that can reliably prevent PML or adequately treat PML if it occurs. Although plasma exchange has not been studied in natalizumab-treated patients with PML, it has been frequently used in the postmarketing setting to enhance natalizumab clearance in patients who develop PML. Results from a study of 12 patients with MS who did not have PML indicate that 3 sessions of plasma exchange over 5–8 days accelerated natalizumab clearance, although α4 integrin receptor binding remained high in the majority of patients.

Prior to initiating natalizumab in MS patients, a baseline MRI scan should be performed since this may be helpful in differentiating subsequent MS symptoms from PML. In patients with Crohn disease, a baseline brain MRI scan may be useful to distinguish preexisting lesions from newly developed lesions, although baseline brain lesions that could cause diagnostic difficulty in patients with Crohn disease who are receiving natalizumab are uncommon.

During natalizumab therapy, patients should be monitored for any new signs or symptoms suggestive of PML. Symptoms associated with PML are diverse, progress over days to weeks, and include progressive weakness on one side of the body or clumsiness of limbs, disturbance of vision, and changes in thinking, memory, and orientation leading to confusion and personality changes; seizures and headache also have been reported rarely. The progression of deficits usually leads to death or severe disability over weeks or months. Natalizumab should be withheld immediately at the first sign or symptom of PML and an appropriate diagnostic evaluation should be performed. The anti-JC virus antibody test should *not* be used to diagnose PML. An evaluation that includes a gadolinium-enhanced MRI brain scan and, when indicated, CSF analysis for JC viral DNA is recommended to diagnose PML. MRI signs of PML may be apparent before clinical manifestations develop; any suspicious findings on MRI should be followed by further evaluation. If clinical suspicion remains despite an initial negative evaluation for PML, natalizumab treatment should not be reinitiated until the evaluation has been repeated and confirmed.

Because of the risk of PML, natalizumab products are available only through a restricted distribution program (Tysabri®: TOUCH® Prescribing Program and Tyruko®: TYRUKO REMS). Any case of PML, serious opportunistic infection, atypical infection, or death should be reported promptly to Biogen for Tysabri® at 800-456-2255 or Sandoz for Tyruko® at 800-525-8747 and to the FDA MedWatch program at 800-332-1088.

Immune reconstitution inflammatory syndrome (IRIS) has been reported in the majority of natalizumab-treated patients who developed PML and subsequently discontinued the drug. IRIS has not been reported to date when natalizumab was discontinued for reasons unrelated to PML.

IRIS is a severe inflammatory response that occurs during or after immune system recovery and presents as a clinical decline (sometimes after apparent clinical improvement) that may progress rapidly and can lead to serious neurologic complications or death. IRIS often is associated with characteristic MRI changes. In MS patients with PML who developed IRIS after discontinuing natalizumab, the inflammatory syndrome occurred within days to several weeks after the patient received plasma exchange or immunoadsorption to enhance natalizumab removal.

Patients should be monitored for the development of IRIS; if IRIS does occur, the associated inflammation should be appropriately treated.

Other Warnings and Precautions

Herpes Infections

Natalizumab increases the risk of developing encephalitis and meningitis caused by herpes simplex and varicella zoster viruses. In the postmarketing setting, serious, life-threatening, and sometimes fatal cases have been reported in patients with MS administered natalizuamb. The duration of natalizumab therapy prior to infection onset ranged from a few months to several years. Patients should be monitored for signs and symptoms of meningitis and encephalitis. If herpes encephalitis or meningitis occurs, natalizumab should be discontinued and appropriate treatment inititated.

Acute retinal necrosis (ARN) is a fulminant viral infection of the retina caused by the family of herpes viruses (e.g., varicella zoster, herpes simplex virus). An increased risk of ARN has occurred in patients administered natalizumab. Patients presenting with eye symptoms, including decreased visual acuity, redness, or eye pain, should be referred for retinal screening for ARN. Some ARN cases occurred in patients with CNS herpes infections (e.g., herpes meningitis or encephalitis). Serious cases have led to blindness in one or both eyes in certain patients. Following ARN diagnosis, discontinuation of natalizumab should be considered.

Hepatotoxicity

During postmarketing experience, clinically important liver dysfunction (e.g., elevated hepatic enzymes, elevated total bilirubin) has been reported as early as 6 days after administration of the first dose of natalizumab and also after multiple doses. In some patients, liver dysfunction recurred upon rechallenge indicating that natalizumab caused the injury. The combination of elevated aminotransferase concentrations and elevated bilirubin (without evidence of obstruction) generally is recognized as an important predictor of severe liver injury.

Natalizumab should be discontinued in patients with jaundice or other evidence of substantial liver injury (e.g., laboratory evidence).

Hypersensitivity/Antibody Formation

Serious hypersensitivity reactions (e.g., anaphylaxis/anaphylactoid reaction) have been reported in less than 1% of patients receiving natalizumab. These reactions usually have occurred within 2 hours after initiation of natalizumab IV infusions and generally were associated with antibodies to the drug.

If hypersensitivity reactions (e.g., anaphylaxis, urticaria, dizziness, fever, rash, rigors, pruritus, nausea, flushing, hypotension, dyspnea, chest pain) occur, the drug should be discontinued immediately and appropriate therapy be initiated.

Natalizumab should not be reinitiated in any patient who experienced a hypersensitivity reaction while receiving the drug. In addition, the possibility of antibodies against natalizumab should be considered in patients who have hypersensitivity reactions.

Patients receiving natalizumab may develop antibodies to the drug. There is in vitro evidence that antibodies against natalizumab can be neutralizing and persistent antibody-positivity may be associated with decreased efficacy and increased risk of infusion-related reactions.

In a clinical study in patients with MS, patients were tested for antibodies against natalizumab every 12 weeks using assays that were unable to detect low to moderate levels (lower limit of detection 0.5 mcg/mL). Data indicate that approximately 9% of those receiving natalizumab developed detectable antibodies at least once during treatment, and approximately 6% had positive antibodies on more than one occasion. Approximately 82% of those who became persistently antibody-positive had developed detectable antibodies by week 12.

The presence of antibodies against natalizumab has been associated with decreased serum concentrations of natalizumab. In a clinical study in MS patients receiving natalizumab, mean serum concentrations of the drug immediately prior to dosing at week 12 were 15 mcg/mL in antibody-negative patients and 1.3 mcg/mL in antibody-positive patients. In addition, persistent antibody-positivity has been associated with substantial decreases in natalizumab efficacy. In studies in MS patients, the risk of increased disability and the annualized relapse rate in those receiving natalizumab who were persistently positive for antibodies against natalizumab were similar to results reported in placebo-treated patients.

In clinical studies evaluating use of natalizumab for Crohn disease, patients were first tested for antibodies against natalizumab at 12 weeks (this was the only test in most patients given the 12-week duration of the placebo-controlled studies). Approximately 10% of those receiving natalizumab developed antibodies at least once during treatment, and 5% had positive antibodies on more than one occasion. Development of persistent antibodies resulted in reduced efficacy and increased infusion-related reactions with symptoms including urticaria, pruritus, nausea, flushing, and dyspnea.

Patients with persistent antibodies against natalizumab are more likely to have an infusion-related reaction compared with those negative for such antibodies. Other adverse events reported more frequently in persistently antibody-positive patients include myalgia, hypertension, dyspnea, anxiety, and tachycardia.

The long-term immunogenicity of natalizumab remains to be determined and the effects of low to moderate levels of antibodies against natalizumab are unknown. Patients who receive natalizumab for a short period (1–2 infusions) followed by an extended period without such treatment may be at higher risk of developing anti-natalizumab antibodies and/or hypersensitivity reactions upon re-exposure than patients who receive regularly scheduled treatment. Testing for presence of antibodies to natalizumab should be considered in patients who wish to resume treatment following an interruption in therapy. Patients who have tested negative for antibodies against natalizumab prior to retreatment have a risk of antibody development with retreatment that is similar to natalizumab-naïve patients.

Antibody testing should be performed if presence of persistent antibodies against natalizumab is suspected. Antibodies may be detected and confirmed with sequential serum antibody tests. Antibodies detected early in the treatment course (e.g., within the first 6 months) may be transient and disappear with continued use of the drug. Therefore, testing should be repeated at 3 months after the initial positive result to confirm that antibodies are persistent. Clinicians should consider the overall benefits and risks of natalizumab in patients who have persistent antibodies.

Immunosuppression and Infections

Natalizumab has immune system effects and may increase the risk of infections, including opportunistic infections.

PML, an opportunistic viral infection of the brain that usually is fatal or associated with severe disability, has been reported in patients receiving natalizumab.

In clinical studies in MS patients, pneumonia, urinary tract infections (sometimes severe), influenza, gastroenteritis, vaginal infections, tooth infections, tonsillitis or pharyngitis, and herpes infections occurred more frequently in patients receiving natalizumab than in those receiving placebo. Most of these infections were considered mild to moderate, and patients generally did not need to interrupt natalizumab therapy. At least 1 case of cryptosporidial gastroenteritis with a prolonged course has been reported in an MS patient receiving natalizumab. The overall incidence of serious infections in the MS1 clinical study was approximately 3% in both natalizumab-treated and placebo-treated patients. In the MS1 and MS2 studies, an increased incidence of infections was observed in patients receiving concurrent therapy with short courses of corticosteroids; however, the incidence was similar to that observed in patients receiving corticosteroids alone.

In clinical studies in patients with Crohn disease, opportunistic infections (e.g., *Pneumocystis jiroveci* [formerly *P. carinii*] pneumonia, *Mycobacterium avium* complex, bronchopulmonary aspergillosis, *Burkholderia cepacia*) were observed in less than 1% of patients receiving natalizumab. In the CD1 and CD2

studies, an increased incidence of infection was observed in patients receiving concurrent therapy with corticosteroids. However, the increase in infections in patients receiving natalizumab concomitantly with corticosteroids was similar to the increase in infections in patients receiving placebo concomitantly with corticosteroids.

Concomitant use of natalizumab and antineoplastic agents, immunosuppressive agents, or immunomodulating agents may further increase the risk of infections, including PML and other opportunistic infections, compared with use of natalizumab alone. Safety and efficacy of natalizumab in combination with antineoplastic agents, immunosuppressive agents, or immunomodulating agents have not been established.

Laboratory Test Abnormalities

Natalizumab induced increases in circulating lymphocytes, monocytes, eosinophils, basophils, and nucleated red blood cells in clinical trials. Observed changes persisted during exposure, but were reversible, returning to baseline levels usually within 16 weeks after the last dose of natalizumab. Natalizumab also induced mild decreases in hemoglobin levels (mean decrease: 0.6 g/dL) that were frequently transient.

Thrombocytopenia

In the postmarketing setting, thrombocytopenia, including immune thrombocytopenic purpura (ITP), has been reported with natalizumab therapy. Symptoms of thrombocytopenia may include easy bruising, abnormal bleeding, and petechiae. If thrombocytopenia is suspected, natalizumab should be discontinued.

Cases of neonatal thrombocytopenia, sometimes associated with anemia, have been reported in newborns with in utero natalizumab exposure. A complete blood cell (CBC) count should be obtained in neonates with in utero exposure.

Immunizations

No data are available on vaccination effects in patients administered natalizumab. No data are available on the secondary transmission of infection by live vaccines in patients administered natalizumab as well.

Specific Populations

Pregnancy

There are no adequate data on the risk of major birth defects, miscarriage, or other adverse maternal outcomes associated with the use of natalizumab during pregnancy; adverse fetal outcomes of neonatal thrombocytopenia, at times associated with anemia, have been reported. A CBC should be obtained in neonates exposed to natalizumab in utero.

Lactation

Natalizumab is distributed into human milk; however, the effects of the drug on nursing infants or on milk production are not known.

The benefits of breastfeeding should be considered along with the woman's clinical need for natalizumab and any potential adverse effects on the breastfed infant from the drug or underlying maternal condition.

Pediatric Use

Safety and efficacy of natalizumab have not been established in MS or Crohn disease patients younger than 18 years of age. Natalizumab is not indicated for use in pediatric patients.

Geriatric Use

Experience with natalizumab in patients 65 years of age or older is insufficient to determine whether they respond differently than younger adults.

Hepatic Impairment

Clinically important liver dysfunction has been reported in patients receiving natalizumab.

Renal Impairment

Natalizumab has not been studied in patients with renal impairment.

● Common Adverse Effects

Adverse effects occurring in 10% or more of patients with MS receiving natalizumab include headache, fatigue, arthralgia, depression, urinary tract infection, lower respiratory tract infection, gastroenteritis, vaginitis, depression, extremity pain, abdominal discomfort, diarrhea, and rash. Adverse effects occurring in 10% or more of patients with Crohn disease receiving the drug include headache, fatigue, upper respiratory tract infections, and nausea.

Approximately 24% of patients with MS receiving natalizumab in clinical studies experienced infusion-related reactions (e.g., headache, dizziness, fatigue, urticaria, pruritus, rigors) within 2 hours after initiation of a natalizumab infusion. Approximately 11% of patients with Crohn disease receiving natalizumab in clinical studies experienced infusion-related reactions (e.g., headache, nausea, urticaria, pruritus, flushing) within 2 hours after initiation of a natalizumab infusion. Patients who had persistent antibodies to natalizumab were more likely to experience an infusion-related reaction than those who were antibody negative.

DRUG INTERACTIONS

● Immunosuppressive Agents

Because of the potential for increased risk of progressive multifocal leukoencephalopathy (PML) and other infections, patients with Crohn disease receiving natalizumab should not be treated concomitantly with immunosuppressants (e.g., mercaptopurine, azathioprine, cyclosporine, methotrexate) or inhibitors of tumor necrosis factor (TNF; TNF-α). Multiple sclerosis (MS) patients receiving chronic immunosuppressant therapy generally should not be treated with natalizumab.

Concomitant use of natalizumab and short courses of corticosteroids was associated with an increased incidence of infection in clinical studies; however, the infection rate reported in those receiving concomitant therapy was similar to that reported in placebo-treated patients receiving corticosteroids. Patients with Crohn disease who initiate natalizumab while receiving chronic oral corticosteroid therapy should start tapering corticosteroid dosage as soon as a therapeutic benefit of natalizumab occurs.

● Interferon Beta

Potential pharmacokinetic interaction (increased serum concentrations and half-life of natalizumab); may not be clinically important. No apparent effect on pharmacokinetics of interferon beta-1a. MS patients receiving chronic immunomodulatory therapy generally should not be treated with natalizumab.

● Vaccines

Data are not available to date on the effects of vaccination in patients receiving natalizumab, including data on secondary transmission of infection from live viral vaccines in those receiving the drug.

DESCRIPTION

Natalizumab is a recombinant humanized anti-α4-integrin monoclonal antibody produced in murine myeloma cells. The drug is an IgG4κ immunoglobulin containing human framework regions and murine complementarity-determining regions. The antibody portion of natalizumab binds specifically to α4-subunits of α4β1 and α4β7 integrins expressed on the surface of all leukocytes (except neutrophils) and inhibits the α4-mediated adhesion of leukocytes to their counterreceptors, including vascular cell adhesion molecule-1 (VCAM-1). In vitro, anti-α4-integrin antibodies also block α4-mediated cell binding to ligands such as osteopontin and CS-1 of fibronectin.

Although the precise mechanism(s) of action of natalizumab has not been fully elucidated, the clinical effect of natalizumab in multiple sclerosis (MS) is thought to be secondary to blockade of α4β1 integrin-mediated leukocyte migration from peripheral blood into the CNS. Inflammatory proteins and other factors released from lymphocytes in the brain during exacerbations of MS are believed to cause lesions that result in progressive disability. Data from an experimental autoimmune encephalitis animal model of MS demonstrate reduction of leukocyte migration into brain parenchyma and reduction of plaque formation detected by magnetic resonance imaging (MRI) following repeated administration of

natalizumab. The clinical relevance of these findings to humans is unknown. However, there is evidence that CSF attained from natalizumab-treated MS patients has decreased levels of all major lymphocyte subsets.

In Crohn disease, the interaction of α4β7 integrin with the endothelial receptor mucosal addressin cell adhesion molecule-1 (MAdCAM-1) has been implicated as an important contributor to the chronic inflammation of the disease. MAdCAM-1 expression has been found to be increased at active sites of inflammation in patients with Crohn's disease, which suggests it may play a role in the recruitment of leukocytes to the mucosa and contribute to the inflammatory response characteristic of Crohn disease. Although the exact mechanism(s) of action of natalizumab has not been fully elucidated, the clinical effect of natalizumab in Crohn disease is thought to be secondary to blockade of the interaction of α4β7 integrin receptor with MAdCAM-1 expressed on the venular endothelium at inflammatory foci. VCAM-1 expression has been found to be upregulated on colonic endothelial cells in a mouse model of inflammatory bowel disease and appears to play a role in leukocyte recruitment to sites of inflammation; however, the role of VCAM-1 in Crohn disease is not clear.

The mean half-life of natalizumab in patients with MS or Crohn disease is approximately 11 days. Clearance of natalizumab increases with body weight in a less than proportional manner. The presence of persistent anti-natalizumab antibodies appears to increase drug clearance approximately 3-fold.

ADVICE TO PATIENTS

- Advise patients to read the FDA-approved patient labeling (medication guide) prior to initiating natalizumab therapy and before each dose of the drug.

- Inform patients that progressive multifocal leukoencephalopathy (PML) has occurred in patients treated with natalizumab and that PML usually leads to death or severe disability over weeks or months.

- Stress importance of promptly informing clinicians of any new or worsening symptoms suggestive of PML (e.g., progressive weakness on one side of the body; clumsiness of limbs; disturbance of vision; changes in thinking, memory, and orientation leading to confusion; personality changes) that have progressed over days to weeks.

- Advise patients that natalizumab is only available through restricted distribution programs under a REMS.

- Advise patients to immediately report any symptoms consistent with a hypersensitivity reaction (e.g., urticaria with or without associated symptoms such as itching or trouble breathing) during or following an infusion of natalizumab.

- Inform patients that natalizumab may lower the ability of their immune system to fight infections and to report any symptoms of infection to their clinican.

- Inform patients that natalizumab increases the risk of developing encephalitis and meningitis, which could be fatal, and acute retinal necrosis, which could lead to blindness, caused by the family of herpes viruses (e.g., herpes simplex and varicella zoster viruses). Instruct patients to immediately report any possible symptoms of encephalitis and meningitis (such as fever, headache, and confusion) or acute retinal necrosis (such as decreased visual acuity, eye redness, or eye pain).

- Inform patients that natalizumab may result in a reduced platelet count, which can cause severe bleeding. Instruct patients to report any related symptoms (e.g., easy bruising, prolonged bleeding, petechiae, abnormally heavy menstrual periods, new bleeding from the nose or gums) to their clinician.

- Inform patients of the risk of liver injury with natalizumab and to contact their clinician if symptoms of hepatotoxicity develop.

- Advise patients to inform their clinicians of existing or contemplated concomitant therapy, including prescription and OTC drugs, and any concomitant illnesses.

- Advise patients to inform their clinicians if they are or plan to become pregnant or plan to breast-feed.

- Inform patients of other important precautionary information.

PREPARATIONS

Natalizumab is available only through a restricted distribution program (TOUCH® Prescribing Program for Tysabri® and TYRUKO REMS for Tyruko®).

Excipients in commercially available drug preparations may have clinically important effects in some individuals; consult specific product labeling for details.

Natalizumab

Parenteral

For injection, concentrate, for IV infusion only	300 mg/15 mL	**Tysabri®**, Biogen

Natalizumab-sztn

Parenteral

For injection, concentrate, for IV infusion only	300 mg/15 mL	**Tyruko®**, Sandoz

† Use is not currently included in the labeling approved by the US Food and Drug Administration.

Selected Revisions September 10, 2024, © Copyright, February 1, 2005, American Society of Health-System Pharmacists, Inc.

Ocrelizumab

90:04.04 · MONOCLONAL ANTIBODIES

■ Ocrelizumab, a recombinant humanized anti-CD20 monoclonal antibody, has immunomodulatory and disease-modifying activity in multiple sclerosis (MS).

USES

● Multiple Sclerosis

Relapsing-remitting Multiple Sclerosis

Ocrelizumab is used in the management of relapsing forms of multiple sclerosis (MS), including clinically isolated syndrome, relapsing-remitting disease, and active secondary progressive disease, in adults.

Clinical Experience

Efficacy and safety of ocrelizumab for the management of relapsing forms of MS were established in 2 identical randomized, double-blind, active-controlled studies (OPERA I and II) that compared ocrelizumab with a standard drug used in the management of MS (interferon beta-1a [Rebif®]). In these studies, ocrelizumab was more effective than interferon beta-1a in reducing relapse rates and progression of disability.

Both studies included adults with relapsing forms of MS who had experienced at least 2 clinical relapses during the previous 2 years or at least 1 clinical relapse during the prior year and had an Expanded Disability Status Scale (EDSS) score of 0–5.5 at baseline. Ocrelizumab was administered by IV infusion at a dosage of 600 mg every 24 weeks (after 2 initial doses of 300 mg were given 14 days apart) and interferon beta-1a was administered subcutaneously at a dosage of 44 mcg 3 times weekly. Neurologic examinations were performed every 12 weeks and at the time of suspected relapse, and MRI scans were performed at baseline and at weeks 24, 48, and 96. The primary efficacy end point in both studies was the annualized relapse rate at 96 weeks. Relapse was defined as new or worsening neurologic symptoms not associated with fever or infection that persisted for at least 24 hours after at least 30 days of clinical stability or improvement, and was confirmed by objective changes on neurologic examination. Secondary outcome measures included MRI findings and the proportion of patients with confirmed disability progression (defined as an increase from baseline of at least 1 EDSS point [or at least 0.5 points for patients with baseline EDSS score greater than 5.5] that was sustained for at least 12 weeks). Baseline characteristics were similar across both studies (mean age was 37 years, 66% were female, mean number of relapses in the previous year was 1.3, mean EDSS score was 2.8, and mean duration of disease was 3.8–4.1 years).

In both studies, ocrelizumab substantially reduced the annualized relapse rate and the proportion of patients with disability progression compared with interferon beta-1a therapy. The annualized relapse rate was 0.16 with ocrelizumab versus 0.29 with interferon beta-1a in both studies, corresponding to a relative risk reduction of 46–47%. The proportion of patients with confirmed disability progression based on pooled data from the 2 studies was 9.8% in the ocrelizumab group compared with 15.2% in the interferon beta-1a group (relative risk reduction of 40%). In addition to these clinical findings, ocrelizumab had a substantial effect on MRI measures of disease activity; patients who received ocrelizumab had substantially fewer T1 gadolinium-enhancing lesions (relative reduction of 94–95%) and new and/or enlarged T2-weighted hyperintense lesions (relative reduction of 77–83%) compared with those who received interferon beta-1a.

In an open-label extension of the OPERA I and II studies, patients were continued on ocrelizumab or switched from interferon beta-1a to ocrelizumab, and treatment was continued for up to 5 years. The cumulative proportion of patients with 24-week confirmed disability progression was lower for patients who continued on ocrelizumab compared to those who switched from interferon beta-1a. New brain MRI lesion activity from years 3–5 was nearly completely suppressed in both groups. Patients continuing on ocrelizumab exhibited less whole brain volume loss at 5 years when assessed from baseline values compared to those who switched from interferon beta-1a.

Clinical Perspective

Ocrelizumab is one of several disease-modifying therapies used in the management of relapsing forms of MS. Although not curative, these therapies have all been shown to modify several measures of disease activity, including relapse rates, new or enhancing magnetic resonance imaging (MRI) lesions, and disability progression. The American Academy of Neurology (AAN) recommends that disease-modifying therapy be offered to patients with relapsing forms of MS who have had recent relapses and/or MRI activity; these experts state that the benefits versus risks (e.g., adverse effects or burden of taking a long-term medication) of treatment in patients who have not had relapses in 2 or more years and do not have active MRI lesions are not known. Because CNS damage occurs early and continues throughout the course of MS, other clinicians recommend that disease-modifying therapy be initiated as soon as possible following diagnosis and continued indefinitely unless there is a clear lack of benefit, adverse effects are intolerable, the patient is unable to adhere to the recommended treatment regimen, or a more appropriate treatment becomes available. Clinicians should consider the adverse effects, tolerability, method of administration, safety, efficacy, and cost of the drugs in addition to patient preferences when selecting an appropriate disease-modifying therapy.

Primary Progressive Multiple Sclerosis

Ocrelizumab is used in the management of primary progressive MS (PPMS) in adults.

Clinical Experience

Efficacy and safety of ocrelizumab for the management of PPMS were established in a randomized, double-blind, placebo-controlled study (ORATORIO) in 732 adults with PPMS who had a baseline EDSS score of 3–6.5 and a score of 2 or greater on the EDSS pyramidal functional scale due to lower extremity findings. Patients were randomized in a 2:1 ratio to receive ocrelizumab 600 mg (administered as two 300-mg IV infusions 14 days apart) or placebo every 24 weeks for at least 5 doses (i.e., 120 weeks) and until a prespecified number of confirmed disability progression events occurred. Neurologic examinations were performed every 12 weeks and MRI scans were performed at baseline and at weeks 24, 48, and 120. The primary efficacy end point was the time to onset of confirmed disability progression (defined as an increase from baseline of at least 1 EDSS point [or at least 0.5 points for patients with baseline EDSS score greater than 5.5] that was sustained for at least 12 weeks, or patient withdrawal from the study due to onset of disability progression). The mean age of patients in this study was 45 years, 49% were female, the mean duration of symptoms was 6.7 years, and the mean EDSS score at baseline was 4.7.

Ocrelizumab substantially delayed the time to onset of disability progression compared with placebo. At the end of the study, the proportion of patients with confirmed disability progression was 32.9% in the ocrelizumab group and 39.3% in the placebo group (relative risk reduction of 24%). Patients who received ocrelizumab also demonstrated substantial improvement in the timed 25-foot walk, a major secondary end point. In addition, a substantial reduction in T2 hyperintense lesion volume was observed with ocrelizumab compared with placebo at 120 weeks; mean T2 lesion volume decreased by 0.39 cm³ from baseline in patients who received ocrelizumab, but increased by 0.79 cm³ in those who received placebo. Results of an exploratory subgroup analysis suggested an apparent lack of treatment effect on the disability progression outcome in women compared with men. However, a gender imbalance was not observed with other clinical and MRI outcome measures (e.g., annualized relapse rate, T2 lesion volume, number of new or enlarging T2 lesions).

In an open-label extension of the ORATORIO study, patients initially assigned to ocrelizumab continued to receive the drug and those receiving placebo were switched to ocrelizumab. Patients who continued ocrelizumab experienced substantial improvement over those who switched to ocrelizumab in several disability progression measures over the 6.5 years of study follow up. MRI outcomes including T2 lesion volume and T1 hypointense lesion volume were also significantly reduced in the continuous ocrelizumab group after 6.5 years of treatment. After 8 years of follow-up, the proportion of patients with 48-week confirmed disability progression (defined as a >20% increase from baseline) was significantly lower in patients who continued ocrelizumab versus those who switched to ocrelizumab at the start of the open-label extension.

Clinical Perspective

PPMS affects approximately 10–15% of patients diagnosed with MS and is characterized by progressive worsening of neurologic function from disease onset. In contrast to relapsing forms of MS, patients with PPMS generally do not experience distinct relapses or remissions, although relapses may occur. Ocrelizumab is currently the only disease-modifying therapy that has been shown to alter disease progression in patients with PPMS; other immunomodulatory agents used for the treatment of relapsing forms of MS generally have not been effective for patients with PPMS, and other drugs that have been used in PPMS (e.g., IV glucocorticoids, methotrexate, cladribine, immune globulin IV, rituximab, mitoxantrone) have only demonstrated limited efficacy in clinical studies. Because of the demonstrated benefits of ocrelizumab, experts recommend that the drug be offered to PPMS patients unless the risks outweigh the benefits.

DOSAGE AND ADMINISTRATION

• *General*

Pretreatment Screening

- Prior to initiating ocrelizumab therapy, screen patients for hepatitis B virus (HBV) infection.

- Perform testing for quantitative serum immunoglobulins. In patients with low serum immunoglobulins, consult an immunology expert before initiating treatment.

- Prior to each infusion, evaluate patients for active infections; delay ocrelizumab therapy in patients with active infection until the infection resolves.

- Patients should complete any necessary immunizations at least 4 weeks prior to initiation of ocrelizumab for live or live attenuated vaccines, and whenever possible, at least 2 weeks prior to initiation of ocrelizumab for inactivated vaccines.

Patient Monitoring

- Monitor patients for infusion-related reactions during and for at least 1 hour after each infusion.

Premedication and Prophylaxis

- To reduce the incidence and/or severity of infusion-related reactions, patients should be premedicated with IV methylprednisolone 100 mg (or an equivalent corticosteroid) 30 minutes prior to each ocrelizumab infusion and an antihistamine (e.g., diphenhydramine) approximately 30–60 minutes prior to each ocrelizumab infusion. In addition, premedication with an antipyretic (e.g., acetaminophen) may be considered.

Dispensing and Administration Precautions

- Ocrelizumab should be administered under close supervision of an experienced clinician and only in settings where appropriate medical support is available for management of serious infusion-related reactions.

- Initial and subsequent doses of ocrelizumab require different rates of administration and durations of infusion; pay special attention to differences in dose titration.

• *Administration*

Ocrelizumab is administered by IV infusion. The first 2 doses of the drug (300 mg) are each administered over approximately 2.5 hours, and subsequent doses (600 mg) are administered over either approximately 2 hours (if no previous reaction with any ocrelizumab infusion), or approximately 3.5 hours. Patients receiving 2-hour infusions of ocrelizumab had similar incidences, intensity, and types of symptoms as patients receiving 3.5-hour infusions in clinical studies. The total duration of infusion may be increased if infusion reactions occur.

Commercially available ocrelizumab injection concentrate should be stored at 2–8°C in the original carton to protect the drug from light; the vials should not be frozen or shaken.

The injection concentrate and diluted solutions of the drug should be inspected visually for particulate matter and discoloration prior to administration. The injection concentrate should be clear or slightly opalescent, and colorless to pale brown; the drug should be discarded if visible particles or discoloration is present. Each vial is intended for single use only; any unused portions should be discarded because the drug contains no preservatives.

Dilution

Prior to administration, ocrelizumab injection concentrate containing 300 mg/10 mL must be diluted in 0.9% sodium chloride injection using proper aseptic technique. No other diluents should be used.

To prepare the solution for IV infusion, the appropriate dose of ocrelizumab should be withdrawn from 1 or 2 vials of the injection concentrate and diluted in 0.9% sodium chloride injection to yield a final concentration of approximately 1.2 mg/mL. To prepare a 300-mg dose, 10 mL of ocrelizumab injection concentrate should be withdrawn and added to an infusion bag containing 250 mL of 0.9% sodium chloride injection; to prepare a 600-mg dose, 20 mL of ocrelizumab injection concentrate should be withdrawn and added to an infusion bag containing 500 mL of 0.9% sodium chloride injection.

Following dilution, ocrelizumab infusion solution should be administered immediately; if not used immediately, the solution may be stored under refrigeration (2–8°C) for up to 24 hours followed by an additional 8 hours (including infusion time) at room temperature (up to 25°C). The diluted solution should be brought to room temperature prior to the start of infusion. In the event that an infusion cannot be completed in the same day, the remaining solution should be discarded.

Ocrelizumab infusion should be administered through a separate IV line using a 0.2- or 0.22-μm inline filter. The manufacturer states that ocrelizumab solution is compatible with polyvinylchloride (PVC) and polyolefin bags and IV administration sets.

Rate of Administration

The first 2 doses of ocrelizumab (300 mg) should be infused at an initial rate of 30 mL/hour; the infusion rate may be increased by 30 mL/hour every 30 minutes to a maximum rate of 180 mL/hour. Subsequent doses of ocrelizumab (600 mg) can be infused over a duration of approximately 2 hours (this shorter infusion option should only be utilized in patients with no prior serious infusion reactions with ocrelizumab), or a duration of approximately 3.5 hours.

For an infusion duration of approximately 3.5 hours, the following infusion rates and durations are recommended by the manufacturer:

- Start at 40 mL/hour

- Increase by 40 mL/hour every 30 minutes to a maximum rate of 200 mL/hour

For an infusion duration of approximately 2 hours, the following infusion rates and durations are recommended by the manufacturer:

- Start at 100 mL/hour for the first 15 minutes

- Increase to 200 mL/hour for the next 15 minutes

- Increase to 250 mL/hour for the next 30 minutes

- Increase to 300 mL/hour for the remaining 60 minutes

Infusion times may take longer if the ocrelizumab infusion is interrupted or slowed.

If infusion-related reactions occur, the infusion rate should be reduced or ocrelizumab therapy should be interrupted depending on the severity of the reaction. In patients experiencing a mild to moderate infusion-related reaction, the infusion rate should be reduced to half the rate at the onset of the infusion reaction, and the reduced rate should be maintained for at least 30 minutes; if this reduced rate is tolerated, the rate may be increased in the usually recommended increments and intervals. In patients experiencing a severe infusion-related reaction, the infusion should be immediately interrupted and appropriate symptomatic and supportive therapy provided; once the reaction has resolved, the infusion may be resumed at half the rate at the onset of the infusion reaction. If this reduced rate is tolerated, the rate may be increased in the usually recommended increments and intervals. If a life-threatening or disabling infusion reaction occurs, ocrelizumab therapy should be immediately and permanently discontinued and appropriate supportive treatment provided.

• *Dosage*

Multiple Sclerosis

For the management of relapsing or primary progressive forms of multiple sclerosis in adults, ocrelizumab therapy should be initiated with two 300-mg infusions administered 2 weeks apart. The recommended maintenance dosage of 600 mg once every 6 months should then be administered (starting 6 months after the first 300-mg dose).

If a dose is missed, the missed dose should be administered as soon as possible rather than waiting until the next scheduled dose. The schedule of administration should be adjusted to maintain the 6-month interval between maintenance doses. Doses must be separated by at least 5 months.

• Special Populations

Hepatic Impairment

The manufacturer makes no special population dosage recommendations for patients with hepatic impairment at this time.

Renal Impairment

The manufacturer makes no special population dosage recommendations for patients with renal impairment at this time.

Geriatric Patients

The manufacturer makes no special population dosage recommendations for geriatric patients at this time.

CAUTIONS

• Contraindications

- Active hepatitis B virus (HBV) infection.
- History of life-threatening infusion reactions to the drug.

• Warnings/Precautions

Infusion Reactions

Infusion-related reactions have been reported in patients receiving ocrelizumab. Such reactions can include pruritus, rash, urticaria, erythema, bronchospasm, throat irritation, oropharyngeal pain, dyspnea, pharyngeal or laryngeal edema, flushing, hypotension, pyrexia, fatigue, headache, dizziness, nausea, and tachycardia. In clinical studies of ocrelizumab for the management of multiple sclerosis (MS), infusion reactions were reported in 34–40% of patients who received the drug despite the use of premedication; serious reactions occurred in 0.3% of ocrelizumab-treated patients, in some cases requiring hospitalization. Infusion reactions occurred most commonly with the first infusion, and decreased in incidence and severity over subsequent doses.

Ocrelizumab should be administered only in settings where appropriate medical support is available for management of serious infusion-related reactions. Patients should receive appropriate premedication with a corticosteroid and an antihistamine, with or without an antipyretic. Patients should be monitored for infusion-related reactions during and for at least 1 hour after completion of each infusion and be advised that infusion reactions can occur up to 24 hours after the infusion. Management of ocrelizumab-induced infusion reactions should be individualized based on the severity of the reaction. The drug should be immediately and permanently discontinued if a life-threatening infusion reaction occurs. For reactions of lesser severity, the infusion rate may be reduced, the infusion may be temporarily interrupted, and/or symptomatic treatment administered.

Infections

Serious, including life-threatening or fatal, bacterial, viral, parasitic and fungal infections have been reported in patients administered ocrelizumab. An increased risk of infections (including serious and fatal bacterial, fungal, and new or reactivated viral infections) has been observed in patients during and following completion of treatment with anti-CD20 B-cell depleting therapies.

In active-controlled studies in patients with relapsing forms of MS, infections were reported in 58% of patients receiving ocrelizumab compared with 52% of those receiving interferon beta-1a. In the placebo-controlled study in patients with primary progressive MS (PPMS), infections were reported in 70% of patients receiving ocrelizumab compared with 68% of those receiving placebo. Ocrelizumab was not associated with an increased risk of serious infection in patients with MS in controlled trials.

When initiating ocrelizumab after an immunosuppressive therapy or initiating an immunosuppressive therapy after ocrelizumab, consider the potential for increased immunosuppressive effects. Ocrelizumab has not been studied in combination with other therapies for MS.

Ocrelizumab may interfere with the safety and effectiveness of vaccines; patients should receive all necessary vaccinations at least 4 weeks prior to initiating ocrelizumab for live or live-attenuated vaccines, and whenever possible at least 2 weeks prior to initiating ocrelizumab for inactivated vaccines.

Respiratory Tract Infections

Respiratory tract infections occurred with greater frequency in ocrelizumab-treated patients than those who received interferon beta-1a or placebo and consisted mostly of mild to moderate upper respiratory infections; such infections were reported in 40 or 49% of patients with relapsing forms of MS or PPMS, respectively, who received the drug.

Herpes Infection

In clinical studies of patients with relapsing forms of MS, herpes infection was reported more frequently in patients receiving ocrelizumab than those receiving interferon beta-1a, and included oral herpes (3 versus 2.2%), herpes zoster (2.1 versus 1%), herpes simplex (0.7 versus 0.1%), and genital herpes (0.1 versus 0%). Among all herpes virus infections reported in the PPMS study, oral herpes occurred more frequently in ocrelizumab-treated patients than those who received placebo (2.7 versus 0.8%).

Serious CNS infections (e.g., encephalitis and meningitis), intraocular infections, and disseminated skin and soft tissue infections caused by herpes simplex virus and varicella zoster virus have been reported in the postmarketing setting with ocrelizumab. If serious herpes infections occur, discontinue or withhold ocrelizumab until the infection is resolved and appropriately treated.

Hepatitis B Virus Reactivation

Reactivation of HBV infection has occurred in the postmarketing setting with ocrelizumab. Reactivation of HBV infection has also been reported in patients receiving other anti-CD20 monoclonal antibodies and has resulted in fulminant hepatitis, hepatic failure, and death. All patients should be screened for HBV infection by testing for hepatitis B surface antigen (HBsAg) and hepatitis B core antibody (anti-HBc) before initiating treatment with ocrelizumab. Ocrelizumab is contraindicated in patients with active HBV infection confirmed by positive HBsAg and anti-HBc tests. Liver disease experts should be consulted prior to initiating and during ocrelizumab therapy in patients with any evidence of HBV infection (HBsAg-negative and anti-HBc-positive, or carriers of HBV [HBsAg-positive]).

Progressive Multifocal Leukoencephalopathy

Progressive multifocal leukoencephalopathy (PML), an opportunistic viral infection of the brain caused by the JC virus (JCV), has been reported in patients treated with ocrelizumab, other anti-CD20 antibodies, and other MS therapies. PML has occurred in ocrelizumab-treated patients who had not been treated previously with natalizumab (which has a known association with PML), were not taking any immunosuppressive or immunomodulatory medications associated with the risk of PML prior to or concomitantly with ocrelizumab, and did not have any known ongoing systemic medical conditions resulting in compromised immune system function. Patients receiving multiple immunosuppressant therapies are at increased risk for PML. Symptoms typically associated with PML are diverse, progress over a period of days to weeks, and include progressive weakness on one side of the body or clumsiness of limbs, vision disturbances, confusion, and changes in cognition, memory, orientation, or personality.

Monitor patients closely for clinical symptoms or MRI findings that maybe suggestive of PML. MRI signs of PML may be apparent before clinical manifestations develop. If PML is suspected, interrupt ocrelizumab therapy until the condition has been excluded. If PML is confirmed, permanently discontinue ocrelizumab.

Reduction in Immunoglobulins

Decreased immunoglobulins have been observed with ocrelizumab treatment. Clinical studies and their open-label extensions (up to 7 years of exposure) have shown an association between decreased levels of immunoglobulin G (less than the lower limit of normal) and an increased rate of serious infections. Monitor immunoglobulins during treatment with ocrelizumab and after discontinuation until B-cell repletion, especially if serious infection occurs. Consider discontinuation of ocrelizumab if recurrent or serious infections occur, or if there is prolonged hypogammaglobulinemia requiring treatment with parenteral immunoglobulin therapy.

Malignancy

Ocrelizumab may increase the risk of malignancies. Malignancies, including breast cancer, were reported more frequently in patients receiving ocrelizumab (6 of 781 women) than those receiving interferon beta-1a or placebo (0 of 668 women) in controlled studies. The manufacturer recommends following standard breast cancer screening guidelines in patients receiving ocrelizumab.

Immune-Mediated Colitis

Immune-mediated colitis, presenting as a severe and acute-onset form of colitis, has been reported during postmarketing experience in patients receiving ocrelizumab. Some cases of colitis were serious, requiring hospitalization, with a few patients requiring surgical intervention; systemic corticosteroids were required in many of these patients. The onset of symptoms after initiation of therapy ranged from a few weeks to years. Monitor patients for signs of immune-mediated colitis during ocrelizumab treatment such as new or persistent diarrhea or other GI symptoms.

Immunogenicity

As with all therapeutic proteins, there is a potential for immunogenicity with ocrelizumab therapy. In controlled studies, anti-drug antibodies were detected in 12 of 1311 (approximately 1%) ocrelizumab-treated patients and neutralizing antibodies were detected in 2 of these patients. Clearance of ocrelizumab was increased and faster B-cell repletion was observed in the patients with neutralizing antibodies; however, antibody development did not appear to affect efficacy or safety of the drug.

Specific Populations

Pregnancy

There are no adequate data regarding use of ocrelizumab in pregnant women; ocrelizumab may cause fetal harm. Increased perinatal mortality, depletion of B-cell populations, and renal, bone marrow, and testicular toxicity were observed in the offspring of monkeys administered ocrelizumab during pregnancy. Women of childbearing potential should use effective contraceptive measures during ocrelizumab therapy and for 6 months following the last dose of the drug.

A pregnancy registry is available to monitor patients exposed to ocrelizumab during pregnancy as well as fetal and neonatal outcomes. Clinicians and patients are encouraged to by calling 1-833-872-4370 or visiting https://www.ocrevus pregnancyregistry.com.

Transient peripheral B-cell depletion and lymphocytopenia have been reported in infants born to women exposed to other anti-CD20 monoclonal antibodies during pregnancy. The effects of maternal exposure to ocrelizumab on infant B-cell levels are not known. However, the possibility that B-cell depletion may occur in infants born to women who received ocrelizumab during pregnancy should be considered; B-cell depletion can affect vaccine immune responses in infants. Prior to administering live- or live--attenuated vaccines to infants born to mothers treated with ocrelizumab during pregnancy, recovery of B-cell counts should be confirmed in these infants as measured by CD19⁺ B cells. Inactivated vaccines may be administered as indicated to these infants prior to recovery from B-cell depletion, but consideration should be given to assessing the vaccine immune response in consultation with a qualified specialist to determine whether a protective immune response was mounted.

Lactation

It is not known whether ocrelizumab is distributed into human milk; the drug is distributed into milk in monkeys. The effects of ocrelizumab on nursing infants or on milk production are not known. Consider the benefits of breast-feeding along with the importance of ocrelizumab to the woman and any potential adverse effects on the breast-fed infant from the drug or the underlying maternal condition.

Females and Males of Reproductive Potential

Women of childbearing potential should use effective contraceptive measures during ocrelizumab therapy and for 6 months following the last dose of the drug.

Pediatric Use

Safety and efficacy of ocrelizumab have not been established in pediatric patients.

Geriatric Use

Clinical studies of ocrelizumab did not include sufficient numbers of patients ≥65 years of age to determine whether they respond differently than younger patients.

Hepatic Impairment

Data from clinical studies indicate that pharmacokinetics of ocrelizumab are not influenced by mild hepatic impairment.

Renal Impairment

Data from clinical studies indicate that pharmacokinetics of ocrelizumab are not influenced by mild renal impairment.

● Common Adverse Effects

Adverse effects reported in ≥10% of patients with relapsing forms of MS receiving ocrelizumab in clinical studies and with an incidence greater than that observed with interferon beta-1a include upper respiratory tract infection and infusion reaction.

Adverse effects reported in ≥10% of patients with PPMS receiving ocrelizumab in clinical studies and with an incidence greater than that observed with placebo include upper respiratory tract infection, infusion reaction, skin infection, and lower respiratory tract infection.

DRUG INTERACTIONS

No formal drug interaction studies have been performed to date. Drug interactions mediated by cytochrome P-450 (CYP) enzymes, other metabolizing enzymes, or transporters are not expected.

● Immunosuppressive or Immunomodulatory Agents

Increased immunosuppression may occur with concomitant use of immunosuppressive or immunomodulatory agents, including immunosuppressant doses of corticosteroids. The risk of additive immune system effects must be considered if these therapies are administered concomitantly with ocrelizumab.

When switching patients from drugs with prolonged immune effects (e.g., fingolimod, mitoxantrone, natalizumab, teriflunomide) to ocrelizumab, the duration and mechanism of action of these drugs must be considered to avoid unintended additive immunosuppressive effects.

Ocrelizumab has not been studied in combination with other therapies for multiple sclerosis.

● Vaccines

Safety and effectiveness of live or live-attenuated vaccines administered concomitantly with ocrelizumab have not been established; therefore, administration of these vaccines is not recommended during ocrelizumab therapy and until B-cell repletion occurs.

Ocrelizumab may interfere with the effectiveness of inactivated vaccines. In a randomized open-label study, patients with relapsing forms of MS who were receiving ocrelizumab therapy at the time of vaccination with an inactivated vaccine (e.g., tetanus toxoid-containing vaccine, pneumococcal polysaccharide or conjugate vaccine, influenza virus vaccine inactivated) experienced attenuated antibody responses to the vaccine; the impact of this finding on vaccine effectiveness is not known.

Any necessary immunizations should be completed at least 4 weeks prior to initiation of ocrelizumab for live or live attenuated vaccines and, whenever possible, at least 2 weeks prior to initiation of ocrelizumab for inactivated vaccines.

DESCRIPTION

Ocrelizumab, a recombinant humanized anti-CD20 monoclonal antibody, has immunomodulatory and disease-modifying activity in multiple sclerosis (MS); the drug is a glycosylated immunoglobulin G_1 (IgG_1). Although the exact mechanism of action of ocrelizumab in the management of MS has not been fully elucidated, the drug's immunomodulatory effects are thought to result from depletion of CD20-expressing B cells. There is increasing evidence suggesting that B cells play an important role in the pathogenesis of MS through various mechanisms (e.g., antigen presentation, autoantibody production, cytokine secretion). Ocrelizumab binds specifically to the large extracellular loop of CD20, a cell-surface antigen expressed on pre-B cells, mature B cells, and memory B cells; binding of ocrelizumab to CD20 triggers a host immune response consisting of antibody-dependent cell-mediated cytotoxicity (ADCC) and complement-dependent cytotoxicity (CDC), resulting in depletion of CD20-expressing B cells. Because CD20 is not expressed on lymphoid stem cells or plasma cells, B-cell reconstitution and preexisting humoral immunity are preserved.

Circulating CD19⁺ B cells (used as a marker for B-cell counts) are depleted within 14 days of ocrelizumab infusion. In clinical studies, B-cell counts increased above baseline or the lower limit of normal (LLN) at least once between infusions of ocrelizumab in 0.3–4.1% of patients. Following completion of ocrelizumab therapy, median time to B-cell recovery to baseline or LLN was 72 weeks (range: 27–175 weeks). B-cell counts returned to baseline or LLN in 90% of patients within 2.5 years of the last infusion.

Ocrelizumab exhibits essentially linear and dose-proportional pharmacokinetics over the dosage range of 400 mg to 2 g. The metabolic pathway of ocrelizumab has not been characterized, but the drug is expected to be cleared principally by catabolism. The terminal half-life of ocrelizumab is 26 days. Pharmacokinetics of ocrelizumab are not substantially affected by gender, race, or body weight.

ADVICE TO PATIENTS

- Advise patients to read the manufacturer's patient information (medication guide).

- Risk of infusion reactions; inform patients that they will need to be monitored for ≥1 hour after each infusion. Advise patients that infusion reactions may occur up to 24 hours after each infusion and to immediately contact their clinician if they experience any manifestations of such a reaction (e.g., rash, urticaria, cough or wheezing, shortness of breath, difficulty breathing, swelling of the throat, flushing, dizziness, tachycardia).

- Risk of infections; advise patients to immediately contact their clinician if they develop any signs or symptoms of infection (e.g., fever, chills, cough, cold sores, shingles, genital sores) during or after ocrelizumab therapy.

- Inform patients that progressive multifocal leukoencephalopathy (PML) has occurred in patients treated with ocrelizumab and other similar drugs and that the condition usually leads to death or severe disability over weeks or months. Advise patients to inform their clinician if they develop any new or worsening neurologic symptoms suggestive of PML such as progressive

weakness on one side of the body or clumsiness of limbs, disturbance of vision, and changes in thinking, memory, and orientation leading to confusion and personality changes.

- Risk of reactivation of HBV infection. Advise patients that monitoring will be required if they are at risk.

- Advise patients that any necessary immunizations should be completed ≥4 weeks prior to initiation of ocrelizumab for live or live attenuated vaccines and, whenever possible, ≥2 weeks prior to initiation of ocrelizumab for inactivated vaccines. Administration of live or live attenuated vaccines is not recommended during ocrelizumab therapy and until B-cell recovery occurs.

- Risk of malignancies, including breast cancer. Advise patients to follow standard breast cancer screening guidelines.

- Advise patients to promptly contact their healthcare provider if they experience any signs and symptoms of colitis, including diarrhea, abdominal pain, and blood in the stool.

- Importance of women informing clinicians if they are or plan to become pregnant or plan to breast-feed. Advise females of childbearing potential of the need for effective contraception during therapy and for 6 months after the last dose of ocrelizumab. Advise patients that if they become pregnant while receiving ocrelizumab to enroll in the Ocrevus® Pregnancy Registry.

- Importance of informing clinicians of recent, existing, or contemplated concomitant therapy, including prescription and OTC drugs and dietary or herbal supplements, as well as any concomitant illnesses (e.g., active infections).

- Inform patients of other important precautionary information.

PREPARATIONS

Ocrelizumab is available through a specialty pharmacy network. Consult the manufacturer's website for additional information.

Excipients in commercially available drug preparations may have clinically important effects in some individuals; consult specific product labeling for details.

Ocrelizumab

Parenteral		
Injection concentrate, for IV Infusion	30 mg/mL (300 mg)	Ocrevus®, Genentech

† Use is not currently included in the labeling approved by the US Food and Drug Administration.

Selected Revisions June 10, 2024, © Copyright, April 10, 2017, American Society of Health-System Pharmacists, Inc.

Baricitinib

90:24.12.92 • JANUS KINASE INHIBITORS, MISCELLANEOUS

- Baricitinib, a Janus kinase (JAK) inhibitor, is an immunomodulating agent and a disease-modifying antirheumatic drug (DMARD).

USES

• Rheumatoid Arthritis

Baricitinib is used for the management of moderately to severely active rheumatoid arthritis in adults who have had an inadequate response to one or more tumor necrosis factor (TNF; TNF-α) blocking agents. Baricitinib has been shown to induce clinical responses and improve physical function in patients with rheumatoid arthritis when administered at the recommended dosage. Safety and efficacy of baricitinib in rheumatoid arthritis were based principally on the results of 2 randomized controlled trials (RA-BUILD and RA-BEACON) in adults with active disease; baricitinib has also been studied in confirmatory clinical trials at a higher dosage of 4 mg once daily†. Guidelines generally support the use of targeted synthetic disease-modifying antirheumatic drugs (DMARDs), including Janus kinase (JAK) inhibitors, such as baricitinib, following failure with first-line methotrexate therapy.

Baricitinib can be used alone or in combination with methotrexate or other nonbiologic DMARDs; examples include hydroxychloroquine, leflunomide, and sulfasalazine. Concomitant use of baricitinib with other JAK inhibitors (e.g., tofacitinib) or biologic DMARDs, such as TNF blocking agents (e.g., adalimumab, certolizumab pegol, etanercept, golimumab, infliximab), interleukin-1 (IL-1) receptor antagonists (e.g., anakinra), anti-CD20 monoclonal antibodies (e.g., rituximab), selective costimulation modulators (e.g., abatacept), and anti-interleukin-6-receptor monoclonal antibodies (e.g., sarilumab, tocilizumab), is not recommended. Concomitant use of baricitinib with potent immunosuppressive agents (e.g., azathioprine, cyclosporine) also is not recommended.

Clinical Experience

Efficacy and safety of baricitinib at a dosage of 2 mg daily have been evaluated in 2 randomized, double-blind, controlled studies (RA-BUILD and RA-BEACON) in adults with active rheumatoid arthritis, as defined by the American College of Rheumatology (ACR)/European League Against Rheumatism (EULAR) 2010 rheumatoid arthritis classification criteria. Patients had moderately to severely active disease with 6 or more tender joints, 6 or more swollen joints, and elevated C-reactive protein (CRP) concentrations at baseline. In RA-BUILD, patients who had an inadequate response or intolerance to at least one conventional nonbiologic DMARD were randomized to receive baricitinib 2 mg daily, baricitinib 4 mg daily, or placebo for 24 weeks either alone or in addition to a stable background regimen of up to 2 nonbiologic DMARDs; most patients were receiving methotrexate with or without another nonbiologic DMARD (23 or 49%, respectively) and only 7% were not receiving any other DMARDs concomitantly with baricitinib. Patients who had received prior biologic DMARD therapy were excluded from RA-BUILD. In RA-BEACON, patients who had an inadequate response or intolerance to at least one TNF blocking agent and were receiving a stable dosage of one or more nonbiologic DMARDs at study entry were randomized to receive baricitinib 2 mg daily, baricitinib 4 mg daily, or placebo for 24 weeks in addition to their existing nonbiologic DMARD therapy; approximately 38% of patients in RA-BEACON also had received prior therapy with at least one biologic DMARD that was not a TNF blocking agent. Patients in RA-BEACON were required to have discontinued biologic DMARDs at least 4 weeks before randomization (or at least 6 months for rituximab). In both studies, those receiving low stable dosages of corticosteroids (equivalent to 10 mg or less of prednisone daily) and/or stable dosages of nonsteroidal anti-inflammatory agents (NSAIAs) or analgesics could continue such agents. Patients who failed to achieve at least 20% reduction in tender and swollen joint counts by week 16 were switched from their assigned treatment to baricitinib 4 mg daily.

The ACR criteria for improvement (ACR response) in measures of disease activity were used as the principal measure of clinical response; an ACR 20 response is achieved if the patient experiences a 20% or greater improvement in tender and swollen joint count and a 20% or greater improvement in at least 3 of the following criteria: patient pain assessment, patient global assessment, physician global assessment, patient self-assessed disability, or laboratory measures of disease activity (i.e., erythrocyte sedimentation rate [ESR] or CRP level). An ACR 50 or ACR 70 response is defined using the same criteria but with a level of improvement of 50 or 70%, respectively. The primary end point in RA-BUILD and RA-BEACON was the proportion of patients who achieved an ACR 20 response at week 12.

In both studies, a substantially greater proportion of patients treated with baricitinib 2 or 4 mg daily achieved an ACR 20 response at weeks 12 and 24 compared with those receiving placebo. ACR 20 response was achieved at 12 weeks by 66, 62, or 39% of patients receiving baricitinib 2 mg daily, baricitinib 4 mg daily, or placebo, respectively, in RA-BUILD and by 49, 55, or 27% of patients receiving these respective treatments in RA-BEACON. ACR 50 and ACR 70 responses also were achieved in a greater proportion of baricitinib-treated patients compared with placebo recipients. In addition, a greater proportion of patients receiving baricitinib 2 or 4 mg daily in both studies achieved a low level of disease activity at week 12, as measured by a 28-joint Disease Activity Score using CRP (DAS 28 [CRP]) of less than 2.6, compared with those receiving placebo. Patients receiving baricitinib also demonstrated greater improvements in physical function as measured by the Health Assessment Questionnaire-Disability Index (HAQ-DI) at week 24.

Because a clear relationship between dosage and ACR response has not been established and because the risk of serious adverse events appears to be dose related, only the 2-mg daily dosage of baricitinib currently is recommended for management of rheumatoid arthritis in FDA-approved labeling. In addition, because of uncertain risk-benefit assessment, baricitinib currently is FDA-labeled only for patients who have had an inadequate response to one or more TNF blocking agents.

In clinical trials (RA-BEGIN and RA-BEAM), baricitinib at a dosage of 4 mg once daily† has been compared with methotrexate and with adalimumab as add-on therapy to methotrexate. Baricitinib 4 mg once daily as monotherapy or in combination with methotrexate has been evaluated in a double-blind, double-dummy, randomized controlled phase 3 trial (RA-BEGIN) in 588 adults with rheumatoid arthritis naive to conventional synthetic or biologic therapies. In this study, patients were randomized in a 4:3:4 ratio to oral methotrexate monotherapy (administered once weekly), baricitinib monotherapy (4 mg administered once daily), or baricitinib in combination with methotrexate. At week 24, noninferiority and superiority of baricitinib to methotrexate monotherapy was demonstrated in ACR 20 response (77 versus 62%, respectively). Substantial improvements in DAS 28, HAQ DI, and SDAI were observed at week 24 in patients receiving baricitinib monotherapy and baricitinib-methotrexate combination therapy compared with patients receiving methotrexate monotherapy. At week 52, baricitinib-treated patients (as monotherapy or in combination with methotrexate) maintained substantial improvement compared with methotrexate monotherapy in all outcomes. In the double-blind, placebo- and active-controlled phase 3 trial (RA-BEAM), 1305 adults with moderate to severe active rheumatoid arthritis who were receiving therapy with methotrexate were randomized to receive placebo (followed by a switch to baricitinib after 24 weeks), baricitinib 4 mg once daily, or adalimumab 40 mg every other week. Open-label rescue therapy (baricitinib 4 mg) was provided at week 16 for patients whose tender and swollen joint counts were reduced by less than 20% at both week 14 and 16. At week 12, the primary ACR 20 response rate was substantially higher in patients receiving baricitinib compared with those receiving placebo (70 versus 40%, respectively). Baricitinib also demonstrated noninferiority to adalimumab (70 versus 61%, respectively). The key secondary end point of change from baseline in modified total Sharp score was also substantially improved in patients receiving baricitinib compared with placebo (least squares mean, 0.41 versus 0.9, respectively); change from baseline with adalimumab was 0.33.

Clinical Perspective

The American College of Rheumatology issued guidelines for the treatment of rheumatoid arthritis in 2021. Disease-modifying treatments for rheumatoid arthritis include conventional DMARDs (e.g., hydroxychloroquine, leflunomide, methotrexate, sulfasalazine), biologic DMARDs (e.g., TNF blocking agents, abatacept, tocilizumab, sarilumab, rituximab), and/or targeted synthetic DMARDs (e.g., JAK inhibitors). Specific agents for rheumatoid arthritis treatment are selected according to current disease activity, prior therapies used, and the presence of comorbidities. A "treat-to-target" approach is typically employed, with the goal of achieving a predefined target of low disease activity or remission.

Targeted synthetic DMARDs used in the treatment of rheumatoid arthritis include the JAK inhibitors baricitinib, tofacitinib, and upadacitinib. Methotrexate monotherapy is strongly recommended over biologic or targeted synthetic DMARD monotherapy in DMARD-naive patients with moderate to high disease activity. Methotrexate monotherapy also is strongly preferred over combined therapy with a non-TNF blocking agent biologic DMARD or targeted synthetic DMARD because of the lack of proven benefit and additional risks and costs associated with combined therapy. Randomized controlled trials evaluating add-on therapy with a biologic or targeted synthetic DMARD or triple therapy (methotrexate, sulfasalazine, and hydroxychloroquine) demonstrated equivalent long-term outcomes in patients receiving add-on therapy with a biologic or targeted synthetic DMARD and those receiving triple therapy; therefore, targeted synthetic DMARDs and biologic DMARDs (including TNF blocking agents) are conditionally recommended as add-on therapy for patients with an inadequate response to maximally tolerated doses of methotrexate. Recommendations for the use and selection of targeted synthetic DMARDs in rheumatoid arthritis vary based on the presence of certain comorbidities (e.g., heart failure, previous serious infection, nontuberculous mycobacterial lung disease). Consult the American College of Rheumatology guidelines for additional details.

● *Treatment of Coronavirus Disease 2019 (COVID-19)*

Baricitinib is used for the treatment of COVID-19 in hospitalized adults requiring supplemental oxygen, non-invasive or invasive mechanical ventilation, or extracorporeal membrane oxygenation (ECMO). Baricitinib was previously used in this setting following FDA issuance of an Emergency Use Authorization (EUA). Baricitinib received approval for this use in 2022. Safety and efficacy of baricitinib for this use were based principally on results of 2 randomized placebo-controlled trials that evaluated baricitinib in hospitalized adults with COVID-19. Guidelines generally recommend the addition of baricitinib to other therapies (e.g., remdesivir, corticosteroids) in adult patients hospitalized with severe COVID-19; clinicians should consult the most recent COVID-19 guidelines available from the National Institutes of Health (NIH) and Infectious Diseases Society of America (IDSA) for additional information.

Baricitinib has been used in the treatment of COVID-19 in hospitalized pediatric patients 2 to less than 18 years of age requiring supplemental oxygen, non-invasive ventilation or invasive mechanical ventilation, or ECMO†. On May 10, 2022, following approval of baricitinib for this use in adults, the EUA was updated to reflect emergency use in pediatric patients.

Baricitinib has been used for the treatment of COVID-19† because the drug inhibits the signaling pathway of cytokines that are elevated in severe COVID-19 (e.g., interleukins, interferons, granulocyte–macrophage colony stimulating factor). Baricitinib also prevents SARS-CoV-2 cellular entry, inhibits viral propagation, and improves lymphocyte counts in patients with COVID-19.

Clinical Experience

Efficacy and safety of baricitinib for the treatment of COVID-19 were evaluated in two phase 3, randomized, double-blind, placebo-controlled trials (ACTT-2 and COV-BARRIER).

The ACTT-2 trial randomized 1033 hospitalized adults with laboratory-confirmed SARS-CoV-2 infection to treatment with baricitinib in combination with remdesivir or to placebo in combination with remdesivir. Patients were required to have at least one of the following to be enrolled in the trial: radiographic infiltrates by imaging, peripheral oxygen saturation (SpO₂) ≤94% on room air, a requirement for supplemental oxygen, or a requirement for mechanical ventilation or ECMO. Patients in the combination group received baricitinib 4 mg orally once daily for 14 days or until hospital discharge and remdesivir 200 mg IV on day 1 followed by a dosage of 100 mg IV once daily beginning on day 2 for a total treatment duration of 10 days or until hospital discharge. The primary efficacy endpoint was time to recovery within 29 days of randomization; the major secondary efficacy endpoint was clinical status on day 15 (based on an 8-point ordinal scale ranging from scores of 1 [not hospitalized and no limitations] to 8 [death]).

In the overall population, mean age was 55 years; 63% of patients were male, 51% were Hispanic or Latino, 48% were white, 15% were Black or African American, and 10% were Asian. Fourteen percent of patients did not require supplemental oxygen, 55% required supplemental oxygen, 21% required non-invasive ventilation or high-flow oxygen, and 11% required invasive mechanical ventilation

or ECMO. The most common comorbidities were obesity (56%), hypertension (52%), and type 2 diabetes (37%).

In the ACTT-2 trial, the median time to recovery was 7 days in patients receiving baricitinib in combination with remdesivir and 8 days in patients receiving placebo in combination with remdesivir (hazard ratio [HR], 1.16; 95% confidence interval [CI], 1.01–1.33). Patients assigned to baricitinib in combination with remdesivir were more likely to have a better clinical status at day 15 (odds ratio [OR], 1.26; 95% CI, 1.01–1.57). The proportion of patients who died or progressed to non-invasive ventilation/high-flow oxygen or invasive mechanical ventilation by day 29 was lower in those receiving baricitinib in combination with remdesivir (23 versus 28%; OR, 0.74; 95% CI, 0.56–0.99). The proportion of patients who died by day 29 was 4.7% in the baricitinib-remdesivir combination group versus 7.1% in the placebo-remdesivir group (estimated difference in day 29 probability of mortality: -2.6%; 95% CI, -5.8 to 0.5%).

The COV-BARRIER trial randomized 1525 hospitalized adults with laboratory-confirmed SARS-CoV-2 infection to baricitinib 4 mg once daily or placebo. Patients were permitted to remain on background standard of care, as defined per local guidelines. The most frequently used background therapies were corticosteroids (79% of patients) and remdesivir (19% of patients). Patients were required to have at least one instance of elevation of at least one inflammatory marker (C-reactive protein, D-dimer, lactate dehydrogenase, ferritin), and at least one of the following: radiographic infiltrates by imaging, SpO₂ ≤94% on room air, evidence of active COVID infection with clinical symptoms including any of the following: fever, vomiting, diarrhea, dry cough, tachypnea, or requirement for supplemental oxygen. The primary efficacy endpoint was the proportion of patients who died or progressed to non-invasive ventilation/high-flow oxygen or invasive mechanical ventilation within 28 days; a key secondary efficacy endpoint was all-cause mortality by day 28. In the overall population, mean age was 58 years; 63% of patients were male, 60% were white, 5% were Black or African American, 11% were Asian. Twelve percent did not require supplemental oxygen, 63% required supplemental oxygen, and 24% required non-invasive ventilation or high-flow oxygen. The most common comorbidities were hypertension (48%), obesity (33%), and type 2 diabetes (29%).

In the COV-BARRIER trial, the estimated proportion of patients who died or progressed to non-invasive ventilation/high-flow oxygen or invasive mechanical ventilation was numerically lower in patients treated with baricitinib compared with those receiving placebo (27.8 versus 30.5%, respectively; OR, 0.85; 95% CI, 0.67–1.08). The mortality rate by day 28 was substantially lower in the baricitinib treatment group compared with the placebo group (8.1 versus 13.3%; estimated difference in day 28 probability of mortality, -4.9%; 95% CI, -8.0 to -1.9%; HR, 0.56; 95% CI, 0.41–0.77). An exploratory trial followed the design of the COV-BARRIER trial and included critically ill patients not enrolled in COV-BARRIER who required invasive mechanical ventilation or ECMO (n=101). This trial demonstrated a lower risk of death by day 28 compared with placebo (39.2 versus 58.0%, respectively; estimated difference, -18.8%; 95% CI, -36.3 to 0.6%).

The RECOVERY trial was a randomized, controlled, open-label platform trial that evaluated the effects of various treatments in patients hospitalized with COVID-19. Among 159 hospitals in the United Kingdom, 8156 patients were randomized to usual care plus baricitinib 4 mg daily for 10 days or until hospital discharge, or to usual care alone. Patients were aged 2 years and older, and were excluded if they had an estimated glomerular filtration rate (eGFR) less than 15 mL/minute per 1.73 m², were on dialysis or hemofiltration, had a neutrophil count of less than 0.5 × 10⁹/L, had evidence of active tuberculosis infection, or were pregnant or breastfeeding. The primary outcome was all-cause mortality at day 28.

In the RECOVERY trial, the mean age of all patients was 58.1 years, 66% were male, 80% were white, and 11–12% were of Black, Asian, and other minority ethnic groups. Approximately 95% were receiving corticosteroids, and 23% were receiving tocilizumab (with another 9% having planned use within the next 24 hours). Approximately 67% were receiving simple oxygen, and 25% were receiving non-invasive ventilation. Forty-two percent of patients had received at least 1 dose of a COVID-19 vaccine.

At 28 days, all-cause mortality occurred in substantially fewer patients treated with baricitinib compared with usual care (12% versus 14%, respectively; risk ratio [RR], 0.87; 95% CI, 0.77–0.99). Key secondary endpoints of discharge from hospital within 28 days (80% versus 78%; RR, 1.10; 95% CI, 1.04–1.15) and receipt of mechanical ventilation or death (16% versus 17%, respectively; RR, 0.89; 95% CI, 0.81–0.98) were also improved with baricitinib.

The ACTT-4 trial was a randomized, double-blind, double-placebo-controlled trial that evaluated the effect of baricitinib plus remdesivir compared with dexamethasone plus remdesivir in hospitalized adults with COVID-19. Overall, 1010 patients were enrolled and randomized to baricitinib, remdesivir, and placebo or dexamethasone, remdesivir, and placebo. Baricitinib was administered at a dosage of 4 mg daily for up to 14 days or until hospital discharge or death. Included patients were hospitalized adults with COVID-19 who required supplemental oxygen administered by low-flow (≤15 L/minute), high-flow (>15 L/minute), or non-invasive mechanical ventilation modalities. The primary outcome was mechanical ventilation-free survival by day 29.

In the ACTT-4 trial, 58–59% of patients were male, 57–59% of patients were white, 18–19% of patients were Black or African American, 32–36% of patients were Hispanic or Latino, 7% were Asian, and 56–58% of patients were age 40–64 years. Overall, 97% of patients were enrolled in North America.

At day 29, mechanical ventilation-free survival was similar between patients assigned to baricitinib plus remdesivir and those assigned to dexamethasone plus remdesivir (87.0% and 87.6%, respectively; risk difference, 0.6%; 95% CI, -3.6 to 4.8). The key secondary outcome of clinical status at day 15 based on an 8-category ordinal scale was also similar between groups (OR for improved status, 1.01; 95% CI, 0.80–1.27).

Clinical Perspective

Based on data available to date, the NIH COVID-19 Treatment Guidelines Panel recommends that in hospitalized adults who require conventional oxygen, oral baricitinib or IV tocilizumab be added to other treatments, including remdesivir with or without dexamethasone, depending on disease severity and clinical scenario. The Panel also recommends that in hospitalized adults who require high-flow nasal cannula (HFNC) oxygen, noninvasive ventilation (NIV), mechanical ventilation (MV), or ECMO, most patients should be treated with either dexamethasone plus oral baricitinib or dexamethasone plus IV tocilizumab. For treatment of children who require oxygen via HFNC, NIV, MV, or ECMO, the Panel recommends consideration of baricitinib or tocilizumab for patients who do not have rapid (e.g., within 24 hours) improvement in oxygenation after initiation of dexamethasone and who are age 2 years and older†. Continuation of baricitinib after hospital discharge is not recommended.

Based on data available to date, the IDSA suggests that in hospitalized adults with severe COVID-19, baricitinib be used with corticosteroids rather than no baricitinib. In hospitalized patients with severe COVID-19 who cannot receive a corticosteroid because of a contraindication, the IDSA suggests use of baricitinib with remdesivir rather than remdesivir alone.

Clinicians should consult the most recent COVID-19 guidelines available from the NIH (https://www.covid19treatmentguidelines.nih.gov/) and IDSA (https://www.idsociety.org/practice-guideline/covid-19-guideline-treatment-and-management/) for additional information.

● *Alopecia Areata*

Baricitinib is used in the treatment of adults with severe alopecia areata. Concomitant use of baricitinib with other JAK inhibitors (e.g., tofacitinib) or biologic DMARDs, such as TNF blocking agents (e.g., adalimumab, certolizumab pegol, etanercept, golimumab, infliximab), IL-1 receptor antagonists (e.g., anakinra), anti-CD20 monoclonal antibodies (e.g., rituximab), selective costimulation modulators (e.g., abatacept), and anti-interleukin-6-receptor monoclonal antibodies (e.g., sarilumab, tocilizumab), is not recommended. Concomitant use of baricitinib with potent immunosuppressive agents (e.g., azathioprine, cyclosporine) also is not recommended. Safety and efficacy of baricitinib for this use were based principally on results from 2 randomized, double-blind, placebo-controlled trials in patients with severe alopecia areata. The specific place in therapy of baricitinib has not been addressed in guidelines; typical treatments include intralesional, topical, and systemic corticosteroids; minoxidil; and other immunomodulators.

Clinical Experience

Safety and efficacy of baricitinib in the treatment of severe alopecia areata are supported by results from 2 randomized, double-blind, placebo-controlled trials (BRAVE-AA1 and BRAVE-AA2). These trials enrolled a total of 1200 patients with alopecia areata, who had at least 50% scalp hair loss as measured by the Severity of Alopecia Tool (SALT) for more than 6 months. The trials enrolled

males 18–60 years of age and females 18–70 years of age. Patients were randomized in a 3:2:2 ratio to baricitinib 4 mg once daily, baricitinib 2 mg once daily, or placebo. The primary outcome was clinical response at week 36, defined as at least 80% scalp hair coverage (SALT score of 20 or less).

Among enrolled patients, 61% were female, 52% were white, 36% were Asian, and 8% were Black. At baseline, 53% of patients had at least 95% scalp hair loss, 34% had a current episode lasting at least 4 years, 69% had significant gaps in eyebrow hair or no notable eyebrow hair, and 58% had significant gaps in eyelashes or no notable eyelashes.

At 36 weeks, clinical response occurred in substantially greater proportions of patients treated with baricitinib 2 mg once daily and baricitinib 4 mg once daily compared with placebo in both BRAVE-AA1 (22, 35, and 5%, respectively) and BRAVE-AA2 (17, 32, and 3%, respectively). Results were consistent in analyses of achievement of 90% scalp hair coverage (SALT score of 10 or less). In AA-2, patients who achieved the primary outcome (SALT score of 20 or less) with baricitinib 4 mg once daily at 52 weeks of treatment entered a randomized downtitration period and received either baricitinib 2 mg once daily or continued baricitinib 4 mg once daily. After an additional 24 weeks of treatment, response was maintained by 75% of patients randomized to baricitinib 2 mg once daily and 98% of patients who remained on baricitinib 4 mg.

Clinical Perspective

Goals of treatment for alopecia areata include inhibition of disease progression and stimulation of hair regrowth. First-line treatment in adults with 1 to 2 small patches typically includes intralesional corticosteroids, which may be repeated every 4–6 weeks, and discontinued if there is lack of response within 3–6 months. Topical corticosteroids are also frequently used in adults and pediatric patients; they should be continued for at least 3 months and discontinued after 6 months if there is lack of response. Systemic corticosteroids may be used for extensive alopecia, particularly during the acute progressive stage of disease. Other options include topical minoxidil, contact immunotherapy, and other immunomodulators. The specific place in therapy of baricitinib has not been addressed in guidelines.

DOSAGE AND ADMINISTRATION

● *General*

Pretreatment Screening

- Evaluate for active or latent tuberculosis infection prior to initiation of therapy; initiate antimycobacterial therapy if indicated prior to use in patients with rheumatoid arthritis or alopecia areata.

- Evaluate for risk of thrombosis and GI perforation prior to initiation of therapy.

- Evaluate for risk of major cardiovascular events prior to initiation of therapy, particularly in patients who are current or past smokers and patients with other cardiovascular risk factors.

- Measure absolute lymphocyte count, absolute neutrophil count (ANC), and hemoglobin prior to initiation of therapy. Do not initiate therapy for rheumatoid arthritis or alopecia areata in patients with an absolute lymphocyte count (ALC) of less than 500/mm³, an ANC of less than 1000/mm³, or hemoglobin concentration of less than 8 g/dL. Do not initiate therapy for COVID-19 in patients with an ALC less than 200/mm³ or if the ANC is less than 500/mm³.

- Screen for viral hepatitis infection before initiating therapy.

- Evaluate renal and liver function tests at baseline.

- Weigh benefits of therapy against risks of all-cause mortality prior to initiating therapy.

- In patients with rheumatoid arthritis or alopecia areata, update immunizations according to current guidelines.

- Weigh benefits of therapy against risks of developing malignancies prior to initiating therapy with baricitinib, particularly in patients with a known malignancy (other than successfully treated nonmelanoma skin cancer), patients who develop a malignancy, and patients who are current or past smokers.

Patient Monitoring

- Monitor patients with positive hepatitis B surface antibody and hepatitis B core antibody, without hepatitis B surface antigen for expression of hepatitis B virus (HBV) DNA. Consult a hepatologist if HBV DNA is detected.

- Monitor closely for signs or symptoms of infection, including the possible development of tuberculosis in patients who tested negative for latent tuberculosis prior to initiating therapy, during, and after treatment with the drug.

- Evaluate for risk of major cardiovascular events during therapy.

- Routinely monitor ANC, lymphocyte count, and hemoglobin concentrations during therapy.

- Perform dermatologic examinations periodically during therapy in patients at increased risk for skin cancer.

- Measure lipids approximately 12 weeks after initiation of therapy in patients with rheumatoid arthritis or alopecia areata.

- Monitor for onset of new abdominal symptoms.

- Monitor for changes in renal and liver function.

- Monitor for thrombosis.

- Weigh benefits of therapy against risk of all-cause mortality prior to continuing therapy with the drug.

- Weigh benefits of therapy against risks of developing malignancies prior to continuing therapy with baricitinib, particularly in patients with a known malignancy (other than successfully treated nonmelanoma skin cancer), patients who develop a malignancy, and patients who are current or past smokers.

Premedication and Prophylaxis

- In studies supporting approval for use in treatment of hospitalized adults with COVID-19, prophylaxis for venous thromboembolic events was recommended or required for all patients unless a major contraindication was present.

Dispensing and Administration Precautions

Handling and Disposal

- The package insert and Emergency Use Authorization (EUA) for baricitinib that permits use of the drug for the treatment of COVID-19 in adults and pediatric patients† state that proper control measures (e.g., ventilated enclosure) or personal protective equipment (i.e., N95 respirator) should be used when crushing baricitinib tablets, since it is not known if powder from crushed tablets is hazardous.

Other General Considerations

- Do not use concomitantly with other Janus kinase (JAK) inhibitors, biologic disease-modifying antirheumatic drugs (DMARDs), or potent immunosuppressive agents.

● Administration

Baricitinib is administered orally without regard to food.

Store baricitinib at 20–25°C; excursions permitted between 15–30°C.

Alternative Administration in Patients Unable to Swallow Tablets

The package insert and the EUA for baricitinib that permits use of the drug for the treatment of COVID-19 in hospitalized pediatric patients 2 years and older requiring supplemental oxygen, non-invasive or invasive mechanical ventilation, or extracorporeal membrane oxygenation (ECMO)† provide information on alternative administration of the drug via oral dispersion, gastrostomy tube, or nasogastric or orogastric tube for patients who are unable to swallow whole tablets. Tablets dispersed in water are stable for up to 4 hours.

Oral Administration of Dispersed Tablets

Tablets (1-mg, 2-mg, or 4-mg tablets, or any combination needed to achieve the desired dose up to 4 mg) may be placed in a container with approximately 10 mL (minimum of 5 mL) of room temperature water; disperse the tablets by gently swirling the container. The resulting solution should be immediately consumed by the patient. Rinse the container with an additional 10 mL (minimum of 5 mL) of room temperature water; the patient should then consume the remaining contents.

Tablets dispersed in water are stable for up to 4 hours.

Administration via Gastrostomy Feeding Tube

Tablets (1-mg, 2-mg, or 4-mg tablets, or any combination needed to achieve the desired dose up to 4 mg) may be placed in a container with approximately 15 mL (minimum of 10 mL) of room temperature water; disperse tablets by gently swirling the container. Ensure the tablet(s) are sufficiently dispersed to allow free passage through the tip of the syringe. Withdraw entire contents from the container into an appropriate syringe and immediately administer through the gastric feeding tube. Rinse container with approximately 15 mL (minimum of 10 mL) of room temperature water, then withdraw solution into the syringe and administer through the gastric feeding tube.

Tablets dispersed in water are stable for up to 4 hours.

Administration via Nasogastric or Orogastric Feeding Tube

Tablets (1-mg, 2-mg, or 4-mg tablets, or any combination needed to achieve the desired dose up to 4 mg) may be placed into a container with approximately 30 mL of room temperature water; disperse tablets by gently swirling the container. Ensure the tablet(s) are sufficiently dispersed to allow free passage through the tip of the syringe. Withdraw the entire contents from the container into an appropriate syringe and immediately administer through the enteral feeding tube. Hold syringe horizontally and shake during administration to avoid clogging small diameter tubes (smaller than 12 Fr). Rinse container with a sufficient amount (minimum of 15 mL) of room temperature water, withdraw solution into the syringe, and administer through the enteral feeding tube.

Tablets dispersed in water are stable for up to 4 hours.

● Dosage

Rheumatoid Arthritis in Adults

For the management of rheumatoid arthritis in adults who have had an inadequate response or intolerance to one or more tumor necrosis factor (TNF; TNF-α) blocking agents, the recommended dosage of baricitinib is 2 mg once daily. Baricitinib dosages of 4 mg once daily† have been evaluated in clinical trials.

Treatment Interruption for Toxicity

If a serious infection develops, baricitinib therapy should be interrupted until the infection has been controlled. Modify the dosage of baricitinib during treatment for rheumatoid arthritis according to Table 1.

TABLE 1. Dosage modifications for cytopenias and anemia in patients with rheumatoid arthritis or alopecia areata.

Laboratory analyte	Value	Recommendation
ALC	≥500 cells/mm³	Maintain dosage
	<500 cells/mm³	Interrupt therapy until ALC ≥500 cells/mm³
ANC	≥1000 cells/mm³	Maintain dosage
	<1000 cells/mm³	Interrupt therapy until ANC ≥1000 cells/mm³
Hemoglobin	≥8 g/dL	Maintain dosage
	<8 g/dL	Interrupt therapy until hemoglobin ≥8 g/dL

Treatment of COVID-19

Adults

For treatment of COVID-19 in hospitalized adults requiring supplemental oxygen, non-invasive or invasive mechanical ventilation, or ECMO, the recommended dosage of baricitinib is 4 mg once daily for a total duration of 14 days or until hospital discharge, whichever occurs first. In studies of hospitalized patients with COVID-19, prophylaxis for venous thromboembolism was recommended unless contraindicated.

Modify the dosage of baricitinib during treatment for COVID-19 in hospitalized adults according to Table 2.

TABLE 2. Dosage modifications for cytopenias in hospitalized adults with COVID-19.

Laboratory analyte	Value	Recommendation
ALC	≥200 cells/mm³	Maintain dosage
	<200 cells/mm³	Interrupt therapy until ALC ≥200 cells/mm³
ANC	≥500 cells/mm³	Maintain dosage
	<500 cells/mm³	Interrupt therapy until ANC ≥500 cells/mm³

Pediatric Patients

Limited data are available regarding baricitinib dosing in hospitalized pediatric patients for the treatment of COVID-19†.

For patients ≥9 years of age requiring supplemental oxygen, non-invasive or invasive mechanical ventilation, or ECMO, EUA permits 4 mg once daily for a total duration of 14 days or until hospital discharge, whichever occurs first.

For patients 2 to <9 years of age requiring supplemental oxygen, non-invasive or invasive mechanical ventilation, or ECMO, EUA permits 2 mg once daily for a total duration of 14 days or until hospital discharge, whichever occurs first.

Treatment Interruption for Toxicity

Dosage modification may be necessary in hospitalized pediatric patients with COVID-19† who develop laboratory abnormalities (see Table 3).

TABLE 3. Recommended Dosage Modification for Laboratory Abnormalities in Pediatric Patients with COVID-19†

Laboratory Abnormality	Dosage Modification
ALC <200 cells/mm³	Consider interrupting baricitinib therapy until ALC ≥200 cells/mm³
ANC <500 cells/mm³	Consider interrupting baricitinib therapy until ANC ≥500 cells/mm³
Increased serum ALT or AST concentrations and drug-induced hepatic injury is suspected	Interrupt baricitinib until diagnosis of drug-induced liver injury is excluded

Alopecia Areata

The recommended dosage of baricitinib for alopecia areata is 2 mg once daily. Increase the dosage to 4 mg once daily if the response to treatment is not adequate. For patients with nearly complete or complete scalp hair loss, with or without substantial eyelash or eyebrow hair loss, consider treating with 4 mg once daily. Once patients achieve an adequate response to treatment with 4 mg, decrease the dosage to 2 mg once daily.

Treatment Interruption for Toxicity

Modify the dosage of baricitinib during treatment for alopecia areata according to Table 1.

Dosage Modifications for Drug Interactions

In patients receiving concomitant therapy with potent inhibitors of organic anion transporter (OAT)3 (e.g., probenecid), reduce the dosage of baricitinib from 4 mg once daily to 2 mg once daily or from 2 mg once daily to 1 mg once daily. If the recommended baricitinib dose is 1 mg once daily, consider discontinuing probenecid.

● Special Populations

Hepatic Impairment

Rheumatoid Arthritis: Dosage adjustment is not necessary in patients with mild or moderate hepatic impairment. Use of the drug in patients with severe hepatic impairment has not been evaluated and is not recommended. Interrupt treatment if increases in ALT or AST are observed and drug-induced liver injury (DILI) is suspected, until DILI is excluded.

COVID-19: Dosage adjustment is not necessary in patients with mild or moderate hepatic impairment. Baricitinib has not been studied in patients with severe hepatic impairment; use in patients with severe hepatic impairment only if the potential benefit outweighs the potential risk. Interrupt treatment if increases in ALT or AST are observed and DILI is suspected, until DILI is excluded.

Alopecia Areata: Dosage adjustment is not necessary in patients with mild or moderate hepatic impairment. Use of the drug in patients with severe hepatic impairment is not recommended. Interrupt treatment if increases in ALT or AST are observed and DILI is suspected, until DILI is excluded.

Renal Impairment

Rheumatoid Arthritis: In patients with mild renal impairment (estimated glomerular filtration rate [eGFR] 60–<90 mL/minute per 1.73 m²), maintain the recommended dosage of baricitinib 2 mg once daily. The recommended dosage of baricitinib in patients with moderate renal impairment (eGFR 30–<60 mL/minute per 1.73 m²) is 1 mg once daily. Baricitinib is not recommended for use in patients with severe renal impairment (eGFR <30 mL/minute per 1.73 m²).

COVID-19: Dosage adjustments based on eGFR may be necessary (see Table 4).

TABLE 4. Recommended Dosage Modification for Renal Impairment in Patients with COVID-19

eGFR Value	Adults	Pediatric Patients ≥9 years of age†	Pediatric Patients 2 to <9 years of age†
60 to <90 mL/min per 1.73 m²	4 mg once daily	4 mg once daily	2 mg once daily
30 to <60 mL/min per 1.73 m²	Reduce initial dosage to 2 mg once daily	Reduce initial dosage to 2 mg once daily	Reduce initial dosage to 1 mg once daily
15 to <30 mL/min per 1.73 m²	Reduce initial dosage to 1 mg once daily	Reduce initial dosage to 1 mg once daily	Use not recommended
<15 mL/min per 1.73 m²	Use not recommended	Use not recommended	Use not recommended

Alopecia Areata: Dosage adjustments based on eGFR may be necessary (see Table 5).

TABLE 5. Recommended Dosage Modification for Renal Impairment in Patients with Alopecia Areata

eGFR Value	Recommendation	
	If the recommended dosage is 2 mg once daily	If the recommended dosage is 4 mg once daily
60 to <90 mL/min per 1.73 m²	Maintain dosage	Maintain dosage
30 to <60 mL/min per 1.73 m²	Reduce to 1 mg once daily	Reduce to 2 mg once daily
<30 mL/min per 1.73 m²	Use not recommended	Use not recommended

Geriatric Patients

Dosage adjustment not required.

CAUTIONS

● Contraindications

None.

● Warnings/Precautions

Warnings

Infectious Complications

A boxed warning regarding the risk of infectious complications is included in the prescribing information for baricitinib. Serious and sometimes fatal infections, including bacterial, mycobacterial, invasive fungal, viral, or other opportunistic infections, have been reported in patients with rheumatoid arthritis receiving baricitinib. The most common serious infections reported in patients receiving baricitinib have included pneumonia, herpes zoster, and urinary tract infection. Tuberculosis may present with pulmonary or extrapulmonary disease. Opportunistic infections (e.g., multidermatomal herpes zoster, esophageal candidiasis, pneumocystosis, histoplasmosis, cryptococcosis, cytomegalovirus [CMV] infection, BK virus infection) have been reported in patients receiving baricitinib. Some patients have presented with disseminated rather than local disease. Most patients who experienced serious infections were receiving concomitant therapy with immunosuppressive agents such as methotrexate or corticosteroids.

In controlled clinical trials in patients with rheumatoid arthritis, the rate of infections during the first 16 weeks of treatment was approximately 99, 100, or 82 events per 100 patient-years in patients receiving baricitinib 2 mg daily, baricitinib 4 mg daily, or placebo, respectively. Serious infections during the first 16 weeks were reported at a rate of 3.6, 3.7, or 4.2 events per 100 patient-years in patients receiving baricitinib 2 mg daily, baricitinib 4 mg daily, or placebo, respectively.

Patients should be closely monitored during and after treatment with baricitinib for the development of signs or symptoms of infection.

Baricitinib therapy should not be initiated in patients with serious active infections, including localized infections. Clinicians should consider potential risks and benefits of the drug prior to initiating therapy in patients with a history of chronic, recurring, serious, or opportunistic infections; patients with underlying conditions that may predispose them to infections; and patients who have been exposed to tuberculosis or who reside or have traveled in regions where tuberculosis or mycoses are endemic. Any patient who develops a new infection while receiving baricitinib should undergo a thorough diagnostic evaluation (appropriate for an immunocompromised patient), appropriate anti-infective therapy should be initiated, and the patient should be closely monitored. Baricitinib therapy should be interrupted in patients who develop an infection that fails to respond to anti-infective therapy, a serious infection, an opportunistic infection, or sepsis and should not be resumed until the infection is controlled.

Because tuberculosis has been reported in patients receiving baricitinib, all patients should be evaluated for active or latent tuberculosis prior to and periodically during therapy with the drug. Patients with active tuberculosis should not receive baricitinib. When indicated, an appropriate antimycobacterial regimen for the treatment of latent tuberculosis infection should be initiated prior to baricitinib therapy. Antimycobacterial therapy also should be considered prior to initiation of baricitinib in individuals with a history of latent or active tuberculosis in whom an adequate course of antimycobacterial therapy cannot be confirmed and in individuals with a negative test for latent tuberculosis who have risk factors for tuberculosis. Consultation with a tuberculosis specialist is recommended when deciding whether antimycobacterial therapy should be initiated. Patients receiving baricitinib, including individuals with a negative test for latent tuberculosis, should be monitored for signs and symptoms of active tuberculosis.

Viral reactivation can occur in patients receiving baricitinib. Herpes zoster reactivation has been reported in patients receiving the drug. If herpes zoster reactivation occurs, baricitinib therapy should be interrupted until the episode has resolved.

The risk of reactivation of chronic viral hepatitis in patients receiving baricitinib is not known. Patients with evidence of active hepatitis B virus (HBV) or hepatitis C virus (HCV) infection were excluded from clinical trials of baricitinib. All patients should be screened for viral hepatitis in accordance with current standards of care before initiation of baricitinib therapy. Patients testing positive for hepatitis C antibody but negative for HCV RNA may receive baricitinib. Patients testing positive for hepatitis B surface antibody (anti-HBs) and hepatitis B core antibody (anti-HBc) but negative for hepatitis B surface antigen (HBsAg) also may receive baricitinib but should be monitored for expression of HBV DNA; consultation with liver disease experts is recommended if HBV DNA is detected.

Mortality

A boxed warning regarding the increased risk of mortality is included in the prescribing information for baricitinib. In a large, randomized, postmarketing safety study of another JAK inhibitor (i.e., tofacitinib) in patients with rheumatoid arthritis who were ≥50 years of age with at least one cardiovascular risk factor, the rate of all-cause mortality, including sudden cardiovascular death, was higher in patients who received the JAK inhibitor compared with those who received a TNF blocking agent.

The risks and benefits of baricitinib should be considered prior to initiating therapy or when considering whether to continue baricitinib therapy.

Malignancies and Lymphoproliferative Disorders

A boxed warning regarding the risk of malignancies, including lymphomas, is included in the prescribing information for baricitinib. Lymphoma and other malignancies have been observed in patients receiving baricitinib.

In controlled clinical trials in patients with moderately to severely active rheumatoid arthritis, malignancies (excluding nonmelanoma skin cancer) were reported during the first 16 weeks of treatment at a rate of 0.7 or 0.3 events per 100 patient-years in patients receiving baricitinib 2 or 4 mg daily, respectively, and at a rate of 0 events per 100 patient-years in placebo recipients. In a long-term extension study, malignancies (excluding nonmelanoma skin cancer) were reported at a rate of 0.6 or 0.7 events per 100 patient-years in patients receiving baricitinib 2 or 4 mg daily, respectively, for up to 52 weeks.

In a large, randomized, postmarketing safety study of another JAK inhibitor in patients with rheumatoid arthritis, a higher rate of malignancies (excluding nonmelanoma skin cancer) was observed in patients treated with the JAK inhibitor compared to those treated with a TNF blocking agent. A higher rate of lymphomas was observed in patients treated with the JAK inhibitor compared to those treated with a TNF blocking agent. A higher rate of lung cancers also was observed in current or past smokers treated with the JAK inhibitor compared to those treated with a TNF blocking agent. In this study, current or past smokers had an additional increased risk of overall malignancies.

The risks and benefits of baricitinib should be considered prior to initiating therapy or when considering whether to continue baricitinib, particularly in patients with a known malignancy (other than successfully treated nonmelanoma skin cancer), in those who develop a malignancy, and those who are current or past smokers.

Because nonmelanoma skin cancers have been reported in patients receiving baricitinib, periodic dermatologic examinations are recommended for patients receiving the drug who are at increased risk for skin cancer.

Major Adverse Cardiovascular Events

A boxed warning regarding the increased risk of major adverse cardiovascular events is included in the prescribing information for baricitinib. In a large randomized safety clinical trial in patients ≥50 years of age with rheumatoid arthritis and at least one cardiovascular risk factor, the risk of major adverse cardiovascular events (i.e., cardiovascular death, nonfatal MI, nonfatal stroke) was increased in patients receiving another JAK inhibitor (i.e., tofacitinib 5 or 10 mg twice daily) compared with those receiving a tumor necrosis factor (TNF) blocking agent. Although the safety profile of other JAK inhibitors, such as baricitinib and upadacitinib, have not been studied in similar large safety clinical trials as tofacitinib, the FDA states that these drugs may also have similar risks based on their mechanisms of action. Based on findings of the postmarketing study, and to ensure the benefits of baricitinib outweigh its risks, use of baricitinib in all approved indications is limited to patients who have not responded to or cannot tolerate one or more TNF blocking agents.

The risks and benefits of baricitinib should be considered prior to initiating therapy or when considering whether to continue baricitinib, particularly in patients who are current or past smokers and in those with other cardiovascular risk factors. Patients receiving baricitinib should be advised to seek immediate medical attention if symptoms of serious cardiovascular events occur. In patients who experience MI or stroke, baricitinib therapy should be discontinued.

Thromboembolic Events

A boxed warning regarding the risk of thrombosis is included in the prescribing information for baricitinib. Serious and sometimes fatal thromboembolic events, including deep-vein thrombosis, pulmonary embolism, and arterial thrombosis in the extremities, have been reported in patients receiving baricitinib in controlled clinical trials. A relationship between platelet count elevation and thromboembolic events has not been established.

In controlled clinical trials in patients with moderately to severely active rheumatoid arthritis, venous thromboembolic events (i.e., deep-vein thrombosis or pulmonary embolism) were reported during the first 16 weeks of treatment at a rate of 1.7 events per 100 patient-years in patients receiving baricitinib 4 mg daily and in none of the patients receiving baricitinib 2 mg daily or placebo. In a long-term extension study, venous thromboembolic events were reported at a rate of 0.6 or 0.8 events per 100 patient-years in patients receiving baricitinib 2 or 4 mg daily, respectively, for up to 52 weeks. Arterial thromboembolic events were reported during the first 16 weeks of treatment at a rate of 1.4 or 0.7 events per 100 patient-years in patients receiving baricitinib 2 or 4 mg daily, respectively, and at a rate of 0.3 events per 100 patient-years in placebo recipients; following treatment for up to 52 weeks, the rate of arterial thromboembolic events was 0.9 or 0.3 events per 100 patient-years in patients receiving baricitinib 2 or 4 mg daily, respectively.

In a postmarketing study evaluating safety of another JAK inhibitor (i.e., tofacitinib) in patients ≥50 years of age with rheumatoid arthritis, analysis revealed higher incidences of thromboembolic events, including pulmonary embolism and deep-vein thrombosis, in patients receiving tofacitinib 10 mg twice daily compared with those receiving either tofacitinib 5 mg twice daily or a TNF blocking agent, each given in combination with methotrexate.

The risks and benefits of baricitinib should be considered prior to initiation of therapy in patients who may be at increased risk of thrombosis; baricitinib should be avoided in patients who may be at increased risk of thrombosis. Patients with signs or symptoms suggestive of thrombosis should discontinue baricitinib therapy and be evaluated promptly and treated appropriately.

Other Warnings and Precautions

Hypersensitivity Reactions

Hypersensitivity reactions (i.e., angioedema, urticaria, rash), sometimes serious, have been reported in patients receiving baricitinib in clinical trials. If a serious hypersensitivity reaction occurs, baricitinib should be discontinued while evaluating for other potential causes.

GI Perforation

Cases of GI perforation have been reported in patients receiving baricitinib in controlled clinical trials. The role of JAK inhibition by baricitinib in these cases is not known. Baricitinib should be used with caution in patients who may be at increased risk for GI perforation (e.g., patients with a history of diverticulitis). Patients with new onset of abdominal symptoms should be evaluated promptly for early identification of GI perforation.

Hematologic Effects

Lymphopenia with absolute lymphocyte count less than 500/mm³ has been reported in patients receiving baricitinib. Lymphocyte counts below the lower limit of normal were associated with infection in patients receiving baricitinib in controlled clinical trials. Lymphocyte counts should be monitored at baseline and periodically during treatment. Baricitinib therapy should not be initiated in patients with rheumatoid arthritis or alopecia areata with lymphocyte counts less than 500/mm³, and treatment should be interrupted if lymphocyte count decreases to less than 500/mm³. In patients with COVID-19, there is limited information on use of baricitinib with absolute lymphocyte counts less than 200/mm³; avoid initiation or interrupt treatment in these patients if absolute lymphocyte count is less than 200/mm³.

Neutropenia with absolute neutrophil count (ANC) less than 1000/mm³ has been reported in patients receiving baricitinib. Neutrophil counts should be monitored at baseline and periodically during treatment. Baricitinib therapy should not be initiated in patients with ANC less than 1000/mm³, and treatment should be interrupted if ANC decreases to less than 1000/mm³. In patients with COVID-19, there is limited information on use of baricitinib with ANC less than 1000/mm³; avoid initiation or interrupt treatment in these patients if ANC is less than 500/mm³.

Anemia with hemoglobin concentration less than 8 g/dL has been reported in patients receiving baricitinib. Hemoglobin concentrations should be monitored at baseline and periodically during treatment. Baricitinib therapy should not be initiated in patients with rheumatoid arthritis or alopecia areata with hemoglobin concentrations less than 8 g/dL, and treatment should be interrupted if hemoglobin concentration decreases to less than 8 g/dL. In patients with COVID-19, there is limited information on use of baricitinib in patients with hemoglobin less than 8 g/dL.

Dose-related increases in platelet count have been reported in patients receiving baricitinib. In controlled clinical trials in patients with rheumatoid arthritis, mean platelet counts at 16 weeks were increased by 15,000 or 23,000/mm³ in patients receiving baricitinib 2 or 4 mg daily, respectively, compared with a mean increase of 3000/mm³ in those who received placebo. A relationship between platelet count elevation and thromboembolic events has not been established.

Hepatic Effects

Baricitinib has been associated with elevated hepatic enzyme concentrations. ALT and AST elevations of at least 5 or 10 times the upper limit of normal (ULN), respectively, have been observed in controlled clinical trials.

Liver function tests should be monitored at baseline and periodically during treatment. In case of elevated hepatic enzyme concentrations, patients should be evaluated promptly for drug-induced hepatotoxicity. If drug-induced hepatic injury is suspected, baricitinib therapy should be interrupted until such diagnosis has been excluded.

Metabolic Effects

Dose-related increases in total cholesterol, low-density lipoprotein (LDL)-cholesterol, high-density lipoprotein (HDL)-cholesterol, and triglyceride concentrations have been observed in patients receiving baricitinib. Increases in these parameters were observed at 12 weeks of baricitinib therapy and concentrations remained stable thereafter. In controlled clinical trials, mean concentrations of LDL-cholesterol and HDL-cholesterol increased by 8 and 7 mg/dL, respectively, in patients receiving baricitinib 2 mg daily and by 14 and 9 mg/dL, respectively, in patients receiving baricitinib 4 mg daily. Mean ratios of LDL-cholesterol to HDL-cholesterol were essentially unchanged. Mean triglyceride concentrations increased by 7 or 15 mg/dL in patients receiving baricitinib 2 or 4 mg daily, respectively.

Lipid concentrations should be monitored approximately 12 weeks after initiation of baricitinib therapy for patients with rheumatoid arthritis or alopecia areata. Dyslipidemia should be managed according to current standards of care.

Immunization

Administration of live vaccines should be avoided during therapy with baricitinib. Immunizations should be updated according to current administration guidelines prior to initiation of baricitinib therapy for patients with rheumatoid arthritis or alopecia areata.

Specific Populations

Pregnancy

Based on findings from animal reproduction studies, baricitinib may cause fetal harm during pregnancy.

Reduced fetal body weight, dose-related increases in skeletal malformations, and embryolethality (in rabbits only) have been observed in rats and rabbits given baricitinib at dosages producing exposures of 11 and 46 times, respectively, the exposure at the maximum recommended human dosage. However, there was no evidence of developmental toxicity in rats and rabbits at exposure levels approximately 2 and 7 times, respectively, the exposure at the maximum recommended human dosage. Consider the association between increased disease activity and risk for adverse pregnancy outcomes in women with rheumatoid arthritis. Report pregnancies to the manufacturer according to instructions in the prescribing information.

Lactation

It is not known whether baricitinib is distributed into human milk; the drug is distributed into milk in rats. The effects of baricitinib on nursing infants or on milk production are not known. Because of the potential for serious adverse reactions to baricitinib in nursing infants, female patients should be advised not to breastfeed while receiving the drug and for 4 days after the last dose.

Females and Males of Reproductive Potential

Baricitinib may cause fetal harm when administered during pregnancy. Consider pregnancy planning and prevention for females of reproductive potential.

Pediatric Use

Safety and efficacy of baricitinib have not been established in pediatric patients with rheumatoid arthritis or alopecia areata.

The Emergency Use Authorization (EUA) permits use of baricitinib for the treatment of COVID-19 in hospitalized pediatric patients ≥2 years old†. Dosing recommendations are based on limited data from ongoing clinical trials evaluating use of baricitinib in pediatric patients with conditions other than COVID-19.

Geriatric Use

In controlled clinical trials of baricitinib in patients with rheumatoid arthritis, 17% of patients were 65 years of age or older, while 2% were 75 years of age and older. No overall differences in safety or efficacy relative to younger adults were observed, but increased sensitivity in some older individuals cannot be ruled out.

In controlled trials of baricitinib in patients with alopecia areata, approximately 2% of patients were 65 years of age or older; this number was insufficient to determine whether these patients respond differently from younger patients.

Dosage in geriatric patients should be selected with caution because of possible age-related decreases in renal function. Monitoring of renal function may be useful in such patients.

Hepatic Impairment

Systemic exposure to baricitinib is not substantially increased in individuals with moderate hepatic impairment. Therefore, no dosage adjustment is recommended in patients with mild or moderate hepatic impairment. Use of baricitinib has not been studied and is not recommended in patients with rheumatoid arthritis or alopecia areata and severe hepatic impairment.

When baricitinib is used for the treatment of COVID-19 in hospitalized adults and treatment of COVID-19 in hospitalized pediatric patients†, the drug should be used in patients with severe hepatic impairment only if the potential benefit outweighs the potential risk; the drug has not been studied in those with severe hepatic impairment.

Renal Impairment

Systemic exposure to baricitinib is increased by 1.41-, 2.22-, or 4.05-fold in individuals with mild, moderate, or severe renal impairment, respectively, and by 2.41-fold in individuals with end-stage renal disease receiving hemodialysis.

In patients with rheumatoid arthritis or alopecia areata and moderate renal impairment (estimated glomerular filtration rate [eGFR] 30 to less than 60 mL/minute per 1.73 m²), the recommended dosage of baricitinib should be reduced by half. Baricitinib is not recommended for these uses in patients with severe impairment (eGFR less than 30 mL/minute per 1.73 m²).

In hospitalized adult patients with COVID-19 and moderate renal impairment (eGFR 30 to less than 60 mL/minute per 1.73 m²) or severe renal impairment (eGFR less than 30 mL/minute per 1.73 m²), the recommended dosage of baricitinib is 2 mg once daily and 1 mg once daily, respectively. Baricitinib is not recommended for this use in patients who are on dialysis, have end-stage renal disease, or have an eGFR less than 15 mL/minute per 1.73 m².

● Common Adverse Effects

Adverse effects occurring in 1% or more of patients receiving baricitinib (2 or 4 mg daily) for the treatment of rheumatoid arthritis include upper respiratory tract infection, nausea, herpes simplex, and herpes zoster.

Adverse effects occurring in 1% or more of patients receiving baricitinib for the treatment of COVID-19 in hospitalized adults and in hospitalized pediatric patients† include increases of liver enzymes, thrombocytosis, creatine phosphokinase increases, neutropenia, deep vein thrombosis, pulmonary embolism, and urinary tract infection.

Adverse effects occurring in 1% or more of patients receiving baricitinib for the treatment of alopecia areata include upper respiratory tract infection, headache, acne, hyperlipidemia, blood creatine phosphokinase increase, urinary tract infection, liver enzyme elevations, folliculitis, fatigue, lower respiratory tract

infections, nausea, genital *Candida* infections, anemia, neutropenia, abdominal pain, herpes zoster, and weight increase.

DRUG INTERACTIONS

In vitro studies suggest that baricitinib is a substrate for organic anion transporter (OAT) 3, P-glycoprotein (P-gp), breast cancer resistance protein (BCRP), and multidrug and toxin extrusion transporter (MATE) 2K.

In vitro studies also suggest that baricitinib is a substrate for cytochrome P-450 (CYP) isoenzyme 3A4; however, concomitant administration of a CYP3A inducer (i.e., rifampin) or CYP3A inhibitors (i.e., fluconazole, ketoconazole) did not result in clinically important changes in the pharmacokinetics of baricitinib.

Baricitinib neither inhibits nor induces CYP isoenzymes 1A2, 2B6, 2C8, 2C9, 2C19, 2D6, or 3A in vitro. Baricitinib also does not inhibit P-gp or organic anion transporting polypeptide (OATP) 1B1 in vitro.

In vitro, baricitinib inhibits OAT1, OAT2, OAT3, organic cation transporter (OCT) 1, OCT2, OATP1B3, BCRP, MATE1, and MATE2K; however clinically important changes in the pharmacokinetics of drugs that are substrates of these transporters is unlikely.

● Drugs Affecting Organic Anion Transport

Concomitant use of baricitinib with potent inhibitors of OAT3 (e.g., probenecid) may result in substantially increased exposure to baricitinib. However, pharmacokinetic simulations using less-potent OAT3 inhibitors (e.g., diclofenac, ibuprofen) predicted minimal effect on the pharmacokinetics of baricitinib.

Rheumatoid arthritis, COVID-19, or Alopecia areata: In patients receiving concomitant therapy with potent inhibitors of OAT3 (e.g., probenecid), dosage of baricitinib should be reduced from 4 mg once daily to 2 mg once daily or from 2 mg once daily to 1 mg once daily. If the recommended baricitinib dose is 1 mg once daily, consider discontinuing probenecid.

● Biologic Antirheumatic Agents

Baricitinib should not be used concomitantly with biologic disease-modifying antirheumatic drugs (DMARDs).

● Immunosuppressive Agents

Concomitant use of baricitinib with other immunosuppressive agents may increase the risk of serious infection. Concomitant use with potent immunosuppressive agents (e.g., azathioprine, cyclosporine) is not recommended.

Concomitant administration of baricitinib and cyclosporine (an inhibitor of P-gp and BCRP) had no clinically important effect on the pharmacokinetics of baricitinib.

● Antifungal Agents

Concomitant administration of baricitinib and ketoconazole (a CYP3A inhibitor) or fluconazole (an inhibitor of CYP3A, 2C9, and 2C19) had no clinically important effects on the pharmacokinetics of baricitinib. Dosage adjustment of baricitinib is not necessary if used concomitantly with ketoconazole or fluconazole.

● Oral Contraceptives

Concomitant administration of baricitinib and an oral contraceptive containing ethinyl estradiol and levonorgestrel (CYP3A substrates) had no clinically important effects on the pharmacokinetics of the oral contraceptive components.

● Digoxin

Concomitant administration of baricitinib and digoxin (a P-gp substrate) had no clinically important effect on the pharmacokinetics of digoxin. Dosage adjustment of digoxin is not necessary with concomitant use.

● Methotrexate

Concomitant administration of baricitinib and methotrexate did not have clinically important effects on the pharmacokinetics of either drug. Dosage adjustments are not necessary if baricitinib is used concomitantly with methotrexate.

● *Omeprazole*

Concomitant administration of baricitinib and omeprazole had no clinically important effects on the pharmacokinetics of baricitinib. Dosage adjustment of baricitinib is not necessary if used concomitantly with omeprazole.

● *Probenecid*

Concomitant administration of baricitinib and probenecid (a potent OAT3 inhibitor) resulted in an approximately twofold increase in the area under the concentration-time curve (AUC) of baricitinib; peak plasma concentration of baricitinib was not affected. Concomitant use of baricitinib and probenecid is not recommended; however, if concomitant use is necessary, consider reducing the dosage of baricitinib.

Rheumatoid arthritis: In patients receiving concomitant therapy with potent inhibitors of OAT3 (e.g., probenecid), reduce dosage of baricitinib to 1 mg once daily.

COVID-19 in hospitalized adults and in hospitalized pediatric patients†: In patients receiving concomitant therapy with potent inhibitors of OAT3 (e.g., probenecid), reduce dosage of baricitinib from 4 mg once daily to 2 mg once daily or from 2 mg once daily to 1 mg once daily. If the recommended baricitinib dosage is 1 mg once daily, consider discontinuing probenecid.

● *Rifampin*

Concomitant administration of baricitinib and rifampin (a CYP inducer) had no clinically important effect on the pharmacokinetics of baricitinib. Dosage adjustment of baricitinib is not necessary if used concomitantly with rifampin.

● *Simvastatin*

Concomitant administration of baricitinib and simvastatin (a CYP3A substrate) had no clinically important effect on the pharmacokinetics of simvastatin. Dosage adjustment of simvastatin is not necessary with concomitant use.

● *Vaccines*

Live vaccines should not be administered to patients receiving baricitinib.

DESCRIPTION

Baricitinib, a Janus kinase (JAK) inhibitor, is an immunomodulating agent and a disease-modifying antirheumatic drug (DMARD). JAKs are a family of intracellular tyrosine kinases consisting of JAK1, JAK2, JAK3, and tyrosine kinase (TYK) 2 that mediate the signaling of cytokines and growth factors that are important for hematopoiesis and immune function. Binding of cytokines to receptors on the cell surface activates pairing of JAKs (e.g., JAK1/JAK2, JAK1/JAK3, JAK1/TYK2, JAK2/JAK2, JAK2/TYK2), which leads to phosphorylation and subsequent localization of signal transducer and activator of transcription (STAT) proteins to the nucleus and modulation of gene expression. Baricitinib modulates the cytokine signaling pathway at the point of JAKs, preventing the phosphorylation and activation of STATs. In vitro, baricitinib has greater inhibitory potency at JAK1 and JAK2 and, to a lesser extent, TYK2 relative to JAK3, and the drug inhibits cytokine-induced STAT phosphorylation mediated by JAK1/JAK2, JAK1/JAK3, JAK1/TYK2, or JAK2/TYK2 combinations with comparable potencies. The relevance of inhibition of specific JAKs to the therapeutic efficacy of baricitinib is not known.

Baricitinib has been shown to cause dose-dependent inhibition of interleukin-6 (IL-6)-induced STAT3 phosphorylation in whole blood of healthy individuals, with maximal inhibition observed approximately 1 hour after dosing and a return to near baseline activity by 24 hours.

In clinical trials, mean serum concentrations of IgG, IgM, and IgA decreased within 12 weeks of initiation of baricitinib and then remained stable through 52 weeks of therapy; changes in concentrations of these immunoglobulins generally occurred within normal reference ranges. Decreases in serum C-reactive protein (CRP) concentrations were observed as early as 1 week in patients with rheumatoid arthritis receiving baricitinib; these decreases were maintained throughout treatment.

Following oral administration, peak plasma concentrations of baricitinib are achieved in approximately 1 hour. Following repeated once-daily dosing, steady-state concentrations of the drug are attained in 2–3 days with minimal accumulation.

Administration with a high-fat meal delays time to peak plasma concentration by 0.5 hours and reduces the area under the concentration-time curve (AUC) and peak plasma concentrations of the drug by 11 and 18%, respectively; these effects on drug exposure are not considered clinically important. The absolute oral bioavailability of baricitinib is approximately 80%. Baricitinib is approximately 50% bound to plasma proteins and 45% bound to serum proteins. Baricitinib is eliminated principally by renal filtration and active secretion. Approximately 69% of an orally administered dose is eliminated in urine as unchanged drug, 15% is eliminated in feces as unchanged drug, and 6% is eliminated as metabolites. Metabolism of the drug is mediated mainly by cytochrome P-450 (CYP) isoenzyme 3A4. The elimination half-life of baricitinib is approximately 12–16 hours in patients with rheumatoid arthritis and alopecia areata. The elimination half-life of baricitinib in hospitalized adults with COVID-19 who are intubated and have baricitinib administered via nasogastric or orogastric tube is 10.8 hours. The pharmacokinetics of baricitinib are not affected by age, gender, body weight, or race.

ADVICE TO PATIENTS

● Importance of advising patients about potential benefits and risks of baricitinib. Importance of patients reading the medication guide prior to initiation of therapy and each time the prescription is refilled.

● Importance of informing clinicians of existing or contemplated concomitant therapy, including prescription and OTC drugs, as well as any concomitant illnesses or any history of cancer, thromboembolism, diverticulitis, gastric or intestinal ulcers, tuberculosis, hepatitis B virus or hepatitis C virus infection, or other chronic or recurring infections.

● Increased susceptibility to infection. Risk of herpes zoster, which may be serious. Importance of promptly informing clinicians if any signs or symptoms of infection (e.g., fever, sweating, chills, myalgia, cough, dyspnea, fatigue, diarrhea, dysuria, erythema) develop.

● Risk of lymphoma and other malignancies. Importance of periodic skin examinations.

● Risk of major adverse cardiovascular events, including MI, stroke, and cardiovascular death. Instruct all patients, especially current or past smokers and those with other cardiovascular risk factors, to monitor for the development of signs and symptoms of cardiovascular events.

● Risk of thromboembolic events. Importance of contacting clinicians if symptoms of thromboembolism (e.g., shortness of breath; chest pain; swelling, pain, or tenderness in the leg) develop.

● Risk of GI perforation. Importance of seeking immediate medical care if abdominal pain, fever, chills, nausea, or vomiting occur.

● Risk of hypersensitivity reactions. Importance of seeking immediate medical attention if signs and symptoms of serious allergic reactions occur.

● Importance of periodic laboratory monitoring.

● Importance of informing clinicians of receipt of baricitinib prior to any potential vaccinations.

● Importance of females informing clinicians if they are or plan to become pregnant or plan to breast-feed.

● Importance of informing patients of other important precautionary information. (See Cautions.)

● Prior to administration of baricitinib for treatment of COVID-19 in hospitalized pediatric patients 2 years of age and older, the patient or their caregiver must be provided with information consistent with the Fact Sheet for Patients, Parents and Caregivers Emergency Use Authorization (EUA) of baricitinib and given a copy of the fact sheet or directed to the manufacturer's website to obtain the fact sheet.

● Inform recipients or their caregivers that FDA authorized the emergency use of the baricitinib for treatment of COVID-19 in hospitalized pediatric patients 2 years of age and older, which is an investigational treatment that has not received FDA approval. In addition, inform the parent/caregiver (and patient if age-appropriate) that they have the option to accept or refuse baricitinib, inform them about important known and potential risks and benefits of baricitinib and the extent to which risks and benefits are unknown, and provide information on available alternative treatments and the risks and benefits of those alternatives.

PREPARATIONS

Distribution of baricitinib is restricted. Consult manufacturer's website for specific information regarding distribution of the drug.

For use of baricitinib under the FDA Emergency Use Authorization (EUA), inpatient pharmacies may obtain baricitinib directly from an Authorized Distributor of Record. Consult the manufacturer's website for a list of Authorized Distributors of Record (https://www.lillytrade.com/) or the EUA for additional information regarding access to the drug.

Excipients in commercially available drug preparations may have clinically important effects in some individuals; consult specific product labeling for details.

Baricitinib

Oral		
Tablets, film-coated	1 mg	Olumiant®, Lilly
	2 mg	Olumiant®, Lilly
	4 mg	Olumiant®, Lilly

† Use is not currently included in the labeling approved by the US Food and Drug Administration.

Selected Revisions May 10, 2024, © Copyright, June 20, 2018, American Society of Health-System Pharmacists, Inc.

Tofacitinib Citrate

90:24.12.92 • JANUS KINASE INHIBITORS, MISCELLANEOUS

■ Tofacitinib citrate, a Janus kinase (JAK) inhibitor, is an immunomodulating agent and a disease-modifying antirheumatic drug (DMARD).

USES

● *Rheumatoid Arthritis*

Tofacitinib citrate (as conventional or extended-release tablets) is used for the management of moderately to severely active rheumatoid arthritis in adults who have had an inadequate response or intolerance to one or more tumor necrosis factor (TNF) blocking agents. Tofacitinib has been shown to induce clinical responses, improve physical function, and inhibit progression of structural damage in patients with rheumatoid arthritis. Safety and efficacy of tofacitinib in the treatment of rheumatoid arthritis in adults is principally based on results from 5 randomized controlled trials. Guidelines generally support use of Janus kinase (JAK) inhibitors, including tofacitinib, as add on therapy to methotrexate in patients who do not meet treatment goals with methotrexate alone.

Tofacitinib can be used alone or in combination with methotrexate or other nonbiologic disease-modifying antirheumatic drugs (DMARDs; examples include hydroxychloroquine, leflunomide, and sulfasalazine). Concomitant use of tofacitinib with biologic DMARDs, such as TNF blocking agents (e.g., adalimumab, certolizumab pegol, etanercept, golimumab, infliximab), interleukin-1 (IL-1) receptor antagonists (e.g., anakinra), anti-CD20 monoclonal antibodies (e.g., rituximab), selective costimulation modulators (e.g., abatacept), and anti-interleukin-6-receptor monoclonal antibodies (e.g., sarilumab, tocilizumab), is not recommended. Concomitant use of tofacitinib with potent immunosuppressive agents (e.g., azathioprine, cyclosporine) also is not recommended.

Clinical Experience

Safety and efficacy of tofacitinib have been evaluated in 6 randomized, double-blind, controlled studies of 6–24 months' duration in adults (18 years of age or older) with moderate to severe active rheumatoid arthritis. In these studies, tofacitinib was administered as monotherapy in patients with an inadequate response to at least one biologic or nonbiologic DMARD, in combination with methotrexate in patients with an inadequate response to methotrexate or at least one TNF blocking agent, or in combination with nonbiologic DMARD(s) in patients with an inadequate response to at least one biologic or nonbiologic DMARD. Patients in these studies generally had 6 or more tender joints and 6 or more swollen joints. Those receiving low stable dosages of corticosteroids (equivalent to 10 mg or less of prednisone daily) and/or stable dosages of nonsteroidal anti-inflammatory agents (NSAIAs) generally could continue such agents. In some studies, patients also were allowed to continue stable dosages of DMARD antimalarial agents. Tofacitinib was administered orally at a dosage of 5 or 10 mg twice daily (as conventional tablets). In all 5 studies, patients randomized to receive placebo were subsequently advanced in a blinded manner to a second predetermined treatment of tofacitinib 5 or 10 mg twice daily. Advancement to tofacitinib therapy occurred at 3 months in clinical studies of 6 months' duration. In studies of at least 12 months' duration, treatment was advanced at 3 months in placebo recipients who were nonresponders and at 6 months in all other placebo recipients.

The principal measures of clinical response in studies evaluating the efficacy of tofacitinib were the American College of Rheumatology criteria for improvement (ACR response) in measures of disease activity, changes in the Health Assessment Questionnaire–Disability Index (HAQ-DI, a measure of physical function and disability), and achievement of a Disease Activity Score (DAS28 [ESR]) of less than 2.6 (i.e., DAS-defined remission) at 3 or 6 months. DAS28 (ESR) is a composite index of 4 weighted variables: swollen and tender counts for 28 joints, patient global assessment, and erythrocyte sedimentation rate (ESR). An ACR 20 response is achieved if the patient experiences a 20% or greater improvement in tender and swollen joint count and a 20% or greater improvement in at least 3 of the following criteria: patient pain assessment, patient global assessment, physician global assessment, patient self-assessed disability, or laboratory measures of disease activity (i.e., ESR or C-reactive protein [CRP] concentrations). An ACR 50 or ACR 70 response is defined using the same criteria but with a level of improvement of 50 or 70%, respectively. Structural damage, as measured by changes in the total modified Sharp/van der Heijde score, a composite measure of radiographically assessed structural damage (i.e., joint erosion and joint space narrowing), also was assessed in the 2-year study.

Clinical evaluations of tofacitinib indicate that, in adults with active rheumatoid arthritis despite therapy with methotrexate or other DMARD(s), administration of tofacitinib (alone or in combination with methotrexate or other nonbiologic DMARDs) at a dosage of 5 or 10 mg twice daily (as conventional tablets) results in higher ACR 20, ACR 50, and ACR 70 response rates at 3 and 6 months compared with placebo. In clinical trials, higher ACR 20 response rates compared with placebo were observed within 2 weeks. In clinical trials with a duration of at least 12 months, ACR response rates and HAQ-DI results were consistent at 6 and 12 months in patients receiving tofacitinib. Across the 5 clinical trials, improvements in HAQ-DI scores for tofacitinib versus placebo were similar.

In a 6-month study evaluating tofacitinib as monotherapy, 610 patients who had an inadequate response to prior DMARD therapy (biologic or nonbiologic) received tofacitinib 5 mg twice daily, tofacitinib 10 mg twice daily, or placebo. An ACR 20 response at 3 months was achieved in 59, 65, or 26% of patients receiving tofacitinib 5 mg twice daily, tofacitinib 10 mg twice daily, or placebo, respectively. The ACR 20 response rate following 6 months of therapy with tofacitinib 5 or 10 mg twice daily was 69 or 70%, respectively. Patients receiving tofacitinib experienced greater improvements in physical functioning (as measured by change in HAQ-DI score) from baseline to 3 months, but were not substantially more likely to achieve DAS-defined remission at 3 months, compared with patients receiving placebo.

In a 12-month clinical study evaluating concomitant therapy with tofacitinib and methotrexate, 717 patients with an inadequate response to prior methotrexate therapy were randomized to receive tofacitinib 5 or 10 mg twice daily, adalimumab 40 mg subcutaneously every other week, or placebo, each given in conjunction with a stable dosage of methotrexate. Patients receiving tofacitinib 5 or 10 mg twice daily demonstrated greater improvement from baseline in physical functioning at 3 months compared with patients receiving placebo. The mean difference from placebo in HAQ-DI improvement from baseline was -0.22 or -0.32 in patients receiving tofacitinib 5 or 10 mg twice daily, respectively. At 6 months, an ACR 20 response was achieved in 52, 53, 47, or 28% and DAS-defined remission was achieved in 6, 13, 7, or 1% of patients assigned to receive tofacitinib 5 mg twice daily, tofacitinib 10 mg twice daily, adalimumab, or placebo, respectively; in these analyses, in order to account for patients who switched from placebo to tofacitinib at 3 months, patients who did not respond by 3 months were considered nonresponders even if they responded after 3 months.

In a 24-month clinical study evaluating concomitant therapy with tofacitinib and methotrexate, 797 patients with an inadequate response to prior methotrexate therapy were randomized to receive tofacitinib 5 or 10 mg twice daily or placebo, each given in conjunction with a stable dosage of methotrexate. Patients receiving tofacitinib 10 mg twice daily, but not those receiving tofacitinib 5 mg twice daily, demonstrated greater improvement from baseline in HAQ-DI scores at 3 months compared with patients receiving placebo. An ACR 20 response at 3 months was achieved in 55, 67, or 27% of patients receiving tofacitinib 5 mg twice daily, tofacitinib 10 mg twice daily, or placebo, respectively; at 6 months, ACR 20 response rates were 50, 62, and 25%, respectively. DAS-defined remission at 6 months was reported in 6, 13, or 1% of patients assigned to receive tofacitinib 5 mg twice daily, tofacitinib 10 mg twice daily, or placebo, respectively. In these analyses, patients who did not achieve a response by month 3 were considered nonresponders even if they achieved a response after month 3. At 6 months, tofacitinib 10 mg twice daily inhibited progression of structural damage, as measured by mean change in the total modified Sharp/van der Heijde score, compared with placebo; the difference between tofacitinib 5 mg twice daily and placebo did not reach statistical significance. At 6 months, 84 or 79% of patients receiving tofacitinib 5 or 10 mg twice daily, respectively, had no progression of structural damage compared with 74% of those receiving placebo. Although radiographic findings from this study suggested that tofacitinib slows progression of joint damage, interpretation of the results is complicated because the proportion of study patients with radiographic progression of structural damage during this time period was small, approximately one-half of placebo recipients were considered nonresponders at 3 months and were advanced to a tofacitinib regimen, and missing data created problems with analysis. Analysis of outcomes at study completion revealed that among 539 patients who completed 24 months of treatment, the proportion of patients who achieved disease remission or low disease activity was maintained from month 12 to month 24 and were similar between tofacitinib 5 or 10 mg twice daily. Similarly, disease progression as measured by changes in Sharp/van der Heijde score, Erosion score, and Joint Space Narrowing score indicated that progression was minimal between month 12 and month 24 and was similar between tofacitinib dosages.

Another 6-month clinical study evaluated concomitant therapy with tofacitinib and methotrexate in 399 patients with an inadequate response to prior therapy with at least one TNF blocking agent; patients were randomized to receive tofacitinib 5 or 10 mg twice daily or placebo, each given in conjunction with a stable dosage of methotrexate. An ACR 20 response at 3 months was achieved in 41, 48, or 24% of patients receiving tofacitinib 5 mg twice daily, tofacitinib 10 mg twice daily, or placebo, respectively. The ACR 20 response rate following 6 months of therapy with tofacitinib 5 or 10 mg twice daily was 51 or 54%, respectively. Patients receiving tofacitinib experienced greater improvements in physical functioning (as measured by change in HAQ-DI score) from baseline to 3 months and were substantially more likely to achieve DAS-defined remission at 3 months compared with patients receiving placebo. DAS-defined remission was reported at 3 months in 7, 9, or 2% of patients receiving tofacitinib 5 mg twice daily, tofacitinib 10 mg twice daily, or placebo, respectively. The DAS-defined remission rate following 6 months of therapy with tofacitinib 5 or 10 mg twice daily was 8 or 15%, respectively.

In a 12-month study in 792 patients with an inadequate response to at least one biologic or nonbiologic DMARD, tofacitinib 5 or 10 mg twice daily or placebo was added to a stable dosage of a nonbiologic DMARD (excluding potent immunosuppressive agents such as azathioprine or cyclosporine). ACR responses and improvements in physical functioning generally were similar to those observed in other clinical studies evaluating tofacitinib for management of rheumatoid arthritis.

A sixth clinical study, which was conducted in 952 adults with moderately to severely active rheumatoid arthritis who had never received methotrexate therapy, provided additional evidence that tofacitinib inhibits progression of joint damage. In this 2-year study, patients were randomized to receive tofacitinib 5 or 10 mg twice daily (as conventional tablets) or methotrexate (initiated at a dosage of 10 mg weekly and increased to 20 mg weekly, if tolerated, by week 8). At 6 and 12 months, tofacitinib 5 or 10 mg twice daily inhibited progression of structural damage, as measured by the mean change from baseline in the total modified Sharp/van der Heijde score, compared with methotrexate. At 6 months, 73 or 77% of patients receiving tofacitinib 5 or 10 mg twice daily, respectively, had no progression of structural damage compared with 55% of patients receiving methotrexate.

Although other dosages of tofacitinib have been studied, the recommended dosage of tofacitinib for the management of rheumatoid arthritis in adults is 5 mg twice daily (as conventional tablets) or 11 mg once daily (as extended-release tablets). A dosage of 10 mg twice daily (as conventional tablets) or 22 mg once daily (as extended-release tablets) is *not* recommended for the management of rheumatoid arthritis.

For further information on the treatment of rheumatoid arthritis, see Uses: Rheumatoid Arthritis, in Methotrexate 10:00.

Clinical Perspective

The American College of Rheumatology issued guidelines for the treatment of rheumatoid arthritis in 2021. Disease-modifying treatments for rheumatoid arthritis include nonbiologic DMARDs (e.g., hydroxychloroquine, leflunomide, methotrexate, sulfasalazine), biologic DMARDs (e.g., TNF blocking agents, abatacept, tocilizumab, sarilumab, rituximab), and/or targeted synthetic DMARDs (e.g., Janus kinase [JAK] inhibitors). Specific agents for rheumatoid arthritis treatment are selected according to current disease activity, prior therapies used, and the presence of comorbidities. A "treat-to-target" approach is typically employed, with the goal of achieving a predefined target of low disease activity or remission.

Targeted synthetic DMARDs used in the treatment of rheumatoid arthritis include the JAK inhibitors baricitinib, tofacitinib, and upadacitinib. Methotrexate monotherapy is strongly recommended over biologic or targeted synthetic DMARD monotherapy in DMARD-naive patients with moderate to high disease activity. Methotrexate monotherapy also is strongly preferred over combined therapy with a non-TNF blocking agent biologic DMARD or targeted synthetic

DMARD because of the lack of proven benefit and additional risks and costs associated with combined therapy. Randomized controlled trials evaluating add-on therapy with a biologic or targeted synthetic DMARD or triple therapy (methotrexate, sulfasalazine, and hydroxychloroquine) demonstrated equivalent long-term outcomes in patients with receiving add-on therapy with a biologic or targeted synthetic DMARD and those receiving triple therapy; therefore, targeted synthetic DMARDs and biologic DMARDs (including TNF blocking agents) are conditionally recommended as add-on therapy for patients with an inadequate response to maximally tolerated doses of methotrexate. Recommendations for the use and selection of targeted synthetic DMARDs in rheumatoid arthritis vary based on the presence of certain comorbidities (e.g., heart failure, previous serious infection, nontuberculous mycobacterial lung disease). Consult the American College of Rheumatology guidelines for additional details.

● *Juvenile Idiopathic Arthritis*

Tofacitinib (as oral solution or conventional tablets) is used for the management of active polyarticular-course juvenile idiopathic arthritis (JIA) in pediatric patients 2 years of age and older who have had an inadequate response or intolerance to one or more TNF blocking agents. Tofacitinib has been shown to reduce disease flares in such patients. Concomitant use of tofacitinib with biologic DMARDs or with potent immunosuppressive agents (e.g., azathioprine, cyclosporine) is not recommended. Safety and efficacy of tofacitinib in polyarticular-course JIA is based principally on the results of a randomized controlled trial.

Clinical Experience

Efficacy and safety of tofacitinib for the management of polyarticular-course JIA has been evaluated in a double-blind, placebo-controlled, randomized-withdrawal study (NCT02592434) in pediatric patients 2–17 years of age with active polyarthritis. The study included patients with rheumatoid factor (RF)-negative polyarthritis (46%), RF-positive polyarthritis (17%), extended oligoarthritis (12%), or systemic JIA with active arthritis but without systemic manifestations (6%) who had an inadequate response or intolerance to one or more DMARDs (methotrexate or biologic agents), as well as pediatric patients with juvenile psoriatic arthritis (9%) or enthesitis-related arthritis (9%) who had an inadequate response to non-steroidal anti-inflammatory agents (NSAIAs). The principal measures of clinical response were the ACR core criteria for juvenile idiopathic arthritis (JIA ACR criteria). A JIA ACR 30 response is achieved if the patient experiences a 30% or greater improvement in at least 3 of the following 6 criteria, with no more than 1 criterion worsening by more than 30%: number of active joints, number of joints with limited range of motion, physician's global assessment of disease activity, parent's or patient's global assessment of overall well-being, physical function, and ESR.

Following an 18-week, run-in period during which 225 patients received open-label treatment with tofacitinib (5 mg twice daily or an equivalent, weight-based, twice-daily dosage), those who achieved a JIA ACR 30 response were randomized to receive tofacitinib (5 mg twice daily or an equivalent, weight-based, twice-daily dosage) or placebo for 26 weeks; tofacitinib was administered as oral solution or conventional tablets. During both treatment periods, approximately one-third of patients received oral corticosteroids and approximately two-thirds received methotrexate concomitantly; concomitant use of biologic agents or DMARDs other than methotrexate was not permitted. A total of 173 patients were entered into the 26-week randomized-withdrawal period. Over this period, a smaller proportion of tofacitinib-treated patients compared with placebo recipients (31 versus 55%) experienced disease flares (defined as worsening of at least 30% from baseline in at least 3 of the 6 JIA ACR core criteria and improvement of at least 30% in no more than 1 of the core criteria).

Clinical Perspective

Polyarticular JIA is characterized by involvement of more than 5 joints. Because of the prolonged course of active disease, children with polyarticular-course JIA are often refractory to treatment compared with children without polyarticular disease, and are at greater risk for joint damage, poor functional outcome, and decreased quality of life.

The American College of Rheumatology and the Arthritis Foundation issued a joint guideline for the treatment of juvenile idiopathic arthritis manifesting as nonsystemic polyarthritis (including polyarticular disease), sacroiliitis, or enthesitis in 2019. Several drug classes are used to treat juvenile idiopathic arthritis, including NSAIAs, systemic and intra-articular corticosteroids, nonbiologic

DMARDs (e.g., methotrexate, sulfasalazine, hydroxychloroquine, leflunomide), and biologic DMARDs (e.g., TNF blocking agents, abatacept, tocilizumab, rituximab). Specific agents for juvenile idiopathic arthritis treatment are selected according to the presence of certain risk factors (e.g., positive anti-cyclic citrullinated peptide antibodies, positive rheumatoid factor, joint damage), level of disease activity, involvement of specific joints, presence of certain comorbidities (e.g., uveitis), and prior therapies used. An individualized "treat-to-target" approach is typically employed, with the goal of achieving remission or minimal/low disease activity.

● Psoriatic Arthritis

Tofacitinib citrate (as conventional or extended-release tablets) is used for the management of active psoriatic arthritis in adults who have had an inadequate response or intolerance to one or more TNF blocking agents. Tofacitinib has been shown to induce clinical responses and improve physical functioning in patients with psoriatic arthritis. Concomitant use of tofacitinib with biologic DMARDs or with potent immunosuppressive agents (e.g., azathioprine, cyclosporine) is not recommended. Safety and efficacy of tofacitinib in treatment of psoriatic arthritis is based principally on the results of 2 randomized controlled trials. Guidelines for the treatment of psoriatic arthritis generally recommend that patients with active disease despite treatment with an oral small molecule or with a TNF blocking agent be switched to a TNF blocking agent, an IL-17 inhibitor, or an IL-12/23 inhibitor instead of switching to tofacitinib. Tofacitinib may also be used if oral administration is preferred by the patient or if the patient has a history of recurrent or severe Candida infection.

Clinical Experience

Efficacy and safety of tofacitinib for the management of psoriatic arthritis in adults have been established in 2 randomized, double-blind studies. OPAL Broaden was a 12-month active-and placebo-controlled study in 422 patients who had not responded adequately to at least one nonbiologic DMARD and had not received prior therapy with a TNF blocking agent. OPAL Beyond was a 6-month placebo-controlled study in 394 patients with a history of inadequate response or intolerance to at least one TNF blocking agent. Patients in both studies had active psoriatic arthritis (with at least 3 tender/painful joints and at least 3 swollen joints) and active plaque psoriasis. In OPAL Broaden, patients were randomized in a 2:2:2:1:1 ratio to receive tofacitinib 5 mg twice daily, tofacitinib 10 mg twice daily, adalimumab 40 mg every 2 weeks, placebo for 3 months followed by tofacitinib 5 mg twice daily, or placebo for 3 months followed by tofacitinib 10 mg twice daily. In OPAL Beyond, patients were randomized in 2:2:1:1 ratio to receive tofacitinib 5 mg twice daily, tofacitinib 10 mg twice daily, placebo for 3 months followed by tofacitinib 5 mg twice daily, or placebo for 3 months followed by tofacitinib 10 mg twice daily. Patients in these studies received tofacitinib as conventional tablets. Patients in both studies received concomitant therapy with a stable dosage of a single nonbiologic DMARD, most commonly methotrexate, throughout the study. The primary measures of efficacy were the proportion of patients achieving an ACR 20 response at 3 months and the change from baseline in HAQ-DI score at 3 months; ACR 50 and ACR 70 responses also were assessed. OPAL Broaden was not designed to evaluate noninferiority or superiority of tofacitinib compared with adalimumab.

Patients enrolled in the 2 studies had various manifestations of psoriatic arthritis: involvement of more than 5 joints (90%), distal interphalangeal joint involvement (61%), involvement of fewer than 5 joints or asymmetric involvement (21%), spondylitis (19%), and arthritis mutilans (8%). Enthesitis or dactylitis was present in 80 or 53% of patients, respectively. The mean duration of the disease prior to enrollment in OPAL Broaden or OPAL Beyond was 6 or 9.4 years, respectively. In OPAL Beyond, 66, 19, or 15% of patients had experienced treatment failure following use of 1, 2, or at least 3 TNF blocking agents, respectively.

A greater proportion of patients receiving tofacitinib (5 or 10 mg twice daily) compared with those receiving placebo achieved ACR 20, ACR 50, and ACR 70 responses at 3 months in OPAL Broaden and ACR 20 and ACR 50 responses in OPAL Beyond. In these 2 studies, ACR 20, ACR 50, and ACR 70 responses were achieved at 3 months in 50, 28–30, and 17%, respectively, of patients receiving tofacitinib 5 mg twice daily; 47–61, 28–40, and 14%, respectively, of patients receiving tofacitinib 10 mg twice daily; 52, 33, and 19%, respectively, of those receiving adalimumab 40 mg every 2 weeks (in OPAL Broaden); and 24–33, 10–15, and 5–10%, respectively, of those receiving placebo. Improvement in ACR 20 response was observed within 2 weeks following initiation of tofacitinib

therapy. ACR responses were maintained through the end of the studies (6 or 12 months), but could not be compared with placebo because of the advancement from placebo to tofacitinib at 3 months. Improvements in dactylitis and enthesitis also were observed in tofacitinib-treated patients.

Improvements in physical function, as measured by change in HAQ-DI score from baseline to 3 months, were greater in both studies for patients receiving tofacitinib 5 or 10 mg twice daily compared with those receiving placebo. In the 2 studies, 50–53 of patients receiving tofacitinib 5 mg twice daily and 41–55% of those receiving tofacitinib 10 mg twice daily achieved a HAQ-DI response (defined as improvement from baseline to 3 months of 0.35 or greater) compared with 28–31% of those receiving placebo.

Although radiographic evaluations were performed at baseline and 12 months in OPAL Broaden, all placebo recipients were advanced to tofacitinib therapy at 3 months and mean change in total modified Sharp/van der Heijde score from baseline to 12 months was minimal in all treatment groups in this study. Comparisons between the tofacitinib groups and the placebo or adalimumab groups were insufficient to establish an effect of tofacitinib on progression of structural damage in patients with psoriatic arthritis.

Although other dosages of tofacitinib have been studied, the recommended dosage of tofacitinib for the management of psoriatic arthritis in adults is 5 mg twice daily (as conventional tablets) or 11 mg once daily (as extended-release tablets). A dosage of 10 mg twice daily (as conventional tablets) or 22 mg once daily (as extended-release tablets) is *not* recommended for the management of psoriatic arthritis.

Clinical Perspective

The American College of Rheumatology and the National Psoriasis Foundation issued a joint guideline for the treatment of psoriatic arthritis in 2018. Nonpharmacologic (e.g., physical therapy, occupational therapy, smoking cessation, weight loss, exercise, massage therapy) and pharmacologic therapy can ameliorate psoriatic arthritis symptoms and can occasionally result in disease remission. Disease-modifying treatments for psoriatic arthritis include nonbiologic DMARDs (e.g., methotrexate, sulfasalazine, cyclosporine, leflunomide, apremilast), biologic DMARDs (e.g., TNF blocking agents, secukinumab, ixekizumab, ustekinumab, brodalumab, abatacept), and/or targeted synthetic DMARDs (e.g., Janus kinase [JAK] inhibitors). Specific agents for psoriatic arthritis treatment are selected according to disease characteristics, including disease severity, as well as patient preferences and comorbidities. A "treat-to-target" approach is typically employed, with the goal of achieving low/minimal disease activity or remission.

Tofacitinib is a targeted synthetic DMARD that is used in the treatment of psoriatic arthritis, generally in patients with disease activity despite treatment. ACR and NPF conditionally recommend switching to a TNF blocking agent, IL-17 inhibitor, or IL-12/23 inhibitor over switching to tofacitinib therapy in adults with active disease despite treatment with nonbiologic DMARDs; however, clinicians should consider patient preferences and characteristics (e.g., administration route, comorbidities, risk of bacterial or fungal infection). Consult the American College of Rheumatology/National Psoriasis Foundation guideline for additional details.

● Ankylosing Spondylitis

Tofacitinib citrate (as conventional or extended-release tablets) is used for the treatment of adults with active ankylosing spondylitis who have had an inadequate response or intolerance to one or more TNF blocking agents. Concomitant use of tofacitinib with biologic DMARDs or with potent immunosuppressive agents (e.g., azathioprine, cyclosporine) is not recommended. Safety and efficacy of tofacitinib for this use is based principally on the results of a placebo-controlled, randomized trial. Guidelines for the treatment of ankylosing spondylitis generally recommend other agents, including conventional synthetic DMARDs, TNF blocking agents, secukinumab, and ixekizumab over treatment with tofacitinib in patients with active disease.

Clinical Experience

Efficacy and safety of tofacitinib in ankylosing spondylitis have been assessed in one placebo-controlled, randomized, double-blind trial. In this study, 269 adults with active ankylosing spondylitis (defined by both Bath Ankylosing Spondylitis Disease Activity Index [BASDAI] and back pain score of 4 or greater despite therapy with an NSAIA, corticosteroid, or DMARD) were randomized to receive tofacitinib 5 mg twice daily for 16 weeks followed by tofacitinib 5 mg twice daily for 32 weeks, or placebo for 16 weeks followed by tofacitinib 5 mg twice daily for 32 weeks. Approximately 7 or 21% of enrolled patients received concomitant methotrexate or sulfasalazine, respectively, from baseline to week 16. The primary endpoint was the proportion of patients who achieved a response (defined as an Assessment of SpondyloArthritis International Society score of at least 20% improvement [ASAS20]) at 16 weeks. The mean age of enrolled patients was approximately 40–42 years; 80–87% of patients were male, 78–81% were white, and 22% did not achieve an adequate response to 1 or 2 TNF blocking agents.

At week 16, patients treated with tofacitinib 5 mg twice daily achieved substantially greater improvements in ASAS20 (56 versus 29%) and ASAS40 (41 versus 13%) responses compared to placebo. In the subgroup of patients who had an inadequate response to TNF blocking agents, ASAS20 and ASAS40 response rates were 41 or 28%, respectively, in patients receiving tofacitinib 5 mg twice daily and 17 or 7%, respectively, in placebo recipients.

Clinical Perspective

The American College of Rheumatology (ACR), the Spondylitis Association of America (SAA), and the Spondyloarthritis Research and Treatment Network (SPARTAN) issued a joint guideline for the treatment of ankylosing spondylitis in 2019. Treatments for ankylosing spondylitis include NSAIAs, nonbiologic DMARDs (e.g., methotrexate, sulfasalazine), biologic DMARDs (e.g., TNF blocking agents, secukinumab, ixekizumab), and/or targeted synthetic DMARDs (e.g., tofacitinib). Specific agents for ankylosing spondylitis treatment are selected according to current disease activity, prior therapies, and the presence of comorbidities. Treatment goals in ankylosing spondylitis include amelioration of symptoms, improved functioning, maintained ability to work, decreased complications, and prevention or slowing of skeletal damage.

Tofacitinib is a targeted synthetic DMARD used in the treatment of ankylosing spondylitis. For adults with active ankylosing spondylitis despite treatment with NSAIAs, ACR/SAA/SPARTAN conditionally recommend secukinumab or ixekizumab over treatment with tofacitinib, and in those who have contraindications to TNF blocking agents, secukinumab or ixekizumab are conditionally recommended over treatment with methotrexate, sulfasalazine, or tofacitinib. Clinicians should consider patients preferences and comorbidities (e.g., iritis, inflammatory bowel disease) when selecting therapy. Consult the joint guideline issued by the American College of Rheumatology, the Spondylitis Association of America, and the Spondyloarthritis Research and Treatment Network for additional details.

● *Ulcerative Colitis*

Tofacitinib citrate (as conventional or extended-release tablets) is used for the management of moderately to severely active ulcerative colitis in adults who have had an inadequate response to or have not tolerated therapy with one or more TNF blocking agents. Tofacitinib has been shown to induce clinical remission, improve endoscopic appearance of the mucosa, and produce sustained corticosteroid-free remission during maintenance therapy in patients with ulcerative colitis. Concomitant use of tofacitinib with biologic therapies for ulcerative colitis or with potent immunosuppressive agents (e.g., azathioprine, cyclosporine) is not recommended. Safety and efficacy of tofacitinib in the management of ulcerative colitis are based principally on the results of 3 randomized controlled trials. Guidelines generally support the use of tofacitinib as an option for induction of remission in patients with moderate to severe ulcerative colitis; continuation of tofacitinib is recommended in patients with previously moderate to severe active disease who are in remission after induction with tofacitinib.

Clinical Experience

Efficacy and safety of tofacitinib for the management of ulcerative colitis in adults have been established in 3 randomized, double-blind, placebo-controlled studies, including 2 identically designed studies (OCTAVE Induction studies 1 and 2) evaluating tofacitinib (as conventional tablets) as induction therapy in a total of 1139 patients and one study (OCTAVE Sustain) evaluating tofacitinib (as conventional tablets) as maintenance therapy in 593 patients who achieved a clinical response upon completion of an OCTAVE Induction study.

Patients enrolled in the induction studies had moderately to severely active ulcerative colitis (as defined by a Mayo score of 6–12 with an endoscopy subscore of at least 2 and rectal bleeding subscore of at least 1) and had a history

of inadequate response or intolerance (i.e., treatment failure) to at least 1 of the following drugs: oral or IV corticosteroids, azathioprine, mercaptopurine, or a TNF blocking agent. The Mayo score ranges from 0–12 and includes 4 subscales (i.e., stool frequency, rectal bleeding, findings on endoscopy, and physician global assessment), each scored from 0–3 (normal to most severe, respectively). An endoscopy subscore of 2 is defined by marked erythema, lack of vascular pattern, friability, and erosions, whereas an endoscopy subscore of 3 is defined by spontaneous bleeding and ulceration. The median baseline Mayo score for the induction studies was 9. Patients were randomized in a 4:1 ratio to receive tofacitinib (10 mg twice daily) or placebo for 8 weeks. Stable dosages of oral aminosalicylates and corticosteroids (up to 25 mg daily of prednisone or equivalent) were permitted during the induction studies, but concomitant therapy with immunosuppressive agents (oral immunomodulators or biologic therapies) was not allowed. In the 2 induction studies combined, 52, 73, or 72% of patients had a history of treatment failure with TNF blocking agents, corticosteroids, or immunosuppressive agents, respectively. During the induction studies, 47% of patients received concomitant therapy with oral corticosteroids and 71% received aminosalicylates.

In the induction studies, the primary measure of efficacy was the proportion of patients achieving clinical remission at 8 weeks; other outcome measures included clinical response and improved or normalized mucosal appearance at 8 weeks. Clinical remission was defined as a Mayo score of 0–2 with no individual subscore exceeding 1 and a rectal bleeding subscore of 0. Clinical response was defined as a decrease in Mayo score of at least 3 points and at least 30% from baseline score, with a reduction in rectal bleeding subscore of at least 1 point or an absolute rectal bleeding subscore of 0 (no blood seen) or 1 (streaks of blood with stool less than half the time). Improved mucosal appearance was defined as a Mayo endoscopy subscore of 0 (normal mucosa or inactive disease) or 1 (erythema, decreased vascular pattern), and normalized mucosal appearance was defined as a Mayo endoscopy subscore of 0.

In both induction studies, clinical remission rates and rates of improved mucosal appearance were higher in patients receiving tofacitinib compared with those receiving placebo. Clinical remission was achieved in 17–18 or 4–8% of patients receiving tofacitinib or placebo, respectively, and improved mucosal appearance was observed in 28–31 or 12–16% of those receiving tofacitinib or placebo, respectively. In addition, clinical response was achieved in 55–60 or 29–33% of patients receiving tofacitinib or placebo, respectively, and mucosal appearance was normalized in 7% of patients receiving tofacitinib and 2% of those receiving placebo in both studies. Decreases in subscores for rectal bleeding and stool frequency were observed as early as 2 weeks in patients receiving tofacitinib.

In OCTAVE Sustain, patients who achieved a clinical response at 8 weeks in OCTAVE Induction study 1 or 2 were re-randomized in a 1:1:1 ratio to receive tofacitinib (5 or 10 mg twice daily) or placebo for 52 weeks. Approximately 30% of patients were in clinical remission at the start of the maintenance study; 49% were receiving oral corticosteroids; and 45, 75, or 70% had a history of treatment failure with TNF blocking agents, corticosteroids, or immunosuppressive agents, respectively. In patients receiving corticosteroids, a corticosteroid-tapering regimen was initiated at the start of the maintenance trial. As in the induction studies, concomitant therapy with oral aminosalicylates was permitted, but concomitant therapy with immunosuppressive agents (oral immunomodulators or biologic therapies) was not allowed. The primary measure of efficacy was the proportion of patients in clinical remission at 52 weeks. Other outcome measures included improved or normalized mucosal appearance at 52 weeks, maintenance of clinical response (i.e., clinical response at both baseline and 52 weeks), maintenance of clinical remission (i.e., clinical remission at both baseline and 52 weeks), and sustained corticosteroid-free remission (i.e., corticosteroid-free remission at baseline, 24 weeks, and 52 weeks).

In the maintenance study, both dosages of tofacitinib were more effective than placebo for achieving remission at 52 weeks, improved mucosal appearance at 52 weeks, and sustained corticosteroid-free remission. Clinical remission was achieved at 52 weeks in 34 or 41% of patients receiving tofacitinib 5 or 10 mg twice daily, respectively, compared with 11% of those receiving placebo. Improved mucosal appearance was observed at 52 weeks in 37 or 46% of patients receiving tofacitinib 5 or 10 mg twice daily, respectively, compared with 13% of those receiving placebo. Sustained corticosteroid-free remission was achieved in 35 or 47% of patients receiving tofacitinib 5 or 10 mg twice daily, respectively, compared with 5% of those receiving placebo. In addition, maintenance of clinical remission or clinical response was observed in 46 or 52%, respectively, of patients receiving tofacitinib 5 mg twice daily; 56 or 62%, respectively, of those receiving tofacitinib 10 mg twice daily, and 10 or 20%, respectively, of those receiving placebo. Mucosal appearance was normalized at 52 weeks in 15, 17, or 4% of patients receiving these respective treatments.

Exploratory subgroup analysis demonstrated treatment effects regardless of prior failure of TNF blocking agent therapy, but suggested that response and remission rates tended to be higher in patients without a history of failed therapy with TNF blocking agents.

Data are available from an open-label extension study for a subset of 291 patients who did not achieve a clinical response upon completion of an OCTAVE Induction study but continued to receive tofacitinib at a dosage of 10 mg twice daily; after a total of 16 weeks of tofacitinib therapy, 149 of these patients (51%) achieved a clinical response and 25 patients (8.6%) achieved clinical remission. Data available at 52 weeks (for 144 of these patients) indicated that 65 patients were in clinical remission following 52 weeks of treatment with tofacitinib 10 mg twice daily.

Clinical Perspective

The American College of Gastroenterology (ACG) and the American Gastroenterological Association (AGA) issued guidelines for the medical treatment of ulcerative colitis in adults in 2019 and 2020. Goals of therapy in ulcerative colitis include achieving and maintaining corticosteroid-free remission and promoting mucosal healing. Specific treatments for ulcerative colitis are selected according to the disease severity, as well as disease location/extent, disease prognosis, and previous therapies used. Drug classes used to treat ulcerative colitis include oral and rectal 5-aminosalicylates, oral and rectal corticosteroids, immunomodulators (e.g., thiopurines, methotrexate), tofacitinib, and biologic agents, including TNF blocking agents, vedolizumab, and ustekinumab. In most cases, if a drug used for induction therapy is effective, it is continued as maintenance of remission.

For adult outpatients with moderate to severe ulcerative colitis, AGA recommends TNF blocking therapies, vedolizumab, tofacitinib, or ustekinumab over no treatment. ACG recommends the use of oral corticosteroids, TNF blocking agents, vedolizumab, or tofacitinib for induction of remission in patients with moderately to severely active ulcerative colitis. Early use of biologic agents with or without immunomodulator therapy is conditionally recommended over gradual step up therapy after failure of 5-aminosalicylates. Patients with mildly active ulcerative colitis and multiple prognostic factors associated with an increased risk of hospitalization or surgery should be treated with therapies for moderately to severely active disease. Consult the American College of Gastroenterology guideline for additional details.

● Other Uses

Psoriasis

Tofacitinib has been investigated for the treatment of plaque psoriasis† in several phase 3 randomized controlled trials. In two similarly designed 16-week trials, patients with moderate to severe chronic plaque psoriasis were randomized to receive tofacitinib 5 or 10 mg twice daily (as conventional tablets) or placebo twice daily. Primary efficacy end points included the proportion of patients achieving Physician's Global Assessment (PGA) score of "clear" or "almost clear" (also referred to as PGA response) and the proportion of patients achieving a 75% or greater reduction in Psoriasis Area and Severity Index (PASI 75) score. In these trials, substantially higher proportions of patients receiving tofacitinib 5 mg (41.9–46%) or 10 mg twice daily (approximately 59%) achieved PGA responses compared with placebo recipients (9–10.9%) at 16 weeks. Similarly, substantially higher PASI 75 rates was observed in patients receiving tofacitinib 5 mg (39.9–46%) or 10 mg twice daily (59.2–59.6%) compared with placebo recipients (6.2–11.4%,).

An additional 12-week phase 3 noninferiority trial randomized adult patients with chronic stable plaque psoriasis to tofacitinib 5 mg twice daily, tofacitinib 10 mg twice daily, etanercept 50 mg twice weekly, or placebo. Primary efficacy end points included the proportion of patients achieving PGA response and the proportion achieving PASI 75. Tofacitinib 10 mg twice daily demonstrated noninferiority compared with etanercept for PGA response and PASI 75 response; however, tofacitinib 5 mg twice daily did not meet the prespecified criteria for noninferiority.

DOSAGE AND ADMINISTRATION

● General

Pretreatment Screening

- Evaluate for latent or active tuberculosis infection prior to initiation of therapy; initiate antimycobacterial therapy if indicated.

- Evaluate for risk of thrombosis prior to initiation of therapy.

- Measure absolute lymphocyte count, absolute neutrophil count (ANC), and hemoglobin prior to initiation of therapy. Do not initiate therapy in patients with an absolute lymphocyte count of <500/mm³, ANC <1000/mm³, or hemoglobin concentration <9 g/dL.

- Screen for viral hepatitis infection before initiating therapy.

Patient Monitoring

- Evaluate for latent or active tuberculosis infection during therapy according to applicable guidelines.

- Monitor closely for signs or symptoms of infection, including the possible development of tuberculosis in patients who tested negative for latent tuberculosis prior to initiating therapy, during and after treatment with tofacitinib.

- Monitor lymphocyte count every 3 months during therapy.

- Monitor ANC and hemoglobin concentrations 4–8 weeks after initial of therapy and then every 3 months.

- Monitor liver enzymes periodically during therapy.

- Perform dermatologic examinations periodically throughout therapy in patients at increased risk for skin cancer.

- Monitor lipids 4–8 weeks after therapy initiation.

Other General Considerations

- Do not use concomitantly with biologic disease-modifying antirheumatic drugs (DMARDs), or potent immunosuppressive agents.

- Concomitant use with potent inducers of cytochrome P-450 (CYP) isoenzyme 3A4 (e.g., rifampin) may result in loss of or reduced clinical response to tofacitinib.

- Update immunizations according to current immunization guidelines prior to initiating therapy.

● Administration

Tofacitinib citrate conventional tablets, oral solution, or extended-release tablets are administered orally without regard to meals. The extended-release tablets should be swallowed intact and should not be crushed, split, or chewed. The oral solution should be administered using the press-in bottle adapter and oral dosing syringe provided by the manufacturer.

Changes between conventional and extended-release tablets should be made by a clinician. Pediatric patients receiving 5 mg as oral solution may be switched to the equivalent dose as conventional tablets. The extended-release tablets and the oral solution are not interchangeable and should not be substituted for each other.

Store tofacitinib (conventional tablets, extended-release tablets, and oral solution) at 20–25°C; excursions permitted between 15–30°C for tofacitinib oral solution . Protect from light. Tofacitinib oral solution must be used within 60 days of opening; discard any remaining oral solution after 60 days.

● Dosage

Dosage of tofacitinib citrate is expressed in terms of tofacitinib.

Dosage recommendations specific to the condition being treated should be followed.

Rheumatoid Arthritis, Psoriatic Arthritis, or Ankylosing Spondylitis in Adults

For the management of rheumatoid arthritis, psoriatic arthritis, or ankylosing spondylitis in adults who have had an inadequate response or intolerance to methotrexate or for the management of psoriatic arthritis in adults who have had an inadequate response or intolerance to one or more tumor necrosis factor (TNF) blocking agents, the recommended dosage of tofacitinib is 5 mg twice daily (as conventional tablets) or 11 mg once daily (as extended-release tablets). Patients receiving tofacitinib 5 mg twice daily (as conventional tablets) may be switched to tofacitinib 11 mg once daily (as extended-release tablets) the day following the last dose of the conventional tablets.

In patients receiving concomitant therapy with potent inhibitors of CYP3A4 (e.g., ketoconazole) and in patients receiving concomitant therapy with a moderate inhibitor of CYP3A4 and potent inhibitor of CYP2C19 (e.g., fluconazole), dosage of tofacitinib (as conventional or extended-release tablets) should be reduced to 5 mg once daily (as conventional tablets).

Dosage Modifications for Toxicity

If a serious infection develops, tofacitinib therapy should be interrupted until the infection has been controlled.

Tofacitinib therapy also should be interrupted or discontinued in patients with lymphopenia, neutropenia, or anemia.

In patients who develop a lymphocyte count of less than 500/mm³ (confirmed by repeat testing), tofacitinib should be discontinued.

In patients with a persistent decrease in ANC to 500–1000/mm³, tofacitinib therapy should be interrupted until the ANC exceeds 1000/mm³; tofacitinib therapy then may be resumed at the usual dosage of 5 mg twice daily (as conventional tablets) or 11 mg once daily (as extended-release tablets). Tofacitinib therapy should be discontinued in patients with an ANC of less than 500/mm³.

In patients with a decrease in hemoglobin concentration of more than 2 g/dL or with a hemoglobin concentration of less than 8 g/dL, tofacitinib therapy should be interrupted until the hemoglobin concentration has normalized.

Juvenile Idiopathic Arthritis

For the management of active polyarticular-course juvenile idiopathic arthritis (JIA) in pediatric patients 2 years of age and older who have had an inadequate response or intolerance to one or more TNF blocking agents, dosage of tofacitinib (as conventional tablets or oral solution) is based on body weight; pediatric patients weighing 10 to less than 20 kg should receive 3.2 mg twice daily (as oral solution), those weighing 20 to less than 40 kg should receive 4 mg twice daily (as oral solution), and those weighing 40 kg or more should receive 5 mg twice daily (as conventional tablets or oral solution).

In pediatric patients receiving concomitant therapy with potent inhibitors of CYP3A4 (e.g., ketoconazole) and in patients receiving concomitant therapy with one or more drugs that result in both moderate inhibition of CYP3A4 and potent inhibition of CYP2C19 (e.g., fluconazole), dosage of tofacitinib should be reduced from 3.2 mg twice daily to 3.2 mg once daily, from 4 mg twice daily to 4 mg once daily, or from 5 mg twice daily to 5 mg once daily.

Dosage Modifications for Toxicity

If a serious infection develops, tofacitinib therapy should be interrupted until the infection has been controlled.

Tofacitinib therapy also should be interrupted or discontinued in patients with lymphopenia, neutropenia, or anemia.

In patients who develop a lymphocyte count of less than 500/mm³ (confirmed by repeat testing), tofacitinib should be discontinued.

In patients with a persistent decrease in ANC to 500–1000/mm³, tofacitinib therapy should be interrupted until the ANC exceeds 1000/mm³. Tofacitinib therapy should be discontinued in patients with an ANC of less than 500/mm³.

In patients with a decrease in hemoglobin concentration of more than 2 g/dL or with a hemoglobin concentration of less than 8 g/dL, tofacitinib therapy should be interrupted until the hemoglobin concentration has normalized.

Ulcerative Colitis

For the management of ulcerative colitis in adults who have had an inadequate response or intolerance to TNF blocking agents, the recommended induction dosage of tofacitinib is 10 mg twice daily (as conventional tablets) or 22 mg once daily (as extended-release tablets) for at least 8 weeks; patients should then be evaluated and, depending on therapeutic response, may begin maintenance

therapy with the drug. If necessary, the induction dosage of 10 mg twice daily (as conventional tablets) or 22 mg once daily (as extended-release tablets) may be administered for a maximum of 16 weeks. If adequate therapeutic benefit is not achieved after 16 weeks of treatment at this dosage, this dosage should be discontinued.

The recommended adult maintenance dosage is 5 mg twice daily (as conventional tablets) or 11 mg once daily (as extended-release tablets). For patients with loss of response during maintenance therapy, a dosage of 10 mg twice daily (as conventional tablets) or 22 mg once daily (as extended-release tablets) may be considered and should be limited to the shortest duration needed, with careful consideration of potential benefits and risks for the individual patient. The lowest effective dosage that maintains response should be used.

Patients may be switched from therapy with tofacitinib conventional tablets to therapy with the extended-release tablets (i.e., from 5 mg twice daily [as conventional tablets] to 11 mg once daily [as extended-release tablets] or from 10 mg twice daily [as conventional tablets] to 22 mg once daily [as extended-release tablets]) the day following the last dose of the conventional tablets.

In patients receiving concomitant therapy with potent inhibitors of CYP3A4 (e.g., ketoconazole) and in patients receiving concomitant therapy with a moderate inhibitor of CYP3A4 and potent inhibitor of CYP2C19 (e.g., fluconazole), dosage of tofacitinib (as conventional tablets) should be reduced from 10 mg twice daily to 5 mg twice daily or from 5 mg twice daily to 5 mg once daily and dosage of tofacitinib (as extended-release tablets) should be reduced from 22 mg once daily to 11 mg once daily or from 11 mg once daily (as extended-release tablets) to 5 mg once daily (as conventional tablets).

Dosage Modifications for Toxicity

If a serious infection develops, tofacitinib therapy should be interrupted until the infection has been controlled.

Tofacitinib therapy also should be interrupted or discontinued in patients with lymphopenia, neutropenia, or anemia.

In patients who develop a lymphocyte count of less than 500/mm³ (confirmed by repeat testing), tofacitinib (as conventional tablets or extended-release tablets) should be discontinued.

In patients receiving tofacitinib (as conventional tablets) who have a persistent decrease in ANC to 500–1000/mm³ on a dosage of 10 mg twice daily, dosage of the drug should be reduced to 5 mg twice daily; when the ANC exceeds 1000/mm³, dosage may be returned to 10 mg twice daily based on clinical response. In patients with a persistent decrease in ANC to 500–1000/mm³ on a dosage of 5 mg twice daily, tofacitinib therapy should be interrupted until the ANC exceeds 1000/mm³; therapy with tofacitinib conventional tablets then may be resumed at a dosage of 5 mg twice daily. Tofacitinib therapy should be discontinued in patients with an ANC of less than 500/mm³.

In patients receiving tofacitinib (as extended-release tablets) who have a persistent decrease in ANC to 500–1000/mm³ on a dosage of 22 mg once daily, dosage of the drug should be reduced to 11 mg once daily; when the ANC exceeds 1000/mm³, dosage may be returned to 22 mg once daily based on clinical response. In patients with a decrease in ANC to 500–1000/mm³ on a dosage of 11 mg once daily, tofacitinib therapy should be interrupted until the ANC exceeds 1000/mm³; therapy with tofacitinib extended-release tablets then may be resumed at a dosage of 11 mg once daily. Tofacitinib therapy should be discontinued in patients with an ANC of less than 500/mm³.

In patients with a decrease in hemoglobin concentration of more than 2 g/dL or with a hemoglobin concentration of less than 8 g/dL, tofacitinib therapy should be interrupted until the hemoglobin concentration has normalized.

Psoriasis†

For the treatment of plaque psoriasis† in adults, tofacitinib 5 or 10 mg twice daily (as conventional tablets) has been used.

● Special Populations

Hepatic Impairment

Dosage reduction may be necessary in patients with hepatic impairment (see Table 1).

TABLE 1. Recommended Dosage Modification for Tofacitinib in Patients with Hepatic Impairment

Severity	Rheumatoid Arthritis, Psoriatic Arthritis, or Ankylosing Spondylitis	Juvenile Idiopathic Arthritis	Ulcerative Colitis
Mild hepatic impairment	No dosage adjustment necessary	No dosage adjustment necessary	No dosage adjustment necessary
Moderate hepatic impairment	*Conventional tablet:* Reduce dosage to 5 mg once daily	*Oral solution:* If current dosage is 3.2 mg twice daily, reduce dosage to 3.2 mg *once* daily If current dosage is 4 mg twice daily, reduce dosage to 4 mg *once* daily If current dosage is 5 mg twice daily, reduce dosage to 5 mg *once* daily	*Conventional tablet:* If current dosage is 10 mg twice daily, reduce dosage to 5 mg twice daily If current dosage is 5 mg twice daily, reduce dosage to 5 mg *once* daily
	Extended-release tablet: Reduce dosage to 5 mg once daily (as conventional tablets)		*Extended-release tablet:* If current dosage is 22 mg once daily, reduce dosage to 11 mg once daily; if current dosage is 11 mg once daily, reduce dosage to 5 mg once daily (as conventional tablets)
Severe hepatic impairment	Do not use	Do not use	Do not use

Renal Impairment

Dosage reduction may be necessary in patients with renal impairment (see Table 2).

TABLE 2. Recommended Dosage Modification for Tofacitinib in Patients with Renal Impairment

Severity	Rheumatoid Arthritis, Psoriatic Arthritis, or Ankylosing Spondylitis	Juvenile Idiopathic Arthritis	Ulcerative Colitis
Mild renal impairment	No dosage adjustment necessary	No dosage adjustment necessary	No dosage adjustment necessary
Moderate or severe renal impairment	*Conventional tablet:* Reduce dosage to 5 mg once daily	*Oral solution:* If current dosage is 3.2 mg twice daily, reduce dosage to 3.2 mg *once* daily If current dosage is 4 mg twice daily, reduce dosage to 4 mg *once* daily If current dosage is 5 mg twice daily, reduce dosage to 5 mg *once* daily	*Conventional tablet:* If current dosage is 10 mg twice daily, reduce dosage to 5 mg twice daily If current dosage is 5 mg twice daily, reduce dosage to 5 mg *once* daily

TABLE 2. Continued

Severity	Rheumatoid Arthritis, Psoriatic Arthritis, or Ankylosing Spondylitis	Juvenile Idiopathic Arthritis	Ulcerative Colitis
	Extended-release tablet: Reduce dosage to 5 mg once daily (as conventional tablets)		*Extended-release tablet:* If current dosage is 22 mg once daily, reduce dosage to 11 mg once daily; if current dosage is 11 mg once daily, reduce dosage to 5 mg once daily (as conventional tablets)
Hemodialysis	Administer after dialysis session; if a dose is taken before the dialysis procedure, administering a supplemental dose after dialysis is not necessary	Administer after dialysis session; if a dose is taken before the dialysis procedure, administering a supplemental dose after dialysis is not necessary	Administer after dialysis session; if a dose is taken before the dialysis procedure, administering a supplemental dose after dialysis is not necessary

Geriatric Patients

The manufacturer makes no specific dosage recommendations for geriatric patients.

CAUTIONS

● Contraindications

The manufacturer states that there are no known contraindications to the use of tofacitinib.

● Warnings/Precautions

Warnings

Infectious Complications

A boxed warning regarding the risk of infectious complications is included in the prescribing information for tofacitinib. Patients receiving tofacitinib are at increased risk of developing serious infections that may require hospitalization or result in death. Serious and sometimes fatal infections caused by bacterial, mycobacterial, invasive fungal, viral, or other opportunistic organisms—including cryptococcosis, pneumocystosis, histoplasmosis, tuberculosis and other mycobacterial infections, esophageal candidiasis, multidermatomal herpes zoster, cytomegalovirus infection, listeriosis, and BK virus infection—have been reported in patients receiving tofacitinib. The most common serious infections reported in patients receiving tofacitinib included pneumonia, cellulitis, herpes zoster, urinary tract infection, diverticulitis, and appendicitis. Other serious infections (e.g., coccidioidomycosis) also may occur. Patients may present with disseminated rather than localized disease. Most patients who developed serious infections were receiving concomitant therapy with immunosuppressive agents such as methotrexate or corticosteroids.

In controlled clinical trials in patients with rheumatoid arthritis, the overall frequency of infections during the first 3 months of treatment was 20, 22, or 18% in patients receiving tofacitinib 5 mg twice daily, tofacitinib 10 mg twice daily, or placebo, respectively. Serious infections were reported at a rate of 1.7 events per 100 patient-years in tofacitinib-treated patients and 0.5 events per 100 patient-years in placebo-treated patients during the first 3 months of therapy. The rate of serious infections during the first 12 months of tofacitinib therapy was 2.7 events per 100 patient-years.

In patients with ulcerative colitis, the risk of serious infections and herpes zoster (including meningoencephalitis and ophthalmologic and disseminated cutaneous infections) was dose dependent, occurring more frequently in patients receiving tofacitinib 10 mg twice daily compared with those receiving tofacitinib 5 mg twice daily.

The risk of infection may be higher with increasing degrees of lymphopenia. Lymphocyte counts should be considered when assessing an individual patient's risk of infection.

Because of the higher incidence of infections generally observed in patients with diabetes mellitus, tofacitinib should be used with caution in diabetic patients. In addition, because patients with a history of chronic lung disease and those who develop interstitial lung disease may be more susceptible to infections, caution is advised in these patients.

Patients should be closely monitored during and after treatment with tofacitinib for the development of signs or symptoms of infection (e.g., fever, malaise, weight loss, sweats, cough, dyspnea, pulmonary infiltrates, serious systemic illness including shock).

Tofacitinib therapy should not be initiated in patients with serious active infections, including localized infections. Tofacitinib should be interrupted in patients who develop a serious infection, opportunistic infection, or sepsis and should not be resumed until the infection is controlled. Clinicians should consider potential risks and benefits of tofacitinib prior to initiating therapy in patients with a history of chronic, recurring, serious, or opportunistic infections; patients with underlying conditions that may predispose them to infections; and patients who have been exposed to tuberculosis or who reside or have traveled in regions where tuberculosis or mycoses are endemic. Any patient who develops a new infection while receiving tofacitinib should undergo a thorough diagnostic evaluation (appropriate for an immunocompromised patient), appropriate anti-infective therapy should be initiated, and the patient should be closely monitored.

Because tuberculosis has been reported in patients receiving tofacitinib, all patients should be evaluated for active or latent tuberculosis and for the presence of risk factors for tuberculosis prior to and periodically during therapy with the drug. When indicated, an appropriate antimycobacterial regimen for the treatment of latent tuberculosis infection should be initiated prior to tofacitinib therapy. Antimycobacterial therapy also should be considered prior to initiation of tofacitinib in individuals with a history of latent or active tuberculosis in whom an adequate course of antimycobacterial therapy cannot be confirmed and in individuals with a negative test for latent tuberculosis who have risk factors for tuberculosis. Consultation with a tuberculosis specialist is recommended when deciding whether antimycobacterial therapy should be initiated. Patients receiving tofacitinib, including individuals with a negative test for latent tuberculosis, should be monitored for signs and symptoms of active tuberculosis, which may present with pulmonary or extrapulmonary disease.

Viral reactivation can occur in patients receiving tofacitinib. Herpes zoster reactivation has been reported in patients receiving the drug. The risk of herpes zoster is increased in patients receiving tofacitinib and appears to be increased in patients treated in Japan or Korea.

Reactivation of hepatitis B virus (HBV) infection also has been reported during postmarketing experience. The effect of tofacitinib on the risk of reactivation of chronic viral hepatitis is not known; patients with serologic evidence of HBV or hepatitis C virus (HCV) infection were excluded from clinical trials of the drug. All patients should be screened for viral hepatitis in accordance with clinical guidelines before initiation of tofacitinib therapy.

Mortality

A boxed warning regarding the increased risk of mortality is included in the prescribing information for tofacitinib. In a postmarketing study (NCT02092467; RA Safety Study 1) evaluating safety of tofacitinib in patients with rheumatoid arthritis, a higher overall mortality rate, including sudden cardiovascular death, in patients receiving tofacitinib 5 or 10 mg twice daily compared with those receiving a tumor necrosis factor (TNF) blocking agent (0.88 and 1.23, respectively, versus 0.69 cases of all-cause mortality per 100 patient-years) was observed. Because the study was designed to assess cardiovascular risks as well as risks of cancer and opportunistic infections, enrolled patients were 50 years of age or older and had at least one cardiovascular risk factor.

The 10-mg twice-daily (as conventional tablets) or 22-mg once-daily (as extended-release tablets) dosage of tofacitinib is FDA-labeled only for the management of ulcerative colitis for use as induction therapy and in limited situations during maintenance therapy. Tofacitinib at a dosage of 10 mg twice daily or

an equivalent weight-based, twice-daily dosage (as conventional tablets or oral solution) or at a dosage of 22 mg once daily (as extended-release tablets) is *not* recommended for the management of rheumatoid arthritis, psoriatic arthritis, ankylosing spondylitis, or polyarticular-course JIA. In patients with ulcerative colitis, tofacitinib should be used at the lowest effective dosage and for the shortest duration needed to achieve and maintain therapeutic response.

Malignancies and Lymphoproliferative Disorders

A boxed warning regarding the risk of malignancies and lymphoproliferative disorders is included in the prescribing information for tofacitinib. Lymphoma and other malignancies (e.g., lung cancer, breast cancer, melanoma, prostate cancer, pancreatic cancer) have been observed in patients receiving tofacitinib. In addition, an increased incidence of Epstein Barr virus (EBV)-associated posttransplant lymphoproliferative disorder has been observed in renal allograft recipients receiving tofacitinib concomitantly with immunosuppressive agents.

Among 3328 patients with rheumatoid arthritis receiving tofacitinib with or without other disease-modifying antirheumatic drugs (DMARDs) in clinical trials, 11 solid tumors and one lymphoma were diagnosed during the first 12 months of treatment compared with no cases of solid tumors or lymphoma in 809 patients receiving placebo with or without other DMARDs. Lymphomas and solid tumors also have been observed in long-term extension studies in patients with rheumatoid arthritis receiving tofacitinib.

In controlled clinical trials in patients with rheumatoid arthritis, malignancies (excluding nonmelanoma skin cancer) were reported at a rate of 0.3 events per 100 patient-years in tofacitinib-treated patients and 0 events per 100 patient-years in placebo-treated patients during the first 3 months of treatment. The rate of malignancies (excluding nonmelanoma skin cancer) during the first 12 months of treatment in patients receiving tofacitinib in clinical trials was 0.6 events per 100 patient-years in patients receiving 10 mg twice daily and 0.4 events per 100 patient-years in patients receiving 5 mg twice daily. The most common malignancies reported, including those reported during long-term extension studies, were lung and breast cancer, followed by gastric, colorectal, renal cell, and prostate cancer, lymphoma, and malignant melanoma.

Initial results from a postmarketing safety study (NCT02092467) in patients with rheumatoid arthritis have suggested a higher incidence of malignancies (excluding nonmelanoma skin cancer) in patients receiving tofacitinib (either 5 or 10 mg twice daily) compared with those receiving a TNF blocking agent. The manufacturer released results indicating that the trial failed to establish noninferiority of tofacitinib for this outcome compared with a TNF blocking agent; the incidence of malignancies (excluding nonmelanoma skin cancer) in patients receiving tofacitinib (both dosages combined) or a TNF blocking agent was 1.13 or 0.77 events per 100 patient-years, respectively. The manufacturer stated that the most frequently reported malignancy (excluding nonmelanoma skin cancer) in patients receiving tofacitinib was lung cancer. FDA is awaiting additional results from the study.

In controlled clinical trials in patients with psoriatic arthritis, 3 malignancies (excluding nonmelanoma skin cancer) were diagnosed in 474 patients receiving tofacitinib with nonbiologic DMARDs for 6–12 months compared with no malignancies in 236 patients receiving placebo with nonbiologic DMARDs for 3 months and no malignancies in 106 patients receiving adalimumab with nonbiologic DMARDs for 12 months. Malignancies also have been observed in a long-term extension study in patients with psoriatic arthritis receiving tofacitinib.

In controlled clinical trials in 1220 patients with ulcerative colitis (including both 8-week induction and 52-week maintenance trials), no cases of solid tumors or lymphoma were diagnosed in tofacitinib-treated patients. In a long-term extension study, malignancies (including solid tumors and lymphoma) were observed more frequently in patients receiving a tofacitinib dosage of 10 mg twice daily. The occurrence of nonmelanoma skin cancer in tofacitinib-treated patients with ulcerative colitis was dose dependent; a tofacitinib dosage of 10 mg twice daily was associated with increased risk.

In the RA Safety Study 1 (NCT02092467), malignancies occurred more frequently in patients with rheumatoid arthritis treated with tofacitinib 5 or 10 mg twice daily compared with those who received a TNF blocking agent. The incidence rate of malignancies (excluding nonmelanoma skin cancer) per 100 patient-years was 1.13 with tofacitinib 5 mg twice daily, 1.13 with tofacitinib 10 mg twice daily, and 0.77 with TNF blocking agents. Lymphomas and lung cancers were observed at a higher rate in patients treated with tofacitinib 5 mg twice a day and tofacitinib 10 mg twice a day compared to those treated with TNF blocking agents. The incidence rate of lymphomas per 100 patient-years was 0.07 for tofacitinib 5 mg twice daily, 0.11 for tofacitinib 10 mg twice daily, and 0.02 for TNF blocking agents. The incidence rate of lung cancers per 100 patient-years among current and past smokers was 0.48 for tofacitinib 5 mg twice a day, 0.59 for tofacitinib 10 mg twice a day, and 0.27 for TNF blocking agents. Based on findings of the postmarketing study, and to ensure the benefits of tofacitinib outweigh its risks, use of tofacitinib in all approved indications is limited to patients who have not responded to or cannot tolerate one or more TNF blocking agents.

EBV-associated posttransplant lymphoproliferative disorder was observed in 5 of 218 patients (2.3%) receiving tofacitinib compared with 0 of 111 patients receiving cyclosporine in dose-ranging trials in de novo renal transplant recipients; all patients had received induction therapy with basiliximab, high-dose corticosteroids, and mycophenolate.

The risks and benefits of tofacitinib should be considered prior to initiating therapy or when considering whether to continue tofacitinib, particularly in patients with a known malignancy (other than successfully treated nonmelanoma skin cancer), in those who develop a malignancy, and those who are current or past smokers.

Because nonmelanoma skin cancers have been reported in patients receiving tofacitinib, periodic dermatologic examinations are recommended for patients receiving the drug who are at increased risk for skin cancer.

Major Adverse Cardiovascular Events

A boxed warning regarding the increased risk of major adverse cardiovascular events is included in the prescribing information for tofacitinib. Major adverse cardiovascular events have occurred in patients receiving tofacitinib. In the RA Safety Study 1 (NCT02092467) in patients ≥50 years of age with rheumatoid arthritis and at least one cardiovascular risk factor, the risk of major adverse cardiovascular events (i.e., cardiovascular death, nonfatal MI, nonfatal stroke) was increased in patients receiving the JAK inhibitor tofacitinib (either 5 or 10 mg twice daily) compared with those receiving a tumor necrosis factor (TNF) blocking agent. The incidence rate of a major adverse cardiovascular event per 100 patient-years was 0.91 for tofacitinib 5 mg twice a day, 1.11 for tofacitinib 10 mg twice a day, and 0.79 for TNF blockers. The incidence rate of fatal or non-fatal MI per 100 patient-years was 0.36 with tofacitinib 5 mg twice daily, 0.39 with tofacitinib 10 mg twice daily, and 0.20 for TNF blocking agents. Patients who are current or past smokers are at additional risk.

The risks and benefits of tofacitinib should be considered prior to initiating therapy or when considering whether to continue tofacitinib, particularly in patients who are current or past smokers and in those with other cardiovascular risk factors. Patients receiving tofacitinib should be advised to seek immediate medical attention if symptoms of serious cardiovascular events occur. In patients who experience MI or stroke, tofacitinib therapy should be discontinued. Tofacitinib dosages of 10 mg twice daily (as conventional tablets or oral solution) or 22 mg once daily of tofacitinib extended-release tablets are not recommended for the treatment of rheumatoid arthritis, psoriatic arthritis, ankylosing spondylitis, or polyarticular-course JIA.

Thromboembolic Events

A boxed warning regarding the risk of thrombosis is included in the prescribing information for tofacitinib. Thromboembolic events, including pulmonary embolism, deep-vein thrombosis, and arterial thrombosis, have occurred in patients receiving tofacitinib and other Janus kinase inhibitors used to treat inflammatory conditions; many events were serious and some were fatal.

In a postmarketing study (NCT02092467; RA Study 1) evaluating safety of tofacitinib in patients with rheumatoid arthritis, analysis revealed higher incidences of thromboembolic events, including pulmonary embolism, deep-vein thrombosis, and arterial thrombosis, in patients receiving tofacitinib 10 mg twice daily compared with those receiving either tofacitinib 5 mg twice daily or a TNF blocking agent, each given in combination with methotrexate. Because the study was designed to assess cardiovascular risks as well as risks of cancer and opportunistic infections, enrolled patients were 50 years of age or older and had at least one cardiovascular risk factor. The incidence rate of deep-vein thrombosis per 100 patient-years was 0.22 with tofacitinib 5 mg twice a day, 0.28 with tofacitinib 10 mg twice a day, and 0.16 with TNF blocking agents. The incidence rate of pulmonary embolism per 100 patient-years was 0.18 with tofacitinib 5 mg twice a day, 0.49 with tofacitinib 10 mg twice a day, and 0.05 for TNF blocking agent. Based on

these findings, patients enrolled in the safety study who were receiving tofacitinib 10 mg twice daily for the management of rheumatoid arthritis were switched to the labeled dosage of 5 mg twice daily.

In a long-term extension study in patients with ulcerative colitis, 5 cases of pulmonary embolism were reported in patients receiving tofacitinib 10 mg twice daily, including one death in a patient with advanced cancer.

Promptly evaluate patients who develop symptoms of thrombosis and discontinue tofacitinib in these patients. Avoid tofacitinib in patients that may be at increased risk of thrombosis. In patients with ulcerative colitis, use tofacitinib at the lowest effective dosage and for the shortest duration needed to achieve and maintain therapeutic response.

Patients receiving tofacitinib should be advised to seek immediate medical attention if symptoms of thrombosis occur. The drug should be discontinued in patients experiencing such symptoms, and the patient should be evaluated promptly. Use of tofacitinib should be avoided in patients who may be at increased risk of thrombosis.

Other Warnings/Precautions

Sensitivity Reactions

Serious hypersensitivity reactions, including angioedema and urticaria, have been reported in patients receiving tofacitinib. If a serious hypersensitivity reaction occurs, tofacitinib should be discontinued promptly while the potential cause is investigated.

GI Perforation

Cases of GI perforation have been reported in patients receiving tofacitinib in clinical trials. In clinical trials in patients with rheumatoid arthritis, many of the patients were receiving concomitant therapy with nonsteroidal anti-inflammatory agents (NSAIAs). In clinical trials in patients with ulcerative colitis, GI perforation appeared to occur at similar frequencies in patients receiving tofacitinib and those receiving placebo; many of the patients with ulcerative colitis were receiving concomitant corticosteroid therapy. The role of Janus kinase (JAK) inhibition by tofacitinib in these cases is not known.

Tofacitinib should be used with caution in patients who may be at increased risk for GI perforation (e.g., patients with a history of diverticulitis or receiving NSAIAs). Patients with new onset of abdominal symptoms should be evaluated promptly for early identification of GI perforation.

Hematologic Effects

Initial lymphocytosis (e.g., at one month following initiation of treatment) followed by gradual development of lymphopenia, with a decrease from baseline lymphocyte count of about 10% at 12 months, has been observed in patients receiving tofacitinib. Confirmed lymphocyte counts below 500/mm^3 were associated with an increased incidence of treated and serious infections. Initiation of tofacitinib therapy should be avoided in patients with lymphocyte counts of less than 500/mm^3. Lymphocyte counts should be monitored at baseline and every 3 months during treatment. Tofacitinib therapy should be interrupted or discontinued based on lymphocyte counts.

Treatment with tofacitinib is associated with an increased incidence of neutropenia (neutrophil count less than 2000/mm^3) compared with placebo. A clear relationship between neutropenia and the occurrence of serious infection has not been demonstrated. Initiation of tofacitinib therapy should be avoided in patients with an ANC of less than 1000/mm^3. Neutrophil counts should be monitored at baseline, at 4–8 weeks after initiation of therapy, and every 3 months thereafter. Tofacitinib therapy should be interrupted or discontinued based on ANC measurements.

Anemia has been reported in patients receiving tofacitinib. Initiation of tofacitinib therapy should be avoided in patients with hemoglobin concentrations of less than 9 g/dL. Hemoglobin concentrations should be monitored at baseline, at 4–8 weeks after initiation of therapy, and every 3 months thereafter. Tofacitinib therapy should be interrupted or discontinued based on hemoglobin concentration.

Hepatic Effects

Tofacitinib has been associated with an increased incidence of elevated hepatic aminotransferase concentrations compared with placebo. These increases, which included elevations exceeding 3 times the upper limit of normal (ULN), were observed predominantly in patients who were receiving concomitant therapy with other DMARDs, primarily methotrexate. Hepatic enzyme elevations were reversible upon modification of the treatment regimen (e.g., dosage reduction of concomitant DMARD or tofacitinib; interruption of tofacitinib therapy). Drug-induced hepatic injury was reported in one patient who received tofacitinib 10 mg twice daily for approximately 2.5 months. The patient developed symptomatic elevations of AST and ALT to greater than 3 times the ULN and elevation of bilirubin concentration to greater than 2 times the ULN; hospitalization and liver biopsy were required.

Hepatic aminotransferase concentrations should be routinely monitored in patients receiving tofacitinib. In case of elevations, patients should be evaluated promptly for drug-induced hepatotoxicity. If drug-induced hepatic injury is suspected, tofacitinib therapy should be interrupted until such diagnosis has been excluded.

Metabolic Effects

Dose-related increases in concentrations of total cholesterol, low-density lipoprotein (LDL)-cholesterol, high-density lipoprotein (HDL)-cholesterol, and triglycerides have been observed in patients receiving tofacitinib. Increases in these parameters were observed following one month of tofacitinib therapy and remained stable thereafter, with maximum increases generally occurring within the first 6 weeks of therapy. The effect of these increases on cardiovascular morbidity and mortality has not been determined.

In controlled clinical trials, mean concentrations of LDL-cholesterol and HDL-cholesterol increased during the first 3 months of therapy by 15 and 10%, respectively, in patients receiving tofacitinib 5 mg twice daily and by 19 and 12%, respectively, in patients receiving tofacitinib 10 mg twice daily. Mean ratios of LDL-cholesterol to HDL-cholesterol were essentially unchanged. In a controlled clinical trial, elevated concentrations of LDL-cholesterol and apolipoprotein B decreased to pretreatment concentrations in response to treatment with a hydroxymethylglutaryl-CoA (HMG-CoA) reductase inhibitor (statin).

Lipid concentrations should be measured approximately 4–8 weeks after initiation of tofacitinib therapy. Hyperlipidemia should be managed according to current standards of care.

Immunizations

Administration of live vaccines should be avoided during therapy with tofacitinib. Immunizations should be updated according to current administration guidelines prior to initiation of tofacitinib therapy.

GI Obstruction

Because symptoms of GI obstruction have been reported rarely following administration of nondeformable extended-release drug formulations in patients with known GI strictures, tofacitinib extended-release tablets should be used with caution in patients with preexisting, severe, pathologic or iatrogenic narrowing of the GI tract.

Specific Populations

Pregnancy

Adequate data are not available regarding use of tofacitinib in pregnant women. Fetocidal and teratogenic effects have been observed in rats and rabbits. In addition, reductions in live litter size, postnatal survival, and pup body weights have been observed in rats. Because the applicability of these findings to women receiving recommended dosages of tofacitinib is uncertain, pregnancy planning and prevention should be considered in females with reproductive potential.

Data suggest that increased disease activity in women with rheumatoid arthritis or ulcerative colitis is associated with an increased risk of adverse pregnancy outcomes (e.g., preterm delivery, low birthweight, small for gestational age at birth).

A pregnancy registry has been established to monitor fetal outcomes of pregnant women exposed to tofacitinib; patients or clinicians may contact the registry at 877-311-8972 to report any exposures to the drug that occur during pregnancy.

Lactation

Tofacitinib is distributed into milk in rats; it is not known whether the drug is distributed into human milk, affects milk production, or affects nursing infants. Because of the serious adverse effects (e.g., serious infections) observed in tofacitinib-treated adults, breast-feeding is not recommended during tofacitinib therapy and for at least 18 hours after the last dose of the drug administered as conventional tablets or 36 hours after the last dose administered as extended-release tablets.

Females and Males of Reproductive Potential

Reproductive planning and prevention should be considered in females with reproductive potential.

Findings of animal studies suggest that tofacitinib may reduce fertility in females; this effect may be irreversible.

Pediatric Use

Safety and efficacy of tofacitinib as conventional tablets and oral solution for the management of active polyarticular-course JIA have been established in pediatric patients 2–17 years of age based on evidence from adequate and well-controlled studies of tofacitinib (as conventional tablets) in adults with rheumatoid arthritis and additional data from a clinical trial of tofacitinib (as conventional tablets or oral solution) in pediatric patients with active polyarthritis (see Uses: Juvenile Idiopathic Arthritis). Adverse reactions observed in pediatric patients receiving tofacitinib generally were consistent with those reported in adults with rheumatoid arthritis. Safety and efficacy have not been established for the management of active polyarticular-course JIA in patients younger than 2 years of age or for uses other than polyarticular-course JIA in pediatric patients.

Safety and efficacy of tofacitinib as extended-release tablets have not been established in pediatric patients.

Geriatric Use

In controlled trials of tofacitinib in patients with rheumatoid arthritis, 15% of patients were 65 years of age or older, while 2% were 75 years of age and older. In these studies, a higher incidence of serious infections was reported in patients 65 years of age or older compared with younger patients. Clinical studies of tofacitinib in patients with ulcerative colitis did not include sufficient numbers of patients 65 years of age or older to determine whether geriatric patients respond differently than younger adults. Tofacitinib should be used with caution in geriatric patients, taking into consideration the higher incidence of infections generally observed in geriatric patients. Age does not substantially alter pharmacokinetics of the drug.

Hepatic Impairment

Use of tofacitinib is not recommended in patients with severe hepatic impairment. Dosage adjustment is recommended in patients with moderate hepatic impairment since increased drug exposure may increase the risk of adverse effects. Systemic exposure to tofacitinib is increased by 3 or 65% in patients with mild or moderate hepatic impairment, respectively.

Safety and efficacy of tofacitinib have not been evaluated in patients with serologic evidence of HBV or HCV infection.

Renal Impairment

Systemic exposure to tofacitinib is increased by 41, 71, or 156% in patients with mild, moderate, or severe renal impairment, respectively. In patients with end-stage renal disease receiving hemodialysis, systemic exposure to tofacitinib is increased by approximately 40%. Dosage adjustment is recommended in patients with moderate to severe renal impairment, including those receiving hemodialysis.

● Common Adverse Effects

Adverse effects occurring in 2% or more of patients with rheumatoid arthritis receiving tofacitinib 5 or 10 mg twice daily monotherapy or in combination with DMARDs and occurring greater than 1% more than placebo include diarrhea, headache, nasopharyngitis, and upper respiratory tract infection. Adverse effects in patients with psoriatic arthritis and ankylosing spondylitis are similar to those observed in patients with rheumatoid arthritis.

Adverse effects occurring in 5% or more of patients with ulcerative colitis receiving tofacitinib for either induction therapy (10 mg twice daily) or maintenance therapy (5 or 10 mg twice daily) and more commonly than in patients receiving placebo include nasopharyngitis, elevated cholesterol concentrations, headache, upper respiratory tract infection, increased blood creatine kinase (CK, creatine phosphokinase, CPK) concentrations, rash, diarrhea, and herpes zoster.

Adverse effects reported in pediatric patients with polyarticular-course JIA receiving tofacitinib generally are consistent with those reported in adults with rheumatoid arthritis.

DRUG INTERACTIONS

● Drugs Affecting Hepatic Microsomal Enzymes

Metabolism of tofacitinib is mediated primarily by cytochrome P-450 (CYP) isoenzyme 3A4, with a minor contribution from CYP2C19.

CYP2C19 and CYP3A4 Inhibitors

Concomitant administration of tofacitinib with a potent inhibitor of CYP3A4 (e.g., ketoconazole) or with one or more drugs that result in both moderate inhibition of CYP3A4 and potent inhibition of CYP2C19 (e.g., fluconazole) results in increased tofacitinib exposure. Concomitant administration of drugs that inhibit only CYP2C19 is unlikely to substantially alter the pharmacokinetics of tofacitinib.

Reduction of tofacitinib dosage is recommended when tofacitinib is used concomitantly with a potent inhibitor of CYP3A4 or with one or more drugs that result in both moderate inhibition of CYP3A4 and potent inhibition of CYP2C19. In adults receiving tofacitinib as conventional tablets, a dosage of 10 mg twice daily should be reduced to 5 mg twice daily and a dosage of 5 mg twice daily should be reduced to 5 mg once daily. In adults receiving tofacitinib as extended-release tablets, a dosage of 22 mg once daily should be reduced to 11 mg once daily and a dosage of 11 mg once daily (as extended-release tablets) should be reduced to 5 mg once daily (as conventional tablets). In pediatric patients, dosage of tofacitinib (as oral solution or conventional tablets) should be reduced from 3.2 mg twice daily to 3.2 mg once daily, from 4 mg twice daily to 4 mg once daily, or from 5 mg twice daily to 5 mg once daily.

CYP3A4 Inducers

Concomitant administration of potent inducers of CYP3A4 (e.g., rifampin) results in decreased tofacitinib exposure and may result in decreased efficacy or loss of efficacy of tofacitinib. Concomitant use of such drugs is not recommended.

● Drugs Metabolized by Hepatic Microsomal Enzymes

Tofacitinib does not substantially inhibit or induce the activity of CYP isoenzymes 1A2, 2B6, 2C8, 2C9, 2C19, 2D6, or 3A4 in vitro at clinically relevant concentrations. In addition, tofacitinib does not appear to normalize CYP enzyme activity over time in patients with rheumatoid arthritis. Therefore, tofacitinib is not expected to alter metabolism of CYP substrates.

● Drugs Metabolized by Uridine Diphosphate-glucuronosyltransferase

In vitro studies indicate that tofacitinib does not substantially inhibit the activity of uridine diphosphate-glucuronosyltransferase (UGT) isoenzymes 1A1, 1A4, 1A6, 1A9, or 2B7.

● Drugs Affecting or Affected by Transport Systems

Pharmacokinetic interactions are unlikely with drugs that inhibit the P-glycoprotein transport system.

In vitro studies indicate that tofacitinib is unlikely to inhibit transporter proteins such as P-glycoprotein or organic anion or cation transport proteins at clinically relevant concentrations.

● Antifungal Agents

In healthy individuals, the potent CYP3A4 inhibitor ketoconazole (400 mg orally once daily for 3 days) increased peak plasma concentrations and area under the concentration-time curve (AUC) of tofacitinib (single oral dose of 10 mg) by 16 and 103%, respectively. Oral administration of fluconazole (a moderate CYP3A4 and potent CYP2C19 inhibitor) under steady-state conditions (400-mg loading dose followed by 200 mg once daily) increased peak plasma concentrations and AUC of tofacitinib (single oral dose of 30 mg) by 27 and 78%, respectively.

● Biologic Antirheumatic Agents

Tofacitinib should not be used concomitantly with biologic disease-modifying antirheumatic drugs (DMARDS). Concomitant use of tofacitinib with such drugs in patients with rheumatoid arthritis, psoriatic arthritis, ankylosing spondylitis, ulcerative colitis, or polyarticular course juvenile idiopathic arthritis has not been studied to date.

● Immunosuppressive Agents

Concomitant use of tofacitinib with potent immunosuppressive agents (e.g., azathioprine, cyclosporine, tacrolimus) increases the risk of immunosuppression and is not recommended. Concomitant use of tofacitinib with such agents in patients with rheumatoid arthritis, psoriatic arthritis, ankylosing spondylitis, ulcerative colitis, or polyarticular course juvenile idiopathic arthritis has not been studied to date.

In healthy individuals, cyclosporine (200 mg orally every 12 hours for 5 days) decreased the clearance of tofacitinib (single oral dose of 10 mg), resulting in a 73% increase in the AUC of tofacitinib, accompanied by a 17% decrease in peak plasma tofacitinib concentrations.

In healthy individuals, tacrolimus (5 mg orally every 12 hours for 7 days) slightly decreased the clearance of tofacitinib (single oral dose of 10 mg), resulting in a 21% increase in the AUC of tofacitinib, accompanied by a 9% decrease in peak plasma tofacitinib concentrations.

● Metformin

Metformin (a substrate of organic cation transporter [OCT] and multidrug and toxin extrusion transporter [MATE] proteins) does not substantially alter peak plasma concentrations or AUC of tofacitinib. No dosage adjustment is required when the drugs are used concomitantly.

● Methotrexate

Tofacitinib pharmacokinetics were not substantially altered by methotrexate administration in patients with rheumatoid arthritis; tofacitinib decreased peak plasma concentrations and AUC of methotrexate by 13 and 10%, respectively. Dosage adjustments are not necessary when tofacitinib is used concomitantly with methotrexate.

● Midazolam

In healthy individuals, tofacitinib (30 mg orally twice daily for 6 days) did not substantially alter peak plasma concentrations or AUC of the CYP3A substrate midazolam (single oral dose of 2 mg). No dosage adjustment is required when the drugs are used concomitantly.

● Oral Contraceptives

In healthy women, tofacitinib (30 mg orally twice daily for 9 days) did not substantially alter exposure to a single dose of an oral contraceptive containing ethinyl estradiol 30 mcg and levonorgestrel 0.15 mg. Tofacitinib increased AUCs of ethinyl estradiol and levonorgestrel by 7 and 1%, respectively; decreased peak plasma concentrations of ethinyl estradiol by 10%; and increased peak plasma concentrations of levonorgestrel by 12%. No dosage adjustment is required.

● Rifampin

In healthy individuals, the CYP3A inducer rifampin (600 mg orally once daily for 7 days) decreased peak plasma concentrations and AUC of tofacitinib (single oral dose of 30 mg) by 74 and 84%, respectively. Concomitant use of rifampin may decrease efficacy of tofacitinib.

● Vaccines

Live vaccines should not be administered to patients receiving tofacitinib. The interval between administration of live vaccines and initiation of tofacitinib therapy should be in accordance with current vaccination guidelines for patients receiving immunosuppressive agents.

Dissemination of the vaccine virus strain from zoster vaccine live (a vaccine containing live, attenuated varicella zoster virus) in a patient initiating tofacitinib therapy has been reported. Dissemination of the vaccine strain occurred 16 days after vaccine administration and 2 days after initiation of tofacitinib therapy (5 mg twice daily). The patient had no history of varicella infection and no anti-varicella antibodies at baseline. Tofacitinib was discontinued and the patient recovered following standard antiviral therapy.

DESCRIPTION

Tofacitinib citrate, a Janus kinase (JAK) inhibitor, is an immunomodulating agent and a disease-modifying antirheumatic drug (DMARD). JAKs are a family of intracellular tyrosine kinases consisting of JAK1, JAK2, JAK3, and tyrosine kinase (TYK) 2 that mediate the signaling of cytokines and growth factors that are important for hematopoiesis and immune function. Binding of cytokines to receptors on the cell surface activates pairing of JAKs (e.g., JAK1/JAK2, JAK1/JAK3, JAK1/TYK2, JAK2/JAK2, JAK2/TYK2), which leads to phosphorylation and subsequent localization of signal transducer and activator of transcription (STAT) proteins to the nucleus and modulation of gene expression. Tofacitinib modulates the signaling pathway at the point of JAKs, preventing the phosphorylation and activation of STATs. Tofacitinib inhibits JAK1 and JAK3 and, to a lesser extent, JAK2. In vitro, tofacitinib inhibited the activity of JAK1/JAK2, JAK1/JAK3, and JAK2/JAK2 combinations with IC_{50} (concentration that inhibits activity by 50%) values of 406, 56, and 1377 nM, respectively. The relevance of inhibition of specific JAK combinations to the therapeutic efficacy of tofacitinib is not known.

Treatment with tofacitinib has been shown to cause dose-dependent decreases in circulating CD16/56$^+$ natural killer cells, with estimated maximum reductions occurring after approximately 8–10 weeks of therapy; these decreases resolved approximately 2–6 weeks following discontinuance of tofacitinib. Dose-dependent increases in B-cell counts also have been observed with tofacitinib therapy; however, changes in circulating T-lymphocyte counts and T-lymphocyte subsets (CD3$^+$, CD4$^+$, and CD8$^+$) were small and inconsistent. The clinical importance of these changes in cell counts is unknown.

After 6 months of treatment, total serum concentrations of IgG, IgM, and IgA were lower in patients with rheumatoid arthritis receiving tofacitinib compared with patients receiving placebo; however, the changes in these concentrations were small and were not dose dependent.

Rapid decreases in serum C-reactive protein (CRP) concentrations have been observed in patients with rheumatoid arthritis receiving tofacitinib; these decreases were maintained throughout dosing. Changes in CRP concentrations are not reversed fully within 2 weeks following discontinuance of tofacitinib, indicating a longer duration of pharmacodynamic activity compared with the pharmacokinetic half-life of the drug.

Similar changes in T-cell and B-cell counts and CRP concentrations have been observed in patients with active psoriatic arthritis although reversibility was not assessed.

The absolute bioavailability of tofacitinib following oral administration as conventional tablets is approximately 74%. Peak plasma concentrations of the drug are achieved within 0.5–1 hour following oral administration as conventional tablets or oral solution and at 4 hours following oral administration as extended-release tablets. Peak concentrations and area under the serum concentration-time curve (AUC) are similar at tofacitinib dosages of 5 mg twice daily as conventional tablets or 11 mg once daily as extended-release tablets and at dosages of 10 mg twice daily as conventional tablets or 22 mg once daily as extended-release tablets. Administration of tofacitinib conventional tablets with a high-fat meal reduces peak plasma concentrations of the drug by 32% but does not substantially alter the AUC. Administration of tofacitinib extended-release tablets with a high-fat meal increases peak plasma concentrations of the drug by 19–27% and delays the time to peak plasma concentrations by approximately 1 hour, but does not alter AUC. The elimination half-life of tofacitinib is approximately 3 hours following oral administration as conventional tablets or oral solution and 6–8 hours following oral administration as extended-release tablets. Tofacitinib is eliminated mainly by hepatic metabolism (70%) and, to a lesser extent, by renal excretion as unchanged drug (30%). Metabolism of the drug is mediated mainly by cytochrome P-450 (CYP) isoenzyme 3A4, with a minor contribution by CYP2C19.

Age, weight, sex, and race do not have clinically important effects on tofacitinib exposure in adults. However, in pediatric patients with polyarticular-course juvenile idiopathic arthritis (JIA), body weight affects systemic exposure to the drug and weight-based dosing is recommended; no additional dosage adjustment is needed based on age, sex, race, or disease severity in this patient population.

ADVICE TO PATIENTS

- Discuss potential risks and benefits of therapy with the patient; importance of the patient reading the medication guide prior to initiation of therapy and each time the prescription is refilled. Importance of providing a copy of the manufacturer's instructions for use of the oral solution when this formulation is prescribed.

- Store tofacitinib conventional or extended-release tablets in the original container.

- Increased susceptibility to infection. Risk of herpes zoster, which may be serious. Importance of not initiating tofacitinib therapy if active infection is present. Importance of promptly informing clinicians if any signs or symptoms of infection (e.g., persistent fever, sweating, chills, myalgia, cough, dyspnea, fatigue, diarrhea, dysuria, erythema) develop.

- Risk of lymphoma and other malignancies. Risk of lymphoproliferative disorder in patients receiving tofacitinib in combination with drugs for prevention of renal allograft rejection.

- Risk of major adverse cardiovascular events, including MI, stroke, and cardiovascular death. Instruct all patients, especially current or past smokers and those with other cardiovascular risk factors, to monitor for the development of signs and symptoms of cardiovascular events.

- Importance of discontinuing tofacitinib therapy and seeking immediate medical attention if signs or symptoms suggestive of thrombosis (e.g., sudden shortness of breath; chest pain exacerbated by breathing; leg pain or tenderness; redness, swelling, or discoloration of a leg or arm) occur.

- Importance of discontinuing tofacitinib therapy and promptly notifying clinician if manifestations of a hypersensitivity reaction (e.g., swelling of the lips, tongue, or throat; urticaria) occur.

- Risk of GI perforation. Importance of promptly notifying clinicians of persistent fever and abdominal pain or changes in bowel function.

- Importance of informing clinicians of existing or contemplated concomitant therapy, including prescription and OTC drugs, as well as any concomitant illnesses or any history of cancer, tuberculosis, hepatitis B virus or hepatitis C virus infection, other chronic or recurring infections, or thrombotic or cardiac disease.

- Importance of periodic laboratory monitoring.

- Importance of women informing clinicians if they are or plan to become pregnant or plan to breast-feed. Women with reproductive potential should be advised of the potential risk to the fetus, and those who become pregnant while receiving tofacitinib should be advised that a pregnancy registry is available. Women should be advised to avoid breast-feeding during tofacitinib therapy and for at least 18 hours after the last dose is given as conventional tablets or 36 hours after the last dose is given as extended-release tablets.

- Potential for tofacitinib to impair fertility in females. It is not known whether this effect is reversible.

- Potential for the inert shell of the extended-release tablets to be eliminated in the stool or via colostomy after the drug has been absorbed.

- Importance of informing patients of other important precautionary information. (See Cautions.)

PREPARATIONS

Excipients in commercially available drug preparations may have clinically important effects in some individuals; consult specific product labeling for details.

Tofacitinib Citrate

Oral

Solution	5 mg (of tofacitinib) per 5 mL	Xeljanz® (with bottle adapter and 5-mL oral dosing syringe), Pfizer
Tablets, extended-release, film-coated	11 mg (of tofacitinib)	Xeljanz® XR, Pfizer
	22 mg (of tofacitinib)	Xeljanz® XR, Pfizer
Tablets, film-coated	5 mg (of tofacitinib)	Xeljanz®, Pfizer
	10 mg (of tofacitinib)	Xeljanz®, Pfizer

† Use is not currently included in the labeling approved by the US Food and Drug Administration.

Selected Revisions May 10, 2024, © Copyright, August 1, 2013, American Society of Health-System Pharmacists, Inc.

Upadacitinib

90:24.12.92 • JANUS KINASE INHIBITORS, MISCELLANEOUS

■ Upadacitinib, a Janus kinase (JAK) inhibitor, is an immunomodulating agent and a disease-modifying antirheumatic drug (DMARD).

USES

● Rheumatoid Arthritis in Adults

Upadacitinib is used for the management of moderately to severely active rheumatoid arthritis in adults who have had an inadequate response or intolerance to one or more tumor necrosis factor (TNF) blocking agents. Upadacitinib has been shown to induce clinical responses, improve physical function, and inhibit progression of joint structural damage in patients with rheumatoid arthritis. Guidelines generally support use of Janus kinase (JAK) inhibitors, including upadacitinib, as add on therapy to methotrexate in patients who do not meet treatment goals with methotrexate alone.

Clinical Experience

Upadacitinib can be used alone or in combination with methotrexate or other nonbiologic (conventional) disease-modifying antirheumatic drugs (DMARDs; examples include hydroxychloroquine, leflunomide, and sulfasalazine). Concomitant use of upadacitinib with other JAK inhibitors, potent immunosuppressants (e.g., azathioprine, cyclosporine), or biologic DMARDs is not recommended.

Efficacy and safety of upadacitinib have been evaluated in 5 randomized, double-blind, controlled studies of 12–48 weeks' duration in adults with moderately to severely active RA. In these studies, upadacitinib was administered as monotherapy in patients who had never received methotrexate (SELECT-EARLY) or who had experienced an inadequate response to methotrexate (SELECT-MONOTHERAPY), in combination with methotrexate in patients who had an inadequate response to methotrexate (SELECT-COMPARE), or in combination with nonbiologic DMARDs in patients who had an inadequate response to nonbiologic DMARD therapy (SELECT-NEXT) or an inadequate response or intolerance to biologic DMARD therapy (SELECT-BEYOND). The monotherapy studies included an active control (methotrexate); 2 of the studies of combination therapy included a placebo control for upadacitinib, and one included both active (adalimumab) and placebo controls. Four of the 5 studies evaluated both 15- and 30-mg daily dosages of upadacitinib, while one study evaluated only the 15-mg daily dosage. Patients in these studies met American College of Rheumatology/European League Against Rheumatism (ACR/EULAR) classification criteria for rheumatoid arthritis, had 6 or more tender joints, 6 or more swollen joints, and evidence of systemic inflammation (i.e., elevated high-sensitivity C-reactive protein [hs-CRP]). Those receiving stable dosages of oral corticosteroids (equivalent to 10 mg or less of prednisone daily), nonsteroidal anti-inflammatory agents (NSAIAs), or acetaminophen could continue these agents.

Clinical response was evaluated at week 12 in all studies except SELECT-MONOTHERAPY (evaluated at week 14). The ACR criteria for improvement in measures of disease activity (ACR responses) were the principal measure of clinical response. An ACR 20 response is achieved if the patient experiences a 20% improvement in tender and swollen joint counts and a 20% or greater improvement in at least 3 of the following criteria: patient pain assessment, patient global assessment, physician global assessment, patient self-assessed disability, and laboratory measures of disease activity (i.e., erythrocyte sedimentation rate [ESR] or CRP). ACR 50 and ACR 70 responses are defined using the same criteria but with a level of improvement of 50 and 70%, respectively. Greater proportions of patients receiving upadacitinib alone or in combination with nonbiologic DMARDs achieved ACR responses compared with those receiving placebo- or methotrexate-based comparator regimens. (See Table 1; results shown in Table 1 for upadacitinib are for the 15-mg daily dosage.) In placebo-controlled studies, higher ACR 20 response rates were observed as early as 1 week following initiation of upadacitinib therapy. Overall results of the clinical studies did not indicate a consistent dose-response effect for upadacitinib or a substantial therapeutic advantage for the 30-mg daily dosage relative to the 15-mg daily dosage.

TABLE 1. Proportion of Patients with Rheumatoid Arthritis Achieving Clinical Responses at 12 or 14 Weeks of Treatment

Study and Treatment	ACR 20	ACR 50	ACR 70
SELECT-EARLY[a]			
Upadacitinib	76%	52%	32%
Methotrexate	54%	28%	14%
SELECT-MONOTHERAPY[b]			
Upadacitinib	68%	42%	23%
Methotrexate	41%	15%	3%
SELECT-COMPARE[c]			
Upadacitinib	71%	45%	25%
Adalimumab	63%	29%	13%
Placebo	36%	15%	5%
SELECT-NEXT[d]			
Upadacitinib	64%	38%	21%
Placebo	36%	15%	6%
SELECT-BEYOND[e]			
Upadacitinib	65%	34%	12%
Placebo	28%	12%	7%

[a] Both treatments used as monotherapy in patients with no history of prior methotrexate therapy.

[b] Both treatments used as monotherapy in patients with a history of inadequate response to methotrexate.

[c] Both treatments used in combination with nonbiologic DMARD therapy in patients with a history of inadequate response to nonbiologic DMARD therapy.

[d] Each treatment used in combination with methotrexate in patients with a history of inadequate response to methotrexate.

[e] Both treatments used in combination with nonbiologic DMARD therapy in patients with a history of inadequate response or intolerance to biologic DMARD therapy.

Greater proportions of patients receiving upadacitinib alone or in combination with nonbiologic DMARDs achieved a Disease Activity Score in 28 joints using CRP (DAS 28 [CRP]) of less than 2.6 (i.e., DAS-defined remission) at week 12 or 14 compared with those receiving placebo- or methotrexate-based comparator regimens.

Patients receiving upadacitinib alone or in combination with conventional DMARDs also had greater improvement in physical function at week 12 or 14, as measured by the Health Assessment Questionnaire Disability Index (HAQ-DI), compared with those receiving placebo- or methotrexate-based comparator regimens.

Progression of joint structural damage, as measured by change in van der Heijde-modified total Sharp score (a composite measure of radiographically assessed structural damage [i.e., joint erosion and joint space narrowing]), was evaluated at week 24 in SELECT-EARLY and at week 26 in SELECT-COMPARE. In SELECT-EARLY, upadacitinib inhibited progression of joint structural damage compared with methotrexate; at week 24, 87% of patients receiving upadacitinib 15 mg daily had no radiographic progression of joint damage compared with 78% of those receiving methotrexate. In SELECT-COMPARE, upadacitinib in combination with methotrexate inhibited progression of joint structural damage compared with placebo in combination with methotrexate; at week 26, 83% of patients receiving upadacitinib 15 mg daily and methotrexate had no radiographic progression of joint damage compared with 76% of those receiving placebo and methotrexate.

In long-term follow-up analyses of the SELECT-BEYOND, SELECT-COMPARE, SELECT-EARLY, and SELECT-MONOTHERAPY studies through 60, 156, 72, and 84 weeks, respectively, clinical response rates and the safety profile of upadacitinib were consistent with previously reported data.

In another double-blind, active-controlled phase 3 study (SELECT-CHOICE), adults with moderate to severe active rheumatoid arthritis who did not achieve an adequate response or tolerate biologic DMARD therapy were randomized to receive upadacitinib 15 mg once daily or abatacept IV. Patients in the study continued stable background therapy with conventional nonbiologic DMARDS, NSAIAs, acetaminophen, or corticosteroids (oral or inhaled). The primary efficacy endpoint of this study was change in DAS28-CRP at week 12. At baseline, DAS28-CRP was 5.70 in the upadacitinib group and 5.88 in the abatacept group; the mean change from baseline to week 12 was -2.52 and -2.00 in the respective treatment groups. Noninferiority of upadacitinib compared with abatacept was demonstrated based on change in DAS28-CRP.

Clinical Perspectice

The American College of Rheumatology issued guidelines for the treatment of rheumatoid arthritis in 2021. Disease-modifying treatments for rheumatoid arthritis include conventional DMARDs (e.g., hydroxychloroquine, leflunomide, methotrexate, sulfasalazine), biologic DMARDs (e.g., TNF blocking agents, abatacept, tocilizumab, sarilumab, rituximab), and/or targeted synthetic DMARDs (e.g., Janus kinase [JAK] inhibitors). Specific agents for rheumatoid arthritis treatment are selected according to current disease activity, prior therapies used, and the presence of comorbidities. A "treat-to-target" approach is typically employed, with the goal of achieving a predefined target of low disease activity or remission.

Targeted synthetic DMARDs used in the treatment of rheumatoid arthritis include the JAK inhibitors baricitinib, tofacitinib, and upadacitinib. Methotrexate monotherapy is strongly recommended over biologic or targeted synthetic DMARD monotherapy in DMARD-naive patients with moderate to high disease activity. Methotrexate monotherapy also is strongly preferred over combined therapy with a non-TNF blocking agent biologic DMARD or targeted synthetic DMARD because of the lack of proven benefit and additional risks and costs associated with combined therapy. Randomized controlled trials evaluating add-on therapy with a biologic or targeted synthetic DMARD or triple therapy (methotrexate, sulfasalazine, and hydroxychloroquine) demonstrated equivalent long-term outcomes in patients receiving add-on therapy with a biologic or targeted synthetic DMARD and those receiving triple therapy; therefore, targeted synthetic DMARDs and biologic DMARDs (including TNF blocking agents) are conditionally recommended as add-on therapy for patients with an inadequate response to maximally tolerated doses of methotrexate. Recommendations for the use and selection of targeted synthetic DMARDs in rheumatoid arthritis vary based on the presence of certain comorbidities (e.g., heart failure, previous serious infection, nontuberculous mycobacterial lung disease). Consult the American College of Rheumatology guidelines for additional details.

● Psoriatic Arthritis

Upadacitinib is used for the management of active psoriatic arthritis in adults and pediatric patients 2 years of age and older who have had an inadequate response or intolerance to one or more TNF blocking agents. Upadacitinib has been shown to induce clinical responses and improve physical functioning in patients with psoriatic arthritis. The specific place in therapy for upadacitinib is not discussed in treatment guidelines for psoriatic arthritis.

Clinical Experience

Upadacitinib can be used alone or in combination with other nonbiologic (conventional) disease-modifying antirheumatic drugs (DMARDs), NSAIAs, or corticosteroids. Concomitant use of upadacitinib with other JAK inhibitors, potent immunosuppressants (e.g., azathioprine, cyclosporine), or biologic DMARDs is not recommended.

Efficacy and safety of upadacitinib for the management of psoriatic arthritis in adults have been established in 2 randomized, double-blind phase 3 studies. Study PsA-1 was a 24-week active- and placebo-controlled study in 1705 patients with a history of inadequate response or intolerance to at least one nonbiologic DMARD. Study PsA-2 was a 24-week placebo-controlled study in 642 patients with a history of inadequate response or intolerance to at least one biologic DMARD. Patients in both studies had active psoriatic arthritis for at least 6 months based upon the Classification Criteria for Psoriatic Arthritis (CASPAR) with at least 3 tender/painful joints and at least 3 swollen joints, and active plaque psoriasis or a history of plaque psoriasis. In Study PsA-1, patients were randomized to receive upadacitinib 15 mg once daily, upadacitinib 30 mg once daily, adalimumab (40 mg every other week), or placebo, alone or concomitantly with a nonbiologic DMARD. In Study PsA-2, patients were randomized to receive upadacitinib 15 mg once daily,

upadacitinib 30 mg once daily, or placebo, alone or concomitantly with a nonbiologic DMARD. In both studies, patients randomized to placebo switched to upadacitinib 15 or 30 mg once daily in a blinded manner at week 24. The primary measure of efficacy was the proportion of patients achieving an ACR 20 response at 12 weeks.

In both studies, a statistically significant greater proportion of patients receiving upadacitinib 15 mg once daily compared with those receiving placebo achieved ACR 20 responses at 12 weeks and a higher proportion of patients receiving upadacitinib 15 mg once daily compared with those receiving placebo achieved ACR 50 and ACR 70 responses at week 12. In these 2 studies, ACR 20, ACR 50, and ACR 70 responses were achieved at 12 weeks in 57–71, 32–38, 9–16%, respectively, of patients receiving upadacitinib 15 mg once daily. Improvements in dactylitis and enthesitis also were observed in patients receiving upadacitinib 15 mg once daily. Although upadacitinib has not been studied for the treatment of plaque psoriasis, upadacitinib 15 mg once daily resulted in improvement in skin manifestations in patients with psoriatic arthritis.

Improvements in physical function, as measured by change in HAQ-DI score from baseline to 12 weeks, were greater in both studies for patients receiving upadacitinib 15 mg once daily compared with those receiving placebo. In the 2 studies, 45–58% of patients receiving upadacitinib 15 mg once daily achieved a HAQ-DI response (defined as improvement of 0.35 or greater from baseline to 12 weeks) compared with 27–33% of those receiving placebo.

In Study PsA-1, radiographic evaluations were performed at baseline and 24 weeks. Treatment with upadacitinib 15 mg once daily inhibited progression of structural joint damage compared to placebo at week 24. Analyses of erosion and joint space narrowing scores were consistent with overall results. The proportion of patients with no radiographic progression (modified total sharp score change of 0 or less) at 24 weeks was 93% in patients receiving upadacitinib 15 mg once daily and 89% in those receiving placebo.

Health-related quality of life was assessed by Short Form Health Survey (SF-36). In both studies, patients receiving upadacitinib 15 mg once daily experienced statistically significant greater improvements in the Physical Component Summary score compared with those receiving placebo at week 12. Improvements in the Mental Component Summary score and all 8 domains of SF-36 also were observed in patients receiving upadacitinib 15 mg once daily compared with those receiving placebo. In both studies, an improvement in fatigue (as measured by FACIT-F score) from baseline to week 12 also was observed in patients receiving upadacitinib 15 mg once daily compared with those receiving placebo.

In long-term follow-up analyses of Study PsA 1 and Study PsA 2 at 104 and 152 weeks, respectively, clinical response rates and the safety profile of upadacitinib were consistent with previously reported data.

Clinical Perspective

The American College of Rheumatology and the National Psoriasis Foundation issued a joint guideline for the treatment of psoriatic arthritis in 2018. Nonpharmacologic (e.g., physical therapy, occupational therapy, smoking cessation, weight loss, exercise, massage therapy) and pharmacologic therapy can ameliorate psoriatic arthritis symptoms and can occasionally result in disease remission. Disease-modifying treatments for psoriatic arthritis include oral small molecule DMARDs (e.g., methotrexate, sulfasalazine, cyclosporine, leflunomide, apremilast), biologic DMARDs (e.g., TNF blocking agents, secukinumab, ixekizumab, ustekinumab, brodalumab, abatacept), and/or targeted synthetic DMARDs (e.g., Janus kinase [JAK] inhibitors). Specific agents for psoriatic arthritis treatment are selected according to disease characteristics, including disease severity, as well as patient preferences and comorbidities. A "treat-to-target" approach is typically employed, with the goal of achieving low/minimal disease activity or remission.

● Atopic Dermatitis

Upadacitinib is used for the treatment of adult and pediatric patients ≥12 years of age with refractory, moderate to severe atopic dermatitis who have had an inadequate response to other systemic therapies or who are not eligible for other systemic therapies. Upadacitinib alone or in combination with topical corticosteroids has been shown to improve vIGA-AD and EASI-75, -90, or -100 score compared with those receiving placebo. Guidelines conditionally recommend the use of oral JAK inhibitors (including upadacitinib) in patients with moderate to severe atopic dermatitis who are refractory to, intolerant of, or unable to use mid- to high-potency topical treatment and systemic treatment inclusive of a recommended biologic agent (dupilumab or tralokinumab).

Clinical Experience

Upadacitinib can be used alone or in combination with topical corticosteroids. Concomitant use of upadacitinib with other JAK inhibitors, immunosuppressants, or biologic immunomodulators is not recommended.

Efficacy and safety of upadacitinib have been evaluated in 3 randomized, double-blind, multicenter phase 3 studies (AD-1, AD-2, and AD-3) in 2584 patients (2240 adults and 344 pediatric patients ≥12 years of age) with moderate to severe atopic dermatitis not adequately controlled by topical therapies. In these studies, upadacitinib was administered as monotherapy (AD-1 and AD-2) or concomitantly with topical corticosteroids (AD-3). Patients enrolled in these studies received upadacitinib once daily (15 or 30 mg) or placebo for 16 weeks. In all 3 studies, the principal measures of efficacy were the proportion of patients with a validated Investigator's Global Assessment (vIGA-AD) score of 0 (clear) or 1 (almost clear) with at least a 2-point improvement and the proportion of patients with Eczema Area and Severity Index (EASI)-75 (defined as an improvement of at least 75% in EASI score from baseline) at week 16. At baseline, 49% of patients had a vIGA-AD score of 3 (moderate atopic dermatitis) and 51% of patients had a vIGA-AD score of 4 (severe atopic dermatitis). The baseline mean EASI score was 29 and the baseline weekly average Worst Pruritus Numerical Rating Score was 7. Approximately 52% of patients received previous therapy for atopic dermatitis.

A greater proportion of patients receiving upadacitinib (15 or 30 mg) alone or concomitantly with topical corticosteroids achieved a vIGA-AD score of 0 or 1 with at least a 2-point improvement and an improvement in EASI-75, -90, or -100 score from baseline compared with those receiving placebo. (See Tables 2, 3, and 4) Subgroup analysis based on age, sex, race, weight, and prior systemic therapy with immunosuppressants did not identify differences in response to upadacitinib monotherapy or concomitant therapy with topical corticosteroids in the AD-1, AD-2, and AD-3 studies. A long-term extension of the AD-3 study found that efficacy and safety of upadacitinib plus topical corticosteroids were maintained through 52 weeks.

TABLE 2. Upadacitinib Monotherapy (AD-1 Study): Proportion of Patients with Atopic Dermatitis Achieving Clinical Response at 16 Weeks of Treatment

Clinical Response	Placebo	Upadacitinib 15 mg once daily	Upadacitinib 30 mg once daily
Adults[a]			
vIGA-AD 0 or 1	8%	48%	62%
EASI-75	16%	70%	80%
EASI-90	8%	53%	66%
EASI-100	2%	17%	27%
≥4-point improvement in Worst Pruritus NRS [b]	12%	52%	60%
≥4-point improvement in Atopic Dermatitis Symptom Scale (ADerm-SS) Skin Pain NRS[c]	15%	54%	63%
Pediatric Patients ≥12 Years of Age[d]			
vIGA-AD 0 or 1	8%	38%	69%
EASI-75	8%	71%	83%
≥4-point improvement in Worst Pruritus NRS [e]	15%	45%	55%

[a] 281, 281, or 285 adults received placebo, upadacitinib 15 mg once daily, or upadacitinib 30 mg once daily, respectively.

[b] 272, 274, or 280 adults in the placebo, upadacitinib 15 mg, or upadacitinib 30 mg treatment groups, respectively, had a Worst Pruritus NRS score of ≥4 at baseline

[c] 233, 237, or 249 adults in the placebo, upadacitinib 15 mg, or upadacitinib 30 mg treatment groups, respectively, had an ADerm-SS Skin Pain NRS score of ≥4 at baseline

[d] 40, 42, or 42 pediatric patients received placebo, upadacitinib 15 mg once daily, or upadacitinib 30 mg once daily, respectively

[e] 39, 40, or 42 pediatric patients in the placebo, upadacitinib 15 mg, or upadacitinib 30 mg treatment groups, respectively, had a Worst Pruritus NRS score of ≥4 at baseline

TABLE 3. Upadacitinib Monotherapy (AD-2 Study): Proportion of Patients with Atopic Dermatitis Achieving Clinical Response at 16 Weeks of Treatment

Clinical Response	Placebo	Upadacitinib 15 mg once daily	Upadacitinib 30 mg once daily
Adults[a]			
vIGA-AD 0 or 1	5%	39%	52%
EASI-75	13%	60%	73%
EASI-90	5%	42%	58%
EASI-100	1%	14%	19%
≥4-point improvement in Worst Pruritus NRS [b]	9%	42%	60%
≥4-point improvement in Atopic Dermatitis Symptom Scale (ADerm-SS) Skin Pain NRS[c]	13%	49%	65%
Pediatric Patients ≥12 Years of Age[d]			
vIGA-AD 0 or 1	3%	42%	62%
EASI-75	14%	67%	74%
≥4-point improvement in Worst Pruritus NRS[e]	3%	33%	50%

[a] 278, 276, or 282 adults received placebo, upadacitinib 15 mg once daily, or upadacitinib 30 mg once daily, respectively.

[b] 274, 270, or 280 adults in the placebo, upadacitinib 15 mg, or upadacitinib 30 mg treatment groups, respectively, had a Worst Pruritus NRS score of ≥4 at baseline

[c] 247, 237, or 238 adults in the placebo, upadacitinib 15 mg, or upadacitinib 30 mg treatment groups, respectively, had an ADerm-SS Skin Pain NRS score of ≥4 at baseline

[d] 36, 33, or 35 pediatric patients received placebo, upadacitinib 15 mg once daily, or upadacitinib 30 mg once daily, respectively

[e] 36, 30, or 34 pediatric patients in the placebo, upadacitinib 15 mg, or upadacitinib 30 mg treatment groups, respectively, had a Worst Pruritus NRS score of ≥4 at baseline

TABLE 4. Concomitant Therapy with Upadacitinib and Topical Corticosteroids (AD-3 Study): Proportion of Patients with Atopic Dermatitis Achieving Clinical Response at 16 Weeks of Treatment

Clinical Response	Placebo plus topical corticosteroid therapy	Upadacitinib 15 mg once daily plus topical corticosteroid therapy	Upadacitinib 30 mg once daily plus topical corticosteroid therapy
Adults[a]			
vIGA-AD 0 or 1	11%	40%	59%
EASI-75	26%	65%	77%
EASI-90	13%	43%	63%
EASI-100	1%	12%	23%
≥4-point improvement in Worst Pruritus NRS [b]	15%	52%	64%

TABLE 4. Continued

Clinical Response	Placebo plus topical corticosteroid therapy	Upadacitinib 15 mg once daily plus topical corticosteroid therapy	Upadacitinib 30 mg once daily plus topical corticosteroid therapy
Pediatric Patients ≥12 Years of Age[c]			
vIGA-AD 0 or 1	8%	31%	65%
EASI-75	30%	56%	76%
≥4-point improvement in Worst Pruritus NRS [d]	13%	42%	55%

[a] 304, 300, or 297 adults received placebo, upadacitinib 15 mg once daily, or upadacitinib 30 mg once daily, respectively.

[b] 294, 288, or 291 adults in the placebo, upadacitinib 15 mg, or upadacitinib 30 mg treatment groups, respectively, had a Worst Pruritus NRS score of ≥4 at baseline

[c] 40, 39, or 37 pediatric patients received topical corticosteroids concomitantly with either placebo, upadacitinib 15 mg once daily, or upadacitinib 30 mg once daily, respectively

[d] 38, 36, or 33 pediatric patients in the placebo, upadacitinib 15 mg, or upadacitinib 30 mg treatment groups, respectively, had a Worst Pruritus NRS score of ≥4 at baseline

Clinical Perspective

Guidelines from the American Academy of Allergy, Asthma, and Immunology and the American College of Allergy, Asthma and Immunology state that topical treatment with moisturizers is first-line for all patients with atopic dermatitis; topical corticosteroids and other topical treatments (e.g., calcineurin inhibitors, crisaborole) are recommended for patients who fail to respond to moisturizers alone. For patients with moderate to severe disease who are refractory to, intolerant of, or unable to use mid- to high-potency topical agents, biologic agents (dupilumab or tralokinumab) are recommended. Oral JAK inhibitors (abrocitinib, baricitinib, and upadacitinib) are conditionally recommended for patients with moderate to severe disease who are refractory to, intolerant of, or unable to use mid- to high-potency topical treatment and systemic treatment inclusive of a recommended biologic agent (dupilumab or tralokinumab). Cyclosporine is suggested as an additional treatment option for this patient population.

• Ulcerative Colitis

Upadacitinib is used for the treatment of moderately to severely active ulcerative colitis in adults who have had an inadequate response or intolerance to one or more TNF blocking agents. Upadacitinib has been shown to induce clinical remission and improve endoscopic findings in patients with ulcerative colitis and inadequate response, loss of response, or intolerance to other therapies. The specific place in therapy for upadacitinib is not discussed in treatment guidelines for ulcerative colitis.

Clinical Experience

Upadacitinib has been used alone or in combination with aminosalicylates, methotrexate, and/or oral corticosteroids. Concomitant use of upadacitinib with other JAK inhibitors, potent immunosuppressants (e.g., azathioprine, cyclosporine), or biologic therapies for ulcerative colitis is not recommended.

Efficacy and safety of upadacitinib have been evaluated in 2 identical, randomized, double-blind, multicenter phase 3 induction studies (U-ACHIEVE induction [UC-1] and U-ACCOMPLISH [UC-2]) and a single maintenance trial (U-ACHIEVE maintenance [UC-3]). In UC-1 and UC-2, adult patients with moderately to severely active ulcerative colitis were randomized to treatment (in a 2:1 ratio) with either upadacitinib 45 mg or placebo once daily for 8 weeks. Patients in both studies had confirmed ulcerative colitis for at least 90 days and active disease with an inadequate response, loss of response, or intolerance to oral aminosalicylates, corticosteroids, immunosuppressants, and/or biologic therapy. Concomitant treatment with stable doses of oral aminosalicylates, methotrexate, ulcerative colitis-related antibiotics, and/or oral corticosteroids (up to 30 mg/day of prednisone or equivalent) was permitted during the study.

Disease activity was assessed using the modified Mayo score (mMS), a 3-component Mayo score consisting of subscores for stool frequency (SFS), rectal bleeding (RBS), and endoscopy findings (ES). The primary measure of efficacy in UC-1 and UC-2 was clinical remission (defined as SFS ≤1 and not greater than baseline, RBS of 0, and ES ≤1 without friability) at week 8. Additional endpoints included clinical response (defined as a decrease in mMS by ≥2 points and ≥30% from baseline with a decrease in RBS ≥1 from baseline or an absolute RBS ≤1); endoscopic improvement (defined as ES ≤1 without friability); and histologic endoscopic mucosal improvement (ES ≤1 without friability and Geboes score ≤3.1).

In UC-1 and UC-2, patients had a median mMS of 7 at baseline; 61% of patients had an mMS of 5–7 and 39% had an mMS of 8–9. Therapies at baseline included aminosalicylates in 68% of patients and corticosteroids in 38% of patients. A total of 51% of patients had previously failed treatment with or were intolerant to at least one biologic therapy.

In UC-1, 473 patients were enrolled; clinical remission at week 8 was achieved in 26 or 5% of patients treated with upadacitinib or placebo, respectively. A clinical response was seen in 73 or 27% of patients given upadacitinib or placebo, respectively, at week 8; endoscopic improvement was observed in 36 or 7% of patients, and histologic endoscopic mucosal improvement was observed in 30 or 7% of patients.

In UC-2, 515 patients were enrolled; clinical remission at week 8 was achieved in 33 or 4% of patients treated with upadacitinib or placebo, respectively. A clinical response was seen in 74 or 25% of patients given upadacitinib or placebo, respectively, at week 8; endoscopic improvement was observed in 44 or 8% of patients, and histologic endoscopic mucosal improvement was observed in 37 or 6% of patients.

In both UC-1 and UC-2, the onset of clinical response (based on RBS and SFS) occurred as early as week 2 among patients receiving upadacitinib. Patients treated with upadacitinib were more likely to achieve endoscopic remission (ES of 0) at week 8 compared to patients receiving placebo, and more patients treated with upadacitinib reported no abdominal pain or bowel urgency at 8 weeks.

Patients who achieved a clinical response on upadacitinib 45 mg daily in UC-1, UC-2, or a phase 2b study were randomized to maintenance treatment (in a 1:1:1 ratio) in study UC-3 with upadacitinib 15 mg, upadacitinib 30 mg, or placebo once daily for up to 52 weeks. The primary endpoint for UC-3 was clinical remission at week 52; secondary outcomes included corticosteroid-free clinical remission (defined as clinical remission with no corticosteroid therapy for ≥90 days immediately preceding week 52), endoscopic improvement, and histologic endoscopic mucosal improvement.

A total of 451 patients enrolled in UC-3. At week 52, clinical remission was achieved in 52, 42, or 12% of patients given upadacitinib 30 mg, upadacitinib 15 mg, or placebo, respectively. Rates for corticosteroid-free clinical remission were 68, 57, or 22% for upadacitinib 30 mg, upadacitinib 15 mg, or placebo, respectively. Endoscopic improvement was observed in 62, 49, or 14% of patients receiving upadacitinib 30 mg, upadacitinib 15 mg, or placebo, respectively; histologic endoscopic mucosal improvement was observed in 50, 35, or 12% of patients receiving upadacitinib 30 mg, upadacitinib 15 mg, or placebo, respectively.

In UC-3, endoscopic remission at week 52 was more common with upadacitinib 15 or 30 mg compared to placebo. More patients treated with upadacitinib 15 or 30 mg reported no abdominal pain or bowel urgency at 52 weeks.

Clinical Perspective

The American College of Gastroenterology (ACG) and the American Gastroenterological Association (AGA) issued guidelines for the medical treatment of ulcerative colitis in adults in 2019 and 2020. Goals of therapy in ulcerative colitis include achieving and maintaining corticosteroid-free remission and promoting mucosal healing. Specific treatments for ulcerative colitis are selected according to the disease severity, as well as disease location/extent, disease prognosis, and previous therapies used. Drug classes used to treat ulcerative colitis include oral and rectal 5-aminosalicylates, oral and rectal corticosteroids, immunomodulators (e.g., thiopurines, methotrexate), tofacitinib, and biologic agents, including TNF blocking agents, vedolizumab, and ustekinumab. In most cases, if a drug used for induction therapy is effective, it is continued as maintenance of remission.

The specific place in therapy for upadacitinib has not been addressed in guidelines. For adult outpatients with moderate to severe ulcerative colitis, AGA recommends TNF blocking therapies, vedolizumab, tofacitinib, or ustekinumab over no treatment. AGA conditionally recommends the use of infliximab or vedolizumab over adalimumab for induction of remission in biologic-naive patients based on evidence from a comparative randomized controlled trial (vedolizumab) and a network meta-analysis (infliximab). ACG recommends the use of oral corticosteroids, TNF blocking agents, vedolizumab, or tofacitinib for induction of remission in patients with moderately to severely active ulcerative colitis. Early use of biologic agents with or without immunomodulator therapy is conditionally recommended over gradual step up therapy after failure of 5-aminosalicylates. Combination therapy with a TNF blocking agent and a thiopurine or methotrexate is conditionally recommended over biologic monotherapy. Patients who achieve remission with TNF blocking therapy should continue such therapy to maintain remission after induction. Patients with primary nonresponse to TNF blocking therapy should be switched to a biologic from a different class; patients who initially respond to one TNF blocking agent and later lose response can be switched to a different TNF blocking agent. Consult the ACG and AGA guidelines for additional details.

● Crohn Disease

Upadacitinib is used for the treatment of moderately to severely active Crohn disease in adults who have had an inadequate response or intolerance to one or more TNF blocking agents. Upadacitinib has been shown to induce clinical remission and improve endoscopic findings in patients with Crohn disease. The specific place in therapy for upadacitinib is not discussed in treatment guidelines for Crohn disease.

Clinical Experience

Upadacitinib has been used alone or in combination with aminosalicylates or methotrexate. Concomitant use of upadacitinib with other JAK inhibitors, potent immunosuppressants (e.g., azathioprine, cyclosporine), or biologic therapies for Crohn disease is not recommended.

Efficacy and safety of upadacitinib have been evaluated in 2 randomized, double-blind, multicenter phase 3 induction studies (U-EXCEED [CD-1] and U-EXCEL [CD-2] and in a single maintenance trial (U-ENDURE [CD-3]). In CD-1 and CD-2, adult patients were randomized to treatment (in a 2:1 ratio) with either upadacitinib 45 mg or placebo once daily for 12 weeks. Patients in both studies had moderately to severely active Crohn disease, with a baseline Crohn Disease Activity Index (CDAI) score ≥220 and a Simple Endoscopic Score for Crohn Disease (SES-CD) ≥6 (or ≥4 for isolated ileal disease). In CD-1, all patients had a history of prior biologic failure (defined as inadequate response or intolerance to at least 1 prior biologic therapy). Patients enrolled in CD-2 had a history of failure with at least 1 conventional or biologic therapy; 45% of patients had a history of prior biologic failure. Stable doses of Crohn disease-related antibiotics, aminosalicylates, and methotrexate were permitted in both studies, and concomitant corticosteroids (up to 30 mg/day prednisone or equivalent) were permitted at enrollment (with tapering initiated at week 4). In CD-1, therapies at baseline included corticosteroids, methotrexate, and aminosalicylates in 36, 7, and 15% of patients, respectively; in CD-2, 37, 3, and 24% of patients were receiving corticosteroids, methotrexate, and aminosalicylates, respectively, at baseline.

The primary measures of efficacy in both induction studies were clinical remission at week 12 (defined as CDAI score <150) and endoscopic response at week 12 (defined as a decrease in SES-CD ≥50% from baseline or a decrease of ≥2 points from baseline for patients with a baseline score of 4). Additional endpoints included clinical response (CR-100; defined as a decrease in CDAI score ≥100 points); endoscopic remission (defined as SES-CD ≤4 and no individual subscore >1 in any individual variable); and corticosteroid-free remission (defined as discontinuation of corticosteroids and achievement of clinical remission for patients on corticosteroids at baseline).

In CD-1, 419 patients were enrolled; at week 12, clinical remission was achieved in 36 or 18% of patients given upadacitinib or placebo, respectively, and endoscopic response was observed in 34 or 3% of patients given upadacitinib or placebo, respectively. Clinical response (CR-100), corticosteroid-free remission (for patients receiving corticosteroids at baseline), and endoscopic remission were achieved in 54, 30, and 19% of patients receiving upadacitinib and 31, 11, and 3% of patients receiving placebo, respectively.

In study CD-2, 438 patients were enrolled; at week 12, clinical remission was achieved in 46 or 23% of patients given upadacitinib or placebo, respectively, and endoscopic response was observed in 46 or 13% of patients given upadacitinib or placebo, respectively. Clinical response (CR-100), corticosteroid-free remission (for patients receiving corticosteroids at baseline), and endoscopic remission were achieved in 64, 40, and 30% of patients receiving upadacitinib and 40, 13, or 8% of patients receiving placebo, respectively.

In both CD-1 and CD-2, onset of clinical response based on CDAI score was seen as early as 2 weeks, with the proportion of patients achieving clinical response at week 2 greater among patients treated with upadacitinib compared to placebo. Reductions in stool frequency and abdominal pain were seen in a greater proportion of patients given upadacitinib compared to placebo at week 12.

Patients who achieved a clinical response on upadacitinib 45 mg daily in CD-1 or CD-2 were randomized to maintenance treatment (in a 1:1:1 ratio) in study CD-3 with upadacitinib 15 mg, upadacitinib 30 mg, or placebo once daily for 52 weeks. The primary endpoints for CD-3 were clinical remission at week 52 and endoscopic response at week 52; secondary outcomes included corticosteroid-free clinical remission (defined as clinical remission with no corticosteroid therapy for ≥90 days immediately preceding week 52), maintenance of clinical remission (defined as achievement of clinical remission at both maintenance study entry and week 52), and endoscopic remission.

A total of 343 patients enrolled in CD-3. Clinical remission at week 52 was achieved in 55, 42, or 14% of patients given upadacitinib 30 mg, upadacitinib 15 mg, or placebo, respectively. Endoscopic response was observed in 41, 28, or 7% of patients given upadacitinib 30 mg, upadacitinib 15 mg, or placebo, respectively. Rates of corticosteroid-free remission were 53, 42, or 14% for upadacitinib 30 mg, upadacitinib 15 mg, or placebo, respectively. Maintenance of clinical remission was achieved in 67, 51, or 22% of patients receiving upadacitinib 30 mg, upadacitinib 15 mg, or placebo, respectively, while endoscopic remission was achieved in 30, 19, or 5% of patients receiving upadacitinib 30 mg, upadacitinib 15 mg, or placebo, respectively. At week 52, a greater proportion of patients given upadacitinib 15 or 30 mg experienced reductions in stool frequency and abdominal pain compared to placebo.

Clinical Perspective

The ACG and AGA have issued guidelines for the medical treatment of Crohn disease. The ACG guideline was issued in 2018, while the AGA issued a guideline on the management of moderate to severe disease in 2021 and a guideline on management after surgical resection in 2017. Medical treatment of Crohn disease is typically divided into 2 phases: induction therapy (where control of inflammation is rapidly achieved) and maintenance therapy (where control of inflammation is sustained for a prolonged period of time). Specific treatments for Crohn disease are selected according to the patient's risk profile and disease severity. Drug classes used to treat Crohn disease include 5-aminosalicylates, antibiotics, corticosteroids, immunomodulators (e.g., thiopurines, methotrexate), and biologic agents including TNF blocking agents, ustekinumab, vedolizumab, and natalizumab.

The specific place in therapy for JAK inhibitors, including upadacitinib, is not addressed in current guidelines. The TNF blocking agents are generally recommended for use as induction and maintenance therapy in adults with moderate to severe Crohn disease. ACG states that TNF blocking agents should be used to treat moderate to severe and/or moderate to high risk Crohn disease that is resistant to treatment with corticosteroids and/or refractory to thiopurines or methotrexate. In adults with moderate to severe Crohn disease who are naive to biologics and immunomodulators, AGA suggests the use of adalimumab in combination with thiopurines for induction and maintenance of remission over adalimumab monotherapy; in addition, combination therapy with adalimumab and methotrexate may be more effective than adalimumab monotherapy based on indirect evidence. Patients with perianal fistulas should be considered for TNF blocking therapy; however, guideline recommendations regarding agent selection differ in this setting.

If a patient with Crohn disease achieves remission with a TNF blocking agent, TNF blocking therapy should be continued to maintain remission; monotherapy with a TNF blocking agent is effective for maintaining remission, but combination therapy with azathioprine/6-mercaptopurine or methotrexate should be considered due to the potential for immunogenicity and loss of response. For patients with surgically induced remission of Crohn disease, AGA suggests TNF blocking agents and/or thiopurines over other agents to prevent recurrence. Similarly, ACG recommends that patients who undergo surgery for Crohn disease and remain at high risk for recurrence should begin therapy with a TNF blocking agent within 4 weeks of surgery to prevent postoperative recurrence.

● Ankylosing Spondylitis

Upadacitinib is used for the treatment of active ankylosing spondylitis in adults who have had an inadequate response or intolerance to one or more TNF blocking agents. Upadacitinib has been shown to induce a clinical response in patients with ankylosing spondylitis refractory to other treatments. The specific place in therapy for upadacitinib is not discussed in treatment guidelines for ankylosing spondylitis.

Clinical Experience

Upadacitinib has been used alone or in combination with conventional DMARDs. Concomitant use of upadacitinib with other JAK inhibitors, potent immunosuppressants (e.g., azathioprine, cyclosporine), or biologic DMARDs is not recommended.

Efficacy and safety of upadacitinib have been evaluated in 2 randomized, double-blind, multicenter phase 3 studies (SELECT-AXIS 1 [AS-1] and SELECT-AXIS 2 [AS-2]). Both studies enrolled adult patients with active ankylosing spondylitis based on Bath Ankylosing Spondylitis Disease Activity Index (BASDAI) score ≥4 and a Patient's Assessment of Total Back Pain score ≥4. In study AS-1, enrolled patients had an inadequate response to ≥2 NSAIAs or intolerance/contraindication to these agents and no previous exposure to biologic DMARDs. In study AS-2, enrolled patients had an inadequate response to 1 or 2 biologic DMARDs. In both studies, patients were randomized to treatment (in a 1:1 ratio) with upadacitinib 15 mg or placebo once daily for 14 weeks. The primary outcome was the proportion of patients achieving an Assessment of Spondyloarthritis International Society 40 (ASAS40) response at week 14. An ASAS40 response was defined as a ≥40% improvement and an absolute improvement of ≥2 units from baseline in at least 3 of the following 4 domains, with no worsening in the remaining domain: patient global assessment of disease activity; patient assessment of back pain; Bath Ankylosing Spondylitis Functional Index [BASFI]; and inflammation (defined as the mean of the BASDAI questions on severity and duration of morning stiffness).

In AS-1, 187 patients were enrolled; approximately 16% were on a concomitant conventional DMARD at baseline. At 14 weeks, ASAS40 response was achieved in 50.5 or 25.5% of patients given upadacitinib or placebo, respectively. An ASAS20 response was achieved in 63.4 or 39.4% of patients given upadacitinib or placebo, respectively.

In AS-2, 420 patients were enrolled; approximately 31% were on a concomitant conventional DMARD at baseline. At 14 weeks, ASAS40 response was achieved in 44.5 or 18.2% of patients given upadacitinib or placebo, respectively. An ASAS20 response was achieved in 65.4 or 38.3% of patients given upadacitinib or placebo, respectively.

At week 14, patients who completed AS-1 or AS-2 entered an open-label treatment phase; patients who were initially randomized to placebo were switched to upadacitinib 15 mg once daily. ASAS40 response rates with upadacitinib were maintained for up to 2 years in AS-1 and up to 1 year in AS-2.

Clinical Perspective

The American College of Rheumatology, the Spondylitis Association of America, and the Spondyloarthritis Research and Treatment Network issued a joint guideline for the treatment of ankylosing spondylitis in 2019. Treatments for ankylosing spondylitis include NSAIAs, conventional DMARDs (e.g., methotrexate, sulfasalazine), biologic DMARDs (e.g., TNF blocking agents, secukinumab, ixekizumab), and/or targeted synthetic DMARDs (e.g., tofacitinib). Continuous NSAIA treatment is typically considered first-line for active ankylosing spondylitis, with other agents used in the treatment of NSAIA-refractory disease. Specific agents for ankylosing spondylitis treatment are selected according to current disease activity, prior therapies, and the presence of comorbidities. Goals of therapy in ankylosing spondylitis are to alleviate symptoms, improve functioning, maintain the ability to work, decrease complications, and prevent or slow skeletal damage.

The specific place in therapy of upadacitinib has not been addressed in guidelines. For adults with active ankylosing spondylitis despite treatment with NSAIAs, treatment with a TNF blocking agent is strongly recommended over no treatment with a TNF blocking agent and conditionally recommended over treatment with tofacitinib, secukinumab, or ixekizumab. No specific TNF blocking agent is recommended over others. In patients with active ankylosing spondylitis despite treatment with a first TNF blocking agent, guidelines conditionally recommend secukinumab or ixekizumab over treatment with a different TNF blocking agent for patients with primary nonresponse to TNF blocking therapy; in patients with secondary nonresponse to TNF blocking therapy, treatment with a different TNF blocking therapy is conditionally recommended over treatment

with a non-TNF blocking biologic agent. In adults with stable ankylosing spondylitis, continuation of biologic monotherapy is conditionally recommended over discontinuation of the biologic or continuation of combination therapy with NSAIAs or conventional DMARDs. Recommendations for treatment selection in ankylosing spondylitis may be influenced by the presence of certain comorbidities (e.g., iritis, inflammatory bowel disease). Consult the joint guideline issued by the American College of Rheumatology, the Spondylitis Association of America, and the Spondyloarthritis Research and Treatment Network for additional details.

● Nonradiographic Axial Spondyloarthritis

Upadacitinib is used for the treatment of active nonradiographic axial spondyloarthritis with objective signs of inflammation in adults who have had an inadequate response or intolerance to TNF blocking agents. Upadacitinib has been shown to induce a clinical response in patients with nonradiographic axial spondyloarthritis refractory to other treatments. The specific place in therapy for upadacitinib is not discussed in treatment guidelines for nonradiographic axial spondyloarthritis.

Clinical Experience

Upadacitinib has been used alone and in combination with conventional DMARDs, NSAIAs, and oral corticosteroids. Concomitant use of upadacitinib with other JAK inhibitors, potent immunosuppressants (e.g., azathioprine, cyclosporine), or biologic DMARDs is not recommended.

Efficacy and safety of upadacitinib have been evaluated in a randomized, double-blind, multicenter phase 3 study (SELECT-AXIS 2). The study enrolled 314 adult patients with active nonradiographic axial spondyloarthritis and intolerance/contraindication to NSAIAs or inadequate response to ≥2 NSAIAs. Active disease was defined as a BASDAI score ≥4 and a Patient's Assessment of Total Back Pain score ≥4. Patients also had objective signs of inflammation (elevated CRP levels) and/or sacroiliitis on MRI, with no definitive radiographic evidence of structural damage on sacroiliac joints. Patients were randomly assigned to treatment (in a 1:1 ratio) with either upadacitinib 15 mg or placebo once daily for 52 weeks. The primary outcome was the proportion of patients achieving an ASAS40 response at week 14.

At baseline, approximately 29.1% of patients were receiving concomitant conventional DMARD therapy; 32.9% of patients had an inadequate response or intolerance to biologic DMARD therapy. At 14 weeks, an ASAS40 response was achieved in 44.9 or 22.3% of patients given upadacitinib or placebo, respectively. An ASAS20 response was seen in 66.7 or 43.3% of patients given upadacitinib or placebo, respectively.

Clinical Perspective

The American College of Rheumatology, the Spondylitis Association of America, and the Spondyloarthritis Research and Treatment Network issued a joint guideline for the treatment of nonradiographic axial spondyloarthritis in 2019. Treatments for nonradiographic axial spondyloarthritis include NSAIAs, conventional DMARDs (e.g., methotrexate, sulfasalazine), biologic DMARDs (e.g., TNF blocking agents, secukinumab, ixekizumab), and/or targeted synthetic DMARDs (e.g., tofacitinib). Continuous NSAIA treatment is typically considered first-line for active nonradiographic axial spondyloarthritis, with other agents being used in the treatment of NSAIA-refractory disease. Specific agents for nonradiographic axial spondyloarthritis treatment are selected according to current disease activity and prior therapies used. Goals of therapy in nonradiographic axial spondyloarthritis are to alleviate symptoms, improve functioning, maintain the ability to work, decrease complications, and prevent or slow skeletal damage.

Recommendations for the treatment of nonradiographic axial spondyloarthritis are largely extrapolated from evidence in the treatment of ankylosing spondylitis, due to a lack of data specific to nonradiographic axial spondyloarthritis. (See Ankylosing Spondylitis under Uses.) The specific place in therapy for upadacitinib has not been addressed in guidelines.

● Polyarticular Juvenile Idiopathic Arthritis

Upadacitinib is used for the treatment of polyarticular juvenile idiopathic arthritis in patients 2 years of age and older who have had an inadequate response or intolerance to TNF blocking agents. Concomitant use of upadacitinib with other JAK inhibitors, potent immunosuppressants (e.g., azathioprine, cyclosporine), or biologic DMARDs is not recommended.

Clinical Experience

The efficacy of upadacitinib in polyarticular juvenile idiopathic arthritis is based on exposure-matched extrapolation of the established efficacy of upadacitinib extended-release tablets in patients with rheumatoid arthritis. Safety and efficacy of upadacitinib were also assessed in a multicenter, open-label, single-arm study in 83 children (2 to < 18 years of age) with this condition. Patient subtypes included in the study were rheumatoid factor negative polyarticular (68.7%), rheumatoid factor positive polyarticular (15.7%), extended oligoarticular (13.3%), and systemic juvenile idiopathic arthritis without systemic manifestations (2.4%). All received upadacitinib dosages based on weight for up to 156 weeks. Efficacy was assessed as supportive endpoints through Week 48; efficacy was generally consistent with responses in patients with rheumatoid arthritis.

Clinical Perspective

The American College of Rheumatology and the Arthritis Foundation issued a joint guideline for the treatment of juvenile idiopathic arthritis manifesting as nonsystemic polyarthritis (including polyarticular disease), sacroiliitis, or enthesitis in 2019. Several drug classes are used to treat juvenile idiopathic arthritis, including NSAIAs, systemic and intra-articular corticosteroids, conventional DMARDs (e.g., methotrexate, sulfasalazine, hydroxychloroquine, leflunomide), and biologic DMARDs (e.g., TNF blocking agents, abatacept, tocilizumab, rituximab). Specific agents for juvenile idiopathic arthritis treatment are selected according to the presence of certain risk factors (e.g., positive anti-cyclic citrullinated peptide antibodies, positive rheumatoid factor, joint damage), level of disease activity, involvement of specific joints, presence of certain comorbidities (e.g., uveitis), and prior therapies used. An individualized "treat-to-target" approach is typically employed, with the goal of achieving remission or minimal/low disease activity.

TNF blocking agents used in the treatment of juvenile idiopathic arthritis include adalimumab, etanercept, golimumab, and infliximab. Methotrexate monotherapy is conditionally recommended as initial therapy for patients with juvenile idiopathic arthritis manifesting as nonsystemic polyarthritis, although initial biologic DMARD therapy may be considered for patients with risk factors and involvement of high-risk joints (e.g., cervical spine, wrist, hip), high disease activity, and/or those judged by their physician to be at high risk of disabling joint damage. In patients with moderate or high disease activity despite methotrexate monotherapy, biologic DMARDs (including TNF blocking agents) are conditionally recommended as add-on therapy. In patients with moderate or high disease activity despite treatment with a first TNF blocking agent (with or without concomitant conventional DMARD therapy), switching to tocilizumab or abatacept is conditionally recommended over switching to a different TNF blocking agent, although a different TNF blocking agent may be appropriate if the patient experienced a good initial response to their first TNF blocking agent. In all patients initiating biologic DMARD therapy, combination therapy with a conventional DMARD is recommended over biologic DMARD monotherapy. Specific choice of biologic DMARD may be influenced by the presence of certain comorbidities (e.g., uveitis). Consult the American College of Rheumatology/Arthritis Foundation guidelines for additional details.

DOSAGE AND ADMINISTRATION

● General

Pretreatment Screening

- Evaluate for active and latent tuberculosis infection prior to initiation of therapy; initiate antimycobacterial therapy if indicated.

- Evaluate for risk of thrombosis prior to initiation of therapy.

- Evaluate for risk of major cardiovascular events prior to initiation of therapy, particularly in patients who are current or past smokers and patients with other cardiovascular risk factors.

- Measure absolute lymphocyte count, absolute neutrophil count (ANC), and hemoglobin prior to initiation of therapy. Do not initiate therapy in patients with an absolute lymphocyte count of <500 cells/mm^3, ANC <1000 cells/mm^3, or hemoglobin concentration <8 g/dL.

- Monitor liver function prior to initiation of therapy. Evaluate for viral hepatitis.

- Verify pregnancy status in females of reproductive potential prior to initiation of therapy.

- Consider benefits and risks of all-cause mortality prior to initiating therapy with upadacitinib.

- Consider benefits and risks of developing malignancies prior to initiating therapy with upadacitinib, particularly in patients with a known malignancy (other than successfully treated nonmelanoma skin cancer [NMSC]), patients who develop a malignancy, and patients who are current or past smokers.

Patient Monitoring

- Monitor closely for signs or symptoms of infection, including the possible development of tuberculosis in patients who tested negative for latent tuberculosis prior to initiating therapy, during and after treatment with upadacitinib.

- Monitor for reactivation of viral hepatitis periodically during therapy.

- Perform dermatologic examinations periodically throughout therapy for patients at increased risk for skin cancer.

- Periodically monitor for thrombosis during therapy.

- Monitor patients at risk of GI perforation for onset of new abdominal symptoms.

- Monitor lymphocyte count, ANC, and hemoglobin concentrations periodically during therapy.

- Monitor lipids approximately 12 weeks after therapy initiation, then periodically thereafter.

- Monitor liver enzymes periodically during therapy.

- Consider benefits and risk of all-cause mortality prior to continuing therapy with the drug.

- Consider benefits and risks of developing malignancies prior to continuing therapy with upadacitinib, particularly in patients with a known malignancy (other than successfully treated NMSC), patients who develop a malignancy, and patients who are current or past smokers.

Other General Considerations

- Upadacitinib can be used in combination with methotrexate or other nonbiologic (conventional) DMARDs.

- Do not use concomitantly with other Janus kinase (JAK) inhibitors, biologic therapies, or potent immunosuppressive agents.

- Update immunizations according to current immunization guidelines prior to initiating therapy.

● Administration

Upadacitinib is commercially available as extended-release tablets and an oral solution. Administer extended-release tablets orally once daily without regard to food. Administer the oral solution twice daily using the provided press-in bottle adapter and oral dosing syringe without regard to food.

The oral solution is not substitutable with the extended-release tablets. Changes between the oral solution and extended-release tablets should be performed by a healthcare provider.

Swallow extended-release tablets whole; do not chew, crush, or split.

Store extended-release tablets at 2–25ºC in original bottle to protect from moisture. Store the oral solution between 2-30ºC; discard remaining solution 60 days after opening the bottle.

● Dosage

Adult Dosage

Rheumatoid Arthritis

For the management of moderately to severely active rheumatoid arthritis in adults who have had an inadequate response or intolerance to one or more TNF blocking agents, the recommended dosage of upadacitinib extended-release tablet is 15 mg once daily.

Psoriatic Arthritis

For the management of active psoriatic arthritis in adults who have had an inadequate response or intolerance to one or more TNF blocking agents, the recommended dosage of upadacitinib extended-release tablet is 15 mg once daily.

Atopic Dermatitis

Adults <65 years of age: For the management of refractory, moderate to severe atopic dermatitis in adults who have had an inadequate response to other systemic therapies or who are not eligible for other systemic therapies, the recommended initial dosage of upadacitinib extended-release tablet is 15 mg once daily. If an adequate response is not achieved, increasing the dosage to 30 mg once daily may be considered; however, if an adequate response is not achieved on a dosage of 30 mg once daily, upadacitinib should be discontinued. The lowest effective dosage should be used to maintain response.

Adults ≥65 years of age: For the management of refractory, moderate to severe atopic dermatitis in adults who have had an inadequate response to other systemic therapies or who are not eligible for other systemic therapies, the recommended dosage of upadacitinib extended-release tablet is 15 mg once daily.

Ulcerative Colitis

For the management of moderately to severely active ulcerative colitis in adults who have had an inadequate response or intolerance to one or more TNF blocking agents, the recommended induction dosage of upadacitinib extended-release tablet is 45 mg once daily for 8 weeks, followed by a maintenance dosage of 15 mg once daily. In patients with refractory, severe, or extensive disease, a maintenance dosage of 30 mg once daily may be considered; however, if an adequate response is not achieved on a dosage of 30 mg once daily, upadacitinib should be discontinued. The lowest effective dosage should be used to maintain response.

Crohn Disease

For the management of moderately to severely active Crohn disease in adults who have had an inadequate response or intolerance to one or more TNF blocking agents, the recommended induction dosage of upadacitinib extended-release tablet is 45 mg once daily for 12 weeks, followed by a maintenance dosage of 15 mg once daily. In patients with refractory, severe, or extensive disease, a maintenance dosage of 30 mg once daily may be considered; however, if an adequate response is not achieved on a dosage of 30 mg once daily, upadacitinib should be discontinued. The lowest effective dosage should be used to maintain response.

Ankylosing Spondylitis

For the management of active ankylosing spondylitis in adults who have had an inadequate response or intolerance to one or more TNF blocking agents, the recommended dosage of upadacitinib extended-release tablet is 15 mg once daily.

Nonradiographic Axial Spondyloarthritis

For the management of active nonradiographic axial spondyloarthritis with objective signs of inflammation in adults who have had an inadequate response or intolerance to TNF blocking agents, the recommended dosage of upadacitinib extended-release tablet is 15 mg once daily.

Pediatric Dosage
Psoriatic Arthritis

For the management of active psoriatic arthritis in pediatric patients 2 to <18 years of age who have had an inadequate response or intolerance to one or more TNF blocking agents, the recommended dosage of upadacitinib is based on body weight and dosage formulation.

The extended-release tablet is *not* recommended for use in pediatric patients 10 to <30 kg. In pediatric patients who weigh ≥30 kg, the extended-release tablet dosage is 15 mg once daily.

The oral solution dosage is 3 mg (3 mL) twice daily in pediatric patients who weigh 10 to <20 kg; 4 mg (4 mL) twice daily in those who weigh 20 to <30 kg; and 6 mg (6 mL) twice daily in those who weigh ≥30 kg.

Atopic Dermatitis

Pediatric patients ≥12 years of age and weighing ≥40 kg: For the management of refractory, moderate to severe atopic dermatitis in pediatric patients who have had an inadequate response to other systemic therapies or who are not eligible for other systemic therapies, the recommended initial dosage of upadacitinib extended-release tablet is 15 mg once daily. If an adequate response is not achieved, increasing the dosage to 30 mg once daily may be considered; however, if an adequate response is not achieved on a dosage of 30 mg once daily,

upadacitinib should be discontinued. The lowest effective dosage should be used to maintain response.

Polyarticular Juvenile Idiopathic Arthritis

For the management of active polyarticular juvenile idiopathic arthritis in pediatric patients ≥2 years of age who have had an inadequate response or intolerance to one or more TNF blocking agents, the recommended dosage of upadacitinib is based on body weight and dosage formulation.

The extended-release tablet is *not* recommended for use in pediatric patients 10 to <30 kg. In pediatric patients who weigh ≥30 kg, the extended-release tablet dosage is 15 mg once daily. The oral solution dosage is 3 mg (3 mL) twice daily in pediatric patients who weigh 10 to <20 kg; 4 mg (4 mL) twice daily in those who weigh 20 to <30 kg; and 6 mg (6 mL) twice daily in those who weigh ≥30 kg.

Dosage Modifications for Drug Interactions

Rheumatoid arthritis, psoriatic arthritis, ankylosing spondylitis, nonradiographic axial spondyloarthritis, polyarticular juvenile idiopathic arthritis: No dosage adjustment is required in patients receiving potent cytochrome P450 (CYP) isoenzyme 3A4 inhibitors.

Atopic dermatitis: The recommended dosage of the extended-release tablet in patients receiving concomitant potent CYP3A4 inhibitors is 15 mg once daily.

Ulcerative colitis: The recommended dosage of the extended-release tablet in patients receiving concomitant potent CYP3A4 inhibitors is 30 mg once daily for 8 weeks for induction and 15 mg once daily for maintenance.

Crohn disease: The recommended dosage of the extended-release tablet in patients receiving concomitant potent CYP3A4 inhibitors is 30 mg once daily for 12 weeks for induction and 15 mg once daily for maintenance.

Treatment Interruption for Toxicity
Infection

If a serious infection, including serious opportunistic infections, develops, upadacitinib therapy should be interrupted until the infection has been controlled.

Hematologic Toxicity

Upadacitinib therapy also should be interrupted in patients with neutropenia, lymphopenia, or anemia. If ANC decreases to less than 1000 cells/mm³, upadacitinib therapy should be interrupted until ANC recovers to greater than 1000 cells/mm³. If absolute lymphocyte count decreases to less than 500 cells/mm³, upadacitinib therapy should be interrupted until lymphocyte count recovers to greater than 500 cells/mm³. If hemoglobin concentration decreases to less than 8 g/dL, upadacitinib therapy should be interrupted until hemoglobin concentration recovers to greater than 8 g/dL.

Hepatic Toxicity

If drug-induced hepatic injury is suspected, upadacitinib therapy should be interrupted until such diagnosis has been excluded.

● Special Populations
Hepatic Impairment

Rheumatoid arthritis, psoriatic arthritis, atopic dermatitis, ankylosing spondylitis, nonradiographic axial spondyloarthritis, polyarticular juvenile idiopathic arthritis: Dosage adjustment is not necessary in patients with mild or moderate hepatic impairment (Child-Pugh class A or B).

Ulcerative colitis: For patients with mild to moderate hepatic impairment (Child-Pugh class A or B), the recommended dosage of the extended-release tablet is 30 mg once daily for 8 weeks for induction and 15 mg once daily for maintenance.

Crohn disease: For patients with mild to moderate hepatic impairment (Child-Pugh class A or B), the recommended dosage of the extended-release tablet is 30 mg once daily for 12 weeks for induction and 15 mg once daily for maintenance.

All indications: Upadacitinib is not recommended in patients with severe hepatic impairment (Child-Pugh class C).

Renal Impairment

Rheumatoid arthritis, psoriatic arthritis, ankylosing spondylitis, nonradiographic axial spondyloarthritis, polyarticular juvenile idiopathic arthritis: No dosage adjustment is necessary in patients with mild, moderate, or severe renal impairment.

Atopic dermatitis: For patients with severe renal impairment (estimated glomerular filtration rate [eGFR] 15 to less than 30 mL/minute/1.73 m²), the recommended dosage of the extended-release tablet is 15 mg once daily. No dosage adjustment is necessary in patients with mild or moderate renal impairment (eGFR exceeding 30 mL/minute/1.73 m²). Not recommended in patients with end-stage renal disease (eGFR less than 15 mL/minute/1.73 m²).

Ulcerative colitis: For patients with severe renal impairment (eGFR 15 to less than 30 mL/minute/1.73 m²), the recommended dosage of the extended-release tablet is 30 mg once daily for 8 weeks for induction and 15 mg once daily for maintenance. No dosage adjustment is necessary in patients with mild or moderate renal impairment (eGFR exceeding 30 mL/minute/1.73 m²). Not recommended in patients with end-stage renal disease (eGFR less than 15 mL/minute/1.73 m²).

Crohn disease: For patients with severe renal impairment (eGFR 15 to less than 30 mL/minute/1.73 m²), the recommended dosage of the extended-release tablet is 30 mg once daily for 12 weeks for induction and 15 mg once daily for maintenance. No dosage adjustment is necessary in patients with mild or moderate renal impairment (eGFR exceeding 30 mL/minute/1.73 m²). Not recommended in patients with end-stage renal disease (eGFR less than 15 mL/minute/1.73 m²).

Geriatric Patients

Atopic dermatitis: For patients ≥65 years of age, the recommended dosage of upadacitinib extended-release tablet is 15 mg once daily.

Other indications: The manufacturer makes no specific dosage recommendations for geriatric patients.

CAUTIONS

● Contraindications

● Known hypersensitivity to upadacitinib or any ingredient in the preparation.

● Warnings/Precautions

Warnings

Serious Infections

A boxed warning regarding the risk of serious infections is included in the prescribing information for upadacitinib. Serious and sometimes fatal infections, including bacterial, mycobacterial, invasive fungal, viral, or other opportunistic infections, have been reported in patients receiving upadacitinib. The most common serious infections reported in patients receiving the drug have included pneumonia and cellulitis. Opportunistic infections (e.g., tuberculosis, multidermatomal herpes zoster, oral or esophageal candidiasis, pneumocystosis, cryptococcosis) have been reported. Tuberculosis may present with pulmonary or extrapulmonary disease. Most patients who experienced serious infections were receiving concomitant therapy with immunosuppressive agents such as methotrexate or corticosteroids. A higher rate of serious infections has been observed with an upadacitinib dosage of 30 mg compared to the 15 mg dosage.

Patients should be closely monitored during and after treatment with upadacitinib for the development of signs or symptoms of infection.

Upadacitinib therapy should not be initiated in patients with serious active infections, including localized infections. Clinicians should consider potential risks and benefits of the drug prior to initiating therapy in patients with a history of chronic, recurring, serious, or opportunistic infections; patients with underlying conditions that may predispose them to infections; and patients who have been exposed to tuberculosis or who reside or have traveled in regions where tuberculosis or mycoses are endemic.

Any patient who develops a new infection while receiving upadacitinib should undergo a thorough diagnostic evaluation (appropriate for an immunocompromised patient), appropriate anti-infective therapy should be initiated, and the patient should be closely monitored. Upadacitinib therapy should be interrupted in patients who develop a serious or opportunistic infection or if an infection fails to respond to initial anti-infective therapy. The drug should not be resumed until the infection is controlled.

Because tuberculosis has been reported in patients receiving upadacitinib, patients should be evaluated for active or latent tuberculosis prior to and periodically during therapy with the drug. Patients with active tuberculosis should not receive upadacitinib. When indicated, an appropriate antimycobacterial regimen for the treatment of latent tuberculosis infection should be initiated prior to upadacitinib therapy. Antimycobacterial therapy should be considered prior to initiation of upadacitinib in individuals with a history of latent or active tuberculosis in whom an adequate course of antimycobacterial therapy cannot be confirmed and in individuals with a negative test for latent tuberculosis who have risk factors for tuberculosis. Consultation with a tuberculosis specialist is recommended when deciding whether antimycobacterial therapy should be initiated. Patients receiving upadacitinib, including individuals with a negative test for latent tuberculosis, should be monitored for signs and symptoms of active tuberculosis.

Viral reactivation, including hepatitis B virus (HBV) reactivation and varicella zoster virus reactivation with development of zoster (shingles), has been reported in patients receiving upadacitinib. The risk of zoster appears to be higher in patients treated with upadacitinib in Japan. If zoster develops, consideration should be given to interrupting upadacitinib therapy until the episode has resolved. Patients testing positive for hepatitis C virus (HCV) antibody and HCV RNA were excluded from clinical trials of upadacitinib, as were those who tested positive for HBV surface antigen or HBV DNA; however, cases of HBV reactivation were still reported. Screening for viral hepatitis and monitoring for reactivation should be performed prior to and during upadacitinib therapy in accordance with current standards of care. Consultation with a hepatologist is recommended if HBV DNA is detected during therapy.

Mortality

A boxed warning regarding the increased risk of mortality is included in the prescribing information for upadacitinib. In a large, randomized, postmarketing safety study of another JAK inhibitor in patients with rheumatoid arthritis who were 50 years of age or older and had at least one cardiovascular risk factor, the rate of all-cause mortality, including sudden cardiovascular death, was higher in patients who received a JAK inhibitor compared with those who received a TNF blocking agent.

The risks and benefits of upadacitinib should be considered prior to initiating therapy or when considering whether to continue upadacitinib therapy.

Malignancies and Lymphoproliferative Disorders

A boxed warning regarding the risk of malignancies, including lymphomas, is included in the prescribing information for upadacitinib. Lymphoma and other malignancies have been observed in patients receiving upadacitinib. In a large, randomized, postmarketing safety study of another JAK inhibitor in patients with rheumatoid arthritis, a higher rate of malignancies (excluding nonmelanoma skin cancer) was observed in patients treated with the JAK inhibitor compared to those treated with a TNF blocking agent. A higher rate of lymphomas was observed in patients treated with the JAK inhibitor compared to those treated with a TNF blocking agent. A higher rate of lung cancers also was observed in current or past smokers treated with the JAK inhibitor compared to those treated with a TNF blocking agent. In this study, current or past smokers had an additional increased risk of overall malignancies.

The risks and benefits of upadacitinib should be considered prior to initiating therapy or when considering whether to continue upadacitinib, particularly in patients with a known malignancy (other than successfully treated nonmelanoma skin cancer), in those who develop a malignancy, and those who are current or past smokers.

Because nonmelanoma skin cancers have been reported in patients receiving upadacitinib, periodic dermatologic examinations are recommended for patients receiving the drug who are at increased risk for skin cancer. Patients should be advised to limit exposure to sunlight and ultraviolet (UV) light by wearing protective clothing and using a broad-spectrum sunscreen.

Major Adverse Cardiovascular Events

A boxed warning regarding the increased risk of major adverse cardiovascular events is included in the prescribing information for upadacitinib. In a large randomized safety clinical trial in patients ≥50 years of age with rheumatoid arthritis and at least one cardiovascular risk factor, the risk of major adverse cardiovascular events (i.e., cardiovascular death, nonfatal MI, nonfatal stroke) was increased in patients receiving another JAK inhibitor (tofacitinib 5 or 10 mg twice daily) compared with those receiving a tumor necrosis factor (TNF) blocking agent. Although the safety profiles of other JAK inhibitors, such as baricitinib and upadacitinib, have not been studied in large safety clinical trials similar to the one with tofacitinib, the FDA states that these drugs may also have similar risks based on their mechanisms of action. Based on findings of the postmarketing study, and to ensure the benefits of upadacitinib outweigh its risks, use of upadacitinib in all approved indications is limited to patients who have not responded to or cannot tolerate one or more TNF blocking agents.

The risks and benefits of upadacitinib should be considered prior to initiating therapy or when considering whether to continue upadacitinib, particularly in patients who are current or past smokers and in those with other cardiovascular risk factors. Patients receiving upadacitinib should be advised to seek immediate medical attention if symptoms of serious cardiovascular events occur. In patients who experience MI or stroke, upadacitinib therapy should be discontinued.

Thrombosis

A boxed warning regarding the risk of thrombosis is included in the prescribing information for upadacitinib. Serious and sometimes fatal thromboembolic events, including deep-vein thrombosis, pulmonary embolism, and arterial thrombosis, have been reported in patients with inflammatory conditions receiving JAK inhibitors, including upadacitinib. In a postmarketing study evaluating safety of another JAK inhibitor in patients ≥50 years of age with rheumatoid arthritis, analysis revealed higher incidences of thromboembolic events, including pulmonary embolism and deep-vein thrombosis, in patients receiving the JAK inhibitor compared with those receiving a TNF blocking agent.

The risks and benefits of upadacitinib should be considered prior to initiation of therapy in patients who may be at increased risk of thrombosis; upadacitinib should be avoided in patients who may be at increased risk of thrombosis. Patients with signs or symptoms suggestive of thrombosis should discontinue upadacitinib therapy and be evaluated promptly and treated appropriately.

Other Warnings and Precautions
Hypersensitivity Reactions

Serious hypersensitivity reactions (e.g., anaphylaxis, angioedema) have been reported in patients receiving upadacitinib in clinical trials. If a clinically significant hypersensitivity reaction occurs, upadacitinib should be discontinued and appropriate therapy should be instituted.

GI Perforation

Cases of GI perforation have been reported in patients receiving upadacitinib.

Monitor patients who may be at increased risk for GI perforation (e.g., patients with a history of diverticulitis or receiving concomitant NSAIAs or corticosteroids). Patients with new onset of abdominal symptoms should be evaluated promptly for early identification of GI perforation.

Hematologic Effects

The incidence of neutropenia with absolute neutrophil count (ANC) less than 1000 cells/mm³ is increased in patients receiving upadacitinib. Neutrophil counts should be monitored at baseline and thereafter in accordance with current standards of care. Upadacitinib therapy should not be initiated in patients with ANC less than 1000 cells/mm³, and treatment should be interrupted if ANC decreases to less than 1000 cells/mm³.

Lymphopenia with absolute lymphocyte count less than 500 cells/mm³ has been reported in patients receiving upadacitinib. Lymphocyte counts should be monitored at baseline and thereafter in accordance with current standards of care. Upadacitinib therapy should not be initiated in patients with lymphocyte counts less than 500 cells/mm³, and treatment should be interrupted if lymphocyte count decreases to less than 500 cells/mm³.

Anemia with hemoglobin concentration less than 8 g/dL has been reported in patients receiving upadacitinib. Hemoglobin concentration should be monitored at baseline and thereafter in accordance with current standards of care. Upadacitinib therapy should not be initiated in patients with hemoglobin concentrations less than 8 g/dL, and treatment should be interrupted if hemoglobin concentration decreases to less than 8 g/dL.

Effects on Serum Lipids

Dose-related increases in concentrations of total cholesterol, low-density lipoprotein (LDL) cholesterol, and high-density lipoprotein (HDL) cholesterol have been observed in patients receiving upadacitinib. Elevations in LDL-cholesterol concentrations decreased to pretreatment levels in response to statin therapy. The effect of upadacitinib-associated lipid elevations on cardiovascular morbidity and mortality has not been determined.

Lipid concentrations should be monitored 12 weeks after initiation of upadacitinib therapy and thereafter in accordance with current standards of care. Dyslipidemia should be managed according to current standards of care.

Hepatic Effects

Elevated hepatic enzyme concentrations have been reported in patients receiving upadacitinib.

Liver function tests should be monitored at baseline and thereafter according to current standards of care. In case of elevated hepatic enzyme concentrations, patients should be evaluated promptly for drug-induced hepatotoxicity. If drug-induced hepatic injury is suspected, upadacitinib therapy should be interrupted until such diagnosis has been excluded.

Fetal/Neonatal Morbidity and Mortality

Limited data regarding use of upadacitinib in pregnant women are not sufficient to evaluate a drug-associated risk for major birth defects or spontaneous abortion; however, based on animal findings, upadacitinib may cause fetal harm. Embryofetal toxicity (e.g., decreased fetal weight, postimplantation loss) and teratogenicity (e.g., cardiovascular and skeletal abnormalities) have been demonstrated in rats and/or rabbits receiving upadacitinib at exposure levels higher than the human exposure at the maximum recommended dosage.

Pregnancy should be avoided during upadacitinib therapy. Verify pregnancy status prior to initiation of upadacitinib, and females of reproductive potential should be advised to use effective methods of contraception during upadacitinib therapy and for 4 weeks following the last dose of the drug. Patients should be apprised of the potential hazard to the fetus if upadacitinib is used during pregnancy.

A pregnancy surveillance program exists to monitor pregnancy outcomes in women exposed to upadacitinib during pregnancy; if exposure occurs during pregnancy, healthcare providers or patients should report the pregnancy by calling 1-800-633-9110.

Immunization

Administration of live attenuated vaccines should be avoided during and immediately prior to therapy with upadacitinib. All indicated immunizations, including immunization against varicella zoster or herpes zoster, should be administered according to current immunization guidelines prior to initiation of upadacitinib therapy.

Medication Residue in Stool

Medication residue in stool or ostomy output has been reported in patients receiving upadacitinib. Most reported cases have described anatomic conditions, including ileostomy, colostomy, and intestinal resection, or functional GI conditions with decreased GI transit times. Patients should be instructed to contact their healthcare provider if medication residue is observed repeatedly. Patients should be clinically monitored and alternative treatments considered if there is an inadequate therapeutic response.

Specific Populations
Pregnancy

Based on animal studies, upadacitinib may cause fetal harm if administered to pregnant women. In order to monitor pregnancy outcomes in women exposed to upadacitinib, healthcare providers or patients should report a pregnancy by calling 1-800-633-9110.

Lactation

It is not known whether upadacitinib is distributed into human milk; the drug is distributed into milk in rats. The effects of upadacitinib on nursing infants or on milk production also are unknown. Following oral administration of a single

10-mg/kg dose of radiolabeled upadacitinib in lactating rats on postpartum day 7 or 8, concentrations of the drug in milk were approximately 30 times greater than maternal plasma concentrations, with 97% present as unchanged drug.

Because of the potential for serious adverse reactions to upadacitinib in nursing infants, breast-feeding is not recommended during upadacitinib therapy and for 6 days following the last dose of the drug.

Females and Males of Reproductive Potential

Verify pregnancy status in females of reproductive potential prior to initiation of upadacitinib. Advise females of reproductive potential to use effective contraception during treatment with upadacitinib and for 4 weeks following the last dose.

Pediatric Use

Atopic dermatitis: Safety and efficacy of upadacitinib for the treatment of atopic dermatitis in pediatric patients ≥12 years of age weighing ≥40 kg is supported by data from clinical trials (AD-1, AD-2 and AD-3) evaluating upadacitinib (15 or 30 mg once daily) or placebo as monotherapy or in combination with topical corticosteroids in 344 pediatric patients (12–17 years of age) with moderate to severe atopic dermatitis. Safety and efficacy were consistent between the pediatric patients and adults. Safety and efficacy of upadacitinib extended-release tablet in pediatric patients <12 years of age with atopic dermatitis have not been established. Safety and efficacy of upadacitinib oral solution in pediatric patients with atopic dermatitis have not been established.

Polyarticular juvenile idiopathic arthritis, psoriatic arthritis: Safety and efficacy of upadacitinib in pediatric patients 2 to <18 years of age is supported by evidence from well-controlled studies of upadacitinib in adults with rheumatoid arthritis and psoriatic arthritis, pharmacokinetic data from adults with rheumatoid arthritis and psoriatic arthritis and 51 pediatric patients with juvenile idiopathic arthritis with active polyarthritis, and safety data from 83 patients 2 to <18 years of age with juvenile idiopathic arthritis with active polyarthritis. Upadacitinib plasma exposures in pediatric patients with polyarticular juvenile idiopathic arthritis and psoriatic arthritis at the recommended dosage are predicted to be comparable to those observed in adults with rheumatoid arthritis and psoriatic arthritis based on population pharmacokinetic modeling and simulation. Safety and efficacy of upadacitinib in pediatric patients <2 years of age with polyarticular juvenile idiopathic arthritis and psoriatic arthritis have not been established.

Ankylosing spondylitis, nonradiographic axial spondyloarthritis: Safety and efficacy of upadacitinib have not been established in pediatric patients with ankylosing spondylitis or nonradiographic axial spondyloarthritis†.

Ulcerative colitis, Crohn disease: Safety and efficacy of upadacitinib have not been established in pediatric patients with ulcerative colitis or Crohn disease†.

Geriatric Use

Rheumatoid arthritis and psoriatic arthritis: In controlled clinical trials of upadacitinib in patients with rheumatoid arthritis or psoriatic arthritis, no differences in efficacy were observed between geriatric patients and younger adults; however, the overall frequency of adverse events, including serious infections, was increased in geriatric patients.

Atopic dermatitis: In controlled clinical trials of upadacitinib in patients with atopic dermatitis, no differences in efficacy were observed between geriatric patients and younger adults; however, serious infections and malignancies occurred at a higher rate in patients ≥65 years of age receiving upadacitinib 30 mg once daily in long-term trials.

Ankylosing spondylitis, nonradiographic axial spondyloarthritis, ulcerative colitis, Crohn disease: In controlled clinical trials of upadacitinib in patients with ankylosing spondylitis, nonradiographic axial spondyloarthritis, ulcerative colitis, or Crohn disease, an insufficient number of patients 65 years of age and older were included to assess differences in response compared to younger adults.

Hepatic Impairment

After administration of a single 15-mg dose of upadacitinib in patients with mild or moderate hepatic impairment (Child-Pugh class A or B), systemic exposure of upadacitinib was increased by 28% or 24%, respectively, compared to individuals with normal hepatic function. Peak plasma concentrations of upadacitinib were unchanged in patients with mild hepatic impairment and increased by 43% on average in those with moderate hepatic impairment when compared to individuals with normal hepatic function. No dosage adjustment is required in

patients with rheumatoid arthritis, psoriatic arthritis, atopic dermatitis, ankylosing spondylitis, nonradiographic axial spondylarthritis, or polyarticular juvenile idiopathic arthritis and mild or moderate hepatic impairment. In patients with mild or moderate hepatic impairment, the recommended dosage of upadacitinib extended-release tablet for ulcerative colitis or Crohn disease is 30 mg once daily for induction and 15 mg once daily for maintenance.

Use of upadacitinib in patients with severe hepatic impairment (Child-Pugh class C) has not been studied and is not recommended.

Renal Impairment

Renal impairment does not increase peak plasma concentrations of upadacitinib compared with patients with normal renal function; however, systemic exposure of upadacitinib increased by 18, 33, or 44% in patients with mild, moderate, or severe renal impairment, respectively. Mild or moderate renal impairment is not expected to have a clinically relevant effect on upadacitinib exposure following 15 mg, 30 mg, or 45 mg daily dosages of the drug. Upadacitinib has not been studied in patients with end-stage renal disease (eGFR less than 15 mL/minute/1.73 m^2).

Rheumatoid arthritis, psoriatic arthritis, ankylosing spondylitis, nonradiographic axial spondyloarthritis, or polyarticular juvenile idiopathic arthritis: No dosage adjustment of upadacitinib is required in patients with mild (eGFR 60 to less than 90 mL/minute/1.73 m^2), moderate (eGFR 30 to less than 60 mL/minute/1.73 m^2), or severe renal impairment (eGFR 15 to less than 30 mL/minute/1.73 m^2).

Atopic dermatitis: For patients with atopic dermatitis and severe renal impairment, the maximum recommended dosage of upadacitinib extended-release tablet is 15 mg once daily. No dosage adjustment is necessary in patients with atopic dermatitis and mild or moderate renal impairment. Use in end-stage renal disease is not recommended for patients with atopic dermatitis.

Ulcerative colitis and Crohn disease: For patients with ulcerative colitis or Crohn disease and severe renal impairment, the recommended dosage of upadacitinib extended-release tablet is 30 mg once daily for induction and 15 mg once daily for maintenance. No dosage adjustment is necessary in patients with ulcerative colitis or Crohn disease and mild or moderate renal impairment. Use in end-stage renal disease is not recommended for patients with ulcerative colitis or Crohn disease.

● Common Adverse Effects

Adverse effects occurring in 1% or more of patients with rheumatoid arthritis, psoriatic arthritis, ankylosing spondylitis, or nonradiographic axial spondyloarthritis receiving upadacitinib include upper respiratory tract infections, herpes zoster infection, herpes simplex infection, bronchitis, nausea, cough, pyrexia, acne, and headache.

Adverse effects occurring in 1% or more of patients with atopic dermatitis receiving upadacitinib include upper respiratory tract infections, acne, herpes simplex infection, headache, increased serum creatine phosphokinase, cough, hypersensitivity, folliculitis, nausea, abdominal pain, pyrexia, increased weight, herpes zoster infection, influenza, fatigue, neutropenia, myalgia, and influenza-like illness.

Adverse effects occurring in 5% or more of patients with ulcerative colitis receiving upadacitinib during induction and maintenance phases include upper respiratory tract infections, increased serum creatine phosphokinase, acne, neutropenia, elevated transaminases, and rash.

Adverse effects occurring in 5% or more of patients with Crohn disease receiving upadacitinib during induction and maintenance phases include upper respiratory tract infections, anemia, pyrexia, acne, herpes zoster, and headache.

DRUG INTERACTIONS

● Drugs Affecting or Metabolized by Hepatic Microsomal Enzymes

Upadacitinib is metabolized in vitro by cytochrome P-450 isoenzyme 3A4 (CYP3A4) and to a minor extent by CYP2D6.

In vitro studies indicate that upadacitinib does not inhibit CYP isoenzymes 1A2, 2B6, 2C8, 2C9, 2C19, 2D6, or 3A4 at clinically relevant concentrations. In vitro, upadacitinib induces CYP3A4 but not CYP2B6 or CYP1A2 at clinically relevant concentrations. Concomitant administration of upadacitinib with bupropion

(CYP2B6 substrate), caffeine (CYP1A2 substrate), dextromethorphan (CYP2D6 substrate), midazolam (CYP3A substrate), omeprazole (CYP2C19 substrate), or warfarin (CYP2C9 substrate) did not result in clinically important effects on the pharmacokinetics of these substrate drugs. Similar effects on CYP1A2, CYP3A, CYP2C9, and CYP2C19, but not CYP2D6 were observed with upadacitinib dosages of 30 mg and 45 mg once daily. A weak induction of CYP3A4 was observed with upadacitinib 30 mg and 45 mg once daily, while a weak inhibition of CYP2D6 was observed with 45 mg once daily, but not 30 mg once daily.

Concomitant administration of upadacitinib and potent CYP3A4 inhibitors (e.g., ketoconazole, clarithromycin, grapefruit) results in increased upadacitinib exposure and possible increased risk of adverse effects. Concomitant administration of ketoconazole (a potent CYP3A4 inhibitor) with upadacitinib increased the peak plasma concentration and area under the plasma concentration-time curve (AUC) of upadacitinib by 70 and 75%, respectively. In patients receiving upadacitinib 15 mg once daily for rheumatoid arthritis, psoriatic arthritis, ankylosing spondylitis, nonradiographic axial spondylarthritis, or polyarticular juvenile idiopathic arthritis, closely monitor for adverse reactions during concomitant use with potent CYP3A4 inhibitors. Patients receiving upadacitinib should avoid food and drink that contains grapefruit during therapy due to possible increased upadacitinib exposure. For patients with atopic dermatitis, coadministration of upadacitinib 30 mg once daily with potent CYP3A4 inhibitors is *not* recommended. Coadministration of potent CYP3A4 inhibitors in patients receiving upadacitinib for ulcerative colitis or Crohn disease necessitates a dosage reduction of upadacitinib to 30 mg once daily for induction and 15 mg once daily for maintenance.

Concomitant administration of upadacitinib and potent CYP3A4 inducers results in decreased upadacitinib exposure and may lead to reduced therapeutic efficacy of upadacitinib. Concomitant administration of rifampin (a potent CYP3A4 inducer) with upadacitinib decreased the peak plasma concentration and AUC of upadacitinib by 51 and 61%, respectively. Concomitant use of upadacitinib and potent CYP3A4 inducers is not recommended.

In population pharmacokinetic analyses, CYP2D6 metabolic phenotype had no effect on upadacitinib pharmacokinetics, indicating that inhibitors of CYP2D6 would have no clinically relevant effect on upadacitinib exposure.

● *Drugs Affecting or Affected by Transport Systems*

In vitro studies indicate that upadacitinib does not inhibit the following transporters at clinically relevant concentrations: P-glycoprotein (P-gp), breast cancer resistance protein (BCRP), organic anion transport polypeptide (OATP) 1B1 or 1B3, organic cation transporter (OCT) 1 or 2, organic anion transporter (OAT) 1 or 3, or multidrug and toxin extrusion transporter (MATE) 1 or 2-K.

● *Drugs Affecting Gastric pH*

Drugs that affect gastric pH (e.g., antacids, proton-pump inhibitors) are not expected to affect systemic exposure to upadacitinib based on in vitro assessments and population pharmacokinetic analyses.

● *Antilipemic Agents*

Concomitant administration of upadacitinib and either atorvastatin or rosuvastatin did not result in clinically important effects on the pharmacokinetics of the antilipemic agent.

● *Disease-modifying Antirheumatic Drugs*

Concomitant administration of methotrexate and upadacitinib did not result in clinically important effects on the pharmacokinetics of either drug.

Concomitant use of upadacitinib and biologic disease-modifying antirheumatic drugs (DMARDs) or other Janus kinase (JAK) inhibitors is not recommended.

● *Hormonal Contraceptives*

Concomitant administration of upadacitinib and an oral contraceptive containing ethinyl estradiol and levonorgestrel did not result in clinically important effects on the pharmacokinetics of either ethinyl estradiol or levonorgestrel.

● *Immunosuppressive Agents*

Concomitant use of potent immunosuppressive agents (e.g., azathioprine, cyclosporine) with upadacitinib is not recommended.

● *Vaccines*

Live, attenuated vaccines should not be administered to patients during or immediately prior to initiating upadacitinib therapy.

DESCRIPTION

Upadacitinib, a Janus kinase (JAK) inhibitor, is an immunomodulating agent and disease-modifying antirheumatic drug (DMARD). JAKs are a family of intracellular tyrosine kinases consisting of JAK1, JAK2, JAK3, and tyrosine kinase (TYK) 2 that mediate the signaling of cytokines and growth factors that are important for hematopoiesis and immune function. Binding of cytokines to receptors on the cell surface activates pairing of JAKs (e.g., JAK1/JAK2, JAK1/JAK3, JAK1/TYK2, JAK2/JAK2, JAK2/TYK2), which leads to phosphorylation and subsequent localization of signal transducer and activator of transcription (STAT) proteins to the nucleus and modulation of gene expression. Upadacitinib modulates the cytokine signaling pathway at the point of JAKs, preventing the phosphorylation and activation of STATs. In a cell-free isolated enzyme assay, upadacitinib had greater inhibitory potency at JAK1 and JAK2 relative to JAK3 and TYK2. In human leukocyte cellular assays, upadacitinib inhibited cytokine-induced STAT phosphorylation mediated by JAK1 and JAK1/JAK3 more potently than JAK2/JAK2-mediated STAT phosphorylation. In healthy individuals, administration of upadacitinib resulted in dose- and concentration-dependent inhibition of interleukin-6 (IL-6)-induced phosphorylation of STAT3 (JAK1/JAK2 dependent) and IL-7-induced phosphorylation of STAT5 (JAK1/JAK3 dependent) in whole blood. The relevance of inhibition of specific JAKs to the therapeutic efficacy of upadacitinib is not known.

Pharmacokinetics of upadacitinib are comparable among patients with rheumatoid arthritis, psoriatic arthritis, atopic dermatitis, ulcerative colitis, Crohn disease, ankylosing spondylitis, and nonradiographic axial spondyloarthritis. Exposure to upadacitinib is proportional to dose over the therapeutic dosage range evaluated. Following repeated once-daily administration, steady-state plasma concentrations are achieved within 4 days with minimal accumulation. Following oral administration of upadacitinib extended-release tablets, peak plasma concentrations of the drug are achieved in approximately 2–4 hours. Following administration of the oral solution (6 mg), the median time to peak plasma concentration is 1 hour. Administration with a high-fat, high-calorie meal increases the area under the concentration-time curve (AUC) and peak plasma concentrations of the drug by 29% and 39—60%, respectively; these effects on drug exposure are not considered clinically important. Coadministration of the oral solution with food is not expected to have a clinically relevant effect on upadacitinib exposure. Upadacitinib is 52% bound to plasma proteins and has a blood to plasma ratio of 1. Upadacitinib is metabolized mainly by cytochrome P-450 isoenzyme 3A4 (CYP3A4) and to a minor extent by CYP2D6. No active metabolites have been identified. Following oral administration of a single dose of radiolabeled upadacitinib as an immediate-release solution, upadacitinib was eliminated principally as unchanged drug in urine (24%) and feces (38%); approximately 34% of the administered dose was excreted as metabolites. The mean terminal elimination half-life of the drug was 8–14 hours. Sex, body weight, and race do not have clinically important effects on the pharmacokinetics of upadacitinib in adult patients. No clinically important differences in upadacitinib exposure have been observed in pediatric patients with atopic dermatitis 12 years of age and older weighing ≥40 kg compared to adult patients. In pediatric patients with juvenile idiopathic arthritis with active polyarthritis, upadacitinib clearance increased with increasing bodyweight. Age (2 to <18 years old) had no additional effect on upadacitinib pharmacokinetics after accounting for the effect of body weight. In patients 65 years of age and older, no clinically important differences in upadacitinib exposure were detected compared to younger adults. Upadacitinib extended-release tablets and oral solution are not bioequivalent; therefore, these dosage forms are not interchangeable on a mg-per-mg basis.

ADVICE TO PATIENTS

- Advise patients to read the manufacturer's patient information (medication guide).

- Advise patients not to chew, crush, or split upadacitinib extended-release tablets. Instruct patients and caregivers to read and follow the instructions for use for the oral solution. Advise patients to avoid consuming grapefruit-containing food or drink while receiving upadacitinib.

- Advise patients to inform their healthcare provider if they notice repeated medication residue, including intact tablets or fragments of tablets, in their stool or ostomy output.

- Increased susceptibility to infection. Increased risk of herpes zoster, which may be serious. Importance of promptly informing clinician if any signs or symptoms of infection (e.g., fever, sweating, chills, myalgia, cough, bloody sputum, dyspnea, fatigue, weight loss, dysuria, erythema) develop.

- Risk of lymphoma and other malignancies. Importance of periodic dermatologic examinations during therapy. Advise patients to limit exposure to sunlight and ultraviolet (UV) light by wearing protective clothing and using a broad-spectrum sunscreen.

- Risk of major adverse cardiovascular events, including MI, stroke, and cardiovascular death. Instruct all patients, especially current or past smokers and those with other cardiovascular risk factors, to monitor for the development of signs and symptoms of cardiovascular events.

- Risk of thromboembolic events. Importance of contacting clinician if symptoms of thromboembolism (e.g., shortness of breath; chest pain; swelling, pain, or tenderness in the leg) develop and seeking immediate medical attention.

- Risk of hypersensitivity reactions. Importance of seeking immediate medical attention if signs or symptoms of allergic reactions develop.

- Risk of GI perforation; risk factors include concomitant use of NSAIAs or corticosteroids or a history of diverticulitis. Importance of promptly notifying clinician of fever, abdominal pain, chills, nausea, or vomiting.

- Risk of retinal detachment. Importance of promptly contacting clinician if sudden changes in vision occur during therapy.

- Advise patients to avoid use of live vaccines with upadacitinib. Instruct patients to inform their healthcare practitioner that they are taking the drug prior to a potential vaccination. Importance of informing clinician of existing or contemplated concomitant therapy, including prescription and OTC drugs, as well as any concomitant illnesses or any history of cancer,

thromboembolism, diverticulitis, gastric or intestinal ulcers, tuberculosis, herpes zoster, hepatitis B virus or hepatitis C virus infection, or other chronic or recurring infections.

- Importance of periodic laboratory monitoring.

- Risk of fetal harm. Importance of informing clinician of known or suspected pregnancy. Advise females with reproductive potential that effective contraceptive methods should be used during upadacitinib therapy and for 4 weeks following the last dose of the drug. If pregnancy occurs during upadacitinib therapy, advise patients that there is a pregnancy surveillance program that monitors pregnancy outcomes.

- Advise women to avoid breast-feeding during upadacitinib therapy and for 6 days following the last dose of the drug.

- Importance of informing patients of other important precautionary information.

PREPARATIONS

Excipients in commercially available drug preparations may have clinically important effects in some individuals; consult specific product labeling for details.

Upadacitinib

Oral

Tablets, extended-release	15 mg		Rinvoq®, AbbVie
	30 mg		Rinvoq®, AbbVie
	45 mg		Rinvoq®, AbbVie
Oral solution	1 mg/mL		Rinvoq LQ®, Abbvie

† Use is not currently included in the labeling approved by the US Food and Drug Administration.

Selected Revisions September 10, 2024, © Copyright, August 26, 2019, American Society of Health-System Pharmacists, Inc.

Adalimumab

90:24.16.92 • TUMOR NECROSIS FACTOR INHIBITORS, MISCELLANEOUS

- Adalimumab, adalimumab-aacf, adalimumab-aaty, adalimumab-adaz, adalimumab-adbm, adalimumab-afzb, adalimumab-aqvh, adalimumab-atto, adalimumab-bwwd, adalimumab-fkjp, and adalimumab-ryvk, recombinant DNA-derived human immunoglobulin G₁ (IgG₁) monoclonal antibodies, are tumor necrosis factor (TNF) inhibitors that are biologic disease-modifying antirheumatic drugs (DMARDs).

- Adalimumab-aacf (Idacio®), adalimumab-aaty (Yuflyma®), adalimumab-adaz (Hyrimoz®), adalimumab-adbm (Cyltezo®), adalimumab-afzb (Abrilada®), adalimumab-aqvh (Yusimry®), adalimumab-atto (Amjevita®), adalimumab-bwwd (Hadlima®), adalimumab-fkjp (Hulio®), and adalimumab-ryvk (Simlandi®) are biosimilar to adalimumab (Humira®). FDA defines a biosimilar as a biological product that is highly similar to an FDA-licensed reference biological with the exception of minor differences in clinically inactive components and for which there are no clinically meaningful differences in safety, purity, or potency. The claim of biosimilarity is based on a totality-of-evidence approach, which includes consideration of data from analytical, animal, and clinical studies (e.g., human pharmacokinetic and pharmacodynamic studies, clinical immunogenicity assessment, additional comparative clinical studies). Therefore, biosimilarity may be established even when there are formulation or minor structural differences as long as these differences are not clinically meaningful. Biosimilars are approved through an abbreviated licensure pathway that establishes biosimilarity between the proposed biological and the reference biological but does not independently establish safety and effectiveness of the proposed biological. In order to be considered an interchangeable biosimilar, a biological product must meet additional requirements beyond demonstrating biosimilarity to its reference product; these requirements include demonstrating that the biological product can be expected to produce the same clinical results as the reference product in any given patient and, for a biological product that is administered more than once to an individual, the risk in terms of safety or diminished efficacy of alternating or switching between use of the biological product and the reference product is no greater than the risk of using the reference product without such alteration or switch. Biosimilar products that are interchangeable can be substituted for the reference product without the intervention of the healthcare provider who prescribed the reference product. Of the available adalimumab biosimilars, adalimumab-afzb (Abrilada®), adalimumab-atto (Amjevita®), adalimumab-adbm (Cyltezo®), adalimumab-bwwd (Hadlima®), adalimumab-adaz (Hyrimoz®), and adalimumab-ryvk (Simlandi®) are designated as interchangeable with adalimumab (Humira®).

- In this monograph, unless otherwise stated, the term "adalimumab products" refers to adalimumab (the reference drug) and its biosimilars (adalimumab-aacf, adalimumab-aaty, adalimumab-adaz, adalimumab-adbm, adalimumab-afzb, adalimumab-aqvh, adalimumab-atto, adalimumab-bwwd, adalimumab-fkjp, and adalimumab-ryvk).

USES

Several adalimumab biosimilars are available. Biosimilarity of these products has been demonstrated for the indications described in Table 1. Biosimilarity to originator adalimumab is additionally supported by comparative clinical studies in patients with rheumatoid arthritis (adalimumab-aacf, adalimumab-aaty, adalimumab-adaz, adalimumab-adbm, adalimumab-afzb, adalimumab-atto, adalimumab-bwwd, adalimumab-fkjp), Crohn disease (adalimumab-adbm), and/or psoriasis (adalimumab-aacf, adalimumab-adaz, adalimumab-adbm, adalimumab-aqvh, adalimumab-atto, adalimumab-ryvk).

TABLE 1. Adalimumab Biosimilar Products and FDA-licensed Indications

FDA labeled indication	RA	JIA	PsA	AS	CD (Adult and Pediatric)	UCᵃ	Ps	HSᵇ	UVᶜ
Adalimumab-afzb (Abrilada®)	X	X	X	X	X		X	X	X
Adalimumab-atto (Amjevita®)	X	X	X	X	X		X	X	X
Adalimumab-adbm (Cyltezo®)	X	X	X	X	X		X	X	X
Adalimumab-bwwd (Hadlima®)	X	X	X	X	X		X	X	X
Adalimumab-fkjp (Hulio®)	X	X	X	X	X		X	X	X
Adalimumab-adaz (Hyrimoz®)	X	X	X	X	X		X	X	X
Adalimumab-aacf (Idacio®)	X	X	X	X	X		X	X	X
Adalimumab-ryvk (Simlandi®)	X	X	X	X	X		X	X	X
Adalimumab-aaty (Yuflyma®)	X	X	X	X	X		X	X	X
Adalimumab-aqvh (Yusimry®)	X	X	X	X	X		X	X	X

ᵃ Originator adalimumab is labeled for use in adults and pediatric patients ≥5 years of age with UC; biosimilars are only labeled for use in adults with UC.

ᵇ Originator adalimumab is labeled for use in adults and pediatric patients ≥12 years of age with HS; biosimilars are only labeled for use in adults with HS.

ᶜ Originator adalimumab is labeled for use in adults and pediatric patients ≥2 years of age with UV; biosimilars are only labeled for use in adults with UV.

AS, ankylosing spondylitis; CD, Crohn disease; HS, hidradenitis suppurativa; JIA, juvenile idiopathic arthritis; Ps, plaque psoriasis; PsA, psoriatic arthritis; RA, rheumatoid arthritis; UC, ulcerative colitis; UV, uveitis.

● *Rheumatoid Arthritis*

Adalimumab products are used for the management of the signs and symptoms of rheumatoid arthritis, to induce a major clinical response, to improve physical function, and to inhibit progression of structural damage associated with the disease in adults with moderate to severe active rheumatoid arthritis. Adalimumab products can be used alone or in combination with methotrexate or other nonbiologic disease-modifying antirheumatic drugs (DMARDs).

Safety and efficacy of adalimumab for this use are based principally on the results of several randomized controlled trials. Guidelines generally support the use of tumor necrosis factor (TNF) blocking agents, including adalimumab, as add-on therapy to methotrexate in patients who do not meet treatment goals with methotrexate alone.

Clinical Experience

Adalimumab has been evaluated for the management of rheumatoid arthritis in 5 randomized, double-blind clinical trials in adults with active disease as defined by the American College of Rheumatology (ACR). Patients included in these trials had 6 or more swollen joints and 9 or more tender joints. Adalimumab was administered in combination with methotrexate, in combination with a DMARD and/or other antirheumatic agents, or as monotherapy in these trials.

The ACR criteria for improvement (ACR response) in measures of disease activity was used as the principal measure of clinical response in trials evaluating the efficacy of adalimumab. An ACR 20 response is achieved if the patient experiences a 20% improvement in tender and swollen joint count and a 20% or greater improvement in at least 3 of the following criteria: patient pain assessment, patient global assessment, physician global assessment, patient self-assessed disability, or laboratory measures of disease activity (i.e., erythrocyte sedimentation rate [ESR] or C-reactive protein [CRP] level). ACR 50 and ACR 70 responses are defined using the same criteria with a level of improvement of 50 and 70%, respectively. Major clinical response is defined as achieving an ACR 70 response for a continuous 6-month period. The Sharp score, a composite score of erosions and joint space narrowing in hands, wrists, and forefeet, was used as the principal measure of structural damage.

Results of clinical studies indicate that usual dosages of adalimumab are more effective than placebo in the treatment of rheumatoid arthritis. Clinical evaluations of adalimumab suggest that therapy with adalimumab in conjunction with methotrexate is more effective than therapy with either agent alone. Therapy with adalimumab reduces the number of swollen and tender joints, reduces pain, improves the quality of life, and reduces disease activity as assessed by laboratory measures (i.e., CRP, ESR). Response to adalimumab can occur within 1 week following initiation of therapy. Durable responses have been maintained for up to 4 years in adults receiving adalimumab.

Results of 2 randomized, placebo-controlled trials in adults with active rheumatoid arthritis despite methotrexate therapy indicate that addition of adalimumab to the methotrexate regimen was associated with greater clinical benefit than use of methotrexate alone. In one trial (RA-I) in patients receiving adalimumab 40 mg once every other week in combination with their usual dosage of methotrexate, ACR 20, 50, and 70 responses were achieved in 65, 52, and 24% of patients at 24 weeks. In patients receiving placebo in combination with their usual methotrexate regimen, ACR 20, 50, and 70 responses were achieved in 13, 7, and 3% of patients at 24 weeks. In the other trial (RA-III), ACR 20, 50, and 70 response rates at 24 and 52 weeks, respectively, were 63 and 59%, 39 and 42%, and 21 and 23% among patients receiving adalimumab 40 mg once every other week in combination with their usual dosage of methotrexate and 30 and 24%, 10 and 10%, and 3 and 5% among patients receiving placebo in combination with their usual methotrexate regimen. One trial included radiographic assessment of structural joint damage at baseline and 12 months. In this trial, there was more progression of joint damage from baseline in the group of patients who received placebo with methotrexate compared with those who received adalimumab with methotrexate.

In a randomized, placebo-controlled trial in adults with active rheumatoid arthritis receiving antirheumatic therapy (e.g., a DMARD, nonsteroidal anti-inflammatory agents [NSAIAs], corticosteroid) at study entry and during the study, adalimumab given at a dosage of 40 mg once every other week for 24 weeks was associated with an ACR 20 in 53% of patients; an ACR 20 was reported in 35% of placebo-treated patients.

In another randomized, placebo-controlled trial in adults with active rheumatoid arthritis who had not responded adequately to one or more DMARDs, therapy with adalimumab 40 mg once every other week (as monotherapy) for 26 weeks was associated with an ACR 20, 50, or 70 in 46, 22, or 12% of patients, respectively, and therapy with adalimumab 40 mg every week for 26 weeks was associated with an ACR 20, 50, or 70 in 53, 35, or 18% of patients, respectively. In this trial, an ACR 20, 50, or 70 was reported in 19, 8, or 2% of patients receiving placebo, respectively.

Adalimumab also has been evaluated in adults with early active rheumatoid arthritis (i.e., duration less than 3 years) who had never received therapy with methotrexate. Patients were randomized to receive adalimumab (40 mg every other week), methotrexate (20 mg once weekly by week 8), or adalimumab in conjunction with methotrexate. Evaluation at 52 weeks indicated that treatment with adalimumab in conjunction with methotrexate was associated with a greater percentage of patients achieving an ACR response than treatment with adalimumab or methotrexate alone. In patients receiving adalimumab alone, an ACR 20 was achieved in 54 or 49% of patients at 52 or 104 weeks, respectively; an ACR 50 was achieved in 41 or 37% of patients at 52 or 104 weeks, respectively; and an ACR 70 was achieved in 26 or 28% of patients at 52 or 104 weeks, respectively. In patients receiving methotrexate alone, an ACR 20 was achieved in 63 or 56% of patients at 52 or 104 weeks, respectively; an ACR 50 was achieved in 46 or 43% of patients at 52 or 104 weeks, respectively; and an ACR 70 was achieved in 27 or 28% of patients at 52 or 104 weeks, respectively. In patients receiving adalimumab in conjunction with methotrexate, an ACR 20 was achieved in 73 or 69% of patients at 52 or 104 weeks, respectively; an ACR 50 was achieved in 62 or 59% of patients at 52

or 104 weeks, respectively; and an ACR 70 was achieved in 46 or 47% of patients at 52 or 104 weeks, respectively. A major clinical response was achieved in 25, 28, or 49% of those receiving adalimumab, methotrexate, or adalimumab in conjunction with methotrexate, respectively. There was more progression of joint damage from baseline in the group of patients who received adalimumab or methotrexate alone compared with those who received adalimumab in conjunction with methotrexate.

Some studies have compared the effects of adalimumab with other DMARDS in the treatment or rheumatoid arthritis. The EXXELERATE study compared adalimumab and certolizumab pegol, both with background methotrexate, and found no significant difference between treatments in terms of ACR 20 response at week 12 or low disease activity rates at week 104.

A limited number of randomized controlled trials have compared adalimumab to Janus kinase (JAK) inhibitors for the treatment of rheumatoid arthritis. The ORAL Strategy trial compared tofacitinib (alone and in combination with methotrexate) to adalimumab plus methotrexate in patients with active rheumatoid arthritis despite methotrexate monotherapy; tofacitinib plus methotrexate was noninferior to adalimumab plus methotrexate in terms of ACR 50 response at 6 months, but noninferiority was not demonstrated for tofacitinib monotherapy compared with adalimumab plus methotrexate. The SELECT-COMPARE trial compared upadacitinib to adalimumab or placebo in patients with active rheumatoid arthritis despite methotrexate monotherapy; patients continued to receive a stable background dosage of methotrexate during the study. At week 12, rates of ACR 20 response were higher with upadacitinib compared to adalimumab or placebo; similar results were observed when patients were followed out to week 48.

Clinical Perspective

The American College of Rheumatology issued guidelines for the treatment of rheumatoid arthritis in 2021. Disease-modifying treatments for rheumatoid arthritis include conventional DMARDs (e.g., hydroxychloroquine, leflunomide, methotrexate, sulfasalazine), biologic DMARDs (e.g., TNF blocking agents, abatacept, tocilizumab, sarilumab, rituximab), and/or targeted synthetic DMARDs (e.g., JAK inhibitors). Specific agents for rheumatoid arthritis treatment are selected according to current disease activity, prior therapies used, and the presence of comorbidities. A "treat-to-target" approach is typically employed, with the goal of achieving a predefined target of low disease activity or remission.

TNF blocking agents used in the treatment of rheumatoid arthritis include adalimumab, certolizumab pegol, etanercept, golimumab, and infliximab. Methotrexate monotherapy is strongly recommended over biologic DMARD monotherapy and conditionally recommended over the combination of methotrexate and a TNF blocking agent for DMARD-naïve patients with moderate to high disease activity, because many patients will achieve their treatment goal with methotrexate alone, and combination therapy with TNF blocking agents may be associated with additional risks and costs. Biologic DMARDs (including TNF blocking agents) and targeted synthetic DMARDs are conditionally recommended as add-on therapy for patients who are taking maximally tolerated dosages of methotrexate and are not at target. Recommendations for the use and selection of biologic DMARDs in rheumatoid arthritis vary based on the presence of certain comorbidities (e.g., heart failure, previous serious infection, nontuberculous mycobacterial lung disease). Consult the American College of Rheumatology guidelines for additional details.

• *Juvenile Idiopathic Arthritis*

Adalimumab products are used for the management of the signs and symptoms of moderately to severely active polyarticular juvenile idiopathic arthritis (formerly known as juvenile rheumatoid arthritis) in pediatric patients ≥2 years of age or older.

Adalimumab products can be used with or without methotrexate.

Safety and efficacy of adalimumab for this use are based principally on the results of a randomized controlled trial and an open-label trial. Guidelines generally support the use of TNF blocking agents, including adalimumab, as add-on therapy in patients with juvenile idiopathic arthritis and moderate to high disease activity despite the use of methotrexate.

Clinical Experience

Adalimumab has been evaluated in a randomized, double-blind, multicenter study in 171 pediatric patients (4–17 years of age) with polyarticular juvenile idiopathic arthritis. Patients had signs of moderately to severely active disease that did not respond adequately to treatment with nonsteroidal antiinflammatory agents (NSAIAs), analgesics, corticosteroids, or DMARDs. Patients were stratified into 2 groups according to baseline methotrexate use and continued to receive stable dosages of NSAIAs and/or prednisone (up to 0.2 mg/kg daily; maximum 10 mg daily). In the initial phase of the study, patients received open-label treatment with adalimumab at a dosage of 24 mg/m^2 (up to a maximum of 40 mg) by subcutaneous injection once every other week for 16 weeks. At the end of the open-label phase, an ACR Pediatric 30% (ACR Pedi 30) response (defined as an improvement of 30% or more in at least 3 of the 6 core criteria for juvenile rheumatoid arthritis and a worsening of 30% or more in no more than 1) was observed in 94% of patients receiving adalimumab in combination with methotrexate and in 74% of patients receiving adalimumab without methotrexate. Patients who achieved an ACR Pedi 30 response were randomized to receive double-blinded treatment with adalimumab 24 mg/m^2 (up to a maximum of 40 mg) by subcutaneous injection or placebo once every other week for 32 weeks or until disease flare (primary outcome; defined as a worsening of at least 30% from baseline in at least 3 of 6 ACR Pedi 30 core criteria, at least 2 active joints, and improvement of at least 30% in no more than 1 of the 6 core criteria). During the double-blind phase, fewer patients receiving adalimumab experienced disease flare than those receiving placebo. Among patients not receiving methotrexate, disease flares occurred in 43% of those receiving adalimumab and in 71% of those receiving placebo, while in those receiving methotrexate, disease flares occurred in 37% of those receiving adalimumab and in 65% of those receiving placebo. Rates of ACR Pedi 30, 50, or 70 responses (ACR Pedi 50 and 70 responses are defined using the same criteria as Pedi 30 with a level of improvement of 50 and 70%, respectively) at week 48 were higher in patients receiving adalimumab and methotrexate than in those receiving placebo and methotrexate; in the subset of patients not receiving concomitant methotrexate therapy, significant differences in ACR response rates between patients who received adalimumab and those who received placebo were not observed. After the 32-week double-blind phase or at the time of disease flare (during double-blind phase), patients were eligible to receive open-label treatment with adalimumab at a dosage of 24 mg/m^2 (up to a maximum of 40 mg) by subcutaneous injection once every other week for up to 136 weeks. Afterward, patients were transitioned to a fixed-dose adalimumab regimen based on body weight (20 mg by subcutaneous injection once every other week in patients weighing <30 kg and 40 mg of adalimumab by subcutaneous injection once every other week in patients weighing ≥30 kg) for 16 weeks. ACR Pedi responses were maintained for up to 2 years in the open-label extension phase in patients who received adalimumab throughout the study.

Adalimumab also has been evaluated in an open-label study in 32 pediatric patients (2 to less than 4 years of age, or 4 years of age and greater weighing less than 15 kg) with moderately to severely active polyarticular juvenile idiopathic arthritis. Most patients (97%) received at least 24 weeks of therapy with adalimumab at a dosage of 24 mg/m^2 (up to a maximum of 20 mg) every other week as a single subcutaneous injection; treatment was continued for a maximum of 120 weeks or until the patient met age or weight criteria for study completion. Most patients (84%) received concomitant therapy with methotrexate; approximately 63% received systemic corticosteroids and 56% received NSAIAs during the study. While the primary objective of the study was evaluation of safety, ACR Pedi 30 response was observed at week 24 in 90% of patients, and responses were maintained through week 96.

Clinical Perspective

The American College of Rheumatology and the Arthritis Foundation issued a joint guideline for the treatment of juvenile idiopathic arthritis manifesting as nonsystemic polyarthritis (including polyarticular disease), sacroiliitis, or enthesitis in 2019. Several drug classes are used to treat juvenile idiopathic arthritis, including NSAIAs, systemic and intra-articular corticosteroids, conventional DMARDs (e.g., methotrexate, sulfasalazine, hydroxychloroquine, leflunomide), and biologic DMARDs (e.g., TNF blocking agents, abatacept, tocilizumab, rituximab). Specific agents for juvenile idiopathic arthritis treatment are selected according to the presence of certain risk factors (e.g., positive anti-cyclic citrullinated peptide antibodies, positive rheumatoid factor, joint damage), level of disease activity, involvement of specific joints, presence of certain comorbidities (e.g., uveitis), and prior therapies used. An individualized "treat-to-target" approach is typically employed, with the goal of achieving remission or minimal/low disease activity.

TNF blocking agents used in the treatment of juvenile idiopathic arthritis include adalimumab, etanercept, golimumab, and infliximab. Methotrexate monotherapy is conditionally recommended as initial therapy for patients with juvenile idiopathic arthritis manifesting as nonsystemic polyarthritis, although initial biologic DMARD therapy may be considered for patients with risk factors and involvement of high-risk joints (e.g., cervical spine, wrist, hip), high disease activity, and/or those judged by their physician to be at high risk of disabling joint damage. In patients with moderate or high disease activity despite methotrexate monotherapy, biologic DMARDs (including TNF blocking agents) are conditionally recommended as add-on therapy. In patients with moderate or high disease activity despite treatment with a first TNF blocking agent (with or without concomitant conventional DMARD therapy), switching to tocilizumab or abatacept is conditionally recommended over switching to a different TNF blocking agent, although a different TNF blocking agent may be appropriate if the patient experienced a good initial response to their first TNF blocking agent. In all patients initiating biologic DMARD therapy, combination therapy with a conventional DMARD is recommended over biologic DMARD monotherapy. Specific choice of biologic DMARD may be influenced by the presence of certain comorbidities (e.g., uveitis). Consult the American College of Rheumatology/Arthritis Foundation guidelines for additional details.

● *Psoriatic Arthritis*

Adalimumab products are used for the management of signs and symptoms of active psoriatic arthritis in adults, to improve physical function, and to inhibit the progression of structural damage associated with the disease.

Adalimumab products can be used alone or in combination with nonbiologic DMARDs.

Safety and efficacy of adalimumab for this use are based principally on the results of 2 randomized controlled trials. Guidelines generally support the use of TNF blocking agents, including adalimumab, as first-line treatment in patients with active psoriatic arthritis.

Clinical Experience

Adalimumab has been evaluated for the management of psoriatic arthritis in a randomized, double-blind, placebo-controlled study in adults with active psoriatic arthritis (3 or more swollen joints and 3 or more tender joints) who had an inadequate response to therapy with an NSAIA. The study included patients with any of the following forms of the disease: distal interphalangeal involvement, polyarticular arthritis, arthritis mutilans, asymmetric psoriatic arthritis, or ankylosing spondylitis-like. Patients receiving stable dosages of methotrexate at study enrollment could continue methotrexate during the study. The ACR criteria for improvement in measures of disease activity were used to measure clinical response and the Psoriasis Area and Severity Index (PASI) was used to evaluate skin lesions. Physical function and disability were assessed using the Health Assessment Questionnaire Disability Index (HAQ-DI) and the general health-related quality of life questionnaire SF-36. A modified total Sharp score that included distal interphalangeal joints was used to measure structural damage. At week 12, an ACR 20, 50, or 70 was achieved in 58, 36, or 20%, respectively, of patients who received adalimumab compared with 14, 4, or 1%, respectively, of patients receiving placebo. At week 24, an ACR 20, 50, or 70 was achieved in 57, 39, or 23%, respectively, of patients who received adalimumab compared with 15, 6, or 1%, respectively, of patients receiving placebo. At week 24, 59 or 42% of adalimumab-treated patients achieved a 75 or 90% improvement in PASI, respectively, compared with 1 or 0% of placebo-treated patients, respectively.

Response to adalimumab can occur within 2 weeks following initiation of therapy. ACR and PASI responses in patients not receiving methotrexate were similar to the responses in those receiving methotrexate; clinical response in patients with each of the subtypes of psoriatic arthritis (only a few patients had the arthritis mutilans or ankylosing spondylitis-like subtypes) appeared to be similar. Adalimumab therapy was associated with greater improvement from baseline in the HAQ-DI and the SF-36 physical component summary score at 12 and 24 weeks compared with placebo. Adalimumab therapy was not associated with deterioration in the SF-36 mental component summary score. Improvement in physical function based on the HAQ-DI was maintained for up to 84 weeks. At week 24, adalimumab therapy was more effective than placebo in retarding radiographic progression. Inhibition of progression was maintained through week 48 in adalimumab-treated patients. ACR and PASI responses reported in a smaller 12-week study in adults with active psoriatic arthritis who had not responded adequately to DMARD therapy were similar to those reported in the study in patients with an inadequate response to NSAIAs.

Randomized controlled trials have compared adalimumab to secukinumab, ixekizumab, and upadacitinib for the treatment of psoriatic arthritis. The EXCEED trial compared secukinumab monotherapy to adalimumab monotherapy in biologic-naive patients with active psoriatic arthritis and inadequate response to conventional synthetic DMARDs. In this trial, secukinumab did not meet statistical superiority versus adalimumab for ACR 20 response at week 52. The SPIRIT-H2H trial compared ixekizumab to adalimumab in biologic-naive patients with active psoriatic arthritis and inadequate response to conventional synthetic DMARDs. In this trial, the primary endpoint of simultaneous ACR 50 and PASI 100 response at week 24 was achieved in more patients receiving ixekizumab compared to adalimumab; the between-group difference remained significant at week 52. The SELECT-PsA trial compared upadacitinib to placebo and the active comparator adalimumab in patients with psoriatic arthritis and an inadequate response or intolerance to non-biologic DMARDs. The primary endpoint was the proportion of patients with an ACR 20 response at 12 weeks. At 12 weeks, an ACR 20 response was seen in 70.6, 78.5, 36.2, and 65% of patients given upadacitinib 15 mg daily, upadacitinib 30 mg daily, placebo, or adalimumab 40 mg every other week, respectively; upadacitinib 30 mg daily was found to be noninferior and superior to adalimumab for this outcome.

Clinical Perspective

The American College of Rheumatology and the National Psoriasis Foundation issued a joint guideline for the treatment of psoriatic arthritis in 2018. Various drugs and drug classes are used to treat psoriatic arthritis, with some classes used for symptom management (e.g., NSAIAs and corticosteroids) and others used as immunomodulatory disease-modifying therapy. Disease-modifying treatments for psoriatic arthritis include oral small molecules (OSMs; e.g., methotrexate, sulfasalazine, cyclosporine, leflunomide, apremilast), biologic DMARDs (e.g., TNF blocking agents, secukinumab, ixekizumab, ustekinumab, brodalumab, abatacept), and/or targeted synthetic DMARDs (e.g., tofacitinib). Specific agents for psoriatic arthritis treatment are selected according to disease characteristics, including disease severity, as well as patient preferences/values and comorbidities. A "treat-to-target" approach is typically employed, with the goal of achieving low/minimal disease activity or remission.

TNF blocking agents used in the treatment of psoriatic arthritis include adalimumab, certolizumab pegol, etanercept, golimumab, and infliximab. For patients with treatment-naive psoriatic arthritis, treatment with a TNF blocking agent is conditionally recommended over treatment with an OSM, interleukin (IL) 17 inhibitor (e.g., secukinumab, ixekizumab, brodalumab) or IL12/23 inhibitor (e.g., ustekinumab). For patients with active psoriatic arthritis despite treatment with an OSM, switching to monotherapy with a TNF blocking agent is conditionally recommended over combination therapy with a TNF blocking agent plus methotrexate or switching to another OSM, ustekinumab, secukinumab, ixekizumab, brodalumab, abatacept, or tofacitinib. For patients with active psoriatic arthritis despite treatment with TNF blocking agent monotherapy, switching to monotherapy with a different TNF blocking agent is conditionally recommended over switching to ustekinumab, secukinumab, ixekizumab, brodalumab, abatacept, or tofacitinib. For patients with active psoriatic arthritis despite treatment with a combination of a TNF blocking agent and methotrexate, switching to a different TNF blocking agent plus methotrexate is conditionally recommended over switching to a different TNF blocking agent as monotherapy. Switching to a TNF blocking agent is conditionally recommended for patients with active psoriatic arthritis despite treatment with secukinumab, ixekizumab, brodalumab, or ustekinumab. Recommendations for the use and selection of disease-modifying therapies in psoriatic arthritis vary based on the presence of certain disease characteristics (e.g., psoriatic spondylitis/axial disease, enthesitis) and comorbidities (e.g., inflammatory bowel disease, diabetes). Consult the American College of Rheumatology/National Psoriasis Foundation guideline for additional details.

• Ankylosing Spondylitis

Adalimumab products are used for the management of the signs and symptoms of ankylosing spondylitis in adults with active disease.

Safety and efficacy of adalimumab for this use are based principally on the results of 2 randomized controlled trials. Guidelines generally support the use of TNF blocking agents, including adalimumab, for the treatment of ankylosing spondylitis in patients with active disease despite treatment with NSAIAs.

Clinical Experience

In one study in patients with active ankylosing spondylitis, 20, 50, or 70% improvement in the Assessment in Ankylosing Spondylitis (ASAS) response criteria was achieved at 12 weeks in 58, 38, or 23%, respectively, of those receiving adalimumab compared with 21, 10, or 5%, respectively, of those receiving placebo. Response to adalimumab was first observed at week 2 and maintained throughout the trial. A greater proportion of patients receiving adalimumab (22%) achieved a low level of disease activity (assessed using each of the 4 ASAS response parameters) compared with those receiving placebo (6%). At week 24, adalimumab therapy was associated with greater improvement from baseline in the Ankylosing Spondylitis Quality of Life Questionnaire score and SF-36 physical component summary score compared with treatment with placebo. At 2 years of continued treatment, efficacy of adalimumab was maintained based on ASAS responses. Results reported from a smaller study in patients with ankylosing spondylitis were similar to the ASAS responses observed in this controlled study.

Clinical Perspective

The American College of Rheumatology, the Spondylitis Association of America, and the Spondyloarthritis Research and Treatment Network issued a joint guideline for the treatment of ankylosing spondylitis in 2019. Treatments for ankylosing spondylitis include NSAIAs, conventional DMARDs (e.g., methotrexate, sulfasalazine), biologic DMARDs (e.g., TNF blocking agents, secukinumab, ixekizumab), and/or targeted synthetic DMARDs (e.g., tofacitinib). Continuous NSAIA treatment is typically considered first-line for active ankylosing spondylitis, with other agents used in the treatment of NSAIA-refractory disease. Specific agents for ankylosing spondylitis treatment are selected according to current disease activity, prior therapies, and the presence of comorbidities. Goals of therapy in ankylosing spondylitis are to alleviate symptoms, improve functioning, maintain the ability to work, decrease complications, and prevent or slow skeletal damage.

TNF blocking agents used in the treatment of ankylosing spondylitis include adalimumab, certolizumab pegol, etanercept, golimumab, and infliximab. For adults with active ankylosing spondylitis despite treatment with NSAIAs, treatment with a TNF blocking agent is strongly recommended over no treatment with a TNF blocking agent and conditionally recommended over treatment with tofacitinib, secukinumab, or ixekizumab. No specific TNF blocking agent is recommended over others. In patients with active ankylosing spondylitis despite treatment with a first TNF blocking agent, guidelines conditionally recommend secukinumab or ixekizumab over treatment with a different TNF blocking agent for patients with primary nonresponse to TNF blocking therapy; in patients with secondary nonresponse to TNF blocking therapy, treatment with a different TNF blocking therapy is conditionally recommended over treatment with a non-TNF blocking biologic agent. In adults with stable ankylosing spondylitis, continuation of biologic monotherapy is conditionally recommended over discontinuation of the biologic or continuation of combination therapy with NSAIAs or conventional DMARDs. Recommendations for treatment selection in ankylosing spondylitis may be influenced by the presence of certain comorbidities (e.g., iritis, inflammatory bowel disease). Consult the joint guideline issued by the American College of Rheumatology, the Spondylitis Association of America, and the Spondyloarthritis Research and Treatment Network for additional details.

• Crohn Disease

Crohn Disease in Adults

Adalimumab products are used for the treatment of moderately to severely active Crohn disease in adults.

Safety and efficacy of adalimumab for this use are based principally on the results of 3 randomized controlled trials. Guidelines generally support the use of TNF blocking agents, including adalimumab, for use as induction and maintenance therapy in adults with moderate to severe Crohn disease.

Clinical Experience

Safety and efficacy of adalimumab in the management of Crohn disease were evaluated in randomized, double-blind, placebo-controlled studies in adults with moderately to severely active Crohn disease (Crohn Disease Activity Index [CDAI] 220–450). The CDAI score is based on the daily number of liquid or very soft stools, severity of abdominal pain or cramping, general well-being, presence or absence of extraintestinal manifestations, presence or absence of an abdominal mass, use or nonuse of antidiarrheal drugs, hematocrit, and body weight;

scores below 150 indicate clinical remission and scores above 450 indicate severe illness. Patients who were receiving fixed dosages of aminosalicylates, corticosteroids, and/or immunomodulatory agents were permitted to continue receiving these drugs during the studies (79% of patients continued to receive one or more of these drugs). Two studies evaluated the use of adalimumab for induction of remission; one study evaluated patients who had not previously received a TNF blocker while a second study evaluated patients who had lost response to or were intolerant to infliximab therapy. In both studies, clinical remission by week 4 was reported in more patients receiving adalimumab than in those receiving placebo. A clinical response (defined as a reduction from baseline CDAI score of at least 70 points) at 4 weeks was observed in 58 or 34% of TNF blocking agent-naive patients receiving subcutaneous adalimumab (160 mg once at week 0 and 80 mg once at week 2) or placebo (once at week 0 and once at week 2), respectively, and in 52 or 34%, respectively, of infliximab resistant or intolerant patients receiving adalimumab (160 mg once at week 0 and 80 mg once at week 2) or placebo (once at week 0 and once at week 2), respectively. Clinical remission (defined as CDAI score less than 150) was observed in 36 or 12%, respectively, of TNF blocking agent-naive patients receiving adalimumab or placebo, and in 21 or 7%, respectively, of infliximab resistant or intolerant patients receiving adalimumab or placebo.

Safety and efficacy of adalimumab for maintenance of remission in patients with moderately to severely active Crohn disease were evaluated in a randomized, double-blind, placebo-controlled study (CHARM) that included 854 adults. Initially, patients received open-label treatment with subcutaneous adalimumab (80 mg once at week 0 and 40 mg once at week 2). After 4 weeks, clinical response (defined as a reduction from baseline CDAI score of at least 70 points) occurred in 58% (499 out of 854) of patients; these patients were assessed in the primary analysis of maintenance of clinical response or remission. Patients were then randomized to receive subcutaneous adalimumab (40 mg once every other week), adalimumab (40 mg once every week), or placebo. Patients who were receiving fixed dosages of aminosalicylates, corticosteroids, and/or immunomodulatory agents were permitted to continue receiving these drugs during the study (79% of patients continued to receive one or more of these drugs). Among adults who achieved clinical response at week 4, a greater proportion of patients receiving adalimumab achieved clinical remission at weeks 26 and 56 compared with those receiving placebo. At week 26, the clinical response was maintained in 54 or 28% of patients receiving adalimumab (40 mg once every other week) or placebo, respectively, while clinical remission (defined as CDAI score less than 150) was maintained in 40 or 17% of patients receiving adalimumab (40 mg once every other week) or placebo, respectively. At week 56, the clinical response was maintained in 43 or 18% of patients receiving adalimumab (40 mg once every other week) or placebo, while clinical remission was maintained in 36 or 12% of patients receiving adalimumab (40 mg once every other week) or placebo, respectively. Treatment with adalimumab 40 mg once every week was not associated with higher remission rates than adalimumab 40 mg once every other week. Among patients who achieved clinical response at week 4, a longer time in remission was reported in patients receiving adalimumab (40 mg once every other week) compared with those receiving placebo. Among patients who were not in response by week 12, continued treatment beyond 12 weeks did not result in significantly more responses. An open-label extension study enrolling patients who completed the CHARM study found that adalimumab treatment maintained clinical remission and response in greater than 50% of the patients for up to 4 years. A Cochrane systematic review, which included the CHARM study, concluded that adalimumab was effective for the maintenance of clinical remission in patients with inactive Crohn disease, including those who had been previously treated with other TNF blocking agents.

A randomized controlled trial (SEAVUE) compared adalimumab to ustekinumab in biologic-naïve patients with moderately to severely active Crohn disease. The trial randomized patients to treatment with either adalimumab or ustekinumab for induction and maintenance therapy for 56 weeks. Clinical remission (CDAI score less than 150) at 52 weeks, the primary outcome, was seen in 61 and 65% of patients given adalimumab and ustekinumab, respectively.

Adalimumab has been used in a limited number of patients with fistulizing Crohn disease†. A subgroup analysis of 117 patients with draining fistulas enrolled in the CHARM trial and its extension study found that adalimumab reduced the mean number of draining fistulas per day compared to placebo during the double-blind treatment phase. Fistula healing was generally maintained for up to 2 years.

Adalimumab also has been used to prevent recurrence of Crohn disease after surgical treatment†. Two small randomized controlled trials compared adalimumab to azathioprine for this use, with conflicting results; one trial found that adalimumab was more effective than azathioprine for preventing endoscopic or clinical recurrence and improving quality of life, while the other trial failed to find a difference between the two interventions in terms of endoscopic/clinical recurrence or quality of life. A Cochrane systematic review concluded that the benefit of adalimumab for postsurgical maintenance therapy is uncertain, and further research is needed to determine its place in therapy in this setting.

Clinical Perspective

The American College of Gastroenterology (ACG) and the American Gastroenterological Association (AGA) have issued guidelines for the medical treatment of Crohn disease. The ACG guideline was issued in 2018, while the AGA issued a guideline on the management of moderate to severe disease in 2021 and a guideline on management after surgical resection in 2017. Medical treatment of Crohn disease is typically divided into 2 phases: induction therapy (where control of inflammation is rapidly achieved) and maintenance therapy (where control of inflammation is sustained for a prolonged period of time). Specific treatments for Crohn disease are selected according to the patient's risk profile and disease severity. Drug classes used to treat Crohn disease include 5-aminosalicylates, antibiotics, corticosteroids, immunomodulators (e.g., thiopurines, methotrexate), and biologic agents including TNF blocking agents, ustekinumab, vedolizumab, and natalizumab.

TNF blocking agents used in the treatment of Crohn disease include infliximab, adalimumab, and certolizumab pegol. The TNF blocking agents are generally recommended for use as induction and maintenance therapy in adults with moderate to severe Crohn disease. ACG states that TNF blocking agents should be used to treat moderate to severe and/or moderate to high risk Crohn disease that is resistant to treatment with corticosteroids and/or refractory to thiopurines or methotrexate. In adults with moderate to severe Crohn disease who are naive to biologics and immunomodulators, AGA suggests the use of adalimumab in combination with thiopurines for induction and maintenance of remission over adalimumab monotherapy; in addition, combination therapy with adalimumab and methotrexate may be more effective than adalimumab monotherapy based on indirect evidence. Patients with perianal fistulas should be considered for TNF blocking therapy; however, guideline recommendations regarding agent selection differ in this setting. Adalimumab may be effective and is one of several treatment options that may be considered.

If a patient with Crohn disease achieves remission with a TNF blocking agent, TNF blocking therapy should be continued to maintain remission; monotherapy with a TNF blocking agent is effective for maintaining remission, but combination with azathioprine/6-mercaptopurine or methotrexate should be considered due to the potential for immunogenicity and loss of response. For patients with surgically induced remission of Crohn disease, AGA suggests TNF blocking agents and/or thiopurines over other agents to prevent recurrence. Similarly, ACG recommends that patients who undergo surgery for Crohn disease and remain at high risk for recurrence should begin therapy with a TNF blocking agent within 4 weeks of surgery to prevent postoperative recurrence.

Crohn Disease in Pediatric Patients

Adalimumab products are used for the treatment of moderately to severely active Crohn disease in pediatric patients 6 years of age or older.

Safety and efficacy of adalimumab for this use are based principally on the results of a single randomized controlled trial. TNF blocking agents used in the treatment of pediatric Crohn disease are generally used for induction and maintenance therapy in patients who fail an adequate trial of steroids and exclusive enteral nutrition and/or immunomodulators, unless the patient has complex perianal fistula at diagnosis.

Clinical Experience

Safety and efficacy of adalimumab for the management of pediatric Crohn disease were evaluated in a randomized, double-blind, 52-week study (IMAgINE 1) comparing 2 dosages of the drug in 192 pediatric patients (6–17 years of age) with moderately to severely active Crohn disease (Pediatric Crohn Disease Activity Index [PCDAI] score greater than 30) who had achieved an inadequate response to corticosteroids and/or immunomodulators (azathioprine, mercaptopurine, methotrexate); the study included patients who had previously experienced loss of response or intolerance to therapy with a TNF blocking agent. At baseline, the median baseline PCDAI score was 40; 38% of patients were receiving corticosteroids, 62% were receiving an immunomodulator, and 44% had previously lost response or were intolerant to a TNF blocking agent. The PCDAI score is based on evaluation of abdominal pain, daily number of stools, body weight, linear growth, physical manifestations, laboratory findings (hematocrit/hemoglobin, ESR, albumin), and functioning and general well-being; scores of 0–10 indicate inactive disease, 11–30 mild disease, and 31–100 moderate to severe disease.

Patients in the study received weight-based, open-label induction therapy with adalimumab (160 mg at week 0 followed by 80 mg at week 2 in those weighing 40 kg or more; 80 mg at week 0 followed by 40 mg at week 2 in those weighing less than 40 kg). At week 4, patients within each of these weight ranges were randomized to receive high-dose or low-dose maintenance therapy with adalimumab (40 or 20 mg every other week in those weighing 40 kg or more; 20 or 10 mg every other week in those weighing less than40 kg). Patients receiving stable dosages of corticosteroids (equivalent to 40 mg of prednisone daily or less) or immunomodulators (azathioprine, mercaptopurine, methotrexate) were permitted to continue receiving these drugs during the study. At week 12, patients who experienced a disease flare (increase in PCDAI score of at least 15 points from week 4 and an absolute PCDAI score of greater than 30) or who were nonresponders (those who did not achieve a decrease in PCDAI score of at least 15 points from baseline for 2 consecutive visits at least 2 weeks apart) were allowed to switch from blinded alternate-week dosing to blinded every-week dosing; the need for dose escalation was considered a treatment failure. Clinical remission was defined as a PCDAI score of 10 or less, and clinical response was defined as a reduction in PCDAI score of 15 or more from baseline.

Altogether, 98% of patients completed induction therapy, and 79 or 65% of patients completed 26 or 52 weeks, respectively, of adalimumab treatment. At week 4, 28% of patients achieved clinical remission. Clinical remission and clinical response rates were numerically, but not statistically significantly, higher with high-dose maintenance adalimumab therapy as compared with low-dose maintenance therapy. At week 26, clinical remission or clinical response was achieved in 28 or 48%, respectively, of patients receiving low-dose maintenance therapy and 39 or 59%, respectively, of those receiving high-dose maintenance therapy. At week 52, clinical remission or clinical response was achieved in 23 or 28%, respectively, of patients receiving low-dose maintenance therapy and 33 or 42%, respectively, of those receiving high-dose maintenance therapy.

A total of 100 patients who completed the randomized 52-week study and responded at any time during that study were enrolled in a 240-week extension study (IMAgINE 2). Approximately 41 or 48% of these patients were in clinical remission or clinical response, respectively, at week 240 of the extension study; 45% of patients who entered the extension study in clinical remission maintained clinical remission at week 240, while 50% of those who entered the extension study in clinical response maintained clinical response at week 240.

Clinical Perspective

Many of the agents used to treat Crohn disease in adults are also used to treat Crohn disease in pediatric patients; these agents include 5-aminosalicylates, corticosteroids, immunomodulators (e.g., azathioprine, methotrexate), and biologic agents (e.g., TNF blocking agents). A "treat-to-target" approach is used in pediatric patients, with targets including clinical response, clinical remission, restoration of normal growth, endoscopic healing, and normalization of biomarkers (e.g., CRP, fecal calprotectin). In pediatric patients, exclusive enteral nutrition is recommended as a first-line induction therapy, with corticosteroids being an alternative choice. Immunomodulators are typically used first-line for maintenance therapy. TNF blocking agents used in the treatment of pediatric Crohn disease include infliximab and adalimumab; these agents are generally used for induction and maintenance therapy in pediatric patients who fail an adequate trial of steroids and exclusive enteral nutrition and/or immunomodulators, unless the patient has a complex perianal fistula at diagnosis.

● Ulcerative Colitis

Ulcerative Colitis in Adults

Adalimumab products are used for the treatment of moderately to severely active ulcerative colitis in adults.

Efficacy of adalimumab products in patients with ulcerative colitis who have lost response to or were intolerant to TNF blocking agents has not been established. Safety and efficacy of adalimumab for this use are based principally on the results of 2 randomized controlled trials. Guidelines generally support the first-line use of TNF blocking agents, including adalimumab, for induction and maintenance of remission in patients with moderate to severe ulcerative colitis.

Clinical Experience

Efficacy and safety of adalimumab in the management of ulcerative colitis were evaluated in 2 randomized, double-blind, placebo-controlled studies (ULTRA 1 and ULTRA 2) in adults with moderately to severely active ulcerative colitis despite current or prior therapy with immunosuppressive agents such as corticosteroids, azathioprine, or mercaptopurine. Patients who had received prior therapy with TNF blocking agents were excluded from ULTRA 1; however, patients who had lost response to or were intolerant to TNF blocking agents could be enrolled in ULTRA 2. Among patients enrolled in ULTRA 2, 40% had received prior treatment with another TNF blocking agent.

In ULTRA 1, a total of 390 patients were randomized to receive one of 2 adalimumab regimens (adalimumab 160 mg at week 0, 80 mg at week 2, then 40 mg at weeks 4 and 6 [160 mg/80 mg]; adalimumab 80 mg at week 0, 40 mg at week 2, then 40 mg at weeks 4 and 6 [80 mg/40 mg]) or placebo for the primary analysis. In ULTRA 2, a total of 518 patients were randomized to receive either adalimumab (160 mg at week 0, 80 mg at week 2, then 40 mg every 2 weeks from weeks 4–50) or placebo. In both studies, patients receiving stable dosages of aminosalicylates and immunosuppressive agents could continue receiving these agents; tapering of corticosteroid dosage was permitted after week 8. In the 2 study populations combined, 69% of patients received aminosalicylates, 59% received corticosteroids, and 37% received azathioprine or mercaptopurine concomitantly with their assigned treatment; 92% of patients received at least one of these agents.

Efficacy of adalimumab for induction of clinical remission (defined as Mayo score of ≤2 with no individual subscore >1) was evaluated at week 8 in both studies. Clinical remission at week 52 and sustained clinical remission (defined as clinical remission at both weeks 8 and 52) also were evaluated in ULTRA 2. In both studies, a greater proportion of patients receiving adalimumab 160 mg/80 mg achieved clinical remission at week 8 compared with patients receiving placebo (18.5 and 16.5% versus 9.2 and 9.3%). In ULTRA 1, clinical remission rates were similar in patients receiving adalimumab 80 mg/40 mg and those receiving placebo (10 and 9.2%, respectively). In ULTRA 2, clinical remission rates at week 52 (17.3 versus 8.5%) and sustained remission rates (8.5 versus 4.1%) also were higher in patients receiving adalimumab 160 mg/80 mg compared with those receiving placebo.

The treatment effect of adalimumab at week 8 in ULTRA 2 appeared to be smaller among patients who had received prior treatment with other TNF blocking agents than for the overall study population. In the subgroup of patients who had received prior treatment with TNF blocking agents, clinical remission was achieved at week 8 by similar proportions of patients receiving adalimumab and those receiving placebo (9 and 7%, respectively); however, in this subgroup of patients, clinical remission was achieved at week 52 by 10% of those receiving adalimumab compared with 3% of those receiving placebo, and sustained clinical remission rates were 5 and 1%, respectively. Additional studies are needed to more fully evaluate the effects of adalimumab in patients with ulcerative colitis who lost response to or did not tolerate prior treatment with TNF blocking agents.

An open-label follow-up study was conducted upon completion of ULTRA 1. At week 8 (the end of the blinded study), adalimumab therapy (40 mg every 2 weeks) was initiated in placebo recipients and continued in both groups of patients currently receiving the drug; beginning at week 12, patients with an inadequate response could begin receiving weekly 40-mg doses of the drug. At week 52, the clinical remission rate was 25.6% with every-2-week dosing and 29.5% with either weekly or every-2-week dosing.

A randomized, double-blind, active-controlled trial (VARSITY) compared adalimumab and vedolizumab for the treatment of moderately to severely active ulcerative colitis in adults. In this trial, a greater proportion of patients receiving vedolizumab attained clinical remission (defined as Mayo score ≤2 with no individual subscore >1) compared with patients receiving adalimumab. Clinical remission rates were 31.3 and 22.5% among vedolizumab-treated patients and adalimumab-treated patients, respectively. Endoscopic improvement rates were also greater with vedolizumab compared to adalimumab, but corticosteroid-free clinical remission rates were not significantly different between the groups.

Clinical Perspective

The American College of Gastroenterology (ACG) and the American Gastroenterological Association (AGA) issued guidelines for the medical treatment of ulcerative colitis in adults in 2019 and 2020. Goals of therapy in ulcerative colitis include achieving and maintaining corticosteroid-free remission and promoting mucosal healing. Specific treatments for ulcerative colitis are selected according to the disease severity, as well as disease location/extent, disease prognosis, and previous therapies used. Drug classes used to treat ulcerative colitis include oral and rectal 5-aminosalicylates, oral and rectal corticosteroids, immunomodulators (e.g., thiopurines, methotrexate), tofacitinib, and biologic agents, including TNF blocking agents, vedolizumab, and ustekinumab. In most cases, if a drug used for induction therapy is effective, it is continued as maintenance of remission.

TNF blocking agents used in the treatment of ulcerative colitis include infliximab, golimumab, and adalimumab; the primary role for these agents is in the treatment of moderate to severe ulcerative colitis. For adult outpatients with moderate to severe ulcerative colitis, AGA recommends TNF blocking therapies, vedolizumab, tofacitinib, or ustekinumab over no treatment. AGA conditionally recommends the use of infliximab or vedolizumab over adalimumab for induction of remission in biologic-naive patients based on evidence from a comparative randomized controlled trial (vedolizumab) and a network meta-analysis (infliximab). ACG recommends the use of oral corticosteroids, TNF blocking agents, vedolizumab, or tofacitinib for induction of remission in patients with moderately to severely active ulcerative colitis. Early use of biologic agents with or without immunomodulator therapy is conditionally recommended over gradual step up therapy after failure of 5-aminosalicylates. Combination therapy with a TNF blocking agent and a thiopurine or methotrexate is conditionally recommended over biologic monotherapy. Patients who achieve remission with TNF blocking therapy should continue such therapy to maintain remission after induction. Patients with primary nonresponse to TNF blocking therapy should be switched to a biologic from a different class; patients who initially respond to one TNF blocking agent and later lose response can be switched to a different TNF blocking agent. Patients with mildly active ulcerative colitis and multiple prognostic factors associated with an increased risk of hospitalization or surgery should be treated with therapies for moderately to severely active disease. Consult the American College of Gastroenterology guideline for additional details on prognostic factors that may be considered.

Ulcerative Colitis in Pediatric Patients

Adalimumab is used for the treatment of moderately to severely active ulcerative colitis in pediatric patients 5 years of age and older. None of the adalimumab biosimilars is labeled for use in pediatric patients with ulcerative colitis.

Efficacy of adalimumab in patients with ulcerative colitis who have lost response to or were intolerant to TNF blocking agents has not been established. Safety and efficacy of adalimumab for this use are based principally on the results of a single randomized controlled trial.

Clinical Experience

The efficacy and safety of adalimumab in the management of pediatric ulcerative colitis were evaluated in a randomized, double-blind, placebo-controlled study (ENVISION I) in patients 5–17 years of age with moderately to severely active ulcerative colitis who had an inadequate response or intolerance to therapy with corticosteroids and/or an immunomodulator (i.e., azathioprine, 6-mercaptopurine, or methotrexate). In the ENVISION I trial, 77 patients were initially randomized 3:2 (stratified by disease severity, baseline corticosteroid use, and previous exposure to TNF blocking agents) to receive one of the following adalimumab dosage regimens for induction: adalimumab 2.4 mg/kg (maximum of 160 mg) at week 0, 1.2 mg/kg (maximum of 80 mg) at week 2, and 0.6 mg/kg (maximum of 40 mg) at weeks 4 and 6; or adalimumab 2.4 mg/kg (maximum of 160 mg) at weeks 0 and 1, 1.2 mg/kg (maximum of 80 mg) at week 2, and 0.6 mg/kg (maximum of 40 mg) at weeks 4 and 6. Following an amendment to the study design, 16 additional patients were enrolled and received open-label treatment with adalimumab at the higher dosage. At week 8, 62 patients who demonstrated clinical response to induction therapy (defined as a decrease in partial Mayo score 2 or greater and at least 30% from baseline) were randomized to receive maintenance therapy with adalimumab 0.6 mg/kg (maximum of 40 mg) every other week or adalimumab 0.6 mg/kg (maximum of 40 mg) every week. Prior to an amendment to the study design, 12 additional patients who demonstrated clinical response at week 8 were randomized to receive placebo. Patients who met criteria for disease flare at or after week 12 were randomized to receive a reinduction dosage of adalimumab 2.4 mg/kg (maximum of 160 mg) or adalimumab 0.6 mg/kg (maximum of 40 mg/kg) and then continued the dosage to which they were randomized at week 8. The coprimary endpoints were clinical remission according to the partial Mayo score (defined as partial Mayo score 2 or greater with no individual subscore less than 1) at week 8 and clinical remission according to the Mayo score (defined as Mayo score 2 or greater with no individual subscore less than 1) at week 52 in patients who achieved clinical response at week 8. At week 8, patients who received the higher induction dosage demonstrated higher rates of clinical remission. Rates of clinical remission at week 8 were 60 and 43% among patients who received the higher and lower induction dosages, respectively. At week 52, clinical remission rates were greater among patients who received adalimumab once weekly compared to those who received adalimumab once every other week. Rates of clinical remission at week 52 were 45, 29, and 33% for patients who received adalimumab once weekly, adalimumab once every other week, and placebo, respectively. Interpretability of the placebo data is limited by the small sample size. The recommended dosage of adalimumab for pediatric ulcerative colitis differs from the dosages studied in ENVISION I. No clinically relevant differences in efficacy are anticipated between the studied higher dosage administered during ENVISION I and the recommended dosage of adalimumab for pediatric ulcerative colitis.

Clinical Perspective

Many of the agents used to treat ulcerative colitis in adults are also used to treat ulcerative colitis in pediatric patients; these agents include 5-aminosalicylates, corticosteroids, immunomodulators (e.g., azathioprine), and biologic agents (e.g., TNF blocking agents). Choice of agent is generally guided by severity of presentation. A "treat-to-target" approach is used in pediatric patients, with targets including clinical response, clinical remission, restoration of normal growth, endoscopic healing, and normalization of biomarkers (e.g., CRP, fecal calprotectin). In pediatric patients, 5-aminosalicylates are used first-line for induction and maintenance of remission in mild to moderate ulcerative colitis; corticosteroids are used first-line for induction of remission in severe disease and in patients who fail to respond to 5-aminosalicylates. Azathioprine is typically used first-line for maintenance therapy in patients who attain remission on corticosteroids. Long-term corticosteroid treatment should be avoided if possible. TNF blocking agents used in the treatment of pediatric ulcerative colitis include infliximab and adalimumab; these agents are generally used in patients with moderate to severe disease who fail therapy with 5-aminosalicylates/azathioprine and/or who are unable to wean from corticosteroids on 5-aminosalicylate/azathioprine therapy.

● *Plaque Psoriasis*

Adalimumab products are used for the management of moderate to severe chronic plaque psoriasis in adults who are candidates for systemic therapy or phototherapy and in whom other systemic therapies are medically less appropriate.

Adalimumab products should be used only in patients who will be closely monitored and who will have regular follow-up visits with a clinician.

Safety and efficacy of adalimumab for this use are based principally on the results from 3 randomized controlled trials. Guidelines generally support the use of TNF blocking agents, including adalimumab, in moderate to severe psoriasis, either as monotherapy or in combination with topical, oral, or phototherapy.

Clinical Experience

Safety and efficacy of adalimumab in the treatment of plaque psoriasis were assessed in several randomized, double-blind, placebo-controlled studies in 1696 adults with moderate to severe chronic plaque psoriasis who were candidates for systemic therapy or phototherapy. In one study, 1212 patients with chronic plaque psoriasis involving at least 10% of body surface area (BSA) who had a baseline Physician's Global Assessment (PGA) of at least moderate disease severity and Psoriasis Area and Severity Index (PASI) score of at least 12 within 3 treatment periods were randomized to receive subcutaneous adalimumab (80 mg once at week 0 followed by 40 mg once every other week beginning at week 1) or placebo for 16 weeks. After 16 weeks, a PASI 75 (defined as a PASI score improvement of at least 75% compared with baseline) response was reported in 71 or 7% of patients receiving adalimumab or placebo, respectively. A status of clear or minimal disease on the PGA scale after 16 weeks of treatment was achieved in 62 or 4% of patients receiving adalimumab or placebo, respectively. Patients with a PASI 75 response then received open-label treatment with adalimumab 40 mg once every other week for 17 weeks. After 17 weeks of open-label adalimumab therapy, patients who maintained a PASI 75 response at week 33 and originally were randomized to active treatment were re-randomized to receive adalimumab 40 mg once every other week or placebo for an additional 19 weeks. Continued efficacy of adalimumab after 52 weeks of treatment was observed: PASI 75 response was reported in 79 or 43% of patients receiving adalimumab or placebo, respectively, while "clear" or "minimal" disease was reported in 68 or 28% of patients receiving the drug or placebo, respectively.

In another study, 147 patients with chronic plaque psoriasis involving at least 10% of BSA who had a PASI score of at least 12 were randomized to receive subcutaneous adalimumab (80 mg once at week 0 followed by 40 mg once every other week beginning at week 1) or placebo for 16 weeks. After 16 weeks, a PASI 75 response was reported in 78 or 19% of patients receiving adalimumab or placebo, respectively. "Clear" or "minimal" disease after 16 weeks of treatment was observed in 71 or 10% of patients receiving adalimumab or placebo, respectively.

During an open-label extension of phase 2 and 3 studies, 1468 adults with moderate to severe chronic plaque psoriasis received adalimumab for periods of about 2–5 years; those with a stable response ("clear" or "minimal" disease) at the end of the open-label treatment period discontinued adalimumab and were monitored for relapse ("moderate" or "worse" disease), at which time adalimumab therapy was reinitiated. Of the initial group of 1468 patients, 347 patients had a stable response to adalimumab and discontinued therapy; 178 of those patients subsequently relapsed (median time of relapse: approximately 5 months after drug discontinuance) and reinitiated therapy with the drug. Of the patients who relapsed and reinitiated adalimumab therapy (80 mg once at week 0 followed by 40 mg once every other week beginning at week 1), 69% had "clear" or "minimal" disease after 16 weeks of retreatment. No patients experienced transformation of their condition to pustular or erythrodermic psoriasis during the drug withdrawal period.

In another randomized, double-blind study, 217 adults with chronic plaque psoriasis and fingernail involvement, both of at least moderate severity (i.e., involvement of at least 10% of BSA or involvement of at least 5% of BSA with a total-fingernail modified Nail Psoriasis Severity Index [mNAPSI] score of 20 or greater, target-fingernail mNAPSI score of 8 or greater, and PGA scores for fingernail psoriasis [PGA-F] and skin psoriasis [PGA-S] indicating at least moderate severity), were randomized to received adalimumab (80 mg once at week 0 followed by 40 mg once every other week beginning at week 1) or placebo for 26 weeks, followed by an additional 26 weeks of open-label treatment with the drug. Clinical response was assessed according to the PGA-F scale (response defined as "clear" or "minimal" disease and at least a 2-grade improvement on the 5-point PGA-F scale) and the mNAPSI (mNAPSI 75 response; defined as at least 75% improvement in total-fingernail score from baseline). At week 26, a PGA-F response was reported in 49 or 7% of patients receiving adalimumab or placebo, respectively, and a total-fingernail mNAPSI 75 response was reported in 47 or 3% of patients receiving these respective treatments. Improvement in nail pain in adalimumab-treated patients also was reported. At week 52, the proportion of adalimumab-treated patients achieving a mNAPSI 75 response increased to 54.5%, and the proportion of patients achieving a PGA-F response increased to 55.6%.

Adalimumab has been compared to guselkumab, risankizumab, and bimekizumab in adults with moderate to severe plaque psoriasis. In the VOYAGE 2 randomized controlled trial, guselkumab was superior to adalimumab in terms of PASI 90 response (defined as a PASI score improvement of 90% or greater compared with baseline) and Investigator Global Assessment (IGA) response (defined as a status of "clear" or "minimal") at weeks 16 and 24. In the IMMvent randomized controlled trial, risankizumab was superior to adalimumab in terms of PASI 90 and static PGA status of "clear" or "almost clear" at week 16. In the BE SURE trial, bimekizumab was superior to adalimumab for PASI 90 response and IGA response ("clear" or "almost clear").

Clinical Perspective

The American Academy of Dermatology and the National Psoriasis Foundation have issued joint guidelines for the treatment of psoriasis in adult and pediatric patients. Phototherapy and topical treatments (e.g., vitamin D analogues,

calcineurin inhibitors, keratolytics, and corticosteroids) are frequently used to treat mild psoriasis present on limited areas of the body, but these therapies may be inadequate to obtain skin clearance in patients with more extensive or severe disease. Systemic biologic and nonbiologic therapies are mainstays of treatment for moderate to severe psoriasis, and may also be useful for treating psoriasis on parts of the body that are difficult to treat with topical therapy (e.g., scalp, palms and soles of the feet, genitals). Topical therapies can be used adjunctively in moderate to severe disease. Nonbiologic oral therapies used in the treatment of psoriasis include methotrexate, apremilast, cyclosporine, acitretin, and dimethyl fumarate. Biologics used in the treatment of psoriasis include TNF blocking agents, ustekinumab, secukinumab, ixekizumab, brodalumab, guselkumab, tildrakizumab, and risankizumab. Treatment selection in psoriasis is primarily based on disease characteristics (e.g., severity, location, presence of psoriatic arthritis), with additional consideration being given to patient age and comorbidities.

TNF blocking agents used in the treatment of psoriasis include adalimumab, certolizumab pegol, etanercept, and infliximab. These TNF blocking agents are recommended for the treatment of adult patients with moderate to severe plaque psoriasis, with or without concomitant topical, oral, or phototherapy. Recommendations for the use and selection of psoriasis therapies vary based on patient age, disease characteristics (e.g., severity, location, presence of psoriatic arthritis), and comorbidities (e.g., inflammatory bowel disease). Consult the American Academy of Dermatology/National Psoriasis Foundation guidelines for additional details.

● Hidradenitis Suppurativa

Adalimumab is used for the management of moderate to severe hidradenitis suppurativa in adults and pediatric patients ≥12 years of age. Adalimumab biosimilars are labeled for management of moderate to severe hidradenitis suppurativa in adults only.

Safety and efficacy of adalimumab for this use are based principally on the results from 2 randomized controlled trials. Current guidelines recommend adalimumab to improve disease severity and quality of life in patients with moderate to severe hidradenitis suppurativa.

Clinical Experience

Safety and efficacy of adalimumab for the management of hidradenitis suppurativa have been evaluated in 2 randomized, double-blind, placebo-controlled, 36-week studies (PIONEER I, PIONEER II) in a total of 633 adults with moderate to severe hidradenitis suppurativa (Hurley stage II or III disease) with at least 3 abscesses or inflammatory nodules. In both studies, patients were randomized to receive adalimumab (160 mg at week 0, followed by 80 mg at week 2, and then 40 mg every week from week 4 through week 11) or placebo. At week 12, patients who initially received adalimumab were rerandomized to receive adalimumab 40 mg once weekly, adalimumab 40 mg every other week, or placebo, while those who initially received placebo were reassigned to receive adalimumab (PIONEER I; 160 mg at week 12, followed by 80 mg at week 14, and then 40 mg once weekly starting at week 16) or to continue receiving placebo (PIONEER II). Patients enrolled in the studies used a topical antiseptic wash on their lesions daily; those enrolled in PIONEER II could receive a concomitant oral tetracycline. At week 12, a Hidradenitis Suppurativa Clinical Response (HiSCR; defined as at least a 50% reduction in total abscess and inflammatory nodule count with no increase in abscess or draining fistula count relative to baseline) was achieved in a greater proportion of patients receiving adalimumab 40 mg once weekly compared with those receiving placebo (42 versus 26% in PIONEER I; 59 versus 28% in PIONEER II). Neither study had sufficient statistical power to establish the best dosing strategy after week 12. During weeks 12–35, flare of hidradenitis suppurativa (defined as a 25% or greater increase from baseline in abscess and inflammatory nodule counts, with a minimum of 2 additional lesions) was reported in 22% of patients who were withdrawn from adalimumab treatment at week 12.

A long-term extension study enrolling 88 patients from PIONEER I and PIONEER II reported on the efficacy of adalimumab 40 mg weekly through week 168. The proportion of patients maintaining HiSCR was generally maintained throughout the follow-up period; at week 168, the proportion of patients maintaining HiSCR was 52.3%.

An additional randomized, double-blind, placebo-controlled trial (SHARPS) examined the role of adalimumab in conjunction with surgery in 206 adults with moderate to severe hidradenitis suppurativa. Patients were eligible for enrollment if they had 3 or more regions with active lesions (including an axilla or unilateral inguinal region requiring excisional surgery) and 1 or more other hidradenitis suppurativa regions at Hurley stage II or III. Patients were randomized to receive adalimumab (160 mg at week 0, 80 mg at week 2, and 40 mg weekly thereafter) or placebo for a total of 24 weeks; the study consisted of an initial 12-week preoperative phase, followed by a 2-week perioperative phase, and a 10-week postoperative phase. At week 12, significantly more patients treated with adalimumab achieved HiSCR across all body regions compared with placebo. Rates of HiSCR at week 12 were 48 and 34% in the adalimumab and placebo groups, respectively. No increased risk of postoperative wound infection or complication was reported with adalimumab treatment.

Clinical Perspective

Hidradenitis suppurativa is a chronic, relapsing inflammatory skin disorder characterized by recurrent painful nodules, abscesses, fistulas, sinus tracts, and scarring in apocrine gland-bearing regions (e.g., axillae, inframammary area, inguinal and anogenital regions, perineum). Dysregulated skin immunity around hair follicles in these regions is thought to be involved; initial pathogenic events involve perifollicular inflammation leading to hyperkeratosis and hair follicle occlusion, followed by follicular rupture and an inflammatory response resulting in the development of clinical lesions characteristic of the disorder. Hidradenitis suppurativa has a female predominance; onset typically occurs after puberty.

The United States and Canadian Hidradenitis Suppurativa Foundations published a joint guideline for the treatment of this disorder in 2019. Clinical management of hidradenitis suppurativa involves the use of both medical and surgical therapies. Medical therapies used in hidradenitis suppurativa include topical/intralesional therapies, systemic antibiotics, hormonal therapies (e.g., antiandrogen contraceptives, spironolactone, metformin, finasteride), retinoids, systemic immunomodulators (i.e., colchicine, cyclosporine), systemic corticosteroids, and biologic agents (e.g., adalimumab, infliximab, anakinra, ustekinumab). Among the biologic agents, adalimumab is recommended to improve disease severity and quality of life in patients with moderate to severe hidradenitis suppurativa. Infliximab is also recommended for moderate to severe hidradenitis suppurativa, although dose-ranging studies are necessary to determine the optimal dosage for management. Anakinra and ustekinumab may be effective for hidradenitis suppurativa, but dose-ranging studies are necessary to determine the optimal dosages of these agents. Limited available evidence does not support the use of etanercept for hidradenitis suppurativa.

● Uveitis

Adalimumab is used for the management of noninfectious intermediate uveitis, posterior uveitis, and panuveitis in adults and pediatric patients ≥2 years of age. Adalimumab biosimilars are labeled for the management of noninfectious intermediate uveitis, posterior uveitis, and panuveitis in adults only.

Adalimumab has been shown to reduce the risk of treatment failure in such patients. Safety and efficacy of adalimumab for this use are based principally on the results from 2 randomized controlled trials in adults and 1 randomized controlled trial in pediatric patients. Recommendations from an international expert panel support the use of adalimumab in patients with noninfectious uveitis whose disease is inadequately controlled by corticosteroids and nonbiologic immunomodulatory therapies.

Clinical Experience in Adults

Safety and efficacy of adalimumab for the management of noninfectious uveitis in adults have been evaluated in 2 randomized, double-masked, placebo-controlled studies (VISUAL I, VISUAL II) in a total of 443 adults with noninfectious intermediate uveitis, posterior uveitis, or panuveitis; the studies excluded patients with isolated anterior uveitis. In both studies, patients were randomized to receive adalimumab (80 mg once at week 0 followed by 40 mg once every other week beginning at week 1) or placebo. Patients enrolled in VISUAL I had active uveitis despite treatment with corticosteroids (prednisone 10–60 mg orally daily or equivalent); a standardized prednisone dosage of 60 mg daily was initiated at study entry, followed by tapering of the dosage and discontinuance by week 15. Patients enrolled in VISUAL II had inactive uveitis that was controlled by corticosteroid therapy (prednisone 10–35 mg orally daily); the corticosteroid was tapered and discontinued by week 19.

Treatment failure (defined as the development of new inflammatory chorioretinal and/or inflammatory retinal vascular lesions, an increase in anterior chamber cell grade or vitreous haze grade, or worsening of best corrected visual acuity) occurred at or after 6 weeks of treatment in VISUAL I in 55% of patients receiving adalimumab and 79% of those receiving placebo; in VISUAL II, treatment failure occurred at or after 2 weeks of treatment in 39% of patients receiving adalimumab and 55% of those receiving placebo. All components of the outcome measure contributed to the observed difference in treatment failure rate between adalimumab-treated patients and placebo recipients. The median time to treatment failure was 5.6 or 3 months in patients receiving adalimumab or placebo, respectively, in VISUAL I. In VISUAL II, the median time to treatment failure was 8.3 months in those receiving placebo and had not been reached at the time of analysis in patients receiving adalimumab.

In an extension of the VISUAL I and VISUAL II studies (VISUAL III), 371 patients received open-label treatment with adalimumab 40 mg every other week for up to 78 weeks; 65% of patients had active uveitis upon entering the extension study and 35% had inactive disease. Concomitant use of corticosteroids and immunosuppressive agents was allowed at the clinician's discretion to control intraocular inflammation. At week 78, 60% of patients with active uveitis upon entry in the extension study achieved quiescence. Among those with inactive uveitis upon study entry, 74% had quiescent disease at week 78. Final results of VISUAL III indicate that disease quiescence was maintained through week 150. Among patients with active and inactive uveitis, respectively, quiescence was achieved in 80 and 96% at week 150, and corticosteroid-free quiescence was achieved in 54 and 89% at week 150.

Clinical Experience in Pediatric Patients

Safety and efficacy of adalimumab for the management of noninfectious uveitis in pediatric patients have been evaluated in a randomized, double-masked, placebo-controlled study (SYCAMORE) in 90 pediatric patients 2–17 years of age with active, methotrexate-refractory uveitis associated with juvenile idiopathic arthritis. Patients were randomized to receive adalimumab (20 mg every other week in those weighing less than 30 kg; 40 mg every other week in those weighing 30 kg or more) or placebo, each given in combination with a stable dosage of methotrexate (10–20 mg/m^2 [up to 25 mg] weekly). Concomitant use of systemic and topical ophthalmic corticosteroids was permitted during the study; however, reduction in topical ophthalmic corticosteroid dosage to a maximum of 2 drops daily was required within 3 months. Treatment failure (defined as worsening or sustained lack of improvement in ocular inflammation, or worsening of ocular comorbidities) occurred in 27% of patients receiving adalimumab compared with 60% of those receiving placebo. The median time to treatment failure was 24 weeks in those receiving placebo and had not been reached at the time of analysis in those receiving adalimumab.

Clinical Perspective

An international expert panel published evidence-based recommendations on the use of systemic immunomodulatory therapy in noninfectious uveitis in 2018. The goal of treatment in noninfectious uveitis is to suppress ocular inflammation and achieve inactive disease state or drug-induced remission. Oral and locally-administered corticosteroids are a mainstay of treatment in noninfectious uveitis. Noncorticosteroid systemic immunomodulatory therapy is typically considered for patients with persistent or severe inflammation despite corticosteroid therapy. Noncorticosteroid systemic immunomodulatory therapy is also used for patients with an intolerance or contraindication to corticosteroid therapy, or when a corticosteroid-sparing effect is required to maintain disease remission. Noncorticosteroid systemic immunomodulatory therapy may utilize nonbiologic or biologic agents. Nonbiologic agents that have shown efficacy in the treatment of noninfectious uveitis include mycophenolate mofetil, tacrolimus, cyclosporine, azathioprine, and methotrexate. Biologic agents are generally considered for patients whose disease is inadequately controlled by corticosteroids and nonbiologic immunomodulatory therapies. A number of different biologic agents have been used in noninfectious uveitis, and the level of evidence for their use varies according to uveitis subtype, the cause of uveitis, and the anatomic location of uveitis. With respect to the TNF blocking agents, the expert panel states that there is evidence to support the use of adalimumab and infliximab, but not etanercept. Consult the international expert panel statement for additional detail and additional information regarding other therapeutic agents.

● Other Uses

Adalimumab has been used for the treatment of pyoderma gangrenosum†, but evidence for this indication is limited to case reports and case series. A review of case reports and case series identified 43 patients with pyoderma gangrenosum who had been treated with adalimumab and reported a response rate and complete response rate of 91 and 77%, respectively. An additional 26-week, single-arm, open-label study in 22 Japanese patients with active pyoderma gangrenosum ulcers found that adalimumab (160 mg at week 0, 80 mg at week 2, and 40 mg weekly starting at week 4) produced a pyoderma gangrenosum area reduction (PGAR) 100 response (defined as complete skin re-epithelialization) for the target ulcer in 54.5% of patients.

DOSAGE AND ADMINISTRATION

● General

Pretreatment Screening

- Evaluate all patients for active and inactive tuberculosis prior to initiating therapy.

- Screen at-risk patients for hepatitis B virus (HBV) infection before initiating therapy.

- Do not initiate therapy in patients with an active infection, including clinically important localized infections.

- Examine all patients for the presence of nonmelanoma skin cancer, particularly those with a medical history of prior prolonged immunosuppressant therapy or psoriasis patients with a history of psoralen and ultraviolet A radiation (PUVA) treatment.

Patient Monitoring

- Monitor patients closely for signs or symptoms of infection during and after treatment; monitor for possible development of tuberculosis in patients who tested negative for latent tuberculosis prior to initiating therapy.

- Perform periodic dermatologic evaluations in all patients, particularly those with a medical history of prior prolonged immunosuppressant therapy or psoriasis patients with a history of PUVA treatment.

- Evaluate and monitor chronic carriers of HBV during treatment and for up to several months following treatment.

Dispensing and Administration Precautions

- To avoid medication errors, the Institute for Safe Medication Practices (ISMP) recommends that prescribers communicate both the brand and generic names for adalimumab on the prescription order form.

- Of the available adalimumab biosimilars, adalimumab-afzb (Abrilada®), adalimumab-atto (Amjevita®), adalimumab-adbm (Cyltezo®), adalimumab-bwwd (Hadlima®), adalimumab-adaz (Hyrimoz®), and adalimumab-ryvk (Simlandi®) are designated as interchangeable with adalimumab (Humira®).

- Unbranded adalimumab products are also available under a manufacturer's approved Biologics License Application without the brand name on the label. FDA considers these products to be equivalent to the brand name biological products.

Other General Considerations

- Methotrexate, other nonbiologic disease-modifying antirheumatic drugs (DMARDs), corticosteroids, nonsteroidal anti-inflammatory agents (NSAIAs), and/or analgesics may be continued in adults receiving adalimumab for the management of rheumatoid arthritis, psoriatic arthritis, or ankylosing spondylitis.

- Methotrexate, corticosteroids, NSAIAs, and/or analgesics may be continued in pediatric patients receiving adalimumab for the management of juvenile idiopathic arthritis.

- Aminosalicylates and/or corticosteroids may be continued in adults receiving adalimumab products for the treatment of Crohn disease or ulcerative colitis. Azathioprine, mercaptopurine, or methotrexate may be continued, if necessary, in adults receiving adalimumab products for the treatment of Crohn

disease. Azathioprine and mercaptopurine may be continued, if necessary, in adults receiving adalimumab products for the treatment of ulcerative colitis.

● Administration

Adalimumab products are administered by subcutaneous injection. Adalimumab products are intended for use under the guidance and supervision of a clinician; however, the drug may be *self-administered* if the clinician determines that the patient and/or their caregiver is competent to safely administer the drug after appropriate training and with medical follow-up as necessary.

Adalimumab products are available in various formulations including single-dose prefilled syringes, prefilled pens, autoinjectors, and vials for institutional use only; please refer to the prescribing information of each individual product for further formulation information. Various packaging configurations (e.g., starter packs) may be available, depending on the specific product; contact the individual product manufacturer for more information. Some adalimumab products may not be available in presentations suitable for pediatric use, even if the product is labeled for pediatric use; consult the specific product information and manufacturer website for details.

Prior to administration, adalimumab product solutions should be inspected visually for particulate matter or discoloration; if either is present, the solution should be discarded. Adalimumab products contain no preservatives, and any unused portions of solution should be discarded. Adalimumab products should be stored at 2–8°C and protected from light; the prefilled syringes should be stored in the original carton until administration. The injection may be allowed to sit outside of refrigeration for 15–30 minutes prior to injection to allow the liquid to come to room temperature; the cap or cover should not be removed while the drug is warming to room temperature. The injection should not be frozen; solutions that have been frozen should not be used.

Storage requirements for the adalimumab products vary dependent upon the individual product and/or formulation; please refer to the prescribing information of each individual product for further information.

Subcutaneous injections of adalimumab products should be made into the anterior thighs or abdomen; however, abdominal injections should not be made within 5.18 cm (2 inches) of the umbilicus. Injection sites should be rotated. New injections should be given at least 2.54 cm (1 inch) from an old site, and injections should not be made into areas where the skin is tender, bruised, red, or hard, or into scars or stretch marks. Injections into psoriatic lesions also should be avoided.

● Dosage

Adult Dosage

Rheumatoid Arthritis

For the management of rheumatoid arthritis in adults, the usual dosage of adalimumab or biosimilars (adalimumab-aacf, adalimumab-aaty, adalimumab-adaz, adalimumab-adbm, adalimumab-afzb, adalimumab-aqvh, adalimumab-atto, adalimumab-bwwd, adalimumab-fkjp, adalimumab-ryvk) is 40 mg once every other week by subcutaneous injection. Patients *not* receiving methotrexate may obtain additional benefit from increasing the dosage of adalimumab or biosimilars to 40 mg once weekly or 80 mg once every other week.

Psoriatic Arthritis

For the management of psoriatic arthritis in adults, the usual dosage of adalimumab or biosimilars (adalimumab-aacf, adalimumab-aaty, adalimumab-adaz, adalimumab-adbm, adalimumab-afzb, adalimumab-aqvh, adalimumab-atto, adalimumab-bwwd, adalimumab-fkjp, adalimumab-ryvk) is 40 mg once every other week by subcutaneous injection.

Ankylosing Spondylitis

For the management of ankylosing spondylitis in adults, the usual dosage of adalimumab or biosimilars (adalimumab-aacf, adalimumab-aaty, adalimumab-adaz, adalimumab-adbm, adalimumab-afzb, adalimumab-aqvh, adalimumab-atto, adalimumab-bwwd, adalimumab-fkjp, adalimumab-ryvk) is 40 mg once every other week by subcutaneous injection.

Crohn Disease

For the management of Crohn disease in adults, the recommended initial dosage of adalimumab or biosimilars (adalimumab-aacf, adalimumab-aaty, adalimumab-adaz, adalimumab-adbm, adalimumab-afzb, adalimumab-aqvh, adalimumab-atto, adalimumab-bwwd, adalimumab-fkjp, adalimumab-ryvk) is 160 mg by subcutaneous injection on day 1 (given in one day or divided over 2 consecutive days), followed by 80 mg once 2 weeks later (on day 15). A maintenance dosage of 40 mg once every other week should be started on day 29 (2 weeks after the 80-mg dose).

Ulcerative Colitis

For the management of ulcerative colitis in adults, the recommended initial dosage of adalimumab or biosimilars (adalimumab-aacf, adalimumab-aaty, adalimumab-adaz, adalimumab-adbm, adalimumab-afzb, adalimumab-aqvh, adalimumab-atto, adalimumab-bwwd, adalimumab-fkjp, adalimumab-ryvk) is 160 mg by subcutaneous injection on day 1 (given in one day or divided over 2 consecutive days), followed by 80 mg once 2 weeks later (on day 15). A maintenance dosage of 40 mg once every other week should be started on day 29 (2 weeks after the 80-mg dose). If clinical remission is not achieved by 8 weeks (day 57), adalimumab or biosimilars should be discontinued.

Plaque Psoriasis

For the management of plaque psoriasis in adults, the recommended initial dosage of adalimumab or biosimilars (adalimumab-aacf, adalimumab-aaty, adalimumab-adaz, adalimumab-adbm, adalimumab-afzb, adalimumab-aqvh, adalimumab-atto, adalimumab-bwwd, adalimumab-fkjp, adalimumab-ryvk) is 80 mg by subcutaneous injection on day 1, followed by 40 mg once every other week starting 1 week after the initial dose. The use of adalimumab products beyond 1 year has not been evaluated in controlled clinical studies in patients with plaque psoriasis.

Hidradenitis Suppurativa

For the management of hidradenitis suppurativa in adults, the recommended initial dosage of adalimumab or biosimilars (adalimumab-aacf, adalimumab-aaty, adalimumab-adaz, adalimumab-adbm, adalimumab-afzb, adalimumab-aqvh, adalimumab-atto, adalimumab-bwwd, adalimumab-fkjp, adalimumab-ryvk) is 160 mg by subcutaneous injection on day 1 (given in one day or divided over 2 consecutive days), followed by 80 mg once 2 weeks later (on day 15). A maintenance dosage of 40 mg once every week or 80 mg once every other week should be started on day 29 (2 weeks after the 80-mg dose).

Uveitis

For the management of noninfectious uveitis in adults, the recommended dosage of adalimumab or biosimilars (adalimumab-aacf, adalimumab-aaty, adalimumab-adaz, adalimumab-adbm, adalimumab-afzb, adalimumab-aqvh, adalimumab-atto, adalimumab-bwwd, adalimumab-fkjp, adalimumab-ryvk) is 80 mg by subcutaneous injection on day 1, followed by 40 mg once every other week starting 1 week after the initial dose.

Pediatric Dosage

Juvenile Idiopathic Arthritis

For the management of polyarticular juvenile idiopathic arthritis in pediatric patients 2 years of age and older, the recommended dosage of adalimumab or biosimilars (adalimumab-aacf, adalimumab-aaty, adalimumab-adaz, adalimumab-adbm, adalimumab-afzb, adalimumab-aqvh, adalimumab-atto, adalimumab-bwwd, adalimumab-fkjp, adalimumab-ryvk) is 10 mg once every other week by subcutaneous injection in patients weighing 10 kg to less than 15 kg, 20 mg once every other week by subcutaneous injection in patients weighing 15 kg to less than 30 kg, and 40 mg once every other week by subcutaneous injection in patients weighing 30 kg or more. Adalimumab products have not been studied in patients with polyarticular juvenile idiopathic arthritis who are less than 2 years of age or who weigh less than 10 kg.

Crohn Disease

For the management of Crohn disease in pediatric patients 6 years of age and older who weigh 17 kg to less than 40 kg, the recommended initial dosage of adalimumab or biosimilars (adalimumab-aacf, adalimumab-aaty, adalimumab-adaz, adalimumab-adbm, adalimumab-afzb, adalimumab-aqvh, adalimumab-atto, adalimumab-bwwd, adalimumab-fkjp, adalimumab-ryvk) is 80 mg by subcutaneous injection on day 1, followed by 40 mg once 2 weeks later (on day 15). A

maintenance dosage of 20 mg once every other week should be started on day 29 (2 weeks after the 40-mg dose).

For the management of Crohn disease in pediatric patients 6 years of age or older who weigh 40 kg or more, the recommended initial dosage of adalimumab or biosimilars (adalimumab-aacf, adalimumab-aaty, adalimumab-adaz, adalimumab-adbm, adalimumab-afzb, adalimumab-aqvh, adalimumab-atto, adalimumab-bwwd, adalimumab-fkjp, adalimumab-ryvk) is 160 mg by subcutaneous injection on day 1 (given in one day or divided over 2 consecutive days), followed by 80 mg once 2 weeks later (on day 15). A maintenance dosage of 40 mg once every other week should be started on day 29 (2 weeks after the 80-mg dose).

Ulcerative Colitis

For the management of ulcerative colitis in pediatric patients 5 years of age or older who weigh 20 kg to less than 40 kg, the recommended initial dosage of adalimumab is 80 mg by subcutaneous injection on day 1, followed by 40 mg once on day 8 (1 week after the 80-mg dose) and 40 mg once on day 15 (1 week after the first 40-mg dose). A maintenance dosage of 40 mg once every other week or 20 mg once every week should be started on day 29 (2 weeks after the second 40-mg dose). For the management of ulcerative colitis in pediatric patients 5 years of age and older who weigh 40 kg or more, the recommended initial dosage of adalimumab is 160 mg by subcutaneous injection on day 1 (given in one day or divided over 2 consecutive days), followed by 80 mg once on day 8 (1 week after the 160-mg dose) and 80 mg once on day 15 (1 week after the first 80-mg dose). A maintenance dosage of 80 mg once every other week or 40 mg once every week should be started on day 29 (2 weeks after the second 80-mg dose). The recommended pediatric dosage should be continued in patients who turn 18 years of age and who are well-controlled on their adalimumab regimen.

Adalimumab biosimilars are not labeled for use in pediatric patients with ulcerative colitis.

Hidradenitis Suppurativa

For the management of hidradenitis suppurativa in adolescents 12 years of age or older who weigh 30 kg to less than 60 kg, the recommended dosage of adalimumab is 80 mg by subcutaneous injection on day 1, followed by 40 mg once on day 8, and then 40 mg once every other week thereafter.

For the management of hidradenitis suppurativa in adolescents 12 years of age or older who weigh 60 kg or more, the recommended initial dosage of adalimumab is 160 mg by subcutaneous injection on day 1 (given in one day or divided over 2 consecutive days), followed by 80 mg once 2 weeks later (on day 15). A dosage of 40 mg once every week or 80 mg once every other week should be started on day 29 (2 weeks after the 80-mg dose).

Adalimumab biosimilars are not labeled for use in pediatric patients with ulcerative colitis.

Uveitis

For the management of noninfectious uveitis in pediatric patients 2 years of age or older, the recommended dosage of adalimumab is 10 mg once every other week by subcutaneous injection in patients weighing 10 kg to less than 15 kg, 20 mg once every other week by subcutaneous injection in patients weighing 15 kg to less than 30 kg, and 40 mg once every other week by subcutaneous injection in patients weighing 30 kg or more. Adalimumab has not been studied in patients with noninfectious uveitis who are less than 2 years of age or who weigh less than 10 kg.

Adalimumab biosimilars are not labeled for use in pediatric patients with uveitis.

● Special Populations

Hepatic Impairment

The manufacturer makes no specific dosage recommendations for patients with hepatic impairment.

Renal Impairment

The manufacturer makes no specific dosage recommendations for patients with renal impairment.

Geriatric Patients

The manufacturer makes no specific dosage recommendations for geriatric patients.

CAUTIONS

● Contraindications
● None.

● Warnings/Precautions

Warnings

Serious Infections

A boxed warning about the risk of serious infections is included in the prescribing information for adalimumab. Patients receiving tumor necrosis factor (TNF) blocking agents, including adalimumab, are at increased risk of developing serious infections involving various organ systems and sites that may require hospitalization or result in death. Opportunistic infections caused by bacterial, mycobacterial, invasive fungal, viral, parasitic, or other opportunistic pathogens—including aspergillosis, blastomycosis, candidiasis, coccidioidomycosis, histoplasmosis, legionellosis, listeriosis, pneumocystosis, and tuberculosis—have been reported in patients receiving TNF blocking agents. Infections frequently have been disseminated rather than localized. Monitor patients closely during and after treatment with TNF blocking agents for the development of signs or symptoms of infection, including the possible development of tuberculosis in patients who tested negative for latent tuberculosis prior to initiating therapy. Most patients who developed serious infections were receiving concomitant therapy with immunosuppressive agents such as methotrexate or corticosteroids.

In controlled trials in adults with rheumatoid arthritis, psoriatic arthritis, ankylosing spondylitis, Crohn disease, ulcerative colitis, plaque psoriasis, noninfectious uveitis, or hidradenitis suppurativa, the rate of serious infection was 4.3 per 100 patient-years in adalimumab-treated patients and 2.9 per 100 patient-years in control patients. Serious infections included pneumonia, septic arthritis, prosthetic infection, postsurgical infection, erysipelas, cellulitis, diverticulitis, and pyelonephritis. Tuberculosis (frequently disseminated or extrapulmonary at clinical presentation), invasive fungal infections, and other opportunistic infections also have occurred in patients receiving adalimumab or other TNF blocking agents. Most of the cases of tuberculosis occurred within the first 8 months following initiation of adalimumab therapy; these cases may reflect recrudescence of latent tuberculosis infection. As of September 2011, the FDA had identified 103 reports of *Legionella* pneumonia associated with TNF blocking agents, including adalimumab. The cases occurred in patients 25–85 years of age, many of whom received concomitant therapy with immunosuppressive agents (e.g., corticosteroids and/or methotrexate); 17 deaths were reported. In 78% of the cases of *Legionella* pneumonia, the median duration of TNF blocker therapy prior to the onset of *Legionella* pneumonia was 10.4 months (range: less than 1 month to 73 months). As of September 2011, FDA also had identified 26 published reports of *Listeria* infections, including meningitis, bacteremia, endophthalmitis, and sepsis, in patients who received TNF blocking agents; 7 deaths were reported. Many of the *Listeria* infections occurred in patients who had received concomitant therapy with immunosuppressive agents. In addition, FDA identified fatal *Listeria* infections during a review of laboratory-confirmed infections that occurred in premarketing clinical studies and during postmarketing surveillance.

An increased incidence of serious infections also was observed in clinical studies in patients with rheumatoid arthritis when a TNF blocking agent was used concomitantly with anakinra (a human interleukin-1 receptor antagonist) or abatacept (a selective costimulation modulator). Concomitant use of adalimumab and other biologic disease-modifying antirheumatic drugs (DMARDs), including abatacept and anakinra, is not recommended.

Do not initiate adalimumab therapy in patients with active infections, including localized infections. Patients >65 years of age, patients with comorbid conditions, and/or patients receiving concomitant therapy with immunosuppressive agents such as corticosteroids or methotrexate may be at increased risk of infection. Consider potential risks and benefits of the drug prior to initiating therapy in patients with a history of chronic, recurring, or opportunistic infections; patients with underlying conditions that may predispose them to infections; and patients who have been exposed to tuberculosis or who have resided or traveled in regions where tuberculosis or mycoses such as histoplasmosis, coccidioidomycosis, and blastomycosis are endemic. Any patient who develops a new infection while receiving adalimumab should undergo a thorough diagnostic evaluation

(appropriate for an immunocompromised patient); appropriate anti-infective therapy should be initiated, and the patient should be closely monitored. Discontinue the drug in patients who develop serious infection or sepsis.

Because tuberculosis has been reported in patients receiving adalimumab, evaluate all patients for active or latent tuberculosis and for the presence of risk factors for tuberculosis prior to and periodically during therapy with the drug. When indicated, initiate an appropriate antimycobacterial regimen for the treatment of latent tuberculosis infection prior to adalimumab therapy. Antimycobacterial treatment lowers the risk of latent tuberculosis infection progressing to active disease (i.e., reactivation) in patients receiving adalimumab. Consider antimycobacterial therapy prior to initiation of adalimumab in individuals with a history of latent or active tuberculosis in whom an adequate course of antimycobacterial treatment cannot be confirmed and in individuals with a negative tuberculin skin test who have risk factors for tuberculosis. Consult a tuberculosis specialist when deciding whether to initiate antimycobacterial therapy. Active tuberculosis has developed in adalimumab-treated patients who previously received antimycobacterial therapy for latent or active tuberculosis. Monitor patients receiving adalimumab, including individuals with a negative tuberculin skin test, for signs and symptoms of active tuberculosis. Strongly consider a diagnosis of tuberculosis in patients who develop new infections while receiving adalimumab, especially in those who previously have traveled to countries where tuberculosis is highly prevalent or who have been in close contact with an individual with active tuberculosis.

If patients develop a serious systemic illness and they reside or travel in regions where mycoses are endemic, consider invasive fungal infection in the differential diagnosis. Antigen and antibody testing for histoplasmosis may be negative in some patients with active infection. Consider empiric antifungal therapy in patients at risk of invasive fungal infections who develop severe systemic illness. Whenever feasible, consider consultation with a specialist in the diagnosis and management of invasive fungal infections.

Malignancies

A boxed warning about the risk of malignancy is included in the prescribing information for adalimumab. Malignancies, some fatal, have been reported in children, adolescents, and young adults who received treatment with TNF blocking agents beginning when they were 18 years of age or younger. These cases were reported postmarketing and were derived from various sources, including registries and spontaneous postmarketing reports. Approximately half of the reported cases were lymphomas, including Hodgkin disease and non-Hodgkin lymphoma. The other cases represented a variety of malignancies, including rare malignancies that are usually associated with immunosuppression and malignancies that are not usually observed in children and adolescents. The malignancies occurred after a median of 30 months (range: 1–84 months) following the first dose of therapy with TNF blocking agents. Most patients were also receiving other immunosuppressive drugs.

Hepatosplenic T-cell lymphoma, a rare, aggressive, usually fatal type of T-cell lymphoma, has been reported during postmarketing experience mainly in adolescents and young adults with Crohn disease or ulcerative colitis who received treatment with TNF blocking agents and/or thiopurine analogs (mercaptopurine or azathioprine). Most of the reported cases of hepatosplenic T-cell lymphoma occurred in patients who had received a combination of immunosuppressive agents, including TNF blocking agents and thiopurine analogs (azathioprine or mercaptopurine). It is not clear whether the occurrence of hepatosplenic T-cell lymphoma was related to use of a TNF blocking agent or use of a TNF blocking agent in conjunction with other immunosuppressive agents. In some cases, potential confounding factors could not be excluded because complete medical histories were not available. As of December 31, 2010, FDA had identified 7 cases of hepatosplenic T-cell lymphoma in patients with Crohn disease, ulcerative colitis, or rheumatoid arthritis who had received adalimumab (2 cases) or both adalimumab and infliximab (5 cases); in 4 of these cases, a thiopurine analog (mercaptopurine or azathioprine) was used concomitantly. These 7 cases of hepatosplenic T-cell lymphoma occurred in patients 21–70 years of age following adalimumab therapy for periods ranging from 3 doses up to 1 year of therapy; most of the patients were men, and 5 of the 7 cases were fatal. Since patients with certain conditions (e.g., rheumatoid arthritis, Crohn disease, ankylosing spondylitis, psoriatic arthritis, plaque psoriasis) may be at increased risk for lymphoma, it may be difficult to measure the added risk of treatment with TNF blocking agents, azathioprine, and/or mercaptopurine.

In clinical studies, lymphoma has been observed more frequently in patients receiving agents that block TNF than in control patients. In controlled and uncontrolled studies evaluating adalimumab in adults with rheumatoid arthritis, psoriatic arthritis, ankylosing spondylitis, Crohn disease, ulcerative colitis, plaque psoriasis, noninfectious uveitis, or hidradenitis suppurativa, the rate of lymphoma in adalimumab-treated patients was approximately 0.11 per 100 patient-years. This rate is approximately threefold higher than the rate expected in the general US population. Patients with rheumatoid arthritis or other chronic inflammatory diseases, especially those with highly active disease and/or chronic exposure to immunosuppressive therapies, may be at increased risk of lymphoma, even in the absence of TNF blocking agent therapy.

In addition to lymphoma, various other malignancies including breast cancer, colorectal cancer, lung cancer, melanoma, nonmelanoma skin cancer, and prostate cancer have been reported in patients receiving adalimumab in clinical trials. In controlled studies evaluating adalimumab in adults with rheumatoid arthritis, psoriatic arthritis, ankylosing spondylitis, Crohn disease, ulcerative colitis, plaque psoriasis, noninfectious uveitis, or hidradenitis suppurativa, the rate of malignancies other than nonmelanoma skin cancer was 0.7 per 100 patient-years in adalimumab-treated patients and in control patients; the rate of nonmelanoma skin cancer was 0.8 per 100 patient-years in adalimumab-treated patients and 0.2 per 100 patient-years in control patients.

In controlled studies of other TNF blocking agents in adults at increased risk of malignancies (e.g., patients with chronic obstructive pulmonary disease [COPD] who have a substantial history of smoking, patients with Wegener's granulomatosis receiving concomitant cyclophosphamide), a greater proportion of malignancies occurred in patients receiving the TNF blocking agent compared with control patients.

Cases of acute and chronic leukemia have been reported during postmarketing surveillance of TNF blocking agents used in the management of rheumatoid arthritis and other conditions. Patients with rheumatoid arthritis may be at increased risk of leukemia, independent of any treatment with TNF blocking agents.

Consider the possibility of and monitor for the occurrence of malignancies during and following treatment with TNF blocking agents. Consider the risks and benefits of TNF blocking agents prior to initiating therapy in patients with a known malignancy (other than a successfully treated nonmelanoma skin cancer) or when considering whether to continue TNF blocking agent therapy in patients who develop a malignancy. Because therapy with TNF blocking agents and/or thiopurine analogs (azathioprine or mercaptopurine) may increase the risk of malignancies, including hepatosplenic T-cell lymphoma, the risks and benefits of these agents should be carefully considered, especially in adolescents and young adults and especially in the treatment of Crohn disease or ulcerative colitis. All patients, but particularly those with a history of prior prolonged immunosuppressive therapy or a history of psoralen and UVA light (PUVA) therapy, should be examined for the presence of nonmelanoma skin cancer prior to and during therapy with adalimumab.

Sensitivity Reactions
Hypersensitivity Reactions

Anaphylaxis, angioedema, and other allergic reactions (e.g., allergic rash, anaphylactoid reactions, fixed drug reaction, nonspecified drug reaction, urticaria) have occurred in patients receiving adalimumab. If a serious allergic reaction or anaphylaxis occurs, discontinue adalimumab immediately and initiate appropriate therapy.

Latex Sensitivity

In certain packaging configurations of reference product adalimumab (injection pens and prefilled syringes containing 40 mg in 0.8 mL), the needle cover may contain dry natural rubber (latex) and should not be handled by individuals sensitive to latex. The needle caps of adalimumab-adbm (Cyltezo®) injection pens and prefilled syringes also contain natural rubber latex.

Other Warnings/Precautions
Hepatitis B Virus Reactivation

Use of TNF blocking agents, including adalimumab, may increase the risk of reactivation of hepatitis B virus (HBV) infection in patients who are chronic carriers of this virus (i.e., hepatitis B surface antigen-positive [HBsAg-positive]). HBV

reactivation has resulted in death in a few individuals receiving TNF blocking agent therapy. Most patients experiencing HBV reactivation were receiving concomitant therapy with other immunosuppressive agents; use of multiple immunosuppressive agents may have contributed to HBV reactivation.

Patients at risk for HBV infection should be screened before initiation of adalimumab therapy. Chronic carriers of HBV should be appropriately evaluated and monitored prior to the initiation of therapy, during treatment, and for up to several months following therapy with adalimumab. Safety and efficacy of antiviral therapy for prevention of viral reactivation in HBV carriers receiving a TNF blocking agent have not been established. Discontinue adalimumab if HBV reactivation occurs and initiate appropriate treatment, including antiviral therapy. It has not been established whether adalimumab can be safely readministered once control of the reactivated HBV infection has been achieved; caution is advised if adalimumab therapy is resumed in such a situation.

Neurologic Reactions

New onset or exacerbation of clinical manifestations and/or radiographic evidence of central or peripheral nervous system demyelinating disorders (e.g., multiple sclerosis, optic neuritis, Guillain-Barré syndrome) has been reported rarely in patients receiving adalimumab or other TNF blocking agents. Clinicians should exercise caution when considering adalimumab therapy in patients with preexisting or recent-onset central or peripheral nervous system demyelinating disorders. Consider discontinuance of adalimumab if any such disorders develop during therapy with the drug. Intermediate uveitis is known to be associated with central demyelinating disorders.

Hematologic Reactions

Pancytopenia including aplastic anemia has been reported rarely in patients receiving agents that block TNF. Adverse hematologic effects, including leukopenia and thrombocytopenia, have occurred rarely in adalimumab-treated patients. Whether these hematologic abnormalities are directly attributable to adalimumab remains to be determined. If substantial hematologic abnormalities occur, consider discontinuance of adalimumab.

Heart Failure

There have been reports of worsening heart failure and new-onset heart failure in patients receiving agents that block TNF, including adalimumab. While adalimumab has not been formally studied in patients with heart failure, other agents that block TNF (i.e., etanercept, infliximab) have been associated with adverse cardiovascular effects in patients with heart failure. If adalimumab is used in patients with heart failure, use caution and carefully monitor the patient.

Autoimmunity

Adalimumab therapy may result in the formation of autoimmune antibodies. In controlled clinical trials in patients with rheumatoid arthritis, 12% of those receiving adalimumab developed new positive antinuclear antibodies (ANA) compared with 7% of those receiving placebo. A lupus-like syndrome has occurred in at least 2 patients receiving adalimumab; symptoms resolved following discontinuance of the drug. If a patient develops manifestations suggestive of a lupus-like syndrome, discontinue adalimumab.

Immunogenicity

Patients receiving adalimumab may develop antibodies to the drug. In clinical studies that evaluated adalimumab in patients with rheumatoid arthritis, approximately 5% of adalimumab-treated patients who were tested for the presence of antibodies at multiple time points over 6–12 months developed low-titer neutralizing antibodies to the drug at least once during therapy. The incidence of antibody formation was lower in patients receiving adalimumab in conjunction with methotrexate than in patients receiving adalimumab monotherapy (1 versus 12%). The incidence of antibody formation may be lower in patients receiving adalimumab (as monotherapy) every week compared with patients receiving the drug every other week. In addition, clinical response (ACR 20) in patients receiving adalimumab (as monotherapy) every other week was achieved in fewer antibody-positive patients than antibody-negative patients. A relationship between the development of antibodies to adalimumab and the incidence of adverse effects has not been observed. The long-term immunogenicity of adalimumab remains to be determined.

In a clinical study in pediatric patients 4–17 years of age receiving adalimumab for the treatment of juvenile idiopathic arthritis, approximately 16% of adalimumab-treated patients developed neutralizing antibodies to the drug at least once during therapy. The incidence of antibody formation was lower in patients receiving adalimumab in conjunction with methotrexate than in patients receiving adalimumab monotherapy (6 versus 26%). Antibodies to the drug were detected in 1 of 15 patients with juvenile idiopathic arthritis who were 2 years to less than 4 years of age or who were 4 years of age or older and weighed less than 15 kg.

In clinical studies that evaluated adalimumab in patients with ankylosing spondylitis, approximately 9% of adalimumab-treated patients developed neutralizing antibodies to the drug at least once during therapy. In clinical studies that evaluated adalimumab in patients with psoriatic arthritis, approximately 13% of adalimumab-treated patients developed neutralizing antibodies to the drug at least once during therapy. The incidence of antibody formation in patients with psoriatic arthritis receiving adalimumab in conjunction with methotrexate was higher than the incidence reported in patients with rheumatoid arthritis receiving adalimumab in conjunction with methotrexate (7 versus 1%).

The incidence of antibody formation to adalimumab was 3% in adults and pediatric patients receiving the drug for Crohn disease and pediatric patients receiving the drug for ulcerative colitis, 5% in adults receiving adalimumab for ulcerative colitis or noninfectious uveitis, 7% in patients receiving adalimumab for hidradenitis suppurativa, and 8% in patients receiving adalimumab monotherapy for plaque psoriasis. However, because of assay limitations, antibodies to adalimumab could be detected only when serum adalimumab concentrations were less than 2 mcg/mL; the incidence of antibody formation in patients with serum adalimumab concentrations of less than 2 mcg/mL (approximately 23–40% of those who were studied) was 21% in those with psoriasis, adult ulcerative colitis, or noninfectious uveitis, 13% in pediatric patients with ulcerative colitis, 10% in pediatric patients with Crohn disease, and 8% in adults with Crohn disease. In patients with hidradenitis suppurativa who interrupted adalimumab therapy and had a reduction in serum concentrations of the drug to less than 2 mcg/mL (approximately 22% of those studied), the incidence of antibody formation was 28%. When adalimumab monotherapy for plaque psoriasis was withdrawn and subsequently reinitiated, the incidence of antibody formation following retreatment was similar to that observed prior to drug withdrawal.

When testing was performed using an assay that could detect antibodies to adalimumab in all patients regardless of serum drug concentration, titers were measured in 40% of adults receiving adalimumab for noninfectious uveitis, 33% of pediatric patients receiving adalimumab for ulcerative colitis, and 61% of those receiving the drug for hidradenitis suppurativa. No association between antibody development and safety or efficacy of adalimumab was observed in adults with noninfectious uveitis. In pediatric patients with ulcerative colitis, development of antibodies to adalimumab was associated with reduced serum adalimumab concentrations, but no association between antibody development and safety was observed; the association between antibody development and efficacy was not assessed due to the limited number of patients in each treatment group. In patients with hidradenitis suppurativa, development of antibodies to adalimumab was associated with reduced serum adalimumab concentrations, but no apparent association between antibody development and safety was observed; the magnitude of the reduction in adalimumab concentration generally was greater with increasing antibody titers.

Immunization

Avoid live vaccines during therapy with adalimumab. Information is not available regarding whether adalimumab would affect the rate of secondary transmission of infection following administration of a live vaccine. Patients receiving adalimumab may receive inactivated vaccines. When use of adalimumab is being considered for pediatric patients, the vaccination status of the child should be reviewed and all age-appropriate vaccines included in current immunization guidelines should be administered. Neonates and infants who were exposed to adalimumab in utero may have impaired immune responses. Consider the risks and benefits of administering live vaccines to infants who were exposed to adalimumab in utero, since the safety of live vaccines in these infants is unknown.

Specific Populations

Pregnancy

Available studies of adalimumab use during pregnancy do not reliably establish an association between the drug and major birth defects. Results of a prospective,

controlled, observational, pregnancy registry cohort study of pregnancy outcomes in adalimumab-treated females with rheumatoid arthritis or Crohn disease indicated that 10% of females in the adalimumab-exposed cohort (8.7% of those with rheumatoid arthritis, 10.5% of those with Crohn disease) delivered a live-born infant with a major birth defect, compared with 7.5% of females with rheumatoid arthritis or Crohn disease who had not been exposed to the drug (6.8% of those with rheumatoid arthritis, 9.4% of those with Crohn disease); however, no pattern of major birth defects was observed, and differences in the cohorts may have affected the observed occurrence rates. All females in the adalimumab-exposed cohort were exposed to the drug for some period of time during the first trimester of pregnancy; 65% were exposed to the drug in all 3 trimesters. The study utilized data from the Organization of Teratology Information Specialists (OTIS)/MotherToBaby pregnancy registry from 2004–2016 and included data for 602 pregnant females, including 257 females with rheumatoid arthritis or Crohn disease who had been exposed to adalimumab during pregnancy, 120 disease-matched unexposed females, and 225 healthy unexposed females. Methodologic limitations of the registry study (e.g., small sample size, voluntary nature of the study, nonrandomized design) preclude drawing definitive conclusions regarding the risk of major birth defects.

In an embryofetal-perinatal development study in cynomolgus monkeys, no fetal harm or malformations were observed at adalimumab exposure levels of up to approximately 373 times the exposure achieved at the maximum recommended human dosage (MRHD) for use without methotrexate.

Data suggest that increased disease activity in females with rheumatoid arthritis or inflammatory bowel disease is associated with an increased risk of adverse pregnancy outcomes (e.g., preterm delivery, low birth weight, small size for gestational age at birth).

As pregnancy progresses, monoclonal antibodies are increasingly transported across the placenta, with the largest amount transferred during the third trimester. Adalimumab is actively transferred across the placenta during the third trimester of pregnancy. Results of a study in 10 pregnant females receiving adalimumab for treatment of inflammatory bowel disease (last dose administered 1–56 days prior to delivery) suggest that adalimumab may be detectable in the serum of infants exposed to the drug in utero for at least 3 months following birth. Adalimumab concentrations in cord blood were higher than maternal serum concentrations in 9 women in this study, and one infant had detectable serum concentrations of the drug measured through 11 weeks of age.

Adalimumab may affect immune response in infants exposed to the drug in utero. Consider the risks and benefits of administering live vaccines to such infants, since the safety of live vaccines in infants exposed to the drug in utero is unknown.

Lactation

Limited data indicate that small amounts of adalimumab distribute into human milk (0.1–1% of maternal serum concentrations) and suggest that systemic exposure to adalimumab in nursing infants is likely to be low since the drug is a large molecule and is degraded in the GI tract. However, the effects of local exposure in the GI tract are unknown. There are no reports of adverse effects of adalimumab on breast-fed infants or effects of the drug on milk production.

Consider the developmental and health benefits of breast-feeding along with the mother's clinical need for adalimumab and any potential adverse effects on the breast-fed child from the drug or underlying maternal condition.

Pediatric Use

Safety and efficacy of adalimumab for uses other than polyarticular juvenile idiopathic arthritis, Crohn disease, ulcerative colitis, and noninfectious uveitis have not been established in pediatric patients. Use of adalimumab for the management of hidradenitis suppurativa in adolescents is supported by clinical trials in adults. For marketing exclusivity reasons, adalimumab biosimilars are not labeled for use in pediatric patients with ulcerative colitis, hidradenitis suppurativa, or noninfectious uveitis.

Use of adalimumab for the management of polyarticular juvenile idiopathic arthritis in pediatric patients 2 years of age or older is supported by results of a safety and efficacy study in pediatric patients 4–17 years of age and additional data from a study in children 2 to <4 years of age indicating that the safety profile in this age group is similar to that in pediatric patients 4–17 years of age. In these studies, the types and frequencies of adverse effects generally were similar to those observed in adults. Safety and efficacy of adalimumab for the management of polyarticular juvenile idiopathic arthritis have not been established in pediatric patients less than 2 years of age or in those who weigh less than 10 kg.

Use of adalimumab for the management of Crohn disease in pediatric patients 6 years of age or older is supported by evidence from adequate and well-controlled studies in adults and additional data from a randomized, double-blind, 52-week clinical study of 2 dosage levels of the drug in 192 pediatric patients 6–17 years of age with moderately to severely active Crohn disease. Safety and efficacy for the management of Crohn disease have not been established in pediatric patients less than 6 years of age.

Use of adalimumab for the management of ulcerative colitis in pediatric patients 5 years of age or older is supported by evidence from adequate and well-controlled studies in adults and additional data from a randomized, double-blind, 52-week clinical study of 2 dosage levels of the drug in 93 pediatric patients 5–17 years of age with moderately to severely active ulcerative colitis. The recommended dosage of adalimumab in pediatric patients with ulcerative colitis is based on modeled dose/exposure-efficacy relationships and pharmacokinetic data; clinically relevant differences between the studied higher dosage administered in the clinical trial and the recommended dosage are not anticipated. Efficacy of adalimumab has not been established in patients who have lost response or were intolerant to TNF blocking agents. Safety and efficacy for the management of ulcerative colitis have not been established in pediatric patients less than 5 years of age.

Use of adalimumab for the management of noninfectious uveitis in pediatric patients 2 years of age or older is supported by evidence from adequate and well-controlled studies in adults and a randomized, controlled study in 90 pediatric patients. Safety and efficacy for the management of noninfectious uveitis have not been established in pediatric patients less than 2 years of age.

Use of adalimumab for the management of hidradenitis suppurativa in pediatric patients 12 years of age or older is supported by evidence from adequate and well-controlled studies in adults. The course of hidradenitis suppurativa in adults and adolescents is sufficiently similar to allow extrapolation of data from adults to adolescents. Population pharmacokinetic modeling and simulation data suggest that weight-based dosing in pediatric patients 12 years of age or older will provide exposure levels that are generally similar to those achieved in adults. Safety and efficacy for the management of hidradenitis suppurativa have not been established in pediatric patients less than 12 years of age.

When use of adalimumab is being considered for pediatric patients, review the vaccination status of the child and administer all age-appropriate vaccines included in current immunization guidelines.

Malignancies, some fatal, have been reported in children and adolescents who received treatment with TNF blocking agents, including adalimumab.

Neonates and infants who were exposed to adalimumab in utero may have impaired immune responses. Data from 8 infants exposed to adalimumab in utero suggest that the drug crosses the placenta; the clinical importance of elevated adalimumab concentrations in infants is unknown. Consider the risks and benefits of administering live vaccines to infants who were exposed to adalimumab in utero, since the safety of live vaccines in these infants is unknown.

Geriatric Use

No substantial differences in efficacy have been observed in geriatric patients with rheumatoid arthritis relative to younger adults. The incidence of serious infection and malignancy in adalimumab-treated patients greater than 65 years of age is higher than the incidence in younger adults receiving the drug. Because the overall incidence of infection and malignancy is higher in the geriatric population in general than in younger adults, consider the risks and benefits of adalimumab in geriatric patients and closely monitor for the development of infection or malignancy if adalimumab is used.

Hepatic Impairment

No pharmacokinetic data are available in patients with hepatic impairment.

Renal Impairment

No pharmacokinetic data are available in patients with renal impairment.

● Common Adverse Effects

Common adverse effects reported in 10% or more of patients receiving adalimumab include infections (e.g., upper respiratory, sinusitis), injection site reactions, headache, and rash.

DRUG INTERACTIONS

● Drugs Metabolized by Hepatic Microsomal Enzymes

Because increased levels of cytokines (e.g., tumor necrosis factor [TNF; TNF-α]) during chronic inflammation may suppress the formation of cytochrome P-450 (CYP) isoenzymes, it is possible that a drug that antagonizes cytokine activity, such as adalimumab, could normalize the formation of CYP enzymes. Following initiation or discontinuance of adalimumab therapy, patients receiving certain drugs metabolized by CYP isoenzymes (i.e., those with a low therapeutic index [e.g., cyclosporine, theophylline, warfarin]) should be monitored for therapeutic effect and/or changes in serum concentrations, and dosages of these drugs may be adjusted as needed.

● Biologic Antirheumatic Agents

Concomitant use of adalimumab and other biologic disease-modifying antirheumatic drugs (DMARDs) is not recommended.

Abatacept

When abatacept and a TNF blocking agent were used concomitantly in patients with rheumatoid arthritis, an increased incidence of infection and serious infection was observed, with no substantial improvement in efficacy. Concomitant use of adalimumab and abatacept is not recommended.

Anakinra

When anakinra (a human interleukin-1 receptor antagonist) and etanercept (another TNF blocking agent) were used concomitantly in patients with rheumatoid arthritis, an increased incidence of serious infection and neutropenia was observed, with no substantial improvement in efficacy over that observed with etanercept alone. Concomitant use of adalimumab and anakinra is not recommended.

Rituximab

An increased risk of serious infection has been observed in patients with rheumatoid arthritis who received rituximab and subsequently received therapy with a TNF blocking agent.

Other TNF Blocking Agents

Concomitant use of adalimumab and other TNF blocking agents is not recommended.

Other Biologic Antirheumatic Agents

The manufacturer states that insufficient data are available regarding the concomitant use of adalimumab and other biologic agents used in the management of rheumatoid arthritis, psoriatic arthritis, ankylosing spondylitis, Crohn disease, ulcerative colitis, plaque psoriasis, noninfectious uveitis, or hidradenitis suppurativa.

● Methotrexate

Methotrexate decreased clearance of adalimumab after single or multiple doses by 29 or 44%, respectively, in patients with rheumatoid arthritis; dosage adjustment is not necessary.

● Vaccines

Live vaccines should not be administered to patients receiving adalimumab. Information is not available regarding whether adalimumab would affect the rate of secondary transmission of infection following administration of a live vaccine.

Patients receiving adalimumab may receive inactivated vaccines. Antibody response to inactivated vaccines (i.e., pneumococcal polysaccharide vaccine, influenza virus vaccine inactivated) has been investigated in patients receiving adalimumab. In patients with rheumatoid arthritis, no difference in antibody response to pneumococcal polysaccharide vaccine was detected between patients receiving adalimumab and patients receiving placebo. Adalimumab-treated rheumatoid arthritis patients receiving influenza virus vaccine inactivated have developed protective antibody titers; however, titers to influenza antigens were lower in patients receiving adalimumab than in placebo-treated patients.

DESCRIPTION

Adalimumab, a human monoclonal antibody specific for human tumor necrosis factor (TNF; TNF-α), is a biologic response modifier. Adalimumab is produced by recombinant DNA technology in a mammalian cell expression system and is purified by a process that includes specific viral inactivation and removal steps.

Adalimumab has high specificity and affinity for TNF (TNF-α); adalimumab does not bind to or inactivate lymphotoxin α (TNF-β). Adalimumab binds to TNF before TNF can interact with the p55 and p75 cell surface tumor necrosis factor receptors (TNFRs). By preventing the binding of TNF to cell surface TNFRs, adalimumab blocks the biologic activity of TNF. In vitro, adalimumab lyses surface TNF-expressing cells in the presence of complement.

TNF, a naturally occurring cytokine, has a broad spectrum of biologic activities; TNF is involved in normal inflammatory and immune responses and also plays a role in a number of autoimmune and inflammatory diseases, including rheumatoid arthritis, juvenile idiopathic arthritis, psoriatic arthritis, and ankylosing spondylitis. While the causes of rheumatoid arthritis have not been fully elucidated, increased concentrations of TNF in the synovial fluid of rheumatoid arthritis patients play a critical role in the progression of inflammatory synovitis and articular matrix degradation in these patients. TNF promotes the synthesis of other proinflammatory cytokines, stimulates endothelial cells to express adhesion molecules that attract leukocytes into affected joints, accelerates the production of metalloproteinases, and inhibits the synthesis of cartilage proteoglycans. Increased concentrations of TNF also are found in psoriatic plaques. Adalimumab treatment may reduce epidermal thickness and infiltration of inflammatory cells in plaque psoriasis. Elevated levels of proinflammatory cytokines, including TNF, also have been observed in hidradenitis suppurativa lesions and in aqueous humor in patients with noninfectious uveitis. Adalimumab modulates responses that are induced or regulated by TNF, including expression of adhesion molecules, serum concentrations of matrix metalloproteinase, and serum concentrations of cytokines.

The bioavailability of subcutaneous adalimumab is approximately 64%, with peak serum concentrations achieved at 131 hours. Adalimumab has been detected in synovial fluid. The elimination route for adalimumab has not been determined. The half-life of adalimumab is approximately 2 weeks, but may range from 10–20 days. Clearance of adalimumab is increased among patients with adalimumab antibodies and decreased among patients over 40 years of age.

ADVICE TO PATIENTS

- Advise patients to read the manufacturer's patient information (medication guide) prior to initiation of therapy and each time the prescription is refilled.

- Instruct patients and/or caregivers regarding proper dosage and administration of adalimumab, including the use of aseptic technique, and proper disposal of needles, syringes, and used pens if it is determined that the patient and/or caregiver is competent to safely administer the drug.

- Advise patients that if a dose is missed, the missed dose should be administered as soon as it is remembered and then the regular dosing schedule should be resumed.

- Increased susceptibility to infection. Advise patients to seek immediate medical attention if signs and symptoms suggestive of infection (e.g., fever; fatigue; cough; warm, red, or painful skin; sores on the body; muscle aches; diarrhea; stomach pain; shortness of breath; weight loss; burning on urination; urinary frequency) develop.

- Risk of lymphoma, including hepatosplenic T-cell lymphoma, leukemia, or other malignancies with use of TNF blocking agents. Counsel patients about the risk of malignancy with adalimumab. Advise patients to inform clinicians if signs and symptoms of malignancies (e.g., unexplained weight loss; abdominal pain; persistent fever; night sweats; hepatomegaly or splenomegaly) occur.

- Advise patients to inform clinicians of any new or worsening medical conditions (e.g., neurologic conditions, heart failure, autoimmune disorders, psoriasis, cytopenias). Advise patients to report symptoms suggestive of a cytopenia (e.g., bruising, bleeding, persistent fever).

- Advise patients to alert their clinician if allergy to latex exists. Advise latex-sensitive patients that the needle cover or cap included in adalimumab-adbm (Cyltezo®) and certain packaging configurations of reference product adalimumab (injection pens and prefilled syringes containing 40 mg in 0.8 mL) may contain natural rubber latex.

- Advise patients to promptly contact a clinician if manifestations of an allergic reaction (e.g., urticaria, facial swelling, difficulty breathing) occur.

- Advise patients to take the drug as prescribed and to not discontinue therapy without first consulting with a clinician.

- Advise females to inform their clinicians if they are or plan to become pregnant or plan to breast-feed.

- Advise patients to inform their clinicians of existing or contemplated concomitant therapy, including prescription and OTC drugs, as well as any concomitant illnesses or any history of cancer, tuberculosis, hepatitis B virus (HBV) infection, or other chronic or recurring infections.

- Inform patients of other important precautionary information.

PREPARATIONS

Excipients in commercially available drug preparations may have clinically important effects in some individuals; consult specific product labeling for details.

Adalimumab

Parenteral

Injection, for subcutaneous use	10 mg/0.1 mL	Humira® (available as disposable prefilled syringes), AbbVie
	20 mg/0.2 mL	Humira® (available as disposable prefilled syringes), AbbVie
	40 mg/0.4 mL	Humira® (available as disposable prefilled syringes and prefilled injection pens), AbbVie
	40 mg/0.8 mL	Humira® (available as disposable prefilled syringes and prefilled injection pens), AbbVie
	80 mg/0.8 mL	Humira® (available as disposable prefilled syringes and prefilled injection pens), AbbVie

Adalimumab-aacf (biosimilar)

Parenteral

Injection, for subcutaneous use	40 mg/0.8 mL	Idacio® (available as disposable prefilled syringes, prefilled injection pens, and vial kit for institutional use only), Fresenius Kabi

Adalimumab-aaty (biosimilar)

Parenteral

Injection, for subcutaneous use	20 mg/0.2 mL	Yuflyma® (available as prefilled syringe), Celltrion
	40 mg/0.4 mL	Yuflyma® (available as disposable prefilled syringe, prefilled syringe with safety guard, and prefilled autoinjectors), Celltrion
	80 mg/0.8 mL	Yuflyma® (available as disposable prefilled syringe, prefilled syringe with safety guard, and prefilled autoinjectors), Celltrion

Adalimumab-adaz (biosimilar)

Parenteral

Injection, for subcutaneous use	10 mg/0.1 mL	Hyrimoz® (available as disposable prefilled syringes), Sandoz
	20 mg/0.2 mL	Hyrimoz® (available as disposable prefilled syringes), Sandoz
	40 mg/0.4 mL	Hyrimoz® (available as disposable prefilled syringes and prefilled injection pens), Sandoz
	80 mg/0.8 mL	Hyrimoz® (available as disposable prefilled syringes and prefilled injection pens), Sandoz

Adalimumab-adbm (biosimilar)

Parenteral

Injection, for subcutaneous use	10 mg/0.2 mL	Cyltezo® (available as prefilled glass syringes), Boehringer Ingelheim
	20 mg/0.4 mL	Cyltezo® (available as prefilled glass syringes), Boehringer Ingelheim
	40 mg/0.4 mL	Cyltezo® (available as prefilled glass syringes and prefilled injection pens), Boehringer Ingelheim
	40 mg/0.8 mL	Cyltezo® (available as prefilled glass syringes and prefilled injection pens), Boehringer Ingelheim

Adalimumab-afzb (biosimilar)

Parenteral

Injection, for subcutaneous use	10 mg/0.2 mL	Abrilada® (available as disposable prefilled syringes), Pfizer
	20 mg/0.4 mL	Abrilada® (available as disposable prefilled syringes), Pfizer
	40 mg/0.8 mL	Abrilada® (available as disposable prefilled syringes, prefilled injection pens, and vial for institutional use only), Pfizer

Adalimumab-aqvh (biosimilar)

Parenteral

Injection, for subcutaneous use	40 mg/0.8 mL	Yusimry® (available as disposable prefilled injection pens), Coherus BioSciences

Adalimumab-atto (biosimilar)

Parenteral

Injection, for subcutaneous use	10 mg/0.2 mL	Amjevita® (available as disposable prefilled syringes), Amgen
	20 mg/0.2 mL	Amjevita® (available as disposable prefilled syringes), Amgen
	20 mg/0.4 mL	Amjevita® (available as disposable prefilled syringes), Amgen
	40 mg/0.4 mL	Amjevita® (available as disposable prefilled syringes and prefilled autoinjectors), Amgen
	40 mg/0.8 mL	Amjevita® (available as disposable prefilled syringes and prefilled autoinjectors), Amgen
	80 mg/0.8 mL	Amjevita® (available as disposable prefilled syringes and prefilled autoinjectors), Amgen

Adalimumab-bwwd (biosimilar)

Parenteral

Injection, for subcutaneous use	40 mg/0.4 mL	Hadlima® (available as disposable prefilled syringes and prefilled autoinjectors), Organon
	40 mg/0.8 mL	Hadlima® (available as disposable prefilled syringes, prefilled autoinjectors, and single-dose vial for institutional use only), Organon

Adalimumab-fkjp (biosimilar)

Parenteral

Injection, for subcutaneous use	20 mg/0.4 mL	Hulio® (available as disposable prefilled syringes), Biocon Biologics
	40 mg/0.8 mL	Hulio® (available as disposable prefilled syringes and prefilled injection pens), Biocon Biologics

Adalimumab-ryvk (biosimilar)

Parenteral

Injection, for subcutaneous use	20 mg/0.2 mL	Simlandi® (available as a single-dose prefilled syringe), Alvotech USA Inc.
	40 mg/0.4 mL	Simlandi® (available as a single-dose autoinjector and prefilled syringe), Alvotech USA Inc.
	80 mg/0.8 mL	Simlandi® (available as a single-dose prefilled syringe), Alvotech USA Inc.

† Use is not currently included in the labeling approved by the US Food and Drug Administration.

Selected Revisions November 10, 2024, © Copyright, September 1, 2003, American Society of Health-System Pharmacists, Inc.

Certolizumab Pegol

90:24.16.92 • TUMOR NECROSIS FACTOR INHIBITORS, MISCELLANEOUS

■ Certolizumab pegol, a pegylated recombinant humanized Fab' fragment of a monoclonal antibody, is a tumor necrosis factor (TNF) inhibitor that is a biologic disease-modifying antirheumatic drug (DMARD).

USES

● Crohn Disease

Certolizumab pegol is used to reduce the signs and symptoms of Crohn disease and to maintain clinical response in adults with moderately to severely active disease who have had an inadequate response to conventional therapies. Safety and efficacy of certolizumab pegol for this use are based principally on the results of 2 randomized controlled trials, with additional data from a long-term extension study. Guidelines generally support the use of tumor necrosis factor (TNF; TNF-α) blocking agents, including certolizumab pegol, for use as induction and maintenance therapy in adults with moderate to severe Crohn disease. However, other TNF blocking agents may be more effective than certolizumab pegol for induction of remission.

Clinical Experience

Efficacy of certolizumab pegol has been evaluated in 2 double-blind, 26-week placebo-controlled, randomized studies in patients with moderately to severely active Crohn disease. In these studies, the Crohn Disease Activity Index (CDAI) was used for clinical assessment. The CDAI score is based on observations by the patient (e.g., the daily number of liquid or very soft stools, severity of abdominal pain, general well-being) and objective evidence (e.g., number of extraintestinal manifestations, presence of an abdominal mass, use or nonuse of antidiarrheal drugs, hematocrit, body weight).

The first study (PRECISE 1) evaluated certolizumab pegol for induction and maintenance therapy in 662 adults with moderately to severely active Crohn disease. To be included in the study, patients were required to have Crohn disease for a minimum of 3 months and a CDAI score of 220–450. Patients receiving stable dosages of 5-aminosalicylates, corticosteroids, azathioprine, 6-mercaptopurine, methotrexate, or anti-infective agents could continue such agents. Patients were randomized to receive certolizumab pegol (400 mg given subcutaneously) or placebo at weeks 0, 2, 4, and then every 4 weeks. Primary end points were response at week 6 and response at both weeks 6 and 26. Clinical response (defined as a reduction from baseline CDAI of at least 100 points) was observed in 35 or 27% of those receiving certolizumab pegol or placebo, respectively, at week 6. At both weeks 6 and 26, clinical response was observed in 23 or 16% of patients receiving certolizumab pegol or placebo, respectively. At week 6 and both weeks 6 and 26, rates of remission (defined as an absolute CDAI score of 150 points or less) did not differ between those receiving certolizumab pegol and those receiving placebo. Remission was observed in 22 or 17% of those receiving certolizumab pegol or placebo, respectively, at week 6 and in 14 or 10% of patients, respectively, at both weeks 6 and 26.

The second study (PRECISE 2) evaluated certolizumab pegol for maintenance therapy in 668 adults with moderately to severely active Crohn disease. To be included in the study, patients were required to have Crohn disease for a minimum of 3 months and a CDAI score of 220–450. Patients receiving stable dosages of 5-aminosalicylates, corticosteroids, azathioprine, 6-mercaptopurine, methotrexate, or anti-infective agents could continue such agents. Patients received induction therapy (i.e., certolizumab pegol 400 mg given subcutaneously at weeks 0, 2, and 4); patients who responded (defined as a reduction from baseline CDAI of at least 100 points) at week 6 were randomized to receive certolizumab pegol (400 mg given subcutaneously) or placebo at weeks 8, 12, 16, 20, and 24. The primary end point was response at week 26. At week 26, response was observed in 63 or 36% of patients receiving certolizumab pegol or placebo, respectively. Remission (defined as an absolute CDAI score of 150 points or less) was observed in 48 or 29% of patients receiving certolizumab pegol or placebo, respectively, at week 26.

Patients who completed the PRECISE 1 or PRECISE 2 studies were eligible for enrollment in a long-term extension study, PRECISE 3. The 595 patients enrolled in PRECISE 3 were treated with open-label certolizumab pegol 400 mg every 4 weeks up to week 362 (7 years). All background therapies for Crohn disease (e.g., 5-aminosalicylates, corticosteroids, azathioprine, 6-mercaptopurine, methotrexate, anti-infective agents) had to remain at or below a stable dosage for the duration of the study. The primary measure of efficacy in PRECISE 3 was remission, defined as a Harvey-Bradshaw Index (HBI) score of ≤4 points. The HBI score is based on 5 parameters including general well-being, abdominal pain, number of liquid stools per day, abdominal mass, and complications. At the end of the 7-year study period, 103 patients remained in the trial; among these patients, the remission rate was 75.7%. In the overall study population, remission rates were 55 and 13% at year 7 when analyzed using last observation carried forward and nonremitter imputation methods, respectively.

Certolizumab pegol has been used in a limited number of patients with fistulizing Crohn disease†. A subgroup analysis of the PRECISE 2 study explored fistula-related outcomes in 58 patients with open, draining fistulas at baseline who responded to initial induction therapy and were randomized to receive maintenance therapy with certolizumab pegol 400 mg every 4 weeks or placebo. Protocol-defined fistula closure (defined as closure of ≥50% of fistulas at any 2 consecutive post-baseline visits at least 3 weeks apart) was not significantly different between treatment groups, with 54 and 43% of certolizumab pegol- and placebo-treated patients, respectively, reporting closure according to this definition. However, at week 26, significantly more patients receiving certolizumab pegol reported 100% fistula closure. The 100% fistula closure rates at week 26 were 36 and 17% in the certolizumab pegol and placebo groups, respectively.

Clinical Perspective

The American College of Gastroenterology (ACG) and the American Gastroenterological Association (AGA) have issued guidelines for the medical treatment of Crohn disease. The ACG guideline was issued in 2018, while the AGA issued a guideline on the management of moderate to severe disease in 2021 and a guideline on management after surgical resection in 2017. Medical treatment of Crohn disease is typically divided into 2 phases: induction therapy (where control of inflammation is rapidly achieved) and maintenance therapy (where control of inflammation is sustained for a prolonged period of time). Specific treatments for Crohn disease are selected according to the patient's risk profile and disease severity. Drug classes used to treat Crohn disease include 5-aminosalicylates, antibiotics, corticosteroids, immunomodulators (e.g., thiopurines, methotrexate), and biologic agents including TNF blocking agents, ustekinumab, vedolizumab, and natalizumab.

TNF blocking agents used in the treatment of Crohn disease include infliximab, adalimumab, and certolizumab pegol. The TNF blocking agents are generally recommended for use as induction and maintenance therapy in adults with moderate to severe Crohn disease. ACG states that TNF blocking agents should be used to treat moderate to severe and/or moderate to high risk Crohn disease that is resistant to treatment with corticosteroids and/or refractory to thiopurines or methotrexate. For induction, AGA recommends other biologic agents (infliximab, adalimumab, and ustekinumab) over certolizumab pegol in adults who are naive to biologic therapy and suggests the use of vedolizumab over certolizumab pegol for induction of remission. Patients with perianal fistulas should be considered for TNF blocking therapy; however, guideline recommendations regarding agent selection differ in this setting. While ACG states that certolizumab pegol may be effective in this setting, AGA states that the drug may not be effective for induction of fistula remission.

If a patient with Crohn disease achieves remission with a TNF blocking agent, TNF blocking therapy should be continued to maintain remission; monotherapy with a TNF blocking agent is effective for maintaining remission, but combination with azathioprine/6-mercaptopurine or methotrexate should be considered due to the potential for immunogenicity and loss of response. For patients with surgically induced remission of Crohn disease, AGA suggests TNF blocking agents and/or thiopurines over other agents to prevent recurrence. Similarly, ACG recommends that patients who undergo surgery for Crohn disease and remain at high risk for recurrence should begin therapy with a TNF blocking agent within 4 weeks of surgery to prevent postoperative recurrence.

● Rheumatoid Arthritis

Certolizumab pegol is used for the management of moderately to severely active rheumatoid arthritis in adults. Certolizumab can be used alone or in combination with methotrexate or other nonbiologic disease-modifying antirheumatic drugs (DMARDs). Safety and efficacy of certolizumab pegol for this use are based on the results of several randomized controlled trials, including 4 pivotal randomized controlled trials. Guidelines generally support the use of TNF blocking agents, including certolizumab pegol, as add-on therapy to methotrexate in patients who do not meet treatment goals with methotrexate alone.

Clinical Experience

Safety and efficacy of certolizumab pegol were evaluated in 4 pivotal randomized, double-blind, placebo-controlled studies in 2068 adults with moderately to severely active rheumatoid arthritis (as defined by the American College of Rheumatology [ACR]) for at least 6 months prior to the start of the study. To be included in these studies, patients were required to have at least 9 swollen and 9 tender joints. Certolizumab pegol was administered in combination with methotrexate (stable dosage of at least 10 mg weekly) in 3 of these studies (studies RA-1, RA-2, and RA-3) and was administered as monotherapy in one study (RA-4). Efficacy data were collected and analyzed through week 24 (studies RA-2, RA-3, and RA-4) or week 52 (study RA-1). Patients receiving stable dosages of low-dose corticosteroids (equivalent to 10 mg of prednisone daily or less), nonsteroidal anti-inflammatory agents (NSAIAs), and/or other analgesics could continue these agents.

In studies RA-1 and RA-2, 1601 patients (982 patients in study RA-1 and 619 patients in study RA-2) who had active rheumatoid arthritis despite receiving methotrexate therapy were randomized to receive one of 2 regimens of certolizumab pegol (400 mg at 0, 2, and 4 weeks, followed by either 200 or 400 mg every 2 weeks thereafter) or placebo, each given in conjunction with a stable methotrexate regimen. Exclusion criteria included, but were not limited to, use of etanercept or anakinra within the previous 3 months or use of another biologic DMARD within the previous 6 months and failure to respond to prior therapy with a TNF blocking agent. Other DMARDs (excluding methotrexate) were discontinued prior to the study. The mean number of prior DMARDs (excluding methotrexate) was 1.2–1.4. In study RA-2, 1.3% of patients had received prior TNF blocking agent therapy.

In study RA-3, 247 patients who had active rheumatoid arthritis despite receiving methotrexate therapy were randomized to receive certolizumab pegol (400 mg every 4 weeks) or placebo, each given in conjunction with a stable methotrexate regimen.

In study RA-4, 220 patients who had not achieved an adequate response to or had not tolerated prior DMARD therapy were randomized to receive certolizumab pegol (400 mg every 4 weeks) or placebo. Exclusion criteria included, but were not limited to, use of a biologic DMARD within the previous 6 months or prior therapy with a TNF blocking agent. Other DMARDs were discontinued prior to the study. Patients had received an average of 2 prior DMARDs; approximately 82% of patients in the study had received prior methotrexate therapy.

The primary outcome measure in studies RA-2, RA-3, and RA-4 was ACR 20 response at 24 weeks; in study RA-1, the primary outcome measures were ACR 20 response at 24 weeks and change from baseline in the modified total Sharp score at 52 weeks. An ACR 20 response is achieved if the patient experiences a 20% improvement in tender and swollen joint count and a 20% or greater improvement in at least 3 of the following criteria: patient pain assessment, patient global assessment, physician global assessment, patient self-assessed disability, or laboratory measures of disease activity (e.g., C-reactive protein [CRP] level). The modified total Sharp score is a composite measure of radiographically assessed structural damage (i.e., joint erosion and joint space narrowing).

In studies RA-1 and RA-2, a greater proportion of patients who received certolizumab pegol in conjunction with methotrexate achieved an ACR 20 response at 24 weeks than did patients who received methotrexate alone. In RA-1, an ACR 20 response at 24 weeks was reported in 59% of patients who received combined therapy with certolizumab pegol 200 mg every 2 weeks and methotrexate, 61% of those who received combined therapy with certolizumab pegol 400 mg every 2 weeks and methotrexate, and 14% of those who received methotrexate and placebo; results were similar in RA-2. Results of study RA-1 also indicated that certolizumab pegol and methotrexate inhibited progression of structural damage, as measured by the modified total Sharp score, to a greater extent than did methotrexate alone. In this study, 69 or 72% of patients receiving combined therapy with certolizumab pegol 200 or 400 mg, respectively, and methotrexate, compared with 52% of those receiving methotrexate and placebo, experienced no radiographic progression at 52 weeks. The mean change in modified total Sharp score from baseline to week 52 was smaller in patients receiving certolizumab pegol 200 or

400 mg (0.4 or 0.2 Sharp units, respectively) in conjunction with methotrexate compared with patients receiving methotrexate and placebo (2.8 Sharp units).

In study RA-4, 46% of patients receiving certolizumab pegol (400 mg every 4 weeks) as monotherapy achieved an ACR 20 response at 24 weeks compared with 9% of patients receiving placebo.

The manufacturer states that responses in study RA-3 were similar to those observed in study RA-4.

In these 4 studies, patients receiving certolizumab pegol, either alone or in conjunction with methotrexate, had greater improvements in physical function, as assessed using the disability index of the Health Assessment Questionnaire (HAQ-DI), from baseline to week 24 (studies RA-2, RA-3, and RA-4) or week 52 (study RA-1) than did control patients receiving placebo or methotrexate.

Extension studies of RA-1 and RA-2 have evaluated the efficacy and safety of up to 5 years of certolizumab pegol therapy in patients with rheumatoid arthritis. These studies found that efficacy of certolizumab pegol was maintained over 5 years, and not affected by a dosage reduction from 400 mg every 2 weeks to 200 mg every 2 weeks. No new safety signals were identified during follow-up. Additional randomized, placebo-controlled trials support the efficacy of certolizumab pegol in various populations of patients with rheumatoid arthritis. The C-EARLY trial found that certolizumab pegol plus methotrexate improved the rate of sustained remission at 52 weeks compared to placebo plus methotrexate in DMARD-naive patients with moderately to severely active rheumatoid arthritis and a disease duration of ≤1 year. The REALISTIC trial, which enrolled adults with active rheumatoid arthritis and inadequate response to at least 1 DMARD, found that certolizumab pegol improved ACR 20 rates compared to placebo at 12 weeks and maintained efficacy up to 28 weeks. Approximately 37% of patients enrolled in the trial had previously used a TNF blocking agent, and most were receiving concomitant DMARDs. The efficacy of certolizumab pegol was consistent across subgroups stratified by prior TNF blocking agent use, concomitant use of methotrexate, and disease duration. The CERTAIN trial found that certolizumab pegol improved remission rates at weeks 20 and 24 compared with placebo among a population of patients with moderately active rheumatoid arthritis receiving concomitant DMARD therapy.

Studies comparing certolizumab pegol with other agents in rheumatoid arthritis are limited. One randomized controlled trial (EXXELERATE) compared certolizumab pegol to adalimumab, both with background methotrexate, and found no significant difference between treatments in terms of ACR 20 response at week 12 or low disease activity rates at week 104. Another randomized controlled trial compared active conventional treatment (oral prednisolone or sulfasalazine combined with hydroxychloroquine plus intraarticular triamcinolone injections) with 3 different biologic treatments (certolizumab pegol, abatacept, or tocilizumab) in patients with early (symptom duration <24 months) moderate to severe rheumatoid arthritis; all patients also received methotrexate therapy. Certolizumab pegol was noninferior to active conventional treatment in terms of remission rate at 24 weeks. Tocilizumab was also noninferior to active conventional treatment in terms of remission rate at 24 weeks, while abatacept was associated with higher rates of remission at 24 weeks compared to active conventional treatment.

Clinical Perspective

The American College of Rheumatology issued guidelines for the treatment of rheumatoid arthritis in 2021. Disease-modifying treatments for rheumatoid arthritis include conventional DMARDs (e.g., hydroxychloroquine, leflunomide, methotrexate, sulfasalazine), biologic DMARDs (e.g., TNF blocking agents, abatacept, tocilizumab, sarilumab, rituximab), and/or targeted synthetic DMARDs (e.g., Janus kinase inhibitors). Specific agents for rheumatoid arthritis treatment are selected according to current disease activity, prior therapies used, and the presence of comorbidities. A "treat-to-target" approach is typically employed, with the goal of achieving a predefined target of low disease activity or remission.

TNF blocking agents used in the treatment of rheumatoid arthritis include adalimumab, certolizumab pegol, etanercept, golimumab, and infliximab. Methotrexate monotherapy is strongly recommended over biologic DMARD monotherapy and conditionally recommended over the combination of methotrexate and a TNF blocking agent for DMARD-naive patients with moderate to high disease activity, because many patients will achieve their treatment goal with methotrexate alone, and combination therapy with TNF blocking agents may be associated with additional risks and costs. Biologic DMARDs (including TNF blocking agents) and targeted synthetic DMARDs are conditionally recommended as add-on therapy for patients who are taking maximally tolerated dosages of methotrexate and are not at target. Recommendations for the use and selection of biologic DMARDs in rheumatoid arthritis vary based on the presence of certain comorbidities (e.g., heart failure, previous serious infection, nontuberculous mycobacterial lung disease). Consult the American College of Rheumatology guidelines for additional details.

● Psoriatic Arthritis

Certolizumab pegol is used for the management of active psoriatic arthritis in adults. Safety and efficacy of certolizumab pegol for this use are based principally on the results of a single randomized controlled trial. Guidelines generally support the use of TNF blocking agents, including certolizumab pegol, as first-line treatment in patients with active psoriatic arthritis.

Clinical Experience

Safety and efficacy of certolizumab pegol were evaluated in a randomized, double-blind, placebo-controlled study (RAPID-PsA) in 409 patients with adult-onset active psoriatic arthritis (as defined by Classification Criteria for Psoriatic Arthritis [CASPAR] criteria, with 3 or more swollen joints and 3 or more tender joints) of at least 6 months' duration who had an inadequate response to treatment with one or more DMARDs. Up to 40% of patients enrolled in the study were allowed to have received prior therapy with a TNF blocking agent. Individuals who had received more than 2 biologic DMARDs or more than one TNF blocking agent for treatment of psoriasis or psoriatic arthritis and those who had not responded to prior therapy with a TNF blocking agent were excluded. Enthesitis or dactylitis was present at baseline in approximately 64 or 26%, respectively, of patients. Patients were randomized to receive one of 2 regimens of certolizumab pegol (400 mg at 0, 2, and 4 weeks, followed by either 200 mg every 2 weeks or 400 mg every 4 weeks) or placebo. Placebo recipients who did not achieve at least 10% improvement from baseline in the number of both tender and swollen joints at weeks 14 and 16 were rerandomized at week 16 to receive one of the 2 certolizumab pegol regimens. Patients receiving stable dosages of a nonbiologic DMARD (methotrexate [25 mg/week or less], sulfasalazine, or leflunomide) and/or oral corticosteroid (equivalent to 10 mg of prednisone daily or less) could continue these agents. Approximately 70% of patients received concomitant DMARD therapy (generally methotrexate), 73% received concomitant NSAIA therapy, and 20% had received prior therapy with a TNF blocking agent.

The primary clinical outcome measure was the proportion of patients achieving an ACR 20 response at week 12. An ACR 20 response was achieved if the patient experienced a 20% improvement in tender and swollen joint count and a 20% or greater improvement in at least 3 of the following criteria: patient pain assessment, patient global assessment, physician global assessment, patient self-assessed disability, or laboratory measures of disease activity (e.g., CRP level). Physical function was assessed using the HAQ-DI; other patient-reported outcomes included fatigue (assessed using the Fatigue Assessment Scale), health status (assessed using the Short Form-36 [SF-36] health survey), and quality of life (assessed using the Psoriatic Arthritis Quality of Life [PsAQOL] scale). Patient work and household productivity were assessed using the Work Productivity Survey (WPS). Structural damage in the hands and feet was assessed radiographically by the change from baseline in the van der Heijde-modified total Sharp score, adapted for assessment of psoriatic arthritis.

A greater proportion of patients who received certolizumab pegol (200 mg every 2 weeks or 400 mg every 4 weeks) achieved an ACR 20 response compared with patients who received placebo. ACR 20 responses were achieved at 12 or 24 weeks by 58 or 64%, respectively, of patients receiving certolizumab pegol 200 mg every 2 weeks; 52 or 56%, respectively, of patients receiving certolizumab pegol 400 mg every 4 weeks; and 24 or 24% of patients receiving placebo. Improved ACR 20 response rates were observed in patients receiving certolizumab pegol compared with those receiving placebo irrespective of concurrent DMARD or prior TNF blocking agent use. ACR 50 responses (defined using the same criteria with a level of improvement of 50%) were achieved at 12 or 24 weeks by 36 or 44%, respectively, of patients receiving certolizumab pegol 200 mg every 2 weeks; 33 or 40%, respectively, of patients receiving certolizumab pegol 400 mg every 4 weeks; and 11 or 13%, respectively, of patients receiving placebo. Both certolizumab pegol dosage regimens were associated with greater improvement from baseline to week 24 in HAQ-DI score, fatigue, SF-36 score, and PsAQOL score compared with placebo. Certolizumab pegol was also associated with improved workplace productivity, reduced absenteeism, and improved household productivity at week

24 compared with placebo. In addition, certolizumab pegol was associated with greater improvement in enthesitis and dactylitis compared with placebo. Certolizumab pegol 200 mg every 2 weeks was more effective than placebo in inhibiting radiographic progression at 24 weeks; however, certolizumab pegol 400 mg every 4 weeks did not demonstrate greater inhibition of radiographic progression compared with placebo at 24 weeks. Results from the RAPID-PsA trial demonstrated that ACR 20 and ACR 50 response rates were generally maintained through the 4-year study period, irrespective of prior exposure to TNF blocking agents or concomitant use of DMARDs.

Although treatment with certolizumab pegol resulted in improvements in skin manifestations in patients with psoriatic arthritis, the manufacturer states that safety and efficacy of the drug in the management of plaque psoriasis have not been established.

Clinical Perspective

The American College of Rheumatology and the National Psoriasis Foundation issued a joint guideline for the treatment of psoriatic arthritis in 2018. Various drugs and drug classes are used to treat psoriatic arthritis, with some classes being used for symptom management (e.g., NSAIAs and corticosteroids) and others being used as immunomodulatory disease-modifying therapy. Disease-modifying treatments for psoriatic arthritis include oral small molecules (OSMs; e.g., methotrexate, sulfasalazine, cyclosporine, leflunomide, apremilast), biologic DMARDs (e.g., TNF blocking agents, secukinumab, ixekizumab, ustekinumab, brodalumab, abatacept), and/or targeted synthetic DMARDs (e.g., tofacitinib). Specific agents for psoriatic arthritis treatment are selected according to disease characteristics, including disease severity, as well as patient preferences/values and comorbidities. A "treat-to-target" approach is typically employed, with the goal of achieving low/minimal disease activity or remission.

TNF blocking agents used in the treatment of psoriatic arthritis include adalimumab, certolizumab pegol, etanercept, golimumab, and infliximab. For patients with treatment-naive psoriatic arthritis, treatment with a TNF blocking agent is conditionally recommended over treatment with an OSM, interleukin (IL) 17 inhibitor (e.g., secukinumab, ixekizumab, brodalumab) or IL12/23 inhibitor (e.g., ustekinumab). For patients with active psoriatic arthritis despite treatment with an OSM, switching to monotherapy with a TNF blocking agent is conditionally recommended over combination therapy with a TNF blocking agent plus methotrexate or switching to another OSM, ustekinumab, secukinumab, ixekizumab, brodalumab, abatacept, or tofacitinib. For patients with active psoriatic arthritis despite treatment with TNF blocking agent monotherapy, switching to monotherapy with a different TNF blocking agent is conditionally recommended over switching to ustekinumab, secukinumab, ixekizumab, brodalumab, abatacept, or tofacitinib. For patients with active psoriatic arthritis despite treatment with a combination of a TNF blocking agent and methotrexate, switching to a different TNF blocking agent plus methotrexate is conditionally recommended over switching to a different TNF blocking agent as monotherapy. Switching to a TNF blocking agent is conditionally recommended for patients with active psoriatic arthritis despite treatment with secukinumab, ixekizumab, brodalumab, or ustekinumab. Recommendations for the use and selection of disease-modifying therapies in psoriatic arthritis vary based on the presence of certain disease characteristics (e.g., psoriatic spondylitis/axial disease, enthesitis) and comorbidities (e.g., inflammatory bowel disease, diabetes). Consult the American College of Rheumatology/National Psoriasis Foundation guideline for additional details.

● Ankylosing Spondylitis

Certolizumab pegol is used for the management of active ankylosing spondylitis in adults. Safety and efficacy of certolizumab pegol for this use are based principally on the results of a single randomized controlled trial. Guidelines generally support the use of TNF blocking agents, including certolizumab pegol, for the treatment of ankylosing spondylitis in patients with active disease despite treatment with NSAIAs.

Clinical Experience

Safety and efficacy of certolizumab pegol were evaluated in a randomized, double-blind, placebo-controlled study (RAPID-axSpA) in 325 patients with adult-onset active axial spondyloarthritis (including 178 patients with ankylosing spondylitis) who had not achieved an adequate response to or had not tolerated prior NSAIA therapy. Patients were excluded if they had received prior treatment with certolizumab pegol or more than 2 other biologic agents (including more than one TNF blocking agent) or had not responded to prior TNF blocking agent therapy. The subset of patients with ankylosing spondylitis met modified New York criteria for ankylosing spondylitis in addition to Assessment of SpondyloArthritis International Society (ASAS) criteria for axial spondyloarthritis. Patients were randomized to receive one of 2 regimens of certolizumab pegol (400 mg at 0, 2, and 4 weeks, followed by either 200 mg every 2 weeks or 400 mg every 4 weeks) or placebo. Placebo recipients who did not achieve an ASAS 20 response at weeks 14 and 16 were rerandomized at week 16 to receive one of the 2 certolizumab pegol regimens. The median duration of symptoms in patients with ankylosing spondylitis was 9.1 years; 91% of patients with ankylosing spondylitis received concomitant therapy with NSAIAs, 35% received concomitant DMARD (sulfasalazine or methotrexate) therapy, and 20% had received prior therapy with a TNF blocking agent.

The primary outcome measure was the proportion of patients achieving an ASAS 20 response at week 12. An ASAS 20 response is achieved if the patient experiences at least a 20% improvement and an absolute improvement of at least 1 unit (on a scale of 0–10) in at least 3 of the following criteria without worsening by at least 20% or 1 unit in the fourth criterion: patient global assessment, pain, function, or inflammation. ASAS 40 response is defined as at least a 40% improvement and an absolute improvement of at least 2 units in at least 3 of these criteria without any worsening in the fourth criterion.

A greater proportion of patients who received certolizumab pegol achieved an ASAS 20 response compared with patients who received placebo; response rates for the 2 certolizumab pegol regimens were similar. ASAS 20 responses were achieved at 12 or 24 weeks by 57 or 68%, respectively, of patients receiving certolizumab pegol 200 mg every 2 weeks; 64 or 70%, respectively, of those receiving certolizumab pegol 400 mg every 4 weeks; and 37 or 33%, respectively, of those receiving placebo. ASAS 40 responses were achieved at 12 or 24 weeks by 40 or 48%, respectively, of patients receiving certolizumab pegol 200 mg every 2 weeks; 50 or 59%, respectively, of those receiving certolizumab pegol 400 mg every 4 weeks; and 19 or 16%, respectively, of those receiving placebo. Patient-reported outcomes, including total back pain, fatigue, and quality of life (as measured by the Ankylosing Spondylitis Quality of Life [ASQOL] measure) were improved from baseline to week 24 in patients treated with certolizumab pegol (either dose) compared to placebo. Final 4-year data from the RAPID-axSpA trial indicate that ASAS 20 and ASAS 40 responses were sustained from week 24 to week 204 among patients with ankylosing spondylitis who were initially randomized to certolizumab pegol (either dose). Imaging results at 4 years also demonstrated sustained reductions in spinal and sacroiliac joint inflammation from week 12 to week 204 in patients treated with certolizumab pegol.

Clinical Perspective

The American College of Rheumatology, the Spondylitis Association of America, and the Spondyloarthritis Research and Treatment Network issued a joint guideline for the treatment of ankylosing spondylitis in 2019. Treatments for ankylosing spondylitis include NSAIAs, conventional DMARDs (e.g., methotrexate, sulfasalazine), biologic DMARDs (e.g., TNF blocking agents, secukinumab, ixekizumab), and/or targeted synthetic DMARDs (e.g., tofacitinib). Continuous NSAIA treatment is typically considered first-line for active ankylosing spondylitis, with other agents used in the treatment of NSAIA-refractory disease. Specific agents for ankylosing spondylitis treatment are selected according to current disease activity, prior therapies, and the presence of comorbidities. Goals of therapy in ankylosing spondylitis are to alleviate symptoms, improve functioning, maintain the ability to work, decrease complications, and prevent or slow skeletal damage.

TNF blocking agents used in the treatment of ankylosing spondylitis include adalimumab, certolizumab pegol, etanercept, golimumab, and infliximab. For adults with active ankylosing spondylitis despite treatment with NSAIAs, treatment with a TNF blocking agent is strongly recommended over no treatment with a TNF blocking agent and conditionally recommended over treatment with tofacitinib, secukinumab, or ixekizumab. No specific TNF blocking agent is recommended over others. In patients with active ankylosing spondylitis despite treatment with a first TNF blocking agent, guidelines conditionally recommend secukinumab or ixekizumab over treatment with a different TNF blocking agent for patients with primary nonresponse to TNF blocking therapy; in patients with secondary nonresponse to TNF blocking therapy, treatment with a different TNF blocking therapy is conditionally recommended over treatment with a non-TNF blocking biologic agent. In adults with stable ankylosing spondylitis, continuation of biologic monotherapy is conditionally recommended over discontinuation of the biologic or continuation of combination therapy with NSAIAs or conventional DMARDs. Recommendations for treatment selection in ankylosing spondylitis may be influenced by the presence of certain comorbidities (e.g., iritis, inflammatory bowel disease). Consult the joint guideline issued by the American College of Rheumatology, the Spondylitis Association of America, and the Spondyloarthritis Research and Treatment Network for additional details.

• Nonradiographic Axial Spondyloarthritis

Certolizumab pegol is used for the management of active nonradiographic axial spondyloarthritis in adults with objective signs of inflammation. Safety and efficacy of certolizumab pegol for this use are based principally on the results of a single randomized controlled trial, with additional supporting data from a previous, mixed-population randomized controlled trial. Guidelines generally support the use of TNF blocking agents, including certolizumab pegol, for the treatment of nonradiographic axial spondyloarthritis in patients with active disease despite treatment with NSAIAs.

Clinical Experience

Safety and efficacy of certolizumab pegol for this indication were evaluated in a randomized, double-blind, placebo-controlled study (C-axSpAnd) in 317 patients with active adult-onset axial spondyloarthritis according to the Assessment of SpondyloArthritis International Society (ASAS) criteria and objective signs of inflammation (i.e., active sacroiliitis on magnetic resonance imaging or CRP above the upper limit of normal) despite treatment with at least 2 NSAIAs. Patients were excluded if they had radiographic sacroiliitis meeting modified New York criteria for ankylosing spondylitis. Patients were randomized to receive certolizumab pegol (400 mg at 0, 2, and 4 weeks, followed by 200 mg every 2 weeks) or placebo. The mean duration of symptoms was 7.8 and 8 years in the certolizumab pegol and placebo groups, respectively. Approximately 87% of patients in each group received concomitant therapy with NSAIAs; 34.6 and 30.4% received concomitant DMARD (sulfasalazine or methotrexate) therapy and 4.4 and 7% had received prior therapy with a TNF blocking agent in the certolizumab pegol and placebo groups, respectively. The primary outcome measure was the proportion of patients achieving an Ankylosing Spondylitis Disease Activity Score-Major Improvement (ASDAS-MI) response at week 52. An ASDAS-MI response was achieved if the patient experienced at least a 2-point decrease from the baseline score in ASDAS or obtained the lowest possible ASDAS value of 0.6. The ASDAS is a composite weighted scoring system that assesses disease activity using 5 elements: patient-reported back pain, patient-reported peripheral pain/swelling in joints, patient-reported duration of morning stiffness, Patient's Global Assessment of Disease Activity score, and CRP level. ASAS 40 was also assessed at weeks 12 and 52. A greater proportion of patients who received certolizumab pegol achieved an ASDAS-MI response compared with patients who received placebo; response rates were 47 and 7% in the certolizumab pegol and placebo groups, respectively. ASAS 40 responses were achieved at 12 and 52 weeks by 47.8 and 56.6%, respectively, of patients receiving certolizumab pegol and 11.4 and 15.8%, respectively, of patients receiving placebo. At week 12, patients receiving certolizumab pegol reported greater improvements in quality of life as measured by the ASQOL compared to those receiving placebo.

The RAPID-axSpA trial included 147 patients with nonradiographic axial spondyloarthritis (see Ankylosing Spondylitis under Uses). The median duration of symptoms in patients with nonradiographic axial spondyloarthritis was 5.5 years; 83.7% received concomitant therapy with NSAIAs, 25.2% received concomitant DMARD (sulfasalazine or methotrexate) therapy, and 10.9% had received prior therapy with a TNF blocking agent. In this trial, the efficacy of certolizumab pegol in patients with nonradiographic axial spondyloarthritis was similar to that observed in patients with ankylosing spondylitis. In the nonradiographic axial spondyloarthritis subpopulation, ASAS 20 responses were achieved at 12 or 24 weeks by 58.7 or 65.2%, respectively, of patients receiving certolizumab pegol 200 mg every 2 weeks; 62.7 or 70.6%, respectively, of those receiving certolizumab pegol 400 mg every 4 weeks; and 40 or 24%, respectively, of those receiving placebo. ASAS 40 responses were achieved at 12 or 24 weeks by 47.8 or 56.5%, respectively, of patients receiving certolizumab pegol 200 mg every 2 weeks; 47.1 or 45.1%, respectively, of those receiving certolizumab pegol 400 mg every 4 weeks; and 16 or 14%, respectively, of those receiving placebo. Patient-reported outcomes, including total back pain, fatigue, and quality of life (as measured by the Ankylosing Spondylitis Quality of Life [ASQOL] measure) were improved from baseline to week 24 in patients treated with certolizumab pegol (either dose) compared to placebo. Final 4-year data from the RAPID-axSpA trial indicate that ASAS 20 and ASAS 40 responses were sustained from week 24 to week 204 among patients with nonradiographic axial spondyloarthritis who were initially randomized to certolizumab pegol (either dose). Imaging results at 4 years also demonstrated sustained reductions in spinal and sacroiliac joint inflammation from week 12 to week 204 in patients treated with certolizumab pegol.

Clinical Perspective

The American College of Rheumatology, the Spondylitis Association of America, and the Spondyloarthritis Research and Treatment Network issued a joint guideline for the treatment of nonradiographic axial spondyloarthritis in 2019. Treatments for nonradiographic axial spondyloarthritis include NSAIAs, conventional DMARDs (e.g., methotrexate, sulfasalazine), biologic DMARDs (e.g., TNF blocking agents, secukinumab, ixekizumab), and/or targeted synthetic DMARDs (e.g., tofacitinib). Continuous NSAIA treatment is typically considered first-line for active nonradiographic axial spondyloarthritis, with other agents being used in the treatment of NSAIA-refractory disease. Specific agents for nonradiographic axial spondyloarthritis treatment are selected according to current disease activity and prior therapies used. Goals of therapy in nonradiographic axial spondyloarthritis are to alleviate symptoms, improve functioning, maintain the ability to work, decrease complications, and prevent or slow skeletal damage. Recommendations for the treatment of nonradiographic axial spondyloarthritis are largely extrapolated from evidence in the treatment of ankylosing spondylitis due to a lack of data specific to nonradiographic axial spondyloarthritis.

TNF blocking agents used in the treatment of ankylosing spondylitis (and, by extension, nonradiographic axial spondyloarthritis) include adalimumab, certolizumab pegol, etanercept, golimumab, and infliximab. For adults with active nonradiographic axial spondyloarthritis despite treatment with NSAIAs, treatment with a TNF blocking agent is strongly recommended over no treatment with a TNF blocking agent and conditionally recommended over treatment with tofacitinib, secukinumab, or ixekizumab. No specific TNF blocking agent is recommended over others. In patients with active nonradiographic axial spondyloarthritis despite treatment with a first TNF blocking agent, guidelines conditionally recommend secukinumab or ixekizumab over treatment with a different TNF blocking agent for patients with primary nonresponse to TNF blocking therapy; in patients with secondary nonresponse to TNF blocking therapy, treatment with a different TNF blocking therapy is conditionally recommended over treatment with a non-TNF blocking biologic agent. In adults with stable nonradiographic axial spondyloarthritis, continuation of biologic monotherapy is conditionally recommended over discontinuation of the biologic or continuation of combination therapy with NSAIAs or conventional DMARDs.

● *Plaque Psoriasis*

Certolizumab pegol is used for the management of moderate to severe plaque psoriasis in adults who are candidates for phototherapy or systemic therapy. Safety and efficacy of certolizumab pegol for this use are based principally on the results from 3 randomized controlled trials. Guidelines generally support the use of TNF blocking agents, including certolizumab pegol, in moderate to severe psoriasis, either as monotherapy or in combination with topical, oral, or phototherapy.

Clinical Experience

The CIMPASI-1, CIMPASI-2, and CIMPACT trials enrolled adults with moderate to severe plaque psoriasis (defined by Physician Global Assessment [PGA] of 3 or greater, Psoriasis Area and Severity Index [PASI] of 12 or greater, and body surface area [BSA] involvement of at least 10%) of at least 6 months' duration who were eligible for phototherapy or systemic therapy. Patients were excluded if they had a history of treatment with more than 2 biologic agents, primary failure with any biologic, or secondary failure with more than 1 biologic.

CIMPASI-1 and CIMPASI-2 were replicate double-blind, placebo-controlled trials enrolling 234 and 227 patients, respectively. Patients in these studies were randomized to receive double-blind treatment with one of 2 regimens of certolizumab pegol (400 mg at 0, 2, and 4 weeks, followed by either 200 or 400 mg every 2 weeks thereafter) or placebo for 16 weeks. Approximately 24% of patients in each group had received 1 previous biologic therapy; 5, 9.7, and 8.6% of patients had received 2 previous biologic therapies in the placebo, certolizumab pegol 200 mg every 2 weeks, and certolizumab pegol 400 mg every 2 weeks groups, respectively.

CIMPACT was a randomized, double-blind placebo-controlled and single-blind active-controlled trial enrolling 559 patients. Patients were randomized 3:3:1:3 to receive one of the following regimens: certolizumab pegol 400 mg every 2 weeks; certolizumab pegol 400 mg at weeks 0, 2, and 4 followed by certolizumab pegol 200 mg every 2 weeks; placebo; or etanercept 50 mg twice weekly. All treatments were continued in a double-blind fashion for 16 weeks, with the exception of etanercept, which was continued in a single-blind fashion for 12 weeks. A total of 28.7, 26.7, 19.3, and 30% of patients had previously received biologic therapy in the certolizumab pegol 400 mg every 2 weeks, certolizumab pegol 200 mg every 2 weeks, placebo, and etanercept groups, respectively.

The coprimary outcome measures in CIMPASI-1 and CIMPASI-2 were PASI 75 response at week 16 and a PGA response of "clear" (0) or "almost clear" (1) with at least a 2-point improvement from baseline at week 16. The primary outcome measure in CIMPACT was PASI 75 response at week 12. A PASI 75 response is achieved if the patient experiences a 75% or greater reduction in PASI from baseline. In CIMPASI-1 and CIMPASI-2, a greater proportion of patients who received certolizumab pegol achieved a PASI 75 response at 16 weeks and a PGA response at 16 weeks than did patients who received placebo. In these 2 studies, a PASI 75 response at 16 weeks was reported in 76.7% of patients who received certolizumab pegol 200 mg every 2 weeks, 82% of patients who received certolizumab pegol 400 mg every 2 weeks, and 9.9% of patients who received placebo. A PGA response at 16 weeks was reported in 56.8% of patients who received certolizumab pegol 200 mg every 2 weeks, 65.3% of patients who received certolizumab pegol 400 mg every 2 weeks, and 2.7% of patients who received placebo. Three-year results from CIMPASI-1 and CIMPASI-2 indicate that PASI 75 responses remained high through week 144 in patients randomized to receive certolizumab pegol 200 mg every 2 weeks or certolizumab pegol 400 mg every 2 weeks. Patients receiving certolizumab pegol 400 mg every 2 weeks had numerically higher PGA responder rates at week 144 than patients receiving certolizumab pegol 200 mg every 2 weeks. In CIMPACT, a greater proportion of patients who received certolizumab pegol achieved a PASI 75 response at 12 weeks than did patients who received placebo. A PASI 75 response at 12 weeks was reported in 61.3% of patients who received certolizumab pegol 200 mg every 2 weeks, 66.7% of patients who received certolizumab pegol 400 mg every 2 weeks, and 5% of patients who received placebo. At 12 weeks, certolizumab pegol 400 mg every 2 weeks was superior to etanercept in terms of PASI 75 response, and certolizumab pegol 200 mg every 2 weeks was noninferior to etanercept in terms of PASI 75 response. The PASI 75 response rate in the etanercept group at week 12 was 53.3%. Three-year results from CIMPACT indicate that PASI 75 response was maintained at week 144 with certolizumab pegol (any dose). PASI 75 response rates decreased when patients receiving certolizumab pegol 400 mg every 2 weeks were switched to certolizumab pegol 200 mg every 2 weeks. A post hoc subgroup analysis of data from all 3 trials found that patients with a body weight of 90 kg or less and patients with lower disease severity may achieve an acceptable response with certolizumab pegol 200 mg every 2 weeks.

Clinical Perspective

The American Academy of Dermatology and the National Psoriasis Foundation issued joint guidelines for the treatment of psoriasis in adult and pediatric patients between 2019 and 2021. Various drugs and drug classes are used to treat psoriasis. Phototherapy and topical treatments (e.g., vitamin D analogues, calcineurin inhibitors, keratolytics, and corticosteroids) are frequently used to treat mild psoriasis present on limited areas of the body, but these therapies may be inadequate to obtain skin clearance in patients with more extensive or severe disease. Systemic biologic and nonbiologic therapies are mainstays of treatment for moderate to severe psoriasis, and may also be useful for treating psoriasis on parts of the body that are difficult to treat with topical therapy (e.g., the scalp, palms and soles of the feet, genitals). Topical therapies can be used adjunctively in moderate to severe disease. Nonbiologic oral therapies used in the treatment of psoriasis include methotrexate, apremilast, cyclosporine, acitretin, and dimethyl fumarate. Biologics used in the treatment of psoriasis include TNF blocking agents, ustekinumab, secukinumab, ixekizumab, brodalumab, guselkumab, tildrakizumab, and risankizumab. Treatment selection in psoriasis is primarily based on disease characteristics (e.g., severity, location, presence of psoriatic arthritis), with additional consideration being given to patient age and comorbidities.

TNF blocking agents used in the treatment of psoriasis include adalimumab, certolizumab pegol, etanercept, and infliximab. These TNF blocking agents are recommended for the treatment of adult patients with moderate to severe plaque psoriasis, with or without concomitant topical, oral, or phototherapy. Although formal recommendations are not made for certolizumab pegol in current guidelines for psoriasis, it is noted that certolizumab pegol is likely to have class characteristics similar to those of the other TNF blocking agents. Recommendations for the use and selection of psoriasis therapies vary based on patient age, disease characteristics (e.g., severity, location, presence of psoriatic arthritis), and comorbidities (e.g., inflammatory bowel disease). Consult the American Academy of Dermatology/National Psoriasis Foundation guidelines for additional details.

DOSAGE AND ADMINISTRATION

● *General*

Pretreatment Screening

- Evaluate all patients for active and inactive tuberculosis prior to initiating therapy using appropriate screening tests (e.g., tuberculin skin test, chest x-ray).

- Screen all patients for hepatitis B virus (HBV) infection before initiating therapy.

- Do not initiate therapy in patients with an active infection, including clinically important localized infections.

Patient Monitoring

- Monitor closely for signs or symptoms of infection (e.g., fever, malaise, weight loss, sweats, cough, dyspnea, pulmonary infiltrates, serious systemic illness including shock) during and after treatment; monitor for possible development of tuberculosis in patients who tested negative for latent tuberculosis prior to initiating therapy.

- Perform periodic dermatologic evaluations in all patients, particularly those with risk factors for skin cancer.

- Evaluate and monitor chronic carriers of HBV during treatment and for up to several months following treatment.

Other General Considerations

- May be used alone or in combination with methotrexate or other nonbiologic disease-modifying antirheumatic drugs (DMARDs); concomitant use with biologic DMARDs, including other TNF blocking agents, is not recommended.

- Corticosteroids, nonsteroidal anti-inflammatory agents (NSAIAs), and/or other analgesics may be continued in adults with rheumatoid arthritis, ankylosing spondylitis, nonradiographic axial spondyloarthritis, or psoriatic arthritis.

- Administered concomitantly with aminosalicylates, corticosteroids, azathioprine, mercaptopurine, methotrexate, or anti-infective agents in patients with Crohn disease.

● *Reconstitution and Administration*

Certolizumab pegol is administered by subcutaneous injection. Commercially available certolizumab pegol lyophilized powder should be reconstituted and administered by a healthcare professional. Certolizumab pegol solution supplied in prefilled syringes may be *self-administered* if the clinician determines that the patient and/or their caregiver is competent to safely administer the drug after appropriate training.

Certolizumab pegol lyophilized powder is supplied in a kit containing components (e.g., diluent, syringes, needles) for reconstitution and administration. Allow the kit to sit at room temperature for 30 minutes prior to reconstitution. Reconstitute the commercially available certolizumab pegol lyophilized powder by adding 1 mL of sterile water for injection (provided by the manufacturer) to the vial labeled as containing 200 mg of the drug to produce a solution containing approximately 200 mg/mL. Direct the sterile water for injection at the vial wall rather than directly on the powder. Gently swirl for about 1 minute to ensure that all of the powder comes into contact with the diluent; to avoid foaming, swirl the vial as gently as possible and do not shake. Full reconstitution may take as long as 30 minutes; continue swirling the vial every 5 minutes as long as non-dissolved particles are observed. The reconstituted solution may be refrigerated at 2–8°C (protect from freezing) for up to 24 hours. The reconstituted solution should be at

room temperature prior to administration, but do not leave reconstituted solution at room temperature for >2 hours prior to administration.

Certolizumab pegol solution in prefilled syringes should be allowed to reach room temperature prior to administration; this may take about 30 minutes.

Solutions of the drug should be a clear to opalescent, colorless to pale yellow liquid and essentially free of particulate matter. Inspect the solution visually for particulate matter and discoloration prior to administration; if either is present, discard the solution. Because the drug contains no preservative, the vials and prefilled syringes are for single use only.

Administer certolizumab pegol subcutaneously into the thighs or abdomen; rotate injection sites. Do not inject into areas where the skin is tender, bruised, red, or hard, or where there are scars or stretch marks. When a dose of 400 mg is given, administer the dose as 2 separate 200-mg injections at different sites.

Store the intact kit containing certolizumab pegol lyophilized powder or certolizumab pegol solution in prefilled syringes at 2–8°C and protect the drug from freezing. Unopened certolizumab pegol vials may also be stored at room temperature up to a maximum of 25°C for 6 months. Prefilled syringes may be stored at room temperature up to a maximum of 25°C in the original carton for a single period of up to 7 days. Vials and prefilled syringes stored at room temperature should not be placed back into refrigeration. Protect certolizumab pegol solutions from light.

● *Dosage*

Crohn Disease

For the treatment of moderately to severely active Crohn disease in adults, the recommended initial dosage of certolizumab pegol is 400 mg (given as 2 divided subcutaneous injections at different sites) at 0, 2, and 4 weeks (induction regimen); patients who respond may receive additional doses every 4 weeks (maintenance regimen).

Rheumatoid Arthritis

For the management of moderately to severely active rheumatoid arthritis in adults, the recommended dosage of certolizumab pegol is 400 mg (given as 2 divided subcutaneous injections at separate sites) at 0, 2, and 4 weeks, followed by 200 mg every 2 weeks. For maintenance therapy, a dosage of 400 mg every 4 weeks may be considered.

Psoriatic Arthritis

For the management of psoriatic arthritis in adults, the recommended dosage of certolizumab pegol is 400 mg (given as 2 divided subcutaneous injections at separate sites) at 0, 2, and 4 weeks, followed by 200 mg every 2 weeks. For maintenance therapy, a dosage of 400 mg every 4 weeks may be considered.

Ankylosing Spondylitis

For the management of ankylosing spondylitis in adults, the recommended dosage of certolizumab pegol is 400 mg (given as 2 divided subcutaneous injections at separate sites) at 0, 2, and 4 weeks, followed by 200 mg every 2 weeks or 400 mg every 4 weeks.

Nonradiographic Axial Spondyloarthritis

For the management of nonradiographic axial spondyloarthritis with objective signs of inflammation in adults, the recommended dosage of certolizumab pegol is 400 mg (given as 2 divided subcutaneous injections at separate sites) at 0, 2, and 4 weeks, followed by 200 mg every 2 weeks or 400 mg every 4 weeks.

Plaque Psoriasis

For the management of moderate to severe plaque psoriasis in adults, the recommended dosage of certolizumab pegol is 400 mg (given as 2 divided subcutaneous injections at separate sites) every 2 weeks.

For patients with a body weight of 90 kg or less, the following dosage regimen can be considered: certolizumab pegol 400 mg (given as 2 divided subcutaneous injections at separate sites) at 0, 2, and 4 weeks, followed by 200 mg every 2 weeks.

● *Special Populations*

The manufacturer makes no special population dosage recommendations at this time. The manufacturer states that there are insufficient data to provide dosage recommendations for patients with moderate or severe renal impairment.

CAUTIONS

● *Contraindications*

- History of hypersensitivity to certolizumab pegol or to any of the excipients. Reactions have included angioedema, anaphylaxis, serum sickness, and urticaria.

● *Warnings/Precautions*

Warnings

Infectious Complications

A boxed warning about the risk of serious infections is included in the prescribing information for certolizumab pegol. Patients receiving tumor necrosis factor (TNF; TNF-α) blocking agents, including certolizumab pegol, are at increased risk of developing serious infections involving various organ systems and sites that may require hospitalization or result in death. Opportunistic infections caused by bacterial, mycobacterial, invasive fungal, viral, parasitic, or other opportunistic pathogens—including aspergillosis, blastomycosis, candidiasis, coccidioidomycosis, histoplasmosis, legionellosis, listeriosis, pneumocystosis, and tuberculosis—have been reported in patients receiving TNF blocking agents. Infections frequently have been disseminated rather than localized. Patients should be closely monitored during and after treatment with TNF blocking agents for the development of signs or symptoms of infection (e.g., fever, malaise, weight loss, sweats, cough, dyspnea, pulmonary infiltrates, serious systemic illness including shock), including the possible development of tuberculosis in patients who tested negative for latent tuberculosis prior to initiating therapy. Most patients who developed serious infections were receiving concomitant therapy with immunosuppressive agents such as methotrexate or corticosteroids.

In placebo-controlled trials in adults with moderately to severely active Crohn disease, the rate of infection was 38 or 30% in patients receiving certolizumab pegol or placebo, respectively; the rate of serious infection was 3 or 1%, respectively. In controlled clinical trials in adults with rheumatoid arthritis, the rate of infection was 0.91 or 0.72 per patient-year in patients receiving certolizumab pegol or placebo, respectively. The rate of serious infection was increased in certolizumab pegol-treated patients compared with placebo-treated patients, with serious infection occurring at a rate of 0.06, 0.04, or 0.02 per patient-year in patients receiving certolizumab pegol 200 mg every 2 weeks, certolizumab pegol 400 mg every 4 weeks, or placebo, respectively. Serious infections in patients with Crohn disease or rheumatoid arthritis have included bacterial and viral infections, pneumonia, pyelonephritis, cellulitis, and tuberculosis. In controlled clinical trials in psoriasis, the rate of infection was similar between the placebo and certolizumab pegol groups. Serious infections in patients with psoriasis have included pneumonia, abdominal abscess, hematoma infection, urinary tract infection, gastroenteritis, and disseminated tuberculosis. Two cases of tuberculosis were reported among 1112 exposed patients. As of September 2011, FDA had identified 103 reports of *Legionella* pneumonia associated with TNF blocking agents. The cases occurred in patients 25–85 years of age, many of whom received concomitant therapy with immunosuppressive agents (e.g., corticosteroids and/or methotrexate); 17 deaths were reported. In 78% of the cases of *Legionella* pneumonia, the median duration of TNF blocker therapy prior to the onset of *Legionella* pneumonia was 10.4 months (range: less than 1 month to 73 months). As of September 2011, FDA also had identified 26 published reports of *Listeria* infections, including meningitis, bacteremia, endophthalmitis, and sepsis, in patients who received TNF blocking agents; 7 deaths were reported. Many of the *Listeria* infections occurred in patients who had received concomitant therapy with immunosuppressive agents. In addition, FDA identified fatal *Listeria* infections during a review of laboratory-confirmed infections that occurred in premarketing clinical studies and during postmarketing surveillance.

An increased incidence of serious infections also was observed in clinical studies in patients with rheumatoid arthritis when a TNF blocking agent was used concomitantly with anakinra (a human interleukin-1 receptor antagonist) or abatacept (a selective costimulation modulator). The use of certolizumab pegol in combination with other biologic DMARDs is not recommended.

Do not initiate certolizumab pegol therapy in patients with active infections, including clinically important localized infections. Patients >65 years of age, patients with comorbid conditions, and/or patients receiving concomitant therapy with immunosuppressive agents such as corticosteroids or methotrexate may be at increased risk of infection. Clinicians should consider potential risks and benefits of the drug prior to initiating therapy in patients with a history of chronic, recurring, or opportunistic infections; patients with underlying conditions that may predispose them to infections; and patients who have been exposed to tuberculosis or who have resided or traveled in regions where tuberculosis or mycoses such as histoplasmosis, coccidioidomycosis, and blastomycosis are endemic. Any patient who develops a new infection while receiving certolizumab pegol should undergo a thorough diagnostic evaluation (appropriate for an immunocompromised patient); initiate appropriate anti-infective therapy and closely monitor the patient. Discontinue the drug in patients who develop serious infection or sepsis.

Because cases of pulmonary and disseminated tuberculosis have been reported in patients receiving certolizumab pegol, all patients should be evaluated for active or latent tuberculosis and for the presence of risk factors for tuberculosis prior to and periodically during therapy with the drug. When indicated, initiate an appropriate antimycobacterial regimen for the treatment of latent tuberculosis infection prior to certolizumab pegol therapy. Antimycobacterial treatment lowers the risk of latent tuberculosis infection progressing to active disease (i.e., reactivation). Also consider antimycobacterial therapy prior to initiation of certolizumab pegol in individuals with a history of latent or active tuberculosis in whom an adequate course of antimycobacterial treatment cannot be confirmed and in individuals with a negative tuberculin skin test who have risk factors for tuberculosis. Despite previous or concomitant treatment for latent tuberculosis, cases of active tuberculosis have occurred in patients treated with certolizumab pegol. Some patients who have been successfully treated for active tuberculosis have redeveloped tuberculosis while receiving certolizumab pegol. Consultation with a tuberculosis specialist is recommended when deciding whether antimycobacterial therapy should be initiated. Monitor patients receiving certolizumab pegol, including individuals with a negative tuberculin skin test, for signs and symptoms of active tuberculosis. Strongly consider a diagnosis of tuberculosis in patients who develop new infections while receiving certolizumab pegol, especially in those who previously have traveled to countries where tuberculosis is highly prevalent or who have been in close contact with an individual with active tuberculosis.

Invasive fungal infections often are not recognized in patients receiving TNF blocking agents; this has led to delays in appropriate treatment. Clinicians should ascertain whether patients receiving TNF blocking agents who present with signs and symptoms suggestive of systemic fungal infection reside or have traveled in regions where mycoses are endemic. Consider empiric antifungal therapy in patients at risk of histoplasmosis or other invasive fungal infections who develop severe systemic illness. Following resolution of an invasive fungal infection, the decision regarding whether to reinitiate TNF blocking agent therapy should involve reevaluation of the risks and benefits of such therapy, particularly in patients who reside in regions where mycoses are endemic. Whenever feasible, decisions regarding initiation and duration of antifungal therapy and reinitiation of TNF blocking agent therapy should be made in consultation with a specialist in the diagnosis and management of fungal infections.

Malignancies and Lymphoproliferative Disorders

A boxed warning about the risk of malignancy is included in the prescribing information for certolizumab pegol. The possibility exists for agents that block TNF, including certolizumab pegol, to affect host defenses against malignancies since TNF mediates inflammation and modulates cellular immune responses.

Malignancies, some fatal, have been reported in children, adolescents, and young adults who received treatment with TNF blocking agents beginning when they were ≤18 years. In August 2009, FDA reported the results of an analysis of reports of lymphoma and other malignancies in children and adolescents who had received TNF blocking agents. These cases were reported postmarketing and were derived from various sources, including registries and spontaneous postmarketing reports. FDA identified 48 cases of malignancies in children and adolescents in the analysis. Approximately 50% were lymphomas, including Hodgkin disease and non-Hodgkin lymphoma. The other cases represented a variety of malignancies, including rare malignancies that are usually associated with immunosuppression and malignancies that are not usually observed in children and adolescents. Other malignancies reported included leukemia, melanoma, and solid organ cancers; malignancies such as leiomyosarcoma, hepatic malignancies, and renal cell carcinoma, which rarely occur in children, also were reported. The malignancies occurred after a median of 30 months (range: 1–84 months) following the first dose of therapy with TNF blocking agents. Of the 48 cases of malignancies, 11 deaths were reported; causes of death included hepatosplenic T-cell lymphoma (9 cases), T-cell lymphoma (1 case), and sepsis following remission of lymphoma (1 case). The reporting rates for cases of malignancy with certolizumab pegol were not calculated during the analysis because of minimal use in pediatric patients. Most of the 48 patients (88%) also were receiving other immunosuppressive drugs such as azathioprine and methotrexate; these agents also are associated with an increased risk of lymphoma. Although there were other contributory factors, the role of TNF blocking agents in the development of malignancies in children and adolescents could not be excluded. Therefore, FDA has concluded that there is an increased risk of malignancy with TNF blocking agents. However, due to the relatively rare occurrence of these cancers, the limited number of pediatric patients who received TNF blocking agents, and the possible role of other immunosuppressive drugs used concomitantly with TNF blocking agents, FDA was unable to fully characterize the strength of the association between use of TNF blocking agents and the development of a malignancy. Additional data are expected from ongoing, long-term, observational, postmarketing studies and registries that are being created by the manufacturers of TNF blocking agents.

Hepatosplenic T-cell lymphoma, a rare, aggressive, usually fatal type of T-cell lymphoma, has been reported during postmarketing experience mainly in adolescents and young adults with Crohn disease or ulcerative colitis who received treatment with TNF blocking agents and/or thiopurine analogs (mercaptopurine or azathioprine). Most of the reported cases of hepatosplenic T-cell lymphoma occurred in patients who had received a combination of immunosuppressive agents, including TNF blocking agents and thiopurine analogs (azathioprine or mercaptopurine). In some cases, potential confounding factors could not be excluded because complete medical histories were not available. As of December 31, 2010, FDA had not identified any cases of hepatosplenic T-cell lymphoma in patients who had received certolizumab pegol. Since patients with certain conditions (e.g., rheumatoid arthritis, Crohn disease) may be at increased risk for lymphoma, it may be difficult to measure the added risk of treatment with TNF blocking agents, azathioprine, and/or mercaptopurine.

In clinical studies, lymphoma has been observed more frequently in patients receiving TNF blocking agents than in control patients. Several cases of lymphoma have been reported during clinical studies in patients receiving certolizumab pegol. Patients with Crohn disease or other diseases requiring long-term treatment with immunosuppressive agents may be at increased risk of lymphoma compared with the general population. Patients with rheumatoid arthritis, especially those with highly active disease, also may be at increased risk of lymphoma.

During controlled and uncontrolled phases of studies evaluating certolizumab pegol in patients with Crohn disease and other diseases, the rate of malignancies other than nonmelanoma skin cancer was 0.5 or 0.6 per 100 patient-years in patients receiving certolizumab pegol or placebo, respectively. During certolizumab pegol studies in patients with psoriasis, the rate of malignancies other than nonmelanoma skin cancer was 0.5 per 100 patient-years in patients receiving certolizumab pegol. The size of the control group and the duration of the controlled phases of these studies were insufficient to draw definitive conclusions regarding an association between certolizumab pegol use and development of malignancies.

Cases of acute and chronic leukemia have been reported during postmarketing surveillance of TNF blocking agents used in the management of rheumatoid arthritis and other conditions. In August 2009, FDA reported the results of a review of 147 cases of leukemia in adults and pediatric patients who received TNF blocking agents; these cases had been identified during postmarketing surveillance. Of the 147 cases, acute myeloid leukemia (44 cases), chronic lymphocytic leukemia (31 cases), and chronic myeloid leukemia (23 cases) were the most frequent types of leukemia reported. Four cases of leukemia were reported in children. Most patients (61%) also were receiving other immunosuppressive drugs. There were a total of 30 deaths reported; leukemia was reported as the cause of 26 of the 30 deaths, and the event was associated with the use of TNF blocking agents. Leukemia generally occurred during the first 2 years of therapy. The interpretation of these findings was complicated by the fact that published epidemiologic studies suggest that patients with rheumatoid arthritis may be at increased risk of leukemia, independent of any treatment with TNF blocking agents. However, based on the available data, FDA has concluded that there is a possible association between treatment with TNF blocking agents and the development of leukemia in patients receiving these drugs.

The role of TNF blocking agents in the development of malignancies has not been fully determined. Clinicians should consider the possibility of and monitor for the occurrence of malignancies during and following treatment with TNF blocking agents. Because melanoma and Merkel cell carcinoma have been reported in patients treated with TNF blocking agents (including certolizumab pegol), periodic dermatologic evaluations are recommended for all patients, but particularly for those with risk factors for skin cancer. Because therapy with TNF blocking agents and/or thiopurine analogs (azathioprine or mercaptopurine) may increase the risk of malignancies, including hepatosplenic T-cell lymphoma, carefully consider the risks and benefits of these agents, especially in adolescents and young adults and especially in the treatment of Crohn disease or ulcerative colitis.

Other Warnings/Precautions

Cardiovascular Effects

There have been reports of worsening heart failure and new-onset heart failure in patients receiving TNF blocking agents, including certolizumab pegol. While certolizumab pegol has not been formally studied in patients with heart failure, other TNF blocking agents have been associated with worsening heart failure and increased mortality due to heart failure. If certolizumab pegol is used in patients with heart failure, use caution and monitor the patient carefully.

Sensitivity Reactions

Allergic reactions (e.g., angioedema, dyspnea, hypotension, rash, serum sickness, urticaria) have been reported rarely in patients receiving certolizumab pegol, sometimes after the first dose of the drug. If an allergic reaction occurs, discontinue certolizumab pegol immediately and initiate appropriate therapy. There are no data on the risks of using certolizumab pegol in patients who have experienced a severe hypersensitivity reaction with another TNF blocking agent; use caution if administering certolizumab pegol to such patients.

The needle shield inside the removable cap of the certolizumab pegol prefilled syringe contains a derivative of natural rubber latex which may cause an allergic reaction in individuals who are sensitive to latex.

Patients Infected with Hepatitis B Virus

Use of TNF blocking agents may increase the risk of reactivation of hepatitis B virus (HBV) infection in patients who are chronic carriers of this virus (i.e., hepatitis B surface antigen-positive [HBsAg-positive]). HBV reactivation has resulted in death in a few individuals receiving TNF blocking agent therapy. Most patients experiencing HBV reactivation were receiving concomitant therapy with other immunosuppressive agents; use of multiple immunosuppressive agents may have contributed to HBV reactivation.

Screen all patients for HBV infection before initiation of certolizumab pegol therapy. In patients who test positive for HBV infection, consultation with an HBV infection specialist is recommended before initiation of TNF blocking agent therapy. Chronic carriers of HBV should be appropriately evaluated and monitored prior to the initiation of therapy, during treatment, and for up to several months following therapy with certolizumab pegol. Safety and efficacy of antiviral therapy for prevention of viral reactivation in HBV carriers receiving a TNF blocking agent have not been established. Discontinue certolizumab pegol if HBV reactivation occurs, and initiate appropriate treatment, including antiviral therapy. It has not been established whether certolizumab pegol can be safely readministered once control of the reactivated HBV infection has been achieved; caution is advised if certolizumab pegol therapy is resumed in such a situation.

Nervous System Effects

New onset or exacerbation of clinical manifestations and/or radiographic evidence of central or peripheral nervous system demyelinating disorders (e.g., multiple sclerosis, Guillain-Barré syndrome) has been reported rarely in patients receiving TNF blocking agents, including certolizumab pegol. Clinicians should exercise caution when considering certolizumab pegol therapy in patients with preexisting or recent-onset central or peripheral nervous system demyelinating disorders.

Seizure disorder, optic neuritis, and peripheral neuropathy also have been reported rarely.

Hematologic Effects

Pancytopenia, including aplastic anemia, has been reported rarely in patients receiving TNF blocking agents. Adverse hematologic effects, including leukopenia, pancytopenia, and thrombocytopenia, have occurred rarely in certolizumab pegol-treated patients. Whether these hematologic abnormalities are directly attributable to certolizumab pegol remains to be determined. If substantial hematologic abnormalities occur, consider discontinuance of certolizumab pegol.

Immunologic Reactions and Antibody Formation

Certolizumab pegol therapy may result in the formation of autoimmune antibodies. In clinical trials in patients with Crohn disease, 4% of those receiving certolizumab pegol developed new positive antinuclear antibodies (ANA) compared with 2% of those receiving placebo; development of ANA also has been reported in patients with rheumatoid arthritis receiving the drug. A lupus-like syndrome has occurred rarely in patients receiving certolizumab pegol. If a patient develops manifestations suggestive of a lupus-like syndrome, certolizumab pegol should be discontinued. The effect of long-term certolizumab pegol treatment on the development of autoimmune diseases remains to be determined.

Antibodies to certolizumab pegol were detected during clinical studies in about 8% of patients with Crohn disease and 7% of patients with rheumatoid arthritis who received the drug. Antibodies with neutralizing activity to certolizumab pegol were detected in about 6% of patients with Crohn disease and 3% of those with rheumatoid arthritis who received the drug. The incidence of antibody formation was lower in patients receiving concomitant therapy with other immunosuppressive agents (e.g., methotrexate) than in those not receiving immunosuppressive agents at baseline (see Drug Interactions: Methotrexate). In patients with rheumatoid arthritis, antibody formation was associated with lower plasma concentrations of certolizumab pegol and reduced efficacy (i.e., American College of Rheumatology [ACR] 20 response). Use of a loading dose of certolizumab pegol (400 mg administered every 2 weeks for 3 doses) and concomitant use of methotrexate were associated with reduced immunogenicity. In patients with Crohn disease, there was no apparent association between antibody development and efficacy or adverse events. In long-term follow-up studies (up to 7 years of exposure) in patients with Crohn disease, antibodies to certolizumab pegol were detected in 23% of patients on at least 1 occasion. Of the patients who developed antibodies, 73% had a persistent reduction in plasma drug concentration, but no association between antibody development and adverse events was observed.

In clinical studies of patients with psoriasis, antibody development was observed in 8% and 19% of patients who received certolizumab pegol 400 mg every 2 weeks and certolizumab pegol 200 mg every 2 weeks, respectively. Of the patients who developed antibodies, 45% developed neutralizing antibodies. Antibody formation was associated with lower plasma concentrations of certolizumab pegol and reduced efficacy.

In clinical studies of patients with nonradiographic axial spondyloarthritis, a more sensitive assay was used to test for antibodies to certolizumab pegol, resulting in a greater proportion of samples having measurable antibodies to certolizumab pegol. After 52 weeks of treatment, 97% of patients were positive for antibodies against certolizumab pegol. Higher antibody titers were associated with reduced plasma concentrations of certolizumab pegol.

Immunization

Live vaccines should be avoided during therapy with certolizumab pegol. Information is not available regarding whether certolizumab pegol would affect the rate of secondary transmission of infection following administration of a live vaccine or regarding the effects of vaccination with live vaccine in patients receiving the drug.

In patients with rheumatoid arthritis, no difference in immune response to pneumococcal polysaccharide vaccine or influenza virus vaccine was detected between patients receiving the vaccines concurrently with certolizumab pegol and those receiving the vaccines with placebo; similar proportions of placebo- and certolizumab pegol-treated patients developed protective antibody titers. However, patients receiving methotrexate concomitantly with certolizumab pegol had a lower immune response to the vaccines than did those receiving certolizumab pegol alone; the clinical importance of this finding is not known.

Immunosuppression

Safety and efficacy of certolizumab pegol in patients with immunosuppression have not been evaluated.

Psoriasis

In controlled clinical studies of certolizumab pegol in patients with plaque psoriasis, changes in psoriasis subtypes (e.g., erythrodermic, pustular, guttate) were observed in less than 1% of patients. Cases of new-onset psoriasis, including pustular and palmoplantar psoriasis, have been reported with the use of TNF blocking agents. In August 2009, FDA reported the results of a review of 69 cases of new-onset psoriasis,

including pustular (17 cases) and palmoplantar (15 cases) psoriasis, in patients receiving TNF blocking agents for the management of autoimmune and rheumatic conditions other than psoriasis and psoriatic arthritis. None of the patients reported having psoriasis prior to initiation of the TNF blocking agent. However, exacerbation of preexisting psoriasis has been reported with the use of TNF blocking agents. Two of the 69 cases of new-onset psoriasis included in FDA's review occurred in pediatric patients. The development of psoriasis during treatment with TNF blocking agents occurred at intervals ranging from weeks to years following initiation of the drug. Twelve of the psoriasis cases resulted in hospitalization, which was the most severe outcome reported. Most patients experienced improvement of their psoriasis following discontinuance of the TNF blocking agent. Due to the number of reported cases and the temporal relationship between the initiation of TNF blocking agents and the development of psoriasis, FDA has concluded that there is a possible association between the development of psoriasis and use of TNF blocking agents. Clinicians should consider the possibility of and monitor for manifestations (e.g., new rash) of new or worsening psoriasis, particularly pustular and palmoplantar psoriasis, during treatment with TNF blocking agents.

Specific Populations

Pregnancy

Limited data from an ongoing pregnancy registry are insufficient to inform a risk of major birth defects or other adverse pregnancy outcomes with use of certolizumab during pregnancy. However, there is some evidence suggesting that placental transfer of the drug is low or negligible in most infants at birth. No adverse developmental effects were observed in animal reproduction studies during which pregnant rats were administered an IV rodent anti-murine TNFα pegylated Fab' fragment similar to certolizumab pegol during organogenesis at up to 2.4 times the recommended human dosage of 400 mg every 4 weeks.

There are risks to the mother and fetus associated with active rheumatoid arthritis or Crohn disease, including increased risks of fetal loss, preterm delivery, low birth weight, and small for gestational age. Certolizumab pegol administered during pregnancy may affect immune responses in the in utero-exposed newborn and infant. Data from an exposed infant suggest that certolizumab pegol may be eliminated at a slower rate in infants than in adults. The safety of administering live or live-attenuated vaccines in exposed infants is unknown. The theoretical risks of live or live-attenuated vaccines to infants exposed to certolizumab pegol in utero should be weighed against the benefits of vaccinations.

A pregnancy registry has been established to monitor fetal outcomes in pregnant women exposed to certolizumab pegol; patients or clinicians may contact the registry at 877-311-8972 or visit https://mothertobaby.org/pregnancy-studies/ to report any exposures to the drug that occur during pregnancy.

Lactation

In a multicenter clinical study of 17 lactating women treated with certolizumab pegol 200 mg every 2 weeks or 400 mg every 4 weeks, minimal drug concentrations were observed in breast milk. No serious adverse reactions were noted in the 17 infants in the study. There are no data on the effects of certolizumab pegol on milk production. In a separate study, certolizumab pegol concentrations were not detected in the plasma of 9 breastfed infants at 4 weeks postpartum.

Consider the developmental and health benefits of breastfeeding along with the mother's clinical need for certolizumab pegol and any potential adverse effects on the breastfed infant from the drug or from the underlying maternal condition.

Pediatric Use

Safety and efficacy of certolizumab pegol have not been established in pediatric patients.

Malignancies, some fatal, have been reported in children and adolescents who received treatment with TNF blocking agents.

Neonates and infants who were exposed to certolizumab pegol in utero may have impaired immune responses. Although certolizumab pegol concentrations were low or negligible in most in utero-exposed infants at birth, the clinical importance of these undetectable or low drug concentrations is unknown. Data from one exposed infant suggested that the drug may be eliminated more slowly in infants than in adults. The safety of administering live or live-attenuated vaccines in exposed infants is unknown. The theoretical risks of live or live-attenuated vaccines to infants exposed to certolizumab pegol in utero should be weighed against the benefits of vaccinations.

Geriatric Use

The manufacturer states that clinical studies of certolizumab pegol did not include a sufficient number of patients ≥65 years of age to determine whether such patients respond differently than younger individuals, but other reported clinical experience has not identified differences in response between geriatric and younger patients. The pharmacokinetic profile in geriatric adults does not appear to differ from that in younger adults. Because the overall incidence of infection is higher in the geriatric population than in younger adults, use certolizumab pegol with caution in geriatric patients.

Renal Impairment

The effect of renal impairment on the pharmacokinetics of certolizumab pegol has not been specifically studied to date; however, the pharmacokinetics of the polyethylene glycol fraction of the drug are expected to be dependent on renal function. The manufacturer states that data are insufficient to provide dosage recommendations for patients with moderate to severe renal impairment.

● Common Adverse Effects

Adverse effects reported in ≥7% of patients receiving certolizumab pegol include upper respiratory infection, rash, and urinary tract infection.

DRUG INTERACTIONS

● Biologic Antirheumatic Agents

Concomitant use of certolizumab pegol and other biologic disease-modifying antirheumatic drugs (DMARDs) is not recommended because of the possibility of an increased risk of infection.

Exercise caution when switching from one biologic DMARD to another, since overlapping biologic activity may further increase the risk of infection.

Abatacept

When abatacept and a tumor necrosis factor (TNF; TNF-α) blocking agent were used concomitantly, an increased incidence of serious infection was observed, with no additional benefit. Concomitant use of certolizumab pegol and abatacept is not recommended.

Anakinra

When anakinra (a human interleukin-1 receptor antagonist) and etanercept (another TNF blocking agent) were used concomitantly in patients with active rheumatoid arthritis, an increased incidence of serious infection and increased risk of neutropenia were observed, with no substantial improvement in efficacy over that observed with etanercept alone. Similar toxicities would be expected with concomitant use of anakinra and other TNF blocking agents, including certolizumab pegol. Concomitant use of certolizumab pegol and anakinra is not recommended.

Rituximab

Formal drug interaction studies between rituximab and certolizumab pegol have not been performed; however, concomitant use of these drugs is not recommended since such use may result in increased risk of serious infection.

● Methotrexate

Methotrexate has been used concomitantly with certolizumab pegol in clinical studies. Methotrexate pharmacokinetics were not altered by certolizumab pegol administration in patients with rheumatoid arthritis; the effect of methotrexate on certolizumab pharmacokinetics was not determined.

In placebo-controlled studies in patients with rheumatoid arthritis, use of methotrexate concomitantly with certolizumab pegol was associated with reduced immunogenicity. The incidence of formation of antibodies to certolizumab pegol was lower in those receiving the drug in conjunction with methotrexate than in those not receiving immunosuppressive agents at baseline. The rate of neutralizing antibody formation also was lower in those receiving certolizumab pegol and methotrexate than in those receiving certolizumab pegol alone. In patients with rheumatoid arthritis, antibody formation was associated with lower plasma concentrations and reduced efficacy of certolizumab.

● Natalizumab

Formal drug interaction studies between natalizumab and certolizumab pegol have not been performed; however, concomitant use may result in increased risk of serious infections and is not recommended.

● Vaccines

Live vaccines should not be administered to patients receiving certolizumab pegol. Information is not available regarding whether certolizumab pegol would affect the rate of secondary transmission of infection following administration of a live vaccine or regarding the effects of vaccination with live vaccine in patients receiving the drug. The safety of administering live or live-attenuated vaccines in exposed infants is unknown. Neonates and infants who were exposed to certolizumab pegol in utero may have impaired immune responses. Although certolizumab pegol concentrations were low or negligible in most in utero-exposed infants at birth, the clinical importance is unknown. The theoretical risks of live or live-attenuated vaccines to infants exposed to certolizumab pegol in utero should be weighed against the benefits of vaccinations.

In patients with rheumatoid arthritis, no difference in immune response to pneumococcal polysaccharide vaccine or influenza virus vaccine was detected between patients receiving the vaccines concurrently with certolizumab pegol and those receiving the vaccines with placebo; similar proportions of placebo- and certolizumab pegol-treated patients developed protective antibody titers. However, patients receiving methotrexate concomitantly with certolizumab pegol had a lower immune response to the vaccines than did those receiving certolizumab pegol alone; the clinical importance of this finding is not known.

● Laboratory Test Interferences

Erroneously elevated activated partial thromboplastin time (aPTT) assay results may be reported in certolizumab pegol-treated patients who do not have coagulation abnormalities; use of certolizumab pegol does not appear to affect thrombin time (TT) or prothrombin time (PT). There is no evidence that certolizumab pegol has any effect on blood coagulation in vivo.

DESCRIPTION

Certolizumab pegol is a recombinant humanized Fab′ fragment of an anti-tumor necrosis factor (TNF; TNF-α) monoclonal antibody conjugated to an approximately 40-kilodalton polyethylene glycol (PEG2MAL40K). Therapeutic use of Fabs have been limited by their short half-lives; attachment of a polyethylene glycol moiety to the Fab′ fragment increases the half-life of certolizumab to a value similar to that of a whole antibody product.

Certolizumab pegol binds with high affinity to TNF-α, a cytokine involved in the regulation of immune response. The drug does not contain a fragment crystallizable (Fc) region; certolizumab pegol does not induce complement activation, antibody-dependent cellular cytotoxicity, apoptosis, or neutrophil degranulation in vitro.

Following subcutaneous administration, the bioavailability of certolizumab pegol is approximately 80%. Peak serum concentrations are achieved between 54 and 171 hours. The route of elimination for certolizumab pegol has not been studied in human subjects, but the polyethylene glycol moiety is principally excreted in urine. The half-life of certolizumab pegol is approximately 14 days. Clearance of certolizumab pegol is increased in patients with certolizumab pegol antibodies.

ADVICE TO PATIENTS

- Importance of advising patients about potential benefits and risks of certolizumab pegol. Importance of patients reading the manufacturer's patient information (medication guide) prior to initiation of therapy and before each injection of the drug.

- Importance of instructing patient and/or caregiver regarding proper dosage and administration of certolizumab pegol, including the use of aseptic technique, and proper disposal of needles and syringes if it is determined that the patient and/or caregiver is competent to safely administer the drug.

- Increased susceptibility to infection. Importance of informing clinicians promptly if any signs or symptoms suggestive of infection (e.g., persistent fever, sweating, cough, dyspnea, fatigue) occur. Importance of informing health care providers about any ongoing active infections.

- Risk of lymphoma, including hepatosplenic T-cell lymphoma, leukemia, and other malignancies with use of TNF blocking agents. Importance of informing patients and caregivers about the increased risk of cancer development in children, adolescents, and young adults, taking into account the clinical utility of TNF blocking agents, the relative risks and benefits of these and other immunosuppressive drugs, and the risks associated with untreated disease. Importance of promptly informing clinicians if signs and symptoms of malignancies (e.g., unexplained weight loss; fatigue; abdominal pain; persistent fever; night sweats; easy bruising or bleeding; swollen lymph nodes in the neck, underarm, or groin; hepatomegaly or splenomegaly) occur.

- Importance of informing clinician of any new or worsening medical conditions (e.g., heart failure, neurologic disease [e.g., demyelinating disorders], autoimmune disorders [e.g., lupus-like syndrome], cytopenias, psoriasis).

- Importance of informing latex-sensitive patients that the needle shield inside the removable cap of the certolizumab pegol prefilled syringe contains a derivative of natural rubber latex.

- Importance of promptly contacting a clinician if manifestations of an allergic reaction (e.g., urticaria, facial swelling, difficulty breathing) occur.

- Importance of taking the drug as prescribed and of not altering or discontinuing therapy without first consulting with a clinician.

- Importance of informing clinicians of existing or contemplated concomitant therapy, including prescription and OTC drugs, as well as any concomitant illnesses or any history of cancer, tuberculosis, HBV infection, or other chronic or recurrent infections.

- Importance of women informing clinicians if they are or plan to become pregnant or plan to breast-feed.

- Importance of informing patients of other important precautionary information. (See Cautions.)

PREPARATIONS

Excipients in commercially available drug preparations may have clinically important effects in some individuals; consult specific product labeling for details.

Certolizumab Pegol

Parenteral		
For injection, for subcutaneous use	200 mg	Cimzia® (available as single-dose vial), UCB
Injection, for subcutaneous use	200 mg/mL	Cimzia® (available as single-dose syringe), UCB

† Use is not currently included in the labeling approved by the US Food and Drug Administration.

Selected Revisions May 10, 2024, © Copyright, December 1, 2008, American Society of Health-System Pharmacists, Inc.

Etanercept

90:24.16.92 • TUMOR NECROSIS FACTOR INHIBITORS, MISCELLANEOUS

■ Etanercept, a recombinant soluble dimeric fusion protein, is a tumor necrosis factor (TNF) inhibitor that is a biologic disease-modifying antirheumatic drug (DMARD).

USES

● Rheumatoid Arthritis

Etanercept is used for the management of the signs and symptoms of rheumatoid arthritis, to induce a major clinical response, to improve physical function, and to inhibit progression of structural damage associated with the disease in adults with moderate to severe active rheumatoid arthritis. Etanercept therapy can be used alone or in combination with methotrexate. Safety and efficacy of etanercept for rheumatoid arthritis are based on the results of several randomized controlled trials and long-term extension studies. Guidelines generally support the use of tumor necrosis factor (TNF; TNF-α) blocking agents, including etanercept, as add-on therapy to methotrexate in patients who do not meet treatment goals with methotrexate alone.

Clinical Experience

Clinical evaluations of etanercept have shown that dosages of 50 mg once weekly or 25 mg twice weekly are more effective than placebo in the treatment of rheumatoid arthritis. In addition, data suggest that etanercept is at least as effective as methotrexate for the management of rheumatoid arthritis in adults. Clinical evaluations of etanercept indicate that combination therapy with methotrexate is more effective than therapy with either agent alone. Response to etanercept can occur within 1–2 weeks following initiation of therapy and maximum improvement usually is achieved within 3 months in adults. Durable responses have been maintained for up to 60 months in adults receiving etanercept, with some patients maintaining response for up to 10 years. Some adults receiving etanercept in conjunction with methotrexate or corticosteroids have maintained clinical response following dosage reduction or discontinuance of concomitant corticosteroid and/or methotrexate therapy. Symptoms of arthritis generally return within 1 month following discontinuance of etanercept; however, in patients who have discontinued etanercept therapy for up to 18 months, reintroduction of the drug has been associated with the same magnitude of symptomatic response as that observed in patients who received continuous therapy. Therapy with etanercept reduces the number of swollen and tender joints, pain, and duration of morning stiffness, improves quality of life, and reduces disease activity as assessed by laboratory measures (i.e., erythrocyte sedimentation rate [ESR], c-reactive protein [CRP]).

Therapy with a Single Disease-modifying Antirheumatic Drug

Etanercept has been evaluated for the management of rheumatoid arthritis in several double-blind, placebo-controlled studies in adults with active disease (American Rheumatism Association criteria for rheumatoid arthritis with American College of Rheumatology [ACR] functional class I, II, or III) who had not responded adequately to one or more disease-modifying antirheumatic drugs (DMARDs) (i.e., hydroxychloroquine, oral or injectable gold, methotrexate, azathioprine, penicillamine, sulfasalazine). Etanercept also has been evaluated in an active-controlled phase 3 study in adults with early active rheumatoid arthritis (i.e., duration 3 years or less) who had never received therapy with methotrexate. Adults included in these studies had 12 or more tender joints, 10 or more swollen joints, and either an ESR of 28 mm/hour or greater, a CRP of 2 mg/dL or greater, or morning stiffness for 45 minutes or longer. Patients receiving stable dosages of nonsteroidal anti-inflammatory agents (NSAIAs) and/or prednisone (10 mg daily or less) at study enrollment could continue such agents during these studies.

The ACR criteria for improvement (ACR response) in measures of disease activity was used as the principal measure of clinical response in studies evaluating the efficacy of etanercept. An ACR 20 response is achieved if the patient experiences a 20% improvement in tender and swollen joint count and a 20% or greater improvement in at least 3 of the following criteria: patient pain assessment, patient global assessment, physician global assessment, patient self-assessed disability, or laboratory measures of disease activity (i.e., ESR or CRP level). ACR 50 and ACR 70 responses are defined using the same criteria with a level of improvement of 50 and 70%, respectively. Major clinical response is defined as achieving an ACR 70 response for a continuous 6-month period. Physical function and disability were assessed using the Health Assessment Questionnaire (HAQ). The Sharp score, a composite score of erosions and joint space narrowing in hands, wrists, and forefeet, was used as the principal measure of structural damage.

In a randomized, placebo-controlled phase 3 study in 234 adults with active rheumatoid arthritis who had not responded adequately to one or more (up to 4) DMARDs, an ACR 20, 50, or 70 was achieved in 62, 41, or 15% of patients, respectively, who received etanercept (25 mg subcutaneously twice weekly) for 3 months, compared with 23, 8, or 4%, respectively, of placebo-treated patients. At 6 months, an ACR 20, 50, or 70 was achieved in 59, 40, or 15%, respectively, of patients who received etanercept compared with 11, 5, or 1%, respectively, of patients who received placebo. Evaluation at 3 months indicated that etanercept therapy was associated with greater decreases in the number of tender joints (from 31.2 at baseline to 10), number of swollen joints (from 23.5 at baseline to 12.6), pain (from 6.9 at baseline to 2.4), HAQ disability index (from 1.6 at baseline to 1), ESR (from 28 mm/hour at baseline to 15.5 mm/hour), and CRP (from 3.5 mg/dL at baseline to 0.9 mg/dL) and greater improvement in physician and patient assessments (from 7 at baseline to 3; sliding scale from 10 [worst] to 0 [best]) than placebo; results at 6 months were essentially the same as those at 3 months. When patients in this study were stratified according to age, results indicated that etanercept was as effective in geriatric patients ≥65 years of age as in younger adults.

In another randomized, placebo-controlled study in 180 adults with active rheumatoid arthritis who had not responded adequately to one or more DMARDs, therapy with etanercept (16 mg/m² subcutaneously twice weekly) for 3 months was associated with an ACR 20 or 50 in 75 or 57% of patients, respectively; an ACR 20 or 50 was reported in 14 or 7%, respectively, of placebo-treated patients.

Efficacy of etanercept compared with methotrexate has been evaluated in a study that included 632 adults with early active rheumatoid arthritis (i.e., duration 3 years or less) who had not previously received methotrexate; patients in this study were randomized to receive etanercept or methotrexate for 12 months. In those receiving etanercept (25 mg subcutaneously twice weekly), an ACR 20, 50, or 70 was achieved in 65, 40, or 21% of patients, respectively, at 6 months and in 72, 49, or 25% of patients, respectively, at 12 months. In patients receiving methotrexate (7.5 mg once weekly initially increased over the first 8 weeks of the study to a maximum of 20 mg once weekly), an ACR 20, 50, or 70 was achieved in 58, 32, or 14% of patients, respectively, at 6 months and in 65, 43, or 22% of patients, respectively, at 12 months. ACR response rates were maintained through 24 months of therapy with etanercept. A major clinical response was achieved in 23% of patients receiving etanercept over the 24-month study period. Etanercept therapy was associated with reductions in the HAQ disability index (from 1.5 at baseline to 0.7 at 6 months). Radiographic analysis at months 6, 12, and 24 indicated that etanercept was at least as effective as methotrexate in delaying joint damage. Inhibition of progression of structural damage was maintained through month 60 in some etanercept-treated patients.

Combination Therapy with Methotrexate

Etanercept can be used in combination with methotrexate for the management of rheumatoid arthritis in adults who have not responded adequately to methotrexate therapy.

Results of a randomized controlled study in adults who had persistently active rheumatoid arthritis despite methotrexate therapy indicated that addition of etanercept to the regimen was associated with greater clinical benefit than use of methotrexate alone. Patients included in the study had received methotrexate for at least 6 months (stable dosage of 12.5–25 mg/week for the preceding 4 weeks) and had 6 or more tender or painful joints. Patients receiving stable dosages of NSAIAs and/or prednisone (10 mg daily or less) at study enrollment could continue such agents during the study. In patients receiving etanercept (25 mg subcutaneously twice weekly) in combination with their usual methotrexate dosage, an ACR 20 was achieved in 66 or 71% of patients at 3 or 6 months, respectively; an ACR 50 was achieved in 42 or 39% at 3 or 6 months, respectively; and an ACR 70 was achieved in 15% of patients at 3 and 6 months. In patients who continued to receive methotrexate alone, an ACR 20 was achieved in 33 or 27% of patients at 3 or 6 months, respectively, and an ACR 50 was attained in 0 or 3% of patients at

3 or 6 months, respectively. At 6 months, the HAQ disability index had decreased from 1.5 at baseline to 0.9 in patients receiving etanercept in combination with methotrexate.

Etanercept also has been evaluated in adults with active rheumatoid arthritis (mean duration: 7 years) who had not responded adequately to at least one DMARD other than methotrexate. Patients were randomized to receive etanercept (25 mg subcutaneously twice weekly), methotrexate (7.5 mg once weekly, increased up to 20 mg once weekly), or etanercept in conjunction with methotrexate. Patients who previously received methotrexate were included in the study provided they had not received the drug within 6 months of study enrollment and had not experienced clinically important toxicity or lack of response to the drug. In this study, treatment with etanercept in conjunction with methotrexate was more effective in reducing disease activity, improving physical function, and slowing radiographic progression than treatment with etanercept or methotrexate alone. At 12 months, an ACR 20, 50, or 70 was achieved in 66, 43, or 22%, respectively, of patients receiving etanercept; in 59, 36, or 17%, respectively, of those receiving methotrexate; and in 75, 63, or 40%, respectively, of those receiving etanercept in conjunction with methotrexate. A major clinical response was achieved in 10, 6, or 24% of those receiving etanercept, methotrexate, or etanercept in conjunction with methotrexate, respectively. All regimens were associated with improvement from baseline in HAQ score. Improvement in HAQ score of at least 1 unit was achieved in 40, 29, or 51% of patients receiving etanercept, methotrexate, or etanercept in conjunction with methotrexate, respectively. There was more progression of joint damage from baseline in the group of patients who received etanercept or methotrexate alone compared with those who received etanercept in conjunction with methotrexate.

Clinical Perspective

The American College of Rheumatology issued guidelines for the treatment of rheumatoid arthritis in 2021. Disease-modifying treatments for rheumatoid arthritis include conventional DMARDs (e.g., hydroxychloroquine, leflunomide, methotrexate, sulfasalazine), biologic DMARDs (e.g., TNF blocking agents, abatacept, tocilizumab, sarilumab, rituximab), and/or targeted synthetic DMARDs (e.g., Janus kinase inhibitors). Specific agents for rheumatoid arthritis treatment are selected according to current disease activity, prior therapies used, and the presence of comorbidities. A "treat-to-target" approach is typically employed, with the goal of achieving a predefined target of low disease activity or remission.

TNF blocking agents used in the treatment of rheumatoid arthritis include adalimumab, certolizumab pegol, etanercept, golimumab, and infliximab. Methotrexate monotherapy is strongly recommended over biologic DMARD monotherapy and conditionally recommended over the combination of methotrexate and a TNF blocking agent for DMARD-naive patients with moderate to high disease activity because many patients will achieve their treatment goal with methotrexate alone, and combination therapy with TNF blocking agents may be associated with additional risks and costs. Biologic DMARDs (including TNF blocking agents) and targeted synthetic DMARDs are conditionally recommended as add-on therapy for patients who are taking maximally tolerated dosages of methotrexate and are not at target. Recommendations for the use and selection of biologic DMARDs in rheumatoid arthritis vary based on the presence of certain comorbidities (e.g., heart failure, previous serious infection, nontuberculous mycobacterial lung disease). Consult the American College of Rheumatology guidelines for additional details.

● Polyarticular Juvenile Idiopathic Arthritis

Etanercept is used for the management of the signs and symptoms of moderate to severe active polyarticular juvenile idiopathic arthritis (formerly known as juvenile rheumatoid arthritis) in pediatric patients ≥2 years of age. Safety and efficacy of etanercept for this use are based principally on the results of a 2-part clinical study and an open-label extension study. Guidelines generally support the use of TNF blocking agents, including etanercept, as add-on therapy in patients with juvenile idiopathic arthritis and moderate to high disease activity despite use of methotrexate.

Clinical Experience

Etanercept was evaluated in pediatric patients 4–17 years of age with juvenile idiopathic arthritis in a 2-part study. Patients enrolled in this study had moderate to severe active polyarticular course juvenile idiopathic arthritis who had not responded adequately to or were intolerant of methotrexate. Methotrexate

was discontinued, but those receiving stable dosages of NSAIAs and/or prednisone (≤0.2 mg/kg daily; maximum 10 mg daily) at study enrollment could continue these drugs during the study. In part 1 (open-label study), patients (median age: 11 years, range: 4–17 years, mean disease duration: 5.9 years, 62% female, 75% white) with juvenile idiopathic arthritis received etanercept 0.4 mg/kg (up to 25 mg per dose) subcutaneously twice weekly for 90 days. In part 2 (placebo-controlled study), patients with a clinical response at day 90 were randomized to continue etanercept or receive placebo for 4 months.

The principal measure of clinical response in part 1 of this study was the juvenile idiopathic arthritis definition of improvement (i.e., 30% or greater improvement in at least 3 of 6 and 30% or greater deterioration in no more than 1 of 6 core set criteria that include physician and patient/parent global assessments, active joint count, limitation of motion, functional assessment, and ESR). In part 2, disease activity was assessed by disease flare (defined as a 30% or greater deterioration in 3 of 6 and a 30% or greater improvement in no more than 1 of 6 core set criteria and a minimum of 2 active joints).

Evaluation at 3 months (i.e., completion of part 1) indicated that clinical response was achieved in 74% of pediatric patients receiving etanercept. Response to etanercept was observed within 2 weeks following initiation of therapy. Of those patients who responded (i.e., study part 2), 24% of patients remaining on etanercept experienced disease flare compared with 77% of patients who switched to placebo. The median time to disease flare was 116 days or longer in patients receiving etanercept or 28 days in placebo-treated patients. Some data suggest that the incidence of flare may be higher in patients with a higher baseline ESR. Each component of the juvenile idiopathic arthritis core set criteria deteriorated in patients receiving placebo and remained stable or improved in patients receiving etanercept. In patients with a clinical response at month 3, continued etanercept therapy was associated with further improvement up to 7 months in some patients while patients receiving placebo did not improve. Durable responses were maintained for up to 48 months in most pediatric patients receiving continuous etanercept treatment, and responses have been maintained for up to 8 years in some patients. In pediatric patients who experienced disease flare while receiving placebo in part 2, reintroduction of etanercept within 4 months was associated with positive clinical response in most patients. The effect of continued etanercept therapy in pediatric patients with polyarticular juvenile idiopathic arthritis who did not respond within 3 months of initiating such therapy has not been determined.

A randomized placebo-controlled trial compared etanercept (0.8 mg/kg per week, up to 50 mg weekly) plus methotrexate (10–15 mg/week) to placebo plus methotrexate in 68 patients 2–17 years of age with polyarticular juvenile idiopathic arthritis. Treatment with etanercept plus methotrexate resulted in a higher response rate than treatment with placebo plus methotrexate.

Clinical Perspective

The American College of Rheumatology and the Arthritis Foundation issued a joint guideline for the treatment of juvenile idiopathic arthritis manifesting as nonsystemic polyarthritis (including polyarticular disease), sacroiliitis, or enthesitis in 2019. Several drug classes are used to treat juvenile idiopathic arthritis, including NSAIAs, systemic and intra-articular corticosteroids, conventional DMARDs (e.g., methotrexate, sulfasalazine, hydroxychloroquine, leflunomide), and biologic DMARDs (e.g., TNF blocking agents, abatacept, tocilizumab, rituximab). Specific agents for juvenile idiopathic arthritis treatment are selected according to the presence of certain risk factors (e.g., positive anti-cyclic citrullinated peptide antibodies, positive rheumatoid factor, joint damage), level of disease activity, involvement of specific joints, presence of certain comorbidities (e.g., uveitis), and prior therapies used. An individualized "treat-to-target" approach is typically employed, with the goal of achieving remission or minimal/low disease activity.

TNF blocking agents used in the treatment of juvenile idiopathic arthritis include adalimumab, etanercept, golimumab, and infliximab. Methotrexate monotherapy is conditionally recommended as initial therapy for patients with juvenile idiopathic arthritis manifesting as nonsystemic polyarthritis, although initial biologic DMARD therapy may be considered for patients with risk factors and involvement of high-risk joints (e.g., cervical spine, wrist, hip), high disease activity, and/or those judged by their physician to be at high risk of disabling joint damage. In patients with moderate or high disease activity despite methotrexate monotherapy, biologic DMARDs (including TNF blocking agents) are conditionally recommended as add-on therapy. In patients with moderate or high disease activity despite treatment with a first TNF blocking agent (with or without concomitant conventional DMARD therapy), switching to tocilizumab or abatacept is conditionally recommended over switching to a different TNF blocking agent, although a different TNF blocking agent may be appropriate if the patient experienced a good initial response to their first TNF blocking agent. In all patients initiating biologic DMARD therapy, combination therapy with a conventional DMARD is recommended over biologic DMARD monotherapy. Specific choice of biologic DMARD may be influenced by the presence of certain comorbidities (e.g., uveitis). Consult the American College of Rheumatology/Arthritis Foundation guidelines for additional details.

● Psoriatic Arthritis

Etanercept is used alone or in combination with methotrexate for the management of the signs and symptoms of active psoriatic arthritis in adults, to improve physical function, and to inhibit progression of structural damage associated with the disease. Safety and efficacy of etanercept for this use are based on the results of randomized controlled trials. Guidelines generally support the use of TNF blocking agents, including etanercept, as first-line treatment in patients with active psoriatic arthritis.

Clinical Experience

Etanercept has been evaluated for the management of psoriatic arthritis in a randomized, double-blind, placebo-controlled study in adults with active psoriatic arthritis (3 or more swollen joints and 3 or more tender joints) in one of the following forms: distal interphalangeal involvement; polyarticular arthritis; arthritis mutilans; asymmetric psoriatic arthritis; or ankylosing spondylitis-like. Patients also had plaque psoriasis with a qualifying target lesion (diameter of 2 cm or greater). Patients receiving stable dosages of methotrexate (25 mg/week or less) at study enrollment could continue receiving the drug during the study. The ACR criteria for improvement in measures of disease activity was used to measure clinical response and the Psoriasis Area and Severity Index (PASI) was used to evaluate skin lesions. Physical function and disability were assessed using the HAQ and the Short Form-36 (SF-36) Survey. A modified total Sharp score which included distal interphalangeal joints was used as the principal measure of structural damage. At 6 months, an ACR 20, 50, or 70 was achieved in 50, 37, or 9%, respectively, of patients who received etanercept (25 mg subcutaneously twice weekly) compared with 13, 4, or 1%, respectively, of patients receiving placebo. At 6 months, 47 or 23% of etanercept-treated patients achieved a 50 or 75% improvement in PASI, respectively, compared with 18 or 3% of placebo-treated patients, respectively. ACR and PASI responses in patients not receiving methotrexate were similar to the responses in those receiving methotrexate; ACR responses in patients with each of the subtypes of psoriatic arthritis (only a few patients had the arthritis mutilans or ankylosing spondylitis-like subtypes) were similar. Etanercept therapy was associated with greater improvement from baseline in the HAQ disability index and the SF-36 physical component summary score at 3 and 6 months compared with placebo. Most patients in this study had little or no change in the modified total Sharp score during the 24-month study. At 12 months, more placebo-treated patients (12%) had increases of 3 or more points in the total Sharp score than etanercept-treated patients (0%). Inhibition of progression of structural damage was maintained during the second year in etanercept-treated patients.

In another double-blind, placebo-controlled study in adults with active psoriatic arthritis, 87% of patients who received etanercept (25 mg subcutaneously twice weekly for 12 weeks) met the Psoriatic Arthritis Response Criteria (a composite measure of patient and clinician global assessments and tender and swollen joint scores) compared with 23% of those who received placebo. An ACR 20 was achieved in 73% of patients who received etanercept for 12 weeks compared with 13% of placebo-treated patients. In addition, etanercept improved psoriasis skin lesions in many patients.

The randomized, double-blind SEAM-PsA trial compared oral methotrexate (target dosage 20 mg weekly) plus subcutaneous etanercept (target dosage 50 mg weekly) to oral methotrexate alone and subcutaneous etanercept in 851 adults with active psoriatic arthritis and an active psoriatic skin lesion. Patients receiving etanercept plus methotrexate or etanercept alone had significantly higher ACR 20 response rates at week 24 compared to patients receiving methotrexate alone. The ACR 20 response rates at week 24 were 65%, 60.9%, and 50.7% among patients receiving combination therapy, etanercept alone, and methotrexate alone, respectively. Patient-reported outcomes (Patient Global Assessments of disease activity and joint pain, SF-36) were also improved with combination therapy or etanercept alone compared with methotrexate alone.

Clinical Perspective

The American College of Rheumatology and the National Psoriasis Foundation issued a joint guideline for the treatment of psoriatic arthritis in 2018. Various drugs and drug classes are used to treat psoriatic arthritis, with some classes used for symptom management (e.g., NSAIAs and corticosteroids) and others used as immunomodulatory disease-modifying therapy. Disease-modifying treatments for psoriatic arthritis include oral small molecules (OSMs; e.g., methotrexate, sulfasalazine, cyclosporine, leflunomide, apremilast), biologic DMARDs (e.g., TNF blocking agents, secukinumab, ixekizumab, ustekinumab, brodalumab, abatacept), and/or targeted synthetic DMARDs (e.g., tofacitinib). Specific agents for psoriatic arthritis treatment are selected according to disease characteristics, including disease severity, as well as patient preferences/values and comorbidities. A "treat-to-target" approach is typically employed, with the goal of achieving low/minimal disease activity or remission.

TNF blocking agents used in the treatment of psoriatic arthritis include adalimumab, certolizumab pegol, etanercept, golimumab, and infliximab. For patients with treatment-naive psoriatic arthritis, treatment with a TNF blocking agent is conditionally recommended over treatment with an OSM, interleukin (IL) 17 inhibitor (e.g., secukinumab, ixekizumab, brodalumab) or IL12/23 inhibitor (e.g., ustekinumab). For patients with active psoriatic arthritis despite treatment with an OSM, switching to monotherapy with a TNF blocking agent is conditionally recommended over combination therapy with a TNF blocking agent plus methotrexate or switching to another OSM, ustekinumab, secukinumab, ixekizumab, brodalumab, abatacept, or tofacitinib. For patients with active psoriatic arthritis despite treatment with TNF blocking agent monotherapy, switching to monotherapy with a different TNF blocking agent is conditionally recommended over switching to ustekinumab, secukinumab, ixekizumab, brodalumab, abatacept, or tofacitinib. For patients with active psoriatic arthritis despite treatment with a combination of a TNF blocking agent and methotrexate, switching to a different TNF blocking agent plus methotrexate is conditionally recommended over switching to a different TNF blocking agent as monotherapy. Switching to a TNF blocking agent is conditionally recommended for patients with active psoriatic arthritis despite treatment with secukinumab, ixekizumab, brodalumab, or ustekinumab. Recommendations for the use and selection of disease-modifying therapies in psoriatic arthritis vary based on the presence of certain disease characteristics (e.g., psoriatic spondylitis/axial disease, enthesitis) and comorbidities (e.g., inflammatory bowel disease, diabetes). Consult the American College of Rheumatology/National Psoriasis Foundation guideline for additional details.

● Ankylosing Spondylitis

Etanercept is used for the management of the signs and symptoms of ankylosing spondylitis in adults with active disease. Safety and efficacy of etanercept for this use are based principally on the results of a randomized controlled trial and an open-label extension study. Guidelines generally support the use of TNF blocking agents, including etanercept, for the treatment of ankylosing spondylitis in patients with active disease despite treatment with NSAIAs.

Clinical Experience

In one randomized controlled study in 277 patients with active ankylosing spondylitis, evaluation at 12 weeks indicated that improvement as assessed by a 20% improvement in the Assessment in Ankylosing Spondylitis response criteria (ASAS 20) was achieved in 60% of those receiving etanercept 25 mg twice weekly compared with 27% of those receiving placebo. Similar ASAS 20 response rates were observed in both groups at week 24. Patients receiving stable dosages of hydroxychloroquine, sulfasalazine, methotrexate, or prednisone (10 mg daily or less) at study entry could continue such agents during the study. Patients who completed this study were eligible to enroll in a long-term extension study, which found that improvements in ankylosing spondylitis signs and symptoms with etanercept treatment were maintained for up to 192 weeks.

Clinical Perspective

The American College of Rheumatology, the Spondylitis Association of America, and the Spondyloarthritis Research and Treatment Network issued a joint guideline for the treatment of ankylosing spondylitis in 2019. Treatments for ankylosing spondylitis include NSAIAs, conventional DMARDs (e.g., methotrexate, sulfasalazine), biologic DMARDs (e.g., TNF blocking agents, secukinumab, ixekizumab), and/or targeted synthetic DMARDs (e.g., tofacitinib). Continuous NSAIA treatment is typically considered first-line for active ankylosing spondylitis, with other agents used in the treatment of NSAIA-refractory disease. Specific agents for ankylosing spondylitis treatment are selected according to current disease activity, prior therapies, and the presence of comorbidities. Goals of therapy in ankylosing spondylitis are to alleviate symptoms, improve functioning, maintain the ability to work, decrease complications, and prevent or slow skeletal damage.

TNF blocking agents used in the treatment of ankylosing spondylitis include adalimumab, certolizumab pegol, etanercept, golimumab, and infliximab. For adults with active ankylosing spondylitis despite treatment with NSAIAs, treatment with a TNF blocking agent is strongly recommended over no treatment with a TNF blocking agent and conditionally recommended over treatment with tofacitinib, secukinumab, or ixekizumab. No specific TNF blocking agent is recommended over others. In patients with active ankylosing spondylitis despite treatment with a first TNF blocking agent, guidelines conditionally recommend secukinumab or ixekizumab over treatment with a different TNF blocking agent for patients with primary nonresponse to TNF blocking therapy; in patients with secondary nonresponse to TNF blocking therapy, treatment with a different TNF blocking therapy is conditionally recommended over treatment with a non-TNF blocking biologic agent. In adults with stable ankylosing spondylitis, continuation of biologic monotherapy is conditionally recommended over discontinuation of the biologic or continuation of combination therapy with NSAIAs or conventional DMARDs. Recommendations for treatment selection in ankylosing spondylitis may be influenced by the presence of certain comorbidities (e.g., iritis, inflammatory bowel disease). Consult the joint guideline issued by the American College of Rheumatology, the Spondylitis Association of America, and the Spondyloarthritis Research and Treatment Network for additional details.

● **Plaque Psoriasis**

Plaque Psoriasis in Adults

Etanercept is used for the management of moderate to severe chronic plaque psoriasis in adults who are candidates for systemic therapy or phototherapy. Safety and efficacy of etanercept for this use are based principally on the results from several randomized controlled trials. Guidelines generally support the use of TNF blocking agents, including etanercept, in moderate to severe psoriasis, either as monotherapy or in combination with topical, oral, or phototherapy.

Clinical Experience

Etanercept has been evaluated for the management of chronic plaque psoriasis in several randomized, placebo-controlled, double-blind studies in adults with chronic stable plaque psoriasis. Efficacy and safety of the drug for this indication were established in 2 of these studies (study 1 and study 2). Patients enrolled in these studies were candidates for or had previously received systemic therapy or phototherapy, had BSA involvement of at least 10%, and a score of 10 or greater (indicating moderate or severe disease) on the Psoriasis Area and Severity Index (PASI; a composite score that takes into consideration both the fraction of body surface area affected and the nature and severity of the psoriatic changes within the affected areas [e.g., induration, erythema, scaling]). Patients were randomized to receive low-dose etanercept (25 mg subcutaneously once weekly), medium-dose etanercept (25 mg subcutaneously twice weekly), high-dose etanercept (50 mg subcutaneously twice weekly), or placebo for 3 months; patients could continue therapy with the same or a different regimen during an open-label phase for an additional 3–9 months. The median baseline PASI score was 15–17; many patients (44–50% in study 1 and 72–73% in study 2) had previously received systemic therapy or phototherapy. Although concomitant use of low- or moderate-potency topical corticosteroids was permitted, use of other therapies for psoriasis was not allowed during the studies.

The primary measure of efficacy in these studies was the proportion of patients achieving a reduction in PASI score of at least 75% (PASI-75) from baseline. In study 1, 14, 32, and 47% of those receiving low-, medium-, and high-dose etanercept, respectively, achieved a PASI-75 at 3 months, compared with 4% of placebo-treated patients. In study 2, 32 and 46% of patients receiving medium- and high-dose etanercept, respectively, achieved a PASI-75 at 3 months, compared with 3% of patients receiving placebo. An additional measure of efficacy was the proportion of patients achieving a status of minimal or clear on the static Physician Global Assessment (sPGA) scale. In study 1, 21, 32, and 47% of patients receiving low-, medium-, and high-dose etanercept, respectively, achieved a status of minimal or clear at 3 months, compared with 5% of patients receiving placebo. In study 2, 37 and 54% of patients receiving medium- and high-dose etanercept, respectively, achieved a status of minimal or clear at 3 months, compared with 3%

of patients receiving placebo. Onset of PASI-75 was observed 2 months after initiation of medium- or high-dose etanercept therapy. The median duration of PASI-75 response following a 6-month course of etanercept therapy was 1–2 months. In one study, retreatment (with the same dosage used in the initial randomized period) of patients who achieved a PASI-75 response during the initial 3-month treatment phase and then discontinued therapy for up to 5 months resulted in a similar proportion of responders as observed during the initial phase of the study. In the other study, most patients (77%) who achieved a PASI-75 response after 3 months of treatment with high-dose etanercept and then received 3 months of medium-dose etanercept maintained their PASI-75 response during therapy with the medium-dose regimen.

Randomized controlled trials have compared etanercept to other TNF blocking agents (certolizumab pegol and infliximab) for the treatment of plaque psoriasis in adults. In the CIMPACT trial, certolizumab pegol 400 mg every 2 weeks was superior to etanercept (50 mg twice weekly) in terms of PASI-75 response at 12 weeks, and certolizumab pegol 200 mg every 2 weeks was noninferior to etanercept in terms of PASI-75 response at 12 weeks. In a small single-blind randomized controlled trial, infliximab (5 mg/kg IV at weeks 0, 2, and 6, then every 8 weeks thereafter) was more effective than etanercept (50 mg twice weekly) in terms of PASI-75 response at week 24.

Randomized controlled trials have also compared etanercept to other biologic agents used in plaque psoriasis. In the UNCOVER-2 and UNCOVER-3 trials, ixekizumab (160 mg once followed by 80 mg every 2 weeks or every 4 weeks) was found to be superior to etanercept (50 mg twice weekly) in terms of PASI-75 response at week 12 and sPGA status of minimal or clear at week 12. In the reSURFACE 2 trial, 2 dosages of tildrakizumab were compared to etanercept (50 mg twice weekly); tildrakizumab 200 mg at weeks 0 and 4 and every 12 weeks thereafter was superior to etanercept in terms of PASI-75 response and sPGA status of minimal or clear at week 12. While tildrakizumab 100 mg at weeks 0 and 4 and every 12 weeks thereafter was superior to etanercept in terms of PASI-75 response at week 12, sPGA status of minimal or clear at week 12 was not significantly different between these treatment groups. The FIXTURE trial compared 2 dosages of secukinumab (300 mg or 150 mg at weeks 0, 1, 2, 3, 4, and then every 4 weeks thereafter) to etanercept (50 mg twice weekly for 12 weeks, then 50 mg once weekly). Both dosages of secukinumab were found to be superior to etanercept in terms of PASI-75 response at week 12, sPGA status of minimal or clear at week 12, and maintenance of PASI-75 response from week 12 to week 52.

Clinical Perspective

The American Academy of Dermatology and the National Psoriasis Foundation have issued joint guidelines for the treatment of psoriasis in adults. Phototherapy and topical treatments (e.g., vitamin D analogues, calcineurin inhibitors, keratolytics, and corticosteroids) are frequently used to treat mild psoriasis present on limited areas of the body, but these therapies may be inadequate to obtain skin clearance in patients with more extensive or severe disease. Systemic biologic and nonbiologic therapies are mainstays of treatment for moderate to severe psoriasis, and may also be useful for treating psoriasis on parts of the body that are difficult to treat with topical therapy (e.g., scalp, palms and soles of the feet, genitals). Nonbiologic oral therapies used in the treatment of psoriasis include methotrexate, apremilast, cyclosporine, acitretin, and dimethyl fumarate. Biologics used in the treatment of psoriasis include TNF blocking agents, ustekinumab, secukinumab, ixekizumab, brodalumab, guselkumab, tildrakizumab, and risankizumab. Treatment selection is primarily based on disease characteristics (e.g., severity, location, presence of psoriatic arthritis), with additional consideration being given to patient age and comorbidities.

TNF blocking agents used in the treatment of psoriasis include adalimumab, certolizumab pegol, etanercept, and infliximab. These TNF blocking agents are recommended for the treatment of adult patients with moderate to severe plaque psoriasis, with or without concomitant topical, oral, or phototherapy. Recommendations for the use and selection of psoriasis therapies vary based on patient age, disease characteristics (e.g., severity, location, presence of psoriatic arthritis), and comorbidities (e.g., inflammatory bowel disease). Consult the American Academy of Dermatology/National Psoriasis Foundation guidelines for additional details.

Plaque Psoriasis in Pediatric Patients

Etanercept is used for the management of moderate to severe chronic plaque psoriasis in pediatric patients ≥4 years of age who are candidates for systemic therapy or phototherapy. Safety and efficacy of etanercept for this use are based principally on the results of a randomized controlled trial and an open-label extension study. Guidelines support the use of etanercept for moderate to severe psoriasis in pediatric patients ≥6 years of age.

Clinical Experience

Etanercept has been evaluated in a randomized, double-blind study in 211 pediatric patients 4–17 years of age with moderate to severe plaque psoriasis (defined as sPGA score ≥3 with BSA involvement ≥10% and PASI score ≥12). Patients enrolled in the study were candidates for systemic therapy or phototherapy, or were inadequately controlled on topical therapy. Patients were randomized to receive etanercept 0.8 mg/kg (up to 50 mg per dose) once weekly or placebo for 12 weeks. After 12 weeks, all patients entered a 24-week open-label treatment phase and received etanercept 0.8 mg/kg (up to 50 mg per dose) once weekly. Following the open-label phase, patients who had achieved a PASI-75 response at week 36 were re-randomized to either etanercept or placebo for 12 additional weeks. The median baseline PASI score was 16.4, and 57% of patients had previously received systemic or phototherapy; the baseline sPGA classifications were moderate, marked, and severe in 65, 31, and 3% of patients, respectively. The primary measure of efficacy in this study was the proportion of patients achieving a PASI-75 response at week 12. At week 12, 57 and 11% of patients receiving etanercept and placebo respectively achieved a PASI-75 response. sPGA status of "clear" or "almost clear" was attained in 52 and 13% of patients receiving etanercept and placebo, respectively. Patients receiving etanercept also experienced greater improvements in health-related quality of life (as measured by the Children's Dermatology Life Quality Index) compared to placebo-treated patients. When patients who attained a PASI-75 response with open-label etanercept were re-randomized to etanercept or placebo at week 36, patients who continued etanercept were more likely to maintain PASI-75 response at week 48 compared with those who were randomized to receive placebo. In an open-label extension study, efficacy of etanercept was maintained for up to 264 weeks.

Clinical Perspective

The American Academy of Dermatology and the National Psoriasis Foundation issued joint guidelines for the treatment of psoriasis in pediatric patients in 2019. Phototherapy and topical treatments (e.g., vitamin D analogues, calcineurin inhibitors, corticosteroids, tazarotene, anthralin, coal tar) are frequently used to treat mild psoriasis present on limited areas of the body, but these therapies may be inadequate to obtain skin clearance in patients with more extensive or severe disease. Systemic biologic and nonbiologic therapies are mainstays of treatment for moderate to severe psoriasis, and may also be useful for treating psoriasis on parts of the body that are difficult to treat with topical therapy (e.g., the scalp, palms and soles of the feet, genitals). Nonbiologic oral therapies used in the treatment of pediatric psoriasis include methotrexate, cyclosporine, acitretin, and fumaric acid esters. Biologics recommended for use in pediatric psoriasis include TNF blocking agents (etanercept, adalimumab, infliximab) and ustekinumab. Other biologic agents used in pediatric psoriasis include secukinumab and ixekizumab. Treatment selection is primarily based on disease characteristics (e.g., severity, location, presence of psoriatic arthritis), with additional consideration being given to patient age and comorbidities.

TNF blocking agents used in the treatment of pediatric psoriasis include adalimumab, etanercept, and infliximab. Etanercept is recommended in clinical practice guidelines for moderate to severe psoriasis in pediatric patients ≥6 years of age. Consult the American Academy of Dermatology/National Psoriasis Foundation guidelines for additional details.

● Juvenile Psoriatic Arthritis

Etanercept is used for the treatment of active juvenile psoriatic arthritis in pediatric patients ≥2 years of age. The efficacy of etanercept for this indication was based on clinical data in adults with psoriatic arthritis; pharmacokinetic data from adults with psoriatic arthritis, rheumatoid arthritis, and psoriasis; and pharmacokinetic data from pediatric patients with juvenile idiopathic arthritis and psoriasis. Safety was established via pediatric trials of etanercept in other approved indications including a study involving 69 pediatric patients (2-17 years of age) with moderately to severely active juvenile idiopathic arthritis, a study enrolling 211 pediatric patients (4-17 years of age) with moderate to severe psoriasis, and an open-label extension involving 182 pediatric patients (4-17 years of age) with moderate to severe psoriasis. The totality of the evidence from these data indicate

comparable trough concentrations between adults with rheumatoid arthritis and psoriatic arthritis and pediatric patients with juvenile idiopathic arthritis as well as similar trough concentrations between adults and pediatric patients with psoriasis. Pharmacokinetic exposure is expected to be similar between adults and pediatric patients with juvenile psoriatic arthritis.

● Other Uses

Nonradiographic Axial Spondyloarthritis

Etanercept may be useful for the management of nonradiographic axial spondyloarthritis†. A randomized controlled trial in 225 adults with active nonradiographic axial spondyloarthritis and inadequate response to at least 2 NSAIAs found that patients receiving etanercept 50 mg weekly were more likely to achieve a 40% improvement in the ASAS response criteria (ASAS 40) at week 12 than patients receiving placebo. At week 12, an ASAS 40 response was achieved in 32 and 16% of patients receiving etanercept and placebo, respectively. An open-label extension of this trial indicated that improvements in the signs and symptoms of nonradiographic axial spondyloarthritis were maintained for up to 104 weeks with continued etanercept treatment.

Acute Graft Versus Host Disease

Etanercept has been used for the management of acute graft versus host disease†. Two small prospective trials evaluated the use of etanercept in conjunction with corticosteroids for the initial treatment of acute graft versus host disease. One of these trials compared complete response rates following treatment with etanercept 0.4 mg/kg (up to 25 mg) twice weekly plus corticosteroids to complete response rates achieved in a contemporaneous cohort of patients receiving corticosteroids alone. Complete response rates at 4 weeks were greater among patients receiving etanercept plus corticosteroids compared with patients receiving corticosteroids alone (69 versus 33%, respectively). The other trial randomized patients to receive etanercept (0.4 mg/kg [up to 25 mg] twice weekly for 4 weeks), mycophenolate mofetil, pentostatin, or denileukin, each in combination with corticosteroids. Although the trial was not designed to compare efficacy across treatment arms, complete response rates were highest in the mycophenolate mofetil arm, followed by denileukin, pentostatin, and etanercept, respectively. Complete response rates with mycophenolate mofetil, denileukin, pentostatin, and etanercept were 67, 65, 55, and 44%, respectively, at day 28, and 82, 76, 74, and 61%, respectively, at day 56. A corticosteroid-only arm was not included in the trial.

Some small retrospective studies have evaluated the efficacy of etanercept in patients with steroid-refractory acute graft versus host disease. Overall response rates in these studies ranged from 46–81%, with the highest response rate attained in a study of patients who also received concomitant antithymocyte globulin. A 2012 guideline from the American Society of Blood and Marrow Transplantation states that monotherapy with corticosteroids remains the standard of care for initial treatment of acute graft versus host disease; for second-line therapy, data were insufficient to recommend the use or avoidance of any specific therapy, including regimens containing etanercept.

Granulomatosis with Polyangiitis

Etanercept has been investigated for the management of granulomatosis with polyangiitis†. Although etanercept was previously designated an orphan drug by the FDA for this use, the designation has since been withdrawn. In an open-label study in a limited number of patients with granulomatosis with polyangiitis who had not responded adequately to standard therapy (i.e., prednisone, cyclophosphamide, methotrexate, azathioprine, cyclosporine), addition of etanercept (25 mg subcutaneously twice weekly) for a mean of 21 weeks resulted in a positive clinical response in most patients, although limited flares and persistent minor features of active disease occurred frequently. In a randomized, placebo-controlled study in patients with granulomatosis with polyangiitis, the rates of sustained remission, sustained periods of low-level disease activity, and time needed to achieve these measures in patients receiving etanercept in combination with standard therapy (corticosteroids plus cyclophosphamide or methotrexate) were similar to those in patients who received standard therapy alone (placebo-treated patients). In addition, the relative risk of disease flares did not differ significantly between the etanercept and placebo groups. Solid malignant tumors developed in 6 of 89 etanercept-treated patients and in none of the 92 patients who received placebo. Based on results of this study and the increased incidence of malignancy associated with etanercept, some clinicians state that use of the drug to induce or maintain remissions in patients with granulomatosis with polyangiitis is not justified. The manufacturer of etanercept states that the drug is not recommended in patients with granulomatosis with polyangiitis who are receiving immunosuppressive therapy.

Crohn Disease

The manufacturer states that etanercept is not effective in the treatment of inflammatory bowel disease†. Etanercept (25 mg subcutaneously twice weekly) was not effective in reducing the signs and symptoms of Crohn disease† in a randomized, double-blind, placebo-controlled study in adults with moderate to severe disease. It is not known whether higher doses or more frequent dosing of etanercept would be effective; however, there is some evidence indicating that different TNF inhibitors may have differential effects on lesional T cells in patients with Crohn disease.

Septic Shock

Etanercept has been investigated in the treatment of septic shock†; however, at single IV infusion doses of 0.15–1.5 mg/kg, treatment with the drug did *not* reduce mortality and higher doses (0.45 and 1.5 mg/kg) appeared to be associated with increased mortality. The manufacturer states that etanercept is contraindicated in patients with sepsis.

Heart Failure

Etanercept has been investigated for the treatment of heart failure† in 2 clinical studies; these studies were terminated early because of a lack of efficacy of the drug. Results of one of the studies suggested that the mortality rate was higher in etanercept-treated patients compared with placebo recipients.

DOSAGE AND ADMINISTRATION

● General

Pretreatment Screening

- Evaluate all patients for active and latent tuberculosis prior to initiating therapy.
- Complete all age-appropriate vaccinations as recommended by current immunization guidelines prior to treatment.
- Screen at-risk patients for hepatitis B virus (HBV) infection before initiating therapy.
- Do not initiate therapy in patients with an active infection, including clinically important localized infections.

Patient Monitoring

- Periodically test all patients for active and latent tuberculosis during therapy.
- Monitor closely for signs or symptoms of infection (e.g., fever, malaise, weight loss, sweats, cough, dyspnea, pulmonary infiltrates, serious systemic illness including shock) during and after treatment.
- Perform periodic dermatologic evaluations in all patients at increased risk for skin cancer.
- Evaluate and monitor chronic carriers of HBV during treatment and for up to several months following treatment.

Dispensing and Administration Precautions

- To avoid medication errors, the Institute for Safe Medication Practices (ISMP) recommends that prescribers communicate both the brand and generic names for etanercept on the prescription order form.

Other General Considerations

- Methotrexate, glucocorticoids, salicylates, nonsteroidal anti-inflammatory agents (NSAIAs), and analgesics may be continued in adults receiving etanercept for the management of rheumatoid arthritis, ankylosing spondylitis, or psoriatic arthritis.
- Glucocorticoids, NSAIAs, and analgesics may be continued in pediatric patients with polyarticular juvenile idiopathic arthritis who are receiving etanercept.

● Administration

Etanercept is administered by subcutaneous injection. The drug is commercially available as a single-dose prefilled syringe, a single-dose prefilled SureClick® auto-injector, single-dose prefilled cartridge for use with an AutoTouch® reusable auto-injector, a single-dose vial, and a multidose vial containing lyophilized powder requiring reconstitution prior to use. The lyophilized powder is used for weight-based dosing. Etanercept is intended for use under the guidance and supervision of a clinician, but may be *self-administered* if the clinician determines that the patient and/or their caregiver is competent to prepare and safely administer the drug after appropriate training and with medical follow-up as necessary. The initial self-administered dose should be made under the supervision of a qualified healthcare provider.

Store all commercially available etanercept preparations at 2–8°C in the original carton for protection from light and physical damage. Avoid storage under conditions of extreme heat or cold, and do not shake or freeze the drug. The manufacturer states that individual single-use prefilled syringes, single-use vials, single-use prefilled cartridges, single-use prefilled auto-injectors, or dose trays containing etanercept powder for injection and diluent may be stored at room temperature (20–25°C) for a maximum single period of 14 days, with protection from light, heat, and humidity (for the powder for injection). Once the drug has been stored at room temperature, it should not be placed back in a refrigerator. If the drug is not used within 14 days when stored at room temperature, it should be discarded. Store the reusable auto-injector device at room temperature (20–25°C) and do not refrigerate.

For greater patient comfort, the etanercept single-use prefilled syringe or the dose tray containing etanercept lyophilized powder and diluent may be kept at room temperature for about 15–30 minutes prior to administration; the etanercept single-use vial may be kept at room temperature for at least 30 minutes prior to administration. The manufacturer states that the single-use prefilled cartridges and the prefilled auto-injector should be kept at room temperature for at least 30 minutes prior to administration. The needle cover should not be removed from the prefilled syringe or auto-injector until immediately prior to administration. The purple cap should not be removed from the single-use prefilled cartridge until the cartridge is inside the reusable autoinjector, immediately prior to administration; the purple cap should not be left off for more than 5 minutes prior to injection.

Reconstitute etanercept lyophilized powder by adding 1 mL of bacteriostatic water for injection (containing 0.9% benzyl alcohol) provided by the manufacturer to a vial labeled as containing 25 mg of the drug to provide a solution containing 25 mg/mL. During reconstitution, slowly add the diluent to the vial and swirl the contents gently to minimize foaming during dissolution; some foaming will occur. To avoid excessive foaming, do not shake the vial and avoid excessive or vigorous agitation. The final volume in the vial will be about 1 mL. Dissolution usually takes less than 10 minutes.

Reconstituted solutions of etanercept may be stored in the original vial at 2–8°C for up to 14 days; discard the solution if it is not used within 14 days of reconstitution. Only the volume of solution corresponding to the correct dose should be withdrawn from the vial into a syringe; some foam or bubbles may remain in the vial. Contents of one vial of etanercept solution should not be mixed with or transferred into the contents of another vial.

If only one dose is being prepared, the vial adapter supplied by the manufacturer may be used to facilitate reconstitution of the drug and withdrawal of the dose from the vial. If multiple doses are being prepared, the manufacturer states that a syringe with a 25-gauge needle should be used to reconstitute the lyophilized powder and withdraw the dose from the vial. A 27-gauge needle should be used to administer the dose.

When preparing a dose of etanercept from a single-use vial of etanercept solution, the manufacturer recommends using a 1-mL Luer-Lock syringe, a 22-gauge needle with Luer-Lock connection for withdrawal of the dose from the vial, and a 27-gauge needle with Luer-Lock connection for administration of the dose. If 2 vials are required to administer the total prescribed etanercept dose, the same syringe should be used for each vial. The single-use vials do not contain preservatives; discard any unused portion of the solution.

Etanercept solutions should not be filtered during preparation or administration. Prior to administration, inspect solutions of etanercept visually for particulate matter or discoloration. The solution may contain small, white, proteinaceous particles. Discard the solution if it is discolored or cloudy, or if foreign particulate matter is present.

Administer subcutaneous injections of etanercept into the thighs, abdomen, or upper arm. Injection sites should be rotated. Do not administer injections into areas where the skin is tender, bruised, red, or hard, or into scars, stretch marks, or psoriatic lesions.

A 50-mg dose of etanercept may be administered as a single subcutaneous injection using the 50-mg/mL prefilled syringe, the prefilled auto-injector, or the single-dose prefilled cartridge for use with a reusable autoinjector. Alternatively, a 50-mg dose may be administered as 2 subcutaneous injections using the 25 mg/0.5 mL single-dose prefilled syringes on the same day once a week or on 2 different days 3–4 days apart; a 50-mg dose can also be obtained using two 25-mg single-dose vials or two 25-mg multidose vials of lyophilized etanercept, when the multidose vials are reconstituted and administered as recommended. To achieve a dose other than 25 mg or 50 mg for a pediatric patient, the single-dose vial or the reconstituted lyophilized powder in the multidose vial may be used.

Patients and/or their caregivers should be cautioned against reuse of syringes and needles, carefully instructed on the proper, safe disposal of needles, syringes, and unused drug, and supplied with a puncture-resistant container for the proper, safe disposal of such equipment after use. For more information on preparation instructions for the various formulations of etanercept, see the prescribing information.

● Dosage

Adult Dosage

Rheumatoid Arthritis

For the management of rheumatoid arthritis in adults, the usual dosage of etanercept is 50 mg once weekly. Etanercept dosages exceeding 50 mg weekly are not recommended because of possible higher incidence of adverse effects and no additional benefit.

Psoriatic Arthritis

For the management of psoriatic arthritis in adults, the usual dosage of etanercept is 50 mg once weekly. Etanercept dosages exceeding 50 mg weekly are not recommended because of possible higher incidence of adverse effects and no additional benefit.

Ankylosing Spondylitis

For the management of ankylosing spondylitis in adults, the usual dosage of etanercept is 50 mg once weekly. Etanercept dosages exceeding 50 mg weekly are not recommended because of possible higher incidence of adverse effects and no additional benefit.

Plaque Psoriasis

For the management of plaque psoriasis in adults, the usual recommended initial dosage of etanercept is 50 mg twice weekly for 3 months. The recommended maintenance dosage is 50 mg once weekly. Initial etanercept dosages of 25 or 50 mg once weekly also have been effective. A dose-related effect was observed in clinical studies.

Pediatric Dosage

Polyarticular Juvenile Idiopathic Arthritis

For the management of polyarticular juvenile idiopathic arthritis in pediatric patients 2–17 years of age, the usual dosage of etanercept is 0.8 mg/kg once weekly (maximum dosage 50 mg once weekly) in patients who weigh <63 kg, and 50 mg once weekly in patients who weigh ≥63 kg. The 50 mg/mL prefilled syringe, prefilled single-use auto-injector, or prefilled single-use auto-injector cartridge can be used for pediatric patients weighing ≥63 kg. The manufacturer states that the 25 mg/0.5 mL prefilled syringe should not be used for pediatric patients weighing <31 kg.

Plaque Psoriasis

For the management of plaque psoriasis in pediatric patients 4–17 years of age, the usual dosage of etanercept is 0.8 mg/kg once weekly (maximum dosage 50 mg once weekly) in patients who weigh <63 kg, and 50 mg once weekly in patients who weigh ≥63 kg. The 50 mg/mL prefilled syringe, prefilled single-use auto-injector, or prefilled single-use auto-injector cartridge can be used for pediatric

patients weighing ≥63 kg. The manufacturer states that the 25 mg/0.5 mL prefilled syringe should not be used for pediatric patients weighing <31 kg.

Juvenile Psoriatic Arthritis

For the management of juvenile psoriatic arthritis in pediatric patients 2–17 years of age, the usual dosage of etanercept is 0.8 mg/kg once weekly (maximum dosage 50 mg once weekly) in patients who weigh <63 kg, and 50 mg once weekly in patients who weigh ≥63 kg. The 50 mg/mL prefilled syringe, prefilled single-use auto-injector, or prefilled single-use auto-injector cartridge can be used for pediatric patients weighing ≥63 kg. The manufacturer states that the 25 mg/0.5 mL prefilled syringe should not be used for pediatric patients weighing <31 kg.

Hepatic Impairment

No specific dosage recommendations for patients with hepatic impairment.

Renal Impairment

No specific dosage recommendations for patients with renal impairment.

Geriatric Patients

No specific dosage recommendations for geriatric patients; however, caution should be used as there is a higher incidence of infections in the geriatric population in general.

Patients with Diabetes

Hypoglycemia has been reported following initiation of etanercept in patients receiving medication for diabetes. A reduction in anti-diabetic medication may be necessary in some patients.

CAUTIONS

● Contraindications

● Sepsis.

● Warnings/Precautions

Warnings

Serious Infections

A boxed warning about the risk of serious infections is included in the prescribing information for etanercept. Patients receiving tumor necrosis factor (TNF) blocking agents, including etanercept, are at increased risk of developing serious infections involving various organ systems potentially resulting in hospitalization or death. Opportunistic infections caused by bacterial, mycobacterial, invasive fungal, viral, parasitic, or other opportunistic pathogens—including aspergillosis, blastomycosis, candidiasis, coccidioidomycosis, histoplasmosis, legionellosis, listeriosis, pneumocystosis, and tuberculosis—have been reported in patients receiving TNF blocking agents. Infections frequently have been disseminated rather than localized. Most patients who developed serious infections were receiving concomitant therapy with immunosuppressive agents such as methotrexate or corticosteroids. Monitor patients closely during and after treatment with TNF blocking agents for the development of signs or symptoms of infection (e.g., fever, malaise, weight loss, sweats, cough, dyspnea, pulmonary infiltrates, serious systemic illness including shock), including the possible development of tuberculosis in patients who tested negative for latent tuberculosis prior to initiating therapy.

Reported incidences of serious infection in controlled trials evaluating etanercept in adults with rheumatoid arthritis, psoriatic arthritis, ankylosing spondylitis, or plaque psoriasis were similar; in these trials, serious infection occurred in 1.4% of patients receiving etanercept alone or in conjunction with methotrexate, 3.6% of those receiving methotrexate, and 0.8% of those receiving placebo. Serious infections have included pyelonephritis, bronchitis, septic arthritis, abscess, cellulitis, osteomyelitis, pneumonia, sepsis, and gastroenteritis.

Tuberculosis (frequently disseminated or extrapulmonary at clinical presentation), invasive fungal infections, and other opportunistic infections also have occurred in patients receiving etanercept or other TNF blocking agents. Opportunistic infections, including atypical mycobacterial infection, herpes zoster, aspergillosis, Pneumocystis jiroveci (formerly Pneumocystis carinii) pneumonia, and other protozoal infections, have been reported during postmarketing surveillance in patients receiving etanercept.

Reactivation of latent tuberculosis and new tuberculosis infections have been reported in patients receiving TNF blocking agents, including etanercept. Although data from clinical and preclinical studies suggest that the risk of reactivation of latent tuberculosis is lower in patients receiving etanercept than in those receiving TNF-blocking monoclonal antibodies, reactivation of latent tuberculosis has been reported. Tuberculosis has developed in patients who tested negative for latent tuberculosis prior to initiation of therapy. As of September 2011, the FDA had identified 103 reports of Legionella pneumonia associated with TNF blocking agents, including etanercept. The 103 cases of Legionella pneumonia occurred in patients 25–85 years of age, many of whom received concomitant therapy with immunosuppressive agents (e.g., corticosteroids and/or methotrexate); 17 deaths were reported. In 78% of the cases of Legionella pneumonia, the median duration of TNF blocker therapy prior to the onset of Legionella pneumonia was 10.4 months (range: less than 1 month to 73 months). As of September 2011, FDA also had identified 26 published reports of Listeria infections, including meningitis, bacteremia, endophthalmitis, and sepsis, in patients who received TNF blocking agents; 7 deaths were reported. Many of the Listeria infections occurred in patients who had received concomitant therapy with immunosuppressive agents. In addition, FDA identified fatal Listeria infections during a review of data regarding laboratory-confirmed infections that occurred in premarketing clinical studies and during postmarketing surveillance. An increased incidence of serious infections was observed when etanercept and anakinra (a human interleukin-1 receptor antagonist) were used concurrently in patients with active rheumatoid arthritis; the incidence of serious infections was 7% among those receiving etanercept and anakinra compared with 0% among those receiving etanercept. The most common infections were bacterial pneumonia and cellulitis; one patient with pulmonary fibrosis and pneumonia died of respiratory failure. In addition, an increased incidence of serious infection was observed when a TNF blocking agent was used concomitantly with abatacept (a selective costimulation modulator) in patients with rheumatoid arthritis. Concomitant use of etanercept and abatacept or anakinra is not recommended.

Do not initiate etanercept therapy in patients with active infections, including clinically important localized infections. Patients >65 years of age, patients with comorbid conditions, and/or patients receiving concomitant therapy with immunosuppressive agents such as corticosteroids or methotrexate may be at increased risk of infection. Clinicians should consider the potential risks and benefits of the drug prior to initiating therapy in patients with a history of chronic, recurring, or opportunistic infections; patients with underlying conditions that may predispose them to infections; and patients who have been exposed to tuberculosis or who reside or have traveled in regions where tuberculosis or mycoses such as histoplasmosis, coccidioidomycosis, and blastomycosis are endemic. Any patient who develops a new infection while receiving etanercept should undergo a thorough diagnostic evaluation (appropriate for an immunocompromised patient); appropriate anti-infective therapy should be initiated, and the patient should be closely monitored. Discontinue the drug in patients who develop a serious infection or sepsis. The manufacturer recommends that etanercept be discontinued temporarily and use of varicella-zoster immune globulin (VZIG) considered in pediatric patients receiving etanercept who are susceptible to varicella and have a significant exposure to varicella virus.

Because tuberculosis has been reported in patients receiving etanercept, all patients should be evaluated for active or latent tuberculosis and for risk factors for tuberculosis prior to and periodically during etanercept therapy. When indicated, an appropriate antimycobacterial regimen for the treatment of latent tuberculosis infection should be initiated prior to etanercept therapy. Antimycobacterial treatment lowers the risk of latent tuberculosis infection progressing to active disease (i.e., reactivation) in patients receiving TNF blocking agents. Antimycobacterial therapy also should be considered prior to initiation of etanercept therapy in individuals with a history of latent or active tuberculosis in whom an adequate course of antimycobacterial treatment cannot be confirmed and in individuals with a negative tuberculin skin test who have risk factors for tuberculosis. Consultation with a tuberculosis specialist is recommended when deciding whether to initiate antimycobacterial therapy. Active tuberculosis has developed in etanercept-treated patients whose latent tuberculosis screening results were negative. Monitor patients receiving etanercept, including individuals with a negative tuberculin skin test, for signs and symptoms of active tuberculosis. Strongly consider the possibility of tuberculosis in patients who develop new infections while receiving etanercept, especially if they previously have traveled to countries where tuberculosis is highly prevalent or have been in close contact with an individual with active tuberculosis.

Invasive fungal infections have occurred in patients receiving TNF blocking agents. Fungal infections often are not recognized in these patients and has led to delays in appropriate treatment. Clinicians should ascertain whether patients who present with signs and symptoms suggestive of systemic fungal infection reside or have traveled to regions where mycoses are endemic. Consider empiric antifungal therapy in patients at risk of histoplasmosis or other invasive fungal infections who develop severe systemic illness. Whenever feasible, consult a specialist in fungal infections when making decisions regarding initiation and duration of antifungal therapy. When deciding whether TNF blocking agent therapy should be re-initiated following resolution of an invasive fungal infection, re-evaluate the risks and benefits of such therapy, particularly in patients who reside in regions where mycoses are endemic.

Malignancies

A boxed warning about the risk of malignancy is included in the prescribing information for etanercept. Malignancies, some fatal, have been reported in children, adolescents, and young adults who received treatment with TNF blocking agents beginning when they were 18 years of age or younger. In August 2009, the FDA reported the results of an analysis of reports of lymphoma and other malignancies in children and adolescents who had received TNF blocking agents. These cases were reported postmarketing and were derived from various sources, including registries and spontaneous postmarketing reports. FDA identified 48 cases of malignancies in children and adolescents in the analysis.

Of the 48 cases reviewed by FDA, approximately 50% were lymphomas, including Hodgkin disease and non-Hodgkin lymphoma. The other cases represented a variety of malignancies, including rare malignancies that are usually associated with immunosuppression and malignancies that are not usually observed in children and adolescents. Other malignancies reported included leukemia, melanoma, and solid organ tumors; malignancies such as leiomyosarcoma, hepatic malignancies, and renal cell carcinoma, which rarely occur in children, also were reported. The malignancies occurred after a median of 30 months (range: 1–84 months) following the first dose of therapy with TNF blocking agents. Of the 48 cases of malignancies, 11 deaths were reported; causes of death included hepatosplenic T-cell lymphoma (9 cases), T-cell lymphoma (1 case), and sepsis following remission of lymphoma (1 case). The observed US reporting rates for cases of malignancy with etanercept in the analysis were higher compared with background rates for lymphomas, but were similar to background rates for all malignancies. The observed reporting rates offer limited inference into the potential differences in risk of malignancy among TNF blocking agents because of uncertainties about actual patient exposure to treatment and the possibility of underreporting of cases of malignancy. Most of the 48 patients (88%) also were receiving other immunosuppressive drugs such as azathioprine and methotrexate; these agents also are associated with an increased risk of lymphoma. Although there were other contributory factors, the role of TNF blocking agents in the development of malignancies in children and adolescents could not be excluded. Therefore, FDA has concluded that there is an increased risk of malignancy with TNF blocking agents. However, due to the relatively rare occurrence of these cancers, the limited number of pediatric patients who received TNF blocking agents, and the possible role of other immunosuppressive drugs used concomitantly with TNF blocking agents, FDA was unable to fully characterize the strength of the association between use of TNF blocking agents and the development of a malignancy.

Hepatosplenic T-cell lymphoma, a rare, aggressive, usually fatal type of T-cell lymphoma, has been reported during postmarketing experience mainly in adolescents and young adults with Crohn disease or ulcerative colitis who received treatment with TNF blocking agents and/or thiopurine analogs (mercaptopurine or azathioprine). Although certain TNF blocking agents (e.g., adalimumab, certolizumab pegol, infliximab) are effective in the management of Crohn disease and/or ulcerative colitis, etanercept is not effective in the management of inflammatory bowel disease. Most of the reported cases of hepatosplenic T-cell lymphoma occurred in patients who had received a combination of immunosuppressive agents, including TNF blocking agents and thiopurine analogs (azathioprine or mercaptopurine). In some cases, potential confounding factors could not be excluded because complete medical histories were not available. As of December 31, 2010, FDA had identified 1 case of hepatosplenic T-cell lymphoma in a patient with psoriasis who had received etanercept; cyclosporine and methotrexate were used concomitantly. Since patients with certain conditions (e.g., rheumatoid arthritis, Crohn disease, ankylosing spondylitis, psoriatic arthritis, plaque psoriasis) may be at increased risk for lymphoma, it may be difficult to measure the added risk of treatment with TNF blocking agents, azathioprine, and/or mercaptopurine.

In clinical studies, lymphoma has been observed more frequently in patients receiving agents that block TNF than in control patients. In clinical studies evaluating etanercept in adults with rheumatoid arthritis, psoriatic arthritis, or ankylosing spondylitis, the rate of lymphoma in etanercept-treated patients was 0.1 per 100 patient-years. This rate is approximately threefold higher than the rate expected for the general population. Patients with rheumatoid arthritis, especially those with highly active disease, may be at increased risk of lymphoma. In clinical studies evaluating etanercept in adults with plaque psoriasis, the rate of lymphoma in etanercept-treated patients was 0.05 per 100 patient-years, which was similar to the rate expected for the general population.

Cases of acute and chronic leukemia have been reported during postmarketing surveillance of TNF blocking agents used in the management of rheumatoid arthritis and other conditions. In August 2009, FDA reported the results of a review of 147 cases of leukemia in adults and pediatric patients who received TNF blocking agents; these cases had been identified during postmarketing surveillance. Of the 147 cases, acute myeloid leukemia (44 cases), chronic lymphocytic leukemia (31 cases), and chronic myeloid leukemia (23 cases) were the most frequent types of leukemia reported.128 Four cases of leukemia were reported in children.128 Most patients (61%) also were receiving other immunosuppressive drugs. There were a total of 30 deaths reported; leukemia was reported as the cause of 26 of the 30 deaths, and the event was associated with the use of TNF blocking agents. Leukemia generally occurred during the first 2 years of therapy. The interpretation of these findings was complicated by the fact that published epidemiologic studies suggest that patients with rheumatoid arthritis may be at increased risk of leukemia, independent of any treatment with TNF blocking agents. However, based on the available data, FDA has concluded that there is a possible association between treatment with TNF blocking agents and the development of leukemia in patients receiving these drugs. In clinical studies evaluating etanercept, the observed rate of leukemia was 0.03 per 100 patient-years.

Melanoma and nonmelanoma skin cancer have been reported in patients receiving TNF blocking agents, including etanercept. In controlled and open-label phases of clinical studies evaluating etanercept, the rate of melanoma was 0.043 per 100 patient-years. In clinical studies evaluating etanercept in adults with rheumatoid arthritis, psoriatic arthritis, or ankylosing spondylitis, the rate of nonmelanoma skin cancer was 0.41 per 100 patient-years in etanercept-treated patients and 0.37 per 100 patient-years in control patients. In clinical studies evaluating etanercept in adults with psoriasis, the rate of nonmelanoma skin cancer was 3.54 per 100 patient-years in etanercept-treated patients and 1.28 per 100 patient-years in control patients. Merkel cell carcinoma has been reported very infrequently during postmarketing surveillance in patients who received etanercept.

In controlled clinical trials evaluating etanercept, there were no differences in exposure-adjusted occurrence rates of malignancies other than lymphoma and nonmelanoma skin cancer between etanercept-treated patients and control patients. Analysis of data from both controlled and uncontrolled phases of clinical studies of etanercept indicate that the types and rates of malignancies are similar to what would be expected in the general population, and the rates do not appear to increase over time. It has not been established whether etanercept influences the development and course of malignancies in adults.

Some immune-related diseases, such as Crohn disease, have been shown to increase the risk of cancer independent of treatment with TNF blocking agents, while for others, such as juvenile idiopathic arthritis, it is unknown whether there is an increased risk of cancer. The role of TNF blocking agents in the development of malignancies has not been fully determined.

In a randomized, placebo-controlled study in patients with granulomatosis with polyangiitis† (previously referred to as Wegener's granulomatosis), solid malignant tumors developed in 6 of 89 patients (adenocarcinoma of the colon occurring in 2 patients and metastatic cholangiocarcinoma, renal cell carcinoma, breast cancer, and recurrent liposarcoma each occurring in one patient) receiving etanercept in conjunction with standard therapy (corticosteroids plus cyclophosphamide or methotrexate) and in none of those who received standard therapy alone. In this study, all of the etanercept-treated patients who developed a solid tumor were receiving cyclophosphamide. Because of the increased incidence of malignancies associated with etanercept and data indicating that use of etanercept in conjunction with standard therapy is not associated with improved clinical benefit for this indication compared with standard therapy alone, some clinicians state that use of the drug in regimens to induce or maintain remissions in patients with granulomatosis with polyangiitis is not justified. The manufacturer of etanercept states that use of etanercept is not recommended in patients with granulomatosis with polyangiitis who are receiving immunosuppressive therapy.

In controlled studies of other TNF blocking agents in adults at increased risk of malignancies (e.g., patients with chronic obstructive pulmonary disease [COPD] who have a substantial history of smoking), a greater proportion of malignancies occurred in patients receiving the TNF blocking agent compared with control patients. Clinicians should consider the possibility of and monitor for the occurrence of malignancies during and following treatment with TNF blocking agents. Because therapy with TNF blocking agents and/or thiopurine analogs (azathioprine or mercaptopurine) may increase the risk of malignancies, including hepatosplenic T-cell lymphoma, carefully consider the risks and benefits of these agents, especially in adolescents and young adults and especially in the treatment of Crohn disease or ulcerative colitis. Although certain TNF blocking agents (e.g., adalimumab, certolizumab pegol, infliximab) are effective in the management of Crohn disease and/or ulcerative colitis, etanercept is not effective in the management of inflammatory bowel disease. Because skin cancer has been reported in patients receiving TNF blocking agents, including etanercept, consider periodic dermatologic examinations in all patients at increased risk.

Other Warnings and Precautions

Neurologic Reactions

New onset or exacerbation of CNS demyelinating disorders (some presenting with mental status changes and some associated with permanent disability) and peripheral nervous system demyelinating disorders have been reported rarely with etanercept or other TNF blocking agents. During postmarketing surveillance, multiple sclerosis, transverse myelitis, optic neuritis, Guillain-Barré syndrome, other peripheral demyelinating neuropathies, and new onset or exacerbation of seizure disorders have been reported in patients receiving etanercept. Clinicians should exercise caution when considering etanercept therapy in patients with preexisting or recent-onset central or peripheral nervous system demyelinating disorders.

New Onset or Worsening of Heart Failure

During postmarketing surveillance, there have been reports describing worsening congestive heart failure (with and without identifiable precipitating factors) and rare reports of new-onset congestive heart failure (including some reports in patients without known cardiovascular disease) in patients receiving etanercept; some of these patients have been younger than 50 years of age. In addition, in one study investigating use of the drug for the treatment of heart failure, there was a suggestion of higher mortality rates in patients receiving etanercept. Etanercept should be used with caution and careful monitoring in patients with heart failure.

Hematologic Reactions

Pancytopenia including aplastic anemia, sometimes with a fatal outcome, has been reported rarely in patients receiving etanercept. Whether this hematologic abnormality is directly attributable to etanercept remains to be determined. Although a high risk group for this adverse effect has not been identified, caution is advised if etanercept is used in patients with a history of substantial hematologic abnormalities. If substantial hematologic abnormalities are confirmed, consider discontinuance of etanercept.

HBV Reactivation

Use of TNF blocking agents, including etanercept, has been associated with reactivation of hepatitis B virus (HBV) infection in patients who were previously infected with this virus. HBV reactivation has resulted in death in a few individuals receiving a TNF blocking agent. Most patients experiencing HBV reactivation were receiving concomitant therapy with other immunosuppressive agents; use of multiple immunosuppressive agents may have contributed to HBV reactivation.

Patients at risk for HBV infection should be screened before initiation of etanercept therapy. Patients who were previously infected with HBV should be appropriately evaluated and monitored prior to the initiation of therapy, during treatment, and for up to several months following therapy with etanercept. Safety and efficacy of antiviral therapy for prevention of viral reactivation in HBV carriers receiving a TNF blocking agent have not been established. Discontinue etanercept if HBV reactivation occurs and initiate appropriate treatment, including antiviral therapy. It has not been established whether etanercept can be safely readministered once control of the reactivated HBV infection has been achieved; use caution if etanercept therapy is resumed in such a situation.

Allergic Reactions

Allergic reactions have been reported in <2% of patients. If serious allergic reaction or anaphylaxis occurs, discontinue etanercept immediately and initiate appropriate therapy.

Immunization

Live vaccines should be avoided during therapy with etanercept. Information is not available regarding whether etanercept affects the rate of secondary transmission of infection following administration of a live vaccine. When use of etanercept is being considered for pediatric patients, review the vaccination status of the patient and administer all age-appropriate vaccines included in current immunization guidelines, if possible, prior to initiation of etanercept therapy. Consider the risks and benefits of administering live vaccines to infants who were exposed to etanercept in utero, since the safety of live vaccines in these infants is unknown.

Patients receiving etanercept may receive inactivated vaccines. An effective B-cell immune response to pneumococcal 23-valent polysaccharide vaccine has been reported in etanercept-treated psoriatic arthritis patients; however, antibody titers in aggregate were moderately lower in these adults compared with adults not receiving the drug, and fewer etanercept-treated adults had twofold increases in antibodies compared with adults not receiving the drug. The clinical importance of these findings remains to be determined.

Autoimmunity

Etanercept therapy may result in the formation of autoimmune antibodies. During postmarketing surveillance, autoimmune hepatitis, cutaneous lupus, or a systemic lupus erythematosus-like syndrome has been reported rarely in patients receiving etanercept. In adults with rheumatoid arthritis who were evaluated for antinuclear antibodies (ANA) in placebo-controlled studies, 11% of those receiving etanercept developed new positive ANA (greater than or equal to 1:40) compared with 5% of those receiving placebo. New positive anti-double stranded DNA antibodies were detected in 15% (radioimmunoassay) or 3% (Crithidia luciliae assay) of those receiving etanercept compared with 4% (radioimmunoassay) or none (Crithidia luciliae assay) of placebo-treated patients. Anticardiolipin antibodies also have been detected in more etanercept-treated than placebo-treated patients. Results of a study comparing etanercept and methotrexate did not reveal a pattern of increased autoantibody development in those receiving etanercept compared with those receiving methotrexate. If a patient develops symptoms and findings suggestive of autoimmune hepatitis or a lupus-like syndrome, discontinue etanercept and carefully evaluate the patient.

Patients receiving etanercept may develop nonneutralizing antibodies to the drug; however, a relationship between development of such antibodies and clinical response or adverse effects (e.g., injection site reactions) has not been observed. In clinical studies evaluating etanercept, patients were tested for the presence of nonneutralizing antibodies at multiple time points and such antibodies were detected at least once in the sera of 6% of etanercept-treated adults with rheumatoid arthritis, psoriatic arthritis, ankylosing spondylitis, or plaque psoriasis; similar results have been obtained in studies in children with juvenile idiopathic arthritis. In patients with plaque psoriasis, nonneutralizing antibodies to the drug were detected at week 24, 48, 72, or 96 of therapy in 3.6–8.7% of patients; the proportion of patients testing positive for antibodies to the drug increased as the duration of therapy increased. The clinical importance of these findings remains to be determined. In pediatric patients with plaque psoriasis, nonneutralizing antibodies to the drug were detected in 10 and 16% of patients at weeks 48 and 264 of therapy, respectively.

No evidence of diminished delayed hypersensitivity, decrease in immunoglobulin concentrations, or change in the enumeration of effector cell populations was observed in a limited number of etanercept-treated rheumatoid arthritis patients.

Patients with Granulomatosis with Polyangiitis Receiving Immunosuppression

Concurrent use of etanercept with immunosuppressive agents in patients with granulomatosis with polyangiitis is not recommended. In a study, the addition of etanercept to standard therapy (including cyclophosphamide) in patients with

this condition was associated with an increased incidence of non-cutaneous solid malignancies without improved clincial outcomes when compared to standard therapy alone.

Increased Mortality in Patients with Moderate to Severe Alcoholic Hepatitis

Because use of etanercept in patients with moderate to severe alcoholic hepatitis has been associated with increased mortality following 6 months of use, etanercept should be used with caution in such patients.

Specific Populations

Pregnancy

Available studies of etanercept use during pregnancy do not reliably establish an association between the drug and major birth defects. Results of a prospective cohort study using data from the Organization of Teratology Information Specialists (OTIS) pregnancy registry indicated that 9.4% of women in the etanercept-exposed cohort delivered a live-born infant with a major birth defect, compared with 3.5% of women with rheumatic diseases or psoriasis who had not been exposed to the drug. Similarly, a Scandinavian study in pregnant women with chronic inflammatory disease indicated that 7% of women in the etanercept-exposed cohort delivered a live-born infant with a major birth defect, compared with 4.7% of women who had not been exposed to the drug. However, no pattern of major birth defects was observed in either study, and differences in the cohorts may have affected the observed occurrence rates.

Reproduction studies in rats and rabbits using etanercept doses 48–58 times higher than the usual human dose have not revealed evidence of harm to the fetus.

Limited data suggest that etanercept crosses the placenta in small amounts; in 3 neonates whose mothers received etanercept during pregnancy, concentrations of the drug in cord blood at the time of delivery were 3–32% of maternal serum concentrations. The clinical implications of in utero exposure to etanercept are unknown. Consider the risks and benefits of administering live vaccines to infants who were exposed to etanercept in utero prior to immunization, since the safety of live vaccines in these infants is unknown.

Lactation

Limited data indicate that etanercept is distributed into human milk in low concentrations and is minimally absorbed by breast-fed infants. No data are available regarding the effects of etanercept on breast-fed infants or on milk production. Consider the benefits of breast-feeding and the importance of etanercept to the woman along with the potential adverse effects on the breast-fed infant from the drug or underlying maternal condition.

Pediatric Use

Use of etanercept for the management of active polyarticular juvenile idiopathic arthritis in pediatric patients ≥2 years of age is supported by the results of a 2-part safety and efficacy study in 69 pediatric patients 2–17 years of age. Safety and efficacy of etanercept for the management of polyarticular juvenile idiopathic arthritis have not been established in pediatric patients <2 years of age.

Use of etanercept for the management of juvenile psoriatic arthritis in pediatric patients ≥2 years of age is supported by the results of studies of etanercept in adults with psoriatic arthritis; pharmacokinetic data from adults with psoriartic arthritis, rheumatoid arthritis, and psoriais; and pharmacokinetic data from pediatric patients with juvenile idiopathic arthritis and psoriasis. The safety of etanercept in juvenile psoriatic arthritis is supported by a clinical study in 69 pediatric patients with juvenile idiopathic arthritis (2 to 17 years of age); a clinical study in 211 pediatric patients with psoriasis (4 to 17 years of age); and an open-label extension study in 182 pediatric patients with psoriasis (4 to 17 years of age). Safety and efficacy of etanercept for the management of juvenile psoriatic arthritis have not been established in pediatric patients <2 years of age.

Use of etanercept for the management of moderate to severe plaque psoriasis in pediatric patients ≥4 years of age is supported by the results of a randomized, double-blind, placebo-controlled trial in 211 pediatric patients 4–17 years of age. Safety and efficacy of etanercept for the management of plaque psoriasis have not been established in pediatric patients <4 years of age.

Malignancies, some fatal, have been reported in children, adolescents, and young adults who received treatment with TNF blocking agents.

Varicella infection associated with septic meningitis has been reported in 2 pediatric patients receiving etanercept; the infection resolved without sequelae. If a varicella-susceptible pediatric patient has a significant exposure to varicella while receiving etanercept, the manufacturer recommends that the drug be discontinued temporarily and use of VZIG considered.

When use of etanercept is being considered for pediatric patients, review the vaccination status of the patient and administer all age-appropriate vaccines included in current immunization guidelines, if possible, prior to initiation of etanercept therapy. Consider the risks and benefits of administering live vaccines to infants who were exposed to etanercept in utero prior to immunization, since the safety of live vaccines in these infants is unknown.

Inflammatory bowel disease has been reported rarely during postmarketing surveillance in patients with juvenile idiopathic arthritis receiving etanercept; the drug is not effective in the management of inflammatory bowel disease.

Geriatric Use

While safety and efficacy of etanercept in geriatric patients have not been studied specifically to date, some patients with rheumatoid arthritis or plaque psoriasis who received the drug in clinical studies have been ≥65 years of age. Etanercept appears to be well tolerated in geriatric patients, and age-related differences in safety or efficacy of the drug have not been observed in clinical studies. However, the manufacturer cautions that clinical studies of the drug in patients with psoriasis did not include sufficient numbers of geriatric patients to determine whether they respond differently than younger adults. Because the geriatric population in general may have a higher incidence of infections than younger adults, etanercept should be used with caution in this age group.

Hepatic Impairment

The pharmacokinetics of etanercept have not been formally studied in patients with hepatic impairment.

Renal Impairment

The pharmacokinetics of etanercept have not been formally studied in patients with renal impairment.

● Common Adverse Effects

Adverse effects reported in >5% of patients receiving etanercept include infections and injection site reactions.

DRUG INTERACTIONS

While specific drug interaction studies evaluating concomitant use of etanercept and other drugs have not been conducted to date, etanercept has been used concomitantly with methotrexate, glucocorticoids, salicylates, nonsteroidal anti-inflammatory agents (NSAIAs), and/or analgesics in clinical studies and the manufacturer of etanercept states that these drugs may be continued in patients receiving etanercept.

● Biologic Antirheumatic Agents

Caution should be exercised when switching from one biologic disease-modifying antirheumatic drug (DMARD) to another, since overlapping biologic activity may further increase the risk of infection.

Abatacept

When abatacept (a selective costimulation modulator) and a tumor necrosis factor (TNF) blocking agent were used concomitantly in patients with rheumatoid arthritis, an increased incidence of infection and serious infection was observed, with no substantial improvement in efficacy over that observed with a TNF blocking agent alone. Concomitant use of etanercept and abatacept is not recommended.

Anakinra

When etanercept and anakinra (a human interleukin-1 receptor antagonist) were used concomitantly in patients with active rheumatoid arthritis, an increased incidence of serious infections was observed, with no substantial improvement

in efficacy over that observed with etanercept alone. Neutropenia was observed in 2% of patients receiving etanercept concomitantly with anakinra. Concomitant use of etanercept with anakinra is not recommended.

Rituximab

An increased risk of serious infection has been observed in patients with rheumatoid arthritis who received rituximab and subsequently received therapy with a TNF blocking agent.

● Cyclophosphamide

In a study in patients with granulomatosis with polyangiitis, addition of etanercept to standard therapy that included cyclophosphamide was associated with a higher incidence of solid malignant tumors compared with standard therapy alone. Concomitant use of etanercept and cyclophosphamide is not recommended.

● Methotrexate

Concomitant use of etanercept and methotrexate in patients with rheumatoid arthritis does not appear to alter the pharmacokinetics of etanercept, result in additive toxicity, or affect the pattern, frequency, or severity of the established toxicities associated with either drug.

● Sulfasalazine

Addition of etanercept to established therapy that included sulfasalazine has resulted in decreases in mean neutrophil counts. The clinical importance of this finding is unknown.

● Vaccines

Live vaccines should not be administered concurrently with etanercept; it is recommended that patients, if possible, be brought up-to-date with all immunizations in accordance with current immunization guidelines prior to initiating etanercept therapy. Information is not available regarding whether etanercept can affect the rate of secondary transmission of infection following administration of a live vaccine.

Patients receiving etanercept may receive inactivated vaccines.

An effective B-cell immune response to pneumococcal 23-valent polysaccharide vaccine has been reported in etanercept-treated psoriatic arthritis patients; however, antibody titers in aggregate were moderately lower in these adults compared with adults not receiving the drug, and fewer etanercept-treated adults had twofold increases in antibodies compared with adults not receiving the drug. The clinical importance of these findings remains to be determined.

Prior to initiating etanercept, review the vaccination status of the patient and administer all age-appropriate vaccines included in current immunization guidelines, if possible. Consider the risks and benefits of administering live or live-attenuated vaccines to infants who were exposed to etanercept in utero.

DESCRIPTION

Etanercept, a biosynthetic tumor necrosis factor receptor fusion protein, is disease-modifying antirheumatic drug (DMARD) of the tumor necrosis factor (TNF) inhibitor class. Etanercept is a recombinant form of the human 75 kilodalton (p75) TNF receptor fused to the Fc fragment of human immunoglobulin G_1 (IgG_1). The drug is prepared from mammalian cells using DNA recombinant technology. Etanercept has high binding affinity for TNF and lymphotoxin-α (TNF-β); each molecule of etanercept can bind to 2 TNF molecules. Etanercept binds to TNF before TNF can interact with cell surface tumor necrosis factor receptors (TNFRs). By preventing the binding of TNF to cell surface TNFRs, etanercept blocks the biologic activity of TNF.

TNF, a naturally occurring cytokine, has a broad spectrum of biologic activity. TNF is involved in the normal inflammatory and immune responses, and also plays a role in the systemic toxicity associated with sepsis and in a number of autoimmune and inflammatory diseases, including rheumatoid arthritis. The biologic activity of TNF is mediated by specific TNF transmembrane receptors. While the causes of rheumatoid diseases or psoriasis have not been fully elucidated, proinflammatory cytokines, particularly TNF (TNF-α), have an important role in the pathogenesis of rheumatoid arthritis, polyarticular course juvenile idiopathic arthritis, ankylosing spondylitis, psoriatic arthritis, and plaque psoriasis. Cytokines such as TNF are mediators involved in the inflammatory, adhesive, angiogenic, and bone-resorbing mechanisms associated with rheumatoid arthritis. TNF induces the release of metalloproteinases (i.e., metalloproteinase-3 [stromelysin-1]) from neutrophils, fibroblasts, and chrondrocytes; induces the expression of endothelial adhesion molecules (intracellular adhesion molecule [ICAM-1], E-selectin) involved in the migration of leukocytes to extravascular sites of inflammation; and stimulates release of other proinflammatory cytokines (i.e., interleukin-1 [IL-1], IL-6). Additional evidence supporting the role of TNF in the pathogenesis of rheumatoid arthritis includes the presence of TNF at the cartilage-pannus junction and increased TNF concentrations in the synovial fluid of patients with active rheumatoid arthritis. In addition, TNF and lymphotoxin-α (TNF-β) are expressed in the synovial fluid of individuals with juvenile idiopathic arthritis or juvenile spondylarthropathy. Increased TNF concentrations have been found in the synovium and psoriatic plaques in patients with psoriatic arthritis. While other proinflammatory cytokines (i.e., IL-1) contribute to the pathogenesis of rheumatoid arthritis, TNF plays a central role because of its prominent role in the cytokine cascade.

While the precise mechanism of action of etanercept in the management of rheumatoid arthritis remains to be determined, the drug inhibits TNF binding to cell surface TNFR, rendering TNF biologically inactive. Etanercept neutralizes circulating TNF, a mechanism of action that differs from that of a receptor antagonist (receptor antagonists block activity by interacting with the receptor but leave the ligand in circulation). Whether etanercept can exert activity through binding to Fc receptors is unknown. In vitro, cells expressing transmembrane TNF that bind etanercept are not lysed in the presence or absence of complement.

Bioavailability following a single subcutaneous dose of etanercept is approximately 60%. Following subcutaneous injection of a single 25-mg dose of etanercept in a limited number of healthy adults or adults with rheumatoid arthritis, peak serum etanercept concentrations were achieved within 51 hours (range: 25–78 hours) or 69 hours, respectively. In another study in patients with rheumatoid arthritis, serum concentrations of etanercept at steady state in patients receiving etanercept 50 mg subcutaneously once weekly were essentially the same as values in patients receiving etanercept 25 mg subcutaneously twice weekly. Based on available data, peak serum concentration of etanercept following repeated dosing is about 2–7 times higher than that achieved with a single dose of the drug and AUC about 4 times higher. Distribution of etanercept into body tissues and fluids, including partition of the drug into synovial fluid, has not been well characterized. Because etanercept is a large molecule, the drug may be eliminated by the reticuloendothelial system. Following subcutaneous administration, mean half-life of the drug was 102 hours. Considerable interindividual variation in clearance has been observed in healthy individuals. Some data indicate that clearance of etanercept is reduced to a small extent in children 4–8 years of age compared with adults. Studies in adults have not revealed differences in the pharmacokinetics of etanercept based on gender or age.

ADVICE TO PATIENTS

- Provide a copy of the manufacturer's patient information (medication guide) for etanercept to all patients with each prescription of the drug. Advise patients about potential benefits and risks of etanercept. Advise patients to read the medication guide prior to initiation of therapy and each time the prescription is refilled.

- If the patient or caregiver is to administer etanercept, provide careful instructions regarding proper dosage and administration, including proper aseptic technique, and proper disposal of needles and syringes.

- Increased susceptibility to infection. Stress importance of seeking immediate medical attention if signs and symptoms suggestive of infection (e.g., fever, chills, flu-like symptoms, cough, burning or pain on urination) develop.

- Risk of lymphoma, including hepatosplenic T-cell lymphoma, leukemia, or other malignancies with TNF blocking agents. Inform patients and caregivers about the increased risk of cancer development in children, adolescents, and young adults, taking into account the clinical utility of TNF blocking agents, the relative risks and benefits of these and other immunosuppressive drugs, and the risks associated with untreated disease. Stress importance of promptly informing clinicians if signs and symptoms of malignancies (e.g., unexplained weight loss; fatigue; abdominal pain; persistent fever; night sweats; easy bruising or bleeding; swollen lymph nodes in the neck, underarm, or groin; easy bruising or bleeding; hepatomegaly or splenomegaly) occur.

- Advise patients to inform their clinician of any new or worsening medical conditions (e.g., neurologic conditions [e.g., demyelinating disorders], heart failure, autoimmune disorders [e.g., lupus-like syndrome, autoimmune hepatitis], psoriasis, cytopenias).

- Advise patients to promptly contact a clinician if manifestations of an allergic reaction (e.g., rash, facial swelling, difficulty breathing) occur.

- Advise patients to take the drug as prescribed and to not alter or discontinue therapy without first consulting with a clinician.

- Advise women to inform their clinicians if they are or plan to become pregnant or plan to breast-feed.

- Advise patients to inform their clinicians of existing or contemplated concomitant therapy, including prescription and OTC drugs, as well as any concomitant illnesses or any history of cancer, tuberculosis, HBV infection, or other chronic or recurring infections.

- Inform patients of other important precautionary information.

PREPARATIONS

Excipients in commercially available drug preparations may have clinically important effects in some individuals; consult specific product labeling for details.

Etanercept

Parenteral		
For injection, for subcutaneous use	25 mg	Enbrel® (multi-dose vial for reconstitution supplied with diluent syringe containing 1 mL sterile bacteriostatic water for injection [with benzyl alcohol 0.9%], 27-gauge ½-inch needle plunger, and vial adapter), Amgen
Injection, for subcutaneous use	25 mg/0.5 mL	Enbrel® (available as single-dose prefilled syringes and single-dose vials), Amgen
	50 mg/mL	Enbrel® (available as single-dose prefilled syringes and single-dose prefilled auto-injectors [SureClick®]), Amgen
		Enbrel Mini® (available as single-dose prefilled cartridges for use with the AutoTouch® reusable autoinjector), Amgen

† Use is not currently included in the labeling approved by the US Food and Drug Administration.

Selected Revisions July 10, 2024, © Copyright, July 1, 2000, American Society of Health-System Pharmacists, Inc.

Golimumab

90:24.16.92 • TUMOR NECROSIS FACTOR INHIBITORS, MISCELLANEOUS

- Golimumab, a human immunoglobulin G_1 kappa (IgG_1) monoclonal antibody, is a tumor necrosis factor (TNF) inhibitor that is a biologic disease-modifying antirheumatic drug (DMARD).

USES

● *Rheumatoid Arthritis*

Golimumab is used in conjunction with methotrexate for the management of moderately to severely active rheumatoid arthritis in adults. Safety and efficacy of golimumab for this use are based principally on the results of several randomized controlled trials and long-term extension studies. Guidelines generally support the use of tumor necrosis factor (TNF; TNF-α) blocking agents, including golimumab, as add-on therapy to methotrexate in patients who do not meet treatment goals with methotrexate alone.

Clinical Experience with Subcutaneous Golimumab

Safety and efficacy of subcutaneous golimumab were evaluated in 3 multicenter, randomized, double-blind studies (RA-1 [GO-AFTER], RA-2 [GO-FORWARD], and RA-3 [GO-BEFORE]) in 1542 adults with moderately to severely active rheumatoid arthritis (as defined by the American College of Rheumatology [ACR]) for at least 3 months prior to administration of the study drug. To be included in these studies, patients were required to have at least 4 swollen and 4 tender joints. Golimumab was administered subcutaneously at dosages of 50 or 100 mg once every 4 weeks. Patients receiving stable dosages of low-dose corticosteroids (equivalent to 10 mg of prednisone daily or less) and/or nonsteroidal anti-inflammatory agents (NSAIAs) could continue such agents, and some patients received oral methotrexate during these studies. Approximately 77 and 57% of patients received concomitant NSAIAs and low-dose corticosteroids, respectively, in the 3 studies.

In study RA-1, 461 patients who previously received one or more doses of a TNF blocking agent (i.e., adalimumab or etanercept discontinued at least 8 weeks or infliximab discontinued at least 12 weeks prior to administration of the study drug) were randomized to receive golimumab (50 or 100 mg once every 4 weeks) or placebo. Patients receiving stable dosages of methotrexate, sulfasalazine, and/or hydroxychloroquine could continue such agents or discontinue the agents prior to study start; the use of other disease-modifying antirheumatic drugs (DMARDs), including cytotoxic agents or other biologic agents, was prohibited. At week 16, patients in certain treatment groups with less than 20% improvement from baseline in the number of both tender and swollen joints entered early escape in which their study drug was adjusted in a double-blind manner (i.e., those meeting the early escape criteria who were receiving golimumab 50 mg had their golimumab dosage increased to 100 mg and those who were receiving placebo began receiving golimumab 50 mg every 4 weeks). At week 24, all remaining patients who had been receiving placebo initiated golimumab 50 mg every 4 weeks. During the unblinded long-term extension period (beginning at week 24 of the 5-year study), golimumab dosage could be adjusted (increased to 100 mg or, after week 160, decreased to 50 mg) at the clinician's discretion. The median duration of rheumatoid arthritis disease prior to study enrollment was 9.4 years, and 99% of patients previously received at least one DMARD.

In study RA-2, 444 patients who had active rheumatoid arthritis despite receiving a stable dosage of methotrexate (15–25 mg/week) and who had not previously been treated with a TNF blocking agent were randomized to receive one of 4 regimens: golimumab 100 mg every 4 weeks and placebo, golimumab 50 mg every 4 weeks and methotrexate, golimumab 100 mg every 4 weeks and methotrexate, or methotrexate and placebo. The use of other DMARDs, including sulfasalazine, hydroxychloroquine, cytotoxic agents, or other biologic agents, was prohibited. At week 16, patients in certain treatment groups with less than 20% improvement from baseline in the number of both tender and swollen joints entered early escape in which their study drug was adjusted in a double-blind manner (i.e., those meeting the early escape criteria who were receiving golimumab 100 mg and placebo

began receiving methotrexate at the same stable dosage at study screening instead of placebo and continued to receive golimumab 100 mg; those meeting the early escape criteria who were receiving golimumab 50 mg and methotrexate had their golimumab dosage increased to 100 mg and continued to receive methotrexate at the same stable dosage; those meeting the early escape criteria who were receiving methotrexate and placebo began receiving golimumab 50 mg every 4 weeks instead of placebo and continued to receive methotrexate at the same stable dosage). At week 24, all remaining patients who had been receiving methotrexate and placebo discontinued placebo, initiated golimumab 50 mg every 4 weeks, and continued to receive methotrexate; patients receiving golimumab 100 mg and placebo, golimumab 50 mg and methotrexate, or golimumab 100 mg and methotrexate continued to receive their originally assigned treatment unless they entered early escape, in which case they continued to receive their modified dosage. Golimumab continued to be administered in a blinded manner every 4 weeks through week 48. During the unblinded long-term extension period (beginning at week 52 of the 5-year study), certain adjustments of golimumab dosage (increase to 100 mg or decrease to 50 mg) and concomitant therapies could be made at the clinician's discretion. The median duration of rheumatoid arthritis disease prior to study enrollment was 5.7 years, and 75% of patients previously received at least one DMARD.

In study RA-3, 637 patients with active rheumatoid arthritis who were methotrexate-naive and had not previously been treated with a TNF blocking agent were randomized to receive one of 4 regimens: golimumab 100 mg every 4 weeks and placebo, golimumab 50 mg every 4 weeks and methotrexate, golimumab 100 mg every 4 weeks and methotrexate, or methotrexate and placebo. In this study, methotrexate was administered at a dosage of 10 mg weekly beginning at week 0 and increased to 20 mg weekly by week 8. The use of other DMARDs, including sulfasalazine, hydroxychloroquine, cytotoxic agents, or other biologic agents, was prohibited. After week 24, patients in certain treatment groups with less than 20% improvement from baseline in the number of both tender and swollen joints entered early escape in which their study drug was adjusted in a blinded manner (i.e., those meeting the early escape criteria who were receiving either golimumab 50 mg and methotrexate or golimumab 100 mg and placebo switched to golimumab 100 mg every 4 weeks and methotrexate, while those receiving placebo and methotrexate switched to golimumab 50 mg every 4 weeks and methotrexate). At week 52, all remaining patients who had been receiving placebo and methotrexate and had at least one tender or swollen joint switched to therapy with golimumab 50 mg every 4 weeks and methotrexate. During the unblinded long-term extension period (beginning at week 52 of the 5-year study), certain adjustments of golimumab dosage (increase from 50 mg to 100 mg) and concomitant therapies could be made at the clinician's discretion. The median duration of rheumatoid arthritis disease prior to study enrollment was 1.2 years, and 54% of patients previously received at least one DMARD.

The primary outcome measures in these 3 studies were the proportion of patients achieving an ACR 20 response at week 14 (studies RA-1 and RA-2) or an ACR 50 response at week 24 (study RA-3) and the change from baseline to week 52 in the van der Heijde-modified Sharp score (study RA-3). An ACR 20 response is achieved if the patient experiences a 20% improvement in tender and swollen joint count and a 20% or greater improvement in at least 3 of the following criteria: patient pain assessment, patient global assessment, physician global assessment, patient self-assessed disability, or laboratory measures of disease activity (e.g., C-reactive protein [CRP] level). ACR 50 responses are defined using the same criteria with a level of improvement of 50%. The van der Heijde-modified Sharp score is a composite measure of radiographically assessed structural damage (i.e., joint erosion and joint space narrowing) in the hands and feet. Physical function was assessed using the disability index of the Health Assessment Questionnaire [HAQ-DI].

In these 3 studies, a greater proportion of patients who received golimumab in conjunction with methotrexate achieved an ACR 20 response at week 14 (studies RA-1 and RA-2) and an ACR 50 response at week 24 (studies RA-2 and RA-3) than patients who received methotrexate alone. The proportion of patients who achieved ACR responses was similar for the golimumab 50- and 100-mg dosage groups. In study RA-1, the difference between the proportion of patients who achieved an ACR 20 response with golimumab as compared with placebo was greater for patients who received concomitant DMARDs than for patients who did not receive concomitant DMARDs. In study RA-1, 40% of patients who received golimumab 50 mg every 4 weeks in conjunction with methotrexate achieved an ACR 20 response at week 14 compared with 17% of patients who received methotrexate and placebo. In study RA-2, 55% of patients who received golimumab 50 mg every 4 weeks in conjunction with methotrexate achieved an ACR 20 response at week 14 compared with 33% of patients who received methotrexate and placebo; the ACR 20 response rates for these 2 groups of patients were 60 and 28%, respectively, at week 24 and 64 and 44%, respectively, at week 52. In study RA-3, 40% of patients who received golimumab 50 mg every 4 weeks in conjunction with methotrexate achieved an ACR 50 response at week 24 compared with 29% of patients who received methotrexate and placebo. In studies RA-2 and RA-3, ACR responses were similar for both the golimumab and methotrexate monotherapy groups. Although a control group was lacking during the extended-treatment periods of these 3 studies, long-term (5 years) follow-up data indicated that ACR responses to golimumab were maintained during continued treatment.

In studies RA-1 and RA-2, patients receiving golimumab 50 mg every 4 weeks had greater improvements in physical function, as assessed using the HAQ-DI, from baseline to week 24 compared with those receiving placebo; a greater proportion of patients receiving golimumab 50 mg every 4 weeks in studies RA-1 (43 versus 27%) and RA-2 (65 versus 35%) also achieved a HAQ-DI response (defined as a change from baseline exceeding 0.22) at week 24.

In study RA-3, progression of structural damage, as measured by change from baseline to week 52 in the total van der Heijde-modified Sharp score, was inhibited in patients who received golimumab in combination with methotrexate but not in those who received golimumab as monotherapy, as compared with those who received methotrexate monotherapy; 71% of patients receiving golimumab 50 mg every 4 weeks and methotrexate had no progression of structural damage as assessed by total van der Heijde-modified Sharp score at week 52, compared with 54% of those receiving methotrexate monotherapy. The 100-mg dosage did not provide benefits over the 50-mg dosage for inhibiting progression of structural damage.

Clinical Experience with IV Golimumab

Safety and efficacy of IV golimumab were evaluated in a randomized, double-blind, controlled study (GO-FURTHER) in 592 adults with moderately to severely active rheumatoid arthritis (as defined by the ACR) despite methotrexate therapy for at least 3 months prior to the study; patients had not received prior therapy with TNF blocking agents. To be included in the study, patients were required to have at least 6 swollen and 6 tender joints. Patients were randomized in a 2:1 ratio to receive either golimumab (2 mg/kg by IV infusion over 30 minutes at weeks 0 and 4 and every 8 weeks thereafter) or placebo, each given in conjunction with a stable methotrexate regimen (15–25 mg weekly). Patients assigned to receive placebo in conjunction with methotrexate were switched to combination therapy with golimumab and methotrexate at week 24 (or at week 16 in those with less than 10% improvement from baseline in the number of tender and swollen joints); however, the study remained blinded until completion of therapy. The final infusion was administered at week 100 and patients were followed for an additional 12 weeks. The median duration of rheumatoid arthritis disease prior to study enrollment was 4.7 years, and 50% of patients had previously received at least one DMARD other than methotrexate. Patients receiving stable dosages of low-dose corticosteroids (equivalent to 10 mg of prednisone daily or less) and/or NSAIAs could continue such agents; after week 52, another DMARD (e.g., sulfasalazine) could be substituted for methotrexate if required for patient tolerance, but use of cytotoxic agents and other biologic agents was prohibited throughout the study. NSAIAs and low-dose corticosteroids were each used in 81% of patients at baseline.

The primary outcome measure was the proportion of patients attaining an ACR 20 response at week 14. Additional measures of clinical response and disease activity included ACR 50 and ACR 70 responses and 28-joint Disease Activity Score using C-reactive protein (DAS 28 [CRP]). A greater proportion of patients receiving golimumab and methotrexate attained an ACR 20 response at weeks 14 and 24 (59 and 63%, respectively, versus 25 and 32%, respectively), an ACR 50 response at weeks 14 and 24 (30 and 35%, respectively, versus 9 and 13%, respectively), and an ACR 70 response at weeks 14 and 24 (12 and 18%, respectively, versus 3 and 4%, respectively) compared with those receiving placebo and methotrexate. Improvements in all components of the ACR response criteria from baseline to week 14 were greater in patients receiving golimumab and methotrexate compared with those receiving placebo and methotrexate. In addition, a greater proportion of patients receiving golimumab and methotrexate attained a low level of disease activity as measured by DAS 28 (CRP) (i.e., score of less than 2.6) at week 14 compared with those receiving placebo and methotrexate (15 versus 5%).

Clinical response to combined therapy with golimumab and methotrexate was maintained during 100 weeks of treatment. At week 100, ACR 20, ACR 50, and ACR 70 response rates for patients receiving combined therapy with golimumab and methotrexate throughout the study were 69, 45, and 23%, respectively; 29% of these patients had a low level of disease activity as measured by DAS 28 (CRP). An exploratory analysis by patient age found that the clinical efficacy of golimumab plus methotrexate was similar in patients <65 years of age and patients ≥65 years of age.

Structural joint damage was assessed radiographically as the change from baseline in the total van der Heijde-modified Sharp score and its component scores (i.e., joint erosion and joint space narrowing). At week 24, progression of structural damage was inhibited in patients who received golimumab and methotrexate compared with those who received placebo and methotrexate; 71% of patients receiving golimumab and methotrexate had no progression of structural damage as assessed by total van der Heijde-modified Sharp score at week 24, compared with 57% of those receiving placebo and methotrexate. Patients who received placebo and methotrexate before crossing over to combined therapy with golimumab and methotrexate at week 16 or 24 exhibited more progression, as measured by change from baseline in total van der Heijde-modified Sharp score, at weeks 52 and 100 than did those who received golimumab and methotrexate throughout the study; however, between weeks 24 and 100, progression was limited in both groups of patients.

Patients receiving golimumab in conjunction with methotrexate also had greater improvements in physical function (as assessed using the HAQ-DI) from baseline to week 14 and in quality-of-life measures (physical component summary score, mental component summary score, and all 8 domains of the Short Form-36 Health Survey [SF-36]) compared with patients receiving placebo in conjunction with methotrexate. Among patients receiving combined therapy with golimumab and methotrexate throughout the study, improvements in physical function and quality of life generally were maintained at weeks 100 and 112, respectively. Patients treated with golimumab and methotrexate additionally demonstrated improved fatigue (as measured by the Functional Assessment of Chronic Illness Therapy-Fatigue [FACIT-F] score).

Clinical Perspective

The American College of Rheumatology issued guidelines for the treatment of rheumatoid arthritis in 2021. Disease-modifying treatments for rheumatoid arthritis include conventional DMARDs (e.g., hydroxychloroquine, leflunomide, methotrexate, sulfasalazine), biologic DMARDs (e.g., TNF blocking agents, abatacept, tocilizumab, sarilumab, rituximab), and/or targeted synthetic DMARDs (e.g., Janus kinase inhibitors). Specific agents for rheumatoid arthritis treatment are selected according to current disease activity, prior therapies used, and the presence of comorbidities. A "treat-to-target" approach is typically employed, with the goal of achieving a predefined target of low disease activity or remission.

TNF blocking agents used in the treatment of rheumatoid arthritis include adalimumab, certolizumab pegol, etanercept, golimumab, and infliximab. Methotrexate monotherapy is strongly recommended over biologic DMARD monotherapy and conditionally recommended over the combination of methotrexate and a TNF blocking agent for DMARD-naive patients with moderate to high disease activity because many patients will achieve their treatment goal with methotrexate alone, and combination therapy with TNF blocking agents may be associated with additional risks and costs. Biologic DMARDs (including TNF blocking agents) and targeted synthetic DMARDs are conditionally recommended as add-on therapy for patients who are taking maximally tolerated dosages of methotrexate and are not at target. Recommendations for the use and selection of biologic DMARDs in rheumatoid arthritis vary based on the presence of certain comorbidities (e.g., heart failure, previous serious infection, nontuberculous mycobacterial lung disease). Consult the American College of Rheumatology guidelines for additional details.

● Psoriatic Arthritis

Psoriatic Arthritis in Adults

Golimumab is used alone or in conjunction with methotrexate for the management of active psoriatic arthritis in adults. Safety and efficacy of golimumab for this use are based principally on the results of 2 randomized controlled trials and a long-term extension study. Guidelines generally support the use of TNF blocking agents, including golimumab, as first-line treatment in adults with active psoriatic arthritis.

Clinical Experience with Subcutaneous Golimumab

Safety and efficacy of subcutaneous golimumab were evaluated in a multicenter, randomized, double-blind, placebo-controlled study (GO-REVEAL) in 405 adults with moderately to severely active psoriatic arthritis (3 or more swollen joints and 3 or more tender joints) who were receiving an NSAIA and/or DMARDs. In addition, patients were required to have a diagnosis of psoriatic arthritis for at least 6 months and plaque psoriasis with a qualifying target lesion (diameter of 2 cm or greater). Patients were randomized to receive golimumab (50 or 100 mg subcutaneously once every 4 weeks) or placebo. The study included patients with any of the following forms of the disease: polyarticular arthritis without rheumatoid nodules, asymmetric peripheral arthritis, distal interphalangeal joint arthritis, spondylitis with peripheral arthritis, or arthritis mutilans. Patients receiving stable dosages of methotrexate (25 mg/week or less), low-dose oral corticosteroids (equivalent to 10 mg of prednisone daily or less), and/or NSAIAs could continue such agents. Previous treatment with a TNF blocking agent was not allowed; the use of other DMARDs, including sulfasalazine, hydroxychloroquine, cytotoxic agents, or other biologic agents, was prohibited. At week 16, patients with less than 10% improvement from baseline in both swollen and tender joint counts entered early escape in which their study drug was adjusted in a double-blind manner (i.e., those meeting the early escape criteria who were receiving golimumab 50 mg had their golimumab dosage increased to 100 mg and those who were receiving placebo began receiving golimumab 50 mg every 4 weeks). At week 24, all remaining patients who had been receiving placebo initiated golimumab 50 mg every 4 weeks. Golimumab continued to be administered in a blinded manner every 4 weeks to week 52. During the unblinded long-term extension period (weeks 52–256), certain adjustments of golimumab dosage (increase to 100 mg or decrease to 50 mg) and concomitant therapies could be made at the clinician's discretion. The median duration of psoriatic arthritis disease prior to study enrollment was 5.1 years, and 78% of patients previously received at least one DMARD; 48, 16, or 72% of patients received stable dosages of methotrexate, low-dose oral corticosteroids, or NSAIAs, respectively, during the blinded study period.

The primary outcome measures were the proportion of patients achieving an ACR 20 response at week 14 and the change from baseline to week 24 in the van der Heijde-Sharp score modified for assessment of psoriatic arthritis. Physical function and health-related quality of life were assessed using the HAQ-DI and SF-36. A greater proportion of patients who received golimumab 50 mg every 4 weeks, with or without methotrexate, achieved an ACR 20 response at week 14 than did patients who received placebo, with or without methotrexate (51 versus 9%, respectively). The proportion of patients who achieved ACR responses was similar for the golimumab 50- and 100-mg dosage groups, as well as for patients who received golimumab with and without methotrexate. At week 24, progression of structural damage, as assessed by the modified van der Heijde-Sharp score, was inhibited in patients who received golimumab 50 mg every 4 weeks compared with those who received placebo. Golimumab therapy also was associated with greater improvements from baseline in the HAQ-DI at week 24 and in the SF-36 physical component summary at week 14 compared with placebo. Although a control group was lacking after week 24, follow-up at 5 years indicated that 63–70% of patients across all randomized groups had ACR 20 responses and the mean change from baseline in the modified van der Heijde-Sharp score was minimal. Concomitant use of golimumab with methotrexate appeared to reduce progression of structural damage compared with use of golimumab without methotrexate.

An additional randomized, double-blind, placebo-controlled trial specifically evaluated the efficacy of golimumab plus methotrexate on dactylitis in psoriatic arthritis. Methotrexate- and biologic DMARD-naive adults with psoriatic arthritis and active dactylitis were randomized to receive subcutaneous golimumab (50 mg every 4 weeks) plus methotrexate or placebo plus methotrexate for 24 weeks. The primary efficacy endpoint was change from baseline to week 24 in Dactylitis Severity Score (DSS), which ranges from 0 to 60 with higher scores representing more severe disease. Study enrollment was halted after 44 patients were randomized based on the results of a pre-planned interim analysis indicating significant benefit with golimumab plus methotrexate. Patients receiving golimumab plus methotrexate had a greater median decrease in DSS from baseline to week 24 compared with patients receiving placebo plus methotrexate (median decrease of 5 versus 2 points, respectively).

Clinical Experience with IV Golimumab

Safety and efficacy of IV golimumab were evaluated in a randomized, double-blind, placebo-controlled study (GO-VIBRANT) in 480 adults with active psoriatic arthritis despite NSAIA and/or DMARD therapy; patients were required to have 5 or more swollen and 5 or more tender joints, and could not have received prior biologic therapy for psoriatic arthritis. Patients were randomized to receive golimumab (2 mg/kg as a 30-minute IV infusion at weeks 0 and 4, then every 8 weeks) or placebo. Those receiving stable dosages of methotrexate (25 mg/week or less), low-dose oral corticosteroids (equivalent to 10 mg of prednisone daily or less), and/or NSAIAs could continue such agents; concomitant use of other DMARDs, including cytotoxic and biologic agents, during the study was prohibited. Patients in the placebo group were switched to golimumab at week 24 (2 mg/kg at weeks 24 and 28, then every 8 weeks through week 52), while patients in the golimumab group continued to receive the drug every 8 weeks through week 52. The median duration of psoriatic arthritis disease prior to study enrollment was 3.5 years; 86% of patients had previously received methotrexate and 35% had received at least one other nonbiologic DMARD. During the study, 70% of patients received concomitant therapy with methotrexate, 71% received NSAIAs, and 28% received oral corticosteroids. The study included patients with any of the following forms of the disease: polyarticular arthritis without rheumatoid nodules (44%), spondylitis with peripheral arthritis (25%), asymmetric peripheral arthritis (19%), distal interphalangeal joint arthritis (8.1%), or arthritis mutilans (4.8%).

The primary outcome measure was the proportion of patients achieving an ACR 20 response at week 14. Physical function and health-related quality of life were assessed using the HAQ-DI and SF-36. Fatigue was assessed using the FAC-IT-F score. A greater proportion of patients receiving golimumab compared with those receiving placebo achieved an ACR 20 response at week 14 (75 versus 22%); ACR 20 response rates at week 24 were similar (77 versus 24%). Greater proportions of patients receiving golimumab compared with those receiving placebo also achieved ACR 50 and ACR 70 responses at weeks 14 and 24. ACR response rates in patients with different forms of psoriatic arthritis were similar, and concomitant use or nonuse of methotrexate did not substantially affect ACR response. Improvements in dactylitis and enthesitis also were observed in golimumab-treated patients. A greater proportion of patients receiving golimumab compared with those receiving placebo had no progression of structural damage, as assessed by the modified van der Heijde-Sharp score, from baseline to week 24 (72 versus 43%) and had clinically meaningful improvements in physical function, as measured by change in HAQ-DI, from baseline to week 14 (69 versus 32%). Golimumab therapy also was associated with greater improvements in the physical and mental component summaries and all 8 domains of the SF-36 compared with placebo, as well as greater improvements in the FACIT-F score. Although a control group was lacking after week 24, follow-up data at week 52 indicated that ACR responses and improvements in health-related quality of life were maintained during continued treatment.

Psoriatic Arthritis in Pediatric Patients

IV golimumab (Simponi Aria®) is used for the management of active psoriatic arthritis in pediatric patients ≥2 years of age. The use of IV golimumab in pediatric patients with psoriatic arthritis is based on pharmacokinetic data and extrapolation of the established efficacy of IV golimumab in adults with psoriatic arthritis.

Clinical Perspective

Psoriatic Arthritis in Adults

The American College of Rheumatology and the National Psoriasis Foundation issued a joint guideline for the treatment of psoriatic arthritis in 2018. Various drugs and drug classes are used to treat psoriatic arthritis, with some classes being used for symptom management (e.g., NSAIAs and corticosteroids) and others being used as immunomodulatory disease-modifying therapy. Disease-modifying treatments for psoriatic arthritis include oral small molecules (e.g., methotrexate, sulfasalazine, cyclosporine, leflunomide, apremilast), biologic DMARDs (e.g., TNF blocking agents, secukinumab, ixekizumab, ustekinumab, brodalumab, abatacept), and/or targeted synthetic DMARDs (e.g., tofacitinib). Specific agents for psoriatic arthritis treatment are selected according to disease characteristics, including disease severity, as well as patient preferences/values and comorbidities. A "treat-to-target" approach is typically employed, with the goal of achieving low/minimal disease activity or remission.

TNF blocking agents used in the treatment of psoriatic arthritis include adalimumab, certolizumab pegol, etanercept, golimumab, and infliximab. For patients with treatment-naive psoriatic arthritis, treatment with a TNF blocking agent is conditionally recommended over treatment with an oral small molecule, interleukin (IL) 17 inhibitor (e.g., secukinumab, ixekizumab, brodalumab) or IL12/23 inhibitor (e.g., ustekinumab). For patients with active psoriatic arthritis despite treatment with an oral small molecule, switching to monotherapy with a TNF blocking agent is conditionally recommended over combination therapy with a TNF blocking agent plus methotrexate or switching to another oral small molecule, ustekinumab, secukinumab, ixekizumab, brodalumab, abatacept, or tofacitinib. For patients with active psoriatic arthritis despite treatment with TNF blocking agent monotherapy, switching to monotherapy with a different TNF blocking agent is conditionally recommended over switching to ustekinumab, secukinumab, ixekizumab, brodalumab, abatacept, or tofacitinib. For patients with active psoriatic arthritis despite treatment with a combination of a TNF blocking agent and methotrexate, switching to a different TNF blocking agent plus methotrexate is conditionally recommended over switching to a different TNF blocking agent as monotherapy. Switching to a TNF blocking agent is conditionally recommended for patients with active psoriatic arthritis despite treatment with secukinumab, ixekizumab, brodalumab, or ustekinumab. Recommendations for the use and selection of disease-modifying therapies in psoriatic arthritis vary based on the presence of certain disease characteristics (e.g., psoriatic spondylitis/axial disease, enthesitis) and comorbidities (e.g., inflammatory bowel disease, diabetes). Consult the American College of Rheumatology/National Psoriasis Foundation guideline for additional details.

Psoriatic Arthritis in Pediatric Patients

Psoriatic arthritis in pediatric patients is classified as a subtype of juvenile idiopathic arthritis. The American College of Rheumatology and the Arthritis Foundation issued a joint guideline for the treatment of juvenile idiopathic arthritis (including psoriatic arthritis) manifesting as nonsystemic polyarthritis, sacroiliitis, or enthesitis in 2019. Guidelines generally support the use of TNF blocking agents, including golimumab, as add-on therapy in pediatric patients with psoriatic arthritis. In patients with psoriatic arthritis manifesting as nonsystemic polyarthritis, TNF blocking agents are recommended if moderate to high disease activity persists despite the use of methotrexate. In patients with psoriatic arthritis manifesting as sacroiliitis or enthesitis, TNF blocking agents, including golimumab, are recommended if active disease persists despite NSAIA use. (See Juvenile Idiopathic Arthritis under Uses.)

In all children and adolescents initiating biologic DMARD therapy, combination therapy with a conventional DMARD is recommended over biologic DMARD monotherapy.

● Ankylosing Spondylitis

Golimumab is used for the management of ankylosing spondylitis in adults with active disease. Safety and efficacy of golimumab for this use are based principally on the results of 2 randomized controlled trials and a long-term extension study. Guidelines generally support the use of TNF blocking agents, including golimumab, for the treatment of ankylosing spondylitis in patients with active disease despite treatment with NSAIAs.

Clinical Experience with Subcutaneous Golimumab

Safety and efficacy of subcutaneous golimumab were evaluated in a multicenter, randomized, double-blind, placebo-controlled study (GO-RAISE) in 356 adults with active ankylosing spondylitis (as defined by the modified New York criteria) for at least 3 months prior to administration of the study drug. To be included in this study, patients were required to have symptoms of active disease (defined as a Bath Ankylosing Spondylitis Disease Activity Index [BASDAI] score of 4 or more and a visual analog scale [VAS] score for total back pain of 4 or more, on scales of 0–10) and an inadequate response to current or previous NSAIA or DMARD therapy. Patients ineligible for participation in the study included, but were not limited to, patients with complete ankylosis of the spine and patients who had previously received treatment with a TNF blocking agent. Patients were randomized to receive golimumab (50 or 100 mg subcutaneously once every 4 weeks) or placebo. Patients receiving stable dosages of methotrexate (25 mg/week or less), sulfasalazine, hydroxychloroquine, low-dose corticosteroids (equivalent to 10 mg of prednisone daily or less), and/or NSAIAs could continue such agents; the use of other DMARDs, including cytotoxic agents or other biologic agents, was prohibited. At week 16, patients with less than 20% improvement from baseline in total back pain and morning stiffness entered early escape in which their study drug was adjusted in a double-blind manner (i.e., those meeting the early escape criteria who were receiving golimumab 50 mg had their golimumab dosage increased to 100 mg and those who were receiving placebo began receiving golimumab 50 mg every 4 weeks). At week 24, all remaining patients who had been receiving placebo

initiated golimumab 50 mg every 4 weeks. Golimumab continued to be administered in a blinded manner every 4 weeks through week 100. During the unblinded long-term extension period (weeks 104–252), certain adjustments of golimumab dosage (increase to 100 mg or decrease to 50 mg) and concomitant therapies could be made at the clinician's discretion. The median duration of ankylosing spondylitis disease prior to study enrollment was 5.6 years, and 55% of patients previously received at least one DMARD; 20, 26, 1, 16, or 90% of patients received stable dosages of methotrexate, sulfasalazine, hydroxychloroquine, low-dose oral corticosteroids, or NSAIAs, respectively, during the blinded study period.

The primary outcome measure was the proportion of patients achieving an Assessment in Ankylosing Spondylitis (ASAS) 20 response at week 14. An ASAS 20 response is achieved if the patient experiences at least a 20% improvement and an absolute improvement of at least 10 units (on a scale of 0–100) in at least 3 of the following criteria without worsening in the fourth criterion: patient global assessment, pain, function, or inflammation. A greater proportion of patients who received golimumab 50 mg every 4 weeks, with or without DMARDs, achieved an ASAS 20 response at week 14 than did patients who received placebo, with or without DMARDs (59 versus 22%, respectively). At week 24, 56% of those receiving golimumab 50 mg every 4 weeks, with or without DMARDs, achieved an ASAS 20 response; 23% of those receiving placebo, with or without DMARDs, achieved an ASAS 20 response. The proportion of patients who achieved ASAS responses was similar for the golimumab 50- and 100-mg dosage groups. Clinical improvements observed in patients receiving golimumab at week 24 were maintained through up to 5 years of treatment.

Clinical Experience with IV Golimumab

Safety and efficacy of IV golimumab were evaluated in a randomized, double-blind, placebo-controlled study (GO-ALIVE) in 208 adults with active ankylosing spondylitis (as defined by the modified New York criteria) who had an inadequate response or intolerance to NSAIAs. Up to 20% of patients enrolled in the study could have received prior therapy with one TNF blocking agent other than golimumab (discontinued for reasons other than lack of efficacy within the first 16 weeks of treatment). To be included in this study, patients were required to have symptoms of active disease, including a BASDAI score of 4 or more and a VAS score for total back pain of 4 or more (on scales of 0–10). Patients were randomized to receive golimumab (2 mg/kg as a 30-minute IV infusion at weeks 0 and 4, then every 8 weeks through week 52) or placebo; at week 16, patients in the placebo group were switched to golimumab (2 mg/kg at weeks 16 and 20, then every 8 weeks through week 52). Patients receiving stable dosages of methotrexate (25 mg/week or less), sulfasalazine, hydroxychloroquine, low-dose corticosteroids (equivalent to 10 mg of prednisone daily or less), and/or NSAIAs could continue such agents; the use of other DMARDs, including cytotoxic and biologic agents, was prohibited during the study. The median duration of ankylosing spondylitis disease prior to study enrollment was 2.8 years, and the median duration of inflammatory back pain was 8 years; 8.2% of patients had undergone prior joint surgery or procedure; 5.8% had complete ankylosis of the spine; 76% had previously received at least one DMARD; and 14% had previously received one other TNF blocking agent. During the study, 88% of patients received concomitant therapy with NSAIAs, 38% received sulfasalazine, 26% received oral corticosteroids, 18% received methotrexate, and less than 1% received hydroxychloroquine.

The primary outcome measure was the proportion of patients achieving an ASAS 20 response at week 16. ASAS 40 response, defined using the same criteria with a level of improvement of 40%, also was assessed. At week 16, greater proportions of patients receiving golimumab compared with those receiving placebo achieved an ASAS 20 response (73 versus 26%), ASAS 40 response (48 versus 8.7%), and ASAS partial remission (i.e., a low level of disease activity defined as a score of less than 2 on a scale of 0–10 in all 4 ASAS domains) (16 versus 4%). Compared with placebo, golimumab therapy also was associated with greater improvements in physical function as measured by the Bath Ankylosing Spondylitis Functional Index (BASFI) and in quality of life as measured by the physical and mental component summaries and all 8 domains of the SF-36 and the Ankylosing Spondylitis Quality of Life [ASQoL] questionnaire. Improvements in disease activity and health-related quality of life were maintained through 52 weeks of follow-up in patients receiving golimumab.

Clinical Perspective

The American College of Rheumatology, the Spondylitis Association of America, and the Spondyloarthritis Research and Treatment Network issued a joint guideline for the treatment of ankylosing spondylitis in 2019. Treatments for ankylosing spondylitis include NSAIAs, conventional DMARDs (e.g., methotrexate, sulfasalazine), biologic DMARDs (e.g., TNF blocking agents, secukinumab, ixekizumab), and/or targeted synthetic DMARDs (e.g., tofacitinib). Continuous NSAIA treatment is typically considered first-line for active ankylosing spondylitis, with other agents used in the treatment of NSAIA-refractory disease. Specific agents for ankylosing spondylitis treatment are selected according to current disease activity, prior therapies, and the presence of comorbidities. Goals of therapy in ankylosing spondylitis are to alleviate symptoms, improve functioning, maintain the ability to work, decrease complications, and prevent or slow skeletal damage.

TNF blocking agents used in the treatment of ankylosing spondylitis include adalimumab, certolizumab pegol, etanercept, golimumab, and infliximab. For adults with active ankylosing spondylitis despite treatment with NSAIAs, treatment with a TNF blocking agent is strongly recommended over no treatment with a TNF blocking agent and conditionally recommended over treatment with tofacitinib, secukinumab, or ixekizumab. No specific TNF blocking agent is recommended over others. In patients with active ankylosing spondylitis despite treatment with a first TNF blocking agent, guidelines conditionally recommend secukinumab or ixekizumab over treatment with a different TNF blocking agent for patients with primary nonresponse to TNF blocking therapy; in patients with secondary nonresponse to TNF blocking therapy, treatment with a different TNF blocking therapy is conditionally recommended over treatment with a non-TNF blocking biologic agent. In adults with stable ankylosing spondylitis, continuation of biologic monotherapy is conditionally recommended over discontinuation of the biologic or continuation of combination therapy with NSAIAs or conventional DMARDs. Recommendations for treatment selection in ankylosing spondylitis may be influenced by the presence of certain comorbidities (e.g., iritis, inflammatory bowel disease). Consult the joint guideline issued by the American College of Rheumatology, the Spondylitis Association of America, and the Spondyloarthritis Research and Treatment Network for additional details.

● Ulcerative Colitis

Golimumab is used in adults with moderately to severely active ulcerative colitis who require continuous corticosteroid therapy or who have had an inadequate response to or were intolerant to conventional therapies (oral aminosalicylates, oral corticosteroids, azathioprine, or mercaptopurine) to induce and maintain clinical response, to improve endoscopic appearance of the mucosa during induction therapy, to induce clinical remission, and to achieve and sustain clinical remission in those who have responded to induction therapy. Safety and efficacy of golimumab for this use are based principally on the results of 2 randomized controlled trials and a long-term extension study. Guidelines generally support the first-line use of TNF blocking agents, including golimumab, for induction and maintenance of remission in patients with moderate to severe ulcerative colitis.

Clinical Experience with Subcutaneous Golimumab

Safety and efficacy of subcutaneous golimumab were established in 2 randomized, double-blind, placebo-controlled studies (PURSUIT-SC and PURSUIT-M) in adults with ulcerative colitis. PURSUIT-SC evaluated golimumab induction therapy and included a dose-finding phase 2 study followed by a dose-confirming phase 3 study. PURSUIT-M evaluated golimumab maintenance therapy in patients who had responded to induction therapy with the drug. Induction therapy with IV† golimumab (single 1-, 2-, or 4-mg/kg induction dose) also has been evaluated (PURSUIT-IV); however, the study failed to establish efficacy of these induction regimens.

Patients enrolled in PURSUIT-SC had moderately to severely active ulcerative colitis (as defined by a Mayo score of 6–12 with an endoscopy subscore of 2 or 3) and were corticosteroid dependent or had an inadequate response or intolerance to one or more conventional therapies (i.e., oral aminosalicylates, oral corticosteroids, azathioprine, mercaptopurine). Those who had received prior therapy with TNF blocking agents were excluded from the study. The Mayo score ranges from 0–12 and includes 4 subscales (i.e., stool frequency, rectal bleeding, findings on endoscopy, and physician global assessment), each scored from 0–3 (normal to most severe, respectively). An endoscopy subscore of 2 is defined by marked erythema, lack of vascular pattern, friability, and erosions, whereas an endoscopy subscore of 3 is defined by spontaneous bleeding and ulceration.

Two of the induction regimens evaluated in the dose-finding phase 2 study (golimumab 400 mg at week 0 and 200 mg at week 2 [400 mg/200 mg], golimumab

200 mg at week 0 and 100 mg at week 2 [200 mg/100 mg]) were selected for further evaluation in the phase 3 study. The phase 3 evaluation included data for 761 patients. Patients receiving stable dosages of oral aminosalicylates, oral corticosteroids (equivalent to 40 mg of prednisone daily or less), azathioprine, mercaptopurine, and/or methotrexate were permitted to continue receiving these drugs throughout the study. The median baseline Mayo score for the phase 2 and 3 studies combined was 8. The primary outcome measure in the phase 3 study was the proportion of patients in clinical response at week 6; clinical response was defined as a decrease in Mayo score of at least 3 points and at least 30% from baseline score, with a reduction in rectal bleeding subscore of at least 1 point or an absolute rectal bleeding subscore of 0 (no blood seen) or 1 (streaks of blood with stool less than half the time). Other outcome measures included clinical remission and improved mucosal appearance. Clinical remission was defined as a Mayo score of 0–2 with no individual subscore exceeding 1. Improved mucosal appearance was defined as a Mayo endoscopy subscore of 0 (normal mucosa or inactive disease) or 1 (erythema, decreased vascular pattern, mild friability). At week 6, clinical response rates (51 versus 30%), clinical remission rates (18 versus 6%), and rates of improved mucosal appearance (42 versus 29%) were higher in patients receiving induction therapy with golimumab 200 mg/100 mg compared with those receiving placebo. Induction therapy with golimumab 400 mg/200 mg provided no additional benefit beyond that provided by a dosage of 200 mg/100 mg.

PURSUIT-M was a randomized-withdrawal study that evaluated 456 patients who had attained clinical response with golimumab induction therapy and had tolerated the drug during either the PURSUIT-SC or PURSUIT-IV study. Approximately 35% of these patients were in clinical remission at the start of the PURSUIT-M maintenance study. Patients who had responded to golimumab induction therapy were randomized to receive maintenance therapy with subcutaneous golimumab (50 or 100 mg every 4 weeks) or placebo. Those receiving stable dosages of oral aminosalicylates, azathioprine, mercaptopurine, and/or methotrexate could continue such agents. At the start of the maintenance study, approximately 52% of patients who had responded to golimumab induction therapy were receiving corticosteroids, 31% were receiving azathioprine or mercaptopurine, less than 1% were receiving methotrexate, and 80% were receiving aminosalicylates. In patients receiving corticosteroids, a corticosteroid-tapering regimen was initiated at the start of the maintenance trial. The primary outcome measure was the proportion of patients maintaining clinical response through week 54. In PURSUIT-M, clinical response was maintained through week 54 in 50, 47, or 31% of those receiving golimumab 100 mg every 4 weeks, golimumab 50 mg every 4 weeks, or placebo, respectively. A greater proportion of patients receiving golimumab 100 mg every 4 weeks, compared with those receiving placebo (28 versus 16%), achieved clinical remission at both weeks 30 and 54 without demonstrating a loss of response at any time point through week 54; although golimumab 50 mg every 4 weeks showed a numerical advantage over placebo for this outcome measure (23% of patients in clinical remission), the difference was not statistically significant.

Patients who completed the PURSUIT-M study were eligible to participate in a long-term extension study if investigators determined that benefit could be derived from continued treatment. Patients enrolled in the long-term extension study received the same treatment that they had received during PURSUIT-M (golimumab or placebo) at the same dosage for up to 3 additional years. Among the 195 patients who continued golimumab treatment in the long-term extension study, treatment efficacy (as measured by Physician's Global Assessment scores and Inflammatory Bowel Disease Questionnaire scores) was maintained through week 216.

Clinical Perspective

The American College of Gastroenterology (ACG) and the American Gastroenterological Association (AGA) issued guidelines for the medical treatment of ulcerative colitis in adults in 2019 and 2020. Goals of therapy in ulcerative colitis include achieving and maintaining corticosteroid-free remission and promoting mucosal healing. Specific treatments for ulcerative colitis are selected according to the disease severity, as well as disease location/extent, disease prognosis, and previous therapies used. Drug classes used to treat ulcerative colitis include oral and rectal 5-aminosalicylates, oral and rectal corticosteroids, immunomodulators (e.g., thiopurines, methotrexate), tofacitinib, and biologic agents, including TNF blocking agents, vedolizumab, and ustekinumab. In most cases, if a drug used for induction therapy is effective, it is continued as maintenance of remission.

TNF blocking agents used in the treatment of ulcerative colitis include infliximab, golimumab, and adalimumab; the primary role for these agents is in the treatment of moderate to severe ulcerative colitis. For adult outpatients with moderate to severe ulcerative colitis, AGA recommends TNF blocking therapies, vedolizumab, tofacitinib, or ustekinumab over no treatment. ACG recommends the use of oral corticosteroids, TNF blocking agents, vedolizumab, or tofacitinib for induction of remission in patients with moderately to severely active ulcerative colitis. Early use of biologic agents with or without immunomodulator therapy is conditionally recommended over gradual step up therapy after failure of 5-aminosalicylates. Combination therapy with a TNF blocking agent and a thiopurine or methotrexate is conditionally recommended over biologic monotherapy. Patients who achieve remission with TNF blocking therapy should continue such therapy to maintain remission after induction. Patients with primary nonresponse to TNF blocking therapy should be switched to a biologic from a different class; patients who initially respond to one TNF blocking agent and later lose response can be switched to a different TNF blocking agent. Patients with mildly active ulcerative colitis and multiple prognostic factors associated with an increased risk of hospitalization or surgery should be treated with therapies for moderately to severely active disease. Consult the American College of Gastroenterology guideline for additional details on prognostic factors that may be considered.

● *Juvenile Idiopathic Arthritis*

IV golimumab (Simponi Aria®) is used for the management of active polyarticular juvenile idiopathic arthritis in pediatric patients ≥2 years of age. Guidelines generally support the use of TNF blocking agents, including golimumab, as add-on therapy in patients with moderate to high disease activity despite the use of methotrexate.

Clinical Experience with IV Golimumab

The use of IV golimumab in pediatric patients with polyarticular juvenile idiopathic arthritis is based on pharmacokinetic data and extrapolation of the established efficacy of IV golimumab in adults with rheumatoid arthritis. Efficacy of IV golimumab for this use was additionally assessed in a single-arm, open-label study. In this study, 127 pediatric patients 2–17 years of age were enrolled. All patients had juvenile idiopathic arthritis and active polyarthritis despite treatment with methotrexate for at least 2 months. Approximately 35% of patients had rheumatoid factor positive disease, and 9, 6, 4, and 3% had enthesitis-related arthritis, oligoarticular extended arthritis, juvenile psoriatic arthritis, and systemic juvenile idiopathic arthritis without systemic manifestations, respectively. All patients received golimumab 80 mg/m² (maximum of 240 mg) as an IV infusion over 30 minutes at week 0, week 4, then every 8 weeks through week 52. Stable dosages of methotrexate were continued through week 28; after week 28, methotrexate dosage changes were permitted. Efficacy endpoints included the proportions of patients achieving a juvenile idiopathic arthritis ACR 30, 50, 70, or 90 response (defined as a 30, 50, 70, or 90% improvement from baseline in at least 3 juvenile idiopathic arthritis core measures without worsening of 30% or more in more than 1 of the remaining core measures). At week 28, the ACR 30, 50, 70, and 90 response rates with golimumab were 83.5, 79.5, 70.1, and 46.5%, respectively. At week 52, the ACR 30, 50, 70, and 90 response rates were 75.6, 74, 65.4, and 48.8%, respectively.

Clinical Experience with Subcutaneous Golimumab

Subcutaneous golimumab also has been used in pediatric patients with active polyarticular juvenile idiopathic arthritis†. The use of subcutaneous golimumab (30 mg/m² based on body surface area, up to a maximum of 50 mg, given every 4 weeks) as add-on therapy to methotrexate was evaluated in a randomized placebo-controlled trial in 173 patients 2–17 years of age with active polyarticular juvenile idiopathic arthritis despite methotrexate therapy. However, the study failed to meet its primary endpoint (proportion of patients with juvenile idiopathic arthritis flares at week 48) and therefore failed to establish efficacy of subcutaneous golimumab in this patient population.

Clinical Perspective

The American College of Rheumatology and the Arthritis Foundation issued a joint guideline for the treatment of juvenile idiopathic arthritis manifesting as nonsystemic polyarthritis (including polyarticular disease), sacroiliitis, or enthesitis in 2019. Several drug classes are used to treat juvenile idiopathic arthritis, including NSAIAs, systemic and intra-articular corticosteroids, conventional DMARDs (e.g., methotrexate, sulfasalazine, hydroxychloroquine, leflunomide),

and biologic DMARDs (e.g., TNF blocking agents, abatacept, tocilizumab, rituximab). Specific agents for juvenile idiopathic arthritis treatment are selected according to the presence of certain risk factors (e.g., positive anti-cyclic citrullinated peptide antibodies, positive rheumatoid factor, joint damage), level of disease activity, involvement of specific joints, presence of certain comorbidities (e.g., uveitis), and prior therapies used. An individualized "treat-to-target" approach is typically employed, with the goal of achieving remission or minimal/low disease activity.

TNF blocking agents used in the treatment of juvenile idiopathic arthritis include adalimumab, etanercept, golimumab, and infliximab. Methotrexate monotherapy is conditionally recommended as initial therapy for patients with juvenile idiopathic arthritis manifesting as nonsystemic polyarthritis, although initial biologic DMARD therapy may be considered for patients with risk factors and involvement of high-risk joints (e.g., cervical spine, wrist, hip), high disease activity, and/or those judged by their physician to be at high risk of disabling joint damage. In patients with moderate or high disease activity despite methotrexate monotherapy, biologic DMARDs (including TNF blocking agents) are conditionally recommended as add-on therapy. In patients with moderate or high disease activity despite treatment with a first TNF blocking agent (with or without concomitant conventional DMARD therapy), switching to tocilizumab or abatacept is conditionally recommended over switching to a different TNF blocking agent, although a different TNF blocking agent may be appropriate if the patient experienced a good initial response to their first TNF blocking agent. In all patients initiating biologic DMARD therapy, combination therapy with a conventional DMARD is recommended over biologic DMARD monotherapy. Specific choice of biologic DMARD may be influenced by the presence of certain comorbidities (e.g., uveitis). Consult the American College of Rheumatology/Arthritis Foundation guidelines for additional details.

● *Nonradiographic Axial Spondyloarthritis*

Subcutaneous golimumab may be useful in the treatment of active nonradiographic axial spondyloarthritis†. A 16-week, randomized, double-blind, placebo-controlled trial (GO-AHEAD) enrolled 198 adults 18–45 years of age with active nonradiographic axial spondyloarthritis and compared subcutaneous golimumab (50 mg at weeks 0, 4, 8, and 12) to placebo. At week 16, more patients receiving golimumab achieved an ASAS 20 response (the primary outcome measure) compared to placebo. Rates of ASAS 20 response at week 16 were 71.1% and 40% among golimumab-treated patients and placebo-treated patients, respectively. Patients who completed this 16-week randomized controlled trial were eligible to enroll in an open-label extension study; all patients received subcutaneous golimumab 50 mg at week 16 and every 4 weeks thereafter until week 48. In the open-label extension study, efficacy responses observed with golimumab at week 16 were maintained at week 52.

DOSAGE AND ADMINISTRATION

● *General*

Pretreatment Screening

- Evaluate all patients for active and inactive tuberculosis prior to initiating therapy.
- Screen all patients for hepatitis B virus (HBV) infection before initiating therapy.
- Do not initiate therapy in patients with an active infection, including clinically important localized infections.

Patient Monitoring

- Monitor closely for signs or symptoms of infection (e.g., fever, malaise, weight loss, sweats, cough, dyspnea, pulmonary infiltrates, serious systemic illness including shock) during and after treatment; monitor for possible development of tuberculosis in patients who tested negative for latent tuberculosis prior to initiating therapy.
- Perform periodic dermatologic evaluations in all patients, particularly those with risk factors for skin cancer.
- Evaluate and monitor chronic carriers of HBV during treatment and for up to several months following treatment.

Dispensing and Administration Precautions

- Efficacy and safety of switching between IV and subcutaneous golimumab formulations and routes of administration have not been established.

Other General Considerations

- Golimumab is used in conjunction with methotrexate for the management of rheumatoid arthritis in adults; the drug may be used with or without methotrexate or other nonbiologic disease-modifying antirheumatic drugs (DMARD) in adults with psoriatic arthritis or ankylosing spondylitis.

- Corticosteroids and nonsteroidal anti-inflammatory agents (NSAIAs) or analgesics may be continued in adults receiving golimumab for the management of rheumatoid arthritis, psoriatic arthritis, or ankylosing spondylitis.

- Aminosalicylates, corticosteroids, azathioprine, mercaptopurine, and/or methotrexate were permitted to be continued during pivotal trials of golimumab in patients with ulcerative colitis. However, the possibility of an increased risk of hepatosplenic T-cell lymphoma with combination immunosuppressive therapy should be considered carefully.

● Administration

Golimumab may be administered by subcutaneous injection in adults with rheumatoid arthritis, psoriatic arthritis, ankylosing spondylitis, or ulcerative colitis. Golimumab may be administered by IV infusion in adults with rheumatoid arthritis, psoriatic arthritis, or ankylosing spondylitis, and in pediatric patients with psoriatic arthritis or polyarticular juvenile idiopathic arthritis.

Golimumab is intended for use under the guidance and supervision of a clinician; however, subcutaneous golimumab may be *self-administered* if the clinician determines that the patient and/or their caregiver is competent to safely administer the drug after appropriate training.

Subcutaneous Administration

For subcutaneous administration, golimumab is commercially available in prefilled syringes and in prefilled auto-injectors (SmartJect®) equipped with a 27-gauge, ½-inch needle. Prior to subcutaneous administration, golimumab solutions should be inspected visually for particulate matter or discoloration; if either is present, the solution should be discarded. Golimumab prefilled syringes and auto-injectors for subcutaneous administration are for single use only; unused portions of the solution should be discarded.

Golimumab injection should be stored at 2–8°C in the original carton until administration and protected from light. The injection should not be frozen or shaken. The golimumab prefilled syringe or auto-injector should be allowed to sit at room temperature outside of the carton for 30 minutes prior to subcutaneous injection; golimumab should *not* be warmed in any other way (e.g., microwave, hot water). The syringe needle cover or auto-injector cap should *not* be removed while the prefilled syringe or auto-injector is warming to room temperature. If necessary, golimumab prefilled syringes and auto-injectors for subcutaneous administration may be stored at room temperature up to 25°C for a maximum single period of 30 days in the original carton protected from light; once a syringe or auto-injector has been stored at room temperature, it should not be returned to the refrigerator and should be discarded if not used within 30 days.

Golimumab is administered subcutaneously into the thighs. Golimumab also may be administered subcutaneously into the lower abdomen below the umbilicus; however, abdominal injections should not be made within 5.08 cm (2 inches) of the umbilicus. Golimumab may be administered subcutaneously into the upper arm by a caregiver. If multiple injections are required to administer a single dose, separate injection sites should be used. Injection sites should be rotated. Injections should not be made into areas where the skin is tender, bruised, red, or hard or into scars or stretch marks.

IV Administration

For IV infusion, golimumab is commercially available as an injection concentrate containing 12.5 mg/mL. IV golimumab should be stored at 2–8°C in the original carton until administration and protected from light. If necessary, golimumab injection concentrate may be stored at room temperature up to 25°C for a maximum single period of 30 days in the original carton protected from light; once the injection concentrate has been stored at room temperature, it should not be

returned to the refrigerator and should be discarded if not used within 30 days. The vials should not be frozen or shaken.

Prior to IV administration, golimumab injection concentrate must be diluted in 0.45 or 0.9% sodium chloride injection to provide a total volume of 100 mL (i.e., if a 100-mL bottle or bag of 0.45 or 0.9% sodium chloride injection is used, a volume of diluent equal to the total required volume of golimumab injection concentrate should be removed from the infusion container prior to addition of the golimumab injection concentrate). The total required volume of golimumab injection concentrate should be added slowly to the infusion container, and the diluted solution gently mixed. Any unused portion of drug should be discarded since the injection concentrate contains no preservative. Golimumab solutions should be inspected visually for particulate matter and discoloration prior to dilution and administration. The injection concentrate should appear colorless to light yellow and should not be used if discoloration or particulates other than a few fine translucent particles are present. The diluted solution may be stored for 4 hours at room temperature. Diluted golimumab solutions should be infused IV over 30 minutes using an inline nonpyrogenic, low-protein-binding filter with a pore size not exceeding 0.22 μm. Golimumab should not be infused simultaneously through the same IV line with any other drug. The diluted solution should not be used if discoloration or particulate matter is present.

● Dosage

Adult Dosage

Rheumatoid Arthritis

For the management of moderately to severely active rheumatoid arthritis in adults, the usual dosage of golimumab is 50 mg once monthly by subcutaneous injection or 2 mg/kg given by IV infusion over 30 minutes at weeks 0 and 4 and then every 8 weeks thereafter; golimumab should be used in conjunction with methotrexate for the management of rheumatoid arthritis.

Psoriatic Arthritis

For the management of active psoriatic arthritis in adults, the usual dosage of golimumab is 50 mg once monthly by subcutaneous injection or 2 mg/kg given by IV infusion over 30 minutes at weeks 0 and 4 and then every 8 weeks thereafter.

Ankylosing Spondylitis

For the management of active ankylosing spondylitis in adults, the usual dosage of golimumab is 50 mg once monthly by subcutaneous injection or 2 mg/kg given by IV infusion over 30 minutes at weeks 0 and 4 and then every 8 weeks thereafter.

Ulcerative Colitis

For the management of moderately to severely active ulcerative colitis in adults, the recommended dosage of golimumab is 200 mg at week 0 followed by 100 mg at week 2 (induction therapy) and then 100 mg every 4 weeks thereafter (maintenance therapy), with all doses given by subcutaneous injection.

Pediatric Dosage

Psoriatic Arthritis

For the management of active psoriatic arthritis in pediatric patients ≥2 years of age, the recommended dosage of golimumab is 80 mg/m² given by IV infusion over 30 minutes at weeks 0 and 4 and then every 8 weeks thereafter. The dosage of golimumab should be calculated based on body surface area.

Juvenile Idiopathic Arthritis

For the management of active polyarticular juvenile idiopathic arthritis in pediatric patients ≥2 years of age, the recommended dosage of golimumab is 80 mg/m² given by IV infusion over 30 minutes at weeks 0 and 4 and then every 8 weeks thereafter. The dosage of golimumab should be calculated based on body surface area.

● Special Populations

Dosage adjustment of subcutaneous golimumab based on weight or gender is not necessary. The manufacturer makes no specific dosage recommendations for geriatric patients or patients with hepatic or renal impairment.

CAUTIONS

● Contraindications

- Manufacturer states none known.

● Warnings/Precautions

Warnings

Infectious Complications

A boxed warning about the risk of serious infections is included in the prescribing information for golimumab. Patients receiving tumor necrosis factor (TNF) blocking agents, including golimumab, are at increased risk of developing serious infections involving various organ systems and sites that may require hospitalization or result in death. Opportunistic infections caused by bacterial, mycobacterial, invasive fungal, viral, or parasitic organisms—including aspergillosis, blastomycosis, candidiasis, coccidioidomycosis, histoplasmosis, legionellosis, listeriosis, pneumocystosis, and tuberculosis—have been reported in patients receiving TNF blocking agents. Infections frequently have been disseminated rather than localized. Patients should be closely monitored during and after treatment with TNF blocking agents for the development of signs or symptoms of infection (e.g., fever, malaise, weight loss, sweats, cough, dyspnea, pulmonary infiltrates, serious systemic illness including shock), including the possible development of tuberculosis in patients who tested negative for latent tuberculosis prior to initiating therapy. Most patients who developed serious infections were receiving concomitant therapy with immunosuppressive agents such as methotrexate or corticosteroids.

In controlled trials evaluating subcutaneous golimumab in adults with rheumatoid arthritis, psoriatic arthritis, or ankylosing spondylitis, infection was reported in 28 or 25% of golimumab-treated or control patients, respectively, following 16 weeks of treatment; the rate of serious infection was 1.4 or 1.3%, respectively. In a controlled trial evaluating IV golimumab in adults with rheumatoid arthritis, infection was reported following 24 weeks of treatment in 27% of patients receiving golimumab and methotrexate compared with 24% of those receiving placebo and methotrexate; the rate of serious infection was 0.9 or 0%, respectively. In controlled trials in patients with ulcerative colitis, rates of infection and serious infection during the induction period (through week 6) were similar in patients receiving subcutaneous golimumab (200 mg at week 0 and 100 mg at week 2) and those receiving placebo; infection was reported in approximately 12% of patients. Among patients who received golimumab induction therapy, rates of infection and serious infection through 60 weeks of treatment were similar in those who received a maintenance regimen of golimumab 100 mg every 4 weeks and those who received placebo.

Serious infections reported in patients receiving golimumab have included sepsis, pneumonia, cellulitis, opportunistic infections, abscess, tuberculosis, invasive fungal infections, and hepatitis B virus (HBV) infection. As of September 2011, FDA had identified 103 reports of *Legionella* pneumonia associated with TNF blocking agents, including golimumab. The 103 cases of *Legionella* pneumonia occurred in patients 25–85 years of age, many of whom received concomitant therapy with immunosuppressive agents (e.g., corticosteroids and/or methotrexate); 17 deaths were reported. In 78% of the cases of *Legionella* pneumonia, the median duration of TNF blocker therapy prior to the onset of *Legionella* pneumonia was 10.4 months (range: less than 1 month to 73 months). As of September 2011, FDA also had identified 26 published reports of *Listeria* infections, including meningitis, bacteremia, endophthalmitis, and sepsis, in patients who received TNF blocking agents; 7 deaths were reported. Many of the *Listeria* infections occurred in patients who had received concomitant therapy with immunosuppressive agents. In addition, FDA identified fatal *Listeria* infections during a review of data regarding laboratory-confirmed infections that occurred in premarketing clinical studies and during postmarketing surveillance.

An increased incidence of serious infections also was observed in clinical studies in patients with rheumatoid arthritis when a TNF blocking agent was used concomitantly with anakinra (a human interleukin-1 receptor antagonist) or abatacept (a selective costimulation modulator). Concomitant use of golimumab and other biologic agents used in the management of rheumatoid arthritis, psoriatic arthritis, ankylosing spondylitis, or polyarticular juvenile idiopathic arthritis (including abatacept and anakinra) is not recommended because of the possibility of an increased risk of infection. Exercise caution when switching from one

biologic disease-modifying antirheumatic drug (DMARD) to another, since overlapping biologic activity may further increase the risk of infection.

Do not initiate golimumab therapy in patients with active infections, including clinically important localized infections. Patients >65 years of age, patients with comorbid conditions, and/or patients receiving concomitant therapy with immunosuppressive agents such as corticosteroids or methotrexate may be at increased risk of infection. Clinicians should consider potential risks and benefits of the drug prior to initiating therapy in patients with a history of chronic, recurring, or opportunistic infections; patients with underlying conditions that may predispose them to infections; and patients who have been exposed to tuberculosis or who reside or have traveled in regions where tuberculosis or mycoses such as histoplasmosis, coccidioidomycosis, and blastomycosis are endemic. Any patient who develops a new infection while receiving golimumab should undergo a thorough diagnostic evaluation (appropriate for an immunocompromised patient), appropriate anti-infective therapy should be initiated, and the patient should be closely monitored. Discontinue the drug in patients who develop a serious infection, an opportunistic infection, or sepsis.

Because tuberculosis has been reported in patients receiving golimumab, including in patients who received golimumab during and following treatment for latent tuberculosis, evaluate all patients for active or latent tuberculosis and for the presence of risk factors for tuberculosis prior to and periodically during therapy with the drug. When indicated, initiate an appropriate antimycobacterial regimen for the treatment of latent tuberculosis infection prior to golimumab therapy. Antimycobacterial treatment lowers the risk of latent tuberculosis infection progressing to active disease (i.e., reactivation) in patients receiving golimumab. Consider antimycobacterial therapy prior to initiating golimumab in individuals with a history of latent or active tuberculosis in whom an adequate course of antimycobacterial treatment cannot be confirmed and in individuals with a negative tuberculin skin test who have risk factors for tuberculosis. Consult a tuberculosis specialist when deciding whether antimycobacterial therapy should be initiated. Monitor patients receiving golimumab, including individuals with a negative tuberculin skin test, patients who are receiving treatment for latent tuberculosis, and patients who previously were treated for tuberculosis infection, for signs and symptoms of active tuberculosis. Consider a diagnosis of tuberculosis in patients who develop new infections while receiving golimumab, especially in those who previously have traveled to countries where tuberculosis is highly prevalent or who have been in close contact with an individual with active tuberculosis.

Failure to recognize invasive fungal infections in patients receiving TNF blocking agents has led to delays in appropriate treatment. Clinicians should ascertain whether patients receiving TNF blocking agents who present with signs and symptoms suggestive of systemic fungal infection reside or have traveled in regions where mycoses are endemic. Consider empiric antifungal therapy in patients at risk of histoplasmosis or other invasive fungal infections who develop severe systemic illness, taking into account both the risk for severe fungal infection and the risks associated with antifungal therapy. Serologic tests for histoplasmosis may be negative in some patients with active infection. Following resolution of an invasive fungal infection, the decision regarding whether to reinitiate TNF blocking agent therapy should involve reevaluation of the risks and benefits of such therapy, particularly in patients who reside in regions where mycoses are endemic. Whenever feasible, decisions regarding initiation and duration of antifungal therapy and reinitiation of TNF blocking agent therapy should be made in consultation with a specialist in the diagnosis and management of fungal infections.

Malignancies and Lymphoproliferative Disorders

A boxed warning about the risk of malignancy is included in the prescribing information for golimumab. Malignancies, some fatal, have been reported in children, adolescents, and young adults who received treatment with TNF blocking agents, including golimumab, beginning when they were 18 years of age or younger. In August 2009, FDA reported the results of an analysis of reports of lymphoma and other malignancies in children and adolescents who had received TNF blocking agents. These cases were reported postmarketing and were derived from various sources, including registries and spontaneous postmarketing reports. Golimumab was not FDA-approved at the time of the analysis and, therefore, was not included in the analysis. The FDA identified 48 cases of malignancies in children and adolescents in the analysis.

Of the 48 cases reviewed by FDA, approximately 50% were lymphomas, including Hodgkin disease and non-Hodgkin lymphoma. The other cases represented a variety of malignancies, including rare malignancies that are usually associated with immunosuppression and malignancies that are not usually observed in children and adolescents. Other malignancies reported included leukemia, melanoma, and solid organ cancers; malignancies such as leiomyosarcoma, hepatic malignancies, and renal cell carcinoma, which rarely occur in children, also were reported. The malignancies occurred after a median of 30 months (range: 1–84 months) following the first dose of therapy with TNF blocking agents. Of the 48 cases of malignancies, 11 deaths were reported; causes of death included hepatosplenic T-cell lymphoma (9 cases), T-cell lymphoma (1 case), and sepsis following remission of lymphoma (1 case). Most of the 48 patients (88%) also were receiving other immunosuppressive drugs such as azathioprine and methotrexate; these agents also are associated with an increased risk of lymphoma. Although there were other contributory factors, the role of TNF blocking agents in the development of malignancies in children and adolescents could not be excluded. Therefore, FDA concluded that there is an increased risk of malignancy with TNF blocking agents. However, due to the relatively rare occurrence of these cancers, the limited number of pediatric patients who received TNF blocking agents, and the possible role of other immunosuppressive drugs used concomitantly with TNF blocking agents, FDA was unable to fully characterize the strength of the association between use of TNF blocking agents and the development of a malignancy.

Hepatosplenic T-cell lymphoma, a rare, aggressive, usually fatal type of T-cell lymphoma, has been reported during postmarketing experience mainly in adolescent and young adult males with Crohn disease or ulcerative colitis who received treatment with TNF blocking agents and/or thiopurine analogs (mercaptopurine or azathioprine). Most of the reported cases of hepatosplenic T-cell lymphoma occurred in patients who had received a combination of immunosuppressive agents, including TNF blocking agents and thiopurine analogs (azathioprine or mercaptopurine), at or prior to diagnosis. In some cases, potential confounding factors could not be excluded because complete medical histories were not available. Since patients with certain conditions (e.g., rheumatoid arthritis, Crohn disease, ankylosing spondylitis, psoriatic arthritis) may be at increased risk for lymphoma, it may be difficult to measure the added risk of treatment with TNF blocking agents, azathioprine, and/or mercaptopurine.

In clinical studies, lymphoma has been observed more frequently in patients receiving TNF blocking agents than in control patients. In controlled studies evaluating golimumab in patients with rheumatoid arthritis, psoriatic arthritis, or ankylosing spondylitis, the incidence of lymphoma was 0.21 per 100 patient-years in golimumab-treated patients and 0 per 100 patient-years in placebo-treated patients. In these studies (including during uncontrolled phases of the studies), the incidence of lymphoma in golimumab-treated patients was approximately 3.8-fold higher than the expected incidence in the general US population. Through week 60 of controlled studies evaluating golimumab in patients with ulcerative colitis, no cases of lymphoma were reported in patients receiving the drug. Patients with rheumatoid arthritis and other chronic inflammatory diseases, especially those with highly active disease and/or long-term exposure to immunosuppressive therapies, may be at increased risk of lymphoma, even in the absence of TNF blocking agent therapy.

Cases of acute and chronic leukemia have been reported in patients receiving TNF blocking agents, including golimumab, for the management of rheumatoid arthritis and other conditions. In August 2009, FDA reported the results of a review of 147 cases of leukemia in adults and pediatric patients who received TNF blocking agents. Of the 147 cases, acute myeloid leukemia (44 cases), chronic lymphocytic leukemia (31 cases), and chronic myeloid leukemia (23 cases) were the most frequent types of leukemia reported. Four cases of leukemia were reported in children. Most patients (61%) also were receiving other immunosuppressive drugs. There were a total of 30 deaths reported; leukemia was reported as the cause of 26 of the 30 deaths, and the event was associated with the use of TNF blocking agents. Leukemia generally occurred during the first 2 years of therapy. The interpretation of these findings was complicated by the fact that published epidemiologic studies suggest that patients with rheumatoid arthritis may be at increased risk of leukemia, independent of any treatment with TNF blocking agents. However, based on the available data, FDA concluded that there is a possible association between treatment with TNF blocking agents and the development of leukemia in patients receiving these drugs.

In a controlled study evaluating IV golimumab in patients with rheumatoid arthritis, one case of malignancy other than lymphoma and nonmelanoma skin cancer was reported in a patient receiving the drug during the 24-week controlled phase of the study; over approximately 92 weeks of treatment (including both controlled and uncontrolled periods of study), the incidence of such malignancies per 100 patient-years of IV golimumab use was 0.31, and the incidence of nonmelanoma skin cancer was 0.1 per 100 patient-years of exposure. In controlled studies evaluating subcutaneous golimumab in patients with rheumatoid arthritis, psoriatic arthritis, or ankylosing spondylitis, the incidence of malignancies other than lymphoma was not increased in golimumab-treated patients compared with placebo-treated patients. In these studies (including during uncontrolled phases of the studies), the incidence of malignancies other than lymphoma in golimumab-treated patients was similar to the expected incidence in the general US population. Through week 60 of controlled studies evaluating golimumab in patients with ulcerative colitis, the incidence of malignancies other than lymphoma and nonmelanoma skin cancer was similar to the expected incidence in the general US population. Short follow-up periods (e.g., 1 year or less) may not accurately reflect the true incidence of malignancies.

Melanoma and Merkel cell carcinoma have been reported in patients receiving TNF blocking agents, including golimumab-treated patients.

In controlled studies of other TNF blocking agents in patients at increased risk of malignancies (e.g., patients with chronic obstructive pulmonary disease [COPD], patients with Wegener's granulomatosis receiving concomitant cyclophosphamide), a greater proportion of malignancies occurred in patients receiving the TNF blocking agent compared with control patients. In a phase 2, dose-ranging, randomized, placebo-controlled study evaluating the safety and efficacy of golimumab (50, 100, or 200 mg once every 4 weeks) in 309 patients with uncontrolled, severe persistent asthma†, malignancies developed in 8 golimumab-treated patients and in none of the control patients; 6 of the 8 golimumab-treated patients developed malignancies other than nonmelanoma skin cancer, and 5 of the 8 golimumab-treated patients received 200-mg doses of the drug. The malignancies in golimumab-treated patients were diagnosed between days 76–448 of the study. Study drug administration was discontinued early as a result of the unfavorable risk-to-benefit profile observed in patients who received golimumab.

Consider the possibility of and monitor for the occurrence of malignancies during and following treatment with TNF blocking agents. Periodic dermatologic evaluations are recommended for all patients receiving TNF blocking agents, but particularly for those with risk factors for skin cancer. Consider the risks and benefits of TNF blocking agents, including golimumab, prior to initiating therapy in patients with a known malignancy (other than a successfully treated nonmelanoma skin cancer) or when considering whether to continue TNF blocking agent therapy in patients who develop a malignancy. Because therapy with TNF blocking agents and/or thiopurine analogs (azathioprine or mercaptopurine) may increase the risk of malignancies, including hepatosplenic T-cell lymphoma, the risks and benefits of these agents should be carefully considered, especially in adolescents and young adults and especially in the treatment of Crohn disease or ulcerative colitis.

Because it remains to be established whether golimumab affects the risk for development of dysplasia or colon cancer, all patients with ulcerative colitis who have a history of dysplasia or colon carcinoma, or are at increased risk for these conditions (e.g., those with long-standing ulcerative colitis or primary sclerosing cholangitis), should be screened for dysplasia at regular intervals, both before therapy and throughout their disease, in accordance with current standards of care. Carefully consider the risks and benefits of continued golimumab therapy in patients with newly diagnosed dysplasia.

Other Warnings/Precautions
Patients Infected with Hepatitis B Virus

Use of TNF blocking agents, including golimumab, may increase the risk of reactivation of hepatitis B virus (HBV) infection in patients who are chronic carriers of this virus (i.e., hepatitis B surface antigen-positive [HBsAg-positive]). HBV reactivation has resulted in death in a few individuals receiving TNF blocking agent therapy. Most patients experiencing HBV reactivation were receiving concomitant therapy with other immunosuppressive agents.

The manufacturer states that all patients should be screened for HBV infection before initiation of golimumab therapy. In patients who test positive for HBsAg, consultation with an HBV infection specialist is recommended before initiation of TNF blocking agent therapy. Chronic carriers of HBV should be appropriately evaluated and monitored prior to the initiation of therapy, during treatment, and for up to several months following therapy with golimumab. Safety and efficacy of antiviral therapy for prevention of viral reactivation in HBV carriers receiving a TNF blocking agent have not been established. Discontinue golimumab if

HBV reactivation occurs, and initiate appropriate treatment. It has not been established whether golimumab can be safely readministered once control of the reactivated HBV infection has been achieved; caution is advised if golimumab therapy is resumed in such a situation.

Cardiovascular Effects

New-onset or worsening heart failure, sometimes fatal, has been reported in patients receiving TNF blocking agents, including golimumab. While golimumab has not been studied in patients with a history of heart failure, other TNF blocking agents have been associated with increased morbidity (exacerbations requiring hospitalization) or mortality in patients with heart failure. If golimumab is used in patients with heart failure, caution and careful monitoring are recommended. Discontinue golimumab if new or worsening symptoms of heart failure occur.

Nervous System Effects

New onset or exacerbation of central or peripheral nervous system demyelinating disorders (e.g., multiple sclerosis, Guillain-Barré syndrome) has been reported rarely in patients receiving golimumab or other TNF blocking agents. Central demyelination, multiple sclerosis, optic neuritis, and peripheral demyelinating polyneuropathy have been reported rarely in patients receiving golimumab. Clinicians should exercise caution when considering therapy with TNF blocking agents, including golimumab, in patients with central or peripheral nervous system demyelinating disorders. Consider discontinuance of golimumab if these disorders develop.

Hematologic Effects

Pancytopenia, leukopenia, neutropenia, agranulocytosis, aplastic anemia, and thrombocytopenia have been reported in patients receiving golimumab. Use TNF blocking agents with caution in patients who have or have had substantial cytopenias.

Immunization and Use of Therapeutic Infectious Agents

Live vaccines and therapeutic infectious agents should be avoided during therapy with golimumab, since such concomitant use could result in infections, including disseminated infections. Limited data are available regarding whether TNF blocking agents would affect the rate of secondary transmission of infection following administration of a live vaccine or regarding the response to live vaccines in patients receiving the drug.

Golimumab may affect immune response in infants exposed in utero. Monoclonal antibodies such as golimumab cross the placenta during the third trimester of pregnancy. Another TNF blocking monoclonal antibody administered during pregnancy was detected for up to 6 months in the serum of infants. Administration of live vaccines to infants who were exposed to golimumab in utero is not recommended for 6 months following the last golimumab dose given to the infant's mother during pregnancy.

Whenever possible, review the patient's vaccination status and administer all appropriate vaccines included in current immunization guidelines prior to starting golimumab therapy. Patients receiving golimumab may receive inactivated vaccines. In a clinical study in patients with psoriatic arthritis, the proportion of patients who had an adequate immune response (at least a twofold increase in antibody titers) to pneumococcal polysaccharide vaccine was similar in golimumab-treated and placebo-treated patients; however, the proportion of patients exhibiting a response to pneumococcal vaccine was lower among patients receiving methotrexate compared with patients not receiving methotrexate in both golimumab-treated and placebo-treated patients. These data suggest that golimumab does not suppress the humoral immune response to pneumococcal polysaccharide vaccine.

Immunologic Reactions and Antibody Formation

The use of TNF blocking agents, including golimumab, has been associated with the formation of antinuclear antibodies (ANA) and, rarely, with the development of a lupus-like syndrome. Discontinue golimumab in patients who develop symptoms suggestive of a lupus-like syndrome. Development of antibodies to double-stranded DNA (anti-dsDNA) also has been reported in patients receiving golimumab.

The original enzyme immunoassay developed to detect antibodies to golimumab detected such antibodies in approximately 3–4% of patients receiving the drug in clinical trials; however, the presence of golimumab in serum samples can interfere with this assay method, and, in a substantial number of patients (e.g., 69% of patients in the ulcerative colitis studies), the assay produced inconclusive results. A subsequently developed enzyme immunoassay (drug-tolerant assay) is approximately 16 times more sensitive than the original assay and is less subject to interference from golimumab present in serum.

In phase 3 clinical trials evaluating subcutaneous golimumab, antibodies to the drug were detected by the drug-tolerant enzyme immunoassay in 23% of golimumab-treated patients, including 16, 28, or 24% of those with rheumatoid arthritis, psoriatic arthritis, or ankylosing spondylitis, respectively. The incidence of antibody formation was lower when golimumab was used concomitantly with methotrexate rather than without methotrexate in patients with rheumatoid arthritis (7 versus 35%), psoriatic arthritis (18 versus 38%), or ankylosing spondylitis (6 versus 29%). Drug concentrations tended to decrease with increasing antibody titers. While development of antibodies to golimumab was not associated with reduced efficacy in these studies, higher antibody titers may be associated with reduced efficacy.

In clinical trials evaluating IV golimumab, antibodies to the drug were detected by the drug-tolerant enzyme immunoassay in 21, 19, 19, or 31% of golimumab-treated patients with rheumatoid arthritis, psoriatic arthritis, ankylosing spondylitis, or polyarticular juvenile idiopathic arthritis, respectively; approximately one-third to one-half of these patients had neutralizing antibodies. Patients who developed anti-golimumab antibodies generally had lower steady-state trough serum concentrations of the drug.

In clinical trials evaluating subcutaneous golimumab in patients with ulcerative colitis, antibodies to the drug were detected by the drug-tolerant enzyme immunoassay in 21% of patients receiving the drug, with the remaining 79% of patients testing negative for antibodies to the drug. The incidence of antibody formation was lower in patients receiving golimumab concomitantly with other immunosuppressive agents (i.e., azathioprine, mercaptopurine, methotrexate) than in patients who received golimumab without such concomitant therapy (12 versus 26%). Drug concentrations tended to decrease with increasing antibody titers. While development of antibodies to golimumab did not preclude clinical response, clinical response rates tended to be lower in patients with antibody development than in those without detectable antibodies to the drug (38 versus 53%).

Psoriasis

Cases of new-onset psoriasis, including pustular and palmoplantar psoriasis, have been reported with the use of TNF blocking agents, including golimumab. In August 2009, FDA reported the results of a review of 69 cases of new-onset psoriasis, including pustular (17 cases) and palmoplantar (15 cases) psoriasis, in patients receiving TNF blocking agents for the management of autoimmune and rheumatic conditions other than psoriasis and psoriatic arthritis. None of the patients reported having psoriasis prior to initiation of the TNF blocking agent. However, exacerbation of preexisting psoriasis has been reported with the use of TNF blocking agents, including golimumab. Two of the 69 cases of new-onset psoriasis occurred in pediatric patients. The development of psoriasis during treatment with TNF blocking agents occurred at intervals ranging from weeks to years following initiation of the drug. Twelve of the psoriasis cases resulted in hospitalization, which was the most severe outcome reported. Most patients experienced improvement of their psoriasis following discontinuation of the TNF blocking agent. Due to the number of reported cases and the temporal relationship between the initiation of TNF blocking agents and the development of psoriasis, FDA concluded that there is a possible association between the development of psoriasis and use of TNF blocking agents. Clinicians should consider the possibility of and monitor for manifestations (e.g., new rash) of new or worsening psoriasis, particularly pustular and palmoplantar psoriasis, during treatment with TNF blocking agents. Discontinuance of golimumab therapy may be considered if new-onset or worsening psoriasis occurs.

Hepatic Effects

Severe hepatic reactions, including acute liver failure, have been reported in patients receiving TNF blocking agents.

In phase 3 clinical studies evaluating subcutaneous golimumab in patients with rheumatoid arthritis, psoriatic arthritis, or ankylosing spondylitis, increased serum ALT and AST concentrations were reported in 4 and 3%, respectively, of golimumab-treated patients, compared with 3 and 2%, respectively, of placebo-treated patients; increases in serum ALT concentrations of ≥3 times the upper limit of normal (ULN) or ≥5 times the ULN occurred in 2 or 0.7%, respectively, of golimumab-treated patients, compared with 2 or 0.2%, respectively, of control patients. In a clinical trial evaluating IV golimumab in patients with rheumatoid arthritis, increases in serum ALT concentrations of ≥3 times the ULN or ≥5 times the ULN occurred during 24 weeks of treatment in 2.3 or 0.8%, respectively, of golimumab-treated patients and in 2.5 or 0%, respectively, of control patients. In a clinical trial evaluating IV golimumab in adult patients with psoriatic arthritis, increases in serum ALT concentrations of 3 to <5 times the ULN or ≥5 times the ULN occurred during 24 weeks of treatment in 2.9 or 1.7%, respectively, of golimumab-treated patients and in less than 1% of control patients. In clinical studies evaluating golimumab in patients with ulcerative colitis, increases in serum ALT concentrations of ≥3 times the ULN or ≥5 times the ULN were reported in 2 or 1%, respectively, of golimumab-treated patients during 46 weeks of follow-up, compared with 1.5 or 1%, respectively, of placebo-treated patients during 18 weeks of follow-up. Because many of the patients in these studies received concomitant therapy with drugs known to increase liver enzyme concentrations (e.g., methotrexate, nonsteroidal anti-inflammatory agents [NSAIAs]), the relationship between golimumab and increased liver enzyme concentrations is not clear.

Sensitivity Reactions

Serious systemic hypersensitivity reactions (e.g., anaphylactic reactions) have been reported during postmarketing surveillance in patients receiving golimumab, sometimes after the first dose of the drug. In patients receiving IV golimumab, hypersensitivity reactions including urticaria, pruritus, dyspnea, and nausea have been reported during and generally within one hour following IV infusion of the drug. If an anaphylactic or other serious allergic reaction occurs, discontinue golimumab immediately and initiate appropriate therapy.

The needle cover of the prefilled syringe and the syringe in the auto-injector contain dry natural rubber; these items should not be handled by individuals sensitive to latex.

Specific Populations

Pregnancy

There are no adequate and well-controlled studies of golimumab in pregnant women. Limited data from observational studies, published case reports, and postmarketing surveillance on the use of golimumab in pregnant women are insufficient to inform a drug-associated risk. Golimumab should be used during pregnancy only if clearly needed.

In an embryofetal development study in cynomolgus monkeys, no evidence of teratogenicity or embryofetal toxicity was observed following subcutaneous administration of golimumab during the period of organogenesis at dosages resulting in exposure levels of up to 360 times the exposure at the maximum recommended human dosage (MRHD) for subcutaneous use. Umbilical cord blood samples collected at the end of the second trimester indicated that fetuses were exposed to golimumab during gestation. In a pre- and postnatal development study in cynomolgus monkeys, no adverse developmental effects were observed in the offspring of monkeys that received subcutaneous golimumab from gestation day 50 to postpartum day 33 at dosages producing peak steady-state maternal blood concentrations of approximately 460 times those observed at the MRHD for subcutaneous use. Golimumab was present in fetal serum at the end of the second trimester and in neonatal serum from the time of birth and for up to 6 months postpartum. No maternal toxicity was observed in these studies.

Golimumab may affect immune response in infants exposed in utero. Monoclonal antibodies such as golimumab cross the placenta during the third trimester of pregnancy. Another TNF blocking monoclonal antibody administered during pregnancy was detected for up to 6 months in the serum of infants. Therefore, infants born to women who received golimumab during their pregnancy may be at increased risk of infection. Administration of live vaccines to infants who were exposed to golimumab in utero is not recommended for 6 months following the last golimumab dose given to the infant's mother during pregnancy.

Lactation

Golimumab is distributed into milk in lactating cynomolgus monkeys; in a pre- and postnatal development study in cynomolgus monkeys, concentrations of golimumab in breast milk were approximately 400-fold lower than maternal serum concentrations. Maternal immunoglobulin G (IgG) distributes into human milk; however, it is not known whether golimumab distributes into human milk, affects breast-fed infants, or affects milk production. Any effects resulting from local exposure in the GI tract or potential limited systemic exposure in the infant also are unknown.

Consider the developmental and health benefits of breast-feeding along with the mother's clinical need for golimumab and any potential adverse effects on the breast-fed infant from the drug or underlying maternal condition.

Pediatric Use

Efficacy of subcutaneous golimumab has not been established in pediatric patients <18 years of age. A placebo-controlled, double-blind, randomized-withdrawal, parallel-group study in 173 pediatric patients 2–17 years of age with active polyarticular juvenile idiopathic arthritis despite methotrexate therapy failed to establish efficacy of subcutaneous golimumab in this patient population; the frequency and type of adverse effects observed in this study were generally similar to those observed in adults. Pediatric patients enrolled in this study received open-label treatment with subcutaneous golimumab 30 mg/m² (maximum 50 mg) every 4 weeks as add-on therapy to their current methotrexate regimen; those who achieved an American College of Rheumatology Pediatric 30% (ACR Pedi 30) response at week 16 were entered into the placebo-controlled, randomized-withdrawal phase of the study. Disease flares occurred during weeks 16–48 in similar proportions of patients receiving golimumab or placebo.

Use of IV golimumab for the management of active polyarticular juvenile idiopathic arthritis and psoriatic arthritis in pediatric patients ≥2 years of age is supported by evidence from adequate and well-controlled studies of IV golimumab in adult patients with rheumatoid arthritis and psoriatic arthritis, pharmacokinetic data from adult patients with rheumatoid arthritis or psoriatic arthritis and pediatric patients with juvenile idiopathic arthritis and active polyarthritis, and safety data from a clinical study in 127 pediatric patients 2–17 years of age with juvenile idiopathic arthritis and active polyarthritis. The observed trough concentrations of golimumab are generally comparable between adults with rheumatoid arthritis or psoriatic arthritis and pediatric patients with juvenile idiopathic arthritis and active polyarthritis. Pharmacokinetic exposure is expected to be comparable between adult patients with psoriatic arthritis and pediatric patients with psoriatic arthritis. Safety and efficacy of IV golimumab for the management of polyarticular juvenile idiopathic arthritis or psoriatic arthritis have not been established in pediatric patients <2 years of age. Safety and efficacy of IV golimumab for the management of conditions other than polyarticular juvenile idiopathic arthritis or psoriatic arthritis have not been established in pediatric patients <18 years of age.

Malignancies, some fatal, have been reported in children and adolescents who received treatment with golimumab and other TNF blocking agents.

Geriatric Use

In phase 3 clinical studies evaluating subcutaneous golimumab in patients with rheumatoid arthritis, psoriatic arthritis, or ankylosing spondylitis, there were no overall differences in serious adverse events, serious infections, and adverse events in those ≥65 years of age compared with younger adults. Clinical studies evaluating subcutaneous golimumab in patients with ulcerative colitis or evaluating IV golimumab in patients with rheumatoid arthritis did not include sufficient numbers of patients ≥65 years of age to determine whether geriatric patients respond differently than younger adults. Because the overall incidence of infection is higher in the geriatric population than in younger adults, use golimumab with caution in geriatric patients.

The pharmacokinetics of subcutaneous golimumab do not appear to be influenced by age in adults. The apparent clearance of subcutaneous golimumab in patients ≥65 years of age appears to be similar to that in younger adults.

Hepatic Impairment

The pharmacokinetics of golimumab have not been formally studied in patients with hepatic impairment.

Renal Impairment

The pharmacokinetics of golimumab have not been formally studied in patients with renal impairment.

Common Adverse Effects

Adverse effects reported in ≥5% of patients receiving subcutaneous golimumab include upper respiratory tract infection, nasopharyngitis, and injection site reactions.

Adverse effects reported in ≥3% of patients receiving IV golimumab include upper respiratory tract infection, increased ALT or AST concentration, viral infection, decreased neutrophil count, bronchitis, hypertension, and rash.

DRUG INTERACTIONS

Drugs Metabolized by Hepatic Microsomal Enzymes

Because increased levels of cytokines (e.g., tumor necrosis factor [TNF]-α) during chronic inflammation may suppress the formation of cytochrome P-450 (CYP) isoenzymes, it is expected that a drug that antagonizes cytokine activity, such as golimumab, could normalize the formation of CYP enzymes. Following initiation or discontinuance of golimumab therapy, patients receiving certain drugs metabolized by CYP isoenzymes (i.e., those with a low therapeutic index [e.g., cyclosporine, theophylline, warfarin]) should be monitored for therapeutic effect and/or changes in serum concentrations, and dosages of these drugs may be adjusted as needed.

Biologic Antirheumatic Agents

Caution should be exercised when switching from one biologic disease-modifying antirheumatic drug (DMARD) to another, since overlapping biologic activity may further increase the risk of infection. Concomitant use of golimumab and other biologic agents used in the management of rheumatoid arthritis, psoriatic arthritis, ankylosing spondylitis, or polyarticular juvenile idiopathic arthritis is not recommended because of the possibility of an increased risk of infection.

Abatacept

When abatacept (a selective costimulation modulator) and a TNF blocking agent were used concomitantly in patients with rheumatoid arthritis, an increased incidence of infection and serious infection was observed, with no substantial improvement in efficacy over that observed with a TNF blocking agent alone. Concomitant use of golimumab and abatacept is not recommended.

Anakinra

When anakinra (a human interleukin-1 receptor antagonist) and etanercept (another TNF blocking agent) were used concomitantly in patients with active rheumatoid arthritis, an increased incidence of serious infection and neutropenia was observed, with no substantial improvement in efficacy over that observed with etanercept alone. Concomitant use of golimumab and anakinra is not recommended.

Rituximab

An increased risk of serious infection has been observed in patients with rheumatoid arthritis who received rituximab and subsequently received therapy with a TNF blocking agent. Concomitant use of golimumab and rituximab is not recommended.

Corticosteroids

Concomitant use of golimumab and oral corticosteroids does not appear to influence the apparent clearance of golimumab.

Methotrexate

For the management of rheumatoid arthritis, golimumab should be used in conjunction with methotrexate.

Since concomitant use or nonuse of methotrexate does not appear to influence the efficacy or safety of golimumab for the management of psoriatic arthritis or ankylosing spondylitis, golimumab may be used with or without methotrexate for the management of psoriatic arthritis or ankylosing spondylitis.

Patients with rheumatoid arthritis, psoriatic arthritis, or ankylosing spondylitis receiving subcutaneous golimumab concomitantly with methotrexate had approximately 52, 36, or 21% higher mean steady-state trough concentrations of golimumab, respectively, than those receiving subcutaneous golimumab without methotrexate. A population pharmacokinetic analysis indicated that concomitant use of methotrexate with IV golimumab in patients with rheumatoid arthritis decreased the clearance of golimumab by about 9%. In addition, methotrexate may decrease clearance of golimumab by reducing the development of antigolimumab antibodies.

Nonsteroidal Anti-inflammatory Agents

Concomitant use of golimumab and nonsteroidal anti-inflammatory agents (NSAIAs) does not appear to influence the apparent clearance of golimumab.

Sulfasalazine

Concomitant use of golimumab and sulfasalazine does not appear to influence the apparent clearance of golimumab.

Vaccines and Therapeutic Infectious Agents

Live vaccines and therapeutic infectious agents (e.g., BCG for intravesical instillation) should not be administered to patients receiving golimumab since such concomitant use could result in infections, including disseminated infections. Limited data are available regarding whether TNF blocking agents would affect the rate of secondary transmission of infection following administration of a live vaccine or regarding the response to live vaccines in patients receiving the drug. Administration of live vaccines to infants who were exposed to golimumab in utero is not recommended for 6 months following the last golimumab dose given to the infant's mother during pregnancy.

Patients receiving golimumab may receive inactivated vaccines. In a clinical study in patients with psoriatic arthritis, the proportion of patients who had an adequate immune response (at least a twofold increase in antibody titers) to pneumococcal polysaccharide vaccine was similar in golimumab-treated and placebo-treated patients; however, the proportion of patients exhibiting a response to pneumococcal vaccine was lower among patients receiving methotrexate compared with patients not receiving methotrexate in both golimumab-treated and placebo-treated patients. These data suggest that golimumab does not suppress the humoral immune response to pneumococcal polysaccharide vaccine.

DESCRIPTION

Golimumab, a human monoclonal antibody specific for human tumor necrosis factor (TNF; TNF-α), is a biologic response modifier and a disease-modifying antirheumatic drug (DMARD). Golimumab is an immunoglobulin G₁ kappa (IgG₁) that was created using genetically engineered mice immunized with human TNF, resulting in an antibody with human-derived antibody variable and constant regions. Golimumab is produced by a recombinant cell line cultured by continuous perfusion and is purified by a process that includes specific viral inactivation and removal steps.

Golimumab binds to both soluble and transmembrane bioactive forms of human TNF-α, which prevents the binding of TNF-α to its receptors. By preventing the binding of TNF-α to its receptors, golimumab inhibits the biologic activity of TNF-α. Golimumab does not appear to bind to other TNF superfamily ligands; golimumab does not bind to or neutralize human lymphotoxin. Golimumab does not lyse human monocytes expressing transmembrane TNF in the presence of complement or effector cells.

Increased concentrations of TNF-α, a cytokine protein, in the blood, synovium, and joints have been implicated in the pathophysiology of several chronic inflammatory diseases such as rheumatoid arthritis, psoriatic arthritis, and ankylosing spondylitis. TNF-α is an important mediator of the articular inflammation that is characteristic of these diseases. In vitro, golimumab modulated the biologic effects mediated by TNF in several bioassays, including the expression of adhesion proteins responsible for leukocyte infiltration and secretion of proinflammatory cytokines. The exact mechanism of action of golimumab in the treatment of ulcerative colitis is unknown.

Golimumab exhibits dose-proportional pharmacokinetics when given IV or subcutaneously within the clinical dosage range. The absolute bioavailability of golimumab following subcutaneous injection is approximately 53%; peak serum concentrations of the drug are attained in approximately 2–6 days in healthy individuals and in patients with active rheumatoid arthritis. Steady-state concentrations of the drug are attained by week 12 in patients with rheumatoid arthritis, psoriatic arthritis, or ankylosing spondylitis receiving the recommended subcutaneous dosage (50 mg every 4 weeks); by week 8 after the first maintenance dose in patients with ulcerative colitis receiving the recommended subcutaneous dosage (induction dosage of 200 mg at week 0 and 100 mg at week 2 and maintenance dosage of 100 mg every 4 weeks thereafter); by week 12 in patients with rheumatoid arthritis receiving the recommended IV dosage (2 mg/kg at weeks 0 and 4 and every 8 weeks thereafter); and by week 12 in patients with juvenile idiopathic arthritis and active polyarthritis receiving the recommended IV dosage (80 mg/m^2 at weeks 0, 4, and every 8 weeks thereafter). Data directly comparing a 2-mg/kg IV dose with a 50-mg subcutaneous dose are not available to date. Patients who developed antigolimumab antibodies generally had lower steady-state serum trough concentrations of the drug. Elimination pathways for golimumab have not been characterized. The terminal half-life of the drug is estimated to be approximately 2 weeks.

ADVICE TO PATIENTS

- A copy of the manufacturer's patient information (medication guide) for golimumab should be provided to all patients with each prescription of the drug. Importance of advising patients about potential benefits and risks of golimumab. Importance of patients reading the medication guide prior to initiation of therapy and each time the prescription is refilled.

- Importance of instructing patient and/or caregiver regarding proper dosage and administration of subcutaneous golimumab, including the use of aseptic technique, and proper disposal of needles and syringes if it is determined that the patient and/or caregiver is competent to safely administer the drug.

- Increased susceptibility to infection. Importance of promptly informing clinicians if any signs or symptoms of infection (e.g., persistent fever, sweating, cough, dyspnea, fatigue, diarrhea, burning upon urination, warm, red, or painful skin) develop.

- Risk of lymphoma, including hepatosplenic T-cell lymphoma, leukemia, and other malignancies with use of TNF blocking agents. Importance of informing patients and caregivers about the increased risk of cancer development in children, adolescents, and young adults, taking into account the clinical utility of TNF blocking agents, the relative risks and benefits of these and other immunosuppressive drugs, and the risks associated with untreated disease. Importance of promptly informing clinicians if signs and symptoms of malignancies (e.g., unexplained weight loss; fatigue; abdominal pain; persistent fever; night sweats; swollen lymph nodes in the neck, underarm, or groin; easy bruising or bleeding; hepatomegaly or splenomegaly; changes in skin appearance or skin growths) occur.

- Importance of alerting clinician if allergy to latex exists.

- Importance of informing clinician of any new or worsening medical conditions (e.g., heart failure, neurologic disease [e.g., demyelinating disorders], autoimmune disorders [e.g., lupus-like syndrome], liver disease, cytopenias, psoriasis).

- Importance of taking the drug as prescribed and of not altering or discontinuing therapy without first consulting with a clinician.

- Importance of informing clinicians of existing or contemplated concomitant therapy, including prescription and OTC drugs, as well as any concomitant illnesses or any history of cancer, tuberculosis, HBV infection, or other chronic or recurring infections.

- Importance of consulting a clinician before receiving any vaccinations. Importance of avoiding live vaccinations while taking golimumab. Importance of informing pregnant women taking golimumab that their infants should not receive live vaccinations for 6 months following the last dose of golimumab during pregnancy.

- Importance of women informing clinicians if they are or plan to become pregnant or plan to breast-feed.

- Importance of informing patients of other important precautionary information. (See Cautions.)

PREPARATIONS

Excipients in commercially available drug preparations may have clinically important effects in some individuals; consult specific product labeling for details.

Golimumab

Parenteral

Injection, for subcutaneous use	50 mg/0.5 mL	**Simponi®** (available as disposable prefilled syringes and prefilled auto-injectors [SmartJect®]), Janssen Biotech
	100 mg/mL	**Simponi®** (available as disposable prefilled syringes and prefilled auto-injectors [SmartJect®]), Janssen Biotech
Concentrate, for Injection, for IV use	12.5 mg/mL (50 mg)	**Simponi Aria®**, Janssen Biotech

† Use is not currently included in the labeling approved by the US Food and Drug Administration.

Selected Revisions May 10, 2024, © Copyright, March 1, 2010, American Society of Health-System Pharmacists, Inc.

inFLIXimab

90:24.16.92 • TUMOR NECROSIS FACTOR INHIBITORS, MISCELLANEOUS

- Infliximab, infliximab-abda, infliximab-axxq, and infliximab-dyyb are chimeric human-murine immunoglobulin G_1 kappa (IgG_1 kappa) monoclonal antibodies that have a high affinity for human tumor necrosis factor (TNF; TNF-α).

- Infliximab-abda, infliximab-axxq, and infliximab-dyyb are biosimilar to infliximab (Remicade®). FDA defines a biosimilar as a biological product that is highly similar to an FDA-licensed reference biological with the exception of minor differences in clinically inactive components and for which there are no clinically meaningful differences in safety, purity, or potency. The claim of biosimilarity is based on a totality-of-evidence approach, which includes consideration of data from analytical, animal, and clinical studies (e.g., human pharmacokinetic and pharmacodynamic studies, clinical immunogenicity assessment, additional comparative clinical studies). Therefore, biosimilarity may be established even when there are formulation or minor structural differences as long as these differences are not clinically meaningful. Biosimilars are approved through an abbreviated licensure pathway that establishes biosimilarity between the proposed biological and the reference biological but does not independently establish safety and effectiveness of the proposed biological. In order to be considered an interchangeable biosimilar, a biological product must meet additional requirements beyond demonstrating biosimilarity to its reference product; these requirements include demonstrating that the biological product can be expected to produce the same clinical results as the reference product in any given patient and, for a biological product that is administered more than once to an individual, the risk in terms of safety or diminished efficacy of alternating or switching between use of the biological product and the reference product is no greater than the risk of using the reference product without such alternation or switch. Biosimilar products that are interchangeable can be substituted for the reference product without the intervention of the healthcare provider who prescribed the reference product. None of the currently available infliximab biosimilars have interchangeable data at this time.

- In this monograph, unless otherwise stated, the term "infliximab products" refers to infliximab (the reference drug) and its biosimilars (infliximab-abda, infliximab-axxq, infliximab-dyyb).

USES

Several infliximab biosimilars are available. Biosimilarity of these products has been demonstrated for the indications described in the table below (see Table 1).

Biosimilarity to originator infliximab is additionally supported by comparative clinical studies in patients with rheumatoid arthritis (infliximab-abda, infliximab-axxq, infliximab-dyyb), Crohn disease (infliximab-dyyb), and/or ankylosing spondylitis (infliximab-dyyb).

A subcutaneous version of infliximab-dyyb (Zymfentra®) is also available for the maintenance treatment of ulcerative colitis and Crohn disease in adults following treatment with IV infliximab.

● Crohn Disease

Crohn Disease in Adults

Infliximab and its biosimilars (infliximab-abda, infliximab-axxq, infliximab-dyyb) are used to reduce the signs and symptoms of Crohn disease and to induce and maintain clinical remission in adults with moderately to severely active disease who have had an inadequate response to conventional therapies. Infliximab and its biosimilars (infliximab-abda, infliximab-axxq, infliximab-dyyb) also are used to reduce the number of draining enterocutaneous and rectovaginal fistulas and to maintain fistula closure in adults with fistulizing Crohn disease. Infliximab has been designated an orphan drug by FDA for these uses.

TABLE 1. Infliximab Biosimilar Products and FDA-licensed Indications

FDA-labeled indication	Infliximab-axxq (Avsola®)	Infliximab-dyyb (Inflectra®)	Infliximab-abda (Renflexis®)
Crohn disease	X	X	X
Pediatric Crohn disease	X	X	X
Ulcerative colitis	X	X	X
Pediatric ulcerative colitis	X	X	X
Rheumatoid arthritis	X	X	X
Ankylosing spondylitis	X	X	X
Psoriatic arthritis	X	X	X
Plaque psoriasis	X	X	X

The subcutaneous formulation of infliximab-dyyb is used for the maintenance treatment of moderately to severely active Crohn disease in adults following IV treatment with an infliximab product.

Safety and efficacy of infliximab for these uses are based principally on the results of randomized controlled trials. Guidelines generally support the use of infliximab for induction and maintenance therapy in adults with moderate to severe Crohn disease or fistulizing Crohn disease.

Clinical Experience

Safety and efficacy of infliximab in the management of active Crohn disease were evaluated in a double-blind, placebo-controlled, dose-ranging study that included 108 adults with moderately to severely active Crohn disease who had an inadequate response to conventional therapies (e.g., corticosteroids, mesalamine, azathioprine, or mercaptopurine). To be included in the study, patients had to have had Crohn disease for a minimum of 6 months and a Crohn Disease Activity Index (CDAI) of 220–400 at the time of study entry. The CDAI score is based on the daily number of liquid or very soft stools, severity of abdominal pain or cramping, general well-being, presence or absence of extraintestinal manifestations, presence or absence of an abdominal mass, use or nonuse of antidiarrheal drugs, the hematocrit, and body weight; scores below 150 indicate clinical remission and scores above 450 indicate severe illness. Patients were randomized to receive placebo or a single dose of 5, 10, or 20 mg/kg of infliximab given by IV infusion over 2 hours. Those who were receiving fixed dosages of oral corticosteroids, oral mesalamine, and/or azathioprine or mercaptopurine continued to receive these drugs during the study (92% continued to receive one or more of these drugs). A clinical response (defined as a reduction from baseline CDAI of 70 points or more at 4 weeks after the dose without an increased need for other Crohn drugs or surgical intervention) was observed in 81, 50, or 64% of patients receiving 5, 10, or 20 mg/kg of infliximab, respectively, compared with 16% of patients receiving placebo. At 4 weeks after the dose, 33% of those who received infliximab and 4% of those who received placebo were in clinical remission based on the CDAI. There was no evidence of a dose-response relationship (doses exceeding 5 mg/kg did not result in a greater response rate) and, at all 3 infliximab dosages, the maximum response was observed within 2–4 weeks after the IV infusion. At 12 weeks after the dose, the overall rate of clinical response or clinical remission based on the CDAI was 41 or 24%, respectively, in those who received infliximab compared with 12 or 8%, respectively, in those who received placebo.

To determine whether patients with moderately or severely active Crohn disease who do not respond to a single dose of infliximab would respond to an additional dose of the drug, the subset of patients in the above study who did not have a clinical response 4 weeks after the initial infliximab or placebo dose were enrolled in an open-label follow-up study and given a single 10-mg/kg dose of infliximab. In those who had received placebo in the original study, the rate of clinical response or remission was 58 or 47%, respectively, 4 weeks following this 10-mg/kg infliximab dose. However, in those who had already received a dose of infliximab in the first phase of the study, the rate of clinical response or remission was only 34 or 17%, respectively, 4 weeks following the second dose of the drug. These results indicate that patients who do not respond to an initial infliximab dose may be less likely to respond to a second dose of the drug.

Safety and efficacy of infliximab for maintenance therapy in patients with moderately or severely active Crohn disease were evaluated in a preliminary study and in a double-blind, multidose, multicenter study (ACCENT I) that included more than 500 adults. The duration of response to infliximab usually ranges from 4–12 weeks in patients who experience a clinical benefit after a single dose of the drug. In one preliminary study, a subset of 73 adults from a double-blind, placebo-controlled study who had maintained a clinical response 8 weeks after an initial placebo or infliximab dose were re-randomized at week 12 to receive 4 doses of placebo or infliximab (10 mg/kg) given by IV infusion at 8-week intervals (i.e., weeks 12, 20, 28, 36). Those who were receiving fixed dosages of oral corticosteroids, oral mesalamine or sulfasalazine, and/or azathioprine or mercaptopurine continued to receive these drugs during the study; patients receiving oral corticosteroids where allowed to taper dosage if they responded to treatment. Patients were assessed every 4 weeks through week 48. The clinical response was maintained through week 44 (8 weeks after the fourth infusion) in 62 or 37% of patients receiving infliximab or placebo, respectively. In those randomized to receive infliximab for maintenance therapy, 37.8% were in clinical remission at week 12 and 52.9% were in clinical remission at week 44. In contrast, 44.4% of those randomized to receive placebo for maintenance therapy were in clinical remission at week 12 and only 20% were in clinical remission at week 44. Although further study is needed to determine the relative benefits of concomitant use of infliximab and azathioprine or mercaptopurine for maintenance of remission, 75% of patients receiving one of these drugs concomitantly with infliximab had a clinical response at 44 weeks compared with 50% of those not receiving one of these drugs concomitantly.

In a double-blind study of 573 adults with moderately to severely active Crohn disease that was designed to compare the safety and efficacy of a maintenance regimen of infliximab to a single dose of the drug (ACCENT I), all patients received an initial 5-mg/kg dose of infliximab; following assessment of clinical response at week 2 (defined as a CDAI decrease of at least 70 points and at least a 25% decrease from baseline CDAI), patients were randomized to receive placebo or an infliximab induction regimen (5-mg/kg doses given at weeks 2 and 6 followed by either 5- or 10-mg/kg maintenance doses given once every 8 weeks) for up to 1 year. Those who were receiving fixed dosages of oral corticosteroids (prednisone 40 mg or less daily or equivalent), oral mesalamine, sulfasalazine, anti-infective agents, azathioprine, mercaptopurine, or methotrexate continued to receive these drugs during the study; patients receiving oral corticosteroids were allowed to taper the dosage after week 6 if they responded to treatment. Among adults who responded to the initial dose of infliximab, 39 or 46% of those receiving 5- or 10-mg maintenance doses of infliximab, respectively, were in clinical remission at week 30 compared with 25% of those receiving maintenance doses of placebo. In addition, among patients receiving corticosteroids at baseline, 25 or 34% of those receiving 5- or 10-mg maintenance doses of infliximab, respectively, were in clinical remission and were able to discontinue corticosteroid use at week 54 compared with 11% of those receiving maintenance doses of placebo. The median time to loss of response in those receiving maintenance doses of infliximab or placebo was 46 or 19 weeks, respectively.

Although the relative benefits of concomitant use of infliximab and an immunosuppressant agent (e.g., methotrexate, azathioprine) for maintenance therapy remain to be determined, 50% of those receiving immunosuppressive therapy at baseline maintained clinical response at week 54 compared with 41% of those not receiving such therapy.

Patients in this study who responded initially but subsequently lost response were eligible to receive infliximab at a higher dose than the dose they had been receiving; these patients were eligible to receive infliximab on an episodic basis at a dose 5 mg/kg higher than the dose they had been receiving in the study. Most patients responded to the higher dose.

Among adults who did not respond to the initial dose of infliximab, 59% of those receiving maintenance doses of infliximab responded by week 14 compared with 51% of those receiving maintenance doses of placebo. In patients who did not respond to infliximab by week 14, additional doses of infliximab did not result in a clinically important response.

In a subset of patients with mucosal ulceration at baseline who participated in an endoscopic study, 13 of 43 patients receiving maintenance doses of infliximab

had endoscopic evidence of mucosal healing at week 10 compared with 1 of 28 patients receiving placebo for maintenance therapy. Nine of 12 patients receiving maintenance doses of infliximab with mucosal healing at week 10 also had mucosal healing at week 54.

Safety and efficacy of infliximab in the management of fistulizing Crohn disease have been evaluated in a double-blind, placebo-controlled study involving 94 adults with one or more cutaneously draining fistulas of at least 3 months' duration (90% had perianal fistulas, 10% had abdominal fistulas, 55% had multiple cutaneously draining fistulas). Patients were randomized to receive placebo or infliximab (5 or 10 mg/kg) given by IV infusion over 2 hours at weeks 0, 2, and 6 and were followed for up to 26 weeks. Those who were receiving fixed dosages of oral corticosteroids, oral mesalamine or sulfasalazine, anti-infectives, and/or methotrexate, azathioprine, or mercaptopurine continued to receive these drugs during the study (83% continued to receive one or more of these drugs). A clinical response (defined as a 50% or greater reduction from baseline in the number of fistulas draining after gentle compression during at least 2 consecutive visits without an increased need for other drugs used for the treatment of Crohn disease or surgical intervention) occurred in 68 or 56% of patients receiving infliximab in a dosage of 5 or 10 mg/kg, respectively, versus 26% of those receiving placebo. Closure of all fistulas was attained in 52% of patients receiving infliximab versus 13% of those receiving placebo. In patients receiving infliximab, the median time to onset of response was 2 weeks and the median duration of response was 12 weeks; there was no evidence of a dose-response relationship. New fistula(s) occurred in approximately 15% of patients receiving infliximab or placebo.

Long-term safety and efficacy of infliximab in the management of fistulizing Crohn disease have been evaluated in a multicenter, double-blind, randomized, placebo-controlled trial (ACCENT II) in adults with at least one draining fistula (e.g., perianal, enterocutaneous, or rectovaginal fistulas) for at least 3 months. In the initial phase of this study, all patients received infliximab (5 mg/kg) at weeks 0, 2, and 6; those with a clinical response (defined as a 50% or greater reduction from baseline in the number of fistulas draining after gentle compression during at least 2 consecutive visits without an increased need for other drugs or surgical intervention) at weeks 10 and 14 were randomized to receive placebo or infliximab 5 mg/kg at week 14 and then every 8 weeks through week 46 (maintenance treatment). Patients who were receiving stable dosages of 5-aminosalicylates, oral corticosteroids, methotrexate, azathioprine, mercaptopurine, mycophenolate mofetil, or anti-infective agents continued to receive these drugs during the study. At week 14, 65% of patients had a clinical response to the initial 3 doses of infliximab; in this group, 87% had perianal fistulas, 14% had abdominal fistulas, and 8% had rectovaginal fistulas. During the maintenance phase of the study, time to loss of clinical response was longer in patients who received infliximab every 8 weeks than those who received placebo (40 versus 14 weeks, respectively). At 54 weeks, 46 or 23% of patients receiving infliximab or placebo, respectively, had a response, while 36 or 19% of patients receiving infliximab or placebo, respectively, had complete response (defined as absence of draining fistulas). There was a trend toward fewer hospitalizations in those receiving infliximab maintenance compared with those receiving placebo. Patients who initially had a clinical response but lost response (defined as recrudescence of draining fistulas, need for a change in a drug, need for additional therapy for persistent or worsening luminal disease activity, need for surgery, or discontinuance of infliximab because of perceived lack of efficacy) were eligible to receive infliximab maintenance treatment using a dosage 5 mg/kg higher than the dosage they originally received; 66% of patients who were originally randomized to placebo responded to infliximab 5 mg/kg and 57% of patients who were originally randomized to infliximab 5 mg/kg responded to infliximab 10 mg/kg. Patients who did not respond to infliximab therapy by week 14 of the study were unlikely to respond to additional doses of the drug. In patients who did not have an initial response to infliximab, 16 (7 out of 44 patients) or 21% (9 out of 43 patients) of those receiving placebo or infliximab, respectively, had a response. At week 22, patients who were receiving placebo and who had a loss of response were eligible to cross over to maintenance therapy with infliximab 5 mg/kg while those who were receiving infliximab 5 mg/kg could cross over to receive infliximab 10 mg/kg. In patients who crossed over from placebo to infliximab, response was reestablished in 61% of individuals. Overall, a similar number of patients in the infliximab or placebo groups developed new fistulas (17%) and new abscesses (15%).

The efficacy and safety of subcutaneous infliximab-dyyb as a maintenance therapy in moderately to severely active Crohn disease following treatment with an IV infliximab product were evaluated in a randomized, double-blind, placebo-controlled trial. All patients were intially administered 3 IV induction doses of 5 mg/kg infliximab-dyyb at weeks 0, 2, and 6. Patients who experienced a clinical response, defined as a decrease from baseline in CDAI of at least 100 points at week 10, were randomly assigned to infliximab-dyyb 120 mg subcutaneously or placebo every 2 weeks. The co-primary endpoints were clinical remission (based on CDAI) and endoscopic response at week 54. Results revealed that maintenance subcutaneous infliximab-dyyb therapy was associated with an improvement in both clinical remission (63% vs. 30%) and endoscopic response (50% vs. 18%) as compared to placebo in the total population.

Clinical Perspective

The American College of Gastroenterology (ACG) and the American Gastroenterological Association (AGA) have issued guidelines for the medical treatment of Crohn disease. Treatment of Crohn disease is typically divided into 2 phases: induction therapy (where control of inflammation is rapidly achieved) and maintenance therapy (where control of inflammation is sustained for a prolonged period of time). Specific treatments for Crohn disease are selected according to the patient's risk profile and disease severity. Drug classes used to treat Crohn disease include 5-aminosalicylates, antibiotics, corticosteroids, immunomodulators (e.g., thiopurines, immunomodulators), and biologic agents, including tumor necrosis factor (TNF; TNF-α) blocking agents, ustekinumab, vedolizumab, and natalizumab.

TNF blocking agents used in the treatment of Crohn disease include infliximab, adalimumab, and certolizumab pegol. The TNF blocking agents are generally recommended for use as induction and maintenance therapy in adults with moderate to severe Crohn disease. The ACG states that TNF blocking agents should be used to treat moderate to severe and/or moderate to high risk Crohn disease that is resistant to treatment with corticosteroids and/or refractory to thiopurines or methotrexate. Combining TNF blocking agents with a thiopurine in the induction setting may be more effective than TNF blocking agent monotherapy in patients who are naïve to these therapies. The AGA suggests combining infliximab or adalimumab with a thiopurine over infliximab or adalimumab monotherapy for induction and maintenance of remission in patients with moderate to severe Crohn disease who are naïve to biologics and immunomodulators. The TNF blocking agents can also be considered to treat severely active Crohn disease, and infliximab may be used to treat fulminant Crohn disease.

Patients with perianal fistulas should be considered for TNF blocking therapy; however, guideline recommendations regarding agent selection differ in this setting. The ACG states that infliximab is effective in this setting, while adalimumab and certolizumab pegol may be effective. The AGA recommends infliximab and suggests adalimumab, ustekinumab, or vedolizumab over no treatment in this setting, and notes that certolizumab pegol may not be effective for induction of fistula remission. In patients with enterocutaneous or rectovaginal fistulas, infliximab may be effective and should be considered. If a patient with Crohn disease achieves remission with a TNF blocking agent, TNF blocking therapy should be continued to maintain remission; monotherapy with a TNF blocking agent is effective for maintaining remission, but combination with azathioprine/6-mercaptopurine or methotrexate should be considered due to the potential for immunogenicity and loss of response. For patients with surgically induced remission of Crohn disease, the AGA suggests TNF blocking agents and/or thiopurines over other agents to prevent recurrence. Similarly, the ACG recommends that patients who undergo surgery for Crohn disease and remain at high risk for recurrence should begin therapy with a TNF blocking agent within 4 weeks of surgery to prevent postoperative recurrence.

Crohn Disease in Pediatric Patients

Infliximab and its biosimilars (infliximab-abda, infliximab-axxq, infliximab-dyyb) are used to reduce the signs and symptoms of Crohn disease and to induce and maintain clinical remission in pediatric patients 6 years of age and older with moderately to severely active disease who have had an inadequate response to conventional therapy. Infliximab has been designated an orphan drug by FDA for this use. Safety and efficacy of infliximab in the treatment of Crohn disease in pediatric patients are based principally on the results of a randomized controlled trial (REACH), with supporting evidence from an open-label extension study and small open-label trials.

Clinical Experience

The REACH study was a randomized, open-label study in 112 pediatric patients 6–17 years of age (median age 13 years) with moderately to severely active Crohn disease who had a median Pediatric Crohn Disease Activity Index (PCDAI) of 40 (on a scale of 0–100) and an inadequate response to conventional therapy. Prior to enrollment in the study, patients were required to be on a stable dosage of mercaptopurine, azathioprine, or methotrexate; 35% of the patients also were receiving corticosteroids at baseline. All patients received infliximab induction therapy with 5 mg/kg administered at weeks 0, 2, and 6. At week 10, 103 patients were randomized to receive maintenance therapy of 5 mg/kg of infliximab every 8 or 12 weeks. At week 10, 88% of patients had clinical response (defined as a decrease in PCDAI score of 15 or more points from baseline and a total PCDAI score of 30 points or less), and 59% of patients were in clinical remission (defined as a PCDAI score of 10 points or less). The proportion of pediatric patients achieving a clinical response at week 10 compared favorably with the rate of clinical response reported in adults with active Crohn disease who received infliximab in a clinical trial. The clinical response rate both at week 30 (73 versus 47%) and week 54 (64 versus 33%) was higher in pediatric patients receiving infliximab every 8 weeks than in those receiving the drug every 12 weeks. In addition, the clinical remission rate both at week 30 (60 versus 35%) and week 54 (56 versus 24%) was higher in patients receiving infliximab every 8 weeks than in those receiving the drug every 12 weeks. Among patients receiving corticosteroids at baseline, 46 or 33% of those receiving maintenance doses of infliximab every 8 or 12 weeks, respectively, were in clinical remission and were able to discontinue corticosteroid use at week 30, while at week 54, 46 or 17% of those receiving maintenance doses of infliximab every 8 or 12 weeks, respectively, were in clinical remission and were able to discontinue corticosteroid use. Patients who completed REACH were eligible to enter an open-label extension study. Patients in the extension study received infliximab 5 mg/kg every 8 or 12 weeks or infliximab 10 mg/kg every 8 weeks, depending on the maintenance regimen they were receiving at the completion of the REACH study. In this study, clinical benefit of infliximab was maintained for up to 3 additional years of treatment.

In another open-label study in 15 pediatric patients 6–18 years of age with medically refractory Crohn disease (unable to tolerate corticosteroid taper; PCDAI score of 30 or greater; no improvement despite use of mercaptopurine, methotrexate, and/or cyclosporine for 4 months or longer), a single 5-mg/kg dose of infliximab was administered by IV infusion. At 4 weeks after the dose, 14/15 (94%) had responded to infliximab with a decrease in the PCDAI score of 25 points or greater; at 10 weeks, 10/15 (67%) were in clinical remission (PCDAI score of 15 or less). All patients continued mercaptopurine or methotrexate therapy during and after the infliximab infusion, but oral corticosteroid dosage was tapered in most patients. During the 52-week follow-up of the 14 responders, 11 (78%) had clinical relapse that required additional drug therapy or surgical intervention. When these children were subdivided based on disease duration, the relapse rate was 50% in those who had been diagnosed with Crohn disease less than 2 years previously; however, the relapse rate was 100% in those who had been diagnosed more than 2 years previously.

In an open-label study in 19 pediatric patients 9–19 years of age with moderately or severely active Crohn disease, 1–3 doses of infliximab (5 mg/kg) were given by IV infusion usually at 4-week intervals. At 4 weeks after the initial dose, all 19 pediatric patients had a clinical response documented by physician global assessment and PCDAI score; at 12 weeks after the initial dose, only 4 patients maintained a clinical response to the drug.

Clinical Perspective

Many of the agents used to treat Crohn disease in adults are also used to treat Crohn disease in pediatric patients; these agents include 5-aminosalicylates, corticosteroids, immunomodulators (e.g., azathioprine, methotrexate), and biologic agents (e.g., TNF blocking agents). A "treat-to-target" approach is used in pediatric patients, with targets including clinical response, clinical remission, restoration of normal growth, endoscopic healing, and normalization of biomarkers (e.g., C-reactive protein [CRP], fecal calprotectin). In pediatric patients, exclusive enteral nutrition is recommended as first-line induction therapy, with corticosteroids as an alternative. Immunomodulators are typically used first-line for maintenance therapy. TNF blocking agents used in the treatment of pediatric Crohn disease include infliximab and adalimumab; these agents are generally used for induction and maintenance therapy in pediatric patients who fail an adequate trial of steroids and exclusive enteral nutrition and/or immunomodulators, unless the patient has a complex perianal fistula at diagnosis.

● Ulcerative Colitis

Ulcerative Colitis in Adults

Infliximab and its biosimilars (infliximab-abda, infliximab-axxq, infliximab-dyyb) are used to reduce signs and symptoms, to induce and maintain clinical remission and mucosal healing, and to eliminate use of corticosteroids in adults with moderately to severely active ulcerative colitis who have had an inadequate response to conventional therapies.

The subcutaneous formulation of infliximab-dyyb is used for the maintenance treatment of moderately to severely active ulcerative colitis in adults following IV treatment with an infliximab product.

Safety and efficacy of infliximab for this use are based principally on the results of 2 randomized controlled trials. Guidelines generally support the first-line use of TNF blocking agents for induction and maintenance of remission in patients with moderate to severe ulcerative colitis.

Clinical Experience

Safety and efficacy of infliximab in the management of ulcerative colitis in adults were evaluated in 2 randomized, double-blind, placebo-controlled studies (the Active Ulcerative Colitis Trials 1 and 2; ACT 1 and ACT 2, respectively) in 728 patients with moderately to severely active ulcerative colitis who had an inadequate response to conventional therapies. In the ACT 1 study, patients had an inadequate response to or were intolerant of corticosteroids alone or in combination with azathioprine or mercaptopurine, while in the ACT 2 study, patients had an inadequate response to or were intolerant of corticosteroids alone or in combination with azathioprine or mercaptopurine and/or to preparations containing 5-aminosalicylates. Patients were randomized to receive placebo or a 5- or 10-mg/kg dose of infliximab at weeks 0, 2, and 6 and then every 8 weeks through week 22 in the ACT 2 study or week 46 in the ACT 1 study. Patients in the ACT 2 study were allowed to continue blinded therapy to week 46 at the investigator's discretion. Those who were receiving fixed dosages of azathioprine or mercaptopurine, and/or 5-aminosalicylates, continued to receive these drugs during the study. Corticosteroids were tapered gradually until discontinuance. In both studies, the proportions of patients who had a clinical response or remission at weeks 8 and 30, and at week 54 in the ACT 1 study, were higher by a factor of 1.7 to more than 2 in patients receiving infliximab than in those receiving placebo. Clinical response (defined as a reduction from baseline Mayo score of at least 3 points and at least 30%, with an accompanying decrease in the subscore for rectal bleeding of at least 1 point or an absolute rectal-bleeding subscore of 0 or 1) at week 30 in the ACT 1 study was reported in 52 or 51% of patients receiving 5 or 10 mg of infliximab, respectively, compared with 30% patients receiving placebo, while in the ACT 2 study such response was observed in 47 or 60% of patients receiving 5 or 10 mg of infliximab, respectively, compared with 26% of patients receiving placebo. At week 54 in the ACT 1 study, clinical response was reported in 46 or 44% of patients receiving 5 or 10 mg of infliximab, respectively, compared with 20% of patients receiving placebo. The rates of clinical response were similar between the subpopulations of patients who were refractory to corticosteroids and those who were not refractory to corticosteroids. In the ACT 1 study, in patients refractory to corticosteroids, clinical response at week 8 was reported in 77 or 68% of those receiving 5 or 10 mg of infliximab, respectively, and in 35% of those receiving placebo, while in patients not refractory to corticosteroids, such response was reported in 67 or 59% of those receiving 5 or 10 mg of infliximab, respectively, and in 38% of those receiving placebo. In the ACT 2 study, in patients refractory to corticosteroids, clinical response at week 8 was reported in 63 or 66% of those receiving 5 or 10 mg of infliximab, respectively, and in 38% of those receiving placebo, while in patients not refractory to corticosteroids, such response was reported in 65 or 70% of those receiving 5 or 10 mg of infliximab, respectively, and in 26% of those receiving placebo. At week 30, clinical remission was reported in 34 and 37% of patients receiving 5 or 10 mg of infliximab, respectively, compared with 16% of those receiving placebo in the ACT 1 study, while such remission was observed in 26 or 36% of patients receiving 5 or 10 mg of infliximab, respectively, compared with 11% of patients receiving placebo. At week 54 in the ACT 1 study, clinical remission was reported in 35 or 34% of patients receiving 5 or 10 mg of infliximab, respectively, compared with 17% of patients receiving placebo. The proportions of patients with a sustained clinical response or sustained remission were significantly higher in patients receiving infliximab than in those receiving placebo. In addition, mucosal healing at weeks 8 and 30 in both studies (ACT 1 and ACT 2) and at week 54 in ACT 1 occurred in significantly more patients receiving infliximab than in those receiving placebo. At baseline, 61 and 51% of patients were receiving corticosteroids in the ACT 1 and ACT 2 studies, respectively. The proportions of patients who were in clinical remission and had discontinued corticosteroids at week 30 in both studies and at week 54 in the ACT 1 study, were higher in those receiving infliximab than in those receiving placebo.

The efficacy and safety of subcutaneous infliximab-dyyb as a maintenance therapy in moderately to severely active ulcerative colitis following treatment with an IV infliximab product were evaluated in a randomized, double-blind, placebo-controlled trial. All patients were initially administered 3 IV induction doses of 5 mg/kg infliximab-dyyb at weeks 0, 2, and 6. Patients who experienced a clinical response, defined as a decrease from baseline in the modified Mayo score of at least 2 points and at least 30%, with an accompanying decrease in the rectal bleeding subscore of at least 1 point or an absolute rectal bleeding subscore of 0 or 1 point at week 10, were randomly assigned to infliximab-dyyb 120 mg subcutaneously or placebo every 2 weeks. The primary endpoint was the proportion of patients in clinical remission at week 54. Results revealed that maintenance subcutaneous infliximab-dyyb therapy was associated with an improvement in clinical remission as compared to placebo (43% vs. 21%) in the total population.

Clinical Perspective

The American College of Gastroenterology (ACG) and the American Gastroenterological Association (AGA) issued guidelines for the medical treatment of ulcerative colitis in adults in 2019 and 2020. Goals of therapy in ulcerative colitis include achieving and maintaining corticosteroid-free remission and promoting mucosal healing. Specific treatments are selected according to disease severity, as well as disease location/extent, disease prognosis, and previous therapies used. Drug classes used to treat ulcerative colitis include oral and rectal 5-aminosalicylates, oral and rectal corticosteroids, immunomodulators (e.g., thiopurines, methotrexate), tofacitinib, and biologic agents, including TNF blocking agents, vedolizumab, and ustekinumab. In most cases, if a drug used for induction therapy is effective, it is continued for maintenance of remission.

TNF blocking agents used in the treatment of ulcerative colitis include infliximab, golimumab, and adalimumab; the primary role for these agents is in the treatment of moderate to severe ulcerative colitis. For adult outpatients with moderate to severe ulcerative colitis, the AGA recommends TNF blocking therapies, vedolizumab, tofacitinib, or ustekinumab over no treatment. AGA conditionally recommends the use of infliximab or vedolizumab over adalimumab for induction of remission in biologic-naïve patients based on evidence from a comparative randomized controlled trial (vedolizumab) and a network meta-analysis (infliximab). ACG recommends the use of oral corticosteroids, TNF blocking agents, vedolizumab, or tofacitinib for induction of remission in patients with moderately to severely active ulcerative colitis.

Early use of biologic agents with or without immunomodulator therapy is conditionally recommended over gradual step up therapy after failure of 5-aminosalicylates. Combination therapy with a TNF blocking agent and a thiopurine or methotrexate is conditionally recommended over biologic monotherapy. Combination therapy with a thiopurine is specifically recommended for patients who receive induction therapy with infliximab. Patients who achieve remission with TNF blocking therapy should continue on TNF blocking therapy to maintain remission after induction. Patients with primary nonresponse to one TNF blocking therapy should be switched to a biologic from a different class; patients who initially respond to TNF blocking therapy and later lose response can be switched to a different TNF blocking agent. Patients with mildly active ulcerative colitis and multiple prognostic factors associated with an increased risk of hospitalization or surgery should be treated with therapies for moderately to severely active disease. Consult the ACG guideline for additional details on prognostic factors that may be considered.

Hospitalized patients with acute severe ulcerative colitis should receive IV corticosteroids to induce remission; if the response to IV corticosteroids is inadequate after 3 to 5 days of therapy, infliximab or cyclosporine should be used as rescue therapy. The choice between infliximab or cyclosporine should be based on provider experience with the agent, history of previous failure of immunomodulator or TNF blocking therapy, and serum albumin.

Ulcerative Colitis in Pediatric Patients

Infliximab and its biosimilars (infliximab-abda, infliximab-axxq, infliximab-dyyb) are used to reduce the signs and symptoms of ulcerative colitis and to induce and maintain clinical remission in pediatric patients 6 years of age and older with moderately to severely active ulcerative colitis who have had an inadequate response to conventional therapy. Infliximab has been designated as an orphan drug by FDA for the treatment of ulcerative colitis in pediatric patients.

Clinical Experience

Efficacy and safety of infliximab for this indication are supported by evidence from controlled clinical studies in adults and by an uncontrolled study in 60 pediatric patients 6–17 years of age with moderately to severely active ulcerative colitis (Mayo score of 6–12, endoscopic subscore of 2 or greater) and an inadequate response to conventional therapies. At the start of the study in pediatric patients, 53% of patients were receiving immunosuppressive therapy with mercaptopurine, azathioprine, or methotrexate, and 62% were receiving corticosteroids; discontinuance of immunosuppressive agents and tapering of corticosteroid dosage was permitted after week 0. All patients received induction therapy with infliximab (5 mg/kg at weeks 0, 2, and 6); those who exhibited a response at week 8 were randomized to receive a maintenance regimen of 5 mg/kg every 8 weeks through week 46 or 5 mg/kg every 12 weeks through week 42. Patients who experienced loss of response during maintenance therapy were allowed to receive higher and/or more frequent doses of the drug.

At week 8 of the pediatric study, approximately 73% of patients exhibited a clinical response (defined as a reduction from baseline Mayo score of at least 3 points and at least 30%, with an accompanying decrease in the subscore for rectal bleeding of at least 1 point or achievement of an absolute rectal-bleeding subscore of 0 or 1); 40% of patients were in clinical remission as defined by Mayo score (2 points or less, with no individual subscore exceeding 1), and approximately 33% of patients were in clinical remission as measured by the Pediatric Ulcerative Colitis Activity Index (PUCAI) (score less than 10 points). Clinical response at 8 weeks was observed in 23 of 32 patients (72%) receiving concomitant immunosuppressive therapy at baseline and in 21 of 28 patients (75%) not receiving such therapy at baseline.

At week 54 of the pediatric study, clinical remission (as measured by PUCAI score) was observed in 8 of 21 patients receiving infliximab every 8 weeks and 4 of 22 patients receiving the drug every 12 weeks. Of the 45 patients randomized to receive maintenance therapy, 23 patients (including 9 patients receiving infliximab every 8 weeks and 14 patients receiving the drug every 12 weeks) required higher and/or more frequent doses of the drug because of loss of response, and 9 of those patients (including 7 patients who received the drug every 8 weeks) achieved remission at week 54. Efficacy of infliximab in inducing and maintaining mucosal healing could not be established because the study was uncontrolled and few patients underwent endoscopy at week 54.

Clinical Perspective

Many of the agents used to treat ulcerative colitis in adults are also used to treat ulcerative colitis in pediatric patients; these agents include 5-aminosalicylates, corticosteroids, immunomodulators (e.g., azathioprine), and biologic agents (e.g., TNF blocking agents). Choice of agent is generally guided by severity of presentation. A "treat-to-target" approach is used in pediatric patients, with targets including clinical response, clinical remission, restoration of normal growth, endoscopic healing, and normalization of biomarkers (e.g., CRP, fecal calprotectin).

In pediatric patients, 5-aminosalicylates are used first-line for induction and maintenance of remission in mild to moderate ulcerative colitis; corticosteroids are used first-line for induction of remission in severe disease and in patients who fail to respond to 5-aminosalicylates. Azathioprine is typically used first-line for maintenance therapy in patients who attain remission on corticosteroids. Long-term corticosteroid treatment should be avoided if possible. TNF blocking agents used in the treatment of pediatric ulcerative colitis include infliximab and adalimumab; these agents are generally used in patients with moderate to severe disease who fail therapy with 5-aminosalicylates/azathioprine and/or who are unable to wean from corticosteroids on 5-aminosalicylate/azathioprine therapy. Hospitalized patients with acute severe colitis are typically treated with corticosteroids first-line, but if adequate response is not attained after 3 to 5 days, infliximab therapy can be used to induce remission.

● Rheumatoid Arthritis

Infliximab and its biosimilars (infliximab-abda, infliximab-axxq, infliximab-dyyb) are used in conjunction with methotrexate to manage signs and symptoms, improve physical function, and inhibit progression of structural damage in adults with moderately to severely active rheumatoid arthritis. Safety and efficacy of infliximab for this use are based principally on the results of several randomized controlled trials. Guidelines generally support the use of TNF blocking agents as add-on therapy to methotrexate in patients who do not meet treatment goals with methotrexate alone.

Clinical Experience

Safety and efficacy of infliximab used in conjunction with methotrexate for the management of rheumatoid arthritis in adults have been evaluated in several open-label and double-blind, placebo-controlled studies in adults with active disease as defined by the American College of Rheumatology (ACR) who had not responded adequately to methotrexate. Infliximab in conjunction with methotrexate also has been evaluated in a controlled study in adults with early active rheumatoid arthritis (i.e., duration of 3 years or less) who had not previously received therapy with methotrexate. Results indicate that addition of infliximab to a methotrexate regimen can result in decreases in the signs and symptoms of rheumatoid arthritis. For patients with early active rheumatoid arthritis, concomitant use of infliximab and methotrexate is more effective than methotrexate (as the sole disease-modifying antirheumatic drug [DMARD]) for the management of rheumatoid arthritis in adults. In addition, infliximab used concomitantly with methotrexate can improve physical function and inhibit the progression of structural damage in patients with rheumatoid arthritis.

Concomitant use of infliximab and methotrexate for the management of rheumatoid arthritis was evaluated in a large double-blind, placebo-controlled, phase III, international study that involved 428 patients (Anti-TNF Trial in Rheumatoid Arthritis with Concomitant Therapy [ATTRACT]). At study entry, patients had active rheumatoid arthritis (defined as 6 or more swollen or tender joints and at least 2 additional manifestations, including morning stiffness for 45 minutes or longer, erythrocyte sedimentation rate [ESR] of 28 mm/hour or greater, or CRP level of 2 mg/dL or greater) despite having received methotrexate (oral or parenteral) and folic acid consistently for at least 3 months. Study patients were a median age of 51 years old, had a median disease duration of 11 years, and previously received treatment with 2.5–2.8 DMARDs other than methotrexate. These patients had median swollen and tender joint counts of 21 and 31, respectively; 77% were rheumatoid factor positive; 37% had undergone a joint surgery; 25% had joint replacement surgery; and approximately 40% were classified as ACR functional class III.

Patients were randomized to receive placebo or 3 or 10 mg/kg of infliximab by IV infusion at weeks 0, 2 and 6, followed by additional doses given once every 4 or 8 weeks. Patients continued to receive stable weekly dosages of methotrexate (median dosage 16 mg once weekly) beginning 4 weeks before and throughout the study. Those who were receiving stable dosages of nonsteroidal anti-inflammatory agents (NSAIAs) and/or oral corticosteroids (oral prednisone 10 mg or less daily or equivalent) for at least 4 weeks prior to study entry were permitted to continue these drugs; patients who had not received such therapy were not permitted to initiate these drugs after entering the study. Patient evaluations were performed every 4 weeks and assessed according to ACR criteria for improvement (ACR response); the primary end point was the proportion of patients at week 30 who experienced a 20% improvement in rheumatoid disease activity (ACR 20 response). The ACR 20 response is achieved if the patient experiences a 20% or greater improvement in both tender and swollen joint counts and a 20% or greater improvement in at least 3 of the following criteria: patient pain assessment, patient global assessment, physician global assessment, patient self-assessed disability, or laboratory indicators of disease activity (i.e., ESR or CRP level). Patients also were evaluated for ACR 50 and 70 responses (these are defined using the same criteria as ACR 20 with a level of improvement of 50 or 70%, respectively); reductions in individual measures of disease activity; and a general health assessment.

At 30 weeks, an ACR 20 response was attained in 50% of patients who received 3 mg/kg of infliximab every 8 weeks concomitantly with weekly methotrexate compared with 20% of patients who received placebo and weekly methotrexate. Similar response rates were observed in patients receiving the higher infliximab dosage (10 mg/kg) and/or more frequent doses (every 4 weeks). At 30 weeks, an ACR 50 response was attained in 26–31% and an ACR 70 response was attained in 8–18% of patients who received infliximab in a dosage of 3 or 10 mg/kg every 4 or 8 weeks concomitantly with once weekly methotrexate; an ACR 50 or 70 response was attained at week 30 in only 5 or 0%, respectively, of patients who received placebo with once weekly methotrexate.

At 54 weeks, 42–59% of those who received 3 or 10 mg/kg of infliximab once every 4 or 8 weeks concomitantly with once weekly methotrexate maintained an ACR 20 response compared with 17% of patients who received placebo concomitantly with once weekly methotrexate. At 54 weeks, an ACR 50 or 70 response was maintained in 21–40% or 11–26%, respectively, of those receiving infliximab concomitantly with once weekly methotrexate compared with only 9 or 2%, respectively, of patients receiving placebo concomitantly with once weekly methotrexate.

Physical function and disability were assessed using the Health Assessment Questionnaire (HAQ) and the general health-related quality-of-life questionnaire SF-36. All 4 dosage regimens of infliximab and weekly methotrexate were associated with greater improvement from baseline in the HAQ and SF-36 physical component summary score averaged over time through week 54 compared with the placebo plus methotrexate regimen; in addition, the infliximab regimens were not associated with deterioration in the SF-36 mental component summary score. Improvements in HAQ and SF-36 were maintained through week 102.

Structural damage in the hands and feet of patients in this study was assessed radiographically at baseline and at weeks 54 and 102 using the van der Heijde-modified Sharp score (a composite score of structural damage that measures the number and size of joint erosions and the degree of joint space narrowing in hands/wrists and feet). At 54 weeks, there was more progression of joint damage from baseline in the group of patients who received placebo with once weekly methotrexate compared with those who received infliximab with once weekly methotrexate. The inhibition of progression of structural damage reported in patients receiving infliximab at week 54 was maintained through week 102. There also was evidence that infliximab had a benefit on both erosions and joint-space narrowing when these scores were examined independently and when the hands and feet were examined separately.

Efficacy of infliximab in conjunction with methotrexate has been evaluated in a study that included 1004 adults with early active rheumatoid arthritis (i.e., duration of 3 years or less) who had not previously received methotrexate. The median age of study patients was 51 years, and the median disease duration was 0.6 years. These patients had median swollen and tender joint counts of 19 and 31, respectively; greater than 80% of these individuals had joint damage at baseline. Patients were randomized to receive placebo or 3 or 6 mg/kg of infliximab by IV infusion at weeks 0, 2, and 6, followed by additional doses given once every 8 weeks. All patients received methotrexate (optimized to a dosage of 20 mg each week by week 8 of the study); patients receiving stable dosages of NSAIAs and/or oral corticosteroids (oral prednisone 10 mg or less daily or equivalent) at study entry were permitted to continue these drugs. Reduction in the signs and symptoms of rheumatoid arthritis were evaluated using ACR criteria, physical function and disability was assessed using HAQ scores, and joint damage was assessed using the van der Heijde-modified Sharp score. At 54 weeks, 62–66% of patients receiving 3 or 6 mg/kg of infliximab with once-weekly methotrexate attained an ACR 20 response compared with 54% of those who received placebo concomitantly with once weekly methotrexate. At 54 weeks, an ACR 50 or 70 response was attained by 46–50 or 33–37%, respectively, of patients receiving infliximab concomitantly with weekly methotrexate compared with 32 or 21%, respectively, of those receiving placebo with once-weekly methotrexate. Both dosage regimens of infliximab and weekly methotrexate were associated with greater improvement from baseline in the HAQ averaged over time through week 54 compared with the placebo plus methotrexate regimen. Radiographic analysis at week 54 indicates that infliximab in conjunction with methotrexate is more effective than methotrexate alone in delaying joint damage.

There are limited data available regarding efficacy of infliximab without concurrent methotrexate for the management of rheumatoid arthritis in adults†.

Results of early open-label and placebo-controlled studies using infliximab as the only DMARD in adults with rheumatoid arthritis indicated that the drug could result in clinical improvement in patients who had not responded adequately to other DMARDs. In one multicenter, placebo-controlled, double-blind study, 73 adults with rheumatoid arthritis were randomized to receive a single dose of placebo or 1 or 10 mg/kg of infliximab given by IV infusion. Patients were not allowed to receive any other DMARDs beginning 4 weeks before the study; however, those receiving stable dosages of oral corticosteroids or NSAIAs were allowed to continue these drugs. At 4 weeks after the dose, a clinical response (defined as a Paulus 20% response) was reported in 44 or 79% of patients who received a 1- or 10-mg/kg infliximab dose, respectively, compared with 8% of those who received placebo. A Paulus 50% response was reported at 4 weeks in 28 or 58% of patients who received 1 or 10 mg/kg of the drug, respectively, compared with 8% of those who received placebo. Although there was no evidence of a dose-response relationship based on results at 2 weeks, the higher dose (10 mg/kg) was associated with significantly higher response rates and greater responses (e.g., improvements in pain score, grip strength, CRP, ESR) than the lower dose (1 mg/kg) at week 4. There also was some evidence that the higher dose resulted in a more prolonged response than the lower dose.

Clinical Perspective

The American College of Rheumatology issued guidelines for the treatment of rheumatoid arthritis in 2021. Disease-modifying treatments for rheumatoid arthritis include conventional DMARDs (e.g., hydroxychloroquine, leflunomide, methotrexate, sulfasalazine), biologic DMARDs (e.g., TNF blocking agents, abatacept, tocilizumab, sarilumab, rituximab), and/or targeted synthetic DMARDs (e.g., Janus kinase inhibitors). Specific agents for rheumatoid arthritis treatment are selected according to current disease activity, prior therapies used, and the presence of comorbidities. A "treat-to-target" approach is typically employed, with the goal of achieving a predefined target of low disease activity or remission.

TNF blocking agents used in the treatment of rheumatoid arthritis include adalimumab, certolizumab pegol, etanercept, golimumab, and infliximab. Methotrexate monotherapy is strongly recommended over biologic DMARD monotherapy and conditionally recommended over the combination of methotrexate and a TNF blocking agent for DMARD-naïve patients with moderate to high disease activity, because many patients will achieve their treatment goal with methotrexate alone, and combination therapy with TNF blocking agents may be associated with additional risks and costs. Biologic DMARDs (including TNF blocking agents) and targeted synthetic DMARDs are conditionally recommended as add-on therapy for patients who are taking maximally tolerated doses of methotrexate and are not at target. Recommendations for the use and selection of biologic DMARDs in rheumatoid arthritis vary based on the presence of certain comorbidities (e.g., heart failure, previous serious infection, nontuberculous mycobacterial lung disease). Consult the American College of Rheumatology guidelines for additional details.

● Ankylosing Spondylitis

Infliximab and its biosimilars (infliximab-abda, infliximab-axxq, infliximab-dyyb) are used to reduce the signs and symptoms of ankylosing spondylitis in patients with active disease. Safety and efficacy of infliximab for this use are based principally on the results of randomized controlled trials in addition to other supporting studies., Guidelines generally support the use of TNF blocking agents for the treatment of ankylosing spondylitis in patients with active disease despite treatment with nonsteroidal antiinflammatory agents (NSAIAs).

Clinical Experience

Safety and efficacy of infliximab for the management of ankylosing spondylitis were assessed in the randomized, double-blind, placebo-controlled ASSERT study. In this study, 279 adults with active ankylosing spondylitis were randomized in a 3:8 ratio to receive placebo or infliximab 5 mg/kg IV at weeks 0, 2, 6, 12, and 18. Patients were not allowed to receive DMARDs or systemic corticosteroids during the study period, but stable dosages of NSAIAs, acetaminophen, and tramadol were permitted. The primary end point was a 20% improvement according to the Assessment in Ankylosing Spondylitis criteria (ASAS 20) at week 24. The ASAS 20 response is achieved if the patient experiences a 20% or greater improvement from baseline and an absolute improvement of at least 1 unit in at least 3 of the following assessment domains: patient global assessment, spinal pain, function according to the Bath Ankylosing Spondylitis Functional Index (BASFI), and morning stiffness. Patients also were evaluated for ASAS 50 and 70 responses (these are defined using the same criteria as ASAS 20 with a level of improvement of 50 or 70%, respectively).

At week 24, the ASAS 20 responder rates were 60 and 18% in the infliximab and placebo groups, respectively. Symptomatic improvements in the infliximab group were observed as early as week 2 and maintained through week 24 of treatment. The ASAS 50 and ASAS 70 responder rates at week 24 were 44 and 28%, respectively, in the infliximab group and 9 and 4%, respectively, in the placebo group. Patients in the infliximab group also experienced improvements in health-related quality of life (measured by the physical component of the Short Form 36 [SF 36]) at week 24. Efficacy and safety of infliximab were maintained for up to 2 years.

In an additional placebo-controlled study in adults with ankylosing spondylitis, 53% of those receiving infliximab (5-mg/kg doses given at 0, 2, and 6 weeks) experienced at least a 50% reduction in disease activity (assessed using the Bath Ankylosing Spondylitis Disease Activity Index [BASDAI]) compared with 9% of those receiving placebo. In addition, infliximab therapy was associated with improvements in physical function and quality of life. Efficacy and safety of infliximab were maintained for up to 5 years of treatment.

An open-label, randomized study compared infliximab to etanercept in 50 DMARD- and biologic-naïve patients with ankylosing spondylitis refractory to oral NSAIAs. Patients were randomized to receive etanercept 50 mg subcutaneously weekly or infliximab 5 mg/kg at weeks 0, 2, and 6, then every 6 weeks thereafter for a period of 102 weeks. At week 12, 75 and 60% of patients receiving infliximab and etanercept, respectively, demonstrated an ASAS 20 response, and 55 and 43% of patients receiving infliximab and etanercept, respectively, demonstrated an ASAS 40 response. For both groups, efficacy was generally maintained up to the end of the observation period (week 104).

Clinical Perspective

The American College of Rheumatology, the Spondylitis Association of America, and the Spondyloarthritis Research and Treatment Network issued a joint guideline for the treatment of ankylosing spondylitis in 2019. Treatments for ankylosing spondylitis include NSAIAs, conventional DMARDs (e.g., methotrexate, sulfasalazine), biologic DMARDs (e.g., TNF blocking agents, secukinumab, ixekizumab), and/or targeted synthetic DMARDs (e.g., tofacitinib). Continuous NSAIA treatment is typically considered first-line for active ankylosing spondylitis, with other agents used in the treatment of NSAIA-refractory disease. Specific agents for ankylosing spondylitis treatment are selected according to current disease activity, prior therapies, and the presence of comorbidities. Goals of therapy in ankylosing spondylitis are to alleviate symptoms, improve functioning, maintain the ability to work, decrease complications, and prevent or slow skeletal damage.

TNF blocking agents used in the treatment of ankylosing spondylitis include adalimumab, certolizumab pegol, etanercept, golimumab, and infliximab. For adults with active ankylosing spondylitis despite treatment with NSAIAs, treatment with a TNF blocking agent is strongly recommended over no treatment with a TNF blocking agent and conditionally recommended over treatment with tofacitinib, secukinumab, or ixekizumab. No specific TNF blocking agent is recommended over others. In patients with active ankylosing spondylitis despite treatment with a first TNF blocking agent, guidelines conditionally recommend secukinumab or ixekizumab for patients with primary nonresponse to TNF blocking therapy and treatment with a different TNF blocking therapy for patients with secondary nonresponse to TNF blocking therapy. In adults with stable ankylosing spondylitis, continuation of biologic monotherapy is conditionally recommended over discontinuation of the biologic or continuation of combination therapy with NSAIAs or conventional DMARDs. Recommendations for treatment selection in ankylosing spondylitis may be influenced by the presence of certain comorbidities (e.g., iritis, inflammatory bowel disease). Consult the joint guideline issued by the American College of Rheumatology, the Spondylitis Association of America, and the Spondyloarthritis Research and Treatment Network for additional details.

● *Psoriatic Arthritis*

Infliximab and its biosimilars (infliximab-abda, infliximab-axxq, infliximab-dyyb) are used to reduce the signs and symptoms of active arthritis, inhibit the progression of structural damage, and improve physical function in adults with psoriatic arthritis. Safety and efficacy of infliximab for this use are based principally on the results from a randomized controlled trial, with supporting data from an additional randomized controlled trial and an open-label extension study. Guidelines generally support the use of TNF blocking agents as first-line treatment in patients with active psoriatic arthritis.

Clinical Experience

Safety and efficacy of infliximab in the management of active psoriatic arthritis (i.e., at least 5 swollen joints and at least 5 tender joints, with one or more of the following subtypes: arthritis involving DIP joints, arthritis mutilans, asymmetric peripheral arthritis, polyarticular arthritis, spondylitis with peripheral arthritis) were evaluated in a multicenter, double-blind, placebo-controlled study in 200 adult patients who had an inadequate response to therapy with DMARDs or NSAIAs (IMPACT 2). Patients also had plaque psoriasis with qualifying target lesion of at least 2 cm in diameter. During the 24-week double-blind phase, patients were randomized to receive infliximab 5 mg/kg by IV infusion (100 patients) or placebo (100 patients) at weeks 0, 2, 6, 14, and 22. Forty-six percent of patients continued to receive stable doses of methotrexate (up to 25 mg weekly). Patient evaluations were assessed according to ACR criteria for improvement (ACR response). Patients receiving placebo, who achieved less than 10% improvement from baseline at week 16, were switched to induction therapy with infliximab (early escape). At week 24, all patients receiving placebo were switched to induction therapy with

infliximab. Infliximab therapy was continued through week 46 for all patients. At 14 weeks, an ACR 20 response was attained in 58% of patients who received infliximab compared with 11% of patients who received placebo. The response was similar regardless of concomitant use with methotrexate. Improvement has been observed in some patients as early as week 2. At 6 months, ACR 20, 50, or 70 response was attained in 54, 41, or 27% of patients, respectively, who received infliximab, compared with 16, 4, or 2% of patients receiving placebo. Similar responses were seen in patients with each of the subtypes of psoriatic arthritis, although few patients were enrolled with arthritis mutilans and spondylitis with peripheral arthritis subtypes. Infliximab therapy resulted in improvements in the components of the ACR response criteria and in dactylitis and enthesopathy compared with placebo. The clinical response was maintained through week 54.

Among the 170 patients who had baseline affected body surface area (BSA) of 3% or more, improvement in the Psoriasis Area and Severity Index (PASI) of at least 75% (PASI 75) from baseline was achieved at week 14 (regardless of concomitant methotrexate use) in 64% of patients receiving infliximab and in 2% of patients receiving placebo. Improvement was observed in some patients as early as week 2. At 6 months, PASI 75 and PASI 90 responses were achieved in 60 and 39%, respectively, of patients receiving infliximab and in 1 and 0%, respectively, of patients receiving placebo. The PASI response generally was maintained through week 54.

Structural damage in the hands and feet was assessed radiographically by the change from baseline in the van der Heijde-Sharp (vdH-S) score, modified by the addition of hand distal interphalangeal (DIP) joints. The total modified vdH-S score was a composite score of structural damage measuring the number and size of joint erosions and the degree of joint space narrowing (JSN) in the hands and feet. At week 24, less radiographic progression (mean change of -0.7 versus 0.82), less progression in erosion scores (-0.56 versus 0.51), and less progression in JSN scores (-0.14 versus 0.31) were observed in patients receiving infliximab compared with those receiving placebo. Continued inhibition of structural damage at week 54 was reported in patients receiving infliximab. A median change of 0 in the vdH-S score was reported during the 12-month study in patients initially randomized to either infliximab or placebo. Readily apparent radiographic progression was observed in a higher percentage of patients receiving placebo than in those receiving infliximab (12 versus 3%).

Patients receiving infliximab experienced substantial improvement in physical function as assessed by the HAQ Disability Index (HAQ-DI), with median improvement of 43% from baseline to week 14 and week 24 in patients receiving infliximab compared with 0% in those receiving placebo. During the 24-week placebo-controlled portion of the trial, a clinically meaningful improvement in HAQ-DI (decrease of at least 0.3 units) was reported in 54% of patients receiving infliximab and in 22% of those receiving placebo. Patients receiving infliximab also achieved a greater improvement in the physical and mental component summary scores of the SF-36 Health Survey compared with patients receiving placebo. These responses were maintained for up to 2 years in an open-label extension study.

An earlier randomized, placebo-controlled study (IMPACT) in 104 adults with psoriatic arthritis and previous failure of at least 1 DMARD therapy additionally evaluated the efficacy and safety of infliximab. Patients were randomized to receive placebo or infliximab 5 mg/kg IV at weeks 0, 2, 6, and 14. Patients who were initially randomized to placebo were crossed over to infliximab beginning at week 16 and received infliximab infusions at weeks 16, 18, 22, 30, 38, and 46. At weeks 16 and 18, patients who were initially randomized to infliximab received placebo infusions to maintain blinding; infliximab infusions were continued in this group at weeks 22, 30, 38, and 46. Concomitant therapy with stable doses of oral corticosteroids, NSAIAs, and/or 1 DMARD (methotrexate, leflunomide, sulfasalazine, hydroxychloroquine, intramuscular gold, penicillamine, or azathioprine) was permitted during the study.

At week 16, an ACR 20 response was achieved in 65 and 10% of patients receiving infliximab and placebo, respectively. Response to infliximab was observed as early as week 2. At week 16, a PASI 75 response was achieved in 68 and 0% of patients who received infliximab and placebo, respectively. Clinical response was maintained for up to 98 weeks of continued infliximab treatment in an open-label extension study. Radiographic progression was inhibited in patients receiving infliximab, with most patients demonstrating no worsening in modified vdH-S scores from baseline at weeks 50 and 98.

Clinical Perspective

The American College of Rheumatology and the National Psoriasis Foundation issued a joint guideline for the treatment of psoriatic arthritis in 2018. Various drugs and drug classes are used to treat psoriatic arthritis, with some classes used for symptom management (e.g., NSAIAs and corticosteroids) and others used as immunomodulatory disease-modifying therapy. Disease-modifying treatments for psoriatic arthritis include oral small molecules (e.g., methotrexate, sulfasalazine, cyclosporine, leflunomide, apremilast), biologic DMARDs (e.g., TNF blocking agents, secukinumab, ixekizumab, ustekinumab, brodalumab, abatacept), and/or targeted synthetic DMARDs (e.g., tofacitinib). Specific agents for psoriatic arthritis treatment are selected according to disease characteristics, including disease severity, as well as patient preferences/values and comorbidities. A "treat-to-target" approach is typically employed, with the goal of achieving low/minimal disease activity or remission.

TNF blocking agents used in the treatment of psoriatic arthritis include adalimumab, certolizumab pegol, etanercept, golimumab, and infliximab. For patients with treatment-naïve psoriatic arthritis, treatment with a TNF blocking agent is conditionally recommended over treatment with an oral small molecule or an interleukin (IL) 17 inhibitor (secukinumab, ixekizumab, brodalumab) or IL12/23 inhibitor (ustekinumab). For patients with active psoriatic arthritis despite treatment with an oral small molecule, switching to monotherapy with a TNF blocking agent is conditionally recommended over combination therapy with a TNF blocking agent plus methotrexate or switching to another oral small molecule, ustekinumab, secukinumab, ixekizumab, brodalumab, abatacept, or tofacitinib. For patients with active psoriatic arthritis despite treatment with TNF blocking agent monotherapy, switching to monotherapy with a different TNF blocking agent is conditionally recommended over switching to ustekinumab, secukinumab, ixekizumab, brodalumab, abatacept, or tofacitinib. For patients with active psoriatic arthritis despite treatment with a combination of a TNF blocking agent and methotrexate, switching to a different TNF blocking agent plus methotrexate is conditionally recommended over switching to a different TNF blocking agent as monotherapy. Switching to a TNF blocking agent is conditionally recommended for patients with active psoriatic arthritis despite treatment with secukinumab, ixekizumab, brodalumab, or ustekinumab. Recommendations for the use and selection of disease-modifying therapies in psoriatic arthritis vary based on the presence of certain disease characteristics (e.g., psoriatic spondylitis/axial disease, enthesitis) and comorbidities (e.g., inflammatory bowel disease, diabetes) Consult the American College of Rheumatology/National Psoriasis Foundation guideline for additional details.

● *Plaque Psoriasis*

Infliximab and its biosimilars (infliximab-abda, infliximab-axxq, infliximab-dyyb) are used for the treatment of chronic, severe (i.e., extensive and/or disabling) plaque psoriasis in adults who are candidates for systemic therapy when other systemic therapies are medically less appropriate. Infliximab products should only be used in patients who will be closely monitored and will have regular follow-up visits with a clinician. Safety and efficacy of infliximab for this use are based principally on the results from 3 randomized controlled trials. Guidelines generally support the use of TNF blocking agents in moderate to severe psoriasis, either as monotherapy or in combination with topical, oral, or phototherapy.

Clinical Experience

Safety and efficacy of infliximab were assessed in 3 randomized, double-blind, placebo-controlled studies (EXPRESS, EXPRESS II, SPIRIT) in adults (18 years of age or older) with chronic, stable plaque psoriasis involving at least 10% of body surface area (BSA), who had a Psoriasis Area and Severity Index (PASI) score of at least 12, and who were candidates for systemic therapy or phototherapy. Patients with guttate, pustular, or erythrodermic psoriasis were excluded from the studies. With the exception of low-dependency topical corticosteroids on the face and groin after week 10, no concomitant psoriasis treatments were allowed during the studies. The primary end point in all 3 studies was the proportion of patients who achieved a reduction in PASI score of at least 75% from baseline to week 10 (PASI 75). Efficacy and safety of infliximab treatment beyond 50 weeks have not been evaluated in patients with plaque psoriasis.

In the EXPRESS study, 378 patients were randomized to receive placebo or a 5-mg/kg dose of infliximab by IV infusion at weeks 0, 2, and 6 (induction therapy) and then every 8 weeks through week 46 (maintenance therapy). At week 24, patients who were randomized to receive placebo were crossed over to receive 5 mg/kg dose of infliximab (induction therapy) by IV infusion and then maintenance therapy (every 8 weeks). Patients had a median baseline PASI score of 21 and a baseline static Physician Global Assessment (sPGA) score ranging from moderate (52% of patients) to marked (36%) to severe (2%). Chronic, stable plaque psoriasis involving at least 20% of BSA was present in 75% of patients. 71 or 82% of patients had received prior systemic therapy or phototherapy, respectively. PASI 75 was achieved in 80 or 3% of patients receiving infliximab or placebo, respectively. Patients also were evaluated by the sPGA score (a 6-category scale ranging from "5=severe" to "0=cleared") according to the physician's overall assessment of the psoriasis severity focusing on induration, erythema, and scaling. "Cleared" or "minimal" score (consisting of none or minimal elevation in plaque, up to faint red coloration in erythema, and none or minimal fine scale over less than 5% of the plaque) was achieved in 80 or 4% of patients receiving the drug or placebo, respectively. In the subgroup of patients with more extensive psoriasis who previously had received phototherapy, PASI 75 was achieved at week 10 in 85% of patients receiving infliximab compared with 4% of those receiving placebo. Health-related quality of life, as measured by Dermatology Life Quality Index (DLQI) and SF 36 scores, was improved with infliximab compared to placebo at weeks 10 and 24.

In the EXPRESS II study, 835 patients (having a median baseline PASI score of 18, 63% having psoriasis involving at least 20% of BSA, and 55 or 64% having received prior systemic or phototherapy, respectively) were randomized to receive placebo or a 3- or 5-mg/kg dose of infliximab at weeks 0, 2, or 6 (induction therapy). At week 14, patients randomized to receive a 3- or 5-mg/kg dose of infliximab were randomized to receive either scheduled (every 8 weeks) or "as needed" maintenance treatment through week 46. At week 16, patients who were randomized to receive placebo were crossed over to receive a 5-mg/kg dose of infliximab induction therapy followed by maintenance therapy every 8 weeks. PASI 75 was achieved in 2, 70, or 75%, respectively, of patients receiving placebo or a dose of 3 or 5 mg/kg of infliximab. Patients also were evaluated by the rPGA score (a 6-category scale ranging from "6=severe" to "1=clear") assessed relative to baseline in which overall lesions were graded with consideration to the percent of body involvement as well as overall induration, scaling, and erythema. "Clear" or "excellent" score (consisting of some residual pinkness or pigmentation to marked improvement [nearly normal skin texture; some erythema may have been present]) was achieved in 1, 69, or 75% of patients receiving placebo or a dose of 3 or 5 mg/kg of infliximab, respectively. In the subgroup of patients with more extensive psoriasis who previously had received phototherapy, PASI 75 was achieved at week 10 in 1, 72, or 77% of patients receiving placebo or a dose of 3 or 5 mg/kg of infliximab, respectively. In the subgroup of patients with more extensive psoriasis who had failed or were intolerant to phototherapy, PASI 75 was achieved at week 10 in 2, 70, or 78% of patients receiving placebo or a dose of 3 or 5 mg/kg of infliximab, respectively. Maintenance of response was studied in 292 (out of 313) patients randomized to receive infliximab 3 mg/kg and in 297 (out of the 314) patients randomized to receive infliximab 5 mg/kg. At week 14, patients were stratified by PASI response at week 10 and by investigational site and were then randomized to receive either scheduled or as needed maintenance therapy. A higher percentage of patients receiving scheduled maintenance therapy (every 8 weeks) appeared to maintain a PASI 75 through week 50 compared with patients receiving as needed maintenance therapy, with the best response maintained with a dosage of 5 mg/kg every 8 weeks. In a subset of patients who had achieved a response at week 10, maintenance of response appeared to be greater in patients receiving infliximab 5 mg/kg every 8 weeks. A decline in response in a subpopulation of patients in each group over time was observed in patients receiving either as needed or scheduled maintenance therapy.

In the SPIRIT study, 249 patients who previously had received either psoralen plus ultraviolet A treatment (PUVA) or other systemic psoriasis therapy were randomized to receive placebo or a 3- or 5-mg/kg dose of infliximab at weeks 0, 2, and 6 (induction therapy). At week 26, patients with an sPGA score of "moderate" or "worse" (a score of at least 3 on a scale of 0–5) received an additional dose of the randomized treatment. Patients had a median baseline PASI score of 19 and a baseline sPGA score of moderate (62% of patients), marked (22%), or severe (3%); BSA of at least 20% was present in 75% of patients. At week 26, 46% of enrolled patients received an additional infliximab dose. At week 10, PASI 75 was achieved in 6, 72, or 88% of patients receiving placebo or a dose of 3 or 5 mg/kg of infliximab, respectively. In addition, a score of "cleared" or "minimal" by the sPGA score was achieved in 10, 72, or 90% of patients receiving placebo or a dose of 3 or 5 mg/kg of infliximab, respectively. Health-related quality of life, as measured by DLQI score, was improved with infliximab compared to placebo at week 10.

A single-blind randomized controlled trial compared infliximab to etanercept for the treatment of moderate to severe plaque psoriasis. In this study, adults were randomized to receive etanercept 50 mg subcutaneously twice weekly or infliximab 5 mg/kg IV at weeks 0, 2, 6, and every 8 weeks thereafter for up to 48 weeks. The primary outcome was PASI 75 response rate at week 24. The PASI 75 response rate at week 24 was significantly higher among patients receiving infliximab compared to patients receiving etanercept. PASI 75 response rates were 72 and 35% in the infliximab and etanercept groups, respectively.

Clinical Perspective

The American Academy of Dermatology and the National Psoriasis Foundation issued joint guidelines for the treatment of psoriasis in adult and pediatric patients between 2019 and 2021. Various drugs and drug classes are used to treat psoriasis. Phototherapy and topical treatments (e.g., vitamin D analogues, calcineurin inhibitors, keratolytics, and corticosteroids) are frequently used to treat mild psoriasis present on limited areas of the body, but these therapies may be inadequate to obtain skin clearance in patients with more extensive or severe disease. Systemic biologic and nonbiologic therapies are mainstays of treatment for moderate to severe psoriasis, and may also be useful for treating psoriasis on parts of the body that are difficult to treat with topical therapy (e.g., the scalp, palms and soles of the feet, genitals). Topical therapies can be used adjunctively in moderate to severe disease. Nonbiologic oral therapies used in the treatment of psoriasis include methotrexate, apremilast, cyclosporine, acitretin, and dimethyl fumarate. Biologics used in the treatment of psoriasis include TNF blocking agents, ustekinumab, secukinumab, ixekizumab, brodalumab, guselkumab, tildrakizumab, and risankizumab. Treatment selection in psoriasis is primarily based on disease characteristics (e.g., severity, location, presence of psoriatic arthritis), with additional consideration being given to patient age and comorbidities.

TNF blocking agents used in the treatment of psoriasis include adalimumab, certolizumab pegol, etanercept, and infliximab. These TNF blocking agents are recommended for the treatment of adult patients with moderate to severe plaque psoriasis, with or without concomitant topical, oral, or phototherapy. Recommendations for the use and selection of psoriasis therapies vary based on patient age, disease characteristics (e.g., severity, location, presence of psoriatic arthritis), and comorbidities (e.g., inflammatory bowel disease). Consult the American Academy of Dermatology/National Psoriasis Foundation guidelines for additional details.

● Other Uses

Juvenile Arthritis

Infliximab has been used in a limited number of pediatric patients with juvenile rheumatoid arthritis† (also known as juvenile idiopathic arthritis); however, further study is needed to evaluate the safety and efficacy of the drug for juvenile rheumatoid arthritis.

Safety and efficacy of infliximab for the management of juvenile rheumatoid arthritis† have been evaluated in children 4–17 years of age with juvenile arthritis who had not responded adequately to methotrexate. Pediatric patients were randomized to receive placebo or 3 mg/kg of infliximab by IV infusion at weeks 0, 2, 6, and 14. Patients continued to receive oral or parenteral methotrexate (10–15 mg/m² per week); study participants also could receive folic acid prophylaxis (required for methotrexate), oral corticosteroids, NSAIAs, and/or other analgesics. At week 14, those who received placebo crossed over to all active treatment; these individuals received 6 mg/kg of infliximab by IV infusion at weeks 14, 16, and 20, followed by additional doses given once every 8 weeks concomitantly with weekly methotrexate through week 44 . Children who received infliximab during the initial 14 weeks of the study continued to receive 3 mg/kg of infliximab once every 8 weeks concomitantly with weekly methotrexate through week 44.

The primary end point of this study was the American College of Rheumatology (ACR) Pediatric 30 (Pedi 30) criteria for improvement (i.e., 30% or greater improvement in at least 3 of 6 and 30% or greater deterioration in no more than 1 of 6 core set criteria that include physician and patient/parent global assessments, active joint count, limitation of motion, functional assessment, and ESR) at week 14. An ACR Pedi 30 was achieved by 63.8% of patients who received infliximab concomitantly with methotrexate compared with 49.2% of patients who received placebo and methotrexate at week 14. Achievement of the primary end point did not differ significantly between infliximab-treated children and placebo-treated children. At week 16 when all study participants were receiving infliximab, an ACR Pedi 30 was achieved by 73.2% of patients. At week 52, an ACR Pedi 50 or 70 (defined using the same criteria as Pedi 30 with a level of improvement of 50 or 70%, respectively) was achieved by 69.6 or 51.8%, respectively, of study participants. Other observations from this study include a higher rate of immunogenic

reactions in study participants than has been observed in infliximab-treated adults.

Behcet Syndrome

Infliximab has been used in a limited number of patients with Behcet syndrome†; however, further study is needed to evaluate safety and efficacy of the drug in this disease. Behcet syndrome is a chronic inflammatory disorder of unknown etiology characterized by recurrent orogenital ulceration, skin lesions, and arthritic symptoms that may be complicated by GI, ocular, and neurologic involvement. Proinflammatory cytokines, including TNF, are produced by monocytes as part of the inflammatory cascade in Behcet disease. Use of infliximab in an adult with Behcet disease who was receiving maintenance therapy with oral prednisone resulted in improvement in GI symptoms and discontinuance of the corticosteroid. In addition, use of infliximab (5-mg/kg doses given at 0, 2, and 6 weeks) resulted in improvements in both oral and genital lesions in an adult with Behcet disease who had recalcitrant orogenital ulceration and a single 5-mg/kg dose of infliximab decreased acute ocular inflammation and improved visual acuity in several adults with panuveitis associated with Behçet disease.

Congestive Heart Failure

Because of evidence that TNF may play a role in progression of heart failure, infliximab has been investigated for the management of congestive heart failure† in patients with moderate to severe (New York Heart Association [NYHA] class III or IV) congestive heart failure. In a phase II, double-blind, placebo-controlled study, patients with stable NYHA class III or IV congestive heart failure (left ventricular ejection fraction 35% or less) were randomized to receive placebo, infliximab 5 mg/kg, or infliximab 10 mg/kg at 0, 2, and 6 weeks. However, there was no evidence that infliximab improved clinical status of these patients and those receiving infliximab (especially those receiving 10 mg/kg) had a higher incidence of mortality and hospitalization for worsening heart failure compared with those receiving placebo.

Pyoderma Gangrenosum

Infliximab has been used in a limited number of patients with pyoderma gangrenosum†. In a single randomized controlled trial, 30 adults with pyoderma gangrenosum were randomized to receive placebo or infliximab 5 mg/kg IV once at week 0; patients were reassessed at week 2 and offered open-label infliximab treatment if no clinical improvement was observed. At week 2, clinical improvement (defined by patient and clinician global assessments) was observed in 46 and 6% of patients who received infliximab and placebo, respectively.

DOSAGE AND ADMINISTRATION

● General

Pretreatment Screening

- Evaluate all patients for active and inactive tuberculosis prior to initiating therapy.
- Screen patients for hepatitis B virus (HBV) infection before initiation of therapy.
- Do not initiate therapy in patients with an active infection, including clinically important localized infections.

Patient Monitoring

- Monitor patients for infusion reactions during and for at least 30 minutes after IV infusion. Ensure that appropriate personnel and medications are available to treat infusion reactions. For patients without a history of acute infusion reactions with prior doses of the drug, monitor vital signs every 30 minutes; for patients with a history of such reactions, monitor every 15 minutes.
- Monitor closely for signs or symptoms of infection (e.g., fever, malaise, weight loss, sweats, cough, dyspnea, pulmonary infiltrates, serious systemic illness including shock), including the possible development of tuberculosis in patients who tested negative for latent tuberculosis prior to initiating therapy, during and after treatment with tumor necrosis factor (TNF; TNF-α) blocking agents.

- Evaluate and monitor chronic carriers of HBV prior to the initiation of infliximab therapy, during treatment, and for several months following treatment.
- Perform periodic dermatologic evaluations in all patients, particularly those with risk factors for skin cancer.
- Monitor patients with psoriasis, particularly those who received prior prolonged phototherapy for their disease, for nonmelanoma skin cancer.
- Perform periodic screening for cervical cancer in females.
- Closely monitor patients during therapy for new or worsening symptoms of heart failure.
- Monitor hepatic enzymes and liver function tests every 3 to 4 months during subcutaneous maintenance therapy with infliximab-dyyb (Zymfentra®).

Premedication and Prophylaxis

- May premedicate patients with histamine-1 receptor antagonists, histamine-2 receptor antagonists, acetaminophen, and/or corticosteroids to prevent IV infusion reactions.

Dispensing and Administration Precautions

- To avoid medication errors, the Institute for Safe Medication Practices (ISMP) recommends that prescribers communicate both the brand and generic names for infliximab products on the prescription order form.

Other General Considerations

- May continue treatment with agents used for the management of Crohn disease or ulcerative colitis (e.g., corticosteroids, mesalamine, sulfasalazine, azathioprine, mercaptopurine, methotrexate, anti-infective agents) in patients receiving infliximab products. However, consider increased risks of hepatosplenic T-cell lymphoma with combination therapy and the observed (in infliximab studies) increase in immunogenicity and hypersensitivity reactions associated with infliximab products given as monotherapy.
- Infliximab products are used in conjunction with methotrexate for the management of rheumatoid arthritis. Other nonbiologic agents used for the management of rheumatoid arthritis (e.g., corticosteroids, nonsteroidal anti-inflammatory agents [NSAIAs]) may be continued in patients receiving infliximab products.
- Infliximab products can be used with or without methotrexate for the management of psoriatic arthritis.

● Administration

IV Admininstration

Infliximab products may be administered by IV infusion. Use an in-line, sterile, nonpyrogenic, low-protein-binding filter with a pore diameter of 1.2 μm or less for administration. Do not admix infliximab products with other drugs or infuse in the same IV line with other drugs.

Store commercially available infliximab lyophilized powders at 2–8°C. Vials of infliximab-axxq should be protected from light. Unopened vials of infliximab or infliximab-abda may be stored at temperatures up to 30°C for a single period of up to 6 months; following removal from refrigerated storage, the drug cannot be returned to refrigerated storage.

Reconstitution

Infliximab products for IV administration are supplied as lyophilized powders that must be reconstituted and diluted prior to administration using proper aseptic technique.

Reconstitute the lyophilized powder by adding 10 mL of sterile water for injection to a vial labeled as containing 100 mg of the infliximab product to provide a solution containing 10 mg/mL. Based on the indicated dosage of the infliximab product, reconstitute the appropriate number of vials of the drug. During reconstitution, direct the sterile water diluent toward the side of the vial using a sterile syringe with a 21-gauge or smaller needle and gently swirl the contents to minimize foaming during dissolution; some foaming will occur. To avoid excessive foaming, do not shake or vigorously agitate the vial. Inspect the reconstituted solution visually for particulate matter. The solution should be colorless to light yellow and opalescent and should not be used if discolored or opaque or if foreign particles other than a few translucent proteinaceous particles are present. Allow the reconstituted solution to stand for 5 minutes before further dilution.

Dilution

Further dilute the reconstituted infliximab solution in 0.9% sodium chloride injection to provide a total volume of 250 mL (i.e., if a 250-mL bottle or bag of 0.9% sodium chloride injection is used, remove a volume of the diluent equal to the total required volume of reconstituted infliximab product solution from the bag or bottle prior to addition of the infliximab product). Add the total required volume of reconstituted infliximab solution slowly to the diluent and gently mix the diluted solution.

The final concentration of the reconstituted and diluted infliximab solution should be 0.4–4 mg/mL. For volumes greater than 250 mL, use a larger infusion bag (e.g., 500 mL) or multiple 250 mL infusion bags to ensure that the concentration of the infusion solution does not exceed 4 mg/mL. Begin the infliximab infusion within 3 hours of reconstitution and dilution of the drug. Discard any unused portions of the reconstituted or diluted solution since the drug does not contain any preservatives or bacteriostatic agents.

Rate of Administration

Infuse diluted infliximab solutions IV over a period of at least 2 hours.

The manufacturer of infliximab states that IV infusions can be given at a rate of 2 mL/minute or, alternatively, a rate titration schedule may be used in an attempt to prevent or ameliorate acute infusion reactions. If a rate titration schedule is used in patients who are receiving an initial infliximab dose or in patients with or without a history of acute infusion reactions to prior doses of the drug, the manufacturer recommends initiating the IV infusion at a rate of 10 mL/hour for the first 15 minutes followed by 20 mL/hour for 15 minutes, 40 mL/hour for 15 minutes, 80 mL/hour for 15 minutes, 150 mL/hour for 30 minutes, and then 250 mL/hour for 30 minutes.

Subcutaneous Administration

Infliximab-dyyb (Zymfentra®) is approved for subcutaneous administration and is intended for use under the supervision of a healthcare provider. After proper training, a patient or a caregiver may be able to administer subcutaneously.

Prior to administration, visually inspect the formulation for particulate matter and discoloration. The formulation should be a clear, colorless to pale brown solution.

Inject infliximab-dyyb (Zymfentra®) into the front of the thighs, the abdomen (except for the 2 inches around the navel), or the outer area of the upper arms (caregiver only). Rotate the injection site each time an injection is administered with at least 1.2 inches between the new and prior injection sites. Do not inject into red, bruised, tender, or indurated skin areas.

If a subcutaneous dose is missed, inject the next dose as soon as possible and then every 2 weeks thereafter.

Store at 2-8°C. Do not freeze. Keep the product in its outer carton until time of administration in order to protect from light.

● Dosage

Adult Dosage

Crohn Disease

The usual adult dosage of infliximab or biosimilars (infliximab-abda, infliximab-axxq, infliximab-dyyb) for the management of moderately or severely active Crohn disease or fistulizing Crohn disease is 5 mg/kg given by IV infusion over a period of at least 2 hours.

The manufacturers recommend that adults with moderately to severely active Crohn disease or with fistulizing Crohn disease receive the initial 3 doses of infliximab at 0, 2, and 6 weeks (induction regimen) and that additional doses be given once every 8 weeks thereafter (maintenance regimen). An increase in infliximab dosage to 10 mg/kg every 8 weeks may be considered in patients who respond initially but subsequently lose response. Patients who do not respond to infliximab by week 14 are unlikely to respond with continued administration; discontinuance of the drug should be considered in these patients.

The usual maintenance dose of infliximab-dyyb (Zymfentra®) in adults with moderately to severely active Crohn disease following treatment with an IV induction regimen with an infliximab product is 120 mg subcutaneously once every 2 weeks. The maintenance dosage should be initiated at week 10.

To switch patients who are responding to maintenance therapy with an infliximab product given IV, administer the initial subcutaneous dose in place of the next scheduled IV infusion and every 2 weeks thereafter.

Ulcerative Colitis

The usual adult dosage of infliximab or biosimilars (infliximab-abda, infliximab-axxq, infliximab-dyyb) for the management of moderately or severely active ulcerative colitis is 5 mg/kg given by IV infusion over a period of at least 2 hours.

The manufacturers recommend that adults with moderately to severely active ulcerative colitis receive the initial 3 doses of infliximab at 0, 2, and 6 weeks (induction regimen) and that additional doses be given once every 8 weeks thereafter (maintenance regimen).

The usual maintenance dose of infliximab-dyyb (Zymfentra®) in adults with moderately to severely active ulcerative colitis following treatment with an IV induction regimen with an infliximab product is 120 mg subcutaneously once every 2 weeks. The maintenance dosage should be initiated at week 10.

To switch patients who are responding to maintenance therapy with an infliximab product given IV, administer the initial subcutaneous dose in place of the next scheduled IV infusion and every 2 weeks thereafter.

Rheumatoid Arthritis

For the management of moderately to severely active rheumatoid arthritis in adults, the usual dosage of infliximab or biosimilars (infliximab-abda, infliximab-axxq, infliximab-dyyb) is 3 mg/kg given by IV infusion over a period of at least 2 hours. The manufacturers recommend that adults with rheumatoid arthritis receive the initial 3 doses of infliximab at 0, 2, and 6 weeks (induction regimen) and that additional doses be given once every 8 weeks thereafter (maintenance regimen). Infliximab should be given in combination with methotrexate. For patients who have an incomplete response to this 3-mg/kg regimen, consideration can be given to increasing the infliximab dosage up to 10 mg/kg every 8 weeks and/or administering infliximab doses as often as once every 4 weeks.

Ankylosing Spondylitis

For the management of ankylosing spondylitis in adults, the usual dosage of infliximab or biosimilars (infliximab-abda, infliximab-axxq, infliximab-dyyb) is 5 mg/kg given by IV infusion over a period of at least 2 hours. The manufacturers recommend that adults with ankylosing spondylitis receive the initial 3 doses of infliximab at 0, 2, and 6 weeks (induction regimen) and that additional doses of 5 mg/kg be given once every 6 weeks thereafter (maintenance regimen).

Psoriatic Arthritis

For the management of psoriatic arthritis in adults, the usual dosage of infliximab or biosimilars (infliximab-abda, infliximab-axxq, infliximab-dyyb) is 5 mg/kg given by IV infusion over a period of at least 2 hours. The manufacturers recommend that adults with psoriatic arthritis receive the initial 3 doses of infliximab at 0, 2, and 6 weeks (induction regimen) and that additional doses of 5 mg/kg be given once every 8 weeks thereafter (maintenance regimen).

Plaque Psoriasis

For the management of chronic severe plaque psoriasis in adults, the usual dosage of infliximab or biosimilars (infliximab-abda, infliximab-axxq, infliximab-dyyb) is 5 mg/kg given by IV infusion over a period of at least 2 hours. The manufacturers recommend that adults with plaque psoriasis receive the initial 3 doses of infliximab at 0, 2, and 6 weeks (induction regimen) and that additional doses of 5 mg/kg be given once every 8 weeks thereafter (maintenance regimen). If maintenance therapy with infliximab for the management of psoriasis is interrupted, itherapy should be reinitiated as a single dose followed by maintenance therapy.

Pediatric Dosage
Crohn Disease

The recommended dosage of infliximab or biosimilars (infliximab-abda, infliximab-axxq, infliximab-dyyb) in pediatric patients 6 years of age or older with moderately to severely active Crohn disease is 5 mg/kg given by IV infusion over a period of at least 2 hours at 0, 2, and 6 weeks (induction therapy) followed by a maintenance regimen of 5 mg/kg every 8 weeks.

Ulcerative Colitis

The recommended dosage of infliximab or biosimilars (infliximab-abda, infliximab-axxq, infliximab-dyyb) in pediatric patients 6 years of age or older with moderately to severely active ulcerative colitis is 5 mg/kg given by IV infusion over a period of at least 2 hours at 0, 2, and 6 weeks (induction regimen) followed by a maintenance regimen of 5 mg/kg every 8 weeks.

● Special Populations
Hepatic Impairment

The manufacturer makes no specific dosage recommendations for patients with hepatic impairment.

Renal Impairment

The manufacturer makes no specific dosage recommendations for patients with renal impairment.

Geriatric Patients

The manufacturer makes no specific dosage recommendations for geriatric patients.

CAUTIONS

● Contraindications

- Prior hypersensitivity reaction to infliximab products or any inactive ingredients in the formulations or any murine proteins.
- Doses greater than 5 mg/kg are contraindicated in patients with moderate or severe heart failure.

● Warnings/Precautions
Warnings
Serious Infections

A boxed warning about the risk of serious infections is included in the prescribing information for infliximab products. Patients receiving tumor necrosis factor (TNF) blocking agents, including infliximab products, are at increased risk of developing serious infections involving various organ systems and sites that may require hospitalization or result in death. Opportunistic infections caused by bacterial, mycobacterial, invasive fungal, viral, or parasitic, or other opportunistic pathogens—including aspergillosis, blastomycosis, candidiasis, coccidioidomycosis, histoplasmosis, legionellosis, listeriosis, pneumocystosis, salmonellosis, and tuberculosis—have been reported in patients receiving TNF blocking agents. Infections frequently have been disseminated rather than localized. Closely monitor patients during and after treatment with TNF blocking agents for the development of signs or symptoms of infection (e.g., fever, malaise, weight loss, sweats, cough, dyspnea, pulmonary infiltrates, serious systemic illness including shock), including the possible development of tuberculosis in patients who tested negative for latent tuberculosis prior to initiating therapy. Most patients who developed serious infections were receiving concomitant therapy with immunosuppressive agents such as corticosteroids or methotrexate.

In clinical studies evaluating infliximab in patients with rheumatoid arthritis, serious infection was reported in 5.3% of patients who received infliximab in conjunction with methotrexate and in 3.4% of those who received methotrexate and placebo (follow-up: 52 weeks for both groups). Serious infections reported in patients receiving infliximab have included pneumonia, cellulitis, abscess, skin ulceration, sepsis, and bacterial infection. Extrapulmonary and disseminated tuberculosis, including fatal miliary tuberculosis, have been reported in patients receiving infliximab products. During clinical trials, tuberculosis was reported in 14 patients receiving infliximab, and there were 4 fatalities related to miliary tuberculosis. During postmarketing surveillance, other cases of tuberculosis have been reported. Reactivation of latent tuberculosis and new tuberculosis infections have been reported in patients receiving infliximab products, including in patients who previously received antimycobacterial therapy for latent or active tuberculosis. Cases of active tuberculosis also have been reported in patients receiving infliximab products while they were receiving antimycobacterial therapy for latent tuberculosis. As of September 2002, FDA had received 335 reports of infliximab-associated tuberculosis. Most of the cases of tuberculosis occurred within the first 2 months following initiation of infliximab therapy; these cases may reflect recrudescence of latent tuberculosis infection. As of September 2011, FDA had identified 103 reports of *Legionella* pneumonia associated with TNF blocking agents, including infliximab. The 103 cases of *Legionella* pneumonia occurred in patients 25–85 years of age, many of whom received concomitant therapy with immunosuppressive agents (e.g., corticosteroids and/or methotrexate); 17 deaths were reported. In 78% of the cases of *Legionella* pneumonia, the median duration of TNF blocker therapy prior to the onset of *Legionella* pneumonia was 10.4 months (range: less than 1 month to 73 months). As of September 2011, FDA also had identified 26 published reports of *Listeria* infections, including meningitis, bacteremia, endophthalmitis, and sepsis, in patients who received TNF blocking agents; 7 deaths were reported. Many of the *Listeria* infections occurred in patients who had received concomitant therapy with immunosuppressive agents. In addition, FDA identified fatal *Listeria* infections during a review of data regarding laboratory-confirmed infections that occurred in premarketing clinical studies and during postmarketing surveillance. Invasive fungal infections have occurred in patients receiving TNF blocking agents. Failure to recognize fungal infections has led to delays in appropriate treatment.

An increased incidence of serious infections also was observed in clinical studies in patients with rheumatoid arthritis when a TNF blocking agent was used concomitantly with anakinra or abatacept . Concomitant use of infliximab products and anakinra, abatacept, or other biological products used to treat the same conditions as infliximab is not recommended.

Do not initiate therapy with infliximab products in patients with active infections, including clinically important localized infections. Patients older than 65 years of age, patients with comorbid conditions, and/or patients receiving concomitant therapy with immunosuppressive agents such as corticosteroids or methotrexate may be at increased risk of infection. Consider the potential risks and benefits of the drug prior to initiating therapy in patients with a history of chronic, recurring, or opportunistic infections; patients with underlying conditions that may predispose them to infections; and patients who have been exposed to tuberculosis or who reside or have traveled in regions where tuberculosis or mycoses such as histoplasmosis, coccidioidomycosis, and blastomycosis are endemic. If a patient develops a new infection while receiving an infliximab product, perform a thorough diagnostic evaluation (appropriate for an immunocompromised patient), initiate appropriate anti-infective therapy, and closely monitor the patient. Discontinue therapy with infliximab products in patients who develop a serious infection or sepsis.

Because tuberculosis has been reported in patients receiving infliximab products, including in patients who received infliximab products during treatment for latent tuberculosis or following treatment for active or latent tuberculosis, evaluate all patients for active or latent tuberculosis and for risk factors for tuberculosis prior to and periodically during therapy with the drug. When indicated, initiate an appropriate antimycobacterial regimen for the treatment of latent tuberculosis prior to therapy with infliximab products. Antimycobacterial treatment lowers the risk of latent tuberculosis infection progressing to active disease (i.e., reactivation) in patients receiving TNF blocking agents. Antimycobacterial therapy also should be considered prior to initiation of infliximab product therapy in individuals with a history of latent or active tuberculosis in whom an adequate course of antimycobacterial treatment cannot be confirmed and in individuals with a negative tuberculin skin test who have risk factors for tuberculosis. Consultation with a tuberculosis specialist is recommended when deciding whether to initiate antimycobacterial therapy. Monitor patients receiving infliximab products, including individuals with a negative tuberculin skin test, for signs and symptoms of active tuberculosis. If active tuberculosis is diagnosed during therapy with infliximab products, discontinue the drug and initiate an appropriate antimycobacterial regimen. The possibility of tuberculosis should be strongly considered in patients who develop new infections while receiving infliximab products, especially if they previously have traveled to countries where tuberculosis is highly prevalent or have been in close contact with an individual with active tuberculosis.

Infection with *Histoplasma capsulatum*, *Coccidioides immitis*, *Legionella*, *Listeria*, *Pneumocystis jiroveci* (formerly *Pneumocystis carinii*) and other bacterial, mycobacterial, or fungal infections have been reported in patients receiving infliximab products. Carefully evaluate the potential risks and benefits of therapy with infliximab products before the drug is initiated in individuals who reside or have traveled in areas where mycoses are endemic. Ascertain if patients receiving TNF blocking agents who present with signs and symptoms suggestive of systemic fungal infection reside or have traveled in regions where mycoses are endemic.

Consider empiric antifungal therapy in patients at risk of histoplasmosis or other invasive fungal infections who develop severe systemic illness, taking into account both the risk for severe fungal infection and the risks associated with antifungal therapy. Serologic tests for histoplasmosis may be negative in some patients with active infection. When deciding whether TNF blocking agent therapy should be reinitiated following resolution of an invasive fungal infection, reevaluate the risks and benefits of such therapy, particularly in patients who reside in regions where mycoses are endemic. Whenever feasible, decisions regarding initiation and duration of antifungal therapy and reinitiation of TNF blocking agent therapy should be made in consultation with a specialist in fungal infections.

Malignancies

A boxed warning about the risk of malignancy is included in the prescribing information for infliximab products. Malignancies, some fatal, have been reported in children, adolescents, and young adults who received treatment with TNF blocking agents beginning when they were 18 years of age or younger. In August 2009, FDA reported the results of an analysis of reports of lymphoma and other malignancies in children and adolescents who had received TNF blocking agents. These cases were reported postmarketing and were derived from various sources, including registries and spontaneous postmarketing reports. FDA identified 48 cases of malignancies in children and adolescents in the analysis.

Of the 48 cases reviewed by FDA, approximately 50% were lymphomas, including Hodgkin's disease and non-Hodgkin's lymphoma. The other cases represented a variety of malignancies, including rare malignancies that are usually associated with immunosuppression and malignancies that are not usually observed in children and adolescents. Other malignancies reported included leukemia, melanoma, and solid organ tumors; malignancies such as leiomyosarcoma, hepatic malignancies, and renal cell carcinoma, which rarely occur in children, also were reported. The malignancies occurred after a median of 30 months (range: 1–84 months) following the first dose of therapy with TNF blocking agents. Of the 48 cases of malignancies, 11 deaths were reported; causes of death included hepatosplenic T-cell lymphoma (9 cases), T-cell lymphoma (1 case), and sepsis following remission of lymphoma (1 case). The observed US reporting rates for cases of malignancy with infliximab were consistently higher compared with expected background rates for lymphomas and all malignancies. The observed reporting rates offer limited inference into the potential differences in risk of malignancy among TNF blocking agents because of uncertainties about actual patient exposure to treatment and the possibility of underreporting of cases of malignancy. Most of the 48 patients (88%) also were receiving other immunosuppressive drugs such as azathioprine and methotrexate, which also are associated with an increased risk of lymphoma. Although there were other contributory factors, the role of TNF blocking agents in the development of malignancies in children and adolescents could not be excluded. Therefore, FDA has concluded that there is an increased risk of malignancy with TNF blocking agents. However, due to the relatively rare occurrence of these cancers, the limited number of pediatric patients who received TNF blocking agents, and the possible role of other immunosuppressive drugs used concomitantly with TNF blocking agents, FDA was unable to fully characterize the strength of the association between use of TNF blocking agents and the development of a malignancy.

Hepatosplenic T-cell lymphoma, a rare, aggressive, usually fatal type of T-cell lymphoma, has been reported during postmarketing experience mainly in adolescent and young adult males with Crohn disease or ulcerative colitis who received treatment with TNF blocking agents and/or thiopurine analogs (mercaptopurine or azathioprine). Most of the reported cases of hepatosplenic T-cell lymphoma occurred in patients who had received a combination of immunosuppressive agents, including TNF blocking agents and thiopurine analogs (azathioprine or mercaptopurine). In some cases, potential confounding factors could not be excluded because complete medical histories were not available. As of December 31, 2010, FDA had identified 25 cases of hepatosplenic T-cell lymphoma in patients with Crohn disease or ulcerative colitis who had received infliximab (20 cases) or both infliximab and adalimumab (5 cases); in 22 of these cases, a thiopurine analog (mercaptopurine or azathioprine) was used concomitantly. These 25 cases of hepatosplenic T-cell lymphoma occurred in patients 12–74 years of age (median age: 29–30 years) following infliximab therapy for periods ranging from 1 dose to 8 years of intermittent therapy; 22 of the patients were males and 21 of the cases were fatal. It is not clear whether the occurrence of hepatosplenic T-cell lymphoma is related to use of TNF blocking agents or use of TNF blocking agents in conjunction with other immunosuppressive agents. Since patients with certain conditions (e.g., rheumatoid arthritis, Crohn disease, ankylosing spondylitis, psoriatic arthritis, plaque psoriasis) may be at increased risk for lymphoma, it may be difficult to measure the added risk of treatment with TNF blocking agents, azathioprine, and/or mercaptopurine.

In clinical studies, lymphoma occurred more frequently in patients receiving TNF blocking agents than in controls. Lymphoproliferative disorders, including lymphoma (e.g., non-Hodgkin's lymphoma, Hodgkin's disease) and myeloma, have been reported in patients receiving infliximab. In the controlled and open-label portions of infliximab clinical trials, 5 out of 5707 patients receiving infliximab (median duration of follow-up: 1 year) developed lymphomas compared with no cases of lymphoma in 1600 control patients (median duration of follow-up: 0.4 years). In rheumatoid arthritis patients, 2 lymphomas were observed for a rate of 0.08 cases per 100 patient-years of follow-up, which is approximately threefold higher than expected in the general population. In the combined clinical trial population for rheumatoid arthritis, Crohn disease, psoriatic arthritis, ankylosing spondylitis, ulcerative colitis, and plaque psoriasis, 5 lymphomas were observed for a rate of 0.1 cases per 100 patient-years of follow-up, which is approximately fourfold higher than expected in the general population. Patients with rheumatoid arthritis, Crohn disease, or plaque psoriasis (especially those with highly active disease and/or chronic exposure to immunosuppressive therapies) may be at increased risk of lymphoma (even in the absence of TNF blocking agent therapy); the role of TNF blocking agents in the development of lymphoma or other malignancies has not been fully determined.

Cases of acute and chronic leukemia have been reported during postmarketing surveillance of TNF blocking agents used in the management of rheumatoid arthritis and other conditions. In August 2009, FDA reported the results of a review of 147 cases of leukemia in adults and pediatric patients who received TNF blocking agents; these cases had been identified during postmarketing surveillance. Of the 147 cases, acute myeloid leukemia (44 cases), chronic lymphocytic leukemia (31 cases), and chronic myeloid leukemia (23 cases) were the most frequent types of leukemia reported. Four cases of leukemia were reported in children. Most patients (61%) also were receiving other immunosuppressive drugs. There were a total of 30 deaths reported; leukemia was reported as the cause of 26 of the 30 deaths, and the event was associated with the use of TNF blocking agents. Leukemia generally occurred during the first 2 years of therapy. The interpretation of these findings was complicated by the fact that published epidemiologic studies suggest that patients with rheumatoid arthritis may be at increased risk of leukemia, independent of any treatment with TNF blocking agents. However, based on the available data, FDA has concluded that there is a possible association between treatment with TNF blocking agents and the development of leukemia in patients receiving these drugs.

Melanoma and Merkel cell carcinoma have been reported in patients receiving TNF blocking agents, including infliximab products.

In a population-based retrospective cohort study using Swedish national health registry data, the incidence of invasive cervical cancer in women with rheumatoid arthritis treated with infliximab was two- to threefold higher compared to biologic-naïve patients or the general population, particularly those over 60 years of age. A causal relationship between infliximab and cervical cancer cannot be excluded.

Other malignancies (basal cell carcinoma, breast cancer, colorectal cancer, rectal adenocarcinoma, squamous cell carcinoma) have also been reported during clinical studies in patients receiving infliximab. In the controlled portions of clinical trials of some TNF blocking agents, including infliximab products, more malignancies (excluding lymphoma and nonmelanoma skin cancer [NMSC]) have been observed in patients receiving TNF blocking agents compared with control patients. During the controlled portions of infliximab trials in patients with moderately to severely active rheumatoid arthritis, Crohn disease, psoriatic arthritis, ankylosing spondylitis, ulcerative colitis, and plaque psoriasis receiving infliximab, 14 of 4019 patients were diagnosed with malignancies (excluding lymphoma and NMSC) compared with 1 patient among 1597 control patients (a rate of 0.52/100 patient-years among patients receiving infliximab compared with a rate of 0.11/100 patient-years among control patients), with a median duration of follow-up of 0.5 years for patients receiving the drug and 0.4 years for control patients. The most common malignancies reported were breast and colorectal cancer and melanoma. The rate of malignancies in patients receiving infliximab was similar to that expected in the general population, while the rate in the control patients was lower than expected in the general population. The role of TNF blocking agents in the development of malignancies has not been fully

determined. Rates of malignancy in clinical trials for infliximab cannot be compared with rates in clinical trials of other TNF blocking agents and such rates may not predict rates in a broader population of patients receiving the drug.

In a randomized, controlled clinical trial investigating the use of infliximab in patients with moderate to severe chronic obstructive pulmonary disease† (COPD) who were or had been heavy smokers, patients received infliximab at dosages similar to those used in rheumatoid arthritis and Crohn disease. Nine (out of 157) patients receiving the drug developed a malignancy, including 1 case of lymphoma, for a rate of 7.67 cases per 100 patient-years of follow-up (median duration of follow-up 0.8 years). One malignancy was reported in 77 control patients, for a rate of 1.63 cases per 100 patient-years of follow-up (median duration of follow-up 0.8 years). The most frequent malignancies were lung or head and neck cancer.

In the maintenance portion of clinical trials evaluating infliximab for treatment of psoriasis, NMSC was more common in patients who had received prior phototherapy.

Consider the possibility of and monitor for the occurrence of malignancies during and following treatment with TNF blocking agents. Exercise caution when considering therapy with infliximab products in patients with a history of malignancy or when deciding whether to continue therapy in patients who develop a malignancy while receiving infliximab. Because therapy with TNF blocking agents and/or thiopurine analogs (azathioprine or mercaptopurine) may increase the risk of malignancies, including hepatosplenic T-cell lymphoma, carefully consider the risks and benefits of these agents, especially in adolescent and young adult males and in the treatment of Crohn disease or ulcerative colitis. When deciding whether infliximab products should be used alone or in combination with other immunosuppressive agents, consider both the possibility of an increased risk of hepatosplenic T-cell lymphoma with combination therapy and the observed (in infliximab studies) increase in immunogenicity and hypersensitivity reactions associated with infliximab given as monotherapy. Because melanoma and Merkel cell carcinoma have been reported in patients receiving infliximab products, periodic skin examination is recommended for all patients, particularly those with risk factors for skin cancer. Because nonmelanoma skin cancer has been reported in patients with psoriasis receiving infliximab, monitor patients with psoriasis who are receiving infliximab products, particularly those who received prior prolonged phototherapy for nonmelanoma skin cancer. Periodically screen women treated with infliximab products for cervical cancer. Because malignancies (mainly lung cancer or head and neck malignancies) were reported more frequently in infliximab-treated than placebo-treated patients with moderate to severe COPD, exercise caution when considering therapy with infliximab in such patients.

Sensitivity Reactions
Acute Sensitivity Reactions

Hypersensitivity reactions have been reported in patients receiving infliximab products; these reactions vary in their time to onset and have required hospitalization in some patients. Most hypersensitivity reactions have occurred during or within 2 hours of infusion; reactions have included anaphylaxis, urticaria, dyspnea, and hypotension.

In clinical studies, infusion reactions were reported in approximately 20% of patients receiving infliximab compared with 10% of patients receiving placebo. In these studies, 27% of patients who experienced an infusion reaction during infliximab induction therapy also experienced an infusion reaction during maintenance therapy with the drug, whereas 9% of patients who had no infusion reactions during infliximab induction therapy experienced an infusion reaction during maintenance therapy. Infusion reaction rates remained stable through 1 year in patients receiving infliximab in the psoriasis EXPRESS study. Infusion reaction rates in the psoriasis EXPRESS II study were variable over time and were somewhat higher following the final infusion than after the initial infusion. In the 3 psoriasis studies, acute infusion reactions were reported in 7, 4, or 1%, respectively, of patients receiving a 3- or 5-mg/kg dose of infliximab or placebo.

Infusion reaction symptoms may include fever, chills, chest pain, hypotension, hypertension, dyspnea, urticaria, and/or pruritus. Most acute infusion reactions have been mild and transient, and symptoms have been controlled by slowing the infusion rate, discontinuing the infusion, or treatment (e.g., with antihistamines). Serious infusion reactions, including anaphylaxis, seizures, erythematous rash, and/or hypotension have been reported in less than 1% of patients receiving infliximab. Anaphylactic reactions, including anaphylactic shock, laryngeal/pharyngeal edema and severe bronchospasm, and seizure have occurred during postmarketing experience in patients receiving infliximab products.

Infusion reactions that were not serious (including nonserious anaphylactoid reactions) were reported in 18% of pediatric patients receiving infliximab for the treatment of Crohn disease. About 13% of pediatric patients receiving infliximab for the treatment of ulcerative colitis experienced one or more nonserious infusion reactions, including 18% of pediatric patients receiving the recommended maintenance regimen of 5 mg/kg every 8 weeks. Infusion reactions were reported in 35 or 18%, respectively, of children receiving 3- or 6-mg/kg doses of infliximab for the treatment of juvenile rheumatoid arthritis. The most frequently reported infusion-related events were vomiting, fever, headache, and hypotension. Serious infusion reactions occurred in a few patients.

In clinical studies in patients with rheumatoid arthritis, Crohn disease, or psoriasis, readministration of infliximab after a period without treatment resulted in a higher incidence of infusion reactions as compared to regular maintenance treatment. In a clinical trial evaluating 2 long-term treatment strategies (i.e., long-term maintenance therapy with infliximab versus retreatment with an induction regimen of infliximab following disease flare) in patients with moderate to severe psoriasis, serious infusion reactions were reported in 4% of patients receiving retreatment following disease flare compared with less than 1% of those receiving long-term maintenance therapy. Patients in this study did not receive other immunosuppressive agents concomitantly with infliximab. Most of the serious infusion reactions occurred during the second infusion at week 2 and manifestations included, but were not limited to, dyspnea, urticaria, facial edema, and hypotension. In all cases, infliximab therapy was discontinued and/or other treatment was instituted with complete resolution of signs and symptoms.

There is some evidence indicating that the incidence of acute infusion reactions to infliximab products is lower in patients who are receiving concomitant therapy with immunosuppressive agents (e.g., azathioprine, mercaptopurine, methotrexate) than in those not receiving such therapy. The manufacturers and some clinicians suggest considering the use of a pretreatment regimen (e.g., acetaminophen, antihistamines, prednisone) prior to each infusion of the drug to prevent or ameliorate these acute infusion reactions. In addition, clinicians may consider the use of a rate titration schedule to administer IV infusions of infliximab. Although safety and efficacy of the procedure have not been established, at least 2 Crohn disease patients with a history of anaphylactic/anaphylactoid reactions to infliximab have received a subsequent dose of the drug using a desensitization procedure that involved dose escalation in an intensive care setting.

Monitor patients closely (including measurement of vital signs) during and for at least 30 minutes after each IV infusion of the drug. Drugs for the treatment of hypersensitivity reactions (e.g., acetaminophen, antihistamines, corticosteroids, and/or epinephrine) should be immediately available. To prevent or ameliorate acute infusion reactions, clinicians can consider the use of a pretreatment regimen (e.g., acetaminophen, antihistamines, prednisone) prior to each infliximab product dose and use of a rate titration schedule to administer IV infusions of the drug. If a patient experiences a clinically important change in vital signs (e.g., diastolic blood pressure drops 15–20 mm Hg) or any symptoms of hypersensitivity (e.g., urticaria, shortness of breath) while receiving an IV infusion of an infliximab product, stop the infusion immediately, evaluate manifestations, and initiate appropriate therapy. The manufacturer of infliximab states that if the infusion is stopped because of an acute infusion reaction but the reaction is not severe and can be controlled with the use of drugs other than epinephrine (e.g., diphenhydramine, acetaminophen, prednisone), then the infusion may be restarted with caution using a rate titration schedule. If the infusion can be completed in these patients, then they may receive additional indicated doses of the infliximab product with caution and in the presence of appropriately trained medical personnel. However, if the acute infusion reaction is more serious and requires treatment with epinephrine or if symptoms increase in severity, then the infusion of the infliximab product should be discontinued.

Delayed Sensitivity Reactions

Infusion reactions that appear to be delayed hypersensitivity or serum sickness-like reactions have occurred after initial therapy with infliximab products (i.e., as early as after the second dose) and when therapy with infliximab products was reinstituted following an extended period without such treatment. Symptoms associated with these reactions included fever, rash, headache, sore throat, myalgia, polyarthralgia, hand/facial edema, and/or dysphagia. These reactions were associated with marked increases in antibodies to infliximab, loss of detectable infliximab concentrations in the serum, and possible loss of drug efficacy.

Delayed infusion reactions to infliximab were first reported in a study in adults with moderately to severely active Crohn disease or fistulizing Crohn disease who were receiving retreatment with infliximab after an interval of 2–4 years. Delayed hypersensitivity reactions (generally reported as serum sickness or a combination of arthralgia and/or myalgia with fever and/or rash) have been reported in about 1% of patients with plaque psoriasis receiving infliximab in clinical studies; these reactions generally occurred within 2 weeks after repeat infusion of the drug.

There is some evidence that patients who have received at least 3 months of therapy with an immunosuppressive agent (e.g., azathioprine, mercaptopurine, methotrexate) prior to administration of infliximab have a lower rate of development of human antichimeric antibodies (HACA) and a lower rate of infusion reactions than patients not receiving such therapy.

Because delayed infusion reactions have occurred 3–12 days after an infliximab dose in patients who received retreatment with the drug after a period of 2–4 years, exercise caution when retreating patients with infliximab products following an extended period of time (e.g., after 1 year or longer).

Carefully consider the risks and benefits of readministration of infliximab products after a period without treatment (especially readministration as a reinduction regimen at 0, 2, and 6 weeks), since such retreatment regimens have resulted in a higher incidence of infusion reactions as compared to regular maintenance treatment. If maintenance therapy with an infliximab product for the management of psoriasis is interrupted, reinitiate the drug as a single dose followed by maintenance therapy.

Other Warnings and Precautions

HBV Reactivation

Use of TNF blocking agents, including infliximab products, has been associated with reactivation of hepatitis B virus (HBV) infection in patients who are chronic carriers of this virus (i.e., hepatitis B surface antigen-positive [HBsAg-positive]). HBV reactivation has resulted in death in a few individuals receiving a TNF blocking agent. Most patients experiencing HBV reactivation were receiving concomitant therapy with other immunosuppressive agents; use of multiple immunosuppressive agents may have contributed to HBV reactivation.

Screen all patients before initiating therapy with infliximab products. Consultation with an expert in the treatment of hepatitis B is recommended for patients who test positive for hepatitis B surface antigen. Appropriately evaluate and monitor chronic carriers of HBV prior to the initiation of therapy, during treatment, and for up to several months following therapy with infliximab products. Safety and efficacy of antiviral therapy for prevention of viral reactivation in HBV carriers receiving a TNF blocking agent have not been established. Discontinue therapy with the infliximab product if HBV reactivation occurs, and initiate appropriate treatment, including antiviral therapy. It has not been established whether an infliximab product can be safely readministered once control of the reactivated HBV infection has been achieved; caution is advised if infliximab products are resumed in such a situation.

Hepatotoxicity

Severe hepatic reactions (e.g., acute liver failure, jaundice, hepatitis, cholestasis) have been reported rarely during postmarketing surveillance in patients receiving infliximab products. These reactions occurred between 2 weeks to longer than 1 year after initiation of therapy with the drug; hepatic aminotransferase elevations were not observed prior to discovery of the liver injury in many of these cases. Some of these cases were fatal or needed liver transplantation.

In clinical trials in patients with rheumatoid arthritis, Crohn disease, ulcerative colitis, ankylosing spondylitis, plaque psoriasis, and psoriatic arthritis, increases in serum AST (SGOT) and/or ALT (SGPT) concentrations were observed in a greater proportion of patients receiving infliximab than in controls, both when infliximab was given as monotherapy and when it was used in combination with other immunosuppressive agents. In these patient populations, increases in serum ALT concentrations of 5 or more times the upper limit of normal (ULN) were observed in less than 1 to 4% of patients receiving infliximab. In general, patients who developed hepatic aminotransferase elevations were asymptomatic, and such increases either decreased or resolved with either continuation or discontinuance of infliximab or modification of concomitant drug therapy.

In clinical trials in adults with rheumatoid arthritis, mild (less than 2 times the ULN) or moderate (2–3 times the ULN) transient increases in serum ALT concentrations have occurred in 34% of patients receiving infliximab in conjunction with methotrexate and in 24% of patients receiving placebo in conjunction with methotrexate. Increases in serum ALT concentrations of 3 or more times the ULN were observed in 4 or 3% of patients receiving infliximab in conjunction with methotrexate or methotrexate without infliximab, respectively (median follow-up 58 weeks).

In clinical trials in patients with Crohn disease (median follow-up 54 weeks), mild to moderate increases in serum ALT concentrations have been observed in 39 or 34% of patients receiving maintenance therapy with infliximab or placebo, respectively. In addition, increases in serum ALT concentrations of 3 or more times the ULN were observed in 5 or 4% of patients receiving maintenance therapy with infliximab or placebo, respectively.

In a clinical trial in pediatric patients with Crohn disease (median follow-up 53 weeks), mild to moderate increases in serum ALT concentrations have been observed in 18% of patients receiving infliximab. In addition, increases in serum ALT concentrations of 3 or more and 5 or more times the ULN were observed in 4 and 1% of patients receiving infliximab, respectively.

In a clinical trial in patients with ankylosing spondylitis, mild to moderate increases in ALT concentrations occurred in 51 or 15% of patients receiving infliximab or placebo, respectively. In addition, increases in serum ALT concentrations of 3 or more times the ULN were observed in 10 or 0% of patients receiving infliximab or placebo, respectively.

In a clinical trial in patients with ulcerative colitis, mild to moderate increases in ALT concentrations have occurred in 17 or 12% of patients receiving infliximab or placebo, respectively. In addition, increases in serum ALT concentrations of 3 or more times the ULN were observed in 2 or 1% of patients receiving infliximab or placebo, respectively.

In a clinical trial in pediatric patients with ulcerative colitis (median follow-up of 49 weeks), increases in serum ALT concentrations of up to 3 times the ULN occurred in 17% of patients receiving infliximab, while increases of 3 or more times the ULN or 5 or more times the ULN occurred in 7 or 2%, respectively, of patients receiving the drug.

In a clinical trial in patients with psoriatic arthritis, mild to moderate increases in ALT concentrations occurred in 50 or 16% of patients receiving infliximab or placebo, respectively. In addition, increases in serum ALT concentrations of 3 or more times the ULN were observed in 7 or 0% of patients receiving infliximab or placebo, respectively.

In clinical trials in patients with plaque psoriasis, mild to moderate increases in ALT concentrations have occurred in 49 or 24% of patients receiving infliximab or placebo, respectively. In addition, increases in serum ALT concentrations of 3 or more times the ULN were observed in 8 or less than 1% of patients receiving infliximab or placebo, respectively.

Evaluate patients with signs or symptoms of hepatic dysfunction for evidence of liver injury. If jaundice and/or marked hepatic aminotransferase elevations (5 or more times the ULN) develop, discontinue infliximab and investigate the hepatic abnormality.

Monitor hepatic enzymes and liver function tests every 3 to 4 months during subcutaneous maintenance treatment with infliximab-dyyb (Zymfentra®). Interrupt this treatment if drug-induced liver injury is suspected, until the diagnosis is excluded.

Heart Failure

Use of infliximab in patients with moderate to severe (New York Heart Association [NYHA] class III or IV) congestive heart failure was associated with higher incidences of mortality and hospitalization for worsening heart failure compared with similar patients receiving placebo. In a phase II study involving use of infliximab (5 or 10 mg/kg given at 0, 2, and 6 weeks) in patients with NYHA class III or IV congestive heart failure, at week 28, 4 of 101 patients receiving infliximab had died versus 0 of 49 patients receiving placebo. At week 28, 14 of 101 patients receiving infliximab had been hospitalized for worsening congestive heart failure versus 5 of 49 patients receiving placebo. Results of this study suggest that infliximab dosages of 10 mg/kg are associated with higher rates of mortality and dosages of 5 and 10 mg/kg are associated with higher rates of adverse cardiovascular effects. There have been postmarketing reports of worsening heart failure, with or without identifiable precipitating factors, in patients receiving infliximab.

If infliximab is used in patients with heart failure, caution and careful monitoring are recommended; if new or worsening symptoms of heart failure occur, discontinue the drug.

Hematologic Reactions

Cases of leukopenia, neutropenia, thrombocytopenia, and pancytopenia, some with fatal outcome, and idiopathic or thrombotic thrombocytopenic purpura have been reported in patients receiving infliximab products. Although a high-risk group for these adverse effects has not been identified, caution is advised if infliximab products are used in patients with a history of substantial hematologic abnormalities. Advise patients receiving infliximab products to seek immediate medical attention if they develop signs and symptoms suggestive of blood dyscrasias or infection (e.g., persistent fever, bruising, bleeding, pallor). If substantial hematologic abnormalities are confirmed, consider discontinuance of the infliximab product.

Cardiovascular and Cerebrovascular Reactions

Serious cerebrovascular accidents, myocardial ischemia/infarction (sometimes fatal), hypotension, hypertension, and arrhythmias have been reported during and within 24 hours of infliximab product infusion. Cases of transient visual loss have also been reported during and within 2 hours of infliximab product infusion. Monitor patients for such events during infusion; if a serious reaction occurs, discontinue the infusion and manage the reaction as dictated by signs and symptoms.

Neurologic Reactions

CNS manifestations of systemic vasculitis, seizure, and new onset or exacerbation of clinical manifestations and/or radiographic evidence of central or peripheral nervous system demyelinating disorders (e.g., multiple sclerosis, optic neuritis, Guillain-Barré syndrome) have been reported rarely in patients receiving infliximab products or other TNF blocking agents.

Exercise caution when considering use of infliximab products in patients with these neurologic disorders and consider discontinuance of infliximab if these disorders develop.

Concurrent Administration with Other Biological Products

Serious infections and neutropenia were seen in clinical studies with concurrent use of anakinra and another TNF blocker, etanercept, with no added clinical benefit compared to etanercept alone. Because of the nature of the adverse reactions seen with the concurrent use of etanercept and anakinra therapy, similar toxicities may also result from the concurrent use of anakinra and other TNF blockers. Therefore, the concurrent use of infliximab and anakinra is not recommended.

In clinical studies, concurrent administration of TNF blockers and abatacept have been associated with an increased risk of infections including serious infections compared with TNF blockers alone, without increased clinical benefit. Therefore, concurrent use of infliximab and abatacept is not recommended.

There is insufficient information regarding the concurrent use of infliximab with other biological products used to treat the same conditions as infliximab. Concurrent use of infliximab with these biological products is not recommended because of the possibility of an increased risk of infection.

Switching Between Biological Disease-Modifying Antirheumatic Drugs (DMARDs)

Care should be taken when switching from one biologic to another, since overlapping biological activity may further increase the risk of infection.

Immunologic Reactions and Antibody Formation

Infliximab therapy may result in the formation of antibodies to infliximab. The presence of infliximab in the serum sample may interfere with enzyme immunoassay (EIA) methods used to measure antibodies to infliximab and result in underestimation of the prevalence of antibody development to the drug. EIA methods were used to assess antibody development in the following studies; however, in pediatric patients with ulcerative colitis, a second assay method, an electrochemiluminescence immunoassay (ECLIA) method (which is 60-fold more sensitive than the original EIA method and permits classification of patient samples as either positive or negative for antibodies to the drug without the need for an inconclusive category) also was used. In patients receiving a 3-dose infliximab induction regimen followed by maintenance therapy who were evaluated over 1–2 years of treatment, 10% of patients were antibody-positive by EIA; most patients had low antibody titers. Patients with Crohn disease who had a drug-free interval longer than 16 weeks were more likely to be antibody-positive than patients who received the usually recommended maintenance regimen of infliximab (i.e., doses every 8 weeks). EIA antibody test results were inconclusive (because infliximab was present in the serum sample) in approximately 77% of pediatric patients receiving infliximab in conjunction with stable dosages of mercaptopurine, azathioprine, or methotrexate for the treatment of Crohn disease; following exclusion of these inconclusive samples, 3 of 24 patients (12.5%) had antibodies to infliximab. Antibodies to infliximab were detected by EIA in 38 or 12%, respectively, of children receiving 3- or 6-mg/kg doses of infliximab for the treatment of juvenile rheumatoid arthritis. In pediatric patients with ulcerative colitis, antibodies to the drug were detected by EIA or ECLIA in 7 or 52%, respectively, of patients. Patients who were antibody-positive were more likely to have higher rates of clearance, have reduced efficacy, and/or experience infusion reactions.

Patients with Crohn disease or rheumatoid arthritis receiving concomitant immunosuppressive therapy (e.g., methotrexate, azathioprine, mercaptopurine) were less likely to be antibody-positive. In patients who received infliximab in a dosage of 1, 3, or 10 mg/kg without concomitant methotrexate, infliximab antibodies were detected by EIA in 53, 21, or 7%, respectively; in those who received the same dosages of infliximab with concomitant methotrexate therapy (7.5 mg once weekly), infliximab antibodies were present in 15, 7, or 0%, respectively. Although further study is needed, it has been suggested that these data indicate that higher infliximab dosages and concomitant methotrexate therapy may induce a degree of immunologic tolerance to infliximab.

In one study, development of antibodies to infliximab was detected by EIA in 15% of 191 patients with psoriatic arthritis receiving infliximab 5 mg/kg with or without methotrexate. In the psoriasis EXPRESS II study in patients who received infliximab for 1 year at a dosage of 5 or 3 mg/kg, antibodies to infliximab were detected by EIA in 36 or 51% of patients, respectively, while in the psoriasis SPIRIT study in patients who received infliximab induction therapy at a dosage of 5 or 3 mg/kg, antibodies to infliximab were detected by EIA in 20 or 27%, respectively. Despite the increase in antibody formation, serious infusion reaction rates in patients receiving infliximab induction therapy at a dosage of 5 mg/kg followed by maintenance therapy every 8 weeks in the psoriasis EXPRESS and EXPRESS II studies and in patients receiving induction therapy at a dosage of 5 mg/kg in the psoriasis SPIRIT study were similar to those observed in other study populations (less than 1%).The effects of the apparent increased immunogenicity in patients with psoriasis on efficacy and infusion reaction rates with chronic infliximab therapy compared with patients with other disease states receiving infliximab products are not known.

No clinically meaningful differences have been found between infliximab biosimilars and infliximab with respect to antidrug antibody response resulting from administration of these drugs. Small numerical differences in antidrug antibody response were noted between infliximab-abda and infliximab; however, these differences were not felt to be clinically meaningful.

Therapy with infliximab products may induce formation of autoantibodies and rarely may result in development of a lupus-like syndrome.

When patients receiving infliximab in clinical studies were evaluated for the presence of antinuclear antibodies (ANA) and antibodies to double stranded DNA (anti-dsDNA), about 50 or 20 % had developed ANA or anti-dsDNA antibodies, respectively, between study entry and final evaluation. In these studies, about 20 or 0% of patients receiving placebo developed ANA or anti-dsDNA antibodies, respectively. When data from several studies in adults with rheumatoid arthritis were combined, approximately 30% of the study population had ANA at the time of study entry and 0% had anti-dsDNA. After infliximab treatment, 53% had ANA and 14% had anti-dsDNA. The mean time to detection of anti-dsDNA following initiation of infliximab therapy was 6.3 weeks (range: 4–10 weeks); in most patients, anti-dsDNA antibodies resolved within 4–6 weeks after induction. With the exception of one patient who had immunoglobulin G (IgG), IgA, and IgM class anti-dsDNA antibodies and who had clinical manifestations suggestive of a drug-induced lupus syndrome, anti-dsDNA antibodies in all other patients were of the IgM class only.

Children receiving infliximab for the treatment of juvenile arthritis have been tested for the presence of ANA and anti-dsDNA antibodies. The 3-mg/kg dose of infliximab was associated with a substantially higher risk of ANAs and anti-dsDNA antibodies than the 6-mg/kg dose. Approximately 14.8 or 13% of children receiving the 3-mg/kg dose of infliximab developed ANA or anti-dsDNA antibodies, respectively, between study entry and final evaluation. Only 2.2% of children

receiving the 6-mg/kg dose of infliximab developed ANA antibodies during the study; 0% of children receiving this dose developed anti-dsDNA antibodies.

Clinical symptoms consistent with a lupus-like syndrome (e.g., rash on face, hands, or forearms, exacerbation of joint pains, fever, dyspnea, pleuropericarditis) have occurred rarely in patients receiving infliximab products; these manifestations improved or resolved following discontinuance of the drug and appropriate medical therapy. One rheumatoid arthritis patient receiving infliximab in a clinical study developed a vasculitic rash and became positive for anti-dsDNA antibodies after the second infliximab dose; however, the rash and antibodies resolved spontaneously 11 weeks later. Current data are insufficient to determine whether induction of anti-dsDNA antibodies is associated with an increased risk of developing a lupus-like syndrome if infliximab therapy is continued for prolonged periods. Discontinue infliximab products in patients who develop a lupus-like syndrome.

Vaccinations and Use of Live Vaccines/Therapeutic Infectious Agents

Avoid live vaccines during therapy with infliximab products. Information is not available regarding whether infliximab would affect the rate of secondary transmission of infection following administration of a live vaccine.

When considering infliximab therapy, review the vaccination status of the patient and administer all age-appropriate vaccines included in current immunization guidelines, if possible, prior to initiation of therapy.

Fatal outcome due to disseminated bacille Calmette-Guérin (BCG) infection has been reported in an infant who received a BCG vaccine after in utero exposure to infliximab. Do not administer live vaccines to infants exposed to infliximab in utero for at least 6 months after birth, as infliximab is known to cross the placenta and has been detected up to 6 months following birth.

Use of therapeutic infectious agents (e.g., BCG bladder instillation for the treatment of cancer) is not recommended with concurrent administration of infliximab products.

Specific Populations

Pregnancy

Available observational studies in pregnant women exposed to infliximab products showed no increased risk of major malformations among live births as compared to those exposed to non-biologics. In a study using data from an inflammatory bowel disease pregnancy registry, infliximab exposure was not associated with increased rates of major congenital malformations, miscarriage/stillbirth, infants of low birth weight, small for gestational age, or infection in the first year of life. In a second study of inflammatory bowel disease patients conducted in Sweden, Finland, and Denmark, exposure to infliximab was not associated with increased rates of congenital anomalies or infant death; however, when infliximab was given in combination with immunosuppressants (e.g., systemic corticosteroids, azathioprine), the combination therapy was associated with increased rates of preterm birth, small for gestational age, low birth weight, and infant hospitalization for infection compared to non-biologic systemic treatment. Methodological limitations may hinder interpretation of these study results. Women with inflammatory bowel disease or rheumatoid arthritis may have an increased risk of adverse pregnancy outcomes (e.g., preterm delivery, low birth weight, small for gestational age at birth) with increased disease activity.

Infliximab crosses the placenta during the third trimester of pregnancy and may affect immune responses in infants who were exposed in utero. Infliximab has been detected for up to 6 months in the serum of infants whose mothers received infliximab products during pregnancy.

Reproduction studies using infliximab products in animals have not been conducted since the drug only binds TNF from humans and other primates and does not cross-react with TNF from other species. In a developmental toxicity study conducted in mice using a murine anti-TNF antibody that selectively inhibits murine TNF, no evidence of maternal toxicity, fetal mortality, or structural abnormalities was observed. In pharmacodynamic animal models using an analogous anti-TNF antibody, doses of 10–15 mg/kg produced maximal pharmacologic effectiveness; in animal reproduction studies, doses up to 40 mg/kg produced no adverse effects.

Lactation

Clinical studies indicate that IV infliximab is present in human milk at low levels. Systemic exposure in a breastfed infant is expected to be low, as infliximab is largely degraded in the GI tract. In a study of 168 women with inflammatory bowel disease treated with infliximab, infants exposed to infliximab through breast milk had no increase in infection rates and demonstrated normal development. There are no data on the effects of infliximab on milk production. Consider the developmental and health benefits of breastfeeding, along with the mother's clinical need for the infliximab product and any potential adverse effects on the breastfed infant from the infliximab product or from the underlying maternal condition.

Pediatric Use

Safety and efficacy of IV infliximab and its biosimilars (infliximab-abda, infliximab-axxq, infliximab-dyyb) have been established in pediatric patients 6 years of age and older with Crohn disease. The manufacturer states that infliximab has been studied in this population only in conjunction with conventional immunosuppressive therapy. Safety and efficacy of long-term therapy (exceeding 1 year) with infliximab products in pediatric patients with Crohn disease have not been established. Use of infliximab products for the management of Crohn disease in pediatric patients 6 years of age or older is supported by the results of a randomized, open-label study in 112 pediatric patients 6 years of age or older. Safety and efficacy for the management of Crohn disease have not been established in pediatric patients younger than 6 years of age.

Safety and efficacy of IV infliximab and its biosimilars (infliximab-abda, infliximab-axxq, infliximab-dyyb) have been established in pediatric patients 6 years of age and older with ulcerative colitis. Safety and efficacy of long-term infliximab therapy (exceeding 1 year) in pediatric patients with ulcerative colitis have not been established. Use of infliximab products for the management of ulcerative colitis in pediatric patients 6 years of age or older is supported by the results of adequate and well-controlled studies in adults with additional safety and pharmacokinetic data from an open-label study in 60 pediatric patients 6 years of age or older. Safety and efficacy for the management of ulcerative colitis have not been established in pediatric patients younger than 6 years of age.

Safety and efficacy of infliximab products in pediatric patients with plaque psoriasis have not been established.

Safety and efficacy of infliximab for the management of juvenile rheumatoid arthritis† have been evaluated in children 4–17 years of age with juvenile arthritis who had not responded adequately to methotrexate. While infliximab in combination with methotrexate produced important and durable clinical effects in children, the primary efficacy end point (i.e., the American College of Rheumatology [ACR] Pediatric 30 [Pedi 30] criteria for improvement) measured at week 14 did not differ between infliximab-treated children and placebo recipients. A 3-mg/kg dose of infliximab was associated with a higher risk of serious adverse events, infusion reactions, and development of antibodies to infliximab, antinuclear antibodies (ANAs), and antibodies to double stranded DNA (anti-ds DNA) compared with a 6-mg/kg dose. Further study is needed to evaluate the safety and efficacy of the drug for juvenile rheumatoid arthritis.

Malignancies, some fatal, have been reported in children and adolescents who received treatment with TNF blocking agents. It is unclear whether reported cases of hepatosplenic T-cell lymphoma in patients receiving infliximab products have been related to use of the TNF blocking agent or use of the TNF blocking agent in conjunction with other immunosuppressive agents. Therefore, carefully assess risks and benefits when deciding whether to use infliximab products alone or in combination with other immunosuppressive agents.

Pharmacokinetic values for infliximab in pediatric patients 6–17 years of age with Crohn disease or ulcerative colitis are similar to values in adults with these diseases.

All pediatric patients should be up to date with their vaccinations prior to initiating therapy with infliximab products.

Infliximab has been detected for up to 6 months in the serum of infants whose mothers received infliximab products during pregnancy. Infants who were exposed to infliximab products in utero may be at increased risk of infection. Fatal disseminated BCG infection has been reported in an infant who received BCG vaccine after having been exposed to infliximab in utero. Do not administer live vaccines to infants exposed to infliximab products in utero for at least 6 months following birth.

The safety and efficacy of infliximab-dyyb (Zymfentra®) in pediatric patients have not been established.

Geriatric Use

Clinical studies evaluating infliximab for the management of Crohn disease, ulcerative colitis, ankylosing spondylitis, and psoriatic arthritis have included an insufficient number of patients 65 years of age and older to make a valid comparison of the drug's safety and efficacy in geriatric patients compared with younger adults. In clinical studies in adults with rheumatoid arthritis or plaque psoriasis, there were no overall differences in the safety and efficacy of infliximab in those 65 years of age or older compared with younger adults; however, the incidence of serious adverse effects was higher in infliximab-treated and control patients 65 years of age or older compared with younger adults. Because serious infectious complications have been reported in some patients receiving infliximab products and because the overall incidence of infection is higher in geriatric adults than in younger individuals, monitor geriatric patients who receive infliximab products closely for the development of serious infections.

Hepatic Impairment

The pharmacokinetics of infliximab have not been formally studied in patients with hepatic impairment.

Renal Impairment

The pharmacokinetics of infliximab have not been formally studied in patients with renal impairment.

● Common Adverse Effects

Adverse effects reported in greater than 10% of patients receiving IV infliximab products include infections (e.g., upper respiratory, sinusitis, pharyngitis), infusion-related reactions, headache, and abdominal pain.

Adverse effects reported in ≥3% of patients receiving subcutaneous infliximab-dyyb for ulcerative colitis include COVID-19, anemia, arthralgia, injection site reaction, increased alanine aminotransferase, and abdominal pain.

Adverse effects reported in ≥3% of patients receiving subcutaneous infliximab-dyyb for Crohn disease include COVID-19, headache, upper respiratory tract infection, injection site reaction, diarrhea, increased blood creatine phosphokinase, arthralgia, increased alanine aminotransferase, hypertension, urinary tract infection, neutropenia, dizziness, and leukopenia.

DRUG INTERACTIONS

Although specific drug interaction studies evaluating concomitant use of infliximab or its biosimilars and other drugs have not been conducted to date, most patients in clinical studies evaluating infliximab received one or more concomitant drugs. Patients with Crohn disease usually received infliximab concomitantly with corticosteroids, mesalamine or sulfasalazine, azathioprine or mercaptopurine, and/or anti-infective agents; patients with rheumatoid arthritis usually received infliximab concomitantly with methotrexate and may also have received corticosteroids, nonsteroidal anti-inflammatory agents (NSAIAs), folic acid, or narcotics.

In patients with Crohn disease, serum concentrations of infliximab do not appear to be affected by baseline use of corticosteroids, 5-aminosalicylates, or anti-infectives (ciprofloxacin, metronidazole). There is some evidence from studies of infliximab that the incidence of some adverse immunologic reactions to infliximab products (e.g., infusion reactions, formation of antibodies to infliximab) is lower in patients receiving infliximab products concomitantly with immunosuppressive agents (e.g., corticosteroids, azathioprine, mercaptopurine, methotrexate) compared with those receiving infliximab products without such agents.

When deciding whether infliximab products should be used alone or in combination with other immunosuppressive agents, clinicians should consider both the possibility of an increased risk of hepatosplenic T-cell lymphoma with combination therapy and the observed (in infliximab studies) increase in immunogenicity and hypersensitivity reactions associated with infliximab products given as monotherapy.

● Drugs Metabolized by Hepatic Microsomal Enzymes

Because increased levels of cytokines (e.g., tumor necrosis factor [TNF]-α, interferon, interleukin-1, interleukin-6, interleukin-10) during chronic inflammation may suppress the formation of cytochrome P-450 (CYP) isoenzymes, it is expected that a drug that antagonizes cytokine activity, such as an infliximab product, could normalize the formation of CYP enzymes. Following initiation or discontinuance of therapy with infliximab products, monitor patients receiving certain drugs metabolized by CYP isoenzymes (i.e., those with a low therapeutic index [e.g., cyclosporine, theophylline, warfarin]) for therapeutic effect and/or changes in serum concentrations, and adjust dosages of these drugs as needed.

● Biologic Agents

Exercise caution when switching from one biologic disease-modifying antirheumatic drug (DMARD) to another, since overlapping biologic activity may further increase the risk of infection.

Insufficient data are available regarding concomitant use of infliximab products with other biologic agents used to treat the same conditions. Concomitant use of infliximab products with these agents is not recommended because of an increased risk of infection.

Abatacept

When abatacept and a TNF blocking agent were used concomitantly, an increased incidence of infection and serious infection was observed, with no substantial improvement in efficacy over that observed with a TNF blocking agent alone. Similar toxicities would be expected with concomitant use of abatacept and infliximab products. Concomitant use of infliximab products and abatacept is not recommended.

Anakinra

When anakinra and etanercept were used concomitantly in patients with rheumatoid arthritis, an increased incidence of serious infection and neutropenia was observed, with no substantial improvement in efficacy over that observed with etanercept alone. Similar toxicities would be expected with concomitant use of anakinra and other agents that block TNF, including infliximab products. Concomitant use of infliximab products and anakinra is not recommended.

Tocilizumab

Avoid concomitant use of tocilizumab and biologic DMARDs such as TNF blocking agents, including infliximab products, because of the possibility of increased immunosuppression and increased risk of infection.

● Methotrexate

Although specific pharmacokinetic interaction studies have not been performed, data from one double-blind, placebo-controlled study in adults with rheumatoid arthritis suggest that concomitant use of methotrexate may affect the pharmacokinetics of infliximab. In this study, patients who received infliximab in a dosage of 1 mg/kg (given by IV infusion over 2 hours at weeks 0, 2, 6, 10, and 14) concomitantly with oral placebo (once weekly) had mean serum infliximab concentrations that decreased to 0.1 mcg/mL (the limits of detection) by the fourth week after the second infusion and by the second week after each subsequent infusion; however, patients who received the same dosage of infliximab concomitantly with oral methotrexate (7.5 mg once weekly) had mean serum infliximab concentrations that were maintained at approximately 2–20 mcg/mL during each interval. Although patients receiving infliximab in a dosage of 3 or 10 mg/kg had serum infliximab concentrations that were similar regardless of whether they were receiving the drug alone or in conjunction with methotrexate (7.5 mg once weekly), serum infliximab concentrations after the final infusion were consistently higher and decreased at a slower rate in those receiving methotrexate than in those receiving placebo.

The mechanisms and clinical importance of this possible pharmacokinetic interaction have not been determined. There is some evidence that development of antibodies to infliximab occurs less frequently in patients receiving infliximab in conjunction with methotrexate than in those receiving infliximab alone. It has been suggested that methotrexate, by decreasing the immunogenic potential of infliximab, may result in a slower rate of clearance of infliximab.

● Vaccines and Therapeutic Infectious Agents

Do not administer live vaccines and other live therapeutic infectious agents (e.g., BCG for intravesical instillation) to patients receiving infliximab products. Use of live vaccines or live therapeutic infectious agents could result in infections, including disseminated infections. Limited data are available regarding whether infliximab products would affect the rate of secondary transmission of infection following administration of a live vaccine or regarding the response to live vaccines in patients receiving the drug. Fatal disseminated BCG infection has been reported in an infant who received BCG vaccine after having been exposed to infliximab in utero. Do not administer live vaccines to infants exposed to infliximab products in utero for at least 6 months following birth.

DESCRIPTION

Infliximab and its biosimilars are chimeric human-murine immunoglobulin G1 kappa (IgG1 kappa) monoclonal antibodies that have a high affinity for tumor necrosis factor (TNF-α). Infliximab products consist of the constant region of human IgG$_1$ kappa coupled to the variable region of a high-affinity neutralizing murine anti-human TNF antibody. Because of the presence of human constant region sequences, the chimeric antibody is less immunogenic, has a longer half-life, and is more potent in binding and neutralizing human TNF compared with the murine antibody.

Infliximab is produced by continuous fermentation of a mouse myeloma cell line that has been transfected with cloned DNA coding for the chimeric antibody. The drug is purified from the culture supernatant using column chromatography and undergoes measures to inactivate and remove viruses.

Infliximab products have a high affinity for and bind specifically to soluble and transmembrane forms of TNF thereby inhibiting binding of TNF to cell surface tumor necrosis factor receptors (TNFRs). By binding to TNF, infliximab and infliximab products neutralize the cytokine. Although the exact mechanism(s) of the anti-inflammatory effects of infliximab products in the management of Crohn disease or rheumatoid arthritis remains to be more fully determined, binding and neutralization of TNF appears to be the principal mechanism. There also is some evidence that infliximab may inhibit expression of TNF by binding soluble TNF attached to TNF receptors present on activated macrophages and T cells.

While it is clear that chronic inflammatory processes are not due solely to overexpression of TNF, the regulatory cytokine plays a critical role in the control of the production of other cytokines involved in the pathogenesis of inflammation of Crohn disease and rheumatoid arthritis. A variety of physiologic and pathologic functions have been ascribed to TNF-TNF receptor interactions and the effects of TNF include induction of proinflammatory cytokines such as interleukin 1(IL-1), IL-6 and IL-8, enhancement of leukocyte migration by increasing endothelial layer permeability and expression of adhesion molecules by endothelial cells and leukocytes, activation of neutrophil and eosinophil functional activity, induction of acute phase proteins (C-reactive protein, serum amyloid A [SAA] haptoglobin, fibrinogen) and tissue degrading enzymes produced by synoviocytes and/or chondrocytes. TNF blocks the action of lipoprotein lipase, causing severe cachexia in experimental models of chronic infection. In addition, TNF induces programmed cell death (apoptosis), stimulates the release matrix metalloproteinases from fibroblasts, chondrocytes, and neutrophils, and upregulates the expression of endothelial adhesion molecules, leading to the migration of leukocytes into extravascular tissues. TNF also mediates pain, fever, shock, and anemia.

The complex interactions of paracrine or autocrine pathways mediated by networks of pro- and anti-inflammatory cytokines are implicated in many chronic inflammatory disorders and TNF plays a prominent role in the pathogenesis of Crohn disease, rheumatoid arthritis, multiple sclerosis, systemic vasculitis, allograft rejection, and graft-versus-host disease. Mucosal biopsies from patients with Crohn disease demonstrate increased TNF concentrations and intestinal mononuclear cell infiltrates in the lamina propria. Increased concentrations of TNF have been measured in fecal samples from Crohn disease patients and in the joints of patients with rheumatoid arthritis and levels correlated with disease manifestations in these patients. Increased concentrations of TNF also have been reported in involved tissues and fluids of patients with ulcerative colitis, ankylosing spondylitis, psoriatic arthritis, and plaque psoriasis.

The ability of infliximab and its biosimilars to inhibit the functional activity of TNF has been demonstrated in a variety of in vitro bioassays utilizing human fibroblasts, endothelial and epithelial cells, neutrophils, and B and T cells. The relationship of these biological response markers to the mechanism(s) of infliximab products' clinical effects is not known. In addition, cell lysis by complement or effector cells has been observed in vitro in cells that express transmembrane TNF and are bound by infliximab. In vivo studies have shown that anti-TNF antibodies reduce GI manifestations in a nonhuman primate model of colitis (cotton-top tamarin) and reduce synovitis and joint erosions in a murine model of collagen-induced arthritis.

In patients with Crohn disease, infliximab products have been shown to reduce inflammatory cell migration, reduce TNF production in areas of intestinal inflammation, and reduce the proportion of lamina propria mononuclear cells able to express TNF and interferon.

In patients with rheumatoid arthritis, infliximab products reduce infiltration of inflammatory cells into inflamed areas of the joint and downregulate expression of molecules that mediate cellular adhesion (E-selectin, intercellular adhesion molecule-1 [ICAM-1], vascular cell adhesion molecule-1 [VCAM-1]), chemoattraction (IL-8 and monocyte chemotactic protein [MCP-1]), and tissue degradation (MMP 1 and 3). Infliximab also has been shown to inhibit pannus neoangiogenesis and proliferation through down-regulation of vascular endothelial growth factor (VEGF). Results of studies in transgenic mice that develop polyarthritis as the result of constitutive expression of TNF indicate that infliximab products can prevent such disease in these mice and, if administered after disease onset, allow eroded joints to heal. There is evidence that infliximab can prevent or inhibit progression of structural damage in patients with rheumatoid arthritis.

In patients with Crohn disease or rheumatoid arthritis, therapy with infliximab products may result in decreases in proinflammatory cytokines (IL-1, IL-6) and decreases in systemic measures of inflammation, including C-reactive protein (CRP) levels and erythrocyte sedimentation rate (ESR). Peripheral blood lymphocytes from patients treated with infliximab products exhibit a normal proliferative response to in vitro mitogenic stimulation and lymphocyte counts are not decreased in patients who receive the drugs.

In patients with psoriatic arthritis, therapy with infliximab products results in a reduction in the number of T-cells and blood vessels in the synovium and psoriatic skin lesions and a reduction of macrophages in the synovium. In patients with plaque psoriasis, therapy with infliximab products may reduce the epidermal thickness and infiltration of inflammatory cells.

Pharmacokinetic similarity between infliximab and its biosimilars has been demonstrated, and FDA considers that the pharmacokinetic data provide support for a totality-of-evidence determination of biosimilarity for infliximab-abda, infliximab-axxq, and infliximab-dyyb.

Data from adults who received single IV infusions of 1–20 mg/kg of infliximab indicate a predictable and linear relationship between the dose administered and the maximum serum concentration and AUC. In one study in adults with rheumatoid arthritis who received single 5-, 10-, or 20-mg/kg doses of infliximab given by IV infusion over 2 hours, peak serum concentrations were achieved 1–4 hours after the start of the infusion; serum concentrations of the drug then decreased exponentially from day 3 through week 12 and were still detectable in most patients at week 10. Systemic accumulation of infliximab does not appear to occur in adults receiving multiple doses of the drug given by IV infusion once every 4 or 8 weeks following an initial 3-dose induction regimen (doses at 0, 2, and 6 weeks). Distribution of infliximab into body tissues and fluids, including joints, has not been characterized. The volume of distribution of infliximab at steady state is independent of dose, indicating that the drug is distributed principally within the vascular compartment. The terminal elimination half-life of infliximab in adults with Crohn disease, rheumatoid arthritis, or plaque psoriasis has been reported to be about 8–12 days. After a single subcutaneous dose of infliximab-dyyb 120 mg in healthy subjects, the median time to maxium serum concentration was 7 days; the mean half-life was 332 hours.

The metabolic fate of infliximab has not been determined to date, but the drug may be eliminated by the reticuloendothelial system. Infliximab is not metabolized by hepatic cytochrome P-450 (CYP) enzymes. While differences in clearance of infliximab have not been observed in patient subgroups defined by age, weight, or gender, clearance of infliximab is increased in patients who have developed antibodies to the drug. Whether renal or hepatic impairment affects infliximab clearance has not been determined.

ADVICE TO PATIENTS

- Advise patients or their caregivers about the potential benefits and risks of receiving infliximab products. Provide a copy of the manufacturer's patient information (Medication Guide) for infliximab products to all patients or their caregivers prior to each infusion session.

- Risk of increased susceptibility to infection. Inform patients or their caregivers to seek immediate medical attention if signs and symptoms suggestive of infection (e.g., fever; fatigue; cough; warm, red, or painful skin; sores on the body) develop.

- Risk of malignancies, including lymphoma, with use of TNF blocking agents in children, adolescents, and young adults. Advise patients to promptly inform clinicians if signs and symptoms of malignancies occur (e.g., unexplained weight loss; fatigue; abdominal pain; persistent fever; night sweats; easy bruising or bleeding; swollen lymph nodes in the neck, underarm, or groin; hepatomegaly or splenomegaly).

- Inform patients or their caregivers to immediately notify their clinician if manifestations of liver dysfunction (e.g., jaundice, dark brown urine, right-sided abdominal pain, fever, fatigue) occur.

- Advise patients or their caregivers to seek immediate medical attention if any new or worsening symptoms of heart failure occur.

- Advise patients or their caregivers to inform their clinician if they develop signs and symptoms suggestive of blood dyscrasias or infection (e.g., persistent fever).

- Advise the patient or their caregivers to seek immediate medical care if they develop symptoms of serious hypersensitivity reactions,

- Advise the patient or their caregivers to seek immediate medical care if they develop symptoms of cardiovascular and cerebrovascular reactions during and within 24 hours of the infliximab infusion.

- Advise the patient or their caregivers to seek medical care if they develop signs or symptoms of neurologic reactions.

- Advise patients or their caregivers of the importance to avoid receiving live vaccines or therapeutic infectious agents. For postpartum women who received infliximab products during pregnancy, inform the infant's clinician of this use since alteration of the infant's vaccination schedule may be indicated.

- Advise women to inform their clinician if they are or plan to become pregnant or plan to breast-feed.

- Advise patients or their caregivers to inform their healthcare provider about all concomitant medications, including prescription medicine, over the counter drugs, vitamins, and herbal products.

- Inform patients or their caregivers of other important precautionary information.

PREPARATIONS

Excipients in commercially available drug preparations may have clinically important effects in some individuals; consult specific product labeling for details.

inFLIXimab

Parenteral		
For injection, for IV infusion	100 mg	Remicade®, Janssen

inFLIXimab-abda (biosimilar)

Parenteral		
For injection, for IV infusion	100 mg	Renflexis®, Organon

inFLIXimab-axxq (biosimilar)

Parenteral		
For injection, for IV infusion	100 mg	Avsola®, Amgen

inFLIXimab-dyyb (biosimilar)

Parenteral		
For injection, for IV infusion	100 mg	Inflectra®, Pfizer
For subcutaneous injection	120 mg/mL	Zymfentra® (available as single-dose prefilled syringe, single-dose prefilled syringe with needle shield, and single-dose prefilled pen)

† Use is not currently included in the labeling approved by the US Food and Drug Administration.

Anakinra

90:24.20.92 • INTERLEUKIN-MEDIATED AGENTS, MISCELLANEOUS

■ Anakinra, a recombinant human interleukin-1 (IL-1) receptor antagonist, is a biologic disease-modifying antirheumatic drug (DMARD).

USES

● Rheumatoid Arthritis

Anakinra is used alone or in combination with disease-modifying antirheumatic drugs (DMARDs) other than tumor necrosis factor (TNF)-blocking agents (e.g., adalimumab, etanercept, infliximab) for the management of signs and symptoms of rheumatoid arthritis and to inhibit progression of structural damage in adults with moderately to severely active disease who have failed one or more DMARDs.

Clinical Experience

Efficacy and safety of anakinra in the management of rheumatoid arthritis are based principally on the results of several randomized, double-blind, placebo-controlled clinical trials in adults with moderately to severely active rheumatoid arthritis. In some trials, anakinra was administered to patients already receiving methotrexate. In another trial, patients either were DMARD-naive or had failed therapy with up to 3 DMARDs prior to receiving anakinra; patients receiving DMARDs had such therapy discontinued 6 weeks prior to entering the study. In the 2 studies evaluating combination therapy with methotrexate, patients had received methotrexate therapy for up to 6 months and had been on a stable dosage of the drug (10–25 mg/week) for at least 2–3 months prior to study entry but were having an inadequate response.

Evaluations of disease activity were performed and assessed at 3 and 6 months according to the American College of Rheumatology criteria for improvement (ACR response). The ACR 20 response is achieved if the patient experiences improvements of ≥20% in tender and swollen joint counts and ≥20% improvement in at least 3 of the following criteria: patient pain assessment, patient global assessment, physician global assessment, patient self-assessed disability, or laboratory indicators of disease activity (i.e., erythrocyte sedimentation rate [ESR] or C-reactive protein [CRP] level). Patients also were evaluated for ACR 50 and 70 responses (defined using the same criteria as ACR 20 but with a level of improvement of 50 or 70%, respectively); reductions in individual measures of disease activity; and general health status.

In these studies, anakinra therapy was associated with greater improvement in the clinical and radiographic manifestations of rheumatoid arthritis than placebo. Most clinical responses occurred within 12 weeks, and improvement with anakinra was dose-related. Some patients who completed the 24-week study in which anakinra monotherapy was administered were maintained on anakinra at the same dosage for an additional 24 weeks. In these patients, improvements in radiographic evidence of rheumatoid arthritis (e.g., joint space narrowing, cartilage degradation) were maintained during the second 24-week treatment period. Although more long-term data with anakinra at the currently recommended dosage are needed to fully elucidate the effects of the drug on structural joint damage and physical function in rheumatoid arthritis, the drug appears to slow radiographic progression of joint damage for up to at least 12 months during continued therapy).

In a randomized, comparative trial in patients concomitantly receiving methotrexate therapy, patients treated with the combination of anakinra and etanercept did not derive additional benefit (as measured by ACR 50 response rate) compared with those given etanercept monotherapy, and serious infections were more frequent with combination therapy.

Clinical Perspective

The American College of Rheumatology issued guidelines for the treatment of rheumatoid arthritis in 2021. Disease-modifying treatments for rheumatoid arthritis include conventional DMARDs (e.g., hydroxychloroquine, leflunomide, methotrexate, sulfasalazine), biologic DMARDs (e.g., TNF blocking agents, abatacept, tocilizumab, sarilumab, rituximab), and/or targeted synthetic DMARDs

(e.g., Janus kinase inhibitors). Specific agents for rheumatoid arthritis treatment are selected according to current disease activity, prior therapies used, and the presence of comorbidities. A "treat-to-target" approach is typically employed, with the goal of achieving a predefined target of low disease activity or remission. The guideline states that anakinra was not included due to infrequent use for patients with rheumatoid arthritis. Consult the American College of Rheumatology guidelines for additional details.

● Cryopyrin-associated Periodic Syndromes

Anakinra is used for the treatment of neonatal-onset multisystem inflammatory disease (NOMID). which is a form of the cryopyrin-associated periodic syndromes (CAPS).

Clinical Experience

Efficacy of anakinra for the treatment of NOMID was demonstrated in an open-label, prospective, uncontrolled study of 43 patients (0.7–46 years of age) who were treated for up to 60 months. Patients were included if they had active disease and at least 2 symptoms (urticaria-like rash, CNS involvement, or epiphyseal and/or patellar overgrowth on radiographs). Patients received an initial anakinra dosage of 1–2.4 mg/kg daily, which was titrated in 0.5–1 mg/kg increments based on disease severity to an average maintenance dosage of 3–4 mg/kg daily. Dosages up to 7.6 mg/kg daily for up to 15 months were administered. In most patients, anakinra was administered as a once-daily dose, but some patients received the drug in divided twice-daily doses. The disease-specific Diary Symptom Sum Score (DSSS) was used to assess NOMID symptoms including fever, rash, joint pain, vomiting, and headache. Serum amyloid A (SAA), high-sensitivity C-reactive protein (hsCRP), and erythrocyte sedimentation rate (ESR) levels were also assessed. DSSS scores and serum markers of inflammation were improved from baseline to months 3–6 with use of anakinra. Improvements occurred across subgroups of patients based on age, gender, presence of CIAS1 mutation, and disease phenotype. Disease symptoms and serum markers of inflammation worsened after drug withdrawal, but promptly responded after treatment was reinitiated.

Clinical Perspective

The American Academy of Allergy, Asthma, and Immunology (AAAAI) and the American College of Allergy, Asthma, and Immunology (ACAAI) issued a practice parameter on the diagnosis and management of primary immunodeficiency, which includes recommendations for cryopyrin-associated periodic syndromes (CAPS); NOMID is part of the spectrum of CAPS diseases characterized by inflammation caused by mutations in the pyrin domain containing 3 (NLRP3) gene. Patients suspected of having CAPS should be screened for systemic signs of inflammation in the absence of demonstrable infection, autoimmune disease, or malignancy. To aid in the diagnosis, a trial of interleukin-1 (IL-1) blockade with anakinra, rilonacept, or canakinumab can be used. The practice parameter recommends IL-1 inhibitors such as anakinra, rilonacept, and canakinumab for all patients with CAPS.

● Deficiency of Interleukin-1 Receptor Antagonist

Anakinra is used for the treatment of deficiency of interleukin-1 receptor antagonist (DIRA).

Clinical Experience

The efficacy of anakinra for this indication is based on a long-term natural history study that included 9 patients with DIRA. Patients ranged from 1 month to 9 years of age at baseline and were treated with anakinra for up to 10 years. Anakinra was administered at an initial dosage of 1–2 mg/kg daily, and then increased as needed to a maximum of 7.5 mg/kg daily. The dosage ranged from 2.2–6.1 mg/kg daily at the last visit of the first treatment period. All 9 patients achieved inflammatory remission with anakinra, defined as CRP level ≤5 mg/L without pustulosis, inflammatory bone disease, or concomitant corticosteroid use.

Clinical Perspective

The AAAAI and ACAAI practice parameter on the diagnosis and management of primary immunodeficiency also includes recommendations for the treatment of DIRA. The practice parameter states that patients with pustular rash, joint swelling, and profound osteopenia and bone lesions at or soon after birth should be suspected of having DIRA. Anakinra or other IL-1 antagonists are recommended for therapeutic use or diagnosis of DIRA. The practice parameter notes that anakinra treatment results in rapid and sustained response, improvement in laboratory abnormalities, resolution of rash, and healing of bone lesions.

● Hidradenitis Suppurativa

Anakinra also has been used in the management of hidradenitis suppurativa†, a chronic, relapsing inflammatory skin disorder characterized by recurrent painful nodules, abscesses, fistulas, sinus tracts, and scarring in apocrine gland-bearing regions (e.g., axillae, inframammary area, inguinal and anogenital regions, perineum).

The United States and Canadian Hidradenitis Suppurativa Foundations published a joint guideline for the treatment of hidradenitis suppurativa in 2019. Clinical management of hidradenitis suppurativa involves the use of both medical and surgical therapies. Medical therapies used for the condition include topical/intralesional therapies, systemic antibiotics, hormonal therapies (antiandrogen contraceptives, spironolactone, metformin, finasteride), retinoids, systemic immunomodulators (e.g., colchicine, cyclosporine, corticosteroids), and biologic agents (e.g., adalimumab, infliximab, anakinra, ustekinumab). The guideline states that anakinra may be effective for hidradenitis suppurativa, but dose-ranging studies are necessary to determine the optimal dosage of these agents.

DOSAGE AND ADMINISTRATION

● General

Pretreatment Screening

- Screen patients for active infections; do not initiate anakinra in patients with an active infection.

- Evaluate for and treat possible latent tuberculosis infections prior to initiating anakinra treatment; follow CDC guidelines.

- Assess absolute neutrophil count (ANC) prior to starting anakinra.

Patient Monitoring

- Monitor patients for hypersensitivity reactions and discontinue anakinra if a severe hypersensitivity reaction occurs. Patients with deficiency of interleukin-1 receptor antagonist (DIRA) may have an increased risk of allergic reactions, particularly in the first several weeks of initiating anakinra; closely monitor patients during this time.

- Assess ANC monthly for 3 months, and then quarterly for up to 1 year during treatment with anakinra.

● Administration

Anakinra is administered by subcutaneous injection using the prefilled syringe. The graduated prefilled syringe allows for doses between 20 mg and 100 mg.

Anakinra is intended for use under the guidance and supervision of a clinician; however, the drug may be self-administered if the clinician determines that the patient and/or their caregiver is competent to safely administer the drug after appropriate training and with medical follow-up as necessary.

Administer the prescribed dose of anakinra using the prefilled syringe and discard any unused portion.

Inspect the injection visually for particulate matter and/or discoloration and discard if either is present.

Allow the prefilled syringe to reach room temperature (about 30 minutes) prior to administration. Do not remove the needle cover until the prefilled syringe has reached room temperature.

Administer subcutaneous injections of anakinra into the thighs, abdomen, outer area of the upper arms, or upper outer areas of the buttocks. Rotate injection sites. Avoid injections into areas where the skin is tender, bruised, red, or hard, or into scars or stretch marks, or close to a vein.

● Dosage

Rheumatoid Arthritis

For the treatment of rheumatoid arthritis, the recommended adult dosage of anakinra is 100 mg once daily given subcutaneously at approximately the same time each day. Higher dosages do not appear to provide additional benefit.

Cryopyrin-associated Periodic Syndromes

For the treatment of cryopyrin-associated periodic syndromes (CAPS), the recommended starting dose of anakinra in patients with neonatal-onset multisystem inflammatory disease (NOMID) is 1–2 mg/kg daily given subcutaneously. Adjust the dosage in 0.5–1 mg/kg increments up to a maximum of 8 mg/kg daily to control active inflammation. Once-daily administration generally is recommended; however, the dose may be split into twice-daily administration.

Each syringe is intended for single use only; a new syringe must be used for each dose and any unused portions should be discarded.

Deficiency of Interleukin-1 Receptor Antagonist

For the treatment of deficiency of interleukin-1 receptor antagonist (DIRA), the recommended starting dosage of anakinra is 1–2 mg/kg daily. Adjust the dosage in 0.5–1 mg/kg increments up to a maximum of 8 mg/kg daily to control active inflammation.

Each syringe is intended for single use only; a new syringe must be used for each dose and any unused portions should be discarded.

● Special Populations

Hepatic Impairment

The manufacturer makes no specific dosage recommendations for patients with hepatic impairment.

Renal Impairment

Since anakinra is eliminated substantially by renal excretion, consideration should be given to administering the prescribed dose every *other* day in patients with severe renal insufficiency or end-stage renal disease (creatinine clearance <30 mL/minute, as estimated from serum creatinine levels). Less than 2.5% of an administered dose is removed by hemodialysis or continuous ambulatory peritoneal dialysis.

Geriatric Patients

The manufacturer makes no specific dosage recommendations for geriatric patients.

CAUTIONS

● Contraindications

- Known hypersensitivity to *Escherichia coli*-derived proteins, anakinra, or any ingredient in the formulation.

● Warnings/Precautions

Serious Infections

In clinical trials in rheumatoid arthritis, anakinra therapy was associated with an increased incidence of serious infections compared with placebo (2% versus <1%, respectively). Opportunistic infections (fungal, mycobacterial, bacterial) have been reported rarely. Patients with asthma may be at a higher risk for developing serious infections.

Do not initiate anakinra therapy in patients with active infections, and discontinue the drug in patients with rheumatoid arthritis who develop a serious infection. In patients with neonatal-onset multisystem inflammatory disease (NOMID) or deficiency of interleukin-1 receptor antagonist (DIRA), weigh the risk of a disease flare when discontinuing anakinra with the potential risk of continued treatment. The safety and efficacy of anakinra in immunosuppressed patients or patients with chronic infections have not been evaluated. It is possible that drugs that block IL-1, such as anakinra, may increase the risk of tuberculosis or other atypical or opportunistic infections. Follow current CDC guidelines to evaluate and treat possible latent tuberculosis infections before initiating anakinra treatment.

Use with TNF Blocking Agents

Concurrent use of anakinra and etanercept in patients with rheumatoid arthritis did not result in higher response rates compared to use of etanercept alone, but combined anakinra and etanercept therapy was associated with an increased rate of serious infections (7 versus 0%) compared to etanercept alone. Use of anakinra concurrently with TNF blocking agents (e.g., adalimumab, etanercept, infliximab) is not recommended.

Hypersensitivity Reactions

Hypersensitivity reactions, including anaphylactic reactions and angioedema, have been reported with anakinra. If a severe hypersensitivity reaction occurs, discontinue anakinra immediately and institute appropriate interventions as indicated.

Patients with DIRA may have an increased risk of allergic reactions, particularly in the first several weeks after initiating anakinra. Closely monitor patients during this time. Initiate appropriate treatment and consider discontinuing anakinra if a severe allergic reaction occurs.

Immunosuppression

The effects of anakinra in patients with active and/or chronic infections or on the subsequent development of malignancies have not been determined.

Immunizations

Do not administer live-virus vaccines to patients receiving anakinra. No data are available on the effects of live vaccination or the secondary transmission of infection by live vaccines in patients receiving anakinra. In a clinical trial, there was no difference in anti-tetanus antibody response between patients receiving anakinra and those receiving placebo after administration of the tetanus/diphtheria toxoid vaccine. No data are available on the effects of vaccination with other inactivated antigens in patients receiving anakinra.

Neutropenia

Patients receiving anakinra may experience a decrease in neutrophil counts. ANC reductions of at least one WHO toxicity grade occurred in 8 or 2% of anakinra- or placebo-treated patients, respectively, in clinical trials. Neutropenia (ANC <1000/mm^3) developed in 0.4% of patients receiving anakinra monotherapy and in 2% of those receiving the drug concomitantly with etanercept. In the clinical trial of patients with NOMID, 2 of 43 patients experienced neutropenia that resolved over time with continued treatment with anakinra.

Evaluate neutrophil counts prior to starting anakinra; after treatment is started, monitor neutrophil counts monthly for 3 months and then quarterly for up to 1 year.

Specific Populations

Pregnancy

The available data from retrospective studies and case reports are insufficient to identify a drug-associated risk of major birth defects, miscarriage, or maternal or fetal adverse events with anakinra; however, no adverse outcomes have been identified with the available human evidence. No evidence of fetal harm was observed in animal studies when anakinra was administered to pregnant rats and rabbits during organogenesis at up to 25 times the maximum recommended human dose (MRHD). Risks to the mother and fetus associated with active rheumatoid arthritis or cryopyrin-associated periodic syndromes (CAPS) include preterm delivery, low birth weight, and the neonate being small for its gestational age at birth.

Lactation

It is not known whether anakinra is distributed into milk or if the drug affects milk production. Available data from a small retrospective study and postmarketing case reports do not establish an association between maternal anakinra use during lactation and adverse effects on breast-fed infants. The limited clinical data preclude a clear determination of the risk of anakinra to an infant during lactation.

Consider the benefits of breastfeeding along with the woman's clinical need for anakinra and any potential adverse effects on the breastfed infant from the drug or underlying maternal condition.

Pediatric Use

Anakinra was evaluated for the treatment of neonatal-onset multisystem inflammatory disease (NOMID) in 36 pediatric patients; these patients included 13 who were <2 years of age, 18 who were 2–11 years of age, and 5 who were 12–17 years of age. Patients received a starting anakinra subcutaneous dosage of 1–2 mg/kg daily and an average maintenance dosage of 3–4 mg/kg daily. Certain patients with severe disease required a higher maintenance dosage. Doses below 20 mg cannot be administered with the prefilled syringe.

Anakinra was evaluated for the treatment of deficiency of interleukin-1 receptor antagonist (DIRA) in 9 pediatric patients 1 month to 9 years of age. Most patients received an initial subcutaneous dosage of 1–2 mg/kg daily, and maintenance dosages up to 7.5 mg/kg daily were administered. Doses below 20 mg cannot be administered with the prefilled syringe.

Anakinra has been evaluated in a limited number of pediatric patients 2–17 years of age with polyarticular course juvenile rheumatoid arthritist†. Clinical response has been observed at week 12 in children receiving anakinra at a dosage of 1 mg/kg (up to a maximum dose of 100 mg) daily by subcutaneous injection. Some children received the drug for up to 1 year in an open-label extension study. Adverse effects reported in pediatric patients with juvenile rheumatoid arthritis were similar to those reported in adults receiving anakinra for rheumatoid arthritis. However, efficacy and safety of the drug have not been established in pediatric patients with juvenile rheumatoid arthritis, and the manufacturer states that such use is not recommended.

Geriatric Use

Available experience in patients ≥65 years of age with rheumatoid arthritis in clinical trials of anakinra suggests that such individuals do not respond differently to the drug compared with younger adults. However, greater sensitivity of some geriatric individuals cannot be ruled out. Because serious infections have been reported in some patients receiving anakinra and because the overall incidence of infection is higher in geriatric adults than in younger individuals, anakinra should be used with caution in geriatric patients.

Because anakinra is substantially excreted by the kidneys, geriatric patients with impaired renal function may be at increased risk of toxic reactions.

Renal Impairment

In patients with renal impairment, plasma clearance of anakinra was reduced by 16–75% depending on the degree of renal insufficiency. Dosage adjustment is recommended for patients with severe renal insufficiency or end-stage renal disease (creatinine clearance <30 mL/minute).

● Common Adverse Effects

Adverse effects reported in ≥5% of patients receiving anakinra for rheumatoid arthritis include injection site reaction, worsening of rheumatoid arthritis, upper respiratory tract infection, headache, nausea, diarrhea, sinusitis, influenza-like symptoms, and abdominal pain.

Adverse effects reported in >10% of patients receiving anakinra for NOMID included injection site reaction, headache, vomiting, arthralgia, pyrexia, and nasopharyngitis.

Adverse effects reported in patients receiving anakinra for DIRA included upper respiratory tract infections, rash, pyrexia, influenza-like illness, and gastroenteritis.

DRUG INTERACTIONS

Anakinra has been used concomitantly with methotrexate, sulfasalazine, hydroxychloroquine, gold, penicillamine, leflunomide, and/or azathioprine in clinical studies of rheumatoid arthritis. Specific drug interactions have not been evaluated in humans.

● TNF Blocking Agents

An increased incidence of serious infections and an increased risk of neutropenia have been observed when anakinra and etanercept were used concomitantly in patients with rheumatoid arthritis. In a 24-week clinical trial, therapy with anakinra and etanercept did not result in additional clinical benefit compared with etanercept alone. Concomitant use of anakinra and TNF blocking agents (e.g., adalimumab, etanercept, infliximab) is not recommended.

● *Abatacept*

Clinical experience is insufficient to establish the safety and efficacy of concomitant use of anakinra and abatacept. Concomitant use of anakinra and abatacept is not recommended.

● *Methotrexate*

Although anakinra has been administered concurrently with methotrexate in clinical studies, specific drug interactions with anakinra have not been evaluated in humans. Studies in rats have not demonstrated any effect on the clearance or toxicologic profile of either anakinra or methotrexate when the 2 drugs were administered concurrently.

● *Vaccines*

Live-virus vaccines should not be administered to patients receiving anakinra. Information is not available regarding whether anakinra would affect the rate of secondary transmission of vaccine virus following administration of a live virus vaccine or regarding the effects of vaccination with live virus vaccine in patients receiving the drug.

In one placebo-controlled study, immunologic response to tetanus toxoid was preserved in individuals receiving anakinra concomitantly with diphtheria and tetanus toxoids. Information is not available regarding the effects of vaccination with other inactivated vaccines in patients receiving anakinra.

DESCRIPTION

Anakinra, a biosynthetic (recombinant DNA origin) form of human interleukin-1 (IL-1) receptor antagonist (IL-1Ra), is a biologic response modifier. Anakinra (rHuIL-1Ra) is prepared from cultures of genetically modified *Escherichia coli* using recombinant DNA technology and differs from native human IL-1Ra by the addition of a single methionine residue at its amino terminus.

Anakinra blocks the biologic activity of naturally occurring IL-1 alpha and beta, including inflammation and cartilage degradation associated with rheumatoid arthritis, by competitively inhibiting the binding of IL-1 to the interleukin-1 type I receptor (IL-1RI), which is expressed in many tissues and organs. IL-1 is produced in response to inflammatory stimuli and mediates various physiologic responses, including inflammatory and immunologic responses. IL-1 also stimulates bone resorption and induces cartilage degradation as a result of loss of proteoglycans. In patients with rheumatoid arthritis, naturally occurring IL-1Ra is not present in adequate concentrations in synovium and synovial fluid to compete with the elevated IL-1 concentrations in these patients.

Most patients with cryopyrin-associated periodic syndromes (CAPS) such as neonatal-onset multisystem inflammatory disease (NOMID) have spontaneous mutations in the CIAS1/NLRP3 gene which encodes for cryopyrin (an inflammasome component). The systemic inflammation and manifestations of NOMID are controlled in part by the activated inflammasome causing proteolytic maturation and IL-1β secretion.

In patients with the autosomal recessive monogenic autoinflammatory disease called deficiency of IL-1 receptor antagonist (DIRA), mutations in the IL1RN gene cause loss of secretion of the IL-1 receptor antagonist. When IL-1 receptor antagonist levels are insufficient, unopposed IL-1α and IL-1β pro-inflammatory signaling causes systemic inflammation, including in the skin and bone.

Following subcutaneous administration of anakinra in healthy subjects, the bioavailability is 95% and peak plasma concentrations are attained within

3–7 hours. No unexpected accumulation after daily subcutaneous dosing has been observed in patients with rheumatoid arthritis who were treated for up to 24 weeks. The terminal half-life of anakinra is 4–6 hours in patients with rheumatoid arthritis. The median half-life of anakinra in NOMID patients is 5.7 hours (range: 3.1–28.2 hours).

ADVICE TO PATIENTS

- Provide patient with a copy of manufacturer's patient information.
- Advise patient to inform clinician about existing or recurrent infections prior to initiating therapy.
- Instruct patient and/or caregiver regarding proper dosage and administration of anakinra. Assess the patient's ability to inject subcutaneously for proper anakinra administration. Discuss proper disposal of and caution against reuse of needles, syringes, and drug product. Provide or advise patient to obtain a puncture-resistant container for disposal of used syringes.
- Advise patient and/or caregiver about recognition and reporting of adverse effects of anakinra (e.g., hypersensitivity reactions, infection). Advise patients with deficiency of interleukin-1 receptor antagonist (DIRA) and their caregivers that patients may have a higher risk of allergic reactions, particularly in the first several weeks of treatment, and that they should be monitored closely.
- Advise patients of the risk of developing an injection-site reaction, which may include pain, erythema, swelling, pruritus, bruising, mass, inflammation, dermatitis, edema, urticaria, vesicles, warmth, and hemorrhage. Advise patients or their caregivers to remove the prefilled syringe from refrigeration and leave at room temperature for 30 minutes before injecting. Advise patients to avoid injecting into areas that are already swollen or red. Advise patients to report any persistent injection-site reaction to their clinician.
- Advise women to inform their clinicians if they are or plan to become pregnant or plan to breast-feed.
- Advise patients to inform their clinicians of existing or contemplated concomitant therapy, including prescription and OTC drugs.
- Inform patients of other important precautionary information. (See Cautions.)

PREPARATIONS

Excipients in commercially available drug preparations may have clinically important effects in some individuals; consult specific product labeling for details.

Anakinra (Recombinant DNA Origin)

Parenteral

Injection, for subcutaneous use	100 mg/0.67 mL	Kineret® (preservative-free; available in prefilled disposable syringes), Swedish Orphan Biovitrum AB

† Use is not currently included in the labeling approved by the US Food and Drug Administration.

Selected Revisions May 10, 2024, © Copyright, March 1, 2002, American Society of Health-System Pharmacists, Inc.

Ixekizumab

90:24.20.92 • INTERLEUKIN-MEDIATED AGENTS, MISCELLANEOUS

■ Ixekizumab, a recombinant humanized immunoglobulin G_4 kappa (IgG_4 kappa) monoclonal antibody, binds specifically to and inhibits the biologic activity of interleukin-17A (IL-17A), a proinflammatory cytokine.

USES

● Plaque Psoriasis

Plaque Psoriasis in Adults

Ixekizumab is used for the management of moderate to severe plaque psoriasis in adult patients who are candidates for phototherapy or systemic therapy. Safety and efficacy of ixekizumab for this use are based principally on the results from 3 randomized controlled trials (UNCOVER-1, UNCOVER-2, and UNCOVER-3), with additional support from other randomized controlled trials and long-term extension studies. Guidelines generally support the use of IL-17 blocking agents as monotherapy for treatment of moderate to severe psoriasis.

Clinical Experience

In 3 randomized, double-blind, placebo-controlled multicenter studies (UNCOVER-1, UNCOVER-2, and UNCOVER-3), 3866 adults were enrolled who had plaque psoriasis with body surface area (BSA) involvement of ≥10%, a static Physician Global Assessment (sPGA) score ≥3, and a Psoriasis Area and Severity (PASI) score ≥12, and who were candidates for phototherapy or systemic therapy. The PASI is a composite score that takes into consideration both the fraction of body surface area affected and the nature and severity of the psoriatic changes within the affected areas (i.e., induration, erythema, scaling); sPGA measures the clinician's impression of disease severity (i.e., plaque thickness/induration, erythema, scaling) at a single time point. Included patients were randomized to receive ixekizumab 80 mg every 2 weeks, ixekizumab 80 mg every 4 weeks, etanercept 50 mg twice weekly (UNCOVER-2 and UNCOVER-3 only), or placebo for 12 weeks. In all 3 studies, those randomized to receive ixekizumab received an initial dose of 160 mg of the drug. Upon completion of the 12-week induction period, patients in UNCOVER-1 and UNCOVER-2 who initially received ixekizumab and had an sPGA score of 0 (clear) or 1 (minimal disease) at week 12 were entered into a randomized withdrawal period (weeks 12–60) and received ixekizumab 80 mg every 4 weeks, ixekizumab 80 mg every 12 weeks, or placebo. In UNCOVER-3, all patients who completed the 12-week induction period were eligible to receive maintenance therapy with ixekizumab every 4 weeks through week 60.

Across the 3 studies, the median baseline PASI score was approximately 17 or 18 in each treatment group, and approximately one-half of patients had a baseline sPGA score of 4 or 5, indicating severe or very severe disease; 23% of patients had a history of psoriatic arthritis. Prior therapy for psoriasis included phototherapy, conventional systemic therapy, or biologic therapy in 44, 49, or 26%, respectively, of patients. Of those who had received prior biologic therapy, 15% had received at least one tumor necrosis factor (TNF; TNF-α) blocking agent, and 9% had received an agent with activity against interleukin-12 (IL-12) and interleukin-23 (IL-23).

Primary measures of efficacy in all 3 studies were the proportion of patients who achieved a reduction in PASI score of at least 75% (PASI 75) and the proportion of patients who attained an sPGA score of 0 or 1 (with a minimum 2-point improvement in the score) from baseline to week 12. Other measures of efficacy assessed the proportion of patients attaining higher levels of response: sPGA score of 0 and a reduction of at least 90% or of 100% in PASI score (PASI 90 or PASI 100, respectively).

A greater proportion of patients receiving ixekizumab (80 mg every 2 or 4 weeks) achieved a PASI 75 response and an sPGA score of 0 or 1 at week 12 compared with those receiving placebo (all 3 studies) or etanercept (UNCOVER-2 and UNCOVER-3). At week 12, PASI 75 response was attained in 87–90, 78–84, 42–53, or 2–7% of those receiving ixekizumab every 2 weeks, ixekizumab every 4 weeks, etanercept, or placebo, respectively, and an sPGA score of 0 or 1 was attained in 81–83, 73–76, 36–42, or 2–7% of patients in these respective treatment groups.

In addition, greater proportions of patients receiving ixekizumab (80 mg every 2 or 4 weeks) achieved a PASI 90 or 100 response or an sPGA score of 0 at week 12 compared with those receiving placebo (all 3 studies) or etanercept (UNCOVER-2 and UNCOVER-3). At week 12, PASI 90 response was attained in 68–71, 60–65, 19–26, or 1–3% of those receiving ixekizumab every 2 weeks, ixekizumab every 4 weeks, etanercept, or placebo, respectively, while PASI 100 response was attained in 35–41, 31–35, 5–7, or 0–1% of patients in these respective treatment groups. An sPGA score of 0 was attained in 37–42, 32–36, 6–9, or 0–1% of patients in these respective treatment groups. Greater proportions of patients receiving ixekizumab also experienced reductions in pruritus compared with those receiving placebo or etanercept.

Subgroup analyses revealed no differences in response to ixekizumab at 12 weeks based on age, gender, race, body weight, or prior therapy with a biologic agent.

Response to ixekizumab generally was maintained over 60 weeks of treatment when the 12-week induction regimen was followed by 48 weeks of maintenance therapy administered every 4 weeks. Analysis of pooled data from UNCOVER-1 and UNCOVER-2 indicated that, among patients who achieved an sPGA score of 0 or 1 upon completion of 12 weeks of ixekizumab induction therapy (every 2 or 4 weeks), 74, 39, or 7% of those who subsequently received maintenance therapy with ixekizumab every 4 weeks, ixekizumab every 12 weeks, or placebo maintained such response at week 60 of the study; response was maintained at week 60 by 78% of those who received ixekizumab 80 mg every 2 weeks for 12 weeks followed by 80 mg every 4 weeks and by 69% of those who received ixekizumab 80 mg every 4 weeks throughout the 60-week study. Patterns of PASI 75 response were similar. Among patients who responded to ixekizumab induction therapy and subsequently received placebo, the median time to relapse (sPGA score of 3 or greater) was 164 days; 66% of these patients regained an sPGA response of 0 or 1 within 12 weeks of reinitiation of therapy with ixekizumab 80 mg every 4 weeks. In UNCOVER-3, PASI 75 and sPGA 0 or 1 responses observed upon completion of ixekizumab induction therapy generally were maintained during an additional 48 weeks of maintenance therapy with ixekizumab 80 mg every 4 weeks. Responses seen in UNCOVER-1, UNCOVER-2, and UNCOVER-3 were sustained through 5 years of treatment. Pooled PASI 75, 90, and 100 responses from UNCOVER-1 and UNCOVER-2 were 90.3, 71.3, and 46.3%, respectively, at 5 years. At 5 years, PASI 75, 90, and 100 responses from UNCOVER-3 were 90.7, 75.9, and 51.9%, respectively.

In a fourth randomized, double-blind, placebo-controlled study (IXORA-Q), 149 adults with moderate to severe overall and genital plaque psoriasis (sPGA and sPGA of Genitalia [sPGA-G] scores of 3 or greater) were randomized to receive ixekizumab (initial dose of 160 mg, followed by 80 mg every 2 weeks) or placebo for 12 weeks; patients enrolled in the study were candidates for phototherapy or systemic therapy and had an inadequate response or intolerance to prior topical therapy for genital psoriasis. The median baseline PASI score was approximately 12, approximately 60% of patients had involvement of at least 10% of the body surface area, 42% had a baseline sPGA-G score indicating severe or very severe genital psoriasis, and 47% had a baseline sPGA score indicating severe or very severe overall psoriasis. At week 12, a score of 0 (clear) or 1 (minimal disease) was attained on the sPGA-G by 73 or 8% of patients receiving ixekizumab or placebo, respectively, and on the sPGA by 73 or 3% of patients receiving these respective treatments. In addition, greater proportions of patients receiving ixekizumab compared with those receiving placebo reported improvement (reduction in score of at least 4 points from baseline) on the 11-point Genital Psoriasis Symptoms Scale (GPSS) Itch numeric rating scale (55 versus 6% of those with a baseline score of at least 4) and reported that genital psoriasis never or rarely limited the frequency of sexual activity (score of 0 or 1 on item 2 of the Genital Psoriasis Sexual Frequency Questionnaire) during the prior week (78 versus 21% of those with a baseline score of at least 2 [sometimes limited the frequency of sexual activity]).

Ixekizumab has been compared to guselkumab and ustekinumab in adults with moderate to severe plaque psoriasis. In the IXORA-R randomized controlled trial, ixekizumab was superior to guselkumab in terms of PASI 100 response (defined as a PASI score improvement of 100% [complete clearance of psoriasis] compared with baseline) at week 12. At 24 weeks, results from IXORA-R showed that ixekizumab was noninferior to guselkumab in regard to the PASI 100 response rate. In the IXORA-S study, ixekizumab was compared to ustekinumab in patients with psoriasis who had previously failed or had a contraindication to a systemic therapy. Ixekizumab was both noninferior and superior to ustekinumab for PASI 90 response at 12 weeks, and was superior to ustekinumab in terms of PASI 90 response at 24 weeks. The superior response with ixekizumab compared to ustekinumab was maintained at week 52.

Clinical Perspective

The American Academy of Dermatology and the National Psoriasis Foundation have issued joint guidelines for the treatment of psoriasis in adults. Various drugs and drug classes are used to treat psoriasis. Phototherapy and topical treatments (e.g., vitamin D analogues, calcineurin inhibitors, keratolytics, and corticosteroids) are frequently used to treat mild psoriasis present on limited areas of the body, but these therapies may be inadequate to obtain skin clearance in patients with more extensive or severe disease. Systemic biologic and nonbiologic therapies are mainstays of treatment for moderate to severe psoriasis, and may also be useful for treating psoriasis on parts of the body that are difficult to treat with topical therapy (e.g., scalp, palms and soles of the feet, genitals). Topical therapies can be used adjunctively in moderate to severe disease. Nonbiologic oral therapies used in the treatment of psoriasis include methotrexate, apremilast, cyclosporine, acitretin, and dimethyl fumarate. Biologics used in the treatment of psoriasis include TNF blocking agents, ustekinumab, secukinumab, ixekizumab, brodalumab, guselkumab, tildrakizumab, and risankizumab. Treatment selection in psoriasis is primarily based on disease characteristics (e.g., severity, location, presence of psoriatic arthritis), with additional consideration being given to patient age and comorbidities.

The interleukin (IL)-17 blocking agents used in the treatment of psoriasis include secukinumab, ixekizumab, and brodalumab. These IL-17 blocking agents are recommended as monotherapy for the treatment of adult patients with moderate to severe plaque psoriasis. Recommendations for the use and selection of psoriasis therapies vary based on patient age, disease characteristics (e.g., severity, location, presence of psoriatic arthritis), and comorbidities (e.g., inflammatory bowel disease). Consult the American Academy of Dermatology/National Psoriasis Foundation guidelines for additional details.

Plaque Psoriasis in Pediatric Patients

Ixekizumab is used for the management of moderate to severe plaque psoriasis in pediatric patients ≥6 years of age who are candidates for phototherapy or systemic therapy. Safety and efficacy of ixekizumab for this use are based principally on the results from a single randomized controlled trial (IXORA-PEDS). Guidelines have not yet incorporated recommendations for use of IL-17 blocking agents, including ixekizumab, for the treatment of pediatric plaque psoriasis.

Clinical Experience

The efficacy and safety of ixekizumab in the management of plaque psoriasis were evaluated in a 108-week randomized, double-blind, multicenter, placebo-controlled study (IXORA-PEDS) conducted in pediatric patients ≥6 years of age with moderate to severe plaque psoriasis (defined as sPGA score ≥3, BSA involvement ≥10%, and PASI score ≥12) who were candidates for systemic therapy or phototherapy, or who failed treatment with topical agents. During the initial 12-week double-blind treatment phase, 171 patients were randomized to placebo or ixekizumab; patients weighing <25 kg received 40 mg of ixekizumab at week 0, then 20 mg every 4 weeks, patients weighing 25–50 kg received ixekizumab 80 mg at week 0, then 40 mg every 4 weeks, and patients weighing >50 kg received 160 mg at week 0, then 80 mg every 4 weeks. Following a protocol amendment, an open-label etanercept reference arm was added; patients in this arm received etanercept 0.8 mg/kg once weekly (maximum 50 mg per dose). After the 12-week double-blind period, patients entered a 48-week maintenance period where all patients received ixekizumab once every 4 weeks.

The primary end points were the proportion of patients who achieved a PASI 75 response and the proportion who achieved an sPGA score of 0 or 1, both measured from baseline to 12 weeks. At baseline, the median PASI score was 17 and 49% of patients had an sPGA score indicating severe or very severe disease; 22% of patients had previously received phototherapy and 32% had received conventional systemic therapy for psoriasis.

At week 12, PASI 75 response rates and sPGA response of 0 or 1, respectively, were significantly higher with ixekizumab dosed every 4 weeks (89 and 81%)

compared to placebo (25 and 11%). Significant improvements were also noted in the PASI 90 and 100 response rate, sPGA response of 0, and itch numeric rating scale for ixekizumab compared to placebo at week 12. PASI 75 and sPGA responses of 0 or 1 were not significantly different between patients treated with etanercept or ixekizumab.

Clinical Perspective

The American Academy of Dermatology and the National Psoriasis Foundation issued joint guidelines for the treatment of psoriasis in pediatric patients in 2019. Various drugs and drug classes are used to treat pediatric psoriasis. Phototherapy and topical treatments (e.g., vitamin D analogues, calcineurin inhibitors, corticosteroids, tazarotene, anthralin, coal tar) are frequently used to treat mild psoriasis present on limited areas of the body, but these therapies may be inadequate to obtain skin clearance in patients with more extensive or severe disease. Systemic biologic and nonbiologic therapies are mainstays of treatment for moderate to severe psoriasis, and may also be useful for treating psoriasis on parts of the body that are difficult to treat with topical therapy (e.g., the scalp, palms and soles of the feet, genitals). Topical therapies can be used adjunctively in moderate to severe disease. Nonbiologic oral therapies used in the treatment of pediatric psoriasis include methotrexate, cyclosporine, acitretin, and fumaric acid esters. Biologics recommended for use in pediatric psoriasis include TNF blocking agents (etanercept, adalimumab, infliximab) and ustekinumab. Other biologic agents used in pediatric psoriasis include secukinumab and ixekizumab. Treatment selection in psoriasis is primarily based on disease characteristics (e.g., severity, location, presence of psoriatic arthritis), with additional consideration being given to patient age and comorbidities.

Current guidelines do not address the place in therapy for IL-17 blocking agents in the treatment of psoriasis in pediatric patients. The current guidelines for pediatric psoriasis are based on literature evaluation through 2017; thus, recommendations for use of IL-17 blocking agents have not yet been incorporated.

• Psoriatic Arthritis

Ixekizumab is used for the management of active psoriatic arthritis in adults. Safety and efficacy of ixekizumab for this use are based principally on the results from 2 randomized controlled trials (SPIRIT-P1 and SPIRIT-P2), with additional support from randomized controlled trials and long-term extension studies. Guidelines generally support the use of the IL-17 blocking agents as second-line therapy after TNF blocking agents for treatment of psoriatic arthritis.

Clinical Experience

Efficacy of ixekizumab for this indication is supported by 2 randomized, double-blind, placebo-controlled studies (SPIRIT-P1, SPIRIT-P2) in adults with active psoriatic arthritis. In SPIRIT-P1, 417 patients who had never received biologic therapy for psoriatic arthritis or plaque psoriasis were randomized to receive ixekizumab (initial dose of 160 mg, followed by 80 mg every 2 or 4 weeks), adalimumab (40 mg every 2 weeks), or placebo. In SPIRIT-P2, 363 patients with active psoriatic arthritis and either active plaque psoriasis or a history of plaque psoriasis who had an inadequate response or intolerance to prior TNF blocking agent therapy were randomized to receive ixekizumab (initial dose of 160 mg, followed by 80 mg every 2 or 4 weeks) or placebo; all patients in SPIRIT-P2 also had received prior therapy with one or more conventional (nonbiologic) DMARDs. Patients in these studies could receive stable dosages of nonsteroidal anti-inflammatory agents (NSAIAs), analgesics, oral corticosteroids, conventional DMARDs, and/or low-potency topical corticosteroids. If response was inadequate at week 16, concomitant therapy was added or modified and those receiving adalimumab or placebo were rerandomized to receive ixekizumab every 2 or 4 weeks; these patients were considered nonresponders to their initially assigned treatment. Approximately 47% of patients in the 2 studies received concomitant methotrexate therapy.

The principal measure of efficacy in both studies was the proportion of patients achieving an American College of Rheumatology (ACR) 20 response at week 24. An ACR 20 response is achieved if the patient experiences a 20% or greater improvement in tender and swollen joint count and a 20% or greater improvement in at least 3 of the following criteria: patient pain assessment, patient global assessment, physician global assessment, patient self-assessed disability, or laboratory measures of disease activity (i.e., erythrocyte sedimentation rate [ESR] or C-reactive protein [CRP] level). An ACR 50 or ACR 70 response is defined using the same criteria but with a level of improvement of 50 or 70%, respectively.

Ixekizumab induced clinical responses, as assessed by ACR criteria, regardless of prior treatment with TNF blocking agents. (See Table 1.) ACR 20 responses were achieved at week 24 in 62 or 58% of patients in SPIRIT-P1 who received ixekizumab every 2 or every 4 weeks, respectively, and in 48 or 53% of patients in SPIRIT-P2 who received ixekizumab every 2 or every 4 weeks, respectively.

TABLE 1. Proportion of Patients with Psoriatic Arthritis Achieving Clinical Responses in the SPIRIT-P1 and SPIRIT-P2 Studies

Response Measure at Week 24	Ixekizumab (80 mg every 4 weeks) vs Placebo in SPIRIT-P1	Ixekizumab (80 mg every 4 weeks) vs Placebo in SPIRIT-P2
ACR 20	58 vs 30%	53 vs 20%
ACR 50	40 vs 15%	35 vs 5%
ACR 70	23 vs 6%	22 vs 0%

In both studies, ixekizumab improved physical functioning, as measured by change in Health Assessment Questionnaire–Disability Index (HAQ-DI) score, from baseline to week 12 and week 24 and improved dactylitis, enthesitis, and psoriatic skin lesions in patients with these manifestations of the disease.

Assessment of the progression of structural joint damage also was performed in SPIRIT-P1 and indicated that ixekizumab inhibited progression, as measured by change in van der Heijde modified total Sharp score (a composite measure of radiographically assessed structural damage [i.e., joint erosion and joint space narrowing]), from baseline to week 16.

Clinical improvements seen in SPIRIT-P1 and SPIRIT-P2 were maintained with continued treatment with ixekizumab over 3 years. In a long-term extension of the SPIRIT-P1 study, ACR 20 responses were sustained in 62.5% of patients who received ixekizumab every 2 weeks and 69.8% of patients who received ixekizumab every 4 weeks. In a long-term extension of the SPIRIT-P2 study, ACR 20 responses were sustained in 84.9 and 83.6% of patients who received ixekizumab every 2 weeks and every 4 weeks, respectively, at 3 years.

A randomized controlled trial has compared ixekizumab to adalimumab for the treatment of psoriatic arthritis. The SPIRIT-H2H trial compared ixekizumab to adalimumab in biologic-naive patients with active psoriatic arthritis and inadequate response to conventional synthetic DMARDs. In this trial, the primary endpoint of simultaneous ACR 50 and PASI 100 response at week 24 was achieved in substantially more patients receiving ixekizumab compared to adalimumab; this between-group difference remained significant at week 52.

Clinical Perspective

The American College of Rheumatology and the National Psoriasis Foundation issued a joint guideline for the treatment of psoriatic arthritis in 2018. Various drugs and drug classes are used to treat psoriatic arthritis, with some classes being used for symptom management (e.g., NSAIAs and corticosteroids) and others being used as immunomodulatory disease-modifying therapy. Disease-modifying treatments for psoriatic arthritis include oral small molecules (OSMs; e.g., methotrexate, sulfasalazine, cyclosporine, leflunomide, apremilast), biologic DMARDs (e.g., TNF blocking agents, secukinumab, ixekizumab, ustekinumab, brodalumab, abatacept), and/or targeted synthetic DMARDs (e.g., tofacitinib). Specific agents for psoriatic arthritis treatment are selected according to disease characteristics, including disease severity, as well as patient preferences/values and comorbidities. A "treat-to-target" approach is typically employed, with the goal of achieving low/minimal disease activity or remission.

The IL-17 blocking agents used in the treatment of psoriatic arthritis are secukinumab, ixekizumab, and brodalumab. For patients with treatment-naive psoriatic arthritis, treatment with a TNF blocking agent or an OSM is conditionally recommended over treatment with secukinumab, ixekizumab, or brodalumab. Secukinumab, ixekizumab, or brodalumab may be considered in place of these therapies in patients with severe psoriasis or psoriatic arthritis, or with contraindications to TNF blocking agents. Treatment with secukinumab, ixekizumab, or brodalumab is conditionally recommended over treatment with ustekinumab for treatment-naive psoriatic arthritis. For patients with active psoriatic arthritis despite treatment with an OSM, switching to a TNF blocking agent

is conditionally recommended over treatment with secukinumab, ixekizumab, or brodalumab. Switching to secukinumab, ixekizumab, or brodalumab monotherapy is conditionally recommended over treatment with a different OSM, ustekinumab, abatacept, or tofacitinib. For patients with active psoriatic arthritis despite treatment with TNF blocking agent monotherapy, switching to monotherapy with a different TNF blocking agent is conditionally recommended over switching to secukinumab, ixekizumab, or brodalumab. Switching to secukinumab, ixekizumab, or brodalumab is conditionally recommended over switching to ustekinumab, abatacept, or tofacitinib. For patients with active psoriatic arthritis despite treatment with a combination of a TNF blocking agent and methotrexate, switching to secukinumab, ixekizumab, or brodalumab monotherapy is conditionally recommended over switching to combination therapy with these agents plus methotrexate. In patients with active psoriatic arthritis despite treatment with secukinumab, ixekizumab, or brodalumab, switching to a TNF blocking agent is conditionally recommended over switching to a different IL-17 blocking agent and over adding methotrexate to an IL-17 blocking agent. In patients with active psoriatic arthritis despite treatment with ustekinumab, switching to a TNF blocking agent is conditionally recommended over switching to secukinumab, ixekizumab, or brodalumab and over adding methotrexate to an IL-17 blocking agent. Recommendations for the use and selection of disease-modifying therapies in psoriatic arthritis vary based on the presence of certain disease characteristics (e.g., psoriatic spondylitis/axial disease, enthesitis) and comorbidities (e.g., inflammatory bowel disease, diabetes). Consult the American College of Rheumatology/National Psoriasis Foundation guideline for additional details.

● **Ankylosing Spondylitis**

Ixekizumab is used for the management of active ankylosing spondylitis (also referred to as radiographic axial spondyloarthritis) in adults. Safety and efficacy of ixekizumab for this use are based principally on the results from 2 randomized controlled trials (COAST-V and COAST-W). Guidelines generally support the use of IL-17 inhibitors as second-line therapy after TNF blocking agents for the treatment of ankylosing spondylitis in patients with active disease despite treatment with NSAIAs.

Clinical Experience

Efficacy of ixekizumab for this indication is supported by 2 randomized, double-blind, placebo-controlled studies (COAST-V, COAST-W) in adults with active ankylosing spondylitis. In COAST-V, 341 patients who had never received biologic therapy for ankylosing spondylitis were randomized to receive ixekizumab (initial dose of 80 or 160 mg, followed by 80 mg every 2 or 4 weeks), adalimumab (40 mg every 2 weeks), or placebo. In COAST-W, 316 patients who had an inadequate response or intolerance to prior therapy with 1 or 2 TNF blocking agents were randomized to receive ixekizumab (initial dose of 80 or 160 mg, followed by 80 mg every 2 or 4 weeks) or placebo. Patients in these studies could receive stable dosages of NSAIAs, analgesics, oral corticosteroids, and conventional DMARDs (sulfasalazine, methotrexate). Approximately 32% of patients in the 2 studies received concomitant therapy with a conventional DMARD.

The primary outcome measure was the proportion of patients achieving an Assessment of Spondyloarthritis International Society (ASAS) 40 response at week 16. An ASAS 40 response is achieved if the patient experiences at least a 40% improvement and an absolute improvement of at least 2 units (on a scale of 0–10) in at least 3 of the following criteria with no worsening in the fourth criterion: patient global assessment, spinal pain, function, and inflammation. An ASAS 20 response is defined using the same criteria but with a level of improvement of at least 20% and an absolute improvement of at least 1 unit in at least 3 of the criteria and with no worsening of 20% or more or 1 or more units in the fourth criterion.

Ixekizumab induced clinical responses, as assessed by ASAS criteria, regardless of concomitant use of conventional DMARDs or prior treatment with TNF blocking agents, although response rates tended to be lower in those with a history of treatment failure with TNF blocking agents. (See Table 2.) ASAS 40 responses were achieved at week 16 in 52 or 48% of patients in COAST-V who received ixekizumab every 2 or every 4 weeks, respectively, and in 31 or 25% of patients in COAST-W who received ixekizumab every 2 or every 4 weeks, respectively. Ixekizumab also improved other secondary measures of disease activity and physical functioning compared with placebo.

TABLE 2. Proportion of Patients with Ankylosing Spondylitis Achieving Clinical Responses in the COAST-V and COAST-W Studies

Response Measure at Week 16	Ixekizumab (80 mg every 4 weeks) vs Placebo in COAST-V	Ixekizumab (80 mg every 4 weeks) vs Placebo in COAST-W
ASAS 20	64 vs 40%	48 vs 30%
ASAS 40	48 vs 18%	25 vs 13%

Results of a double-blind extension of COAST-V and COAST-W, in which patients who had received ixekizumab for 16 weeks continued their assigned treatment and those who had received adalimumab or placebo were rerandomized to receive ixekizumab every 2 or 4 weeks, indicated that responses generally were maintained through up to 52 weeks of treatment with the drug.

Clinical Perspective

The American College of Rheumatology, the Spondylitis Association of America, and the Spondyloarthritis Research and Treatment Network issued a joint guideline for the treatment of ankylosing spondylitis in 2019. Treatments for ankylosing spondylitis include NSAIAs, conventional DMARDs (e.g., methotrexate, sulfasalazine), biologic DMARDs (e.g., TNF blocking agents, secukinumab, ixekizumab), and/or targeted synthetic DMARDs (e.g., tofacitinib). Continuous NSAIA treatment is typically considered first-line for active ankylosing spondylitis, with other agents used in the treatment of NSAIA-refractory disease. Specific agents for ankylosing spondylitis treatment are selected according to current disease activity, prior therapies, and the presence of comorbidities. Goals of therapy in ankylosing spondylitis are to alleviate symptoms, improve functioning, maintain the ability to work, decrease complications, and prevent or slow skeletal damage.

The IL-17 blocking agents used in the treatment of ankylosing spondylitis are secukinumab and ixekizumab. For adults with active ankylosing spondylitis despite treatment with NSAIAs, treatment with a TNF blocking agent is conditionally recommended over treatment with secukinumab or ixekizumab. In these patients, secukinumab or ixekizumab is strongly recommended over no treatment with these drugs, and conditionally recommended over treatment with tofacitinib. In adults with active ankylosing spondylitis despite treatment with NSAIAs and contraindications to treatment with a TNF blocking agent, secukinumab or ixekizumab is conditionally recommended over treatment with sulfasalazine, methotrexate, or tofacitinib. In adults with active ankylosing spondylitis despite treatment with a first TNF blocking agent, guidelines conditionally recommend secukinumab or ixekizumab over treatment with a different TNF blocking agent in patients with primary nonresponse to TNF blocking therapy. In adults with stable ankylosing spondylitis, continuation of biologic monotherapy is conditionally recommended over discontinuation of the biologic or continuation of combination therapy with NSAIAs or conventional DMARDs. Recommendations for treatment selection in ankylosing spondylitis may be influenced by the presence of certain comorbidities (e.g., iritis, inflammatory bowel disease). Consult the joint guideline issued by the American College of Rheumatology, the Spondylitis Association of America, and the Spondyloarthritis Research and Treatment Network for additional details.

● *Nonradiographic Axial Spondyloarthritis*

Ixekizumab is used for the management of active nonradiographic axial spondyloarthritis in adults with objective signs of inflammation. Safety and efficacy of ixekizumab for this use are based principally on the results from a single randomized controlled trial (COAST-X). Guidelines generally support the use of IL-17 inhibitors as second-line therapy after TNF blocking agents for the treatment of nonradiographic axial spondyloarthritis in patients with active disease despite treatment with NSAIAs.

Clinical Experience

Safety and efficacy of ixekizumab for this indication were evaluated in a multicenter randomized, double-blind, placebo-controlled, 52-week study (COAST-X) in 303 adults with active axial spondyloarthritis according to ASAS criteria and objective signs of inflammation (i.e., active sacroiliitis on magnetic resonance imaging [MRI] and/or C-reactive protein [CRP] >5 mg/L) despite treatment with at least 2 NSAIAs. Included patients were also required to have symptoms of active disease, which were defined by a Bath Ankylosing Spondylitis Disease Activity Index (BASDAI) score of ≥4 and a score of ≥4 for spinal pain on a 0 to 10 scale.

Patients were randomized at week 0 (stratified by country, MRI status, and CRP status) to receive subcutaneous ixekizumab 80 mg every 2 weeks†, ixekizumab 80 mg every 4 weeks, or matching placebo every 2 weeks. Patients assigned to receive ixekizumab were also randomly assigned to a starting dose of 80 mg or 160 mg of ixekizumab at week 0. After 16 weeks, patients with residual disease could have their nonbiologic background medications adjusted or could be switched to received open-label ixekizumab 80 mg every 2 weeks or TNF blockers at the investigators' discretion.

At baseline, patients had symptoms of nonradiographic axial spondyloarthritis for an average of 11 years and 39% were taking concomitant conventional DMARDs. The primary outcome measure was the proportion of patients achieving an ASAS 40 response at week 52. ASAS 40 was also assessed at week 16. At week 52, a greater proportion of patients who received ixekizumab achieved an ASAS 40 response compared with patients who received placebo; response rates were 30.2 and 13.3% in the ixekizumab every 4 weeks and placebo groups, respectively. ASAS 40 responses were also significantly higher at 52 weeks for ixekizumab given every 2 weeks compared to placebo. Substantially higher proportions of patients treated with ixekizumab every 2 weeks† or every 4 weeks achieved ASAS 40 response at 16 weeks compared to placebo.

Clinical Perspective

The American College of Rheumatology, the Spondylitis Association of America, and the Spondyloarthritis Research and Treatment Network issued a joint guideline for the treatment of nonradiographic axial spondyloarthritis in 2019. Treatments for nonradiographic axial spondyloarthritis include NSAIAs, conventional DMARDs (e.g., methotrexate, sulfasalazine), biologic DMARDs (e.g., TNF blocking agents, secukinumab, ixekizumab), and/or targeted synthetic DMARDs (e.g., tofacitinib). Continuous NSAIA treatment is typically considered first-line for active nonradiographic axial spondyloarthritis, with other agents being used in the treatment of NSAIA-refractory disease. Specific agents for nonradiographic axial spondyloarthritis treatment are selected according to current disease activity and prior therapies used. Goals of therapy in nonradiographic axial spondyloarthritis are to alleviate symptoms, improve functioning, maintain the ability to work, decrease complications, and prevent or slow skeletal damage.

Recommendations for the treatment of nonradiographic axial spondyloarthritis are largely extrapolated from evidence in the treatment of ankylosing spondylitis, due to a lack of data specific to nonradiographic axial spondyloarthritis. IL-17 blocking agents used in the treatment of ankylosing spondylitis (and, by extension, nonradiographic axial spondyloarthritis) are secukinumab and ixekizumab. (See Ankylosing Spondylitis under Uses.) Consult the joint guideline issued by the American College of Rheumatology, the Spondylitis Association of America, and the Spondyloarthritis Research and Treatment Network for additional details.

DOSAGE AND ADMINISTRATION

● *General*

Pretreatment Screening

* Evaluate for tuberculosis infection prior to initiation of ixekizumab. Do not administer to patients with active tuberculosis infection. Initiate antimycobacterial therapy of latent tuberculosis prior to administering ixekizumab. Consider antimycobacterial therapy prior to initiating ixekizumab in patients with a past history of latent or active tuberculosis in whom an adequate course of treatment cannot be confirmed.

* Administer all age-appropriate vaccines as recommended by current immunizaton guidelines prior to starting ixekizumab therapy.

Patient Monitoring

* Monitor closely for signs or symptoms of infection or active tuberculosis during and after treatment with ixekizumab.

* Monitor for signs and symptoms of inflammatory bowel disease during treatment.

Other General Considerations

- Ixekizumab may be used alone or in combination with conventional DMARDs (e.g., methotrexate) for the treatment of psoriatic arthritis.

● Administration

Administer ixekizumab by subcutaneous injection.

Ixekizumab is intended for use under the guidance and supervision of a clinician; however, the drug may be *self-administered* in adults if the clinician determines that the patient and/or their caregiver is competent to safely administer the drug after appropriate training. A caregiver may also administer ixekizumab to pediatric patients weighing >50 kg after appropriate training.

Administer subcutaneous injections into the upper arms, thighs, or any quadrant of the abdomen; avoid injections within 1 inch of the navel and rotate injection sites. Administration of ixekizumab into the upper outer arm may be performed by a caregiver or clinician. Administration of ixekizumab into the thigh has resulted in higher bioavailability compared with other injection sites, including the arm and abdomen. Do not administer injections into areas where the skin is tender, bruised, erythematous, indurated, or affected by psoriasis.

Ixekizumab injection is commercially available in prefilled autoinjectors and prefilled syringes. Ixekizumab injection is a clear, colorless to slightly yellow solution. Prior to administration, inspect the ixekizumab solution visually for particulate matter or discoloration; discard the solution if it is cloudy, discolored, or contains particulates. Ixekizumab autoinjectors and prefilled syringes are for single use only; discard any unused portions. The full amount (1 mL) of solution contained within the autoinjector or prefilled syringe, providing 80 mg of ixekizumab, should be injected.

Protect ixekizumab injection from light and store refrigerated at 2–8°C in the original carton prior to use; do not freeze or shake the injection. If necessary, ixekizumab injection may be stored at room temperature (up to 30°C) in the original carton for up to 5 days prior to use; after storage at room temperature, the injection should not be returned to a refrigerator and should be discarded if not used within 5 days. When packages containing multiple autoinjectors are used, only a single autoinjector should be removed from the package at one time; the remaining autoinjectors should be left in the original carton in the refrigerator.

Allow the autoinjector or prefilled syringe to sit at room temperature protected from light for 30 minutes prior to subcutaneous injection. The solution should not be warmed in a microwave, by running hot water over the autoinjector or syringe, or by exposing the injection to direct sunlight. Do not remove the base cap of the autoinjector or the needle cap of the syringe while the autoinjector or prefilled syringe is warming to room temperature.

Dose Preparation for Pediatric Patients Weighing ≤50 kg

Pediatric doses of ixekizumab must be prepared and administered by a healthcare professional. Use the 80 mg/1 mL prefilled syringe only to prepare the dose. The following supplies will also be needed: a 0.5 mL or 1 mL disposable syringe, a sterile needle for withdrawal of the drug, a 27-gauge sterile needle for administration, and a sterile, clear glass vial.

Expel the entire contents of the prefilled syringe into the sterile vial; do not shake or swirl the vial. Do not add any other drugs to the ixekizumab solution. Withdraw the appropriate dose of ixekizumab (0.25 mL for a 20-mg dose or 0.5 mL for a 40-mg dose) from the sterile vial using the disposable syringe and sterile needle. Remove the sterile needle from the syringe and replace it with the 27-gauge sterile needle prior to administration. If needed, the prepared dose of ixekizumab may be stored at room temperature for a maximum of 4 hours after first puncturing the sterile vial.

● Dosage

Adult Dosage

Plaque Psoriasis

For the management of moderate to severe plaque psoriasis in adults who are candidates for phototherapy or systemic therapy, the recommended dosage of ixekizumab is 160 mg (administered as two 80-mg subcutaneous injections) at week 0, followed by 80 mg at weeks 2, 4, 6, 8, 10, and 12, and then 80 mg every 4 weeks thereafter.

Psoriatic Arthritis

For the management of active psoriatic arthritis in adults, the recommended dosage of ixekizumab is 160 mg (administered as two 80-mg subcutaneous injections) at week 0, followed by 80 mg every 4 weeks thereafter.

Patients with coexisting psoriatic arthritis and moderate to severe plaque psoriasis should receive the dosage recommended for plaque psoriasis.

Ankylosing Spondylitis

For the management of active ankylosing spondylitis in adults, the recommended dosage of ixekizumab is 160 mg (administered as two 80-mg subcutaneous injections) at week 0, followed by 80 mg every 4 weeks thereafter.

Nonradiographic Axial Spondyloarthritis

For the management of active nonradiographic axial spondyloarthritis in adults, the recommended dosage of ixekizumab is 80 mg by subcutaneous injection every 4 weeks.

Pediatric Dosage

Plaque Psoriasis

For the management of moderate to severe plaque psoriasis in pediatric patients ≥6 years of age who weigh <25 kg, the recommended dosage of ixekizumab is 40 mg at week 0, followed by 20 mg once every 4 weeks by subcutaneous injection.

For the management of moderate to severe plaque psoriasis in pediatric patients ≥6 years of age who weigh 25–50 kg, the recommended dosage of ixekizumab is 80 mg at week 0, followed by 40 mg once every 4 weeks by subcutaneous injection.

For the management of moderate to severe plaque psoriasis in pediatric patients ≥6 years of age who weigh greater than 50 kg, the recommended dosage of ixekizumab is 160 mg (administered as two 80-mg subcutaneous injections) at week 0, followed by 80 mg once every 4 weeks by subcutaneous injection.

● Special Populations

Hepatic Impairment

The manufacturer makes no specific dosage recommendations for patients with hepatic impairment.

Renal Impairment

The manufacturer makes no specific dosage recommendations for patients with renal impairment.

Geriatric Patients

The manufacturer makes no specific dosage recommendations for geriatric patients.

CAUTIONS

● Contraindications

- History of serious hypersensitivity reactions (e.g., anaphylaxis) to ixekizumab or any ingredient in the formulation.

● Warnings/Precautions

Sensitivity Reactions

Hypersensitivity Reactions

Serious hypersensitivity reactions, including angioedema, urticaria, and anaphylaxis, have been reported in patients receiving ixekizumab. If a serious hypersensitivity reaction occurs, discontinue ixekizumab immediately and initiate appropriate supportive treatment.

Infectious Complications

Patients receiving ixekizumab may be at an increased risk of developing infections. During the 12-week, placebo-controlled period of clinical studies in adults with plaque psoriasis, higher rates (27 versus 23%) of infections (e.g., upper respiratory tract infections, oral candidiasis, conjunctivitis, tinea infections) were observed in patients receiving ixekizumab compared with those receiving placebo. An increased risk of infection also was observed in patients with pediatric psoriasis, psoriatic arthritis or ankylosing spondylitis, or nonradiographic axial spondyloarthritis receiving ixekizumab in placebo-controlled clinical studies.

During the 12-week, placebo-controlled period of clinical studies in patients with plaque psoriasis, no difference in the rate of serious infections (0.4%) was observed between ixekizumab-treated patients and placebo recipients. During weeks 13–60 (maintenance treatment period) of these studies, infections occurred in 57 or 32% of patients who received ixekizumab or placebo, respectively, and serious infections were reported in 0.9 or 0% of patients in these respective groups. Over the entire treatment period (weeks 0–60), infections occurred in 38 or 23% of patients with plaque psoriasis who received ixekizumab or placebo, respectively, and serious infections occurred in 0.7 or 0.4% of patients in these respective groups. Although neutropenia was reported in these studies in 11% of patients receiving ixekizumab compared with 3% of those receiving placebo, most cases of neutropenia were grade 1 or 2 in severity and neutropenia in ixekizumab-treated patients was not associated with an increased frequency of infection compared with that in placebo recipients.

If a serious infection develops or if an infection fails to respond to standard therapy, closely monitor the patient and discontinue ixekizumab until the infection has resolved.

Evaluate patients for tuberculosis prior to initiation of ixekizumab therapy. Do not administer the drug to patients with active tuberculosis infection; when indicated, an appropriate antimycobacterial regimen for treatment of latent tuberculosis should be initiated prior to administration of ixekizumab. Antimycobacterial therapy also should be considered prior to initiation of ixekizumab in patients with a history of latent or active tuberculosis in whom an adequate course of antimycobacterial treatment for these indications cannot be confirmed. Monitor patients closely for signs and symptoms of active tuberculosis during and after treatment with ixekizumab.

Inflammatory Bowel Disease

Crohn disease and ulcerative colitis, including exacerbations of these diseases, were reported more frequently in adults with plaque psoriasis receiving ixekizumab 80 mg every 2 weeks compared with those receiving placebo (0.1–0.2% versus 0%) during the 12-week, placebo-controlled period of clinical studies. Crohn disease occurred in 0.9% of pediatric patients with plaque psoriasis receiving ixekizumab, compared to none of the patients who received placebo in clinical studies. In addition, Crohn disease or ulcerative colitis, including exacerbations of these diseases, occurred in 3 patients receiving ixekizumab 80 mg every 4 weeks and in 1 patient receiving placebo during the 16-week, placebo-controlled period of clinical studies in adults with ankylosing spondylitis; these events were considered serious in 1 patient receiving ixekizumab and 1 patient receiving placebo.

Monitor patients for onset or exacerbation of inflammatory bowel disease. If inflammatory bowel disease occurs, discontinue ixekizumab and provide appropriate medical management.

Immunization

Administration of all age-appropriate vaccines recommended by current immunization guidelines should be considered prior to initiation of ixekizumab therapy. Live vaccines should be avoided during therapy with the drug. There are no available data to date regarding response to live vaccines in patients receiving ixekizumab.

Immunogenicity

As with all therapeutic proteins, there is potential for immunogenicity in patients who receive ixekizumab. In clinical studies in adults with plaque psoriasis, antibodies to ixekizumab were detected by week 12 of treatment in approximately 9% of patients receiving ixekizumab every 2 weeks and in approximately 22% of patients receiving the drug at the recommended dosage during the 60-week treatment period. Higher antibody titers were associated with decreasing drug concentrations and decreased clinical response. Neutralizing antibodies were detected during the 60-week treatment period in approximately 2% of patients receiving the drug at the recommended dosage (approximately 10% of those who tested positive for antibodies to the drug); neutralizing antibodies were associated with a reduction in drug concentrations and loss of efficacy. In clinical studies in

pediatric patients with plaque psoriasis, antibodies to ixekizumab were detected by week 12 of treatment in 18% of patients; neutralizing antibodies associated with low concentrations of ixekizumab were detected in 4% of patients. No conclusive evidence could be obtained on the potential association of neutralizing antibodies and clinical response and/or adverse events due to small number of pediatric patients in the study.

In patients with psoriatic arthritis receiving ixekizumab 80 mg every 4 weeks for up to 52 weeks, antibodies to the drug were detected in 11% of patients; neutralizing antibodies were detected in 8% of patients receiving the drug. In patients with ankylosing spondylitis receiving ixekizumab 80 mg every 4 weeks for up to 16 weeks, antibodies to the drug were detected in 5.2% of patients; neutralizing antibodies were detected in 1.5% of patients receiving the drug. In patients with nonradiographic axial spondyloarthritis receiving ixekizumab 80 mg every 4 weeks for up to 52 weeks, antibodies to the drug were detected in 8.9% of patients; no neutralizing antibodies were detected.

Specific Populations

Pregnancy

There are insufficient data from the published literature and the pharmacovigilance database to evaluate the risks of ixekizumab in pregnant women. Human immunoglobulin G (IgG) is known to cross the placenta, and ixekizumab crossed the placenta in monkeys. Thus, the potential exists for fetal exposure to the drug. An embryofetal development study in cynomolgus monkeys revealed no evidence of adverse developmental effects; however, when ixekizumab administration was continued until parturition, an increase in neonatal deaths was observed. No ixekizumab-related effects on functional or immunologic development were observed in the offspring from birth through 6 months of age.

Pregnant women exposed to ixekizumab are encouraged to enroll in the TALTZ Pregnancy Registry by calling 1-800-284-1695 or accessing the website at https://www.taltz.com.

Lactation

It is not known whether ixekizumab is distributed into human milk, affects milk production, or affects the breast-fed infant. Ixekizumab is distributed into milk in cynomolgus monkeys; when a drug is present in animal milk, it is likely to also be present in human milk. Consider the benefits of breast-feeding and the importance of ixekizumab to the woman along with potential adverse effects on the breast-fed infant from the drug or from the underlying maternal condition.

Pediatric Use

Safety and efficacy of ixekizumab in pediatric patients <6 years of age with plaque psoriasis have not been established. Safety and efficacy of ixekizumab in pediatric patients <18 years of age have not been established for other indications.

Geriatric Use

Of the 4204 adult patients with psoriasis who received ixekizumab in clinical trials, 7% were ≥65 years of age, while <1% were ≥75 years of age. Although no overall differences in efficacy or safety between geriatric patients and younger adults were observed, the clinical trials did not include sufficient numbers of patients ≥65 years of age to determine whether geriatric patients respond differently than younger adults.

In a population pharmacokinetic analysis, clearance of ixekizumab was similar in patients ≥65 years of age and younger adults.

Hepatic Impairment

The pharmacokinetics of ixekizumab have not been formally studied in patients with hepatic impairment.

Renal Impairment

The pharmacokinetics of ixekizumab have not been formally studied in patients with renal impairment.

● Common Adverse Effects

Adverse effects reported in ≥1% of patients receiving ixekizumab include injection site reactions, upper respiratory tract infections (including nasopharyngitis and rhinovirus infection), nausea, and tinea infections.

DRUG INTERACTIONS

● Drugs Metabolized by Hepatic Microsomal Enzymes

In patients with plaque psoriasis who were administered a single dose of ixekizumab 160 mg or multiple doses of 80 mg every 2 weeks and were receiving concomitant caffeine (a cytochrome P-450 [CYP]1A2 substrate), warfarin (a CYP2C9 substrate), omeprazole (a CYP2C19 substrate), or midazolam (a CYP3A substrate), no clinically significant changes to exposure of caffeine, warfarin, omeprazole, or midazolam were observed.

The manufacturer states that a potential effect of ixekizumab on CYP2D6 activity cannot be ruled out, based on an approximately twofold variability in exposure to dextromethorphan and its metabolite dextrorphan, which is metabolized by CYP2D6, in patients with psoriasis treated with ixekizumab.

● Corticosteroids

Analysis of population pharmacokinetic data indicates that clearance of ixekizumab is not affected by concomitant use of oral corticosteroids in patients with ankylosing spondylitis and nonradiographic axial spondyloarthritis.

● Disease-modifying Antirheumatic Drugs

Analysis of population pharmacokinetic data indicates that clearance of ixekizumab is not affected by concomitant use of methotrexate or by prior use of methotrexate or adalimumab in patients with psoriatic arthritis or by concomitant use of sulfasalazine or methotrexate in patients with ankylosing spondylitis and nonradiographic axial spondyloarthritis.

● Nonsteroidal Anti-inflammatory Agents

Analysis of population pharmacokinetic data indicates that clearance of ixekizumab is not affected by concomitant use of nonsteroidal anti-inflammatory agents (NSAIAs) in patients with ankylosing spondylitis and nonradiographic axial spondyloarthritis.

● Vaccines

Live vaccines should *not* be administered to patients receiving ixekizumab. There are no available data regarding response to live vaccines in patients receiving ixekizumab.

DESCRIPTION

Ixekizumab is a recombinant humanized immunoglobulin G_4 kappa (IgG_4 kappa) monoclonal antibody that is specific for interleukin-17A (IL-17A); it is produced in a recombinant mammalian cell line. IL-17A is a subtype of the IL-17 family of proinflammatory cytokines secreted principally by T-helper 17 (Th17) cells. Elevated levels of IL-17A have been found in psoriatic lesions and blood of individuals with psoriasis. Ixekizumab binds to IL-17A and inhibits its interaction with the IL-17 receptor, thus neutralizing the biologic activity of IL-17A and inhibiting the release of proinflammatory cytokines and chemokines.

The metabolic pathway of ixekizumab has not been characterized. As a human IgG_4 kappa monoclonal antibody, the drug is expected to be degraded into small peptides and amino acids via catabolic pathways in the same manner as endogenous IgG. Ixekizumab exhibited dose-proportional pharmacokinetics in patients with plaque psoriasis over a subcutaneous dose range of 5–160 mg. In patients with plaque psoriasis, bioavailability of subcutaneous ixekizumab ranged from 60–81%. Higher bioavailability was attained when the drug was injected subcutaneously into the thigh compared with other injection sites, including the arm and abdomen. In patients with psoriasis, peak plasma concentrations of the drug were achieved by approximately 4 days after a single subcutaneous 160-mg dose of ixekizumab. In patients initiating ixekizumab therapy with an initial 160-mg dose followed by doses of 80 mg every 2 weeks, steady-state concentrations of the drug

were attained by week 8 of therapy; after the dosage was changed to 80 mg every 4 weeks at week 12 of therapy, a new steady state was achieved in approximately 10 weeks. The mean half-life of ixekizumab is 13 days in patients with plaque psoriasis. Clearance and volume of distribution of the drug increase as body weight increases, and age does not substantially alter the drug's clearance. The pharmacokinetics of ixekizumab are similar in adults with plaque psoriasis, psoriatic arthritis, ankylosing spondylitis, or nonradiographic axial spondyloarthritis.

ADVICE TO PATIENTS

- Provide all patients and/or caregivers with a copy of the manufacturer's patient information (medication guide) and instructions for use for ixekizumab with each prescription of the drug. Importance of reading the medication guide and instructions for use prior to initiation of therapy and each time the prescription is refilled.

- Instruct patient and/or caregiver regarding proper storage, dosage, and administration of ixekizumab, including the use of aseptic technique, as well as proper disposal of needles and syringes if it is determined that the patient and/or caregiver is competent to safely administer the drug.

- If a dose of ixekizumab is missed, instruct patient to administer the missed dose as soon as possible and then resume the regular dosing schedule.

- Increased susceptibility to infection. Advise patient to promptly inform their clinician if any signs or symptoms of infection (e.g., fever, sweats, or chills; muscle aches; cough, shortness of breath, or blood in the phlegm; weight loss; warm, red, or painful sores on the body; diarrhea or stomach pain; burning upon urination or increased urination) occur.

- Advise patient to inform their clinician if new or worsening symptoms of inflammatory bowel disease (e.g., abdominal pain, diarrhea, weight loss) occur.

- Advise patient to review their vaccination status with clinician and receive all appropriate vaccines prior to initiation of ixekizumab.

- Advise patient to immediately seek medical attention if symptoms of a serious allergic reaction (e.g., feeling of faintness; swelling of eyelids, face, lips, mouth, tongue, or throat; dyspnea or throat tightness; chest tightness; rash) occur.

- Advise patients to inform their clinician of existing or contemplated concomitant therapy, including prescription and OTC drugs, as well as any concomitant illnesses (e.g., active infection, inflammatory bowel disease) or any history of tuberculosis or other infections.

- Advise women to inform their clinicians if they are or plan to become pregnant or plan to breast-feed. Encourage women who have been exposed to ixekizumab during pregnancy to enroll in the pregnancy registry at 1-800-284-1695 or by visiting online at https://www.taltz.com.

- Inform patients of other important precautionary information.

PREPARATIONS

Excipients in commercially available drug preparations may have clinically important effects in some individuals; consult specific product labeling for details.

Ixekizumab

Parenteral

Injection, for subcutaneous use	80 mg/mL	Taltz® (available as single-use prefilled autoinjector and single-use prefilled syringe), Lilly

† Use is not currently included in the labeling approved by the US Food and Drug Administration.

Selected Revisions May 10, 2024, © Copyright, September 13, 2016, American Society of Health-System Pharmacists, Inc.

Sarilumab

90:24.20.92 • INTERLEUKIN-MEDIATED AGENTS, MISCELLANEOUS

■ Sarilumab, a recombinant human immunoglobulin G_1 (IgG_1) kappa monoclonal antibody specific for the interleukin-6 (IL-6) receptor, is a biologic response modifier and a disease-modifying antirheumatic drug (DMARD).

USES

● Rheumatoid Arthritis

Sarilumab is used for the management of moderately to severely active rheumatoid arthritis in adults who have had an inadequate response or intolerance to one or more disease-modifying antirheumatic drugs (DMARDs). Sarilumab may be used alone or in combination with methotrexate or other nonbiologic DMARDs (e.g., hydroxychloroquine, leflunomide, sulfasalazine). Sarilumab has been shown to induce clinical responses, improve physical function, and inhibit progression of structural damage in adults with rheumatoid arthritis. Safety and efficacy of sarilumab for this use are based principally on the results of 2 randomized controlled trials. Guidelines generally support the use of interleukin-6 (IL-6) inhibitors, including sarilumab, as add-on therapy to methotrexate in patients who do not meet treatment goals with methotrexate alone.

Clinical Experience

Efficacy of sarilumab in patients with rheumatoid arthritis has been evaluated primarily in 2 randomized, double-blind, placebo-controlled, multicenter studies in adults (18 years of age or older) with moderately to severely active rheumatoid arthritis (as defined by the American College of Rheumatology [ACR]). In these studies, sarilumab was administered in combination with methotrexate in patients with an inadequate response to this drug (MOBILITY study) or in combination with methotrexate and/or other nonbiologic DMARDs (hydroxychloroquine, leflunomide, and/or sulfasalazine) in patients who had an inadequate response to, or had not tolerated, one or more TNF blocking agents (TARGET study). Patients included in these studies had 8 or more tender joints and 6 or more swollen joints. Those receiving low stable dosages of corticosteroids (equivalent to 10 mg or less of prednisone daily) could continue such therapy. Sarilumab was administered subcutaneously at a dosage of 150 or 200 mg once every 2 weeks.

The ACR criteria for improvement (ACR response) in measures of disease activity were used as the principal measure of clinical response in studies evaluating the efficacy of sarilumab. An ACR 20 response is achieved if the patient experiences a 20% or greater improvement in tender and swollen joint count and a 20% or greater improvement in at least 3 of the following criteria: patient pain assessment, patient global assessment, physician global assessment, patient self-assessed disability, or laboratory measures of disease activity (i.e., erythrocyte sedimentation rate [ESR] or C-reactive protein [CRP] level). An ACR 70 response is defined using the same criteria but with a level of improvement of 70%. The proportion of patients who achieved an ACR 20 response at week 24 was the primary end point in the studies of sarilumab. In addition, the total van der Heijde-modified Sharp score (a composite score of erosions and joint space narrowing in hands and feet) was used as the principal measure of joint damage and the Health Assessment Questionnaire Disability Index (HAQ-DI) was used to assess physical function and disability.

In the MOBILITY study, 1197 patients who had active rheumatoid arthritis for at least 3 months despite receiving a stable dosage of methotrexate (10–25 mg/week) were randomized to receive 1 of 3 regimens: sarilumab 150 mg every 2 weeks, sarilumab 200 mg every 2 weeks, or placebo, each given in combination with methotrexate for 52 weeks. At week 16, patients previously randomized to receive sarilumab 150 mg every 2 weeks or placebo who achieved less than 20% improvement from baseline in the number of tender or swollen joints were permitted to cross over to open-label therapy with sarilumab 200 mg every 2 weeks. Approximately 20% of patients in the study had previously received a biologic DMARD; patients with a history of nonresponse to prior biologic DMARD therapy were excluded from the study.

In the MOBILITY study, ACR 20 responses were achieved at 24 weeks in 58, 66.4, or 33.4% of patients receiving sarilumab 150 mg and methotrexate, sarilumab 200 mg and methotrexate, or placebo and methotrexate, respectively, while ACR 70 responses were achieved at 24 weeks in 19.8, 24.8, or 7.3% of patients receiving these respective treatment regimens. ACR responses observed at 24 weeks were maintained through 1 year. At 1 year, 12.8, 14.8, or 3% of patients receiving sarilumab 150 mg and methotrexate, sarilumab 200 mg and methotrexate, or placebo and methotrexate, respectively, had achieved major clinical responses (defined as ACR 70 responses for a continuous 24-week period). At 24 weeks, a greater proportion of patients receiving sarilumab 150 or 200 mg (27.8 or 34.1%, respectively) had a low level of disease activity, as defined by a 28-joint Disease Activity Score using CRP (DAS 28 [CRP]) of less than 2.6, compared with patients who received placebo (10.1%). However, this criterion does not preclude residual disease activity, and 33.1, 37.8, or 20% of patients in these respective treatment groups who achieved a DAS 28 (CRP) of less than 2.6 still had 3 or more active joints. Findings at 1 year indicated that treatment with sarilumab 150 or 200 mg inhibited progression of structural damage compared with placebo. At 1 year, 47.8 or 55.6% of patients receiving sarilumab 150 or 200 mg, respectively, exhibited no radiographic progression, as determined by change in the total van der Heijde-modified Sharp score, compared with 38.7% of patients receiving placebo. Patients receiving sarilumab 150 or 200 mg also experienced greater improvements in physical function and disability, as assessed using HAQ-DI scores, at 16 weeks compared with those who received placebo. An open-label extension study (EXTEND) enrolling patients who completed the MOBILITY study found that treatment with sarilumab maintained clinical efficacy for up to 5 years.

In the TARGET study, 546 patients who had active rheumatoid arthritis for at least 6 months and who had an inadequate response to, or had not tolerated, one or more TNF blocking agents were randomized to receive 1 of 3 regimens: sarilumab 150 mg every 2 weeks, sarilumab 200 mg every 2 weeks, or placebo, each given in combination with methotrexate and/or other nonbiologic DMARDs for 24 weeks. At week 12, patients with less than 20% improvement from baseline in the number of both tender or swollen joints were permitted to cross over to open-label therapy with sarilumab 200 mg every 2 weeks. ACR 20 responses were achieved at 24 weeks in 55.8, 60.9, or 33.7% of patients receiving sarilumab 150 mg, sarilumab 200 mg, or placebo, respectively, while ACR 70 responses were achieved at 24 weeks in 19.9, 16.3, or 7.2% of patients receiving these respective treatment regimens. At 24 weeks, a greater proportion of patients receiving sarilumab 150 or 200 mg (24.9 or 28.8%, respectively) had a low level of disease activity, as defined by a DAS 28 (CRP) of less than 2.6, compared with patients who received placebo (7.2%). Patients receiving sarilumab 150 or 200 mg also experienced greater improvements in physical function and disability, as assessed using HAQ-DI scores, at 12 weeks compared with those who received placebo. An open-label extension study (EXTEND) enrolling patients who completed the TARGET study found that treatment with sarilumab maintained clinical efficacy for up to 5 years.

In a randomized, double-blind, double-dummy, multicenter trial (MONARCH study), 369 adults who had active rheumatoid arthritis for at least 3 months and were not candidates for methotrexate or had an inadequate response or intolerance to methotrexate were randomized to receive subcutaneous administration of sarilumab 200 mg every 2 weeks or adalimumab 40 mg every 2 weeks. After week 16, dose escalation to weekly administration of adalimumab or matching placebo in the sarilumab group was permitted for patients who did not achieve a 20% or greater improvement in tender and swollen joint count. The primary measure of efficacy was change in the 28-joint Disease Activity Score using ESR (DAS28 [ESR]) from baseline to week 24. At 24 weeks, patients receiving sarilumab 200 mg had significantly greater reductions in DAS28 (ESR) compared to patients treated with adalimumab 40 mg. Secondary endpoints, including remission of DAS28 (ESR), ACR20, ACR50, and ACR 70 responses, and HAQ-DI scores, were also significantly improved at 24 weeks in patients treated with sarilumab compared with those treated with adalimumab.

Subgroup analysis of the MOBILITY, TARGET, and MONARCH studies found that improvements in clinical, radiographic, and physical function seen in patients treated with sarilumab were generally consistent across a variety of subgroups (e.g., based on age, sex, duration of rheumatoid arthritis, and prior treatment).

Clinical Perspective

The American College of Rheumatology issued guidelines for the treatment of rheumatoid arthritis in 2021. Disease-modifying treatments for rheumatoid arthritis include conventional DMARDs (e.g., methotrexate, hydroxychloroquine, sulfasalazine), biologic DMARDs (e.g., TNF blocking agents, abatacept, tocilizumab, sarilumab, rituximab), and/or targeted synthetic DMARDs (e.g., Janus kinase inhibitors). Specific agents for rheumatoid arthritis treatment are selected according to current disease activity, prior therapies used, and the presence of comorbidities. A "treat-to-target" approach is typically employed, with the goal of achieving low disease activity or remission.

The IL-6 inhibitors used in the treatment of rheumatoid arthritis are tocilizumab and sarilumab. Methotrexate monotherapy is strongly recommended over biologic DMARD monotherapy for DMARD-naïve patients with moderate to high disease activity, because it is less costly and has established safety and efficacy. Add-on therapy with biologic DMARDs (including IL-6 inhibitors) and targeted synthetic DMARDs is conditionally recommended over triple therapy (i.e., addition of sulfasalazine and hydroxychloroquine) for patients who are taking maximally tolerated doses of methotrexate and are not at target. Recommendations for the use and selection of biologic DMARDs in rheumatoid arthritis vary based on the presence of certain comorbidities (e.g., heart failure, previous serious infection, nontuberculous mycobacterial lung disease). Consult the American College of Rheumatology guidelines for additional details.

● Polymyalgia Rheumatica

Sarilumab is used for the management of polymyalgia rheumatica in adult patients who have had an inadequate response to corticosteroids or who cannot tolerate tapering of corticosteroids. Sarilumab is used in combination with corticosteroids during the taper and and then as monotherapy following discontinuation of the corticosteroids.

Sarilumab has been shown to achieve sustained remission and reduce the cumulative glucocorticoid dose in patients with a relapse of polymyalgia rheumatica during glucocorticoid tapering.

Clinical Experience

The efficacy of sarilumab in patients with polymyalgia rheumatica has been evaluated in a randomized, double-blind, placebo-controlled, 52-week, multicenter study in adults with polymyalgia rheumatica as defined by the American College of Rheumatology/European Union League against Rheumatism (ACR/EULAR) classification criteria. Patients selected for this study, had at least one episode of unequivocal polymyalgia rheumatica flare while attempting to taper corticosteroids. In this study, patients with active polymyalgia rheumatica were randomized to receive sarilumab 200 mg every 2 weeks with a pre-established 14-week taper of prednisone or placebo every 2 weeks with an established 52-week taper of prednisone. Patients experiencing a disease flare or unable to adhere to the assigned prednisone tapering schedule could receive corticosteroids as rescue therapy.

The primary endpoint of this study was the proportion of patients with sustained remission at week 52. Sustained remission was defined as achievement of disease remission no later than week 12, absence of disease flare from week 12 through week 52, sustained reduction of C-reactive protein (to <10 mg/L from week 12 through week 52, and successful adherence to prednisone taper from week 12 through week 52. An additional endpoint was total cumulative corticosteroid dose over 52 weeks.

Sarilumab exhibited improvement in achieving sustained remission and reducing the cumulative corticosteroid dose in patients with a relapse of polymyalgia rheumatica during corticosteroid tapering. At 52 weeks, a higher proportion of patients receiving sarilumab achieved each component of the sustained remission endpoint (28.3%) compared to those patients receiving placebo (10.3%). Additionally, the total actual cumulative corticosteroid dose including all corticosteroids taken during the study (i.e., prednisone taper regimen per protocol, add-on prednisone prior to week 12, corticosteroid use due to rescue, or corticosteroid used during the treatment period to manage an adverse reaction not related to polymyalgia rheumatica) was 777 mg in those patients receiving sarilumab compared with 2044 mg in those receiving placebo.

DOSAGE AND ADMINISTRATION

● General

Pretreatment Screening

- Evaluate for tuberculosis infection prior to initiation of sarilumab; initiate antimycobacterial therapy if indicated.

- Evaluate neutrophil and platelet counts prior to initiation of sarilumab. Do not initiate therapy in patients with an absolute neutrophil count (ANC) of <2000/mm³ or platelet count of <150,000/mm³.

- Evaluate ALT/AST concentrations prior to initiation of sarilumab. Do not initiate sarilumab if the ALT or AST concentration is >1.5 times the upper limit of normal (ULN).

- Evaluate lipoprotein concentrations (total cholesterol, LDL cholesterol, HDL cholesterol and/or triglycerides) prior to initiation of sarilumab.

- Evaluate patient for any active infections.

Patient Monitoring

- Monitor closely for signs or symptoms of infection.

- Evaluate for tuberculosis infection periodically during therapy; initiate antimycobacterial therapy if indicated.

- Monitor platelet counts after therapy initiation, and then every 3 months.

- Monitor neutrophil counts 4–8 weeks after therapy initiation, and then every 3 months; however, assess neutrophil counts at the end of the 2-week dosing interval because the neutrophil nadir generally occurs 3–4 days following sarilumab administration.

- Monitor ALT/AST concentrations 4–8 weeks after therapy initiation, and then every 3 months. Monitor other liver function tests (e.g., bilirubin) when clinically indicated.

- Monitor lipoprotein concentrations 4–8 weeks after therapy initiation, then approximately every 6 months.

Other General Considerations

- May continue methotrexate, other nonbiologic disease-modifying antirheumatic drugs (DMARDs), and corticosteroids in adults receiving sarilumab for the management of rheumatoid arthritis.

- Do not use concomitantly with other biologic DMARDs, such as tumor necrosis factor (TNF; TNF-α) blocking agents, interleukin-1 (IL-1) receptor antagonists, anti-CD20 monoclonal antibodies, and selective costimulation modulators.

● Administration

Sarilumab is administered by subcutaneous injection only. Sarilumab is intended for use under the guidance and supervision of a clinician; however, the drug may be self-administered if the clinician determines that the patient and/or their caregiver is competent to safely administer the drug after appropriate training.

Sarilumab is commercially available in single-use prefilled syringes and single-use prefilled pens. Each syringe or pen delivers 150 or 200 mg of sarilumab in 1.14 mL. The entire contents of the prefilled syringe or pen should be administered as a single dose.

Sarilumab injection is a clear and colorless to pale yellow solution. Prior to administration, sarilumab solution should be inspected visually for particulate matter or discoloration; if the syringe or pen appears to be damaged or the solution contains particulates or is cloudy or discolored, the solution should be discarded. Sarilumab prefilled syringes and pens should be stored at 2–8°C in the original carton until administration and protected from light. The injection should not be frozen or shaken. If refrigeration is not available, the prefilled syringes and pens may be stored at room temperature up to 25°C in the original carton for a period of up to 14 days. At least 30 minutes prior to administration, the prefilled syringe should be removed from the refrigerator and allowed to reach room temperature; the prefilled pen should be removed from refrigeration at least 60 minutes prior to administration. The syringe or pen should not be warmed in any other way (e.g., microwave, hot water).

Sarilumab is administered subcutaneously into the anterior thigh or abdomen (except for the 2-inch area around the umbilicus). Sarilumab may be administered subcutaneously into the upper arm by a caregiver or clinician. Injection sites should be rotated. Injections should not be made into areas where the skin is tender, bruised, or damaged or into scars.

● Dosage

Rheumatoid Arthritis

For the management of moderately to severely active rheumatoid arthritis in adults who have had an inadequate response or intolerance to one or more

DMARDs, the recommended dosage of sarilumab is 200 mg by subcutaneous injection once every 2 weeks. Sarilumab may be used as monotherapy or in combination with methotrexate or other conventional DMARDs.

Polymyalgia Rheumatica

For the management of polymyalgia rheumatica in adults who have had an inadequate response to corticosteroids or who cannot tolerate corticosteroid taper, the recommended dosage of sarilumab is 200 mg by subcutaneous injection once every 2 weeks, in combination with a tapering course of systemic corticosteroids. Sarilumab can be used as monotherapy following discontinuation of corticosteroids.

Dosage Modifications or Discontinuance due to Toxicity in Patients with Rheumatoid Arthritis

If a serious infection or an opportunistic infection develops, sarilumab should be interrupted until the infection is controlled.

If certain dose-related laboratory changes (i.e., neutropenia, thrombocytopenia, elevated liver enzyme concentrations) occur, reduction in sarilumab dosage to 150 mg every 2 weeks or temporary interruption or discontinuance of sarilumab therapy is recommended (see Tables 1-3).

TABLE 1. Recommended Dosage Adjustment Based on Absolute Neutrophil Count (ANC) in Adults with Rheumatoid Arthritis.

ANC (cells/mm³)	Recommendation
>1000	Maintain current dosage
500–1000	Interrupt sarilumab therapy until ANC is >1000; resume sarilumab at 150 mg every 2 weeks and increase to 200 mg every 2 weeks as clinically indicated
<500	Discontinue sarilumab

TABLE 2. Recommended Dosage Adjustment Based on Platelet Count in Adults with Rheumatoid Arthritis.

Platelet Count (cells/mm³)	Recommendation
50,0000–100,000	Interrupt sarilumab therapy until platelet count is >100,000; resume sarilumab at 150 mg every 2 weeks and increase to 200 mg every 2 weeks as clinically indicated
<50,000	Repeat platelet count; discontinue sarilumab if results are confirmed

TABLE 3. Recommended Dosage Adjustment Based on Changes in Liver Enzyme Laboratory Value in Adults with Rheumatoid Arthritis.

ALT or AST Value	Recommendation
>1 to 3 times ULN	Modify dosage of concomitant DMARDs if appropriate
>3 to 5 times ULN	Interrupt sarilumab therapy until ALT or AST values are <3 times ULN; resume sarilumab at 150 mg every 2 weeks and increase to 200 mg every 2 weeks as clinically indicated
>5 times ULN	Discontinue sarilumab

Dosage Modification or Discontinuance for Toxicity in Patients with Polymyalgia Rheumatica

If a serious infection or an opportunistic infection develops, sarilumab should be interrupted until the infection is controlled.

If certain dose-related laboratory changes (i.e., neutropenia, thrombocytopenia, elevated liver enzyme concentrations) occur, discontinuance of sarilumab therapy is recommended. (See Tables 4-6.) Dosage modifications have not been studied in patients with polymyalgia rheumatica with these conditions.

TABLE 4. Recommended Dosage Adjustment Based on Absolute Neutrophil Count (ANC) in Adults with Polymyalgia Rheumatica.

ANC (cells/mm³)	Recommendation
<1000 at the end of the dosing interval	Discontinue sarilumab

TABLE 5. Recommended Dosage Adjustment Based on Platelet Count in Adults with Polymyalgia Rheumatica.

Platelet Count (cells/mm³)	Recommendation
<100,000	Discontinue sarilumab

TABLE 6. Recommended Dosage Adjustment Based on Changes in Liver Enzyme Laboratory Value in Adults with Polymyalgia Rheumatica.

AST or ALT	Recommendation
>3 times ULN	Discontinue sarilumab

● **Special Populations**

Hepatic Impairment

Sarilumab is not recommended in patients with hepatic impairment.

Renal Impairment

Dosage adjustment is not necessary in patients with mild or moderate renal impairment.

Sarilumab has not been studied in patients with severe renal impairment.

Geriatric Patients

The manufacturer makes no specific dosage recommendations for geriatric patients.

CAUTIONS

● **Contraindications**

- Known hypersensitivity to the drug or any ingredient in the formulation.

● **Warnings/Precautions**

Warnings

Infectious Complications

A boxed warning about the risk of serious infections is included in the prescribing information for sarilumab. Serious and sometimes fatal infections, including bacterial, mycobacterial, invasive fungal, viral, or other opportunistic infections, have been reported in patients with rheumatoid arthritis receiving immunosuppressive agents including sarilumab. The most common serious infections reported in patients with rheumatoid arthritis receiving sarilumab have included pneumonia and cellulitis. Opportunistic infections (e.g., tuberculosis, candidiasis, pneumocystosis) also have been reported in patients receiving sarilumab. Other serious infections (e.g., aspergillosis, cryptococcal infection, histoplasmosis) may occur. Patients have presented with disseminated rather than local disease; patients often were receiving concomitant therapy with immunosuppressive agents (e.g., methotrexate, corticosteroids) that, in addition to their underlying condition, could have predisposed them to infections.

Closely monitor patients during treatment with sarilumab for the development of signs or symptoms of infection.

Sarilumab therapy should not be initiated in patients with active infections, including localized infections. Clinicians should consider potential risks and benefits of the drug prior to initiating therapy in patients with a history of chronic, recurring, serious, or opportunistic infections; patients with underlying conditions that may predispose them to infections; and patients who have been exposed to tuberculosis or who reside or have traveled in regions where tuberculosis or mycoses are endemic. Any patient who develops a new infection while receiving sarilumab should undergo a thorough diagnostic evaluation (appropriate for an immunocompromised patient), appropriate anti-infective therapy should be initiated, and the patient should be closely monitored. If a serious or opportunistic infection develops, sarilumab should be interrupted until the infection is controlled.

All patients should be evaluated for latent tuberculosis and for the presence of risk factors for tuberculosis prior to and periodically during therapy with sarilumab. When indicated, an appropriate antimycobacterial regimen for the treatment of latent tuberculosis infection should be initiated prior to sarilumab therapy. Antimycobacterial therapy should be considered prior to initiation of sarilumab in individuals with a history of latent or active tuberculosis in whom an adequate course of antimycobacterial treatment cannot be confirmed and in individuals with a negative test for latent tuberculosis who have risk factors for tuberculosis. Consultation with a tuberculosis specialist is recommended when deciding whether antimycobacterial therapy should be initiated. Patients receiving sarilumab, including individuals with a negative test for latent tuberculosis, should be monitored for signs and symptoms of active tuberculosis.

Viral reactivation can occur in patients receiving immunosuppressive therapies. Herpes zoster exacerbation has been reported in patients receiving sarilumab. The risk of reactivation of hepatitis B virus (HBV) infection in patients receiving sarilumab is not known.

Other Warnings and Precautions

Hypersensitivity Reactions

Hypersensitivity reactions (e.g., injection site rash or erythema, rash, pruritus, urticaria) have been reported in patients receiving sarilumab. During clinical trials of sarilumab, hypersensitivity reactions requiring treatment discontinuance have been reported.

Patients receiving sarilumab should be advised to seek medical attention if they experience symptoms of a hypersensitivity reaction. If a hypersensitivity reaction occurs, administration of the drug should be stopped immediately. Sarilumab is contraindicated in patients with known hypersensitivity to the drug.

Hematologic Effects

Neutropenia and thrombocytopenia have been reported during clinical trials in patients receiving sarilumab, but decreases in neutrophil counts were not associated with infection, including serious infection, and decreases in platelet counts were not associated with bleeding.

Neutrophil and platelet counts should be evaluated prior to initiation of sarilumab therapy, 4–8 weeks after initiation of therapy, and every 3 months thereafter. In patients with neutropenia or thrombocytopenia, dosage adjustment, treatment interruption, or discontinuance of the drug may be necessary. Neutrophil counts should be evaluated at the end of the 2-week dosing interval because the neutrophil nadir generally occurs 3–4 days following sarilumab administration and the neutrophil count then recovers toward baseline.

Hepatic Effects

Sarilumab has been associated with elevated aminotransferase concentrations. In clinical trials, these changes were reversible following reduction of the sarilumab dosage or interruption of sarilumab therapy and were not associated with clinical evidence of hepatic injury. The incidence and magnitude of aminotransferase elevations were increased when sarilumab was used in conjunction with a hepatotoxic drug (e.g., methotrexate).

Serum ALT and AST concentrations should be evaluated prior to initiation of sarilumab therapy, 4–8 weeks after initiation of therapy, and every 3 months thereafter. Other liver function tests (e.g., bilirubin) should be monitored when clinically indicated. In patients with elevated aminotransferase concentrations, dosage adjustment, treatment interruption, or discontinuance of sarilumab or concomitantly administered disease-modifying antirheumatic drugs (DMARDs) may be necessary.

Effects on Serum Lipids

Increased serum concentrations of total cholesterol, triglycerides, low-density lipoprotein (LDL)-cholesterol, and/or high-density lipoprotein (HDL)-cholesterol have been reported in patients receiving sarilumab.

Evaluate lipoprotein concentrations (total cholesterol, LDL cholesterol, HDL cholesterol and/or triglycerides) prior to initiation of sarilumab. Lipoprotein concentrations should be monitored 4–8 weeks after initiation of sarilumab therapy and approximately every 6 months thereafter. Lipid disorders should be managed according to clinical guidelines.

GI Perforation

GI perforation has been reported in patients receiving sarilumab, usually as a complication of diverticulitis. Most patients who experienced GI perforation were receiving concomitant therapy with nonsteroidal anti-inflammatory agents (NSAIAs) or corticosteroids. The relative contribution of these agents versus sarilumab to the occurrence of GI perforation remains to be determined.

Patients who experience new-onset abdominal symptoms should be promptly evaluated.

Malignancies

Immunosuppressive therapy may increase the risk of malignancies. Whether treatment with sarilumab affects development of malignancies remains to be determined. Malignancies were reported in clinical trials of the drug.

Immunization

Live vaccines should be avoided during therapy with sarilumab.

Immunogenicity

As with all therapeutic proteins, there is potential for immunogenicity in patients who receive sarilumab. In clinical studies in patients with rheumatoid arthritis, antibodies to sarilumab were detected in approximately 4, 5.7, or 1.9% of patients receiving sarilumab 200 mg every 2 weeks, 150 mg every 2 weeks, or placebo, respectively, in combination with a DMARD. Neutralizing antibodies were detected in 1% of patients receiving sarilumab 200 mg, 1.6% of patients receiving sarilumab 150 mg, and 0.2% of patients receiving placebo in combination with a DMARD. Antibodies to sarilumab were detected in approximately 9.2% of patients receiving sarilumab alone; neutralizing antibodies developed in about 6.9% of such patients. Prior to administration of sarilumab monotherapy, 2.3% of patients had neutralizing antibodies. In clinical studies in patients with polymyalgia rheumatica, antibodies to sarilumab were detected in one patient receiving sarilumab 200 mg every 2 weeks in combination with a corticosteroid taper; this patient did not exhibit a clinical response. Population pharmacokinetic analysis suggested that clearance of sarilumab was increased in patients with neutralizing antibodies. However, no relationship between antibody development and adverse effects or loss of clinical response was observed.

Specific Populations

Pregnancy

There are no adequate data regarding use of sarilumab in pregnant women. As pregnancy progresses, monoclonal antibodies are increasingly transported across the placenta, with the largest amount transferred during the third trimester. However, there was no evidence of embryotoxicity or fetal malformations in cynomolgus monkeys following administration of sarilumab during organogenesis at dosages producing exposures up to 84 times the exposure at the maximum recommended human dosage. Because interleukin-6 (IL-6) is increased in cervical and myometrial tissues during parturition, sarilumab may delay parturition by interfering with cervical ripening and myometrial contractions. Sarilumab should be used during pregnancy only when the potential benefits to the woman justify the potential risk to the fetus.

Infants exposed to sarilumab in utero may have impaired immune responses. Consider the risks and benefits of administering live vaccines to such infants.

A pregnancy registry has been established to monitor fetal outcomes of pregnant women exposed to sarilumab; patients or clinicians may contact the registry at 877-311-8972.

Lactation

It is not known whether sarilumab is distributed into milk or is absorbed from the GI tract in breast-fed infants. Because immunoglobulin G (IgG) is distributed into human milk, it is possible that sarilumab is distributed into milk. Potential effects of the drug on milk production or on breast-fed infants are unknown. Consider the benefits of breast-feeding and the importance of sarilumab to the woman along with potential adverse effects on the breast-fed infant from the drug or from the underlying maternal condition.

Pediatric Use

Safety and efficacy of sarilumab in pediatric patients <18 years of age have not been established.

Neonates and infants who were exposed to sarilumab in utero may have impaired immune responses; consider the risks and benefits of administering live vaccines to such infants.

Geriatric Use

Of the total number of patients with rheumatoid arthritis studied in clinical trials of sarilumab, 15% were ≥65 years of age while 1.6% were ≥75 years of age. Of the total number of patients with polymyalgia rheumatica studied in the clinical trials, 55.9% were 65 to 75 years of age and 17% were ≥75 years of age. Although no overall differences in safety and efficacy were observed between geriatric and younger patients, serious infections occurred more frequently in those ≥65 years of age. Because the geriatric population in general may have a higher incidence of infections than younger adults, use sarilumab with caution in this age group.

Hepatic Impairment

Safety and efficacy of sarilumab have not been established in patients with hepatic impairment, including those with serologic evidence of hepatitis B virus (HBV) or hepatitis C virus (HCV) infection. Use of the drug in patients with active hepatic disease or hepatic impairment is not recommended.

Renal Impairment

The effect of renal impairment on the pharmacokinetics of sarilumab has not been specifically studied to date. Although population pharmacokinetic data suggest an increase in exposure to sarilumab in patients with mild to moderate renal impairment (creatinine clearance of 30 to <90 mL/minute), sarilumab is not expected to undergo substantial renal elimination and dosage adjustment is not necessary. Sarilumab has not been evaluated in patients with severe renal impairment.

● Common Adverse Effects

Adverse effects reported in 3% or more of patients with rheumatoid arthritis receiving sarilumab include neutropenia, increased ALT concentrations, injection site reactions (e.g., erythema, pruritus), upper respiratory tract infection, and urinary tract infection.

Adverse effects reported in 5% or more of patients with polymyalgia rheumatica receiving sarilumab include neutropenia, leukopenia, constipation, rash, myalgia, fatigue, and injection site reaction (pruritus).

DRUG INTERACTIONS

● Drugs Metabolized by Hepatic Microsomal Enzymes

Because increased levels of cytokines including interleukin-6 (IL-6) in inflammatory conditions such as rheumatoid arthritis may suppress the formation of cytochrome P-450 (CYP) enzymes, inhibition of IL-6 activity by sarilumab may restore CYP enzyme activity to higher levels. Effects of sarilumab on CYP enzyme activity may persist for several weeks after the drug is discontinued. Following initiation or discontinuance of sarilumab therapy, patients receiving certain drugs metabolized by CYP isoenzymes (i.e., those with a low therapeutic index that require individualized dosing [e.g., theophylline, warfarin]) should be monitored for therapeutic effect and/or changes in serum concentrations, and dosages

of these drugs should be adjusted as needed. Caution also is advised when sarilumab is used concomitantly with CYP3A4 substrates (e.g., oral contraceptives, atorvastatin, lovastatin) for which a reduction in efficacy would be undesirable.

Simvastatin

Subcutaneous administration of a single 200-mg dose of sarilumab one week prior to oral administration of a single 40-mg dose of simvastatin (a substrate of CYP3A4 and organic anion transport protein [OATP] 1B1) in patients with rheumatoid arthritis reduced systemic exposures to simvastatin and simvastatin acid by 45 and 36%, respectively, compared with administration of simvastatin alone.

● Antirheumatic Drugs

Concomitant use of methotrexate does not appear to affect clearance of sarilumab. Sarilumab has not been studied in conjunction with biologic disease-modifying antirheumatic drugs (DMARDs), including tumor necrosis factor (TNF; TNF-α) blocking agents, or with Janus kinase (JAK) inhibitors (e.g., tofacitinib). Concomitant use of sarilumab with biologic DMARDs should be avoided.

● Vaccines

Safety of live vaccines in patients receiving sarilumab has not been established and there is a possibility of increased risk of infection with concomitant use. Live vaccines should be avoided during therapy with sarilumab. The interval between administration of live vaccines and initiation of sarilumab therapy should be in accordance with current vaccination guidelines regarding immunosuppressive agents. Information is not available regarding secondary transmission of infection from individuals receiving live vaccines to patients receiving sarilumab.

DESCRIPTION

Sarilumab, a recombinant human monoclonal antibody specific for the interleukin-6 (IL-6) receptor, is a biologic response modifier and a disease-modifying antirheumatic drug (DMARD). Sarilumab is an IgG$_1$ kappa immunoglobulin that binds specifically to both soluble and membrane-bound IL-6 receptors and inhibits IL-6-mediated signaling through these receptors, thereby resulting in a reduction in inflammatory mediator production.

IL-6, a pleiotropic proinflammatory cytokine, is produced by various cell types, including T cells, B lymphocytes, monocytes, fibroblasts, synoviocytes, and endothelial cells, and has a broad spectrum of biologic activities. IL-6 is involved in T-cell activation, induction of immunoglobulin secretion, initiation of hepatic acute phase protein synthesis, stimulation of hematopoietic precursor cell proliferation and differentiation, and induction of osteoclast differentiation and activation. While the causes of rheumatoid arthritis have not been fully elucidated, proinflammatory cytokines, including IL-6, appear to play critical roles in the disease process. IL-6 is overexpressed in synovial tissue in patients with rheumatoid arthritis and is thought to contribute to synovial proliferation and joint destruction in patients with the disease. Elevated levels of IL-6 in serum and synovial fluid have been shown to correlate with clinical and laboratory measures of disease activity in patients with rheumatoid arthritis.

The absolute bioavailability of sarilumab following subcutaneous injection is approximately 80%. Following repeated subcutaneous administration of sarilumab 150 or 200 mg every 2 weeks in patients with rheumatoid arthritis, peak serum concentrations of the drug are attained in approximately 2–4 days and steady-state concentrations of the drug are attained within 14–16 weeks; systemic accumulation of the drug is 2- to -fold.3 With an increase in dosage from 150 mg every 2 weeks to 200 mg every 2 weeks in patients with rheumatoid arthritis, steady-state concentrations of the drug increase by approximately 2-fold. The median time to steady state in patients with polymyalgia rheumatica is estimated to be 28 weeks and there was accumulation following subcutaneous administration of sarilumab 200 mg, with an accumulation ratio of approximately 6-fold. In general, pharmacokinetic exposures were higher in patients with polymyalgia rheumatica when compared to patients with rheumatoid arthritis. Although systemic exposure to sarilumab tends to decrease as body weight increases, differences in exposure based on body weight are not associated with clinically important effects on efficacy or safety of the drug in patients with rheumatoid arthritis. The metabolic pathway of sarilumab has not been characterized; as with other therapeutic proteins, the drug is expected to be catabolized into peptides and amino acids in the same manner as endogenous IgG. Sarilumab exhibits concentration-dependent clearance. At low sarilumab concentrations, target-mediated nonlinear clearance plays a major role in determining total drug clearance; at higher concentrations, the nonlinear pathway is saturated and clearance is determined mainly by linear clearance. The apparent steady-state half-life of sarilumab in adults with rheumatoid arthritis is up to 8 or 10 days following subcutaneous administration of sarilumab 150 or 200 mg, respectively, every 2 weeks. Patients who developed anti-sarilumab antibodies generally had increased clearance of the drug. The pharmacokinetics of sarilumab are not affected by age, gender, or race.

ADVICE TO PATIENTS

- A copy of the manufacturer's patient information (medication guide and instructions for use) for sarilumab should be provided to all patients. Importance of patients and/or caregivers reading the patient information prior to initiation of therapy and each time the prescription is refilled.

- Instruct patients regarding proper dosage and administration of sarilumab, including the use of aseptic technique, and proper disposal of the prefilled syringes and pens if it is determined that the patient is competent to safely administer the drug.

- Risk of increased susceptibility to infection. Inform clinician immediately if any signs or symptoms suggestive of infection (e.g., fever, sweating, or chills; cough, dyspnea, or blood in the phlegm; diarrhea; weight loss; burning upon urination or increased frequency of urination; warm, red, or painful skin) develop.

- Risk of GI perforation, usually as a complication of diverticulitis and more commonly in those receiving concomitant therapy with nonsteroidal anti-inflammatory agents (NSAIAs) or corticosteroids. Inform a clinician immediately if severe, persistent abdominal pain occurs.

- Risk of hypersensitivity reactions. Contact a clinician prior to administering the next dose if manifestations of an allergic reaction (e.g., urticaria, rash, flushing) occur; seek immediate medical attention if manifestations of a serious allergic reaction (e.g., difficulty breathing, chest pain, feelings of faintness or dizziness, abdominal pain or vomiting, swelling of the lips, tongue, or face) occur.

- Importance of patients informing clinicians that they are receiving sarilumab therapy before scheduling any surgery or medical procedures.

- Inform clinicians of existing or contemplated concomitant therapy, including prescription (e.g., biologic antirheumatic drugs, immunizations) and OTC drugs and dietary or herbal supplements, as well as any concomitant illnesses (e.g., active infection, liver disease, diverticulitis, stomach ulcers) or any history of tuberculosis or other chronic or recurring infections.

- Importance of women informing clinicians if they are or plan to become pregnant or plan to breast-feed. Importance of clinicians informing women about the existence of and encouraging enrollment in the pregnancy registry for sarilumab.

- Inform patients of other important precautionary information.

PREPARATIONS

Excipients in commercially available drug preparations may have clinically important effects in some individuals; consult specific product labeling for details.

Sarilumab

Parenteral		
Injection, for subcutaneous use	150 mg/1.14 mL	Kevzara® (available as single-use prefilled syringes and prefilled injection pens), Sanofi-Aventis and Regeneron
	200 mg/1.14 mL	Kevzara® (available as single-use prefilled syringes and prefilled injection pens), Sanofi-Aventis and Regeneron

† Use is not currently included in the labeling approved by the US Food and Drug Administration.

Selected Revisions May 10, 2024, © Copyright, June 5, 2017, American Society of Health-System Pharmacists, Inc.

Secukinumab

90:24.20.92 • INTERLEUKIN-MEDIATED AGENTS, MISCELLANEOUS

■ Secukinumab is a recombinant human immunoglobulin G$_1$ kappa (IgG$_1$ kappa) monoclonal antibody that binds specifically to interleukin-17A (IL-17A).

USES

● Plaque Psoriasis

Secukinumab is used for the management of moderate to severe plaque psoriasis in adults and pediatric patients 6 years of age and older who are candidates for phototherapy or systemic therapy.

Clinical Experience
Plaque Psoriasis in Adults

Efficacy and safety of secukinumab in the treatment of moderate to severe plaque psoriasis in adults were demonstrated in 4 randomized, double-blind, placebo-controlled studies (ERASURE, FIXTURE, FEATURE, and JUNCTURE). The 4 trials enrolled 2403 adults who had moderate to severe plaque psoriasis, body surface area (BSA) involvement of 10% or greater, a Psoriasis Area and Severity Index (PASI) score of 12 or greater, and who were candidates for phototherapy or systemic therapy. Patients were randomized to treatment with either secukinumab 150 mg, secukinumab 300 mg, etanercept 50 mg (FIXTURE study only), or placebo.

In each study, the assigned dose of secukinumab was administered subcutaneously once weekly for 5 weeks followed by once every 4 weeks. In the FIXTURE study, etanercept was administered subcutaneously at a dosage of 50 mg twice weekly for 12 weeks followed by 50 mg once weekly. In both the ERASURE and FIXTURE studies, placebo recipients who did not achieve a reduction in PASI score of 75% or greater (PASI 75 response) from baseline to week 12 were rerandomized to receive either the 150- or 300-mg regimen of secukinumab beginning at week 12. Each study included a 12-week induction period followed by a 40-week maintenance period.

The pivotal studies were ERASURE and FIXTURE, with a combined enrollment of 2044 patients. FEATURE and JUNCTION were smaller studies (combined enrollment of 359 patients) that evaluated efficacy and safety of secukinumab self-administered by prefilled syringe and injection pen, respectively. Of the 2403 patients included in the 4 placebo-controlled studies, 79% received no prior biologic therapy, and 8 or 45% had experienced treatment failure following prior biologic or nonbiologic therapy, respectively. Approximately 15–25% of patients had a history of psoriatic arthritis.

Primary end points in all 4 studies were the proportion of patients who achieved a PASI 75 response from baseline to week 12 and the proportion who achieved an Investigator's Global Assessment (IGA; a 5-point scale for rating the clinician's impression of the overall severity of psoriasis based on induration, erythema, and scaling: 0 [clear], 1 [almost clear], 2 [mild disease], 3 [moderate disease], and 4 [severe disease]) response of clear or almost clear at week 12.

Across all treatment groups, the median baseline PASI score was 20 (range, 11–72), with a baseline IGA score ranging from moderate (62%) to severe (38%). Among 2077 patients enrolled in placebo-controlled trials, 79% were biologic treatment-naïve and 45% were non-biologic failures. Among biologic treatment-experienced patients, over one-third were biologic treatment failures.

A greater proportion of patients who received secukinumab achieved a PASI 75 response and IGA response of clear or almost clear at week 12 than did those who received placebo (all 4 studies) or etanercept (FIXTURE).

In the ERASURE trial, among patients receiving secukinumab 150 or 300 mg, PASI 75 response rates at week 12 were 71 or 82%, respectively, compared to 4% with placebo. An IGA score of clear or almost clear was achieved by 65, 51, or 2% of patients given secukinumab 300, 150 mg, or placebo, respectively.

In the FIXTURE trial, PASI 75 response rates were 76, 67, or 5% for secukinumab 300 mg, 150 mg, or placebo, respectively. For the etanercept group in the FIXTURE trial, the PASI 75 response rate was 44%. An IGA score of clear or almost clear was achieved by 62, 51, or 3% of patients receiving secukinumab 300 mg, 150 mg, or placebo. In the etanercept group, the IGA response rate was 27.2%.

In the FEATURE study, PASI 75 response rates were 75, 69, or 0% for secukinumab 300 mg, 150 mg, or placebo, respectively. The corresponding PASI 75 response rates in the JUNCTURE study were 87, 70, or 3%, respectively. An IGA score of clear or almost clear was achieved by 68 or 53% of patients given secukinumab 300 or 150 mg, respectively, in the FEATURE trial and by 73 or 52% of patients given secukinumab 300 or 150 mg, respectively, in the JUNCTURE trial. No patients given placebo in either the FEATURE or JUNCTURE trial achieved an IGA response of clear or almost clear.

A PASI 90 response at week 12 was seen in 59, 39, or 1% of patients given secukinumab 300 mg, 150 mg, or placebo, respectively, in the ERASURE trial. In the FIXTURE trial, PASI 90 response rates were 54, 42, or 2% for secukinumab 300 mg, 150 mg, or placebo, respectively; in the etanercept group, the PASI 90 response rate was 20.7%. The PASI 90 response rates at week 12 in the FEATURE trial were 60.3, 45.8, or 0% for secukinumab 300 mg, 150 mg, or placebo, respectively. In the JUNCTURE trial, a PASI 90 response was seen in 55, 40, or 0% of patients receiving secukinumab 300 mg, 150 mg, or placebo, respectively.

Clinical improvements were maintained with continued treatment over 52 weeks. In ERASURE, 72 or 81% of patients who received secukinumab 150 or 300 mg, respectively, and achieved a PASI 75 response at week 12 maintained their responses at week 52, and 59 or 74% of patients who received secukinumab 150 or 300 mg, respectively, and achieved a response of clear or almost clear on the IGA at week 12 also maintained their responses. Similarly, in FIXTURE, PASI 75 responses were maintained at week 52 in 82 or 84% of patients who received secukinumab 150 or 300 mg, respectively, and IGA responses of clear or almost clear were maintained in 68 or 80% of patients receiving these respective treatments. Among patients in the FEATURE study who received secukinumab 150 or 300 mg and achieved a PASI 75 response at week 12, 63.5 and 83.5% of patients, respectively, maintained those responses at week 52. Among those who received secukinumab 150 or 300 mg and achieved an IGA response of clear or almost clear at week 12, 43.6 or 71.5% of patients, respectively, maintained those responses at week 52. In JUNCTURE, 75.2 or 81.4% of patients who received secukinumab 150 or 300 mg, respectively, and achieved a PASI 75 response at week 12 maintained their responses at week 52. Among patients who received secukinumab 150 or 300 mg and achieved a response of clear or almost clear on the IGA at week 12, 60.2 or 69.6%, respectively, also maintained their responses.

Efficacy of secukinumab in scalp psoriasis was evaluated in a randomized, placebo-controlled trial (Trial PsO5) of 102 patients with moderate to severe psoriasis lesions of the scalp. Patients had a Psoriasis Scalp Severity Index (PSSI) score of 12 or greater, an IGA scalp score of 3 or greater, and 30% or more scalp involvement. A total of 102 patients were randomized in a 1:1 ratio to either secukinumab 300 mg or placebo. The primary outcome assessed was the percent of patients achieving a 90% improvement from baseline in PSSI score (PSSI 90), and the key secondary outcome was the percent of patients with an IGA score of clear or almost clear at 12 weeks. At 12 weeks, PSSI 90 response was 52.9 or 2% with secukinumab or placebo, respectively, with an IGA response of 56.9 or 5.9%, respectively.

Several other randomized controlled trials have shown improvements with secukinumab when used for treatment of psoriasis affecting specific areas of the body, including: palmoplantar psoriasis (GESTURE) and nail psoriasis (TRANSFIGURE). These trials found significant improvements in modified versions of the PASI with use of secukinumab compared to placebo; trials evaluating secukinumab for treatment of palmoplantar psoriasis also found significant improvements in a modified version of the IGA with the drug compared to placebo.

A limited number of randomized controlled trials have compared secukinumab to alternate therapies for treatment of plaque psoriasis, including the IL-23 inhibitors guselkumab and risankizumab, and the IL-12 and IL-23 inhibitor ustekinumab. The CLEAR and CLARITY studies compared secukinumab to ustekinumab in patients with psoriasis that was not controlled with topical treatments, phototherapy, and/or previous systemic therapy. In the CLEAR study, secukinumab was superior to ustekinumab for the primary endpoint of PASI 90 response at week 16. In the CLARITY study, secukinumab was superior to ustekinumab for the co-primary endpoints of PASI 90 response at week 12 and the proportion of patients who achieved a response of clear or almost clear on the IGA at week 12. In extension studies of CLEAR and CLARITY, a greater proportion of patients assigned to secukinumab achieved a PASI 90 response and IGA response of clear or almost clear compared to ustekinumab at 52 weeks. A 2-year extension study of CLEAR found that PASI 90 and IGA response rates in patients treated with secukinumab from week 16 were maintained at 2 years. The ECLIPSE study compared secukinumab to guselkumab in patients with moderate to severe plaque psoriasis who were candidates for phototherapy or systemic therapy; at 48 weeks, a significantly greater proportion of patients treated with guselkumab achieved the primary endpoint of PASI 90 response compared to those treated with secukinumab. The IMMerge trial was a randomized, open-label, efficacy-assessor-blinded trial that compared secukinumab to risankizumab in patients with moderate to severe plaque psoriasis who were candidates for systemic therapy. The IMMerge trial found that risankizumab was superior to secukinumab for the co-primary endpoints, which assessed noninferiority and superiority, respectively, for achievement of PASI 90 at week 16 and week 52.

Two additional trials (Trial PsO6, ALLURE; and Trial PsO7, MATURE) evaluated the efficacy and safety of secukinumab 300 mg when administered subcutaneously with a single 300 mg/2 mL prefilled syringe (ALLURE; N=214) or with a single 300 mg/2 mL UnoReady® pen (MATURE; N=122) compared to 2 injections using a 150 mg/1 mL prefilled syringe. The co-primary outcomes were the percent of patients achieving a PASI 75 response and IGA score of clear or almost clear response with a 2-grade or more reduction from baseline at week 12. In ALLURE, a PASI 75 response was seen in 89% of patients using the single 300 mg/2 mL prefilled syringe, compared to 82 or 2% of patients using two 1 mL prefilled syringes or placebo, respectively. The IGA response was 76, 69, or 1% for the single 300 mg/2 mL prefilled syringe, two 1 mL prefilled syringes, or placebo, respectively. In MATURE, PASI 75 response rates were 95, 83, or 10% for the 2 mL pen, two 1 mL prefilled syringes, or placebo, respectively. The IGA response was 76, 68, or 8% for the 2 mL pen, two 1 mL prefilled syringes, or placebo, respectively.

Plaque Psoriasis in Pediatric Patients

The efficacy of secukinumab in the management of severe, chronic plaque psoriasis was evaluated in a 52-week randomized, double-blind, placebo- and active-controlled study (Trial PsO8) comparing 2 dosages of the drug in pediatric patients 6 years of age and older with BSA involvement of 10% and greater and PASI score of 20 or more who were candidates for systemic therapy. A total of 162 patients were randomized to receive 12 weeks of induction therapy with secukinumab 75, 150, or 300 mg; etanercept (0.8 mg/kg, up to a maximum of 50 mg); or placebo. Patients randomized to secukinumab treatment arms (high-dose and low-dose) received a dose based on their weight category: patients weighing ≥50 kg received 150 mg (low-dose group) or 300 mg (high-dose group), those weighing 25 to <50 kg received 75 mg (low-dose group) or 150 mg (high-dose group), and patients weighing <25 kg received 75 mg for both dose groups. After the induction period, patients underwent a 40-week maintenance period. Placebo recipients who did not achieve a PASI 75 response from baseline to week 12 were rerandomized to receive either a low- or high-dose regimen of secukinumab beginning at week 12. The primary end points were the proportion of patients who achieved a PASI 75 response from baseline to week 12 and the proportion who achieved an IGA response of clear or almost clear at week 12.

At week 12, PASI 75 response rates and IGA response of clear or almost clear, respectively, were significantly higher in the low-dose (70 and 56%) secukinumab group compared to placebo (15 and 5%). Significant improvements were also noted in the PASI 90 response rate from baseline to week 12 for low-dose secukinumab compared to placebo (60 and 2%, respectively). High-dose secukinumab was also superior to placebo for PASI 75, IGA response of clear or almost clear, and PASI 90 at week 12. Compared to etanercept, PASI 90 and IGA responses of clear or almost clear were significantly higher among patients treated with secukinumab (low- or high-dose) at 12 weeks; PASI 75 responses were numerically, but not significantly higher with secukinumab compared to etanercept at 12 weeks. Clinical improvements were maintained with continued treatment over 52 weeks.

Clinical Perspective

The American Academy of Dermatology and the National Psoriasis Foundation have issued joint guidelines for the treatment of psoriasis in adults. Phototherapy and topical treatments (e.g., vitamin D analogues, calcineurin inhibitors, keratolytics, and corticosteroids) are frequently used to treat mild psoriasis present on limited areas of the body, but these therapies may be inadequate to obtain skin clearance in patients with more extensive or severe disease. Systemic biologic and nonbiologic therapies are mainstays of treatment for moderate to severe psoriasis, and may also be useful for treating psoriasis on parts of the body that are difficult to treat with topical therapy (e.g., scalp, palms and soles of the feet, genitals). Topical therapies can be used adjunctively in moderate to severe disease. Nonbiologic oral therapies used in the treatment of psoriasis include methotrexate, apremilast, cyclosporine, acitretin, and dimethyl fumarate. Biologics used in the treatment of psoriasis include tumor necrosis factor (TNF) blocking agents, ustekinumab, secukinumab, ixekizumab, brodalumab, guselkumab, tildrakizumab, and risankizumab.

The IL-17 blocking agents used in the treatment of psoriasis include secukinumab, ixekizumab, and brodalumab. These IL-17 blocking agents are recommended as monotherapy for the treatment of adult patients with moderate to severe plaque psoriasis. Recommendations for the use and selection of psoriasis therapies vary based on patient age, disease characteristics (e.g., severity, location, presence of psoriatic arthritis), and comorbidities (e.g., inflammatory bowel disease). Consult the American Academy of Dermatology/National Psoriasis Foundation guidelines for additional details.

The American Academy of Dermatology/National Psoriasis Foundation issued joint guidelines for the treatment of psoriasis in pediatric patients in 2019. Phototherapy and topical treatments (e.g., vitamin D analogues, calcineurin inhibitors, corticosteroids, tazarotene, anthralin, coal tar) are frequently used to treat mild psoriasis present on limited areas of the body, but these therapies may be inadequate to obtain skin clearance in patients with more extensive or severe disease. Systemic biologic and nonbiologic therapies are mainstays of treatment for moderate to severe psoriasis, and may also be useful for treating psoriasis on parts of the body that are difficult to treat with topical therapy (e.g., the scalp, palms and soles of the feet, genitals). Topical therapies can be used adjunctively in moderate to severe disease. Nonbiologic oral therapies used in the treatment of pediatric psoriasis include methotrexate, cyclosporine, acitretin, and fumaric acid esters. Biologics recommended for use in pediatric psoriasis include TNF blocking agents (etanercept, adalimumab, infliximab) and ustekinumab. Other biologic agents that can be used for pediatric psoriasis include secukinumab and ixekizumab. Treatment selection is primarily based on disease characteristics (e.g., severity, location, presence of psoriatic arthritis), with additional consideration being given to patient age and comorbidities.

Current guidelines do not address the place in therapy for IL-17 blocking agents in the treatment of psoriasis in pediatric patients. The current guidelines for pediatric psoriasis are based on literature evaluation through 2017; thus, recommendations for use of IL-17 blocking agents have not yet been incorporated.

● Psoriatic Arthritis

Secukinumab is used for the management of active psoriatic arthritis in patients 2 years of age and older.

Clinical Experience

Psoriatic Arthritis in Adults

Secukinumab has been evaluated for the management of psoriatic arthritis in 3 randomized, double-blind, placebo-controlled studies (FUTURE 1, FUTURE 2, and FUTURE 5) in 1999 adults with active psoriatic arthritis (3 or more swollen joints and 3 or more tender joints), despite treatment with antirheumatic drugs (e.g., non-steroidal anti-inflammatory agents [NSAIAs], corticosteroids, or disease modifying antirheumatic drugs [DMARDs]). In all 3 trials, patients were classified as being either TNF blocking agent-naïve or having experienced inadequate response after prior TNF blocking agent use; randomization was stratified based on past use of TNF blocking agents.

In the FUTURE 1 study, patients received an initial dosage of secukinumab 10 mg/kg IV at weeks 0, 2, and 4, followed by a subcutaneous dose of 75 mg or 150 mg once every 4 weeks. In FUTURE 2, patients were administered subcutaneous secukinumab 300 mg, 150 mg, 75 mg, or placebo once weekly for 5 weeks followed by once every 4 weeks. Patients in FUTURE 5 received 1 of the following 4 treatment options subcutaneously by self-injection: secukinumab 300 mg with loading dose (once weekly for 5 weeks and then once every 4 weeks thereafter), secukinumab 150 mg with loading dose, secukinumab 150 mg without loading dose (once every 4 weeks starting at baseline), or placebo.

In all 3 studies, placebo recipients were classified as responders (those with improvement in the number of tender or swollen joints by at least 20%) or nonresponders at week 16; nonresponders in FUTURE 2 and FUTURE 5 were rerandomized to receive either 150 mg or 300 mg of secukinumab beginning at week

16 and nonresponders in FUTURE 1 were rerandomized to receive either 75 mg or 150 mg of secukinumab at week 16. Responders in each trial received the same dosages as nonresponders, but at week 24.

Of the 1999 patients included in the 3 placebo-controlled studies at baseline, 61% had enthesitis, 42% had dactylitis, 31% had a previously discontinued use of a TNF blocking agent, and 53% reported concomitant use of methotrexate. The following subtypes of psoriatic arthritis were included: polyarticular arthritis without rheumatoid nodules (80%), asymmetric peripheral arthritis (63%), distal interphalangeal involvement (58%), spondylitis with peripheral arthritis (20%), and arthritis mutilans (7%).

The American College of Rheumatology (ACR) criteria for improvement (ACR response) in measures of disease activity were used as the primary efficacy endpoint in all 3 trials; ACR 20 response was measured at 24 weeks in FUTURE 1 and FUTURE 2, and at 16 weeks in FUTURE 5. An ACR 20 response is achieved if the patient experiences a 20% improvement in tender and swollen joint count and a 20% or greater improvement in at least 3 of the following criteria: patient pain assessment, patient global assessment, physician global assessment, patient self-assessed disability, or laboratory measures of disease activity (i.e., erythrocyte sedimentation rate [ESR] or C-reactive protein [CRP] level).

In all 3 trials, a significantly greater proportion of patients who received secukinumab achieved an ACR 20 response compared to those who received placebo. Among patients in FUTURE 1, 50 and 50.5% of patients who were treated with secukinumab 150 or 300 mg, respectively, achieved an ACR 20 response, compared to 17.3% of patients treated with placebo by week 24. In FUTURE 2, 51%, 54%, and 15% of patients treated with secukinumab 150 mg, 300 mg, or placebo, respectively, achieved an ACR 20 response by week 24. By week 16 in the FUTURE 5 study, ACR20 responses occurred in the following proportions: 62.6% in patients who received secukinumab 300 mg with a loading dose, 55.5 and 59.5% in patients who received secukinumab 150 mg with and without a loading dose, respectively, and 27.4% in patients who received placebo. In FUTURE 1 and FUTURE 2, post hoc and subgroup analyses generally showed ACR 20 responses to secukinumab regardless of prior exposure to TNF blocking agents or concomitant use of methotrexate. FUTURE 5 also found ACR 20 responses among patients treated with secukinumab, regardless of prior TNF blocking agent exposure; however, response rates were generally higher among patients who were naïve to treatment with TNF blocking agents at baseline.

Clinical improvements were maintained with continued treatment over 2 years. In the FUTURE 1 study, ACR 20 responses were sustained in 66.8% of patients who received secukinumab 150 mg and 58.6% of patients who received secukinumab 75 mg at 2 years. Similarly, 69.4, 64.4, and 50.3% of patients in FUTURE 2 who received secukinumab 300 mg, 150 mg, and 75 mg, respectively, maintained ACR 20 responses at 2 years. In FUTURE 5, 75.3, 74, and 72.2% of patients treated with secukinumab 300 mg with loading dose, 150 mg with loading dose, and 150 mg without loading dose, respectively, maintained ACR 20 responses at 2 years.

Another randomized, double blind, placebo-controlled trial was conducted to assess the efficacy of secukinumab 150 mg and 300 mg, self-administered subcutaneously via autoinjector, compared to placebo for the treatment of active psoriatic arthritis in 414 adults (FUTURE 3 study). In FUTURE 3, patients self-administered secukinumab 300 mg, 150 mg, or placebo via auto-injector weekly for 5 weeks, then every 4 weeks thereafter. The primary outcome, ACR 20 response at week 24, was significantly greater among patients treated with secukinumab compared to placebo; response occurred in 48.2, 42.0, and 16.1% of patients who received secukinumab 300 mg, secukinumab 150 mg, and placebo, respectively.

An additional randomized, double-blind, placebo-controlled study (FUTURE 4) was conducted to compare efficacy of the following treatment groups in patients with active psoriatic arthritis: subcutaneous secukinumab 150 mg with loading dose, subcutaneous secukinumab 150 mg without loading dose, and placebo. Inclusion criteria in FUTURE 4 were the same as the other FUTURE trials (1, 2, 3, and 5) previously described. The primary endpoint of ACR 20 response at week 16 was met in both the secukinumab 150 mg with loading dose group (41.2%) and the secukinumab 150 mg without loading dose group (39.8%), compared to placebo (18.4%). Clinical responses were sustained for up to 2 years.

Secukinumab has been directly compared to adalimumab, a TNF blocking agent, in a single randomized controlled trial. The EXCEED trial compared secukinumab monotherapy to adalimumab monotherapy in biologic-naïve patients with active psoriatic arthritis and inadequate response to conventional synthetic DMARDs. In this trial, secukinumab was not superior to adalimumab for the primary end point of ACR 20 response at week 52.

The effectiveness of IV secukinumab in the treatment of active psoriatic arthritis in adults was extrapolated from the established effectiveness of subcutaneous secukinumab in adults with active psoriatic arthritis based on pharmacokinetic exposure.

Juvenile Psoriatic Arthritis in Pediatric Patients

Safety and efficacy of secukinumab in the treatment of juvenile psoriatic arthritis in pediatric patients were evaluated in a randomized, double-blind, phase 3 trial in biologic-naïve patients (2 to <18 years of age). Patients with juvenile idiopathic arthritis (enthesitis-related or psoriatic arthritis) underwent open-label treatment with secukinumab (75 mg for weight <50 kg; 150 mg for weight ≥50 kg) for up to 12 weeks, followed by randomization of ACR 30 responders to treatment with either secukinumab or placebo up to week 100. Patients who experienced a flare of disease during the randomized phase entered open-label secukinumab treatment up to week 104. The primary outcome was time to disease flare (30% or greater worsening of ≥3 of 6 juvenile idiopathic arthritis ACR [JIA ACR] criteria and 30% or greater improvement in ≤1 of 6 JIA ACR criteria and a minimum of 2 active joints) in the randomized phase.

Of 86 patients enrolled, 34 had psoriatic arthritis. The mean age of patients with juvenile psoriatic arthritis was 12.2 years of age; 47.1% were male and 91.2% were white, with a baseline Juvenile Arthritis Disease activity score of 15.5. Concomitant methotrexate was used by 67.6% of patients with juvenile psoriatic arthritis.

At weeks 12, JIA ACR 30, 50, 70, or 90 response rates were seen in 91, 91, 71, or 47% of patients with juvenile psoriatic arthritis treated with secukinumab. In the randomized phase, 11 and 4 patients with juvenile psoriatic arthritis who received placebo and secukinumab, respectively, experienced a flare event. Flare risk was reduced by 85% for patients who received secukinumab compared to those who received placebo.

Clinical Perspective

The American College of Rheumatology and the National Psoriasis Foundation issued a joint guideline for the treatment of psoriatic arthritis in 2018. Various drugs and drug classes are used to treat psoriatic arthritis, with some classes being used for symptom management (e.g., NSAIAs and corticosteroids) and others being used as immunomodulatory disease-modifying therapy. Disease-modifying treatments for psoriatic arthritis include oral small molecules (OSMs; e.g., methotrexate, sulfasalazine, cyclosporine, leflunomide, apremilast), biologic DMARDs (e.g., TNF blocking agents, secukinumab, ixekizumab, ustekinumab, brodalumab, abatacept), and/or targeted synthetic DMARDs (e.g., tofacitinib). Specific agents for psoriatic arthritis treatment are selected according to disease characteristics, including disease severity, as well as patient preferences/values and comorbidities. A "treat-to-target" approach is typically employed, with the goal of achieving low/minimal disease activity or remission.

The IL-17 blocking agents used in the treatment of psoriatic arthritis are secukinumab, ixekizumab, and brodalumab. For patients with treatment-naïve psoriatic arthritis, treatment with a TNF blocking agent or an OSM is conditionally recommended over treatment with secukinumab, ixekizumab, or brodalumab. Secukinumab, ixekizumab, or brodalumab may be considered in place of these therapies in patients with severe psoriasis or psoriatic arthritis, or with contraindications to TNF blocking agents. Treatment with secukinumab, ixekizumab, or brodalumab is conditionally recommended over treatment with ustekinumab for treatment-naïve psoriatic arthritis. For patients with active psoriatic arthritis despite treatment with an OSM, switching to a TNF blocking agent is conditionally recommended over treatment with secukinumab, ixekizumab, or brodalumab. Switching to secukinumab, ixekizumab, or brodalumab monotherapy is conditionally recommended over treatment with a different OSM, ustekinumab, abatacept, or tofacitinib. For patients with active psoriatic arthritis despite treatment with TNF blocking agent monotherapy, switching to monotherapy with a different TNF blocking agent is conditionally recommended over switching to secukinumab, ixekizumab, or brodalumab. Switching to secukinumab, ixekizumab, or brodalumab is conditionally recommended over switching to ustekinumab, abatacept, or tofacitinib. For patients with active psoriatic arthritis despite treatment with a combination of a TNF blocking agent and methotrexate, switching to secukinumab, ixekizumab, or brodalumab monotherapy is conditionally recommended over switching to combination therapy with these agents plus methotrexate. In patients with active psoriatic arthritis despite treatment with secukinumab, ixekizumab, or brodalumab, switching to a TNF blocking agent is conditionally recommended over switching to a different IL-17 blocking agent and over adding methotrexate to an IL-17 blocking agent. In patients with active psoriatic arthritis despite treatment with ustekinumab, switching to a TNF blocking agent is conditionally recommended over switching to secukinumab, ixekizumab, or brodalumab and over adding methotrexate to an IL-17 blocking agent. Recommendations for the use and selection of disease-modifying therapies in psoriatic arthritis vary based on the presence of certain disease characteristics (e.g., psoriatic spondylitis/axial disease, enthesitis) and comorbidities (e.g., inflammatory bowel disease, diabetes). Consult the American College of Rheumatology/National Psoriasis Foundation guideline for additional details.

Psoriatic arthritis in pediatric patients is classified as a subtype of juvenile idiopathic arthritis. The American College of Rheumatology and the Arthritis Foundation issued a joint guideline for the treatment of juvenile idiopathic arthritis (including psoriatic arthritis) manifesting as nonsystemic polyarthritis, sacroiliitis, or enthesitis in 2019. Medications recommended for children and adolescents with juvenile idiopathic arthritis and polyarthritis include NSAIAs, non-biologic DMARDs (methotrexate, leflunomide, sulfasalazine), glucocorticoids, and biologic DMARDs (infliximab, etanercept, adalimumab, golimumab, abatacept, or tocilizumab, with combination therapy with a non-biologic DMARD recommended over biologic monotherapy).

For initial therapy for all patients with juvenile idiopathic arthritis and polyarthritis, a non-biologic DMARD is strongly recommended over NSAIA monotherapy, and methotrexate monotherapy is conditionally recommended over triple DMARD therapy. Initial therapy with a biologic DMARD may be considered for patients with risk factors and involvement of high-risk joints, high disease activity, or at high risk for disability joint damage. Subsequent therapy for low disease activity in patients receiving a DMARD and/or a biologic may include escalation of therapy with intraarticular glucocorticoids, optimization of DMARD dose, a trial of methotrexate, and adding/changing biologic. Subsequent therapy for moderate/high disease activity may include addition of a biologic to DMARD monotherapy; switching from a TNF inhibitor to a non-TNF inhibitor (tocilizumab or abatacept); or if using a second biologic, using a TNF inhibitor, abatacept, or tocilizumab. The guideline does not address the specific place in therapy of IL-17 blocking agents; however, the guideline predates published clinical trials of secukinumab in pediatric patients.

● *Ankylosing Spondylitis*

Secukinumab is used for the management of adults with active ankylosing spondylitis.

Clinical Experience

Secukinumab has been evaluated for the management of ankylosing spondylitis in 3 randomized, double-blind, placebo-controlled studies (MEASURE 1, MEASURE 2, and MEASURE 3), which were conducted in a total of 816 adults with active ankylosing spondylitis (as defined by the modified New York criteria) who had an inadequate response to NSAIAs, corticosteroids, or DMARDs. Patients were also required to have active disease, which was defined by a Bath Ankylosing Spondylitis Disease Activity Index (BASDAI) score of 4 or more and visual analog scale (VAS) for total back pain of 4 or more, on scales of 0–10.

Patients in the MEASURE 1 and MEASURE 3 studies received secukinumab or placebo; patients randomized to secukinumab received an initial IV dosage of secukinumab 10 mg/kg at weeks 0, 2, and 4, followed by a subcutaneous dosage of 75 mg or 150 mg (MEASURE 1) or 150 mg or 300 mg (MEASURE 3) once every 4 weeks, starting on week 8. Patients in MEASURE 3 received subcutaneous secukinumab via auto-injector. In MEASURE 2, patients were administered subcutaneous secukinumab 150 mg, secukinumab 75 mg, or placebo once weekly for 5 weeks followed by once every 4 weeks. In MEASURE 2 and MEASURE 3, placebo recipients were rerandomized at week 16 to receive secukinumab, administered once every 4 weeks with the same dosages as the active treatment groups. Patients in MEASURE 2 who received placebo were categorized as responders or nonresponders at week 16 based on the Assessment of Spondyloarthritis International Society 20 (ASAS 20) criteria; an ASAS 20 response is achieved if the patient experiences ≥20% improvement and an absolute improvement of ≥10 units (on a scale of 0–100) in at least 3 of the following criteria without worsening in the fourth criterion: patient global assessment, pain, function, or inflammation.

Nonresponders were rerandomized to subcutaneous secukinumab 150 mg or 75 mg at week 16 and responders were rerandomized to the same dosages at week 24.

Among the 816 patients included in the 3 trials, at baseline, approximately 13% used concomitant methotrexate, 25% used concomitant sulfasalazine, and 29% of patients previously discontinued TNF blocking agents due to intolerance or lack of efficacy. The primary endpoint in all 3 trials was the proportion of patients who achieved ASAS 20 response at week 16.

A significantly greater proportion of patients treated with secukinumab in all 3 trials achieved ASAS 20 response compared to placebo at week 16. In MEASURE 1, ASAS 20 response was achieved in 61, 60, and 29% of patients treated with secukinumab 150 mg, secukinumab 75 mg, and placebo, respectively. In MEASURE 2, ASAS 20 response rates were 61, 41, and 28% with secukinumab 150 mg, secukinumab 75 mg, and placebo, respectively; only the comparison between secukinumab 150 mg and placebo was significant. Among patients treated with secukinumab 300 mg, secukinumab 150 mg, and placebo, ASAS 20 response was achieved in 60.5, 58.1, and 36.8%, respectively. Similarly, ASAS 40 response (improvement of at least 40% and absolute improvement of at least 2 units [on a 10-unit scale] in at least 3 of the 4 criteria previously described without worsening of the fourth criterion) occurred in a significantly greater proportion of patients treated with secukinumab in all 3 trials; this was true for both dosages in MEASURE 1 and MEASURE 3 and the 150-mg dosage only in MEASURE 2. Clinical responses were maintained from week 16 through 52 weeks in all 3 trials.

Extension studies have generally shown that clinical improvements from the initial trials were maintained long-term. At 5 years, 77.6 and 64.5% of patients from the MEASURE 1 trial who received secukinumab 150 mg maintained ASAS 20 and ASAS 40 responses. Patients initially assigned to secukinumab 75 mg in MEASURE 1 were allowed to escalate their dose to 150 mg at or after 156 weeks based on clinician judgment; however, 2-year results also showed sustained ASAS 20 and ASAS 40 responses in patients treated with either secukinumab 75 mg or 150 mg in the initial trial. At 3 years, clinical responses from MEASURE 2 were maintained; ASAS 20 rates were 70.1 and 54.3%, respectively, in patients treated with secukinumab 150 mg and secukinumab 75 mg, and ASAS 40 rates were 60.9 and 37.0%, respectively.

An additional randomized, double-blind, placebo-controlled study (MEASURE 4) was conducted to compare efficacy among the following treatment groups of patients with active ankylosing spondylitis: subcutaneous secukinumab 150 mg with loading dose (once weekly for 5 weeks and then once every 4 weeks thereafter), subcutaneous secukinumab 150 mg without loading dose (once every 4 weeks starting at baseline), and placebo. Inclusion criteria in MEASURE 4 were the same as the other MEASURE trials (1, 2, and 3) previously described. The primary endpoint of ASAS 20 response at week 16 was not met with either secukinumab treatment group compared to placebo.

The effectiveness of IV secukinumab in the treatment of active ankylosing spondylitis in adults was extrapolated from the established effectiveness of subcutaneous secukinumab in adults with active ankylosing spondylitis based on pharmacokinetic exposure.

Clinical Perspective

The American College of Rheumatology, the Spondylitis Association of America, and the Spondyloarthritis Research and Treatment Network issued a joint guideline for the treatment of ankylosing spondylitis in 2019. Treatments for ankylosing spondylitis include NSAIAs, conventional DMARDs (e.g., methotrexate, sulfasalazine), biologic DMARDs (e.g., TNF blocking agents, secukinumab, ixekizumab), and/or targeted synthetic DMARDs (e.g., tofacitinib). Continuous NSAIA treatment is typically considered first-line for active ankylosing spondylitis, with other agents used in the treatment of NSAIA-refractory disease. Specific agents for ankylosing spondylitis treatment are selected according to current disease activity, prior therapies, and the presence of comorbidities. Goals of therapy in ankylosing spondylitis are to alleviate symptoms, improve functioning, maintain the ability to work, decrease complications, and prevent or slow skeletal damage.

The IL-17 blocking agents used in the treatment of ankylosing spondylitis are secukinumab and ixekizumab. For adults with active ankylosing spondylitis despite treatment with NSAIAs, treatment with a TNF blocking agent is conditionally recommended over treatment with secukinumab or ixekizumab. In these patients, secukinumab or ixekizumab is strongly recommended over no treatment with these drugs, and conditionally recommended over treatment with tofacitinib. In patients with active ankylosing spondylitis despite treatment with

NSAIAs and contraindications to treatment with a TNF blocking agent, secukinumab or ixekizumab is conditionally recommended over treatment with sulfasalazine, methotrexate, or tofacitinib. In patients with active ankylosing spondylitis despite treatment with a first TNF blocking agent, guidelines conditionally recommend secukinumab or ixekizumab over treatment with a different TNF blocking agent in patients with primary nonresponse to TNF blocking therapy. In adults with stable ankylosing spondylitis, continuation of biologic monotherapy is conditionally recommended over discontinuation of the biologic or continuation of combination therapy with NSAIAs or conventional DMARDs. Recommendations for treatment selection in ankylosing spondylitis may be influenced by the presence of certain comorbidities (e.g., iritis, inflammatory bowel disease). Consult the joint guideline issued by the American College of Rheumatology, the Spondylitis Association of America, and the Spondyloarthritis Research and Treatment Network for additional details.

● Nonradiographic Axial Spondyloarthritis

Secukinumab is used for the management of active nonradiographic axial spondyloarthritis in adults with objective signs of inflammation.

Clinical Experience

Safety and efficacy of secukinumab for this indication were evaluated in a randomized, double-blind, placebo-controlled study (PREVENT) in 555 patients with active adult-onset axial spondyloarthritis according to ASAS criteria and objective signs of inflammation (i.e., active sacroiliitis on magnetic resonance imaging and/or CRP above the upper limit of normal) despite treatment with NSAIAs. Included patients were also required to have symptoms of active disease, which were defined by a BASDAI score of ≥4 and VAS for total back pain of ≥40 on scales of 0–10 and 0–100 mm, respectively. Patients were excluded if they had radiographic sacroiliitis meeting modified New York criteria for ankylosing spondylitis. Patients were randomized (stratified based on signs of inflammation) to self-administer subcutaneous secukinumab 150 mg with a loading dose (weekly for 5 weeks, then once every 4 weeks thereafter), secukinumab 150 mg without a loading dose (given once every 4 weeks starting week 0), or placebo. After 20 weeks, nonresponders were permitted to switch to open-label treatment with subcutaneous secukinumab 150 mg or standard of care. Approximately 10% of patients received concomitant methotrexate and 15% of patients received concomitant sulfasalazine, and 10% of patients were previously treated with TNF blocking agents but discontinued use due to intolerance or lack of efficacy. The primary outcome measure was the proportion of patients achieving an ASAS 40 response at week 52. ASAS 40 was also assessed at week 16.

At week 52, a greater proportion of patients who received secukinumab 150 mg without a loading dose achieved an ASAS 40 response compared with patients who received placebo; response rates were 34, 38, and 19% in the secukinumab with a loading dose, secukinumab without a loading dose, and placebo groups, respectively. Similarly, ASAS 40 responses were achieved in 40, 41, and 28% of patients in the secukinumab with loading dose, secukinumab without loading dose, and placebo groups, respectively, at week 16. At week 16, patients receiving secukinumab (both with and without a loading dose) reported greater improvements in quality of life as measured by the Ankylosing Spondylitis Quality of Life (ASQOL) measure compared to those receiving placebo.

Clinical response to secukinumab was consistent across a variety of subgroups, including patients grouped by CRP status, MRI status, human leukocyte antigen (HLA)-B27 status, and sex. The largest differences in treatment response between those treated with secukinumab and placebo were seen in patients who had both an elevated CRP and MRI evidence of sacroiliitis.

The effectiveness of IV secukinumab in the treatment of active nonradiographic axial spondyloarthritis in adults was extrapolated from the established effectiveness of subcutaneous secukinumab in adults with active nonradiographic axial spondyloarthritis based on pharmacokinetic exposure.

Clinical Perspective

The American College of Rheumatology, the Spondylitis Association of America, and the Spondyloarthritis Research and Treatment Network issued a joint guideline for the treatment of nonradiographic axial spondyloarthritis in 2019. Treatments for nonradiographic axial spondyloarthritis include NSAIAs, conventional DMARDs (e.g., methotrexate, sulfasalazine), biologic DMARDs (e.g., TNF blocking agents, secukinumab, ixekizumab), and/or targeted synthetic DMARDs (e.g., tofacitinib). Continuous NSAIA treatment is typically considered first-line for

active nonradiographic axial spondyloarthritis, with other agents being used in the treatment of NSAIA-refractory disease. Specific agents for nonradiographic axial spondyloarthritis treatment are selected according to current disease activity and prior therapies used. Goals of therapy in nonradiographic axial spondyloarthritis are to alleviate symptoms, improve functioning, maintain the ability to work, decrease complications, and prevent or slow skeletal damage.

Recommendations for the treatment of nonradiographic axial spondyloarthritis are largely extrapolated from evidence in the treatment of ankylosing spondylitis, due to a lack of data specific to nonradiographic axial spondyloarthritis. IL-17 blocking agents used in the treatment of ankylosing spondylitis (and, by extension, nonradiographic axial spondyloarthritis) are secukinumab and ixekizumab. Consult the joint guideline issued by the American College of Rheumatology, the Spondylitis Association of America, and the Spondyloarthritis Research and Treatment Network for additional details.

● Enthesitis-related Arthritis

Secukinumab is used for the management of active enthesitis-related arthritis in pediatric patients ≥4 years of age.

Clinical Experience

Efficacy of secukinumab in the treatment of enthesitis-related arthritis in pediatric patients was evaluated in a randomized, double-blind, phase 3 trial in biologic-naïve patients (2 to <18 years of age). Patients with juvenile idiopathic arthritis (enthesitis-related or psoriatic arthritis) underwent open-label treatment with secukinumab (75 mg for weight <50 kg; 150 mg for weight ≥50 kg) for up to 12 weeks, followed by randomization of ACR 30 responders to treatment with either secukinumab or placebo up to week 100. Patients who experienced a flare of disease during the randomized phase entered open-label secukinumab treatment up to week 104. The primary outcome was time to disease flare (≥30% worsening of ≥3 of 6 JIA ACR criteria and ≥30% improvement in ≤1 of 6 JIA ACR criteria and a minimum of 2 active joints) in the randomized phase.

Of 86 patients enrolled, 52 had enthesitis-related arthritis. The mean age of patients with enthesitis-related arthritis was 13.7 years of age; 78.8% were male and 98.1% were white, with a baseline Juvenile Arthritis Disease activity score of 14.8. Concomitant methotrexate was used by 63.5% of patients with enthesitis-related arthritis.

At week 12, JIA ACR 30, 50, 70, or 90 response rates were seen in 85, 79, 65, or 33% of patients with enthesitis-related arthritis given open-label secukinumab. In the randomized phase, 10 and 6 patients with enthesitis-related arthritis who received placebo and secukinumab, respectively, experienced a flare event. Flare risk was reduced by 53% for patients who received secukinumab compared to those who received placebo.

Clinical Perspective

Enthesitis-related arthritis in pediatric patients is classified as a subtype of juvenile idiopathic arthritis. The American College of Rheumatology and the Arthritis Foundation issued a joint guideline for the treatment of juvenile idiopathic arthritis manifesting as nonsystemic polyarthritis, sacroiliitis, or enthesitis in 2019. In children and adolescents with juvenile idiopathic arthritis and active enthesitis, NSAIA treatment is strongly recommended over no NSAIA treatment. For active enthesitis despite NSAIA treatment, a TNF inhibitor (e.g., etanercept, adalimumab, infliximab, golimumab) is conditionally recommended over methotrexate or sulfasalazine. Oral glucocorticoids as bridging therapy can be used for a limited course (<3 months) during initiation or escalation of therapy for patients with juvenile idiopathic arthritis and chronic active enthesitis despite use of NSAIAs, especially in the case of high disease activity, limited mobility, and/or significant symptoms. The guideline does not address the use of IL-17 blocking agents.

● Hidradenitis Suppurativa

Secukinumab is used for the management of moderate to severe hidradenitis suppurativa in adults.

Clinical Experience

Efficacy of secukinumab for the treatment of hidradenitis suppurativa in adults was evaluated in 2 randomized, double-blind, phase 3 trials (SUNSHINE and SUNRISE). In both trials, adult patients with moderate to severe hidradenitis suppurativa were randomly assigned to treatment with placebo or secukinumab

300 mg by subcutaneous injection at weeks 0, 1, 2, 3, 4 followed by 300 mg every 2 or every 4 weeks. At week 16, patients initially randomized to placebo were reassigned to treatment with secukinumab 300 mg at weeks 16, 17, 18, 19, and 20, followed by secukinumab 300 mg every 2 or every 4 weeks. The primary outcome in both trials was the percent of patients with a hidradenitis suppurativa clinical response (HiSCR50), defined as ≥50% decrease in abscess and inflammatory nodule count with no increase in the number of abscesses and/or number of draining fistulae at week 16 compared to baseline.

A total of 1084 patients were enrolled in both trials. In SUNSHINE and SUNRISE, respectively, 13% and 11% of patients received concomitant stable dose of systemic antibiotics, and 24% and 23% of patients were previously treated with a biologic and discontinued the biologic for either intolerance or lack of efficacy.

In SUNSHINE, at week 16, HiSCR50 was achieved in 29.4, 41.3, or 44.5% of patients given placebo, secukinumab 300 every 4 weeks, or secukinumab 300 mg every 2 weeks, respectively. In SUNRISE, at week 16, HiSCR50 was achieved in 26.1, 42.5, or 38.3% of patients given placebo, secukinumab 300 mg every 4 weeks, or secukinumab 300 mg every 2 weeks, respectively. Improvements were observed for the primary outcome regardless of previous or concomitant antibiotic treatment or previous biologic exposure.

Clinical Perspective

Hidradenitis suppurativa is a chronic, relapsing inflammatory skin disorder characterized by recurrent painful nodules, abscesses, fistulas, sinus tracts, and scarring in apocrine gland-bearing regions (e.g., axillae, inframammary area, inguinal and anogenital regions, perineum). Dysregulated skin immunity around hair follicles in these regions is thought to be involved; initial pathogenic events involve perifollicular inflammation leading to hyperkeratosis and hair follicle occlusion, followed by follicular rupture and an inflammatory response resulting in the development of clinical lesions characteristic of the disorder. Hidradenitis suppurativa has a female predominance; onset typically occurs after puberty.

The United States and Canadian Hidradenitis Suppurativa Foundations published a joint guideline for the treatment of this disorder in 2019. Clinical management of hidradenitis suppurativa involves the use of both medical and surgical therapies. Medical therapies used in hidradenitis suppurativa include topical/intralesional therapies, systemic antibiotics, hormonal therapies (e.g., antiandrogen contraceptives, spironolactone, metformin, finasteride), retinoids, systemic immunomodulators (i.e., colchicine, cyclosporine), systemic corticosteroids, and biologic agents (e.g., adalimumab, infliximab, anakinra, ustekinumab). Immunomodulation is increasingly becoming the cornerstone of therapy for moderate to severe hidradenitis suppurativa; there is interest in targeting the TNF and interleukin pathways. The specific place in therapy for secukinumab has not yet been established.

DOSAGE AND ADMINISTRATION

● General

Pretreatment Screening

- Evaluate for active or latent tuberculosis infection prior to initiation of secukinumab; start antimycobacterial therapy if indicated.
- Administer all age-appropriate vaccines prior to starting secukinumab therapy.

Patient Monitoring

- Monitor closely for signs or symptoms of infection or active tuberculosis during and after treatment with secukinumab.
- Monitor for signs and symptoms of inflammatory bowel disease during treatment.

Other General Considerations

- Secukinumab may be used alone or in combination with methotrexate for the treatment of psoriatic arthritis (including juvenile psoriatic arthritis).

● Administration

Secukinumab is commercially available as an IV injection containing 125 mg/5 mL solution in a single-dose vial. Secukinumab is also commercially available as a subcutaneous injection containing 300 mg/2 mL solution in a single-dose pen

(UnoReady®) or single-dose prefilled syringe; 150 mg/mL solution in a single-dose pen (Sensoready®) or single-dose prefilled syringe; and 75 mg/0.5 mL solution in a single-dose prefilled syringe (for pediatric patients). Secukinumab injection pens (Sensoready®, UnoReady®) and prefilled syringes are supplied with a 27-gauge, ½-inch needle.

Administer secukinumab by IV infusion or subcutaneous injection. Secukinumab is intended for use under the guidance and supervision of a clinician.

IV Administration

The IV infusion is intended for administration by a healthcare professional in a healthcare setting.

Secukinumab may be administered as an IV infusion only in adults with active psoriatic arthritis, ankylosing spondylitis, or non-radiographic axial spondyloarthritis.

Store the unused IV injection at 2–8°C. Store in the original carton to protect from light until time of use; do not freeze or shake the injection.

Dilute secukinumab solution using proper aseptic technique prior to IV administration.

Calculate the total volume (in mL) of secukinumab required based on the patient's actual body weight as follows: 0.24 mL/kg for loading dose (6 mg/kg), and 0.07 mL/kg for maintenance dose (1.75 mg/kg). Use the number of vials based on total volume needed.

Following dilution, discard unused secukinumab in vials because it does not contain preservatives.

Administer the diluted solution for infusion as soon as possible. If not administered immediately, store the diluted solution either at: a) at room temperature (20–25°C) for ≤4.5 hours from the start of the preparation (piercing the first vial) to the completion of infusion, or b) under refrigeration (2–8°C) for ≤24 hours from the start of the time of the preparation to the completion of infusion. This time includes the refrigeration of the diluted solution and time to allow the diluted solution to warm to room temperature. Protect the diluted solution from light during storage under refrigeration.

Use only an infusion set with a sterile, in-line, nonpyrogenic, low protein-binding, 0.2 micron filter for administration. Information on physical and/or chemical compatibility of secukinumab with other drugs is not available; the manufacturer recommends that secukinumab not be infused through the same IV line as other drugs. When administration of the secukinumab infusion is complete, flush the infusion line with ≥50 mL of 0.9% sodium chloride.

Dilution

Prior to dilution, allow secukinumab vials to sit at room temperature (20-25°C) for approximately 20 minutes.

For patients who weigh >52 kg at the time of dosing, dilute secukinumab loading and maintenance dose in a 100 mL infusion bag of 0.9% sodium chloride.

For patients who weigh ≤52 kg at the time of dosing, dilute secukinumab loading dose in a 100 mL infusion bag of 0.9% sodium chloride, and dilute the maintenance dose in a 50 mL infusion bag of 0.9% sodium chloride. If a 50 mL infusion bag is not available to dilute the maintenance dose, use a 100 mL infusion bag and withdraw and discard 50 mL of saline using aseptic technique, and continue to follow the preparation and administration steps.

From the infusion bag, withdraw and discard a volume of 0.9% sodium chloride equal to the calculated volume of secukinumab solution required for the patient's dose. From the secukinumab vial(s), withdraw the calculated volume (mL) of secukinumab solution and add slowly into the 0.9% sodium chloride infusion bag. To mix the secukinumab solution, gently invert the bag to avoid foaming; do not shake.

Rate of Administration

Administer secukinumab infusion at a flow rate of about 3.3 mL/minute for a 100 mL bag or 1.7 mL/minute for a 50 mL bag. Administer the IV infusion over 30 minutes.

Subcutaneous Administration

Secukinumab may be self-administered subcutaneously by adults if the clinician determines that the patient and/or caregiver is competent to safely administer the drug after appropriate training. Pediatric patients are not eligible for self-administration of secukinumab; however, an adult caregiver can administer secukinumab to a pediatric patient after proper training on subcutaneous injection technique.

Administer subcutaneous injections into the upper arms, thighs, or any quadrant of the abdomen; avoid injections within 2 inches of the navel. Rotate injection sites. Administration in the upper, outer arm may be performed by a caregiver or clinician. Do not administer into areas where the skin is tender, bruised, erythematous, indurated, or affected by psoriasis.

Secukinumab is a clear to slightly opalescent, colorless to slightly yellow solution. Prior to administration, visually inspect the secukinumab solution for particulate matter or discoloration; discard the solution if it is cloudy, discolored, or contains particulates.

Secukinumab injection pens and prefilled syringes are for single use only; discard any unused portions.

Store the injection pens (300 mg/2 mL, 150 mg/mL) and prefilled syringes (150 mg/mL, 75 mg/0.5 mL) at 2–8°C. Store in the original carton to protect from light until time of use; do not freeze or shake the injection. If removed from refrigeration, secukinumab injection pens (150 mg/mL) and prefilled syringes (150 mg/mL, 75 mg/0.5 mL) may be stored at room temperature (not to exceed 30°C) for up to 4 days. If these conditions are met and the product is not used within 4 days, it may be returned to the refrigerator but only 1 time. Discard secukinumab if the drug has been stored outside of refrigeration for more than 4 days.

Allow the injection pen (150 mg/mL) or prefilled syringe (150 mg/mL, 75 mg/0.5 mL) to sit at room temperature in the unopened carton for 15–30 minutes prior to subcutaneous injection. For the 300 mg/2 mL injection pen or prefilled syringe (300 mg/2 mL), allow to sit at room temperature for 30–45 minutes prior to subcutaneous injection. Do not remove the needle cap while the pen or prefilled syringe is warming to room temperature. The removable cap of the injection pen (150 mg/mL) and the prefilled syringe (150 mg/mL, 75 mg/0.5 mL) contains natural rubber latex and should not be handled by latex-sensitive individuals.

Refer to the instructions for use in the prescribing information for more detailed instructions on the preparation and administration of each presentation and strength of secukinumab.

● Dosage

IV dosage for secukinumab is based on actual body weight.

Adult Dosage

Plaque Psoriasis

For subcutaneous use in the management of moderate to severe plaque psoriasis in adults who are candidates for phototherapy or systemic therapy, the recommended dosage of secukinumab is 300 mg at weeks 0, 1, 2, 3, and 4, followed by 300 mg every 4 weeks. Each 300-mg dose can be administered as 2 injections of 150 mg or one 300-mg injection. For some patients (e.g., those with lower body weight and less severe disease), doses of 150 mg may be acceptable.

Psoriatic Arthritis

For subcutaneous use in the management of active psoriatic arthritis in adults, the recommended dosage of secukinumab is 150 mg. This dosage can be administered with a loading dose (150 mg administered at weeks 0, 1, 2, 3, and 4, followed by 150 mg every 4 weeks thereafter), or without a loading dose (150 mg administered once every 4 weeks). Consider dosage escalation to 300 mg once every 4 weeks in patients who continue to experience psoriatic arthritis; each 300-mg dose can be administered as 2 injections of 150 mg or one 300-mg injection.

The recommended subcutaneous dosage of secukinumab in adults with psoriatic arthritis and coexisting moderate to severe plaque psoriasis is 300 mg by subcutaneous injection at weeks 0, 1, 2, 3, and 4, followed by 300 mg every 4 weeks. Each 300-mg dose is administered as 2 injections of 150 mg or one 300-mg injection. For some patients (e.g., those with lower body weight and less severe disease), doses of 150 mg may be acceptable.

For IV use in the management of active psoriatic arthritis in adults, the recommended dosage of secukinumab can be administered with a loading dose (6 mg/kg administered at week 0, followed by 1.75 mg/kg every 4 weeks thereafter), or without a loading dose (1.75 mg/kg administered once every 4 weeks). For

maintenance doses of 1.75 mg/kg, total doses exceeding 300 mg per infusion are not recommended.

For the management of active psoriatic arthritis, secukinumab may be administered with or without methotrexate.

Ankylosing Spondylitis

For subcutaneous use in the management of active ankylosing spondylitis in adults, the recommended dosage of secukinumab is 150 mg. This dosage can be administered with a loading dose (150 mg administered at weeks 0, 1, 2, 3, and 4, followed by 150 mg every 4 weeks thereafter), or without a loading dose (150 mg administered once every 4 weeks). If the patient continues to have active ankylosing spondylitis, consider a dosage of 300 mg every 4 weeks; each 300-mg dose can be administered as 2 injections of 150 mg or one 300-mg injection.

For IV use in the management of active ankylosing spondylitis in adults, the recommended dosage of secukinumab can be administered with a loading dose (6 mg/kg administered at week 0, followed by 1.75 mg/kg every 4 weeks thereafter), or without a loading dose (1.75 mg/kg administered once every 4 weeks). For maintenance doses of 1.75 mg/kg, total doses exceeding 300 mg per infusion are not recommended..

Nonradiographic Axial Spondyloarthritis

For subcutaneous use in the management of active nonradiographic axial spondyloarthritis with objective signs of inflammation in adults, the recommended dosage of secukinumab is 150 mg. This dosage can be administered with a loading dose (150 mg administered at weeks 0, 1, 2, 3, and 4, followed by 150 mg every 4 weeks thereafter), or without a loading dose (150 mg administered once every 4 weeks).

For IV use in the management of active nonradiographic axial spondyloarthritis with objective signs of inflammation in adults, the recommended dosage of secukinumab can be administered with a loading dose (6 mg/kg administered at week 0, followed by 1.75 mg/kg every 4 weeks thereafter), or without a loading dose (1.75 mg/kg administered once every 4 weeks). For maintenance doses of 1.75 mg/kg, total doses exceeding 300 mg per infusion are not recommended.

Hidradenitis Suppurativa

For the management of moderate to severe hidradenitis suppurativa in adults, the recommended dosage of secukinumab is 300 mg by subcutaneous injection at weeks 0, 1, 2, 3, and 4, followed by 300 mg once every 4 weeks. Consider a dosage of 300 mg once every 2 weeks in patients who continue to experience hidradenitis suppurativa. Each 300-mg dose is administered as 2 injections of 150 mg or one 300-mg injection.

Pediatric Dosage

Plaque Psoriasis

For the management of moderate to severe plaque psoriasis in pediatric patients ≥6 years of age who are candidates for phototherapy or systemic therapy and weigh <50 kg, the recommended dosage of secukinumab is 75 mg by subcutaneous injection at weeks 0, 1, 2, 3, and 4, followed by 75 mg once every 4 weeks. In pediatric patients ≥6 years of age who weigh ≥50 kg, the recommended dosage of secukinumab is 150 mg by subcutaneous injection at weeks 0, 1, 2, 3, and 4, followed by 150 mg once every 4 weeks.

Juvenile Psoriatic Arthritis

For the management of juvenile psoriatic arthritis in pediatric patients ≥2 years of age who weigh ≥15 kg and <50 kg, the recommended dosage of secukinumab is 75 mg by subcutaneous injection at weeks 0, 1, 2, 3, and 4, followed by 75 mg once every 4 weeks. In pediatric patients ≥2 years of age who weigh ≥50 kg, the recommended dosage of secukinumab is 150 mg by subcutaneous injection at weeks 0, 1, 2, 3, and 4, followed by 150 mg once every 4 weeks.

For the management of juvenile psoriatic arthritis, secukinumab may be administered with or without methotrexate.

Enthesitis-related Arthritis

For the management of active enthesitis-related arthritis in pediatric patients ≥4 years of age who weigh ≥15 kg and <50 kg, the recommended dosage of secukinumab is 75 mg by subcutaneous injection at weeks 0, 1, 2, 3, and 4, followed by

75 mg once every 4 weeks. In pediatric patients ≥4 years of age who weigh ≥50 kg, the recommended dosage of secukinumab is 150 mg by subcutaneous injection at weeks 0, 1, 2, 3, and 4, followed by 150 mg once every 4 weeks.

• Special Populations

Hepatic Impairment

The manufacturer makes no specific dosage recommendations for patients with hepatic impairment.

Renal Impairment

The manufacturer makes no specific dosage recommendations for patients with renal impairment.

Geriatric Patients

The manufacturer makes no specific dosage recommendations for geriatric patients.

CAUTIONS

• Contraindications

- Serious hypersensitivity to secukinumab or any excipients in the formulation.

• Warnings/Precautions

Sensitivity Reactions

Hypersensitivity Reactions

Anaphylaxis and urticaria were reported in patients who received secukinumab in clinical studies. If an anaphylactic or other serious allergic reaction occurs, secukinumab should be discontinued immediately and appropriate supportive treatment initiated.

Latex Sensitivity

Some packaging components (i.e., removable cap) of the 150 mg/mL injection pen and the 1 mL and 0.5 mL prefilled syringes contain natural latex proteins in the form of natural rubber latex, which may cause a hypersensitivity reaction by individuals sensitive to latex. Some individuals may be hypersensitive to natural latex proteins found in a wide range of medical devices, including such packaging components, and the level of sensitivity may vary depending on the form of natural rubber present; rarely, hypersensitivity reactions to natural latex proteins have been fatal. The manufacturer states that the safety of using the 150 mg/mL injection pen or 1 mL and 0.5 mL prefilled syringes in latex-sensitive individuals has not been established.

Infectious Complications

Patients receiving secukinumab may be at an increased risk of developing infections. In placebo-controlled clinical studies, higher rates of common infections (e.g., nasopharyngitis [11.4 versus 8.6%], upper respiratory tract infections [2.5 versus 0.7%], and mucocutaneous candidiasis [1.2 versus 0.3%]) were observed in patients with moderate to severe plaque psoriasis receiving secukinumab compared with those receiving placebo. Similar increases in infection risk were observed in placebo-controlled trials of secukinumab for treatment of psoriatic arthritis, ankylosing spondylitis, and nonradiographic axial spondyloarthritis. Serious and some fatal infections have also been reported in the postmarketing setting. The incidence of some types of infections (including fungal infections) appeared to be dose dependent.

In the placebo-controlled phase of clinical studies (up to 12 weeks) in plaque psoriasis, a higher rate of infections was reported in individuals receiving secukinumab (28.7%) compared with those receiving placebo (18.9%). Over the entire treatment period (up to 52 weeks for most patients), infections were reported in 47.5% of individuals receiving secukinumab (0.9 per patient-year of follow-up), and serious infections were reported in 1.2% of patients receiving the drug (0.015 per patient-year of follow-up). In open-label extensions of the clinical studies of secukinumab for plaque psoriasis, with a median follow-up of 3.9 years, 74% of patients treated with secukinumab reported infections, and 4.5% of subjects reported serious infections. Clinical trials of secukinumab for its other approved

indications had similar findings. Infection rates for patients treated with secukinumab compared to placebo, respectively, were 29 and 26% in psoriatic arthritis trials and 31 and 18% in ankylosing spondylitis trials. In a clinical trial of secukinumab for nonradiographic axial spondyloarthritis, the incidence of infections and infestations was 92 per 100 patient-years for secukinumab with a loading dose compared to 72 per 100 patient-years for secukinumab without a loading dose.

Secukinumab-associated neutropenia was reported in the controlled portion of clinical studies; however, most cases were transient and reversible, and no serious neutropenia-associated infections were reported. In 2 open-label extensions of psoriatic arthritis studies, neutropenia was reported in 1% of secukinumab-treated patients (0.3 per 100 patient-years). Although some cases of serious infections were reported with neutropenia, a causal relationship was not established.

Clinicians should exercise caution when considering use of secukinumab in patients with a chronic infection or history of recurrent infections. If a serious infection develops, closely monitor the patient and discontinue secukinumab until the infection resolves.

Evaluate patients for active or latent tuberculosis prior to initiation of secukinumab therapy. Do not administer the drug to patients with active tuberculosis infection; when indicated, initiate an appropriate antimycobacterial regimen for treatment of latent tuberculosis prior to administration of secukinumab. Antimycobacterial therapy also should be considered prior to initiation of secukinumab in patients with a history of latent or active tuberculosis in whom an adequate course of antimycobacterial treatment for these indications cannot be confirmed. Monitor patients closely for signs and symptoms of active tuberculosis during and after treatment with secukinumab.

Inflammatory Bowel Disease

Exacerbation of inflammatory bowel disease, which was serious in some cases and/or leading to secukinumab discontinuation, occurred in patients treated with secukinumab during clinical trials in plaque psoriasis, psoriatic arthritis, ankylosing spondylitis, nonradiographic axial spondyloarthritis, and hidradenitis suppurativa. In adults with hidradenitis suppurativa, the incidence of inflammatory bowel disease was higher in patients who received secukinumab 300 mg every 2 weeks compared to those who received secukinumab 300 mg every 4 weeks.

Cases of new onset inflammatory bowel disease have also been reported in clinical trials. A randomized, placebo-controlled phase 2a study evaluating secukinumab in patients with active Crohn disease was terminated early because of lack of efficacy, with the results suggesting an adverse effect on disease activity in patients with objective evidence of inflammation. Secukinumab was associated with higher rates of serious adverse effects, including drug-related worsening of Crohn disease, and higher rates of infection compared with placebo. Secukinumab is not approved for the treatment of Crohn disease.

Use secukinumab with caution in patients with inflammatory bowel disease. Monitor for signs and symptoms of inflammatory bowel disease in patients treated with secukinumab.

Eczematous Eruptions

Severe eczematous eruptions (including atopic dermatitis-like eruptions, dyshidrotic eczema, and erythroderma), some resulting in hospitalization, have been reported in the postmarketing setting. The onset of eczematous eruptions was variable, and ranged from days to months after initiation of secukinumab.

Treatment discontinuation may be required to manage the eczematous eruption, although some patients have been successfully treated for eczematous eruption without discontinuation of secukinumab.

Immunization

Consider administration of all age-appropriate vaccines recommended by current immunization guidelines prior to initiation of secukinumab therapy. Secukinumab may alter the immune response to live vaccinations. Avoid live vaccines during therapy with secukinumab.

Immunogenicity

As with all therapeutic proteins, there is potential for immunogenicity in patients who receive secukinumab. In clinical studies in patients with plaque psoriasis, psoriatic arthritis, ankylosing spondylitis, nonradiographic axial spondyloarthritis, hidradenitis suppurativa, juvenile psoriatic arthritis, or enthesitis-related arthritis, antibodies to secukinumab were detected in <1% of patients receiving secukinumab for periods of up to 52 weeks. Of the patients who developed antibodies to secukinumab, approximately 8% developed neutralizing antibodies. The effect of these neutralizing antibodies on the pharmacokinetics, pharmacodynamics, safety, or efficacy of secukinumab is not known.

Specific Populations

Pregnancy

Limited data regarding use of secukinumab in pregnant females are insufficient to inform a drug-associated risk of adverse developmental outcomes. Reproductive and developmental toxicity studies in monkeys at secukinumab exposure levels of up to 30 times the human exposure at the maximum recommended subcutaneous dosage revealed no evidence of adverse developmental effects on fetuses or neonatal offspring.

Lactation

It is not known whether secukinumab is distributed into human milk or if the drug is absorbed systemically after ingestion. Potential effects of the drug on milk production or on breast-fed infants are unknown. Consider the benefits of breast-feeding and the importance of secukinumab to the female along with potential adverse effects on the breast-fed infant from the drug or from the underlying maternal condition.

Pediatric Use

Safety and efficacy of secukinumab have been established for the treatment of moderate to severe plaque psoriasis in pediatric patients ≥6 years of age who are candidates for systemic therapy or phototherapy. Safety and efficacy of secukinumab in pediatric patients <6 years of age with plaque psoriasis have not been established.

Safety and efficacy of secukinumab have been established for the treatment of active juvenile psoriatic arthritis in pediatric patients ≥2 years of age who weigh ≥15 kg. Safety and efficacy of secukinumab in pediatric patients with juvenile psoriatic arthritis <2 years of age or who weigh <15 kg have not been established.

Safety and efficacy of secukinumab have been established for the treatment of active ethesitis-related arthritis in pediatric patients ≥4 years of age who weigh ≥15 kg. Safety and efficacy of secukinumab in pediatric patients with ethesitis-related arthritis <4 years of age or who weigh <15 kg have not been established.

Safety and efficacy of secukinumab in pediatric patients with hidradenitis suppurativa have not been established.

Safety and efficacy of IV secukinumab in pediatric patients have not been established.

Geriatric Use

Of the 3430 patients with plaque psoriasis who received subcutaneous secukinumab in clinical trials, 7% were ≥65 years of age, while 1% were ≥75 years of age. Although no overall differences in efficacy or safety between geriatric patients and younger adults were observed, the clinical trials did not include sufficient numbers of patients ≥65 years of age to determine whether geriatric patients respond differently than younger adults.

Of the 1060 patients with hidradenitis suppurativa who received secukinumab in clinical trials, 1.3% were ≥65 years of age. Clinical trials in hidradenitis suppurativa did not include a sufficient number of patients ≥65 years of age to assess differences in response compared to younger adults.

Population pharmacokinetic analysis indicated that clearance of secukinumab was not significantly influenced by age in adults with plaque psoriasis, psoriatic arthritis, and ankylosing spondylitis. The apparent clearance of secukinumab appears to be similar in patients ≥65 years of age and patients <65 years of age.

Hepatic Impairment

The pharmacokinetics of secukinumab have not been formally studied in patients with hepatic impairment.

Renal Impairment

The pharmacokinetics of secukinumab have not been formally studied in patients with renal impairment.

• Common Adverse Effects

Adverse effects reported in >1% of patients receiving secukinumab include nasopharyngitis, diarrhea, and upper respiratory tract infection.,

DRUG INTERACTIONS

No formal drug interaction studies have been performed to date.

• Drugs Metabolized by Hepatic Microsomal Enzymes

Increased concentrations of cytokines (e.g., interleukin-17) during chronic inflammation associated with certain diseases including plaque psoriasis, psoriatic arthritis, ankylosing spondylitis, nonradiographic axial spondyloarthritis, enthesitis-related arthritis, and hidradenitis suppurativa may suppress the formation of cytochrome P-450 (CYP) isoenzymes.

In adults with plaque psoriasis, the pharmacokinetics of midazolam (CYP3A4 substrate) was similar when administered alone, or when administered following either a single or 5 weekly subcutaneous administrations of secukinumab 300 mg.

Upon initiation or discontinuance of secukinumab in patients who are receiving concomitant CYP substrates, especially those where minimal decreases in the concentration could reduce the CYP substrate efficacy or minimal increases in the concentration could increase CYP substrate adverse reactions, the clinician should consider monitoring for therapeutic effect or concentration of the CYP substrate and consider dosage adjustment of the CYP substrate as necessary.

• Vaccines

Live Vaccines

Do not administer live vaccines to patients receiving secukinumab.

Inactivated Vaccines

Antibody responses to a meningococcal (group C) oligosaccharide diphtheria CRM$_{197}$ conjugate vaccine (not commercially available in the US) and to an inactivated seasonal influenza virus vaccine (non-US preparation) were similar in healthy individuals who received secukinumab (single 150-mg dose) and those who received placebo 2 weeks prior to immunization. Clinical effectiveness of meningococcal and influenza vaccines in patients receiving secukinumab therapy has not been established.

DESCRIPTION

Secukinumab is a recombinant human immunoglobulin G$_1$ kappa (IgG$_1$ kappa) monoclonal antibody that is specific for interleukin-17A (IL-17A); it is produced in a recombinant Chinese hamster ovary cell line. IL-17A is a subtype of the IL-17 family of proinflammatory cytokines secreted principally by T-helper 17 (Th17) cells. Elevated levels of IL-17A have been found in psoriatic lesions and blood of individuals with psoriasis. Increased numbers of IL-17A-producing lymphocytes and innate immune cells and increased levels of IL-17A have been observed in the blood of patients with psoriatic arthritis and ankylosing spondylitis. Increased numbers of IL-17A-producing lymphocytes also have been observed in patients with nonradiographic axial spondyloarthritis. Secukinumab binds to IL-17A and inhibits its interaction with the IL-17 receptor, thus neutralizing the biologic activity of IL-17A and inhibiting the release of proinflammatory cytokines, chemokines, and mediators of tissue damage.

Following IV administration of the secukinumab maintenance dose of 1.75 mg/kg every 4 weeks (with or without a loading dose of 6 mg/kg at day 0), drug plasma concentrations are estimated to be within the range of steady state concentrations attained following subcutaneous administration of 150 mg and 300 mg secukinumab doses administered every 4 weeks.

The pharmacokinetics of secukinumab administered subcutaneously in patients with plaque psoriasis, psoriatic arthritis, ankylosing spondylitis, and nonradiographic axial spondyloarthritis are similar. The pharmacokinetics of secukinumab are also similar in pediatric patients with enthesitis-related arthritis and plaque psoriasis for the same weight-tiered dosing regimen. In patients with hidradenitis suppurativa, mean steady- state trough concentrations are approximately 26% lower than observed in patients with plaque psoriasis.

Secukinumab exhibited dose-proportional pharmacokinetics in patients with plaque psoriasis over a subcutaneous dosage range of 25–300 mg. In patients with plaque psoriasis, peak plasma concentrations of the drug were achieved by approximately 6 days after subcutaneous administration of secukinumab 150 or 300 mg. Trough concentrations achieved following secukinumab administration by Sensoready® injection pen may be approximately 30% higher than those achieved following administration by prefilled syringe. Following multiple subcutaneous doses of 300 mg administered using the 300 mg/2 mL UnoReady® pen, mean trough concentrations were generally similar to those delivered in a study using the Sensoready® pen to administer 300 mg. Steady-state concentrations of secukinumab were achieved by 24 weeks following the every-4-week secukinumab dosing regimens.

In healthy individuals and patients with plaque psoriasis, bioavailability ranged from 55–77% following a subcutaneous dose of 150 or 300 mg (administered as two 150-mg injections). In clinical trials of individuals with hidradenitis suppurativa, following subcutaneous administration of secukinumab 300 mg at weeks 0, 1, 2, 3, and 4 and then every 2 weeks thereafter, steady-state concentrations of secukinumab were achieved by 24 weeks.

Concentrations of the drug in interstitial fluid in lesional and nonlesional skin of patients with plaque psoriasis were 27–40% of serum concentrations at 1 and 2 weeks following a single 300-mg subcutaneous dose (administered as two 150-mg injections). The metabolic pathway of secukinumab has not been characterized. As a human IgG1 kappa monoclonal antibody, the drug is expected to be degraded into small peptides and amino acids via catabolic pathways in the same manner as endogenous IgG. The mean half-life of secukinumab ranged from 22–31 days in patients with plaque psoriasis following IV or subcutaneous administration. Based on a population pharmacokinetic analysis, the estimated mean elimination half-life of secukinumab is 23 days in patients with hidradenitis suppurativa. Secukinumab clearance and volume of distribution increase as body weight increases.

ADVICE TO PATIENTS

- Advise patients to read the FDA-approved patient labeling (medication guide and instructions for use).

- Instruct patients and/or caregivers regarding proper storage, dosage, and subcutaneous administration of secukinumab prefilled syringes or injection pens, including the use of aseptic technique, and proper disposal of needles and syringes if it is determined that the patient and/or caregiver is competent to safely administer the drug.

- Inform patients and/or caregivers that pediatric patients should not self-administer secukinumab using the prefilled syringe or injection pen.

- Advise patients on the increased susceptibility to infection. Advise patients to promptly inform their clinician if any signs or symptoms of infection (e.g., fever, sweats, or chills; muscle aches; cough or shortness of breath; blood in phlegm; weight loss; warm, red or painful sores on the body; diarrhea or stomach pain; burning upon urination or increased urination) occur.

- Advise patients to inform their clinician if they develop new or worsening symptoms of inflammatory bowel disease (e.g., stomach pain, diarrhea) during secukinumab therapy.

- Inform patients that skin reactions that resemble eczema may occur while taking secukinumab, and that they should seek medical advice if signs or symptoms of eczema occur.

- Advise patients to review their vaccination status with clinicians and receive all appropriate vaccinations prior to initiation of secukinumab. Advise patients that vaccination with live vaccines is not recommended during secukinumab therapy. Instruct patients to inform their clinician that they are taking secukinumab prior to a potential vaccination.

- Advise patients to alert their clinician if allergy to latex exists. Advise latex-sensitive patients that the removal caps of some secukinumab preparations contain natural rubber latex, which may cause an allergic reaction.

- Advise patients to seek immediate medical attention if symptoms of a serious allergic reaction (e.g., feeling faint; swelling of eyelids, face, lips, mouth, tongue, or throat; dyspnea or throat tightness; chest tightness; rash) occur.

- Advise patients to inform their clinicians of existing or contemplated therapy, including prescription or OTC drugs, as well as any concomitant illnesses (e.g., active infection, inflammatory bowel disease) or any history of tuberculosis or other infections.

- Advise females of childbearing age to inform clinicians if they are or plan to become pregnant or plan to breast-feed.

- Inform patients of other important precautionary information.

PREPARATIONS

Excipients in commercially available drug preparations may have clinically important effects in some individuals; consult specific product labeling for details.

Secukinumab

Parenteral

Injection, for subcutaneous use	300 mg/2 mL	Cosentyx® (available as single-dose prefilled syringes and UnoReady® pens), Novartis
	150 mg/mL	Cosentyx® (available as single-dose prefilled syringes and single-use Sensoready® pens), Novartis
	75 mg/0.5 mL	Cosentyx® (available as single-use prefilled syringes), Novartis
For injection, for intravenous use	125 mg/5 mL	Cosentyx® (available as single-dose vial), Novartis

† Use is not currently included in the labeling approved by the US Food and Drug Administration.

Selected Revisions July 10, 2024, © Copyright, July 15, 2015, American Society of Health-System Pharmacists, Inc.

Tocilizumab

90:24.20.92 • INTERLEUKIN-MEDIATED AGENTS, MISCELLANEOUS

■ Tocilizumab, a recombinant humanized immunoglobulin G_1 (IgG_1) monoclonal antibody specific for the interleukin-6 (IL-6) receptor, is a biologic response modifier and a disease-modifying antirheumatic drug (DMARD).

USES

Tocilizumab is used alone or in combination with methotrexate or other nonbiologic disease-modifying antirheumatic drugs (DMARDs) for the management of moderately to severely active rheumatoid arthritis in adults who have had an inadequate response to one or more DMARDs and also is used alone or in combination with methotrexate for the management of active systemic or polyarticular juvenile idiopathic arthritis (JIA). The drug is used in the management of giant cell arteritis (GCA) in adults. Tocilizumab is also used in the management of chimeric antigen receptor (CAR) T cell-induced severe or life-threatening cytokine release syndrome (CRS). Tocilizumab is also used in adults with systemic sclerosis-associated interstitial lung disease (SSc-ILD) to slow the rate of decline in pulmonary function. In addition, the drug is used in the management of coronavirus disease 2019 (COVID-19) in hospitalized patients.

• Rheumatoid Arthritis in Adults

Tocilizumab is used for the management of moderately to severely active rheumatoid arthritis in adults who have had an inadequate response to one or more DMARDs. Tocilizumab can be used alone or in combination with methotrexate or other nonbiologic DMARDs (e.g., hydroxychloroquine, leflunomide, minocycline, sulfasalazine). Concomitant use of tocilizumab with other biologic DMARDs, such as tumor necrosis factor (TNF; TNF-α) blocking agents (e.g., adalimumab, certolizumab pegol, etanercept, golimumab, infliximab), interleukin-1 (IL-1) receptor antagonists (e.g., anakinra), anti-CD20 monoclonal antibodies (e.g., rituximab), and selective costimulation modulators (e.g., abatacept), should be avoided. Concomitant use of these biologic agents with tocilizumab has not been studied, and there is a possibility of increased immunosuppression and increased risk of infection with concomitant use. Tocilizumab has been shown to induce clinical responses, improve physical function, and inhibit progression of structural damage in adults with rheumatoid arthritis.

Although use of tocilizumab is not FDA-approved for treatment-naive patients with rheumatoid arthritis, several studies have been published demonstrating potential efficacy of IV and subcutaneous tocilizumab for treatment-naive patients† with recent onset rheumatoid arthritis.

Clinical Experience with IV Tocilizumab

Safety and efficacy of IV tocilizumab have been evaluated in 5 randomized, double-blind studies in adults (≥18 years of age) with moderate to severe active rheumatoid arthritis. In these studies, tocilizumab was administered as monotherapy, in combination with methotrexate or other nonbiologic DMARDs in patients with an inadequate response to these drugs, or in combination with methotrexate in patients with an inadequate response to TNF blocking agents. Patients included in these studies had 8 or more tender joints and 6 or more swollen joints. Those receiving low stable dosages of corticosteroids (equivalent to 10 mg or less of prednisone daily) and/or stable dosages of nonsteroidal anti-inflammatory agents (NSAIAs) could continue such agents. Tocilizumab was administered IV at a dosage of 4 or 8 mg/kg once every 4 weeks.

The American College of Rheumatology (ACR) criteria for improvement (ACR response) in measures of disease activity were used as the principal measure of clinical response in studies evaluating the efficacy of tocilizumab. An ACR 20 response is achieved if the patient experiences a 20% improvement in tender and swollen joint count and a 20% or greater improvement in at least 3 of the following criteria: patient pain assessment, patient global assessment, physician global assessment, patient self-assessed disability, or laboratory measures of disease activity (i.e., erythrocyte sedimentation rate [ESR] or C-reactive protein

[CRP] level). An ACR 70 response is defined using the same criteria but with a level of improvement of 70%. The proportion of patients who achieved an ACR 20 response at week 24 was the primary end point in the studies of tocilizumab. In one longer-term study, the total Sharp-Genant score (a composite score of erosions and joint space narrowing in hands, wrists, and forefeet) was used as the principal measure of joint damage, and the Health Assessment Questionnaire Disability Index (HAQ-DI) was used to assess physical function and disability.

Clinical evaluations of tocilizumab indicate that, in adults with active rheumatoid arthritis despite therapy with methotrexate or other nonbiologic DMARD(s), the addition of tocilizumab to the DMARD regimen is associated with greater efficacy than use of the nonbiologic DMARD(s) alone. In addition, therapy with tocilizumab in conjunction with methotrexate has been more effective than methotrexate alone in patients with an inadequate response to prior therapy with TNF blocking agents. In patients with an inadequate response to prior therapy with nonbiologic DMARDs or TNF blocking agents, response rates were higher in those receiving tocilizumab 8 mg/kg IV every 4 weeks compared with those receiving 4 mg/kg IV every 4 weeks. When tocilizumab was compared with methotrexate as monotherapy in patients with active rheumatoid arthritis, tocilizumab was more effective than methotrexate. Response to tocilizumab can occur 2–4 weeks following initiation of therapy in some patients.

In the study evaluating efficacy of tocilizumab as monotherapy (AMBITION), patients were randomized to receive either tocilizumab (8 mg/kg IV every 4 weeks) or methotrexate (7.5 mg weekly, increased up to 20 mg weekly). Patients were excluded if they had received methotrexate in the past 6 months, had previously discontinued methotrexate because of lack of response or clinically important toxicity, or had previously discontinued therapy with a TNF blocking agent because of inadequate response. About two-thirds of the patients in the study had never received methotrexate therapy. An ACR 20 response was achieved in 70% of patients receiving tocilizumab and 53% of those receiving methotrexate for 24 weeks.

In 2 studies (OPTION and LITHE), therapy with tocilizumab given in combination with methotrexate was evaluated in patients who had not responded adequately to methotrexate; patients in these studies were randomized to receive tocilizumab 4 mg/kg IV every 4 weeks, tocilizumab 8 mg/kg IV every 4 weeks, or placebo, each given in conjunction with a stable dosage of methotrexate (10–25 mg weekly). Patients who had been treated unsuccessfully with a TNF blocking agent were excluded from these studies. In one study (OPTION), ACR 20 responses were achieved at 24 weeks in 59, 48, or 27% of those receiving tocilizumab 8 mg/kg and methotrexate, tocilizumab 4 mg/kg and methotrexate, or placebo and methotrexate, respectively. The other study (LITHE) was longer term (2 years with an optional 3-year extension phase) and was designed to assess changes in signs and symptoms of rheumatoid arthritis at 24 weeks, with subsequent assessments of joint damage and physical functioning at 1 and 2 years of treatment. Following 1 year of treatment with the randomly assigned regimen, patients received open-label treatment with tocilizumab 8 mg/kg for an additional year or had the option to continue their double-blind treatment if improvement in swollen and tender joint count was maintained above 70%. Planned interim analyses indicated that ACR 20 responses were achieved at 24 weeks in 56, 51, or 27% and at 1 year in 56, 47, or 25% of those receiving tocilizumab 8 mg/kg and methotrexate, tocilizumab 4 mg/kg and methotrexate, or placebo and methotrexate, respectively. At 1 year, 7, 4, or 1% of patients receiving tocilizumab 8 mg/kg and methotrexate, tocilizumab 4 mg/kg and methotrexate, or placebo and methotrexate, respectively, had achieved major clinical responses (defined as ACR 70 responses for a continuous 24-week period). Findings at 1 year also indicated that treatment with tocilizumab 4 or 8 mg/kg and methotrexate inhibited progression of structural damage compared with placebo and methotrexate. At 1 year, 78 or 83% of patients receiving tocilizumab 4 or 8 mg/kg and methotrexate, respectively, exhibited no radiographic progression, as determined by change in total Sharp-Genant score, compared with 66% of patients receiving placebo and methotrexate. Patients receiving tocilizumab 4 or 8 mg/kg and methotrexate also experienced greater improvements in physical function and disability, as assessed using HAQ-DI scores, at 1 year compared with those who received placebo and methotrexate. By the end of the 2-year study, most patients in the placebo and methotrexate group had crossed over to tocilizumab and methotrexate treatment.

In one study (TOWARD) in patients who had not responded adequately to treatment with one or more nonbiologic DMARDs, tocilizumab (8 mg/kg IV weekly) or placebo was added to the stable background DMARD regimen. For 76% of patients in the study, the background regimen contained one DMARD, most commonly methotrexate (mean dosage of 15 mg weekly). Patients who had been treated unsuccessfully with a TNF blocking agent or had previously received any cell-depleting therapy were excluded. At 24 weeks, an ACR 20 response was achieved in 61 or 24% of those receiving tocilizumab or placebo, respectively, in conjunction with the nonbiologic DMARD(s).

Tocilizumab, given in combination with methotrexate, also was evaluated in one study (RADIATE) in patients with rheumatoid arthritis who had not responded adequately to, or who had not tolerated, one or more TNF blocking agents. Patients in this study were randomized to receive tocilizumab 4 mg/kg IV every 4 weeks, tocilizumab 8 mg/kg IV every 4 weeks, or placebo, each given in combination with methotrexate 10–25 mg weekly; tocilizumab was initiated following discontinuance of any other DMARDs and stabilization of the methotrexate dosage. At 24 weeks, an ACR 20 response was achieved in 50, 30, or 10% of those receiving tocilizumab 8 mg/kg and methotrexate, tocilizumab 4 mg/kg and methotrexate, or placebo and methotrexate, respectively.

Analysis of long-term data from the 5 studies showed that improvements from baseline in clinical measures of efficacy generally were sustained through at least 4.2 years of tocilizumab therapy.

General health status was assessed by the Short Form Health Survey (SF-36) in these 5 studies. Patients receiving tocilizumab demonstrated greater improvement from baseline compared with placebo in the physical and mental component summaries and in all 8 domains of the SF-36.

A phase 4, multicenter, open-label randomized trial evaluated the efficacy of tocilizumab compared to rituximab in 161 patients with rheumatoid arthritis who demonstrated an inadequate response to TNF-blocking agents. In this study, 161 patients were stratified based on results of synovial B-cell status determined by biopsy, and randomized to receive two 1000-mg rituximab infusions 2 weeks apart or 8 mg/kg tocilizumab monthly infusions; baseline synovial biopsies from all participants were also subjected to RNA sequencing. In patients who were histologically classified as B-cell rich, no statistically significant difference between treatments was observed in the number of patients who achieved the primary outcome (50% improvement from baseline in the Clinical Disease Activity Index [CDAI]). However, in patients who were classified as having poor B-cell status based on RNA sequencing, a significantly higher response rate for the primary outcome was observed in those who received tocilizumab (63%) than those who received rituximab (36%).

Clinical Experience with Subcutaneous Tocilizumab

Efficacy and safety of subcutaneous tocilizumab have been evaluated in 2 double-blind, controlled studies in adults with moderate to severe active rheumatoid arthritis. One study was a noninferiority study that compared tocilizumab 162 mg subcutaneously every week with tocilizumab 8 mg/kg IV every 4 weeks. The other study was a placebo-controlled superiority study evaluating tocilizumab 162 mg subcutaneously every other week. In these studies, the effects of subcutaneously administered tocilizumab on clinical response and progression of joint damage were consistent with the effects observed in studies evaluating IV administration of the drug.

In the active-control study (SUMMACTA), 1262 patients with moderate to severe active rheumatoid arthritis were randomized in a 1:1 ratio to receive subcutaneous tocilizumab (162 mg every week) or IV tocilizumab (8 mg/kg every 4 weeks) for 24 weeks in conjunction with a stable dosage of one or more nonbiologic DMARDs. To be included in the study, patients were required to have at least 4 tender and 4 swollen joints and to have had an inadequate response to at least one DMARD. Patients receiving stable dosages of NSAIAs and/or low stable dosages of corticosteroids (equivalent to 10 mg or less of prednisone daily) could continue such agents. Approximately 21% of patients included in the study had experienced an inadequate response to prior TNF-blocking agent therapy. ACR 20 response at 24 weeks (the primary measure of efficacy) was observed in 69 or 73% of patients receiving subcutaneous or IV tocilizumab, respectively, establishing noninferiority of the subcutaneous regimen. ACR 50 and ACR 70 responses were observed in 47 and 24%, respectively, of those receiving subcutaneous tocilizumab and 49 and 28%, respectively, of those receiving IV tocilizumab. At 24 weeks, similar proportions of patients receiving subcutaneous or IV tocilizumab (38 or 37%, respectively) had a low level of disease activity, as defined by a Disease Activity Score in 28 joints (DAS 28) of less than 2.6. The mean decrease in HAQ-DI score from baseline to week 24 was 0.6 in both treatment groups, and similar proportions of patients receiving subcutaneous or IV tocilizumab (65 or

67%, respectively) achieved clinically important improvement in HAQ-DI score (change from baseline of at least 0.3 units).

Following the 24-week double-blind period in the SUMMACTA study, patients who had received subcutaneous tocilizumab were randomized in an 11:1 ratio to receive subcutaneous or IV tocilizumab, while those who had received IV tocilizumab were randomized in a 2:1 ratio to receive IV or subcutaneous tocilizumab in a 72-week open-label extension of the study. The proportions of patients who achieved ACR responses, DAS 28 score indicating a low level of disease activity, and clinically important improvement in HAQ-DI score were maintained through week 72 (97 weeks of tocilizumab treatment) and were similar across treatment groups.

In the placebo-controlled study (BREVACTA), 656 patients with moderate to severe active rheumatoid arthritis were randomized in a 2:1 ratio to receive subcutaneous tocilizumab (162 mg every other week) or placebo for 24 weeks in conjunction with a stable dosage of one or more nonbiologic DMARDs. To be included in the study, patients were required to have at least 8 tender and 6 swollen joints and to have had an inadequate response to at least one DMARD. Patients receiving stable dosages of NSAIAs and/or low stable dosages of corticosteroids (equivalent to 10 mg or less of prednisone daily) could continue such agents. Approximately 21% of patients included in the study had experienced an inadequate response to prior TNF-blocking agent therapy. ACR 20 response at 24 weeks (the primary measure of efficacy) was observed in 61% of patients receiving tocilizumab compared with 32% of those receiving placebo. In addition, ACR 50 and ACR 70 responses were observed at 24 weeks in 40 and 20%, respectively, of tocilizumab-treated patients compared with 12 and 5%, respectively, of placebo recipients. At 24 weeks, 32 or 4% of patients receiving tocilizumab or placebo, respectively, had a low level of disease activity, as defined by a DAS 28 score of less than 2.6. Less progression of joint damage, as assessed radiographically by the change in van der Heijde-modified Sharp score (a composite score of structural damage that measures joint erosions and joint space narrowing in the hands, wrists, and feet), was observed in patients receiving tocilizumab compared with those receiving placebo. The mean decrease in HAQ-DI score from baseline to week 24 was 0.4 or 0.3, and the proportion of patients who achieved clinically important improvement in HAQ-DI score (change from baseline of at least 0.3 units) was 58 or 47% for patients receiving tocilizumab or placebo, respectively. In an open-label continuation of this study, efficacy and safety of tocilizumab were maintained for up to 2 years in patients receiving tocilizumab every 2 weeks. Escalation to weekly dosing demonstrated response and tolerability in prior nonresponders.

In the SUMMACTA study, the proportion of patients achieving responses (ACR responses and DAS 28 scores indicating low disease activity) to either IV tocilizumab (8 mg/kg every 4 weeks) or subcutaneous tocilizumab (162 mg every week) generally were similar regardless of body weight, but tended to be lower and more variable in the small subset of patients weighing 100 kg or more. However, in the BREVACTA study, patients weighing 100 kg or more had poorer ACR responses to subcutaneous tocilizumab (162 mg every *other* week) than did patients in 2 lower-weight categories.

Other randomized clinical studies have also demonstrated efficacy of weekly dosing of subcutaneous tocilizumab in patients with inadequate response to every-other-week dosing. Additionally, maintenance of efficacy has been shown in studies of tocilizumab alone (after discontinuation of methotrexate) in patients with low disease activity on methotrexate plus tocilizumab.

Clinical Perspective

The American College of Rheumatology issued guidelines for the treatment of rheumatoid arthritis in 2021. Recommendations for disease-modifying treatments for rheumatoid arthritis include conventional DMARDs (e.g., hydroxychloroquine, leflunomide, methotrexate, sulfasalazine), biologic DMARDs (e.g., TNF blocking agents, abatacept, tocilizumab, sarilumab, rituximab), and/or targeted synthetic DMARDs (e.g., Janus kinase inhibitors). Specific agents for rheumatoid arthritis treatment are selected according to current disease activity, prior therapies used, and the presence of comorbidities. A "treat-to-target" approach is typically employed, with the goal of achieving low disease activity or remission.

IL-6 inhibitors used in the treatment of rheumatoid arthritis include tocilizumab and sarilumab. Methotrexate monotherapy is strongly recommended over biologic DMARD monotherapy for DMARD-naive patients with moderate to high disease activity, because of its established safety and efficacy and lower cost.

Add-on therapy with biologic DMARDs (including IL-6 inhibitors) and targeted synthetic DMARDs is conditionally recommended over triple therapy (i.e., addition of sulfasalazine and hydroxychloroquine) for patients who are taking maximally tolerated doses of methotrexate and are not at target. Recommendations for the use and selection of biologic DMARDs in rheumatoid arthritis vary based on the presence of certain comorbidities (e.g., heart failure, previous serious infection, nontuberculous mycobacterial lung disease).

● Juvenile Idiopathic Arthritis

Tocilizumab is used for the treatment of active systemic or polyarticular juvenile idiopathic arthritis (JIA) in patients ≥2 years of age. Tocilizumab can be used alone or in combination with methotrexate. Concomitant use of tocilizumab with other biologic DMARDs should be avoided. Such concomitant use has not been studied, and there is a possibility of increased immunosuppression and increased risk of infection with concomitant use. Tocilizumab has been shown to produce clinical improvement in patients 2–17 years of age with active polyarticular JIA. Tocilizumab also has been shown to produce clinical improvement and improve physical function in patients 2–17 years of age with active systemic JIA.

Clinical Experience with IV Tocilizumab in Polyarticular Juvenile Idiopathic Arthritis

IV tocilizumab has been evaluated in a randomized, double-blind treatment-withdrawal study (CHERISH) in patients 2–17 years of age with active polyarticular JIA who had not responded adequately to or had not tolerated treatment with methotrexate. Patients included in this study had at least 6 months of active disease, with at least 5 joints with active arthritis (swollen or limitation of movement with pain and/or tenderness) and limitation of motion in at least 3 of the active joints. Disease subtypes included rheumatoid factor-positive or -negative polyarticular JIA and extended oligoarticular JIA. Patients receiving low stable dosages of corticosteroids (equivalent to 0.2 mg/kg or less [maximum of 10 mg] of prednisone daily) and/or a stable dosage of NSAIAs or methotrexate (10–20 mg/m² per week) could continue such therapy; however, concomitant use of other nonbiologic or biologic DMARDs was not permitted. Approximately 32% of patients had received prior biologic DMARD therapy.

During a 16-week lead-in period, all 188 patients enrolled in the study received IV tocilizumab; those weighing 30 kg or more received a dosage of 8 mg/kg every 4 weeks, while those weighing less than 30 kg were randomized to receive a dosage of either 8 or 10 mg/kg every 4 weeks. At week 16, all patients with JIA-ACR 30 response were randomly assigned in a 1:1 ratio (stratified by concomitant methotrexate and corticosteroid use) to continue receiving tocilizumab at the previously assigned dosage or to receive placebo for 24 weeks. JIA-ACR responses are defined as the percentage improvement (e.g., 30, 50, 70, or 90%) in 3 of any 6 core outcome variables compared with baseline, with worsening in no more than 1 of the remaining variables by 30% or more. Core outcome variables consist of physician global assessment, parent or patient global assessment, number of joints with active arthritis, number of joints with limitation of movement, erythrocyte sedimentation rate (ESR), and physical function (as assessed using the disability index of the Childhood Health Assessment Questionnaire [CHAQ-DI]).

At the end of the lead-in period, 91% of patients receiving tocilizumab in combination with methotrexate and 83% of those receiving tocilizumab monotherapy (a total of 163 patients) achieved a JIA-ACR 30 response and entered the treatment-withdrawal period; JIA-ACR 50 and JIA-ACR 70 responses were observed at the end of the lead-in period in 84 and 64%, respectively, of patients receiving tocilizumab in combination with methotrexate and 80 and 55%, respectively, of those receiving tocilizumab monotherapy. Response rates for children weighing less than 30 kg and receiving the 8-mg/kg dose were numerically lower than those for the other 2 treatment groups.

During the treatment-withdrawal period, a greater proportion of patients receiving placebo (48%) compared with those receiving tocilizumab (26%) experienced a JIA-ACR 30 flare (the primary measure of efficacy). JIA-ACR 30 flare was defined as 3 or more of the 6 core outcome variables worsening by at least 30% with no more than 1 of the remaining variables improving by more than 30% relative to the start of the treatment-withdrawal period. At the end of the treatment-withdrawal evaluation period, JIA-ACR 30, 50, and 70 responses were observed in a greater proportion of patients receiving tocilizumab compared with those receiving placebo.

Follow-up of patients in a subsequent open-label extension period is ongoing.

Clinical Experience with Subcutaneous Tocilizumab in Polyarticular Juvenile Idiopathic Arthritis

Subcutaneous tocilizumab was evaluated in pediatric patients with polyarticular JIA in a 52-week, open-label, multicenter, pharmacokinetic, pharmacodynamic, and safety study to determine the appropriate subcutaneous dosage of tocilizumab that achieves comparable pharmacokinetic/pharmacodynamic profiles as the IV tocilizumab regimen. Polyarticular JIA patients 1–17 years of age with an inadequate response to or inability to tolerate methotrexate, including patients with well-controlled disease on IV tocilizumab therapy and tocilizumab-naive patients with active disease, were treated with subcutaneous tocilizumab based on their body weight. Patients weighing 30 kg or more (25 patients) received 162 mg of tocilizumab given subcutaneously every 2 weeks and patients weighing less than 30 kg (27 patients) received 162 mg of tocilizumab subcutaneously every 3 weeks for 52 weeks. Of these 52 patients, 71% were naive to tocilizumab and 29% had been receiving IV tocilizumab and were switched to subcutaneous tocilizumab at baseline. The manufacturer states that the efficacy of subcutaneous tocilizumab in pediatric patients 2–17 years of age is based on pharmacokinetic exposure and extrapolation of the established efficacy of IV tocilizumab in pediatric patients with polyarticular JIA and subcutaneous tocilizumab in adults with rheumatoid arthritis.

Clinical Experience with IV Tocilizumab in Systemic Juvenile Idiopathic Arthritis

Tocilizumab has been evaluated in a 12-week randomized, double-blind, placebo-controlled study in 112 patients 2–17 years of age with active systemic JIA that had not responded adequately to treatment with NSAIAs and corticosteroids. Patients included in this study had at least 6 months of active disease, with either 5 or more active joints or 2 or more active joints and fever. Patients were randomized in a 2:1 ratio to receive tocilizumab (administered IV every 2 weeks at a weight-adjusted dosage [8 mg/kg in those weighing 30 kg or more, 12 mg/kg in those weighing less than 30 kg]) or placebo and were stratified according to body weight, disease duration, corticosteroid dosage, and methotrexate use. Those receiving stables dosages of NSAIAs, corticosteroids (equivalent to 0.5 mg/kg or less [maximum of 30 mg] of prednisone daily), and methotrexate (20 mg/m² or less per week) could continue such therapy; however, concomitant use of other nonbiologic or biologic DMARDs was not permitted. Approximately 82% of patients had received prior biologic DMARD therapy. Tapering of the corticosteroid dosage was permitted beginning at week 6 in patients who achieved a JIA-ACR 70 response. At week 12, the combined primary end point of JIA-ACR 30 response and absence of fever was observed in 85% of patients receiving tocilizumab compared with 24% of those receiving placebo. JIA-ACR 30, 50, and 70 responses were observed at week 12 in 91, 85, and 71%, respectively, of patients receiving tocilizumab, compared with 24, 11, and 8%, respectively, of those receiving placebo. Tocilizumab therapy also was associated with improvement in systemic manifestations (fever and rash). A greater proportion of patients receiving tocilizumab reduced their corticosteroid dosage by at least 20% without experiencing a subsequent occurrence of systemic symptoms or JIA-ACR 30 flare, compared with placebo recipients (24 versus 3%). In addition, a greater proportion of patients receiving tocilizumab had clinically important improvements in physical function, as assessed using the CHAQ-DI, from baseline to week 12, compared with those receiving placebo (77 versus 19%).

A total of 110 patients subsequently were entered into a long-term, single-group, open-label extension study. At 44 weeks of follow-up, responses to tocilizumab therapy (absence of fever, JIA-ACR response rates, systemic symptoms) were similar to those observed in the 12-week randomized study. By week 44, 43% of patients had discontinued oral corticosteroid therapy; about 50% of these patients had discontinued corticosteroid use for 18 weeks or longer. At 52 weeks of follow-up, 80% of patients had JIA-ACR 70 response and no fever, 59% had JIA-ACR 90 response and no fever, 48% had no joints with active arthritis, and 52% had discontinued oral corticosteroid therapy; the proportion of patients with moderate or severe functional impairment was 38%, compared with 82% at study baseline.

Clinical Experience with Subcutaneous Tocilizumab in Systemic Juvenile Idiopathic Arthritis

Subcutaneous tocilizumab was evaluated in pediatric patients with systemic JIA in a 52-week, open-label, multicenter, pharmacokinetic, pharmacodynamic, and safety study to determine the appropriate subcutaneous dosage of tocilizumab that achieves comparable pharmacokinetic/pharmacodynamic profiles as the IV tocilizumab regimen. Eligible patients received tocilizumab subcutaneously dosed according to body weight, with patients weighing 30 kg or more (26 patients) treated with 162 mg of tocilizumab every week and patients weighing less than 30 kg (25 patients) treated with 162 mg of tocilizumab every 10 days (8 patients) or every 2 weeks (17 patients) for 52 weeks. Of these patients, 51% were naive to subcutaneous tocilizumab and 49% had been receiving IV tocilizumab and were switched to subcutaneous tocilizumab at baseline. Efficacy of subcutaneous tocilizumab in pediatric patients 2–17 years of age is based on pharmacokinetic exposure and extrapolation of the established efficacy of IV tocilizumab in pediatric patients with systemic JIA.

Clinical Perspective

The American College of Rheumatology and the Arthritis Foundation issued a joint guideline in 2019 for the treatment of juvenile idiopathic arthritis manifesting as nonsystemic polyarthritis (including polyarticular disease), sacroiliitis, or enthesitis. Several drug classes are used to treat juvenile idiopathic arthritis, including NSAIAs, systemic and intra-articular corticosteroids, conventional DMARDs (e.g., methotrexate, sulfasalazine, hydroxychloroquine, leflunomide), and biologic DMARDs (e.g., TNF blocking agents, abatacept, tocilizumab, rituximab). Specific agents for juvenile idiopathic arthritis treatment are selected according to the presence of certain risk factors (e.g., positive anti-cyclic citrullinated peptide antibodies, positive rheumatoid factor, joint damage), level of disease activity, involvement of specific joints, presence of certain comorbidities (e.g., uveitis), and prior therapies received. An individualized "treat-to-target" approach is typically employed, with the goal of achieving remission or minimal/low disease activity.

Biologic DMARDs, including tocilizumab, are conditionally recommended as an initial therapy option in patients with risk factors and involvement of high-risk joints such as the cervical spine, wrist, or hip; high disease activity; and/or those at high risk of disabling joint disease. Use of tocilizumab is also conditionally recommended as subsequent therapy in patients with moderate/high disease activity as an add-on therapy to a DMARD or when switching from a TNF blocking agent. In patients receiving a second biologic DMARD, the guideline conditionally recommends tocilizumab, abatacept, or a TNF blocking agent over rituximab.

● Giant Cell Arteritis

Tocilizumab is used for the management of giant cell arteritis (GCA) in adults. The drug can be used in combination with a tapering course of corticosteroids or alone following discontinuance of corticosteroids.

Clinicians treating patients with GCA should be aware that monitoring CRP concentrations is not a reliable method to detect active disease or relapse of GCA in patients who are receiving IL-6 inhibitors such as tocilizumab since they may suppress CRP levels regardless of disease activity.

Clinical Experience with Subcutaneous Tocilizumab

Efficacy and safety of subcutaneous tocilizumab in the treatment of GCA were demonstrated in a randomized, double-blind, multicenter study of 1 year's duration (the Giant-Cell Arteritis Actemra [GiACTA] trial; NCT01791153) in adults with active GCA. In this study, 251 patients with new-onset or relapsing GCA were randomized in a 2:1:1:1 ratio to one of four treatment arms; 2 subcutaneous dosages of tocilizumab (162 mg every week and 162 mg every other week) with a prespecified 26-week prednisone taper regimen were compared with 2 different placebo control groups (prespecified prednisone taper regimen over 26 weeks and 52 weeks). The study consisted of a 52-week, blinded period followed by a 104-week, open-label extension. All patients concurrently received corticosteroid therapy (i.e., prednisone). Both tocilizumab treatment groups and one of the placebo groups followed a prespecified prednisone taper regimen with the aim to reach 0 mg by 26 weeks, while the second placebo group followed a prespecified prednisone taper regimen with the aim to reach 0 mg by 52 weeks, which was designed to be more in line with standard clinical practice. The primary efficacy end point was the proportion of patients achieving sustained corticosteroid-free remission at 52 weeks. Sustained remission was defined by a patient attaining a sustained absence of GCA signs and symptoms from week 12 through week 52, normalization of the erythrocyte sedimentation rate (ESR) from week 12 through week 52, normalization of CRP from week 12 through week 52, and successful adherence to the prednisone taper defined by not more than 100 mg of excess prednisone from week 12 through week 52.

In the GiACTA trial (NCT01791153), tocilizumab 162 mg weekly and 162 mg every other week plus a 26-week prednisone taper both showed superiority in achieving sustained remission from week 12 through week 52 (56 and 53% of patients, respectively) compared with placebo plus a 26-week prednisone taper (14%) or placebo plus a 52-week prednisone taper (18%). In addition, the estimated annual cumulative prednisone dose was lower in the 2 tocilizumab treatment groups (medians of 1887 and 2207 mg in the once-weekly and every-2-week tocilizumab treatment groups, respectively) compared with the placebo groups (medians of 3804 and 3902 mg in the placebo plus 26-week prednisone taper and the placebo plus 52-week prednisone taper groups, respectively). The overall tolerability profile of tocilizumab in the treatment of GCA was found to be similar to its tolerability profile in other indications. A post-hoc analysis of this study demonstrated sustained remission and a reduction in flares with tocilizumab compared to placebo in subgroups of patients who had either cranial symptoms only, polymyalgia rheumatica symptoms only, or a combination of both at baseline evaluation.

In a 2-year extension study (part 2) of GiACTA, data from 215 of the original 251 randomized patients were analyzed. Participants who were in clinical remission at the end of the 52-week, double-blind period received no further treatment and those not in clinical remission received therapy at the clinician's discretion, which could include tocilizumab and/or corticosteroids. A higher proportion of patients who were originally assigned to receive tocilizumab were treatment-free during this period (with a higher proportion of treatment-free patients among those who received the drug once weekly compared with every 2 weeks) compared with those originally assigned to receive placebo. Retreatment with tocilizumab with or without corticosteroids restored clinical remission in patients who experienced a disease flare. In addition, cumulative corticosteroid doses were lower in patients originally assigned to tocilizumab than in patients originally assigned to placebo. No new safety concerns emerged in the tocilizumab-treated patients during the 3-year study.

Clinical Experience with IV Tocilizumab

IV tocilizumab for the treatment of GCA was assessed in an open-label pharmacokinetic-pharmacodynamic (PK-PD) and safety study (WP41152; NCT03923738) to determine the appropriate IV dose of tocilizumab that would achieve comparable PK-PD profiles to subcutaneous tocilizumab. A total of 24 patients who had received ≥5 doses of tocilizumab 8 mg/kg IV every 4 weeks and achieved remission were enrolled in the study. In period 1 of the study, all patients received tocilizumab 7 mg/kg IV every 4 weeks for 20 weeks. After completion of period 1, 22 patients remained in remission and continued in period 2 to receive tocilizumab 6 mg/kg IV every 4 weeks for 20 weeks. Both dosages of tocilizumab were generally well tolerated. The efficacy of IV tocilizumab 6 mg/kg in adults with GCA is based on pharmacokinetic exposure and extrapolation to the efficacy established for subcutaneous tocilizumab in patients with GCA.

Clinical Perspective

Giant cell arteritis (GCA) is a systemic vasculitis that primarily involves medium-sized and large arteries; the condition can cause a variety of clinical manifestations, including headaches, ischemic visual symptoms (with a risk of vision loss), limb or jaw claudication, polymyalgia rheumatica, aortic aneurysm, myocardial infarction, and stroke. The condition mainly occurs in adults older than 50 years of age and is 2–3 times more likely to occur in women than in men. Corticosteroids are considered standard first-line initial therapy for GCA and can help control headaches and reduce systemic inflammation, normalize inflammatory markers such as C-reactive protein (CRP), and prevent vision loss. However, long-term corticosteroid therapy can cause severe adverse effects in patients with GCA.

Because concentrations of CRP and other acute-phase reactants increase with elevated serum concentrations of interleukin-6 (IL-6), tocilizumab has been studied as a treatment for GCA. Clinical experience with tocilizumab in GCA to date indicates that the drug can produce sustained remission and allow for reductions in corticosteroid doses (i.e., steroid-sparing effect) that are used to control the disease and to maintain remission. Further study is needed to determine the optimal role of tocilizumab therapy in the management of GCA and to evaluate its efficacy when used alone without corticosteroids. Tocilizumab has been shown to be an effective glucocorticoid-sparing agent for GCA. Therefore, some clinicians recommend that tocilizumab therapy be considered in patients who are experiencing adverse effects from corticosteroid therapy, patients with clinically important preexisting medical conditions that could be adversely affected by long-term corticosteroid therapy (e.g., diabetes mellitus, hypertension, psychiatric conditions, pancreatitis), and patients whose disease is refractory to corticosteroid therapy (i.e., patients who didn't achieve remission or who experienced flares during a corticosteroid taper).

The American College of Rheumatology and Vasculitis Foundation issued a joint guideline in 2021 for the management of GCA. Medications used to treat GCA include systemic glucocorticoids, non-biologic immunosuppressants (e.g., azathioprine, leflunomide, methotrexate, mycophenolate mofetil, cyclophosphamide), and biologic DMARDs (e.g., TNF blocking agents, abatacept, tocilizumab). Specific drug regimens are recommended according to the degree of organ involvement. The guideline conditionally recommends the use of tocilizumab with oral glucocorticoids over oral glucocorticoids alone in patients with newly diagnosed GCA. A conditional recommendation is also given for adding tocilizumab and increasing the dose of glucocorticoids over adding methotrexate and increasing the dose of glucocorticoids in patients who experience disease relapse with cranial symptoms while receiving glucocorticoids alone. Choice of therapy should be based on the physician's experience and the patient's clinical condition, values, and preferences.

• Cytokine Release Syndrome Associated with Chimeric Antigen Receptor T-cell Therapy

Tocilizumab is used in the management of chimeric antigen receptor (CAR) T cell-induced severe or life-threatening cytokine release syndrome (CRS) in adults and pediatric patients ≥2 years of age. Tocilizumab can be used alone or in combination with corticosteroids in the treatment of this condition. CRS is a clinically important adverse effect of CAR T-cell therapies used in the treatment of malignancies. Clinical manifestations may include fever, fatigue, coagulopathy, nausea, capillary leak, and multiorgan dysfunction.

Efficacy of IV tocilizumab in the treatment of CRS was assessed in a retrospective analysis of pooled outcome data from clinical trials of CAR T-cell therapies for hematologic malignancies. Evaluable patients had been treated with tocilizumab 8 mg/kg (12 mg/kg for patients weighing less than 30 kg) with or without additional high-dose corticosteroids for severe or life-threatening CRS; only the first episode of CRS was included in the analysis. The study population included 24 males and 21 females (total 45 patients) of a median age of 12 years (range: 3–23 years); 82% were Caucasian. The median time from the onset of CRS to the first dose of tocilizumab was 4 days (range: 0–18 days). Resolution of CRS was defined as lack of fever and off of vasopressors for at least 24 hours. Patients were considered responders if CRS resolved within 14 days of the first dose of tocilizumab, if no more than 2 doses of tocilizumab were needed, and if no drugs other than tocilizumab and corticosteroids were used for treatment. Thirty-one patients (69%) achieved a response. Achievement of resolution of CRS within 14 days was confirmed in a second study using an independent cohort that included 15 patients (range: 9–75 years old) with CAR T cell-induced CRS.

Clinical Perspective

The American Society of Clinical Oncology (ASCO) issued a guideline in 2021 for the management of immune-related adverse events in patients treated with CAR T-cell therapy. Specific agents are selected according to grading of fever, hypoxia, and hypotension based on the American Society of Transplantation and Cellular Therapy (ASTCT) consensus grading system. Management of CRS begins with supportive care (e.g., antipyretics, IV hydration, broad-spectrum antibiotics, granulocyte-colony stimulating factor), but may require pharmacologic treatment for prolonged or severe CRS. Tocilizumab with or without a corticosteroid is recommended in patients with prolonged or severe CAR T-cell-associated CRS.

• Systemic Sclerosis-Associated Interstitial Lung Disease (SSc-ILD)

Tocilizumab is used for the management of adults with systemic sclerosis-associated interstitial lung disease to slow the rate of pulmonary function decline.

Clinical Experience with Subcutaneous Tocilizumab

Efficacy of tocilizumab in SSc-ILD was evaluated in a phase 3, multicenter, randomized, double-blind, placebo-controlled study (focuSSced) in 212 adults with SSc as defined by the 2013 ACR/EULAR criteria with onset of disease of 5 years or less, modified Rodnan Skin Score (mRSS) of 10–35 units at screening, increased inflammatory markers (or platelets), and active disease. Criteria for active disease included at least one of the following: disease duration 18 months or less, increase

in mRSS of 3 or more units over 6 months, involvement of one new body area and an increase in mRSS of at least 2 units over 6 months, or involvement of 2 new body areas within the previous 6 months, or presence of at least one tendon friction rub. Use of biologic agents, alkylating agents, or cyclophosphamide was not permitted.

Patients were randomized to tocilizumab 162 mg or placebo administered weekly by subcutaneous injection for 48 weeks, followed by open-label tocilizumab 162 mg administered subcutaneously every week for another 48 weeks. Rescue treatment was allowed after 16 weeks if there was more than a 10% decline in predicted forced vital capacity (FVC) or after 24 weeks for worsening skin fibrosis. The primary efficacy endpoint was change in mRSS from baseline to week 48. Change from baseline in FVC at week 48 was a secondary endpoint.

Sixty-seven percent of patients in the tocilizumab group and 64% in the placebo group had SSc-ILD. Primary and secondary endpoints were evaluated in the overall population and a post-hoc analysis evaluated outcomes in the subgroup of patients with and without SSc-ILD. No statistically significant difference in the primary outcome of change in mRSS was observed in the overall population or in the subgroup of patients with SSc-ILD. The change from baseline in predicted FVC and observed FVC was substantially improved in the overall population and in SSc-ILD subgroup.

A phase 2/3 multicenter, randomized, double-blind, placebo-controlled study provides supportive information on the efficacy of tocilizumab in adult patients with SSc. Results in terms of mRSS and FVC outcomes were similar to those observed in the principal phase 3 study.

• Coronavirus Disease 2019 (COVID-19)

Tocilizumab is used in the management of coronavirus disease 2019 (COVID-19) in hospitalized adult patients who are receiving systemic corticosteroids and require supplemental oxygen, noninvasive or invasive mechanical ventilation, or extracorporeal membrane oxygenation (ECMO). Tocilizumab is also used in the management of COVID-19 in hospitalized pediatric patients 2–18 years of age.

The rationale for tocilizumab's use in this infection is related to its specificity for the interleukin-6 (IL-6) receptor, which may help to relieve symptoms of CRS (e.g., fever, organ failure, death) in severely ill patients with COVID-19.

Clinical Experience with IV Tocilizumab

Efficacy of tocilizumab for the treatment of COVID-19 was evaluated in a randomized, controlled, open-label, multicenter study (RECOVERY; NCT04381936) in 4116 hospitalized adult patients with severe COVID-19-related pneumonia. The primary efficacy endpoint was time to death through day 28. Patients were randomized to receive either standard of care or IV tocilizumab at a weight-tiered dosing comparable to the recommended dosage in addition to standard of care. At baseline, 0.2% of patients were not on supplemental oxygen, 45% of patients required low flow oxygen, 41% required non-invasive ventilation or high-flow oxygen, and 14% required invasive mechanical ventilation. Initially, 82% of patients were reported to be receiving systemic corticosteroids. Tocilizumab improved survival and clinical outcomes at 28 days. In patients who received tocilizumab, the mortality rate was 31% compared with a mortality rate of 35% in those who received standard of care. Reduction in mortality was observed in a larger proportion of patients receiving systemic corticosteroids compared with those not receiving a systemic corticosteroid at randomization; however, this may have been a chance finding. Patients receiving tocilizumab were also more likely to be discharged from the hospital within 28 days and less likely to require invasive mechanical ventilation.

Efficacy of tocilizumab for the treatment of COVID-19 was additionally supported in a randomized, double-blind, placebo-controlled, multicenter study (EMPACTA; NCT04372186) in 377 hospitalized patients with confirmed COVID-19-related pneumonia who were not receiving mechanical ventilation; the study enrolled a substantial proportion of patients from high-risk and racial and ethnic minority groups. The primary efficacy endpoint was time to progression to mechanical ventilation or death through day 28. At baseline, 9% of patients were not on supplemental oxygen, 64% of patients required low flow oxygen, 27% of patients required high-flow oxygen, and 73% were on corticosteroids. Patients were randomized to receive standard of care plus 1 or 2 doses of IV tocilizumab 8 mg/kg (maximum dose 800 mg) or placebo. The cumulative proportion of patients who required mechanical ventilation or died by day 28 was 12% in those receiving tocilizumab and 19.3% in those receiving placebo. Mortality from any cause at day 28 was 10.4% in those receiving tocilizumab compared to 8.6% in those receiving placebo.

In a phase 3 randomized, double-blind, placebo-controlled, multicenter study (COVACTA trial; NCT04320615), 452 adults hospitalized with severe COVID-19-related pneumonia were randomized 2:1 to receive either a single dose of tocilizumab 8 mg/kg or placebo. The primary efficacy end point was improved clinical status, which was measured using a 7-point ordinal scale to assess clinical status based on the need for intensive care and/or ventilator use and the requirement for supplemental oxygen over a 4-week period. The trial failed to meet its primary end point or several key secondary end points. Key secondary end points included 4-week mortality. Differences in the primary end points between the tocilizumab and placebo groups were not statistically significant. At week 4, mortality rates did not differ between the tocilizumab and placebo groups (19.7 versus 19.4%, respectively).

In a double-blind, placebo-controlled, multicenter study (REMDACTA; NCT04 409262). 649 hospitalized patients with severe COVID-19 pneumonia were randomized 2:1 to receive IV tocilizumab and remdesivir or placebo and remdesivir. Tocilizumab was given as a single IV dose of 8 mg/kg along with IV remdesivir 200 mg on day 1 followed by remdesivir 100 mg once daily for a total of 10 days. The primary efficacy endpoint was time from randomization to hospital discharge or "ready for discharge" up to Day 28. At baseline, 7% of patients were on low flow oxygen, 80% were on non-invasive ventilation or high flow oxygen, 14% were on invasive mechanical ventilation, and 84% were on corticosteroids. At day 28, there was no statistically significant difference between the study groups with respect to time to hospital discharge or "ready for discharge" through Day 28. Mortality at day 28 was 18.1% in the tocilizumab and remdesivir study population compared to 19.5% in the placebo and remdesivir study population.

A meta-analysis of the EMPACTA, COVACTA, REMDACTA and RECOVERY studies evaluated the risk difference through Day 28, estimated by the Kaplan-Meier method, in the subgroup of patients receiving baseline corticosteroids. Patients from the RECOVERY trial represent 78.8% of the total sample size in this meta-analysis. The combined risk difference showed that tocilizumab treatment (n=2261) resulted in a 4.61% absolute reduction in the risk of death at Day 28 compared to standard of care.

Emergency Use Authorization in Pediatric Patients

FDA has issued an emergency use authorization (EUA) that permits use of tocilizumab for treatment of COVID-19 in hospitalized pediatric patients 2–18 years of age who are receiving systemic corticosteroids and require supplemental oxygen, non-invasive or invasive mechanical ventilation, or extracorporeal membrane oxygenation (ECMO). FDA states that, based on review of data from an open-label, controlled, platform trial (NCT04381936; RECOVERY); a double-blind, placebo-controlled trial (NCT04320615; COVACTA); a double-blind, placebo-controlled trial (NCT04372186; EMPACTA); and a double-blind, placebo-controlled trial (NCT04409262; REMDACTA]), it is reasonable to believe that tocilizumab may be effective for the treatment of COVID-19 in the pediatric patient population specified in the tocilizumab EUA and, when used under the conditions described in the EUA, the known and potential benefits of tocilizumab when used to treat COVID-19 in such patients outweigh the known and potential risks.

For additional information about the EUA, the tocilizumab EUA letter of authorization (https://www.fda.gov/media/150319/download), EUA fact sheet for healthcare providers (https://www.fda.gov/media/150321/download), and EUA fact sheet for patients, parents and caregivers (https://www.fda.gov/media/150320/download) should be consulted.

For further information on the use of tocilizumab in the treatment of pediatric patients with COVID-19, clinicians also may consult the most recent COVID-19 treatment guidelines from NIH (https://www.covid19treatmentguidelines.nih.gov/).

DOSAGE AND ADMINISTRATION

● General

Pretreatment Screening

- Consider potential risks and benefits of tocilizumab prior to initiating therapy in patients with chronic infection or history of recurrent infection. Do not administer in patients with an active infection until the infection resolves or is appropriately treated.

- Evaluate for active or inactive tuberculosis prior to initiation of tocilizumab therapy. Do not administer to patients with active tuberculosis.

- Administer all age-appropriate vaccines prior to starting tocilizumab therapy.

- Measure absolute neutrophil count (ANC), platelet count, ALT, and AST prior to initiating therapy. In patients with rheumatoid arthritis, giant cell arteritis (GCA), systemic sclerosis-associated interstitial lung disease (SSc-ILD), polyarticular juvenile idiopathic arthritis (PJIA), or systemic juvenile idiopathic arthritis (SJIA), do not initiate therapy if ANC <2000/mm³, platelet count <100,000/mm³, or ALT or AST >1.5 times the upper limit of normal (ULN). In patients with COVID-19, do not initiate therapy if ANC <1000/mm³, platelet count <50,000/mm³, or ALT or AST >10 times ULN.

- Perform a pregnancy test prior to initiating therapy in females of reproductive potential; if positive, enroll patients in manufacturer's pregnancy registry.

Patient Monitoring

- Monitor patients for signs and symptoms of bacterial, viral, or fungal infections.

- Evaluate for active tuberculosis infection during treatment, even if initial latent tuberculosis test is negative.

- Monitor patients who present with new-onset abdominal symptoms for signs of GI perforation.

- Monitor lipid parameters approximately 4 to 8 weeks after start of therapy, and manage according to clinical guidelines.

- Monitor patients for signs and symptoms of infusion-related and hypersensitivity reactions during and after infusions.

- Monitor patients for signs and symptoms indicative of demyelinating disorders.

- In patients with rheumatoid arthritis, GCA, or SSc-ILD: obtain a liver test panel (alkaline phosphatase, total bilirubin, ALT and AST levels) every 4 to 8 weeks after start of therapy for the first 6 months of treatment and every 3 months thereafter.

- In patients with rheumatoid arthritis, GCA, or SSc-ILD: monitor ANC and platelet count 4 to 8 weeks after start of therapy and every 3 months thereafter.

- In patients with PJIA: monitor liver test panel (alkaline phosphatase, total bilirubin, ALT and AST levels), ANC, and platelet count at the time of second administration and every 4 to 8 weeks thereafter.

- In patients with SJIA: monitor liver test panel (alkaline phosphatase, total bilirubin, ALT and AST levels), ANC, and platelet count at the time of second administration and every 2 to 4 weeks thereafter.

Dispensing and Administration Precautions

- IV infusions of tocilizumab should only be administered by a healthcare professional with appropriate medical support to manage anaphylaxis. If anaphylaxis or other hypersensitivity reaction occurs, stop administration of tocilizumab immediately and permanently discontinue therapy.

Other General Considerations

- Patients with severe or life-threatening chimeric antigen receptor (CAR) T cell-induced cytokine release syndrome (CRS) frequently have cytopenias or elevated ALT or AST concentrations due to lymphodepleting chemotherapy or the CRS itself. Consider the potential benefit of treating the CRS versus the risks of short-term therapy with the drug.

- For the management of rheumatoid arthritis, tocilizumab may be used as monotherapy or concomitantly with methotrexate or other nonbiologic disease-modifying antirheumatic drugs (DMARDs). Tocilizumab may be used alone or in combination with methotrexate in patients with systemic or polyarticular JIA.

- For the management of GCA, administer tocilizumab initially in combination with a tapering course of corticosteroids. Once corticosteroids are discontinued, continue tocilizumab alone.

- Do not use tocilizumab concomitantly with other biologic DMARDs, such as tumor necrosis factor (TNF) blocking agents, interleukin-1 (IL-1) receptor antagonists, anti-CD20 monoclonal antibodies, and selective costimulation modulators.

● Administration

For the management of rheumatoid arthritis, GCA, and systemic or polyarticular JIA, tocilizumab may be administered either by IV infusion over 60 minutes or by subcutaneous injection. The drug should *not* be administered by rapid IV injection (e.g., IV push or bolus).

For the management of SSc-ILD, tocilizumab is administered by subcutaneous injection. The drug currently is not FDA-labeled for IV administration for this indications. The use of the prefilled pen has not been studied in patients with SSc-ILD.

For the management of CAR T cell-induced CRS, tocilizumab is administered only by IV infusion over 60 minutes. The drug should *not* be administered by rapid IV injection (e.g., IV push or bolus). Tocilizumab currently is not FDA-labeled for subcutaneous use for this indication.

IV Administration

Tocilizumab injection concentrate is commercially available in single-dose vials (containing 20 mg/mL) and must be diluted prior to IV administration. The appropriate dose of the injection concentrate should be diluted in 0.9 or 0.45% sodium chloride injection to provide a final volume of 50 mL for administration in patients who weigh less than 30 kg and to a final volume of 100 mL for administration in patients who weigh 30 kg or more. A volume of diluent equal to the total required volume of tocilizumab injection concentrate should be removed from the bag or bottle of 0.9 or 0.45% sodium chloride injection prior to the addition of tocilizumab injection concentrate. The total required volume of tocilizumab injection concentrate (0.2, 0.3, 0.4, 0.5, or 0.6 mL/kg for a dose of 4, 6, 8, 10, or 12 mg/kg, respectively) should be added slowly to the diluent, and the bag or bottle should be inverted gently to mix the solution and avoid foaming.

The manufacturer states that tocilizumab infusion solutions are compatible with polypropylene, polyethylene, and polyvinyl chloride infusion bags and polypropylene, polyethylene, and glass infusion bottles. Prior to administration, tocilizumab infusion solutions should be inspected visually for particulate matter and discoloration; if either is present, the solution should be discarded. Tocilizumab infusion solutions using 0.9% sodium chloride injection may be stored at 2–8°C or room temperature for up to 24 hours and should be protected from light. Tocilizumab infusion solutions using 0.45% sodium chloride injection may be stored at 2–8°C for up to 24 hours or at room temperature for up to 4 hours and should be protected from light. Any unused portion remaining in the vial should be discarded since the injection concentrate contains no preservative.

Tocilizumab infusion solutions should be allowed to reach room temperature prior to administration. Tocilizumab should not be infused simultaneously through the same IV line with other drugs.

Subcutaneous Administration

Tocilizumab is administered by subcutaneous injection. Tocilizumab is intended for use under the guidance of a clinician; however, the drug may be *self-administered* or the patient's caregiver may administer the injection if the clinician determines that the patient and/or their caregiver is competent to safely administer the drug after appropriate training. Polyarticular and systemic JIA patients may *self-administer* tocilizumab if both the clinician and the parent/legal guardian determine it is appropriate. Patients or caregivers should be instructed to follow the instructions for use for detailed information on administration of the drug.

Tocilizumab for subcutaneous use is commercially available in prefilled single-use syringes or as prefilled single-use autoinjectors. Each syringe or autoinjector delivers 162 mg of tocilizumab in 0.9 mL. The entire contents of the prefilled syringe or autoinjector should be administered as a single dose. Prior to administration, tocilizumab solutions should be inspected visually for particulate matter or discoloration; if the syringe or autoinjector appears to be damaged or the solution contains particulates or is cloudy or discolored, the solution should be discarded.

Tocilizumab injection for subcutaneous use should be protected from light and stored at 2–8°C in the original carton until administration. The injection should not be frozen and the prefilled syringes and autoinjectors should be kept dry. The prefilled syringe or autoinjector should be allowed to sit at room temperature outside of the carton for 30 minutes or 45 minutes, respectively, prior to subcutaneous injection; tocilizumab should not be warmed in any other way (e.g., microwave, hot water). After removal from the refrigerator, the prefilled syringe and autoinjector can be stored up to 2 weeks at or below 30°C. The commercially available subcutaneous injection should *not* be used for IV administration.

Tocilizumab is administered subcutaneously into the anterior thigh or abdomen (except for the 2-inch area around the umbilicus). Tocilizumab also may be administered subcutaneously into the upper arm by a caregiver. Injection sites should be rotated. Injections should not be made into areas where the skin is tender, bruised, red, hard, or nonintact or into scars or moles.

● Dosage

Rheumatoid Arthritis in Adults

For the management of rheumatoid arthritis in adults who have had an inadequate response to one or more DMARDs, the recommended initial dosage of tocilizumab is 4 mg/kg by IV infusion once every 4 weeks; the dosage can be increased to 8 mg/kg by IV infusion once every 4 weeks based on clinical response. Doses exceeding 800 mg per infusion are not recommended.

Alternatively, adults with rheumatoid arthritis who weigh less than 100 kg may receive tocilizumab 162 mg subcutaneously every other week; the dosage can be increased to 162 mg every week based on clinical response. Patients who weigh 100 kg or more may receive tocilizumab 162 mg subcutaneously every week.

When switching from IV to subcutaneous administration, the first subcutaneous dose may be administered in place of the next scheduled IV dose.

Treatment Interruptions or Discontinuance for Toxicity

If certain dose-related laboratory changes (i.e., elevated liver enzyme concentrations, neutropenia, thrombocytopenia) occur in patients with rheumatoid arthritis receiving IV or subcutaneous tocilizumab, interruption of tocilizumab therapy, dose reduction, or discontinuance of therapy may be required (see Tables 1–3).

Juvenile Idiopathic Arthritis

Tocilizumab is administered IV in a weight-adjusted dosage once every 4 weeks in patients with polyarticular JIA and once every 2 weeks in those with systemic JIA. For the management of polyarticular JIA in patients ≥2 years of age, the recommended IV dosage of tocilizumab is 10 mg/kg by IV infusion once every 4 weeks in those weighing <30 kg and 8 mg/kg by IV infusion once every 4 weeks in those weighing 30 kg or more. For the management of systemic JIA in patients ≥2 years of age, the recommended dosage of tocilizumab is 12 mg/kg by IV infusion once every 2 weeks in those weighing <30 kg and 8 mg/kg by IV infusion once every 2 weeks in those weighing ≥30 kg.

Alternatively, tocilizumab may be administered by subcutaneous injection in a weight-adjusted dosage for the management of polyarticular JIA. In patients ≥2 years of age, the recommended subcutaneous dosage of tocilizumab is 162 mg once every 3 weeks in those weighing less than 30 kg and 162 mg once every 2 weeks in those weighing 30 kg or more. For the management of systemic JIA in patients ≥2 years of age, the recommended subcutaneous dosage of tocilizumab is 162 mg once every 2 weeks in those weighing less than 30 kg and 162 mg once weekly in those weighing 30 kg or more.

Because the patient's weight may fluctuate, dosage should not be adjusted based solely on the patient's weight as measured at a single visit. If certain dose-related laboratory changes (i.e., elevated liver enzyme concentrations, neutropenia, thrombocytopenia) occur, interruption of therapy may be required.

When switching from IV to subcutaneous administration, the first subcutaneous dose may be administered in place of the next scheduled IV dose.

Treatment Interruptions or Discontinuance for Toxicity

Tocilizumab dosage reductions have not been evaluated in patients with polyarticular or systemic JIA. However, interruption of tocilizumab therapy is recommended for certain dose-related laboratory changes (i.e., elevated liver enzyme concentrations, neutropenia, thrombocytopenia) at values similar to those considered in adults with rheumatoid arthritis (see Tables 1–3). If clinically appropriate, dosage reduction or discontinuance of concomitant therapy with methotrexate and/or other agents should be considered and tocilizumab withheld pending clinical evaluation. The decision to discontinue tocilizumab therapy because of a laboratory abnormality should be individualized.

Giant Cell Arteritis in Adults

For the management of giant cell arteritis (GCA), the recommended IV dosage of tocilizumab in adults is 6 mg/kg by IV infusion once every 4 weeks in combination with a tapering course of glucocorticoids. Doses >600 mg per infusion are not recommended. Tocilizumab can be used alone following discontinuation of glucocorticoids.

The recommended subcutaneous dosage of tocilizumab in adults with GCA is 162 mg subcutaneously once every week in combination with a tapering course of glucocorticoids. A dosage of 162 mg given once every other week as a subcutaneous injection in combination with a tapering course of corticosteroids also may be prescribed based on clinical considerations. Tocilizumab may be used alone following discontinuance of glucocorticoids.

When switching from tocilizumab IV to subcutaneous administration, the first subcutaneous dose may be administered in place of the next scheduled IV dose.

Treatment Interruptions or Discontinuance for Toxicity

If certain dose-related laboratory changes (i.e., elevated liver enzyme concentrations, neutropenia, thrombocytopenia) occur in patients with GCA receiving IV or subcutaneous tocilizumab, interruption of tocilizumab therapy, dose reduction, or discontinuance of therapy may be required (see Tables 1–3).

Cytokine Release Syndrome Associated with Chimeric Antigen Receptor-T cell Therapy

For the management of CAR T cell-induced severe or life-threatening CRS, tocilizumab should only be given IV as an infusion over 60 minutes. Subcutaneous administration is *not* labeled by the FDA for the treatment of CRS. Tocilizumab may be used alone or in combination with corticosteroids.

In patients 2 years of age or older who weigh less than 30 kg, the manufacturer recommends a tocilizumab dosage of 12 mg/kg given by IV infusion over 60 minutes. In adults and pediatric patients 2 years of age or older who weigh 30 kg or more, the manufacturer recommends a tocilizumab dosage of 8 mg/kg given by IV infusion over 60 minutes.

If clinical improvement in the signs and symptoms of CRS does not occur following the first dose of tocilizumab, up to 3 additional doses may be administered. The interval between consecutive doses should be at least 8 hours. Doses exceeding 800 mg per infusion are not recommended.

Systemic Sclerosis-Associated Interstitial Lung Disease

The recommended dosage of tocilizumab in adults with SSc-ILD is 162 mg subcutaneously every week.

Tocilizumab is not FDA-labeled for IV administration in patients with SSc-ILD. The use of the prefilled pen has not been evaluated in patients with SSc-ILD.

Treatment Interruptions or Discontinuance for Toxicity

If certain dose-related laboratory changes (i.e., elevated liver enzyme concentrations, neutropenia, thrombocytopenia) occur in patients with SSc-ILD receiving IV or subcutaneous tocilizumab, interruption of tocilizumab therapy, dose reduction, or discontinuance of therapy may be required (see Tables 1–3).

Coronavirus Disease 2019 (COVID-19)

The recommended dosage of tocilizumab in adult patients with COVID-19 is 8 mg/kg given as a single IV infusion over 60 minutes. If clinical signs or symptoms worsen or do not improve after the first dose, one additional infusion may be administered at least 8 hours after the initial infusion. Doses >800 mg per infusion are not recommended.

The FDA EUA permits administration of tocilizumab for treatment of COVID-19 in hospitalized pediatric patients† (2–18 years of age weighing less than 30 kg) in a dosage of 12 mg/kg (maximum of 800 mg per infusion) given as a single 60-minute IV infusion; one additional IV infusion may be administered at least 8 hours after the first infusion if clinical signs or symptoms worsen or do not improve after the initial dose. In hospitalized pediatric patients 2–18 years of age weighing 30 kg or more, the FDA EUA permits administration of tocilizumab in a dosage of 8 mg/kg (maximum of 800 mg per infusion) given as a single 60-minute IV infusion; one additional IV infusion may be administered at least 8 hours after the first infusion if clinical signs or symptoms worsen or do not improve after the initial dose.

Tocilizumab is not authorized by the EUA or FDA-label for subcutaneous administration for treatment of COVID-19.

Dosage Modification for Serious Infections or Laboratory Abnormalities

If a serious infection, an opportunistic infection, or sepsis develops, tocilizumab should be discontinued until the infection is controlled.

TABLE 1. Recommended Dosage Adjustment Based on Liver Enzyme Abnormalities in Adults with Rheumatoid Arthritis, SSc-ILD, or GCA

ALT or AST Value	Recommendation for RA and SSc-ILD	Recommendation for GCA
>1 to 3 times ULN	Modify dosage of concomitant DMARDs if appropriate	Modify dosage of concomitant immunomodulatory agents if appropriate
	For persistent increases within this range in patients receiving IV tocilizumab, reduce dose of tocilizumab to 4 mg/kg or withhold therapy until ALT/AST values normalize	For persistent increases within this range in patients receiving IV tocilizumab, withhold therapy until ALT/AST values normalize
	For persistent increases within this range in patients receiving sub-Q tocilizumab, reduce frequency of tocilizumab administration to every other week or withhold therapy until ALT/AST values normalize; resume tocilizumab at every other week and increase frequency to every week as clinically indicated	For persistent increases within this range in patients receiving sub-Q tocilizumab, reduce frequency of tocilizumab administration to every other week or withhold therapy until ALT/AST values normalize; resume tocilizumab at every other week and increase frequency to every week as clinically indicated
>3 to 5 times ULN (confirmed by repeat testing)	Interrupt tocilizumab therapy until ALT/AST <3 times ULN and follow recommendations for ALT/AST >1 to 3 times ULN	Interrupt tocilizumab therapy until ALT/AST <3 times ULN and follow recommendations for ALT/AST >1 to 3 times ULN
	For persistent increases of >3 times ULN, discontinue tocilizumab	For persistent increases of >3 times ULN, discontinue tocilizumab
>5 times ULN	Discontinue tocilizumab	Discontinue tocilizumab

TABLE 2. Recommended Dosage Adjustment Based on Absolute Neutrophil Count (ANC) in Adults with Rheumatoid Arthritis, GCA, or SSc-ILD

ANC (cells/mm³)	Recommendation for RA and SSc-ILD	Recommendation for GCA
>1000	Maintain current dosage	Maintain current dosage
500–1000	Interrupt tocilizumab therapy	Interrupt tocilizumab therapy
	When ANC >1000/mm³ in patients receiving IV tocilizumab, resume tocilizumab at a dose of 4 mg/kg and increase to 8 mg/kg as clinically indicated	When ANC >1000/mm³ in patients receiving IV tocilizumab, resume tocilizumab at a dose of 6 mg/kg
	When ANC >1000/mm³ in patients receiving sub-Q tocilizumab, resume tocilizumab at every other week and increase frequency to every week as clinically indicated	When ANC >1000/mm³ in patients receiving sub-Q tocilizumab, resume tocilizumab at every other week and increase frequency to every week as clinically indicated
<500	Discontinue tocilizumab	Discontinue tocilizumab

TABLE 3. Recommended Dosage Adjustment Based on Platelet Count in Adults with Rheumatoid Arthritis, GCA, or SSc-ILD

Platelet Count (cells/mm³)	Recommendation for RA and SSc-ILD	Recommendation for GCA
50,000–100,000	Interrupt tocilizumab therapy	Interrupt tocilizumab therapy
	When platelet count >100,000/mm³ in patients receiving IV tocilizumab, resume tocilizumab at a dose of 4 mg/kg and increase to 8 mg/kg as clinically indicated	When platelet count >100,000/mm³ in patients receiving IV tocilizumab, resume tocilizumab at a dose of 6 mg/kg
	When platelet count >100,000/mm³ in patients receiving sub-Q tocilizumab, resume tocilizumab at every other week and increase frequency to every week as clinically appropriate	When platelet count >100,000/mm³ in patients receiving sub-Q tocilizumab, resume tocilizumab at every other week and increase frequency to every week as clinically appropriate
<50,000	Discontinue tocilizumab	Discontinue tocilizumab

● Special Populations

Hepatic Impairment

Use of the drug in patients with active hepatic disease or hepatic impairment is not recommended.

Renal Impairment

Dosage adjustment is not necessary in patients with mild or moderate renal impairment; use of tocilizumab in patients with severe renal impairment has not been evaluated.

Geriatric Patients

The manufacturer makes no specific dosage recommendations for geriatric patients.

CAUTIONS

● Contraindications

- Tocilizumab is contraindicated in patients with known hypersensitivity to the drug.

● Warnings/Precautions

Warnings

Risk of Serious Infections

A boxed warning regarding the risk of serious infections is included in the prescribing information for tocilizumab. Patients treated with tocilizumab are at an increased risk for developing serious infections that may lead to hospitalization or death. Reported infections include active tuberculosis, invasive fungal infections including candidiasis, aspergillosis, and pneumocystis, bacterial, viral, and other infections due to opportunistic pathogens.

The most common serious infections reported in patients receiving tocilizumab have included pneumonia, urinary tract infection, cellulitis, herpes zoster, gastroenteritis, diverticulitis, sepsis, and septic (bacterial) arthritis. Opportunistic infections (e.g., tuberculosis, cryptococcus, aspergillosis, candidiasis, pneumocystosis) also have been reported in patients receiving tocilizumab. Other serious infections may occur. Patients have presented with disseminated rather than local disease; patients often were receiving concomitant therapy with immunosuppressive agents (e.g., methotrexate, corticosteroids) that, in addition to their underlying condition, could have predisposed them to infections.

The risks and benefits of treatment with tocilizumab should be carefully considered prior to initiating therapy in patients with chronic or recurrent infection.

Patients should be closely monitored for the development of signs and symptoms of infection during and after treatment with tocilizumab, including the possible development of tuberculosis in patients who tested negative for latent tuberculosis infection prior to initiating therapy.

Tocilizumab therapy should not be initiated in patients with active infections, including localized infections. Clinicians should consider potential risks and benefits of the drug prior to initiating therapy in patients with a history of chronic, recurring, serious, or opportunistic infections; patients with underlying conditions that may predispose them to infections; and patients who have been exposed to tuberculosis or who reside or have traveled in regions where tuberculosis or mycoses are endemic. Any patient who develops a new infection while receiving tocilizumab should undergo a thorough diagnostic evaluation (appropriate for an immunocompromised patient), appropriate anti-infective therapy should be initiated, and the patient should be closely monitored. If a serious infection, an opportunistic infection, or sepsis develops, tocilizumab should be discontinued until the infection is controlled. There is limited information regarding the use of tocilizumab in patients with COVID-19 and concomitant active serious infections; consider the risks and benefits of treatment with tocilizumab in COVID-19 patients with other concurrent infections

Patients, except for those with COVID-19, should be evaluated for latent tuberculosis and for the presence of risk factors for tuberculosis prior to and periodically during therapy with tocilizumab. When indicated, an appropriate antimycobacterial regimen for the treatment of latent tuberculosis infection should be initiated prior to tocilizumab therapy. Antimycobacterial therapy should be considered prior to initiation of tocilizumab in individuals with a history of latent or active tuberculosis in whom an adequate course of antimycobacterial treatment cannot be confirmed and in individuals with a negative test for latent tuberculosis who have risk factors for tuberculosis. Consultation with a tuberculosis specialist is recommended when deciding whether antimicrobial therapy should be initiated. Patients receiving tocilizumab, including individuals with a negative test for latent tuberculosis, should be monitored for signs and symptoms of active tuberculosis.

Viral reactivation can occur in patients receiving immunosuppressive therapies. Herpes zoster exacerbation has been reported in patients receiving tocilizumab. No cases of hepatitis B reactivation were observed in clinical trials of tocilizumab; however, patients who screened positive for hepatitis were excluded from these studies.

Other Warnings and Precautions

GI Perforation

GI perforation has been reported in patients receiving tocilizumab in clinical trials, usually as a complication of diverticulitis. Most patients who experienced GI perforation were receiving concomitant therapy with nonsteroidal anti-inflammatory agents (NSAIAs), corticosteroids, or methotrexate. The relative contribution of these agents versus IV tocilizumab to the occurrence of GI perforation remains to be determined.

Caution is advised if tocilizumab is used in patients at risk for GI perforation. Patients who experience new-onset abdominal symptoms should be promptly evaluated for GI perforation.

Hepatotoxicity

Serious hepatic injury has been observed in patients receiving IV or subcutaneous tocilizumab. Some of these cases have resulted in a liver transplantation or death. The time to onset for these cases ranged from months to years after initiation of tocilizumab therapy. While most cases presented with marked elevations of aminotransferase concentrations (exceeding 5 times the upper limit of normal [ULN]), some cases presented with signs or symptoms of hepatic dysfunction and only mildly elevated aminotransferases. In randomized controlled studies, tocilizumab treatment was associated with a higher incidence of aminotransferase elevations compared with placebo. The incidence and magnitude of aminotransferase elevations were increased when tocilizumab was used in conjunction with a potentially hepatotoxic drug (e.g., methotrexate).

In adults with rheumatoid arthritis, giant cell arteritis (GCA), or systemic sclerosis-associated interstitial lung disease (SSc-ILD), perform liver function tests (i.e., serum ALT and AST, alkaline phosphatase, and total bilirubin concentrations) before initiating tocilizumab therapy and then monitor every 4–8 weeks after initiation of therapy for the first 6 months of treatment and every 3 months thereafter. The manufacturer recommends that tocilizumab therapy not be initiated in rheumatoid arthritis, GCA, or SSc-ILD patients with elevated aminotransferase concentrations greater than 1.5 times the ULN. In patients who develop elevated ALT or AST concentrations exceeding 5 times the ULN, tocilizumab should be discontinued. A similar pattern of serum aminotransferase elevations has been observed with tocilizumab therapy in patients with polyarticular or systemic JIA. In such patients, liver function tests should be monitored at the time of the second infusion and every 4–8 weeks thereafter in patients with polyarticular JIA and every 2–4 weeks thereafter in patients with systemic JIA.

In patients hospitalized with COVID-19, perform liver function tests (i.e., serum ALT and AST) before initiating tocilizumab therapy and during treatment. The manufacturer recommends tocilizumab therapy should not be initiated in COVID-19 patients with elevated ALT or AST above 10 times the ULN. Multi-organ failure with involvement of the liver is recognized as a complication of severe COVID-19. The decision to administer tocilizumab should balance the potential benefit of treating COVID-19 against the potential risks of acute treatment with tocilizumab.

In patients with symptoms indicative of possible liver injury (e.g., fatigue, anorexia, right upper abdominal discomfort, dark urine, jaundice), liver function tests should be performed promptly. If the patient is found to have abnormal liver function tests (e.g., ALT greater than 3 times the ULN, total bilirubin greater than 2 times the ULN), tocilizumab therapy should be interrupted and the patient evaluated to determine the probable cause. Therapy should only be restarted in patients with another explanation for their liver function test abnormalities after normalization of the liver function test results.

Hematologic Effects

Treatment with tocilizumab has been associated with a higher incidence of neutropenia. Reduction in neutrophil count to less than 1000/mm³ has been reported during clinical trials in patients receiving tocilizumab. Infections have been infrequently reported in association with treatment-related neutropenia in long-term extension studies and postmarketing clinical experience.

Reductions in platelet counts also have been reported in patients receiving tocilizumab. In clinical trials of the drug, decreases in platelet counts were not associated with severe bleeding.

Tocilizumab should not be initiated in RA, GCA, and SSc-ILD patients with an absolute neutrophil count less than 2000/mm³. Treatment should be discontinued in patients who developed an absolute neutrophil count less than 500/mm³.

Neutrophil and platelet counts should be monitored 4–8 weeks after initiation of tocilizumab therapy and every 3 months thereafter in adults with rheumatoid arthritis, GCA, or SSc-ILD. Monitor neutrophils and platelet counts at the time of the second administration and every 4–8 weeks thereafter in patients with PJIA and every 2–4 weeks thereafter in patients with SJIA. In patients with neutropenia or thrombocytopenia, dosage adjustment, treatment interruption, or discontinuance of the drug may be necessary.

It is not recommended to initiate tocilizumab treatment in COVID-19 patients with an absolute neutrophil count less than 1000/mm³ or a platelet count less than 50,000/mm³. Neutrophil and platelet counts should be monitored.

Effects on Serum Lipids

Increased serum concentrations of total cholesterol, triglycerides, low-density lipoprotein (LDL)-cholesterol, and/or high-density lipoprotein (HDL)-cholesterol have been reported in patients receiving tocilizumab.

Lipoprotein concentrations should be monitored approximately 4–8 weeks after initiation of tocilizumab therapy. Lipid disorders should be managed as clinically appropriate.

Because tocilizumab may adversely affect lipid profiles and also elevate blood pressure in some patients, a postmarketing, randomized, open-label, multicenter cardiovascular outcomes study was conducted in patients with moderate to severe rheumatoid arthritis. This cardiovascular safety study was designed to exclude a moderate increase in cardiovascular risk in patients treated with tocilizumab compared with the TNF blocking agent etanercept. The study included 3,080 seropositive rheumatoid arthritis patients with active disease and an inadequate response to nonbiologic DMARDs who were 50 years of age or older with at least one additional cardiovascular risk factor beyond rheumatoid arthritis. Patients were randomized in a 1:1 ratio to either IV tocilizumab 8 mg/kg every 4 weeks or

subcutaneous etanercept 50 mg every week and then followed for an average of 3.2 years. The primary end point was the comparison of the time-to-first occurrence of any component of a composite of major adverse cardiovascular events (e.g., nonfatal myocardial infarction, nonfatal stroke, cardiovascular death); the final intent-to-treat analysis was based on a total of 161 confirmed cardiovascular events (83 [5.4%] for tocilizumab and 78 [5.1%] for etanercept) reviewed by an independent and blinded adjudication committee. Non-inferiority of tocilizumab to etanercept for cardiovascular risk was determined by excluding a more than 80% relative increase in the risk of major adverse cardiovascular events. The estimated hazard ratio for this risk comparing tocilizumab to etanercept was 1.05 (95% confidence interval [0.77, 1.43]).

Malignancies

Immunosuppressive therapy may increase the risk of malignancies. Whether treatment with tocilizumab affects development of malignancies remains to be determined. Malignancies were reported in clinical trials of the drug.

Sensitivity Reactions

Hypersensitivity reactions, including anaphylaxis, have been reported in patients receiving tocilizumab; fatal anaphylactic reactions have occurred in those receiving IV infusions of the drug. During clinical trials of tocilizumab, hypersensitivity reactions requiring treatment discontinuance (e.g., anaphylaxis, generalized erythema, rash, urticaria) have been reported in various patient populations and with either IV or subcutaneous therapy. During postmarketing experience, hypersensitivity reactions, including anaphylaxis and death, have occurred in patients receiving various IV dosages, either with or without concomitant therapy, including in patients who received premedication. Hypersensitivity reactions, including anaphylaxis, have occurred both with and without prior hypersensitivity reactions and as early as the first IV infusion of the drug.

Appropriate agents and equipment should be available for immediate use in case a serious hypersensitivity reaction occurs during IV infusion of the drug. Patients receiving subcutaneous therapy with tocilizumab should be advised to seek immediate medical attention if they experience symptoms of a hypersensitivity reaction. If a hypersensitivity reaction occurs, administration of the drug should be stopped immediately and the drug should be permanently discontinued. Tocilizumab is contraindicated in patients with known hypersensitivity to the drug.

Demyelinating Disorders

The effect of tocilizumab on demyelinating disorders remains to be determined. Multiple sclerosis and chronic inflammatory demyelinating polyneuropathy have been reported rarely in patients with rheumatoid arthritis receiving tocilizumab in clinical trials. Patients receiving tocilizumab should be monitored for signs and symptoms suggestive of a demyelinating disorder. Clinicians should exercise caution when considering tocilizumab therapy in patients with preexisting or recent-onset demyelinating disorders.

Immunization

Live vaccines should be avoided in patients receiving tocilizumab. Vaccinations should be brought up to date prior to initiation of the drug.

Immunogenicity

In clinical trials evaluating IV tocilizumab in patients with rheumatoid arthritis, antibodies to the drug were detected in about 2% of tocilizumab-treated patients; about 11% of these patients experienced hypersensitivity reactions resulting in drug discontinuance. Neutralizing antibodies developed in about 1% of such patients receiving the drug IV. In clinical trials evaluating subcutaneous tocilizumab in patients with rheumatoid arthritis, antibodies to the drug were detected in 0.9% of patients receiving the drug; neutralizing antibodies developed in about 0.8% of patients receiving subcutaneous tocilizumab. No relationship between antibody development and adverse effects or loss of clinical response was observed, and detection rates were similar with IV or subcutaneous therapy.

In clinical trials evaluating subcutaneous tocilizumab in patients with SSc-ILD, antibodies to tocilizumab were detected in about 1.8% of patients. Antibodies were neutralizing, and none of the patients experienced hypersensitivity reactions.

In clinical trials evaluating IV tocilizumab in patients with polyarticular JIA, one patient developed antibodies to the drug without developing a hypersensitivity reaction. In clinical trials evaluating subcutaneous tocilizumab in patients with polyarticular JIA, 3 patients developed neutralizing antibodies without developing a serious or clinically important hypersensitivity reaction. In clinical trials evaluating IV tocilizumab in patients with systemic JIA, 2 patients (2%) developed neutralizing antibodies, with urticaria and angioedema occurring in one of the patients and macrophage activation syndrome while on escape therapy reported in the other patient.

Specific Populations

Pregnancy

A pregnancy exposure registry has been established by the manufacturer that monitors pregnancy outcomes in women receiving tocilizumab. Clinicians or pregnant patients can register at 877-311-8972.

Limited data regarding tocilizumab use in pregnant women are not sufficient to determine whether there is a drug-associated risk for major birth defects and miscarriage. Monoclonal antibodies such as tocilizumab are actively transported across the placenta during the third trimester of pregnancy and may affect immune response in infants exposed to the drugs in utero.

In animal reproduction studies, IV administration of tocilizumab to cynomolgus monkeys during organogenesis caused abortion/embryofetal death at dosages of 1.25 (or more) times the maximum recommended human IV dosage of 8 mg/kg every 2–4 weeks. Evidence in animals suggests that inhibition of interleukin-6 (IL-6) signaling may interfere with cervical ripening and dilatation and myometrial contractile activity, which could potentially result in parturition delays. Based on animal data, there may be a potential risk to the fetus.

As pregnancy progresses, monoclonal antibodies are increasingly transported across the placenta, with the largest amount transferred during the third trimester. The risks and benefits of administering live or live attenuated vaccines to infants exposed to tocilizumab in utero should be considered, since the safety of such vaccines in infants exposed to the drug in utero is unknown.

Lactation

It is not known whether tocilizumab is distributed into milk, and the effects of the drug on the breast-fed infant and on milk production also are not known. Maternal immunoglobulin G (IgG) is distributed into human milk. If tocilizumab is distributed into human milk, the effects of local exposure in the GI tract and potential limited systemic exposure in the infant are unknown. The lack of clinical data during lactation precludes a clear determination of the risk of tocilizumab exposure to nursing infants. Therefore, the manufacturer states that the developmental and health benefits of breast-feeding should be considered along with the mother's clinical need for tocilizumab and any potential adverse effects on the breast-fed child from the drug or from the underlying maternal condition.

Pediatric Use

Safety and efficacy of IV and subcutaneous tocilizumab for the management of active polyarticular or systemic JIA and safety and efficacy of IV tocilizumab for the management of severe or life-threatening chimeric antigen receptor (CAR) T cell-induced cytokine release syndrome (CRS) have been established in pediatric patients 2 years of age and older. Safety and efficacy of the drug in children younger than 2 years of age or for the management of conditions other than polyarticular or systemic JIA and CAR T cell-induced CRS in children have not been established.

A multicenter, open-label, single-arm study to evaluate the pharmacokinetics, safety, pharmacodynamics, and efficacy of tocilizumab over 12 weeks in 11 patients with systemic JIA under 2 years of age was conducted. Patients received IV tocilizumab 12 mg/kg every 2 weeks, and concurrent use of stable background treatment with corticosteroids, methotrexate, and/or nonsteroidal anti-inflammatory agents was permitted. Patients who completed the 12-week phase of the study could continue to an optional extension phase for a total of 52 weeks or until the age of 2 years, whichever was longer. The primary pharmacokinetic parameters (peak and trough concentrations and AUC) of tocilizumab at steady state in these patients under 2 years of age were within the ranges of these parameters observed in patients 2–17 years of age with systemic JIA. In patients under 2 years of age with systemic JIA, serious adverse effects, adverse effects leading to drug discontinuance, and infectious adverse effects were reported in 27.3, 36.4, and 81.8% of patients, respectively. Six patients (54.5%) experienced hypersensitivity reactions and 3 of these patients experienced serious hypersensitivity

reactions and were withdrawn from the study. Three of the patients who developed hypersensitivity reactions (two with serious hypersensitivity reactions) developed treatment-induced anti-tocilizumab antibodies after the event. There were no cases of macrophage activation syndrome (MAS) based on the study protocol-specified criteria, but there were 2 cases of suspected MAS based on Ravelli criteria.

In a retrospective analysis of pooled outcome data for patients treated with IV tocilizumab for CAR T cell-induced CRS, 25 patients were children (2–12 years of age) and 17 patients were adolescents (12–18 years of age). There were no differences in safety or efficacy between the pediatric patients and the adults.

Geriatric Use

Approximately 16% of patients with rheumatoid arthritis who received IV tocilizumab in clinical trials were ≥65 years of age and about 2% were ≥75 years of age. Approximately 28% of patients with rheumatoid arthritis who received subcutaneous tocilizumab in clinical trials were ≥65 years of age and about 4% were ≥75 years of age. Serious infection occurred with greater frequency in those ≥65 years of age relative to younger adults. Because the geriatric population in general may have a higher incidence of infections than younger adults, tocilizumab should be used with caution in this age group.

Clinical studies that evaluated tocilizumab for CAR T cell-induced CRS did not include sufficient numbers of patients ≥65 years of age to determine whether they respond differently than younger adults.

Population pharmacokinetic analyses indicate that age does not affect the pharmacokinetics of tocilizumab.

Hepatic Impairment

Safety and efficacy of tocilizumab have not been established in patients with hepatic impairment, including those with serologic evidence of hepatitis B virus (HBV) or hepatitis C virus (HCV) infection. Use of the drug in patients with active hepatic disease or hepatic impairment is not recommended.

The pharmacokinetics of tocilizumab have not been formally studied in patients with hepatic impairment.

Renal Impairment

The pharmacokinetics of tocilizumab have not been formally studied in patients with renal impairment. Most of the patients with rheumatoid arthritis, GCA, and SSc-ILD in the population pharmacokinetic analysis had normal renal function or mild renal impairment. Mild renal impairment (creatinine clearance less than 80 mL/minute but not less than 50 mL/minute) did not appear to affect the pharmacokinetics of the drug. About one-third of the patients in the GCA trial had moderate renal impairment at baseline (creatinine clearance 30–59 mL/minute); no effect on tocilizumab exposure was noted in these patients.

No dosage adjustment is required in patients with mild or moderate renal impairment. Tocilizumab has not been evaluated in patients with severe renal impairment to date.

● Common Adverse Effects

Adverse effects reported in 5% or more of patients receiving tocilizumab include upper respiratory tract infection, nasopharyngitis, headache, hypertension, increased ALT concentrations, and injection site reactions (e.g., erythema, pruritus, pain, hematoma).

DRUG INTERACTIONS

● Drugs Metabolized by Hepatic Microsomal Enzymes

Possible increased metabolism of drugs that are metabolized by cytochrome P-450 (CYP) isoenzymes. Because cytokines such as interleukin-6 (IL-6) may down-regulate CYP enzymes, inhibition of IL-6 by tocilizumab in patients with rheumatoid arthritis may restore CYP enzyme activity to higher levels. In vitro studies indicate that tocilizumab may alter expression of CYP isoenzymes including 1A2, 2B6, 2C9, 2C19, 2D6, and 3A4; effects of the drug on CYP2C8 or transporters (e.g., P-glycoprotein) have not been elucidated. Effects of tocilizumab on CYP enzyme activity may persist for several weeks after the drug is discontinued.

Following initiation or discontinuance of tocilizumab therapy, patients receiving certain drugs metabolized by CYP isoenzymes (i.e., those with a low therapeutic index that require individualized dosing [e.g., cyclosporine, theophylline, warfarin]) should be monitored for therapeutic effect and/or changes in serum concentrations, and dosages of these drugs should be adjusted as needed. Caution also is advised when tocilizumab is used concomitantly with CYP3A4 substrates (e.g., oral contraceptives, atorvastatin, lovastatin) for which a reduction in efficacy would be undesirable.

Dextromethorphan

Pharmacokinetic interaction (possible decreased exposure to dextromethorphan and/or dextrorphan). In patients with rheumatoid arthritis who are not receiving tocilizumab, administration of dextromethorphan 30 mg results in systemic exposure to dextromethorphan (a substrate of CYP2D6 and CYP3A4) that is similar to that observed in healthy individuals; however, exposure to the dextrorphan metabolite (a substrate of CYP3A4) is substantially reduced in rheumatoid arthritis patients. One week following IV administration of a single 8-mg/kg dose of tocilizumab, exposures to dextromethorphan and dextrorphan were decreased by 5 and 29%, respectively.

Omeprazole

Pharmacokinetic interaction (possible decreased exposure to omeprazole following initiation of tocilizumab therapy). In patients with rheumatoid arthritis who are not receiving tocilizumab, administration of omeprazole 10 mg results in systemic exposure to omeprazole (a substrate of CYP2C19 and CYP3A4) that is approximately twofold higher than values observed in healthy individuals. In patients with rheumatoid arthritis who received 10 mg of omeprazole before and one week after IV administration of an 8-mg/kg dose of tocilizumab, systemic exposure to omeprazole (as measured by area under the plasma concentration–time curve [AUC]) decreased by 12% in poor and intermediate metabolizers of the drug and by 28% in extensive metabolizers; AUC values for omeprazole observed following the tocilizumab dose were slightly higher than values observed after omeprazole administration in healthy individuals.

Simvastatin

Pharmacokinetic interaction (possible decreased exposure to simvastatin and simvastatin acid following initiation of tocilizumab therapy). In patients with rheumatoid arthritis who are not receiving tocilizumab, administration of simvastatin 40 mg results in systemic exposures to simvastatin (a substrate of CYP3A4 and organic anion transporter [OATP] 1B1) and its metabolite, simvastatin acid, that are approximately fourfold to tenfold higher and twofold higher, respectively, than values observed in healthy individuals. One week after rheumatoid arthritis patients received a single 10-mg/kg IV dose of tocilizumab, systemic exposures to simvastatin and simvastatin acid decreased by 57 and 39%, respectively, and values in the tocilizumab-treated patients were similar to or slightly higher than values observed after simvastatin administration in healthy individuals. Following discontinuance of tocilizumab in rheumatoid arthritis patients, systemic exposure to simvastatin and simvastatin acid increased. When selecting simvastatin dosages for patients with rheumatoid arthritis, clinicians should consider the potential for altered systemic exposure to the drug following initiation or discontinuance of tocilizumab therapy.

● Antirheumatic Drugs

In rheumatoid arthritis patients, population pharmacokinetic analyses indicated that concomitant use of methotrexate, corticosteroids, or nonsteroidal antiinflammatory agents (NSAIAs) does not appear to affect clearance of tocilizumab. Concomitant use of methotrexate (10–25 mg once weekly) and tocilizumab (single 10-mg/kg IV dose) did not substantially affect exposure to methotrexate. An increased incidence and magnitude of serum aminotransferase elevations were observed when potentially hepatotoxic drugs such as methotrexate were used in combination with tocilizumab.

Tocilizumab has not been studied in conjunction with biologic disease-modifying antirheumatic drugs (DMARDs), including tumor necrosis factor (TNF; TNF-α) blocking agents, interleukin-1 (IL-1) receptor antagonists, anti-CD20 monoclonal antibodies, and selective costimulation modulators. Because of the possibility of increased immunosuppression and an increased risk of infection, concomitant use of tocilizumab with biologic DMARDs should be avoided.

● Vaccines

Live vaccines should not be administered to patients receiving tocilizumab. Because inhibition of interleukin-6 (IL-6) may interfere with the normal immune response to new antigens, all patients (particularly pediatric and geriatric patients) should receive all appropriate vaccines recommended by current immunization guidelines prior to initiation of tocilizumab therapy, if possible. The interval between administration of live vaccines and initiation of tocilizumab therapy should be in accordance with current vaccination guidelines regarding immunosuppressive agents. Information is not available regarding immune response to vaccines in patients receiving tocilizumab, nor is information available regarding secondary transmission of infection from individuals receiving live vaccines to patients receiving tocilizumab.

DESCRIPTION

Tocilizumab, a recombinant humanized monoclonal antibody specific for interleukin-6 (IL-6) receptor, is a biologic response modifier and a disease-modifying antirheumatic drug (DMARD). Tocilizumab is an IgG₁ kappa immunoglobulin that binds to both soluble and membrane-bound IL-6 receptors and inhibits IL-6-mediated signaling through these receptors, thereby resulting in a reduction in inflammatory mediator production. The drug is produced in mammalian (Chinese hamster ovary) cells.

IL-6, a pleiotropic proinflammatory cytokine, is produced by various cell types, including T-cells, B-lymphocytes, monocytes, fibroblasts, synoviocytes, and endothelial cells, and has a broad spectrum of biologic activities. IL-6 is involved in T-cell activation, induction of immunoglobulin secretion, initiation of hepatic acute phase protein synthesis, stimulation of hematopoietic precursor cell proliferation and differentiation, and induction of osteoclast differentiation and activation. While the causes of rheumatoid arthritis have not been fully elucidated, proinflammatory cytokines, including IL-6, appear to play critical roles in the disease process. IL-6 is overexpressed in synovial tissue in patients with rheumatoid arthritis and is thought to contribute to synovial proliferation and joint destruction in patients with the disease. Elevated levels of IL-6 in serum and synovial fluid have been shown to correlate with clinical and laboratory measures of disease activity in patients with rheumatoid arthritis. IL-6 also is elevated in serum and synovial fluid in patients with polyarticular or systemic juvenile idiopathic arthritis (JIA), and the elevated levels of IL-6 have been correlated with disease activity.

The pharmacokinetics of tocilizumab are characterized by nonlinear elimination that is a combination of linear clearance and Michaelis-Menten elimination. The nonlinear part of the drug's elimination leads to an increase in drug exposure that is more than dose proportional. The pharmacokinetics of tocilizumab do not change with time. Because of the dependence of total clearance on tocilizumab serum concentrations, the half-life of the drug is also concentration dependent and varies depending on the serum concentration. Population pharmacokinetic analyses in patient populations tested to date do not suggest any relationship between clearance of tocilizumab and the presence of anti-drug antibodies. The apparent steady-state half-life of tocilizumab in adults with rheumatoid arthritis is up to 11 or up to 13 days following IV administration of tocilizumab 4 or 8 mg/kg, respectively, every 4 weeks and up to 13 or up to 5 days after subcutaneous administration of tocilizumab 162 mg every week or every other week, respectively. In patients with giant cell arteritis (GCA), the effective half-life of tocilizumab at steady state was 18.3–18.9 days in patients receiving 162 mg subcutaneously once weekly and 4.2–7.9 days in those receiving 162 mg subcutaneously every other week. For intravenous administration in GCA patients, the effective half-life of tocilizumab at steady state was 13.2 days in patients receiving 6 mg/kg every 4 weeks. The reported half-life in pediatric patients with polyarticular or systemic juvenile idiopathic arthritis (JIA) following IV administration is up to 17 or up to 16 days, respectively, at steady state. Population pharmacokinetic analyses in adult rheumatoid arthritis and GCA patients indicate that age, gender, and race do not affect the pharmacokinetics of tocilizumab. However, linear clearance was found to increase with body size. In rheumatoid arthritis patients, systemic drug exposure was substantially greater (86%) in patients weighing more than 100 kg than in those weighing less than 60 kg following administration of a weight-based IV dose of 8 mg/kg (see Dosage and Administration: Dosage). At a fixed subcutaneous dosage, tocilizumab exposure is inversely related to body weight.

ADVICE TO PATIENTS

- Advise patients and/or caregivers about potential benefits and risks of tocilizumab. Advise patients and/or caregivers to read the medication guide.

- Instruct the patient and/or caregiver regarding proper dosage and administration of tocilizumab, including the use of aseptic technique, and proper disposal of prefilled syringes and autoinjectors if it is determined that the patient and/or caregiver is competent to safely administer subcutaneous injections of the drug.

- Inform patients to consult clinician if the subcutaneous injection does not deliver the full dose.

- Risk of increased susceptibility to infection. Instruct patients to inform their clinician immediately if any signs or symptoms suggestive of infection (e.g., fever or chills; sweating; cough; dyspnea; fatigue; diarrhea; burning or pain upon urination; warm, red, or painful skin) develop to assure rapid evaluation and appropriate treatment.

- Risk of GI perforation. Instruct patients to inform their clinician immediately if severe, persistent abdominal pain occurs.

- Risk of liver injury. Inform patients to notify their clinician if they develop right-sided abdominal swelling or pain, fatigue, lack of appetite for several days, yellowing of the skin or whites of the eyes, light-colored stools, weakness, nausea and vomiting, confusion, or dark colored urine.

- Risk of hypersensitivity and serious allergic reactions, including anaphylaxis. Instruct patient to contact their clinician prior to administering the next dose if manifestations of an allergic reaction (e.g., urticaria, rash, flushing) occur; importance of seeking immediate medical attention if manifestations of a serious allergic reaction (e.g., difficulty breathing, chest pain, feelings of faintness or dizziness, abdominal pain or vomiting, swelling of the lips, tongue, or face) occur.

- Importance of informing clinicians of existing or contemplated concomitant therapy, including prescription (e.g., biologic antirheumatic drugs, immunizations) and OTC drugs, vitamins, and herbal supplements, as well as any concomitant illnesses or any history of tuberculosis or other chronic or recurring infections.

- Advise patients of periodic laboratory monitoring.

- Advise women to inform their clinicians if they are or plan to become pregnant or plan to breast-feed. Inform women about the existence of and encourage enrollment in the pregnancy registry for tocilizumab.

- Inform patients of other important precautionary information.

PREPARATIONS

Tocilizumab is obtained through designated specialty pharmacies. Contact manufacturer for specific availability information.

Excipients in commercially available drug preparations may have clinically important effects in some individuals; consult specific product labeling for details.

Tocilizumab (recombinant)

Parenteral

Injection, for subcutaneous use	162 mg/0.9 mL	Actemra® (available as single-use prefilled syringe), Genentech
	162 mg/0.9 mL	Actemra® ACTPen® (available as single-use prefilled autoinjector), Genentech
Injection concentrate, for IV infusion	20 mg/mL (80 mg, 200 mg, 400 mg)	Actemra®, Genentech

† Use is not currently included in the labeling approved by the US Food and Drug Administration.

Selected Revisions May 10, 2024, © Copyright, July 1, 2010, American Society of Health-System Pharmacists, Inc.

Ustekinumab

90:24.20.92 • INTERLEUKIN-MEDIATED AGENTS, MISCELLANEOUS

- Ustekinumab and ustekinumab-auub, human immunoglobulin G_1 kappa (IgG_1) monoclonal antibodies directed against the p40 subunit of interleukin-12 (IL-12) and interleukin-23 (IL-23), are immunosuppressive agents.

- Ustekinumab-auub is biosimilar to ustekinumab (Stelara®). FDA defines a biosimilar as a biological product that is highly similar to an FDA-licensed reference biological with the exception of minor differences in clinically inactive components and for which there are no clinically meaningful differences in safety, purity, or potency. The claim of biosimilarity is based on a totality-of-evidence approach, which includes consideration of data from analytical, animal, and clinical studies (e.g., human pharmacokinetic and pharmacodynamic studies, clinical immunogenicity assessment, additional comparative clinical studies). Therefore, biosimilarity may be established even when there are formulation or minor structural differences as long as these differences are not clinically meaningful. Biosimilars are approved through an abbreviated licensure pathway that establishes biosimilarity between the proposed biological and the reference biological but does not independently establish safety and effectiveness of the proposed biological. In order to be considered an interchangeable biosimilar, a biological product must meet additional requirements beyond demonstrating biosimilarity to its reference product; these requirements include demonstrating that the biological product can be expected to produce the same clinical results as the reference product in any given patient and, for a biological product that is administered more than once to an individual, the risk in terms of safety or diminished efficacy of alternating or switching between use of the biological product and the reference product is no greater than the risk of using the reference product without such alternation or switch. Biosimilar products that are interchangeable can be substituted for the reference product without the intervention of the healthcare provider who prescribed the reference product. The currently available evidence demonstrates that the ustekinumab biosimilar (Wezlana®) is interchangeable with Stelera® at the pharmacy level.

- In this monograph, unless otherwise stated, the term "ustekinumab products" refers to ustekinumab (the reference drug) and its biosimilar (ustekinumab-auub).

USES

● Plaque Psoriasis

Ustekinumab and its biosimilar (ustekinumab-auub) are used for the management of moderate to severe plaque psoriasis in adults and pediatric patients ≥6 years of age who are candidates for systemic therapy or phototherapy. Safety and efficacy of ustekinumab for this use are based principally on the results of 2 randomized controlled trials in adults, one randomized controlled trial in adolescent patients 12–17 years of age, and one single-arm study in pediatric patients 6–11 years of age. Guidelines generally support the use of ustekinumab in adults and pediatric patients with moderate-to-severe plaque psoriasis.

Clinical Experience in Adults

Ustekinumab has been evaluated in 2 multicenter, randomized, double-blind, placebo-controlled studies (PHOENIX 1 and PHOENIX 2) in adults 18 years of age or older who had plaque psoriasis for at least 6 months with involvement of at least 10% of the body surface area, had a Psoriasis Area and Severity Index (PASI) score of at least 12, and were candidates for systemic therapy or phototherapy. PASI is a composite score that takes into consideration both the fraction of body surface area affected and the nature and severity of the psoriatic changes within the affected areas (i.e., induration, erythema, scaling). Patients with guttate, erythrodermic, or pustular psoriasis were excluded from these studies. Both studies were conducted

in 3 phases. For the first phase (weeks 0–12), patients were randomized in equal proportions, stratified by body weight, to receive ustekinumab 45 mg, ustekinumab 90 mg, or placebo. Treatment was initiated with 2 doses of the drug administered 4 weeks apart; subsequent doses were administered at 12-week intervals. In the second phase (weeks 12–40 in PHOENIX 1 and weeks 12–28 in PHOENIX 2), patients assigned to placebo crossed over to active treatment. The third phase of PHOENIX 1 (weeks 40–76) was a randomized withdrawal phase during which long-term responders (i.e., patients originally assigned to receive ustekinumab who achieved at least 75% improvement from baseline in PASI score [PASI-75] at weeks 28 and 40) were rerandomized to continue receiving the drug or to receive placebo until loss of response. In PHOENIX 2, the third phase (weeks 28–52) was a randomized dose-intensification phase during which partial responders (i.e., patients originally assigned to receive ustekinumab who achieved at least 50 but less than 75% improvement from baseline in PASI score) were rerandomized to continue receiving the drug every 12 weeks or to begin receiving the drug every 8 weeks.

In the PHOENIX 1 and 2 studies, the primary outcome measure was the proportion of patients who achieved a PASI-75 response at week 12. In these 2 studies, a PASI-75 response at 12 weeks was achieved in 67, 66–76, or 3–4% of patients who received ustekinumab 45 mg, ustekinumab 90 mg, or placebo, respectively. In addition, a status of cleared or minimal disease on the Physician's Global Assessment (PGA) scale was achieved at 12 weeks in 59–68, 61–73, or 4% of patients who received ustekinumab 45 mg, ustekinumab 90 mg, or placebo, respectively. Onset of response, as measured by PASI-75 response, was observed by 4 weeks after initiation of therapy. In patients who weighed less than 100 kg, response rates were similar for both the 45- and 90-mg doses of ustekinumab; however, in patients who weighed more than 100 kg, higher response rates were observed with 90-mg doses compared with 45-mg doses of ustekinumab. In these 2 studies, a PASI-75 response at 12 weeks was achieved in 73–74 or 65–78% of patients weighing 100 kg or less who received ustekinumab 45 or 90 mg, respectively; however, a PASI-75 response at 12 weeks was achieved in 49–54 or 68–71% of patients weighing more than 100 kg who received ustekinumab 45 or 90 mg, respectively. In PHOENIX 1, 89% of long-term responders who were rerandomized to ustekinumab at week 40 maintained a PASI-75 response at week 52, compared with 63% of those rerandomized to placebo. The median time to loss of PASI-75 response among long-term responders rerandomized to placebo was 16 weeks.

Ustekinumab also has been evaluated in a multicenter, randomized, active comparator study (ACCEPT) in adults 18 years of age or older who had plaque psoriasis for at least 6 months with involvement of at least 10% of the body surface area, had a PASI score of at least 12, had a PGA score of at least 3, and were candidates for systemic therapy or phototherapy. Patients were randomized to receive ustekinumab (45 or 90 mg at weeks 0 and 4) or etanercept (50 mg twice weekly for 12 weeks), a tumor necrosis factor (TNF; TNF-α) blocking agent. Patients in the etanercept group who did not have a response (i.e., patients who had moderate, marked, or severe psoriasis) at week 12 received 90 mg of ustekinumab at weeks 16 and 20, and patients who did not have a response to ustekinumab received one additional dose of ustekinumab at week 16. Treatment was interrupted starting at week 12 in all patients with cleared, minimal, or mild psoriasis; patients were retreated with ustekinumab if psoriasis recurred and was classified as moderate, marked, or severe. The primary outcome measure (i.e., proportion of patients who achieved a PASI-75 response at week 12) was achieved in 68 or 74% of patients who received ustekinumab 45 or 90 mg, respectively, compared with 57% of those who received etanercept. In addition, a status of cleared or minimal disease on the PGA scale at 12 weeks was achieved in 65 or 71% of patients receiving ustekinumab 45 or 90 mg, respectively, compared with 49% of those receiving etanercept. Among patients who did not respond to 12 weeks of etanercept therapy, 49% achieved a PASI-75 response and 40% had cleared or minimal disease at 12 weeks after initiating ustekinumab therapy. Retreatment of patients who experienced a recurrence of their disease after ustekinumab discontinuance resulted in responses (cleared, minimal, or mild disease) in 84% of the patients.

A limited number of randomized controlled trials have compared ustekinumab to anti-interleukin 17A monoclonal antibodies (secukinumab and ixekizumab) for the treatment of moderate-to-severe plaque psoriasis. The CLEAR and CLARITY studies compared ustekinumab to secukinumab in patients with psoriasis that was not controlled with topical treatments, phototherapy, and/or previous systemic therapy. In the CLEAR study, secukinumab was superior to ustekinumab for the primary endpoint of PASI 90 response at week 16. In the CLARITY study, secukinumab was superior to ustekinumab for the co-primary endpoints of PASI 90 response at week 12 and the proportion of patients who achieved modified Investigator's Global Assessment (IGA) score of 0 (clear) or

1 (almost clear) at week 12. In an extension study of the CLARITY study, a greater proportion of patients assigned to secukinumab achieved a PASI 90 response and IGA score of 0 or 1 compared to ustekinumab at 52 weeks. In the IXORA-S study, ustekinumab was compared to ixekizumab in patients with psoriasis who had previously failed or had a contraindication to systemic therapy. Ixekizumab was both noninferior and superior to ustekinumab for PASI 90 response at 12 weeks, and was superior to ustekinumab at 24 weeks. Clinical benefit of ixekizumab was maintained at week 52.

Two randomized, placebo-controlled trials (UltIMMa-1 and UltIMMa-2) have also compared risankizumab and ustekinumab in patients with moderate-to-severe plaque psoriasis. The co-primary endpoints of PASI 90 response and sPGA of 0 (clear) or 1 (almost clear) were superior with risankizumab compared to both ustekinumab or placebo at week 16.

Clinical Experience in Pediatric Patients

Ustekinumab has been shown to induce clinical responses in pediatric patients with moderate to severe plaque psoriasis. The drug was studied in 2 pediatric trials, one in adolescent patients 12–17 years of age and one in pediatric patients 6–11 years of age.

Ustekinumab was evaluated in a randomized, double-blind, placebo-controlled study (CADMUS) in 110 adolescents 12–17 years of age who had plaque psoriasis (with involvement of at least 10% of the body surface area, a PASI score of at least 12, and a PGA score of at least 3) that was inadequately controlled by topical therapy and who were candidates for systemic therapy or phototherapy. Patients were randomized to receive ustekinumab (either the recommended dose or one-half the recommended dose by subcutaneous injection at weeks 0 and 4 and then every 12 weeks) or placebo. The recommended ustekinumab dose was 0.75 mg/kg for patients weighing less than 60 kg, 45 mg for those weighing 60–100 kg, and 90 mg for those weighing more than 100 kg. At week 12, placebo recipients crossed over to receive ustekinumab at either the recommended dosage or one-half the recommended dosage. Approximately 63% of patients had previously received phototherapy or conventional systemic therapy and approximately 11% had received biologic agents. Greater proportions of patients receiving ustekinumab compared with those receiving placebo achieved PASI and PGA responses at week 12 (see Table 1). Responses to the drug were maintained through week 52 of treatment. Beyond week 12, clinical response rates generally were higher and responses were better sustained throughout each 12-week dosing interval in patients receiving the recommended ustekinumab dosage rather than one-half the recommended dosage.

TABLE 1. Proportion of Adolescents with Psoriasis Responding to Assigned Treatment at Week 12

Response Measure	Ustekinumab (at recommended dosage)	Ustekinumab (at one-half recommended dosage)	Placebo
PGA score 0 or 1 (clear or minimal disease)	69.4%	67.6%	5.4%
PASI 75 response	80.6%	78.4%	10.8%
PASI 90 response	61.1%	54.1%	5.4%

The efficacy, safety and pharmacokinetics of ustekinumab were evaluated in an open-label, single-arm, multicenter study (CADMUS Jr.) in 44 pediatric patients 6–11 years of age with moderate to severe plaque psoriasis. Patients were required to have body surface area (BSA) involvement ≥10%, a PASI score ≥12, and PGA score ≥3, and were candidates for systemic therapy, phototherapy, or have psoriasis that was not controlled with topical therapy. The recommended ustekinumab dose was 0.75 mg/kg for patients weighing less than 60 kg, 45 mg for those weighing 60–100 kg, and 90 mg for those weighing more than 100 kg. Approximately 34% of patients had previously received phototherapy, 18% had previously received conventional systemic agents, and 5% had previously received biologic agents. At week 12, 77% (95% confidence interval [CI], 62.2–88.5) of patients achieved a PGA score of 0 or 1, 84% (95% CI, 69.9–93.4) achieved a PASI 75 response, and 64% (95% CI, 47.8–77.6) achieved a PASI 90 response. Responses

to the drug were maintained or increased through week 52. In the pharmacokinetic analysis, median trough serum concentrations were maintained at steady-state levels from week 28 to 52 without evidence of ustekinumab accumulation.

Clinical Perspective

The American Academy of Dermatology and the National Psoriasis Foundation have issued joint guidelines for the treatment of psoriasis in adult and pediatric patients. Various drugs and drug classes are used to treat psoriasis. Phototherapy and topical treatments (e.g., vitamin D analogues, calcineurin inhibitors, keratolytics, and corticosteroids) are frequently used to treat mild psoriasis present on limited areas of the body, but these therapies may be inadequate to obtain skin clearance in patients with more extensive or severe disease. Systemic biologic and nonbiologic therapies are mainstays of treatment for moderate to severe psoriasis, and may also be useful for treating psoriasis on parts of the body that are difficult to treat with topical therapy (e.g., scalp, palms and soles of the feet, genitals). Topical therapies can be used adjunctively in moderate to severe disease. Nonbiologic oral therapies used in the treatment of psoriasis include methotrexate, apremilast, cyclosporine, acitretin, and dimethyl fumarate. Biologics used in the treatment of psoriasis include TNF blocking agents, ustekinumab, secukinumab, ixekizumab, brodalumab, guselkumab, tildrakizumab, and risankizumab.

The IL-12/IL-23 inhibitor, ustekinumab, is recommended as monotherapy in adult patients with moderate-to-severe plaque psoriasis, including in patients with psoriasis affecting the palms and soles, nails, scalp, and patients with other subtypes of psoriasis (palmoplantar, pustular, or erythrodermic). However, the guideline notes there is limited evidence for its use in inverse and guttate psoriasis. Ustekinumab is recommended for psoriasis of all severity when associated with psoriatic arthritis. Ustekinumab can be used in combination with several agents to treat moderate-to-severe plaque psoriasis in adults, including topical products (i.e., high-potency corticosteroids) with or without a vitamin D analogue, acitretin, methotrexate, apremilast, cyclosporine, and narrowband ultraviolet phototherapy.

In pediatric patients, ustekinumab is recommended based on good-quality evidence in patients ≥12 years of age with moderate-to-severe plaque psoriasis. The guideline states that based on consensus, opinion, case studies, or disease-oriented evidence, ustekinumab can also be used in pediatric patients <12 years of age. Ustekinumab can be used in combination with topical steroids, with or without a vitamin D analogue in pediatric patients.

Recommendations for the use and selection of psoriasis therapies vary based on patient age, disease characteristics (e.g., severity, location, presence of psoriatic arthritis), and comorbidities (e.g., inflammatory bowel disease). Consult the American Academy of Dermatology/National Psoriasis Foundation guidelines for additional details.

● Psoriatic Arthritis

Ustekinumab and its biosimilar (ustekinumab-auub) are used for the management of active psoriatic arthritis in adults and pediatric patients ≥6 years of age. Safety and efficacy of ustekinumab for this use is based principally on the results of 2 randomized controlled trials. Guidelines generally support the use of ustekinumab for psoriatic arthritis, although other agents such as a TNF blocking agent, oral small molecule (OSM), or IL-17 inhibitor are typically preferred.

Clinical Experience

Ustekinumab has been evaluated for the management of active psoriatic arthritis (5 or more swollen joints and 5 or more tender joints) in 2 randomized, double-blind, placebo-controlled studies (PSUMMIT 1 and PSUMMIT 2) in 927 adults who had an inadequate response to therapy with disease-modifying antirheumatic drugs (DMARDs) or nonsteroidal anti-inflammatory agents (NSAIAs). The studies included patients with any of the following forms of the disease: polyarticular arthritis without rheumatoid nodules, spondylitis with peripheral arthritis, asymmetric peripheral arthritis, distal interphalangeal joint arthritis, or arthritis mutilans. Patients in these studies were required to have had active psoriatic arthritis for at least 6 months. Enthesitis or dactylitis was present at baseline in more than 70 or 40%, respectively, of patients. Patients were randomized to receive ustekinumab 45 or 90 mg or placebo at weeks 0 and 4 and then every 12 weeks thereafter. At week 16, patients with less than 5% improvement from baseline in the number of both tender and swollen joints entered early escape in which their assigned treatment was adjusted in a blinded manner; among patients meeting the early escape criteria, those receiving placebo began receiving ustekinumab 45 mg, those receiving ustekinumab 45 mg began receiving ustekinumab 90 mg, and those receiving ustekinumab 90 mg continued receiving this dosage. At 24 weeks, all patients still receiving placebo began receiving ustekinumab 45 mg. Patients receiving stable dosages of methotrexate (25 mg/week or less), oral corticosteroids (equivalent to 10 mg or less of prednisone daily), or NSAIAs could continue receiving these agents during the studies. In PSUMMIT 1, 80% of patients had received prior DMARD therapy; prior treatment with TNF blocking agents was not allowed. In PSUMMIT 2, 86% of patients had received prior treatment with DMARDs, including one or more TNF blocking agents in 58% of patients; more than 70% of these patients had discontinued treatment with TNF blocking agents because of inadequate efficacy or intolerance. About 50% of patients received stable dosages of methotrexate during the 2 studies.

The primary outcome measure was the proportion of patients achieving an American College of Rheumatology (ACR) 20 response at week 24. An ACR 20 response is achieved if the patient experiences a 20% or greater improvement in tender and swollen joint count and a 20% or greater improvement in at least 3 of the following criteria: patient pain assessment, patient global assessment, physician global assessment, patient self-assessed disability, or laboratory measures of disease activity (e.g., C-reactive protein [CRP] level). ACR 50 responses are defined using the same criteria with a level of improvement of 50%. Physical function was assessed using the disability index of the Health Assessment Questionnaire (HAQ-DI). Structural damage in the hands and feet was assessed radiographically by the change from baseline in the van der Heijde-Sharp score modified for assessment of psoriatic arthritis.

In both studies, a greater proportion of patients who received ustekinumab 45 or 90 mg achieved an ACR 20 response compared with patients who received placebo. ACR 20 responses were achieved at 24 weeks by 50 or 44% of patients receiving ustekinumab 90 mg, 42 or 44% of those receiving ustekinumab 45 mg, and 23 or 20% of those receiving placebo in PSUMMIT 1 and PSUMMIT 2, respectively. ACR 20 response was maintained through week 52. ACR 50 responses were achieved at 24 weeks by 28 or 23% of patients receiving ustekinumab 90 mg, 25 or 17% of those receiving ustekinumab 45 mg, and 9 or 7% of those receiving placebo in PSUMMIT 1 and PSUMMIT 2, respectively. In both studies, treatment with ustekinumab 45 or 90 mg was associated with greater improvement from baseline to week 24 in HAQ-DI score compared with placebo; improvements were maintained through week 52. In addition, ustekinumab was associated with greater improvement in enthesitis and dactylitis compared with placebo.

ACR responses were observed regardless of prior therapy with TNF blocking agents, although response rates tended to be lower among those who had received prior TNF blocking therapy. Among patients in PSUMMIT 2 who had received prior therapy with one or more TNF blocking agents, ACR 20 response was achieved at 24 weeks by 34, 37, or 14% of those receiving ustekinumab 90 mg, ustekinumab 45 mg, or placebo, respectively; among those who had not received prior therapy with TNF blocking agents, corresponding ACR 20 response rates were 55, 54, and 29%, respectively.

Analysis of combined radiographic data from the 2 studies indicated less progression of structural damage at 24 weeks in patients receiving ustekinumab 45 or 90 mg compared with those receiving placebo; continued inhibition of structural damage at week 52 was reported in patients receiving ustekinumab. The treatment effect observed in the combined data analysis was derived from PSUMMIT 1. Differences in treatment effect between the 2 studies may be related to the smaller size and the heterogeneity of the patient population in PSUMMIT 2 or the higher rate of missing data due to early treatment discontinuance in PSUMMIT 2, especially among placebo recipients who had received prior treatment with TNF blocking agents. Further study is needed to determine the effect of ustekinumab on progression of structural damage in patients with psoriatic arthritis who have received prior treatment with TNF blocking agents.

Use of ustekinumab in pediatric patients 6–17 years of age with psoriatic arthristis is supported by pharmacokinetic data from adults with psoriasis, adults and pediatric patients with psoriatic arthritis, and safety data from 2 clinical studies in 44 pediatric patients 6–11 years of age with psoriasis and 110 pediatric patients 12–17 years of age with psoriasis. The observed trough concentrations are generally comparable between adults with psoriasis, adults with psoriatic arthritis, and pediatric patients with psoriasis; drug exposure is also expected to be comparable between adults and pediatric patients with psoriatic arthritis.

Clinical Perspective

The American College of Rheumatology and the National Psoriasis Foundation issued a joint guideline for the treatment of psoriatic arthritis in 2018. Various drugs and drug classes are used to treat psoriatic arthritis, with some classes being used for symptom management (e.g., nonsteroidal anti-inflammatory agents [NSAIAs] and corticosteroids) and others being used as immunomodulatory disease-modifying therapy. Disease-modifying treatments for psoriatic arthritis include oral small molecules (OSMs; e.g., methotrexate, sulfasalazine, cyclosporine, leflunomide, apremilast), biologic DMARDs (e.g., TNF blocking agents, secukinumab, ixekizumab, ustekinumab, brodalumab, abatacept), and/or targeted synthetic DMARDs (e.g., tofacitinib). Specific agents for psoriatic arthritis treatment are selected according to disease characteristics, including disease severity, as well as patient preferences/values and comorbidities. A "treat-to-target" approach is typically employed, with the goal of achieving low/minimal disease activity or remission.

For patients with treatment-naive psoriatic arthritis, treatment with a TNF blocking agent, OSM, or IL-17 inhibitor (e.g., secukinumab, ixekizumab, brodalumab) is conditionally recommended over treatment with ustekinumab. For patients with active psoriatic arthritis despite treatment with an OSM, TNF blocking agents are conditionally recommended over ustekinumab, while use of ustekinumab is conditionally recommended over a different OSM, abatacept, or tofacitinib.

In patients with active psoriatic arthritis despite use of TNF blocking agent monotherapy, switching to a different TNF blocking agent is conditionally recommended over ustekinumab, while switching to ustekinumab is conditionally recommended over abatacept and tofacitinib. Ustekinumab monotherapy is recommended over combination treatment with methotrexate. Similarly, ustekinumab monotherapy is conditionally recommended over combination therapy with ustekinumab and methotrexate in patients with active psoriatic arthritis despite treatment with a TNF blocking agent and methotrexate.

In patients who have active psoriatic arthritis despite treatment with IL-17 inhibitor monotherapy, switching to ustekinumab is recommended over switching to a different IL-17 inhibitor or adding methotrexate. Switching to a TNF blocking agent is conditionally recommended over switching to ustekinumab.

Recommendations for the use and selection of disease-modifying therapies in psoriatic arthritis vary based on the presence of certain disease characteristics (e.g., psoriatic spondylitis/axial disease, enthesitis) and comorbidities (e.g., inflammatory bowel disease, diabetes). Consult the American College of Rheumatology/National Psoriasis Foundation guideline for additional details.

● Crohn Disease

Ustekinumab and ustekinumab-auub are used for the treatment of moderately to severely active Crohn disease in adults. The drug has been shown to induce and maintain clinical response and remission in patients with moderately to severely active Crohn disease. Safety and efficacy of ustekinumab for Crohn disease is based on the results of 3 randomized controlled trials. Guidelines generally recommend use of ustekinumab in patients with moderate-to-severe Crohn disease compared to no treatment or in those who have failed previous treatments.

Clinical Experience

Ustekinumab has been evaluated in 3 phase 3, double-blind, placebo-controlled clinical studies, including two 8-week randomized induction studies followed by a 44-week randomized-withdrawal maintenance study in adults with moderately to severely active Crohn's disease. One induction study (UNITI-1) included 741 patients who had not responded to or had not tolerated therapy with one or more TNF blocking agents, while the other induction study (UNITI-2) included 627 patients who had not tolerated or had not responded to corticosteroid or immunomodulator (azathioprine, mercaptopurine, or methotrexate) therapy but had no history of treatment failure with TNF blocking agents. Patients in these studies were randomized to receive ustekinumab (single IV dose of either 130 mg or approximately 6 mg/kg) or placebo. Patients who had a clinical response 8 weeks following ustekinumab induction (either dose) were then entered into the maintenance study (IM-UNITI); a total of 388 patients were randomized to receive maintenance therapy with subcutaneous ustekinumab (90 mg every 8 or 12 weeks) or placebo. Patients who did not achieve a clinical response were eligible to receive a 90-mg dose at the start of the maintenance trial but were not included in the primary efficacy analysis of the maintenance trial.

In UNITI-1, 29% of patients had a history of inadequate initial response to one or more TNF blocking agents, 69% responded but subsequently lost response, and 36% had not tolerated these agents; 52% had a history of intolerance or nonresponse to 2 or 3 TNF blocking agents. In UNITI-2, 81, 68, or 49% of patients had not responded to or had not tolerated prior therapy with corticosteroids, at least one immunomodulator (azathioprine, mercaptopurine, or methotrexate), or an agent from both drug classes, respectively; 69% had never received a TNF blocking agent. Patients were allowed to continue receiving stable dosages of aminosalicylates and immunomodulators throughout the studies; oral corticosteroids were maintained at a stable dosage during the induction studies but were tapered at the start of the maintenance study.

In these induction and maintenance studies, disease assessment was based on the Crohn's Disease Activity Index (CDAI; score range of 0–600, with higher scores indicating more severe disease). Clinical remission was defined as a CDAI score of less than 150; clinical response was defined as an absolute CDAI score of less than 150 or a reduction of at least 100 points from baseline. Mean baseline CDAI scores ranged from 319–327 in UNITI-1 and 302–304 in UNITI-2.

In these studies, ustekinumab was more effective than placebo in inducing and maintaining clinical response and remission (see Table 2 and Table 3). Clinical response and remission were observed as early as week 3 in patients receiving ustekinumab induction. Among patients who did not achieve a clinical response to the induction dose and received a 90-mg subcutaneous dose of the drug at the start of the maintenance study, 47% achieved a clinical response 8 weeks later. Clinical response and remission rates tended to be higher following an induction dose of 6 mg/kg rather than 130 mg. In addition, administration of maintenance doses every 8 weeks rather than every 12 weeks appeared to provide greater clinical benefit.

TABLE 2. Proportion of Patients with Crohn's Disease Responding to Induction Therapy

Response Measure	Ustekinumab (6-mg/kg dose) vs Placebo in UNITI-1	Ustekinumab (6-mg/kg dose) vs Placebo in UNITI-2
Clinical response, week 6	34 vs 21%	56 vs 29%
Clinical remission, week 8	21 vs 7%	40 vs 20%
Clinical response, week 8	38 vs 20%	58 vs 32%
CDAI 70-point reduction, week 6	44 vs 30%	65 vs 39%
CDAI 70-point reduction, week 3	41 vs 27%	51 vs 32%

TABLE 3. Proportion of Patients with Crohn's Disease Responding at Week 44 of Maintenance Therapy

Response Measure	Ustekinumab (90 mg every 8 weeks)	Placebo
Clinical remission	53%	36%
Clinical response	59%	44%
Corticosteroid-free clinical remission	47%	30%
Clinical remission at week 44 in those in remission at start of maintenance therapy	67%	46%

Induction therapy with ustekinumab was more effective than placebo in both the UNITI-1 and UNITI-2 study populations, although the proportion of patients achieving each efficacy end point tended to be higher in UNITI-2 (i.e., patients with a history of failed therapy with conventional agents but not with TNF blocking agents). At weeks 0 and 44 of the maintenance study, remission rates in the subgroup of patients enrolled from UNITI-1 were 61 and 41%, respectively, in those receiving ustekinumab every 8 weeks and 44 and 26%, respectively, in those receiving placebo. In the subgroup of patients enrolled from UNITI-2, the respective remission rates were 64 and 63% for those receiving ustekinumab every 8 weeks and 71 and 44% for those receiving placebo.

Results of a long-term extension of IM-UNITI indicated that clinical response and remission generally were maintained up to 92 weeks of ustekinumab maintenance therapy. Among patients who initially responded to ustekinumab induction therapy, clinical response and remission generally were maintained up to 152 weeks.

Clinical Perspective

The American College of Gastroenterology (ACG) and the American Gastroenterological Association (AGA) have issued guidelines for the medical treatment of Crohn disease. The ACG guideline was issued in 2018, while the AGA issued a guideline on the management of moderate to severe disease in 2021 and a guideline on management after surgical resection in 2017. Medical treatment of Crohn disease is typically divided into 2 phases: induction therapy (where control of inflammation is rapidly achieved) and maintenance therapy (where control of inflammation is sustained for a prolonged period of time). Specific treatments for Crohn disease are selected according to the patient's risk profile and disease severity. Drug classes used to treat Crohn disease include 5-aminosalicylates, antibiotics, corticosteroids, immunomodulators (e.g., thiopurines, methotrexate), and biologic agents including TNF blocking agents, ustekinumab, vedolizumab, and natalizumab.

The ACG states that ustekinumab is recommended for patients with moderate-to-severe Crohn disease who have failed prior therapy with corticosteroids, thiopurines, methotrexate, or TNF blocking agents with no previous exposure to TNF blocking agents. In addition, ustekinumab should be used to maintain remission in patients with a response to the drug. The AGA recommends use of ustekinumab over no therapy for induction and maintenance of remission of moderate-to-severe Crohn disease. It also recommends use of infliximab, adalimumab, or ustekinumab over certolizumab for induction of remission in patients who are naïve to biologic agents. Ustekinumab is also recommended for patients who have never responded to TNF blocking agents and for those who have previously responded to infliximab.

Patients with Crohn disease and perianal fistulas should be considered for ustekinumab therapy; however, recommended agent selection may vary in guidelines.

● Ulcerative Colitis

Ustekinumab and ustekinumab-auub are used for the treatment of moderately to severely active ulcerative colitis in adults. The drug has been shown to induce and maintain clinical remission in patients with moderately to severely active ulcerative colitis. Safety and efficacy of the drug for this indication are based primarily on results from a randomized controlled trial. Guidelines generally recommend ustekinumab for adult outpatients with moderate to severe ulcerative colitis.

Clinical Experience

Ustekinumab has been evaluated in a phase 3, double-blind, placebo-controlled clinical study (UNIFI) that included an 8-week randomized induction phase followed by a 44-week randomized-withdrawal maintenance phase in adults with moderately to severely active ulcerative colitis who had not responded to or had not tolerated therapy with biologic agents (i.e., TNF blocking agent and/or vedolizumab), corticosteroids, and/or mercaptopurine or azathioprine. Most patients had moderate disease at baseline (mean Mayo score of 8.9). A total of 961 patients were randomized to receive induction therapy with ustekinumab (single IV dose of either 130 mg or approximately 6 mg/kg) or placebo; 523 patients who had a clinical response 8 weeks following ustekinumab induction therapy (either dose) were then randomized to receive maintenance therapy with subcutaneous ustekinumab (90 mg every 8 or 12 weeks) or placebo. Patients who did not achieve a clinical response were eligible to receive a 90-mg dose at week 8 but were not included in the primary efficacy analysis in the maintenance phase.

In 51% of patients, prior therapy with one or more biologic agents had failed, and both a TNF blocking agent and vedolizumab had failed in 17% of patients; 46% of patients had a history of corticosteroid or immunomodulator (azathioprine, mercaptopurine, or methotrexate) failure but had not received a biologic agent. Patients were allowed to continue receiving stable dosages of aminosalicylates and immunomodulators throughout the study; oral corticosteroids were maintained at a stable dosage during the induction phase but were tapered at the start of the maintenance phase.

In this study, ustekinumab was more effective than placebo in inducing and maintaining clinical remission and achieving other secondary end points (see

Table 4 and Table 5). Decreases in rectal bleeding and stool frequency occurred as early as week 2 in patients receiving ustekinumab induction. Among patients who did not achieve a clinical response to the 6-mg/kg IV induction dose and received a 90-mg subcutaneous dose of the drug at week 8, 54% achieved a clinical response at week 16. Ustekinumab was effective in patients who had not received prior biologic therapy as well as in those with a history of biologic treatment failure, although the proportion of patients achieving each efficacy end point tended to be lower for those with a history of biologic treatment failure. The clinical response rate appeared to be higher following an induction dose of 6 mg/kg rather than 130 mg. In addition, administration of maintenance doses every 8 weeks rather than every 12 weeks appeared to provide greater clinical benefit on more objective and stringent end points (e.g., endoscopic improvement, combined histologic and endoscopic mucosal improvement, corticosteroid-free remission, discontinuance of corticosteroids at least 90 days prior to the end of the maintenance phase). The relationship between combined histologic and endoscopic mucosal improvement at the end of the induction and maintenance phases and disease progression or long-term outcomes was not assessed.

TABLE 4. Proportion of Patients with Ulcerative Colitis Responding to Induction Therapy at Week 8

Response Measure	Ustekinumab (6-mg/kg dose)	Placebo
Clinical remission	19%	7%
Endoscopic improvement	25%	13%
Clinical response	58%	31%
Histologic and endoscopic mucosal improvement	17%	8%
Endoscopic normalization	8%	4%

TABLE 5. Proportion of Patients with Ulcerative Colitis Responding at Week 44 of Maintenance Therapy

Response Measure	Ustekinumab (90 mg every 8 weeks)	Placebo
Clinical remission	45%	26%
Corticosteroid-free clinical remission	43%	26%
Maintenance of clinical remission at week 44 in those who achieved clinical remission 8 weeks after induction	66%	36%
Maintenance of clinical response through week 44	74%	48%
Endoscopic improvement	47%	27%
Histologic and endoscopic mucosal improvement	44%	23%
Endoscopic normalization	29%	18%

In this study, disease assessment was based on the Mayo scale, which includes 4 subscales (i.e., stool frequency, rectal bleeding, findings on endoscopy, physician global assessment), each scored from 0–3 (normal to most severe, respectively). Clinical remission and response rates in Table 4 and Table 5 reflect the FDA definitions for remission (score of 0 or 1 on the stool frequency subscale, 0 on the rectal bleeding subscale, and 0 or 1 on the endoscopy subscale [modified so that 1 does not include friability]) and response (decrease from baseline in the Mayo score [modified to exclude the physician global assessment subscale] of at least 2 points and at least 30%, with a reduction in rectal bleeding subscore of at least 1 point or an absolute rectal bleeding subscore of 0 or 1). Endoscopic

improvement was defined as an endoscopy subscore of 0 or 1 (modified so that 1 does not include friability), and histologic improvement of colon tissue was defined as neutrophil infiltration in less than 5% of crypts, no crypt destruction, and no erosions, ulcerations, or granulation tissue.

Results of a long-term extension of UNIFI indicated that clinical response and symptomatic remission generally were maintained through up to 92 weeks of ustekinumab therapy.

Clinical Perspective

The American College of Gastroenterology (ACG) and the American Gastroenterological Association (AGA) issued guidelines for the medical treatment of ulcerative colitis in adults in 2019 and 2020, respectively. Goals of therapy in ulcerative colitis include achieving and maintaining corticosteroid-free remission and promoting mucosal healing. Specific treatments for ulcerative colitis are selected according to the disease severity, as well as disease location/extent, disease prognosis, and previous therapies used. Drug classes used to treat ulcerative colitis include oral and rectal 5-aminosalicylates, oral and rectal corticosteroids, immunomodulators (e.g., thiopurines, methotrexate), tofacitinib, and biologic agents including TNF blocking agents, vedolizumab, and ustekinumab. In most cases, if a drug used for induction therapy is effective, it is continued as maintenance of remission. The AGA includes ustekinumab in its guideline, but the ACG does not include ustekinumab in its recommendations.

For adult outpatients with moderate to severe ulcerative colitis, the AGA strongly recommends TNF blocking therapies, vedolizumab, tofacitinib, or ustekinumab over no treatment. Ustekinumab or tofacitinib is conditionally recommended over vedolizumab or adalimumab for induction of remission in patients previously exposed to infliximab with a primary nonresponse. Biologic agents (TNF blocking agents, vedolizumab, or ustekinumab) or tofacitinib are conditionally recommended over thiopurine monotherapy for induction of remission; combination therapy with a thiopurine or methotrexate is conditionally recommended over biologic monotherapy.

DOSAGE AND ADMINISTRATION

● General

Pretreatment Screening

- Consider potential risks and benefits of the drug prior to initiating therapy in patients with chronic infection or history of recurrent infection. Do not administer in patients with a clinically important active infection until the infection resolves or is appropriately treated.

- Evaluate for active or inactive tuberculosis prior to initiation of ustekinumab therapy. Do not administer to patients with active tuberculosis.

- Administer all age-appropriate vaccines prior to starting ustekinumab therapy. Do not administer live vaccines during ustekinumab therapy. Do not administer BCG vaccine during ustekinumab therapy or for 1 year before or after ustekinumab therapy.

Patient Monitoring

- Monitor for signs and symptoms of infection or active tuberculosis during and after treatment.

- Monitor patients for signs and symptoms of nonmelanoma skin cancer, particularly those >60 years of age, those with a history of prolonged immunosuppressive therapy, and those with a history of psoralen and UVA radiation (PUVA).

- Monitor all patients for signs and symptoms of posterior reversible encephalopathy syndrome (PRES), a neurologic disorder characterized by headaches, seizures, confusion, visual disturbances, and imaging changes.

Premedication and Prophylaxis

- Administer an appropriate antimycobacterial regimen for the treatment of latent tuberculosis if indicated prior to initiating ustekinumab therapy.

● Administration

Administer ustekinumab products by subcutaneous injection or IV infusion depending on indication for use.

Ustekinumab products are intended for use under the supervision of a clinician, but may be *self-administered* if the clinician determines that the patient and/or their caregiver is competent to prepare and safely administer the drug by subcutaneous injection after appropriate training. When the drug is used in pediatric patients, the manufacturer recommends that subcutaneous doses be administered by a clinician. IV infusions of ustekinumab products must be administered by a clinician. Ustekinumab products should only be administered to patients who will be closely monitored and have regular follow-up visits with a clinician.

Subcutaneous Administration

For subcutaneous administration, ustekinumab products are commercially available as a 90-mg/mL solution in 0.5- or 1-mL prefilled syringes and 0.5-mL single-dose vials. The solution is colorless to light yellow and may contain a few small translucent or white particles. Store ustekinumab vials and prefilled syringes at 2–8°C in the original carton to protect the solution from light until administration. Ustekinumab injection should not be frozen or shaken. The individual pre-filled syringes may be stored at room temperature (up to 30°C) for one single period that does not exceed 30 days or more. Do not return the syringe to the refrigerator following storage at room temperature. If the drug has not been used within 30 days, discard the syringe. Discard any unused portion remaining in the vial or syringe since the drug contains no preservative.

The manufacturers recommend that each subcutaneous injection be administered at a different anatomic site (such as upper arms, gluteal regions, thighs, or any quadrant of the abdomen) than the previous injection, and not into areas where the skin is tender, bruised, erythematous, or indurated. Prior to administration, visually inspect the commercially available ustekinumab injection for particular matter and discoloration; if either is present, discard the solution. The manufacturer recommends use of a 1-mL syringe with a 27-gauge, ½-inch needle to administer ustekinumab supplied in single-dose vials.

IV Administration

For IV infusion, ustekinumab products are commercially available as a 5-mg/mL injection concentrate in 26-mL (130-mg) single-dose vials. The vials should be stored at 2–8°C in the original carton for protection from light. Ustekinumab injection concentrate should not be frozen or shaken. Any unused portions should be discarded since the injection concentrate contains no preservative.

Prior to IV administration, dilute the appropriate volume of ustekinumab injection concentrate in 0.9% sodium chloride injection to provide a total volume of 250 mL (i.e., remove a volume of diluent equal to the total required volume of ustekinumab injection from a 250-mL infusion bag prior to addition of the drug). A 250 mL infusion bag of 0.45% sodium chloride may be used as an alternative. Gently mix the diluted solution. Inspect the diluted solution visually for particulate matter and discoloration prior to administration and do not use if opaque particles, discoloration, or foreign particles are observed. The diluted solution may be stored for up to 7 hours at room temperature (up to 25°C) prior to administration. Complete administration of the infusion within 8 hours of dilution in the infusion bag.

Diluted ustekinumab solutions should be infused IV over at least 1 hour using an inline, nonpyrogenic, low-protein-binding 0.2-μm filter. Do not infuse ustekinumab simultaneously through the same IV line with any other drug.

● Dosage

The patient's current weight at the time of dosing should be used to determine the appropriate weight-based dose of ustekinumab.

Adult Dosage

Plaque Psoriasis

For the management of moderate to severe plaque psoriasis, the recommended dose of ustekinumab or its biosimilar (ustekinumab-auub) in adults weighing 100 kg or less is 45 mg by subcutaneous injection at weeks 0 and 4, then every 12 weeks thereafter. The recommended dose of ustekinumab or its biosimilar in adults weighing more than 100 kg is 90 mg by subcutaneous injection at weeks 0 and 4, then every 12 weeks thereafter. In patients weighing more than 100 kg, 45-mg doses were effective in clinical studies, but not as effective as 90-mg doses.

Psoriatic Arthritis

For the management of active psoriatic arthritis, the recommended dose of ustekinumab or its biosimilar (ustekinumab-auub) in adults is 45 mg by subcutaneous injection at weeks 0 and 4, then every 12 weeks thereafter. The recommended dose of ustekinumab products in patients with coexisting moderate-to-severe plaque psoriasis who weigh more than 100 kg is 90 mg by subcutaneous injection at 0 and 4 weeks, followed by 90 mg by subcutaneous injection every 12 weeks.

Crohn Disease or Ulcerative Colitis

For the management of moderately to severely active Crohn disease or ulcerative colitis in adults, the recommended induction dose of ustekinumab or its biosimilar (ustekinumab-auub) is a single IV infusion of 260 mg in patients weighing ≤55 kg, 390 mg in those weighing >55 to 85 kg, and 520 mg in those weighing >85 kg. The recommended maintenance dose of ustekinumab products is 90 mg administered by subcutaneous injection every 8 weeks; maintenance therapy should be initiated 8 weeks after the initial IV induction dose.

Pediatric Dosage

Plaque Psoriasis

For the management of moderate to severe plaque psoriasis in pediatric patients 6–17 years of age, the recommended weight-based dose of ustekinumab or its biosimilar (ustekinumab-auub) is 0.75 mg/kg in those weighing <60 kg, 45 mg in those weighing 60–100 kg, or 90 mg in those weighing >100 kg); the dose should be administered by subcutaneous injection at weeks 0 and 4, and every 12 weeks thereafter.

For pediatric patients weighing <60 kg, see the prescribing information for recommended injection volumes for the recommended dose (0.75 mg/kg).

Psoriatic Arthritis

For the management of active psoriatic arthritis in pediatric patients 6–17 years of age, the recommended weight-based dose of ustekinumab or its biosimilar (ustekinumab-auub) is 0.75 mg/kg in those weighing <60 kg, 45 mg in those weighing ≥60 kg, or 90 mg in those weighing >100 kg with co-existing moderate-to-severe plaque psoriasis; the dose should be administered by subcutaneous injection at weeks 0 and 4, and every 12 weeks thereafter.

For pediatric patients weighing <60 kg, see the prescribing information for recommended injection volumes for the recommended dose (0.75 mg/kg).

● Special Populations

The manufacturer makes no specific dosage recommendations for geriatric patients or patients with hepatic or renal impairment.

CAUTIONS

● Contraindications

- History of clinically important hypersensitivity to the drug or any ingredient in the formulation.

● Warnings/Precautions

Infectious Complications

Risk of infection, including reactivation of latent infections, may be increased in patients receiving ustekinumab products. Serious bacterial, mycobacterial, fungal, and viral infections have been observed in patients receiving ustekinumab products. Serious or clinically important infections (e.g., requiring hospitalization) including cellulitis, diverticulitis, osteomyelitis, viral infections, gastroenteritis, appendicitis, cholecystitis, sepsis, pneumonia, and urinary tract infections occurred during clinical studies in patients with psoriasis. In clinical studies in patients with psoriatic arthritis, serious or clinically important infections included cholecystitis. Anal abscess, gastroenteritis, ophthalmic herpes zoster, pneumonia, listeriosis, and listeria meningitis have been reported in clinical studies in patients with Crohn disease or ulcerative colitis.

In placebo-controlled portions of clinical studies in patients with psoriasis (mean follow-up of approximately 13 weeks), infections and serious infections occurred in 27 and 0.3%, respectively, of patients receiving ustekinumab, compared with 24 and 0.4%, respectively, of those receiving placebo. In the controlled and uncontrolled portions of clinical studies in patients with psoriasis (median follow-up of 3.2 years), infections and serious infections were reported in 72.3 and 2.8%, respectively, of patients receiving ustekinumab.

Individuals genetically deficient in interleukin-12 (IL-12)/interleukin-23 (IL-23) are particularly vulnerable to disseminated infections caused by mycobacteria (including nontuberculous environmental mycobacteria), salmonella (including nontyphi strains), and BCG vaccine; serious, sometimes fatal, infections have been reported in such individuals. It is not known whether patients with ustekinumab-induced blockade of IL-12/IL-23 may be susceptible to these types of infections. Consider appropriate diagnostic testing for these infections (e.g., tissue culture, stool culture) as dictated by clinical circumstances.

Do not initiate ustekinumab products in patients with any clinically important active infection until the infection resolves or is adequately treated. If a serious or clinically important infection develops, consider discontinuing ustekinumab until the infection resolves or is adequately treated. Consider potential risks and benefits of the drug prior to initiating therapy in patients with a chronic infection or a history of recurrent infection.

Evaluate patients for active or latent tuberculosis prior to initiation of ustekinumab therapy. Do not administer ustekinumab products to patients with active tuberculosis. When indicated, an appropriate antimycobacterial regimen for the treatment of latent tuberculosis should be initiated prior to ustekinumab therapy. Consider antimycobacterial therapy prior to initiation of ustekinumab products in individuals with a history of latent or active tuberculosis in whom an adequate course of antimycobacterial treatment for these indications cannot be confirmed. Closely monitor patients receiving ustekinumab products for signs and symptoms of active tuberculosis during and after treatment.

Malignancies

Ustekinumab products are immunosuppressants and may increase the risk of malignancy. Malignancies have been reported in patients who received the drug in clinical studies.

In the controlled and uncontrolled portions of clinical studies evaluating ustekinumab in patients with psoriasis (median follow-up of 3.2 years), nonmelanoma skin cancer or other malignancies were reported in 1.5 or 1.7%, respectively, of patients receiving the drug. The most frequently observed malignancies other than nonmelanoma skin cancer included prostate cancer, melanoma, colorectal cancer, and breast cancer. The incidence of malignancies other than nonmelanoma skin cancer in ustekinumab-treated patients with psoriasis was similar to the expected incidence in the general US population.

In clinical studies of up to one year's duration in patients with Crohn disease, nonmelanoma skin cancer or other malignancies were each reported in 0.2% of patients receiving the drug and in 0.2 or 0%, respectively, of those receiving placebo. In clinical studies of up to one year's duration in patients with ulcerative colitis, nonmelanoma skin cancer or other malignancies were reported in 0.4 or 0.5%, respectively, of patients receiving ustekinumab and in 0 or 0.2%, respectively, of those receiving placebo.

In animals, inhibition of the p40 subunit of IL-12/IL-23 increased the risk of malignancy. Ultraviolet (UV) radiation-induced skin cancers developed earlier and more frequently in mice genetically manipulated to be deficient in both IL-12 and IL-23 or IL-12 alone. The relevance of these experimental data to risk of malignancy in humans is unknown.

The rapid appearance of multiple cutaneous squamous cell carcinomas has been reported in ustekinumab-treated patients with preexisting risk factors for nonmelanoma skin cancer. All patients receiving ustekinumab products should be monitored for the appearance of nonmelanoma skin cancer. Monitor patients >60 years of age, those with a history of prolonged immunosuppressive therapy, and those with a history of psoralen and UVA radiation (PUVA) closely.

The safety of ustekinumab products has not been evaluated in patients with a history of malignancy or a known malignancy.

Sensitivity Reactions

Hypersensitivity Reactions

Hypersensitivity reactions, including anaphylaxis, angioedema, rash, and urticaria, have been reported in patients receiving ustekinumab products. If an anaphylactic or other clinically important hypersensitivity reaction occurs, discontinue ustekinumab and initiate appropriate therapy.

Latex Sensitivity

The needle cover of the Stelara® prefilled syringe contains dry natural rubber and should not be handled by individuals sensitive to latex. The Wezlana® prefilled syringe does not contain dry natural rubber.

Posterior Reversible Encephalopathy Syndrome

Posterior reversible encephalopathy syndrome (PRES), also known as reversible posterior leukoencephalopathy syndrome (RPLS), is a neurologic syndrome characterized by reversible vasogenic subcortical edema. PRES was reported in two patients in clinical trials. Cases have also been reported in postmarketing experience in patients with psoriasis, psoriatic arthritis, and Crohn disease. Patients experienced headaches, seizures, confusion, visual disturbances, and imaging changes. After starting ustekinumab, signs and symptoms typically occurred within a few days to several months, although some cases reported latency of a year or more. Patients recovered after stopping ustekinumab and receiving supportive care.

Monitor all patients for signs and symptoms of PRES. If PRES is suspected, discontinue ustekinumab and initiate appropriate treatment.

Immunization

Prior to initiation of ustekinumab therapy, patients should receive all age-appropriate vaccines as recommended by current immunization guidelines. Do not administer live vaccines to patients receiving ustekinumab. Do not administer BCG vaccine during ustekinumab therapy or for 1 year before or after ustekinumab therapy.

Noninfectious Pneumonia

Interstitial pneumonia, eosinophilic pneumonia, and cryptogenic organizing pneumonia have been reported during postmarketing experience in patients receiving ustekinumab products. Manifestations have included the onset of cough, dyspnea, and interstitial infiltrates following 1–3 doses of the drug; serious outcomes, including respiratory failure and prolonged hospitalization, have occurred. Patients have improved following discontinuance of ustekinumab therapy and, in some cases, administration of corticosteroids. If a diagnosis of interstitial pneumonia, eosinophilic pneumonia, or cryptogenic organizing pneumonia is confirmed, discontinue ustekinumab and initiate appropriate treatment.

Immunogenicity

Antibodies to ustekinumab have been detected, generally in low titers, in approximately 6–12.4% of patients with psoriasis or psoriatic arthritis receiving the drug. In patients with psoriasis, antibodies to ustekinumab were associated with reduced or undetectable serum ustekinumab concentrations and reduced efficacy. Neutralizing antibodies were detected in a majority of patients with psoriasis who tested positive for anti-ustekinumab antibodies. Antibodies to ustekinumab also have been detected in 2.9 or 4.6% of patients with Crohn disease or ulcerative colitis, respectively, receiving the drug for approximately one year. No apparent association between antibody development and injection site reactions has been observed.

Specific Populations

Pregnancy

Reproductive and developmental toxicity studies in monkeys at ustekinumab exposure levels of more than 100 times the human exposure at the maximum recommended subcutaneous dosage revealed no evidence of adverse developmental effects on fetuses or neonatal offspring. Limited data regarding use of ustekinumab products in pregnant women are insufficient to inform a drug-associated risk.

Lactation

It is not known whether ustekinumab is distributed into human milk or affects breast-fed infants or milk production. Ustekinumab is distributed into milk in lactating monkeys, and maternal immunoglobulin G (IgG) is distributed into human milk. If ustekinumab is distributed into human milk, the effects on the infant from local exposure in the GI tract are unknown. Systemic exposure to ustekinumab in breast-fed infants is expected to be low since the drug is a large molecule and is degraded in the GI tract. Consider the developmental and health benefits of breast-feeding along with the mother's clinical need for the ustekinumab product and any potential adverse effects on the breast-fed infant from the drug or underlying maternal condition.

Pediatric Use

Safety and efficacy of ustekinumab and its biosimilar (ustekinumab-auub) have been established in pediatric patients 6–17 years of age with moderate to severe plaque psoriasis. Use of ustekinumab in adolescent patients 12–17 years of age is based on evidence from a randomized clinical trial in this age group. Use of ustekinumab in pediatric patients 6–11 years of age with moderate to severe plaque psoriasis is based on evidence from an open-label, single-arm, efficacy, safety, and pharmacokinetics study. The safety profile of ustekinumab products in pediatric patients with psoriasis is similar to that in adults with psoriasis.

Safety and efficacy of ustekinumab and its biosimilar (ustekinumab-auub) have been established in pediatric patients 6–17 years of age with psoriatic arthritis. Use of ustekinumab in this age group is based on evidence from randomized clinical trials in adults with psoriasis and psoriatic arthritis, pharmacokinetic data from adults and pediatric patients with psoriasis, pharmacokinetic data from adults with psoriatic arthritis, and safety data from two clinical studies in 44 pediatric patients 6–11 years of age with psoriasis and 110 pediatric patients 12–17 years of age with psoriasis. The observed pre-dose (trough) concentrations are generally comparable between adult patients with psoriasis and psoriatic arthritis and pediatric patients with psoriasis, and the pharmacokinetic exposure is expected to be comparable between adult and pediatric patients with psoriatic arthritis.

Safety and efficacy of ustekinumab products have not been established in pediatric patients Crohn disease or ulcerative colitis or in pediatric patients <6 years of age with psoriasis or psoriatic arthritis.

Geriatric Use

In clinical trials evaluating ustekinumab in patients with psoriasis, psoriatic arthritis, Crohn disease, or ulcerative colitis, approximately 5.1% of patients receiving ustekinumab were ≥65 years of age and about 0.6% were ≥75 years of age. Although no differences in safety and efficacy relative to younger adults were observed, the number of patients ≥65 years of age is insufficient to determine whether they respond differently than younger adults.

About 5.5% of patients with psoriasis included in a population pharmacokinetic analysis of ustekinumab were ≥ 65 years of age; there were no apparent changes in pharmacokinetic parameters (clearance and volume of distribution) in those ≥65 years of age.

● Common Adverse Effects

Adverse effects reported in ≥3% of patients with psoriasis receiving ustekinumab products in clinical studies include nasopharyngitis, upper respiratory tract infection, headache, and fatigue. Adverse effects in patients with psoriatic arthritis are similar to those in patients with psoriasis.

Adverse effects reported in ≥3% of patients with Crohn disease receiving ustekinumab products in clinical studies include vomiting during induction therapy and nasopharyngitis, injection site erythema, vulvovaginal candidiasis/mycotic infection, bronchitis, pruritus, urinary tract infection, and sinusitis during maintenance therapy.

Adverse effects reported in ≥3% of patients with ulcerative colitis receiving ustekinumab products in clinical studies include nasopharyngitis during induction therapy and nasopharyngitis, headache, abdominal pain, influenza, fever, diarrhea, sinusitis, fatigue, and nausea during maintenance therapy.

DRUG INTERACTIONS

No formal drug interaction studies have been performed to date.

● Drugs Metabolized by Hepatic Microsomal Enzymes

Because increased levels of cytokines (e.g., interleukin-1 [IL-1], interleukin-6 [IL-6], interleukin-10 [IL-10], tumor necrosis factor [TNF; TNF-α], interferon [IFN]) during chronic inflammation may suppress the formation of cytochrome P-450 (CYP) isoenzymes, ustekinumab could normalize the formation of CYP

enzymes. Although IL-12 and/or IL-23 at concentrations of 10 ng/mL did not alter the activity of CYP isoenzymes 1A2, 2B6, 2C9, 2C19, 2D6, or 3A4 in human hepatocytes in vitro, the clinical relevance of these data has not been established. Following initiation of ustekinumab therapy in patients who are receiving concomitant therapy with drugs metabolized by CYP isoenzymes , particularly those with a narrow therapeutic index (e.g., cyclosporine, warfarin), monitoring for therapeutic effect and/or changes in serum drug concentrations should be considered, and the dosage of the drug adjusted as needed.

● Allergy Immunotherapy

Ustekinumab products have not been evaluated in patients who have undergone allergy immunotherapy. The drug may decrease the protective effect of allergy immunotherapy (i.e., decrease tolerance), which may increase the risk of an allergic reaction to a dose of allergen immunotherapy. Exercise caution in patients who are receiving or who have received allergy immunotherapy, particularly for anaphylaxis.

● Biologic Agents

Analysis of population pharmacokinetic data for patients with psoriatic arthritis indicated that prior use of TNF blocking agents does not alter clearance of ustekinumab.

● Corticosteroids

Ustekinumab products have been used concomitantly with corticosteroids in patients with psoriatic arthritis; analysis of population pharmacokinetic data indicated that concomitant use of corticosteroids does not alter clearance of ustekinumab.

In clinical studies of ustekinumab induction therapy in patients with Crohn's disease or ulcerative colitis, corticosteroids were used concomitantly in approximately 40–50% of patients and did not appear to affect the overall safety or efficacy of ustekinumab; analysis of population pharmacokinetic data indicated that concomitant use of corticosteroids does not alter clearance or serum concentrations of ustekinumab.

● Immunosuppressive or Immunomodulatory Agents

The safety of ustekinumab products in combination with other immunosuppressive agents in patients with psoriasis has not been established.

Ustekinumab products have been used concomitantly with methotrexate in patients with psoriatic arthritis. Concomitant use of methotrexate in patients with psoriatic arthritis does not appear to alter the safety or efficacy of ustekinumab. Analysis of population pharmacokinetic data indicated that concomitant use of methotrexate does not alter clearance of ustekinumab.

In clinical studies of ustekinumab induction therapy in patients with Crohn disease or ulcerative colitis, immunomodulators (azathioprine, mercaptopurine, or methotrexate) were used concomitantly in approximately 30% of patients and did not appear to affect the overall safety or efficacy of ustekinumab; analysis of population pharmacokinetic data indicated that concomitant use of these agents does not alter clearance or serum concentrations of ustekinumab.

● Nonsteroidal Anti-inflammatory Agents

Ustekinumab products have been used concomitantly with nonsteroidal anti-inflammatory agents (NSAIAs) in patients with psoriatic arthritis; analysis of population pharmacokinetic data indicated that concomitant use of NSAIAs does not alter clearance of ustekinumab.

● Phototherapy

The safety of ustekinumab products in combination with phototherapy in patients with psoriasis has not been established. Ultraviolet (UV) radiation-induced skin cancers developed earlier and more frequently in mice genetically manipulated to be deficient in both IL-12 and IL-23 or IL-12 alone.

● Vaccines

Live vaccines should not be administered to patients receiving ustekinumab products. Patients receiving ustekinumab products should not be given live vaccines. BCG vaccine should not be administered during therapy with the drug for one year before or after ustekinumab therapy. Caution is advised when administering live vaccines to household contacts of patients receiving ustekinumab because of the potential risk for shedding the vaccine organism from the household contact and transmission to the patient.

Inactivated vaccines administered during a course of ustekinumab therapy may not elicit an immune response sufficient to prevent disease.

DESCRIPTION

Ustekinumab and its biosimilar are human monoclonal antibodies directed against the p40 subunit of interleukin-12 (IL-12) and interleukin-23 (IL-23) are immunosuppressive agents. Ustekinumab products are produced in a murine cell line using recombinant DNA technology.

Ustekinumab and its biosimilar are immunoglobulin G₁ kappa (IgG₁) monoclonal antibodies that bind with high affinity and specificity to the p40 subunit of both IL-12 and IL-23. IL-12 and IL-23 are naturally occurring cytokines that are involved in inflammatory and immune responses, such as natural killer cell activation and CD4⁺ T-cell differentiation and activation. IL-12 and IL-23 contribute to the chronic inflammation associated with Crohn's disease and ulcerative colitis; in animal models of colitis, genetic absence or antibody blockade of the p40 subunit of IL-12 and IL-23 was shown to be protective. Studies using in vitro models indicate that ustekinumab disrupts IL-12- and IL-23-mediated signaling and cytokine cascades by disrupting the interaction of these cytokines with a shared cell-surface receptor chain, IL-12 β1.

The metabolic pathway of ustekinumab products has not been characterized. As a human IgG₁ kappa monoclonal antibody, the drug is expected to be degraded into small peptides and amino acids via catabolic pathways in the same manner as endogenous IgG. Across all psoriasis studies, the mean half-life of ustekinumab following subcutaneous administration was 14.9–45.6 days. The estimated median terminal half-life of ustekinumab in patients with Crohn's disease or ulcerative colitis is approximately 19 days. Administration of 90-mg doses of ustekinumab products in patients with psoriasis or psoriatic arthritis who weigh more than 100 kg results in median trough serum concentrations of the drug that are comparable to those achieved following administration of 45-mg doses in patients weighing 100 kg or less.

ADVICE TO PATIENTS

- Instruct patients to read the manufacturer's patient information (medication guide) prior to initiation of therapy and each time the prescription is refilled.

- Instruct patient and/or caregiver regarding proper dosage and administration of ustekinumab products, including the use of aseptic technique, and proper disposal of needles and syringes if it is determined that the patient and/or caregiver is competent to safely administer the drug.

- Inform patients that ustekinumab products may lower the ability of their immune system to fight infections. Importance of contacting clinicians if any signs or symptoms of infection develop.

- Risk of malignancies while receiving ustekinumab products.

- Advise patients to discontinue use of ustekinumab products and seek immediate medical attention if they experience any symptoms of serious allergic reactions.

- Advise patients that the needle cover of the prefilled syringe Stelara® brand contains dry natural rubber, which may cause allergic reactions in individuals sensitive to latex. The prefilled syringe needle cover of Wezlana® brand does not contain dry natural rubber.

- Advise patients that ustekinumab products can interfere with the usual response to immunizations and that they should avoid receiving live vaccines during ustekinumab therapy.

- Advise patients to inform their clinicians of existing or contemplated concomitant therapy, including prescription and OTC drugs and dietary or herbal supplements (e.g., St. John's wort), as well as any concomitant illnesses.

- Advise women to inform their clinicians if they are or plan to become pregnant or plan to breast-feed.

- Inform patients of other important precautionary information.

PREPARATIONS

Excipients in commercially available drug preparations may have clinically important effects in some individuals; consult specific product labeling for details.

Ustekinumab

Parenteral

Injection concentrate, for IV infusion	5 mg/mL	Stelara®, Janssen Biotech
Injection, for subcutaneous use	45 mg/0.5 mL	Stelara® (available as single-use prefilled syringes and single-use vials), Janssen Biotech
	90 mg/mL	Stelara® (available as single-use prefilled syringes), Janssen Biotech

Ustekinumab-auub (biosimilar)

Parenteral

Injection concentrate, for IV infusion	5 mg/mL	Wezlana®, Amgen
Injection, for subcutaneous use	45 mg/0.5 mL	Wezlana® (available as single-use prefilled syringes and single-use vials), Amgen
	90 mg/mL	Wezlana® (available as single-use prefilled syringes), Amgen

† Use is not currently included in the labeling approved by the US Food and Drug Administration.

Selected Revisions May 10, 2024, © Copyright, July 29, 2011, American Society of Health-System Pharmacists, Inc.

Apremilast

90:24.24.92 · PDE4 INHIBITORS, MISCELLANEOUS

■ Apremilast, a selective phosphodiesterase type 4 (PDE4) inhibitor, is a disease-modifying antirheumatic drug (DMARD).

USES

● Psoriatic Arthritis

Apremilast is used for the management of active psoriatic arthritis in adults. The drug has been shown to reduce the signs and symptoms of active psoriatic arthritis and to improve physical function in patients with the disease.

Clinical Experience

Safety and efficacy of apremilast for this indication were evaluated in 3 randomized, double-blind, placebo-controlled studies (PALACE-1, PALACE-2, and PALACE-3) in 1493 adults with active psoriatic arthritis (as defined by the Classification Criteria for Psoriatic Arthritis [CASPAR], with 3 or more swollen joints and 3 or more tender joints) who had an inadequate response to therapy with biologic and/or nonbiologic disease-modifying antirheumatic drugs (DMARDs). Patients were required to have a diagnosis of psoriatic arthritis for at least 6 months and, in PALACE-3, to have plaque psoriasis with a qualifying skin lesion (diameter ≥2 cm). Patients were randomized to receive apremilast 20 or 30 mg twice daily (initiated at 10 mg daily and titrated to the assigned dosage) or placebo and were stratified by use of a DMARD at baseline. Patients receiving stable dosages of methotrexate (≤25 mg/week), leflunomide (<20 mg/day), sulfasalazine (<2 g/day), low-dose oral corticosteroids (equivalent to ≤10 mg of prednisone daily), and/or nonsteroidal anti-inflammatory agents (NSAIAs) could continue such agents during the studies. Prior DMARD therapy included only nonbiologic agents in 76% of patients; 22% of patients received prior therapy with biologic DMARDs. Patients who had experienced treatment failure following use of more than 3 biologic or nonbiologic DMARDs or more than 1 tumor necrosis factor (TNF; TNF-α) blocking agent were excluded, and no more than 10% of patients enrolled in the studies were permitted to have a history of TNF blocker failure. During the studies, 65% of patients received concomitant therapy with at least one DMARD (e.g., methotrexate, leflunomide, sulfasalazine); in addition, 14 or 71% of patients received stable dosages of low-dose oral corticosteroids or NSAIAs, respectively. The median duration of psoriatic arthritis was 5 years; most patients had either the symmetric polyarthritis (62%) or asymmetric oligoarthritis (27%) form of the disease.

The primary outcome measure in all 3 studies was the proportion of patients achieving an American College of Rheumatology (ACR) 20 response (modified for psoriatic arthritis) at week 16. An ACR 20 response was achieved if the patient experienced a 20% improvement in tender and swollen joint count and a 20% or greater improvement in at least 3 of the following criteria: patient pain assessment, patient global assessment, physician global assessment, patient self-assessed disability, or laboratory measures of disease activity (i.e., C-reactive protein [CRP] level). ACR 50 and 70 responses were also evaluated and were defined as a level of improvement of 50 or 70%, respectively. Physical function was assessed using the Health Assessment Questionnaire Disability Index (HAQ-DI).

In all 3 studies, a greater proportion of patients who received apremilast achieved an ACR 20 response at week 16 than those who received placebo. Among patients receiving apremilast 20 or 30 mg twice daily, ACR 20 response rates at week 16 were 30 or 38%, respectively, in PALACE-1; 37 or 32%, respectively, in PALACE-2; and 28 or 41%, respectively, in PALACE-3; in comparison, 18–19% of patients receiving placebo in the 3 studies attained ACR 20 responses at week 16. The response data indicated a small numerical advantage for the 30-mg dosage over the 20-mg dosage, but results of the 3 studies did not show a clear, consistent statistical or clinical advantage for the higher dosage.

ACR 50 and 70 responses at week 16 generally supported the primary efficacy results. ACR 50 response rates at week 16 for patients receiving apremilast 20 or 30 mg twice daily were 16 or 16%, respectively, in PALACE-1; 15 or 11%, respectively,

in PALACE-2; and 12 or 15%, respectively, in PALACE-3; in comparison, 5–8% of patients receiving placebo in the 3 studies attained ACR 50 responses at week 16. ACR 70 response rates at week 16 for patients receiving apremilast 20 or 30 mg twice daily were 6 or 4%, respectively, in PALACE-1; 4 or 1%, respectively, in PALACE-2; and 5 or 4%, respectively, in PALACE-3; in comparison, 1–2% of patients receiving placebo in the 3 studies attained ACR 70 responses at week 16. Apremilast also improved dactylitis and enthesitis in patients with these manifestations of the disease.

Improvements in physical function (as measured by change in HAQ-DI score) from baseline to week 16 were greater in all 3 studies for patients receiving apremilast 30 mg twice daily compared with those receiving placebo and also were greater in 2 of the 3 studies (PALACE-1 and PALACE-2) for patients receiving apremilast 20 mg twice daily compared with those receiving placebo.

Results of these studies suggested a sustained ACR20 response up to 52 weeks with use of apremilast. A long-term extension study including patients in PALACE-1, PALACE-2, and PALACE-3 reported ACR20, ACR50, and ACR70 response rates of 67.2%, 44.4%, and 27.4% at week 260, respectively.

Clinical Perspective

The American College of Rheumatology (ACR) and the National Psoriasis Foundation issued a joint guideline for the treatment of psoriatic arthritis in 2018. Various drugs and drug classes are used to treat psoriatic arthritis, with some classes being used for symptom management (e.g., NSAIAs and corticosteroids) and others being used as immunomodulatory disease-modifying therapy. Disease-modifying treatments for psoriatic arthritis include oral small molecules (OSMs; e.g., methotrexate, sulfasalazine, cyclosporine, leflunomide, apremilast), biologic DMARDs (e.g., TNF blocking agents, secukinumab, ixekizumab, ustekinumab, brodalumab, abatacept), and/or targeted synthetic DMARDs (e.g., tofacitinib). Specific agents for psoriatic arthritis treatment are selected according to disease characteristics, including disease severity, as well as patient preferences/values and comorbidities. A "treat-to-target" approach is typically employed, with the goal of achieving low/minimal disease activity or remission.

The guideline recommends the use of TNF blocking agents over OSMs in treatment-naive patients with active psoriatic arthritis, but gives this a conditional recommendation based on low- to very-low-quality evidence. An OSM such as apremilast may be considered in treatment-naive patients without severe psoriasis or psoriatic arthritis, in those who prefer oral over parenteral therapy, and those with contraindications to TNF blocking therapy (e.g., congestive heart failure, previous serious infection, recurrent infections, demyelinating disease). TNF blocking agents and OSMs are conditionally recommended over interleukin (IL) 17 inhibitors (secukinumab, ixekizumab, brodalumab) and IL12/23 inhibitors (ustekinumab). In patients who are not responding to treatment with an OSM, switching to another OSM is generally recommended over adding another OSM to the current regimen except in the case of apremilast since evidence of benefit with this drug is mostly with combination therapy. Switching to apremilast monotherapy may be considered instead of apremilast combination therapy if the patient has intolerable adverse events with the current OSM. In patients with active psoriatic arthritis and predominant enthesitis who are naive to OSMs and biologics, the guideline conditionally recommends use of oral NSAIAs, TNF blocking agents, and tofacitinib over apremilast; however, apremilast may be considered if the patient prefers an oral treatment or has contraindications to the recommended therapy. Recommendations for the use and selection of disease-modifying therapies in psoriatic arthritis vary based on the presence of certain disease characteristics (e.g., psoriatic spondylitis/axial disease, enthesitis) and comorbidities (e.g., inflammatory bowel disease, diabetes). Consult the ACR/National Psoriasis Foundation guideline for additional details.

● Plaque Psoriasis

Apremilast is used for the management of plaque psoriasis in adults who are candidates for phototherapy or systemic therapy. Apremilast has been shown to reduce disease activity, as measured by the Psoriasis Area and Severity Index (PASI) and the static Physician Global Assessment (sPGA) score. PASI is a composite score that takes into consideration both the fraction of body surface area affected and the nature and severity of the psoriatic changes within the affected areas (i.e., induration, erythema, scaling); the sPGA measures the clinician's impression of disease severity at a single time point.

Clinical Experience

Efficacy and safety of apremilast for moderate to severe plaque psoriasis have been established in 2 randomized, double-blind, placebo-controlled studies (ESTEEM 1 and ESTEEM 2). A total of 1257 adults who had moderate to severe plaque psoriasis, with body surface area (BSA) involvement ≥10%, an sPGA score ≥3, and a PASI score ≥12, and who were candidates for phototherapy or systemic therapy were randomized to receive apremilast 30 mg twice daily or placebo. Patients could receive concurrent therapy with certain topical treatments (i.e., low-potency topical corticosteroids on the face, axilla, and groin; coal tar shampoo and/or salicylic acid preparations for psoriatic scalp lesions). The primary outcome measure was the proportion of patients achieving a PASI score of ≥ 75% from baseline (PASI 75 response) at week 16. Approximately 30% of patients enrolled in these studies had received prior phototherapy and 54% had received prior conventional systemic and/or biologic therapy for psoriasis; approximately one-third of the patients had received no prior phototherapy or systemic or biologic therapy. The mean baseline PASI score was 19.07, and approximately 70 or 30% of patients had baseline sPGA scores of 3 (indicating moderate disease) or 4 (indicating severe disease), respectively. In both studies, a greater proportion of patients receiving apremilast achieved a PASI 75 response compared to placebo. Among patients receiving apremilast 30 mg twice daily, 33.1% of patients in ESTEEM 1 and 28.8% of patients in ESTEEM 2 achieved a PASI 75 response at week 16; in comparison, 5.3 and 5.8% of patients receiving placebo in the 2 studies achieved a PASI 75 response. In addition, 21.7% (ESTEEM 1) and 20.4% (ESTEEM 2) of patients receiving apremilast achieved a status of clear (0) or almost clear (1), respectively, on the sPGA scale at week 16, compared with 3.9 and 4.4%, respectively, of those receiving placebo. Among patients who responded to apremilast and were rerandomized at week 32 to receive placebo, the median time to loss of PASI 75 response following treatment withdrawal was 5.1 weeks. Most of the patients in the original placebo group who were rerandomized to apremilast at week 32 had improvements in PASI 75 response at week 52.

Another randomized, double-blind, placebo-controlled study (STYLE) enrolled 303 adults with moderate to severe plaque psoriasis of the scalp. Patients included in the study had a Scalp Physician Global Assessment (ScPGA) score ≥3, Scalp Surface Area (SSA) involvement ≥20%, BSA involvement ≥10%, sPGA score ≥3, and PASI score ≥12. Patients also were required to have an inadequate response or intolerance to at least 1 topical treatment for plaque psoriasis of the scalp. Patients were excluded if they used topical therapies (e.g., medicated shampoos, coal tar, and salicylic acid), intralesional corticosteroids, phototherapy, or biologic agents for a predefined period prior to trial enrollment. Patients were randomized to apremilast 30 mg twice daily or placebo for 16 weeks. The primary outcome measure was the proportion of patients who achieved an ScPGA score of 0 (clear) or 1 (almost clear) with at least a 2-point reduction from baseline to week 16. At baseline, the mean age of patients was 46.9 years; 61.7% were men, 75.6% were White, 76.9% had moderate scalp psoriasis, 23.1% had severe scalp psoriasis, 71.6% were naive to biologic agents, and 58.8% had failed 1 or 2 topical agents. At week 16, a greater percentage of patients achieved a ScPGA response with apremilast (43.3%) compared to placebo (13.7%). An improvement in Whole Body Itch Numerical Rating Scale (NRS) response and Scalp Itch NRS response was also greater with apremilast compared to placebo.

A randomized, double-blind, placebo-controlled study (LIBERATE) enrolled 250 adults with moderate to severe plaque psoriasis. Patients included in the study had plaque psoriasis for ≥12 months (BSA involvement ≥10%, sPGA score ≥3, and a PASI score ≥12) and no prior exposure to a biologic therapy for psoriasis or psoriatic arthritis. Patients had an inadequate response, intolerance, or contraindication to at least one conventional systemic agent used for psoriasis. Patients were allowed to use topical therapies (low-potency corticosteroids, coal tar shampoo, salicylic acid) except for 24 hours prior to study visits. Patients were randomized to receive apremilast 30 mg orally twice daily, etanercept 50 mg by subcutaneous injection once a week, or placebo for 16 weeks; after 16 weeks, patients in the etanercept and placebo groups were switched to apremilast 30 mg twice daily for the apremilast extension phase. The primary outcome measure was the proportion of patients who achieved a PASI 75 response at week 16. At baseline, the mean duration of psoriasis was 18.2 years, mean baseline PASI score was 19.6, approximately 59–70% of patients were men, mean age was approximately 43–47 years, and approximately 90–95% of patients were White. At week 16, a greater percentage of patients achieved a PASI 75 response with apremilast (39.8%) and etanercept (48.2%) compared to placebo (11.9%). Compared to placebo, use of apremilast resulted in improvement in sPGA score of 0–1 and achievement of PASI 50 response. In the apremilast extension phase (weeks 16–104), patients

experienced continued achievement of PASI 75 response, ranging from 45.9–51.9% across treatment groups. In addition, switching from etanercept to apremilast did not result in any clinically important safety findings.

A randomized, double-blind, placebo-controlled, multicenter study (ADVANCE) enrolled 595 adults with chronic mild to moderate plaque psoriasis (sPGA 2-3, BSA involvement 2-15%, and a PASI score of 2-15) for ≥6 months. Patients included in the study were inadequately controlled with, or intolerant to, at least 1 topical psoriatic therapy and had not received prior biologic therapy. Patients were randomly assigned to apremilast 30 mg or placebo orally twice daily for 16 weeks. At week 16, all patients were administered apremilast 30 mg orally twice daily for an additional 16 weeks (until week 32). The primary endpoint was the proportion of patients achieving a sPGA response of 0 (clear) or 1 (almost clear) with at least a 2-point reduction from baseline at week 16. At baseline, the median age of patients was 50 years; the mean baseline BSA involvement was 6.4%, mean PASI score was 6.5, and the proportions of patients with an sPGA score of 2 (mild) or 3 (moderate) were 30.6% or 69.4%, respectively. Results revealed a greater improvement in the percentage of patients with a sPGA response at week 16 in the apremilast group as compared to placebo (21.6 versus 4.1%).

Clinical Perspective

The American Academy of Dermatology and the National Psoriasis Foundation have issued joint guidelines for the treatment of psoriasis in adult and pediatric patients. Various drugs and drug classes are used to treat psoriasis. Phototherapy and topical treatments (e.g., vitamin D analogues, calcineurin inhibitors, keratolytics, and corticosteroids) are frequently used to treat mild psoriasis on limited areas of the body, but these therapies may be inadequate to obtain skin clearance in patients with more extensive or severe disease. Systemic biologic and nonbiologic therapies are mainstays of treatment for moderate to severe psoriasis, and may also be useful for treating psoriasis on parts of the body that are difficult to treat with topical therapy (e.g., scalp, palms and soles of the feet, genitals). Topical therapies can be used adjunctively in moderate to severe disease. Nonbiologic oral therapies used in the treatment of psoriasis include methotrexate, apremilast, cyclosporine, acitretin, and dimethyl fumarate. Biologics used in the treatment of psoriasis include TNF blocking agents, ustekinumab, secukinumab, ixekizumab, brodalumab, guselkumab, tildrakizumab, and risankizumab. Treatment selection in psoriasis is primarily based on disease characteristics (e.g., severity, location, presence of psoriatic arthritis), with additional consideration being given to patient age and comorbidities.

Apremilast is recommended for adults with moderate to severe psoriasis, and may be used to augment the efficacy of certain biologic agents (e.g., adalimumab, etanercept, infliximab, ustekinumab). The guideline notes that higher quality evidence supporting use of apremilast in combination with other agents, such as biologics, is lacking; however, some benefit has been observed in case reports and case series.

Recommendations for the use and selection of psoriasis therapies vary based on patient age, disease characteristics (e.g., severity, location, presence of psoriatic arthritis), and comorbidities (e.g., inflammatory bowel disease). Consult the American Academy of Dermatology/National Psoriasis Foundation guidelines for additional details.

● *Oral Ulcers Associated with Behçet Disease*

Apremilast is used for the treatment of oral ulcers associated with Behçet disease in adults.

Clinical Experience

A randomized, placebo-controlled study enrolled 207 adults with Behçet disease and active oral ulcers (at least 2 oral ulcers at screening and randomization), which occurred at last 3 times in the past year. Patients were previously treated with at least 1 nonbiologic therapy for Behçet disease and were candidates for systemic therapy. Patients with major organ involvement related to Behçet disease that required treatment were excluded. Patients were randomized to receive apremilast 30 mg twice daily or placebo for 12 weeks. At baseline, patients had active skin lesions (56%) and a history of skin lesions (99%), genital ulcers (90.3%), musculoskeletal involvement (72.5%), ocular involvement (17.4%), CNS involvement (9.7%), GI involvement (9.2%), and vascular involvement (1.4%).

Pain related to oral ulcers as measured by a visual analog scale (VAS) from 0 (no pain) to 100 (worst pain), number of oral ulcers, and percentage of patients who achieved a complete response (oral ulcer-free) were improved with apremilast compared to placebo at week 12. The mean decrease from baseline in oral ulcer pain as measured by VAS was 42.7 with apremilast compared with 18.7 with placebo. The proportion of patients who achieved complete freedom from oral ulcers was 52.9% and 22.3% in the apremilast and placebo groups, respectively. The daily average number of ulcers during treatment in the 12-week study was 1.5 with apremilast and 2.6 with placebo.

Clinical Perspective

Behçet disease is an inflammatory multisystem disease that typically includes recurrent oral ulcers, genital ulcers, uveitis, arthritis, CNS disease, vascular disease, and GI disease. Treatment of Behçet disease is determined by the involved organs, the severity and duration of disease, age, gender, frequency of attacks, and patient preferences. The European Alliance of Associations for Rheumatology (EULAR) has issued guidelines for the management of Behçet disease. Topical treatments (such as steroids) and colchicine are recommended for mucocutaneous lesions. Apremilast can be considered as an alternative to colchicine in selected patients who have recurrent lesions despite colchicine use; other options include azathioprine, thalidomide, interferon-alpha, or TNF blockers.

DOSAGE AND ADMINISTRATION

● General

Pretreatment Screening

- Evaluate renal function prior to starting apremilast; dosage reductions are recommended for severe renal impairment.
- Weigh the risks and benefits of apremilast therapy in patients with a history of depression and/or suicidal thoughts or behaviors.

Patient Monitoring

- Monitor patients for the potential development of serious hypersensitivity reactions including anaphylaxis and angioedema.
- Monitor patients for diarrhea, nausea, and vomiting.
- Monitor for emergence or worsening of depression, suicidal thoughts or other mood changes.
- Monitor weight regularly; consider discontinuing apremilast if unexplained or clinically significant weight loss occurs.

● Administration

Administer apremilast orally without regard to meals. Do not crush, split, or chew tablets.

● Dosage

Psoriatic Arthritis

For the management of active psoriatic arthritis in adults, the recommended maintenance dosage of apremilast is 30 mg twice daily. Therapy should be initiated at a dosage of 10 mg daily and increased gradually (over 5 days in increments of 10 mg daily) to reduce the risk of GI symptoms. The recommended titration schedule is as follows:

- 10 mg in the morning on day 1
- 10 mg in the morning and 10 mg in the evening on day 2
- 10 mg in the morning and 20 mg in the evening on day 3
- 20 mg in the morning and 20 mg in the evening on day 4
- 20 mg in the morning and 30 mg in the evening on day 5, and 30 mg twice daily thereafter

Plaque Psoriasis

For the management of plaque psoriasis in adults, the recommended maintenance dosage of apremilast is 30 mg twice daily. Therapy should be initiated at a dosage of 10 mg daily and increased gradually (over 5 days in increments of 10 mg daily) to reduce the risk of GI symptoms. The recommended titration schedule is as follows:

- 10 mg in the morning on day 1
- 10 mg in the morning and 10 mg in the evening on day 2
- 10 mg in the morning and 20 mg in the evening on day 3
- 20 mg in the morning and 20 mg in the evening on day 4
- 20 mg in the morning and 30 mg in the evening on day 5, and 30 mg twice daily thereafter

Oral Ulcers Associated with Behçet Disease

For the management of oral ulcers associated with Behçet disease in adults, the recommended maintenance dosage of apremilast is 30 mg twice daily. Therapy should be initiated at a dosage of 10 mg daily and increased gradually (over 5 days in increments of 10 mg daily) to reduce the risk of GI symptoms. The recommended titration schedule is as follows.

- 10 mg in the morning on day 1
- 10 mg in the morning and 10 mg in the evening on day 2
- 10 mg in the morning and 20 mg in the evening on day 3
- 20 mg in the morning and 20 mg in the evening on day 4
- 20 mg in the morning and 30 mg in the evening on day 5, and 30 mg twice daily thereafter

● Special Populations

Hepatic Impairment

Dosage adjustments are not necessary in patients with hepatic impairment.

Renal Impairment

In adults with severe renal impairment (creatinine clearance <30 mL/minute), a reduced maintenance apremilast dosage of 30 mg once daily is recommended for the management of psoriatic arthritis, plaque psoriasis, or oral ulcers associated with Behçet disease; the recommended dosage titration schedule for initiation of therapy in adults with severe renal impairment is as follows:

- 10 mg in the morning for 3 days (days 1, 2, and 3)
- 20 mg in the morning for 2 days (days 4 and 5)
- 30 mg once daily thereafter

Geriatric Patients

The manufacturer makes no specific dosage recommendations for geriatric patients.

CAUTIONS

● Contraindications

Patients with known hypersensitivity to the drug or any ingredient in the formulation.

● Warnings/Precautions

Hypersensitivity

During postmarketing surveillance, apremilast therapy was associated with hypersensitivity reactions including cases of angioedema and anaphylaxis. Avoid use of apremilast in patients with a known hypersensitivity to the drug of any of its excipients. Discontinue apremilast if signs or symptoms of serious hypersensitivity reactions occur and initiate appropriate therapy.

GI Effects

Apremilast has been associated with postmarketing reports of severe diarrhea, nausea, and vomiting, including cases resulting in hospitalization. Most cases occurred within the first few weeks of treatment. A higher risk was seen in patients ≥65 years of age and those taking medications that can cause volume depletion or hypotension.

Monitor patients who are more susceptible to complications of diarrhea or vomiting. Consider dosage reduction or temporary discontinuation of therapy if diarrhea, nausea, or vomiting occurs.

Depression and Suicidality

Apremilast therapy is associated with an increase in depression. In clinical trials in patients with psoriatic arthritis, depression or depressed mood was reported in 1% of patients receiving apremilast compared with 0.8% of those receiving placebo and resulted in discontinuance of the assigned treatment in 0.3% of those receiving the drug compared with none of those receiving placebo; depression was considered serious in 0.2% of apremilast-treated patients and no placebo recipients. In clinical trials in patients with moderate to severe psoriasis, depression was reported in 1.3% of patients receiving apremilast compared with 0.4% of those receiving placebo and resulted in discontinuance of the assigned treatment in 0.1% of patients receiving the drug and none of those receiving placebo; depression was considered serious in 0.1% of apremilast-treated patients and none of the patients who received. In the clinical trial in patients with Behçet disease, depression or depressed mood was reported in 1% of patients in both treatment groups; none of the reports were considered serious or led to study discontinuation.

Suicidal ideation and behavior, including completed suicide, also have been observed in clinical trials of apremilast. In studies in patients with psoriatic arthritis, suicidal ideation and behavior were observed in 3 patients (0.2%) receiving apremilast and in no patients receiving placebo; completed suicide was reported in no patients receiving apremilast but in 2 patients receiving placebo. In clinical trials in patients with psoriasis, suicidal behavior was observed in 1 patient (0.1%) receiving apremilast and in 1 patient (0.2%) receiving placebo; 1 patient receiving apremilast attempted suicide and 1 patient receiving placebo completed suicide. In the clinical trial in patients with Behçet disease, no cases of suicidal ideation or behavior were reported.

Carefully weigh the risks and benefits of apremilast therapy prior to using the drug in patients with a history of depression and/or suicidal thoughts or behavior. In addition, carefully evaluate the risks and benefits of continuing therapy with apremilast if such effects occur.

Weight Loss

Weight loss has been reported in patients receiving recommended dosages of apremilast. In clinical trials in patients with psoriatic arthritis, weight loss of 5–10% of body weight was reported in 10% of patients receiving apremilast (30 mg twice daily) compared with 3.3% of those receiving placebo. In clinical trials in patients with moderate to severe psoriasis, weight loss of 5–10% of body weight was reported in 12% of patients receiving apremilast (30 mg twice daily) compared with 5% of those receiving placebo, while loss of ≥10% of body weight was reported in 2% of patients receiving apremilast (30 mg twice daily) and 1% of those receiving placebo. In the clinical trial in patients with Behçet disease, loss of >5% body weight was reported in 4.9% of patients receiving apremilast (30 mg twice daily) and 3.9% of those receiving placebo.

Monitor patient's weight regularly during apremilast therapy. If unexplained or clinically important weight loss occurs, evaluate and consider discontinuation of the drug.

Interactions

Concomitant use of cytochrome P-450 (CYP) enzyme inducers (e.g., carbamazepine, phenobarbital, phenytoin, rifampin) with apremilast is not recommended because loss of apremilast efficacy may occur.

Specific Populations

Pregnancy

In animal reproduction studies, administration of apremilast to cynomolgus monkeys during organogenesis resulted in dose-related increases in spontaneous abortion and embryofetal death at doses equivalent to 2.1 times the maximum recommended human dose.

To monitor pregnancy outcomes in women who have been exposed to apremilast, a pregnancy registry has been established. Information about the registry can be obtained by calling 877-311-8972 or visiting https://mothertobaby.org/ongoing-study/otezla/.

Lactation

Apremilast is distributed into milk in mice; it is not known whether the drug is distributed into human milk. Consider the benefits of breast-feeding and the importance of apremilast to the patient along with potential adverse effects on the breast-fed infant from the drug or from the underlying maternal condition.

Pediatric Use

Safety and efficacy of apremilast have not been established in pediatric patients <18 years of age.

Geriatric Use

In controlled clinical trials evaluating apremilast for the management of psoriatic arthritis, about 10% of patients were ≥65 years of age, and about 1% were ≥75 years of age. No overall differences in safety were observed between geriatric and younger adults.

Similarly, no overall differences in efficacy and safety were observed between geriatric and younger adults in two placebo-controlled plaque psoriasis trials.

Following oral administration of a single 30-mg dose of apremilast, AUC and peak plasma concentrations of the drug were approximately 13 and 6% higher, respectively, in patients 65–85 years of age compared with those 18–55 years of age.

Patients ≥65 years of age should be monitored closely for volume depletion or hypotension resulting from treatment-related severe diarrhea, nausea, or vomiting.

Hepatic Impairment

Moderate or severe hepatic impairment (Child-Pugh class B or C) does not alter the pharmacokinetics of apremilast. No dosage adjustment is necessary in these patients.

Renal Impairment

Following administration of a single 30-mg dose of apremilast in patients with severe renal impairment (creatinine clearance < 30 mL/minute), AUC and peak plasma concentrations of the drug were increased by approximately 88 and 42%, respectively. Dosage adjustment is recommended in patients with severe renal impairment (creatinine clearance <30 mL/minute). Mild or moderate renal impairment did not affect the pharmacokinetics of apremilast.

● Common Adverse Effects

Adverse effects reported in ≥5% of patients receiving apremilast for active psoriatic arthritis include diarrhea, nausea, and headache.

Adverse effects reported in ≥5% of patients receiving apremilast for plaque psoriasis include diarrhea, nausea, upper respiratory tract infection, and headache, including tension headache.

Adverse effects reported in ≥10% of patients receiving apremilast for Behçet disease include diarrhea, nausea, headache, and upper respiratory tract infection.

DRUG INTERACTIONS

Apremilast undergoes cytochrome P-450 (CYP)-mediated oxidative metabolism, with subsequent glucuronidation, and non-CYP-mediated hydrolysis. In vitro, oxidative metabolism is mediated principally by CYP3A4, with minor contributions from CYP1A2 and CYP2A6.

In vitro, apremilast does not inhibit CYP isoenzyme 1A2, 2A6, 2B6, 2C8, 2C9, 2C19, 2D6, 2E1, or 3A4, nor does apremilast induce CYP isoenzyme 1A2, 2B6, 2C9, 2C19, or 3A4.

In vitro data indicate that apremilast is a substrate but not an inhibitor of P-glycoprotein (P-gp) and that the drug is neither a substrate nor an inhibitor of organic anion transporters (OAT) 1 and 3, organic anion transporting polypeptides (OATP) 1B1 and 1B3, organic cation transporter (OCT) 2, or breast cancer resistance protein (BCRP).

● Drugs Affecting Hepatic Microsomal Enzymes

Systemic exposure of apremilast is reduced when the drug is used concomitantly with potent CYP inducers. Concomitant use of apremilast with potent CYP inducers (e.g., carbamazepine, phenobarbital, phenytoin, rifampin) may result in loss of apremilast efficacy and is not recommended.

● Estrogens/Progestins

In healthy women, concomitant administration of apremilast (30 mg twice daily) with an oral contraceptive containing the CYP3A4 substrates ethinyl estradiol and norgestimate did not substantially affect the pharmacokinetics of the oral contraceptive components; pharmacokinetics of apremilast also were unchanged.

● Ketoconazole

In healthy individuals, concomitant administration of ketoconazole (400 mg daily for 7 days) (an inhibitor of both CYP3A and P-gp) with apremilast (single 20-mg dose) appeared to have some effects on apremilast disposition, but overall did not result in clinically important effects on exposure to the drug.

● Methotrexate

In patients receiving stable weekly methotrexate therapy, concomitant use of apremilast (30 mg twice daily) with methotrexate (15 or 20 mg once weekly) did not substantially affect the pharmacokinetics of either drug.

● Rifampin

When the potent CYP inducer rifampin (600 mg once daily for 15 days) was administered concomitantly with apremilast (single 30-mg dose) in healthy individuals, AUC and peak plasma concentration of apremilast were reduced by 72 and 43%, respectively. Concomitant use of rifampin may result in loss of apremilast efficacy and is not recommended.

DESCRIPTION

Apremilast, a selective inhibitor of phosphodiesterase type 4 (PDE4), is a disease-modifying antirheumatic drug (DMARD). PDE4 is the dominant phosphodiesterase expressed in immune cells and a major enzyme involved in metabolism of cyclic adenosine-3′,5′-monophosphate (cAMP). Thus, selective inhibition of PDE4 results in accumulation of intracellular cAMP, a modulator of inflammatory responses, which can down-regulate inflammatory responses by increasing expression of anti-inflammatory mediators and partially inhibiting expression of inflammatory cytokines that are thought to play a role in the pathogenesis of psoriasis and active psoriatic arthritis. The exact mechanism(s) of action of apremilast in the management of these conditions has not been fully elucidated.

Following oral administration, apremilast has an absolute bioavailability of approximately 73%. Administration with food does not alter the extent of absorption. Apremilast is extensively metabolized; up to 23 metabolites have been identified in plasma, urine, and feces. The major circulating forms of the drug are apremilast (45%) and the inactive glucuronide conjugate M12 (39%). Apremilast undergoes cytochrome P-450 (CYP)-mediated oxidative metabolism, with subsequent glucuronidation, and non-CYP-mediated hydrolysis; in vitro, oxidative metabolism is mediated principally by CYP3A4, with minor contributions from CYP1A2 and CYP2A6. The terminal elimination half-life of apremilast is approximately 6–9 hours. Following oral administration of radiolabeled apremilast, approximately 58% of radioactivity was recovered in urine and 39% was recovered in feces; unchanged drug in urine and feces accounted for only 3 and 7%, respectively, of the radiolabeled dose.

ADVICE TO PATIENTS

- Importance of taking apremilast only as prescribed.
- Advise patients to *not* crush, split, or chew apremilast tablets.
- Inform patients that apremilast may be taken without regard to meals.
- Advise patients of the potential for serious allergic reactions following administration and to contact a clinician if symptoms of an allergic reaction occur.
- Advise patients to contact a clinician if they experience severe diarrhea, nausea, or vomiting.
- Risk of emergence or worsening of depression. Instruct patients and their caregivers or families to be alert for the emergence or worsening of depression, suicidal thoughts, or other mood changes and to contact a clinician if such changes occur.
- Risk of weight loss. Importance of regularly monitoring for weight loss; advise patients to inform clinician if substantial or unexplained weight loss occurs.
- Risk of interactions with potent CYP inducers (e.g., carbamazepine, phenobarbital, phenytoin, rifampin). Advise patients to inform their clinician of existing or contemplated concomitant therapy, including prescription and OTC drugs and dietary and herbal supplements, as well as any concomitant illnesses.
- Advise women to inform their clinician if they are or plan to become pregnant or plan to breast-feed.
- Advise patients of other important precautionary information. (See Cautions.)

PREPARATIONS

Excipients in commercially available drug preparations may have clinically important effects in some individuals; consult specific product labeling for details.

Apremilast

Oral		
Kit	4 tablets, film-coated, apremilast 10 mg	
	4 tablets, film-coated, apremilast 20 mg	
	19 tablets, film-coated, apremilast 30 mg	Otezla® 2-Week Starter Pack (available as blister pack containing tablets for first 2 weeks of therapy), Amgen
	4 tablets, film-coated, apremilast 10 mg	
	4 tablets, film-coated, apremilast 20 mg	
	47 tablets, film-coated, apremilast 30 mg	Otezla® 28-Day Starter Pack (available as blister pack containing tablets for first 28 days of therapy), Amgen
	28 tablets, film-coated, apremilast 30 mg	Otezla® 28-Count Carton (available as 2 blister cards), Amgen
Tablets, film-coated	30 mg	Otezla® Amgen

† Use is not currently included in the labeling approved by the US Food and Drug Administration.

Selected Revisions May 10, 2024, © Copyright, March 9, 2015, American Society of Health-System Pharmacists, Inc.

Abatacept

90:24.92 • DISEASE-MODIFYING ANTIRHEUMATIC DRUGS, MISCELLANEOUS

■ Abatacept, a recombinant fusion protein, is a selective costimulation modulator that inhibits T-cell activation and is a biologic disease-modifying antirheumatic drug (DMARD).

USES

● Rheumatoid Arthritis

Abatacept is used for the management of moderately to severely active rheumatoid arthritis in adults. Safety and efficacy of abatacept for this use are based on the results of several randomized controlled trials and further supported by long-term extension studies and comparative clinical trials. Guidelines generally support the use of abatacept as add-on therapy to methotrexate in patients who do not meet treatment goals with methotrexate alone.

Clinical Experience with IV Abatacept

Clinical evaluations of abatacept indicate that recommended IV dosages of the drug are more effective than placebo for improving clinical manifestations of rheumatoid arthritis. In adults with persistently active rheumatoid arthritis despite methotrexate therapy, addition of IV abatacept to the methotrexate regimen has been associated with greater efficacy than use of methotrexate alone. In patients with early rheumatoid arthritis and poor prognostic factors who had not previously received methotrexate, therapy with IV abatacept in conjunction with methotrexate has been more effective than methotrexate alone. In addition, therapy with IV abatacept in conjunction with at least one other disease-modifying antirheumatic drug (DMARD) has been effective in patients who had an inadequate response to therapy with a tumor necrosis factor (TNF) blocking agent. Response to abatacept can occur within 15 days following initiation of therapy in some patients; response has been maintained for up to 5–7 years in some studies.

Evidence of clinical benefit of IV abatacept in the management of rheumatoid arthritis is based principally on the results of several randomized, double-blind, placebo-controlled clinical trials in adults with the disease. Patients in these trials were randomized to receive abatacept or placebo by IV infusion at weeks 0, 2, and 4, followed by additional doses given once every 4 weeks. In one study, abatacept was administered as monotherapy after therapy with at least one other DMARD had failed; patients in this study were randomized to receive 0.5, 2, or 10 mg/kg of abatacept or placebo. In another study (AIM trial), abatacept was added to a stable methotrexate regimen in patients who had not responded adequately to methotrexate alone; patients in this study were randomized to receive abatacept at a dosage of approximately 10 mg/kg (500 mg, 750 mg, or 1 g of abatacept in patients who weighed less than 60, 60–100, or more than 100 kg, respectively) or placebo. In another study (AGREE trial), patients with early rheumatoid arthritis (duration of 2 years or less) and poor prognostic factors who had not previously received methotrexate were randomized to receive abatacept or placebo in conjunction with methotrexate; abatacept was given at a dosage of approximately 10 mg/kg (500 mg, 750 mg, or 1 g of abatacept in patients who weighed less than 60, 60–100, or more than 100 kg, respectively). In this study, addition of a non-biologic DMARD was permitted after month 6. Abatacept also was evaluated in patients who had an inadequate response to therapy with one or more TNF blocking agents (ATTAIN trial). Patients in this study received abatacept or placebo in conjunction with at least one other DMARD following discontinuance of the TNF blocking agent; abatacept was given at a dosage of approximately 10 mg/kg (500 mg, 750 mg, or 1 g of abatacept in patients who weighed less than 60, 60–100, or more than 100 kg, respectively). Patients included in these studies had 12 or more tender joints and 10 or more swollen joints at study entry.

The American College of Rheumatology (ACR) criteria for improvement (ACR response) in measures of disease activity was used as the principal measure of clinical response in these studies. An ACR 20 response is achieved if the patient experiences a 20% improvement in tender and swollen joint count and a 20% or greater improvement in at least 3 of the following criteria: patient pain

assessment, patient global assessment, physician global assessment, patient self-assessed disability, or laboratory measures of disease activity (i.e., C-reactive protein [CRP] level). ACR 50 and ACR 70 responses are defined using the same criteria with a level of improvement of 50 and 70%, respectively. Major clinical response is defined as achieving an ACR 70 response for a continuous 6-month period. In one study, disease activity based on the 28-joint Disease Activity Score using C-reactive protein (DAS 28 [CRP]) was the principal measure of clinical benefit. Physical function and disability were assessed using the Health Assessment Questionnaire Disability Index (HAQ-DI) and the health-related quality-of-life questionnaire SF-36. The Genant-modified total Sharp score was used as the principal measure of structural damage.

In the study that evaluated abatacept as monotherapy after therapy with at least one other DMARD had failed, an ACR 20, 50, or 70 response was achieved at 3 months in 53, 16, or 6 %, respectively, of patients who received abatacept 10 mg/kg and in 31, 6, or 0%, respectively, of those who received placebo.

Results of the AIM trial indicated that the addition of abatacept to a methotrexate regimen was associated with greater clinical benefit than use of methotrexate alone. An ACR 20 response was achieved in 62, 68, or 73% of patients receiving abatacept at a dosage of approximately 10 mg/kg (i.e., 500 mg, 750 mg, or 1 g depending on the patient's weight) in conjunction with methotrexate at 3, 6, or 12 months, respectively; an ACR 50 response was achieved in 32, 40, or 48% of these patients at 3, 6, or 12 months, respectively; and an ACR 70 response was achieved in 13, 20, or 29% of these patients at 3, 6, or 12, months, respectively. In patients who continued their usual methotrexate dosage, an ACR 20 response was achieved in 37, 40, or 40% of patients at 3, 6, or 12 months, respectively; an ACR 50 response was achieved in 8, 17, or 18% of patients at 3, 6, or 12 months, respectively; and an ACR 70 response was achieved in 3, 7, or 6% of patients at 3, 6, or 12, months, respectively. A major clinical response was achieved in 14% of those who received abatacept in conjunction with methotrexate and in 2% of those who continued their usual methotrexate dosage. Patients receiving abatacept in conjunction with methotrexate experienced greater improvement from baseline in HAQ-DI and SF-36 scores at 1 year than did patients who continued to receive their usual methotrexate dosage. There was more progression of joint damage from baseline in the group of patients who received methotrexate alone compared with those who received abatacept in conjunction with methotrexate. In a long-term extension of the AIM trial, clinical response and radiographic benefit were maintained through up to 5 years of abatacept treatment.

In the AGREE trial, a greater proportion of patients receiving abatacept in conjunction with methotrexate achieved a low level of disease activity, as measured by a DAS 28 (CRP) score of less than 2.6, at 12 months compared with those receiving methotrexate alone (41 versus 23%). Among abatacept- and methotrexate-treated patients who achieved such response, 54% had no tender or swollen (active) joints, 17% had 1 active joint, 7% had 2 active joints, and 22% had 3 or more active joints. An ACR 20 response was achieved at 3, 6, or 12 months in 64, 75, or 76%, respectively, of patients receiving abatacept in conjunction with methotrexate compared with 53, 62, or 62%, respectively, of those receiving methotrexate alone. ACR 50 response rates at these respective time points were 40, 53, or 57% in patients receiving abatacept in conjunction with methotrexate compared with 23, 38, or 42% in those receiving methotrexate alone. ACR 70 response rates at these respective time points were 19, 32, or 43% in patients receiving abatacept in conjunction with methotrexate compared with 10, 20, or 27% in those receiving methotrexate alone. In patients receiving abatacept in conjunction with methotrexate, improvement in the ACR 20 response rate over that observed with methotrexate alone was observed within 29 days following initiation of therapy. A major clinical response was achieved in 27% of those receiving abatacept in conjunction with methotrexate compared with 12% of those receiving methotrexate alone. After one year of treatment, patients receiving abatacept in conjunction with methotrexate had less progression of joint damage and greater improvement from baseline in HAQ-DI and SF-36 scores than did patients receiving methotrexate alone. The improvements in disease activity, ACR response, and physical function initially seen in the AGREE trial were sustained over a 2-year period.

When abatacept was evaluated in conjunction with at least one other DMARD in patients who had responded inadequately to prior TNF blocking agent therapy (ATTAIN study), an ACR 20 response was achieved in 46 or 50% of patients receiving abatacept in conjunction with other DMARD therapy (75.6% received methotrexate) at 3 or 6 months, respectively; an ACR 50 response was achieved in 18 or 20% of these patients at 3 or 6 months, respectively, and an ACR 70 response was achieved in 6 or 10% of these patients at 3 or 6 months, respectively. An ACR

20 response was achieved in 18 or 20% of patients receiving placebo in conjunction with other DMARD therapy (82% received methotrexate) at 3 or 6 months, respectively; an ACR 50 response was achieved in 6 or 4% of these patients at 3 or 6 months, respectively; and an ACR 70 response was achieved in 1 or 2% of these patients at 3 or 6 months, respectively. At 6 months, more patients receiving abatacept in conjunction with other DMARD therapy had clinically meaningful improvement in physical function, as reflected by improvement in HAQ-DI and SF-36 scores, than patients receiving placebo with DMARD therapy.

A limited number of clinical trials have compared abatacept to alternative biologic agents, including upadacitinib and adalimumab, for the treatment of rheumatoid arthritis. The double-blind SELECT-CHOICE trial assessed the noninferiority of oral upadacitinib 15 mg once daily to IV abatacept, both in combination with nonbiologic DMARDs, in adults with moderately to severely active rheumatoid arthritis and inadequate response or intolerance to biologic DMARD therapy. The primary outcome of this study assessed the change in DAS28-CRP at week 12. Noninferiority of upadacitinib compared to abatacept with regard to change in DAS28-CRP at week 12 was met as a primary endpoint, and superiority (a secondary endpoint) was also achieved. Another randomized trial (AMPLE) assessed noninferiority of adalimumab compared to abatacept in patients with active rheumatoid arthritis and an inadequate response to methotrexate. Patients were administered subcutaneous abatacept weekly or subcutaneous adalimumab every other week in combination with methotrexate therapy. After 1 year of treatment, the primary outcome of ACR 20 response met criteria for noninferiority. After 2 years of treatment, observed ACR 20 responses remained comparable between the two groups.

Clinical Experience with Subcutaneous Abatacept

Evidence of efficacy of subcutaneous abatacept in the management of rheumatoid arthritis is based principally on the results of a randomized, double-blind, noninferiority study comparing subcutaneous and IV abatacept regimens in 1457 adults with moderately to severely active rheumatoid arthritis despite methotrexate therapy; to be enrolled in the study, patients were required to have at least 10 swollen and 12 tender joints and an elevated CRP level. Patients were randomized to receive abatacept by subcutaneous injection (125 mg on days 1 and 8 and weekly thereafter) or IV infusion (approximately 10 mg/kg [i.e., 500 mg, 750 mg, or 1 g of abatacept in patients who weighed less than 60, 60–100, or more than 100 kg, respectively] on days 1, 15, and 29 and every 4 weeks thereafter) in combination with their usual methotrexate dosage; those receiving subcutaneous abatacept also received an initial IV loading dose of the drug of approximately 10 mg/kg (i.e., 500 mg, 750 mg, or 1 g depending on the patient's weight) on day 1. Patients receiving stable dosages of low-dose corticosteroids (equivalent to 10 mg of prednisone daily or less) could continue such therapy, and patients could receive up to 2 courses of high-dose corticosteroids during the study; corticosteroid use was similar in the two treatment groups.

ACR 20 response was achieved at 6 months in 76% of patients receiving either subcutaneous or IV abatacept, indicating that the subcutaneous regimen was noninferior to IV therapy; ACR 50 and ACR 70 response rates at 6 months also were similar with subcutaneous (52 and 26%, respectively) or IV therapy (50 and 25%, respectively). Within each of the 3 body weight ranges, ACR responses were achieved in similar proportions of patients receiving subcutaneous or IV abatacept. The time course for ACR response was similar regardless of administration route. In addition, improvements in physical function, as measured by the HAQ-DI, were similar in patients receiving subcutaneous or IV abatacept, and similar proportions of patients receiving subcutaneous or IV abatacept achieved a low level of disease activity as measured by a DAS 28 (CRP) score of less than 2.6. During an open-label extension period, efficacy of subcutaneous abatacept was maintained during treatment periods of up to 5 years.

Clinical Perspective

The American College of Rheumatology issued updated guidelines in 2021 for the treatment of rheumatoid arthritis. Disease-modifying treatments for rheumatoid arthritis include conventional disease-modifying antirheumatic drugs (DMARDs; e.g., methotrexate, hydroxychloroquine, sulfasalazine), biologic DMARDs (e.g., TNF blocking agents, abatacept, tocilizumab, sarilumab, rituximab), and/or targeted synthetic DMARDs (e.g., Janus kinase inhibitors). Specific agents for rheumatoid arthritis treatment are selected according to current disease activity, prior therapies used, and the presence of comorbidities. A "treat-to-target" approach is typically employed, with the goal of achieving low disease activity or remission.

Methotrexate monotherapy is strongly recommended over biologic DMARD monotherapy in DMARD-naive patients with moderate to high disease activity. Methotrexate monotherapy is also strongly recommended over the combination of methotrexate and a non-TNF blocking biologic DMARD in such patients, because of a lack of proven benefit and additional risks and costs of combination therapy over monotherapies. Biologic DMARDs and targeted synthetic DMARDs are conditionally recommended as add-on therapy for patients who are taking maximally tolerated doses of methotrexate and are not at target. Recommendations for the use and selection of biologic DMARDs in rheumatoid arthritis vary based on the presence of certain comorbidities (e.g., heart failure, previous serious infection, nontuberculous mycobacterial lung disease). Consult the American College of Rheumatology guidelines for additional details.

● Juvenile Idiopathic Arthritis

Abatacept is used for the management of moderately to severely active polyarticular juvenile idiopathic arthritis in pediatric patients ≥2 years of age. Safety and efficacy of abatacept for this use are based principally on the results of a 2-part, open-label clinical study and its long-term extension. The 2019 American College of Rheumatology/Arthritis Foundation guidelines generally support the use of abatacept as add-on therapy in patients with juvenile idiopathic arthritis and moderate to high disease activity despite the use of methotrexate.

Clinical Experience with IV Abatacept

IV abatacept has been evaluated for the management of polyarticular juvenile idiopathic arthritis in pediatric patients 6–17 years of age in a 3-part study. Patients enrolled in this study included those with moderate to severe active polyarticular juvenile idiopathic arthritis who had not responded adequately to one or more DMARDS (e.g., methotrexate, TNF blocking agents). Those receiving stable dosages of methotrexate and/or prednisone (0.2 mg or less/kg daily) at study enrollment could continue these drugs during the study. In part 1 (open-label study), pediatric patients (median age: 12.4 years, mean disease duration: 4 years, 72% female, 77% white) with juvenile arthritis received abatacept 10 mg/kg (maximum dose 1 g) given by IV infusion on days 1, 15, 29, 57, and 85. In part 2 (placebo-controlled study), patients with a clinical response at month 4 were randomized to continue IV abatacept or receive placebo at 28-day intervals for 6 months or until disease flare. Part 3 was an open-label extension study for patients who participated in parts 1 and 2.

The principal measure of clinical response in part 1 of this study was the ACR pediatric 30 definition of improvement (i.e., 30% or greater improvement in at least 3 of 6 and 30% or greater deterioration in no more than 1 of 6 core set criteria that include physician and patient/parent global assessments, active joint count, limitation of motion, functional assessment, and erythrocyte sedimentation rate). In part 2, the primary end point was time to disease flare (defined as a 30% or greater deterioration in 3 of 6 and a 30% or greater improvement in no more than 1 of 6 core set criteria).

Evaluation at month 4 (i.e., completion of part 1) indicated that 65% of patients had improved by 30% or more according to the ACR pediatric response criteria. Pediatric ACR 30 response was similar in patients with different disease subtypes. Of those patients who responded (i.e., study part 2), 20% of patients remaining on IV abatacept experienced disease flare compared with 53% of those switched to placebo. Durable responses have been maintained for up to 7 years in pediatric patients receiving IV abatacept.

Clinical Experience with Subcutaneous Abatacept

Subcutaneous abatacept has been evaluated for the management of polyarticular juvenile idiopathic arthritis in 205 pediatric patients 2–17 years of age in a 2-part, open-label, noncomparative study. During the first 4 months of the study (part 1), patients received once-weekly, weight-based, subcutaneous doses of abatacept (50 mg in those weighing 10 kg to less than 25 kg, 87.5 mg in those weighing 25 kg to less than 50 kg, or 125 mg in those weighing 50 kg or more) without an IV loading dose. At month 4, patients with a pediatric ACR 30 response could be enrolled in a 20-month extension (part 2) and continue receiving open-label subcutaneous abatacept therapy. Patients enrolled in the study included those with active disease (mean of 11.9 active joints and 10.4 joints with loss of motion, elevated CRP levels) and an inadequate response to one or more nonbiologic or biologic DMARDs. Most patients (79%) had polyarticular disease; 14% had extended and persistent oligoarthritis. Those receiving methotrexate and/or oral corticosteroids at study enrollment could continue these drugs during the study; 80%

of patients received concomitant therapy with methotrexate during the study. While the primary objective of the study was evaluation of the pharmacokinetics of subcutaneous abatacept, pediatric ACR responses at 4 months were consistent with responses observed with IV abatacept in pediatric patients 6–17 years of age. Responses were maintained in pediatric patients receiving subcutaneous therapy with the drug for periods of up to 24 months.

Clinical Perspective

The American College of Rheumatology and the Arthritis Foundation issued a joint guideline in 2019 for the treatment of juvenile idiopathic arthritis manifesting as nonsystemic polyarthritis (including polyarticular disease), sacroiliitis, or enthesitis. Several medication classes are used to treat juvenile idiopathic arthritis, including NSAIAs, systemic and intra-articular corticosteroids, conventional DMARDs (e.g., methotrexate, sulfasalazine, hydroxychloroquine, leflunomide), and biologic DMARDs (e.g., TNF blocking agents, abatacept, tocilizumab, rituximab). Specific agents for juvenile idiopathic arthritis treatment are selected according to the presence of certain risk factors (e.g., positive anti-cyclic citrullinated peptide antibodies, positive rheumatoid factor, joint damage), level of disease activity, involvement of specific joints, presence of certain comorbidities (e.g., uveitis), and prior therapies used. An individualized "treat-to-target" approach is typically employed, with the goal of achieving remission or minimal/low disease activity.

Methotrexate monotherapy is conditionally recommended as initial therapy for patients with juvenile idiopathic arthritis manifesting as nonsystemic polyarthritis, although initial biologic DMARD therapy may be considered for patients with risk factors and involvement of high risk joints (e.g., cervical spine, wrist, hip), high disease activity, and/or those judged by their physician to be at high risk of disabling joint damage. In patients with moderate or high disease activity despite methotrexate monotherapy, biologic DMARDs are conditionally recommended as add-on therapy. In patients with moderate or high disease activity despite treatment with a first TNF blocking agent (with or without concomitant conventional DMARD therapy), switching to tocilizumab or abatacept is conditionally recommended over switching to a different TNF blocking agent. In all patients initiating biologic DMARD therapy, combination therapy with a conventional DMARD is recommended over biologic DMARD monotherapy. Specific choice of biologic DMARD may be influenced by the presence of certain comorbidities (e.g., uveitis). Consult the American College of Rheumatology/Arthritis Foundation guidelines for additional details.

• Psoriatic Arthritis

Abatacept is used for the management of adults and pediatric patients ≥2 years of age with active psoriatic arthritis. Safety and efficacy of abatacept for this use are principally based on the results of 2 randomized controlled trials. Guidelines generally recommend alternative therapies (e.g., TNF blocking agents, secukinumab, ixekizumab, brodalumab, ustekinumab) for treatment of psoriatic arthritis before treatment with abatacept; abatacept may be considered in patients with failure to respond to first-line therapies or with other comorbidities.

Clinical Experience with IV Abatacept

Evidence of efficacy of IV abatacept in the management of psoriatic arthritis is based principally on the results of a randomized, double-blind, placebo-controlled phase 2 study in 170 adults with active psoriatic arthritis despite DMARD therapy; to be enrolled in the study, patients were required to have at least 3 swollen and 3 tender joints, active plaque psoriasis with at least one qualifying skin lesion, and inadequate response or intolerance to at least one DMARD. Patients were randomized to receive placebo or 1 of 3 different doses of abatacept administered as an IV infusion on days 1, 15, and 29 and every 28 days thereafter for a total treatment period of 24 weeks: abatacept 3 mg/kg, weight-based abatacept doses of approximately 10 mg/kg (i.e., 500 mg, 750 mg, or 1 g of abatacept in patients who weighed less than 60, 60–100, or more than 100 kg, respectively), or abatacept 30 mg/kg on days 1 and 15 followed by weight-based doses of approximately 10 mg/kg thereafter. After 24 weeks of randomized treatment, patients received 18 months of open-label therapy with the weight-based 10-mg/kg dosage of abatacept. Approximately 37% of patients in this study had received prior therapy with TNF blocking agents. Patients receiving stable dosages of methotrexate, low-dose corticosteroids (equivalent to 10 mg of prednisone daily or less), and/or nonsteroidal anti-inflammatory agents (NSAIAs) could continue such agents during the study; approximately 60 or 20% of patients received concomitant methotrexate or corticosteroid therapy, respectively.

The primary outcome measure in this study was the proportion of patients achieving an ACR 20 response at 24 weeks. Physical function and health-related quality of life were assessed using the HAQ-DI and SF-36; a decrease in HAQ-DI score of at least 0.3 was considered to be a clinically important difference.

Overall results of the study supported use of IV abatacept at doses of approximately 10 mg/kg in the management of psoriatic arthritis; response rates tended to be higher with this dosage than with the other dosages that were studied. ACR 20, ACR 50, or ACR 70 response was achieved at 24 weeks in 48, 25, or 13%, respectively, of patients receiving abatacept 10 mg/kg compared with 19, 2, or 0% of those receiving placebo. ACR 20 responses were observed as early as day 29 and were maintained through 24 weeks of abatacept treatment. ACR 20 responses were observed regardless of prior therapy with TNF blocking agents or concomitant use of nonbiologic DMARDs. Improvements in dactylitis and enthesitis also were observed in abatacept-treated patients. Clinically meaningful improvements in physical function, as measured by change in HAQ-DI score from baseline to 24 weeks, were observed in a greater proportion of patients receiving abatacept 10 mg/kg compared with those receiving placebo (45 versus 19%). Abatacept therapy also was associated with greater improvements in the physical and mental component summaries of the SF-36 compared with placebo.

Clinical Experience with Subcutaneous Abatacept

Evidence of efficacy of subcutaneous abatacept in the management of psoriatic arthritis is based principally on the results of a randomized, double-blind, placebo-controlled phase 3 study (ASTRAEA) in 424 adults with active psoriatic arthritis despite DMARD therapy; to be enrolled in the study, patients were required to have at least 3 swollen and 3 tender joints, active plaque psoriasis with at least one qualifying skin lesion, and inadequate response or intolerance to at least one nonbiologic DMARD. Patients were randomized to receive abatacept (125 mg once weekly by subcutaneous injection without an IV loading dose) or placebo. Most patients (61%) had received prior therapy with one or more TNF blocking agents. Those receiving stable dosages of conventional (nonbiologic) DMARDs (methotrexate, leflunomide, sulfasalazine, hydroxychloroquine), low-dose oral corticosteroids (equivalent to 10 mg of prednisone daily or less), and/or NSAIAs could continue such agents during the study; approximately 61, 13, or 26% of patients in the treatment group received concomitant therapy with methotrexate, other nonbiologic DMARDs, or corticosteroids, respectively. At week 16, patients with less than 20% improvement from baseline in both swollen and tender joint counts entered early escape and were switched to open-label treatment with once-weekly abatacept. At week 24, all remaining patients were switched to open-label abatacept treatment, which was continued until week 52. At that time, patients could enter an optional 1-year open-label treatment extension.

The primary outcome measure in this study was the proportion of patients achieving an ACR 20 response at week 24. Progression of radiographically assessed structural damage was evaluated using the van der Heijde-Sharp score modified for assessment of psoriatic arthritis. Physical function was assessed using the HAQ-DI.

ACR 20 response was achieved at 24 weeks in a greater proportion of patients receiving subcutaneous abatacept compared with those receiving placebo (39 versus 22%); responses were observed regardless of prior therapy with TNF blocking agents or concomitant use of nonbiologic DMARDs. ACR 50 or ACR 70 response was achieved at week 24 in 19 or 10%, respectively, of those receiving abatacept and 12 or 7%, respectively, of those receiving placebo. Improvements in dactylitis and enthesitis also were observed in abatacept-treated patients. Although abatacept was associated with a numerically higher HAQ-DI response rate (31 versus 24%; defined as a reduction from baseline of 0.35 or more) at week 24, the difference between the abatacept and placebo groups was not significant; nominal improvements in the adjusted mean change in HAQ-DI score from baseline to week 24 were observed in abatacept-treated patients compared with placebo recipients. In this study, 43% of patients receiving abatacept and 33% of those receiving placebo had no progression of structural damage, as assessed by the modified van der Heijde-Sharp score, from baseline to week 24. ACR responses observed at week 24 were maintained during treatment periods of up to 1 year.

Clinical Perspective

The American College of Rheumatology and the National Psoriasis Foundation issued a joint guideline for the treatment of psoriatic arthritis in 2018. Various agents and medication classes are used to treat psoriatic arthritis, with some classes being used for symptom management (e.g., NSAIAs, corticosteroids) and others being used as immunomodulatory disease-modifying therapy. Disease-modifying treatments for psoriatic arthritis include oral small molecules (e.g., methotrexate, sulfasalazine, cyclosporine, leflunomide, apremilast), biologic DMARDs (e.g., TNF blocking agents, secukinumab, ixekizumab, ustekinumab, brodalumab, abatacept), and/or targeted synthetic DMARDs (e.g., tofacitinib). Specific agents for psoriatic arthritis treatment are selected according to disease characteristics, including disease severity, as well as patient preferences/values and comorbidities. A "treat-to-target" approach is typically employed, with the goal of achieving low/minimal disease activity or remission.

For patients with treatment-naive psoriatic arthritis, TNF blocking agents, oral small molecules, and secukinumab, ixekizumab, or brodalumab are conditionally recommended as initial treatment options. For patients with active psoriatic arthritis despite treatment with an oral small molecule, switching to monotherapy with a TNF blocking agent, secukinumab, ixekizumab, brodalumab, or ustekinumab is conditionally recommended over switching to abatacept. For patients with active psoriatic arthritis despite treatment with TNF blocking agent monotherapy, switching to monotherapy with a different TNF blocking agent, secukinumab, ixekizumab, brodalumab, or ustekinumab is conditionally recommended over switching to abatacept. Abatacept may be considered in place of these therapies based on patient-specific factors including contraindications to the use of TNF blocking agents, serious or recurrent infections, desire for IV dosing, or demyelinating disease. Recommendations for the use and selection of disease-modifying therapies in psoriatic arthritis vary based on the presence of certain disease characteristics (e.g., psoriatic spondylitis/axial disease, enthesitis) and comorbidities (e.g., inflammatory bowel disease, diabetes). Consult the American College of Rheumatology/National Psoriasis Foundation guideline for additional details.

● Acute Graft-Versus-Host Disease Prophylaxis

Abatacept is used in combination with a calcineurin inhibitor and methotrexate for the prophylaxis of acute graft-versus-host disease (GVHD) in adults and pediatric patients ≥2 years of age undergoing hematopoietic stem cell transplantation (HSCT) from a matched or 1 allele-mismatched unrelated donor. Safety and efficacy of abatacept for this use are based principally on the results of a 2-cohort multicenter clinical study, with support from an additional clinical study. The place in therapy for abatacept for prophylaxis of GVHD in patients undergoing HSCT from an unrelated donor has not yet been defined.

Clinical Experience with IV Abatacept

Evidence of clinical benefit of IV abatacept for the prophylaxis of acute GVHD is based principally on the results of a multicenter clinical study (GVHD-1 or ABA2) that included 2 strata of patients ≥6 years of age who underwent HSCT from an unrelated donor: 1) a single-arm, open-label study that enrolled 43 patients who underwent 7 of 8 human leukocyte antigen (HLA)-matched HSCT and 2) a randomized, double-blind, placebo-controlled stratum that enrolled 142 patients who underwent 8 of 8 HLA-matched HSCT. Patients in both strata received IV abatacept 10 mg/kg per dose (maximum dose 1 g) on the day before HSCT and on days 5, 14, and 28 after HSCT, in combination with methotrexate on days 1, 3, 6, and 11 after HSCT and a calcineurin inhibitor (cyclosporine or tacrolimus). Myeloablative regimens for pretransplant conditioning included busulfan/fludarabine, busulfan/cyclophosphamide, total body irradiation/cyclophosphamide, or fludarabine/melphalan. Patients from the single-arm, open-label study were compared to a prespecified control group from the Center for International Blood and Marrow Transplant Research; the randomized double-blinded trial compared abatacept to placebo. In the 7 of 8 HLA-matched single arm cohort at baseline, the median age was 38 years (range: 6–76); 63% of patients were male, and 72% were white. In the 8 of 8 HLA-matched randomized cohort, the median age of patients in the abatacept and placebo groups was 44 years (range: 6–71) and 40 years (range: 7–74), respectively; 56 and 54% of patients were male, and 86 and 88% were white in the respective treatment groups.

The primary outcome measure in both strata of the study was the cumulative incidence of severe (grade 3–4) acute GVHD at day 100 post-transplantation; grade 2–4 acute GVHD at day 180 post-transplantation and overall survival were assessed as secondary outcomes.

In the 7/8 HLA-matched cohort at day 180, the rates of grade 3–4 acute GVHD-free survival, grade 2–4 acute GVHD-free survival, and overall survival were 95, 53, and 98%, respectively. In the 8/8 HLA-matched cohort, no difference in grade 3–4 acute GVHD at day 100 was found between abatacept and placebo. However, secondary outcomes were improved with abatacept compared to

placebo at 180 days: the grade 2–4 acute GVHD-free survival rate was 50 versus 32% among patients treated with abatacept and placebo respectively, and the overall survival rate was 97 and 84%, respectively.

A second clinical study (GVHD-2) was conducted using data from the Center for International Blood and Marrow Transplant Research to compare outcomes between patients ≥6 years of age who underwent HSCT from a 1-allele mismatched unrelated donor. The study included 54 patients treated with abatacept plus a calcineurin inhibitor and methotrexate comprised of 42 patients from the GVHD-1 study and 12 additional patients. Patients were compared to a control group of 162 patients who were treated with a calcineurin inhibitor plus methotrexate alone. At 180 days post-HSCT, overall survival was 98% in the abatacept group compared to 75% in the control group.

Clinical Perspective

Prophylactic treatment of GVHD is necessary in patients undergoing allogeneic HSCT to ensure viability of the graft. Prophylaxis of GVHD in patients undergoing HLA-matched HSCT consists of T-cell suppression with calcineurin inhibitors (i.e., tacrolimus, cyclosporine) in combination with antimetabolites (i.e., methotrexate, mycophenolate mofetil). Recombinant anti-thymocyte globulin is also recommended as part of the conditioning regimen to prevent GVHD in patients undergoing matched HSCT from an unrelated donor. The place in therapy for abatacept for prophylaxis of GVHD in patients undergoing HSCT from an unrelated donor has not yet been defined.

DOSAGE AND ADMINISTRATION

● General

Pretreatment Screening

- Evaluate for active and latent tuberculosis infection prior to initiation of therapy; initiate antimycobacterial therapy, if indicated.

- Evaluate for viral hepatitis infection prior to initiating abatacept.

Patient Monitoring

- Monitor patients for infections, including Epstein-Barr virus (EBV) reactivation and cytomegalovirus (CMV) infection or reactivation, during treatment with abatacept for prophylaxis of graft-versus-host disease (GVHD) following hematopoietic stem cell transplantation (HSCT).

- Perform periodic skin examinations during treatment with abatacept, particularly in patients at risk for skin cancer.

Premedication and Prophylaxis

- Prior to initiation of abatacept for GVHD and for 6 months following HSCT, administer appropriate prophylaxis for EBV reactivation and consider additional prophylaxis for CMV infection or reactivation.

Other General Considerations

- Abatacept may be used as monotherapy or in combination with certain other drugs when used to treat rheumatoid arthritis, juvenile idiopathic arthritis, or psoriatic arthritis; must be used in combination with a calcineurin inhibitor and methotrexate when used for prophylaxis of acute GVHD.

- Concomitant use of abatacept and other potent immunosuppressants (e.g., biologic disease-modifying antirheumatic drugs [DMARDs], Janus kinase inhibitors) is not recommended.

- Update immunizations according to current immunization guidelines in adults and pediatric patients prior to initiating therapy.

● Administration

Administer abatacept by IV infusion or subcutaneous injection for the management of rheumatoid arthritis or psoriatic arthritis in adults and for the management of polyarticular juvenile idiopathic arthritis in pediatric patients ≥6 years of age; administer abatacept by subcutaneous injection only in children 2 to less than 6 years of age with polyarticular juvenile idiopathic arthritis.

Administer abatacept by subcutaneous injection only in children ≥2 years of age with psoriatic arthritis.

Administer abatacept by IV infusion only for prophylaxis of GVHD in adults and pediatric patients ≥2 years of age.

IV Administration

For IV infusion, abatacept is commercially available as a lyophilized powder that must be reconstituted and diluted prior to administration using proper aseptic technique. Complete IV infusion of the drug within 24 hours of reconstitution of abatacept lyophilized powder.

Use a sterile, nonpyrogenic, low-protein-binding filter with a pore diameter of 0.2–1.2 μm for administration. Visually inspect diluted solutions of the drug for particulate matter and discoloration prior to administration and discard if either is present. Information on physical and/or chemical compatibility of abatacept with other drugs is not available; the manufacturer recommends that abatacept not be infused through the same IV line as other drugs.

Reconstitution

Reconstitute commercially available abatacept lyophilized powder by adding 10 mL of sterile water for injection to a vial labeled as containing 250 mg of the drug to produce a solution containing 25 mg/mL. Reconstitute the appropriate number of vials of the drug based on the indicated dosage of abatacept. Use vials containing lyophilized abatacept only if a vacuum is present. During reconstitution, direct the sterile water for injection toward the side of the vial using the **silicone-free disposable syringe** provided by the manufacturer and an 18- to 21-gauge needle; gently swirl the contents to minimize foaming during dissolution. Do not shake the vial, and avoid prolonged or vigorous agitation. If abatacept lyophilized powder is inadvertently reconstituted using a siliconized syringe, the solution may develop translucent particles and should be discarded. If the silicone-free disposable syringe is dropped or becomes contaminated, use a new silicone-free disposable syringe; additional silicone-free syringes may be obtained from the manufacturer by calling 800-673-6242 (800-ORENCIA). Upon complete dissolution, insert a vent needle into the vial to dissipate any foam that may be present. The reconstituted solution should be colorless to pale yellow; do not use if opaque particles, discoloration, or other foreign particles are present.

Dilution

Further dilute reconstituted abatacept with 0.9% sodium chloride injection to provide a total volume of 100 mL (i.e., if a 100-mL bottle or bag of 0.9% sodium chloride injection is used, remove a volume of diluent equal to the total required volume of reconstituted abatacept solution from the bag or bottle prior to addition of the abatacept solution). Slowly add the total required volume of reconstituted solution to the diluent using the same **silicone-free disposable syringe** used for reconstitution and gently mix the diluted solution. Do not shake the infusion solution. The final concentration of the abatacept infusion solution depends on the amount of abatacept added but will not exceed 10 mg/mL. Immediately discard any unused portion of abatacept reconstituted solution. Diluted solutions of the drug may be stored at room temperature or refrigerated at 2–8°C; discard the infusion solution if not used within 24 hours of reconstitution.

Rate of Administration

Infuse diluted abatacept solution IV over 30 minutes when used to treat rheumatoid arthritis, juvenile idiopathic arthritis, or adults with psoriatic arthritis. Infuse diluted abatacept solution over 60 minutes when used for prophylaxis of GVHD.

Subcutaneous Administration

For subcutaneous administration, abatacept is commercially available as a clear to slightly opalescent, colorless to pale yellow solution in single-use prefilled syringes equipped with a 29-gauge, ½-inch needle and in single-use prefilled auto-injectors equipped with a 27-gauge, ½-inch needle. Abatacept in prefilled syringes and auto-injectors is *not* intended for IV administration.

Abatacept is intended for subcutaneous use under the guidance and supervision of a clinician; however, abatacept may be *self-administered* by subcutaneous injection if the clinician determines that the patient and/or their caregiver is competent to safely administer the drug after appropriate training and with medical follow-up as necessary. Pediatric patients may self-administer the subcutaneous formulation if both the clinician and caregiver determine that self-administration is appropriate. The manufacturer states that the ability of pediatric patients to self-administer the drug using the auto-injector has not been tested.

Prior to subcutaneous administration, visually inspect abatacept injection for particulate matter and discoloration; do not use if the solution is cloudy or discolored or contains particulates. Store abatacept injection at 2–8°C in the original carton until administration and protect from light. Do not freeze the injection. During travel, store abatacept prefilled syringes and auto-injectors in a cool carrier at 2–8°C.

Allow the abatacept prefilled syringe or auto-injector to sit at room temperature for 30 minutes prior to administration; do not warm the solution in any other way (e.g., microwave, immersion in warm water). Do not remove the syringe or auto-injector needle cover while the drug is warming to room temperature.

Inject abatacept subcutaneously into the anterior thigh or abdomen; abdominal injections should not be made within 5.08 cm (2 inches) of the umbilicus. Abatacept may be administered into the upper outer arm by a caregiver. Inject the full amount of solution in the prefilled syringe or auto-injector. Rotate injection sites. Do not inject into areas where the skin is tender, bruised, red, scaly, or hard, or into scars or stretch marks.

● Dosage

Rheumatoid Arthritis

For IV use in the management of rheumatoid arthritis in adults, dosage of abatacept is based on the patient's weight. Individuals weighing less than 60 kg should receive doses of 500 mg, those weighing 60–100 kg should receive doses of 750 mg, and those weighing more than 100 kg should receive doses of 1 g. Administer abatacept by IV infusion over 30 minutes at 0, 2, and 4 weeks and once every 4 weeks thereafter.

For subcutaneous use in the management of rheumatoid arthritis in adults, the recommended dosage of abatacept is 125 mg administered once weekly by subcutaneous injection. A single optional loading dose may be administered by IV infusion within one day prior to the initial subcutaneous dose; if an IV loading dose is used, the recommended dose is 500 mg in individuals weighing less than 60 kg, 750 mg in those weighing 60–100 kg, and 1 g in those weighing more than 100 kg. In patients being switched from IV to subcutaneous therapy, give the initial subcutaneous dose of abatacept in place of the next scheduled IV dose of the drug.

Juvenile Idiopathic Arthritis

For IV use in the management of polyarticular juvenile idiopathic arthritis in pediatric patients *≥6 years of age* who weigh less than 75 kg, the usual dosage of abatacept is 10 mg/kg administered by IV infusion over 30 minutes at 0, 2, and 4 weeks and once every 4 weeks thereafter. Pediatric patients weighing 75 kg or more may receive the adult IV dosage (maximum dose 1 g).

For subcutaneous use in the management of polyarticular juvenile idiopathic arthritis in pediatric patients *2 years of age or older*, dosage of abatacept is based on the patient's weight. Pediatric patients weighing 10 kg to less than 25 kg should receive doses of 50 mg, those weighing 25 kg to less than 50 kg should receive doses of 87.5 mg, and those weighing 50 kg or more should receive doses of 125 mg. Administer doses once weekly by subcutaneous injection *without* an IV loading dose.

Psoriatic Arthritis

For IV use in the management of psoriatic arthritis in adults, dosage of abatacept is based on the patient's weight. Individuals weighing less than 60 kg should receive doses of 500 mg, those weighing 60–100 kg should receive doses of 750 mg, and those weighing more than 100 kg should receive doses of 1 g. Administer abatacept by IV infusion over 30 minutes at 0, 2, and 4 weeks and once every 4 weeks thereafter.

For subcutaneous use in the management of psoriatic arthritis in adults, the recommended dosage of abatacept is 125 mg administered once weekly by subcutaneous injection. An IV loading dose is *not* required. In patients being switched from IV to subcutaneous therapy, give the initial subcutaneous dose of abatacept in place of the next scheduled IV dose of the drug.

For subcutaneous use in the management of psoriatic arthritis in pediatric patients *2 years of age or older*, dosage of abatacept is based on the patient's weight. Pediatric patients weighing 10 kg to less than 25 kg should receive doses of 50 mg, those weighing 25 kg to less than 50 kg should receive doses of 87.5 mg, and those weighing 50 kg or more should receive doses of 125 mg. Administer doses once weekly.

Acute Graft-Versus-Host Disease Prophylaxis

For prophylaxis of acute GVHD in patients ≥6 years of age undergoing hematopoietic stem cell transplantation (HSCT), the usual dosage of abatacept is 10 mg/kg (maximum dose 1 g) administered by IV infusion over 60 minutes on the day before HSCT and on days 5, 14, and 28 after HSCT.

For prophylaxis of acute GVHD in patients 2 to <6 years of age undergoing HSCT, administer abatacept 15 mg/kg by IV infusion over 60 minutes on the day before HSCT, followed by 12 mg/kg on days 5, 14, and 28 after HSCT.

● Special Populations

Hepatic Impairment

The manufacturer makes no specific dosage recommendations at this time for patients with hepatic impairment.

Renal Impairment

The manufacturer makes no specific dosage recommendations at this time for patients with renal impairment.

Geriatric Patients

The manufacturer makes no specific dosage recommendations at this time for geriatric patients.

CAUTIONS

● Contraindications

● None.

● Warnings/Precautions

Hypersensitivity Reactions

Hypersensitivity reactions (e.g., anaphylaxis, angioedema), including life-threatening or fatal events, have occurred in patients receiving abatacept. Fatal anaphylaxis has occurred after the initial IV infusion of the drug, and angioedema has occurred after the initial dose or with subsequent doses of the drug; the onset of angioedema has occurred within hours of administration but also has been delayed (i.e., by days) in some cases. Other events (e.g., hypotension, urticaria, dyspnea) potentially associated with hypersensitivity to abatacept have been reported.

Have appropriate treatment measures readily available for use in the event of a hypersensitivity reaction. If an anaphylactic or other serious allergic reaction occurs, immediately stop administration of the drug, and permanently discontinue therapy.

Infectious Complications

The possibility exists for agents that inhibit T-cell activation, including abatacept, to affect host defenses against infection because T cells mediate cellular immune responses. Serious and sometimes fatal infections have been reported in patients receiving abatacept. Serious infections have occurred in 3 or 1.9% of patients with rheumatoid arthritis receiving IV abatacept or placebo, respectively, in clinical trials. Serious infections reported in clinical trials include sepsis, pneumonia, cellulitis, urinary tract infection, bronchitis, diverticulitis, and acute pyelonephritis. Patients often were receiving concomitant therapy with immunosuppressive agents that, in addition to their underlying condition, could have predisposed them to infection.

Data from clinical trials indicate that the risk of infection and of serious infection is increased in patients with rheumatoid arthritis receiving concomitant therapy with abatacept and a tumor necrosis factor (TNF; TNF-α) blocking agent (e.g., adalimumab, etanercept, infliximab) compared with those receiving a TNF blocking agent alone. The rate of infection or serious infection was 63 or 4.4%, respectively, in those receiving concomitant therapy with abatacept and a TNF blocking agent and 43 or 0.8%, respectively, in those receiving a TNF blocking agent alone. In addition, concomitant therapy with abatacept and a TNF blocking agent did not demonstrate enhanced clinical benefit relative to the TNF blocking agent alone. Concomitant use of abatacept and a TNF blocking agent is not recommended. Monitor patients being switched from a TNF blocking agent to abatacept

for infection. In addition, concomitant use of abatacept with other biologic antirheumatic therapies or with Janus kinase (JAK) inhibitors is not recommended.

Exercise caution when considering abatacept therapy in patients with a history of recurring infections, underlying conditions that may predispose them to infections, or chronic, latent, or localized infections. Closely monitor any patient who develops a new infection while receiving abatacept; discontinue the drug in patients who develop a serious infection.

Evaluate all patients for latent tuberculosis prior to initiation of abatacept therapy. Abatacept has not been evaluated in patients with latent tuberculosis infection, and safety of therapy with the drug in such individuals is unknown. When indicated, initiate an appropriate antimycobacterial regimen for the treatment of latent tuberculosis infection prior to abatacept therapy.

Use of antirheumatic drugs has been associated with reactivation of hepatitis B virus (HBV) infection in patients who are carriers of the virus (i.e., hepatitis B surface antigen-positive [HBsAg-positive]). Prior to initiation of abatacept therapy, patients should be tested for chronic HBV infection according to recommendations from published guidelines. Individuals with chronic HBV infection were excluded from clinical studies that evaluated abatacept.

Cytomegalovirus and Epstein-Barr Virus Reactivation in Acute GVHD Prophylaxis after Hematopoietic Stem Cell Transplantation

Posttransplant lymphoproliferative disorder (PTLD) has occurred in patients who received abatacept for prophylaxis of acute graft-versus-host disease (GVHD) during hematopoietic stem cell transplantation (HSCT) from an unrelated donor. Four of 116 patients (3.4%) who received abatacept in the GVHD-1 clinical trial developed PTLD; all PTLD events were related to infection with Epstein-Barr virus (EBV). Of the four patients who developed a PTLD, three were seropositive for EBV at baseline and one was seronegative for EBV at baseline with an unknown donor EBV serology. Three of the 4 patients discontinued EBV prophylaxis by posttransplantation day 30; onset of PTLD occurred between 49–89 days posttransplantation. Monitor patients for evidence of EBV reactivation according to institutional guidance and provide EBV prophylaxis for 6 months after HSCT to prevent EBV-related PTLD.

Invasive cytomegalovirus (CMV) disease has also occurred in patients who received abatacept for prophylaxis of acute GVHD during unrelated HSCT. Of 116 patients who received abatacept in the GVHD-1 trial, 7% experienced invasive CMV diseases through posttransplantation day 225; most cases involved the gastrointestinal tract. The median time to onset was 91 days after HSCT. All patients who developed invasive CMV disease were seropositive at baseline. Monitor patients for evidence of CMV infection or reactivation for 6 months posttransplantation, regardless of donor and recipient CMV serology prior to transplantation, and consider initiation of CMV prophylaxis.

Immunization

Do not administer live virus vaccines to patients receiving abatacept or within 3 months after discontinuance of the drug. No data are available on the secondary transmission of infection by live virus vaccines in abatacept-treated patients. Patients receiving abatacept may receive inactivated vaccines. However, because abatacept interferes with the immune response to antigens, vaccine efficacy may be reduced in patients receiving the drug.

It is not known if abatacept can cross the placenta when administered to a pregnant woman or whether the immune response of an infant exposed to abatacept in utero and subsequently administered a live vaccine is affected. Consider the risks and benefits prior to administering live vaccines in such infants.

Immunizations should be updated according to current administration guidelines prior to initiation of abatacept therapy.

Exacerbation of Chronic Obstructive Pulmonary Disease

In a controlled clinical trial in patients with rheumatoid arthritis, adverse effects including exacerbations of chronic obstructive pulmonary disease (COPD), cough, rhonchi, and dyspnea were reported more frequently in patients with COPD who received abatacept compared with those who received placebo; serious adverse events were reported in 27% of patients with COPD receiving abatacept compared with 6% of those receiving placebo. Caution and careful monitoring for worsening of respiratory function are advised if abatacept is used in patients with coexisting COPD.

Malignancies and Lymphoproliferative Disorders

The possibility exists for agents that inhibit T-cell activation, including abatacept, to affect host defenses against malignancies because T cells mediate cellular immune responses. Lymphoma has occurred in patients with rheumatoid arthritis receiving IV abatacept in clinical trials; the rate of lymphoma was approximately 3.5-fold higher than the rate expected in the general population. Patients with rheumatoid arthritis, especially those with highly active disease, may be at increased risk of lymphoma. In clinical trials in patients with rheumatoid arthritis, lung cancer has been reported more frequently in abatacept-treated patients than placebo-treated patients. Other malignancies (myelodysplastic syndrome, melanoma, breast, bile duct, bladder, cervical, endometrial, ovarian, prostate, renal, thyroid, uterine, and nonmelanoma skin cancer) also have occurred. The effect of abatacept on the development and course of malignancies has not been fully determined.

Because skin cancer has been reported in patients receiving abatacept, periodic dermatologic evaluations are recommended for all patients receiving the drug, particularly for those who are at increased risk for skin cancer.

Blood Glucose Testing

Parenteral preparations containing maltose, including abatacept lyophilized powder for IV infusion, may cause falsely elevated results in blood glucose determinations that use nonspecific methods based on glucose dehydrogenase pyrroloquinolinequinone (GDH-PQQ). Only glucose-specific test methods that are not affected by maltose (e.g., methods that use glucose dehydrogenase nicotine adenine dinucleotide [GDH-NAD], glucose oxidase, glucose hexokinase) should be used to measure blood glucose concentrations in patients receiving this formulation of abatacept.

Because abatacept injection for subcutaneous use does not contain maltose, special glucose monitoring precautions are not required in patients receiving this formulation of the drug.

Immunogenicity

Development of binding antibodies to abatacept or its cytotoxic T-lymphocyte-associated antigen 4 (CTLA-4) component has been reported in 1–2% of adults with rheumatoid arthritis receiving IV or subcutaneous therapy with abatacept. Because trough concentrations of abatacept can interfere with assay results, antibody development was assessed in a subset of patients who had discontinued IV abatacept therapy for more than 56 days; in this subset of patients, binding antibodies to the CTLA-4 component were confirmed in 9 patients (6%), and 6 of the 9 patients had neutralizing antibodies.

In a study of the immunogenicity of subcutaneous abatacept (used in conjunction with methotrexate) in adults with rheumatoid arthritis, development of antibodies to abatacept or its CTLA-4 component was reported at the end of the 9-month study in 3% of patients regardless of whether abatacept was given continuously for 9 months or the 9-month treatment period included a 3-month interruption (during months 4–6) in abatacept administration. At month 6, antibodies to abatacept or its CTLA-4 component were detected in 0% of those who had received abatacept continuously for 6 months and in 10% of those who had received the drug for only the first 3 months of the 6-month period.

Development of binding antibodies to abatacept or its CTLA-4 component has been reported in pediatric patients with juvenile idiopathic arthritis receiving IV abatacept. Antibodies generally were transient and present in low titers. Antibodies to the CTLA-4 component of the drug were detected in 41% of patients who discontinued abatacept for periods of up to 6 months and in 13% of those who received continuous abatacept therapy; neutralizing antibodies were detected in 8 of 20 patients (40%) with samples evaluable for neutralizing activity.

No apparent effect of antibody development on the safety, efficacy, or pharmacokinetics of abatacept has been observed. No serious acute infusion-related reactions were observed in pediatric patients with juvenile idiopathic arthritis who resumed abatacept therapy following treatment interruption for periods of up to 6 months.

In clinical trials of patients undergoing HSCT who were treated with a 4-dose regimen of abatacept for prophylaxis of acute GVHD, no patients developed antibodies to abatacept during the 28-day treatment period. During the off-treatment period (days 29–180 after transplantation), 6.6% of 91 immunogenicity evaluable subjects were positive for antibodies to the CTLA-4 component of the drug; 4 of the 6 positive patients had at least 1 sample positive for neutralization activity.

Since patients positive for immunogenicity only had samples positive for anti-drug antibodies during the off-treatment period, the impact of these findings on the pharmacokinetics, safety, and efficacy of abatacept are not known.

Specific Populations

Pregnancy

There are no adequate and well-controlled studies of abatacept in pregnant women. Available data on use of the drug in pregnant women are insufficient to inform a drug-associated risk. It is not known if abatacept can cross the placenta when administered to a pregnant woman or whether the immune response of infants exposed to abatacept in utero and subsequently administered a live vaccine is affected.

The safety of administering live vaccines to infants who were exposed to abatacept in utero is unknown, and the risks and benefits should be considered prior to vaccinating such infants.

In reproductive toxicology studies in rats and rabbits, no embryotoxicity or fetal malformations were observed at abatacept exposure levels of approximately 29 times the exposure at the maximum recommended human dosage (MRHD) of 10 mg/kg per month. However, in a prenatal and postnatal development study in rats, effects on immune function (i.e., 9-fold increase in T-cell-dependent antibody response, thyroiditis) were observed in female offspring at abatacept exposure levels of 11 times the MRHD. It is unknown whether immunologic effects in rats are indicative of a risk for autoimmune disease development in humans who were exposed to abatacept in utero. Exposure to abatacept in juvenile rats, which may be more representative of the fetal human immune system, resulted in immune system abnormalities including inflammation of the thyroid and pancreas.

Lactation

It is not known whether abatacept is distributed into milk in humans; the drug is distributed into milk in rats. Effects of abatacept on nursing infants and on milk production also are unknown.

Pediatric Use

Safety and efficacy of abatacept for the management of moderately to severely active polyarticular juvenile idiopathic arthritis have been established in pediatric patients ≥2 years of age; the drug may be used as monotherapy or in combination with methotrexate. Safety and efficacy of abatacept used in combination with a calcineurin inhibitor and methotrexate for prophylaxis of acute GVHD in patients undergoing HSCT from a matched or 1-allele mismatched unrelated donor have been established in pediatric patients ≥2 years of age. Safety and efficacy of abatacept for the treatment of psoriatic arthritis have been established in pediatric patients ≥2 years of age; the drug may be used as monotherapy or in combination with methotrexate. Safety and efficacy of abatacept have not been established in pediatric patients younger than 2 years of age or for pediatric uses other than polyarticular juvenile idiopathic arthritis, acute GVHD, and psoriatic arthritis.

Use of IV abatacept (in combination with a calcineurin inhibitor and methotrexate) for the prophylaxis of acute GVHD in pediatric patients ≥6 years of age undergoing HSCT from a matched or 1-allele mismatched unrelated donor is supported by controlled trials in adults and pediatric patients ≥6 years who were administered a dosage of 10 mg/kg on the day prior to transplantation and days 5, 14, and 28 posttransplantion. Use of IV abatacept for the prophylaxis of acute GVHD in pediatric patients 2 to less than 6 years of age is supported by pharmacokinetic modeling and simulations of drug exposure in such patients administered a dose of 15 mg/kg one day prior to HSCT, followed by a 12-mg/kg dose on days 5, 14, and 28 posttransplantation. The course of disease among patients <6 years of age and those ≥6 years of age is sufficiently similar to allow for this extrapolation of data.

Use of IV abatacept for the management of polyarticular juvenile idiopathic arthritis is supported by results of a randomized-withdrawal study evaluating efficacy, safety, and pharmacokinetics of IV abatacept in 190 pediatric patients 6–17 years of age; IV administration has not been evaluated in children younger than 6 years of age.

Use of subcutaneous abatacept for the management of polyarticular juvenile idiopathic arthritis is supported by results of an open-label pharmacokinetic and safety study of subcutaneous abatacept in 205 pediatric patients 2–17 years of age and evidence of efficacy for IV abatacept in pediatric patients with polyarticular juvenile idiopathic arthritis and for subcutaneous abatacept in adults with rheumatoid arthritis.

Use of subcutaneous abatacept for the treatment of psoriatic arthritis in pediatric patients ≥2 years of age is supported by results from well-controlled studies in adults with psoriatic arthritis; pharmacokinetic data from adults with rheumatoid arthritis or psoriatic arthritis and pediatric patients with polyarticular juvenile idiopathic arthritis; and safety data from pediatric studies of patients with polyarticular juvenile idiopathic arthritis using subcutaneous abatacept. The efficacy and safety of IV abatacept in pediatric patients with psoriatic arthritis have not been established.

Population pharmacokinetic analyses indicate that clearance of abatacept increases with body weight in pediatric patients 6–17 years of age receiving the drug by IV infusion. Consistent with these data for IV administration, population pharmacokinetic analyses of subcutaneous administration in pediatric patients 2–17 years of age indicate a trend toward higher clearance with increasing body weight.

In juvenile rats, administration of abatacept prior to immune system maturity (from day 4 to day 94) was associated with an increased incidence of fatal infections compared with that observed in control animals. Changes in T-cell subsets (e.g., increased T-helper cells, decreased T-regulatory cells) and inhibition of T-cell-dependent antibody responses also were observed. In addition, lymphocytic inflammation of the thyroid and pancreatic islets was observed once these animals reached adulthood. The relevance of these findings to humans is unknown since the immune system of rats is undeveloped in the first few weeks after birth. In studies in adult mice and monkeys, inhibition of T-cell-dependent antibody responses was observed, but increased rates of infection and mortality, altered T-helper cells, and inflammation of the thyroid and pancreas were not observed.

It is not known if abatacept can cross the placenta when administered to a pregnant woman or whether the immune response of infants exposed to abatacept in utero and subsequently administered a live vaccine is affected.

Geriatric Use

A total of 323 patients ≥65 years of age, including 53 patients ≥75 years of age, have received abatacept in clinical trials of patients with rheumatoid arthritis. Although no overall differences in safety or efficacy were observed between geriatric patients ≥65 years of age and younger adults, and other clinical experience has revealed no evidence of age-related differences in responses, the possibility that some older patients may exhibit increased sensitivity to the drug cannot be ruled out.

The incidence of serious infection and malignancy in abatacept-treated patients older than 65 years of age is higher than the incidence in younger adults receiving the drug. Because the overall incidence of infection and malignancy is higher in the geriatric population in general than in younger adults, abatacept should be used with caution in geriatric patients.

Among patients who received abatacept at a dosage of 10 mg/kg for acute GVHD prophylaxis in the GVHD-1 trial, 10% were ≥65 years of age and 2% were ≥75 years of age. Experience with abatacept for prophylaxis of acute GVHD in geriatric patients is insufficient to determine whether efficacy and safety of the drug are similar to those in younger adults.

Hepatic Impairment

Formal studies evaluating the effect of hepatic impairment on the pharmacokinetics of abatacept are lacking.

Renal Impairment

Formal studies evaluating the effect of renal impairment on the pharmacokinetics of abatacept are lacking.

● Common Adverse Effects

Adverse effects reported in ≥10% of patients receiving abatacept for rheumatoid arthritis include headache, upper respiratory tract infection, nasopharyngitis, and nausea. Adverse effects generally are similar following IV infusion or subcutaneous injection for patients receiving abatacept for rheumatoid arthritis.

In general, adverse events in pediatric patients with polyarticular juvenile idiopathic arthritis treated with IV abatacept were similar in frequency and type to those seen in adult patients with rheumatoid arthritis treated with IV abatacept. The adverse effect profile in patients with juvenile idiopathic arthritis treated with subcutaneous abatacept were consistent with the adverse effect profile in patients with IV abatacept.

The safety profile of abatacept was comparable when given IV or subcutaneously for the treatment of psoriatic arthritis, and also consistent with the safety profile of abatacept in patients with rheumatoid arthritis.

Adverse effects reported in ≥10% of patients receiving abatacept for prophylaxis of acute GVHD include anemia, hypertension, CMV reactivation or infection, pyrexia, pneumonia, epistaxis, decreased CD4 lymphocyte count, hypermagnesemia, and acute kidney injury.

DRUG INTERACTIONS

● Antirheumatic Drugs

Concomitant use of methotrexate, corticosteroids, or nonsteroidal anti-inflammatory agents (NSAIAs) does not affect clearance of abatacept.

Biologic Antirheumatic Drugs

An increased incidence of infection and serious infection, with no substantial increase in efficacy, was observed when abatacept and a tumor necrosis factor (TNF; TNF-α) blocking agent were used concomitantly. Clinical experience is insufficient to establish the safety and efficacy of concomitant use of abatacept and other biologic antirheumatic drugs. Concomitant use of abatacept and a TNF blocking agent or other biologic antirheumatic drug is not recommended.

Janus Kinase Inhibitors

Clinical experience is insufficient to establish the safety and efficacy of concomitant use of abatacept and Janus kinase (JAK) inhibitors. Concomitant use of abatacept and JAK inhibitors is not recommended.

● Vaccines

Live virus vaccines should not be administered to patients receiving abatacept or within 3 months following discontinuance of the drug.

DESCRIPTION

Abatacept, a recombinant fusion protein, consists of the extracellular domain of human cytotoxic T-lymphocyte-associated antigen 4 (CTLA-4) linked to a modified Fc portion of human immunoglobulin G_1 (IgG_1). The Fc component contains the hinge region, the C_H2 domain, and the C_H3 domain of IgG_1.

Evidence suggests that activation of T cells may play an important role in the immunopathology of rheumatoid arthritis, psoriatic arthritis, and polyarticular juvenile idiopathic arthritis. One of the first steps in T-cell activation is antigen recognition. Following antigen recognition, T cells require costimulation to become fully active. One of the costimulatory pathways involves interaction between CD28 on the T cell and CD80 or CD86 on the surface of the antigen-presenting cell. After T cell activation has occurred, expression of the inhibitory molecule CTLA-4 on the surface of the T cell is increased; CTLA-4 downregulates T-cell activation and has a much higher affinity for CD80 and CD86 than does CD28. Abatacept, like CTLA-4, competes with CD28 for CD80 and CD86 binding; by binding to CD80 and CD86 on antigen-presenting cells, abatacept prevents these molecules from engaging CD28 on T cells and thereby prevents delivery of the second costimulatory signal required for optimum activation of T cells.

In vitro, abatacept decreases T-cell proliferation and inhibits production of tumor necrosis factor (TNF, TNF-α), interferon gamma, and interleukin-2.

Following administration of multiple IV doses of abatacept in adults with rheumatoid arthritis, systemic exposure and peak serum concentrations of the drug are dose proportional over the dose range of 2–10 mg/kg; at a dosage of 10 mg/kg administered IV on days 1, 15, and 30 and then monthly thereafter, steady-state concentrations were achieved by day 60 and no systemic accumulation was observed with continued administration. In adults with psoriatic arthritis receiving abatacept at recommended IV weight-based dosages or as weekly 125-mg subcutaneous doses, steady-state concentrations were achieved by day 57. Following subcutaneous administration, abatacept exhibits linear pharmacokinetics and an absolute bioavailability of approximately 79%. Estimates of the terminal half-life of abatacept in adults with rheumatoid arthritis are similar following IV or subcutaneous administration (approximately 13–14 days). In patients ≥6 years of age undergoing hematopoietic stem cell transplantation (HSCT) from a matched or 1-allele mismatched unrelated donor who received abatacept 10 mg/kg IV, the terminal half-life was approximately 20 days. Clearance of abatacept tends to increase with increasing body weight, but age and sex (when corrected for body weight) do not affect clearance. Clearance of abatacept was reduced by 29% in patients who underwent 7/8 human leukocyte antigen (HLA)-matched HSCT compared to those who underwent 8/8 HLA-matched HSCT in population pharmacokinetic analyses.

ADVICE TO PATIENTS

- Advise patients to read the manufacturer's patient information.

- Advise patients that concomitant use of abatacept and other potent immunosuppressive agents (e.g., biologic DMARDs, JAK inhibitors) is not recommended.

- Immediately inform a clinician if signs or symptoms of an allergic reaction (e.g., urticaria, difficulty breathing, swelling of the face, eyelids, or lips) occur on the day of or the day after abatacept administration.

- Risk of serious infectious complications. Inform clinicians promptly if any signs or symptoms of infection occur.

- Inform patients to avoid live vaccines during abatacept therapy and for 3 months following discontinuance of the drug.

- Advise patients that the IV formulation of abatacept contains maltose and may cause falsely elevated glucose readings when blood glucose monitoring systems based on glucose dehydrogenase pyrroloquinolinequinone (GDH-PQQ) are used; importance of using glucose-specific test methods not affected by maltose.

- Stress importance of women informing clinicians if they are or plan to become pregnant or plan to breast-feed.

- Instruct the patient and/or caregiver regarding proper dosage and administration of abatacept, including the use of aseptic technique, and proper disposal of prefilled syringes and auto-injectors if it is determined that the patient and/or caregiver is competent to safely administer subcutaneous injections of the drug.

- Inform clinicians of existing or contemplated concomitant therapy, including prescription and OTC drugs, as well as any other illnesses (e.g., COPD; concomitant or recurrent infections; history of cancer, tuberculosis, or HBV infection).

- Inform patients of other important precautionary information.

PREPARATIONS

Excipients in commercially available drug preparations may have clinically important effects in some individuals; consult specific product labeling for details.

Abatacept

Parenteral		
For injection, for IV infusion	250 mg	Orencia® (available as a single-dose vial with a silicone-free disposable syringe), Bristol-Myers Squibb
Injection, for subcutaneous use	50 mg/0.4 mL	Orencia® (available as disposable prefilled syringe), Bristol-Myers Squibb
	87.5 mg/0.7 mL	Orencia® (available as disposable prefilled syringe), Bristol-Myers Squibb
	125 mg/mL	Orencia® (available as disposable prefilled syringe and prefilled auto-injector [ClickJect]®), Bristol-Myers Squibb

† Use is not currently included in the labeling approved by the US Food and Drug Administration.

Selected Revisions August 10, 2024, © Copyright, May 1, 2006, American Society of Health-System Pharmacists, Inc.

azaTHIOprine, azaTHIOprine Sodium

90:28.08.92 • ANTIMETABOLITES, IMMUNOSUPPRESSIVE THERAPY, MISCELLANEOUS

On 4/29/24, FDA alerted healthcare professionals of the rare risk of intrahepatic cholestasis of pregnancy (ICP) associated with the use of thiopurines (azathioprine, 6-mercaptopurine, and 6-thioguanine). Reported cases of ICP occurred among pregnant patients using azathioprine or 6-mercaptopurine primarily to treat inflammatory bowel disease (IBD), including Crohn's disease (CD) and ulcerative colitis (UC), or systemic lupus erythematosus (SLE). Thiopurines are not FDA-approved to treat these conditions; however, the American Gastroenterological Association and the American College of Rheumatology have published guidelines indicating that these drugs may be appropriate to continue on an individualized basis for the management of some immunologic conditions during pregnancy. Pregnant patients should stop using thiopurines if they develop ICP. FDA is requiring manufacturers to update labeling to include additional warning information on the risk of ICP associated with thiopurines. For additional information, see https://www.fda.gov/drugs/drug-safety-and-availability/fda-alerts-health-care-professionals-pregnancy-problems-associated-thiopurines

■ Azathioprine, a chemical analog of the physiologic purines adenine, guanine, and hypoxanthine, is a purine antagonist antimetabolite and an immunosuppressive agent.

USES

● Renal Allotransplantation

Azathioprine is used as an adjunct for prevention of the rejection of kidney allografts. The drug is usually used in conjunction with other immunosuppressive therapy including local radiation therapy, corticosteroids, and other cytotoxic agents.

The maximum effectiveness of azathioprine occurs when the drug is administered during the induction period of the antibody response, starting either at the time of antigenic stimulation or within 2 days following. Under certain conditions of pretreatment with mercaptopurine, followed by an interval of at least 5 days before administration of the antigen and no subsequent treatment, a paradoxical enhancement of antibody formation has been observed. The effects of azathioprine and its active metabolite, mercaptopurine, may not be observed until several days after initiation of therapy and may persist for several days after clearance of the compounds is completed.

● Rheumatoid Arthritis

Azathioprine is used for the management of the signs and symptoms of rheumatoid arthritis in adults. Azathioprine is one of several disease modifying antirheumatic drugs (DMARDs) that can be used when DMARD therapy is appropriate. (For further information on the treatment of rheumatoid arthritis, see Uses: Rheumatoid Arthritis, in Methotrexate 10:00.) Nonsteroidal anti-inflammatory agents (NSAIAs), including aspirin, and/or corticosteroids may be continued when treatment with azathioprine is initiated. The manufacturers state that combined use of azathioprine and other DMARDS has not been studied and is not recommended.

● Crohn's Disease

Azathioprine has been used in the management of moderately to severely or chronically active Crohn's disease†, and to maintain clinical remission in corticosteroid-dependent patients, and to provide benefit in patients with fistulizing Crohn's disease†.

Azathioprine (e.g., 2–3 mg/kg daily) has been used in conjunction with corticosteroids to induce remission in patients with mildly to severely active refractory Crohn's disease; however, onset of action of azathioprine is slow and several months usually are required to achieve clinical response. Therefore, the role, if any, of azathioprine in the management of acute disease activity is uncertain. Azathioprine is used in patients with chronically active corticosteroid-dependent Crohn's disease. Results of several placebo-controlled trials indicate that azathioprine may be effective in maintaining remission in patients with corticosteroid-induced clinical remissions and in allowing reduction of oral corticosteroid therapy in corticosteroid-dependent patients. In several studies, frequency of relapse associated with azathioprine has been substantially lower than that associated with placebo. Results of long-term follow-up studies indicate that treatment with azathioprine may be effective for up to 4 years. Limited data indicate that relapse rates after 4 years of immunosuppressive therapy may be similar whether therapy has been maintained or discontinued; however, further larger studies are needed to confirm such data.

Azathioprine also has been found effective in the management of fistulizing Crohn's disease. Current clinical practice concerning use of azathioprine is based on a point analysis of 5 controlled trials in which fistula closure was considered a secondary end point and on several uncontrolled case studies. Data from these studies indicate that long-term (several years) therapy with azathioprine may be effective in the management of fistulizing Crohn's disease. However, because there currently are no controlled studies employing fistula closure as a primary end point, additional study is needed to more clearly establish efficacy.

Azathioprine (1.5–2 mg/kg daily) has been used effectively in pediatric patients with refractory or corticosteroid-dependent Crohn's disease†. In these patients, therapy with azathioprine may result in improvement of disease symptoms and reduction of corticosteroid dosage, and frequency of hospitalization.

Risks and benefits of azathioprine therapy should be carefully considered in patients with inflammatory bowel disease†, especially in adolescents and young adults with the disease. Cases of hepatosplenic T-cell lymphoma have been reported in patients receiving azathioprine for the management of inflammatory bowel disease. (See Cautions: Malignancies and Lymphoproliferative Disorders.)

For more information on the management of Crohn's disease, see Uses: Crohn's Disease, in Mesalamine 56:36.

DOSAGE AND ADMINISTRATION

● Reconstitution and Administration

Azathioprine is usually administered orally. Following renal transplantation, azathioprine may initially be given IV to patients unable to tolerate oral medication. Oral therapy should replace parenteral therapy as soon as possible.

Since azathioprine is an antimetabolite, the manufacturer states that consideration should be given to handling and disposal according to guidelines issued for hazardous drugs (see the ASHP Guidelines on Handling Hazardous Drugs at http://www.ahfsdruginformation.com), although there is no general agreement that all of the procedures recommended in such guidelines are necessary or appropriate.

Azathioprine sodium powder for injection is reconstituted by adding 10 mL of sterile water for injection to a vial labeled as containing 100 mg of the drug. The resultant solution contains 10 mg/mL, and may be given by direct IV injection or further diluted in 0.9% sodium chloride or 5% dextrose injection for IV infusion. IV infusions of the drug are usually administered over 30–60 minutes; however, infusions have been given over periods ranging from 5 minutes to 8 hours.

Reconstituted solutions of azathioprine should be inspected visually prior to administration, whenever solution and container permit.

● Dosage

Dosage of azathioprine must be carefully adjusted and individualized according to the patient's response and tolerance. Dosage may need to be reduced in patients with impaired renal function. (See Cautions: Precautions and Contraindications.) Dosage of azathioprine sodium is expressed in terms of azathioprine. Azathioprine may be given as a single daily dose or in divided doses.

The manufacturers and some clinicians recommend that thiopurine methyl transferase (TPMT) phenotype or genotype be determined prior to initiation of azathioprine therapy, since risk of hematologic toxicity may be increased in patients with intermediate, low, or absent activity of the enzyme and decreased dosage or alternative therapy should be considered in these individuals. (See Pharmacokinetics: Elimination and see Cautions: Precautions and Contraindications.)

Renal Allotransplantation

The usual oral dosage of azathioprine in adults undergoing renal transplantation is 3–5 mg/kg daily beginning on the day of (and in some cases 1–3 days before) transplantation. Following transplantation, the drug may be given IV in the same dosage until the patient can tolerate oral therapy (usually 1–4 days). Dosage reduction to maintenance levels of 1–3 mg/kg daily is usually possible. When severe hematologic or other toxicity occurs, discontinuance of azathioprine therapy may be required even if rejection of the allograft may be a consequence of drug withdrawal.

Rheumatoid Arthritis

For the treatment of severe, active rheumatoid arthritis, the usual initial oral adult dosage of azathioprine is 1 mg/kg (approximately 50–100 mg) daily. If the initial response is unsatisfactory and no serious adverse effects occur after 6–8 weeks of therapy, daily dosage may be increased by 0.5 mg/kg; daily dosage may then be increased as necessary at 4-week intervals by 0.5 mg/kg up to a maximum of 2.5 mg/kg. A therapeutic response usually occurs after 6–8 weeks of therapy; an adequate trial should be a minimum of 12 weeks. Patients who do not respond after 12 weeks can be considered unresponsive to the drug. Therapy may be continued in patients who respond, but patients must be closely monitored and gradual dosage reduction to the lowest possible effective level should be attempted. Daily maintenance dosage may be reduced to the lowest possible effective level in increments of 0.5 mg/kg (or approximately 25 mg) every 4 weeks, while keeping other therapy constant. The optimum duration of maintenance therapy has not been determined. Azathioprine may be administered in a single or twice-daily doses.

Crohn's Disease

For the management of Crohn's disease†, adults have received an oral azathioprine dosage of 2–4 mg/kg daily, while pediatric patients have received 1.5–2 mg/kg daily.

CAUTIONS

• Malignancies and Lymphoproliferative Disorders

Chronic immunosuppression with azathioprine increases the risk of malignancy. Patients receiving immunosuppressive drugs, including azathioprine, are at increased risk of developing lymphoma and other malignancies, particularly of the skin. Malignancies, including posttransplant lymphoma and hepatosplenic T-cell lymphoma in patients with inflammatory bowel disease, have been reported. (See Cautions: Precautions and Contraindications.)

Renal transplant recipients have an increased risk of developing malignancy (e.g., skin cancer, reticulum cell sarcoma, lymphomas). The risk of posttransplant lymphomas may be increased in patients who receive aggressive treatment with immunosuppressive drugs, including azathioprine. Therefore, therapy with immunosuppressive drugs should be maintained at the lowest effective dosage.

The incidence of lymphoproliferative disease in patients with rheumatoid arthritis appears to be substantially higher than that in the general population. The precise risk of malignancy associated with azathioprine is unknown; however, evidence suggests that the risk may be elevated in patients with rheumatoid arthritis, although to a lesser extent than in renal transplant patients. Limited data are available on the incidence and risk of malignancy in patients with rheumatoid arthritis receiving azathioprine. In one study, the incidence of lymphoproliferative disease in patients with rheumatoid arthritis receiving higher-than-recommended doses of azathioprine was 1.8 cases per 1000 patient-years of follow-up compared with 0.8 cases per 1000 patient-years of follow-up in those not receiving the drug. However, the proportion of risk attributable to the azathioprine dosage or to other therapies (e.g., alkylating agents) in these patients has not been determined. Acute myelogenous leukemia and solid tumors have been reported in patients with rheumatoid arthritis who received the drug. Patients with rheumatoid arthritis who have previously been treated with alkylating agents (e.g., cyclophosphamide, chlorambucil, melphalan) may have a prohibitive risk of malignancy if treated with azathioprine.

Hepatosplenic T-cell lymphoma, a rare, aggressive, usually fatal type of T-cell lymphoma, has been reported during postmarketing experience mainly in adolescent and young adult males with Crohn's disease or ulcerative colitis who received treatment with thiopurine analogs (azathioprine or mercaptopurine) and/or

tumor necrosis factor (TNF) blocking agents. Although most of the reported cases occurred in patients who had received a combination of immunosuppressive agents, including TNF blocking agents and thiopurine analogs (azathioprine or mercaptopurine), cases have been reported in patients receiving azathioprine or mercaptopurine alone. As of December 31, 2010, the US Food and Drug Administration (FDA) had identified 12 cases of hepatosplenic T-cell lymphoma in patients with Crohn's disease or ulcerative colitis who had received azathioprine without concomitant or sequential immunosuppressive therapy. These 12 cases of hepatosplenic T-cell lymphoma occurred mostly in patients 15–45 years of age (median age: 21 years) following 4–17 years of azathioprine therapy; most of the patients were males, and 10 of the 12 cases were fatal. In addition, FDA identified 25 cases of hepatosplenic T-cell lymphoma in patients with Crohn's disease or ulcerative colitis who had received a TNF blocking agent (infliximab or both infliximab and adalimumab); in 22 of these cases, a thiopurine analog (azathioprine or mercaptopurine) was used concomitantly. In some cases, potential confounding factors could not be excluded because complete medical histories were not available. Since patients with certain conditions (e.g., Crohn's disease, rheumatoid arthritis) may be at increased risk for lymphoma, it may be difficult to measure the added risk of treatment with TNF blocking agents, azathioprine, and/or mercaptopurine. (See Cautions: Precautions and Contraindications.)

• Hematologic Effects

The principal toxic effect of azathioprine is bone marrow depression manifested by leukopenia, anemias including macrocytic anemia, pancytopenia, and thrombocytopenia, which may result in prolongation of clotting time and eventual hemorrhage. Hematologic effects are dose related and may be more severe in renal transplant patients whose allograft is undergoing rejection. Delayed hematologic suppression may occur. Hematologic status must be carefully monitored. (See Cautions: Precautions and Contraindications.)

When receiving usual dosages of azathioprine, patients with intermediate levels of thiopurine methyl transferase (TPMT) activity (about 10–11% of the population) may be at increased risk of developing myelotoxicity, while those with low or absent levels of the enzyme (0.3% of the population) are at increased risk of life-threatening myelotoxicity. Reduced dosage is recommended in patients with intermediate TPMT activity, while alternative therapy may be considered in those with low or absent levels of TPMT.

• GI Effects

Nausea, vomiting, anorexia, and diarrhea may occur in patients receiving large doses of azathioprine. Adverse GI effects may be minimized by giving the drug in divided doses and/or after meals. Vomiting with abdominal pain may occur rarely with a hypersensitivity pancreatitis.

A GI hypersensitivity reaction characterized by severe nausea and vomiting has been reported. This reaction also may be accompanied by diarrhea, rash, fever, malaise, myalgias, elevations in liver enzymes, and, occasionally, hypotension. Symptoms of GI toxicity most often develop within the first several weeks of azathioprine therapy and are reversible upon discontinuance of the drug. The reaction can occur within several hours after rechallange with a single dose of the drug.

Other adverse GI effects include ulceration of the mucous membranes of the mouth, esophagitis with possible ulceration, and steatorrhea.

• Hepatic Effects

Hepatotoxicity manifested by increased serum alkaline phosphatase, bilirubin, and/or aminotransferase concentrations may occur in patients receiving azathioprine, principally in allograft recipients. Azathioprine-induced hepatotoxicity following transplantation occurs most frequently within 6 months of transplantation and is generally reversible following discontinuance of the drug. Rare, but life-threatening hepatic veno-occlusive disease has occurred during chronic azathioprine therapy in several renal allograft recipients and in a patient with panuveitis; serious complications, including progressive portal hypertension, progressive liver failure requiring a portacaval shunt, progressive chronic liver failure with portal hypertension and esophageal varices, and/or rapid deterioration resulting in death, occurred in most of these patients. Veno-occlusive disease was associated with cytomegalovirus infection in some of these patients and with use of azathioprine but not with dosage of the drug, type or duration of renal allograft, or type of underlying renal disease. Reports to date suggest that the onset of hepatic veno-occlusive disease generally occurs after 1–2 years of therapy and that the disease occurs principally in males. The clinical syndrome is usually manifested initially by jaundice, often followed by the development of ascites and other signs of portal hypertension. Serum alkaline phosphatase and bilirubin concentrations are usually elevated. Prognosis is poor. Because hepatic veno-occlusive disease may result in rapid clinical deterioration, prompt diagnosis and therapeutic intervention are necessary. Many clinicians suggest that liver biopsy to diagnose veno-occlusive disease should be performed in renal allograft recipients receiving azathioprine at the first sign of mild hepatic dysfunction. If veno-occlusive disease is evident, azathioprine therapy should be promptly and permanently discontinued; alternative immunosuppressive therapy should be considered and, if liver failure is progressive, anticoagulation, a portacaval shunt, or hepatic allotransplantation should be considered.

Hepatotoxicity occurs in less than 1% of patients with rheumatoid arthritis who receive azathioprine.

● Other Adverse Effects

Azathioprine may also cause rash, infection, drug fever, serum sickness, alopecia, arthralgia, retinopathy, Raynaud's disease, reversible interstitial pneumonitis, and pulmonary edema. Some of these adverse effects can occur as manifestations of rare hypersensitivity reactions. Azathioprine-induced hypersensitivity reactions are often characterized by a combination of symptoms, including fever, rigors, musculoskeletal symptoms (arthralgias, myalgias), and/or cutaneous effects (generalized erythematous or maculopapular rash with nonspecific inflammatory changes demonstrated on biopsy); pulmonary manifestations (e.g., cough and/or dyspnea) and hypotension (which may be severe and, in the presence of fever, mimic septic shock) may also occur. Sweet's syndrome (acute febrile neutrophilic dermatosis) also has been reported.

● Precautions and Contraindications

Azathioprine is a toxic drug and must be used only under close medical supervision. Clinicians using azathioprine should be thoroughly familiar with the risks for development of malignancy, the mutagenic potential of the drug in female and male patients, and the possible hematologic toxicities associated with the immunosuppressant. Other immunosuppressive therapy given concomitantly with azathioprine therapy may increase the toxic potential of the drug.

Patients who have received azathioprine therapy should be monitored for the occurrence of malignancies since these patients are at increased risk for developing lymphoma and other malignancies, particularly of the skin. Because therapy with thiopurine analogs (azathioprine or mercaptopurine) and/or TNF blocking agents may increase the risk of malignancies, including hepatosplenic T-cell lymphoma, the risks and benefits of these agents should be carefully considered, especially in adolescents and young adults with Crohn's disease or ulcerative colitis. Patients and caregivers should be informed of the increased risk of malignancy associated with azathioprine, including the potential increased risk of hepatosplenic T-cell lymphoma, especially in adolescents and young adults with inflammatory bowel disease who receive treatment with thiopurine analogs (azathioprine or mercaptopurine) and/or TNF blocking agents, and should be advised of the relative risks and benefits of these and other immunosuppressive agents. Patients and caregivers should be informed of the signs and symptoms of malignancies such as hepatosplenic T-cell lymphoma (e.g., splenomegaly, hepatomegaly, abdominal pain, persistent fever, night sweats, weight loss) and advised to contact a clinician if such signs or symptoms occur. Patients should be advised not to discontinue therapy without consulting a clinician. Because therapy with azathioprine increases the risk for skin cancer, patients receiving the drug should be advised to limit exposure to sunlight and UV light by wearing protective clothing and using a sunscreen with a high protection factor. (See Cautions: Malignancies and Lymphoproliferative Disorders.)

Because patients with intermediate levels of thiopurine methyl transferase (TPMT; an enzyme involved in the methylation of 6-mercaptopurine, a metabolite of azathioprine) may be at increased risk of developing hematologic toxicity and those with low or absent levels of the enzyme are at increased risk of life-threatening hematologic toxicity, the manufacturers and some clinicians recommend that TPMT phenotype or genotype be determined prior to initiation of azathioprine therapy. (See Pharmacokinetics: Elimination.) TPMT testing should be considered in patients with abnormal complete blood cell count (CBC) results that persist despite dosage reduction of azathioprine.

Hematologic status must be carefully monitored in patients receiving azathioprine. When azathioprine therapy is initiated, patients should be informed of the need for periodic blood counts while receiving the drug and encouraged to report any unusual bleeding or bruising to their clinician. Complete blood counts, including platelet counts, should be monitored weekly during the first month of therapy, twice monthly for the second and third months of therapy, and monthly thereafter (or more frequently if dosage alterations or other therapy changes are necessary). Since the drug effect may continue for several days after the last dose of azathioprine, to avoid irreversible depression of the bone marrow, dosage of azathioprine should be reduced or therapy interrupted from the first sign of abnormal depression of the bone marrow until the count stabilizes. Since azathioprine-induced leukopenia does not correlate with therapeutic effect, dosage of the drug should not be increased intentionally to decrease the leukocyte count.

Hepatic function must be carefully monitored in patients receiving azathioprine. Serum alkaline phosphatase, bilirubin, and aminotransferase concentrations should be determined periodically for early detection of possible hepatotoxicity. Consideration should be given to discontinuing the drug if jaundice occurs. If hepatic veno-occlusive disease is clinically suspected, azathioprine therapy should be promptly and permanently discontinued; appropriate diagnostic and therapeutic measures should be initiated. (See Cautions: Hepatic Effects.) In patients with preexisting liver dysfunction, azathioprine should be administered with caution.

Despite the use of immunosuppressive therapy, the successful outcome of renal transplantation is largely dependent on careful donor selection. Although acute rejection of kidney transplants may be prevented or treated by the use of immunosuppressive therapy, signs of chronic rejection of the organ may occur; these changes may not be apparent until several months or years after transplantation.

Infection, which may be fatal, is a common hazard during therapy with immunosuppressive agents. Fungal, protozoal, viral, and uncommon bacterial infections may occur. Patients receiving azathioprine should be advised of the danger of infection during therapy with the drug and encouraged to report signs and symptoms of infection to their clinician. When infection occurs, dosage of azathioprine and/or other drugs used to prevent rejection should be reduced, and appropriate therapy for the infection instituted.

Patients receiving azathioprine, particularly those with impaired renal function or those receiving allopurinol concomitantly, should be given careful dosage instructions. (See Drug Interactions: Allopurinol.) Only small initial doses of azathioprine should be administered to patients with renal impairment, since the drug and its metabolites may be excreted more slowly in these patients and result in a greater cumulative effect. Because cadaveric kidneys often develop tubular necrosis and delayed onset of adequate function, clearance of azathioprine and mercaptopurine may be impaired; dosage should be appropriately reduced in these patients.

Persistent negative nitrogen balance and/or muscle wasting have been reported in some patients receiving prolonged therapy with azathioprine and corticosteroids; dosage should be reduced if this occurs.

Azathioprine is contraindicated in patients who are hypersensitive to the drug. If severe, continuous rejection occurs, it is probably preferable to allow the allograft to be rejected than to increase the dosage of azathioprine to very toxic levels.

● Pediatric Precautions

Safety and efficacy of azathioprine have not been established in pediatric patients.

Cases of hepatosplenic T-cell lymphoma have been reported in adolescents receiving azathioprine for the management of inflammatory bowel disease. (See Cautions: Malignancies and Lymphoproliferative Disorders.)

● Mutagenicity and Carcinogenicity

Chronic immunosuppression with azathioprine increases the risk of malignancy in humans; malignancies, including posttransplant lymphoma and hepatosplenic T-cell lymphoma in patients with inflammatory bowel disease, have been reported. (See Cautions: Malignancies and Lymphoproliferative Disorders.)

Azathioprine is mutagenic in humans. Chromosomal abnormalities have been documented in humans receiving azathioprine, but the abnormalities were reversed following discontinuance of the drug.

● *Pregnancy, Fertility, and Lactation*

Pregnancy

Azathioprine is teratogenic in rabbits and mice when given in dosages equivalent to the human dosage (5 mg/kg daily). Abnormalities included skeletal malformations and visceral anomalies.

Azathioprine can cause fetal harm when administered to a pregnant woman. Limited immunologic and other abnormalities have occurred in some infants born to renal transplant recipients who received azathioprine. Lymphopenia, decreased IgG and IgM concentrations, cytomegalovirus infection, and a decreased thymic shadow were observed in one infant whose mother had received 150 mg of azathioprine and 30 mg of prednisone daily throughout pregnancy; most of these findings had apparently normalized by 10 weeks of age. Pancytopenia and severe immunodeficiency were reported in a premature infant whose mother received 125 mg of azathioprine and 12.5 mg of prednisone throughout pregnancy. Preaxial polydactyly was observed in one infant whose mother received 200 mg of azathioprine daily and 20 mg of prednisone every other day during pregnancy, while a large myelomeningocele in the upper lumbar region and bilateral lower limb deformities were reported in another infant whose father was receiving long-term azathioprine therapy. Azathioprine should not be used during pregnancy unless the potential benefits outweigh the possible risks; whenever possible, use of the drug during pregnancy should be avoided. If azathioprine is used during pregnancy or if the patient becomes pregnant while taking the drug, the patient should be informed about the potential hazard to the fetus. Women of childbearing potential should be advised to avoid becoming pregnant. The manufacturer states that azathioprine should not be used for the treatment of rheumatoid arthritis in pregnant women. Some clinicians state that, because of the potential for carcinogenesis and unknown long-term effects on fetal immunosuppression, use of azathioprine in pregnancy should be limited to women with severe or life-threatening rheumatoid arthritis. If azathioprine is administered during pregnancy, serious neonatal leukopenia and thrombocytopenia may be prevented by reducing the azathioprine dosage at 32 weeks' gestation; close prenatal monitoring for growth and long-term follow-up of offspring are essential.

Fertility

Azathioprine has been reported to cause temporary depression in spermatogenesis and reduction in sperm viability and sperm count in mice at doses 10 times the usual human dose; a reduced percentage of fertile matings occurred when animals received 5 mg/kg.

Lactation

Azathioprine or its metabolites are distributed into milk. Because of the potential for tumorigenicity associated with the drug, a decision should be made whether to discontinue nursing or the drug taking into account the importance of the drug to the woman.

DRUG INTERACTIONS

● *Allopurinol*

Allopurinol inhibits one of the metabolic pathways of azathioprine (i.e., the oxidative metabolism of mercaptopurine by xanthine oxidase), thus increasing the possibility of toxic effects of azathioprine, particularly bone marrow depression. When azathioprine and allopurinol are administered concomitantly, dosage of azathioprine should be reduced to 25–33% of the usual dosage, and subsequent dosage adjusted according to the patient response and toxic effects.

● *Angiotensin-converting Enzyme Inhibitors*

Anemia and severe leukopenia may occur when angiotensin-converting enzyme (ACE) inhibitors are administered concomitantly with azathioprine.

● *Aminosalicylates*

In vitro, aminosalicylates (mesalamine, olsalazine, sulfasalazine) have been shown to inhibit the enzyme thiopurine methyl transferase (TPMT), an enzyme involved in the methylation of 6-mercaptopurine (a metabolite of azathioprine). Caution should be used during concomitant administration of azathioprine with aminosalicylates.

● *Drugs affecting Myelopoiesis*

Concomitant use of drugs affecting myelopoiesis (e.g., co-trimoxazole) with azathioprine may result in severe leukopenia, especially in patients who have undergone renal transplantation.

● *Ribavirin*

Use of ribavirin for the treatment of hepatitis C virus (HCV) infection in patients receiving azathioprine has been reported to result in severe pancytopenia and may increase the risk of azathioprine-related myelotoxicity. Ribavirin inhibits inosine monophosphate dehydrogenase, an enzyme required for one of the metabolic pathways of azathioprine; this leads to accumulation of an azathioprine metabolite, 6-methylthiopurine ribonucleoside-5′-phosphate (6-methylthioinosine monophosphate), that is associated with myelotoxicity (e.g., neutropenia, thrombocytopenia, anemia). Patients receiving azathioprine concomitantly with ribavirin should have complete blood counts, including platelet counts, monitored weekly for the first month of therapy, twice monthly for the second and third months of therapy, and monthly thereafter (or more frequently if dosage or other therapy changes are necessary).

● *Warfarin*

Azathioprine may inhibit the anticoagulant effect of warfarin.

PHARMACOLOGY

Azathioprine mainly exhibits immunosuppressive activity. The exact mechanism of immunosuppressive activity of the drug has not been determined. The action of azathioprine probably depends on several factors. Azathioprine, which is an antagonist to purine metabolism, may inhibit RNA and DNA synthesis. The drug may also be incorporated into nucleic acids resulting in chromosome breaks, malfunctioning of the nucleic acids, or synthesis of fraudulent proteins. The drug may also inhibit coenzyme formation and functioning, thereby interfering with cellular metabolism. Mitosis may also be inhibited by the drug.

In patients who undergo renal transplantation, azathioprine suppresses hypersensitivities of the cell-mediated type and causes variable alterations in antibody production. Suppression of T-cell effects depends on the temporal relationship to antigenic stimulus and engraftment; azathioprine has little effect on established transplant rejections or secondary responses. In animal models of autoimmune disease, the drug suppresses disease manifestations and underlying pathology.

PHARMACOKINETICS

● *Absorption*

Azathioprine is readily absorbed from the GI tract. Following oral administration of usual doses of azathioprine, blood concentrations of the drug are usually less than 1 mcg/mL; however, because purine antagonists rapidly enter into anabolic and catabolic pathways of purines, blood measurements actually represent several compounds and the importance of blood concentrations is questionable.

● *Distribution*

Distribution of azathioprine has not been fully characterized, but the drug is rapidly cleared from blood. Both mercaptopurine and azathioprine are approximately 30% bound to serum proteins, but both appear to be dialyzable. Azathioprine and its metabolites have been shown to cross the placenta.

● *Elimination*

Azathioprine is metabolized in vivo to 6-mercaptopurine, apparently by sulfhydryl compounds such as glutathione. The metabolites of azathioprine are excreted by the kidneys; only small amounts of azathioprine and mercaptopurine are excreted intact. 6-Mercaptopurine is metabolized by 2 major competing metabolic pathways in erythrocytes and liver or, alternatively, 6-mercaptopurine is incorporated as cytotoxic 6-thioguanine nucleotides into DNA. The proportion of metabolites varies among individuals. 6-Mercaptopurine is oxidized to 6-thiouric acid by the enzyme xanthine oxidase. In addition, the sulfhydryl group of 6-mercaptopurine undergoes methylation, catalyzed by thiopurine methyl transferase (TPMT) to form the inactive metabolite methyl-6-mercaptopurine. The degree of activity of TPMT is under genetic control and is subject to individual variation. The most common nonfunctional alleles associated with reduced TPMT activity are TPMT*2, TPMT*3A, and TPMT*3C. Approximately 10% of Caucasians and African Americans inherit 1 nonfunctional allele (heterozygous) and have intermediate TPMT activity while about 0.3% of such populations inherit 2 nonfunctional alleles (homozygous) and have low or absent TPMT activity. Nonfunctional alleles are less common in the Asian population. There is an inverse relationship between TPMT activity and 6-thioguanine nucleotide concentrations in erythrocytes and, possibly, other hematopoietic tissues, because these cells have negligible amounts of xanthine oxidase (the enzyme involved in the other [oxidative] metabolism of 6-mercaptopurine), leaving TPMT methylation as the only inactivation pathway in these cells. Patients who have low TPMT activity have increased concentrations of the immunosuppressive 6-thiogunanine nucleotides in erythrocytes and, therefore, they may develop myelotoxicity. (See Cautions: Hematologic Effects and see Cautions: Precautions and Contraindications.) The fate of the nitromethylimidazole portion of azathioprine has not been completely elucidated. Small amounts of azathioprine are also split to give 1-methyl-4-nitro-5-thioimidazole. azathioprine is only partially dialyzable.

CHEMISTRY AND STABILITY

● Chemistry

Azathioprine is a chemical analog of the physiologic purines—adenine, guanine, and hypoxanthine. Azathioprine, like mercaptopurine and thioguanine, is a purine antagonist antimetabolite. The drug is used mainly for its immunosuppressive activity. Azathioprine occurs as a pale yellow, odorless powder and is insoluble in water and very slightly soluble in alcohol. Azathioprine sodium powder for injection is a sterile, bright yellow, amorphous mass or cake prepared by lyophilization of an aqueous solution of azathioprine and sodium hydroxide. Some manufacturers may add hydrochloric acid to the commercially available azathioprine sodium powder for injection to adjust the pH. Following reconstitution of azathioprine sodium powder for injection with sterile water for injection to a concentration of 10 mg/mL, the solution has a pH of approximately 9.6.

● Stability

Azathioprine tablets should be protected from light and stored in well-closed containers, usually at 15–25°C; one manufacturer states that the tablets should be stored at a controlled room temperature between 20–25°C. Azathioprine sodium powder for injection should be protected from light and stored at 15–25°C in the carton until time of use.

Azathioprine is stable in solution at neutral or acid pH but is hydrolyzed to mercaptopurine at alkaline pH. Hydrolysis to mercaptopurine also occurs in the presence of sulfhydryl compounds such as cysteine, glutathione, or hydrogen sulfide. Following reconstitution of azathioprine sodium powder for injection with sterile water for injection to a concentration of 10 mg/mL, the solution is reportedly stable for approximately 2 weeks at room temperature; however, the reconstituted solution contains no preservatives, and it is recommended that the solution be used within 24 hours after reconstitution.

An oral suspension of azathioprine containing 50 mg/mL has been prepared extemporaneously from the commercially available tablets. The tablets were crushed, mixed with a volume of suspending agent (Cologel®) equal to one-third the final volume, and then the suspension was brought to the final volume with a 2:1 mixture of simple syrup and wild cherry syrup. The resulting suspension was stable for at least 56 or 84 days when stored in an amber glass bottle at room temperature or 5°C, respectively.

PREPARATIONS

Excipients in commercially available drug preparations may have clinically important effects in some individuals; consult specific product labeling for details.

azaTHIOprine

Oral			
Tablets	50 mg*		azaTHIOprine Tablets (scored)
			Imuran® (scored), Prometheus
	75 mg		Azasan® (scored), Salix
	100 mg		Azasan® (scored), Salix

* available from one or more manufacturer, distributor, and/or repackager by generic (nonproprietary) name

azaTHIOprine Sodium

Parenteral			
For injection, for IV use	100 mg (of azathioprine)*		azaTHIOprine Sodium for Injection

* available from one or more manufacturer, distributor, and/or repackager by generic (nonproprietary) name

† Use is not currently included in the labeling approved by the US Food and Drug Administration.

Selected Revisions June 10, 2024. © Copyright, December 1, 1968, American Society of Health-System Pharmacists, Inc.

Mycophenolate Mofetil, Mycophenolate Sodium

90:28.08.92 • ANTIMETABOLITES, IMMUNOSUPPRESSIVE THERAPY, MISCELLANEOUS

■ Mycophenolate mofetil and mycophenolate sodium are used as immunosuppressive agents. Mycophenolate mofetil is a prodrug that has little pharmacologic activity until hydrolyzed in vivo to mycophenolic acid, the pharmacologically active metabolite. Mycophenolate sodium delayed-release tablets release the active moiety, mycophenolic acid, in the small intestine.

USES

Mycophenolate mofetil (CellCept®) is used for the prevention of rejection of kidney, heart, or liver allografts. The manufacturer recommends that mycophenolate mofetil be used in conjunction with cyclosporine and corticosteroid therapy. Mycophenolate mofetil also has been used in the management of Crohn's disease†.

Mycophenolate sodium (Myfortic®) is used in conjunction with cyclosporine and corticosteroid therapy for the prevention of rejection of kidney allografts.

Mycophenolate mofetil and mycophenolate sodium have been used in conjunction with other immunosuppressants for the prevention of rejection of lung allografts†.

Mycophenolate mofetil and mycophenolate sodium have been used in the management of systemic sclerosis (often called scleroderma)†.

● Renal Allotransplantation

Adult Patients

Mycophenolate mofetil is used for the prevention of rejection of renal allografts in adults and pediatric patients 3 months to 18 years of age. In clinical trials in renal transplant patients, a regimen consisting of mycophenolate mofetil, cyclosporine, and corticosteroids was more effective than regimens consisting of either azathioprine or placebo in combination with cyclosporine and corticosteroids in preventing acute rejection, graft loss, or death at 6 months following transplantation.

Efficacy and safety of mycophenolate mofetil has been evaluated in 3 randomized, double-blind, multicenter trials in adults undergoing cadaveric renal transplantation. In each trial, mycophenolate mofetil was given in 2 different dosages (1 or 1.5 g twice daily) in immunosuppressive regimens that included cyclosporine, corticosteroids, and (in one study) antithymocyte globulin. Mycophenolate mofetil was compared with azathioprine (1–2 mg/kg daily or 100–150 mg daily) in 2 studies and with placebo in a third study; patients receiving azathioprine or placebo in these studies also received cyclosporine and corticosteroids. In these trials, the primary efficacy end point was the rate of treatment failure, defined as the first occurrence of an acute episode of biopsy-proven acute rejection, death, graft loss, or early termination of the study for any reason without a prior biopsy-proven acute rejection episode, in the first 6 months after transplantation. Results of these studies indicate that mycophenolate mofetil was more effective than azathioprine or placebo in reducing the incidence of treatment failure at 6 months following transplantation. When mycophenolate mofetil was compared with azathioprine, the treatment failure rates at 6 months for mycophenolate mofetil 2 g, mycophenolate mofetil 3 g, azathioprine (1–2 mg/kg daily), and azathioprine (100–150 mg daily) were 31.1–38.2, 31.3–34.8, 47.6, and 50%, respectively. When mycophenolate mofetil was compared with placebo, treatment failure rates at 6 months for mycophenolate mofetil 2 g, mycophenolate mofetil 3 g, and placebo were 30.3, 38.8, and 56%, respectively. The cumulative incidence of combined 1-year graft loss or patient death for mycophenolate mofetil 2 g, mycophenolate mofetil 3 g, and control (placebo or azathioprine), were 8.5–11.7%, 10–11.5, and 11.5–13.6%, respectively.

Mycophenolate sodium is used for the prevention of rejection of renal allografts in adults and pediatric patients 5–16 years of age. In clinical trials in *de novo* or stable renal transplant patients, a regimen consisting of mycophenolate sodium, cyclosporine, and/or corticosteroids was as effective as a regimen consisting of mycophenolate mofetil, cyclosporine, and corticosteroids in preventing acute rejection, graft loss, or death.

Mycophenolate mofetil therapy has been associated with a high incidence of adverse GI effects and a high proportion of patients receiving the drug required dosage reductions, interruptions in therapy, or discontinuance of the immunosuppressant due to adverse effects. Such changes in drug therapy have a negative impact on transplant outcomes (higher incidence of acute rejection, decreased graft survival). Mycophenolate sodium delayed-release tablets were designed to improve GI tolerance by delaying release of mycophenolic acid until the drug reaches the small intestine. However, results of comparative clinical studies have shown that incidence of adverse GI effects reported in patients receiving mycophenolate sodium have been similar to those in patients receiving mycophenolate mofetil.

Safety and efficacy of mycophenolate sodium delayed-release tablets have been evaluated in 2 multicenter, randomized, double-blind, comparative trials. In one 12-month study, 423 *de novo* renal transplant patients (18–75 years of age) who were receiving their first cadaveric (84%), living- unrelated, or human leukocyte antigen (HLA)-mismatched living-related donor kidney transplant, were randomized to receive (within 24–48 hours of transplantation) mycophenolate sodium (mycophenolic acid 720 mg twice daily) or mycophenolate mofetil (1 g twice daily) in conjunction with cyclosporine and corticosteroids. Patients undergoing transplantation at centers that routinely used induction therapy with antithymocyte or antilymphocyte antibody preparations (about 41%) were allowed to receive such therapy. The primary efficacy end point was the rate of treatment failure, defined as the first occurrence of acute rejection episode (biopsy-proven), graft loss, death, or loss to follow-up, in the first 6 months after transplantation. Mycophenolate sodium was as effective as mycophenolate mofetil in reducing the incidence of treatment failure rates at 6 and 12 months following transplantation. The treatment failure rates at 6 months for mycophenolate sodium and mycophenolate mofetil in this study were 25.8 and 26.2%, respectively, while at 12 months, treatment failure rates were 28.6 and 28.1%, respectively.

In the other 12-month study, maintenance therapy with mycophenolate sodium delayed-release tablets has been evaluated in 322 renal transplant patients (18–75 years of age) who had undergone primary or secondary cadaveric or living donor kidney transplantation, were at least 6 months posttransplant, and were receiving immunosuppressive regimens that included mycophenolate mofetil and cyclosporine, with or without corticosteroids, for at least 2 weeks before study entry. Patients were randomized to continue mycophenolate mofetil (1 g twice daily) or to switch to mycophenolate sodium (mycophenolic acid 720 mg twice daily). The incidence of treatment failure (defined as the first occurrence of acute rejection episode [biopsy-proven], graft loss, death, or loss to follow-up) at 6 and 12 months in patients receiving mycophenolate sodium was similar to that in patients receiving mycophenolate mofetil. The treatment failure rates at 6 months for mycophenolate sodium and mycophenolate mofetil in this study were 4.4 and 6.7%, respectively, while at 12 months, treatment failure rates were 7.5 and 12.3%, respectively. Results of this and other studies indicate that mycophenolate sodium can be substituted for mycophenolate mofetil without loss of efficacy.

Pediatric Patients

In an open-label multicenter study in pediatric patients 3 months to 18 years of age who underwent cadaveric renal transplantation, mycophenolate mofetil was administered by oral suspension in a dosage of 600 mg/m² twice daily (maximum daily dosage 1 g twice daily) in conjunction with cyclosporine and corticosteroids. In this study, the overall biopsy-proven rejection rate at 6 months was comparable to that reported in adults. In addition, the rate of biopsy-proven rejection was similar across the various age groups (i.e., 3 months to younger than 6 years of age, 6 years to younger than 12 years of age; 12–18 years of age). At 12 months, the combined incidence of graft loss (5%) and patient death (2%) in children was similar to that observed in adults.

Safety and efficacy of mycophenolate sodium have been established in stable renal transplant pediatric patients 5–16 years of age. Use of mycophenolate sodium in this age group is supported by evidence from adequate and well controlled studies in stable adult renal transplant patients (who received mycophenolate sodium therapy) and limited pharmacokinetic data in stable renal transplant pediatric patients 5–16 years of age. Safety and efficacy of mycophenolate sodium in pediatric *de novo* renal transplant patients have not been established .

● *Cardiac Allotransplantation*

Mycophenolate mofetil is used in adults for the prevention of rejection of cardiac allografts. This indication for mycophenolate mofetil is based on the results of one double-blind, randomized, multicenter active-controlled trial that enrolled 650 adults (578 of whom received at least one dose of either study drug) undergoing their first cardiac transplantation. Patients were randomized to receive oral mycophenolate mofetil (1.5 g twice daily) or oral azathioprine (1.5–3 mg/kg daily) in immunosuppressive regimens that included cyclosporine and corticosteroids. In this study, there were 2 primary efficacy end points; the first one was defined as the proportion of patients who had at least one endomyocardial biopsy-proven rejection with hemodynamic compromise after transplantation, underwent retransplantation, or died within the first 6 months, while the second primary efficacy end point was defined as the proportion of patients who died or underwent retransplantation during the first 12 months after the original transplantation. At 6 months, the incidence of biopsy-proven rejection accompanied by hemodynamic compromise in patients receiving mycophenolate mofetil (35%) was similar to that seen in patients receiving azathioprine (32%). At 12 months, mycophenolate mofetil was at least as effective as azathioprine in preventing death or retransplantation (6.2 vs 11.4%, respectively).

Use of an immunosuppressive regimen consisting of mycophenolate mofetil in conjunction with sirolimus and a corticosteroid following 12 weeks of therapy with a regimen consisting of mycophenolate mofetil, cyclosporine or tacrolimus, and a corticosteroid was investigated in the Heart Spare the Nephron (HSN) clinical trial in patients undergoing cardiac transplantation. The trial was designed to investigate whether switching from cyclosporine or tacrolimus to sirolimus at 12 weeks after transplantation would be associated with beneficial effects on renal function. The study was terminated early due to a higher than expected incidence of acute rejection in patients switched to sirolimus.

● *Hepatic Allotransplantation*

Mycophenolate mofetil is used in adults for the prevention of rejection of liver allografts. This indication for mycophenolate mofetil is based on the results of one double-blind, randomized, active-controlled, multicenter trial that enrolled 565 adults undergoing primary hepatic allotransplantation. Patients were randomized to receive mycophenolate mofetil (1 g IV twice daily for up to 14 days, followed by 1.5 g given orally twice daily) or azathioprine (1–2 mg/kg IV daily followed by the same dosage orally) in immunosuppressive regimens that included cyclosporine and corticosteroids. In this study, there were 2 primary efficacy end points; the first was defined as the proportion of patients who had one or more biopsy-proven and treated rejection, who underwent retransplantation, or who died, while the second primary efficacy point was defined as the proportion of patients who experienced graft loss (by death or undergoing retransplantation) during the first 12 months after the primary transplantation. At 6 months, the incidence of one or more episodes of biopsy-proven and treated rejection, retransplantation, or death was 38.5 or 47.7% in those receiving mycophenolate mofetil or azathioprine, respectively. At 12 months, mycophenolate mofetil and azathioprine were similarly effective in preventing retransplantation or death.

● *Lung Allotransplantation*

Mycophenolate mofetil and mycophenolate sodium have been used for the prevention of rejection of lung allografts† in patients who have undergone lung transplantation. Following lung transplantation, acute allograft rejection and chronic lung allograft dysfunction, including bronchiolitis obliterans syndrome (BOS), are major complications affecting long-term graft and patient survival. Conventional maintenance immunosuppression commonly consists of triple drug therapy with a calcineurin inhibitor (e.g., tacrolimus or cyclosporine), either mycophenolate or azathioprine, and corticosteroids; either sirolimus or everolimus is used much less commonly as an alternative to mycophenolate or azathioprine. According to data from the International Society for Heart and Lung Transplantation (ISHLT) registry, among adults who underwent lung transplantation between 2005 and 2018, the most common maintenance immunosuppressive regimen at 1 year posttransplantation was tacrolimus, mycophenolate, and corticosteroids. Approximately 80% of adult lung transplant recipients were receiving mycophenolate mofetil or mycophenolate sodium at 1 year posttransplantation.

Several clinical trials and clinical experience to date indicate that mycophenolate used in combination with other immunosuppressants is effective in the prevention of allograft rejection following lung transplantation. The comparative efficacy of mycophenolate mofetil and azathioprine in maintenance immunosuppression following lung transplantation was evaluated in a randomized, open-label, multicenter study in 315 adults who underwent lung transplantation. Patients in this study received mycophenolate mofetil (1.5 g twice daily for the first 3 months, followed by 1 g twice daily) or azathioprine (2 mg/kg daily) in combination with cyclosporine and corticosteroids; all patients also received induction therapy with antithymocyte globulin. At 3 years posttransplantation, there were no significant differences between the 2 treatment groups in overall survival, incidence of acute rejection, or the incidence, severity, or time to acquisition of BOS. Although both immunosuppressants generally were well tolerated in this study, more patients withdrew from azathioprine than from mycophenolate mofetil; this resulted in a shorter observation period for patients in the azathioprine group. An earlier randomized, open-label, 2-center study in 81 adult lung transplant recipients also found no difference between mycophenolate mofetil and azathioprine in acute rejection rates or overall survival at 6 months. In this study, mycophenolate mofetil (1 g twice daily) or azathioprine (2 mg/kg daily) was used in combination with cyclosporine and corticosteroids without antilymphocyte induction therapy.

● *Crohn's Disease*

Mycophenolate mofetil has been used in the management of Crohn's disease†. The comparative efficacy of mycophenolate mofetil versus azathioprine has been investigated in several studies. In a randomized, comparative, prospective trial that included 70 patients with moderately to severely active Crohn's disease, efficacy of mycophenolate mofetil was evaluated in the management of corticosteroid-dependent chronically active Crohn's disease. In this study, the Crohn's Disease Activity Index (CDAI) was used for clinical assessment. The CDAI score is based on subjective observations by the patient (e.g., the daily number of liquid or very soft stools, severity of abdominal pain, general well-being) and objective evidence (e.g., number of extraintestinal manifestations, presence of an abdominal mass, use or nonuse of antidiarrheal drugs, the hematocrit, body weight). Patients with a CDAI score of 150 to greater than 300 were randomized to receive prednisolone (50 mg daily initially and tapered to a maintenance dosage of 5 mg daily) concomitantly with mycophenolate mofetil (15 mg/kg daily; approximately 1.5 g daily) or azathioprine (2.5 mg/kg daily). One month after randomization, efficacy of mycophenolate mofetil was similar to that of azathioprine (median reduction of 120 points for mycophenolate mofetil versus 97 points for azathioprine) in patients with moderately active disease (CDAI of 150–300), while in patients with severely active disease (CDAI exceeding 300), use of mycophenolate mofetil was associated with substantially greater reduction in CDAI scores than azathioprine (median reduction of 265 points for mycophenolate mofetil versus 117 points for azathioprine). During 2–6 months of therapy, CDAI scores remained stable and at comparable levels in mycophenolate-treated patients with moderately and severely active disease. However, after 6 months of therapy, there was a clear trend for a continuous decrease in CDAI scores in patients with severely active disease who were receiving azathioprine.

Efficacy of mycophenolate mofetil also has been evaluated in several small uncontrolled trials in patients with refractory Crohn's disease. While results of some clinical studies have indicated that mycophenolate mofetil may be beneficial in some patients with chronically active disease (including those with fistulizing disease) who did not respond or were intolerant of other immunosuppressants, results of other clinical trials in patients with chronically active disease refractory to corticosteroids, mercaptopurine, or azathioprine have not demonstrated such benefit. Although mycophenolate has been well tolerated in many of these studies, it should be considered that the drug has been associated rarely with an increased incidence of adverse GI effects (e.g., ulceration, hemorrhage, perforation) and mycophenolate should be used with caution in patients with active serious GI disease. In general, mycophenolate mofetil should be reserved for patients with Crohn's disease who are refractory to or intolerant of azathioprine, mercaptopurine, methotrexate, or infliximab. Additional well-controlled studies are needed to define the role, if any, of mycophenolate mofetil in the management of refractory Crohn's disease.

For further information on the management of Crohn's disease, see Uses: Crohn's Disease, in Mesalamine 56:36.

● *Systemic Sclerosis*

Mycophenolate mofetil and mycophenolate sodium have been used in the management of systemic sclerosis (often called scleroderma)†. Systemic sclerosis is a rare and heterogeneous autoimmune connective tissue disease and fibrosing disorder; the disease most commonly affects women and often develops during middle age. Systemic sclerosis is characterized by immune dysregulation, microvascular disease, and excess collagen deposition. The disease can impair organ function, reduce physical function, decrease quality of life, and result in premature mortality. Although sclerosis of the skin (i.e., fibrosis and thickening) is a hallmark of the diffuse cutaneous form of the disease and skin involvement is usually extensive, progressive, and debilitating, cardiopulmonary involvement, particularly interstitial lung disease (ILD) and pulmonary arterial hypertension (PAH), accounts for most of the increased mortality in patients with this condition. The etiology of systemic sclerosis is not fully understood at this time.

Treatment of systemic sclerosis should be individualized and usually is based on the disease comorbidities (i.e., clinical manifestations, organ involvement). Prevention of progression of the disease is an important goal of treatment, and early diagnosis and intervention appear to be essential in achieving this goal. Because of the clinical complexity in diagnosing and treating systemic sclerosis, some experts state that referral to a specialized treatment center with expertise in treating systemic sclerosis should be strongly considered. A variety of immunosuppressants have been used in the clinical management of skin and lung involvement associated with systemic sclerosis to date, including azathioprine, cyclophosphamide, methotrexate, mycophenolate mofetil or mycophenolate sodium, rituximab, and corticosteroids. However, because of the heterogeneity and variable course of this rare disease, it is difficult to fully assess the relative clinical efficacy of various therapeutic interventions, including immunosuppressant therapy.

Based on encouraging results in a number of uncontrolled clinical studies and case series as well as a randomized, controlled clinical trial, which are summarized below, many experts currently recommend mycophenolate (i.e., mycophenolate mofetil and mycophenolate sodium) as one of several immunosuppressants that can be used as first-line therapy in the initial management (i.e., induction therapy) of patients with systemic sclerosis, particularly for those with early and active systemic sclerosis and with active skin involvement or ILD. Longer-term mycophenolate therapy also is used and recommended by some experts to maintain improvement and prevent progression of skin involvement and/or ILD in patients with systemic sclerosis. Although mycophenolate mofetil and mycophenolate sodium are considered therapeutically equivalent, some clinicians consider mycophenolate sodium to be better tolerated than mycophenolate mofetil, particularly in terms of adverse GI effects. Some clinicians feel more comfortable and have greater experience prescribing mycophenolate mofetil in patients with systemic sclerosis but would consider switching to mycophenolate sodium in patients who are unable to tolerate mycophenolate mofetil at the recommended target dosage while other clinicians prefer to initiate and maintain therapy with mycophenolate sodium because of its potential for improved tolerability.

In a randomized, double-blind, multicenter clinical trial (the Scleroderma Lung Study II [SLS-II]), efficacy and tolerability of oral cyclophosphamide and mycophenolate mofetil therapy were compared in 126 adults with scleroderma-associated ILD. Mycophenolate mofetil therapy was initiated at a dosage of 500 mg given twice daily and the dosage was increased over time up to a maximum target dosage of 1.5 g twice daily; therapy was continued for 2 years. In the other treatment arm, cyclophosphamide therapy was initiated at a dosage of 50–150 mg once daily (based on weight) and was titrated up to a target dosage of 2 mg/kg (range: 1.8–2.3 mg/kg) once daily for 12 months followed by matching placebo for the next 12 months. The principal study end point was the change in forced vital capacity (FVC) from baseline as a percentage of the predicted normal value (FVC %) over the 24-month course of the study. Although no significant difference was noted between the treatment groups for the primary end point in post-hoc analyses, both 24-month mycophenolate mofetil treatment and 12-month cyclophosphamide treatment produced substantial improvement in lung function (as assessed by the adjusted FVC %) over 24 months. Both mycophenolate and cyclophosphamide therapy also resulted in significant improvements in skin scores and dyspnea over the 2-year course of the study. Responses to therapy occurred mainly between 9 and 24 months, suggesting slow onset of the potential disease-modifying effects of these drugs in patients with scleroderma-associated lung disease. Overall, mycophenolate mofetil therapy appeared to be better tolerated and resulted in fewer withdrawals from therapy than oral cyclophosphamide.

Mycophenolate therapy (given as either mycophenolate mofetil or mycophenolate sodium) also has been evaluated in the treatment of systemic sclerosis in a number of prospective and retrospective observational studies and case series to date. The results from these studies suggest that mycophenolate therapy may help improve skin involvement and stabilize or improve pulmonary function and fibrosis in patients with the disease. Mycophenolate therapy generally has been well tolerated in these clinical studies and case series and appears to be better tolerated than some other immunosuppressants that have been used to treat systemic sclerosis (e.g., cyclophosphamide, azathioprine).

In an observational study evaluating the long-term efficacy and tolerability of mycophenolate mofetil in the management of skin disease in a cohort of 42 adults with diffuse scleroderma from the Australian Scleroderma Cohort Study, mycophenolate therapy (mean dosage of 1.9 g daily) for a minimum of 12 months was associated with modest improvements in modified Rodnan skin score (mRSS). After 1 year of therapy, 43% of the patients demonstrated clinically important improvement (defined as a reduction in mRSS of 5 or more from baseline); 92% of the patients demonstrated such improvement after 4 years of mycophenolate therapy. In a retrospective study, data from 12 patients with scleroderma-associated ILD who did not adequately respond to IV cyclophosphamide and who were treated with mycophenolate mofetil therapy for 2 years were reviewed. Overall, pulmonary function tests improved in approximately 42% of these patients following mycophenolate mofetil therapy; 25% of the patients demonstrated improved FVC values and about 17% of the patients demonstrated improved diffusing capacity of the lung for carbon monoxide (DLCO) values.

In a retrospective study in 98 patients with diffuse cutaneous systemic sclerosis who received long-term mycophenolate mofetil therapy (i.e., 12 months), improvement in skin disease (as assessed by the mRSS) was observed as early as 3 months after initiating therapy and continued throughout the 12-month follow-up period. Improved general and muscle severity scores as well as improved subjective quality-of-life measures and stable pulmonary disease were also observed in the mycophenolate-treated patients. In a prospective, open-label study in 15 adults with early diffuse systemic sclerosis who received mycophenolate mofetil therapy (500 mg twice daily for week 1, then 1 g twice daily for week 2, and, if tolerated, 1.5 g twice daily by week 4 and thereafter) for over 12 months, significantly improved mRSS and Medsger severity scores in the general, peripheral vascular, and skin organ system categories were reported. In addition, pulmonary function did not worsen in the mycophenolate-treated patients and showed a trend toward improvement.

In a retrospective study, 109 patients with systemic sclerosis who were treated with mycophenolate mofetil therapy for 5 years were compared to a cohort of 63 patients receiving other immunosuppressants. A substantially lower frequency of clinically important pulmonary fibrosis and substantially higher 5-year survival from disease onset and from initiation of therapy were observed in the mycophenolate-treated cohort compared with the cohort receiving other immunosuppressants. There was no significant difference in the change in mRSS or FVC between the 2 treatment cohorts. In another retrospective study in 13 patients with recent-onset scleroderma-associated ILD who had received mycophenolate mofetil in dosages higher than 1 g daily for at least 6 months, a small but statistically significant improvement in vital capacity (VC) was observed (a mean increase of 4% of the predicted normal value after 12 months of treatment). These patients had demonstrated a substantial decline in VC (mean decrease of 5% of the predicted normal value) in the 12 months prior to initiation of mycophenolate mofetil therapy. DLCO did not change significantly during mycophenolate therapy (mean increase of 1% of the predicted normal value after 12 months of treatment) but had decreased significantly in the 12 months prior to mycophenolate treatment (a mean decrease of 5% of the predicted normal value).

In a prospective, observational study of mycophenolate mofetil in 25 previously untreated patients with diffuse progressive cutaneous systemic sclerosis of recent onset (i.e., within 24 months), patients treated with a median mycophenolate mofetil dosage of 2 g daily for an average of about 8 months demonstrated substantial improvement in skin involvement (as measured by the mRSS and affected body surface area) and stabilization of pulmonary function. In addition, skin biopsies from 3 of the patients revealed histopathological improvement and decreased expression of fibrosis-related genes.

Further controlled clinical studies are needed to more clearly determine the optimal role of mycophenolate therapy and other immunosuppressants in the clinical management of patients with systemic sclerosis-associated skin and lung disease.

DOSAGE AND ADMINISTRATION

• Reconstitution and Administration

Mycophenolate mofetil and mycophenolate sodium are administered orally; mycophenolate mofetil hydrochloride is administered by IV infusion. When mycophenolate is used for the prevention of rejection of organ allographs, the drug usually is used concomitantly with an immunosuppressive regimen that includes cyclosporine and corticosteroids; other immunosuppressive agents, including antithymocyte globulin, antilymphocyte globulin, muromonab-CD3, basiliximab, or daclizumab (no longer commercially available in the US), also have been used.

The US Food and Drug Administration (FDA) currently requires that the manufacturer's patient information (medication guide) for mycophenolate mofetil or mycophenolate sodium be distributed to every patient each time the drug is dispensed. Because of the teratogenic potential of the drug, mycophenolate oral and parenteral preparations should be handled and prepared with care. Mycophenolate mofetil tablets should not be crushed and capsules should not be opened or crushed. Mycophenolate sodium delayed-release tablets should not be crushed, chewed, or cut. Inhalation of mycophenolate mofetil powder contained in the oral capsules or in the oral suspension (before and after reconstitution) and contact with the skin or mucous membranes should be avoided. In addition, contact with mycophenolate mofetil hydrochloride IV solution should be avoided. In case of accidental skin or mucous membrane contact, the affected area should be washed thoroughly with soap and water. If contact with the eyes occurs, they should be washed with water. The manufacturer recommends wiping up any spilled drug with a wet paper towel.

IV mycophenolate mofetil hydrochloride, which should be initiated within 24 hours following transplantation, generally is reserved for patients who cannot tolerate or are unable to take an oral dosage form. The drug can be administered IV for up to 14 days. Oral therapy should replace parenteral therapy as soon as possible.

Mycophenolate mofetil hydrochloride powder for injection is reconstituted by adding 14 mL of 5% dextrose injection to a vial labeled as containing 500 mg of mycophenolate mofetil; the vial should be gently shaken. The reconstituted solution is slightly yellow. For a 1-g infusion dose, the contents of 2 such reconstituted vials are added to 140 mL of 5% dextrose injection while for a 1.5-g infusion dose, the contents of 3 such reconstituted vials are added to 210 mL of 5% dextrose injection; the concentration of mycophenolate mofetil in the resulting solutions is 6 mg/mL. IV administration of mycophenolate mofetil hydrochloride should be started within 4 hours of reconstitution and dilution of the drug; solutions should be stored at 25°C with excursions of 15–30°C permitted. Strict aseptic technique must be observed since the drug contains no preservative. Mycophenolate mofetil hydrochloride should not be admixed with other drugs nor should other drugs be infused simultaneously through the same IV line. Prior to administration, reconstituted and diluted solutions of mycophenolate mofetil hydrochloride should be inspected visually for particulate matter and discoloration; if particulate matter or discoloration is evident, the solution should be discarded.

Mycophenolate mofetil hydrochloride should be infused IV over at least 2 hours by either a peripheral or central vein; the drug should *not* be administered by rapid IV ("bolus") injection or rapid IV infusion.

Oral mycophenolate mofetil should be administered as soon as possible following renal, cardiac, or hepatic transplantation.

Administration of mycophenolate mofetil with food does not affect the area under the plasma concentration-time curve (AUC) of mycophenolic acid; however, decreases (by about 40%) of peak plasma concentrations of mycophenolic acid have been observed. Therefore, the manufacturer recommends that mycophenolate mofetil tablets, capsules, and oral suspension be administered on an empty stomach (e.g., 1 hour before or 2 hours after a meal); however, in stable renal transplant recipients, the drug may be given with food, if necessary. If a dose is missed, the dose should be taken as soon as it is remembered unless it is time for the next dose; a double dose should not be taken to make up for a missed dose.

Mycophenolate sodium may be administered as soon as possible following renal transplantation in adults.

Mycophenolate sodium delayed-release tablets are administered on an empty stomach, 1 hour before or 2 hours after food. If a dose is missed, the dose should be taken as soon as it is remembered unless it is time for the next dose; a double dose should not be taken to make up for a missed dose. Administration of mycophenolate sodium with food does not affect the AUC of mycophenolic acid; however, decreases in peak plasma concentration (by about 33%) and delay in time to peak plasma concentrations (from 1.5–2.75 hours to 5 hours) have been observed. To reduce variability in mycophenolic acid absorption between doses, mycophenolate sodium should be taken on an empty stomach.

It is recommended that mycophenolate mofetil powder for oral suspension be reconstituted at the time of dispensing by adding 94 mL of water (about 47 mL initially followed by another 47 mL after vigorous shaking for 1 minute) to provide a suspension containing 200 mg/mL. The bottle should be shaken well again for 1 minute to suspend the powder. Mycophenolate mofetil oral suspension also can be administered by a nasogastric tube (minimum 1.7 mm in interior diameter; minimum French size number 8).

● General Dosage

Dosage of mycophenolate mofetil and mycophenolate mofetil hydrochloride are both expressed in terms of mycophenolate mofetil. Dosage of mycophenolate sodium is expressed in terms of mycophenolic acid.

Commercially available mycophenolate mofetil tablets, capsules, and oral suspension reportedly are bioequivalent. Mycophenolate sodium delayed-release tablets should not be used interchangeably with mycophenolate mofetil tablets, capsules, or oral suspension without supervision of a clinician, because absorption of the drug from these preparations is not equivalent. In a study in stable renal transplant recipients, administration of single oral doses of mycophenolate sodium delayed-release tablets (mycophenolic acid 720 mg) or mycophenolate mofetil 1-g oral preparations resulted in bioequivalent mycophenolic acid exposure.

Adults

Renal Allotransplantation

For the prevention of renal allograft rejection in adults, the usual dosage of mycophenolate mofetil is 1 g administered IV or orally twice daily. Although 2- and 3-g daily dosages of mycophenolate mofetil have been used in clinical trials, no efficacy advantage could be shown for the higher dosage in the overall renal transplant patient population. In addition, 2-g daily dosages of mycophenolate mofetil were associated with a superior safety profile when compared with the 3-g daily dosage.

When mycophenolate sodium delayed-release tablets are used for the prevention of renal allograft rejection in adults, the usual dosage is 720 mg of mycophenolic acid twice daily.

Cardiac Allotransplantation

For the prevention of cardiac allograft rejection in adults, the usual dosage of mycophenolate mofetil is 1.5 g administered IV or orally twice daily (3 g total daily dosage).

Hepatic Allotransplantation

For the prevention of hepatic allograft rejection in adults, the usual dosage of mycophenolate mofetil hydrochloride is 1 g administered IV twice daily or 1.5 g administered orally twice daily.

Lung Allotransplantation

For the prevention of lung allograft rejection† in adults, mycophenolate mofetil dosages of 1–1.5 g administered IV or orally twice daily have been used.

When mycophenolate sodium delayed-release tablets have been used for the prevention of lung allograft rejection† in adults, a dosage of 1.08 g of mycophenolic acid twice daily has been used.

Crohn's Disease

For the management of Crohn's disease† in adults who do not respond to or were intolerant of other immunosuppressants (e.g., azathioprine, mercaptopurine), mycophenolate mofetil dosages of 1–2 g daily have been used.

Systemic Sclerosis

For the treatment of systemic sclerosis† in adults, an initial mycophenolate mofetil dosage of 500 mg given orally twice daily (1 g total daily dosage) for the first 1–4 weeks has been used. The dosage has then been gradually increased up to a target maintenance dosage of 1–1.5 g given orally twice daily (total daily dosage of 2–3 g) based on clinical response and tolerability. Although many patients can tolerate a total daily dosage of 3 g, some patients may require somewhat lower maintenance dosages because of adverse effects, particularly adverse GI effects (see Cautions).

When mycophenolate sodium delayed-release tablets have been used for the treatment of systemic sclerosis† in adults, initial dosages of 360 mg of mycophenolic acid once or twice daily have been used. The dosage has then been increased to 720 or 1080 mg of mycophenolic acid twice daily if tolerated.

Although the optimal duration of mycophenolate therapy in the treatment of systemic sclerosis is not fully known, the drug has been used for up to 5 years in some patients with the disease. Some clinical experience to date suggests that long-term immunosuppressant therapy may be necessary to stabilize and prevent progression of the disease.

Pediatric Patients

Renal Allotransplantation

For the prevention of renal allograft rejection in pediatric patients 3 months to 18 years of age, the usual dosage of mycophenolate mofetil (as the oral suspension) is 600 mg/m² administered orally twice daily, up to a maximum dosage of 1 g twice daily. Children with a body surface area of 1.25–1.5 m² can receive 750 mg (as capsules) twice daily for a total daily mycophenolate mofetil dosage of 1.5 g, while children with a body surface area greater than 1.5 m² can receive a dosage of 1 g (as capsules or tablets) twice daily for a total daily mycophenolate mofetil dosage of 2 g.

Mycophenolate sodium should be administered as maintenance therapy *only* in stable pediatric renal transplant recipients; safety and efficacy of the drug in *de novo* pediatric renal transplant recipients have not been established.

For the prevention of renal allograft rejection in pediatric patients 5–16 years of age, the usual dosage of mycophenolic acid (administered as mycophenolate sodium delayed-release tablets) is 400 mg/m² twice daily (up to a maximum of 720 mg twice daily). Pediatric patients with a body surface area of 1.19–1.58 m² may receive a daily dosage of 1080 mg (administered as three 180-mg tablets or one 180-mg tablet and one 360-mg tablet twice daily). Pediatric patients with a body surface area greater than 1.58m² may receive a daily dosage of 1440 mg (administered as four 180-mg tablets or two 360-mg tablets twice daily). A mycophenolate sodium dosage form suitable for providing an appropriate dosage for pediatric patients with a body surface area less than 1.19 m² is not commercially available in the US.

● Special Populations

Dosage adjustment of mycophenolate mofetil preparations or mycophenolic acid (administered as mycophenolate sodium delayed-release tablets) is not necessary in renal transplant recipients experiencing postoperative delayed graft function. No dosage adjustment is necessary in renal transplant recipients with severe hepatic parenchymal disease; however, it is not known whether dosage adjustment is needed in hepatic impairment of other etiologies.

Mycophenolate mofetil dosages exceeding 1 g twice daily should be avoided in renal transplant recipients with severe chronic renal impairment (GFR less than 25 mL/minute per 1.73 m²) beyond the immediate posttransplant period.

If neutropenia (absolute neutrophil count [ANC] of less than 1300/mm³) develops, mycophenolate therapy should be temporarily discontinued or the dosage reduced, suitable diagnostic tests be performed, and appropriate patient management be instituted.

Mycophenolate mofetil dosage adjustment based solely on age is not necessary in geriatric patients 65 years of age or older.

When mycophenolate sodium is used in geriatric adults, the maximum recommended dosage is mycophenolic acid 720 mg twice daily.

CAUTIONS

● Contraindications

Known hypersensitivity to mycophenolate mofetil, mycophenolate sodium, mycophenolic acid, or any ingredient in the formulation. Mycophenolate mofetil hydrochloride for IV injection contains polysorbate (Tween®) 80 and should not be used in patients with known severe hypersensitivity to the surfactant.

● Warnings/Precautions

Warnings

Mycophenolate shares the toxic potentials of currently available immunosuppressive agents. Immunosuppression with the drug may result in increased susceptibility to infection (e.g., infectious complications) and the possible development of lymphoma. Such risk appears to be related to the intensity and duration of immunosuppression rather than to the use of any specific immunosuppressive agent. Mycophenolate mofetil and mycophenolate sodium should be used by clinicians experienced in immunosuppressive therapy and the management of patients receiving these drugs. Patients receiving the drug should be managed in facilities equipped with adequate laboratory and supportive medical resources, and the clinician responsible for maintenance therapy should have complete information requisite for follow-up of the patients. Patients should be advised to read the medication guide for mycophenolate mofetil or mycophenolate sodium that is provided each time the drug is dispensed.

Carcinogenicity

Potential for the development of lymphoma and other malignancies, particularly of the skin, which may result from immunosuppression. Because of the increased risk for skin cancer, patients should be advised to limit their exposure to sunlight or other UV light by wearing protective clothing and using sunscreen with a high protection factor.

Lymphoproliferative disease or lymphoma occurred in 0.4–1.3% of allograft recipients receiving mycophenolate in conjunction with other immunosuppressive agents in clinical studies. Non-melanoma skin carcinoma was reported in 0.9–4.2% of patients while other types of malignancy were reported in 0.5–2.1% of patients.

Fetal/Neonatal Morbidity and Mortality

Mycophenolate may cause fetal toxicity when administered to pregnant women. Use of mycophenolate mofetil has been associated with increased risk of first-trimester pregnancy loss and serious congenital malformations. Information on pregnancy outcome in transplant recipients has been compiled by the National Transplantation Pregnancy Registry (NTPR). Information on 33 pregnancies in transplant recipients who received mycophenolate mofetil during pregnancy has been reported to the registry; there were 15 spontaneous abortions (45%) and 18 live-born infants; 4 of these infants had structural abnormalities (22%). NTPR data indicate that congenital abnormalities have occurred in 4–5% of neonates born to transplant recipients receiving other immunosuppressive agents. Postmarketing data are available on 77 women exposed to mycophenolate mofetil during pregnancy; 25 had a spontaneous abortion and 14 had a malformed infant or fetus. Fetal anomalies reported include ear abnormalities (43%, from postmarketing data), other orofacial deformities (e.g., cleft lip, cleft palate), and malformations of the limbs, heart, esophagus, and kidneys.

Teratogenic and embryocidal effects have been observed in animals receiving mycophenolate at doses 0.02–0.9 times the recommended human dose. Fetal anomalies have included anophthalmia, agnathia, and hydrocephaly in rats, and ectopia cordis, ectopic kidneys, diaphragmatic hernia, and umbilical hernia in rabbits.

Mycophenolate should be used during pregnancy only when the potential benefits justify the possible risks to the fetus. Women of childbearing potential should be informed of the potential risks of fetal toxicity prior to the initiation of therapy. A reliable blood or urine pregnancy test (i.e., having a sensitivity of at least 25 mIU/mL for human chorionic gonadotropin [HCG]) should be performed within 1 week prior to beginning mycophenolate therapy, and therapy with the drug should not be initiated until a report of the pregnancy test is available indicating that results are negative. Women of childbearing potential should use 2 reliable forms of contraception for at least 4 weeks prior to, throughout, and for at least 6 weeks after discontinuance of mycophenolate, unless the patient commits to continuous abstinence from heterosexual contact. Concomitant use of mycophenolate and certain oral hormonal contraceptives may result in decreased concentrations of the oral hormonal contraceptive. (See Drug Interactions: Oral Contraceptives.)

If mycophenolate is administered during pregnancy or if a patient becomes pregnant while receiving the drug, the patient should be informed of the potential hazard to the fetus. In certain situations, maternal benefits may outweigh the risks to the fetus. Women exposed to mycophenolate during pregnancy should be encouraged to enroll in the NTPR.

Infectious Complications

Use of immunosuppressive agents, including mycophenolate, may result in increased susceptibility to infection (i.e., opportunistic infections, sepsis, life-threatening/fatal infections). In clinical studies, serious infections (e.g., sepsis, fatal infections) occurred in 2% of renal and cardiac allograft recipients and in 5% of hepatic allograft recipients receiving mycophenolate mofetil. In one clinical study, the overall incidence of opportunistic infections in cardiac allograft recipients receiving mycophenolate mofetil was about 10% higher than in those receiving azathioprine; however, such difference was not associated with excess mortality associated with the infection or sepsis in patients receiving mycophenolate mofetil. Viral infections (e.g., cytomegalovirus [CMV] infections, herpes simplex, herpes zoster) have been reported more frequently in cardiac transplant recipients receiving mycophenolate mofetil than in those receiving azathioprine. Meningitis, infectious endocarditis, tuberculosis, and atypical mycobacterial infections have been reported during postmarketing surveillance of the drug.

Latent Viral Infections

Immunosuppressed patients are at an increased risk for opportunistic infections, including reactivation of latent viral infections. These include BK virus-associated nephropathy (BKVN), which has been reported in patients receiving immunosuppressants, including mycophenolate mofetil, cyclosporine, sirolimus, and tacrolimus. Primary infection with polyoma BK virus typically occurs in childhood; following initial infection, the virus remains latent, but reactivation may occur in immunocompromised patients. BKVN has principally been observed in renal transplant patients (usually within the first year posttransplantation), and may result in serious outcomes, including deterioration of kidney function and renal allograft loss. Risk of BK virus reactivation appears to be related to the degree of overall immunosuppression rather than use of any specific immunosuppressive agent; patients receiving a maintenance immunosuppressive regimen of at least 3 drugs appear to be at highest risk. Patients should be monitored for possible signs of BKVN, including deterioration in renal function, during therapy with mycophenolate mofetil or mycophenolate sodium; screening assays for polyomavirus replication also have been recommended by some clinicians. Early intervention in patients who develop BKVN is critical; a reduction in immunosuppressive therapy should initially be considered in such patients. Although a variety of other treatment approaches have been used anecdotally in patients with BKVN, including antiviral therapy (e.g., cidofovir), leflunomide, IV immunoglobulins, and fluoroquinolone antibiotics, additional experience and well-controlled studies are necessary to more clearly establish the optimal treatment of such patients.

Progressive multifocal leukoencephalopathy (PML), an opportunistic viral infection of the brain, has been reported during postmarketing experience with mycophenolate mofetil (CellCept®). PML is caused by the JC virus and typically occurs in immunocompromised patients. At least 17 cases (10 confirmed, 7 possible) of PML have been reported in patients receiving mycophenolate mofetil; death occurred in at least 7 patients. Most reported cases of PML have occurred in patients who were receiving mycophenolate mofetil for the prevention of rejection of a solid organ transplant or for the management of systemic lupus erythematosus (SLE)†. These patients also were receiving other immunosuppressants (i.e., corticosteroids, cyclosporine, tacrolimus, and azathioprine in transplant recipients; corticosteroids, cyclophosphamide, and cyclosporine in SLE patients) or had compromised immune function. Hemiparesis, apathy, confusion, cognitive impairment, and ataxia were the most common manifestations of PML observed in these patients.

To date, no cases of PML have been reported in patients receiving mycophenolate sodium (Myfortic®). Because mycophenolate sodium is converted to the same active metabolite (mycophenolic acid) as mycophenolate mofetil, use of mycophenolate sodium is expected to be associated with the same risk of PML as use of mycophenolate mofetil.

The possible diagnosis of PML should be considered in immunocompromised patients receiving mycophenolate who experience neurologic manifestations. Consultation with a neurologist is advised as clinically indicated. Decreasing total immunosuppression may improve the outcome of PML, but also may increase the risk of graft rejection in transplant recipients. Clinicians should consider the potential risks versus benefits of reduced immunosuppression.

Hematologic Effects

Severe neutropenia (i.e., absolute neutrophil counts [ANC] of less than 500/mm³) has been reported in up to 2, 2.8, or 3.6% of renal, cardiac, or hepatic allograft recipients, respectively, receiving 3-g daily dosages of mycophenolate mofetil.

Neutropenia has been observed most frequently between 31–180 days posttransplant in patients receiving immunosuppressive therapy for the prevention of

rejection of kidney, heart, or liver allograft. Neutropenia may be related to mycophenolate, concomitant therapies, viral infection, or a combination of these causes.

Complete blood cell counts (CBCs) should be performed weekly during the first month of therapy, twice monthly during the second and third month, and then monthly thereafter, during the first year. If neutropenia (ANC of less than 1300/mm³) develops, mycophenolate therapy should be temporarily discontinued or the dosage reduced, suitable diagnostic tests should be performed, and appropriate patient management should be instituted.

Pure red cell aplasia (PRCA), a condition in which red blood cell precursors in the bone marrow are absent or nearly absent, has been reported in patients receiving immunosuppressive regimens containing mycophenolate mofetil. At least 41 cases of PRCA have been reported in patients receiving mycophenolate mofetil. Some of these patients also were receiving other immunosuppressants, including alemtuzumab, azathioprine, and tacrolimus. Because these patients were receiving multiple immunosuppressive agents, the relative contribution of mycophenolate mofetil and other immunosuppressants to the development of PRCA is not known. Risk of PRCA also should be considered in patients receiving mycophenolate sodium, because this drug is converted to the same active metabolite (mycophenolic acid) as mycophenolate mofetil. PRCA can produce varying degrees of anemia from subclinical to severe; manifestations may include fatigue, lethargy, pallor, weakness, tachycardia, and/or dyspnea. Although the mechanism for mycophenolate-induced PRCA has not been determined, immunosuppression may play a role. In some cases, PRCA was found to be reversible with dosage reduction or discontinuance of mycophenolate mofetil. However, clinicians should consider the possibility of graft rejection if immunosuppression is reduced in transplant patients; any changes in immunosuppressive therapy should be implemented under appropriate medical supervision.

● Major Toxicities

GI Effects

Severe GI bleeding (requiring hospitalization) has occurred in 3, 1.7, or 5.4% of renal, cardiac, or hepatic transplant recipients, respectively, receiving 3-g daily dosages of mycophenolate mofetil in clinical studies. In studies evaluating safety of mycophenolate sodium, severe GI bleeding was reported in 1% of de novo renal transplant patients and 1.3% of those receiving maintenance therapy. Mycophenolate mofetil therapy is associated with a high incidence of adverse GI effects; mycophenolate sodium delayed-release tablets were developed to improve GI tolerance. However, adverse GI effects in patients receiving mycophenolate sodium in comparative clinical studies have been similar to those in patients receiving mycophenolate mofetil. Because mycophenolate mofetil and mycophenolate sodium have been associated with adverse GI effects and rarely with serious GI effects (ulceration, hemorrhage, or perforation), the drugs should be administered with caution in patients with active serious GI disease.

General Precautions

Hypoxanthine Phosphoribosyltransferase Deficiency

Because mycophenolic acid inhibits inosine monophosphate dehydrogenase, mycophenolate mofetil and mycophenolate sodium should be avoided, on theoretical grounds, in patients with rare hereditary deficiency of hypoxanthine-guanine phosphoribosyltransferase (HGPRT), including Kelley-Seegmiller or Lesch-Nyhan syndrome.

Phenylketonuria

Individuals with phenylketonuria and those who must restrict their intake of phenylalanine should be warned that mycophenolate mofetil oral suspension contains aspartame (NutraSweet®), which is metabolized in the GI tract to provide about 0.56 mg of phenylalanine per 5 mL of the suspension.

Specific Populations

Pregnancy

Category D. (see Users Guide), and see Fetal/Neonatal Morbidity and Mortality under Warnings/Precautions: Warnings, in Cautions.

Lactation

Mycophenolic acid is distributed into milk in rats; not known whether this drug is distributed into milk in humans. Discontinue nursing or the drug, taking into account the importance of the drug to the woman. Women should not breast-feed for at least 6 weeks after discontinuance of mycophenolate sodium therapy.

Pediatric Use

Safety of mycophenolate mofetil for the prevention of rejection of renal allografts in children 3 months to 18 years of age is based on data from a pediatric pharmacokinetic and safety study. The manufacturer states that safety and efficacy of mycophenolate mofetil in pediatric patients younger than 3 months of age receiving renal allografts have not been established. In addition, safety and efficacy have not been established in pediatric patients younger than 18 years of age receiving allogenic cardiac or hepatic transplants.

Limited data are available concerning use of mycophenolate mofetil in pediatric patients. In one study in children 1–18 years of age receiving mycophenolate mofetil 600 mg/m^2 (oral suspension) twice daily following renal transplantation, pharmacokinetic parameters, including the area under the plasma concentration-time curve (AUC), were similar to those reported in adult renal transplant recipients receiving mycophenolate mofetil 1 g twice daily. Results of several pediatric studies and analysis of an open-label study in children 3 months to 18 years of age undergoing renal transplantation suggest that the safety profile in children generally is similar to that in adults, although a difference in the incidence of certain adverse effects (e.g. abdominal pain, fever, infection, pain, sepsis, diarrhea, vomiting, pharyngitis, respiratory tract infection, hypertension, and anemia) has been higher in pediatric patients than in adults. In clinical studies in pediatric patients, lymphoproliferative malignancies have been reported rarely (about 1.4%), while other types of malignancies were not observed in children in these studies. Severe GI bleeding (requiring hospitalization) has been reported in 3.4% of pediatric patients undergoing renal transplantation.

Safety and efficacy of mycophenolate sodium in stable renal transplant pediatric patients 5–16 years of age is based on evidence from adequate and well controlled studies in stable adult renal transplant patients receiving mycophenolate sodium and limited pharmacokinetic data in stable renal transplant pediatric patients 5–16 years of age. Safety and efficacy of mycophenolate sodium have not been established in pediatric de novo renal transplant patients.

Limited data are available concerning use of mycophenolate sodium in pediatric patients. Following administration of a single dose of mycophenolate sodium (mycophenolic acid 450 mg/m^2) in stable pediatric renal transplant patients 5–16 years of age, peak plasma concentrations and AUC of mycophenolic acid were 33 and 18% higher, respectively, than those reported in adults receiving the same dose based on body surface area (720 mg). The clinical importance of these findings remains to be determined. Pharmacokinetic data are not available in pediatric patients younger than 5 years of age.

Geriatric Use

Clinical studies of mycophenolate did not include sufficient numbers of patients 65 years of age or older to determine whether they respond differently than younger adults. While other clinical experience has not revealed differences in response, drug dosages should be selected cautiously in geriatric patients. The greater frequency of decreased hepatic, renal, and/or cardiac function and of concomitant diseases and drug therapy observed in the elderly also should be considered. Geriatric patients may be at increased risk of developing GI hemorrhage, pulmonary edema, or certain infections (e.g., invasive CMV infection) than younger patients.

Hepatic Impairment

No dosage adjustment for mycophenolate preparations is necessary for renal transplant recipients with severe hepatic parenchymal disease; not known whether dosage adjustment is needed for other hepatic diseases. No data are available for cardiac transplant recipients with severe hepatic parenchymal disease.

Renal Impairment

Administration of a single dose of mycophenolate mofetil in individuals with severe long-term renal impairment (glomerular filtration rate less than 25 mL/minute per 1.73 m^2) has resulted in higher AUC values for mycophenolic acid and the phenolic glucuronide of mycophenolic acid than values in individuals with less severe impairment or no impairment.

Patients receiving mycophenolate mofetil who experience posttransplant delay in graft function generally have AUC values for mycophenolic acid that are similar to those not experiencing graft function delay; however, the AUC for the phenolic glucuronide of mycophenolic acid is increased twofold to threefold in patients experiencing delayed graft function compared with those not experiencing delayed function. Dosage adjustment does not appear to be necessary in these patients; however, patients should be carefully observed.

No data are available on the use of mycophenolate mofetil in cardiac or hepatic transplant recipients with severe chronic renal impairment; mycophenolate mofetil may be used in these patients if the potential benefits outweigh the potential risks.

Studies evaluating the pharmacokinetics of mycophenolate sodium have not been conducted in patients with renal impairment. AUC values for mycophenolic acid in patients with renal impairment receiving mycophenolate sodium are not expected to increase appreciably relative to values in patients with normal renal function; however, AUC values for the phenolic glucuronide metabolite of mycophenolic acid are expected to increase substantially with decreased renal function. Plasma concentrations of mycophenolic acid and the phenolic glucuronide of mycophenolic acid may be increased in patients with severe renal impairment (glomerular filtration rate less than 25 mL/minute per 1.73 m^2) compared with plasma concentrations of healthy individuals and those with mild to moderate renal impairment. Patients with severe renal impairment should be carefully observed for possible adverse effects associated with increased plasma concentrations of free (unbound) mycophenolic acid and the phenolic glucuronide of mycophenolic acid. Safety of long-term exposure to increased concentrations of the phenolic glucuronide of mycophenolic acid remains to be determined.

● Common Adverse Effects

The most frequently reported adverse effects associated with mycophenolate mofetil therapy are diarrhea, leukopenia, sepsis, vomiting, higher frequency of infections, including opportunistic infections (e.g., CMV infections, herpes zoster, herpes simplex, candidal infections, aspergillosis, and Pneumocystis carinii pneumonia). Adverse reactions occurring in 20% or more of patients receiving mycophenolate mofetil include pain (e.g., abdominal, chest, back), fever, headache, anemia (e.g., hypochromic), thrombocytopenia, leukocytosis, urinary tract infection, abnormal renal function, hypertension, hypotension, cardiovascular disorder, tachycardia, edema (e.g., peripheral) hypercholesterolemia, hypokalemia, hyperkalemia, hyperglycemia, increases in blood urea nitrogen (BUN) and serum creatinine concentration, increased lactic dehydrogenase, hypomagnesemia, hypocalcemia, constipation, dyspepsia, nausea, vomiting, anorexia, abnormal liver function test results, cough, dyspnea, lung disorder, sinusitis, pleural effusion, rash, tremor, insomnia, dizziness, anxiety, and paresthesia.

The adverse effect profile in patients receiving IV mycophenolate mofetil hydrochloride is similar to that in patients receiving oral mycophenolate mofetil; phlebitis and thrombosis have been reported in 4% of patients receiving IV infusion of the drug.

In controlled studies in patients undergoing renal transplantation, the overall safety profile in those receiving mycophenolate mofetil 2 g daily was better than in those receiving 3 g daily. The types of adverse effects reported in renal, cardiac, or hepatic transplant studies generally are similar (except for those unique to the specific organ involved).

The most frequent adverse effects reported in patients receiving mycophenolate sodium include constipation, nausea, diarrhea, urinary tract infection, and nasopharyngitis. Adverse reactions occurring in 20% or more of patients receiving mycophenolate sodium include leukopenia, vomiting, dyspepsia, CMV infections, insomnia, and postoperative pain. In controlled studies in patients undergoing renal transplantation, the incidence of adverse effects reported in patients receiving mycophenolate sodium was similar to that reported in patients receiving mycophenolate mofetil.

DRUG INTERACTIONS

● Immunosuppressants

In clinical trials in patients undergoing transplant procedures, mycophenolate mofetil has been administered concurrently with cyclosporine, antithymocyte globulin (equine), muromonab-CD3, and/or corticosteroids; the manufacturer states that safety and efficacy of mycophenolate mofetil in combination with immunosuppressive agents other than these agents have not been determined.

In clinical trials in patients undergoing renal transplantation, mycophenolate sodium has been administered concurrently with cyclosporine, antithymocyte globulin, antilymphocyte globulin, muromonab-CD3, basiliximab, daclizumab (no longer commercially available in the US), and/or corticosteroids; the manufacturer states that safety and efficacy of mycophenolate sodium in combination with immunosuppressive agents other than these agents have not been determined.

Potential pharmacodynamic interaction (bone marrow suppression) with azathioprine. Concomitant use not recommended.

Concomitant use of mycophenolate mofetil with mycophenolate sodium is not recommended. Potential pharmacodynamic interaction (bone marrow suppression).

Concomitant use of mycophenolate mofetil without cyclosporine results in increased systemic exposure to mycophenolic acid compared with use of mycophenolate mofetil with cyclosporine. The lower systemic exposure to mycophenolic acid when mycophenolate mofetil is used with cyclosporine has been attributed to cyclosporine-induced inhibition of multidrug-resistance-associated protein 2 transporter in the biliary tract; inhibition of this transporter prevents excretion of the phenolic glucuronide of mycophenolic acid into bile (the phenolic glucuronide of mycophenolic acid is converted to mycophenolic acid via enterohepatic recirculation). Use of mycophenolate mofetil or mycophenolate sodium with or without cyclosporine does not affect plasma cyclosporine concentrations.

● **Anti-infective Agents**

Pharmacokinetic interaction with co-trimoxazole unlikely.

Potential pharmacokinetic interaction with concomitant use of rifampin with mycophenolate mofetil (decreased systemic exposure to mycophenolic acid). Concomitant use of mycophenolate mofetil and rifampin not recommended unless benefit outweighs risk.

Concomitant use of mycophenolate mofetil and the anti-infective combination of norfloxacin and metronidazole not recommended due to potential pharmacokinetic interaction (decreased systemic exposure to mycophenolic acid); however, no substantial effect on systemic exposure to mycophenolic acid was observed when mycophenolate mofetil was administered with norfloxacin or metronidazole.

Concomitant administration of mycophenolate mofetil and oral ciprofloxacin or amoxicillin plus clavulanic acid decreased median trough concentrations of mycophenolic acid (active metabolite of mycophenolate mofetil) by approximately 50% in 3 days following initiation of antibiotic therapy in one study in renal transplant recipients. The potential mechanism for this drug interaction may be an antibiotic-induced reduction in glucuronidase-possessing enteric bacteria resulting in decreased enterohepatic recirculation of mycophenolic acid. Because changes in mycophenolic acid concentrations did not necessarily correlate with overall drug exposure, the clinical importance of these findings is not clear.

● **Antiviral Agents**

Potential pharmacokinetic interaction with concomitant use of acyclovir with mycophenolate mofetil (increased plasma concentrations of acyclovir and the phenolic glucuronide of mycophenolic acid). Potential pharmacokinetic interaction with ganciclovir and valganciclovir in patients with renal impairment (increased plasma concentrations of the metabolites of the drugs). If acyclovir or ganciclovir is used in patients receiving mycophenolate sodium, blood cell counts should be monitored during treatment with the antiviral agent.

● **Antacids**

Potential pharmacokinetic interaction (decreased plasma concentrations of mycophenolic acid) with antacids containing aluminum and magnesium hydroxides. Mycophenolate mofetil or mycophenolate sodium may be used in patients receiving these antacids; however, the immunosuppressant should not be administered simultaneously with the antacids.

● **Salicylates**

Potential pharmacokinetic interaction based on in vitro data (increased free fraction of mycophenolic acid).

● **Cholestyramine**

Potential pharmacokinetic interaction (decreased plasma concentrations of mycophenolic acid). Administration of mycophenolate mofetil or mycophenolate sodium with cholestyramine or other agents that interfere with enterohepatic recirculation of the drug is not recommended.

● **Oral Contraceptives**

Potential pharmacokinetic interaction with concomitant use of levonorgestrel with mycophenolate mofetil (decreased plasma concentrations of levonorgestrel). Pharmacokinetic interaction unlikely with concomitant use of mycophenolate mofetil with ethinyl estradiol, desogestrel, or gestodene. Pharmacokinetic interaction unlikely with mycophenolate sodium. Oral contraceptives should be administered with caution in patients receiving mycophenolate and additional methods of birth control methods should be used.

● **Phosphate Binders**

Potential pharmacokinetic interaction with concomitant administration of sevelamer and mycophenolate mofetil (decreased plasma concentrations of mycophenolic acid). The manufacturer recommends that sevelamer or other non-calcium-containing phosphate binders be given 2 hours after the administration of mycophenolate mofetil.

● **Probenecid and other Inhibitors of Tubular Secretion**

Potential pharmacokinetic interaction based on animal data (increased plasma concentrations of mycophenolic acid and the phenolic glucuronide of mycophenolic acid).

● **Drugs that Alter Intestinal Flora**

Drugs that alter intestinal flora may interfere with mycophenolate mofetil or mycophenolate sodium by disrupting enterohepatic recirculation; interference with the hydrolysis of the phenolic glucuronide metabolite of mycophenolic acid to mycophenolic acid may decrease the amount of mycophenolic acid available for absorption.

● **Vaccines**

Potential interaction with live virus vaccine (decreased response to vaccination). Avoid use of live virus vaccine in patients receiving mycophenolate mofetil or mycophenolate sodium. Vaccination with influenza virus vaccine inactivated may be of value.

PHARMACOKINETICS

● **Absorption**

Mycophenolate mofetil is rapidly absorbed following oral administration; bioavailability is 94%. Following oral and IV administration, mycophenolate mofetil undergoes rapid and complete metabolism to mycophenolic acid, the active metabolite. Mycophenolate mofetil tablets, capsules, and oral suspension are bioequivalent.

Following oral administration of the delayed-release tablets (mycophenolate sodium), mycophenolic acid is released in the small intestine; bioavailability is 72%.

Mycophenolate sodium delayed-release tablets cannot be used interchangeably with mycophenolate mofetil tablets, capsules, or oral suspension without clinician supervision. Single oral doses of mycophenolate sodium delayed-release tablets (mycophenolic acid 720 mg) and mycophenolate mofetil 1 g result in bioequivalent mycophenolic acid exposure.

Food decreases peak plasma concentrations of mycophenolic acid (by 33–40%); no effect on the mycophenolic acid AUC.

Plasma concentrations of free (unbound) mycophenolic acid and total mycophenolic acid glucuronide have increased in nontransplant individuals with severe chronic renal impairment (GFR <25 mL/minute per 1.73 m^2). Plasma mycophenolic acid concentrations in patients with delayed graft function similar to values in patients not experiencing delayed graft function.

Pharmacokinetic parameters, including AUC, in children 1–18 years of age receiving mycophenolate mofetil 600 mg/m² (oral suspension) twice daily following renal transplantation, are similar to values in adult renal transplant recipients receiving 1 g twice daily. Peak plasma concentrations and AUC of mycophenolic acid in stable pediatric renal transplant patients 5–16 years of age receiving a single dose of mycophenolate sodium (mycophenolic acid 450 mg/m²) increased (33 and 18%, respectively) relative to adults receiving the same dose based on body surface area. Clinical importance not determined.

● *Distribution*

Mycophenolic acid is ≥97–98% bound to plasma protein (mainly albumin).

● *Elimination*

Mycophenolate mofetil undergoes complete metabolism to mycophenolic acid; metabolism occurs presystemically following oral administration. Mycophenolic acid is metabolized by glucuronyl transferase to the phenolic glucuronide of mycophenolic acid. The phenolic glucuronide is converted to mycophenolic acid via enterohepatic recirculation.

Mycophenolate mofetil is excreted in urine (93%) as the phenolic glucuronide of mycophenolic acid (87%) and in feces (6%). Mycophenolate sodium is excreted principally in urine as phenolic glucuronide of mycophenolic acid (>60%) and as unchanged mycophenolic acid (3%).

The half-life of mycophenolic acid is 8–17.9 hours.

Plasma concentrations of mycophenolic acid glucuronide are higher in nontransplant subjects with severe renal impairment than in those with mild impairment or normal renal function. Plasma concentrations of mycophenolic acid glucuronide are higher in transplant patients with delayed renal graft function than in patients not experiencing delayed graft function. Dialysis does not remove mycophenolic acid. Pharmacokinetic studies in patients with alcoholic cirrhosis indicate that hepatic mycophenolic acid glucuronidation is not affected by hepatic parenchymal disease; hepatic disease with other etiologies (e.g., biliary cirrhosis) may show a different effect.

DESCRIPTION

Mycophenolate mofetil, the 2-morpholinoethyl ester of mycophenolic acid, is an immunosuppressive agent. Mycophenolate mofetil is a prodrug that has little pharmacologic activity until it is rapidly and completely hydrolyzed in vivo to the pharmacologically active metabolite, mycophenolic acid. Mycophenolate mofetil differs structurally and pharmacologically from other immunosuppressive agents.

Mycophenolate sodium also is an immunosuppressive agent. Following oral administration of mycophenolate sodium delayed-release tablets, mycophenolic acid (the active moiety) is released in the small intestine.

Acute rejection episodes occur in up to 60% or more of patients who have undergone renal transplantation and result in a substantial reduction in long-term (5 years or longer) graft survival. Although the exact mechanism of the immunosuppressive effect of action of mycophenolic acid has not been fully elucidated, it appears to be related to inhibition of lymphocyte production. Mycophenolic acid is a potent, selective, noncompetitive, reversible inhibitor of inosine monophosphate dehydrogenase (IMPDH), an essential enzyme in *de novo* guanosine synthesis. Because T- and B-cells are dependent on *de novo* synthesis of purines (e.g., guanosine), mycophenolic acid selectively inhibits proliferation of T- and B-cells. The drug inhibits proliferative responses of T- and B-cells to both mitogenic and allospecific stimulation. Mycophenolic acid suppresses antibody formation by B-cells. By preventing glycosylation of lymphocyte and monocyte glycoproteins involved in intercellular adhesion to endothelial cells, mycophenolic acid may inhibit recruitment of leukocytes to sites of inflammation and graft rejection.

Mycophenolate mofetil is well absorbed following oral administration, having an absolute bioavailability of approximately 94% (based on mycophenolic acid). The absolute bioavailability of mycophenolic acid following oral administration of mycophenolate sodium delayed-release tablets in stable renal transplant patients has been reported to be approximately 72%. Following oral administration of mycophenolate sodium delayed-release (enteric-coated) tablets, the median time to peak plasma concentrations of the drug is 1.5–2.75 hours compared with 0.5–1 hour reported with conventional preparations of mycophenolate mofetil. Administration of mycophenolate sodium (as delayed-release tablets) or mycophenolate mofetil with food does not affect the AUC of mycophenolic acid; however, decreases by about 33 or 40% of the peak plasma concentrations of mycophenolic acid have been observed, respectively.

The pharmacologically active metabolite, mycophenolic acid, is metabolized principally by glucuronyl transferase to form the phenolic glucuronide metabolite of mycophenolic acid, which is not pharmacologically active. In vivo, the phenolic glucuronide metabolite is converted back to mycophenolic acid via enterohepatic recirculation; concurrent administration of drugs that interfere with such recirculation may decrease plasma concentrations of mycophenolic acid. (See Drug Interactions: Cholestyramine.) Ninety-three percent of an orally administered dose of mycophenolate mofetil is excreted in urine (mainly [about 87%] as the phenolic glucuronide of mycophenolic acid) and 6% is excreted in feces. Following administration of mycophenolate sodium, most of the dose (greater than 60%) of mycophenolic acid is excreted in urine as the phenolic glucuronide of mycophenolic acid and 3% is excreted in urine as mycophenolic acid. Mycophenolic acid and the phenolic glucuronide of mycophenolic acid usually are not removed by dialysis.

ADVICE TO PATIENTS

Importance of taking mycophenolate as directed. Importance of reading manufacturer's patient information (medication guide) before initiating therapy and each time drug is refilled. Importance in following patient instructions for administration, handling, and storage of mycophenolate mofetil oral suspension.

Patients should be informed about the risk of lymphoproliferative disease and other malignancies (particularly skin cancer). Importance of informing clinician of any unexplained fever, prolonged tiredness, weight loss, swelling of lymph nodes, or unusual skin changes (e.g., new lesions or bumps, discoloration, brown or black lesions with uneven borders). Importance of limiting sunlight or other UV light exposure by wearing protective clothing and using sunscreens with a high protection factor; importance of avoiding tanning beds or sunlamps.

Patients receiving mycophenolate should be informed of the necessity of routine laboratory testing (e.g., complete blood cell count).

Importance of informing a clinician immediately of any evidence of infection (e.g., temperature elevations of 100.5°F or greater, cold or flu symptoms, earache, headache, pain on urination, white patches in the mouth or throat), unexpected bruising, bleeding, or other manifestations of bone marrow depression. Importance of also informing a clinician of any unusual tiredness, lack of energy, dizziness, or fainting.

Inform women of childbearing potential of possible risk to fetus prior to initiating therapy. Importance of women informing clinicians if they are or plan to become pregnant or plan to breast-feed. Advise women of childbearing potential to avoid pregnancy and to use 2 methods of effective contraception for at least 4 weeks before, during, and for at least 6 weeks after discontinuance of the drug. Advise such women that mycophenolate may decrease effectiveness of certain oral contraceptives. When the drug is administered during pregnancy, or if the patient becomes pregnant while receiving the drug, the patient should be informed of the potential hazard to the fetus and the potential risk for loss of the pregnancy, especially in the first trimester.

Women receiving mycophenolate sodium should avoid breast-feeding for at least 6 weeks after discontinuance of the drug.

Importance of patients informing a clinician if they plan on receiving any vaccines while taking mycophenolate; patients should be instructed to avoid live virus vaccines.

Importance of informing clinicians of concomitant conditions (e.g., ulcers, Lesch-Nyhan or Kelley-Seegmiller syndrome, phenylketonuria) and existing or contemplated concomitant therapy, including prescription and OTC drugs.

Importance of informing patients of other important precautionary information. (See Cautions.)

PREPARATIONS

Excipients in commercially available drug preparations may have clinically important effects in some individuals; consult specific product labeling for details.

Mycophenolate Mofetil

Oral

Capsules	250 mg	**CellCept®**, Roche
For oral suspension	200 mg/mL	**CellCept®**, Roche
Tablets	500 mg	**CellCept®**, Roche

Mycophenolate Mofetil Hydrochloride

Parenteral

For injection, for IV infusion only	500 mg (of mycophenolate mofetil)	**CellCept® Intravenous**, Roche

Mycophenolate Sodium

Oral

Tablets, delayed-release, (enteric-coated) film-coated	180 mg (of mycophenolic acid)	**Myfortic®**, Novartis
	360 mg (of mycophenolic acid)	**Myfortic®**, Novartis

† Use is not currently included in the labeling approved by the US Food and Drug Administration.

Selected Revisions May 10, 2024, © Copyright, January 1, 2004, American Society of Health-System Pharmacists, Inc.

cycloSPORINE (Systemic)

90:28.28.92 • CALCINEURIN INHIBITORS, MISCELLANEOUS

■ Cyclosporine is a cyclosporin immunosuppressive agent and disease-modifying antirheumatic drug.

USES

Cyclosporine is used for the prevention of rejection of kidney, liver, or heart allografts. The manufacturers and some clinicians recommend that cyclosporine be used in conjunction with corticosteroid therapy, at least initially. Cyclosporine is also used for the treatment of chronic allograft rejection in patients previously treated with other immunosuppressive agents (e.g., azathioprine).

● Renal Allotransplantation

Cyclosporine is used to prolong graft survival of allogeneic renal transplants. Therapy with cyclosporine alone has achieved graft survival rates ranging from 71–91% 1 year after renal transplantation. In a retrospective study, patient and graft survival rates were 86 and 70%, respectively, 4 years after transplantation in cyclosporine-treated patients.

Concomitant administration of cyclosporine and corticosteroids in some studies has resulted in reduction of cyclosporine dosage and decreased frequency of cyclosporine's nephrotoxic effects while continuing to optimally prolong graft survival; however, some clinicians suggest that concomitant administration of cyclosporine and corticosteroids does not increase effectiveness and may increase the frequency of adverse systemic effects (e.g., lymphoma). In a study in renal allograft recipients receiving cyclosporine alone or in combination with corticosteroids, graft survival rates after 1 year were 88 vs 84%, respectively; infectious complications and hypertension occurred more frequently in patients receiving combined therapy with cyclosporine and a corticosteroid than in those receiving cyclosporine alone. Concomitant administration of cyclosporine and corticosteroids did not improve renal function and was associated with increased frequency of lymphoma, probably resulting from excessive immunosuppression. Although the manufacturers recommend that cyclosporine be used in conjunction with corticosteroid therapy, at least initially, further study is needed to determine the role of concomitant therapy in renal allograft recipients.

When immunosuppressive therapy with cyclosporine alone or combined with corticosteroids has been compared with combined azathioprine and corticosteroid therapy, graft survival rates generally were equivalent or higher in patients receiving cyclosporine with or without corticosteroids. In patients with renal allografts, the 1-year actuarial graft survival rates for cyclosporine vs combined azathioprine and corticosteroid therapy have been reported to be 72–77 vs 52–62%, respectively; the 1-year patient survival rates for cyclosporine vs combined azathioprine and corticosteroid therapy were 88–94 vs 76–92%, respectively. Some cyclosporine-treated patients also received periodic corticosteroid therapy for acute rejection episodes. The 4-year actuarial graft survival rates for these therapies have been reported to be 76 vs 62%, respectively, and the 4-year actuarial patient survival rates were 86 vs 70%, respectively. In one study, graft survival rate in cyclosporine-treated patients was higher in patients receiving first renal allografts than in those receiving second ones and in patients receiving HLA-A and/or B mismatched allografts than in those receiving allografts matched at HLA-A and B loci; there was no correlation in graft survival with warm or cold ischemia or with anti-HLA antibodies. Cyclosporine-treated patients generally have had higher serum creatinine concentrations than those receiving combined azathioprine and corticosteroid therapy. The relative effects of prophylactic immunosuppressive regimens containing cyclosporine and/or equine antithymocyte globulin (ATG) on graft survival rates remain to be determined. Results of several comparative studies indicate that the effects on graft survival rates of prophylactic immunosuppressive regimens containing cyclosporine or equine antilymphocyte globulin (ALG) are similar.

Although cyclosporine prolongs graft survival, the drug may not prevent acute episodes of renal allograft rejection. The number of patients experiencing acute episodes of renal allograft rejection and the median time to onset of these episodes (about 1 week) have been reported to be similar for cyclosporine- or combined azathioprine/corticosteroid-treated patients. However, in one study, first acute episodes of rejection were substantially less severe in patients receiving cyclosporine than in those receiving combined azathioprine and corticosteroid therapy. In some cyclosporine-treated patients, renal graft losses resulting from irreversible acute graft rejection may be associated with persistently low trough serum concentrations of the drug; however, optimum therapeutic trough concentrations have not been determined. The occurrence of graft rejection is difficult to differentiate from cyclosporine-induced nephrotoxicity. (See Cautions: Renal Effects.) Rapid increases in serum creatinine concentration that occur simultaneously with low blood or plasma cyclosporine concentrations may indicate graft rejection.

Some clinicians recommend that cyclosporine generally be discontinued and combined therapy with azathioprine and corticosteroids be initiated in patients who do not tolerate cyclosporine (e.g., nephrotoxicity) or in whom intractable rejection occurs. In one study, the 1-year actuarial graft survival rate in patients switched from cyclosporine to combined azathioprine and corticosteroid therapy was 60%. Conversion to immunosuppressive therapy with azathioprine and corticosteroids usually results in decreased serum creatinine concentrations; however, complications, including acute rejection episodes, serious infections, or azathioprine-induced leukopenia, may occur. In one study, the need to switch from cyclosporine to combined azathioprine and corticosteroid therapy because of cyclosporine-induced nephrotoxicity or intractable rejection was eliminated when routine (3 times weekly) monitoring of trough serum cyclosporine concentrations was initiated; however, optimum trough concentrations have not been determined.

● Hepatic Allotransplantation

Cyclosporine is used to prolong graft and patient survival in hepatic allograft recipients. Administration of cyclosporine and low-dose prednisone has resulted in 1-year actuarial patient survival rates of 60–80% in a limited number of hepatic allograft recipients. However, response rates may be variable and may depend on the underlying condition of the patient or the immunosuppressive regimen used. Cyclosporine's effectiveness in hepatic allotransplantation has been shown in children and adults. Decreased frequency of postoperative infectious complications may be observed in hepatic allograft recipients who have received cyclosporine compared with those treated with other immunosuppressive therapy.

● Cardiac Allotransplantation

Cyclosporine is used to prolong graft and patient survival in cardiac allograft recipients. The drug has been used concomitantly with low-dose corticosteroid therapy to decrease the frequency and clinical severity of rejection episodes, reduce infectious complications compared with other immunosuppressive agents, and facilitate early patient rehabilitation following cardiac transplantation. Two-year actuarial patient survival rates for cardiac allograft recipients receiving cyclosporine vs combined azathioprine and corticosteroid therapy have been reported to be 77 vs 58%, respectively, in a limited number of patients.

Cyclosporine has also been used in a limited number of patients with combined heart-lung transplantation†.

● Bone Marrow Allotransplantation

The value of cyclosporine in the prevention of acute graft-vs-host disease following bone marrow transplantation† remains to be clearly established. Results of studies to date suggest that prophylaxis with cyclosporine is comparable to, but not more effective than, prophylaxis with methotrexate for the prevention or amelioration of acute graft-vs-host disease or improving survival in patients undergoing bone marrow transplantation for leukemias. Limited data suggest that prophylactic combination therapy with cyclosporine and methotrexate is more effective for the prevention or amelioration of acute graft-vs-host disease and possibly improves survival compared with cyclosporine alone. Cyclosporine has also been used with some success for the treatment of moderate to severe, acute graft-vs-host disease following bone marrow transplantation. Limited data suggest that cyclosporine may be as effective as corticosteroid therapy. Corticosteroids are generally considered the initial therapy of choice for the treatment of acute graft-vs-host disease.

● Rheumatoid Arthritis

Oral cyclosporine is used in the management of the active stage of severe rheumatoid arthritis in selected adults who have an inadequate therapeutic response to methotrexate; the drug may be used in combination with methotrexate in those who do not respond adequately to methotrexate monotherapy. Oral cyclosporine also has been useful in the treatment of rheumatoid arthritis in adults who had an insufficient therapeutic response to, or who did not tolerate nonsteroidal anti-inflammatory agents† (NSAIAs) and other† disease-modifying antirheumatic drugs (DMARDs) (e.g., gold compounds, penicillamine). Cyclosporine is one of several DMARDs that can be used when DMARD therapy is appropriate. (For further information on the treatment of rheumatoid arthritis, see Uses: Rheumatoid Arthritis, in Methotrexate 10:00.)

In a placebo-controlled study, cyclosporine administered for 6 months was more effective than placebo in decreasing the number of painful and tender or swollen joints. Results of an uncontrolled clinical study of patients treated with cyclosporine for a median of 29 months showed in comparison to baseline articular index that at 18 months pain (as rated on a visual analog scale) and the duration of morning stiffness were decreased, while functional capacity (as rated on a visual analog scale) was improved. After 24 months of therapy, articular index, pain, and duration of morning stiffness remained decreased. Although few comparative studies with other DMARDs have been published, cyclosporine appears to be as effective as azathioprine, chloroquine, or methotrexate in the management of rheumatoid arthritis. Cyclosporine, azathioprine, and methotrexate did not differ in global assessment of efficacy based on the number of clinical and laboratory variables that improved after 1 year of therapy. The decrease in the number of swollen joints did not differ between cyclosporine and chloroquine after 24 weeks of therapy with either drug as the initial DMARD. The difference between groups in radiologic evidence of progression of disease, as indicated by the increase in the number of target joints with juxtaarticular erosions at 12 months compared with baseline, favored patients who were receiving cyclosporine over the controls who were receiving another DMARD (e.g., chloroquine, hydroxychloroquine, sulfasalazine, auranofin, parenteral gold compounds, penicillamine).

Combined use of cyclosporine and methotrexate appears to improve therapeutic response in patients with rheumatoid arthritis that had improved partially with methotrexate alone. After 6 months of therapy, improvement in the tender-joint count was greater with combined cyclosporine (mean dosage: 3 mg/kg daily) and methotrexate than with methotrexate alone. In addition, more patients treated with cyclosporine and methotrexate had improvement in rheumatoid arthritis, based on criteria of the American College of Rheumatology (i.e., improvement by at least 20% in the number of tender joints, number of swollen joints, and in 3 of 5 other clinical measures including pain, physician's global assessment, patient's global assessment, degree of disability, erythrocyte sedimentation rate). Complete blood cell count and liver function should be monitored at least monthly in patients receiving cyclosporine and methotrexate therapy concomitantly.

● Psoriasis

Oral cyclosporine is used in immunocompetent adults with severe (i.e., extensive and/or disabling), recalcitrant plaque psoriasis that is not adequately responsive to at least one systemic therapy (e.g., retinoids, methotrexate, psoralen and UVA light [PUVA therapy]) or in patients for whom other systemic therapy is contraindicated or cannot be tolerated. Discontinuance of therapy with cyclosporine, as with other therapies, will result in relapse of psoriasis in most patients, while rebound occurs rarely.

● Crohn's Disease

Cyclosporine has been used in the management of refractory inflammatory, fistulizing, and chronically active Crohn's disease.†

Efficacy of cyclosporine has been evaluated in several uncontrolled studies in patients with refractory (e.g., to corticosteroids, anti-infective agents, mercaptopurine, azathioprine, surgery) inflammatory or fistulizing Crohn's disease†. In these studies, a limited number of patients with inflammatory or fistulizing disease (who continued to receive anti-infective agents, corticosteroids, azathioprine, mercaptopurine, and/or mesalamine) initially received a continuous IV infusion of cyclosporine over 24 hours (4 mg/kg daily for about 2–10 days) until clinical response (complete response in inflammatory disease usually was defined as resolution of diarrhea and abdominal pain, while partial response was defined as

a decrease in stool frequency and/or abdominal pain; complete response in fistulizing disease was defined as closure of the fistulas and cessation of drainage, while partial response was defined as reduction in the size, drainage, and discomfort associated with fistulas) was achieved. About 78–88% of patients responded while receiving IV cyclosporine and most of those who responded were switched to oral cyclosporine (5–8 mg/kg daily) for a mean duration of about 2.5–12.2 (range: 0.5–37 months) months. However, only about 29–71% of the patients who responded to IV cyclosporine, continued to respond while receiving oral cyclosporine and in 1 study (patients receiving oral cyclosporine for a median of 10.5 weeks), 71% of patients who responded to IV cyclosporine, relapsed after discontinuance of cyclosporine therapy. Some clinicians suggest, however, that a short course (about 4–6 months) of therapy with cyclosporine (administered as an IV infusion initially and followed by an oral course of the drug) given concomitantly with mercaptopurine or azathioprine (drugs associated with long-term improvement in fistulizing Crohn's disease) may be effective in some patients with refractory inflammatory or fistulizing Crohn's disease. Because both mercaptopurine and azathioprine have a slow onset of action (17 weeks or more) and cyclosporine has a faster onset, such an overlap of therapies (for about 4 months) may be beneficial in the fistulizing disease; however, additional well-controlled studies are needed to evaluate the clinical efficacy of these combinations. It also should be considered, that IV administration of cyclosporine may be associated with severe adverse effects and many clinicians state that the drug should be reserved for the management of severe refractory disease.

Results of several uncontrolled and some placebo-controlled trials indicate that oral cyclosporine (5–15 mg/kg daily) has not been consistently effective for inducing or maintaining remission in refractory chronically active Crohn's disease†. In a placebo-controlled, double-blind, randomized trial in patients with refractory, chronically active Crohn's disease, clinical improvement has been reported in more patients receiving oral cyclosporine (5–7.5 mg/kg daily) than in those receiving placebo (59% for cyclosporine versus 32% for placebo) at the end of a 3-month treatment period. However, during a subsequent 3-month tapering period, 36 or 55% of patients receiving cyclosporine or placebo, respectively, whose disease improved during the initial 3-month therapy, have relapsed; no substantial difference in disease improvement between cyclosporine therapy and placebo has been observed during the 6-month follow-up period.

For further information about the management of Crohn's disease, see Uses: Crohn's Disease, in Mesalamine 56:36.

● Ophthalmic Uses

For ophthalmic uses of cyclosporine, see 52:08.92.

● Other Uses

Cyclosporine potentially may be useful for the treatment of various other conditions that have an immunologic basis†.

Cyclosporine also has been used to decrease the frequency of pancreatic† or corneal allograft rejection†.

DOSAGE AND ADMINISTRATION

● Administration

Cyclosporine is administered orally as conventional (nonmodified) or modified formulations; the drug also is administered by IV infusion.

Oral Administration

Cyclosporine may be administered orally as the conventional liquid-filled capsules or the conventional oral solution. Alternatively, the drug may be administered orally as modified, liquid formulations (Gengraf®, Neoral®) that form emulsions in aqueous fluids; the modified formulations are available as oral solutions for emulsion and as oral liquid-filled capsules. When exposed to an aqueous environment, Neoral® oral solution forms a homogenous transparent emulsion with a droplet size smaller than 100 nm in diameter, which has been referred to as a microemulsion. Gengraf® also is described as forming a microemulsion when exposed to an aqueous environment. The 2 commercially available modified oral formulations of cyclosporine, Neoral® and Gengraf®, have been demonstrated to be bioequivalent to each other.

Modified formulations of cyclosporine (Gengraf®, Neoral®), both as the solution and in the liquid-filled capsules, have increased oral bioavailability compared with the conventional oral solution and liquid-filled capsules of the drug, and therefore the conventional (nonmodified) and modified formulations are *not* bioequivalent and cannot be used interchangeably without appropriate medical supervision. (See Pharmacokinetics: Absorption.) Patients should be informed that any change in the formulation of cyclosporine that they are receiving should be performed under the supervision of a clinician since adjustment of the dosage may be necessary and caution should be observed during such a transition.

Patients should be advised that oral formulations of cyclosporine should be administered on a consistent schedule with regard to time of day and in relation to meals. When an oral solution formulation is used, doses of cyclosporine should be measured carefully. A graduated oral syringe is provided for proper measurement of a dose of cyclosporine oral solution formulations. When measuring a dose of an oral solution formulation, the protective cover of the oral syringe should be removed, if present, and the prescribed dose of the drug withdrawn from the bottle of oral solution and transferred to a glass (not plastic) container of suitable beverage to enhance palatability. To increase the palatability of the conventional (nonmodified) oral solution, the measured dose of cyclosporine may be mixed with milk, chocolate milk, or orange juice, preferably at room temperature but not hot. To increase palatability of the modified oral solution of Gengraf® or Neoral®, the measured dose of the oral cyclosporine solution preferably should be mixed with orange or apple juice at room temperature; milk should *not* be used for dilution of the solution since the resultant mixture can be unpalatable. The manufacturers recommend that frequent changing of the diluting beverage be avoided. The diluted solution or emulsion containing cyclosporine should be stirred well and administered immediately, not allowing the mixture to stand before administration. Use of a glass container may minimize adherence of the drug to the walls of the container; styrofoam containers should *not* be used because they are porous and may absorb the drug. After the initial diluted solution or emulsion has been administered, the container should be rinsed with additional diluent (e.g., juice) and the remaining mixture administered to ensure that the entire dose of the drug has been given. After use of Neoral® oral solution, the manufacturer states that the outside of the dosing syringe should be dried with a clean, dry towel and the syringe replaced in its protective cover. After use of Gengraf® oral solution, the manufacturer states that the outside of the dosing syringe should be dried with a clean, dry towel and the syringe stored in a clean, dry place. To avoid turbidity, the dosing syringes for Gengraf® and Neoral® oral solution should not be rinsed with water, alcohol, or other cleaning agents. If the syringes require cleaning, they must be completely dry before reuse. Introduction of water into the product by any means will cause variation in dose.

Concomitant oral administration of cyclosporine conventional (nonmodified) or modified capsules or solutions with grapefruit juice should be avoided since unpredictable but potentially clinically important increases in oral bioavailability of the drug can result. Although some evidence suggested that patients who wished to continue consumption of grapefruit juice during cyclosporine therapy could do so if at least 90 minutes elapsed between administration of the drug and such consumption, other evidence indicates that such separation in timing may not be adequate, and additional study is needed. (See Drugs and Foods Affecting Hepatic Microsomal Enzymes: Grapefruit Juice, in Drug Interactions.)

IV Infusion

Because of the risk of anaphylaxis, IV administration of cyclosporine should be reserved for patients in whom oral administration of the drug is not tolerated or is contraindicated. (See Cautions: Precautions and Contraindications.)

Cyclosporine concentrate for injection must be diluted prior to IV infusion. For IV infusion, each mL of the concentrate should be diluted in 20–100 mL of 0.9% sodium chloride or 5% dextrose injection immediately before administration. Diluted solutions that have not been administered within 24 hours should be discarded. The required dose of diluted solution is infused over 2–6 hours.

Cyclosporine concentrate for injection and the diluted solution for infusion should be inspected visually for particulate matter and discoloration prior to administration whenever solution and container permit.

• Dosage

Transplant Recipients

Dosage of cyclosporine should be individualized. Monitoring blood or plasma, but preferably whole blood, concentrations of cyclosporine has an essential role in individualizing dosage and managing transplant recipients during therapy with the drug. However, optimum concentrations have not been precisely defined, and suggested ranges vary depending on the assay method and body fluid employed as well as the patient population treated and therapeutic regimen used. Therefore, the type of assay used (See Pharmacokinetics), organ transplanted, time since transplantation, other immunosuppressive agents administered concurrently, and other factors are important considerations in the assessment of cyclosporine blood concentrations. The clinical evaluation of rejection and toxicity, adjustment of dosage, and assessment of compliance may be assisted by monitoring blood concentrations of cyclosporine; however, recommended ranges of cyclosporine concentrations that are consistent with optimum efficacy for *all* patients currently cannot be defined. Therefore, it is preferable that patients be managed using a center experienced in the use and interpretation of cyclosporine concentrations and their application to dosage adjustment.

Laboratory Monitoring

Most clinicians currently base monitoring on trough (predose) concentrations of the drug. It is important that the sampling time for a given patient be standardized and that consideration be given to the effect of once- versus twice-daily dosing of cyclosporine. While most recent experience has been with assays that are specific for unchanged cyclosporine (See Pharmacokinetics), data are accumulating on the use of total drug (both cyclosporine and metabolites) concentrations, and some centers may have switched to such monitoring methods. The frequency of monitoring depends in part on the time that has elapsed since transplantation, intercurrent illness, and concomitant drugs. While there are no hard and fast rules, and monitoring should be performed whenever clinical manifestations suggest that dosage adjustment might be necessary, some clinicians generally monitor frequently (e.g., 3 or 4 times weekly to daily) during the early posttransplantation period, reducing monitoring to once monthly by 6 months to 1 year after transplantation. Timing of determinations also should take into account the time to pharmacokinetic reequilibration following recent dosage changes; in general, determinations made within 3 days of a dosage change (2 days for children) will not reflect steady state. If management with a center experienced in therapeutic drug monitoring of cyclosporine is not possible, specialized references can be consulted for general monitoring and dosing guidelines. Results obtained with various methods are not interchangeable, and specialized references and/or the assay manufacturer's labeling should be consulted for interpretive guidelines.

If plasma assay methods are used, the possibility that concentrations may vary with temperature at the time of plasma separation from whole blood and that cyclosporine plasma concentrations may be about 20–50% of cyclosporine blood concentrations should be considered. In addition, monitoring of blood or plasma cyclosporine concentrations does not obviate monitoring of renal function (e.g., serum creatinine and creatinine clearance determination) or tissue biopsies in patients receiving the drug. Periodic determination of blood or plasma cyclosporine concentrations and adjustment in dosage, when necessary, are especially important in patients, particularly hepatic allograft recipients, receiving long-term oral therapy since absorption of the drug may be erratic.

In one suggested regimen employing a highly specific assay (high-pressure liquid chromatography [HPLC]), dosage of cyclosporine in renal allograft recipients was adjusted to achieve trough blood concentrations determined just prior to the next dose (24 hours after the previous dose) of 100–200 ng/mL. Blood concentrations determined by HPLC are unchanged cyclosporine alone, and they have been shown to correlate directly to those determined by monoclonal specific radioimmunoassays (m-RIA-sp). Nonspecific assay methods that detect both unchanged drug and its metabolites also are available, and such assay methods generally were employed in older studies; blood cyclosporine concentrations determined by these methods were about twice those reported with specific assay methods. Therefore, comparing concentrations reported in the published literature with those for a given patient using current assays must employ a detailed knowledge of the assay method used. Although several assays and assay matrices are available, the current consensus is that assays specific for unchanged cyclosporine correlate best with clinical events. Such assays include HPLC, monoclonal antibody RIAs, monoclonal antibody FPIA, and EMIT, which have sensitivity and are reproducible and convenient.

Usual Dosage

For prevention of allograft rejection in adults and children, the usual initial oral dose of conventional (nonmodified) formulations of cyclosporine is 15 mg/kg administered as a single dose 4–12 hours before transplantation. Although this initial dose varied from 14–18 mg/kg in most clinical studies, the highest dose continues to be used in only a few transplant centers, while doses at the lower end of the range have been favored. Administration of even lower initial dosages (e.g., 10–14 mg/kg daily) is the trend for renal allotransplantation. Postoperatively, the usual dosage of 15 mg/kg (range: 14–18 mg/kg) daily, administered as a single daily dose, is continued for 1–2 weeks and then tapered by 5% per week (over about 6–8 weeks) to a maintenance dosage of 5–10 mg/kg daily. In several studies, pediatric patients have required and tolerated higher dosages. Some clinicians have successfully tapered maintenance dosage to as low as 3 mg/kg daily in selected renal allograft recipients without an apparent increase in graft rejection rate.

Therapy with modified oral cyclosporine formulations (Gengraf®, Neoral®) can be started with an initial dose given 4–12 hours before transplantation or postoperatively. The initial dosage of the modified formulations varies depending on the organ transplanted and the other immunosuppressive agents included in the immunosuppressive protocol. Newly transplanted patients may receive a modified oral formulation at the same initial dose as for the conventional (nonmodified) oral formulation. A survey conducted in 1994 on the use of the conventional oral formulation in American transplant centers provides additional information on suggested initial dosages. Renal allograft recipients received an average initial dosage of 9 mg/kg in 2 equally divided doses daily at 75 centers. Hepatic allograft recipients received an average initial dosage of 8 mg/kg in 2 equally divided doses daily at 30 centers, and cardiac allograft recipients received an average initial dosage of 7 mg/kg in 2 equally divided doses daily at 24 centers. The dosage of the modified oral formulation subsequently is adjusted to attain a predefined blood cyclosporine concentration. The therapeutic range of *trough* blood concentrations of cyclosporine is the same for both the modified oral formulations and the conventional oral formulations. However, attainment of therapeutic trough blood concentrations of cyclosporine with the modified oral formulations will result in greater exposure (AUC) to the drug than would occur with conventional oral formulations. Titration of dosage should be based on clinical evaluation of rejection and patient tolerability. Lower maintenance dosages may be possible with the modified oral formulations.

If consideration is given to conversion of an allograft recipient from a conventional oral formulation of cyclosporine to a modified oral one, therapy with the modified oral formulation should be initiated at the same dosage that the patient is receiving of the conventional oral formulation (1:1 conversion). After conversion to the modified oral formulation, the increase in trough blood concentrations may be more pronounced and clinically important in some patients. The initial dosage subsequently should be adjusted to attain trough blood concentrations that are similar to those achieved with the conventional oral formulation. However, attainment of therapeutic trough blood concentrations will result in greater exposure (AUC) to cyclosporine than would occur with the conventional oral formulation. Monitoring of trough blood cyclosporine concentrations every 4–7 days after conversion to the modified oral formulation is recommended strongly until this measure is the same as it was with the conventional oral formulation. Safety of the patient also should be monitored with evaluation of such measures as the serum creatinine concentration and blood pressure every 2 weeks for the first 2 months after conversion to the modified oral formulation. The dosage must be adjusted appropriately if trough blood concentrations are outside of the range desired and/or if the measures of safety worsen.

Different strategies in dosage with the modified oral formulations are required for patients suspected of having poor absorption of cyclosporine from the conventional oral formulation. When trough blood concentrations are lower than expected relative to the dosage of the conventional oral formulation, the patient may have poor or inconsistent absorption of cyclosporine from this formulation. Patients tend to have higher blood cyclosporine concentrations after conversion to the modified oral formulations. The higher bioavailability of cyclosporine from the modified oral formulations (may result in excessive trough blood concentrations after conversion to these formulations. Clinicians should be particularly cautious with conversional dosages exceeding 10 mg/kg daily. Individual titration of

the dosage should be guided by trough blood concentrations, tolerability, and clinical response. After conversion to the modified oral formulation in patients who may have poor absorption of cyclosporine from the conventional oral formulation, trough blood concentrations should be measured more frequently, at least twice weekly, while such monitoring should be done daily in patients receiving more than 10 mg/kg daily, until the trough blood cyclosporine concentration is maintained in the desired range.

In patients unable to take the drug orally, cyclosporine may be administered by IV infusion at about one-third the recommended oral dosage. The usual initial IV dose of cyclosporine for adults and children is 5–6 mg/kg administered as a single dose 4–12 hours before transplantation. Postoperatively, the usual IV dosage of 5–6 mg/kg once daily is continued until the patient is able to tolerate oral administration of the drug. Pediatric patients may require higher dosages. Patients should be switched to an oral formulation of cyclosporine as soon as possible after surgery.

Concomitant Corticosteroid Therapy

For the prevention of allograft rejection, the manufacturer states that corticosteroid therapy should always be used concomitantly with IV cyclosporine. For the prevention of allograft rejection, the manufacturers recommend that corticosteroid therapy be administered concomitantly with conventional (nonmodified) oral formulations and be administered concomitantly, at least initially, with the modified oral formulations. Dosage of corticosteroids should be adjusted individually according to the clinical situation. Various schedules to taper corticosteroid dosage appear to yield similar results. Prednisone may be administered orally at an initial dosage of 2 mg/kg daily for 4 days and then tapered to 1 mg/kg daily by day 7, to 0.6 mg/kg daily by day 14, to 0.3 mg/kg daily by the end of the first month, and to a maintenance dosage of 0.15 mg/kg daily by the end of the second month. Corticosteroid dosage may be tapered further based on individual consideration of patient status and allograft function. Alternatively, an initial oral prednisone dose of 200 mg may be given and then tapered by 40 mg daily until a maintenance dosage of 20 mg daily is achieved; this maintenance dosage is then continued for 60 days and tapered to 10 mg daily during subsequent months.

Some clinicians believe that routine concomitant use of corticosteroids during cyclosporine therapy is not necessary and that their use should be reserved for acute periods of allograft rejection. Some clinicians suggest that if an acute rejection episode occurs in renal allograft recipients, 1 g of methylprednisolone be administered IV daily for 3 days; this dosage may be continued for an additional 3 days if rejection does not resolve following the initial course. If rejection continues after two 3-day courses of therapy, switching the patient to therapy with azathioprine and corticosteroids should be considered. Alternatively, some clinicians suggest that methylprednisolone be administered IV in a dosage of 0.5 or 1 g daily for 3 days for the management of an acute rejection reaction in renal allograft recipients. If necessary, courses of methylprednisolone therapy may be repeated until a total dosage of 6 g has been administered. If rejection continues, cyclosporine should be discontinued and switching the patient to therapy with azathioprine and corticosteroids should be considered.

Rheumatoid Arthritis

For the management of rheumatoid arthritis in adults and children 18 years of age and older, the usual initial dosage of a modified oral cyclosporine formulation (e.g., Gengraf®, Neoral®) is 2.5 mg/kg daily given in 2 divided doses. Therapeutic response in patients with rheumatoid arthritis generally is apparent after 4–8 weeks of therapy. In patients with insufficient therapeutic response who have good tolerance to the drug (including serum creatinine concentration less than 30% above baseline), the dosage may be increased by 0.5–0.75 mg/kg daily after 8 weeks and, again, after 12 weeks to a maximum of 4 mg/kg daily. Lack of benefit by the 16th week of therapy should be considered a therapeutic failure and cyclosporine should be discontinued. Therapy with salicylates, other nonsteroidal antiinflammatory agents (NSAIAs), or oral corticosteroids may be continued during cyclosporine therapy. To control adverse effects (e.g., hypertension, elevations in serum creatinine concentration to 30% above baseline, clinically important laboratory test abnormalities) that occur at any time during cyclosporine therapy, the cyclosporine dosage should be decreased by 25–50%. Cyclosporine should be discontinued if adverse effects are severe or do not respond to reduction of dosage.

When cyclosporine is used concomitantly with methotrexate for the management of rheumatoid arthritis, cyclosporine should be administered at the same initial dosage and range of adjustment as when administered alone. Administration of a modified oral cyclosporine formulation at 3 mg/kg daily or less generally is applicable in patients also receiving methotrexate at up to 15 mg weekly. There currently is only limited experience with long-term treatment of rheumatoid arthritis with the modified oral cyclosporine formulations. Following discontinuance of the drug, control of rheumatoid arthritis usually wanes within 4 weeks.

Use of cyclosporine for rheumatoid arthritis should be preceded by careful physical examination of the patient, including measurement of blood pressure on at least 2 occasions and determination of serum creatinine concentration twice for a baseline. During the first 3 months of therapy with cyclosporine, blood pressure and serum creatinine concentration should be evaluated every 2 weeks; thereafter, patients should be evaluated monthly if they are stable. Hypertension that develops during therapy with cyclosporine should elicit reduction of the dosage by 25–50%. Persistent hypertension should be managed by further reduction of the dosage of cyclosporine or use of antihypertensive agents. Withdrawal of cyclosporine generally results in return of blood pressure to baseline. Serum creatinine concentration and blood pressure should always be monitored after concomitant NSAIA therapy is modified by an increase in dosage and after initiation of new NSAIA therapy during cyclosporine therapy. Monthly evaluation with complete blood cell count and liver function tests is recommended in patients who also are receiving methotrexate concomitantly with cyclosporine.

Psoriasis

For the management of psoriasis in adults and children 18 years of age and older, the usual initial dosage of a modified oral cyclosporine formulation (e.g., Gengraf®, Neoral®) is 1.25 mg/kg twice daily. This dosage should be continued for at least 4 weeks unless prohibited by adverse effects. Some improvement in clinical manifestations of psoriasis generally is observed after 2 weeks of therapy. If the initial cyclosporine dosage does not produce substantial clinical improvement within 4 weeks, dosage should be increased by approximately 0.5 mg/kg daily once every 2 weeks. Dosage may be increased in these increments to a maximum of 4 mg/kg daily based on the patient's tolerance and response.

Cyclosporine may not produce satisfactory control and stabilization of psoriasis until after 12–16 weeks of therapy. In a clinical study that evaluated titration of the dosage of cyclosporine, improvement of psoriasis by at least 75%, as indicated by scores on the Psoriasis Area and Severity Index, was observed in 51 or 79% of patients after 8 or 16 weeks of therapy, respectively. Lack of satisfactory response after patients receive 6 weeks of cyclosporine at the maximum dosage tolerated, up to 4 mg/kg daily, should lead to discontinuance of therapy.

In patients whose disease is controlled adequately and who appear stable, the regimen of cyclosporine should be adjusted so that the patient receives the lowest dosage that maintains an adequate response, which would not necessarily be total clearance of psoriasis. A satisfactory response was maintained in 60% of patients in clinical studies with dosages at the lower end of the recommended range. Dosages less than 2.5 mg/kg daily also may be equally effective.

To control adverse effects (e.g., hypertension, elevations in serum creatinine concentration to 25% or more above baseline, clinically important laboratory test abnormalities) that occur at any time during cyclosporine therapy, the dosage should be decreased by 25–50%. Cyclosporine should be discontinued if adverse effects are severe or do not respond to reduction of the dosage.

Discontinuance of cyclosporine therapy will result in relapse after several weeks, with approximately 50 or 75% of patients experiencing relapse within 6 or 16 weeks of discontinuance, respectively. Rebound does not occur in most patients after withdrawal of cyclosporine. Transformation of chronic plaque psoriasis to more severe forms of psoriasis that included pustular and erythrodermic psoriasis reportedly has occurred in some patients. There currently is only limited experience with the long-term treatment of psoriasis with modified oral cyclosporine formulations, and the manufacturers do not recommend continuous therapy with the drug for extended periods exceeding 1 year. Strategies in the long-term management of psoriasis should include consideration of alternation of cyclosporine with other therapies.

Use of cyclosporine for psoriasis should be preceded by careful dermatologic and physical examination of the patient, including measurement of blood pressure on at least 2 occasions. Physical examination should include evaluation for the presence of occult infection because cyclosporine is an immunosuppressive agent. The patient also should be evaluated for the presence of tumors at this initial examination and throughout therapy with cyclosporine. A biopsy should be obtained from dermatologic lesions that do not typify psoriasis before therapy

with cyclosporine commences. Cyclosporine should be administered only after malignant or premalignant dermatologic lesions have been treated appropriately and only if other therapies for psoriasis are not an option.

During the first 3 months of therapy with cyclosporine in the management of psoriasis, blood pressure should be evaluated every 2 weeks; thereafter, patients should be evaluated monthly if they are stable or more frequently if their dosage is adjusted. Hypertension may occur at recommended dosages, with risk increased as the dosage and duration of therapy with the drug increases. If hypertension develops during therapy with cyclosporine, dosage should be reduced by 25–50% in patients without a history of hypertension prior to receiving the drug. Cyclosporine should be withdrawn if hypertension fails to respond to multiple reductions in dosage. Antihypertensive therapy of patients being managed for hypertension prior to initiation of cyclosporine therapy should be adjusted for effectiveness during cyclosporine therapy. When adequate adjustment of antihypertensive therapy is not possible or is not tolerated, cyclosporine should be withdrawn.

Measurements that should be obtained for baseline include serum creatinine concentration determined on 2 occasions, BUN, complete blood cell count, and serum concentrations of magnesium, potassium, uric acid, and lipoproteins. Serum creatinine must be monitored frequently. During the first 3 months of therapy with cyclosporine in the management of psoriasis, serum creatinine concentration and BUN should be evaluated every 2 weeks; thereafter, stable patients should be evaluated monthly. When the serum creatinine concentration exceeds baseline by 25% or more, repeated measurement should be obtained within 2 weeks. The dosage of cyclosporine should be reduced by 25–50% if the serum creatinine concentration on repeated measurement continues to exceed baseline by 25% or more. Such reduction of the dosage also is necessary if serum creatinine concentration exceeds baseline by 50% or more at *any time*. If the serum creatinine concentration does not decrease to within 25% of baseline after the dosage was modified twice, the drug should be withdrawn. Serum creatinine concentration also should be monitored after concomitant therapy with a NSAIA is modified by an increase in dosage and after initiation of new NSAIA therapy.

Complete blood cell count and serum concentrations of magnesium, potassium, uric acid, and lipids should be monitored every 2 weeks during the first 3 months of therapy with cyclosporine in the management of psoriasis; thereafter, these values should be monitored monthly in stable patients or more frequently when the dosage is adjusted. Mild hypomagnesemia and hyperkalemia that are asymptomatic and increases in the serum concentration of uric acid may occur with cyclosporine. Serum concentrations of triglycerides or cholesterol may be increased modestly during therapy with cyclosporine. The dosage of cyclosporine should be reduced by 25–50% in response to any abnormality of clinical concern.

Patients receiving cyclosporine to treat psoriasis should be warned about appropriate protection from the sun and avoidance of excessive solar exposure.

Crohn's Disease

For the management of refractory, inflammatory or fistulizing Crohn's disease†, cyclosporine has been administered initially in a dosage of 4 mg/kg daily for about 2–10 days, as a continuous IV infusion over 24 hours. Most of those who responded were switched to oral cyclosporine (5–8 mg/kg daily) for a mean duration of about 2.5–12.2 (range: 0.5–37 months) months.

CAUTIONS

Patients who experienced adverse effects during treatment with cyclosporine for rheumatoid arthritis were affected principally by renal dysfunction, hypertension, headache, hirsutism/hypertrichosis, and GI disturbances. Therapy with cyclosporine was discontinued in clinical studies because of elevated serum creatinine concentration or hypertension in about 7 or 5% of patients, respectively, treated with the drug for rheumatoid arthritis at dosages within the recommended range. Reversibility of these changes generally occurred with timely reduction of the dosage or withdrawal of cyclosporine. Elevation of serum creatinine concentration increases in frequency and severity as the dosage of cyclosporine and its duration of administration increase. Maintenance of the regimen is likely to result in more pronounced increases in serum creatinine concentration.

Patients who experienced adverse effects during treatment with cyclosporine for psoriasis were affected principally by renal dysfunction, hypertension, headache, paresthesia or hyperesthesia, hirsutism/hypertrichosis, abdominal discomfort, diarrhea, nausea/vomiting, influenza-like symptoms, hypertriglyceridemia, lethargy, and musculoskeletal or joint pain. Therapy with cyclosporine was discontinued in clinical studies because of elevated serum creatinine concentration or hypertension in about 5 or 1% of patients, respectively, treated with the drug for psoriasis at dosages within the range recommended. Elevation of blood pressure or serum creatinine concentration in patients receiving cyclosporine for the management of psoriasis generally was reversible after dosage reduction or withdrawal of the drug. Elevation of serum creatinine concentration increases in frequency and severity as the dosage of cyclosporine and its duration of therapy increase. Maintenance of the regimen is likely to result in more pronounced increases in serum creatinine concentration that may lead to irreversible renal damage. Progressive renal failure led to the death of a patient who developed renal deterioration while receiving cyclosporine for the treatment of psoriasis and continued to receive the drug.

● Renal Effects

The most frequent and clinically important adverse effect of cyclosporine is nephrotoxicity. Nephrotoxic effects (usually manifested as increased BUN and serum creatinine concentrations) of cyclosporine have been observed in 25–32, 38, or 37% of patients receiving the drug for kidney, heart, or liver allografts, respectively. Elevations of BUN and serum creatinine concentrations resulting from cyclosporine therapy appear to be dose related, may be associated with high trough concentrations of the drug, and are usually reversible upon discontinuance of the drug. Clinical manifestations of cyclosporine-induced nephrotoxicity may include fluid retention, dependent edema, and, in some cases, a hyperchloremic, hyperkalemic metabolic acidosis. The risk of cyclosporine-induced nephrotoxicity may be increased in patients receiving other potentially nephrotoxic agents. (See Drug Interactions: Nephrotoxic Drugs.) Mild cyclosporine-induced nephrotoxicity generally occurs within 2–3 months after transplantation. Although some decline from preoperative levels generally occurs in patients with mild nephrotoxicity, the BUN and serum creatinine concentrations reportedly become stabilized in the range of 35–45 mg/dL and 2–2.5 mg/dL, respectively, in these patients; however, these elevations often respond to dosage reduction. In some patients, more severe nephrotoxic effects have been observed early after transplantation and have been characterized by rapid increases in BUN and serum creatinine concentrations; these elevations usually respond to dosage reduction.

Differentiation of Nephrotoxicity and Allograft Rejection

In patients with renal allografts, acute episodes of allograft rejection must be differentiated from nephrotoxic effects of cyclosporine. When increased serum creatinine concentrations occur without the usual symptoms of renal allograft rejection (e.g., fever, graft tenderness or enlargement), cyclosporine-induced nephrotoxicity is likely. Although reliable and sensitive differentiation of cyclosporine-induced nephrotoxicity from renal allograft rejection through specific diagnostic criteria currently is not possible, and nephrotoxicity and rejection may coexist in up to 20% of patients, either adversity has been associated with various parameters (e.g., history, clinical, laboratory, biopsy, aspiration cytology, urine cytology, manometry, ultrasonography, magnetic resonance imagery, radionuclide scan, and response to therapy) that can be used in an attempt to differentiate between the two. For example, nephrotoxicity from cyclosporine has been associated with a history of having undergone a transplant involving prolonged kidney preservation time or prolonged anastomosis time, having received concomitant therapy with nephrotoxic drugs (e.g., an aminoglycoside, a nonsteroidal anti-inflammatory agent), or having received an organ from a donor who was older than 50 years of age or who was hypotensive, whereas renal allograft rejection has been associated with a history of antidonor immune response or previous renal allotransplantation. Nephrotoxicity often becomes apparent clinically more than 6 weeks postoperatively in patients whose allograft functioned initially or as prolonged initial nonfunction of the allograft that resembles acute tubular necrosis, whereas renal allograft rejection often becomes apparent clinically less than 4 weeks postoperatively and manifests with signs such as fever exceeding 37.5°C, swelling and tenderness of the graft, weight gain exceeding 0.5 kg, and a decrease in daily urine volume by more than 500 mL or 50%.

In some studies, patients with nephrotoxicity had high trough concentrations of cyclosporine in biologic fluid, as measured with a nonspecific (e.g., polyclonal radioimmunoassay [RIA] now obsolete) or a specific (e.g., high-performance liquid chromatography [HPLC]) assay for cyclosporine. The manufacturers state that a trough serum concentration of cyclosporine, as measured by polyclonal RIA, exceeding 200 ng/mL has been associated with the occurrence of nephrotoxicity. However, the relationship between nephrotoxicity and trough or other concentrations of cyclosporine in biologic fluid (e.g., whole blood) measured with specific monoclonal RIA or HPLC has not been fully established. (See Pharmacokinetics.) By comparison, allograft rejection has been associated with low trough concentrations of cyclosporine in biologic fluid, as measured with a nonspecific (e.g., polyclonal RIA) or a specific (e.g., monoclonal RIA, HPLC) assay for cyclosporine. The manufacturers state that a trough serum concentration of cyclosporine, as measured by polyclonal RIA, of less than 150 ng/mL has been associated with the occurrence of rejection. Other concentrations of the drug in biologic fluid (e.g., whole blood) at which rejection occurred have been reported with the use of specific assays for cyclosporine.

Common laboratory findings associated with cyclosporine-induced nephrotoxicity include a gradual increase in serum creatinine concentration (e.g., less than 0.15 mg/dL daily) that reaches a plateau of less than 25% above baseline, and a ratio of blood urea nitrogen (BUN) to serum creatinine of at least 20. By comparison, laboratory findings associated with allograft rejection include a rapid increase in serum creatinine concentration (e.g., exceeding 0.3 mg/dL daily) that reaches a plateau exceeding 25% above baseline, or a BUN to creatinine ratio of less than 20.

The histologic features of allograft biopsies in patients with cyclosporine-induced nephrotoxicity include effects on the arterioles, tubules, and interstitium. Such findings include arteriolopathy manifested as medial hypertrophy and hyalinosis, nodular deposits, intimal thickening, endothelial vacuolization, and progressive scarring. Renal tubular effects of nephrotoxicity include atrophy, isometric vacuolization, and isolated calcifications. Interstitial effects of nephrotoxicity include minimal edema, mild focal infiltrates of mononuclear cells, and diffuse interstitial fibrosis that often is the striped form. The histologic features of allograft biopsies in patients with rejection include effects on the arterioles and arteries, tubules, interstitium, and glomeruli. Such findings include endovasculitis manifested as arteriolar and arterial endothelial cell proliferation, intimal arteritis, fibrinoid necrosis, and sclerosis. Renal tubular effects of rejection include tubulitis with erythrocyte and leukocyte casts and some irregular vacuolization. Interstitial effects of rejection include a diffuse moderate to severe infiltrate of mononuclear cells, edema, and hemorrhage. Glomerulitis, manifested as infiltration of glomerular capillaries by mononuclear cells, is associated with rejection. Histologic changes, including thromboses of arteriolar and glomerular capillaries and mesangial sclerosis, also have occurred in cyclosporine-treated patients with renal dysfunction following bone marrow transplantation.

With cyclosporine-induced nephrotoxicity, renal allograft evaluation with aspiration cytology reveals deposits of the drug in tubular and endothelial cells and fine isometric vacuolization of tubular cells; urine cytology reveals tubular cells with vacuolization of cytoplasm and granularization. Manometry shows an intracapsular pressure of less than 40 mm Hg, and ultrasonography shows the renal cross-sectional area to be unchanged. With rejection, aspiration cytology shows that the graft generally is affected by an inflammatory infiltrate of mononuclear cells that includes phagocytes, macrophages, lymphoblastoid cells, and activated T-cells; HLA-DR antigens are expressed strongly by these mononuclear cells. Urine cytology in rejection may show degenerative renal tubular cells, plasma cells, and lymphocyturia exceeding 20% of the urinary sediment. Intrarenal manometry shows an intracapsular pressure exceeding 40 mm Hg in many patients with rejection, and ultrasonography shows an increase in graft cross-sectional area; the anteroposterior diameter is equal to or greater than the transverse diameter.

In most patients with nephrotoxicity, magnetic resonance imagery shows normal renal appearance, and radionuclide scans performed with technetium Tc 99m pentetate (DTPA) and iodohippurate sodium I 131 to evaluate renal perfusion and tubular function, respectively, show renal perfusion to be normal (although a generally decreased perfusion is observed occasionally) and tubular function to be decreased. While the decrease in tubular function is a deteriorative effect, renal perfusion is not decreased to a deleterious extent. With rejection, findings of magnetic resonance imagery include loss of distinct corticomedullary junction, swelling of the allograft, image intensity of parenchyma that approaches the image intensity of psoas, and loss of hilar fat; radionuclide scans may show patchy arterial flow. Evaluation of renal perfusion and tubular function with technetium Tc 99m pentetate or iodohippurate sodium I 131, respectively, shows that renal perfusion is decreased to a greater extent than is tubular function in patients with rejection; uptake of indium In 111-labeled platelets or technetium Tc 99m in colloid is increased.

Limited data suggest that some of the variables associated with nephrotoxicity actually may be risk factors for the development of nephrotoxicity from cyclosporine. The number of episodes of acute deterioration of renal function induced by cyclosporine (e.g., increase in serum creatinine concentration corrected by a decrease in the dose of cyclosporine), trough concentrations of cyclosporine during the second and third months after transplantation, the number of episodes of unexplained acute deterioration of renal function (e.g., increase in serum creatinine concentration unresponsive to a decrease in the dose of cyclosporine), and the number of treatments for rejection (e.g., corticosteroids) were correlated with chronic nephrotoxicity (e.g., arteriolopathy, striped form of interstitial fibrosis, tubular atrophy). The variables that were discriminative of nephrotoxicity included the number of episodes of acute deterioration of renal function induced by cyclosporine, the number of episodes of unexplained acute deterioration of renal function, the number of episodes of rejection, and the number of treatments for rejection, with patients with nephrotoxicity having experienced more episodes of acute deterioration of renal function, whether induced by the drug or unexplained, than patients with rejection, and those with rejection exhibiting a stronger history of multiple episodes of rejection and being treated for such more often. Some patients with chronic nephrotoxicity did not exhibit acute cyclosporine-induced deterioration of renal function. Poor primary function of the allograft occurred more often in these patients than in patients who had both acute deterioration of renal function induced by cyclosporine and chronic nephrotoxicity.

Response to a reduction in cyclosporine dosage generally can distinguish nephrotoxicity from rejection since the renal function of patients with nephrotoxicity usually recovers with such dosage modification. By comparison, response (e.g., in renal function) to an increase in dosage of concomitant corticosteroids or to antithymocyte globulin generally indicates the presence of rejection rather than nephrotoxicity.

A form of cyclosporine-associated nephropathy that is characterized by serial deterioration in renal function and changes in renal morphology also has been described. In this nephropathy, the rise in serum creatinine concentration does not diminish in response to a decrease in the dosage of, or discontinuance of therapy with, cyclosporine in 5–15% of allograft recipients. Renal biopsy in such patients will show one or more morphologic changes, none of which is entirely specific to structural nephrotoxicity associated with cyclosporine, although diagnosis of such nephropathy requires evidence of these changes. The morphologic changes include renal tubular vacuolization, tubular microcalcifications, peritubular capillary congestion, arteriolopathy, and a striped form of interstitial fibrosis with tubular atrophy. Of interest in the consideration of the development of cyclosporine-associated nephropathy is that the appearance of interstitial fibrosis reportedly is associated with higher cumulative doses of cyclosporine or persistently high circulating trough concentrations of the drug, particularly during the first 6 months after transplantation when dosages tend to be highest. Furthermore, renal allografts appear to be most vulnerable to the toxic effects of cyclosporine during this time. Other factors that contribute to the development of interstitial fibrosis include prolonged perfusion time, warm ischemia time, and episodes of acute toxicity and acute or chronic rejection. Whether interstitial fibrosis is reversible and its correlation to renal function are not known. Arteriolopathy reportedly was reversible when the dosage of cyclosporine was decreased or therapy with the drug was discontinued.

Management of Nephrotoxicity

Gradual reduction of cyclosporine dosage is recommended for the management of nephrotoxicity, with careful patient assessment for several days to weeks. When patients are unresponsive to reduction of cyclosporine dosage and the possibility of allograft rejection has been excluded, switching from cyclosporine to therapy with alternative immunosuppressants (e.g., azathioprine and prednisone) should be considered. Concomitant use of corticosteroids with cyclosporine does not appear to improve renal function.

Other Renal Effects

Hyperkalemia (that may be associated with hyperchloremic metabolic acidosis), hypomagnesemia, and decreased serum bicarbonate concentration have been reported frequently in patients receiving cyclosporine; these effects may result from nephrotoxic effects of the drug. Hyperuricemia also occurs commonly in cyclosporine-treated patients, particularly in those receiving diuretics concurrently, and may result in gout in some patients. Although not clearly established, hyperuricemia appears to result at least in part from decreased renal clearance of uric acid. Hematuria has occurred rarely in patients receiving cyclosporine.

Impairment of renal function (e.g., increased BUN and serum creatinine concentrations, decreased glomerular filtration rate (GFR) and effective renal plasma flow) and morphologic evidence of renal injury (e.g., renal tubular atrophy, interstitial fibrosis, arteriolar hyalinosis) have been observed in some patients who received short- or long-term treatment with cyclosporine for psoriasis. Elevated serum creatinine concentrations occurred in about 20% of patients. Elevations of BUN and serum creatinine concentrations resulting from cyclosporine at dosages used for psoriasis may be associated with relatively high trough concentrations of the drug but usually are reversible after discontinuance of the drug. Although limited data suggested the reversibility of decreases in GFR and effective renal plasma flow resulting from cyclosporine therapy for psoriasis, these manifestations of renal impairment may persist despite discontinuance of the drug. In patients who developed nephrotoxicity, as indicated by a decrease of more than 20% in GFR or a decrease of more than 25% in total renal blood flow, after 3 months of treatment with cyclosporine, evaluation at 3 months subsequent to discontinuance of the drug showed recovery of GFR but not of renal blood flow. GFR and effective renal plasma flow continued to be decreased below baseline 4 months after discontinuance of cyclosporine in patients who received the drug for a median of 12 months at a dosage of 5 mg/kg daily for 3 months that was then reduced by 0.35 mg/kg daily every month until the minimum effective dose was achieved. In some patients who received cyclosporine for an average of 30 months at a dosage of up to 5 mg/kg daily, GFR and renal plasma flow rate were below the lower 2.5 percentile of normal compared with the renal function of healthy individuals matched for age and gender 1 month after discontinuance of the drug. Biopsies occasionally showed kidneys with structural damage manifested as renal tubular atrophy, interstitial fibrosis, and hyaline arteriolopathy that were graded as moderate. Mild tubulointerstitial scarring and glomerulosclerosis were observed in the other patients but a relationship to cyclosporine was not certain. A correlation between severity of renal injury and severity of recurrent acute nephrotoxicity was found, which suggests recurrent severe acute nephrotoxicity (i.e., serum creatinine increased by more than 90% above baseline) to be a risk factor for chronic nephrotoxicity from cyclosporine. Histologic evidence of renal tubular atrophy, arteriolar hyalinosis, and increases above normal in interstitium and obsolescent glomeruli have been observed in patients who received cyclosporine at a mean dosage of 3 mg/kg daily for an average of 5 years.

Cyclosporine administered to treat rheumatoid arthritis resulted in serum creatinine concentrations increasing by at least 30 or 50% in up to 43–48 or 18–24% of patients, respectively. Maintenance of the regimen is likely to result in more pronounced increases in serum creatinine concentration that may lead to irreversible renal damage. The maximal increase in serum creatinine concentration may be a predictor of nephropathy from cyclosporine. Features suggesting nephropathy were observed in the renal biopsies of some patients with rheumatoid arthritis treated with cyclosporine for an average of 19 months. The dosage was 4 mg/kg daily or less in one of the patients. Dosage reduction or withdrawal of cyclosporine resulted in improvement in serum creatinine concentrations in most of these patients. Morphologic features that are identified with nephropathy induced by cyclosporine generally were not observed in renal biopsies from patients who had mostly completed 6 months of therapy with the drug and who did not appear to have renal dysfunction. Renal biopsies obtained by the 20th month of therapy with cyclosporine for rheumatoid arthritis and after 30–46 months of treatment showed morphologic changes compared with baseline that were not considered to be specific to nephropathy induced by the drug. In a limited study, differences in renal biopsies were not observed between patients with rheumatoid arthritis treated with cyclosporine at dosages less than 5 mg/kg daily for an average of 26 months and controls derived from autopsies of patients with rheumatoid arthritis. In the patients treated with cyclosporine, creatinine clearance that was measured or calculated was decreased from baseline by 26 or 24%, respectively, after 24 months of therapy. Cyclosporine administered to treat rheumatoid arthritis resulted in elevated BUN in 1% to less than 3% of patients.

Renal tubular atrophy and interstitial fibrosis was observed in 21% of patients with psoriasis who received cyclosporine dosages of 1.2–7.6 mg/kg daily for an average of 23 months. Such structural damage to the kidney was shown on repeated biopsy in some of the patients who were maintained on various dosages of cyclosporine for an additional period averaging 2 years, so that 30% of patients were affected overall. Most of these patients were receiving at least 5 mg/kg daily of cyclosporine, which exceeds the highest dosage recommended, had been taking the drug for more than 15 months, and/or had a clinically important increase in serum creatinine concentration for more than 1 month. Discontinuance of therapy with cyclosporine resulted in normalization of serum creatinine concentration in most patients. Quantitative digital morphometric analysis showed an increase in the percentage of fibrotic area in the tubular interstitium after 3.5 years of therapy with 3–6 mg/kg daily of cyclosporine compared with evaluation 1 year earlier. After 2 years of receiving cyclosporine generally at a dosage of 2.5–6 mg/kg daily, all patients had abnormal renal morphology, although the renal biopsy was normal at baseline in many of the patients. Evaluation of biopsies for focal interstitial fibrosis and arteriolar hyaline wall thickening showed increases compared with baseline. The percentage of sclerotic glomeruli was increased compared with baseline after 4 years of therapy with cyclosporine.

● **Cardiovascular Effects**

The manufacturers state that mild to moderate hypertension occurs in about 50% of renal transplant recipients who receive cyclosporine and in most cardiac transplant patients receiving the drug. In one study in renal allograft recipients, hypertension occurred in about 40% of cyclosporine-treated patients; 2 of these patients developed malignant hypertension with associated seizures. In some patients with cardiac allografts who developed hypertension while receiving cyclosporine, therapy with hypotensive agents has been required.

Hypertension generally develops within a few weeks after beginning cyclosporine therapy and affects both the systolic and diastolic blood pressure. Although the mechanism has not been clearly established, there is some evidence that hypertension may result from the renal vasoconstrictive effects of the drug. The manufacturers state that hypertension associated with cyclosporine therapy may respond to dosage reduction and/or antihypertensive therapy. However, some evidence from clinical studies suggests that response to antihypertensive therapy may be variable and that elevations in diastolic blood pressure may be more resistant to treatment than elevations in systolic pressure.

Myocardial infarction has occurred rarely in patients receiving the drug.

Cyclosporine administered to treat rheumatoid arthritis resulted in hypertension in up to about 26% of patients. Systolic hypertension (i.e., measurement of systolic blood pressure that twice exceeded 140 mm Hg) and diastolic hypertension (i.e., measurement of diastolic blood pressure that twice exceeded 90 mm Hg) developed in 33 and 19% of patients, respectively. Arrhythmia occurred in up to about 5% of patients. Abnormal heart sounds, cardiac failure, myocardial infarction, and peripheral ischemia each occurred in 1% to less then 3% of patients.

Cyclosporine administered to treat psoriasis resulted in the development of hypertension (i.e., systolic blood pressure of 160 mm Hg or greater and/or diastolic blood pressure of 90 mm Hg or greater) in about 28% of patients.

● **Nervous System Effects**

Adverse nervous system effects occur frequently in patients receiving cyclosporine. Tremor reportedly occurs in 12–21, 31, or 55% of patients with kidney, heart, or liver allografts, respectively, who receive cyclosporine. In one study in renal allograft recipients, however, tremor occurred in about 40% of cyclosporine-treated patients. Cyclosporine-induced tremor may be manifested as a fine hand tremor, usually is mild in severity, may improve despite continued therapy, and/or may be alleviated by a decrease in dosage of the drug.

Seizures (particularly when cyclosporine was used in combination with high-dose corticosteroids), headache, paresthesia, hyperesthesia, flushing, and confusion have been reported occasionally in patients receiving cyclosporine. There is some evidence that cyclosporine-induced seizures and other neurotoxicity may be associated with high blood or plasma concentrations of the drug, concurrent high-dose corticosteroid therapy, hypertension, and/or hypomagnesemia. Encephalopathy, manifested by impaired consciousness, seizures, visual changes (e.g., blindness), loss of motor function, movement disorders, and psychiatric disturbances, has been described in patients receiving cyclosporine; in many cases, such manifestations were accompanied by white-matter changes (documented by imaging procedures and pathologic findings). Adverse neurologic effects in most cases are reversible upon discontinuance of the drug or in some patients following dosage reduction.

Optic disc edema with possible visual impairment secondary to benign intracranial hypertension has been reported rarely in patients receiving cyclosporine; this complication occurred more frequently in transplant recipients than in patients receiving the drug for other indications.

Psychiatric disorders including anxiety, flat affect, and depression have occurred rarely in patients receiving the drug.

Cyclosporine administered to treat rheumatoid arthritis resulted in headache in up to about 25% of patients. Tremor or paresthesia occurred in up to about 13 or 11% of patients, respectively. Dizziness, depression, flushing, insomnia, or migraine occurred in up to about 8, 6, 5, 4, or 3% of patients, respectively. Hypoesthesia, neuropathy, and vertigo each occurred in 1% to less than 3% of patients. Psychiatric disorders that occurred in 1% to less than 3% of patients include anxiety, impaired concentration, confusion, emotional lability, decreased libido, increased libido, nervousness, paroniria, and somnolence.

Cyclosporine administered to treat psoriasis resulted in adverse effects of the central and peripheral nervous system in about 26% of patients. Headache occurred in about 16% of patients. Paresthesia occurred in about 7% of patients. Dizziness, flushes, insomnia, nervousness, and vertigo each occurred in 1% to less than 3% of patients. Adverse psychiatric effects occurred in about 5% of patients.

● **Dermatologic Effects**

Adverse dermatologic effects including hirsutism and gingival hyperplasia have occurred frequently during cyclosporine therapy. The manufacturers state that hirsutism occurs in 21, 28, or 45% of patients with kidney, heart, or liver allografts, respectively, who received cyclosporine; however, hirsutism reportedly has been observed in 30–45% of renal allograft recipients in some studies. Hirsutism usually develops within 2–4 weeks after transplantation, is mild, and involves the face, arms, eyebrows, and back. Although most patients can tolerate cyclosporine-induced hirsutism, occasionally it can be severe and some patients may prefer cosmetic alleviation of the excess hair (e.g., by shaving or use of depilatories). In addition, although development of hirsutism does not appear to be dose related, improvement may occur following a decrease in dosage of the drug.

Gingival hyperplasia reportedly occurs in 4–9, 5, or 16% of cyclosporine-treated patients with kidney, heart, or liver allografts, respectively, although in one study, gingival hyperplasia occurred in 30% of cyclosporine-treated patients. Cyclosporine-induced gingival hyperplasia is clinically similar to that observed with phenytoin therapy and appears to occur more frequently in pediatric patients. To reduce the risk of developing cyclosporine-induced gingival hyperplasia, careful oral hygiene should be maintained before and following transplantation. Gingival hyperplasia generally resolves 1–2 months following discontinuance of the drug; gingivectomy has been required rarely in patients with severe hyperplasia.

Acne and brittle and abnormal fingernails occur occasionally in patients receiving cyclosporine.

Cyclosporine administered to treat rheumatoid arthritis resulted in hypertrichosis or rash in up to about 19 or 12% of patients. Alopecia, gingival hyperplasia, or gingivitis each occurred in up to about 4% of patients. Bullous eruption or skin ulceration each occurred in up to about 1% of patients. Angioedema, dermatitis, dry skin, eczema, folliculitis, gingival bleeding, nail disorder, abnormal pigmentation, pruritus, skin disorder, and urticaria each occurred in 1% to less than 3% of patients.

Cyclosporine administered to treat psoriasis resulted in adverse effects of the skin and appendages in about 18% of patients. Hypertrichosis occurred in about 7% of patients. Gingival hyperplasia occurred in about 4% of patients. Acne, dry skin, folliculitis, gingival bleeding, keratosis, pruritus, and rash each occurred in 1% to less than 3% of patients.

● **Hepatic Effects**

Hepatotoxicity has reportedly occurred in 4 or less, 7, or 4% of patients with kidney, heart, or liver allografts, respectively, usually during the first month of therapy with cyclosporine when higher dosages of the drug are used. Abnormalities of liver function test results (e.g., increased serum aminotransferase [transaminase] and gamma-glutamyl transferase concentrations) and increased serum bilirubin concentration are signs of cyclosporine hepatotoxicity. Reduction of cyclosporine dosage usually reverses the hepatotoxic effects of the drug; in one study, hepatotoxicity was associated with trough serum concentrations (determined by RIA) greater than 1000 ng/mL. Although increased serum alkaline phosphatase concentration has also been reported, it appears to be from bone rather than liver origin.

Hyperbilirubinemia occurred in 1% to less than 3% of patients with psoriasis receiving cyclosporine. Hyperbilirubinemia that was minor and related to dosage has been observed without evidence of hepatocellular damage.

● **GI Effects**

Adverse GI effects, including diarrhea, nausea and vomiting, anorexia, and abdominal discomfort have occurred frequently during cyclosporine therapy. Gastritis, hiccups, and peptic ulcer have occurred less frequently. Constipation, difficulty in swallowing, and upper GI bleeding have been reported rarely in patients receiving the drug.

Cyclosporine administered to treat rheumatoid arthritis resulted in nausea, abdominal pain, diarrhea, or dyspepsia in up to about 23, 15, 13, or 12% of patients, respectively. Vomiting, flatulence, or GI disorder that was not otherwise specified occurred in up to about 9, 5, or 4% of patients, respectively. Anorexia or rectal hemorrhage each occurred in up to about 3% of patients. Stomatitis occurred in up to about 7% of patients. Constipation, dysphagia, eructation, esophagitis, gastritis, gastroenteritis, glossitis, salivary gland enlargement, tongue disorder, tooth disorder, gastric ulcer, and peptic ulcer each occurred in 1% to less than 3% of patients.

Cyclosporine administered to treat psoriasis resulted in adverse GI effects in about 20% of patients. Nausea, diarrhea, abdominal pain, or dyspepsia occurred in about 6, 5, 3, or 2% of patients. Abdominal distention, increased appetite, and constipation each occurred in 1% to less than 3% of patients.

● **Infectious Complications**

Infectious complications, including pneumonia, septicemia, abscesses, and urinary tract, viral, local and systemic fungal, and skin and wound infections, have occurred frequently during cyclosporine therapy. When infectious complications occurring during cyclosporine therapy were compared with those occurring during combined azathioprine and corticosteroid therapy in one study, the frequency of bacterial, viral, and fungal infections was similar in both groups. However, in another study, septicemia, abscesses, and cytomegalovirus infections occurred less frequently in patients receiving cyclosporine than in those receiving azathioprine and corticosteroids; the frequency of other viral infections, local fungal infections, urinary tract infections, pneumonia, and wound and skin infections was similar in both groups.

Cyclosporine administered to treat rheumatoid arthritis resulted in respiratory infection that was not otherwise specified, influenza-like symptoms, urinary tract infection, or pneumonia in up to about 9, 6, 3 or 1% of patients, respectively. Abscess, bacterial infection, cellulitis, fungal infection, herpes simplex, herpes zoster, moniliasis, renal abscess, and viral infection each occurred in 1% to less than 3% of patients.

Cyclosporine administered to treat psoriasis resulted in infection or potential infection in about 25% of patients. Influenza-like symptoms or upper respiratory tract infections occurred in about 10 or 8% of patients, respectively. In addition, respiratory infection or viral and other infections of the respiratory system occurred in 1% to less than 3% of patients.

● **Hematologic Effects**

Adverse hematologic effects of cyclosporine reportedly occurring occasionally include leukopenia, anemia, and thrombocytopenia. Renal and other (e.g., bone marrow) allograft recipients who received cyclosporine as well as some patients who received the drug for other conditions (e.g., uveitis) have developed a syndrome of thrombocytopenia and microangiopathic hemolytic anemia. This vasculopathy is pathologically similar to the hemolytic uremic syndrome, with manifestations that include thrombosis of the renal microvasculature with platelet-fibrin thrombi occluding glomerular capillaries and afferent arterioles, microangiopathic hemolytic anemia, thrombocytopenia and decreased renal function, and such findings are generalizable to other immunosuppressive agents used after transplantation. Although graft failure can result from this syndrome, rejection is not conditional to such vasculopathy, which occurs with avid platelet consumption within the allograft, as shown by indium-111 labeled platelet studies.

Neither the pathogenesis nor optimal management of the syndrome are clear. Although resolution has occurred after reduction of the dosage or discontinuance of cyclosporine, and therapy with streptokinase and heparin or with plasmapheresis, the efficacy of such interventions appears to depend on early detection with indium-111 labeled platelet scans. Lymphoma has also occurred occasionally. (See Cautions: Mutagenicity and Carcinogenicity.) Evidence from animal studies and clinical studies in humans indicates that cyclosporine does not appear to depress bone marrow function. In one study, bone marrow depression occurred in 12% of patients receiving azathioprine and corticosteroids but did not occur in cyclosporine-treated patients. In another study, leukopenia (leukocyte count less than 2000/mm³) occurred in only one cyclosporine-treated patient while it occurred in about 10% of patients receiving azathioprine and corticosteroids.

Cyclosporine administered to treat rheumatoid arthritis resulted in anemia, leukopenia, or lymphadenopathy in 1% to less than 3% of patients.

Cyclosporine administered to treat psoriasis resulted in adverse effects related to leukocytes and the reticuloendothelial system in about 4% of patients. Platelet, bleeding, and clotting disorders or red blood cell disorder occurred in 1% to less than 3% of patients.

● **Sensitivity Reactions**

Sensitivity reactions (including anaphylaxis) have reportedly occurred in 2% or less of patients receiving cyclosporine. Anaphylaxis has been reported in 0.1% of patients receiving the drug IV. There have been no reports to date of anaphylaxis following administration of cyclosporine as conventional (nonmodified) liquid-filled capsules or oral solution (which do *not* contain polyoxyl 35 castor oil); in addition, some patients who developed anaphylaxis while receiving the drug IV subsequently received the conventional oral solution without unusual adverse effect. Anaphylactic reactions to IV cyclosporine include flushing of the face and upper thorax, acute respiratory distress with dyspnea and wheezing, hypotension, tachycardia, and, rarely, death. Although the exact mechanism of these reactions is not known, an association with polyoxyl 35 castor oil in the vehicle of the commercially available concentrate for injection has been suggested. Polyoxyl 35 castor oil has been shown to cause anaphylactoid reactions in animals, including stimulation of histamine release and a hypotensive effect; death has occurred in some animals. An immunologic mechanism (e.g., antibody production, complement activation) has been suggested in some studies and case reports; it has also been suggested that polyoxyl 35 castor oil may enhance the immunogenicity of other agents such as drugs. Anaphylactic reactions have been associated with administration of other drugs in a polyoxyl 35 castor oil-containing vehicle; other reactions (e.g., severe edema, abnormal liver function test results, hyperlipidemia, decreased plasma viscosity) have also been associated with IV use of polyoxyl 35 castor oil-containing preparations. Although IV cyclosporine-induced anaphylactic reactions may subside in some patients when IV infusion of the drug is stopped, death resulting from respiratory arrest and aspiration pneumonia has occurred in at least one patient.

Allergic reactions occurred in 1% to less than 3% of patients who received cyclosporine to treat rheumatoid arthritis.

● **Other Adverse Effects**

Hyperlipidemia and abnormalities in electrophoresis may occur in patients receiving IV cyclosporine, since the vehicle in the commercially available cyclosporine concentrate for injection (polyoxyl 35 castor oil) has been associated with the development of these effects. Although hyperlipidemia and lipoprotein abnormalities are reversible following discontinuance of the drug, their occurrence during cyclosporine therapy usually does not require discontinuance of the drug.

Benign fibroadenoma of the breast has been reported in a few renal allograft recipients receiving cyclosporine alone. Although a definite causal relationship to the drug has not been established, fibroadenoma resolved in one patient following dosage reduction of cyclosporine.

Other adverse effects reportedly occurring in at least 3% of patients receiving cyclosporine include sinusitis and gynecomastia. Conjunctivitis, edema, fever, hearing loss, hyperglycemia (possibly induced by concomitant corticosteroid therapy), muscle pain, and tinnitus have occurred in 2% or less of patients receiving the drug. Chest pain, hair breaking, joint pain, aseptic necrosis, lethargy, mouth sores, night sweats, pancreatitis, visual disturbances, weakness, musculoskeletal abnormalities, and weight loss have been reported rarely in patients receiving cyclosporine.

Cyclosporine administered to treat rheumatoid arthritis resulted in increases in nonprotein nitrogen (NPN) in up to about 19% of patients. Edema that was not otherwise specified, pain, or leg cramps/involuntary muscle contractions occurred in up to about 14, 13, or 12% of patients, respectively. Upper respiratory tract disorders occurred in up to 14% of patients, respectively. Fatigue, chest pain, or hypomagnesemia each occurred in up to about 6% of patients. Arthropathy, coughing, dyspnea, ear disorder that was not otherwise specified, or pharyngitis each occurred in up to about 5% of patients. Micturition frequency, purpura, sinusitis, or accidental trauma each occurred in up to 4% of patients. Bronchitis, fever, rhinitis, or rigors each occurred in up to about 3% of patients. Menstrual disorder or leukorrhea occurred in up to about 3 or 1% of female patients; breast fibroadenosis, breast pain, and uterine hemorrhage each occurred in 1% to less than 3% of patients. Dysuria occurred in up to about 1% of patients. Other adverse effects that occurred in 1% to less than 3% of patients include arthralgia, asthenia, bilirubinemia, bone fracture, bronchospasm, bursitis, cataract, abnormal chest sounds, conjunctivitis, deafness, diabetes mellitus, dry mouth, enanthema, epistaxis, ocular pain, goiter, hematuria, hot flushes, hyperkalemia, hyperuricemia, hypoglycemia, joint dislocation, malaise, micturition urgency, myalgia, nocturia, overdose, polyuria, procedure not otherwise specified, pyelonephritis, stiffness, increased sweating, synovial cyst, taste perversion, tendon disorder, tinnitus, tonsillitis, urinary incontinence, abnormal urine, vestibular disorder, abnormal vision, weight decrease, and weight increase.

Cyclosporine administered to treat psoriasis resulted in adverse effects in the body as a whole in about 29% of patients. Pain occurred in about 4% of patients. Chest pain, fever, and hot flushes each occurred in 1% to less than 3% of patients. Adverse effects of the urinary system occurred in about 24% of patients. Micturition frequency occurred in 1 to less than 3% of patients. Adverse effects related to resistance mechanism occurred in about 19% of patients. Serum concentrations of triglycerides increased to more than 750 mg/dL in about 15% of patients and serum concentrations of cholesterol increased to more than 300 mg/dL in less than 3% of patients. Elevated serum concentrations of triglycerides or cholesterol generally are reversible after dosage reduction or discontinuance of cyclosporine. Adverse effects of the musculoskeletal system occurred in about 13% of patients. Arthralgia occurred in about 6% of patients. Adverse metabolic and nutritional effects occurred in about 9% of patients. Adverse reproductive effects occurred in about 9% of female patients. Adverse effects of the respiratory system (e.g., bronchospasm, coughing, dyspnea, rhinitis) occurred in about 5% of patients. Abnormal vision occurred in 1% to less than 3% of patients. Uric acid may increase in concentration and attacks of gout occurred rarely with cyclosporine.

● *Precautions and Contraindications*

Cyclosporine should be used for therapeutic applications other than transplantation only by clinicians experienced in such use of immunosuppressive therapy. The risks and benefits of cyclosporine in the management of psoriasis should be weighed carefully since the drug is a potent immunosuppressive agent with a number of potentially serious adverse effects. At dosages used in organ transplant recipients, cyclosporine should be used only under the supervision of a clinician experienced in immunosuppressive therapy and the management of organ transplant patients. Management of patients during initiation of, or any major change in, cyclosporine therapy should be performed in facilities equipped with adequate laboratory and supportive medical equipment and staffed with adequate medical personnel. Although patients who are stabilized on cyclosporine may receive the drug as outpatients, periodic laboratory monitoring is required. The clinician responsible for cyclosporine maintenance therapy should have complete information necessary for appropriate follow-up of the patient.

Immunosuppression with cyclosporine may result in increased susceptibility to infection, including serious infections with fatal outcomes, and the possible development of lymphoma. (See Cautions: Mutagenicity and Carcinogenicity.) The increased risk of developing lymphomas and other malignancies, especially of the skin, associated with cyclosporine or other immunosuppressive therapy appears to be related to the degree and duration of immunosuppression irrespective of the specific drugs. Because of the increased risk for skin cancer, patients should be advised to limit ultraviolet light exposure. The manufacturer cautions that, although cyclosporine should be administered with corticosteroids, conventional (nonmodified) oral formulations of the drug and the concentrate for injection should not be administered concomitantly with other

immunosuppressive agents since increased susceptibility to infection and risk of lymphoma may result. However, the manufacturers of the modified oral formulations (Gengraf®, Neoral®) state that these modified formulations may be administered with other immunosuppressives, although the degree of immunosuppression produced may result in an increased risk of lymphoma and other neoplasms and in susceptibility to infection. In addition, such potential danger for oversuppression of the immune system requires that the benefits versus risks of therapeutic regimens containing multiple immunosuppressive agents be weighed carefully.

Comparative risk remains to be elucidated as to whether the risk of developing lymphomas is greater, in general, in patients with rheumatoid arthritis receiving cyclosporine than in rheumatoid arthritis patients who are untreated or being treated with cytotoxic agents. Before therapy with cyclosporine for rheumatoid arthritis is initiated, as well as during its course, patients should be evaluated thoroughly for the presence of malignancies. The risk for malignancies may be increased with concurrent use of cyclosporine and other immunosuppressive agents through induction of excessive immunosuppression.

The risk of developing malignancies of the skin and lymphoproliferative disorders is increased in patients receiving cyclosporine to treat psoriasis, although the relative risk of such occurrence with cyclosporine or other immunosuppressive agents is comparable. In addition, previous therapy with PUVA and, to a lesser extent, with methotrexate or other immunosuppressive agents, coal tar, UVB light, or other radiation increases the risk of developing malignancies of the skin. Before therapy with cyclosporine is initiated, as well as during its course, patients should be evaluated thoroughly for the presence of malignancies with consideration that psoriatic plaques may obscure malignant lesions. A biopsy should be obtained from dermatologic lesions that do not typify psoriasis, before therapy with cyclosporine commences. Cyclosporine should be administered only after suspicious lesions resolve completely and only if other therapies are not an option. Because excessive immunosuppression is possible that would place the patient at risk for malignancies to develop, therapy with methotrexate or other immunosuppressive agents, PUVA, UVB, or other radiation should *not* be administered concurrently with cyclosporine in the management of psoriasis. In addition, therapy with coal tar should not be administered concurrently with cyclosporine.

Immunosuppressed patients are at an increased risk for opportunistic infections, including reactivation of latent viral infections. These include BK virus-associated nephropathy (BKVN), which has been reported in patients receiving immunosuppressants, including cyclosporine, mycophenolate, sirolimus, and tacrolimus. Primary infection with polyoma BK virus typically occurs in childhood; following initial infection, the virus remains latent, but reactivation may occur in immunocompromised patients. BKVN has principally been observed in renal transplant patients (usually within the first year posttransplantation) and may result in serious outcomes, including deterioration of kidney function and renal allograft loss. Risk of BK virus reactivation appears to be related to the degree of overall immunosuppression rather than use of any specific immunosuppressive agent; patients receiving a maintenance immunosuppressive regimen of at least 3 drugs appear to be at highest risk. Patients should be monitored for possible signs of BKVN, including deterioration in renal function, during therapy with cyclosporine; screening assays for polyomavirus replication also have been recommended by some clinicians. Early intervention in patients who develop BKVN is critical; a reduction in immunosuppressive therapy should initially be considered in such patients. Although a variety of other treatment approaches have been used anecdotally in patients with BKVN, including antiviral therapy (e.g., cidofovir), leflunomide, IV immunoglobulins, and fluoroquinolone antibiotics, additional experience and well-controlled studies are necessary to more clearly establish the optimal treatment of such patients.

Cyclosporine should not be administered as therapy for psoriasis in patients with abnormal renal function, hypertension that is uncontrolled, or malignancies because such conditions may increase the risk for nephrotoxicity and hypertension. The presence of these conditions also contraindicates therapy with cyclosporine to manage rheumatoid arthritis.

Because of the risk of anaphylaxis (see Cautions: Sensitivity Reactions), IV cyclosporine should be reserved for patients unable to tolerate oral formulations of the drug. Patients receiving IV cyclosporine should be under continuous observation for at least the first 30 minutes following initiation of the IV infusion and should be closely monitored at frequent intervals thereafter for possible allergic manifestations. Appropriate equipment for maintenance of an adequate airway and other supportive measures and agents for the treatment of anaphylactic reactions (e.g., epinephrine, oxygen) should be readily available whenever cyclosporine is administered IV. If anaphylaxis occurs, IV infusion of cyclosporine should be discontinued immediately and the patient given appropriate therapy (e.g., epinephrine, oxygen) as indicated.

Any cyclosporine preparation is contraindicated in patients with known hypersensitivity to the drug, and the concentrate for injection or modified oral formulations also are contraindicated in those with known hypersensitivity to any ingredient in the formulation (e.g., polyoxyl 35 castor oil [Cremophor® EL] or polyoxyl 40 hydrogenated castor oil [Cremophor® RH40]).

Blood or plasma concentrations of the drug should be monitored periodically in patients receiving conventional (nonmodified) oral formulations of cyclosporine (liquid-filled capsules or oral solution), since absorption of orally administered cyclosporine is reportedly erratic during long-term therapy. Because of the highly variable GI absorption of cyclosporine and the accumulation of data relating trough concentrations with efficacy, predose (trough) concentrations should be monitored. However, monitoring of blood or plasma concentrations of cyclosporine is not a substitute for renal function monitoring or tissue biopsies. When necessary (e.g., because of changes in oral absorption of the drug), dosage adjustment should be made to avoid toxicity resulting from high blood or plasma concentrations of the drug or to prevent possible organ rejection resulting from low concentrations. Monitoring of blood or plasma cyclosporine concentrations may be especially important in hepatic allograft recipients, since absorption of the drug in these patients may be erratic, especially during the first few weeks of the posttransplantation period because of surgical techniques (e.g., bile duct management) or surgically induced liver dysfunction. In addition, patients with GI malabsorption syndromes may have difficulty in achieving therapeutic blood or plasma concentrations when the drug is administered orally. Blood or plasma concentrations of cyclosporine also should be monitored routinely in allograft recipients receiving modified oral formulations and periodically in patients with rheumatoid arthritis being treated with these preparations of cyclosporine so that toxicity secondary to high concentrations of the drug is avoided.

Patients receiving cyclosporine should be informed of the necessity of routine laboratory testing (e.g., BUN and serum creatinine, bilirubin, and liver enzyme concentrations) for the assessment of renal and hepatic function. Patients should also be given careful dosage instructions, advised of the potential risks during pregnancy, and informed of the increased risk of neoplasia during cyclosporine therapy. In addition, they should be advised that oral formulations of cyclosporine should be administered on a consistent schedule with regard to time of day and in relation to meals, and that any change in oral formulation of the drug requires the supervision of a clinician and should be done cautiously.

At high dosages, cyclosporine may cause nephrotoxicity and/or hepatotoxicity. Renal allograft recipients who develop increased BUN and serum creatinine concentrations should be carefully evaluated before adjustment of cyclosporine dosage is initiated, since these increases do not necessarily indicate that organ rejection has occurred. The development of renal dysfunction at any time during the course of cyclosporine therapy requires close monitoring of the patient and frequent dosage adjustment may be required. In patients with persistently high elevations of BUN and serum creatinine concentrations who are unresponsive to adjustment of cyclosporine dosage, switching to other immunosuppressive therapy should be considered. (See Cautions: Renal Effects.) If severe, intractable renal allograft rejection occurs and does not respond to rescue therapy with corticosteroids and monoclonal antibodies, it may be preferable to switch to alternative immunosuppressive therapy or to allow the kidney to be rejected and removed rather than to increase cyclosporine dosage to an excessive level in an attempt to reverse the rejection episode.

During therapy with cyclosporine in the management of psoriasis, renal function must be monitored since renal dysfunction and structural damage to the kidney are potential adverse effects. Nephrotoxicity may occur at recommended dosages, with increasing risk as the dosage and duration of therapy with the drug increases. The serum creatinine concentration and BUN may increase in patients receiving cyclosporine, reflecting a decrease in the glomerular filtration rate. The maximal increase in serum creatinine concentration may be a predictive factor for cyclosporine-induced nephropathy. Structural damage to the kidney and persistent renal dysfunction may result from cyclosporine when patients are monitored inadequately and adjustment of the dosage is improper. Geriatric

patients should be monitored with particular care because renal function also decreases with age. Monitoring the serum creatinine concentration regularly and reducing the dosage when values exceed baseline by 25% or more help to lower the risk of nephropathy from cyclosporine. Elevated serum creatinine concentrations generally reverse upon timely cyclosporine dosage reduction or discontinuance. The risk of nephropathy from cyclosporine in patients with psoriasis also is decreased by initiating therapy with the drug at 2.5 mg/kg daily and not exceeding a maximum dosage of 4 mg/kg daily.

● *Pediatric Precautions*

Although there are no adequate and controlled studies to date in children, cyclosporine has been used in children as young as 6 months of age without unusual adverse effects; the modified oral formulations have been used in children as young as 1 year of age. Cyclosporine has been used in hepatic and renal allograft recipients 7.5 months to 18 years of age. Children receiving cyclosporine and low-dose corticosteroid therapy have shown increased patient and graft survival rates and fewer adverse systemic effects on growth and development than those receiving therapy with other immunosuppressive agents; however, some clinicians have reported an increased frequency of seizures, possibly related to concomitant hypertension or high-dose corticosteroid therapy, in children receiving cyclosporine. The possibility that serious nephrotoxicity, hypertension, and/or seizures may occur in children receiving the drug should be considered.

The safety and efficacy of cyclosporine for the management of juvenile rheumatoid arthritis or psoriasis in children younger than 18 years of age have not been established.

● *Geriatric Precautions*

Although safety and efficacy of cyclosporine have not been specifically studied in geriatric patients, 17.5% of patients treated with the drug for rheumatoid arthritis in clinical studies were 65 years of age and older. Patients 65 years of age or older were more likely to develop systolic hypertension while receiving cyclosporine to treat rheumatoid arthritis in clinical studies. This age group also was more likely to have elevated serum creatinine concentrations that were 50% or more above baseline after 3–4 months of receiving cyclosporine.

● *Mutagenicity and Carcinogenicity*

Various tests have not shown cyclosporine to be mutagenic. No evidence of cyclosporine-induced mutagenesis or genotoxicity was observed with the Ames microbial mutagen test, the V-79-HGPRT test, the micronucleus assay in mice and Chinese hamsters, chromosome-aberration tests in Chinese hamster bone marrow, the mouse dominant lethal assay, or the DNA-repair test in sperm from mice treated with the drug. However, in an in vitro study that used human lymphocytes, high concentrations of cyclosporine appeared to induce sister chromatid exchange.

In a long-term study, the frequency of lymphocytic lymphomas was increased in female mice and that of hepatocellular adenomas was increased in male mice receiving 4 mg/kg daily. Following long-term administration in rats, the frequency of pancreatic islet cell adenomas was higher than the control rate in rats receiving 0.5 mg/kg of cyclosporine daily. In these studies, cyclosporine was administered in doses 0.01–0.16 times the maintenance dose for humans. The development of hepatocellular carcinomas and pancreatic islet cell adenomas in mice and rats did not appear to be dose related.

An increase in the incidence of malignancy is a recognized complication of immunosuppression in allograft recipients and patients with psoriasis or rheumatoid arthritis. Skin cancers and non-Hodgkin's lymphoma develop most commonly. Lesions may regress after reduction or discontinuance of immunosuppression. Patients treated with cyclosporine are at greater risk for the development of malignancies than is the normal, healthy population, although such risk is similar to patients treated with other immunosuppressive therapies.

Lymphomas have developed in patients receiving cyclosporine alone or in combination with other immunosuppressive agents, and some patients have developed a lymphoproliferative disorder that resolved following discontinuance of the drug. The lymphomas and lymphoproliferative disorders appear to be associated with Epstein-Barr virus (EBV) infections. It has been suggested that cyclosporine may cause alteration of the antibody for EBV or may inhibit the cell-mediated response to EBV, resulting in the development of lymphoma. With the exception of corticosteroids, the manufacturer states that conventional (nonmodified) oral formulations of cyclosporine or the concentrate for injection should not be used concomitantly with other immunosuppressive agents, since the risk of lymphoma may be increased. However, the manufacturers of the modified oral formulations (Gengraf®, Neoral®) state that these modified formulations may be administered with other immunosuppressives, although the degree of immunosuppression produced may result in an increased risk of lymphoma and other neoplasms and in susceptibility to infection. In addition, such potential danger for oversuppression of the immune system requires that the benefits versus risks of therapeutic regimens containing multiple immunosuppressive agents be weighed carefully.

Although the risk of lymphoma appears to be greatest when there is substantial immunosuppression (i.e., concomitant use of multiple immunosuppressive agents), all immunosuppressed patients should be considered at risk for developing lymphoma. The nature and optimum management of posttransplant lymphomas and lymphoproliferative disorders in allograft recipients remain to be clearly established, and clinicians should consult specialized references for current methods of evaluation and management. Some clinicians suggest that immunosuppressive therapy with cyclosporine and corticosteroids should be reduced or discontinued in patients who develop posttransplant lymphomas or lymphoproliferative disorders. In one study, reduction of cyclosporine and/or prednisone dosage resulted in resolution of lymphomas but was not associated with allograft rejection. Squamous cell carcinoma occurred in one patient receiving cyclosporine following renal transplantation but has not been directly attributed to the drug.

Lymphoma developed in several patients who received cyclosporine to treat rheumatoid arthritis. Epidemiologic analyses indicated a relationship between cyclosporine and lymphoma, but no relationship to other malignancies that have been reported, including skin cancers, diverse types of solid tumors, and multiple myeloma. Carcinoma or tumor not otherwise specified each occurred in 1% to less than 3% of patients who received cyclosporine.

Patients receiving cyclosporine to treat psoriasis have developed malignancies, especially of the skin. Squamous cell carcinoma or basal cell carcinoma occurred in 0.9 or 0.4% of patients, respectively, who received the drug. In another aggregate of clinical studies, tumors were reported in about 2% of patients who received the drug. Malignancies of the skin that included squamous cell and basal cell carcinomas were reported in about 1% of patients who received cyclosporine. Most of these patients had been treated previously with PUVA and some had received prior therapy with methotrexate, coal tar, or UVB. A history of previous cancer of the skin or a lesion that was a potential predisposition to such cancer was present in some of the patients before therapy with cyclosporine began. The lymphoproliferative disorders that developed in patients receiving cyclosporine for psoriasis included in one patient each non-Hodgkin's lymphoma that required chemotherapy and mycosis fungoides that regressed spontaneously after withdrawal of cyclosporine. Benign lymphocytic infiltration occurred in some patients with spontaneous regression occurring after withdrawal of cyclosporine or, in one patient, while administration of the drug continued. Malignancies that involved various organs accounted for the rest of the patients affected to yield an incidence of about 1%. During postmarketing surveillance, several more patients were reported to have developed tumors while receiving cyclosporine for psoriasis. Cervical intraepithelial neoplasia developed in a patient with chronic plaque psoriasis treated for over 3 years with 3 mg/kg daily of cyclosporine.

● Pregnancy, Fertility, and Lactation

Pregnancy

Although there are no adequate and well-controlled studies using cyclosporine in pregnant women, the drug has been shown to be embryotoxic and fetotoxic in rats and rabbits when administered orally at maternally toxic doses. Fetal toxicity was observed in these animals at doses 0.8–5.4 times (corrected for body surface area) the human maintenance dose of 6 mg/kg. Cyclosporine caused increased prenatal and postnatal mortality and reduced fetal weight with related skeletal retardation in these rats and rabbits. In women who received cyclosporine therapy throughout pregnancy, premature birth (gestational age of 28–36 weeks) and reduced neonatal weight occurred consistently. Most of the pregnancies also were complicated by growth retardation (which may be severe), fetal loss, preeclampsia, eclampsia, premature labor, abruptio placentae, oligohydramnios, Rh incompatibility, and fetoplacental dysfunction. Premature

birth was the most frequent complication, while being small for gestational age and neonatal complications were less common. Malformations occurred in some neonates and in a few cases of fetal loss. A full-term neonate was born to a woman who underwent a renal transplant prior to conception and received 450 mg of cyclosporine alone daily throughout pregnancy, and other successful pregnancies have been reported in allograft recipients who received the drug daily during pregnancy. Abnormalities in renal function or blood pressure were not observed in a limited number of children 7 years of age or younger exposed to cyclosporine in utero.

Cyclosporine should be used during pregnancy only when the potential benefits justify the possible risks to the fetus. In patients with psoriasis, the risks and benefits of therapy with cyclosporine during pregnancy should be evaluated carefully, with discontinuance of therapy considered seriously because of possible disruption of the interaction between the mother and fetus.

Fertility

Reproduction studies in rats receiving cyclosporine have not revealed evidence of impaired fertility.

Lactation

Since cyclosporine is distributed into milk, nursing should be avoided in women receiving the drug.

DRUG INTERACTIONS

● Nephrotoxic Drugs

Interactions that may potentiate renal dysfunction are well substantiated between cyclosporine and various drugs, including aminoglycosides, vancomycin, co-trimoxazole, ciprofloxacin, melphalan, amphotericin B, ketoconazole, certain nonsteroidal anti-inflammatory agents (NSAIAs) (e.g., azapropazon [not commercially available in the US], diclofenac, naproxen, sulindac), cimetidine, ranitidine, fibric acid derivatives (e.g., fenofibrate, bezafibrate), methotrexate, colchicine, and tacrolimus; in some cases, the resultant potentiation of renal dysfunction resulted from the nephrotoxic potential of the interacting drug while in others it resulted from accumulation of cyclosporine induced by the interacting drug. If concomitant use of cyclosporine with such drugs is unavoidable, renal function should be monitored carefully.

Since nephrotoxic effects may be additive, concomitant use of cyclosporine with potentially nephrotoxic drugs (e.g., acyclovir, aminoglycoside antibiotics, amphotericin B) should be avoided.

Concomitant administration of cyclosporine and amphotericin B has produced additive nephrotoxicity. In bone marrow allograft recipients receiving cyclosporine alone, cyclosporine and amphotericin B, or amphotericin B and methotrexate, increases in serum creatinine concentration were substantially greater in patients receiving cyclosporine and amphotericin B compared with those receiving cyclosporine alone or amphotericin B and methotrexate. Since it may be dangerous (i.e., risk of allograft rejection) to completely discontinue cyclosporine therapy when serum creatinine increases in allograft recipients, it has been suggested that if concomitant amphotericin B therapy is necessary in these patients, cyclosporine be temporarily withheld until the trough serum cyclosporine concentration (determined by RIA) is less than 150 ng/mL and that subsequent dosage be adjusted accordingly; this reduction in cyclosporine dosage may decrease the risk of nephrotoxicity while maintaining adequate immunosuppression.

Concomitant administration of cyclosporine and gentamicin has resulted in an increased risk of acute tubular necrosis in renal allograft recipients when compared with concomitant administration of ampicillin and cyclosporine or gentamicin alone. Therefore, administration of aminoglycosides should be avoided in renal allograft recipients who are receiving cyclosporine.

Concomitant administration of cyclosporine and co-trimoxazole has resulted in increases in serum creatinine concentrations. Concomitant administration of cyclosporine and melphalan has resulted in renal failure, and plasma creatinine concentrations and BUN were within normal limits or did not deteriorate in patients treated with melphalan without subsequent administration of cyclosporine.

In patients with rheumatoid arthritis, the combination of cyclosporine and naproxen or sulindac resulted in additive decreases in renal function, as determined with technetium Tc 99m pentatate (DTPA) and iodohippurate sodium I 131 or p-aminohippuric acid (PAH) clearances. However, calculated creatinine clearance did not distinguish NSAIAs from acetaminophen in patients receiving cyclosporine in a dosage stabilized to treat rheumatoid arthritis and 4 weeks of concomitant therapy with 200 mg daily of indomethacin, 200 mg daily of ketoprofen, 400 mg daily of sulindac, or 4 g daily of acetaminophen. Creatinine clearance differed between indomethacin and acetaminophen but the increase of 6% observed with acetaminophen compared with indomethacin was not considered clinical in magnitude.

Concomitant administration of cyclosporine and diclofenac may increase the nephrotoxic potential of cyclosporine. In addition to increases in serum creatinine concentration, increased serum potassium concentrations and/or blood pressure have occurred in some patients receiving the drugs concomitantly. In patients with rheumatoid arthritis, concomitant administration of cyclosporine and diclofenac resulted in elevation of the AUC of diclofenac but did not affect blood concentrations of cyclosporine. Because blood concentrations of diclofenac have been observed to increase by approximately double with concomitant administration of cyclosporine and diclofenac, a lower dosage in the therapeutic range of diclofenac should be used in patients receiving this combination. Pharmacokinetic interactions of clinical importance have not been observed between cyclosporine and aspirin, indomethacin, ketoprofen, or piroxicam. However, because of the risk of additive decreases in renal function, patients with rheumatoid arthritis who are receiving concurrent therapy with cyclosporine and any NSAIA should be monitored with close attention to clinical status and serum creatinine concentration.

Concomitant administration of cyclosporine and colchicine may increase concentrations of cyclosporine, resulting in additive nephrotoxic effects. Cyclosporine also may reduce clearance of colchicine increasing the potential for enhanced colchicine toxicity (myopathy, neuropathy), particularly in patients with renal impairment. Patients should be monitored closely for colchicine toxicity during concurrent administration with cyclosporine; colchicine should be discontinued or dosage of the drug reduced if toxicity occurs.

Immunosuppressive and Antineoplastic Agents

With the exception of corticosteroids, the manufacturer states that conventional (nonmodified) oral formulations of cyclosporine or the concentrate for injection should not be used concomitantly with other immunosuppressive agents since the risk of lymphoma (see Cautions: Mutagenicity and Carcinogenicity) and susceptibility to infection may be increased. However, the manufacturers of the modified oral formulations (Gengraf®, Neoral®) state that these modified formulations may be administered with other immunosuppressives, although the degree of immunosuppression produced may result in an increased risk of lymphoma and other neoplasms and in susceptibility to infection. In addition, such potential danger for oversuppression of the immune system requires that the benefits versus risks of therapeutic regimens containing multiple immunosuppressive agents be weighed carefully. The manufacturers state that patients with psoriasis should not receive cyclosporine concomitantly with other immunosuppressive agents since excessive immunosuppression may result.

Concomitant administration of cyclosporine and sirolimus substantially increases blood sirolimus concentrations. Sirolimus should be given 4 hours following cyclosporine administration to minimize the effect on sirolimus concentrations. Elevated serum creatinine concentrations also have been reported in patients receiving sirolimus and full dosages of cyclosporine concurrently; such increases generally are reversible following cyclosporine dosage reduction.

Concomitant administration of cyclosporine and methotrexate resulted in elevation of the AUC of methotrexate in patients with rheumatoid arthritis. In a limited study, the AUC of methotrexate increased by approximately 30% and the AUC of the metabolite, 7-hydroxymethotrexate, decreased by approximately 80% during coadministration of cyclosporine and methotrexate to patients with rheumatoid arthritis. However, the clinical importance of these observations is not known. Blood concentrations of cyclosporine did not appear to be affected by coadministration of cyclosporine and methotrexate.

Potassium-sparing Drugs

Because cyclosporine may cause hyperkalemia, the manufacturers state that the drug should not be used concomitantly with potassium-sparing diuretics. Caution is advised and control of potassium concentrations recommended when cyclosporine is administered concomitantly with potassium-sparing drugs (e.g., angiotensin-converting enzyme [ACE] inhibitors, angiotensin II receptor antagonists) or potassium-containing drugs or in patients receiving a potassium-rich diet.

Drugs and Foods Affecting Hepatic Microsomal Enzymes

Because cyclosporine is extensively metabolized, the concentration of drug in biologic fluid (e.g., plasma, blood) may be altered by drugs or foods (e.g., grapefruit juice) that affect hepatic microsomal enzymes, especially cytochrome P-450 isoenzyme subfamily CYP3A. Drugs and foods that inhibit hepatic microsomal enzymes could decrease the metabolism of cyclosporine and increase its concentration in biologic fluid. This potential interaction has been well substantiated to occur between cyclosporine and diltiazem, nicardipine, verapamil, mibefradil, fluconazole, itraconazole, ketoconazole, voriconazole, clarithromycin, erythromycin, quinupristin/dalfopristin, methylprednisolone, allopurinol, amiodarone, bromocriptine, colchicine, imatinib, danazol, oral contraceptives, or metoclopramide. Drugs that induce cytochrome P-450 activity could increase the metabolism of cyclosporine and decrease its concentration in biologic fluid. This potential interaction has been well substantiated to occur between cyclosporine and nafcillin, rifampin, carbamazepine, oxcarbazepine, phenobarbital, phenytoin, octreotide, sulfinpyrazone, terbinafine, or ticlopidine. In addition, clinicians should be cautious about concurrent administration of cyclosporine with rifabutin. Although the effect of rifabutin on the metabolism of cyclosporine has not been studied, the metabolism of other drugs by the cytochrome P-450 system has increased with rifabutin. Concomitant administration of cyclosporine with drugs that affect its metabolism requires monitoring of the concentration of cyclosporine in biologic fluid with appropriate adjustment of cyclosporine dosage.

Azole-derivative Antifungal Agents

Concomitant administration of cyclosporine and ketoconazole has been reported to increase plasma concentrations of cyclosporine and serum creatinine concentrations. It has been suggested that ketoconazole may interfere with the metabolism of cyclosporine via hepatic microsomal enzyme inhibition, although other mechanisms may also be involved. When ketoconazole therapy is initiated in patients receiving cyclosporine, renal function and blood or plasma cyclosporine concentrations should be monitored; some clinicians also recommend that reduction in cyclosporine dosage or replacement of cyclosporine with another immunosuppressive agent be considered. Patients stabilized on both drugs may require an increase in cyclosporine dosage when ketoconazole is discontinued.

Concomitant administration of cyclosporine and fluconazole has been reported to increase whole blood concentrations of cyclosporine, and such increase may be associated with nephrotoxic effects. Serum creatinine concentration increased in at least one patient receiving cyclosporine following initiation of fluconazole therapy at a dosage of 200 mg every other day. However, such changes were not observed in several other patients receiving fluconazole 100 or 200 mg daily. Increases in trough cyclosporine concentrations and serum creatinine concentration also occurred when fluconazole dosage was increased from 100 to 300 mg daily. Evidence suggests that fluconazole interferes with the metabolism of cyclosporine via hepatic microsomal enzyme inhibition.

Concomitant administration of cyclosporine and itraconazole has been reported to increase whole blood or serum concentrations of cyclosporine and serum creatinine concentrations. Evidence indicates that itraconazole competitively inhibits the hydroxylation of cyclosporine via hepatic microsomal enzyme inhibition.

Concomitant administration of cyclosporine and voriconazole also may increase blood or plasma cyclosporine concentrations.

Macrolides

Concomitant use of cyclosporine and erythromycin may result in substantial increases in blood or plasma concentrations of cyclosporine and subsequent signs of cyclosporine toxicity (e.g., nephrotoxicity). Studies in healthy adults indicate that erythromycin can substantially decrease plasma clearance of cyclosporine, presumably by inhibiting hepatic metabolism of the drug, although the exact mechanism remains to be clearly determined. Cyclosporine and erythromycin should be used concomitantly with caution, and patients should be monitored for evidence of cyclosporine toxicity. Renal function and blood or plasma concentrations of cyclosporine should be monitored when erythromycin therapy is administered or discontinued in patients receiving cyclosporine or vice versa, and cyclosporine dosage adjusted appropriately as necessary.

Concomitant use of cyclosporine and clarithromycin has resulted in increases in the whole blood concentration of cyclosporine. Elevation in serum creatinine concentration was uncommon.

Corticosteroids

Concomitant administration of prednisolone with cyclosporine may result in decreased plasma clearance of prednisolone, and plasma concentrations of cyclosporine may be increased during concomitant therapy with cyclosporine and methylprednisolone. In addition, seizures have reportedly occurred in adult and pediatric patients receiving cyclosporine and high-dose corticosteroid therapy concurrently with cyclosporine. The mechanism for this interaction may involve competitive inhibition of hepatic microsomal enzymes. The potential drug interaction between cyclosporine and prednisolone or methylprednisolone and the possibility of exacerbated toxicity, as well as the need for appropriate dosage adjustment, should be considered when these drugs are administered concomitantly.

Calcium-Channel Blocking Agents

Mibefradil (no longer commercially available in the US) inhibits the metabolism of cyclosporine, with resultant increased blood concentrations of the immunosuppressive agent; the possible need for cyclosporine dosage adjustment should be considered during concomitant mibefradil therapy. In addition, when cyclosporine is used in combination with mibefradil and an HMG-CoA reductase inhibitor (e.g., lovastatin, simvastatin), increased blood concentrations of cyclosporine and the HMG-CoA reductase inhibitor also may occur which potentially could lead to HMG-CoA reductase inhibitor-induced rhabdomyolysis; therefore, concomitant use of the drugs should be avoided.

Concomitant administration of cyclosporine and verapamil has resulted in increased whole blood concentrations of cyclosporine. It has been suggested that verapamil may interfere with metabolism of cyclosporine via hepatic microsomal enzyme inhibition. However, evaluation of the effect of verapamil on the pharmacokinetics of the major metabolites of cyclosporine indicated that the interaction between cyclosporine and verapamil was not secondary to interference with N-demethylation.

Concomitant administration of cyclosporine and nicardipine has resulted in increased whole blood or plasma cyclosporine concentrations. Concomitant administration of cyclosporine and nifedipine resulted in more frequent occurrence of gingival hyperplasia compared with cyclosporine alone.

Concomitant administration of cyclosporine and diltiazem has resulted in increased blood cyclosporine concentrations and consequent cyclosporine-induced nephrotoxicity. Although further study is needed, it has been suggested that diltiazem may interfere with metabolism of cyclosporine via hepatic microsomal enzyme inhibition.

Other Drugs Affecting Hepatic Microsomal Enzymes

Concomitant administration of cyclosporine and rifampin, phenytoin, phenobarbital, or a combination of IV sulfamethazine and trimethoprim (co-trimoxazole) reportedly has resulted in decreased cyclosporine concentrations, probably by increasing hepatic metabolism of the drug. Monitoring of plasma or blood cyclosporine concentrations and appropriate dosage adjustment are necessary when any of these drugs is used concomitantly with cyclosporine.

Concomitant administration of cyclosporine and cimetidine has resulted in increased serum creatinine concentrations, although some evidence suggests that renal function may not be adversely affected despite a decrease in creatinine clearance. An increase in whole blood concentrations of cyclosporine occurred with concomitant administration of cyclosporine, cimetidine, and metronidazole. Concomitant administration of cyclosporine and ranitidine also has resulted in an increase in serum creatinine concentrations. However, some evidence indicates that serum creatinine concentration, creatinine clearance, and inulin clearance are affected minimally by the combination of cyclosporine and ranitidine.

Clearance of lovastatin reportedly was reduced with concomitant administration of cyclosporine, and such alterations could result in toxic effects of the antilipemic agent. Adverse effects observed during concomitant cyclosporine and lovastatin therapy have included myositis, myolysis, or rhabdomyolysis. Manifestations of such myopathy included myalgia and/or muscle weakness and increases in serum creatine kinase concentration. Acute renal failure has occurred concurrently with myopathy.

Combined use of mibefradil (no longer commercially available in the US), cyclosporine, and an HMG-CoA reductase inhibitor (e.g., lovastatin, simvastatin) can result in a potentially serious interaction and therefore should be avoided. (See Drugs and Foods Affecting Hepatic Microsomal Enzymes: Calcium-Channel Blocking Agents, in Drug Interactions.)

Concomitant use of cyclosporine and allopurinol has resulted in increases in the whole blood concentration of cyclosporine. Serum creatinine concentration may also be elevated. Concomitant administration of cyclosporine and danazol also has resulted in increased blood cyclosporine concentrations and serum creatinine concentrations.

Concomitant administration of cyclosporine and carbamazepine has resulted in decreased concentrations of cyclosporine in biologic fluid (e.g., whole blood) that were subtherapeutic in adults. In children whose dosage of cyclosporine was stabilized, trough concentrations of cyclosporine in whole blood were lower compared with control in patients treated concurrently with carbamazepine.

Grapefruit Juice

Concomitant oral administration of grapefruit juice with cyclosporine has been reported to increase bioavailability of the drug. The interaction does *not* appear to occur with sweet ("common") orange juice, but some evidence indicates that it is likely with sour (Seville) orange juice.

In several studies in healthy adults or renal transplant recipients receiving cyclosporine as conventional (nonmodified) oral capsules with 175–250 mL of oral grapefruit juice, oral bioavailability of the drug increased by about 20–200%. Although it has been suggested that separating oral administration of cyclosporine and the juice by at least 90 minutes may minimize the effect on bioavailability, peak serum cyclosporine concentrations still may be increased, and other evidence suggests that the effect of grapefruit juice on drug bioavailability may persist much longer (e.g., for at least 10 hours), possibly secondary to a prolonged effect of the interacting constituent(s) on enzymes in the gut wall. Therefore, additional study is needed to determine whether separation of cyclosporine and grapefruit juice administration during the day can adequately minimize the potential interaction.

The interaction between grapefruit juice and cyclosporine bioavailability appears to result from inhibition, probably prehepatic, of the cytochrome P-450 enzyme system by some constituent(s) in the juice; grapefruit juice does not interfere appreciably with metabolism following IV drug administration. Both fresh and frozen grapefruit juice have been shown to inhibit first-pass metabolism of drugs metabolized by various cytochrome P-450 isoenzymes, including CYP1A2, CYP2A6, and the CYP3A subfamily (e.g., CYP3A4); these enzymes are present in the liver and/or extrahepatic tissues such as intestinal mucosa. Following oral administration of cyclosporine, certain benzodiazepines (e.g., midazolam, triazolam), and certain calcium-channel blocking agents (e.g., 1,4-dihydropyridine derivatives), such prehepatic inhibition of drug metabolism by grapefruit juice appears mainly to involve the CYP3A4 isoenzyme, principally within the small intestinal wall (e.g., in the jejunum), thus increasing systemic availability of these drugs. The magnitude of this interaction may be particularly notable for drugs such as cyclosporine that exhibit poor oral bioavailability when administered alone and in individuals in whom oral bioavailability is already relatively low.

The constituent(s) of grapefruit juice principally responsible for this interaction has not been elucidated fully. In addition, the composition of grapefruit juice is variable depending on natural and commercial factors. Such factors influencing individual concentrations of various grapefruit constituents include fruit variety, environmental conditions (e.g., temperature, humidity, location), fruit maturity, and juicing procedures (e.g., extraction pressure, method and extent of debittering, final adjustments of the juice product such as addition of essential oils and pulp). Grapefruit juice contains high concentrations of bioflavonoids, which have been shown to inhibit cytochrome P-450 microsomal enzymes. Although naringin, a bioflavonoid that gives grapefruit its characteristic bitter taste, has been a principal suspect because of the relatively high concentrations present in the fruit, in vitro and in vivo evidence indicates that this bioflavonoid probably has little or no effect on the inhibition of cytochrome P-450 enzymes. Naringenin, the aglycone metabolite of naringin, is a more potent inhibitor of cytochrome enzymes, but recent evidence suggests that this constituent may only contribute to, not be principally responsible for, grapefruit juice-induced drug interactions. Complicating interpretation of these data, however, are methodologic limitations of human studies that currently cannot elucidate the extent to which these or other flavonoids may contribute to the metabolic interactions. Further complicating interpretation are potential problems with extrapolating results obtained with hepatic microsomes to extrahepatic cytochromes since the interaction probably is prehepatic (i.e., involving the small intestine). In addition, the effects of flavonoids on metabolic reactions can be complex and, in some cases, the same flavonoid or possibly a metabolite can inhibit one reaction and stimulate another or even the same reaction in a concentration-dependent manner. Alternatively, some evidence indicates that 6′,7′-dihydroxybergamottin, a furanocoumarin (psoralen) compound present in grapefruit juice but not in sweet orange juice, may be the main constituent responsible for such drug interactions involving cytochrome P-450 enzymes.

Cyclosporine concentrations ideally are maintained in a relatively narrow range to prevent transplant rejection and minimize toxicity. Because concomitant oral administration of cyclosporine and grapefruit juice can result in clinically important increases in systemic concentrations of the drug, such administration should be avoided. Although some clinicians have suggested that grapefruit juice may provide a nontoxic and inexpensive alternative to drugs that have been used to improve oral bioavailability of cyclosporine and thus reduce the required dose of this expensive drug, others have cautioned that the resultant effects would be unpredictable since the composition of this juice is not standardized. The effect of grapefruit juice on oral bioavailability of the drug from the more bioavailable modified oral formulations (i.e., Gengraf®, Neoral®) remains to be established, but the manufacturers recommend that concomitant use of these formulations and the juice also be avoided.

• St. John's Wort (Hypericum perforatum)

Concomitant use of cyclosporine and St. John's wort (Hypericum perforatum) has resulted in marked reduction in the blood concentrations of cyclosporine, leading to subtherapeutic levels, rejection of transplanted organs, and graft loss.

• Vaccines

The possibility that the immune response to vaccination may be diminished in patients receiving cyclosporine should be considered. In addition, because of the immunosuppressive effects of cyclosporine, the manufacturers recommend that live vaccines be avoided during therapy with the drug.

• Other Drugs

Concomitant administration of cyclosporine and metoclopramide has resulted in increased area under the blood concentration-time curve of cyclosporine. It has been suggested that absorption of cyclosporine increased through acceleration of gastric emptying of the drug stimulated by metoclopramide. Concomitant use of cyclosporine and orlistat should be avoided because of the potential for decreased cyclosporine absorption.

Concomitant use of bosentan and cyclosporine has resulted in decreased plasma cyclosporine concentrations by approximately 50% and increased steady-state plasma bosentan concentrations by about 3- to 4-fold. The manufacturer of bosentan states that concomitant use of bosentan and cyclosporine is contraindicated.

Concomitant administration of cyclosporine and digoxin has resulted in decreases in apparent volume of distribution and serum clearance of digoxin. Cardiac glycoside toxicity (e.g., bidirectional ventricular tachycardia, anorexia, nausea, vomiting, diarrhea) occurred and serum digoxin concentrations were increased within a few days after patients already receiving digoxin began receiving cyclosporine. The mechanism of this interaction may involve the decrease in glomerular filtration rate induced by cyclosporine, since in dogs concomitant administration of cyclosporine and digoxin resulted in acute decreases in the renal clearance of the glycoside, glomerular filtration, and renal perfusion.

For information on potential interactions between cyclosporine and NSAIAs, see Drug Interactions: Nephrotoxic Drugs.

ACUTE TOXICITY

• Pathogenesis

Limited information is available on the acute toxicity of cyclosporine. The oral LD_{50} of cyclosporine is about 2.3, 1.5, or greater than 1 g/kg in mice, rats, and rabbits, respectively. The IV LD_{50} is 148, 104, or 46 mg/kg in mice, rats, and rabbits, respectively.

• Manifestations

Overdosage of cyclosporine is likely to produce symptoms that are mainly extensions of common adverse reactions. Transient hepatotoxicity and nephrotoxicity may occur but should resolve following elimination or discontinuance of the drug.

• Treatment

In acute oral cyclosporine overdose, the stomach should be emptied by inducing emesis. Induction of emesis is probably useful up to 2 hours after ingestion. If the patient is comatose, having seizures, or lacks the gag reflex, gastric lavage may be performed if an endotracheal tube with cuff inflated is in place to prevent aspiration of gastric contents. Supportive and symptomatic treatment should be initiated. Hemodialysis and charcoal hemoperfusion reportedly are not useful for enhancing the elimination of cyclosporine following overdosage. When overdosage occurs in patients prescribed cyclosporine therapy, the drug may be withheld for a few days or alternate-day therapy may be initiated until the patient is stabilized.

PHARMACOLOGY

• Immunosuppressive Effects

Cyclosporine mainly exhibits immunosuppressive activity. In vivo studies in animals have shown that cyclosporine inhibits cell-mediated immune responses such as allograft rejection, delayed hypersensitivity (e.g., tuberculin-induced), experimental allergic encephalomyelitis, Freund's adjuvant-induced arthritis, and graft-vs-host disease. Cyclosporine has also been shown to inhibit primary and secondary responses to T cell-dependent antigens (e.g., xenogeneic [heterologous]erythrocytes) in animals. The drug may also inhibit humoral immune responses to some extent. Increased survival of allogeneic (homologous) transplants involving skin, heart, kidney, liver, pancreas, bone marrow, small intestine, and lung has been shown in animals receiving the drug.

The exact mechanism(s) of immunosuppressive action of cyclosporine has not been fully elucidated but appears to mainly involve inhibition of lymphocytic proliferation and function. It has been suggested that the immunosuppressive action of cyclosporine results from specific and reversible inhibition of immunocompetent T cells (T-lymphocytes) in the G_0 (resting) or G_1 (first "gap," postmitotic, or presynthetic) phase of the cell cycle. Cyclosporine mainly inhibits T-helper (inducer) cells; some inhibition of T-suppressor cells may also be involved. The drug also inhibits T-cytotoxic cells and interleukin-2-producing T cells. Cyclosporine inhibits production and/or release of lymphokines including interleukin-2 (T-cell growth factor) and interleukin-1 (lymphocyte-activating factor). Cyclosporine inhibits the release of interleukin-2 from activated T cells and also inhibits interleukin-2-induced activation of resting T cells; the drug does not appear to inhibit activation of resting T cells that is induced by exogenous interleukin-2.

There is conflicting evidence to date whether cyclosporine affects B cells (B-lymphocytes). In some studies, cyclosporine inhibited B-cell responses to macrophage-processed antigens and directly suppressed B cells in the blastogenic phase. In other studies, cyclosporine did not inhibit B-cell antibody production. In animals, cyclosporine does not affect the function of phagocytic cells (enzyme secretion, chemotactic migration of granulocytes, macrophage migration, in vivo carbon clearance) or that of tumor cells (growth rate, metastasis).

Unlike other currently available immunosuppressive agents (e.g., azathioprine), cyclosporine lacks clinically important myelosuppressive activity. In one study following administration of high dosages of cyclosporine, bone marrow cell counts (i.e., granulocytes, monocytes, stem cells) showed only slight reductions in cell numbers; proliferation of bone marrow stem cells was normal or enhanced.

● **Renal Effects**

Cyclosporine produces nephrotoxic effects which generally appear to be dose dependent and reversible. (See Cautions: Renal Effects.) Increased BUN and/or serum creatinine concentrations have been observed during therapy with the drug. In some patients following bone marrow or renal transplantation, histologic evidence of nephrotoxicity has been observed including arteriolar and glomerular thrombi, marked tubular injury, and interstitial fibrosis. Ischemically injured kidneys may be particularly sensitive to the nephrotoxic effects of the drug. Hypertension, hyperkalemia, and hyperuricemia frequently result from therapy with cyclosporine and may be caused directly by the drug's nephrotoxic effects. Increased plasma renin activity has been reported in animals receiving cyclosporine and may contribute to the development of hypertension.

● **Other Effects**

There is some evidence that cyclosporine may have antimalarial, antineoplastic, and antischistosomal activity; however, the clinical importance of these findings has not been determined.

PHARMACOKINETICS

Cyclosporine as unchanged drug is chiefly responsible for immunosuppressive activity, although certain metabolites (e.g., AM1, AM9, AM4N) appear to contribute, at least in part, to this activity. Determination of the pharmacokinetics of cyclosporine appears to be biologic fluid dependent (blood vs plasma or serum) and assay-method dependent (radioimmunoassay vs high-pressure liquid chromatography). Because of these apparent differences, interpretation of pharmacokinetic data and determination of a relationship between biologic fluid concentrations and therapeutic and/or toxic effects of the drug are difficult. Although the most appropriate biologic fluid and assay method for determining cyclosporine concentrations have not been fully established, most experts currently recommend that whole blood preferably be used since the higher cyclosporine concentrations present in this fluid (relative to plasma or serum) can be measured more precisely and accurately than with these other fluids. In addition, there is some evidence from renal allograft recipients that whole blood rather than plasma determinations may be a more useful guide to efficacy and/or toxicity of cyclosporine, although precise relationships remain to be established. In addition, these experts currently recommend that an assay method with high specificity for unchanged cyclosporine preferably be used. Some laboratories may continue to report, and clinicians to use, cyclosporine concentrations determined in plasma or serum, and, while the benefits remain unclear,some centers advocate the use of both nonspecific and specific assays in order to gain insight into the proportion of immunoreactivity resulting from metabolites of the drug. In addition, interpretation of results can be difficult, in part because of the complex pharmacokinetics of the drug, variety of assay methods used, and the broad range of acceptable values, depending on the clinical indication for cyclosporine use and time since transplantation. Therefore, all values for cyclosporine concentration must be qualified by the biologic fluid and assay method used, and any guidance regarding possible dosage adjustment should include information on appropriate reference ranges and be tailored to the patient population being treated and any associated treatment protocols.

Distribution of cyclosporine into erythrocytes is temperature and concentration dependent; therefore, reported plasma concentrations are affected by temperature during the separation of plasma and may also be affected by concentration of the drug. Variability of plasma cyclosporine concentrations may be minimized by allowing the sample to equilibrate at room temperature for at least 1 hour prior to centrifugation. Determinations of drug concentration using anticoagulated, hemolyzed whole blood may avoid the problem of temperature-dependent redistribution of the drug between plasma and erythrocytes. Plasma concentrations of the drug may also be affected by the patient's lipoprotein concentration and hematocrit. Following administration of the same dose, blood concentrations of cyclosporine are higher than plasma concentrations since the drug is distributed into erythrocytes. Plasma and serum cyclosporine concentrations are comparable.

Although both RIA and HPLC have been used to determine biologic fluid cyclosporine concentrations, RIA has been used most extensively since HPLC determination of cyclosporine concentrations is technically difficult and variable; the 2 assays do not yield comparable results. Both specific (for unchanged drug) and nonspecific RIA methods are available. When RIA methods that employ nonspecific monoclonal or polyclonal antibodies are used for monitoring cyclosporine concentrations, cross-reactivity of the antisera with circulating metabolites of cyclosporine has resulted in higher cyclosporine concentrations than when HPLC is used. The ratio of specific (either RIA or HPLC) to nonspecific assays of blood cyclosporine concentrations has varied from 1:1 to 1:8; however, for nonspecific immunoassays, the ratio usually is 1:2 to 1:3 for stable renal allograft patients several months after surgery but is 1:3 to 1:4 for cardiac or hepatic allograft recipients, and may be as great as 1:19 in hepatic allograft recipients with severe cholestasis. The ratio may remain constant for fixed points of comparison during the dosing interval. Additional study is needed to determine whether a similar constancy for these fixed-point ratios exists in patients with impaired hepatic function, especially during the early posttransplantation period in hepatic allograft recipients, since cyclosporine is metabolized principally in the liver and undergoes substantial biliary elimination. In addition to RIA, immunoassay methods currently employed include a nonspecific or specific fluorescence polarization immunoassay (FPIA) and a specific enzyme multiplied immunoassay technique (EMIT). Even with specific immunoassays, some cross-reactivity with cyclosporine metabolites may exist, resulting in slightly different reference ranges for cyclosporine concentrations. Therefore, it is important that consistent laboratories and methods be used and that the reference ranges for each group of organ transplant recipients and method of assay be known; in addition, any attempt at comparing these ranges with other institutions generally should be limited to circumstances in which the same assay method and therapeutic regimens are employed.

At present, use of any of the currently available specific immunoassays (RIA, FPIA, FPIA) is acceptable for routine monitoring of whole blood trough cyclosporine concentrations. Although use of HPLC also may be appropriate for determining trough cyclosporine concentrations, differences in the results obtained with this assay method relative to immunoassays should be considered when monitoring cyclosporine therapy.

● **Absorption**

Following oral administration, cyclosporine is variably and incompletely absorbed. The extent of absorption depends on the individual patient, patient population (e.g., transplant type), posttransplantation time (e.g., increasing during the early posttransplantation period in renal transplant recipients), bile flow (micellar absorption of the drug involving bile), GI state (e.g., decreased with diarrhea), and the formulation administered. Absorption of orally administered cyclosporine from conventional (nonmodified) oral formulations reportedly is erratic during long-term therapy. In hepatic allograft recipients, GI absorption of cyclosporine also may be erratic, especially during the first few weeks of the posttransplantation period because of surgical techniques (e.g., bile duct management with resultant reductions in bile flow) or surgically induced liver dysfunction.

Peak blood and plasma cyclosporine concentrations occur at about 3.5 hours following oral administration of conventional (nonmodified) formulations of the drug. Following oral administration, cyclosporine is metabolized on first pass through the liver. (See Pharmacokinetics: Elimination.) Although oral bioavailability of cyclosporine administered as conventional oral formulations averages 30% across various allograft recipients, it exhibits considerable interindividual variation, ranging from 2–89%, depending on numerous variables including organ transplant type; in hepatic or renal allograft recipients, estimates range from less than 10% to as high as 89%, respectively. Following oral administration of a single 600-mg dose of cyclosporine as a conventional solution in one study, the mean absolute bioavailability was about 30% (range: 10–60%) and a mean peak plasma concentration of about 540 ng/mL (range: 240–1250 ng/mL) was reached at about 3–4 hours. Limited data indicate that the bioavailability of the conventional liquid-filled capsules of cyclosporine is equivalent to that of the conventional oral solution. In a small number of renal transplant patients who received a mean daily cyclosporine dosage of 3.9 mg/kg (range: 2.2–6.6 mg/kg), given as the conventional oral solution for 1 week followed by the same dosage as the capsules for 1 week, the relative bioavailability of the conventional liquid-filled capsules was 111% (based on the area under the blood concentration-time curve from 0–12 hours) of the oral solution. The manufacturer states that peak plasma or blood concentrations of cyclosporine (as determined by HPLC) are approximately 1 or 1.4–2.7 ng/mL per mg of an orally administered dose from a conventional formulation, respectively, in healthy adults.

Although the absolute oral bioavailability of cyclosporine administered as the modified oral formulations (Gengraf®, Neoral®) has not been determined in adults, these formulations have greater bioavailability than the conventional (non-modified) oral formulations of cyclosporine. In addition, while the peak blood or plasma concentration and area under the concentration-time curve (AUC) of cyclosporine increase with the dose administered, with a curvilinear (parabolic) relationship observed at doses between 0–1.4 g of conventional (nonmodified) oral formulations when the biologic fluid used is blood, the AUC of cyclosporine is linearly related to usual doses of the drug administered as the modified oral formulations; a linear relationship also has been described for conventional oral formulations when plasma and HPLC were used. Despite the increased AUC and peak blood concentrations of cyclosporine associated with the modified oral formulations, dose-normalized trough concentrations of the drug are similar for both the conventional and modified formulations. The AUC of cyclosporine differed between individuals by a percent coefficient of variation of approximately 20–50% in renal transplant patients administered cyclosporine as the conventional (nonmodified) oral formulation or a modified oral formulation. Such a factor makes individualization of dosage necessary for optimal therapy. Intraindividual variability in the AUC of cyclosporine and time to peak blood concentration of the drug is reduced with the modified oral formulations compared with the conventional oral formulation. Some evidence indicates that intraindividual variability in peak and trough blood concentrations of cyclosporine also is less with the modified oral formulations. In renal allograft recipients, the percent coefficients of variation within individuals in the AUC of cyclosporine for modified and conventional (nonmodified) oral formulations were 9–21 and 19–26%, respectively. Intraindividual variabilities in the trough concentration of cyclosporine from modified and conventional oral formulations were 17–30 and 16–38%, respectively, in these patients. Limited data in children also show that the bioavailability of cyclosporine is higher with the modified oral formulations. The modified oral capsules of Neoral® are bioequivalent with Neoral® oral solution. The modified oral capsules of Gengraf® also are bioequivalent with the modified oral solution of Gengraf®. In addition, the 2 commercially available modified oral formulations of cyclosporine, Neoral® and Gengraf®, have been demonstrated to be bioequivalent to each other.

The higher bioavailability of the modified oral formulations relative to the conventional (nonmodified) oral formulation varies across patient populations. The mean relative AUC of cyclosporine for a modified oral formulation (Neoral®) compared with the conventional oral formulation ranged from 1.2–1.5 in crossover studies of stable renal transplant patients. In de novo renal transplant patients administered either formulation of cyclosporine, the dose-normalized AUC was 23% greater with the modified oral formulation. In de novo hepatic allograft recipients administered either formulation of cyclosporine 28 days after transplantation, the dose-normalized AUC was 50% greater with the modified oral formulation. The absolute oral bioavailability of cyclosporine was 43% (range: 30–68%) from the modified oral formulation compared with 28% (range: 17–42%) from the conventional oral formulation in de novo hepatic transplant patients aged 1.4–10 years old. In a limited number of hepatic allograft recipients with external biliary diversion, the oral bioavailability of cyclosporine was 6.5 times greater with the modified oral formulation (Neoral®) administered during the first month after transplantation than with the conventional oral formulation. In a limited number of cardiac allograft recipients, the AUC of cyclosporine was greater with the modified oral formulation (Neoral®) relative to the conventional oral formulation. In a limited number of patients with rheumatoid arthritis, the AUC of cyclosporine was about 20% greater with the modified oral formulation (Neoral®) compared with the conventional oral formulation. Peak blood concentrations are increased by 40–106% in renal transplant patients and by approximately 90% in hepatic transplant patients. Peak blood concentrations of cyclosporine from 1.5–2 hours following oral administration of the modified formulations to renal transplant patients.

Food decreases the AUC and peak blood concentration of cyclosporine attained with the modified oral formulations. In healthy individuals, the AUC and peak blood concentration of cyclosporine were decreased by 15 and 26%, respectively, when the oral formulation of Neoral® was administered 30 minutes after the start of consumption of a high-fat meal (e.g., 960 calories, 54.4 g of fat). In another study, the AUC and peak blood concentration of cyclosporine decreased by 13 and 33%, respectively, when a high-fat meal (e.g., 669 calories, 45 g of fat) was eaten within 30 minutes before administration of this modified oral formulation. Similar effects occurred with a low-fat meal (e.g., 667 calories, 15 g of fat). However, other data have not shown the AUC of cyclosporine from the modified oral

formulation of Neoral® to be affected by a high-fat meal (45 g) or a low-fat meal (15 g). Similar discordance of data on the effect of food on cyclosporine absorption with conventional formulations has been described, although high-fat meals and meals given early postoperatively appear most likely to enhance absorption.

External biliary diversion in de novo hepatic transplant patients had very little effect on the absorption of cyclosporine from the oral formulation of Neoral®. The change from the trough to the maximal blood concentration of cyclosporine when the T-tube was closed differed by 6.9% from when it was open. In adult de novo renal transplant patients being treated with this modified oral formulation at a dosage of 597 mg (7.95 mg/kg) daily, the AUC over one dosing interval of cyclosporine was 8772 ng •h/mL at 4 weeks. The peak and trough (obtained prior to the morning dose, approximately 12 hours after last dose) blood concentrations of cyclosporine were 1802 and 361 ng/mL, respectively, as determined by specific monoclonal fluorescence polarization immunoassay. In stable adult renal transplant patients being treated with this modified oral formulation at a dosage of 344 mg (4.1 mg/kg) daily, the AUC over one dosing interval was 6035 ng•h/mL. The peak and trough blood concentrations of cyclosporine in these patients were 1333 and 251 ng/mL, respectively, as determined by specific monoclonal fluorescence polarization immunoassay. In adult de novo hepatic transplant patients being treated with this formulation at a dosage of 458 mg (6.9 mg/kg) daily, the AUC over one dosing interval was 7187 ng•h/mL at 4 weeks. The peak and trough blood concentrations of the drug in these patients were 1555 and 268 ng/mL, respectively, as determined by specific monoclonal RIA.

In stable hepatic transplant patients 2–8 years of age being treated with the oral formulation of Neoral® at a dosage of 101 mg (5.95 mg/kg) in 3 divided doses daily, the peak blood concentration of cyclosporine was 629 ng/mL, as determined by specific monoclonal RIA, and the AUC over one dosing interval was 2163 ng•h/mL. In stable hepatic transplant patients 8–15 years of age being treated with this modified formulation at a dosage of 188 mg (4.96 mg/kg) in 2 divided doses daily, the peak blood concentration of the drug was 975 ng/mL, as determined by specific monoclonal RIA, and the AUC over one dosing interval was 4272 ng•h/mL. In a stable hepatic transplant patient 3 years of age being treated with this modified formulation at a dosage of 120 mg (8.3 mg/kg) in 2 divided doses daily, the peak blood concentration was 1050 ng/mL, as determined by specific monoclonal fluorescence polarization immunoassay, and the AUC over one dosing interval was 5832 ng•h/mL. In stable hepatic transplant patients 8–15 years of age being treated with this modified formulation at a dosage of 158 mg (5.5 mg/kg) in 2 divided doses daily, the peak blood cyclosporine concentration was 1013 ng/mL, as determined by specific monoclonal fluorescence polarization immunoassay, and the AUC over one dosing interval was 4452 ng•h/mL. In stable renal transplant patients 7–15 years of age being treated with the modified oral formulation at a dosage of 328 mg (7.4 mg/kg) in 2 divided doses daily, the peak blood concentration was 1827 ng/mL, as determined by specific monoclonal fluorescence polarization immunoassay, and the AUC over one dosing interval was 6922 ng•h/mL.

Blood or plasma concentrations of cyclosporine required for therapeutic effect or associated with toxicity have not been established precisely. (See introductory paragraphs in Pharmacokinetics.) Organ rejection has reportedly occurred less frequently when trough blood concentrations of the drug (determined by HPLC) were greater than 100 ng/mL. Although optimum trough cyclosporine concentrations have not been determined, trough blood or plasma concentrations (i.e., at 24 hours) of 250–800 or 50–300 ng/mL, respectively, as determined by RIA, appear to minimize the frequency of graft rejection and cyclosporine-induced adverse effects. An association between trough serum concentrations (determined by RIA) greater than 500 ng/mL and cyclosporine-induced nephrotoxicity has been reported.

● **Distribution**

Cyclosporine is widely distributed into body fluids and tissues, with most of the drug being distributed outside the blood volume. Following oral administration of a single 600-mg dose as a conventional formulation in adults with normal renal and hepatic function, the apparent volume of distribution (V_d) of cyclosporine has been reported to be 13 L/kg. The drug has a volume of distribution at steady-state (V_{ss}) of 3–5 L/kg following IV administration in solid organ allograft recipients. In one study following IV administration of cyclosporine in patients with severely impaired renal function (i.e., creatinine clearance less than 5 mL/minute), V_{ss} ranged from 1.45–7.26 L/kg.

Approximately 90–98% of cyclosporine in plasma is protein bound, mainly to lipoproteins (85–90% of total protein binding). Of lipoprotein binding, 43–57% is to high-density lipoproteins (HDLs), 25% to low-density lipoproteins (LDLs), and 2% to very-low-density lipoproteins (VLDLs). Distribution of the drug in blood is dose dependent; in vitro in blood, 33–47% of the drug is distributed into plasma, 4–9% into lymphocytes, 4–12% into granulocytes, and 41–58% into erythrocytes. At high concentrations, distribution of cyclosporine into leukocytes and erythrocytes becomes saturated. Concentrations of the drug achieved in mononuclear cells have been reported to be 1000 times greater than those achieved in erythrocytes.

Cyclosporine crosses the placenta in animals and humans. In a renal allograft recipient who received 450 mg of cyclosporine daily throughout pregnancy, the drug was not present in amniotic fluid at 36 weeks or at amniotomy, but maternal and cord blood concentrations at delivery were 86 and 54 mcg/L, respectively.

Cyclosporine is distributed into milk. Cyclosporine concentrations in milk reportedly were 101, 109, and 263 mcg/L on the second, third, and fourth days of the postpartum period, respectively, in a patient who received 450 mg of the drug daily throughout pregnancy and the postpartum period. Studies in animals have shown that cyclosporine is distributed into milk at a maximum concentration of 2% of the maternal dose.

● Elimination

Blood concentrations of cyclosporine generally appear to decline in a biphasic manner, although a triphasic disposition also has been described. In adults with normal renal and hepatic function, the half-life in the initial phase ($t_{\frac{1}{2}\alpha}$) has been reported to average 1.2 hours and the half-life in the terminal elimination phase ($t_{\frac{1}{2}\beta}$) has averaged 8.4–27 hours (range: 4–50 hours). In one study following IV administration of cyclosporine in patients with severely impaired renal function (i.e., creatinine clearance less than 5 mL/minute), $t_{\frac{1}{2}\beta}$ averaged 15.8 or 16.5 hours based on blood cyclosporine concentrations determined by HPLC or RIA, respectively.

Clearance of cyclosporine from blood following IV administration is approximately 5–7 mL/minute per kg as determined with data (using HPLC) from adult renal or hepatic transplant patients. Clearance of the drug in infants may be up to severalfold higher and in older children twice as high as that in adults. Cardiac transplant patients appear to have slightly slower blood cyclosporine clearance.

The apparent clearance of cyclosporine administered as a modified oral formulation was 593 mL/minute (7.8 mL/minute per kg) after 4 weeks of therapy and 492 mL/minute (5.9 mL/minute per kg) as determined with data (using monoclonal fluorescence polarization immunoassay) from adult de novo renal transplant patients who received a dosage of 597 mg (7.95 mg/kg) daily and from stable adult renal transplant patients who received a dosage of 344 mg (4.1 mg/kg) daily, respectively; after 4 weeks of therapy clearance was 577 mL/minute (8.6 mL/minute per kg) as determined with data (using monoclonal RIA) from de novo hepatic transplant patients who received a dosage of 458 mg (6.89 mg/kg) daily. Limited data are available for pediatric patients. Clearance of cyclosporine from blood averaged 10.6 mL/minute per kg in a study (using specific monoclonal RIA) of renal transplant patients 3–16 years of age administered the drug IV. The range in cyclosporine clearance was 9.8–15.5 mL/minute per kg in a study of renal transplant patients 2–16 years old. Data (using HPLC) from hepatic transplant patients 0.6–5.6 years of age revealed an average clearance of 9.3 mL/minute per kg. The clearance of cyclosporine administered as a modified oral formulation was 285 mL/minute (16.6 mL/minute per kg) or 378 mL/minute (10.2 mL/minute per kg) as determined with data (specific monoclonal RIA used) from stable hepatic transplant patients 2–8 or 8–15 years of age, respectively, who received a dosage of 101 mg (5.95 mg/kg) or 188 mg (4.96 mg/kg) daily, respectively; clearance was 171 mL/minute (11.9 mL/minute per kg) and 328 mL/min (11 mL/minute per kg) as determined with data (using specific monoclonal fluorescence polarization immunoassay) from stable hepatic transplant patients 3 years of age or 8–15 years old, respectively, who received a dosage of 120 mg (8.3 mg/kg) or 158 mg (5.5 mg/kg) daily, respectively. In stable renal transplant patients 7–15 years of age who received cyclosporine as a modified oral formulation at a dosage of 328 mg (7.4 mg/kg) daily, clearance of the drug was 418 mL/minute (8.7 mL/minute per kg) as determined with specific monoclonal fluorescence polarization immunoassay. The clearance of cyclosporine reportedly is not changed substantially by renal failure or dialysis.

Cyclosporine is extensively metabolized in the liver via the cytochrome P-450 enzyme system, principally by the CYP3A isoenzyme, and less extensively in the GI tract and the kidney to at least 30 metabolites found in bile, feces, blood, and urine. The pharmacologic and toxicologic activities of cyclosporine's metabolites are considerably less than those of the parent drug. The drug undergoes extensive first-pass metabolism following oral administration. Several major metabolic pathways, including hydroxylation of the C_γ-carbon of 2 leucine residues, C_λ-carbon hydroxylation and cyclic ether formation (with oxidation of the double bond) in the side chain of the amino acid 3-hydroxyl-N,4-dimethyl-l-2-amino-6-octenoic acid, and N-demethylation of N-methyl leucine residues, are involved. Conjugation of these metabolites or hydrolysis of the cyclic peptide chain does not appear to be an important pathway for cyclosporine metabolism. Oxidation of cyclosporine at its 1-λ, 4-N-desmethylated, and 9-γ positions yields the major metabolites known as AM1 (M17), AM4N (M21), and AM9 (M1), respectively. The AUCs at steady state of AM1, AM4N, and AM9 were approximately 70, 7.5, and 21%, respectively, of the blood AUC for cyclosporine in renal transplant patients treated with a conventional oral formulation of the drug. The manufacturers state that the percentages of a dose present as AM1, AM4N, and AM9 are similar after administration of the conventional (nonmodified) oral formulation or the modified oral formulations, as indicated by blood or biliary concentrations in stable renal or de novo hepatic transplant patients, respectively. In stable renal transplant patients, the ratio of AUC at steady state for AM1 and AM9 to that for cyclosporine did not differ between the conventional oral formulation and the modified oral formulation.

Cyclosporine is principally excreted via bile, almost entirely as metabolites. Only about 6% of a dose of the drug is excreted in urine, with 0.1% of a dose being excreted unchanged. However, urinary excretion of unchanged drug may be increased in certain patient populations (e.g., early posttransplant period in bone marrow allograft recipients) and in younger patients.

CHEMISTRY AND STABILITY

● Chemistry

Cyclosporine (cyclosporin A) is a cyclosporin immunosuppressive agent produced as a metabolite of the fungus species Aphanocladium album or Beauveria nivea. The drug is a nonpolar, cyclic polypeptide antibiotic consisting of 11 amino acids. Cyclosporine is one of several biologically active antibiotics (cyclosporins) produced by these fungi; cyclosporin A and C are the major metabolites.

Cyclosporine occurs as a white or essentially white, finely crystalline powder. The drug is relatively insoluble in water, having an aqueous solubility of 0.04 mg/mL at 25°C, and is generally soluble in lipids and organic solvents, having a solubility of more than 80 mg/mL in alcohol at 25°C. The potency of cyclosporine is determined on the anhydrous basis; each mcg of cyclosporine is defined as the activity (potency) contained in 1.0173 mcg of the FDA's cyclosporine master standard.

Commercially available cyclosporine conventional (nonmodified) oral solution has a clear, yellow, oily appearance. Cyclosporine conventional oral solution contains the drug in an olive oil and peglicol 5 oleate (Labrafil® M 1944CS) vehicle with 12.5% (v/v) alcohol. Commercially available cyclosporine concentrate for injection occurs as a clear, faintly brownish-yellow solution. Cyclosporine concentrate for injection is a sterile solution of the drug in polyoxyl 35 castor oil (Cremophor® EL, polyethoxylated castor oil) with 32.9% (v/v) alcohol. At the time of manufacture, the air in the ampuls of cyclosporine concentrate for injection is replaced with nitrogen. The concentrate for injection contains no more than 42 USP endotoxin units per mL. Cyclosporine also is commercially available as 25-, 50-, and 100-mg conventional (nonmodified) liquid-filled, soft gelatin capsules.

Cyclosporine also is commercially available as a modified, nonaqueous liquid formulation (Neoral®) of the drug that immediately forms an emulsion in aqueous fluids; the formulation is available as an oral solution for emulsion and as oral 25- and 100-mg liquid-filled soft gelatin capsules containing the oral solution for emulsion. When exposed to an aqueous environment, the oral solution for emulsion forms a homogenous transparent emulsion with a droplet size smaller than 100 nm in diameter; as a result, the formulation has been referred to as an oral solution for microemulsion. In this formulation, the molecular structure of cyclosporine is unaltered, and aqueous dilution results in formation of an emulsion without reprecipitation of the drug. Cyclosporine is dispersed in a mixture of propylene glycol (hydrophilic solvent) and corn oil monoglycerides, diglycerides, and triglycerides (lipophilic solvent); when dispersed, polyoxyl 40 hydrogenated castor oil serves as a surfactant, and d,l-α-tocopherol is present as an antioxidant. Neoral® oral solution and liquid-filled capsules also contains dehydrated alcohol in a maximum concentration of 11.9% (v/v).

In addition, cyclosporine is commercially available as a modified liquid formulation (Gengraf®) of the drug that forms an aqueous dispersion (also referred to as a microemulsion) of the drug in an aqueous environment; this formulation is available as both an oral solution and as oral 25- and 100-mg liquid-filled capsules. Cyclosporine is dispersed in a mixture of propylene glycol, sorbitan monooleate, and either polyoxyl 40 hydrogenated castor oil (in the oral solution) or polyoxyl 35 castor oil and polyethylene glycol (in the capsules). Gengraf® liquid-filled capsules also contain alcohol 12.8% (v/v).

The modified oral formulations of cyclosporine (Neoral® and Gengraf®), both as the oral solution and the oral capsules, have increased oral bioavailability compared with the conventional (nonmodified) oral solution and liquid-filled capsules of the drug (i.e., Sandimmune®). Therefore, the conventional (nonmodified) and modified formulations are *not* bioequivalent and cannot be used interchangeably without appropriate medical supervision. (See Pharmacokinetics: Absorption.)

● **Stability**

Cyclosporine conventional (nonmodified) oral solution should be stored in the original container at temperature less than 30°C and protected from freezing; refrigeration should be avoided since coalescence and separation of the oral solution could occur. Opened containers of cyclosporine conventional oral solution must be used within 2 months. Cyclosporine concentrate for injection should be stored at a temperature less than 30°C and protected from freezing and light. Cyclosporine conventional liquid-filled capsules should be stored in their original unit-dose container at a controlled room temperature of 25°C but may be exposed to temperatures ranging from 15–30°C. When stored as directed, the capsules have an expiration date of 3 years from the date of manufacture. An odor may be detected when the unit-dose container is opened, which will dissipate shortly thereafter, but this odor does not affect the quality of the preparation.

Cyclosporine (modified) liquid-filled, soft gelatin capsules (commercially available as Neoral®) should be stored in their original unit-dose packaging at 20–25°C, and Neoral® oral solution also should be stored in the original container at 20–25°C. At temperatures less than 20°C, Neoral® oral solution may gel, and light flocculation and/or the formation of a light sediment also may occur; however, such changes do not affect dosing with the syringe provided or efficacy and can be reversed by allowing the solution to warm to a room temperature of 25°C. Neoral® oral solution should not be refrigerated, and once opened, containers of the oral solution must be used within 2 months.

Cyclosporine (modified) liquid-filled capsules commercially available as Gengraf® should be stored in their original unit-dose packaging at 15–30°C, and Gengraf® oral solution also should be stored in the original container at 15–30°C. At temperatures less than 20°C, Gengraf® oral solution may gel, and light flocculation and/or the formation of a light sediment also may occur; however, such changes do not affect dosing with the syringe provided or efficacy and can be reversed by allowing the solution to warm to a room temperature of 15–30°C. Gengraf® oral solution should not be refrigerated, and once opened, containers of the oral solution must be used within 2 months.

Cyclosporine concentrate for injection that has been diluted to a final concentration of approximately 2 mg/mL is stable for 24 hours in 5% dextrose or 0.9% sodium chloride injection in glass or PVC containers. Diluted solutions of the drug in 5% dextrose or 0.9% sodium chloride injection do not require protection from light. There is some evidence that substantial amounts of cyclosporine may be lost during infusion through plastic tubing in IV administration sets. Because of combined loss during storage and administration via plastic IV tubing, it has been suggested that dilutions in 0.9% sodium chloride injection be considered stable for no longer than 6 or 12 hours in PVC or glass containers, respectively. Polyoxyl 35 castor oil can cause leaching of bis(2-ethylhexyl) phthalate (BEHP, DEHP) from PVC containers and, following dilution of cyclosporine concentrate for injection in PVC containers, substantial leaching of DEHP occurs in a time-dependent manner. The manufacturer makes no specific recommendations regarding the compatibility of the concentrate for injection with plastic containers; however, to minimize exposure of the patient to leached DEHP, some clinicians recommend that diluted solutions of the drug in PVC containers be administered immediately after preparation.

PREPARATIONS

Excipients in commercially available drug preparations may have clinically important effects in some individuals; consult specific product labeling for details.

cycloSPORINE

Oral		
Capsules, liquid-filled (nonmodified)	25 mg	SandIMMUNE®, Novartis
	50 mg	SandIMMUNE®, Novartis
	100 mg	SandIMMUNE®, Novartis
Capsules, liquid-filled, for emulsion (modified)	25 mg	Gengraf®, Abbott Neoral®, Novartis
	100 mg	Gengraf®, Abbott Neoral®, Novartis
For emulsion, solution (modified)	100 mg/mL	Gengraf®, Abbott Neoral®, Novartis
For solution, concentrate (nonmodified)	100 mg/mL	SandIMMUNE®, Novartis
Parenteral		
For injection, concentrate for IV infusion only	50 mg/mL	SandIMMUNE® I.V., Novartis

† Use is not currently included in the labeling approved by the US Food and Drug Administration.

Selected Revisions May 10, 2024, © Copyright, July 1, 1984, American Society of Health-System Pharmacists, Inc.

Tacrolimus

90:28.28.92 • CALCINEURIN INHIBITORS, MISCELLANEOUS

■ Tacrolimus, a calcineurin inhibitor, is a potent immunosuppressive agent.

USES

Tacrolimus immediate-release oral preparations (conventional capsules, granules for oral suspension) are used in combination with other immunosuppressants for the prevention of organ rejection in adult and pediatric patients receiving kidney, liver, heart, or lung allografts. A parenteral preparation of tacrolimus is available for IV use in patients who cannot tolerate oral formulations; patients should be converted from IV to oral therapy as soon as oral therapy is tolerated. Tacrolimus also is available as extended-release capsule and tablet formulations for the prevention of rejection of kidney allografts.

Because of differences in pharmacokinetic properties, extended-release capsule and tablet formulations are not interchangeable with each other or with tacrolimus immediate-release formulations. Medication errors, including substitution and dispensing errors, between tacrolimus immediate-release products and tacrolimus extended-release products have been reported outside the US.

● Renal Transplantation

Tacrolimus is used in combination with other immunosuppressants for the prevention of rejection of renal allografts. Immediate-release oral preparations of tacrolimus and the IV formulation are indicated for the prophylaxis of organ rejection in adult and pediatric kidney transplant patients. Tacrolimus extended-release capsules (Astagraf XL®) are indicated for the prophylaxis of organ rejection in adult and pediatric kidney transplant patients who are able to swallow capsules intact. Tacrolimus extended-release tablets (Envarsus XR®) are indicated for the prophylaxis of organ rejection in de novo adult kidney transplant patients or patients who are converting from tacrolimus immediate-release formulations.

Efficacy and safety of tacrolimus in renal allograft transplantation were evaluated in a randomized, multicenter, non-blinded, prospective study that compared tacrolimus-based immunosuppression with a cyclosporine-based regimen in 412 patients ≥6 years of age. Treatment with study medication was initiated when post-transplant renal function was stable (i.e., serum creatinine ≤4 mg/dL), which was a median of 4 days after transplant (range: 1–14 days). All patients received combination immunosuppressive induction therapy with steroids, azathioprine, and an antilymphocyte antibody. One-year patient survival rates were 95.6% in the tacrolimus group and 96.6% in the cyclosporine group, and one-year graft survival rates were 91.2% and 87.9% in the respective treatment groups.

Efficacy and safety of tacrolimus in conjunction with mycophenolate mofetil (MMF), corticosteroids, and induction therapy were evaluated in a randomized, open-label, multicenter trial (ELITE-Symphony) in 1589 adult kidney transplant patients. Patients received standard-dose cyclosporine, MMF, and corticosteroids, or daclizumab induction, MMF, and corticosteroids in combination with low-dose cyclosporine, low-dose tacrolimus, or low-dose sirolimus. The initial dosage of tacrolimus used in the study was 0.1 mg/kg per day divided into 2 daily doses; the dosage was then adjusted to achieve a target trough level of 3–7 ng/mL. At 12 months, the overall survival rate was similar between all groups and was more than 96%. Patients who received tacrolimus had improved kidney function (as evidenced by higher estimated creatinine clearance rates), lower rates of biopsy-proven acute rejection, and higher allograft survival than those in the other treatment groups, but were more likely to develop diarrhea and diabetes after transplantation.

In another randomized, open-label, multicenter trial, 424 kidney transplant patients received tacrolimus or cyclosporine in combination with MMF (1 g twice daily), basiliximab induction, and corticosteroids. In this trial, the rate for the combined endpoint of biopsy-proven acute rejection, graft failure, death, and/or lost to follow-up at 12 months in the tacrolimus/MMF group was similar to the rate in the cyclosporine/MMF group. Mortality at 12 months in patients receiving tacrolimus in combination with MMF was 4% compared to 2% in those receiving cyclosporine in combination with MMF, including cases attributed to over-immunosuppression.

Other studies evaluating tacrolimus in kidney transplant recipients have reported one-year graft and patient survival rates of 82–99% and 93–100%, respectively. Numerous randomized controlled studies and meta analyses have shown that tacrolimus is superior to cyclosporine for preventing acute rejection and improving allograft survival after kidney transplantation, but increases post-transplant diabetes, neurological, and GI adverse effects.

Efficacy and safety of tacrolimus extended-release capsules (Astagraf XL®) for the prevention of rejection of renal allografts in kidney transplant patients were evaluated in 2 multicenter randomized studies (an open-label study that included induction therapy with basiliximab, and a double-blind study without induction) of 12 months' duration that compared extended-release tacrolimus with immediate-release tacrolimus in combination with MMF and corticosteroids. In both studies, the overall rate of treatment failure (i.e., biopsy-proven acute rejection, graft loss, death, or loss to follow-up) at 12 months was not substantially different between the groups and mean estimated glomerular filtration rates were similar at the end of the study. Follow-up of the open-label study that included induction therapy with basiliximab continued to have similar safety and efficacy results through 4 years.

Efficacy and safety of tacrolimus extended-release tablets (Envarsus XR®) for prevention of transplant rejection in de novo kidney transplant patients were evaluated in a 12-month randomized, double-blind study and an open-label phase 2 study; both studies compared tacrolimus extended-release tablets once daily to tacrolimus immediate-release capsules twice daily. All patients received only IL-2 receptor antagonist induction therapy and concomitant treatment with MMF and corticosteroids. At 12 months, the overall rate of treatment failure (i.e., biopsy-proven acute rejection, graft loss, death, or loss to follow-up) was not substantially different between patients who received tacrolimus extended-release tablets versus those who received the immediate-release capsules. There were no deaths or graft failures in the open-label study. Follow-up of this study at 24 months continued to report comparable safety and efficacy results between immediate-release and extended-release tacrolimus.

An additional randomized, open-label multinational study evaluated the use of tacrolimus extended-release tablets administered once daily as a replacement for tacrolimus immediate-release capsules administered twice daily as maintenance immunosuppression to prevent acute allograft rejection in stable adult kidney transplant patients. Patients received a kidney transplant 3 months to 5 years before study entry; mycophenolate mofetil or mycophenolate sodium, azathioprine, and/or corticosteroids were allowed as concomitant immunosuppressants during the study period. At 12 months, the overall rate of treatment failure (i.e., biopsy-proven acute rejection, graft loss, death, or loss to follow-up) was not substantially different between patients who received tacrolimus extended-release tablets versus those who received the immediate-release capsules. Additionally, kidney function (as assessed by mean estimated glomerular filtration rates) was similar in the two treatment groups.

● Liver Transplantation

Tacrolimus (as immediate-release and IV preparations) is used in combination with other immunosuppressants for the prevention of organ rejection in adults and pediatric patients receiving liver transplant.

Efficacy of tacrolimus immediate-release formulations in hepatic allograft transplantation is based on data from 2 prospective, randomized, open-label multicenter studies. One of the studies was conducted in the US; this study excluded patients with renal dysfunction, fulminant hepatic failure with stage IV encephalopathy, and cancers but included pediatric patients aged ≤12 years. The other study was conducted in Europe and excluded pediatric patients but did allow enrollment of patient groups excluded from the first study (other than patients who had primary hepatic cancers with metastases). Patients in both studies received an immunosuppressive regimen that included corticosteroids and either tacrolimus or cyclosporine; the majority of patients treated with cyclosporine also received azathioprine. Tacrolimus and cyclosporine were comparably effective in these patients in terms of patient survival and graft survival 1 year after transplantation. In the US study, patient and graft survival rates for both groups combined were 88 and 81%, respectively. In the European study, patient and graft survival rates for both groups combined were 78 and 73%, respectively.

Efficacy of tacrolimus immediate-release granules for oral suspension in pediatric liver transplant patients is based on data from a prospective, randomized, open-label multicenter study involving de novo hepatic allograft recipients ≤16 years of age. In this study, 181 patients received an immunosuppressive regimen containing corticosteroids and either tacrolimus granules for suspension or cyclosporine with azathioprine, starting 6 hours after conclusion of allotransplantation surgery. Tacrolimus dosing was adjusted throughout the study to maintain whole blood trough levels in the range of 5–20 ng/mL. The overall failure rate (i.e., biopsy-proven acute rejection, graft loss, death, or loss to follow-up) was comparable for tacrolimus-based and cyclosporine-based immunosuppression regimens (52.7 versus 61.1%, respectively).

The use of sirolimus with tacrolimus in studies of de novo liver transplant patients was associated with an excess mortality, graft loss, and hepatic artery thrombosis (HAT), and is therefore not recommended.

● Cardiac Transplantation

Tacrolimus (as immediate-release and IV preparations) is used in combination with other immunosuppressants for the prevention of organ rejection in adults and pediatric patients receiving cardiac transplant.

Efficacy of tacrolimus immediate-release formulations in cardiac allograft transplantation is based on data from 2 open-label, randomized, multicenter studies comparing the safety and efficacy of tacrolimus-based immunosuppression and cyclosporine-based immunosuppression in primary orthotopic heart transplantation.

In the first study, which was conducted in Europe, 314 adults received a regimen of antibody induction therapy, corticosteroids, and azathioprine in combination with either tacrolimus or modified cyclosporine for 18 months. The incidence of biopsy-proven acute rejection at 6 months was substantially lower in the tacrolimus-based group of patients than in those receiving the cyclosporine-based regimen (ISHLT grade 1B acute rejection or greater: 54 versus 66%, respectively; grade 3A or greater: 28 versus 42%, respectively). Tacrolimus and cyclosporine were comparably effective in the treatment groups in terms of patient survival and graft survival 18 months after transplantation (92 and 90%, respectively).

In the second study, which was conducted in the US and consisted of 3 treatment arms, 331 adults undergoing de novo cardiac transplantation received an immunosuppressive regimen containing corticosteroids and either tacrolimus with sirolimus, tacrolimus with mycophenolate mofetil, or modified cyclosporine with mycophenolate mofetil for 1 year; antibody induction therapy also was allowed. The incidence of biopsy-proven acute rejection (ISHLT grade 3A or greater) or hemodynamic compromise requiring treatment was lower in the tacrolimus-treated patients at 6 months (22–24 versus 32%, respectively) and was significantly lower at 1 year in patients treated with tacrolimus and mycophenolate mofetil compared with patients treated with cyclosporine and mycophenolate mofetil (23 versus 37%, respectively). Similar patient and graft survival rates 1 year after transplantation were evident in the 2 mycophenolate mofetil-treated groups with approximately 93% survival reported in the tacrolimus plus mycophenolate mofetil group and 86% survival in the modified cyclosporine plus mycophenolate mofetil group. However, patients in the tacrolimus and sirolimus group exhibited an increased risk of wound healing complications, renal impairment, and insulin-dependent posttransplant diabetes mellitus; the manufacturer states that this combination is therefore not recommended.

● Lung Transplantation

Tacrolimus (as immediate-release and IV preparations) is used in combination with other immunosuppressants for the prevention of organ rejection in adults and pediatric patients receiving lung transplantation.

Efficacy of tacrolimus immediate-release formulations in lung transplantation is based on observational data from the U.S. Scientific Registry of Transplant Recipients (SRTR). Outcomes were evaluated for 19,741 adult and 522 pediatric lung transplant patients receiving tacrolimus in combination with either mycophenolate mofetil or azathioprine at the time of hospital discharge. The 1-year graft survival estimates were similar for adults receiving tacrolimus plus mycophenolate mofetil or tacrolimus plus azathioprine (90.9 and 90.8%, respectively). In pediatric patients, the 1-year graft survival rates were 91.7 and 84.7% for tacrolimus plus mycophenolate mofetil and tacrolimus plus azathioprine, respectively.

● Transplantation - Clinical Perspective

The Kidney Disease: Improving Global Outcomes (KDIGO) clinical practice guideline on the monitoring, management, and treatment of kidney transplant recipients states that immunosuppressive medication recommendations in this setting are complex as combinations of multiple drug classes are utilized and choices between varying regimens are determined through an evaluation of benefits (e.g., reduced risk of rejection) and harms (e.g., increased risk of infection and malignancy). For initial maintenance immunosuppression, KDIGO recommends a combination of immunosuppressive medications including a calcineurin inhibitor (tacrolimus – first line) and an antiproliferative agent (mycophenolate – first line), with or without corticosteroids. KDIGO states that there is no reason to delay initiation of calcineurin inhibitor therapy and no evidence that delaying such therapy prevents or ameliorates delayed graft function. Additionally, the guideline notes that tacrolimus reduces the risk of acute rejection and improves graft survival as compared to cyclosporine during the first year of transplantation, that low-dose tacrolimus therapy reduces the risk of new onset diabetes after transplant as compared to higher doses, and that the earlier that therapeutic calcineurin inhibitor blood levels can be attained, the more effective the medication will be in preventing acute rejection.

In 2022, consensus recommendations for the use of maintenance immunosuppression in solid organ transplantation were developed and endorsed by the American College of Clinical Pharmacy (ACCP), American Society of Transplantation (AST), and the International Society for Heart and Lung Transplantation (ISHLT). These recommendations state there is no standardized approach to maintenance immunosuppression management in solid organ transplantation. A variety of factors may impact choice of agents including the transplanted organ, center-specific protocols, provider expertise, insurance and cost issues, and patient characteristics and tolerability of therapy. The consensus recommendations note that tacrolimus is superior to cyclosporine for the prevention of acute rejection in various solid organ transplants. Tacrolimus is also superior to cyclosporine with regard to reducing the severity of rejection in kidney and pancreas transplants and is associated with improved allograft survival in kidney, pancreas, and liver transplantation. Tacrolimus may offer an advantage over cyclosporine in lung transplant regarding prevention of bronchiolitis obliterans syndrome.

● Crohn's Disease

Tacrolimus has been used in the management of fistulizing Crohn's disease†. Administration of oral tacrolimus has been effective for fistula improvement, but not for fistula remission in patients with perianal Crohn's disease. Efficacy of tacrolimus in the management of fistulizing Crohn's disease has been evaluated in a randomized, double-blind, placebo-controlled study involving 48 patients (≥12 years of age) with one or more open draining enterocutaneous fistulas that had not closed with administration of at least one anti-infective agent. Patients were randomized to receive placebo (26 patients) or oral tacrolimus (22 patients) 200 mcg/kg daily for 10 weeks. Those who were receiving stable dosages of corticosteroids, oral or rectal 5-aminosalicylic acid derivatives, oral anti-infective agents, azathioprine, mercaptopurine, methotrexate, or mycophenolate mofetil continued to receive these drugs during the study. The primary outcome was fistula improvement (defined as closure of 50% or more of particular fistulas that were open and draining at baseline and maintenance of such closures for at least 4 weeks), while secondary outcome was fistula remission (defined as closure of all fistulas and maintenance of such closures for at least 4 weeks). Fistula improvement was attained in 43% of patients receiving tacrolimus versus 8% of those receiving placebo, while fistula remission was attained in 10 or 8% of patients receiving tacrolimus or placebo, respectively; the difference in fistula remission was not considered statistically significant. Some clinicians state that because of the potential for tacrolimus-associated nephrotoxicity (especially at high doses) and because complete fistula remission has not been achieved with the drug, tacrolimus should be reserved for patients who do not respond to or are intolerant of all other therapies used for the management of fistulizing Crohn's disease (e.g., ciprofloxacin and/or metronidazole, azathioprine or mercaptopurine, infliximab).

For topical uses of tacrolimus, see 84:06.28.

Clinical Perspective

The American College of Gastroenterology guideline on the management of Crohn's disease in adults strongly recommends that tacrolimus should not be used for moderate-to-severe/moderate-to-high-risk Crohn's disease. However, for perianal and cutaneous fistulizing disease, tacrolimus can be administered short-term; significant toxicity precludes the use of tacrolimus on a long-term basis.

Pancreas Transplantation

Some studies have evaluated the role of tacrolimus in the setting of prevention of rejection of pancreas allografts† (often performed simultaneously with a kidney transplant). The 2022 ACCP, AST, and ISHLT consensus recommendations for use of maintenance immunosuppression in solid organ transplantation state that tacrolimus is superior to cyclosporine for the prevention of allograft rejection and is also superior for reducing the severity of rejection in pancreas transplantation. The recommendations also note that tacrolimus is associated with improved allograft survival compared to cyclosporine in pancreas transplant.

Intestinal Transplantation

Several studies have evaluated the role of tacrolimus in the prevention of rejection of intestinal allografts†. The 2022 ACCP, AST, and ISHLT consensus recommendations for use of maintenance immunosuppression in solid organ transplantation state that tacrolimus is superior to cyclosporine for the prevention of allograft rejection in intestinal transplantation.

Other Uses

Tacrolimus has also been used to prevent rejection of vascular composite allografts†.

DOSAGE AND ADMINISTRATION

General

Pretreatment Screening

- Evaluate immunizations and give complete complement of needed vaccines before transplantation and treatment.

- Assess patients for a history of cardiac arrhythmias, symptomatic bradycardia, hypokalemia, or hypomagnesemia that could increase the risk of torsades de pointes and/or sudden death with tacrolimus use.

Patient Monitoring

- Therapeutic drug monitoring is recommended for all patients.

- Continuously observe patients receiving IV tacrolimus for at least the first 30 minutes following the start of the infusion and at frequent intervals thereafter. If signs or symptoms of anaphylaxis occur, stop the infusion.

- Examine patients for skin changes periodically.

- Monitor patients for signs and symptoms of infection.

- Perform routine laboratory testing (e.g., for assessment of renal and hepatic function, for monitoring of glucose and potassium concentrations).

- Monitor patients for neurologic changes.

- Check blood pressure periodically.

Dispensing and Administration Precautions

- Tacrolimus should only be used under the supervision of a provider with experience managing immunosuppressive therapy. Changes between tacrolimus immediate-release and extended-release dosage forms must occur under physician supervision.

- When IV tacrolimus is administered, emergency drugs and equipment such as epinephrine and oxygen should be available at the bedside.

- Wearing disposable gloves is recommended during dilution of the injection or when preparing the oral suspension in the hospital and when wiping any spills.

- Avoid inhalation or direct contact with skin or mucous membranes of the powder or granules contained in tacrolimus capsules and tacrolimus granules, respectively. If such contact occurs, wash the skin thoroughly with soap and water; if ocular contact occurs, rinse eyes with water. If a spill occurs, wipe the surface with a wet paper towel.

Other General Considerations

- Do not use simultaneously with cyclosporine. Tacrolimus or cyclosporine should be discontinued at least 24 hours before initiating the other drug. In the presence of elevated tacrolimus or cyclosporine concentrations, dosing with the other drug usually should be further delayed.

Administration

Tacrolimus is administered orally as immediate-release capsules, granules for oral suspension, or extended-release capsules and tablets; tacrolimus also may be administered by IV infusion. Because of the risk of anaphylaxis, IV administration of the drug should be reserved for patients who cannot tolerate oral administration. If therapy is initiated with the IV formulation, substitute oral therapy as soon as tolerated. Extended-release formulations of the drug are indicated only in kidney transplant patients.

Because of differences in pharmacokinetic properties, extended-release preparations are not interchangeable with each other or with tacrolimus immediate-release capsules or granules for suspension. When converting between immediate-release capsules and granules for suspension, the total daily dosage should remain the same; therapeutic drug monitoring is recommended when switching between tacrolimus formulations.

Store tacrolimus capsules and granules for oral suspension at 20 to 25°C and extended-release capsules and extended-release tablets at 25°C; with excursions permitted between 15 to 30°C. Store tacrolimus injection between 5 to 25°C.

Oral Administration

Immediate-release Capsules

Tacrolimus immediate-release capsules should be administered every 12 hours at consistent times of day to minimize variability in systemic exposure. Tacrolimus immediate-release capsules can be taken with or without food, but because food affects absorption of tacrolimus from the gastrointestinal tract, it should be taken in the same way for each dose. Do not open or crush capsules.

In liver, heart, or lung transplant patients, administer the initial dose of immediate-release capsules no sooner than 6 hours after transplantation. In kidney transplant patients, the initial dose of immediate-release capsules may be administered within 24 hours of transplantation, but should be delayed until renal function has recovered.

Granules for Oral Suspension

Tacrolimus granules for oral suspension may be used in patients who have difficulty swallowing capsules. To minimize variability in systemic exposure to tacrolimus, the suspension should be administered every 12 hours at consistent times of day. Tacrolimus suspension can be taken with or without food, but because food affects absorption of tacrolimus from the gastrointestinal tract, it should be taken in the same way for each dose.

Tacrolimus granules for oral suspension must be mixed with water to form a suspension prior to administration. Do not sprinkle tacrolimus granules on food for administration. To prepare tacrolimus suspension, empty the entire contents of the packet or packets needed for the prescribed dose into an empty glass drinking container; check that no granules remain in the packet or packets. Add 15–30 mL of room temperature drinking water to the glass, and mix; the granules will not dissolve completely. Administer the suspension immediately, then rinse the glass with an additional 15–30 mL of room temperature water, and administer this additional volume to the patient. Do not prepare tacrolimus suspension in a plastic (PVC-containing) cup or use plastic tubing, syringes, or other equipment during administration, as tacrolimus granules will adhere to plastic items; use glass or metal materials when preparing tacrolimus suspension. A non-PVC oral syringe may be used for administration to younger patients. Do not prepare tacrolimus suspension in advance or store after mixing with water. The manufacturer's labeling and instructions for use should be consulted for detailed information on preparing and administering tacrolimus granules for oral suspension.

Extended-release Capsules (Astagraf XL®)

Tacrolimus extended-release capsules should be administered every morning on an empty stomach, at least 1 hour before a meal, or at least 2 hours after a meal, at a consistent time each day to minimize variability in systemic exposure. Swallow extended-release capsules whole with liquid; do not chew, divide, or crush the capsules.

If a dose of tacrolimus extended-release capsules is missed by up to 14 hours, administer the missed dose as soon as possible. If a dose is missed by longer than 14 hours, the regular schedule should be resumed the following morning; the missed dose should not be administered later in the day and an extra dose should not be administered to make up for the missed dose.

Extended-release Tablets (Envarsus XL®)

Tacrolimus extended-release tablets should be administered every morning on an empty stomach, at least 1 hour before a meal, or at least 2 hours after a meal, at a consistent time each day to minimize variability in systemic exposure. Swallow extended-release tablets whole with liquid (preferably water); do not chew, divide, or crush the tablets.

If a dose of tacrolimus extended-release tablets is missed by up to 15 hours, administer the missed dose as soon as possible. If a dose is missed by longer than 15 hours, the regular schedule should be resumed the following morning; the missed dose should not be administered later in the day and an extra dose should not be administered to make up for the missed dose.

Standardize 4 Safety

Standardized concentrations for an extemporaneously prepared oral liquid formulation of tacrolimus have been established through Standardize 4 Safety (S4S), a national patient safety initiative to reduce medication errors, especially during transitions of care. Multidisciplinary expert panels were convened to determine recommended standard concentrations. Because recommendations from the S4S panels may differ from the manufacturer's prescribing information, caution is advised when using concentrations that differ from labeling, particularly when using rate information from the label. For additional information on S4S (including updates that may be available), see https://www.ashp.org/standardize4safety.

TABLE 1. Standardize 4 Safety Compounded Oral Liquid Standards for Tacrolimus.

Concentration Standard
1 mg/mL

IV Administration

Prepare infusion solutions in glass or polyethylene containers; avoid use of PVC containers. Use PVC-free tubing for administration of more dilute solutions (e.g., those for pediatric patients).

Tacrolimus injection should not be mixed or co-infused with solutions of pH 9 or greater (e.g., ganciclovir or acyclovir) due to the chemical instability of tacrolimus in alkaline media.

Continuously observe patient for ≥30 minutes following initiation of the IV infusion and then at frequent intervals thereafter for possible allergic manifestations. In addition, appropriate equipment and agents for the management of anaphylactic reactions (e.g., epinephrine, oxygen) should be readily available. If anaphylaxis occurs, IV infusion of the drug should be discontinued and appropriate therapy instituted. The oral formulation of tacrolimus does not contain polyoxyl 60 hydrogenated castor oil, and therefore a history of anaphylaxis with the parenteral formulation does not necessarily preclude oral therapy with the drug.

Dilution

Must be diluted with 0.9% sodium chloride or 5% dextrose injection to a concentration of 4–20 mcg (0.004–0.02 mg) per mL prior to administration.

Rate of Administration

Administer daily dose over 24 hours by continuous IV infusion.

Standardize 4 Safety

Standardized concentrations for IV tacrolimus have been established through Standardize 4 Safety (S4S), a national patient safety initiative to reduce medication errors, especially during transitions of care. Multidisciplinary expert panels were

convened to determine recommended standard concentrations. Because recommendations from the S4S panels may differ from the manufacturer's prescribing information, caution is advised when using concentrations that differ from labeling, particularly when using rate information from the label. For additional information on S4S (including updates that may be available), see https://www.ashp.org/standardize4safety.

TABLE 2. Standardize 4 Safety Continuous Infusion Standards for IV Tacrolimus.

Patient Population	Concentration Standard	Dosing Units
Pediatric patients (<50 kg)	0.02 mg/mL	mg/kg/day

● Dosage

Available as anhydrous tacrolimus; dosage expressed in terms of anhydrous drug.

Individualize dosage based on clinical assessments of organ rejection and patient tolerability.

Dosage requirements generally decline with continued therapy; long-term administration is necessary to prevent rejection.

Adult Oral Dosage

Dosage requirements generally decline with continued therapy, and long-term administration is necessary to prevent rejection.

Kidney Transplantation

Immediate-release oral preparations in combination with azathioprine: The usual initial adult oral tacrolimus dosage is 200 mcg/kg (0.2 mg/kg) daily, administered in 2 divided daily doses every 12 hours. Patients receiving this tacrolimus dosage should have typical trough whole blood tacrolimus concentrations of 7–20 ng/mL and 5–15 ng/mL when measured at months 1–3 and 4–12 post-transplant, respectively.

Immediate-release oral preparations in combination with mycophenolate mofetil/interleukin 2 receptor antagonist: The usual initial adult oral tacrolimus dosage is 100 mcg/kg (0.1 mg/kg) daily, administered in 2 divided daily doses every 12 hours. Patients receiving this tacrolimus dosage should have typical trough whole blood tacrolimus concentrations of 4–11 ng/mL when measured at months 1–12 post-transplant. Alternatively, in a small clinical trial, the initial dose of tacrolimus *in combination with mycophenolate mofetil/interleukin 2 receptor antagonist* was 150–200 mcg/kg (0.15-0.2 mg/kg) daily and observed tacrolimus concentrations were 6–16 ng/mL and 5–12 ng/mL during months 1–3 and months 4–12, respectively.

Extended-release capsules (Astagraf XL®) in combination with basiliximab, mycophenolate mofetil, and steroids: The usual initial dosage is 150–200 mcg/kg (0.15 to 0.2 mg/kg) once daily prior to reperfusion or within 48 hours of completion of transplant. Patients receiving this tacrolimus dosage should have typical whole blood tacrolimus concentrations of 7–15 ng/mL, 5–15 ng/mL, and 5–10 ng/mL when measured at month 1, months 2–6, or ≥6 months post-transplant, respectively.

Extended-release capsules (Astagraf XL®) in combination with mycophenolate mofetil and steroids (without basiliximab induction): The usual initial dosage is a first dose (pre-operative) of 100 mcg/kg (0.1 mg/kg), within 12 hours prior to reperfusion. Subsequent doses postoperatively are 200 mcg/kg (0.2 mg/kg) once daily at least 4 hours after pre-operative dose and within 12 hours after reperfusion. Patients receiving this tacrolimus dosage regimen should have typical trough whole blood tacrolimus concentrations of 10–15 ng/mL, 5–15 ng/mL, and 5–10 ng/mL when measured at month 1, months 2–6, or ≥6 months post-transplant, respectively.

Extended-release tablets (Envarsus XR®): The usual initial dosage of tacrolimus extended-release tablets is 140 mcg/kg (0.14 mg/kg) once daily. Patients receiving this tacrolimus dosage should have typical trough whole blood tacrolimus concentrations of 6–11 ng/mL in the first month and 4–11 ng/mL when measured after the first month. To convert from a tacrolimus immediate-release product to tacrolimus extended-release tablets, administer tacrolimus extended-release tablets once daily at a dose that is 80% of the total daily dose of the tacrolimus immediate-release product. Monitor tacrolimus trough whole blood concentrations and titrate tacrolimus extended-release tablet dosage to achieve trough whole blood concentrations of 4 to 11 ng/mL.

Liver Transplantation

Immediate-release oral preparations: The usual initial oral tacrolimus dosage *in combination with corticosteroids only* in hepatic transplant patients is 100–150 mcg/kg (0.1–0.15 mg/kg) daily, administered in 2 divided daily doses every 12 hours. In hepatic transplant patients, the typical trough whole blood tacrolimus concentrations should be 5–20 ng/mL when measured at months 1–12 post-transplant.

Cardiac Transplantation

Immediate-release oral preparations: The usual initial oral tacrolimus dosage *in combination with azathioprine or mycophenolate mofetil* in cardiac transplant patients is 75 mcg/kg (0.075 mg/kg) daily, administered in 2 divided daily doses every 12 hours. Patients receiving this tacrolimus dosage should have typical trough whole blood tacrolimus concentrations of 10–20 ng/mL and 5–15 ng/mL when measured at months 1–3 and from ≥4 months post-transplant, respectively.

Lung Transplantation

Immediate-release oral preparations: The usual initial oral tacrolimus dosage *in combination with azathioprine or mycophenolate mofetil* in lung transplant patients is 75 mcg/kg (0.075 mg/kg) daily, administered in 2 divided daily doses every 12 hours. Patients receiving this tacrolimus dosage should have typical trough whole blood tacrolimus concentrations of 10–15 ng/mL and 8–12 ng/mL when measured at months 1–3 and from 4-12 months post-transplant, respectively. Cystic fibrosis patients may have a reduced bioavailability of orally administered tacrolimus resulting in the need for higher doses in lung transplantation to achieve target tacrolimus trough concentrations. Monitor tacrolimus trough concentrations and adjust the dose accordingly.

Crohn's Disease

If tacrolimus is used for the management of fistulizing Crohn's disease†, an oral dosage of 200 mcg/kg daily administered in 2 divided daily doses for 10 weeks was used in one study in patients ≥12 years of age.

Adult IV Dosage

If an adult patient is unable to receive an oral formulation, the patient may be started on tacrolimus injection as a continuous IV infusion *only*.

Adults should generally receive initial dosages at the lower end of the following ranges.

Kidney Transplantation

The usual initial starting dose of tacrolimus injection is 30-50 mcg/kg (0.03–0.05 mg/kg) daily in renal transplant patients, administered as a continuous infusion.

Liver Transplantation

The usual initial starting dose of tacrolimus injection is 30-50 mcg/kg (0.03–0.05 mg/kg) daily in hepatic transplant patients, administered as a continuous infusion.

Cardiac Transplantation

The usual initial starting dose of tacrolimus injection is 10 mcg/kg (0.01 mg/kg) daily in heart transplant patients, administered as a continuous infusion.

Lung Transplantation

The usual initial starting dose of tacrolimus injection is 10-30 mcg/kg (0.01–0.03 mg/kg) daily in lung transplant patients, administered as a continuous infusion.

Pediatric Oral Dosage

Generally, children require and tolerate higher tacrolimus maintenance dosages than adults.

To convert pediatric patients from tacrolimus granules to tacrolimus capsules or from tacrolimus capsules to tacrolimus granules, the total daily dose should remain the same. Perform therapeutic drug monitoring after conversion of one tacrolimus formulation to another.

Kidney Transplantation

The usual initial oral immediate-release tacrolimus dosage in pediatric kidney transplant patients is 300 mcg/kg (0.3 mg/kg) daily, administered in 2 divided daily doses every 12 hours. In pediatric kidney transplant patients, the typical trough whole blood tacrolimus concentrations should be 5–20 ng/mL when measured at months 1–12 post-transplant.

The usual initial oral tacrolimus dosage for tacrolimus extended-release capsules *in combination with basiliximab, mycophenolate mofetil, and steroids* is 300 mcg/kg (0.3 mg/kg) once daily within 24 hours of reperfusion. Patients receiving this tacrolimus dosage should have typical whole blood tacrolimus concentrations of 10–20 ng/mL in the first month and 5–15 ng/mL when measured after the first month.

Liver Transplantation

The usual initial oral tacrolimus dosage in pediatric liver transplant patients is 150–200 mcg/kg (0.15–0.2 mg/kg) daily, administered in 2 divided daily doses every 12 hours as an immediate-release formulation. In pediatric liver transplant patients, the typical trough whole blood tacrolimus concentrations should be 5–20 ng/mL when measured at months 1–12 post-transplant.

Cardiac Transplantation

The usual initial oral tacrolimus dosage in pediatric heart transplant patients is 300 mcg/kg (0.3 mg/kg) daily, administered in 2 divided daily doses every 12 hours as an immediate-release formulation. If antibody induction treatment is administered, a dose of 100 mcg/kg (0.1 mg/kg) daily, administered in 2 divided daily doses every 12 hours should be given. In pediatric heart transplant patients, the typical trough whole blood tacrolimus concentrations should be 5–20 ng/mL when measured at months 1–12 post-transplant.

Lung Transplantation

The usual initial oral tacrolimus dosage in pediatric lung transplant patients is 300 mcg/kg (0.3 mg/kg) daily, administered in 2 divided daily doses every 12 hours as an immediate-release preparation. If antibody induction treatment is administered, a dose of 100 mcg/kg (0.1 mg/kg) daily, administered in 2 divided daily doses every 12 hours should be given. In pediatric lung transplant patients, the typical trough whole blood tacrolimus concentrations should be 10-20 ng/mL at weeks 1-2 and 10-15 ng/mL for week 2 to month 12 post-transplant.

Cystic fibrosis patients may have a reduced bioavailability of orally administered tacrolimus resulting in the need for higher doses in lung transplantation to achieve target tacrolimus trough concentrations. Monitor tacrolimus trough concentrations and adjust the dose accordingly.

Pediatric IV Dosage

If a pediatric patient is unable to receive an oral formulation, the patient may be started on tacrolimus injection as a continuous intravenous infusion *only*. Discontinue the infusion as soon as the patient can tolerate oral administration with the first dose of oral tacrolimus given 8–12 hours after discontinuing the intravenous infusion.

Liver Transplantation

The usual intravenous dose is 0.03–0.05 mg/kg/day.

Therapeutic Drug Monitoring

Monitoring blood tacrolimus concentrations is essential for assessing organ rejection and toxicity, adjusting dosage, and determining compliance. Factors influencing frequency of monitoring include, but are not limited to, hepatic or renal dysfunction, the addition or discontinuance of potentially interacting drugs, and the time since transplant. The manufacturer states that therapeutic drug monitoring is not a replacement for renal and hepatic function monitoring and tissue biopsies. The relative risk of drug toxicity (e.g., nephrotoxicity, post-transplant diabetes mellitus) appears to be increased with higher trough concentrations. Therefore, the monitoring of trough whole blood concentrations is recommended to assist in the clinical evaluation of toxicity. Methods commonly used for assaying tacrolimus concentrations include high-performance liquid chromatography with tandem mass spectrometric detection (HPLC/MS/MS) and immunoassays. Specialized sources should be consulted for further discussion of the clinical utility of therapeutic monitoring of tacrolimus.

Pharmacogenomic Considerations in Dosing

Enzymes in the cytochrome P450 (CYP) 3A family are responsible for the oxidative metabolism of tacrolimus. Variations in these genes responsible for tacrolimus metabolism may affect tacrolimus dosage requirements. Blood concentrations of tacrolimus are strongly influenced by CYP3A5 genotype. In kidney, heart, and lung transplant patients, over 50 clinical studies have found that individuals with the CYP3A5*1/*1 or CYP3A5*1/*3 genotype have significantly lower dose-adjusted trough concentrations of tacrolimus as compared to those with the CYP3A5*3/*3 genotype, with *1 carriers requiring 1.5–2 times the dose to achieve similar blood concentrations. CPIC guidelines recommend that individuals that are extensive or intermediate metabolizers (CYP3A5 expressers) should increase the recommended starting dose of tacrolimus by 1.5–2 times (total dose not to exceed 0.3 mg/kg daily). Poor metabolizers (CYP3A5 nonexpressers) should initiate therapy with the standard recommended dose. Therapeutic drug monitoring should be used to guide dosage adjustments.

If genotype information is known at the initiation of therapy, it may be used to individualize initial tacrolimus dosing and more rapidly achieve therapeutic drug concentrations. However, initiation of tacrolimus therapy should not be delayed to await genotyping test results.

● Special Populations

Hepatic Impairment

Initiate therapy with the lowest dosage in the recommended range.

Further dosage reduction may be required (e.g., in patients with severe hepatic impairment [Child-Pugh score ≥10]).

The use of tacrolimus in liver transplant recipients experiencing post-transplant hepatic impairment may be associated with increased risk of developing renal insufficiency related to high whole blood concentrations of tacrolimus. These patients should be monitored closely, and dosage adjustments should be considered.

Renal Impairment

Initiate therapy with the lowest dosage in the recommended range. Further dosage reduction may be required.

In patients who develop postoperative oliguria, the initial dose of tacrolimus should be administered no sooner than 6 hours and within 24 hours of transplantation, but may be delayed until renal function shows evidence of recovery.

Race or Ethnicity

Black patients may need to be titrated to higher dosages to attain comparable trough concentrations compared to white patients.

CAUTIONS

● Contraindications

● Known hypersensitivity to tacrolimus or any ingredient in the formulation (e.g., polyoxyl 60 hydrogenated castor oil [HCO-60] in the IV formulation). Dyspnea, rash, pruritus, and acute respiratory distress syndrome have been reported.

● Warnings/Precautions

Warnings

Lymphomas and Other Malignancies

Possible increased development of lymphoma or other malignancies, particularly of the skin, has been reported in patients receiving immunosuppressive therapies, such as tacrolimus. This risk may be related to the intensity and duration of immunosuppression. A boxed warning about the risk for developing serious malignancies has been included in the prescribing information.

Post-transplant lymphoproliferative disorder (PTLD), which appears to be associated with Epstein-Barr virus (EBV) infection, has been reported in immunosuppressed organ transplant patients. Risk of this disorder appears greatest in patients who are seronegative, including many young children who are at risk for primary EBV infections while immunosuppressed or whose immunosuppressive regimen is changed to tacrolimus following long-term immunosuppressive therapy. Monitoring of EBV serology during treatment is recommended.

Serious Infections

Patients receiving immunosuppressant therapy, including tacrolimus, have an increased risk of susceptibility to viral, fungal and protozoal infection, including opportunistic infections, that may be serious or fatal. A boxed warning about the risk for developing serious infections has been included in the prescribing information for tacrolimus.

Serious viral infections reported with use of tacrolimus include polyomavirus-associated nephropathy (PVAN), mostly due to BK virus infection or reactivation of latent viral infections. These infections are principally observed in renal transplant patients (usually within the first year post-transplantation) and may result in severe allograft dysfunction and/or graft loss. Risk appears to correlate with the degree of overall immunosuppression rather than the use of a specific immunosuppressant. Monitor closely for signs of PVAN (e.g., deterioration of renal function); if PVAN develops, institute early treatment, and consider reducing immunosuppressive therapy.

Progressive multifocal leukoencephalopathy (PML), an opportunistic viral infection of the brain caused by the JC virus has also been reported with tacrolimus use. Use of multiple immunosuppressive agents may contribute to risk of PML. Consider possible diagnosis of PML in any immunocompromised patient who develops progressive neurologic deficits. If PML develops, consider decreasing total immunosuppression.

Cytomegalovirus (CMV)-seronegative transplant patients who receive an organ from a CMV-seropositive donor are at higher risk of developing CMV infection and CMV disease during treatment with tacrolimus. Monitor for development of infection and consider changing immunosuppressant dosage to balance the risk of infection with the organ rejection risk.

Increased Mortality in Female Liver Transplant Patients (Extended-release Capsules [Astagraf XL®])

Increased mortality has been reported in female patients who received tacrolimus extended-release capsules (Astagraf XL®) for the prevention of liver allotransplantation rejection. A boxed warning about this risk has been included in the prescribing information for the extended-release capsules. Mortality occurred in 18 and 8% of female liver transplant patients who received tacrolimus extended-release capsules (Astagraf XL®) and tacrolimus immediate-release product (Prograf®), respectively. Tacrolimus extended-release capsules (Astagraf XL®) are not labeled for use in prophylaxis of organ rejection in liver transplantation.

Other Warnings and Precautions

Anaphylaxis

Risk of anaphylaxis associated with IV tacrolimus therapy; reserve for patients who cannot accommodate oral administration.

Have appropriate equipment and agents for the treatment of anaphylactic reactions readily available whenever tacrolimus is administered IV and monitor patients during administration of the infusion. If anaphylaxis occurs, immediately discontinue the IV infusion and institute appropriate therapy (e.g., epinephrine, oxygen).

Interchangeability of Extended-release Products

Outside the U.S., medication errors were reported, including substitution and dispensing errors, between tacrolimus immediate-release products and tacrolimus extended-release products; these errors led to serious adverse reactions, including graft rejection, or other adverse reactions due to under- or over-exposure to tacrolimus. Interchange or substitution between tacrolimus extended-release products and tacrolimus immediate-release products must occur only under physician supervision. Instruct patients and caregivers to recognize the appearance of their prescribed dosage form and to confirm with the healthcare provider if a different product is dispensed or if dosing instructions have changed.

New-onset Diabetes

Increased risk of hyperglycemia or new-onset, insulin-dependent, post-transplant diabetes mellitus was reported with tacrolimus use in clinical studies for heart, lung, kidney, and liver transplantation. Black and Hispanic renal transplant patients are most at risk for development of post-transplant diabetes mellitus.

Development of insulin-dependent diabetes mellitus reported in 20% of renal transplant patients receiving tacrolimus; insulin resistance was reversible in 15 and 50% of these patients at 1 and 2 years post-transplant, respectively.

Development of insulin-dependent diabetes mellitus also reported in 11–18% of hepatic transplant patients receiving the drug; insulin resistance was reversible in 31–45% of these patients at 1 year post-transplant.

Monitor fasting blood glucose concentrations regularly in patients receiving tacrolimus.

Nephrotoxicity

Nephrotoxicity is among the most common adverse effects of tacrolimus in transplant patients due to its vasoconstrictive effect on renal vasculature, toxic tubulopathy, and tubular-interstitial effects. Nephrotoxicity occurred in approximately 36–40%, 52%, and 59% of patients receiving the drug following hepatic, renal, and cardiac transplantation, respectively, in clinical trials. Increased serum creatinine concentration occurred in 24–45% and increased BUN in 12–30% of patients receiving tacrolimus in clinical trials. Nephrotoxicity may be dose related and may respond to dosage reduction or temporary interruption of tacrolimus administration.

The risk for nephrotoxicity may increase when tacrolimus is concomitantly administered with CYP3A inhibitors or drugs associated with nephrotoxicity.

Monitor S_{cr} and tacrolimus blood concentrations regularly during tacrolimus treatment and adjust dosage or discontinue tacrolimus, as needed.

Neurotoxicity

Risk of neurotoxicity (e.g., tremor, headache, other changes in motor function, mental status, or sensory function) in patients receiving tacrolimus, especially at high doses.

Closely monitor neurologic function and status. Consider dosage reduction or discontinue treatment if neurotoxicity occurs.

Hyperkalemia

Possible hyperkalemia (sometimes severe) reported in patients receiving tacrolimus during clinical studies.

Monitor serum potassium concentrations regularly; carefully consider concomitant use of potassium-sparing diuretics, ACE inhibitors, or angiotensin receptor blockers.

If hyperkalemia occurs, institute appropriate management (e.g., restriction of potassium intake, administration of potassium-binding resin or mineralocorticoid).

Hypertension

Development of hypertension reported commonly; generally is mild to moderate. Antihypertensive therapy may be required, but should be selected to carefully consider use of antihypertensive agents associated with hyperkalemia (e.g., potassium-sparing diuretics, ACE inhibitors, angiotensin receptor blockers).

Concomitant Use with Sirolimus

The use of sirolimus with tacrolimus immediate-release products in studies of de novo liver transplant patients was associated with an excess mortality, graft loss, and hepatic artery thrombosis (HAT). The use of sirolimus (at a dose of 2 mg per day) with tacrolimus in heart transplant patients in a U.S. clinical trial was associated with increased risk of renal function impairment, wound healing complications, and insulin-dependent post-transplant diabetes mellitus. The use of sirolimus concomitantly with tacrolimus is not recommended. The use of sirolimus with tacrolimus may also increase the risk of thrombotic microangiopathy.

QT Prolongation

Tacrolimus may prolong the QT interval and increase the risk of causing torsades de pointes. Use of tacrolimus should be avoided in patients with known QT interval prolongation. Consider obtaining electrocardiograms and monitoring electrolytes (magnesium, potassium, calcium) periodically during treatment for those who have congestive heart failure or bradyarrhythmias; those who are receiving drugs known to prolong the QT interval (e.g., class IA and III

antiarrhythmic agents); and in those with electrolyte disturbances such as hypokalemia, hypocalcemia, or hypomagnesemia.

When co-administering tacrolimus with other substrates and/or inhibitors of CYP3A4 that also have the potential to prolong the QT interval, a reduction in tacrolimus dose, frequent monitoring of tacrolimus whole blood concentrations, and monitoring for QT prolongation is recommended.

Myocardial Hypertrophy

Myocardial hypertrophy has been reported in infants, children, and adults, particularly those with high tacrolimus trough concentrations; this effect is generally reversible following dosage reduction or drug discontinuance.

Consider performing echocardiographic evaluation if renal failure or clinical manifestations of ventricular dysfunction occur.

If myocardial hypertrophy is diagnosed, consider decreasing dosage or discontinuing therapy.

Immunizations

Tacrolimus may interfere with the safety and effectiveness of vaccines. Avoid use of live vaccines during treatment with tacrolimus. Inactivated vaccines noted to be safe for administration after transplantation may not be sufficiently immunogenic during treatment with tacrolimus. When possible, administer the complete complement of vaccines before transplantation and treatment with tacrolimus.

Pure Red Cell Aplasia

Pure red cell aplasia (PRCA) has been reported in patients treated with tacrolimus. Although a mechanism has not been confirmed, all patients who developed PRCA reported risk factors such as parvovirus B19 infection, underlying disease, or concomitant medications associated with PRCA. If PRCA is diagnosed, discontinuation of tacrolimus should be considered.

Thrombotic Microangiopathy

Cases of thrombotic microangiopathy, including hemolytic uremic syndrome (HUS) and thrombotic thrombocytopenic purpura (TTP), have been reported in patients treated with tacrolimus. Risk factors for thrombotic microangiopathy that can occur in transplant patients include severe infections, graft-versus-host disease (GVHD), HLA mismatch, and calcineurin inhibitor and mTOR inhibitor use. These risk factors may, either alone or combined, contribute to the risk of thrombotic microangiopathy.

Cannabidiol Drug Interactions

Patients should be closely monitored for an increase in tacrolimus levels and adverse reactions suggestive of toxicity when tacrolimus is administered with cannabidiol. Dosage reduction of tacrolimus should be considered as needed.

Specific Populations

Pregnancy

Tacrolimus may cause fetal harm if administered to pregnant females. Data from postmarketing surveillance and The Transplantation Pregnancy Registry International (TPRI) suggest that infants exposed to tacrolimus in utero are at a risk of prematurity, birth defects/congenital anomalies, low birth weight, and fetal distress. Females of reproductive potential should use effective birth control prior to intitation and during tacrolimus treatment. Males who have female partners who are able to become pregnant should also use effective birth control before and during treatment with tacrolimus.

TPRI is a voluntary pregnancy exposure registry that monitors outcomes of pregnancy in female transplant recipients and those fathered by male transplant recipients exposed to immunosuppressants including tacrolimus; clinicians are encouraged to advise their patients to register by contacting the TPRI at 1-877-955-6877 or their website https://www.transplantpregnancyregistry.org/.

Tacrolimus may increase hyperglycemia in pregnant females with diabetes; monitor blood glucose levels regularly. Tacrolimus also may exacerbate hypertension in pregnant females and increase the risk of pre-eclampsia, therefore blood pressure should be monitored and controlled.

Lactation

Tacrolimus has been reported to be distributed into human milk; however, the effects on the infant or milk production has not been assessed. Consider the benefits of breast-feeding along with the importance of tacrolimus to the mother and any potential adverse effects on the breast-fed infant from the drug or the underlying maternal condition.

Females and Males of Reproductive Potential

Tacrolimus can cause fetal harm when administered to pregnant females. Advise female and male patients of reproductive potential to speak to their healthcare provider to discuss family planning options including appropriate contraception prior to starting treatment with tacrolimus. Females of reproductive potential should use effective birth control prior to intitation and during tacrolimus treatment. Males who have female partners who are able to become pregnant should also use effective birth control before and during treatment with tacrolimus.

Based on findings in animals, male and female fertility may be compromised by treatment with tacrolimus.

Pediatric Use

Safety and effectiveness have been established in pediatric liver, kidney, heart, and lung transplant patients in clinical studies. Clinical experience in children suggests that the safety and efficacy of tacrolimus are similar to those in adults.

A randomized, active-controlled study of tacrolimus in primary liver transplantation of pediatric patients ≤16 years of age included 91 patients who were randomized to tacrolimus-based therapy and 90 patients receiving cyclosporine-based therapy. At 12 months, the incidence rate of biopsy-proven acute rejection, graft loss, death, or loss to follow-up was 52.7% in the tacrolimus group and 61.1% in the cyclosporine group.

Efficacy and safety of tacrolimus immunosuppression in pediatric lung transplation were also established in 450 patients receiving tacrolimus immediate-release products in combination with mycophenolate mofetil or 72 patients receiving tacrolimus immediate-release products in combination with azathioprine; one-year graft survival estimates from time of discharge were 91.7% and 84.7%, respectively.

Pharmacokinetic studies have been conducted in pediatric patients, with dosage adjustments made based on clinical status and whole blood concentrations. Pediatric patients generally require higher doses of tacrolimus to maintain trough whole blood concentrations similar to adult patients.

Geriatric Use

Insufficient experience in patients ≥65 years of age to determine whether geriatric patients respond differently than younger adults; select dosage with caution.

If evidence of renal impairment exists or develops, adjust dosage.

Hepatic Impairment

Decreased clearance in patients with severe hepatic impairment; adjust dosage and closely monitor blood concentrations in these patients.

Hepatic transplant patients experiencing post-transplant hepatic impairment may be at increased risk of renal impairment secondary to high blood tacrolimus concentrations; monitor such patients closely and consider dosage adjustment.

Renal Impairment

Patients with renal impairment had similar pharmacokinetic profiles of tacrolimus compared to that in healthy volunteers with normal renal function. Consideration should be given to dosing tacrolimus at the lower end of the therapeutic dosing range in patients who have received a liver or heart transplant and have pre-existing renal impairment; further dosage reductions below the targeted range may be required.

Potential for nephrotoxicity; monitor patient closely. Dosage adjustments recommended.

Race

Black renal transplant patients may require higher doses than patients of other races to maintain comparable whole blood trough drug concentrations.

Black and Hispanic patients are at increased risk for new onset diabetes posttransplantion. Monitor blood glucose concentrations and treat appropriately.

Common Adverse Effects

Kidney Transplantation

The most common adverse reactions reported in ≥30% of patients receiving immediate-release products were: infection, tremor, hypertension, abnormal renal function, constipation, diarrhea, headache, abdominal pain, insomnia, nausea, hypomagnesemia, urinary tract infection, hypophosphatemia, peripheral edema, asthenia, pain, hyperlipidemia, hyperkalemia, and anemia. The most common adverse reactions reported in ≥30% of patients receiving tacrolimus extended-release capsules were: diarrhea, constipation, nausea, peripheral edema, tremor, and anemia. The most common adverse reactions reported in ≥30% of patients receiving tacrolimus extended-release tablets were: infection and diarrhea.

Liver Transplantation

The most common adverse reactions reported in ≥40% of patients receiving immediate-release products were: tremor, headache, diarrhea, hypertension, nausea, abnormal renal function, abdominal pain, insomnia, paresthesia, anemia, pain, fever, asthenia, hyperkalemia, hypomagnesemia, and hyperglycemia.

Heart Transplantation

The most common adverse reactions reported in ≥15% of patients receiving immediate-release products were: abnormal renal function, hypertension, diabetes mellitus, CMV infection, tremor, hyperglycemia, leukopenia, infection, anemia, bronchitis, pericardial effusion, urinary tract infection, and hyperlipidemia.

Lung Transplantation

Adverse reactions reported in lung tranplant patients receiving immediate-release products were similar to those in kidney, heart, or liver transplant patients treated with tacrolimus.

DRUG INTERACTIONS

Tacrolimus is metabolized by CYP isoenzymes, principally CYP3A.

● Drugs Affecting or Metabolized by Hepatic Microsomal Enzymes

Strong CYP3A Inducers

Concomitant use of tacrolimus and strong CYP3A4 inducers such as antimycobacterials (e.g., rifampin, rifabutin), anticonvulsants (e.g., phenytoin, carbamazepine, and phenobarbital), and St. John's wort may decrease tacrolimus whole blood trough concentrations and increase the risk of rejection. When these drugs are used together, increase tacrolimus dose and monitor tacrolimus whole blood trough concentrations.

Strong CYP3A Inhibitors

Concomitant use of tacrolimus and strong CYP3A4 inhibitors such as protease inhibitors (e.g, nelfinavir, ritonavir), azole antifungals (e.g., voriconazole, posaconazole, itraconazole, ketoconazole), antibiotics (e.g., clarithromycin, troleandomycin, chloramphenicol), nefazodone, cobicistat, letermovir, and Schisandra sphenanthera extracts may increase tacrolimus whole blood trough concentrations and increase the risk of serious adverse reactions (e.g., neurotoxicity, QT prolongation). A rapid, sharp rise in tacrolimus levels may occur early with coadministration, despite an immediate reduction of tacrolimus dose. When these drugs are used together, reduce the tacrolimus dose (for voriconazole and posaconazole, give one third of the original dose) and adjust the dose based on tacrolimus whole blood trough concentrations. Early and frequent monitoring of tacrolimus whole blood trough levels should start within 1–3 days and continue monitoring as necessary when these drugs are used concomitantly.

Mild or Moderate CYP3A4 Inhibitors

Concomitant use of tacrolimus and mild to moderate CYP3A4 inhibitors such as clotrimazole, antibiotics (e.g., erythromycin, fluconazole), calcium channel blockers (e.g., verapamil, diltiazem, nifedipine, nicardipine), amiodarone, danazol, ethinyl estradiol, cimetidine, lansoprazole and omeprazole, may increase tacrolimus whole blood trough concentrations and increase the risk of serious adverse reactions (e.g., neurotoxicity, QT prolongation). Monitor tacrolimus whole blood trough concentrations and adjust tacrolimus dose if needed when these drugs are used concomitantly.

Mild or Moderate CYP3A4 Inducers

Concomitant use of tacrolimus and mild to moderate CYP3A4 inducers such as methylprednisolone or prednisone may decrease tacrolimus whole blood trough concentrations. Monitor tacrolimus whole blood trough concentrations and adjust tacrolimus dose if needed.

● Mycophenolic Acid

When tacrolimus is used concomitantly with a given dose of a mycophenolic acid (MPA) product, exposure to MPA is higher than with cyclosporine co-administration with MPA, because cyclosporine interrupts the enterohepatic recirculation of MPA while tacrolimus does not. Monitor for MPA-associated adverse reactions and reduce the dose of concomitantly administered mycophenolic acid products as needed.

● Antacids

Concomitant use of magnesium and aluminum hydroxide antacids may increase tacrolimus whole blood trough concentrations and increase the risk of serious adverse reactions (e.g., neurotoxicity, QT prolongation). Monitor tacrolimus whole blood trough concentrations throughout therapy and reduce the tacrolimus dose if necessary.

● Metoclopramide

Concomitant use of metoclopramide may increase tacrolimus whole blood trough concentrations and increase the risk of serious adverse reactions (e.g., neurotoxicity, QT prolongation). Monitor tacrolimus whole blood trough concentrations throughout therapy and reduce the tacrolimus dose if necessary.

● Immunosuppressants

Because of the risk of oversuppression of the immune system and associated susceptibility to infection and risk of lymphoma, the manufacturer recommends that combination immunosuppressant therapy be used with caution.

Concomitant use of tacrolimus and sirolimus in de novo liver transplant recipients has been associated with an increased risk of hepatic artery thrombosis (HAT), graft loss, and death. Most cases of HAT occurred within 30 days post-transplantation and led to graft loss or death. In one study reporting excess mortality and graft loss in association with combined use of sirolimus and tacrolimus in de novo liver transplant recipients, many of the patients had evidence of infection at or near the time of death. In addition, concomitant use of tacrolimus and sirolimus in cardiac transplant recipients in one arm of a US clinical trial was associated with an increased risk of wound healing complications, renal function impairment, and insulin-dependent post-transplant diabetes mellitus. Therefore, the manufacturer states that concurrent administration of tacrolimus and sirolimus is not recommended.

● Nephrotoxic Drugs

Because of the potential for additive or synergistic impairment of renal function, tacrolimus should be used with caution in patients receiving other nephrotoxic drugs (e.g., aminoglycoside antibiotics, amphotericin B, cisplatin, ganciclovir, nucleotide reverse transcriptase inhibitors, protease inhibitors). Monitor renal function and consider dosage reduction if nephrotoxicity occurs with concomitant use of these drugs.

● Cyclosporine

Concomitant administration of tacrolimus and cyclosporine has resulted in additive/synergistic nephrotoxicity. To avoid excessive nephrotoxicity, tacrolimus should not be used concomitantly with cyclosporine. The manufacturer

recommends delaying initiation of tacrolimus or cyclosporine therapy for at least 24 hours after discontinuance of the other therapy. Initiation of tacrolimus or cyclosporine therapy may be further delayed in the presence of elevated cyclosporine or tacrolimus levels.

● Direct Acting Antiviral (DAA) Therapy

The pharmacokinetics of tacrolimus may be affected by changes in liver function during DAA therapy, related to clearance of HCV virus. Monitor tacrolimus whole blood trough concentrations throughout therapy and adjust tacrolimus dose if necessary.

● Alcohol

When taken with tacrolimus extended-release capsules or extended-release tablets, alcohol may modify the rate of release of tacrolimus and increase the risk of serious adverse reactions (e.g., neurotoxicity, QT prolongation). Patients should be instructed to avoid alcoholic beverages.

● Grapefruit and Grapefruit Juice

Because grapefruit and grapefruit juice affect CYP3A-mediated metabolism of tacrolimus, it may increase tacrolimus whole blood trough concentrations and increase the risk of serious adverse reactions (e.g., neurotoxicity, QT prolongation). Patients should be instructed to avoid grapefruit-containing foods and beverages.

● Potassium-sparing Diuretics

Concomitant use of tacrolimus and potassium-sparing diuretics ACE inhibitors, or angiotensin receptor blockers may result in potentially severe hyperkalemia and should be carefully considered.

● ACE inhibitors

Concomitant use of tacrolimus and ACE inhibitors may result in potentially severe hyperkalemia and should be carefully considered.

● Angiotensin Receptor Blockers

Concomitant use of tacrolimus and angiotensin receptor blockers may result in potentially severe hyperkalemia and should be carefully considered.

● Calcium Channel Blocking Agents

Concomitant use of tacrolimus and calcium channel blocking agents may increase tacrolimus blood concentrations. Monitor tacrolimus whole blood trough concentrations throughout therapy and reduce tacrolimus dose if necessary.

● Vaccines

The possibility that the immune response to vaccination may be diminished in patients receiving tacrolimus should be considered. Inactivated vaccines noted to be safe for administration after transplantation may not be sufficiently immunogenic during treatment with tacrolimus. In addition, the manufacturer recommends that live vaccines (e.g., measles, mumps, rubella, oral polio, BCG, yellow fever, TY21a typhoid) be avoided during therapy with the drug. Administer the complete complement of vaccines before transplantation and treatment with tacrolimus when possible.

● Cannabidiol

Tacrolimus blood levels may increase upon concomitant use with cannabidiol. Closely monitor for an increase in tacrolimus blood levels and for adverse reactions suggestive of tacrolimus toxicity with concomitant administration. A dose reduction of tacrolimus should be considered as needed.

DESCRIPTION

Tacrolimus is a macrolide antibiotic produced by *Streptomyces tsukubaensis*. The drug is a potent immunosuppressive agent that is pharmacologically but *not* structurally related to cyclosporine and that exhibits only limited antimicrobial activity. Tacrolimus is approximately 10- to 200-fold more potent than cyclosporine on a weight basis in various in vitro T-cell test systems of immune function.

In animals, tacrolimus inhibits cell-mediated immune responses such as allograft rejection, delayed hypersensitivity, collagen-induced arthritis, experimental allergic encephalomyelitis, and graft-vs-host disease while humoral immunity is inhibited to a lesser extent. Increased survival of the host and of the transplanted graft of liver, kidney, heart, bone marrow, small bowel, pancreas, lung, trachea, skin, cornea, and limb has been shown in animals receiving the drug.

The exact mechanism(s) of immunosuppressive action of tacrolimus has not been elucidated but appears to involve inhibition of the activation and proliferation of T cells, as well as T helper cell dependent B-cell response. Studies suggest that tacrolimus binds to an intracellular protein, FKBP-12. Binding of the complex of tacrolimus and FKBP-12 with calcium, calmodulin, and calcineurin inhibits the phosphatase activity of calcineurin, which may prevent the dephosphorylation and translocation of nuclear factor of activated T cells (NF-AT). NF-AT putatively initiates gene transcription for the formation of lymphokines (e.g., interleukin-2, gamma interferon) involved in the activation of T cells.

ADVICE TO PATIENTS

- Advise patients and/or caregivers about potential benefits and risks of tacrolimus. Advise patients and/or caregivers to read the medication guide.
- Advise patients to inspect their tacrolimus medicine when they receive a new prescription and before taking it. If the appearance of the product is not the same as usual, or if dosage instructions have changed they should contact their healthcare provider to make sure that they have the right medicine.
- Risk of lymphomas and other malignancies, particularly of the skin. Advise patients to limit exposure to sunlight and ultraviolet (UV) light by wearing protective clothing and using a broad spectrum sunscreen with a high protection factor.
- Risk of infections, including opportunistic infections; advise patients to inform their clinician if they develop fever, sweats, chills, or flu-like symptoms, muscle aches, or warm, red, painful areas on the skin.
- Risk of new onset diabetes mellitus; advise patients to inform their clinician if frequent urination or increased thirst or hunger develops.
- Risk of nephrotoxicity; advise patients of the importance of monitoring renal function.
- Risk of neurotoxicity; advise patients to contact their physician if vision changes, delirium, or tremors develop.
- Risk of hypertension developing or worsening during therapy. Advise patients of the importance of regular monitoring of blood pressure during treatment.
- Risk of myocardial hypertrophy; advise patients to inform their clinician if they develop symptoms of tiredness, swelling, and/or shortness of breath.
- Inform patients that any necessary immunizations should be completed prior to transplantation and initiation of tacrolimus. Avoid administration of live vaccines during treatment and consider decreased immunogenic response of inactivated vaccines.
- Risk of thrombotic microangiopathy; advise patients that blood clotting problems may occur with therapy. This risk may increase when patients take tacrolimus and sirolimus or everolimus together, or when certain infections develop. Advise patients to seek immediate medical care if they develop fever,

petequiae or bruises, fatigue, confusion, yellowing of the skin or eyes, or low urine output.

- Advise patients of the importance of routine laboratory testing (e.g., for assessment of renal and hepatic function, for monitoring of glucose and potassium concentrations).
- Advise patient to inform their clinician of existing or contemplated concomitant therapy, including prescription and OTC drugs and dietary or herbal supplements.
- Advise patients to avoid grapefruit products during treatment with tacrolimus. Also advise patients to avoid alcohol with use of extended-release products.
- Advise females to inform their clinician if they are or plan to become pregnant or plan to breast-feed. Advise females of childbearing potential and male patients with female partners of childbearing potential of the need for effective contraception during therapy. Advise patients if they become pregnant or father a pregnancy to enroll in the in the voluntary Transplantation Pregnancy Registry International. To enroll or register, patients can call the toll free number 1-877-955-6877 or visit https://www.transplantpregnancyregistry.org.
- Advise patients of the potential for tacrolimus use to affect male and female fertility.
- Inform patients of other important precautionary information.

PREPARATIONS

Excipients in commercially available drug preparations may have clinically important effects in some individuals; consult specific product labeling for details.

Tacrolimus

Oral

Capsules	0.5 mg (of anhydrous tacrolimus)	**Prograf®**, Astellas
	1 mg (of anhydrous tacrolimus)	**Prograf®**, Astellas
	5 mg (of anhydrous tacrolimus)	**Prograf®**, Astellas
Capsules, extended-release	0.5 mg (of anhydrous tacrolimus)	**Astagraf XL**, Astellas
	1 mg (of anhydrous tacrolimus)	**Astagraf XL**, Astellas
	5 mg (of anhydrous tacrolimus)	**Astagraf XL**, Astellas
Granules, for suspension	0.2 mg (of anhydrous tacrolimus)	**Prograf**, Astellas
	1 mg (of anhydrous tacrolimus)	**Prograf**, Astellas
Tablets, extended-release	0.75 mg (of anhydrous tacrolimus)	**Envarsus XR**, Veloxis
	1 mg (of anhydrous tacrolimus)	**Envarsus XR**, Veloxis
	4 mg (of anhydrous tacrolimus)	**Envarsus XR**, Veloxis

Parenteral

For injection, concentrate, for IV infusion only	5 mg (of anhydrous tacrolimus) per mL	**Prograf®**, Astellas

† Use is not currently included in the labeling approved by the US Food and Drug Administration.

Selected Revisions July 10, 2024, © Copyright, January 1, 1995, American Society of Health-System Pharmacists, Inc.

Table of Contents

91:00 ANTIDOTE THERAPEUTICS

§ Omitted from the print version of *AHFS Drug Information*® because of space limitations. This monograph is available on the *AHFS Drug Information*® website, http://ahfsdruginformation.com.

Acetylcysteine, Acetylcysteine Lysine

91:04.04 • ACETAMINOPHEN ANTIDOTES

■ Acetylcysteine, the *N*-acetyl derivative of the naturally occurring amino acid, L-cysteine, is an antidote for acetaminophen overdosage as well as a mucolytic agent and sulfhydryl donor.

USES

● Antidote for Acetaminophen Overdosage

Acetylcysteine is used orally or by IV infusion as an antidote to prevent or lessen hepatic injury, which may occur following the ingestion of a potentially hepatotoxic quantity of acetaminophen. Acetylcysteine injection is designated an orphan drug by FDA for the treatment of moderate to severe acetaminophen overdosage.

When administered within 8 hours of acetaminophen ingestion, oral or IV acetylcysteine can effectively prevent or minimize hepatotoxicity associated with acute overdosage of acetaminophen. The effectiveness of *oral* acetylcysteine depends on early administration, with benefits seen principally in patients treated within 16 hours of overdose. The manufacturer of oral acetylcysteine states that it is essential to initiate treatment as soon as possible after the overdose, with treatment beginning within 24 hours of ingestion. According to the manufacturer of acetylcysteine *injection*, the critical ingestion-treatment interval for maximal protection against severe hepatic injury is between 0 and 8 hours. Efficacy diminishes progressively after 8 hours and treatment initiation between 15 and 24 hours after ingestion of acetaminophen yields limited efficacy. However, acetylcysteine does not appear to worsen the patient's condition and should not be withheld, particularly since the reported time of ingestion may be incorrect.

Clinical studies have clearly demonstrated efficacy of orally administered acetylcysteine, and oral administration may result in higher intrahepatic concentrations of the drug than IV administration. However, oral administration often produces nausea and vomiting, and administration of antiemetic agents may be needed to complete therapy; IV administration obviates potential difficulties associated with administration of an antiemetic. Intravenous administration achieves higher plasma concentrations compared with oral administration; it has been suggested that higher plasma concentrations may exert useful extrahepatic effects. However, anaphylactoid reactions have been reported following IV administration.

In all cases of suspected acetaminophen overdosage, a regional poison control center (800-222-1222) may be contacted immediately for assistance in diagnosis and for directions in the use of acetylcysteine as an antidote. Consult the manufacturer's labeling for information on appropriate acetaminophen assay methodology and supportive treatment for acetaminophen overdosage.

● Mucolytic Uses

Acetylcysteine is used by oral inhalation or intratracheal instillation as a mucolytic agent in the adjunctive treatment of patients with abnormal, viscid, or inspissated mucous secretions in such conditions as acute and chronic bronchopulmonary disorders (e.g., pneumonia, bronchitis, emphysema, tracheobronchitis, chronic asthmatic bronchitis, tuberculosis, bronchiectasis, primary amyloidosis of the lung); atelectasis caused by mucus obstruction; pulmonary complications of cystic fibrosis; pulmonary complications of surgery; and post-traumatic chest conditions. Acetylcysteine is also used during anesthesia and in the preparation of patients for bronchograms, bronchospirometry, bronchial wedge catheterization, and other diagnostic bronchial studies. The drug also is used in tracheostomy care to prevent endotracheal crusting and to reduce or eliminate the need for bronchoscopy.

● Prevention of Nephropathy Associated with Radiographic Contrast Media

Acetylcysteine has been used to prevent radiographic contrast media-induced nephropathy†. The most important risk factor for contrast-induced acute kidney injury (CI-AKI) is preexisting severe renal insufficiency. Other risk factors may include diabetes mellitus, older age, low hematocrit, hemodynamic instability, or conditions resulting in low effective circulating blood volume (e.g., heart failure, left ventricular systolic dysfunction). In addition, the risk of contrast media-induced decreases in renal function depends on contrast media properties (high osmolality, ionic compound, increased viscosity) and administration of a larger volume of contrast media.

Various strategies have been investigated for prophylaxis of contrast media-induced nephropathy. Available evidence supports use of hydration as a prophylactic measure. Several pharmacologic agents, including acetylcysteine, have been evaluated for prophylaxis of contrast media-induced nephropathy.

Some controlled studies and meta-analyses have suggested benefit of acetylcysteine for prevention of CI-AKI; however, a large amount of unexplained heterogeneity among the studies has been observed. Two large randomized controlled trials including a total of >7000 patients undergoing angiography showed no effect of oral acetylcysteine for prevention of CI-AKI. Homogeneous results indicating no benefit of acetylcysteine for prevention of CI-AKI were seen when only large studies (with ≥500 patients) were included. In an analysis of randomized clinical trials of any size in which mortality (41 trials) or need for kidney replacement (45 trials) was assessed, no benefit of acetylcysteine on these clinical outcomes was reported. The proposed mechanism of the drug's effects in preventing CI-AKI has been called into question, and the possibility that reductions in creatinine associated with acetylcysteine are due to analytical interference rather than an effect on kidney function has been suggested, highlighting the limitations of using creatinine measurements as a surrogate for clinical outcomes.

Based on insufficient evidence of its effectiveness, use of acetylcysteine for prevention of CI-AKI is not recommended in the 2021 American College of Cardiology/American Heart Association/Society for Cardiovascular Angiography & Interventions (ACC/AHA/SCAI) Guideline for Coronary Artery Revascularization. In addition, the 2023 American College of Radiology (ACR) Manual on Contrast Media does not recommend acetylcysteine for prevention of CI-AKI in patients receiving IV contrast media.

DOSAGE AND ADMINISTRATION

● General

Pretreatment Screening

Acetaminophen Overdosage

- Because the reported or estimated amount of acetaminophen ingestion often is inaccurate and is not a reliable guide to the therapeutic management of the overdose, the preferred method to assess the risk of toxicity after acute acetaminophen ingestion usually is measurement of plasma or serum acetaminophen concentrations.

- Determine plasma or serum acetaminophen concentrations as soon as possible (but no sooner than 4 hours) after ingestion. May be appropriate to obtain an additional sample at 4–6 hours after initial sample (or 8–10 hours after ingestion) if an extended-release acetaminophen preparation was ingested.

- Also obtain baseline liver transaminases, bilirubin, international normalized ratio/prothrombin time (INR/PT), creatinine, blood urea nitrogen (BUN), blood glucose, and electrolytes.

- Use plasma or serum acetaminophen concentrations in conjunction with a nomogram (https://www.merckmanuals.com/professional/multimedia/image/rumack-matthew-nomogram-for-single-acute-acetaminophen-ingestions) to estimate potential for hepatotoxicity and necessity of acetylcysteine therapy. A full course of acetylcysteine therapy is indicated if initial plasma or serum acetaminophen concentrations fall on or above the dashed line on the nomogram.

- Assistance is available from a regional poison center at 800-222-1222 or an assistance line for acetaminophen overdosage at 800-525-6115.

- If plasma or serum acetaminophen concentrations cannot be obtained, assume that the overdosage is potentially toxic and initiate acetylcysteine therapy.

- Regardless of the quantity of acetaminophen reported to have been ingested, administer acetylcysteine immediately if ≤24 hours have elapsed from the reported time of ingestion of an overdose of acetaminophen. Do not await results of assays for acetaminophen levels before initiating treatment with acetylcysteine.

- In the event that a loading dose of acetylcysteine is administered before plasma or serum acetaminophen concentrations are available, the initial plasma or serum concentration (obtained ≥4 hours after ingestion) is used in conjunction with the nomogram to determine the necessity of completing a full course of acetylcysteine therapy. In such situations, administration of a full course of therapy is indicated if the initial plasma or serum acetaminophen concentration falls on or above the dashed line on the nomogram; acetylcysteine therapy is discontinued if the initial acetaminophen concentration falls below the dashed line on the nomogram.

- Because acetylcysteine therapy may be useful even when instituted >24 hours after an overdose, a full course of acetylcysteine therapy is recommended for patients presenting ≥24 hours postingestion with measurable plasma or serum acetaminophen concentrations or biochemical evidence of hepatic injury.

- The nomogram may underestimate the hepatotoxicity risk in patients with chronic alcoholism or malnutrition and in those receiving CYP2E1 enzyme-inducing drugs (e.g., isoniazid); consider treating such patients even if the acetaminophen concentrations are in the nontoxic range.

- Since oral administration of acetylcysteine may result in vomiting or aggravate vomiting associated with acetaminophen overdosage, evaluate patients at risk of gastric hemorrhage (e.g., those with esophageal varices or peptic ulcers) with regard to the relative risks of upper GI hemorrhage and acetaminophen-induced hepatotoxicity and treat with acetylcysteine accordingly.

Multiple Supratherapeutic Acetaminophen Doses

- Guidelines for the treatment of ingestions involving multiple, higher-than-recommended acetaminophen doses over an extended period of time currently are not available. Plasma transaminase concentrations (along with other laboratory tests to monitor hepatic and renal function and electrolyte and fluid balance, e.g., bilirubin, INR, creatinine, BUN, blood glucose, electrolytes) and plasma or serum acetaminophen concentrations have been used to estimate potential for hepatotoxicity and necessity of acetylcysteine therapy.

- Assistance is available from a regional poison center at 800-222-1222 or an assistance line for acetaminophen overdosage at 800-525-6115.

Patient Monitoring

- Closely monitor patients with asthma during initiation of and throughout acetylcysteine therapy.

Acetaminophen Overdosage

- Monitor hepatic and renal function and electrolytes throughout the detoxification process in patients receiving acetylcysteine as an antidote for acetaminophen overdosage.

- If the initial acetaminophen concentration was in the non-toxic range, but time of ingestion was unknown or <4 hours, obtain a second sample for acetaminophen concentration and consider the patient's clinical status to decide whether or not to continue acetylcysteine treatment beyond the loading dose.

- In cases of suspected massive overdose, or with concomitant ingestion of other substances, or in patients with preexisting liver disease, the absorption and/or the half-life of acetaminophen may be prolonged. In such cases, consider the need for continued treatment with IV acetylcysteine beyond a total of 3 separate doses over a 21-hour infusion period. Obtain acetaminophen levels, ALT/AST, and INR following the last maintenance dose. If acetaminophen levels are still detectable, or if the ALT/AST are still increasing or the INR remains elevated, continue dosing and consult a regional poison center at 800-222-1222 or an assistance line for acetaminophen overdosage at 800-525-6115.

● Administration

As an antidote for acetaminophen overdosage, acetylcysteine is administered as an oral solution or by IV infusion. As a mucolytic agent, acetylcysteine, usually in a 10–20% solution, may be administered by nebulization, direct instillation, or intratracheal instillation.

Acetylcysteine has been administered orally or by IV infusion for prevention of radiographic contrast media-induced nephropathy†.

Oral

For the treatment of acetaminophen overdosage, acetylcysteine may be administered orally as a 5% solution prepared from the commercially available 20% solution. To prepare the solution, dilute the 20% solution 1:3 with a diet cola soft drink or other diet soft drink; if administered via a gastric tube or Miller-Abbott tube, water may be used as the diluent. Diluted solutions should be freshly prepared and used within 1 hour. Store the solution at 20–25°C (excursions permitted to 15–30°C). Store opened vials of undiluted solution in the refrigerator and use within 96 hours. Do not store admixtures.

Alternatively, an oral solution may be prepared from commercially available packets containing 500 mg or 2.5 g of acetylcysteine (available as acetylcysteine lysine [Legubeti®]). To prepare the oral solution, dissolve the appropriate number of packets in the volume of caffeine-free diet cola or other diet soft drink, as indicated in dosing tables provided in the prescribing information. The Legubeti® preparation is for oral administration only and should not be used for nebulization or intratracheal instillation.

Store the packets at 20–25°C (excursions permitted to 15–30°C). Use the prepared solution within 1 hour after preparation.

If the patient is persistently unable to retain orally administered acetylcysteine, the drug may be administered via a duodenal or nasoduodenal tube; alternatively, an IV formulation may be considered.

IV Infusion

Acetylcysteine injection concentrate must be diluted in 5% dextrose injection, 0.45% sodium chloride injection, or sterile water for injection prior to IV infusion. Acetylcysteine solution for inhalation or oral administration should *not* be administered by injection.

Store the injection concentrate at 20–25°C. Do not use previously opened vials of acetylcysteine injection concentrate.

Dilution

The appropriate dose of acetylcysteine should be withdrawn from the required number of vials and added to an appropriate volume of 5% dextrose, 0.45% sodium chloride injection, or sterile water for injection (see Table 1). The total volume administered should be adjusted for patients weighing <40 kg or requiring fluid restriction. In patients weighing ≤20 kg, the recommended volume of diluent is 3, 7, and 14 mL/kg for the loading, second, and third doses, respectively.

TABLE 1. Recommended Volumes of Diluent for Dilution of IV Acetylcysteine Doses

Patient's Weight (kg)	Volume of Diluent for Indicated Dose		
	Loading Dose	First Maintenance Dose	Second Maintenance Dose
≥41	200 mL	500 mL	1 L
21–40	100 mL	250 mL	500 mL
20	60 mL	140 mL	280 mL
15	45 mL	105 mL	210 mL
10	30 mL	70 mL	140 mL
5	15 mL	35 mL	70 mL

Dilution in the 3 compatible diluents results in different osmolarity of the solution for IV administration (see Table 2). Adjust osmolarity to a physiologically safe level (generally ≥150 mOsmol/L in pediatric patients).

TABLE 2. Examples of Acetylcysteine Concentration and Osmolarity in Different Diluents

Acetylcysteine Concentration	Osmolarity in Sterile Water for Injection	Osmolarity in 0.45% Sodium Chloride Injection	Osmolarity in 5% Dextrose Injection
7 mg/mL	91 mOsmol/L	245 mOsm/L	343 mOsm/L
24 mg/mL	312 mOsmol/L	466 mOsmol/L	564 mOsmol/L

Following dilution with 5% dextrose, 0.45% sodium chloride injection, or sterile water for injection, solutions are stable at controlled room temperature for 24 hours. The presence of a light pink to purple color in the diluted solution does not affect the quality of the product.

Rate of Administration

When acetylcysteine is used for the treatment of acetaminophen overdosage, the manufacturer recommends that diluted solutions of the drug be infused IV as a loading dose given over 1 hour, followed by a first maintenance dose given over 4 hours, and then a second maintenance dose given over 16 hours.

Oral Inhalation and Intratracheal Instillation

When used as a mucolytic agent by oral inhalation or intratracheal instillation, the commercially available 20% solution of acetylcysteine may be administered undiluted or may be diluted with sodium chloride injection, sodium chloride inhalation solution, sterile water for injection, or sterile water for inhalation. The 10% solution of acetylcysteine may be used undiluted. Solutions of acetylcysteine do not contain a preservative and care should be taken to minimize contamination of the sterile solution.

The presence of a light purple color in acetylcysteine sodium oral inhalation solutions does not appreciably affect potency of the drug; however, it is best to utilize equipment constructed with plastic or glass and with stainless steel or another nonreactive metal when administering acetylcysteine by nebulization. The manufacturer states that solutions of acetylcysteine sodium are physically and/or chemically incompatible with solutions containing amphotericin B, tetracyclines, erythromycin lactobionate, or ampicillin sodium. When one of these anti-infectives is to be administered by aerosol inhalation, it should be nebulized separately. Acetylcysteine solutions are also physically incompatible with iodized oil, trypsin, chymotrypsin, and hydrogen peroxide. Consult the manufacturer's prescribing information for additional information on the physical and chemical compatibility of acetylcysteine solutions with other drugs.

When acetylcysteine is used as a mucolytic agent, the method of administration depends on the condition being treated and the equipment available. When administered by nebulization, compressed air should be used to provide pressure. Oxygen may also be used but the usual precautions in patients with severe respiratory disease and CO_2 retention should be observed. Ultrasonic nebulizers may also be used to administer acetylcysteine. Hand-bulb nebulizers are not recommended because the output is usually too small and the particle size is often too large. Acetylcysteine may be administered using conventional nebulizers made of plastic or glass; however, certain materials used in nebulization equipment react with acetylcysteine (e.g., iron, copper, rubber), and any part of the equipment that may come in contact with acetylcysteine should be made of glass, plastic, or a metal that does not react with the drug. The nebulized solution may be breathed directly or a plastic face mask, face tent, mouthpiece, oxygen tent, or head tent may be used. Nebulizers may also be fitted to intermittent positive pressure breathing (IPPB) machines. Acetylcysteine solutions should not be placed directly into the chamber of heated (hot-pot) nebulizers. A heated nebulizer may be part of the nebulizer assembly to provide a warm saturated atmosphere if acetylcysteine is introduced by means of a separate unheated nebulizer and the usual precautions for administration of warm saturated nebulae are observed. When acetylcysteine is nebulized continuously with a dry gas, the solution may become

over-concentrated and nebulization may be impaired; after three-fourths of the initial volume has been nebulized, it is advisable to dilute the remaining solution with an approximately equal volume of sterile water for injection. Nebulizing equipment should be cleaned immediately after use since residues may occlude fine orifices or corrode metal parts.

Store the solution at 15–30°C. Store opened vials of undiluted solution in the refrigerator and use within 96 hours. Do not store admixtures.

The manufacturer's labeling should be consulted for detailed information on equipment requirements and recommendations for nebulization of acetylcysteine.

● Dosage

Antidote for Acetaminophen Overdosage

When indicated, initiate acetylcysteine therapy as soon as possible with an IV or oral loading dose in adults and pediatric patients.

Oral

When acetylcysteine is administered orally for the treatment of acetaminophen overdose, a loading dose of 140 mg/kg is recommended in adults and pediatric patients. To complete a full course of therapy, the loading dose is followed by oral maintenance doses of 70 mg/kg every 4 hours for 17 doses. If a patient receiving oral acetylcysteine vomits within 1 hour of administration of a loading or maintenance dose, the dose should be repeated.

IV

Alternatively, acetylcysteine can be administered by IV infusion. Acetylcysteine is administered as a loading dose of 150 mg/kg infused over 1 hour, followed by a first maintenance dose of 50 mg/kg infused over 4 hours, and then a second maintenance dose of 100 mg/kg infused over 16 hours (for a full course consisting of 300 mg/kg administered IV over 21 hours). Dosage of IV acetylcysteine for patients weighing <5 kg or >100 kg has not been studied.

An IV regimen that delivers a total dose of 980 mg/kg over 48 hours† also has been used. This regimen involves IV administration of a loading dose of 140 mg/kg over 1 hour, followed by IV maintenance doses of 70 mg/kg every 4 hours for 12 additional doses. Each maintenance dose is infused over 1 hour.

Mucolytic Uses
Nebulization

When nebulized into a face mask, mouthpiece, or tracheostomy, as in the treatment of bronchopulmonary disease or cystic fibrosis, the usual adult or pediatric dosage of acetylcysteine is 3–5 mL of the 20% solution or 6–10 mL of the 10% solution 3 or 4 times daily; however, 1–10 mL of the 20% solution or 2–20 mL of the 10% solution may be given every 2–6 hours. When a closed tent or croupette is used, maintenance of a heavy mist may require up to 300 mL of the 10 or 20% solution for a single, continuous treatment. The volume of acetylcysteine solution should be sufficient to maintain a very heavy mist in the tent or croupette for the desired period. Administration for intermittent or continuous prolonged periods, including overnight, may be desirable.

Direct Instillation

When acetylcysteine is administered by direct instillation in adults or pediatric patients, 1–2 mL of a 10–20% solution may be given as often as every hour.

Intratracheal Instillation

When acetylcysteine is administered by instillation through a percutaneous intratracheal catheter in adults or pediatric patients, 1–2 mL of the 20% solution or 2–4 mL of the 10% solution may be given every 1–4 hours via a syringe attached to the catheter.

When acetylcysteine is administered by instillation through a catheter into the trachea in adults or pediatric patients, 2–5 mL of the 20% solution may be given via a syringe attached to the catheter.

Diagnostic Bronchial Studies

Prior to diagnostic bronchial studies in adults or pediatric patients, 2 or 3 doses of 1–2 mL of the 20% solution or 2–4 mL of the 10% solution may be administered by nebulization or intratracheal instillation.

Tracheostomy Care

When acetylcysteine is used in adults or pediatric patients for tracheostomy care, 1–2 mL of a 10–20% solution may be instilled into the tracheostomy every 1–4 hours.

Prevention of Contrast Media-induced Nephropathy

For the prevention of nephropathy associated with administration of radiographic contrast media† in adults, an oral acetylcysteine dosage of 600 mg twice daily, given the day before and on the day of the administration of contrast media, has been used, for a total of 4 doses. Other oral dosages have been investigated. IV administration of acetylcysteine also has been investigated.

● Special Populations

Hepatic Impairment

Limited data in subjects with hepatic impairment suggest no clinically meaningful effects of hepatic impairment on acetylcysteine pharmacokinetics. The manufacturers make no specific dosage recommendations for patients with hepatic impairment.

Renal Impairment

The manufacturers make no specific dosage recommendations for patients with renal impairment. Hemodialysis may remove some acetylcysteine.

CAUTIONS

● Contraindications

- Acetylcysteine injection is contraindicated in patients with known hypersensitivity or previous anaphylactoid reaction to acetylcysteine or any ingredient in the formulation.

- Acetylcysteine solution for oral inhalation or intratracheal instillation is contraindicated in patients with known hypersensitivity to the drug.

- When administered orally as an antidote, no contraindications.

● Warnings/Precautions

Encephalopathy Due to Hepatic Failure

If encephalopathy resulting from hepatic failure occurs during oral acetylcysteine therapy, discontinue the drug to avoid further administration of nitrogenous substances. There are no available data indicating that acetylcysteine adversely affects hepatic failure; however, this remains a theoretical possibility.

Respiratory Effects

An increased volume of liquefied bronchial secretions may develop following oral inhalation or intratracheal instillation and the airway may become occluded. If cough is inadequate to maintain an open airway, institute mechanical suction or endotracheal aspiration (with or without bronchoscopy). Observe asthmatic patients closely.

Irritation of the tracheal and bronchial tracts and hemoptysis have occurred following administration of acetylcysteine; however, such findings are not uncommon in patients with bronchopulmonary disease and a causal relationship has not been established.

Chest tightness and bronchoconstriction have been reported with acetylcysteine. Clinically overt acetylcysteine-induced bronchospasm occurs rarely and unpredictably, even in patients with asthmatic bronchitis or bronchitis complicating bronchial asthma. Occasionally, patients receiving oral inhalation of acetylcysteine develop increased airway obstruction of varying and unpredictable severity. Patients who have had such reactions to previous therapy with acetylcysteine may not react during subsequent therapy with the drug, and patients who have had inhalation treatments with acetylcysteine without incident may react to subsequent therapy.

If bronchospasm occurs, give a bronchodilator by nebulization. If bronchospasm progresses, discontinue acetylcysteine immediately.

When administered by IV infusion, use with caution in patients with asthma or history of bronchospasm.

Hypersensitivity Reactions

Serious hypersensitivity reactions (e.g., rash, hypotension, wheezing, dyspnea), including death in a patient with asthma, have been reported in patients receiving IV acetylcysteine.

Acute flushing and erythema also have been reported; these reactions generally occur 30–60 minutes after initiation of the infusion and resolve despite continued infusion. Reactions to acetylcysteine that involve symptoms other than flushing and erythema should be considered anaphylactoid reactions and treated accordingly.

If a severe hypersensitivity reaction occurs during IV acetylcysteine therapy, immediately discontinue IV acetylcysteine and initiate appropriate treatment. If less severe hypersensitivity reactions occur, manage according to the severity; management may include temporary interruption of acetylcysteine infusion and/or administration of antihistamines. Once treatment of the hypersensitivity reaction has been initiated, carefully reinstitute IV acetylcysteine. If the hypersensitivity reaction recurs or increases in severity, discontinue IV acetylcysteine and consider alternative management.

Closely monitor patients with asthma during initiation of and throughout IV acetylcysteine therapy.

Generalized urticaria has been reported rarely in patients receiving oral acetylcysteine for acetaminophen overdosage. If urticaria or other allergic symptoms occur during oral therapy, discontinue the drug unless it is considered essential and allergic symptoms can be otherwise controlled.

Acquired sensitization to acetylcysteine has been reported rarely. Sensitization has not been confirmed by patch testing. Sensitization to acetylcysteine and dermal eruptions have been reported by several inhalation therapists after frequent and extended exposure to the drug.

GI Effects

Oral administration may result in vomiting or may aggravate vomiting associated with acetaminophen overdosage. Administration of dilute acetylcysteine solutions may minimize the tendency of the drug to aggravate vomiting. Acetylcysteine solutions have a slight, disagreeable odor.

Evaluate patients at risk of gastric hemorrhage (e.g., those with esophageal varices or peptic ulcers) with regard to relative risks of upper GI hemorrhage and acetaminophen-induced hepatotoxicity; provide acetylcysteine treatment accordingly.

Fluid Overload

IV administration of acetylcysteine can cause fluid overload, possibly resulting in hyponatremia, seizures, and death. To avoid fluid overload, follow recommendations for dilution and reduce the volume of diluent as needed.

Nebulization Administration Precautions

A slight disagreeable odor that tends to become unnoticeable, and stickiness on the face with use of a face mask (easily removed with water) can occur with administration by nebulization.

An increased concentration of the drug in the nebulizer due to evaporation of the solvent occurs with continued nebulization of acetylcysteine solution with a dry gas. If extreme concentration impedes nebulization and efficient delivery of the drug, dilute the nebulizing solution with appropriate amounts of sterile water for injection as concentration occurs to resolve this problem.

Specific Populations

Pregnancy

Reproductive studies in rabbits using oral acetylcysteine dosages of 500 mg/kg daily (2.6 times the human mucolytic dose) on days 6 through 16 of gestation revealed no teratogenicity. Studies in rabbits exposed for 30–35 minutes twice daily to a nebulized solution containing acetylcysteine and isoproterenol hydrochloride on days 6 through 18 of pregnancy revealed no teratogenicity. Perinatal and postnatal studies in rats exposed to a nebulized solution containing acetylcysteine and isoproterenol did not reveal harm to the fetus or newborns. Acetylcysteine has been reported to cross the placenta in humans following oral or IV administration. However, there are no adequate and controlled studies to date using acetylcysteine in pregnant women, and the drug should be used during pregnancy only when clearly needed.

Limited published case reports and case series of pregnant women exposed to acetylcysteine during various trimesters are not sufficient to inform any drug-associated risk. Delaying treatment of acetaminophen overdose may increase the risk of maternal or fetal morbidity and mortality. Reproduction studies in rats and rabbits following oral administration of acetylcysteine during the period of organogenesis at doses similar to the total IV dose (based on body surface area) did not result in any adverse effects to the fetus.

Lactation

It is not known whether acetylcysteine is distributed into human milk; the drug's effects on the breast-fed infant or on milk production also are not known. Consider the developmental and health benefits of breast-feeding along with the mother's need for acetylcysteine and any potential adverse effects on the breast-fed child from acetylcysteine or from the underlying maternal condition. Use acetylcysteine with caution in nursing women.

Based on pharmacokinetic data, acetylcysteine should be nearly completely cleared 30 hours after IV administration of the drug. Breast-feeding women may consider pumping and discarding their milk for 30 hours after administration.

Pediatric Use

Efficacy of IV acetylcysteine as an antidote for acetaminophen overdosage in pediatric patients appears to be similar to that in adults. Safety and efficacy of IV acetylcysteine in pediatric patients have not been established by adequate and well-controlled studies; use of IV acetylcysteine as an antidote for acetaminophen overdosage in pediatric patients ≥5 kg is based on clinical practice.

Geriatric Use

Insufficient experience with IV acetylcysteine in patients 65 years of age or older in order to determine whether these patients respond differently than younger adults.

● Common Adverse Effects

Common adverse effects following oral administration of acetylcysteine include nausea, vomiting, and other GI symptoms.

Common adverse effects following IV administration of acetylcysteine reported in >2% of patients include rash, urticaria/facial flushing, and pruritus.

Common adverse effects following oral inhalation or intratracheal instillation of acetylcysteine include stomatitis, nausea, vomiting, fever, rhinorrhea, drowsiness, clamminess, chest tightness, and bronchoconstriction.

DRUG INTERACTIONS

● Activated Charcoal

Possible interference with absorption of oral acetylcysteine; however, usual dosage of acetylcysteine is appropriate in patients given activated charcoal (higher dosages not necessary). The manufacturer recommends that if activated charcoal has been administered, lavage should be performed before administering oral acetylcysteine treatment.

DESCRIPTION

The exact mechanism(s) by which acetylcysteine prevents or minimizes acetaminophen-induced hepatotoxicity has not been fully determined. Acetylcysteine may protect the liver following acetaminophen overdosage by maintaining or restoring glutathione levels or by acting as an alternate substrate for conjugation with (and detoxification of) a toxic intermediate metabolite of acetaminophen.

Acetylcysteine reduces the viscosity of purulent and nonpurulent pulmonary secretions and facilitates their removal by coughing, postural drainage, or mechanical means. The mucolytic effect of the drug has been shown to depend on the free sulfhydryl group, which is thought to reduce disulfide linkages of mucoproteins.

The exact mechanism(s) by which acetylcysteine might prevent radiographic contrast media-associated nephrotoxicity is unclear. It has been suggested that since radiographic contrast media-induced renal toxicity may be related to

formation of reactive oxygen species or to reduced antioxidant activity; acetylcysteine, a thiol-containing antioxidant, may reduce the ability of the generated oxygen free radicals to damage cells by acting as an oxygen free-radical scavenger. In addition, the drug also may increase the biologic effects of nitric oxide by combining with the oxide to form *S*-nitrosothiol, a potent vasodilator. The interaction of acetylcysteine and nitric oxide may limit the production of the damaging peroxinitrate radical, because acetylcysteine would compete with the superoxide radical for nitric oxide. Acetylcysteine also increases the expression of nitric oxide synthase and therefore may improve blood flow. Evidence suggesting the possibility that decreases in serum creatinine associated with acetylcystine may occur in the absence of any actual effect on kidney function has been observed.

Following oral administration (e.g., when used as an antidote for acetaminophen overdosage), acetylcysteine is absorbed from the GI tract, with peak plasma concentrations achieved within 1–2 hours. The drug is 50–87% bound to plasma proteins. Acetylcysteine is deacetylated to cysteine and oxidized to yield diacetylcysteine; cysteine is further metabolized to form glutathione and other metabolites. Following oral administration of acetylcysteine, a mean elimination half-life of 6.25 hours has been reported. Following IV administration of acetylcysteine, a mean elimination half-life of 5.6 hours has been reported in adults. Elimination of acetylcysteine is principally (70%) nonrenal. Following IV administration of acetylcysteine in subjects with mild (Child-Pugh class A), moderate (Child-Pugh class B), or severe (Child-Pugh class C) hepatic impairment, mean elimination half-life is increased by 80% compared with normal subjects. Mean clearance is decreased by 30% and systemic exposure increased 1.6-fold in subjects with hepatic impairment compared to subjects with normal hepatic function. These changes are not considered clinically meaningful. Hemodialysis may remove some of total acetylcysteine.

ADVICE TO PATIENTS

- Advise patients and caregivers that hypersensitivity reactions, including hypotension, wheezing, shortness of breath, and bronchospasm, may occur during or after acetylcysteine treatment.

- Advise women to inform their clinician if they are or plan to become pregnant or plan to breast-feed. Breast-feeding women may consider pumping and discarding their milk for 30 hours after administration.

- Advise patients to inform their clinician of existing or contemplated concomitant therapy, including prescription and OTC drugs and dietary or herbal supplements, as well as any concomitant illnesses.

- Inform patients of other important precautionary information.

PREPARATIONS

Excipients in commercially available drug preparations may have clinically important effects in some individuals; consult specific product labeling for details.

Acetylcysteine

Oral-inhalation-intratracheal-install-oral		
Solution	100 mg/mL (10%)*	Acetylcysteine Solution
	200 mg/mL (20%)*	Acetylcysteine Solution
Parenteral		
For injection concentrate, for IV infusion	200 mg/mL	Acetadote®, Cumberland

* available from one or more manufacturer, distributor, and/or repackager by generic (nonproprietary) name

Acetylcysteine Lysine

Oral		
For oral solution	500 mg (of acetylcysteine)	Legubeti®, Galephar
	2.5 g (of acetylcysteine)	Legubeti®, Galephar

† Use is not currently included in the labeling approved by the US Food and Drug Administration.

Glucarpidase

91:04.12 · CHEMOTHERAPY ANTIDOTES/PROTECTANTS

■ Glucarpidase (also known as carboxypeptidase G_2 [$CPDG_2$]) is a recombinant bacterial enzyme that is used as an antidote for methotrexate toxicity.

USES

● Methotrexate Toxicity

Glucarpidase is used as an adjunct to leucovorin rescue for the treatment of toxic plasma methotrexate concentrations (exceeding 0.454 mcg/mL [1 µmol/L]) in patients with delayed methotrexate clearance due to renal impairment. Glucarpidase is designated an orphan drug by the US Food and Drug Administration (FDA) for this use. Because of the potential for subtherapeutic concentrations of methotrexate, glucarpidase should *not* be used in patients who exhibit the expected clearance of methotrexate (plasma methotrexate concentrations within 2 standard deviations of the mean methotrexate excretion curve specific for the methotrexate dose administered) or in those with normal or mildly impaired renal function.

Treatment of methotrexate toxicity traditionally has included leucovorin rescue and supportive measures (IV hydration, urinary alkalinization). However, leucovorin rescue alone does not reduce systemic (i.e., extracellular) methotrexate concentrations and does not completely reverse toxicity when methotrexate concentrations are sustained above 10 µmol/L. Extracorporeal procedures (e.g., hemodialysis) have been used, although such procedures are invasive, have variable efficacy in removing systemic methotrexate, and often are associated with rebound methotrexate concentrations. Because methotrexate is excreted principally by the kidneys, high systemic concentrations of the drug (e.g., following high-dose methotrexate therapy) may cause acute renal impairment in some patients (i.e., by pH-dependent precipitation of methotrexate and its metabolites in renal tubules or by causing direct injury to the renal tubular epithelium); this causes further delay in methotrexate clearance, resulting in subsequent severe systemic toxicities (e.g., myelosuppression, mucositis, hepatotoxicity). Glucarpidase converts circulating methotrexate to inactive metabolites that are primarily eliminated hepatically, thus providing an alternative, nonrenal route for methotrexate elimination in patients with renal impairment.

The current indication for glucarpidase is based principally on data from a subset of 22 treatment-evaluable patients enrolled in a single-arm, open-label study that involved 184 patients with markedly delayed methotrexate clearance (defined as more than 2 standard deviations greater than the mean excretion curve for methotrexate) and toxic plasma methotrexate concentrations (exceeding 0.454 mcg/mL [1 µmol/L]) due to renal impairment. The primary measure of efficacy was the proportion of patients who achieved a rapid and sustained clinically important reduction (RSCIR) in plasma methotrexate concentration (defined as an attainment of plasma methotrexate concentration of 0.454 mcg/mL [1 µmol/L] or less within 15 minutes of glucarpidase administration that was sustained for up to 8 days). The median age of patients was 15.5 years (range: 5–84 years); the most common types of malignancies were osteogenic sarcoma (50%) and leukemia or lymphoma (45%). In this study, all patients received glucarpidase 50 units/kg by IV injection over 5 minutes; a second dose of glucarpidase was administered 48 hours after the initial dose in patients with pre-glucarpidase plasma methotrexate concentrations exceeding 45.4 mcg/mL (100 µmol/L). Patients continued to receive IV hydration, urinary alkalinization, and leucovorin rescue. Following administration of the first dose of glucarpidase, 10 of the 22 patients (45%) achieved RSCIR. Of the remaining 12 patients who failed to achieve RSCIR, 5 patients (23%) achieved a *transient* plasma methotrexate concentration of 0.454 mcg/mL (1 µmol/L) or less; in these 5 patients, the median increase in plasma methotrexate concentration from nadir was 0.636 mcg/mL (1.4 µmol/L). Methotrexate concentrations were reduced by at least 97% within 15 minutes in all 22 patients and were maintained at a greater than 95% reduction for up to 8 days in 20 of the 22 patients. Based on results of exploratory analyses, patients with lower pre-glucarpidase plasma methotrexate concentrations were more likely to achieve RSCIR compared with patients with higher pre-glucarpidase plasma methotrexate concentrations; RSCIR was achieved in 10 of 13 patients (77%) with pre-glucarpidase methotrexate concentrations of 22.7 mcg/mL (50 µmol/L) or less and in 0 of 9 patients (0%) with pre-glucarpidase methotrexate concentrations exceeding 22.7 mcg/mL (50 µmol/L). Despite this observation, all 9 patients with pre-glucarpidase plasma methotrexate concentrations exceeding 22.7 mcg/mL (50 µmol/L) were able to achieve a greater than 95% reduction in plasma methotrexate concentration for up to 8 days following glucarpidase administration.

There currently are no controlled trials comparing efficacy of glucarpidase plus supportive care with supportive care alone in patients with toxic plasma methotrexate concentrations due to renal impairment. Therefore, effects of glucarpidase on survival or on the risk of death associated with methotrexate toxicity have not been established. Glucarpidase did not prevent fatal methotrexate toxicity in 3% of patients receiving the drug in clinical safety studies.

Administration of a second dose of glucarpidase has *not* been shown to provide additional benefit. In the pivotal single-arm, open-label study in which patients with pre-glucarpidase methotrexate concentrations exceeding 45.4 mcg/mL (100 µmol/L) received a second dose of glucarpidase (50 units/kg administered 48 hours after the first dose), RSCIR was not achieved in any patient with pre-second-dose concentrations exceeding 0.454 mcg/mL (1 µmol/L). In other studies, administration of a second dose of glucarpidase did not result in further reduction in plasma methotrexate concentrations. (See Methotrexate Toxicity under Dosage and Administration: Dosage.) This lack of efficacy following the second dose may be due to the presence of high concentrations of the methotrexate inactive metabolite 4-deoxy-4-amino-N^{10}-methylpteroic acid (DAMPA), which inhibits hydrolysis of methotrexate, and/or the presence of antiglucarpidase antibodies. (See Antibody Formation under Cautions: Warnings/Precautions.)

DOSAGE AND ADMINISTRATION

● General

Glucarpidase should be used only in patients who exhibit delayed methotrexate clearance (plasma methotrexate concentrations exceeding 2 standard deviations above the mean methotrexate excretion curve specific for the methotrexate dose administered) due to renal impairment. Early recognition of delayed methotrexate clearance and renal impairment (i.e., an increase in serum creatinine concentration and/or oliguria) and urgent intervention are essential to prevent development of severe methotrexate-induced toxicities.

Glucarpidase should be used in conjunction with leucovorin rescue and supportive measures (i.e., IV hydration, urinary alkalinization with sodium bicarbonate). Because the pharmacokinetics of leucovorin and levoleucovorin are similar, the manufacturer of glucarpidase states that levoleucovorin may be substituted for leucovorin.

● Reconstitution and Administration

Glucarpidase is administered by direct IV injection over 5 minutes. The IV line should be flushed before and after administration of the drug.

Prior to administration, glucarpidase powder for injection should be reconstituted by adding 1 mL of sterile 0.9% sodium chloride for injection to the vial labeled as containing 1000 units of glucarpidase. The contents should be mixed by gently rolling and tilting the vial; the vial should *not* be shaken. The reconstituted solution should be inspected visually and should be discarded if the solution is not clear, colorless, and free of particulate matter. Reconstituted glucarpidase solution may be used immediately or stored at 2–8°C for up to 4 hours; unused portions of the solution should be discarded.

Unreconstituted glucarpidase powder for injection should be stored at 2–8°C and should *not* be frozen.

● Dosage

Dosage of glucarpidase is expressed in terms of units; a unit of glucarpidase activity is defined as the quantity of enzyme needed to catalyze the hydrolysis of 0.454 mcg/mL (1 µmol/L) of methotrexate per minute at 37°C.

Methotrexate Toxicity

The recommended dosage of glucarpidase for the treatment of toxic plasma methotrexate concentrations (exceeding 0.454 mcg/mL [1 μmol/L]) in adults and pediatric patients with delayed methotrexate clearance due to renal impairment is a single IV injection of 50 units/kg.

Following administration of glucarpidase, rescue therapy with leucovorin (or levoleucovorin) should be continued. During the first 48 hours after glucarpidase administration, leucovorin (or levoleucovorin) should be administered at the same dosage administered prior to glucarpidase administration; beyond 48 hours, dosage should be based on the measured methotrexate concentration. (See Drug Interactions: Reduced Folates and also see Leucovorin Calcium 92:12.) Therapy with leucovorin (or levoleucovorin) should be continued until the methotrexate concentration has been maintained below the threshold for such treatment for at least 3 days.

Because of the lack of efficacy observed with the second dose, use of more than one dose of glucarpidase is *not* recommended. (See Uses: Methotrexate Toxicity.)

- ### Special Populations

There are no special population dosage recommendations at this time. (See Specific Populations under Cautions: Warnings/Precautions.)

CAUTIONS

- ### Contraindications

The manufacturer states there are no known contraindications to the use of glucarpidase.

- ### Warnings/Precautions

Sensitivity Reactions

Serious hypersensitivity reactions, including anaphylaxis, may occur. In clinical studies, serious hypersensitivity reactions occurred in less than 1% of patients receiving glucarpidase.

Monitoring of Methotrexate Concentrations and Assay Interference

Glucarpidase converts methotrexate to 4-deoxy-4-amino-N^{10}-methylpteroic acid (DAMPA), an inactive metabolite that interferes with immunoassays and causes an overestimation of plasma methotrexate concentrations. Because of the long half-life of DAMPA (approximately 9 hours), plasma methotrexate concentrations measured by immunoassay within 48 hours following glucarpidase administration are unreliable. Therefore, the manufacturer recommends using a chromatographic method to obtain reliable measurements of plasma methotrexate concentrations within 48 hours following glucarpidase administration.

Continuation of Adjunctive Therapy

Following administration of glucarpidase, rescue therapy with leucovorin (or levoleucovorin) should be continued until the methotrexate concentration has been maintained below the threshold for such treatment for at least 3 days. (See Methotrexate Toxicity under Dosage and Administration: Dosage and also see Drug Interactions: Reduced Folates.) IV hydration and urinary alkalinization should be continued as indicated.

Antibody Formation

Antiglucarpidase antibodies have been detected in 16 of 96 (17%) patients receiving the drug in clinical studies. Antiglucarpidase antibodies were detected between 7 days to 7 months following exposure to glucarpidase. The incidence of antiglucarpidase antibody formation appeared to be similar in patients receiving either 1 or 2 doses of glucarpidase (12 of 78 patients [15%] or 4 of 18 patients [22%], respectively).

The development of antiglucarpidase antibodies is not expected to be clinically important considering the rapid time to maximum pharmacodynamic effect (15 minutes) and the recommended dosage regimen (i.e., single dose).

Specific Populations

Pregnancy

Category C. (See Users Guide.)

Lactation

It is not known whether glucarpidase is distributed into human milk. Caution is advised when glucarpidase is administered in nursing women.

Pediatric Use

Efficacy of glucarpidase as adjunctive therapy for the treatment of toxic plasma methotrexate concentrations (exceeding 0.454 mcg/mL [1 μmol/L]) in pediatric patients with delayed methotrexate clearance due to renal impairment has been established in one study that included 12 patients 5–16 years of age. In this study, 3 of the 6 pediatric patients with pre-glucarpidase plasma methotrexate concentrations of 0.454–22.7 mcg/mL (1–50 μmol/L) achieved rapid and sustained clinically important reductions (RSCIR) in plasma methotrexate concentrations, while none of the remaining 6 patients with pre-glucarpidase plasma methotrexate concentrations exceeding 22.7 mcg/mL (50 μmol/L) achieved RSCIR.

In an analysis of pooled clinical safety data in 147 patients 1 month to 17 years of age, no overall difference in safety was observed between pediatric and adult patients.

Geriatric Use

In clinical studies, 15% of patients were 65 years of age or older and 4% were 75 years of age or older. No overall differences in safety or efficacy were observed between geriatric patients and younger adults.

Hepatic Impairment

Glucarpidase has not been studied in patients with hepatic impairment.

Renal Impairment

Following IV administration of glucarpidase 50 units/kg in 4 patients with severe renal impairment (creatinine clearance less than 30 mL/minute), mean pharmacokinetic parameters of glucarpidase (as assessed by enzymatic assay) were similar to those observed in healthy individuals except for a prolonged half-life (8.2 hours compared with 5.6 hours in healthy individuals).

- ### Common Adverse Effects

Adverse effects reported in 1% or more of patients receiving glucarpidase include paresthesia, flushing, nausea and/or vomiting, hypotension, and headache.

DRUG INTERACTIONS

- ### Reduced Folates

Leucovorin is a substrate of glucarpidase. In patients receiving high-dose methotrexate therapy with leucovorin rescue, administration of glucarpidase 2 hours before a leucovorin dose reduced peak plasma concentrations and area under the plasma concentration-time curve (AUC) of leucovorin by 52 and 33%, respectively, and of its active metabolite (5-methyltetrahydrofolate) by 93 and 92%, respectively. Similar effects would be expected with levoleucovorin. Therefore, leucovorin or levoleucovorin should not be administered within 2 hours before or after glucarpidase administration. During the first 48 hours after glucarpidase administration, dosage adjustment of the continuing leucovorin or levoleucovorin regimen is not necessary since dosage is based on the patient's methotrexate concentration prior to glucarpidase administration. (See Methotrexate Toxicity under Dosage and Administration: Dosage.)

- ### Other Substrates of Glucarpidase

Concomitant use with other drugs that are substrates of glucarpidase (including folic acid antagonists [e.g., pyrimethamine, trimethoprim]) may result in decreased peak plasma concentrations and AUC of the glucarpidase substrate.

DESCRIPTION

Glucarpidase (also known as carboxypeptidase G$_2$ [CPDG$_2$]) is a bacterial enzyme produced by recombinant DNA technology. Glucarpidase was isolated from the *Pseudomonas* strain RS-16 and cloned, purified, and sequenced in genetically modified *Escherichia coli*. Glucarpidase rapidly hydrolyzes the carboxyl-terminal glutamate residue of folic acid, folic acid derivatives, and classic antifolates (e.g., methotrexate, leucovorin); the drug converts methotrexate to its inactive metabolites 4-deoxy-4-amino-N^{10}-methylpteroic acid (DAMPA) and glutamate, which are metabolized principally by the liver. Following administration of glucarpidase (50 units/kg) in the pivotal single-arm, open-label study, plasma methotrexate concentrations (measured by chromatographic method) were reduced by at least 97% within 15 minutes in all 22 treatment-evaluable patients and were maintained at a greater than 95% reduction for up to 8 days in 20 of the 22 patients.

Because of the large molecular size of glucarpidase, the drug is distributed primarily in the intravascular (i.e., extracellular) compartment and does not directly reduce intracellular concentrations (or interfere with intracellular antineoplastic effects) of methotrexate; therefore, rescue therapy with leucovorin must be continued following administration of glucarpidase. (See Methotrexate Toxicity under Dosage and Administration: Dosage and also see Drug Interactions: Reduced Folates.) Reductions in plasma methotrexate concentrations produced by glucarpidase are expected to cause redistribution (i.e., efflux) of intracellular methotrexate back into plasma, resulting in a rise in plasma methotrexate concentrations; as such, small rebound increases in plasma methotrexate concentrations have been observed in patients receiving glucarpidase in clinical studies.

The mean elimination half-life of glucarpidase is 5.6 hours (as assessed by enzymatic assay) or 9 hours (as assessed by enzyme-linked immunosorbent assay [ELISA]).

ADVICE TO PATIENTS

Risk of hypersensitivity reactions, including anaphylaxis.

Risk of infusion reactions. Importance of immediately reporting signs and symptoms of such reactions, including fever, chills, flushing, feeling hot, rash, hives, itching, throat tightness or breathing difficulty, tingling, numbness, or headache.

Importance of continued monitoring of plasma methotrexate concentrations and renal function after discharge from the hospital.

Importance of women informing clinicians if they are or plan to become pregnant or plan to breast-feed.

Importance of informing clinicians of existing or contemplated concomitant therapy, including prescription and OTC drugs, as well as any concomitant illnesses.

Importance of informing patients of other important precautionary information. (See Cautions.)

PREPARATIONS

Excipients in commercially available drug preparations may have clinically important effects in some individuals; consult specific product labeling for details.

Glucarpidase

Parenteral		
For injection, for IV use only	1000 units	**Voraxaze®**, BTG

† Use is not currently included in the labeling approved by the US Food and Drug Administration.

Selected Revisions May 10, 2024, © Copyright, December 13, 2012, American Society of Health-System Pharmacists, Inc.

Leucovorin Calcium

91:04.12 • CHEMOTHERAPY ANTIDOTES/PROTECTANTS

■ Leucovorin calcium is the calcium salt of folinic acid, an active metabolite of folic acid.

USES

● Prevention and Treatment of Toxicity Associated with Folic Acid Antagonists

Leucovorin is used as an antidote to diminish the toxicity and counteract the effect of unintentional overdosage of folic acid antagonists, such as methotrexate, trimethoprim, and pyrimethamine. Leucovorin also is used in conjunction with these folic acid antagonists for the prevention and treatment of undesired hematopoietic effects of the drugs. When used in the treatment of accidental overdosage of folic acid antagonists, leucovorin therapy should be initiated as soon as possible since the effectiveness of leucovorin in counteracting hematologic toxicity diminishes as the time period between antifolate (e.g., methotrexate) administration and leucovorin rescue increases.

Methotrexate Toxicity

Leucovorin rescue has been administered in conjunction with high-dose methotrexate therapy in an effort to control the duration of exposure of sensitive cells to methotrexate. This regimen has been more effective than methotrexate alone in inducing and maintaining remissions in osteogenic sarcoma, head and neck cancer, refractory acute leukemia, and lung carcinoma; the superiority of this combination in other neoplastic diseases has not been demonstrated. Generally, leucovorin should not be administered simultaneously with systemic methotrexate because the therapeutic effect as well as the toxicity of the antimetabolite may be nullified; however, leucovorin can generally be administered 6–24 hours after methotrexate infusion. When methotrexate is administered by intra-arterial (regional perfusion) or intrathecal injection, leucovorin can be given IM, IV, or orally concomitantly to offset systemic methotrexate toxicity without abolishing the local activity of the antineoplastic drug.

Leucovorin has been used in conjunction with methotrexate in the treatment of psoriasis; however, results have been conflicting. Some investigators reported small doses of leucovorin increased the number, size, and activity of psoriasiform lesions when administered orally 24–72 hours after oral methotrexate. Other investigators have found leucovorin to decrease the adverse effects of methotrexate without decreasing the effects of the antimetabolite when leucovorin was administered IM 2 hours after IM methotrexate.

Trimetrexate Glucuronate Toxicity

Leucovorin is administered concomitantly with trimetrexate glucuronate and continued for 72 hours after the last dose to prevent potentially serious or life-threatening toxicities (e.g., bone marrow suppression) associated with the drug.

Pyrimethamine Toxicity

Protozoa are unable to utilize leucovorin, apparently because they require *p*-aminobenzoic acid (PABA) for biosynthesis of an active cofactor. For this reason, therapeutic doses of leucovorin have been administered at the same time as pyrimethamine to decrease the hematologic toxicity of pyrimethamine in the treatment of toxoplasmosis, *Pneumocystis carinii* pneumonia, or *Plasmodium falciparum* malaria, without nullifying the effect of pyrimethamine on the parasite.

Trimethoprim Toxicity

Leucovorin has been used to antagonize the hematologic toxicity of trimethoprim without interfering with the drug's antibacterial effectiveness.

● Megaloblastic Anemia

Leucovorin is used in the treatment of folate deficient megaloblastic anemias of infancy, pregnancy, sprue, and nutritional deficiencies when oral folic acid therapy is not feasible. However, since the ability to convert folic acid to tetrahydrofolic acid is not impaired in these anemias, leucovorin has no advantage over folic acid injection.

In contrast to folic acid, leucovorin is also effective in the treatment of megaloblastic anemia produced by congenital dihydrofolate reductase deficiency. Leucovorin is *not* effective in and should not be used for the treatment of pernicious anemia and other megaloblastic anemias secondary to lack of vitamin B_{12}. (See Cautions: Precautions and Contraindications.)

● Combined Therapy with Fluorouracil for Advanced Colorectal Carcinoma

Leucovorin calcium is used to potentiate the antineoplastic activity of, and thus improve response to, fluorouracil in the palliative treatment of advanced colorectal carcinoma. Leucovorin calcium is designated an orphan drug by the US Food and Drug Administration (FDA) for such use. Such combined therapy is employed in an attempt to prolong survival relative to fluorouracil alone in patients with advanced disease. In vitro studies and clinical evidence have shown that the cytotoxicity of fluorouracil may be enhanced by leucovorin; it appears that elevated intracellular concentrations of reduced folates (e.g., leucovorin) may stabilize the covalent ternary complex formed by fluorodeoxyuridylic acid, 5,10-methylenetetrahydrofolate, and thymidylate synthase, enhancing inhibition of this enzyme and thereby increasing the efficacy of fluorouracil.

Analysis of pooled data from several randomized studies in patients with advanced colorectal carcinoma indicates that combined therapy with IV fluorouracil and IV leucovorin calcium produces higher objective response rates (i.e., tumor responses) than does IV fluorouracil alone. However, despite the superiority in objective tumor response with combined therapy, overall survival rates were not improved appreciably compared with fluorouracil alone. In this analysis, overall objective response rates were about 23% for combined fluorouracil and leucovorin therapy and 11% for fluorouracil alone, with only 3 and 2.6%, respectively, exhibiting complete responses; median durations of survival were 11.5 months for combined therapy and 11 months for fluorouracil alone. It remains unclear why the higher response rate did not result in improved survival with combination therapy. It was suggested that the low rates of response, particularly complete responses, for such advanced disease observed both in patients receiving combined therapy and in those receiving monotherapy may have been insufficient to affect overall survival. In addition, the large number of nonresponders to fluorouracil alone who subsequently received combined therapy may have obscured any potential difference in survival; however, a survival benefit also was not apparent when trials with crossovers were excluded. While it remains to be established, the possibility exists that survival differences may be more apparent with less advanced stages of disease.

Combination therapy in randomized studies in patients with advanced colorectal carcinoma consisted of regimens in which courses of IV fluorouracil and IV leucovorin calcium therapy were repeated at approximately monthly intervals and those in which courses were repeated weekly. The approximately monthly regimens included 5-day courses of fluorouracil 370 mg/m^2 and leucovorin calcium 200 or 500 mg/m^2 daily, fluorouracil 425 mg/m^2 and leucovorin calcium 20 mg/m^2 daily, or fluorouracil 400 mg/m^2 and leucovorin calcium 200 mg/m^2 daily, repeated at intervals of 4–5 weeks. Weekly dosage schedules of the combination included 600 mg/m^2 of fluorouracil and 25, 200, or 500 mg/m^2 of leucovorin administered once weekly, usually for 6 weeks. Fluorouracil alone was administered in various dosage regimens, including 5-day courses of 370, 400, or 500 mg/m^2 or 13.5 mg/kg daily, repeated at intervals of 4–5 weeks. Other dosage regimens of IV fluorouracil without leucovorin (i.e., fluorouracil 12 mg/kg daily for 5 days [total daily dosage did not exceed 800 mg] followed by fluorouracil 15 mg/kg once weekly, with dosage being increased by 10% weekly until dose-limiting toxicity or the desired degree of myelosuppression occurred) or 600 mg every 7 days also were used.

While analysis of almost all individual randomized studies in patients with advanced disease also failed to reveal a survival benefit, a tendency toward improved survival was observed with combined fluorouracil and leucovorin therapy in a few of these studies; however, this tendency may be lost with continued follow-up. In one study (the NCCTG/Mayo Clinic Trial) in which patients were followed for a median of 21 months (range: 14—41 months), improved survival was associated with combined regimens of fluorouracil and either high- (200 mg/m^2 daily for 5 days) or low- (20 mg/m^2 daily for 5 days) dose leucovorin; however, the survival benefit was limited to those with nonmeasurable disease. In this study, no advantage was apparent for the high-dose leucovorin regimen, but study and analysis of possible dose-response differences are continuing.

IV fluorouracil also has been used in combination with orally administered leucovorin in a limited number of patients with advanced colorectal carcinoma.

The combination of fluorouracil and leucovorin with methotrexate or cisplatin also is being studied in the treatment of advanced colorectal carcinoma. In patients with advanced colorectal carcinoma, combined therapy with fluorouracil and leucovorin was associated with higher objective response rates and longer median durations of survival than therapy with sequential methotrexate, fluorouracil, and leucovorin; objective response rates were 31–33% and median durations of survival were 402–418 days in patients receiving combined therapy with fluorouracil and leucovorin compared with objective response rates of 4% and a median duration of survival of 223 days in patients receiving sequential methotrexate, fluorouracil, and leucovorin therapy.

In addition to possible therapeutic potentiation, leucovorin may potentiate the risk of fluorouracil-induced toxicity (especially GI toxicity, including diarrhea, nausea, stomatitis, and vomiting, and, to a lesser degree, myelosuppression). A syndrome characterized by progression from mild to severe GI symptoms and rarely to potentially fatal enterocolitis has been reported in several studies of patients with advanced colorectal carcinoma receiving combined therapy with the drugs; in these studies, adverse GI effects (e.g., severe diarrhea, stomatitis) were the dose-limiting toxicity. (See Cautions: GI Effects, in Fluorouracil 10:00). Limited data suggest that once-weekly administration of fluorouracil plus leucovorin may be associated with a higher risk of developing serious adverse GI effects than 5-day regimens administered at approximately monthly intervals. Severe diarrhea appears to be the dose-limiting toxicity associated with once-weekly administration of the combination, while diarrhea and/or mucositis appear to be the dose-limiting toxicities associated with the 5-day regimens. Combined therapy with fluorouracil and leucovorin should *not* be initiated or continued in patients with symptomatic GI toxicity until such symptoms have completely resolved. Close monitoring is particularly important in patients who develop diarrhea with such combined therapy since rapid clinical deterioration and death can occur. Death secondary to severe enterocolitis, diarrhea, and dehydration has occurred in geriatric patients receiving the combination.

DOSAGE AND ADMINISTRATION

● *Reconstitution and Administration*

Leucovorin calcium is administered orally or by IM or IV injection. The drug should be given parenterally rather than orally in patients with GI toxicity, nausea, or vomiting and when individual doses greater than 25 mg are to be administered. Parenteral administration generally is preferred when leucovorin is administered following chemotherapy with a folic acid antagonist and there is a possibility that the patient may vomit and not absorb oral leucovorin. Leucovorin calcium should *not* be administered intrathecally.

Leucovorin calcium powder for injection should be reconstituted by adding 5 or 10 mL of sterile water for injection or bacteriostatic water for injection containing benzyl alcohol to a vial labeled as containing 50 or 100 mg of leucovorin, respectively; the resultant solutions contain 10 mg/mL. Leucovorin calcium vials of the powder for injection labeled as containing 350 mg of leucovorin should be reconstituted by adding 17 mL of sterile water for injection or bacteriostatic water for injection containing benzyl alcohol to the vial; the resultant solution contains 20 mg/mL. When parenteral doses greater than 10 mg/m² are necessary, leucovorin calcium powder for injection reconstituted with sterile water for injection should be used; leucovorin calcium powder for injection reconstituted with bacteriostatic water containing benzyl alcohol should be used only when parenteral doses of 10 mg/m² or lower are required. Since parenteral leucovorin calcium doses exceeding 10 mg/m² are used in combination with fluorouracil for the treatment of advanced colorectal carcinoma, leucovorin calcium *powder for injection* (reconstituted with *sterile water for injection*) should be used for this indication. When leucovorin is administered by IV infusion, the infusion rate should not exceed 16 mL (160 mg of leucovorin) per minute because of the calcium concentration of the solution.

● *Dosage*

Dosage of leucovorin calcium is expressed in terms of leucovorin.

Prevention and Treatment of Hematologic Toxicity Associated with Folic Acid Antagonists

As an antidote for inadvertent overdosage of folic acid antagonists, the manufacturers recommend that leucovorin be administered IM or IV in amounts equal to the weight of the antagonist given, as soon as the overdosage is detected and preferably within the first hour. When large doses or overdoses of methotrexate are given, leucovorin can be administered by IV infusion in doses up to 75 mg within 12 hours, followed by 12 mg IM every 6 hours for 4 doses. When average doses of methotrexate appear to have an adverse effect, 6–12 mg of leucovorin may be given IM every 6 hours for 4 doses. Prompt administration of leucovorin calcium is essential.

Methotrexate Toxicity

As part of a high-dose methotrexate regimen in cancer chemotherapy, leucovorin rescue therapy must begin within 24 hours of methotrexate administration. Dosage of leucovorin is approximately twice that of levoleucovorin (the active levorotatory [*l*] isomer). (See Levoleucovorin Calcium 92:12.)

The manufacturers of leucovorin calcium state that a typical leucovorin rescue dosage schedule is 10 mg/m² usually administered parenterally followed by 10 mg/m² orally (if there is adequate GI function) every 6 hours until the serum methotrexate concentration has declined to less than 10^{-8} M. If at 24 hours following methotrexate administration the patient's serum creatinine has increased to 50% or more above the serum creatinine prior to methotrexate or the serum methotrexate concentration is greater than 5×10^{-6} M, or if at 48 hours following methotrexate administration the serum methotrexate concentration is greater than 9×10^{-7} M, leucovorin dosage should be increased immediately to 100 mg/m² every 3 hours until the serum methotrexate concentration is less than 10^{-8} M. Use of high-dose methotrexate and leucovorin rescue therapy in treating certain cancers is an evolving science, and the optimum dosage and sequence of methotrexate and leucovorin calcium have not been established. Patients should not be given such therapy unless a specific formal protocol is being followed; the clinician should consult published protocols for the dosage of leucovorin calcium and the duration of methotrexate therapy before leucovorin calcium is administered.

In one study utilizing methotrexate in the treatment of psoriasis, the toxic effects of methotrexate were usually overcome by 4–8 mg of leucovorin administered IM 2 hours after IM methotrexate.

Trimetrexate Glucuronate Toxicity

The usual leucovorin dosage for the prevention of potentially serious and life-threatening toxicities in immunocompromised patients receiving trimetrexate glucuronate for the treatment of *Pneumocystis carinii* pneumonia is 20 mg/m² every 6 hours (total daily dose of 80 mg/m²). Leucovorin may be administered orally or IV (over 5–10 minutes) in these patients; if leucovorin is administered orally, the calculated dose should be rounded up to the next 25-mg increment. Leucovorin should be continued for at least 72 hours after the last trimetrexate dose. For the treatment of moderate to severe *Pneumocystis carinii* pneumonia in adults, the usual dosage of trimetrexate is 45 mg/m² given once daily. The recommended course of trimetrexate therapy is 21 days and that of leucovorin is 24 days.

Dosage of trimetrexate and leucovorin must be adjusted according to the hematologic tolerance of the patient. For patients with neutrophil counts exceeding 1000/ mm³ and platelet counts exceeding 75,000/ mm³ (grade 1 toxicity), the usual dosages of trimetrexate and leucovorin can be used. For those with neutrophil counts of 750–1000/ mm³ and platelet counts of 50,000–75,000/ mm³ (grade 2 toxicity), the usual trimetrexate dosage should be used but leucovorin dosage should be increased to 40 mg/m² every 6 hours. Trimetrexate dosage should be reduced to 22 mg/ mm² once daily and leucovorin dosage should be increased to 40 mg/m² every 6 hours for neutrophil and platelet counts of 500–749 and 25,000–49,999 per mm³ (grade 3 toxicity), respectively. When using these dosage guidelines, dosage should be modified based on the *worst* of the two blood cell counts. For patients with lower neutrophil or platelet counts (grade 4 toxicity), leucovorin dosage should be increased to 40 mg/m² every 6 hours, and trimetrexate therapy should be discontinued if such changes occur prior to day 10 of therapy, continuing the higher dosage of leucovorin for an additional 72 hours. If such low counts develop during days 10–21 of trimetrexate therapy, the drug may be withheld up to 96 hours to permit recovery of the blood count(s) to a minimum of grade 3 toxicity before reinstituting trimetrexate; dosage should be adjusted according to the grade of hematologic toxicity achieved at the time of recovery. If hematologic toxicity does not improve to a minimum of grade 3 toxicity after 96 hours, trimetrexate therapy should be discontinued; leucovorin should be continued at the higher dosage for 72 hours after the last dose of trimetrexate.

Pyrimethamine Toxicity

The dosage of leucovorin necessary to prevent hematologic toxicity associated with pyrimethamine varies depending on the dosage of the folic acid antagonist and the clinical status of the patient.

In adults or children receiving pyrimethamine in a dosage of 25–100 mg daily or 1–2 mg/kg daily for the *treatment* of toxoplasmosis, some clinicians suggest that 10–25 mg of leucovorin be administered with each dose of pyrimethamine.

When a regimen containing pyrimethamine (50 or 75 mg once weekly) and dapsone is used for the prevention of initial episodes (*primary prophylaxis*) of *P. carinii* pneumonia or *Toxoplasma gondii* infections or prevention of recurrence (*chronic maintenance therapy of secondary prophylaxis*) of *P. carinii* pneumonia in adults or adolescents with human immunodeficiency virus (HIV) infection, some clinicians recommend that oral leucovorin be administered concomitantly in a dosage of 25 mg once weekly. If adults or adolescents are receiving a regimen that contains a higher dosage of pyrimethamine (25–50 mg once daily) with clindamycin or sulfadiazine for *secondary prophylaxis* of toxoplasmosis, the dosage of leucovorin necessary to prevent hematologic toxicity may range from 10–25 mg once daily. When a regimen containing pyrimethamine 25 mg once daily and atovaquone is used for *primary* or *secondary* prophylaxis against toxoplasmosis in adults and adolescents with HIV infection, some clinicians recommend that oral leucovorin be administered concomitantly in a dosage of 10 mg daily.

In HIV-infected children receiving a regimen that contains pyrimethamine (1 mg/kg once daily) with dapsone or clindamycin for *primary or secondary prophylaxis*, respectively, of toxoplasmosis, some clinicians recommend a leucovorin dosage of 5 mg once every 3 days.

Megaloblastic Anemia

In the treatment of folate deficient megaloblastic anemias, up to 1 mg of leucovorin may be given IM daily. Although doses of 10 mg daily have been recommended in the past, the manufacturers state there is no evidence that IM doses greater than 1 mg daily are more effective. The duration of leucovorin therapy for megaloblastic anemia depends on the hematologic response to the drug, as evidenced in both peripheral blood and bone marrow. In general, patient response to therapy depends on the degree and nature of the folate deficiency, but once proper corrective measures are undertaken, deficient patients will generally respond rapidly. During the first 24 hours of treatment, the patient experiences an improved sense of well-being; the bone marrow begins to become normoblastic within 48 hours. Reticulocytosis generally begins within 2–5 days after the start of therapy.

In the treatment of megaloblastic anemia resulting from a congenital deficiency of dihydrofolate reductase, 3–6 mg of leucovorin has been given IM daily.

Combined Therapy with Fluorouracil for Advanced Colorectal Carcinoma

For potentiation of the antineoplastic effects of fluorouracil in the palliative treatment of advanced colorectal carcinoma, optimum dosage of leucovorin has not been clearly established. Current evidence indicates that an IV leucovorin dose of 20 mg/m² followed by an IV fluorouracil dose of 425 mg/m² can be used. Alternatively, a leucovorin dose of 200 mg/m² administered by slow IV injection (over a minimum of 3 minutes) followed by an IV fluorouracil dose of 370 mg/m² can be used, but there currently is no evidence of superiority with this leucovorin dosage. Either selected regimen is administered daily for 5 days and may be repeated at 4-week intervals for 2 additional courses; thereafter, the regimen may be repeated at intervals of 4–5 weeks provided toxicity from the previous course of combined therapy has subsided. Dosage of fluorouracil in subsequent courses of therapy should be adjusted according to patient tolerance of the prior treatment course; dosage of leucovorin in subsequent courses generally is not adjusted according to toxicity. Daily fluorouracil dosage generally is reduced by 20% in patients who experienced moderate hematologic or GI toxicity in the prior course and by 30% in those patients who experienced severe toxicity. If no toxicity occurs,

fluorouracil dosage may be increased by 10%. Other combination dosage regimens also have been used. (See Uses: Combined Therapy with Fluorouracil for Advanced Colorectal Carcinoma.)

CAUTIONS

● Adverse Effects

Leucovorin appears to be nontoxic in therapeutic doses, although thrombocytosis has been reported in patients receiving leucovorin during intra-arterial infusion of methotrexate. In addition, hypersensitivity reactions, including anaphylactoid reactions and urticaria, have been reported with both oral and parenteral use of leucovorin. While leucovorin can potentiate the toxic effects of fluorouracil, potentially resulting in increased severity and frequency of certain effects, the observed toxicity is that generally associated with fluorouracil. (See Uses: Combined Therapy with Fluorouracil for Advanced Colorectal Carcinoma and also see the Cautions section in the monograph on Fluorouracil 10:00.)

● Precautions and Contraindications

Since allergic reactions have been reported following oral and parenteral administration of folic acid, the possibility of allergic reactions to leucovorin should be considered.

There is a potential danger in administering leucovorin to patients with undiagnosed anemia, as leucovorin may obscure the diagnosis of pernicious anemia by alleviating hematologic manifestations of the disease while allowing neurologic complications to progress. This may result in severe nervous system damage before the correct diagnosis is made. Adequate doses of vitamin B₁₂ may prevent, halt, or improve neurologic changes caused by pernicious anemia.

When leucovorin rescue is used in conjunction with high-dose methotrexate therapy, the drugs should be administered only by physicians experienced in cancer chemotherapy, in centers where facilities for measuring blood methotrexate concentrations are available. Leucovorin is usually effective in counteracting severe methotrexate toxicity in these regimens, but toxic reactions to methotrexate may occur despite leucovorin therapy, especially when the half-life of methotrexate is increased (e.g., renal dysfunction). Therefore, it is extremely important that leucovorin be administered until the blood concentration of methotrexate declines to nontoxic concentrations.

Since leucovorin calcium enhances the toxicity of fluorouracil, adjunctive therapy with leucovorin calcium and fluorouracil should be given only by, or under the supervision of, physicians experienced in cancer chemotherapy and in the use of antimetabolites. Hematologic indices (complete blood cell counts with differential, and quantitative platelet count) should be performed before each course of therapy with fluorouracil and leucovorin and repeated weekly during the first 2 courses of therapy and once during each subsequent course of therapy (when anticipated leukocyte nadir occurs). Determinations of serum electrolyte concentrations and liver function tests should be performed before each course of therapy for the first 3 courses of therapy and then prior to each other course of therapy. Dosage of fluorouracil should be reduced in patients who experienced moderate or severe hematologic or GI toxicity. (See Dosage and Administration: Dosage.) Therapy should be interrupted until the leukocyte count is 4000/mm³ and the platelet count is 130,000/mm³. If these counts do not increase to these levels within 2 weeks, therapy should be discontinued. Patients should be followed up with physical examinations before each course of therapy, and appropriate radiographic examinations should be performed as needed. Therapy should be discontinued if there is clear evidence of tumor progression.

There is some evidence to suggest that the risk of fluorouracil-induced GI toxicity may be increased in patients receiving leucovorin concomitantly with the drug. Death secondary to severe enterocolitis, diarrhea, and dehydration has occurred in geriatric patients receiving the drugs concomitantly. Concomitant granulocytopenia and fever were present in some but not all cases. (See Cautions: GI Effects, in Fluorouracil 10:00.) Combined leucovorin and fluorouracil therapy should be used with extreme caution in geriatric or debilitated patients since such patients are more likely to develop serious toxicity from fluorouracil.

• Pregnancy, Fertility, and Lactation

Pregnancy

Animal reproduction studies have not been performed with leucovorin. It is also not known whether leucovorin can cause fetal harm when administered to pregnant women. Leucovorin should be used during pregnancy only when clearly needed.

Lactation

Since it is not known if leucovorin is distributed into milk, the drug should be used with caution in nursing women.

PHARMACOLOGY

Leucovorin is a derivative of tetrahydrofolic acid, the reduced form of folic acid, which is involved as a cofactor for 1-carbon transfer reactions in the biosynthesis of purines and pyrimidines of nucleic acids. Impairment of thymidylate synthesis in patients with folic acid deficiency is thought to account for the defective DNA synthesis that leads to megaloblast formation and megaloblastic and macrocytic anemias. Because of its ready conversion to other tetrahydrofolic acid derivatives, leucovorin is a potent antidote for both the hematopoietic and reticuloendothelial toxic effects of folic acid antagonists (e.g., methotrexate, pyrimethamine, trimethoprim). It is postulated that in some cancers leucovorin enters and "rescues" normal cells from the toxic effects of folic acid antagonists, in preference to tumor cells, because of a difference in membrane transport mechanisms; this principle is the basis of high-dose methotrexate therapy with "leucovorin rescue."

PHARMACOKINETICS

• Absorption and Distribution

In vivo, leucovorin calcium is rapidly and extensively converted to other tetrahydrofolic acid derivatives including 5-methyl tetrahydrofolate, which is the major transport and storage form of folate in the body.

Normal total serum folate concentrations have been reported to range from 0.005–0.015 mcg/mL. Folate is actively concentrated in CSF, and normal CSF concentrations are reported to be about 0.016–0.021 mcg/mL. Normal erythrocyte folate concentrations range from 0.175–0.316 mcg/mL. In general, serum folate concentrations less than 0.005 mcg/mL indicate folate deficiency and concentrations less than 0.002 mcg/mL usually result in megaloblastic anemia. Following IM administration of a 15-mg (7.5 mg/m²) dose in healthy men, mean peak serum folate concentrations of 0.241 mcg/mL occur within about 40 minutes. Following oral administration of a 15-mg (7.5 mg/m²) dose in healthy men, mean peak serum folate concentrations of 0.268 mcg/mL occur within about 1.72 hours. Areas under the serum folate concentration-time curves (AUCs) are reported to be about 8% less following IM injection in the gluteal region than in the deltoid region and about 12% less following IM injection in the gluteal region than following IV or oral administration.

Tetrahydrofolic acid and its derivatives are distributed to all body tissues; the liver contains about one-half of total body folate stores. In a small number of patients, biliary concentration of folates was about 4.5 times the plasma folate concentration after oral administration of a 2-mg dose of leucovorin; this is believed to represent the hepatic folate pool rather than excretion of the administered dose.

• Elimination

Leucovorin is excreted in urine, mainly as 10-formyl tetrahydrofolate and 5,10-methenyl tetrahydrofolate. There is some evidence that 5-methyl tetrahydrofolate may be conserved by the kidneys in preference to 5-formyl tetrahydrofolate (leucovorin). Loss of folate in the urine becomes approximately logarithmic as the amount of leucovorin administered exceeds 1 mg.

CHEMISTRY AND STABILITY

• Chemistry

Leucovorin calcium is the calcium salt of folinic acid, an active metabolite of folic acid. Leucovorin consists of equal amounts of d- and l-isomers; the l-isomer (levoleucovorin) is the pharmacologically active isomer. (See Levoleucovorin Calcium 92:12.) Leucovorin calcium occurs as a yellowish white or yellow, odorless powder and has solubilities of more than 500 mg/mL in water and less than 1 mg/mL in alcohol. The pK$_a$s of leucovorin are 3.1, 4.8, and 10.4.

• Stability

Leucovorin calcium powder for injection and tablets should be stored at 15–30°C and protected from light.

When leucovorin calcium powder for injection is reconstituted as directed, resultant solutions should be used immediately when reconstituted with sterile water for injection or within 7 days when reconstituted with bacteriostatic water for injection containing benzyl alcohol.

Leucovorin calcium solutions that have been admixed with 10% dextrose injection, 10% dextrose and 0.9% sodium chloride injection, Ringer's injection, or lactated Ringer's injection are stable for 24 hours when stored at room temperature protected from light. Although some former manufacturers of leucovorin calcium powder for injection have recommended that reconstituted solutions of the drug be protected from light, there is evidence that solutions of the drug are not adversely affected by exposure to room light. Reconstituted solutions of leucovorin calcium that have been further diluted with 50 mL of 5% dextrose injection and stored in Viaflex® or glass containers unprotected from light retain at least 90% potency for 24 hours at room temperature.

PREPARATIONS

Excipients in commercially available drug preparations may have clinically important effects in some individuals; consult specific product labeling for details.

Leucovorin Calcium

Oral		
Tablets	5 mg (of leucovorin)*	Leucovorin Calcium Tablets (scored)
	10 mg (of leucovorin)*	Leucovorin Calcium Tablets (scored)
	15 mg (of leucovorin)*	Leucovorin Calcium Tablets (scored)
	25 mg (of leucovorin)*	Leucovorin Calcium Tablets (scored)
Parenteral		
For injection	50 mg (of leucovorin)*	Leucovorin Calcium for Injection
	100 mg (of leucovorin)*	Leucovorin Calcium for Injection
	200 mg (of leucovorin)*	Leucovorin Calcium for Injection (preservative-free)
	350 mg (of leucovorin)*	Leucovorin Calcium for Injection
	500 mg (of leucovorin)*	Leucovorin Calcium for Injection (preservative-free)
Injection	10 mg (of leucovorin) per mL (500 mg)*	Leucovorin Calcium Injection (preservative-free)

* available from one or more manufacturer, distributor, and/or repackager by generic (nonproprietary) name

† Use is not currently included in the labeling approved by the US Food and Drug Administration.

LEVOleucovorin Calcium

91:04.12 • CHEMOTHERAPY ANTIDOTES/PROTECTANTS

■ Levoleucovorin calcium, the levorotatory (*l*) isomer of racemic *d,l*-leucovorin, is one of several active, chemically reduced derivatives of folic acid.

USES

● Toxicity Associated with Folic Acid Antagonists

Levoleucovorin calcium rescue is used after high-dose methotrexate therapy (to control the duration of exposure of sensitive cells to methotrexate for treatment of osteosarcoma. Levoleucovorin also is used as an antidote to diminish the toxicity and counteract the effects of unintentional overdosage of methotrexate (e.g., resulting from impaired elimination) and other folic acid antagonists. Levoleucovorin is designated an orphan drug by the US Food and Drug Administration (FDA) for these uses.

Safety and efficacy of levoleucovorin rescue were evaluated in an analysis of data from 2 open-label studies and other unpublished trials in a limited number of patients (6–21 years of age) with osteogenic sarcoma. Of the 16 patients evaluated, 13 received levoleucovorin 7.5 mg every 6 hours for 60 hours or longer beginning 24 hours after completion of methotrexate (12 g/m^2 IV over 4 hours), and 3 received levoleucovorin 7.5 mg every 3 hours for 18 doses beginning 12 hours after completion of methotrexate (12.5 g/m^2 IV over 6 hours). Patients received a mean of 18.2 doses of levoleucovorin and a mean total dose of 350 mg per methotrexate course. Efficacy of levoleucovorin was determined by comparing its ability to prevent methotrexate-related toxicity with that of racemic leucovorin. In the first open-label study, 3 patients receiving a total of 22 courses of levoleucovorin following high-dose methotrexate therapy experienced fewer serious adverse events (0% of the 22 courses) compared with 6 historical control patients receiving a total of 24 courses of racemic leucovorin (10% of the 24 courses). In the second open-label study in which 15 patients received a total of 90 courses of levoleucovorin, severe adverse events were reported in 4% of the 90 courses. However, it should be noted that interpretation of these results is limited by the statistical limitations of the studies (e.g., small sample size, reliance on retrospective review of records for historical control data).

Although levoleucovorin may ameliorate the hematologic toxicity associated with high-dose methotrexate, the drug has no effect on other established toxicities of methotrexate such as the nephrotoxicity resulting from drug and/or metabolite precipitation in the kidney.

● Colorectal Cancer

Combined Therapy with Fluorouracil for Advanced-stage Colorectal Cancer

Levoleucovorin calcium is used in combination with fluorouracil for the palliative treatment of advanced-stage colorectal cancer. Use of levoleucovorin calcium in combination with fluorouracil and other agents (i.e., irinotecan, oxaliplatin)† also has been studied for the treatment of advanced-stage colorectal cancer†; however, use of levoleucovorin in regimens containing fluorouracil and either irinotecan or oxaliplatin currently is not fully established for this indication because of inadequate data and/or experience.

Levoleucovorin and Fluorouracil

The current indication for use of levoleucovorin in combination with fluorouracil for the palliative treatment of advanced-stage colorectal cancer is based principally on the results of a phase 3, open-label, randomized study. In this study, 926 patients with advanced-stage (i.e., unresectable) colorectal cancer were randomized to receive levoleucovorin 100 mg/m^2 by IV injection, racemic leucovorin 125 mg/m^2 orally at 1-hour intervals for 4 doses, or racemic leucovorin 200 mg/m^2 by IV injection; fluorouracil (370 mg/m^2 given as an IV injection) was administered immediately following the IV dose of leucovorin or levoleucovorin or 1 hour after the fourth oral dose of leucovorin. The drugs were administered daily on days 1–5 of the treatment cycle, with dosages adjusted as needed based on

toxicity and response; treatment cycles were repeated at 4 and 8 weeks and every 5 weeks thereafter until disease progression or unacceptable toxicity occurred. Overall response rates for the 3 groups did not differ significantly; 1-year survival was approximately 40% for all treatment groups. There were no substantial differences in toxicity between levoleucovorin and racemic leucovorin when used in conjunction with fluorouracil.

In a second phase 3, open-label, randomized trial in 248 patients with metastatic and/or recurrent colorectal cancer, levoleucovorin was compared with racemic leucovorin to determine if a twofold increase in leucovorin dosage (given as levoleucovorin) would result in differences in overall response rate, toxicity, and survival. Patients received either levoleucovorin (100 mg/m^2) or racemic leucovorin (100 mg/m^2) by IV injection, followed immediately by fluorouracil (400 mg/m^2 as a 2-hour IV infusion), on days 1–5 of each 4-week treatment cycle, with dosages adjusted as needed based on toxicity and response. A slight improvement in overall response rate was reported for levoleucovorin/fluorouracil compared with racemic leucovorin/fluorouracil; the overall response rate was 32% (5% complete and 27% partial responses) for patients receiving levoleucovorin/fluorouracil compared with 25% (3% complete and 21% partial responses) for those receiving racemic leucovorin/fluorouracil. Median time to progression was 8 or 6.25 months with levoleucovorin/fluorouracil or racemic leucovorin/fluorouracil treatment, respectively; overall survival (14.5 versus 15 months), 1-year survival (58.3 versus 60.6%), and estimated 2-year survival (15.3 versus 23%) for patients receiving racemic leucovorin/fluorouracil or levoleucovorin/fluorouracil, respectively, did not differ significantly. The discontinuance rates were similar (34%) for both groups. Severe adverse events were slightly more common in patients receiving racemic leucovorin/fluorouracil compared with those receiving levoleucovorin/fluorouracil (18 versus 13%). Increased incidences of granulocytopenia (all grades; 39 versus 21%), grade 3 or 4 granulocytopenia (8 versus 2%), grade 3 or 4 leukopenia (5 versus 0%), and grade 3 or 4 diarrhea (10 versus 7%) were reported with racemic leucovorin/fluorouracil compared with levoleucovorin/fluorouracil treatment; however, the investigators acknowledged that the increased incidence of granulocytopenia observed with racemic leucovorin/fluorouracil treatment may be of limited clinical importance based on a lack of complications (e.g., febrile/neutropenic events) and the low incidence of granulocytopenia overall for the study population. The incidences of grade 1 or 2 stomatitis and diarrhea were similar for both groups.

In a third study (OPTIMOX1; a study that evaluated alternative dosing sequences and regimens as a means for reducing the incidence of oxaliplatin-induced sensory neuropathy), one of the treatment regimens, the simplified de Gramont regimen, consisted of IV levoleucovorin or racemic leucovorin in combination with fluorouracil (as a continuous IV infusion). However, neither response nor toxicity results based on the leucovorin formulation used have been reported to date.

Levoleucovorin/Fluorouracil in Combination with Other Agents

Levoleucovorin has been used as a component of irinotecan/fluorouracil/levoleucovorin (FOLFIRI) or oxaliplatin/fluorouracil/levoleucovorin (FOLFOX) regimens for treatment of advanced-stage colorectal cancer; however, data are not available from randomized studies directly comparing safety and efficacy of levoleucovorin versus racemic leucovorin in such regimens. Randomized studies evaluating different schedules of various FOLFOX regimens (i.e., FOLFOX4, FOLFOX6, modified FOLFOX6, FOLFOX7), as well as the FOLFIRI regimen, have allowed use of either IV levoleucovorin or racemic leucovorin in these regimens, although the basis for selection of one leucovorin formulation over the other is unclear. Available response and toxicity data from these studies reflect the treatment schedules and sequences evaluated; analyses based on the leucovorin formulation used have not been reported.

In the FOCUS (Fluorouracil, Oxaliplatin, and CPT11 [irinotecan]–Use and Sequencing) study in patients with poor-prognosis, advanced-stage colorectal cancer, levoleucovorin was used exclusively as the leucovorin component of the fluorouracil-, irinotecan-, and oxaliplatin-based regimens evaluated for first- or second-line therapy. Safety and response data have been reported from this study for the various chemotherapy sequences and combinations studied; however, the specific effects attributable to levoleucovorin have not been fully characterized.

Data are not available from randomized studies directly comparing safety and efficacy of levoleucovorin and racemic leucovorin in combination with fluorouracil and either irinotecan or oxaliplatin in patients with advanced-stage colorectal cancer. Published data describing the use of levoleucovorin as a component of combination therapy with a fluorouracil-based regimen (i.e., FOLFOX or

FOLFIRI) and bevacizumab are not available; therefore, the safety of levoleucovorin in such combination regimens has not been fully established.

DOSAGE AND ADMINISTRATION

● Reconstitution and Administration

Levoleucovorin calcium is administered by IV administration; the drug should *not* be administered intrathecally. When administered by IV injection, the injection rate should not exceed 160 mg of levoleucovorin per minute (16 mL per minute as a 10-mg/mL solution) because of the calcium concentration (4.26 mg Ca^{++} per 64 mg of levoleucovorin calcium pentahydrate) of the solution. Levoleucovorin has been administered by IV infusion in various published studies.

Levoleucovorin calcium is commercially available as a powder for injection and as an injection solution. Strict aseptic technique must be observed since the drug contains no preservative.

Levoleucovorin calcium powder for injection is reconstituted by adding 5.3 mL of 0.9% sodium chloride injection to a vial labeled as containing 50 mg of levoleucovorin to provide a solution containing 10 mg/mL. The manufacturer states that reconstitution with sodium chloride solutions containing preservatives (e.g., benzyl alcohol) has not been studied and is not recommended. Following reconstitution, levoleucovorin solution may be administered by IV injection or further diluted, immediately, in an appropriate volume of 0.9% sodium chloride injection or 5% dextrose injection to yield a concentration of 0.5–5 mg/mL. Following reconstitution or further dilution using 0.9% sodium chloride injection, levoleucovorin is stable for up to 12 hours when stored at room temperature. Following dilution in 5% dextrose injection, the drug is stable for up to 4 hours when stored at room temperature.

The commercially available levoleucovorin 10-mg/mL injection may be further diluted in an appropriate volume of 0.9% sodium chloride injection or 5% dextrose injection to yield a concentration of 0.5 mg/mL. Following dilution in 0.9% sodium chloride injection or 5% dextrose injection, the drug is stable for up to 4 hours when stored at room temperature.

Reconstituted and diluted solutions of levoleucovorin should be inspected visually for particulate matter and discoloration prior to administration whenever solution and container permit; the solutions should not be used if cloudiness or a precipitate is observed.

Because of the risk of precipitation, levoleucovorin should not be combined with other agents in the same admixture.

● Dosage

Levoleucovorin is commercially available as the calcium pentahydrate; dosage of the drug is expressed in terms of levoleucovorin (i.e., 64 mg of levoleucovorin calcium pentahydrate is equivalent to 50 mg of levoleucovorin).

Levoleucovorin is dosed at one-half the usual dosage of racemic leucovorin. (See Description.) The manufacturer makes no specific recommendations regarding dosage in pediatric patients; however, safety and efficacy of levoleucovorin have been evaluated in 16 patients 6–21 years of age. (See Uses: Toxicity Associated with Folic Acid Antagonists.)

Toxicity Associated with Folic Acid Antagonists
Rescue after High-dose Methotrexate Therapy

Dosage recommendations for levoleucovorin are based on a methotrexate dosage of 12 g/m^2 administered by IV infusion over 4 hours; the prescribing information for methotrexate should be consulted for additional information. Dosage and duration of levoleucovorin rescue therapy should be adjusted based on the elimination pattern of methotrexate and the patient's renal function (see Table 1).

Serum creatinine and methotrexate concentrations should be monitored at least once daily. Levoleucovorin therapy should be continued, and adequate hydration and urinary alkalinization (pH of 7 or greater) maintained, until serum methotrexate concentration declines to less than 0.05 micromolar (5×10^{-8} M). Patients who experience delayed early methotrexate elimination are likely to develop reversible renal failure; therefore, fluid and electrolyte status also should be closely monitored in such patients until serum methotrexate concentration declines to less than 0.05 micromolar (5×10^{-8} M) and renal failure has resolved.

TABLE 1. Guidelines for Levoleucovorin Dosage Adjustment in Patients with Normal or Delayed Methotrexate Elimination

Clinical Situation	Serum Methotrexate Concentration[a]	Levoleucovorin Dosage and Monitoring
Normal methotrexate elimination[b]	Approximately 10 micromolar (10^{-5} M) at 24 hours, 1 micromolar (10^{-6} M) at 48 hours, and less than 0.2 micromolar (2×10^{-7} M) at 72 hours after methotrexate administration	7.5 mg (approximately 5 mg/m^2) IV every 6 hours for 60 hours (10 doses), starting at 24 hours after initiation of methotrexate infusion[b]
Delayed late methotrexate elimination	Greater than 0.2 micromolar (2×10^{-7} M) at 72 hours and greater than 0.05 micromolar (5×10^{-8} M) at 96 hours after methotrexate administration	Continue levoleucovorin 7.5 mg IV every 6 hours until methotrexate concentration declines to less than 0.05 micromolar (5×10^{-8} M)
Delayed early methotrexate elimination and/or evidence of acute renal injury	50 micromolar (5×10^{-5} M) or greater at 24 hours or 5 micromolar (5×10^{-6} M) or greater at 48 hours after methotrexate administration, *or* a 100% or greater increase in serum creatinine concentration at 24 hours after methotrexate administration (e.g., an increase from 0.5 to 1 mg/dL or more)	75 mg IV every 3 hours until methotrexate concentration declines to less than 1 micromolar (10^{-6} M), then 7.5 mg IV every 3 hours until methotrexate concentration declines to less than 0.05 micromolar (5×10^{-8} M)

[a] The possibility that the patient is receiving other drugs that interact with methotrexate (e.g., by decreasing methotrexate elimination, binding to serum albumin) should always be considered when laboratory abnormalities or clinical toxicities are observed.

[b] In patients with mild abnormalities in methotrexate elimination or renal function who experience clinically important toxicity, levoleucovorin rescue should be extended for an additional 24 hours (i.e., 14 doses over 84 hours) for subsequent methotrexate courses.

Methotrexate Overdosage

Levoleucovorin rescue should begin as soon as possible following unintentional overdosage and within 24 hours of methotrexate administration if delayed elimination is detected; delayed administration of levoleucovorin may reduce its effectiveness in counteracting toxicity associated with folic acid antagonists.

The usual levoleucovorin dosage for management of methotrexate overdosage is 7.5 mg (approximately 5 mg/m^2) IV every 6 hours until serum methotrexate concentration declines to less than 0.01 micromolar (10^{-8} M). Serum creatinine and serum methotrexate concentrations should be determined at 24-hour intervals. If the 24-hour serum creatinine concentration increases 50% over baseline, the 24-hour methotrexate concentration is greater than 5 micromolar (5×10^{-6} M), or the 48-hour methotrexate concentration is greater than 0.9 micromolar (9×10^{-7} M), levoleucovorin dosage should be increased to 50 mg/m^2 IV every 3 hours until serum methotrexate concentration declines to less than 0.01 micromolar (10^{-8} M). Hydration (3 L daily) and urinary alkalinization with sodium bicarbonate (to maintain a urinary pH of 7 or greater) should be employed concomitantly.

Colorectal Cancer
Combined Therapy with Fluorouracil for Advanced-stage Colorectal Cancer

Regimens of levoleucovorin and fluorouracil that historically have been used for the palliative treatment of advanced-stage colorectal cancer include a levoleucovorin dose of 100 mg/m^2 administered by slow IV injection (over a minimum of 3 minutes) followed by an IV fluorouracil dose of 370 mg/m^2, or a levoleucovorin dose of 10 mg/m^2 administered by IV injection followed by an IV fluorouracil dose of 425 mg/m^2. Either regimen is administered daily for 5 days and may be repeated at 4-week intervals for 2 additional courses; thereafter, the regimen may be repeated at intervals of 4–5 weeks provided toxicity from the previous course of combined therapy has resolved completely.

Dosage of fluorouracil in subsequent courses of therapy should be adjusted according to patient tolerance of the prior treatment course; dosage of levoleucovorin in subsequent courses is not adjusted because of toxicity. Daily fluorouracil dosage generally is reduced by 20% in patients who experienced moderate hematologic or GI toxicity in the prior course and by 30% in those patients who experienced severe toxicity. If no toxicity occurs, fluorouracil dosage may be increased by 10%.

Other levoleucovorin and fluorouracil dosage regimens also have been used. (See Levoleucovorin and Fluorouracil under Colorectal Cancer: Combined Therapy with Fluorouracil for Advanced-stage Colorectal Cancer, in Uses.)

- **Special Populations**

Patients with Delayed Methotrexate Elimination

Higher dosages and extended duration of levoleucovorin therapy may be required if delayed methotrexate excretion is caused by third space fluid accumulation (i.e., ascites, pleural effusion), renal impairment, or inadequate hydration.

CAUTIONS

- **Contraindications**

Pernicious anemia or other megaloblastic anemias secondary to lack of vitamin B_{12}; such use may obscure the diagnosis of pernicious anemia by alleviating hematologic manifestations while allowing neurologic complications to progress.

Hypersensitivity to folic acid or folinic acid.

- **Warnings/Precautions**

Rate of Administration

The injection rate should not exceed 160 mg of levoleucovorin per minute (16 mL per minute as a 10-mg/mL solution) because of the calcium concentration of the solution.

Toxicity Potentiation with Concomitant Therapy

Levoleucovorin potentiates the toxicity of fluorouracil; therefore, fluorouracil dosage must be reduced when levoleucovorin is used concomitantly in the treatment of advanced-stage colorectal cancer. Although toxicities in patients receiving levoleucovorin in combination with fluorouracil are qualitatively similar to those in patients receiving fluorouracil alone, GI toxicities (particularly stomatitis and diarrhea) occur more frequently and may be more severe or prolonged in patients receiving combined therapy. Deaths from severe enterocolitis, diarrhea, and dehydration have been reported in geriatric patients receiving weekly racemic leucovorin concomitantly with fluorouracil. In addition, in a study evaluating higher weekly dosages of fluorouracil and racemic leucovorin, an increased risk of severe GI toxicity was observed in geriatric and/or debilitated patients.

In several clinical trials in patients with advanced-stage colorectal cancer, treatment-related toxicity occurred more frequently in patients receiving a low dose of racemic leucovorin (20 mg/m²) in combination with fluorouracil (425 mg/m²) than in patients receiving a higher dose of racemic leucovorin (200 mg/m²) in combination with fluorouracil (370 mg/m²). In one study, 20% of patients receiving fluorouracil in combination with racemic leucovorin 20 mg/m² experienced toxicity (primarily GI toxicity) requiring hospitalization, compared with 7% of those receiving fluorouracil alone or in combination with racemic leucovorin 200 mg/m². In another study, 11% of patients receiving fluorouracil in combination with racemic leucovorin 20 mg/m² required hospitalization for treatment-related toxicity, compared with 3% of those receiving fluorouracil in combination with racemic leucovorin 200 mg/m².

Combined therapy with fluorouracil and levoleucovorin should not be initiated or continued in patients with symptomatic GI toxicity until such symptoms have resolved completely. Patients who develop diarrhea should be monitored with particular care until the diarrhea has resolved, since rapid clinical deterioration and death can occur. (See Cautions: Precautions and Contraindications, in Leucovorin Calcium 92:12.)

Concomitant use of racemic leucovorin with co-trimoxazole for treatment of *Pneumocystis jiroveci* (formerly *P. carinii*) pneumonia in patients with HIV infection has been associated with increased rates of treatment failure and morbidity.

Seizures and/or syncope have occurred rarely in cancer patients receiving racemic leucovorin, usually in conjunction with fluoropyrimidine therapy; cases have occurred most commonly in patients with other predisposing factors (e.g.,

CNS metastasis). A causal relationship to racemic leucovorin has not been fully established.

Sensitivity Reactions

Allergic reactions have been reported in patients receiving levoleucovorin.

Specific Populations

Pregnancy

Category C. (See Users Guide.)

Lactation

It is not known whether levoleucovorin is distributed into milk; because of the potential for serious adverse reactions to levoleucovorin in nursing infants, a decision should be made whether to discontinue nursing or the drug, taking into account the importance of the drug to the woman.

Pediatric Use

Safety and efficacy of levoleucovorin have been evaluated in 16 patients 6–21 years of age. (See Uses: Toxicity Associated with Folic Acid Antagonists.) The manufacturer makes no specific recommendations regarding use in pediatric patients.

Geriatric Use

Clinical studies of levoleucovorin in the treatment of osteosarcoma did not include patients 65 years of age and older to determine whether geriatric patients respond differently than younger patients.

In a clinical trial evaluating levoleucovorin in combination with fluorouracil for the treatment of advanced-stage colorectal cancer, adverse reactions were consistent with known toxicities of fluorouracil; no overall differences in adverse effects were observed between geriatric patients (65 years of age or older) and younger adults. However, deaths from severe enterocolitis, diarrhea, and dehydration have been reported in geriatric patients receiving weekly racemic leucovorin concomitantly with fluorouracil. (See Cautions: Precautions and Contraindications, in Leucovorin Calcium 92:12.)

Renal Impairment

Renal impairment may cause delayed methotrexate elimination; higher dosages and extended duration of levoleucovorin therapy may be required in patients with renal impairment. (See Dosage and Administration: Special Populations.)

- **Common Adverse Effects**

Adverse effects reported in more than 15% of patients receiving levoleucovorin rescue following high-dose methotrexate therapy include vomiting, stomatitis, and nausea. Less frequently reported adverse effects, occurring in less than 10% of patients, include diarrhea, dyspepsia, typhlitis, dyspnea, dermatitis, confusion, neuropathy, abnormal renal function, and taste perversion.

Adverse effects reported in more than 50% of patients with advanced-stage colorectal cancer receiving levoleucovorin in combination with fluorouracil include diarrhea, nausea, and stomatitis. Other frequently reported adverse effects, occurring in 20–40% of patients, include vomiting, asthenia/fatigue/malaise, anorexia/decreased appetite, dermatitis, and alopecia. The incidence of adverse effects is similar to that reported in patients receiving an equipotent dosage of racemic leucovorin in combination with fluorouracil.

DRUG INTERACTIONS

- **Anticonvulsants**

Folic acid in large amounts may counteract the anticonvulsant effect of phenobarbital, phenytoin, and primidone and increase the frequency of seizures in susceptible children. Racemic leucovorin has been shown to increase hepatic metabolism and decrease plasma concentrations of phenytoin in rats. Therefore, caution is advised when levoleucovorin is used concomitantly with anticonvulsants.

- **Co-trimoxazole**

Concomitant use of racemic leucovorin with co-trimoxazole for treatment of *Pneumocystis jiroveci* (formerly *P. carinii*) pneumonia in patients with HIV infection has been associated with increased rates of treatment failure and morbidity.

● *Fluorouracil*

Levoleucovorin potentiates the toxicity of fluorouracil. (See Toxicity Potentiation with Concomitant Therapy under Cautions: Warnings/Precautions.)

● *Glucarpidase*

In patients receiving high-dose methotrexate therapy with leucovorin rescue, administration of glucarpidase (an enzyme that converts methotrexate to inactive metabolites) 2 hours before a racemic leucovorin dose reduced systemic exposure and peak plasma concentrations of leucovorin and its active metabolite, 5-methyltetrahydrofolate. Similar effects would be expected with levoleucovorin. In addition, methotrexate concentrations measured by immunoassay within 48 hours following glucarpidase administration are unreliable. Racemic leucovorin or levoleucovorin should not be administered within 2 hours before or after glucarpidase administration. Dosage adjustment of the continuing racemic leucovorin or levoleucovorin regimen is not necessary since dosage is based on the patient's methotrexate concentration prior to glucarpidase administration. During the first 48 hours after glucarpidase administration, racemic leucovorin or levoleucovorin should be administered at the same dosage administered prior to glucarpidase administration; beyond 48 hours, dosage should be based on the measured methotrexate concentration. Therapy with racemic leucovorin or levoleucovorin should be continued until the methotrexate concentration has been maintained below the threshold for such treatment for at least 3 days.

● *Methotrexate*

High dosages of racemic leucovorin may reduce the efficacy of intrathecally administered methotrexate.

DESCRIPTION

Levoleucovorin is the levorotatory (*l*) isomer of racemic *d,l*-leucovorin. Levoleucovorin is the pharmacologically active isomer and constitutes approximately 50% of racemic leucovorin; therefore, the effects of levoleucovorin are observed at half the dose of racemic leucovorin. Because levoleucovorin is a reduced derivative of folic acid and does not require reduction by dihydrofolate reductase to participate in reactions utilizing folates, the drug counteracts the therapeutic and toxic effects of folic acid antagonists (e.g., methotrexate). The drug also enhances the efficacy and toxicity of fluoropyrimidines (e.g., fluorouracil) by stabilizing binding of the fluorouracil metabolite 5-fluoro-2′-deoxyuridine-5′-monophosphate (FdUMP) to thymidylate synthase (an enzyme responsible for DNA repair and replication), thus enhancing inhibition of this enzyme.

Levoleucovorin is actively and passively transported across cell membranes. In vivo, levoleucovorin is converted to 5-methyltetrahydrofolic acid (5-methyl-THF), the primary circulating form of active reduced folate. Levoleucovorin and 5-methyl-THF are polyglutamated intracellularly by the enzyme folylpolyglutamate synthetase. Folylpolyglutamates are active and participate in numerous biochemical pathways that require reduced folate.

Following IV administration of a single 15-mg dose of levoleucovorin in healthy male volunteers, peak serum concentrations of (6*S*)-5-methyl-5,6,7,8-tetrahydrofolate (the *l*-isomer of 5-methyl-THF) were reached within 0.9 hours. The mean terminal half-life of total tetrahydrofolate and (6*S*)-5-methyl-5,6,7,8-tetrahydrofolate were 5.1 and 6.8 hours, respectively. Levoleucovorin and its metabolites are excreted in urine.

Data from several crossover studies in healthy individuals and patients with colorectal cancer have shown no substantial differences in exposure to the *l*-isomer of leucovorin or to 5-methyltetrahydrofolate regardless of whether IV racemic leucovorin or an equipotent dose of IV levoleucovorin is administered.

ADVICE TO PATIENTS

Risk of diarrhea, vomiting, stomatitis, and nausea.

Importance of women informing clinicians immediately if they are or plan to become pregnant or plan to breast-feed.

Importance of informing clinicians of existing or contemplated concomitant therapy, including prescription and OTC drugs, as well as any concomitant illnesses (e.g., renal impairment).

Importance of informing patients of other important precautionary information. (See Cautions.)

PREPARATIONS

Excipients in commercially available drug preparations may have clinically important effects in some individuals; consult specific product labeling for details.

LEVOleucovorin Calcium

Parenteral		
For injection, for IV use	50 mg (of levoleucovorin)	Fusilev®, Spectrum
Injection, for IV use	10 mg (of levoleucovorin) per mL (175 and 250 mg)	Fusilev®, Spectrum

† Use is not currently included in the labeling approved by the US Food and Drug Administration.

Selected Revisions May 10, 2024, © Copyright, January 1, 2009, American Society of Health-System Pharmacists, Inc.

Pralidoxime Chloride

91:04.20 • ORGANOPHOSPHATE ANTIDOTE

USES

● Organophosphate Pesticide Poisoning

Pralidoxime chloride is used concomitantly with atropine and supportive measures (e.g., removal of secretions, maintenance of an adequate airway, and artificial ventilation) to reverse muscle paralysis (particularly of respiratory muscles) associated with toxic exposure to organophosphate anticholinesterase pesticides and chemicals. Pralidoxime appears to be most effective when given soon after exposure; the drug may still be effective if more than 48 hours have elapsed. Clinical cases in which atropine and pralidoxime have been used include toxic exposure to azodrin, bidrin, carbophenthion, coumaphos (Co-ral), DFP, diazinon, dichlorvos, dichlorvos with chlordane, dicrotophos, dimethoate, disulfoton, EPN, guthion, isoflurophate, Metasystox 1® and fenthion, methyl demeton, methyl parathion, mevinphos, OMPA, parathion, parathion and mevinphos, phosdrin, phosphamidon, sarin, Systox®, trithion, and TEPP. Results of animal studies indicate that pralidoxime may be an effective antidote in toxic exposure to various other organophosphates possessing anticholinesterase activity, but the drug appears to be ineffective or only marginally effective against toxic exposure to Ciodrin®, dimefox, dimethoate, methyl diazinon, methyl phencapton, mipafox, phorate, schradan, and Wepsyn®. Pralidoxime is not effective in the treatment of toxic exposure to phosphorus, inorganic phosphates, or organophosphates which do not possess anticholinesterase activity.

● Chemical Warfare Agent Poisoning

Pralidoxime chloride is used concomitantly with atropine for the treatment of nerve agent poisoning in the context of chemical warfare or terrorism. Pralidoxime chloride must be administered within minutes to hours following exposure to nerve agents to be effective.

The most toxic of the known chemical warfare agents are the nerve agents. Most nerve agents are liquid at room temperature (although most are volatile at ambient temperatures, the term nerve gas is a misnomer); nerve agents are readily absorbed after inhalation of aerosols (e.g., following an explosion), ingestion, or dermal contact. Nerve agents (e.g., sarin, soman, tabun, VX [methylphosphonothioic acid]) are chemically similar to the organophosphate pesticides and exert their biologic effects by inhibiting acetylcholinesterase enzymes. Nerve agents alter cholinergic synaptic transmission at neuroeffector junctions (muscarinic effects), at skeletal myoneural junctions and autonomic ganglia (nicotinic effects), and in the CNS. Manifestations of nerve agent exposure include rhinorrhea, chest tightness, pinpoint pupils, dyspnea, excessive salivation and sweating, nausea, vomiting, abdominal cramps, involuntary defecation and/or urination, muscle twitching, confusion, seizures, flaccid paralysis, coma, respiratory failure, and death. While initial effects of nerve agent exposure depend on the dose and route of exposure, signs and symptoms generally are similar regardless of the route of exposure. Manifestations may not be apparent until as long as 18 hours following dermal exposure, and CNS effects (e.g., fatigue, irritability, nervousness, memory impairment) may persist as long as 6 weeks following recovery from the acute effects of nerve agent exposure.

Initial management of nerve agent poisoning includes aggressive airway control and ventilation (administration of nebulized β-adrenergic agonist [e.g., albuterol] and antimuscarinics [e.g., ipratropium bromide] may be necessary), and administration of atropine and pralidoxime chloride. Diazepam may be needed for seizure control. Rapid decontamination using standard hazardous materials (HAZMAT) procedures is important to prevent further absorption by the victim and to prevent contamination of others (e.g., emergency personnel, health-care workers) by direct contact or off-gassing of nerve agents from contaminated clothing. Following initial therapy and decontamination, additional treatment with atropine and supportive measures in a hospital setting are likely to be necessary.

● Other Uses

Atropine is generally used alone in the treatment of muscarinic toxicity resulting from exposure to carbamate insecticides; pralidoxime is not generally used. Pralidoxime is contraindicated in the treatment of toxic exposure to carbaryl since it appears to increase the toxicity of carbaryl.

Pralidoxime has been used for the management of overdosage of drugs that carbamylate cholinesterase, such as ambenonium, neostigmine, and pyridostigmine, particularly in the treatment of cholinergic crisis in patients with myasthenia gravis. However, pralidoxime is reportedly less effective against these agents than against organophosphate anticholinesterases and may precipitate a myasthenic crisis in these patients. (See Cautions: Precautions and Contraindications.)

DOSAGE AND ADMINISTRATION

● Reconstitution and Administration

Pralidoxime chloride is usually administered IV, preferably as an infusion given over 15–30 minutes. (See Cautions: Adverse Effects.) In patients with pulmonary edema or if IV infusion is not practical or a more rapid effect is desired, pralidoxime chloride solutions containing 50 mg/mL may be administered by slow IV injection over a period of at least 5 minutes. Pralidoxime chloride may also be administered by IM injection.

Pralidoxime chloride sterile powder for injection is reconstituted by adding 20 mL of sterile water for injection to the vial labeled as containing 1 g of the drug to provide a solution containing approximately 50 mg/mL. Because of the relatively large volume of diluent required, sterile water for injection containing preservatives should not be used to reconstitute pralidoxime chloride sterile powder for injection. Following reconstitution, pralidoxime chloride solutions should be used within a few hours. For IV infusion, the calculated dose of the reconstituted solution is further diluted in 100 mL with 0.9% sodium chloride injection.

To facilitate out-of-hospital IM administration in the event of pesticide or nerve agent poisoning, pralidoxime chloride injection is available as an auto-injector (pralidoxime chloride injection auto-injector). In addition, pralidoxime chloride is available in an auto-injector that also contains atropine (DuoDote® auto-injector, ATNAA auto-injector). Each prefilled DuoDote® auto-syringe and each prefilled ATNAA auto-syringe provides a single IM dose of atropine 2.1 mg and pralidoxime chloride 600 mg. When activated, the auto-injector sequentially administers atropine and pralidoxime chloride through a single needle. For self-administration or administration by a partner or civilian emergency responder in an out-of-hospital setting, the contents of a pralidoxime chloride auto-injector or atropine and pralidoxime chloride auto-injector (DuoDote®) should be injected IM into the anterolateral aspect of the thigh. In an out-of-hospital setting, the contents of an atropine and pralidoxime chloride auto-injector (ATNAA) should be injected IM into the anterolateral aspect of the thigh or into the buttock.

For IM administration, some authorities suggest that pralidoxime chloride sterile powder for injection be reconstituted by adding 3 mL of sterile water for injection or 0.9% sodium chloride for injection to the vial labeled as containing 1 g of the drug to provide a solution containing 300 mg/mL.

● Dosage

Organophosphate Pesticide Poisoning

For the treatment of toxic exposure to organophosphate cholinesterase inhibitors, pralidoxime therapy should be initiated at the same time as atropine. The usual initial IV dose of pralidoxime chloride is 1–2 g given over 15 to 30 minutes for adults, or 20–40 mg/kg given over 30 minutes for children. Dosage of pralidoxime chloride should be reduced in patients with renal insufficiency. The dose of pralidoxime chloride may be repeated in about 1 hour if muscle weakness has not been relieved. Additional doses may be administered cautiously if muscle weakness continues. Alternatively, some clinicians recommend continuous IV infusion of 500 mg of the drug per hour. In severe cases, especially after ingestion of the poison, the manufacturer recommends electrocardiographic monitoring because the anticholinesterase may cause heart block. Continued absorption of the anticholinesterase from the lower bowel constitutes new exposure; in such cases, additional doses of pralidoxime may be needed every 3–8 hours. As in all cases of organophosphate poisoning, the patient should be observed closely for at least 24 hours.

To facilitate out-of-hospital administration, pralidoxime is available in a pre-filled auto-injector containing atropine 2.1 mg and pralidoxime chloride 600 mg (e.g., DuoDote®); the auto-injector should be used by emergency medical service personnel. For administration in an out-of-hospital setting, the dose of pralidoxime and atropine (DuoDote®) is based on severity of symptoms. For the treatment of adults with 2 or more mild symptoms of pesticide exposure (e.g., miosis or blurred vision, tearing, runny nose, hypersalivation or drooling, wheezing, muscle fasciculations, nausea/vomiting), administer contents of one auto-injector (atropine 2.1 mg and pralidoxime chloride 600 mg) by IM injection. If the patient develops any severe symptoms (behavioral changes, severe breathing difficulty, severe respiratory secretions, severe muscle twitching, involuntary defecation or urination, seizures, unconsciousness), administer contents of two additional auto-injectors IM in rapid succession. For the treatment of adults who present with any severe symptoms, administer contents of three auto-injectors (total dose: atropine 6.3 mg and pralidoxime chloride 1800 mg) IM in rapid succession. Additional doses should not be administered unless definitive medical care is available.

Chemical Warfare Agents

The dose and route of administration of pralidoxime chloride for the treatment of nerve agent (e.g., sarin, soman, tabun, VX [methylphosphonothiotic acid]) poisoning in the context of chemical warfare or terrorism is based on the severity of symptoms (i.e., mild/moderate or severe), the victim's age, and the treatment setting. Mild to moderate symptoms include localized sweating, muscle fasciculations, nausea, vomiting, weakness, and/or dyspnea; severe symptoms include apnea, flaccid paralysis, seizures, and/or unconsciousness. Pralidoxime chloride must be administered within minutes to hours following exposure to nerve agents to be effective. Pralidoxime is administered concomitantly with atropine.

For the immediate treatment of nerve agent poisoning in an out-of-hospital setting, pralidoxime chloride usually is administered IM. The usual out-of-hospital IM adult dose is 600 mg for those with mild to moderate symptoms and 1800 mg for those with severe symptoms; frail geriatric adults with mild to moderate symptoms may receive 10 mg/kg and those with severe symptoms may receive 25 mg/kg. In an out-of-hospital setting, the usual IM dose of pralidoxime chloride for children 0–10 years of age and adolescents older than 10 years of age with mild to moderate symptoms is 15 mg/kg, and the usual dose for children 0–10 years of age and adolescents older than 10 years of age with severe symptoms is 25 mg/kg.

To facilitate out-of-hospital administration, pralidoxime chloride injection is available in a prefilled auto-injector; the auto-injector should be used by individuals who have received adequate training in the recognition and treatment of nerve agent poisoning. For the initial treatment of adults with symptoms of nerve agent poisoning, one 600-mg IM dose of pralidoxime chloride should be administered; pralidoxime is administered after atropine. If symptoms are still present after 15 minutes, another dose of atropine and another 600-mg dose of pralidoxime chloride should be administered. If symptoms persist after an additional 15 minutes, another dose of atropine and another 600-mg dose of pralidoxime chloride should be administered. If symptoms persist after the third doses, medical care should be sought.

Another option for out-of-hospital administration is to administer atropine and pralidoxime using a prefilled auto-injector containing atropine 2.1 mg and pralidoxime chloride 600 mg (e.g., DuoDote®, ATNAA). For the treatment of adults with 2 or more mild symptoms of nerve agent poisoning (e.g., miosis or blurred vision, tearing, runny nose, hypersalivation or drooling, muscle fasciculations, nausea/vomiting), the contents of one auto-injector (atropine 2.1 mg and pralidoxime chloride 600 mg) should be administered by IM injection. If the patient develops any severe symptoms (behavioral changes, severe breathing difficulty, severe respiratory secretions, severe muscle twitching, involuntary defecation or urination, seizures, unconsciousness), the contents of 2 additional auto-injectors should be administered by IM injection in rapid succession. For the treatment of adults who present with any severe symptoms, the contents of 3 auto-injectors (total dose: atropine 6.3 mg and pralidoxime chloride 1800 mg) should be administered by IM injection in rapid succession. Additional doses should not be administered unless definitive medical care is available.

In an emergency department or similar setting, pralidoxime chloride generally is administered by slow IV injection. When pralidoxime chloride is administered IV in such a setting for the treatment of nerve agent poisoning, the usual adult dose is 15 mg/kg (maximum 1 g) for those with mild to moderate or severe symptoms; frail geriatric adults with mild to moderate or severe symptoms may receive 5–10 mg/kg. In an emergency department setting, the usual IV dose of pralidoxime chloride for children 0–10 years of age and adolescents older than 10 years of age with mild to moderate or severe symptoms is 15 mg/kg. Atropine is administered concomitantly with pralidoxime.

Diazepam may be administered for seizure control.

Other Uses

As an antagonist to carbamate anticholinesterase agents used in the treatment of myasthenia gravis (e.g., ambenonium, neostigmine, pyridostigmine), 1–2 g of pralidoxime chloride has been given IV initially, followed by 250 mg every 5 minutes.

CAUTIONS

● Adverse Effects

Although pralidoxime is generally well-tolerated, dizziness, blurred vision, diplopia and impaired accommodation, headache, drowsiness, nausea, tachycardia, hyperventilation, maculopapular rash, and muscular weakness have been reported following administration of the drug. However, it is difficult to differentiate the toxic effects produced by atropine or organophosphates from those of pralidoxime, and the condition of patients suffering from organophosphate intoxication will generally mask minor signs and symptoms reported in normal subjects who receive pralidoxime. When atropine and pralidoxime are used concomitantly, signs of atropinism may occur earlier than when atropine is used alone, especially if the total dose of atropine is large and administration of pralidoxime is delayed. Excitement, confusion, manic behavior, and muscle rigidity have been reported following recovery of consciousness, but these symptoms have also occurred in patients who were not treated with pralidoxime.

Rapid IV injection of pralidoxime has produced tachycardia, laryngospasm, muscle rigidity, and transient neuromuscular blockade; therefore, the drug should be administered slowly, preferably by IV infusion. IV administration of pralidoxime reportedly may also cause hypertension which is related to the dose and rate of infusion. Some clinicians recommend that the patient's blood pressure be monitored during pralidoxime therapy. For adults, IV administration of 5 mg of phentolamine mesylate reportedly quickly reverses pralidoxime-induced hypertension.

IM administration of pralidoxime may produce mild pain at the injection site.

● Precautions and Contraindications

Pralidoxime should always be used under close medical supervision.

Pralidoxime should be used with caution in patients with myasthenia gravis who are receiving anticholinesterase agents, since the drug may precipitate a myasthenic crisis.

Pralidoxime should be used with caution and in reduced dosage in patients with impaired renal function.

The use of succinylcholine, theophylline, aminophylline, reserpine, and respiratory depressants (e.g., barbiturates, morphine, phenothiazines) should be avoided in patients with toxic exposure to anticholinesterase compounds.

● Pregnancy, Fertility, and Lactation

Pregnancy

Safe use of pralidoxime during pregnancy has not been established.

PHARMACOLOGY

The principal pharmacologic effect of pralidoxime is reactivation of cholinesterase which has been recently inactivated by phosphorylation as the result of exposure to certain organophosphates. Pralidoxime removes the phosphoryl group from the active site of the inhibited enzyme by nucleophilic attack, regenerating active cholinesterase and forming an oxime complex. Pralidoxime also detoxifies certain organophosphates by direct chemical reaction and probably also reacts directly with cholinesterase to protect it from inhibition. Pralidoxime must be administered before aging of the inhibited enzyme occurs; after aging is completed, phosphorylated cholinesterase cannot be reactivated, and newly synthesized cholinesterase must replace the inhibited enzyme. Pralidoxime is not equally antagonistic to all anticholinesterases, partly because the time period required for aging of the inhibited enzyme varies and depends on the specific organophosphate bound to the cholinesterase.

Pralidoxime also reactivates cholinesterase which has been inactivated by carbamylation. However, carbamylated cholinesterase has a much faster rate of spontaneous reactivation than does phosphorylated cholinesterase.

Cholinesterase reactivation produced by pralidoxime occurs principally at the neuromuscular junction and results in reversal of anticholinesterase-induced paralysis of respiratory and other skeletal muscles. The drug also reactivates cholinesterase at autonomic effector sites and, to a lesser degree, within the CNS. Pralidoxime is effective against nicotinic manifestations of anticholinesterase poisoning (e.g., muscular twitching, fasciculation, cramps, weakness, pallor, tachycardia, elevated blood pressure). The drug does not substantially influence muscarinic effects (e.g., bronchoconstriction, dyspnea, cough, increased bronchial secretion, nausea, vomiting, abdominal cramps, diarrhea, increased sweating, salivation, lacrimation, bradycardia, fall in blood pressure, miosis, blurred vision, urinary frequency, and incontinence). Therefore, pralidoxime is used in conjunction with atropine, which ameliorates muscarinic symptoms and directly blocks the effects of accumulation of excess acetylcholine at various sites including the respiratory center.

Other reported pharmacologic effects of pralidoxime include depolarization at the neuromuscular junction, anticholinergic action, mild inhibition of cholinesterase, sympathomimetic effects, potentiation of the depressor action of acetylcholine in nonatropinized animals, and potentiation of the pressor action of acetylcholine in atropinized animals. However, the contribution of these effects to the therapeutic action of the drug has not been established.

PHARMACOKINETICS

● Absorption

Absorption of pralidoxime chloride is variable and incomplete following oral administration (oral tablets of the drug are no longer commercially available in the US). Based on results of animal studies, the minimum therapeutic plasma concentration of pralidoxime is considered to be 4 mcg/mL. Peak plasma oxime concentrations are reached 5–15 minutes after IV administration and 10–20 minutes after IM administration of pralidoxime chloride. In a study in healthy adults, IV pralidoxime chloride doses of 7.5–10 mg/kg were needed to produce plasma oxime concentrations of 4 mcg/mL or greater at 1 hour after administration; IM doses of 7.5–10 mg/kg were needed to achieve initial plasma concentrations of 4 mcg/mL or greater, and only IM doses of 10 mg/kg maintained plasma oxime concentrations at 4 mcg/mL or greater for 1 hour.

● Distribution

Pralidoxime is distributed throughout the extracellular water. Because of its quaternary ammonium structure, the drug is not generally believed to enter the CNS, but recent animal studies and human clinical responses observed by some investigators have raised some controversy on this point. Pralidoxime does not readily penetrate the cornea following systemic or topical administration, but therapeutic concentrations are reportedly achieved in the eye following subconjunctival injection. Pralidoxime is not appreciably bound to plasma proteins.

It is not known if pralidoxime is distributed into milk.

● Elimination

Although the exact metabolic fate of pralidoxime has not been completely elucidated, the drug is believed to be metabolized in the liver. The half-life of pralidoxime in patients with normal renal function varies and has been reported to range from 0.8–2.7 hours. Pralidoxime is rapidly excreted in urine as unchanged drug and as a metabolite. Approximately 80–90% of an IV or IM dose of pralidoxime chloride is excreted unchanged within 12 hours after administration. A recent study has suggested that active tubular secretion may be involved, although the specific mechanism has not been identified.

CHEMISTRY

Pralidoxime chloride, a quaternary ammonium oxime, is a cholinesterase reactivator. The drug occurs as a white to pale yellow, crystalline powder and is freely soluble in water. Following reconstitution with sterile water for injection, pralidoxime chloride solutions containing 50 mg/mL have a pH of 3.5–4.5. The pK_a of pralidoxime is 7.8–8.

PREPARATIONS

Pralidoxime chloride injection auto-injector is supplied through the Directorate of Medical Materiel, Defense Supply Center Philadelphia or other local, state, or federal agency. ATNAA is supplied through the Directorate of Medical Material, Defense Supply Center Philadelphia. Duodote® is available for hospitals and emergency responders through Meridian Medical Technology (800-638-8093).

Excipients in commercially available drug preparations may have clinically important effects in some individuals; consult specific product labeling for details.

Pralidoxime Chloride

Parenteral		
For injection	1 g	Protopam® Chloride, Baxter
Injection	600 mg*	Pralidoxime Chloride Injection Auto-Injector

* available from one or more manufacturer, distributor, and/or repackager by generic (nonproprietary) name

Pralidoxime Chloride and Atropine

Parenteral		
Injection	600 mg/2 mL Pralidoxime Chloride and 2.1 mg/ 0.7 mL Atropine	ATNAA Auto-Injector each drug is in a separate chamber, Meridian
	600 mg/2 mL Pralidoxime Chloride and 2.1 mg/ 0.7 mL Atropine	DuoDote® Auto-Injector each drug is in a separate chamber, Meridian

† Use is not currently included in the labeling approved by the US Food and Drug Administration.

Sugammadex Sodium

91:04.28 • NEUROMUSCULAR BLOCKING AGENT ANTIDOTES

■ Sugammadex sodium, a modified γ-cyclodextrin, is a selective relaxant binding agent.

USES

● Reversal of Neuromuscular Blockade

Sugammadex is used for the reversal of neuromuscular blockade induced by rocuronium bromide or vecuronium bromide in adults undergoing surgery. The drug substantially decreases the time to recovery from *moderate* or *deep* neuromuscular blockade induced by these steroidal neuromuscular blocking agents. At the highest recommended dose of 16 mg/kg, sugammadex also demonstrated efficacy for *rapid* reversal of profound neuromuscular blockade induced by high-dose (1.2 mg/kg) rocuronium bromide when given shortly (approximately 3 minutes) after the onset of the neuromuscular block. Sugammadex is an effective reversal agent for rocuronium and vecuronium only and should *not* be used to reverse the effects of *nonsteroidal* neuromuscular blocking agents (e.g., succinylcholine, benzylisoquinolinium compounds [atracurium, mivacurium]).

It is important that the effects of neuromuscular blocking agents are quickly and effectively terminated after surgery to prevent postoperative residual neuromuscular blockade. Incomplete neuromuscular recovery can cause prolonged weakness of the upper airway muscles and associated complications (e.g., airway obstruction, aspiration, hypoxemia, pneumonia, atelectasis, respiratory failure). Risk of postoperative pulmonary complications may be further increased based on certain patient- and procedure-related factors. Therefore, residual neuromuscular block is an important patient safety issue that requires appropriate management. The available data indicate that reversal of neuromuscular blockade should be a standard practice unless there is quantitative evidence that no reversal is needed (train-of-four [TOF] >0.9). Cholinesterase inhibitors (e.g., neostigmine, edrophonium, pyridostigmine) have been traditionally used for reversal of nondepolarizing neuromuscular agents. Sugammadex is another option that may be considered for reversing the effects of rocuronium or vecuronium.

Efficacy of sugammadex for reversal of *moderate* neuromuscular blockade induced by rocuronium or vecuronium was evaluated in a randomized, multicenter, active-controlled study in 189 adults (median age 50–51 years, median body weight 72–76 kg, 54% male) undergoing elective surgery under general anesthesia that required endotracheal intubation and maintenance of neuromuscular blockade. Surgical procedures were mainly endocrine, ocular, ENT (ear, nose, and throat), abdominal (gynecologic, colorectal, urologic), orthopedic, vascular, or dermatologic. Patients were first randomized to receive either rocuronium bromide (initial intubating dose of 0.6 mg/kg followed by 0.1–0.2 mg/kg as needed during surgery) or vecuronium bromide (initial intubating dose of 0.1 mg/kg followed by 0.02–0.03 mg/kg as needed during surgery) for neuromuscular blockade. The reversal agent (sugammadex 2 mg/kg or neostigmine methylsulfate 50 mcg/kg plus glycopyrrolate 10 mcg/kg) was then given at the reappearance of the second twitch (T$_2$) in a TOF stimulation (indicating recovery to moderate neuromuscular blockade) after the last dose of rocuronium or vecuronium was administered. The primary measure of efficacy was time to recovery of the TOF twitch ratio to 0.9, which is the currently accepted standard for adequate recovery of neuromuscular function following use of neuromuscular blocking agents. Time to recovery of neuromuscular function was substantially faster following administration of sugammadex compared with neostigmine. In patients with rocuronium- or vecuronium-induced neuromuscular blockade, median time to recovery was 1.4 or 2.1 minutes, respectively, with sugammadex compared with 21.5 or 29 minutes, respectively, with neostigmine.

Efficacy of sugammadex for reversal of *deep* neuromuscular blockade induced by rocuronium or vecuronium was evaluated in a similarly designed randomized, active-controlled study in 157 adults (median age 54–56 years, median body weight 81–84 kg, 45% male) undergoing elective surgery under general anesthesia that required endotracheal intubation and maintenance of neuromuscular blockade. In this study, the surgical procedures were mainly abdominal (i.e., gynecologic, colorectal, urologic), orthopedic, reconstructive, or neurologic. Patients

were randomized to receive rocuronium bromide (initial intubating dose of 0.6 mg/kg followed by 0.15 mg/kg as needed during surgery) or vecuronium bromide (initial intubating dose of 0.1 mg/kg followed by 0.015 mg/kg as needed during surgery) to maintain neuromuscular blockade. The reversal agent (sugammadex 4 mg/kg or neostigmine methylsulfate 70 mcg/kg plus glycopyrrolate 14 mcg/kg) was given at the reappearance of 1–2 posttetanic counts (indicating deep neuromuscular blockade) after the last dose of rocuronium or vecuronium was administered. The primary efficacy measure in this study also was time to recovery of the TOF twitch ratio to 0.9, although neostigmine was not expected to have an effect on recovery time since anticholinesterase agents are not effective in reversing deep neuromuscular blockade. Time to recovery of neuromuscular function was substantially faster following sugammadex administration compared with neostigmine; median time to recovery in patients receiving sugammadex was 2.7 or 3.3 minutes in the rocuronium or vecuronium groups, respectively, while time to recovery in patients receiving neostigmine was 49–50 minutes. A wider range of recovery times was observed with sugammadex in this study compared with recovery times in the study evaluating reversal from moderate neuromuscular blockade.

Efficacy of sugammadex for *rapid* reversal of rocuronium-induced neuromuscular blockade was evaluated in a randomized, active-controlled study that compared time to recovery from a profound rocuronium-induced neuromuscular block after administration of sugammadex with time to spontaneous recovery from succinylcholine. In this study, 110 patients (median age 43 years, median weight 70 kg, 42% male) undergoing elective surgery (mainly gynecologic, orthopedic, or reconstructive) that required endotracheal intubation and a short duration of neuromuscular blockade were randomized to receive high-dose rocuronium bromide (1.2 mg/kg) or succinylcholine chloride (1 mg/kg). Sugammadex was administered 3 minutes after the start of rocuronium. The primary measure of efficacy in this study was time from the start of administration of the neuromuscular blocking agent to recovery of the first twitch (T$_1$) in a TOF to 10% of the baseline value. Time to recovery of the TOF ratio to 0.9 was evaluated as a secondary end point. Mean time to recovery of T$_1$ to 10% of baseline was substantially faster with rocuronium/sugammadex than with spontaneous recovery from succinylcholine (4.4 and 7.1 minutes, respectively). In patients who received sugammadex, mean time to recovery of the TOF ratio to 0.9 was 2.2 minutes.

Because of its pharmacology and mechanism of action, sugammadex may provide potential clinical benefits over the cholinesterase inhibitors, including fast and predictable reversal of any degree of block, less potential for adverse effects (due to lack of effect on the acetylcholinesterase receptor system), and reduced incidence of residual block on recovery. In a Cochrane meta-analysis that included 41 randomized controlled studies comparing neostigmine and sugammadex for reversal of rocuronium-induced neuromuscular blockade in adults, sugammadex 2 mg/kg was 10.22 minutes (6.6 times) faster than neostigmine 0.05 mg/kg in reversing moderate paralysis, and sugammadex 4 mg/kg was 45.78 minutes (16.8 times) faster than neostigmine 0.07 mg/kg in reversing deep paralysis.

Sugammadex has not been studied for reversal of rocuronium- or vecuronium-induced neuromuscular blockade in the intensive care unit (ICU) setting.

DOSAGE AND ADMINISTRATION

● General

Patient Monitoring

- Monitor patients for adequate ventilation and maintenance of a patent airway from the time of sugammadex administration until complete recovery of neuromuscular function. (See Respiratory Function Monitoring under Cautions.)

- To ensure adequate reversal from the neuromuscular block, an objective (quantitative) method of monitoring is recommended in conjunction with qualitative monitoring (e.g., with a peripheral nerve stimulator) and other clinical assessments (e.g., observation of skeletal muscle tone, respiratory measurements).

- Adequate recovery of neuromuscular function generally is defined as a train-of-four (TOF) ratio of ≥0.9 in addition to the patient's ability to maintain satisfactory ventilation and a patent airway.

Dispensing and Administration Precautions

- Administer sugammadex only by trained clinicians experienced in the use of neuromuscular blocking agents and their reversal agents.

● Administration

Sugammadex is administered by direct IV ("bolus") injection over 10 seconds into an existing IV line. The manufacturer states that the drug has only been administered as a single direct IV injection in clinical trials.

Sugammadex injection should be inspected visually for particulate matter and discoloration prior to administration. The drug may be administered through an existing IV line containing the following solutions: 5% dextrose, 0.9% sodium chloride, 5% dextrose and 0.9% sodium chloride, 2.5% dextrose and 0.45% sodium chloride, Isolyte® P in 5% dextrose, Ringer's injection, or lactated Ringer's injection. The IV administration line should be adequately flushed (e.g., with 0.9% sodium chloride injection) between administration of sugammadex and other drugs. Sugammadex should not be mixed with other drugs.

Prior to use, sugammadex injection should be stored at room temperature (25°C) but may be exposed to temperatures of 15–30°C. The drug should be protected from light; if not protected from light, the vial should be used within 5 days.

● Dosage

Dosage of sugammadex sodium is expressed in terms of sugammadex.

The appropriate dose and timing of sugammadex should be based on twitch response monitoring and the extent of spontaneous recovery that has occurred. Recommended doses are based on actual body weight (ABW) and not on the anesthetic regimen used. Use of lower than recommended doses of sugammadex may lead to an increased risk of recurrence of neuromuscular blockade and is therefore not recommended.

No clinically relevant differences in pharmacokinetic parameters have been observed between obese patients and the general population when the drug is dosed according to ABW. The current evidence therefore supports the use of ABW-based dosing for sugammadex in patients who are morbidly obese (body mass index [BMI] ≥40 kg/m²) irrespective of the depth of neuromuscular blockade.

If readministration of a steroidal neuromuscular blocking agent is required (e.g., for intubation) after reversal with sugammadex, a minimum wait time should be observed. (See Readministration of Neuromuscular Blocking Agents under Cautions.)

Routine Reversal of Rocuronium- or Vecuronium-induced Neuromuscular Blockade

For reversal of rocuronium- or vecuronium-induced *moderate* neuromuscular blockade (i.e., spontaneous recovery has reached the reappearance of the second twitch [T_2] in response to TOF stimulation), the recommended adult dose of sugammadex is 2 mg/kg.

For reversal of rocuronium- or vecuronium-induced *deep* neuromuscular blockade (i.e., spontaneous recovery of the twitch response has reached 1–2 posttetanic counts and there are no twitch responses to TOF stimulation), the recommended adult dose of sugammadex is 4 mg/kg.

Immediate Reversal of Rocuronium-induced Neuromuscular Blockade

If there is a clinical need for reversal of neuromuscular blockade immediately (i.e., approximately 3 minutes) following administration of a single 1.2-mg/kg dose of rocuronium bromide, the recommended adult dose of sugammadex is 16 mg/kg. Efficacy of sugammadex 16 mg/kg for immediate reversal of *vecuronium*-induced neuromuscular blockade has not been established.

● Special Populations

Renal Impairment

No dosage adjustment is necessary in patients with mild or moderate renal impairment. Sugammadex is not recommended in patients with severe renal impairment, including those requiring dialysis. (See Renal Impairment under Cautions.)

Geriatric Patients

No dosage adjustment is necessary in geriatric patients with normal organ function. However, because sugammadex is substantially excreted by the kidneys and geriatric patients are more likely to have decreased renal function, the risk of adverse effects may be greater in such patients; careful dosage selection and monitoring of renal function are advised. (See Geriatric Use under Cautions.)

Other Special Populations

No dosage adjustment is necessary in patients with preexisting cardiac (e.g., ischemic heart disease, heart failure, arrhythmia) or pulmonary conditions, or those assessed as having an American Society of Anesthesiologists (ASA) physical status class of 3 or 4.

CAUTIONS

● Contraindications

- Known hypersensitivity to the drug or any ingredient in the formulation. (See Anaphylaxis and Hypersensitivity under Cautions.)

● Warnings/Precautions

Anaphylaxis and Hypersensitivity

Serious, potentially fatal, hypersensitivity reactions (including anaphylaxis) have been reported with sugammadex in premarketing clinical trials, postmarketing reports, and the medical literature. Such reactions have occurred in patients with no prior exposure to the drug. Manifestations have ranged from isolated skin reactions (e.g., flushing, urticaria, erythematous rash) to more severe systemic reactions (e.g., anaphylaxis or anaphylactic shock with manifestations such as severe hypotension, tachycardia, swelling of the tongue or pharynx, bronchospasm, and pulmonary obstructive events). In some cases, severe hypersensitivity reactions required the use of vasopressors, prolonged hospitalization, and/or additional respiratory support (e.g., intubation, prolonged intubation, assisted ventilation). Although the risk of anaphylaxis appears to increase with higher doses, anaphylactic reactions have occurred at sugammadex doses less than 16 mg/kg in the postmarketing setting.

In a double-blind, placebo-controlled repeat-dose study evaluating hypersensitivity reactions to sugammadex, healthy individuals were randomized to receive repeat IV injections of sugammadex 4 mg/kg, sugammadex 16 mg/kg, or placebo separated by an approximate 5-week period between doses to allow potential sensitization to develop. Of the 299 individuals who received sugammadex, anaphylaxis was reported in one patient (0.3%) in the 16-mg/kg group; manifestations including conjunctival edema, urticaria, erythema, swelling of the uvula, and reduction in peak expiratory flow occurred within 5 minutes after the first dose was administered. Nausea, pruritus, and urticaria were the most common non-anaphylactic hypersensitivity reactions reported in this study and appeared to be dose related; the overall incidence of hypersensitivity was 1, 7, or 9% in individuals receiving placebo, sugammadex 4 mg/kg, or sugammadex 16 mg/kg, respectively. In another study in healthy individuals, anaphylaxis occurred in 3 of 298 individuals (1%) receiving sugammadex 16 mg/kg.

Patients should be observed closely for possible hypersensitivity reactions after administration of sugammadex. Clinicians should be prepared for the possibility of such reactions and take necessary precautions.

Bradycardia

Marked bradycardia, sometimes resulting in cardiac arrest, has been reported within minutes after administration of sugammadex. Patients should be closely monitored for hemodynamic changes during and after reversal of neuromuscular blockade; anticholinergic agents (e.g., atropine) should be administered if clinically important bradycardia is observed.

Respiratory Function Monitoring

In clinical studies, a small number of patients experienced delayed or minimal reversal of neuromuscular blockade following sugammadex administration. Recurrence of neuromuscular blockade also is possible following extubation. Therefore, ventilatory support must be provided for all patients until adequate spontaneous respiration is restored and the ability to maintain a patent airway is assured. Ventilatory support may still be required after complete recovery of neuromuscular function because residual respiratory depression may occur due to other drugs used perioperatively or postoperatively.

If neuromuscular blockade persists after sugammadex is administered or recurs following extubation, appropriate steps should be taken to provide adequate ventilation. (See General under Dosage and Administration.)

Readministration of Neuromuscular Blocking Agents

If readministration of a steroidal neuromuscular blocking agent is necessary (e.g., for intubation) after reversal with sugammadex, a minimum wait time should be observed before the neuromuscular blocking agent is administered.

Following administration of sugammadex (2 or 4 mg/kg), at least 5 minutes should elapse before administration of rocuronium bromide 1.2 mg/kg, and at least 4 hours should elapse before administration of rocuronium bromide 0.6 mg/kg or vecuronium bromide 0.1 mg/kg. If rocuronium bromide 1.2 mg/kg is administered within 30 minutes after reversal with sugammadex, the onset of neuromuscular blockade may be delayed up to approximately 4 minutes and the duration of blockade shortened by approximately 15 minutes. In patients with mild or moderate renal impairment, a minimum wait time of 24 hours is recommended between administration of sugammadex (2 or 4 mg/kg) and readministration of rocuronium bromide 0.6 mg/kg or vecuronium bromide 0.1 mg/kg; if a shorter wait time is necessary, a rocuronium bromide dose of 1.2 mg/kg should be used for a new blockade.

Following reversal of rocuronium-induced neuromuscular blockade with sugammadex 16 mg/kg, a wait time of 24 hours is recommended before readministration of rocuronium or administration of vecuronium.

If neuromuscular blockade is required before the recommended wait times have elapsed, the manufacturer states that a nonsteroidal neuromuscular blocking agent should be used. However, the onset of neuromuscular blockade may be delayed with use of a depolarizing neuromuscular blocking agent such as succinylcholine in this setting.

Recurrence of Neuromuscular Blockade

The risk of recurrence of neuromuscular blockade may be increased with concurrent use of certain drugs (i.e., drugs that displace rocuronium or vecuronium from sugammadex binding sites) or use of lower than recommended doses of sugammadex. Risk also may be increased when drugs that potentiate neuromuscular blockade are used during the postoperative period; the manufacturer states that the prescribing information for rocuronium or vecuronium should be consulted for specific drugs that may potentiate neuromuscular blockade. (See Drugs that Displace Rocuronium or Vecuronium under Drug Interactions.)

Mechanical ventilation may be required if recurrence of neuromuscular blockade occurs.

Coagulopathy and Bleeding

Sugammadex may alter coagulation parameters and increase the risk of bleeding. In healthy individuals, sugammadex increased activated partial thromboplastin time (aPTT), prothrombin time (PT), and the international normalized ratio (INR) by up to 25% for up to 1 hour. In vitro, sugammadex in combination with vitamin K antagonists (e.g., warfarin), unfractionated heparin, low molecular weight heparins, rivaroxaban, or dabigatran resulted in additional increases in aPTT and PT/INR of up to 25 or 50% at peak plasma concentrations of sugammadex corresponding to 4 or 16 mg/kg doses, respectively.

In a study in patients undergoing major orthopedic surgery who were receiving thromboprophylaxis with heparin or a low molecular weight heparin, increases in aPTT and PT/INR of 5.5 and 3%, respectively, were observed within 1 hour following administration of sugammadex 4 mg/kg; however, a corresponding increase in the incidence of bleeding or anemia was not observed.

The risk of bleeding has not been evaluated with sugammadex 16 mg/kg in patients receiving thromboprophylaxis drugs. Bleeding risk also has not been evaluated in patients with known coagulopathies and those receiving therapeutic anticoagulation or thromboprophylaxis with drugs other than heparin and low molecular weight heparin; coagulation parameters should be carefully monitored in such patients.

Light Anesthesia

When neuromuscular blockade was reversed intentionally during anesthesia in clinical trials, signs of light anesthesia (e.g., movement, coughing, grimacing, suckling of the tracheal tube) were occasionally noted.

Specific Populations

Pregnancy

There are no clinical trial data regarding use of sugammadex in pregnant women. Data from a pharmacovigilance safety database and published literature in pregnant women are insufficient to inform a drug-associated risk. Animal studies revealed no evidence of malformations when sugammadex was administered during the period of organogenesis in rats and rabbits at maternal exposures up to 6 and 8 times, respectively, the maximum recommended human dose. However, incomplete ossification and reduced fetal body weight were observed in rabbits at sugammadex doses 8 times the maximum recommended human dose, which corresponds to a dose level that also produced maternal toxicity.

Lactation

It is not known whether sugammadex is distributed into human milk or if the drug has any effect on milk production or the nursing infant. The drug is distributed into milk in rats. The benefits of breast-feeding and the importance of sugammadex to the woman should be considered along with the potential adverse effects on the breast-fed infant from the drug or underlying maternal condition.

Pediatric Use

The manufacturer states that safety and efficacy of sugammadex have not been established in pediatric patients; however, the drug has been used for reversal of moderate rocuronium-induced neuromuscular blockade in pediatric patients.

In a study evaluating sugammadex for reversal of rocuronium-induced neuromuscular blockade in pediatric and adult patients undergoing surgery, similar recovery times were observed in pediatric patients 2–17 years of age and adults. Sugammadex plasma concentrations were similar in the different age groups, and no overall difference in safety was observed.

Animal studies have demonstrated increased sugammadex bone deposition in juvenile rats compared with adult rats. Decreased bone length and tooth abnormalities (i.e., discoloration and disturbance of enamel formation) were observed in juvenile rats receiving IV sugammadex daily for 28 days at doses approximately 0.1–3 times the maximum recommended human dose; these effects were not observed with once-weekly sugammadex doses up to 1.2 times the maximum recommended human dose.

Geriatric Use

In a study evaluating use of sugammadex in geriatric patients, median time to recovery of the train-of-four (TOF) ratio to 0.9 following administration of sugammadex 2 mg/kg at the reappearance of T_2 was 2.5 and 3.6 minutes in patients 65–74 years of age and those 75 years of age or older, respectively, compared with 2.2 minutes in younger adults (18–64 years of age). Across all clinical trials, geriatric patients 65 years of age or older who received sugammadex 4 mg/kg at 1–2 posttetanic counts had a median time to recovery of 2.5 minutes compared with 2 minutes in younger adults.

Hepatic Impairment

The pharmacokinetics of sugammadex have not been studied in patients with hepatic impairment. The manufacturer states that caution should be exercised if sugammadex is used in patients with hepatic impairment accompanied by coagulopathy or severe edema.

In a small observational study in patients undergoing hepatic surgery, the mean time to recovery from rocuronium-induced neuromuscular blockade following sugammadex 2 or 4 mg/kg was not substantially different in patients with hepatic impairment compared with those with normal hepatic function.

Renal Impairment

Sugammadex is principally eliminated by renal excretion; clearance is decreased and half-life prolonged in patients with renal impairment, resulting in increased systemic exposure of the drug.

Restricted Distribution Program

Uridine triacetate (as Vistogard®) can only be obtained through a specialty pharmacy. For inpatient use, clinicians may contact the specialty pharmacy at 844-293-0007. For outpatient use and information on the case management program, clinicians may contact the specialty pharmacy at 844-374-0604. Ordering information also is available on the Vistogard® website (https://www.vistogard.com/Resources/How-to-Order).

Uridine triacetate (as Xuriden®) also can only be obtained through a specialty pharmacy. Clinicians may contact the manufacturer at 800-914-0071 for availability and ordering information.

● *Administration*

Uridine triacetate is administered orally as granules (e.g., Vistogard®, Xuriden®) and may be given without regard to meals (see Description).

Opened packets or mixtures of uridine triacetate with food, milk, or infant formula should not be stored. Packets of the drug are for single use only; any unused portions should be discarded. Any granules left in an open packet should not be used for subsequent dosing.

Vistogard® Granules

Uridine triacetate (Vistogard®) treatment should begin as soon as possible following overdosage or early-onset toxicity of fluorouracil or capecitabine and should be given within 96 hours following the end of fluorouracil or capecitabine administration.

Pediatric doses of uridine triacetate should be weighed using a scale accurate to at least 0.1 g or measured using a graduated teaspoon accurate to one-fourth teaspoonful. For patients requiring 10-g doses of uridine triacetate, the contents of a full packet may be administered without weighing or measuring.

Each Vistogard® dose should be mixed with 3–4 ounces of soft food (e.g., applesauce, pudding, yogurt) and ingested within 30 minutes. The drug may be given without regard to meals. The granules should *not* be chewed. Patients should drink at least 120 mL (4 ounces) of water after each dose.

Nausea and vomiting may occur during Vistogard® therapy because of capecitabine or fluorouracil toxicity and, less commonly, because of the slightly bitter taste of the uridine triacetate granules. If a patient vomits within 2 hours after receiving a dose of uridine triacetate, another full dose should be administered as soon as possible after the vomiting episode. The next dose should be administered at the regularly scheduled time. Use of an antiemetic (e.g., a type 3 serotonin [5-HT$_3$] receptor antagonist) also may be helpful in such cases.

If a dose of uridine triacetate is missed, the missed dose should be administered as soon as possible and the next dose should be administered at the regularly scheduled time.

Nasogastric Tube or Gastrostomy Tube

Uridine triacetate (Vistogard®) may be administered via nasogastric or gastrostomy tube when necessary (e.g., severe mucositis, coma). About 100 mL (approximately 4 fluid ounces) of a food starch-based thickening product in water should be prepared and stirred briskly until the thickener has dissolved. The contents of one 10-g packet of Vistogard® granules should be crushed to a fine powder and then added to about 100 mL (4 ounces) of reconstituted food starch-based thickening product. For pediatric patients receiving doses of less than 10 g, the mixture should be prepared in a ratio not exceeding 1 g of uridine triacetate to 10 mL of reconstituted food starch-based thickening product and mixed thoroughly.

Following administration of the mixture using the nasogastric or gastrostomy tube, the tube should be flushed with water.

Xuriden® Granules

Doses of uridine triacetate (Xuriden®) should be weighed using a scale accurate to at least 0.1 g or measured using a graduated teaspoon accurate to the fraction of the dose to be administered. For patients requiring doses of uridine triacetate in multiples of 2 g (i.e., three-fourths teaspoonful), the contents of the required number of 2-g packets may be administered without weighing or measuring.

Doses of uridine triacetate should be administered orally immediately after mixing with 3–4 ounces of applesauce, pudding, or yogurt. The granules should *not* be chewed. Administration of each dose should be followed with at least 120 mL (4 ounces) of water.

Xuriden® granules may be mixed with 5 mL of milk or infant formula instead of soft foods for patients receiving up to 2 g (three-fourths teaspoonful) of uridine triacetate granules. The manufacturer's instructions for preparing such doses using a medicine cup and an oral syringe in the Xuriden® prescribing information should be consulted. Doses that are mixed in milk or infant formula should be administered using an oral syringe placed between the patient's cheek and gum at the back of the mouth. A bottle of milk or infant formula may be given after administration of the drug, if desired.

● *Dosage*

Dosage of uridine triacetate is expressed in terms of the salt.

Fluorouracil or Capecitabine Overdosage or Toxicity

For the emergency treatment of patients following fluorouracil or capecitabine overdosage (regardless of the presence of symptoms) or patients who exhibit early onset, severe or life-threatening cardiac or CNS toxicity and/or early onset, unusually severe adverse reactions (e.g., GI toxicity, neutropenia), the recommended dosage of uridine triacetate (Vistogard®) in adults is 10 g (one packet) orally every 6 hours for a total of 20 doses for a full course of treatment.

In pediatric patients with such fluorouracil or capecitabine overdosage or toxicity, the recommended dosage of uridine triacetate is 6.2 g/m^2 of body surface area (not exceeding 10 g/dose) orally every 6 hours for a total of 20 doses for a full course of treatment. (See Table 1.)

TABLE 1. Uridine Triacetate (Vistogard®) Pediatric Dosing Based on Body Surface Area.

Body Surface Area (m^2)	Vistogard® 6.2 g/m^2 per dose	
	Dose (g)	Dose (graduated teaspoonful)
0.34–0.44	2.1–2.7	1
0.45–0.55	2.8–3.4	1¼
0.56–0.66	3.5–4.1	1½
0.67–0.77	4.2–4.8	1¾
0.78–0.88	4.9–5.4	2
0.89–0.99	5.5–6.1	2¼
1–1.1	6.2–6.8	2½
1.11–1.21	6.9–7.5	2¾
1.22–1.32	7.6–8.1	3
1.33–1.43	8.2–8.8	3¼
1.44 or greater	10	1 full 10-g packet[a]

Note: One packet of Vistogard® granules contains 10 g of uridine triacetate. Dose by body surface area in this table was rounded to achieve the approximate dose. Each dose is administered every 6 hours for 20 doses.

[a] One entire 10-g packet may be used without weighing or measuring.

Hereditary Orotic Aciduria

The recommended initial dosage of uridine triacetate (Xuriden®) for the treatment of adult and pediatric patients with hereditary orotic aciduria is 60 mg/kg orally once daily. (See Table 2.)

TABLE 2. *Initial* Uridine Triacetate (Xuriden®) 60 mg/kg Daily Dosage Based on Body Weight.

| Patient Weight (in kg) | Xuriden® 60 mg/kg Daily Dosage | |
	Dose (in grams using a scale)	Dose (in teaspoonsful)
Up to 5	0.4	1/8
6–10	0.4–0.6	¼
11–15	0.7–0.9	½
16–20	1–1.2	½
21–25	1.3–1.5	½
26–30	1.6–1.8	¾[a]
31–35	1.9–2.1[a]	¾[a]
36–40	2.2–2.4	1
41–45	2.5–2.7	1
46–50	2.8–3	1
51–55	3.1–3.3	1¼
56–60	3.4–3.6	1¼
61–65	3.7–3.9[b]	1½[b]
66–70	4–4.2[b]	1½[b]
71–75	4.3–4.5	1½[b]
greater than 75	6[c]	2[c]

Note: One packet of Xuriden® granules contains 2 g (approximately three-fourths teaspoon) of uridine triacetate. Total daily dosages by weight category in this table were rounded to achieve the approximate dosage level.

[a] One entire 2-g packet may be used without weighing or measuring.

[b] Two entire 2-g packets may be used without weighing or measuring.

[c] Three entire 2-g packets may be used without weighing or measuring.

Dosage of uridine triacetate may be increased to 120 mg/kg (not to exceed 8 g) orally once daily for insufficient response. (See Table 3.) Signs of insufficient response may include urinary concentrations of orotic acid that are above normal or are increased above the usual or expected range for the patient, worsening of laboratory parameters affected by the condition (e.g., red or white blood cell indices), or worsening of other manifestations of the condition.

TABLE 3. *Increased* Uridine Triacetate (Xuriden®) 120 mg/kg Daily Dosage for Insufficient Response Based on Body Weight.

| Patient Weight (in kg) | Xuriden® 120 mg/kg Daily Dosage | |
	Dose (in grams using a scale)	Dose (in teaspoonsful)
Up to 5	0.8	¼
6–10	0.8–1.2	½
11–15	1.4–1.8	¾
16–20	2–2.4	1
21–25	2.6–3	1
26–30	3.2–3.6	1¼

TABLE 3. Continued

| Patient Weight (in kg) | Xuriden® 120 mg/kg Daily Dosage | |
	Dose (in grams using a scale)	Dose (in teaspoonsful)
31–35	3.8–4.2[a]	1½[a]
36–40	4.4–4.8	1¾
41–45	5–5.4	2[b]
46–50	5.6–6	2[b]
51–55	6.2–6.6	2¼
56–60	6.8–7.2	2½
61–65	7.4–7.8	2½
66–70	8[c]	2¾[c]
71–75	8[c]	2¾[c]
greater than 75	8[c]	2¾[c]

Note: One packet of Xuriden® granules contains 2 g (approximately three-fourths teaspoon) of uridine triacetate. Total daily dosages by weight category in this table were rounded to achieve the approximate dosage level.

[a] Two entire 2-g packets may be used without weighing or measuring.

[b] Three entire 2-g packets may be used without weighing or measuring.

[c] Four entire 2-g packets may be used without weighing or measuring.

● *Special Populations*

No dosage adjustment is necessary based on age, body size, race, or gender in adults.

CAUTIONS

● *Contraindications*

The manufacturer states that there are no known contraindications to the use of uridine triacetate.

● *Warnings/Precautions*

Warnings and Precautions

The manufacturer states that there are no warnings or precautions associated with uridine triacetate therapy.

Specific Populations

Pregnancy

Limited case reports of uridine triacetate (Vistogard®) use during pregnancy are inadequate to inform a drug-associated risk of birth defects and miscarriage. There are no data regarding use of uridine triacetate (Xuriden®) in pregnant women to inform a drug-associated risk.

Animal studies have not revealed evidence of teratogenicity or fetal harm at uridine triacetate dosages of about one-half the maximum recommended human dosage of Vistogard® or 2.7 times the maximum recommended human dosage of Xuriden® administered to pregnant rats during the period of organogenesis.

Lactation

It is not known whether uridine triacetate is distributed into human milk; effects of the drug on breast-fed infants or milk production also are not known. The benefits of breast-feeding and the woman's clinical need for uridine triacetate should be considered along with any potential adverse effects on the breast-fed infant from the drug or from the underlying maternal condition.

Pediatric Use

Safety and efficacy of uridine triacetate (Vistogard®) for emergency treatment following fluorouracil or capecitabine overdosage or early-onset, severe or life-threatening toxicity have been established in pediatric patients. Such use is supported by an open-label study that included 6 pediatric patients 1–16 years of age. Four of these pediatric patients were 1–7 years of age and received a body surface area-adjusted dosage of the drug.

Safety and efficacy of uridine triacetate (Xuriden®) for treatment of hereditary orotic aciduria have been established in a single open-label study in 4 pediatric patients 3 years of age or older and based on case reports of 18 pediatric patients who began uridine triacetate treatment at 2 months to 12 years of age.

Clinical response and safety of uridine triacetate in adults and pediatric patients are similar; however, data are limited. (See Uses.)

Geriatric Use

In clinical studies evaluating uridine triacetate (Vistogard®) for treatment of fluorouracil or capecitabine overdosage or toxicity, 30% of patients were 65 years of age or older and 11% were 75 years of age or older. Clinical studies did not include sufficient numbers of patients 65 years of age or older to determine whether they respond differently than younger adults.

In a population pharmacokinetic analysis, patient age (range: 20–83 years) did not substantially affect uridine pharmacokinetics.

● Common Adverse Effects

The most common adverse effects occurring in more than 2% of patients receiving uridine triacetate (Vistogard®) for emergency treatment of fluorouracil or capecitabine overdosage or toxicity in clinical trials were vomiting, nausea, and diarrhea.

No adverse effects were reported in patients receiving uridine triacetate (Xuriden®) for the treatment of hereditary orotic aciduria in the principal efficacy study.

DRUG INTERACTIONS

Clinically important drug interactions with uridine triacetate have not been identified to date.

In vitro studies indicate that uridine triacetate and uridine do not have clinically important inhibitory effects on cytochrome P-450 (CYP) isoenzymes 3A4, 1A2, 2C8, 2C9, 2C19, 2D6, or 2E1. In vitro studies also indicate that uridine triacetate and uridine do not induce CYP isoenzymes 1A2, 2B6, or 3A4.

● Drugs Affecting or Metabolized by Hepatic Microsomal Enzymes

Clinically important drug interactions between uridine triacetate and drugs that affect or are metabolized by CYP isoenzymes appear unlikely.

● Drugs Affecting or Affected by P-glycoprotein Transport System

In vitro studies indicate that uridine triacetate is a weak substrate for P-glycoprotein (P-gp). Uridine triacetate inhibited the transport of digoxin (a P-gp substrate) with an IC_{50} (concentration that inhibits activity by 50%) of 344 μM. Potential pharmacokinetic interaction of uridine triacetate with orally administered substrates of P-gp cannot be ruled out due to the potential for locally increased (gut) concentrations of uridine triacetate.

● Drugs Affecting GI Absorption

The manufacturer states that the expanded access protocol for uridine triacetate (Vistogard®) initially contained instructions to avoid drugs that could potentially interfere with the GI absorption of uridine triacetate (e.g., bismuth subsalicylate, cholestyramine, sucralfate). However, there currently is no evidence that these drugs can slow the absorption of uridine or uridine triacetate. In addition, formal drug interaction studies have confirmed the lack of such an interaction. Therefore, the instruction to avoid drugs that may interfere with absorption of uridine triacetate was removed from the expanded access protocol and also was not included in the Vistogard® prescribing information.

● Antineoplastic Agents

The effect of uridine triacetate on the antitumor activity of fluorouracil is not known. However, concomitant use of uridine triacetate potentially may result in decreased fluorouracil or capecitabine efficacy. The manufacturer states that use of uridine triacetate is *not* recommended for the *nonemergency* treatment of adverse reactions associated with fluorouracil or capecitabine.

DESCRIPTION

Uridine triacetate is an acetylated prodrug of uridine and a pyrimidine analog. In fluorouracil or capecitabine overdosage or toxicity, uridine triacetate is a direct biochemical antagonist of fluorouracil. Excess circulating uridine derived from uridine triacetate is converted into uridine triphosphate (UTP), which competes with 5-fluorouridine triphosphate (FUTP; a cytotoxic intermediate metabolite of fluorouracil) for incorporation into RNA, thereby inhibiting cell damage and cell death.

In hereditary orotic aciduria, uridine triacetate provides an exogenous source of uridine for replacement therapy in patients who are unable to synthesize adequate quantities of uridine. Uridine can be used for the synthesis of uridine nucleotides by essentially all cells. Restoration of intracellular uridine nucleotide concentrations to within the normal range reduces the overproduction of orotic acid by feedback inhibition, thereby also reducing the urinary excretion of orotic acid.

Following oral administration, uridine triacetate is deacetylated by nonspecific esterases present throughout the body to form uridine. Uridine triacetate has a substantially higher oral bioavailability than uridine, providing fourfold to sixfold more uridine into the systemic circulation than equimolar oral doses of uridine. Uridine triacetate crosses the intestinal mucosa much more readily than uridine, and peak plasma concentrations of uridine following single-dose oral administration of uridine triacetate are generally achieved within 2–3 hours. Administration of a slightly different formulation of uridine triacetate granules with food in healthy adults did not affect the overall rate and extent of uridine exposure compared with those observed following administration of the drug in the fasted state. Uridine crosses the blood-brain barrier. Circulating uridine is taken up by mammalian cells via specific nucleoside transporters. Uridine can be excreted by the kidneys or metabolized by normal pyrimidine catabolic pathways present in most tissues. The elimination half-life of uridine is approximately 2–2.5 hours.

ADVICE TO PATIENTS

Importance of providing patients or their caregivers with a copy of the manufacturer's patient information (Vistogard®) or instructions for use (Xuriden®).

For Vistogard® or Xuriden® doses less than the entire contents of a packet, importance of weighing or measuring the prescribed dose using appropriate equipment (e.g., a scale accurate to at least 0.1 g, a graduated teaspoon accurate to one-fourth teaspoonful or the fraction of the dose to be administered).

Uridine triacetate granules should *not* be chewed. Vistogard® and Xuriden® granules may be mixed with food (e.g., applesauce, pudding, yogurt). Xuriden® also may be mixed in milk or infant formula. Any unused portion of uridine triacetate granules remaining in the single-use packets after measuring out the appropriate dose should be discarded.

Importance of patients completing the full course of treatment (i.e., 20 doses) of Vistogard® even if they feel well. If a patient vomits within 2 hours after receiving a dose of Vistogard®, another full dose should be administered as a replacement as soon as possible after the vomiting episode; the next dose should be administered at the regularly scheduled time. If a dose of Vistogard® is missed, the missed dose should be administered as soon as possible and the next dose should be administered at the regularly scheduled time.

Importance of informing clinicians of existing or contemplated concomitant therapy, including prescription and OTC drugs and dietary or herbal supplements, as well as any concomitant illnesses.

Importance of advising women receiving uridine triacetate to inform clinicians if they are or plan to become pregnant or plan to breast-feed.

Importance of informing patients of other important precautionary information. (See Cautions.)

PREPARATIONS

Distribution of uridine triacetate (Vistogard® and Xuriden®) is restricted. (See Restricted Distribution Program under Dosage and Administration: General.)

Excipients in commercially available drug preparations may have clinically important effects in some individuals; consult specific product labeling for details.

Uridine Triacetate

Oral

Granules	2 g (of uridine triacetate) per packet	**Xuriden®**, Wellstat
	10 g (of uridine triacetate) per packet	**Vistogard®**, Wellstat (marketed by BTG)

† Use is not currently included in the labeling approved by the US Food and Drug Administration.

Selected Revisions May 10, 2024, © Copyright, April 13, 2017, American Society of Health-System Pharmacists, Inc.

Flumazenil

91:32.04 • GABA-MEDIATED BENZODIAZEPINE ANTIDOTES

■ Flumazenil, a 1,4-imidazobenzodiazepine derivative, is a benzodiazepine antagonist.

USES

Flumazenil is used in adults for the complete or partial reversal of benzodiazepine-induced sedation when benzodiazepines are used for induction or maintenance of general anesthesia or for diagnostic or therapeutic procedures (i.e., conscious sedation) and for the management of benzodiazepine intoxication. Flumazenil also is used in children 1–17 years of age for the reversal of benzodiazepine-induced sedation when benzodiazepines are used for diagnostic or therapeutic procedures. The manufacturer states that the safety and efficacy of flumazenil have *not* been established in pediatric patients for reversal of benzodiazepine-induced sedation when benzodiazepines are used for induction of general anesthesia, for the management of benzodiazepine intoxication, nor for the resuscitation of neonates. (See Special Populations: Pediatric Use.)

● Reversal of General Anesthesia

Flumazenil has been shown to be effective in reversing sedation and restoring psychomotor function in adults who received midazolam for induction or maintenance of general anesthesia. Efficacy was established in 4 clinical studies in adults who received 5–80 mg of midazolam alone or in conjunction with skeletal muscle relaxants, nitrous oxide, regional or local anesthetics, opiates, and/or inhalational anesthetics. A 0. 2-mg dose of flumazenil was administered, followed by additional 0. 2-mg doses as needed to reach a complete response (up to a maximum of 1 mg). In these studies, 81% of patients became completely alert or remained only slightly drowsy following total flumazenil doses of 0.4–0.6 mg (36%) or 0.8–1 mg (64%). However, resedation occurred in 10–15% of patients who responded to flumazenil. (See Warnings: Resedation.) Flumazenil failed to restore memory completely as tested by picture recall. In addition, flumazenil was not as effective in the reversal of sedation in patients who received multiple anesthetic agents in addition to benzodiazepines.

● Reversal of Conscious Sedation

Flumazenil has been shown to be effective in reversing the sedative and psychomotor effects of benzodiazepines when these drugs are used for diagnostic or therapeutic procedures but was less effective in completely and consistently reversing benzodiazepine-induced amnesia. Efficacy was established in 4 clinical studies in adults who received an average of 30 mg of diazepam or 10 mg of midazolam for sedation (with or without an opiate) for both inpatient and outpatient diagnostic or surgical procedures. Flumazenil was administered as an initial dose of 0.4 mg (2 doses of 0.2 mg each), with additional 0. 2-mg doses administered as needed to achieve complete awakening, up to a maximum of 1 mg. In these studies, 78% of patients receiving flumazenil achieved complete consciousness, but approximately 50% of these patients required 2–3 additional doses of the drug in order to achieve this level of consciousness. In addition, while most patients remained alert throughout the 3-hour postprocedure observation period, resedation occurred in 3–9% of these patients.

Pediatric Considerations

The safety and efficacy of flumazenil for the reversal of benzodiazepine-induced conscious sedation have been established in children 1 year of age and older. In one uncontrolled clinical trial involving 107 children 1–17 years of age who had received midazolam for conscious sedation, flumazenil was administered at doses of 0.01 mg/kg (maximum of 0.2 mg) up to a maximum of 5 doses or a total dose of 1 mg. In this study, 56% of the children achieved complete consciousness within 10 minutes of flumazenil administration, but 51% of them required the maximum number of doses of the drug allowed for initial treatment in order to achieve this level of consciousness. In addition, approximately 12% of the patients (all of whom were 1–5 years of age) who achieved complete consciousness following flumazenil administration experienced resedation within 19–50 minutes of initial

administration of the drug. Episodes of resedation were reversed by additional doses of flumazenil. However, the manufacturer states that the safety and efficacy of repeated flumazenil administration in pediatric patients experiencing resedation have *not* been established.

● Benzodiazepine Overdosage

Flumazenil is used in adults for the management of benzodiazepine overdosage. The drug is an adjunct to, not a replacement for, appropriate supportive and symptomatic measures (e.g., ventilatory and circulatory support) in the management of benzodiazepine overdosage. Because patients admitted to hospitals for drug overdoses may have ingested multiple substances and/or are being treated for concomitant illnesses (e.g., depression, substance abuse), the presence of contraindications or precautions, which may limit the use of flumazenil therapy, should be considered. (See Contraindications under Warnings/Precautions, in Cautions.) Flumazenil has no known benefit other than reversal of benzodiazepine-induced sedation in seriously ill patients with multiple-drug overdosage, and the drug should *not* be used in cases where seizures (from any cause) are likely. In addition, the manufacturer warns that flumazenil should *not* be used in patients with serious cyclic depressant overdosage. (See Drug Interactions: Cyclic Antidepressants.) For information on the pathogenesis, manifestations, and treatment of benzodiazepine overdosage, see Acute Toxicity in the Benzodiazepines General Statement 28:24.08.

Efficacy of flumazenil has been established in 2 studies in patients who were presumed to have taken an overdose of a benzodiazepine, either alone or in combination with a variety of other agents. In these studies, of patients who were proven to have taken a benzodiazepine, 80% of those who received flumazenil responded with an improvement in level of consciousness. Of those who responded to flumazenil, 75% responded to a total dose of 1–3 mg. However, reversal of sedation was associated with an increased frequency of symptoms of CNS excitation, and 1–3% of patients who received flumazenil were treated for agitation or anxiety.

● Other Uses

The manufacturer states that the safety and efficacy of flumazenil for the treatment of benzodiazepine dependence or for the management of protracted benzodiazepine abstinence syndrome have not been established and therefore such use currently is not recommended.

DOSAGE AND ADMINISTRATION

● General

Flumazenil is administered by rapid (over 15–30 seconds) IV injection through a freely flowing IV infusion into a large vein. Because of the risk of local irritation, the drug is recommended for IV use only, and extravasation into perivascular tissues should be avoided. Patients should have a secure airway and established IV access prior to administration of the drug.

While flumazenil dosages exceeding the minimally effective dose may be tolerated by most adults, such dosages can complicate the management of patients who are physically dependent on benzodiazepines or in whom the therapeutic benefit of the drugs is needed (e.g., for seizure control in cyclic antidepressant overdosage). Therefore, flumazenil dosage should be titrated carefully using the smallest effective dosage. Currently recommended flumazenil dosing regimens involve multiple small doses rather than large bolus doses in order to provide better control of sedation reversal while minimizing the risk of adverse effects.

Reversal of General Anesthesia and Conscious Sedation in Adults

When flumazenil is used to reverse benzodiazepine-induced sedative effects after anesthesia or conscious sedation in adults, the usual initial dose is 0.2 mg given IV over 15 seconds; if the desired consciousness level is not achieved after waiting 45 seconds, additional 0.2-mg doses may be administered at 1-minute intervals until an adequate response is achieved or a maximum of 4 additional doses is administered (i.e., maximum cumulative dose of 1 mg during an initial 5-minute dosing period). If resedation occurs, the initial dosing regimen (i.e., up to 1 mg given in divided 0.2-mg doses at 1-minute intervals) may be repeated no more frequently than every 20 minutes up to a maximum of 3 mg in any 1-hour period. In certain high risk patients (consult the manufacturer's labeling), it may be necessary to reduce the dose and/or increase the interval between doses to longer than 1 minute. Most patients respond to cumulative flumazenil doses of 0.6–1 mg, but individual requirements may vary considerably depending on the dose and duration of effect of the benzodiazepine administered and patient characteristics. In clinical situations where resedation is not yet apparent but must be prevented, the initial dosing regimen can be repeated at 30 and possibly repeated at 60 minutes despite the current absence of manifestations of recurrence.

Reversal of Conscious Sedation in Children

When flumazenil is used in children to reverse benzodiazepine-induced sedative effects after conscious sedation, the usual initial dose is 0.01 mg/kg (up to 0.2 mg) given IV over 15 seconds; if the desired consciousness level is not achieved after waiting 45 seconds, additional 0.01-mg/kg (up to 0.2 mg) doses may be administered at 1-minute intervals until an adequate response is achieved or a maximum of 4 additional doses is administered (i.e., maximum cumulative dose of 0.05 mg/kg or 1 mg, whichever is lower). In the pediatric clinical trial of flumazenil, a mean total dose of 0.65 mg (range: 0.08–1 mg) was administered to children 1–17 years of age with approximately 50% of children requiring the maximum of 5 injections. The safety and efficacy of repeated flumazenil administration in pediatric patients experiencing resedation have not been established.

Management of Benzodiazepine Overdosage in Adults

When flumazenil is used for known or suspected benzodiazepine overdosage in adults, the usual initial dose is 0.2 mg given IV over 30 seconds; if the desired consciousness level is not achieved after waiting 30 seconds, an additional 0.3-mg dose may be administered over 30 seconds. If an adequate response still is not achieved, further additional 0.5-mg doses may be administered over 30 seconds at 1-minute intervals up to a cumulative dose of 3 mg. Most patients respond to cumulative flumazenil doses of 1–3 mg, and cumulative doses exceeding 3 mg have not been shown reproducibly to provide additional benefit. However, some patients who exhibit a partial response after a 3-mg cumulative dose rarely may require additional doses up to a total of 5 mg. If no response is observed within 5 minutes after administration of an initial 5-mg cumulative dose of flumazenil, the major cause of sedation may not be a benzodiazepine and additional flumazenil doses likely will provide little if any beneficial effect. If resedation occurs, the initial dosing regimen (i.e., up to 1 mg given in divided 0.5-mg doses at 1-minute intervals) may be repeated no more frequently than every 20 minutes up to a maximum dose of 3 mg in any 1-hour period.

● *Special Populations*

Patients with hepatic impairment have decreased clearance of flumazenil. While the initial dose of flumazenil for reversal of benzodiazepine effects is not affected, repeat doses of the drug should be reduced in size or frequency in patients with hepatic impairment.

CAUTIONS

● *Contraindications*

Flumazenil is contraindicated in patients receiving a benzodiazepine for control of a potentially life-threatening condition (e.g., control of intracranial pressure or status epilepticus) and in those exhibiting manifestations of serious cyclic antidepressant overdosage. (See Warnings: Seizures.) Flumazenil also is contraindicated in patients with known hypersensitivity to the drug or benzodiazepines.

● *Warnings/Precautions*

Warnings

Seizures

Use of flumazenil for the reversal of benzodiazepine effects may be associated with the onset of seizures in certain high-risk patients. Seizures are most frequent in patients who have been receiving benzodiazepines for long-term sedation or in patients with manifestations of serious cyclic antidepressant overdose. Other risk factors for seizures following flumazenil administration include major sedative-hypnotic drug withdrawal, recent therapy with repeated doses of parenteral benzodiazepines, myoclonic jerking or seizure activity prior to flumazenil administration in overdose cases, or concurrent cyclic antidepressant poisoning. Most convulsions associated with flumazenil administration require treatment, and have been successfully managed with anticonvulsants such as phenytoin,

barbiturates, or benzodiazepines. However, if benzodiazepines are used to treat flumazenil-associated seizures, higher dosages than usual may be required.

Hypoventilation

The manufacturer states that the efficacy of flumazenil in reversing benzodiazepine-induced hypoventilation has not been established, and the drug may not fully reverse postoperative airway problems or ventilatory insufficiency associated with benzodiazepine administration. In addition, even if initial efficacy is observed, the ventilatory effects of flumazenil may subside prior to those of the benzodiazepine; therefore, facilities and equipment for immediate ventilatory support should be readily available for any patient receiving the drug. In patients with serious pulmonary disease who experience serious benzodiazepine-induced respiratory depression, primary therapy should be appropriate ventilatory support rather than flumazenil therapy.

General Precautions

Return of Sedation

Resedation may occur in patients who have responded to flumazenil. Resedation is most likely to occur in cases where a large single or cumulative dose of a benzodiazepine (e.g., midazolam dosages exceeding 10 mg) has been administered in the course of a long procedure (e.g., longer than 60 minutes) along with neuromuscular blocking agents and multiple anesthetic agents and least likely to occur in cases where flumazenil is administered to reverse a low dose of a short-acting benzodiazepine (less than 10 mg of midazolam). In clinical studies, resedation was observed in 1–3% of adults and in about 12% of children. Therefore, patients should be carefully monitored for an adequate period of time (i.e., up to 2 hours) based on the dose and duration of effect of the benzodiazepine employed for signs of resedation, respiratory depression, or other residual benzodiazepine effects. Although the safety and efficacy of repeated flumazenil administration in pediatric patients experiencing resedation have not been established, repeated doses of flumazenil may be administered to adult patients when necessary. (See Dosage and Administration: Dosage.)

Withdrawal Reactions

Flumazenil may precipitate dose-dependent manifestations of withdrawal in patients with established physical dependence on benzodiazepines. An acute withdrawal syndrome characterized by dizziness, mild confusion, emotional lability, agitation (with signs and symptoms of anxiety), and mild sensory distortions has occurred in adults receiving flumazenil, particularly at doses above 1 mg. However, such reactions rarely required treatment other than reassurance and were usually short-lived. When treatment was necessary, patients were successfully treated with usual doses of barbiturates, benzodiazepines, or other sedative agents. Because benzodiazepine tolerance and dependence is frequently observed in patients with alcoholism and other drug dependencies, clinicians should assume that flumazenil administration may complicate the management of withdrawal syndromes for alcohol, barbiturates, and cross-tolerant sedatives. Seizures also may occur following flumazenil administration in patients with established physical dependence on benzodiazepines. (See Warnings: Seizures.)

Intensive Care Setting

The manufacturer states that use of flumazenil in an intensive care setting to define CNS depression as being benzodiazepine induced is *not* recommended because of the risk of precipitating potentially serious manifestations of withdrawal (e.g., seizures) in cases of unrecognized benzodiazepine dependence and because of the prognostic uncertainty of failure to respond to flumazenil in cases confounded by a metabolic disorder, traumatic injury, effects of other drugs, or any other factor not associated with benzodiazepine-receptor occupancy.

Head Injury

Because flumazenil may precipitate seizures or alter cerebral blood flow in patients receiving benzodiazepines, the drug should be used with caution and only by clinicians who are prepared to manage such complications in patients with head injury.

Panic Disorders

Flumazenil has been reported to provoke panic attacks in patients with a history of panic disorder.

Pulmonary Disease

Because the efficacy of flumazenil in reversing benzodiazepine-induced alterations in ventilatory drive has not been established, the primary treatment of patients with serious lung disease who experience serious respiratory depression secondary to benzodiazepines should be appropriate ventilatory support (see Warnings: Hypoventilation) rather than the administration of flumazenil.

Cardiovascular Disease

Use of flumazenil alone had no clinically important effects on cardiovascular parameters when administered to patients with stable ischemic heart disease to reverse the effects of benzodiazepines.

Specific Populations

Pregnancy

Category C. (See Users Guide.) Use during labor and delivery is not recommended since the effects of flumazenil on the neonate are not known.

Lactation

It is not known whether flumazenil is distributed in milk. Caution is advised if the drug is administered in nursing women.

Pediatric Use

Safety and efficacy of flumazenil in the reversal of conscious sedation in infants younger than 1 year of age have not been established. In addition, the manufacturer states that safety and efficacy of flumazenil, including the potential risks, benefits, and appropriate dosages, have not been established for the management of benzodiazepine overdosage, for neonatal resuscitation, nor for the reversal of sedation when benzodiazepines are used for induction of general anesthesia. However, published anecdotal reports discussing the use of flumazenil in pediatric patients for these indications have reported similar safety profiles and dosing guidelines to those described for the reversal of conscious sedation. The risks associated with flumazenil use in the adult population also apply to pediatric patients. (See Cautions: Warnings/Precautions.)

Geriatric Use

No substantial differences in safety or efficacy relative to younger adults, but increased sensitivity to flumazenil cannot be ruled out.

● Common Adverse Effects

Adverse effects occurring in 3–9% of patients receiving flumazenil include dizziness, injection site pain, increased sweating, headache, and abnormal or blurred vision. In addition, serious adverse effects such as cardiac arrhythmias (e.g., junctional or ventricular tachycardias), seizures, and deaths have occurred. Most deaths occurred in patients with serious underlying disease or in patients who had ingested large amounts of non-benzodiazepine drugs (usually cyclic antidepressants) as part of an overdose. (See Warnings: Seizures in Cautions.)

DRUG INTERACTIONS

● Cyclic Antidepressants

Potential pharmacodynamic interactions. (See Warnings: Seizures.) Flumazenil should *not* be used in patients exhibiting manifestations of serious concurrent cyclic antidepressant overdosage, such as motor abnormalities (e.g., twitching, rigidity, focal seizures), arrhythmias (e.g., wide QRS complexes, ventricular arrhythmias, heart block), anticholinergic effects (e.g., mydriasis, dry mucosa, hypoperistalsis), or cardiovascular collapse. In such cases, the patient should be managed with ventilatory and circulatory supportive measures as needed until the signs of antidepressant toxicity have subsided. For information on the pathogenesis, manifestations, and treatment of cyclic antidepressant overdosage, see Acute Toxicity in the Tricyclic Antidepressants General Statement 28:16.04.28.

● Benzodiazepines

Pharmacokinetic interaction unlikely. However, flumazenil may precipitate dose-dependent manifestations of withdrawal in patients with established physical dependence on benzodiazepines.

● Other Drugs

Interactions of flumazenil with CNS depressants other than benzodiazepines have not been studied. However, no deleterious interactions have been observed when flumazenil was administered after opiates, inhalational anesthetics, skeletal muscle relaxants, or muscle relaxant antagonists administered in conjunction with sedation or anesthesia. Flumazenil should not be administered until the effects of neuromuscular blockade have been fully reversed.

DESCRIPTION

Flumazenil, a 1,4-imidazobenzodiazepine derivative, is a benzodiazepine antagonist. Flumazenil antagonizes the CNS effects (e.g., sedation, impaired recall, psychomotor impairment, respiratory depression) of benzodiazepines by competitively inhibiting the activity of the drugs at the benzodiazepine recognition site on the γ-aminobutyric acid (GABA)/benzodiazepine receptor complex. Reversal of benzodiazepine-induced effects usually is evident within 1–2 minutes following completion of IV injection of flumazenil, with an 80% response occurring within 3 minutes, and the peak effect occurring at 6–10 minutes. The duration and degree of reversal of benzodiazepine-induced effects appear to be related to the dose and plasma concentrations of flumazenil. However, because the elimination half-life of flumazenil (0.7–1.3 hours) is shorter than that of benzodiazepines, repeat doses of the drug may be needed to prevent resedation. The half-life of flumazenil appears to be shorter (averaging 40 minutes; range: 20–75 minutes) and more variable in children 1–17 years of age compared with that of adults.

Flumazenil is extensively metabolized in the liver with less than 1% of an administered dose excreted unchanged in urine. Ingestion of food during an IV infusion of the drug results in a 50% increase in clearance, most likely because of the increased hepatic blood flow that accompanies a meal.

ADVICE TO PATIENTS

Impairment of memory and judgment may occur. Importance of avoiding activities that require complete alertness, and not operating hazardous machinery or a motor vehicle until at least 18–24 hours after discharge and it is certain that no residual sedative effects of the benzodiazepine remain. Importance of avoiding alcohol or nonprescription drugs for 18–24 hours following flumazenil administration or in the presence of persistent benzodiazepine effects.

Importance of informing clinicians of existing or contemplated concomitant therapy, including prescription and OTC drugs.

Importance of women informing clinicians if they are or plan to become pregnant or to breast-feed.

PREPARATIONS

Excipients in commercially available drug preparations may have clinically important effects in some individuals; consult specific product labeling for details.

Flumazenil

Parenteral		
Injection, for IV use	0.1 mg/mL (0.5 and 1 mg)*	Flumazenil Injection
		Romazicon®, Roche

* available from one or more manufacturer, distributor, and/or repackager by generic (nonproprietary) name

† Use is not currently included in the labeling approved by the US Food and Drug Administration.

Table of Contents

92:00 MISCELLANEOUS THERAPEUTIC AGENTS

§ Omitted from the print version of *AHFS Drug Information*® because of space limitations. This monograph is available on the *AHFS Drug Information*® website, http://ahfsdruginformation.com. See the Preface for details on accessing this site.

Allopurinol

92:16 • ANTIGOUT AGENTS

- Allopurinol, a structural isomer of hypoxanthine, is a xanthine oxidase inhibitor.

USES

● Gout

Allopurinol is used to lower serum and urinary uric acid concentrations in the management of primary and secondary gout. The drug is indicated in patients with frequent disabling attacks of gout. Because therapy with allopurinol is not without some serious risks, the drug is *not* recommended for the management of asymptomatic hyperuricemia; however, some clinicians have suggested that therapy should be initiated when serum urate concentrations exceed 9 mg/dL (by the colorimetric method) because these concentrations are often associated with increased joint changes and renal complications. Allopurinol is used for the management of gout when uricosurics cannot be used because of adverse effects, allergy, or inadequate response; when there are visible tophi or radiographic evidence of uric acid deposits and stones; or when serum urate concentrations are greater than 8.5–9 mg/dL and a family history of tophi and low urate excretion exists. Allopurinol also is used for the management of primary or secondary gouty nephropathy with or without secondary oliguria. The goal of therapy is to lower serum urate concentration to about 6 mg/dL. Allopurinol will often promote resolution of tophi and uric acid crystals by decreasing serum urate concentrations.

Since allopurinol has no analgesic or anti-inflammatory activity, it is of no value in the treatment of acute gout attacks and will prolong and exacerbate inflammation during the acute phase. Allopurinol may increase the frequency of acute attacks during the first 6–12 months of therapy, even when normal or subnormal serum urate concentrations have been maintained. Therefore, prophylactic doses of colchicine should generally be administered concurrently during the first 3–6 months of allopurinol therapy. Acute attacks may occur in spite of such therapy, but usually become less severe and are of briefer duration after several months of allopurinol therapy. During these acute attacks, allopurinol should be continued without changing dosage and full therapeutic doses of colchicine or other anti-inflammatory agents should be administered.

In early uncomplicated gout, either allopurinol or a uricosuric agent may be used. Since uricosuric agents tend to increase urinary uric acid concentrations and the risk of stone formation, allopurinol is preferred in patients with urinary uric acid excretion of greater than 900 mg daily or with gouty nephropathy, urinary tract stones or obstruction, or azotemia. The activity of allopurinol and uricosurics is additive and, when administered concomitantly, smaller doses of each drug can be used. Combined use of the two types of drugs is especially effective in the presence of tophaceous deposits.

● Chemotherapy-induced Hyperuricemia

Allopurinol and allopurinol sodium are used for the management of patients with leukemia, lymphoma, and solid tumor malignancies who are undergoing chemotherapy expected to result in tumor lysis and subsequent elevations of serum and urinary uric acid concentrations. For patients unable to tolerate oral therapy, allopurinol sodium for injection may be used. Allopurinol is especially useful in preventing hyperuricemia and uric acid nephropathy resulting from tissue breakdown after cancer chemotherapy or radiation therapy. Allopurinol therapy should be discontinued when the potential for hyperuricemia is no longer present.

In one compassionate treatment program in patients undergoing chemotherapy for the management of malignancies, administration of IV allopurinol sodium was shown to reduce serum uric acid concentrations in 93% of patients with hyperuricemia (68% of whom achieved normal serum urate concentrations) and to maintain normal serum uric acid concentrations in 97% of those patients in whom the drug was initiated while having normal serum urate concentrations. However, because of study design, clinical outcome associated with IV allopurinol sodium therapy could not be assessed.

Results of a randomized, open-labeled comparative study in pediatric patients 4 months to 17 years of age with leukemia or lymphoma and a high risk for developing tumor lysis suggest that oral allopurinol may be slower and less effective in decreasing plasma uric acid concentrations than IV rasburicase. (See Uses:

Chemotherapy-induced Hyperuricemia, in Rasburicase 44:00.) At the time of this study, IV allopurinol was unavailable. However, the different routes of administration for the drugs (i.e., oral versus IV) are not believed to account for the differences that were observed. Further study is needed to determine whether the more rapid control and reduction of plasma uric acid concentrations that is achieved with rasburicase therapy than is achieved with allopurinol therapy also will result in substantial decreases in metabolic complications and morbidity associated with tumor lysis syndrome, or the need for additional renal support (dialysis or hemofiltration).

● Recurrent Renal Calculi

Allopurinol is used in the management of recurrent calcium oxalate renal calculi in males whose urinary urate excretion exceeds 800 mg daily and in females whose urinary urate excretion exceeds 750 mg daily. Therapy with the drug has reduced the rate of calculus events (passage of a new calculus or radiographic evidence of a new or enlarged calculus) and has prolonged the time to recurrence in patients with hyperuricosuria and normocalciuria and a history of recurrent calcium oxalate renal calculi. The use of allopurinol for this disorder must be carefully evaluated initially and reevaluated periodically to determine that therapy with the drug is beneficial and outweighs the risks. Clinical experience suggests that patients with recurrent calcium oxalate renal calculi may also benefit from dietary changes such as reductions in animal protein, sodium, refined sugars, oxalate-rich foods, and excessive calcium intake, as well as increases in oral fluids and dietary fiber. Allopurinol is also used for the prevention of uric acid renal calculi in patients with a history of recurrent stone formation.

● Other Uses

Allopurinol has been used to reduce hyperuricemia secondary to glucose-6-phosphate dehydrogenase deficiency†, Lesch-Nyhan syndrome†, polycythemia vera†, sarcoidosis†, and secondary to the administration of thiazides† or ethambutol†.

DOSAGE AND ADMINISTRATION

● Administration

Allopurinol is administered orally. Allopurinol also has been administered rectally†. Allopurinol sodium is administered by IV infusion. IV therapy with the drug generally is used in patients who do not tolerate oral therapy.

In all patients receiving allopurinol, fluid intake should be sufficient to yield a daily urine output of at least 2 L and maintenance of a neutral or, preferably, alkaline urine is desirable.

Pharmacogenetic Testing

Because of a strong association between the presence of the variant human leukocyte antigen (HLA)-B*5801 allele and risk of developing allopurinol-induced severe hypersensitivity reactions, pharmacogenetic testing for HLA-B*5801 should be considered prior to initiation of allopurinol therapy in certain high-risk populations in which this allele is known to be highly prevalent. The American College of Rheumatology (ACR) and some clinicians state that screening for HLA-B*5801 should be considered prior to initiation of allopurinol therapy in populations in which both the HLA-B*5801 allele frequency is increased and HLA-B*5801-positive patients have a very high risk of experiencing severe hypersensitivity reactions (e.g., individuals of Korean ancestry with stage 3 or worse chronic kidney disease, individuals of Han Chinese or Thai ancestry irrespective of renal function). Genotyping results are considered positive if 1 or 2 copies of HLA-B*5801 are detected and negative if no copies of the variant allele are detected. Experts state that allopurinol therapy should be avoided in patients who have tested positive for HLA-B*5801. If use of allopurinol cannot be avoided and the benefits are considered to outweigh the risks, more intensive monitoring for manifestations of hypersensitivity reactions is required. (See Pharmacogenomics of Allopurinol-induced Serious Hypersensitivity Reactions under Cautions: Dermatologic and Sensitivity Reactions.)

Application of HLA genotyping as a screening tool has important limitations and must never substitute for appropriate clinical vigilance and patient management. Many HLA-B*5801-positive patients who are treated with allopurinol will never develop severe cutaneous reactions, and such reactions may develop in HLA-B*5801-negative patients. (See Cautions: Dermatologic and Sensitivity Reactions.) For additional information and guidance on how to interpret and apply the results of HLA-B*5801 testing, the Clinical Pharmacogenetics Implementation Consortium (CPIC) guideline for HLA genotype and allopurinol dosing should be consulted.

Oral Administration

Oral allopurinol usually is administered in a single daily dose. The manufacturers recommend that oral doses greater than 300 mg be administered in divided doses. Administration of the drug after meals may minimize adverse GI effects.

IV Infusion

Allopurinol sodium powder for injection is reconstituted by adding 25 mL of sterile water for injection to a vial labeled as containing allopurinol sodium equivalent to 500 mg of allopurinol to provide a solution containing 20 mg of allopurinol per mL. Reconstituted solutions should be further diluted prior to administration with 0.9% sodium chloride injection or 5% dextrose injection to a final concentration not exceeding 6 mg of allopurinol per mL Allopurinol solutions should be inspected visually for particulate matter and discoloration whenever solution and container permit. The injection should be discarded if discoloration or particulate matter is present.

Rectal Administration

Extemporaneously prepared allopurinol suppositories† have been given rectally in patients unable to tolerate oral medications, particularly during cancer chemotherapy, but pharmacokinetic studies indicate that little if any of the drug is absorbed systemically following this route of administration.

● Dosage

Dosage of allopurinol varies with the severity of the disease and should be adjusted according to the response and tolerance of the patient. Dosage of allopurinol also may be adjusted according to results of serum uric acid concentrations, which should be maintained within the normal range.

Gout

In patients with gout, allopurinol therapy should be initiated at a low dosage to reduce the possibility of early flare-up of acute gouty attacks and also because some data suggest that higher initial dosages may be associated with increased risk of severe hypersensitivity reactions. Dosage should be gradually increased to achieve target serum urate concentrations (less than 6 mg/dL), or until the maximum recommended dosage is reached.

The manufacturers recommend that patients be started on oral allopurinol dosages of 100 mg daily and that the daily dose of the drug be increased by 100 mg at weekly intervals until the serum urate concentration falls to 6 mg/dL or less, or until the maximum recommended dosage of 800 mg daily is reached. The manufacturers state that the usual dosage may range from 200–300 mg daily in adults with mild gout and from 400–600 mg daily in those with moderately severe tophaceous gout. Serum urate concentrations are often reduced more slowly with allopurinol than with uricosuric drugs and minimum concentrations may not be reached for 1–3 weeks. After serum urate concentrations are controlled, it may be possible to reduce dosage; the manufacturers state that the minimum effective dosage is 100–200 mg daily. Allopurinol therapy should be continued indefinitely; irregular dosage schedules may lead to increased serum urate concentrations.

Some experts recommend that allopurinol therapy be initiated at a dosage of 100 mg daily or less in adults with gout and that dosage be increased every 2–5 weeks in increments of 100 mg daily to achieve target serum urate concentrations or until a maximum recommended dosage of 800–900 mg daily is reached. Although a dosage of 300 mg daily is commonly used, up to one-half of patients with normal renal function will not achieve target serum urate concentrations at this dosage. In some studies utilizing dosages up to 600–800 mg daily, target serum urate concentrations were achieved in 75–80% of patients.

When allopurinol is added to a therapeutic regimen of colchicine, uricosuric agents, and/or anti-inflammatory agents, a transition period of several months may be necessary before the latter drugs can be discontinued. During this period, the drugs should be administered concomitantly, and allopurinol dosage should be adjusted until serum urate concentrations are normal and freedom from acute gouty attacks is maintained for several months. When the uricosuric agent is being withdrawn, dosage of the uricosuric agent should be gradually reduced over several weeks.

Chemotherapy-induced Hyperuricemia
Oral Dosage

For the prevention of acute uric acid nephropathy in patients with leukemia, lymphoma, and solid tumor malignancies who are undergoing chemotherapy that is expected to result in tumor lysis and subsequent elevations of serum and urinary uric acid concentrations, adults may receive 600–800 mg of allopurinol daily for 2–3 days; most clinicians recommend that this therapy begin 1–2 days before initiating chemotherapy. When allopurinol is used with mercaptopurine or azathioprine, dosage of the latter drugs must be reduced. (See Drug Interactions: Antineoplastic Agents.) In the initial management of hyperuricemia secondary to neoplastic disease, children younger than 6 years of age may receive 150 mg of allopurinol daily and children 6–10 years of age may receive 300 mg daily. After about 48 hours of therapy, dosage should be adjusted according to the response of the patient.

IV Dosage

Dosage of allopurinol sodium is expressed in terms of allopurinol.

For patients who cannot tolerate oral allopurinol therapy, the manufacturer of allopurinol sodium for injection recommends that adults and children older than 10 years of age receive an allopurinol dosage of 200–400 mg/m² daily and children 10 years and younger receive an initial dosage of 200 mg/m² daily (both by continuous infusion or in equally divided intermittent IV infusions administered at 6-, 8-, or 12-hour intervals) beginning 24–48 hours before initiation of chemotherapy. In adults and children greater than 10 years of age daily IV allopurinol dosages should not exceed 600 mg since higher dosages do not appear to provide additional benefit.

Recurrent Calcium Oxalate Renal Calculi

For the management of recurrent calcium oxalate renal calculi in patients with hyperuricosuria, the recommended initial dosage of allopurinol is 200–300 mg daily. Subsequent dosage may be increased or decreased depending on control of hyperuricosuria assessed by 24-hour urinary urate excretion determinations.

● Dosage in Renal Impairment

Various approaches to dosing allopurinol in patients with renal impairment have been recommended in an attempt to minimize the risk of allopurinol-induced hypersensitivity reactions. Use of a low initial dosage has been recommended to reduce the risk of such reactions; the relationship between hypersensitivity reactions and the maintenance dosage used in renal impairment is more controversial. This uncertainty is reflected in the lack of consensus on allopurinol dosage in patients with renal impairment. (See Cautions: Dermatologic and Sensitivity Reactions.)

In patients with impaired renal function, allopurinol and particularly its metabolite oxypurinol may accumulate and, thus, dosage should be reduced. Initial dosages in these patients should be lower than those used in patients with normal renal function.

The manufacturers and some experts recommend that maximum dosages of allopurinol be adjusted according to creatinine clearance. For oral dosing, the manufacturers recommend 200 mg of allopurinol daily when creatinine clearance is 10–20 mL/minute and state that dosage should not exceed 100 mg daily in patients with creatinine clearances less than 10 mL/minute. In patients with severely impaired renal function (i.e., creatinine clearance less than 3 mL/minute), the manufacturers state that use of longer dosing intervals also may be required.

Some clinicians have recommended alternative maintenance dosages of allopurinol based on the patient's creatinine clearance (see Table 1). Although such creatinine clearance-based dosing was widely adopted, this dosing strategy frequently fails to reduce serum urate concentrations to target levels, and evidence that this strategy reduces the risk of allopurinol-induced hypersensitivity reactions in patients who tolerate low initial dosages of the drug is lacking. More recent data suggest that dosage can be increased safely beyond these creatinine clearance-based maintenance dosages, with greater reduction of serum urate concentrations.

TABLE 1. Creatinine Clearance-based Maintenance Dosages of Allopurinol in Renal Impairment

Creatinine Clearance (mL/minute)	Maintenance Dosage
0	100 mg every 3 days
10	100 mg every 2 days
20	100 mg daily
40	150 mg daily
60	200 mg daily
80	250 mg daily

Based on data suggesting that initial dosage is a risk factor for allopurinol-induced hypersensitivity reactions, the American College of Rheumatology (ACR) and some clinicians recommend that allopurinol therapy be initiated at a reduced dosage of 50 mg daily in patients with stage 4 or worse chronic kidney disease (creatinine clearance less than 30 mL/minute). Dosage may be adjusted in increments of 50–100 mg every 2–5 weeks to achieve target serum urate concentrations. The ACR and some other clinicians state that dosage may be increased to levels exceeding 300 mg daily, even in patients with renal impairment, provided patients receive appropriate education and are monitored regularly for evidence of hypersensitivity reactions or other adverse effects.

Other experts and clinicians recommend use of even lower initial dosages (based on estimated glomerular filtration rate [eGFR]) in patients with renal impairment (see Table 2), followed by a gradual increase in dosage (e.g., in 50-mg increments at intervals of approximately every 4 weeks); although these experts state that maximum dosage in patients with renal impairment should be lower than in patients without renal impairment, target serum urate concentrations should be the same.

TABLE 2. GFR-based Dosages for Initiation of Allopurinol Therapy in Renal Impairment

Estimated GFR (mL/minute per 1.73 m^2)	Initial Dosage
Less than 5	50 mg weekly
5–15	50 mg twice weekly
16–30	50 mg every 2 days
31–45	50 mg daily
46–60	50 and 100 mg on alternating days
61–90	100 mg daily

For IV dosing, the manufacturer states that patients with creatinine clearances of 10–20 mL/minute can receive 200 mg daily, those with creatinine clearances of 3–10 mL/minute can receive 100 mg daily, and those with creatinine clearances less than 3 mL/minute may receive 100 mg daily at extended intervals.

CAUTIONS

Results of early clinical studies and experience suggested that some allopurinol-induced adverse effects (e.g., acute attacks of gout, rash) occurred in more than 1% of patients, but current experience suggests that adverse effects of the drug occur in less than 1% of patients. The reduced incidence in adverse effects observed with more recent experience may have resulted in part from initiating therapy with the drug more gradually and following current prescribing precautions and recommendations.

● Dermatologic and Local Effects

The most common adverse effect of oral allopurinol is a pruritic maculopapular rash. Dermatitides of the exfoliative, urticarial, erythematous, eczematoid, hemorrhagic, and purpuric types have also occurred. Alopecia, fever, and malaise may also occur alone or in conjunction with dermatitis. In addition, severe furunculoses of the nose, cellulitis, and ichthyosis have been reported. The incidence of rash may be increased in patients with renal insufficiency. Skin reactions may be delayed and have been reported to occur as long as 2 years after initiating allopurinol therapy. Rarely, skin rash may be followed by severe hypersensitivity reactions which may sometimes be fatal. (See Cautions: Dermatologic and Sensitivity Reactions.) Some patients who have developed severe dermatitis have also developed cataracts (including a case of toxic cataracts), but the exact relationship between allopurinol and cataracts has not been established. Pruritus, onycholysis, and lichen planus have also occurred rarely in patients receiving allopurinol. Facial edema, sweating, and skin edema have also occurred rarely, but a causal relationship to the drug has not been established.

Local injection site reactions have been reported in patients receiving allopurinol sodium IV.

● Dermatologic and Sensitivity Reactions

Serious and sometimes fatal hypersensitivity reactions have been reported in approximately 0.1–0.4% of patients receiving allopurinol. The reactions include a spectrum of cutaneous reactions and systemic manifestations, including toxic epidermal necrolysis (TEN), Stevens-Johnson syndrome (SJS), drug reaction with eosinophilia and systemic symptoms (DRESS), and allopurinol hypersensitivity syndrome; systemic manifestations may include fever, leukocytosis, atypical circulating lymphocytes, eosinophilia, lymphadenopathy, vasculitis, and organ system involvement such as hepatitis and acute renal failure. The reactions also have been referred to as severe cutaneous adverse reactions (SCARs). These reactions have similar clinical presentations, and some of the terms have been used interchangeably in published literature to describe the clinical syndromes. Onset typically occurs within weeks or months following initiation of allopurinol therapy, but may occur later. The mortality rate of severe allopurinol-induced hypersensitivity reactions is up to 20–30%. If such reactions occur, allopurinol should be discontinued immediately, since early diagnosis and drug discontinuance may improve prognosis.

Serious and fatal cases of hypersensitivity angiitis and allergic vasculitis involving erythematous maculopapular rash with desquamation, severe exfoliative dermatitis, vesicular bullous dermatitis, arterial nephrosclerosis, oliguria, congestive heart failure, and acute onset of permanent deafness have been reported during therapy with the drug. Allopurinol-induced hepatotoxicity may also be a hypersensitivity reaction to the drug. (See Cautions: Hepatic Effects.) A generalized hypersensitivity vasculitis has rarely led to irreversible hepatotoxicity and death.

Presence of human leukocyte antigen (HLA)-B*5801, an inherited allelic variant of the HLA-B gene, is strongly associated with severe hypersensitivity reactions to allopurinol, particularly in certain Asian populations. (See Pharmacogenomics of Allopurinol-induced Serious Hypersensitivity Reactions under Cautions: Dermatologic and Sensitivity Reactions.) However, other genetic or nongenetic factors (e.g., renal impairment, thiazide diuretic use, recent initiation of allopurinol therapy, high initial allopurinol dosage) also have been associated with an increased risk of such reactions. The magnitude of risk associated with these factors is uncertain because of the low incidence of severe allopurinol-associated hypersensitivity reactions. The frequency of allopurinol-induced hypersensitivity reactions may be increased in patients with decreased renal function who receive allopurinol and a thiazide diuretic concomitantly. (See Cautions: Precautions and Contraindications and see Drug Interactions: Diuretics.)

Some of the reported nongenetic risk factors (e.g., renal impairment, diuretic therapy, higher allopurinol dosage) are associated with increased plasma concentrations of oxypurinol, the active metabolite of allopurinol. Oxypurinol has been shown to bind to the peptide-binding groove of HLA-B*5801 and activate T cells in a dose-dependent manner, and some reports suggest that increased oxypurinol concentrations may be associated with poorer prognosis in patients who experience hypersensitivity reactions. However, evidence of a clear relationship between oxypurinol concentration and development of allopurinol-induced hypersensitivity is lacking.

There are conflicting data regarding allopurinol dosage. Some data suggest that high initial dosages are associated with increased risk of hypersensitivity reactions and that initiating allopurinol therapy at a low dosage adjusted for renal function may reduce the risk of such reactions. However, the relationship between allopurinol maintenance dosage, particularly in individuals with renal impairment, and hypersensitivity is more controversial, and this uncertainty is reflected in the lack of consensus on allopurinol dosage in renal impairment. (See Dosage and Administration: Dosage in Renal Impairment.)

Allopurinol should not be administered to patients who have previously shown hypersensitivity to it or who have had a serious reaction to the drug. (See Cautions: Precautions and Contraindications.)

Pharmacogenomics of Allopurinol-induced Serious Hypersensitivity Reactions

Studies have demonstrated a strong association, particularly in certain Asian populations, between the risk of developing allopurinol-induced severe hypersensitivity reactions (SJS, TEN, DRESS, allopurinol hypersensitivity syndrome) and the presence of HLA-B*5801, an inherited allelic variant of the HLA-B gene. The HLA-B*5801 allele is found most commonly in individuals of Han Chinese, Korean, or Thai ancestry, with some estimates indicating that up to 20%, approximately 12%, or 6–15% of individuals in these respective ethnic groups may be

HLA-B*5801-positive. Studies conducted in Japan and Europe suggest that 1–2% of these populations may be HLA-B*5801-positive. In the US, the allele reportedly is present in approximately 7% of individuals of Asian ancestry, 3–6% of African-Americans, and less than 2% of Caucasians and Hispanics. The strength of the association between HLA-B*5801 and hypersensitivity reactions appears to vary among ethnic groups according to the frequency of HLA-B*5801 expression. In one study in Taiwan, HLA-B*5801 was present in 100% of Han Chinese patients with allopurinol-induced hypersensitivity syndrome, SJS, or TEN, compared with 15% of allopurinol-tolerant patients and 20% of population controls. Strong associations also have been reported in Thai and Korean populations. More modest associations have been observed in Japanese and European Caucasian populations, with HLA-B*5801 present in approximately 36–56 and 55–64%, respectively, of patients with severe hypersensitivity reactions to allopurinol.

Presence of the HLA-B*5801 allele has not been found to be predictive of less severe dermatologic reactions (e.g., simple or mild rash, maculopapular eruption) associated with allopurinol.

Pharmacogenetic testing for HLA-B*5801 should be considered prior to initiation of allopurinol therapy in certain high-risk populations in which this allele is known to be highly prevalent. The American College of Rheumatology (ACR) and some clinicians state that screening for HLA-B*5801 should be considered prior to initiation of allopurinol therapy in populations in which both the HLA-B*5801 allele frequency is increased and HLA-B*5801-positive patients have a very high risk of experiencing severe hypersensitivity reactions (e.g., individuals of Korean ancestry with stage 3 or worse chronic kidney disease, individuals of Han Chinese or Thai ancestry irrespective of renal function). Experts state that allopurinol therapy should be avoided in patients who have tested positive for HLA-B*5801. If use of allopurinol cannot be avoided and the benefits of allopurinol are considered to outweigh the risks, more intensive monitoring for manifestations of hypersensitivity reactions is required.

Severe hypersensitivity reactions can occur in allopurinol-treated patients who are negative for HLA-B*5801 regardless of their ethnicity, and a substantial number of patients with the variant allele will not develop severe hypersensitivity reactions if they receive allopurinol therapy. Results of cost-effectiveness analyses conducted for some populations (mostly in Asia) suggest that screening for HLA-B*5801 prior to initiation of allopurinol therapy would be cost-effective in certain populations (e.g., Taiwanese and Thai populations, Korean patients with chronic renal insufficiency), and prospective studies evaluating HLA-B*5801 screening in Taiwanese individuals of Han Chinese ancestry and in Korean patients with chronic renal insufficiency suggest that screening these populations for HLA-B*5801 reduces the incidence of allopurinol-induced severe adverse cutaneous reactions below historically predicted rates. Additional studies are needed to assess the role of screening in other populations with lower or ill-defined frequencies of the allele. Based on estimated allele frequency and health-care costs in the US, some clinicians suggest that screening of African-Americans prior to initiation of allopurinol therapy also may be cost-effective.

Application of HLA genotyping as a screening tool has important limitations and must never substitute for appropriate clinical vigilance and patient management. Regardless of genotyping results, patients receiving allopurinol should be monitored closely.

● Hepatic Effects

Alterations in liver function test results, including transient elevations of serum alkaline phosphatase, urinary urobilinogen, AST, and ALT, and decreases in sulfobromophthalein excretion have occurred in some patients. Reversible hepatomegaly, hepatocellular damage (including necrosis), granulomatous changes, liver failure, hepatitis, hyperbilirubinemia, and jaundice have also occurred. The mechanism of some hepatotoxic reactions to allopurinol has been described as a hypersensitivity reaction, since fever, rash, peripheral eosinophilia, and liver biopsy findings of eosinophilia and noncaseating granulomas occurred; however, other mechanisms may also have been involved.

● Hematologic Effects

Leukocytosis, leukopenia, eosinophilia, thrombocytopenia, blast crisis, hemorrhage, bone marrow aplasia, neutropenia, ecchymosis, disseminated intravascular coagulation, and fatal bone marrow suppression and granulocytopenia have been reported rarely in patients receiving allopurinol. Most patients in whom bone marrow suppression was reported during allopurinol therapy were also receiving other drugs with myelosuppressive potential concomitantly. Bone marrow suppression may occur as early as 6 weeks and as late as 6 years after initiation of

allopurinol. Mild reticulocytosis, lymphocytosis, agranulocytosis, pancytopenia, anemia, hemolytic anemia, aplastic anemia, decreased prothrombin levels, and eosinophilic fibrohistiocytic bone marrow lesions have also occurred rarely, but a causal relationship to allopurinol has not been established.

● GI Effects

Adverse GI effects of allopurinol may include nausea, vomiting, diarrhea, intermittent abdominal pain, enlarged abdomen, constipation, flatulence, intestinal obstruction, proctitis, alteration or loss of taste, gastritis, and dyspepsia. Anorexia, GI bleeding, hemorrhagic pancreatitis, stomatitis, mucositis, salivary gland swelling, and tongue edema have also occurred rarely in patients receiving allopurinol, but a causal relationship to the drug has not been established.

● Nervous System Effects

Peripheral neuropathy, neuritis, paresthesia, headache, generalized seizure, status epilepticus, myoclonus, hypotonia, twitching, agitation, changes in mental status, cerebral infarction, coma, dystonia, paralysis, tremor, and somnolence have occurred rarely in patients receiving allopurinol. Optic neuritis, dizziness, vertigo, depression, confusion, amnesia, insomnia, asthenia, and foot drop have also occurred rarely in patients receiving allopurinol, but a causal relationship to the drug has not been established.

● Other Adverse Effects

Other reported adverse effects of allopurinol include fever, diaphoresis, myopathy, arthralgias, and epistaxis. Renal failure, decreased renal function, hematuria, increased creatinine, oliguria, hyperuricemia, and urinary tract infection also have been reported. Patients receiving allopurinol also have developed lactic acidosis, metabolic acidosis, water intoxication, hyperphosphatemia, hypomagnesemia, hyponatremia, hypernatremia, hypokalemia, hyperkalemia, hypercalcemia, and other electrolyte abnormalities. Tumor lysis syndrome, sepsis, septic shock, and other infections also have been reported.

Other adverse effects reported with allopurinol include respiratory failure/insufficiency, acute respiratory distress syndrome (ARDS), increased respiratory rate, and apnea. Hypervolemia, heart failure, cardiorespiratory arrest, hypotension, hypertension, pulmonary embolism, decreased venous pressure, flushing, stroke, ECG abnormalities, ventricular fibrillation, splenomegaly, hyperglycemia, glycosuria, and uremia also have been reported. Malaise, pericarditis, peripheral vascular disease, thrombophlebitis, bradycardia, vasodilation, hypercalcemia, hyperlipidemia, gynecomastia in males, lymphadenopathy, myalgia, bronchospasm, pharyngitis, rhinitis, asthma, macular retinitis, iritis, conjunctivitis, amblyopia, tinnitus, nephritis, albuminuria, primary hematuria, and decreased libido have occurred rarely in patients receiving allopurinol, but a causal relationship to the drug has not been established.

Patients with renal disease have shown either an increase or a decrease in BUN concentrations, pyelonephritis, renal colic, bilateral ureteral obstruction, xanthine stones, and oxypurinol stones and sludge during allopurinol therapy. In cancer patients who develop hyperuricemia, changes in renal function may be associated with the underlying malignancy, rather than with administration of allopurinol. In several patients in whom renal function deteriorated during allopurinol therapy, concurrent conditions (e.g., multiple myeloma, congestive myocardial disease) were present before initiation of allopurinol therapy.

One study in rats indicated that the concentration of iron stored in the liver was increased during administration of allopurinol. This disturbance in iron storage has not been demonstrated clinically. In another study, however, a reversible rise in serum iron concentrations and decrease in total iron binding capacity occurred in patients receiving 500–600 mg of allopurinol daily; these effects reverted to normal when dosage was reduced to 300 mg daily.

● Precautions and Contraindications

Allopurinol should be discontinued at the first appearance of rash or any sign that may indicate an allergic reaction, since severe hypersensitivity reactions that may be fatal have been reported following appearance of rash. Although, in some patients with rash, allopurinol may be reinstated at a lower dosage without untoward incident, the drug should *not* be reinstituted in patients who have had a severe reaction. Patients initiating allopurinol therapy should be informed of the potential for severe hypersensitivity reactions to occur and should be advised to immediately discontinue the drug and seek medical attention at the first appearance of any signs or symptoms of hypersensitivity (e.g., rash, pruritus). Pharmacogenetic testing should be considered prior to initiation of therapy in certain high-risk patients who may have a genetic predisposition to severe allopurinol-induced hypersensitivity reactions. (See Pharmacogenetic Testing under Dosage and Administration: Administration.)

Allopurinol may increase the frequency of acute gouty attacks during the first 6–12 months of therapy; therefore, prophylactic doses of colchicine should generally be administered concurrently during the first 3–6 months of allopurinol therapy. (See Uses: Gout.)

Patients should be warned that drowsiness may occur during allopurinol therapy and may impair their ability to perform activities requiring mental alertness. Patients should also be warned to discontinue the drug and consult their physician immediately at the first sign of rash, painful urination, blood in the urine, irritation of the eyes, or swelling of the lips or mouth.

Liver function tests (particularly in patients with preexisting liver disease), renal function tests (particularly in patients with impaired renal function or concurrent illness that can affect renal function such as hypertension or diabetes mellitus), and complete blood cell counts should be performed before initiating allopurinol and periodically during therapy, especially during the first few months. If patients receiving allopurinol develop anorexia, weight loss, or pruritus, assessment of liver function should be part of the diagnostic evaluation.

Patients with impaired renal function must be carefully observed while receiving allopurinol (particularly during the early stages of therapy) and the dosage decreased or the drug discontinued if evidence of deterioration in renal function occurs and persists. Patients with impaired renal function require lower dosages of allopurinol than those with normal renal function. (See Dosage and Administration: Dosage in Renal Impairment.) The usual initial dosage of allopurinol should be reduced in patients with impaired renal function. Since concomitant therapy with allopurinol and a thiazide diuretic in patients with decreased renal function may increase the risk of allopurinol-induced hypersensitivity reactions, concomitant therapy with the drugs should be used with caution in such patients and the patients should be observed closely. (See Drug Interactions: Diuretics.)

● Pediatric Precautions

Pending further accumulation of data, the manufacturers state that allopurinol is rarely indicated in children except in those with hyperuricemia secondary to neoplastic disease, cancer chemotherapy, or genetic disorders of purine metabolism. Clinical experience in about 200 pediatric patients suggests that safety and efficacy of allopurinol sodium for injection are similar to those in adults.

● Geriatric Precautions

The manufacturer of allopurinol sodium for injection states that clinical studies of parenteral allopurinol sodium did not include a sufficient number of patients 65 years of age or older to determine whether such patients respond differently than younger individuals, but that other reported clinical experience has not identified differences in response between geriatric and younger patients. In a pharmacokinetic study, peak plasma concentrations and area under the plasma concentration-time curve (AUC) of oxypurinol (active metabolite of allopurinol) were about 50–60% higher in geriatric individuals than in younger individuals following single oral allopurinol dosing. (See Pharmacokinetics: Absorption.) Since these differences appear to be related to changes in renal function in geriatric patients, some clinicians state that adjustments in allopurinol dosage may be necessary in geriatric patients based on the degree of renal impairment. (See Dosage and Administration: Dosage in Renal Impairment.) In addition, appropriate dosage of allopurinol in geriatric patients should be selected with caution because of the greater frequency of decreased hepatic, renal, or cardiac function and of concomitant disease and drug therapy in these patients.

● Pregnancy, Fertility, and Lactation
Pregnancy

Although there are no adequate and controlled studies to date using allopurinol in pregnant women, the drug has been shown to be teratogenic in mice using intraperitoneal allopurinol doses of 50 or 100 mg/kg (0.3 or 0.75 times the recommended human dose on a mg/m² basis) on gestation days 10 or 13. Allopurinol should be used during pregnancy only when clearly needed.

Fertility

Reproduction studies in rats and rabbits using dosages up to 20 times the usual human dosage have not revealed evidence of impaired fertility. Infertility in human males and impotence have occurred rarely during allopurinol therapy, but a causal relationship to the drug has not been established.

Lactation

Since allopurinol and oxypurinol are distributed into milk, allopurinol should be used with caution in nursing women.

DRUG INTERACTIONS

The following drug interactions were observed in patients receiving oral allopurinol therapy. Although many patients received long-term oral administration of allopurinol (e.g., those with gout or renal calculi), these interactions may be relevant to allopurinol sodium for injection therapy as well.

● Drugs that Increase Serum Urate Concentration

Many drugs may increase serum urate concentrations, including most diuretics, pyrazinamide, diazoxide, alcohol, and mecamylamine. If these drugs are administered during allopurinol therapy, dosage of allopurinol may need to be increased.

● Ampicillin and Amoxicillin

An increased incidence of rash reportedly occurs in patients with hyperuricemia who are receiving allopurinol and concomitant ampicillin or amoxicillin as compared with those receiving allopurinol, ampicillin, or amoxicillin alone. Some clinicians suggest that either allopurinol or hyperuricemia may potentiate aminopenicillin allergenicity. However, other clinicians state that the rash reported in patients receiving allopurinol and aminopenicillins concomitantly is generally the delayed aminopenicillin rash that appears to be nonimmunologic. The clinical importance of this effect has not been determined; however, some clinicians suggest that concomitant use of the drugs should be avoided if possible.

● Anticoagulants

Allopurinol inhibits the hepatic microsomal drug metabolism of dicumarol. In one study, the half-life of dicumarol was increased from 51 to 152 hours when the anticoagulant was taken concurrently with allopurinol. Although the clinical importance of this effect may vary, patients taking allopurinol with dicumarol should be observed for increased anticoagulant effects and prothrombin time should be monitored periodically in these patients. Allopurinol has *not* been shown to substantially potentiate the anticoagulant effect of warfarin except in one case when warfarin, allopurinol, and indomethacin were administered concurrently.

● Antineoplastic Agents

In dosages of 300–600 mg daily, allopurinol inhibits the oxidative metabolism of azathioprine and mercaptopurine by xanthine oxidase, thus increasing the possibility of toxic effects from these drugs, particularly bone marrow depression. When allopurinol is administered concomitantly with mercaptopurine or azathioprine, the doses of the antineoplastic agents should initially be reduced to 25–33% of the usual dose and subsequent dosage adjusted according to the patient response and toxic effects. Substitution of thioguanine for mercaptopurine has also been suggested.

Concomitant administration of allopurinol with cyclophosphamide may increase the incidence of bone marrow depression as compared with cyclophosphamide alone, but the mechanism for this interaction is not known. However, results of a well-controlled study in patients with lymphoma have shown that concomitant use of allopurinol with cyclophosphamide, doxorubicin, bleomycin, procarbazine, and/or mechlorethamine did not increase the incidence of bone marrow depression in these patients.

● Chlorpropamide

Allopurinol and chlorpropamide cause adverse hepatorenal reactions. Although the combination does not enhance the occurrence of these reactions, caution is indicated if these 2 drugs are administered concomitantly. Because allopurinol or its metabolites may compete with chlorpropamide for renal tubular secretion, patients who receive these drugs concomitantly (especially those with renal insufficiency) should be observed for signs of excessive hypoglycemia.

● Cyclosporine

Increased blood concentrations of cyclosporine have been reported in patients receiving allopurinol and cyclosporine concomitantly. Therefore, blood cyclosporine concentrations should be monitored and dosage adjustments of cyclosporine should be considered when these drugs are used concomitantly.

● Didanosine

In 2 patients with renal impairment, concomitant use of allopurinol (300 mg daily) and buffered didanosine (single 200-mg dose) increased peak plasma concentrations and area under the concentration-time curve (AUC) of didanosine by 232 and 312%, respectively. In 14 healthy individuals who received allopurinol (300 mg daily) and buffered didanosine (single 400-mg dose), peak plasma concentrations and AUC of didanosine were increased by 69 and 113%, respectively. The manufacturer of didanosine states that concomitant use of allopurinol and didanosine is contraindicated since increased didanosine exposure may result in increased didanosine-associated toxicity.

● **Diuretics**

Diuretics such as thiazides, furosemide, and ethacrynic acid, when given with allopurinol, may increase serum oxypurinol concentrations and may thereby increase the risk of serious allopurinol toxicity, including hypersensitivity reactions (particularly in patients with decreased renal function); however, allopurinol has been used safely with thiazides to reduce hyperuricemia induced by the diuretics†. A review of reports of allopurinol toxicity in patients who were receiving concomitant therapy with allopurinol and a thiazide indicated that patients were principally receiving a thiazide for hypertension and that tests to rule out decreased renal function secondary to hypertensive nephropathy were not often performed; however, in patients in whom renal insufficiency was documented, dosage of allopurinol was not appropriately reduced. Although a causal mechanism and relationship have not been definitely established, the evidence suggests that renal function should be monitored (even in the absence of renal failure) in patients receiving allopurinol and a thiazide concomitantly and that dosage of allopurinol in such patients should be adjusted even more conservatively than usual if decreased renal function is detected. Consideration should be given to the indication for concomitant diuretic use and whether alternative agents (e.g., other antihypertensive agents) might appropriately be used. When diuretics (particularly thiazides) and allopurinol are used concomitantly, especially in patients with chronic renal impairment, more intensive monitoring for manifestations of hypersensitivity reactions is required. (See Cautions: Dermatologic and Sensitivity Reactions.)

● **Uricosuric Agents**

Uricosurics promote urinary excretion of oxypurinol (which also inhibits xanthine oxidase) and may thereby reduce the inhibition of xanthine oxidase produced by allopurinol therapy; however, the effects of allopurinol and a uricosuric are generally additive, and the combination is usually used to therapeutic advantage. Renal precipitation of oxypurines has not occurred to date in patients receiving allopurinol alone or in combination with a uricosuric, but the possibility should be kept in mind.

PHARMACOLOGY

Allopurinol inhibits xanthine oxidase, the enzyme that catalyzes the conversion of hypoxanthine to xanthine and of xanthine to uric acid. Oxypurinol, a metabolite of allopurinol, also inhibits xanthine oxidase. By inhibiting xanthine oxidase, allopurinol and its metabolite block conversion of the oxypurines (hypoxanthine and xanthine) to uric acid, thus decreasing serum and urine concentrations of uric acid. The drug differs, therefore, from uricosuric agents which lower serum urate concentrations by promoting urinary excretion of uric acid. Xanthine oxidase concentrations are not altered by long-term administration of the drug.

Allopurinol does not directly interfere with purine nucleotide or nucleic acid synthesis. The drug, however, indirectly increases oxypurine and allopurinol ribonucleotide concentrations and decreases phosphoribosylpyrophosphate concentrations, thus decreasing *de novo* purine biosynthesis by pseudofeedback inhibition. In addition, allopurinol increases the incorporation of hypoxanthine and xanthine into DNA and RNA, thereby further decreasing serum urate concentrations. Allopurinol may produce a deficit of total purines (uric acid and oxypurines) amounting to several hundred mg daily.

Accompanying the decrease in uric acid produced by allopurinol is an increase in serum and urine concentrations of hypoxanthine and xanthine. Plasma concentrations of these oxypurines do not, however, rise commensurately with the fall in serum urate concentrations and are often 20–30% less than would be expected in view of urate concentrations prior to allopurinol therapy. This discrepancy occurs because renal clearance of the oxypurines is at least 10 times greater than that of uric acid. In addition, normal urinary purine output is almost exclusively uric acid, but after treatment with allopurinol, it is composed of uric acid, xanthine, and hypoxanthine, each having independent solubility. Thus, the risk of crystalluria is reduced. Alkalinization of the urine increases the solubility of the purines, further minimizing the risk of crystalluria. Decreased tubular

transport of uric acid also results in increased renal reabsorption of calcium and decreased calcium excretion.

Allopurinol also interferes with *de novo* pyrimidine nucleotide synthesis by inhibiting orotidine 5′-phosphate decarboxylase. Secondary orotic aciduria and orotidinuria result. Orotic acid is highly insoluble and could form a heavy sediment of urinary crystals; however, the increased excretion of orotic acid and orotidine rarely exceeds 10% of the total pyrimidines synthesized by the body. In addition, enhanced conversion of uridine to uridine 5′-monophosphate usually occurs and, therefore, this partial inhibition of pyrimidine synthesis is considered innocuous.

In rats, allopurinol reportedly increases liver storage of iron by inhibiting the ferritin-xanthine oxidase system responsible for mobilization of iron from the liver; however, this effect has not been demonstrated clinically.

Allopurinol may also inhibit hepatic microsomal enzymes. Allopurinol is not cytotoxic and has no effect on transplantable tumors. The drug has no analgesic, anti-inflammatory, or uricosuric activity.

PHARMACOKINETICS

● **Absorption**

Following oral administration, approximately 80–90% of a dose of allopurinol is absorbed from the GI tract. Peak plasma concentrations of allopurinol are reached 2–6 hours after a usual dose.

Following oral administration of single 100- or 300-mg dose of allopurinol in healthy adult males in one study, peak plasma allopurinol concentrations of about 0.5 or 1.4 μg/mL, respectively, occurred in about 1–2 hours, while peak oxypurinol (the active metabolite of allopurinol) concentrations of about 2.4 and 6.4 μg/mL, respectively, were reached within about 3–4 hours. In the same study, following IV infusion over 30 minutes of a single 100- or 300-mg dose of allopurinol (as allopurinol sodium), peak plasma concentrations of about 1.6 and 5.1 μg/mL, respectively, occurred in about 30 minutes, while peak oxypurinol concentrations of about 2.2 and 6.2 μg/mL, respectively, were reached within about 4 hours.

Peak plasma concentrations and the area under the plasma concentration-time curve (AUC) of oxypurinol following oral administration of allopurinol 200 mg as a single dose have been reported to be about 50–60% higher in geriatric patients (71–93 years of age) than in younger adults (24–35 years of age); these differences appear to be related to changes in renal function in geriatric patients. Some clinicians state that adjustments in allopurinol dosage may be necessary in geriatric patients based on the degree of renal impairment. (See Dosage and Administration: Dosage in Renal Impairment.)

Because allopurinol concentrations are difficult to determine and because serum concentrations may not adequately reflect the amount of drug bound to xanthine oxidase in the tissues, serum urate concentrations should be used to monitor therapy. After beginning allopurinol therapy, serum urate concentrations begin to decrease slowly within 24–48 hours and reach a nadir after 1–3 weeks of therapy. During allopurinol therapy, serum urate concentrations remain relatively constant; however, serum urate concentrations usually return to pretreatment levels within 1–2 weeks after discontinuing the drug. Because of the continued mobilization of urate deposits, substantial reduction of uric acid may be delayed 6–12 months or may not occur in some patients, particularly in those with tophaceous gout and in those who are underexcretors of uric acid.

Allopurinol is absorbed poorly following rectal administration of the drug as suppositories (in a cocoa butter or polyethylene glycol base). Plasma allopurinol or oxypurinol concentrations have been minimal or undetectable following such rectal administration.

● **Distribution**

Allopurinol is uniformly distributed in total tissue water with the exception of the brain, where concentrations of the drug are approximately 50% those of other tissues. Small amounts of oxypurinol and allopurinol crystals have been found in muscle. Allopurinol and oxypurinol are not bound to plasma proteins. Allopurinol and oxypurinol are distributed into milk.

● **Elimination**

Allopurinol and allopurinol sodium are rapidly metabolized by xanthine oxidase to oxypurinol, which is pharmacologically active. Rapid metabolism of allopurinol to oxypurinol does not seem to be affected substantially during multiple dosing. Pharmacokinetic parameters (e.g., AUC, plasma elimination half-lives) of oxypurinol appear to be similar following oral administration of allopurinol and IV administration of allopurinol sodium. The half-lives of allopurinol and oxypurinol are about 1–3 hours and 18–30 hours, respectively, in patients with normal renal function and are increased in patients with renal impairment. Patients genetically deficient in xanthine oxidase are unable to convert allopurinol to oxypurinol. Both allopurinol and oxypurinol are conjugated and form their respective ribonucleosides.

About 5–7% of an oral allopurinol dose is excreted in urine unchanged within 6 hours after ingestion and about 12% of an IV dose of the drug is excreted unchanged 5 hours after administration. After this time, the drug is excreted by the kidneys as oxypurinol and in small amounts as allopurinol and oxypurinol ribonucleosides. Unlike allopurinol, a large part of oxypurinol is reabsorbed by the renal tubules; therefore, its renal clearance is much lower than that of allopurinol. About 70% of the administered daily dose is excreted in urine as oxypurinol and an additional 20% appears in feces as unchanged drug within 48–72 hours.

Allopurinol and oxypurinol are dialyzable.

CHEMISTRY AND STABILITY

● Chemistry

Allopurinol, a structural isomer of hypoxanthine, is a xanthine oxidase inhibitor used in the treatment of gout and selected hyperuricemias. The drug occurs as a fluffy white to off-white powder having a slight odor and is very slightly soluble in water and in alcohol. The apparent pK_a of allopurinol is 9.4 and its active oxidative metabolite, oxypurinol (alloxanthine), has an apparent pK_a of 7.7.

Allopurinol sodium occurs as a white amorphous mass and has a pK_a of 9.31. Following reconstitution of the commercially available allopurinol sodium lyophilized powder with sterile water for injection to a concentration of 20 mg/mL, the solution is clear and almost colorless with no more than a slight opalescence and has a pH of 11.1–11.8.

● Stability

Allopurinol tablets should be stored in well-closed containers at 15–30°C. Commercially available allopurinol sodium lyophilized powder for injection should be stored at a controlled room temperature of 20–25°C. Following reconstitution of allopurinol sodium for injection with sterile water for injection, the solutions contain approximately 20 mg/mL and should be further diluted with 0.9% sodium chloride injection or 5% dextrose injection. These further diluted allopurinol sodium solutions, containing no more than 6 mg/mL, should be stored

at 20–25°C and should be used within 10 hours of reconstitution. Reconstituted and/or diluted solutions should not be refrigerated.

Allopurinol sodium injection has been reported to be incompatible with various drugs (e.g., sodium bicarbonate), but the compatibility depends on several factors (e.g., concentrations of the drugs, resulting pH, temperature). Specialized references should be consulted for specific compatibility information.

An oral suspension of allopurinol containing 20 mg/mL has been prepared extemporaneously from the commercially available tablets. The tablets were crushed, mixed with a volume of suspending agent (Cologel®) equal to one-third the final volume, and then the suspension was brought to the final volume with a 2:1 mixture of simple syrup and wild cherry syrup. The resulting suspension was stable for at least 14 days when stored in an amber glass bottle at room temperature or 5°C.

PREPARATIONS

Excipients in commercially available drug preparations may have clinically important effects in some individuals; consult specific product labeling for details.

Allopurinol

Oral

Tablets	100 mg*	**Allopurinol Tablets**
		Zyloprim® (scored), Prometheus
	300 mg*	**Allopurinol Tablets**
		Zyloprim® (scored), Prometheus

* available from one or more manufacturer, distributor, and/or repackager by generic (nonproprietary) name

Allopurinol Sodium

Parenteral

| For injection, for IV infusion only | 500 mg (of allopurinol)* | **Allopurinol Sodium for Injection** Aloprim®, Mylan |

* available from one or more manufacturer, distributor, and/or repackager by generic (nonproprietary) name

† Use is not currently included in the labeling approved by the US Food and Drug Administration.

Zoledronic Acid

92:24 • BONE RESORPTION INHIBITORS

- Zoledronic acid, a synthetic imidazole bisphosphonate analog of pyrophosphate, is a bone resorption inhibitor.

USES

• Hypercalcemia Associated with Malignancy

Zoledronic acid is used in conjunction with achievement and maintenance of adequate hydration for the treatment of hypercalcemia (albumin-corrected serum calcium concentration of 12 mg/dL or greater) associated with malignant neoplasms. For the treatment of mild or asymptomatic hypercalcemia, measures more conservative (e.g., hydration alone or combined with loop diuretics) than therapy with agents such as zoledronic acid generally are used.

Controlled clinical studies have shown that single-dose IV zoledronic acid (4 mg infused over 5 minutes) is more effective in the treatment of moderate to severe malignancy-associated hypercalcemia (albumin-corrected serum calcium concentration of 12 mg/dL or greater) than single-dose IV pamidronate disodium (90 mg infused over 2 hours). In these studies, patients received zoledronic acid or pamidronate disodium in conjunction with IV hydration (750 mL of fluid, of which 250 mL was administered prior to study drug administration). Normocalcemia (corrected serum calcium concentrations not exceeding 10.8 mg/dL) was attained more quickly and maintained for a longer period of time in patients receiving zoledronic acid than in those receiving pamidronate. Analysis of pooled data from these studies indicates that 70 or 88% of patients receiving pamidronate disodium or zoledronic acid, respectively, achieved a normal serum calcium concentration within 10 days of treatment. For responders, the median duration of complete response (defined as the time from onset of normocalcemia until the last corrected serum calcium concentration of 10.8 mg/dL or less) following a single dose was approximately 32 or 18 days for zoledronic acid or pamidronate, respectively. The median time to recurrence (defined as the time from drug administration until the last corrected serum calcium concentration of less than 11.6 mg/dL) was longer with zoledronic acid (30 days) than with pamidronate (17 days). Subgroup analysis indicates that complete response rates were not affected by cancer type, the presence or absence of bone metastases, baseline blood parathyroid hormone-related protein concentrations, baseline BUN-to-creatinine ratio, age, sex, or race.

Retreatment with zoledronic acid may be considered in patients with recurrent or refractory hypercalcemia of malignancy. Data from a limited number of patients indicate that a second course of IV zoledronic acid therapy can normalize serum calcium concentrations when malignancy-associated hypercalcemia is refractory to or recurs following an adequate response to an initial course of therapy. A second course of therapy with zoledronic acid at a higher than recommended dose (8 mg) returned corrected serum calcium concentrations to normal within 10 days after retreatment in 52% of patients whose hypercalcemia was refractory to or recurred following an adequate response to an initial dose of zoledronic acid 4 mg. For responders, the median duration of complete response following retreatment was 11 days. The median time to recurrence following retreatment was 8 days.

• Bone Metastases of Solid Tumors and Osteolytic Lesions of Multiple Myeloma

Zoledronic acid is used as an adjunct to antineoplastic therapy for the treatment of bone metastases of solid tumors and osteolytic lesions of multiple myeloma. In patients with bone metastases associated with prostate cancer, zoledronic acid should be used as second-line therapy and is reserved for those with disease progression following one or more hormonal therapies.

The efficacy of zoledronic acid in combination with antineoplastic therapy (e.g., chemotherapy or hormonal therapy) for the treatment of bone metastases in patients with advanced solid tumors or osteolytic bone lesions associated with multiple myeloma has been demonstrated in several large clinical trials. In a long-term (12 months' duration) comparative study in patients with breast cancer and bone metastases or with stage III multiple myeloma and at least one osteolytic bone lesion, combined zoledronic acid (4 mg, administered as a 5- or 15-minute IV infusion once every 3–4 weeks) and antineoplastic therapy (chemotherapy or hormonal therapy) was as effective as combined pamidronate disodium (90 mg, administered as a

2-hour IV infusion once every 3–4 weeks) and antineoplastic therapy in reducing the incidence of bone-related complications (e.g., fractures or spinal cord compression, bone deterioration requiring radiotherapy or orthopedic surgery) and in delaying the development of such complications. The median time to the first bone-related complication was 373 days in patients receiving zoledronic acid and 363 days in patients receiving pamidronate. Patients with pain experienced a decrease in pain during adjunctive zoledronic acid or pamidronate therapy, while the need for supplemental analgesic therapy decreased or remained relatively unchanged. Secondary end points such as change in performance status or median time to overall disease progression or death did not differ between the treatment groups.

In a long-term (10.5 months' duration) placebo-controlled trial, patients with hormone-refractory prostate cancer and bone metastases who were receiving combined zoledronic acid (4 mg, administered as a 5- or 15-minute IV infusion once every 3 weeks) and hormonal therapy showed a decrease in the incidence and a delay in the development of bone-related complications (e.g., fractures or spinal cord compression, bone deterioration requiring radiotherapy or orthopedic surgery, bone pain necessitating a change in hormonal therapy) compared with those receiving hormonal therapy alone. The incidence of bone-related complications was lower in patients receiving adjunctive zoledronic acid (33%) than in those receiving hormonal therapy alone (44%). The first bone-related complication was observed at 321 days in those receiving hormonal therapy alone and such complications were not observed at that time in those receiving adjunctive zoledronic acid.

Data from a long-term placebo-controlled trial in patients with bone metastases and solid tumors other than breast or prostate cancer showed no appreciable difference in the incidence of bone-related complications (e.g., fractures or spinal cord compression, bone deterioration requiring radiotherapy or orthopedic surgery, bone pain necessitating a change in antineoplastic therapy) in patients receiving combined zoledronic acid (4 mg, administered as a 15-minute IV infusion once every 3 weeks) and antineoplastic therapy compared with those receiving antineoplastic therapy alone; however, there was a median delay of 67 days in the development of such complications in the group receiving zoledronic acid. Bone-related complications were observed in 38% of patients receiving adjunctive zoledronic acid compared with 44% of those receiving antineoplastic therapy alone. The median time to the first bone-related complication was 230 or 163 days, respectively, in patients receiving adjunctive zoledronic acid or antineoplastic therapy alone. More than two-thirds of the patients had preexisting bone-related complications; the median survival of patients enrolled in the trial (6 months) was less than the planned trial duration (9 months).

• Osteoporosis

Zoledronic acid is used for the prevention and treatment of postmenopausal osteoporosis; the drug also is used to increase bone mass in men with osteoporosis.

In addition to adequate intake of calcium/vitamin D and other lifestyle modifications (e.g., exercise, avoidance of excessive alcohol and tobacco use), experts recommend that pharmacologic therapy for osteoporosis be considered in postmenopausal women and in men 50 years of age or older who are at high risk of fractures (generally those who have experienced a previous hip or vertebral fracture or who have low bone mineral density [BMD]); pharmacologic therapy also may be considered in postmenopausal women and in men 50 years of age or older who have low bone mass, although there is less evidence supporting overall fracture risk reduction in such patients. When selecting an appropriate pharmacologic agent, use of a drug with proven antifracture efficacy is recommended. Available options include bisphosphonates (e.g., alendronate, risedronate, zoledronic acid, ibandronate), denosumab, raloxifene, calcitonin, or teriparatide with varying levels of recommendation given in expert guidelines based on the available evidence supporting fracture risk reduction for each drug. Choice of therapy should be individualized based on the potential benefits and adverse effects of therapy as well as patient preferences, comorbidities, and risk factors. For additional information on the prevention and treatment of osteoporosis, see Uses: Osteoporosis, in Alendronate 92:24.

Prevention in Postmenopausal Women

Zoledronic acid is used for the prevention of osteoporosis in postmenopausal women. Risk factors for postmenopausal osteoporosis and related fractures include early menopause, decreased BMD, low body mass index (BMI), previous fracture or family history of fracture/osteoporosis, excessive alcohol intake, smoking, inadequate physical activity, low calcium and vitamin D intake, certain drugs (e.g., glucocorticoids), and medical conditions or diseases (e.g., rheumatoid arthritis, diabetes mellitus, Cushing syndrome, hyperparathyroidism).

In a 2-year, double-blind, placebo-controlled study in postmenopausal women 45 years of age or older with osteopenia, treatment with zoledronic acid resulted in a substantial increase in total hip and lumbar spine BMD compared with placebo at 2 years. In this study, zoledronic acid 5 mg was administered as a once-yearly IV infusion (total of 2 doses) or as a single IV infusion at study randomization (total of 1 dose); both dosage regimens were effective in preventing bone loss over the 2-year study period. Levels of bone turnover markers were reduced at all time points in both zoledronic acid treatment groups, but the effect was more sustained with the once-yearly regimen.

Treatment in Postmenopausal Women

Zoledronic acid is used for the treatment of osteoporosis in postmenopausal women. Efficacy of zoledronic acid given as a once-yearly IV infusion has been established in 2 long-term (3 years' duration) randomized, double-blind, placebo-controlled, multinational studies in postmenopausal women with osteoporosis (diagnosed by BMD with or without vertebral fracture[s]). In each study, zoledronic acid was given as a single 5-mg dose by IV infusion over at least 15 minutes. In these studies, the incidence of new fractures (hip, vertebral, non-vertebral fractures) was reduced among patients receiving zoledronic acid compared with that observed with placebo with or without background therapies for osteoporosis (excluding bisphosphonates). Bone histology studies of patients from one of the studies indicated that the bone formed during therapy with zoledronic acid had normal architecture and mineralization. In patients at high risk of fractures (defined as those with a history of a recent, low-trauma hip fracture), zoledronic acid reduced the incidence of subsequent fractures.

Treatment in Men

Zoledronic acid is used to increase bone mass in men with osteoporosis. Efficacy of zoledronic acid given as a once-yearly IV infusion was established in a long-term (2 years' duration) randomized, double-blind, active-controlled, multicenter study in men with osteoporosis or osteoporosis secondary to hypogonadism. Zoledronic acid was given as a single 5-mg dose by IV infusion over at least 15 minutes; this dose could be repeated once. The active control was an oral bisphosphonate administered once weekly for up to 2 years. All patients received elemental calcium 1 g and vitamin D 800–1000 international units (IU, units) daily. In this study, once-yearly zoledronic acid by IV infusion was noninferior to the once-weekly oral bisphosphonate based on the percent change in lumbar spine BMD at month 24 compared with baseline (6.1 versus 6.2% increase in BMD with zoledronic acid versus oral bisphosphonate, respectively).

• Glucocorticoid-induced Osteoporosis

Zoledronic acid is used in the treatment and prevention of glucocorticoid-induced osteoporosis. The manufacturer recommends use of zoledronic acid in men and women who are either initiating or receiving long-term (at least 12 months) systemic glucocorticoid therapy in a daily dosage equivalent to at least 7.5 mg of prednisone.

The American College of Rheumatology (ACR) recommends optimizing calcium and vitamin D intake and lifestyle modifications (e.g., diet, smoking cessation, weight-bearing or resistance-training exercise) in all patients receiving long-term glucocorticoid therapy; in addition, pharmacologic therapy with an oral bisphosphonate is recommended in patients who are considered to be at moderate-to-high risk of fracture. Oral bisphosphonates generally are preferred because of their anti-fracture benefits as well as their safety and low cost; other options include IV bisphosphonates, teriparatide, denosumab, and raloxifene (for postmenopausal women if no other therapy is appropriate). For additional information on the use of bisphosphonates for prevention and treatment of glucocorticoid-induced osteoporosis, see Uses: Glucocorticoid-induced Osteoporosis, in Alendronate 92:24.

Safety and efficacy of zoledronic acid for the treatment and prevention of glucocorticoid-induced osteoporosis were evaluated in a randomized, double-blind, active-controlled study in men and women receiving glucocorticoid therapy (daily dosage of at least 7.5 mg of prednisone or equivalent). Patients were stratified according to their duration of glucocorticoid use: up to 3 months (prevention group) or more than 3 months (treatment group). In this study, zoledronic acid was administered in a single 5-mg dose by IV infusion over 15–20 minutes, and the active control (risedronate) was administered orally in a dosage of 5 mg once daily. At 12 months, zoledronic acid increased lumbar spine BMD to a greater extent than risedronate; lumbar BMD increased by an average of 4.1 versus 2.7%, respectively, in the treatment group and by an average of 2.6 versus 0.6%,

respectively, in the prevention group. Qualitative histology assessments in a subset of patients who received zoledronic acid revealed normal architecture with no evidence of mineralization defects. However, there was an apparent reduction in activation frequency and bone remodeling rates when compared with histomorphometry results seen with zoledronic acid in the postmenopausal osteoporosis population; the long-term consequences of such effects are unknown.

• Paget Disease of Bone

Zoledronic acid is used for the management of moderate-to-severe Paget disease of bone (osteitis deformans). Efficacy of the drug in the treatment of Paget disease of bone has been established in 2 randomized, double-blind studies of 6 months' duration, in which zoledronic acid 5 mg as a single dose by IV infusion produced a more rapid and effective therapeutic response (as defined by either normalization of serum alkaline phosphatase concentrations or a reduction of at least 75% from baseline in total serum alkaline phosphatase excess [i.e., "excess" being defined as the difference between the measured concentration and the midpoint of the normal range] at the end of 6 months) than risedronate 30 mg orally once daily for 2 months. Most patients achieved a response to zoledronic acid by day 63 of the study.

Treatment with zoledronic acid should be considered in patients with serum alkaline phosphatase concentrations of at least twice the age-specific upper limit of normal, in those who are symptomatic, or in those at risk for future complications from their disease. After a single treatment of zoledronic acid in patients with Paget disease of bone, an extended remission period is observed. Specific data on retreatment of the disease are not available. However, retreatment may be considered in patients who have relapsed based on increases in serum alkaline phosphatase concentrations, in those who failed to achieve normalization of serum alkaline phosphatase concentrations, or in patients who are symptomatic, according to current standards of medical care.

• Prevention of Aromatase Inhibitor-associated Bone Loss

Zoledronic acid has been studied for the prevention of aromatase inhibitor-associated bone loss in women receiving adjuvant hormonal therapy for early-stage breast cancer†.

Prevention in Postmenopausal Women

Efficacy and safety of zoledronic acid for the prevention of aromatase inhibitor-associated bone loss in women receiving adjuvant hormonal therapy for early-stage breast cancer† have been studied in several phase 3, open-label, randomized studies (Zometa-Femara Adjuvant Synergy Trial [Z-FAST], ZO-FAST, E-ZO-FAST, and North Central Cancer Treatment Group [NCCTG]-N03CC study). The Z-FAST, ZO-FAST, and E-ZO-FAST studies included postmenopausal women with stage I–IIIa estrogen receptor-positive and/or progesterone receptor-positive breast cancer; patients had a baseline T-score of −2 standard deviations (SD) from normal or better and did not have a history of a low-intensity fracture or evidence of an existing fracture. Patients enrolled in these studies were randomized to receive upfront or delayed zoledronic acid. Women in the upfront group received zoledronic acid following randomization; women in the delayed group did not begin treatment with zoledronic acid until their T-score declined to less than −2 standard deviations or after occurrence of a nontraumatic fracture or evidence of an asymptomatic fracture. Patients received zoledronic acid 4 mg by IV infusion over 15 minutes every 6 months for 5 years in addition to oral calcium and vitamin D. All patients received letrozole 2.5 mg orally daily for 5 years. Patients enrolled in these studies were not permitted to receive other drugs known to affect the skeleton (e.g., IV bisphosphonates, chronic corticosteroids) during the study or for a specified period of time prior to study entry.

In the Z-FAST study, BMD in both the lumbar spine and total hip sites was improved at 61 months for the upfront group but declined in the delayed group in women still remaining in the study at that time (approximately 60% of those initially enrolled), regardless of baseline T-score, clinically important risk factors, or chemotherapy status. A decline in BMD of at least 8% in the lumbar spine in women with a normal BMD at baseline (defined as T-score better than −1 SD from normal) occurred more frequently in those receiving delayed treatment than in those receiving upfront treatment (20 versus 1.7%, respectively, based on intent-to-treat analysis). In women with preexisting mild to moderate osteopenia (i.e., a decline to a T-score between −1 and −2 SD), a BMD decrease of at least 8% in the lumbar spine occurred in 5.7 and 0.3% of patients in the delayed and upfront treatment groups, respectively, based on intent-to-treat analysis. At 61 months, upfront administration of zoledronic acid reduced progression to mild to moderate osteopenia in women with a normal BMD at baseline compared with delayed administration of the drug (2 versus 11%, respectively), and reduced progression to severe osteopenia (i.e., a decline to a T-score below −2 SD) in women with preexisting mild to moderate osteopenia (0 versus 4.9%, respectively). The 2-year fracture rate was similar (4.3 and 4%) for both treatment groups, with an increase at 5 years to 9.3 and 11% in the upfront and delayed groups, respectively. The mean difference in percentage change from baseline BMD for the lumbar spine and total hip sites at 61 months was 8.9 and 6.7%, respectively, between the upfront treatment and delayed treatment groups. At the time of the final analysis at a follow-up of 61 months, 24.6% of the women in the delayed group had begun treatment with zoledronic acid; 66.2% of these women had met protocol-defined criteria to receive zoledronic acid. Bone turnover marker analysis at 61 months revealed lower serum N-telopeptide (NTx) and bone-specific alkaline phosphatase (BSAP) concentrations in the upfront group than those in the delayed group. Renal impairment occurred at a similar rate in both treatment groups; however, potential osteonecrosis of the jaw occurred more frequently in women receiving upfront therapy than in those receiving delayed therapy (2 versus 0 cases).

Data from the ZO-FAST study also demonstrated improvement of BMD in both the lumbar spine and total hip sites at 60 months for the upfront group but BMD declined in the delayed group. Upfront administration of zoledronic acid increased BMD in the lumbar spine by 3.9% in women with a normal BMD at baseline, but a 7.1% decrease occurred in those receiving delayed administration of the drug. Upfront zoledronic acid substantially improved BMD in the lumbar spine by 5.3% compared with delayed administration, which resulted in a 4.2% decrease in women with established (natural) postmenopausal status. In women who were newly (induced) postmenopausal, a decrease of 0.3 or 9.3% in BMD in the lumbar spine was reported in the upfront or delayed treatment groups, respectively. At the time of the final analysis, the mean difference in percentage change from baseline BMD in the lumbar spine and total hip sites was 9.7 and 5.8%, respectively, between the upfront treatment and delayed treatment groups. At the time of the final analysis at a follow-up of 60 months, 27% of the women in the delayed group had met criteria to receive zoledronic acid. Renal impairment occurred at a similar rate in both treatment groups, and 9 potential osteonecrosis of the jaw events were reported in the overall study population.

Data from the E-ZO-FAST study were consistent with the Z-FAST and ZO-FAST studies. Improvement of BMD at both the lumbar spine and total hip sites was observed at 12 months for the upfront group, but BMD declined in the delayed group regardless of baseline T-score, postmenopausal status, or chemotherapy status. At 12 months, 13% of the women in the delayed group had met criteria to receive zoledronic acid. In this study, upfront administration of zoledronic acid reduced progression to osteopenia in women with a normal BMD at baseline compared with delayed administration of the drug (2.1 versus 12.5%, respectively). In women with preexisting osteopenia, improvement to a normal BMD occurred more frequently in women receiving upfront administration of zoledronic acid compared with those receiving delayed administration of the drug (18.3 versus 8%, respectively), and maintenance of a normal BMD in women with a normal BMD at baseline occurred more frequently in those receiving upfront therapy than in those receiving delayed therapy (71.1 versus 57.2%, respectively). The 1-year fracture rate was 0.8 and 1.9% in the upfront and delayed groups, respectively. At 12 months, the mean difference in percentage change from baseline BMD in the lumbar spine and total hip sites was 5.4 and 3.3%, respectively, between the upfront and delayed treatment groups. Among women with established postmenopausal status and those who were recently (induced) menopausal, the percentage change from baseline BMD between the upfront and delayed treatment groups was 5.2 and 6.8%, respectively. Adverse effects generally were similar in both treatment groups, although bone pain (8.3 versus 4.1%), pyrexia (6.7 versus 0%), and influenza-like illness (6 versus 1.1%) occurred more frequently in women in the upfront group compared with those in the delayed group. Osteonecrosis of the jaw occurred in 0.4% of women receiving upfront therapy compared with none of those receiving delayed therapy.

Data from a similarly designed study (NCCTG-N03CC) also demonstrated an improvement in lumbar spine BMD in postmenopausal women treated with letrozole who had received prior tamoxifen therapy and were randomized to receive upfront zoledronic acid therapy. At the time of the final analysis at a follow-up of 60 months, 42% of women initially enrolled in the study were evaluable for the primary BMD end point and 14.7% of women in the delayed group crossed over to receive zoledronic acid. Clinically important lumbar spine bone loss (i.e., BMD decrease of 5% or greater from baseline) occurred more frequently in women receiving delayed therapy compared with those receiving upfront therapy (41.2 versus 10.2%), and clinically important total hip and femoral neck bone loss was reported in 45.8 or 7.6% of those receiving delayed or upfront therapy, respectively; a BMD decrease of

10% from baseline in the lumbar spine occurred in 16.8 and 5.1% of women in the delayed and upfront treatment groups, respectively. The mean difference in BMD for the lumbar spine was 9.4% between the upfront treatment and delayed treatment groups. However, there was no difference between the groups in the 5-year fracture rate. Adverse effects generally were similar between both treatment groups, although pyrexia (9 versus 3%) and elevated serum creatinine concentrations (9 versus 5%) occurred more frequently in women receiving upfront therapy compared with those receiving delayed therapy. Osteonecrosis of the jaw occurred in 2 or 1% of women receiving upfront or delayed therapy, respectively.

Although longer-term follow-up of the 3 companion Zometa-Femara Adjuvant Synergy Trials (Z-FAST, ZO-FAST, E-ZO-FAST) and NCCTG-N03CC study is needed to further clarify between-treatment differences in fracture incidence, upfront administration of zoledronic acid in postmenopausal women receiving aromatase inhibitor therapy significantly prevented lumbar spine and total hip BMD losses compared with those whose therapy was delayed until a decline in T-score to less than −2 SD or nontraumatic fracture, or evidence of an asymptomatic fracture occurred. Based on current evidence, use of zoledronic acid in postmenopausal women receiving aromatase inhibitor therapy may be considered a reasonable choice (accepted, with possible conditions); factors that should be considered when determining the optimal time to initiate therapy are baseline BMD and history of prior fractures.

Prevention in Premenopausal Women

Efficacy and safety of zoledronic acid for the prevention of aromatase inhibitor-associated bone loss in premenopausal women receiving adjuvant hormonal therapy plus a gonadotropin-releasing hormone (GnRH, luteinizing hormone-releasing hormone) agonist (e.g., goserelin) for stage I or II estrogen receptor-positive or progesterone receptor-positive breast cancer† were studied in a BMD substudy of a phase 3, open-label, randomized study (Austrian Breast and Colorectal Cancer Study Group-12 [ABCSG-12]). The ABCSG-12 study included premenopausal women with early-stage estrogen receptor-positive and/or progesterone receptor-positive breast cancer. In this substudy, 401 patients were randomized in a 1:1:1:1 ratio to receive hormonal therapy with tamoxifen (20 mg orally daily) or anastrozole (1 mg orally daily) plus a GnRH agonist (goserelin acetate 3.6 mg by subcutaneous injection every 28 days) to induce ovarian suppression with or without zoledronic acid. An initial zoledronic acid dosage of 8 mg IV every 6 months was used; the protocol was subsequently amended to reduce the dosage to 4 mg by IV infusion over 15 minutes every 6 months following reports of increased toxicity (e.g., nephrotoxicity) with the higher dose. Therapy was continued for a duration of 3 years in all treatment groups.

A lower rate of decline in bone loss after 3 years of treatment was reported in those premenopausal women still remaining in the study at that time (about one-third of those initially enrolled) who were receiving zoledronic acid with anastrozole-goserelin or tamoxifen-goserelin compared with those receiving anastrozole-goserelin or tamoxifen-goserelin alone. The incidence of osteopenia at 3 years in the lumbar spine was 44 or 54% in patients receiving zoledronic acid-anastrozole-goserelin or anastrozole-goserelin alone, respectively. Osteoporosis was not reported in patients receiving zoledronic acid-anastrozole-goserelin, but 25% of women receiving anastrozole-goserelin alone became osteoporotic. Two years after the completion of the study treatment, partial improvement in BMD at both the lumbar spine and trochanter sites was observed in those receiving anastrozole-goserelin or tamoxifen-goserelin alone, although BMD had not fully recovered to the baseline measurement; in contrast, an improvement in BMD was reported in those receiving zoledronic acid with anastrozole-goserelin or tamoxifen-goserelin. Although not specific for the anastrozole-goserelin regimen, no fractures were reported in patients receiving zoledronic acid at 5 years; 2 fractures occurred in women receiving anastrozole-goserelin or tamoxifen-goserelin alone.

Improvements in BMD were observed in premenopausal women with early-stage breast cancer when zoledronic acid was administered concurrently with an aromatase inhibitor and GnRH agonist. However, longer-term follow-up of this study is needed, especially as these women enter menopause, to further clarify lasting clinical efficacy (i.e., clinically important fracture reduction) and late adverse effects of zoledronic acid therapy. Based on current evidence, use of zoledronic acid for the prevention of aromatase inhibitor-associated bone loss in premenopausal women is not fully established because of unclear risk/benefit.

● Breast Cancer

Efficacy and safety of zoledronic acid in combination with adjuvant systemic therapy in postmenopausal women with early or locally advanced breast cancer† have been studied in 2 open-label, randomized phase 3 studies (Austrian Breast and Colorectal Cancer Study Group-12 [ABCSG-12] and Adjuvant Zoledronic Acid to Reduce Recurrence [AZURE]-BIG 01/04 study), with supportive data from a meta-analysis and 3 open-label, randomized phase 3 studies evaluating the use of zoledronic acid for the prevention of aromatase inhibitor-associated bone loss†.

In the ABCSG-12 study, 1803 premenopausal women with estrogen receptor-positive and/or progesterone receptor-positive stage I or II breast cancer were randomized in a 1:1:1:1 ratio to receive hormonal therapy with tamoxifen (20 mg orally daily) or anastrozole (1 mg orally daily) plus a GnRH agonist (goserelin acetate 3.6 mg by subcutaneous injection every 28 days) to induce ovarian suppression with or without zoledronic acid. An initial zoledronic acid dosage of 8 mg IV every 6 months was used; the protocol was subsequently amended to reduce the dosage to 4 mg by IV infusion over 15 minutes every 6 months following reports of increased toxicity (e.g., nephrotoxicity) with the higher dose. Therapy was continued for a duration of 3 years in all treatment groups. In this study, the primary measure of efficacy was disease-free survival. The median age of patients enrolled in the study was 45 years (range: 25–58); 31% had positive lymph node involvement and 85% did not receive neoadjuvant chemotherapy. All patients enrolled in the study had hormone receptor-positive tumors. At a median follow-up of 62 months, addition of zoledronic acid to hormonal therapy improved the rate of disease-free survival compared with hormonal therapy alone (92 versus 88%; hazard ratio of 0.68). Similar results were observed but predefined statistical significance was not achieved at a median follow-up of 94.4 months. Zoledronic acid administered concurrently with hormonal therapy was associated with numerically, but not significantly, improved overall survival compared with hormonal therapy alone (96.7 versus 94.5%). A subset analysis of disease-free survival and overall survival based on clinically relevant baseline patient and disease characteristics demonstrated consistent treatment benefit with zoledronic acid regardless of lymph node status and disease stage (T1 or T2/3), but no difference in disease-free survival or overall survival was apparent in patients 40 years of age or younger receiving zoledronic acid compared with those receiving hormonal therapy alone. Adverse effects generally were consistent with known safety profiles of each agent, although arthralgia (24 versus 18%), bone pain (35 versus 25%), nausea/vomiting (8.6 versus 6.1%), pyrexia (8.9 versus 2.2%), dermatologic effects (6.5 versus 4.3%), peripheral nerve disease (5.7 versus 3.4%), tachycardia (2.1 versus 0.8%), cognitive disorder (1.4 versus 0.3%), and hypocalcemia (0.4 versus 0%) occurred more frequently in women receiving zoledronic acid concurrently with hormonal therapy compared with those receiving hormonal therapy alone. No confirmed cases of osteonecrosis of the jaw were reported.

In the AZURE-BIG 01/04 study, 3360 patients with stage II or III invasive breast cancer were randomized to receive zoledronic acid in addition to adjuvant antineoplastic therapy (i.e., hormonal therapy, chemotherapy, or both) or adjuvant antineoplastic therapy alone. Patients randomized to receive zoledronic acid received 4 mg by IV infusion every 3–4 weeks for 6 doses, then every 3 months for 8 doses, followed by every 6 months for 5 doses (for a total duration of 5 years). The majority of patients had positive lymph node involvement (98%), 78% had estrogen receptor-positive tumors, 45% were premenopausal, 31% had been postmenopausal for greater than 5 years, and 15% had been postmenopausal for 5 years or less. Most patients (74%) enrolled in the study planned to receive hormonal therapy in combination with chemotherapy. The majority of patients enrolled in the study planned to receive an anthracycline-containing regimen (93%) and 23% planned to receive a taxane-containing regimen. In this study, the primary measure of efficacy was disease-free survival. At median follow-up times of 59 and 84 months, no significant difference in disease-free survival (hazard ratios of 0.98 and 0.94, respectively) or overall survival (hazard ratios of 0.85 and 0.93, respectively) was observed between patients receiving zoledronic acid and antineoplastic therapy and those receiving antineoplastic therapy alone; however, zoledronic acid substantially reduced the incidence of bone fractures and bone metastasis by 31 and 19–22%, respectively, compared with antineoplastic therapy alone. A preplanned subset analysis of invasive disease-free survival based on menopausal status suggested a treatment benefit, primarily a reduction in extraskeletal invasive disease-free events, with the addition of zoledronic acid to antineoplastic therapy in women who had experienced menopause at least 5 years before study entry (hazard ratio of 0.77), but not in women in other menopausal groups (e.g., premenopausal, perimenopausal, unknown menopausal status) (hazard ratio of 1.03). Adverse effects were similar between both treatment groups, although 33 cases (confirmed in 26 cases) of potential osteonecrosis of the jaw occurred in women receiving zoledronic acid plus antineoplastic therapy compared with no cases in those receiving antineoplastic therapy alone.

Use of zoledronic acid in combination with adjuvant endocrine therapy in postmenopausal women also has been evaluated in several phase 3, open-label, randomized bone mineral density (BMD) studies (Z-FAST, ZO-FAST, and E-ZO-FAST).

(See Prevention in Postmenopausal Women under Uses: Prevention of Aromatase Inhibitor-associated Bone Loss.) Women enrolled in these studies were postmenopausal with stage I to IIIa estrogen receptor-positive and/or progesterone receptor-positive breast cancer. Patients enrolled in these studies were randomized to receive zoledronic acid as either upfront therapy or delayed therapy (based on decline in BMD). Patients received zoledronic acid 4 mg by IV infusion over 15 minutes every 6 months for 5 years. All patients received letrozole 2.5 mg orally daily for 5 years. In the E-ZO-FAST study at a median follow-up of 12 months, no difference in disease-free survival rate was observed between women receiving upfront or delayed zoledronic acid (97.2 versus 98.1%, respectively). Although no difference in disease-free survival was observed between the 2 treatment groups in the Z-FAST study at a median follow-up of 61 months (absolute difference of 0.7%), upfront administration of zoledronic acid therapy prolonged disease-free survival compared with delayed administration of the drug (hazard ratio of 0.66) in the ZO-FAST study. In the ZO-FAST study, breast cancer-related events in patients receiving upfront administration versus delayed administration of zoledronic acid included locoregional recurrence (0.9 versus 2.3%), distant recurrence (5.5 versus 7.7%), and bone metastases (2.6 versus 4.5%). No difference in overall survival was observed between the 2 treatment groups in the Z-FAST and ZO-FAST studies. At the time of analysis in the Z-FAST, ZO-FAST, and E-ZO-FAST studies, 25, 27, and 13%, respectively, of women in the delayed treatment group had begun treatment with zoledronic acid.

The Early Breast Cancer Trialists' Collaborative Group (EBCTCG) conducted a meta-analysis of individual patient data from 26 randomized clinical trials evaluating addition of bisphosphonate (any drug, dose, and schedule) therapy to standard adjuvant systemic therapy in women with early-stage breast cancer. This meta-analysis indicated that addition of bisphosphonate therapy to standard systemic therapy (median duration of therapy of 3.4 years) modestly reduced the risk of bone recurrence (rate ratio of 0.83) and bone fractures (rate ratio of 0.85) at 10 years compared with standard systemic therapy alone. Addition of bisphosphonate therapy to adjuvant systemic therapy also resulted in small reductions in the risk of recurrence (rate ratio of 0.94, which corresponded to an absolute difference in recurrence rate of 1.1% at 10 years), distant recurrence (rate ratio of 0.92, which corresponded to an absolute difference in rate of distance recurrence of 1.4% at 10 years), and breast cancer mortality (rate ratio 0.91, which corresponded to an absolute difference in breast cancer mortality rate of 1.7% at 10 years). However, consistent with data from the ABCSG-12 and AZURE-BIG 01/04 studies, subset analysis based on menopausal status suggested clinical benefit with adjuvant bisphosphonate therapy in postmenopausal women but not in premenopausal women. In postmenopausal women, the addition of bisphosphonate therapy to adjuvant systemic therapy reduced the risk of bone recurrence (rate ratio of 0.72, which corresponded to an absolute difference in bone recurrence rate of 2.2% at 10 years) and breast cancer mortality (rate ratio of 0.82, which corresponded to an absolute difference in breast cancer mortality rate of 3.3% at 10 years).

Based on current evidence, use of zoledronic acid in combination with adjuvant systemic therapy may be considered a reasonable choice (accepted) in postmenopausal women with early or locally advanced breast cancer. The American Society of Clinical Oncology (ASCO) and Cancer Care Ontario (CCO) state that postmenopausal women who are candidates for adjuvant systemic therapy for the treatment of breast cancer should consider receiving a bisphosphonate (i.e., zoledronic acid) during the course of adjuvant therapy for up to 5 years. Although some clinicians state that any bone-modifying agent that has demonstrated a reduction in the risk of fragility fractures in at-risk populations (e.g., postmenopausal women, drug-induced osteoporosis) may be effective as adjuvant therapy for breast cancer, sufficient data are only available from clinical trials evaluating zoledronic acid or clodronate (not commercially available in the US); additional data are needed to further elucidate clinical benefit of other bone-modifying agents. The optimal time for initiating bisphosphonates is not known; however, bisphosphonate therapy was generally initiated soon after surgery or chemotherapy in most clinical trials. The optimal duration of adjuvant bisphosphonate therapy is not known; however, the duration should not exceed 5 years since toxicity of long-term (e.g., beyond 5 years) use of bisphosphonates, including zoledronic acid, has not been determined. ASCO states that clinicians should consider patient and disease characteristics (e.g., risk of recurrence) and adverse effects when deciding whether bisphosphonate therapy should be added to adjuvant systemic therapy.

DOSAGE AND ADMINISTRATION

● General

Hypocalcemia and other disturbances of bone and mineral metabolism must be corrected before zoledronic acid therapy is initiated for the management of osteoporosis or Paget disease.

Renal function should be evaluated (with creatinine clearance or serum creatinine concentrations) prior to each dose of zoledronic acid; more frequent monitoring is recommended in patients at high risk of acute renal failure (e.g., geriatric patients, those receiving diuretic therapy). (See Renal Effects under Cautions: Warnings/Precautions.) Zoledronic acid should not be administered for prevention or treatment of osteoporosis or for treatment of Paget disease of bone in patients who have severe renal impairment (creatinine clearance less than 35 mL/minute) or evidence of acute renal impairment.

● Administration

Zoledronic acid is administered by IV infusion over *no less than* 15 minutes. (See Renal Effects under Cautions: Warnings/Precautions.)

Zoledronic acid is commercially available as a *solution concentrate* containing 4 mg of the drug per 5 mL (Zometa® concentrate or generic equivalents) and as a *ready-to-use injection* containing 4 mg of the drug per 100 mL (Zometa® ready-to-use or generic equivalents) for use in patients with cancer-related indications. Zoledronic acid also is available as a *ready-to-use injection* containing 5 mg of the drug per 100 mL (Reclast® or generic equivalents) for use in the prevention or treatment of osteoporosis or for treatment of Paget disease of bone.

Zoledronic acid should be administered through separate vented infusion lines apart from other drugs and should not be allowed to come in contact with any solutions containing calcium or other divalent cations.

Zoledronic Acid for Cancer-related Indications

The concentrated zoledronic acid solution (Zometa® concentrate or generic equivalents) must be diluted in 100 mL of 0.9% sodium chloride or 5% dextrose injection prior to IV administration. The commercially available 5-mL vial of injection concentrate is formulated to provide the full labeled dose of zoledronic acid (4 mg) when diluted as directed for patients with normal renal function (baseline creatinine clearance exceeding 60 mL/minute). For preparation of reduced doses in patients with mild to moderate renal impairment (baseline creatinine clearance of 30–60 mL/minute), the appropriate volume of drug concentrate should be withdrawn from the vial and *further diluted* as directed. For patients with a baseline creatinine clearance of 50–60 mL/minute, 4.4 mL of the concentrated drug solution should be withdrawn from the 5-mL vial to obtain a dose of 3.5 mg (for subsequent dilution). For patients with a baseline creatinine clearance of 40–49 mL/minute, 4.1 mL of the concentrated drug solution should be withdrawn to obtain a dose of 3.3 mg (for subsequent dilution). For patients with a baseline creatinine clearance of 30–39 mL/minute, 3.8 mL of the concentrated drug solution should be withdrawn to obtain a dose of 3 mg (for subsequent dilution). The withdrawn amount of drug concentrate should then be diluted in 100 mL of 0.9% sodium chloride or 5% dextrose injection. (See Bone Metastases of Solid Tumors and Osteolytic Lesions of Multiple Myeloma under Dosage and Administration: Dosage.) *To avoid inadvertent injection of the concentrated solution, the undiluted drug concentrate should not be stored in a syringe.*

The ready-to-use 4-mg/100-mL formulation of zoledronic acid (Zometa® ready-to-use or generic equivalents) may be administered directly without further dilution in patients with normal renal function (baseline creatinine clearance greater than 60 mL/minute). For preparation of reduced doses of the drug for patients with mild to moderate renal impairment (baseline creatinine clearance of 30–60 mL/minute), the appropriate volume of the drug solution should be withdrawn from the 100-mL bottle and replaced with an equal volume of 0.9% sodium chloride or 5% dextrose injection. For patients with a baseline creatinine clearance of 50–60 mL/minute, 12 mL of the drug solution should be withdrawn from the 100-mL bottle (and replaced with 12 mL of 0.9% sodium chloride or 5% dextrose injection) to obtain the recommended dose of 3.5 mg. For patients with a baseline creatinine clearance of 40–49 mL/minute, 18 mL of the drug solution should be withdrawn (and replaced with 18 mL of 0.9% sodium chloride or 5% dextrose injection) to obtain the recommended dose of 3.3 mg. For patients with a baseline creatinine clearance of 30–39 mL/minute, 25 mL of the drug solution should be withdrawn (and replaced with 25 mL of 0.9% sodium chloride or 5% dextrose injection) to obtain the recommended dose of 3 mg.

Zoledronic acid should *not* be mixed or diluted with calcium-containing solutions (e.g., lactated Ringer's solution).

Strict adherence to administration recommendations for diluted zoledronic acid concentrate (Zometa® concentrate or generic equivalents) is important, since smaller infusion volumes (e.g., 50 mL) and rapid (over 5 minutes) IV infusion rates have been associated with an increased risk of renal impairment, which may progress to renal failure.

Prior to initiating zoledronic acid therapy in the treatment of malignancy-associated hypercalcemia, it is important to establish adequate hydration and urinary output in order to increase renal excretion of calcium; adequate hydration should be maintained throughout therapy with the drug. Overhydration should be avoided, especially in those with heart failure. An attempt should be made to achieve and maintain a urinary output of 2 L per day throughout therapy with zoledronic acid.

Zoledronic Acid for Osteoporosis and Paget Disease of Bone

To minimize risk of renal toxicity, patients receiving zoledronic acid for prevention or treatment of osteoporosis or for treatment of Paget disease of bone must be appropriately hydrated prior to administration of the drug. Zoledronic acid therapy should be withheld in such patients with evidence of dehydration and may be resumed once normovolemic status has been achieved. Each dose of zoledronic acid should be followed by a flush with 10 mL of 0.9% sodium chloride.

Administration of acetaminophen following zoledronic acid administration may reduce the incidence of acute-phase inflammatory reactions (e.g., fever, myalgia, flu-like symptoms, headache, arthralgia).

● Dosage

Dosage of zoledronic acid, which is commercially available for parenteral use as the monohydrate, is calculated on the anhydrous basis.

Hypercalcemia Associated with Malignancy

For the treatment of hypercalcemia (albumin-corrected serum calcium concentration of at least 12 mg/dL) associated with malignancy in adults, the manufacturer recommends that zoledronic acid (Zometa®) be infused IV as a single dose of 4 mg over no less than 15 minutes.

Single doses of the drug should not exceed 4 mg since renal impairment, which may progress to renal failure has occurred following administration of zoledronic acid in recommended or higher than recommended dosages.

After a post-treatment observation period of at least 7 days, a second course of zoledronic acid *at the same dosage* may be considered if there is evidence of recurrence of the disease process or if the initial treatment fails to normalize serum calcium concentrations. If patients with hypercalcemia of malignancy experience a deterioration of renal function during therapy with zoledronic acid, the possible risk of renal failure with subsequent doses of the drug must be carefully weighed against the potential benefits of treatment. No data are available to date on the safety and efficacy of more than one course of retreatment with zoledronic acid or of the recommended retreatment dosage of 4 mg of zoledronic acid in patients with hypercalcemia of malignancy.

Bone Metastases of Solid Tumors and Osteolytic Lesions of Multiple Myeloma

For the treatment of bone metastases associated with solid tumors or the treatment of osteolytic lesions associated with multiple myeloma in adults, the manufacturer-recommended dosage of zoledronic acid is 4 mg given IV over no less than 15 minutes once every 3–4 weeks. Single doses of the drug should not exceed 4 mg since renal impairment, which may progress to renal failure has occurred following administration of zoledronic acid in recommended or higher than recommended dosages. The optimum duration of such therapy is not known.

In patients with bone metastases of solid tumors and osteolytic lesions of multiple myeloma and mild to moderate renal impairment (baseline creatinine clearance of 30–60 mL/minute), lower initial dosages of zoledronic acid are recommended. The following dosages are recommended:

TABLE 1. Initial Dosage of Zoledronic Acid in Adults with Bone Metastases of Solid Tumors and Osteolytic Lesions of Multiple Myeloma Based on Renal Function

Calculated Creatinine Clearance (mL/minute)	IV Dosage (Infused over no less than 15 minutes)
>60	4 mg every 3–4 weeks
50–60	3.5 mg every 3–4 weeks
40–49	3.3 mg every 3–4 weeks
30–39	3 mg every 3–4 weeks

If patients with bone metastases associated with solid tumors or with osteolytic lesions associated with multiple myeloma experience a deterioration of renal function during therapy with zoledronic acid (defined as an increase in serum creatinine concentration of at least 0.5 or 1 mg/dL, respectively, in patients with normal [less than 1.4 mg/dL] or elevated [1.4 mg/dL or greater] baseline serum creatinine concentrations), the drug should be withheld until serum creatinine concentrations return to within 10% of baseline concentrations. Zoledronic acid should be reinitiated at the same dosage that was used prior to the treatment interruption. Studies in this patient population included individuals with serum creatinine concentrations up to 3 mg/dL.

Patients with multiple myeloma or bone metastases associated with solid tumors who are receiving zoledronic acid therapy should receive supplemental therapy with oral calcium (500 mg of elemental calcium daily) and a multivitamin containing vitamin D (400 international units [IU, units] daily).

Osteoporosis in Postmenopausal Women

For *prevention* of osteoporosis in postmenopausal women, the recommended dosage of zoledronic acid is 5 mg by IV infusion over no less than 15 minutes every 2 years in patients with a creatinine clearance of at least 35 mL/minute. (See Renal Impairment under Warnings/Precautions: Specific Populations, in Cautions.) Patients must receive supplemental calcium and vitamin D if dietary intake is inadequate; postmenopausal women generally require at least 800–1000 units of vitamin D and 1.2 g of calcium daily.

For *treatment* of osteoporosis in postmenopausal women, the manufacturer recommends that zoledronic acid be infused IV as a single 5-mg dose over no less than 15 minutes once yearly in patients with a creatinine clearance of at least 35 mL/minute. (See Renal Impairment under Warnings/Precautions: Specific Populations, in Cautions.) For treatment of osteoporosis and to reduce the risk of hypocalcemia, patients must receive supplemental calcium and vitamin D if dietary intake is inadequate; generally, women older than 50 years of age require 800–1000 units of vitamin D daily and at least 1.2 g of elemental calcium daily.

The optimal duration of bisphosphonate treatment for osteoporosis has not been established. Safety and efficacy of zoledronic acid for the treatment of osteoporosis is based on clinical data supporting fracture reduction over 3 years of treatment. Some evidence suggests that increased durations of bisphosphonate use may be associated with an increased risk of some adverse effects (e.g., atypical fractures, jaw osteonecrosis). All patients receiving a bisphosphonate should have periodic evaluations to determine the need for continued therapy with the drug. Discontinuance of bisphosphonate therapy may be considered after 3–5 years of use for patients who are assessed to be at low risk of fracture. Patients who discontinue therapy should have their risk for fracture evaluated periodically.

Osteoporosis in Men

For the treatment of osteoporosis or osteoporosis secondary to hypogonadism in men, the manufacturer recommends that zoledronic acid be infused IV as a single 5-mg dose over no less than 15 minutes once yearly in patients with a creatinine clearance of at least 35 mL/minute. (See Renal Impairment under Warnings/Precautions: Specific Populations, in Cautions.) For treatment of osteoporosis and to reduce the risk of hypocalcemia, patients must receive supplemental calcium and vitamin D if dietary intake is inadequate; generally, 800–1000 units of vitamin D daily and at least 1.2 g of elemental calcium daily is recommended.

The optimal duration of bisphosphonate treatment for osteoporosis has not been established. Some evidence suggests that bisphosphonate therapy for more than 3 years (median 7 years in one analysis of available data) in patients with osteoporosis may be associated with an increased risk of atypical fracture of the femur. (See Atypical Fracture of the Femur under Cautions: Warnings/Precautions.) All patients receiving a bisphosphonate should have periodic evaluations to determine the need for continued therapy with the drug.

Glucocorticoid-induced Osteoporosis

For the treatment or prevention of glucocorticoid-induced osteoporosis, the manufacturer recommends that zoledronic acid be infused IV as a single 5-mg dose over no less than 15 minutes once yearly in patients with a creatinine clearance of at least 35 mL/minute. (See Renal Impairment under Warnings/Precautions: Specific Populations, in Cautions.) Patients must receive supplemental calcium and vitamin D if dietary intake is inadequate; an average of at least 800–1000 units of vitamin D and 1.2 g of calcium daily is recommended.

Paget Disease of Bone

For the treatment of Paget disease of bone, the initial adult dosage of zoledronic acid is 5 mg, infused IV over at least 15 minutes, in patients with a creatinine clearance of at least 35 mL/minute. (See Renal Impairment under Warnings/Precautions: Specific Populations, in Cautions.) Retreatment with zoledronic acid may be considered if relapse occurs based on increases in serum alkaline phosphatase, if initial treatment failed to normalize serum alkaline phosphatase concentrations, or if the patient is symptomatic, according to current standards of medical care. However, no data are available to date on the safety and efficacy of more than one course of treatment with zoledronic acid in patients with Paget disease of bone. To reduce the risk for hypocalcemia, all patients with Paget disease of bone should receive 1.5 g of elemental calcium daily in divided doses (750 mg twice daily or 500 mg 3 times daily) and 800 units of vitamin D daily, particularly in the first 2 weeks following zoledronic acid administration.

Prevention of Aromatase Inhibitor-associated Bone Loss in Postmenopausal Women

When zoledronic acid has been used for prevention of bone loss associated with use of aromatase inhibitor therapy in postmenopausal women†, zoledronic acid 4 mg has been administered by IV infusion over 15 minutes every 6 months for 5 years. In clinical trials, patients were encouraged to take supplemental oral calcium (500 mg to 1.2 g daily) and vitamin D (400–800 units daily). (See Prevention in Postmenopausal Women under Uses: Prevention of Aromatase Inhibitor-associated Bone Loss.)

Adjuvant Therapy for Early or Locally Advanced Breast Cancer

When zoledronic acid has been used in combination with adjuvant systemic therapy in postmenopausal women with early or locally advanced breast cancer†, zoledronic acid 4 mg has been administered by IV infusion over 15 minutes every 6 months for 3–5 years. In clinical trials, patients were encouraged to take supplemental oral calcium (400 mg to 1.2 g daily) and vitamin D (200–800 units daily). (See Uses: Breast Cancer.)

● Special Populations

The manufacturer states that dosage adjustments of zoledronic acid are not necessary in patients with hypercalcemia of malignancy who have mild to moderate renal impairment (serum creatinine concentrations less than 4.5 mg/dL) prior to initiation of therapy.

In patients with bone metastases of solid tumors and osteolytic lesions of multiple myeloma and mild to moderate renal impairment (baseline creatinine clearance of 30–60 mL/minute), lower initial dosages of zoledronic acid are recommended. (See Bone Metastases of Solid Tumors and Osteolytic Lesions of Multiple Myeloma under Dosage and Administration: Dosage.)

The manufacturer states that dosage adjustments of zoledronic acid are not necessary in patients receiving the drug for prevention or treatment of osteoporosis or for treatment of Paget's disease of bone who have a creatinine clearance of 35 mL/minute or greater.

CAUTIONS

● Contraindications

Known hypersensitivity to zoledronic acid, other bisphosphonates, or any ingredient in the formulations.

Hypocalcemia.

Use of zoledronic acid for prevention or treatment of osteoporosis or for treatment of Paget disease of bone is contraindicated in patients with creatinine clearance of less than 35 mL/minute or those with evidence of acute renal impairment.

● Warnings/Precautions
Osteonecrosis of the Jaw

Osteonecrosis and osteomyelitis of the jaw have been reported in patients receiving bisphosphonates. Most of these patients had neoplasms and were receiving IV bisphosphonates and concurrent chemotherapy, head and neck radiation therapy, or corticosteroids, and most cases have been associated with dental procedures such as tooth extraction. Some cases also have occurred in patients with postmenopausal osteoporosis treated with oral or IV bisphosphonate therapy. Other risk factors for the development of osteonecrosis of the jaw may include coexisting infection(s), anemia, coagulation disorders, preexisting oral disease, and/or trauma. Risk also may be increased with increased duration of bisphosphonate use.

A dental examination (panoramic jaw radiograph) to detect dental and periodontal infections with appropriate preventive dentistry (e.g., removal of abscessed and nonrestorable teeth and involved periodontal tissues, rehabilitation of salvageable dentition, dental prophylaxis, caries control, restorative dental care) should be considered prior to treatment with bisphosphonates in patients with risk factors (e.g. cancer; concomitant chemotherapy, corticosteroids, angiogenesis inhibitors, or radiation therapy; poor oral hygiene). Follow-up hard and soft tissue oral assessment should be performed every 3–4 months, depending on risk, and oncologists should briefly inspect the oral cavity of prospective candidates for bisphosphonate therapy at baseline and at every follow-up visit. If bisphosphonate therapy can be briefly delayed without risk of a skeletal-related complication, teeth with a poor prognosis should be extracted and other dental surgeries should be completed prior to initiation of bisphosphonate therapy. The benefit or risk of withholding bisphosphonate therapy in cancer patients requiring dental surgery has not been evaluated to date. The decision to withhold bisphosphonate therapy in such patients must be made by an oncologist in consultation with an oral maxillofacial surgeon or another dental specialist. During treatment with bisphosphonates in cancer patients with risk factors for osteonecrosis, dentists should check and adjust removable dentures for potential soft-tissue injury, especially tissue overlying bone. Such patients should avoid invasive dental procedures if possible during treatment with bisphosphonates, as dental surgery may exacerbate the condition. In patients requiring dental procedures during bisphosphonate treatment or patients with established osteonecrosis, no data are available to suggest whether discontinuance of therapy reduces the risk of osteonecrosis of the jaw or disease progression, respectively. Management of patients requiring dental treatment should be based on an individual assessment of risks and benefits. Dental infections should be managed aggressively nonsurgically with root canal treatment if possible or with minimal surgical intervention.

In patients with established osteonecrosis requiring dental surgery, cessation or interruption of therapy may be considered taking into account the potential risk of further osteonecrosis versus the risk of skeletal complication or hypercalcemia of malignancy. The decision to withdraw bisphosphonate therapy may be coordinated between the oncologist and an oral surgeon.

Atypical Fracture of the Femur

Findings from several case reports and case series suggest that therapy with bisphosphonates, particularly when used for more than 3 years (median 7 years in this analysis), may be associated with an increased risk of atypical fractures of the femur. The magnitude of this risk with bisphosphonate therapy is unclear, although such fractures appear to be rare; in addition, causality has not been established since atypical fractures also have occurred in patients not receiving bisphosphonates. Most cases of atypical femoral fractures with bisphosphonate therapy have been reported in individuals receiving treatment for osteoporosis.

Atypical femoral fractures represent a subset of femoral fractures occurring in the subtrochanteric region (i.e. below the lesser trochanter) or femoral diaphysis (or shaft) of the femur, which are *not* common sites associated with osteoporosis-related hip fractures. Such fractures often occur with minimal or no trauma, are referred to as low-energy or low-trauma fractures (i.e., equivalent to a fall from a standing height or less), and may be associated with activities of normal daily living. Radiographically, these fractures have unique characteristics described as a transverse or short oblique configuration and often lack evidence of comminution; both complete (extension through both cortices) and incomplete (involving only the lateral cortex) fractures have been reported with bisphosphonate therapy.

The pathophysiology of bisphosphonate-associated atypical femoral fractures is not fully known; however, severely suppressive (or oversuppressive) effects on both bone turnover and bone remodeling, leading to accumulation of localized microdamage and a subsequent impairment in bone repair have been proposed as possible mechanisms. Reports of atypical fractures in the general population and in individuals receiving bisphosphonate therapy are rare, accounting for less than 1% of all reported hip and femur fractures.

In a report published by the Task Force of the American Society for Bone and Mineral Research (ASBMR), 310 cases of bisphosphonate-associated atypical femoral fractures were identified through case reports/series; the majority (286 of 310) of reported cases involved the use of bisphosphonate therapy for an osteoporosis-related condition. The age range of individuals was 36–92 years; the median duration of bisphosphonate therapy at the time of fracture was 7 years (range: 1.3–17 years). Most individuals, including 70% of cases reported in the ASBMR analysis, reported prodromal symptoms presenting as a dull, aching thigh pain, weeks to months prior to occurrence of an atypical fracture. Bilateral involvement, either as a confirmed fracture (i.e., a simultaneous or sequential fracture) or the presence of a radiographic

change in the contralateral limb, also may be present at the time of diagnosis of an atypical femoral fracture and was reported in 28% (60 of 215) of cases in the ASBMR analysis. Delayed healing of the fracture site, possibly related to suppressive effects on bone turnover associated with bisphosphonate therapy, has been described with atypical femoral fractures and was reported in 26% (29 of 112) of cases in the ASBMR analysis. Concomitant use of glucocorticoid, estrogen, and proton-pump inhibitor therapy may increase the risk of an atypical fracture. In the ASBMR analysis, 34% of cases occurred in individuals receiving concomitant glucocorticoids (i.e., prednisone) at the time of fracture; in one series, the risk of subtrochanteric fracture was increased in individuals receiving concomitant bisphosphonate and glucocorticoid therapy. Use of concomitant proton-pump inhibitor therapy was reported in 39% of evaluable cases. Vitamin D deficiency, defined as a serum 25-hydroxyvitamin D (25-OHD) concentration of 20 ng/mL or less, also has been identified as a risk factor in some patients experiencing a bisphosphonate-related fracture.

The safety and efficacy of zoledronic acid for the treatment of osteoporosis are based on clinical data supporting fracture reduction over 3 years of treatment. The optimal duration of bisphosphonate treatment for osteoporosis has not been established. The US Food and Drug Administration (FDA) is continuing to collect data on the safety and efficacy of long-term bisphosphonate use (i.e., greater than 3 to 5 years) when used for the prevention and treatment of osteoporosis. FDA and some experts recommend reevaluation of the need for continued bisphosphonate therapy in individuals receiving treatment for 5 years or longer, taking into consideration bone mineral density (particularly in the hip region), fracture history, and possible risk factors (i.e., a co-morbid condition and/or use of concomitant drugs known to adversely affect bone integrity); some experts recommend an annual evaluation in such patients. Because atypical fractures also have been reported in some individuals receiving bisphosphonate therapy in combination with other drugs known to affect bone integrity and/or bone remodeling (i.e., glucocorticoids, proton pump inhibitors, estrogen, tamoxifen), some experts recommend performing a risk-benefit assessment in individuals determined to have a low or slightly elevated fracture risk, to determine the need for continued bisphosphonate therapy in light of the potential increased risk associated with the use of required concomitant therapy.

Individuals with a history of bisphosphonate exposure presenting with new thigh or groin pain should be evaluated for possible atypical femur fracture; an assessment of the contralateral limb also should be performed to rule out possible bilateral involvement (i.e., presence of a radiographic change or fracture). Interruption of bisphosphonate therapy should be considered in individuals presenting with symptoms suggestive of a possible femoral fracture following completion of a comprehensive risk-benefit assessment performed on an individualized basis. Bisphosphonate therapy should be *discontinued* if a femoral shaft fracture is confirmed.

Musculoskeletal Pain

Severe, occasionally incapacitating bone, joint, and/or muscle pain have been reported infrequently through postmarketing experience in patients receiving bisphosphonates, including zoledronic acid. The time to the onset of symptoms varied from 1 day to years after treatment initiation. Musculoskeletal pain has improved following discontinuance of the drug in some patients, whereas other patients have reported slow or incomplete resolution of such pain. In some patients, musculoskeletal pain recurred upon subsequent rechallenge with the same drug or another bisphosphonate. The risk factors for and incidence of severe musculoskeletal pain associated with bisphosphonates are unknown. The association between bisphosphonates and severe musculoskeletal pain may be overlooked by clinicians, which may delay diagnosis, prolong pain and/or impairment, and necessitate the use of analgesics. Clinicians should evaluate whether bisphosphonate use might be responsible for severe musculoskeletal pain in patients who present with these symptoms; temporary or permanent discontinuance of therapy should be considered in such cases.

Fetal/Neonatal Morbidity and Mortality

Although no data are available on the fetal risk of bisphosphonates in humans, these drugs do cause fetal harm in animals. Data from animals suggest that uptake of bisphosphonates into fetal bone is greater than that into maternal bone. A theoretical risk to the fetus (e.g., skeletal and other abnormalities) exists if a woman becomes pregnant after completing a course of bisphosphonate therapy. The impact of variables such as time between cessation of bisphosphonate therapy to conception, the particular bisphosphonate used, and the route of administration (IV versus oral) on this risk has not been established.

Renal Effects

Bisphosphonates, including zoledronic acid, have been associated with renal toxicity, manifested as deterioration of renal function and potential renal failure. Acute renal failure requiring dialysis and sometimes resulting in hospitalization and/or death, has occurred rarely in patients receiving zoledronic acid (Reclast®), mostly for osteoporosis indications. At least 24 cases of renal impairment and acute renal failure were identified in an FDA postmarketing safety review of Reclast® in 2009; 7 deaths were reported. Since the initial safety review, additional reports of renal toxicity associated with the use of Reclast® have been received by the FDA. The time to onset of renal toxicity was approximately 11 days following infusion of the drug. More than half of the patients in these reports also experienced a transient increase in serum creatinine concentrations following infusion of zoledronic acid; the median increase in serum creatinine concentration was 4 mg/dL. Many of the patients had underlying renal disease or other risk factors (e.g., dehydration, advanced age, concomitant use of nephrotoxic agents) that may have contributed to their risk of renal impairment. Renal function deterioration progressing to renal failure and dialysis also has been observed in clinical trials and during postmarketing experience in patients receiving Zometa®. Such renal function deterioration has occurred following administration of higher than recommended doses, but also after administration of the usual dose of 4 mg infused over the recommended infusion period (15 minutes). In some cases, renal impairment occurred after administration of the initial zoledronic acid dose.

Renal function should be evaluated (with creatinine clearance or serum creatinine concentrations) prior to administering each dose of zoledronic acid and more frequently in patients at high risk of acute renal failure, including geriatric patients and those receiving diuretic therapy. Interim monitoring of renal function also should be considered in patients receiving concomitant drugs (e.g., digoxin) that are primarily eliminated by the kidneys. (See Drug Interactions: Drugs Eliminated by Renal Excretion.) Use of zoledronic acid for prevention or treatment of osteoporosis or for treatment of Paget disease of bone is contraindicated in patients with creatinine clearance less than 35 mL/minute and in those with evidence of acute renal impairment; the drug should be used with caution in patients with chronic renal impairment. Risk factors predisposing patients to renal deterioration, such as dehydration (e.g., secondary to fever, sepsis, GI loss, or diuretic therapy) or use of other nephrotoxic agents, should be identified and managed. To help prevent renal impairment, patients should be appropriately hydrated prior to administration of zoledronic acid, especially geriatric patients and those receiving concomitant diuretic therapy. Transient increases in serum creatinine concentrations during therapy may be corrected with administration of IV fluids.

Administration of zoledronic acid 4 mg by IV infusion over a period of 5 minutes has been shown to increase the risk of renal toxicity (i.e., increases in serum creatinine), which can progress to renal failure. The incidence of renal toxicity and renal failure is reduced when the same dose is administered IV over a period of 15 minutes. *Zoledronic acid should be administered by IV infusion over no less than 15 minutes.* (See Dosage and Administration: Administration.)

Metabolic Effects

Hypocalcemia and other factors affecting bone and mineral metabolism (e.g., hypoparathyroidism, thyroid surgery, parathyroid surgery, malabsorption syndromes, excision of small intestine) must be corrected before zoledronic acid therapy is initiated in patients with Paget's disease of bone or postmenopausal osteoporosis. Serum calcium, phosphorus, and magnesium concentrations should be monitored in such patients. Standard hypercalcemia-related metabolic parameters, including serum concentrations of calcium, phosphate, magnesium, potassium, and other electrolytes, should be monitored carefully following initiation of zoledronic acid therapy in patients with hypercalcemia of malignancy. If hypocalcemia, hypophosphatemia, or hypomagnesemia occurs, short-term supplemental therapy may be necessary.

Respiratory Effects

Bisphosphonates have been associated with bronchoconstriction in aspirin-sensitive asthmatic patients. Zoledronic acid should be used with caution in such patients.

Atrial Fibrillation

While data are conflicting, a possible increased risk of atrial fibrillation has been identified with use of bisphosphonates. In 1 of the 2 pivotal preapproval studies in women with postmenopausal osteoporosis, an increased incidence of serious (i.e., events resulting in hospitalization or disability or considered life-threatening) atrial fibrillation was observed in patients receiving zoledronic acid compared with that in placebo recipients. Most of these cases occurred more than 1 month after infusion of zoledronic acid. However, an increased incidence of serious atrial fibrillation with zoledronic acid was not confirmed in a second preapproval study in women with osteoporosis or in a study in men with osteoporosis. Among patients with postmenopausal osteoporosis with or without vertebral fractures who received alendronate, another bisphosphonate drug, in 2 randomized, placebo-controlled trials, the incidence of atrial fibrillation was numerically higher in the alendronate-treated groups compared with that observed in the placebo-treated groups.

To further evaluate the potential for increased risk of atrial fibrillation with certain bisphosphonates, the FDA reviewed data from long-term (6 months' to 3 years' duration) placebo-controlled clinical trials from the sponsors of alendronate, ibandronate, risedronate, and zoledronic acid. Analysis of data from approximately 19,700 patients receiving bisphosphonates and approximately 18,300 patients receiving placebo indicated a difference in event rates of 0–3 events per 1000 patients between bisphosphonates and placebo. The occurrence of atrial fibrillation was rare in each study; 2 or fewer instances of atrial fibrillation occurred in most studies. Across all studies reviewed, no clear association was observed between overall bisphosphonate exposure, dosage, or duration of bisphosphonate therapy and the rate of atrial fibrillation. FDA is continuing to monitor postmarketing adverse event reports of atrial fibrillation and is exploring the feasibility of conducting additional epidemiologic studies to examine the incidence and clinical course of atrial fibrillation in patients exposed to bisphosphonates.

Formulation Considerations

Patients receiving Zometa® should not receive Reclast® or other bisphosphonates, nor should patients receiving Reclast® be treated concomitantly with Zometa® or other bisphosphonates.

Specific Populations

Pregnancy

Category D. (See Users Guide and see Fetal/Neonatal Morbidity and Mortality under Cautions: Warnings/Precautions.)

Lactation

It is not known whether zoledronic acid is distributed into milk; because of the potential for serious adverse effects in nursing infants from zoledronic acid, a decision should be made whether to discontinue nursing or the drug, taking into account the importance of the drug to the woman. It is also important to consider that zoledronic acid is retained by bone for prolonged periods and may be released over weeks to years, possibly affecting nursing infants.

Pediatric Use

Zoledronic acid is not indicated for use in children.

Geriatric Use

No overall differences in safety and efficacy of zoledronic acid relative to younger adults; however, the incidence of acute-phase inflammatory reactions was less in geriatric patients with osteoporosis or Paget disease of bone than in younger adults. Because of the greater frequency of impaired renal function in geriatric patients, the manufacturer states that renal function should be monitored with particular care in this age group.

Renal Impairment

In clinical studies of zoledronic acid in patients with multiple myeloma or bone metastases associated with solid tumors or in those with hypercalcemia associated with malignancy, individuals with severe renal impairment (serum creatinine concentrations exceeding 3 or 4.5 mg/dL, respectively) were excluded. Limited data are available in patients with a baseline serum creatinine concentration exceeding 2 mg/dL or with a creatinine clearance of less than 30 mL/minute. The drug should be used in patients with hypercalcemia of malignancy and severe renal impairment only after consideration of other treatment options and only when the potential benefit from the drug outweighs the possible risk of worsening renal function. Zoledronic acid is not recommended in patients with bone metastases associated with solid tumors or multiple myeloma and severe renal impairment. Use of zoledronic acid for prevention or treatment of osteoporosis or for treatment of Paget disease of bone is contraindicated in patients who have severe renal impairment (creatinine clearance of less than 35 mL/minute); the drug should be used with caution in such patients with chronic renal impairment.

Common Adverse Effects

Hypercalcemia of Malignancy

Fever, nausea, constipation, anemia, dyspnea, diarrhea, progression of cancer, abdominal pain, insomnia, vomiting, urinary tract infection, anxiety, hypophosphatemia, confusion, agitation, moniliasis, hypokalemia, skeletal pain, cough, hypotension, hypomagnesemia.

Bone Metastases of Solid Tumors and Osteolytic Lesions of Multiple Myeloma

Nausea, fatigue, anemia, vomiting, fever, constipation, dyspnea, diarrhea, myalgia, cough, edema of the lower extremities, arthralgia, headache, dizziness, weight loss, paresthesia, back pain, depression, abdominal pain, dehydration, limb pain, decreased appetite, neutropenia, urinary tract infection, hypoesthesia, anxiety, alopecia, dermatitis, rigors, thrombocytopenia, dyspepsia, upper respiratory tract infection.

Osteoporosis Treatment in Postmenopausal Women

Arthralgia, fever, headache, hypertension, myalgia, extremity pain, flu-like illness, dizziness, shoulder pain, diarrhea, bone pain, fatigue, chills, asthenia.

Osteoporosis Prevention in Postmenopausal Women

Headache, dizziness, hypoesthesia, hypertension, nausea, diarrhea, vomiting, dyspepsia, abdominal pain, constipation, arthralgia, myalgia, back pain, extremity pain, muscle spasms, musculoskeletal pain, bone pain, neck pain, generalized pain, pyrexia, chills fatigue, asthenia, peripheral edema, non-cardiac chest pain.

Osteoporosis Treatment in Men

Myalgia, fatigue, headache, musculoskeletal pain, pain (unspecified), chills, flu-like illness, abdominal pain, malaise, dyspnea.

Glucocorticoid-induced Osteoporosis

Adverse effects are generally similar to those reported in the postmenopausal osteoporosis population. Common adverse effects that were either not observed in the postmenopausal osteoporosis treatment trial or reported more frequently in the corticosteroid-induced osteoporosis trial included abdominal pain, musculoskeletal pain, back pain, bone pain, extremity pain, nausea, and dyspepsia.

Paget Disease of Bone

Headache, nausea, dizziness, arthralgia, bone pain, influenza/flu-like illness, fever, fatigue, rigors, myalgia, diarrhea, constipation, lethargy, dypsnea, dyspepsia, pain.

DRUG INTERACTIONS

Drugs Eliminated by Renal Excretion

When zoledronic acid is used concomitantly with drugs eliminated renally (e.g., digoxin), increased exposure of the concomitantly administered drug is possible.

Loop Diuretics

Pharmacologic interaction (increased risk of hypocalcemia) is possible when zoledronic acid is used with loop diuretics. Caution is advised.

Aminoglycosides

Pharmacologic interaction (additive effect in lowering serum calcium concentrations for prolonged periods) is possible when zoledronic acid is used with aminoglycosides. Caution is advised.

Nephrotoxic Agents

Pharmacologic interaction (increased risk of renal dysfunction) is possible when zoledronic acid is used with nephrotoxic agents. The drugs should be used concomitantly with caution.

Thalidomide

No substantial changes in pharmacokinetics of zoledronic acid or in creatinine clearance were observed with concomitant administration of thalidomide. Dosage adjustments are not necessary.

DESCRIPTION

Zoledronic acid, a synthetic imidazole bisphosphonate analog of pyrophosphate, is an inhibitor of osteoclast-mediated bone resorption. Zoledronic acid is structurally and pharmacologically related to alendronate, risedronate, and pamidronate.

Zoledronic acid inhibits increased osteoclastic activity and skeletal calcium release induced by tumors. In patients with hypercalcemia of malignancy, zoledronic acid decreases serum calcium and phosphorus and increases urinary calcium and phosphorus excretion.

Zoledronic acid is eliminated in urine as unchanged drug. In patients with cancer and bone metastases, an average of 39% of an IV dose of zoledronic acid was excreted in urine within 24 hours. Nonrenal clearance is believed to result from uptake of the drug by bone; subsequently, the drug is released systemically via bone turnover. Results of in vitro studies indicate that zoledronic acid does not inhibit the cytochrome P-450 (CYP) enzyme system.

ADVICE TO PATIENTS

Importance of calcium and vitamin D supplementation for maintenance of serum calcium concentrations in patients with Paget's disease of bone, multiple myeloma and bone metastasis of solid tumors, or osteoporosis. Importance of contacting a clinician promptly if symptoms of hypocalcemia (e.g., numbness or tingling feeling [especially in or around the mouth], muscle spasms) occur.

Importance of informing a clinician if severe bone pain, joint pain, muscular pain, or jaw disease develops.

Importance of informing a clinician if new thigh or groin pain develops.

Importance of informing patients that zoledronic acid should not be used for prevention or treatment of osteoporosis or for treatment of Paget's disease of bone in patients with severe renal impairment. Patients should be advised of the importance of monitoring kidney function during therapy.

Importance of informing clinicians of existing or contemplated concomitant therapy, including prescription and OTC drugs (e.g., diuretics, nonsteroidal anti-inflammatory agents, antibiotics), as well as any concomitant conditions (e.g., kidney disease, aspirin sensitivity). Importance of women informing clinicians if they are or plan to become pregnant or plan to breast-feed. Advise women of childbearing potential to avoid pregnancy. Apprise pregnant patients of potential fetal hazard. Importance of advising patients of other important precautionary information. (See Cautions.)

PREPARATIONS

Excipients in commercially available drug preparations may have clinically important effects in some individuals; consult specific product labeling for details.

Zoledronic Acid

Parenteral		
For injection, concentrate, for IV infusion	0.8 mg (of anhydrous zoledronic acid) per mL*	Zoledronic Acid Injection Zometa®, Novartis
For injection, for IV infusion	0.05 mg (of anhydrous zoledronic acid) per mL*	Zoledronic Acid Injection Reclast®, Novartis
	0.04 mg (of anhydrous zoledronic acid) per mL*	Zoledronic Acid Injection Zometa®, Novartis

* available from one or more manufacturer, distributor, and/or repackager by generic (nonproprietary) name

† Use is not currently included in the labeling approved by the US Food and Drug Administration.

Selected Revisions November 25, 2019, © Copyright, July 1, 2002, American Society of Health-System Pharmacists, Inc.

Index

Boldface type is used for the title of the monograph and the proprietary (trade, brand) names. In some index entries, "tall man" (mixed case) lettering is used for drug names or synonyms (e.g., diazePAM) when recommended by FDA or the Institute for Safe Medication Practices (ISMP).

The monograph title listed in boldface type following *"see"* usually is the corresponding nonproprietary (generic) name for the index entry (e.g., **Abelcet®**, *see* **Amphotericin B**); however, the monograph title may indicate that information about a drug can be found in a monograph about a group of drugs (e.g., **Colace®**, *see* **Stool Softeners** [Colace® is a proprietary name for

docusate sodium, which is described in the monograph titled Stool Softeners]).

Some monographs have been omitted from the print edition of *AHFS Drug Information®* because of space limitations. Copies of these monographs are available on the "For Subscribers" page of the *AHFS Drug Information®* website, www.ahfsdruginformation.com, in the "Electronic Only Monographs" section. (Username: ahfs2025; Password: ASHP46360.) Associated index entries for these monographs are followed by a symbol ("§") rather than by a page number. This symbol refers the user to a footnote that also provides the above username and password for the 2025 edition.

A

aMILoride 40:28.16 §

Aminess®, *see* Amino Acid Injections §

Amino Acid Injections 40:20 §

Aminocaproic Acid 20:28.16 §

Aminoglycosides General Statement 8:12.02 §

Aminolevulinic Acid 84:18 §

Aminopenicillins General Statement 8:12.16.08 §

Aminophylline DF®, *see* Theophyllines §

Aminosalicylic Acid 8:16.04 §

Aminosyn®, *see* Amino Acid Injections §

Amiodarone 24:04.04.20, 1679

Amisulpride 56:22.12 §

Amitiza®, *see* Lubiprostone, 2715

Amitriptyline 28:16.04.28, 2372

Amivantamab-vmjw 10:00 §

Amjevita®, *see* Adalimumab, 3215

amLODIPine 24:28.08, 1844

Ammonia Spirit, Aromatic 28:20.32 §

Ammonul®, *see* Sodium Phenylacetate and Sodium Benzoate §

Amnesteem®, *see* ISOtretinoin §

Amobarbital 28:24.04 §

Amondys 45®, *see* Casimersen §

Amoply®, *see* Ammonia Spirit, Aromatic §

Amoxapine 28:16.04.28 §

Amoxicillin 8:12.16.08, 174

Amoxicillin and Clavulanate 8:12.16.08, 178

Amoxil®, *see* Amoxicillin, 174

Amphetamine 28:20.04 §

Amphetamines General Statement 28:20.04 §

Amphojel®, *see* Antacids, 2688

Amphotericin B 8:14.28, 460

Ampicillin 8:12.16.08, 187

Ampicillin and Sulbactam 8:12.16.08, 190

Ampyra®, *see* Dalfampridine §

Amrix®, *see* Cyclobenzaprine, 1454

Amtagvi®, *see* Lifileucel §

Amvuttra®, *see* Vutrisiran §

Amyl Nitrite 24:08.08 §

Amytal® *see* Amobarbital §

Amzeeq®, *see* Minocycline §

Anacaine®, *see* Benzocaine §

Anacaulase-bcdb 84:28 §

Anacin®, *see* Aspirin, 2073

Anafranil®, *see* clomiPRAMINE §

Anagrelide 20:12.14 §

Anakinra 90:24.20.92, 3287

Analpram-HC®, *see* Hydrocortisone §

Anaprox®, *see* Naproxen, 2028

Anascorp®, *see* Centruroides (Scorpion) Immune F(ab')2 (Equine) §

Anaspaz®, *see* Hyoscyamine §

Anastrozole 68:16.08 §

Anavip®, *see* Crotalidae Immune F(ab')2 (Equine) §

Anbesol®, *see* Benzocaine §

Ancobon®, *see* Flucytosine, 481

Andexxa®, *see* Factor Xa (Recombinant), Inactivated-zhzo §

Androderm®, *see* Testosterone, 2861

AndroGel®, *see* Testosterone, 2861

Android®, *see* methylTESTOSTERone, 2857

Anectine®, *see* Succinylcholine, 1472

Angeliq®, *see* Estradiol, 2909

Angiotensin II Acetate 68:44, 3150

Anidulafungin 8:14.16, 442

Anifrolumab-fnia 90:24.28 §

Anjeso®, *see* Meloxicam, 2021

Anktiva®, *see* Nogapendekin Alfa Inbakicept-pmln §

Anoro®, *see* Umeclidinium and Vilanterol §

Ansuvimab-zykl 8:18.24 §

Antabuse®, *see* Disulfiram §

Antacid Double Strength®, *see* Antacids, 2688

Antacids 56:04, 2688

Antagon®, *see* Ganirelix §

Antara®, *see* Fenofibrate §

Anthim®, *see* Obiltoxaximab §

Anthraquinone Laxatives 56:12 §

Anthrasil®, *see* Anthrax Immune Globulin IV (Human) §

Anthrax Immune Globulin IV (Human) 80:04 §

Anthrax Vaccine Adsorbed 80:12 §

Antibiotic Otic®, *see* Hydrocortisone §

Anticonvulsants General Statement 28:12 §

Antidote Therapeutics 91:00, 3394

Antihemophilic Factor (Human) 20:28.16 §

Antihemophilic Factor (Recombinant) 20:28.16 §

Antihemophilic Factor (Recombinant), Fc Fusion Protein 20:28.16 §

Antihemophilic Factor (Recombinant), Fc-VWF-XTEN Fusion Protein-ehtl 20:28.16 §

Antihemophilic Factor (Recombinant), Glycopegylated-exei 20:28.16 §

Antihemophilic Factor (Recombinant), PEGylated 20:28.16 §

Antihemophilic Factor (Recombinant), PEGylated-aucl 20:28.16 §

Antihemophilic Factor (Recombinant), Porcine Sequence 20:28.16 §

Antihistamine Drugs 4:00, 1

Antihistamines General Statement 4:00, 2

Anti-infective Agents 8:00, 20

Anti-inhibitor Coagulant Complex 20:28.16 §

Antimuscarinics/Antispasmodics General Statement 12:08.08 §

Antineoplastic Agents 10:00, 773

Antithrombin alfa 20:12.04.20 §

Antithrombin III (Human) 20:12.04.20 §

Antithymocyte Globulin (Equine) 90:28.04.92 §

Antithymocyte Globulin (Rabbit) 90:28.04.92 §

Antitoxins, Immune Globulins, Toxoids, and Vaccines 80:00 §

Antituberculosis Agents General Statement 8:16.04 §

Antivenin (Latrodectus mactans) (Equine) 80:04 §

Antivenin (Micrurus fulvius) (Equine) 80:04 §

Antivert®, *see* Meclizine, 2725

Antizol®, *see* Fomepizole §

Anucort-HC®, *see* Hydrocortisone §

Anu-Med®, *see* Hydrocortisone §

Anusert®, *see* Hydrocortisone §

Anusol-HC®, *see* Hydrocortisone §

Anx®, *see* hydrOXYzine, 2548

Anzemet®, *see* Dolasetron §

Apalutamide 10:00, 799

Aphexda®, *see* Motixafortide §

Apidra®, *see* Insulin Glulisine §

Apixaban 20:12.04.14, 1546

Aplenzin®, *see* Bupropion, 2374

Aplisol®, *see* Tuberculin §

Apokyn®, *see* Apomorphine §

Apomorphine 28:36.20.08 §

Apraclonidine 52:40.04 §

Apremilast 90:24.24.92, 3336

Aprepitant, Fosaprepitant 56:22.32, 2733

Apretude®, *see* Cabotegravir Sodium, 494

Apri®, *see* Estrogen-Progestin Combinations, 2874

Azilsartan 24:32.08 §

Azithromycin 8:12.12.08 § *and* 52:04.04 §

Azmacort®, *see* Triamcinolone, 2854

Azo-Dine®, *see* Phenazopyridine §

Azo-Gesic®, *see* Phenazopyridine §

Azo-Natural®, *see* Phenazopyridine §

Azopt®, *see* Brinzolamide §

Azor®, *see* amLODIPine, 1844 *and see* Olmesartan, 1922

Azo-Standard®, *see* Phenazopyridine §

Azstarys®, *see* Dexmethylphenidate §

Aztreonam 8:12.07.16, 128

Azulfidine®, *see* sulfaSALAzine §

B

BabyBIG®, *see* Botulism Immune Globulin IV §

Bacid®, *see* Lactobacillus Acidophilus §

Bacitracin 52:04.04 § *and* 84:04.04 §

Bacitraycin Plus®, *see* Bacitracin §

Baclofen 12:20.12, 1461

Bactrim®, *see* Co-trimoxazole, 296

Bactroban®, *see* Mupirocin §

Bafiertam®, *see* Monomethyl Fumarate §

BAL in Oil®, *see* Dimercaprol §

Balnetar®, *see* Coal Tar Preparations §

Baloxavir 8:18.30, 632

Balsalazide 56:36 §

Balversa®, *see* Erdafitinib, 1024

Bamlanivimab and Etesevimab 8:18.24 §

Banzel®, *see* Rufinamide §

Baraclude®, *see* Entecavir, 663

Barbiturates General Statement 28:24.04 §

Barhemsys®, *see* Amisulpride §

Baricitinib 90:24.12.92, 3180

Baridium®, *see* Phenazopyridine §

Basaglar®, *see* Insulin Glargine, 3033

Basaljel®, *see* Antacids, 2688

Basiliximab 90:28.16.92 §

Bavencio®, *see* Avelumab §

Baxdela®, *see* Delafloxacin Meglumine, 250

Bayer®, *see* Aspirin, 2073 *and see* diphenhydrAMINE Hydrochloride, 12

Bazedoxifene 68:16.12 §

BC®, *see* Aspirin, 2073 *and see* Salicylamide §

BCG Vaccine 80:12 §

B-D Glucose®, *see* Dextrose §

Bebtelovimab 8:18.24 §

Bebulin®, *see* Factor IX (Human) §

Becaplermin 84:16 §

Beclomethasone 52:08.08 § *and* 68:04 §

Beconase AQ®, *see* Beclomethasone §

Bedaquiline Fumarate 8:16.04 §

Belatacept 90:28.12.92 §

Belbuca®, *see* Buprenorphine, 2172

Beleodaq®, *see* Belinostat §

Belimumab 90:24.28 §

Belinostat 10:00 §

Belrapzo®, *see* Bendamustine §

Belsomra®, *see* Suvorexant §

Belumosudil 92:92 §

Belzutifan 10:00 §

Bempedoic Acid 24:06.07 §

Benadryl®, *see* diphenhydrAMINE, 12

Benazepril 24:32.04, 1864

Bendamustine 10:00 §

Bendeka®, *see* Bendamustine §

BeneFIX®, *see* Factor IX (Recombinant) §

Benicar®, *see* hydroCHLOROthiazide, 2649 *and see* Olmesartan, 1922

Benlysta®, *see* Belimumab §

Benralizumab 48:10.20 §

Bensulfoid®, *see* Sulfur §

Bentyl®, *see* Dicyclomine §

BenzaClin®, *see* Clindamycin §

Benzalkonium Chloride 84:04.16 §

Benzamycin®, *see* Erythromycin §

Benzedrex®, *see* Propylhexedrine §

Benzgalantamine 12:04 §

Benznidazole 8:30.16.04 §

Benzocaine 52:16 § *and* 84:08 §

Benzocol®, *see* Benzocaine §

Benzodiazepines General Statement 28:24.08, 2497

Benzonatate 48:08 §

Benzphetamine 28:20.04 §

Benztropine 28:36.08 §

Beovu®, *see* Brolucizumab-dbll §

Bepotastine 52:02 §

Bepreve®, *see* Bepotastine §

Beqvez®, *see* Fidanacogene Elaparvovec-dzkt §

Beractant 48:36 §

Berdazimer 84:04.06 §

Beremagene Geperpavec-svdt 26:12 §

Berinert®, *see* C1-Esterase Inhibitor (Human) §

Berotralstat 24:48.08 §

Besifloxacin 52:04.04 §

Besivance®, *see* Besifloxacin §

Besponsa®, *see* Inotuzumab §

Besremi®, *see* Ropeginterferon Alfa-2b-njft §

Beta Carotene 88:04 §

Betagan®, *see* Levobunolol §

Betaine 92:92 §

Betamethasone 68:04 § *and* 84:06.08 §

Betapace®, *see* Sotalol, 1837

Betasept®, *see* Chlorhexidine §

Betaseron®, *see* Interferon Beta §

Betatrex®, *see* Betamethasone §

Beta-Val®, *see* Betamethasone §

Betaxolol 24:20 § *and* 52:40.08 §

Bethanechol Chloride 12:04 §

Betibeglogene Autotemcel 26:12 §

Betimol®, *see* Timolol §

Betoptic S®, *see* Betaxolol §

Bevacizumab 10:00, 817

Bevespi®, *see* Formoterol Fumarate, 1405 *and see* Glycopyrrolate §

Bexagliflozin 68:20.18 §

Bexarotene 10:00 § *and* 84:18 §

Bexsero®, *see* Meningococcal Group B Vaccine §

Beyaz®, *see* Estrogen-Progestin Combinations, 2874

Beyfortus®, *see* Nirsevimab-alip §

Bezlotoxumab 80:04 §

Biaxin®, *see* Clarithromycin §

Bicalutamide 10:00, 825

Bicillin®, *see* Penicillin G Benzathine, 147 *and see* Penicillin G Procaine, 163

Bicitra®, *see* Citrates, 2581

BiCNU®, *see* Carmustine §

BiCOZENE®, *see* Benzocaine §

Bictegravir, Emtricitabine, and Tenofovir Alafenamide Fumarate 8:18.08.12, 487

BiDil®, *see* hydrALAZINE § *and see* Isosorbide, 1755

Biktarvy®, *see* Bictegravir Sodium, Emtricitabine, and Tenofovir Alafenamide Fumarate, 487

Biltricide®, *see* Praziquantel §

Bimatoprost 52:40.28 §

Bimekizumab-bkzx 84:06.28 §

Bimzelx®, *see* Bimekizumab-bkzx §

Binimetinib 10:00, 828

Binosto®, *see* Alendronate §

Biopatch®, *see* Chlorhexidine §

Biothrax®, *see* Anthrax Vaccine Adsorbed §

Birch Triterpenes 84:92 §

Candida Albicans Skin Test Antigen 36:32 §

Candin®, *see* Candida Albicans Skin Test Antigen §

Cangrelor 20:12.18 §

Cannabidiol 28:12.92 §

Cantharidin 84:04.06 §

Capecitabine 10:00, 879

Capex®, *see* Fluocinolone Acetonide §

Capital®, *see* Acetaminophen, 2199

Capivasertib 10:00 §

Caplacizumab-yhdp 20:12.10 §

Caplyta®, *see* Lumateperone §

Capmatinib Hydrochloride 10:00 §

Caprelsa®, *see* Vandetanib, 1322

Capsaicin 84:08 §

Captopril 24:32.04, 1869

Carac®, *see* Fluorouracil §

Carafate®, *see* Sucralfate §

Carbachol 52:40.20 §

Carbaglu®, *see* Carglumic Acid §

carBAMazepine 28:12.92 §

Carbamide Peroxide 52:04.24 §

Carbastat®, *see* Carbachol §

Carbatrol®, *see* carBAMazepine §

Carbidopa, *see* Levodopa/Carbidopa 28:36.16, 2567

Carbinoxamine Maleate 4:04 §

Carbocaine®, *see* Mepivacaine §

Carbol-Fuchsin Topical Solution 36:32 §

Carbonic Anhydrase Inhibitors General Statement 52:40.12 §

CARBOplatin 10:00, 887

Carboprost 76:00 §

Carboptic®, *see* Carbachol §

Cardene®, *see* niCARdipine §

Cardio-Green®, CG®, *see* Indocyanine Green §

Cardiovascular Drugs 24:00, 1642

Cardizem®, *see* dilTIAZem, 1712

Cardura®, *see* Doxazosin, 1771

Carfilzomib 10:00 §

Carglumic Acid 40:10 §

Carimune®, *see* Immune Globulin §

Cariprazine 28:16.08.04, 2407

Carisoprodol 12:20.04 §

Carmol®, *see* Hydrocortisone § *and see* Urea §

Carmustine 10:00 §

Carnexiv®, *see* carBAMazepine §

Carnitor®, *see* levOCARNitine §

CaroSpir®, *see* Spironolactone, 1942

Carter's Little Pills®, *see* Bisacodyl §

Cartia®, *see* dilTIAZem, 1712

Carvedilol 24:20, 1795

Carvykti®, *see* Ciltacabtagene Autoleucel §

Casgevy®, *see* Exagamglogene Autotemcel §

Casimersen 92:18 §

Casirivimab and Imdevimab 8:18.24 §

Casodex®, *see* Bicalutamide, 825

Caspofungin Acetate 8:14.16, 447

Casporyn®, *see* Neomycin § *and see* Polymyxin B §

Castor Oil 56:12 §

Catapres®, *see* cloNIDine §

Cathartics and Laxatives General Statement 56:12, 2702

Cathflo®, Activase®, *see* Alteplase, 1632

Caverject®, *see* Alprostadil §

Cayston®, *see* Aztreonam, 128

CeeNU®, *see* Lomustine §

Cefaclor 8:12.06.08 §

Cefadroxil 8:12.06.04, 22

ceFAZolin Sodium 8:12.06.04, 24

Cefdinir 8:12.06.12 §

Cefepime Hydrochloride 8:12.06.16, 99

Cefepime Hydrochloride and Enmetazobactam 8:12.06.16 §

Cefiderocol 8:12.06.28, 118

Cefixime 8:12.06.12 §

Cefotaxime 8:12.06.12, 44

cefoTEtan 8:12.07.12 §

cefOXitin 8:12.07.12 §

Cefpodoxime 8:12.06.12 §

Cefprozil 8:12.06.08 §

Ceftaroline 8:12.06.20, 107

cefTAZidime 8:12.06.12, 56

cefTAZidime and Avibactam 8:12.06.12, 68

Ceftin®, *see* Cefuroxime, 32

Ceftolozane and Tazobactam 8:12.06.20, 112

cefTRIAXone 8:12.06.12, 74

Cefuroxime 8:12.06.08, 32

Cefzil®, *see* Cefprozil §

CeleBREX®, *see* Celecoxib, 2040

Celecoxib 28:08.04.08, 2040

Celestone®, *see* Betamethasone §

CeleXA®, *see* Citalopram, 2302

CellCept®, *see* Mycophenolate, 3355

Cellular and Gene Therapy 26:00, §

Celontin®, *see* Methsuximide §

Cemiplimab-rwlc 10:00, 898

Cenegermin-bkbj 52:08 §

Cenestin®, *see* Estrogens, Conjugated, 2915

Cenobamate 28:12.24 §

Centany®, *see* Mupirocin §

Central Nervous System Agents 28:00, 1954

Centruroides (Scorpion) Immune F(ab')2 (Equine) 80:04 §

Ceo-Two®, *see* Saline Laxatives §

Cepacol®, *see* Benzocaine §

Cephalexin 8:12.06.04, 29

Cephalosporins General Statement 8:12.06 §

Ceprotin®, *see* Protein C (Human) §

Cerdelga®, *see* Eliglustat §

Cerebyx®, *see* Fosphenytoin §

Cerezyme®, *see* Imiglucerase §

Cerliponase Alfa 44:00 §

Certain Dri®, *see* Aluminum Chloride Hexahydrate §

Certolizumab Pegol 90:24.16.92, 3232

Cerubidine®, *see* DAUNOrubicin §

Cervidil®, *see* Dinoprostone §

Cesamet®, *see* Nabilone §

Cetacaine®, *see* Benzocaine §

Cetacort®, *see* Hydrocortisone §

Cetirizine 4:08 § *and* 52:02 §

Cetraxal®, *see* Ciprofloxacin §

Cetrorelix 68:18.04 §

Cetrotide®, *see* Cetrorelix §

Cetuximab 10:00, 908

Cevimeline Hydrochloride 12:04 §

Chantix®, *see* Varenicline §

CharcoAid®, *see* Charcoal, Activated §

Charcoal, Activated 56:04 §

CharcoCaps®, *see* Charcoal, Activated §

Chemet®, *see* Succimer §

Chenodal®, *see* Chenodiol §

Chenodiol 56:14 §

Cheracol D®, *see* Dextromethorphan, 2659

Cheratussin®, *see* Codeine, 2657 *and see* guaiFENesin, 2684

Chiggerex®, *see* Benzocaine §

Chiggertox®, *see* Benzocaine §

Chikungunya Vaccine Live 80:12 §

Chlorambucil 10:00 §

Chloramphenicol 8:12.08, 137

Chloraseptic®, *see* Benzocaine §

chlordiazePOXIDE 28:24.08 §

Chlorhexidine 52:04.24 § *and* 84:04.16 §

Chloroprocaine 52:16 § *and* 72:00 §

Chloroquine 8:30.08 §

Contrave®, *see* Naltrexone and Bupropion §

Conzip®, *see* traMADol, 2163

Copanlisib 10:00 §

Copaxone®, *see* Glatiramer §

Cope®, *see* Aspirin, 2073

Copegus®, *see* Ribavirin §

Copiktra®, *see* Duvelisib §

Cordarone®, *see* Amiodarone, 1679

Cordran®, *see* Flurandrenolide §

Coreg®, *see* Carvedilol, 1795

Corgard®, *see* Nadolol §

Coricidin®, *see* Chlorpheniramine § *and see* Dextromethorphan, 2659

Corifact®, *see* Factor XIII (Human) §

Corlanor®, *see* Ivabradine, 1743

Corlopam®, *see* Fenoldopam §

Cormax®, *see* Clobetasol §

Correctol®, *see* Anthraquinone Laxatives § *and see* Bisacodyl § *and see* Stool Softeners §

CortaGel®, *see* Hydrocortisone §

Cortaid®, *see* Hydrocortisone §

Cortef®, *see* Hydrocortisone §

Corticaine®, *see* Hydrocortisone §

Corticosteroids General Statement 68:04, 2814

Corticotropin 68:28 §

Cortifoam®, *see* Hydrocortisone §

Cortisone Acetate 68:04 §

Cortisporin®, *see* Bacitracin § *and see* Hydrocortisone § *and see* Neomycin § *and see* Polymyxin B §

Cortizone®, *see* Hydrocortisone §

Cortrosyn®, *see* Cosyntropin §

Corvert®, *see* Ibutilide, 1706

Corzide®, *see* Nadolol §

Cosela®, *see* Trilaciclib §

Cosentyx®, *see* Secukinumab, 3304

Cosmegen®, *see* DACTINomycin §

Cosopt®, *see* Dorzolamide § *and see* Timolol §

Cosyntropin 36:04 §

Cotellic®, *see* Cobimetinib Fumarate, 935

Cotempla XR-ODT®, *see* Methylphenidate Hydrochloride §

Co-trimoxazole 8:12.20, 296

Covaryx®, *see* Estropipate §

COVID-19 Vaccine, Adjuvanted (Novavax) 80:12 §

COVID-19 Vaccine, mRNA (Moderna) 80:12 §

COVID-19 Vaccine, mRNA (Pfizer-BioNTech) 80:12 §

Cozaar®, *see* Losartan, 1917

Creon®, *see* Pancrelipase §

Cresemba®, *see* Isavuconazonium Sulfate, 412

Crestor®, *see* Rosuvastatin §

Crinone®, *see* Progesterone, 3128

Crisaborole 84:06.12 §

Crizanlizumab-tmca 20:92 §

Crizotinib 10:00, 941

CroFab®, *see* Crotalidae Polyvalent Immune Fab (Ovine) §

Crofelemer 56:08 §

Crolom®, *see* Cromolyn §

Cromolyn 48:10.32 § *and* 52:02 §

Crotalidae Immune F(ab´)2 (Equine) 80:04 §

Crotalidae Polyvalent Immune Fab (Ovine) 80:04 §

Crotamiton 84:04.12 §

Crovalimab-akkz 90:20 §

Cryselle®, *see* Estrogen-Progestin Combinations, 2874

Crysvita®, *see* Burosumab-twza §

Cubicin®, *see* Daptomycin, 320

Cuprimine®, *see* penicillAMINE §

Curad®, *see* Salicylic Acid §

Curosurf®, *see* Poractant Alfa §

Cutaquig®, *see* Immune Globulin §

Cutar®, *see* Coal Tar Preparations §

Cuvitru®, *see* Immune Globulin §

Cuvposa®, *see* Glycopyrrolate §

Cuvrior®, *see* Trientine §

Cyanokit®, *see* Vitamin B12 §

Cyclessa®, *see* Estrogen-Progestin Combinations, 2874

Cyclobenzaprine 12:20.04, 1454

Cyclocort®, *see* Amcinonide §

Cyclogyl®, *see* Cyclopentolate §

Cyclomydril®, *see* Cyclopentolate § *and see* Phenylephrine §

Cyclopentolate 52:24 §

Cyclophosphamide 10:00, 949

cycloSERINE 8:16.04 §

Cycloset®, *see* Bromocriptine §

cycloSPORINE 52:08 § *and* 90:28.28.92, 3365

Cyklokapron®, *see* Tranexamic Acid §

Cylate®, *see* Cyclopentolate §

Cyltezo®, *see* Adalimumab, 3215

Cymbalta®, *see* DULoxetine, 2293

Cyproheptadine 4:04 §

Cyramza®, *see* Ramucirumab, 1246

Cystadane®, *see* Betaine §

Cystagon®, *see* Cysteamine §

Cystaran®, *see* Cysteamine §

Cysteamine 52:44 § *and* 92:92 §

Cystospaz®, *see* Hyoscyamine §

Cytarabine 10:00 §

Cytogam®, *see* Cytomegalovirus Immune Globulin IV §

Cytomegalovirus Immune Globulin IV 80:04 §

Cytomel®, *see* Liothyronine §

Cytosar-U®, *see* Cytarabine §

Cytotec®, *see* Misoprostol, 2754

Cytovene®, *see* Ganciclovir, 674

Cytoxan®, *see* Cyclophosphamide, 949

D

D.H.E. 45®, *see* Dihydroergotamine §

Dabigatran 20:12.04.12, 1536

Dabrafenib 10:00, 956

Dacarbazine 10:00 §

Dacogen®, *see* Decitabine §

Dacomitinib 10:00 §

DACTINomycin 10:00 §

Dalbavancin 8:12.28.16, 325

Dalfampridine 92:56 §

Daliresp®, *see* Roflumilast §

Dalteparin 20:12.04.16 §

Dalvance®, *see* Dalbavancin, 325

Danazol 68:08 §

Danicopan 90:20 §

Dantrium®, *see* Dantrolene §

Dantrolene 12:20.08 §

Danyelza®, *see* Naxitamab-gqgk §

Dapagliflozin 68:20.18, 3046

Daprodustat 20:16 §

Dapsone 8:16.08 § *and* 84:04.04 §

Daptacel®, *see* Diphtheria and Tetanus Toxoids and Acellular Pertussis Vaccine Adsorbed/Tetanus Toxoid, Reduced Diphtheria Toxoid and Acellular Pertussis Vaccine Adsorbed §

Daptomycin 8:12.28.12, 320

Daranide®, *see* Dichlorphenamide §

Daraprim®, *see* Pyrimethamine §

Daratumumab 10:00 §

Darbepoetin Alfa 20:16 §

Daridorexant 28:24.40 §

Darifenacin 86:12.04 §

F

G

H

Hyftor®, *see* Sirolimus §

Hyoscyamine 12:08.08 §

Hyosyne®, *see* Hyoscyamine §

Hypercare®, *see* Aluminum Chloride Hexahydrate §

HyperHEP B®, *see* Hepatitis B Immune Globulin §

Hyperosmotic Laxatives 56:12 §

HyperRAB®, *see* Rabies Immune Globulin §

HyperRHO®, *see* Rho(D) Immune Globulin §

HyperTET®, *see* Tetanus Immune Globulin §

HypoKit®, *see* Glucagon, 3090

Hyqvia®, *see* Immune Globulin §

Hyrimoz®, *see* Adalimumab, 3215

Hysingla®, *see* HYDROcodone, 2118

Hytinic®, *see* Iron Preparations, Oral, 1498

Hytone®, *see* Hydrocortisone §

Hyzaar®, *see* hydroCHLOROthiazide, 2649 *and see* Losartan, 1917

I

Ibalizumab-uiyk 8:18.08.04 §

Ibandronate 92:24 §

Ibrance®, *see* Palbociclib, 1203

Ibrexafungerp Citrate 8:14.20 §

Ibritumomab Tiuxetan 10:00 §

Ibrutinib 10:00, 1062

Ibsrela®, *see* Tenapanor §

IBU®, *see* Ibuprofen, 1996

Ibuprofen 28:08.04.04, 1996

Ibutab®, *see* Ibuprofen, 1996

Ibutilide 24:04.04.20, 1706

Icar®, *see* Iron Preparations, Oral, 1498

Icatibant 24:48.04 §

Iclusig®, *see* PONATinib §

Icosapent Ethyl 24:06.12 §

Idacio®, *see* Adalimumab, 3215

Idamycin PFS®, *see* IDArubicin Hydrochloride §

IDArubicin Hydrochloride 10:00 §

idaruCIZUmab 20:28.92 §

Idecabtagene Vicleucel 26:12 §

Idelalisib 10:00 §

Idelvion®, *see* Factor IX (Recombinant), Albumin Fusion Protein §

Idhifa®, *see* Enasidenib Mesylate, 1000

Idursulfase 44:00 §

Ifex®/Mesnex®, *see* Ifosfamide §

Ifosfamide 10:00 §

Igalmi®, *see* Dexmedetomidine §

Iheezo®, *see* Chloroprocaine §

Ilaris®, *see* Canakinumab, 2665

Ilopan®, *see* Pantothenic Acid §

Iloperidone 28:16.08.04 §

Iloprost 24:08.92 § *and* 48:48.28 §

Ilumya®, *see* Tildrakizumab-asmn §

Imatinib Mesylate 10:00, 1070

Imbruvica®, *see* Ibrutinib, 1062

Imcivree®, *see* Setmelanotide §

Imdelltra®, *see* Tarlatamab-dlle §

Imdur®, *see* Isosorbide, 1755

Imetelstat Sodium 10:00 §

Imfinzi®, *see* Durvalumab §

Imiglucerase 44:00 §

Imipenem and Cilastatin Sodium 8:12.07.08 §

Imipenem, Cilastatin Sodium, and Relebactam 8:12.07.08 §

Imipramine 28:16.04.28 §

Imiquimod 84:18 §

Imitrex®, *see* SUMAtriptan §

Imjudo®, *see* Tremelimumab-actl §

Imlygic®, *see* Talimogene Laherparepvec §

Immune Globulin 80:04 §

Immunomodulatory Agents 90:00, 3167

Imodium®, *see* Loperamide, 2698 *and see* Simethicone §

Imogam®, *see* Rabies Immune Globulin §

Imovax®, Rabies, *see* Rabies Vaccine §

Impavido®, *see* Miltefosine §

Implanon®, *see* Progestins, 2893

Imuran®, *see* azaTHIOprine, 3350

Inapsine®, *see* Droperidol §

Inbrija®, *see* Levodopa Carbidopa, 2567

Inclisiran 24:06.92 §

IncobotulinumtoxinA 12:20.20.24 §

Increlex®, *see* Mecasermin §

Incruse®, Ellipta®, *see* Umeclidinium §

Inderal®, *see* Propranolol, 1826

Indigotindisulfonate 36:40 §

Indocin®, *see* Indomethacin §

Indocyanine Green 36:18 § *and* 36:44 §

Indomethacin 28:08.04.04 §

Inebilizumab-cdon 90:12.04 §

Infanrix®, *see* Diphtheria and Tetanus Toxoids and Acellular Pertussis Vaccine Adsorbed/Tetanus Toxoid, Reduced Diphtheria Toxoid and Acellular Pertussis Vaccine Adsorbed §

INFeD®, *see* Iron Dextran, 1494

Infigratinib Phosphate 10:00 §

Inflamase®, *see* prednisoLONE §

Inflectra®, *see* inFLIXimab, 3268

inFLIXimab 90:24.16.92, 3268

Influenza Vaccine Live Intranasal (Seasonal) 80:12 §

Influenza Vaccine Recombinant (Seasonal) 80:12 §

Influenza Virus Vaccine Inactivated (Seasonal) 80:12 §

Infumorph®, *see* Morphine, 2142

Ingrezza®, *see* Valbenazine §

Injectafer®, *see* Ferric Carboxymaltose §

Inlyta®, *see* Axitinib §

Inmazeb®, *see* Atoltivimab, Maftivimab, and Odesivimab-ebgn §

Innopran®, *see* Propranolol, 1826

INOmax®, *see* Nitric Oxide §

Inotersen Sodium 92:18 §

Inotuzumab Ozogamicin 10:00 §

Inpefa®, *see* Sotagliflozin §

Inpersol®, *see* Peritoneal Dialysis Solutions §

Inqovi®, *see* Decitabine and Cedazuridine §

Inrebic®, *see* Fedratinib Hydrochloride §

Inspra®, *see* Eplerenone §

Insta-Char®, *see* Charcoal, Activated §

Insta-Glucose®, *see* Dextrose §

Insulin Aspart 68:20.08.04, 3013

Insulin Degludec 68:20.08.16, 3027

Insulin Glargine 68:20.08.16, 3033

Insulin Glulisine 68:20.08.04 §

Insulin Human 68:20.08.08, 3023

Insulin Lispro 68:20.08.04, 3017

Insulins General Statement 68:20.08, 3000

Intal®, *see* Cromolyn §

Integrilin®, *see* Eptifibatide, 1606

Intelence®, *see* Etravirine §

Interferon Alfa 8:18.20 § *and* 10:00 §

Interferon Beta 90:04.12 §

Interferon Gamma 92:20 §

Intestinex®, *see* Lactobacillus Acidophilus §

Intralipid®, *see* Fat Emulsions §

Intrarosa®, *see* Prasterone §

Intron®, *see* Interferon Alfa § *and see* Interferon Alfa §

INVanz®, *see* Ertapenem Sodium §

Invega®, *see* Paliperidone, 2466

Invokamet®, *see* Canagliflozin, 3038 *and see* metFORMIN, 2918

Invokana®, *see* Canagliflozin, 3038

Iobenguane I 131 10:00 §

Iodine 84:04.16 §

Iodoquinol 8:30.04 § *and* 84:04.16 §

Ionamin®, *see* Phentermine §

Ionil T®, *see* Coal Tar Preparations §

Iopidine®, *see* Apraclonidine §

Iosat®, *see* Potassium Iodide, 3141

Ipilimumab 10:00, 1079

IPOL®, *see* Poliovirus Vaccine Inactivated §

Ipratropium 12:08.08, 1372 *and* 52:92 §

Iptacopan 90:20 §

Iqirvo®, *see* Elafibranor §

Irbesartan 24:32.08, 1912

Ircon®, *see* Iron Preparations, Oral, 1498

Iressa®, *see* Gefitinib §

Irinotecan Hydrochloride 10:00, 1083

Iris®, *see* Fluorides §

Iron Dextran 20:04.04, 1494

Iron Preparations, Oral 20:04.04, 1498

Iron Sucrose 20:04.04, 1507

Irrigating Solutions 40:36 §

Isatuximab-irfc 10:00 §

Isavuconazonium 8:14.08, 412

Isentress®, *see* Raltegravir Potassium, 553

Ismo®, *see* Isosorbide, 1755

Isoniazid 8:16.04 §

Isoproterenol Hydrochloride 12:12.08.04 §

Isopto®, *see* Atropine § *and see* Carbachol § *and see* Homatropine § *and see* Pilocarpine § *and see* Scopolamine §

Isordil®, *see* Isosorbide, 1755

Isosorbide 24:08.08, 1755

ISOtretinoin 84:28 §

Isradipine 24:28.08 §

Istalol®, *see* Timolol §

Istodax®, *see* romiDEPsin §

Istradefylline 28:36.24 §

Isturisa®, *see* Osilodrostat §

Itch-X®, *see* Pramoxine §

Itraconazole 8:14.08 §

Ivabradine 24:04.08, 1743

Ivacaftor 48:14.12 §

Ivarest®, *see* Benzocaine §

Ivermectin 8:08 § *and* 84:04.12 §

Ivosidenib 10:00 §

Iwilfin®, *see* Eflornithine §

Ixabepilone 10:00 §

Ixazomib Citrate 10:00 §

Ixchiq®, *see* Chikungunya Vaccine Live §

Ixekizumab 90:24.20.92, 3291

Ixempra®, *see* Ixabepilone §

Ixiaro®, *see* Japanese Encephalitis Vaccine §

Izervay®, *see* Avacincaptad Pegol §

J

Jadenu®, *see* Deferasirox §

Jakafi®, *see* Ruxolitinib §

Jalyn®, *see* Dutasteride §

Jantoven®, *see* Warfarin, 1514

Janumet®, *see* metFORMIN, 2918 *and see* SITagliptin, 2952

Januvia®, *see* SITagliptin, 2952

Japanese Encephalitis Vaccine 80:12 §

Jardiance®, *see* Empagliflozin, 3054

Jay-Phyl®, *see* Theophyllines §

Jaypirca®, *see* Pirtobrutinib §

Jemperli®, *see* Dostarlimab-gxly §

Jentadueto®, *see* Linagliptin, 2941 *and see* Metformin , 2918

Jesduvroq®, *see* Daprodustat §

Jetrea®, *see* Ocriplasmin §

Jeuveau®, *see* PrabotulinumtoxinA-xvfs §

Jevtana®, *see* Cabazitaxel, 866

Jivi®, *see* Antihemophilic Factor (Recombinant), PEGylated-aucl §

Joenja®, *see* Leniolisib §

Jornay PM®, *see* Methylphenidate §

Jublia®, *see* Efinaconazole §

Juluca®, *see* Dolutegravir and Rilpivirine, 526

Just for Kids®, *see* Fluorides §

Juxtapid®, *see* Lomitapide §

Jynneos®, *see* Smallpox and Mpox Vaccine Live §

K

K+®, *see* Potassium Supplements, 2602

Kabiven®, *see* Amino Acid Injections §

Kadcyla®, *see* Ado-Trastuzumab Emtansine §

Kalbitor®, *see* Ecallantide §

Kaletra®, *see* Lopinavir and Ritonavir §

Kalydeco®, *see* Ivacaftor §

Kank-A®, *see* Benzocaine §

Kanuma®, *see* Sebelipase Alfa §

Kaochlor®, 10%, *see* Potassium Supplements, 2602

Kaon®, *see* Potassium Supplements, 2602

Kaopectate®, *see* Bismuth Salts, 2694

Kao-Tin®, *see* Bismuth Salts, 2694

Kariva®, *see* Estrogen-Progestin Combinations, 2874

Kay Ciel®, *see* Potassium Supplements, 2602

Kazano®, *see* Alogliptin, 2936 *and see* metFORMIN, 2918

Kcentra®, *see* Prothrombin Complex Concentrate (Human) §

K-Dur®, *see* Potassium Supplements, 2602

Keflex®, *see* Cephalexin, 29

Kenalog®, *see* Triamcinolone, 2854 *and* §

Kengreal®, *see* Cangrelor §

Kepivance®, *see* Palifermin §

Keppra®, *see* levETIRAcetam, 2261

Keralyt®, *see* Salicylic Acid §

Kerasal®, *see* Salicylic Acid §

Kerendia®, *see* Finerenone §

Kerydin®, *see* Tavaborole §

Kesimpta®, *see* Ofatumumab §

Ketalar®, *see* Ketamine, 1960

Ketamine 28:04.08, 1960

Ketoconazole 8:14.08 § *and* 84:04.08.08 §

Ketoprofen 28:08.04.04 §

Ketorolac 28:08.04.04, 2009 *and* 52:08.20 §

Ketotifen 52:02 §

Keveyis®, *see* Dichlorphenamide §

Kevzara®, *see* Sarilumab, 3298

Keygesic-10®, *see* Salicylate Salts §

Keytruda®, *see* Pembrolizumab, 1216

Kidkare®, *see* Dextromethorphan, 2659 *and see* Pseudoephedrine §

Kimmtrak®, *see* Tebentafusp-tebn §

Kineret®, *see* Anakinra, 3287

Kinevac®, *see* Sincalide §

Kinrix®, *see* Diphtheria and Tetanus Toxoids and Acellular Pertussis Vaccine Adsorbed/Tetanus Toxoid, Reduced Diphtheria Toxoid and Acellular Pertussis Vaccine Adsorbed § *and see* Poliovirus Vaccine Inactivated §

Kionex®, *see* Sodium Polystyrene Sulfonate, 2610

Kisqali® Femara® Co-Pack, *see* Letrozole § *and see* Ribociclib Succinate §

Kisunla®, *see* Donanemab-azbt §

Klisyri®, *see* Tirbanibulin §

KlonoPIN®, *see* clonazePAM, 2228

K-Lor®, *see* Potassium Supplements, 2602

Klor-Con®, *see* Potassium Supplements, 2602

Klotrix®, *see* Potassium Supplements, 2602

Kloxxado®, *see* Naloxone, 2211

K-Lyte/CL®, *see* Potassium Supplements, 2602

K-Lyte®, *see* Potassium Supplements, 2602

Koate®, *see* Antihemophilic Factor (Human) §

Kogenate®, *see* Antihemophilic Factor (Recombinant) §

Kolephrin®, *see* Chlorpheniramine §

Kolorz®, *see* Fluorides §

Kombiglyze®, *see* metFORMIN, 2918 *and* *see* sAXagliptin, 2946

Kondremul®, *see* Mineral Oil §

Konsyl®, *see* Bulk-Forming Laxatives §

Korlym®, *see* Mifepristone, 3153

Korsuva®, *see* Difelikefalin Acetate §

Koselugo®, *see* Selumetinib Sulfate §

Krazati®, *see* Adagrasib §

Krintafel®, *see* Tafenoquine Succinate (Krintafel) §

Kristalose®, *see* Lactulose, 2588

Krystexxa®, *see* Pegloticase §

K-Tab®, Filmtab®, *see* Potassium Supplements, 2602

Kudrox®, *see* Antacids, 2688

Kuvan®, *see* Sapropterin Dihydrochloride §

Ku-Zyme®, *see* Pancrelipase §

Kybella®, *see* Deoxycholic Acid §

Kymriah®, *see* Tisagenlecleucel §

Kyo-Dophilus®, *see* Lactobacillus Acidophilus §

Kyprolis®, *see* Carfilzomib §

Kytril®, *see* Granisetron §

L

Labetalol 24:20, 1802

Lacosamide 28:12.24 §

LactiCare®, *see* Hydrocortisone §

Lactinex®, *see* Lactobacillus Acidophilus §

Lactobacillus Acidophilus 56:08 §

Lactulose 40:10, 2588

LaMICtal®, *see* lamoTRIgine, 2250

LamISIL®, *see* Terbinafine §

lamiVUDine 8:18.08.20, 595

lamoTRIgine 28:12.92, 2250

Lampit®, *see* Nifurtimox §

Lamprene®, *see* Clofazimine §

Lamzede®, *see* Velmanase Alfa-tycv §

Lanacort®, *see* Hydrocortisone §

Lanadelumab-flyo 24:48.08 §

Lanoxin®, *see* Digoxin, 1733

Lanreotide 68:29.04 §

Lansoprazole 56:28.36, 2771

Lanthanum 40:18.19 §

Lantidra®, *see* Donislecel-jujn §

Lantus®, *see* Insulin Glargine, 3033

Lapatinib Ditosylate 10:00, 1091

Lariam®, *see* Mefloquine Hydrochloride §

Laronidase 44:00 §

Larotid®, *see* Amoxicillin, 174

Larotrectinib Sulfate 10:00, 1096

Lartruvo®, *see* Olaratumab §

Lasix®, *see* Furosemide, 2621

Lasmiditan 28:32.28 §

Lastacaft®, *see* Alcaftadine §

Latanoprost 52:40.28 §

Latanoprostene Bunod 52:40.28 §

Latisse®, *see* Bimatoprost §

Latuda®, *see* Lurasidone, 2432

Lazcluze®, *see* Lazertinib §

LazerSporin-C®, *see* Hydrocortisone §

Lazertinib Mesylate 10:00 §

Lebrikizumab-lbkz 84:06.28 §

Lecanemab 90:10.04 §

Ledipasvir and Sofosbuvir 8:18.40.24, 736

Lefamulin Acetate 8:12.28.26 §

Leflunomide 90:24.04 §

Legubeti®, *see* Acetylcysteine, 3395

Lemborexant 28:24.40 §

Lemtrada®, *see* Alemtuzumab §

Lenacapavir Sodium 8:18.08.24 §

Lenalidomide 10:00, 1101

Leniolisib 92:20 §

Lenmeldy®, *see* Atidarsagene Autotemcel §

Lenvatinib Mesylate 10:00, 1111

Lenvima®, *see* Lenvatinib Mesylate, 1111

Leqembi®, *see* Lecanemab §

Leqselvi®, *see* Deuruxolitinib §

Leqvio®, *see* Inclisiran §

Lescol®, *see* Fluvastatin §

Lessina®, 28, *see* Estrogen-Progestin Combinations, 2874

Letairis®, *see* Ambrisentan §

Letermovir 8:18.44 §

LetibotulinumtoxinA-wlbg 12:20.20.24 §

Letrozole 68:16.08 §

Leucovorin 91:04.12, 3403

Leukeran®, *see* Chlorambucil §

Leukine®, *see* Sargramostim §

Leuprolide 68:18.08 §

Levacetylleucine 92:92 §

Levamlodipine 24:28.08 §

Levaquin®, *see* levoFLOXacin, 256

Levbid®, *see* Hyoscyamine, Hyoscyamine Sulfate §

levETIRAcetam 28:12.92, 2261

Levitra®, *see* Vardenafil §

Levlen®, *see* Estrogen-Progestin Combinations, 2874

Levlite®, 28, *see* Estrogen-Progestin Combinations, 2874

Levobunolol 52:40.08 §

levOCARNitine 92:92 §

Levocetirizine 4:08 §

Levodopa/Carbidopa 28:36.16, 2567

levoFLOXacin 8:12.18, 256 *and* 52:04.04 §

Levoketoconazole 68:04 §

LEVOleucovorin 91:04.12, 3407

Levomilnacipran 28:16.04.16 §

Levophed®, *see* Norepinephrine, 1445

Levora®, *see* Estrogen-Progestin Combinations, 2874

Levorphanol 28:08.08 §

Levothroid®, *see* Levothyroxine, 3137

Levothyroxine Sodium 68:36.04, 3137

Levoxyl®, *see* Levothyroxine, 3137

Levsin®, *see* Hyoscyamine §

Levsinex®, *see* Hyoscyamine §

Levulan®, *see* Aminolevulinic Acid §

Lexapro®, *see* Escitalopram, 2322

Lexiscan®, *see* Regadenoson §

Lexiva®, *see* Fosamprenavir §

L-Glutamine 92:92 §

Lialda®, *see* Mesalamine §

Librax®, *see* chlordiazePOXIDE § *and see* Clidinium §

Libtayo®, *see* Cemiplimab-rwlc, 898

Licart®, *see* Diclofenac, 1982

Licide®, *see* Pyrethrins with Piperonyl Butoxide §

Lidex®, *see* Fluocinolone Acetonide §

Lidocaine 24:04.04.08, 1650 *and* 72:00 § *and* 84:08 §

Lidoderm®, *see* Lidocaine §

Lifileucel 26:04 §

Lifitegrast 52:08 §

Mandelamine®, *see* Methenamine §
Mannitol 36:40 § *and* 40:28.12, 2629
Mantadil®, *see* Hydrocortisone §
Maralixibat 56:14 §
Maraviroc 8:18.08.04 §
Marblen®, *see* Antacids, 2688
Marcaine®, *see* Bupivacaine §
Mar-Cof®, *see* Codeine, 2657
Margenza®, *see* Margetuximab-cmkb §
Margetuximab-cmkb 10:00 §
Maribavir 8:18.44 §
Marinol®, *see* Dronabinol §
Marqibo®, *see* vinCRIStine Sulfate, 1343
Massengill®, *see* Hydrocortisone §
Matulane®, *see* Procarbazine §
Matzim®, *see* dilTIAZem, 1712
Mavacamten 24:04.92 §
Mavenclad®, *see* Cladribine §
Mavik®, *see* Trandolapril §
Mavorixafor 20:16 §
Mavyret®, *see* Glecaprevir and
    Pibrentasvir, 714
Maxalt®, *see* Rizatriptan §
Maxidex®, *see* Dexamethasone §
Maxipime®, *see* Cefepime Hydrochloride,
    99
Maxitrol®, *see* Dexamethasone § *and see*
    Neomycin § *and see* Polymyxin B §
Maxivate®, *see* Betamethasone §
Maxzide®, *see* hydroCHLOROthiazide,
    2649 *and see* Triamterene, 2632
Mayzent®, *see* Siponimod §
M-Clear®, *see* Codeine, 2657
Measles Virus Vaccine Live 80:12 §
Mebendazole 8:08 §
Mecasermin 68:30.04 §
Mechlorethamine 84:18 §
Meclizine 56:22.08, 2725
Meclofenamate 28:08.04.04 §
Medrol®, *see* methylPREDNISolone §
medroxyPROGESTERone 68:32, 3119
Mefenamic Acid 28:08.04.04 §
Mefloquine Hydrochloride 8:30.08 §
Mefoxin®, *see* cefOXitin Sodium §
Megace®, *see* Megestrol §
Megestrol 68:32 §
Mekinist®, *see* Trametinib, 1293
Mektovi®, *see* Binimetinib, 828
Melanex®, *see* Hydroquinone §
Melfiat®, *see* Phendimetrazine §
Meloxicam 28:08.04.04, 2021
Melpaque®, *see* Hydroquinone §

Melphalan 10:00 §
Melquin®, *see* Hydroquinone §
Memantine 28:92, 2576
Menactra®, *see* Meningococcal Groups A,
    C, Y, and W-135 Vaccine §
Menest®, *see* Estropipate §
Meni-D®, *see* Meclizine, 2725
Meningococcal Group B Vaccine 80:12 §
Meningococcal Groups A, B, C, W, and Y
    Vaccine 80:12 §
Meningococcal Groups A, C, Y, and
    W-135 Vaccine 80:12 §
Menopur®, *see* Menotropins §
Menostar®, *see* Estradiol, 2909
Menotropins 68:18.08 §
MenQuadfi®, *see* Meningococcal Groups
    A, C, Y, and W-135 Vaccine §
Mentax®, *see* Butenafine Hydrochloride §
Menveo®, *see* Meningococcal Groups A, C,
    Y, and W-135 Vaccine §
Meperidine 28:08.08 §
Mephyton®, *see* Phytonadione §
Mepivacaine 72:00 §
Mepolizumab 48:10.20 §
Meprobamate 28:24.12 §
Mepron®, *see* Atovaquone §
Mepsevii®, *see* Vestronidase alfa-vjbk §
Mercaptopurine 10:00 §
Meropenem 8:12.07.08 §
Meropenem and Vaborbactam 8:12.07.08,
    124
Merrem®, *see* Meropenem §
Mesalamine 56:36 §
Mesna 91:04.12 §
Mesnex®, *see* Mesna §
Mestinon®, *see* Pyridostigmine Bromide §
Metaglip®, *see* glipiZIDE, 3069
Metamucil®, *see* Bulk-Forming Laxatives §
Metaxalone 12:20.04 §
Meted®, *see* Sulfur §
metFORMIN 68:20.04, 2918
Methadone 28:08.08, 2130
Methadose®, *see* Methadone, 2130
Methamphetamine 28:20.04 §
methazolAMIDE 52:40.12 §
Methenamine 8:36 §
Methergine®, *see* Ergonovine §
methIMAzole 68:36.08 §
Methitest®, *see* methylTESTOSTERone,
    2857
Methocarbamol 12:20.04 §
Methohexital 28:04.04 §

Methotrexate 10:00, 1126
Methoxsalen 84:50.06 §
Methoxy Polyethylene Glycol-epoetin
    Beta 20:16 §
Methscopolamine Bromide 12:08.08 §
Methsuximide 28:12.20 §
Methyldopa 24:24 §
Methylene Blue 91:04.16 §
Methylin®, *see* Methylphenidate §
Methylnaltrexone 56:18.04 §
Methylphenidate 28:20.32 §
methylPREDNISolone 68:04 §
methylTESTOSTERone 68:08, 2857
Metoclopramide 56:32, 2798
metOLazone 40:28.24 §
Metopirone®, *see* metyraPONE §
Metoprolol 24:20, 1813
Metreleptin 68:40 §
MetroCream®, *see* metroNIDAZOLE §
MetroGel®, *see* metroNIDAZOLE §
MetroLotion®, *see* metroNIDAZOLE §
metroNIDAZOLE 8:30.16.92 § *and*
    84:04.04 §
metyraPONE 36:66 §
metyroSINE 36:64 §
Mexiletine 24:04.04.08 §
Mexitil®, *see* Mexiletine §
MG 217®, *see* Coal Tar Preparations § *and*
    see Salicylic Acid § *and see* Sulfur §
Miacalcin®, *see* Calcitonin §
Micafungin Sodium 8:14.16, 454
Micardis®, *see* hydroCHLOROthiazide,
    2649 *and see* Telmisartan §
Micatin®, *see* Miconazole §
Miconazole 84:04.08.08 §
Micrainin®, *see* Aspirin, 2073
MICRhoGAM®, *see* Rho(D) Immune
    Globulin §
Microgestin®, *see* Estrogen-Progestin
    Combinations, 2874
Micro-K®, *see* Potassium Supplements,
    2602
Micronor®, *see* Progestins, 2893
Microzide®, *see* hydroCHLOROthiazide,
    2649
Midazolam 28:24.08, 2519
Midodrine 12:12.04 §
Midol®, *see* Acetaminophen, 2199
Midostaurin 10:00 §
Miebo®, *see* Perfluorohexyloctane §
Mifeprex®, *see* Mifepristone, 3153
Mifepristone 76:00, 3153

N

O

P

Plendil®, *see* Felodipine §

Plerixafor 20:16 §

Pletal®, *see* Cilostazol §

Pneumococcal Vaccine 80:12 §

Pneumovax®, 23, *see* Pneumococcal
Vaccine §

Podocon-25®, *see* Podophyllum Resin §

Podofilox 84:28 §

Podophyllum Resin 84:28 §

Polatuzumab Vedotin-piiq 10:00 §

Polidocanol 24:12 §

Poliovirus Vaccine Inactivated 80:12 §

Polivy®, *see* Polatuzumab Vedotin-piiq §

Polocaine®, *see* Mepivacaine §

Polymyxin B 8:12.28.28, 376 *and*
52:04.04 §

Poly-Pred®, *see* prednisoLONE §

Poly-Rx®, *see* Polymyxin B, 376

Polysporin®, *see* Bacitracin §

Polytar®, *see* Coal Tar Preparations §

Polytrim®, *see* Polymyxin B §

Pomalidomide 10:00, 1240

Pomalyst®, *see* Pomalidomide, 1240

Pombiliti®, *see* Cipaglucosidase alfa-atga §

PONATinib 10:00 §

Ponesimod 90:04.16 §

Pontocaine®, *see* Tetracaine §

Ponvory®, *see* Ponesimod §

Poractant Alfa 48:36 §

Portia®, *see* Estrogen-Progestin
Combinations, 2874

Portrazza®, *see* Necitumumab §

Posaconazole 8:14.08, 419

Posture®, *see* Calcium Salts, 2591

Posture-D®, *see* Calcium Salts, 2591

Potassium Iodide 68:36.08, 3141

Potassium Supplements 40:12, 2602

Poteligeo®, *see* Mogamulizumab-kpkc §

Pozelimab-bbfg 92:32 §

PrabotulinumtoxinA-xvfs 12:20.20.24 §

Pradaxa®, *see* Dabigatran, 1536

PRALAtrexate 10:00 §

Pralidoxime 91:04.20, 3411

Pralsetinib 10:00 §

Praluent®, *see* Alirocumab §

PrameGel®, *see* Pramoxine §

Pramipexole 28:36.20.08 §

Pramlintide 68:20.03 §

Pramosone®, *see* Hydrocortisone §

Pramoxine 84:08 §

Prasterone 68:04 §

Prasugrel 20:12.18, 1614

Pravastatin 24:06.08 §

Prax®, *see* Pramoxine §

Praxbind®, *see* idaruCIZUmab §

Praziquantel 8:08 §

Prazosin 24:16, 1776

Precedex®, *see* Dexmedetomidine
Hydrochloride §

Pred Mild®, *see* prednisoLONE §

Pred-G®, *see* Gentamicin § *and see*
prednisoLONE §

Prednicarbate 84:06.08 §

prednisoLONE 52:08.08 § *and* 68:04 §

predniSONE 68:04 §

Preface to the Penicillins 8:12.16, 145

Prefest®, *see* Estradiol, 2909

Pregabalin 28:12.28, 2242

Pregnyl®, *see* Gonadotropin, Chorionic §

Prelone®, *see* prednisoLONE §

Premarin®, *see* Estrogens, Conjugated, 2915

Premasol®, *see* Amino Acid Injections §

Premphase®, *see* Estrogens,
Conjugated, 2915 *and see*
medroxyPROGESTERone, 3119

Prempro®, *see* Estrogens,
Conjugated, 2915 *and see*
medroxyPROGESTERone, 3119

Premsyn PMS®, *see* Acetaminophen, 2199

Preparation H®, *see* Hydrocortisone § *and*
see Phenylephrine, 1390

Prepidil®, *see* Dinoprostone §

Prestalia®, *see* amLODIPine, 1844 *and see*
Perindopril §

Pretomanid 8:16.04 §

Prevacid®, *see* Lansoprazole, 2771

Prevalite®, *see* Cholestyramine Resin §

PreviDent®, *see* Fluorides §

Prevnar 20®, *see* Pneumococcal Vaccine §

Prevpac®, *see* Clarithromycin § *and see*
Lansoprazole, 2771

Prevymis®, *see* Letermovir §

Prezcobix®, *see* Darunavir §

Prezista®, *see* Darunavir §

Prialt®, *see* Ziconotide §

Priftin®, *see* Rifapentine §

Prilocaine 72:00 §

Priloprim®, *see* Trimethoprim §

PriLOSEC®, *see* Omeprazole, 2780

Primaquine Phosphate 8:30.08 §

Primatene®, *see* Ephedrine, 1429 *and see*
guaiFENesin, 2684

Primaxin®, *see* Imipenem and Cilastatin
Sodium §

Primidone 28:12.04 §

Primlev®, *see* Acetaminophen, 2199 *and*
see Oxycodone, 2156

Primsol®, *see* Trimethoprim §

Prinivil®, *see* Lisinopril, 1901

Prinzide®, *see* hydroCHLOROthiazide,
2649 *and see* Lisinopril, 1901

Pristiq®, *see* Desvenlafaxine, 2287

Privigen®, *see* Immune Globulin §

Privine®, *see* Naphazoline §

Proactiv®, *see* Salicylic Acid §

ProAir®, *see* Albuterol §

Proamatine®, *see* Midodrine §

Probenecid 40:40 §

Probiata®, *see* Lactobacillus Acidophilus §

ProBiotic®, *see* Lactobacillus
Acidophilus §

Probuphine®, *see* Buprenorphine, 2172

Procainamide 24:04.04.04, 1644

Procalamine®, *see* Amino Acid
Injections §

Procarbazine Hydrochloride 10:00 §

Procardia®, *see* NIFEdipine, 1854

Prochlorperazine 28:16.08.24 § *and*
56:22.08, 2726

Procrit®, *see* Epoetin Alfa §

Proctocort®, *see* Hydrocortisone §

proctocream®, *see* Hydrocortisone §

Proctofoam®, *see* Hydrocortisone § *and*
see Pramoxine §

Procysbi®, *see* Cysteamine §

Prodium®, *see* Phenazopyridine §

Profasi®, *see* Gonadotropin, Chorionic §

Profilnine®, *see* Factor IX (Human) §

Progesterone 68:32, 3128

Progestins 68:12, 2893

Progestins General Statement 68:32, 3117

Proglycem®, *see* Diazoxide §

Prograf®, *see* Tacrolimus, 3384

Prolastin®, *see* alpha-1-Proteinase
Inhibitor (Human) §

Proleukin®, *see* Aldesleukin §

Prolia®, *see* Denosumab §

Prolixin®, *see* fluPHENAZine §

Promacta®, *see* Eltrombopag §

Prometh®, *see* Promethazine, 16 *and* 2551

Promethazine 4:04, 16 *and* 28:24.92, 2551

Promethegan®, *see* Promethazine, 16 *and*
2551

Prometrium®, *see* Progesterone, 3128

Pronto®, *see* Pyrethrins with Piperonyl
Butoxide §

RelCof-C®, *see* Codeine, 2657

Relenza®, *see* Zanamivir, 626

Releuko®, *see* Filgrastim §

Relief®, *see* Phenylephrine §

Relistor®, *see* Methylnaltrexone §

Relpax®, *see* Eletriptan §

Relugolix 68:18.04 §

Relugolix, Estradiol, and Norethindrone 68:18.04 §

Remdesivir 8:18.32 §

Remeron®, *see* Mirtazapine §

Remicade®, *see* inFLIXimab, 3268

Remifentanil 28:08.08 §

Remimazolam 28:24.08 §

Remodulin®, *see* Treprostinil §

Renagel®, *see* Sevelamer §

Renamin®, *see* Amino Acid Injections §

Renflexis®, *see* inFLIXimab, 3268

Renova®, *see* Tretinoin §

Renvela®, *see* Sevelamer §

Repaglinide 68:20.16 §

Repatha®, *see* Evolocumab §

Repotrectinib 10:00 §

Reprexain®, *see* HYDROcodone, 2118

Requip®, *see* rOPINIRole §

Rescon®, *see* guaiFENesin, 2684

Reslizumab 48:10.20 §

Resmetirom 56:92 §

Respiratory Syncytial Virus Vaccine 80:12 §

Respiratory Syncytial Virus Vaccine, Adjuvanted 80:12 §

Respiratory Syncytial Virus Vaccine (mRNA) 80:12 §

Respiratory Tract Agents 48:00, 2656

Restasis®, *see* cycloSPORINE §

Restoril®, *see* Temazepam §

Retacrit®, *see* Epoetin Alfa §

Retapamulin 84:04.04 §

Retavase®, *see* Reteplase §

Reteplase 20:12.20 §

Retevmo®, *see* Selpercatinib §

Retifanlimab 10:00 §

Retin-A®, *see* Tretinoin §

Retisert®, *see* Fluocinolone §

Retrovir®, *see* Zidovudine, 604

Revatio®, *see* Sildenafil §

Revcovi®, *see* Elapegademase-lvlr §

Revefenacin 12:08.08 §

Revex®, *see* Nalmefene §

ReVia®, *see* Naltrexone, 2217

Revlimid®, *see* Lenalidomide, 1101

Revonto®, *see* Dantrolene §

Rexulti®, *see* Brexpiprazole, 2400

Reyataz®, *see* Atazanavir Sulfate §

Reyvow®, *see* Lasmiditan §

Rezafungin Acetate 8:14.16 §

Rezamid®, *see* Sulfur §

Rezdiffra®, *see* Resmetirom §

Rezira®, *see* HYDROcodone, 2663

Rezlidhia®, *see* Olutasidenib §

Rezurock®, *see* Belumosudil §

Rezzayo®, *see* Rezafungin Acetate §

R-Gene®, *see* Arginine §

Rheomacrodex®, *see* Dextran 40 §

Rheumatrex®, *see* Methotrexate 1126

Rhinocort®, *see* Budesonide §

Rho(D) Immune Globulin 80:04 §

Rhofade®, *see* Oxymetazoline §

RhoGAM®, *see* Rho(D) Immune Globulin §

Rhophylac®, *see* Rho(D) Immune Globulin §

Rhopressa®, *see* Netarsudil §

Rhulicream®, *see* Benzocaine §

RiaSTAP®, *see* Fibrinogen (Human) §

Ribasphere®, *see* Ribavirin §

Ribavirin 8:18.32 §

Ribociclib Succinate 10:00 §

Riboflavin 88:08 §

RID®, *see* Pyrethrins with Piperonyl Butoxide §

Ridaura®, *see* Auranofin §

Rifabutin 8:16.04 §

Rifadin®, *see* rifAMPin §

Rifamate®, *see* Isoniazid § *and see* rifAMPin §

rifAMPin 8:16.04 §

Rifamycin Sodium 8:12.28.30 §

Rifapentine 8:16.04 §

Rifater®, *see* Isoniazid § *and see* Pyrazinamide § *and see* rifAMPin §

rifAXIMin 8:12.28.30, 382

Rilonacept 48:10.20 §

Rilpivirine Hydrochloride 8:18.08.16, 567

Rilutek®, *see* Riluzole §

Riluzole 28:44 §

RimabotulinumtoxinB 12:20.20.24 §

Rimactane®, *see* rifAMPin §

riMANTADine Hydrochloride 8:18.04 §

Rimegepant 28:32.12 §

Rinvoq®, *see* Upadacitinib, 3202

Riociguat 48:48.92 §

Riomet®, *see* metFORMIN, 2918

Riopan Plus®, *see* Antacids, 2688

Ripretinib 10:00 §

Risankizumab-rzaa 84:06.28 §

Risdiplam 92:92 §

Risedronate 92:24 §

RisperDAL®, *see* risperiDONE, 2478

risperiDONE 28:16.08.04, 2478

Ritalin®, *see* Methylphenidate §

Ritlecitinib 84:06.16 §

Ritonavir 8:18.08.08 §

Rituxan®, *see* riTUXimab, 1257

riTUXimab 10:00, 1257

Rivaroxaban 20:12.04.14, 1562

Rivastigmine 12:04 §

Rivfloza®, *see* Nedosiran Sodium §

Rixubis®, *see* Factor IX (Recombinant) §

Rizatriptan 28:32.28 §

Robafen®, *see* Codeine, 2657 *and see* guaiFENesin, 2684

Robaxin®, *see* Methocarbamol §

Robinul®, *see* Glycopyrrolate §

Robitussin®, *see* Dextromethorphan, 2659 *and see* guaiFENesin, 2684

Rocaltrol®, *see* Calcitriol §

Rocklatan®, *see* Latanoprost § *and see* Netarsudil §

Roctavian®, *see* Valoctocogene Roxaparvovec-rvox §

Rocuronium 12:20.20 §

Roflumilast 48:32 § *and* 84:06.12 §

Rogaine®, *see* Minoxidil §

Rohto®, *see* Naphazoline § *and see* Tetrahydrozoline §

Rolaids®, *see* Antacids, 2688

Rolapitant 56:22.32, 2742

Rolvedon®, *see* Eflapegrastim-xnst §

Romazicon®, *see* Flumazenil, 3423

romiDEPsin 10:00 §

romiPLOStim 20:16 §

Romosozumab-aqqg 90:16 §

Ropeginterferon Alfa-2b-njft 10:00 §

rOPINIRole 28:36.20.08 §

Ropivacaine 72:00 §

Rosiglitazone 68:20.28, 3085

Rosuvastatin 24:06.08 §

Rotarix®, *see* Rotavirus Vaccine Live Oral §

RotaTeq®, *see* Rotavirus Vaccine Live Oral §

Rotavirus Vaccine Live Oral 80:12 §

Rotigotine 28:36.20.08 §

Rowasa®, *see* Mesalamine §

T

U

Ublituximab-xiiy 90:04.04 §
Ubrelvy®, *see* Ubrogepant §
Ubrogepant 28:32.12 §
Udenyca®, *see* Pegfilgrastim §
Uliprista 68:12 §
Uloric®, *see* Febuxostat §
Ultiva®, *see* Remifentanil §
Ultomiris®, *see* Ravulizumab §
Ultra Mide®, *see* Urea §
Ultracet®, *see* Acetaminophen, 2199
UltraSal®, *see* Salicylic Acid §
Ultrase®, *see* Pancrelipase §
Umeclidinium 12:08.08 §
Umeclidinium and Vilanterol 12:08.08 §
Unasyn®, *see* Ampicillin and Sulbactam, 190
Undecylenic Acid and Undecylenate Salts 84:04.16 §
Uniphyl®, *see* Theophyllines §
Uniretic®, *see* hydroCHLOROthiazide, 2649
Unisom®, *see* diphenhydrAMINE, 12 *and see* Doxylamine §
Unithroid®, *see* Levothyroxine Sodium, 3137
Unituxin®, *see* Dinutuximab §
Upadacitinib 90:24.12.92, 3202
Uplinza®, *see* Inebilizumab-cdon §
Uptravi®, *see* Selexipag §
Urea 40:28.12 § *and* 84:28 §
Ureacin®, *see* Urea §
Urex®, *see* Methenamine §
Uridine Triacetate 91:04.32, 3418
Urispas®, *see* flavoxATE §
Uro-Mag®, *see* Antacids, 2688
Uroxatral®, *see* Alfuzosin §
Urso Forte®, *see* Ursodiol §
Ursodiol 56:14 §
Ustekinumab 90:24.20.92, 3327
UTI Relief®, *see* Phenazopyridine §
Utibron®, *see* Glycopyrrolate §

V

Vabomere®, *see* Meropenem and Vaborbactam, 124
Vabysmo®, *see* Faricimab-svoa §
Vaccinia Immune Globulin IV 80:04 §
Vadadustat 20:16 §

Vafseo®, *see* Vadadustat §
Vagifem®, *see* Estradiol, 2909
Vagisil®, *see* Pramoxine §
Vagistat®, *see* Tioconazole §
valACYclovir 8:18.32, 691
Valbenazine 28:56 §
Valchlor®, *see* Mechlorethamine §
Valcyte®, *see* valGANciclovir, 697
valGANciclovir 8:18.32, 697
Valium®, *see* diazePAM, 2510
Valoctocogene Roxaparvovec-rvox 26:12 §
Valproate 28:12.28 §
Valrubicin 10:00 §
Valsartan 24:32.08, 1927
Valstar®, *see* Valrubicin §
Valtrex®, *see* valACYclovir, 691
Vamorolone 68:04 §
Vancocin®, *see* Vancomycin, 337
Vancomycin 8:12.28.16, 337
Vandazole®, *see* metroNIDAZOLE §
Vandetanib 10:00, 1322
Vanflyta®, *see* Quizartinib §
Vanquish®, *see* Acetaminophen, 2199 *and see* Aspirin, 2073
Vantas®, *see* Histrelin §
Vantin®, *see* Cefpodoxime §
Vaprisol®, *see* Conivaptan §
Vaqta®, *see* Hepatitis A Virus Vaccine Inactivated §
Vardenafil 24:08.12 §
Varenicline 12:02 § *and* 52:92 §
Varicella Virus Vaccine Live 80:12 §
Varicella Zoster Immune Globulin 80:04 §
Varivax®, *see* Varicella Virus Vaccine Live §
Varizig®, *see* Varicella Zoster Immune Globulin §
Varubi®, *see* Rolapitant, 2742
Vascepa®, *see* Icosapent Ethyl §
Vaseretic®, *see* Enalaprilat, 1884 *and see* hydroCHLOROthiazide, 2649
Vasocidin®, *see* prednisoLONE §
Vasopressin 68:28, 3112
Vasostrict®, *see* Vasopressin, 3112
Vasotec®, *see* Enalaprilat, 1884
Vaxchora®, *see* Cholera Vaccine Live Oral §
Vaxneuvance®, *see* Pneumococcal Vaccine §
Vazculep®, *see* Phenylephrine, 1390

Vectibix®, *see* Panitumumab §
Vecuronium 12:20.20, 1476
Vedolizumab 90:24.92 §
Veinamine®, *see* Amino Acid Injections §
Veklury®, *see* Remdesivir §
Velaglucerase Alfa 44:00 §
Velcade®, *see* Bortezomib, 834
Veletri®, *see* Epoprostenol §
Velmanase Alfa-tycv 44:00 §
Velphoro®, *see* Sucroferric Oxyhydroxide §
Velsipity®, *see* Etrasimod §
Veltassa®, *see* Patiromer, 2608
Vemlidy®, *see* Tenofovir Alafenamide Fumarate, 686
Vemurafenib 10:00, 1327
Venclexta®, *see* Venetoclax, 1333
Venetoclax 10:00, 1333
Venlafaxine 28:16.04.16 §
Venofer®, *see* Iron Sucrose, 1507
Ventavis®, *see* Iloprost §
Ventolin®, *see* Albuterol §
Veopoz®, *see* Pozelimab-bbfg §
Veozah®, *see* Fezolinetant §
VePesid®, *see* Etoposide, 1035
Verapamil 24:04.04.24, 1723
Veregen®, *see* Sinecatechins §
Verelan®, *see* Verapamil, 1723
Vericiguat 24:08.10, 1763
Vermox®, *see* Mebendazole §
Verquvo®, *see* Vericiguat, 1763
Versacloz®, *see* cloZAPine, 2413
Versiclear®, *see* Sodium Thiosulfate §
Verteporfin 52:44 §
Verzenio®, *see* Abemaciclib, 775
Vesicare®, *see* Solifenacin §
Vestronidase alfa-vjbk 44:00 §
Vfend®, *see* Voriconazole, 430
Viactiv®, *see* Calcium Salts, 2591
Viagra®, *see* Sildenafil §
Vibativ®, *see* Telavancin Hydrochloride, 332
Vibegron 86:12.08.12 §
Viberzi®, *see* Eluxadoline §
Vibramycin®, *see* Doxycycline §
Vibra-Tabs®, *see* Doxycycline §
Vicks Sinex®, *see* Oxymetazoline § *and see* Phenylephrine §
Vicks®, *see* Dextromethorphan, 2659 *and see* guaiFENesin, 2684 *and see* Phenylephrine 1390

---

§ Electronic-only monographs at ahfsdruginformation.com. Username: ahfs2025; Password: ASHP46360

W

X

Y

Z